Martindale

The complete drug reference

Thirty-third edition

Edited by

Sean C Sweetman

BPharm, MRPharmS

London • Chicago **Pharmaceutical Press**

Published by the Pharmaceutical Press

Publications division of the Royal Pharmaceutical Society of Great Britain

1 Lambeth High Street, London SE1 7JN, UK
100 South Atkinson Road, Suite 206, Grayslake, IL 60030-7820, USA

© Pharmaceutical Press 2002

First edition of *Martindale: The Extra Pharmacopoeia* was published in 1883.
Squire's Companion was incorporated in the twenty-third edition in 1952.

Thirty-third edition published 2002

Printed in Great Britain by The Bath Press

ISBN 0 85369 499 0

ISSN 0263-5364

A catalogue record for this book is available from the British Library

Contents

Part 1 • Monographs on drugs and ancillary substances

Part 2 • Supplementary drugs and other substances

Part 3 • Preparations

Directory of Manufacturers

General Index

Preface

The aim of Martindale is to provide practising pharmacists and physicians with unbiased evaluated information on drugs and medicines used throughout the world. It therefore has to develop as the body of knowledge on existing drugs grows, new drugs emerge, new preparations are launched, old preparations abandoned, reformulated, or redefined, and the information needs of those practising pharmacy and medicine continue to evolve. We have tried to ensure that the new edition continues to meet these needs.

All the drug monographs from the last edition have been revised, more than 160 having been deleted and more than 175 added, and organised into chapters that reflect the uses of the drugs being described. A new Neuromuscular Blockers chapter draws together drugs that were formerly described in the Muscle Relaxants chapter and whose main uses are in Anaesthesia and Intensive Care. The chapter on Lipid Regulating Drugs and its associated disease reviews on Hyperlipidaemias has been incorporated into the chapter on Cardiovascular Drugs.

The disease treatment reviews, 634 in all and generally located in the chapter introductions, have also been thoroughly revised in order to reflect current trends and provide key references. Cross-references to these reviews appear in the monographs of the drugs cited; the reviews can also be accessed via the general index. It is hoped that these reviews will be of use to readers who want an overview of a particular disease and its drug treatment and will provide a useful starting point for those who want to pursue particular aspects further.

The information on proprietary preparations, an important feature of Martindale, has been updated and a much wider range of countries has been covered for this edition.

Martindale is based on published information and more than 32 000 selected references are included. Since the last printed edition of Martindale appeared a significant amount of information on drugs is now additionally being published in various electronic formats, including on the Internet as web pages. The reader will therefore note that this edition of Martindale now carries citations to online publications as well as to traditional printed sources.

Our aim is to evaluate the literature, covering important studies, guidelines, and useful reviews and placing them in context. Multicentre studies, meta-analyses, and systematic reviews play an important role in the study of drug treatment, and their findings and conclusions are considered in many of our chapters. However, there is also a place for the anecdotal report and the small study, and information from such sources is included where appropriate. A clearer acknowledgement is now also given to information referenced from a number of authoritative sources including the *British National Formulary*, the *British Pharmacopoeia*, the *European Pharmacopoeia*, the *United States National Formulary*, and the *United States Pharmacopeia*.

Once again strenuous editorial efforts have been made to produce a book of manageable size without sacrificing content. The use of more headings and other changes to the typography and layout have been introduced to improve readability.

Possibly one of the most noticeable changes apparent to the reader will be in the new monograph titles resulting from the preferential use of International Nonproprietary Names (INN) for drugs and radicals (for further information see below under Nomenclature). Anatomical Therapeutic Chemical (ATC) classification codes have also been added to many monographs for this edition.

Martindale is not a book of standards. Inclusion of a substance or a preparation is not to be considered as a recommendation for use, nor does it confer any status on the substance or preparation. While considerable efforts have been made to check the material in Martindale, the publisher cannot accept any responsibility for errors and omissions. Also the reader is assumed to possess the necessary knowledge to interpret the information that Martindale provides.

Arrangement

PART 1 (pages 1–1570) contains 4293 monographs arranged in 51 chapters. These chapters generally bring together monographs on drugs and groups of drugs that have similar uses or actions. The introductions of those chapters that describe drugs used in the management of disease contain disease treatment reviews—descriptions of those diseases together with reviews of the choice of treatments.

PART 2 (pages 1571–1682) consists of a series of 852 short monographs arranged in the alphabetical order of their main titles. It includes monographs on some new drugs, on drugs not easily classified, on herbals, and on drugs no longer used clinically but still of interest. There are also monographs on toxic substances, the effects of which may require drug therapy.

PART 3 (pages 1683–2180) contains proprietary preparations from a range of countries. For this edition we have covered Australia, Austria, Belgium, Brazil, Canada, Denmark, Finland, France, Germany, Hong Kong, Ireland, Israel, Italy, Mexico, the Netherlands, New Zealand, Norway, Portugal, Singapore, South Africa, Spain, Sweden, Switzerland, Thailand, the United Arab Emirates, UK, and USA. We have also included some proprietary preparations from Japan. The information provided includes the proprietary name, the manufacturer or distributor, the active ingredients with cross-references to the drug monographs, and a summary of the indications as given by the manufacturer.

Indexes

DIRECTORY OF MANUFACTURERS. In Martindale the names of manufacturers and distributors are abbreviated. Their full names are given in this directory together with the full address if it is available. This directory contains some 7800 entries.

GENERAL INDEX. To make fullest use of the contents of Martindale the general index should always be consulted. The exhaustive index includes entries for drugs (approved names, synonyms, and chemical names), preparations, pharmacological and therapeutic groups, and clinical uses (disease treatment reviews). As in previous editions, the index is arranged alphabetically 'word-by-word' rather than 'letter-by-letter'. The index indicates the column in which the relevant entry appears as well as the page.

Nomenclature

MARTINDALE IDENTITY NUMBERS. Each monograph title is followed by an identity number in brackets which consists of a maximum of 6 figures followed by a check character. These numbers are used in the Martindale database and their purpose is to identify each substance and its associated records.

TITLES AND SYNONYMS. The title of each monograph is in English, with preference usually being given to International Nonproprietary Names (INN), British Approved Names (BAN), and United States Adopted Names (USAN). These 3 authorities are shown where appropriate. A European Directive (92/27/EEC) requires the use of Recommended International Nonproprietary Names (rINNs) in the labelling of medicinal products throughout member states of the European Community and where the BAN and INN differed in the past the BAN has been changed to accord with the rINN. In the UK, a proposed system of dual labelling for those drugs where a change of name was considered to pose the highest risk to public health has yet to be adopted. However, in recognition of this risk, this edition of Martindale has retained the original BAN for those substances on the proposed list and whenever one of these drugs is referred to, its name will be appended by the new rINN printed in square brackets. In some approved names it is now general policy to use 'f' for 'ph' in sulpha, 't' for 'th', and 'i' for 'y'; for this reason entries in alphabetical lists and indexes should be sought in alternative spellings if the expected spellings are not found. Inevitably there may be some inconsistencies of style with older approved names but wherever possible the names used for drugs or radicals in Martindale have been altered in accordance with the guidelines on the use of INNs for pharmaceutical substances. A table of contracted names for ions and groups used in approved names and titles is given on page ix.

This section also includes names given as synonyms such as commonly used abbreviated names; Latin versions of *Ph. Eur.* titles; English, American, and Latin synonyms; names used in other languages when these may not be readily identifiable; manufacturers' code numbers; and chemical names.

CAS REGISTRY NUMBERS. Chemical Abstracts Service (CAS) registry numbers are provided, where available, for each monograph substance to help readers refer to other information systems. Numbers for various forms of the monograph substance are listed with the variation in form given in parentheses.

ATC CODES. Codes from the Anatomical Therapeutic Chemical (ATC) classification system have been provided, where available, for each monograph substance to help readers refer to other information systems.

Atomic and Molecular Weights

Atomic weights are based on the table of Atomic Weights as revised in 1999 by the Commission on Atomic Weights and Isotopic Abundance, International Union of Pure and Applied Chemistry (IUPAC) and based on the ^{12}C scale (see page x). Molecular weights are given corrected to one place of decimals or to four significant figures for relative weights of less than 100.

Pharmacopoeias

The selected pharmacopoeias in which each substance appears are listed. Current copies of the pharmacopoeias and their addenda should be consulted for confirmation and for details of standards.

The pharmacopoeias covered include: Austrian, Belgian, *British, British Veterinary,* Chinese, *European,* French, *German,* International, Italian, *Japanese,* Netherlands, Polish, Portuguese, *Swiss,* and *United States* (including the *Formulary*). Those *italicised* in the above list either appeared as new editions or were revised by supplements since the last edition of Martindale, and have been examined for this 33rd edition.

The abbreviations for these pharmacopoeias are included in the list of abbreviations used in Martindale, see page vii which also includes details of the edition and/or supplement(s) consulted.

Several countries are parties to the Convention on the Elaboration of a European Pharmacopoeia. This means that they must adopt the standards of the European Pharmacopoeia. These countries are currently Austria, Belgium, Bosnia-Herzegovina, Croatia, Cyprus, Czech Republic, Denmark, Finland, France, Germany, Greece, Hungary, Iceland, Ireland, Italy, Luxembourg, the Netherlands, Norway, Portugal, Slovakia, Slovenia, Spain, Sweden, Switzerland, Turkey, the United Kingdom of Great Britain and Northern Ireland, Yugoslavia, and the Former Yugoslav Republic of Macedonia. Hence the European Pharmacopoeia is cited in the drug monograph lists of pharmacopoeias rather than these individual national pharmacopoeias.

Official preparations, mainly from the current British and US Pharmacopoeias, are listed at the end of drug monographs.

Pharmaceutical Information

Information on the chemical and physical properties of each substance is given when it is likely to be of use or interest, but only when it is certain that it applies to the form of substance being described in the monograph.

PERCENTAGE STRENGTHS. Unless otherwise stated, solutions of solids in liquids are expressed as percentage w/v, of liquids in liquids as percentage v/v, and of gases in liquids as percentage w/w.

SOLUBILITY. The figures given for solubility in each monograph have generally been obtained from the major pharmacopoeias in which the substance is described, but should not be considered absolute. Unless otherwise indicated in the text, the figures are for solubility at temperatures between 15° and 25°. The information usually relates to w/v solubilities but in some cases is v/v if the monograph substance itself is a liquid. Where solubilities are given in words, the following terms describe the indicated solubility ranges:

solubility

very soluble	1 in less than 1
freely soluble	1 in 1 to 1 in 10
soluble	1 in 10 to 1 in 30
sparingly soluble	1 in 30 to 1 in 100
slightly soluble	1 in 100 to 1 in 1000
very slightly soluble	1 in 1000 to 1 in 10 000
practically insoluble	1 in more than 10 000

STORAGE. Substances and preparations should be stored under conditions which prevent contamination and diminish deterioration, and the conditions of storage given in the text indicate the precautions recommended in specific cases. The term 'a cool place' is generally used to describe a place in which the temperature is between 8° and 15°. In general, the storage conditions apply to the monograph substance and not its solutions or preparations.

TEMPERATURE. Temperatures are expressed in degrees Celsius (centigrade) unless otherwise indicated.

Pharmacological and Therapeutic Information

Information on adverse effects, treatment of adverse effects, precautions (including contra-indications), interactions, pharmacokinetics, and uses and administration of each substance is provided by concise statements and these may be elaborated and expanded by referenced reviews and abstracts from papers and other publications. This edition contains about 11 750 such abstracts or reviews based on information in an ever widening range of publications.

Much information has been found in sources such as World Health Organization publications, government reports and legislation, and other official and standard publications. Manufacturers' literature has been considered in the light of other available information.

The risks of administering drugs in pregnancy are well known and the general principle is to give a drug only when the benefit to the individual mother outweighs the risk to the fetus. Where there is a clear risk it is noted under the Precautions or Adverse Effects heading but safety should not be inferred from the absence of a statement for any drug.

Doses

Doses are described under the Uses and Administration heading with as much detail as is necessary and available. Unless otherwise stated the doses represent the average range of quantities which are generally regarded as suitable for adults when administered by mouth. More information on doses and drug administration may be given in the abstracts or reviews. Unless otherwise specified, glucose injection is 5% w/v and sodium chloride injection is 0.9% w/v.

When doses for children are expressed as a range of quantities within specified age limits, the lower dose applies at the lower age and the higher dose at the higher age.

Acknowledgements

The Editor gratefully acknowledges the advice and assistance of the many experts who have suggested amendments to the text of Martindale. Thanks are due to DN Bateman, SJD Brecker, S Cottam, PR Jackson, PM Mason, S O'Halloran, K Parfitt, T Pullar, LE Ramsay, J Schofield, SJ Shankie, M Summerhayes, C Taylor, and W Watkins for reading and commenting on drafts of this edition. Thanks are also due to Sian Harding for advice and comments on specific issues during revision.

The Editor is grateful to the many organisations that have helped in providing information, including the World Health Organization and the British Pharmacopoeia Commission.

Martindale staff have been able to call freely on the expertise of other members of the Royal Pharmaceutical Society's staff. In particular the Editor is grateful to DK Mehta and the editorial staff of the British National Formulary, and the staff of the library and information department. Thanks are due to M Davis, EJ Laughton, and SJ Shankie for work on the Preparations database and for other editorial tasks, and also to C Graham, RH Jolley, M Joshi, LC Litman, R McLarney, and GC Sweetman who contributed to this edition. Thanks are also due to C Fry the Society's Director of Publications and to the staff of the Pharmaceutical Press for their support.

The contents of this 33rd edition were planned, written, checked, indexed, keyed, proofed, and processed by the Martindale staff. The Editor is pleased to acknowledge the skills and commitment of all the Martindale staff and to record his gratitude: to Christine Iskandar and Claire Ryan for clerical assistance; to the Staff Editors Bosede Abe, Alison Brayfield, Catherine Cadart, Kathleen Eager, Jennifer Flatman, Prakash Gotecha, Sue Handy, Rhoda Lee, Valerie Lee, Gail Neathercoat, Keith Riley, Louise Sheridan, and Gerda Viedge; to the Assistant Editors Julie McGlashan and Anne Parsons; and to the Senior Assistant Editor Paul Blake.

London   January 2002

Abbreviations

For abbreviations of the names of manufacturers or their distributors, see Directory of Manufacturers, p.2181.

≈—approximately equals.

ACE—angiotensin-converting enzyme.

agg.—aggregate (in botanical names), including 2 or more species which resemble each other closely.

AIDS—acquired immunodeficiency syndrome.

a.m.—ante meridiem, 'before noon'.

ARC—AIDS-related complex.

ATC—Anatomical Therapeutic Chemical classification.

Aust.—Austria.

Aust. P.—Austrian Pharmacopoeia 1990 (Österreichisches Arzneibuch) including Addenda 1990 and 1991.

Austral.—Australia.

BAN—British Approved Name.

BANM—British Approved Name Modified.

Belg. P.—Belgian Pharmacopoeia 1980 (Pharmacopée Belge, Sixième Edition) and Supplements to 1988.

BMA—British Medical Association.

b.p.—boiling point.

BP—British Pharmacopoeia. Unless otherwise specified, BP references are to the 2001 edition including Amendments No. 1.

BP(Vet)—British Pharmacopoeia (Veterinary) 2001 including Amendments No. 1.

BPC—British Pharmaceutical Codex.

Br.—British.

Braz.—Brazil.

BUN—Blood-urea-nitrogen.

°C—degrees Celsius (centigrade). Unless otherwise indicated in the text, temperatures are expressed in this thermometric scale.

C.—*Campylobacter*, *Candida*, *Chlamydia*, or *Corynebacterium*.

Canad.—Canada.

CAPD—continuous ambulatory peritoneal dialysis.

CAS—Chemical Abstracts Service.

CCPD—continuous cycle peritoneal dialysis.

CDC—Centers for Disease Control (USA).

Chin. P.—Chinese Pharmacopoeia 1990.

CI—Colour Index.

CNS—central nervous system.

cP—centipoise(s).

CPMP—Committee on Proprietary Medicinal Products of the European Union.

CRM—the former Committee on the Review of Medicines (UK).

CSF—cerebrospinal fluid.

CSM—Committee on Safety of Medicines (UK).

cSt—centistokes.

D & C—designation applied in USA to dyes permitted for use in drugs and cosmetics.

d.c.—direct current.

Denm.—Denmark.

DHSS—the former Department of Health and Social Security (UK).

dL—decilitre(s).

DNA—deoxyribonucleic acid.

DoH—Department of Health (UK).

DTF—Drug Tariff Formulary.

ECG—electrocardiogram.

ECT—electroconvulsive therapy.

Ecuad.—Ecuador.

ed.—editor(s) *or* edited by *or* edition.

EEC—European Economic Community, now the European Union.

EEG—electro-encephalogram.

e.g.—*exempli gratia* 'for example'.

ENL—erythema nodosum leprosum.

ESRD—end-stage renal disease.

et al.—*et alii*, 'and others': for three or more co-authors or co-workers.

et seq.—and what follows.

EU—European Union.

Eur. P.—see Ph. Eur.

Ext. D & C—designation applied in USA to dyes permitted for use in external drug and cosmetic preparations.

°F—degrees Fahrenheit.

FAC—Food Additives and Contaminants Committee of the Ministry of Agriculture, Fisheries and Food (UK).

FAO—Food and Agriculture Organization of the United Nations.

FAO/WHO—Food and Agriculture Organization of the United Nations *and the* World Health Organization.

FDA—Food and Drug Administration of USA.

FdAC—Food Advisory Committee of the Ministry of Agriculture, Fisheries and Food (UK).

FD & C—designation applied in USA to dyes permitted for use in foods, drugs, and cosmetics.

FEV$_1$—forced expiratory volume in 1 second.

Fin.—Finland.

FIP—Fédération Internationale Pharmaceutique.

f.p.—freezing point.

FPA—Family Planning Association (UK).

Fr.—France.

Fr. P.—French Pharmacopoeia 1982 (Pharmacopée Francaise, Xe Edition) and Supplements 1 to 13.

g—gram(s).

Ger.—Germany.

Ger. P.— German Pharmacopoeia (Deutsches Arzneibuch, 1999).

GFR—glomerular filtration rate.

Hb— haemoglobin.

Hib—*Haemophilus influenzae* type b.

HIV—human immunodeficiency virus.

HLA—human lymphocyte antigens.

HLB—hydrophilic-lipophilic balance.

HRT—hormone replacement therapy.

HSE—Health and Safety Executive (UK).

Hung.—Hungary.

IARC—International Agency for Research on Cancer.

ibid.—*ibidem*, 'in the same place (journal or book)'.

idem—'the same': used for the same authors and titles.

i.e.—*id est*, 'that is'.

Ig—immunoglobulin.

INN—International Nonproprietary Name.

Int. P.—International Pharmacopoeia 3rd ed., Volume 1, 1979; Volume 2, 1981; Volume 3, 1988; and Volume 4, 1994.

IPCS—International Programme on Chemical Safety.

IQ—intelligence quotient.

Irl.—Ireland.

It. P.—Italian Pharmacopoeia 1985 (Farmacopea Ufficiale della Repubblica Italiana, Edizione Nona) and Supplements 1 to 3.

Ital.—Italy.

iu—international unit(s).

IUD—intra-uterine device.

IUPAC—International Union of Pure and Applied Chemistry.

J—joule(s).

Jpn—Japan.

Jpn P.—The Pharmacopoeia of Japan, 13th ed., 1996 and Supplements 1 and 2.

K—kelvin.

kcal—kilocalorie(s).

kg—kilogram(s).

kJ—kilojoule(s).

lb—pound(s) avoirdupois.

LD$_{50}$—a dose lethal to 50% of the specified animals or micro-organisms.

m—metre(s).

m^2—square metre(s).

m^3—cubic metre(s).

M—molar.

MAFF—Ministry of Agriculture, Fisheries and Food (UK).

MAOI—monoamine oxidase inhibitor.

max.—maximum.

MBC—minimum bactericidal concentration.

MCA—Medicines Control Agency (UK).

mEq—milliequivalent(s).

Mex.—Mexico.

mg—milligram(s).

MIC—minimum inhibitory concentration.

min—minute.

min.—minimum.

MJ—megajoule(s).

mL—millilitre(s).

mm—millimetre(s).

mm^2—square millimetre(s).

mm^3—cubic millimetre(s).

mmHg—millimetre(s) of mercury.

mmol—millimole.

mol—mole.

mol. wt—molecular weight.

Mon.—Monaco.

mosmol—milliosmole.

m.p.—melting point.

MRC—Medical Research Council (UK).

µg—microgram(s).

µL—microlitre(s).

µm—micrometre(s).

Neth.—The Netherlands.

Neth. P.—Netherlands Pharmacopoeia 1983 (Nederlandse Farmacopee, Negende Uitgave) and Supplements to 1993.

ng—nanogram(s).

NIH—National Institutes of Health (USA).

nm—nanometre(s).

Norw.—Norway.

NSAID—nonsteroidal anti-inflammatory drug.

NZ—New Zealand.

OP—over proof.

o/w—oil-in-water.

P—probability.

Pa—pascal(s).

pCO$_2$—plasma partial pressure (concentration) of carbon dioxide.

p$_a$CO$_2$—arterial plasma partial pressure (concentration) of carbon dioxide.

pg—picogram(s).

pH—the negative logarithm of the hydrogen ion concentration.

Ph. Eur.—European Pharmacopoeia, 4th ed., 2002 and Supplement 4.1.

Pharm. Soc. Lab. Rep.—Royal Pharmaceutical Society's Laboratory Report.

PHLS—Public Health Laboratory Service (UK).

pINN—Proposed International Nonproprietary Name.

pINNM—Proposed International Nonproprietary Name Modified.

pK$_a$—the negative logarithm of the dissociation constant.

p.m.—*post meridiem*, 'afternoon'.

pO$_2$—plasma partial pressure (concentration) of oxygen.

p$_a$O$_2$—arterial plasma partial pressure (concentration) of oxygen.

Pol.—Poland.

Pol. P.—Polish Pharmacopoeia (Farmakopea Polska) 5th ed., Volume 1, 1990; Volume 2, 1993; Supplement 1, 1995; Volume 3, 1996.

Port.—Portugal.

Port. P.—Portuguese Pharmacopoeia 1986 (Farmacopoeia Portuguesa V) and Supplements to 1991.

ppm—parts per million.

PSGB—The Pharmaceutical Society of Great Britain. Now the Royal Pharmaceutical Society of Great Britain.

q.s.—*quantum sufficit*, 'as much as suffices'.

q.v.—*quod vide*, 'which see'.

RCGP—Royal College of General Practitioners (UK).

RIMA—reversible inhibitor of monoamine oxidase type A.

rINN—Recommended International Nonproprietary Name.

rINNM—Recommended International Nonproprietary Name Modified.

RNA—ribonucleic acid.

RPSGB—The Royal Pharmaceutical Society of Great Britain.

S. Afr.—South Africa.

SGOT—serum glutamic oxaloacetic transaminase (serum aspartate aminotransferase *now preferred*).

SGPT—serum glutamic pyruvic transaminase (serum alanine aminotransferase *now preferred*).

SI—Statutory Instrument *or* Système International d'Unités (International System of Units).

sic—written exactly as it appears in the original.

SLE—systemic lupus erythematosus.

sp.—species (plural spp.).

sp. gr.—specific gravity.

SSRI—selective serotonin reuptake inhibitor.

St—stokes.

subsp.—subspecies.

suppl—supplement(s).

Swed.—Sweden.

Swiss P.—Swiss Pharmacopoeia 1997 (Pharmacopoea Helvetica, 8e édition, Edition Française) and Supplement 1998.

Switz.—Switzerland.

Thai.—Thailand.

TPN—total parenteral nutrition.

UAE—United Arab Emirates.

UK—United Kingdom.

UNICEF—United Nations Children's Fund.

UP—under proof.

US and *USA*—United States of America.

USAN—United States Adopted Name.

USNF—The United States 'National Formulary 20', 2002.

USP—The United States Pharmacopeia 25, 2002.

UV—ultraviolet.

var.—variety.

vol.—volume(s).

v/v—volume in volume.

v/w—volume in weight.

WHO—World Health Organization.

w/o—water-in-oil.

wt—weight.

wt per mL—weight per millilitre.

w/v—weight in volume.

w/w—weight in weight.

Contracted Names for Ions and Groups

Contracted Name	Chemical Name
acetonide	isopropylidene ether of a dihydric alcohol
aceturate	*N*-acetylglycinate
acistrate	2′-acetate (ester) and stearate (salt)
acoxil	acetoxymethyl
amsonate	4,4′-diaminostilbene-2,2′-disulphonate
anisatil	2-(4-methoxyphenyl)-2-oxoethyl
axetil	1-acetoxyethyl
besilate (besylate)	benzenesulphonate
bezomil	(benzoyloxy)methyl
buciclate	*trans*-4-butylcyclohexanecarboxylate
bunapsilate	3,7-di-*tert*-butylnaphthalene-1,5-disulphonate
buteprate	17-(1-oxobutoxy) (ester) and 21-(1-oxopropoxy) (ester)
camsilate (camsylate)	camphor-10-sulphonate
caproate	hexanoate
carbesilate	4-carboxybenzenesulphonate
ciclotate (cyclotate)	4-methylbicyclo[2.2.2]oct-2-ene-l-carboxylate
cilexetil	(*RS*)-1-{[(cyclohexyloxy)carbonyl]oxy}ethyl
cipionate (cypionate)	3-cyclopentylpropionate
closilate (closylate)	4-chlorobenzenesulphonate
crobefate	(±)-(*E*)-6-hydroxy-4′-methoxy-3-(*p*-methoxybenzylidene)flavone phosphate ion (2−)
cromacate	[(6-hydroxy-4-methyl-2-oxo-2*H*-chromen-7-yl)oxy]acetate
cromesilate	6,7-dihydroxycoumarin-4-methanesulphonate
deanil	2-dimethylaminoethyl
dibudinate	2,6-di-*tert*-butylnaphthalene-1,5-disulphonate
dibunate	2,6-di-*tert*-butyl-l-naphthalenesulphonate
digolil	2-(2-hydroxyethoxy)ethyl
diolamine	diethanolamine
dofosfate	octadecyl hydrogen phosphate
edamine	ethylenediamine
edetate	ethylenediamine-*NNN′N′*-tetra-acetate
edisilate (edisylate)	ethane-1,2-disulphonate
embonate	4,4′-methylenebis(3-hydroxy-2-naphthoate) (=pamoate)
enantate (enanthate)	heptanoate
epolamine	1-pyrrolidineethanol
erbumine	*tert*-butylamine
esilate (esylate)	ethanesulphonate
estolate	propionate dodecyl sulphate
etabonate	(ethoxycarbonyl)oxy (=ethyl carbonate)
farnesil	(2*E*,6*E*)-3,7,11-trimethyl-2,6,10-dodecatrienyl
fendizoate	2-[(2′-hydroxy-4-biphenylyl)carbonyl]benzoate

Contracted Name	Chemical Name
fostedate	tetradecyl hydrogen phosphate
gluceptate	glucoheptonate
hibenzate (hybenzate)	2-(4-hydroxybenzoyl)benzoate
hyclate	monohydrochloride hemi-ethanolate hemihydrate
isetionate (isethionate)	2-hydroxyethanesulphonate
laurilsulfate (lauryl sulphate)	dodecyl sulphate
megallate	3,4,5-trimethoxybenzoate
meglumine	*N*-methylglucamine
mesilate (mesylate)	methanesulphonate
metembonate	4,4′-methylenebis(3-methoxy-2-naphthoate)
mofetil	2-(morpholino)ethyl
napadisilate (napadisylate)	naphthalene-1,5-disulphonate
napsilate (napsylate)	naphthalene-2-sulphonate
olamine	ethanolamine
oxoglurate	2-oxoglutarate
pamoate	4,4′-methylenebis(3-hydroxy-2-naphthoate) (=embonate)
pendetide	N^6-{*N*-[2-({2-[bis(carboxymethyl)amino]-ethyl}(carboxymethyl)amino)ethyl]-*N*-(carboxymethyl)glycyl}-N^2-(*N*-glycyl-L-tyrosyl)-L-lysine
pentexil	1-hydroxyethyl pivalate
phenpropionate	3-phenylpropionate
pivalate	trimethylacetate
pivoxetil	1-(2-methoxy-2-methylpropionyloxy)ethyl
pivoxil	(2,2-dimethyl-1-oxopropoxy)methyl or (pivaloyloxy)methyl
polistirex	sulphonated styrene-divinylbenzene copolymer complex
probutate	17-(1-oxobutoxy) (ester) and 21-(1-oxopropoxy) (ester)
proxetil	1-[(isopropoxycarbonyl)oxy]ethyl
soproxil	[(isopropoxycarbonyl)oxy]methyl
steaglate	stearoyloxyacetate
suleptanate	sodium 7-[methyl(2-sulphonatomethyl)carbamoyl]heptanoyl
tebutate	*tert*-butylacetate
tenoate	2-thiophenecarboxylate
teoclate (theoclate)	8-chlorotheophyllinate
teprosilate	3-(theophyllin-7-yl)propanesulphonate
tofesilate	2-(theophyllin-7-yl)ethanesulphonate
tosilate (tosylate)	toluene-4-sulphonate
triclofenate	2,4,5-trichlorophenolate
triflutate	trifluoroacetate
trolamine	triethanolamine
troxundate	3,6,9-trioxaundecanoate
xinafoate	1-hydroxy-2-naphthoate

Atomic Weights of the Elements— $^{12}C=12$

Atomic Number	Name	Symbol	Atomic Weight
89	Actinium	Ac	*
13	Aluminium	Al	26.981538
95	Americium	Am	*
51	Antimony	Sb	121.760
18	Argon	Ar	39.948
33	Arsenic	As	74.92160
85	Astatine	At	*
56	Barium	Ba	137.327
97	Berkelium	Bk	*
4	Beryllium	Be	9.012182
83	Bismuth	Bi	208.98038
107	Bohrium	Bh	*
5	Boron	B	10.811
35	Bromine	Br	79.904
48	Cadmium	Cd	112.411
55	Caesium	Cs	132.90545
20	Calcium	Ca	40.078
98	Californium	Cf	*
6	Carbon	C	12.0107
58	Cerium	Ce	140.116
17	Chlorine	Cl	35.453
24	Chromium	Cr	51.9961
27	Cobalt	Co	58.933200
29	Copper	Cu	63.546
96	Curium	Cm	*
105	Dubnium	Db	*
66	Dysprosium	Dy	162.50
99	Einsteinium	Es	*
68	Erbium	Er	167.259
63	Europium	Eu	151.964
100	Fermium	Fm	*
9	Fluorine	F	18.9984032
87	Francium	Fr	*
64	Gadolinium	Gd	157.25
31	Gallium	Ga	69.723
32	Germanium	Ge	72.64
79	Gold	Au	196.96655
72	Hafnium	Hf	178.49
108	Hassium	Hs	*
2	Helium	He	4.002602
67	Holmium	Ho	164.93032
1	Hydrogen	H	1.00794
49	Indium	In	114.818
53	Iodine	I	126.90447
77	Iridium	Ir	192.217
26	Iron	Fe	55.845
36	Krypton	Kr	83.80
57	Lanthanum	La	138.9055
103	Lawrencium	Lr	*
82	Lead	Pb	207.2
3	‡Lithium	Li	6.941
71	Lutetium	Lu	174.967
12	Magnesium	Mg	24.3050
25	Manganese	Mn	54.938049
109	Meitnerium	Mt	*
101	Mendelevium	Md	*
80	Mercury	Hg	200.59
42	Molybdenum	Mo	95.94
60	Neodymium	Nd	144.24
10	Neon	Ne	20.1797
93	Neptunium	Np	*
28	Nickel	Ni	58.6934
41	Niobium	Nb	92.90638
7	Nitrogen	N	14.0067

Atomic Number	Name	Symbol	Atomic Weight
102	Nobelium	No	*
76	Osmium	Os	190.23
8	Oxygen	O	15.9994
46	Palladium	Pd	106.42
15	Phosphorus	P	30.973761
78	Platinum	Pt	195.078
94	Plutonium	Pu	*
84	Polonium	Po	*
19	Potassium	K	39.0983
59	Praseodymium	Pr	140.90765
61	Promethium	Pm	*
91	†Protactinium	Pa	231.03588
88	Radium	Ra	*
86	Radon	Rn	*
75	Rhenium	Re	186.207
45	Rhodium	Rh	102.90550
37	Rubidium	Rb	85.4678
44	Ruthenium	Ru	101.07
104	Rutherfordium	Rf	*
62	Samarium	Sm	150.36
21	Scandium	Sc	44.955910
106	Seaborgium	Sg	*
34	Selenium	Se	78.96
14	Silicon	Si	28.0855
47	Silver	Ag	107.8682
11	Sodium	Na	22.989770
38	Strontium	Sr	87.62
16	Sulfur	S	32.065
73	Tantalum	Ta	180.9479
43	Technetium	Tc	*
52	Tellurium	Te	127.60
65	Terbium	Tb	158.92534
81	Thallium	Tl	204.3833
90	†Thorium	Th	232.0381
69	Thulium	Tm	168.93421
50	Tin	Sn	118.710
22	Titanium	Ti	47.867
74	Tungsten	W	183.84
112	Ununbium	Uub	*
116	Ununhexium	Uuh	*
110	Ununnilium	Uun	*
118	Ununoctium	Uuo	*
114	Ununquadium	Uuq	*
111	Unununium	Uuu	*
92	†Uranium	U	238.02891
23	Vanadium	V	50.9415
54	Xenon	Xe	131.293
70	Ytterbium	Yb	173.04
39	Yttrium	Y	88.90585
30	Zinc	Zn	65.39
40	Zirconium	Zr	91.224

Elements marked (*) have no stable nuclides and IUPAC states "there is no general agreement on which of the isotopes of the radioactive elements is, or is likely to be judged 'important' and various criteria such as 'longest half-life', 'production in quantity', 'used commercially', etc., have been applied in the Commission's choice." However, atomic weights are given for radioactive elements marked (†) as they do have a characteristic terrestrial isotopic composition. Commercially available lithium (‡) materials have atomic weights ranging from 6.939 to 6.996; if a more accurate value is required, it must be determined for the specific material.

Part I

Monographs on Drugs and Ancillary Substances

Analgesics Anti-inflammatory Drugs and Antipyretics

The compounds described in this chapter are used mainly in the relief of pain, inflammation and, sometimes, fever. They can be grouped broadly into one of the categories briefly described below.

Aspirin and other Salicylates
Aspirin and other salicylates have analgesic, anti-inflammatory, and antipyretic properties. Like other NSAIDs (see below) they are inhibitors of the enzyme cyclo-oxygenase; however, aspirin (though not the non-acetylated salicylates) irreversibly acetylates the enzyme whereas other NSAIDs compete with arachidonic acid for the active site. Salicylates are used for the relief of mild to moderate pain, minor febrile conditions, and for acute and chronic inflammatory disorders such as osteoarthritis, rheumatoid arthritis, juvenile idiopathic arthritis, and ankylosing spondylitis. Some salicylates are applied topically in rubefacient preparations for the relief of muscular and rheumatic pain. Aspirin also inhibits platelet aggregation and is used in cardiovascular disorders. Non-acetylated salicylates do not have antiplatelet activity.

For further discussion of the actions and uses of salicylates, see Aspirin, p.14.

Described in this chapter are

Disease-modifying Antirheumatic Drugs
Disease-modifying antirheumatic drugs (DMARDs) have anti-inflammatory properties thought to be mediated, in some cases, by the inhibition of the release or activity of cytokines. They are used in the treatment of rheumatoid arthritis and juvenile idiopathic arthritis; some are also of benefit in psoriatic arthritis. Many DMARDs also possess other therapeutic properties and are use in a wide variety of non-rheumatic conditions. The DMARD gold is referred to below; DMARDs discussed in other chapters include the antimalarials chloroquine (p.432) and hydroxychloroquine (p.437), sulfasalazine (p.1251), penicillamine (p.1017), and the immunosuppressants azathioprine (p.509), ciclosporin

(p.518), cyclophosphamide (p.527), etanercept (p.1608), infliximab (p.1228), leflunomide (p.549) and methotrexate (p.553).

Gold compounds. Gold compounds are used mainly for their anti-inflammatory effect in active progressive rheumatoid arthritis and progressive juvenile idiopathic arthritis; they may also be beneficial in psoriatic arthritis. The mechanism of action of gold compounds in rheumatic disorders is as yet unknown.

For further discussion of the actions and uses of gold compounds, see Sodium Aurothiomalate, p.82.

Described in this chapter are

Nonsteroidal Anti-inflammatory Drugs
Nonsteroidal anti-inflammatory drugs (NSAIDs) are a group of unrelated organic acids that have analgesic, anti-inflammatory, and antipyretic properties (see p.63). NSAIDs are inhibitors of the enzyme cyclo-oxygenase, and so directly inhibit the biosynthesis of prostaglandins and thromboxanes from arachidonic acid (see p.1438). There are 2 forms of cyclo-oxygenase, COX-1, which is the constitutive form of the enzyme, and COX-2, which is the form induced in the presence of inflammation. Inhibition of COX-2 is therefore thought to be responsible for at least some of the analgesic, anti-inflammatory, and antipyretic properties of NSAIDs whereas inhibition of COX-1 is thought to produce some of their toxic effects, particularly those on the gastrointestinal tract. Most of the NSAIDs currently available for clinical use inhibit both COX-1 and COX-2, although selective COX-2 inhibitors such as celecoxib and rofecoxib are becoming available.

NSAIDs are used for the relief of mild to moderate pain, minor febrile conditions, and for acute and chronic inflammatory disorders such as osteoarthritis, rheumatoid arthritis, juvenile idiopathic arthritis, and ankylosing spondylitis. Indometacin and some other NSAIDs are used to close patent ductus arteriosus in premature neonates. Some NSAIDs are applied topically for the relief of muscular and rheumatic pain, and some are used in ophthalmic preparations for ocular inflammatory disorders. Aspirin (see above) is considered to be an NSAID, although it has other properties.

Described in this chapter are

Opioid Analgesics
Opioid analgesics include the opium alkaloids morphine and codeine and their derivatives as well as synthetic substances with agonist, partial agonist, or mixed agonist and antagonist activity at opioid receptors (see p.66). The term opiate analgesics refers only to those opioids derived from opium, or their semisynthetic congeners. The term narcotic analgesics has legal connotations and is no longer used pharmacologically or clinically.

The majority of opioids are used as analgesics, and morphine is the standard against which all other opioid analgesics are compared. Opioids such as codeine or dextropropoxyphene are used in the treatment of less severe pain, and are often combined with non-opioid analgesics such as aspirin, other NSAIDs, or paracetamol. More potent opioids such as morphine are used in severe acute and chronic pain, including cancer pain. Some opioids such as codeine, morphine, and diamorphine are also used as antitussives, although the latter two are usually reserved for use in terminal lung disease. Some opioid analgesics such as fentanyl and its congeners are used mainly as adjuncts to anaesthesia; some of these may also be used in higher doses as the sole anaesthetic drug.

Some opioids are not used as analgesics and are described elsewhere; they include the antitussives dextromethorphan (p.1087) and pholcodine (p.1099), and the antidiarrhoeals diphenoxylate (p.1222) and loperamide (p.1231).

Opioids can produce physical dependence and withdrawal symptoms on sudden discontinuation. They are also subject to abuse.

Described in this chapter are

Paracetamol and other Para-aminophenols

Paracetamol is the principal para-aminophenol derivative in use. Acetanilide and phenacetin have generally been replaced by safer analgesics. Propacetamol is hydrolysed to paracetamol in the plasma.

Paracetamol has analgesic and antipyretic properties and weak anti-inflammatory activity. The mechanism of analgesic action remains to be fully elucidated, but may be due to inhibition of prostaglandin synthesis both centrally and peripherally. Paracetamol is used for the relief of mild to moderate pain and minor febrile conditions.

Described in this chapter are

Analgesia and Pain

Pain is defined by the International Association for the Study of Pain as 'an unpleasant sensory and emotional experience associated with actual or potential tissue damage, or described in terms of such damage.'

Under normal circumstances pain is the result of stimulation of peripheral receptors which transmit impulses through pain pathways to the brain. Pain receptors or nociceptors are of two basic types: mechanoheat and polymodal receptors. *Mechanoheat receptors* have a high stimulation threshold and respond to intense or potentially damaging noxious stimuli. These receptors are associated with rapidly conducting thinly myelinated Aδ fibres and their stimulation produces rapid sharp localised pain that serves to activate withdrawal reflexes. The other type of receptors are referred to as *polymodal nociceptors* as they respond to mechanical, thermal, or chemical insults. These receptors are also activated by cellular components that are released following tissue damage. Their impulses are transmitted slowly along unmyelinated C type fibres and produce dull, aching, and poorly localised pain with a slower onset.

Nerve fibres from nociceptors terminate in the dorsal root of the spinal cord before transmission by ascending pathways to the brain. There have been many theories on the processing of pain signals at the spinal level but the 'gate theory' proposed by Melzack and Wall is one of the best known. This theory postulates that the transmission of impulses to the brain is modulated by a gate mechanism in the substantia gelatinosa. Stimulation of small fibres opens the gate and facilitates transmission whereas stimulation of large fibres, which normally carry non-painful sensory input, can close the gate and inhibit transmission. Transmission also appears to be modulated by several other mechanisms which can influence the sensitivity of the gate.

Inflammatory mediators such as bradykinin, histamine, serotonin, and prostaglandins produced in response to tissue damage can produce peripheral sensitisation so that receptors respond to low intensity or innocuous stimuli; central sensitisation also occurs. Pain associated with tissue damage hence results in increased sensitivity of the sensory system so that the pain can occur in the absence of a clear stimulus. There may be a reduction in the pain threshold (*allodynia*) resulting in an exaggerated response (*hyperalgesia*) or a prolonged effect (*hyperpathia*).

Pain is often classified as being acute or chronic in nature. **Acute pain** is associated with trauma or disease and usually has a well-defined location, character, and timing. It is accompanied by symptoms of autonomic hyperactivity such as tachycardia, hypertension, sweating, and mydriasis. **Chronic pain** is usually regarded as pain lasting more than a few months and is not necessarily readily associated with trauma or disease; its localisation, character, and timing are more vague than with acute pain. Furthermore, as the autonomic nervous system adapts, the signs of autonomic hyperactivity associated with acute pain disappear. Some forms of pain regarded as being chronic may consist of intermittent attacks of pain followed by relatively long pain-free periods. Patients with chronic pain experience physical, psychological, social, and functional deterioration which contributes towards exacerbation of the pain.

Physiologically, pain may be divided into nociceptive pain and neuropathic pain. **Nociceptive pain** follows activation of nociceptors by noxious stimuli as described above but is not associated with injury to peripheral nerves or the CNS. It may be somatic or visceral, depending on which receptors or nerves are involved. *Somatic pain* is usually well localised and may be described as deeply located, sharp or dull, nagging, stabbing, throbbing, or pressure-like. *Visceral pain* is generally less localised and more diffuse than somatic pain and may be referred to remote areas of the body. Depending on the structure involved it is variously described as deeply located, aching, nagging, cramping, or pressing and may be accompanied by nausea and vomiting. Nociceptive pain usually responds to treatment with conventional analgesics.

Pain resulting from damage or dysfunction of peripheral nerves/receptors or of the CNS is known as **neuropathic pain** (or neurogenic pain). The term covers *sympathetically maintained pain* including causalgia and reflex sympathetic dystrophy, and painful conditions such as postherpetic and trigeminal neuralgia, and diabetic neuropathy. Neuropathic pain associated with central nervous tissue, such as in central post-stroke pain (the thalamic syndrome) is referred to as *central pain*. The clinical signs of neuropathic pain can vary greatly. Some of the more common features include heightened pain sensitivity and sensations of superficial burning or stabbing (lancinating) pain. The pain may be associated with areas of sensory deficit or some form of autonomic instability. Neuropathic pain responds poorly to conventional analgesics and can be difficult to treat.

Early **treatment** of pain is important as unrelieved pain can have profound psychological effects on the patient, and acute pain that is poorly managed initially can degenerate into chronic pain, which may prove to be much more difficult to treat. It is also important to assess and treat the mental and emotional aspects of the pain as well as its physical aspects. Although drug therapy is the mainstay of pain treatment (see below) other methods that may be tried include physical methods such as physiotherapy and surgery; physiotherapy may include massage and the application of heat and cold in many forms. A number of other physical methods are also used in the management of pain; these include nervous system stimulation techniques such as acupuncture and transcutaneous electrical nerve stimulation (TENS).

◊ General references to pain and its management.

1. Melzack R, Wall PD. Pain mechanisms: a new theory. *Science* 1965; **150:** 971–9.
2. International Association for the Study of Pain. Classification of chronic pain: descriptions of chronic pain syndromes and definitions of pain terms. *Pain* 1986; (suppl 3): S1–S225.
3. Lewis KS, *et al.* Effect of analgesic treatment on the physiological consequences of acute pain. *Am J Hosp Pharm* 1994; **51:** 1539–54.
4. Justins DM. Chronic pain management. *Br J Hosp Pharm* 1994; **52:** 12–16.
5. Reidenberg MM, Portenoy RK. The need for an open mind about the treatment of chronic nonmalignant pain. *Clin Pharmacol Ther* 1994; **55:** 367–9.
6. American Pain Society Quality of Care Committee. Quality improvement guidelines for the treatment of acute pain and cancer pain. *JAMA* 1995; **274:** 1874–80.
7. Anonymous. Pain: under-recognized and undertreated? *WHO Drug Inf* 1996; **10:** 36–8.
8. Markenson JA. Mechanisms of chronic pain. *Am J Med* 1996; **101** (suppl 1A): 6S–18S.
9. Katz WA. Approach to the management of nonmalignant pain. *Am J Med* 1996; **101** (suppl 1A): 54S–63S.
10. McQuay H, *et al.* Treating acute pain in hospital. *BMJ* 1997; **314:** 1531–5.
11. American Academy of Pain Medicine and the American Pain Society. The use of opioids for the treatment of chronic pain: a consensus statement. *Clin J Pain* 1997; **13:** 6–8.
12. American Society of Anesthesiologists Task Force on Pain Management, Chronic Pain Section. Practice guidelines for chronic pain management. *Anesthesiology* 1997; **86:** 995–1004.
13. Barnes J, White A. Acupuncture. *Pharm J* 1998; **260:** 664–7.
14. Loeser JD, Melzack R. Pain: an overview. Available at: http://www.thelancet.com/journal/vol357/iss1/full/llan.357.s1.pain_series.15830.1 (accessed 06/09/01).
15. Ashburn MA, Staats PS. Management of chronic pain. Available at: http://www.thelancet.com/journal/vol357/iss1/full/llan.357.s1.pain_series.15831.1 (accessed 06/09/01).
16. Woolf CJ, Mannion RJ. Neuropathic pain: aetiology, symptoms, mechanisms, and management. Available at: http://www.thelancet.com/journal/vol357/iss1/full/llan.357.s1.pain_series.15832.1 (accessed 06/09/01).
17. Carr DB, Goudas LC. Acute pain. Available at: http://www.thelancet.com/journal/vol357/iss1/full/llan.357.s1.pain_series.15828.1 (accessed 06/09/01).
18. Cervero F, Laird JMA. Visceral pain. Available at: http://www.thelancet.com/journal/vol357/iss1/full/llan.357.s1.pain_series.15834.1 (accessed 06/09/01).

Choice of Analgesic

Paracetamol and **aspirin** and **other NSAIDs** are the first choice analgesics for treating mild or moderate pain and are also used in moderate or severe pain to potentiate the effects of opioids. They are suitable for use in acute or chronic pain. Aspirin and paracetamol are of similar potency in most types of pain but paracetamol only has a weak anti-inflammatory effect. NSAIDs are particularly effective in bone pain of malignant origin and pain due to inflammation. Dependence and tolerance are not a problem with non-opioid analgesics but as the dose is increased, their efficacy reaches a ceiling. Most NSAIDs have a greater analgesic effect than aspirin or paracetamol in single doses but it has not been established whether this is true when used repeatedly in chronic pain. Aspirin and other NSAIDs inhibit blood platelet function, adversely affect the gastrointestinal tract, and can precipitate hypersensitivity reactions including asthma. Paracetamol does not have the haematological or gastrointestinal adverse effects of aspirin but large doses can produce severe or sometimes fatal hepatotoxicity.

For the treatment of moderate or moderate to severe opioid-sensitive pain **codeine** is the traditional choice; alternatives include **dextropropoxyphene** and **dihydrocodeine**. They are often given together with non-opioid analgesics. Combinations of codeine with paracetamol produce a small but significant increase in analgesia compared with paracetamol alone and might be appropriate for occasional pain relief, but the incidence of adverse effects increases with repeated use. Combinations of dextropropoxyphene with paracetamol are no more effective than paracetamol alone for acute pain; efficacy in chronic pain is unclear and adverse effects may become troublesome.

More potent opioids such as **morphine** are mainly used in the treatment of severe acute non-malignant pain and cancer pain (see below). Their use in chronic non-malignant pain is somewhat controversial because of fears of psychological dependence and respiratory depression. However, in practice such problems rarely occur and those fears should not prevent patients being given effective analgesic therapy.

Morphine is the opioid of choice in severe pain. It is well absorbed when given orally and has a short half-life so that administration of an immediate-release oral preparation offers a flexible means of dosage titration. Once initial pain relief has been achieved, administration of modified-release morphine tablets every 12 hours is more convenient for maintenance of analgesia in severe chronic pain. Other routes may be used such as intramuscular or intravenous injection for emergency pain control or intermittent infusion for patient-controlled analgesia (see also below). Alternative routes should also be used where there would be problems with oral administration as in patients with persistent vomiting or at risk of vomiting, or with dysphagia, malabsorption, delayed gastric emptying, or intestinal obstruction.

Occasionally **other opioids** may be useful as an alternative to morphine. Methadone, levorphanol, or oxycodone have a longer duration of action than morphine, but it should be noted that methadone and levorphanol, which have long half-lives, may accumulate and therefore should not be used long term because of progressive CNS effects. A rapid onset of action is provided by pethidine, alfentanil, and fentanyl, and dextromoramide is useful if a short action is needed. Diamorphine may be preferred to morphine when the parenteral route has to be used because it is more soluble and can be given in a smaller volume.

Adverse effects of opioids include sedation, nausea, vomiting, constipation, and, most seriously, respiratory depression. Tolerance generally develops to all of these effects except constipation, which may be prevented by regular use of laxatives.

A number of other groups of drugs have significant roles in pain management either alone or as **analgesic adjuvants**.

Subantidepressant doses of tricyclic **antidepressants** (usually amitriptyline) are considered to be useful in refractory chronic pain, including neuropathic pain of the burning, dysaesthetic type such as postherpetic neuralgia and diabetic neuropathy; shooting pain has also been reported to respond. They may be used in addition to conventional analgesics, notably in the treatment of cancer pain of mixed aetiology. There is little evidence for benefit in acute pain although musculoskeletal pain has sometimes responded. Amitriptyline has also been found to be useful for tension-type headache and for the prophylaxis of migraine. The role of other antidepressants in the treatment of neuropathic pain is less clear.

Antiepileptics (often carbamazepine and, more recently, gabapentin) have also been found useful in the relief of neuropathic pain especially when there is a stabbing (lancinating) element, as in trigeminal neuralgia; there have also been reports of efficacy in the treatment of diabetic neuropathy and for migraine prophylaxis.

Benzodiazepines and **other muscle relaxants** such as baclofen or dantrolene are useful for relieving painful muscle spasm in acute or chronic conditions.

Bone modulating drugs such as calcitonin and bisphosphonates may be useful in cancer pain arising from bone metastases (see below) but have a slow onset of action and are second choice to NSAIDs. Bisphosphonates may cause an initial transient increase in bone pain.

Caffeine has been used with the aim of enhancing the effects of non-opioid and opioid analgesics but is of debatable benefit. There are similar doubts about whether caffeine enhances the effect of ergotamine in the treatment of migraine (see Pharmacokinetics, p.453); it may also add to gastrointestinal adverse effects and in large doses can itself cause headache.

Corticosteroids have produced improvement, often substantial, in neuropathic pain. They can also relieve headache caused by raised intracranial pressure and refractory pain caused by bone metastases, and have the added benefits of increasing well-being and appetite.

Some **inhalational anaesthetics** are employed in subanaesthetic doses as inhalation analgesics for acute pain. In particular, nitrous oxide is given with oxygen for pain relief in obstetrics and during dental and other procedures, and in emergency management. Isoflurane, enflurane, and in some countries methoxyflurane or trichloroethylene have been used similarly.

Miscellaneous drugs. Following the discovery that epidural or intrathecal injection of opioids can produce effective analgesia many other drugs have been tried by these routes, either alone or with opioids or local anaesthetics, but their role, if any, in the management of pain remains to be determined. Some of these drugs, such as clonidine and ketamine, also appear to have analgesic properties when given by other routes. Some antiarrhythmics may be effective in chronic neuropathic pain, but must be used with extreme caution. The use of antipsychotics, such as the phenothiazines, as adjuvant analgesics is controversial; methotrimeprazine [levomepromazine] is sometimes used as an adjunct in palliative care.

See below for discussions of the use of nerve blocks, patient-controlled analgesia, and rubefacients and topical analgesics.

References.
1. Pon D, Hart LL. IV lidocaine as an analgesic. *DICP Ann Pharmacother* 1989; **23:** 602–4.
2. American Pain Society. Principles of analgesic use in the treatment of acute pain and chronic cancer pain, 2nd edition. *Clin Pharm* 1990; **9:** 601–11.
3. Bushnell TG, Justins DM. Choosing the right analgesic: a guide to selection. *Drugs* 1993; **46:** 394–408.
4. Rummans TA. Nonopioid agents for treatment of acute and subacute pain. *Mayo Clin Proc* 1994; **69:** 481–90.
5. Patt RB, et al. The neuroleptics as adjuvant analgesics. *J Pain Symptom Manage* 1994; **9:** 446–53.
6. Sawynok J. Pharmacological rationale for the clinical use of caffeine. *Drugs* 1995; **49:** 37–50.
7. McQuay H, et al. Anticonvulsant drugs for management of pain: a systematic review. *BMJ* 1995; **311:** 1047–52.
8. McQuay HJ, et al. A systematic review of antidepressants in neuropathic pain. *Pain* 1996; **68:** 217–27.
9. McQuay HJ, Moore RA. Antidepressants and chronic pain: effective analgesia in neuropathic pain and other syndromes. *BMJ* 1997; **314:** 763–4.
10. Anonymous. Drugs for pain. *Med Lett Drugs Ther* 1998; **40:** 79–84.
11. Tremont-Lukats IW, et al. Anticonvulsants for neuropathic pain syndrome: mechanisms of action and place in therapy. *Drugs* 2000; **60:** 1029–52.

Choice of analgesics in children

Pain has often been undertreated in infants and children because of fears of respiratory depression, cardiovascular collapse, depressed levels of consciousness, and addiction with potent opioid analgesics. Assessment of pain is also a problem in children of all ages and it is not that long since it was widely believed that neonates were incapable of feeling pain.

INFANTS AND CHILDREN

In infants and children **opioids** are still the mainstay of analgesia for moderate to severe pain and morphine is the standard against which the others are compared. Continuous intravenous infusion with or without initial loading doses has become popular for postoperative pain relief, but titration of the infusion rate is necessary to achieve a balance between analgesia and respiratory depression (particular care is needed in neonates, see below). Subcutaneous infusions of morphine have also been used, mostly for the relief of terminal cancer pain in children. Intramuscular injections can provide excellent analgesia but are painful and therefore probably only suitable for short-term use. Fentanyl has also been widely used for short-term analgesia in surgical procedures. Other opioid analgesics used in infants and children have included codeine, buprenorphine, meptazinol, nalbuphine, papaveretum, and pethidine. Patient-controlled analgesia using morphine has been tried in children (see below).

Morphine has also been given to children by the epidural route; experience with the intrathecal route is more limited. Other methods of opioid drug delivery of possible value in paediatric analgesia include transmucosal, nasal, and transdermal administration.

Local anaesthetics are especially suitable for the management of acute pain in day-care situations. Single injections given by the epidural route are often used to provide analgesia during and after surgery. Continuous epidural infusions of local anaesthetics have also been used. However, simpler techniques such as wound infiltration or peripheral nerve blocks can also provide effective analgesia for some procedures and are free of the problems of lower limb weakness or urinary retention associated with caudal blocks. Application of eutectic creams (see p.1316) containing lignocaine [lidocaine] with prilocaine to intact skin, to produce surface anaesthesia, may be sufficient for some minor painful procedures in children, although use in those under 1 year of age is not recommended.

Non-opioid analgesics are used in children, either alone for minor pain or as an adjunct to opioid analgesics in severe pain. Paracetamol is frequently employed but it lacks any anti-inflammatory effect. NSAIDs are useful for pain associated with inflammation. The use of aspirin is greatly restricted by its association with Reye's syndrome.

Cancer pain in children may be treated using the analgesic ladder scheme described under Cancer Pain (see below).

Ketamine is used in outpatients for brief, painful procedures such as fracture reduction and to provide immobility for repair of facial lacerations in young children. The emergence reactions that limit its use in adults are less common in children.

NEONATES

Most neonates requiring analgesia and receiving respiratory support can be managed with an infusion of morphine but in neonates who are breathing spontaneously there is a substantial risk of respiratory depression. Morphine has been used in such neonates but should be limited to those under intensive care, as for example after major surgery (see also Intensive Care under Sedation, p.652). Fentanyl citrate and codeine phosphate have also been used in neonates. **Sucrose** and other sweet tasting solutions have been shown to reduce physiologic and behavioural indicators of stress and pain in neonates undergoing painful procedures although there had been some doubt expressed over whether this indicates effective analgesia.

References.
1. Lloyd-Thomas AR. Pain management in paediatric patients. *Br J Anaesth* 1990; **64:** 85–104.
2. Commission on the provision of surgical services. *Report of the working party on pain after surgery.* London: Royal College of Surgeons of England and Anaesthetists, 1990.
3. Schecter NL, et al. Report on the consensus conference on the management of pain in childhood cancer. *Pediatrics* 1990; **86:** 813–34.
4. Gaukroger PB. Paediatric analgesia: which drug? which dose? *Drugs* 1991; **41:** 52–9.
5. Bhatt-Mehta V, Rosen DA. Management of acute pain in children. *Clin Pharm* 1991; **10:** 667–85.
6. Selbst SM. Analgesia in children: why is it underused in emergency departments? *Drug Safety* 1992; **7:** 8–13.
7. Burrows FA, Berde CB. Optimal pain relief in infants and children. *BMJ* 1993; **307:** 815–16.
8. Anonymous. Treating moderate and severe pain in infants. *Drug Ther Bull* 1994; **32:** 21–4.
9. Anonymous. Managing acute pain in children. *Drug Ther Bull* 1995; **33:** 41–4 and 79.
10. Anonymous. Managing chronic pain in children. *Drug Ther Bull* 1995; **33:** 52–5.
11. Bhatt-Mehta V. Current guidelines for the treatment of acute pain in children. *Drugs* 1996; **51:** 760–76.
12. Ball AJ, Ferguson S. Analgesia and analgesic drugs in paediatrics. *Br J Hosp Med* 1996; **55:** 586–90.
13. Anderson BJ, et al. Size, myths and the clinical pharmacokinetics of analgesia in paediatric patients. *Clin Pharmacokinet* 1997; **33:** 313–27.
14. Morton NS. Prevention and control of pain in children. *Br J Anaesth* 1999; **83:** 118–29.
15. American Academy of Pediatrics and Canadian Paediatric Society. Prevention and management of pain and stress in the neonate. *Pediatrics* 2000; **105:** 454–61.
16. Krauss B, Green SM. Sedation and analgesia for procedures in children. *N Engl J Med* 2000; **342:** 938–45.

Nerve blocks

Nerve blocks produce analgesia by interrupting the nervous transmission of pain signals either by temporary inhibition of conduction or by destruction of the nerve. Nerve blocks may be used alone or with analgesics in the management of acute or chronic pain associated with a well-defined anatomical site, especially when the pain is unresponsive to or not adequately controlled by conventional therapy. The route of administration and method employed depend on the site to be blocked but may include peripheral nerve block, autonomic nerve blocks such as sympathetic nerve blocks and coeliac plexus block, and central nerve blocks such as epidural (including caudal) and spinal block. **Local anaesthetics** are used when a temporary effect is required. **Neurolytics** such as phenol or alcohol or freezing of the nerve (cryoanalgesia) produce more prolonged block, but even so the effects may last no more than a few months, and the variable and non-selective neural damage produced correlates poorly with pain relief; some consider the risk of complications to outweigh the benefits obtained.[1]

The use of nerve blocks in the management of cancer has declined following the refinement of the use of conventional analgesics. Some consider that their value may be limited to patients with a life expectancy of 3 months or less[2] and that the main benefit of nerve blocks in cancer is to produce maximum pain relief rapidly. However, others consider that chemical and thermal neurolysis can provide long-term control of severe cancer pain without a substantial incidence of adverse effects.[3] Neurolytic blocks may be of particular value in cancer pain syndromes involving the viscera or the torso, but are rarely applicable in the management of extremity pain.[4] Neuropathic pain is rarely helped by somatic neural block and may even be aggravated,[1] but block of the splanchnic nerves or coeliac plexus with alcohol or phenol is reputed to be effective in relieving severe intractable pain caused by cancer of the pancreas, stomach, small intestine, gallbladder, or other abdominal viscera, especially when the cancer has not spread to the parietal peritoneum.[5] Similar neurolytic blocks preceded by a local anaesthetic have also been used in patients with severe intractable pain of chronic pancreatitis, postcholecystectomy syndrome, or other chronic abdominal visceral diseases unrelieved by medical or surgical therapy.

Central nerve blocks using local anaesthetics with or without **opioids** are used for the management of acute pain such as labour pain during childbirth and postoperative pain; they are also sometimes used for cancer pain.[1,6]

Sympathetic nerve blocks using repeated injections of local anaesthetics or neurolytics have been used for sympathetically maintained pain. Intravenous regional sympathetic block is an alternative when a single limb is involved;[1] guanethidine is one of the drugs that has been used.[7]

Injections of local anaesthetics with or without **corticosteroids** are often used for blocks of localised painful joints. Nerve blocks are also used to block localised painful trigger areas[8] such as postoperative or post-traumatic neuroma formation and for focal muscle pain.

1. Hanks GW, Justins DM. Cancer pain: management. *Lancet* 1992; **339:** 1031–4.
2. WHO. Cancer pain relief and palliative care: report of a WHO expert committee. *WHO Tech Rep Ser 804*, 1990.

3. American Society of Anesthesiologists Task Force on Pain Management, Cancer Pain Section. Practice guidelines for cancer pain management. *Anesthesiology* 1996; **84:** 1243–7.
4. Marshall KA. Managing cancer pain: basic principles and invasive treatments. *Mayo Clin Proc* 1996; **71:** 472–7.
5. Bonica JJ. Management of pain with regional analgesia. *Postgrad Med J* 1984; **60:** 897–904.
6. Hunt R, Massolino J. Spinal bupivacaine for the pain of cancer. *Med J Aust* 1989; **150:** 350.
7. Hannington-Kiff JG. Relief of causalgia in limbs by regional intravenous guanethidine. *BMJ* 1979; **2:** 367–8.
8. Foley KM. The treatment of cancer pain. *N Engl J Med* 1985; **313:** 84–95.

Patient-controlled analgesia

Patient-controlled analgesia involves the use of automated delivery systems that enable patients to administer doses of an analgesic to themselves on demand. Doses of **opioids** are usually given intravenously, their frequency being controlled by each patient within the safety limits of the delivery system. The technique is useful for the control of pain from a variety of causes including postoperative pain[1,2] and has been used successfully by children as young as 5 years of age[3,4] and by the elderly.[5]

The safety and efficacy of patient-controlled opioid analgesia largely depends on the availability of adequately trained staff and reliable pumps designed to minimise the possibility of programming errors or tampering by patients or visitors. There have been isolated reports of patients receiving very large doses through deliberate operation of the system by relatives,[6] electrical interference,[7] or incorrect use by the patient or staff.[8,9]

In the simplest type of patient-controlled analgesia the patient is able to self-administer a fixed bolus dose on demand; further doses are not then permitted until a pre-programmed lockout interval has expired. Bolus doses are adjusted to prevent overdosage but maintain analgesic blood concentrations. Variable-dose patient-controlled analgesia has also been tried in which the patient selects one of several doses, although this method offered no advantage over fixed-dose systems in one study.[10] Some devices allow the dose to be administered as a short infusion to reduce adverse effects associated with high peak concentrations of opioids. In another commonly used method, sometimes described as patient-augmented analgesia, the patient is given a continuous background infusion which is supplemented by self-administered bolus doses. However, with this method patients may receive more opioids without any improvement in analgesia;[11,12] they may also experience more adverse effects such as nausea and vomiting, respiratory depression, drowsiness, and pruritus,[12,13] although this may depend on the size of the dose used for the background infusion.[14] It remains to be seen if there is any advantage with the more sophisticated devices that can be programmed to adjust the background infusion according to the frequency of the bolus demands.

Morphine or pethidine are the most commonly used opioids for patient-controlled analgesia but consideration should be given to the risks from the accumulation of the pethidine metabolite, norpethidine. Oxymorphone or hydromorphone may be useful alternatives, and the agonist-antagonist nalbuphine has been used because of its ceiling effect on respiratory depression. The use of buprenorphine and methadone is limited by their long half-lives, while the action of drugs such as fentanyl and its analogues may be too short.

Most experience has been with the intravenous route, but the intramuscular, subcutaneous, epidural, and intrathecal routes have also been used. Epidural or intrathecal administration may allow the use of smaller doses but the development of respiratory depression can be delayed when using the epidural route; a greater degree of patient monitoring may be required when using either of these routes.[15] Epidural administration of the **local anaesthetic** bupivacaine with an opioid analgesic such as fentanyl has been tried for use in patient-controlled analgesia, and may allow reduced opioid doses, although whether this confers any clinical benefit is questionable.[16]

Other routes are also being investigated.

Inhaled **nitrous oxide** in oxygen has a long history of effective use in patient-controlled analgesia during childbirth; patient-controlled opioid analgesia may not be suitable for such pain.[17]

1. Mitchell RWD, Smith G. The control of acute postoperative pain. *Br J Anaesth* 1989; **63:** 147–58.
2. Rowbotham DJ. The development and safe use of patient-controlled analgesia. *Br J Anaesth* 1992; **68:** 331–2.
3. Berde CB, *et al.* Patient-controlled analgesia in children and adolescents: a randomized, prospective comparison with intramuscular administration of morphine for postoperative analgesia. *J Pediatr* 1991; **118:** 460–6.

4. Irwin M, *et al.* Evaluation of a disposable patient-controlled analgesia device in children. *Br J Anaesth* 1992; **68:** 411–13.
5. Egbert AM, *et al.* Randomized trial of postoperative patient-controlled analgesia vs intramuscular narcotics in frail elderly men. *Arch Intern Med* 1990; **150:** 1897–1903.
6. Lam FY. Patient-controlled analgesia by proxy. *Br J Anaesth* 1993; **70:** 113.
7. Notcutt WG, *et al.* Overdose of opioid from patient-controlled analgesia pumps. *Br J Anaesth* 1992; **69:** 95–7.
8. Farmer M, Harper NJN. Unexpected problems with patient-controlled analgesia. *BMJ* 1992; **304:** 574.
9. Johnson T, Daugherty M. Oversedation with patient controlled analgesia. *Anaesthesia* 1992; **47:** 81–2.
10. Love DR, *et al.* A comparison of variable-dose patient-controlled analgesia with fixed-dose patient-controlled analgesia. *Anesth Analg* 1996; **83:** 1060–4.
11. Parker RK, *et al.* Patient-controlled analgesia: does a concurrent opioid infusion improve pain management after surgery? *JAMA* 1991; **266:** 1947–52.
12. Doyle E, *et al.* Comparison of patient-controlled analgesia with and without a background infusion after lower abdominal surgery in children. *Br J Anaesth* 1993; **71:** 670–3.
13. Smythe MA, *et al.* Patient-controlled analgesia versus patient-controlled analgesia plus continuous infusion after hip replacement surgery. *Ann Pharmacother* 1996; **30:** 224–7.
14. Doyle E, *et al.* Patient-controlled analgesia with low dose background infusions after lower abdominal surgery in children. *Br J Anaesth* 1993; **71:** 818–22.
15. Hill HF, Mather LE. Patient-controlled analgesia: pharmacokinetic and therapeutic considerations. *Clin Pharmacokinet* 1993; **24:** 124–40.
16. Cooper DW, *et al.* Patient-controlled extradural analgesia with bupivacaine, fentanyl, or a mixture of both, after Caesarean section. *Br J Anaesth* 1996; **76:** 611–15.
17. McIntosh DG, Rayburn WF. Patient-controlled analgesia in obstetrics and gynecology. *Obstet Gynecol* 1991; **78:** 1129–35.

Postoperative analgesia

Pain relief following surgery has often been inadequate and it is now recognised that pain control should be adjusted for each patient and each situation. Where it can be done safely, the pain control should be established on a preventative basis (pre-emptive analgesia), but caution is necessary since any residual respiratory depression is liable to be enhanced by injection of an opioid post-operatively.

Opioid analgesics, in particular the pure opioid agonist morphine, are still the mainstay of the treatment of postoperative pain. Opioids can control most postoperative pain, but the desired degree of analgesia needs to be balanced against adverse effects such as nausea, vomiting, and respiratory depression. Alternatives to morphine include alfentanil, fentanyl, papaveretum, and remifentanil. Partial opioid agonists or mixed agonist-antagonists such as buprenorphine, nalbuphine, and meptazinol, although less likely to produce respiratory depression, have a weaker analgesic action than morphine and they are rarely used for postoperative pain. The traditional method of giving a fixed intramuscular dose of an opioid on an 'as required' basis is painful, demanding of nursing time, and can produce widely fluctuating plasma concentrations (with associated risk of sudden respiratory depression). The intravenous route is more satisfactory and is now widely used; an effective means of providing opioid-induced analgesia intravenously in the immediate postoperative period is to administer a variable rate intravenous infusion with an initial bolus dose and subsequent top-up boluses if necessary. Patient-controlled analgesia (see above) has also proved popular by the intravenous route.

Opioids injected centrally via the epidural and intrathecal routes provide excellent analgesia; a catheter can be inserted during surgery to permit continuous infusion or bolus injections; however, there is a high incidence of nausea, vomiting, urinary retention, pruritus, and respiratory depression (which may be delayed, calling for close monitoring of respiratory function). Morphine is the opioid most commonly given centrally, but an opioid such as fentanyl, which is more lipid soluble, may be preferable in the case of epidural injection. The epidural and intrathecal routes have also been used for patient-controlled analgesia. For co-administration of opioids with local anaesthetics, see below.

The oral route is not suitable for opioid administration in the immediate postoperative period, but may be convenient later, when gastrointestinal function has recovered. Opioids have also been given in the treatment of postoperative pain by the rectal, subcutaneous, sublingual, buccal, transdermal, and intranasal routes, but, because of unreliable absorption and/or slow onset of action, these routes are not usually suitable for use immediately after surgery.

The lack of sedative effects with **NSAIDs** makes them of particular value in the management of acute pain after day-case surgery, but they are usually considered to be unsuitable as sole analgesics immediately after major surgery. They can, however, be used effectively with other drugs, and concomitant use of an NSAID with an opioid enables the dose of the opioid to be reduced without loss of analgesic effect. However, the risk of gastric ulceration, impaired coagulation, and reduced renal function may limit the use of NSAIDs in some patients. Diclofenac, flurbiprofen, ketoprofen, and ketorolac are among the NSAIDs used for postoperative pain. Diclofenac, ketoprofen, and ketorolac may be given by injection.

Nerve blocks with **local anaesthetics** carried out during surgery often produce profound analgesia in the immediate postoperative period. However, effects are only temporary and repeated administration may be impractical. Local infiltration of anaesthetic at the site of operation is a simple method of preventing postoperative wound pain. Central nerve blocks obtained with epidural or intrathecal administration of local anaesthetics produce excellent analgesia and use of a long-acting drug such as bupivacaine can produce prolonged pain relief. Insertion of a catheter during the operation allows subsequent administration by infusion or bolus injection. Hypotension is a potentially serious problem with central nerve blocks and necessitates constant monitoring of blood pressure. Administration of mixtures of opioids and local anaesthetics epidurally or intrathecally has permitted good postoperative analgesia to be obtained in some situations using relatively smaller doses of each drug. A wide range of **other drugs** such as clonidine has also been tried by these routes, either alone or with opioids or local anaesthetics, but their role, if any, remains to be determined.

References.

1. Commission on the provision of surgical services. *Report of the working party on pain after surgery.* London: Royal College of Surgeons of England and College of Anaesthetists, 1990.
2. Anonymous. Managing postoperative pain. *Drug Ther Bull* 1993; **31:** 11–12.
3. Nuutinen LS, *et al.* A risk-benefit appraisal of injectable NSAIDs in the management of postoperative pain. *Drug Safety* 1993; **9:** 380–93.
4. Howard R. Preoperative and postoperative pain control. *Arch Dis Child* 1993; **69:** 699–703.
5. Katz J. Preop analgesia for postop pain. *Lancet* 1993; **342:** 65–6.
6. Kehlet H. Postoperative pain relief—what is the issue? *Br J Anaesth* 1994; **72:** 375–8.
7. Leith S, *et al.* Extradural infusion analgesia for postoperative pain relief. *Br J Anaesth* 1994; **73:** 552–8.
8. Chrubasik S, Chrubasik J. Selection of the optimum opioid for extradural administration in the treatment of postoperative pain. *Br J Anaesth* 1995; **74:** 121–2.
9. Cashman J, McAnulty G. Nonsteroidal anti-inflammatory drugs in perisurgical pain management: mechanisms of action and rationale for optimum use. *Drugs* 1995; **49:** 51–70.
10. American Society of Anesthesiologists Task Force on Pain Management, Acute Pain Section. Practice guidelines for acute pain management in the perioperative setting. *Anesthesiology* 1995; **82:** 1071–81.
11. McQuay HJ. Pre-emptive analgesia: a systematic review of clinical studies. *Ann Med* 1995; **27:** 249–56.
12. Raja SN. Is an ounce of preoperative local anesthetic better than a pound of postoperative analgesic? *Reg Anesth* 1996; **21:** 277–80.
13. Follin SL, Charland SL. Acute pain management: operative or medical procedures and trauma. *Ann Pharmacother* 1997; **31:** 1068–76.
14. Kehlet H, *et al.* Balanced analgesia: what is it and what are its advantages in postoperative pain? *Drugs* 1999; **58:** 793–7.

Rubefacients and topical analgesia

Rubefacients or counter-irritants can relieve superficial or deep-seated pain probably by producing counter stimulation, which according to the 'gate theory' of pain (see Analgesia and Pain, above) helps to inhibit the transmission of pain signals. Their topical application produces hyperaemia or irritation of the skin and they are used alone or as an adjunct to massage in the management of a variety of painful musculoskeletal conditions. Some are also traditionally used in preparations for the symptomatic relief of minor peripheral vascular disorders such as chilblains. Substances commonly used in **rubefacient** preparations include nicotinate and salicylate compounds, essential oils, capsicum, solutions of ammonia, camphor, and nonivamide. **Capsaicin**, which is one of the active ingredients of capsicum, is used alone as a topical analgesic in a range of painful conditions, including neuropathic pain and rheumatic disorders. It does not rely on vasodilatation in the skin and it is therefore not considered to be a traditional counter-irritant.

Some **NSAIDs** have been used topically in the treatment of soft-tissue injuries and inflammatory musculoskeletal conditions, although this route does not necessarily avoid the adverse effects of systemic treatment. There is some evidence[1] to suggest that topical NSAIDs might be more effective than placebo but without comparative studies against other forms of treatment some[2] consider that their therapeutic role is unclear.

Other agents used as topical analgesics include compounds such as ethyl chloride and the halogenated hydrocarbon propellants; their evaporation produces an intense cold that numbs the tissues.

Local anaesthetics are sometimes included in topical preparations used for the relief of painful skin and musculoskeletal disorders.

Application of heat to the skin can also help to relieve pain and melted hard paraffin has been used in wax baths as an adjunct to physiotherapy for painful joints and sprains. Warm kaolin poultices have also been used as a means of applying heat for pain relief.

1. Moore RA, *et al.* Quantitative systematic review of topically applied non-steroidal anti-inflammatory drugs. *BMJ* 1998; **316:** 333–8.
2. Duerden M, *et al.* Topical NSAIDs are better than placebo. *BMJ* 1998; **317:** 280–1.

Specific pain states

Biliary and renal colic. Gallstones (see Ursodeoxycholic Acid, p.1678) or other biliary disorders that result in obstruction of the bile ducts may produce **biliary colic.** Morphine may relieve the accompanying pain, but as it can also produce spasm of the sphincter of Oddi it can raise intrabiliary pressure and exacerbate the pain. It is therefore usually recommended that morphine and its derivatives should either be avoided in patients with biliary disorders or that they should be given with an antispasmodic. Pethidine or phenazocine, which have less smooth muscle activity than morphine, may be more suitable. Prostaglandins have also been implicated in the aetiology of biliary colic and NSAIDs have been successfully used to relieve the pain. Antimuscarinics have been tried for their action on biliary smooth muscle and the sphincter of Oddi.

Ureteral obstruction, such as in the formation and passage of renal calculi (see p.910), produces painful **renal** or **ureteral colic.** The acute pain of renal or ureteral colic may be relieved using opioid analgesics such as pethidine that have a minimal effect on smooth muscle. NSAIDs or antimuscarinics may also be of use. Diclofenac sodium given intramuscularly or rectally appears to be of similar efficacy to pethidine. The use of intranasal desmopressin is being studied.

Cancer pain. The pain cancer patients experience may be acute, chronic, or intermittent. It may result from tumour involvement of the viscera and extension into soft tissues, tumour-induced nerve compression and injury, raised intracranial pressure, or bone metastases. Pain may also arise as a result of side-effects of treatment, or from a concurrent disease, and may be exacerbated by emotional or mental changes. Many patients will have more than one type of pain. There may also be exacerbations due to movement (incident pain) or worsening of cancer.

Pain relief involves the treatment of the cause of the pain as well as treatment of the pain itself, together with explanation, reassurance, and supportive care to improve any mental and social complicating factors. The mainstay of cancer pain management is drug treatment with non-opioid or opioid analgesics, or both together, plus adjuvant analgesics if necessary. A small proportion of patients (about 10 to 20%) may experience pain that responds poorly or not at all to opioid analgesics given at tolerable doses, e.g. neuropathic pain resulting from nerve destruction or compression, incident bone pain, pancreatic pain, and muscle spasm.

In the management of cancer pain the aim is to achieve adequate continuous pain relief with the minimum of side-effects and this calls for regular monitoring of the treatment. Guidelines for the relief of cancer pain, published by WHO in 1986[1] and revised in 1996,[2] are widely endorsed by specialists in pain relief and the care of the terminally ill.[3-19] Specific guidelines for the relief of cancer pain in children have also been published.[20] Regardless of age, patients need to be assessed individually and, wherever possible, treatment is given by mouth. It should be given regularly and should follow the accepted three-step **'analgesic ladder'.**[1,2] This approach is often described as treatment 'by mouth, by the clock, and by the ladder'. Regular dosage rather than treatment as required aims to prevent pain re-emerging and to minimise the expectation of pain. The analgesic ladder consists of 3 stages, treatment beginning at step 1 and progressing to step

3 if pain is uncontrolled or increases. The stages are as follows:

1. a non-opioid analgesic such as aspirin, other NSAIDs, or paracetamol; an adjuvant (see below) may also be given if necessary to tackle specific pain or associated symptoms
2. an opioid analgesic such as codeine or dihydrocodeine plus a non-opioid analgesic; an adjuvant may also be given
3. a potent opioid analgesic such as oral morphine; a non-opioid analgesic may also be given, as may an adjuvant.

Using analgesics with different pharmacological actions together can produce additive or synergistic increases in analgesia but only one analgesic from each of the 3 groups (non-opioid, less potent opioid, potent opioid) should be used at the same time.

Unmanageable adverse effects of one analgesic may be eliminated by changing to another. Any sedation should be assessed, for while it may be useful in the management of acute pain, it is undesirable in patients with chronic pain. Although tolerance, physical dependence, and withdrawal symptoms can occur with continued use of opioids, this does not prevent their effective use for cancer pain. Withdrawal symptoms may be avoided by gradually tapering doses on discontinuing a drug. Psychological dependence and addictive behaviour do not occur when opioids are used in cancer patients, so fears of their development should not restrict use of these analgesics, and opioid-sensitive pain appears to protect against respiratory depression, although it may occur if the source of opioid-sensitive pain is removed (e.g. by surgery) without adequate reduction in opioid dosage.

The opioid of choice for moderate to severe pain is morphine. It is given by mouth as a solution or tablets every 4 hours or as modified-release formulations every 12 to 24 hours. Individualisation of dosage by gradual adjustment is important; doses have ranged from 2.5 to over 2500 mg of morphine sulfate every 4 hours, although most patients need far less than 100 mg every 4 hours. In patients receiving modified-release preparations the oral solution or standard tablets are used for breakthrough pain pending an increase in modified-release dosage (for further details see under Uses and Administration of Morphine, p.59). Patients vary in their response to opioids and sequential trials may be needed to identify the drug which yields the most favourable balance between analgesia and adverse effects. Alternatives to morphine include hydromorphone, oxycodone, and fentanyl. 'Brompton Cocktail' mixtures or elixirs, which contained diamorphine or morphine and cocaine with or without chlorpromazine, are now obsolete.

Although the oral route is generally preferred, other routes, such as rectal administration, may be necessary if, for example, there is intractable vomiting, inability to swallow, or unconsciousness. When injections become necessary a continuous subcutaneous infusion may be preferable to repeated subcutaneous or intramuscular injections. In the UK diamorphine hydrochloride is often preferred to morphine sulfate for parenteral administration because it is more soluble and allows a smaller dose volume; hydromorphone hydrochloride is an alternative to diamorphine. Morphine has also been given intravenously by bolus injection or infusion.

Epidural or intrathecal administration of opioids, either by injection or infusion, has been used when conventional routes have failed. Some advocate the use of these routes because smaller doses may produce analgesia equivalent to that of larger doses given by mouth or parenterally, although there has been little conclusive evidence for a lower incidence of side-effects or a better quality of analgesia.

Other routes of administration that have been investigated include buccal, sublingual, and nebulised routes, but these are not recommended for morphine because there is no current evidence of clinical advantage over conventional routes.[15] However, buprenorphine is administered sublingually and may be a useful alternative in patients with dysphagia, although experience of long-term use in cancer pain is limited. Fentanyl can be administered via a transdermal system that provides continuous and controlled delivery for 72 hours. A lozenge-on-a-stick-lollipop dosage form of fentanyl is also available for the management of breakthrough cancer pain.

Automated delivery systems for self-administration of parenteral analgesics (patient-controlled analgesia) have been used to administer opioid analgesics (see above).

Adjuvant drugs that may be necessary at any stage include antidepressants, antiepileptics, and class I antiarrhythmics for neuropathic pain, corticosteroids for nerve compression and headache resulting from raised intracranial pressure, and muscle relaxants for muscle spasm. Radiotherapy and radioisotopes such as strontium-89 may be of use when the bone pain of metastases is unresponsive to NSAIDs alone. Bone modulating drugs such as calcitonin and bisphosphonates may be of additional benefit but have a slow onset of action and bisphosphonates may cause an initial transient increase in pain. Corticosteroids have been used as an alternative to NSAIDs in refractory bone pain but long-term use should be avoided. Nerve blocks with local anaesthetics or neurolytic solutions may benefit a few patients, in particular those with sympathetically maintained pain or specific localised pain (see above). Physiotherapy and relaxation techniques may be useful for painful muscle spasm. Adjuvant therapy should be fully explored before moving on to the next 'rung' of the treatment ladder or increasing the dosage of an opioid analgesic. For further details of analgesic adjuvants, see Choice of Analgesic, above.

1. WHO. *Cancer pain relief.* Geneva: WHO, 1986.
2. WHO. *Cancer pain relief.* 2nd ed. Geneva: WHO, 1996.
3. Hillier R. Control of pain in terminal cancer. *Br Med Bull* 1990; **46:** 279–91.
4. American Pain Society. Principles of analgesic use in the treatment of acute pain and chronic cancer pain, 2nd edition. *Clin Pharm* 1990; **9:** 601–11.
5. WHO. Cancer pain relief and palliative care: report of a WHO expert committee. *WHO Tech Rep Ser 804* 1990.
6. Schechter NL, *et al.* Report of the consensus conference on the management of pain in childhood cancer. *Pediatrics* 1990; **86:** 813–34.
7. Hanks GW, Justins DM. Cancer pain: management. *Lancet* 1992; **339:** 1031–6.
8. Davis CL, Hardy JR. Palliative care. *BMJ* 1994; **308:** 1359–62.
9. Hammack JE, Loprinzi CL. Use of orally administered opioids for cancer-related pain. *Mayo Clin Proc* 1994; **69:** 384–90.
10. Lamer TJ. Treatment of cancer-related pain: when orally administered medications fail. *Mayo Clin Proc* 1994; **69:** 473–80.
11. US Agency for Health Care Policy and Research. Management of cancer pain: adults. *Am J Hosp Pharm* 1994; **51:** 1643–56.
12. American Society of Anesthesiologists Task Force on Pain Management, Cancer Pain Section. Practice guidelines for cancer pain management. *Anesthesiology* 1996; **84:** 1243–57.
13. Marshall KA. Managing cancer pain: basic principles and invasive treatments. *Mayo Clin Proc* 1996; **71:** 472–7.
14. Levy MH. Pharmacologic treatment of cancer pain. *N Engl J Med* 1996; **335:** 1124–32.
15. Expert Working Group of the European Association for Palliative Care. Morphine in cancer pain: modes of administration. *BMJ* 1996; **312:** 823–6.
16. Thürlimann B, de Stoutz ND. Causes and treatment of bone pain of malignant origin. *Drugs* 1996; **51:** 383–98.
17. O'Neill B, Fallon M. ABC of palliative care. Principles of palliative care and pain control. *BMJ* 1997; **315:** 801–4.
18. Sykes J, *et al.* ABC of palliative care. Difficult pain problems. *BMJ* 1997; **315:** 867–9.
19. Portenoy RK, Lesage P. Management of cancer pain. *Lancet* 1999; **353:** 1695–1700.
20. WHO. *Cancer pain relief and palliative care in children.* Geneva: WHO, 1998.

Central post-stroke pain. Central pain is a neuropathic pain arising from lesions of the CNS. Pain following a cerebrovascular accident has been referred to as thalamic syndrome but is now commonly known as central post-stroke pain and may arise not only from classical stroke but also from surgery or trauma to the head. The pain, which has been described as burning, stabbing, and aching, may be mild to intolerable and occurs spontaneously or in response to a mild stimulus.

As for other types of neuropathic pain, opioid analgesics are ineffective and management of central post-stroke pain involves the use of antidepressants such as amitriptyline and antiepileptics including lamotrigine. Early peripheral sympathetic blockade may produce temporary relief in some cases. Mexiletine may be of use in patients with refractory pain. Transcutaneous electrical nerve stimulation (TENS) may occasionally be of help but some advocate brain or spinal cord stimulation. Surgical treatment generally gives disappointing results.

References.
1. Illis LS. Central pain. *BMJ* 1990; **300:** 1284–6.
2. Bowsher D. Cerebrovascular disease: sensory consequences of stroke. *Lancet* 1993; **341:** 156.
3. Bowsher D. The management of central post-stroke pain. *Postgrad Med J* 1995; **71:** 598–604.

Diabetic neuropathy. Sensory polyneuropathy, a complication of diabetes mellitus, is the commonest of the neuropathies producing neuropathic pain. The pain is mainly experienced as a burning sensation, sometimes accompanied by shooting, or aching pain. Painful neuropathy benefits from optimal diabetic control (see p.317). Non-opioid analgesics such as aspirin or other NSAIDs, or paracetamol may be tried, although neuropathic pain is often resistant to conventional analgesics, and the treatment of painful diabetic neuropathy is generally as for postherpetic neuralgia (see below). Relief may be obtained using tricyclic antidepressants with or without a phenothiazine. SSRIs have been tried but studies suggest that they are ineffective or less effective than tricyclic antidepressants. Antiepileptics such as carbamazepine, gabapentin, and phenytoin can be used to control any shooting or stabbing components of the pain. Antiarrhythmics such as lignocaine [lidocaine] given intravenously or mexiletine given orally have been shown to be effective against some components of the pain. Topical application of capsaicin may have some effect.

References.
1. Bowsher D. Neurogenic pain syndromes and their management. *Br Med Bull* 1991; **47**: 644–66.
2. Fedele D, Giugliano D. Peripheral diabetic neuropathy: current recommendations and future prospects for its prevention and management. *Drugs* 1997; **54**: 414–21.
3. Collins SL, *et al.* Antidepressants and anticonvulsants for diabetic neuropathy and postherpetic neuralgia: a quantitative systematic review. *J Pain Symptom Manage* 2000; **20**: 449–58.

Dysmenorrhoea. Dysmenorrhoea is painful menstruation, and in the more common primary form arises from uterine contractions produced by release of prostaglandins from the endometrium in the luteal phase of the menstrual cycle. For this reason, drugs that inhibit ovulation or prostaglandin production are often effective treatments.[1] NSAIDs inhibit cyclo-oxygenase (prostaglandin synthetase) and are usually the drugs of first choice. They are taken at the onset of discomfort and continued for a few days while symptoms persist. Those most commonly used have included aspirin, diflunisal, flurbiprofen, ibuprofen, indometacin, ketoprofen, mefenamic acid, naproxen, and piroxicam. Theoretically, mefenamic acid has the advantage of inhibiting both the synthesis and the peripheral action of prostaglandins, but clinical studies have not consistently shown fenamates to be more effective than other cyclo-oxygenase inhibitors. Paracetamol has also been given for pain relief. A systematic review[2] comparing several of these drugs concluded that ibuprofen appeared to have the best risk-benefit ratio in dysmenorrhoea and was the preferred analgesic; naproxen, mefenamic acid, and aspirin were also effective, but the limited data on paracetamol did not demonstrate such clear benefits.

Patients who fail to respond to analgesics may benefit from the use of progestogens either alone for part of the cycle or more usually together with oestrogens in the form of oral contraceptive preparations.

Antispasmodic drugs such as hyoscine butylbromide are included in some preparations promoted for the relief of spasm associated with dysmenorrhoea but do not generally provide significant relief.

Secondary dysmenorrhoea is associated with various other disorders such as endometriosis, and treatment is primarily aimed at the underlying cause.

1. Shapiro SS. Treatment of dysmenorrhoea and premenstrual syndrome with non-steroidal anti-inflammatory drugs. *Drugs* 1988; **36**: 475–90.
2. Zhang WY, Li Wan Po A. Efficacy of minor analgesics in primary dysmenorrhoea: a systematic review. *Br J Obstet Gynaecol* 1998; **105**: 780–9.

Headache. Aspirin and other NSAIDs, or paracetamol are often tried first for the symptomatic treatment of various types of headache including migraine (p.449) and tension-type headache (p.450). NSAIDs may also be effective for the prophylaxis of migraine, although they are not considered first-line options.

Opioid analgesics such as codeine are sometimes included in oral compound analgesic preparations used in the initial treatment of migraine or tension-type headache, but are best avoided, especially in patients who experience frequent attacks.

Labour pain. It is important to assess the adverse effects, on both the mother and the fetus, when selecting any method for the management of labour pain. Non-drug measures such as relaxation and massage, and warm baths are often advocated, but pharmacological methods of analgesia are requested by the majority of women in labour.[1,2]

The inhalational anaesthetic **nitrous oxide**, given with oxygen, is suitable for self-administration and is commonly used to relieve labour pain. It is relatively safe and can produce substantial analgesia in most patients. Other inhalational analgesics are also sometimes used (see above).

Opioid analgesics have been given systemically in the management of labour pain for many years, although they do not appear to provide adequate analgesia in most patients at a tolerable dosage.[3] Pethidine tends to be the most commonly used drug. Unfortunately, like all

opioids, it can cross the placenta and produce respiratory depression in the fetus and, when given by intramuscular injection, the onset of action can be unpredictable. Intravenous administration by intermittent doses or continuous infusion or patient-controlled intravenous analgesia has been tried in an attempt to improve pain control, but such techniques are thus far not considered superior to epidural blocks (see below) and do not appear to be widely used.[1]

Epidural analgesia with a *local anaesthetic* provides the most effective pain relief during labour.[2] It is considered to be beneficial to both mother and baby, particularly in high-risk cases,[1,4] although it does require management by suitably experienced staff and the availability of resuscitation facilities to avoid maternal complications. In the mother epidural analgesia prevents many of the adverse physiological responses associated with the stress of pain and general anaesthesia. Neonates appear to do better after maternal epidural block than after non-epidural opioid analgesics or general anaesthesia, and the incidence of neonatal mortality may be lower, particularly in low birth-weight neonates.[4]

Epidural block has few contra-indications. In the absence of coagulopathy it may be of particular value in pre-eclampsia as it produces beneficial haemodynamic changes.[4] Serious adverse events are rare and usually arise from administration errors.[1,4] Nonetheless, epidural analgesia has been associated with an increased risk of prolonged labour, forceps delivery, and caesarean section[5] (although meta-analysis[3] refutes the latter), and may not improve maternal experience of childbirth. Profound hypotension can occur as a result of sympathetic block.[6] Other effects may include diminished patient awareness of uterine contractions and of giving birth, sensations of weakness, numbness and paraesthesia of the lower limbs, impaired mobility, bladder distension, and pyrexia or uncontrollable shivering.[1,4] Many of these effects are associated with motor block and can be reduced by using doses of local anaesthetic lower than those required for surgery. Epidural analgesia can also prolong the second stage of labour and the use of oxytocin may be required.[4] However, since a request for epidural analgesia is most likely from women experiencing a slow, complicated, painful labour it is difficult to quantify the effect of the epidural itself.[7,8] Further details of the adverse effects and precautions for epidural block can be found under Central Block on p.1302 and p.1303 respectively. Occasionally epidural administration of local anaesthetics does not produce adequate analgesia due to patchy or incomplete block.[6]

Bupivacaine is one of the local anaesthetics most commonly used in epidural analgesia.

Opioid analgesics have been given epidurally but are not particularly effective for labour pain when used alone.[6,9] Adequate analgesia is usually only obtained with doses that are associated with nausea, sedation, and disorientation.[1] Severe pruritus can also be a problem with some opioids such as morphine. Delayed respiratory depression is also a potential hazard, but may be less of a problem with drugs such as pethidine or fentanyl.[1,6] Epidural opioids are considered to be most useful when given with epidural local anaesthetics. The addition of small doses of opioid analgesics to bupivacaine provides additional pain relief and reduces the amount of local anaesthetic required as well as the degree of motor block.[2,6,9] The addition of an opioid can also control epidural-induced shivering.[9] Several opioids have been tried epidurally with bupivacaine but it has not yet been determined which is the most suitable for pain relief during labour; favourable results have been obtained with drugs such as fentanyl or sufentanil. The use of drugs such as clonidine with local anaesthetics or opioids is also being studied.

Once the initial block is established additional analgesia can be provided through a catheter by intermittent 'top-up' doses or by a continuous epidural infusion;[1,10] a combination of the two methods forms the basis of patient-controlled epidural analgesia.[10-12]

A spinal block given before the epidural block reduces the degree of motor block associated with epidural analgesia and allows the patient to be ambulatory during labour.[11,13-16] Combined **spinal-epidural analgesia** provides the rapid onset of spinal block and the flexibility of continuous epidural block,[7,10] and may have advantages when analgesia is requested late in labour, where maternal distress is severe, and in situations where epidural analgesia has proved unsatisfactory.[12]

Although there is renewed interest in the use of **spinal blocks** in labour[11] they do not appear to have been widely

used alone for the relief of labour pain and it is considered[7] that no single drug or combination of drugs by this route reliably provides adequate analgesia for the duration of labour. The use of spinal blocks in obstetrics has been more commonly associated with anaesthesia and management of postoperative pain in caesarean section.[1,2] Spinal blocks with local anaesthetics have a greater tendency to produce hypotension and headache than epidural blocks, and this appears to be particularly so in pregnant patients.[17] Although spinal block using opioids may control labour pain, some consider that they are unsuitable for use alone because they also produce a greater incidence of adverse effects in pregnant patients.[17] Further details of the adverse effects and precautions for spinal block can be found under Central Block on p.1302 and p.1303 respectively.

Pudendal nerve blocks with lignocaine [lidocaine] followed by administration of a local anaesthetic into the perineum provides pain relief during labour.[2] However, the technique of paracervical local anaesthetic block has been largely abandoned in labour pain[1] because of the high incidence of fetal arrhythmias, acidosis, and asphyxia and isolated reports of fetal death.

1. Brownridge P. Treatment options for the relief of pain during childbirth. *Drugs* 1991; **41**: 69–80.
2. Findley I, Chamberlain G. ABC of labour care. Relief of pain. *BMJ* 1999; **318**: 927–30.
3. Halpern SH, *et al.* Effect of epidural vs parenteral opioid analgesia in the progress of labor. *JAMA* 1998; **280**: 2105–10.
4. Reynolds F. Epidural analgesia in obstetrics. *BMJ* 1989; **299**: 751–2.
5. Thorp JA, *et al.* The effect of intrapartum epidural analgesia on nulliparous labor: a randomized, controlled, prospective trial. *Am J Obstet Gynecol* 1993; **169**: 851–8.
6. Anonymous. Pain relief in labour: old drugs, new route. *Lancet* 1991; **337**: 1446–7.
7. Eberle RL, Norris MC. Labour analgesia: a risk-benefit analysis. *Drug Safety* 1996; **14**: 239–51.
8. McGrady EM. Extradural analgesia: does it affect progress and outcome in labour? *Br J Anaesth* 1997; **78**: 115–17.
9. Reynolds F. Extradural opioids in labour. *Br J Anaesth* 1989; **63**: 251–3.
10. Collis RE. Regional analgesia in labour: a new look. *Hosp Med* 1998; **59**: 388–92.
11. Reynolds F, Hughes SC. Recent developments in analgesia during labour. *Drugs* 1995; **50**: 417–22.
12. Paech M. New epidural techniques for labour analgesia: patient-controlled epidural analgesia and combined spinal-epidural analgesia. *Baillieres Clin Obstet Gynaecol* 1998; **12**: 377–95.
13. Collis RE. Combined spinal epidural analgesia with ability to walk throughout labour. *Lancet* 1993; **341**: 767–8. Correction *ibid.*; 1038.
14. Camann W, Abouleish A. Spinal epidural analgesia and walking throughout labour. *Lancet* 1993; **341**: 1095.
15. Collis RE, *et al.* Randomised comparison of combined spinal-epidural and standard epidural analgesia in labour. *Lancet* 1995; **345**: 1413–16.
16. Nageotte MP, *et al.* Epidural analgesia compared with combined spinal-epidural analgesia during labor in nulliparous women. *N Engl J Med* 1997; **337**: 1715–19.
17. Kestin IG. Spinal anaesthesia in obstetrics. *Br J Anaesth* 1991; **66**: 596–607.

Low back pain. Low back pain (sometimes referred to as lumbago), is a common complaint but only a small percentage of patients suffer from a recognised organic disease, the most frequent identifiable cause being disc disease. In patients with a herniated or prolapsed disc, the rupture of one of the fibrocartilagenous intervertebral discs can exert pressure on spinal nerves and produce a condition characterised by severe and often acute pain radiating from the back along the distribution of the nerves affected. In lumbar disc herniation the sciatic nerve may be involved and patients experience pain (sciatica), usually in one leg along the typical distribution of the nerve.

Treatment for **acute back pain** should be given early to prevent the condition becoming chronic. For simple back pain in the absence of nerve root symptoms or signs of serious spinal pathology paracetamol is tried and if this fails to give relief an NSAID is substituted. If neither of these drugs controls the pain adequately, paracetamol may be combined with an opioid such as codeine; more potent opioid analgesics such as morphine should be avoided if possible. Analgesics should be given regularly rather than when required. A short course of a muscle relaxant such as diazepam or baclofen may also be considered. Unless patients are in severe pain or unable to stand or walk, bed rest is no longer recommended; if it is necessary, bed rest should be limited to up to 3 days. Early physical activity, even if it causes some discomfort, improves the rate of recovery. Specific exercises do not appear to be useful for acute back pain but manipulation may be considered during the first weeks after onset.

Bed rest was often advocated in the treatment of **sciatica** but it has subsequently been found to be no more useful than watchful waiting. Epidural injections of corticosteroids with or without local anaesthetics, using either the caudal or lumbar route, may facilitate recovery. Manipulation should not be used for patients with evidence of nerve root entrapment as it may exacerbate the lesion. Surgery is indicated in patients with herniated disc if conservative treatment fails or if there is severe nerve compression. Dissolution of the disc by injection of enzymes (chemonucleolysis) such as chymopapain or collagenase appears to be an effective alternative to surgery, but anaphylactic reactions may occur.

The prevalence of **chronic or recurrent back problems** is high, and in the majority of cases, the source of the pain cannot be identified. Chronic pain is not necessarily the same as prolonged acute back pain and treatment is difficult. Surgery may be indicated for disc disease (see above) or spondylosis, and local injections of corticosteroids, sclerosant injections into ligaments, or cryotherapy to facet joints have all been tried, but the success rate of these procedures is low. Rehabilitation programmes combining physical and psychological approaches to managing back pain, transcutaneous electrical nerve stimulation (TENS), acupuncture, and neurolytic nerve blocks are other methods that have been tried for intractable chronic back pain.

References.
1. Bush K. Lower back pain and sciatica: how best to manage them. *Br J Hosp Med* 1994; **51**: 216–22.
2. Royal College of General Practitioners. *Clinical guidelines for the management of acute low back pain: low back pain evidence review.* London: Royal College of General Practitioners, 1996.
3. Jayson MIV. Back pain. *BMJ* 1996; **313**: 355–8.
4. Deyo RA. Acute low back pain: a new paradigm for management. *BMJ* 1996; **313**: 1343–4.
5. Jayson MIV. Why does acute back pain become chronic? *BMJ* 1997; **314**: 1639–40.
6. van Tulder MW, *et al.* Conservative treatment of acute and chronic nonspecific low back pain: a systematic review of randomized controlled trials of the most common interventions. *Spine* 1997; **22**: 2128–56.
7. Anonymous. Managing acute low back pain. *Drug Ther Bull* 1998; **12**: 93–5.
8. Vroomen PCAJ, *et al.* Lack of effectiveness of bed rest for sciatica. *N Engl J Med* 1999; **340**: 418–23.
9. Jenner JR, Barry M. Low back pain. In: Snaith ML, ed. *ABC of rheumatology.* 2nd ed. London: BMJ Publishing Group, 1999: 10–13.
10. Malanga GA, Nadler SF. Nonoperative treatment of low back pain. *Mayo Clin Proc* 1999; **74**: 1135–48.
11. Deyo RA, Weinstein JN. Low back pain. *N Engl J Med* 2001; **344**: 363–70.

Myocardial infarction pain. The severe pain of acute myocardial infarction is located in the retrosternal area with radiation to the arms, neck, jaw, and epigastrium. Pain relief is of benefit not only in its own right but also because pain may cause adverse haemodynamic effects such as increases in blood pressure, heart rate, and stroke volume. Although early treatment of the myocardial infarction (p.805) may relieve pain dramatically, opioid analgesics are the first-line treatment for pain and should be given intravenously as soon as possible, that is before hospital admission, to patients with suspected infarction. Opioids can also help to reduce anxiety. An inhaled mixture of nitrous oxide and oxygen has sometimes been used to provide pain relief before arrival in hospital; sublingual glyceryl trinitrate or an alternative fast-acting nitrate may also be given.

Diamorphine or morphine given by slow intravenous injection have generally been the opioids of choice, partly because of a more advantageous haemodynamic profile, but pethidine has also been used. An antiemetic such as metoclopramide or, if left ventricular function is not compromised, cyclizine, by intravenous injection should also be given. The intramuscular route should only be used if venous access is unobtainable since it is relatively ineffective in shocked patients, complicates the enzymatic assessment of the infarction, and may result in large haematomas when patients are given thrombolytics. Alternative analgesics include nalbuphine or buprenorphine, although the latter may not produce pain relief as quickly as diamorphine. The cardiovascular effects of pentazocine make it unsuitable for use during or after myocardial infarction.

References.
1. Herlitz J. Analgesia in myocardial infarction. *Drugs* 1989; **37**: 939–44.
2. Wyllie HR, Dunn FG. Pre-hospital opiate and aspirin administration in patients with suspected myocardial infarction. *BMJ* 1994; **308**: 760–1.
3. Weston CFM, *et al.* Guidelines for the early management of patients with myocardial infarction. *BMJ* 1994; **308**: 767–71.

Neuropathic pain syndromes. The definition and characteristics of neuropathic pain are described under Analgesia and Pain, above. Treatment can be difficult and is best undertaken in specialist pain clinics, since neuropathic pain responds poorly to conventional analgesics.[1] The painful disorders characterised by neuropathic pain (either as the predominant form of pain or as one component of the overall pain) discussed in this

section are Central Post-stroke Pain, Diabetic Neuropathy, Phantom Limb Pain, Postherpetic Neuralgia, Sympathetic Pain Syndromes such as reflex sympathetic dystrophy and causalgia, and Trigeminal Neuralgia.
1. Anonymous. Drug treatment of neuropathic pain. *Drug Ther Bull* 2000; **38**: 89–93.

Orofacial pain. Orofacial pain may arise from a wide range of disorders so its effective management depends very much on the correct identification and treatment of any underlying cause, which may include dental disease, cluster headache (p.449), migraine (p.449), trigeminal neuralgia (see below), sinusitis (p.139), ear disease such as otitis media (p.132), giant cell arteritis (p.1050), aneurysms, and neoplasms. In the treatment of dental pain analgesics are used judiciously as a temporary measure until the underlying cause has been effectively managed. Paracetamol or aspirin or other NSAIDs are adequate for most purposes. Opioid analgesics are relatively ineffective and are rarely needed.

In addition, a large number of patients have a type of facial pain of unknown cause which is typically exacerbated by stress and can develop into a chronic debilitating disorder. Many patients with such idiopathic facial pain respond to non-opioid analgesics, explanation, and reassurance. Antidepressants such as the tricyclics are often of value. Treatment needs to be continued for several months if pain recurrence on withdrawal is to be avoided. Psychological treatments can also be helpful. Botulinum A toxin has been tried for the relief of facial pain associated with some disorders of the orofacial muscles.

References.
1. Hunter S. The management of "psychogenic" orofacial pain. *BMJ* 1992; **304**: 329–30.
2. Feinmann C, Peatfield R. Orofacial neuralgia: diagnosis and treatment guidelines. *Drugs* 1993; **46**: 263–8.

Pancreatic pain. Pain in pancreatitis (p.1646) can be severe and may require the administration of opioid analgesics. Unfortunately, morphine and its derivatives can produce spasm of the sphincter of Oddi, and therefore they need to be given with an antispasmodic. Pethidine has a minimal effect on smooth muscle and may be given intravenously for pain relief in acute pancreatitis; phenazocine is another suitable opioid analgesic.

Concerns over the long-term use of opioids in non-malignant pain should not prevent the patient being given effective analgesia which may be achieved by following the general principles recommended by the WHO for treatment of cancer pain (see above). Mild attacks of pain may be treated using non-opioid analgesics with or without antispasmodics such as antimuscarinics. Patients experiencing inadequate pain relief may progress to opioids such as codeine and then if necessary to more potent opioids such as morphine. Analgesics are given before meals to alleviate the postprandial exacerbation of pain. Administration should be on a regular basis and doses titrated for each patient. Pancreatic extracts may ease the pain but are otherwise reserved for those with symptomatic malabsorption. Coeliac plexus block has been used for the relief of severe intractable pain in some patients with chronic pancreatitis; it has also been used similarly in patients with cancer of the pancreas. However, the benefits of such a block are unclear.

References.
1. Trewby PN. Chronic pancreatitis. *Prescribers' J* 1991; **31**: 111–17.
2. Caraceni A, Portenoy RK. Pain management in patients with pancreatic carcinoma. *Cancer* 1996; **78**: 639–53.
3. Mergener K, Baillie J. Chronic pancreatitis. *Lancet* 1997; **350**: 1379–85.

Phantom limb pain. Phantom limb pain is associated with an amputated limb and is more common when there has been severe pre-amputation pain. It is frequently a mixture of neuropathic and other types of pain. Management may be difficult[1,2] and in a survey of war veteran amputees, for those who took any form of treatment for phantom limb pain, conventional analgesics such as NSAIDs or paracetamol with or without opioid analgesics were reported as being satisfactory.[2] Transcutaneous electrical nerve stimulation (TENS) was another method used by some and considered to be at least as effective as other therapies.[2] Tricyclic antidepressants and antiepileptics may be of help for the neuropathic components of the pain[1,3] and some relief may be obtained with sympathetic blocks.[1] From a review[4] of studies investigating the effect of regional anaesthesia in preventing phantom limb pain in patients undergoing lower-limb amputation it appeared that epidural blockade started before and continuing for the duration of surgery or for several days after amputation conferred more protection from long-term

pain than blockade commenced late intra-operatively or postoperatively. However, a randomised, double-blind, controlled trial[5] failed to demonstrate any beneficial effect of pre-emptive analgesia using epidural blockade in such patients.
1. Stannard CF. Phantom limb pain. *Br J Hosp Med* 1993; **50**: 583–7.
2. Wartan SW, *et al.* Phantom pain and sensation among British veteran amputees. *Br J Anaesth* 1997; **78**: 652–9.
3. Ward A, *et al.* Phantom limb pain—a pain beyond reach? *Hosp Pharm* 1998; **5**: 241–6.
4. Katz J. Prevention of phantom limb pain by regional anaesthesia. *Lancet* 1997; **349**: 519–20.
5. Nikolajsen L, *et al.* Randomised trial of epidural bupivacaine and morphine in prevention of stump and phantom pain in lower-limb amputation. *Lancet* 1997; **350**: 1353–7.

Postherpetic neuralgia. About 10% of patients who have had acute herpes zoster still experience neuropathic pain resulting from peripheral nerve injury one or more months after the rash has healed. The elderly are the most susceptible. The affected area (commonly head, neck, and limbs) is extremely sensitive to any stimuli; even the pressure of clothing can produce unbearable pain. Spontaneous remission of postherpetic neuralgia occurs in many patients within a few months. In a small percentage of patients the pain can last for several years.

Attempts have been made to prevent the development of postherpetic neuralgia. A meta-analysis[1] concluded that, if started within 72 hours of the onset of rash, aciclovir might reduce the incidence of residual pain at 6 months in some patients. A more recent analysis[2] considered that there was only marginal evidence of a decreased incidence of postherpetic neuralgia with aciclovir treatment and that there was no reduction in incidence with either famciclovir or valaciclovir treatments. It is, however, generally agreed that antiviral treatment does reduce the duration of postherpetic neuralgia.[2-4] Other drugs such as corticosteroids and local and regional anaesthesia have also been tried but without noted success in the prevention of postherpetic neuralgia,[5] although corticosteroids may reduce its duration.

Various treatments have been tried once neuralgia develops.[2-10] The value of conventional analgesics is limited because of the neuropathic character of the pain but tricyclic antidepressants appear to help some patients. The early use of low-dose amitriptyline during the acute phase of the disease may also reduce the duration of the neuralgia. Where amitriptyline fails to control the pain an antiepileptic (alone or in combination with a tricyclic) may be helpful. Topical application of capsaicin or lignocaine [lidocaine] may produce some benefit. Nerve blocks and surgical techniques may provide temporary pain relief, but results have generally been disappointing. Transcutaneous electrical nerve stimulation (TENS) has also been tried. Topical preparations of aspirin or indometacin, have shown some promise.
1. 7. Jackson JL, *et al.* The effect of treating herpes zoster with oral acyclovir in preventing postherpetic neuralgia: a meta-analysis. *Arch Intern Med* 1997; **157**: 909–12.
2. Alper BS, Lewis PR. Does treatment of acute herpes zoster prevent or shorten postherpetic neuralgia? *J Fam Pract* 2000; **49**: 255–64.
3. Lee JJ, Gauci CAG. Postherpetic neuralgia: current concepts and management. *Br J Hosp Med* 1994; **52**: 565–70.
4. Kost RG, Straus SE. Postherpetic neuralgia—pathogenesis, treatment, and prevention. *N Engl J Med* 1996; **335**: 32–42.
5. Robertson DRC, George CF. Treatment of post herpetic neuralgia in the elderly. *Br Med Bull* 1990; **46**: 113–123.
6. Anonymous. Postherpetic neuralgia. *Lancet* 1990; **336**: 537–8.
7. Bowsher D. Neurogenic pain syndromes and their management. *Br Med Bull* 1991; **47**: 644–66.
8. Bowsher D. The management of postherpetic neuralgia. *Postgrad Med J* 1997; **73**: 623–9.
9. Collins SL, *et al.* Antidepressants and anticonvulsants for diabetic neuropathy and postherpetic neuralgia: a quantitative systematic review. *J Pain Symptom Manage* 2000; **20**: 449–58.
10. Kanazi GE, *et al.* Treatment of postherpetic neuralgia: an update. *Drugs* 2000; **59**: 1113–26.

Sickle-cell crisis. The management of pain of sickle-cell crisis (p.717) is similar to that of other forms of acute pain. The pain of mild crises may be controlled using analgesics such as paracetamol, an NSAID, codeine, or dihydrocodeine. Partial agonist and antagonist opioids such as buprenorphine are not recommended to treat acute pain before transfer to hospital.[1] Crises severe enough to necessitate hospital admission usually require the use of more potent opioid analgesics such as morphine but NSAIDs may be useful as an adjunct for bone pain. Some patients appear to prefer pethidine to morphine but many workers[2-4] avoid its use if possible as control of pain may be inadequate and doses of pethidine commonly used to manage crises may lead to accumulation of its neuroexcitatory metabolite norpethidine and precipitate seizures (see also Effects on the Nervous System, p.75). Diamorphine has been used as an alternative to morphine. As the dose of opioid required to control the pain can vary considerably, not only during each episode but also from one episode to another and between individual patients, patient-controlled analgesia (see above) may be of help to manage the pain once initial pain relief has been obtained with loading doses of parenteral opioids;[3,5] opioids used have included morphine and fentanyl. The use of continuous epidural analgesia with local anaesthetics alone or in combination with opioids has been tried. A randomised trial[6] of morphine for the management of severe painful sickle-cell crises in children showed that oral modified-release morphine was a safe and effective alternative to continuous intravenous morphine. Inhalation of a mixture of nitrous oxide and oxygen may be a useful analgesic during transfer to hospital.[1]

1. Report of a working party of the Standing Medical Advisory Committee on sickle cell, thalassaemia and other haemoglobinopathies. London: HMSO, 1993.
2. Davies SC, Oni L. Management of patients with sickle cell disease. *BMJ* 1997; 315: 656–60.
3. Vijay V, *et al.* The anaesthetist's role in acute sickle cell crisis. *Br J Anaesth* 1998; 80: 820–8.
4. Pryle BJ, *et al.* Toxicity of norpethidine in sickle cell crisis. *BMJ* 1992; 304: 1478–9.
5. Grundy R, *et al.* Practical management of pain in sickling disorders. *Arch Dis Child* 1993; 69: 256–9.
6. Jacobson SJ, *et al.* Randomised trial of oral morphine for painful episodes of sickle-cell disease in children. *Lancet* 1997; 350: 1358–61.

Sympathetic pain syndromes. Reflex sympathetic dystrophy and causalgia are neuropathic pain syndromes, with apparent involvement of the sympathetic nervous system.

Reflex sympathetic dystrophy (also referred to as complex regional pain syndrome type I, algodystrophy, Sudeck's atrophy, post-traumatic osteoporosis, or shoulder-hand syndrome) is a severely painful syndrome of the limbs. Patients with reflex sympathetic dystrophy who respond to a sympatholytic procedure (see below) have been described as having 'sympathetically maintained pain' while those who do not as having 'sympathetic-independent pain'. Reflex sympathetic dystrophy is usually precipitated by injury or follows lack of use of the affected limb. There may be accompanying autonomic hyperactivity and trophic changes of skin and bone.

Causalgia (complex regional pain syndrome type II) may be regarded as a specific type of reflex sympathetic dystrophy which follows damage to a peripheral nerve. The pain is continuous, diffuse, and burning, and is easily exacerbated. Its onset can be within days or weeks of an initial injury.

Management of reflex sympathetic dystrophy involves treating the causative injury and easing the acute pain, followed by sympathetic nerve block with a local anaesthetic and aggressive physiotherapy. Neurolytic nerve block with phenol has also been tried. Intravenous regional sympathetic block with guanethidine has been used, although opinions as to its efficacy vary.

Stimulation techniques such as transcutaneous electrical nerve stimulation (TENS) have been employed in some patients. Alpha blockers such as phenoxybenzamine or high doses of corticosteroids might produce some improvement. In refractory patients antidepressants, antiepileptics, and other drugs used in the general treatment of neuropathic pain (see under Postherpetic Neuralgia, above) may be tried. Application of capsaicin has also been tried and preliminary data suggest that bisphosphonates may be beneficial in some patients.

References.

1. Schott GD. An unsympathetic view of pain. *Lancet* 1995; 345: 634–6.
2. Murray P, Atkinson R. Reflex sympathetic dystrophy. *Br J Hosp Med* 1995; 53: 35–40.
3. Paice E. Reflex sympathetic dystrophy. *BMJ* 1995; 310: 1645–8.
4. Lloyd-Thomas AR, Lauder G. Reflex sympathetic dystrophy in children. *BMJ* 1995; 310: 1648–9.
5. Jadad AR, *et al.* Intravenous regional sympathetic blockade for pain relief in reflex sympathetic dystrophy: a systematic review and a randomized, double-blind crossover study. *J Pain Symptom Manage* 1995; 10: 13–20.
6. Kingery WS. A critical review of controlled clinical trials for peripheral neuropathic pain and complex regional pain syndromes. *Pain* 1997; 73: 123–39.
7. Schott GD. Bisphosphonates for pain relief in reflex sympathetic dystrophy? *Lancet* 1997; 350: 1117. Correction. *ibid.* 1998; 351: 682.
8. Schott GD. Interrupting the sympathetic outflow in causalgia and reflex sympathetic dystrophy: a futile procedure for many patients. *BMJ* 1998; 316: 792.
9. Schott GD. Reflex sympathetic dystrophy. *J Neurol Neurosurg Psychiatry* 2001; 71: 291–5.

Trigeminal neuralgia. Trigeminal neuralgia (tic douloureux) is a neuropathic pain characterised by sudden, brief, sharp, agonising, episodic pain in the distribution of one or more branches of the fifth cranial nerve. There may be several episodes (lasting several seconds or minutes) a day over a number of weeks, followed by a pain-free interval which may last for weeks or years. Trigeminal neuralgia generally has a 'trigger zone' in which even a very light stimulus such as a draught of air produces pain. In some cases firm pressure applied around but not to the zone itself may help to relieve pain. Trigeminal neuralgia may be idiopathic or may be secondary to nerve compression (such as that caused by a tumour), facial injury, or multiple sclerosis.

Carbamazepine is the drug of choice for the management of trigeminal neuralgia and initially may produce satisfactory pain relief in 70% or more of patients, although increasingly large doses may be required. If pain relief is inadequate phenytoin or baclofen may be added to carbamazepine therapy; these drugs may also be used alone or together in patients intolerant of carbamazepine. Other antiepileptics such as valproate and clonazepam have also been used in carbamazepine-intolerant patients.

In some patients drug therapy eventually fails to control the pain or produces unacceptable side-effects and invasive procedures become necessary. One method frequently used is the selective destruction of pain bearing nerve fibres with radiofrequency thermocoagulation; instillation of glycerol has also been used to achieve the same effect but the efficacy and safety of the procedure is debatable. Microvascular decompression of the trigeminal nerve root has also been used in intractable cases.

References.

1. Sweet WH. The treatment of trigeminal neuralgia (tic douloureux). *N Engl J Med* 1986; 315: 174–7.
2. Bowsher D. Neurogenic pain syndromes and their management. *Br Med Bull* 1991; 47: 644–66.
3. Green MW, Selman JE. Review article: the medical management of trigeminal neuralgia. *Headache* 1991; 31: 588–92.
4. Zakrzewska JM. Trigeminal neuralgia. *Prim Dent Care* 1997; 4: 17–19.

Increased Body Temperature

The hypothalamus is the centre of the thermoregulatory system and is responsible for maintaining the body temperature at a set point (known as the set-point temperature) which is normally 37°. Mechanisms which produce or conserve body heat include passive heat absorption from the environment, peripheral vasoconstriction, and thermogenic processes such as metabolic reactions and shivering. Heat loss is achieved mainly through sweating and peripheral vasodilatation. Various states may lead to an abnormal increase in body temperature.

Fever and hyperthermia

Fever (pyrexia) is defined as an increase in body temperature due to an elevated set-point temperature. Common causes of fever include infections, inflammatory disorders, neoplastic disease, and some drug treatment. The term hyperthermia (hyperpyrexia) has been used when there is a disturbance of thermoregulatory control. This may be caused by injury to the hypothalamus, or heat stroke following defective heat loss as occurs in dehydration or excessive heat production following strenuous activities; it may also be caused by excessive dosage of some drugs or a reaction to certain drugs such as anaesthetics (malignant hyperthermia, p.1329) or antipsychotics (neuroleptic malignant syndrome, p.662). Underlying thermoregulatory defects may be a particular problem in sedentary elderly subjects.

Whenever possible the underlying cause of **fever** should be identified and treated.[1] Apart from pregnant women or patients who are already dehydrated or malnourished or those with cardiac, respiratory, or neurological diseases, body temperatures up to 41° are relatively harmless.[1] It is not clear if there is any value in treating fever at lower temperatures.

Methods for reducing body temperature in fever include the use of antipyretics and/or physical means. Maintaining an adequate fluid intake is important. Fanning and tepid sponging are often employed,[1-4] but cold baths should not be used as they may actually increase body temperature by inducing vasoconstriction, and the risks of a cold-induced pressor response should be borne in mind. Antipyretics appear to promote the return of the set-point temperature to normal by inhibiting central synthesis and release of prostaglandins that mediate the effect of endogenous pyrogens in the hypothalamus. They cannot lower the body temperature below normal and are ineffective against raised body temperature not associated with fever.

Paracetamol is usually the antipyretic of choice in children; salicylates (including aspirin) are generally contra-indicated because of the possible link between their use and the development of Reye's syndrome. Ibuprofen appears to be as effective as paracetamol.[5,6] Antipyretic treatment of febrile children does not necessarily improve their comfort[7] and might even prolong any infection.[2] It has also been suggested[8] that in severe infection the use of antipyretics might increase mortality; the WHO recommend that in developing countries antipyretics should not be given routinely to children with fever but should be reserved for those with severe discomfort or high fever. In the UK, antipyretic therapy is recommended to treat post-immunisation fever developing after some vaccines.[9] However, if the fever persists after the second dose of antipyretic medical advice should be sought. Antipyretics have also been given as prophylaxis against febrile convulsions, especially in those with a previous history of such seizures or in those with epilepsy. However, antipyretic therapy does not appear to prevent recurrence of febrile convulsions (p.341).[1,3,10] There is also little to support the use of antipyretics for prophylaxis of post-immunisation fever although some suggest offering it to infants at higher risk of seizures receiving diphtheria-tetanus-pertussis or polio immunisation.[9]

Hyperthermia may produce body temperatures greater than 41°. These high temperatures are life-threatening and need to be lowered immediately. Antipyretics are ineffective since the high temperatures are a result of thermoregulatory failure. One of the most rapid and effective means of cooling is to immerse the patient in very cold water but core temperature should be monitored to avoid inducing hypothermia.[11] Some consider evaporative cooling methods to be more efficient.[12] Intravenous or intraperitoneal administration of cool fluids, gastric lavage or enemas with ice water have also been used.[11,13]

When hyperthermia is associated with muscle rigidity and fulminant hypermetabolism of skeletal muscle, as in the neuroleptic malignant syndrome and malignant hyperthermia, temperature reductions may be obtained using the muscle relaxant dantrolene. There is also anecdotal evidence that dantrolene may produce beneficial effects for the treatment of similar symptoms resulting from poisoning with various agents. However, the manufacturers have warned that dantrolene is not an effective treatment for all types of hyperthermia and rigidity accompanying poisoning. Although experience in a small number of patients suggests that dantrolene can hasten cooling in patients with heat stroke when used with conventional cooling methods, there is no evidence that it affects outcome.[14] In severe cases of hyperthermia when neuromuscular hyperactivity may also impair ventilation, a neuromuscular blocker has been used, although suxamethonium is best avoided as it can itself precipitate malignant hyperthermia.

1. Drwal-Klein LA, Phelps SJ. Antipyretic therapy in the febrile child. *Clin Pharm* 1992; 11: 1005–21.
2. Plaisance KI, Mackowiak PA. Antipyretic therapy: physiologic rationale, diagnostic implications, and clinical consequences. *Arch Intern Med* 2000; 160: 449–56.
3. Joint Working Group of the Research Unit of the Royal College of Physicians and the British Paediatric Association. Guidelines for the management of convulsions with fever. *BMJ* 1991; 303: 634–6.
4. Kinmonth A-L, *et al.* Management of feverish children at home. *BMJ* 1992; 305: 1134–6.
5. McIntyre J, Hull D. Comparing efficacy and tolerability of ibuprofen and paracetamol in fever. *Arch Dis Child* 1996; 74: 164–7.
6. Anonymous. Junifen suspension—ibuprofen for febrile children. *Drug Ther Bull* 1991; 29: 11–12.
7. Kramer MS, *et al.* Risks and benefits of paracetamol antipyresis in young children with fever of presumed viral origin. *Lancet* 1991; 337: 591–4.
8. Shann F. Antipyretics in severe sepsis. *Lancet* 1995; 345: 338.
9. Anonymous. Prophylactic paracetamol with childhood immunisation? *Drug Ther Bull* 1990; 28: 73–4.
10. Uhari M, *et al.* Effect of acetaminophen and of low intermittent doses of diazepam on prevention of recurrences of febrile seizures. *J Pediatr* 1995; 126: 991–5.
11. Simon HB. Hyperthermia. *N Engl J Med* 1993; 329: 483–7.
12. Slovis CM. Hyperthermia. *N Engl J Med* 1994; 330: 218–19.
13. Duthie DJR. Heat-related illness. *Lancet* 1998; 352: 1329–30.
14. Channa AB, *et al.* Is dantrolene effective in heat stroke patients? *Crit Care Med* 1990; 18: 290–2.

Musculoskeletal and Joint Disorders

The **rheumatic disorders** are a wide range of painful disorders affecting primarily the joints and related structures of the musculoskeletal system, but there may also be widespread involvement of other systems. The term arthritis is used when the disease is largely confined to the joints. Some of the most common forms of arthritis are discussed in this section and these include rheumatoid arthritis, osteoarthritis, juvenile idiopathic arthritis, and the spondyloarthropathies such as ankylosing spondylitis. Other conditions that are associated with arthritis and which are discussed elsewhere include gout (p.397) and systemic lupus erythematosus (p.1059).

The names **soft-tissue rheumatism** (see below) and **non-articular rheumatism**, have been used to describe a number of painful conditions associated with disease of the structures that surround a joint. For a discussion of the management of **low back pain**, see above.

Juvenile idiopathic arthritis

Juvenile idiopathic arthritis (juvenile chronic arthritis) is a term used to describe a clinically heterogeneous group of idiopathic arthritides occurring in children under 16 years of age.

Methods of treatment are generally the same as for rheumatoid arthritis in adults (see below), although for some drugs there is limited experience of their use in children. Juvenile idiopathic arthritis is one of the limited number of indications for the use of aspirin in children, although other NSAIDs are preferred.

References.
1. Malleson PN. Management of childhood arthritis. Part 2: chronic arthritis. *Arch Dis Child* 1997; **76**: 541–4.
2. Schaller JG. Juvenile rheumatoid arthritis. *Pediatr Rev* 1997; **18**: 337–49.
3. Woo P, Wedderburn LR. Juvenile chronic arthritis. *Lancet* 1998; **351**: 969–73. Correction. *ibid.*; 1292.
4. Dolezalova P, Southwood TR. Arthritis in children. In: Snaith ML, ed. *ABC of rheumatology*. 2nd ed. London: BMJ Publishing Group, 1999: 52–6.
5. Cron RQ, *et al.* Current treatment by United States and Canadian pediatric rheumatologists. *J Rheumatol* 1999; **26**: 2036–8.
6. Cassidy JT. Medical management of children with juvenile rheumatoid arthritis. *Drugs* 1999; **58**: 831–50.

Osteoarthritis

Osteoarthritis is a diverse collection of diseases also known as osteoarthrosis, degenerative joint disease, or joint failure. It is characterised by progressive disintegration of articular cartilage, usually accompanied by new bone formation at joint margins and beneath the involved cartilage. There may be synovial inflammation, particularly in advanced disease, but it is different in nature from that seen with rheumatoid arthritis and is usually only a minor component of the disease. Osteoarthritis may be a sequel to trauma, inflammation, or metabolic disorders, but usually the underlying origin is not apparent.

Despite claims based largely on *animal* studies, there is no evidence from controlled studies in humans that any treatment affects disease progression. Management is therefore aimed at relief of pain and maintenance of joint function.

Physical methods of treatment include physiotherapy, heat and cold therapy, exercises, splinting, and weight reduction in the obese. Acupuncture and transcutaneous electrical nerve stimulation (TENS) may also be tried.

For pain relief, paracetamol is often sufficient and should be used first. A low-dose NSAID may be tried when paracetamol is ineffective or when there is a significant inflammatory component but there is the risk of adverse effects with prolonged use of NSAIDs, especially in the elderly. There has also been concern that NSAIDs such as indometacin may accelerate osteoarthritis. UK guidelines recommend that treatment with NSAIDs such as celecoxib and rofecoxib that are selective inhibitors of cyclo-oxygenase-2 is limited to those patients considered to be at high risk of developing serious gastrointestinal problems if given a non-selective NSAID (see p.63). If pain relief is inadequate, paracetamol may be combined with an NSAID; opioids such as codeine or dihydrocodeine are sometimes also used in combination with paracetamol. The use of dietary supplements such as glucosamine and chondroitin in osteoarthritis is being investigated.

Topical analgesics such as NSAIDs, or capsaicin or rubefacients, may provide some relief of pain.

Systemic corticosteroids have no place in the management of osteoarthritis. Intra-articular or peri-articular injections of corticosteroids are somewhat controversial but may be of help in some patients with localised inflammation, although if used they should only be given infrequently and as adjunctive therapy. Intra-articular injections of hyaluronic acid may improve the viscosity and elasticity of the synovial fluid; they may be useful in osteoarthritis of the knee.

Surgery, including joint replacement, is of great benefit to patients with severe osteoarthritis that cannot be effectively managed by physical or medical therapy.

References.
1. Ghosh P. Nonsteroidal anti-inflammatory drugs and chondroprotection: a review of the evidence. *Drugs* 1993; **46**: 834–46.
2. Puett DW, Griffin MR. Published trials of nonmedicinal and noninvasive therapies for hip and knee osteoarthritis. *Ann Intern Med* 1994; **121**: 133–40.
3. Brandt KD. Toward pharmacologic modification of joint damage in osteoarthritis. *Ann Intern Med* 1995; **122**: 874–5.
4. Wollheim FA. Current pharmacological treatment of osteoarthritis. *Drugs* 1996; **52** (suppl 3): 27–38.
5. Anonymous. What can be done about osteoarthritis? *Drug Ther Bull* 1996; **34**: 33–5.
6. Creamer P, Hochberg MC. Osteoarthritis. *Lancet* 1997; **350**: 503–9.
7. Eccles M, *et al.* North of England evidence based guideline development project: summary guideline for non-steroidal anti-inflammatory drugs versus basic analgesia in treating the pain of degenerative arthritis. *BMJ* 1998; **317**: 526–30.
8. LaPrade RF, Swiontkowski MF. New horizons in the treatment of osteoarthritis of the knee. *JAMA* 1999; **281**: 876–8.
9. Jones A, Doherty M. Osteoarthritis. In: Snaith ML, ed. *ABC of rheumatology*. 2nd ed. London: BMJ Publishing Group, 1999: 28–31.
10. American College of Rheumatology Subcommittee on Osteoarthritis Guidelines. Recommendations for the medical management of osteoarthritis of the hip and knee: 2000 update. *Arthritis Rheum* 2000; **43**: 1905–15. Also available at http://www.rheumatology.org/research/guidelines/oa-mgmt/oa-mgmt.html
11. Walker-Bone K, *et al.* Medical management of osteoarthritis. *BMJ* 2000; **321**: 936–40.
12. Felson DT, *et al.* Osteoarthritis: new insights. Part 1: the disease and its risk factors. *Ann Intern Med* 2000; **133**: 635–46.
13. Felson DT, *et al.* Osteoarthritis: new insights. Part 2: treatment approaches. *Ann Intern Med* 2000; **133**: 726–37.
14. Manek NJ. Medical management of osteoarthritis. *Mayo Clin Proc* 2001; **76**: 533–9.
15. National Institute for Clinical Excellence. Guidance on the use of cyclo-oxygenase (Cox) II selective inhibitors, celecoxib, rofecoxib, meloxicam and etodolac for osteoarthritis and rheumatoid arthritis (issued July 2001). Available at: http://www.nice.org.uk/Docref.asp?d=18034

Rheumatoid arthritis

Rheumatoid arthritis is a common chronic systemic inflammatory disease that predominantly affects the synovial joints and results in progressive disability and increased mortality. Early rheumatoid arthritis is characterised primarily by inflammation of the synovium; as the disease progresses the patient suffers destruction of cartilage and bone. Extra-articular features commonly include general malaise, fatigue, weight loss, fever, and anaemia. Features associated with more severe forms of the disease include vasculitis, pericarditis, pleurisy, pleural effusion, pulmonary interstitial fibrosis, peripheral neuropathies, subcutaneous and pulmonary nodules, scleritis, and Sjögren's syndrome. Palindromic rheumatism is characterised by repeated episodes of arthritis and periarthritis without fever; the joints appear normal between attacks.

The severity and course of rheumatoid arthritis varies greatly between patients. Some experience brief attacks with little or no disease progression, but the majority will have intermittent relapses and remissions with an overall pattern of slowly progressive joint destruction and deformity; a few patients may have very severe and rapidly progressive disease.

Since there is no curative treatment for rheumatoid arthritis, management is aimed at alleviating pain and improving or maintaining joint function. This is accomplished through physiotherapy as well as the use of drugs. In some cases surgery may be required.

The choice of **drugs for relief of pain** depends upon the severity of symptoms. In mild cases an analgesic such as paracetamol may be all that is required but most patients need the additional anti-inflammatory effect provided by an NSAID. Although there is little apparent difference between the various NSAIDs in terms of anti-inflammatory activity, patient responses vary widely. When starting an NSAID the dose is gradually increased to the recommended maximum over one to two weeks; if the response is inadequate after a total of about four weeks, or if adverse effects are intolerable, other NSAIDs are tried. Treatment with NSAIDs such as celecoxib and rofecoxib that are selective inhibitors of cyclo-oxygenase-2 is limited to those patients considered to be at high risk of developing serious gastrointestinal problems if given a non-selective NSAID[1] (see p.63). Topical analgesics such as NSAIDs or capsaicin, or rubefacients may provide slight relief of pain but their role, if any, is unclear.

Although NSAIDs provide symptomatic relief they do not affect the course of the disease. The use of **disease-modifying antirheumatic drugs** (DMARDs) (also referred to as second-line drugs) had conventionally been delayed until there was overt evidence of progressive disease but it is now clear that irreversible joint damage

commonly occurs early in the disease and rheumatologists now generally add a DMARD shortly after rheumatoid arthritis has been diagnosed.[2] There is some evidence[3,4] that early aggressive treatment can improve prognosis but whether it should be given to all patients with very early disease remains to be determined.[5] It is also unclear whether early use of DMARDs will reduce long-term disability[2] but data from 2888 patients with rheumatoid arthritis followed up for an average of 9 years indicated that consistent use of DMARDs was associated with an improvement in long-term functional outcomes.[6]

DMARDs include antimalarials (chloroquine, hydroxychloroquine), sulfasalazine, gold compounds (auranofin, sodium aurothiomalate), penicillamine, and immunosuppressants (methotrexate, azathioprine, ciclosporin, cyclophosphamide, etanercept, infliximab, and leflunomide). It is thought that most DMARDs inhibit the release or activity of cytokines involved in maintaining the inflammatory process, although other actions may also contribute.[7] Any therapeutic effect may not be apparent for 4 to 6 months.

Intramuscular *gold* has long been used for the treatment of rheumatoid arthritis, but although it is still prescribed, its toxicity and poor long-term efficacy have led to debate over its place in antirheumatic therapy.[8,9] Oral gold is less toxic but is also much less effective. Early enthusiasm for *penicillamine* has also been curtailed by a high incidence of adverse effects although better tolerability than gold or antimalarials has been reported if the dose is limited to 500 mg daily or less.[10] The *antimalarials* are less effective than most other DMARDs but as they are generally less toxic and better tolerated they may be preferred in patients with milder forms of the disease. Hydroxychloroquine is generally preferred to chloroquine. *Sulfasalazine* is often one of the DMARDs of first choice.[2,11] About 60% of patients given the drug are still taking it after 3 years.[12] *Immunosuppressants* are also used in rheumatoid arthritis. Methotrexate can improve disease activity when given once weekly in doses too small to produce systemic immunosuppression, and when used in this manner adverse effects are usually mild. In a recent long-term study[13] almost two-thirds of patients were still taking methotrexate after 5 years. Concomitant use of folic acid or folinic acid can reduce the toxicity of methotrexate without reducing efficacy,[14,15] but the timing of administration may be important. The risk of hepatotoxicity remains a concern, but many rheumatologists[2,16,17] nevertheless consider methotrexate to be a first choice DMARD. Improvement generally begins earlier with methotrexate than with other DMARDs. The use of other immunosuppressants is more debatable but azathioprine and cyclophosphamide are used in some patients with severe disease who have failed to respond to other drugs. Ciclosporin is effective but, because of concern over nephrotoxicity, it is reserved for refractory disease; the use of low-dose regimens may help to minimise adverse effects.[18,19] Leflunomide, etanercept, and infliximab are immunosuppressants recently introduced for the treatment of rheumatoid arthritis.[20,21] Leflunomide is said to be equivalent in efficacy to sulfasalazine; comparative data with methotrexate is, however, conflicting. Long-term data on these new drugs is lacking and they are usually reserved for second-line DMARD therapy.

At present, data from comparative studies are insufficient to allow more than a crude ranking of DMARDs with regard to efficacy and toxicity, but a number of reviews and analyses have been published to aid rational selection.[2,11,12,16,17,22-28] Some meta-analyses[22,24] of generally short-term comparative studies suggest that methotrexate, intramuscular gold (sodium aurothiomalate), sulfasalazine, and penicillamine are more or less equivalent in efficacy, while the antimalarials and oral gold (auranofin) appear to be somewhat less effective. Intramuscular gold exhibited the highest toxicity while the antimalarials and oral gold had relatively low toxicity rates.[22] Another meta-analysis[23] considered that antimalarials and methotrexate had the best ratio of toxicity to efficacy.

The long-term use of DMARDs is limited by toxicity and loss of efficacy and many patients do not continue to take a particular drug for more than one or two years. Discontinuation of therapy in a patient who has shown improvement may initiate a relapse but, drug withdrawal may be considered on an empirical basis by some clinicians for patients in complete remission.[29] In a randomised, placebo-controlled study[30] of stopping DMARDs in rheumatoid arthritis, the risk of synovitis was doubled in patients who discontinued active therapy but 62% of the placebo group went for a full year without experiencing a rheumatoid flare. In a further study[31] in patients who had discontinued DMARDs, restarting therapy with the same antirheumatic drug when the disease flared up again was effective in most cases.

As adverse reactions with DMARDs may be life threatening, all patients require careful monitoring.[32,33] Patients who relapse during treatment with one DMARD may gain benefit when a different one is substituted. Treatment with more than one DMARD in various regimens is being tried but there is little available evidence to assess benefit.[2,12] A meta-analysis[34] of 5 different combinations of DMARDs found that although efficacy might be greater, toxicity was also increased. However some combinations have produced favourable results.[20,35]

The use of **corticosteroids** in rheumatoid arthritis is controversial. Although systemic corticosteroids can suppress the symptoms of the disease, their value is limited by adverse effects. They are usually reserved for patients with severe rapidly progressing disease that has failed to respond to other antirheumatics or when there are severe extra-articular effects, or to control disease activity temporarily during initiation of DMARDs. However, it has been suggested that, in line with current thinking on the earlier use of more aggressive therapy, early use of short-term corticosteroids might also be appropriate.[36] Although corticosteroids are associated with bone loss,[37] this appears to be dose-related[38] and, at low doses, the benefits of corticosteroid therapy on inflammation and mobility might result in a reduced loss of bone in patients with rheumatoid arthritis. The rate of joint destruction may be substantially reduced by corticosteroids in low doses (such as prednisolone 7.5 mg daily) in patients with moderate to severe rheumatoid arthritis of less than 2 years duration;[39] the corticosteroid should be gradually discontinued after 2 to 4 years to avoid long-term adverse effects. Reduction in joint destruction should be distinguished from symptomatic improvement, which, at low corticosteroid doses, lasts only for 6 to 12 months. Such symptomatic benefits have been confirmed by two recent meta-analyses.[40,41] The authors considered that the short-term, intermittent use of low-dose corticosteroids (not exceeding the equivalent of 15 mg of prednisolone per day) may be justified, particularly in patients not controlled by other means,[40] and that benefit persisted in moderate-term use (at least 3 months).[41] Intra-articular injections of corticosteroids may be used when there are acute flares affecting one or a few individual joints[42] but they should be used with care.

A wide range of **other drugs** has been tried in rheumatoid arthritis,[25,28,43,44] but for most there is little clearcut evidence of efficacy. Studies[45,46] indicate that minocycline can produce modest beneficial effects in patients with advanced rheumatoid arthritis, but the clinical significance of these improvements has been questioned.[47] Greater symptomatic improvements have been obtained with minocycline when it is used in patients with early rheumatoid arthritis;[48] continued treatment with minocycline may also reduce the need for DMARDs.[49] Testosterone has also produced clinical improvement in male and postmenopausal female patients. Much research has been conducted into immunomodulators and immunotherapy. Interferons have produced results similar to conventional DMARDs but the need for repeated injections is a drawback. Other drugs that have been tried[50-52] include amiprilose, mycophenolate mofetil, zileuton, oral desensitisation with collagen, and immunoglobulins. Tumour necrosis factor (TNF) is involved in the inflammatory process and inhibitors of TNF-α under investigation include tumour necrosis factor receptor fusion protein, as well as interleukin antagonists.[53,54] A CD4 antibody (IDEC-CE9.1) and matrix metalloprotease inhibitors have also been studied. Other methods of treatment that are under investigation include gene therapy and autologous bone marrow transplantation. A rheumatoid arthritis vaccine is also in clinical trials. Some studies suggest that addition of fish oils and/or evening primrose oil to standard antirheumatic therapy might help to reduce pain and joint swelling.

Findings that significant skeletal bone loss occurs early in the disease have raised the question of the need for general measures to prevent osteoporosis in patients with rheumatoid arthritis.[36] Some[36] consider the use of oestrogen therapy in postmenopausal women with rheumatoid arthritis to be appropriate but it appears to have little effect on disease activity.[55] The use of bisphosphonates is being studied.[56]

The treatment of rheumatoid arthritis during **pregnancy** presents its own problems; the rational selection of suitable drugs has been discussed in a number of reviews.[57,58]

1. National Institute for Clinical Excellence. Guidance on the use of cyclo-oxygenase (Cox) II selective inhibitors, celecoxib, rofecoxib, meloxicam and etodolac for osteoarthritis and rheumatoid arthritis (issued July 2001). Available at: http://www.nice.org.uk/Docref.asp?d=18034
2. Anonymous. Modifying disease in rheumatoid arthritis. Drug Ther Bull 1998; 36: 3–6.
3. van der Heide A, et al. The effectiveness of early treatment with "second-line" antirheumatic drugs: a randomized, controlled trial. Ann Intern Med 1996; 124: 699–707.
4. Egsmose C, et al. Patients with rheumatoid arthritis benefit from early 2nd line therapy: 5 year followup of a prospective double blind placebo controlled study. J Rheumatol 1995; 22: 2208–13.
5. Wollheim FA. Disease modifying drugs in rheumatoid arthritis. BMJ 1997; 314: 766–7.
6. Fries JF, et al. Reduction in long-term disability in patients with rheumatoid arthritis by disease-modifying antirheumatic drug-based treatment strategies. Arthritis Rheum 1996; 39: 616–22.
7. Choy E, Kingsley G. How do second-line agents work? Br Med Bull 1995; 51: 472–92.
8. Anonymous. Gold therapy in rheumatoid arthritis. Lancet 1991; 338: 19–20.
9. Pincus T, Wolfe F. Treatment of rheumatoid arthritis: challenges to traditional paradigms. Ann Intern Med 1991; 115: 825–7.
10. Jessop JD, et al. A long-term five year randomized controlled trial of hydroxychloroquine, sodium aurothiomalate, auranofin and penicillamine in the treatment of patients with rheumatoid arthritis. Br J Rheumatol 1998; 37: 992–1002.
11. Jackson CG, Williams HJ. Disease-modifying antirheumatic drugs: using their clinical pharmacological effects as a guide to their selection. Drugs 1998; 56: 337–44.
12. Akil M, Amos RS. Rheumatoid arthritis: treatment. In: Snaith ML, ed. ABC of rheumatology. 2nd ed. London: BMJ Publishing Group, 1999: 44–7.
13. Weinblatt ME, et al. Methotrexate in rheumatoid arthritis: a five-year prospective multicenter study. Arthritis Rheum 1994; 37: 1492–8.
14. Shiroky JB, et al. Low-dose methotrexate with leucovorin (folinic acid) in the management of rheumatoid arthritis: results of a multicenter randomized, double-blind, placebo-controlled trial. Arthritis Rheum 1993; 36: 795–803.
15. Morgan SL, et al. Supplementation with folic acid during methotrexate therapy for rheumatoid arthritis: a double-blind, placebo-controlled trial. Ann Intern Med 1994; 121: 833–41.
16. Cash JM, Klippel JH. Second-line drug therapy for rheumatoid arthritis. N Engl J Med 1994; 330: 1368–75.
17. Anonymous. Drugs for rheumatoid arthritis. Med Lett Drugs Ther 2000; 42: 57–64.
18. Tugwell P. International consensus recommendations on cyclosporin use in rheumatoid arthritis. Drugs 1995; 50: 48–56.
19. Cush JJ, et al. US consensus guidelines for the use of cyclosporin A in rheumatoid arthritis. J Rheumatol 1999; 26: 1176–86.
20. Kremer JM. Rational use of new and existing disease-modifying agents in rheumatoid arthritis. Ann Intern Med 2001; 134: 695–706.
21. Luong BT, et al. Treatment options for rheumatoid arthritis: celecoxib, leflunomide, etanercept, and infliximab. Ann Pharmacother 2000; 34: 743–60.
22. Felson DT, et al. The comparative efficacy and toxicity of second-line drugs in rheumatoid arthritis. Arthritis Rheum 1990; 33: 1449–61.
23. Felson DT, et al. Use of short-term efficacy/toxicity tradeoffs to select second-line drugs in rheumatoid arthritis: a metaanalysis of published clinical trials. Arthritis Rheum 1992; 35: 1117–25.
24. Capell HA, et al. Second line (disease modifying) treatment in rheumatoid arthritis: which drug for which patient? Ann Rheum Dis 1993; 52: 423–8.
25. Brooks PM. Clinical management of rheumatoid arthritis. Lancet 1993; 341: 286–90.
26. Porter DR, Sturrock RD. Medical management of rheumatoid arthritis. BMJ 1993; 307: 425–8.
27. Kalla AA, et al. A risk-benefit assessment of slow-acting antirheumatic drugs in rheumatoid arthritis. Drug Safety 1994; 11: 21–36.
28. Luqmani R, et al. Clinical pharmacology and modification of autoimmunity and inflammation in rheumatoid disease. Drugs 1994; 47: 259–85.
29. Gómez-Reino JJ. Long-term therapy for rheumatoid arthritis. Lancet 1996; 347: 343–4.
30. ten Wolde S, et al. Randomised placebo-controlled study of stopping second-line drugs in rheumatoid arthritis. Lancet 1996; 347: 347–52.
31. ten Wolde S, et al. Effect of resumption of second line drugs in patients with rheumatoid arthritis that flared up after treatment discontinuation. Ann Rheum Dis 1997; 56: 235–9.
32. Wijnands MJH, van Riel PLCM. Management of adverse effects of disease-modifying antirheumatic drugs. Drug Safety 1995; 13: 219–27.
33. Lehmann T, et al. Toxicity of antirheumatic drugs. Med J Aust 1997; 116: 378–83.
34. Felson DT, et al. The efficacy and toxicity of combination therapy in rheumatoid arthritis: a meta-analysis. Arthritis Rheum 1994; 37: 1487–91.
35. Möttönen T, et al. FIN-RACo trial group. Comparison of combination therapy with single-drug therapy in early rheumatoid arthritis: a randomised trial. Lancet 1999; 353: 1568–73.
36. Sambrook PN. Osteoporosis in rheumatoid arthritis: what is the role of antirheumatic therapy? Lancet 1994; 344: 3–4.
37. Laan RFJM, et al. Low-dose prednisone induces rapid reversible axial bone loss in patients with rheumatoid arthritis: a randomized, controlled study. Ann Intern Med 1993; 119: 963–8.
38. Saag KG, et al. Low dose long-term corticosteroid therapy in rheumatoid arthritis: an analysis of serious adverse effects. Am J Med 1994; 96: 115–23.
39. Kirwan JR. The Arthritis and Rheumatism Council Low-dose Glucocorticoid Study Group. The effect of glucocorticoids on joint destruction in rheumatoid arthritis. N Engl J Med 1995; 333: 142–6.
40. Gotzsche PC, Johansen HK. Short-term low-dose corticosteroids vs placebo and nonsteroidal antiinflammatory drugs in rheumatoid arthritis (updated 29 August 2001). Available in The Cochrane Library; Issue 4. Oxford: Update Software; 2001.
41. Criswell LA, et al. Moderate-term, low-dose corticosteroids for rheumatoid arthritis (updated 29 August 2001). Available in The Cochrane Library; Issue 4. Oxford: Update Software, 2001.
42. Hunter JA, Blyth TH. A risk-benefit assessment of intra-articular corticosteroids in rheumatic disorders. Drug Safety 1999; 21: 353–65.
43. Capell HA, Brzeski M. Slow drugs: slow progress? Use of slow acting antirheumatic drugs (SAARDs) in rheumatoid arthritis. Ann Rheum Dis 1992; 51: 424–9.
44. Miller-Blair DJ, Robbins DL. Rheumatoid arthritis: new science, new treatment. Geriatrics 1993; 48: 28–38.
45. Kloppenburg M, et al. Minocycline in active rheumatoid arthritis. Arthritis Rheum 1994; 37: 629–36.
46. Tilley BC, et al. Minocycline in rheumatoid arthritis: a 48-week, double-blind, placebo-controlled trial. Ann Intern Med 1995; 122: 81–9.
47. McKendry RJR. Is rheumatoid arthritis caused by an infection? Lancet 1995; 345: 1319–20.
48. O'Dell JR, et al. Treatment of early rheumatoid arthritis with minocycline or placebo. Arthritis Rheum 1997; 40: 842–8.
49. O'Dell JR, et al. Treatment of early seropositive rheumatoid arthritis with minocycline: four-year followup of a double-blind, placebo-controlled trial. Arthritis Rheum 1999; 42: 1691–5.
50. Panush RS, Arend WP. Rheumatology. JAMA 1997; 277: 1899–1900.
51. Choy EHS, Scott DL. Drug treatment of rheumatic diseases in the 1990s: achievements and future developments. Drugs 1997; 53: 337–48.
52. Schiff M. Emerging treatments for rheumatoid arthritis. Am J Med 1997; 102 (suppl 1A): 11S–15S.
53. Buckley CD. Treatment of rheumatoid arthritis. BMJ 1997; 315: 236–8.
54. Koopman WJ, Moreland LW. Rheumatoid arthritis: anticytokine therapies on the horizon. Ann Intern Med 1998; 128: 231–3.
55. Bijlsma JW. Can we use steroid hormones to immunomodulate rheumatic diseases? Rheumatoid arthritis as an example. Ann N Y Acad Sci 1999; 876: 366–7.
56. Maillefert JF, et al. Bisphosphonates in rheumatoid arthritis (osteoporosis excluded). Rev Rhum Engl Ed 1999; 66: 442–5.
57. Witter FR. Clinical pharmacokinetics in the treatment of rheumatoid arthritis in pregnancy. Clin Pharmacokinet 1993; 25: 444–9.
58. Østensen M, Ramsey-Goldman R. Treatment of inflammatory rheumatic disorders in pregnancy: what are the safest treatment options? Drug Safety 1998; 19: 389–410.

Soft-tissue rheumatism

Soft-tissue rheumatism includes a number of conditions such as fibromyalgia (fibrositis, muscular rheumatism, myofascial pain), humeral epicondylitis (e.g. tennis or golfer's elbow), frozen shoulder, Tietze's syndrome, fascitis, tendinitis, tenosynovitis, bursitis (e.g. housemaid's knee), and sprains and strains. Inflamed or displaced tissue may also impinge on nearby nerves and produce compression neuropathies such as carpal tunnel syndrome.

Some forms of soft-tissue rheumatism will respond to selective rest of the affected region and splinting where appropriate. Gentle exercise, massage, application of heat, cold, or rubefacients can also be of benefit. Many soft tissue lesions respond to local injection of a corticosteroid given with a local anaesthetic. Short-term use of oral NSAIDs may help to relieve pain and reduce inflammation of soft-tissue trauma. The role of topical NSAIDs is unclear. Capsaicin has also been tried as a topical analgesic.

Patients with fibromyalgia have a number of other somatic symptoms including disturbed sleep and depression, in addition to their musculoskeletal pain. Pain and sleep quality may both be improved by low doses of amitriptyline with fluoxetine. If these drugs are ineffective after a trial of 4 to 6 weeks dothiepin [dosulepin] may be tried; if there is still no response after a month, further drug treatment is probably best avoided. Exercise has also been shown to be of benefit.

References.

1. Dawson DM. Entrapment neuropathies of the upper extremities. N Engl J Med 1993; 329: 2013–18.
2. Campbell P, Lawton JO. Heel pain: diagnosis and management. BMJ 1994; 52: 380–5.
3. Muhammed N, et al. Peripheral nerve entrapment syndromes: diagnosis and management. Br J Hosp Med 1995; 53: 141–6.
4. Caldwell JR. Intra-articular corticosteroids. Drugs 1996; 52: 507–14.
5. Reveille JD. Soft-tissue rheumatism: diagnosis and treatment. Am J Med 1997; 102 (suppl 1A): 23S–29S.
6. Shipley M. Pain in the hand and wrist. In: Snaith ML, ed. ABC of rheumatology. 2nd ed. London: BMJ Publishing Group, 1999: 1–5.
7. Barry M, Jenner JR. Pain in the neck, shoulder, and arm. In: Snaith ML, ed. ABC of rheumatology. 2nd ed. London: BMJ Publishing Group, 1999: 6–9.
8. Doherty M, Jones A. Fibromyalgia syndrome. In: Snaith ML, ed. ABC of rheumatology. 2nd ed. London: BMJ Publishing Group, 1999: 24–7.
9. Leventhal LJ. Management of fibromyalgia. Ann Intern Med 1999; 131: 850–8.
10. Goldenberg DL. Fibromyalgia syndrome a decade later: what have we learned? Arch Intern Med 1999; 159: 777–85.

Spondyloarthropathies

The spondyloarthropathies are a group of seronegative arthritides which include ankylosing spondylitis, psoriatic arthritis, arthritis associated with inflammatory bowel disorders (enteropathic arthritis), and arthritis associated with infection as in reactive arthritis (aseptic arthritis).

Ankylosing spondylitis is characterised by arthritis of the spine and sacroiliac joints and sometimes there is also asymmetrical peripheral involvement. Males under 40 years of age are predominantly affected. The aim of management of the disease is to reduce pain and stiffness and to prevent spine and joint deformity, which is accomplished using a combination of active physical therapy and drug therapy. Exercises are used to strengthen muscles and to maintain a good posture and range of movement in joints. NSAIDs are used to relieve pain and inflammation, thus allowing the exercises to be performed; they do not influence the progression of the disease. Some patients may require concomitant treatment with other non-opioid analgesics such as paracetamol for additional pain control. Phenylbutazone is sometimes used when other drugs are unsuitable but in the UK its use is limited to hospital rheumatology departments because of the risk of serious adverse effects. Systemic corticosteroids are rarely indicated but intra-articular injections of corticosteroids may be beneficial when one or two peripheral joints are severely affected. The disease-modifying antirheumatic drug (DMARD) sulfasalazine, which has proven efficacy in ankylosing spondylitis (mainly in patients with peripheral involvement), may help to control severe or refractory disease; the efficacy of other DMARDs used in rheumatoid arthritis (see above) remains to be demonstrated.

Psoriatic arthritis (or psoriatic arthropathy) is an inflammatory seronegative arthritis occurring in patients with psoriasis. In some patients the spine may be involved when the condition may be indistinguishable from ankylosing spondylitis. Less frequently some patients have a form of symmetrical arthritis resembling rheumatoid arthritis (see above). The psoriasis (p.1106) and the arthritis usually require separate treatment. Treatment of the arthritis is initially as for ankylosing spondylitis with NSAIDs and physical therapy. If these methods fail treatment with a DMARD may be instituted, although chloroquine and hydroxychloroquine should be avoided since they may precipitate skin reactions (see p.434). Systemic corticosteroids have little or no place in the management of psoriatic arthritis.

Reactive arthritis is characterised by sterile synovitis following 1 to 4 weeks after an infection most commonly of the gastrointestinal or genito-urinary tract. Extra-articular features involving the skin, eyes, or genito-urinary tract may or may not be present. Reactive arthritis is also a feature of Reiter's syndrome. Reactive arthritis is treated with physical therapy and NSAIDs and, if indicated, intra-articular injections of corticosteroids; the role of antibacterials is less certain (see under Bone and Joint Infections, p.116).

References.
1. Gran JT, Husby G. Ankylosing spondylitis: current drug treatment. *Drugs* 1992; **44**: 585–603.
2. Svenungsson B. Reactive arthritis. *BMJ* 1994; **308**: 671–2.
3. Toussirot E, Wendling D. Current guidelines for the drug treatment of ankylosing spondylitis. *Drugs* 1998; **56**: 225–40.
4. Keat A. Spondyloarthropathies. In: Snaith ML, ed. *ABC of rheumatology.* 2nd ed. London: BMJ Publishing Group, 1999: 48–51.
5. Jones G, *et al.* Interventions for psoriatic arthritis (updated 28 October 1999). Available in The Cochrane Library; Issue 1. Oxford: Update Software; 2000.

Still's disease

Still's disease is characterised by a high fever, polyarthritis, and an evanescent pink macular rash that is most prominent during bouts of fever; patients are seronegative for rheumatoid factor. Onset is usually in children under 5 years of age, but can occur in adults. Treatment is usually with NSAIDs or corticosteroids.

The name Still's disease has also been used rather inconsistently to describe some types of juvenile idiopathic arthritis (above).

References.
1. Evans RH. Pyrexia of unknown origin. *BMJ* 1997; **314**: 583–6.
2. Watts RA, Scott DGI. Rashes and vasculitis. In: Snaith ML, ed. *ABC of rheumatology.* 2nd ed. London: BMJ Publishing Group, 1999: 69–73.

Aceclofenac (2545-k)

Aceclofenac (BAN, rINN).

Aceclofenacum. [o-(2,6-Dichloroanilino)phenyl]acetate glycolic acid ester; 2-(2,6-Dichloroanilino)phenylacetoxyacetic acid.
$C_{16}H_{13}Cl_2NO_4 = 354.2.$
$CAS — 89796-99-6.$
$ATC — M01AB16.$
Pharmacopoeias. In *Eur.* (see p.vi).

Pharmacopoeial description

Ph. Eur.: A white or almost white, crystalline powder. Practically insoluble in water; soluble in alcohol; freely soluble in acetone. Store in airtight containers. Protect from light.

The symbol † denotes a preparation no longer actively marketed

Adverse Effects

As for NSAIDs in general, p.63.

Hypersensitivity. Leukocytoclastic vasculitis, a type III hypersensitivity reaction, with lung haemoptysis has been reported in a patient following therapy with aceclofenac.[1]

1. Epelde F, Boada L. Leukocytoclastic vasculitis and hemoptysis after treatment with aceclofenac. *Ann Pharmacother* 1995; **29**: 1168.

Precautions

As for NSAIDs in general, p.64.

Aceclofenac should be avoided in patients with moderate to severe renal impairment.

Interactions

For interactions associated with NSAIDs, see p.65.

Pharmacokinetics

Aceclofenac is well absorbed from the gastrointestinal tract; peak plasma concentrations are reached 1 to 3 hours after an oral dose. Aceclofenac is more than 99% bound to plasma proteins. The plasma-elimination half-life is approximately 4 hours. About two-thirds of a dose is excreted in the urine, mainly as hydroxymetabolites.

Uses and Administration

Aceclofenac, a phenylacetic acid derivative, is an NSAID (see p.65) related to diclofenac (p.31). It is used in the management of osteoarthritis, rheumatoid arthritis, and ankylosing spondylitis.

The usual dose of aceclofenac is 100 mg given twice daily by mouth. The initial dose should be reduced to 100 mg daily in patients with hepatic impairment.

◊ Reviews.
1. Dooley M, *et al.* Aceclofenac: a reappraisal of its use in the management of pain and rheumatic disease. *Drugs* 2001; **61**: 1351–78.

Preparations

Proprietary Preparations (details are given in Part 3)
Aust.: Beofenac; *Belg.:* Air-Tal; Biofenac; *Braz.:* Proflam; *Denm.:* Barcan; *Fin.:* Barcan; *Ger.:* Beofenac; *Irl.:* Airtal†; *Mex.:* Bristaflam; *Neth.:* Biofenac; *Norw.:* Barcan; *Port.:* Airtal; Biofenac; *Spain:* Airtal; Airtal Difucrem; Falcol; Gerbin; Sanein; *Swed.:* Barcan; *Switz.:* Locomin; *UAE:* Aceclofar; *UK:* Preservex.

Acemetacin (12308-x)

Acemetacin (BAN, rINN).

Bay-f-4975; TVX-1322. O-[(1-p-Chlorobenzoyl-5-methoxy-2-methylindol-3-yl)acetyl]glycolic acid.
$C_{21}H_{18}ClNO_6 = 415.8.$
$CAS — 53164-05-9.$
$ATC — M01AB11.$

Profile

Acemetacin, a glycolic acid ester of indometacin, is an NSAID (p.63). Its pharmacological activity is due to both acemetacin and its major metabolite indometacin (p.44). Acemetacin is used in rheumatoid arthritis, osteoarthritis, and low back pain, and for postoperative pain and inflammation. Usual daily doses are 120 to 180 mg by mouth in divided doses. Acemetacin is eliminated by both hepatic and renal routes, although pharmacokinetics are not affected by moderate renal or hepatic impairment and appear to be unchanged in the elderly.

◊ References.
1. Jones RW, *et al.* Comparative pharmacokinetics of acemetacin in young subjects and elderly patients. *Br J Clin Pharmacol* 1991; **31**: 543–5.
2. Hazleman B, Bernstein RM. Acemetacin in the long-term therapy of rheumatoid arthritis. *Curr Med Res Opin* 1993; **13**: 119–26.

Preparations

Proprietary Preparations (details are given in Part 3)
Aust.: Rheutrop; *Ger.:* Acemetadoc; Acephlogont; Peran; Rantudil; *Ital.:* Acemix; Solart; *Mex.:* Rantudil; *Port.:* Rantudil; *Singapore:* Rantudil; *Spain:* Espledol; Oldan; *Switz.:* Tilur; *UK:* Emflex.

Acetanilide (2603-e)

Antifebrin. N-Phenylacetamide.
$C_8H_9NO = 135.2.$
$CAS — 103-84-4.$
Pharmacopoeias. In *Fr.*

Profile

Acetanilide, a para-aminophenol derivative related to paracetamol (p.71), has analgesic and antipyretic properties. It was replaced by safer analgesics.

Actarit (13756-g)

Actarit (rINN).

(p-Acetamidophenyl)acetic acid.
$C_{10}H_{11}NO_3 = 193.2.$
$CAS — 18699-02-0.$

Profile

Actarit is reported to be an immunomodulator. It is given by mouth in the treatment of rheumatoid arthritis in a usual dose of 100 mg three times daily.

◊ References.
1. Nobunaga M. Long term administration study of a new DMARD actarit on rheumatoid arthritis. *Rinsho Iyaku* 1994; **10**: 947–62.

Preparations

Proprietary Preparations (details are given in Part 3)
Jpn: Mover; Orcl.

Alclofenac (2605-y)

Alclofenac (BAN, USAN, rINN).

W-7320. (4-Allyloxy-3-chlorophenyl)acetic acid.
$C_{11}H_{11}ClO_3 = 226.7.$
$CAS — 22131-79-9.$
$ATC — M01AB06.$

Profile

Alclofenac, a phenylacetic acid derivative related to diclofenac (p.30), is an NSAID (p.63). It was used in musculoskeletal and joint disorders but following reports of toxicity, especially skin reactions, it was withdrawn from the market. It was also used as the aminoethanol derivative.

Alfentanil Hydrochloride (12339-b)

Alfentanil Hydrochloride (BANM, USAN, rINN).

Alfentanili Hydrochloridum; R-39209. N-{1-[2-(4-Ethyl-5-oxo-2-tetrazolin-1-yl)ethyl]-4-(methoxymethyl)-4-piperidyl}propionanilide hydrochloride.
$C_{21}H_{32}N_6O_3,HCl = 453.0.$
$CAS — 71195-58-9$ (alfentanil); $69049-06-5$ (anhydrous alfentanil hydrochloride); $70879-28-6$ (alfentanil hydrochloride, monohydrate).
Pharmacopoeias. In *Eur.* (see p.vi) and US.

Alfentanil hydrochloride 109 µg is approximately equivalent to 100 µg of alfentanil.

Pharmacopoeial description

Ph. Eur.: A white or almost white powder. Freely soluble in water, in alcohol, and in methyl alcohol. Protect from light.

USP 25: A white to almost white powder. Soluble in water; freely soluble in alcohol, in chloroform, and in methyl alcohol; sparingly soluble in acetone.

◊ CAUTION. *Avoid contact with the skin and the inhalation of particles of alfentanil hydrochloride.*

Dependence and Withdrawal

As for Opioid Analgesics, p.66.

Adverse Effects and Treatment

As for Opioid Analgesics in general, p.67, and for Fentanyl, p.37.

Effects on the cardiovascular system. A report of 2 cases of sinus arrest during intubation following administration of alfentanil 30 µg per kg body-weight.[1]

1. Maryniak JK, Bishop VA. Sinus arrest after alfentanil. *Br J Anaesth* 1987; **59**: 390–1.

Effects on mental function. Like fentanyl, alfentanil 7.5 or 15 µg per kg body-weight intravenously had no effect on memory in healthy subjects.[1] In another study impairment of memory for new facts did occur 2 hours after operation in patients anaesthetised with alfentanil 7.5 µg per kg, but not in those given fentanyl;[2] methohexital might have contributed to the impairment.

1. Scamman FL, *et al.* Ventilatory and mental effects of alfentanil and fentanyl. *Acta Anaesthesiol Scand* 1984; **28**: 63–7.
2. Kennedy DJ, Ogg TW. Alfentanil and memory function: a comparison with fentanyl for day case termination of pregnancy. *Anaesthesia* 1985; **40**: 537–40.

Effects on the respiratory system. Alfentanil, like other opioid agonists, causes dose-related respiratory depression; it is significant with doses of more than 1 mg. Recovery has been reported to be faster after alfentanil than after fentanyl (see p.37),[1,2] possibly reflecting the shorter elimination half-life of alfentanil. Even so, accumulation of alfentanil is possible with large doses over a prolonged period. Profound analgesia is accompanied by marked respiratory depression which may persist or recur postoperatively.

After an initial rapid recovery from anaesthesia, 2 patients suffered sudden respiratory arrest about an hour after the end of alfentanil infusion;[3] both responded to treatment with naloxone. Close monitoring of respiration in the initial postoperative period was recommended and this was reinforced by the manufacturers;[4] factors such as hyperventilation and the use of opioid premedication might enhance or prolong the respiratory depressant effects of alfentanil.

1. Andrews CJH, *et al.* Ventilatory effects during and after continuous infusion of fentanyl or alfentanil. *Br J Anaesth* 1983; **55**: 211S–16S.

2. Scamman FL, *et al.* Ventilatory and mental effects of alfentanil and fentanyl. *Acta Anaesthesiol Scand* 1984; **28**: 63–7.
3. Sebel PS, *et al.* Respiratory depression after alfentanil infusion. *BMJ* 1984; **289**: 1581–2.
4. Waldron HA, Cookson RF. Respiratory depression after alfentanil infusion. *BMJ* 1985; **290**: 319.

Precautions

As for Opioid Analgesics in general, p.68.

Children. Alfentanil given to preterm infants undergoing paralysis and mechanical ventilation for respiratory distress syndrome resulted in a rapid and significant fall in heart rate and blood pressure, emphasising that proper evaluation of the pharmacological and clinical effects was necessary.[1]

1. Marlow N. Hazards of analgesia for newborn infants. *Arch Dis Child* 1988; **63**: 1293.

The elderly. Elderly patients had increased brain sensitivity to alfentanil as demonstrated by EEG changes,[1] and lower doses might be indicated in older patients for pharmacodynamic rather than pharmacokinetic reasons. See also under Pharmacokinetics, below.

1. Scott JC, Stanski DR. Decreased fentanyl and alfentanil dose requirements with age: a simultaneous pharmacokinetic and pharmacodynamic evaluation. *J Pharmacol Exp Ther* 1987; **240**: 159–66.

Inflammatory bowel disease. Patients with Crohn's disease required higher doses of alfentanil than control patients[1] although there were no differences in alfentanil pharmacokinetics between the 2 groups of patients.

1. Gesink-van der Veer BJ, *et al.* Influence of Crohn's disease on the pharmacokinetics and pharmacodynamics of alfentanil. *Br J Anaesth* 1993; **71**: 827–34.

Pregnancy. The UK manufacturers contra-indicate the use of alfentanil in labour or before clamping of the cord during caesarean section because placental transfer means there is a risk of neonatal respiratory depression.

Interactions

For interactions associated with opioid analgesics, see p.68.

Drugs that depress the heart or increase vagal tone, such as beta blockers and anaesthetic drugs, may predispose patients given alfentanil to develop bradycardia and hypotension. Concomitant administration of alfentanil and non-vagolytic neuromuscular blockers may produce bradycardia and possibly asystole.

The metabolism of alfentanil is inhibited by ketoconazole resulting in a risk of prolonged or delayed respiratory depression. A similar effect has been reported with fluconazole.

Antibacterials. The elimination half-life of alfentanil was increased and clearance decreased when given after a 7-day course of *erythromycin* by mouth in healthy subjects.[1] Other hepatic enzyme inhibitors and drugs interfering with hepatic blood flow might also affect the clearance of alfentanil.

1. Bartkowski RR, *et al.* Inhibition of alfentanil metabolism by erythromycin. *Clin Pharmacol Ther* 1989; **46**: 99–102.

Antifungals. Azole antifungals such as *ketoconazole* or *fluconazole* can inhibit the metabolism of alfentanil. In one study, administration of alfentanil one hour after intravenous or oral fluconazole decreased the clearance of alfentanil by 60 and 55% respectively and increased the mean half-life of alfentanil from 1.5 hours to 2.7 and 2.5 hours respectively.[1]

1. Palkama VJ, *et al.* The effect of intravenous and oral fluconazole on the pharmacokinetics and pharmacodynamics of intravenous alfentanil. *Anesth Analg* 1998; **87**: 190–4.

Pharmacokinetics

After parenteral administration alfentanil hydrochloride has a rapid onset and short duration of action. Alfentanil is highly protein bound (about 90%) and has a small volume of distribution. Its terminal elimination half-life is about 1 to 2 hours. It is metabolised in the liver by oxidative *N*- and *O*-dealkylation to inactive metabolites which are excreted in the urine. Alfentanil crosses the blood-brain barrier and the placenta and has been detected in colostrum.

◊ Alfentanil is less lipid-soluble than fentanyl, but more than morphine. It is highly bound to plasma protein, principally to α_1-acid glycoprotein. Decreased lipid solubility can be expected to limit penetration of the blood-brain barrier when compared with fentanyl, but the majority of unbound alfentanil is unionised and can rapidly gain access to the CNS. It has a smaller volume of distribution than fentanyl. The elimination half-life of alfentanil is shorter than that of fentanyl. The manufacturers have given values for a three-compartment pharmacokinetic model with a distribution half-life of 0.4 to 3.1 minutes, a redistribution half-life of 4.6 to 21.6 minutes, and a terminal elimination half-life of 64.1 to 129.3 minutes following single bolus injections of 50 or 125 µg per kg body-weight. Accumulation is less likely than with fentanyl, but can occur following repeated or continuous administration especially in

patients with reduced clearance. The mean elimination half-life reported is usually about 90 minutes, but this is reduced in children and increased in the elderly, in hepatic impairment, in the obese, and during cardiopulmonary bypass (see below).

◊ Reviews.

1. Hull CJ. The pharmacokinetics of alfentanil in man. *Br J Anaesth* 1983; **55**: 157S–64S.
2. Mather LE. Clinical pharmacokinetics of fentanyl and its newer derivatives. *Clin Pharmacokinet* 1983; **8**: 422–46.
3. Davis PJ, Cook DR. Clinical pharmacokinetics of the newer intravenous anaesthetic agents. *Clin Pharmacokinet* 1986; **11**: 18–35.
4. Bodenham A, Park GR. Alfentanil infusions in patients requiring intensive care. *Clin Pharmacokinet* 1988; **15**: 216–26.
5. Scholz J, *et al.* Clinical pharmacokinetics of alfentanil, fentanyl and sufentanil. *Clin Pharmacokinet* 1996; **31**: 275–92.

Administration. CONTINUOUS INTRAVENOUS INFUSION. Small studies of alfentanil given by continuous intravenous infusion[1-3] have found pharmacokinetic parameters to be similar to those after a single bolus injection, but with some conflicting results. In 29 patients undergoing orthopaedic surgery an initial bolus intravenous injection of alfentanil 50 µg per kg body-weight was followed by intravenous infusion of 1 µg per kg per minute, continued for 44 to 445 minutes; a second bolus injection of 50 µg per kg was given immediately before incision and an additional bolus injection of 1 mg given if necessary.[4] The time course of the plasma-alfentanil concentration fitted a two-compartmental model in 26 patients. Terminal half-lives varied widely from 56 to 226 minutes (mean 106 minutes), the highest values being mainly in patients over 60 years. There was no significant correlation between pharmacokinetic parameters and the duration of the infusion or the total dose. Plasma clearance and volumes of distribution did not correlate significantly with body-weight although steady-state volume of distribution was enlarged with increasing age. The mean estimated steady-state concentration was 293 nanograms per mL (range 147 to 636 nanograms per mL).

1. Fragen RJ, *et al.* Pharmacokinetics of the infusion of alfentanil in man. *Br J Anaesth* 1983; **55**: 1077–81.
2. Shafer A, *et al.* Pharmacokinetics and pharmacodynamics of alfentanil infusions during general anesthesia. *Anesth Analg* 1986; **65**: 1021–8.
3. Reitz JA, *et al.* The pharmacokinetics of alfentanil in gynecologic surgical patients. *J Clin Pharmacol* 1986; **26**: 60–4.
4. van Beem H, *et al.* Pharmacokinetics of alfentanil during and after a fixed rate infusion. *Br J Anaesth* 1989; **62**: 610–15.

INTRAMUSCULAR. See under the Elderly, below.

Burns. The volume of distribution and total clearance of alfentanil were reduced and its elimination half-life prolonged in patients with burns.[1] This was due, in part, to raised concentrations of α_1-acid glycoprotein leading to increased protein binding.

1. Macfie AG, *et al.* Disposition of alfentanil in burns patients. *Br J Anaesth* 1992; **69**: 447–50.

Cardiopulmonary bypass. The elimination half-life of alfentanil increased from 72 minutes before bypass to 195 minutes afterwards in 5 patients undergoing cardiopulmonary bypass.[1] This was attributed to an increase in volume of distribution, based in part on a dilution-induced decrease in plasma protein binding. Others[2,3] found that on starting cardiopulmonary bypass total serum concentrations of alfentanil were halved, mainly because of dilution of α_1-acid glycoprotein and an increase in unbound alfentanil.

1. Hug CC, *et al.* Alfentanil pharmacokinetics in patients before and after cardiopulmonary bypass. *Anesth Analg* 1983; **62**: 266.
2. Kumar K, *et al.* The effect of cardiopulmonary bypass on plasma protein binding of alfentanil. *Eur J Clin Pharmacol* 1988; **35**: 47–52.
3. Hynynen M, *et al.* Plasma concentration and protein binding of alfentanil during high-dose infusion for cardiac surgery. *Br J Anaesth* 1994; **72**: 571–6.

Children. Alfentanil has been shown to have a shorter elimination half-life (about 40 minutes) and a smaller volume of distribution in children than in adults.[1] See also under Hepatic Impairment, below.

1. Meistelman C, *et al.* A comparison of alfentanil pharmacokinetics in children and adults. *Anesthesiology* 1987; **66**: 13–16.

The elderly. Plasma clearance of alfentanil following 50 µg per kg body-weight as a single intravenous dose was reduced in elderly patients aged more than 65 years when compared with that in healthy young adults.[1] Mean elimination half-life was 137 minutes in the elderly and 83 minutes in the young adults. Volumes of distribution were similar and it was considered that reduced clearance might be due to decreased hepatic metabolism in the elderly. In a study in male patients the terminal elimination half-life of alfentanil increased with age, although clearance was not significantly affected.[2] In patients given alfentanil 1 µg per kg per minute by continuous intravenous infusion during orthopaedic surgery,[3] terminal half-life increased linearly with age in those older than 40 years and steady-state volume of distribution was enlarged with increasing age; clearance did not correlate significantly with age and was thought to be more variable during a continuous infusion in long-term surgery than after a single bolus injection. Others have reported[4] that the effects of age on alfentanil pharmacokinetics are dependent on gender. In this study total plasma clearance decreased and terminal half-life increased with increasing age in women, but not in men. It has been suggested that this effect in

women may be more dependent on menopausal status than on age.[5]

In a study[6] in elderly patients plasma concentrations of alfentanil were greater and the maximum concentration occurred earlier when alfentanil was injected into the deltoid muscle compared with injection into the gluteal muscle.

1. Helmers H, *et al.* Alfentanil kinetics in the elderly. *Clin Pharmacol Ther* 1984; **36**: 239–43.
2. Scott JC, Stanski DR. Decreased fentanyl and alfentanil dose requirements with age: a simultaneous pharmacokinetic and pharmacodynamic evaluation. *J Pharmacol Exp Ther* 1987; **240**: 159–66.
3. van Beem H, *et al.* Pharmacokinetics of alfentanil during and after a fixed rate infusion. *Br J Anaesth* 1989; **62**: 610–15.
4. Lemmens HJM, *et al.* Influence of age on the pharmacokinetics of alfentanil: gender dependence. *Clin Pharmacokinet* 1990; **19**: 416–22.
5. Rubio A, Cox C. Sex, age and alfentanil pharmacokinetics. *Clin Pharmacokinet* 1991; **21**: 81.
6. Virkkilä M, *et al.* Pharmacokinetics and effects of im alfentanil as premedication for day-case ophthalmic surgery in elderly patients. *Br J Anaesth* 1993; **71**: 507–11.

Hepatic impairment. Total plasma clearance and protein binding of alfentanil were decreased in patients with alcoholic cirrhosis when compared with control subjects. Elimination half-life was prolonged from 90 to 219 minutes in the cirrhotic patients following a single intravenous dose of 50 µg per kg body-weight and was attributed in part to alterations in binding sites of α_1-acid glycoprotein.[1] There might be different effects on alfentanil disposition in patients with non-alcoholic cirrhosis or other liver disorders.[2] The pharmacokinetics of alfentanil were apparently not affected in children with cholestatic hepatic disease whereas clearance was reduced postoperatively in 3 patients who had undergone liver transplantation.[3]

1. Ferrier C, *et al.* Alfentanil pharmacokinetics in patients with cirrhosis. *Anesthesiology* 1985; **62**: 480–4.
2. Bower S, *et al.* Effects of different hepatic pathologies on disposition of alfentanil in anaesthetized patients. *Br J Anaesth* 1992; **68**: 462–5.
3. Davis PJ, *et al.* Effects of cholestatic hepatic disease and chronic renal failure on alfentanil pharmacokinetics in children. *Anesth Analg* 1989; **68**: 579–83.

Obesity. The pharmacokinetics of alfentanil are reportedly altered in obesity.[1] Elimination half-life was 172 minutes in 6 obese patients compared with 92 minutes in 7 who were not obese. Plasma clearance of alfentanil was also decreased, although others[2] found that obesity had no effect on clearance, but it did have a direct relationship with the volume of the central compartment.

1. Bentley JB, *et al.* Obesity and alfentanil pharmacokinetics. *Anesth Analg* 1983; **62**: 251.
2. Maitre PO, *et al.* Population pharmacokinetics of alfentanil: the average dose-plasma concentration relationship and interindividual variability in patients. *Anesthesiology* 1987; **66**: 3–12.

Renal impairment. The pharmacokinetics of alfentanil were not affected significantly in adults[1] or children[2] with chronic renal failure. In another study[3] increased volume of distribution of alfentanil at steady-state was associated with decreased plasma protein binding in patients with chronic renal failure.

1. Van Peer A, *et al.* Alfentanil kinetics in renal insufficiency. *Eur J Clin Pharmacol* 1986; **30**: 245–7.
2. Davis PJ, *et al.* Effects of cholestatic hepatic disease and chronic renal failure on alfentanil pharmacokinetics in children. *Anesth Analg* 1989; **68**: 579–83.
3. Chauvin M, *et al.* Pharmacokinetics of alfentanil in chronic renal failure. *Anesth Analg* 1987; **66**: 53–6.

Uses and Administration

Alfentanil is a short-acting opioid analgesic (p.68) related to fentanyl (p.38).

Alfentanil is used in surgical procedures as an analgesic and adjunct to general anaesthetics or as a primary anaesthetic. It is also used as an analgesic and respiratory depressant in the management of mechanically ventilated patients under intensive care.

Alfentanil is administered intravenously as the hydrochloride. Doses are expressed in terms of alfentanil base. A peak effect may be seen within 1.5 to 2 minutes of an injection and analgesia can be expected to last for up to 10 minutes; dose supplements are therefore required if it is to be used for more prolonged surgical procedures. It may be given by continuous intravenous infusion in ventilated patients.

The dosage of alfentanil employed depends on whether the patient has spontaneous respiration or assisted ventilation and on the expected duration of anaesthesia. When used as an adjunct in the **maintenance of general anaesthesia** the recommended initial dose in the UK is as follows:

- in adults with *spontaneous respiration*, up to 500 µg given slowly over about 30 seconds; supplementary doses of 250 µg may be given.
- *Ventilated* adults and children may be given 30 to 50 µg per kg body-weight with supplements of 15 µg per kg. When given by infusion to ventilated

adults and children there is an initial loading dose of 50 to 100 µg per kg given as a bolus or by infusion over 10 minutes, and this is followed by infusion at a rate of 0.5 to 1 µg per kg per minute.

Typical doses that have been used in the USA are as follows:

- for procedures lasting *less than 30 minutes* in adults with spontaneous respiration or assisted ventilation, the dose is 8 to 20 µg per kg body-weight followed by supplementary doses of 3 to 5 µg per kg every 5 to 20 minutes or an infusion of 0.5 to 1 µg per kg per minute.

- When the expected duration of anaesthesia is *longer than 30 minutes*, the initial dose for adults with assisted ventilation is 20 to 75 µg per kg followed by supplementary doses of 5 to 15 µg per kg or an infusion of 0.5 to 3 µg per kg per minute. If alfentanil has been given in anaesthetic doses (see below) for the induction of anaesthesia, infusion rates may need to be reduced by 30 to 50% during the first hour of maintenance. Maintenance infusions of alfentanil should be discontinued 10 to 30 minutes before the anticipated end of surgery.

The dose for the **induction of anaesthesia** in patients with assisted ventilation undergoing procedures of at least 45 minutes is 130 to 245 µg per kg followed by an inhalation anaesthetic or maintenance doses of alfentanil of 0.5 to 1.5 µg per kg per minute.

In **intensive care** ventilated adults may be given alfentanil initially at an infusion rate of 2 mg per hour or a loading dose of 5 mg may be given in divided doses over 10 minutes or more slowly if hypotension or bradycardia occur. Thereafter a suitable rate of infusion should be determined for each patient (rates of 0.5 to 10 mg per hour have been used); patients should be carefully monitored and the duration of treatment should not generally exceed 4 days. During continuous infusion additional bolus injections of 0.5 to 1 mg may be given if required to provide analgesia for short painful procedures that may be carried out in intensive care.

Doses are adjusted according to the needs of the patient. Children may require higher or more frequent doses than adults, whereas the elderly or debilitated patients may require lower or less frequent doses.

◊ Reviews.
1. Larijani GE, Goldberg ME. Alfentanil hydrochloride: a new short-acting narcotic analgesic for surgical procedures. *Clin Pharm* 1987; **6:** 275–82.
2. Clotz MA, Nahata MC. Clinical uses of fentanyl, sufentanil, and alfentanil. *Clin Pharm* 1991; **10:** 581–93.

Administration. Alfentanil is usually given by intravenous injection or infusion, but has also been given intramuscularly[1,2] or epidurally (see under Pain, below).
1. Arendt-Nielsen L, *et al.* Analgesic efficacy of im alfentanil. *Br J Anaesth* 1990; **65:** 164–8.
2. Virkkilä M, *et al.* Pharmacokinetics and effects of im alfentanil as premedication for day-case ophthalmic surgery in elderly patients. *Br J Anaesth* 1993; **71:** 507–11.

Anaesthesia. Alfentanil, like fentanyl (p.39), appears to produce fewer circulatory changes than morphine and may be preferred for anaesthetic use, especially in cardiovascular surgery. It is generally considered to have a shorter duration of action than fentanyl. It has been used in conjunction with propofol to facilitate intubation, and for total intravenous anaesthesia.

For a discussion of the drugs used to facilitate intubation and of opioids such as alfentanil used to control the pressor response and the rise of intra-ocular pressure associated with intubation, see under Anaesthesia, p.1331. For reference to a study indicating that pretreatment with alfentanil can reduce the pain associated with injection of propofol, see p.1266.

CAESAREAN SECTION. The UK manufacturers contra-indicate the use of alfentanil before clamping the cord during caesarean section because of the risk of respiratory depression in the neonate. A study of alfentanil 30 µg per kg body-weight in women undergoing caesarean section was abandoned after massive respiratory depression had occurred in 4 of 5 neonates.[1] However, alfentanil has been used successfully to minimise haemodynamic responses to intubation and surgery in patients with severe cardiovascular disorders undergoing caesarean section.[2,3] A baby delivered after the successful use of alfentanil 35 µg per kg in a mother with severe aortic stenosis[2] was apnoeic and unresponsive with poor muscle tone; it responded rapidly to naloxone. Alfentanil 10 µg per kg immediately before induction attenuated the cardiovascular response to intubation in patients with severe pregnancy-induced hypertension[3] and was considered a suitable alternative to fentanyl 2.5 µg per kg; no effect on neonatal mortality could be attributed to anaesthetic technique. However, it has been suggested that the use of smaller doses of alfentanil of 7.5 µg per kg with magnesium sulfate 30 mg per kg may provide better cardiovascular control.[4]
1. Leuwer M, *et al.* Pharmacokinetics and pharmacodynamics of an equipotent fentanyl and alfentanil dose in mother and infant during caesarean section. *Br J Anaesth* 1990; **64:** 398P–9P.
2. Redfern N, *et al.* Alfentanil for caesarean section complicated by severe aortic stenosis: a case report. *Br J Anaesth* 1987; **59:** 1309–12.
3. Rout CC, Rocke DA. Effects of alfentanil and fentanyl on induction of anaesthesia in patients with severe pregnancy-induced hypertension. *Br J Anaesth* 1990; **65:** 468–74.
4. Ashton WB, *et al.* Attenuation of the pressor response to tracheal intubation by magnesium sulphate with and without alfentanil in hypertensive proteinuric patients undergoing caesarean section. *Br J Anaesth* 1991; **67:** 741–7.

PHAEOCHROMOCYTOMA. Alfentanil does not release histamine and was of value in the anaesthetic management of patients with phaeochromocytoma.[1] It has a rapid onset of action, good vasodilating properties, and a relatively short elimination half-life. These patients are often very somnolent for the first 48 hours after surgery and postoperative opioid dosage requirements may be less than expected. Alfentanil infusion continued into the postoperative period allows careful titration of dosage.
1. Hull CJ. Phaeochromocytoma: diagnosis, preoperative preparation and anaesthetic management. *Br J Anaesth* 1986; **58:** 1453–68.

Pain. POSTOPERATIVE ANALGESIA. Continuous on-demand epidural infusions of alfentanil 200 µg per hour or fentanyl 20 µg per hour provided comparable analgesia to morphine 200 µg per hour in the early postoperative period;[1] alfentanil (16 minutes) and fentanyl (13 minutes) had the advantage of more rapid onset of analgesia than morphine (44 minutes). However, some considered that there was no overall advantage of epidural over intravenous administration in patients receiving alfentanil either as patient-controlled analgesia[2] or as a continuous infusion.[3]
1. Chrubasik J, *et al.* Relative analgesic potency of epidural fentanyl, alfentanil, and morphine in treatment of postoperative pain. *Anesthesiology* 1988; **68:** 929–33.
2. Chauvin M, *et al.* Equivalence of postoperative analgesia with patient-controlled intravenous or epidural alfentanil. *Anesth Analg* 1993; **76:** 1251–8.
3. van den Nieuwenhuyzen MCO, *et al.* Epidural vs intravenous infusion of alfentanil in the management of postoperative pain following laparotomies. *Acta Anaesthesiol Scand* 1996; **40:** 1112–18.

Preparations

USP 25: Alfentanil Injection.

Proprietary Preparations (details are given in Part 3)
Aust.: Rapifen; *Austral.:* Rapifen; *Belg.:* Rapifen; *Braz.:* Rapifen; *Canad.:* Alfenta; *Denm.:* Rapifen; *Fin.:* Rapifen; *Fr.:* Rapifen; *Ger.:* Rapifen; *Hong Kong:* Rapifen; *Irl.:* Rapifen; *Israel:* Rapifen; *Ital.:* Fentalim; *Mex.:* Rapifen; *Neth.:* Rapifen; *Norw.:* Rapifen; *NZ:* Rapifen; *S.Afr.:* Rapifen; *Spain:* Fanaxal; Limifen; *Swed.:* Rapifen; *Switz.:* Rapifen; *UK:* Rapifen; *USA:* Alfenta.

Alminoprofen (16021-j)

Alminoprofen *(rINN).*
4-[(2-Methylallyl)amino]hydratropic acid.
$C_{13}H_{17}NO_2 = 219.3.$
$CAS — 39718-89-3.$
$ATC — M01AE16.$

Profile

Alminoprofen, a propionic acid derivative related to ibuprofen (p.43), is an NSAID (p.63). It has been used in inflammatory and rheumatic disorders in doses of up to 900 mg daily by mouth.

Preparations

Proprietary Preparations (details are given in Part 3)
Fr.: Minalfene.

Aloxiprin (2607-z)

Aloxiprin *(BAN, rINN).*
$CAS — 9014-67-9.$
$ATC — B01AC15; N02BA02.$
Pharmacopoeias. In Br.

Aloxiprin 600 mg is approximately equivalent to 500 mg of aspirin.

Pharmacopoeial description

BP 2001: A polymeric condensation product of aluminium oxide and aspirin. A fine, white or slightly pink powder, odourless or almost odourless. It contains not less than 7.5% and not more than 8.5% of aluminium, Al, and not less than 79.0% and not more than 87.4% of total salicylates, calculated as aspirin, $C_9H_8O_4$, both calculated with reference to the dried substance. Practically insoluble in water, in alcohol, and in ether; slightly soluble in chloroform.

Adverse Effects, Treatment, and Precautions

As for Aspirin, p.14.

Aloxiprin, like aspirin, should not generally be given to children under the age of 12 years because of the risk of Reye's syndrome.

Interactions

For interactions associated with salicylates, see Aspirin, p.16.

Pharmacokinetics

Aloxiprin is hydrolysed in the gastrointestinal tract to salicylate, the rate of breakdown being low in the acid conditions of the stomach and greater at the higher pH values of the intestine.

Uses and Administration

Aloxiprin, a polymeric condensation product of aluminium oxide and aspirin, has actions similar to those of aspirin (p.16) and has been used as an analgesic and anti-inflammatory in musculoskeletal and joint disorders. A usual dose was 600 mg to 1.2 g three times daily by mouth taken 30 minutes before food. Aloxiprin has also been used in the treatment and prevention of thromboembolic disorders.

Preparations

BP 2001: Aloxiprin Tablets.

Proprietary Preparations (details are given in Part 3)
Aust.: Palaprin; *Switz.:* Thrombace†.
Multi-ingredient: *UK:* Askit.

Aluminium Aspirin (2608-c)

Aluminum Acetylsalicylate; Aluminum Aspirin; Aspirin Aluminium. Bis(2-acetoxybenzoato-*O'*)hydroxyaluminium.
$C_{18}H_{15}AlO_9 = 402.3.$
$CAS — 23413-80-1.$
Pharmacopoeias. In Jpn.

Profile

Aluminium aspirin is a salicylic acid derivative (see Aspirin, p.14) that has been given by mouth in the management of fever, pain, and musculoskeletal and joint disorders.

Preparations

Proprietary Preparations (details are given in Part 3)
Ital.: Alupir; *Port.:* Aluprim†.
Multi-ingredient: *Aust.:* Kratofin†; *S.Afr.:* Analgen-SA; *Spain:* Meridol†.

Aminophenazone (2609-k)

Aminophenazone *(rINN).*
Amidazofen; Amidopyrine; Amidopyrine-Pyramidon; Aminopyrine; Dimethylaminoantipyrine; Dimethylaminophenazone. 4-Dimethylamino-1,5-dimethyl-2-phenyl-4-pyrazolin-3-one.
$C_{13}H_{17}N_3O = 231.3.$
$CAS — 58-15-1.$
$ATC — N02BB03.$
Pharmacopoeias. In Aust., It., and Port.

Profile

Aminophenazone, a pyrazolone derivative, is an NSAID (p.63), but the risk of agranulocytosis is sufficiently great to render it unsuitable for use. Onset of agranulocytosis may be sudden and unpredictable. Aminophenazone has been used in the form of a variety of salts or complexes including topically as the salicylate.

Precautions. CARCINOGENICITY. Some[1] consider that aminophenazone should be regarded as a potential carcinogen because it reacted readily with nitrous acid to form dimethylnitrosamine. The reaction was catalysed by thiocyanate present in the saliva particularly in smokers.
1. Boyland E, Walker SA. Catalysis of the reaction of aminopyrine and nitrite by thiocyanate. *Arzneimittelforschung* 1974; **24:** 1181–4.

PORPHYRIA. Aminophenazone has been associated with acute attacks of porphyria and is considered unsafe in porphyric patients.

Preparations

Proprietary Preparations (details are given in Part 3)
Multi-ingredient: *Braz.:* Gineburno; *Ital.:* Virdex; *Switz.:* Thermocutan.

Aminopropylone (14142-q)

Aminopropylon. *N*-(2,3-Dihydro-1,5-dimethyl-3-oxo-2-phenyl-1*H*-pyrazol-4-yl)-2-(dimethylamino)propanamide.
$C_{16}H_{22}N_4O_2 = 302.4.$
$CAS — 3690-04-8.$

Profile

Aminopropylone is an NSAID (p.63) used in topical preparations, usually in a concentration of 5% with a heparinoid, for the local treatment of pain and inflammatory conditions. The hydrochloride has been used similarly.

Preparations

Proprietary Preparations (details are given in Part 3)
Multi-ingredient: *Ital.:* Artrocur; Vessiflex.

Ammonium Salicylate (12370-m)

$C_7H_9NO_3 = 155.2$.
CAS — 528-94-9.

Profile
Ammonium salicylate is a salicylic acid derivative used topically in rubefacient preparations similarly to methyl salicylate (p.55) for the relief of pain in musculoskeletal and joint disorders.

Preparations
Proprietary Preparations (details are given in Part 3)
Multi-ingredient: *Austral.:* Radian-B; *Irl.:* Radian-B; *UK:* Aspellin; Radian-B.

Ampiroxicam (2484-x)

Ampiroxicam (BAN, rINN).
CP-65703. 4-[1-(Ethoxycarbonyloxy)ethoxy]-2-methyl-N^2-pyridyl-2H-1,2-benzothiazine-3-carboxamide 1,1-dioxide.
$C_{20}H_{21}N_3O_7S = 447.5$.
CAS — 99464-64-9.

Profile
Ampiroxicam is an NSAID (p.63) that is reported to be metabolised to piroxicam (p.79). Photosensitivity has been reported with its use.

Amtolmetin Guacil (15445-q)

Amtolmetin Guacil (rINN).
MED-15; ST-679. *N*-[(1-Methyl-5-*p*-toluoylpyrrol-2-yl)acetyl]glycine *o*-methoxyphenyl.
$C_{24}H_{24}N_2O_5 = 420.5$.
CAS — 87344-06-7.

Profile
Amtolmetin guacil is an NSAID (p.63). It is an ester prodrug of tolmetin (p.88) used in painful and inflammatory disorders. It is given by mouth in daily doses of 600 to 1200 mg.

Preparations
Proprietary Preparations (details are given in Part 3)
Ital.: Artromed; Eufans.

Amyl Salicylate (16508-j)

Isoamyl Salicylate; Isopentyl Salicylate. 3-Methylbutyl 2-hydroxybenzoate.
$C_{12}H_{16}O_3 = 208.3$.
CAS — 87-20-7.
Pharmacopoeias. In Fr.

Profile
Amyl salicylate is a salicylic acid derivative used topically in rubefacient preparations similarly to methyl salicylate (p.55) for its analgesic and anti-inflammatory actions. It has also been used in perfumery.

Preparations
Proprietary Preparations (details are given in Part 3)
Multi-ingredient: *Fr.:* Baume Dalet†; Baume Saint-Bernard†; Sedartryl; *Spain:* Balsamo Analgesic Karmel†; Linimento Klari.

Anileridine (6204-v)

Anileridine (BAN, rINN).
Ethyl 1-(4-aminophenethyl)-4-phenylpiperidine-4-carboxylate.
$C_{22}H_{28}N_2O_2 = 352.5$.
CAS — 144-14-9.
ATC — N01AH05.
Pharmacopoeias. In US.

Pharmacopoeial description
USP 25: A white to yellowish-white, odourless or practically odourless, crystalline powder. When exposed to light and air it oxidises and darkens in colour. It exhibits polymorphism, and of two crystalline forms observed, one melts at about 80° and the other at about 89°. Very slightly soluble in water; soluble 1 in 2 of alcohol and 1 in 1 of chloroform; soluble in ether but solutions may be turbid. Store in airtight containers. Protect from light.

Anileridine Hydrochloride (6205-g)

Anileridine Hydrochloride (BANM, rINNM).
$C_{22}H_{28}N_2O_2,2HCl = 425.4$.
CAS — 126-12-5.
Pharmacopoeias. In US.

Anileridine hydrochloride 30 mg is approximately equivalent to 25 mg of anileridine.

Pharmacopoeial description
USP 25: A white and nearly white odourless crystalline powder. Soluble 1 in 5 of water and 1 in 80 of alcohol; practically insoluble in chloroform and in ether. pH of a 5% solution in water is 2.5 to 3.0. Store in airtight containers. Protect from light.

Anileridine Phosphate (6206-q)

Anileridine Phosphate (BANM, rINNM).
$C_{22}H_{28}N_2O_2,H_3PO_4 = 450.5$.
CAS — 4268-37-5.

Anileridine phosphate 32 mg is approximately equivalent to 25 mg of anileridine.

Profile
Anileridine, a phenylpiperidine derivative, is an opioid analgesic (p.66) chemically related to pethidine (p.75) and with similar actions. It is used in the management of moderate to severe pain, including labour pain, and as an adjunct to anaesthesia. Anileridine is used as the hydrochloride and phosphate with doses expressed as anileridine base.

The usual dose of anileridine by mouth is 25 to 50 mg every 6 hours given as the hydrochloride.

The usual subcutaneous or intramuscular dose of anileridine for pain is 25 to 50 mg every 4 to 6 hours given as the phosphate, although for severe pain single doses of 75 to 100 mg may be given. The total daily dosage should not exceed 200 mg.

As an adjunct to anaesthesia, 50 to 100 mg of anileridine (as the phosphate) is added to 500 mL of glucose injection (5%) and the equivalent of 5 to 10 mg of anileridine is given by slow intravenous injection followed by slow intravenous infusion of the solution at a rate of about 600 µg of anileridine per minute.

Preparations
USP 25: Anileridine Hydrochloride Tablets; Anileridine Injection.
Proprietary Preparations (details are given in Part 3)
Canad.: Leritine.

Aspirin (2601-s)

Aspirin (BAN).
Acetylsal. Acid; Acetylsalicylic Acid; Acidum Acetylsalicylicum; Polopiryna; Salicylic Acid Acetate. *O*-Acetylsalicylic acid; 2-Acetoxybenzoic acid.
$C_9H_8O_4 = 180.2$.
CAS — 50-78-2.
ATC — A01AD05; B01AC06; N02BA01.

NOTE. The use of the name Aspirin is limited; in some countries it is a trade-mark.
Compounded preparations of aspirin may be represented by the following names:

• Co-codaprin (*BAN*)—aspirin 50 parts and codeine phosphate 1 part (w/w)

• Co-codaprin (*USP 25*)—aspirin and codeine phosphate.

Pharmacopoeias. In Chin., Eur. (see p.vi), Int., Jpn, Pol., and US.

Pharmacopoeial description
Ph. Eur.: White, crystalline powder or colourless crystals. Slightly soluble in water; freely soluble in alcohol; soluble in ether. Store in airtight containers.
USP 25: White crystals, commonly tubular or needle-like, or white crystalline powder; odourless or has a faint odour. Is stable in dry air; in moist air it gradually hydrolyses to salicylic and acetic acids. Soluble 1 in 300 of water, 1 in 5 of alcohol, 1 in 17 of chloroform, and 1 in 10 to 15 of ether; sparingly soluble in absolute ether. Store in airtight containers.

Adverse Effects and Treatment
Aspirin has many properties in common with the non-aspirin NSAIDs, the adverse effects of which are described on p.63.

The most common adverse effects occurring with therapeutic doses of aspirin are gastrointestinal disturbances such as nausea, dyspepsia, and vomiting. Gastrointestinal symptoms may be minimised by giving aspirin with food. Irritation of the gastric mucosa with erosion, ulceration, haematemesis, and melaena may occur. Histamine H_2-antagonists, proton pump inhibitors, and prostaglandin analogues such as misoprostol may be used in the management of aspirin-induced mucosal damage (see under Peptic Ulcer Disease, p.1208). Slight blood loss, which is often asymptomatic, may occur in about 70% of patients; it is not usually of clinical significance but may, in a few patients, cause iron-deficiency anaemia during long-term therapy. Such occult blood loss is not affected by administration of aspirin with food but may be reduced by use of enteric-coated or other modified-release tablets, H_2-antagonists, or high doses of antacids. Major upper gastrointestinal bleeding occurs rarely.

Some persons, especially those with asthma, chronic urticaria, or chronic rhinitis, exhibit notable hypersensitivity to aspirin (see also below), which may pro-voke various reactions including urticaria and other skin eruptions, angioedema, rhinitis, and severe, even fatal, paroxysmal bronchospasm and dyspnoea. Persons sensitive to aspirin often exhibit cross-sensitivity to other NSAIDs.

Aspirin increases bleeding time, decreases platelet adhesiveness, and, in large doses, may cause hypoprothrombinaemia. It may cause other blood disorders, including thrombocytopenia.

Aspirin and other salicylates may cause hepatotoxicity, particularly in patients with juvenile idiopathic arthritis or other connective tissue disorders. In children the use of aspirin has been implicated in some cases of Reye's syndrome, thus leading to severe restrictions on the indications for aspirin therapy in children. For further details see under Reye's Syndrome, below.

Aspirin given rectally may cause local irritation; anorectal stenosis has been reported.

Mild chronic salicylate intoxication, or salicylism, usually occurs only after repeated use of large doses. Salicylism can also occur following excessive topical application of salicylates. Symptoms include dizziness, tinnitus, deafness, sweating, nausea and vomiting, headache, and mental confusion, and may be controlled by reducing the dosage. Tinnitus can occur at the plasma concentrations of 150 to 300 µg per mL required for optimal anti-inflammatory activity; more serious adverse effects occur at concentrations above 300 µg per mL. Symptoms of more severe intoxication or of acute poisoning following overdosage include hyperventilation, fever, restlessness, ketosis, and respiratory alkalosis and metabolic acidosis. Depression of the CNS may lead to coma; cardiovascular collapse and respiratory failure may also occur. In children drowsiness and metabolic acidosis commonly occur; hypoglycaemia may be severe.

In acute oral salicylate overdosage repeated doses of activated charcoal may be given by mouth if the patient is suspected of ingesting more than 250 mg of salicylate per kg body-weight. The administration of activated charcoal not only prevents the absorption of any salicylate remaining in the stomach but also aids the elimination of any that has been absorbed.

Measurement of plasma-salicylate concentration should be carried out in patients who have ingested more than 120 mg of salicylate per kg, although the severity of poisoning cannot be estimated from plasma concentrations alone. Absorption of aspirin can be delayed due to reduced gastric emptying, formation of concretions in the stomach, or as a result of ingestion of enteric-coated preparations. In consequence, plasma concentrations should be measured at least 2 hours after ingestion and repeated 2 hours later. Patients who overdose with enteric preparations require continual monitoring of plasma concentrations.

Fluid and electrolyte management is essential to correct acidosis, hyperpyrexia, hypokalaemia, and dehydration. Intravenous sodium bicarbonate is given to enhance urinary salicylate excretion if plasma salicylate concentrations exceed 500 µg per mL (350 µg per mL in children). Haemodialysis or haemoperfusion are also effective methods of removing salicylate from the plasma. The *British National Formulary* considers haemodialysis the method of choice in severe poisoning; it should be seriously considered when the plasma salicylate concentration is greater than 700 µg per mL. Vulnerable patients such as children or the elderly may require dialysis at an earlier stage.

◊ References to salicylate toxicity and its management.
1. Notarianni L. A reassessment of the treatment of salicylate poisoning. *Drug Safety* 1992; **7:** 292–303.
2. Woods D, *et al.* Acute toxicity of drugs: salicylates. *Pharm J* 1993; **250:** 576–8.
3. Collee GG, Hanson GC. The management of acute poisoning. *Br J Anaesth* 1993; **70:** 562–73.
4. Watson JE, Tagupa ET. Suicide attempt by means of aspirin enema. *Ann Pharmacother* 1994; **28:** 467–9.

Effects on the blood. In addition to its beneficial effects on platelets aspirin can cause adverse blood effects. An indication of this toxicity is given by an early reference[1] to reports submitted to the UK Committee on Safety of Medicines (CSM). There were 787 reports of adverse reactions to aspirin reported to the CSM between June 1964 and January 1973. These included 95 reports of blood disorders (17 fatal) including thrombocytopenia (26; 2 fatal), aplastic anaemia (13; 7 fatal), and agranulocytosis or pancytopenia (10; 2 fatal). Aspirin has also been associated with haemolytic anaemia in patients with glucose-6-phosphate dehydrogenase deficiency.[2]

1. Cuthbert MF. Adverse reactions to non-steroidal antirheumatic drugs. Curr Med Res Opin 1974; 2: 600–9.
2. Magee P, Beeley L. Drug-induced blood dyscrasias. Pharm J 1991; 246: 396–7.

Effects on blood pressure. For reference to the effects of aspirin on blood pressure compared with other NSAIDs, see Effects on the Cardiovascular System, p.63.

Effects on the gastrointestinal tract. Clinical and epidemiological evidence suggests that aspirin produces dose-related gastrointestinal toxicity[1,2] that is sometimes, but rarely, fatal.[2] Meta-analysis[3] suggests that the risk of gastrointestinal bleeding is not significantly lowered with the use of low-dose aspirin (less than 300 mg daily). Although it was suggested that very small doses of aspirin can produce prophylactic benefits in cardiovascular disease without the risk of gastrointestinal toxicity,[4] others have reported gastric injury even with doses of 10 mg daily.[5] There appears to be no convincing evidence that the risk of major gastrointestinal bleeding associated with a 75-mg dose is reduced by using enteric-coated or modified-release formulations rather than soluble aspirin,[3,6] although individual studies have reported a reduction in acute mucosal injury with enteric coating.[7] All known NSAIDs have the potential for causing acute damage to the gastric mucosa (see p.63), and comparative studies of acute gastric mucosal damage caused by such drugs consistently associate aspirin with the most severe lesions.[1] Gastric mucosal injury can occur even with cutaneous application.[8]

1. Graham DY, Smith JL. Aspirin and the stomach. Ann Intern Med 1986; 104: 390–8.
2. Roderick PJ, et al. The gastrointestinal toxicity of aspirin: an overview of randomised controlled trials. Br J Clin Pharmacol 1993; 35: 219–26.
3. Derry S, Loke YK. Risk of gastrointestinal haemorrhage with long term use of aspirin: meta-analysis. BMJ 2000; 321: 1183–7.
4. Lee M, et al. Dose effects of aspirin on gastric prostaglandins and stomach mucosal injury. Ann Intern Med 1994; 120: 184–9.
5. Cryer B, Feldman M. Effects of very low dose daily, long-term aspirin therapy on gastric, duodenal, and rectal prostaglandin levels and on mucosal injury in healthy humans. Gastroenterology 1999; 117: 17–25.
6. Anonymous. Which prophylactic aspirin? Drug Ther Bull 1997; 35: 7–8.
7. Cole AT, et al. Protection of human gastric mucosa against aspirin—enteric coating or dose reduction? Aliment Pharmacol Ther 1999; 13: 187–93.
8. Cryer B, et al. Effects of cutaneous aspirin on the human stomach and duodenum. Proc Assoc Am Physicians 1999; 111: 448–56.

Effects on hearing. Studies have indicated that tinnitus develops at serum-salicylate concentrations above 200 μg per mL.[1] However, there appears to be considerable intersubject variation in the response of the ear to salicylate;[2] tinnitus may occur at lower concentrations, whereas patients with pre-existing hearing loss may not experience tinnitus despite serum-salicylate concentrations of 311 to 677 μg per mL.[1] A graded increase in intensity of ototoxicity with increasing salicylate dose and plasma concentration has been demonstrated.[2] For example, at an average total plasma-salicylate concentration of 110 μg per mL, the hearing loss at any given frequency was about 12 decibels; such a deficit might be relevant to patients with pre-existing hearing impairment.[2]

1. Mongan E, et al. Tinnitus as an indication of therapeutic serum salicylate levels. JAMA 1973; 226: 142–5.
2. Day RO, et al. Concentration-response relationships for salicylate-induced ototoxicity in normal volunteers. Br J Clin Pharmacol 1989; 28: 695–702.

Effects on the heart. Salicylate poisoning may result in cardiovascular collapse but details of such cases have not been widely reported. In 2 patients with salicylate intoxication asystole developed following the intravenous administration of diazepam.[1] It was suggested that diazepam-induced respiratory depression affected the acid-base balance so that the concentration of non-ionised membrane-penetrating fraction of salicylate was increased.

1. Berk WA, Andersen JC. Salicylate-associated asystole: report of two cases. Am J Med 1989; 86: 505–6.

Effects on the kidneys. Although abuse of combined analgesic preparations containing aspirin has been implicated in the development of analgesic nephropathy, kidney damage associated with the therapeutic use of aspirin alone appears to be comparatively rare. Many studies have failed to find an increased risk of renal damage in patients taking aspirin.[1-8]

1. New Zealand Rheumatism Association Study. Aspirin and the kidney. BMJ 1974; 1: 593–6.
2. Walker BR, et al. Aspirin and renal function. N Engl J Med 1977; 297: 1405.
3. Akyol SM, et al. Renal function after prolonged consumption of aspirin. BMJ 1982; 284: 631–2.
4. Bonney SL, et al. Renal safety of two analgesics used over the counter: ibuprofen and aspirin. Clin Pharmacol Ther 1986; 40: 373–7.

5. Sandler DP, et al. Analgesic use and chronic renal disease. N Engl J Med 1989; 320: 1238–43.
6. Pommer W, et al. Regular analgesic intake and the risk of end-stage renal failure. Am J Nephrol 1989; 9: 403–12.
7. Dubach UC, et al. An epidemiological study of abuse of analgesic drugs: effects of phenacetin and salicylate on mortality and cardiovascular morbidity (1968 to 1987). N Engl J Med 1991; 324: 155–60.
8. Perneger TV, et al. Risk of kidney failure associated with the use of acetaminophen, aspirin, and nonsteroidal antiinflammatory drugs. N Engl J Med 1994; 331: 1675–9.

Effects on the liver. Aspirin-induced hepatic injury is generally mild and manifests as a mild to moderate elevation in aminotransferase values; however, there is a risk of severe liver injury.[1] One review[2] reported an increase in aminotransferase values in 59 of 439 patients given aspirin; the increase was considered to be probably related to aspirin in 23 of the 59 patients. Hepatotoxicity appears to be correlated with serum-salicylate concentrations greater than 150 μg per mL and with active rheumatoid disease. Aspirin-induced liver injury is usually reversible on discontinuing the drug.[2]
See also under Reye's Syndrome, below.

1. Lewis JH. Hepatic toxicity of nonsteroidal anti-inflammatory drugs. Clin Pharm 1984; 3: 128–38.
2. Freeland GR. Hepatic safety of two analgesics used over the counter: ibuprofen and aspirin. Clin Pharmacol Ther 1988; 43: 473–9.

Effects on the mouth. Aspirin burn (ulceration of the mucosal layer of the lips) developed in a 26-year-old woman after taking an aspirin-containing powder for a migraine.[1] The woman had swallowed the powder undissolved rather than adding to water before administering.

1. Dellinger TM, Livingston HM. Aspirin burn of the oral cavity. Ann Pharmacother 1998; 32: 1107.

Hypersensitivity. The main clinical features of patients who have aspirin hypersensitivity include middle-age, female sex, diagnoses of asthma or rhinitis, a personal or family history of atopy, and a history of nasal polyps.[1,2] The occurrence of aspirin sensitivity in patients with asthma and nasal polyps has been referred to in some reports as the 'aspirin triad'. Other sensitivities often found concomitantly include allergy to food dyes such as tartrazine and to other drugs such as other NSAIDs. The response to individual NSAIDs is believed to be closely linked to the extent to which they inhibit prostaglandin synthesis.[3,4] There may be a dose threshold below which no detectable symptoms occur and patients who may be tolerant of regular low-dose aspirin may develop symptoms when they take larger doses.[4] Some[4] use a formal challenge with a 300-mg dose of aspirin by mouth to confirm a diagnosis of NSAID sensitivity but others[5] consider this to be a dangerous technique and use inhalation of lysine aspirin which they consider to be a safer and more predictable alternative.

1. Kwoh CK, Feinstein AR. Rates of sensitivity reactions to aspirin: problems in interpreting the data. Clin Pharmacol Ther 1986; 40: 494–505.
2. Schiavino D, et al. The aspirin disease. Thorax 2000; 55 (suppl 2): S66–S69.
3. Power I. Aspirin-induced asthma. Br J Anaesth 1993; 71: 619–11.
4. Frew A. Selected side-effects: 13. non-steroidal anti-inflammatory drugs and asthma. Prescribers' J 1994; 34: 74–7.
5. Davies BH. NSAIDs and asthma. Prescribers' J 1994; 34: 163–4.

DESENSITISATION. Successful desensitisation has been achieved using various oral aspirin challenge protocols.[1,2] Incremental doses of aspirin (starting at 30 mg) are given until an allergic response is obtained; aspirin is readministered at the dose that caused the response and again incremental doses are given until finally a 650-mg dose is tolerated. After desensitisation, an interruption of continuous aspirin administration results in the reappearance of sensitivity.

1. Asad SI, et al. Effect of aspirin in "aspirin sensitive" patients. BMJ 1984; 288: 745–8.
2. Stevenson DD. Desensitization of aspirin-sensitive asthmatics: a therapeutic alternative? J Asthma 1983; 20: 31–8.

Hypoglycaemia. A review of the literature[1] on drug-induced hypoglycaemia has highlighted the fact that overdosage with salicylates can produce hypoglycaemia in children. Although it is recognised[1,2] that therapeutic doses of salicylates in adults can lower blood-glucose concentrations in diabetic and non-diabetic subjects alike, opinion on the clinical significance of this effect varies. Salicylates have been implicated in a few cases of hypoglycaemia in adults[1] and some[2] suggest that patients with renal impairment or those receiving large doses, such as in the treatment of rheumatoid arthritis, may be at risk. Hypoglycaemia has been reported in a patient with renal failure following excessive application of a topical preparation containing salicylic acid.[3]

1. Seltzer HS. Drug-induced hypoglycemia: a review of 1418 cases. Endocrinol Metab Clin North Am 1989; 18: 163–83.
2. Pandit MK, et al. Drug-induced disorders of glucose tolerance. Ann Intern Med 1993; 118: 529–39.
3. Raschke R, et al. Refractory hypoglycemia secondary to topical salicylate intoxication. Arch Intern Med 1991; 151: 591–3.

Reye's syndrome. Reye's syndrome is a disorder characterised by acute encephalopathy and fatty degeneration of the liver. It occurs almost exclusively in children although cases have been seen[1] in patients over the age of 12. Many factors may be involved in its aetiology but it typically occurs after a viral infection such as chickenpox or influenza and may be precipitated by a chemical trigger. Several large studies, as well as indi-

vidual case reports, have found an association between Reye's syndrome and the prior ingestion of aspirin.[2-5] The evidence for other salicylates could not be adequately evaluated.[4] Although the role of aspirin and possibly other salicylates in the pathogenesis of Reye's syndrome remains to be determined, the use of aspirin and other acetylated salicylates as analgesics or antipyretics is generally considered contra-indicated in children under the age of 12 years and, in some countries, in teenagers. Some authorities also extend this precaution to non-acetylated salicylates. Most authorities consider one of the few acceptable indications remaining for the use of aspirin in children to be juvenile idiopathic arthritis. One group of workers[6] who re-examined some of the original studies suggested that there might also be a link between Reye's syndrome and the use of antiemetics, phenothiazines, and some other antihistamines, but their conclusions have been criticised.[7]

1. Hall SM, Lynn R. Reye's syndrome. N Engl J Med 1999; 341: 845–6.
2. Waldman RJ, et al. Aspirin as a risk factor in Reye's syndrome. JAMA 1982; 247: 3089–94.
3. Halpin TJ, et al. Reye's syndrome and medication use. JAMA 1982; 248: 687–91.
4. Hurwitz ES, et al. Public health service study of Reye's syndrome and medications: report of the main study. JAMA 1987; 257: 1905–11.
5. Hall SM, et al. Preadmission antipyretics in Reye's syndrome. Arch Dis Child 1988; 63: 857–66.
6. Casteels-Van Daele M, Eggermont E. Reye's syndrome. BMJ 1994; 308: 919–20.
7. Hall SM. Reye's syndrome. BMJ 1994; 309: 411.

Precautions

Aspirin has many properties in common with the non-aspirin NSAIDs, the precautions of which are described on p.64.

Aspirin should be cautiously employed, if at all, in patients prone to dyspepsia or known to have a lesion of the gastric mucosa. It should not be administered to patients with haemophilia or other haemorrhagic disorders, or to treat patients with gout since low doses increase urate concentrations.

Aspirin should be used with caution in patients with asthma or allergic disorders. It should not be given to patients with a history of sensitivity reactions to aspirin or other NSAIDs, which includes those in whom attacks of asthma, angioedema, urticaria, or rhinitis have been precipitated by such drugs (for further details of risk factors see Hypersensitivity under Adverse Effects, above).

Caution is necessary when renal or hepatic function is impaired; aspirin should be avoided in severe renal or hepatic impairment. Aspirin should be used cautiously in dehydrated patients and in the presence of uncontrolled hypertension.

High doses may precipitate acute haemolytic anaemia in patients with glucose 6-phosphate dehydrogenase deficiency. Aspirin may interfere with insulin and glucagon control in diabetics (see Hypoglycaemia under Adverse Effects, above).

The use of aspirin in children under the age of 12 years is extremely limited because of the risk of Reye's syndrome (see under Adverse Effects, above, and under Uses and Administration, below).

Although low-dose aspirin might be used in some pregnant patients, analgesic doses of aspirin should not be used at term as it may be associated with delayed onset and prolongation of labour and with maternal and neonatal bleeding. High doses may cause closure of fetal ductus arteriosus before birth and possibly persistent pulmonary hypertension in the newborn (but see under Pregnancy, below); kernicterus may occur in jaundiced neonates. Mothers who are breast feeding their infants should not take aspirin.

Continuous prolonged use of aspirin should be avoided in the elderly because of the risk of gastrointestinal bleeding.

Aspirin should be discontinued several days before scheduled surgical procedures (see below).

Aspirin and other salicylates can interfere with thyroid function tests.

Pregnancy. The potential adverse effects of aspirin when used during pregnancy have been reviewed.[1] Salicylates readily cross the placenta in animals. Although some studies and anecdotal reports have implicated aspirin in the formation of congenital abnormalities, most large studies[2-4] have failed to find any significant risk or evidence of teratogenicity. Analysis of data collected by the Slone Epidemiology Unit Birth Defects Study suggests that use of aspirin during the early months of pregnancy, when the fetal heart is developing, is not associated with an increased risk of cardiac defects.[5] The ability of aspirin, however, to alter platelet function may be a potential risk. There have been a few reports of haemorrhagic disorders in infants whose mothers had consumed aspirin during pregnancy[6] and of salicylate-associated haemorrhagic complications in mothers.[7] However, no clinically significant adverse effects on maternal or neonatal bleeding or on fetal ductus flow were reported in 6 controlled studies which evaluated low-dose aspirin (less than 325 mg daily) in pregnancy-induced hypertension.[8] It appeared that the degree of cyclo-oxygenase inhibition produced by aspirin was unlikely to be great enough to cause premature closure of the ductus arteriosus or to affect the pulmonary blood vessels.[1] However, in some studies in patients considered to have high-risk pregnancies the risk of abruptio placentae[9] or consequent perinatal death[10] was increased by maternal administration of aspirin. For reference to a possible association between aspirin and other NSAIDs and persistent pulmonary hypertension of the newborn, see under NSAIDs, p.65.

Although aspirin has the potential to inhibit uterine contractions of labour it was considered that intermittent or low dose aspirin therapy was unlikely to inhibit cyclo-oxygenase for long enough to prolong pregnancy or labour.[1]

1. de Swiet M, Fryers G. The use of aspirin in pregnancy. *J Obstet Gynaecol* 1990; **10:** 467–82.
2. Slone D, *et al.* Aspirin and congenital malformations. *Lancet* 1976; **1:** 1373–5.
3. Shapiro S, *et al.* Perinatal mortality and birth-weight in relation to aspirin taken during pregnancy. *Lancet* 1976; **i:** 1375–6.
4. Winship KA, *et al.* Maternal drug histories and central nervous system anomalies. *Arch Dis Child* 1984; **59:** 1052–60.
5. Werler MM, *et al.* The relation of aspirin use during the first trimester of pregnancy to congenital cardiac defects. *N Engl J Med* 1989; **321:** 1639–42.
6. Bleyer WA, Breckenridge RT. Studies on the detection of adverse drug reactions in the newborn II: the effects of prenatal aspirin on newborn hemostasis. *JAMA* 1970; **213:** 2049–53.
7. Collins E, Turner G. Maternal effects of regular salicylate ingestion in pregnancy. *Lancet* 1975; **ii:** 335–7.
8. Imperiale TF, Petrulis AS. A meta-analysis of low-dose aspirin for the prevention of pregnancy-induced hypertensive disease. *JAMA* 1991; **266:** 261–4.
9. Sibai BM, *et al.* Prevention of preeclampsia with low-dose aspirin in healthy, nulliparous pregnant women. *N Engl J Med* 1993; **329:** 1213–18.
10. Hamid R, *et al.* Low dose aspirin in women with raised maternal serum alpha-fetoprotein and abnormal Doppler waveform patterns from the uteroplacental circulation. *Br J Obstet Gynaecol* 1994; **101:** 481–4.

Surgical procedures. Aspirin prolongs bleeding time, mainly by inhibiting platelet aggregation. This effect is irreversible and new platelets must be released into the circulation before bleeding time can return to normal. Therefore aspirin therapy should be discontinued several days before surgical procedures. In some clinical situations, aspirin may have been given shortly before a surgical procedure. When emergency coronary bypass surgery is required following myocardial infarction, most patients would have received aspirin as part of the initial treatment for infarction. Perioperative bleeding, transfusion requirements, and surgical re-exploration rates may be increased when aspirin is given.[1] Administration of desmopressin acetate may reduce the risk of perioperative bleeding (see under Haemorrhagic Disorders, p.1282).

Aspirin is sometimes given during the second and third trimester for the prevention of pregnancy-induced hypertensive disease (see under Hypertension, p.802). Studies indicate that when given in a dose of 325 mg daily or less, clinically significant effects on maternal or neonatal bleeding do not occur.[2] Some have suggested that aspirin therapy may increase the risk of formation of extradural haematoma thus making epidural anaesthesia inadvisable[3] but a subsequent study[4] found that low-dose aspirin during pregnancy did not increase the risk of bleeding complications during epidural anaesthesia.

Patients on low-dose aspirin, in whom tourniquets are used for nerve blocks or other procedures, may be at increased risk of developing purpuric rash.[5]

It has been suggested that in patients undergoing dermatological surgery, aspirin need only be stopped before surgery in those patients with a prolonged bleeding time, whereas patients with a normal bleeding time could continue therapy.[6]

1. Goldman S, *et al.* Improvement in early saphenous vein graft patency after coronary artery bypass surgery with antiplatelet therapy: results of a Veterans Administration Cooperative Study. *Circulation* 1988; **77:** 1324–32.
2. Imperiale TF, Petrulis AS. A meta-analysis of low-dose aspirin for the prevention of pregnancy-induced hypertensive disease. *JAMA* 1991; **266:** 260–4.
3. Macdonald R. Aspirin and extradural blocks. *Br J Anaesth* 1991; **66:** 1–3.
4. Sibai BM, *et al.* Low-dose aspirin in nulliparous women: safety of continuous epidural block and correlation between bleeding time and maternal-neonatal bleeding complications. *Am J Obstet Gynecol* 1995; **172:** 1553–7.
5. Runcie CJ, *et al.* Aspirin and intravenous regional blocks. *Br J Hosp Med* 1990; **43:** 229–30.
6. Lawrence C, *et al.* Effect of aspirin and nonsteroidal antiinflammatory drug therapy on bleeding complications in dermatologic surgical patients. *J Am Acad Dermatol* 1994; **31:** 988–92.

Interactions

Aspirin has many properties in common with the non-aspirin NSAIDs, the interactions of which are described on p.65.

Some of the effects of aspirin on the gastrointestinal tract are enhanced by alcohol. Concurrent use of aspirin and dipyridamole may result in an increase in plasma-salicylate concentrations. Administration of drugs such as metoclopramide in patients with migraine headache results in earlier absorption of aspirin and higher peak plasma-salicylate concentrations. Metoprolol may increase peak plasma-salicylate concentrations. Salicylate intoxication has occurred in patients on high-dose salicylate regimens and carbonic anhydrase inhibitors. Plasma-salicylate concentrations may be reduced by concurrent use of corticosteroids. This interaction is likely to be important in patients receiving high-dose long-term salicylate treatment. Conversely, salicylate toxicity may occur if corticosteroids are withdrawn. Also the risk of gastrointestinal bleeding and ulceration associated with aspirin is increased when used with corticosteroids. Antacids and adsorbents may increase the excretion of aspirin in alkaline urine. Administration of gold compounds with aspirin may exacerbate aspirin-induced liver damage. Aspirin may enhance the activity of coumarin anticoagulants, sulfonylurea hypoglycaemic drugs, zafirlukast, methotrexate, phenytoin, and valproate. Aspirin diminishes the effects of uricosurics such as probenecid and sulfinpyrazone. The concomitant use of aspirin and other NSAIDs should be avoided because of the increased risk of adverse effects. Aspirin may decrease the plasma concentration of some other NSAIDs, for example, fenbufen, indometacin, and piroxicam. The manufacturer of mifepristone advises that aspirin or NSAIDs should be avoided for 8 to 12 days after mifepristone use because of a theoretical risk that these prostaglandin synthetase inhibitors may alter the efficacy of mifepristone.

◊ A review[1] of potential drug interactions related to aspirin.

1. Miners JO. Drug interactions involving aspirin (acetylsalicylic acid) and salicylic acid. *Clin Pharmacokinet* 1989; **17:** 327–44.

ACE inhibitors. For a discussion of aspirin and other NSAIDs reducing the activity of ACE inhibitors, see p.823.

Antifungals. Plasma-salicylate concentrations in an 8-year-old child receiving long-term aspirin therapy for rheumatic heart disease were markedly reduced when treatment with griseofulvin was started.[1] It was suggested that griseofulvin might interfere with absorption of aspirin.

1. Phillips KR, *et al.* Griseofulvin significantly decreases serum salicylate concentrations. *Pediatr Infect Dis J* 1993; **12:** 350–2.

Calcium-channel blockers. The antiplatelet effects of aspirin and calcium-channel blockers may be increased when they are used together; there have been isolated reports[1,2] of disturbed haemostasis including abnormal bruising, prolonged bleeding times and ecchymosis in patients taking aspirin and verapamil concurrently.

1. Ring ME, *et al.* Clinically significant antiplatelet effects of calcium-channel blockers. *J Clin Pharmacol* 1986; **26:** 719–20.
2. Verzino E, *et al.* Verapamil-aspirin interaction. *Ann Pharmacother* 1994; **28:** 536–7.

General anaesthetics. For the effect of aspirin on thiopental anaesthesia, see p.1269.

Spironolactone. For the effect of aspirin in patients taking spironolactone, see p.974.

Pharmacokinetics

Aspirin and other salicylates are absorbed rapidly from the gastrointestinal tract but absorption following rectal administration is less reliable than after oral administration. Aspirin and other salicylates can also be absorbed through the skin.

Following oral administration, absorption of non-ionised aspirin occurs in the stomach and intestine. Some aspirin is hydrolysed to salicylate in the gut wall. After absorption aspirin is rapidly converted to salicylate but during the first 20 minutes following oral administration, aspirin is the predominant form of the drug in the plasma. Aspirin is 80 to 90% bound to plasma proteins and is widely distributed; its volume of distribution is reported to be 170 mL per kg bodyweight in adults. As plasma-drug concentrations increase, the binding sites on the proteins become satu-

rated and the volume of distribution increases. Both aspirin and salicylate have pharmacological activity; only aspirin has an anti-platelet effect. Salicylate is extensively bound to plasma proteins and is rapidly distributed to all body parts. Salicylate appears in breast milk and crosses the placenta.

Salicylate is mainly eliminated by hepatic metabolism; the metabolites include salicyluric acid, salicyl phenolic glucuronide, salicylic acyl glucuronide, gentisic acid, and gentisuric acid. The formation of the major metabolites, salicyluric acid and salicyl phenolic glucuronide, is easily saturated and follows Michaelis-Menten kinetics; the other metabolic routes are first-order processes. As a result, steady-state plasma-salicylate concentrations increase disproportionately with dose. Following a 325-mg aspirin dose, elimination is a first-order process and the plasma-salicylate half-life is about 2 to 3 hours; at high aspirin doses, the half-life increases to 15 to 30 hours. Salicylate is also excreted unchanged in the urine; the amount excreted by this route increases with increasing dose and also depends on urinary pH, about 30% of a dose being excreted in alkaline urine compared with 2% of a dose in acidic urine. Renal excretion involves glomerular filtration, active renal tubular secretion, and passive tubular reabsorption.

Salicylate is removed by haemodialysis.

◊ References.

1. Needs CJ, Brooks PM. Clinical pharmacokinetics of the salicylates. *Clin Pharmacokinet* 1985; **10:** 164–77.

Uses and Administration

Aspirin is a salicylate NSAID and has many properties in common with non-aspirin NSAIDs (p.65). Aspirin and other salicylates have analgesic, anti-inflammatory, and antipyretic properties; they act as inhibitors of the enzyme cyclo-oxygenase, which results in the direct inhibition of the biosynthesis of prostaglandins and thromboxanes from arachidonic acid (see p.1438). Aspirin also inhibits platelet aggregation; non-acetylated salicylates do not.

Aspirin is used for the relief of mild to moderate pain such as headache, dysmenorrhoea, myalgias, and dental pain. It has also been used in the management of pain and inflammation in acute and chronic rheumatic disorders such as rheumatoid arthritis, juvenile idiopathic arthritis, osteoarthritis, and ankylosing spondylitis. In the treatment of minor febrile conditions, such as colds or influenza, aspirin is of value for the reduction of temperature and relief of the headache and the joint and muscle pains.

Aspirin is also used for its antiplatelet activity in the initial treatment of cardiovascular disorders such as angina pectoris and myocardial infarction and for the prevention of cardiovascular events in a variety of conditions or procedures for patients at risk. For further details see under Antiplatelet Therapy, below.

Aspirin is usually taken by mouth. Gastric irritation may be reduced by taking doses after food. Various dosage forms are available including plain uncoated tablets, buffered tablets, dispersible tablets, enteric-coated tablets, and modified-release tablets. In some instances aspirin may be administered rectally by suppository.

The usual oral dose of aspirin as an analgesic and antipyretic is 0.3 to 0.9 g, repeated every 4 to 6 hours according to clinical needs, to a maximum of 4 g daily. The dose of suppositories is 0.6 to 0.9 g every 4 hours to a maximum of 3.6 g daily.

Plasma-salicylate concentrations of 150 to 300 μg per mL are required for optimal anti-inflammatory activity (but see also Adverse Effects, above). Doses need to be adjusted individually to achieve optimum concentrations. Generally doses of about 4 to 8 g daily in divided doses are used for acute rheumatic disorders such as rheumatoid arthritis or osteoarthritis. Doses of up to 5.4 g daily in divided doses may be sufficient in chronic conditions.

Indications for aspirin therapy in children are extremely limited because of the risk of Reye's syndrome (see under Adverse Effects, above), and include juvenile idiopathic arthritis and Still's disease. Suggested doses for children are 80 to 100 mg per kg body-weight daily in 5 or 6 divided doses with up to 130 mg per kg daily used in acute exacerbations if necessary.

Sodium aspirin has also been used for the treatment of pain and fever.

Antiplatelet therapy. Aspirin's antiplatelet activity has led to its use or investigation in a variety of disorders.[1-4] It is used as part of the initial treatment of unstable *angina* (p.791) and is given in the early treatment of *myocardial infarction* (p.805); it is also of some benefit in the initial treatment of acute *ischaemic stroke* (p.813). It is of value for the *secondary prevention* of cardiovascular events in patients with stable or unstable angina or those with current or previous myocardial infarction. Similarly, aspirin reduces the risk of future serious vascular events, including stroke, in patients who have already suffered an ischaemic stroke or transient ischaemic attack and it has been used in the long-term management of atrial fibrillation (see under Cardiac Arrhythmias, p.794) for the prevention of stroke in patients with contra-indications to warfarin or if there are no other risk factors for stroke. The value of aspirin for *primary prevention* of myocardial infarction and stroke is considered to depend upon the accurate estimation of coronary event risk.[13]

Although aspirin may prevent *venous thromboembolism* (p.817) following surgery other treatments have been preferred. However, it is recommended for use in preventing thrombotic complications associated with procedures such as angioplasty and coronary bypass grafting (see under Reperfusion and Revascularisation Procedures, p.812). Aspirin is often given as an adjunct to patients with *peripheral arterial thromboembolism* (p.808) to prevent propagation of the clot and also to prevent post-operative complications. It may have some effect in delaying disease progression and reducing vascular events in patients with *peripheral arterial disease* (p.809) but an analysis[5] concluded that there was insufficient evidence to support its prophylactic use in patients with intermittent claudication but no additional cardiovascular risk factors. Similarly, the benefit of aspirin for the primary prevention of cardiovascular events in patients with *diabetes mellitus* (see under Diabetic Complications, p.317) and who have no other cardiovascular risk factors remains to be determined. The value of adding aspirin to anticoagulants for the prophylaxis of thromboembolism in patients with *artificial heart valves* (see p.816) is still to be firmly established. It is usually recommended as an adjunct in patients with other risk factors. Aspirin alone may be considered in patients with bioprosthetic valves who do not require anticoagulation.

Aspirin's range of activities, including its antiplatelet activity, is put to use in the treatment of *Kawasaki disease* (see below). It is also used to treat thrombotic symptoms associated with *antiphospholipid syndrome*, such as occurs in patients with systemic lupus erythematosus (p.1059), and has been recommended for prophylactic use in pregnant patients with antiphospholipid antibodies who are at risk of fetal loss. Aspirin has also been tried in *pregnancy-induced hypertension* (see under Hypertension, p.802) for the prevention of pre-eclampsia and intra-uterine growth retardation but it appears that its use may be justified only in women at high risk.

Aspirin is an inhibitor of the enzyme cyclo-oxygenase, the **action** being considered to be due to an irreversible acetylation process. In blood platelets such enzyme inhibition prevents the synthesis of thromboxane A$_2$, a compound which is a vasoconstrictor, causes platelet aggregation and is thus potentially thrombotic. In blood vessel walls the enzyme inhibition prevents the synthesis of prostacyclin, which is a vasodilator, has anti-aggregating properties and is thus potentially anti-thrombotic. Aspirin therefore appears to have paradoxical biological effects. The duration of these effects, however, may be somewhat different with the effects on the vascular tissue generally being shorter lived than the effects on the platelets (although the animal species studied, the type of blood vessel employed, and the prevailing experimental conditions may alter the results). The differing duration of effects may be explained by the fact that vascular cells regain the ability to regenerate prostacyclin in a few hours but platelets are unable to re-synthesise cyclo-oxygenase thus resulting in no new thromboxane A$_2$ being produced until, after about 24 hours, more platelets are released by the bone marrow; as platelet activity in bone marrow may also be affected by aspirin it is generally considered that aspirin need not be given more frequently than once daily for inhibition of platelet aggregation to occur. The inhibitory effect on thromboxane is rapid and unrelated to serum concentrations of aspirin, this probably being due to inactivation of cyclo-oxygenase in platelets in the presystemic circulation. Since the effect is unrelated to systemic bioavailability modified-release and dermal delivery preparations which do not achieve high systemic concentrations of aspirin are being developed to limit extraplatelet effects of aspirin. Inhibition is cumulative on repeat administration and it has been estimated that a daily dose of 20 to 50 mg will result in virtually complete suppression of platelet thromboxane synthesis within a few days. Large doses can produce maximum suppression almost instantaneously.

Several pharmacological studies have attempted to find a **dose** of aspirin that would inhibit synthesis of platelet thromboxane A$_2$ while sparing the effect on prostacyclin production[6-8] but it has been pointed out[4] that in patients with vascular disease accompanying or caused by endothelial dysfunction, such as in atherosclerosis, a selective sparing of vascular prostacyclin production may not be obtained at any effective antiplatelet dose. However, Hirsh *et al.*[9] have suggested that the clinical relevance of inhibiting the synthesis of prostacyclin has been exaggerated. Experimental evidence indicates that aspirin is thrombogenic only at extremely high doses (200 mg per kg body-weight), far exceeding the minimum dose required to inhibit prostacyclin production. Also aspirin is clinically effective as an antithrombotic drug at doses that inhibit the synthesis of prostacyclin. Further support for the lack of importance of inhibition of prostacyclin synthesis comes from epidemiological studies in patients with arthritis given large doses of aspirin and patients with congenital cyclo-oxygenase deficiency; neither of these groups of patients have experienced an excess of thrombotic episodes.

In the series of meta-analyses conducted by the Antiplatelet Trialists' Collaboration[10-12] doses of 75 to 325 mg were the most commonly tested; doses in this range appeared to be equally effective for their antiplatelet effect; larger doses did not appear to be superior and caused more gastrointestinal adverse effects. Whether lower doses offer the same efficacy with reduced gastrointestinal toxicity remains to be determined (see Effects on the Gastrointestinal Tract, above). A more recent analysis[5] concluded that a dose of 75 mg daily should be effective for secondary prophylaxis of vascular events although for patients with suspected or proven myocardial infarction a suitable dose may be 150 mg daily for the first month followed by 75 mg thereafter. Because doses in the order of 75 mg daily take a few days to exert a full antiplatelet effect treatment should be initiated with a loading dose such as 150 to 300 mg if immediate suppression is desirable as in the initial treatment of acute myocardial infarction and unstable angina. Aspirin should be chewed or dispersed in water; chewing a tablet of aspirin ensures that some buccal absorption occurs.

1. Patrono C. Aspirin as an antiplatelet drug. *N Engl J Med* 1994; **330:** 1287–94.
2. Lutomski DM, *et al.* Pharmacokinetic optimisation of the treatment of embolic disorders. *Clin Pharmacokinet* 1995; **28:** 67–92.
3. Catella-Lawson F, Fitzgerald GA. Long term aspirin in the prevention of cardiovascular disorders: recent developments and variations on a theme. *Drug Safety* 1995; **13:** 69–75.
4. Schrör K. Antiplatelet drugs: a comparative review. *Drugs* 1995; **50:** 7–28.
5. Eccles M, *et al.* North of England evidence based guideline development project: guideline on the use of aspirin as secondary prophylaxis for vascular disease in primary care. *BMJ* 1998; **316:** 1303–9.
6. Patrignani P, *et al.* Selective cumulative inhibition of platelet thromboxane production by low-dose aspirin in healthy subjects. *J Clin Invest* 1982; **69:** 1366–72.
7. Weksler BB, *et al.* Differential inhibition by aspirin of vascular and platelet prostaglandin synthesis in atherosclerotic patients. *N Engl J Med* 1983; **308:** 800–5.
8. McLeod LJ, *et al.* The effects of different doses of some acetyl-salicylic acid formulations on platelet function and bleeding times in healthy subjects. *Scand J Haematol* 1986; **36:** 379–84.
9. Hirsh J, *et al.* Aspirin and other platelet active drugs: relationship among dose, effectiveness, and side effects. *Chest* 1989; **95** (suppl 2): 12S–18S.
10. Antiplatelet Trialists' Collaboration. Collaborative overview of randomised trials of antiplatelet therapy—I: prevention of death, myocardial infarction, and stroke by prolonged antiplatelet therapy in various categories of patients. *BMJ* 1994; **308:** 81–106. Correction. *ibid.* : 1540.
11. Antiplatelet Trialists' Collaboration. Collaborative overview of randomised trials of antiplatelet therapy—II: maintenance of vascular graft or arterial patency by antiplatelet therapy. *BMJ* 1994; **308:** 159–68.
12. Antiplatelet Trialists' Collaboration. Collaborative overview of randomised trials of antiplatelet therapy—III: reduction in venous thrombosis and pulmonary embolism by antiplatelet prophylaxis among surgical and medical patients. *BMJ* 1994; **308:** 235–46.
13. Sanmuganathan PS, *et al.* Aspirin for primary prevention of coronary heart disease: safety and absolute benefit related to coronary risk derived from meta-analysis of randomised trials. *Heart* 2001; **85:** 265–71.

Behçet's syndrome. For reference to a recommendation that aspirin may be used with colchicine to prevent acute exacerbations of Behçet's syndrome, see p.1047.

Cataract. It has been suggested that some anti-inflammatory drugs might have beneficial effects against cataract formation but evidence to support or disprove the hypothesis that aspirin has a protective effect against cataract formation is considered inconclusive.[1,2] One study in the US in over 22 000 males concluded that low-dose aspirin (325 mg on alternate days) for 5 years was unlikely to have a major effect on cataract formation but that a slightly decreased risk for cataract extraction could not be excluded.[3] In a later study[4] in the UK ophthalmic examination of over 1800 patients who were receiving 300 to 1200 mg of aspirin daily for transient ischaemic attacks failed to confirm any protective effect. Re-analysis[5] of the results of the original US study identified additional cases of cataract formation or extraction although these cases did not affect the overall conclusions of the original study. However, when the study patients were followed up over 15 years, observational data[6] suggested that the use of low-dose aspirin may, in fact, increase the risk of cataract development. It was considered

that further trials were needed to establish the role of long-term aspirin in cataract prevention.

1. Cheng H. Aspirin and cataract. *Br J Ophthalmol* 1992; **76:** 257–8.
2. Anonymous. Preventing cataract. *Lancet* 1992; **340:** 883–4.
3. Seddon JM, *et al.* Low dose aspirin and risks of cataract in a randomised trial of US physicians. *Arch Ophthalmol* 1991; **109:** 252–5.
4. UK-TIA Study Group. Does aspirin affect the rate of cataract formation? Cross-sectional results during a randomised double-blind placebo controlled trial to prevent serious vascular events. *Br J Ophthalmol* 1992; **76:** 259–61.
5. Christen WG, *et al.* Low-dose aspirin and risk of cataract and subtypes in a randomized trial of U.S. physicians. *Ophthalmic Epidemiol* 1998; **5:** 133–42.
6. Christen WG, *et al.* Aspirin use and risk of cataract in posttrial follow-up of Physicians' Health Study I. *Arch Ophthalmol* 2001; **119:** 405–12.

Dysmenorrhoea. Drugs such as aspirin and other NSAIDs that inhibit prostaglandin production through inhibition of cyclo-oxygenase are effective drugs in the treatment of dysmenorrhoea (p.6).

Fever. Methods for controlling fever (see p.8) include the use of antipyretics and/or physical cooling methods. Paracetamol, salicylates such as aspirin and some other NSAIDs are the main antipyretics used. However, salicylates are generally contra-indicated for the management of fever in children because of the possible link between their use and the development of Reye's syndrome (see under Adverse Effects, above).

Headache. Aspirin is often used for the symptomatic treatment of various types of headache including migraine (see p.449) and tension-type headache (see p.450). Aspirin given at the onset of symptoms can successfully treat an acute attack of migraine. However, absorption may be poor due to gastric stasis which is commonly present in migraine. For this reason dispersible and effervescent preparations and compound preparations containing drugs such as metoclopramide which relieve gastric stasis have been advocated.
References.

1. Tfelt-Hansen P, Olesen J. Effervescent metoclopramide and aspirin (Migravess) versus effervescent aspirin or placebo for migraine attacks: a double-blind study. *Cephalalgia* 1984; **4:** 107–11.
2. Buring JE, *et al.* Low-dose aspirin for migraine prophylaxis. *JAMA* 1990; **264:** 1711–13.
3. The Oral Sumatriptan and Aspirin plus Metoclopramide Comparative Study Group. A study to compare oral sumatriptan with oral aspirin plus oral metoclopramide in the acute treatment of migraine. *Eur Neurol* 1992; **32:** 177–84.
4. Tfelt-Hansen P, *et al.* The effectiveness of combined oral lysine acetylsalicylate and metoclopramide compared with oral sumatriptan for migraine. *Lancet* 1995; **346:** 923–6.

Kawasaki disease. Aspirin has been given in regimens with normal immunoglobulins to children with Kawasaki disease (p.1554) because of its anti-inflammatory, antipyretic, and antiplatelet activity.[1-5]

The optimum dose and duration of treatment with aspirin have not yet been established but the usual practice is to use an anti-inflammatory regimen until the fever has settled and then convert to an antithrombotic regimen. Usual initial doses used have ranged from 30 to 120 mg per kg body-weight daily. Some clinicians recommend administration of aspirin in a dose of 80 to 100 mg per kg daily in 4 divided doses until the patient is afebrile or for the first 14 days after the onset of symptoms. Once fever and signs of inflammatory disease resolve, the aspirin dose is reduced to 3 to 5 mg per kg daily as a single dose for its antiplatelet effect. Aspirin may be discontinued 6 to 8 weeks after the onset of illness but is usually continued for at least one year if coronary abnormalities are present and is continued indefinitely if coronary aneurysms persist.

It has been noted[6] that aspirin has never been demonstrated in a prospective study to reduce the prevalence of coronary artery abnormalities in children with Kawasaki disease and recent studies[3,5] indicate that the incidence of such abnormalities following treatment was similar for regimens using high or low doses of aspirin. In view of the potential risks and lack of obvious cardiac benefits of high-dose aspirin some[6] consider that an argument could be made for use of a low dose such as 3 to 5 mg per kg daily to prevent thrombosis, with other drugs such as paracetamol or ibuprofen being added for fever control or severe arthritis.

1. Dajani AS, *et al.* Diagnosis and therapy of Kawasaki disease in children. *Circulation* 1993; **87:** 1776–80.
2. Dajani AS, *et al.* Guidelines for long-term management of patients with Kawasaki disease: report from the Committee on Rheumatic Fever, Endocarditis, and Kawasaki Disease, Council on Cardiovascular Disease in the Young, American Heart Association. *Circulation* 1994; **89:** 916–22.
3. Durongpisitkul K, *et al.* The prevention of coronary artery aneurysm in Kawasaki disease: a meta-analysis on the efficacy of aspirin and immunoglobulin treatment. *Pediatrics* 1995; **96:** 1057–61.
4. Samuel J, O'Sullivan J. Kawasaki disease. *Br J Hosp Med* 1996; **55:** 9–14.
5. Terai M, Shulman ST. Prevalence of coronary artery abnormalities in Kawasaki disease is highly dependent on gamma globulin dose but independent of salicylate dose. *J Pediatr* 1997; **131:** 888–93.
6. Newburger JW. Treatment of Kawasaki disease. *Lancet* 1996;

Leg ulcers. A 4-month placebo controlled study[1] in 20 patients suggested that aspirin 300 mg daily aided healing of chronic venous leg ulcers; the mechanism of action was unclear.[2] However, the validity of the findings has been challenged.[3] The management of leg ulcers is discussed on p.1108.

1. Layton AM, *et al.* Randomised trial of oral aspirin for chronic venous leg ulcers. *Lancet* 1994; **344:** 164–5.
2. Ibbotson SH, *et al.* The effect of aspirin on haemostatic activity in the treatment of chronic venous leg ulceration. *Br J Dermatol* 1995; **132:** 422–6.
3. Ruckley CV, Prescott RJ. Treatment of chronic leg ulcers. *Lancet* 1994; **344:** 1512–13.

Malignant neoplasms. For references to studies suggesting that regular use of aspirin and other NSAIDs may reduce the risk of developing malignant neoplasms of the gastrointestinal tract, see under NSAIDs, p.66.

Myeloproliferative disorders. Aspirin in low doses may be used to provide symptomatic relief for erythromelalgia (burning pain and erythema of the hands and feet) in patients with polycythaemia vera (p.486) and primary thrombocythaemia (p.486).

Pain. Aspirin and other salicylates are used in the management of mild to moderate pain (for details see p.2).

Rheumatic disorders. Aspirin was once widely used in the treatment of rheumatoid arthritis (p.9) but has been superseded by better tolerated NSAIDs; however, juvenile chronic arthritis (p.9) and Still's disease (p.11) are among the limited number of indications for aspirin use in children.

Preparations

BP 2001: Aspirin and Caffeine Tablets; Aspirin Tablets; Co-codaprin Tablets; Dispersible Aspirin Tablets; Dispersible Co-codaprin Tablets; Effervescent Soluble Aspirin Tablets; Enteric-coated Aspirin Tablets;
USP 25: Acetaminophen and Aspirin Tablets; Acetaminophen, Aspirin, and Caffeine Tablets; Aspirin and Codeine Phosphate Tablets; Aspirin Capsules; Aspirin Delayed-release Capsules; Aspirin Delayed-release Tablets; Aspirin Effervescent Tablets for Oral Solution; Aspirin Extended-release Tablets; Aspirin Suppositories; Aspirin Tablets; Aspirin, Alumina, and Magnesia Tablets; Aspirin, Alumina, and Magnesium Oxide Tablets; Buffered Aspirin Tablets; Butalbital and Aspirin Tablets; Butalbital, Aspirin, and Caffeine Capsules; Butalbital, Aspirin, and Caffeine Tablets; Butalbital, Aspirin, Caffeine, and Codeine Phosphate Capsules; Carisoprodol and Aspirin Tablets; Carisoprodol, Aspirin, and Codeine Phosphate Tablets; Oxycodone and Aspirin Tablets; Pentazocine Hydrochloride and Aspirin Tablets; Propoxyphene Hydrochloride, Aspirin, and Caffeine Capsules; Propoxyphene Napsylate and Aspirin Tablets.

Proprietary Preparations (details are given in Part 3)

Aust.: Acekapton; Acimetten†; Algobene; Aspiricor; Aspro; ASS; Colfarit†; Corsalbene; Thrombo ASS; *Austral.:* Aspro; Astrix; Bex; Cardiprin; Cartia; Disprin; Disprin Direct; Ecotrin†; Solprin; Spren; Vincent's Powders; Winsprin†; *Belg.:* Acenterine; Asaflow; Asarid; Aspirine; Aspro; Cardioaspirine; Catalgix†; Dispril; Rhodine†; Rhonal†; Sedergine; Therasa; *Braz.:* AAS; Aceticil; Acetin; Alidor; Aspirina; Aspisin; Aspylin; Buferin; Caas; Doloxene-A; Ecasil; Endosalil; Melhoral Infantil; Ronal; Somalgin; *Canad.:* Asaphen; Aspergum; Aspirin with Stomach Guard; Bufferin; Coryphen; Entrophen; Headache Tablets; Novasen; *Denm.:* Acetard†; Albyl†; Hjertealbyl†; Hjertemagnyl; Idotyl; Iskaemyl†; Magnyl; *Fin.:* Aspirin Cardio; Disperin; Primaspan; *Fr.:* Aspirine; Aspirine pH8; Aspirisucre; Aspro; Catalgine; Claragine; Juvepirine†; Rhonal†; Sargepirine†; *Ger.:* Acesal; Acesal Calcium†; Acetylin; Aspro; ASS; Godamed; Hermes ASS; HerzASS; Micristin†; Miniasal; Neuralgin ASS; Romigal; Santasal N; Spalt†; Thomapyrin akut; Togal ASS; *Hong Kong:* Ascriptin; Aspilets; Aspro; Astrix; Cardiprin; Cartia; Disprin; Ecotrin; *Irl.:* Ascriptin†; Aspro; Caprin; Clonteric; Disprin; Lowasa; Nu-Seals; Resprin; *Israel:* Acetosal; Alka-Seltzer; Ascriptin; Cartia; Ecoprin; Micropirin; Rhonal; *Ital.:* Acesal; Ascriptin; Aspiglicina; Aspirina; Aspirina 03 and 05; Aspirina 05; Aspirinetta; Aspro; Bufferin; Cardioaspirin; Cemirit; Kilios; Upsalgina; *Mex.:* Aciben; Adiro; Antacsal; ASA; Asawin; Ascriptin; Aspirina; Axal; Dolmex; Ecotrin; Labysal; Mejoral; Midolen; Rhonal. *Neth.:* Aspirine Protect; Aspro; Rhonal†; *Norw.:* Albyl-E; Bamycor; Dispril; Globentyl; Globoid; Novid; *NZ:* Aspec; Aspro; Cardiprin; Cartia; Disprin; Ecotrin; Pharmacare Aspec; *Port.:* AAS; ASP; Aspirina; Aspro; Cartia; Melhoral Infantil; Salycilina; Sedergine†; Toldex; *S.Afr.:* ASAtard; Aspirin†; Disprin; Ecotrin; Myoprin; *Singapore:* Aspro; Astrix; Cardiprin; Disprin; Dusil; *Spain:* AAS; Adiro; Algho†; Aspinfantil; Aspirina; Aspro†; Bioplak; Calmantina; Helver Sal; Lafena; Mejoral; Okal Infantil; Orravina; Rhonal; Saspryl; Sedergine; Tromalyt; Upsalgina†; *Swed.:* Albyl minor; Bamycor; Bamyl; Bamyl S; Dispril†; Magnecyl; Trombyl; *Switz.:* Aspro; ASS; Demoprin nouvelle formule; Thrombace Neo; Tiatral 100 SR; Togal ASS; *Thai.:* Aspent; Cardiprin; Comoprin; Entrarin; Seferin; *UAE:* Jusprin; *UK:* Angettes; Aspro; Beechams Lemon Tablets; Caprin; Disprin; Disprin CV†; Disprin Direct; Enprin; Fynnon Calcium Aspirin†; Gencardia; Micropirin; Nu-Seals; Platet†; PostMI; *USA:* 8-Hour Bayer Timed-Release†; Adprin-B; Arthritis Foundation Pain Reliever†; Arthritis Pain Formula; Arthritis Pain Tablets†; Ascriptin; Aspergum; Asprimox; Bayer Low Adult Strength; Bufferin; Buffex; Cama Arthritis Pain Reliever; Easprin; Ecotrin; Empirin; Extra Strength Bayer Plus; Genprin; Halfprin; Heartline; Magnaprin; Norwich Extra Strength; Regular Strength Bayer; St. Joseph Adult Chewable; ZORprin.

Multi-ingredient: numerous preparations are listed in Part 3.

Auranofin   (5293-j)

Auranofin *(BAN, USAN, rINN).*
SKF-39162; SKF-D-39162. (1-Thio-β-D-glucopyranosato)(triethylphosphine)gold 2,3,4,6-tetra-acetate.
$C_{20}H_{34}AuO_9PS = 678.5$.
CAS — 34031-32-8.
ATC — M01CB03.

Auranofin has a gold content of about 29%.

Adverse Effects and Treatment

The most common adverse effects of auranofin involve the gastrointestinal tract with nausea, abdominal pain, and sometimes vomiting, but most often diarrhoea which can affect up to 50% of patients and may be severe enough to cause patients to withdraw from treatment. Other adverse effects are similar to those experienced with sodium aurothiomalate (p.82), although they appear to be less troublesome in that fewer patients have been reported to discontinue treatment with auranofin than with injectable gold. As with other gold salts, treatment of adverse effects is generally symptomatic (see p.83). A bulking agent such as bran or modifying the diet to increase bulk or a temporary reduction in dosage may help the diarrhoea.

◊ Reviews.
1. Tozman ECS, Gottlieb NL. Adverse reactions with oral and parenteral gold preparations. *Med Toxicol* 1987; **2:** 177–89.

Effects on the gastrointestinal tract. Diarrhoea and abdominal pain are frequent adverse effects in patients taking auranofin. The mechanism of gastrointestinal toxicity has not been established but may be associated with a reversible defect in intestinal permeability.[1] Colitis and eosinophilia have been reported in a patient taking auranofin.[2]

1. Behrens R, *et al.* Investigation of auranofin-induced diarrhoea. *Gut* 1986; **27:** 59–65.
2. Michet CJ, *et al.* Auranofin-associated colitis and eosinophilia. *Mayo Clin Proc* 1987; **62:** 142–4.

Effects on the kidneys. In a retrospective review[1] of 1283 patients who had received auranofin for treatment of rheumatoid arthritis 41 were found to have developed proteinuria. Treatment of proteinuria in the majority of patients consisted of discontinuing auranofin therapy. Long-term follow-up of 36 patients indicated that proteinuria had resolved in 31 patients within 2 years and in 29 patients within 1 year. Seven of 8 patients later rechallenged with auranofin had no relapses. In a further review of 2 comparative double-blind studies using gold compounds in the treatment of rheumatoid arthritis, proteinuria was found to have developed in 27% (23 of 85) of patients treated with sodium aurothiomalate, in 17% (42 of 247) of those treated with auranofin, and in 17% (36 of 210) of those receiving placebo. All patients were receiving NSAIDs.

1. Katz WA, *et al.* Proteinuria in gold-treated rheumatoid arthritis. *Ann Intern Med* 1984; **101:** 176–9.

Precautions

As for Sodium Aurothiomalate, p.83. Urine and blood tests should be carried out monthly; the manufacturer advises that auranofin should be withdrawn if the platelet count falls below 100 000 per m³ or if signs and symptoms suggestive of thrombocytopenia occur. Auranofin should be administered with caution to patients with inflammatory bowel disease.

Porphyria. Auranofin has been associated with acute attacks of porphyria and is considered unsafe in porphyric patients.

Interactions

As for Sodium Aurothiomalate, p.83.

Pharmacokinetics

Auranofin is incompletely absorbed from the gastrointestinal tract, only about 25% of the gold being absorbed. Gold from auranofin is bound to plasma proteins as well as to red blood cells. After 2 to 3 months of treatment the steady-state concentration of gold in the blood is reported to be about 0.7 µg per mL. The average terminal plasma half-life of gold at steady state is about 26 days while the biological half-life is 81 days. Tissue retention and total gold accumulation in the body are less than with intramuscular gold. Gold from auranofin penetrates into synovial fluid.

Most of a dose of auranofin appears in the faeces due to its poor absorption. About 60% of the absorbed gold is excreted in the urine and the remainder in the faeces.

◊ Reviews.
1. Blocka KLN, *et al.* Clinical pharmacokinetics of oral and injectable gold compounds. *Clin Pharmacokinet* 1986; **11:** 133–43.

Uses and Administration

Auranofin has similar actions and uses to those of sodium aurothiomalate (p.83). It is given by mouth in active progressive rheumatoid arthritis (p.9); such oral treatment is less toxic than intramuscular gold but is also much less effective. The usual initial dose of auranofin is 6 mg daily either as a single dose or in two divided doses. Treatment should be continued for at least 6 months to assess the response; the dose may be increased after 6 months, if the response is inadequate, to 3 mg three times daily. If the response is still inadequate after 3 months at this dosage, then treatment should be discontinued.

Asthma. Auranofin is not usually used in the management of asthma (p.757) but studies[1] indicate that it can have a corticosteroid-sparing effect.

1. Bernstein IL, *et al.* A placebo-controlled multicenter study of auranofin in the treatment of patients with corticosteroid-dependent asthma. *J Allergy Clin Immunol* 1996; **98:** 317–24.

Lupus. Since the introduction of less toxic drugs gold salts are now rarely used in the treatment of systemic lupus erythematosus, however, there have been anecdotal reports suggesting that auranofin may still be of use in patients with discoid lupus erythematosus[1] or cutaneous lupus erythematosus[2] refractory to conventional treatment.

1. Dalziel K, *et al.* Treatment of chronic discoid lupus erythematosus with an oral gold compound (auranofin). *Br J Dermatol* 1986; **115:** 211–16.
2. Farrell AM, Bunker CB. Oral gold therapy in cutaneous lupus erythematosus (revisited). *Br J Dermatol* 1996; **135** (suppl 47): 41.

Psoriasis. Although efficacy for topical auranofin in the treatment of plaque-type psoriasis (p.1106) has been demonstrated in a placebo-controlled study,[1] the high incidence of adverse skin reactions, such as contact dermatitis, was thought to outweigh any benefit.

1. Helm KF, *et al.* Topical auranofin ointment for the treatment of plaque psoriasis. *J Am Acad Dermatol* 1995; **33:** 517–19.

Preparations

Proprietary Preparations (details are given in Part 3)
Aust.: Ridaura; *Austral.:* Ridaura; *Belg.:* Ridaura; *Braz.:* Ridaura; *Canad.:* Ridaura; *Denm.:* Ridaura; *Fin.:* Ridaura; *Fr.:* Ridaura; *Ger.:* Ridaura; *Hong Kong:* Ridaura; *Irl.:* Ridaura; *Israel:* Ridaura; *Ital.:* Ridaura; *Mex.:* Ridaura; *Neth.:* Ridaura; *Norw.:* Ridaura; *NZ:* Ridaura; *S.Afr.:* Ridaura; *Singapore:* Ridaura; *Spain:* Crisinor†; Ridaura; *Swed.:* Ridaura; *Switz.:* Ridaura; *Thai.:* Ridaura; *UK:* Ridaura; *USA:* Ridaura.

Aurothioglucose   (5294-z)

1-Aurothio-D-glucopyranose; (D-Glucosylthio)gold; Gold Thioglucose. (1-Thio-D-glucopyranosato)gold.
$C_6H_{11}AuO_5S = 392.2$.
CAS — 12192-57-3.
ATC — M01CB04.
Pharmacopoeias. In US.

Aurothioglucose has a gold content of about 50%.

Pharmacopoeial description

USP 25: A yellow odourless or practically odourless powder. An aqueous solution is unstable on long standing. It is stabilised by the addition of a small amount of sodium acetate. pH of a 1% solution in water is about 6.3. Freely soluble in water; practically insoluble in alcohol, in acetone, in chloroform, and in ether. Store in airtight containers. Protect from light.

Adverse Effects, Treatment, and Precautions
As for Sodium Aurothiomalate, p.82.

Interactions
As for Sodium Aurothiomalate, p.83.

Pharmacokinetics
As for Sodium Aurothiomalate, p.83; absorption is slower and more irregular.

Uses and Administration
Aurothioglucose has similar actions and uses to those of sodium aurothiomalate (p.83). It is used in the treatment of active rheumatoid arthritis (p.9) and juvenile idiopathic arthritis (p.9). Aurothioglucose is administered intramuscularly as a suspension in oil in arthritic disorders in an initial weekly dose of 10 mg increasing gradually to 50 mg weekly. Therapy is continued at weekly intervals until a total dose of 0.8 to 1 g has been given; if improvement has occurred at this stage with no signs of toxicity 50 mg may then be given at intervals of 3 or 4 weeks. Children, 6 to 12 years, may be given one-quarter the adult dose, to a maximum of 25 mg per dose.

Preparations

USP 25: Aurothioglucose Injectable Suspension.

Proprietary Preparations (details are given in Part 3)
Austral.: Gold-50; **Canad.:** Solganal; **Ger.:** Aureotan†; **Israel:** Solganal; **Neth.:** Auromyose; **USA:** Solganal.

Aurotioprol (12407-d)

Sodium 3-aurothio-2-hydroxypropane-1-sulphonate.
$C_3H_6AuNaO_4S_2 = 390.2.$
$CAS — 27279-43-2.$
$ATC — M01CB05.$

Aurotioprol has a gold content of about 50%.

Profile
Aurotioprol is a gold compound with similar actions and uses to those of sodium aurothiomalate (p.82). It is given by intramuscular injection for the treatment of rheumatoid arthritis (p.9). The initial dose is 25 mg weekly, increased to 50 to 100 mg weekly, until a total dose of 1.2 to 1.5 g has been given. If improvement has occurred at this stage with no signs of toxicity, this may be followed by a dose of 50 to 100 mg intramuscularly every month.

Preparations

Proprietary Preparations (details are given in Part 3)
Belg.: Allochrysine; **Fr.:** Allochrysine.

Azapropazone (2610-w)

Azapropazone (BAN, rINN).
AHR-3018; Apazone (USAN); Mi85; NSC-102824. 5-Dimethylamino-9-methyl-2-propylpyrazolo[1,2-a][1,2,4]benzotriazine-1,3(2H)-dione.
$C_{16}H_{20}N_4O_2 = 300.4.$
$CAS — 13539-59-8.$
$ATC — M01AX04.$
Pharmacopoeias. Br. includes the dihydrate, $C_{16}H_{20}N_4O_2,2H_2O = 336.4.$

Azapropazone dihydrate 300 mg is approximately equivalent to 268 mg of azapropazone.

Pharmacopoeial description

BP 2001: Azapropazone dihydrate is a white to pale yellow crystalline powder. Very slightly soluble in water and in chloroform; soluble in alcohol; dissolves in solutions of alkali hydroxides.

Adverse Effects
As for NSAIDs in general, p.63. Some adverse effects appear to be more common with azapropazone than with other NSAIDs (see below).

◊ Analysis of spontaneous reporting of adverse reactions to the UK Committee on Safety of Medicines revealed that azapropazone had been associated with the highest risk of gastrointestinal reactions compared with 6 other NSAIDs, as well as with a relatively high frequency of renal, hepatic, allergic, and haematological reactions.[1]

1. Committee on Safety of Medicines/Medicines Control Agency. Current Problems 1994; **20:** 9–11.

Effects on the blood. The UK Committee on Safety of Medicines (CSM) had received 6 reports of Coombs positive haemolytic anaemia associated with azapropazone between January 1984 and March 1985 and the manufacturers 6 reports of auto-immune haemolysis over 10 years.[1] One group of workers[2] who reported haemolytic anaemia and reversible pulmonary infiltration, suggestive of an allergic or immune reaction in 3 patients, noted that since 1976 the CSM had received 18 reports of haemolytic anaemia and 11 reports of allergic alveolitis, pulmonary fibrosis, or fibrosing alveolitis. Fatal haemolytic anaemia has subsequently been reported in one patient.[3]

1. Chan-Lam D, et al. Red cell antibodies and autoimmune haemolysis after treatment with azapropazone. BMJ 1986; **293:** 1474.
2. Albbazaz MK, et al. Alveolitis and haemolytic anaemia induced by azapropazone. BMJ 1986; **293:** 1537–8.
3. Montgomery RD, Babb RG. Alveolitis and haemolytic anaemia induced by azapropazone. BMJ 1987; **294:** 375.

Effects on the gastrointestinal tract. In a review[1] of the relative safety of 7 oral NSAIDs, the UK Committee on Safety of Medicines commented that azapropazone was associated with the highest risk of gastrointestinal reactions in both epidemiological studies and an analysis of spontaneous reporting of adverse reactions. Although it appeared that some patients over 60 years of age had received doses exceeding those recommended for this age group it was considered that even when this was taken into account a marked difference remained between gastrointestinal reactions for azapropazone compared with other NSAIDs. *The Committee recommended that azapropazone should be restricted to use in rheumatoid arthritis, ankylosing spondylitis, and acute gout and only when other NSAIDs have been ineffective. Its use in patients with a history of peptic ulceration was contra-indicated. It was also recommended that when used in patients over 60 years of age for*

rheumatoid arthritis or ankylosing spondylitis the dose should be restricted to a maximum of 600 mg daily.

1. Committee on Safety of Medicines/Medicines Control Agency. Current Problems 1994; **20:** 9–11.

Effects on the lungs. See under Effects on the Blood, above.

Effects on the skin. Of 917 reports of adverse reactions associated with azapropazone forwarded to the WHO Collaborating Centre for International Drug Monitoring[1] before September 1984, 190 (21%) were of photosensitivity. Of 154 reports of photosensitivity evaluated a causal relationship to use of azapropazone was considered certain in 6, probable in 138, and possible in 10. In May 1994 the UK Committee on Safety of Medicines stated[2] that since 1976 they had received 464 reports of photosensitivity reactions associated with azapropazone and commented that, when corrected for prescription volume, reporting of this reaction was 50 times greater than with other commonly prescribed NSAIDs. They recommended that patients should be advised to avoid direct exposure to sunlight or to use sunblock preparations.

1. Olsson S, et al. Photosensitivity during treatment with azapropazone. BMJ 1985; **291:** 939.
2. Committee on Safety of Medicines/Medicines Control Agency. Photosensitivity associated with azapropazone (Rheumox). Current Problems 1994; **20:** 6.

Precautions
As for NSAIDs in general, p.64. Azapropazone is also contraindicated in patients with a history or evidence of peptic ulceration, inflammatory bowel disorders, or blood disorders. Reduced doses should be given to elderly patients and patients with renal impairment; its use should be avoided in patients with severe renal impairment. Its use should also be avoided in breast-feeding mothers.

Patients should be advised to avoid direct exposure to sunlight or to use sunblock preparations.

Porphyria. Azapropazone is considered to be unsafe in patients with porphyria because it has been shown to be porphyrinogenic in *animals.*

Interactions
For interactions associated with NSAIDs, see p.65. Like phenylbutazone, azapropazone may be particularly likely to cause interactions with oral anticoagulants such as warfarin.

Pharmacokinetics
Azapropazone is absorbed from the gastrointestinal tract and peak plasma concentrations are reached about 4 hours after administration. It is highly protein bound. A half-life of 12 to 24 hours has been reported. Azapropazone is excreted in the urine as unchanged drug (about 65%), 8-hydroxyazapropazone, and glucuronide or sulfate metabolites. Very small amounts are distributed into breast milk.

◊ References.
1. Bald R, et al. Excretion of azapropazone in human breast milk. Eur J Clin Pharmacol 1990; **39:** 271–3.

Uses and Administration
Azapropazone is an NSAID (see p.65), structurally related to phenylbutazone (p.78). It also has uricosuric properties. Because azapropazone appears to be associated with a higher incidence of adverse effects than with some other NSAIDs its use in the UK is restricted to the treatment of rheumatoid arthritis, ankylosing spondylitis, and acute gout in patients for whom other NSAIDs have been ineffective.

Azapropazone is used as the dihydrate. For the treatment of rheumatoid arthritis or ankylosing spondylitis the usual dose in the UK is 1.2 g of azapropazone dihydrate daily in 2 or 4 divided doses by mouth. Patients *over 60 years of age* or those with *reduced renal function* may be given 300 mg twice daily but azapropazone should be avoided in patients with severe renal impairment.

Usually uricosuric drugs should not be given during an acute attack of gout as they may prolong its duration, but azapropazone appears to be suitable for the treatment of acute gout. In acute gout 1.8 g of the dihydrate may be given daily in divided doses until the attack is resolving (usually by the fourth day), then reduced to 1.2 g daily until symptoms have disappeared. An adequate fluid intake should be maintained. If symptoms persist appropriate alternative treatment (see p.397) should be considered. For patients with mildly *reduced renal function,* as long as they have a creatinine clearance of 60 mL or more per minute, the dose is 1.8 g daily in divided doses for the first 24 hours only, followed by 1.2 g daily. This should be reduced as soon as possible to a maximum of 600 mg daily. The same regimen may be used in the *elderly,* provided their renal function is normal; azapropazone should not be used to treat gout in elderly patients with even mild renal impairment.

Azapropazone has been given intravenously in some countries.

Preparations

BP 2001: Azapropazone Capsules; Azapropazone Tablets.

Proprietary Preparations (details are given in Part 3)
Aust.: Prolixan; **Ger.:** Tolyprin; **Irl.:** Rheumox; **Neth.:** Prolixan; **Port.:** Prolixan; **S.Afr.:** Rheumox†; **Swed.:** Prolixana†; **Switz.:** Prolixan†; **UK:** Rheumox.

Multi-ingredient: Aust.: Algo-Prolixan; **Switz.:** Dolo-Prolixan†.

Bendazac (2614-j)

Bendazac (BAN, USAN, rINN).
AF-983; Bindazac. (1-Benzyl-1H-indazol-3-yloxy)acetic acid.
$C_{16}H_{14}N_2O_3 = 282.3.$
$CAS — 20187-55-7.$
$ATC — M02AA11; S01BC07.$

Bendazac Lysine (16536-a)

Bendazac Lysine (BANM, rINNM).
AF-1934. L-Lysine-(1-benzyl-1H-indazol-3-yloxy)acetic acid.
$C_{22}H_{28}N_4O_5 = 428.5.$
$CAS — 81919-14-4.$

Profile
Bendazac is an NSAID (p.63) structurally related to indometacin (p.44). It has been used topically in preparations containing 1 or 3% for the treatment of various inflammatory skin disorders.

Bendazac lysine has been used in the management of cataract, 2 drops of a 0.5% solution being instilled three times daily. It has also been given by mouth for similar purposes.

◊ References.
1. Balfour JA, Clissold SP. Bendazac lysine: a review of its pharmacological properties and therapeutic potential in the management of cataracts. Drugs 1990; **39:** 575–96.

Preparations

Proprietary Preparations (details are given in Part 3)
Aust.: Versus; **Ital.:** Bendalina; Versus; **Port.:** Bendalina; Benzum.

Benorilate (2611-e)

Benorilate (BAN, rINN).
Benorylate; FAW-76; Fensasprate; Win-11450. 4-Acetamidophenyl O-acetylsalicylate.
$C_{17}H_{15}NO_5 = 313.3.$
$CAS — 5003-48-5.$
$ATC — N02BA10.$
Pharmacopoeias. In Br.

Pharmacopoeial description

BP 2001: A white or almost white, odourless or almost odourless, crystalline powder. Practically insoluble in water; sparingly soluble in alcohol and in methyl alcohol; soluble in acetone and in chloroform.

Adverse Effects, Treatment, and Precautions
As for Aspirin, p.14, and Paracetamol, p.71.

Benorilate may cause nausea, indigestion, heartburn, and constipation; drowsiness, diarrhoea, and skin rashes have also been reported. Some patients have experienced dizziness, tinnitus, and deafness associated with high blood-salicylate concentrations.

Benorilate, like aspirin (see p.15), should not generally be given to children under the age of 12 years because of the risk of Reye's syndrome.

When an overdose of benorilate is suspected, it has been suggested that plasma concentrations of both salicylate and paracetamol should be measured since a normal plasma-paracetamol concentration cannot necessarily be assumed from a normal plasma-salicylate measurement.

◊ References.
1. Aylward M. Toxicity of benorylate. BMJ 1973; **2:** 118.
2. Symon DNK, et al. Fatal paracetamol poisoning from benorylate therapy in child with cystic fibrosis. Lancet 1982; **ii:** 1153–4.

Interactions
For the interactions associated with aspirin, see p.16, and for those associated with paracetamol, see p.73.

Pharmacokinetics
Benorilate is slowly absorbed virtually unchanged from the gastrointestinal tract. Following absorption, benorilate is rapidly metabolised to salicylate and paracetamol. It is excreted mainly as metabolites of salicylic acid and paracetamol in the urine.

Uses and Administration
Benorilate is an aspirin-paracetamol ester with analgesic, anti-inflammatory, and antipyretic properties. It is used in the treatment of mild to moderate pain (p.2) and fever (p.8). It is also used in osteoarthritis (p.9), rheumatoid arthritis (p.9), and soft-tissue rheumatism (p.10). Benorilate is given by mouth, preferably after food, in doses of 2 g twice daily for mild to moderate pain and fever. Doses for osteoarthritis, quiescent rheumatoid arthritis, and soft-tissue rheumatism are up to 6 g daily in divided doses. In active rheumatoid arthritis 4 g twice daily may be required. In elderly patients reduced doses of 2 g twice daily or possibly 2 g in the morning and 4 g at night should be given; a maximum daily dose of 6 g should not be exceeded.

Preparations

BP 2001: Benorilate Oral Suspension; Benorilate Tablets.

Proprietary Preparations (details are given in Part 3)
Belg.: Duvium; **Fr.:** Longalgic†; Salipran; **Irl.:** Benoral; **Spain:** Doline†; Vetedol†; **Switz.:** Duvium; **UK:** Benoral.

The symbol † denotes a preparation no longer actively marketed

Benoxaprofen   (2612-I)

Benoxaprofen (BAN, USAN, rINN).

Compound 90459; LRCL-3794. 2-[2-(4-Chlorophenyl)benzoxazol-5-yl]propionic acid.

$C_{16}H_{12}ClNO_3 = 301.7$.
CAS — 51234-28-7.
ATC — M01AE06.

Profile

Benoxaprofen is an NSAID (p.63) structurally related to ibuprofen (p.43). It was formerly given by mouth in rheumatoid arthritis and osteoarthritis but because of reports of adverse reactions and fatalities the manufacturers halted worldwide marketing of the preparation known as Opren in the early 1980s. Side-effects that have occurred with benoxaprofen include skin disorders, notably photosensitivity reactions but also erythema multiforme and the Stevens-Johnson syndrome, onycholysis and other nail disorders, gastrointestinal disturbances including peptic ulceration and bleeding, blood disorders such as thrombocytopenia, cholestatic jaundice and other liver or biliary disorders, and renal failure.

Benzydamine Hydrochloride   (2613-y)

Benzydamine Hydrochloride (BANM, USAN, rINNM).

AF-864; Benzindamine Hydrochloride. 3-(1-Benzyl-1H-indazol-3-yloxy)-NN-dimethylpropylamine hydrochloride.

$C_{19}H_{23}N_3O$, HCl = 345.9.
CAS — 642-72-8 (benzydamine); 132-69-4 (benzydamine hydrochloride).
Pharmacopoeias. In Br. and Pol.

Pharmacopoeial description

BP 2001: A white crystalline powder. Very soluble in water; freely soluble in alcohol and in chloroform; practically insoluble in ether. A 10% solution in water has a pH of 4.0 to 5.5.

Adverse Effects

Following topical application to the skin local reactions such as erythema or rash may occur and photosensitivity has been reported. Following use as mouth and throat preparations, numbness or stinging sensations of the oral mucosa have been reported.

Effects on the kidneys. A 57-year-old woman who had used 400 g of a topical cream containing benzydamine hydrochloride 3% over a period of 4 months was found to have raised plasma concentrations of creatinine and urea consistent with a substantial reduction in glomerular filtration rate.[1]

1. O'Callaghan CA, et al. Renal disease and use of topical nonsteroidal anti-inflammatory drugs. BMJ 1994; 308: 110–11.

Overdose. A 6-year old girl experienced hallucinations[1] after receiving 500 mg of benzydamine orally; it had been intended for administration as a vaginal douche for pruritus vulvae. She recovered spontaneously.

1. Gómez-López L, et al. Acute overdose due to benzydamine. Hum Exp Toxicol 1999; 18: 471–3.

Uses and Administration

Benzydamine hydrochloride is an NSAID (p.65). It is used topically on the skin in concentrations of 3 to 5% in painful musculoskeletal and soft-tissue disorders. Benzydamine hydrochloride is also used as a mouthwash or spray in concentrations of 0.15% for the relief of inflammatory conditions of the mouth and throat. It has also been given by mouth, rectally, or by intramuscular or intravenous injection for the relief of painful and inflammatory conditions, and as a topical solution for vaginal irrigation.

Benzydamine salicylate (benzasal) has been used topically on the skin as a 6% cream or spray.

Mouth disorders. Results of a randomised placebo-controlled study in patients undergoing radiotherapy for oropharyngeal cancer indicated that benzydamine as an oral rinse was effective in reducing the area and severity of mucositis.[1] Benzydamine is used locally for the management of mouth ulcers (p.1206) although one study[2] found it no more useful than placebo.

1. Epstein JB, et al. Prevention of oral mucositis in radiation therapy: a controlled study with benzydamine hydrochloride rinse. Int J Radiat Oncol Biol Phys 1989; 16: 1571–5.
2. Matthews RW, et al. Clinical evaluation of benzydamine, chlorhexidine, and placebo mouthwashes in the management of recurrent aphthous stomatitis. Oral Surg Oral Med Oral Pathol 1987; 63: 189–91.

Preparations

BP 2001: Benzydamine Cream; Benzydamine Mouthwash; Benzydamine Oromucosal Spray.

Proprietary Preparations (details are given in Part 3)
Aust.: Tantum; Austral.: Difflam; Difflam Anti-Inflammatory Solution; Difflam Anti-Inflammatory Throat Spray; Braz.: Benflogin; Benziflex; Benzitrat; Ciclinalgin; Ciflogex; Eridamin; Flogi-Ped; Flogo Rosa; Flogoral; Neoflogin; Panflogin; Petiflog; Canad.: Sun-Benz; Tantum; Denm.: Andolex; Fr.: Opalgyne; Ger.: Tantum Verde; Hong Kong: Difflam; Verax; Irl.: Difflam; Israel: Easy gel; Ital.: Afloben; Benzirin; Ginesal; Lagin; Mul-

tum; Saniflor Dentifricio; Saniflor Vena; Tantum; Verax; Mex.: Lonol; Vantal; Neth.: Tantum†; NZ: Difflam; Port.: Flogoral; Rosalgin; Tantum; Tantum Verde; S.Afr.: Andolex; Tantum†; Singapore: Difflam; Spain: Fulgium; Rosalgin; Tantum; Tantum Verde; Swed.: Andolex; Switz.: Bucco-Tantum; Thai.: Difflam; UK: Difflam.

Multi-ingredient: Austral.: Difflam Anti-Inflammatory Lozenges; Difflam Anti-Inflammatory Lozenges with Cough Suppressant; Difflam Mouth Gel; Difflam-C; Logicin Rapid Relief; Fr.: Hexo-Imotryl†; Hong Kong: Difflam-C; Ital.: Algolisina; Leucorsan†; Linea F; Mediplus; Mex.: Lonol Sport; NZ: Difflam Anti-inflammatory Antibacterial Lozenges; Difflam Anti-inflammatory Cough Lozenges; Difflam Mouth Gel; Difflam-C; Port.: Tantum Rosa; Tantum Verde; S.Afr.: Andolex-C; Singapore: Difflam Mouth Gel; Difflam-C; Spain: Bristaciclina Dental; Dolosarto; Etermol Antitusivo; Mentamida; Prosturol; Tantum; Tantum Ciclina; Vinciseptil Otico.

Benzyl Nicotinate   (9212-g)

Benzyl pyridine-3-carboxylate.

$C_{13}H_{11}NO_2 = 213.2$.
CAS — 94-44-0.
Pharmacopoeias. In Ger.

Profile

Benzyl nicotinate is used in topical preparations as a rubefacient.

Preparations

Proprietary Preparations (details are given in Part 3)
Ger.: Pernionin Teil-Bad; Pykaryl T; Rheubalmin Bad Nico†; Rubriment.

Multi-ingredient: Aust.: Ambenat; Bayolin; Derivon; Expectal-Balsam; Forapin†; Igitur-antirheumatische; Menthoneurin; Mobilisin plus; Pelvichthol†; Rheumex; Rubizon-Rheumagel; Rubriment; Thermo-Rheumon; Thrombophob; Tifenso; Belg.: Forapin†; Braz.: Etrat; Pergalen; Trombofob; Fr.: Bayoline†; Lumbalgine; Ger.: ABC Warme-Salbe; Akrotherm; Ambene N; Arthrodestal N; Auroanalin; Bartelin nico; Brachialin percutan N†; Brachont†; Camphopin†; Capsamol; Caye Balsam; Contrheuma; Cor-Select; Cuxaflex N†; Cuxaflex Thermo†; Dolo-Menthoneurin CreSa†; Dolo-Rubriment; Dolorgiet†; DoloVisano Salbe; Emasex-N; exrheudon OPT; Fibraflex; Fibraflex-W-Creme N†; Fibraflex†; Flexocutan N; Forapin E; Heilit; Hot Thermo; Intradermi Fluid N†; Lomazell forte N; Marament Balsam W†; Menthoneurin-Vollbad N†; Myalgol N; Mylagon N; Nitro-Praecordin N†; Ortholan mit Salicylester†; Ostochont; Pelvichthol N; Percutase N†; Pernionin; Pernionin Voll-Bad N; Phardol Rheuma; Phlogont-Thermal; Praecordin S; Reumaless†; Rheubalmin Thermo; Rheubalmin†; Rheuma-Bad; Rheuma-Liquidum; Rheuma-Salbe; Rheumasalbe; Rheumasan N; Rheumasit; Rosarthron forte; Rubriment; Rubriment-N; Salhumin Gel N†; Segmentocut Thermo†; Tachynerg N; Thermo Mobilisin; thermo-loges; Thermo-Menthoneurin; Thermo-Menthoneurin Bad†; Thermo-Rheumon; Thermosenex; Togal Mobil Rheuma-Bad; Togal Mobil-Gel; Warme-Gel; zuk thermo; Ital.: Lasoreuma†; Salonpas; Sloan; Neth.: Menthoneurin; Sloan's balsem; Port.: Adrinex; DM Termo; Medalginan; S.Afr.: Thrombophob†; Swed.: Remysal N†; Switz.: Artragel; Assan-Thermo; Demotherm Pommade contre le rhumatisme; Dolo Demotherm; Forapin; Histalgane; Incutin; Marament-N; Roliwol S†; Thermocutan; UK: Salonair.

Beta-aminopropionitrile   (4266-m)

Aminopropionitrile; β-Aminopropionitrile; BAPN. 3-Aminopropionitrile.

$C_3H_6N_2 = 70.09$.
CAS — 151-18-8.

Profile

Beta-aminopropionitrile, a lysyl oxidase inhibitor, is an anti-inflammatory used as the fumarate in veterinary medicine for the treatment of tendinitis.

Bezitramide   (6208-s)

Bezitramide (BAN, rINN).

R-4845. 4-[4-(2,3-Dihydro-2-oxo-3-propionyl-1H-benzimidazol-1-yl)piperidino]-2,2-diphenylbutyronitrile.

$C_{31}H_{32}N_4O_2 = 492.6$.
CAS — 15301-48-1.
ATC — N02AC05.

Profile

Bezitramide is an opioid analgesic (p.66) that has been given by mouth in usual daily doses of 5 to 15 mg in the treatment of severe pain. Its action is slow in onset, but prolonged.

◊ References.

1. Meijer DKF, et al. Pharmacokinetics of the oral narcotic analgesic bezitramide and preliminary observations on its effect on experimentally induced pain. Eur J Clin Pharmacol 1984; 27: 615–18.

Preparations

Proprietary Preparations (details are given in Part 3)
Belg.: Burgodin†; Neth.: Burgodin†.

Bornyl Salicylate   (11271-z)

Borneol Salicylate. 2-Hydroxybenzoic acid 1,7,7-trimethylbicyclo[2.2.1]hept-2-yl ester.

$C_{17}H_{22}O_3 = 274.4$.
CAS — 560-88-3.

Profile

Bornyl salicylate is a salicylic acid derivative that is used topically in rubefacient preparations similarly to methyl salicylate (p.55) for the relief of pain in musculoskeletal and joint disorders.

Preparations

Proprietary Preparations (details are given in Part 3)

Multi-ingredient: Aust.: Forapin†; Belg.: Forapin†; Ger.: Contrheuma-Gel forte N†; Forapin E; Switz.: Acidodermil†; Forapin; Hygiodermil; Sedodermil†.

Bromfenac Sodium   (2896-k)

Bromfenac Sodium (USAN, rINNM).

AHR-10282; AHR-10282B. Sodium [2-amino-3-(p-bromobenzoyl)phenyl]acetate sesquihydrate.

$C_{15}H_{11}BrNNaO_3, 1\frac{1}{2}H_2O = 383.2$.
CAS — 91714-94-2 (bromfenac); 91714-93-1 (bromfenac sodium); 120638-55-3 (bromfenac sodium).

Profile

Bromfenac sodium, a phenylacetic acid derivative related to diclofenac (p.30), is an NSAID (p.63). It was withdrawn from the market following reports of severe and sometimes fatal hepatic failure.

Preparations

Proprietary Preparations (details are given in Part 3)
USA: Duract†.

Bufexamac   (2618-a)

Bufexamac (BAN, rINN).

Bufexamacum. 2-(4-Butoxyphenyl)acetohydroxamic acid.

$C_{12}H_{17}NO_3 = 223.3$.
CAS — 2438-72-4.
ATC — M01AB17; M02AA09.
Pharmacopoeias. In Eur. (see p.vi) and Jpn.

Pharmacopoeial description

Ph. Eur.: A white or almost white, crystalline powder. Practically insoluble in water; soluble in dimethylformamide; slightly soluble in ethyl acetate and in methyl alcohol. Protect from light.

Profile

Bufexamac is an NSAID (p.63) that is applied topically in concentrations of 5% in various skin disorders. Stinging and burning may occur after application; hypersensitivity reactions have been reported.

Preparations

Proprietary Preparations (details are given in Part 3)
Aust.: Bufexan; Droxaryl; Parfenac; Austral.: Paraderm; Belg.: Bufexine; Droxaryl; Canad.: Norfemac; Fr.: Bufal†; Calmaderm; Parfenac; Ger.: Allergipuran N†; Bufederm; duradermal; Ekzemase; Haemo-Exhirud Bufexamac Zapfchen; Jomax; Logomed Ekzem-Salbe†; Malipuran; Parfenac; Windol; Ital.: Parfenal; Viafen; Neth.: Droxaryl†; Parfenac; Port.: Parfenac; S.Afr.: Parfenac†; Switz.: Flogocid; Parfenac; Thai.: Droxaryl.

Multi-ingredient: Austral.: Fungo; Paraderm Plus; Belg.: Flogocid; Ger.: Bufeproct†; Faktu akut; Haemomact†; Hamoagil plus; Logomed Hamorrhoiden†; Mastu S; Proctoparf; Hong Kong: Mastu S; Switz.: Flogocid NN†.

Bumadizone Calcium   (2619-t)

Bumadizone Calcium (rINNM).

Calcium 2-(1,2-diphenylhydrazinocarbonyl)hexanoate hemihydrate.

$(C_{19}H_{21}N_2O_3)_2Ca, \frac{1}{2}H_2O = 699.8$.
CAS — 3583-64-0 (bumadizone); 34461-73-9 (bumadizone calcium).

Profile

Bumadizone calcium is an NSAID (p.63) that is reported to be metabolised to phenylbutazone (p.78) and oxyphenbutazone (p.71). Its use was limited by the risk of agranulocytosis and other haematological adverse effects.

Preparations

Proprietary Preparations (details are given in Part 3)
Braz.: Eumotol; Mex.: Desflam; Dibilan F.

Buprenorphine (19995-d)

Buprenorphine (BAN, rINN).

Buprenorphinum; RX-6029-M. (6R,7R,14S)-17-Cyclopropyl-methyl-7,8-dihydro-7-[(1S)-1-hydroxy-1,2,2-trimethylpropyl]-6-O-methyl-6,14-ethano-17-normorphine; (2S)-2-[(−)-(5R,6R,7R,14S)-9a-Cyclopropylmethyl-4,5-epoxy-3-hydroxy-6-methoxy-6,14-ethanomorphinan-7-yl]-3,3-dimethylbutan-2-ol.

$C_{29}H_{41}NO_4$ = 467.6.
CAS — 52485-79-7.
ATC — N02AE01.
Pharmacopoeias. In Eur. (see p.vi).

Pharmacopoeial description

Ph. Eur.: A white or almost white crystalline powder. Very slightly soluble in water; freely soluble in acetone; slightly soluble in cyclohexane; soluble in methyl alcohol. It dissolves in dilute solutions of acids. Protect from light.

Buprenorphine Hydrochloride (6209-w)

Buprenorphine Hydrochloride (BANM, USAN, rINNM).

Buprenorphini Hydrochloridum; CL-112302; NIH-8805; UM-952.

$C_{29}H_{41}NO_4,HCl$ = 504.1.
CAS — 53152-21-9.
Pharmacopoeias. In Eur. (see p.vi) and US.

Buprenorphine hydrochloride 107.8 µg is approximately equivalent to 100 µg of buprenorphine.

Pharmacopoeial description

Ph. Eur.: A white or almost white crystalline powder. Sparingly soluble in water; soluble in alcohol; practically insoluble in cyclohexane; freely soluble in methyl alcohol. Protect from light.

USP 25: pH of a 1% solution in water is between 4.0 and 6.0. Store in airtight containers. Protect from light.

Dependence and Withdrawal

As for Opioid Analgesics, p.66.

Buprenorphine may have a lower potential for producing dependence than pure agonists such as morphine. However, it has been subject to abuse. Abrupt withdrawal of buprenorphine is said to produce only a mild abstinence syndrome.

Adverse Effects and Treatment

As for Opioid Analgesics in general, p.67.

Treatment of adverse effects is similar to that for other opioid analgesics (p.68). The effects of buprenorphine are only partially reversed by naloxone (see under Effects on the Respiratory System, below) but use of the latter is still recommended.

◊ Adverse effects reported[1] following administration of buprenorphine injection in 8187 patients were nausea (8.8%), vomiting (7.4%), drowsiness (4.3%), sleeping (1.9%), dizziness (1.2%), sweating (0.98%), headache (0.55%), confusion (0.53%), lightheadedness (0.38%), blurred vision (0.28%), euphoria (0.27%), dry mouth (0.11%), depression (0.09%), and hallucinations (0.09%). Some studies have reported nausea, vomiting, and dizziness to be more troublesome with buprenorphine than with morphine.[2,3]

In a trial of sublingual buprenorphine 50 of 141 cancer patients withdrew because of side-effects, especially dizziness, nausea, vomiting, and drowsiness; constipation was not reported.[4] One woman developed a painless ulcer on the upper surface of her tongue after she had put sublingual buprenorphine tablets on rather than under her tongue.[5]

Shock occurred[6] in 2 patients 2 hours after receiving epidural buprenorphine 300 µg; treatment with naloxone was unsuccessful but symptoms disappeared spontaneously after 2 to 3 hours.

1. Harcus AW, et al. Methodology of monitored release of a new preparation: buprenorphine. BMJ 1979; 2: 163–5.
2. Sear JW, et al. Buprenorphine for postoperative analgesia. Br J Anaesth 1979; 51: 71.
3. Kjaer M, et al. A comparative study of intramuscular buprenorphine and morphine in the treatment of chronic pain of malignant origin. Br J Clin Pharmacol 1982; 13: 487–92.
4. Robbie DS. A trial of sublingual buprenorphine in cancer pain. Br J Clin Pharmacol 1979; 7 (suppl 3): 315S–17S.
5. Lockhart SP, Baron JH. Tongue ulceration after lingual buprenorphine. BMJ 1984; 288: 1346.
6. Christensen FR, Andersen LW. Adverse reaction to extradural buprenorphine. Br J Anaesth 1982; 54: 476.

Effects on the heart. For a report of myocardial infarction associated with abuse of buprenorphine, see Abuse under Precautions, below.

Effects on mental function. Psychotomimetic effects have been relatively uncommon with buprenorphine. Hallucinations were reported[1] in only 7 of 8147 patients (0.09%) given bup-

renorphine by injection. There have been reports of hallucinations following sublingual[2] or epidural[3] administration.

1. Harcus AW, et al. Methodology of monitored release of a new preparation: buprenorphine. BMJ 1979; 2: 163–5.
2. Paraskevaides EC. Near fatal auditory hallucinations after buprenorphine. BMJ 1988; 296: 214.
3. MacEvilly M, O'Carroll C. Hallucinations after epidural buprenorphine. BMJ 1989; 298: 928–9.

Effects on the respiratory system. There have been varying reports on the occurrence of respiratory depression in association with buprenorphine. It might be subject to a 'ceiling effect' in that respiratory depression does not necessarily increase proportionately with dose. However, high doses of 30 or 40 µg per kg body-weight given as sole intravenous analgesic in balanced anaesthesia have been associated with significant and severe respiratory depression.[1]

Respiratory depression may be delayed in onset and more prolonged than that seen with morphine and is only partially reversed by naloxone, possibly because buprenorphine is very firmly bound to opioid receptors. A study of sublingual buprenorphine for postoperative pain relief was abandoned when 3 of the first 16 patients showed signs of late-onset respiratory depression after the second dose of buprenorphine; the respiratory depression did not respond to naloxone.[2] Successful reversal has been demonstrated in healthy subjects with buprenorphine-induced respiratory depression given large doses of naloxone 5 or 10 mg, but not with 1 mg; reversal was gradual in onset and decreased the duration of the normally prolonged respiratory depression.[3] The respiratory depressant and analgesic effects of buprenorphine were decreased by the concomitant administration of naloxone.[4]

1. Schmidt JF, et al. Postoperative pain relief with naloxone: severe respiratory depression and pain after high dose buprenorphine. Anaesthesia 1985; 40: 583–6.
2. Thörn S-E, et al. Prolonged respiratory depression caused by sublingual buprenorphine. Lancet 1988; i: 179–80.
3. Gal TJ. Naloxone reversal of buprenorphine-induced respiratory depression. Clin Pharmacol Ther 1989; 45: 66–71.
4. Lehmann KA, et al. Influence of naloxone on the postoperative analgesic and respiratory effects of buprenorphine. Eur J Clin Pharmacol 1988; 34: 343–52.

Precautions

As for Opioid Analgesics in general, p.68.

Buprenorphine has opioid antagonist actions and may precipitate withdrawal symptoms if given to patients physically dependent on opioids.

Respiratory depression, if it occurs, is relatively slow in onset and of prolonged duration; it may be only partially reversed by naloxone.

◊ There is a risk that, with opioid agonist-antagonists such as buprenorphine, their antagonistic effects might impair more effective analgesic therapy. This appeared to happen in 2 cancer patients both of whom were given sublingual buprenorphine that was later substituted by morphine.[1] Conventional doses of morphine were inadequate and in one patient raising the dose of morphine proved fatal.

1. Overweg-van Kints J, Stricker BHC. Falende pijnbestrijding tijdens sublinguaal gebruik van buprenorfine. Ned Tijdschr Geneeskd 1987; 131: 1973–4.

Abuse. A 22-year-old man experienced chest pains on each of two occasions after he had inhaled crushed buprenorphine tablets. An ECG taken after the second episode suggested that the patient had suffered a myocardial infarction.

1. Cracowski J-L, et al. Myocardial infarction associated with buprenorphine. Ann Intern Med 1999; 130: 537.

Breast feeding. Some authorities consider that the amount of buprenorphine distributed into breast milk is probably too small to be harmful to a breast-fed infant. From a study[1] of one breast-feeding mother who was receiving buprenorphine 4 mg daily it was estimated that at the age of 4 weeks the total amount ingested by the infant during a 24-hour period was 3.28 µg for buprenorphine and 0.33 µg for norbuprenorphine.

1. Marquet P, et al. Buprenorphine withdrawal syndrome in a newborn. Clin Pharmacol Ther 1997; 62: 569–71.

Pregnancy and the neonate. An infant born to a mother who was being treated with buprenorphine 4 mg daily for diamorphine addiction suffered a minor withdrawal syndrome 2 days after birth.[1] The infant rapidly recovered without any treatment. No further signs of withdrawal occurred when breast feeding was abruptly stopped at the age of 8 weeks.

1. Marquet P, et al. Buprenorphine withdrawal syndrome in a newborn. Clin Pharmacol Ther 1997; 62: 569–71.

Interactions

For interactions associated with opioid analgesics, see p.68. Buprenorphine is metabolised by the cytochrome P450 isoenzyme CYP3A4. Therefore use with other drugs that induce or inhibit this isoenzyme may result in changes in plasma concentrations of buprenorphine and, possibly adverse effects.

Pharmacokinetics

Following intramuscular injection, buprenorphine rapidly reaches peak plasma concentrations. Absorption also takes place through the buccal mucosa following sublingual administration and peak plasma concentrations are achieved after 90 minutes. Buprenorphine is about 96% bound to plasma proteins. Plasma elimination half-lives have ranged from 1.2 to 7.2 hours; there is a lack of correlation between plasma concentrations and analgesic activity. Some is metabolised in the liver to N-dealkylbuprenorphine (norbuprenorphine) and conjugated metabolites, but buprenorphine is excreted predominantly unchanged in the faeces; there is some evidence for enterohepatic recirculation. The terminal elimination half-life is 20 to 25 hours. Metabolites are excreted in the urine, but very little unchanged drug. Buprenorphine is subject to considerable first-pass metabolism following oral administration. Small amounts of buprenorphine are distributed into breast milk.

Administration. BUCCAL ROUTE. Absorption of sublingual buprenorphine is relatively slow. In a 10-hour study[1] plasma concentrations following 400 or 800 µg sublingually peaked at about 200 minutes (range 90 to 360 minutes) and buprenorphine was still detected in plasma at the end of the study. Systemic availability was about 55% (range 16 to 94%) and absorption was more or less complete 5 hours after a dose. However, the authors of a subsequent study[2] considered that this was an overestimation, possibly due to methodological flaws. The later study results indicated that the bioavailability of sublingual buprenorphine is about 30% and that sublingual holding times between 3 and 5 minutes are bioequivalent. Another study found that the bioavailability of sublingual buprenorphine was 50% less from a tablet than from a liquid formulation.[3]

1. Bullingham RES, et al. Sublingual buprenorphine used postoperatively: ten hour plasma drug concentration analysis. Br J Clin Pharmacol 1982; 13: 665–73.
2. Mendelson J, et al. Bioavailability of sublingual buprenorphine. J Clin Pharmacol 1997; 37: 31–7.
3. Nath RP, et al. Buprenorphine pharmacokinetics: relative bioavailability of sublingual tablet and liquid formulations. J Clin Pharmacol 1999; 39: 619–23.

Children. The terminal elimination half-life of buprenorphine was only about 1 hour in small children aged 4 to 7 years given 3 µg per kg body-weight intravenously as premedication, but could not be estimated reliably because of the rapid decline in plasma-buprenorphine concentrations.[1] Clearance values did however appear higher than in adults; steady-state volume of distribution was similar. Premature neonates (gestational age 27 to 32 weeks) given a similar dose followed by an infusion of 0.72 µg per kg per hour had a considerably lower clearance rate and had a mean elimination half-life of 20 hours.[2] Although this dosing regimen appeared to be safe, sedation was judged to be inadequate in 4 of the 12 neonates studied. It was suggested that as buprenorphine given by infusion might not produce consistent sedation and analgesia in premature neonates, it could not be recommended for use in neonatal care.

1. Olkkola KT, et al. Pharmacokinetics of intravenous buprenorphine in children. Br J Clin Pharmacol 1989; 28: 202–4.
2. Barrett DA, et al. The pharmacodynamics and physiological effect of buprenorphine infusion in premature neonates. Br J Clin Pharmacol 1993; 36: 215–19.

Renal impairment. Buprenorphine clearance appears to occur mainly by hepatic extraction and metabolism and would not be expected to be related to renal function, whereas metabolites are excreted in urine. Buprenorphine kinetics were similar in a study in anaesthetised healthy patients and those with renal impairment, with a mean elimination half-life of 398 and 239 minutes respectively.[1] Plasma concentrations of the metabolites norbuprenorphine and buprenorphine-3-glucuronide were increased about 4 times and 15 times respectively in patients with renal impairment,[1] but significant pharmacological activity was unlikely since norbuprenorphine has little analgesic activity compared with the parent compound and buprenorphine-3-glucuronide has none.

1. Hand CW, et al. Buprenorphine disposition in patients with renal impairment: single and continuous dosing, with special reference to metabolites. Br J Anaesth 1990; 64: 276–82.

Uses and Administration

Buprenorphine is an opioid analgesic (p.68) classified as an opioid agonist and antagonist. It is used for the relief of moderate to severe pain and as an adjunct to anaesthesia. Buprenorphine is also used in the treatment of opioid dependence.

Buprenorphine has a relatively slow onset but prolonged duration of action. Following intramuscular injection analgesia is apparent within 30 minutes and lasts up to 6 hours. A slower more prolonged response is achieved following sublingual administration.

Buprenorphine is used as the hydrochloride but doses are expressed in terms of the equivalent amount of the base.

The dose by intramuscular or slow intravenous injection for moderate to severe **pain** is 300 to 600 µg repeated every 6 to 8 hours as required. Children over 6 months may be given 3 to 6 µg per kg body-weight by injection every 6 to 8 hours; up to 9 µg per kg may be given if required in refractory cases.

By the sublingual route, doses of 200 to 400 µg are given every 6 to 8 hours. Suggested sublingual doses for children over 6 months are: 16 to 25 kg body-weight, 100 µg; 25 to 37.5 kg, 100 to 200 µg; and 37.5 to 50 kg, 200 to 300 µg.

When used in balanced **anaesthesia** 300 µg may be given intramuscularly or 400 µg sublingually for premedication; 300 to 450 µg may be given intravenously as a perioperative analgesic supplement.

In the treatment of **opioid dependence**, buprenorphine is given in an initial dose of 0.8 to 4 mg sublingually once daily. The dose may be increased as necessary but maintenance doses should not exceed 32 mg daily. Once the patient has been stabilised, the dosage should be reduced gradually to a lower maintenance dose; treatment may eventually be discontinued if appropriate. For addicts who have not undergone opioid withdrawal before starting buprenorphine, the first dose of buprenorphine should not be given until the first signs of craving appear or until at least 4 hours after the last opioid use. In those already receiving methadone replacement, the dose of methadone should be reduced to a maximum of 30 mg daily before starting buprenorphine therapy.

Action. Buprenorphine is generally described as a mixed agonist-antagonist acting mainly as a partial agonist at µ opioid receptors, with some antagonist activity at κ receptors. It has also been shown to bind at μ, δ, and κ opioid binding sites and to have high affinity for the μ and δ receptor and lesser affinity for the κ receptor.[1] Buprenorphine, like fentanyl, has high lipid solubility, but has a lower intrinsic activity than fentanyl. Differences between buprenorphine and pure μ opioid agonists such as fentanyl, including relatively slow onset of action, prolonged duration of action, resistance to antagonism by naloxone, and lack of correlation between plasma concentrations and analgesic effects, have been explained by differences in the way buprenorphine binds to opioid receptors. In a study *in vitro* buprenorphine had slow rates of association and dissociation from the opioid receptor when compared with fentanyl.[2]

1. Bovill JG. Which potent opioid? Important criteria for selection. *Drugs* 1987; **33**: 520–30.
2. Boas RA, Villiger JW. Clinical actions of fentanyl and buprenorphine: the significance of receptor binding. *Br J Anaesth* 1985; **57**: 192–6.

Anaesthesia. Buprenorphine may be used for premedication and as an adjunct to anaesthesia. It has also been used after anaesthesia with fentanyl; in one study[1] buprenorphine antagonised the respiratory rate depression following fentanyl as effectively as naloxone.

1. Boysen K, *et al.* Buprenorphine antagonism of ventilatory depression following fentanyl anaesthesia. *Acta Anaesthesiol Scand* 1988; **32**: 490–2.

Opioid dependence. Buprenorphine is used in the treatment of opioid dependence (p.66). Its agonist-antagonist properties may mean that it has a lower potential for dependence and a lower risk of respiratory depression in overdose than pure agonists such as methadone. However, its place in clinical practice as an alternative to methadone remains to be proven and abuse of the preparation, as with other substitution therapies, may be a problem. In patients dependent on high doses of opioids buprenorphine may precipitate withdrawal due to its partial antagonist properties; the daily opioid dose should be reduced gradually in such patients before beginning buprenorphine.

In some countries buprenorphine is available in combination with naloxone for the treatment of opioid dependence.

References.

1. Fudala PJ, *et al.* Use of buprenorphine in the treatment of opioid addiction: II physiologic and behavioural effects of daily and alternate-day administration and abrupt withdrawal. *Clin Pharmacol Ther* 1990; **47**: 525–34.
2. Ling W, *et al.* A controlled trial comparing buprenorphine and methadone maintenance in opioid dependence. *Arch Gen Psychiatry* 1996; **53**: 401–407.
3. O'Connor PG, *et al.* A randomized trial of buprenorphine maintenance for heroin dependence in a primary care clinic for substance users versus a methadone clinic. *Am J Med* 1998; **105**: 100–105.
4. Gowing L, *et al.* Buprenorphine for the management of opioid withdrawal (updated 29 August 2001). Available in The Cochrane Library; Issue 4. Oxford: Update Software, 2001.

Pain. ACUTE PAIN. Buprenorphine can be given intramuscularly, intravenously, or sublingually for the control of *postoperative* pain although the intravenous route may be preferred for acute pain relief. The epidural route has also been used.[1] Patient-controlled analgesia with intravenous[2] and intramuscular[3] buprenorphine has been effective although its long half-life may limit such use.

Buprenorphine had no adverse cardiovascular effects when given intravenously after open-heart surgery,[4] suggesting that it was a suitable analgesic for patients with unstable circulation. Epidural analgesia with buprenorphine has also been used after cardiac surgery.[5] Buprenorphine was also considered suitable for the relief of pain in *myocardial infarction*.[6]

1. Miwa Y, *et al.* Epidural administered buprenorphine in the perioperative period. *Can J Anaesth* 1996; **43**: 907–13.
2. Gibbs JM, *et al.* Patient administration of iv buprenorphine for postoperative pain relief using the 'Cardiff' demand analgesia apparatus. *Br J Anaesth* 1982; **54**: 279–84.
3. Harmer M, *et al.* Intramuscular on demand analgesia: double blind controlled trial of pethidine, buprenorphine, morphine, and meptazinol. *BMJ* 1983; **286**: 680–2.
4. Rosenfeldt FL, *et al.* Haemodynamic effects of buprenorphine after heart surgery. *BMJ* 1978; **2**: 76–3.
5. Mehta Y, *et al.* Lumbar versus thoracic epidural buprenorphine for postoperative analgesia following coronary artery bypass graft surgery. *Acta Anaesthesiol Scand* 1999; **43**: 388–93.
6. Hayes MJ, *et al.* Randomised trial comparing buprenorphine and diamorphine for chest pain in suspected myocardial infarction. *BMJ* 1979; **2**: 300–2.

Preparations

Proprietary Preparations (details are given in Part 3)
Aust.: Temgesic; **Austral.:** Subutex; Temgesic; **Belg.:** Temgesic; **Braz.:** Temgesic; **Denm.:** Anorfin; Subutex; Temgesic; **Fin.:** Subutex; Temgesic; **Fr.:** Subutex; Temgesic; **Ger.:** Temgesic; **Hong Kong:** Temgesic; **Irl.:** Temgesic; **Israel:** Nopan; **Ital.:** Subutex; Temgesic; **Mex.:** Temgesic; **Neth.:** Temgesic; **Norw.:** Subutex; **NZ:** Temgesic; Temgesic; **Port.:** Buprex; Subutex; **S.Afr.:** Temgesic; **Singapore:** Temgesic; **Spain:** Buprex; Prefin; **Swed.:** Subutex; Temgesic; **Switz.:** Subutex; Temgesic; **Thai.:** Buprine; Temgesic; **UK:** Subutex; Temgesic; **USA:** Buprenex.

Butibufen Sodium (12475-I)

Butibufen Sodium (*rINNM*).
FF-106 (butibufen). Sodium 2-(4-isobutylphenyl)butyrate.
$C_{14}H_{19}NaO_2 = 242.3$.
CAS — 55837-18-8 (butibufen); 60682-24-8 (butibufen sodium).

Profile
Butibufen sodium is an NSAID (p.63) that has been used by mouth in inflammatory and rheumatic disorders.

Preparations

Proprietary Preparations (details are given in Part 3)
Spain: Mijal.

Butorphanol Tartrate (6210-m)

Butorphanol Tartrate (BANM, USAN, rINNM).
levo-BC-2627 (butorphanol). (−)-17-(Cyclobutylmethyl)morphinan-3,14-diol hydrogen tartrate.
$C_{21}H_{29}NO_2, C_4H_6O_6 = 477.5$.
CAS — 42408-82-2 (butorphanol); 58786-99-5 (butorphanol tartrate).
Pharmacopoeias. In US.

Pharmacopoeial description
USP 25: A white powder. Its solutions are slightly acidic. Sparingly soluble in water; insoluble in alcohol, in chloroform, in ether, in ethyl acetate, and in hexane; slightly soluble in methyl alcohol; soluble in dilute acids. Store in airtight containers.

Dependence and Withdrawal
As for Opioid Analgesics, p.66.
Butorphanol may have a lower potential for producing dependence than pure agonists such as morphine. However, it has been subject to abuse. Abrupt discontinuation of chronic butorphanol administration has produced a less severe withdrawal syndrome than with morphine.

Adverse Effects and Treatment
As for Opioid Analgesics in general, p.67, and for Pentazocine, p.74.
Headache, and feelings of floating may also occur. Hallucinations and other psychotomimetic effects are rare and have been reported less frequently than with pentazocine. In addition insomnia and nasal congestion may occur frequently when butorphanol is given intranasally.

Because butorphanol has opioid agonist and antagonist activity, naloxone is the recommended antagonist for the treatment of overdosage.

Effects on the respiratory system. Butorphanol 2 mg produces a similar degree of respiratory depression to morphine 10 mg, but a ceiling effect is apparent with higher doses of butorphanol.[1] It has been reported to be a less potent respiratory depressant than fentanyl,[2] but more potent than nalbuphine.[3]

1. Nagashima H, *et al.* Respiratory and circulatory effects of intravenous butorphanol and morphine. *Clin Pharmacol Ther* 1976; **19**: 738–45.

2. Dryden GE. Voluntary respiratory effects of butorphanol and fentanyl following barbiturate induction: a double-blind study. *J Clin Pharmacol* 1986; **26**: 203–7.
3. Zucker JR, *et al.* Respiratory effects of nalbuphine and butorphanol in anesthetized patients. *Anesth Analg* 1987; **66**: 879–81.

Precautions
As for Opioid Analgesics in general, p.68.
Although cardiovascular effects may be less than with pentazocine, butorphanol should generally be avoided after myocardial infarction.

Butorphanol may precipitate withdrawal symptoms if given to patients physically dependent on opioids. The dosage regimen of butorphanol may need to be adjusted in the elderly and in patients with hepatic or renal impairment.

Abuse. There has been a report of fibrous myopathy associated with chronic intramuscular abuse of butorphanol.[1]

1. Wagner JM, Cohen S. Fibrous myopathy from butorphanol injections. *J Rheumatol* 1991; **18**: 1934–5.

Pregnancy. Two instances of sinusoidal fetal heart rate pattern were noted out of 188 consecutive cases of butorphanol administration in active-phase labour.[1]

1. Welt SI. Sinusoidal fetal heart rate and butorphanol administration. *Am J Obstet Gynecol* 1985; **152**: 362–3.

Interactions
For interactions associated with opioid analgesics, see p.68.

Pharmacokinetics
Butorphanol is absorbed from the gastrointestinal tract but it undergoes extensive first-pass metabolism. Peak plasma concentrations occur 0.5 to 1 hour after intramuscular and nasal administration and 1 to 1.5 hours after oral administration. Butorphanol has a plasma elimination half-life of about 3 hours. About 80% is bound to plasma proteins.

Butorphanol is extensively metabolised in the liver through hydroxylation, N-dealkylation, and conjugation, only 5% being excreted unchanged. Excretion is mainly in the urine; about 11 to 14% of a parenteral dose is excreted in the bile. It crosses the placenta and is distributed into breast milk.

◊ References.

1. Shyu WC, *et al.* Multiple-dose phase I study of transnasal butorphanol. *Clin Pharmacol Ther* 1993; **54**: 34–41.
2. Shyu WC, *et al.* The absolute bioavailability of transnasal butorphanol in patients experiencing rhinitis. *Eur J Clin Pharmacol* 1993; **45**: 559–62.
3. Shyu WC, *et al.* The effects of age and sex on the systemic availability and pharmacokinetics of transnasal butorphanol. *Eur J Clin Pharmacol* 1994; **47**: 57–60.

Uses and Administration
Butorphanol tartrate, a phenanthrene derivative, is an opioid analgesic (p.68) with opioid agonist and antagonist properties; it is pharmacologically similar to pentazocine (p.74). Butorphanol is used for the relief of moderate to severe pain and as an adjunct to anaesthesia. Onset of analgesia is reported within 10 to 15 minutes of intramuscular injection and may last for 3 to 4 hours. With intranasal administration, onset of action is also within 10 to 15 minutes but duration of action is longer and can be up to 5 hours.

For the relief of moderate to severe pain, butorphanol tartrate is given in doses of 1 to 4 mg by intramuscular injection or in doses of 0.5 to 2 mg by intravenous injection every 3 to 4 hours. It may also be given as a nasal spray, in usual doses of 1 mg (1 spray in 1 nostril), repeated after 60 to 90 minutes, if necessary. This sequence may be repeated after 3 to 4 hours as needed. An initial dose of 2 mg (1 spray in each nostril) may be given for severe pain, but should not be repeated until 3 to 4 hours later.

For premedication 2 mg may be given intramuscularly 60 to 90 minutes before surgery. For use in balanced anaesthesia a usual dose is 2 mg given intravenously shortly before induction followed by 0.5 to 1 mg intravenously in increments during anaesthesia.

The dosage of butorphanol may need to be adjusted in the elderly and in patients with hepatic or renal impairment. When given by injection the initial dose for pain should be half the usual initial adult dose. Subsequent doses should be determined by the patient's response; a dosage interval of 6 to 8 hours has been recommended. For nasal administration the initial dose should be limited to 1 mg followed by 1 mg after 90 to 120 minutes if necessary; subsequent doses if required should generally be given at intervals of not less than 6 hours.

◊ References.

1. Atkinson BD, *et al.* Double-blind comparison of intravenous butorphanol (Stadol) and fentanyl (Sublimaze) for analgesia during labor. *Am J Obstet Gynecol* 1994; **171**: 993–8.
2. Gillis JC. Transnasal butorphanol: a review of its pharmacodynamic and pharmacokinetic properties, and therapeutic potential in acute pain management. *Drugs* 1995; **50**: 157–75.

Headache. Butorphanol has been advocated for use as a nasal spray in the treatment of migraine, but its place in therapy, if any, remains to be established.

References.

1. Freitag FG. The acute treatment of migraine with transnasal butorphanol (TNB). *Headache Q* 1993; **4** (suppl 3): 22–8.
2. Hoffert MJ, *et al.* Transnasal butorphanol in the treatment of acute migraine. *Headache* 1995; **35**: 65–9.
3. Melanson SW, *et al.* Transnasal butorphanol in the emergency department management of migraine headache. *Am J Emerg Med* 1997; **15**: 57–61.

Pruritus. Preliminary results from a small study[1] of 6 patients with severe opioid-induced pruritus unresponsive to diphenhydramine indicated that intranasal butorphanol 2 mg administered every 4 to 6 hours may be an effective treatment.

1. Dunteman E, *et al.* Transnasal butorphanol for the treatment of opioid-induced pruritus unresponsive to antihistamines. *J Pain Symptom Manage* 1996; **12:** 255–60.

Preparations

USP 25: Butorphanol Tartrate Injection.

Proprietary Preparations (details are given in Part 3)
Canad.: Stadol; **Israel:** Stadol; **Mex.:** Stadol; **Spain:** Verstadol†; **USA:** Stadol.

Capsaicin   (9679-a)

(E)-8-Methyl-N-vanillylnon-6-enamide.
$C_{18}H_{27}NO_3 = 305.4$.
CAS — 404-86-4.
ATC — N01BX04.

NOTE. Do not confuse capsaicin with capsicin (p.1591) which is capsicum oleoresin.

Pharmacopoeias. In *US.*

The active principle of the dried ripe fruits of *Capsicum* spp.

Pharmacopoeial description

USP 25: An off-white powder. M.p. 57° to 66°. Practically insoluble in cold water; soluble in alcohol, in chloroform, and in benzene; slightly soluble in carbon disulfide. Store in a cool place in airtight containers. Protect from light.

◊ CAUTION. *Capsaicin should be handled with care. Particles should not be inhaled nor come into contact with any part of the body.*

Adverse Effects

A warm, stinging, or burning sensation may be experienced at the site of application; this usually disappears after a few days of use but may persist longer if applications are less frequent than recommended (see Uses and Administration, below). Coughing, sneezing, or respiratory irritation may occur if dried residue from topical preparations is inhaled.

Precautions

Contact with eyes and broken or irritated skin should be avoided. The hands should be washed after application of the cream, unless the hands are the treated areas, in which case, they should be washed 30 minutes after application. If bandages are used to cover treated areas they should not be wound too tightly. Heating pads should not be used with capsaicin, and patients should avoid taking a hot bath or shower immediately before or after application, as the burning sensation may be exacerbated. Thick applications of the cream should be avoided.

Uses and Administration

Capsaicin is used as a topical analgesic (p.4) in painful conditions such as postherpetic neuralgia after the lesions have healed, diabetic neuropathy, osteoarthritis, and rheumatoid arthritis. Capsaicin is usually applied sparingly 3 or 4 times daily as a 0.025% or 0.075% cream; in the UK it is only licensed for use over 12 years of age, but in the USA it may be used in children over 2 years of age. A more concentrated cream containing 0.25% capsaicin is available in some countries for adults and children over 12 years of age, and is applied sparingly twice daily. Capsaicin cream should be rubbed well into the skin until little or no residue is left on the surface. Therapeutic response may not be evident for 1 to 2 weeks for arthritic disorders, or 2 to 4 weeks for neuralgias (or even longer if the head or neck are involved). The UK manufacturer recommends that for the management of painful diabetic neuropathy, capsaicin should only be used under specialist supervision and that treatment should be reviewed after the first 8 weeks and regularly re-evaluated thereafter. Although not a counter-irritant itself, capsaicin has been included in rubefacient preparations for the relief of muscular and rheumatic pain.

Action. The analgesic effect following topical application of capsaicin is attributed to its ability to deplete the neuropeptide substance P from local sensory C-type nerve fibres.[1-5] Its action in depleting substance P, after repeated applications, serves to reduce the transmission of pain impulses to the CNS. Since the effect of capsaicin does not rely on vasodilatation in the skin it is therefore not considered to be a traditional counter-irritant. A vanilloid receptor, activated not only by capsaicin and related substances but also by heat and acids, has been identified.[6]

1. Rumsfield JA, West DP. Topical capsaicin in dermatologic and peripheral pain disorders. *DICP Ann Pharmacother* 1991; **25:** 381–7.
2. Cordell GA, Araujo OE. Capsaicin: identification, nomenclature, and pharmacotherapy. *Ann Pharmacother* 1993; **27:** 330–6.
3. Winter J, *et al.* Capsaicin and pain mechanisms. *Br J Anaesth* 1995; **75:** 157–68.
4. Del Bianco E, *et al.* The effects of repeated dermal application of capsaicin to the human skin on pain and vasodilatation induced by intradermal injection of acid and hypertonic solutions. *Br J Clin Pharmacol* 1996; **41:** 1–6.
5. Fusco BM, Giacovazzo M. Peppers and pain: the promise of capsaicin. *Drugs* 1997; **53:** 909–14.
6. Szallasi A, Blumberg PM. Vanilloid (capsaicin) receptors and mechanisms. *Pharmacol Rev* 1999; **51:** 159–211.

Cluster headache. Prevention of occurrence of attacks of cluster headache (p.449) using repeated applications of capsaicin to the nasal mucosa has been reported.[1]

1. Fusco BM, *et al.* Preventative effect of repeated nasal applications of capsaicin in cluster headache. *Pain* 1994; **59:** 321–5.

Micturition disorders. Intravesical capsaicin has been tried for painful bladder disorders and to treat bladder detrusor hyperreflexia.[1-4] Results have been variable, and the characteristic sensory effects of capsaicin make blinding of studies impossible, but some patients have reported benefit. Instillation into the ureter has also been tried in the management of the loin pain/haematuria syndrome.[5]

1. Nitti VW. Intravesical capsaicin for treatment of neurogenic bladder. *Lancet* 1994; **343:** 1448.
2. Lazzeri M, *et al.* Intravesical capsaicin for treatment of severe bladder pain: a randomized placebo controlled study. *J Urol (Baltimore)* 1996; **156:** 947–52.
3. de Sèze M, *et al.* Capsaicin and neurogenic detrusor hyperreflexia: a double-blind placebo-controlled study in 20 patients with spinal cord lesions. *Neurourol Urodyn* 1998; **17:** 513–23.
4. Petersen T, *et al.* Intravesical capsaicin in patients with detrusor hyper-reflexia: a placebo-controlled cross-over study. *Scand J Urol Nephrol* 1999; **33:** 104–10.
5. Bultitude MI. Capsaicin in treatment of loin pain/haematuria syndrome. *Lancet* 1995; **345:** 921–2.

Neuropathic pain. Capsaicin has been tried topically in various types of pain that may be mediated by the neurotransmitter, substance P, including neuropathic pain, which does not generally respond to conventional systemic analgesics. Topical capsaicin is used in the management of diabetic neuropathy (p.5) and postherpetic neuralgia (p.7), but while a meta-analysis[1] of randomised, double-blind, placebo-controlled studies and later studies[2] suggested that it is effective in painful diabetic neuropathy the evidence for efficacy in postherpetic neuralgia was considered[1] to be less convincing. Another meta-analysis suggested that capsaicin was of benefit in neuropathic pain,[3] but noted the difficulty of blinding in placebo-controlled trials of this substance, because of the burning sensation it produces. Other types of neuropathic pain that capsaicin has been tried in include reflex sympathetic dystrophy[4] (p.8), postmastectomy neuroma,[5,6] and stump pain.[7]

1. Zhang WY, Li Wan Po A. The effectiveness of topically applied capsaicin. *Eur J Clin Pharmacol* 1994; **46:** 517–22.
2. Biesbroeck R, *et al.* A double-blind comparison of topical capsaicin and oral amitriptyline in painful diabetic neuropathy. *Adv Therapy* 1995; **12:** 111–20.
3. Kingery WS. A critical review of controlled clinical trials for peripheral neuropathic pain and complex regional pain syndromes. *Pain* 1997; **73:** 123–39.
4. Cheshire WP, Snyder CR. Treatment of reflex sympathetic dystrophy with topical capsaicin: case report. *Pain* 1990; **42:** 307–11.
5. Watson CPN, Evans RJ. The postmastectomy pain syndrome and topical capsaicin: a randomized trial. *Pain* 1992; **51:** 375–9.
6. Dini D, *et al.* Treatment of the post-mastectomy pain syndrome with topical capsaicin. *Pain* 1993; **54:** 223–6.
7. Rayner HC, *et al.* Relief of local stump pain by capsaicin cream. *Lancet* 1989; **ii:** 1276–7.

Pruritus. Substance P is a possible mediator of itch sensations and capsaicin has been tried in the relief of pruritus (p.1106) associated with various diseases and haemodialysis.[1-4] It has also been tried to provide relief from pruritus induced by hetastarch[5] and for the itch and pain associated with PUVA therapy.[6,7]

1. Breneman DL, *et al.* Topical capsaicin for treatment of hemodialysis-related pruritus. *J Am Acad Dermatol* 1992; **26:** 91–4.
2. Leibsohn E. Treatment of notalgia paresthetica with capsaicin. *Cutis* 1992; **49:** 335–6.
3. Fölster-Holst R, Brasch J. Effect of topically applied capsaicin on pruritus in patients with atopic dermatitis. *J Dermatol Treat* 1996; **7:** 13–15.
4. Hautmann G, *et al.* Aquagenic pruritus, PUVA and capsaicin treatments. *Br J Dermatol* 1994; **131:** 920–1.
5. Szeimies R-M, *et al.* Successful treatment of hydroxyethyl starch-induced pruritus with topical capsaicin. *Br J Dermatol* 1994; **131:** 380–2.
6. Burrows NP, Norris PG. Treatment of PUVA-induced skin pain with capsaicin. *Br J Dermatol* 1994; **131:** 584–5.
7. Kirby B, Rogers S. Treatment of PUVA itch with capsaicin. *Br J Dermatol* 1997; **137:** 152.

Psoriasis. Since substance P has been implicated in the pathophysiology of several inflammatory dermatological processes, capsaicin has been tried in a number of skin disorders including psoriasis.[1,2]

The usual management of psoriasis is discussed on p.1106.

1. Bernstein JE, *et al.* Effects of topically applied capsaicin on moderate and severe psoriasis vulgaris. *J Am Acad Dermatol* 1986; **15:** 504–7.
2. Ellis CN, *et al.* A double-blind evaluation of topical capsaicin in pruritic psoriasis. *J Am Acad Dermatol* 1993; **29:** 438–42.

Rheumatic disorders. Topical capsaicin is used for the temporary relief of the pain of arthritis. From the results of a meta-analysis[1] of randomised, double-blind, placebo-controlled studies and later studies[2] it appears that capsaicin is effective in easing the pain of osteoarthritis (p.9) but its role, if any, is unclear; published evidence[3] for efficacy in rheumatoid arthritis (p.9) appears to be limited. Capsaicin may be a useful therapy for pain associated with primary fibromyalgia,[4] which responds poorly to conventional treatment.

1. Zhang WY, Li Wan Po A. The effectiveness of topically applied capsaicin. *Eur J Clin Pharmacol* 1994; **46:** 517–22.

2. Altman RD, *et al.* Capsaicin cream 0.025% as monotherapy for osteoarthritis: a double-blind study. *Semin Arthritis Rheum* 1994; **23** (suppl 3): 25–33.
3. Deal CL, *et al.* Treatment of arthritis with topical capsaicin: a double-blind trial. *Clin Ther* 1991; **13:** 383–95.
4. McCarty DJ, *et al.* Treatment of pain due to fibromyalgia with topical capsaicin: a pilot study. *Semin Arthritis Rheum* 1994; **23** (suppl 3): 41–7.

Preparations

Proprietary Preparations (details are given in Part 3)
Austral.: Zostrix; **Canad.:** Antiphlogistine Rub A-535 Capsaicin; Arthritic Pain Relief; Axsain†; Capzasin-P†; Zostrix; **Irl.:** Axsain; Zacin; **Israel:** Zostrix; **Spain:** Capsidol; Gelcen; Katrum; Priltam; **Swed.:** Capsina; **UK:** Axsain; Zacin; **USA:** Capsin; Capzasin-P; Dolorac; Doublecap; No Pain-HP; R-Gel; Theragen; Zostrix.

Multi-ingredient: **Aust.:** Rubizon-Rheumagel; **Braz.:** Infrarub; **Canad.:** Arthricare Odor Free; Arthricare Ultra; Heet; Methacin; Midalgan; **Fr.:** Capzasin-P†; Zostrix-P†; **Ger.:** Capsamol; **Irl.:** Algipan; Radian-B; **Ital.:** Disalgil; **UK:** NatraFlex; **USA:** Arthricare Odor Free; Heet; Menthacin; Pain Doctor; Pain X†; Ziks.

Carbasalate Calcium   (2620-l)

Carbasalate Calcium (BAN, rINN).

Calcium Acetylsalicylate Carbamide; Calcium Carbaspirin; Carbasalatum Calcicum; Carbasalatum Calcium; Carbaspirin Calcium (USAN). Calcium bis[2-(acetoxy)benzoate]—urea.
$C_{19}H_{18}CaN_2O_9 = 458.4$.
CAS — 5749-67-7.
ATC — B01AC08; N02BA15.

Pharmacopoeias. In *Eur.* (see p.vi).

A 1:1 complex of calcium acetylsalicylate and urea.

Pharmacopoeial description

Ph. Eur.: A white crystalline powder. It contains not less than 99.0% and not more than the equivalent of 101.0% of an equimolecular compound of calcium di[2-(acetyloxy)benzoate] and urea, calculated with reference to the anhydrous substance. Freely soluble in water and in dimethylformamide; practically insoluble in acetone and in anhydrous methyl alcohol. Store in airtight containers.

Adverse Effects, Treatment, and Precautions
As for Aspirin, p.14.

Carbasalate calcium, like aspirin, should not generally be given to children under the age of 12 years because of the risk of Reye's syndrome.

Interactions
For interactions associated with aspirin, see p.16.

Uses and Administration
Carbasalate calcium is metabolised to aspirin following absorption; it thus has the actions of aspirin (p.16). Carbasalate calcium is given in doses equivalent to 500 mg to 1 g of aspirin (maximum 3 g daily) for pain or fever and in doses equivalent to 0.5 to 2 g of aspirin every 4 hours (maximum 6 g daily) for rheumatic disorders. Carbasalate calcium has also been used in the management of thromboembolic disorders.

Preparations

Proprietary Preparations (details are given in Part 3)
Aust.: Iromin; **Belg.:** Solupsa; Upsalgine; **Fr.:** Cardiosolupsan; Solupsan; **Neth.:** Ascal; **Spain:** Ascal; Alcacyl.

Multi-ingredient: **Aust.:** Irocopar cC; Irocophan; Iromin Chinin C; **Braz.:** Gripefin; **Fr.:** Cephalgan; **Switz.:** Alca-C; Calonat.

Carfentanil Citrate   (18911-a)

Carfentanil Citrate (USAN, rINNM).

R-33799. Methyl 1-phenethyl-4-(N-phenylpropionamido)isonipecotate citrate.
$C_{24}H_{30}N_2O_3,C_6H_8O_7 = 586.6$.
CAS — 59708-52-0 (carfentanil); 61380-27-6 (carfentanil citrate).

Profile
Carfentanil citrate is an opioid analgesic related to fentanyl (p.37). It is used in veterinary medicine.

Carprofen   (12531-b)

Carprofen (BAN, USAN, rINN).

C-5720; Ro-20-5720/000. (±)-2-(6-Chlorocarbazol-2-yl)propionic acid.
$C_{15}H_{12}ClNO_2 = 273.7$.
CAS — 53716-49-7.

Profile
Carprofen, a propionic acid derivative, is an NSAID (p.63) that is used in veterinary medicine.

The symbol † denotes a preparation no longer actively marketed

Celecoxib (3624-n)

Celecoxib (BAN, USAN, rINN).
SC-58635. *p*-[5-*p*-Tolyl-3-(trifluoromethyl)pyrazol-1-yl]benzenesulfonamide.
$C_{17}H_{14}F_3N_3O_2S = 381.4$.
CAS — 169590-42-5.
ATC — M01AH01.

Adverse Effects and Precautions

As for NSAIDs in general, p.63. Celecoxib should not be used in patients with severe hepatic impairment. Therapy should be withdrawn if signs or symptoms of hepatic toxicity develop. Celecoxib should not be given to patients with a history of hypersensitivity to sulfonamides. It is also contra-indicated in patients with severe heart failure, inflammatory bowel disease, and renal impairment associated with a creatinine clearance of less than 30 mL per minute.

Effects on the cardiovascular system. The UK Committee on Safety of Medicines had received a small number of reports[1] of myocardial infarction or ischaemia in association with the selective cyclo-oxygenase-2 (COX-2) inhibitors as of February 2001. COX-2 inhibitors such as celecoxib do not possess the intrinsic antiplatelet activity associated with aspirin and possibly other non-selective NSAIDs and consequently do not provide protection against ischaemic cardiac events.

For a comparison of the hypertensive effects of celecoxib and rofecoxib, see p.81.

1. Committee on Safety of Medicines/Medicines Control Agency. COX-2 selective NSAIDs lack antiplatelet activity. *Current Problems* 2001; **27:** 7.

Effects on the gastrointestinal tract. It is generally accepted that the inhibition of cyclo-oxygenase-1 (COX-1) results in the adverse gastrointestinal effects of the NSAIDs, and that the selective inhibition of the other isoform, COX-2, by NSAIDs such as celecoxib may cause less gastrotoxicity than that seen with the non-selective inhibition of the traditional NSAIDs.

Results from controlled trials confirm that NSAIDs selective for COX-2 are associated with a lower incidence of serious gastrointestinal effects. In a placebo-controlled trial[1] the incidence of endoscopically determined gastroduodenal ulcers in patients taking celecoxib for rheumatoid arthritis (dose range 200 to 800 mg daily) was not significantly different to that seen with the placebo group. Another study[2] in patients taking celecoxib at supratherapeutic doses (800 mg daily) concluded that there was a lower combined incidence of symptomatic gastrointestinal ulcers and ulcer complications (bleeding, perforation, and obstruction) when compared with non-selective NSAIDs (ibuprofen 2.4 g daily or diclofenac 150 mg daily). However, the incidence of ulcer complications alone was not significantly different to that seen with other NSAIDs. The study also found that the risk of ulcer complications was significantly increased in celecoxib users taking concomitant low-dose aspirin. It has been noted that the use of aspirin appears to nullify any potential protective effect of COX-2 selectivity by celecoxib.[3,4] There have been individual case reports of gastrotoxicity with celecoxib.[5,6]

1. Simon LS, *et al.* Anti-inflammatory and upper gastrointestinal effects of celecoxib in rheumatoid arthritis: a randomized controlled trial. *JAMA* 1999; **282:** 1921–8.
2. Silverstein FE, *et al.* Gastrointestinal toxicity with celecoxib vs nonsteroidal anti-inflammatory drugs for osteoarthritis and rheumatoid arthritis. The CLASS study: a randomized controlled trial. *JAMA* 2000; **284:** 1247–55.
3. Lichtenstein DR, Wolfe MM. COX-2-selective NSAIDs: new and improved? *JAMA* 2000; **284:** 1297–9.
4. Bates DE, Lemaire JB. Possible celecoxib-induced gastroduodenal ulceration. *Ann Pharmacother* 2001; **35:** 782–3.
5. Mohammed S, Croom DW. Gastropathy due to celecoxib, a cyclooxygenase-2 inhibitor. *N Engl J Med* 1999; **340:** 2005–6.
6. Anonymous. Celecoxib: early Australian reporting experience. *Aust Adverse Drug React Bull* 2000; **19:** 6–7.

Effects on the kidneys. Limited evidence of the renal toxicity of the selective cyclo-oxygenase-2 (COX-2) inhibitors such as celecoxib suggests that such NSAIDs appear to have effects on renal function similar to those of the non-selective NSAIDs (see p.64).

Some references to the adverse renal effects of celecoxib.

1. Boyd IW, *et al.* COX-2 inhibitors and renal failure: the triple whammy revisited. *Med J Aust* 2000; **173:** 274.
2. Perazella MA, Tray K. Selective cyclooxygenase-2 inhibitors: a pattern of nephrotoxicity similar to traditional nonsteroidal anti-inflammatory drugs. *Am J Med* 2001; **111:** 64–7.
3. Graham MG. Acute renal failure related to high-dose celecoxib. *Ann Intern Med* 2001; **135:** 69–70.

Pancreatitis. Acute hepatitis and pancreatitis developed in an elderly patient with a reported history of hypersensitivity to sulfonamides who was given celecoxib.[1] Symptoms resolved on discontinuation of the drug. Pancreatitis has also been reported in a patient known to be tolerant of sulfonamides.[2]

1. Carrillo-Jimenez R, Nurnberger M. Celecoxib-induced acute pancreatitis and hepatitis: a case report. *Arch Intern Med* 2000; **160:** 553–4.
2. Baciewicz AM, *et al.* Acute pancreatitis associated with celecoxib. *Ann Intern Med* 2000; **132:** 680.

Interactions

The metabolism of celecoxib is mediated mainly by the cytochrome P450 isoenzyme CYP2C9. Concomitant administration of other drugs that inhibit or are metabolised by this isoenzyme may result in changes in plasma concentration of celecoxib; co-administration of fluconazole has resulted in increased plasma concentrations of celecoxib. Celecoxib is an inhibitor of the isoenzyme CYP2D6 and the potential therefore exists for an effect on drugs metabolised by this enzyme.

For interactions associated with NSAIDs in general, see p.65.

Pharmacokinetics

Celecoxib is absorbed from the gastrointestinal tract, peak plasma concentrations being achieved after about 3 hours. Protein binding is approximately 97%. Celecoxib is metabolised predominantly by the cytochrome P450 isoenzyme CYP2C9; the three identified metabolites are inactive as inhibitors of COX-1 or COX-2 enzymes. It is eliminated mainly as metabolites in the faeces and urine; less than 3% is recovered as unchanged drug. The effective terminal half-life is about 11 hours.

◊ References.

1. Davies NM, *et al.* Clinical pharmacokinetics and pharmacodynamics of celecoxib: a selective cyclo-oxygenase-2 inhibitor. *Clin Pharmacokinet* 2000; **38:** 225–42.

Uses and administration

Celecoxib is an NSAID (p.65) reported to be a selective inhibitor of cyclo-oxygenase-2 (COX-2). It is used in the treatment of rheumatoid arthritis and osteoarthritis and in the adjunctive treatment of adenomatous colorectal polyps. Celecoxib is also used in the management of acute pain and dysmenorrhoea.

For osteoarthritis the recommended dose is 200 mg daily given by mouth as a single dose or in 2 divided doses. If necessary a dose of 200 mg twice daily may be used. For rheumatoid arthritis the dose is 100 to 200 mg given twice daily. In elderly patients and those of Afro-Caribbean origin treatment should be initiated at the lowest recommended dose.

In the treatment of pain and dysmenorrhoea, an initial dose of 400 mg followed by an additional dose of 200 mg, if necessary, is recommended on the first day; thereafter the dose is 200 mg twice daily.

Celecoxib is also used as an adjunct to standard therapy to reduce the number of adenomatous colorectal polyps in patients with familial adenomatous polyposis. For this purpose it may be given in doses of 400 mg twice daily with food.

The manufacturers recommend that doses of celecoxib should be reduced by 50% in patients with moderate hepatic impairment.

◊ Reviews.

1. Clemett D, Goa KL. Celecoxib: a review of its use in osteoarthritis, rheumatoid arthritis and acute pain. *Drugs* 2000; **59:** 957–80.

Familial adenomatous polyposis. Celecoxib is used in the treatment of familial adenomatous polyposis, an inherited syndrome known to predispose sufferers to the development of colonic cancer (see Malignant Neoplasms of the Gastrointestinal Tract, p.493). A randomised trial[1] found that treatment with celecoxib reduced the number of colonic polyps; the authors considered celecoxib to be a useful adjunct to the standard therapy of colectomy.

1. Steinbach G, *et al.* The effect of celecoxib, a cyclooxygenase-2 inhibitor, in familial adenomatous polyposis. *N Engl J Med* 2000; **342:** 1946–52.

Musculoskeletal and joint disorders. Celecoxib is used in the treatment of the musculoskeletal disorders osteoarthritis (p.9) and rheumatoid arthritis (p.9). However, in the UK it is recommended that the use of celecoxib and other selective cyclo-oxygenase-2 (COX-2) inhibitors be limited to those patients considered to be at high risk of developing serious gastrointestinal problems if given a non-selective NSAID. High-risk patients include the elderly, those already receiving gastrotoxic drugs, and those with existing gastrointestinal disorders. Celecoxib has also been tried in the treatment of ankylosing spondylitis.

References.

1. Bensen WG, *et al.* Treatment of osteoarthritis with celecoxib, a cyclooxygenase-2 inhibitor: a randomized controlled trial. *Mayo Clin Proc* 1999; **74:** 1095–1105.

2. Anonymous. Celecoxib for arthritis. *Med Lett Drugs Ther* 1999; **41:** 11–12.
3. Simon LS, *et al.* Anti-inflammatory and upper gastrointestinal effects of celecoxib in rheumatoid arthritis: a randomized controlled trial. *JAMA* 1999; **282:** 1921–28.
4. Emery P, *et al.* Celecoxib versus diclofenac in long-term management of rheumatoid arthritis: randomised double-blind comparison. *Lancet* 1999; **354:** 2106–11.
5. Dougados M, *et al.* Efficacy of celecoxib, a cyclooxygenase 2-specific inhibitor, in the treatment of ankylosing spondylitis: a six-week controlled study with comparison against placebo and against a conventional nonsteroidal antiinflammatory drug. *Arthritis Rheum* 2001; **44:** 180–5.

Preparations

Proprietary Preparations (details are given in Part 3)
Austral.: Celebrex; *Canad.:* Celebrex; *Denm.:* Celebra; *Fr.:* Celebrex; *Irl.:* Celebrex; *NZ:* Celebrex; *S.Afr.:* Celebrex; *Singapore:* Celebrex; *Switz.:* Celebrex; *Thai.:* Celebrex; *UK:* Celebrex; *USA:* Celebrex.

Choline Magnesium Trisalicylate (2624-c)

CAS — 64425-90-7.

Adverse Effects, Treatment, and Precautions

As for Aspirin, p.14.

The use of aspirin and other acetylated salicylates is generally not recommended for children under the age of 12 years unless specifically indicated, because of the risk of Reye's syndrome. Some authorities also extend this precaution to non-acetylated salicylates.

Effects on the liver. References.

1. Cersosimo RJ, Matthews SJ. Hepatotoxicity associated with choline magnesium trisalicylate: case report and review of salicylate-induced hepatotoxicity. *Drug Intell Clin Pharm* 1987; **21:** 621–5.

Interactions

For interactions associated with salicylates, see Aspirin, p.16.

Uses and Administration

Choline magnesium trisalicylate is a combination of the salicylic acid derivatives choline salicylate (p.24) and magnesium salicylate (p.50). It has analgesic, anti-inflammatory, and antipyretic actions similar to those of aspirin (p.16). Following oral administration, choline magnesium trisalicylate dissociates and the salicylate moiety is rapidly absorbed. Each unit dose of 500 mg of salicylate is provided by approximately 293 mg of choline salicylate with 362 mg of magnesium salicylate (anhydrous). Choline magnesium trisalicylate is used in osteoarthritis, rheumatoid arthritis, and other arthritides in doses equivalent to 1 or 1.5 g of salicylate twice daily by mouth; doses may also be given as a single daily dose if required. A dose of 750 mg given three times daily may be more suitable for elderly patients. Choline magnesium trisalicylate is also used in similar doses in the general management of other forms of pain and for fever.

Preparations

Proprietary Preparations (details are given in Part 3)
Canad.: Trilisate; *USA:* Tricosal†; Trilisate.

Choline Salicylate (2625-k)

Choline Salicylate (BAN, USAN, rINN).
(2-Hydroxyethyl)trimethylammonium salicylate.
$C_{12}H_{19}NO_4 = 241.3$.
CAS — 2016-36-6.
ATC — N02BA03.
Pharmacopoeias. Br. includes Choline Salicylate Solution.

Choline salicylate 1 g is approximately equivalent to 750 mg of aspirin.

Pharmacopoeial description

BP 2001: Choline Salicylate Solution is an aqueous solution containing 47.5 to 52.5% of choline salicylate. It is a clear colourless liquid. It may contain a suitable antimicrobial preservative.

Profile

Choline salicylate is a salicylic acid derivative (see Aspirin, p.14) used in the treatment of pain and fever, and in the management of rheumatic disorders. It is given by mouth in doses of 435 to 870 mg every four hours as necessary for pain and fever, and in doses of 4.8 to 7.2 g daily in divided doses for rheumatic disorders.

Choline salicylate is also used as a local analgesic. Solutions containing up to about 20% choline salicylate are used in ear disorders such as the relief of pain in otitis media and externa but are considered to be of doubtful value; they are also used to soften ear wax as an aid to removal (see p.1223). An 8.7% gel is used for lesions of the mouth (p.1206). Choline salicylate has also been applied topically in a rubefacient preparation for the relief of muscular and rheumatic pain.

Choline salicylate is also given in the form of choline magnesium trisalicylate (see above).

Adverse effects. There has been a report[1] of a 21-month-old boy who developed salicylate poisoning after his mother had rubbed the contents of 3 tubes of 'Bonjela' teething ointment (containing a total of 2.61 g of choline salicylate) on his gums over 48 hours.

1. Paynter AS, Alexander FW. Salicylate intoxication caused by teething ointment. *Lancet* 1979; **ii**: 1132.

Preparations

BP 2001: Choline Salicylate Ear Drops; Choline Salicylate Oromucosal Gel.

Proprietary Preparations (details are given in Part 3)
Austral.: Applicaine; Herron Baby Teething Gel; Ora-Sed Jel; **Belg.:** Teejel; **Canad.:** Teejel; **Ger.:** Audax; Rheumavincin†; **Hong Kong:** Ora-Sed; **Irl.:** Audax; Teejel; **Israel:** Teejel; **NZ:** Applicaine; Orased; **S.Afr.:** Audax†; **Singapore:** Ora-Sed; **UK:** Audax; Dinnefords Teejel; **USA:** Arthropan.
Multi-ingredient: Aust.: Mundisal; Tifenso; **Austral.:** Bonjela; Seda-Gel; **Belg.:** Givalex; **Fr.:** Givalex; Pansoral; **Ger.:** Givalex; Mundisal; **Hong Kong:** Bonjela; Dermojela; **Irl.:** Bonjela; **Israel:** Bonjela; **NZ:** Bonjela; **Port.:** Bucagel; **S.Afr.:** Bonjela; **Singapore:** Bonjela; **Spain:** Aldo Otico; **Switz.:** Mundisal; Pansoral†; **Thai.:** Bonjela; **UK:** Bonjela; Earex Plus.

Cinchophen (2627-t)

Cinchophen (BAN, rINN).
Acifenokinolin; Phenylcinchoninic Acid; Quinophan. 2-Phenylquinoline-4-carboxylic acid.
$C_{16}H_{11}NO_2 = 249.3$.
CAS — 132-60-5.
ATC — M04AC02.

Profile

Cinchophen and its derivatives were formerly used in the treatment of gout but were associated with severe and unpredictable hepatotoxicity.

Clofexamide (12585-a)

Clofexamide (rINN).
ANP-246. 2-(4-Chlorophenoxy)-*N*-(2-diethylaminoethyl)acetamide.
$C_{14}H_{21}CIN_2O_2 = 284.8$.
CAS — 1223-36-5.

Profile

Clofexamide has been used topically as the hydrochloride in preparations for musculoskeletal, joint, and soft-tissue disorders.

Preparations

Proprietary Preparations (details are given in Part 3)
Multi-ingredient: Fr.: Perclusone†.

Clofezone (2628-x)

Clofezone (rINN).
ANP-3260. An equimolar combination of clofexamide and phenylbutazone.
$C_{14}H_{21}CIN_2O_2,C_{19}H_{20}N_2O_2,2H_2O = 629.2$.
CAS — 60104-29-2.
ATC — M01AA05; M02AA03.

Profile

Clofezone, a combination molecule containing clofexamide (above) and phenylbutazone (p.78), has been used topically in preparations for musculoskeletal, joint, and soft-tissue disorders.

Preparations

Proprietary Preparations (details are given in Part 3)
Multi-ingredient: Fr.: Perclusone†.

Clonixin (2630-j)

Clonixin (USAN, rINN).
CBA-93626; Sch-10304. 2-(3-Chloro-o-toluidino)nicotinic acid.
$C_{13}H_{11}CIN_2O_2 = 262.7$.
CAS — 17737-65-4.

Profile

Clonixin is an NSAID (p.63). It has been used as the lysine salt in doses of up to 250 mg four times daily by mouth for the relief of pain. Clonixin has also been given as the lysine salt by intramuscular or intravenous injection and as a rectal suppository.

◊ References.

1. Eberhardt R, *et al.* Analgesic efficacy and tolerability of lysineclonixinate versus ibuprofen in patients with gonarthrosis. *Curr Ther Res* 1995; **56**: 573–80.

Preparations

Proprietary Preparations (details are given in Part 3)
Braz.: Dolamin; **Mex.:** Disinal; Donodol; Dorixina; Firac; **Port.:** Algimate; Clonix; **Spain:** Dolalgial.

Multi-ingredient: Mex.: Donodol Compuesto; Espacil Compuesto; Firac Plus; Plidan Compuesto.

Codeine (6211-b)

Codeine (BAN).
Codeinum; Methylmorphine; Metilmorfina; Morphine Methyl Ether. 7,8-Didehydro-4,5-epoxy-3-methoxy-17-methylmorphinan-6-ol monohydrate.
$C_{18}H_{21}NO_3,H_2O = 317.4$.
CAS — 76-57-3 (anhydrous codeine); 6059-47-8 (codeine monohydrate).
ATC — R05DA04.
Pharmacopoeias. In Eur. (see p.vi), Int., and US.

Codeine is obtained from opium or made by methylating morphine.

Pharmacopoeial description

Ph. Eur.: White crystalline powder or colourless crystals. Soluble in boiling water and in ether; freely soluble in alcohol. A 0.5% solution in water has a pH of more than 9. Protect from light.
USP 25: Colourless or white crystals or white crystalline powder. It effloresces slowly in dry air. Soluble 1 in 120 of water, 1 in 2 of alcohol, 1 in 0.5 of chloroform, and 1 in 50 of ether. Its saturated solution in water is alkaline to litmus. Store in airtight containers. Protect from light.

Codeine Hydrochloride (6212-v)

Codeine Hydrochloride (BANM).
Codeini Hydrochloridum Dihydricum.
$C_{18}H_{21}NO_3,HCl,2H_2O = 371.9$.
CAS — 1422-07-7 (anhydrous codeine hydrochloride).
Pharmacopoeias. In Eur. (see p.vi).

Pharmacopoeial description

Ph. Eur.: Small colourless crystals or a white crystalline powder. Soluble in water; slightly soluble in dehydrated alcohol; practically insoluble in cyclohexane. Protect from light.

Codeine Phosphate (6213-g)

Codeine Phosphate (BANM).
Codeine Phosphate Hemihydrate; Codeini Phosphas; Codeinii Phosphas Hemihydricus; Codeinii Phosphas; Methylmorphine Phosphate.
$C_{18}H_{21}NO_3,H_3PO_4,\frac{1}{2}H_2O = 406.4$.
CAS — 52-28-8 (anhydrous codeine phosphate); 41444-62-6 (codeine phosphate hemihydrate); 5913-76-8 (codeine phosphate sesquihydrate).

NOTE. Compounded preparations of codeine phosphate may be represented by the following names:

• Co-codamol x/y (BAN)—where x and y are the strengths in milligrams of codeine phosphate and paracetamol respectively
• Co-codAPAP (USP 25)—codeine phosphate and paracetamol
• Co-codaprin (BAN)—codeine phosphate 1 part and aspirin 50 parts (w/w)
• Co-codaprin (USP 25)—codeine phosphate and aspirin.

Pharmacopoeias. In Chin., Eur. (see p.vi), Int., Jpn, Pol., and US. Chin. specifies 1½ H_2O. Int. permits 1½H_2O or ½H_2O. Eur. also has a monograph for Codeine Phosphate Sesquihydrate ($C_{18}H_{21}NO_3,H_3PO_4,1\frac{1}{2}H_2O = 424.4$).

Pharmacopoeial description

Ph. Eur.: The hemihydrate and the sesquihydrate occur as a white, crystalline powder or small, colourless crystals. Solubilities for the hemihydrate or sesquihydrate are: freely soluble in water; slightly soluble in alcohol; practically insoluble in ether. A 4% solution in water has a pH of 4.0 to 5.0. Protect from light.
USP 25: Fine, white, needle-shaped crystals or white crystalline powder; odourless. Soluble 1 in 2.5 of water, 1 in 0.5 of water at 80°, 1 in 325 of alcohol, and 1 in 125 of boiling alcohol. Its solutions are acid to litmus. Store in airtight containers. Protect from light.

Incompatibility. Acetylation of codeine phosphate by aspirin has occurred in solid dosage forms containing the two drugs, even at a low moisture level.[1] Animal work suggested that the analgesic activity of codeine was not affected by acetylation.[2]

1. Galante RN, *et al.* Solid-state acetylation of codeine phosphate by aspirin. *J Pharm Sci* 1979; **68**: 1494–8.
2. Buckett WR, *et al.* The analgesic properties of some 14-substituted derivatives of codeine and codeinone. *J Pharm Pharmacol* 1964; **16**: 174–82.

Codeine Sulfate (6214-q)

Codeine Sulphate (BANM).
$(C_{18}H_{21}NO_3)_2,H_2SO_4,3H_2O = 750.9$.
CAS — 1420-53-7 (anhydrous codeine sulfate); 6854-40-6 (codeine sulfate trihydrate).
Pharmacopoeias. In US.

Pharmacopoeial description

USP 25: White crystals, usually needle-like, or white crystalline powder. Soluble 1 in 30 of water, 1 in 6.5 of water at 80°, and 1 in 1300 of alcohol; insoluble in chloroform and in ether. Store in airtight containers. Protect from light.

Stability. Codeine sulfate solutions appear to be intrinsically more stable than codeine phosphate solutions.[1]

1. Powell MF. Enhanced stability of codeine sulfate: effect of pH, buffer, and temperature on the degradation of codeine in aqueous solution. *J Pharm Sci* 1986; **75**: 901–3.

Dependence and Withdrawal

As for Opioid Analgesics, p.66. Codeine is subject to abuse (see under Precautions, below), but produces less euphoria and sedation than morphine.

Neonatal abstinence syndrome. Some of the symptoms characteristic of the neonatal abstinence syndrome were seen in a neonate whose mother had taken about 90 mg of codeine daily during the last 2 months of pregnancy.[1]

1. Khan K, Chang J. Neonatal abstinence syndrome due to codeine. *Arch Dis Child* 1997; **76**: F59–F60.

Adverse Effects and Treatment

As for Opioid Analgesics in general, p.67.
In therapeutic doses codeine is much less liable than morphine to produce adverse effects, although constipation may be troublesome with long-term use. Following large doses of codeine, excitement and convulsions may occur.

Codeine, like morphine, has a dose-related histamine-releasing effect. Anaphylactic reactions following intravenous administration have been reported, rarely.

Effects on mental function. Central effects of codeine phosphate appeared to be limited, but dose-related, in subjects given 30, 60, or 90 mg; visuo-motor coordination was altered with doses of 60 and 90 mg and dynamic visual acuity with 90 mg.[1] Drowsiness reported by subjects receiving 90 mg of codeine phosphate could not be linked with impaired performance whereas nausea could.

1. Bradley CM, Nicholson AN. Effects of a μ-opioid receptor agonist (codeine phosphate) on visuo-motor coordination and dynamic visual acuity in man. *Br J Clin Pharmacol* 1986; **22**: 507–12.

Effects on the pancreas. A 26-year-old woman developed acute pancreatitis on 2 separate occasions a few hours after taking a single, 40-mg dose of codeine.[1] There was no history of alcohol consumption and her recovery was uneventful.

1. Hastier P, *et al.* Pancreatitis induced by codeine: a case report with positive rechallenge. *Gut* 1997; **41**: 705–6.

Effects on the skin. Pruritus and burning erythemato-vesicular plaques that developed in a patient in response to oral codeine were attributed to a fixed drug eruption.[1]

1. Gonzalo-Garijo MA, Revenga-Arranz F. Fixed drug eruption due to codeine. *Br J Dermatol* 1996; **135**: 498–9.

Overdosage. Acute codeine intoxication in 430 children, due to accidental ingestion of antitussive preparations, was analysed.[1] The children were nearly all between 1 and 6 years old. Symptoms in decreasing order of frequency included somnolence, rash, miosis, vomiting, itching, ataxia, and swelling of the skin. Respiratory failure occurred in 8 children and 2 died; all 8 had taken 5 mg or more per kg body-weight. Infants are at special risk and there have been reports of fatality[2,3] or near fatality[4] following inappropriate treatment in infants given mixtures containing codeine.

Opioid toxicity, in addition to severe salicylate toxicity, has occurred in adults following overdoses of aspirin and codeine tablets.[5]

1. von Mühlendahl KE, *et al.* Codeine intoxication in childhood. *Lancet* 1976; **ii**: 303–5.
2. Ivey HH, Kattwinkel J. Danger of Actifed-C. *Pediatrics* 1976; **57**: 164–5.
3. Magnani B, Evans R. Codeine intoxication in the neonate. Abstract: *Pediatrics* 1999; **104**: 1379. Full version: http://www.pediatrics.org/cgi/content/full/104/6/e75
4. Wilkes TCR, *et al.* Apnoea in a 3-month-old baby prescribed compound linctus containing codeine. *Lancet* 1981; **i**: 1166–7.
5. Leslie PJ, *et al.* Opiate toxicity after self poisoning with aspirin and codeine. *BMJ* 1986; **292**: 96.

Precautions

As for Opioid Analgesics in general, p.68.

Abuse. Although the risk of dependence on codeine is low with normal use,[1] it is the subject of deliberate abuse. In the UK linctuses containing codeine are particularly liable to abuse. Reports in the literature include the use in New Zealand of codeine-containing preparations to produce demethylated products known as "Homebake" containing variable amounts of morphine[2] and abuse of co-codaprin tablets for their codeine content.[3-5]

1. Rowden AM, Lopez JR. Codeine addiction. *DICP Ann Pharmacother* 1989; **23**: 475–7.
2. Shaw JP. Drug misuse in New Zealand. *Pharm J* 1987; **238**: 607.
3. Sakol MS, Stark CR. Codeine abuse. *Lancet* 1989; **ii**: 1282.
4. Paterson JR, *et al.* Codeine abuse from co-codaprin. *Lancet* 1990; **335**: 224.
5. Sakol MS, Stark CR. Codeine abuse from co-codaprin. *Lancet* 1990; **335**: 224.

Children. See under Overdosage, above, and under Uses and Administration, below.

Driving. Codeine phosphate 50 mg alone and in combination with alcohol had a deleterious effect on driving skills in a simulated driving test.[1]

1. Linnoila M, Häkkinen S. Effects of diazepam and codeine, alone and in combination with alcohol, on simulated driving. *Clin Pharmacol Ther* 1974; **15:** 368–73.

Interactions

For interactions associated with opioid analgesics, see p.68.

Quinidine. For reference to a suggestion that quinidine can inhibit the analgesic effect of codeine, see under Metabolism in Pharmacokinetics, below.

Pharmacokinetics

Codeine and its salts are absorbed from the gastrointestinal tract. Rectal absorption of codeine phosphate has been reported. Ingestion of codeine phosphate produces peak plasma-codeine concentrations in about one hour. Codeine is metabolised by *O*- and *N*-demethylation in the liver to morphine, norcodeine, and other metabolites including normorphine and hydrocodone. Codeine and its metabolites are excreted almost entirely by the kidney, mainly as conjugates with glucuronic acid.

The plasma half-life has been reported to be between 3 and 4 hours after administration by mouth or intramuscular injection.

◊ References.

1. Guay DR, *et al.* Pharmacokinetics of codeine after single- and multiple-oral-dose administration to normal volunteers. *J Clin Pharmacol* 1987; **27:** 983–7.
2. Persson K, *et al.* The postoperative pharmacokinetics of codeine. *Eur J Clin Pharmacol* 1992; **42:** 663–6.
3. Lafolie P, *et al.* Urine and plasma pharmacokinetics of codeine in healthy volunteers: implications for drugs-of-abuse testing. *J Anal Toxicol* 1996; **20:** 541–6.

Administration. In a comparative study[1] codeine had an oral/intramuscular analgesic relative potency ratio of 6:10. This was high compared with that of morphine and was attributed to protection from rapid first-pass metabolism rather than more efficient absorption following oral administration.

1. Beaver WT, *et al.* Analgesic studies of codeine and oxycodone in patients with cancer I: comparisons of oral with intramuscular codeine and of oral with intramuscular oxycodone. *J Pharmacol Exp Ther* 1978; **207:** 92–100.

Metabolism. The analgesic effect of codeine may be partly due to its metabolite morphine and it has been suggested that its efficacy may be impaired in patients who are poor metabolisers of codeine[1-3] or in those who are also receiving drugs such as quinidine which impair its metabolism.[1] However, patients unable to demethylate codeine to produce detectable plasma concentrations of morphine obtained a similar analgesic effect to patients with detectable plasma morphine concentrations.[4] A study[5] involving infants aged 6 to 10 months has indicated that children were capable of demethylating codeine to morphine at the age of 6 months although glucuronidation of the morphine appeared to be impaired when compared with older children.

1. Desmeules J, *et al.* Impact of environmental and genetic factors on codeine analgesia. *Eur J Clin Pharmacol* 1991; **41:** 23–6.
2. Chen ZR, *et al.* Disposition and metabolism of codeine after single and chronic doses in one poor and seven extensive metabolisers. *Br J Clin Pharmacol* 1991; **31:** 381–90.
3. Sindrup SH, *et al.* Codeine increases pain thresholds to copper vapor laser stimuli in extensive but not poor metabolizers of sparteine. *Clin Pharmacol Ther* 1991; **49:** 686–93.
4. Quiding H, *et al.* Analgesic effect and plasma concentrations of codeine and morphine after two dose levels of codeine following oral surgery. *Eur J Clin Pharmacol* 1993; **44:** 319–23.
5. Quiding H, *et al.* Infants and young children metabolise codeine to morphine: a study after single and repeated rectal administration. *Br J Clin Pharmacol* 1992; **33:** 45–9.

Uses and Administration

Codeine, a phenanthrene derivative, is an opioid analgesic (p.68). It is much less potent as an analgesic than morphine and has relatively mild sedative effects.

Codeine or its salts, especially the phosphate, are administered by mouth in the form of linctuses for the relief of cough, and as tablets for the relief of mild to moderate pain, often in association with a non-opioid analgesic such as aspirin or paracetamol. The phosphate is also given by intramuscular or subcutaneous injection, in doses similar to those by mouth, for the relief of pain; the intravenous route has also been used in adults.

For the relief of pain codeine phosphate may be given in doses of 30 to 60 mg every 4 hours to a usual maximum of 240 mg daily. Children aged 1 to 12 years

may be given 500 µg per kg body-weight 4 to 6 times daily.

To allay unproductive cough codeine phosphate may be given in doses of 15 to 30 mg three or four times daily. Children aged 5 to 12 years may be given 7.5 to 15 mg three or four times daily and those aged 1 to 5 years, 3 mg three or four times daily (but see below). Codeine phosphate is also used as tablets or in mixtures for the symptomatic relief of acute diarrhoea in adult doses of 30 mg given 3 or 4 times daily.

Other codeine salts used include the hydrochloride, sulfate, acephyllinate, camsilate, and hydrobromide. Codeine polistirex (a codeine and sulfonated diethenylbenzene-ethenylbenzene copolymer complex) is used in modified-release preparations.

◊ Systematic reviews[1,2] comparing paracetamol-codeine combinations versus paracetamol alone concluded that in single dose studies addition of codeine to paracetamol produced a comparatively small but statistically significant increase in analgesic effect; however, there was an increased incidence of side-effects with the combination.

1. de Craen AJM, *et al.* Analgesic efficacy and safety of paracetamol-codeine combinations versus paracetamol alone: a systematic review. *BMJ* 1996; **313:** 321–5.
2. Moore A, *et al.* Single dose paracetamol (acetaminophen), with and without codeine, for postoperative pain (updated 30 August 2001). Available in The Cochrane Library; Issue 4. Oxford: Update Software; 2001.

Administration in children. Dosage recommendations for codeine in the treatment of *pain* or cough are generally restricted to those over 1 year of age. However, some have considered codeine to be an effective analgesic in neonates and children.[1] With a single dose of codeine phosphate 1 mg per kg body-weight by mouth or by intramuscular injection there was a relatively small risk of respiratory depression in neonates, but significant respiratory depression has occurred with multiple doses and patients should be observed closely.[1] Case reports of adverse reactions such as vasodilatation, severe hypotension, and apnoea in infants and children after intravenous administration of codeine have precluded its use by this route in children of all ages.[2]

Antimotility drugs such as codeine should not be used in infants and young children with acute *diarrhoea*.[3,4]

Cough suppressants containing codeine or similar opioids are generally not recommended for administration to children and should be avoided in those under 1 year of age.

1. Lloyd-Thomas AR. Pain management in paediatric patients. *Br J Anaesth* 1990; **64:** 85–104.
2. Marsh DF, *et al.* Opioid systems and the newborn. *Br J Anaesth* 1997; **79:** 787–95.
3. Anonymous. Drugs in the management of acute diarrhoea in infants and young children. *Bull WHO* 1989; **67:** 94–6.
4. Cimolai N, Carter JE. Antimotility agents for paediatric use. *Lancet* 1990; **336:** 874.

Preparations

BP 2001: Co-codamol Tablets; Co-codaprin Tablets; Codeine Linctus; Codeine Phosphate Oral Solution; Codeine Phosphate Tablets; Dispersible Co-codaprin Tablets; Paediatric Codeine Linctus;
USP 25: Acetaminophen and Codeine Phosphate Capsules; Acetaminophen and Codeine Phosphate Oral Solution; Acetaminophen and Codeine Phosphate Oral Suspension; Acetaminophen and Codeine Phosphate Tablets; Aspirin and Codeine Phosphate Tablets; Butalbital, Aspirin, Caffeine, and Codeine Phosphate Capsules; Carisoprodol, Aspirin, and Codeine Phosphate Tablets; Codeine Phosphate Injection; Codeine Phosphate Tablets; Codeine Sulfate Tablets; Guaifenesin and Codeine Phosphate Syrup; Terpin Hydrate and Codeine Elixir.

Proprietary Preparations (details are given in Part 3)
Aust.: Codipertussin; Tricodein; *Austral.:* Actacode; *Belg.:* Bromophar; Bronchodine; Bronchosedal; Codocalyptol†; Eulyptan; Glottyl; Toularynx; *Fr.:* Codedrill; Codenfan; Neo-Codion; Paderyl; Pneumogenol; *Ger.:* Antitussivum Burger; Bronchicum Mono Codein; codi OPT; Codicaps mono; Codicaps N; Codicompren; Codiforton†; Codipront mono; Dicton; Melrosum Codein Hustensirup; Neo-Codion NN; Optipect Kodein; Tricodein; Tryasol; Tussamag Codeintropfen†; Tussoret; *Irl.:* Codant; *Israel:* Codical; Rekod; *Port.:* Codeisan†; *Spain:* Analgiol; Bisoltus; Codeisan; Fludan Codeina; Histaverin; Perduretas Codeina; Toseina NF; *Switz.:* Tricodein; *UK:* Evacode; Galcodine.

Multi-ingredient: numerous preparations are listed in Part 3.

Cymene (2631-z)

p-Cymene; *p*-Cymol. 4-Isopropyl-1-methylbenzene; 4-Isopropyltoluene.

$C_{10}H_{14} = 134.2$.
CAS — 25155-15-1; 99-87-6 (*p*-cymene).

Profile

Cymene has been used as a topical local analgesic for the relief of pain in rheumatic conditions.

Preparations

Proprietary Preparations (details are given in Part 3)
Multi-ingredient: *Fr.:* Neuriplege†.

Devil's Claw Root (3082-w)

Harpagophyti Radix; Harpagophyton; Harpagophytum; Harpagophytum Procumbens; Teufelskrallenwurzel.

Pharmacopoeias. In *Eur.* (see p.vi).

Pharmacopoeial description

Ph. Eur.: The cut and dried tuberous, secondary roots of *Harpagophytum procumbens* D.C. Greyish-brown to dark brown with a bitter taste. Contains not less than 1.2% harpagoside ($C_{24}H_{30}O_{11} = 494.5$), calculated with reference to the dried drug. Protect from light.

Profile

Devil's claw root is used in herbal remedies for musculoskeletal and joint disorders.

Preparations

Proprietary Preparations (details are given in Part 3)
Austral.: Doloteffin; *Fr.:* Algophytum†; Harpadol; Harpagocid; *Ger.:* ALLYA; Arthrosetten H; Arthrotabs; Cefatec; Defencid†; Dolo-Arthrodynat; Dolo-Arthrosetten H; Doloteffin; flexi-loges; Harpagoforte Asmedic; HarpagoMega; Herbadon; Jucurba N†; Pargo; Rheuferm Phyto; Rheuma-Sern; Rheuma-Teufelskralle HarpagoMega†; Rivoltan; Salus†; Sogoon; Teltonal; *Spain:* Harpagofito Orto; Hartiosen.

Multi-ingredient: *Austral.:* Arthriforte; Arthritic Pain Herbal Formula 1; Bioglan Arthri Plus; Devils Claw Plus; Extralife Arthri-Care; Harpagophytum Complex; Herbal Arthritis Formula; Lifesystem Herbal Formula 1 Arthritic Aid; Lifesystem Herbal Formula 12 Willowbark†; Prost-1; Willowbark Plus Herbal Formula 11†; *Fr.:* Actisane Douleurs Articulaires†; Arkophytum; Artrosan†; *Ger.:* Dr Wiemanns Rheumatonikum; *Ital.:* Artoxan†; Bodyguard; Pik-Gel; *UK:* Arthrotone.

Dextromoramide (6215-p)

Dextromoramide (BAN, pINN).

Dextrodiphenopyrine; *d*-Moramid; Pyrrolamidol. (+)-1-(3-Methyl-4-morpholino-2,2-diphenylbutyryl)pyrrolidine.
$C_{25}H_{32}N_2O_2 = 392.5$.
CAS — 357-56-2.
ATC — N02AC01.

Dextromoramide Tartrate (6216-s)

Dextromoramide Tartrate (BANM, pINNM).

Bitartrate de Dextromoramide; Dextromoramide Acid Tartrate; Dextromoramide Hydrogen Tartrate; Dextromoramidi Tartras.
$C_{25}H_{32}N_2O_2,C_4H_6O_6 = 542.6$.
CAS — 2922-44-3.
Pharmacopoeias. In *Eur.* (see p.vi).

Dextromoramide tartrate 6.9 mg is approximately equivalent to 5 mg of dextromoramide.

Pharmacopoeial description

Ph. Eur.: A white crystalline or amorphous powder. Soluble in water; sparingly soluble in alcohol; very slightly soluble in ether. A 1% solution in water has a pH of 3.0 to 4.0.

Dependence and Withdrawal

As for Opioid Analgesics, p.66. Dextromoramide is subject to abuse.

Adverse Effects, Treatment, and Precautions

As for Opioid Analgesics, p.67. It is reported to be less sedating than morphine.

Interactions

For interactions associated with opioid analgesics, see p.68.

Uses and Administration

Dextromoramide is an opioid analgesic (p.68) structurally related to methadone (p.54) and is used in the treatment of severe pain. It is not recommended for use in obstetric analgesia because of an increased risk of neonatal depression.

Dextromoramide is given as the tartrate by mouth or by rectum. It has also been given by subcutaneous or intramuscular injection and similar analgesic effects have been claimed for the same dose whether given by mouth or by injection. The analgesic effect begins after about 20 to 30 minutes, but its duration of action is only about 2 to 3 hours.

The usual dose is the equivalent of dextromoramide 5 mg by mouth increased if necessary up to a maximum of 20 mg as a single dose, repeated as necessary. Dextromoramide has been given rectally as suppositories of 10 mg.

An initial oral dose equivalent to not more than 80 µg per kg body-weight has been suggested by the manufacturers for use in children.

Preparations

BP 2001: Dextromoramide Tablets.

Proprietary Preparations (details are given in Part 3)
Austral.: Palfium; *Belg.:* Palfium†; *Fr.:* Palfium†; *Irl.:* Palfium; *Neth.:* Palfium; *UK:* Palfium.

Dextropropoxyphene (13408-s)

Dextropropoxyphene (BAN, pINN).

Propoxyphene. (+)-(1S,2R)-1-Benzyl-3-dimethylamino-2-methyl-1-phenylpropyl propionate.

$C_{22}H_{29}NO_2 = 339.5$.

CAS — 469-62-5.

ATC — N02AC04.

Dextropropoxyphene Hydrochloride (6217-w)

Dextropropoxyphene Hydrochloride (BANM, pINNM).

Dextropropoxypheni Hydrochloridum; Propoxyphene Hydrochloride (USAN).

$C_{22}H_{29}NO_2,HCl = 375.9$.

CAS — 1639-60-7.

NOTE. Compounded preparations of dextropropoxyphene hydrochloride may be represented by the following names:

- Co-proxamol (BAN)—dextropropoxyphene hydrochloride 1 part and paracetamol 10 parts (w/w).

Pharmacopoeias. In Eur. (see p.vi) and US.

Pharmacopoeial description

Ph. Eur.: A white or almost white crystalline powder. Very soluble in water; freely soluble in alcohol; practically insoluble in ether. Protect from light.

USP 25: A white odourless crystalline powder. Freely soluble in water; soluble in alcohol, in acetone, and in chloroform; practically insoluble in ether and in benzene. Store in airtight containers.

Dextropropoxyphene Napsilate (6218-e)

Dextropropoxyphene Napsilate (BANM, pINNM).

Dextropropoxyphene Napsilate; Propoxyphene Napsylate (USAN). Dextropropoxyphene naphthalene-2-sulphonate monohydrate.

$C_{22}H_{29}NO_2,C_{10}H_8O_3S,H_2O = 565.7$.

CAS — 17140-78-2 (anhydrous dextropropoxyphene napsilate); 26570-10-5 (dextropropoxyphene napsilate monohydrate).

NOTE. Compounded preparations of dextropropoxyphene napsilate may be represented by the following names:

- Co-proxAPAP (USP 25)—dextropropoxyphene napsilate and paracetamol.

Pharmacopoeias. In Br. and US.

Dextropropoxyphene napsilate 100 mg is approximately equivalent to 66 mg of dextropropoxyphene hydrochloride.

Pharmacopoeial description

BP 2001: An odourless or almost odourless white powder. It exhibits polymorphism. Practically insoluble in water; soluble in alcohol; freely soluble in chloroform.

USP 25: A white powder having essentially no odour. Very slightly soluble in water; soluble 1 in 15 of alcohol and 1 in 10 of chloroform; soluble in acetone and in methyl alcohol. Store in airtight containers.

Dependence and Withdrawal

As for Opioid Analgesics, p.66. Dextropropoxyphene has been subject to abuse (see under Precautions, below).

◊ Reports of dextropropoxyphene dependence and its treatment.

1. Wall R, et al. Addiction to Distalgesic (dextropropoxyphene). BMJ 1980; 280: 1213–14.
2. D'Abadie NB, Lenton JD. Propoxyphene dependence: problems in management. South Med J 1984; 77: 299–301.

Adverse Effects

As for Opioid Analgesics in general, p.67. In the recommended dosage the adverse effects of dextropropoxyphene are less marked than those of morphine. Gastrointestinal effects, dizziness, and drowsiness are the most common. Liver impairment has been reported.

There are a disturbing number of fatalities from either accidental or intentional overdose with dextropropoxyphene. Many reports emphasise the rapidity with which death ensues; death within an hour of overdosage is considered by some not to be uncommon and can occur within 15 minutes. Overdosage is often complicated by patients also taking alcohol and using mixed preparations such as dextropropoxyphene with paracetamol or aspirin.

Symptoms of overdosage are similar to those of opioid poisoning in general, but in addition patients may experience psychotic reactions. There may be cardiac conduction abnormalities and arrhythmias.

Dextropropoxyphene injections are painful and have had a very destructive effect on soft tissues and veins

when dextropropoxyphene has been abused in this way.

Anorectal reactions have followed the prolonged use of suppositories containing dextropropoxyphene; the reactions appear to be dose dependent.

Effects on the blood. A 12-year history of haemolysis and subsequent significant haemolytic anaemia in an elderly woman[1] was associated with chronic, periodic, and occasionally excessive intake of co-proxamol.

1. Fulton JD, McGonigal G. Steroid responsive haemolytic anaemia due to dextropropoxyphene paracetamol combination. J R Soc Med 1989; 82: 228.

Effects on the ears. A report of complete nerve deafness associated with chronic abuse of co-proxamol was made to the UK Committee on Safety of Medicines.[1] The Committee had received 2 other reports of permanent hearing loss attributed to co-proxamol abuse; transient hearing loss had also been reported in 2 patients taking usual doses; 7 further reports described tinnitus.

1. Ramsay BC. Complete nerve deafness after abuse of co-proxamol. Lancet 1991; 338: 446–7.

Effects on the liver. There have been occasional reports of jaundice in patients taking dextropropoxyphene without paracetamol. Many of the 49 suspected hepatic reactions with dextropropoxyphene reported to the UK Committee on Safety of Medicines by 1985[1] had involved dextropropoxyphene in association with paracetamol; clinical features including malaise, jaundice, raised serum transaminases, and sometimes fever, were however generally characteristic of dextropropoxyphene alone. Relapsing jaundice mimicking biliary disease was attributable to the dextropropoxyphene component of co-proxamol in 3 patients,[2] whereas there was no abnormality of liver function in 11 patients on long-term co-proxamol analgesia.[3] Another report of 9 cases also found that the hepatotoxic effects of dextropropoxyphene mimicked symptoms of large bile duct obstruction, and suggested that such toxicity might be misdiagnosed.[4]

1. Committee on Safety of Medicines. Hepatotoxicity with dextropropoxyphene. Current Problems 17 1986.
2. Bassendine MF, et al. Dextropropoxyphene induced hepatotoxicity mimicking biliary tract disease. Gut 1986; 27: 444–9.
3. Hutchinson DR, et al. Liver function in patients on long-term paracetamol (co-proxamol) analgesia. J Pharm Pharmacol 1986; 38: 242–3.
4. Rosenberg WMC, et al. Dextropropoxyphene induced hepatotoxicity: a report of nine cases. J Hepatol 1993; 19: 470–4.

Effects on the lungs. Hypersensitivity pneumonitis and skin rash has been reported in a patient taking co-proxamol (dextropropoxyphene and paracetamol).[1] No such reaction occurred when the patient was subsequently given paracetamol alone.

1. Matusiewicz SP, et al. Hypersensitivity pneumonitis associated with co-proxamol (paracetamol + dextropropoxyphene) therapy. Postgrad Med J 1999; 75: 475–6.

Hypoglycaemia. References to a hypoglycaemic effect of dextropropoxyphene.[1-3]

1. Wiederholt IC, et al. Recurrent episodes of hypoglycemia induced by propoxyphene. Neurology 1967; 11: 703–4.
2. Almirall J, et al. Propoxyphene-induced hypoglycemia in a patient with chronic renal failure. Nephron 1989; 53: 273–5.
3. Lowenstein W, et al. Hypoglycémie au dextropropoxyphène: une urgence chez le toxicomane. Presse Med 1993; 22: 133.

Overdosage. There have been several reviews or retrospective studies of acute self-poisoning with dextropropoxyphene.[1-4] At a symposium on the safety and efficacy of dextropropoxyphene[5] many of the participants dealt with the problems of dextropropoxyphene overdosage, often in conjunction with paracetamol and sometimes with alcohol. Profound and even fatal CNS depression can develop rapidly as a result of the dextropropoxyphene content and in many cases death has occurred within an hour;[6] it was suggested that as few as 15 to 20 tablets of co-proxamol might be fatal.[7,8] In the USA[9] the incidence of dextropropoxyphene-associated deaths reached a peak in 1977 and has then fallen at a rate that was not matched by a decline in prescribing. However, the number of deaths associated with dextropropoxyphene poisoning continues to be high in some countries.[4] It is not clear whether the metabolite nordextropropoxyphene plays an important role in fatalities.[9] However, nordextropropoxyphene, like dextropropoxyphene, is considered to have local anaesthetic activity and the membrane stabilising activity of dextropropoxyphene has been implicated as a major factor responsible for its severe cardiac depressant effect.[10]

1. Young RJ. Dextropropoxyphene overdosage: pharmacological considerations and clinical management. Drugs 1983; 26: 70–9.
2. Madsen PS, et al. Acute propoxyphene self-poisoning in 222 consecutive patients. Acta Anaesthesiol Scand 1984; 28: 661–5.
3. Segest E. Poisoning with dextropropoxyphene in Denmark. Hum Toxicol 1987; 6: 203–7.
4. Jonasson U, et al. Correlation between prescription of various dextropropoxyphene preparations and their involvement in fatal poisonings. Forensic Sci Int 1999; 103: 125–32.
5. Bowen D, et al. (ed). Distalgesic; safety and efficacy. Hum Toxicol 1984; 3 (suppl): 1S–238S.
6. Proudfoot AT. Clinical features and management of Distalgesic overdose. Hum Toxicol 1984; 3 (suppl): 85S–94S.
7. Whittington RM. Dextropropoxyphene deaths: coroner's report. Hum Toxicol 1984; 3 (suppl): 175S–85S.
8. Young RJ, Lawson AAH. Distalgesic poisoning—cause for concern. BMJ 1980; 280: 1045–7.

9. Finkle BS. Self-poisoning with dextropropoxyphene and dextropropoxyphene compounds: the USA experience. Hum Toxicol 1984; 3 (suppl): 115S–34S.
10. Henry JA, Cassidy SL. Membrane stabilising activity: a major cause of fatal poisoning. Lancet 1986; i: 1414–17.

Treatment of Adverse Effects

As for Opioid Analgesics in general, p.68.

Rapid treatment of overdosage with naloxone and assisted respiration is essential. Cardiac effects may not be reversed by naloxone. Gastric lavage and administration of activated charcoal may be of value if performed within 1 hour of ingestion, but dialysis is of little use.

Convulsions may require control with an anticonvulsant, bearing in mind that the CNS depressant effects of dextropropoxyphene might be exacerbated (see also under Interactions, below). Stimulants should not be used because of the risk of inducing convulsions.

Patients taking overdoses of dextropropoxyphene with paracetamol will also require treatment for paracetamol poisoning (p.71). Mixtures of dextropropoxyphene and aspirin may be involved; the treatment of aspirin poisoning is described on p.14.

◊ Reviews.

1. Proudfoot AT. Clinical features and management of Distalgesic overdose. Hum Toxicol 1984; 3 (suppl): 85S–94S.

Precautions

As for Opioid Analgesics in general, p.68.

Abuse. There have been reports of the abuse of dextropropoxyphene,[1] and some[2] considered that the ready availability of dextropropoxyphene made it liable to abuse although it was a relatively weak opioid analgesic. However, others[3] thought there was no evidence that dextropropoxyphene was frequently associated with abuse, or concluded that, although there was abuse potential, it was of relatively low importance in terms of the community as a whole.[4]

A severe withdrawal syndrome has been reported[5] in one elderly patient who covertly consumed a daily dose of dextropropoxyphene of 1 to 3 g for at least 12 months. The patient was treated by a gradually decreasing dosage schedule of dextropropoxyphene over 9 weeks.

1. Tennant FS. Complications of propoxyphene abuse. Arch Intern Med 1973; 132: 191–4.
2. Lader M. Abuse of weak opioid analgesics. Hum Toxicol 1984; 3 (suppl): 229S–36S.
3. Finkle BS. Self-poisoning with dextropropoxyphene and dextropropoxyphene compounds: the USA experience. Hum Toxicol 1984; 3 (suppl): 115S–34S.
4. Turner P. Final remarks. Hum Toxicol 1984; 3 (suppl): 237S–8S.
5. Hedenmalm K. A case of severe withdrawal syndrome due to dextropropoxyphene. Ann Intern Med 1995; 123: 473.

Breast feeding. See under Pharmacokinetics, below.

Porphyria. Dextropropoxyphene has been associated with acute attacks of porphyria and is considered unsafe in porphyric patients.

Interactions

For interactions associated with opioid analgesics, see p.68.

Plasma concentrations of dextropropoxyphene are increased by ritonavir, with a resultant risk of toxicity; concomitant administration should be avoided.

CNS depressants, including alcohol, may contribute to the hazards of dextropropoxyphene. The convulsant action of high doses of dextropropoxyphene may be enhanced by CNS stimulants.

Dextropropoxyphene interacts with several other drugs through inhibition of liver metabolism. Drugs reported to be affected include antidepressants, benzodiazepines, beta blockers, carbamazepine (see p.344), phenobarbital (see p.355), phenytoin (see p.359), and warfarin.

Antimuscarinics. A suggested interaction between orphenadrine and dextropropoxyphene has been questioned (see p.471).

Pharmacokinetics

Dextropropoxyphene is readily absorbed from the gastrointestinal tract, the napsilate tending to be more slowly absorbed than the hydrochloride, but both are subject to considerable first-pass metabolism. Peak plasma concentrations occur about 1 to 2 hours after ingestion. It is rapidly distributed and concentrated in the liver, lungs, and brain. About 80% of dextropropoxyphene and its metabolites are reported to be bound to plasma proteins. Dextropropoxyphene crosses the placenta. It has been detected in breast milk but some authorities consider that the amount is too small to be harmful to a breast-fed infant.

Dextropropoxyphene is *N*-demethylated to nordextropropoxyphene (norpropoxyphene) in the liver. It is excreted in the urine mainly as metabolites. It is now recognised that dextropropoxyphene and nordextropropoxyphene have prolonged elimination half-lives; values of 6 to 12 hours and 30 to 36 hours, respectively, have been reported. Accumulation of dextropropoxyphene and its metabolites may occur with repeated doses and nordextropropoxyphene may contribute to the toxicity seen with overdosage.

◊ Reviews.
1. Pearson RM. Pharmacokinetics of propoxyphene. *Hum Toxicol* 1984; **3** (suppl): 37S–40S.

The elderly. The elimination half-lives of dextropropoxyphene and its metabolite nordextropropoxyphene were prolonged in healthy elderly subjects when compared with young controls.[1] After multiple dosing median half-lives of dextropropoxyphene and nordextropropoxyphene were 36.8 and 41.8 hours respectively in the elderly compared with 22.0 and 22.1 hours in the young subjects. In this study[1] there was a strong correlation between half-life of nordextropropoxyphene and estimated creatinine clearance.
1. Flanagan RJ, *et al.* Pharmacokinetics of dextropropoxyphene and nordextropropoxyphene in young and elderly volunteers after single and multiple dextropropoxyphene dosage. *Br J Clin Pharmacol* 1989; **28:** 463–9.

Hepatic impairment. Plasma concentrations of dextropropoxyphene were higher in patients with cirrhosis given the drug than in healthy controls whereas concentrations of nordextropropoxyphene were lower.[1]
1. Giacomini KM, *et al.* Propoxyphene and norpropoxyphene plasma concentrations after oral propoxyphene in cirrhotic patients with and without surgically constructed portacaval shunt. *Clin Pharmacol Ther* 1980; **28:** 417–24.

Renal impairment. Higher and more persistent plasma concentrations of dextropropoxyphene and nordextropropoxyphene in anephric patients when compared with healthy subjects[1] were attributed to decreased first-pass metabolism of dextropropoxyphene and decreased renal excretion of nordextropropoxyphene in the anephric patients.
1. Gibson TP, *et al.* Propoxyphene and norpropoxyphene plasma concentrations in the anephric patient. *Clin Pharmacol Ther* 1980; **27:** 665–70.

Uses and Administration

Dextropropoxyphene is an opioid analgesic (p.68) structurally related to methadone (p.54). It has mild analgesic activity and is administered by mouth as the hydrochloride or napsilate to alleviate mild to moderate pain. Unlike the laevo-isomer (levopropoxyphene, p.1094), dextropropoxyphene has little antitussive activity.

Dextropropoxyphene is mainly used in conjunction with other analgesics with anti-inflammatory and antipyretic effects, such as aspirin or paracetamol. In the UK the usual dose is 65 mg of the hydrochloride or 100 mg of the napsilate given three or four times daily. In the USA similar doses are given every 4 hours up to a maximum total daily dose of 390 mg of the hydrochloride and 600 mg of the napsilate.

Pain. A detailed review[1] of the analgesic effectiveness of dextropropoxyphene suggested that with respect to single oral doses, recommended doses of dextropropoxyphene were no more (and probably less) than usual doses of paracetamol, aspirin, or other NSAIDs. However, the comparative effectiveness may vary substantially depending on the cause of the pain. When it comes to comparative studies involving combinations of dextropropoxyphene with other analgesics, findings are even less clear-cut.[2] The effectiveness of co-proxamol has long been a matter of controversy yet despite this a survey[3] conducted in 30 UK teaching hospitals found that co-proxamol was the most widely used paracetamol-containing analgesic. It was suggested that the popularity of co-proxamol was purely down to prescribing habits passed on to new medical staff, rather than hard evidence regarding efficacy. This view has been refuted by others[4] who say that a large number of studies have demonstrated clear analgesic effects for dextropropoxyphene. However, any assumption that the combination was widely used because it was more effective than paracetamol alone was not supported by a systematic review of single-dose studies.[5] This concluded that while co-proxamol was indeed an effective analgesic it was no better than paracetamol alone. While the evidence from this and other systematic reviews indicate that co-proxamol

should be replaced by paracetamol alone for acute pain the position for chronic use is considered to be not so clear.[6]
1. Beaver WT. Analgesic efficacy of dextropropoxyphene and dextropropoxyphene-containing combinations: a review. *Hum Toxicol* 1984; **3** (suppl): 191S–220S.
2. Collins SL, *et al.* Single dose dextropropoxyphene, alone and with paracetamol (acetaminophen), for postoperative pain (updated 30 August 2001). Available in The Cochrane Library; Issue 4. Oxford: Update Software; 2001.
3. Haigh S. 12 Years on: co-proxamol revisited. *Lancet* 1996; **347:** 1840–1. Correction. *ibid.*; **348:** 346.
4. Sykes JV, *et al.* Coproxamol revisited. *Lancet* 1996; **348:** 408.
5. Li Wan Po A, Zhang WY. Systematic overview of co-proxamol to assess analgesic effects of addition of dextropropoxyphene to paracetamol. *BMJ* 1997; **315:** 1565–71. Correction *ibid.* 1998; **316:** 116 and 656.
6. Anonymous. Co-proxamol or paracetamol for acute pain? *Drug Ther Bull* 1998; **36:** 80.

Preparations

BP 2001: Co-proxamol Tablets; Dextropropoxyphene Capsules; **USP 25:** Propoxyphene Hydrochloride and Acetaminophen Tablets; Propoxyphene Hydrochloride Capsules; Propoxyphene Hydrochloride, Aspirin, and Caffeine Capsules; Propoxyphene Napsylate and Acetaminophen Tablets; Propoxyphene Napsylate Aspirin Tablets; Propoxyphene Napsylate Oral Suspension; Propoxyphene Napsylate Tablets.

Proprietary Preparations (details are given in Part 3)
Austral.: Doloxene; **Belg.:** Depronal; **Braz.:** Doloxene-A; **Canad.:** 642; Darvon-N; Novo-Propoxyn†; **Denm.:** Abalgin; Doloxene; **Fin.:** Abalgin; **Fr.:** Antalvic†; **Ger.:** Develin; **Hong Kong:** Doloxene; **Irl.:** Doloxene; **Ital.:** Liberen; **Mex.:** Darvon Simple; Darvon-N; Dibagesic; Troliber; **Neth.:** Depronal; **NZ:** Doloxene; **Port.:** Algifene; **S.Afr.:** Doloxene; Doxypol; **Spain:** Darvon; Deprancol; **Swed.:** Dexofen; Dolotard; **Switz.:** Depronal; **UK:** Doloxene; **USA:** Darvon; Darvon-N; Dolene†; PP-Cap†.

Multi-ingredient: **Aust.:** Algo-Prolixan; APA; Contraforte; Sigmalin B6 forte; **Austral.:** Capadex; Di-Gesic; Paradex; **Belg.:** Algophene; Distalgic; Yamalen; **Braz.:** Algafan; **Canad.:** 692†; **Fin.:** Paraflex comp; **Fr.:** Di Dolko; Di-Antalvic; Dialgirex; Dioalgo; Propofan; Starem; **Hong Kong:** Cosalgesic; Dologesic; Doloxene Compound; Dolpocetmol; **Irl.:** Cosalgesic; Distalgesic; Doloxene Compound; **Israel:** Algolysin; Proxol; Rogaan; **Norw.:** Aporex; **NZ:** Apo-Paradex; Capadex; Di-Gesic; Paradex; **Port.:** Algifene; **S.Afr.:** Distalgesic; Doloxene Co; Doxyfene; Lentogesic; Synap; **Swed.:** Dexodon; Distalgesic; Doleron; Paraflex comp; **Switz.:** Distalgesic; Dolo-Prolixan†; **UK:** Cosalgesic; Distalgesic; Doloxene Compound†; **USA:** Darvocet-N; Darvon Compound; Genagesic†; PC-Cap; Propacet; Wygesic.

Dezocine (12637-j)

Dezocine *(USAN, rINN).*

Wy-16225. (–)-13β-Amino-5,6,7,8,9,10,11α,12-octahydro-5α-methyl-5,11-methanobenzocyclodecen-3-ol.
$C_{16}H_{23}NO = 245.4.$
CAS — 53648-55-8.
ATC — N02AX03.

Dependence and Withdrawal
As for Opioid Analgesics, p.66.

◊ According to a WHO expert committee[1] the potential for physical dependence on dezocine was low in *animals* and had not been studied in humans. In the absence of reports of actual abuse of dezocine up to 1989, WHO rated its likelihood as moderate and considered that international control was not warranted.
1. WHO. WHO expert committee on drug dependence: twenty-fifth report. *WHO Tech Rep Ser* 775 1989.

Adverse Effects and Treatment
As for Opioid Analgesics in general, p.67.

Effects on mental function. At high doses symptoms suggestive of psychotomimetic effects were more frequent after dezocine than after morphine,[1] but a WHO expert committee[2] considered that, although dezocine produced miosis and other opioid effects such as euphoria, there was no evidence for the dysphoric sedative and hallucinogenic effects seen with pentazocine.
1. Romagnoli A, Keats AS. Ceiling respiratory depression by dezocine. *Clin Pharmacol Ther* 1984; **35:** 367–73.
2. WHO. WHO expert committee on drug dependence: twenty-fifth report. *WHO Tech Rep Ser* 775 1989.

Precautions
As for Opioid Analgesics in general, p.68.

Dezocine may precipitate withdrawal symptoms if given to patients who are physically dependent on opioids (see below).

Abuse. Opioid-dependent subjects maintained on oral methadone in a daily dose of 30 mg were challenged with different doses of intramuscular dezocine ranging from 7.5 to 60 mg.[1] Dezocine produced primarily antagonist-like effects and precipitated a withdrawal syndrome which was not directly dose-related in magnitude. The greatest withdrawal effects were seen in the mid-dose range and the least with the higher doses. These results suggest that lower doses of dezocine should have a relatively low abuse liability in opioid-dependent patients. Assessment of the morphine-like subjective and miotic effects of dezocine indicated that it had the potential to be abused, but

suggested that its abuse potential was less than that of morphine.[2]
1. Strain EC, *et al.* Opioid antagonist effects of dezocine in opioid-dependent humans. *Clin Pharmacol Ther* 1996; **60:** 206–17.
2. Jasinski DR, Preston KL. Assessment of dezocine for morphine-like subjective effects and miosis. *Clin Pharmacol Ther* 1985; **38:** 544–8.

Interactions
For interactions associated with opioid analgesics, see p.68.

Pharmacokinetics
Dezocine is readily absorbed following intramuscular administration. It appears to be metabolised in the liver and excreted mainly as the glucuronide conjugate in the urine.

Uses and Administration
Dezocine is an opioid analgesic (p.68). It is structurally related to pentazocine (p.74) and, likewise, has mixed opioid agonist and antagonist actions. Dezocine has been given by injection for the relief of moderate to severe pain.

Preparations
Proprietary Preparations (details are given in Part 3)
USA: Dalgan†.

Diacerein (1729-k)

Diacerein *(rINN).*

Diacerhein; Diacetylrhein; Rhein Diacetate; SF-277. 9,10-Dihydro-4,5-dihydroxy-9,10-dioxo-2-anthroic acid diacetate.
$C_{19}H_{12}O_8 = 368.3.$
CAS — 13739-02-1.
ATC — M01AX21.

Profile
Diacerein is an anthraquinone derivative that has been used in osteoarthritis (p.9) in doses of 50 mg twice daily by mouth. Doses should be halved in patients with creatinine clearance less than 30 mL per minute. Its active metabolite, rhein, a constituent of rhubarb (p.1248), is reported to act as an interleukin-1 inhibitor. Diarrhoea is a common side-effect with diacerein.

◊ References.
1. Debord P, *et al.* Influence of renal function on the pharmacokinetics of diacerein after a single oral dose. *Eur J Drug Metab Pharmacokinet* 1994; **19:** 13–19.
2. Spencer CM, Wilde MI. Diacerein. *Drugs* 1997; **53:** 98–106.
3. Nicolas P, *et al.* Clinical pharmacokinetics of diacerein. *Clin Pharmacokinet* 1998; **35:** 347–59.

Preparations
Proprietary Preparations (details are given in Part 3)
Fr.: Art; Zondar; **Israel:** Art; **Ital.:** Artrodar†; Fisiodar; **Port.:** Artrolyt; Cartivix.

Diamorphine Hydrochloride (6219-l)

Diamorphine Hydrochloride *(BANM).*

Diacetylmorphine Hydrochloride; Heroin Hydrochloride. 4,5-Epoxy-17-methylmorphinan-3,6-diyl diacetate hydrochloride monohydrate.
$C_{21}H_{23}NO_5,HCl,H_2O = 423.9.$
CAS — 561-27-3 (diamorphine); 1502-95-0 (diamorphine hydrochloride).

Pharmacopoeias. In *Br.* and *Swiss.* *Swiss* also includes the anhydrous form.

Pharmacopoeial description
BP 2001: A white or almost white crystalline powder, odourless when freshly prepared but develops an odour characteristic of acetic acid on storage. Freely soluble in water and in chloroform; soluble in alcohol; practically insoluble in ether. Protect from light.

Incompatibility. Diamorphine hydrochloride is incompatible with mineral acids and alkalis and with chlorocresol.[1]
Cyclizine may precipitate from mixtures with diamorphine hydrochloride at concentrations of cyclizine greater than 10 mg per mL, or in the presence of sodium chloride, or as the concentration of diamorphine relative to cyclizine increases; mixtures of diamorphine and cyclizine are also liable to precipitate after 24 hours.
Mixtures of diamorphine and haloperidol are liable to precipitate after 24 hours if the haloperidol concentration is above 2 mg per mL. Under some conditions mixtures of metoclopramide and diamorphine may become discoloured and should be discarded.
1. McEwan JS, Macmorran GH. The compatibility of some bactericides. *Pharm J* 1947; **158:** 260–2.

Stability. Diamorphine is relatively unstable in aqueous solution and is hydrolysed to 6-O-monoacetylmorphine and then morphine to a significant extent at room temperature; 3-O-mono-acetylmorphine is only occasionally detected. The rate of decomposition is at a minimum at about pH 4.[1,2]
Cooper *et al.*[3] studied the stability of aqueous solutions of diamorphine in chloroform water and concluded that such solutions should be used within 3 weeks of preparation when stored at room temperature. Twycross[4] commented that the degradation products of diamorphine were not devoid of analgesic ac-

tivity. Using a more sensitive analytical method Beaumont[5] reported that although the pH range of maximum stability of diamorphine in aqueous solution was 3.8 to 4.4, the addition of buffers reduced stability. Simple unbuffered chloroform water gave maximum stability, the shelf-life of such a solution being 4 weeks at room temperature.

The BP 2001 recommends that solutions for injection be prepared immediately before use by dissolving Diamorphine Hydrochloride for Injection in Water for Injections. This may pose a problem with solutions for subcutaneous infusion when concentrated solutions may remain in infusion pump reservoirs for some time.[6] Investigation of 9 concentrations of diamorphine stored at 4 different temperatures for 8 weeks[7] revealed instability under conditions of concentration, time, and temperature prevalent during subcutaneous infusion. Degradation of diamorphine occurred at all concentrations (0.98 to 250 mg per mL) at temperatures of 4° and above; the effect of temperature was significant at 21° and 37°. The percentage fall in diamorphine concentration was directly related to initial concentration and was accompanied by a corresponding increase in 6-O-monoacetylmorphine and, to a lesser extent, morphine; other possible breakdown products such as 3-O-monoacetylmorphine were not present in detectable quantities. Diamorphine degradation was associated with a fall in pH and the development of a strong acetic acid-like odour. Precipitation and a white turbidity was seen in solutions of 15.6 mg per mL and above after incubation for 2 weeks at 21° and 37°. Omar et al.[7] noted that solutions for infusion are generally freshly prepared and used within 24 hours, but advised that signs of precipitation should be watched for, especially when using longer-term infusions and high concentrations of diamorphine.

In another stability study[8] diamorphine hydrochloride in concentrations of both 1 and 20 mg per mL in sodium chloride 0.9% was stable for a minimum of 15 days at room temperature (23° to 25°) and 4° when stored in a PVC container. In one type of disposable infusion device (Infusor) similar solutions were stable for 15 days even at 31°. In another infusion device (Intermate 200) diamorphine was stable for a minimum of 15 days at both concentrations and all temperatures except for the 1 mg per mL solution kept at 31° when stability was only maintained for a minimum of 2 days. When stored in glass syringes both strengths of diamorphine hydrochloride were stable for 15 days at 4° and at room temperature the 1 mg per mL solution was stable for a minimum of 7 days and the 20 mg per mL solution was stable for a minimum of 12 days. There were no substantial changes in physical appearance or pH.

1. Davey EA, Murray JB. Hydrolysis of diamorphine in aqueous solutions. *Pharm J* 1969; **203:** 737.
2. Davey EA, Murray JB. Determination of diamorphine in the presence of its degradation products using gas liquid chromatography. *Pharm J* 1971; **207:** 167.
3. Cooper H, et al. Stability of diamorphine in chloroform water mixture. *Pharm J* 1981; **226:** 682–3.
4. Twycross RG. Stability of diamorphine in chloroform water. *Pharm J* 1981; **227:** 218.
5. Beaumont IM. Stability of diamorphine in chloroform water. *Pharm J* 1981; **227:** 41.
6. Jones VA, et al. Diamorphine stability in aqueous solution for subcutaneous infusion. *Br J Clin Pharmacol* 1987; **23:** 651P.
7. Omar OA, et al. Diamorphine stability in aqueous solution for subcutaneous infusion. *J Pharm Pharmacol* 1989; **41:** 275–7.
8. Kleinberg ML, et al. Stability of heroin hydrochloride in infusion devices and containers for intravenous administration. *Am J Hosp Pharm* 1990; **47:** 377–81.

Dependence and Withdrawal

As for Opioid Analgesics, p.66. Diamorphine is subject to abuse (see under Adverse Effects, Treatment, and Precautions, below).

Diamorphine is used for substitution therapy in the management of opioid dependence (see under Uses and Administration, below).

Adverse Effects, Treatment, and Precautions

As for Opioid Analgesics in general, p.67.

Pulmonary oedema after overdosage is a common cause of fatalities among diamorphine addicts. Nausea and hypotension are claimed to be less common than with morphine.

There are many reports of adverse effects associated with the abuse of diamorphine, usually obtained illicitly in an adulterated form.

Abuse. Most of the reports of adverse effects with diamorphine involve its abuse. In addition to the central effects, there are effects caused by the administration methods and by the adulterants.[1] Thus in many instances it is difficult to identify the factor causing the toxicity. Most body systems are involved including the immune system,[2] kidneys,[3] liver,[4] respiratory system,[5,6] and the nervous system.[7-10]

Other aspects of the illicit use of diamorphine include fatal overdose[11] and smuggling by swallowing packages of drug[12] or other methods of internal bodily concealment.

1. Hendrickse RG, et al. Aflatoxins and heroin. *BMJ* 1989; **299:** 492–3.

2. Husby G, et al. Smooth muscle antibody in heroin addicts. *Ann Intern Med* 1975; **83:** 801–5.
3. Cunningham EE, et al. Heroin-associated nephropathy. *JAMA* 1983; **250:** 2935–6.
4. Weller IVD, et al. Clinical, biochemical, serological, histological and ultrastructural features of liver disease in drug abusers. *Gut* 1984; **25:** 417–23.
5. Anderson K. Bronchospasm and intravenous street heroin. *Lancet* 1984; **i:** 1208.
6. Hughes S, Calverley PMA. Heroin inhalation and asthma. *BMJ* 1988; **297:** 1511–12.
7. Sempere AP, et al. Spongiform leucoencephalopathy after inhaling heroin. *Lancet* 1991; **338:** 320.
8. Roulet Perez E, et al. Toxic leucoencephalopathy after heroin ingestion in a 2½-year-old child. *Lancet* 1992; **340:** 729.
9. Zuckerman GB. Neurologic complications following intranasal administration of heroin in an adolescent. *Ann Pharmacother* 1996; **30:** 778–81.
10. Kriegstein AR, et al. Heroin inhalation and progressive spongiform leukoencephalopathy. *N Engl J Med* 1997; **336:** 589–90.
11. Kintz P, et al. Toxicological data after heroin overdose. *Hum Toxicol* 1989; **8:** 487–9.
12. Stewart A, et al. Body packing—a case report and review of the literature. *Postgrad Med J* 1990; **66:** 659–61.

Administration. Although generally free from complications, sterile abscess formation was reported in 2 patients with advanced cancer receiving diamorphine by continuous *subcutaneous* infusions.[1] Acute dysphoric reactions have been reported after the use of *epidural* diamorphine.[2]

1. Hoskin PJ, et al. Sterile abscess formation by continuous subcutaneous infusion of diamorphine. *BMJ* 1989; **296:** 1605.
2. Holder KJ, Morgan BM. Dysphoria after extradural diamorphine. *Br J Anaesth* 1994; **72:** 728.

Breast feeding. See under Opioid Dependence in Uses and Administration, below.

Phaeochromocytoma. Diamorphine can liberate endogenous histamine which may in turn stimulate release of catecholamines. Its use provoked hypertension and tachycardia in a patient with phaeochromocytoma.[1]

1. Chaturvedi NC, et al. Diamorphine-induced attack of paroxysmal hypertension in phaeochromocytoma. *BMJ* 1974; **2:** 538.

Pregnancy and the neonate. Some references to diamorphine dependence in pregnant women and the effects on the fetus and neonate.

1. Fricker HS, Segal S. Narcotic addiction, pregnancy, and the newborn. *Am J Dis Child* 1978; **132:** 360–6.
2. Ostrea EM, Chavez CJ. Perinatal problems (excluding neonatal withdrawal) in maternal drug addiction: a study of 830 cases. *J Pediatr* 1979; **94:** 292–5.
3. Lifschitz MH, et al. Fetal and postnatal growth of children born to narcotic-dependent women. *J Pediatr* 1983; **102:** 686–91.
4. Klenka HM. Babies born in a district general hospital to mothers taking heroin. *BMJ* 1986; **293:** 745–6.
5. Gregg JEM, et al. Inhaling heroin during pregnancy: effects on the baby. *BMJ* 1988; **296:** 754.
6. Little BB, et al. Maternal and fetal effects of heroin addiction during pregnancy. *J Reprod Med* 1990; **35:** 159–62.

Interactions

For interactions associated with opioid analgesics, see p.68.

Pharmacokinetics

Diamorphine hydrochloride is well absorbed from the gastrointestinal tract and following subcutaneous or intramuscular injection. Following injection it is rapidly converted to the active metabolite 6-O-monoacetylmorphine (6-acetylmorphine) in the blood and then to morphine. Orally administered diamorphine is subject to extensive first-pass metabolism to morphine; neither diamorphine nor 6-acetylmorphine have been detected in the blood following administration of diamorphine by this route. Both diamorphine and 6-acetylmorphine readily cross the blood-brain barrier. Morphine glucuronides are the main excretion products in the urine.

◊ Reviews and studies of the pharmacokinetics of diamorphine.

1. Boerner U, et al. The metabolism of morphine and heroin in man. *Drug Metab Rev* 1975; **4:** 39–73.
2. Inturrisi CE, et al. The pharmacokinetics of heroin in patients with chronic pain. *N Engl J Med* 1984; **310:** 1213–17.
3. Moore RA, et al. Opiate metabolism and excretion. *Baillieres Clin Anaesthesiol* 1987; **1:** 829–58.
4. Barrett DA, et al. Morphine kinetics after diamorphine infusion in premature neonates. *Br J Clin Pharmacol* 1991; **32:** 31–7.

Administration. Diamorphine is much more lipid-soluble and has a more rapid onset and shorter duration of action than morphine. Although deacetylation to morphine occurs rapidly in the blood it occurs only slowly in the CSF following intraspinal injection of diamorphine.[1] After intrathecal injection diamorphine was removed from the CSF much more rapidly than morphine.[2] Peak plasma concentrations of morphine following epidural diamorphine injection were significantly higher and were achieved significantly faster than after epidural injection of morphine.[3]

1. Morgan M. The rational use of intrathecal and extradural opioids. *Br J Anaesth* 1989; **63:** 165–88.

2. Moore A, et al. Spinal fluid kinetics of morphine and heroin. *Clin Pharmacol Ther* 1984; **35:** 40–5.
3. Watson J, et al. Plasma morphine concentrations and analgesic effects of lumbar extradural morphine and heroin. *Anesth Analg* 1984; **63:** 629–34.

Children. Loading doses of diamorphine of either 50 µg per kg body-weight or 200 µg per kg were given as an infusion over 30 minutes to 19 ventilated neonates followed by a continuous infusion of 15 µg per kg per hour, and the pharmacokinetics of the products of diamorphine metabolism (morphine, morphine-6-glucuronide, and morphine-3-glucuronide) studied.[1] Although the overall elimination of morphine was reduced compared with adults, the relative contributions of the various metabolic routes of morphine remained similar between neonates and adults. Data from this study did not indicate any advantage for the higher loading dose (see also under Uses and Administration, below).

1. Barrett DA, et al. Morphine, morphine-6-glucuronide and morphine-3-glucuronide pharmacokinetics in newborn infants receiving diamorphine infusions. *Br J Clin Pharmacol* 1996; **41:** 531–7.

Uses and Administration

Diamorphine hydrochloride is an acetylated morphine derivative and is a more potent opioid analgesic (p.68) than morphine (p.58). Diamorphine is used for the relief of severe pain especially in palliative care. It is also used similarly to morphine for the relief of dyspnoea due to pulmonary oedema resulting from left ventricular failure. Diamorphine has a powerful cough suppressant effect and has been given as Diamorphine Linctus (BPC 1973) to control cough associated with terminal lung cancer although morphine is now preferred.

In the treatment of acute pain standard doses of diamorphine hydrochloride by subcutaneous or intramuscular injection are 5 to 10 mg every 4 hours. Doses equivalent to one-quarter to one-half of the corresponding intramuscular dose may be given by slow intravenous injection. For the pain of myocardial infarction diamorphine hydrochloride is given in doses of 5 mg by slow intravenous injection at a rate of 1 mg per minute with a further dose of 2.5 to 5 mg if required; doses may be reduced by one-half for elderly or frail patients. Doses of 2.5 to 5 mg may be given intravenously at the same rate for acute pulmonary oedema. For chronic pain 5 to 10 mg may be given by mouth or by subcutaneous or intramuscular injection every 4 hours; the dose may be increased according to needs. Diamorphine hydrochloride may also be administered by continuous subcutaneous infusion or intraspinally.

For the treatment of cough in terminal disease, doses of diamorphine hydrochloride 1.5 to 6 mg by mouth every 4 hours have been given.

◊ Because of its abuse potential, supply of diamorphine is carefully controlled and in many countries it is not available for clinical use; morphine can provide equivalent analgesia by dose adjustment. There has been much debate regarding the relative merits of analgesia with diamorphine or morphine. Many now regard oral morphine to be the opioid analgesic of choice although diamorphine hydrochloride may be preferred for administration by injection because it is more soluble in water thus allowing the use of smaller dose volumes. Diamorphine hydrochloride may also be preferred to morphine salts for intraspinal administration because it is more lipid-soluble.

As a guide to relative potency diamorphine hydrochloride 5 mg intramuscularly is approximately equivalent to 10 mg by mouth which in turn is approximately equivalent to morphine sulfate 15 mg by mouth.

Administration in children. In a study[1] of the effects of diamorphine in 34 premature infants (gestational age 26 to 40 weeks), a loading dose of 50 µg per kg body-weight given as an intravenous infusion over 30 minutes followed by a continuous infusion at a rate of 15 µg per kg per hour was considered to be safe and resulted in plasma concentrations of morphine comparable with those that usually produce adequate analgesia in children and adults; the duration of the infusion ranged from 14 to 149 hours. Small but significant reductions in heart rate and mean blood pressure were noted but these were not associated with any clinical deterioration. The fall in respiration rate reflected the desired intention to encourage synchronisation of the infants' breathing with the ventilator. The authors concluded that intravenous diamorphine could be given safely to neonates and would provide adequate analgesia. A later study[2] indicated that the use of a 200 µg per kg loading dose conferred no benefit over a 50 µg per kg dose and might produce undesirable physiological effects. In a comparative study[3] with morphine (200 µg per kg loading dose over 2 hours, followed by maintenance infusion of 25 µg per kg per hour) in ventilated preterm neonates requiring sedation, diamorphine (120 µg per kg over 2 hours and then 15 µg per kg per hour) was as effective as morphine in producing sedation and also had a faster onset of action. The small but significant drop in blood pressure noted during morphine infusions was not seen with diamorphine infusions. Continuous intravenous infusions of 7 µg per kg per hour have been used in neonates not requiring ventilation.[4]

The subcutaneous route appeared to be as effective and safe as the intravenous route for administration of diamorphine infusions in children for postoperative pain relief following elective abdominal surgery.[5] The dose of diamorphine used in both groups of children was 40 µg per kg body-weight administered at a rate of 20 µg per kg per hour.

1. Elias-Jones AC, et al. Diamorphine infusion in the preterm neonate. Arch Dis Child 1991; 66: 1155–7.
2. Barker DP, et al. Randomised, double blind trial of two loading dose regimens of diamorphine in ventilated newborn infants. Arch Dis Child 1995; 73: F22–F26.
3. Wood CM, et al. Randomised double blind trial of morphine versus diamorphine for sedation of preterm neonates. Arch Dis Child Fetal Neonatal Ed 1998; 79: F34–F39.
4. Blanchard S. Analgesic use in neonatal necrotising enterocolitis. Pharm J 1992; 248: 52.
5. Semple D, et al. Comparison of iv and sc diamorphine infusions for the treatment of acute pain in children. Br J Anaesth 1996; 76: 310–12.

Opioid dependence. Many opiate misusers have expressed a preference for withdrawal using diamorphine rather than methadone. In a comparative study stabilisation was achieved using either diamorphine or methadone 1 mg per mL oral solutions;[1] patients could not identify which they had been given. Whenever signs of physical withdrawal were observed 10 mL of either solution was given and the total amount over the first 24 hours taken as the patient's daily requirement. The mean dose of diamorphine required for stabilisation was 55 mg compared with 36 mg for methadone. Some centres have administered diamorphine in the form of reefers.
Breast feeding has been used to treat diamorphine dependence in the offspring of dependent mothers but this is no longer considered to be the best method and some authorities recommend that breast feeding should be stopped.

1. Ghodse AH, et al. Comparison of oral preparations of heroin and methadone to stabilise opiate misusers as inpatients. BMJ 1990; 300: 719–20.

Pain. ACUTE PAIN. Rapid pain relief may be obtained with the intravenous injection of diamorphine. Other routes include the intraspinal route for which diamorphine is well suited because of its lipid solubility and pharmacokinetics. Epidural doses of diamorphine have ranged from 0.5 to 10 mg.[1] One study[2] found that diamorphine 5 mg produced rapid analgesia whether given intramuscularly (in 1 mL of 0.9% sodium chloride) or epidurally (in 10 mL of 0.9% sodium chloride) for pain following caesarean section, but analgesia was significantly more prolonged and more intense following epidural injection; itching was reported by 50% of patients undergoing epidural analgesia. Continuous epidural infusion of diamorphine 0.5 mg per hour in 15 mL of 0.125% bupivacaine provided postoperative analgesia superior to that with either drug alone in patients undergoing major abdominal gynaecological surgery.[3] Continuous epidural infusion of diamorphine 0.4 to 0.6 mg per hour in 0.15% bupivacaine produced analgesia superior to that with either epidural bolus injection of diamorphine 3.6 mg in 9 mL of 0.9% saline or patient-controlled intravenous administration of diamorphine at a maximum rate of 1 mg per 5 minutes in patients undergoing total abdominal hysterectomy.[4] However, more patients receiving the continuous epidural infusion were hypoxaemic in the other 2 groups. Diamorphine 5 mg in 8 mL of 0.9% sodium chloride produced comparable analgesia to 8 mL of 0.375% bupivacaine when given epidurally during labour but the duration was longer with diamorphine; addition of adrenaline [epinephrine] appeared to improve the quality and duration of analgesia with diamorphine.[5] The addition of diamorphine 5 mg to 10 mL of 0.25% bupivacaine also enhanced pain relief when given epidurally in the first stage of labour.[6] In a similar study addition of diamorphine to bupivacaine produced a high incidence of pruritus and drowsiness.[7] Diamorphine has also been given intrathecally for postoperative analgesia and should be effective at lower doses than with the epidural route because of greater CSF concentrations. Diamorphine 0.25 or 0.5 mg administered intrathecally with bupivacaine spinal anaesthesia both provided greater postoperative analgesia than bupivacaine alone,[8] but the incidence of adverse effects, especially nausea, vomiting, and urinary retention, was still high with either dose and routine use of this technique was not recommended. Intrathecal administration of diamorphine with bupivacaine has also been used for analgesia during labour.[9]

Diamorphine has been extensively used by cardiologists in the UK for the management of pain in acute left ventricular failure, unstable angina, and myocardial infarction. It has been theorised that diamorphine may offer benefits over morphine because its stimulatory effects at opioid δ receptors on the myocardium may reduce the extent of myocardial damage.[10] Evidence to support this theory is, however, lacking.

1. Morgan M. The rational use of intrathecal and extradural opioids. Br J Anaesth 1989; 63: 165–88.
2. Macrae DJ, et al. Double-blind comparison of the efficacy of extradural diamorphine, extradural phenoperidine and im diamorphine following caesarean section. Br J Anaesth 1987; 59: 354–9.

3. Lee A, et al. Postoperative analgesia by continuous extradural infusion of bupivacaine and diamorphine. Br J Anaesth 1988; 60: 845–50.
4. Madej TH, et al. Hypoxaemia and pain relief after lower abdominal surgery: comparison of extradural and patient-controlled analgesia. Br J Anaesth 1992; 69: 554–7.
5. Keenan GMA, et al. Extradural diamorphine with adrenaline in labour: comparison with diamorphine and bupivacaine. Br J Anaesth 1991; 66: 242–6.
6. McGrady EM, et al. Epidural diamorphine and bupivacaine in labour. Anaesthesia 1989; 44: 400–3.
7. Bailey CR, et al. Diamorphine-bupivacaine mixture compared with plain bupivacaine for analgesia. Br J Anaesth 1994; 72: 58–61.
8. Reay BA, et al. Low-dose intrathecal diamorphine analgesia following major orthopaedic surgery. Br J Anaesth 1989; 62: 248–52.
9. Kestin IG, et al. Analgesia for labour and delivery using incremental diamorphine and bupivacaine via a 32-gauge intrathecal catheter. Br J Anaesth 1992; 68: 244–7.
10. Poullis M. Diamorphine and British cardiology: so we are right! Heart 1999; 82: 645–6.

CHRONIC PAIN. Patients with chronic opioid-sensitive pain are often treated with diamorphine given by continuous subcutaneous infusion using a small battery-operated syringe driver. The following technique has been described.[1] Diamorphine hydrochloride 1 g can be dissolved in 1.6 mL of water to give a solution with a volume of 2.4 mL (415 mg per mL), but the maximum suggested concentration is 250 mg per mL. If the analgesic requirement is not known the following protocol is recommended:

• Start injections every 4 hours of 2.5 or 5 mg diamorphine or, if the patient has already been taking opioids, a dose that is equivalent to the last dose
• If this is unsatisfactory increase this dose in 50% increments until the patient reports even a little pain relief
• Calculate the 24-hour requirement by multiplying by six, and start the infusion at this level
• Increase the 24-hour dosage in the pump by 50% increments until the pain is controlled. Note that requirements may vary from less than 20 mg to more than 5 g per 24 hours.

When starting an infusion it is important not to allow any breakthrough pain. This may be achieved either by starting the infusion more than 2 hours before the previous oral dose wears off or by giving a loading dose injection of the 4-hourly requirement.

Although generally free from complications, sterile abscess formation was reported in 2 patients with advanced cancer receiving diamorphine by continuous subcutaneous infusions.[2]
The intraventricular route was used successfully in 2 patients with intractable cancer pain.[3]

1. Dover SB. Syringe driver in terminal care. BMJ 1987; 294: 553–5.
2. Hoskin PJ, et al. Sterile abscess formation by continuous subcutaneous infusion of diamorphine. BMJ 1988; 296: 1605.
3. Reeve WG, Todd JG. Intraventricular diamorphine via an Ommaya shunt for intractable cancer pain. Br J Anaesth 1990; 65: 544–7.

Preparations

BP 2001: Diamorphine Injection;
BPC 1973: Diamorphine Linctus.

Proprietary Preparations (details are given in Part 3)
UK: Diagesil; Diamorf.

Diclofenac (13409-w)

Diclofenac (BAN, rINN).
[2-(2,6-Dichloroanilino)phenyl]acetic acid.
$C_{14}H_{11}Cl_2NO_2 = 296.1$.
CAS — 15307-86-5.
ATC — M01AB05; M02AA15; S01BC03.

Diclofenac Diethylamine (11328-c)

Diclofenac Diethylamine (BANM).
$C_{18}H_{22}Cl_2N_2O_2 = 369.3$.
CAS — 78213-16-8.
Pharmacopoeias. In Br.

Pharmacopoeial description

BP 2001: A white to light beige, crystalline powder. Sparingly soluble in water and in acetone; freely soluble in alcohol and in methyl alcohol; practically insoluble in 1M sodium hydroxide. The pH of a 1% solution in alcohol (10%) is between 6.4 and 8.4. Store in airtight containers. Protect from light.

Diclofenac Potassium (15163-x)

Diclofenac Potassium (BANM, USAN, rINNM).
CGP-45840B; Diclofenacum Kalicum. Potassium [o-(2,6-dichloroanilino)phenyl]acetate.
$C_{14}H_{10}Cl_2KNO_2 = 334.2$.
CAS — 15307-81-0.
Pharmacopoeias. In Eur. (see p.vi).

Pharmacopoeial description

Ph. Eur.: A white or slightly yellowish, slightly hygroscopic, crystalline powder. Sparingly soluble in water; soluble in alcohol; slightly soluble in acetone; freely soluble in methyl alcohol. Store in airtight containers. Protect from light.

Diclofenac Sodium (2632-c)

Diclofenac Sodium (BANM, USAN, rINNM).
Diclofenacum Natricum; Diclophenac Sodium; GP-45840. Sodium [2-(2,6-dichloroanilino)phenyl]acetate.
$C_{14}H_{10}Cl_2NNaO_2 = 318.1$.
CAS — 15307-79-6.

NOTE. DICL is a code approved by the BP 2001 for use on single unit doses of eye drops containing diclofenac sodium where the individual container may be too small to bear all the appropriate labelling information.
Pharmacopoeias. In Eur. (see p.vi), Jpn, and US.

Pharmacopoeial description

Ph. Eur.: A white to slightly yellowish, slightly hygroscopic, crystalline powder. Sparingly soluble in water; soluble in alcohol; slightly soluble in acetone; practically insoluble in ether; freely soluble in methyl alcohol. Store in airtight containers. Protect from light.
USP 25: A white to off-white, hygroscopic, crystalline powder. Sparingly soluble in water; soluble in alcohol; practically insoluble in chloroform and in ether; freely soluble in methyl alcohol. pH of a 1% solution in water is between 7.0 and 8.5. Store in airtight containers. Protect from light.

Adverse Effects

As for NSAIDs in general, p.63.

There may be pain and, occasionally, tissue damage at the site of injection when diclofenac is given intramuscularly. Diclofenac suppositories may cause local irritation. Transient burning and stinging may occur with diclofenac ophthalmic solution; more serious corneal adverse effects have occurred (see Effects on the Eyes, below).

◊ A review of worldwide clinical studies with diclofenac[1] has reported the incidence of drug-associated adverse effects to be about 12%; about 16% of patients who experienced adverse effects discontinued treatment (a figure corresponding to about 2% of the entire patient sample). The most frequently reported adverse effects were gastrointestinal and were reported in 7.6% of patients. CNS-related adverse effects were reported in 0.7% of patients and allergy or local reactions in 0.4%. This and other reviews[2] have shown that adverse effects associated with diclofenac are usually mild and transient and appear to be unrelated to the dose of drug given.

1. Willkens RF. Worldwide clinical safety experience with diclofenac. Semin Arthritis Rheum 1985; 15 (suppl 1): 105–10.
2. Small RE. Diclofenac sodium. Clin Pharm 1989; 8: 545–8.

Effects on the blood. Results of a large survey undertaken to assess the relation between agranulocytosis, aplastic anaemia, and drug exposure indicated that diclofenac was significantly associated with aplastic anaemia, providing an estimated tenfold increase in risk.[1] There are reports of other haematological abnormalities including haemolytic anaemia,[2] thrombocytopenia,[3-5] neutropenia,[5] and agranulocytosis[6] occurring in patients given diclofenac.
Localised spontaneous bleeding,[7,8] bruising,[9,10] inhibition of platelet aggregation,[7,8] and prolonged bleeding time[10] have been reported.

1. The International Agranulocytosis and Aplastic Anemia Study. Risks of agranulocytosis and aplastic anemia: a first report of their relation to drug use with special reference to analgesics. JAMA 1986; 256: 1749–57.
2. López A, et al. Autoimmune hemolytic anemia induced by diclofenac. Ann Pharmacother 1995; 29: 787.
3. Kramer MR, et al. Severe reversible autoimmune haemolytic anaemia and thrombocytopenia associated with diclofenac therapy. Scand J Haematol 1986; 36: 118–20.
4. George S, Rahi AHS. Thrombocytopenia associated with diclofenac therapy. Am J Health-Syst Pharm 1995; 52: 420–1.
5. Kim HL, Kovacs MJ. Diclofenac-associated thrombocytopenia and neutropenia. Ann Pharmacother 1995; 29: 713–15.
6. Colomina P, Garcia S. Agranulocytosis caused by diclofenac. DICP Ann Pharmacother 1989; 23: 507.
7. Michalevicz R, Seligsohn U. Clinical bleeding due to diclofenac (Voltaren). Arthritis Rheum 1982; 25: 599.
8. Price AJ, Obeid D. Spontaneous non-gastrointestinal bleeding associated with diclofenac. Lancet 1989; ii: 1520.
9. Parapia L, Cox JA. Spontaneous platelet aggregation after diclofenac treatment. BMJ 1984; 289: 368.
10. Khazan U, et al. Diclofenac sodium and bruising. Ann Intern Med 1990; 112: 472–3.

Effects on electrolytes. There have been case reports of diclofenac being associated with the development of symptoms resembling the syndrome of inappropriate antidiuretic hormone secretion in elderly women.[1,2] Also the UK Committee on Safety of Medicines had received a report of fatal hyponatraemia in another elderly woman.[2]

1. Petersson I, et al. Water intoxication associated with non-steroidal anti-inflammatory drug therapy. Acta Med Scand 1987; 221: 221–3.
2. Cheung NT, et al. Syndrome of inappropriate secretion of antidiuretic hormone induced by diclofenac. BMJ 1993; 306: 186.

Effects on the eyes. A patient who had been taking oral diclofenac for several years and had increasingly complained of dry, gritty eyes noticed that eye irritation disappeared within 3 days when diclofenac had to be discontinued because of gastrointestinal effects.[1]

Ocular diclofenac has been implicated in reports of corneal toxicity. Ulceration of the conjunctiva or cornea, corneal or scleral melts, and perforations have been reported in patients using diclofenac eye drops, particularly after cataract surgery.[2-4] Keratitis and perforations were also reported with ketorolac eye drops,[4] although less frequently.

1. Reid ALA, Henderson R. Diclofenac and dry, irritable eyes. *Med J Aust* 1994; **160:** 308.
2. Lin JC, *et al.* Corneal melting associated with use of topical nonsteroidal anti-inflammatory drugs after ocular surgery. *Arch Ophthalmol* 2000; **118:** 1129–32.
3. Congdon NG, *et al.* Corneal complications associated with topical ophthalmic use of nonsteroidal antiinflammatory drugs. *J Cataract Refract Surg* 2001; **27:** 622–31.
4. Guidera AC, *et al.* Keratitis, ulceration, and perforation associated with topical nonsteroidal anti-inflammatory drugs. *Ophthalmology* 2001; **108:** 936–44.

Effects on the gastrointestinal tract. The most frequent adverse effects reported in patients given diclofenac systemically are gastrointestinal in nature. Typical reactions include epigastric pain, nausea, vomiting, and diarrhoea. Rarely peptic ulcer and gastrointestinal bleeding have occurred. Diclofenac has also been implicated as the causative agent in colonic ulceration,[1] small bowel perforation,[2] and pseudomembranous colitis.[3] Rectal administration of diclofenac suppositories may cause local reactions such as itching, burning, or exacerbation of haemorrhoids.

1. Carson J, *et al.* Colonic ulceration and bleeding during diclofenac therapy. *N Engl J Med* 1990; **323:** 135.
2. Deakin M, *et al.* Small bowel perforation associated with an excessive dose of slow release diclofenac sodium. *BMJ* 1988; **297:** 488–9.
3. Gentric A, Pennec YL. Diclofenac-induced pseudomembranous colitis. *Lancet* 1992; **340:** 126–7.

Effects on the kidneys. Renal papillary necrosis[1] and nephrotic syndrome[2-4] have been reported in patients taking diclofenac. See also under Effects on Electrolytes, above.

1. Scott SJ, *et al.* Renal papillary necrosis associated with diclofenac sodium. *BMJ* 1986; **292:** 1050.
2. Beun GDM, *et al.* Isolated minimal change nephropathy associated with diclofenac. *BMJ* 1987; **295:** 182–3.
3. Yinnon AM, *et al.* Nephrotic syndrome associated with diclofenac sodium. *BMJ* 1987; **295:** 556.
4. Tattersall J, *et al.* Membranous nephropathy associated with diclofenac. *Postgrad Med J* 1992; **68:** 392–3.

Effects on the liver. Elevations of serum aminotransferase activity and clinical hepatitis,[1-6] including fatal fulminant hepatitis[2,5] have occurred in patients taking diclofenac. There has also been a case report of hepato-renal damage attributed to diclofenac.[7] Analysis[8] of 180 of the cases of diclofenac-associated hepatic injury received by the FDA between November 1988 and June 1991 suggested an increased risk of hepatotoxicity in female patients and those taking diclofenac for osteoarthritis. Hepatotoxicity had been detected within 6 months of starting diclofenac in 85% of the patients. The biochemical pattern of injury was hepatocellular or mixed hepatocellular in 66% of patients and cholestatic injury was found in 8% of patients. Signs of hypersensitivity were uncommon and it was considered that the mechanism of hepatic injury was likely to be a metabolic idiosyncratic reaction rather than due to intrinsic toxicity of diclofenac.

1. Dunk AA, *et al.* Diclofenac hepatitis. *BMJ* 1982; **284:** 1605–6.
2. Breen EG, *et al.* Fatal hepatitis associated with diclofenac. *Gut* 1986; **27:** 1390–3.
3. Schapira D, *et al.* Diclofenac-induced hepatotoxicity. *Postgrad Med J* 1986; **62:** 63–5.
4. Ryley NG, *et al.* Diclofenac associated hepatitis. *Gut* 1989; **30:** A708.
5. Helfgott SM, *et al.* Diclofenac-associated hepatotoxicity. *JAMA* 1990; **264:** 2660–2.
6. Purcell F, *et al.* Diclofenac hepatitis. *Gut* 1991; **32:** 1381–5.
7. Diggory P, *et al.* Renal and hepatic impairment in association with diclofenac administration. *Postgrad Med J* 1989; **64:** 507–8.
8. Banks AT, *et al.* Diclofenac-associated hepatotoxicity: analysis of 180 cases reported to the Food and Drug Administration as adverse reactions. *Hepatology* 1995; **22:** 820–7.

Effects on the skin. Self-limiting skin reactions such as rash or pruritus may occur in patients given diclofenac. More serious skin reactions attributed to diclofenac include bullous dermatitis[1] and erythema multiforme.[2] Local irritation and necrosis has occurred on intramuscular injection of diclofenac.[3,4]

1. Gabrielsen TØ, *et al.* Drug-induced bullous dermatosis with linear IgA deposits along the basement membrane. *Acta Derm Venereol (Stockh)* 1981; **61:** 439–41.
2. Morris BAP, Remtulla SS. Erythema multiforme major following use of diclofenac. *Can Med Assoc J* 1985; **133:** 665.
3. Stricker BHC, van Kasteren BJ. Diclofenac-induced isolated myonecrosis and the Nicolau syndrome. *Ann Intern Med* 1992; **117:** 1058.
4. Pillans PI, O'Connor N. Tissue necrosis and necrotising fasciitis after intramuscular administration of diclofenac. *Ann Pharmacother* 1995; **29:** 264–6.

Hypersensitivity. Aspirin-sensitive asthmatic patients have developed reactions (rhinorrhoea, tightness of chest, wheezing, dyspnoea) when challenged with diclofenac in doses of 10 to 25 mg[1] and the UK Committee on Safety of Medicines has received a report of one aspirin-sensitive patient who died from acute asthma 4 hours after a single 25-mg dose of diclofenac.[2] Anaphylactic shock has been reported.[3]

1. Szczeklik A, *et al.* Asthmatic attacks induced in aspirin-sensitive patients by diclofenac and naproxen. *BMJ* 1977; **2:** 231–2.

The symbol † denotes a preparation no longer actively marketed

2. Committee on Safety of Medicines/Medicines Control Agency. Avoid all NSAIDs in aspirin-sensitive patients. *Current Problems* 1993; **19:** 8.
3. Dux S, *et al.* Anaphylactic shock induced by diclofenac. *BMJ* 1983; **286:** 1861.

Precautions

As for NSAIDs in general, p.64.

Ophthalmic preparations containing diclofenac should not be used by patients who wear soft contact lenses.

Administration of intravenous diclofenac is contraindicated in patients with moderate or severe renal impairment, hypovolaemia, or dehydration; in patients with a history of haemorrhagic diathesis, cerebrovascular bleeding (including suspected), or asthma; and in patients undergoing surgery with a high risk of haemorrhage.

Breast feeding. See under Pharmacokinetics, below.

Porphyria. Diclofenac sodium has been associated with acute attacks of porphyria and is considered unsafe in porphyric patients.

Interactions

For interactions associated with NSAIDs, see p.65.

Diclofenac should not be administered intravenously to patients already receiving other NSAIDs or anticoagulants including low-dose heparin.

Ciclosporin. Deterioration in renal function has been attributed to the concomitant use of diclofenac with ciclosporin.[1] Increased concentrations of diclofenac were also noted with concomitant administration of ciclosporin;[2] the manufacturer of ciclosporin recommends that the dosage of diclofenac should be reduced by about one-half when diclofenac is used with ciclosporin.

1. Branthwaite JP, Nicholls A. Cyclosporin and diclofenac interaction in rheumatoid arthritis. *Lancet* 1991; **337:** 252.
2. Kovarik JM, *et al.* Cyclosporine and nonsteroidal antiinflammatory drugs: exploring potential drug interactions and their implications for the treatment of rheumatoid arthritis. *J Clin Pharmacol* 1997; **37:** 336–43.

Diuretics. Deterioration in renal function has been attributed to the concomitant use of diclofenac with *triamterene*.[1]

1. Härkönen M, Ekblom-Kullberg S. Reversible deterioration of renal function after diclofenac in patient receiving triamterene. *BMJ* 1986; **293:** 698–9.

Gastrointestinal drugs. A decrease in the plasma concentration of diclofenac has been reported[1] following administration of diclofenac after pretreatment with *sucralfate*.

1. Pedrazzoli J, *et al.* Short-term sucralfate administration alters potassium diclofenac absorption in healthy male volunteers. *Br J Clin Pharmacol* 1997; **43:** 104–108.

Lipid regulating drugs. *Colestyramine* appears substantially to reduce the bioavailability of diclofenac when the two drugs are given together;[1] *colestipol* produces a similar but smaller effect.

1. Al-balla SR, *et al.* The effects of cholestyramine and colestipol on the absorption of diclofenac in man. *Int J Clin Pharmacol Ther* 1994; **32:** 441–5.

Misoprostol. The plasma concentration of diclofenac was reduced when it was administered as a 100-mg daily in the form of a modified-release preparation to subjects receiving misoprostol 800 µg daily.[1] Concomitant administration was also associated with an increase in the incidence and severity of gastrointestinal effects. Studies by the manufacturer[2] had failed to find any significant pharmacokinetic interactions between diclofenac and misoprostol when administered in a formulation containing diclofenac 50 mg and misoprostol 200 µg.

1. Dammann HG, *et al.* Differential effects of misoprostol and ranitidine on the pharmacokinetics of diclofenac and gastrointestinal symptoms. *Br J Clin Pharmacol* 1993; **36:** 345–9.
2. Karim A. Pharmacokinetics of diclofenac and misoprostol when administered alone or as a combination product. *Drugs* 1993; **45** (suppl 1): 7–14.

Parasympathomimetics. The manufacturer of acetylcholine ophthalmic preparations has stated that there have been reports that *acetylcholine* and *carbachol* have been ineffective when used in patients treated with topical (ophthalmic) NSAIDs.

Pharmacokinetics

Diclofenac is rapidly absorbed when given as an oral solution, rectal suppository, or by intramuscular injection. It is absorbed more slowly when given as enteric-coated tablets, especially when this dosage form is given with food. Although orally-administered diclofenac is almost completely absorbed, it is subject to first-pass metabolism so that about 50% of the drug reaches the systemic circulation in the unchanged form. Diclofenac is also absorbed percutaneously. At therapeutic concentrations it is more than 99% bound

to plasma proteins. Diclofenac penetrates synovial fluid where concentrations may persist even when plasma concentrations fall; diclofenac is distributed into breast milk but the amount is considered by some authorities to be too small to be harmful to a breastfed infant. The terminal plasma half-life is about 1 to 2 hours. Diclofenac is metabolised to 4′-hydroxydiclofenac, 5-hydroxydiclofenac, 3′-hydroxydiclofenac and 4′,5-dihydroxydiclofenac. It is then excreted in the form of glucuronide and sulfate conjugates, mainly in the urine (about 65%) but also in the bile (about 35%).

◊ References.
1. Fowler PD, *et al.* Plasma and synovial fluid concentrations of diclofenac sodium and its major hydroxylated metabolites during long-term treatment of rheumatoid arthritis. *Eur J Clin Pharmacol* 1983; **25:** 389–94.
2. Maggi CA, *et al.* Comparative bioavailability of diclofenac hydroxyethylpyrrolidine vs diclofenac sodium in man. *Eur J Clin Pharmacol* 1990; **38:** 207–8.
3. Davies NM, Anderson KE. Clinical pharmacokinetics of diclofenac: therapeutic insights and pitfalls. *Clin Pharmacokinet* 1997; **33:** 184–213.

Uses and Administration

Diclofenac, a phenylacetic acid derivative, is an NSAID (p.65). It is used mainly as the sodium salt for the relief of pain and inflammation in various conditions: musculoskeletal and joint disorders such as rheumatoid arthritis, osteoarthritis, and ankylosing spondylitis; peri-articular disorders such as bursitis and tendinitis; soft-tissue disorders such as sprains and strains; and other painful conditions such as renal colic, acute gout, dysmenorrhoea, migraine, and following some surgical procedures. It has also been used in some countries for the management of actinic keratoses and fever. Eye drops of diclofenac sodium are used for the prevention of intra-operative miosis during cataract extraction, for the treatment of postoperative inflammation following cataract extraction, and for pain in corneal epithelial defects following photorefractive keratectomy.

The usual dose of diclofenac sodium **by mouth** or **rectally** is 75 to 150 mg daily in divided doses. Modified-release preparations of diclofenac sodium are available for oral use. Diclofenac has also been given in equivalent doses by mouth as the free acid in dispersible preparations for short-term treatment up to 3 months long. Diclofenac is also given by mouth as the potassium salt. Doses of the potassium salt are similar to those for diclofenac sodium. Diclofenac potassium is also used in the treatment of migraine in an initial dose of 50 mg taken at the first signs of an attack; an additional dose of 50 mg may be taken after 2 hours if symptoms persist. If necessary further doses of 50 mg may be taken every 4 to 6 hours to a maximum daily dose of 200 mg.

Diclofenac sodium may also be given by deep intramuscular **injection** into the gluteal muscle in a dose of 75 mg once daily or, if required in severe conditions, 75 mg twice daily. Diclofenac sodium may also be given as a continuous or intermittent intravenous infusion in glucose 5% or sodium chloride 0.9% (both previously buffered with sodium bicarbonate). For the treatment of postoperative pain a dose of 75 mg may be given over 30 to 120 minutes. The dose may be repeated if necessary after 4 to 6 hours. To prevent postoperative pain, 25 to 50 mg diclofenac sodium may be given after surgery over 15 to 60 minutes followed by 5 mg per hour to a maximum of 150 mg daily. The maximum period recommended for parenteral use is 2 days. Diclofenac sodium is also used intramuscularly in renal colic in a dose of 75 mg repeated once after 30 minutes if necessary.

In children 1 to 12 years old the dose by mouth or rectally for juvenile idiopathic arthritis is 1 to 3 mg per kg body-weight daily in divided doses.

Diclofenac sodium is used as a 0.1% **ophthalmic solution** in cataract extraction and after laser keratectomy. For the prevention of intra-operative miosis, it is instilled in the appropriate eye 4 times during the 2 hours before surgery and for the treatment of postoperative inflammation, it is instilled 4 times daily for up to 28 days starting 24 hours after surgery. For the control of post-photorefractive keratectomy pain, it is instilled twice in the hour before surgery, then one drop twice at 5-minute intervals immediately after the procedure, and then every 2 to 5 hours during the waking hours for up to 24 hours.

Diclofenac diethylamine is used **topically** as a gel containing the equivalent of 1% of diclofenac sodium for the local symptomatic relief of pain and inflammation; it is applied to the affected site 3 or 4 times daily; treatment should be reviewed after 14 days or after 28 days if used for osteoarthritis. A topical solution of diclofenac sodium 1.5% is also available for the treatment of osteoarthritis; it is applied in small aliquots to achieve a total of 20 to 40 drops, repeated four times daily. Diclofenac is also used in the management of actinic keratoses; it is applied twice daily as diclofenac sodium gel 3%. Diclofenac epolamine (diclofenac hydroxyethylpyrrolidine; DHEP) is also used topically.

Diclofenac is available in combination with misoprostol (see p.1446) for patients at risk of NSAID-induced peptic ulceration.

◊ Reviews.
1. Todd PA, Sorkin EM. Diclofenac sodium: a reappraisal of its pharmacodynamic and pharmacokinetic properties, and therapeutic efficacy. *Drugs* 1988; **35:** 244–85.
2. Small RE. Diclofenac sodium. *Clin Pharm* 1989; **8:** 545–8.

Administration. TOPICAL. Some references to the use of plasters providing sustained topical release of diclofenac epolamine.
1. Galeazzi M, Marcolongo R. A placebo-controlled study of the efficacy and tolerability of a nonsteroidal anti-inflammatory drug, DHEP plaster, in inflammatory peri- and extra-articular rheumatological diseases. *Drugs Exp Clin Res* 1993; **19:** 107–15.
2. Dreiser RL, Tisne-Camus M. DHEP plasters as a topical treatment of knee osteoarthritis—a double-blind placebo-controlled study. *Drugs Exp Clin Res* 1993; **19:** 117–23.

Actinic keratoses. Diclofenac sodium 3% in hyaluronic acid gel is used[1] in the treatment of actinic keratoses (see Basal Cell and Squamous Cell Carcinoma, p.498) despite previous concerns that the preparation may not be significantly more effective than hyaluronic acid gel alone.[2]
1. Rivers JK, McLean DI. An open study to assess the efficacy and safety of topical 3% diclofenac in a 2.5% hyaluronic acid gel for the treatment of actinic keratoses. *Arch Dermatol* 1997; **133:** 1239–42.
2. McEwan LE, Smith JG. Topical diclofenac/hyaluronic acid gel in the treatment of solar keratoses. *Australas J Dermatol* 1997; **38:** 187–9.

Headache. Diclofenac potassium may provide rapid relief in the treatment of acute migraine (p.449).[1]
1. McNeely W, Goa KL. Diclofenac-potassium in migraine. *Drugs* 1999; **57:** 991–1003.

Preparations

BP 2001: Diclofenac Gel; Diclofenac Tablets; Slow Diclofenac Tablets;
USP 25: Diclofenac Sodium Delayed-release Tablets.

Proprietary Preparations (details are given in Part 3)
Aust.: Algefit; Arthrotec; Dedolor; Deflamat; Deflamm; Diclac; Diclobene; Diclomelan; Diclostad; Diclosyl; Fenaren; Magluphen; Tratul; Voltaren; *Austral.:* Arthrotec; Dichlohexal; Dinac; Fenac; Voltaren; Voltaren Ophtha; *Belg.:* Cataflam; Motifene; Voltaren; *Braz.:* Ana-Flex; Artren; Benevran; Biofenac; Cataflam; Cataren; Clofenak; Deltaflogin; Deltaren; Diclofen; Dorgen; Doriflan; Dorpiren; Fenaflan; Fenaren; Fenburil; Flanaren; Flogan; Flogiren; Gezon; Infladoren; Inflaren; Ortoflan; Reumadil; Reumaren; Still; Voltaflex; Voltaren; Voltrix; *Canad.:* Apo-Diclo; Arthrotec; Diclotec; Novo-Difenac; Nu-Diclo; Voltaren; Voltaren Ophtha; *Denm.:* Arthrotec; Diclon; Difenet; Modifenac; Voltaren; Vostar; *Fin.:* Arthrotec; Diclomentin; Diclomex; Motifene; Trabona; Voltaren; *Fr.:* Artotec; Flector; Voldal; Voltarene; Xenid; *Ger.:* Allvoran; Arthotec; Arthrex; Arthrex Duo; Benfofen; Delphinac; Diclac; Diclo; Diclo-Divido; Diclo-Puren; Diclo-saar; Diclo-Spondyril; Diclo-Tablinen†; Diclo-Wolff; Diclo†; Diclodoc; Diclofenbeta; Diclogrun; Diclomerck†; Diclophlogont; Diclorektal†; Dolgit-Diclo; duravolten; Effekton; Jenafenac; Lexobene; Monoflam; Myogit; Rewodina; Sigafenac; Toryxil; Voltaren; Voltaren Ophtha; *Hong Kong:* Abitren; Almiral; Analpan; Apo-Diclo; Arthrotec; Cataflam; Clofec; Diclo-Denk; Diclofen; Difena; Difenac; Flector; Grofenac; Inflanac; Olfen; Remafen; Remethan R; Rhemofenax; Voltaren; Voltaren Ophtha; *Irl.:* Arthrotec; Cataflam; Diclac; Diclo; Diclomel; Difene; Vologen; Voltarol; Voltarol Ophtha; *Israel:* Abitren; Arthrotec; Betaren; Cataflam; Dicloplast; Diclorengel; Voltaren; Voltaren Ophtha; *Ital.:* Artrotec; Cataflam†; Dealgic; Deflamat; Diclocular; Diclodol; Diclofan; Dicloftil; Dicloreum; Dolaut; Fenadol; Flector; Flogofenac; Forgenac; Misofenac; Molfenac; Novapirina; Ribex Flu; Voltaren; Voltfast; *Mex.:* 3-A; Algenac; Alsidexten; Artrenac; Artrenac Pro; Artrotec; Cataflam; Clonodifen; Deflox; Dicloran; Dolaren; Dolflam; Dolofenac; Ehlifena; Evadol; Flogoken; Fustaren; Galedol; Lifenac; Liroken; Logesic; Mafena; Merxil; Practiser; Precifenac; Selectofen; Volfenac; Voltaren; Cataflam; Modifenac; Voltaren; Voltaren Ophtha; *NZ:* Anfenax; Apo-Diclo; Cataflam; Diclax; Flameril; Voltaren; Voltaren Ophtha; *Port.:* Arthrotec; Cataflam; Diclotec; Difnan†; Dorcafer; Fenil-V; Flameril; Olfen; Painex; Voltaren; *S.Afr.:* Arcanafenac†; Arthrotec; Athru-Derm; Brovaflamp†; Cataflam; Cliniflam†; Di-

clofam; Diclohexal; Difenac; Flexagen; Fortfen; Infla-Ban; Naclof; Panamor; Pharmaflam†; Sodiclo†; Veltex; Voltaren; *Singapore:* Almiral; Arthrotec; Biclopan; Cataflam; Clofenac; Diclowal; Difenac; Difnal; Inac; Inflanac; Neo-Pyrazon; Olfen; Remafen; Remethan; Rhewlin; Uniren; Voltaren; Voltaren Ophta; Zolterol; *Spain:* Artrotec; Di Retard; Dolo Nervobion; Dolo-Voltaren; Dolotren; Liberalgium; Luase; Voltaren; Voltaren Emulgel; *Swed.:* Arthrotec; Nacloff†; Voltaren; Voltaren Ophtha; Voltaren T; *Switz.:* Agofenac; Arthrotec; Diclo; diclo-basan; Diclosifar; Ecofenac; Flector; Fortenac; Grofenac; Inflamac; Olfen; Primofenac; Rheufenac; Traumasport; Vifenac; Voltaren Emulgel; Voltaren Ophtha; Voltarene; Voltarene Rapide; *Thai.:* Abitren; Almiral; Arclonac; Arthrotec; Cataflam; Catanac; Clofec; Clofon; Demac; Diclofen; Diclogel; Diclolan; Diclomol; Diclosian; Difelene; Difenac; Difeno; Dinac; Dinefec; Dosanac; Fenac; Inflanac; Lofenac; Masaren; Medaren; Myonac; Naclof; Olfen; Ostaren; Posnac; Putaren; Remethan; Rhumanol; Rumatab; Silflam; Taks; Tarjen; Tarjena; Uniren; Veenac; Volfenac; Volnac; Voltanac; Voltaren; Volverac; Voren; Votamed; *UK:* Clofen; Arthrotec; Dicloflex; Diclomax; Diclotard; Diclovol; Diclozip; Digenact†; Econac; Flamatak; Flamrase; Flexotard; Isclofen; Lofensaid; Motifene; Pennsaid; Rheumatac; Rhumalgan; Slofenac; Solaraze; Volraman; Volsaid; Voltarol; Voltarol Ophtha; *USA:* Arthrotec; Cataflam; Solaraze; Voltaren.

Multi-ingredient: *Aust.:* Diclovit; Dolo-Neurobion; Neodolpasse; Neurofenac; *Braz.:* Dorpinol; Tandrilax; *Fr.:* Voltamicine; *Ger.:* Combaren; *Hong Kong:* Neurofenac; *Ital.:* Voltamicin; *Mex.:* Dolo-Neurobion; Trazinac; *Spain:* Ocubrax; *Switz.:* Tobrafen; Voltamicin; *UK:* Dexomon.

Diethylamine Salicylate   (2633-k)

$C_{11}H_{17}NO_3 = 211.3.$
CAS — 4419-92-5.

Pharmacopoeias. In Br.

Pharmacopoeial description

BP 2001: White or almost white, odourless or almost odourless crystals. Very soluble in water; freely soluble in alcohol and in chloroform. Protect from light. Avoid contact with iron or iron salts.

Profile

Diethylamine salicylate is a salicylic acid derivative used topically in rubefacient preparations similarly to methyl salicylate (p.55) for rheumatic and muscular pain.

Preparations

BP 2001: Diethylamine Salicylate Cream.

Proprietary Preparations (details are given in Part 3)
Belg.: Algesal; *Canad.:* Algesal†; Physiogesic; *Fin.:* Algesal; *Ital.:* Algesal; Algoflex Same†; *Neth.:* Algesal; *Norw.:* Algesal; *Port.:* Algiderma; Massagim; *Spain:* Algoderm†; Artrogota; *Swed.:* Algesal; *UK:* Algesal; Lloyd's Cream.

Multi-ingredient: *Aust.:* Algesal; Derivon; Dolo-Menthoneurin; Igitur-antirheumatische; Kalisyl†; Latesyl; Pasta rubra salicylata; Reparil; Rheugesal; Thermal; *Austral.:* Rubesal; *Belg.:* Reparil; *Braz.:* Reparil; *Fr.:* Algesal Suractive; Reparil; Traumalgyl; *Ger.:* ABC Warme-Salbe; Algesal; Algesalona; Bartelin N; Bartelin nico; Brachialin percutan N†; Contrheuma V + T Bad N†; Dolo-Menthoneurin; Doloneuro; Fibraflex†; Reparil-Gel N, Reparil-Sportgel; Rheubalmin†; Rheuma V + T Bad N; Rheuma-Bad; Rheumasan Moor-Bad; Rheumichthol Bad†; *Hong Kong:* Reparil; Rubesal; *Ital.:* Aspercreme†; Reparil; Sedalpan; Via Mal Trauma Gel; *Neth.:* Algesal Forte; *Norw.:* Thermal; *Port.:* Latesil; Medalginan; Venoparil; *S.Afr.:* Reparil; *Spain:* Algesal; Contusin; Doctomitil; Dolmitin; Feparil; Radio Salil; *Swed.:* Remysal N†; *Switz.:* Algesal; Algesalona; Proctalgen; Reparil; Reparil N†; Roliwol B†; *Thai.:* Reparil; *UAE:* Rubicalm; *UK:* Fiery Jack; Transvasin Heat Spray.

Diflunisal   (2635-t)

Diflunisal (BAN, USAN, rINN).

Diflunisalum; MK-647. 5-(2,4-Difluorophenyl)salicylic acid.
$C_{13}H_8F_2O_3 = 250.2.$
CAS — 22494-42-4.
ATC — N02BA11.

Pharmacopoeias. In Eur. (see p.vi) and US.

Pharmacopoeial description

Ph. Eur.: A white or almost white, crystalline powder. Practically insoluble in water; soluble in alcohol and in ether; dissolves in dilute solutions of alkali hydroxides. Protect from light.

USP 25: A white to off-white, practically odourless, powder. Insoluble in water and in hexane; freely soluble in alcohol and in methyl alcohol; soluble in acetone and in ethyl acetate; slightly soluble in carbon tetrachloride, in chloroform, and in dichloromethane.

Adverse Effects and Treatment

As for NSAIDs in general, p.63. The commonest side-effects occurring with diflunisal are gastrointestinal disturbances, headache, and rash. Peptic ulceration and gastrointestinal bleeding have been reported. Dizziness, drowsiness, insomnia, and tinnitus may also occur.

Effects on the blood. Haematological adverse effects associated with diflunisal therapy appear to be infrequent. Throm-

bocytopenia associated with diflunisal-induced peripheral platelet destruction has been reported in a patient with rheumatoid arthritis.[1] Heinz-body haemolytic anaemia has also been reported, see under Hypersensitivity, below.
1. Bobrove AM. Diflunisal-associated thrombocytopenia in a patient with rheumatoid arthritis. *Arthritis Rheum* 1988; **31:** 148–9.

Effects on the kidneys. Acute interstitial nephritis, presenting as acute oliguric renal failure, erythroderma, and eosinophilia has followed the use of diflunisal.[1]
1. Chan LK, *et al.* Acute interstitial nephritis and erythroderma associated with diflunisal. *BMJ* 1980; **280:** 84–5.

Effects on the lungs. For reference to pneumonitis associated with diflunisal therapy, see under Hypersensitivity, below.

Effects on the skin. Reports of Stevens-Johnson syndrome associated with diflunisal.[1,2] See also under Hypersensitivity, below.
1. Hunter JA, *et al.* Diflunisal and Stevens-Johnson syndrome. *BMJ* 1978; **2:** 1088.
2. Grom JA, *et al.* Diflunisal-induced erythema multiforme major. *Hosp Formul* 1986; **21:** 353–4.

Hypersensitivity. Three cases of hypersensitivity to diflunisal in which the main clinical features were fever, elevated liver enzyme values, erythroderma, and eosinophilia, have been reported.[1] Heinz-body haemolytic anaemia occurred in one of the patients. Other hypersensitivity reactions associated with diflunisal therapy have included pneumonitis[2] and fulminant necrotising fasciitis.[3]
1. Cook DJ, *et al.* Three cases of diflunisal hypersensitivity. *Can Med Assoc J* 1988; **138:** 1029–30.
2. Rich MW, Thomas RA. A case of eosinophilic pneumonia and vasculitis induced by diflunisal. *Chest* 1997; **111:** 1767–9.
3. Krige JEJ, *et al.* Necrotising fasciitis after diflunisal for minor injury. *Lancet* 1985; **ii:** 1432–3.

Overdosage. Diflunisal poisoning has sometimes been fatal.[1,2] A dose of 15 g has been reported to have caused death when no other drugs were involved but a dose of 7.5 g has also been fatal when taken with other drugs.
1. Court H, Volans GN. Poisoning after overdose with non-steroidal anti-inflammatory drugs. *Adverse Drug React Acute Poisoning Rev* 1984; **3:** 1–21.
2. Levine B, *et al.* Diflunisal related fatality: a case report. *Forensic Sci Int* 1987; **35:** 45–50.

Precautions

As for NSAIDs in general, p.64. Diflunisal may need to be given in reduced dosage in patients with renal impairment and should not be given when renal impairment is severe.

Interactions

For interactions associated with NSAIDs, see p.65.

Aspirin may produce a small decrease in the plasma concentration of diflunisal. Diflunisal has been reported to increase the plasma concentrations of indometacin and paracetamol; the concomitant administration of diflunisal and indometacin has been associated with fatal gastrointestinal haemorrhage and therefore the combination should not be used. Antacids may reduce the absorption of diflunisal.

Benzodiazepines. For the effect of diflunisal on plasma concentrations of *oxazepam*, see p.677.

Probenecid. Average steady state plasma concentrations of diflunisal were increased by 65% when it was administered with probenecid.[1] This was due mainly to reduced formation of the phenolic and acyl glucuronides. However, plasma concentrations of these glucuronides and the sulfate conjugate were also increased even more because probenecid also reduced their renal clearance.
1. Macdonald JI, *et al.* Effect of probenecid on the formation and elimination kinetics of the sulphate and glucuronide conjugates of diflunisal. *Eur J Clin Pharmacol* 1995; **47:** 519–23.

Pharmacokinetics

Diflunisal is well absorbed from the gastrointestinal tract and peak plasma concentrations occur about 2 to 3 hours after ingestion of a single dose. It is extensively bound (more than 99%) to plasma protein and has a plasma half-life of about 8 to 12 hours. Diflunisal exhibits non-linear pharmacokinetics so that doubling the dose produces a greater than doubling of drug accumulation. Due to the long half-life and non-linear kinetics, several days are required to reach steady-state plasma concentrations following multiple dosing. The time to steady-state concentrations can be reduced by giving an initial loading dose. Concentrations of diflunisal in synovial fluid reach about 70% of those in plasma. Diflunisal is excreted in the urine mainly as glucuronide conjugates. Some biliary recycling may also occur. Diflunisal is distributed into breast milk with concentrations reported to be about 2 to 7% of those in plasma.

◊ References.
1. Loewen GR, *et al.* Effect of dose on the glucuronidation and sulphation kinetics of diflunisal in man: single dose studies. *Br J Clin Pharmacol* 1988; **26**: 31–9.
2. Eriksson L-O, *et al.* Influence of renal failure, rheumatoid arthritis and old age on the pharmacokinetics of diflunisal. *Eur J Clin Pharmacol* 1989; **36**: 165–74.
3. Verbeeck RK, *et al.* The effect of multiple dosage on the kinetics of glucuronidation and sulphation of diflunisal in man. *Br J Clin Pharmacol* 1990; **29**: 381–9.
4. Macdonald JI, *et al.* Sex-difference and the effects of smoking and oral contraceptive steroids on the kinetics of diflunisal. *Eur J Clin Pharmacol* 1990; **38**: 175–9.
5. Nuernberg B, *et al.* Pharmacokinetics of diflunisal in patients. *Clin Pharmacokinet* 1991; **20**: 81–9.

Uses and Administration

Diflunisal is a salicylic acid derivative (see Aspirin, p.16) but it is not hydrolysed to salicylate and its clinical effects are considered to resemble more closely those of propionic acid derivative NSAIDs (p.65). Diflunisal is used in the acute or long-term management of mild to moderate pain, pain and inflammation associated with osteoarthritis and rheumatoid arthritis, and symptoms of primary dysmenorrhoea. The usual initial dose for pain relief is 1000 mg followed by a maintenance dose of 500 mg every 12 hours. In some patients 250 mg every 8 to 12 hours may be sufficient but some may require 500 mg every 8 hours. Maintenance doses greater than 1500 mg daily are not recommended. The usual dose for arthritis is 500 to 1000 mg daily; this dose may be given as a single dose or as 2 divided doses.

Diflunisal may need to be given in reduced dosage in patients with renal impairment and should not be given when renal impairment is severe.

Diflunisal arginine has been used similarly given by mouth or by intramuscular or intravenous injection.

Preparations

BP 2001: Diflunisal Tablets;
USP 25: Diflunisal Tablets.

Proprietary Preparations (details are given in Part 3)
Aust.: Fluniget; *Austral.:* Dolobid; *Belg.:* Biartac; Diflusal; *Braz.:* Dorbid; *Canad.:* Dolobid; *Denm.:* Diflonid†; Donobid; *Fin.:* Donobid; *Fr.:* Dolobis; *Ger.:* Fluniget†; *Hong Kong:* Dolobid; *Irl.:* Dolobid; *Israel:* Dolobid; *Ital.:* Aflogos; Artrodol; Difludol; Dolobid; Fluodonid†; *Mex.:* Dolocid; *Neth.:* Dolocid; *Norw.:* Diflonid†; Donobid; *Port.:* Dolobid; Flunidor†; *S.Afr.:* Dolobid; *Spain:* Dolobid; *Swed.:* Donobid; *Switz.:* Unisal; *Thai.:* Dolobid; *UK:* Dolobid; *USA:* Dolobid.

Dihydrocodeine Phosphate (6221-g)

Dihydrocodeine Phosphate (BANM, rINNM).
Hydrocodeine Phosphate.
$C_{18}H_{23}NO_3,H_3PO_4 = 399.4$.
CAS — 24204-13-5.
Pharmacopoeias. In Jpn.

Dihydrocodeine Tartrate (6222-q)

Dihydrocodeine Tartrate (BANM, rINNM).
Dihydrocodeine Acid Tartrate; Dihydrocodeine Bitartrate; Drocode Bitartrate; Hydrocodeine Bitartrate. 4,5-Epoxy-3-methoxy-17-methylmorphinan-6-ol hydrogen tartrate.
$C_{18}H_{23}NO_3,C_4H_6O_6 = 451.5$.
CAS — 125-28-0 (dihydrocodeine); 5965-13-9 (dihydrocodeine tartrate).

NOTE. Compounded preparations of dihydrocodeine tartrate may be represented by the following names:
• Co-dydramol (*BAN*)—dihydrocodeine tartrate 1 part and paracetamol 50 parts (w/w).
Pharmacopoeias. In Aust., Br., Ger., Pol., and US.

Pharmacopoeial description

BP 2001: Odourless, or almost odourless, colourless crystals or white crystalline powder. Freely soluble in water; sparingly soluble in alcohol; practically insoluble in ether. A 10% solution in water has a pH of 3.2 to 4.2. Protect from light.
USP 25: pH of a 10% solution in water is between 3.2 and 4.2. Store in airtight containers.

Dependence and Withdrawal

As for Opioid Analgesics, p.66. Dihydrocodeine has been subject to abuse (see under Precautions, below).

Adverse Effects and Treatment

As for Opioid Analgesics in general, p.67; side-

---

effects from dihydrocodeine are less pronounced than those from morphine.

◊ For reference to increased postoperative pain associated with the use of dihydrocodeine, see under Pain in Uses and Administration, below.

Overdosage. A 29-year-old man who had taken 2.1 g of dihydrocodeine had biochemical evidence of acute renal and hepatic impairment when admitted 13 hours after the overdose.[1] Severe life-threatening respiratory depression subsequently developed 36 hours after the overdose and only responded to treatment with naloxone after large doses (a total of 46.6 mg of naloxone) over a long period (106 hours). Commenting on this report some questioned the evidence for hepatic impairment and considered that the raised liver enzyme values were of muscular origin as a result of rhabdomyolysis.[2-4] Rhabdomyolysis might also have contributed to renal failure.

An anaphylactoid reaction following an overdose of an unspecified number of dihydrocodeine tablets[5] appeared to respond to intravenous naloxone.
1. Redfern N. Dihydrocodeine overdose treated with naloxone infusion. *BMJ* 1983; **287**: 751–2.
2. Buckley BM, Vale JA. Dihydrocodeine overdose treated with naloxone infusion. *BMJ* 1983; **287**: 1547.
3. Blain PG, Lane RJM. Dihydrocodeine overdose treated with naloxone infusion. *BMJ* 1983; **287**: 1547.
4. Wen P. Dihydrocodeine overdose treated with naloxone infusion. *BMJ* 1983; **287**: 1548.
5. Panos MZ, *et al.* Use of naloxone in opioid-induced anaphylactoid reaction. *Br J Anaesth* 1988; **61**: 371.

Precautions

As for Opioid Analgesics in general, p.68.

Abuse. Dihydrocodeine has been reported to be widely abused by opiate addicts.[1-3]
1. Swadi H, *et al.* Misuse of dihydrocodeine tartrate (DF 118) among opiate addicts. *BMJ* 1990; **300**: 1313.
2. Robertson JR, *et al.* Misuse of dihydrocodeine tartrate (DF 118) among opiate addicts. *BMJ* 1990; **301**: 119.
3. Strang J, *et al.* Misuse of dihydrocodeine tartrate (DF 118) among opiate addicts. *BMJ* 1990; **301**: 119.

The elderly. Despite some impaired renal function an elderly group of patients[1] appeared to handle dihydrocodeine similarly to healthy young subjects. There was marked variability in all measurements and on the basis of this study no clear conclusions on guidelines for dosage in elderly patients could be drawn. However, the recommendation that small doses be given initially with subsequent doses according to response was endorsed.
1. Davies KN, *et al.* The effect of ageing on the pharmacokinetics of dihydrocodeine. *Eur J Clin Pharmacol* 1989; **37**: 375–9.

Renal impairment. Caution is necessary when giving dihydrocodeine to patients with severe renal impairment. Severe narcosis occurred in a patient with anuria and on maintenance haemodialysis after she had received dihydrocodeine by mouth for 4 days.[1] She responded to treatment with naloxone.
See also under Pharmacokinetics, below.
1. Barnes JN, Goodwin FJ. Dihydrocodeine narcosis in renal failure. *BMJ* 1983; **286**: 438–9.

Interactions

For interactions associated with opioid analgesics, see p.68.

Quinidine. Like codeine (p.26) dihydrocodeine is metabolised via the cytochrome P450 isoenzyme CYP2D6 to active metabolites, which it has been suggested may play a role in its analgesic activity in extensive metabolisers; quinidine impairs this metabolism, but a study in 11 healthy subjects did not demonstrate any reduced analgesic activity when dihydrocodeine and quinidine were given concomitantly, despite a three- to fourfold reduction in plasma concentrations of the metabolite dihydromorphine.[1]
1. Wilder-Smith CH, *et al.* The visceral and somatic antinociceptive effects of dihydrocodeine and its metabolite, dihydromorphine: a cross-over study with extensive and quinidine-induced poor metabolizers. *Br J Clin Pharmacol* 1998; **45**: 575–81.

Pharmacokinetics

◊ There have been few pharmacokinetic studies of dihydrocodeine. In one study[1] peak plasma concentrations were achieved 1.6 and 1.8 hours after an oral dose of 30 and 60 mg, respectively; elimination half-lives varied between about 3.5 and 4.5 hours. The rate of absorption was independent of dose and oral bioavailability was only about 20%, possibly because of substantial first-pass metabolism in the gut wall or liver.
1. Rowell FJ, *et al.* Pharmacokinetics of intravenous and oral dihydrocodeine and its acid metabolites. *Eur J Clin Pharmacol* 1983; **25**: 419–24.

Renal impairment. The pharmacokinetics of dihydrocodeine tartrate, given by mouth as a single 60-mg dose, were affected in 9 patients with chronic renal failure treated with haemodialysis when compared with 9 healthy subjects.[1] Time to peak plasma concentration in those with renal failure was 3 hours compared with 1 hour in healthy subjects; the area under the plasma concentration/time curve was greater in those with renal failure; and after 24 hours dihydrocodeine was still de-

---

tectable in the plasma of all renal failure patients, but in only 3 of the healthy subjects.
1. Barnes JN, *et al.* Dihydrocodeine in renal failure: further evidence for an important role of the kidney in the handling of opioid drugs. *BMJ* 1985; **290**: 740–2.

Uses and Administration

Dihydrocodeine is an opioid analgesic (p.68). It is related to codeine (p.26) and has similar analgesic activity. Dihydrocodeine is used for the relief of moderate to severe pain, often in combination with paracetamol. It has also been used as a cough suppressant.

For analgesia the usual dose of dihydrocodeine tartrate by mouth is 30 mg after food every 4 to 6 hours; up to 240 mg daily may be given for severe pain. Children over 4 years of age may be given 0.5 to 1 mg per kg body-weight every 4 to 6 hours. Modified-release preparations are available for twice daily administration in adults with chronic severe pain.

Dihydrocodeine tartrate may also be given by deep subcutaneous or intramuscular injection in doses of up to 50 mg every 4 to 6 hours. Doses equivalent to those used orally in children may be given parenterally to children over 4 years of age.

As a cough suppressant dihydrocodeine tartrate may be given by mouth in doses of 10 to 30 mg up to three times daily.

Dihydrocodeine phosphate has also been used. Other salts of dihydrocodeine used, mainly for their antitussive effects, include the hydrochloride and the thiocyanate. Dihydrocodeine polistirex has been used in modified-release preparations.

Dyspnoea. Dihydrocodeine has been reported[1] to have produced benefit in normocapnic patients severely disabled by breathlessness due to chronic airflow obstruction. A dose of 15 mg was taken 30 minutes before exercise up to three times a day.
1. Johnson MA, *et al.* Dihydrocodeine for breathlessness in 'pink puffers'. *BMJ* 1983; **286**: 675–7.

Pain. Dihydrocodeine is used in the management of moderate to severe pain. However, dose-related increase in postoperative pain has been seen[1] in patients given 25 or 50 mg dihydrocodeine tartrate intravenously following dental surgery, and it has been proposed that dihydrocodeine might act as an antagonist in situations where acute pain was accompanied by high opioid activity.[2] Systematic review of the use of single oral doses of dihydrocodeine has indicated that these are insufficient to provide adequate relief of post-operative pain, and that dihydrocodeine is less effective than ibuprofen.[3]
1. Seymour RA, *et al.* Dihydrocodeine-induced hyperalgesia in postoperative dental pain. *Lancet* 1982; **i**: 1425–6.
2. Henry JA. Dihydrocodeine increases dental pain. *Lancet* 1982; **ii**: 223.
3. Edwards JE, *et al.* Single dose dihydrocodeine for acute postoperative pain (updated 30 August 2001). Available in The Cochrane Library; Issue 4. Oxford: Update Software; 2001.

Preparations

BP 2001: Co-dydramol Tablets; Dihydrocodeine Injection; Dihydrocodeine Oral Solution; Dihydrocodeine Tablets.

Proprietary Preparations (details are given in Part 3)
Aust.: Codidol; Paracodin; *Austral.:* Paracodin; Rikodeine; *Belg.:* Codicontin; Paracodine; *Fr.:* Dicodin; *Ger.:* DHC; Paracodin N; Remedacen; Tiamon Mono; *Hong Kong:* DF 118; *Irl.:* DF 118; DHC Continus; Hydol; Paracodin; *Israel:* DHC Continus; *Ital.:* Paracodin; *NZ:* DHC Continus; *Port.:* Didor; Paracodina; *S.Afr.:* DF 118; Paracodin; *Spain:* Contugesic; Paracodina; Tosidrin; *Switz.:* Codicontin; Hydrocodeinon; Paracodin; *UK:* DF 118; DHC Continus.

Multi-ingredient: *Aust.:* Paracodin; *Austral.:* Codox; *Belg.:* Paracodine; *Ger.:* Antitussivum Burger N; Makatussin Tropfen forte; Paracodin retard; *Irl.:* Paramol; *Ital.:* Cardiazol-Paracodina; *Spain:* Traquivan; *Switz.:* Escotussin; Makatussin forte; Neo Makatussin N; Paracodin retard; *UK:* Boots Dental Pain Relief; Galake; Paramol; Remedeine; *USA:* DHC Plus; Panlor DC; Synalgos-DC; Vanex Grape†.

Dipipanone Hydrochloride (6224-s)

Dipipanone Hydrochloride (BANM, rINNM).
Phenylpiperone Hydrochloride; Piperidyl Methadone Hydrochloride; Piperidylamidone Hydrochloride. (±)-4,4-Diphenyl-6-piperidinoheptan-3-one hydrochloride monohydrate.
$C_{24}H_{31}NO,HCl,H_2O = 404.0$.
CAS — 467-83-4 (dipipanone); 856-87-1 (dipipanone hydrochloride).
Pharmacopoeias. In Br.

Pharmacopoeial description

BP 2001: An odourless or almost odourless, white, crystalline powder. Sparingly soluble in water; freely soluble in alcohol and in acetone; practically insoluble in ether. A 2.5% solution in water has a pH of 4.0 to 6.0.

Profile
Dipipanone hydrochloride is an opioid analgesic (p.66) structurally related to methadone (p.53). Used alone it is reported to be less sedating than morphine. It is used in the treatment of moderate to severe pain.

Dipipanone hydrochloride is usually administered with cyclizine hydrochloride in order to reduce the incidence of nausea and vomiting, but the use of opioid preparations containing an antiemetic is not recommended for the management of chronic pain as an antiemetic is usually only required for the first few days of treatment. The usual dose of dipipanone hydrochloride given by mouth is 10 mg, repeated every 6 hours. The dose may be increased if necessary in increments of 5 mg; it is seldom necessary to exceed a dose of 30 mg. Following administration by mouth the effect begins within an hour and lasts about 4 to 6 hours.

Preparations of dipipanone hydrochloride with cyclizine hydrochloride are subject to abuse.

Preparations
BP 2001: Dipipanone and Cyclizine Tablets.
Proprietary Preparations (details are given in Part 3)
Multi-ingredient: *Hong Kong:* Wellconal; *Irl.:* Diconal; *S.Afr.:* Wellconal; *UK:* Diconal.

Diproqualone (16607-k)
Diproqualone *(rINN).*
3-(2,3-Dihydroxypropyl)-2-methyl-4(3H)-quinazolinone.
$C_{12}H_{14}N_2O_3 = 234.3.$
CAS — 36518-02-2.

Profile
Diproqualone is an analgesic that has been given by mouth as the camsilate.

Preparations
Proprietary Preparations (details are given in Part 3)
Multi-ingredient: *Switz.:* Algopriv.

Dipyrone (2638-f)
Dipyrone *(BAN, USAN).*
Metamizole Sodium (pINN); Aminopyrine-sulphonate Sodium; Analginum; Metamizole; Metamizolum Natricum; Methampyrone; Methylmelubrin; Natrium Novaminsulfonicum; Noramidazophenum; Noraminophenazonum; Novamidazofen; NSC-73205; Sodium Noramidopyrine Methanesulphonate; Sulpyrine. Sodium N-(2,3-dimethyl-5-oxo-1-phenyl-3-pyrazolin-4-yl)-N-methylaminomethanesulphonate monohydrate.
$C_{13}H_{16}N_3NaO_4S,H_2O = 351.4.$
CAS — 68-89-3 (anhydrous dipyrone); 5907-38-0 (dipyrone monohydrate).
ATC — N02BB02.

NOTE. Dipyrone is referred to in some countries by the colloquial name 'Mexican aspirin'.

Pharmacopoeias. In *Chin., Eur.* (see p.vi), *Jpn,* and *Pol.*

Pharmacopoeial description
Ph. Eur.: A white or almost white crystalline powder. Very soluble in water; soluble in alcohol. Protect from light.

Adverse Effects and Precautions
Administration of dipyrone is associated with an increased risk of agranulocytosis and with shock.

Effects on the blood. Data collected from 8 population groups in Europe and Israel by the International Agranulocytosis and Aplastic Anemia Study[1] revealed that there was a significant regional variability in the rate-ratio estimate for agranulocytosis and dipyrone (0.9 in Budapest to 33.3 in Barcelona). Although a large relative increase in risk between agranulocytosis and use of dipyrone was found, the incidence was less than some previous reports had suggested.

1. The International Agranulocytosis and Aplastic Anemia Study. Risks of agranulocytosis and aplastic anemia: a first report of their relation to drug use with special reference to analgesics. *JAMA* 1986; **256:** 1749–57.

Effects on the skin. Dipyrone has been considered responsible for a case of drug-induced toxic epidermal necrolysis.[1]

1. Roujeau J-C, *et al.* Sjögren-like syndrome after drug-induced toxic epidermal necrolysis. *Lancet* 1985; **i:** 609–11.

Hypersensitivity. Cross-sensitivity between aspirin and dipyrone occurred in one patient.[1] Dipyrone produced an exacerbation of dyspnoea, cyanosis, and respiratory arrest.

1. Bartoli E, *et al.* Drug-induced asthma. *Lancet* 1976; **i:** 1357.

Porphyria. Dipyrone has been associated with acute attacks of porphyria and is considered unsafe in porphyric patients.

Pharmacokinetics
Following oral administration dipyrone is rapidly hydrolysed in gastric juice to the active metabolite 4-methyl-amino-antipyrine which after absorption undergoes metabolism to 4-formyl-amino-antipyrine and other metabolites. Dipyrone is also rapidly undetectable in plasma following intravenous administra-

tion. None of the metabolites of dipyrone are extensively bound to plasma proteins. Most of a dose is excreted in the urine as metabolites. Dipyrone metabolites are also distributed into breast milk.

◊ References.
1. Heinemeyer G, *et al.* The kinetics of metamizol and its metabolites in critical-care patients with acute renal dysfunction. *Eur J Clin Pharmacol* 1993; **45:** 445–50.
2. Levy M, *et al.* Clinical pharmacokinetics of dipyrone and its metabolites. *Clin Pharmacokinet* 1995; **28:** 216–34.
3. Zylber-Katz E, *et al.* Dipyrone metabolism in liver disease. *Clin Pharmacol Ther* 1995; **58:** 198–209.

Uses and Administration
Dipyrone is the sodium sulfonate of aminophenazone (p.13) and has similar properties. Because of the risk of serious adverse effects its use is justified only in severe pain where no alternative is available or suitable. Dipyrone has been given by mouth in doses of 0.5 to 4 g daily in divided doses. It has also been given by intramuscular or intravenous injection and rectally as a suppository.

A magnesium congener of dipyrone, metamizole magnesium has been used similarly to dipyrone as has the calcium congener metamizole calcium.

Preparations
Proprietary Preparations (details are given in Part 3)
Aust.: Inalgon Neu; Novalgin; Spasmo Inalgon Neu; *Belg.:* Novalgine; *Braz.:* Anador; Analgex; Analgina; Baralgin M; Cefaldina; Conmel; Debela; Doran; Evergin; Febralgin; Magnopyrol; Nevralgina; Novalgina; Toloxin; *Fr.:* Novalgine; Pyrethane†; *Ger.:* Analgin; Analgit†; Baralgin; Berlosin; Novalgin; Novaminsulfon; *Hong Kong:* Metilon; Novaminsulfon; Sulpyrin; *Israel:* Novalgin; Optalgin; Phanalgin; V-Talgin; *Ital.:* Novalgina; Trisalgina; *Mex.:* Alnex; Anaprol; Avafontan; Ayoral F; Conmel; Dalmasin; Dipiraxil; Dipydol; Dolgan; Dolofur; Exalgin; Exodalina; Fandall; Fardolpin; Farlin; Mach-2; Macodin; Magnil; Magnol; Magnopyrol; Magsons; Mayopirina; Mecoten; Medipirol; Mermid; Metapirona; Midelin; Minoral; Neo-Melubrina; Nesol; Odon-Pyr; Paleodina; Pifrol; Piramagno; Pirandall; Pirawil; Pirinovag; Piromebrina; Pironal; Pirongil; Poloren; Precidona; Prodolina; Profelina; Propiral; Pyranol; Pyril; Pyron; Sesalgin; Suprim; Termonil; Therma Ayoral; Tredol; Utidol; Vegal; Zolidin; *Neth.:* Novalgin; *Port.:* Conmel†; Dolocalma; Nolotil; Novalgina; *Spain:* Adolkin†; Afebrin†; Algi; Dolemicin; Lasain; Neo Melubrina; Nolotil; Optalgin; *Swed.:* Novalgin; *Switz.:* Minalgin; Novalgine; *Thai.:* Acodon; Genergin; Invoigin; Medalgin; Nivagin; Nominfone; Novalgin; Olan-Gin.

Multi-ingredient: *Aust.:* Buscopan Compositum; Spasmium comp; *Belg.:* Buscopan Compositum; Visceralgine Compositum; *Braz.:* Adegrip; Adegripan; Algice; Algiflex; Aminocid; Analgex C; Analgin C-R; Analgosedan; Analverin; Anapirol; Apracur; Beserol; Bicavine; Bioscina; Bipasmin Composto; Bromalgina; Broncopirol; Buscopan Composto; Cafalena; Cefaliv; Cortagrip; Cortagrip D; Cortegripan; Dexalgen; Diarona; Dilubrin; Dimex; Doralon; Dorflex; Doricin; Dorscopena; Dorspan; Espasmobel; Espasmodid Composto; Espasmosan Composto; Eucaliptol; Eucaliptol Composto; Flenalgin; Flexdor; Fluviral; Gripefago C; Gripion; Gripol C; Gripol Capuride; Gripol Composto; Gripomatine; Griponia; Gripsay; Inatrex Balsamico; Killgrip; Lisador; Melpaz; Metilsedor; Mio-Citalgan; Mionevrix; Napiro; Neosaldina; Novalgrip; Par; Plenocedan; Plenogripe; Pulmodex-C; Resfrialgina; Rielex; Sedalene; Sedobion; Somaflex; Spasmotropin; Sulindor; Tebasedan; Tetrapulmo; Tropinal; *Fin.:* Litalgin; *Fr.:* Avafortan; Cefaline-Pyrazole; Optalidon a la Noramidopyrine; Salgydal a la noramidopyrine; Visceralgine Forte; *Hung.:* Quarelin; *Ital.:* Soma Complex; *Mex.:* Ayoral; Bipasmin Compuesto; Buscapina Compositum; Busconet; Busprina; Colepren; Dolnefort; Dolo-Tiaminal; Retodol Compositum; Selpiran; *S.Afr.:* Baralgan†; Buscopan Compositum; Norifortan†; Scopex Co†; *Spain:* Buscapina Compositum; Nolotil Compositum; Vapin Complex; *Thai.:* Butarion; Novapam.

Droxicam (2737-h)
Droxicam *(rINN).*
5-Methyl-3-(2-pyridyl)-2H,5H-1,3-oxazino[5,6-c]-[1,2]benzothiazine-2,4(3H)-dione 6,6-dioxide.
$C_{16}H_{11}N_3O_5S = 357.3.$
CAS — 90101-16-9.
ATC — M01AC04.

Profile
Droxicam is an NSAID (p.63) reported to act as a prodrug for piroxicam (p.79). It has been given by mouth for pain and inflammation associated with musculoskeletal, joint, and soft-tissue disorders but marketing was suspended in December 1994 because it was associated with adverse liver effects.

Effects on the liver. Up to October 1993 the Spanish National System of Pharmacovigilance had received 82 spontaneous reports of hepatic damage associated with droxicam[1] and in December 1994 the European Union Committee for Proprietary Medicinal Products recommended that marketing authorisation for droxicam should be suspended pending further studies. An industry sponsored study[1] (submitted in December 1994) of 8910 patients who had taken droxicam identified one patient whose hepatic damage was considered to be attributable to droxicam, a figure comparable with the base-line estimate observed for NSAIDs in general (see p.64).

1. García-Rodríguez LA, *et al.* Acute liver injury and droxicam use in the region of Friuli-Venezia Giulia. *Br J Clin Pharmacol* 1995; **40:** 103–6.

Preparations
Proprietary Preparations (details are given in Part 3)
Braz.: Ombolan.

Eltenac (2797-j)
Eltenac *(rINN).*
4-(2,6-Dichloroanilino)-3-thiopheneacetic acid.
$C_{12}H_9Cl_2NO_2S = 302.2.$
CAS — 72895-88-6.

Profile
Eltenac is an NSAID (p.63) used in veterinary medicine.

Embutramide (12687-n)
Embutramide *(BAN, USAN, rINN).*
Hoe-18-680. N-(β,β-Diethyl-m-methoxyphenethyl)-4-hydroxybutyramide.
$C_{17}H_{27}NO_3 = 293.4.$
CAS — 15687-14-6.

Profile
Embutramide is an opioid analgesic used in veterinary medicine for euthanasia.

Enadoline Hydrochloride (17326-c)
Enadoline Hydrochloride *(USAN, rINNM).*
CI-977. N-Methyl-N-[(5R,7S,8S)-7-(1-pyrrolidinyl)-1-oxaspiro[4.5]dec-8-yl]-4-benzofuranacetamide monohydrochloride.
$C_{24}H_{32}N_2O_3,HCl = 433.0.$
CAS — 124378-77-4 (enadoline); 124439-07-2 (enadoline hydrochloride).

Profile
Enadoline hydrochloride is under investigation for its opioid analgesic properties (p.66). It is reported to have selective κ agonist activity.

◊ References.
1. Reece PA, *et al.* Diuretic effects, pharmacokinetics, and safety of a new centrally acting kappa-opioid agonist (CI-977) in humans. *J Clin Pharmacol* 1994; **34:** 1126–32.
2. Pande AC, *et al.* Analgesic efficacy of enadoline versus placebo or morphine in postsurgical pain. *Clin Neuropharmacol* 1996; **19:** 451–6.

Enoxolone (1608-p)
Enoxolone *(BAN, rINN).*
Enoxolonum; Glycyrrhetic Acid; Glycyrrhetinic Acid. 3β-Hydroxy-11-oxo-olean-12-en-30-oic acid.
$C_{30}H_{46}O_4 = 470.7.$
CAS — 471-53-4.
Pharmacopoeias. In *Eur.* (see p.vi).

Pharmacopoeial description
Ph. Eur.: A white or almost white, crystalline powder. It exhibits polymorphism. Practically insoluble in water; soluble in dehydrated alcohol; sparingly soluble in dichloromethane. Protect from light.

Profile
Enoxolone is a complex triterpene prepared from glycyrrhizinic acid, a constituent of liquorice. Enoxolone is used locally in preparations for the treatment of non-infective inflammatory disorders of the skin, mouth, throat, and rectum.

Derivatives of enoxolone, including its aluminium salt (p.1225) and carbenoxolone (p.1215) are used in the treatment of benign peptic ulcer disease and other gastrointestinal disorders.

◊ Enoxolone is a potent inhibitor of the enzyme 11β-hydroxysteroid dehydrogenase which inactivates cortisol and concomitant application of enoxolone with hydrocortisone has been shown in *animal* studies to potentiate the activity of hydrocortisone in skin.[1] Whether this also increases the systemic absorption and toxicity of hydrocortisone remains to be determined.[2]

1. Teelucksingh S, *et al.* Potentiation of hydrocortisone activity in skin by glycyrrhetinic acid. *Lancet* 1990; **335:** 1060–3.
2. Greaves MW. Potentiation of hydrocortisone activity in skin by glycyrrhetinic acid. *Lancet* 1990; **336:** 876.

Preparations
Proprietary Preparations (details are given in Part 3)
Fr.: Arthrodont; P.O. 12.

Multi-ingredient: *Fr.:* Dermeol; Hexalyse; Lelong Irritations†; Phlebocreme; Phlebosup; Pyreflor; Sedorrhoide; Tiq'Aouta; Valda Septol†; Vocadys; *Hong Kong:* Hexalyse; *Ital.:* Acnesan; Eudent con Glysan; Lenipasta; Lenirose; Lisomucil Gola; Neo-Stomygen; Pastiglie Valda; Valda F3†; Viderm; *Port.:* Hyseke; *Spain:* Angileptol; Anginovag; Pentalmicina†; Roberfarin; *UK:* Gelclair.

Epirizole (2640-c)

Epirizole (USAN, pINN).
DA-398; Mepirizole. 4-Methoxy-2-(5-methoxy-3-methylpyrazol-1-yl)-6-methylpyrimidine.
$C_{11}H_{14}N_4O_2 = 234.3$.
CAS — 18694-40-1.
Pharmacopoeias. In Jpn.

Profile
Epirizole is an NSAID (p.63) that has been used by mouth in a usual dose of 150 to 450 mg daily in divided doses.

Preparations
Proprietary Preparations (details are given in Part 3)
Braz.: Mebron; Jpn: Mebron.

Ethenzamide (2641-k)

Ethenzamide (BAN, rINN).
Aethoxybenzamidum; Etenzamide; Ethoxybenzamide; Ethylsalicylamide; HP-209. 2-Ethoxybenzamide.
$C_9H_{11}NO_2 = 165.2$.
CAS — 938-73-8.
ATC — N02BA07.
Pharmacopoeias. In Aust. and Jpn.

Profile
Ethenzamide is a salicylic acid derivative (see Aspirin, p.14) given by mouth in painful and inflammatory conditions and to reduce fever.

Preparations
Proprietary Preparations (details are given in Part 3)
Belg.: Simil NF†.
Multi-ingredient: Aust.: Coldadolin; Dolmix; Helopyrin; Neuro-Europan†; Nisicur; Seltoc; Braz.: Recilugo; Ger.: Antifohnon-N; Glutisal; Kolton grippale N; Port.: Cephyl; Katagrip; Switz.: Algopriv; Ergosanol a la cafeine; Ergosanol special a la cafeine; Ergosanol special†; Nicaphlogyl; Seranex sans codeine.

Ethoheptazine Citrate (6225-w)

Ethoheptazine Citrate (BANM, rINNM).
Wy-401. Ethyl 1-methyl-4-phenylperhydroazepine-4-carboxylate dihydrogen citrate.
$C_{16}H_{23}NO_2, C_6H_8O_7 = 453.5$.
CAS — 77-15-6 (ethoheptazine); 6700-56-7 (ethoheptazine citrate); 2085-42-9 ((±)-ethoheptazine citrate).

Profile
Ethoheptazine citrate is an opioid analgesic (p.66) structurally related to pethidine (p.75). It is employed as an analgesic in the short-term treatment of mild to moderate pain, usually in conjunction with other compounds such as aspirin and meprobamate.

Preparations
Proprietary Preparations (details are given in Part 3)
Multi-ingredient: Canad.: Equagesic†; S.Afr.: Equagesic†; UK: Equagesic.

Ethyl Nicotinate (9231-s)

$C_8H_9NO_2 = 151.2$.
CAS — 614-18-6.

Profile
Ethyl nicotinate is used in concentrations of up to 2% in topical rubefacient preparations for the relief of pain in musculoskeletal, joint, and soft-tissue disorders. It has also been used as suppositories in anorectal disorders.

Preparations
Proprietary Preparations (details are given in Part 3)
Aust.: Mucotherm.
Multi-ingredient: Aust.: Thermal; Belg.: Transvane†; Ger.: Striatidin; Irl.: Transvasin; Norw.: Thermal; NZ: Transvasin; Swed.: Transvasin†; Switz.: Baume Esco Forte; Sloan Baume†; Thermocutan; UK: PR Heat Spray; Transvasin Heat Rub.

Ethyl Salicylate (12707-l)

Ethyl 2-hydroxybenzoate.
$C_9H_{10}O_3 = 166.2$.
CAS — 118-61-6.

Profile
Ethyl salicylate is a salicylic acid derivative that is used similarly to methyl salicylate (p.55) in concentrations of up to 5% in topical rubefacient preparations for the relief of pain in musculoskeletal, joint, and soft-tissue disorders.

Preparations
Proprietary Preparations (details are given in Part 3)
Multi-ingredient: Austral.: Deep Heat; Radian-B; Belg.: Rado-Salil; Ger.: Contrheuma-Gel forte N†; Israel: Deep Heat Spray; Ital.: Remy; Singapore: Deep Heating Spray; Switz.: Alginex; UK: Aspellin; Deep Heat Spray; Dubam; Ralgex.

Ethylmorphine Hydrochloride (6226-e)

Ethylmorphine Hydrochloride (BANM).
Aethylmorphinae Hydrochloridum; Aethylmorphini Hydrochloridum; Chlorhydrate de Codéthyline; Ethylmorphini Hydrochloridum; Ethylmorphinium Chloride. 3-O-Ethylmorphine hydrochloride dihydrate; 7,8-Didehydro-4,5-epoxy-3-ethoxy-17-methylmorphinan-6-ol hydrochloride dihydrate.
$C_{19}H_{23}NO_3, HCl, 2H_2O = 385.9$.
CAS — 76-58-4 (ethylmorphine); 125-30-4 (ethylmorphine hydrochloride).
Pharmacopoeias. In Chin., Eur. (see p.vi), Jpn, and Pol.

Pharmacopoeial description
Ph. Eur.: A white or almost white crystalline powder. Soluble in water and in alcohol; practically insoluble in ether. A 2% solution in water has a pH of 4.3 to 5.7. Protect from light.

Profile
Ethylmorphine hydrochloride is an opioid analgesic (p.66) and has properties similar to those of codeine (p.25). It is used mainly as a cough suppressant. It has also been used for its analgesic and antidiarrhoeal properties and has been given in eye drops as a lymphagogue.
Ethylmorphine free base and the camphorate and camsilate have also been used.

◊ References.
1. Aasmundstad TA, et al. Biotransformation and pharmacokinetics of ethylmorphine after a single oral dose. Br J Clin Pharmacol 1995; 39: 611–20.

Preparations
Proprietary Preparations (details are given in Part 3)
Belg.: Codethyline†; Fin.: Cocillana; Fr.: Codethyline†; Trachyl†; UK: Collins Elixir.
Multi-ingredient: Aust.: Modiscop; Belg.: Solucamphre†; Theralene Pectoral†; Tux; Denm.: Cosylan†; Fin.: Indalgin; Fr.: Bronpax†; Ephydion; Eubispasme Codethyline†; Humex; Marrubene Codethyline†; Peter's Sirop†; Sedophon; Sirop Pectoral adulte†; Sirop Pectoral enfant†; Thiosedal†; Tussipax; Tussipax a l'Euquinine†; Vegetoserum; Ital.: Codetilina-Eucaliptolo He†; Mindol-Merck; Norw.: Cosylan; Solvipect comp; Sterk hostesirup†; Port.: Bronquiasmol; Calmarum; Diacol; Fluidin Nocturno†; Gotas Zimaia; Xarope Antigripal; Spain: Demusin; Sedalmerck; Swed.: Cocillana-Etyfin; Cosylan†; Lepheton; Switz.: Ipeca; Phol-Tux; Saintbois nouvelle formule; Sano Tuss; Solucamphre†.

Etodolac (12717-j)

Etodolac (BAN, USAN, rINN).
AY-24236; Etodolacum; Etodolic Acid. 1,8-Diethyl-1,3,4,9-tetrahydropyrano[3,4-b]indol-1-ylacetic acid.
$C_{17}H_{21}NO_3 = 287.4$.
CAS — 41340-25-4.
ATC — M01AB08.
Pharmacopoeias. In Eur. (see p.vi) and US.

Pharmacopoeial description
Ph. Eur.: A white or almost white crystalline powder. Practically insoluble in water; freely soluble in dehydrated alcohol and in acetone.
USP 25: Store in airtight containers.

Adverse Effects and Precautions
As for NSAIDs in general, p.63.
The presence of phenolic metabolites of etodolac in the urine may give rise to a false-positive reaction for bilirubin.

Effects on the blood. A report[1] of a patient who had agranulocytosis associated with the use of etodolac.
1. Cramer RL, et al. Agranulocytosis associated with etodolac. Ann Pharmacother 1994; 28: 458–60.

Effects on the gastrointestinal tract. Etodolac may produce less gastric toxicity than naproxen.[1,2]
1. Taha AS, et al. Effect of repeated therapeutic doses of naproxen and etodolac on gastric and duodenal mucosal prostaglandins (PGs) in rheumatoid arthritis (RA). Gut 1989; 30: A751.
2. Bianchi Porro G, et al. A double-blind gastroscopic evaluation of the effects of etodolac and naproxen on the gastrointestinal mucosa of rheumatic patients. J Intern Med 1991; 229: 5–8.

Interactions
For interactions associated with NSAIDs, see p.65.

Pharmacokinetics
Etodolac is a chiral compound given as the racemate. Peak plasma concentrations of the active (S)-enantiomer and of the inactive (R)-enantiomer are usually obtained within about 2 hours of administration by mouth but plasma concentrations of the (R)-enantiomer have been reported to greatly exceed those of the (S)-enantiomer. Both enantiomers are highly bound to plasma protein. Both are also distributed to the synovial fluid, although the difference in their concentra-

tions may not be as marked as the difference in plasma concentrations. The plasma half-life of total etodolac has been reported to be about 7 hours; excretion is predominantly in the urine mainly as hydroxylated metabolites and glucuronide conjugates; some may be excreted in the bile.

◊ References.
1. Brocks DR, et al. Stereoselective disposition of etodolac enantiomers in synovial fluid. J Clin Pharmacol 1991; 31: 741–6.
2. Brocks DR, et al. The stereoselective pharmacokinetics of etodolac in young and elderly subjects, and after cholecystectomy. J Clin Pharmacol 1992; 32: 982–9.
3. Brocks DR, Jamali F. Etodolac clinical pharmacokinetics. Clin Pharmacokinet 1994; 26: 259–74.
4. Boni J, et al. Pharmacokinetic and pharmacodynamic action of etodolac in patients after oral surgery. J Clin Pharmacol 1999; 39: 729–37.

Uses and Administration
Etodolac, a pyrano-indoleacetic acid derivative, is an NSAID (p.65) reported to be a preferential inhibitor of cyclo-oxygenase 2 (COX-2). It is used for rheumatoid arthritis and osteoarthritis and for the treatment of acute pain.

For the treatment of rheumatoid arthritis and osteoarthritis, the recommended dose is initially 600 to 1000 mg daily in divided doses adjusted according to response to a maximum of 1200 mg daily. Modified-release preparations are available for once daily administration in the treatment of rheumatoid arthritis or osteoarthritis.

For the treatment of acute pain, the recommended dose is 200 to 400 mg every 6 to 8 hours to a usual maximum of 1000 mg daily although some patients have been given up to 1200 mg daily.

Preparations
BP 2001: Etodolac Capsules; Etodolac Tablets;
USP 25: Etodolac Capsules; Etodolac Tablets.
Proprietary Preparations (details are given in Part 3)
Aust.: Lodine; Canad.: Ultradol; Denm.: Todolac; Fr.: Lodine; Hong Kong: Elderin; Lodine; Israel: Etopan; Ital.: Lodine; Jpn: Hypen; Mex.: Lodine; Port.: Acudor; Articulan; Dualgan; Lodine; Metazin; Sodolac†; Switz.: Lodine; Thai.: Etonox; UK: Lodine; USA: Lodine.

Etofenamate (2644-x)

Etofenamate (BAN, USAN, rINN).
B-577; Bay-d-1107; Etofenamatum; TV-485; TVX-485; WHR-5020. 2-(2-Hydroxyethoxy)ethyl N-(ααα-trifluoro-m-tolyl)anthranilate.
$C_{18}H_{18}F_3NO_4 = 369.3$.
CAS — 30544-47-9.
ATC — M02AA06.
Pharmacopoeias. In Eur. (see p.vi).

Pharmacopoeial description
Ph. Eur.: A yellowish viscous liquid. Practically insoluble in water; miscible with alcohol and with ethyl acetate.

Profile
Etofenamate is an NSAID (p.63) that has been applied topically in a concentration of 5 or 10% for the relief of pain and inflammation associated with musculoskeletal, joint, and soft-tissue disorders. It has also been given by deep intramuscular injection in single doses of 1 g.

Preparations
Proprietary Preparations (details are given in Part 3)
Aust.: Rheumon; Traumon; Belg.: Flexium; Braz.: Bayro; Ger.: Algesalona E; Rheuma-Gel; Rheumon; Traumon; Ital.: Bayro; Mex.: Bayro; Reumagel; Port.: Fenogel; Reumon; Spain: Afrolate†; Bayro; Flogoprofen; Zenavan; Switz.: Activon; Etofen; Rheumon; Traumalix.
Multi-ingredient: Aust.: Thermo-Rheumon; Ger.: Thermo-Rheumon.

Etorphine Hydrochloride (6227-l)

Etorphine Hydrochloride (BANM, rINNM).
M-99; 19-Propylorvinol Hydrochloride. (6R,7R,14R)-7,8-Dihydro-7-(1R-1-hydroxy-1-methylbutyl)-6-O-methyl-6,14α-ethenomorphine hydrochloride; (2R)-2-[(−)-(5R,6R,7R,14R)-4,5-Epoxy-3-hydroxy-6-methoxy-9α-methyl-6,14-ethenomorphinan-7-yl]pentan-2-ol hydrochloride.
$C_{25}H_{33}NO_4, HCl = 448.0$.
CAS — 14521-96-1 (etorphine); 13764-49-3 (etorphine hydrochloride).
Pharmacopoeias. In BP(Vet).

Pharmacopoeial description
BP(Vet) 2001: A white or almost white microcrystalline powder. Sparingly soluble in water and in alcohol; very slightly sol-

---

The symbol † denotes a preparation no longer actively marketed

uble in chloroform; practically insoluble in ether. A 2% solution in water has a pH of 4.0 to 5.5. Protect from light.

Dependence and Withdrawal
As for Opioid Analgesics, p.66.

Adverse Effects and Treatment
As for Opioid Analgesics in general, p.67. Etorphine is not used therapeutically in humans.

Etorphine hydrochloride is highly potent and rapid acting; minute amounts can exert serious effects leading to coma. It may be absorbed through skin and mucous membranes. It is thus advisable to inject an antagonist *immediately* following contamination of skin or mucous membranes with preparations containing etorphine hydrochloride and to wash the affected areas copiously. Accidental injection or needle scratch should also be treated immediately by injecting an antagonist. Naloxone is preferred as the antagonist in medical treatment. However, veterinary preparations of etorphine are supplied with a preparation containing diprenorphine hydrochloride (Revivon) and this should be used for immediate first-aid antagonism if naloxone is not available.

Uses and Administration
Etorphine hydrochloride is a highly potent opioid analgesic (p.68) used for reversible neuroleptanalgesia (see under Anaesthetic Techniques, p.1256) in veterinary medicine. It is given with acepromazine maleate or methotrimeprazine [levomepromazine] (Immobilon) to restrain animals and prior to minor veterinary surgery. The duration of action of etorphine is up to about 45 to 90 minutes depending on the species but it may be longer in man, especially if the large animal preparation is involved.

Famprofazone (2645-r)
Famprofazone (BAN, rINN).
4-Isopropyl-2-methyl-3-[methyl(α-methylphenethyl)aminomethyl]-1-phenyl-3-pyrazolin-5-one.
$C_{24}H_{31}N_3O = 377.5$.
CAS — 22881-35-2.

Profile
Famprofazone has analgesic and antipyretic properties and has been given by mouth, usually in conjunction with other analgesics.

Preparations
Proprietary Preparations (details are given in Part 3)
Multi-ingredient: *Ger.:* Gewodin.

Felbinac (2491-t)
Felbinac (BAN, USAN, rINN).
CL-83544; LJC-10141. Biphenyl-4-ylacetic acid.
$C_{14}H_{12}O_2 = 212.2$.
CAS — 5728-52-9.
ATC — M02AA08.
Pharmacopoeias. In Br.

Pharmacopoeial description
BP 2001: A fine white, crystalline powder. Practically insoluble in water; sparingly soluble in dehydrated alcohol; freely soluble in dimethylformamide.

Adverse Effects and Precautions
Mild local reactions such as erythema, dermatitis, and pruritus have occurred in patients using felbinac topically. Bronchospasm or wheeziness has also been reported. Gastrointestinal disturbances may occur.

Felbinac preparations should be avoided in patients with a history of hypersensitivity reactions to aspirin or other NSAIDs.

◊ The UK Committee on Safety of Medicines had received 49 reports of adverse reactions associated with felbinac by October 1989, about 11 months after it was released on the UK market.[1] Bronchospasm or wheeziness was reported in 8 patients using felbinac gel. Four of these patients had a history of asthma of whom 3 were reported to have had a similar reaction to aspirin or other NSAIDs. Other reported reactions included skin rashes (17 cases), local application site reactions (7), and dyspepsia (6).
1. Committee on Safety of Medicines. Felbinac (Traxam) and bronchospasm. *Current Problems* 27 1989.

Uses and Administration
Felbinac, an active metabolite of fenbufen (p.36), is an NSAID (p.65). It is used topically in the symptomatic treatment of musculoskeletal pain including that due to soft-tissue injuries. It is applied as a 3% gel or a 3.17% foam to unbroken skin over affected areas 2 to 4 times daily. The total daily dose of gel or foam should not exceed 25 g regardless of the size or number of affected areas. Therapy should be reviewed after 14 days.

Diisopropanolamine felbinac has been used similarly.

◊ References.
1. Hosie GAC. The topical NSAID, felbinac, versus oral ibuprofen: a comparison of efficacy in the treatment of acute lower back injury. *Br J Clin Res* 1993; **4:** 5–17.

Preparations
BP 2001: Felbinac Cutaneous Foam; Felbinac Gel.
Proprietary Preparations (details are given in Part 3)
Aust.: Target; *Belg.:* Flexfree†; *Denm.:* Dolinac†; *Ger.:* Dolinac†; Spalt Schmerz-Gel; Target; *Irl.:* Traxam; *Ital.:* Dolinac; Traxam; *Jpn:* Napageln†; Seltouch; *S.Afr.:* Dolinac†; *Switz.:* Dolo Target; Target†; *UK:* Traxam.

Fenbufen (2646-f)
Fenbufen (BAN, USAN, rINN).
CL-82204; Fenbufenum. 4-(Biphenyl-4-yl)-4-oxobutyric acid.
$C_{16}H_{14}O_3 = 254.3$.
CAS — 36330-85-5.
ATC — M01AE05.
Pharmacopoeias. In Eur. (see p.vi) and Jpn.

Pharmacopoeial description
Ph. Eur.: A white fine crystalline powder. Very slightly soluble in water; slightly soluble in alcohol, in acetone, and in dichloromethane.

Adverse Effects and Precautions
As for NSAIDs in general, p.63, although the commonest side-effects of fenbufen are skin rashes, particularly in women and in patients with seronegative rheumatoid arthritis or psoriatic arthritis. Disorders such as erythema multiforme and Stevens-Johnson syndrome have also been reported. A small number of patients who develop rash may go on to develop a severe illness characterised by a pulmonary eosinophilia or an allergic alveolitis. Treatment with fenbufen should be discontinued immediately if a rash appears.

The UK manufacturer advises that fenbufen should be avoided in breast-feeding mothers, because of the presence of its metabolites in breast milk.

Effects on the blood. Haemolytic anaemia[1] and aplastic anaemia[2] have been reported in patients receiving fenbufen.
1. Martland T, Stone WD. Haemolytic anaemia associated with fenbufen. *BMJ* 1988; **297:** 921.
2. Andrews R, Russell N. Aplastic anaemia associated with a nonsteroidal anti-inflammatory drug: relapse after exposure to another such drug. *BMJ* 1990; **301:** 38.

Effects on the lungs. In January 1989 the UK Committee on Safety of Medicines reported that it had received 7 reports of a suspected association between rash and an allergic interstitial lung disorder in patients receiving fenbufen.[1] In 5 patients, the lung disorder was diagnosed as pulmonary eosinophilia; in the 2 other patients the pulmonary component of the reaction was described as allergic alveolitis. Several of these reactions have been reported in the literature.[2,3]
1. Committee on Safety of Medicines. Fenbufen, rash and pulmonary eosinophilia. *Current Problems* 24 1989.
2. Swinburn CR. Alveolitis and haemolytic anaemia induced by azapropazone. *BMJ* 1987; **294:** 375.
3. Burton GH. Rash and pulmonary eosinophilia associated with fenbufen. *BMJ* 1990; **300:** 82–3.

Effects on the skin. In September 1988 the UK Committee on Safety of Medicines reported[1] that it was still receiving large numbers of reports of adverse reactions to fenbufen when such reports were expected to have declined. Fenbufen was the most commonly reported suspect drug in 1986 and 1987. At the time of the report more than 6000 such reports had been received, 80% concerning mucocutaneous reactions and most involving a generalised florid erythematous rash, often with pruritus. There were 178 reports of erythema multiforme, 30 of Stevens-Johnson syndrome, and 2 fatalities.
1. Committee on Safety of Medicines. Fenbufen and mucocutaneous reactions. *Current Problems* 23 1988.

Hypersensitivity. See under Effects on the Lungs (above).

Interactions
For interactions associated with NSAIDs, see p.65.
Concomitant administration of fenbufen and aspirin may result in decreased serum concentrations of fenbufen and its metabolites.

Pharmacokinetics
Fenbufen is absorbed from the gastrointestinal tract and peak plasma concentrations are reached in about 70 minutes. Fenbufen is over 99% bound to plasma proteins. It is metabolised in the liver to active metabolites. Fenbufen and its metabolites are reported to have plasma half-lives of about 10 hours and are mainly eliminated as conjugates in the urine. Metabolites of fenbufen have been detected in breast milk.

Uses and Administration
Fenbufen, a propionic acid derivative, is an NSAID (p.65). It is given by mouth for the relief of pain and inflammation associated with musculoskeletal and joint disorders such as rheumatoid arthritis, osteoarthritis, and ankylosing spondylitis in doses of 900 mg daily by mouth; the dose may be either 450 mg in the morning and evening or 300 mg in the morning with 600 mg in the evening.

Preparations
BP 2001: Fenbufen Capsules; Fenbufen Tablets.
Proprietary Preparations (details are given in Part 3)
Aust.: Lederfen; *Denm.:* Cinopal†; *Fr.:* Cinopal†; *Irl.:* Lederfen; *Israel:* Lederfen; *Ital.:* Cinopal†; *Port.:* Reugast; *S.Afr.:* Cinopal†; *Spain:* Cincopal; *Thai.:* Cepal; Cinopal; *UK:* Lederfen.

Fenoprofen Calcium (2649-h)
Fenoprofen Calcium (BANM, USAN, rINNM).
69323; 53858 (acid). Lilly-61169 (sodium salt). Calcium (±)-2-(3-phenoxyphenyl)propionate dihydrate.
$(C_{15}H_{13}O_3)_2Ca, 2H_2O = 558.6$.
CAS — 31879-05-7 (fenoprofen); 34597-40-5 (anhydrous fenoprofen calcium); 53746-45-5 (fenoprofen calcium dihydrate).
Pharmacopoeias. In Br. and US.

Fenoprofen calcium (dihydrate) 1.1 g is approximately equivalent to 1 g of fenoprofen.

Pharmacopoeial description
BP 2001: A white or almost white odourless or almost odourless crystalline powder. Slightly soluble in water and in chloroform; soluble in alcohol.

USP 25: A white crystalline powder. Slightly soluble in water, in methyl alcohol, and in n-hexanol; practically insoluble in chloroform. Store in airtight containers.

Adverse Effects and Precautions
As for NSAIDs in general, p.63. Dysuria, cystitis, haematuria, interstitial nephritis, and renal failure have been reported with fenoprofen. Nephrotic syndrome, which may be preceded by fever, rash, arthralgia, oliguria, azotaemia, and anuria, has also occurred. Upper respiratory-tract infection and nasopharyngitis have been reported. There have been reports of severe hepatic reactions, including jaundice and fatal hepatitis.

Effects on the blood. Haematological adverse effects including agranulocytosis,[1] aplastic anaemia,[2] and thrombocytopenia[3,4] have been reported in patients taking fenoprofen; the manufacturers also report haemolytic anaemia.
1. Simon SD, Kosmin M. Fenoprofen and agranulocytosis. *N Engl J Med* 1978; **299:** 490.
2. Ashraf M, *et al.* Aplastic anaemia associated with fenoprofen. *BMJ* 1982; 284: 1301–2.
3. Simpson RE, *et al.* Acute thrombocytopenia associated with fenoprofen. *N Engl J Med* 1978; **298:** 629–30.
4. Katz ME, Wang P. Fenoprofen-associated thrombocytopenia. *Ann Intern Med* 1980; **92:** 262.

Effects on the kidneys. References to reversible renal failure and nephrotic syndrome in patients taking fenoprofen.[1-4]
1. Brezin JH, *et al.* Reversible renal failure and nephrotic syndrome associated with nonsteroidal anti-inflammatory drugs. *N Engl J Med* 1979; **301:** 1271–3.
2. Curt GA, *et al.* Reversible rapidly progressive renal failure with nephrotic syndrome due to fenoprofen calcium. *Ann Intern Med* 1980; **92:** 72–3.
3. Handa SP. Renal effects of fenoprofen. *Ann Intern Med* 1980; **93:** 508–9.
4. Lorch J, *et al.* Renal effects of fenoprofen. *Ann Intern Med* 1980; **93:** 509.

Effects on the liver. Cholestatic jaundice and hepatitis developed in a 68-year-old woman after receiving fenoprofen 600 mg four times daily for 7 weeks. Subsequent use of naproxen and indometacin did not result in hepatotoxicity.[1] However, there has been a report of cross-hepatotoxicity between fenoprofen and naproxen.[2]
1. Stennett DJ, *et al.* Fenoprofen-induced hepatotoxicity. *Am J Hosp Pharm* 1978; **35:** 901.
2. Andrejak M, *et al.* Cross hepatotoxicity between non-steroidal anti-inflammatory drugs. *BMJ* 1987; **295:** 180–1.

Effects on the skin. Toxic epidermal necrolysis was associated with fenoprofen in 2 patients.[1]
1. Stotts JS, *et al.* Fenoprofen-induced toxic epidermal necrolysis. *J Am Acad Dermatol* 1988; **18:** 755–7.

Overdosage. A report of coma, respiratory depression, hypotension, and metabolic acidosis in a patient who had ingested between 24 and 36 g of fenoprofen.[1] The patient responded to gastric lavage and activated charcoal and intensive supportive care.

1. Kolodzik JM, *et al.* Nonsteroidal anti-inflammatory drugs and coma: a case report of fenoprofen overdose. *Ann Emerg Med* 1990; **19**: 378–81.

Interactions
For interactions associated with NSAIDs, see p.65.

Aspirin is reported to reduce plasma concentrations of fenoprofen.

Antiepileptics. *Phenobarbital* might increase the rate of metabolism of fenoprofen.[1]

1. Helleberg L, *et al.* A pharmacokinetic interaction in man between phenobarbitone and fenoprofen, a new anti-inflammatory agent. *Br J Clin Pharmacol* 1974; **1**: 371–4.

Pharmacokinetics
Fenoprofen is readily absorbed from the gastrointestinal tract; bioavailability is about 85% but food and milk may reduce the rate and extent of absorption. Peak plasma concentrations occur 1 to 2 hours after a dose. The plasma half-life is about 3 hours. Fenoprofen is 99% bound to plasma proteins. About 90% of a dose is excreted in the urine in 24 hours, chiefly as the glucuronide and the glucuronide of hydroxylated fenoprofen. Fenoprofen is distributed into breast milk but the amount is considered by some authorities to be too small to be harmful to a breast-fed infant.

Uses and Administration
Fenoprofen, a propionic acid derivative, is an NSAID (p.65). It is used as the calcium salt in the management of mild to moderate pain and for the relief of pain and inflammation associated with disorders such as osteoarthritis, rheumatoid arthritis, and ankylosing spondylitis. A usual initial dose is the equivalent of 300 to 600 mg of fenoprofen three or four times daily, adjusted thereafter according to response. It has been recommended that the total daily dose should not exceed 3 g (UK) or 3.2 g (USA). In the USA, lower doses of 200 mg every 4 to 6 hours are recommended for mild to moderate pain.

Preparations
BP 2001: Fenoprofen Tablets;
USP 25: Fenoprofen Calcium Capsules; Fenoprofen Calcium Tablets.

Proprietary Preparations (details are given in Part 3)
Aust.: Nalfon; *Braz.:* Trandor; *Canad.:* Nalfon; *Denm.:* Nalfon; *Fr.:* Nalgesic; *Hong Kong:* Fenopron; *Irl.:* Fenopron; *Ital.:* Fepron; *Mex.:* Nalfon; *Neth.:* Fepron†; *S.Afr.:* Fenopron; *UK:* Fenopron; *USA:* Nalfon.

Fentanyl   (12127-z)

Fentanyl *(BAN, rINN)*.

Fentanylum. N-(1-Phenethyl-4-piperidyl) propionanilide.
$C_{22}H_{28}N_2O = 336.5$.
CAS — 437-38-7.
ATC — N01AH01; N02AB03.
Pharmacopoeias. In Eur. (see p.vi).

Pharmacopoeial description
Ph. Eur.: A white or almost white polymorphic powder. Practically insoluble in water; freely soluble in alcohol and in methyl alcohol. Protect from light.

Fentanyl Citrate   (6228-y)

Fentanyl Citrate *(BANM, USAN, rINNM)*.

Fentanyli Citras; McN-JR-4263-49; Phentanyl Citrate; R-4263. N-(1-Phenethyl-4-piperidyl)propionanilide dihydrogen citrate.
$C_{22}H_{28}N_2O,C_6H_8O_7 = 528.6$.
CAS — 990-73-8.
Pharmacopoeias. In Chin., Eur. (see p.vi), Jpn, Pol., and US.

Fentanyl citrate 157 µg is approximately equivalent to 100 µg of fentanyl.

Pharmacopoeial description
Ph. Eur.: White or almost white powder. Soluble in water; sparingly soluble in alcohol; freely soluble in methyl alcohol. Protect from light.

USP 25: A white crystalline powder or white glistening crystals. Sparingly soluble in water; slightly soluble in chloroform; soluble in methyl alcohol. Protect from light.

◊ CAUTION. *Avoid contact with skin and the inhalation of particles of fentanyl citrate.*

Incompatibility. Fentanyl citrate is incompatible with thiopental sodium and methohexital sodium.

The symbol † denotes a preparation no longer actively marketed

---

A thick white precipitate formed in the intravenous tubing when fentanyl citrate with droperidol was given shortly after nafcillin sodium. There was no precipitate when fentanyl citrate alone was mixed with nafcillin sodium.[1]

Fentanyl citrate underwent rapid and extensive loss when admixed with fluorouracil in PVC containers.[2] The loss was due to sorption of fentanyl to the PVC containers as a result of the alkaline pH of the admixture, and presumably could occur from admixture of fentanyl citrate with any sufficiently alkaline drug.

See also under Stability, below.

1. Jeglum EL, *et al.* Nafcillin sodium incompatibility with acidic solutions. *Am J Hosp Pharm* 1981; **38**: 462, 464.
2. Xu QA, *et al.* Rapid loss of fentanyl citrate admixed with fluorouracil in polyvinyl chloride containers. *Ann Pharmacother* 1997; **31**: 297–302.

Stability. In a 48-hour study fentanyl citrate was stable when stored at room temperature under usual light conditions in glass or PVC containers of 5% glucose or 0.9% sodium chloride solution;[1] the concentration of fentanyl delivered by a patient-controlled system was relatively constant throughout a 30-hour study period. Fentanyl citrate injection diluted to 20 µg per mL with 0.9% sodium chloride was stable for 30 days at 3° or 23° in PVC reservoirs for portable infusion pumps.[2] An admixture of fentanyl citrate and bupivacaine in 0.9% sodium chloride[3] appeared compatible and stable when stored for up to 30 days at 3° or 23° in a portable infusion pump. In another study[4] the stability of solutions containing fentanyl, bupivacaine, and adrenaline [epinephrine], alone and in combination was studied over a period of 56 days which varied as to temperatures in the light or in the dark in PVC bags. Both fentanyl and bupivacaine were adsorbed from solution onto the PVC for the first 3 days but thereafter concentrations of these drugs remained relatively stable; freezing appeared to slow the concentration change for bupivacaine but not for fentanyl. Solutions containing adrenaline [epinephrine] became more acidic during the study as the adrenaline [epinephrine] progressively deteriorated but this was greatly reduced by freezing. Autoclaving produced a further reduction in the concentration of all drugs. There was no sign of precipitation from any of the solutions studied. Fentanyl is potentially unstable in PVC containers when admixed with alkaline drugs (see under Incompatibility, above).

1. Kowalski SR, Gourlay GK. Stability of fentanyl citrate in glass and plastic containers and in a patient-controlled delivery system. *Am J Hosp Pharm* 1990; **47**: 1584–7.
2. Allen LV, *et al.* Stability of fentanyl citrate in 0.9% sodium chloride solution in portable infusion pumps. *Am J Hosp Pharm* 1990; **47**: 1572–4.
3. Tu Y-H, *et al.* Stability of fentanyl citrate and bupivacaine hydrochloride in portable pump reservoirs. *Am J Hosp Pharm* 1990; **47**: 2037–40.
4. Dawson PJ, *et al.* Stability of fentanyl, bupivacaine and adrenaline solutions for extradural infusion. *Br J Anaesth* 1992; **68**: 414–17.

Dependence and Withdrawal
As for Opioid Analgesics, p.66. Fentanyl and illicitly manufactured analogues are subject to abuse (see under Precautions, below).

◊ Movement disorders, extreme irritability, and symptoms characteristic of opioid abstinence syndrome have been reported in children after withdrawal of prolonged fentanyl infusions.[1] One group of workers reported that plasma concentrations required to produce satisfactory sedation increased steadily in neonates receiving continuous infusions suggesting the development of tolerance to the sedating effects of fentanyl.[2]

Acute opioid withdrawal syndrome has also been seen in cancer patients switched from modified-release oral morphine to transdermal fentanyl despite adequate analgesia being maintained.[3]

1. Lane JC, *et al.* Movement disorder after withdrawal of fentanyl infusion. *J Pediatr* 1991; **119**: 649–51.
2. Arnold JH, *et al.* Changes in the pharmacodynamic response to fentanyl in neonates during continuous infusion. *J Pediatr* 1991; **119**: 639–43.
3. Anonymous. Opiate withdrawal with transdermal fentanyl. *Pharm J* 1995; **255**: 680.

Adverse Effects and Treatment
As for Opioid Analgesics in general, p.67.

Respiratory depression which occurs especially with high doses of fentanyl responds to naloxone (see also under Effects on the Respiratory System, below). Atropine may be used to block the vagal effects of fentanyl such as bradycardia. Unlike morphine, fentanyl is reported not to cause significant histamine release. Transient hypotension may follow intravenous administration. Muscle rigidity may occur and may require administration of neuromuscular blockers.

Local reactions such as rash, erythema, and itching have been reported with the transdermal patches.

Effects on the cardiovascular system. For a reference to the effects of fentanyl on histamine release compared with some other opioids, see under Pethidine, p.75.

Effects on mental function. Fentanyl had some dose-related effects on mental function and motor activity in healthy subjects,[1] but immediate and delayed recall were not affected. See also under Alfentanil (p.11).

Acute toxic delirium has been reported following treatment with transdermal fentanyl.[2]

1. Scamman FL, *et al.* Ventilatory and mental effects of alfentanil and fentanyl. *Acta Anaesthesiol Scand* 1984; **28**: 63–7.
2. Kuzma PJ, *et al.* Acute toxic delirium: an uncommon reaction to transdermal fentanyl. *Anesthesiology* 1995; **83**: 869–71.

Effects on the nervous system. There have been reports of seizures with low and high doses of fentanyl or sufentanil.[1] There was, however, no EEG evidence of cortical seizure activity in a patient who had seizure-like muscle movements during a fentanyl infusion;[2] the muscle movements might have been due to myoclonus produced by depression of higher CNS inhibitory centres or to a pronounced form of opioid-induced muscle rigidity.

For a report of encephalopathy associated with prolonged use of fentanyl and midazolam in infants in intensive care, see under Encephalopathy in the Adverse Effects of Diazepam, p.676.

1. Zaccara G, *et al.* Clinical features, pathogenesis and management of drug-induced seizures. *Drug Safety* 1990; **5**: 109–51.
2. Scott JC, Sarnquist FH. Seizure-like movements during a fentanyl infusion with absence of seizure activity in a simultaneous EEG recording. *Anesthesiology* 1985; **62**: 812–14.

Effects on the respiratory system. Fentanyl, like other opioid agonists, causes dose-related respiratory depression; it is significant with *intravenous* fentanyl doses of more than 200 µg and may be more prolonged than analgesia. Anaesthesia with fentanyl may result in either prolonged or delayed respiratory depression postoperatively.[1] If present at the end of operation it should be reversed by an opioid antagonist such as naloxone; alternatively a respiratory stimulant such as doxapram that does not reverse analgesia has been given. Buprenorphine has also been tried for the reversal of respiratory depression induced by fentanyl (see Anaesthesia, p.22). Because of the risk of delayed respiratory depression patients should continue to be monitored postoperatively until spontaneous breathing has been re-established. Severe respiratory depression in a 14-month-old child following intravenous sedation with fentanyl and midazolam has highlighted the necessity for careful monitoring when giving respiratory depressants concurrently.[2]

Rigidity of the respiratory muscles (chest wall rigidity) may occur during fentanyl anaesthesia. The effects can be minimised by using a slow intravenous injection but administration of a neuromuscular blocker may be required to allow artificial ventilation; rigidity has been reversed postoperatively by naloxone. Similar muscle rigidity induced by alfentanil could be attenuated by pretreatment with a benzodiazepine whereas small doses of neuromuscular blockers appeared to be ineffective.[3]

The risk of respiratory depression associated with *epidural* administration of fentanyl, a highly lipid-soluble opioid, has been considered relatively small and only slight ventilatory depression was noted[4] following a dose of 50 µg. However, profound delayed respiratory depression has been reported in 2 women 100 minutes[5] and 80 minutes[6] respectively after fentanyl 100 µg had been administered epidurally for caesarean section. No adverse effects on neonatal respiration or neurobehaviour were detected in a study[7] of neonates of mothers given epidural infusions of bupivacaine and fentanyl during labour.

Respiratory depression is also a risk with *topically* applied fentanyl preparations. Severe hypoventilation with some fatalities has occurred in patients receiving fentanyl through a transdermal patch for minor painful conditions.[8]

1. Bennett MRD, Adams AP. Postoperative respiratory complications of opiates. *Clin Anaesthesiol* 1983; **1**: 41–56.
2. Yaster M, *et al.* Midazolam-fentanyl intravenous sedation in children: case report of respiratory arrest. *Pediatrics* 1990; **86**: 463–7.
3. Sanford TJ, *et al.* Pretreatment with sedative-hypnotics, but not with nondepolarizing muscle relaxants, attenuates alfentanil-induced muscle rigidity. *J Clin Anesth* 1994; **6**: 473–80.
4. Morisot P, *et al.* Ventilatory response to carbon dioxide during extradural anaesthesia with lignocaine and fentanyl. *Br J Anaesth* 1989; **63**: 97–102.
5. Brockway MS, *et al.* Profound respiratory depression after extradural fentanyl. *Br J Anaesth* 1990; **64**: 243–5.
6. Wang CY. Respiratory depression after extradural fentanyl. *Br J Anaesth* 1992; **69**: 544.
7. Porter J, *et al.* Effect of epidural fentanyl on neonatal respiration. *Anesthesiology* 1998; **89**: 79–85.
8. FDC Reports Pink Sheet 1994; January 24: 12.

Effects on the skin. Report of a patient[1] who developed a macular rash covering the whole body, except for the face and scalp, while using transdermal fentanyl patches.

1. Stoukides CA, Stegman M. Diffuse rash associated with transdermal fentanyl. *Clin Pharm* 1992; **11**: 222.

Precautions

As for Opioid Analgesics in general, p.68.

Caution is advised in patients with myasthenia gravis; the effects of muscular rigidity on respiration may be particularly pronounced in these patients.

Absorption of fentanyl from transdermal patches may be increased as the temperature rises and patients should therefore avoid exposing the patch to external heat; similarly, patients with fever may require monitoring because of increased absorption. It may take 17 hours or longer for plasma concentrations of fentanyl to decrease by 50% after removal of a patch; patients who have experienced side-effects should be monitored for up to 24 hours and those requiring replacement opioid therapy should initially receive low doses increased gradually thereafter.

Abuse. Several synthetic analogues of fentanyl, so-called 'designer drugs' have been manufactured illicitly for recreational use, particularly in the USA. They are highly potent and respiratory depression and death may occur very rapidly.[1] The 'fentanyls' have been smoked or snorted as well as injected intravenously.

Fentanyl analogues identified by WHO[2,3] as being subject to street abuse or likely to be abused include: alpha-methylfentanyl (also known as 'China white' or 'synthetic heroin'), 3-methylfentanyl, acetyl-alpha-methylfentanyl, alpha-methylthiofentanyl, para-fluorofentanyl, beta-hydroxyfentanyl, beta-hydroxy-3-methylfentanyl, thiofentanyl, and 3-methylthiofentanyl.

Fentanyl itself is also subject to illicit use. It is chemically unrelated to morphine and therefore not reactive to screening tests for morphine-related opioids. It has therefore been recommended[4] that fentanyl should be tested for specifically in cases with suspected opioid misuse.

Used fentanyl transdermal patches may contain significant amounts of fentanyl[5] and have been subject to abuse. The manufacturers advise that used patches should be folded firmly in half, adhesive side inwards to conceal the release membrane, and disposed of safely.

1. Buchanan JF, Brown CR. 'Designer drugs': a problem in clinical toxicology. *Med Toxicol* 1988; **3:** 1–17.
2. WHO. WHO expert committee on drug dependence: twenty-fourth report. *WHO Tech Rep Ser 761* 1988.
3. WHO. WHO expert committee on drug dependence: twenty-sixth report. *WHO Tech Rep Ser 787* 1989.
4. Berens AIL, et al. Illicit fentanyl in Europe. *Lancet* 1996; **347:** 1334–5.
5. Marquardt KA, et al. Fentanyl remaining in a transdermal system following three days of continuous use. *Ann Pharmacother* 1995; **29:** 969–71.

Administration. Fentanyl is much more lipid-soluble than morphine and after standard single intravenous doses has a rapid onset and short duration of action. However, fentanyl is rapidly redistributed in the body and has a longer elimination half-life than morphine (see Pharmacokinetics, below). Hence with high or repeated doses fentanyl becomes a relatively long-acting drug and to avoid accumulation patients should be monitored and doses adjusted accordingly.

Repeated intra-operative doses of fentanyl should be given with care, since not only may the respiratory depression persist into the postoperative period but it may become apparent for the first time postoperatively when the patient is away from immediate nursing attention.

Interactions

For interactions associated with opioid analgesics, see p.68.

Antivirals. *Ritonavir* might prolong fentanyl-induced respiratory depression. The plasma clearance of fentanyl was decreased, and the elimination half-life and area under the plasma concentration-time curve increased, when given concomitantly with ritonavir in a study in healthy subjects.[1]

1. Olkkola KT, et al. Ritonavir's role in reducing fentanyl clearance and prolonging its half-life. *Anesthesiology* 1999; **91:** 681–5.

Benzodiazepines. For the effects of concomitant use of opioids such as fentanyl with benzodiazepines, see under Analgesics in the Interactions of Diazepam, p.677.

Propofol. For reference to the effect that concomitant administration of fentanyl has on blood concentrations of propofol, see p.1266.

Pharmacokinetics

After parenteral administration fentanyl citrate has a rapid onset and short duration of action. It is metabolised in the liver by *N*-dealkylation and hydroxylation. Metabolites and some unchanged drug are excreted mainly in the urine. The short duration of action is probably due to rapid redistribution into the tissues rather than metabolism and excretion. An elimination half-life of about 4 hours reflects slower

release from tissue depots. About 80% has been reported to be bound to plasma proteins. Fentanyl appears in the cerebrospinal fluid. It crosses the placenta and small amounts have been detected in breast milk.

◊ Marked differences in results of pharmacokinetic studies of fentanyl have been attributed[1] to differences in assay methods. The need for sensitive assay methods has been emphasised because the potency of fentanyl means that small doses are used. However, there are differences in pharmacokinetic parameters that occur between bolus administration and prolonged infusion with highly lipophilic drugs such as fentanyl.[2] Terminal half-lives ranging from 2 to 7 hours have been reported in healthy subjects and surgical patients. However, the duration of action of fentanyl after a single intravenous dose of up to 100 µg may be only 30 to 60 minutes as a result of rapid redistribution into the tissues. The manufacturers have given values for a three-compartment pharmacokinetic model with a distribution time of 1.7 minutes, a redistribution time of 13 minutes, and a terminal elimination half-life of 219 minutes. Administration of repeated or large doses, or continuous infusions, may result in accumulation and a more prolonged action.

The clinical significance of secondary peak plasma-fentanyl concentrations and the possible role of entero-systemic recirculation[3] has been controversial, but some[4] considered that irregular decay curves were not unlikely for lipophilic compounds such as fentanyl, especially in patients undergoing operations and subject to large changes in blood flow. Unexpectedly high plasma-fentanyl concentrations in a patient following epidural administration were thought to be a result of aortic clamping and might reflect the effect of changes in blood flow.[5]

The main metabolites of fentanyl excreted in the urine have been identified as 4-*N*-(*N*-propionylanilino) piperidine and 4-*N*-(*N*-hydroxypropionylanilino) piperidine; 1-(2-phenethyl)-4-*N*-(*N*-hydroxypropionylanilino) piperidine is a minor metabolite.[6] According to Moore et al.[4] fentanyl has no active or toxic metabolites.

1. Mather LE. Clinical pharmacokinetics of fentanyl and its newer derivatives. *Clin Pharmacokinet* 1983; **8:** 422–46.
2. Scholz J, et al. Clinical pharmacokinetics of alfentanil, fentanyl and sufentanil: an update. *Clin Pharmacokinet* 1996; **31:** 275–92.
3. Bennett MRD, Adams AP. Postoperative respiratory complications of opiates. *Clin Anaesthesiol* 1983; **1:** 41–56.
4. Moore RA, et al. Opiate metabolism and excretion. *Baillieres Clin Anaesthesiol* 1987; **1:** 829–58.
5. Bullingham RES, et al. Unexpectedly high plasma fentanyl levels after epidural use. *Lancet* 1980; **i:** 1361–2.
6. Goromaru T, et al. Identification and quantitative determination of fentanyl metabolites in patients by gas chromatography-mass spectrometry. *Anesthesiology* 1984; **61:** 73–7.

Administration. Some references to the pharmacokinetics of fentanyl following constant rate intravenous infusion,[1] transdermal application,[2] use of the oral transmucosal route,[3] intranasal administration,[4] subcutaneous infusion,[5] and epidural administration.[6,7]

1. Duthie DJR, et al. Pharmacokinetics of fentanyl during constant rate iv infusion for the relief of pain after surgery. *Br J Anaesth* 1986; **58:** 950–6.
2. Grond S, et al. Clinical pharmacokinetics of transdermal opioids: focus on transdermal fentanyl. *Clin Pharmacokinet* 2000; **38:** 59–89.
3. Streisand JB, et al. Absorption and bioavailability of oral transmucosal fentanyl citrate. *Anesthesiology* 1991; **75:** 223–9.
4. Walter SH, et al. Pharmacokinetics of intranasal fentanyl. *Br J Anaesth* 1993; **70** (suppl 1): 108.
5. Miller RS, et al. Plasma concentrations of fentanyl with subcutaneous infusion in palliative care patients. *Br J Clin Pharmacol* 1995; **40:** 553–6.
6. Gourlay GK, et al. Pharmacokinetics of fentanyl in lumbar and cervical CSF following lumbar epidural and intravenous administration. *Pain* 1989; **38:** 253–9.
7. Bader AM, et al. Maternal and neonatal fentanyl and bupivacaine concentrations after epidural infusion during labor. *Anesth Analg* 1995; **81:** 829–32.

Cardiopulmonary bypass. The pharmacokinetics of fentanyl during cardiopulmonary bypass.[1,2] In general, studies indicate that serum concentrations of fentanyl decrease initially and then remain stable during the bypass procedure. The fall in concentrations has been attributed to haemodilution although adsorption to the bypass apparatus has also been demonstrated.

1. Buylaert WA, et al. Cardiopulmonary bypass and the pharmacokinetics of drugs: an update. *Clin Pharmacokinet* 1989; **17:** 10–26.
2. Gedney JA, Ghosh S. Pharmacokinetics of analgesics, sedatives and anaesthetic agents during cardiopulmonary bypass. *Br J Anaesth* 1995; **75:** 344–51.

Children. The disposition of intravenous fentanyl 10 to 50 µg per kg body-weight in 14 neonates undergoing various major surgical procedures was highly variable.[1] The mean elimination half-life of 317 minutes and other pharmacokinetic parameters including volume of distribution and total body clearance were greater than reported in adults, but both pharmacodynamic and pharmacokinetic mechanisms appeared responsible for the very prolonged respiratory depression that can occur in neonates after fentanyl administration. In 9 premature neonates given fentanyl 30 µg per kg intravenously for induction of anaesthesia[2] the elimination half-life ranged from 6 to 32

hours, but cautious interpretation was advised because of the method of calculation.

1. Koehntop DE, et al. Pharmacokinetics of fentanyl in neonates. *Anesth Analg* 1986; **65:** 227–32.
2. Collins C, et al. Fentanyl pharmacokinetics and hemodynamic effects in preterm infants during ligation of patent ductus arteriosus. *Anesth Analg* 1985; **64:** 1078–80.

The elderly. Bentley et al.[1] reported the elimination half-life of fentanyl to be increased from 265 minutes in patients with a mean age of 36 years to 945 minutes in those with a mean age of 67 years. Scott and Stanski[2] were critical of the relatively short sampling time used and in contrast to Bentley et al. they found that major fentanyl pharmacokinetic parameters did not correlate with age. However, elderly patients had increased brain sensitivity to fentanyl, as demonstrated by EEG changes[2] and lower doses might be indicated in older patients for pharmacodynamic rather than pharmacokinetic reasons.

1. Bentley JB, et al. Age and fentanyl pharmacokinetics. *Anesth Analg* 1982; **61:** 968–71.
2. Scott JC, Stanski DR. Decreased fentanyl and alfentanil dose requirements with age: a simultaneous pharmacokinetic and pharmacodynamic evaluation. *J Pharmacol Exp Ther* 1987; **240:** 159–66.

Hepatic impairment. The pharmacokinetics of fentanyl were not affected significantly in surgical patients with cirrhosis of the liver.[1] A 1987 review[2] considered that fentanyl had not been associated with clinical problems when given to patients with liver dysfunction.

1. Haberer JP, et al. Fentanyl pharmacokinetics in anaesthetized patients with cirrhosis. *Br J Anaesth* 1982; **54:** 1267–70.
2. Moore RA, et al. Opiate metabolism and excretion. *Baillieres Clin Anaesthesiol* 1987; **1:** 829–58.

Renal impairment. Clearance of fentanyl from plasma was reported to be enhanced in surgical patients with end-stage renal disease,[1] although clearance was reduced and elimination half-life increased in patients with renal failure undergoing transplantation,[2] possibly because of the influence of uraemia on metabolism in the liver. Nevertheless, a 1987 review[2] noted that fentanyl had no active or toxic metabolites and had not been associated with clinical problems when given to patients with renal dysfunction.

1. Corall IM, et al. Plasma concentrations of fentanyl in normal surgical patients and those with severe renal and hepatic disease. *Br J Anaesth* 1980; **52:** 101P.
2. Moore RA, et al. Opiate metabolism and excretion. *Baillieres Clin Anaesthesiol* 1987; **1:** 829–58.

Uses and Administration

Fentanyl, a phenylpiperidine derivative, is a potent opioid analgesic (p.68) chemically related to pethidine (p.76) and is primarily a µ-opioid agonist.

Fentanyl is used as an analgesic, an adjunct to general anaesthetics, and as an anaesthetic for induction and maintenance. It is also used as a respiratory depressant in the management of mechanically ventilated patients under intensive care. When used with an antipsychotic such as droperidol it can induce a state of neuroleptanalgesia in which the patient is calm and indifferent to his surroundings and is able to cooperate with the surgeon.

Fentanyl is usually administered by intramuscular or intravenous injection as the citrate or in transdermal patches as the base. It has also been given by epidural injection or by the transmucosal route as the citrate. Doses are expressed in terms of the base.

It is more lipid soluble than morphine and following an intravenous injection of 100 µg the effects of fentanyl begin almost immediately, although maximum analgesia and respiratory depression may not occur for several minutes; the duration of action of fentanyl depends on the dose and the intensity of the pain involved, and may vary from 10 minutes to several hours.

For **premedication** 50 to 100 µg of fentanyl may be given *intramuscularly* 30 to 60 minutes before the induction of anaesthesia.

As an **adjunct** to general anaesthesia, fentanyl is usually given by *intravenous* injection. Dosage recommendations show a wide range depending on the technique.

- *Patients with spontaneous respiration* may be given 50 to 200 µg of fentanyl as an initial dose with supplements of 50 µg. In the USA it is recommended that doses above 2 µg per kg body-weight should be used in conjunction with assisted ventilation. Significant respiratory depression follows doses of more than 200 µg.
- *Patients whose ventilation is assisted* may be given 300 to 3500 µg (up to 50 µg per kg) as an initial

dose with supplements of 100 to 200 μg or higher depending on the patient's response. High doses have been reported to moderate or attenuate the response to surgical stress (see under Anaesthesia, below).

- Reduced doses are used in *the elderly*.
- In the UK recommended initial doses for use as an adjunct to general anaesthesia for *children* above 2 years of age range from 3 to 5 μg per kg intravenously for those with *spontaneous respiration*; supplements of 1 μg per kg may be given. When *ventilation* is *assisted*, the initial recommended dose is 15 μg per kg, with supplements of 1 to 3 μg per kg. In the USA doses as low as 2 to 3 μg per kg are employed in children between the ages of 2 and 12 years. See also under Administration in Children, below.

Similar doses to those used for premedication may also be given by *intramuscular* injection **postoperatively**, and by *intramuscular* or *slow intravenous injection* as an adjunct to **regional anaesthesia**.

For the treatment of intractable **chronic pain** in adults when opioid analgesia is indicated *transdermal* patches delivering amounts of fentanyl ranging from 25 to 100 μg per hour are available.

- Doses should be individually titrated for each patient according to previous opioid usage. Initial dosages should not exceed 25 μg per hour in *opioid-naive* patients.
- For *patients who have been receiving a strong opioid analgesic* the initial dose of the fentanyl patch should be based on the previous 24-hour opioid requirement. Use of a patch providing 25 μg of fentanyl per hour is approximately equivalent to oral administration of 90 mg of morphine sulfate daily. During transfer to treatment with fentanyl patches previous opioid analgesic therapy should be phased out gradually in order to allow for the gradual increase in plasma-fentanyl concentrations.
- Patches should be replaced every 72 hours with the new patch being applied to a different site; use of the same area of the skin should be avoided for several days. More than one patch may be applied if doses greater than 100 μg per hour are required (applied at the same time to avoid confusion); additional or alternative analgesic therapy should be considered if doses greater than 300 μg per hour are required. Elderly or debilitated patients should be observed carefully for signs of toxicity and the dose reduced if necessary. Fentanyl patches are not appropriate for acute or postoperative pain.

A lozenge-on-a-stick lollipop dosage form of fentanyl citrate for *transmucosal* delivery is used as a premedicant and analgesic in anaesthesia and as an analgesic in the management of breakthrough cancer pain in those already receiving and tolerant to opioid treatment. Lozenges containing the equivalent of 100 μg to up to 1600 μg of fentanyl base are available.

- In *anaesthesia*, adults may receive up to a maximum of 5 μg per kg (2.5 to 5 μg per kg in the elderly); children weighing more than 10 kg may receive up to 15 μg per kg. The maximum dose for adults and children, regardless of weight, is 400 μg. Patients receiving the lozenges in this setting require constant supervision, including monitoring of respiratory function.
- In *cancer* patients, an initial unit dose of 200 μg may be taken over 15 minutes for an episode of breakthrough pain and repeated if necessary after a further 15 minutes. Doses are subsequently titrated according to response, up to a unit dose of 1600 μg if necessary. Once the patient has been stabilised on an effective dose, no more than 4 doses should be taken daily.

◊ References.
1. Clotz MA, Nahata MC. Clinical uses of fentanyl, sufentanil, and alfentanil. *Clin Pharm* 1991; **10**: 581–93.

Administration. INHALATION ROUTE. A study indicating that inhaled fentanyl can provide plasma concentrations similar to those after intravenous administration and that it can be used for patient-controlled analgesia.
1. Mather LE, *et al.* Pulmonary administration of aerosolised fentanyl: pharmacokinetic analysis of systemic delivery. *Br J Clin Pharmacol* 1998; **46**: 37–43.

INTRANASAL ROUTE. Studies[1-3] indicating that intranasal administration of fentanyl is as effective as intravenous administration for postoperative pain management and that it can be used in a patient-controlled analgesia system.
1. Striebel HW, *et al.* Intranasal fentanyl titration for postoperative pain management in an unselected population. *Anaesthesia* 1993; **48**: 753–7.
2. Striebel HW, *et al.* Patient-controlled intranasal analgesia: a method for noninvasive postoperative pain management. *Anesth Analg* 1996; **83**: 548–51.
3. Toussaint S, *et al.* Patient-controlled intranasal analgesia: effective alternative to intravenous PCA for postoperative pain relief. *Can J Anaesth* 2000; **47**: 299–302.

TRANSDERMAL ROUTE. Transdermal fentanyl is used for chronic intractable cancer pain in adults.[1] Its use in children with cancer pain is not recommended by the manufacturers although a small study[2] has shown that transdermal fentanyl is well tolerated in this group; the authors have suggested that further trials are warranted.

Transdermal fentanyl has also been used successfully in chronic non-cancer pain;[3] however the manufacturers state that its use is contra-indicated in the management of acute or postoperative pain because the problems of dose titration in the short term increase the possibility of development of significant respiratory depression (see also under Adverse Effects, above).
1. Jeal W, Benfield P. Transdermal fentanyl: a review of its pharmacological properties and therapeutic efficacy in pain control. *Drugs* 1997; **53**: 109–38.
2. Collins JJ, *et al.* Transdermal fentanyl in children with cancer pain: feasibility, tolerability, and pharmacokinetic correlates. *J Pediatr* 1999; **134**: 319–23.
3. Allan L, *et al.* Randomised crossover trial of transdermal fentanyl and sustained release oral morphine for treating chronic non-cancer pain. *BMJ* 2001; **322**: 1154–8.

TRANSMUCOSAL ROUTE. A lozenge-on-a-stick lollipop dosage form of fentanyl for transmucosal administration has been given for sedation and analgesia before anaesthesia or painful procedures in children[1,2] and in adults.[3] The formulation is also used for breakthrough cancer pain in opioid-tolerant patients.[4,5] It has been noted[6] that this route of administration can cause all the adverse effects of parenteral opioids; nausea and vomiting are common and potentially lethal respiratory depression can occur.
1. Nelson PS, *et al.* Comparison of oral transmucosal fentanyl citrate and an oral solution of meperidine, diazepam, and atropine for premedication in children. *Anesthesiology* 1989; **70**: 616–21.
2. Schechter NL, *et al.* The use of oral transmucosal fentanyl citrate for painful procedures in children. *Pediatrics* 1995; **95**: 335–9.
3. Macaluso AD, *et al.* Oral transmucosal fentanyl citrate for pre-medication in adults. *Anesth Analg* 1996; **82**: 158–61.
4. Farrar JT, *et al.* Oral transmucosal fentanyl citrate: randomized, double-blinded, placebo-controlled trial for treatment of breakthrough pain in cancer patients. *J Natl Cancer Inst* 1998; **15**: 611–16.
5. Christie JM, *et al.* Dose-titration, multicenter study of oral transmucosal fentanyl citrate for the treatment of breakthrough pain in cancer patients using transdermal fentanyl for persistent pain. *J Clin Oncol* 1998; **16**: 3238–45.
6. Anonymous. Oral transmucosal fentanyl citrate. *Med Lett Drugs Ther* 1994; **36**: 24–5.

Administration in children. Satisfactory anaesthesia has been reported[1] with high-dose fentanyl citrate (30 to 50 μg per kg body-weight) in premature infants when used as sole anaesthetic, in conjunction with pancuronium, for ligation of patent ductus arteriosus; cardiovascular stability was maintained throughout the procedure. However, others[2] found significant hypotension in preterm infants given either fentanyl 20 μg per kg, isoflurane, halothane, or ketamine; systolic arterial pressure was best maintained with the ketamine technique. The surgical stress response in preterm babies was abolished by the addition of fentanyl 10 μg per kg intravenously to an anaesthetic regimen of nitrous oxide and tubocurarine.[3] Dose responses of fentanyl in neonatal anaesthesia have been discussed.[4] For sedation and analgesia during intensive care an infusion rate of 2 to 4 μg per kg per hour has been useful and associated with cardiovascular stability.[5] Although the use of fentanyl for prolonged sedation of infants and children during ventilatory support is reported to be widespread there is a lack of evidence of its safety and efficacy for this use.[6] In one double-blind placebo-controlled study[7] investigating the use of a continuous fentanyl infusion for 5 days in premature neonates receiving mechanical ventilation for respiratory distress syndrome, it was noted that although fentanyl was effective in reducing physiological indicators of pain and stress, there was an increased need for ventilatory support associated with the use of fentanyl compared with placebo. Fentanyl was infused initially in a dose of 5 μg per kg over 20 minutes, and thereafter in a decreasing dosage schedule over 120 hours from a rate of 2 μg per kg per hour to 0.5 μg per kg per hour. The authors pointed out that the results of this study could not assess the effects of fentanyl on long-term outcome and a larger multicentre study was required. There have also been reports of possible tolerance and withdrawal symptoms associated with prolonged administration of fentanyl (see under Dependence and Withdrawal, above).

See also under Transdermal Route and Transmucosal Route, above, and Postoperative Pain, below.
1. Robinson S, Gregory GA. Fentanyl-air-oxygen anesthesia for ligation of patent ductus arteriosus in preterm infants. *Anesth Analg* 1981; **60**: 331–4.
2. Friesen RH, Henry DB. Cardiovascular changes in preterm neonates receiving isoflurane, halothane, fentanyl, and ketamine. *Anesthesiology* 1986; **64**: 238–42.
3. Anand KJS, *et al.* Randomised trial of fentanyl anaesthesia in preterm neonates undergoing surgery: effects on the stress response. *Lancet* 1987; **i**: 243–8.
4. Yaster M. The dose response of fentanyl in neonatal anesthesia. *Anesthesiology* 1987; **66**: 433–5.
5. Lloyd-Thomas AR. Pain management in paediatric patients. *Br J Anaesth* 1990; **64**: 85–104.
6. Kauffman RE. Fentanyl, fads, and folly: who will adopt the therapeutic orphans? *J Pediatr* 1991; **119**: 588–9.
7. Orsini AJ, *et al.* Routine use of fentanyl infusions for pain and stress reduction in infants with respiratory distress syndrome. *J Pediatr* 1996; **129**: 140–5.

Anaesthesia. Fentanyl and its newer congeners alfentanil and sufentanil are shorter-acting than morphine and appear to produce fewer circulatory changes; they may be preferred for use as supplements during anaesthesia with inhalational or intravenous drugs.

In a comparative study of opioid supplements to nitrous oxide anaesthesia fentanyl and sufentanil were equally preferable to morphine or pethidine in terms of haemodynamic changes to stress and rates of recovery.[1] For further comparisons between fentanyl and its congeners, see under alfentanil (p.13) and under sufentanil (p.85). The cardiovascular stress response to intubation was attenuated by the use of fentanyl 3 μg per kg body-weight intravenously as an adjunct to thiopental induction in elderly patients,[2] and fentanyl 2.5 μg per kg or alfentanil 10 μg per kg decreased intra-ocular pressure and reduced the haemodynamic responses associated with intubation when given at induction to adults undergoing ophthalmic operations[3] or women with severe pregnancy-induced hypertension undergoing caesarean section.[4] For a discussion of the use of opioids such as fentanyl to attenuate these responses to intubation, see under Anaesthesia, p.1331.

High doses of fentanyl are used in an attempt to reduce the cardiovascular, endocrine, and metabolic changes that may accompany surgery. When attenuation of surgical stress is especially important, for example in cardiac surgery, intravenous fentanyl 50 to 100 μg per kg in conjunction with oxygen and a neuromuscular blocker, and sometimes up to 150 μg per kg, may be used for general anaesthesia.

Attenuation of metabolic and endocrine responses has been achieved with high-dose fentanyl (at least 50 μg per kg) given before the onset of surgery,[5] but appeared to have little effect on established responses when given after the start of surgery.[6] Supplementation with fentanyl 15 μg per kg at induction of anaesthesia with nitrous oxide-oxygen suppressed β-endorphin, ACTH, growth hormone, cortisol, and glucose response to pelvic surgery.[7]

Stanley and Webster[8] found that fentanyl up to 50 μg per kg as sole anaesthetic produced minimal changes in cardiovascular dynamics in patients undergoing mitral valvular replacement, although Wynands *et al.*[9] were unable to confirm stable haemodynamics using a loading dose of 75 μg per kg, sometimes followed by an infusion of 0.75 μg per kg per minute up to a total dose of about 160 μg per kg. Induction of anaesthesia with an intravenous bolus of fentanyl 100 μg per kg prevented the increased plasma-catecholamine concentrations associated with perioperative stress and attenuated circulatory responses in patients undergoing cholecystectomy when compared with those who underwent a balanced technique of anaesthesia with fentanyl 5 μg per kg at induction followed by continuous infusion of 3 μg per kg per hour.[10] Total intravenous anaesthesia with fentanyl and propofol has been successful.[11]

For the use of fentanyl for anaesthesia in neonates and children, see under Administration in Children, above.

Neuroleptanalgesia. An injection of short-acting fentanyl 50 μg per mL with the longer-acting antipsychotic droperidol 2.5 mg per mL is available and has been used for neuroleptanalgesia, premedication, and as an adjunct to anaesthesia. However, such a fixed-ratio combination has been criticised as irrational and having the potential to cause distressing and possibly lethal adverse effects.[12]
1. Ghoneim MM, *et al.* Comparison of four opioid analgesics as supplements to nitrous oxide anaesthesia. *Anesth Analg* 1984; **63**: 405–12.
2. Chung F, Evans D. Low-dose fentanyl: haemodynamic response during induction and intubation in geriatric patients. *Can Anaesth Soc J* 1985; **32**: 622–8.
3. Sweeney J, *et al.* Modification by fentanyl and alfentanil of the intraocular pressure response to suxamethonium and tracheal intubation. *Br J Anaesth* 1989; **63**: 688–91.
4. Rout CC, Rocke DA. Effects of alfentanil and fentanyl on induction of anaesthesia in patients with severe pregnancy-induced hypertension. *Br J Anaesth* 1990; **65**: 468–74.
5. Hall, GM. Fentanyl and the metabolic response to surgery. *Br J Anaesth* 1980; **52**: 561–2.
6. Bent JM, *et al.* Effects of high-dose fentanyl anaesthesia on the established metabolic and endocrine response to surgery. *Anaesthesia* 1984; **39**: 19–23.
7. Lacoumenta S, *et al.* Fentanyl and the β-endorphin, ACTH and glucoregulatory hormonal response to surgery. *Br J Anaesth* 1987; **59**: 713–20.
8. Stanley TH, Webster LR. Anesthetic requirements and cardiovascular effects of fentanyl-oxygen and fentanyl-diazepam-oxygen anesthesia in man. *Anesth Analg* 1978; **57**: 411–16.

9. Wynands JE, *et al.* Blood pressure response and plasma fentanyl concentrations during high- and very high-dose fentanyl anesthesia for coronary artery surgery. *Anesth Analg* 1983; **62:** 661–5.
10. Klingstedt C, *et al.* High- and low-dose fentanyl anesthesia: circulatory and plasma catecholamine responses during cholecystectomy. *Br J Anaesth* 1987; **59:** 184–8.
11. Jenstrup M, *et al.* Total iv anaesthesia with propofol-alfentanil or propofol-fentanyl. *Br J Anaesth* 1990; **64:** 717–22.
12. Anonymous. Innovar: a follow-up. *Med Lett Drugs Ther* 1981; **23:** 74–5.

PHAEOCHROMOCYTOMA. Unlike morphine and some other opioids, fentanyl and alfentanil do not release histamine and may be used safely in the anaesthetic management of patients with phaeochromocytoma.[1]

1. Hull CJ. Phaeochromocytoma: diagnosis, preoperative preparation and anaesthetic management. *Br J Anaesth* 1986; **58:** 1453–68.

POSTOPERATIVE SHIVERING. As pethidine appears to be effective in the treatment of postoperative shivering a number of other opioids including fentanyl have also been tried but not all opioids are necessarily effective. Fentanyl was reported to be effective in one study.[1]

1. Alfonsi P, *et al.* Fentanyl, as pethidine, inhibits post anaesthesia shivering. *Br J Anaesth* 1993; **70** (suppl 1): 38.

Intensive care. Despite the short duration of action of fentanyl after single doses, rapid redistribution in the body results in an elimination half-life longer than that of morphine. Consequently fentanyl is not a short-acting drug when used for analgesia in intensive care, and may offer little advantage over morphine.[1]

See also under Administration in Children, above.

1. Aitkenhead AR. Analgesia and sedation in intensive care. *Br J Anaesth* 1989; **63:** 196–206.

Pain. CANCER PAIN. Transdermal fentanyl is used in the management of chronic intractable cancer pain; for references see Administration, Transdermal Route, above. For references to the use of transmucosal fentanyl in the management of breakthrough cancer pain, see Administration, Transmucosal Route, above.

LABOUR PAIN. Fentanyl has been reported to be an effective analgesic during active labour. An intravenous dose of 50 or 100 µg was given every hour on request to a mean cumulative dose of 140 µg (range 50 to 600 µg). Temporary analgesia and mild sedation were apparent in each treated woman when compared with controls. Onset of analgesia was within 5 minutes of a dose and was sustained for about 45 minutes.[1] In a non-blinded comparative study[2] equivalent analgesia was obtained during early and late labour with intravenous fentanyl 50 to 100 µg every hour or pethidine 25 to 50 mg every 2 to 3 hours; there were fewer maternal and immediate neonatal side-effects with fentanyl.

Opioids have also been given epidurally in labour and, although fentanyl is unreliable when used alone,[3] it does enhance the epidural analgesia achieved with the local anaesthetic bupivacaine when given as a bolus epidural injection[4] or by continuous epidural infusion[5] and may increase overall maternal satisfaction with labour.[6] However, profound respiratory depression was reported 100 minutes after the use of bupivacaine and fentanyl epidural analgesia and it was strongly advised that patients be observed continuously for 2 to 3 hours after such treatment.[7] Excellent analgesia has been reported with low-dose bupivacaine and fentanyl by continuous epidural infusion,[8,9] and some have considered that local anaesthetic-opioid combinations might be the way ahead.[10,11] The reduction in the minimum local analgesic concentration of epidural bupivacaine for labour pain increased with increasing dose of fentanyl added to bupivacaine.[12] However, the incidence of pruritus increased significantly with fentanyl in a dose of 4 µg per mL and therefore the optimum dose of fentanyl may be 3 µg per mL for bupivacaine-sparing epidural analgesia during labour.

1. Rayburn W, *et al.* Fentanyl citrate analgesia during labor. *Am J Obstet Gynecol* 1989; **161:** 202–6.
2. Rayburn WF, *et al.* Randomized comparison of meperidine and fentanyl during labor. *Obstet Gynecol* 1989; **74:** 604–6.
3. Reynolds F. Extradural opioids in labour. *Br J Anaesth* 1989; **63:** 251–3.
4. Lirzin JD, *et al.* Controlled trial of extradural bupivacaine with fentanyl, morphine or placebo for pain relief in labour. *Br J Anaesth* 1989; **62:** 641–4.
5. Jones G, *et al.* Comparison of bupivacaine and bupivacaine with fentanyl in continuous extradural analgesia during labour. *Br J Anaesth* 1989; **63:** 254–9.
6. Murphy JD, *et al.* Bupivacaine versus bupivacaine plus fentanyl for epidural analgesia: effect on maternal satisfaction. *BMJ* 1991; **302:** 564–7.
7. McClure JH, Jones G. Comparison of bupivacaine and bupivacaine with fentanyl in continuous extradural analgesia during labour. *Br J Anaesth* 1989; **63:** 637–40.
8. Chestnut DH, *et al.* Continuous infusion epidural analgesia during labor: a randomized, double-blind comparison of 0.0625% bupivacaine/0.0002% fentanyl versus 0.125% bupivacaine. *Anesthesiology* 1988; **68:** 754–9.
9. Chestnut DH, *et al.* Continuous epidural infusion of bupivacaine-fentanyl during the second stage of labor. *Anesthesiology* 1989; **71:** A841.
10. Reynolds F. Extradural opioids in labour. *Br J Anaesth* 1990; **64:** 529.
11. Herman NL, *et al.* Extradural opioids in labour. *Br J Anaesth* 1990; **64:** 528–9.
12. Lyons G, *et al.* Extradural pain relief in labour: bupivacaine sparing by extradural fentanyl is dose dependent. *Br J Anaesth* 1997; **78:** 493–7.

POSTOPERATIVE PAIN. Small intravenous bolus doses of opioid analgesic may be injected immediately after surgery for postoperative analgesia and faster acting opioids such as fentanyl may be preferable to morphine.[1] Fentanyl has also been given by epidural injection in doses of 100 or 200 µg or by continuous epidural infusion in doses of 20 to 80 µg per hour; patient-controlled systems have been used.[2]

Epidural fentanyl or sufentanil provided effective postoperative analgesia following caesarean section with comparable adverse effect profiles.[3] The suggested optimal dose of fentanyl was 100 µg. For references comparing epidural fentanyl with alfentanil, see under Postoperative Pain in Uses and Administration of Alfentanil, p.13. In a review[4] of postoperative pain management epidural opioids were considered to provide superior analgesia to systemically administered opioids. Fentanyl may be administered through a lumbar epidural catheter that is often inserted immediately postoperatively. After an initial loading dose of 1 to 1.5 µg per kg body-weight of fentanyl, infusion at the rate of 0.7 to 2 µg per kg per hour is begun and continued for about 48 hours on average. Some prefer to use intermittent injection.

Combined opioid and local anaesthetic epidural infusions have also proved effective, for example fentanyl 1 µg per mL with bupivacaine 0.1%; both could be infused at lower rates than either drug alone. Although a study[5] comparing bupivacaine-fentanyl combinations with each drug alone for epidural analgesia following caesarean section confirmed an additive analgesic effect for the combination, there was no demonstrable clinical benefit compared with fentanyl alone in this patient group who expect early mobilisation. However, the combination may be of greater benefit in patients for whom early ambulation is not routine.

Fentanyl has also been given by epidural injection to children for postoperative analgesia.[6]

Fentanyl has been tried by intrathecal injection for postoperative pain.[7]

1. Mitchell RWD, Smith G. The control of acute postoperative pain. *Br J Anaesth* 1989; **63:** 147–58.
2. Morgan M. The rational use of intrathecal and extradural opioids. *Br J Anaesth* 1989; **63:** 165–88.
3. Grass JA, *et al.* A randomized, double-blind, dose-response comparison of epidural fentanyl versus sufentanil analgesia after caesarean section. *Anesth Analg* 1997; **85:** 365–71.
4. Lutz LJ, Lamer TJ. Management of postoperative pain: review of current techniques and methods. *Mayo Clin Proc* 1990; **65:** 584–96.
5. Cooper DW, *et al.* Patient-controlled extradural analgesia with bupivacaine, fentanyl, or a mixture of both, after caesarean section. *Br J Anaesth* 1996; **76:** 611–15.
6. Lejus C, *et al.* Postoperative extradural analgesia in children: comparison of morphine with fentanyl. *Br J Anaesth* 1994; **72:** 156–9.
7. Sudarshan G, *et al.* Intrathecal fentanyl for post-thoracotomy pain. *Br J Anaesth* 1995; **75:** 19–22.

Preparations

BP 2001: Fentanyl Injection;
USP 25: Fentanyl Citrate Injection.

Proprietary Preparations (details are given in Part 3)
Aust.: Durogesic; *Austral.:* Durogesic; Sublimaze; *Belg.:* Durogesic; *Canad.:* Duragesic; Sublimaze†; *Denm.:* Durogesic; Haldid; *Fin.:* Durogesic; *Fr.:* Durogesic; *Ger.:* Durogesic; *Hong Kong:* Durogesic; *Irl.:* Durogesic; Sublimaze; *Israel:* Durogesic; *Ital.:* Durogesic; Fentanest; *Mex.:* Durogesic; Fentanest; *Neth.:* Durogesic; *Norw.:* Durogesic; Leptanal; *NZ:* Durogesic; Sublimaze; *Port.:* Durogesic; *S.Afr.:* Durogesic; Sublimaze; Tanyl; *Singapore:* Durogesic; *Spain:* Durogesic; Fentanest; *Swed.:* Durogesic; Leptanal; *Switz.:* Durogesic; Sintenyl; *UK:* Actiq; Durogesic; Sublimaze; *USA:* Actiq; Duragesic; Sublimaze.

Multi-ingredient: *Aust.:* Thalamonal; *Austral.:* Marcain with Fentanyl; Naropin with Fentanyl; *Belg.:* Thalamonal; *Braz.:* Inoval; *Ger.:* Thalamonal; *Ital.:* Leptofen; *Neth.:* Thalamonal; *NZ:* Marcain with Fentanyl; *USA:* Innovar†.

Fentiazac (12747-x)

Fentiazac (BAN, USAN, rINN).
BR-700; Wy-21894. [4-(4-Chlorophenyl)-2-phenylthiazol-5-yl]acetic acid.
$C_{17}H_{12}ClNO_2S = 329.8.$
CAS — 18046-21-4.
ATC — M01AB10; M02AA14.

Profile
Fentiazac is an NSAID (p.63) that has been used for the relief of pain and inflammation associated with musculoskeletal, joint, peri-articular, and soft-tissue disorders. It has also been used in the treatment of fever. Fentiazac has been given in usual doses of 100 to 200 mg once or twice daily by mouth. Fentiazac has also been applied topically as a 5% cream and has been given rectally as the calcium salt.

Preparations
Proprietary Preparations (details are given in Part 3)
Aust.: Norvedan; *Braz.:* Atilan; *Ital.:* Flogene; O-Flam; *Port.:* Donorest†; IDR†; Norvedan; *Spain:* Donorest; Riscalon†.

Fenyramidol Hydrochloride (2690-m)

Fenyramidol Hydrochloride (BANM, rINNM).
IN-511; MJ-505; NSC-17777; Phenyramidol Hydrochloride (USAN). 1-Phenyl-2-(2-pyridylamino)ethanol hydrochloride; α-(2-Pyridylaminomethyl)benzyl alcohol hydrochloride.
$C_{13}H_{14}N_2O,HCl = 250.7.$
CAS — 553-69-5 (fenyramidol); 326-43-2 (fenyramidol hydrochloride).

Profile
Fenyramidol hydrochloride has analgesic and skeletal muscle relaxant properties and was used by mouth in the treatment of muscular pain and stiffness. It may enhance the effects of coumarin anticoagulants (p.994) and of phenytoin (p.359).

Preparations
Proprietary Preparations (details are given in Part 3)
Ger.: Cabral†.

Fepradinol (3788-r)

Fepradinol (rINN).
(±)-α-{[(2-Hydroxy-1,1-dimethylethyl)amino]methyl}benzyl alcohol.
$C_{12}H_{19}NO_2 = 209.3.$
CAS — 63075-47-8.

Profile
Fepradinol is an NSAID (p.63) that has been used topically in a concentration of 6% for the relief of pain and inflammation. The hydrochloride has been used similarly.

Preparations
Proprietary Preparations (details are given in Part 3)
Spain: Dalgen; Flexidol.

Feprazone (2650-a)

Feprazone (BAN, rINN).
DA-2370; Phenylprenazone; Prenazone. 4-(3-Methylbut-2-enyl)-1,2-diphenylpyrazolidine-3,5-dione.
$C_{20}H_{20}N_2O_2 = 320.4.$
CAS — 30748-29-9 (feprazone); 57148-60-4 (feprazone piperazine salt 1:1).
ATC — M01AX18; M02AA16.

Profile
Feprazone, a phenylbutazone (p.78) derivative, is an NSAID (p.63). It has been given by mouth in the treatment of mild to moderate pain, fever, and inflammation associated with musculoskeletal and joint disorders. Feprazone has also been given rectally and used topically as a 5% cream.

Pinazone, the piperazine salt of feprazone, has been used similarly.

Preparations
Proprietary Preparations (details are given in Part 3)
Aust.: Zepelin; *Braz.:* Metrazone; Zepelan; *Ital.:* Zepelin; *Spain:* Brotazona; Reuflodol†.

Floctafenine (2651-t)

Floctafenine (BAN, USAN, rINN).
R-4318; RU-15750. 2,3-Dihydroxypropyl N-(8-trifluoromethyl-4-quinolyl)anthranilate.
$C_{20}H_{17}F_3N_2O_4 = 406.4.$
CAS — 23779-99-9.
ATC — N02BG04.
Pharmacopoeias. In Jpn.

Adverse Effects and Precautions
As for NSAIDs in general, p.63. Anaphylactic shock has been reported in patients given floctafenine; anaphylactic reactions may be preceded by minor allergic manifestations, therefore floctafenine should be discontinued in any who develops signs suggestive of allergy (such as pruritus or urticaria). Reactions may also involve the liver. Floctafenine may cross-react with glafenine (p.42) and should not be given to patients who have experienced glafenine-associated reactions.

Porphyria. Floctafenine is considered to be unsafe in patients with porphyria because it has been shown to be porphyrinogenic in *in-vitro* systems.

Interactions
For interactions associated with NSAIDs, see p.65.

Pharmacokinetics
Floctafenine is absorbed from the gastrointestinal tract; peak plasma concentrations are obtained 1 to 2 hours after ingestion. Its plasma half-life is about 8 hours. It is metabolised in the liver to floctafenic acid. It is excreted mainly as glucuronide conjugates in the urine and bile.

Uses and Administration
Floctafenine, an anthranilic acid derivative related to glafenine (p.42), is an NSAID (p.65) used in doses of up to 1.2 g daily, in divided doses, by mouth for the short-term relief of pain.

Preparations

Proprietary Preparations (details are given in Part 3)
Belg.: Idarac†; **Braz.:** Idarac; **Canad.:** Idarac; **Fr.:** Idarac; **Irl.:** Idarac; **Ital.:** Idarac†; **Neth.:** Idalon; **Spain:** Idarac; **Thai.:** Idarac.

Flufenamic Acid (2652-x)

Flufenamic Acid (BAN, USAN, rINN).
CI-440; CN-27554; INF-1837; NSC-82699. N-(ααα-Trifluoro-m-tolyl)anthranilic acid.
$C_{14}H_{10}F_3NO_2 = 281.2$.
CAS — 530-78-9.
ATC — M01AG03.

Adverse Effects and Precautions
As for NSAIDs in general, p.63.

Effects on the gastrointestinal tract. Acute proctocolitis associated with oral flufenamic acid in a patient.[1]
1. Ravi S, et al. Colitis caused by non-steroidal anti-inflammatory drugs. Postgrad Med J 1986; 62: 773–6.

Porphyria. Flufenamic acid has been associated with acute attacks of porphyria and is considered unsafe in porphyric patients.

Uses and Administration
Flufenamic acid, an anthranilic acid derivative related to mefenamic acid (p.51), is an NSAID (p.65). Flufenamic acid is mainly used topically in a concentration of 2.5 to 3.5% for the relief of pain and inflammation associated with musculoskeletal, joint, and soft-tissue disorders. It has also been given by mouth.

Preparations
Proprietary Preparations (details are given in Part 3)
Ger.: Dignodolin; Rheuma Lindofluid.
Multi-ingredient: **Aust.:** Mobilisin; Mobilisin plus; Rheugesal; **Belg.:** Mobilisin; **Braz.:** Mobilisin Composto; **Ger.:** Algesalona; Flexocutan N; Mobilisin; Thermo Mobilisin; **Hong Kong:** Movilisin; **Ital.:** Mobilisin; **Port.:** Latesil; Mobilisin; **Spain:** Movilisin; **Switz.:** Algesalona; Assan; Assan-Thermo; Mobilisin.

Flunixin Meglumine (16811-r)

Flunixin Meglumine (BANM, USAN, rINNM).
Sch-14714 (flunixin). 2-{[2-Methyl-3-(trifluoromethyl)phenyl]amino}-3-pyridinecarboxylic acid compounded with 1-deoxy-1-(methylamino)-D-glucitol (1:1); 2-(α³,α³,α³-Trifluoro-2,3,-xylidino)nicotinic acid compounded with 1-deoxy-1-(methylamino)-D-glucitol (1:1).
$C_{14}H_{11}F_3N_2O_2,C_7H_{17}NO_5 = 491.5$.
CAS — 38677-85-9 (flunixin); 42461-84-7 (flunixin meglumine).
Pharmacopoeias. In BP(Vet). Also in US for veterinary use only.

Pharmacopoeial description
BP(Vet) 2001: A white to almost white powder. Freely soluble in water, in alcohol, and in methyl alcohol; practically insoluble in ethyl acetate. A 5% solution in water has a pH of 7.0 to 8.5. Store in airtight containers at a temperature not exceeding 25°.

USP 25: A white to off-white crystalline powder. Soluble in water, in alcohol, in methyl alcohol, and in ethyl acetate. pH of a 5% solution in water is between 7.0 and 9.0.

Profile
Flunixin meglumine is an NSAID (p.63) used in veterinary medicine for relief of pain and inflammation in acute and chronic disorders and as adjunctive therapy in the treatment of endotoxic or septic shock and mastitis.

Flunoxaprofen (16812-f)

Flunoxaprofen (rINN).
RV-12424. (+)-2-(p-Fluorophenyl)-α-methyl-5-benzoxazole-acetic acid.
$C_{16}H_{12}FNO_3 = 285.3$.
CAS — 66934-18-7.
ATC — G02CC04; M01AE15.

Profile
Flunoxaprofen, a propionic acid derivative, is an NSAID (p.63) that has been given for the relief of painful and inflammatory conditions by mouth, as a rectal suppository, and as a 5% topical gel. It has also been used as a vaginal irrigation.

Preparations
Proprietary Preparations (details are given in Part 3)
Ital.: Priaxim.

Flupirtine Maleate (18644-z)

Flupirtine Maleate (BANM, USAN, rINNM).
D-9998; W-2964M. Ethyl 2-amino-6-(4-fluorobenzylamino)-3-pyridylcarbamate maleate.
$C_{15}H_{17}FN_4O_2,C_4H_4O_4 = 420.4$.
CAS — 56995-20-1 (flupirtine); 75507-68-5 (flupirtine maleate).

The symbol † denotes a preparation no longer actively marketed

---

Profile
Flupirtine maleate is an analgesic that has been given for the relief of pain (p.2) in usual doses of 100 mg three or four times daily by mouth or in doses of 150 mg three or four times daily as a rectal suppository; daily doses of up to 600 mg by mouth or 900 mg rectally have been used where necessary.

◊ References.
1. Friedel HA, Fitton A. Flupirtine: a review of its pharmacological properties, and therapeutic efficacy in pain states. Drugs 1993; 45: 548–69.

Preparations
Proprietary Preparations (details are given in Part 3)
Braz.: Katadolon; **Ger.:** Katadolon; Trancopal Dolo; **Port.:** Metanor.

Flurbiprofen (2653-r)

Flurbiprofen (BAN, USAN, rINN).
BTS-18322; Flurbiprofenum; U-27182. 2-(2-Fluorobiphenyl-4-yl)propionic acid.
$C_{15}H_{13}FO_2 = 244.3$.
CAS — 5104-49-4.
ATC — M01AE09; M02AA19; S01BC04.
Pharmacopoeias. In Eur. (see p.vi), Jpn, and US.

Pharmacopoeial description
Ph. Eur.: A white or almost white crystalline powder. Practically insoluble in water; freely soluble in alcohol and in dichloromethane; dissolves in aqueous solutions of alkali hydroxides and carbonates.

USP 25: A white crystalline powder. Practically insoluble in water; freely soluble in dehydrated alcohol, in acetone, in ether, and in methyl alcohol; soluble in acetonitrile. Store in airtight containers.

Flurbiprofen Sodium (11385-h)

Flurbiprofen Sodium (BANM, rINNM).
Sodium (±)-2-(2-fluoro-4-biphenylyl)propionate dihydrate.
$C_{15}H_{12}FNaO_2,2H_2O = 302.3$.
CAS — 56767-76-1.
Pharmacopoeias. In Br. and US.

Pharmacopoeial description
BP 2001: A white to creamy-white, crystalline powder. Sparingly soluble in water; soluble in alcohol; practically insoluble in dichloromethane.

Adverse Effects
As for NSAIDs in general, p.63.

Minor symptoms of ocular irritation including transient burning and stinging have been reported following the instillation of flurbiprofen sodium eye drops; there may be increased bleeding from ocular surgery and wound healing may be delayed. Local irritation may occur following rectal administration of flurbiprofen. Similar effects may be seen after administration of flurbiprofen lozenges.

◊ Reports from the manufacturers on the range and incidence of the side-effects of flurbiprofen.[1,2]
1. Sheldrake FE, et al. A long-term assessment of flurbiprofen. Curr Med Res Opin 1977; 5: 106–16.
2. Brooks CD, et al. Clinical safety of flurbiprofen. J Clin Pharmacol 1990; 30: 342–51.

Effects on the CNS. A severe symmetrical parkinsonian syndrome developed in a 52-year-old man who had taken flurbiprofen for 7 days.[1]
1. Enevoldson TP, et al. Acute parkinsonism associated with flurbiprofen. BMJ 1990; 300: 540–1.

Effects on the kidneys. Renal papillary necrosis has been described in one patient associated with the use of flurbiprofen for many years.[1] Acute flank pain and reversible renal dysfunction, similar to that seen with suprofen (see p.87) has been reported in 2 patients treated with flurbiprofen.[2,3]
1. Nafría EC, et al. Renal papillary necrosis induced by flurbiprofen. DICP Ann Pharmacother 1991; 25: 870–1.
2. Kaufhold J, et al. Flurbiprofen-associated tubulointerstitial nephritis. J Am Nephrol 1991; 11: 144–6.
3. McIntire SC, et al. Acute flank pain and reversible renal dysfunction associated with nonsteroidal anti-inflammatory drug use. Pediatrics 1993; 92: 459–60.

Effects on the liver. A case of cholestatic jaundice probably due to flurbiprofen has been reported.[1]
1. Kotowski KE, Grayson MF. Side effects of non-steroidal anti-inflammatory drugs. BMJ 1982; 285: 377.

Effects on the skin. Cutaneous vasculitis apparently due to flurbiprofen occurred in a 59-year-old woman with long-standing rheumatoid arthritis.[1]
1. Wei N. Flurbiprofen and cutaneous vasculitis. Ann Intern Med 1990; 112: 550–1.

Precautions
As for NSAIDs in general, p.64.

Breast feeding. See under Pharmacokinetics, below.

Herpes simplex keratitis. Animal studies investigating the pro-infectious effects of flurbiprofen in the treatment of ocular herpes simplex infections are contradictory,[1,2] but the manufacturer of flurbiprofen sodium eye drops recommends that they should not be used in patients with active epithelial herpes simplex keratitis. Patients with a history of herpes simplex keratitis should also be monitored closely when undergoing treatment with these eye drops.
1. Trousdale MD, et al. Effect of flurbiprofen on herpes simplex keratitis in rabbits. Invest Ophthalmol Vis Sci 1980; 19: 267–70.
2. Hendricks RL, et al. The effect of flurbiprofen on herpes simplex virus type 1 stromal keratitis in mice. Invest Ophthalmol Vis Sci 1990; 31: 1503–11.

Interactions
For interactions associated with NSAIDs, see p.65.

Parasympathomimetics. The manufacturer of acetylcholine chloride ophthalmic preparations has stated that there have been reports that acetylcholine and carbachol have been ineffective when used in patients treated with topical (ophthalmic) NSAIDs.

Pharmacokinetics
Flurbiprofen is readily absorbed from the gastrointestinal tract with peak plasma concentrations occurring about 1 to 2 hours after ingestion. It is about 99% bound to plasma proteins and has a plasma half-life of about 3 to 6 hours. It is metabolised mainly by hydroxylation and conjugation in the liver and excreted in urine. Flurbiprofen is distributed into breast milk in amounts considered by some authorities to be too small to be harmful to a breast-fed infant.

Flurbiprofen is a chiral compound given as the racemate and the above pharmacokinetic characteristics refer to the racemic mixture. Allowance may have to be made for the different activities of the enantiomers.

◊ References.
1. Aarons L, et al. Plasma and synovial fluid kinetics of flurbiprofen in rheumatoid arthritis. Br J Clin Pharmacol 1986; 21: 155–63.
2. Smith IJ, et al. Flurbiprofen in post-partum women: plasma and breast milk disposition. J Clin Pharmacol 1989; 29: 174–84.
3. Kean WF, et al. The pharmacokinetics of flurbiprofen in younger and elderly patients with rheumatoid arthritis. J Clin Pharmacol 1992; 32: 41–8.
4. Davies NM. Clinical pharmacokinetics of flurbiprofen and its enantiomers. Clin Pharmacokinet 1995; 28: 100–14.

Uses and Administration
Flurbiprofen, a propionic acid derivative, is an NSAID (p.65). It is used in musculoskeletal and joint disorders such as ankylosing spondylitis, osteoarthritis, and rheumatoid arthritis, in soft-tissue disorders such as sprains and strains, for postoperative pain, and in mild to moderate pain including dysmenorrhoea and migraine. Flurbiprofen is also used as lozenges in the symptomatic relief of sore throat. Flurbiprofen sodium is used in eye drops to inhibit intra-operative miosis and to control postoperative inflammation of the anterior segment of the eye.

Flurbiprofen is given in usual doses of 150 to 200 mg daily by mouth in divided doses, increased to 300 mg daily in acute or severe conditions if necessary. A modified-release preparation for once daily administration is also available. Patients with dysmenorrhoea may be given an initial dose of 100 mg followed by 50 to 100 mg every four to six hours to a maximum total daily dose of 300 mg. Doses given rectally as suppositories are similar to those given by mouth.

For the relief of sore throat, a lozenge containing 8.75 mg of flurbiprofen may be sucked or allowed to dissolve slowly in the mouth every 3 to 6 hours to a maximum daily dose of 5 lozenges. It is recommended that treatment should be limited to a maximum of 3 days.

To inhibit intra-operative miosis during ocular surgery one drop of flurbiprofen sodium 0.03% is instilled into the eye every 30 minutes beginning 2 hours before surgery and ending not less than 30 minutes before surgery. To control postoperative inflammation the same dosage regimen is used before ocular surgery followed 24 hours after surgery by the instillation of one drop 4 times daily for 1 to 3 weeks. Flurbiprofen sodium eye drops have also been used in the topical treatment of cystoid macular oedema.

Flurbiprofen axetil has been given in some countries by intravenous injection for severe pain.

Preparations

BP 2001: Flurbiprofen Eye Drops; Flurbiprofen Suppositories; Flurbiprofen Tablets;
USP 25: Flurbiprofen Sodium Ophthalmic Solution; Flurbiprofen Tablets.

Proprietary Preparations (details are given in Part 3)
Aust.: Froben; Ocuflur; *Austral.:* Ocufen; Strepfen; *Belg.:* Froben; Ocuflur; *Braz.:* Evril; Ocufen; *Canad.:* Ansaid; Froben; Novo-Flurprofen; Ocufen; *Denm.:* Flurofen; Ocufen; *Fr.:* Cebutid; Ocufen; *Ger.:* Froben; Ocuflur; *Hong Kong:* Froben; Ocufen; *Irl.:* Fenomel; Froben; Ocufen; *Ital.:* Benactiv; Froben; Ocufen; Transact Lat; *Mex.:* Ansaid; Froben; Ocufen; *Mon.:* Antadys; *Neth.:* Froben; Ocufen; Strepfen; *Port.:* Edolfene; Froben; Ocuflur; Reupax; Transact Lat; *S.Afr.:* Froben; Ocufen; Transact; *Singapore:* Froben; Ocufen; Spain: Froben; Neo Artrol; Ocuflur; Tulip; *Switz.:* Froben; Ocuflur; *Thai.:* Flurozin; Ocufen; *UK:* Froben; Ocufen; Strefen; *USA:* Ansaid; Ocufen.

Fosfosal (15322-t)

Fosfosal (*rINN*).

UR-1521. 2-Phosphono-oxybenzoic acid.

$C_7H_7O_6P = 218.1$.
CAS — 6064-83-1.

Profile

Fosfosal is a salicylic acid derivative (see Aspirin, p.14). It has been given in usual doses of up to 3.6 g daily by mouth for the treatment of pain.

Preparations

Proprietary Preparations (details are given in Part 3)
Spain: Aydolid; Disdolen; Protalgia.

Multi-ingredient: *Spain:* Aydolid Codeina; Disdolen Codeina.

Furprofen (19751-m)

4-(2-Furanylcarbonyl)-α-methylbenzeneacetic acid.

$C_{14}H_{12}O_4 = 244.2$.
CAS — 66318-17-0.

Profile

Furprofen, a propionic acid derivative, is an NSAID (p.63) that has been given by mouth in doses of 200 to 400 mg daily for the relief of pain.

Preparations

Proprietary Preparations (details are given in Part 3)
Ital.: Dolex.

Glafenine (2654-f)

Glafenine (*rINN*).

Glaphenine. 2,3-Dihydroxypropyl *N*-(7-chloro-4-quinolyl)anthranilate.

$C_{19}H_{17}ClN_2O_4 = 372.8$.
CAS — 3820-67-5.
ATC — N02BG03.
Pharmacopoeias. In Fr.

Profile

Glafenine, an anthranilic acid derivative, is an NSAID (p.63) that was used for the relief of all types of pain. However, its high incidence of anaphylactic reactions has led to its withdrawal from the market in most countries. Glafenine hydrochloride was also used.

Adverse effects and precautions. Glafenine is a common cause of anaphylaxis. There may be hepatotoxicity (which may be fatal), nephrotoxicity, and gastrointestinal disturbances. It should be discontinued at the first sign of any allergic reaction. Crystallisation of glafenine in the urinary tract has also occurred. Cross-reactivity with floctafenine has been reported.

Glucametacin (2655-d)

Glucametacin (*rINN*).

2-{2-[1-(4-Chlorobenzoyl)-5-methoxy-2-methylindol-3-yl]acetamido}-2-deoxy-D-glucose.

$C_{25}H_{27}ClN_2O_8 = 518.9$.
CAS — 52443-21-7.

Profile

Glucametacin, a derivative of indometacin (p.44), is an NSAID (p.63) that has been given by mouth in musculoskeletal, joint, peri-articular, and soft-tissue disorders.

Preparations

Proprietary Preparations (details are given in Part 3)
Braz.: Teoremin; *Mex.:* Teoremac.

Glycol Salicylate (2656-n)

Ethylene Glycol Monosalicylate; Hydroxyethylis Salicylas. 2-Hydroxyethyl salicylate.

$C_9H_{10}O_4 = 182.2$.
CAS — 87-28-5.

Pharmacopoeias. In Eur. (see p.vi).

Pharmacopoeial description

Ph. Eur.: An oily, colourless or almost colourless liquid or colourless crystals. M.p. about 21°. Sparingly soluble in water; freely soluble in alcohol; very soluble in acetone and in dichloromethane. Protect from light.

Profile

Glycol salicylate is a salicylic acid derivative used similarly to methyl salicylate (p.55) in topical rubefacient preparations in usual concentrations of 5 to 15% for the relief of muscular and rheumatic pain.

Preparations

Proprietary Preparations (details are given in Part 3)
Ger.: Dolo-Arthrosenex N; Kytta; Lumbinon; Phardol mono; Phlogont; Phlogont Rheuma; Rheubalmin N; Salhumin Gel; Traumasenex; zuk rheuma.

Multi-ingredient: *Aust.:* Ambenat; Bayolin; Dolex; Etrat; Menthoneurin; Mobilisin; Moviflex; Rheumex; Rubizon-Rheumagel; Rubriment; Sportino Akut; Venosin; *Austral.:* Deep Heat; Goanna Analgesic Ice; *Belg.:* Algipan; Mobilisin; Percutalgine; Rado-Salil; *Braz.:* Etrat; Infrarub; Mobilisin Composto; Venostasin Composto; *Canad.:* Midalgan; *Fin.:* Moviflex; *Fr.:* Algipan; Bayoline†; Lao-Dal†; Le Thermogene; Lumbalgine; Percutaline; *Ger.:* Ambene N; Arthrodental N; Auroanalin; Brachont†; Caye Balsam; Contrheuma; Contrheuma V + T Bad N†; Cuxaflex N†; Cuxaflex Thermo†; Dolo Mobilat; Dolo-Menthoneurin CreSa†; Dolo-Rubriment; Doloneuro; Dolorgiet†; DoloVisano Salbe; Essaven Sport; Etrat Sportgel; exrheudon OPT; Fibraflex; Fibraflex-W-Creme N†; Flexocutan N; Hot Thermo; Infrotto Ultra; Li-iL Rheuma-Bad; Menthoneurin-Salbe; Menthoneurin-Vollbad N†; Midysalb†; mikanil N; Mobilisin; Myalgol N; Ortholan mit Salicylester†; Ostochont; Percutase N†; Phardol Rheuma; Phlogont-Thermal; Rheubalmin Thermo; Rheuma V + T Bad N; Rheuma-Bad; Rheuma-Liquidum; Rheuma-Salbe; Rheumichthol Bad†; Rubriment-N; Salhumin Gel N†; Sangenstocut Thermo†; Sportino Akut; Thermo-Menthoneurin; Thermo-Menthoneurin Bad†; Thermosenex; Togal Mobil-Gel; Trauma-Puren; Venoplant AHS; Venostasin; Vertebralon N; Warme-Gel; zuk thermo; *Hong Kong:* Movilisin; New Patecs A; Prelloran; *Irl.:* Algipan; *Israel:* Deep Heat Spray; *Ital.:* Balsamo Sifcamina; Disalgil; Lasoreuma†; Mobilisin; Salonpas; Sloan; *Neth.:* Menthoneurin; Sloan's balsem; *Port.:* DM Creme; DM Gel; DM Termo; Etrat†; Midalgan; *Singapore:* Deep Heating Spray; *Spain:* Movilisin; Percutalin†; *Switz.:* Artragel; Assan; Assan-Thermo; Demotherm Pommade contre le rhumatisme; Dolo Demotherm; Dolo-Arthrosenex; Dolo-Arthrosenex sine Heparino; Dolo-Veniten; Dolorex Neo†; Dolorex†; Histalgane; Histalgane mite; Incutin; Midalgan; Mobilisin; Moviflex†; Phlebostasin compositum; Prelloran; Radalgin; Remexal; Roliwol B†; Roliwol S†; Sportusal; Sportusal Spray sine heparino; Venoplant comp; Venucreme; Venugel; *Thai.:* Percutalgine; *UK:* Algipan; Cremalgin; Deep Heat Spray; Dubam; Fiery Jack; Ralgex; Ralgex Freeze Spray; Ralgex Heat Spray (low-odour); Ralgex†; Salonair; Salonpas; Transvasin Heat Spray.

Hexyl Nicotinate (9240-w)

n-Hexyl nicotinate.

$C_{12}H_{17}NO_2 = 207.3$.
CAS — 23597-82-2.

Profile

Hexyl nicotinate is used in topical preparations as a rubefacient.

Preparations

Proprietary Preparations (details are given in Part 3)
Multi-ingredient: *Belg.:* Transvane†; *Irl.:* Transvasin; *NZ:* Transvasin; *Port.:* Hipodor; *Swed.:* Transvasin†; *UK:* Transvasin Heat Rub.

Hydrocodone Hydrochloride (6229-j)

Hydrocodone Hydrochloride (*BANM, rINNM*).

$C_{18}H_{21}NO_3,HCl,2\frac{1}{2}H_2O = 380.9$.
CAS — 25968-91-6 (anhydrous hydrocodone hydrochloride).

Hydrocodone Tartrate (6231-p)

Hydrocodone Tartrate (*BANM, rINNM*).

Dihydrocodeinone Acid Tartrate; Hydrocodone Acid Tartrate; Hydrocodone Bitartrate (*USAN*); Hydrocodoni Bitartras; Hydrocone Bitartrate. 6-Deoxy-3-*O*-methyl-6-oxomorphine hydrogen tartrate hemipentahydrate; (−)-(5R)-4,5-Epoxy-3-methoxy-9a-methylmorphinan-6-one hydrogen tartrate hemipentahydrate.

$C_{18}H_{21}NO_3,C_4H_6O_6,2\frac{1}{2}H_2O = 494.5$.
CAS — 125-29-1 (hydrocodone); 143-71-5 (anhydrous hydrocodone tartrate); 34195-34-1 (hydrocodone tartrate hemipentahydrate).

NOTE. Compounded preparations of hydrocodone tartrate may be represented by the following names:

- Co-hycodAPAP (*USP 25*)—hydrocodone tartrate and paracetamol.

Pharmacopoeias. In Aust., Belg., Ger., Swiss, and US.

Pharmacopoeial description

USP 25: Fine, white crystals or crystalline powder. Soluble in water; slightly soluble in alcohol; insoluble in chloroform and in ether. pH of a 2% solution in water is between 3.2 and 3.8. Store in airtight containers. Protect from light.

Profile

Hydrocodone, a phenanthrene derivative, is an opioid analgesic (p.66) related to codeine (p.25) and has similar actions, but is more potent on a weight for weight basis. Hydromorphone (below) is one of the metabolites of hydrocodone.

Hydrocodone is used chiefly as the tartrate for the relief of irritant cough, though it has no particular advantage over codeine. It is also used for the relief of moderate to moderately severe pain, sometimes in combination with paracetamol.

Hydrocodone tartrate is taken by mouth in doses of 5 to 10 mg every 4 to 6 hours.

Hydrocodone hydrochloride is given by injection. The polistirex (a hydrocodone and sulfonated diethenylbenzene-ethenylbenzene copolymer complex) is used in modified-release preparations.

Hydrocodone has also been used in the treatment of dyspnoea.

Effects on the ears. Sensorineural hearing loss in 12 patients has been associated with the overuse or abuse of the hydrocodone and paracetamol preparation, Vicodin.[1] Cochlear implants improved the hearing loss in some of the patients.

1. Friedman RA, *et al.* Profound hearing loss associated with hydrocodone/acetaminophen abuse. *Am J Otol* 2000; **21:** 188–91.

Preparations

USP 25: Hydrocodone Bitartrate and Acetaminophen Tablets; Hydrocodone Bitartrate Tablets.

Proprietary Preparations (details are given in Part 3)
Belg.: Biocodone; *Canad.:* Hycodan; Robidone; *Ger.:* Dicodid; *Switz.:* Dicodid.

Multi-ingredient: *Austral.:* Hycomine†; *Canad.:* Caldomine-DH; Calmydone; Coristex-DH; Coristine-DH; Dalmacol; Dimetane Expectorant DC; Hycomine; Mercodol with Decapryn; Novahistex DH; Novahistex DH Expectorant; Novahistine DH; Triaminic Expectorant DH†; Tussaminic DH†; *USA:* Alor; Amacodone†; Anaplex HD; Anexsia; Atuss EX; Atuss G; Atuss HD; Bancap HC; Ceta Plus; Chlorgest-HD†; Co-Gesic; Co-Tuss V; Codal-DH; Codamine†; Codiclear DH; Codimal DH; Cophene XP; Cyndal HD; Cytuss HC; Damason-P; Deconamine CX; Dolacet; Donatussin DC; Duocet; Duratuss HD; ED Tuss HC; ED-TLC; Endagen-HD; Endal-HD; Endal-HD Plus; Entex HC; Entuss Expectorant; Entuss-D; Entuss-D Jr; H-Tuss-D; Histex HC; Histinex D; Histinex HC; Histinex HY; Histussin D; Histussin HC; Hy-Phen; Hyco-Pap†; HycoClear Tuss; Hycodan; Hycomine Compound; Hycomine†; Hycotuss; Hydro PC; Hydro-Tussin HD; Hydrocet; Hydrocodone CP; Hydrocodone GF; Hydrocodone HD; Hydrocodone PA†; Hydrogesic; Hydromet; Hydron KGS; Hydropane; Hydrophene DH†; Hyphed; Iodal; Iotussin HC; Kwelcof; Levall; Lorcet 10/650; Lorcet Plus; Lorcet-HD; Lortab; Lortab ASA; Marcof; Margesic H; Maxidone; Medipain†; Nalex DH; Nasatuss†; Norco; Oncet; P-V-Tussin; Panacet; Panasal; Pancof XP; Pancof-HC; Pancof-XL; Para-Hist HD; Pneumotussin HC; Protuss; Protuss-D; Rolatuss with Hydrocodone†; Ru-Tuss with Hydrocodone†; S-T Forte 2; S-T Forte†; SRC Expectorant; Stagesic; Statuss Green†; Su-Tuss HD; T-Gesic; Triaminic Expectorant DH†; Tussafed HC; Tussafin Expectorant; Tussanil DH; Tussend; Tussgen†; Tussigon; Tussionex Pennkinetic; Tyrodone; Unituss HC; Vanex Expectorant; Vanex-HD; Vetuss HC†; Vicodin; Vicodin Tuss; Vicoprofen; Vitussin; Zydone.

Hydromorphone Hydrochloride (6233-w)

Hydromorphone Hydrochloride (*BANM, rINNM*).

Dihydromorphinone Hydrochloride. 6-Deoxy-7,8-dihydro-6-oxomorphine hydrochloride; (−)-(5R)-4,5-Epoxy-3-hydroxy-9a-methylmorphinan-6-one hydrochloride.

$C_{17}H_{19}NO_3,HCl = 321.8$.
CAS — 466-99-9 (hydromorphone); 71-68-1 (hydromorphone hydrochloride).

Pharmacopoeias. In Aust., Ger., and US.

Pharmacopoeial description

USP 25: A fine white, or practically white, odourless, crystalline powder. Soluble 1 in 3 of water; sparingly soluble in alcohol; practically insoluble in ether. Store in airtight containers. Protect from light.

Incompatibility. Colour change from pale yellow to light green occurred when solutions of minocycline hydrochloride or tetracycline hydrochloride were mixed with hydromorphone hydrochloride in 5% glucose injection.[1] Mixtures of hydromorphone hydrochloride and dexamethasone sodium phosphate exhibited concentration-dependent incompatibility.[2] White cloudiness, haziness, or precipitation developed 4 hours after mixing thiopental sodium and hydromorphone hydrochloride.[3] Stability of mixtures of fluorouracil and hydromorphone hydrochloride in 0.9% sodium chloride or 5% glucose was dependent on the concentration of fluorouracil present.[4] Hydromorphone hydrochloride 0.5 mg per mL with fluorouracil 1 mg per mL was stable for at least 7 days at 32° and for at least 35 days at 23°, 4°, or −20°. When the concentration of fluorouracil was increased to 16 mg per mL, hydromorphone was noted to decompose incurring unacceptable losses after 3 days at 32° or after 7 days at 23°, but was stable for at least 35 days at 4° or −20°.

1. Nieves-Cordero AL, et al. Compatibility of narcotic analgesic solutions with various antibiotics during simulated Y-site injection. Am J Hosp Pharm 1985; 42: 1108–9.
2. Walker SE, et al. Compatibility of dexamethasone sodium phosphate with hydromorphone hydrochloride or diphenhydramine hydrochloride. Am J Hosp Pharm 1991; 48: 2161–6.
3. Chiu MF, Schwartz ML. Visual compatibility of injectable drugs used in the intensive care unit. Am J Health-Syst Pharm 1997; 54: 64–5.
4. Xu QA, et al. Stability and compatibility of fluorouracil with morphine sulfate and hydromorphone hydrochloride. Ann Pharmacother 1996; 30: 756–61.

Dependence and Withdrawal
As for Opioid Analgesics, p.66.

Adverse Effects, Treatment, and Precautions
As for Opioid Analgesics in general, p.67.

Interactions
For interactions associated with opioid analgesics, see p.68.

Pharmacokinetics
Hydromorphone hydrochloride is rapidly but incompletely absorbed from the gastrointestinal tract following oral administration. Oral bioavailability is about 50%. A plasma elimination half-life of about 2.5 hours has been reported after oral and intravenous administration. Hydromorphone appears to be widely distributed in the tissues and it crosses the placenta. It is metabolised in the liver and excreted in the urine mainly as conjugated hydromorphone, dihydroisomorphine, and dihydromorphine.

◊ References.
1. Vallner JJ, et al. Pharmacokinetics and bioavailability of hydromorphone following intravenous and oral administration to human subjects. J Clin Pharmacol 1981; 21: 152–6.

Uses and Administration
Hydromorphone hydrochloride, a phenanthrene derivative, is an opioid analgesic (p.68). It is related to morphine (p.58) but with a greater analgesic potency. It is a useful alternative to morphine sulfate for subcutaneous administration since its greater solubility in water allows a smaller dose volume. Following injection onset of action usually occurs within 15 minutes and analgesia is reported to last for about 3 to 5 hours; after oral administration onset of analgesia is usually within 30 minutes.

Hydromorphone hydrochloride is used for the relief of moderate to severe pain. It is administered by subcutaneous or intramuscular injection in initial doses of 1 to 2 mg every 4 to 6 hours as necessary. It may also be given by slow intravenous injection or by intravenous or subcutaneous infusion, with doses adjusted according to individual requirements. Higher parenteral doses may be given to opioid-tolerant patients using a highly concentrated solution containing 10 mg per mL that allows smaller dose volumes. In the UK, the initial dose of hydromorphone hydrochloride by mouth is 1.3 mg every 4 hours; thereafter the dose may be increased as necessary. In the USA doses of 2 mg may be given by mouth every 4 to 6 hours; doses may be increased to 4 mg or more for severe pain. Modified-release formulations of hydromorphone hydrochloride are available for twice-daily administration. By rectum, the usual dose is 3 mg every 6 to 8 hours.

Hydromorphone hydrochloride is given, as a syrup, in doses of 1 mg repeated every 3 to 4 hours for the relief of non-productive cough.

◊ References.
1. Searle NR, et al. Hydromorphone patient-controlled analgesia (PCA) after coronary artery bypass surgery. Can J Anaesth 1994; 41: 198–205.
2. Hays H, et al. Comparative clinical efficacy and safety of immediate release and controlled release hydromorphone for chronic severe cancer pain. Cancer 1994; 74: 1808–16.
3. Bruera E, et al. A randomized, double-blind, double-dummy, crossover trial comparing the safety and efficacy of oral sustained-release hydromorphone with immediate-release hydromorphone in patients with cancer pain. J Clin Oncol 1996; 14: 1713–17.

Preparations
USP 25: Hydromorphone Hydrochloride Injection; Hydromorphone Hydrochloride Tablets.

Proprietary Preparations (details are given in Part 3)
Aust.: Hydal; Austral.: Dilaudid; Canad.: Dilaudid; Hydromorph; Denm.: Opidol; Fin.: Opidol; Fr.: Sophidone; Ger.: Dilaudid; Palladon; Irl.: Palladone; Israel: Palladone; Swed.: Opidol; Switz.: Opidol; UK: Palladone; USA: Dilaudid; HydroStat IR†; Palladone.

Multi-ingredient: Ger.: Dilaudid-Atropin; Swed.: Dilaudid-Atropin; Switz.: Dilaudid-Atropin; USA: Dilaudid Cough.

Ibuprofen (2657-h)

Ibuprofen (BAN, USAN, rINN).

Ibuprofenum; RD-13621; U-18573. 2-(4-Isobutylphenyl)propionic acid.

$C_{13}H_{18}O_2 = 206.3$.

CAS — 15687-27-1.
ATC — G02CC01; M01AE01; M02AA13.

Pharmacopoeias. In Chin., Eur. (see p.vi), Int., Jpn, Pol., and US.

Pharmacopoeial description
Ph. Eur.: A white crystalline powder or colourless crystals. Practically insoluble in water; freely soluble in acetone, in dichloromethane, in ether, and in methyl alcohol; it dissolves in dilute solutions of alkali hydroxides and carbonates.

USP 25: A white to off-white crystalline powder having a slight characteristic odour. Practically insoluble in water; very soluble in alcohol, in acetone, in chloroform, and in methyl alcohol; slightly soluble in ethyl acetate. Store in airtight containers.

Adverse Effects, Treatment, and Precautions
As for NSAIDs in general, p.63. Ibuprofen may be better tolerated than other NSAIDs.

Symptoms of nausea, vomiting, and tinnitus have been reported after ibuprofen overdosage. More serious toxicity is uncommon, but gastric emptying followed by supportive measures is recommended if the quantity ingested within the previous hour exceeds 400 mg per kg body-weight.

◊ An analysis[1] of the outcome of treatment of 83 915 children found that the risk of hospitalisation for gastrointestinal bleeding, renal failure, or anaphylaxis was no greater in children given ibuprofen than in those given paracetamol.
1. Lesko SM, Mitchell AA. An assessment of the safety of pediatric ibuprofen. JAMA 1995; 273: 929–33.

Breast feeding. The amount of ibuprofen distributed into breast milk is considered by some authorities to be too small to be harmful to a breast-fed infant although some manufacturers recommend that breast feeding should be avoided during ibuprofen treatment, including topical application. A recent study[1] estimated that a breast-fed infant would ingest about 0.0008% of the maternal dose.
1. Walter K, Dilger C. Ibuprofen in human milk. Br J Clin Pharmacol 1997; 44: 211–12.

Effects on the blood. Blood disorders including agranulocytosis,[1] aplastic anaemia,[1] pure white-cell aplasia,[2] and thrombocytopenia[3] have been reported in patients taking ibuprofen. Fatal haemolytic anaemia occurred in a man taking ibuprofen and oxazepam.[4]
1. Gryfe CI, Rubenzahl S. Agranulocytosis and aplastic anemia possibly due to ibuprofen. Can Med Assoc J 1976; 114: 877.
2. Mamus SW, et al. Ibuprofen-associated pure white-cell aplasia. N Engl J Med 1986; 314: 624–5.
3. Jain S. Ibuprofen-induced thrombocytopenia. Br J Clin Pract 1994; 48: 51.
4. Guidry JB, et al. Fatal autoimmune hemolytic anemia associated with ibuprofen. JAMA 1979; 242: 68–9.

Effects on the CNS. Aseptic meningitis has occurred in patients taking NSAIDs. A review[1] of NSAID-related CNS adverse effects summarised 23 literature reports of NSAID-associated aseptic meningitis; 17 reports involved ibuprofen, 4 sulindac, 1 naproxen, and 1 tolmetin. Of the 23 reports, 11 involved patients with a diagnosis of systemic lupus erythematosus. Typically the reaction is seen in patients who have just recommenced NSAID treatment after a gap in their treatment. Within a few hours of restarting the NSAID the patient experiences fever, headache, and a stiff neck; abdominal pain may be present. The patient may become lethargic and eventually comatose. Symptoms resolve if the NSAID is stopped. It is believed to be a hypersensitivity reaction but there does not appear to be cross-reactivity between NSAIDs. More recently, a 56-year-old man with rheumatoid arthritis developed symptoms of aseptic meningitis 2 hours after ingesting ibuprofen.[2] The authors believed this to be the first reported case of ibuprofen-induced aseptic meningitis in a patient with rheumatoid arthritis.
1. Hoppmann RA, et al. Central nervous system side effects of nonsteroidal anti-inflammatory drugs: aseptic meningitis, psychosis, and cognitive dysfunction. Arch Intern Med 1991; 151: 1309–13.
2. Horn AC, Jarrett SW. Ibuprofen-induced aseptic meningitis in rheumatoid arthritis. Ann Pharmacother 1997; 31: 1009–11.

Effects on electrolytes. A patient with pre-existing renal disease developed severe hyponatraemia and symptoms of severe water intoxication after receiving ibuprofen.[1] All symptoms resolved on discontinuation of ibuprofen.
1. Blum M, Aviram A. Ibuprofen induced hyponatraemia. Rheumatol Rehabil 1980; 19: 258–9.

Effects on the eyes. Reversible amblyopia has been reported in patients receiving ibuprofen.[1,2] For reference to effects on the optic nerve associated with ibuprofen, see p.63.
1. Collum LMT, Bowen DI. Ocular side-effects of ibuprofen. Br J Ophthalmol 1971; 55: 472–7.
2. Palmer CAL. Toxic amblyopia from ibuprofen. BMJ 1972; 3: 765.

Effects on the gastrointestinal tract. Ibuprofen may be associated with a lower risk of upper gastrointestinal effects than some other NSAIDs, but nonetheless it, like other NSAIDs, can cause dyspepsia, nausea and vomiting, gastrointestinal bleeding, and peptic ulcers and perforation. Colitis and its exacerbation have occurred.[1,2]
1. Ravi S, et al. Colitis caused by non-steroidal anti-inflammatory drugs. Postgrad Med J 1986; 62: 773–6.
2. Clements D, et al. Colitis associated with ibuprofen. BMJ 1990; 301: 987.

Effects on the kidneys. Reports of adverse renal effects with ibuprofen include an increase in serum creatinine concentration,[1] acute renal failure,[2-5] and nephrotic syndrome.[6] Cystitis, haematuria, and interstitial nephritis may occur. Acute flank pain and reversible renal dysfunction, similar to that seen with suprofen (p.87), have been reported in some patients treated with ibuprofen.[7,8] See also under Effects on Electrolytes, above.
1. Whelton A, et al. Renal effects of ibuprofen, piroxicam, and sulindac in patients with asymptomatic renal failure: a prospective, randomized, crossover comparison. Ann Intern Med 1990; 112: 568–76.
2. Brandstetter RD, Mar DD. Reversible oliguric renal failure associated with ibuprofen treatment. BMJ 1978; 2: 1194–5.
3. Kimberly RP, et al. Apparent acute renal failure associated with therapeutic aspirin and ibuprofen administration. Arthritis Rheum 1979; 22: 281–5.
4. Spierto RJ, et al. Acute renal failure associated with the use of over-the-counter ibuprofen. Ann Pharmacother 1992; 26: 714.
5. Fernando AHN, et al. Renal failure after topical use of NSAIDs. BMJ 1994; 308: 533.
6. Justiniani FR. Over-the-counter ibuprofen and nephrotic syndrome. Ann Intern Med 1986; 105: 303.
7. McIntire SC, et al. Acute flank pain and reversible renal dysfunction associated with nonsteroidal anti-inflammatory drug use. Pediatrics 1993; 92: 459–60.
8. Wattad A, et al. A unique complication of nonsteroidal anti-inflammatory drug use. Pediatrics 1994; 93: 693.

Effects on the liver. Raised liver transaminase levels were noted in 3 patients with chronic hepatitis C infection after taking ibuprofen.[1] Levels returned to normal on discontinuation of the drug; the effect recurred in one patient who was re-exposed.
1. Riley TR, Smith JP. Ibuprofen-induced hepatotoxicity in patients with chronic hepatitis C: a case series. Am J Gastroenterol 1998; 93: 1563–5.

Effects on the skin. Skin rashes may occur during hypersensitivity reactions. Erythema multiforme bullosum, including the Stevens-Johnson syndrome and toxic epidermal necrolysis have been reported in patients taking ibuprofen.[1]
1. Sternlieb P, Robinson RM. Side effects of ibuprofen. Ann Intern Med 1980; 92: 570.

Hypersensitivity. A fatal asthma attack occurred in a 65-year-old-woman with adult-onset asthma, 30 minutes after ingestion of ibuprofen 800 mg.[1]

For other hypersensitivity reactions or possible reactions see also under Effects on the CNS and under Effects on the Skin, above.
1. Ayres JG, et al. Asthma death due to ibuprofen. Lancet 1987; i: 1082.

Meningitis. For reports of aseptic meningitis following administration of ibuprofen, see under Effects on the CNS, above.

Overdosage. There has been a review[1] of cases of ibuprofen overdose reported to the National Poisons Information Service of the UK in the 2 years following its introduction as an 'over-the-counter' medication. Although there was a substantial increase in the number of cases reported, no concurrent increase in severity of poisoning was demonstrated and in only 1 of 203 cases was ibuprofen thought to have caused serious problems. It was concluded that ibuprofen appeared to be much less toxic in acute overdose than either aspirin or paracetamol. However, subsequent reports illustrate the complexity of major overdosage with ibuprofen. A syndrome of coma, hyperkalaemia with cardiac arrhythmias, metabolic acidosis, pyrexia, and respiratory and renal failure was reported[2] in a 17-year-old man following major overdosage with ibuprofen and minor overdosage with doxepin. Hyperkalaemia was not evident until 14 hours after hospital admission and was thought to be due to a combination of potassium replacement for initial hypokalaemia, acidosis, muscle damage, and ibuprofen-induced renal failure. A 6-year-old child developed shock, coma, and metabolic acidosis following ingestion of a dose of ibuprofen equivalent to 300 mg per kg body-weight.[3] Treatment consisting of intubation, mechanical ventilation, fluid resuscitation, gastric lavage, and activated charcoal proved successful. In another report,[4] in which a 21-month-old child had ingested the equivalent of 500 mg per kg of ibuprofen, the presenting symptoms were acute renal failure with severe metabolic acidosis. The child developed tonic-clonic seizures 46 hours after ingestion, with significant hypocalcaemia and hypomagnesaemia, which may have been exacerbated by the administration of sodium polystyrene sulfonate and frusemide [furosemide]. The seizures, which could not be controlled with diazepam, phenytoin, and phenobarbital, ceased following correction of electrolyte balance.

1. Perry SJ, *et al.* Ibuprofen overdose: the first two years of over-the-counter sales. *Hum Toxicol* 1987; **6:** 173–8.
2. Menzies DG, *et al.* Fulminant hyperkalaemia and multiple complications following ibuprofen overdose. *Med Toxicol Adverse Drug Exp* 1989; **4:** 468–71.
3. Zuckerman GB, Uy CC. Shock, metabolic acidosis, and coma following ibuprofen overdose in a child. *Ann Pharmacother* 1995; **29:** 869–71.
4. Al-Harbi NN, *et al.* Hypocalcemia and hypomagnesemia after ibuprofen overdose. *Ann Pharmacother* 1997; **31:** 432–4.

Interactions
For interactions associated with NSAIDs, see p.65. Moclobemide enhances the effects of ibuprofen.

Lipid regulating drugs. For a report of rhabdomyolysis and renal failure attributed to an interaction between ibuprofen and *ciprofibrate*, see p.858.

Pharmacokinetics
Ibuprofen is absorbed from the gastrointestinal tract and peak plasma concentrations occur about 1 to 2 hours after ingestion. Ibuprofen is also absorbed following rectal administration. There is some absorption following topical application to the skin. For example, one manufacturer reports that percutaneous absorption from one topical dose form is about 5% of that obtained following administration of an oral dose form. Ibuprofen is 90 to 99% bound to plasma proteins and has a plasma half-life of about 2 hours. It is rapidly excreted in the urine mainly as metabolites and their conjugates. About 1% is excreted in urine as unchanged ibuprofen and about 14% as conjugated ibuprofen. There appears to be little if any distribution into breast milk.

The above figures refer to racemic ibuprofen. However, ibuprofen's disposition is stereoselective and there is some metabolic conversion of the inactive *R*-(–)-enantiomer to the active *S*-(+)-enantiomer (dexibuprofen).

◊ References.

1. Davies NM. Clinical pharmacokinetics of ibuprofen: the first 30 years. *Clin Pharmacokinet* 1998; **34:** 101–54.

Uses and Administration
Ibuprofen, a propionic acid derivative, is an NSAID (p.65). Its anti-inflammatory properties may be weaker than those of some other NSAIDs.

Ibuprofen is used in the management of mild to moderate pain and inflammation in conditions such as dysmenorrhoea, headache including migraine, postoperative pain, dental pain, musculoskeletal and joint disorders such as ankylosing spondylitis, osteoarthritis, and rheumatoid arthritis including juvenile idiopathic arthritis, peri-articular disorders such as bursitis and tenosynovitis, and soft-tissue disorders such as sprains and strains. It is also used to reduce fever.

Ibuprofen has also been used as an alternative to indometacin in the treatment of patent ductus arteriosus.

The usual dose by mouth for painful conditions in adults is 1.2 to 1.8 g daily in divided doses although maintenance doses of 0.6 to 1.2 g daily may be effective in some patients. If necessary the dose may be increased; in the UK the maximum recommended dose is 2.4 g daily whereas in the USA it is 3.2 g daily. Modified-release preparations of ibuprofen are available for once- or twice daily dosing, although actual dosages vary with different preparations. Patients with rheumatoid arthritis generally require higher doses of ibuprofen than those with osteoarthritis. The recommended dose for fever reduction in adults is 200 to 400 mg every 4 to 6 hours to a maximum of 1.2 g daily.

In the UK the usual dose by mouth for the treatment of pain or fever in children is 20 to 30 mg per kg body-weight daily in divided doses. Alternatively, total daily doses to be given in divided doses may be expressed in terms of age and are: 6 to 12 months, 150 mg; 1 to 2 years, 150 to 200 mg; 3 to 7 years, 300 to 400 mg; and 8 to 12 years, 600 to 800 mg. Up to 40 mg per kg may be given daily in juvenile idiopathic arthritis if necessary. Ibuprofen is not generally recommended for children weighing less than 7 kg or

some manufacturers suggest a maximum daily dose of 500 mg in those weighing less than 30 kg.

In the USA, suggested doses for children are: for fever, 5 to 10 mg per kg (depending on the severity of the fever) and for pain, 10 mg per kg; doses may be given every 6 to 8 hours up to a maximum daily dose of 40 mg per kg. A usual daily dose in the USA for juvenile idiopathic arthritis is 30 to 40 mg per kg in divided doses.

Ibuprofen is also applied topically as a 5% cream, foam, gel, or spray solution; a 10% gel is also available.

Ibuprofen is usually given as the base but various salts, esters, and other complexes are also used. These include lysine and sodium salts, guaiacol and pyridoxine esters, and mabuprofen (ibuprofen aminoethanol), isobutanolammonium, and meglumine derivatives.

Ibuprofen is usually administered as a racemic mixture but preparations containing only the *S*-(+)-isomer (dexibuprofen) are available in some countries.

Cachexia. For reference to the use of ibuprofen in combination with megestrol to treat cancer cachexia, see p.1481.

Cystic fibrosis. In patients with cystic fibrosis (see p.117), the inflammatory response to chronic pulmonary infection with *Pseudomonas* organisms contributes to lung destruction. Ibuprofen and other NSAIDs are being studied in patients with cystic fibrosis as an alternative to corticosteroids to reduce pulmonary inflammation, but despite some evidence of benefit their place in therapy is yet to be established.[1] A study[2] in patients with cystic fibrosis and mild lung disease indicated that ibuprofen given in high doses for four years slowed the progression of the lung disease without serious adverse effects. Initial doses were in the region of 20 to 30 mg per kg body-weight to a maximum of 1600 mg but were then adjusted individually to achieve peak plasma concentrations of 50 to 100 µg per mL.

1. Dezateux C, Crighton A. Oral non-steroidal anti-inflammatory drug therapy for cystic fibrosis (updated 27 February 2001). Available in The Cochrane Library; Issue 4. Oxford: Update Software; 2001.
2. Konstan MW, *et al.* Effect of high-dose ibuprofen in patients with cystic fibrosis. *N Engl J Med* 1995; **332:** 848–54.

Patent ductus arteriosus. For a suggestion that ibuprofen might be a better choice than indometacin for the treatment of patent ductus arteriosus, see p.46.

Preparations
BP 2001: Ibuprofen Cream; Ibuprofen Gel; Ibuprofen Oral Suspension; Ibuprofen Tablets;
USP 25: Ibuprofen and Pseudoephedrine Hydrochloride Tablets; Ibuprofen Oral Suspension; Ibuprofen Tablets.

Proprietary Preparations (details are given in Part 3)
Aust.: Actifen; Avallone; Brufen; Dismenol Neu; Dolgit; Dolibu; Dolofort; Doloren†; Duafen; Ibudol; Ibugel†; Ibumetin; Ibupron†; Iburem†; Ibutop; Imbun; Kratalgin; Nurofen†; Seractil; Tabcin; **Austral.:** ACT-3; Actiprofen; Brufen; Nurofen; Rafen; Tri-Profen; **Belg.:** Advil Mono; Brufen; Bufedon†; Decontractyl New; Ibu-Slow; Ibumed; Ibutop; Inabrin†; Junifen; Malafene; Motrin†; Nurofen; Perviam; Siprofen; Spidifen; **Braz.:** Actiprofen; Advil; Artril; Danilon; Doretrim AP; Motrin; Parartrin; **Canad.:** Actiprofen; Advil; Motrin; Novo-Profen; **Denm.:** Apain; Brufen; Ibumetin; Ibunet†; Ibureumin; Ibutop; Ipren; Nurofen†; Solpaflex†; **Fin.:** Brufen; Burana; Dexit; Ibumax; Ibumetin; Ibusal; Ibuxin; **Fr.:** Advil; Algifene; Anadvil; Antarene; Brufen; Doctril; Dolgit; Ergix; Expanfen; Gelufene; Hemagene Tailleur; Ibualgic; Ibutop; Intralgis; Nureflex; Nurofen; Oralfene; Solufen; Syntofene; Tiburon†; Upfen; **Ger.:** Aktren; Anco; Brufen; Cesra†; Contraneural; Dentigoat†; Dignoflex†; Dismenol N; Dolgit; Dolo neos†; Dolo-Puren; Dolodoc; Dolormin; dura-Ibu†; duraIbuprofen; Esprenit; Exneural; Fibraflex; Gyno-Neuralgin; Gynofug; Ibu; Ibu-ratiopharm; Ibu-Vivimed†; Ibubest†; Ibubeta; Ibudolor; Ibuflam; Ibufug; Ibuhexal; Ibumerck; Ibuphlogont; Ibuprof; Ibutad; Ibutop; Ilvico grippal; Imbun; Jenaprofen; Kontagripp Mono; Logomed Schmerz†; Mensoton; Mobilat†; Novogent; Nurofen; Optalidon; Opturem; Parsal; Pfeil; ratioDolor; Schmerz-Dolgit; Seclodin†; Tabalon; Tempil; Tispol Ibu-DD; Togal N; Trauma-Dolgit; Urem; **Hong Kong:** Advil; Brufen; Ibuslow; Nurofen; Rupan; **Irl.:** Actiprofen†; Advil; Brufen; Bufigen; Cunil; Ibugel; Melfen; Nurofen; Phorpain; Proflex; Solfen; **Israel:** Adex; Artofen; Ibufen; Ibuleve; Nurofen; **Ital.:** Aciril; Algofen; Antalgil; Antalisin; Arfen; Asepsal†; Benfast; Benflogin; Brufen; Brufort; Calmine; Cibalgina Due Fast; Dolocyl; Edenil; Faspic; Flubenil†; Gineflor; Ginenorm; Kost†; Moment; Neo-Mindol†; Nurofen; Zafen; **Mex.:** Advidon; Advil; Ainex; Algidol; Butacortelone; Citalgan; Days; Dibufen; Dipofen; Diprodol; Dolver; Eufenil; Flexafen; Gobrosan; Ibuflex; Ibupril; Medifen; Mejorultra; Micarzin; Motrin; Natiken; Proartrinal; Quadrax; Realdrax; Ribufen; Tabalon; **Neth.:** Advil; Brufen; Femapirint; Nerofent; Nurofen; Zafen; **Norw.:** Brufen; Ibumetin; Ibux; **NZ:** ACT-3; Anafen; Brufen; Nurofen; Panafen; **Port.:** Arfen; Belep; Brufen; Dolocyl; Ibupax; Inabrin†; Motrin†; Nuprilan†; Ozonol; Trifene; **S.Afr.:** Adfen†; Antiflam; Betagesic; Betaprofen; Brufen; Brugesic; Clinofen†; Dynofen; Ibopaint†; Ibufarm†; Ibuleve; Ibumed; Inza; Magnatex†; Norflam T; Nurofen; Ranfen; Rolab-Antiflam; Solufen†; **Singapore:** Ampifen; Bifen; Brufen; Ibufen; Ibuloid; Nurofen; **Spain:** Actimidol; Advil; Aldospray Analgesico; Algiasdin; Algisan†; Altior; Dalsy; Doctril; Dolocyl†; Dorival; Ediluna†; Espidifen; Faspic†; Femaprin;

Femidol; Feminalin; Ibenon; Ibuscent; Isdol; Kalma; Leonal; Narfent; Neobrufen; Noalgil†; Nodolfen; Nureflex; Nurofen; Pocyl; Sadefen; Saetil; Solufena; Solvium; Todalgil†; **Swed.:** Alindrin; Brufen; Duobrus†; Ibumetin; Ipren; Nurofen†; **Switz.:** Algifor; Brufen; Bufeno†; DexOptifen; Dismenol N; Dolgit; Dolo-Dismenol; Dolo-Spediden; Dolocyl; Dologel†; Ecoprofen; Faspic; Grefen; Ibufen-L; Ibugel†; Ibumed†; Ibusifar; Iproben; Iprogel; Irfen; Motrin†; Nurofen; Optifen; Panax N; Redufen; Serviprofen†; Solufen; Spedifen; **Thai.:** Aprofen; Brufen; Brumed; Bruprin; Brusil; Bumed; Cefen; Duran; G-Fen; Greatofen; Ibrufen; Ibu; Ibufac; Ibufen; Ibugan; Ibulan; Iburen; Junifen; Mafen; Nurofen; Ostofen; P-Fen; Perofen; Pippen; Probufen; Profena; Rheumanox; Rumasian; Rumatifen; Rupan; Schufen; Serviprofen; Skelan IB; Tofen; Trofen; **UAE:** Profinal; **UK:** Advil; Anadin Ibuprofen; Anadin Ultra; Apsifen†; Arthrofen; Brufen; Cuprofen; Ebufac; Femafen†; Fenbid; Galprofen; Hedex Ibuprofen; Ibrufhalal; Ibufac; Ibufem; Ibugel; Ibular; Ibuleve; Ibumousse; Ibuspray; Ibutop Cuprofen; Ibutop Ralgex; Inoven; Isisfen; Junifen†; Librofem; Lidifen; Manorfen; Mentholatum Ibuprofen; Migrafen; Motrin; Novaprin; Nurofen; Nurofen Advance; Obifen; Orbifen; Pacifene; Phensic Ibuprofen; Phor Pain; Proflex; Relcofen; Rimafen; **USA:** Advil; Arthritis Foundation Ibuprofen†; Bayer Select Pain Relief Formula†; Dynafed IB†; Genpril; Haltran; Ibifon†; Ibu; Ibu-Tab; Ibu-4, -6, -8; Ibuprin†; Ibuprohm†; Menadol; Midol IB†; Motrin; Nuprin; Saleto-200.

Multi-ingredient: **Austral.:** Nurofen Cold & Flu; Tri-Profen Cold & Flu; **Belg.:** Nurofen + Codeine; **Braz.:** Algi-Danilon; Algifen; Fymnal; Reuplex; **Canad.:** Advil Cold & Sinus; Dayquil Sinus with Pain Relief†; Dristan Sinus; **Fin.:** Ardinex; Burana-C; **Fr.:** Cliptol; Nurofen Rhume; Rhinadvil; Rhinureflex; Vicks Rhume; **Irl.:** Advil Cold & Flu; Codafen Continus; Nurofen Cold & Flu; **Ital.:** Solviflu; **Mex.:** Carbager-Plus; Dolocibal; **NZ:** Nurofen Cold & Flu; Nurofen Plus; **S.Afr.:** Advil CS; Lotem; Mypaid; Myprodol; Nurofen Cold & Flu; **Spain:** Nurogrip; Salvarina; **Swed.:** Ardinex; **Switz.:** Ibufen-L; **Thai.:** Brustan; Cetan; Dologen; Rumatifen-Plus; Skelan; **UK:** Advil Cold & Sinus; Codafen Continus; Deep Relief; Lemsip Pharmacy Powercaps; Lemsip Power +†; Non-Drowsy Sudafed Dual Relief Max; Nurofen Cold & Flu; Nurofen Plus; Radian-B Ibuprofen; Solpaflex; Vicks Action†; **USA:** Advil Cold & Sinus; Childrens Motrin Cold; Dimetapp Sinus; Dristan Sinus; Motrin IB Sinus; Sine-Aid IB; Vicoprofen.

Ibuproxam (12841-a)

Ibuproxam (rINN).

4-Isobutylhydratropohydroxamic acid.
$C_{13}H_{19}NO_2 = 221.3.$
CAS — 53648-05-8.
ATC — M01AE13.

Profile
Ibuproxam is an NSAID (p.63) that has been used in musculoskeletal, joint, and soft-tissue disorders.

Preparations
Proprietary Preparations (details are given in Part 3)
Ital.: Ibudros; **Spain:** Nialen.

Imidazole Salicylate (16848-e)

Imidazole Salicylate (rINN).

Imidazole compounded with salicylic acid.
$C_{10}H_{10}N_2O_3 = 206.2.$
CAS — 36364-49-5.
ATC — N02BA16.

Profile
Imidazole salicylate is a salicylic acid derivative (see Aspirin, p.14) that has been used in the treatment of fever and inflammatory respiratory-tract and otorhinolaryngeal disorders. Imidazole salicylate has been given in doses of up to 2.25 g daily in divided doses by mouth. It has also been given as a rectal suppository and has been applied topically as a 5% gel for the relief of muscular and rheumatic pain.

Preparations
Proprietary Preparations (details are given in Part 3)
Ital.: Flogozen; Fluenzen; Selezen.

Indometacin (2658-m)

Indometacin (BAN, rINN).

Indometacinum; Indomethacin (USAN). [1-(4-Chlorobenzoyl)-5-methoxy-2-methylindol-3-yl]acetic acid.
$C_{19}H_{16}ClNO_4 = 357.8.$
CAS — 53-86-1.
ATC — C01EB03; M01AB01; M02AA23; S01BC01.
Pharmacopoeias. In Chin., Eur. (see p.vi), Int., Jpn, and US.

Indometacin is unstable in alkaline solution.

Pharmacopoeial description
Ph. Eur.: A white or yellow, crystalline powder. Practically insoluble in water; sparingly soluble in alcohol. Protect from light.

USP 25: A pale yellow to yellow-tan, crystalline powder having not more than a slight odour. It exhibits polymorphism. Practically insoluble in water; soluble 1 in 50 of alcohol, 1 in 30 of chloroform, and 1 in 40 of ether. Protect from light.

Indometacin Sodium (19343-w)

Indometacin Sodium (BANM, rINNM).

Indomethacin Sodium (USAN); Indometacin Sodium Trihydrate. Sodium 1-(4-chlorobenzoyl)-5-methoxy-2-methylindole-3-acetate, trihydrate.

$C_{19}H_{15}ClNNaO_4,3H_2O = 433.8$.

CAS — 74252-25-8.

Pharmacopoeias. In US.

Pharmacopoeial description

USP 25: Protect from light.

Incompatibility. Indometacin sodium injection is reconstituted with preservative-free sodium chloride for injection or water for injection. Preparations containing glucose should not be used; reconstitution at a pH below 6 may cause precipitation of indometacin. Visual incompatibility has been reported between indometacin sodium injection and tolazoline hydrochloride,[1] 7.5 and 10% glucose injection, calcium gluconate, dobutamine, dopamine, cimetidine,[2] gentamicin sulfate, levofloxacin,[3] and tobramycin sulfate.[4] A pH below 6 may account for the visual incompatibility of indometacin sodium and several of these drugs.

1. Marquardt ED. Visual compatibility of tolazoline hydrochloride with various medications during simulated Y-site injection. *Am J Hosp Pharm* 1990; **47**: 1802–3.
2. Ishisaka DY, *et al.* Visual compatibility of indomethacin sodium trihydrate with drugs given to neonates by continuous infusion. *Am J Hosp Pharm* 1991; **48**: 2442–3.
3. Saltsman CL, *et al.* Compatibility of levofloxacin with 34 medications during simulated Y-site administration. *Am J Health-Syst Pharm* 1999; **56**: 1458–90.
4. Thompson DF, Heflin NR. Incompatibility of injectable indomethacin with gentamicin sulfate or tobramycin sulfate. *Am J Hosp Pharm* 1992; **49**: 836–8.

Stability. A reconstituted solution of indometacin sodium 500 µg per mL was stable for 14 days when stored at 2° to 6° in either the manufacturer's original glass vial or in a polypropylene syringe.[1]

1. Walker SE, *et al.* Stability of reconstituted indomethacin sodium trihydrate in original vials and polypropylene syringes. *Am J Health-Syst Pharm* 1998; **55**: 154–8.

Adverse Effects

As for NSAIDs in general, p.63.

Adverse effects are more frequent with indometacin than with many other NSAIDs, the most common being gastrointestinal disturbances, headache, vertigo, dizziness, and lightheadedness. Gastrointestinal perforation, ulceration, and bleeding may also occur; rarely, intestinal strictures have been reported. Other adverse effects include depression, drowsiness, tinnitus, confusion, insomnia, psychiatric disturbances, syncope, convulsions, coma, peripheral neuropathy, blurred vision, corneal deposits and other ocular effects, oedema and weight gain, hypertension, haematuria, skin rashes, pruritus, urticaria, stomatitis, alopecia, and hypersensitivity reactions. Leucopenia, purpura, thrombocytopenia, aplastic anaemia, haemolytic anaemia, agranulocytosis, epistaxis, hyperglycaemia, hyperkalaemia, and vaginal bleeding have been reported. There have also been reports of hepatitis, jaundice, and renal failure. Hypersensitivity reactions may also occur in aspirin-sensitive patients. Rectal irritation and bleeding has been reported occasionally in patients who have received indometacin suppositories.

Adverse effects associated with the use of indometacin in premature **neonates** also include haemorrhagic, renal, gastrointestinal, metabolic, and coagulation disorders; pulmonary hypertension, intracranial bleeding, fluid retention, and exacerbation of infection may also occur.

Effects on the blood. There were 1261 reports of adverse reactions to indometacin reported to the UK Committee on Safety of Medicines between June 1964 and January 1973. These included 157 reports of blood disorders (25 fatal) including thrombocytopenia (35; 5 fatal), aplastic anaemia (17; no fatalities), and agranulocytosis or leucopenia (21; 3 fatal).[1] Subsequently, the First Report from the International Agranulocytosis and Aplastic Anemia Study confirmed a significant relationship between the use of indometacin and agranulocytosis and aplastic anaemia.[2]

Although use of indometacin in 20 women being treated for premature labour did not affect maternal prothrombin or activated partial thromboplastin time, maternal bleeding time during therapy was increased.[3] However, no cases of neonatal intraventricular haemorrhage or maternal postpartum haemorrhage were seen.

1. Cuthbert MF. Adverse reactions to non-steroidal antirheumatic drugs. *Curr Med Res Opin* 1974; **2**: 600–10.

The symbol † denotes a preparation no longer actively marketed

2. The International Agranulocytosis and Aplastic Anemia Study. Risks of agranulocytosis and aplastic anemia: a first report of their relation to drug use with special reference to analgesics. *JAMA* 1986; **256**: 1749–57.
3. Lunt CC, *et al.* The effect of indomethacin tocolysis on maternal coagulation status. *Obstet Gynecol* 1994; **84**: 820–2.

Effects on cerebral blood flow. See under Patent Ductus Arteriosus in Uses and Administration, below.

Effects on electrolytes. Hyporeninaemia, hypoaldosteronism, and hyperkalaemia have been associated with the use of indometacin.[1-5] See also under Effects on the Kidneys, below.

1. Zimran A, *et al.* Incidence of hyperkalaemia induced by indomethacin in a hospital population. *BMJ* 1985; **291**: 107–8.
2. Tan SY, *et al.* Indomethacin-induced prostaglandin inhibition with hyperkalaemia: a reversible cause of hyporeninemic hypoaldosteronism. *Ann Intern Med* 1979; **90**: 783–5.
3. MacCarthy EP, *et al.* Indomethacin-induced hyperkalaemia. *Med J Aust* 1979; **1**: 550.
4. Beroniade V, *et al.* Indomethacin-induced inhibition of prostaglandin with hyperkalemia. *Ann Intern Med* 1979; **91**: 499–500.
5. Findling JW, *et al.* Indomethacin-induced hyperkalemia in three patients with gouty arthritis. *JAMA* 1980; **244**: 1127–8.

Effects on the eyes. Severe and irreversible retinopathy, presumably due to long-term ingestion of high doses of indometacin occurred in a 33-year-old man.[1] A summary of previous literature reports of indometacin-induced ocular effects indicated that indometacin was retinotoxic, although to what degree was uncertain. For reference to effects on the optic nerve associated with indometacin, see p.63.

1. Graham CM, Blach RK. Indomethacin retinopathy: case report and review. *Br J Ophthalmol* 1988; **72**: 434–8.

Effects on the gastrointestinal tract. Nausea, vomiting, dyspepsia, gastrointestinal lesions, and serious reactions including gastrointestinal bleeding, ulceration, and perforation have occurred in patients receiving indometacin. Although it is well established that NSAIDs can produce adverse effects on the upper gastrointestinal tract, indometacin and other NSAIDs can also affect the large intestines.[1]

Between January 1965 and 1985 the UK Committee on Safety of Medicines had recorded 12 cases of intestinal perforation (7 deaths), 5 cases of intestinal ulceration (1 death), and 2 cases of intestinal ulceration and perforation (no deaths).[2]

Intestinal perforation has been observed in **neonates** following enteral administration of indometacin.[3] However, intravenous administration appears to be associated with a lower incidence of adverse effects.[4] Of 2482 preterm neonates given indometacin intravenously 146 were reported as having experienced adverse effects.[4] Half of the reports (73 cases) were rated as being possibly, probably, or definitely related to the drug treatment by the reporting physician. There were 18 reports of gastrointestinal bleeding and 13 reports of necrotising enterocolitis.

1. Oren R, Ligumsky M. Indomethacin-induced colonic ulceration and bleeding. *Ann Pharmacother* 1994; **28**: 883–5.
2. Stewart JT, *et al.* Anti-inflammatory drugs and bowel perforations and haemorrhage. *BMJ* 1985; **290**: 787–8.
3. Alpan G, *et al.* Localized intestinal perforations after enteral administration of indomethacin in premature infants. *J Pediatr* 1985; **106**: 277–81.
4. Walters M. Tolerance of intravenous indomethacin treatment for premature infants with patent ductus arteriosus. *BMJ* 1988; **297**: 773–4.

Effects on the joints. For references to concern that NSAIDs such as indometacin may accelerate the rate of cartilage destruction in patients with osteoarthritis, see under NSAIDs, p.64.

Effects on the kidneys. Acute renal failure,[1-3] nephrotic syndrome,[4] and renal papillary necrosis[5] have been reported in patients given indometacin. There have been suggestions that misoprostol might reduce the risk of indometacin-induced renal toxicity.[6,7]

Renal dysfunction has also occurred in **neonates** given indometacin intravenously for patent ductus arteriosus. Of 2482 neonates treated in the UK between 1980 and 1988, indometacin-associated adverse effects reported to the manufacturer[8] included renal failure or shutdown (10 neonates), fall in urea concentration (12), hyponatraemia (16), and increase in creatinine concentration (5). The renal impairment was not usually sustained or serious, but in neonates with pre-existing renal impairment, indometacin therapy may lead to serious deterioration. Autopsy of 6 neonates who had had prolonged exposure to indometacin *in utero* and had died of persistent anuria showed cystic dilatation of the superficial nephrons, ischaemia of the inner renal cortex, and interstitial fibrosis.[9]

1. Walshe JJ, Venuto RC. Acute oliguric renal failure induced by indomethacin: possible mechanism. *Ann Intern Med* 1979; **91**: 47–9.
2. Bernheim JL, Korzets Z. Indomethacin-induced renal failure. *Ann Intern Med* 1979; **91**: 792.
3. Chan X. Fatal renal failure due to indomethacin. *Lancet* 1987; **ii**: 340.
4. Boiskin I, *et al.* Indomethacin and the nephrotic syndrome. *Ann Intern Med* 1987; **106**: 776–7.
5. Mitchell H, *et al.* Indomethacin-induced renal papillary necrosis in juvenile chronic arthritis. *Lancet* 1982; **ii**: 558–9.
6. Weir MR, *et al.* Minimization of indomethacin-induced reduction in renal function by misoprostol. *J Clin Pharmacol* 1991; **31**: 729–35.
7. Wong F, *et al.* The effect of misoprostol on indomethacin-induced renal dysfunction in well-compensated cirrhosis. *J Hepatol* 1995; **23**: 1–7.

8. Walters M. Tolerance of intravenous indomethacin treatment for premature infants with patent ductus arteriosus. *BMJ* 1988; **297**: 773–4.
9. van der Heijden BJ, *et al.* Persistent anuria, neonatal death, and renal microcystic lesions after prenatal exposure to indomethacin. *Am J Obstet Gynecol* 1994; **171**: 617–23.

Effects on the liver. Cholestasis occurred in a 52-year-old woman several days after starting indometacin;[1] liver function values returned to normal once indometacin was discontinued.

1. Cappell MS, *et al.* Indomethacin-associated cholestasis. *J Clin Gastroenterol* 1988; **10**: 445–7.

Hypersensitivity. Hypersensitivity reactions including acute asthma have been reported following the use of indometacin suppositories,[1] eye drops,[2] or capsules[3] by patients who were aspirin-sensitive or had a history of asthma.

1. Timperman J. A fatal asthmatic attack following administration of an indomethacin suppository. *J Forensic Med* 1971; **18**: 30–2.
2. Sheehan GJ, *et al.* Acute asthma attack due to ophthalmic indomethacin. *Ann Intern Med* 1989; **111**: 337–8.
3. Johnson NM, *et al.* Indomethacin-induced asthma in aspirin-sensitive patients. *BMJ* 1977; **2**: 1291.

Precautions

As for NSAIDs in general, p.64.

Indometacin should be administered with caution to patients with epilepsy, parkinsonism, or psychiatric disorders. Dizziness may affect the performance of skilled tasks such as driving. Patients on long-term indometacin therapy should be examined regularly for adverse effects, and some authorities particularly recommend periodic blood and ophthalmic examinations. Rectal administration should be avoided in patients with proctitis and haemorrhoids.

In addition indometacin should not be given to **neonates** with untreated infection, with significantly impaired renal function, or with necrotising enterocolitis. Infants who are bleeding (especially gastrointestinal bleeding or intracranial haemorrhage) or who have thrombocytopenia or coagulation defects should not be given indometacin and those receiving indometacin should be monitored during treatment for signs of bleeding. Electrolytes and renal function should also be monitored and if anuria or marked oliguria is evident at the time of a scheduled second or third dose, administration should be delayed until renal function has returned to normal.

False-negative results in the dexamethasone suppression test have been reported in patients taking indometacin.

Breast feeding. Convulsions in a one-week old breast-fed infant appeared to be associated with ingestion of indometacin by the mother;[1] the child had normal motor and mental development at the age of 1 year and seizures had not recurred. Indometacin has been detected in breast milk, but some workers[2] consider that the amount is so small that it should not constitute a contra-indication to breast feeding.

1. Eeg-Olofsson O, *et al.* Convulsions in a breast-fed infant after maternal indomethacin. *Lancet* 1978; **ii**: 215.
2. Beaulac-Baillargeon L, Allard G. Distribution of indomethacin in human milk and estimation of its milk to plasma ratio in vitro. *Br J Clin Pharmacol* 1993; **36**: 413–16.

The elderly. Following a study[1] of the pharmacokinetics of indometacin in the elderly it was suggested that the maintenance dose of indometacin in elderly patients should be reduced by 25%. The total clearance of indometacin in elderly subjects had been reduced when compared with that in young subjects; this was thought to be due to reduced hepatic metabolism in the elderly.

1. Oberbauer R, *et al.* Pharmacokinetics of indomethacin in the elderly. *Clin Pharmacokinet* 1993; **24**: 428–34.

Pregnancy. See under Premature Labour in Uses and Administration, below.

Interactions

For interactions associated with NSAIDs, see p.65.

Concurrent administration of anti-inflammatory doses of aspirin decreases indometacin blood concentrations by about 20%. Administration of diflunisal with indometacin decreases the renal clearance and increases plasma concentrations of indometacin. Combined use of diflunisal and indometacin has resulted in fatal gastrointestinal haemorrhage; therefore, these drugs should not be used concurrently. Plasma concentrations of indometacin are likely to be increased in patients receiving probenecid.

Antibacterials. Concomitant administration of indometacin has been reported to increase plasma concentrations of *aminoglycoside antibiotics*.

Antipsychotics. A report[1] of severe drowsiness and confusion in patients given *haloperidol* with indometacin.

1. Bird HA, *et al.* Drowsiness due to haloperidol/indomethacin in combination. *Lancet* 1983; **i:** 830–1.

Bone modulating drugs. Concomitant administration of indometacin has been reported to increase the bioavailability of *tiludronate*.

Desmopressin. Concomitant administration of indometacin has been reported to enhance the effect of desmopressin.

Parasympathomimetics. The manufacturer of acetylcholine chloride ophthalmic preparations has stated that there have been reports that *acetylcholine* and *carbachol* have been ineffective when used in patients treated with topical (ophthalmic) NSAIDs.

Pharmacokinetics

Indometacin is readily absorbed from the gastrointestinal tract in adults; peak plasma concentrations are reached about 2 hours after a dose. Absorption may be slowed by food or by aluminium or magnesium containing antacids. In premature neonates, absorption of oral indometacin is poor and incomplete. The bioavailability of rectal suppositories in adults has been reported to be comparable with or slightly less than the bioavailability with oral dosage forms.

Indometacin is about 99% bound to plasma proteins. It is distributed into synovial fluid, the CNS, and placenta. Low concentrations have been distributed into breast milk. The terminal plasma half-life has been reported to range from 2.6 to 11.2 hours in adults. The terminal half-life in neonates has been reported to be between 15 and 30 hours. Indometacin is metabolised in the liver to its glucuronide conjugate and to desmethylindometacin, desbenzoylindometacin, desmethyl-desbenzoylindometacin, and to their glucuronides. Some indometacin undergoes N-deacylation. Indometacin and its conjugates undergo enterohepatic circulation. Excretion of indometacin and its metabolites is predominantly in the urine with lesser amounts appearing in the faeces.

◊ References.

1. Moise KJ, *et al.* Placental transfer of indometacin in the human pregnancy. *Am J Obstet Gynecol* 1990; **162:** 549–54.
2. Lebedevs TH, *et al.* Excretion of indometacin in breast milk. *Br J Clin Pharmacol* 1991; **32:** 751–4.
3. Wiest DB, *et al.* Population pharmacokinetics of intravenous indomethacin in neonates with symptomatic patent ductus arteriosus. *Clin Pharmacol Ther* 1991; **49:** 550–7.
4. Beaulac-Baillargeon L, Allard G. Distribution of indometacin in human milk and estimation of its milk to plasma ratio in vitro. *Br J Clin Pharmacol* 1993; **36:** 413–16.

Uses and Administration

Indometacin, an indole acetic acid derivative, is an NSAID (p.65).

It is used in musculoskeletal and joint disorders including ankylosing spondylitis, osteoarthritis, rheumatoid arthritis, and acute gout, and in peri-articular disorders such as bursitis and tendinitis. It may also be used in inflammation, pain, and oedema following orthopaedic procedures, in mild to moderate pain in conditions such as dysmenorrhoea, and it has been used in the management of postoperative pain as an adjunct to opioids, and in the treatment of fever. Indometacin is also used as the sodium salt to close patent ductus arteriosus in premature infants (see below).

The usual initial dose by mouth in chronic musculoskeletal and joint disorders is 25 mg two or three times daily increased, if required, by 25 to 50 mg daily at weekly intervals to 150 to 200 mg daily. To alleviate night pain and morning stiffness, up to 100 mg of the total daily dose may be administered by mouth, or rectally as a suppository, on retiring. Alternatively, the total daily dose may be administered by rectum as 100 mg in the morning and at night. The total daily combined dose by mouth and by rectum should not exceed 200 mg. In acute gout the daily dose is 150 to 200 mg in divided doses until all symptoms and signs subside; in dysmenorrhoea up to 75 mg daily has been suggested.

Modified-release preparations of indometacin are available for administration once or twice daily.

Indometacin has been used topically as 0.5 or 1% eye drops to prevent miosis during cataract surgery; the

usual dose is one drop instilled 4 times daily, beginning on the day before surgery, and one drop 45 minutes before surgery. The eye drops may then be instilled 4 times daily for up to 10 to 12 weeks postoperatively to prevent cystoid macular oedema.

When used to close patent ductus arteriosus in premature infants indometacin sodium is given as a short course of therapy of three intravenous doses given at 12- to 24-hour intervals; each dose should be infused over 20 to 30 minutes. Indometacin sodium injection is reconstituted with preservative-free sodium chloride for injection or water for injection; glucose solutions should not be used. The dose of indometacin sodium (expressed as indometacin) depends upon the age of the neonate and the following doses have been suggested based upon the age at the first dose: less than 48 hours old, 200 µg per kg body-weight initially followed by two further doses of 100 µg per kg each; 2 to 7 days old, three doses of 200 µg per kg each; over 7 days old, 200 µg per kg initially followed by two further doses of 250 µg per kg each. If, 48 hours after this course of therapy the ductus remains open or re-opens a second course of therapy may be employed, but if this produces no response surgery may be necessary.

Meglumine indometacin and a lipid soluble ester of indometacin, indometacin farnesil ($C_{34}H_{40}ClNO_4 = 562.1$), have also been used for painful and inflammatory conditions. A complex of indometacin and L-arginine, known as indoarginine, has been used in pain, inflammation, and febrile conditions.

Bartter's syndrome. The treatment of Bartter's syndrome can often be difficult (see p.1183). Blocking the kinin-prostaglandin axis with a cyclo-oxygenase inhibitor such as indometacin improves hypokalaemia and other clinical features (including growth retardation) in children with the syndrome.[1-3]

1. Littlewood JM, *et al.* Treatment of childhood Bartter's syndrome with indomethacin. *Lancet* 1976; **ii:** 795.
2. Seidel C, *et al.* Pre-pubertal growth in the hyperprostaglandin E syndrome. *Pediatr Nephrol* 1995; **9:** 723–8.
3. Craig JC, Falk MC. Indomethacin for renal impairment in neonatal Bartter's syndrome. *Lancet* 1996; **347:** 550.

Diabetes insipidus. Indometacin and other prostaglandin synthetase inhibitors have been reported to decrease urine volume in all types of nephrogenic diabetes insipidus (p.1273).

References.

1. Rosen GH, *et al.* Indomethacin for nephrogenic diabetes insipidus in a four-week-old infant. *Clin Pharm* 1986; **5:** 254–6.
2. Libber S, *et al.* Treatment of nephrogenic diabetes insipidus with prostaglandin synthesis inhibitors. *J Pediatr* 1986; **108:** 305–11.
3. Allen HM, *et al.* Indomethacin in the treatment of lithium-induced nephrogenic diabetes insipidus. *Arch Intern Med* 1989; **149:** 1123–6.
4. Martinez EJ, *et al.* Lithium-induced nephrogenic diabetes insipidus treated with indomethacin. *South Med J* 1993; **86:** 971–3.

Malignant neoplasms. Some NSAIDs such as indometacin may be of value both for the differential diagnosis and the management of neoplastic fever as they appear to be more effective in reducing this type of fever than against fever associated with infections.[1] Indometacin has also been tried for the treatment of fever and flu-like symptoms associated with interleukin-2 therapy although there has been concern over exacerbation of renal toxicity (see p.548). It has been suggested that indometacin might also possess some antineoplastic activity.[2]

1. Engervall P, *et al.* Antipyretic effect of indomethacin in malignant lymphoma. *Acta Med Scand* 1986; **219:** 501–6.
2. Mertens WC, *et al.* Effect of indomethacin plus ranitidine in advanced melanoma patients on high-dose interleukin-2. *Lancet* 1992; **340:** 397–8.

Neonatal intraventricular haemorrhage. Indometacin is one of a number of drugs that has been tried prophylactically to prevent the development of intraventricular haemorrhage in neonates at risk (see p.723). Several mechanisms have been proposed for its possible action including reduction of cerebral flow as a result of vasoconstriction, reduction of oxygen free-radical damage, and accelerated maturation of blood vessels around the ventricles. Early studies[1-3] of the use of indometacin for prevention of intraventricular haemorrhage produced conflicting results. A subsequent large multicentre study[4] suggested that indometacin could reduce the incidence and severity of intraventricular haemorrhage, especially for the more severe forms. Neonates who received indometacin were given a dose of 100 µg per kg body-weight intravenously at 6 to 12 hours after delivery and then every 24 hours for 2 additional doses. Despite concern[5] that an unusually large number of neonates with severe intraventricular haemorrhage in the control group might have biased the findings, a systematic review came to similar conclusions about the benefit.[6] A concern with the use of indometacin is the possibility that it may produce cerebral ischaemia due to its vasoconstrictor action and therefore increase the risk of developmental handicaps. A review[6] of stud-

ies of prophylactic indometacin concluded that more studies of possible adverse effects and long-term outcome are needed before indometacin can be recommended for routine use. However, follow-up at 3 years of age[7] and at 4 ½ years of age[8] of the infants included in the multicentre study reported no adverse effects on cognitive or motor development.

Another study[9] has indicated that indometacin does not prevent the progression of existing low grade intraventricular haemorrhage.

1. Ment LR, *et al.* Randomized indomethacin trial for prevention of intraventricular hemorrhage in very low birth weight infants. *J Pediatr* 1985; **107:** 937–43.
2. Rennie JM, *et al.* Early administration of indomethacin to preterm infants. *Arch Dis Child* 1986; **61:** 233–8.
3. Bada HS, *et al.* Indomethacin reduces the risks of severe intraventricular hemorrhage. *J Pediatr* 1989; **115:** 631–7.
4. Ment LR, *et al.* Low-dose indomethacin and prevention of intraventricular hemorrhage: a multicenter randomized trial. *Pediatrics* 1994; **93:** 543–50.
5. Volpe JJ. Brain injury caused by intraventricular hemorrhage: is indomethacin the silver bullet for prevention? *Pediatrics* 1994; **93:** 673–7.
6. Fowlie PW. Intravenous indomethacin for preventing mortality and morbidity in very low birth weight infants (updated 29 May 2001). Available in The Cochrane Library; Issue 4. Oxford: Update Software; 2001.
7. Ment LR, *et al.* Neurodevelopmental outcome at 36 months' corrected age of preterm infants in the multicenter indomethacin intraventricular hemorrhage prevention trial. *Pediatrics* 1996; **98:** 714–18.
8. Mint LR, *et al.* Outcome of children in the indomethacin intraventricular hemorrhage prevention trial. *Pediatrics* 2000; **105:** 485–91.
9. Ment LR, *et al.* Low-dose indomethacin therapy and extension of intraventricular hemorrhage: a multicenter randomized trial. *J Pediatr* 1994; **124:** 951–5.

Patent ductus arteriosus. In the fetal circulation the ductus arteriosus connects the pulmonary artery and the descending aorta. After birth, various mechanisms, including a fall in prostaglandin concentration, trigger its closure but in some infants the ductus arteriosus fails to close, a condition known as persistent patent ductus arteriosus. This condition may be found in infants with congenital heart defects but is more commonly seen in premature neonates, especially those with respiratory distress syndrome. Some infants may be asymptomatic or have only slight clinical symptoms and no immediate intervention is required. In many cases spontaneous closure will occur after several months, or else surgical ligation may be performed if clinical symptoms persist. In some infants a patent ductus arteriosus is necessary for maintaining some oxygenation of the blood, for example in pulmonary artery atresia or transposition of the great arteries. These infants require treatment with a prostaglandin such as alprostadil or dinoprostone to maintain patency of the ductus arteriosus until surgery can be performed to correct the malformation. Infants with haemodynamically significant ductus arteriosus, signs of heart failure, and who require ventilation should undergo treatment.

Initial management of persistent patent ductus arteriosus involves fluid restriction, diuretics, correction of anaemia, and support of respiration. If this fails to control symptoms after 24 to 48 hours then indometacin is generally given to promote closure of the ductus.[1-4] Some workers[5] advocate treatment with indometacin as soon as symptoms become apparent rather than delaying treatment until signs of congestive failure develop. Early treatment may significantly reduce the morbidities arising from a persistent patent ductus arteriosus. Chlorothiazide and frusemide [furosemide] are common diuretics used. There has been concern that frusemide [furosemide] may promote delayed ductus closure in infants with respiratory distress syndrome,[2,6] although the concurrent use of frusemide [furosemide] does not seem to inhibit closure during treatment with indometacin[7] and may reduce adverse renal effects of indometacin.[7,8] Indometacin probably leads to closure of the ductus through inhibition of prostaglandin synthesis. It is usually given intravenously as the sodium salt. The current practice is to give 3 doses at usual intervals of 12 to 24 hours with the amount depending on the age of the neonate. Indometacin has been given by mouth where the injection is unavailable, but absorption of oral indometacin is poor and incomplete in premature neonates. A second course of injections may be given 48 hours after the first course if the ductus remains open or has re-opened. Should that fail (which may be the case in 25% of infants treated[1,9]) then surgery is required.

A decreased need for surgical closure and reduced recurrences were seen in neonates in whom standard intravenous indometacin therapy was followed by maintenance therapy (intravenous indometacin 200 µg per kg body-weight per day for an additional 5 days). Similar beneficial findings were reported[10] in infants given prolonged low-dose indometacin therapy (100 µg per kg per day for 6 days). An additional benefit was a lower incidence of adverse effects; fewer infants experienced a rise in serum creatinine or urea concentrations. However, a later study[11] has suggested that prolonged administration of low-dose indometacin (100 µg per kg per day for 7 days) is less effective than standard therapy and may be associated with more adverse effects. Prophylactic administration of indometacin reduces the chance of developing symptomatic patent ductus arteriosus,[5,12,13] but not morbidity, and more data are needed on the incidence of possible adverse effects and neurodevelopmental outcomes before routine use of this strategy can be recommended.[13] Indeed, a more recent study[14] has found that although prophylactic indometacin did reduce the frequency of patent ductus arteriosus it did not improve the rate of survival without neurosensory impairment at 18 months in extremely low birth-weight infants.

Ibuprofen also appears to be effective in closing a patent ductus arteriosus,[15-19] and it has been suggested that ibuprofen might be a better choice than indometacin as, unlike indometacin, it does not have adverse effects on renal, mesenteric, and cerebral haemodynamics, and oxygenation.[15,16,18,20] However, some workers[21] found that when indometacin was given by continuous intravenous infusion, rather than by rapid injection, the usual fall in cerebral blood flow velocity was avoided.

1. Silove ED. Pharmacological manipulation of the ductus arteriosus. *Arch Dis Child* 1986; **61:** 827–9.
2. Bhatt V, Nahata MC. Pharmacologic management of patent ductus arteriosus. *Clin Pharm* 1989; **8:** 17–33.
3. Barst RJ, Gersony WM. The pharmacological treatment of patent ductus arteriosus: a review of the evidence. *Drugs* 1989; **38:** 249–66.
4. Archer N. Patent ductus arteriosus in the newborn. *Arch Dis Child* 1993; **69:** 529–32.
5. Clyman RI. Recommendations for the postnatal use of indomethacin: an analysis of four separate treatment strategies. *J Pediatr* 1996; **128:** 601–7.
6. Anonymous. Delayed closure of the ductus. *Lancet* 1983; **ii:** 436.
7. Yeh TF, *et al.* Furosemide prevents the renal side effects of indomethacin therapy in premature infants with patent ductus arteriosus. *J Pediatr* 1982; **101:** 433–7.
8. Nahata MC, *et al.* Furosemide can prevent decline in urine output in infants receiving indomethacin for patent ductus closure: a multidose study. *Infusion* 1988; **12:** 11–12 and 15.
9. Gersony WM, *et al.* Effects of indomethacin in premature infants with patent ductus arteriosus: results of a national collaborative study. *J Pediatr* 1983; **102:** 895–906.
10. Rennie JM, Cooke RWI. Prolonged low dose indomethacin for persistent ductus arteriosus of prematurity. *Arch Dis Child* 1991; **66:** 55–8.
11. Tammela O, *et al.* Short versus prolonged indomethacin therapy for patent ductus arteriosus in preterm infants. *J Pediatr* 1999; **134:** 552–7.
12. Couser RJ, *et al.* Prophylactic indomethacin therapy in the first twenty-four hours of life for the prevention of patent ductus arteriosus in preterm infants treated prophylactically with surfactant in the delivery room. *J Pediatr* 1996; **128:** 631–7.
13. Fowlie PW. Intravenous indomethacin for preventing mortality and morbidity in very low birth weight infants (updated 29 May 2001). Available in The Cochrane Library; Issue 4. Oxford: Update Software; 2001.
14. Schmidt B, *et al.* Long-term effects of indomethacin prophylaxis in extremely-low-birth-weight infants. *N Engl J Med* 2001; **344:** 1966–72.
15. Patel J, *et al.* Randomized double-blind controlled trial comparing the effects of ibuprofen with indomethacin on cerebral hemodynamics in preterm infants with patent ductus arteriosus. *Pediatr Res* 2000; **47:** 36–42.
16. Van Overmeire B, *et al.* Treatment of patent ductus arteriosus with ibuprofen. *Arch Dis Child* 1997; **76:** F179–F184.
17. Varvarigou A, *et al.* Early ibuprofen administration to prevent patent ductus arteriosus in premature newborn infants. *JAMA* 1996; **275:** 539–44.
18. Mosca F, *et al.* Comparative evaluation of the effects of indomethacin and ibuprofen on cerebral perfusion and oxygenation in preterm infants with patent ductus arteriosus. *J Pediatr* 1997; **131:** 549–54.
19. Hammerman C, Kaplan M. Comparative tolerability of pharmacological treatments for patent ductus arteriosus. *Drug Safety* 2001; **24:** 537–51.
20. Pezzati M, *et al.* Effects of indomethacin and ibuprofen on mesenteric and renal blood flow in preterm infants with patent ductus arteriosus. *J Pediatr* 1999; **135:** 733–8.
21. Hammerman C, *et al.* Continuous versus multiple rapid infusions of indomethacin: effects on cerebral blood flow velocity. *Pediatrics* 1995; **95:** 244–8.

Polyhydramnios. Reports[1,2] of the beneficial effects of indometacin in the management of polyhydramnios (an excessive accumulation of amniotic fluid).

1. Kirshon B, *et al.* Indomethacin therapy in the treatment of symptomatic polyhydramnios. *Obstet Gynecol* 1990; **75:** 202–5.
2. Ash K, *et al.* TRAP sequence—successful outcome with indomethacin treatment. *Obstet Gynecol* 1990; **76:** 960–2.

Premature labour. The most common approach to postponing premature labour (p.773) with drugs is with a selective beta$_2$ agonist. However, as prostaglandins have a role in uterine contraction and cervical ripening and dilatation, prostaglandin synthetase inhibitors such as indometacin have also been used. Comparative studies[1,2] have demonstrated that indometacin and ritodrine are equally effective in inhibiting uterine contractions and delaying delivery in patients in preterm labour who have intact membranes and in whom the gestational age is less than or equal to 34 weeks. In one study[2] an initial oral loading dose of indometacin 50 mg was given, followed by 25 to 50 mg orally every 4 hours until contractions stopped and then by a maintenance dose of 25 mg every 4 to 6 hours. In the other comparative study[1] indometacin was given as a 100-mg rectal suppository followed by 25 mg orally every 4 hours for 48 hours; if regular uterine contractions persisted 1 to 2 hours after the initial suppository, an additional 100-mg suppository was given before beginning oral therapy. Terbutaline was given for maintenance therapy.

Unfortunately indometacin can adversely affect the fetus. Reported adverse effects include: constriction of the ductus arteriosus,[3,4] which may lead to pulmonary hypertension,[2] bronchopulmonary dysplasia,[5] reduced volume of amniotic fluid (oligohydramnios)[2,4] and possible renal damage.[6] Another complication is that prenatal indometacin exposure may increase both the incidence and severity of patent ductus arteriosus in premature infants,[7,8] as shown by the increased need for post-natal indometacin therapy and surgical ligation in such in-

fants. However, some consider the benefits to outweigh the potential risks.[9] As a result of the risks associated with indometacin it is generally reserved as a second-line tocolytic or for combination with an intravenous tocolytic when an additive effect is required.

1. Morales WJ, *et al.* Efficacy and safety of indomethacin versus ritodrine in the management of preterm labor: a randomized study. *Obstet Gynecol* 1989; **74:** 567–72.
2. Besinger RE, *et al.* Randomized comparative trial of indomethacin and ritodrine for the long-term treatment of preterm labor. *Am J Obstet Gynecol* 1991; **164:** 981–8.
3. Moise KJ, *et al.* Indomethacin in the treatment of premature labor: effects on the fetal ductus arteriosus. *N Engl J Med* 1988; **319:** 327–31.
4. Hallak M, *et al.* Indomethacin for preterm labor: fetal toxicity in a dizygotic twin gestation. *Obstet Gynecol* 1991; **78:** 911–13.
5. Eronen M, *et al.* Increased incidence of bronchopulmonary dysplasia after antenatal administration of indomethacin to prevent preterm labour. *J Pediatr* 1994; **124:** 782–8.
6. van der Heijden BJ, *et al.* Persistent anuria, neonatal death, and renal microcystic lesions after prenatal exposure to indomethacin. *Am J Obstet Gynecol* 1994; **171:** 617–23.
7. Norton ME, *et al.* Neonatal complications after the administration of indomethacin for preterm labor. *N Engl J Med* 1993; **329:** 1602–7.
8. Hammerman C, *et al.* Indomethacin tocolysis increases post-natal patent ductus arteriosus severity. Abstract: *Pediatrics* 1998; **102:** 1202–3. Full version: http://www.pediatrics.org/cgi/content/full/102/5/e56
9. Macones GA, Robinson CA. Is there justification for using indomethacin in preterm labor? An analysis of neonatal risks and benefits. *Am J Obstet Gynecol* 1997; **177:** 819–24.

Preparations

BP 2001: Indometacin Capsules; Indometacin Suppositories; **USP 25:** Indomethacin Capsules; Indomethacin Extended-release Capsules; Indomethacin for Injection; Indomethacin Oral Suspension; Indomethacin Suppositories.

Proprietary Preparations (details are given in Part 3)
Aust.: Flexidin; Indo; Indobene; Indocid; Indocollyre; Indohexal; Indomelan; Indoptol; Liometacen; Luiflex; Ralicid; *Austral.:* Arthrexin; Hicin†; Indocid; Indocid PDA; Indomed†; Indoptol; Indospray; *Belg.:* Indocid; Indoptol; Luiflex; *Braz.:* Agilisin; Indocid; Indocid Colirio; *Canad.:* Indocid; Indocid PDA; Indocollyre†; Indotec; Novo-Methacin; Nu-Indo; Rhodacine; *Denm.:* Confortid; Indocid; Indonet†; *Fin.:* Confortid; Indocid; Indometin; *Fr.:* Ainscrid†; Chrono-Indocid; Indocid; Indocollyre; *Ger.:* Amuno; Chibro-Amuno 3; Confortid; Elmetacin; Indo; Indo Top; Indo-paed; Indo-Phlogont; Indo-Tablinen†; Indocontin; Indomet; Indometratiopharm; Indomet-ratiopharm m; Indometacinum-mp; Indomisal; Indorektal†; Inflam; Jenatacin†; Mobilat; Rheubalmin Indo; Sigadoc; *Hong Kong:* Imbrilon; Indocid; Indocid PDA; Indocollyre; *Irl.:* Cidomel; Flexin Continus; Idomed†; Imbrilon†; Indocid; Indocid PDA; Indomod†; *Israel:* Idomed; Indocollyre; Indotard; Indovis; *Ital.:* Imet; Indocid; Indocollirio; Indom Collirio; Indoxen; Liometacen; Metacen; *Jpn:* Infree; *Mex.:* Antalgin; Endacil; Indocarsil; Indocid; Indoman; Indosan; Indotrin; Labymetacyn; Malival; Mefazil; Reumin; *Neth.:* Indocid; Indocid PDA; Indoptol; *Norw.:* Confortid; Indocid; *NZ:* Arthrexin; Elmetacin; Indocid; Indocid PDA; Rheumacin; *Port.:* Autritis; Dolovin; Elmetacin; Indocid; Indocollyre; *S.Afr.:* Acuflex†; Aflamin; Arthrexin; Articulen; Betacin; Dynametcin†; Elmetacin†; Famethacin; Flamaret; Flamecid†; Indocid; Indoflam†; Indoflex†; Indomed†; Indotal†; Mediflex; Methabid†; Methamax†; Methocaps; Nisaid; Restameth-SR; Rumitard†; *Singapore:* Bonidon; Indocollyre; Indoflam; Methacin; *Spain:* Aliviosin; Artrinovo; Flogoter; Inacid; Indo Framan; Indocaf; Indoftol; Indolgina; Indonilo; Medereumol; Neo Decabutin; Reumo; Reusin; *Swed.:* Confortid; Indomee; *Switz.:* Bonidon; Elmetacin; Helvecin; Indo-Mepha; Indocid; Indophtal; Indoptic; *Thai.:* Bucin; Elmetacin; Idc; Indocid; Indocollyre; Indomed; Inflamate; Inthacine; Liometacen; Metindo; Putatone; Servindomet; *UAE:* Rothacin; *UK:* Artracin; Flexin Continus; Imbrilon†; Indocid; Indocid PDA; Indolar SR; Indomax; Indomod; Indotard†; Maximet SR; Pardelprin; Rheumacin; Rimacid; Slo-Indo; *USA:* Indochron†; Indocin.

Multi-ingredient: *Aust.:* Vonum; *Fin.:* Indalgin; *Fr.:* Indobiotic; *Ger.:* Inflam; *Ital.:* Difmetre; *Mex.:* Malival Compuesto; *Spain:* Artri; Betartrinovo†; Fiacin; *Switz.:* Ralur; *Thai.:* Sancago.

Isonixin   (12870-d)

Isonixin *(rINN).*

2-Hydroxy-*N*-(2,6-dimethylphenyl)nicotinamide.
$C_{14}H_{14}N_2O_2 = 242.3.$
CAS — 57021-61-1.

Profile

Isonixin is an NSAID (p.63) that has been used in the management of pain and inflammation associated with musculoskeletal and joint disorders. Isonixin has been used in doses of 400 mg two to four times daily by mouth or by rectal suppository. It has also been applied topically as a 2.5% cream.

Preparations

Proprietary Preparations (details are given in Part 3)
Spain: Nixyn.

Multi-ingredient: *Spain:* Nixyn.

Kebuzone   (2661-r)

Kebuzone *(rINN).*

Ketophenylbutazone.   4-(3-Oxobutyl)-1,2-diphenylpyrazolidine-3,5-dione.
$C_{19}H_{18}N_2O_3 = 322.4.$
CAS — 853-34-9.
ATC — M01AA06.

Profile

Kebuzone, a phenylbutazone derivative, is an NSAID (p.63). It has been used in musculoskeletal, joint, and soft-tissue disorders in doses of up to 1.5 g daily in divided doses by mouth. Kebuzone has also been given as the sodium salt by intramuscular injection in doses equivalent to 1 g of base.

Porphyria. Kebuzone is considered to be unsafe in patients with porphyria because it has been shown to be porphyrinogenic in *animals* or *in-vitro* systems.

Preparations

Proprietary Preparations (details are given in Part 3)
Aust.: Ketazon; *Ger.:* Ketazon.

Multi-ingredient: *Aust.:* Rheumesser.

Ketobemidone   (6234-e)

Ketobemidone *(BAN, rINN).*

Cetobemidone.   1-(4-*m*-Hydroxyphenyl)-1-methyl-4-piperidyl)propan-1-one.
$C_{15}H_{21}NO_2 = 247.3.$
CAS — 469-79-4.
ATC — N02AB01.

Profile

Ketobemidone is an opioid analgesic (p.66). It has been given as the hydrochloride by mouth, by injection, or rectally, sometimes with an antispasmodic.

◊ References.
1. Anderson P, *et al.* Clinical pharmacokinetics of ketobemidone: its bioavailability after rectal administration. *Eur J Clin Pharmacol* 1981; **19:** 217–23.

Preparations

Proprietary Preparations (details are given in Part 3)
Denm.: Ketodur; *Norw.:* Ketodur; Ketorax; *Swed.:* Ketodur; Ketogan Novum.

Multi-ingredient: *Denm.:* Ketogan; *Norw.:* Ketogan; *Swed.:* Ketogan.

Ketoprofen   (2662-f)

Ketoprofen *(BAN, USAN, rINN).*

Ketoprofenum; RP-19583. (*RS*)-2-(3-Benzoylphenyl)propionic acid.
$C_{16}H_{14}O_3 = 254.3.$
CAS — 22071-15-4 (ketoprofen); 57469-78-0 (ketoprofen lysine); 57495-14-4 (ketoprofen sodium).
ATC — M01AE03; M02AA10.

Pharmacopoeias. In *Eur.* (see p.vi), *Jpn,* and *US.*

Pharmacopoeial description

Ph. Eur.: A white or almost white, crystalline powder. M.p. 94° to 97°. Practically insoluble in water; freely soluble in alcohol, in acetone, and in dichloromethane.

USP 25: Store in airtight containers.

Dexketoprofen Trometamol   (20259-b)

Dexketoprofen Trometamol *(BANM, rINNM).*
CAS — 22161-81-5 (dexketoprofen).

Adverse Effects and Precautions

As for NSAIDs in general, p.63.

When ketoprofen is administered intramuscularly there may be pain at the injection site and occasionally tissue damage. Ketoprofen suppositories may cause local irritation. Ketoprofen and dexketoprofen should be used with caution in patients with renal or hepatic impairment. In some countries ketoprofen is considered to be contra-indicated in patients with heart failure; however, evidence that ketoprofen is any more likely than other NSAIDs to precipitate or aggravate heart failure (see p.63) seems to be lacking.

Hypersensitivity. Life-threatening asthma, urticaria, and angioedema developed in 2 aspirin-sensitive patients after taking ketoprofen 50 mg by mouth.[1] Cardiac and respiratory arrest occurred in an asthmatic patient shortly after taking ketoprofen.[2] There was a report[3] of delayed skin hypersensitivity in a patient who used a topical gel containing ketoprofen. The reaction recurred on rechallenge to ketoprofen gel but not to a similar gel containing diclofenac. The authors of the report noted that the UK Committee on Safety of Medicines had received 15 reports of skin reactions to ketoprofen gel, including two each of dermatitis and urticaria.

1. Frith P, *et al.* Life-threatening asthma, urticaria, and angioedema after ketoprofen. *Lancet* 1978; **ii:** 847–8.
2. Schreuder G. Ketoprofen: possible idiosyncratic acute bronchospasm. *Med J Aust* 1990; **152:** 332–3.
3. Oh VMS. Ketoprofen gel and delayed hypersensitivity dermatitis. *BMJ* 1994; **309:** 512.

Myasthenia gravis. There has been a brief report[1] of a single dose of ketoprofen 50 mg by mouth precipitating a cholinergic crisis in a patient with well-controlled myasthenia gravis. The patient had previously noted a similar but milder reaction with aspirin, but not with paracetamol.[1]

1. McDowell IFW, McConnell JB. Cholinergic crisis in myasthenia gravis precipitated by ketoprofen. *BMJ* 1985; **291**: 1094.

Pancreatitis. A report of pancreatitis associated with ketoprofen.[1]

1. Cobb TK, Pierce JR. Acute pancreatitis associated with ketoprofen. *South Med J* 1992; **85**: 430–1.

Photosensitivity. Ketoprofen has been reported to cause photosensitivity reactions.[1]

1. Anonymous. Drugs that cause photosensitivity. *Med Lett Drugs Ther* 1986; **28**: 51–2.

Renal impairment. The elimination half-life and unbound plasma concentrations of dexketoprofen are increased in patients with impaired renal function given racemic ketoprofen;[1] this appears to be principally attributable to impaired renal clearance of the acyl-glucuronide conjugates in a stereoselective fashion, with subsequent hydrolysis of the unstable conjugate back to the aglycone producing increased plasma-ketoprofen concentrations.[2] It has been suggested[2] that dosage adjustments of racemic ketoprofen are indicated only for patients with moderately severe renal failure (creatinine clearance of less than 20 mL per minute). For general precautions regarding the administration of NSAIDs in patients with renal impairment, see p.65.

1. Hayball PJ, et al. The influence of renal function on the enantioselective pharmacokinetics and pharmacodynamics of ketoprofen in patients with rheumatoid arthritis. *Br J Clin Pharmacol* 1993; **36**: 185–93.
2. Skeith KJ, et al. The influence of renal function on the pharmacokinetics of unchanged and acyl-glucuroconjugated ketoprofen enantiomers after 50 and 100 mg racemic ketoprofen. *Br J Clin Pharmacol* 1996; **42**: 163–9.

Interactions

For interactions associated with NSAIDs, see p.65. Probenecid delays the excretion of ketoprofen and decreases its extent of protein binding resulting in increased plasma-ketoprofen concentrations.

Pharmacokinetics

Ketoprofen is readily absorbed from the gastrointestinal tract; peak plasma concentrations occur about 0.5 to 2 hours after a dose. When ketoprofen is given with food, the bioavailability is not altered but the rate of absorption is slowed. Ketoprofen is well absorbed from the intramuscular and rectal routes; only a small amount of ketoprofen is absorbed following topical application. Ketoprofen is 99% bound to plasma proteins and substantial concentrations of drug are found in the synovial fluid. The elimination half-life in plasma is about 1.5 to 4 hours. Ketoprofen is metabolised mainly by conjugation with glucuronic acid, and is excreted mainly in the urine.

Ketoprofen possesses a chiral centre. It is usually given as the racemate but its pharmacological actions appear to be due largely to the (*S*)-enantiomer, dexketoprofen. The pharmacokinetics of ketoprofen appear to exhibit little stereoselectivity (but see under Renal Impairment, above).

◊ References.

1. Debruyne D, et al. Clinical pharmacokinetics of ketoprofen after single intravenous administration as a bolus or infusion. *Clin Pharmacokinet* 1987; **12**: 214–21.
2. Flouvat B, et al. Pharmacokinetics of ketoprofen in man after repeated percutaneous administration. *Arzneimittelforschung* 1989; **39**: 812–15.
3. Jamali F, Brocks DR. Clinical pharmacokinetics of ketoprofen and its enantiomers. *Clin Pharmacokinet* 1990; **19**: 197–217.
4. Geisslinger G, et al. Pharmacokinetics of ketoprofen enantiomers after different doses of the racemate. *Br J Clin Pharmacol* 1995; **40**: 73–5.
5. Barbanoj MJ, et al. Pharmacokinetics of dexketoprofen trometamol in healthy volunteers after single and repeated oral doses. *J Clin Pharmacol* 1998; **38**: 33S–40S.
6. Kokki H, et al. Pharmacokinetics of ketoprofen syrup in small children. *J Clin Pharmacol* 2000; **40**: 354–9.
7. Barbanoj M-J, et al. Clinical pharmacokinetics of dexketoprofen. *Clin Pharmacokinet* 2001; **40**: 245–62.

Uses and Administration

Ketoprofen, a propionic acid derivative, is an NSAID (p.65). Its anti-inflammatory properties may be weaker than those of some other NSAIDs. Ketoprofen is a racemic mixture; in *animal* studies the S-(+) enantiomer, dexketoprofen, has approximately twice the analgesic activity of ketoprofen by weight.

Ketoprofen is used in musculoskeletal and joint disorders such as ankylosing spondylitis, osteoarthritis, and rheumatoid arthritis, and in peri-articular disorders such as bursitis and tendinitis. It is also used in

dysmenorrhoea, postoperative pain, in painful and inflammatory conditions such as acute gout or soft-tissue disorders, and to reduce fever. Dexketoprofen is used in the treatment of mild to moderate pain such as musculoskeletal pain, dysmenorrhoea, or dental pain.

In the treatment of rheumatic disorders a usual daily dose of *ketoprofen* by mouth is 100 to 200 mg in 2 to 4 divided doses; modified-release formulations taken once daily may also be used. In the USA some manufacturers suggest initial oral doses of 75 mg three times daily or 50 mg four times daily increased as needed to a maximum of 300 mg daily in divided doses. Ketoprofen may also be administered rectally as suppositories in a usual dose of 100 mg at night. In the UK, it is recommended that the total daily combined dose by mouth and by rectum should not exceed 200 mg. The dose by mouth for the treatment of other painful conditions including dysmenorrhoea is 25 to 50 mg every 6 to 8 hours.

Ketoprofen may be given by deep intramuscular injection into the gluteal muscle for acute exacerbations of musculoskeletal, joint, peri-articular and soft-tissue disorders and in the management of pain following orthopaedic surgery. Doses of 50 to 100 mg may be given every 4 hours, up to a maximum dose of 200 mg in 24 hours for up to 3 days. Ketoprofen may be applied as a 2.5% gel for local pain relief. Doses vary slightly between preparations: a typical regimen is application 2 or 3 times daily for up to 10 days.

Dexketoprofen is given by mouth as the trometamol salt; doses are expressed in terms of the base. Usual doses are 12.5 mg every 4 to 6 hours or 25 mg every 8 hours; the total daily dose should not exceed 75 mg. Patients with mild to moderate hepatic impairment or mild renal impairment or elderly patients should be started on a total daily dose not exceeding 50 mg. Dexketoprofen should not be used in those with severe hepatic impairment or moderate to severe renal impairment.

Ketoprofen has also been used as the lysine and as the sodium salt.

◊ Reviews.

1. Mauleón D, et al. Preclinical and clinical development of dexketoprofen. *Drugs* 1996; **52**: 24–46.

Preparations

BP 2001: Ketoprofen Capsules; Ketoprofen Gel.

Proprietary Preparations (details are given in Part 3)
Aust.: Actron; Keprodol; Profenid; Toprek; **Austral.:** Orudis; Oruvail; **Belg.:** Birofenid†; Fastum; Rofenid; Toprek; **Braz.:** Algiprofen; Artrinid; Keduril; Profenid; **Canad.:** Apo-Keto; Novo-Keto; Orafen; Orudis; Oruvail; Rhodis; Rhovail; **Denm.:** Orofen; Orudis; **Fin.:** Keto; Ketofen; Ketomex; Ketorin; Orudis; **Fr.:** Actroneffix; Bi-Profenid; Ketum; Profenid; Topfena; Toprec; **Ger.:** Alrheumun†; Gabrilen; Ketolist; Orudis; Spondylon; Sympal; **Hong Kong:** Apo-Keto; Fastum; Orudis; Oruvail; **Irl.:** Fastum; Keral; Orudis; Orugesic; Oruvail; **Israel:** Ketonal; Oruvail; Profenid; **Ital.:** Alket; Artrosilene; Desketo; Enantyum; Fastum; Flexen; Ketalgesic; Ketartrium; Ketesse; Ketodol; Ketofen†; Ketoplus; Meprofen; Oki; Orudis; Reuprofen; Sinketol†; Toprek; Zepelindue; **Mex.:** K-Profen; Keduril; Kezer; Orudis; Piketofen; Profenid; Neth.: Oscorel; Orudis or; **N.Z.:** Kefen; Orudis; Oruvail; **Port.:** Artrofene; Deflogix; Fastum; Ketesse; Ketofene; Profenid; **S.Afr.:** Fastum; Ketoflam; Myproflam; Orucote; Oruject; Oruvail; **Singapore:** Apo-Keto; Fastum; Kefentech; Kenhancer; Ketotop; Oruvail; Provail; **Spain:** Arcental; Arcental Topica; Enantyum; Extraplus; Fastum; Ketesse; Ketosolan; Orudis; Quiralam; Reumoquin†; **Swed.:** Orudis; Prodon; Siduro; Zon; **Switz.:** Fastum; Orudis†; **Thai.:** Fastum; Oruvail; Profenid; Rofepain; **UK:** Fenoket; Jomethid; Keral; Ketil; Ketocid; Ketotard; Ketovail†; Ketozip; Larafen; Orudis; Oruvail; Powergel; Solpaflex†; **USA:** Actron†; Orudis; Oruvail.

Multi-ingredient: Mex.: Bifebral; Reumophan.

Ketorolac Trometamol   (16867-j)

Ketorolac Trometamol (*BANM, rINNM*).

Ketorolac Tromethamine (*USAN*); RS-37619-00-31-3. (±)-5-Benzoyl-2,3-dihydro-1*H*-pyrrolizine-1-carboxylic acid compound with 2-amino-2-(hydroxymethyl)-1,3-propanediol (1 : 1).

$C_{19}H_{24}N_2O_6 = 376.4$.

CAS — 74103-06-3 (ketorolac); 74103-07-4 (ketorolac trometamol).

Pharmacopoeias. In US.

Pharmacopoeial description

USP 25: A white to off-white, crystalline powder. Freely soluble in water and in methyl alcohol; slightly soluble in alcohol,

in dehydrated alcohol, and in tetrahydrofuran; practically insoluble in acetone, in acetonitrile, in butyl alcohol, in dichloromethane, in dioxan, in ethyl acetate, in hexane, and in toluene. pH of a 1% solution in water is between 5.7 and 6.7. Store in airtight containers and protect from light.

Adverse Effects

As for NSAIDs in general, p.63.

Concern over the high incidence of reported adverse effects with ketorolac trometamol has led to its withdrawal from the market in some countries while in others its permitted dosage and maximum duration of treatment have been reduced. Adverse effects reported include gastrointestinal disturbances including gastrointestinal bleeding (especially in the elderly), perforation, and peptic ulceration. Hypersensitivity reactions such as anaphylaxis, rash, bronchospasm, laryngeal oedema, and hypotension have also occurred. Other adverse effects reported include drowsiness, dizziness, headache, mental and sensory changes, psychotic reactions, sweating, dry mouth, thirst, fever, convulsions, myalgia, aseptic meningitis, hypertension, dyspnoea, pulmonary oedema, bradycardia, chest pain, palpitations, fluid retention, increases in blood urea and creatinine, acute renal failure, oedema, hyponatraemia, hyperkalaemia, urinary frequency or retention, nephrotic syndrome, flank pain with or without haematuria, purpura, thrombocytopenia, epistaxis, inhibition of platelet aggregation, increased bleeding time, postoperative wound haemorrhage, haematoma, flushing or pallor, and pancreatitis. Severe skin reactions including Stevens-Johnson syndrome and Lyell's syndrome have been reported. Liver function changes may occur; hepatitis and liver failure have been reported. There may be pain at the site of injection.

Administration of ketorolac eye drops has resulted in transient stinging and other minor symptoms of ocular irritation. As with some other NSAIDs used in the eye, ketorolac has been implicated in reports of corneal toxicity (see p.30).

◊ Adverse effects reported with ketorolac are mainly those common to all NSAIDs with gastrointestinal reactions being the most frequent followed by haematological, renal, hypersensitivity, and then neurological reactions. Since the launch of ketorolac in 1990, 97 reactions with a fatal outcome had been reported worldwide up to 1993.[1] The causes of death were as follows: gastrointestinal bleeding or perforation (47 cases); renal impairment or insufficiency (20 cases); anaphylaxis or asthma (7 cases); haemorrhagic reactions (4 cases); and unexplained or miscellaneous causes (19 cases). Concern over the safety of ketorolac has led to adverse reactions being monitored closely and to the implementation of restrictions on dose and duration of treatment (see under Uses and Administration, below). A postmarketing surveillance study,[2] led by Dr B Strom for the US manufacturer, has examined the risks of parenteral ketorolac in 9 900 patients who received 10 272 courses of ketorolac. Gastrointestinal bleeding and operative site bleeding were expected to be the major risks of ketorolac, and were the major focus of this study. The results of the study indicated a dose-response relationship with average daily ketorolac dose for both gastrointestinal bleeding and operative site bleeding, and an association with duration of therapy beyond 5 days for gastrointestinal bleeding. The risk of serious gastrointestinal bleeding and operative site bleeding was higher for elderly patients [the manufacturer recommends that the elderly should not receive daily parenteral doses greater than 60 mg]. Although the overall associations between ketorolac use and both gastrointestinal bleeding and operative site bleeding are small, the risk becomes clinically important as doses increase, in elderly patients, and, for gastrointestinal bleeding only, when used for longer than 5 days. The US manufacturer has consequently emphasised that ketorolac is a potent NSAID and is indicated only for the short-term management of moderate to severe pain and not for minor or chronic painful conditions; its administration carries many risks and related adverse effects can be serious especially when used inappropriately. After examining data from the Strom study the EU Committee for Proprietary Medicinal Products adopted the opinion that ketorolac had a narrow therapeutic margin but that it was indicated for the short-term management of moderate to severe acute postoperative pain.

Further references to ketorolac's adverse effects are given below.[3-12]

1. Committee on Safety of Medicines/Medicines Control Agency. Ketorolac: new restrictions on dose and duration of treatment. *Current Problems* 1993; **19**: 5–6.
2. Strom BL, et al. Parenteral ketorolac and risk of gastrointestinal and operative site bleeding: a postmarketing surveillance study. *JAMA* 1996; **275**: 376–82.

3. Rotenberg FA, Giannini VS. Hyperkalemia associated with ketorolac. *Ann Pharmacother* 1992; **26:** 778–9.
4. Boras-Uber LA, Brackett NC. Ketorolac-induced acute renal failure. *Am J Med* 1992; **92:** 450–2. Correction *ibid.*; **93:** 117.
5. Schoch PH, *et al.* Acute renal failure in an elderly woman following intramuscular ketorolac administration. *Ann Pharmacother* 1992; **26:** 1233–6.
6. Goetz CM, *et al.* Anaphylactoid reaction following ketorolac tromethamine administration. *Ann Pharmacother* 1992; **26:** 1237–8.
7. Randi ML, *et al.* Haemolytic uraemic syndrome during treatment with ketorolac trometamol. *BMJ* 1993; **306:** 186.
8. Fong J, Gora ML. Reversible renal insufficiency following ketorolac therapy. *Ann Pharmacother* 1993; **27:** 510–12.
9. Corelli RL, Gericke KR. Renal insufficiency associated with intramuscular administration of ketorolac tromethamine. *Ann Pharmacother* 1993; **27:** 1055–7.
10. Buck ML, Norwood VF. Ketorolac-induced acute renal failure in a previously healthy adolescent. *Pediatrics* 1996; **98:** 294–6.
11. Feldman HI, *et al.* Parenteral ketorolac: the risk for acute renal failure. *Ann Intern Med* 1997; **126:** 193–9.
12. Reinhart DJ, *et al.* Minimising the adverse effects of ketorolac. *Drug Safety* 2000; **22:** 487–97.

Precautions

As for NSAIDs in general, p.64.

In light of the concern over the toxicity of ketorolac it has been recommended that ketorolac should not be used during pregnancy or labour and that it should not be given to mothers who are breast feeding.

Ketorolac is contra-indicated in patients with a history of hypersensitivity to aspirin or other NSAIDs, a history of asthma, nasal polyps, bronchospasm, or angioedema, a history of peptic ulceration or gastrointestinal bleeding, in patients with moderate or severe renal impairment, and in those with hypovolaemia or dehydration. Ketorolac should not be given to patients with coagulation or haemorrhagic disorders or those with confirmed or suspected cerebrovascular bleeding. It is contra-indicated as a prophylactic analgesic before surgery because of its inhibitory effects on platelets and for intraoperative use; it should not be given postoperatively to those who have undergone procedures with a high risk of haemorrhage.

The dose of ketorolac should be reduced in the elderly and in patients weighing less than 50 kg. It is recommended that patients with mild renal impairment should receive a reduced dose of ketorolac and undergo close monitoring of renal function. Ketorolac should be used with caution in heart failure, hepatic impairment and conditions leading to reduction in blood volume or in renal blood flow. Ketorolac should be withdrawn if clinical symptoms of liver disease develop.

Dizziness may affect the performance of skilled tasks such as driving.

Interactions

For interactions associated with NSAIDs, see p.65.

Ketorolac should not be given to patients already receiving anticoagulants or to those who will require prophylactic anticoagulant therapy, including low-dose heparin. The risk of ketorolac-associated bleeding is increased by other NSAIDs or aspirin and by oxpentifylline [pentoxifylline] and concomitant use should be avoided. Probenecid increases the half-life and plasma concentrations of ketorolac and the two drugs should not be given together.

Parasympathomimetics. The manufacturer of acetylcholine chloride ophthalmic preparations has stated that there have been reports that acetylcholine and carbachol have been ineffective when used in patients treated with topical (ophthalmic) NSAIDs.

Pharmacokinetics

Ketorolac trometamol is absorbed following intramuscular or oral administration. At physiological pH ketorolac trometamol dissociates to form an anionic ketorolac molecule which is less hydrophilic than the trometamol salt. The peak plasma concentration of ketorolac is reached within about 30 to 60 minutes; absorption following intramuscular administration may be slower than that following oral administration in some individuals. Ketorolac is over 99% bound to plasma protein. It does not readily penetrate the blood-brain barrier. Ketorolac crosses the placenta and small amounts of drug are distributed into breast milk. The terminal plasma half-life is about 4 to 6

hours, but is about 6 to 7 hours in the elderly and 9 to 10 hours in patients with renal dysfunction. The major metabolic pathway is glucuronic acid conjugation; there is some *para*-hydroxylation. About 90% of a dose is excreted in urine as unchanged drug and conjugated and hydroxylated metabolites, the remainder is excreted in the faeces.

Uses and Administration

Ketorolac, a pyrrolizine carboxylic acid derivative structurally related to indometacin (p.46), is an NSAID (p.65). It is used principally as an analgesic.

Ketorolac is used intramuscularly, intravenously, or orally as the trometamol salt in the short-term management of moderate to severe **postoperative pain**. However, it should be noted that because of concerns over the high incidence of reported adverse effects with ketorolac its dosage and maximum duration of use are restricted. The recommended maximum duration for parenteral therapy is 2 days in the UK, and patients should be transferred to oral therapy as soon as possible. In the USA it is recommended that the maximum combined duration of use of parenteral and oral ketorolac should not exceed 5 days.

- In the UK the recommended initial dose by the *parenteral* route is 10 mg of ketorolac trometamol followed by 10 to 30 mg every 4 to 6 hours as required, although ketorolac may be given as often as every 2 hours in the initial postoperative period if required. The total maximum daily dose is 90 mg (60 mg in the elderly, patients with mild renal impairment, and in those weighing less than 50 kg). Intravenous injections should be administered over at least 15 seconds. During transfer from parenteral to oral therapy the combined daily dose on the day of converting for all forms of ketorolac trometamol should not exceed 90 mg (60 mg in the elderly, patients with mild renal impairment, and in those weighing less than 50 kg) of which no more than 40 mg should be given orally.

- Regimens in use in the USA include a single intramuscular dose of 60 mg or a single intravenous dose of 30 mg, or a multiple-dose regimen comprising 30 mg every 6 hours intramuscularly or intravenously, up to a maximum of 120 mg daily. These doses should be halved in the elderly, those with renal impairment, and those weighing less than 50 kg.

- The recommended *oral* dose in the UK is 10 mg every 4 to 6 hours (every 6 to 8 hours in the elderly) to a maximum of 40 mg daily for a maximum duration of 7 days.

- In the USA the recommended oral dose is 20 mg (10 mg in the elderly, the renally impaired, or those weighing under 50 kg), followed by 10 mg every 4 to 6 hours.

Ketorolac trometamol is also used as 0.5% eye drops to relieve **ocular itching** associated with seasonal allergic conjunctivitis. Ketorolac trometamol eye drops 0.5% have also been used for the topical treatment of **cystoid macular oedema** and for the prevention and reduction of **inflammation** associated with ocular surgery.

◊ Reviews.
1. Gillis JC, Brogden RN. Ketorolac: a reappraisal of its pharmacodynamic and pharmacokinetic properties and therapeutic use in pain management. *Drugs* 1997; **53:** 139–88.

Preparations

USP 25: Ketorolac Tromethamine Injection; Ketorolac Tromethamine Tablets.

Proprietary Preparations (details are given in Part 3)
Aust.: Acular; *Austral.:* Acular; Toradol; *Belg.:* Aculare; Taradyl; *Canad.:* Acular; Toradol; *Denm.:* Acular; Toradol; *Fin.:* Acular; Toradol; *Fr.:* Acular; *Ger.:* Acular; Toradol; *Hong Kong:* Acular; Toradol; *Irl.:* Acular; *Israel:* Topadol; *Ital.:* Acular; Lixidol; Tora-Dol; *Mex.:* Acularen; Alidol; Dolac; Dolotor; Findol; Supradol; *Neth.:* Acular†; *Norw.:* Toradol; *NZ:* Acular; Toradol; *Port.:* Acular; Toradol; *S.Afr.:* Acular; Tora-Dol; *Singapore:* Acular; Toradol; *Spain:* Acular; Algikey; Droal; Tonum; Toradol; *Swed.:* Toradol; *Switz.:* Acular; Tora-Dol; *UK:* Acular; Toradol; *USA:* Acular; Toradol.

Lefetamine Hydrochloride (19403-g)

Lefetamine Hydrochloride (*rINNM*).
(−)-N,N-Dimethyl-1,2-diphenylethylamine hydrochloride.
$C_{16}H_{19}N,HCl = 261.8$.
CAS — 7262-75-1 (*lefetamine*); 14148-99-3 (*lefetamine hydrochloride*).

Profile
Lefetamine hydrochloride has analgesic properties and has been given by intramuscular or subcutaneous injection.

Preparations
Proprietary Preparations (details are given in Part 3)
Ital.: Santenol.

Levacetylmethadol (6235-I)

Levacetylmethadol (*rINN*).
l-α-Acetylmethadol; LAAM; LAM; Levomethadyl Acetate (*USAN*); l-Methadyl Acetate. (−)-4-Dimethylamino-1-ethyl-2,2-diphenylpentyl acetate.
$C_{23}H_{31}NO_2 = 353.5$.
CAS — 1477-40-3 (*levomethadyl*); 34433-66-4 (*levacetylmethadol*); 43033-72-3 (*levacetylmethadol hydrochloride*).
ATC — N02AC06.

NOTE. Levacetylmethadol Hydrochloride is *USAN*.

Dependence and Withdrawal
As for Opioid Analgesics in general, p.66.
As it may take 2 to 3 days before the effects of levacetylmethadol become apparent after intravenous injection its potential for abuse is considered to be very low.

Adverse Effects, Treatment, and Precautions
As for opioid analgesics in general, p.67.
Prolongation of the QT interval, torsade de pointes, and sudden death have been associated with levacetylmethadol use. These proarrhythmic effects have led to the use of levacetylmethadol being suspended in the European Union and restricted in the USA.

Clearly, when levacetylmethadol is prescribed it should not be given to patients with known or suspected prolongation of the QT interval, to those patients with conditions known to prolong the QT interval or to those with electrolyte imbalance. Concomitant administration of other drugs that prolong the QT interval or induce hypokalaemia or hypomagnesaemia should be avoided. An ECG should be performed before starting levacetylmethadol, 12 to 14 days later, and periodically thereafter to detect any alterations in the QT interval. Treatment with levacetylmethadol should be discontinued in patients who experience symptoms suggestive of severe arrhythmia and the patient evaluated for QT prolongation and arrhythmias.

Interactions
For interactions associated with opioid analgesics, see p.68. Levacetylmethadol should not be given with drugs that prolong the QT interval or induce hypokalaemia or hypomagnesaemia. Levacetylmethadol is metabolised to active metabolites by the cytochrome P450 isoenzyme CYP3A4. Therefore concomitant administration of other drugs that induce or inhibit this isoenzyme may result in changes in plasma concentrations of levacetylmethadol or its active metabolites, and, possibly adverse effects.

Pharmacokinetics
Levacetylmethadol is absorbed from the gastrointestinal tract. It has a slow onset and long duration of action. It undergoes first-pass metabolism and is metabolised to compounds which have morphine-like activity and a long half-life. The primary route of metabolism is demethylation, mediated by the cytochrome P450 isoenzyme CYP3A4, to l-α-noracetylmethadol and l-α-dinoracetylmethadol. The minor metabolites methadol and normethadol have been identified in urine.

◊ References.
1. Kaiko RF, Inturrisi CE. Disposition of acetylmethadol in relation to pharmacologic action. *Clin Pharmacol Ther* 1975; **18:** 96–103.
2. Henderson GL, *et al.* Plasma l-α-acetylmethadol (LAAM) after acute and chronic administration. *Clin Pharmacol Ther* 1977; **21:** 16–25.

Uses and Administration
Levacetylmethadol, a diphenylheptane derivative, is an opioid analgesic (p.68); it is a derivative of methadone (p.54). It has been used in the management of opioid dependence. The proarrhythmic effects of levacetylmethadol (see Adverse Effects, above) have led to its use being suspended in the European Union and restricted in the USA to patients who have failed to respond to other appropriate treatments of dependence.

When levacetylmethadol is prescribed, the longer duration of action of levacetylmethadol allows intermittent administration. It is given as the hydrochloride by mouth three times a week or on alternate days as maintenance treatment. However, it has a slow onset of action and supplements of other short-acting opiates or a non-opioid withdrawal suppressant may be required to prevent withdrawal symptoms during the first three days of treatment. The usual initial dose is between 20 and 40 mg of levacetylmethadol hydrochloride, although patients dependent on methadone may require higher initial doses. Subsequent doses are given at 48- or 72-hour intervals, and may be adjusted in increments of 5 to 10 mg until an acceptable maintenance dose is achieved which should generally not exceed 140 mg. Doses should not be given on consecutive days.

◊ References.
1. Eissenberg T, *et al.* Dose-related efficacy of levomethadyl acetate for treatment of opioid dependence: a randomized clinical trial. *JAMA* 1997; **277:** 1945–51.

Preparations

Proprietary Preparations (details are given in Part 3)
Denm.: OrLAAM†; *Spain:* OrLAAM†; *UK:* OrLAAM†; *USA:* OrLAAM.

Levomethadone Hydrochloride (9871-a)

Levomethadone Hydrochloride *(rINNM)*.
(–)-Methadone Hydrochloride. (–)-6-Dimethylamino-4,4-diphenylheptan-3-one hydrochloride.
$C_{21}H_{27}NO,HCl = 345.9$.
CAS — 125-58-6 *(levomethadone)*; 5967-73-7 *(levomethadone hydrochloride)*.

Profile
Levomethadone is an opioid analgesic (p.66). It is the active isomer of racemic methadone (p.53) and is used similarly as the hydrochloride in the treatment of severe pain.

◊ References.
1. Olsen GD, *et al.* Clinical effects and pharmacokinetics of racemic methadone and its optical isomers. *Clin Pharmacol Ther* 1977; **21:** 147–57.

Preparations

Proprietary Preparations (details are given in Part 3)
Ger.: L-Polamidon.

Levorphanol Tartrate (6236-y)

Levorphanol Tartrate *(BANM, rINNM)*.
Levorphan Tartrate; Levorphanol Bitartrate; Methorphinan Tartrate. (–)-9a-Methylmorphinan-3-ol hydrogen tartrate dihydrate.
$C_{17}H_{23}NO,C_4H_6O_6,2H_2O = 443.5$.
CAS — 77-07-6 *(levorphanol)*; 125-72-4 *(levorphanol tartrate, anhydrous)*; 5985-38-6 *(levorphanol tartrate dihydrate)*.
Pharmacopoeias. In It. and US.

Pharmacopoeial description
USP 25: A practically white, odourless, crystalline powder. Soluble 1 in 50 of water and 1 in 120 of alcohol; insoluble in chloroform and in ether.

Profile
Levorphanol tartrate, a phenanthrene derivative, is a potent opioid analgesic (p.66) used in the management of moderate to severe pain and for premedication. The analgesic effect usually begins about 10 to 60 minutes after oral administration and lasts up to about 8 hours.

In the management of pain a usual initial dose of levorphanol tartrate by mouth is 2 mg repeated in 6 to 8 hours if necessary. The maximum initial daily dose in non-opioid tolerant patients should not exceed 12 mg.

Levorphanol tartrate may be given by intramuscular or subcutaneous injection in initial doses of 1 or 2 mg, repeated in 6 to 8 hours if necessary. Levorphanol tartrate may also be given by slow intravenous injection in an initial dose of up to 1 mg in divided doses, repeated in 3 to 6 hours if necessary. The maximum initial daily dose by the parenteral route in non-opioid tolerant patients should not exceed 8 mg.

For premedication, a usual dose is 1 or 2 mg by intramuscular or subcutaneous injection given 60 to 90 minutes before surgery.

Elderly or debilitated patients may require lower doses.

Preparations

USP 25: Levorphanol Tartrate Injection; Levorphanol Tartrate Tablets.

Proprietary Preparations (details are given in Part 3)
USA: Levo-Dromoran.

Lithium Salicylate (2663-d)

$C_7H_5LiO_3 = 144.1$.
CAS — 552-38-5.

Profile
Lithium salicylate is a salicylic acid derivative (see Aspirin, p.14) that has been used in rheumatic disorders, but its use cannot be recommended because of the pharmacological effect of the lithium ion.

Preparations

Proprietary Preparations (details are given in Part 3)
Multi-ingredient: *Fr.:* Antigoutteux Rezall†.

Lonazolac Calcium (11435-t)

Lonazolac Calcium *(rINNM)*.
Calcium 3-(4-chlorophenyl)-1-phenylpyrazol-4-ylacetate.
$C_{34}H_{24}CaCl_2N_4O_4 = 663.6$.
CAS — 53808-88-1 *(lonazolac)*; 75821-71-5 *(lonazolac calcium)*.

Profile
Lonazolac calcium is an NSAID (p.63). It has been used in pain, inflammation, and musculoskeletal and joint disorders in usual doses of up to 600 mg daily, in divided doses, by mouth. Suppositories have also been employed in doses of 400 mg twice daily.

Preparations

Proprietary Preparations (details are given in Part 3)
Aust.: Irritren; *Ger.:* Argun; arthro akut; Irritren†; *Hong Kong:* Irritren; *Port.:* Atrilon.

Lornoxicam (6486-p)

Lornoxicam *(BAN, USAN, rINN)*.
Chlortenoxicam; Chlortenoxicam; CTX; Ro-13-9297. 6-Chloro-4-hydroxy-2-methyl-N-2-pyridyl-2H-thieno[2,3-e][1,2]-thiazine-3-carboxamide 1,1-dioxide.
$C_{13}H_{10}ClN_3O_4S_2 = 371.8$.
CAS — 70374-39-9.
ATC — M01AC05.

Adverse Effects and Precautions
As for NSAIDs in general, p.63. Lornoxicam should not be used in patients with severe renal impairment.

Interactions
For interactions associated with NSAIDs, see p.65. Increased plasma concentrations of lornoxicam have occurred when given concomitantly with cimetidine.

Pharmacokinetics
Lornoxicam is almost completely absorbed from the gastrointestinal tract with peak concentrations reached in 1 to 2 hours. It is 99% bound to plasma proteins. Lornoxicam is metabolised to its inactive hydroxylated metabolite. About one-third of a dose is excreted via the urine as inactive metabolites. The mean elimination half-life is 3 to 4 hours.

Uses and Administration
Lornoxicam, an oxicam derivative, is an NSAID (p.65). It is used in musculoskeletal and joint disorders such as osteoarthritis and rheumatoid arthritis; it is also used in the treatment of other painful conditions including postoperative pain.

In the treatment of osteoarthritis and rheumatoid arthritis lornoxicam is given by mouth in a daily dose of 12 mg in two or three divided doses.

Lornoxicam is given in doses of 8 to 16 mg daily by mouth for the treatment of pain. Doses above 8 mg should be given in divided doses. Similar doses may be given by intravenous or intramuscular injection, although in rare cases the maximum initial daily dose may be increased to 24 mg; treatment by injection should be limited to 2 days.

◊ References.
1. Balfour JA, *et al.* Lornoxicam: a review of its pharmacology and therapeutic potential in the management of painful and inflammatory conditions. *Drugs* 1996; **51:** 639–57.
2. Skjodt NM, Davies NM. Clinical pharmacokinetics of lornoxicam: a short half-life oxicam. *Clin Pharmacokinet* 1998; **34:** 421–8.
3. Staunstrup H, *et al.* Efficacy and tolerability of lornoxicam versus tramadol in postoperative pain. *J Clin Pharmacol* 1999; **39:** 834–41.

Preparations

Proprietary Preparations (details are given in Part 3)
Aust.: Xefo; *Denm.:* Xefo; *Fin.:* Xefo; *Ger.:* Telos; *Port.:* Acabel; *S.Afr.:* Xefo; *Spain:* Acabel; Bosporon; *Swed.:* Xefo; *Thai.:* Xefo; *UK:* Xefo.

Loxoprofen Sodium (11675-l)

Loxoprofen Sodium *(rINNM)*.
CS-600 *(loxoprofen)*. Sodium (±)-p-[(2-oxocyclopentyl)methyl]hydratropate dihydrate.
$C_{15}H_{17}O_3Na,2H_2O = 304.3$.
CAS — 68767-14-6 *(loxoprofen)*; 80382-23-6 *(loxoprofen sodium dihydrate)*.
Pharmacopoeias. In Jpn.

Anhydrous loxoprofen sodium 10 mg is approximately equivalent to 11.3 mg of loxoprofen sodium dihydrate.

Profile
Loxoprofen sodium is an NSAID (p.63) given by mouth for the management of pain and inflammation associated with musculoskeletal and joint disorders or operative procedures. Loxoprofen sodium is given as the dihydrate in a usual dose equivalent to 60 mg of the anhydrous form by mouth three times daily.

Preparations

Proprietary Preparations (details are given in Part 3)
Jpn: Lobu; Loxonin; *Thai.:* Loxonin.

Lysine Aspirin (9560-m)

Aspirin DL-Lysine; Lysine Acetylsalicylate; DL-Lysine Acetylsalicylate.
$C_{15}H_{22}N_2O_6 = 326.3$.
CAS — 62952-06-1.
Pharmacopoeias. In Fr.

Lysine aspirin 900 mg is approximately equivalent to 500 mg of aspirin.

Adverse Effects, Treatment, and Precautions
As for Aspirin, p.14. Shock has been reported in patients given lysine aspirin by injection.

Lysine aspirin, like aspirin, should not generally be given to children under the age of 12 years because of the risk of Reye's syndrome.

Interactions
For interactions associated with aspirin, see p.16.

Uses and Administration
Lysine aspirin has analgesic, anti-inflammatory, and antipyretic actions similar to those of aspirin (see p.16). Following administration, lysine aspirin dissociates into lysine and aspirin; aspirin is then hydrolysed to salicylic acid. Lysine aspirin is used in the treatment of pain, fever, and rheumatic disorders. It is given by mouth in doses equivalent to 0.5 to 1 g of aspirin, repeated every 4 hours as needed up to a maximum of 3 g of aspirin daily (2 g daily in the elderly) for pain and fever. The dose for rheumatic disorders is equivalent to 4 to 6 g of aspirin daily in 3 or 4 divided doses. Lysine aspirin is also given intramuscularly or intravenously in similar doses; the maximum daily parenteral dose is equivalent to 4 g of aspirin for very severe pain and to 6 g of aspirin for rheumatic disorders.

Lysine aspirin is also used in combination with metoclopramide in the treatment of migraine.

Lysine aspirin has also been used in the management of thromboembolic disorders.

◊ References.
1. Tfelt-Hansen P, *et al.* The effectiveness of combined oral lysine acetylsalicylate and metoclopramide compared with oral sumatriptan for migraine. *Lancet* 1995; **346:** 923–6.

◊ For a suggestion that lysine aspirin might be more suitable than aspirin for the diagnosis of sensitivity to NSAIDs, see under Hypersensitivity on p.15.

Preparations

Proprietary Preparations (details are given in Part 3)
Belg.: Aspegic; Cardegic; *Fr.:* Aspegic; Kardegic; *Ger.:* Aspisol; *Israel:* Lysoprin; *Ital.:* Aspegic; Cardirene; Flectadol; *Mex.:* Coraspir; *Neth.:* Aspegic; Cardegic; *Port.:* Aspegic; Evasprin; Lisaspin; Tiplac; *Spain:* ASL; Aspegic†; Inyesprin; Lysinotol; Solusprin; *Switz.:* Alcacyl instant; Aspegic; Kardegic.

Multi-ingredient: *Belg.:* Migpriv; *Denm.:* Migpriv; *Fin.:* Migpriv; *Fr.:* Migpriv; *Ital.:* Migpriv; Migraprim; *Neth.:* Migrafin; *Spain:* Fluxal; Neurodif†; Neurogobens†; *Swed.:* Migpriv; *Switz.:* Migpriv; *UK:* Migramax.

Magnesium Salicylate (2664-n)

$C_{14}H_{10}MgO_6,4H_2O = 370.6$.
CAS — 18917-89-0 *(anhydrous magnesium salicylate)*; 18917-95-8 *(magnesium salicylate tetrahydrate)*.
Pharmacopoeias. In US.

Anhydrous magnesium salicylate 1 g is approximately equivalent to 1.2 g of aspirin.

Pharmacopoeial description
USP 25: A white, odourless, efflorescent, crystalline powder. Soluble in water and in alcohol; slightly soluble in ether; freely soluble in methyl alcohol. Store in airtight containers.

Adverse Effects, Treatment, and Precautions
As for Aspirin, p.14.

The use of aspirin and other acetylated salicylates is generally not recommended for children under the age of 12 years because of the risk of Reye's syndrome, unless specifically indicated. Some authorities also extend this precaution to non-acetylated salicylates such as magnesium salicylate.

There is an additional caution in renal impairment because of the risk of hypermagnesaemia.

Interactions
For interactions associated with salicylates, see Aspirin, p.16.

Uses and Administration
Magnesium salicylate has analgesic, anti-inflammatory, and antipyretic actions similar to those of aspirin (see p.16). It is used in the treatment of pain and fever and in the management of inflammatory conditions such as osteoarthritis, rheumatoid arthritis, and other arthritides. Usual doses of magnesium salicylate, expressed in terms of anhydrous magnesium salicylate, are about 300 to 600 mg by mouth every 4 hours for pain or fever. A total daily dose of about 3.5 g should not be exceeded. A dose of 545 mg to 1.2 g given 3 or 4 times daily is used for arthritic disorders.

Preparations

USP 25: Magnesium Salicylate Tablets.

Proprietary Preparations (details are given in Part 3)
Canad.: Back-Ese M; Doans Backache Pills; Herbogesic; *USA:* Backache Maximum Strength Relief; Bayer Select Maximum Strength Backache; Doans; Magan; Mobidin; Momentum Muscular Backache Formula; Nuprin Backache.

Multi-ingredient: *USA:* Extra Strength Doans PM; Magsal; Maximum Strength Arthriten†; Mobigesic; Myogesic†; Tetra-Mag.

Meclofenamic Acid (2717-r)

Meclofenamic Acid *(BAN, USAN, rINN)*.
CI-583; INF-4668. *N*-(2,6-Dichloro-*m*-tolyl)anthranilic acid.
$C_{14}H_{11}Cl_2NO_2 = 296.1$.
CAS — 644-62-2.
ATC — M01AG04; M02AA18.
Pharmacopoeias. In BP(Vet).

Pharmacopoeial description

BP(Vet) 2001: A white or almost white, odourless or almost odourless, crystalline powder. Practically insoluble in water; slightly soluble in alcohol and in chloroform; sparingly soluble in ether; soluble in dimethylformamide and in 1M sodium hydroxide.

Meclofenamate Sodium (2665-h)

Meclofenamate Sodium *(BANM, USAN, rINNM)*.
$C_{14}H_{10}Cl_2NNaO_2,H_2O = 336.1$.
CAS — 6385-02-0.
Pharmacopoeias. In US.

Pharmacopoeial description

USP 25: A white to creamy white, odourless to almost odourless, crystalline powder. Freely soluble in water, the solution sometimes being somewhat turbid due to partial hydrolysis and absorption of carbon dioxide; the solution is clear above pH 15. Slightly soluble in chloroform; practically insoluble in ether; soluble in methyl alcohol. Store in airtight containers. Protect from light.

Adverse Effects and Precautions

As for NSAIDs in general, p.63.

◊ The commonest adverse effect in 2500 patients who received meclofenamate sodium in double-blind or long-term studies was gastrointestinal disturbance.[1] Diarrhoea occurred in 11.2% of patients in double-blind studies and 32.8% of patients in long-term studies (up to 3 years). Ulcers were detected in 22 patients during therapy and skin rashes occurred in 4% of patients. Transient increases in serum aminotransferases and BUN occurred in some patients.

1. Preston SN. Safety of sodium meclofenamate (Meclomen™). *Curr Ther Res* 1978; **23** (suppl 4S): S107–12.

Effects on the blood. Case reports of agranulocytosis[1] and thrombocytopenia[2] associated with meclofenamate therapy.

1. Wishner AJ, Milburn PB. Meclofenamate sodium-induced agranulocytosis and suppression of erythropoiesis. *J Am Acad Dermatol* 1985; **13:** 1052–3.
2. Rodriguez J. Thrombocytopenia associated with meclofenamate. *Drug Intell Clin Pharm* 1981; **15:** 999.

Interactions

For interactions associated with NSAIDs, see p.65.

Pharmacokinetics

Meclofenamate sodium is readily absorbed when given by mouth. Peak plasma concentrations occur about 0.5 to 1 hour after ingestion. Meclofenamate is over 99% bound to plasma proteins. The plasma elimination half-life of meclofenamate sodium is about 2 to 4 hours. It is metabolised by oxidation, hydroxylation, dehalogenation, and conjugation with glucuronic acid and excreted in urine mainly as glucuronide conjugates of the metabolites. About 20 to 30% is recovered in the faeces. One of the metabolites, a 3-hydroxymethyl compound, is reported to be active.

◊ References.

1. Koup JR, *et al.* A single and multiple dose pharmacokinetic and metabolism study of meclofenamate sodium. *Biopharm Drug Dispos* 1990; **11:** 1–15.

Uses and Administration

Meclofenamic acid, an anthranilic acid derivative similar to mefenamic acid (below), is an NSAID (p.65). It is given by mouth as the sodium salt in musculoskeletal and joint disorders such as osteoarthritis and rheumatoid arthritis, in mild to moderate pain, and in dysmenorrhoea and menorrhagia.

Doses of meclofenamate sodium are expressed in terms of the equivalent amount of meclofenamic acid. In arthritic conditions it is given in doses of 200 to 400 mg daily; daily doses are usually given in 3 or 4 divided doses. For relief of mild to moderate pain doses are 50 to 100 mg every 4 to 6 hours; the daily dose should not exceed 400 mg. The dose in the treatment of dysmenorrhoea and menorrhagia is 100 mg three times daily for up to 6 days during menstruation.

Meclofenamic acid has also been given as a rectal suppository and is also used in veterinary medicine.

The symbol † denotes a preparation no longer actively marketed

---

Preparations

USP 25: Meclofenamate Sodium Capsules.

Proprietary Preparations (details are given in Part 3)
Aust.: Meclomen; *Hong Kong:* Meclomen; *Ital.:* Lenidolor; Meclodol; Movens; *S.Afr.:* Meclomen†; *Spain:* Meclomen.

Mefenamic Acid (2666-m)

Mefenamic Acid *(BAN, USAN, rINN)*.
Acidum Mefenamicum; CI-473; CN-35355; INF-3355. *N*-(2,3-Xylyl)anthranilic acid.
$C_{15}H_{15}NO_2 = 241.3$.
CAS — 61-68-7.
ATC — M01AG01.
Pharmacopoeias. In Eur. (see p.vi), Jpn, Pol., and US.

Pharmacopoeial description

Ph. Eur.: A white to almost white, microcrystalline powder. Practically insoluble in water; slightly soluble in alcohol and in dichloromethane; dissolves in dilute solutions of alkali hydroxides.

USP 25: A white to off-white, crystalline powder. Practically insoluble in water; slightly soluble in alcohol and in methyl alcohol; sparingly soluble in chloroform; soluble in solutions of alkali hydroxides. Store in airtight containers. Protect from light.

Adverse Effects and Precautions

As for NSAIDs in general, p.63. Treatment should be discontinued if diarrhoea and rashes occur. Other effects reported include drowsiness, thrombocytopenia, occasionally haemolytic anaemia, and rarely aplastic anaemia. Convulsions are a prominent feature of overdosage with mefenamic acid.

Mefenamic acid is contra-indicated in patients with inflammatory bowel disease. The UK manufacturers recommend that blood counts and liver function should be monitored during long-term therapy. Drowsiness may affect the performance of skilled tasks.

Mefenamic acid may give a false positive in tests for the presence of bile in the urine.

Effects on the blood. References to haematological reactions in patients taking mefenamic acid including haemolytic anaemia,[1] leucopenia,[2] neutropenia,[3] and agranulocytosis.[4]

1. Scott GL, *et al.* Autoimmune haemolytic anaemia and mefenamic acid therapy. *BMJ* 1968; **3:** 534–5.
2. Burns A, Young RE. Mefenamic acid induced leucopenia in the elderly. *Lancet* 1984; **ii:** 46.
3. Handa SI, Freestone S. Mefenamic acid-induced neutropenia and renal failure in elderly females with hypothyroidism. *Postgrad Med J* 1990; **66:** 557–9.
4. Muroi K, *et al.* Treatment of drug-induced agranulocytosis with granulocyte-colony stimulating factor. *Lancet* 1989; **ii:** 55.

Effects on the gastrointestinal tract. Reversible steatorrhoea has occurred[1] and mefenamic acid may provoke colitis in patients without a past history of this condition.[2]

1. Marks JS, Gleeson MH. Steatorrhoea complicating therapy with mefenamic acid. *BMJ* 1975; **4:** 442.
2. Ravi S, *et al.* Colitis caused by non-steroidal anti-inflammatory drugs. *Postgrad Med J* 1986; **62:** 773–6.

Effects on the kidneys. Nonoliguric renal failure has occurred in elderly patients who had experienced diarrhoea and vomiting while taking mefenamic acid and had continued to take the drug. It is normally recommended that mefenamic acid be discontinued in the event of diarrhoea and it was suggested that in these patients the gastrointestinal toxicity had led to fluid and electrolyte depletion, thus predisposing these patients to mefenamic acid's nephrotoxicity.[1] There has been a subsequent report[2] of nonoliguric renal failure in elderly patients given mefenamic acid for musculoskeletal pain.

1. Taha A, *et al.* Non-oliguric renal failure during treatment with mefenamic acid in elderly patients: a continuing problem. *BMJ* 1985; **291:** 661–2.
2. Grant DJ, MacConnachie AM. Mefenamic acid is more dangerous than most. *BMJ* 1995; **311:** 392.

Effects on the skin. Bullous pemphigoid, together with haemolytic anaemia and diarrhoea,[1] and fixed drug eruptions[2,3] have been associated with the use of mefenamic acid. Additionally, Stevens-Johnson syndrome, together with cholestatic hepatitis and haemolytic anaemia, in one patient has been attributed to mefenamic acid therapy.[4] It is generally recommended that mefenamic acid should be withdrawn if skin reactions develop.

1. Shepherd AN, *et al.* Mefenamic acid-induced bullous pemphigoid. *Postgrad Med J* 1986; **62:** 67–8.
2. Wilson CL, Otter A. Fixed drug eruption associated with mefenamic acid. *BMJ* 1986; **293:** 1243.
3. Long CC, *et al.* Fixed drug eruption to mefenamic acid: a report of three cases. *Br J Dermatol* 1992; **126:** 409–11.
4. Chan JCN, *et al.* A case of Stevens-Johnson syndrome, cholestatic hepatitis and haemolytic anaemia associated with use of mefenamic acid. *Drug Safety* 1991; **6:** 230–4.

Overdosage. Mefenamic acid overdose has been associated with CNS toxicity, especially with convulsions.[1] Coma[2,3] has also been reported.

1. Court H, Volans GN. Poisoning after overdose with non-steroidal anti-inflammatory drugs. *Adverse Drug React Acute Poisoning Rev* 1984; **3:** 1–21.
2. Gössinger H, *et al.* Coma in mefenamic acid poisoning. *Lancet* 1982; **ii:** 384.
3. Hendrickse MT. Mefenamic acid overdose mimicking brainstem stroke. *Lancet* 1988; **ii:** 1019.

Pancreatitis. A report of pancreatitis associated with mefenamic acid.[1]

1. van Walraven AA, *et al.* Pancreatitis caused by mefenamic acid. *Can Med Assoc J* 1982; **126:** 894.

Porphyria. Mefenamic acid is considered to be unsafe in patients with porphyria although there is conflicting experimental evidence of porphyrinogenicity.

Interactions

For interactions associated with NSAIDs, see p.65.

Pharmacokinetics

Mefenamic acid is absorbed from the gastrointestinal tract. Peak plasma concentrations occur about 2 to 4 hours after ingestion. The plasma elimination half-life is reported to be 2 to 4 hours. Mefenamic acid is extensively bound to plasma proteins. Mefenamic acid is distributed into breast milk but the amount is considered by some authorities to be too small to be harmful to a breast-fed infant. Over 50% of a dose may be recovered in the urine, as unchanged drug or conjugates of mefenamic acid and its metabolites.

Uses and Administration

Mefenamic acid, an anthranilic acid derivative, is an NSAID (p.65), although its anti-inflammatory properties are considered to be minor.

It is used in mild to moderate pain including headache, dental pain, postoperative and postpartum pain, and dysmenorrhoea, in musculoskeletal and joint disorders such as osteoarthritis and rheumatoid arthritis, in menorrhagia, and in children with fever and juvenile idiopathic arthritis. The usual dose by mouth is up to 500 mg three times daily. A suggested dose for children over 6 months of age is 25 mg per kg bodyweight daily in divided doses. Alternatively, doses in children may be given according to age: 6 months to under 2 years, 50 mg; 2 years to under 5 years, 100 mg; 5 years to under 9 years, 150 mg; 9 years to 12 years, 200 mg. These doses may be repeated as necessary, up to three times daily. In the USA, where mefenamic acid is only licensed for the treatment of moderate pain in adults, it is recommended that it should not be given for longer than 7 days at a time, but in the UK this restriction is only applied to children unless they are receiving mefenamic acid for juvenile chronic arthritis.

Preparations

BP 2001: Mefenamic Acid Capsules;
USP 25: Mefenamic Acid Capsules.

Proprietary Preparations (details are given in Part 3)
Aust.: Parkemed; *Austral.:* Mefic; Ponstan; *Braz.:* Ponstan; *Canad.:* Ponstan; *Fin.:* Ponstan; *Fr.:* Ponstyl; *Ger.:* Parkemed; Ponalar; *Hong Kong:* Dyspen; Medicap; Mefacap; Mefic; Napan; Ponstan; *Irl.:* Mefac; Pinalgesic; Ponalgic; Ponmel; Ponstan; *Ital.:* Lysalgo; *Mex.:* Artriden; Namifen; Ponstan; *NZ:* Ponstan; *Port.:* Ponstan; *S.Afr.:* Clinstan†; Fenamin; Mefalgic; Ponac; Ponstan; Ponstel; *Singapore:* Mefacap; Mefenix; Ponstan; Pontyl; *Spain:* Coslan; *Switz.:* Mefenacide; Ponstan; Spiralgin; *Thai.:* Conamic; Dyspen; Fenamic; Gandin; Manic; Mednil; Mefenan; Mefenix; Namic; Painnox; Ponnac; Ponnesia; Ponstan; Pontalon; Prostan; Pynamic; Sefmic; *UK:* Contraflam†; Dysman; Meflam; Opustan; Ponstan; *USA:* Ponstel.

Multi-ingredient: *Thai.:* Difemic; Mainnox; Med-Anspasmic.

Meloxicam (2751-d)

Meloxicam *(BAN, USAN, rINN)*.
UH-AC-62; UH-AC-62XX. 4-Hydroxy-2-methyl-*N*-(5-methyl-2-thiazolyl)-2*H*-1,2-benzothiazine-3-carboxamide 1,1-dioxide.
$C_{14}H_{13}N_3O_4S_2 = 351.4$.
CAS — 71125-38-7.
ATC — M01AC06.
Pharmacopoeias. In BP.

Pharmacopoeial description

BP 2001: A pale yellow powder. Practically insoluble in water; very slightly soluble in alcohol and in methyl alcohol; slightly soluble in acetone; soluble in dimethylformamide.

Adverse Effects

As for NSAIDs in general, p.63.

◊ Between September 1996, when meloxicam was first marketed in the UK, and mid June 1998 the UK Committee on Safety of Medicines had received a total of 773 reports of 1339 suspected adverse reactions for meloxicam.[1] Of all the reactions 41% were gastrointestinal and of these 18% involved gastrointestinal perforation, ulceration and/or bleeding; the mean age of the patients involved had been 64 years. Although most patients recovered after withdrawal of meloxicam and/or treatment, 5 had died. A total of 193 reactions involved the skin, the most common being pruritus, rash, and urticaria. There were also reports of angioedema (25), photosensitivity (12), and bullous dermatoses, including erythema multiforme and Stevens Johnson syndrome (5). No patients died from skin reactions and most recovered after meloxicam was withdrawn. Other frequently reported reactions were neurological (mostly headache), cardiovascular (oedema and palpitations) dizziness, flushing, and fatigue. A prescription event monitoring study has also analysed events reported with meloxicam use.[2] In a cohort of 19 087 patients who had received meloxicam some time between December 1996 and March 1997, 203 patients had experienced 252 events considered to be suspected adverse reactions. The majority of reactions were not serious or were labelled side-effects of meloxicam. Rare, serious suspected adverse reactions included 2 reports of thrombocytopenia and 1 each of interstitial nephritis and idiosyncratic liver abnormality. The most frequent gastrointestinal event was dyspepsia; other more serious gastrointestinal events occurring during meloxicam exposure included upper gastrointestinal bleeding (33 reports) and peptic ulcer (19 reports). However it was considered that the incidence of gastrointestinal disturbance was low in the absence of gastrointestinal risk factors. Adverse drug reactions reported during the first year of marketing of meloxicam to the Swedish Medical Products Agency suggested a similar safety profile to other NSAIDs.[3] Of the 15 reports, 6 were for gastrointestinal disturbances and 5 involved skin reactions.

It has been proposed that preferential inhibitors of cyclo-oxygenase-2, such as meloxicam, might produce fewer adverse effects than other NSAIDs but there has been little convincing evidence that the risk of severe gastrointestinal events is lower with meloxicam than with other NSAIDs at equi-effective doses.[4] Two recent large multicentre studies[5,6] have reported a lower incidence of gastrointestinal adverse effects with meloxicam than with non-selective cyclo-oxygenase inhibitors (diclofenac[5] or piroxicam[6]) but in one of these[5] the dose of meloxicam given also appeared to be less effective than the reference drug.

1. Committee on Safety of Medicines/Medicines Control Agency. Meloxicam (Mobic): gastrointestinal and skin reactions. *Current Problems* 1998; **24:** 13.
2. Martin RM, *et al.* The incidence of adverse events and risk factors for upper gastrointestinal disorders associated with meloxicam use amongst 19 087 patients in general practice in England: cohort study. *Br J Clin Pharmacol* 2000; **50:** 35–42.
3. Anonymous. Meloxicam safety similar to other NSAIDs. *WHO Drug Information* 1998; **12:** 147.
4. Anonymous. Meloxicam—a safer NSAID? *Drug Ther Bull* 1998; **36:** 62–4.
5. Hawkey C, *et al.* Gastrointestinal tolerability of meloxicam compared to diclofenac in osteoarthritis patients. *Br J Rheumatol* 1998; **37:** 937–45.
6. Dequeker J, *et al.* Improvement in gastrointestinal tolerability of the selective cyclooxygenase (COX)-2 inhibitor, meloxicam, compared with piroxicam: results of the safety and efficacy large-scale evaluation of COX-inhibiting therapies (SELECT) trial in osteoarthritis. *Br J Rheumatol* 1998; **37:** 946–51.

Precautions

As for NSAIDs in general, p.64.

Meloxicam should be avoided in severe hepatic impairment, in bleeding disorders, and in patients with renal failure unless receiving dialysis. Rectal administration should be avoided in patients with a history of proctitis, haemorrhoids, or rectal bleeding.

Renal impairment. The pharmacokinetics of meloxicam were not substantially altered in patients with a creatinine clearance of 41 to 60 mL per minute compared with those with normal renal function.[1] In those with a creatinine clearance of 20 to 40 mL per minute, total plasma-meloxicam concentrations were lower but meloxicam free fractions were higher. Such free meloxicam concentrations were similar to the other groups. On the basis of these results, it was suggested that it was not necessary to reduce meloxicam doses in patients with a creatinine clearance greater than 20 mL per minute.

1. Boulton-Jones JM, *et al.* Meloxicam pharmacokinetics in renal impairment. *Br J Clin Pharmacol* 1997; **43:** 35–40.

Interactions

For interactions associated with NSAIDs, see p.65.

There may be an increased risk of bleeding during concomitant use of meloxicam and oxpentifylline [pentoxifylline].

Pharmacokinetics

Meloxicam is well absorbed following oral administration. It is 99% bound to plasma proteins. Meloxicam has a plasma-elimination half-life of approximately 20 hours. It is extensively metabolised mainly by oxidation and excreted in similar amounts in the urine and in the faeces; less than 3% of a dose is excreted unchanged. The volume of distribution is increased in severe renal failure.

◊ References.
1. Narjes H, *et al.* Pharmacokinetics and tolerability of meloxicam after i.m. administration. *Br J Clin Pharmacol* 1996; **41:** 135–9.
2. Türck D, *et al.* Clinical pharmacokinetics of meloxicam. *Arzneimittelforschung* 1997; **47:** 253–8.
3. Davies NM, Skjodt NM. Clinical pharmacokinetics of meloxicam: a cyclooxygenase-2 preferential nonsteroidal anti-inflammatory drug. *Clin Pharmacokinet* 1999; **36:** 115–26.

Renal impairment. For reference to the pharmacokinetics of meloxicam in renal impairment, see under Precautions, above.

Uses and Administration

Meloxicam, an oxicam derivative, is an NSAID (p.65). It is reported to be a preferential inhibitor of cyclo-oxygenase-2 (COX-2). Meloxicam is used in the management of rheumatoid arthritis, for the short-term symptomatic treatment of acute exacerbations of osteoarthritis, and for the symptomatic treatment of ankylosing spondylitis.

In the treatment of rheumatoid arthritis and ankylosing spondylitis, meloxicam is given by mouth in a usual dose of 15 mg daily as a single dose. Those with an increased risk of adverse reactions should be started on 7.5 mg daily. A dose of 7.5 mg daily is recommended for long-term treatment in the elderly. In the treatment of acute exacerbations of osteoarthritis the usual dose of meloxicam by mouth is 7.5 mg, increased if necessary to a maximum of 15 mg daily given as a single dose.

The recommended maximum daily dose in dialysis patients is 7.5 mg.

Meloxicam may be given by rectal suppository in doses similar to those used orally but use should be limited to the shortest time possible.

Preparations

Proprietary Preparations (details are given in Part 3)

Aust.: Mobic; Movalis; *Belg.:* Mobic; *Braz.:* Movatec; *Denm.:* Mobic; *Fin.:* Mobic; *Fr.:* Mobic; *Ger.:* Mobic; *Hong Kong:* Mobic; *Irl.:* Mobic; *Ital.:* Leutrol; Mobic; *Mex.:* Masflex; Mobicox; *Neth.:* Movicox; *Norw.:* Mobic; *Port.:* Movalis; *S.Afr.:* Mobic; *Singapore:* Mobic; *Spain:* Movalis; Parocin; Uticox; *Swed.:* Latonid; Mobic; *Switz.:* Mobicox; Zilutrol; *Thai.:* Mobic; *UK:* Mobic; *USA:* Mobic.

Meptazinol Hydrochloride   (12932-r)

Meptazinol Hydrochloride (BANM, USAN, rINNM).

IL-22811 (meptazinol); Wy-22811 (meptazinol). 3-(3-Ethyl-1-methylperhydroazepin-3-yl)phenol hydrochloride.

$C_{15}H_{23}NO,HCl = 269.8$.

CAS — 54340-58-8 (meptazinol); 59263-76-2 (meptazinol hydrochloride); 34154-59-1 (±-meptazinol hydrochloride).

Pharmacopoeias. In Br.

Meptazinol hydrochloride 115.6 mg is approximately equivalent to 100 mg of meptazinol.

Pharmacopoeial description

BP 2001: A white or almost white powder. Very soluble in water and in methyl alcohol; freely soluble in alcohol; very slightly soluble in acetone; dissolves in dilute solutions of alkali hydroxides. Store at a temperature not exceeding 25°.

Dependence and Withdrawal

As for Opioid Analgesics, p.66.

◊ In assessing the dependence potential of meptazinol, a WHO expert committee[1] noted in 1989 that abrupt discontinuation of chronic meptazinol administration precipitated only slight withdrawal signs in *animals* and that meptazinol did not suppress opioid withdrawal signs and symptoms in humans dependent on morphine. Abuse had not been reported. They considered that the likelihood of abuse was moderate and that international control was not warranted at that time.

1. WHO. WHO expert committee on drug dependence: twenty-fifth report. *WHO Tech Rep Ser 775* 1989.

Adverse Effects, Treatment, and Precautions

As for Opioid Analgesics in general, p.67.

Meptazinol is claimed to have a low incidence of respiratory depression. There have been occasional reports of psychiatric disorders such as hallucinations, confusion, and depression. As meptazinol has both antagonist and agonist properties its effects may be only partially reversed by naloxone, but use of the latter is still recommended in overdosage.

Meptazinol has the potential to precipitate withdrawal symptoms if given to patients who are physically dependent on opioids.

Effects on the respiratory system. Meptazinol is said to have a relatively low potential for respiratory depression and in healthy subjects was reported to produce substantially less respiratory depression than morphine or pentazocine at usual analgesic doses.[1] Respiratory depression does occur in anaesthetised patients.[2] When compared with pethidine in anaesthetised patients meptazinol 1 mg per kg body-weight intravenously

produced less respiratory depression than pethidine 1 mg per kg, but more than pethidine 0.5 mg per kg.[3] Ventilatory depressant effects were similar in another study,[4] although a second injection produced a further decrease in ventilation only with pethidine. Compensatory mechanisms may come into play following repeated doses of meptazinol but the authors[4] considered that intravenous administration of meptazinol during anaesthesia should be viewed with as much caution as with any other opioid. In a comparison with morphine[5] similar effects on ventilation were seen with meptazinol by intravenous infusion postoperatively when patients were monitored continuously. In another postoperative study[6] respiratory rate fell following meptazinol or morphine, although their effects on central regulation of respiration differed; CO_2 sensitivity seemed to be impaired by morphine but not meptazinol.

Respiratory arrest occurred after an overdose of 50 meptazinol 200-mg tablets and a quarter of a bottle of whisky.[7] Full recovery eventually followed supportive measures although spontaneous respiration was not re-established by naloxone intravenously to a cumulative total dose of 10 mg.

1. Jordan C, *et al.* A comparison of the respiratory effects of meptazinol, pentazocine and morphine. *Br J Anaesth* 1979; **51:** 497–502.
2. Hardy PAJ. Meptazinol and respiratory depression. *Lancet* 1983; **ii:** 576.
3. Wilkinson DJ, *et al.* Meptazinol— a cause of respiratory depression in general anaesthesia. *Br J Anaesth* 1985; **57:** 1077–84.
4. Lee A, Drummond GB. Ventilatory effects of meptazinol and pethidine in anaesthetised patients. *Br J Anaesth* 1987; **59:** 1127–33.
5. Frater RAS, *et al.* Analgesia-induced respiratory depression: comparison of meptazinol and morphine in the postoperative period. *Br J Anaesth* 1989; **63:** 260–5.
6. Verborgh C, Camu F. Post-surgical pain relief with zero-order intravenous infusions of meptazinol and morphine: a double-blind placebo-controlled evaluation of their effects on ventilation. *Eur J Clin Pharmacol* 1990; **38:** 437–42.
7. Davison AG, *et al.* Meptazinol overdose producing near fatal respiratory depression. *Hum Toxicol* 1987; **6:** 331.

Hepatic impairment. See under Pharmacokinetics, below.

Interactions

For interactions associated with opioid analgesics, see p.68.

Pharmacokinetics

Following oral administration of meptazinol peak plasma concentrations have been achieved within 0.5 to 2 hours, but bioavailability is low since it undergoes extensive first-pass metabolism. Systemic availability is improved after rectal administration. Peak plasma concentrations have been achieved 30 minutes after rectal or intramuscular administration. Plasma protein binding has averaged only about 27%. Elimination half-lives of about 2 hours have been reported. Meptazinol is extensively metabolised in the liver and is excreted mainly in the urine as the glucuronide conjugate. Less than 10% of a dose has been recovered from the faeces. Meptazinol crosses the placenta.

◊ References.
1. Franklin RA, *et al.* Studies on the metabolism of meptazinol, a new analgesic drug. *Br J Clin Pharmacol* 1976; **3:** 497–502.
2. Franklin RA, *et al.* Studies on the absorption and disposition of meptazinol following rectal administration. *Br J Clin Pharmacol* 1977; **4:** 163–7.
3. Davies G, *et al.* Pharmacokinetics of meptazinol in man following repeated intramuscular administration. *Eur J Clin Pharmacol* 1982; **23:** 535–8.
4. Norbury HM, *et al.* Pharmacokinetics of the new analgesic, meptazinol, after oral and intravenous administration to volunteers. *Eur J Clin Pharmacol* 1983; **25:** 77–80.
5. Murray GR, *et al.* The systemic availability of meptazinol in man after oral and rectal doses. *Eur J Clin Pharmacol* 1989; **36:** 279–82.

The elderly. A lower clearance and longer elimination half-life has been reported for meptazinol in elderly patients, but dosage reduction was not considered warranted on pharmacokinetic grounds. Mean half-lives in elderly and young subjects were 3.39 and 1.94 hours respectively following single oral doses[1] and 2.93 and 2.06 hours respectively following intravenous administration.[2]

1. Norbury HM, *et al.* Pharmacokinetics of meptazinol after single and multiple oral administration to elderly patients. *Eur J Clin Pharmacol* 1984; **27:** 223–6.
2. Murray GR, *et al.* Pharmacokinetics of meptazinol after parenteral administration in the elderly. *Eur J Clin Pharmacol* 1987; **31:** 733–6.

Hepatic impairment. Oral bioavailability of meptazinol appeared to be enhanced in patients with liver disease. Mean peak plasma concentrations of 184 nanograms per mL, 131 nanograms per mL, and 53 nanograms per mL were measured in cirrhotic patients, patients with non-cirrhotic liver disease, and patients with normal liver function, respectively, after a single oral dose of meptazinol, although there was no evidence of accumulation after chronic dosing.[1] There were no significant differences in plasma clearance after an intravenous dose. Reduced oral doses of meptazinol might be advisable in cirrhotic patients.

1. Birnie GG, *et al.* Enhanced oral bioavailability of meptazinol in cirrhosis. *Gut* 1987; **28:** 248–54.

Pregnancy. In women given an intramuscular injection of 100 to 150 mg during labour, meptazinol was found to cross the placenta readily but was rapidly eliminated from the neonate.[1] This contrasted with pethidine which was known to be excreted very slowly from neonates. As in the adult, elimination of meptazinol by the neonate appeared to take place mainly by conjugation with glucuronic acid.[2] A half-life of 3.4 hours, similar to that in adults, has been reported in the neonate,[3] in contrast to 22.7 hours for pethidine in neonates.

Disposition of meptazinol appears not to be significantly affected by pregnancy. Mean half-lives of 1.36 and 1.68 hours were reported in pregnant and non-pregnant women, respectively,[4] compared with 2.06 hours in men.

1. Franklin RA, *et al.* Preliminary studies on the disposition of meptazinol in the neonate. *Br J Clin Pharmacol* 1981; **12:** 88–90.
2. Dowell PS, *et al.* Routes of meptazinol conjugation in the neonate. *Br J Clin Pharmacol* 1982; **14:** 748–9.
3. Jackson MBA, Robson PJ. Preliminary clinical and pharmacokinetic experiences in the newborn when meptazinol is compared with pethidine as an obstetric analgesic. *Postgrad Med J* 1983; **59** (suppl 1): 47–51.
4. Murray GR, *et al.* The disposition of meptazinol after single and multiple intravenous administration to pregnant and non-pregnant women. *Eur J Clin Pharmacol* 1989; **36:** 273–7.

Uses and Administration

Meptazinol is a mixed opioid agonist and antagonist with partial opioid agonist activity at the μ_1 opioid receptor (see p.68); it also has cholinergic activity. Meptazinol is used in the treatment of moderate to severe pain. It has a shorter duration of action than morphine.

Meptazinol hydrochloride is given by mouth or by intramuscular or intravenous injection; doses are expressed in terms of the base. For the short-term treatment of moderate pain meptazinol is given by mouth in a dose of 200 mg every 3 to 6 hours. The intramuscular dose is 75 to 100 mg given every 2 to 4 hours; for obstetric pain a dose of 2 mg per kg body-weight (100 to 150 mg) may be used. Meptazinol is also given by slow intravenous injection in doses of 50 to 100 mg every 2 to 4 hours.

Administration. EPIDURAL ROUTE. Epidural administration of meptazinol 90 mg for postoperative pain was reported to be superior to intramuscular administration of 90 mg.[1] Others[2,3] tried epidural meptazinol for analgesia after caesarean section, but discouraged its use. In one study[2] a 30-mg dose was ineffective with an unacceptable incidence of adverse effects and in the other[3] a 60-mg dose was ineffective because of its short duration of action.

The manufacturers in the UK state that the injectable formulation is not suitable for epidural or intrathecal use.

1. Verborgh C, *et al.* Meptazinol for postoperative pain relief in man: comparison of extradural and im administration. *Br J Anaesth* 1987; **59:** 1134–9.
2. Francis RI, Lockhart AS. Epidural meptazinol. *Anaesthesia* 1986; **41:** 88–9.
3. Birks RJS, Marsh DRG. Epidural meptazinol. *Anaesthesia* 1986; **41:** 883.

Preparations

BP 2001: Meptazinol Injection; Meptazinol Tablets.

Proprietary Preparations (details are given in Part 3)
Aust.: Meptidol; *Ger.:* Meptid; *Irl.:* Meptid; *UK:* Meptid.

Methadone Hydrochloride (6237-j)

Methadone Hydrochloride (BANM, pINNM).

Amidine Hydrochloride; Amidone Hydrochloride; (±)-Methadone Hydrochloride; Methadoni Hydrochloridum; Phenadone. (±)-6-Dimethylamino-4,4-diphenylheptan-3-one hydrochloride.

$C_{21}H_{27}NO,HCl = 345.9$.

CAS — 76-99-3 (methadone); 297-88-1 (methadone, ±); 1095-90-5 (methadone hydrochloride); 125-56-4 (methadone hydrochloride, ±).

Pharmacopoeias. In Chin., Eur. (see p.vi), and US.

Pharmacopoeial description

Ph. Eur.: White crystalline powder. Soluble in water; freely soluble in alcohol; practically insoluble in ether. Protect from light.

USP 25: Odourless colourless crystals or white crystalline powder. Soluble in water; freely soluble in alcohol and in chloroform; practically insoluble in ether and in glycerol. pH of a 1% solution in water is between 4.5 and 6.5. Store in airtight containers. Protect from light.

Incompatibility. There appears to be adequate evidence that stable solutions containing methadone hydrochloride and hydroxybenzoate esters can be formulated but the risk of precipitation exists if syrup preserved with hydroxybenzoates is used to extemporaneously prepare a methadone mixture 1 mg per mL to the DTF formula.[1] An oral formulation of methadone hydrochloride 5 mg per mL containing methyl hydroxybenzoate 0.1% as preservative rather than chloroform has been reported stable for at least 4 months at room temperature.[2]

1. *PSGB Lab Report P/80/1* 1980.
2. Ching MS, *et al.* Stability of methadone mixture with methyl hydroxybenzoate as a preservative. *Aust J Hosp Pharm* 1989; **19:** 159–61.

Dependence and Withdrawal

As for Opioid Analgesics, p.66. Methadone withdrawal symptoms are similar to, but more prolonged, than those produced by morphine or diamorphine. They develop more slowly and do not usually appear until 24 to 48 hours after the last dose.

Methadone is used for substitution therapy in the management of opioid dependence (see under Uses and Administration, below).

Adverse Effects and Treatment

As for Opioid Analgesics in general, p.67.

Methadone is subject to accumulation in the body and has a more prolonged effect than morphine. It may have a relatively greater respiratory depressant effect than morphine and, although reported to be less sedating, repeated administration of methadone may result in marked sedation. After gross overdosage symptoms are similar to those of morphine poisoning. Pulmonary oedema after overdosage is a common cause of fatalities among addicts.

Methadone causes pain at injection sites; subcutaneous injection causes local tissue irritation and induration.

◊ It has been pointed out[1] that most cases of methadone poisoning occurred in persons not on maintenance, who were often children or family members of maintenance patients. Methadone is highly toxic to anyone who is not tolerant to opioids; 50 to 100 mg can be life-threatening in non-tolerant adults and 10 mg can be fatal in a young child.

A group[2] in Australia has found that the risk of death from methadone toxicity is greatest during the first 2 weeks of maintenance therapy. This has been attributed to the difficulty in determining a safe and effective starting dose of methadone and unreliable accounts of a patient's recent drug use.

1. Harding-Pink D. Opioid toxicity: methadone: one person's maintenance dose is another's poison. *Lancet* 1993; **341:** 665–6.
2. Caplehorn JRM, Drummer OH. Mortality associated with New South Wales methadone programs in 1994: lives lost and saved. *Med J Aust* 1999; **170:** 104–9.

Effects on the endocrine system. Hypoadrenalism has been demonstrated in chronic methadone addicts. Findings consistent with deficient ACTH production and subsequent secondary hypoadrenalism have been reported[1] although others[2] found evidence of methadone-induced primary adrenal cortical hypofunction.

1. Dackis CA, *et al.* Methadone induced hypoadrenalism. *Lancet* 1982; **ii:** 1167.
2. Pullan PT, *et al.* Methadone-induced hypoadrenalism. *Lancet* 1983; **i:** 714.

Effects on the nervous system. Choreic movements in a patient on long-term methadone maintenance treatment for diamorphine addiction disappeared when methadone was discontinued.[1]

1. Wasserman S, Yahr MD. Choreic movements induced by the use of methadone. *Arch Neurol* 1980; **37:** 727–8.

Effects on sexual function. Sexual performance was impaired in 29 male diamorphine addicts receiving methadone maintenance therapy.[1] The function of secondary sex organs was markedly suppressed when compared with untreated diamorphine addicts or controls and serum-testosterone concentrations were 43% lower in those on methadone.

1. Cicero TJ, *et al.* Function of the male sex organs in heroin and methadone users. *N Engl J Med* 1975; **292:** 882–7.

Precautions

As for Opioid Analgesics in general, p.68.

Administration. Methadone has a long half-life and accumulation may occur with repeated doses, especially in elderly or debilitated patients.[1] An 81-year-old woman given methadone 5 mg three times a day by mouth for 2 days became deeply unconscious but awoke immediately when given naloxone 400 µg intravenously.[2]

Sudden death in 10 diamorphine addicts occurred between 2 and 6 days after starting a methadone maintenance programme.[3] The mean prescribed dose of methadone at the time of death had been about 60 mg. There was evidence of chronic

---

persistent hepatitis in all cases and liver disease could have reduced methadone clearance resulting in higher than expected blood concentrations. Liver function tests and urine testing for the presence of drugs prior to entry into methadone maintenance programmes and lower starting doses might decrease the likelihood of such deaths. Like dextropropoxyphene, methadone has membrane stabilising activity and can block nerve conduction, and it was suggested[4] that the sudden deaths were mainly due to accumulation of methadone over several days resulting in complications such as cardiac arrhythmias or cardiovascular collapse. See also under Adverse Effects, above.

For the effects of hepatic impairment and renal impairment on the disposition of methadone, see under Pharmacokinetics, below.

1. Twycross RG. A comparison of diamorphine-with-cocaine and methadone. *Br J Clin Pharmacol* 1977; **4:** 691–3.
2. Symonds P. Methadone and the elderly. *BMJ* 1977; **i:** 512.
3. Drummer OH, *et al.* Deaths of heroin addicts starting on a methadone maintenance programme. *Lancet* 1990; **335:** 108.
4. Wu C, Henry JA. Deaths of heroin addicts starting on methadone maintenance. *Lancet* 1990; **335:** 424.

Breast feeding. Methadone is distributed into breast milk and death of the 5-week-old infant of a mother on methadone maintenance was attributed to methadone received via his mother's milk.[1] Others have suggested that the amount of methadone in breast milk was unlikely to have any pharmacological effect on the infant.[2,3]

1. Smialek JE, *et al.* Methadone deaths in children. *JAMA* 1977; **238:** 2516–17.
2. Anonymous. Methadone in breast milk. *Med Lett Drugs Ther* 1979; **21:** 52.
3. Wojnar-Horton RE, *et al.* Methadone distribution and excretion into breast milk of clients in a methadone maintenance programme. *Br J Clin Pharmacol* 1997; **44:** 543–7.

Pregnancy. Methadone is not recommended for use in labour because its prolonged duration of action increases the risk of neonatal respiratory depression.

Neonatal withdrawal syndrome and low birth-weight are immediate problems in the infants born to women receiving methadone for the management of opioid addiction; increased stillbirth rates have also been noted.[1-3] In the neonatal period moderate to severe opioid abstinence syndrome occurred in 75% of infants in one study,[2] as well as reduced head circumference and raised systolic blood pressure. At follow-up over 18 months these children had a higher incidence of otitis media, of reduced head circumference, and of abnormal eye findings when compared with drug-free controls. Neurobehavioural abnormalities and lower scores on mental and motor developmental indices were thought to be possible predictors of later learning and behavioural problems. However, no specific effect of methadone or diamorphine has been noted on intra-uterine and postnatal growth.[4]

1. Blinick G, *et al.* Methadone maintenance, pregnancy, and progeny. *JAMA* 1973; **225:** 477–9.
2. Rosen TS, Johnson HL. Children of methadone-maintained mothers: follow-up to 18 months of age. *J Pediatr* 1982; **101:** 192–6.
3. Kalter H, Warkany J. Congenital malformations. *N Engl J Med* 1983; **308:** 491–7.
4. Lifschitz MH, *et al.* Fetal and postnatal growth of children born to narcotic-dependent women. *J Pediatr* 1983; **102:** 686–91.

Interactions

For interactions associated with opioid analgesics, see p.68.

◊ Drugs that *acidify* or *alkalinise* the urine may have an effect on methadone pharmacokinetics since body clearance is increased at acidic pH and decreased at alkaline pH.[1]

1. Nilsson M-I, *et al.* Effect of urinary pH on the disposition of methadone in man. *Eur J Clin Pharmacol* 1982; **22:** 337–42.

Antibacterials. Methadone is metabolised in the liver to inactive metabolites by the mixed-function oxidase system and thus interactions are likely with enzyme inducers. Withdrawal symptoms have been reported in patients maintained on methadone when they were given *rifampicin*.[1-3]

1. Kreek MJ, *et al.* Rifampin-induced methadone withdrawal. *N Engl J Med* 1976; **294:** 1104–6.
2. Bending MR, Skacel PO. Rifampicin and methadone withdrawal. *Lancet* 1977; **i:** 1211.
3. Raistrick D, *et al.* Methadone maintenance and tuberculosis treatment. *BMJ* 1996; **313:** 925–6.

Antidepressants. *SSRIs* such as fluoxetine[1] and fluvoxamine[1,2] may enhance the effects of some opioid analgesics; such interactions may lead to methadone toxicity.

1. Eap CB, *et al.* Fluvoxamine and fluoxetine do not interact in the same way with the metabolism of the enantiomers of methadone. *J Clin Psychopharmacol* 1997; **17:** 113–17.
2. Bertschy G, *et al.* Probable metabolic interaction between methadone and fluvoxamine in addict patients. *Ther Drug Monit* 1994; **16:** 42–5.

Antiepileptics. Withdrawal symptoms have been reported in patients maintained on methadone when they were given *phenobarbital*[1] or *phenytoin*.[2,3]

1. Liu S-J, Wang RIH. Case report of barbiturate-induced enhancement of methadone metabolism and withdrawal syndrome. *Am J Psychiatry* 1984; **141:** 1287–8.
2. Finelli PF. Phenytoin and methadone tolerance. *N Engl J Med* 1976; **294:** 227.
3. Tong TG, *et al.* Phenytoin-induced methadone withdrawal. *Ann Intern Med* 1981; **94:** 349–51.

The symbol † denotes a preparation no longer actively marketed

Antifungals. Concomitant administration of methadone and *fluconazole* has been reported[1] to result in increased serum concentrations of methadone although the authors of the study considered that for patients being treated for opioid dependence the interaction was unlikely to require adjustment of the methadone dose.

1. Cobb MN, *et al.* The effect of fluconazole on the clinical pharmacokinetics of methadone. *Clin Pharmacol Ther* 1998; **63**: 655–62.

Antivirals. Methadone possibly increases plasma concentrations of *zidovudine* (see p.646). There is limited evidence[1] that *nelfinavir* or *ritonavir* may reduce plasma concentrations of methadone; *indinavir* and *saquinavir* had no effect on plasma-methadone. *Nevirapine* has been reported to reduce plasma-methadone concentrations and withdrawal symptoms have occurred when it was given to patients receiving methadone.[2] A similar interaction has occurred when *efavirenz* has been taken concomitantly with methadone.[3,4]

1. Beauverie P, *et al.* Therapeutic drug monitoring in HIV-infected patients receiving protease inhibitors. *AIDS* 1998; **12**: 2510–11.
2. Altice FL, *et al.* Nevirapine induced opiate withdrawal among injection drug users with HIV infection receiving methadone. *AIDS* 1999; **13**: 957–62.
3. Pinzani V, *et al.* Methadone withdrawal symptoms with nevirapine and efavirenz. *Ann Pharmacother* 2000; **34**: 405–7.
4. Clarke SM, *et al.* The pharmacokinetics of methadone in HIV-positive patients receiving the non-nucleoside reverse transcriptase inhibitor efavirenz. *Br J Clin Pharmacol* 2001; **51**: 213–17.

Gastrointestinal drugs. Histamine H_2-antagonists such as *cimetidine* (see p.68) may enhance the effects of some opioid analgesics; such interactions may lead to methadone toxicity.

Pharmacokinetics

Methadone hydrochloride is readily absorbed from the gastrointestinal tract and following subcutaneous or intramuscular injection. It is widely distributed in the tissues, diffuses across the placenta, and is distributed into breast milk. It is extensively protein bound. Methadone is metabolised in the liver, mainly by *N*-demethylation and cyclisation, and the metabolites are excreted in the bile and urine. Metabolism is primarily catalysed by CYP3A4, although other cytochrome P450 isoenzymes also play a role. It has a prolonged half-life and is subject to accumulation.

◊ In reviews of the pharmacokinetics of methadone[1,2] particular reference has been made to its long elimination half-life, accumulation following repeated doses, and wide interindividual variations.

Methadone is rapidly absorbed after administration by mouth and has high oral bioavailability. Peak plasma concentrations have been reported 1 to 5 hours after oral administration of a single dose in tablet form. It undergoes considerable tissue distribution and protein binding is reported to be 60 to 90% with α_1-acid glycoprotein being the main binding protein in plasma. Metabolism to the major metabolite 2-ethylidine-1,5-dimethyl-3,3-diphenylpyrrolidine and the minor metabolite 2-ethyl-3,3-diphenyl-5-methylpyrrolidine, both of them inactive, occurs in the liver. These metabolites are excreted in the faeces and urine together with unchanged methadone. Other metabolites, including methadol and normethadol, have also been described. The liver may also serve as a major storage site of unchanged methadone which is taken up, bound non-specifically by the liver, and released again mainly unchanged. Urinary excretion of methadone is pH-dependent, the lower the pH the greater the clearance.

In addition to marked interindividual variations there are differences in the pharmacokinetics of methadone following single or multiple doses. Elimination half-lives vary considerably (a range of 15 to 60 hours has been quoted) and may be much longer than the 18 hours reported following a single dose. Careful adjustment of dosage is necessary with repeated administration.

Most studies have been in addicts. Plasma concentrations have been found to vary widely during methadone maintenance therapy with large differences between patients and wide fluctuations in individual patients. Interindividual variations in kinetics have also been seen in cancer patients.

1. Säwe J. High-dose morphine and methadone in cancer patients: clinical pharmacokinetic considerations of oral treatment. *Clin Pharmacokinet* 1986; **11**: 87–106.
2. Moore RA, *et al.* Opiate metabolism and excretion. *Baillieres Clin Anaesthesiol* 1987; **1**: 829–58.

Administration. Methadone is considerably more lipid-soluble than morphine. A study of plasma concentrations and analgesia following their intramuscular injection indicated that more rapid and greater relief of pain might be achieved if lipid-soluble opioid analgesics were injected into the deltoid rather than the gluteal muscle; there was no significant difference in absorption of morphine from the two sites.[1]

Other routes of administration investigated in pharmacokinetic studies include continuous intravenous infusion[2] and continuous epidural infusion.[3]

1. Grabinski PY, *et al.* Plasma levels and analgesia following deltoid and gluteal injections of methadone and morphine. *J Clin Pharmacol* 1983; **23**: 48–55.

2. Denson DD, *et al.* Pharmacokinetics of continuous intravenous infusion of methadone in the early post-burn period. *J Clin Pharmacol* 1990; **30**: 70–5.
3. Shir Y, *et al.* Plasma concentrations of methadone during postoperative patient-controlled extradural analgesia. *Br J Anaesth* 1990; **65**: 204–9.

Hepatic impairment. Overall hepatic dysfunction does not seem unduly to disrupt methadone metabolism[1] and it has been suggested[2] that maintenance dosage of methadone need not be changed in stable chronic liver disease, although abrupt changes in hepatic status might result in substantial alterations in methadone disposition requiring dosage adjustments.

In a study of patients on methadone maintenance therapy[2] apparent terminal half-life of methadone was prolonged from a mean of 18.8 hours in those with healthy livers to 35.5 hours in patients with severe chronic liver disease. However plasma concentrations were not increased in such patients, possibly because the storage capacity of the liver was decreased.

1. Moore RA, *et al.* Opiate metabolism and excretion. *Baillieres Clin Anaesthesiol* 1987; **1**: 829–58.
2. Novick DM, *et al.* Methadone disposition in patients with chronic liver disease. *Clin Pharmacol Ther* 1981; **30**: 353–62.

Pregnancy. Plasma concentrations of methadone were reduced in methadone-maintained pregnant women, probably due to enhanced metabolism.[1] It was suggested that the dose of methadone might need to be increased in such patients.

1. Pond SM, *et al.* Altered methadone pharmacokinetics in methadone-maintained pregnant women. *J Pharmacol Exp Ther* 1985; **233**: 1–6.

Renal impairment. The urinary excretion of methadone was reduced in renal failure,[1] but plasma concentrations were within the usual range and faecal excretion accounted for the majority of the dose. Very little methadone was removed by peritoneal dialysis or haemodialysis.

1. Kreek MJ, *et al.* Methadone use in patients with chronic renal disease. *Drug Alcohol Depend* 1980; **5**: 197–205.

Uses and Administration

Methadone hydrochloride, a diphenylheptane derivative, is an opioid analgesic (p.68) that is primarily a μ opioid agonist. Single doses of methadone have a less marked sedative action than single doses of morphine. Methadone is a racemic mixture and levomethadone (p.50) is the active isomer. Methadone hydrochloride is used in the treatment of severe pain; it may be of use for those patients who experience excitation or exacerbation of pain with morphine. It is also used in the management of opioid dependence. Methadone has a depressant action on the cough centre and has been used as a cough suppressant in terminal illness, although some authorities discourage this use because of the risks of accumulation.

The analgesic effect of methadone begins about 10 to 20 minutes after parenteral injection and about 30 to 60 minutes after administration by mouth, the effect of a single dose usually lasting about 4 hours. As accumulation occurs following repeated doses, the effects become more prolonged.

The analgesic dose of methadone hydrochloride ranges from 2.5 to 10 mg given at intervals of 3 to 8 hours depending on the pain. A commonly used range is 5 to 10 mg every 6 to 8 hours initially, adjusted according to response. To avoid the risk of accumulation and opioid overdosage it is recommended that in prolonged use methadone should not be administered more than twice daily. It may be given by mouth or by subcutaneous or intramuscular injection; if repeated injections are required the intramuscular route is preferred to the subcutaneous.

Methadone hydrochloride is used as part of the treatment of dependence on opioids, although prolonged use of methadone itself may result in dependence. In the treatment of opioid withdrawal, or detoxification, methadone is given initially in doses sufficient to suppress withdrawal symptoms. A mixture containing 1 mg per mL of methadone hydrochloride is used in the UK for opioid dependent persons. A daily dose of 10 to 20 mg of methadone hydrochloride by mouth may be given initially and increased as necessary by 10 to 20 mg daily until there are no signs of withdrawal or intoxication. After stabilisation, which can often be achieved with a daily dose of 40 to 60 mg, the dose of methadone is gradually decreased until total withdrawal is achieved. Similar doses may also be given by subcutaneous or intramuscular injection. Some treatment schedules for opioid dependence involve prolonged maintenance therapy with metha-

done where the daily dose is adjusted carefully for the individual; there have been reports of some patients receiving 120 mg or more daily.

For the control of intractable cough associated with terminal lung cancer, methadone hydrochloride is usually given in the form of a linctus in a dose of 1 to 2 mg every 4 to 6 hours, but reduced to twice daily on prolonged use.

Levomethadone is used similarly in the treatment of severe pain.

Administration. Although duration of action following single doses of methadone is similar to that with morphine it increases considerably with multiple dosing of methadone because of the long elimination half-life (see Pharmacokinetics, above). The minimum effective dose of methadone can be difficult to titrate for the individual patient. A fixed 10-mg oral dose with a flexible patient-controlled dosage interval has been used in patients with chronic cancer pain.[1] Dosage not more frequently than every 4 hours during the first 3 to 5 days, followed by a fixed dose every 8 to 12 hours depending on the patient's requirements, was advised.

A suggested dose for patients who need to switch from oral morphine to methadone because of poor pain control is one tenth of the total daily dose of morphine, but not greater than 100 mg given at intervals determined by the patient and not more frequently than every 3 hours.[2]

When switching from oral to parenteral administration it was suggested[3] that the dose of methadone should be halved and adjusted thereafter as necessary.

Apart from subcutaneous or intramuscular injection methadone has also been given intravenously or intraspinally. Evidence of the prolonged effect of methadone was demonstrated when a single intravenous bolus dose of 20 mg resulted in postoperative analgesia lasting about 25 hours.[4] Methadone has also been tried intravenously in children to prevent postoperative pain; a dose of 200 µg per kg body-weight was given perioperatively followed postoperatively by 50 µg per kg every 10 minutes until the patient was both comfortable and adequately alert.[5] An initial 2-hour loading intravenous infusion of methadone 100 to 200 µg per kg body-weight per hour to provide rapid analgesia followed by infusion at a lower maintenance rate of 10 to 20 µg per kg per hour for continuous pain relief has been used in burn patients.[6] Epidural methadone has been used successfully in doses of up to 5 mg for analgesia in association with bupivacaine.[7,8]

1. Säwe J, *et al.* Patient-controlled dose regimen of methadone for chronic cancer pain. *BMJ* 1981; **282**: 771–3.
2. Morley JS, *et al.* Methadone in pain uncontrolled by morphine. *Lancet* 1993; **342**: 1243.
3. Säwe J. High-dose morphine and methadone in cancer patients: clinical pharmacokinetic considerations of oral treatment. *Clin Pharmacokinet* 1986; **11**: 87–106.
4. Gourlay GK, *et al.* Methadone produces prolonged postoperative analgesia. *BMJ* 1982; **284**: 630–1.
5. Berde CB, *et al.* Comparison of morphine and methadone for prevention of postoperative pain in 3- to 7-year-old children. *J Pediatr* 1991; **119**: 136–41.
6. Denson DD, *et al.* Pharmacokinetics of continuous intravenous infusion of methadone in the early post-burn period. *J Clin Pharmacol* 1990; **30**: 70–5.
7. Drenger B, *et al.* Extradural bupivacaine and methadone for extracorporeal shock-wave lithotripsy. *Br J Anaesth* 1989; **62**: 82–6.
8. Martin CS, *et al.* Extradural methadone and bupivacaine in labour. *Br J Anaesth* 1990; **65**: 330–2.

Opioid dependence. The treatment of opioid dependence is discussed on p.66. The following formula is not official but is that formerly listed in the Drug Tariff Formulary (DTF) for Methadone Mixture 1 mg per mL. The preparation is 2.5 times the strength of Methadone Linctus (BP 2001) and is intended only for drug-dependent persons.

Methadone Mixture 1 mg/mL

methadone hydrochloride 10 mg
Green S and Tartrazine Solution (BP 1980) 0.02 mL
Compound Tartrazine Solution (BP 1980) 0.08 mL
syrup, unpreserved 5 mL
chloroform water, double-strength to 10 mL.

An official preparation of methadone has also recently been introduced: Methadone Oral Solution (1 mg per mL) (BP 2001) is available as a ready-to-use solution or may be prepared from Methadone Hydrochloride Oral Concentrate. However, most commercially available preparations in the UK still follow the DTF formula.

Some commercially available forms of DTF Methadone Mixture 1 mg per mL employ a preservative system based on hydroxybenzoate esters rather than chloroform; however, syrup preserved with hydroxybenzoate esters may be unsuitable for extemporaneous dispensing (see under Incompatibility, above).

References.

1. Ghodse AH, *et al.* Comparison of oral preparations of heroin and methadone to stabilise opiate misusers as inpatients. *BMJ* 1990; **300**: 719–20.
2. Wolff K, *et al.* Measuring compliance in methadone maintenance patients: use of a pharmacologic indicator to "estimate" methadone plasma levels. *Clin Pharmacol Ther* 1991; **50**: 199–207.
3. Wilson P, *et al.* Methadone maintenance in general practice: patients, workload, and outcomes. *BMJ* 1994; **309**: 641–4.

4. Farrell M, *et al.* Methadone maintenance treatment in opiate dependence: a review. *BMJ* 1994; **309:** 997–1001.
5. Henry JA. Methadone: where are we now? *Hosp Med* 1999; **60:** 161–4.

Preparations

BP 2001: Methadone Injection; Methadone Linctus; Methadone Oral Solution (1 mg per mL); Methadone Tablets;
USP 25: Methadone Hydrochloride Injection; Methadone Hydrochloride Oral Concentrate; Methadone Hydrochloride Oral Solution; Methadone Hydrochloride Tablets.

Proprietary Preparations (details are given in Part 3)
Aust.: Heptadon; *Austral.:* Biodone Forte; Physeptone; *Fin.:* Dolmed; *Ger.:* Methaddict; *Hong Kong:* Physeptone; *Irl.:* Phymet DTF; Physeptone; Pinadone DTF; *Israel:* Adolan; *Ital.:* Eptadone; *Neth.:* Symoron; *NZ:* Biodone; Pallidone; *S.Afr.:* Physeptone; *Singapore:* Physeptone; *Spain:* Metasedin; Sedo†; *Switz.:* Ketalgine; *UK:* Martindale Methadone Mixture DTF; Methadose; Methex; Physeptone; Synastone; *USA:* Dolophine; Methadose.

Methyl Butetisalicylate (12947-v)

Methyl Diethylacetylsalicylate. Methyl *O*-(2-ethylbutyryl)salicylate.
$C_{14}H_{18}O_4 = 250.3$.

Profile
Methyl butetisalicylate is a salicylic acid derivative that has been used similarly to methyl salicylate (p.55) as a 30% rubefacient cream for the relief of musculoskeletal, joint, and soft-tissue pain.

Preparations
Proprietary Preparations (details are given in Part 3)
Fr.: Dolöderm; *Ital.:* Dolöderm.

Methyl Gentisate (14229-j)

2,5-Dihydroxybenzoic acid methyl ester.
$C_8H_8O_4 = 168.1$.
CAS — 2150-46-1.

Profile
Methyl gentisate has been used topically for the relief of musculoskeletal and joint pain.

Preparations
Proprietary Preparations (details are given in Part 3)
Multi-ingredient: *Ital.:* Reumacort.

Methyl Nicotinate (9253-z)

Methyl Nicotinate (*USAN*).
Methyl pyridine-3-carboxylate.
$C_7H_7NO_2 = 137.1$.
CAS — 93-60-7.
Pharmacopoeias. In *Br.*

Pharmacopoeial description
BP 2001: White or almost white crystals or crystalline powder with a characteristic odour; m.p. 40° to 42°. Very soluble in water, in alcohol, and in chloroform; freely soluble in ether.

Profile
Methyl nicotinate is used in topical preparations as a rubefacient.

Preparations
Proprietary Preparations (details are given in Part 3)
Austral.: Vas†; *UK:* Pickles Chilblain Cream.
Multi-ingredient: *Aust.:* Berggeist; Forapin†; *Austral.:* Deep Heat; *Belg.:* Algipan; Decontractyl†; Percutalgine; *Braz.:* Ateroide; Infrarub; *Canad.:* Arthricare Odor Free; Arthricare Triple Medicated; Decontractyl†; Midalgan; *Fr.:* Algipan; Capsic; Decontractyl; Percutalgine; Sedartyl; *Ger.:* Contrheuma-Gel forte N†; Doloneuro; Forapin E; Kytta-Balsam f; Menthoneurin-Vollbad N†; Midysalb†; Pernionin; Pernionin Voll-Bad N; Rheumasan N; Spondylon; Thermo-Menthoneurin Bad†; *Irl.:* Algipan; *Israel:* Deep Heat Spray; *Ital.:* Aspercreme†; Balsamo Sifcamina; Relaxar; Sedalpan; *Port.:* Midalgan; *S.Afr.:* Sportsman Rub; *Singapore:* Deep Heating Spray; *Spain:* Balsamo Midalgan; Doctofril Antiinflamat; Doctomitil; Percutalin†; Radio Salil; *Switz.:* Kytta Baume†; Midalgan; Radalgin; Roliwol†; *Thai.:* Percutalgine; *UK:* Algipan; Cremalgin; Deep Heat Spray; Dubam; Fiery Jack; Ralgex; Ralgex Heat Spray (low-odour); Ralgex†; Red Oil; Transvasin Heat Spray; *USA:* Arthricare Odor Free; Arthricare Triple Medicated; Musterole.

Methyl Salicylate (2667-b)

Methyl Sal.; Methylis Salicylas. Methyl 2-hydroxybenzoate.
$C_8H_8O_3 = 152.1$.
CAS — 119-36-8.
Pharmacopoeias. In *Eur.* (see p.vi), *Jpn*, and *Pol.* Also in *USNF*, which allows in addition to synthetic methyl salicylate, that obtained from the leaves of *Gaultheria procumbens* (Ericaceae) and the bark of *Betula lenta* (Betulaceae). The source of the methyl salicylate must be indicated on the label.

Certain plastic containers, such as those made from polystyrene, are unsuitable for liniments or ointments containing methyl salicylate.

NOTE. The BP 2001 directs that methyl salicylate be dispensed or supplied when Oil of Wintergreen, Wintergreen, or Wintergreen Oil is prescribed or demanded, unless it is ascertained that Methyl Salicylate Liniment (BP 2001) is required. Wintergreen Oil has also been known as Sweet Birch Oil.

Pharmacopoeial description
Ph. Eur.: A colourless or slightly yellow liquid. Very slightly soluble in water; miscible with alcohol, and with fatty and essential oils. Protect from light.
USNF 20: Methyl salicylate is produced synthetically or is obtained from the leaves of *Gaultheria procumbens* (Ericaceae) or from the bark of *Betula lenta* (Betulaceae).
A colourless, yellowish, or reddish liquid having the characteristic odour of wintergreen. Slightly soluble in water; soluble in alcohol and in glacial acetic acid. Store in airtight containers.

Adverse Effects, Treatment, and Precautions
Salicylate intoxication can occur following ingestion or topical application of methyl salicylate (see Adverse Effects of Aspirin, p.14).

◊ Ingestion of methyl salicylate poses the threat of severe, rapid-onset salicylate poisoning because of its liquid concentrated form and lipid solubility.[1] It is readily absorbed from the gastrointestinal tract and most is rapidly hydrolysed to free salicylate. The symptoms, which may appear within 2 hours of ingestion, are similar to those of salicylate poisoning in general (see Adverse Effects of Aspirin, p.14), although methyl salicylate is expected to be more toxic because of its lipid solubility. There have been reports of fatalities following ingestion of as little as 4 mL in a child and 6 mL in an adult, although the adult lethal dose is estimated to be 30 mL.[1] Topical Chinese herbal medicinal oils may contain methyl salicylate in variable amounts, and salicylate poisoning has been reported in a woman who had attempted suicide by taking such a preparation, Red Flower Oil.[2] The authors also noted that some patients took small amounts of this preparation orally in an attempt to enhance its analgesic effects.

Like other salicylates, methyl salicylate may be absorbed through intact skin.[1] Percutaneous absorption is enhanced by exercise, heat, occlusion, or disruption of the integrity of the skin. The amount absorbed will also be increased by application to large areas of skin. Results from a study in healthy subjects demonstrated that a considerable amount of salicylic acid may be absorbed through the skin after topical application of products containing methyl salicylate.[3] Both the rate and extent of absorption increased after repeated application; the bioavailability of the ointment preparation used in the study increased from 15% after the second dose to 22% after the third to eighth dose. The authors recommend that topical analgesic preparations containing methyl salicylate or other salicylates should be used with caution in patients at increased risk of developing salicylate adverse effects (see Precautions of Aspirin, p.15). Results from another study[4] demonstrating high tissue to plasma ratios following topical application of a methyl salicylate formulation suggest that direct penetration and not recirculation in the blood is responsible for the salicylate concentrations found. The results also demonstrated that methyl salicylate is extensively metabolised to salicylic acid in the dermal and subcutaneous tissues following topical administration.

1. Chan TYK. Potential dangers from topical preparations containing methyl salicylate. *Hum Exp Toxicol* 1996; **15:** 747–50.
2. Chan TH, *et al.* Severe salicylate poisoning associated with the intake of Chinese medicinal oil ('Red Flower Oil'). *Aust N Z J Med* 1995; **25:** 57.
3. Morra P, *et al.* Serum concentrations of salicylic acid following topical applied salicylate derivatives. *Ann Pharmacother* 1996; **30:** 935–40.
4. Cross SE, *et al.* Is there tissue penetration after application of topical salicylate formulations? *Lancet* 1997; **350:** 636.

Interactions
Absorption of methyl salicylate through the skin can occur following excessive topical application (see above), and interactions would be expected to be as for other salicylates (see Interactions of Aspirin, p.16).

Anticoagulants. Potentiation of warfarin anticoagulation has been reported[1,2] following topical application of methyl salicylate preparations.

1. Littleton F. Warfarin and topical salicylates. *JAMA* 1990; **263:** 2888.
2. Tam LS, *et al.* Warfarin interactions with Chinese traditional medicines: danshen and methyl salicylate medicated oil. *Aust N Z J Med* 1995; **25:** 258.

Uses and Administration
Methyl salicylate is a salicylic acid derivative that is irritant to the skin and is used topically in rubefacient preparations for the relief of pain in musculoskeletal, joint, and soft-tissue disorders. It is also used for minor peripheral vascular disorders such as chilblains and as an ingredient in inhalations for the symptomatic relief of upper respiratory-tract disorders.

Preparations
BP 2001: Kaolin Poultice; Methyl Salicylate Liniment; Methyl Salicylate Ointment; Surgical Spirit.
Proprietary Preparations (details are given in Part 3)
Austral.: Linsal; Metsal Liniment; *Ger.:* Rheumax†; *Mex.:* Tolan; *Port.:* Balsamo Analgesico Labesfal; *S.Afr.:* Thermo-Rub; *Thai.:* Mygesal; *USA:* Argesic; Exocaine; Gordogesic.
Multi-ingredient: *Aust.:* Aciforin; Carl Baders Divinal; DDD; Derivon; Embrocation; Erkaltungsbalsam; Leukona-Rheuma-Bad; Mayfit akut†; Mayfit chronisch†; Medizinalbad; Neo-Phlogicid; Onycho Phytex; Pasta rubra salicylata; Phytex; Red Point; Tineafax†; Trauma-kuhlend; Trauma-warmend; Traumasalbe; *Austral.:* Alcusal Sport†; Analgesic Rub†; APR Cream; Arthrirub; Austral-Balm; Biosal; Bosisto's Eucalyptus Rub; Deep Heat; Dencorub; Dencorub Extra Strength; Goanna Heat Cream; Goanna Liniment; Goanna Salve; Liniment Balm; Methyl Salicylate Compound Liniment; Metsal; Metsal AR Heat Rub; Metsal Heat Rub; PC Arthri-Spray†; Radian-B; Vicks Inhaler; *Belg.:* Baume Dalet†; Dencorub; Dencorub Extra Strength; Goanna Heat Cream; Goanna Liniment; Goanna Salve; Liniment Balm; Methyl Salicylate Compound Liniment; *Braz.:* Aliviador; Analgen; Antiphlogistine; Axol; Benegel; Calminex S; Capiloton; Cardec; Friccex; Frixodon; Frixopel; Gelflex; Gelofrix; Gelogel; Gelol; Gelonevral; Inalador Vick; Lenidor; Massageol; Massubal; Mialgex; Oleo Eletrico; Pomalgex; Prontoalivio; Rubi-Dex; Salimetin; Sanador; Traumac; Traumagel; Untigex; *Canad.:* Absorbine Analgesic; Alsirub; Analgesic Balm; Antiphlogistine Rub A-535; Arthricare Triple Medicated; Artritol; Baume Analgesique; Baume Analgesique Medicamente; Ben-Gay Original, Ben-Gay Extra Strength; Ben-Gay Ultra; Buckley's White Rub; Buckleys Pain Relief; Cal Mo Dol; Calmomusc; Carboseptol; Carmatis†; Corn Salve†; Deep Heating; Extra Strength Analgesic; Flex-All; Heat Rub; Heet; Inarub†; Infraline†; Instant Rub; Kiro Rub; Kwan Loong Oil; Medicated Analgesic Cream; Nasal Jelly; Obus Form Therapeutic Heat; Pain Buster; Penetrating Heat†; Physio-Rub; Pommade au Thé des Bois; Rheumalan; Rhumatisme; SJ Liniment; Therapeutic Soothing Ice; Thermo Rub; Thuna Salve for Rheumatic Pains; Tiger Liniment; *Fr.:* Baume Aroma; Baume Bengue; Capsic; Disalgyl; Eutalgic; Inongan; Kamol; Lao-Dal†; *Ger.:* Brachialin percutan N†; Camphopin†; Cuxaflex N†; Dalet Med Balsam; DDD†; Dolorsan-Balsam; Finalgon N Schmerzpflaster†; Heilit; Heilit Rheuma-Olbad; Hewedolor; Hoemarin Rheuma†; Hoevenol†; Kneipp Rheuma-Bad; Leukona-Rheuma-Bad N; Li-iL Rheuma-Bad; Marament Balsam W†; Olbas; Pernionin; Pernionin N; Psoriasis-Salbe M†; Reumaless†; Rheubalmin Bad; Rheuma-Pasc N†; Rosarthron forte; Schupps Heilkrauter Rheumabad; Trauma-Salbe Rodler 301 N; Vipratox; *Hong Kong:* Counterpain; Metsal; Saliment; *Irl.:* Bengue's Balsam; Germolene; Listerine†; Monphytol†; Phytex; Radian-B; *Israel:* Antiseptic Foot Balm; Ben-Gay; Ben-Gay Ultra; Deep Heat Rub; Deep Heat Spray; Gargol; Mentholatum Balm; Mentholatum Nasal Inhaler; Mento-O-Cap; Radian-B; Rublex D; Rublex Massage Cream; Vicks Inhaler; *Ital.:* Balsamo Italstadium; Salonpas; Soluzione Composta Alcoolica Saponosa di Coaltar†; Vegetallumina; Vicks Inalante; *Mex.:* Lonol Sport; Power Rub; *NZ:* DP Warm Up; Metsal; Vicks Inhaler; *Port.:* Analgil; Balsamo Analgesico; Balsamo Analgesico Sanitas; Dologel; Freimax; Hipodor; Lauromentol; Linimento de Sloan; Listerine; *S.Afr.:* Chisi†; Counterpain; Docrub; Radian; Sportsman Rub; Warm-Up†; *Singapore:* Begesic; Ben-Gay; Deep Heating Rub; Deep Heating Spray; Flanil; Icy Hot; Metsal; *Spain:* Arnicon; Artrodesmol Extra; Balsamo Midalgan; Buco Regis; Carbocaina; Dologex; Dolokey; Embrocacion Gras; Halogedol; Inhalador†; Liderflex; Linimento Naion; Linimento Sloan; Masagil; Mentobox; Mitiderma; Nixyn; Odontocromil c Sulfamida; Piorlis; Pomada Balsamica†; Pomada Revulsiva†; Radio Salil; Reflex; Regal†; Termosan; *Swed.:* Sloan's liniment†; *Switz.:* Antiphlogistine; Baby Liberol†; Baume Esco; Baume Esco Forte; Embropax; Emplatre Croix D; Fortalis; Huile analgesique "Polar-Bar"; Incutin; Kernosan Huile de Massage†; Liberol†; Marament-N; Massorax; Neo-Decongestine; Olbas; Pasta boli; Pirom; Roliwol†; Sedasept; Sloan Baume†; Sloan Liniment†; Vicks Inhaler N; *Thai.:* Ammeltz; Begesic; Buta Pee Dee; Cibis; Counterpain; Dexalin; Flanil; Heat Cream; Masa Balm; Masaga; Muscalax; Neotica; Olympic Balm; Painza; Reduxpain; St Luke's Oil; St Luke's Sports Oil; Stopain; *UK:* Aezodent; Antiseptic Foot Balm; Aspellin; Balmosa; Bengue's Balsam†; Boots Medicated Pain Relief Plaster; Chymol; DDD; Deep Heat Massage; Deep Heat Maximum Strength; Deep Heat Rub; Deep Heat Spray; Dermacreme; Dubam; Eftab†; Germolene; Gonne Balm; Kleer Cream; Listerine Antiseptic Mouthwash; Massage Balm Arnica; Medicated Extract of Rosemary; Mentholatum Nasal Inhaler; Mentholatum Rub; Modern Herbals Muscular Pain; Monphytol; Nasal Inhaler; Nasciodine; Nine Rubbing Oils; Olbas; Phytex; PR Heat Spray; Psorin; Radian-B; Ralgex; Salonair; Salonpas; TCP; Tea Tree & Witch Hazel Cream; Vadarex; Vapour Rub; *USA:* Analgesic Balm; Arthricare Triple Medicated; Arthritis Hot Creme; Astring-O-Sol†; Banalg; Ben-Gay; Ben-Gay Ultra; Betuline; Cool-Mint Listerine; Deep Heating Lotion†; Deep Heating Rub†; Deep-Down Rub; Dermal-Rub†; Dermolin; Flex-all 454; FreshBurst Listerine; Gordobalm; Heet; Icy Hot; Improved Analgesic; Infrarub; Iodex with Methyl Salicylate; Ivy-Chex; Listerine; Massengill; Maximum Strength Flex-all 454; Methagual; Methalgen; Minit-Rub; Muscle Rub†; Musterole; Musterole Extra; Pain Bust-R II; Pain Doctor; Panalgesic Gold; Paralgesic†; Pharmacists Creme; Pharmacists Lotion; Phylorinol; Soltice; Thera-gesic; Ziks.

Mofebutazone (2670-f)

Mofebutazone (*rINN*).
Monobutazone; Monophenylbutazone. 4-Butyl-1-phenylpyrazolidine-3,5-dione.
$C_{13}H_{16}N_2O_2 = 232.3$.
CAS — 2210-63-1.
ATC — M01AA02; M02AA02.

Profile
Mofebutazone, a derivative of phenylbutazone (p.78), is an NSAID (p.63). It has been used in the management of musculoskeletal and joint disorders. Mofebutazone has been given by mouth, by rectal suppository, and by intramuscular injection of the sodium salt.

Preparations
Proprietary Preparations (details are given in Part 3)
Ger.: Diadin M; Mofesal; Mofesal N.
Multi-ingredient: *Aust.:* Clinit†; *Ger.:* Vasotonin forte†.

The symbol † denotes a preparation no longer actively marketed

Mofezolac (5515-I)

Mofezolac (rINN).

3,4-Bis(p-methoxyphenyl)-5-isoxazoleacetic acid.
$C_{19}H_{17}NO_5 = 339.3$.
CAS — 78967-07-4.

Profile
Mofezolac is an NSAID (p.63).

Morniflumate (3845-j)

Morniflumate (USAN, rINN).

UP-164.   2-Morpholinoethyl   2-(α,α,α-trifluoro-m-toluidi-no)nicotinate.
$C_{19}H_{20}F_3N_3O_3 = 395.4$.
CAS — 65847-85-0.
ATC — M01AX22.

Profile
Morniflumate, the morpholinoethyl ester of niflumic acid (p.62), is an NSAID (p.63). It has been used in inflammatory conditions in doses of 700 mg given twice daily by mouth or rectally as suppositories.

Preparations
Proprietary Preparations (details are given in Part 3)
Fr.: Nifluril; **Ital.:** Flomax; Morniflu; Niflam; **Spain:** Niflactol; **Switz.:** Nifluril.

Morphine (6239-c)

Morphine (BAN).

7,8-Didehydro-4,5-epoxy-17-methylmorphinan-3,6-diol.
$C_{17}H_{19}NO_3 = 285.3$.
CAS — 57-27-2 (anhydrous morphine); 6009-81-0 (morphine monohydrate).
ATC — N02AA01.

Morphine is the chief alkaloid of opium (p.69). It is now commonly obtained from whole opium poppies (Papaver somniferum) which are harvested as poppy straw; a concentrate of poppy straw is known as CPS.

Morphine Hydrochloride (6241-w)

Morphine Hydrochloride (BANM).

Morphini Hydrochloridum; Morphinii Chloridum; Morphinum Chloratum.
$C_{17}H_{19}NO_3,HCl,3H_2O = 375.8$.
CAS — 52-26-6 (anhydrous morphine hydrochloride); 6055-06-7 (morphine hydrochloride trihydrate).
Pharmacopoeias. In Chin., Eur. (see p.vi), Int., Jpn, and Pol.

Pharmacopoeial description
Ph. Eur.: Colourless, silky needles, cubical masses or a white or almost white, crystalline powder. It is efflorescent in a dry atmosphere. Soluble in water and in glycerol; slightly soluble in alcohol. Protect from light.

Incompatibility. See under Morphine Sulfate, below.

Morphine Sulfate (6242-e)

Morphine Sulphate (BANM); Morphini Sulfas.
$(C_{17}H_{19}NO_3)_2,H_2SO_4,5H_2O = 758.8$.
CAS — 64-31-3 (anhydrous morphine sulfate); 6211-15-0 (morphine sulfate pentahydrate).
Pharmacopoeias. In Eur. (see p.vi), Int., and US.

Pharmacopoeial description
Ph. Eur.: A white or almost white, crystalline powder. Soluble in water; very slightly soluble in alcohol; practically insoluble in toluene. Protect from light.

USP 25: White, feathery, silky crystals, cubical masses of crystals, or a white crystalline powder. Is odourless and when exposed to air it gradually loses water of hydration. It darkens on prolonged exposure to light. Soluble 1 in 16 of water and 1 in 1 of water at 80°; soluble 1 in 570 of alcohol and 1 in 240 of alcohol at 60°; insoluble in chloroform and in ether. Store in airtight containers. Protect from light.

Incompatibility. Morphine salts are sensitive to changes in pH and morphine is liable to be precipitated out of solution in an alkaline environment. Compounds incompatible with morphine salts include aminophylline and sodium salts of barbiturates and phenytoin. Other incompatibilities, sometimes attributed to particular formulations, have included:

- aciclovir sodium—precipitate noted two hours after admixture with morphine sulfate solution;[1]
- chlorpromazine hydrochloride injection—precipitation was considered to be due to chlorocresol present in the morphine sulfate injection;[2]
- doxorubicin—addition of morphine sulfate 1 mg per mL to doxorubicin hydrochloride liposomal injection 0.4 mg per mL in dextrose 5% resulted in turbidity changes;[3]
- fluorouracil—immediate precipitate formed after admixture of fluorouracil 1 or 16 mg per mL with morphine sulfate 1 mg per mL in dextrose 5% or sodium chloride 0.9%;[4]

- frusemide [furosemide]—precipitate noted one hour after admixture with morphine sulfate solution;[1]
- heparin sodium—incompatibility has been reported from straightforward additive studies.[5] A more recent study[6] indicated that morphine sulfate and heparin sodium were only incompatible at morphine sulfate concentrations greater than 5 mg per mL and that this incompatibility could be prevented by using 0.9% sodium chloride solution as the admixture diluent rather than water;
- pethidine hydrochloride—incompatibility has been noted following admixture with morphine sulfate;[5,7]
- prochlorperazine edisilate—immediate precipitation was attributed to phenol in the morphine sulfate injection formulation;[8,9]
- promethazine hydrochloride—cloudiness was reported to develop when 12.5 mg of promethazine hydrochloride was drawn into a syringe containing morphine sulfate 8 mg.[10] Others[7] have noted no incompatibility;
- tetracyclines—colour change from pale yellow to light green occurred when solutions of minocycline hydrochloride or tetracycline hydrochloride were mixed with morphine sulfate in 5% glucose injection.[11]

1. Pugh CB, et al. Visual compatibility of morphine sulphate and meperidine hydrochloride with other injected drugs during simulated Y-site injection. Am J Hosp Pharm 1991; 48: 123–5.
2. Crapper JB. Mixing chlorpromazine and morphine. BMJ 1975; i: 33.
3. Trissel LA, et al. Compatibility of doxorubicin hydrochloride liposome injection with selected other drugs during simulated Y-site administration. Am J Health-Syst Pharm 1997; 54: 2708–13.
4. Xu QA, et al. Stability and compatibility of fluorouracil with morphine sulfate and hydromorphone hydrochloride. Ann Pharmacother 1996; 30: 756–61.
5. Patel JA, Phillips GL. A guide to physical compatibility of intravenous drug admixtures. Am J Hosp Pharm 1966; 23: 409–11.
6. Baker DE, et al. Compatibility of heparin sodium and morphine sulfate. Am J Hosp Pharm 1985; 42: 1352–5.
7. Parker WA. Physical compatibilities of preanesthetic medications. Can J Hosp Pharm 1976; 29: 91–2.
8. Stevenson JG, Patriarca C. Incompatibility of morphine sulfate and prochlorperazine edisylate in syringes. Am J Hosp Pharm 1985; 42: 2651.
9. Zuber DEL. Compatibility of morphine sulfate injection and prochlorperazine edisylate injection. Am J Hosp Pharm 1987; 44: 67.
10. Fleischer NM. Promethazine hydrochloride—morphine sulfate incompatibility. Am J Hosp Pharm 1973; 30: 665.
11. Nieves-Cordero AL, et al. Compatibility of narcotic analgesic solutions with various antibiotics during simulated Y-site injection. Am J Hosp Pharm 1985; 42: 1108–9.

Stability. Solutions of morphine sulfate for intravenous infusion appear to be relatively stable. In one study[1] 0.04 mg per mL and 0.4 mg per mL solutions retained more than 90% of their initial concentration of morphine sulfate when stored at 4° or 23° for 7 days, whether or not they were protected from light. Solutions prepared from commercially available injection or from powder, in 0.9% sodium chloride or 5% glucose, and stored in polyvinyl chloride bags or glass bottles did not differ in stability from one another. In a further study[2] 10 mg per mL or 5 mg per mL solutions of morphine sulfate in glucose or sodium chloride and stored in portable infusion pump cassettes retained more than 95% of their initial concentration when kept at 23° for 30 days. A 0.9% solution of sodium chloride containing morphine sulfate 2 mg per mL was stable for 6 weeks when stored in polypropylene syringes at ambient temperatures in the light or dark but a similar solution which also contained 0.1% sodium metabisulfite lost 15% of its potency during the same period.[3] Stability of such a solution with or without sodium metabisulfite was considered to be unacceptable when stored in glass syringes in the dark.[4]

1. Vecchio M, et al. The stability of morphine intravenous infusion solutions. Can J Hosp Pharm 1988; 41: 5–9, 43.
2. Walker SE, et al. Hydromorphone and morphine stability in portable infusion pump cassettes and minibags. Can J Hosp Pharm 1988; 41: 177–82.
3. Grassby PF. The stability of morphine sulphate in 0.9 per cent sodium chloride stored in plastic syringes. Pharm J 1991; 248: HS24–HS25.
4. Grassby PF, Hutchings L. Factors affecting the physical and chemical stability of morphine sulphate solutions stored in syringes. Int J Pharm Pract 1993; 2: 39–43.

◊ References to the stability of morphine in Kaolin and Morphine Mixture (BP).

1. Helliwell K, Game P. Stability of morphine in kaolin and morphine mixture BP. Pharm J 1981; 227: 128–9.
2. Helliwell K, Jennings P. Kaolin and morphine mixture BP: effects of containers on the stability of morphine. Pharm J 1984; 232: 682.

Morphine Tartrate (6243-I)

Morphine Tartrate (BANM).
$(C_{17}H_{19}NO_3)_2,C_4H_6O_6,3H_2O = 774.8$.
CAS — 302-31-8 (anhydrous morphine tartrate); 6032-59-3 (morphine tartrate trihydrate).

Incompatibility. See under Morphine Sulfate, above.

Dependence and Withdrawal
As for Opioid Analgesics, p.66.

Dependence associated with morphine and closely related μ-agonists appears to result in more severe with-

drawal symptoms than that associated with κ-receptor agonists. With morphine, withdrawal symptoms usually begin within a few hours, reach a peak within 36 to 72 hours, and then gradually subside.

Adverse Effects and Treatment
As for Opioid Analgesics in general, p.67.

Effects on the cardiovascular system. For a reference to the effects of morphine on histamine release compared with some other opioids, see under Pethidine, p.75.

Effects on the muscles. There has been a report of severe rectovaginal spasms in a patient following intrathecal administration of morphine.[1] The spasms were successfully controlled with midazolam.

1. Littrell RA, et al. Muscle spasms associated with intrathecal morphine therapy: treatment with midazolam. Clin Pharm 1992; 11: 57–9.

Effects on the nervous system. Myoclonus has been reported in patients with advanced malignant disease receiving high doses of morphine.[1] It was unrelated to plasma-morphine concentrations and was attributed in part to the concurrent use of other drugs including antidepressants, antipsychotics, and NSAIDs. The diagnosis of myoclonus and the role of morphine in this case has been questioned;[2] others[3] also criticised the importance attached to myoclonus and considered it probably the least common and least important of all the side-effects of morphine.

Myoclonus was also reported[4] in 2 cancer patients with renal impairment on high stable doses of morphine; the metabolite normorphine, found in the plasma of both patients, might have been responsible.

It has been reported that myoclonus induced by morphine may be successfully controlled using a benzodiazepine such as midazolam.[5]

1. Potter JM, et al. Myoclonus associated with treatment with high doses of morphine: the role of supplemental drugs. BMJ 1989; 299: 150–3.
2. Quinn N. Myoclonus associated with high doses of morphine. BMJ 1989; 299: 683–4.
3. McQuay HJ, et al. Myoclonus associated with high doses of morphine. BMJ 1989; 299: 684.
4. Glare PA, et al. Normorphine, a neurotoxic metabolite? Lancet 1990; 335: 725–6.
5. Holdsworth MT, et al. Continuous midazolam infusion for the management of morphine-induced myoclonus. Ann Pharmacother 1995; 29: 25–9.

Precautions
As for Opioid Analgesics in general, p.68.

Biliary-tract disorders. See under Precautions of Opioid Analgesics, p.68.

Hepatic impairment. In view of its hepatic metabolism, caution is generally advised when giving morphine to patients with impaired liver function (but see under Pharmacokinetics, below). Some advise that administration should be avoided or the dose reduced because of the risk of precipitating a coma. Twycross and Lack[1] considered that moderate hepatic insufficiency does not affect morphine metabolism whereas severe hepatic impairment may.

The mean elimination half-life of morphine in 12 patients with cirrhosis was almost twice that in 10 healthy subjects after administration of a modified-release oral morphine preparation (MST-Continus) and peak serum concentrations were almost three times as high.[2] Patients with cirrhosis exhibited a greater degree of sedation but none developed encephalopathy. It was recommended that the dose for modified-release preparations should be reduced and the frequency of administration prolonged for patients with cirrhosis.

1. Twycross RG, Lack SA. Oral morphine in advanced cancer. 2nd ed. Beaconsfield: Beaconsfield Publishers, 1989.
2. Kotb HIM, et al. Pharmacokinetics of controlled release morphine (MST) in patients with liver cirrhosis. Br J Anaesth 1997; 79: 804–6.

Phaeochromocytoma. Morphine and some other opioids can induce the release of endogenous histamine and thereby stimulate catecholamine release making them unsuitable for use in patients with phaeochromocytoma. For further details, see p.68.

Renal impairment. Severe and prolonged respiratory depression has occurred in patients with renal impairment given morphine. Toxicity in 3 such patients was attributed to the accumulation of the active metabolite morphine-6-glucuronide. Plasma concentrations of this metabolite were found[2] to be ten times higher than normal in a 7-year-old girl with haemolytic uraemic syndrome given morphine intravenously although the half-life of morphine was also prolonged. Plasma concentrations of morphine-6-glucuronide were also reported[3] to be persistently increased 19 days after stopping morphine by intravenous infusion in a 17-year-old girl with normal renal function. The authors of the report suggested that alterations in bowel flora following antibiotic therapy or inhibition of morphine-3-glucuronidation by lorazepam might be responsible. It has also been reported[4] that accumulation of morphine can occur in renal failure, although to a lesser extent than accumulation of metabolites (see also under Pharmacokinetics, below).

1. Osborne RJ, *et al.* Morphine intoxication in renal failure: the role of morphine-6-glucuronide. *BMJ* 1986; **292:** 1548–9.
2. Hasselström J, *et al.* Long lasting respiratory depression induced by morphine-6-glucuronide? *Br J Clin Pharmacol* 1989; **27:** 515–18.
3. Calleja MA, *et al.* Persistently increased morphine-6-glucuronide concentrations. *Br J Anaesth* 1990; **64:** 649.
4. Osborne R, *et al.* The pharmacokinetics of morphine and morphine glucuronides in kidney failure. *Clin Pharmacol Ther* 1993; **54:** 158–67.

Interactions

For interactions associated with opioid analgesics, see p.68.

◊ For references to myoclonus associated with morphine and the concurrent use of other drugs, see Effects on the Nervous System under Adverse Effects, above.

Antibacterials. There is some evidence[1] that the potent enzyme inducer *rifampicin* can reduce the serum concentration of morphine and decrease its analgesic effect; induction of the enzymes responsible for conversion of morphine to the active glucuronide metabolite did not seem to occur.

1. Fromm MF, *et al.* Loss of analgesic effect of morphine due to coadministration of rifampin. *Pain* 1997; **72:** 261–7.

Benzodiazepines. An additive sedative effect is to be expected between opioid analgesics and benzodiazepines and has been reported with morphine and *midazolam*.[1]

For reference to a suggestion that *lorazepam* may inhibit morphine-3-glucuronide glucuronidation, see Renal Impairment under Precautions, above.

1. Tverskoy M, *et al.* Midazolam-morphine sedative interaction in patients. *Anesth Analg* 1989; **68:** 282–5.

Cisapride. Plasma concentrations of morphine have been increased following concomitant oral use of cisapride.[1]

1. Rowbotham DJ, *et al.* Effect of cisapride on morphine absorption after oral administration of sustained-release morphine. *Br J Anaesth* 1991; **67:** 421–5.

Histamine H$_2$-antagonists. See under Opioid Analgesics, p.68.

Local anaesthetics. Prior use of epidural *chloroprocaine* has been reported[1] to reduce the duration of epidural morphine analgesia.

1. Eisenach JC, *et al.* Effect of prior anesthetic solution on epidural morphine analgesia. *Anesth Analg* 1991; **73:** 119–23.

Metoclopramide. Reports on the effects of metoclopramide on morphine have included an increased rate of onset and degree of sedation when metoclopramide was given by mouth with modified-release morphine[1] and antagonism of the effects of morphine on gastric emptying by intravenous metoclopramide.[2]

1. Manara AR, *et al.* The effect of metoclopramide on the absorption of oral controlled release morphine. *Br J Clin Pharmacol* 1988; **25:** 518–21.
2. McNeill MJ, *et al.* Effect of iv metoclopramide on gastric emptying after opioid premedication. *Br J Anaesth* 1990; **64:** 450–2.

Tricyclic antidepressants. Both *clomipramine* and *amitriptyline* significantly increased the plasma availability of morphine when given to cancer patients taking oral morphine solution.[1] It was noted however that the potentiation of the analgesic effects of morphine by these drugs might not be confined to increased bioavailability of morphine; the dose of tricyclic to use with morphine in the treatment of cancer pain should be decided by clinical evaluation rather than by pharmacokinetic data.

1. Ventafridda V, *et al.* Antidepressants increase bioavailability of morphine in cancer patients. *Lancet* 1987; **i:** 1204.

Pharmacokinetics

Morphine salts are well absorbed from the gastrointestinal tract but have poor oral bioavailability since they undergo extensive first-pass metabolism in the liver and gut. After subcutaneous or intramuscular injection morphine is readily absorbed into the blood. The majority of a dose of morphine is conjugated with glucuronic acid in the liver and gut to produce morphine-3-glucuronide and morphine-6-glucuronide. The latter is considered to contribute to the analgesic effect of morphine, especially when repeated doses are given by mouth. Morphine-3-glucuronide on the other hand may antagonise the analgesic action of morphine and morphine-6-glucuronide and it has been suggested that it might be responsible for the paradoxical pain observed in some patients given morphine. Other active metabolites include normorphine, codeine, and morphine ethereal sulfate. Enterohepatic circulation probably occurs. Morphine is distributed throughout the body but mainly in the kidneys, liver, lungs, and spleen, with lower concentrations in the brain and muscles. Morphine crosses the blood-brain barrier less readily than more lipid-soluble opioids such as diamorphine, but it has been detected in the CSF as have its highly polar metabolites morphine-3-glucuronide and morphine-6-glucuronide. Morphine diffuses across the placenta and traces also appear in breast milk and sweat. About 35% is protein bound. Mean plasma elimination half-lives of 1.7 hours for morphine and 2.4 to 6.7 hours for morphine-3-glucuronide have been reported.

Up to 10% of a dose of morphine may eventually be excreted, as conjugates, through the bile into the faeces. The remainder is excreted in the urine, mainly as conjugates. About 90% of total morphine is excreted in 24 hours with traces in urine for 48 hours or more.

◊ Much has been published on the metabolism and disposition of morphine and its relevance to the clinical use of morphine, in particular the analgesic effect of repeated oral doses and the relative potency of oral to parenteral doses. There has been uncertainty as to the contributions in man of first-pass metabolism in the liver and gut,[1-4] the possible role of renal metabolism,[2,3,5,6] the analgesic activity and clinical importance of the metabolite morphine-6-glucuronide,[2,7-18] and enterohepatic circulation.[2,9] There has also been interest in the effects of the metabolite morphine-3-glucuronide.[19-21]

1. Hanks GW, Aherne GW. Morphine metabolism: does the renal hypothesis hold water? *Lancet* 1985; **i:** 221–2.
2. Hanks GW, *et al.* Explanation for potency of repeated oral doses of morphine? *Lancet* 1987; **ii:** 723–5.
3. Bodenham A, *et al.* Extrahepatic morphine metabolism in man during the anhepatic phase of orthotopic liver transplantation. *Br J Anaesth* 1989; **63:** 380–4.
4. Moore RA, *et al.* Opiate metabolism and excretion. *Baillieres Clin Anaesthesiol* 1987; **1:** 829–58.
5. McQuay H, Moore A. Metabolism of narcotics. *BMJ* 1984; **288:** 237.
6. Moore A, *et al.* Morphine kinetics during and after renal transplantation. *Clin Pharmacol Ther* 1984; **35:** 641–5.
7. McQuay HJ, *et al.* Potency of oral morphine. *Lancet* 1987; **ii:** 1458–9.
8. Hanks GW, *et al.* Enterohepatic circulation of morphine. *Lancet* 1988; **i:** 469.
9. Osborne R, *et al.* Analgesic activity of morphine-6-glucuronide. *Lancet* 1988; **i:** 828.
10. Hanks GW, Wand PJ. Enterohepatic circulation of opioid drugs: is it clinically relevant in the treatment of cancer patients? *Clin Pharmacokinet* 1989; **17:** 65–8.
11. Paul D, *et al.* Pharmacological characterization of morphine-6β-glucuronide, a very potent morphine metabolite. *J Pharmacol Exp Ther* 1989; **251:** 477–83.
12. Hanna MH, *et al.* Analgesic efficacy and CSF pharmacokinetics of intrathecal morphine-6-glucuronide: comparison with morphine. *Br J Anaesth* 1990; **64:** 547–50.
13. Osborne R, *et al.* Morphine and metabolite behavior after different routes of morphine administration: demonstration of the importance of the active metabolite morphine-6-glucuronide. *Clin Pharmacol Ther* 1990; **47:** 12–19.
14. McQuay HJ, *et al.* Oral morphine in cancer pain: influences on morphine and metabolite concentration. *Clin Pharmacol Ther* 1990; **48:** 236–44.
15. Hanna MH, *et al.* Disposition of morphine-6-glucuronide and morphine in healthy volunteers. *Br J Anaesth* 1991; **66:** 103–7.
16. Portenoy RK, *et al.* The metabolite morphine-6-glucuronide contributes to the analgesia produced by morphine infusion in patients with pain and normal renal function. *Clin Pharmacol Ther* 1992; **51:** 422–31.
17. Thompson PI, *et al.* Respiratory depression following morphine and morphine-6-glucuronide in normal subjects. *Br J Clin Pharmacol* 1995; **40:** 145–52.
18. Lötsch J, Geisslinger G. Morphine-6-glucuronide: an analgesic of the future? *Clin Pharmacokinet* 2001; **40:** 485–99.
19. Smith MT, *et al.* Morphine-3-glucuronide—a potent antagonist of morphine analgesia. *Life Sci* 1990; **47:** 579–85.
20. Morley JS, *et al.* Paradoxical pain. *Lancet* 1992; **340:** 1045.
21. Morley JS, *et al.* Methadone in pain uncontrolled by morphine. *Lancet* 1993; **342:** 1243.

Administration. There have been many studies on the pharmacokinetics of morphine following administration by various routes and methods. They include administration by the buccal route (see below), modified-release oral preparations,[1,2] the rectal route,[3,4] the pulmonary route,[5,6] continuous subcutaneous compared with intravenous infusion,[7] and the intraspinal route.[8-12]

Slow dural transfer of morphine and its prolonged presence in the CSF appear to correlate with its slow onset and long duration of action by epidural and intrathecal injection.[13] More lipid-soluble opioids, such as diamorphine and pethidine, enter and leave the CSF more rapidly than morphine.

The pharmacokinetics of morphine administered by 5 different routes—intravenous bolus injection and oral, sublingual, buccal, and modified-release buccal tablets—were studied[14] with particular reference to morphine-6-glucuronide, the active metabolite. This metabolite occurred in large quantities after intravenous administration and plasma concentrations rapidly exceeded those of morphine. Following oral administration morphine-6-glucuronide and morphine-3-glucuronide were present in quantities similar to those seen after intravenous morphine; morphine concentrations in plasma were very low and the mean morphine-6-glucuronide to morphine area under the curve ratio was 9.7 to 1. There was delayed absorption with attenuation and delay of peak morphine and metabolite plasma concentrations following sublingual or buccal administration. Compared with oral administration, concentrations of morphine were higher and those of its glucuronides lower when morphine was given rectally,[15] suggesting avoidance of first-pass metabolism.

1. Pinnock CA, *et al.* Absorption of controlled release morphine sulphate in the immediate postoperative period. *Br J Anaesth* 1986; **58:** 868–71.
2. Savarese JJ, *et al.* Steady-state pharmacokinetics of controlled release oral morphine sulphate in healthy subjects. *Clin Pharmacokinet* 1986; **11:** 505–10.
3. Moolenaar F, *et al.* Drastic improvement in the rectal absorption profile of morphine in man. *Eur J Clin Pharmacol* 1985; **29:** 119–21.
4. Cole L, *et al.* Further development of a morphine hydrogel suppository. *Br J Clin Pharmacol* 1990; **30:** 781–6.
5. Ward ME, *et al.* Morphine pharmacokinetics after pulmonary administration from a novel aerosol delivery system. *Clin Pharmacol Ther* 1997; **62:** 596–609.
6. Masood AR, Thomas SHL. Systemic absorption of nebulized morphine compared with oral morphine in healthy subjects. *Br J Clin Pharmacol* 1996; **41:** 250–2.
7. Waldmann CS, *et al.* Serum morphine levels: a comparison between continuous subcutaneous infusion and continuous intravenous infusion in postoperative patients. *Anaesthesia* 1984; **39:** 768–71.
8. Gustafsson LL, *et al.* Disposition of morphine in cerebrospinal fluid after epidural administration. *Lancet* 1982; **i:** 796.
9. Moore A, *et al.* Spinal fluid levels of morphine and heroin. *Clin Pharmacol Ther* 1984; **35:** 40–5.
10. Max MB, *et al.* Epidural and intrathecal opiates: cerebrospinal fluid and plasma profiles in patients with chronic cancer pain. *Clin Pharmacol Ther* 1985; **38:** 631–41.
11. Nordberg G, *et al.* Extradural morphine: influence of adrenaline admixture. *Br J Anaesth* 1986; **58:** 598–604.
12. Ionescu TI, *et al.* The pharmacokinetics of intradural morphine in major abdominal surgery. *Clin Pharmacokinet* 1988; **14:** 178–86.
13. Morgan M. The rational use of intrathecal and extradural opioids. *Br J Anaesth* 1989; **63:** 165–88.
14. Osborne R, *et al.* Morphine and metabolite behavior after different routes of morphine administration: demonstration of the importance of the active metabolite morphine-6-glucuronide. *Clin Pharmacol Ther* 1990; **47:** 12–19.
15. Babul N, Darke AC. Disposition of morphine and its glucuronide metabolites after oral and rectal administration: evidence of route specificity. *Clin Pharmacol Ther* 1993; **54:** 286–92.

BUCCAL ROUTE. Conflicting results from studies on buccal administration of morphine may reflect differences in formulation[1] and hence absorption. Some[2] reported equivalent analgesia with buccal and intramuscular morphine although others[3] found marked interindividual variability with mean peak serum concentrations of morphine some eight times lower after a buccal tablet than after an intramuscular injection and occurring a mean of 4 hours later. Morphine sulfate in aqueous solution has been reported to be moderately well absorbed from the buccal mucosa.[4] Absolute bioavailability for morphine was estimated to be 23.8% after an oral solution, 22.4% after a modified-release oral tablet (MST Continus), and 20.2% after a modified-release buccal tablet, with maximum plasma-morphine concentrations at 45 minutes, 2.5 hours, and 6 hours respectively; mean ratios of area under the plasma concentration-time curve for morphine-6-glucuronide to morphine in plasma were 11:1 after buccal and oral morphine compared with 2:1 for intravenous morphine.[5] There was considerable inter-subject variation in plasma concentrations of the morphine metabolites, morphine-3-glucuronide and morphine-6-glucuronide, following buccal administration of morphine as a modified-release formulation[6] and lack of pain relief was subsequently reported with this buccal formulation.[7] Poor absorption of morphine from modified-release buccal tablets when compared with intramuscular injection was also reported;[8] bitterness of the tablets, leading to their premature removal, and poor dissolution may have contributed.

1. Calvey TN, Williams NE. Pharmacokinetics of buccal morphine. *Br J Anaesth* 1990; **64:** 256.
2. Bell MDD, *et al.* Buccal morphine—a new route for analgesia? *Lancet* 1985; **i:** 71–3.
3. Fisher AP, *et al.* Serum morphine concentrations after buccal and intramuscular morphine administration. *Br J Clin Pharmacol* 1987; **24:** 685–7.
4. Al-Sayed-Omar O, *et al.* Influence of pH on the buccal absorption of morphine sulphate and its major metabolite, morphine-3-glucuronide. *J Pharm Pharmacol* 1987; **39:** 934–5.
5. Hoskin PJ, *et al.* The bioavailability and pharmacokinetics of morphine after intravenous, oral and buccal administration in healthy volunteers. *Br J Clin Pharmacol* 1989; **27:** 499–505.
6. Manara AR, *et al.* Pharmacokinetics of morphine following administration by the buccal route. *Br J Anaesth* 1989; **62:** 498–502.
7. Manara AR, *et al.* Analgesic efficacy of perioperative buccal morphine. *Br J Anaesth* 1990; **64:** 551–5.
8. Simpson KH, *et al.* An investigation of premedication by morphine given by the buccal or intramuscular route. *Br J Clin Pharmacol* 1989; **27:** 377–80.

Children. The pharmacokinetics of morphine in children are generally considered similar to those in adults;[1-3] in both an elimination half-life of about 2 hours has been reported following intravenous administration of morphine. Pharmacokinetic differences have however been observed in neonates given morphine by intravenous infusion. An elimination half-life of 13.9 ± 6.4 hours was reported in 8 neonates aged 1 to 30 days.[4] In another study 7 neonates aged 1 to 4 days had a mean elimination half-life of 6.81 hours compared with 3.91 hours in 4 infants aged 17 to 65 days; clearance of morphine was also significantly reduced in the newborn group.[5] The metabolism of morphine in 12 children aged 1 to 16 years was compared with that in 9 premature infants aged 2 to 12 days.[6] As expected, plasma clearance was lower in the neonates than in the children, probably due to a reduction in the metabolism of morphine in the neonates, as well as to immature renal function.

Morphine-3-glucuronide and morphine-6-glucuronide were however detected in plasma or urine from children and neonates indicating that preterm infants can metabolise morphine by glucuronidation, although capacity to do so was enhanced after the neonatal period. However, some[7] have reported that while morphine-3-glucuronide could be measured in plasma samples from premature neonates obtained at 2 hours and 24 hours morphine-6-glucuronide could only be measured in samples obtained at 24 hours. Also in another study of 16 acutely ill infants of less than 32 weeks gestational age 6 did not conjugate morphine at all and eliminated it in the urine unchanged.[8] The pharmacokinetics of morphine were very variable in preterm and term neonates given a single intravenous dose in the first week of life;[9] nearly 80% of morphine remained unbound. The 10 preterm infants with a gestational age of up to 30 weeks had a mean elimination half-life of 10.0 hours compared with 6.7 hours in 3 term neonates.

1. Dahlström B, et al. Morphine kinetics in children. Clin Pharmacol Ther 1979; 26: 354–65.
2. Stanski DR, et al. Kinetics of high-dose intravenous morphine in cardiac surgery patients. Clin Pharmacol Ther 1976; 19: 752–6.
3. Olkkola KT, et al. Clinical pharmacokinetics and pharmacodynamics of opioid analgesics in infants and children. Clin Pharmacokinet 1995; 5: 385–404.
4. Koren G, et al. Postoperative morphine infusion in newborn infants: assessment of disposition characteristics and safety. J Pediatr 1985; 107: 963–7.
5. Lynn AM, Slattery JT. Morphine pharmacokinetics in early infancy. Anesthesiology 1987; 66: 136–9.
6. Choonara IA, et al. Morphine metabolism in children. Br J Clin Pharmacol 1989; 28: 599–604.
7. Hartley R, et al. Morphine pharmacokinetics of morphine infusion in premature neonates. Arch Dis Child 1993; 69: 55–8.
8. Bhat R, et al. Morphine metabolism in acutely ill preterm newborn infants. J Pediatr 1992; 120: 795–9.
9. Bhat R, et al. Pharmacokinetics of a single dose of morphine in preterm infants during the first week of life. J Pediatr 1990; 117: 477–81.

The elderly. The pharmacokinetics of morphine were compared in 7 elderly (60 to 69 years) and 13 young (24 to 28 years) subjects, all of them healthy, following a single intravenous injection of morphine sulfate 10 mg per 70 kg body-weight.[1] Although the terminal rate of drug disappearance from plasma was faster in the elderly group, apparent volume of distribution at steady state was about half that of the young group and plasma clearance was reduced.

1. Owen JA, et al. Age-related morphine kinetics. Clin Pharmacol Ther 1983; 34: 364–8.

Hepatic impairment. The liver is a major site of morphine metabolism and therefore impaired liver function could be expected to affect elimination. There is some evidence that in cirrhosis glucuronidation might be relatively spared compared with other metabolic processes and that some extrahepatic metabolism may occur. Several studies have served to illustrate these points; hepatic extraction of morphine was impaired in cirrhotic patients, but less than expected;[1] morphine metabolism was minimal during the anhepatic phase of liver transplantation, but increased markedly when the new liver was reperfused;[2] morphine metabolism was virtually complete following liver transplantation with only 4.5% unchanged morphine being excreted in the urine 24 hours after administration;[3] morphine elimination was reduced when hepatic blood flow was impaired.[4]

1. Crotty B, et al. Hepatic extraction of morphine is impaired in cirrhosis. Eur J Clin Pharmacol 1989; 36: 501–6.
2. Bodenham A, et al. Extrahepatic morphine metabolism in man during the anhepatic phase of orthotopic liver transplantation. Br J Anaesth 1989; 63: 380–4.
3. Shelly MP, et al. Pharmacokinetics of morphine in patients following orthotopic liver transplantation. Br J Anaesth 1989; 63: 375–9.
4. Manara AR, et al. Morphine elimination and liver blood flow: a study in patients undergoing distal splenorenal shunt. Br J Hosp Med 1989; 42: 148 (abstract).

Renal impairment. Only a small amount of morphine is excreted unchanged in the urine. There are conflicting reports of morphine accumulation; some for,[1,2] others against.[3-5] It does seem clear though that morphine metabolites accumulate in patients with renal impairment;[5-9] the half-life of the active metabolite morphine-6-glucuronide was reported to be prolonged and its clearance reduced when morphine-6-glucuronide was administered to patients with renal impairment.[10] Opioid intoxication[11] and a prolonged opioid effect[12] in patients with renal failure has been associated with morphine-6-glucuronide (see also under Precautions, above).

1. Ball M, et al. Renal failure and the use of morphine in intensive care. Lancet 1985; i: 784–6.
2. Osborne R, et al. The pharmacokinetics of morphine and morphine glucuronides in kidney failure. Clin Pharmacol Ther 1993; 54: 158–67.
3. Säwe J, et al. Kinetics of morphine in patients with renal failure. Lancet 1985; ii: 211.
4. Woolner DF, et al. Renal failure does not impair the metabolism of morphine. Br J Clin Pharmacol 1986; 22: 55–9.
5. Chauvin M, et al. Morphine pharmacokinetics in renal failure. Anesthesiology 1987; 66: 327–31.
6. Säwe J, Odar-Cederlöf I. Kinetics of morphine in patients with renal failure. Eur J Clin Pharmacol 1987; 32: 377–82.
7. Wolff J, et al. Influence of renal function on the elimination of morphine and morphine glucuronides. Eur J Clin Pharmacol 1988; 34: 353–7.
8. Sear JW, et al. Studies on morphine disposition: influence of renal failure on the kinetics of morphine and its metabolites. Br J Anaesth 1989; 62: 28–32.

9. Peterson GM, et al. Plasma levels of morphine and morphine glucuronides in the treatment of cancer pain: relationship to renal function and route of administration. Eur J Clin Pharmacol 1990; 38: 121–4.
10. Hanna MH, et al. Morphine-6-glucuronide disposition in renal impairment. Br J Anaesth 1993; 70: 511–14.
11. Osborne RJ, et al. Morphine intoxication in renal failure: the role of morphine-6-glucuronide. BMJ 1986; 292: 1548–9.
12. Bodd E, et al. Morphine-6-glucuronide might mediate the prolonged opioid effect of morphine in acute renal failure. Hum Exp Toxicol 1990; 9: 317–21.

Uses and Administration

Morphine, a phenanthrene derivative and the principal alkaloid of opium, is an opioid analgesic (p.68) with agonist activity mainly at μ opioid receptors and perhaps at κ and δ receptors. It acts mainly on the CNS and smooth muscle. Although morphine is predominantly a CNS depressant it has some central stimulant actions which result in nausea and vomiting and miosis. Morphine generally increases smooth muscle tone, especially the sphincters of the gastrointestinal and biliary tracts.

Morphine may produce both physical and psychological dependence (see p.66) and should therefore be used with discrimination. Tolerance may also develop.

Morphine is used for the relief of moderate to severe pain, especially in pain associated with cancer, myocardial infarction, and surgery. In addition to relieving pain, morphine also alleviates the anxiety associated with severe pain and it is useful as a hypnotic where sleeplessness is due to pain.

Morphine reduces intestinal motility but its role, if any, in the symptomatic treatment of diarrhoea is very limited. It also relieves dyspnoea associated with various conditions, including that due to pulmonary oedema resulting from left ventricular failure. It is an effective cough suppressant, but codeine is usually preferred as there is less risk of dependence; morphine may however be necessary to control intractable cough associated with terminal lung cancer. Morphine has been used pre-operatively as an adjunct to anaesthesia for pain relief and to allay anxiety. It has also been used in high doses as a general anaesthetic in specialised procedures.

Morphine is usually **administered** as the sulfate, although the hydrochloride and the tartrate are used in similar doses. Routes of administration include the oral, subcutaneous, intramuscular, intravenous, intraspinal, and rectal routes. Subcutaneous injections are considered unsuitable for oedematous patients. Parenteral doses may be intermittent injections or continuous or intermittent infusions adjusted according to individual analgesic requirements.

Doses should generally be reduced in the elderly or debilitated or in patients with hepatic or renal impairment (see also under Precautions, above).

Doses by mouth for **pain** are usually in the range of 5 to 20 mg every 4 hours and may be given as an aqueous solution of the hydrochloride or sulfate, as modified-release granules, or as tablets. With modified-release preparations the 24-hour dose may be given as a single dose or in 2 divided doses (additional doses of a conventional formulation may also be needed if breakthrough pain occurs). As with the other routes, high oral doses may be required for effective analgesia in palliative care.

Morphine is sometimes administered rectally generally as suppositories in doses of 10 to 30 mg every 4 hours. A modified-release suppository of morphine sulfate for once daily administration is also available.

The usual dose by subcutaneous or intramuscular injection is 10 mg every 4 hours but may range from 5 to 20 mg. Children up to 1 month of age may be given 150 μg per kg body-weight every 4 hours; those aged 1 to 12 months, 200 μg per kg; 1 to 5 years, 2.5 to 5 mg; 6 to 12 years, 5 to 10 mg. See also under Administration in Children, below.

Doses of up to 15 mg have been given by slow intravenous injection, sometimes as a loading dose for continuous or patient-controlled infusion. For continuous intravenous administration maintenance doses

have generally ranged from 0.8 to 80 mg per hour, although some patients have required and been given much higher doses. Similar doses have been given by continuous subcutaneous infusion.

For myocardial infarction 10 mg may be given by intravenous injection at a rate of 2 mg per minute followed by a further 5 to 10 mg if necessary; half this dose should be used in elderly or debilitated patients.

Intraspinal doses are in the region of 5 mg for an initial epidural injection; if pain relief is unsatisfactory after one hour, further doses of 1 to 2 mg may be given up to a total dose of 10 mg per 24 hours. The recommended initial dose for continuous epidural infusion is 2 to 4 mg per 24 hours increased if necessary by further 1 to 2 mg increments. Intrathecal administration of morphine and its salts has tended to be less common than epidural administration. Doses of 0.2 to 1 mg have been injected intrathecally on a single occasion.

In **acute pulmonary oedema** 5 to 10 mg may be given by intravenous injection at a rate of 2 mg per minute.

For the control of intractable **cough** associated with terminal lung cancer, morphine hydrochloride oral solution is given in an initial dose of 5 mg every 4 hours.

Administration. CONTINUOUS INFUSION. Both acute and chronic pain have been controlled satisfactorily by continuous intravenous or subcutaneous infusions of morphine sulfate[1-3] but diamorphine hydrochloride or hydromorphone hydrochloride may be preferred for subcutaneous infusion because their greater solubility in water allows a smaller dose volume. Continuous subcutaneous infusions may be preferred to continuous intravenous infusions.[4] Although one group of workers[5] found continuous subcutaneous infusion to be less effective then epidural administration for relief of postoperative pain, it was still considered to provide simple and relatively effective analgesia with a low rate of adverse effects.

See also under Patient-controlled Analgesia, below.

1. Waldmann CS, et al. Serum morphine levels: a comparison between continuous subcutaneous infusion and continuous intravenous infusion in postoperative patients. Anaesthesia 1984; 39: 768–71.
2. Goudie TA, et al. Continuous subcutaneous infusion of morphine for postoperative pain relief. Anaesthesia 1985; 40: 1086–92.
3. Stuart GJ, et al. Continuous intravenous morphine infusions for terminal pain control: a retrospective review. Drug Intell Clin Pharm 1986; 20: 968–72.
4. Drexel H. Long-term continuous subcutaneous and intravenous opioid infusions. Lancet 1991; 337: 979.
5. Hindsholm KB, et al. Continuous subcutaneous infusion of morphine—an alternative to extradural morphine for postoperative pain relief. Br J Anaesth 1993; 71: 580–2.

INTRA-ARTICULAR ROUTE. Intra-articular injection of morphine into the knee at the end of arthroscopy has been reported to provide some degree of postoperative pain relief;[1,2] such pain relief may be more pronounced than that produced by the same dose given intravenously.[1] The effect appears to be due to the action of morphine on peripheral opioid receptors.[3] However, there have been conflicting results on whether addition of morphine to intra-articular bupivacaine improves analgesia.[4,5] Doses of morphine reported to have been injected intra-articularly have ranged from 1 to 5 mg.

1. Stein C, et al. Analgesic effect of intra-articular morphine after arthroscopic knee surgery. N Engl J Med 1991; 325: 1123–6.
2. Joshi GP, et al. Intra-articular morphine for pain relief after anterior cruciate ligament repair. Br J Anaesth 1993; 70: 87–8.
3. Stein C, et al. Local analgesic effect of endogenous opioid peptides. Lancet 1993; 342: 321–4.
4. Laurent SC, et al. Addition of morphine to intra-articular bupivacaine does not improve analgesia after day-case arthroscopy. Br J Anaesth 1994; 72: 170–3.
5. Heine MF, et al. Intra-articular morphine after arthroscopic knee operation. Br J Anaesth 1994; 73: 413–15.

INTRASPINAL ROUTE. Morphine is given epidurally and intrathecally to relieve both acute and chronic pain. However, reviews on the role of spinal opioids have generally concluded that they should be reserved for pain not controlled by more conventional methods of administration.[1-3] When converting from more conventional routes of administration McQuay[3] suggested that 1% of the total daily dose could be tried as the daily intrathecal dose and 10% as the epidural dose.

Intrathecal morphine may be delivered continuously via an implanted programmable infusion pump for the long-term management of chronic non-malignant and cancer pain.

See also under Patient-controlled Analgesia, below.

1. Anonymous. Spinal opiates revisited. Lancet 1986; i: 655–6.
2. Gustafsson LL, Wiesenfeld-Hallin Z. Spinal opioid analgesia: a critical update. Drugs 1988; 35: 597–603.
3. McQuay HJ. Opioids in chronic pain. Br J Anaesth 1989; 63: 213–26.

PATIENT-CONTROLLED ANALGESIA. Morphine is one of the most frequently used opioid analgesics for patient-controlled analgesia (see p.4). Most experience has been with the intravenous route, but the intramuscular, subcutaneous, oral, pulmonary, and epidural[1] routes have also been used. Reasonable initial settings recommended for intravenous administration have been a demand dose of 1 mg of morphine sulfate (or its equivalent) and a lockout interval of 5 to 10 minutes.[2]

1. Sjöström S, *et al.* Patient-controlled analgesia with extradural morphine or pethidine. *Br J Anaesth* 1988; **60**: 358–66.
2. Anonymous. Patient-controlled analgesia. *Med Lett Drugs Ther* 1989; **31**: 104.

PULMONARY ROUTE. For reference to the use of nebulised morphine see under Dyspnoea, below.

Administration in children. The management of pain in children is discussed on p.3. Morphine is widely used[1] and may be given to *neonates* who require analgesia as a result of surgery, invasive procedures, or intensive care. They do however have enhanced susceptibility to the respiratory depression associated with opioids although those already receiving respiratory support are at less risk; a transient drop in blood pressure may also be noted on initiation of the infusion in preterm neonates.[2] Allowance also has to be made for morphine's altered pharmacokinetics in this group (see above). Most neonates receiving respiratory support can be managed with an infusion of morphine 10 μg per kg body-weight per hour; the dose should not exceed 15 μg per kg per hour. In neonates who are breathing spontaneously there is a substantial risk of respiratory depression with powerful opioid analgesics such as morphine, and its administration to such neonates should be limited to those under intensive care. Morphine 5 to 7 μg per kg per hour by intravenous infusion allows adequate analgesia without respiratory depression, but the infusion rate should be titrated against response. Suggested infusion rates range from 5 to 15 μg per kg per hour. Bolus injections should be avoided. The use of opioids for sedation and analgesia in neonates in intensive care is mentioned on p.652; morphine is considered to be a more rational choice than fentanyl in such a setting where long-term infusions are required.

In *infants and children* opioids are still the mainstay of analgesia and morphine is the standard against which the others are compared. Techniques of continuous intravenous infusion have become popular for postoperative pain relief. From the age of 5 to 6 months morphine metabolism appears to conform to an adult pattern; in younger infants the regimens for neonates (see above) should be followed. Titration of infusion rate against patient response minimises the risks and most have found 10 to 30 μg per kg per hour to be satisfactory with minimal respiratory depression; if required a loading dose of morphine 100 to 200 μg per kg may be given initially with bolus top-up doses of 50 to 100 μg per kg every 4 hours. Subcutaneous infusions of morphine 30 to 60 μg per kg per hour have been used for the relief of terminal cancer pain in children, but for postoperative analgesia the dose needed should be similar to that for intravenous infusion. An intramuscular injection of morphine 100 to 200 μg per kg provides excellent short-term analgesia. Patient-controlled analgesia using morphine has been tried in children as young as 5 years of age.

Some spinal doses of morphine in children are as follows: caudal epidural block, 100 μg per kg; thoracic or lumbar epidural block, 50 μg per kg. Intrathecal doses of 20 or 30 μg per kg have provided satisfactory postoperative pain relief, but respiratory depression occurred in 10 and 25%, respectively.

Guidelines[3] for the control of pain associated with *major trauma* in children recommend that after resuscitation a bolus dose of 25 μg per kg body-weight of morphine should be given intravenously with further doses of 10 μg per kg at intervals of 10 minutes titrated against the patient's response. However, it should be noted that opioid analgesics should not be given to patients with appreciable head injuries whose conscious level is depressed or fluctuating.

1. Lloyd-Thomas AR. Pain management in paediatric patients. *Br J Anaesth* 1990; **64**: 85–104.
2. Wood CM, *et al.* Randomised double blind trial of morphine versus diamorphine for sedation of preterm neonates. *Arch Dis Child Fetal Neonatal Ed* 1998; **79**: F34–F39.
3. Lloyd-Thomas AR, Anderson I. Paediatric trauma: secondary survey. *BMJ* 1990; **301**: 433–7.

Cancer pain. The starting dose of morphine in cancer pain depends on the type of analgesic previously taken; 5 to 10 mg by mouth every 4 hours is enough to replace a non-opioid or a less potent opioid analgesic whereas 10 to 20 mg or more may be necessary to replace an opioid of equivalent strength to morphine. Doses should be increased gradually until the lowest effective analgesic dose is reached, taking into account any 'rescue' doses that have been administered to relieve breakthrough pain. There are no 'standard' doses; they have ranged from 2.5 to over 2500 mg of morphine sulfate every 4 hours, although most patients need far less than 100 mg every 4 hours. For patients on 4-hourly regimens, a double dose may be taken at bedtime to avoid waking up in the night.

Modified-release preparations are also used and, depending on the preparation, can be given either twice daily or as a single daily dose. The initial dose of a modified-release preparation is 10 to 20 mg every 12 hours if replacing paracetamol or no previous analgesic, but 20 to 30 mg every 12 hours if replacing a less potent opioid. The dose and not the frequency of administration should be altered if required. Some argue that dose titration should always be carried out with immediate-release preparations, only transferring to modified-release formulations

once the optimum analgesic dose has been achieved. When transferring a patient, the same total 24-hour immediate-release dose is given as two equal 12-hourly modified-release doses, with the first dose given 4 hours after the last immediate-release dose. Any breakthrough pain during titration or as a result of loss of analgesic control should be managed with immediate-release formulations.

If the patient is unable to swallow, parenteral morphine may be given. The equivalent intramuscular dose of morphine is half the oral dose; if a modified-release preparation has been given the total 24-hour dose should be halved to give the intramuscular daily dose, which is given in 6 divided doses, at 4-hourly intervals.

References.
1. Expert Working Group of the European Association for Palliative Care. Morphine in cancer pain: modes of administration. *BMJ* 1996; **312**: 823–6.

Dyspnoea. In the treatment of dyspnoea, doses of morphine tend to be smaller than those used for pain relief. Morphine hydrochloride or sulfate may be given as an oral solution in carefully titrated doses, starting at a dose of 5 mg every 4 hours; as little as 2.5 mg every 4 hours may be sufficient for opioid-naive patients.[1] In acute pulmonary oedema, 5 to 10 mg may be given by slow intravenous injection. In incurable malignant chest disease a test dose of 5 mg by mouth should be repeated every 4 hours with 5 to 10 mg at bedtime; if necessary the dose may be increased gradually up to 15 to 20 mg every 4 hours. If the patient is already receiving morphine for pain a 50% increase in dose may be tried.[2] Patients have also obtained relief from subcutaneous injection.[3]

Although one group of workers[4] reported that a low dose of nebulised morphine (mean dose 1.7 mg) improved exercise endurance in patients with dyspnoea due to advanced chronic lung disease, several subsequent studies[5-7] have failed to obtain significant improvements with doses up to 40 mg. It is considered that current evidence does not support the use of nebulised morphine for breathlessness.[1] Furthermore, bronchospasm, particularly at high doses can be a problem and there is no consensus on the optimal dose, schedule of administration, or method of dose titration.

1. Davis CL. ABC of palliative care: breathlessness, cough, and other respiratory problems. *BMJ* 1997; **315**: 931–4.
2. Twycross RG, Lack SA. *Oral morphine in advanced cancer.* 2nd ed. Beaconsfield: Beaconsfield Publishers, 1989.
3. Bruera E, *et al.* Subcutaneous morphine for dyspnea in cancer patients. *Ann Intern Med* 1993; **119**: 906–7.
4. Young IH, *et al.* Effect of low dose nebulised morphine on exercise endurance in patients with chronic lung disease. *Thorax* 1989; **44**: 387–90.
5. Beauford W, *et al.* Effects of nebulized morphine sulfate on the exercise tolerance of the ventilatory limited COPD patients. *Chest* 1993; **104**: 175–8.
6. Noseda A, *et al.* Disabling dyspnoea in patients with advanced disease: lack of effect of nebulized morphine. *Eur Respir J* 1997; **10**: 1079–83.
7. Jankelson D, *et al.* Lack of effect of high doses of inhaled morphine on exercise endurance in chronic obstructive pulmonary disease. *Eur Respir J* 1997; **10**: 2270–4.

Intensive care. When used to provide analgesia for patients in intensive care, morphine has a relatively slow onset of action, but longer term rather than rapid-onset analgesia can be achieved by a loading dose of 10 to 15 mg, in adults, followed by an infusion of 2 to 3 mg per hour; the dose must be individually titrated.

Preparations

BP 2001: Chloroform and Morphine Tincture; Morphine and Atropine Injection; Morphine Sulphate Injection; Morphine Suppositories; Morphine Tablets; Prolonged-release Morphine Tablets; **USP 25:** Morphine Sulfate Injection; Morphine Sulfate Suppositories.

Proprietary Preparations (details are given in Part 3)
Aust.: Kapanol; M-Dolor; Morapid; Mundidol; Oramorph; Substitol; Vendal; ***Austral.:*** Anamorph; Kapanol; MS Contin; MS Mono; Ordine; ***Belg.:*** Kapanol; MS Contin; MS Direct; Skenan; Stellorphinad; Stellorphine; ***Braz.:*** Dimorf; MS-Long; MST Continus; ***Canad.:*** Kadian; M-Eslon; Morphitec; MOS; MS Contin; MSIR; Oramorph; Statex; ***Denm.:*** Contalgin; Depolan; Doltard; Duralgin; Kapanol†; Malfin†; Repriadol†; ***Fin.:*** Depolan; Dolcontin; ***Fr.:*** Actiskenan; Kapanol; Moscontin; Sevredol; Skenan; ***Ger.:*** Capros; Kapanol; M-beta; M-Dolor; M-long; M-Stada; Mogetic; MSI; MSR; MST; Onkomorphin; Sevredol; ***Hong Kong:*** MST Continus; ***Irl.:*** Morstel; MST Continus; MXL; Oramorph; Sevredol; Slo-Morph; ***Israel:*** Kapanol; MCR; MIR; MSP; ***Ital.:*** MS Contin; Skenan; ***Mex.:*** Analfin; Duralmor; Graten; Kapanol; MST Continus; ***Neth.:*** Kapanol; MS Contin; Noceptin; Sevredol; Skenan; ***Norw.:*** Dolcontin; Kapanol†; ***NZ:*** Kapanol; LA Morph; MST Continus; RA Morph; RMS; Sevredol; ***Port.:*** MST; ***S.Afr.:*** MST Continus; SRM-Rhotard; ***Singapore:*** MST Continus; SRM-Rhotard; Statex; ***Spain:*** MST Continus; Oblioser†; Oglos; Sevredol; Skenan; Uni Mist; ***Swed.:*** Depolan; Dolcontin; Loceptin†; Maxidon; Oramorph; ***Switz.:*** Kapanol; MST Continus; Sevre-Long; Sevredol; ***UK:*** Moraxen; Morcap; MST Continus; MXL; Oramorph; Sevredol; Zomorph; ***USA:*** Astramorph PF; Duramorph; Infumorph; Kadian; MS Contin; MS/L†; MS/S†; MSIR; OMS Concentrate†; Oramorph; RMS; Roxanol.

Multi-ingredient: ***Aust.:*** Modiscop; ***Austral.:*** Morphalgin; ***Belg.:*** Spasma; ***Irl.:*** Cyclimorph; Diocalm†; ***Ital.:*** Cardiostenol; ***S.Afr.:*** Chloropect; Collodyne†; Cyclimorph; Diastat†; Enterodyne; Pectrolyte; ***Swed.:*** Spasmofen; ***Switz.:*** Spasmosol; ***UK:*** Collis Browne's; Cyclimorph; Diocalm Dual Action; Enterosan†; Opazimes.

The symbol † denotes a preparation no longer actively marketed

Morpholine Salicylate (9591-w)

2-Hydroxybenzoic acid compounded with morpholine (1 : 1).
$C_{11}H_{15}NO_4 = 225.2$.
CAS — 147-90-0.
ATC — N02BA08.

Profile
Morpholine salicylate is a salicylic acid derivative (see Aspirin, p.14) that has been used by mouth or topically for musculoskeletal disorders.

Preparations
Proprietary Preparations (details are given in Part 3)
Israel: Dolical.

Nabumetone (12990-p)

Nabumetone (BAN, USAN, rINN).
BRL-14777; Nabumetonum. 4-(6-Methoxy-2-naphthyl)butan-2-one.
$C_{15}H_{16}O_2 = 228.3$.
CAS — 42924-53-8.
ATC — M01AX01.
Pharmacopoeias. In *Eur.* (see p.vi).

Pharmacopoeial description
Ph. Eur.: A white or almost white crystalline powder. Practically insoluble in water; freely soluble in acetone; slightly soluble in methyl alcohol. Protect from light.

Adverse Effects and Precautions
As for NSAIDs in general, p.63.

Effects on the gastrointestinal tract. Like other NSAIDs nabumetone can produce adverse effects on the gastrointestinal tract, although some studies have produced favourable comparisons with ibuprofen[1] or naproxen.[2] It has been suggested[3] that nabumetone may be a preferential inhibitor of cyclo-oxygenase-2 (COX-2) but the significance of this in determining its adverse effects is uncertain.

1. Roth SH, *et al.* A controlled study comparing the effects of nabumetone, ibuprofen, and ibuprofen plus misoprostol on the upper gastrointestinal tract mucosa. *Arch Intern Med* 1993; **153**: 2565–71.
2. Roth SH, *et al.* A longterm endoscopic evaluation of patients with arthritis treated with nabumetone vs naproxen. *J Rheumatol* 1994; **21**: 1118–23.
3. Davies NM. Clinical pharmacokinetics of nabumetone: the dawn of selective cyclo-oxygenase-2 inhibition? *Clin Pharmacokinet* 1997; **33**: 403–16.

Effects on the lungs. Pulmonary fibrosis developed in a 68-year-old woman receiving nabumetone 1500 mg; symptoms appeared after 2 weeks of therapy and worsened during the next 6 weeks.[1] There was rapid resolution on withdrawal of nabumetone and treatment with oral corticosteroids.

1. Morice A, *et al.* Pulmonary fibrosis associated with nabumetone. *Postgrad Med J* 1991; **67**: 1021–2.

Effects on the skin. Pseudoporphyria characterised by blistering on the neck and hands developed in a 36-year-old woman taking nabumetone and auranofin for rheumatoid arthritis.[1] Stopping auranofin had no effect on the blistering which only resolved once nabumetone was withdrawn. The authors of the report stated that the UK Committee on Safety of Medicines had received 3 additional reports of pseudoporphyria suspected to be caused by nabumetone.

1. Varma S, Lanigan SW. Pseudoporphyria caused by nabumetone. *Br J Dermatol* 1998; **138**: 549–50. Correction. *ibid.* **139**: 759. [dose]

Interactions
For interactions associated with NSAIDs, see p.65.

Pharmacokinetics
Although nabumetone is well absorbed from the gastrointestinal tract, plasma concentrations following oral administration are too small to be measured as it undergoes rapid and extensive first-pass metabolism in the liver to the principal active compound 6-methoxy-2-naphthylacetic acid (6-MNA) and other inactive metabolites. 6-MNA is more than 99% bound to plasma proteins. 6-MNA diffuses into synovial fluid. It crosses the placenta and is distributed into breast milk. There is considerable interindividual variation in the plasma elimination half-life of 6-MNA, especially in the elderly; some reported mean values at steady state include 22 to about 27 hours for young adults and about 25 and 34 hours in elderly patients. 6-MNA eventually undergoes further metabolism by *O*-methylation and conjugation. About 80% of a dose is excreted in the urine as inactive or conjugated metabolites and less than 1% as unchanged 6-MNA.

◊ References.
1. Brier ME, *et al.* Population pharmacokinetics of the active metabolite of nabumetone in renal dysfunction. *Clin Pharmacol Ther* 1995; **57**: 622–7.
2. Davies NM. Clinical pharmacokinetics of nabumetone: the dawn of selective cyclo-oxygenase-2 inhibition? *Clin Pharmacokinet* 1997; **33**: 403–16.

Uses and Administration
Nabumetone is a non-active prodrug whose major metabolite is an NSAID (p.65) structurally similar to naproxen (p.61). It is used for the relief of pain and inflammation associated with osteoarthritis and rheumatoid arthritis in a usual dose of 1 g by

mouth taken as a single dose in the evening; if necessary 0.5 to 1 g may be given additionally in the morning. It has been recommended that a dose of 1 g daily should not be exceeded in elderly patients and that 500 mg daily may be satisfactory in some cases.

◊ References.
1. Anonymous. Nabumetone—a new NSAID. *Med Lett Drugs Ther* 1992; **34:** 38–40.
2. Friedel HA, *et al.* Nabumetone: a reappraisal of its pharmacology and therapeutic use in rheumatic diseases. *Drugs* 1993; **45:** 131–56.
3. Proceedings of a symposium: continuing developments with nabumetone: an investigators' update. *Am J Med* 1993; 95 (suppl 2A): 1S–45S.
4. Dahl SL. Nabumetone: a "nonacidic" nonsteroidal antiinflammatory drug. *Ann Pharmacother* 1993; **27:** 456–63.

Preparations

BP 2001: Nabumetone Oral Suspension; Nabumetone Tablets.

Proprietary Preparations (details are given in Part 3)
Braz.: Relifex; *Canad.:* Relafen; *Denm.:* Relifex; *Fin.:* Relifex; *Fr.:* Nabucox; *Ger.:* Arthaxan†; *Hong Kong:* Relifex; *Irl.:* Relifex; *Israel:* Relifex; *Ital.:* Artaxan; Nabuser; *Mex.:* Relifex; *Neth.:* Mebutan; *Norw.:* Relifex; *Port.:* Balmox; *S.Afr.:* Relifen; Relisan; Relitone; *Singapore:* Relifex; *Spain:* Dolsinal; Listran; Relif; *Swed.:* Relifex; *Switz.:* Balmox; *Thai.:* Nabone; Nametone; Relifex; *UK:* Relifex; *USA:* Relafen.

Nalbuphine Hydrochloride (6244-y)

Nalbuphine Hydrochloride *(BANM, USAN, rINNM)*.
EN-2234A. 17-Cyclobutylmethyl-7,8-dihydro-14-hydroxy-17-normorphine hydrochloride; (−)-(5R,6S,14S)-9a-Cyclobutylmethyl-4,5-epoxymorphinan-3,6,14-triol hydrochloride.
$C_{21}H_{27}NO_4,HCl = 393.9$.
CAS — 20594-83-6 (nalbuphine); 23277-43-2 (nalbuphine hydrochloride).

Incompatibility. Incompatibility has been reported between injections of nalbuphine hydrochloride and nafcillin sodium,[1] diazepam,[2] pentobarbital sodium,[2] or thiethylperazine maleate.[2]
1. Jeglum EL, *et al.* Nafcillin sodium incompatibility with acidic solutions. *Am J Hosp Pharm* 1981; **38:** 462–4.
2. Jump WG, *et al.* Compatibility of nalbuphine hydrochloride with other preoperative medications. *Am J Hosp Pharm* 1982; **39:** 841–3.

Dependence and Withdrawal

As for Opioid Analgesics, p.66.

◊ A WHO expert committee considered in 1989 that the likelihood of nalbuphine abuse was low to moderate and was not great enough to warrant international control.[1] Abuse had been reported infrequently and the withdrawal syndrome produced when naloxone was given after continuous nalbuphine administration was less severe than that in morphine dependence. There have been later reports of abuse among athletes.[2,3]
1. WHO. WHO expert committee on drug dependence: twenty-fifth report. *WHO Tech Rep Ser* 775 1989.
2. McBride AJ, *et al.*. Three cases of nalbuphine hydrochloride dependence associated with anabolic steroid use. *Br J Sports Med* 1996; **30:** 69–70.
3. Wines JD, *et al.*. Nalbuphine hydrochloride dependence in anabolic steroid users. *Am J Addict* 1999; **8:** 161–4.

Adverse Effects and Treatment

As for Opioid Analgesics in general, p.67.

Headache may occur. Nausea and vomiting occur less than with other opioids. Hallucinations and other psychotomimetic effects are rare and have been reported much less frequently than with pentazocine. As nalbuphine has both antagonist and agonist activity its effects may be only partially reversed by naloxone, but use of the latter is still recommended in nalbuphine overdose.

Effects on the respiratory system. Nalbuphine produces similar respiratory depression to morphine at equianalgesic doses, but there is a ceiling effect with nalbuphine and, unlike morphine, respiratory depression does not increase appreciably with higher doses.[1] In a cumulative-dose study[2] a plateau effect was seen with nalbuphine above a total dose of 30 mg per 70 kg body-weight intravenously. Similar ventilatory depression has been noted[3] with single intravenous doses of nalbuphine of 15, 30, or 60 mg per 70 kg; naloxone failed to reverse the depression at the highest dose.
1. Klepper ID, *et al.* Respiratory function following nalbuphine and morphine in anaesthetized man. *Br J Anaesth* 1986; **58:** 625–9.
2. Romagnoli A, Keats AS. Ceiling effect for respiratory depression by nalbuphine. *Clin Pharmacol Ther* 1980; **27:** 478–85.
3. Pugh GC, *et al.* Effect of nalbuphine hydrochloride on the ventilatory and occlusion pressure responses to carbon dioxide in volunteers. *Br J Anaesth* 1989; **62:** 601–9.

Precautions

As for Opioid Analgesics in general, p.68.

Nalbuphine may precipitate withdrawal symptoms if given to patients physically dependent on opioids.

The dose of nalbuphine should be reduced in patients with hepatic or renal impairment.

Abuse. See under Dependence and Withdrawal, above.

Pregnancy. When nalbuphine is used for analgesia during labour there is more placental transfer and sedation in mothers and their infants than with pethidine.[1] There have also been reports of bradycardia and respiratory depression in neonates whose mothers received nalbuphine during labour.[2,3] It was considered that nalbuphine should be given with caution during labour, especially by the intravenous route. Some[2] have recommended subcutaneous administration and advised that nalbuphine should not be given around the expected time of delivery. Further references on the transplacental transfer of nalbuphine are given under Pharmacokinetics, below.
1. Wilson CM, *et al.* Transplacental gradient of pethidine and nalbuphine in labour. *Br J Clin Pharmacol* 1986; **21:** 571P–2P.
2. Guillonneau M, *et al.* Perinatal adverse effects of nalbuphine given during parturition. *Lancet* 1990; **335:** 1588.
3. Sgro C, *et al.* Perinatal adverse effects of nalbuphine given during labour. *Lancet* 1990; **336:** 1070.

Interactions

For interactions associated with opioid analgesics, see p.68.

Pharmacokinetics

Following intramuscular injection nalbuphine has been reported to produce peak plasma concentrations after 30 minutes. It is metabolised in the liver and is excreted in the urine and faeces as unchanged drug and conjugates.

Nalbuphine crosses the placenta.

There appears to be considerable first-pass metabolism of nalbuphine following oral administration.

◊ References.
1. Aitkenhead AR, *et al.* The pharmacokinetics of oral and intravenous nalbuphine in healthy volunteers. *Br J Clin Pharmacol* 1988; **25:** 264–8.
2. Sear JW, *et al.* Disposition of nalbuphine in patients undergoing general anaesthesia. *Br J Anaesth* 1987; **59:** 572–5.
3. Kay B, *et al.* Pharmacokinetics of oral nalbuphine in postoperative patients. *Br J Anaesth* 1987; **59:** 1327P.
4. Jaillon P, *et al.* Pharmacokinetics of nalbuphine in infants, young healthy volunteers, and elderly patients. *Clin Pharmacol Ther* 1989; **46:** 226–33.

Pregnancy. References.
1. Wilson CM, *et al.* Transplacental gradient of pethidine and nalbuphine in labour. *Br J Clin Pharmacol* 1986; **21:** 571P–2P.
2. Dadabhoy ZP, *et al.* Transplacental transfer of nalbuphine in patients undergoing cesarean section: a pilot study. *Acta Anaesthesiol Ital* 1988; **39:** 227–32.
3. Nicolle E, *et al.* Therapeutic monitoring of nalbuphine: transplacental transfer and estimated pharmacokinetics in the neonate. *Eur J Clin Pharmacol* 1996; **49:** 485–9.

Uses and Administration

Nalbuphine hydrochloride, a phenanthrene derivative, is an opioid analgesic (p.68). It has mixed opioid agonist and antagonist activity. It is used for the relief of moderate to severe pain, including that associated with myocardial infarction, and as an adjunct to anaesthesia. Nalbuphine hydrochloride is reported to act within 15 minutes of subcutaneous or intramuscular injection or within 2 to 3 minutes of intravenous injection and generally to produce analgesia for 3 to 6 hours. It is given subcutaneously, intramuscularly, or intravenously; intravenous infusion as part of a patient-controlled analgesia system is also permitted.

The dose of nalbuphine hydrochloride for pain relief is 10 to 20 mg every 3 to 6 hours as required. Doses of 10 to 30 mg have been given by slow intravenous injection in myocardial infarction; a second dose of 20 mg may be given after 30 minutes if necessary. Children may be given up to 300 µg per kg body-weight initially, repeated once or twice as necessary.

Premedication has been carried out using doses of 100 to 200 µg per kg. As an adjunct to anaesthesia a usual dose is 0.3 to 1 mg per kg given intravenously over 10 to 15 minutes at induction; in the USA doses of up to 3 mg per kg have been used. Maintenance doses of 250 to 500 µg per kg are given at half-hourly intervals.

◊ Nalbuphine is generally described as a mixed agonist and antagonist acting mainly as an agonist at κ opioid receptors and

as an antagonist or partial agonist at µ receptors. It has shown antagonist activity similar to that seen with naloxone in opioid-dependent subjects.[1] Nalbuphine is structurally related to naloxone and oxymorphone. Pharmacologically nalbuphine is qualitatively similar to pentazocine, but nalbuphine is a more potent antagonist at µ opioid receptors, is less likely to produce psychotomimetic effects such as hallucinations, and is reported to produce no significant cardiovascular effects in patients with ischaemic heart disease. It differs from pure µ agonists such as morphine in that its analgesic, sedative, and respiratory depressant actions are subject to a 'ceiling' effect and may not increase proportionately with dose.
1. Preston KL, *et al.* Antagonist effects of nalbuphine in opioid-dependent human volunteers. *J Pharmacol Exp Ther* 1989; **248:** 929–37.

Pain. ACUTE PAIN. Although nalbuphine has the possible advantage of a 'ceiling' effect for respiratory depression this effect may also be applicable to analgesia. When nalbuphine was used for *postoperative* pain relief following abdominal surgery there was an apparent reversal of analgesic effect at high doses.[1] In comparative studies of pain relief following various types of surgery nalbuphine has been reported to be inferior to morphine following hip replacement,[2] but of longer duration and with fewer complications than pethidine.[3] Nalbuphine has been administered postoperatively in patient-controlled analgesia and has been found to be as effective as pethidine[4] or morphine.[5] Because of its µ-opioid antagonist properties nalbuphine has been used to reverse the side-effects of µ agonists without reducing analgesia[6] although increased pain has sometimes been reported.
Labour. Nalbuphine given intravenously in a patient-controlled device was preferred to pethidine given similarly for labour pain,[7] whereas no advantage has been found[8] with intramuscular nalbuphine over pethidine for labour pain. More recently, severe respiratory depression has been reported in neonates following the use of nalbuphine; subcutaneous administration and avoidance of the expected delivery time was advised (see Pregnancy under Precautions, above).
1. Pugh GC, Drummond GB. A dose-response study with nalbuphine hydrochloride for pain in patients after upper abdominal surgery. *Br J Anaesth* 1987; **59:** 1356–63.
2. Fee JPH, *et al.* Analgesia after hip replacement surgery: comparison of nalbuphine with morphine. *Br J Anaesth* 1989; **63:** 756–8.
3. Brock-Utne JG, *et al.* A comparison of nalbuphine and pethidine for postoperative pain relief after orthopaedic surgery. *S Afr Med J* 1985; **68:** 391–3.
4. Sprigge JS, Otton PE. Nalbuphine versus meperidine for postoperative analgesia: a double-blind comparison using the patient controlled analgesic technique. *Can Anaesth Soc J* 1983; **30:** 517–21.
5. Christiansen S. Nalbuphine in patient-controlled analgesia: a comparison with morphine. *Curr Ther Res* 1987; **41:** 933–45.
6. Chalmers PC, *et al.* Double-blind comparison of intravenous nalbuphine and placebo in the amelioration of side-effects of epidural narcotics. *Pain Clin* 1988; **2:** 49–56.
7. McAteer EJ, *et al.* Patient controlled analgesia in labour: a comparison of nalbuphine and pethidine. *Br J Anaesth* 1986; **58:** 122P.
8. Wilson CM, *et al.* A double-blind comparison of intramuscular pethidine and nalbuphine in labour. *Anaesthesia* 1986; **41:** 1207–13.

CHRONIC PAIN. Using subcutaneous administration nalbuphine was found[1] to provide equivalent analgesia to morphine in chronic cancer pain and with fewer complications, but it has been noted[2] that a ceiling of analgesic efficacy (equivalent to morphine 30 mg) appeared to restrict the value of nalbuphine in chronic pain.
1. Stambaugh JE. Evaluation of nalbuphine: efficacy and safety in the management of chronic pain associated with advanced malignancy. *Curr Ther Res* 1982; **31:** 393–401.
2. McQuay HJ. Opioids in chronic pain. *Br J Anaesth* 1989; **63:** 213–26.

Preparations

Proprietary Preparations (details are given in Part 3)
Aust.: Nubain; *Canad.:* Nubain; *Fr.:* Azerty; *Ger.:* Nubain; *Hong Kong:* Intapan; Nubain; *Israel:* Nubain; *Mex.:* Bufigen; Bufilem; Nalbu; Nalcryn; Nubain; *NZ:* Nubain; *S.Afr.:* Nubain†; *Singapore:* Nubain; *Switz.:* Nubain; *Thai.:* Nubain; *UK:* Nubain; *USA:* Nubain.

Naproxen (2672-n)

Naproxen *(BAN, USAN, rINN)*.
Naproxenum; RS-3540. (+)-2-(6-Methoxy-2-naphthyl)propionic acid.
$C_{14}H_{14}O_3 = 230.3$.
CAS — 22204-53-1.
ATC — G02CC02; M01AE02; M02AA12.
Pharmacopoeias. In Chin., Eur. (see p.vi), Jpn, and US.

Pharmacopoeial description

Ph. Eur.: A white or almost white, crystalline powder. Practically insoluble in water; soluble in alcohol and in methyl alcohol; sparingly soluble in ether. Protect from light.

USP 25: A white to off-white, practically odourless, crystalline powder. Practically insoluble in water; soluble in alcohol; freely soluble in dehydrated alcohol and in chloroform; sparingly soluble in ether. Store in airtight containers.

Naproxen Sodium (2673-h)

Naproxen Sodium (BANM, USAN, rINNM).
RS-3650.
$C_{14}H_{13}NaO_3 = 252.2$.
CAS — 26159-34-2.
Pharmacopoeias. In *US*.

Each 550 mg of naproxen sodium is approximately equivalent to 500 mg of naproxen.

Pharmacopoeial description
USP 25: A white to creamy crystalline powder. Soluble in water and in methyl alcohol; sparingly soluble in alcohol; very slightly soluble in acetone; practically insoluble in chloroform and in toluene. Store in airtight containers.

Adverse Effects and Precautions

As for NSAIDs in general, p.63.

Administration of suppositories containing naproxen may cause rectal irritation and occasional bleeding.

◊ Reviews.
1. Bansal V, *et al.* A look at the safety profile of over-the-counter naproxen sodium: a meta-analysis. *J Clin Pharmacol* 2001; **41:** 127–38.

Breast feeding. The amount of naproxen distributed into breast milk is considered by some authorities to be too small to be harmful to a breast-fed infant although some manufacturers recommend that breast feeding should be avoided during naproxen therapy. In a study[1] of one breast-fed infant only 0.26% of the mother's dose was recovered from the infant.
1. Jamali F, Stevens DRS. Naproxen excretion in milk and its uptake by the infant. *Drug Intell Clin Pharm* 1983; **17:** 910–11.

Effects on the blood. Haematological adverse effects reported in patients receiving naproxen include haemolytic anaemia,[1,2] aplastic anaemia,[3] and agranulocytosis.[4]
1. Hughes JA, Sudell W. Hemolytic anemia associated with naproxen. *Arthritis Rheum* 1983; **26:** 1054.
2. Lo TCN, Martin MA. Autoimmune haemolytic anaemia associated with naproxen suppositories. *BMJ* 1986; **292:** 1430.
3. McNeil P, *et al.* Naproxen-associated aplastic anaemia. *Med J Aust* 1986; **145:** 53–4.
4. Nygard N, Starkebaum G. Naproxen and agranulocytosis. *JAMA* 1987; **257:** 1732.

Effects on the CNS. Aseptic meningitis has been associated with naproxen therapy.[1] Details of a patient who suffered recurrent attacks have been published.[1]

There has been a report[2] of a patient with Parkinson's disease whose symptoms had previously been well controlled but who deteriorated when she was given naproxen. She improved on withdrawal of naproxen and the effect was confirmed by re-challenge. It was noted that the UK Committee on Safety of Medicines had records of one case of parkinsonism associated with a combined preparation of naproxen and misoprostol and 12 other reports of tremor or ataxia precipitated by naproxen.
1. Weksler BB, Lehany AM. Naproxen-induced recurrent aseptic meningitis. *DICP Ann Pharmacother* 1991; **25:** 1183–4.
2. Shaunak S, *et al.* Exacerbation of idiopathic Parkinson's disease by naproxen. *BMJ* 1995; **311:** 422.

Effects on the eyes. Keratopathy, characterised by whorl-like corneal opacities, occurred in a woman receiving naproxen; complete regression occurred after discontinuation of naproxen.[1] There has also been a report of exacerbation of glaucoma in a 65-year-old woman given naproxen.[2]
For reference to effects on the optic nerve associated with naproxen, see p.63.
1. Szmyd L, Perry HD. Keratopathy associated with the use of naproxen. *Am J Ophthalmol* 1985; **99:** 598.
2. Fincham JE. Exacerbation of glaucoma in an elderly female taking naproxen sodium: a case report. *J Geriatr Drug Ther* 1989; **3:** 139–43.

Effects on the gastrointestinal tract. Gastrointestinal adverse effects are among the most frequently reported during short- and long-term treatment with naproxen. Rectal proctocolitis associated with the use of naproxen has been reported[1] in one patient. Oesophageal ulceration reported in 7 patients[2] may have arisen due to incorrect consumption (such as taking the dosage without fluids or lying down after administration) but other causes could not be dismissed.
1. Ravi S, *et al.* Colitis caused by non-steroidal anti-inflammatory drugs. *Postgrad Med J* 1986; **62:** 773–6.
2. Kahn LH, *et al.* Over-the-counter naproxen sodium and esophageal injury. *Ann Intern Med* 1997; **126:** 1006.

Effects on the kidneys. Acute renal failure,[1] renal papillary necrosis,[2] interstitial nephritis,[3] and hyperkalaemia[1] have been reported in patients receiving naproxen. As with other NSAIDs, renal adverse effects occur more frequently in patients with certain risk factors such as volume depletion, diuretic therapy, heart failure, and pre-existing renal dysfunction.[1]
1. Todd PA, Clissold SP. Naproxen: a reappraisal of its pharmacology, and therapeutic use in rheumatic diseases and pain states. *Drugs* 1990; **40:** 91–137.
2. Caruana RJ, Semble EL. Renal papillary necrosis due to naproxen. *J Rheumatol* 1984; **11:** 90–1.
3. Quigley MR, *et al.* Concurrent naproxen- and penicillamine-induced renal disease in rheumatoid arthritis. *Arthritis Rheum* 1982; **25:** 1016–19.

Effects on the liver. There have been a few reports[1,2] of moderate to severe jaundice attributed to naproxen including one in which the patient also had a similar reaction with fenoprofen.[2]
1. Victorino RMM, *et al.* Jaundice associated with naproxen. *Postgrad Med J* 1980; **56:** 368–70.
2. Andrejak M, *et al.* Cross hepatotoxicity between non-steroidal anti-inflammatory drugs. *BMJ* 1987; **295:** 180–1.

Effects on the lungs. See under Hypersensitivity, below.

Effects on the salivary glands. For reference to salivary gland swelling associated with naproxen therapy, see under Hypersensitivity, below.

Effects on the skin. Cutaneous reactions reported in patients receiving naproxen include erythema nodosum,[1] lichen planus,[2] toxic pustular skin eruption,[3] and bullous dermatosis.[4]
Photodermatitis, characterised by vesicle formation or increased skin fragility on sun-exposed skin, has been reported in adults[5-7] and children.[8,9]
Relapse of subacute cutaneous lupus erythematosus has been reported in one patient to be possibly associated with the administration of naproxen.[10]
For reference to facial scars of unknown origin developing in children receiving NSAIDs, and in particular naproxen, see under NSAIDs, p.64.
1. Grattan CEH, Kennedy CTC. Naproxen induced erythema nodosum. *BMJ* 1984; **288:** 114.
2. Heymann WR, *et al.* Naproxen-induced lichen planus. *J Am Acad Dermatol* 1984; **10:** 299–301.
3. Page SR, Grattan CEH. Pustular reaction to naproxen with cholestatic jaundice. *BMJ* 1986; **293:** 510.
4. Bouldin MB, *et al.* Naproxen-associated linear IgA bullous dermatosis: case report and review. *Mayo Clin Proc* 2000; **75:** 967–70.
5. Howard AM, *et al.* Pseudoporphyria due to naproxen. *Lancet* 1985; **i:** 819–20.
6. Rivers JK, Barnetson RS. Naproxen-induced bullous photodermatitis. *Med J Aust* 1989; **151:** 167–8.
7. Levy ML, *et al.* Naproxen-induced pseudoporphyria: a distinctive photodermatitis. *J Pediatr* 1990; **117:** 660–4.
8. Parodi A, *et al.* Possible naproxen-induced relapse of subacute cutaneous lupus erythematosus. *JAMA* 1992; **268:** 51–2.
9. Lang BA, Finlayson LA. Naproxen-induced pseudoporphyria in patients with juvenile rheumatoid arthritis. *J Pediatr* 1994; **124:** 639–42.
10. Cox NH, Wilkinson DS. Dermatitis artefacta as the presenting feature of auto-erythrocyte sensitization syndrome and naproxen-induced pseudoporphyria in a single patient. *Br J Dermatol* 1992; **126:** 86–9.

Hypersensitivity. All of 11 aspirin-sensitive asthmatic patients developed reactions (rhinorrhoea, tightness of chest, wheezing, dyspnoea) after taking naproxen in doses of 40 to 80 mg.[1] Hypersensitivity to individual NSAIDs is believed to be closely linked to the extent to which these drugs inhibit prostaglandin (see under Aspirin, p.15). There may therefore be a dose threshold below which no detectable symptoms occur. Such an effect has been reported[2] in a patient previously stabilised on naproxen for about one year who had a hypersensitivity reaction following a dosage increase.
A hypersensitivity reaction characterised by pulmonary infiltrates with eosinophilia[3,4] has been reported in patients taking naproxen. There has also been a report of a generalised hypersensitivity reaction with acute eosinophilic colitis in a 57-year-old woman treated with naproxen for osteoarthritis.[5]
Bilateral swelling of the major salivary glands, a generalised rash, and eosinophilia suggestive of a hypersensitivity response has been reported in a patient following use of naproxen.[6]
1. Szczeklik A, *et al.* Asthmatic attacks induced in aspirin-sensitive patients by diclofenac and naproxen. *BMJ* 1977; **2:** 231–2.
2. Briscoe-Dwyer L, Etzel JV. Dyspnea and periorbital edema following an increase in naproxen dose. *Ann Pharmacother* 1994; **28:** 1110.
3. Nader DA, Schillaci RF. Pulmonary infiltrates with eosinophilia due to naproxen. *Chest* 1983; **83:** 280–2.
4. Buscaglia AJ, *et al.* Pulmonary infiltrates associated with naproxen. *JAMA* 1984; **251:** 65–6.
5. Bridges AJ, *et al.* Acute eosinophilic colitis and hypersensitivity reaction associated with naproxen therapy. *Am J Med* 1990; **89:** 526–7.
6. Knulst AC, *et al.* Salivary gland swelling following naproxen therapy. *Br J Dermatol* 1995; **133:** 647–9.

Parkinsonism. For a report of a patient whose symptoms of Parkinson's disease were exacerbated by naproxen, see under Effects on the CNS, above.

Interactions

For interactions associated with NSAIDs, see p.65.

The excretion of naproxen is delayed by probenecid resulting in raised plasma concentrations of naproxen.

Antiepileptics. For the effect of naproxen on the protein binding of valproic acid, see p.368.

Pharmacokinetics

Naproxen and naproxen sodium are readily absorbed from the gastrointestinal tract. Peak plasma concentrations are attained about 1 to 2 hours after ingestion of naproxen sodium and in about 2 to 4 hours after ingestion of naproxen. Food reduces the rate but not the extent of absorption. Naproxen and naproxen so-

dium are also well absorbed following rectal administration but absorption is slower compared with the oral route. At therapeutic concentrations naproxen is more than 99% bound to plasma proteins. Plasma concentrations of naproxen increase proportionally with dose up to about 500 mg daily; at higher doses there is an increase in clearance caused by saturation of plasma proteins. Naproxen diffuses into synovial fluid; it crosses the placenta and is distributed into breast milk in small amounts. Naproxen has a plasma elimination half-life of about 13 hours. Approximately 95% of a dose is excreted in urine as naproxen and 6-O-desmethylnaproxen and their conjugates. Less than 5% of a dose has been recovered in the faeces.

◊ References.
1. Bruno R, *et al.* Naproxen kinetics in synovial fluid of patients with osteoarthritis. *Br J Clin Pharmacol* 1988; **26:** 41–4.
2. Bertin P, *et al.* Sodium naproxen: concentration and effect on inflammatory response mediators in human rheumatoid synovial fluid. *Eur J Clin Pharmacol* 1994; **46:** 3–7.
3. Davies NM, Anderson KE. Clinical pharmacokinetics of naproxen. *Clin Pharmacokinet* 1997; **32:** 268–93.

Uses and Administration

Naproxen, a propionic acid derivative, is an NSAID (p.65).

Naproxen is used in musculoskeletal and joint disorders such as ankylosing spondylitis, osteoarthritis, and rheumatoid arthritis including juvenile idiopathic arthritis. It is also used in dysmenorrhoea, headache including migraine, postoperative pain, soft-tissue disorders, acute gout, and to reduce fever. Naproxen is usually given by mouth as the free acid or as the sodium salt.

In the treatment of rheumatic disorders, the usual dose of naproxen or naproxen sodium is the equivalent of 500 mg to 1 g of naproxen daily either as a single dose or in 2 divided doses. A dose of 10 mg per kg body-weight daily of naproxen in 2 divided doses has been used in children over 5 years of age with juvenile idiopathic arthritis.

In other painful conditions such as dysmenorrhoea and acute musculoskeletal disorders the usual initial dose is the equivalent of 500 mg of naproxen followed by 250 mg every 6 to 8 hours, up to a maximum daily dose of 1250 mg after the first day.

In acute gout an initial dose equivalent to 750 mg of naproxen followed by 250 mg every 8 hours is used.

Modified-release preparations are available in some countries for once daily administration.

For the treatment of migraine, the equivalent of 750 mg of naproxen can be given at the first symptom of an impending attack and, if necessary, this may be followed after at least half an hour by further doses of 250 to 500 mg throughout the day to a total maximum daily dose of 1250 mg. See below for a suggested dose for the prophylaxis of migraine.

Rectal administration of naproxen in doses of 500 mg once or twice daily is sometimes employed.

Naproxen has also been used as the piperazine, aminobutanol, and lysine salts and as naproxen cetrimonium. Naproxen is available in combination with misoprostol (p.1446) for patients at risk of NSAID-induced peptic ulceration.

◊ Reviews.
1. Todd PA, Clissold SP. Naproxen: a reappraisal of its pharmacology, and therapeutic use in rheumatic diseases and pain states. *Drugs* 1990; **40:** 91–137.

Headache. An NSAID such as naproxen is among the drugs tried first for the symptomatic treatment of various types of headache including migraine (p.449) and tension-type headache (p.450). An NSAID given at the onset of symptoms can successfully treat an acute attack of migraine.[1] NSAIDs also appear to be effective for the prophylaxis of migraine, although propranolol or pizotifen are generally preferred. Studies have indicated that naproxen sodium 550 mg [equivalent to 500 mg of naproxen] given twice daily may be useful for reducing the number of attacks suffered.[2-5]
1. Treves TA, *et al.* Naproxen sodium versus ergotamine tartrate in the treatment of acute migraine attacks. *Headache* 1992; **32:** 280–2.
2. Sargent J, *et al.* A comparison of naproxen sodium to propranolol hydrochloride and a placebo control for the prophylaxis of migraine headache. *Headache* 1985; **25:** 320–4.

3. Welch KMA, *et al.* Successful migraine prophylaxis with naproxen sodium. *Neurology* 1985; **35:** 1304–10.
4. Sances G, *et al.* Naproxen sodium in menstrual migraine prophylaxis: a double-blind placebo controlled study. *Headache* 1990; **30:** 705–9.
5. Bellavance AJ, Meloche JP. A comparative study of naproxen sodium, pizotyline and placebo in migraine prophylaxis. *Headache* 1990; **30:** 710–15.

Malignant neoplasms. Some NSAIDs such as naproxen may be of value both for the differential diagnosis and the management of neoplastic fever[1,2] as they appear to be more effective in reducing this type of fever than against fever associated with infections.

1. Chang JC, Gross HM. Neoplastic fever responds to the treatment of an adequate dose of naproxen. *J Clin Oncol* 1985; **3:** 552–8.
2. Azeemuddin SK, *et al.* The effect of naproxen on fever in children with malignancies. *Cancer* 1987; **59:** 1966–8.

Preparations

BP 2001: Naproxen Oral Suspension; Naproxen Suppositories; Naproxen Tablets;
USP 25: Naproxen Oral Suspension; Naproxen Sodium Tablets; Naproxen Tablets.

Proprietary Preparations (details are given in Part 3)
Aust.: Miranax; Naprobene; Nycopren; Proxen; Xenopan†; *Austral.:* Aleve; Anaprox; Crysanal; Inza; Naprogesic; Naprosyn; Proxen; *Belg.:* Apra-Gel; Apranax; Naprosyne; *Braz.:* Flanax; Naprosyn; *Canad.:* Anaprox; Apo-Napro-Na; Naprosyn; Naxen; Novo-Naprox; Nu-Naprox; Rhodiaprox; Roche†; Synflex; *Denm.:* Alpoxen; Bonyl; Daprox; Miranax; Napronet†; Naprosyn; Nycopren†; *Fin.:* Alpoxen; Miranax; Naprometin; Napromex; Naprosyn; Naxopren; Nycopren; Pronaxen; *Fr.:* Aleve; Apranax; Naprosyne; *Ger.:* Aleve; Apranax†; Dysmenalgit; Malexin; Napro-Dorsch; Proxen; Synflex; *Hong Kong:* Ap-Napro-Na; Genoxen; Inza; Naprosyn; Noflam-N; Proxen; Soren; Synflex; *Irl.:* Genoxen†; Gerinap; Napmel; Naprex; Naprosyn; Synflex; *Israel:* Aponacin; Naprex; Naproxi; Narocin; Naxyn; Point; *Ital.:* Akudol; Aleve; Aperdan; Artroxent†; AS/85; Axer; D/N PR; Floginax; Flogogin†; Floxalin; Gibinap; Gibixen; Gynestrel; Laser; Leniantril; Momendol; Naprius; Naprocet; Naprodol; Naprorex; Naprosyn; Natrixen†; Neo Eblimon; Nitens; Numidan; Piproxen; Prexan; Primeral†; Proxine†; Synalgo; Synflex; Ticoflex; Xenar; *Mex.:* Actiquim; Alexan; Anaflin; Artron; Atiflan; Bioxan; Dafloxen; Dartrox; Dolnaxen; Doloatrixen; Dolxen; Donaprox; Faraxen; Flanax; Flexen; Flogen; Fuxen; Genalgen; Kenaprox; Lixogan; Lorexen; Naprodil; Nasocan; Navixen; Naxen; Naxil; Neonaxil; Nixal; Novadex; Novaxen; Pactens; Patxen; Pronat; Pronax-P; Pronaxil; Pronoxen; Proxalin; Sertrixen; Sodixen; Tandax; Velsay; *Neth.:* Aleve; Femex; Naprocoat; Naprosyne; Naprovite; Nycopren; *Norw.:* Alpoxen; Ledox; Napren; Naprosyn; *NZ:* Naprogesic; Naprosyn; Naxen; Noflam; Synflex; *Port.:* Naprosyn; Reuxen; *S.Afr.:* Acusprain†; Aleve; Clinosyn†; Fibroxyn; Nafasol; Napflam; Naprel; Naprosript; Naprosyn; Naxen; Pranoxen†; Proxen†; Synflex; Traumox; *Singapore:* Anax; Apo-Napro-Na; Bipronyl; Gesiprox; Inza; Naprosyn; Noflam-N; Soden; Soproxen; Sunprox; Synflex; Zynal; *Spain:* Aleve; Alviomas; Anaprox; Antalgin; Denaxpren; Ilagane†; Lundiran; Naprokes; Naprosyn; Naproval; Proxen; Tacron; *Swed.:* Alpoxen; Miranax†; Naprelan†; Naprosyn; Pronaxen; *Switz.:* Apranax; Naprosyn; Nycopren; Proxen; Servinaprox†; *Thai.:* Annoxen; Artagen; Flexin; Naprosian; Naprosyn; Naprosyn; Napxen; Narzen; Polyxen; Proxen; Roxen; Serviproxan; Soproxen; Synflex; Synogin; U-Proxyn; Vinsen; *UK:* Arthroxin; Arthroxen; Condrotec†; Laraflex; Napratec; Naprosyn; Nycopren; Prosaid†; Rimoxyn; Synflex; Timpron; *USA:* Aleve; Anaprox; Naprelan; Naprosyn.

Multi-ingredient: *Ital.:* Flogogin†; *Mex.:* Bifardol S; Dafloxen F; Dolotandex; Farxen; Febrax; Grifed; Naxodol; Somalgesic.

Narceine   (14234-e)

6-({6-[2-(Dimethylamino)ethyl]-2-methoxy-3,4-(methylenedioxy)phenyl}acetyl)-o-veratric acid; 6-({6-[2-(Dimethylamino)ethyl]-4-methoxy-1,3-benzodioxol-5-yl}acetyl)-2,3-dimethoxybenzoic acid.
$C_{23}H_{27}NO_8 = 445.5$.
CAS — 131-28-2.

Profile
Narceine is an opioid analgesic (p.66) that was used in cough preparations for its antitussive action; the phosphate was used similarly.

Nefopam Hydrochloride   (2674-m)

Nefopam Hydrochloride (*BANM, USAN, rINNM*).
Benzoxazocine; Fenazoxine; R-738. 3,4,5,6-Tetrahydro-5-methyl-1-phenyl-1*H*-2,5-benzoxazocine hydrochloride.
$C_{17}H_{19}NO,HCl = 289.8$.
CAS — 13669-70-0 (nefopam); 23327-57-3 (nefopam hydrochloride).

Adverse Effects and Treatment
Side-effects occurring with nefopam include nausea, vomiting, sweating, drowsiness, insomnia, urinary retention, lightheadedness, nervousness, mental confusion, blurred vision, headache, dry mouth, and tachycardia. Euphoria, hallucinations, and convulsions have occasionally been reported, as has temporary pink discoloration of the urine. Symptoms of over-

dosage have included CNS and cardiovascular toxicity.

Effects on the urinary tract. In January 1989, the UK Committee on Safety of Medicines[1] reported that it had received 53 reports in which nefopam was associated with the development of urinary retention or symptoms of hesitancy, poor stream, or dribbling. In one case there was a history of prostatism.

1. Committee on Safety of Medicines. Nefopam hydrochloride (Acupan). *Current Problems* 24 1989.

Overdosage. There have been two reported cases of fatal overdoses with nefopam.[1,2] The earlier report[1] also provided details of 9 other patients who recovered with routine supportive treatment.

1. Piercy DM, *et al.* Death due to overdose of nefopam. *BMJ* 1981; **283:** 1508–9.
2. Urwin SC, Smith HS. Fatal nefopam overdose. *Br J Anaesth* 1999; **83:** 501–2.

Precautions
Nefopam is contra-indicated in patients with a history of convulsive disorders. It should be used with caution in the elderly and in patients with glaucoma, urinary retention, or impaired hepatic or renal function.

Interactions
It has been recommended that nefopam should not be given to patients receiving MAOIs and should be used cautiously in those receiving tricyclic antidepressants. The adverse effects of nefopam may be additive to those of other drugs with antimuscarinic or sympathomimetic activity.

Pharmacokinetics
Nefopam is absorbed from the gastrointestinal tract. Peak plasma concentrations occur 1 to 3 hours after administration by mouth and about 1.5 hours after intramuscular injection. About 73% is bound to plasma proteins. Nefopam is distributed into breast milk. It has an elimination half-life of about 4 hours. It is extensively metabolised and excreted mainly in urine, in which less than 5% of a dose is excreted unchanged. About 8% of a dose is excreted via the faeces.

Distribution into breast milk. Studies in 5 healthy nursing mothers given nefopam for post-episiotomy pain indicated that nefopam was present in human milk in an equivalent concentration to that in plasma.[1] It was calculated that on a body-weight basis a breast-fed infant would receive less than 3% of the maternal dose.

1. Liu DTY, *et al.* Nefopam excretion in human milk. *Br J Clin Pharmacol* 1987; **23:** 99–101.

Uses and Administration
Nefopam hydrochloride is a non-opioid analgesic considered to act centrally, although its mechanism of action is unclear. It also has some antimuscarinic and sympathomimetic actions. Nefopam hydrochloride is used for the relief of moderate acute and chronic pain. The usual dose range by mouth is 30 to 90 mg three times daily; the recommended initial dose is 60 mg (or 30 mg in elderly patients) three times daily. Nefopam hydrochloride may also be given in doses of 20 mg by intramuscular injection, repeated every 6 hours if necessary; it is recommended that the patient should always be lying down when receiving the injection and should remain so for 15 to 20 minutes afterwards. It has also been given by slow intravenous injection in similar doses.

Preparations
Proprietary Preparations (details are given in Part 3)
Belg.: Acupan; *Fr.:* Acupan; *Ger.:* Ajan; Silentan; *Irl.:* Acupan; *Israel:* Acupan; *Ital.:* Nefadol†; Nefam; Oxadol; *NZ:* Acupan; *S.Afr.:* Acupan†; *Spain:* Acupan†; *Switz.:* Acupan; *UK:* Acupan.

Nicoboxil   (9216-w)

Nicoboxil (*rINN*).
Butoxyethyl Nicotinate. 2-Butoxyethyl nicotinate.
$C_{12}H_{17}NO_3 = 223.3$.
CAS — 13912-80-6.

Profile
Nicoboxil is a nicotinate used in topical preparations as a rubefacient. It is also included in some topical preparations used for the treatment of acne vulgaris.

Preparations
Proprietary Preparations (details are given in Part 3)
Multi-ingredient: *Aust.:* Finalgon; *Austral.:* Finalgon; *Canad.:* Actinac; Finalgon; *Ger.:* Finalgon; *Irl.:* Actinac; *Ital.:* Anti-Acne; *NZ:* Finalgon; *Port.:* Finalgon; *Spain:* Finalgon; *UK:* Actinac.

Nicomorphine Hydrochloride   (13012-l)

Nicomorphine Hydrochloride (*BANM, rINNM*).
3,6-Di-*O*-nicotinoylmorphine hydrochloride; (−)-(5*R*,6*S*)-4,5-Epoxy-9a-methylmorphin-7-en-3,6-diyl dinicotinate hydrochloride.
$C_{29}H_{25}N_3O_5,HCl = 532.0$.
CAS — 639-48-5 (nicomorphine); 12040-41-4 (nicomorphine hydrochloride); 35055-78-8 (nicomorphine xHCl).

Profile
Nicomorphine hydrochloride is an opioid analgesic (p.66) used in the treatment of moderate to severe pain. It is given by mouth in initial doses of 5 to 10 mg daily or by intramuscular, slow intravenous, or subcutaneous injection in usual doses of 10 to 20 mg; it may also be given rectally.

◊ References.
1. Koopman-Kimenai PM, *et al.* Pharmacokinetics of intramuscular nicomorphine and its metabolites in man. *Eur J Clin Pharmacol* 1991; **41:** 375–8.

Preparations
Proprietary Preparations (details are given in Part 3)
Aust.: Vilan; *Denm.:* Vilan; *Neth.:* Vilan; *Switz.:* Vilan.

Nifenazone   (2676-v)

Nifenazone (*BAN, rINN*).
N-(2,3-Dimethyl-5-oxo-1-phenyl-3-pyrazolin-4-yl)nicotinamide.
$C_{17}H_{16}N_4O_2 = 308.3$.
CAS — 2139-47-1.
ATC — N02BB05.

Profile
Nifenazone is an NSAID (p.63) that has been used in musculoskeletal and joint disorders given by mouth or rectally.

Preparations
Proprietary Preparations (details are given in Part 3)
Ital.: Reumatosil.

Niflumic Acid   (2677-g)

Niflumic Acid (*rINN*).
UP-83. 2-(ααα-Trifluoro-m-toluidino)nicotinic acid.
$C_{13}H_9F_3N_2O_2 = 282.2$.
CAS — 4394-00-7.
ATC — M01AX02; M02AA17.
Pharmacopoeias. In Fr.

Adverse Effects and Precautions
As for NSAIDs in general, p.63. Fluoride-associated osteosis has been reported with prolonged use. Niflumic acid should be discontinued if hypersensitivity skin reactions appear.

Uses and Administration
Niflumic acid, a nicotinic acid derivative, is an NSAID (p.65). It has been used in inflammatory and musculoskeletal and joint disorders in usual doses of about 250 mg three or four times daily by mouth; up to 1500 mg daily has been used in severe disorders. It has also been used topically as a 3% cream or ointment or 2.5% gel. The morpholinoethyl ester morniflumate (p.56) has similar uses.
Niflumic acid glycinamide has been used topically in inflammatory mouth disorders.

Preparations
Proprietary Preparations (details are given in Part 3)
Aust.: Actol; *Belg.:* Niflugel; Nifluril; *Fr.:* Flunir; Niflugel; Nifluril; *Ger.:* Actol†; *Hong Kong:* Nifluril; Niflam; *Port.:* Nifluril; *Spain:* Niflactol; *Switz.:* Niflugel; Nifluril.

Multi-ingredient: *Fr.:* Nifluril†; *Port.:* Nifluril†.

Nimesulide   (13017-k)

Nimesulide (*BAN, rINN*).
Nimesulidum; R-805. 4′-Nitro-2′-phenoxymethanesulphonanilide.
$C_{13}H_{12}N_2O_5S = 308.3$.
CAS — 51803-78-2.
ATC — M01AX17.
Pharmacopoeias. In Eur. (see p.vi).

Pharmacopoeial description
Ph. Eur.: A yellowish crystalline powder. It exhibits polymorphism. Practically insoluble in water; slightly soluble in dehydrated alcohol; freely soluble in acetone.

Profile
Nimesulide is an NSAID (p.63) reported to be a selective inhibitor of cyclo-oxygenase-2 (COX-2). It has been given in doses

of up to 200 mg twice daily by mouth or rectally for inflammatory conditions, fever, and pain. Nimesulide betadex (nimesulide betacyclodextrin complex) has been used similarly.

◊ References.

1. Bennett A, *et al*. Nimesulide: a multifactorial therapeutic approach to the inflammatory process? a 7-year clinical experience. *Drugs* 1993; **46**: (suppl 1): 1–283.
2. Davis R, Brogden RN. Nimesulide: an update of its pharmacodynamic and pharmacokinetic properties, and therapeutic efficacy. *Drugs* 1994; **48**: 431–54.
3. Senna GE, *et al*. Nimesulide in the treatment of patients intolerant of aspirin and other NSAIDs. *Drug Safety* 1996; **14**: 94–103.
4. Vizzardi M, *et al*. Nimesulide beta cyclodextrin (nimesulidebetadex) versus nimesulide in the treatment of pain after arthroscopic surgery. *Curr Ther Res* 1998; **59**: 162–71.
5. Bernareggi A. Clinical pharmacokinetics of nimesulide. *Clin Pharmacol* 1998; **35**: 247–74.
6. Shah AA, *et al*. Selective inhibition of COX-2 in humans is associated with less gastrointestinal injury: a comparison of nimesulide and naproxen. *Gut* 2001; **48**: 339–46.

Adverse effects. Although *thrombocytopenia* is a common feature in patients infected with HIV one group of workers considered that thrombocytopenia in one of their patients was related to the use of nimesulide.[1]

There has been a report[2] of a patient who developed *fulminant hepatic failure* after treatment with nimesulide.

Irreversible *end-stage renal failure* has been reported in a neonate born to a mother who received nimesulide as a tocolytic from the 26th to the 32nd week of pregnancy.[3] Others have also reported neonatal renal failure associated with nimesulide use.[4]

1. Pasticci MB, *et al*. Nimesulide, thrombocytopenic purpura, and human immunodeficiency virus (HIV) infection. *Ann Intern Med* 1990; **112**: 233–4.
2. McCormick PA, *et al*. COX 2 inhibitor and fulminant hepatic failure. *Lancet* 1999; **353**: 40–1.
3. Peruzzi L, *et al*. Neonatal end-stage renal failure associated with maternal ingestion of cyclo-oxygenase-type-2 selective inhibitor nimesulide as tocolytic. *Lancet* 1999; **354**: 1615. Correction. *ibid*. 2000; **355**: 238.
4. Balasubramaniam J. Nimesulide and neonatal renal failure. *Lancet* 1999; **355**: 575.

Premature labour. Nimesulide has been tried as an alternative to indometacin to delay labour in a patient with a history of preterm delivery.[1] Nimesulide was given from 16 to 34 weeks of gestation and a successful delivery started 6 days after withdrawal. There appeared to be no adverse effect on fetal renal function or the ductus arteriosus. The authors suggested that fetal prostaglandin synthesis might be mainly mediated through cyclo-oxygenase-1 and that a relatively selective cyclo-oxygenase-2 inhibitor such as nimesulide might produce fewer adverse effects on the fetus than other non-selective NSAIDs. However, adverse renal effects have been reported in some neonates whose mothers received nimesulide for premature labour, see above.

1. Sawdy R, *et al*. Use of a cyclo-oxygenase type-2-selective nonsteroidal anti-inflammatory agent to prevent preterm delivery. *Lancet* 1997; **350**: 265–6.

Preparations

Proprietary Preparations (details are given in Part 3)
Belg.: Mesulid; *Braz.*: Antiflogil; Deglogen; Nisulid; Scaflam; Scalid; Sintalgin; *Fin.*: Nimed; *Fr.*: Nexen; *Hong Kong*: Nidol; *Irl.*: Aulin; Mesulid; *Israel*: Mesulid; *Ital.*: Algimesil; Algolider; Antalgo; Areuma; Aulin; Biosal; Domes; Edemax; Efridol; Eudolene; Fansidol; Fenisal; Flolid; Isodol; Laidor; Ledoren; Mesid†; Mesulid; MF 110†; Nerelid; Nide; Nidol†; Nimedex; Nimesil; Nimesulene; Nimexan; Nims; Nisal†; Noalgos; Noxalide; Remov; Resulin; Solving; Sulidamor; Sulide; Teonim; *Mex.*: Apolide; Eskaflam; Mesulid; Redaflam; Severin; *Port.*: Aulin; Donulide; Jabasulide; Nimed; Sulimed; *Spain*: Antifloxil; Guaxan; *Switz.*: Aulin; Nisulid; *Thai.*: Nidol.

Nonivamide (9265-t)

Nonivamide (rINN)

Nonylvanillamide. *N*-Vanillylnonamide; *N*-[(4-Hydroxy-3-methoxyphenyl)methyl]nonanamide.
$C_{17}H_{27}NO_3 = 293.4$.
CAS — 2444-46-4.

NOTE. Use of the term 'synthetic capsaicin' to describe nonivamide has arisen from the use of nonivamide as an adulterant for capsaicin and capsicum oleoresin.

Profile
Nonivamide is used in topical preparations as a rubefacient.

Preparations

Proprietary Preparations (details are given in Part 3)
Ger.: ABC Warme-Pflaster Sensitive; Gothaplast Capsicum-Warmepflaster.

Multi-ingredient: *Aust.*: Finalgon; Forapin†; Rubriment; *Austral.*: Finalgon; *Belg.*: Forapin†; *Canad.*: Finalgon; *Ger.*: ABC Warme-Salbe; Akrotherm; Finalgon; Histapodol N; Infrotto Ultra; Lomazell forte N; Ostochont; Rheuma-Liquidum; Rheumasalbe; Rubriment; Vertebralon N; *NZ*: Finalgon; *Port.*: Finalgon; *Spain*: Finalgon; *Switz.*: Forapin; Histalgane; Radalgin; Roliwol S†; Thermocutan.

Nonsteroidal Anti-inflammatory Drugs (2600-p)

NSAIDs.

Adverse Effects and Treatment

The commonest side-effects occurring during therapy with NSAIDs are generally gastrointestinal disturbances, such as gastrointestinal discomfort, nausea, and diarrhoea; these are usually mild and reversible but in some patients peptic ulceration and severe gastrointestinal bleeding may occur. It is generally agreed that the gastrointestinal effects of NSAIDs are due to inhibition of cyclo-oxygenase-1 (COX-1); the selective inhibition of COX-2 improves gastrointestinal tolerance.

CNS-related side-effects include headache, vertigo, dizziness, nervousness, tinnitus, depression, drowsiness, and insomnia. Hypersensitivity reactions may occur occasionally and include fever, angioedema, bronchospasm, and rashes. Hepatotoxicity and aseptic meningitis, which occur rarely, may also be hypersensitivity reactions. Some patients may experience visual disturbances.

Haematological adverse effects of NSAIDs include anaemias, thrombocytopenia, neutropenia, eosinophilia, and agranulocytosis. Unlike aspirin, inhibition of platelet aggregation is reversible with other NSAIDs.

Some NSAIDs have been associated with nephrotoxicity such as interstitial nephritis and nephrotic syndrome; renal failure may be provoked by NSAIDs especially in patients with pre-existing renal impairment. Haematuria has also occurred. Fluid retention may occur, rarely precipitating heart failure in elderly patients. Long-term use or abuse of analgesics, including NSAIDs, has been associated with nephropathy. Other adverse effects include photosensitivity. Alveolitis, pulmonary eosinophilia, pancreatitis, Stevens-Johnson syndrome, and toxic epidermal necrolysis are other rare adverse effects. Induction or exacerbation of colitis has also been reported.

Further details concerning the adverse effects of the individual NSAIDs may be found under their respective monographs.

◊ The relative toxicity of NSAIDs is a continuing subject of debate.[1] Attempts have been made to rank these drugs according to their toxicity on various body systems.[2] For further details see below under individual headings.

1. Skeith KJ, *et al*. Differences in NSAID tolerability profiles: fact or fiction? *Drug Safety* 1994; **10**: 183–95.
2. Committee on Safety of Medicines/Medicines Control Agency. Relative safety of oral non-aspirin NSAIDs. *Current Problems* 1994; **20**: 9–11.

Effects on the blood. The UK Committee on Safety of Medicines has provided data on the reports it had received between July 1963 and January 1993 on agranulocytosis and neutropenia.[1] Several groups of drugs were commonly implicated, among them NSAIDs for which there were 133 reports of agranulocytosis (45 fatal) and 187 of neutropenia (15 fatal). The most frequently implicated NSAID was phenylbutazone with 74 reports of agranulocytosis (39 fatal) and 40 of neutropenia (4 fatal).

1. Committee on Safety of Medicines/Medicines Control Agency. Drug-induced neutropenia and agranulocytosis. *Current Problems* 1993; **19**: 10–11.

Effects on the cardiovascular system. A meta-analysis[1] of 50 randomised trials studying the effects of NSAIDs on *blood pressure* in a total of 771 patients found that NSAIDs had elevated mean supine blood pressure by 5 mmHg. Piroxicam, indometacin, and ibuprofen had produced the greatest increase but the effect was only found to be statistically significant for piroxicam. Aspirin, sulindac, and flurbiprofen produced the smallest elevation in blood pressure while the effect of tiaprofenic acid, diclofenac, and naproxen was intermediate. The increase was more marked in studies in which patients had received antihypertensive therapy than in those where such treatment had not been used. NSAIDs had antagonised all antihypertensive therapy but the effect had been greater against beta blockers and vasodilators than against diuretics. An earlier meta-analysis of intervention studies had produced similar results.[2] Of the 1324 patients who had received NSAIDs, increases in mean arterial pressure were greatest in hypertensive patients who had taken either indometacin, naproxen, or piroxicam, although results were only significant for indometacin and naproxen. Sulindac and aspirin had minimal effects on mean arterial pressure.

It has been suggested that the use of NSAIDs in the elderly may increase the risk of the need for antihypertensive therapy.[3] A study[3] of 9411 patients aged 65 years or older who had just started treatment with antihypertensives found that 41% had used NSAIDs in the previous year compared with 26% of 9629 control patients not being treated with antihypertensives.

The recent use of NSAIDs has also been associated with an increased risk of developing *heart failure* in elderly patients. A case-control study[4] found that the use of an NSAID in the previous week doubled the odds of being admitted to hospital with heart failure; this risk was increased tenfold in those with a history of heart disease. The study also suggested an association between both high-dose and long drug plasma half-life and an increased risk of heart failure.

For mention of the cardiovascular effects of the selective cyclo-oxygenase-2 inhibitors including their lack of antiplatelet activity, see under Rofecoxib, p.81.

1. Johnson AG, *et al*. Do nonsteroidal anti-inflammatory drugs affect blood pressure? *Ann Intern Med* 1994; **121**: 289–300.
2. Pope JE, *et al*. A meta-analysis of the effects of nonsteroidal anti-inflammatory drugs on blood pressure. *Arch Intern Med* 1993; **153**: 477–84.
3. Gurwitz JH, *et al*. Initiation of antihypertensive treatment during nonsteroidal anti-inflammatory drug therapy. *JAMA* 1994; **272**: 781–6.
4. Page J, Henry D. Consumption of NSAIDs and the development of congestive heart failure in elderly patients: an underrecognised public health problem. *Arch Intern Med* 2000; **160**: 777–84.

Effects on the CNS. A literature review[1] revealed that headache, hearing loss, and tinnitus are the most frequent CNS adverse effects in patients taking NSAIDs. Aseptic meningitis has occurred rarely in patients using NSAIDs such as naproxen, sulindac, or tolmetin, but the most common reports are in patients with systemic lupus erythematosus who were receiving ibuprofen (see also p.43). Reports of psychosis appear to be rare and have involved indometacin or sulindac, but in the reviewers' experience it is probably under-reported and is typically seen in elderly patients given indometacin. The role of NSAIDs in the development of cognitive decline in the elderly is unclear. They have been associated with memory impairment and attention deficits in elderly patients,[1,2] especially when given in high doses;[3] however some authors have also reported that long-term NSAID use may reduce the rate of cognitive decline[3,4] or the risk of developing Alzheimer's disease.[5]

1. Hoppmann RA, *et al*. Central nervous system side effects of nonsteroidal anti-inflammatory drugs: aseptic meningitis, psychosis, and cognitive dysfunction. *Arch Intern Med* 1991; **151**: 1309–13.
2. Saag KG, *et al*. Nonsteroidal antiinflammatory drugs and cognitive decline in the elderly. *J Rheumatol* 1995; **22**: 2142–7.
3. Karplus TM, Saag KG. Nonsteroidal anti-inflammatory drugs and cognitive function - do they have a beneficial or deleterious effect? *Drug Safety* 1998; **19**: 427–33.
4. Rozzini R, *et al*. Protective effect of chronic NSAID use on cognitive decline in older persons. *J Am Geriatr Soc* 1996; **44**: 1025–9.
5. Stewart WF, *et al*. Risk of Alzheimer's disease and duration of NSAID use. *Neurology* 1997; **48**: 626–32.

Effects on electrolytes. See under Effects on the Kidneys, below.

Effects on the eyes. Ocular effects such as blurred vision occur rarely in patients taking NSAIDs. Other more serious effects on the eyes associated with NSAIDs also appear to be rare. In the USA the National Registry of Drug-Induced Ocular Side Effects analysed 144 reports they received of possible adverse optic nerve reactions associated with the use of NSAIDs.[1] Of the 24 cases of papilloedema with or without pseudotumour cerebri more than half were associated with propionic acid derivatives, but it was considered that the data indicated that, on rare occasions, most NSAIDs could cause this effect; the number of reports for individual drugs was: 7 for ibuprofen, 5 each for indometacin and naproxen, 3 for meclofenamate, and 1 each for diflunisal, ketoprofen, sulindac, and fenoprofen. Almost two-thirds of the 120 cases of optic or retrobulbar neuritis were also associated with propionic acid derivatives; the number of reports for individual drugs was: ibuprofen 43, naproxen 17, indometacin 9, benoxaprofen 8, phenylbutazone 8, piroxicam 8, zomepirac 7, sulindac 6, fenoprofen 5, oxyphenbutazone 3, meclofenamate 2, tolmetin 2, diflunisal 1, and ketoprofen 1.

There have been reports of severe corneal toxicity associated with the use of some topical NSAIDs, such as diclofenac and ketorolac, in the eye (see p.30).

1. Fraunfelder FT, *et al*. Possible optic nerve side effects associated with nonsteroidal anti-inflammatory drugs. *J Toxicol Cutan Ocul Toxicol* 1994; **13**: 311–16.

Effects on the gastrointestinal tract. NSAIDs can cause clinically important damage of the gastrointestinal tract. The complex mechanisms involved are not fully understood, although it is generally accepted that the inhibition of cyclo-oxygenase-1 (COX-1) results in gastrointestinal toxicity and that the selective COX-2 inhibitors may be less gastrotoxic than the traditional NSAIDs (see below).[1-5] The gastric mucosa is damaged both by local and systemic effects of NSAIDs.[2] The local effect is pH-dependent and varies between individual drugs. The systemic effect is pH-independent, can occur with any route of administration, and is less drug specific; it is this effect that is thought to involve COX-1 inhibition.

NSAIDs may increase the incidence of bleeding in the upper gastrointestinal tract and of perforation, but serious complications are relatively infrequent. Although the effects of NSAIDs on the upper gastrointestinal tract are well recognised they have also been associated with damage to the distal small intestine and colon.[6-8] Risk factors continue to be studied and so far the most important patient-related factors for upper gastrointestinal toxicity are old age, a history of peptic ulcers or bleeding of the gastrointestinal tract, and concomitant use of corticosteroids. A pilot study has also suggested that NSAIDs can produce a high degree of gastrointestinal toxicity in children.[9] Whether infection with *Helicobacter pylori* affects the risk for NSAID-induced peptic ulcers is unclear.[10] Duration of therapy is not thought to influence the risk for serious events; a recent cohort study[11] has found that the risk of gastrointestinal bleeding or perforation with NSAIDs is constant throughout treatment.

Several studies[12-14] have been conducted on the relative toxicity of oral NSAIDs on the upper gastrointestinal tract and various rankings of these drugs have been discussed.[15-17] The UK Committee on Safety of Medicines (CSM)[17] examined 10 epidemiological studies for 7 oral non-aspirin NSAIDs and also examined the spontaneous reports they had received of gastrointestinal effects associated with NSAIDs. The CSM concluded that **azapropazone** was associated with the *highest* risk of gastrointestinal reactions and **ibuprofen** with the *lowest* risk. **Piroxicam, ketoprofen, indometacin, naproxen,** and **diclofenac** had an *intermediate* risk; it was considered that the risk for piroxicam might be higher than for the other NSAIDs with intermediate toxicity. In a systematic review[18] of controlled epidemiological studies that found a relation between NSAID use and hospital admission for gastric haemorrhage or perforation, the low risk of serious gastric toxicity with ibuprofen appeared to be attributable mainly to the low doses used clinically; higher doses of ibuprofen were associated with a similar risk to indometacin and naproxen. For reference to an association between aspirin and the most severe gastric lesions compared with other NSAIDs, see p.15. Results from controlled trials have confirmed that the selective COX-2 inhibitors are associated with a lower incidence of serious gastrointestinal effects, such as bleeding, perforation, and obstruction, than the traditional NSAIDs[19] (see also Celecoxib, p.24 and Rofecoxib, p.81 for further details). However, since the risk of such effects is inherently low in those with no history of peptic ulcer disease, the general prescribing of selective COX-2 inhibitors to all patients requiring an NSAID is questioned. Indeed, in the UK, the use of selective COX-2 inhibitors is limited to those at high risk of developing serious gastrointestinal problems if given a non-selective NSAID. High-risk patients include the elderly, those already receiving gastrotoxic drugs, and those with existing gastrointestinal disorders.

There has been concern that topical use of NSAIDs may also be associated with gastrointestinal toxicity but a case-controlled study[20] concluded that topical administration was not associated with significant upper gastrointestinal bleeding or perforation.

Apart from the selection of an NSAID with a lower risk for gastrointestinal toxicity, other methods used for the prevention or treatment of NSAID-associated ulceration are discussed under the treatment of peptic ulcer disease on p.1208.

1. Hayllar J, Bjarnason I. NSAIDs, Cox-2 inhibitors, and the gut. *Lancet* 1995; **346**: 521–2.
2. Bjorkman DJ. Nonsteroidal anti-inflammatory drug-induced gastrointestinal injury. *Am J Med* 1996; **101** (suppl 1A): 25S–32S.
3. Soll A. Pathogenesis of nonsteroidal anti-inflammatory drug-related upper gastrointestinal toxicity. *Am J Med* 1998; **105** (suppl 5A): 10S–16S.
4. Hawkey CJ. COX-2 inhibitors. *Lancet* 1999; **353**: 307–14. Correction. *ibid.* 1440. [dose]
5. Wolfe MM, et al. Gastrointestinal toxicity of nonsteroidal anti-inflammatory drugs. *N Engl J Med* 1999; **340**: 1888–99.
6. Kwo PY, Tremaine WJ. Nonsteroidal anti-inflammatory drug-induced enteropathy: case discussion and review of the literature. *Mayo Clin Proc* 1995; **70**: 55–61.
7. Gleeson MH, et al. Non-steroidal anti-inflammatory drugs, salicylates, and colitis. *Lancet* 1996; **347**: 904–5.
8. Evans JMM, et al. Non-steroidal anti-inflammatory drugs are associated with emergency admission to hospital for colitis due to inflammatory bowel disease. *Gut* 1997; **40**: 619–22.
9. Mulberg AE, et al. Identification of nonsteroidal antiinflammatory drug-induced gastroduodenal injury in children with juvenile rheumatoid arthritis. *J Pediatr* 1993; **122**: 647–9.
10. Marshall B. NSAIDs and Helicobacter pylori: therapeutic options. *Lancet* 1998; **352**: 1001–3.
11. MacDonald TM, et al. Association of upper gastrointestinal toxicity of non-steroidal anti-inflammatory drugs with continued exposure: cohort study. *BMJ* 1997; **315**: 1333–7.
12. Kaufman DW, et al. Nonsteroidal anti-inflammatory drug use in relation to major upper gastrointestinal bleeding. *Clin Pharmacol Ther* 1993; **53**: 485–94.
13. García Rodríguez LA, Jick H. Risk of upper gastrointestinal bleeding and perforation associated with individual non-steroidal anti-inflammatory drugs. *Lancet* 1994; **343**: 769–72.
14. Langman MJS, et al. Risks of bleeding peptic ulcer associated with individual non-steroidal anti-inflammatory drugs. *Lancet* 1994; **343**: 1075–8.
15. Bateman DN. NSAIDs: time to re-evaluate gut toxicity. *Lancet* 1994; **343**: 1051–2.
16. Smith CC, et al. NSAIDs and gut toxicity. *Lancet* 1994; **344**: 56–7.
17. Committee on Safety of Medicines/Medicines Control Agency. Relative safety of oral non-aspirin NSAIDs. *Current Problems* 1994; **20**: 9–11.

18. Henry D, et al. Variability in risk of gastrointestinal complications with individual non-steroidal anti-inflammatory drugs: results of a collaborative meta-analysis. *BMJ* 1996; **312**: 1563–6.
19. Fitzgerald GA, Patrono C. The coxibs, selective inhibitors of cyclooxygenase-2. *N Engl J Med* 2001; **345**: 433–42.
20. Evans JMM, et al. Topical non-steroidal anti-inflammatory drugs and admission to hospital for upper gastrointestinal bleeding and perforation: a record linkage case-control study. *BMJ* 1995; **311**: 22–6.

Effects on the joints. There is concern that NSAIDs such as indometacin may accelerate the rate of cartilage destruction in patients with osteoarthritis.[1,2]

1. Rashad S, et al. Effect of non-steroidal anti-inflammatory drugs on the course of osteoarthritis. *Lancet* 1989; **ii**: 519–22.
2. Huskisson EC, et al. Effects of antiinflammatory drugs on the progression of osteoarthritis of the knee. *J Rheumatol* 1995; **22**: 1941–6.

Effects on the kidneys. NSAIDs can produce a number of different renal disorders following systemic or topical administration,[1] some of which are due to their inhibition of prostaglandin synthesis.[2,3] Under normal conditions prostaglandins appear to have little effect on renal homoeostasis but in the presence of renal vasoconstriction their vasodilator action increases renal blood flow and thereby helps to maintain renal function.[4,5] Patients whose renal function is being maintained by prostaglandins are therefore at risk from NSAIDs. Such patients include those with impaired circulation, the elderly, those on diuretics, and those with heart failure or renal vascular disease.[2,4] Other risk factors for renal impairment with NSAIDs include dehydration, cirrhosis, surgery, sepsis,[6] and a history of gout or hyperuricaemia.[6,7] The half-life of an NSAID may be a more important determinant of the risk of developing functional renal impairment than the ingested dose.[7] Evidence of renal toxicity of the cyclo-oxygenase-2 (COX-2) selective inhibitors is less extensive; however such NSAIDS appear to have effects on renal function similar to those of the non-selective NSAIDs.[8]

ACE inhibitors can also produce renal impairment and combined use with NSAIDs should be undertaken with great care. Prostaglandin inhibition may also lead to salt and water retention particularly when there is pre-existing hypertension or sodium depletion.[4] NSAIDs, therefore, tend to counteract the action of diuretics and antihypertensives.[2,4] There have been isolated reports of severe hyponatraemia and other symptoms resembling the syndrome of inappropriate antidiuretic hormone secretion in patients taking NSAIDs.[9,10]

Potassium homoeostasis is less dependent on prostaglandins and hyperkalaemia occurs infrequently with NSAIDs.[3] It is more likely to occur in patients with specific risk factors such as those receiving potassium supplements or potassium-sparing diuretics.[3] Indometacin appears to be the main NSAID implicated (see also Effects on Electrolytes, p.45).

NSAIDs may cause acute interstitial nephritis, perhaps involving an allergic response,[2,3,11] and it may progress to interstitial fibrosis or papillary necrosis.[3,12]

Analgesic abuse or prolonged excessive use can produce nephropathy, a condition characterised by renal papillary necrosis and chronic interstitial nephritis, and, eventually, renal failure.[13] Phenacetin, a para-aminophenol derivative, has long been recognised as being one of the main drugs responsible for analgesic nephropathy,[14,15] but nephropathy has also been associated with the long-term use of NSAIDs and paracetamol without phenacetin.[16]

1. O'Callaghan CA, et al. Renal disease and use of topical nonsteroidal anti-inflammatory drugs. *BMJ* 1994; **308**: 110–11.
2. Kendall MJ, Horton RC. Clinical pharmacology and therapeutics. *Postgrad Med J* 1990; **66**: 186–.
3. Whelton A, Hamilton CW. Nonsteroidal anti-inflammatory drugs: effects on kidney function. *J Clin Pharmacol* 1991; **31**: 588–98.
4. Harris K. The role of prostaglandins in the control of renal function. *Br J Anaesth* 1992; **69**: 233–5.
5. Kenny GNC. Potential renal, haematological and allergic adverse effects associated with nonsteroidal anti-inflammatory drugs. *Drugs* 1992; **44** (suppl 5): 31–7.
6. MacDonald TM. Selected side-effects: 14. non-steroidal anti-inflammatory drugs and renal damage. *Prescribers' J* 1994; **34**: 77–80.
7. Henry D, et al. Consumption of non-steroidal anti-inflammatory drugs and the development of functional renal impairment in elderly subjects: results of a case-control study. *Br J Clin Pharmacol* 1997; **44**: 85–90.
8. Perazella MA, Tray K. Selective cyclooxygenase-2 inhibitors: a pattern of nephrotoxicity similar to traditional nonsteroidal anti-inflammatory drugs. *Am J Med* 2001; **111**: 64–7.
9. Petersson I, et al. Water intoxication associated with non-steroidal anti-inflammatory drug therapy. *Acta Med Scand* 1987; **221**: 221–3.
10. Cheung NT, et al. Syndrome of inappropriate secretion of antidiuretic hormone induced by diclofenac. *BMJ* 1993; **306**: 186.
11. Ravnskov U. Glomerular, tubular and interstitial nephritis associated with non-steroidal anti-inflammatory drugs. Evidence of a common mechanism. *Br J Clin Pharmacol* 1999; **47**: 203–10.
12. Sandler DP, et al. Nonsteroidal anti-inflammatory drugs and the risk for chronic renal disease. *Ann Intern Med* 1991; **115**: 165–72.
13. De Broe ME, Elseviers MM. Analgesic nephropathy. *N Engl J Med* 1998; **338**: 446–52.
14. Dubach UC, et al. Analgesic use and chronic renal disease. *N Engl J Med* 1989; **320**: 1238–43.
15. Dubach UC, et al. An epidemiologic study of abuse of analgesic drugs: effects of phenacetin and salicylate on mortality and cardiovascular morbidity (1968 to 1987). *N Engl J Med* 1991; **324**: 155–60.
16. Perneger TV, et al. Risk of kidney failure associated with the use of acetaminophen, aspirin, and nonsteroidal antiinflammatory drugs. *N Engl J Med* 1994; **331**: 1675–9.

Effects on the liver. A retrospective study involving over 220 000 adults who were either using, or had used, NSAIDs identified a small excess risk of serious, acute non-infectious liver injury; in current users there was a twofold increase in risk and there was a predominance of the cholestatic type of liver injury among such patients. Nonetheless, admissions to hospital for liver injury had been rare.[1] In a review[2] of cohort and case-control studies describing an association between NSAIDs and liver disease, the strongest evidence emerged for sulindac. There were also a significant number of reports of hepatotoxicity on rechallenge with diclofenac. Evidence of hepatotoxicity for other NSAIDs was weak, although the risk appeared to be high when they were used with other hepatotoxic drugs. However, the overall incidence of liver disease with NSAIDs was very low.

1. García Rodríguez LA, et al. The role of non-steroidal anti-inflammatory drugs in acute liver injury. *BMJ* 1992; **305**: 865–8. Correction. *ibid.*: 920.
2. Manoukian AV, Carson JL. Nonsteroidal anti-inflammatory drug-induced hepatic disorders. *Drug Safety* 1996; **15**: 64–71.

Effects on the lungs. Adverse pulmonary effects such as pneumonitis, alveolitis, pulmonary infiltrates, and pulmonary fibrosis, often suggestive of an allergic or immune reaction, have been reported with a number of NSAIDs. For references, see under individual monographs.

Effects on the pancreas. A review[1] of drug-induced pancreatitis considered that sulindac was amongst the drugs for which a definite association with pancreatitis had been established. There had been isolated reports of pancreatitis with ketoprofen, mefenamic acid, and piroxicam but any association was considered to be questionable. For further references see under individual monographs.

1. Underwood TW, Frye CB. Drug-induced pancreatitis. *Clin Pharm* 1993; **12**: 440–8.

Effects on the skin. The diverse cutaneous reactions to NSAIDs have been reviewed.[1] Of 250 children attending a rheumatology clinic 34 (13.6%) were found to have 4 or more facial scars of unknown origin.[2] This number of scars was found in 22.2% of the 116 children who had received naproxen and in 9.2% of the 87 who had received other NSAIDs. Children affected were more likely to have light skin and blue or green eyes. It was not known whether this was a form of phototoxic reaction but pseudoporphyria-like eruptions associated with NSAIDs, and naproxen in particular (see p.61), have been reported.

See also under Hypersensitivity, below.

1. Bigby M, Stern R. Cutaneous reactions to nonsteroidal anti-inflammatory drugs. *J Am Acad Dermatol* 1985; **12**: 866–76.
2. Wallace CA, et al. Increased risk of facial scars in children taking nonsteroidal antiinflammatory drugs. *J Pediatr* 1994; **125**: 819–22.

Hypersensitivity. NSAIDs have produced a wide range of hypersensitivity reactions in susceptible individuals; the most common include skin rashes, urticaria, rhinitis, angioedema, bronchoconstriction, and anaphylactic shock. Hypersensitivity to NSAIDs appears to occur more frequently in patients with asthma or allergic disorders but other risk factors have been identified (for further details see under Aspirin, p.15). The occurrence of aspirin sensitivity in patients with asthma and nasal polyps has been referred to as the 'aspirin triad'. There is considerable cross-reactivity between aspirin and other NSAIDs and it is generally recommended that patients who have had a hypersensitivity reaction to aspirin or any other NSAID should avoid all NSAIDs. For references to hypersensitivity reactions associated with NSAIDs, see under individual monographs.

Overdosage. The clinical signs and symptoms following acute overdosage of NSAIDs and methods of treatment have been reviewed.[1] In general, symptoms of NSAID poisoning are mild, and usually include nausea and vomiting, headache, drowsiness, blurred vision, and dizziness. There have been isolated case reports of more serious toxicity, including seizures, hypotension, apnoea, coma, and renal failure, although usually after ingestion of substantial quantities. Seizures are a particular problem with mefenamic acid overdosage.

Treatment of NSAID overdosage is entirely supportive. Gastric lavage and activated charcoal may be of benefit within 1 hour of ingestion. Multiple doses of activated charcoal may be useful in enhancing elimination of NSAIDs with long half-lives such as piroxicam and sulindac. Forced diuresis, haemodialysis, or haemoperfusion are unlikely to be of benefit for NSAID overdosage, although haemodialysis may be required if oliguric renal failure develops.

1. Smolinske SC, et al. Toxic effects of nonsteroidal anti-inflammatory drugs in overdose: an overview of recent evidence on clinical effects and dose-response relationships. *Drug Safety* 1990; **5**: 252–74.

Precautions

NSAIDs should not be given to patients with peptic ulceration and should be used with caution, if at all, in patients with a history of such disorders. To reduce the risk of gastrointestinal effects, NSAIDs may be taken with or after food or milk. Histamine H$_2$-antagonists, omeprazole, or misoprostol may be used for a similar purpose in high-risk patients (see under Peptic Ulcer Disease, p.1208). However, food, milk, and such measures may reduce the rate and extent of drug absorption. UK authorities recommend that NSAIDs associated with the lowest risk of gastrointestinal toxicity (see Effects on the Gastrointestinal Tract, under Adverse Effects, above) should be tried first in the lowest recommended dose, and not more than one oral NSAID should be used at a time; selective inhibitors of cyclo-oxygenase-2 (COX-2) are reserved for patients at highest risk.

NSAIDs should be used with caution in patients with infections, since symptoms such as fever and inflammation may be masked, and also used with caution in patients with asthma or allergic disorders. NSAIDs (including topical NSAIDs) are contra-indicated in patients with a history of hypersensitivity reactions to such drugs, including those in whom attacks of asthma, angioedema, urticaria, or rhinitis have been precipitated by aspirin or any other NSAID.

Other general precautions to be observed include administration to patients with haemorrhagic disorders, hypertension, and impaired renal, hepatic, or cardiac function. Patients undergoing therapy with some NSAIDs may need to be monitored for the development of blood, kidney, liver, or eye disorders. NSAIDs should be used with caution in the elderly and may need to be given in reduced doses.

Regular use of NSAIDs during the third trimester of pregnancy may result in closure of fetal ductus arteriosus *in utero*, and possibly in persistent pulmonary hypertension of the newborn. The onset of labour may be delayed and its duration increased.

Some NSAIDs can interfere with thyroid function tests by lowering serum-thyroid hormone concentrations.

Further details concerning the precautions of the individual NSAIDs may be found under their respective monographs.

Pregnancy. Results from a case-control interview study[1] suggested that prenatal ingestion of aspirin or other NSAIDs might be implicated in persistent pulmonary hypertension of the newborn. The authors suggested that these drugs may be responsible for gestational structural or functional alterations of the pulmonary vasculature. However, the primary cause might also have been the underlying disorder for which the NSAIDs or aspirin were ingested. They were unable to pinpoint in which trimester the drugs might have their proposed action, and concluded that further evaluation was necessary. A more recent study[2] has found that persistent pulmonary hypertension of the newborn is significantly associated with *in utero* NSAID exposure, particularly to aspirin, ibuprofen, and naproxen. Fetal exposure to an NSAID was confirmed by meconium analysis.

Another study[3] has suggested that the risk of miscarriage is increased with NSAID use; however, the authors pointed out that the observation remained to be confirmed. The same study also found no association between NSAID use and congenital abnormalities, low birth weight, or preterm birth.

Most manufacturers recommend avoidance of NSAIDs during pregnancy, unless the proposed benefit outweighs the risks, but in many cases published data on use of the drugs in pregnancy is scanty or absent, making an informed decision difficult.

1. Van Marter LJ, *et al.* Persistent pulmonary hypertension of the newborn and smoking and aspirin and nonsteroidal antiinflammatory drug consumption during pregnancy. *Pediatrics* 1996; **97:** 658–63.
2. Alano MA, *et al.* Analysis of nonsteroidal antiinflammatory drugs in meconium and its relation to persistent pulmonary hypertension of the newborn. *Pediatrics* 2001; **107:** 519–23.
3. Nielsen GL, *et al.* Risk of adverse birth outcome and miscarriage in pregnant users of non-steroidal anti-inflammatory drugs: population based observational study and case-control study. *BMJ* 2001; **322:** 266–70.

Renal impairment. The *British National Formulary* recommends that NSAIDs in general should be given at the lowest effective dose in patients with mild renal impairment and that renal function should be carefully monitored; they should be avoided if possible in patients with moderate to severe renal impairment.

See also under individual monographs.

Thyroid function tests. References to the interference with thyroid function tests by some NSAIDs.

1. Bishnoi A, *et al.* Effect of commonly prescribed nonsteroidal anti-inflammatory drugs on thyroid hormone measurements. *Am J Med* 1994; **96:** 235–8.

Interactions

Notable interactions involving NSAIDs include enhancement of the effects of oral anticoagulants (especially by azapropazone and phenylbutazone) and in-

creased plasma concentrations of lithium, methotrexate, and cardiac glycosides. The risk of nephrotoxicity may be increased if given with ACE inhibitors, ciclosporin, tacrolimus, or diuretics. Effects on renal function may lead to reduced excretion of some drugs. There may also be an increased risk of hyperkalaemia with ACE inhibitors and potassium-sparing diuretics. The antihypertensive effects of some antihypertensives including ACE inhibitors, beta blockers, and diuretics may be reduced. Convulsions may occur due to an interaction with quinolones. NSAIDs may enhance the effects of phenytoin and sulfonylurea antidiabetics. The effects of NSAIDs might be enhanced by use with moclobemide. The concomitant use of more than one NSAID (including aspirin) should be avoided because of the increased risk of adverse effects. The risk of gastrointestinal bleeding and ulceration associated with NSAIDs is increased when used with corticosteroids, the antiplatelets clopidogrel and ticlopidine, or, possibly, alcohol, bisphosphonates, or oxpentifylline [pentoxifylline]. There may be an increased risk of haematotoxicity during concomitant use of zidovudine and NSAIDs; blood counts 1 to 2 weeks after starting use together are recommended. Ritonavir may increase the plasma concentrations of NSAIDs. The manufacturer of mifepristone advises that NSAIDs or aspirin should be avoided for 8 to 12 days after mifepristone use because of a theoretical risk that these prostaglandin synthetase inhibitors may alter the efficacy of mifepristone. There have been occasional reports of increased adverse effects when NSAIDs were given with misoprostol although such combinations have sometimes been employed to *decrease* the gastrointestinal toxicity of NSAIDs.

Further details concerning the interactions of the individual NSAIDs may be found under their respective monographs.

◊ References.

1. Brouwers JRBJ, de Smet PAGM. Pharmacokinetic-pharmacodynamic drug interactions with nonsteroidal anti-inflammatory drugs. *Clin Pharmacokinet* 1994; **27:** 462–85.

Antihypertensives. For reference to the relative effects of NSAIDs in antagonising different types of antihypertensive drugs, see Effects on the Cardiovascular System under Adverse Effects, above.

Pharmacokinetics

Details of the pharmacokinetics of individual NSAIDs may be found under their respective monographs.

◊ General reviews.

1. Woodhouse KW, Wynne H. The pharmacokinetics of non-steroidal anti-inflammatory drugs in the elderly. *Clin Pharmacokinet* 1987; **12:** 111–22.
2. Walson PD, Mortensen ME. Pharmacokinetics of common analgesics, anti-inflammatories and antipyretics in children. *Clin Pharmacokinet* 1989; **17** (suppl 1): 116–37.
3. Simkin PA, *et al.* Articular pharmacokinetics of protein-bound antirheumatic agents. *Clin Pharmacokinet* 1993; **25:** 342–50.
4. Lapicque F, *et al.* Protein binding and stereoselectivity of nonsteroidal anti-inflammatory drugs. *Clin Pharmacokinet* 1993; **25:** 115–25.
5. Day RO, *et al.* Pharmacokinetics of nonsteroidal anti-inflammatory drugs in synovial fluid. *Clin Pharmacokinet* 1999; **36:** 191–210.

Uses and Administration

Administered as single doses or in short-term intermittent therapy NSAIDs can relieve mild to moderate pain. However, it may take up to 3 weeks of use before their anti-inflammatory effects become evident. The combined analgesic and anti-inflammatory effects make them particularly useful for the symptomatic relief of painful and/or inflammatory conditions including rheumatic disorders such as rheumatoid arthritis, osteoarthritis, and the spondyloarthropathies, and also in peri-articular disorders, and soft-tissue rheumatism. Some NSAIDs are used in the management of postoperative pain. Some NSAIDs, but not aspirin or other salicylates, are also used to treat acute gouty arthritis.

Generally, it is felt that there are only small differences in anti-inflammatory activity between the various NSAIDs and choice is largely empirical. Responses

of individual patients vary widely. Thus, if a patient fails to respond to one NSAID, another drug may be successful. However, it has been recommended that NSAIDs associated with a low risk of gastrointestinal toxicity should generally be preferred and the lowest effective dose used. Treatment with NSAIDs such as celecoxib and rofecoxib that are selective inhibitors of cyclo-oxygenase-2 is limited in the UK to those patients considered to be at high risk of developing serious gastrointestinal problems if given a non-selective NSAID (see Effects on the Gastrointestinal Tract, above).

NSAIDs are usually given by mouth, with or after food, although some such as diclofenac, ketoprofen, ketorolac, piroxicam, and tenoxicam can be given by intramuscular injection; diclofenac, ketorolac, and tenoxicam can also be given intravenously. Some NSAIDs are applied topically or given rectally as suppositories.

Several NSAIDs are used in ophthalmic preparations for the inhibition of intra-operative miosis, control of postoperative ocular inflammation, and prevention of cystoid macular oedema.

Action. Cyclo-oxygenases play an important role in the biosynthesis of prostaglandins (p.1438). NSAIDs inhibit cyclo-oxygenase-1 (COX-1) and cyclo-oxygenase-2 (COX-2) and it is thought that inhibition of COX-1 is associated with adverse gastrointestinal effects while inhibition of COX-2 is associated with anti-inflammatory activity,[1-6] hence the interest[7] in preferential or selective inhibitors of COX-2. COX-2 inhibitors may also have a potential use in other diseases in which COX-2 might be implicated.[4] Meloxicam and nimesulide are preferential inhibitors of COX-2, that is they have a higher selectivity for COX-2 than COX-1 but are not exclusive COX-2 inhibitors; etodolac and nabumetone are also claimed to have preference for COX-2 although there is less evidence for this. Drugs with a very high selectivity for COX-2 have also been developed. Celecoxib and rofecoxib are two examples. Although the selective inhibition of COX-2 may be associated with reduced gastrointestinal toxicity, adverse effects associated with such inhibition have been noted in other body systems, see Effects on the Cardiovascular System and Effects on the Kidneys, above.

There is evidence that NSAIDs may also have a central mechanism of action that augments the peripheral mechanism.[6]

Many NSAIDs possess centres of chirality within their molecular structure, with different chiral forms (enantiomers) having different degrees of pharmacological activity.[8,9] For example, indometacin, its analogues, and some arylpropionic acids are chiral drugs with the S(+)-enantiomer in most cases showing the dominant pharmacological activity. However, the ratio of S/R activity varies between drugs and between animal species. NSAIDs are generally administered clinically as the racemate with only a few currently being given as the (S)-enantiomer (for example, dexketoprofen). The chirality of a drug may have subtle effects on its toxicity and interactions, and it may be more desirable to administer a drug as its active enantiomer.[9]

1. Hayllar J, Bjarnason I. NSAIDs, Cox-2 inhibitors, and the gut. *Lancet* 1995; **346:** 521–2.
2. Bennett A, Tavares IA. NSAIDs, Cox-2 inhibitors, and the gut. *Lancet* 1995; **346:** 1105.
3. Vane JR. NSAIDs, Cox-2 inhibitors, and the gut. *Lancet* 1995; **346:** 1105–6.
4. Jouzeau J-Y, *et al.* Cyclo-oxygenase isoenzymes: how recent findings affect thinking about nonsteroidal anti-inflammatory drugs. *Drugs* 1997; **53:** 563–82.
5. Richardson C, Emery P. The clinical implications of inhibition of the inducible form of cyclo-oxygenase. *Drug Safety* 1996; **15:** 249–60.
6. Cashman JN. The mechanisms of action of NSAIDs in analgesia. *Drugs* 1996; **52** (suppl 5): 13–23.
7. Hawkey CJ. COX-2 inhibitors. *Lancet* 1999; **353:** 307–14. Correction. *ibid.* 1440. [dose]
8. Kean WF, *et al.* Chirality in antirheumatic drugs. *Lancet* 1991; **338:** 1565–8.
9. Hayball PJ. Chirality and nonsteroidal anti-inflammatory drugs. *Drugs* 1996; **52** (suppl 5): 47–58.

Colic pain. Prostaglandins have been implicated in the aetiology of biliary colic (p.5), and some NSAIDs such as diclofenac, indometacin, and ketoprofen have been used to relieve such pain.

Ectopic ossification. NSAIDs are an effective alternative to radiotherapy for prevention of ectopic ossification (p.744) after surgery or trauma. Indometacin is widely used for this purpose. References.

1. Pagnani MJ, *et al.* Effect of aspirin on heterotopic ossification after total hip arthroplasty in men who have osteoarthrosis. *J Bone Joint Surg Am* 1991; **73A:** 924–9.
2. Knelles D, *et al.* Prevention of heterotopic ossification after total hip replacement: a prospective, randomised study using acetyl-salicylic acid, indomethacin and fractional or single-dose irradiation. *J Bone Joint Surg Br* 1997; **79B:** 596–602.
3. Moore KD, *et al.* Indomethacin versus radiation therapy for prophylaxis against heterotopic ossification in acetabular fractures: a randomised, prospective study. *J Bone Joint Surg Br* 1998; **80:** 259–63.

4. Kolbi O, *et al.* Preoperative irradiation versus the use of nonster-oidal anti-inflammatory drugs for prevention of heterotopic ossi-fication following total hip replacement: the results of a rand-omized trial. *Int J Radiat Oncol Biol Phys* 1998; **42:** 397–401.
5. Sell S, *et al.* The suppression of heterotopic ossifications: radia-tion versus NSAID therapy–a prospective study. *J Arthroplasty* 1998; **13:** 854–9.
6. Kienapfel H, *et al.* Prevention of heterotopic bone formation af-ter total hip arthroplasty: a prospective randomised study com-paring postoperative radiation therapy with indomethacin medi-cation. *Arch Orthop Trauma Surg* 1999; **119:** 296–302.
7. Neal B, *et al.* Non-steroidal anti-inflammatory drugs for prevent-ing heterotopic bone formation after hip arthroplasty (updated 30 August 2001). Available in The Cochrane Library; Issue 4. Ox-ford: Update Software: 2001.

Eye disorders. Miosis resistant to conventional mydriatics of-ten develops during ocular surgery, possibly due to release of prostaglandins and other substances associated with trauma. NSAIDs, which are prostaglandin synthetase inhibitors, are therefore used prophylactically as eye drops before ocular sur-gery to ameliorate intra-operative miosis but there has been some doubt that the effect they produce is of clinical signifi-cance. Those commonly used include diclofenac, indometacin, flurbiprofen, and suprofen. These drugs do not possess intrinsic mydriatic properties.

Some NSAIDs are used topically or systemically in a number of inflammatory ocular disorders, including inflammation and cystoid macular oedema following ocular surgery (see below). However, their role in the treatment of macular oedema associ-ated with uveitis (p.1060) is less clear. NSAIDs are also used in the treatment of scleritis (see p.1058).

References.
1. Flach AJ. Cyclo-oxygenase inhibitors in ophthalmology. *Surv Ophthalmol* 1992; **36:** 259–84.
2. Koay P. The emerging roles of topical non-steroidal anti-inflam-matory agents in ophthalmology. *Br J Ophthalmol* 1996; **80:** 480–5.

POSTOPERATIVE INFLAMMATORY OCULAR DISORDERS. Corticoster-oids are used topically for the control of **postoperative ocular inflammation** but caution is required as they can delay wound healing and mask postoperative infection. They should only be used for short periods as they can cause glaucoma in suscepti-ble individuals. Topical NSAIDs have also been tried. Despite some doubts over efficacy several studies have found eye drops containing diclofenac sodium to be effective in controlling signs of inflammation after ocular surgery,[1-3] but there has been some concern about reports of corneal toxicity (see p.30).

Cystoid macular oedema may follow cataract or retinal de-tachment surgery due to a disturbance of the blood-retinal bar-rier. A number of NSAIDs,[3-6] including diclofenac, flurbipro-fen, indometacin, and ketorolac are used topically with or without corticosteroids to prevent or relieve cystoid macular oedema. NSAIDs such as indometacin are also used systemi-cally in its management.
1. Kraff MC, *et al.* Inhibition of blood-aqueous humor barrier breakdown with diclofenac: a fluorophotometric study. *Arch Ophthalmol* 1990; **108:** 380–3.
2. Wright M, *et al.* Comparison of the efficacy of diclofenac and betamethasone following strabismus surgery. *Br J Ophthalmol* 1997; **81:** 299–301.
3. Italian Diclofenac Study Group. Efficacy of diclofenac eyedrops in preventing postoperative inflammation and long-term cystoid macular edema. *J Cataract Refract Surg* 1997; **23:** 1183–9.
4. Jampol LM. Pharmacologic therapy of aphakic and pseudophak-ic cystoid macular edema. *Ophthalmology* 1985; **92:** 807–10.
5. Flach AJ, *et al.* Effectiveness of ketorolac tromethamine 0.5% ophthalmic solution for chronic aphakic and pseudophakic cyst-oid macular edema. *Am J Ophthalmol* 1987; **103:** 479–86.
6. Jampol LM, *et al.* Nonsteroidal anti-inflammatory drugs and cat-aract surgery. *Arch Ophthalmol* 1994; **112:** 891–4.

Fever. Paracetamol, salicylates and some other NSAIDs are the main antipyretics used to control fever (p.8). Paracetamol is usually the antipyretic of choice in infants and children but ibu-profen appears to be an effective alternative; salicylates are generally contra-indicated in these patients because of the pos-sible link between their use and the development of Reye's syn-drome (see under Adverse Effects of Aspirin, p.15).

Gout. NSAIDs are the drugs usually used first for the treat-ment of acute attacks of gout (p.397). Since the treatment of chronic gout can lead to the mobilisation of urate crystals from established tophi to produce acute attacks, NSAIDs may also be used for the prophylaxis of acute gout during the first few months of antihyperuricaemic therapy.

Headache. An NSAID is often tried first for the symptomatic treatment of various types of headache including migraine (p.449) and tension-type headache (p.450). NSAIDs may also be effective prophylactic drugs for migraine, although pro-pranolol or pizotifen are generally preferred. Chronic paroxys-mal hemicrania, a rare variant of cluster headache (p.449), re-sponds to indometacin.

Kidney disorders. Although NSAIDs can produce adverse effects on the kidney (see above) they may have a role in the management of some types of glomerular kidney disease (p.1051). They may be of use for the control of proteinuria due to nephrotic syndrome except when there is overt renal failure.

Malignant neoplasms. Results of a study by the American Cancer Society[1] have suggested that regular use of aspirin may reduce the risk of developing fatal cancer of the oesophagus, stomach, colon, or rectum. Death rates due to other gastroin-testinal cancers did not appear to be affected. Other studies[2-7] ap-

pear to support the reduced risk of colorectal cancer (p.493) in regular users of aspirin or other NSAIDs. However, a 1998 study[8] found no evidence of an association between the use of aspirin and the incidence of colorectal cancer, although the au-thors suggest that these results may be explained by the short treatment period and the low dose of aspirin used. Long-term use of aspirin may itself be associated with an increased risk of certain other diseases.

Treatment with sulindac (p.86) has been found to reduce the number of polyps in patients with familial adenomatous poly-posis, a condition which predisposes to development of color-ectal cancer. Celecoxib is now indicated for use in such pa-tients.
1. Thun MJ, *et al.* Aspirin use and the risk of fatal cancer. *Cancer Res* 1993; **53:** 1322–7.
2. Rosenberg L, *et al.* A hypothesis: nonsteroidal anti-inflammatory drugs reduce the incidence of large-bowel cancer. *J Natl Cancer Inst* 1991; **83:** 355–8.
3. Logan RFA, *et al.* Effect of aspirin and non-steroidal anti-inflam-matory drugs on colorectal cancer: case-control study of sub-jects participating in the Nottingham faecal occult blood screen-ing programme. *BMJ* 1993; **307:** 285–9.
4. Giovannucci E, *et al.* Aspirin use and the risk for colorectal can-cer and adenoma in male health professionals. *Ann Intern Med* 1994; **121:** 241–6.
5. Giovannucci E, *et al.* Aspirin and the risk of colorectal cancer in women. *N Engl J Med* 1995; **333:** 609–14.
6. Sandler RS, *et al.* Aspirin and nonsteroidal anti-inflammatory agents and risk for colorectal adenomas. *Gastroenterology* 1998; **114:** 441–7.
7. Smalley W, *et al.* Use of nonsteroidal anti-inflammatory drugs and incidence of colorectal cancer: a population-based study. *Arch Intern Med* 1999; **159:** 161–6.
8. Stürmer T, *et al.* Aspirin use and colorectal cancer: post-trial fol-low-up data from the Physicians' Health Study. *Ann Intern Med* 1998; **128:** 713–20.

Menstrual disorders. Menorrhagia (p.1490) is thought to be associated with abnormalities of prostaglandin production. Treatment with NSAIDs such as ibuprofen, mefenamic acid, or naproxen during menstruation, can reduce uterine blood loss by an average of 30% in women with menorrhagia. There does not appear to be any evidence that one NSAID is more effective than another.

NSAIDs are usually the first choice for the pain of dysmenor-rhoea (p.6). Mefenamic acid may have a theoretical advantage over other NSAIDs in being able to inhibit both the synthesis and the peripheral action of prostaglandins, but clinical studies have not shown fenemates to be more effective, and systematic review has suggested that ibuprofen may have the best risk/benefit ratio.

Migraine. See under Headache, above.

Orthostatic hypotension. Fludrocortisone is usually the first drug tried in the treatment of orthostatic hypotension (p.1070) when nonpharmacological treatment has failed. NSAIDs such as flurbiprofen, ibuprofen, or indometacin may be used alone or added to treatment if the response is inade-quate.

Pain. NSAIDs have a similar analgesic effect to aspirin and paracetamol in single doses but, in regular full dosage, they have both a lasting analgesic and an anti-inflammatory effect. They are used in the management of mild to moderate pain (p.2) and are of particular value in pain due to inflammation. NSAIDs may be of benefit for inflammatory pain in infants and children (p.3), although paracetamol is generally the preferred non-opioid analgesic in this age group. NSAIDs may be used in the treatment of acute low back pain (p.6) if paracetamol fails to provide adequate pain relief. NSAIDs may also be used as an adjunct to opioids in the management of severe pain such as cancer pain (p.5) and are particularly effective in bone pain of malignant origin. NSAIDs may be used for postoperative an-algesia (p.4), and are of particular value following day-case surgery because of their lack of sedative effects. They are not usually considered to be strong enough as the sole analgesic following major surgery, but may be used with stronger analge-sics and may allow dosage reduction of concomitant opioids. The pain of mild sickle-cell crises (p.7) may be controlled by analgesics such as NSAIDs or less potent opioids, for example codeine or dihydrocodeine; NSAIDs may be used with more potent opioids such as morphine for severe crises.

Dependence and tolerance are not a problem with non-opioid analgesics such as NSAIDs, but there is a ceiling of efficacy, above which, increasing the dose has no further therapeutic ef-fect.

Rheumatic disorders. NSAIDs provide symptomatic relief for rheumatic disorders such as rheumatoid arthritis (p.9) and spondyloarthropathies (p.10), but they do not alter the course of the disease and additional antirheumatic drugs may need to be given to prevent irreversible joint damage. NSAIDs may also be used as an alternative to paracetamol for osteoarthritis (p.9). Short-term use of oral NSAIDs may help to relieve pain and reduce inflammation of soft-tissue rheumatism (p.10); topical formulations of some NSAIDs are also used but their therapeu-tic role, if any, is unclear.

Opioid Analgesics (6200-n)

Dependence and Withdrawal
Repeated administration of opioids is associated with the development of psychological and physical de-pendence. Although this is less of a problem with le-gitimate therapeutic use, dependence may develop rapidly when opioids are regularly abused for their euphoriant effects. Drug dependence of the opioid type is characterised by an overwhelming need to keep taking the drug (or one with similar properties), by a physical requirement for the drug in order to avoid withdrawal symptoms, and by a tendency to in-crease the dose owing to the development of toler-ance.

Abrupt withdrawal of opioids from persons physical-ly dependent on them precipitates a withdrawal syn-drome, the severity of which depends on the individ-ual, the drug used, the size and frequency of the dose, and the duration of drug use. Withdrawal symptoms may also follow the administration of an opioid an-tagonist such as naloxone or a mixed agonist and an-tagonist such as pentazocine to opioid-dependent per-sons. Neonatal abstinence syndrome may occur in the offspring of opioid-dependent mothers and these in-fants can suffer withdrawal symptoms at birth.

Opioid analgesics can be classified according to the receptors at which they act (see under Uses and Ad-ministration, below) and withdrawal syndromes are characteristic for a receptor type. Cross-tolerance and cross-dependence can be expected between opioids acting at the same receptors. Dependence associated with morphine and closely related μ-agonists appears to result in more severe withdrawal symptoms than that associated with κ-receptor agonists. Onset and duration of withdrawal symptoms also vary according to the duration of action of the specific drug. With morphine and diamorphine *withdrawal symptoms* usually begin within a few hours, reach a peak within 36 to 72 hours, and then gradually subside; they de-velop more slowly with methadone. Withdrawal symptoms include yawning, mydriasis, lachrymation, rhinorrhoea, sneezing, muscle tremor, weakness, sweating, anxiety, irritability, disturbed sleep or in-somnia, restlessness, anorexia, nausea, vomiting, loss of weight, diarrhoea, dehydration, leucocytosis, bone pain, abdominal and muscle cramps, gooseflesh, vas-omotor disturbances, and increases in heart rate, res-piratory rate, blood pressure, and temperature. Some physiological values may not return to normal for several months following the acute withdrawal syn-drome.

Withdrawal symptoms may be terminated by a suita-ble dose of the original or a related opioid. Tolerance diminishes rapidly after withdrawal so that a previ-ously tolerated dose may prove fatal.

For a discussion of the treatment of opioid depend-ence and neonatal abstinence syndrome, see below.

◊ Review.
1. Van Ree JM, *et al.* Opioids, reward and addiction: an encounter of biology, psychology, and medicine. *Pharmacol Rev* 1999; **51:** 341–96.

Diagnosis. Naloxone (p.1015) and other opioid antagonists have been used to diagnose opioid dependence.

Treatment of opioid dependence. The treatment of opioid dependence has been the subject of a number of reviews and discussions.[1-7]
Planned withdrawal (**detoxification**) may be effected slowly or rapidly. The usual method in many countries is to replace the drug of dependence with *methadone* given as a liquid oral prep-aration, and then gradually withdraw the methadone if possi-ble. Methadone is suitable for withdrawal therapy because it can be given orally and its long half-life allows once daily ad-ministration. Oral *diamorphine* has been used similarly to methadone; reefers containing diamorphine have also been used in some centres. *Dihydrocodeine* tablets have been used successfully. *Buprenorphine* given sublingually is another al-ternative to methadone in the treatment of opioid dependence. The methadone derivative *levacetylmethadol* was a more recent introduction but its proarrhythmic effects have led to its use being suspended or severely restricted.

Iatrogenic opioid dependence may occur in patients receiving μ-agonists such as morphine, fentanyl, or pethidine for the management of acute pain or in an intensive care setting for more than 5 to 10 days. Methadone has been used successfully to manage opioid withdrawal in adult intensive care patients.[8] However, some[9] avoid using methadone to manage withdrawal in children because of the stigma of its associations with managing withdrawal in drug addicts. In physically dependent but non-addicted patients, gradual weaning using the same opioid that was used therapeutically is preferred where possible, although in some cases, it may be necessary to change to a different opioid because of ease of administration, duration of action, and ability to taper the dose; virtually any opioid can be used.[9]

Other drugs used in the management of opioid withdrawal include alpha$_2$-adrenoceptor agonists such as *clonidine* and opioid antagonists such as *naltrexone* and *naloxone*. Clonidine may help to suppress symptoms of opioid withdrawal, such as anxiety, insomnia, and muscle aches. It appears to be more effective when used in the control of symptoms following abrupt withdrawal than when used during gradual withdrawal of methadone. Hypotension may limit its usefulness in some patients. The clonidine analogue *lofexidine* may produce similar results to those obtained with clonidine and appears to be less sedating and hypotensive.

Naltrexone and naloxone block the euphoriant effects of opioids although their use in detoxification as monotherapy is limited by unacceptable opioid withdrawal effects. Naltrexone may be used with clonidine and some workers have reported that withdrawal can be achieved within a few days using combined therapy.[10,11] Moreover, naloxone and naltrexone are being used in the relatively new technique of rapid or ultra rapid opioid detoxification,[12,13] which is achieved while the patient is heavily sedated or under *general anaesthesia* and hence unaware of any unpleasant withdrawal symptoms. However, although detoxification may be achieved within 24 hours and has a high initial success rate, the technique itself is not without risks and it does not obviate the need for maintenance treatment (see below).

Concomitant counselling and other psychosocial services have been shown to be important in the outcome of withdrawal therapy.[14] Detoxification alone does not ensure long-term abstinence.

A number of other drugs may be of use as *adjuncts* in the management of withdrawal symptoms. *Diphenoxylate* with atropine or *loperamide* may be used for the control of diarrhoea. *Promethazine* has been used for its antiemetic and sedative actions. Beta blockers such as *propranolol* may be of use for patients with pronounced somatic anxiety symptoms. *Benzodiazepines* or *clomethiazole* can be given to relieve anxiety and associated insomnia but only short courses should be used in order to minimise the risk of dependence and abuse.

Long-term **maintenance** treatment (stabilisation treatment) with an opioid is sometimes used, in conjunction with psychosocial support, to enable the patient to acquire some form of social stability. *Methadone* is most commonly used; the use of *diamorphine* although feasible[15] is controversial[16] and is advocated by only a few individual centres. The use of methadone for maintenance has been reviewed.[17,18] *Naltrexone* can be effective in maintaining abstinence in opioid addicts following detoxification, especially after rapid or ultra rapid detoxification. It is considered that naltrexone would probably be of most use in highly motivated addicts with good sociological and psychological support to discourage impulsive use of opioids.[1,19,20]

The problems associated with the **pregnant** patient with opioid dependence have been discussed.[21] The aim should be to stabilise the patient first using *methadone* since acute withdrawal can result in fetal death. Drug withdrawal is best done slowly during the second trimester. It has been suggested that if patients present during the final trimester and cannot be detoxified, maintenance with *diamorphine* might be preferable to the use of methadone as it might produce less severe withdrawal symptoms in the neonate.[22] The management of neonatal abstinence syndrome is discussed below.

1. Herridge P, Gold MS. Pharmacological adjuncts in the treatment of opioid and cocaine addicts. *J Psychoactive Drugs* 1988; **20**: 233–42.
2. Guthrie SK. Pharmacologic interventions for the treatment of opioid dependence and withdrawal. *DICP Ann Pharmacother* 1990; **24**: 721–34.
3. DOH. *Drug misuse and dependence: guidelines on clinical management.* London: The Stationery Office, 1999.
4. Wodak A. Managing illicit drug use: a practical guide. *Drugs* 1994; **47**: 446–57.
5. Mattick RP, Hall W. Are detoxification programmes effective? *Lancet* 1996; **347**: 97–100.
6. Seivewright NA, Greenwood J. What is important in drug misuse treatment? *Lancet* 1996; **347**: 373–6.
7. National Concensus Development Panel on Effective Medical Treatment of Opiate Addiction. Effective medical treatment of opiate addition. *JAMA* 1998; **280**: 1936–43.
8. Böhrer H, *et al.* Methadone treatment of opioid withdrawal in intensive care patients. *Lancet* 1993; **341**: 636–7.
9. Yaster M, *et al.* The management of opioid and benzodiazepine dependence in infants, children, and adolescents. *Pediatrics* 1996; **98**: 135–40.
10. Charney DS, *et al.* The combined use of clonidine and naltrexone as a rapid, safe, and effective treatment of abrupt withdrawal from methadone. *Am J Psychiatry* 1986; **143**: 831–7.
11. Brewer C, *et al.* Opioid withdrawal and naltrexone induction in 48–72 hours with minimal drop-out, using a modification of the naltrexone-clonidine technique. *Br J Psychiatry* 1988; **153**: 340–3.
12. Justins D. Rapid opioid detoxification under anaesthesia. *Hosp Med* 1998; **59**: 180.

13. Cook TM, Collins PD. Rapid opioid detoxification under anaesthesia. *Hosp Med* 1998; **59**: 245–7.
14. McLellan AT, *et al.* The effects of psychosocial services in substance abuse treatment. *JAMA* 1993; **269**: 1953–9.
15. Perneger TV, *et al.* Randomised trial of heroin maintenance programme for addicts who fail in conventional drug treatments. *BMJ* 1998; **317**: 13–18.
16. Farrell M, Hall W. The Swiss heroin trials: testing alternative approaches. *BMJ* 1998; **316**: 639.
17. Farrell M, *et al.* Methadone maintenance treatment in opiate dependence: a review. *BMJ* 1994; **309**: 997–1001.
18. Ward J, *et al.* Role of maintenance treatment in opioid dependence. *Lancet* 1999; **353**: 221–6.
19. Ginzburg HM, MacDonald MG. The role of naltrexone in the management of drug abuse. *Med Toxicol* 1987; **2**: 83–92.
20. Gonzalez JP, Brogden RN. Naltrexone: a review of its pharmacodynamic and pharmacokinetic properties and therapeutic efficacy in the management of opioid dependence. *Drugs* 1988; **35**: 192–213.
21. Gerada C, *et al.* Management of the pregnant opiate user. *Br J Hosp Med* 1990; **43**: 138–41.
22. Thomas CS, Osborn M. Inhaling heroin during pregnancy. *BMJ* 1988; **296**: 1672.

NEONATAL ABSTINENCE SYNDROME. Infants born to opioid-dependent mothers may suffer withdrawal, with signs including CNS hyperirritability, gastrointestinal dysfunction, respiratory distress, yawning, sneezing, mottling, and fever. Onset of symptoms is partly dependent on the drug abused and varies from shortly after birth to 2 weeks of age, although most symptoms appear within 72 hours. Some symptoms may persist for 3 months or more.

The American Academy of Pediatrics[1] recommended that treatment of the neonate with abstinence syndrome should be primarily supportive and considered that many infants manifesting signs of drug withdrawal could be managed in this way. They advised adoption of abstinence scoring methods to judge the need for drug therapy, although such systems do not appear to have been validated. Drugs that have been used for opioid withdrawal include paregoric (a USP preparation containing opium), diluted tincture of opium, morphine, methadone, diazepam, chlorpromazine, phenobarbital, and clonidine. Naloxone should not routinely be given to infants of opioid-dependent mothers because of the risk of seizures with abrupt opioid withdrawal. The Committee[1] made no hard and fast recommendations but considered that, when appropriate, specific drug therapy should be used for treatment of withdrawal symptoms. Thus for opioid withdrawal, tincture of opium was the preferred drug. Others favour treatment with oral morphine solution.[2]

Practice varies widely and evidence for the efficacy of particular drugs in the management of neonatal abstinence syndrome is scanty and difficult to compare.[3] It has been suggested that diazepam may be less useful than phenobarbital or paregoric but the use of paregoric (which contains both camphor and alcohol) has been questioned. In the UK, chlorpromazine has also been widely used.[4]

1. American Academy of Pediatrics, Committee on Drugs. Neonatal drug withdrawal. *Pediatrics* 1998; **101**: 1079–88. Correction. *ibid.*; **102**: 660 [dosage error].
2. Gregg JEM, *et al.* Maternal narcotic abuse and the newborn. *Arch Dis Child* 1988; **63**: 684.
3. Theis JGW, *et al.* Current management of the neonatal abstinence syndrome: a critical analysis of the evidence. *Biol Neonate* 1997; **71**: 345–56.
4. Morrison CL, Siney C. A survey of the management of neonatal opiate withdrawal in England and Wales. *Eur J Pediatr* 1996; **155**: 323–6.

Adverse Effects

In normal doses the commonest side-effects of opioid analgesics are nausea, vomiting, constipation, drowsiness, and confusion; tolerance to these (except constipation) generally develops with long-term use. Micturition may be difficult and there may be ureteric or biliary spasm; there is also an antidiuretic effect. Dry mouth, dizziness, sweating, facial flushing, headache, vertigo, bradycardia, tachycardia, palpitations, orthostatic hypotension, hypothermia, restlessness, changes of mood, decreased libido or potency, hallucinations, and miosis also occur. These effects tend to occur more commonly in ambulant patients than in those at rest in bed and in those without severe pain. Raised intracranial pressure occurs in some patients. Muscle rigidity has been reported following high doses. The euphoric activity of opioids has led to their abuse. For a discussion of opioid dependence, see above.

Larger doses of opioids produce respiratory depression and hypotension, with circulatory failure and deepening coma. Convulsions may occur, especially in infants and children. Rhabdomyolysis progressing to renal failure has been reported in overdosage. Death may occur from respiratory failure. Toxic doses of specific opioids vary considerably with the individual and regular users may tolerate large doses. The triad of coma, pinpoint pupils, and respiratory depression is considered indicative of opioid overdosage;

dilatation of the pupils occurs as hypoxia develops. Pulmonary oedema after overdosage is a common cause of fatalities among opioid addicts.

Morphine and some other opioids have a dose-related histamine-releasing effect which may be responsible in part for reactions such as urticaria and pruritus as well as hypotension and flushing. Contact dermatitis has been reported and pain and irritation may occur on injection. Anaphylactic reactions following intravenous injection have been reported rarely.

◊ The adverse effects associated with individual opioid analgesics may reflect to some extent their activity at specific opioid receptors (see Uses and Administration, below) or may result from a direct toxic effect.[1,2] Some adverse effects of pure opioid agonists, such as the respiratory depressant effect of morphine, are dose-related, whereas agonist-antagonists such as buprenorphine, butorphanol, and nalbuphine exhibit a 'ceiling effect' as the dose increases.

The type and extent of side-effects experienced in practice may depend on whether or not opioid-sensitive pain is present, whether the opioid analgesic is being given for the control of chronic severe pain or acute pain, and the route of administration. In reviewing the use of opioids in *chronic pain* McQuay[3] commented that, despite worries to the contrary, respiratory depression and dependence liability are not generally a problem when appropriate doses are used to treat opioid-sensitive pain. In fact the presence of opioid-sensitive pain appears to protect against the respiratory depressant effect, although it may occur if the source of opioid-sensitive pain is removed (e.g. by surgery) without adequate reduction in opioid dosage. The side-effects of opioid analgesics when used in advanced cancer have been put into context by Twycross and Lack.[4] They considered constipation to be the most troublesome adverse effect and stated that significant respiratory depression was rarely seen with their suggested regimens, since pain antagonises the central depressant effects of morphine.

In the context of *acute postoperative pain* opioid-induced respiratory depression is of concern but short-term postoperative use is unlikely to cause dependence (although see under Treatment of Opioid Dependence, above for references to iatrogenic physical dependence).[5] It was hoped that administration of opioids by the *spinal route* would result in fewer side-effects, especially respiratory depression. In postoperative pain relief with spinal opioids, the incidence of side-effects is said to be low when patients are properly monitored.[6] However, some[7] have reported pruritus, nausea and vomiting, and urinary retention to be common and respiratory depression to occur; more seriously the appearance of respiratory depression could be considerably delayed. These effects were more common with morphine, but all opioid analgesics had the propensity to produce respiratory depression when given spinally.[7] Delayed respiratory depression has been attributed to the poor lipid solubility of morphine, but does occur after other opioids. Some have considered that despite earlier worries, potentially fatal late respiratory depression was as rare with the spinal route as postoperative respiratory depression with the conventional route.[8,9] Disputes regarding the frequency of respiratory depression associated with even conventional methods of administration of opioid analgesics might be due to the methods used for measuring respiratory effects.[10] The incidence of ventilatory depression has been reported to be higher following intrathecal than epidural administration of morphine.[11]

1. Duthie DJR, Nimmo WS. Adverse effects of opioid analgesic drugs. *Br J Anaesth* 1987; **59**: 61–77.
2. Schug SA, *et al.* Adverse effects of systemic opioid analgesics. *Drug Safety* 1992; **7**: 200–13.
3. McQuay HJ. Opioids in chronic pain. *Br J Anaesth* 1989; **63**: 213–26.
4. Twycross RG, Lack SA. *Oral morphine in advanced cancer.* 2nd ed. Beaconsfield: Beaconsfield Publishers, 1989.
5. Mitchell RWD, Smith G. The control of acute postoperative pain. *Br J Anaesth* 1989; **63**: 147–58.
6. Lutz LJ, Lamer TJ. Management of postoperative pain: review of current techniques and methods. *Mayo Clin Proc* 1990; **65**: 584–96.
7. Morgan M. The rational use of intrathecal and extradural opioids. *Br J Anaesth* 1989; **63**: 165–88.
8. Anonymous. Spinal opiates revisited. *Lancet* 1986; **i**: 655–6.
9. McQuay HJ. Spinal opiates. *Br J Hosp Med* 1987; **37**: 354–5.
10. Wheatley RG, *et al.* Postoperative hypoxaemia: comparison of extradural, i.m. and patient-controlled opioid analgesia. *Br J Anaesth* 1990; **64**: 267–75.
11. Gustafsson LL, *et al.* Adverse effects of extradural and intrathecal opiates: report of a nationwide survey in Sweden. *Br J Anaesth* 1982; **54**: 479–85.

Effects on the biliary tract and liver. Opioids may cause spasm of the sphincter of Oddi (see also below), and this may be associated with raised serum concentrations of amylase and hydroxybutyric acid dehydrogenase.[1] Serum-aspartate aminotransferase (SGOT) and serum-alanine aminotransferase (SGPT) concentrations can be raised by opioids and they could induce an increase in serum-lactic dehydrogenase concentration of hepatic origin by increasing intrabiliary pressure.[1]

1. Clark F. Drugs and enzymes. *Adverse Drug React Bull* 1977; (Oct.): 232–5.

Effects on the cardiovascular system. For reference to histamine release and cardiovascular effects following the intravenous administration of some opioids see under Pethidine, p.75.

Effects on the endocrine system. Endogenous opioid peptides may have a role in the regulation of endocrine function. Like endorphin and enkephalins, morphine has been found to stimulate prolactin release[1] and synthetic analogues of morphine are reported to have similar properties. Opioids such as morphine are also part of a large group of drugs implicated in causing hyperglycaemia.[2]

1. Hell K, Wernze H. Drug-induced changes in prolactin secretion: clinical implications. *Med Toxicol* 1988; **3:** 463–98.
2. O'Byrne S, Feely J. Effects of drugs on glucose tolerance in non-insulin-dependent diabetics (part II). *Drugs* 1990; **40:** 203–19.

Treatment of Adverse Effects

Activated charcoal may be given by mouth in conscious patients if a substantial overdose has been ingested within 1 hour or so; it should be considered in all patients if a substantial amount of a sustained release preparation has been ingested. Gastric lavage has been used. A laxative may be given to aid peristalsis.

Intensive supportive therapy may be required to correct respiratory failure and shock. In addition, the specific antagonist naloxone is used for rapid reversal of the severe respiratory depression and coma produced by excessive doses of opioid analgesics (see p.1015). Since naloxone has a shorter duration of action than many opioids patients who have already responded should be kept under close observation for signs of relapse and repeated injections given according to the respiratory rate and depth of coma. Alternatively, in situations where one of the longer acting opioids is known or suspected to be the cause of symptoms, a continuous intravenous infusion of naloxone, adjusted according to response, may be used.

The use of opioid antagonists such as naloxone in persons physically dependent on opioids may induce withdrawal symptoms.

Constipation. For reference to the use of naloxone to relieve opioid-induced constipation without compromising analgesic control in patients receiving long-term therapy with opioids, see under Reversal of Opioid Effects in the Uses and Administration of Naloxone, p.1015.

Precautions

Opioid analgesics are generally contra-indicated in respiratory depression and obstructive airways disease, although opioids such as morphine are used in some forms of dyspnoea (see below). They are also contra-indicated or should be used with great caution in acute alcoholism, convulsive disorders, head injuries, and conditions in which intracranial pressure is raised. They should not be given to comatose patients.

Opioid analgesics should be given with caution or in reduced doses to patients with hypothyroidism, adrenocortical insufficiency, asthma, renal or hepatic impairment, prostatic hyperplasia, hypotension, shock, inflammatory or obstructive bowel disorders, or myasthenia gravis. Dosage should be reduced in elderly or debilitated patients.

Opioid analgesics should be given with great care to infants, especially neonates. Their administration during labour may cause respiratory depression in the newborn infant. Babies born to opioid-dependent mothers may suffer withdrawal symptoms (see under Neonatal Abstinence Syndrome, above).

Discontinuation of therapy with opioid analgesics should be carried out gradually in patients who may have developed physical dependence, to avoid precipitating withdrawal symptoms (see Dependence, above). Opioid analgesics with some antagonist activity, such as buprenorphine, butorphanol, nalbuphine, or pentazocine, may precipitate withdrawal symptoms in physically dependent patients who have recently used pure agonists such as morphine.

Drowsiness may affect the ability to perform skilled tasks; those so affected should not drive or operate machinery.

Asthma. Opioids are usually contra-indicated in asthma.[1] However it has been suggested that they are safe in controlled asthma, but should be avoided during acute exacerbations.[2]
1. Gorchein A. Difficult asthma. *BMJ* 1989; **299:** 1031.
2. Barnes PJ, Chung KF. Difficult asthma. *BMJ* 1989; **299:** 1031–2.

Biliary-tract disorders. It is usually recommended that opioids such as morphine should either be avoided in patients with biliary disorders or that they should be given with an antispasmodic. Morphine can cause an increase in intrabiliary pressure as a result of effects on the sphincter of Oddi[1] and might therefore be expected to exacerbate rather than relieve pain in patients with biliary colic (p.5) or other biliary-tract disorders. Biliary-type pain has also been induced in patients given morphine after cholecystectomy.[2]

Morphine caused a more marked delay in gallbladder emptying than pethidine, pentazocine, or butorphanol in a study[3] in healthy subjects; this was considered confirmation that morphine should be avoided in biliary disorders. Others[4] found that fentanyl and sufentanil do not constrict the common bile duct like morphine and therefore may be suitable for perioperative pain control in patients in whom spasm of the common bile duct is undesirable. Phenazocine also has less tendency to increase biliary pressure than other opioids.

1. Helm JF, *et al.* Effects of morphine on the human sphincter of Oddi. *Gut* 1988; **29:** 1402–7.
2. Roberts-Thomson IC, *et al.* Sympathetic activation: a mechanism for morphine induced pain and rises in liver enzymes after cholecystectomy? *Gut* 1990; **31:** 217–21.
3. Hahn M, *et al.* The effect of four narcotics on cholecystokinin octapeptide stimulated gall bladder contraction. *Aliment Pharmacol Ther* 1988; **2:** 129–34.
4. Vieira ZEG, *et al.* Evaluation of fentanyl and sufentanil on the diameter of the common bile duct by ultrasonography in man: a double blind, placebo controlled study. *Int J Clin Pharmacol Ther* 1994; **32:** 274–7.

Children. There is some evidence to suggest that children under 6 months of age are more sensitive to opioids; neonates in particular may be more sensitive to respiratory depression with morphine than adults. Pharmacokinetic differences may contribute to this increased sensitivity. Nonetheless, neonates can be treated with opioids such as morphine if receiving respiratory support.

Older infants and children can be treated effectively with morphine or other opioid analgesics and from the age of 5 or 6 months morphine metabolism follows the course seen in adults. For a discussion of the choice of analgesic in children see p.3. The use of opioids for sedation and analgesia in neonates in intensive care is mentioned on p.652.

References.
1. Choonara IA. Pain relief. *Arch Dis Child* 1989; **64:** 1101–2.
2. Lloyd-Thomas AR. Pain management in paediatric patients. *Br J Anaesth* 1990; **64:** 85–104.
3. Bhatt-Mehta V. Current guidelines for the treatment of acute pain in children. *Drugs* 1996; **51:** 760–76.
4. Marsh DF, *et al.* Opioid systems and the newborn. *Br J Anaesth* 1997; **79:** 787–95.

Hepatic impairment. Although some patients with hepatic dysfunction have been reported to be particularly sensitive to opioids, many patients with liver impairment have been reported to tolerate opioids normally.[1] See also under the individual monographs.
1. Hanks GW, Aherne GW. Morphine metabolism: does the renal hypothesis hold water? *Lancet* 1985; **i:** 221–2.

Phaeochromocytoma. Morphine and some other opioids can induce the release of endogenous histamine and thereby stimulate catecholamine release. Both diamorphine[1] and pethidine[2] have been reported to cause hypertension when given to patients with phaeochromocytoma and histamine-releasing opioids should be avoided in such patients. Alfentanil, like fentanyl, does not release histamine and may be the opioid of choice in the anaesthetic management of patients with phaeochromocytoma.[3]
1. Chaturvedi NC, *et al.* Diamorphine-induced attack of paroxysmal hypertension in phaeochromocytoma. *BMJ* 1974; **2:** 538.
2. Lawrence CA. Pethidine-induced hypertension in phaeochromocytoma. *BMJ* 1978; **1:** 149–50.
3. Hull CJ. Phaeochromocytoma: diagnosis, preoperative preparation and anaesthetic management. *Br J Anaesth* 1986; **58:** 1453–68.

Interactions

As serious and sometimes fatal reactions have occurred following administration of pethidine to patients receiving MAOIs (including moclobemide), pethidine and related drugs are contra-indicated in patients taking MAOIs or within 14 days of stopping such treatment; other opioid analgesics should be avoided or given with extreme caution (for further details, see p.305). Life-threatening reactions have also been reported when selegiline, a selective inhibitor of monoamine oxidase type B, has been given with pethidine. The depressant effects of opioid analgesics are enhanced by other CNS depressants such as alcohol, anaesthetics, anxiolytics, hypnotics, tricyclic antidepressants, and antipsychotics. Cyclizine may counteract the haemodynamic benefits of opioids. Cimetidine inhibits the metabolism of some opioids, especially pethidine.

The actions of opioids may in turn affect the activities of other compounds. For instance, their gastrointesti-

nal effects may delay absorption as with mexiletine or may be counteractive as with cisapride, metoclopramide, or domperidone. Opioid premedicants such as papaveretum have been reported to reduce serum concentrations of ciprofloxacin when given concomitantly.

Antivirals. Interactions between opioid analgesics and ritonavir, other *HIV-protease inhibitors*, or *non-nucleoside reverse transcriptase inhibitors* are complex, and the results of the limited number of studies and reports *in vivo* have not always borne out predictions about the nature of potential interactions.

• Substantial **decreases** in the area under the plasma concentration-time curve (AUC) and in the plasma concentration have been reported for both methadone and for pethidine when given with *ritonavir*. In the case of pethidine, however, plasma concentrations of the toxic metabolite norpethidine are greatly **increased**, and the manufacturers of ritonavir counsel against such combined use. Patients requiring methadone may need an increase in the dose of this drug if given with ritonavir; *nelfinavir* reduces plasma-methadone concentrations similarly, but *indinavir* or *saquinavir* do not appear to do so. *Nevirapine* may also reduce methadone concentrations and can provoke withdrawal symptoms in dependent patients. A similar interaction has occurred when *efavirenz* has been taken with methadone. Ritonavir is predicted to reduce plasma concentrations of morphine.

• In contrast, an **increase** in AUC and in elimination half-life has been reported in subjects given fentanyl with ritonavir. The manufacturers of *ritonavir* also consider that increased plasma concentrations of dextropropoxyphene and tramadol, with an increased likelihood of opioid toxicity, may occur if either drug is given during ritonavir treatment.

Histamine H2-antagonists. Histamine H_2-antagonists may enhance the effects of some opioid analgesics. *Cimetidine* was reported to alter the clearance and volume of distribution of pethidine[1] whereas *ranitidine* did not.[2] Morphine has been considered less likely to interact with cimetidine than pethidine because of differences in metabolism. However, although cimetidine did not affect the disposition of morphine in healthy subjects in one study[3] there have been isolated reports of possible interactions between morphine and H_2-antagonists; apnoea, confusion, and muscle twitching have been associated with concomitant cimetidine and morphine,[4] and confusion associated with concomitant ranitidine and morphine.[5] There has also been a report[6] of a patient receiving regular analgesia with oral methadone and subcutaneous morphine who became unresponsive 6 days after starting cimetidine for prophylaxis of peptic ulcer; treatment with naloxone was required.

1. Guay DRP, *et al.* Cimetidine alters pethidine disposition in man. *Br J Clin Pharmacol* 1984; **18:** 907–14.
2. Guay DRP, *et al.* Ranitidine does not alter pethidine disposition in man. *Br J Clin Pharmacol* 1985; **20:** 55–9.
3. Mojaverian P, *et al.* Cimetidine does not alter morphine disposition in man. *Br J Clin Pharmacol* 1982; **14:** 809–13.
4. Fine A, Churchill DN. Potentially lethal interaction of cimetidine and morphine. *Can Med Assoc J* 1981; **124:** 1434, 1436.
5. Martinez-Abad M, *et al.* Ranitidine-induced confusion with concomitant morphine. *Drug Intell Clin Pharm* 1988; **22:** 914–15.
6. Sorkin EM, Ogawa GS. Cimetidine potentiation of narcotic action. *Drug Intell Clin Pharm* 1983; **17:** 60–1.

Uses and Administration

Opioid analgesics possess some of the properties of naturally occurring or **endogenous opioid peptides**. Endogenous opioid peptides are widely distributed in the CNS and are also found in other parts of the body. They appear to function as neurotransmitters, modulators of neurotransmission, or neurohormones. Their presence in the hypothalamus suggests a role in the regulation of endocrine function. Opioids have been shown to stimulate the release of some pituitary hormones, including prolactin and growth hormone, and to inhibit the release of others, including corticotropin.

Endogenous peptides include the enkephalins, endorphins, and dynorphins; their polypeptide precursors may also be precursors for non-opioid peptides. Pro-enkephalin is the precursor of met- and leu-enkephalin; pro-opiomelanocortin is the precursor of beta-endorphin, beta-lipotrophin, melanocyte-stimulating hormone, and corticotropin; and prodynorphin is the precursor of dynorphins and neoendorphins.

Pharmacologically the opioid analgesics are broadly similar; qualitative and quantitative differences may be dependent on their interaction with **opioid receptors**. There are several types of opioid receptor and they are distributed in distinct patterns through the central and peripheral nervous systems. The three main types in the CNS were originally designated μ (mu), κ (kappa), and δ (delta) although they have more recently been reclassified as OP_3, OP_2, and OP_1 respectively. Activities attributed to the stimulation of these receptors have been as follows:

- μ—analgesia (mainly at supraspinal sites), respiratory depression, miosis, reduced gastrointestinal motility, and euphoria; $μ_1$ (supraspinal analgesia) and $μ_2$ (respiratory depression and gastrointestinal activity) subtypes have been postulated;

- κ—analgesia (mainly in the spinal cord); less intense miosis and respiratory depression, dysphoria and psychotomimetic effects;

- δ—less certain in man, but probably analgesia; selective for enkephalins.

- Other receptors include σ (sigma) and ε (epsilon) receptors. The psychotomimetic effects of agonist-antagonists such as pentazocine that are poorly antagonised by naloxone have been thought by some to be mediated by σ receptors.

Opioids act at one or more of these receptors as full or partial agonists, or as antagonists. Morphine and similar opioid agonists (sometimes called μ agonists) are considered to act primarily at μ and perhaps at κ and δ receptors. Opioid agonist-antagonists such as pentazocine appear to act as κ agonists and μ antagonists whereas buprenorphine is a partial agonist at μ receptors with some antagonist activity at κ receptors. The opioid antagonist naloxone acts at μ, κ, and δ receptors.

In addition to differing affinities for particular receptors the degree of activation once bound also differs. The full agonist morphine produces maximum activation at the μ receptor and its effects increase with dose, whereas partial agonists and agonist-antagonists may demonstrate a 'ceiling effect' in that above a certain level their effects do not increase proportionately with dose.

Other differences between opioid analgesics may relate to their lipid solubility and pharmacokinetics; speed of onset and duration of action may influence the choice of analgesic.

Opioid analgesics were traditionally classified as weak opioids or strong opioids; however this classification has largely been replaced by the one used in the WHO three-step analgesic ladder (see Cancer Pain, p.5). In this system opioids are divided into those that are used for **mild to moderate pain** and those that are used for **moderate to severe pain**. Examples of opioids in the first group include codeine, dextropropoxyphene, and dihydrocodeine; such opioids are distinguished by the existence of a ceiling effect and are often used with non-opioid analgesics. The principal opioid for the treatment of moderate to severe pain is morphine. Others include: diamorphine, fentanyl, methadone, and pethidine.

In addition to being used for the relief of pain opioids are used in anaesthesia for premedication, induction, or maintenance. In balanced anaesthesia they are used in conjunction with an anaesthetic and a neuromuscular blocker. When used with a compound such as droperidol they can produce a state of mild sedation with analgesia called neuroleptanalgesia.

Some opioids are used for analgesia, sedation, and suppression of respiration in the management of mechanically ventilated patients under intensive care (p.652).

Codeine is used for the suppression of cough; for intractable cough in terminal illness morphine may be used.

Opioids may relieve some forms of dyspnoea; morphine and diamorphine are probably the most commonly used in the UK, but dihydrocodeine and hydrocodone have also been tried.

Methadone and buprenorphine are used in the treatment of opioid dependence (see above).

◊ References.
1. Cherny NI. Opioid analgesics: comparative features and prescribing guidelines. *Drugs* 1996; **51:** 713–37.
2. Upton RN, *et al.* Pharmacokinetic optimisation of opioid treatment in acute pain therapy. *Clin Pharmacokinet* 1997; **33:** 225–44.

Action. Some references to opioid receptors.
1. Pleuvry BJ. Opioid receptors and their ligands: natural and unnatural. *Br J Anaesth* 1991; **66:** 370–80.
2. Pleuvry BJ. Opioid receptors and awareness of the Greek alphabet. *Br J Hosp Med* 1992; **48:** 678–81.
3. Atcheson R, Lambert DG. Update on opioid receptors. *Br J Anaesth* 1994; **73:** 132–4.
4. Dhawan BN, *et al.* International Union of Pharmacology. XII. Classification of opioid receptors. *Pharmacol Rev* 1996; **48:** 567–86.
5. Lambert DG. Recent advances in opioid pharmacology. *Br J Anaesth* 1998; **81:** 1–2.

Administration in children. See under Precautions, above.

Anaesthesia. Opioid analgesics have been given intravenously as supplements during general anaesthesia with inhalational or intravenous drugs. They have also been widely used as premedication before surgery to reduce anxiety, for smooth induction of anaesthesia, to reduce overall anaesthetic requirements, and to provide postoperative pain relief. Such use of opioids is now rare and is restricted to patients already in pain or to those who will experience pain before induction of anaesthesia. Very high doses of morphine have been infused intravenously to produce anaesthesia for cardiac surgery, but shorter acting drugs such as fentanyl and related opioids are generally used now; some may prefer agonist-antagonist opioids. Sedation and respiratory depression may be prolonged necessitating assisted ventilation; reversal of these effects can be achieved by opioid antagonists such as naloxone. For a discussion of the various drugs used to achieve and maintain conditions suitable for surgery, including the use of opioids in the induction and maintenance of anaesthesia, see p.1256. Opioid analgesics, most commonly fentanyl, have been used with a neuroleptic to induce a state known as neuroleptanalgesia in which the patient is calm and indifferent to the surroundings yet is responsive to commands. For a brief discussion of neuroleptanalgesia and similar anaesthetic techniques, see p.1256.

References.
1. Sear JW. Recent advances and developments in the clinical use of i.v. opioids during the perioperative period. *Br J Anaesth* 1998; **81:** 38–50.

POSTOPERATIVE SHIVERING. Pethidine appears to be effective in the treatment of postoperative shivering (see p.1255) but not all opioids are necessarily effective.

Cough. Opioids are used to suppress cough (p.1082). Pholcodine (p.1099) and dextromethorphan (p.1087), which lack any intrinsic analgesic activity are the most commonly used opioids. Of the analgesic opioids, codeine is the most widely used as a cough suppressant. However, these opioids are seldom sufficiently potent to be effective in severe cough. Morphine and diamorphine are used for the relief of intractable cough in terminal illness, although morphine is now preferred. Methadone has also been used but should be avoided as it has a long duration of action and tends to accumulate. Cough suppressants containing codeine or similar opioids are not recommended for use in children, and should be avoided in those under 1 year of age.

Diarrhoea. Oral rehydration therapy, which is the treatment of choice for acute diarrhoea (p.1203), prevents dehydration, but it does not necessarily shorten the duration of the diarrhoea. Preparations containing morphine or other opioids have therefore been used for their antimotility action as adjuncts in the management of acute diarrhoea. However, the WHO considers that such antidiarrhoeal drug therapy is of limited value, may delay the expulsion of causative organisms, and should never be given to children. Furthermore opioids should not be used in conditions where inhibition of peristalsis should be avoided, where abdominal distension develops, or in diarrhoeal conditions such as severe ulcerative colitis or antibiotic-associated colitis.

Dyspnoea. Dyspnoea (a subjective feeling of abnormally uncomfortable, difficult, or laboured breathing) is associated with diseases that interfere with oxygenation of the blood. Dyspnoea is best relieved by treatment of the underlying disorder: the treatment of dyspnoea associated with asthma and chronic obstructive pulmonary disease is discussed on p.757 and p.759 respectively. However, many patients may remain symptomatic.
Oxygen may reduce dyspnoea in some patients even if dyspnoea is not related to hypoxia. Also a flow of air directed across the face by a fan can be effective. Despite the hazards of the administration of benzodiazepines to patients with any form of respiratory depression or pulmonary insufficiency (see Precautions for Diazepam, p.677), they may be helpful in patients with advanced cancer who have rapid shallow respiration, especially when this is associated with anxiety.[1,2] Diazepam, lorazepam, and midazolam are benzodiazepines that have been tried in such patients. Methotrimeprazine [levomepromazine] is occasionally used as an alternative.
Opioids may relieve some forms of dyspnoea[2] especially that due to acute left ventricular failure, pulmonary oedema, and malignant chest disease. The cause of dyspnoea should be established since the use of opioids is generally not advised, or only with extreme caution, in patients with obstructive airways disease whose dyspnoea may be relieved by other means. In the UK morphine and diamorphine are probably the most commonly used opioids for dyspnoea, but dihydrocodeine, hydrocodone, and oxymorphone have also been tried.

Nebulised morphine, hydromorphone, or fentanyl have been tried for the management of dyspnoea, and there are anecdotal reports of benefit, especially in palliative care, but evidence from controlled studies to date does not support such use.[2,3]
In patients with advanced cancer and intractable dyspnoea unresponsive to the above measures, chlorpromazine may be useful to relieve air hunger and sedate dying patients who have unrelieved distress;[1] midazolam may be used as an alternative. Promethazine has also been used. High doses of a corticosteroid such as dexamethasone may help to relieve dyspnoea in patients with airways obstruction due to a tumour by reducing oedema around the tumour.
1. Walsh D. Dyspnoea in advanced cancer. *Lancet* 1993; **342:** 450–1.
2. Davis CL. ABC of palliative care: breathlessness, cough, and other respiratory problems. *BMJ* 1997; **315:** 931–4.
3. Chandler S. Nebulized opioids to treat dyspnea. *Am J Hosp Palliat Care* 1999; **16:** 418–22.

Pain. Opioid analgesics are used for the relief of acute and chronic pain (p.2). Not every type of pain responds; neuropathic pain, for example, is not alleviated by opioid therapy. For further discussion of specific pain states and the role of opioid analgesics in their treatment see p.5 onwards.
There has also been interest in the local analgesic effects of opioids themselves.[1,2]
1. Thompson DF, Pierce DR. Local analgesia with opioid drugs. *Ann Pharmacother* 1995; **29:** 189–90.
2. Stein C. The control of pain in peripheral tissue by opioids. *N Engl J Med* 1995; **332:** 1685–90.

HEADACHE. Opioid analgesics such as codeine are sometimes included in oral compound analgesic preparations used in the initial treatment of migraine (see p.449) or tension-type headache (see p.450), but are best avoided, especially in patients who experience frequent attacks.

Restless legs syndrome. Some opioids may be beneficial in the treatment of restless legs syndrome (see Parasomnias, p.653), although evidence is scanty.

Sedation. In addition to their analgesic action opioids have been used in a variety of procedures for their sedative properties. Mention of this use of opioids can be found in the discussions of anaesthesia (p.1256), endoscopy (p.652), and intensive care (p.652).

Tetanus. Opioid analgesics can be used to provide analgesia and additional sedation in patients undergoing treatment for tetanus (p.142 and p.1332). Morphine has also been given to control the sympathetic overactivity in such patients.[1]
1. Rocke DA, *et al.* Morphine in tetanus—the management of sympathetic nervous system overactivity. *S Afr Med J* 1986; **70:** 666–8.

Opium   (6246-z)

Gum Opium; Opium Crudum; Raw Opium.
ATC — A07DA02; N02AA02.
Pharmacopoeias. In Chin., Eur. (see p.vi), *and US.*
Aust., Chin., Ger., It., Neth., and US also include a monograph for Prepared Opium. Jpn includes only Prepared Opium. Jpn also includes a diluted opium powder containing 1% of anhydrous morphine.

Opium is the air-dried latex obtained by incision from the unripe capsules of *Papaver somniferum* (Papaveraceae). It contains morphine, codeine, and thebaine and a variable mixture of other alkaloids including noscapine and papaverine.
The exuded latex is dried and manipulated to form cakes of uniform composition, variously shaped according to the country of origin, and known in commerce as Turkish, Indian, or European opium.
Prepared Opium (Opium Titratum; Powdered Opium; Pulvis Opii; Standardised Opium Powder) is opium, dried, powdered, and adjusted in strength. The BP 1988 included a similar preparation containing 9.5 to 10.5% of anhydrous morphine.

Pharmacopoeial description

Ph. Eur.: The air-dried latex obtained by incision from the unripe capsules of *Papaver somniferum* L. It has a characteristic odour and a blackish-brown colour. It should contain not less than 10% of anhydrous morphine, not less than 2% of anhydrous codeine, and not more than 3% of anhydrous thebaine. Protect from light.
NOTE. Opium is intended only as the starting material for the manufacture of galenical preparations and is not dispensed as such.
USP 25: The air-dried milky exudate obtained by incising the unripe capsules of *Papaver somniferum* (Papaveraceae). Externally it is pale olive-brown or olive-grey; internally it is reddish-brown. It has a very characteristic odour and a very bitter taste. It yields not less than 9.5% of anhydrous morphine.
Powdered Opium is a light brown or moderately yellowish-brown powder that yields not less than 10% and not more than 10.5% of anhydrous morphine. It may contain any of the permitted diluents with the exception of starch.

Profile

Opium has the properties of opioid analgesics (p.66). Its analgesic and sedative actions are due mainly to its content of morphine (p.58). It acts less rapidly than morphine since opium appears to be more slowly absorbed; the relaxing action of the papaverine and noscapine on intestinal muscle makes it more constipating than morphine.

Opium is used as prepared opium, as Opium Tincture (BP 2001) or (USP 25), or as Camphorated Opium Tincture (BP 2001) or Paregoric (USP 25) in various oral preparations. These have included Opiate Squill Linctus (BP 2001) (Gee's linctus) for cough.

Paregoric (USP 25) has been advocated in the USA for the treatment of neonatal opioid dependence.

◊ Reports of squill-associated cardiac toxicity resulting from the abuse of opiate squill linctus (Gee's linctus).[1,2]
1. Thurston D, Taylor K. Gee's linctus. *Pharm J* 1984; **233**: 63.
2. Smith W, *et al.* Wenckebach's phenomenon induced by cough linctus. *BMJ* 1986; **292**: 868.

Preparations
BP 2001: Camphorated Opium Tincture; Concentrated Camphorated Opium Tincture; Opium Tincture;
USP 25: Opium Tincture; Paregoric.

Proprietary Preparations (details are given in Part 3)
Multi-ingredient: *Braz.:* Camomila; Elixir de Marinheiro; Elixir Paregorico; *Canad.:* Diban; Donnagel-PG; *Denm.:* Pectyl; *Fin.:* Tannopon; *Fr.:* Colchimax; Eubispasme Codethyline†; Lamaline; Paregorique; *Israel:* Doveri; *S.Afr.:* Stilpane; *Spain:* Digestovital; Tanagel; *Switz.:* Bromocod N; Pectocalmine; *USA:* B & O Supprettes No. 15A; B & O Supprettes No. 16A.

Hydrochlorides of Mixed Opium Alkaloids
(15940-f)

Alkaloidosum Opii Hydrochloridum; Extractum Concentratum Opii; Omnoponum; Opialum; Opium Concentratum.

Pharmacopoeias. Preparations of the hydrochlorides of mixed opium alkaloids are included in *Jpn.*

Papaveretum (6250-e)
Papaveretum *(BAN).*

A mixture of 253 parts of morphine hydrochloride, 23 parts of papaverine hydrochloride, and 20 parts of codeine hydrochloride.
CAS — 8002-76-4.
ATC — N02AA10.

NOTE. Do not confuse papaveretum with papaverine (p.1648).
Pharmacopoeias. In *Br.*

15.4 mg of Papaveretum (BP 2001) contains the equivalent of approximately 10 mg of the major component, anhydrous morphine.

Pharmacopoeial description
BP 2001: Papaveretum contains 80.0 to 88.4% of anhydrous morphine hydrochloride, 8.3 to 9.2% of papaverine hydrochloride, and 6.6 to 7.4% of anhydrous codeine hydrochloride. A white or almost white crystalline powder. Soluble in water, sparingly soluble in alcohol. A 1.5% solution in water has a pH of 3.7 to 4.7. Protect from light.

Profile
Hydrochlorides of mixed opium alkaloids have the properties of opioid analgesics (p.66). In the UK, papaveretum formerly contained the hydrochlorides of morphine, codeine, noscapine, and papaverine. However, because of concern over the potential genotoxicity of noscapine (p.1096) UK preparations containing papaveretum were reformulated to exclude the noscapine component and the name papaveretum was redefined in the BP 1993 to reflect this change of formulation. It is possible that in other countries the term papaveretum is still being used to describe a mixture containing noscapine.

Mixtures of opium alkaloids such as papaveretum have the analgesic and sedative properties of morphine (p.58) and are used in the treatment of moderate to severe pain and for pre-operative sedation.

In adults papaveretum is generally administered by subcutaneous or intramuscular injection in doses of 7.7 to 15.4 mg every 4 hours. The initial dose in the elderly should not exceed 7.7 mg. Children aged 1 to 5 years may be given 1.93 to 3.85 mg and those 6 to 12 years, 3.85 to 7.7 mg. In infants, dosage is calculated by body-weight: infants aged up to 1 month may be given 115.5 µg per kg and infants aged up to 1 year, 154 µg per kg.

Papaveretum may also be given intravenously in doses of one-quarter to one-half the corresponding subcutaneous or intramuscular dose.

For pre-operative medication papaveretum is given intramuscularly or subcutaneously sometimes in conjunction with hyoscine hydrobromide.

Papaveretum has also been given by mouth with aspirin for the management of moderate to severe pain.

◊ Papaveretum has been confused with papaverine (p.1648) and in one such case[1] a patient became unconscious after self-injection of papaveretum in mistake for papaverine.
1. Robinson LQ, Stephenson TP. Self injection treatment for impotence. *BMJ* 1989; **299**: 1568.

Preparations
BP 2001: Papaveretum Injection.
Proprietary Preparations (details are given in Part 3)
S.Afr.: Omnopon; *USA:* Pantopon†.
Multi-ingredient: *UK:* Aspav.

Oxaprozin (13055-d)
Oxaprozin *(BAN, USAN, rINN).*
Wy-21743. 3-(4,5-Diphenyloxazol-2-yl)propionic acid.
$C_{18}H_{15}NO_3 = 293.3.$
CAS — 21256-18-8.
ATC — M01AE12.
Pharmacopoeias. In *Jpn.*

Adverse Effects and Precautions
As for NSAIDs in general, p.63.

Diagnosis and testing. False-positive results for testing of benzodiazepines in urine have been reported in patients taking oxaprozin.[1] The manufacturer[2] has commented that the interaction occurs with some immunoassay tests and that thin-layer chromatography can successfully discriminate between benzodiazepines and oxaprozin. False-positive results for a fluorescence polarisation immunoassay for phenytoin have also been reported in patients receiving oxaprozin.[3]
1. Pulini M. False-positive benzodiazepine urine test due to oxaprozin. *JAMA* 1995; **273**: 1905.
2. Raphan H, Adams MH. False-positive benzodiazepine urine test due to oxaprozin. *JAMA* 1995; **273**: 1905–6.
3. Patel T, *et al.* Assay interaction between oxaprozin and phenytoin. *Ann Pharmacother* 1997; **31**: 254.

Effects on the liver. A report[1] of fatal fulminant hepatitis in a 56-year-old woman who had received 600 to 1200 mg of oxaprozin daily for about 6 weeks. In another patient symptomatic hepatitis developing during oxaprozin use resolved on discontinuation of the drug.[2]
1. Purdum PP, *et al.* Oxaprozin-induced fulminant hepatitis. *Ann Pharmacother* 1994; **28**: 1159–61.
2. Kethu SR, *et al.* Oxaprozin-induced symptomatic hepatotoxicity. *Ann Pharmacother* 1999; **33**: 942–4.

Interactions
For interactions associated with NSAIDs, see p.65.

Pharmacokinetics
Oxaprozin is slowly but extensively absorbed from the gastrointestinal tract and is highly bound to plasma proteins. Peak plasma concentrations are reached after 3 to 5 hours. At steady state, which may take several days to achieve, the accumulation half-life is about 25 hours after 600 mg daily and 21 hours after 1200 mg daily. Oxaprozin is metabolised mainly in the liver by microsomal oxidation and conjugation with glucuronic acid to form inactive metabolites which are excreted in the urine and faeces.

◊ References.
1. Karim A. Inverse nonlinear pharmacokinetics of total and protein unbound drug (oxaprozin): clinical and pharmacokinetic implications. *J Clin Pharmacol* 1996; **36**: 985–97.
2. Karim A, *et al.* Oxaprozin and piroxicam, nonsteroidal antiinflammatory drugs with long half-lives: effect of protein-binding differences on steady-state pharmacokinetics. *J Clin Pharmacol* 1997; **37**: 267–78.
3. Davies NM. Clinical pharmacokinetics of oxaprozin. *Clin Pharmacokinet* 1998; **35**: 425–36.

Uses and Administration
Oxaprozin, a propionic acid derivative, is an NSAID (p.65). It is used in the treatment of osteoarthritis and rheumatoid arthritis in a usual dose of 1200 mg given once daily by mouth, although in osteoarthritis, patients with low body-weight or mild disease may respond to an initial dose of 600 mg daily. The recommended maximum daily dose is 1800 mg or 26 mg per kg body-weight, whichever is the lower.

◊ References.
1. Miller LG. Oxaprozin: a once-daily nonsteroidal anti-inflammatory drug. *Clin Pharm* 1992; **11**: 591–603.
2. Anonymous. Oxaprozin for arthritis. *Med Lett Drugs Ther* 1993; **35**: 15–16.

Preparations
Proprietary Preparations (details are given in Part 3)
Canad.: Daypro; *S.Afr.:* Deflam; *USA:* Daypro.

Oxycodone Hydrochloride (6248-k)
Oxycodone Hydrochloride *(BANM, USAN, rINNM).*
7,8-Dihydro-14-hydroxycodeinone hydrochloride; Dihydrone Hydrochloride; NSC-19043 (oxycodone); Oxycone Hydrochloride; Thecodine. 6-Deoxy-7,8-dihydro-14-hydroxy-3-O-methyl-6-oxomorphine hydrochloride; (−)-(5R,6S,14S)-4,5-Epoxy-14-hydroxy-3-methoxy-9a-methylmorphinan-6-one hydrochloride.
$C_{18}H_{21}NO_4,HCl = 351.8.$
CAS — 76-42-6 (oxycodone); 124-90-3 (oxycodone hydrochloride).

NOTE. Compounded preparations of oxycodone may be represented by the following names:
• Co-oxycodAPAP (*USP 25*)—oxycodone and paracetamol.
Pharmacopoeias. In *Aust., Belg., Fr., Jpn,* and *US* (some specify the trihydrate).

Pharmacopoeial description
USP 25: A white to off-white, odourless, hygroscopic crystals or powder. Soluble in water; slightly soluble in alcohol. Store in airtight containers.

Oxycodone Terephthalate (18469-c)
4,5α-Epoxy-14-hydroxy-3-methoxy-17-methylmorphinan-6-one 1,4-benzenedicarboxylate (2:1) salt.
$(C_{18}H_{21}NO_4)_2,C_8H_6O_4 = 796.9.$
CAS — 64336-55-6.
Pharmacopoeias. In *US.*

Pharmacopoeial description
USP 25: Store in airtight containers.

Dependence and Withdrawal
As for Opioid Analgesics in general, p.66.

Adverse Effects, Treatment, and Precautions
As for Opioid Analgesics in general, p.67.

Abuse. Oxycodone hydrochloride modified-release tablets have been subject to abuse. The crushed tablets have been inhaled or injected by addicts and in some cases this has resulted in fatalities.

Effects on the respiratory system. References to respiratory depression occurring in children given oxycodone.
1. Olkkola KT, *et al.* Pharmacokinetics and ventilatory effects of intravenous oxycodone in postoperative children. *Br J Clin Pharmacol* 1994; **38**: 71–6.
2. Kalso E. Pharmacokinetics and ventilatory effects of intravenous oxycodone in postoperative children. *Br J Clin Pharmacol* 1995; **39**: 214.

Hepatic impairment. The clearance and elimination of oxycodone were shown to be prolonged in 6 female patients with end-stage liver cirrhosis awaiting liver transplantations.[1] Significant ventilatory depression was also observed. Pharmacokinetic values after successful transplantation were similar to those previously reported for healthy adults. It was recommended that, when administering oxycodone to patients with end-stage liver disease, the dosing frequency should be reduced and the dose lowered.
1. Tallgren M, *et al.* Pharmacokinetics and ventilatory effects of oxycodone before and after liver transplantation. *Clin Pharmacol Ther* 1997; **61**: 655–61.

Porphyria. Oxycodone is considered to be unsafe in patients with porphyria because it has been shown to be porphyrinogenic in *animals.*

Interactions
For interactions associated with opioid analgesics, see p.68.

Antidepressants. For reference to a possible case of serotonin syndrome when *sertraline* was given with high doses of oxycodone, see p.287.

Pharmacokinetics
Oxycodone is absorbed from the gastrointestinal tract. It is metabolised to noroxycodone and, to a lesser extent, oxymorphone (p.71). Both metabolites undergo glucuronidation and are excreted with unchanged drug in urine. The elimination half-life of oxycodone is reported to be 2 to 3 hours. Oxycodone is distributed into breast milk.

◊ References.
1. Pöyhiä R, *et al.* The pharmacokinetics of oxycodone after intravenous injection in adults. *Br J Clin Pharmacol* 1991; **32**: 516–18.
2. Leow KP, *et al.* Single-dose and steady-state pharmacokinetics and pharmacodynamics of oxycodone in patients with cancer. *Clin Pharmacol Ther* 1992; **52**: 487–95.
3. Olkkola KT, *et al.* Pharmacokinetics and ventilatory effects of intravenous oxycodone in postoperative children. *Br J Clin Pharmacol* 1994; **38**: 71–6.
4. Mandema JW, *et al.* Characterization and validation of a pharmacokinetic model for controlled-release oxycodone. *Br J Clin Pharmacol* 1996; **42**: 747–56.
5. Kaiko RF, *et al.* Pharmacokinetic-pharmacodynamic relationships of controlled-release oxycodone. *Clin Pharmacol Ther* 1996; **59**: 52–61.

Uses and Administration
Oxycodone, a phenanthrene derivative, is an opioid analgesic (p.68). Oxycodone hydrochloride is given by mouth for the relief of moderate to severe pain. A usual starting dose for severe pain is 5 mg every 4 to 6 hours increased thereafter as necessary according to response. Combined preparations containing oxycodone hydrochloride and aspirin or paracetamol are also used. Oxycodone hydrochloride may also be given by mouth as a modified-release preparation every 12 hours.

Oxycodone has been given rectally every 6 to 8 hours in suppositories containing 30 mg of oxycodone (as the pectinate) or 10 to 40 mg of oxycodone hydrochloride.

Oxycodone terephthalate is also used by mouth.

◊ References.
1. Kalso E, Vainio A. Morphine and oxycodone hydrochloride in the management of cancer pain. *Clin Pharmacol Ther* 1990; **47**: 639–46.

2. Sunshine A, *et al.* Analgesic efficacy of controlled-release oxycodone in postoperative pain. *J Clin Pharmacol* 1996; **36:** 595–603.
3. Curtis GB, *et al.* Relative potency of controlled-release oxycodone and controlled-release morphine in a postoperative pain model. *Eur J Clin Pharmacol* 1999; **55:** 425–9.

Preparations

USP 25: Oxycodone and Acetaminophen Capsules; Oxycodone and Acetaminophen Tablets; Oxycodone and Aspirin Tablets; Oxycodone Hydrochloride Oral Solution; Oxycodone Hydrochloride Tablets.

Proprietary Preparations (details are given in Part 3)
Austral.: Endone; Oxycontin; Oxynorm; Proladone; **Canad.:** Oxycontin; Supeudol; **Denm.:** Oxycontin; Oxynorm; **Fin.:** Oxanest; Oxycontin; Oxynorm; **Fr.:** Eubine; **Ger.:** Oxygesic; **Irl.:** Oxycontin; Oxynorm; **Israel:** Oxycod; Oxycontin; **Mex.:** Oxycontin; **NZ:** Proladone; Oxynorm; **Swed.:** Oxycontin; Oxynorm; **UK:** Oxycontin; Oxynorm; **USA:** Endocodone; Oxycontin; Oxyfast; OxyIR; Percolone; Roxicodone.

Multi-ingredient: Canad.: Endocet; Endodan; Oxycocet; Oxycodan; Percocet; Percodan; Roxicet†; **Israel:** Percocet; Percodan; **USA:** Percocet; Percodan; Roxicet; Roxilox; Roxiprin; Tylox.

Oxymorphone Hydrochloride (6249-a)

Oxymorphone Hydrochloride (BANM, rINNM).
7,8-Dihydro-14-hydroxymorphinone hydrochloride; Oximorphone Hydrochloride. 6-Deoxy-7,8-dihydro-14-hydroxy-6-oxomorphine hydrochloride; (−)-(5R,6S,14S)-4,5-Epoxy-3,14-dihydroxy-9a-methylmorphinan-6-one hydrochloride.
$C_{17}H_{19}NO_4,HCl = 337.8$.
CAS — 76-41-5 (oxymorphone); 357-07-3 (oxymorphone hydrochloride).
Pharmacopoeias. In US.

Pharmacopoeial description

USP 25: A white or slightly off-white odourless powder, darkening on exposure to light. Its aqueous solutions are slightly acidic. Soluble 1 in 4 of water, 1 in 100 of alcohol, and 1 in 25 of methyl alcohol; very slightly soluble in chloroform and in ether. Store in airtight containers. Protect from light.

Uses and Administration

Oxymorphone hydrochloride, a phenanthrene derivative, is an opioid analgesic (p.66) with actions and uses similar to those of morphine (p.56), apart from a lack of cough suppressant activity. Oxymorphone is used in the treatment of moderate to severe pain, including pain in obstetrics, and is reported to provide analgesia for 3 to 6 hours. It may also be used as an adjunct to anaesthesia and to relieve dyspnoea due to pulmonary oedema resulting from left ventricular failure.

Oxymorphone hydrochloride is given in initial doses of 1 to 1.5 mg, repeated every 4 to 6 hours as necessary, by intramuscular or subcutaneous injection; 500 µg may be given by intravenous injection. The usual dose for analgesia during labour is 0.5 to 1 mg intramuscularly.

Oxymorphone hydrochloride is given rectally as a suppository in a dose of 5 mg every 4 to 6 hours.

Preparations

USP 25: Oxymorphone Hydrochloride Injection; Oxymorphone Hydrochloride Suppositories.

Proprietary Preparations (details are given in Part 3)
Canad.: Numorphan; **USA:** Numorphan.

Oxyphenbutazone (2678-q)

Oxyphenbutazone (BAN, rINN).
G-27202; Hydroxyphenylbutazone; Oxifenbutazona; Oxyphenbutazonum. 4-Butyl-1-(4-hydroxyphenyl)-2-phenylpyrazolidine-3,5-dione monohydrate.
$C_{19}H_{20}N_2O_3,H_2O = 342.4$.
CAS — 129-20-4 (anhydrous oxyphenbutazone); 7081-38-1 (oxyphenbutazone monohydrate).
ATC — M01AA03; M02AA04; S01BC02.
Pharmacopoeias. In Eur. (see p.vi).

Pharmacopoeial description

Ph. Eur.: A white crystalline powder. Practically insoluble in water; freely soluble in alcohol; soluble in ether; it dissolves in dilute solutions of alkali hydroxides. Protect from light.

Adverse Effects and Precautions

As for Phenylbutazone, p.78. Adverse effects on the blood may be more frequent with oxyphenbutazone than with phenylbutazone.

Porphyria. Oxyphenbutazone has been associated with acute attacks of porphyria and is considered unsafe in porphyric patients.

Interactions

For interactions associated with NSAIDs, see p.65.

Uses and Administration

Oxyphenbutazone, a metabolite of phenylbutazone (p.78), is an NSAID (p.63). It has been applied topically to the eye as an anti-inflammatory ointment (usually 10%) in conditions such as episcleritis. Oxyphenbutazone was used systemically in disorders such as ankylosing spondylitis, osteoarthritis, and rheu-

---

matoid arthritis but such use is no longer considered justified owing to the risk of severe haematological adverse effects. The piperazine salt has also been used.

Preparations

BP 2001: Oxyphenbutazone Eye Ointment.

Proprietary Preparations (details are given in Part 3)
Aust.: Tanderil; **Braz.:** Tandrex; **Ger.:** Phlogont†; **Mex.:** Butafen; Edefen; Maderil; Oxabenal; Redolet; Tandorene; **Spain:** Diflamil.

Multi-ingredient: Braz.: Algi-Peralgin; Algi-Reumac; Algiflamanil; Algizolin; Analtrix; Febupen; Flamanan; Reumazine; Tandrex A; **Ger.:** Phlogase†.

Paracetamol (2679-p)

Paracetamol (BAN, rINN).
Acetaminophen; N-Acetyl-p-aminophenol; Paracetamolum. 4'-Hydroxyacetanilide; N-(4-Hydroxyphenyl)acetamide.
$C_8H_9NO_2 = 151.2$.
CAS — 103-90-2.
ATC — N02BE01.

NOTE. Compounded preparations of paracetamol may be represented by the following names:

*   Co-bucafAPAP (*USP 25*)—butalbital, paracetamol, and caffeine
*   Co-codamol *x/y* (*BAN*)—where *x* and *y* are the strengths in milligrams of codeine phosphate and paracetamol respectively
*   Co-codAPAP (*USP 25*)—paracetamol and codeine phosphate
*   Co-dydramol (*BAN*)—dihydrocodeine tartrate 1 part and paracetamol 50 parts (w/w)
*   Co-hycodAPAP (*USP 25*)—hydrocodone tartrate and paracetamol
*   Co-methiamol *x/y* (*BAN*)—where *x* and *y* are the strengths in milligrams of DL-methionine and paracetamol respectively
*   Co-oxycodAPAP (*USP 25*)—oxycodone and paracetamol
*   Co-proxamol (*BAN*)—dextropropoxyphene hydrochloride 1 part and paracetamol 10 parts (w/w)
*   Co-proxAPAP (*USP 25*)—dextropropoxyphene napsilate and paracetamol.

Pharmacopoeias. In Chin., Eur. (see p.vi), Int., Jpn, Pol., and US.

Pharmacopoeial description

Ph. Eur.: A white crystalline powder. Sparingly soluble in water; freely soluble in alcohol; very slightly soluble in dichloromethane and in ether. Protect from light.

USP 25: A white odourless crystalline powder. Soluble 1 in 20 of boiling water, 1 in 10 of alcohol, and 1 in 15 of 1N sodium hydroxide. Store in airtight containers. Protect from light.

Adverse Effects and Treatment

Side-effects of paracetamol are rare and usually mild, although haematological reactions including thrombocytopenia, leucopenia, pancytopenia, neutropenia, and agranulocytosis have been reported. Skin rashes, and other hypersensitivity reactions occur occasionally.

Overdosage with paracetamol can result in severe liver damage and sometimes acute renal tubular necrosis. Prompt treatment with acetylcysteine or methionine is essential and is discussed under Overdosage, below.

Effects on the kidneys. For reference to evidence that abuse or prolonged excessive use of analgesics, including paracetamol, can produce nephropathy, see under NSAIDs, p.64.
See also under Overdosage, below.

Effects on the respiratory tract. The results of a case-control study[1] have suggested that the frequent (daily or weekly) use of paracetamol may be associated with asthma. However, the UK Committee on Safety of Medicines has commented that the results of this study do not alter any advice regarding the use of paracetamol and that it remains a safe and effective pain killer for many patients including asthmatics.

1. Shaheen SO, *et al.* Frequent paracetamol use and asthma in adults. *Thorax* 2000; **55:** 266–70.

Hypersensitivity. Reactions, characterised by urticaria, dyspnoea, and hypotension, have occurred following the administration of paracetamol to adults[1-3] and children.[4] Angioedema has also been reported.[5] Fixed drug eruptions, confirmed by rechallenge, have been described,[6-9] and toxic epidermal necrolysis has occurred.[10]

1. Stricker BHC, *et al.* Acute hypersensitivity reactions to paracetamol. *BMJ* 1985; **291:** 938–9.
2. Van Diem L, Grilliat JP. Anaphylactic shock induced by paracetamol. *Eur J Clin Pharmacol* 1990; **38:** 389–90.
3. Kumar RK, Byard I. Paracetamol as a cause of anaphylaxis. *Hosp Med* 1999; **60:** 66–7.
4. Ellis M, *et al.* Immediate adverse reactions to acetaminophen in children: evaluation of histamine release and spirometry. *J Pediatr* 1989; **114:** 654–6.

---

5. Idoko JA, *et al.* Angioneurotic oedema following ingestion of paracetamol. *Trans R Soc Trop Med Hyg* 1986; **80:** 175.
6. Thomas RHM, Munro DD. Fixed drug eruption due to paracetamol. *Br J Dermatol* 1986; **115:** 357–9.
7. Cohen HA, *et al.* Fixed drug eruption caused by acetaminophen. *Ann Pharmacother* 1992; **26:** 1596–7.
8. Harris A, Burge SM. Fixed drug eruption due to paracetamol. *Br J Dermatol* 1995; **133:** 790–1.
9. Hern S, *et al.* Bullous fixed drug eruption due to paracetamol with an unusual immunofluorescence pattern. *Br J Dermatol* 1998; **139:** 1129–31.
10. Halevi A, *et al.* Toxic epidermal necrolysis associated with acetaminophen ingestion. *Ann Pharmacother* 2000; **34:** 32–4.

Overdosage. Acute overdosage with paracetamol, whether accidental or deliberate, is relatively common and can be extremely serious because of the narrow margin between therapeutic and toxic doses. Ingestion of as little as 10 to 15 g of paracetamol by adults may cause severe hepatocellular necrosis and, less often, renal tubular necrosis. Indeed, any patient should be considered at risk of severe liver damage if they have ingested more than 150 mg per kg body-weight of paracetamol or 12 g or more in total, whichever is the smaller.

Early features of overdosage such as nausea and vomiting usually settle within 24 hours; other early symptoms may include lethargy and sweating. Abdominal pain may be the first indication of liver damage, which is not usually apparent for 24 to 48 hours and sometimes may be delayed for up to 4 to 6 days after ingestion. Liver damage is generally at a maximum 72 to 96 hours after ingestion. Hepatic failure, encephalopathy, coma, and death may result. Complications of hepatic failure include acidosis, cerebral oedema, haemorrhage, hypoglycaemia, hypotension, infection, and renal failure. An increasing prothrombin time is a reliable indicator of deteriorating liver function and it is recommended by some that the prothrombin time should be measured regularly. Measurement of serum concentrations of aspartate aminotransferase and alanine aminotransferase is also considered to be of value.[1] Patients receiving enzyme-inducing drugs or those with a history of alcohol abuse are at special risk of hepatic damage, as may be patients suffering from malnutrition such as those with anorexia or AIDS. It has also been suggested that fasting may predispose to hepatotoxicity.[2]

Acute renal failure with acute tubular necrosis may develop, even in the absence of severe liver damage. Other non-hepatic symptoms that have been reported following paracetamol overdosage include myocardial abnormalities and pancreatitis.

Toxicity following overdosage with paracetamol has been attributed to the production of a minor but highly reactive metabolite, N-acetyl-p-benzoquinoneimine (NABQI) by mixed function oxidase enzymes in the liver and kidney. The amount of NABQI produced after normal doses of paracetamol is usually completely detoxified by conjugation with glutathione and excreted as mercaptopurine and cysteine conjugates. In paracetamol overdosage, tissue stores of glutathione become depleted, allowing NABQI to accumulate and bind to sulfhydryl groups within hepatocytes causing cell damage. Substances capable of replenishing depleted stores of glutathione, such as acetylcysteine or methionine, are thus used as antidotes in paracetamol overdosage. Acetylcysteine may also be involved in the repair of damaged tissue.

Treatment of paracetamol overdosage. The management of paracetamol overdosage as practised in the UK and US has been the subject of several reviews.[3-13] Guidelines have also been issued in the UK by the Paracetamol Information Centre.

Prompt treatment is essential, even when there are no obvious symptoms, and all patients should be admitted to hospital; full supportive measures should also be instituted. Activated charcoal may be given to reduce gastrointestinal absorption, if it can be given within 1 hour of the overdose, and if more than 150 mg per kg of paracetamol has been ingested. However, if acetylcysteine or methionine is to be given by mouth the charcoal is best cleared from the stomach to prevent it reducing the absorption of the antidote. There is little evidence that gastric lavage is of benefit in those who have overdosed solely with paracetamol.

In order to assess the risk of liver damage, the plasma-paracetamol concentration should be determined as soon as possible, but not within 4 hours of ingestion, to ensure that peak concentrations are recorded. The patient's plasma-paracetamol concentration is compared against a standard nomogram reference line on a plot of plasma-paracetamol concentration against hours after ingestion. A semi-logarithmic plot or a linear plot may be used, see Figure 1 (p.72) and Figure 2 (p.72). Generally, antidote treatment is required if the patient's plasma-paracetamol concentration is higher than this line (but see below). Plasma-paracetamol concentrations measured more than 16 hours after ingestion are not reliable indicators of hepatic toxicity. Furthermore, the nomogram may not be suitable for use when patients have taken modified-release preparations of paracetamol.[14,15] Some suggestions for modified strategies for the use of the Rumack-Matthew nomogram in the face of overdosage with modified-release preparations have been made.[16-18] Deaths from liver failure have occurred in patients presenting with plasma-paracetamol concentrations below the treatment line: suggested explanations include inadequate patient histories and a need for a lower treatment threshold.[19] However if there is any doubt about timing or the need to treat, then a patient should be treated with an antidote. In some centres, patients who have ingested 150 mg per kg or more of paracetamol

Figure 1. A semi-logarithmic plot of plasma-paracetamol concentration against hours after ingestion.

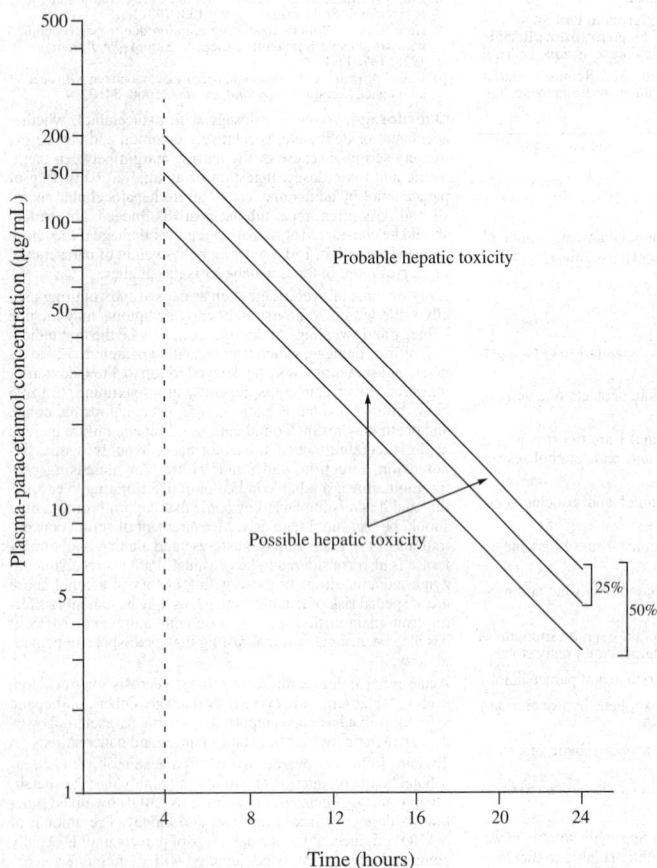

Figure 2. A linear plot of plasma-paracetamol concentration against hours after ingestion.

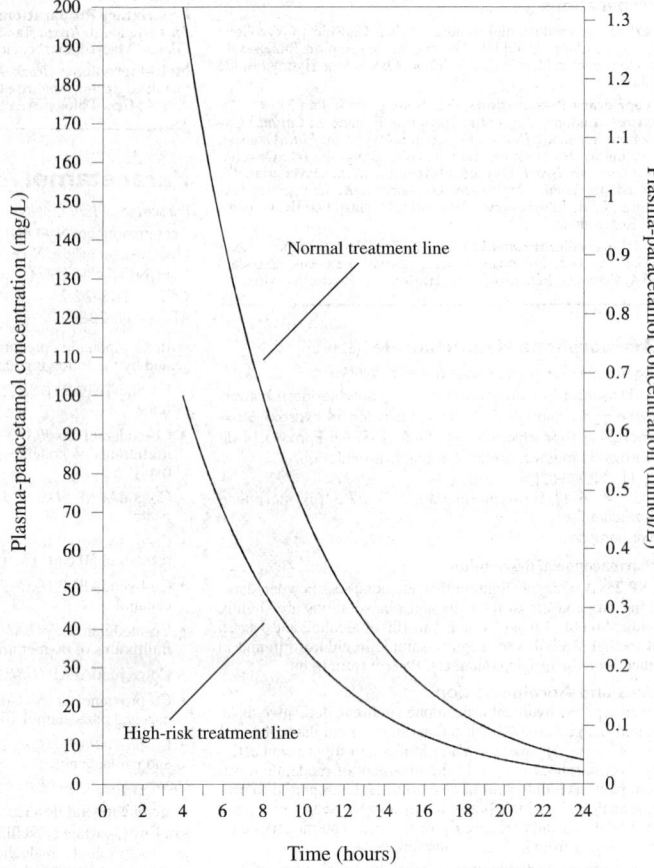

Adapted from Rumack BH, Matthew HJ. Acetaminophen poisoning and toxicity. *Pediatrics* 1975; **55**: 871–6.

Notes for the use of this chart:
1. The time coordinates refer to time after ingestion.
2. Plasma-paracetamol concentrations drawn before 4 hours may not represent peak concentrations.
3. The graph should be used only in relation to a single acute ingestion.
4. The solid line 25% below the standard nomogram is included to allow for possible errors in plasma assays and estimated time from ingestion of an overdose.
5. The solid line 50% below the standard nomogram is to assess the possible hepatic toxicity in patients receiving enzyme-inducing drugs or with malnutrition or a history of alcohol abuse.

Courtesy of P A Routledge.

Notes for the use of this chart:
1. The time coordinates refer to time after ingestion.
2. Plasma-paracetamol concentrations drawn before 4 hours may not represent peak concentrations.
3. The graph should be used only in relation to a single acute ingestion.
4. Patients whose plasma-paracetamol concentrations are above the normal treatment line should be treated.
5. Patients on enzyme-inducing drugs or with malnutrition or a history of alcohol abuse should be treated if their plasma-paracetamol concentrations are above the high-risk treatment line.

are treated regardless of plasma-paracetamol concentrations.[20] Plasma-paracetamol concentrations are also of little value in patients who have taken several overdoses of paracetamol over a short period of time: such patients should be considered as at serious risk and given antidote treatment.

Antidote treatment should be started as soon as possible after suspected paracetamol ingestion and should not be delayed while awaiting the results of plasma assays. Once the results become available, treatment may be stopped if the initial concentration is below the nomogram reference line. However, if the initial concentration is above the reference line, the full course of antidote must be administered and should not be discontinued when subsequent plasma concentrations fall below the reference line. Patients receiving enzyme-inducing drugs such as carbamazepine, phenytoin, phenobarbital, rifampicin, or those with malnutrition or a history of alcohol abuse should receive an antidote even if their plasma-paracetamol concentrations are up to 50% below the standard reference line.

Choice of antidote. Acetylcysteine (p.1082) is usually the antidote of choice but the route of administration varies. Although intravenous administration has been associated with anaphylactic reactions it is the preferred route in the UK because of concerns over the effects of vomiting and activated charcoal on oral absorption. Nausea and vomiting are amongst the most common early symptoms of paracetamol overdosage and may be exacerbated by the extremely disagreeable taste and odour of oral acetylcysteine. However, oral administration is the usual route of choice in the USA and experience there suggests that

it is effective and that the outcome of treatment is not adversely affected by the use of activated charcoal.

An alternative used in the UK is methionine (p.1012) by mouth, which is cheaper and easier to administer than intravenous acetylcysteine. It may also be used in situations where a patient cannot be transferred to hospital, provided it is given within 10 to 12 hours of the overdose and the patient is not vomiting. Methionine absorption is impaired if activated charcoal has been administered or in patients who are vomiting.

Acetylcysteine is most effective when administered during the first 8 hours following ingestion of the overdose and the effect diminishes progressively thereafter. It used to be believed that starting treatment more than 15 hours after overdosage was of no benefit and might possibly aggravate the risk of hepatic encephalopathy. However, late administration has now been shown to be safe,[21] and studies of patients treated up to 36 hours after ingestion suggest that beneficial results may be obtained up to and possibly beyond 24 hours.[22,23] Furthermore, administration of intravenous acetylcysteine to patients who had already developed fulminant hepatic failure has been shown to reduce morbidity and mortality.[24]

In the UK, an initial dose of 150 mg per kg body-weight of acetylcysteine in 200 mL of glucose 5% is given intravenously over 15 minutes, followed by an intravenous infusion of 50 mg per kg in 500 mL of glucose 5% over the next 4 hours and then 100 mg per kg in one litre over the next 16 hours. Sodium chloride 0.9% may be used where glucose 5% is unsuitable. The volume of intravenous fluids should be modified for children. If an anaphylactoid reaction develops, the infusion should be

stopped and an antihistamine administered; it may be possible to continue the acetylcysteine infusion at a slower rate. In the USA, acetylcysteine is given by mouth in an initial dose of 140 mg per kg as a 5% solution followed by 70 mg per kg every 4 hours for an additional 17 doses. Some[25] have suggested using a larger loading dose of acetylcysteine when it is given orally with activated charcoal whereas others[26] have found that the efficacy of acetylcysteine is not adversely affected by prior administration of activated charcoal and consider that increasing the acetylcysteine dose appears to be unwarranted.

Methionine is an alternative to acetylcysteine and, likewise, is most effective when given as early as possible following paracetamol overdosage. However, it is not as effective in late presentation[6,27-29] and the incidence and severity of hepatic damage is greater if treatment with methionine is started more than 10 hours after ingestion; it may also precipitate hepatic encephalopathy.[6]

The usual dose of methionine is 2.5 g by mouth every 4 hours for 4 doses starting less than 10 to 12 hours after ingestion of the paracetamol and provided the patient is not vomiting. It has also been given intravenously. The literature relating to the use of methionine in paracetamol poisoning is, in general, imprecise as to the form of methionine used. In the UK, the doses quoted above refer to DL-methionine. Preparations containing both methionine and paracetamol (co-methiamol) have been formulated for use in situations where overdosage may occur. However, the issue of whether methionine should be routinely added to paracetamol preparations is contentious for medical and ethical reasons.

Histamine H2-antagonists. It has been suggested that since cimetidine blocks the hepatic cytochrome P450 mixed function oxidase system, it might be of use as an adjunct to acetylcysteine for patients whose production of the toxic metabolite of paracetamol is increased due to enzyme induction. Although there have been several anecdotal reports claiming benefit for cimetidine in patients with paracetamol poisoning, there is no current evidence to support these claims.[12,13,30]

Liver transplantation may be considered as a last recourse in some patients.

1. Routledge P, *et al.* Paracetamol (acetaminophen) poisoning. *BMJ* 1998; **317:** 1609–10.
2. Whitcomb DC, *et al.* Association of acetaminophen hepatotoxicity with fasting and ethanol use. *JAMA* 1994; **272:** 1845–50.
3. Keays R, Williams R. Paracetamol poisoning and liver failure. *Prescribers' J* 1989; **29:** 155–62.
4. Scott DK, Vale JA. Paracetamol poisoning. *Pharm J* 1990; **245:** 95–7.
5. Lewis RK, Paloucek FP. Assessment and treatment of acetaminophen overdose. *Clin Pharm* 1991; **10:** 765–74.
6. Janes J, Routledge PA. Recent developments in the management of paracetamol (acetaminophen) poisoning. *Drug Safety* 1992; **7:** 170–7.
7. Bray GP. Liver failure induced by paracetamol. *BMJ* 1993; **306:** 157–8.
8. Ferner R. Paracetamol poisoning—an update. *Prescribers' J* 1993; **33:** 45–50.
9. Collee GG, Hanson GC. The management of acute poisoning *Br J Anaesth* 1993; **70:** 562–73.
10. Makin AJ, *et al.* Management of severe cases of paracetamol overdosage. *Br J Hosp Med* 1994; **52:** 210–13.
11. Vale JA, Proudfoot AT. Paracetamol (acetaminophen) poisoning. *Lancet* 1995; **346:** 547–52.
12. Prescott LF. Paracetamol overdose. In: *Paracetamol (acetaminophen): a critical bibliographic review.* London: Taylor & Francis, 1996: 401–73.
13. Zed PJ, Krenzelok EP. Treatment of acetaminophen overdose. *Am J Health-Syst Pharm* 1999; **56:** 1081–91.
14. Graudins A, *et al.* Overdose of extended-release acetaminophen. *N Engl J Med* 1995; **333:** 196.
15. Vassallo S, *et al.* Use of the Rumack-Matthew nomogram in cases of extended-release acetaminophen toxicity. *Ann Intern Med* 1996; **125:** 940.
16. Temple AR, Mrazik TJ. More on extended-release acetaminophen. *N Engl J Med* 1995; **333:** 1508.
17. Graudins A, *et al.* More on extended-release acetaminophen. *N Engl J Med* 1995; **333:** 1508–9.
18. Cetaruk EW, *et al.* Extended-release acetaminophen overdose. *JAMA* 1996; **275:** 686.
19. Bridger S, *et al.* Deaths from low dose paracetamol poisoning. *BMJ* 1998; **316:** 1724–5.
20. Aujla KS, *et al.* Nomogram does not show absolute concentration for treatment. *BMJ* 1998; **317:** 1655.
21. Parker D, *et al.* Safety of late acetylcysteine treatment in paracetamol poisoning. *Hum Exp Toxicol* 1990; **9:** 25–7.
22. Smilkstein MJ, *et al.* Efficacy of oral N-acetylcysteine in the treatment of acetaminophen overdose: analysis of the National Multicenter Study (1976 to 1985). *N Engl J Med* 1988; **319:** 1557–62.
23. Harrison PM, *et al.* Improved outcome of paracetamol-induced fulminant hepatic failure by late administration of acetylcysteine. *Lancet* 1990; **335:** 1572–3.
24. Keays R, *et al.* Intravenous acetylcysteine in paracetamol induced fulminant hepatic failure: a prospective controlled trial. *BMJ* 1991; **303:** 1026–9.
25. Chamberlain JM, *et al.* Use of activated charcoal in a simulated poisoning with acetaminophen: a new loading dose for N-acetylcysteine? *Ann Emerg Med* 1993; **22:** 1398–1402.
26. Spiller HA, *et al.* A prospective evaluation of the effect of activated charcoal before oral N-acetylcysteine in acetaminophen overdose. *Ann Emerg Med* 1994; **23:** 519–23.
27. Vale JA, *et al.* Intravenous N-acetylcysteine: the treatment of choice in paracetamol poisoning? *BMJ* 1979; **2:** 1435–6.
28. Vale JA, *et al.* Treatment of acetaminophen poisoning: the use of oral methionine. *Arch Intern Med* 1981; **141:** 394–6.
29. Tee LGB, *et al.* N-Acetylcysteine for paracetamol overdose. *Lancet* 1986; **i:** 331–2.
30. Kaufenberg AJ, Shepherd MF. Role of cimetidine in the treatment of acetaminophen poisoning. *Am J Health-Syst Pharm* 1998; **55:** 1516–19.

Pancreatitis. A review of drug-induced pancreatitis reported that pancreatitis associated with paracetamol had only occurred in patients taking more than recommended doses and even then it had been a rare reaction.[1]

1. Underwood TW, Frye CB. Drug-induced pancreatitis. *Clin Pharm* 1993; **12:** 440–8.

Precautions

Paracetamol should be given with care to patients with impaired kidney or liver function. It should also be given with care to patients with alcohol dependence.

Breast feeding. The amount of paracetamol distributed into breast milk is considered by some authorities to be too small to be harmful to a breast-fed infant. Pharmacokinetic studies in 12 nursing mothers given a single dose of paracetamol showed that peak paracetamol concentrations in breast milk of 10 to 15 µg per mL were achieved in 1 to 2 hours. Plasma concentrations were determined in 2 mothers; a breast milk/plasma ratio of about 1 was reported.[1] Similar findings were reported from another study.[2]

1. Berlin CM, *et al.* Disposition of acetaminophen in milk, saliva, and plasma of lactating women. *Pediatr Pharmacol* 1980; **1:** 135–41.
2. Hurden EL, *et al.* Excretion of paracetamol in human breast milk. *Arch Dis Child* 1980; **55:** 969–72.

Renal impairment. Caution is recommended when giving paracetamol to patients with renal impairment. Plasma concentrations of paracetamol and its glucuronide and sulfate conjugates are increased in patients with moderate renal failure and in patients on dialysis.[1-3] It has been suggested that paracetamol itself may be regenerated from these metabolites.[1,2] There are conflicting data on whether the conjugates of paracetamol accumulate in patients with renal impairment receiving multiple doses.[2,3]

1. Prescott LF, *et al.* Paracetamol disposition and metabolite kinetics in patients with chronic renal failure. *Eur J Clin Pharmacol* 1989; **36:** 291–7.
2. Martin U, *et al.* The disposition of paracetamol and the accumulation of its glucuronide and sulphate conjugates during multiple dosing in patients with chronic renal failure. *Eur J Clin Pharmacol* 1991; **41:** 43–6.
3. Martin U, *et al.* The disposition of paracetamol and its conjugates during multiple dosing in patients with end-stage renal failure maintained on haemodialysis. *Eur J Clin Pharmacol* 1993; **45:** 141–5.

Interactions

The risk of paracetamol toxicity may be increased in patients receiving other potentially hepatotoxic drugs or drugs that induce liver microsomal enzymes. The absorption of paracetamol may be accelerated by drugs such as metoclopramide. Excretion may be affected and plasma concentrations altered when administered with probenecid. Colestyramine reduces the absorption of paracetamol if given within one hour of paracetamol administration.

Antibacterials. The plasma-paracetamol concentrations considered an indication for antidote treatment (see under Overdosage, above) should be halved in patients receiving enzyme-inducing drugs such as *rifampicin*. Severe hepatotoxicity at therapeutic doses or moderate overdoses of paracetamol has been reported in patients receiving *isoniazid*, alone[1-3] or with other drugs for tuberculosis.[4]

For the effects of paracetamol on chloramphenicol, see p.180.

1. Murphy R, *et al.* Severe acetaminophen toxicity in a patient receiving isoniazid. *Ann Intern Med* 1990; **113:** 799–800.
2. Moulding TS, *et al.* Acetaminophen, isoniazid, and hepatic toxicity. *Ann Intern Med* 1991; **114:** 431.
3. Crippin JS. Acetaminophen hepatotoxicity: potentiation by isoniazid. *Am J Gastroenterol* 1993; **88:** 590–2.
4. Nolan CM, *et al.* Hepatotoxicity associated with acetaminophen usage in patients receiving multiple drug therapy for tuberculosis. *Chest* 1994; **105:** 408–11.

Anticoagulants. For the effects of paracetamol on oral anticoagulants, see under Warfarin, p.994.

Antiepileptics. The plasma-paracetamol concentrations considered an indication for antidote treatment (see under Overdosage, above) should be halved in patients receiving enzyme-inducing drugs such as *carbamazepine, phenobarbital, phenytoin,* or *primidone.*

For the effects of paracetamol on *lamotrigine*, see p.352.

Antivirals. For reports of adverse effects on the liver associated with concomitant use of paracetamol and antiviral drugs, see under Interferons, p.629 and Zidovudine, p.646.

Probenecid. Pretreatment with probenecid can decrease paracetamol clearance and increase its plasma half-life.[1] Although urinary excretion of the sulfate and glucuronide conjugates of paracetamol are reduced, that of paracetamol is unchanged.

1. Kamali F. The effect of probenecid on paracetamol metabolism and pharmacokinetics. *Eur J Clin Pharmacol* 1993; **45:** 551–3.

Pharmacokinetics

Paracetamol is readily absorbed from the gastrointestinal tract with peak plasma concentrations occurring about 10 to 60 minutes after oral administration. Paracetamol is distributed into most body tissues. It crosses the placenta and is present in breast milk. Plasma-protein binding is negligible at usual therapeutic concentrations but increases with increasing concentrations. The elimination half-life of paracetamol varies from about 1 to 3 hours.

Paracetamol is metabolised predominantly in the liver and excreted in the urine mainly as the glucuronide and sulfate conjugates. Less than 5% is excreted as unchanged paracetamol. A minor hydroxylated metabolite (*N-acetyl-p-benzoquinoneimine*), which is usually produced in very small amounts by mixed-function oxidases in the liver and kidney and which is usually detoxified by conjugation with glutathione, may accumulate following paracetamol overdosage and cause tissue damage.

Absorption. The absorption of paracetamol was slow and incomplete in vegetarian subjects compared with non-vegetarian subjects.[1]

1. Prescott LF, *et al.* Impaired absorption of paracetamol in vegetarians. *Br J Clin Pharmacol* 1993; **36:** 237–40.

Uses and Administration

Paracetamol, a para-aminophenol derivative, has analgesic and antipyretic properties and weak anti-inflammatory activity. Paracetamol is given by mouth or as a rectal suppository for mild to moderate pain and for fever (p.8). Paracetamol is often the analgesic or antipyretic of choice especially in patients in whom salicylates or other NSAIDs are contra-indicated. Such patients include asthmatics or those with a history of peptic ulcer, or children. Its use is also generally preferred in elderly patients.

The usual adult dose by mouth is 0.5 to 1 g every 4 to 6 hours up to a maximum of 4 g daily. Usual doses in children are: under 3 months, 10 mg per kg bodyweight (reduce to 5 mg per kg if jaundiced); 3 months to 1 year, 60 to 120 mg; 1 to 5 years, 120 to 250 mg; 6 to 12 years, 250 to 500 mg. These doses may be given every 4 to 6 hours when necessary up to a maximum of 4 doses in 24 hours. For post-immunisation pyrexia, a dose of 60 mg has been recommended for children 2 to 3 months of age. A second dose may be given after four to six hours; if the pyrexia persists after that dose, medical advice should be sought.

Rectal doses for adults and children over 12 years of age are 0.5 to 1 g. Rectal doses in younger children are: 1 to 5 years, 125 to 250 mg; 6 to 12 years, 250 to 500 mg. Doses may be administered up to 4 times daily.

◊ References.

1. Prescott LF. *Paracetamol (acetaminophen): a critical bibliographic review.* London: Taylor & Francis, 1996.

Administration in children. It has been suggested[1] that the recommended doses of paracetamol for children may result in subtherapeutic blood concentrations, and that an initial loading dose should be given, followed by regular doses up to the recommended maximum daily dose. However, the appropriate maximum daily dose remains controversial, and there is obvious concern given the risks of overdosage. For recommended doses in children see above.

1. Zacharias M, Watts D. Pain relief in children. *BMJ* 1998; **316:** 1552.

Headache. Non-opioid analgesics such as paracetamol, aspirin, and other NSAIDs are often tried first for the symptomatic treatment of various types of headache including migraine (see p.449) and tension-type headache (see p.450). These drugs given at the onset of symptoms can successfully treat an acute attack of migraine. However, absorption may be poor due to gastric stasis which is commonly present in migraine. For this reason dispersible and effervescent preparations and compound preparations containing drugs such as metoclopramide which relieve gastric stasis have been advocated.

Pain. Paracetamol is used in the management of mild to moderate pain (p.2). It is of similar potency to aspirin, but with weak anti-inflammatory activity. Paracetamol may also be used as an adjunct to opioids in the management of severe pain such as cancer pain (p.5). Paracetamol is the preferred choice for pain in children (p.3) because of the association of aspirin with Reye's syndrome in this age group (see p.15). In the treatment of rheumatic disorders, a weak anti-inflammatory effect limits the role of paracetamol. However, it may be of benefit for simple pain control in rheumatoid arthritis (p.9) and ankylosing spondylitis (see under Spondyloarthropathies, p.10), although these patients usually require the additional anti-inflammatory effects provided by NSAIDs. Synovial inflammation is usually only a minor component of osteoarthritis (p.9), and paracetamol is generally recommended as first choice of treatment before NSAIDs are tried. Paracetamol is useful for the relief of acute low back pain (p.6).

Dependence and tolerance are not a problem with non-opioid analgesics such as paracetamol, but there is a ceiling of efficacy, above which increasing the dose has no further therapeutic effect.

Preparations

BP 2001: Co-codamol Tablets; Co-dydramol Tablets; Co-proxamol Tablets; Dispersible Paracetamol Tablets; Paediatric Paracetamol Oral Solution; Paracetamol Oral Suspension; Paracetamol Suppositories; Paracetamol Tablets; Soluble Paracetamol Tablets; *USP 25:* Acetaminophen and Aspirin Tablets; Acetaminophen and Caffeine Tablets; Acetaminophen and Codeine Phosphate Capsules; Acetaminophen and Codeine Phosphate Oral Solution; Acetaminophen and Codeine Phosphate Oral Suspension; Acetaminophen and Codeine Phosphate Tablets; Acetaminophen and Diphenhydramine Citrate Tablets; Acetaminophen and Pseudoephedrine Hydrochloride Tablets; Acetaminophen Capsules; Acetaminophen for Effervescent Oral Solution; Acetaminophen Oral Solution; Acetaminophen Oral Suspension; Acetaminophen Suppositories; Acetaminophen Tablets; Acetaminophen, Aspirin, and Caffeine Tablets; Acetaminophen, Diphenhydramine Hydrochloride, and Pseudoephedrine Hydrochloride Tablets; Acetaminophen, Dextromethorphan Hydrobromide, Doxylamine Succinate, and Pseudoephedrine Hydrochloride Oral Solution; Acetaminophen, Diphenhydramine Hydrochloride, and Pseudoephedrine Hydrochloride Tablets; Butalbital, Acetaminophen, and Caffeine Capsules; Butalbital,

---

The symbol † denotes a preparation no longer actively marketed

Acetaminophen, and Caffeine Tablets; Hydrocodone Bitartrate and Acetaminophen Tablets; Isometheptene Mucate, Dichloralphenazone, and Acetaminophen Capsules; Oxycodone and Acetaminophen Capsules; Oxycodone and Acetaminophen Tablets; Propoxyphene Hydrochloride and Acetaminophen Tablets; Propoxyphene Napsylate and Acetaminophen Tablets.

Proprietary Preparations (details are given in Part 3)
Aust.: Apacet; Ben-u-ron; Duaneo; Enelfa; Kratofin simplex; Mexalen; Momentum; Parakapton; Peinfort; Tylenol; *Austral.:* Chemists Own Pain & Fever; Childrens Panadol; Dymadon; Febridol; Lemsip; Lemsip Headcold; Lemsip Max; Ordov Febrigesic; Panadol; Panamax; Parahexal; Paralgin; Setamol; Tempra; Tylenol; *Belg.:* Curpol; Dafalgan; Dolprone; Efferalgan; Lemgrip; Lonarid Mono; Neuridon†; Panadol; Pe-Tam; Perdolan Mono; Sanicopyrine; Tempra; *Braz.:* Acetamol; Acetofen; Anatyl; Baicurina; Calpol; Dordendril; Dorico; Gripeonil; Pacemol; Parador; Piramin; Tylenol; Tylephen; *Canad.:* 222 AF; Abenol; Acet; Acetab; AF Anacin†; Alsiphene; Artritol; Atasol; Cephanol; Childrens Feverhalt; Novo-Gesic; Pain Aid Free; Panadol; Pediatrix; Robigesic; Rounox; Tantaphen; Tempra; Tylenol; *Denm.:* Pamol; Panodil; Pinex; *Fin.:* Panadol; Para-Suppo; Para-Tabs; *Fr.:* Aferadol†; Claradol; Compralsol; Dafalgan; Dolflash†; Doliprane; Dolitabs; Dolko; Dolotec; Efferalgan; Expandox; Febrectol; Geluprane; Gynospasmine†; Oralgan†; Panadol; Paralyoc; *Ger.:* Anti-Algos†; Antipanin N; Antipanin P; Ben-u-ron; Captin; Contac Erkaltungs-Trunk; Doloreduct; Dorocoff-Paracetamol; duracetamol; Enelfa; Fensum; Finiweh; Grippostad Heissgetrank; Larylin Heissgetrank gegen Schmerzen und Fieber†; Logomed Schmerz-/Fieber†; Mandrogripp†; Momentum Analgetikum†; Mono Pracimed; NeoCitran†; NilnOcen; Paedialgon; Pyromed S; RubieMol; Togal; Treupel mono; Vivimed†; *Hong Kong:* Afebrin; Apap; Arfen; Ben-u-ron; Biogesic; Calpol; Cortal for Children; Dhamol; Fortolin; Panadol; Progesic; Tiffy; Tylenol; Uni-Febrin; *Irl.:* Calpol; Disprol; Hedex; Panadol; Paralief; Paralink; Parapaed; Tylenol; *Israel:* Abrol; Abrolet; Acamol; Acamoli; Aldolor; Dexamol; Dexamol Kid; Liqiprin; Paramolan; Rokamol; Supramol; Vimoli; *Ital.:* Acetamol; Efferalgan; Levadol; Neo-Fepramol; Panadol; Puernol; Tachipirina; *Mex.:* Acetafen; Acetif; Alpirex; Amolgen; Analmex; Andopan; Andox; Antidol; Brontonyl; Calinofen; Calpol; Carofril; Colderina; Coriver; Datril; Dolviran NF; Farpik; Febrim; Febronyl; Ifutemp; Infalgina; Magnidol-Plus; Masferol; Minofen; Minomex; Neodol; Neodolito; Panadol; Parengesico; Pharmacen; Piraldin; Precifen; Resfin; Sedalito; Sinedol; Sons Piral; Temperal; Tempra; Temprin; Termotrin; Terol; Tylenol; Tylex; Verbalem; Wifibrin; Winasorb; *Neth.:* Daro†; Darocet†; Hedex†; Kinder Finimal; Momentum; Panadol; Sinaspril-Paracetamol; *Norw.:* Alvedon†; Pamol; Panodil; Paracet; Pinex; *NZ:* Disprol; Lemsip Cold & Flu Original, Cold & Flu Max; Pamol; Panadol; Paracare; Parasorbe; Paramolan; Parsel; Supofen; Tylenol; Zaramol; *S.Afr.:* Antalgic; Arcanagesic†; Brunomol; Calpol; Cetapon†; Compu-Pain†; Dolorol; Doxypol; Dynadol; Empaped; Entalgic; Farmacetamol†; Fevamol; Lyteca†; Maxadol-P; Medpramol†; Merck-Gesic; Napamol; Pacimol; Painamol; Pamol†; Panado; Prolief; Pyradol; Pyragesic†; Temol; Tylenol; Winpain; *Singapore:* Acet; Biogesic; Calpol; Dhamol; Milidon; Naprex; Pacemol; Panadol; Rapidol; Remedol; Setamol; Tempra; *Spain:* Acertol; Actron; Akindol†; Analter; Antidol; Apiretal; Aspac; Asplin†; Bandol; Calmanticold; Cupanol; Dafalgan; Dolgesic; Dolostop; Duorol; Efferalgan; Febranine; Febrectal; Gelocatil; Hedex; Melabon Infantil; Nofedol; Panadol; Pediapirin†; Pirinasol; Sinmol; Stopain; Temperal; Tempra; Termalgin; Tylenol; Zatinol†; Zolben†; *Swed.:* Alvedon; Curadon; Lemsip†; Panodil; Reliv; *Switz.:* Acetalgine; Becetamol; Ben-u-ron; Comprimes analgesiques no 534; Contre-Douleurs P; Dafalgan; Democyl; Demogripal; Dolprone; Fortalidon P; Influbene N; Nina; Ortensan†; Panadol; Spalt N; Termalgin; Treupel N†; Treuphadol; Tylenol; Zolben; *Thai.:* Aceta-P; Acetasil; Algogen; Biogesic; Calpol; Daga; Detamol; Nutamol; Panadol; Paracap; Paracet; Paramol; Paramol TP; Paramol TP without Lignocaine; Paranal; Paranal-L; Parat; Paratol; Partamol; Pyracon; Pyretal; Ramol; Sara; Saridon; Temolan; Tempra; Tumdi; Tylenol; Tymol; Unimol; Vemol; *UAE:* Adol; *UK:* Alvedon; Anadin Paracetamol; Calpol; Disprol; Elkamol; Fanalgic; Fennings Children's Powders; Galpamol; Hedex; Infadrops; Mandanol; Medinol; Miradol; Obimol; Pain Relief Syrup for Children; Paldesic; Panadol; Panaleve; Paracets; Paraclear; Paramin; Parapaed; Placidex; Salzone; Tixymol; Tramil†; *USA:* Acephen; Aceta; AlbaTemp†; Apacet; Apap; Arthritis Foundation Pain Reliever, Aspirin Free†; Arthritis Pain Formula Aspirin Free; Aspirin Free Anacin; Aspirin Free Pain Relief; Bromo Seltzer; Childrens Dynafed Jr; Childrens Mapap; Dapa†; Dolanex†; Dolono; Dorcol Children's Fever & Pain Reducer†; Dynafed EX; Feverall; Genapap; Genebs; Halenol; Liquiprin; Mapap; Maranox; Meda; Myapap†; Neopap; Oraphen-PD; Panadol; Panex†; Panitone; Redutemp; Ridenol; Silapap; Snaplets-FR†; St. Joseph Aspirin-Free for Children†; Suppap†; Tapanol; Tempra; Tylenol; Uni-Ace.

Multi-ingredient: numerous preparations are listed in Part 3.

Parecoxib Sodium (20432-n)

Parecoxib Sodium *(BANM, USAN, rINNM)*.
SC-69124A. N-{[p-(5-Methyl-3-phenyl-4-isoxazolyl)phenyl]sulfonyl}propionamide sodium.
$C_{19}H_{17}N_2NaO_4S = 392.4$.
CAS — 198470-84-7 (parecoxib); 197502-82-2 (parecoxib sodium).

Profile
Parecoxib is an NSAID (p.63) reported to be a selective inhibitor of cyclo-oxygenase-2 (COX-2). It has been given by injection in the treatment of postoperative pain.

◊ References.
1. Cheer SM, Goa KL. Parecoxib (parecoxib sodium). *Drugs* 2001; **61:** 1133–41.

Pentazocine (6251-l)

Pentazocine *(BAN, USAN, rINN)*.
NIH-7958; NSC-107430; Pentazocinum; Win-20228. (2R*,6R*,11R*)-1,2,3,4,5,6-Hexahydro-6,11-dimethyl-3-(3-methylbut-2-enyl)-2,6-methano-3-benzazocin-8-ol.
$C_{19}H_{27}NO = 285.4$.
CAS — 359-83-1.
ATC — N02AD01.
Pharmacopoeias. In Eur. (see p.vi), Jpn, and US.

Pentazocine 100 mg is approximately equivalent to 112.8 mg of pentazocine hydrochloride or 131.6 mg of pentazocine lactate.

Pharmacopoeial description
Ph. Eur.: A white or almost white powder. It shows polymorphism. Practically insoluble in water; soluble in alcohol; freely soluble in dichloromethane. Protect from light.
USP 25: A white or very pale, tan-coloured powder. Practically insoluble in water; soluble 1 in 11 of alcohol, 1 in 2 of chloroform, and 1 in 42 of ether; soluble in acetone; sparingly soluble in ethyl acetate and in benzene. Store in airtight containers. Protect from light.

Pentazocine Hydrochloride (6252-y)

Pentazocine Hydrochloride *(BANM, USAN, rINNM)*.
Pentazocini Hydrochloridum.
$C_{19}H_{27}NO,HCl = 321.9$.
CAS — 2276-52-0; 64024-15-3.
Pharmacopoeias. In Eur. (see p.vi) and US.

Pharmacopoeial description
Ph. Eur.: A white or almost white powder. It shows polymorphism. Sparingly soluble in water and in dichloromethane; soluble in alcohol. A 1% solution in water has a pH of 4.0 to 6.0. Protect from light.
USP 25: A white crystalline powder. It exhibits polymorphism, one form melting at about 254° and the other at about 218°. Soluble 1 in 30 of water, 1 in 20 of alcohol, and 1 in 4 of chloroform; very slightly soluble in acetone and in ether; practically insoluble in benzene. Store in airtight containers. Protect from light.

Pentazocine Lactate (6253-j)

Pentazocine Lactate *(BANM, USAN, rINNM)*.
$C_{19}H_{27}NO,C_3H_6O_3 = 375.5$.
CAS — 17146-95-1.
Pharmacopoeias. Br. includes Pentazocine Injection and Pentazocine Suppositories which contain pentazocine lactate. US includes Pentazocine Lactate Injection.

Incompatibility. Commercial injections of pentazocine lactate are reported to be incompatible with soluble barbiturates and other alkaline substances including sodium bicarbonate. Diazepam and chlordiazepoxide have also been reported to be incompatible, as have glycopyrronium bromide[1] and nafcillin sodium.[2]

1. Ingallinera TS, *et al.* Compatibility of glycopyrrolate injection with commonly used infusion solutions and additives. *Am J Hosp Pharm* 1979; **36:** 508–10.
2. Jeglum EL, *et al.* Nafcillin sodium incompatibility with acidic solutions. *Am J Hosp Pharm* 1981; **38:** 462, 464.

Dependence and Withdrawal
As for Opioid Analgesics, p.66. Pentazocine is subject to abuse.

◊ Pentazocine does produce physical dependence, but withdrawal symptoms are substantially less severe than with morphine. It does not typically produce drug-seeking behaviour of the same degree or intensity as morphine or other prototypic μ agonists, nor does it substitute for morphine in dependent subjects.[1] Pentazocine injection has been abused,[2] but street abuse, especially in the USA, has more often involved the intravenous use of crushed tablets of pentazocine and tripelennamine ('T's and Blues').[3-5] A decreased incidence of pentazocine abuse in the USA appeared to coincide with the introduction of oral tablets incorporating naloxone,[1] the rationale being that naloxone antagonises the effect of pentazocine if illicitly injected, but has no effect when taken by mouth. Some continued to abuse the new pentazocine/naloxone formulation;[6] intravenous abuse in one woman, who was unaware of the reformulation, resulted in opioid withdrawal symptoms and severe hypertension.[7] A 1989 report from the WHO committee[1] rated the likelihood of abuse of pentazocine as moderate, based on its pharmacological profile, dependence potential, and actual abuse. The committee considered that it should continue to be scheduled as a psychotropic substance rather than a narcotic drug.

1. WHO. WHO expert committee on drug dependence: twenty-fifth report. *WHO Tech Rep Ser* 775 1989.
2. Hunter R, Ingram IM. Intravenous pentazocine abuse by a nurse. *Lancet* 1983; **ii:** 227.
3. Poklis A, Whyatt PL. Current trends in the abuse of pentazocine and tripelennamine: the metropolitan St. Louis experience. *J Forensic Sci* 1980; **25:** 72–8.
4. Senay EC. Clinical experience with T's and B's. *Drug Alcohol Depend* 1985; **14:** 305–11.
5. Jackson C, *et al.* Fatal intracranial hemorrhage associated with phenylpropanolamine, pentazocine, and tripelennamine overdose. *J Emerg Med* 1985; **3:** 127–32.

6. Reed DA, Schnoll SH. Abuse of pentazocine-naloxone combination. *JAMA* 1986; **256:** 2562–4.
7. Reinhart S, Barrett SM. An acute hypertensive response after intravenous use of a new pentazocine formulation. *Ann Emerg Med* 1985; **14:** 591–3.

Adverse Effects
As for Opioid Analgesics in general, p.67.
Pentazocine may cause hallucinations and other psychotomimetic effects such as nightmares and thought disturbances. High doses may result in hypertension and tachycardia; increased aortic and pulmonary artery pressure with an increase in cardiac work has followed intravenous administration in patients with myocardial infarction. Like morphine it causes respiratory depression, but pentazocine is said to have a 'ceiling' effect in that the depth of respiratory depression does not increase proportionately with higher doses.
Rare adverse effects with pentazocine have included agranulocytosis and toxic epidermal necrolysis.
Pentazocine injections may be painful. Local tissue damage may occur at injection sites particularly after subcutaneous injection or multiple doses; there have been reports of muscle fibrosis associated with intramuscular injections.

Effects on the blood. There have been reports of agranulocytosis associated with pentazocine.[1-3]
1. Marks A, Abramson N. Pentazocine and agranulocytosis. *Ann Intern Med* 1980; **92:** 433.
2. Haibach H, *et al.* Pentazocine-induced agranulocytosis. *Can Med Assoc J* 1984; **130:** 1165–6.
3. Sheehan M, *et al.* Pentazocine-induced agranulocytosis. *Can Med Assoc J* 1985; **132:** 1401.

Effects on the CNS. A report of oculogyric crisis associated with the use of pentazocine.[1]
1. Burstein AH, Fullerton T. Oculogyric crisis possibly related to pentazocine. *Ann Pharmacother* 1993; **27:** 874–6.

Effects on the skin. Toxic epidermal necrolysis in a 62-year-old man was attributed to pentazocine;[1] he had taken 50 to 75 mg every 4 hours for 8 days. His severe uraemia was attributed to fluid loss through the skin.
1. Hunter JAA, Davison AM. Toxic epidermal necrolysis associated with pentazocine therapy and severe reversible renal failure. *Br J Dermatol* 1973; **88:** 287–90.

Treatment of Adverse Effects
As for Opioid Analgesics in general, p.68. As pentazocine has both opioid agonist and antagonist activity its effects may not be completely reversed by naloxone, but use of the latter is still recommended in pentazocine overdosage.

Precautions
As for Opioid Analgesics in general, p.68.
Pentazocine has weak opioid antagonist actions and may precipitate withdrawal symptoms if given to patients who are physically dependent on opioids. It should generally be avoided after myocardial infarction and in patients with heart failure or arterial or pulmonary hypertension.
When frequent injections are needed, pentazocine should be given intramuscularly rather than subcutaneously and the injection sites should be varied.

Abuse. See under Dependence and Withdrawal, above.

Porphyria. Pentazocine has been associated with acute attacks of porphyria and is considered unsafe in porphyric patients.

Interactions
For interactions associated with opioid analgesics, see p.68.

Tobacco smoking. Smokers metabolised about 40% more pentazocine than non-smokers, although there was large intersubject variation;[1] tobacco smoking might induce liver enzymes responsible for drug oxidation.[1]
1. Vaughan DP, *et al.* The influence of smoking on the inter-subject variation in pentazocine elimination. *Br J Clin Pharmacol* 1976; **3:** 279–83.

Pharmacokinetics
Pentazocine is absorbed from the gastrointestinal tract; following administration by mouth, peak plasma concentrations are reached in 1 to 3 hours and the half-life is reported to be about 4 hours. After intramuscular injection, peak plasma concentrations are reached in 15 minutes to 1 hour. About 60% has been reported to be bound to plasma protein. Pentazocine undergoes extensive first-pass metabolism in the liver; oral bioavailability is low with only about half of a dose reaching the systemic circulation. Metabolites and a small amount of unchanged drug are excreted in the urine. It diffuses across the placenta.

Hepatic impairment. Clearance of pentazocine was significantly reduced and terminal half-life and oral bioavailability increased in cirrhotic patients when compared with healthy subjects.[1]
1. Neal EA, *et al.* Enhanced bioavailability and decreased clearance of analgesics in patients with cirrhosis. *Gastroenterology* 1979; **77:** 96–102.

Uses and Administration
Pentazocine, a benzomorphan derivative, is an opioid analgesic (p.68) that has mixed opioid agonist and antagonist actions. Agonist activity is thought to be predominantly at κ opioid receptors (with possibly some σ receptor activity); it acts as a weak antagonist or partial agonist at μ receptors. Pentazocine is used for the relief of moderate to severe pain. Combined preparations with paracetamol or aspirin may also be used in the treatment of moderate pain. It may also be used for pre-opera-

tive sedation and as an adjunct to anaesthesia. Its analgesic effect declines more rapidly than that of morphine.

Pentazocine is administered by mouth as the hydrochloride. A usual dose is the equivalent of 50 to 100 mg of pentazocine or pentazocine hydrochloride every 3 to 4 hours after food. Children aged 6 to 12 years may be given 25 mg every 3 to 4 hours.

Pentazocine is also administered by subcutaneous, intramuscular, and intravenous injection as the lactate. The usual dose is the equivalent of pentazocine 30 to 60 mg every 3 to 4 hours; it should not be necessary to exceed 360 mg daily. Also if frequent injections are needed, the intramuscular route should be used rather than the subcutaneous route, and the injection sites should be varied. In the USA single intravenous doses of not more than 30 mg are advised.

Pentazocine is also given rectally as the lactate in suppositories usually in a dose equivalent to pentazocine 50 mg up to 4 times daily.

As a deterrent to abuse a combined oral preparation of pentazocine hydrochloride and naloxone hydrochloride is available in some countries.

Preparations

BP 2001: Pentazocine Capsules; Pentazocine Injection; Pentazocine Suppositories; Pentazocine Tablets;
USP 25: Pentazocine and Naloxone Hydrochlorides Tablets; Pentazocine Hydrochloride and Aspirin Tablets; Pentazocine Lactate Injection.

Proprietary Preparations (details are given in Part 3)
Aust.: Fortral†; *Austral.:* Fortral; *Belg.:* Fortal; *Canad.:* Talwin; *Denm.:* Fortral; *Fr.:* Fortal; *Ger.:* Fortral; *Irl.:* Fortral; *Israel:* Rafazocine; Talwin; Talwin NX; *Ital.:* Pentafen†; Pentalgina†; Talwin; Talwin-Tab; *Jpn:* Peltazon; Pentagin; Sosegon; *Neth.:* Fortral; *Norw.:* Fortralin; *NZ:* Fortral; *Port.:* Sosegon; *S.Afr.:* Ospronim; Sosenol; *Singapore:* Talwin; *Spain:* Sosegon; *Swed.:* Fortalgesic†; *Switz.:* Fortalgesic; *Thai.:* Fortwin; Pangon; Sosegon; *UK:* Fortral; *USA:* Talwin; Talwin NX.

Multi-ingredient: *Irl.:* Fortagesic; *Israel:* Rafazocine X; *USA:* Emergent-Ez; Talacen; Talwin Compound.

Pethidine Hydrochloride (6254-z)

Pethidine Hydrochloride (BANM, rINNM).
Meperidine Hydrochloride; Pethidini Hydrochloridum. Ethyl 1-methyl-4-phenylpiperidine-4-carboxylate hydrochloride.
$C_{15}H_{21}NO_2,HCl = 283.8$.
CAS — 57-42-1 (pethidine); 50-13-5 (pethidine hydrochloride).
Pharmacopoeias. In Chin., Eur. (see p.vi), Int., Jpn, Pol., and US.

Pharmacopoeial description

Ph. Eur.: A white crystalline powder. Very soluble in water; freely soluble in alcohol. Store in airtight containers. Protect from light.

USP 25: A fine white odourless crystalline powder. Very soluble in water; soluble in alcohol; sparingly soluble in ether. pH of a 5% solution in water is about 5. Protect from light.

Incompatibility. Solutions of pethidine hydrochloride are acidic. They are incompatible with barbiturate salts and loss of clarity was also observed in an early additive study[1] with other drugs including aminophylline, heparin sodium, meticillin sodium, morphine sulfate, nitrofurantoin sodium, phenytoin sodium, sodium iodide, sulfadiazine sodium, and sulfafurazole diolamine. Colour change from pale yellow to light green occurred when solutions of minocycline hydrochloride or tetracycline hydrochloride were mixed with pethidine hydrochloride in 5% glucose injection.[2] In the same study an immediate precipitate occurred on admixture with cefoperazone sodium or mezlocillin sodium; with nafcillin sodium an immediate cloudy appearance cleared on agitation. Incompatibility has also been observed between pethidine hydrochloride and aciclovir sodium, imipenem, frusemide [furosemide],[3] liposomal doxorubicin hydrochloride,[4] and idarubicin.[5] Solutions of cefazolin sodium[6] and pethidine hydrochloride mixed in 5% glucose injection turned light yellow after 5 days storage at 25°; the admixture was stable for at least 20 days at 4°.

1. Patel JA, Phillips GL. A guide to physical compatibility of intravenous drug admixtures. *Am J Hosp Pharm* 1966; **23:** 409–11.
2. Nieves-Cordero AL, et al. Compatibility of narcotic analgesic solutions with various antibiotics during simulated Y-site injection. *Am J Hosp Pharm* 1985; **42:** 1108–9.
3. Pugh CB, et al. Visual compatibility of morphine sulfate and meperidine hydrochloride with other injectable drugs during simulated Y-site injection. *Am J Hosp Pharm* 1991; **48:** 123–5.
4. Trissel LA, et al. Compatibility of doxorubicin hydrochloride liposome injection with selected other drugs during simulated Y-site administration. *Am J Health-Syst Pharm* 1997; **54:** 2708–13.
5. Turowski RC, Durthaler JM. Visual compatibility of idarubicin hydrochloride with selected drugs during simulated Y-site injection. *Am J Hosp Pharm* 1991; **48:** 2181–4.
6. Lee DKT, et al. Stability of cefazolin sodium and meperidine hydrochloride. *Am J Health-Syst Pharm* 1996; **53:** 1608–10.

Stability. Pethidine hydrochloride injection 100 mg per mL was stable for at least 24 hours at room temperature when diluted to a concentration of 300 mg per mL in glucose 5% and 4% and in sodium chloride injection (0.9%) and sodium chloride injection (0.9%) diluted 1 in 5.[1]

The symbol † denotes a preparation no longer actively marketed

Accelerated stability studies using elevated temperatures and humidities to simulate tropical conditions classified pethidine hydrochloride as a 'less stable drug substance'.[2] It was suggested that during quality assurance of preparations containing pethidine hydrochloride particular attention should be paid to their stability.

1. Rudd L, Simpson P. Pethidine stability in intravenous solutions. *Med J Aust* 1978; **2:** 34.
2. WHO. WHO expert committee on specifications for pharmaceutical preparations: thirty-first report. *WHO Tech Rep Ser 790* 1990.

Dependence and Withdrawal

As for Opioid Analgesics, p.66. Doses of pethidine as large as 3 or 4 g daily have been taken by addicts. As tolerance to the CNS stimulant and antimuscarinic effects is not complete with these very large doses, muscle twitching, tremor, mental confusion, dilated pupils, and sometimes convulsions may be present.

Withdrawal symptoms appear more rapidly than with morphine and are of shorter duration.

For the abuse of pethidine analogues, see under Precautions, below.

Adverse Effects and Treatment

As for Opioid Analgesics in general, p.67.

The effects on smooth muscle may be relatively less intense than with morphine and constipation occurs less frequently. After overdosage, symptoms are generally similar to those of morphine poisoning. However, stimulation of the CNS and convulsions may also occur, especially in tolerant individuals or following toxic doses by mouth; these have been attributed mainly to the metabolite norpethidine. Local reactions often follow injection of pethidine; general hypersensitivity reactions occur rarely. The intravenous administration of pethidine may result in increased heart rate.

◊ The incidence of adverse effects in hospitalised patients receiving pethidine was monitored by the Boston Collaborative Drug Surveillance Program.[1] Following pethidine by mouth adverse reactions were reported in 16 of 366 patients and mainly involved the gastrointestinal tract. Following pethidine by injection 102 of 3268 patients had adverse effects, the CNS being involved in 38.

1. Miller RR, Jick H. Clinical effects of meperidine in hospitalized medical patients. *J Clin Pharmacol* 1978; **18:** 180–9.

Effects on the cardiovascular system. Histamine release was more frequent after pethidine than after morphine, fentanyl, or sufentanil administered intravenously for the induction of anaesthesia.[1] Increased plasma-histamine concentrations occurred in 5 of 16 patients given pethidine in a mean dose of 4.3 mg per kg body-weight and were generally accompanied by hypotension, tachycardia, erythema, and increased plasma-adrenaline concentrations. Only 1 of 10 given morphine and none of those receiving fentanyl or sufentanil showed evidence of histamine release. All of the histamine releasers were young women.

1. Flacke JW, et al. Histamine release by four narcotics: a double-blind study in humans. *Anesth Analg* 1987; **66:** 723–30.

Effects on the nervous system. CNS excitatory effects of pethidine such as tremors, muscle twitches, and convulsions have been associated with toxic doses and have been attributed to the metabolite norpethidine. Accumulation of norpethidine may occur if large doses of pethidine are repeated at short intervals (including for patient-controlled analgesia) and is especially likely when renal function is impaired.[1-12]

1. Kaiko RF, et al. Central nervous system excitatory effects of meperidine in cancer patients. *Ann Neurol* 1983; **13:** 180–5.
2. Lieberman AN, Goldstein M. Reversible parkinsonism related to meperidine. *N Engl J Med* 1985; **312:** 509.
3. Mauro VF, et al. Meperidine-induced seizure in a patient without renal dysfunction or sickle cell anemia. *Clin Pharm* 1986; **5:** 837–9.
4. Morisy L, Platt D. Hazards of high-dose meperidine. *JAMA* 1986; **255:** 467–8.
5. Armstrong PJ, Bersten A. Normeperidine toxicity. *Anesth Analg* 1986; **65:** 536–8.
6. Eisendrath SJ, et al. Meperidine-induced delirium. *Am J Psychiatry* 1987; **144:** 1062–5.
7. Kyff JV, Rice TL. Meperidine-associated seizures in a child. *Clin Pharm* 1990; **9:** 337–8.
8. Pryle BJ, et al. Toxicity of norpethidine in sickle cell crisis. *BMJ* 1992; **304:** 1478–9.
9. Hagmeyer KO, et al. Meperidine-related seizures associated with patient-controlled analgesia pumps. *Ann Pharmacother* 1993; **27:** 29–32.
10. Stone PA, et al. Norpethidine toxicity and patient controlled analgesia. *Br J Anaesth* 1993; **71:** 738–40.
11. Marinella MA. Meperidine-induced generalized seizures with normal renal function. *South Med J* 1997; **90:** 556–8.
12. McHugh GJ. Norpethidine accumulation and generalized seizure during pethidine patient-controlled analgesia. *Anaesth Intensive Care* 1999; **27:** 289–91.

Precautions

As for Opioid Analgesics in general, p.68. Pethidine should also be given cautiously to patients with a history of convulsive disorders.

Abuse. A synthetic analogue of pethidine, MPPP (1-methyl-4-phenyl-4-propionoxypiperidine), manufactured illicitly for recreational use, achieved notoriety when it was accidentally contaminated with MPTP (1-methyl-4-phenyl-1,2,3,6-tetrahydropyridine) leading to an epidemic of parkinsonism among intravenous drug abusers.[1] WHO has also identified another analogue, PEPAP (1-phenylethyl-4-phenyl-4-acetoxypiperidine) as being liable to abuse.[2]

1. Buchanan JF, Brown CR. 'Designer drugs': a problem in clinical toxicology. *Med Toxicol* 1988; **3:** 1–17.
2. WHO. WHO expert committee on drug dependence: twenty-fourth report. *WHO Tech Rep Ser 761* 1988.

The elderly. Pethidine had a slower elimination rate in elderly compared with young patients and a reduction in total daily dose might be necessary in elderly patients receiving repeated doses of pethidine.[1] Another study concluded that age-related changes in disposition were not sufficient to warrant modification of pethidine dosage regimens.[2]

1. Holmberg L, et al. Comparative disposition of pethidine and norpethidine in old and young patients. *Eur J Clin Pharmacol* 1982; **22:** 175–9.
2. Herman RJ, et al. Effects of age on meperidine disposition. *Clin Pharmacol Ther* 1985; **37:** 19–24.

Phaeochromocytoma. Pethidine provoked episodes of hypertension in a patient with phaeochromocytoma; the effect was suppressed by labetalol.[1] Like other histamine-releasing opioids, pethidine should be used with caution in such patients.

1. Lawrence CA. Pethidine-induced hypertension in phaeochromocytoma. *BMJ* 1978; **1:** 149–50.

Pregnancy and the neonate. Pethidine is widely used for analgesia during labour. It rapidly crosses the placenta and like other opioid analgesics may cause respiratory depression in the neonate although this may be less than with morphine. Respiratory depression varies according to the timing and size of the maternal dose.

Fetal depression was not apparent when delivery occurred within 1 hour of pethidine administration, but was present in 6 of 24 infants delivered 1 to 3 hours after injection and in all of 5 infants delivered 3 to 6 hours after injection.[1] Higher blood concentrations of pethidine were seen in infants delivered within 1 hour of a single dose of pethidine 150 mg intramuscularly when compared with those born following administration 1 to 4 hours before delivery. The role of pethidine metabolites was not certain, but relatively little of a dose might have been metabolised by the mother within 1 hour. Others[2] reported that neonates appeared able to metabolise pethidine although probably more slowly than adults. They also showed that the amounts of pethidine and norpethidine excreted by the neonate increased significantly with the maternal dose-delivery interval for intervals of up to 5 hours and considered that most of the placentally transferred pethidine should be excreted by the third day. Elimination of pethidine took up to 6 days in the neonates in one study.[3] In another study,[4] depressed neonatal responses persisted for the first 2 days of life; depression was dose-related being greatest with the highest dose of pethidine (75 to 150 mg within 4 hours of delivery).

Further references on the transplacental transfer of pethidine can be found under Pregnancy in Pharmacokinetics, below.

Neither psychological nor physical effects were found in 5-year-old children of mothers who had received pethidine during labour.[5] Neonatal behaviour does not appear to have been affected significantly by pethidine, although it has been acknowledged that the relationship between maternal analgesia in labour and subsequent infant behaviour is by no means simple.[6] The results of early studies which suggested an excess of cases of cancer in children whose mothers received pethidine during labour have been refuted by a later and larger study.[7]

1. Morrison JC, et al. Metabolites of meperidine related to fetal depression. *Am J Obstet Gynecol* 1973; **115:** 1132–7.
2. Hogg MIJ, et al. Urinary excretion and metabolism of pethidine and norpethidine in the newborn. *Br J Anaesth* 1977; **49:** 891–9.
3. Cooper LV, et al. Elimination of pethidine and bupivacaine in the newborn. *Arch Dis Child* 1977; **52:** 638–41.
4. Hodgkinson R, et al. Double-blind comparison of the neurobehaviour of neonates following the administration of different doses of meperidine to the mother. *Can Anaesth Soc J* 1978; **25:** 405–11.
5. Buck C. Drugs in pregnancy. *Can Med Assoc J* 1975; **112:** 1285.
6. Anonymous. To measure life. *Lancet* 1981; **ii:** 291–2.
7. Golding J, et al. Childhood cancer, intramuscular vitamin K, and pethidine given during labour. *BMJ* 1992; **305:** 341–6.

Renal impairment. Caution is necessary when pethidine is given to patients with renal impairment. Evidence of CNS excitation, including seizures and twitches, in 2 patients with renal insufficiency receiving multiple doses of pethidine was attributed to accumulation of the metabolite norpethidine; they both had high norpethidine : pethidine plasma concentration ratios.[1]

See also under Pharmacokinetics, below.

1. Szeto HH, et al. Accumulation of normeperidine, an active metabolite of meperidine, in patients with renal failure or cancer. *Ann Intern Med* 1977; **86:** 738–41.

Interactions

For interactions associated with opioid analgesics, see p.68.

Very severe reactions, including coma, severe respiratory depression, cyanosis, and hypotension have occurred in patients receiving MAOIs (including moclobemide and selegiline) and given pethidine. There are also reports of hyperexcitability, convulsions, tachycardia, hyperpyrexia, and hypertension. Pethidine should not be given to patients receiving MAOIs or within 14 days of their discontinuation. Concurrent administration of pethidine and phenothiazines has produced severe hypotensive episodes and may prolong the respiratory depression due to pethidine.

Plasma concentrations of norpethidine are increased by ritonavir, with a resultant risk of toxicity; concomitant administration should be avoided (see also p.68).

Barbiturates. Opioid analgesics and barbiturates can be expected to have additive CNS depressant effects. Prolonged sedation with pethidine in the presence of phenobarbital has also been attributed to induction of N-demethylation of pethidine, resulting in the enhanced formation of the potentially neurotoxic metabolite norpethidine.[1,2]

1. Stambaugh JE, *et al.* A potentially toxic drug interaction between pethidine (meperidine) and phenobarbitone. *Lancet* 1977; i: 398–9.
2. Stambaugh JE, *et al.* The effect of phenobarbital on the metabolism of meperidine in normal volunteers. *J Clin Pharmacol* 1978; 18: 482–90.

Histamine H₂-antagonists. Cimetidine reduced the clearance and volume of distribution of pethidine in healthy subjects,[1] whereas ranitidine did not.[2]

1. Guay DRP, *et al.* Cimetidine alters pethidine disposition in man. *Br J Clin Pharmacol* 1984; 18: 907–14.
2. Guay DRP, *et al.* Ranitidine does not alter pethidine disposition in man. *Br J Clin Pharmacol* 1985; 20: 55–9.

MAOIs. Some of the most serious interactions involving pethidine have been with non-selective MAOIs and have been manifest as enhanced depressant effects or hyperexcitability (see above). However, a life-threatening interaction has also been reported between pethidine and selegiline, a selective monoamine oxidase type B inhibitor.[1] Also, symptoms suggestive of a mild serotonin syndrome developed in a 73-year-old woman taking moclobemide (a reversible inhibitor of monoamine oxidase type A), nortriptyline, and lithium after she was given pethidine intravenously.[2]

1. Zornberg GL, *et al.* Severe adverse interaction between pethidine and selegiline. *Lancet* 1991; 337: 246. Correction. *ibid.*; 440.
2. Gillman PK. Possible serotonin syndrome with moclobemide and pethidine. *Med J Aust* 1995; 162: 554.

Phenothiazines. Prochlorperazine prolonged the respiratory depressant effect of pethidine in healthy subjects.[1] Enhanced CNS depression and hypotension were reported when healthy subjects were given chlorpromazine in addition to pethidine; there was evidence of increased N-demethylation of pethidine.[2]

1. Steen SN, Yates M. Effects of benzquinamide and prochlorperazine, separately and combined with meperidine, on the human respiratory center. *Clin Pharmacol Ther* 1972; 13: 153.
2. Stambaugh JE, Wainer IW. Drug interaction: meperidine and chlorpromazine, a toxic combination. *J Clin Pharmacol* 1981; 21: 140–6.

Phenytoin. The hepatic metabolism of pethidine appears to be enhanced by phenytoin. Concomitant administration resulted in reduced half-life and bioavailability in healthy subjects; blood concentrations of norpethidine were increased.[1]

1. Pond SM, Kretschzmar KM. Effect of phenytoin on meperidine clearance and normeperidine formation. *Clin Pharmacol Ther* 1981; 30: 680–6.

Pharmacokinetics

Pethidine hydrochloride is absorbed from the gastrointestinal tract, but only about 50% of the drug reaches the systemic circulation because of first-pass metabolism. Absorption following intramuscular injection is variable. Peak plasma concentrations have been reported 1 to 2 hours after oral administration. It is about 60 to 80% bound to plasma proteins.

Pethidine is metabolised in the liver by hydrolysis to pethidinic acid (meperidinic acid) or demethylation to norpethidine (normeperidine) and hydrolysis to norpethidinic acid (normeperidinic acid), followed by partial conjugation with glucuronic acid. Norpethidine is pharmacologically active and its accumulation may result in toxicity. Pethidine is reported to have a plasma elimination half-life of about 3 to 6 hours in healthy subjects; the metabolite norpethidine is eliminated more slowly, with a half-life reported to be up to about 20 hours. Both pethidine and norpethidine appear in the CSF. At the usual values of urinary pH or if the urine is alkaline, only a small amount of

pethidine is excreted unchanged; urinary excretion of pethidine and norpethidine is enhanced by acidification of the urine. Pethidine crosses the placenta and is distributed into breast milk.

◊ Reviews.
1. Edwards DJ, *et al.* Clinical pharmacokinetics of pethidine: 1982. *Clin Pharmacokinet* 1982; 7: 421–33.
2. Moore RA, *et al.* Opiate metabolism and excretion. *Baillieres Clin Anaesthesiol* 1987; 1: 829–58.

Administration. The elimination half-life of pethidine was prolonged and plasma clearance decreased when given perioperatively compared with postoperatively.[1]

During labour the pharmacokinetics of pethidine may depend on the method of administration. In a comparison of intramuscular injection at different sites, absorption of pethidine from the gluteus muscle was impaired and the deltoid muscle was preferred.[2]

No statistically significant differences were found in pharmacokinetic parameters for deltoid and gluteal intramuscular injections in elderly postoperative patients.[3] However, substantial interpatient variability was noted for both sites, and the authors suggested that more rapid and predictable routes such as intravenous injection may be more appropriate for postoperative use in the elderly.

1. Tamsen A, *et al.* Patient-controlled analgesic therapy, part 1: pharmacokinetics of pethidine in the per- and postoperative periods. *Clin Pharmacokinet* 1982; 7: 149–63.
2. Lazebnik N, *et al.* Intravenous, deltoid, or gluteus administration of meperidine during labor? *Am J Obstet Gynecol* 1989; 160: 1184–9.
3. Erstad BL, *et al.* Site-specific pharmacokinetics and pharmacodynamics of intramuscular meperidine in elderly postoperative patients. *Ann Pharmacother* 1997; 31: 23–8.

Hepatic impairment. The terminal half-life of pethidine was prolonged to about 7 hours in cirrhotic patients compared with 3 hours in healthy subjects and was attributed to impairment of the drug-metabolising activity of the liver.[1] Another study concluded that although impaired hepatic metabolism might confer relative protection from norpethidine toxicity in patients with cirrhosis, there might be an increased risk of cumulative toxicity because of slow elimination of the metabolite.[2]

1. Klotz U, *et al.* The effect of cirrhosis on the disposition and elimination of meperidine in man. *Clin Pharmacol Ther* 1974; 16: 667–75.
2. Pond SM, *et al.* Presystemic metabolism of meperidine to normeperidine in normal and cirrhotic subjects. *Clin Pharmacol Ther* 1981; 30: 183–8.

Pregnancy. Some references to the pharmacokinetics of pethidine during labour are given below.

1. Tomson G, *et al.* Maternal kinetics and transplacental passage of pethidine during labour. *Br J Clin Pharmacol* 1982; 13: 653–9.
2. Kuhnert BR, *et al.* Disposition of meperidine and normeperidine following multiple doses during labor: I mother. *Am J Obstet Gynecol* 1985; 151: 406–9.
3. Kuhnert BR, *et al.* Disposition of meperidine and normeperidine following multiple doses during labor: II fetus and neonate. *Am J Obstet Gynecol* 1985; 151: 410–15.

Renal impairment. Plasma protein binding of pethidine was reported to be decreased in renal disease and ranged from 58.2% in healthy subjects to 31.8% in anuric patients.[1] The same workers also reported impaired elimination of pethidine in patients with renal dysfunction.[2]

See also under Precautions, above.

1. Chan K, *et al.* Plasma protein binding of pethidine in patients with renal disease. *J Pharm Pharmacol* 1983; 35: 94P.
2. Chan K, *et al.* The influence of renal dysfunction on the disposition of pethidine in man. *Br J Clin Pharmacol* 1984; 17: 198P.

Uses and Administration

Pethidine, a phenylpiperidine derivative, is a synthetic opioid analgesic (p.68) that acts mainly as a μ opioid agonist. Pethidine is used for the relief of most types of moderate to severe acute pain including the pain of labour. It is more lipid soluble than morphine and has a less potent and shorter lasting analgesic effect; analgesia usually lasts for 2 to 4 hours. Its short duration of action and accumulation of its potentially neurotoxic metabolite norpethidine on repeated administration make it unsuitable for the management of chronic pain. Pethidine has a weaker action on smooth muscle than morphine and its lower potential to increase biliary pressure makes it suitable when opioid analgesics are required to manage pain associated with biliary colic and pancreatitis. It is also used as pre-operative medication and as an adjunct to anaesthesia. It has been given with phenothiazines such as promethazine to achieve basal narcosis. Pethidine has little effect on cough or on diarrhoea.

For the relief of **pain**, pethidine hydrochloride is given in doses of 50 to 150 mg by mouth every 4 hours. It may also be given by intramuscular or subcutaneous injection in doses of 25 to 100 mg and by slow

intravenous injection in doses of 25 to 50 mg repeated after 4 hours. For *postoperative* pain the subcutaneous or intramuscular doses may be given every 2 to 3 hours if necessary. In children, doses of 0.5 to 2 mg per kg body-weight may be given by mouth or by intramuscular injection.

In *obstetric analgesia* 50 to 100 mg may be given by intramuscular or subcutaneous injection as soon as contractions occur at regular intervals. This dose may be repeated after 1 to 3 hours if necessary up to a maximum of 400 mg in 24 hours.

For *pre-operative* medication 25 to 100 mg may be given intramuscularly or subcutaneously about 1 hour before surgery; children may be given 0.5 to 2 mg per kg. As an adjunct to nitrous oxide-oxygen anaesthesia 10 to 25 mg may be given by slow intravenous injection.

Administration. In addition to conventional routes of administration pethidine has been given epidurally[1-4] and intrathecally.[5] It has also been given intravenously[6,7] and intranasally[8] by a patient-controlled system. However, some consider that the use of pethidine should be avoided for patient-controlled analgesia because of the increased risk of norpethidine-induced seizures[9] (see also under Effects on the Nervous System, above).

1. Perriss BW. Epidural pethidine in labour: a study of dose requirements. *Anaesthesia* 1980; 35: 380–2.
2. Husemeyer RP, *et al.* A study of pethidine kinetics and analgesia in women in labour following intravenous, intramuscular and epidural administration. *Br J Clin Pharmacol* 1982; 13: 171–6.
3. Perriss BW, *et al.* Analgesia following extradural and im pethidine in post-caesarean section patients. *Br J Anaesth* 1990; 64: 355–7.
4. Blythe JG, *et al.* Continuous postoperative epidural analgesia for gynecologic oncology patients. *Gynecol Oncol* 1990; 37: 307–10.
5. Acalovschi I, *et al.* Saddle block with pethidine for perineal operations. *Br J Anaesth* 1986; 58: 1012–16.
6. Tamsen A, *et al.* Patient-controlled analgesic therapy, part II: individual analgesic demand and analgesic plasma concentrations of pethidine in postoperative pain. *Clin Pharmacokinet* 1982; 7: 164–75.
7. Rayburn W, *et al.* Intravenous meperidine during labor: a randomized comparison between nursing- and patient-controlled administration. *Obstet Gynecol* 1989; 74: 702–6.
8. Striebel WH, *et al.* Intranasal meperidine titration for postoperative pain relief. *Anesth Analg* 1993; 76: 1047–51.
9. Hagmeyer KO, *et al.* Meperidine-related seizures associated with patient-controlled analgesia pumps. *Ann Pharmacother* 1993; 27: 29–32.

Eclampsia and pre-eclampsia. See Lytic Cocktails under Sedation, below.

Pain. Pethidine may be preferred to morphine when rapid control of acute pain is required. It is widely used in obstetrics to control the pain of labour and for postoperative pain relief following caesarean section or other surgical procedures.

In a study of patients with intractable pain the minimum effective analgesic blood concentration ranged from 100 to 820 nanograms per mL (median 250 nanograms per mL) in 15 of 16; the remaining patient failed to obtain analgesia with pethidine. Additional measures were considered necessary[1] if the minimum effective concentration exceeded 400 nanograms per mL.

Pethidine has traditionally been given by intermittent intramuscular injection in the treatment of acute pain, but inconsistent pain relief can be expected because of fluctuating blood-pethidine concentrations;[2] continuous intravenous infusion might be more effective for acute pain. For reference to various routes of administration, see Administration, above.

1. Mather LE, Glynn CJ. The minimum effective analgesic blood concentration of pethidine in patients with intractable pain. *Br J Clin Pharmacol* 1982; 14: 385–90.
2. Edwards DJ, *et al.* Clinical pharmacokinetics of pethidine: 1982. *Clin Pharmacokinet* 1982; 7: 421–33.

SICKLE-CELL CRISIS. Concern has been expressed over the continued use of pethidine for analgesia in painful crises in sickle-cell disease. Control of pain may be inadequate and doses commonly used to manage crises may lead to accumulation of the neuroexcitatory metabolite of pethidine and precipitate seizures.[1,2] See also under Effects on the Nervous System, above.

1. Pryle BJ, *et al.* Toxicity of norpethidine in sickle cell crisis. *BMJ* 1992; 304: 1478–9.
2. Harrison JFM, *et al.* Pethidine in sickle cell crisis. *BMJ* 1992; 305: 182.

Sedation. Some references to the use of pethidine for endoscopy are given below.

1. Chokhavatia S, *et al.* Sedation and analgesia for gastrointestinal endoscopy. *Am J Gastroenterol* 1993; 88: 393–6.
2. Bahal-O'Mara N, *et al.* Sedation with meperidine and midazolam in pediatric patients undergoing endoscopy. *Eur J Clin Pharmacol* 1994; 47: 319–23.

LYTIC COCKTAILS. Lytic cocktails consisting of chlorpromazine, pethidine, and/or promethazine have been given intravenously in some countries for the management of pre-eclampsia and imminent eclampsia. However, the use of phenothiazines is generally not recommended late in pregnancy, and other treatments are preferred for hypertension (see Hypertension in

Pregnancy, under Hypertension, p.802); the management of eclampsia, which is the convulsive phase, is discussed on p.341.

Lytic cocktails have also been used for sedation and analgesia in paediatric patients, by intramuscular or occasionally intravenous injection. However, there is a high rate of therapeutic failure as well as serious adverse effects with such combinations, and the American Academy of Pediatrics[1] has recommended that alternative sedatives and analgesics should be considered; guidelines have been drawn up should it be appropriate to use a lytic cocktail. Lytic cocktails are not the most appropriate means of sedation for short procedures since patients must be monitored for approximately one hour before the procedure while the drugs take effect, and for even longer during the recovery period.[2]

1. American Academy of Pediatrics Committee on Drugs. Reappraisal of Lytic cocktail/Demerol, Phenergan, and Thorazine (DPT) for the sedation of children. *Pediatrics* 1995; **95**: 598–602.
2. Barst SM, et al. A comparison of propofol and Demerol-Phenergan-Thorazine for brief, minor, painful procedures in a pediatric hematology-oncology clinic. *Int J Pediatr Hematol/Oncol* 1995; **1**: 587–91.

Shivering. For reference to the use of pethidine in the management of shivering associated with anaesthesia, see under Adverse Effects of General Anaesthetics, p.1255. Pethidine has also been used to treat amphotericin B-induced shaking chills.[1]

1. Burks LC, et al. Meperidine for the treatment of shaking chills and fever. *Arch Intern Med* 1980; **140**: 483–4.

Preparations

BP 2001: Pethidine Injection; Pethidine Tablets;
USP 25: Meperidine Hydrochloride Injection; Meperidine Hydrochloride Syrup; Meperidine Hydrochloride Tablets.

Proprietary Preparations (details are given in Part 3)
Aust.: Alodan; *Belg.:* Dolantine; *Braz.:* Demerol; Dolantina; Dolosal; *Canad.:* Demerol; *Fr.:* Dolosal; *Ger.:* Dolantin; *Israel:* Dolestine; *Spain:* Dolantina; *Switz.:* Centralgine†; *USA:* Demerol.

Multi-ingredient: *Austral.:* Marcain with Pethidine; *NZ:* Marcain with Pethidine; *UK:* Pamergan P100; *USA:* Atropine and Demerol; Mepergan.

Phenacetin (2681-h)

Phenacetin (rINN).

Aceto-p-phenetidide; Acetophenetidin; Acetylphenetidin; Fenacetina; Paracetophenetidin; Phenacetinum. p-Acetophenetidide; 4′-Ethoxyacetanilide; N-(4-Ethoxyphenyl)acetamide.

$C_{10}H_{13}NO_2 = 179.2$.
CAS — 62-44-2.
ATC — N02BE03.

Pharmacopoeias. In Jpn and Pol.

Adverse Effects and Precautions

Phenacetin may cause methaemoglobinaemia, sulfhaemoglobinaemia, and haemolytic anaemia.

Prolonged administration of large doses of analgesic mixtures containing phenacetin has been associated with the development of renal papillary necrosis (see Effects on the Kidneys, p.64) and transitional-cell carcinoma of the renal pelvis.

Porphyria. Phenacetin is considered to be unsafe in patients with porphyria because it has been shown to be porphyrinogenic in *animals*.

Uses and Administration

Phenacetin, a para-aminophenol derivative, has analgesic and antipyretic properties. It was usually given with aspirin, caffeine, or codeine but is now little used because of adverse haematological effects and nephrotoxicity.

Phenazocine Hydrobromide (6256-k)

Phenazocine Hydrobromide (BANM, rINNM).

1,2,3,4,5,6-Hexahydro-6,11-dimethyl-3-phenethyl-2,6-methano-3-benzazocin-8-ol hydrobromide hemihydrate.

$C_{22}H_{27}NO,HBr,\frac{1}{2}H_2O = 411.4$.
CAS — 127-35-5 (phenazocine); 1239-04-9 (anhydrous phenazocine hydrobromide).

Profile

Phenazocine hydrobromide is an opioid analgesic (p.66). It is considered to be less sedating than morphine and has a weaker action on smooth muscle; its lower potential to increase biliary pressure makes it suitable when opioid analgesics are required for pain associated with biliary colic and pancreatitis.

Phenazocine hydrobromide may be given for the relief of severe pain. It acts within 20 minutes after administration by mouth and the analgesic effect may last up to 6 hours. The usual oral or sublingual dose is 5 mg every 4 to 6 hours, though single doses of up to 20 mg may be given.

Preparations

Proprietary Preparations (details are given in Part 3)
UK: Narphen†.

Phenazone (2684-v)

Phenazone (BAN, rINN).

Analgésine; Antipyrin; Antipyrine; Azophenum; Fenazona; Phenazonum; Phenyldimethylpyrazolone. 1,5-Dimethyl-2-phenyl-4-pyrazolin-3-one.

$C_{11}H_{12}N_2O = 188.2$.
CAS — 60-80-0.
ATC — N02BB01.

Pharmacopoeias. In Eur. (see p.vi), Jpn, and US.

Pharmacopoeial description

Ph. Eur.: White or almost white crystalline powder or colourless crystals. Very soluble in water, in alcohol, and in dichloromethane; sparingly soluble in ether. Protect from light.

USP 25: Colourless crystals or white crystalline powder. Is odourless. Very soluble in water; freely soluble in alcohol and in chloroform; sparingly soluble in ether. Solutions are neutral to litmus. Store in airtight containers.

Phenazone and Caffeine Citrate (2683-b)

Antipyrino-Coffeinum Citricum; Migrenin; Phenzone and Caffeine Citrate.

Pharmacopoeias. In Aust. and Jpn.

A powder usually containing phenazone 90%, caffeine 9%, and citric acid monohydrate 1%.

Phenazone Salicylate (2682-m)

Antipyrin Salicylate; Salipyrin.

$C_{11}H_{12}N_2O,C_7H_6O_3 = 326.3$.
CAS — 520-07-0.

Pharmacopoeias. In Aust. and Fr.

Adverse Effects and Precautions

Phenazone is liable to give rise to skin eruptions and in susceptible individuals even small doses may have this effect. Hypersensitivity reactions and nephrotoxicity have been reported. Large doses by mouth may cause nausea, drowsiness, coma, and convulsions.

Effects on the blood. Phenazone had been shown to cause haemolytic anaemia in certain individuals with a deficiency of glucose-6-phosphate dehydrogenase.[1] Episodes of agranulocytosis were reported[2] in 6 women using a cream containing phenazone; all recovered on withdrawal.

1. Prankerd TAJ. Hemolytic effects of drugs and chemical agents. *Clin Pharmacol Ther* 1963; **4**: 334–50.
2. Delannoy A, Schmit J-C. Agranulocytosis after cutaneous contact with phenazone. *Eur J Haematol* 1993; **50**: 124.

Effects on the kidneys. Phenazone is considered nephrotoxic but only limited clinical information on phenazone is available because it has been mainly used in association with phenacetin.[1]

1. Prescott LF. Analgesic nephropathy: a reassessment of the role of phenacetin and other analgesics. *Drugs* 1982; **23**: 75–149.

Effects on the skin. In a summary[1] of 77 cases of fixed drug eruption phenazone derivatives were considered to be the causative agent in 9 of the 14 cases that were severe generalised reactions.

1. Stubb S, et al. Fixed drug eruptions: 77 cases from 1981 to 1985. *Br J Dermatol* 1989; **120**: 583.

Hypersensitivity. Immediate allergic reactions to phenazone have been reported.[1,2] In one patient leucopenia was detected 8 weeks later.[1]

1. Kadar D, Kalow W. Acute and latent leukopenic reaction to antipyrine. *Clin Pharmacol Ther* 1980; **28**: 820–22.
2. McCrea JB, et al. Allergic reaction to antipyrine, a marker of hepatic enzyme activity. *DICP Ann Pharmacother* 1989; **23**: 38–40.

Porphyria. Phenazone is considered to be unsafe in patients with porphyria because it has been shown to be porphyrinogenic in *animals*.

Interactions

Phenazone affects the metabolism of some other drugs and its metabolism is affected by other drugs that increase or reduce the activity of liver enzymes.

Pharmacokinetics

Phenazone is absorbed from the gastrointestinal tract and peak plasma concentrations are obtained within 1 to 2 hours of ingestion. It is distributed throughout the body fluids with concentrations in the saliva and breast milk reaching about the same levels as those in plasma. Less than 10% is bound to plasma proteins and it has an elimination half-life of about 12 hours. Phenazone is metabolised in the liver to 3 major metabolites 3-hydroxymethylphenazone, 4-hydroxyphenazone and norphenazone. Phenazone, 3-hydroxymethylphenazone, and glucuronidated metabolites are all excreted in the urine. A small portion may be eliminated via the bile.

Uses and Administration

Phenazone is an NSAID (p.65) and has been given by mouth; phenazone and caffeine citrate and phenazone salicylate have similarly been given by mouth as analgesics.

Solutions containing about 5% of phenazone have been used topically as ear drops in disorders such as acute otitis media (but see below).

Phenazone is used as a test for the activity of drug-metabolising enzymes in the liver.

Diagnosis and testing. A review[1] of normal plasma-phenazone pharmacokinetics, urinary metabolite disposition, and total body clearances of phenazone in the presence of cirrhosis, fatty liver, hepatitis, and cholestatis.

1. St Peter JV, Awni WM. Quantifying hepatic function in the presence of liver disease with phenazone (antipyrine) and its metabolites. *Clin Pharmacokinet* 1991; **20**: 50–65.

Otitis media. There seems to be no justification[1] for the inclusion of phenazone in topical preparations used in treating acute otitis media (p.132). It is presumably included in such preparations because it is believed to have a local anti-inflammatory and, therefore, analgesic action. It would, however, seem unlikely that phenazone would have any action on the skin of the intact tympanic membrane and, therefore, on the pain which is due primarily to the stretching and distention of the membrane.

In general, no topical treatment is considered effective in acute otitis media.

1. Carlin WV. Is there any justification for using phenazone in a local application prescribed for the treatment of acute otitis media? *BMJ* 1987; **294**: 1333.

Preparations

USP 25: Antipyrine and Benzocaine Otic Solution; Antipyrine, Benzocaine, and Phenylephrine Hydrochloride Otic Solution.

Proprietary Preparations (details are given in Part 3)
Austral.: Erasol; *Ger.:* Aequiton-P; Eu-Med†; Migrane-Kranit mono; *Irl.:* Tropex; *S.Afr.:* Aurone; Oto-Phen; *Swed.:* Spalt N†.

Multi-ingredient: *Aust.:* Asthma Efeum; Asthma-Frenon†; Bellasthman†; Coffo Selt; Otalgan; Spalt; *Austral.:* Auralgan; *Belg.:* Otalgan; Otipax; Otocalmine; Ouate Hemostatique; Parmentier†; Tympalgine; *Braz.:* Anestesiol; Auditol; Espasmalgon; Espasmocron; *Canad.:* Auralgan; *Denm.:* Koffisal; *Fr.:* Brulex; HEC; Otipax; Ovules Sedo-Hemostatiques du Docteur Jouve; *Ger.:* Coffeemed N; Felsol Neo; Migranin; Otalgan; Otodolor; Titralgan; *Israel:* Anaesthetic Ear Drops; Otidin; *Ital.:* Otalgan; Otomidone; Otopax; *Norw.:* Antineuralgica; Codalgin†; Fanalgin; *NZ:* Degest 2; *Port.:* Otalgan; Otipax; Otocalma; Profrin-A†; *S.Afr.:* Auralgicin; Aurasept; Aurone Forte; Covancaine; Ilvico; Otised; Oto-Phen Forte; Universal Earache Drops; *Singapore:* HEC; Tropex; *Spain:* AB FE; Epistaxol; Hemostatico Antisep Asen†; Otalgan; Otosedol; Pomada Heridas; Quimpedor; Tabletas Quimpe; *Swed.:* Doleron; Koffazon; *Switz.:* Otalgan; Otipax; Otosan; Otothricinol; Seranex sans codeine; Spedralgin sans codeine; Spirogel†; *Thai.:* Auralgan; *USA:* Allergen; Analgesic Otic Solution†; Auralgan; Auroto; Benzotic†; Cy-Gesic; Otocalm; Tympagesic.

Phenazopyridine Hydrochloride (2685-g)

Phenazopyridine Hydrochloride (BANM, USAN, rINNM).

Chloridrato de Fenazopiridina; NC-150; NSC-1879; W-1655. 3-Phenylazopyridine-2,6-diyldiamine hydrochloride.

$C_{11}H_{11}N_5,HCl = 249.7$.
CAS — 94-78-0 (phenazopyridine); 136-40-3 (phenazopyridine hydrochloride).

Pharmacopoeias. In Pol. and US.

REMOVAL OF STAINS. Phenazopyridine stains may be removed from fabric by soaking in a solution of sodium dithionite 0.25%.

Pharmacopoeial description

USP 25: A light or dark red to dark violet crystalline powder. Is odourless or with a slight odour. Soluble 1 in 300 of cold water, 1 in 20 of boiling water, 1 in 59 of alcohol, 1 in 331 of chloroform, and 1 in 100 of glycerol; very slightly soluble in ether. Store in airtight containers.

Adverse Effects

Phenazopyridine hydrochloride has caused gastrointestinal side-effects, headache, and rashes. Hepatotoxicity, haemolytic anaemia, methaemoglobinaemia, and acute renal failure have also been reported, generally associated with overdosage or with therapeutic doses in patients with impaired renal function. Crystal deposits of phenazopyridine have formed in the urinary tract.

Abnormal coloration of body tissues or fluids may occur. Staining of contact lenses has occurred.

Effects on the CNS. A case of aseptic meningitis, with distinct episodes of fever and confusion, was associated with the administration of phenazopyridine.[1]

1. Herlihy TE. Phenazopyridine and aseptic meningitis. *Ann Intern Med* 1987; **106**: 172–3.

Precautions

Phenazopyridine hydrochloride is contra-indicated in patients with impaired renal function or severe hepatitis or those with glucose-6-phosphate dehydrogenase deficiency. Treatment should be discontinued if the skin or sclerae become discoloured; this may indicate accumulation as a result of impaired renal excretion. Phenazopyridine may interfere with urinalysis based on colour reactions or spectrometry.

Pharmacokinetics

Phenazopyridine hydrochloride is absorbed from the gastrointestinal tract. It is excreted mainly in the urine; up to 65% may be excreted as unchanged phenazopyridine and 18% as paracetamol.

The symbol † denotes a preparation no longer actively marketed

Uses and Administration

Phenazopyridine is an azo dye that exerts an analgesic effect on the mucosa of the urinary tract and is used to provide symptomatic relief of pain and irritability in conditions such as cystitis and prostatitis (see under Urinary-tract Infections, p.146), and urethritis (p.146). It has been given by mouth as the hydrochloride in usual doses of about 200 mg three times daily after food. It may be given in conjunction with an antibacterial for the treatment of urinary-tract infections, usually for up to 2 days, although lower doses have been given as part of a combined preparation for at least a week. During administration the urine is tinged either orange or red and underclothes are apt to be stained.

Urinary-tract infections. There is currently no well-substantiated role for phenazopyridine in the treatment of urinary-tract infections and its adverse effects are potentially serious.[1]

1. Zelenitsky SA, Zhanel GG. Phenazopyridine in urinary tract infections. *Ann Pharmacother* 1996; **30:** 866–8.

Preparations

USP 25: Phenazopyridine Hydrochloride Tablets.

Proprietary Preparations (details are given in Part 3)
Belg.: Uropyrine; ***Braz.:*** Pyridium; Urologin; ***Canad.:*** Phenazo; Pyridium; ***Hong Kong:*** Phenazo; Pyridium; ***Israel:*** Sedural; ***Mex.:*** Bioferina; Umizan; ***S.Afr.:*** Azodine†; Pyridium; ***Singapore:*** Urogesic; ***Thai.:*** Anazo; Phendiridine; Sumedium; ***USA:*** Azo-Standard; Baridium; Geridium†; Prodium; Pyridiate; Pyridium; Re-Azo; Uro-Trac†; Urodine†; Urogesic.

Multi-ingredient: ***Aust.:*** Gastrotest; ***Braz.:*** Azo-Wintomylon; Mictrex; Uretil; Urizal; Uro Bac Septin; Uro Bactrim; Uro Batrox; Uro Duoctrim; Uro Heractrim; Uro Septoprin; Uro-Bacteracin; Uro-Baxapril; Uro-Leotrim; Uro-Septolan; Uro-Teutrim; Urobactrex; Urobioctrin; Urobiotic; Uroctrim; Urofar; Urofen; Uromix; Uroneotrim; Uropac; Uropielon; Uropirite; Uropol; Uroseptin; Urotril; Uroxazol; Ultrer; ***Ger.:*** Urospasmon; ***Mex.:*** Azo-Wintomylon; Nalixone; Naxilan-Plus; Pirifur; ***S.Afr.:*** Azo-Mandelamine†; ***Spain:*** Micturol Sedante; Urogobens Antiespasmo†; ***USA:*** Pyridium Plus; Urobiotic-250.

Phenicarbazide (2689-w)

Phenicarbazide (*rINN*).

Phenylsemicarbazide. 1-Phenylsemicarbazide.
$C_7H_9N_3O = 151.2$.
CAS — 103-03-7.

Profile

Phenicarbazide has analgesic properties. It has been given by mouth and rectally.

Phenoperidine Hydrochloride (6257-a)

Phenoperidine Hydrochloride (*BANM, rINNM*).

R-1406. Ethyl 1-(3-hydroxy-3-phenylpropyl)-4-phenylpiperidine-4-carboxylate hydrochloride.
$C_{23}H_{29}NO_3,HCl = 403.9$.
CAS — 562-26-5 (phenoperidine); 3627-49-4 (phenoperidine hydrochloride).

Incompatible with propanidid and solutions of methohexital sodium and thiopental sodium.

Profile

Phenoperidine hydrochloride is an opioid analgesic (p.66) related to pethidine (p.75) that produces surgical analgesia and has also been used with an antipsychotic such as droperidol, to induce neuroleptanalgesia. It has also been given as an analgesic and respiratory depressant in patients requiring long-term assisted ventilation in intensive care. It was usually given intravenously.

Preparations

Proprietary Preparations (details are given in Part 3)
Austral.: Operidine†; ***Fr.:*** R 1406†; ***Swed.:*** Lealgin†.

Phenylbutazone (2686-q)

Phenylbutazone (*BAN, rINN*).

Butadione; Fenilbutazona; Phenylbutazonum. 4-Butyl-1,2-diphenylpyrazolidine-3,5-dione.
$C_{19}H_{20}N_2O_2 = 308.4$.
CAS — 50-33-9 (phenylbutazone); 129-18-0 (phenylbutazone sodium); 4985-25-5 (phenylbutazone piperazine).
ATC — M01AA01; M02AA01.

Pharmacopoeias. In Chin., Eur. (see p.vi), Jpn, Pol., and US.

Pharmacopoeial description

Ph. Eur.: A white or almost white, crystalline powder. Practically insoluble in water; sparingly soluble in alcohol; soluble in ether; it dissolves in alkaline solutions. Protect from light.

USP 25: A white to off-white, odourless, crystalline powder. Very slightly soluble in water; soluble in alcohol; freely soluble in acetone and in ether. Store in airtight containers.

Adverse Effects

Nausea, vomiting, epigastric distress, diarrhoea, oedema due to salt retention, skin rashes, dizziness, drowsiness, headache, and blurred vision may occur with phenylbutazone. More serious reactions include gastric irritation with ulceration and gastrointestinal bleeding, ulcerative stomatitis, hepatitis, jaundice, haematuria, nephritis, renal failure, pancreatitis, ocular toxicity, and goitre. Phenylbutazone may precipitate heart failure and may also cause an acute pulmonary syndrome with dyspnoea and fever. Salivary gland enlargement (parotitis), hypersensitivity reactions including asthma, and severe generalised reactions including lymphadenopathy, erythema multiforme, Stevens-Johnson syndrome, toxic epidermal necrolysis, and exfoliative dermatitis have been reported.

The most serious adverse effects of phenylbutazone are related to bone-marrow depression and include agranulocytosis and aplastic anaemia. Leucopenia, pancytopenia, haemolytic anaemia, and thrombocytopenia may also occur. These adverse haematological reactions have resulted in the indications for use of phenylbutazone being restricted (see under Uses and Administration, below). Blood disorders may develop soon after starting treatment or may occur suddenly after prolonged treatment, and regular haematological monitoring should be carried out as discussed under Precautions, below.

The adverse effects of NSAIDs in general are described on p.63.

Effects on the blood. Both phenylbutazone[1-3] and oxyphenbutazone[1,3] are well known for their adverse effects on the blood and especially for fatal agranulocytosis and aplastic anaemia. The UK Committee on Safety of Medicines[4] noted that between July 1963 and January 1993 it had received 74 reports of agranulocytosis (39 fatal) associated with phenylbutazone and 40 reports of neutropenia (4 fatal). Up-to-date figures were not provided on oxyphenbutazone, but it is considered to be more toxic to the bone marrow than phenylbutazone.[1]

1. Anonymous. Phenylbutazone and oxyphenbutazone: time to call a halt. *Drug Ther Bull* 1984; **22:** 5–6.
2. Böttiger LE, Westerholm B. Drug-induced blood dyscrasias in Sweden. *BMJ* 1973; **3:** 339–43.
3. The International Agranulocytosis and Aplastic Anemia Study. Risks of agranulocytosis and aplastic anemia: a first report of their relation to drug use with special reference to analgesics. *JAMA* 1986; **256:** 1749–57.
4. Committee on Safety of Medicines/Medicines Control Agency. Drug-induced neutropenia and agranulocytosis. *Current Problems* 1993; **19:** 10–11.

Precautions

Phenylbutazone is contra-indicated in patients with blood disorders or active gastrointestinal disorders such as peptic ulcer or inflammatory bowel disease and in those with a history of such disorders. It is also contra-indicated in patients with cardiovascular, pulmonary, or thyroid disease, severe impairment of hepatic or renal function, or a history of hypersensitivity to aspirin or other NSAIDs. It is further contra-indicated in patients with salivary gland disorders or Sjögren's syndrome. It may aggravate systemic lupus erythematosus.

Blood-cell counts should be performed before and regularly during therapy in patients receiving the drug for more than 1 week but should not be relied upon to predict dysplasia; monitoring of hepatic and renal function is also recommended. Patients or their carers should be told to discontinue the drug at the first signs of toxic effects and to report at once the appearance of symptoms such as fever, sore throat, stomatitis, skin rashes, bruising, and weight gain or oedema. Treatment should also be withdrawn if symptoms of the acute pulmonary syndrome, including dyspnoea and fever, develop.

It should be used with caution in elderly patients who may require reduced doses. The use of phenylbutazone in breast-feeding patients should be avoided.

Courses of treatment should be kept as short as possible. Dizziness or drowsiness may affect the performance of skilled tasks such as driving.

The precautions to be taken with NSAIDs in general are described on p.64.

Porphyria. Phenylbutazone has been associated with acute attacks of porphyria and is considered unsafe in porphyric patients.

Interactions

For interactions associated with NSAIDs, see p.65. Like azapropazone, phenylbutazone may be particularly likely to cause interactions with oral anticoagulants such as warfarin. The elimination half-life of phenylbutazone is reduced in patients pretreated with drugs that increase liver microsomal enzyme activity. Concurrent administration of methylphenidate or anabolic steroids and phenylbutazone may increase the serum concentration of the metabolite oxyphenbutazone. Colestyramine reduces the absorption of phenylbutazone.

Misoprostol. A report[1] in 2 patients of side-effects including headaches, dizziness, ambulatory instability, tingles, and transient diplopia suggesting a potentiation of neurological adverse effects attributed to concomitant administration of phenylbutazone and misoprostol.

1. Jacquemier JM, *et al.* Neurosensory adverse effects after phenylbutazone and misoprostol combined treatment. *Lancet* 1989; **ii:** 1283.

Pharmacokinetics

Phenylbutazone is readily absorbed from the gastrointestinal tract with peak plasma concentrations occurring about 2 hours after ingestion. It is also readily absorbed when administered rectally. Phenylbutazone is widely distributed throughout body fluids and tissues; it diffuses into the synovial fluid, crosses the placenta, and small amounts enter the CNS and breast milk. It is 98% bound to plasma proteins. It is extensively metabolised in the liver by oxidation and by conjugation with glucuronic acid. Oxyphenbutazone, γ-hydroxyphenbutazone, and *p*,γ-dihydroxyphenylbutazone are formed by oxidation but only small amounts appear in urine, the remainder being further metabolised. It is mainly excreted in the urine as metabolites although about a quarter of a dose may be excreted in the faeces. The plasma elimination half-life is about 70 hours but it is subject to large interindividual variations.

Uses and Administration

Phenylbutazone, a pyrazolone derivative, is an NSAID (p.65). However, because of its toxicity it is not employed as a general analgesic or antipyretic. Although phenylbutazone is effective in almost all musculoskeletal and joint disorders including ankylosing spondylitis, acute gout, osteoarthritis, and rheumatoid arthritis, it should only be used in acute conditions where less toxic drugs have failed. In the UK the use of phenylbutazone is restricted to the hospital treatment of ankylosing spondylitis unresponsive to other drugs, when the recommended initial dose is 200 mg given by mouth two or three times daily for 2 days. The dose is then reduced to the minimum effective amount, which is usually 200 to 300 mg daily given in divided doses. Treatment should be given for the shortest period possible. Elderly patients may require reduced doses.

In some countries phenylbutazone has also been given as a rectal suppository and applied topically for musculoskeletal pain and in soft-tissue injury. It has also been given intramuscularly as the sodium salt. Other salts of phenylbutazone that have been used in musculoskeletal, joint, and soft-tissue disorders include the calcium, megallate, and piperazine salts.

Preparations

USP 25: Phenylbutazone Tablets.

Proprietary Preparations (details are given in Part 3)
Aust.: Butazolidin; ***Austral.:*** Butazolidin; ***Belg.:*** Butazolidin; ***Braz.:*** Butazolidina; Butazolon; Butazona; Butazonil; Peralgin; ***Canad.:*** Novo-Butazone†; ***Fr.:*** Butazolidine; Carudol†; ***Ger.:*** Ambene; Butazolidin; Demoplas; exrheudon OPT; ***Ital.:*** Kadol; ***Mex.:*** Aflamina; Bresal; Butazolidina; Delbulasa; Feniben; Fezona; Rudesol; Tisatin; ***Neth.:*** Butazolidin; ***Port.:*** Basireuma; ***S.Afr.:*** Butrex†; Inflazone; Scriptozone†; ***Spain:*** Butazolidina; Carudol†; ***Switz.:*** Butadion; Butazolidine†; ***Thai.:*** Buta; ***UK:*** Butacote; Butazone.

Multi-ingredient: ***Aust.:*** Ambene; Ambene N; Delta-Tomanol†; ***Braz.:*** Algiflan; Betazon; Butapirin; Butazil; Mioflex; Reumix; ***Fr.:*** Dextrarine Phenylbutazone; ***Ger.:*** Ambene Comp; ***Hong Kong:*** Trabit; ***Spain:*** Artrodesmol Extra; Doctofril Antiinflamat; ***Switz.:*** Butaparin; Carudol†; Hepabuzone; ***Thai.:*** Alaxan; Asialax; Buta Pee Dee; Butarion; Myophen; Trabit.

Picolamine Salicylate (9592-e)

NOTE. Picolamine is *rINN*.

Profile

Picolamine salicylate is a salicylic acid derivative that has been used similarly to methyl salicylate (p.55) in concentrations of 10% in topical rubefacient preparations for the treatment of musculoskeletal, joint, peri-articular, and soft-tissue disorders.

Preparations

Proprietary Preparations (details are given in Part 3)
Fr.: Reflex†; ***Spain:*** Algiospray†.

Piketoprofen (19662-h)

Piketoprofen (*rINN*).

m-Benzoyl-N-(4-methyl-2-pyridyl)hydratropamide.
$C_{22}H_{20}N_2O_2 = 344.4$.
CAS — 60576-13-8.

Profile

Piketoprofen is an NSAID (p.63) that has been used topically as the hydrochloride in concentrations of about 2% in musculoskeletal, joint, peri-articular, and soft-tissue disorders.

Preparations

Proprietary Preparations (details are given in Part 3)
Port.: Picalm; ***Spain:*** Calmatel; Triparsean.

Piritramide (6259-x)

Piritramide (*BAN, rINN*).

Pirinitramide; R-3365. 1-(3-Cyano-3,3-diphenylpropyl)-4-piperidinopiperidine-4-carboxamide.
$C_{27}H_{34}N_4O = 430.6$.
CAS — 302-41-0.
ATC — N02AC03.

Profile

Piritramide is an opioid analgesic (p.66).

It is used for the management of severe pain including postoperative pain, for premedication, and to provide analgesia during anaesthesia. It is given by intramuscular, subcutaneous, or slow intravenous injection as the tartrate in doses equivalent of up to about 30 mg of the base.

◊ Reviews.
1. Kumar N, Rowbotham DJ. Piritramide. *Br J Anaesth* 1999; **82**: 3–5.

Porphyria. Piritramide is considered to be unsafe in patients with porphyria because it has been shown to be porphyrinogenic in *animals* or *in vitro* systems.

Preparations

Proprietary Preparations (details are given in Part 3)
Aust.: Dipidolor; **Belg.:** Dipidolor; **Ger.:** Dipidolor; **Neth.:** Dipidolor.

Piroxicam (2692-v)

Piroxicam *(BAN, USAN, rINN)*.
CP-16171; Piroxicamum. 4-Hydroxy-2-methyl-*N*-(2-pyridyl)-2*H*-1,2-benzothiazine-3-carboxamide 1,1-dioxide.
$C_{15}H_{13}N_3O_4S = 331.3$.
CAS — 36322-90-4.
ATC — M01AC01; M02AA07; S01BC06.
Pharmacopoeias. In Eur. (see p.vi) and *US.*

Pharmacopoeial description

Ph. Eur.: A white or slightly yellow, crystalline powder. It shows polymorphism. Practically insoluble in water; slightly soluble in dehydrated alcohol; soluble in dichloromethane. Store in airtight containers. Protect from light.
USP 25: An off-white to light tan or light yellow, odourless powder. It forms a monohydrate that is yellow. Very slightly soluble in water, in dilute acids, and in most organic solvents; slightly soluble in alcohol and in aqueous alkaline solutions. Store in airtight containers. Protect from light.

Piroxicam Betadex (5561-a)

Piroxicam Betadex *(USAN, rINNM)*.
CHF-1194; Piroxicam Beta Cyclodextrin; Piroxicam Beta Cyclodextrin Complex.
$(C_{15}H_{13}N_3O_4S)_{2}.-(C_{42}H_{70}O_{35})_{5} = 6337.6$.
CAS — 96684-40-1.

Piroxicam betadex 191.3 mg is approximately equivalent to 20 mg of piroxicam.

Adverse Effects

As for NSAIDs in general, p.63.

Local irritation and occasionally bleeding may occur with piroxicam suppositories and there may be pain and occasionally tissue damage at the injection site on intramuscular administration.

Piroxicam is considered to be associated with an intermediate risk of gastrointestinal effects although there is some suggestion that the risk may be higher than for other intermediate-risk NSAIDs (p.63). At present there is little evidence to support the manufacturer's claim that piroxicam betadex has improved gastrointestinal tolerability.

◊ A report[1] of the adverse reactions associated with piroxicam in South Africa during 1981-86 including two reactions, paraesthesia and hair loss, not previously recorded in the literature.
1. Gerber D. Adverse reactions of piroxicam. *Drug Intell Clin Pharm* 1987; **21**: 707–10.

Effects on the blood. Decreases in haemoglobin and haematocrit not associated with obvious gastrointestinal bleeding, have occurred in patients taking piroxicam. Thrombocytopenia, thrombocytopenic purpura,[1] and aplastic anaemia[2] have been described in patients on piroxicam.
1. Bjørnstad H, Vik Ø. Thrombocytopenic purpura associated with piroxicam. *Br J Clin Pract* 1986; **40**: 42.
2. Lee SH, *et al.* Aplastic anaemia associated with piroxicam. *Lancet* 1982; **i:** 1186.

Effects on electrolytes. Reversible hyperkalaemic hyperchloraemic acidosis has been reported[1,2] in patients receiving piroxicam. Severe hyponatraemia and symptoms resembling the syndrome of inappropriate antidiuretic hormone secretion have also been associated with piroxicam.[3]
See also under Effects on the Kidneys, below.
1. Grossman LA, Moss S. Piroxicam and hyperkalemic acidosis. *Ann Intern Med* 1983; **99**: 282.
2. Miller KP, *et al.* Severe hyperkalemia during piroxicam therapy. *Arch Intern Med* 1984; **144**: 2414–15.
3. Petersson I, *et al.* Water intoxication associated with non-steroidal anti-inflammatory drug therapy. *Acta Med Scand* 1987; **221**: 221–3.

Effects on the kidneys. Acute nephropathy with characteristic features of Henoch-Schönlein purpura,[1] acute renal failure,[2] uraemia with hyperkalaemia, and acute interstitial nephritis[3] have been associated with systemic administration of piroxicam. Nephrotic syndrome and interstitial nephritis have been reported in a patient following topical application of piroxicam gel.[4]
1. Goebel KM, Mueller-Brodmann W. Reversible overt nephropathy with Henoch-Schönlein purpura due to piroxicam. *BMJ* 1982; **284**: 311–12.

2. Frais MA, *et al.* Piroxicam-induced renal failure and hyperkalemia. *Ann Intern Med* 1983; **99**: 129–30.
3. Mitnick PD, Klein WJ. Piroxicam-induced renal disease. *Arch Intern Med* 1984; **144**: 63–4.
4. O'Callaghan CA, *et al.* Renal disease and use of topical non-steroidal anti-inflammatory drugs. *BMJ* 1994; **308**: 110–11.

Effects on the liver. Necrosis of the liver has been associated with piroxicam. Details have been supplied on 3 patients,[1,2] of whom 2 died.
1. Lee SM, *et al.* Subacute hepatic necrosis induced by piroxicam. *BMJ* 1986; **293**: 540–1.
2. Paterson D, *et al.* Piroxicam induced submassive necrosis of the liver. *Gut* 1992; **33;** 1436–8.

Effects on the skin. As with other NSAIDs, rash has occurred in patients taking piroxicam. Phototoxic reactions have been described.[1] Serious skin reactions attributed to piroxicam therapy include toxic epidermal necrolysis[2] and pemphigus vulgaris.[3]
1. Stern RS. Phototoxic reactions to piroxicam and other nonsteroidal antiinflammatory agents. *N Engl J Med* 1983; **309**: 186–7.
2. Chosidow O, *et al.* Intestinal involvement in drug-induced toxic epidermal necrolysis. *Lancet* 1991; **337**: 928.
3. Martin RL. Fatal pemphigus vulgaris in a patient taking piroxicam. *N Engl J Med* 1983; **309**: 795–6.

Overdosage. Details of 16 patients who were considered to have taken an overdosage of piroxicam alone were reported[1] to the National Poisons Information Service of the UK. Thirteen patients (including 5 children) experienced no symptoms after doses estimated to be up to 300 to 400 mg; 2 patients complained of dizziness and blurred vision after 200 to 300 mg; the last patient who claimed to have taken 600 mg presented in coma, regained consciousness within one hour, and had recovered fully within 24 hours. Severe multisystem toxicity has been reported in a 2-year-old child after ingestion of 100 mg of piroxicam.[2]
1. Court H, Volans GN. Poisoning after overdose with non-steroidal anti-inflammatory drugs. *Adverse Drug React Acute Poisoning Rev* 1984; **3**: 1–21.
2. MacDougall LG, *et al.* Piroxicam poisoning in a 2-year-old child: a case report. *S Afr Med J* 1984; **66**: 31–3.

Pancreatitis. A report[1] of pancreatitis associated with piroxicam.
1. Haye OL. Piroxicam and pancreatitis. *Ann Intern Med* 1986; **104**: 895.

Precautions

As for NSAIDs in general, p.64.

Breast feeding. See under Pharmacokinetics, below.

Porphyria. Piroxicam has been associated with acute attacks of porphyria and is considered unsafe in porphyric patients.

Interactions

For interactions associated with NSAIDs, see p.65.
Concurrent administration of aspirin and piroxicam results in decreased plasma concentrations of piroxicam to about 80% of normal. The UK manufacturer of ritonavir suggests that concomitant administration of piroxicam and ritonavir may result in increased plasma concentrations of piroxicam and an increased risk of toxicity; they recommend that use together should be avoided.

Pharmacokinetics

Piroxicam is well absorbed from the gastrointestinal tract; peak plasma concentrations are reached 3 to 5 hours after an oral dose. Piroxicam is also absorbed to some degree following topical application. Piroxicam is 99% bound to plasma proteins. It has been detected in breast milk in concentrations of 1 to 3% of those in maternal plasma, but such amounts are considered by some authorities to be too small to be harmful to a breast-fed infant. Piroxicam has a long plasma elimination half-life of approximately 50 hours. Because of this, steady-state concentrations are not reached for 7 to 12 days. It is metabolised in the liver by hydroxylation and conjugation with glucuronic acid and excreted predominantly in the urine with smaller amounts in the faeces. Enterohepatic recycling occurs. Less than 5% of the dose is excreted unchanged in the urine.

Piroxicam betadex dissociates in the gastrointestinal tract to piroxicam and beta-cyclodextrin. Piroxicam absorption from piroxicam betadex is more rapid than that of unmodified piroxicam; peak plasma concentrations of piroxicam are reached 30 to 60 minutes after an oral dose. Beta-cyclodextrin is not absorbed but is metabolised in the colon to various sugars.

◊ References.
1. Østensen M. Piroxicam in human breast milk. *Eur J Clin Pharmacol* 1983; **25**: 829–30.

2. Richardson CJ, *et al.* Piroxicam and 5′-hydroxypiroxicam kinetics following multiple dose administration of piroxicam. *Eur J Clin Pharmacol* 1987; **32**: 89–91.
3. Mäkelä A-L, *et al.* Steady state pharmacokinetics of piroxicam in children with rheumatic diseases. *Eur J Clin Pharmacol* 1991; **41**: 79–81 (higher clearance and shorter half-life in children).
4. Rudy AC, *et al.* The pharmacokinetics of piroxicam in elderly persons with and without renal impairment. *Br J Clin Pharmacol* 1994; **37**: 1–5.
5. Deroubaix X, *et al.* Oral bioavailability of CHF1194, an inclusion complex of piroxicam and β-cyclodextrin, in healthy subjects under single dose and steady-state conditions. *Eur J Clin Pharmacol* 1995; **47**: 531–6.
6. Karim A, *et al.* Oxaprozin and piroxicam, nonsteroidal antiinflammatory drugs with long half-lives: effect of protein-binding differences on steady-state pharmacokinetics. *J Clin Pharmacol* 1997; **37**: 267–78.
7. Wang D, *et al.* Comparative population pharmacokinetic-pharmacodynamic analysis for piroxicam-β-cyclodextrin and piroxicam. *J Clin Pharmacol* 2000; **40**: 1257–66.

Uses and Administration

Piroxicam, an oxicam derivative, and piroxicam betadex are NSAIDs (p.65). Piroxicam betadex may have a more rapid onset of therapeutic effect due to its enhanced solubility (see Pharmacokinetics above). Both are used in musculoskeletal and joint disorders such as ankylosing spondylitis, osteoarthritis, rheumatoid arthritis including juvenile idiopathic arthritis, in soft-tissue disorders, and in acute gout.

In rheumatic disorders a usual initial dose of piroxicam by mouth is 20 mg daily as a single dose. Daily maintenance doses may vary between 10 and 30 mg given in single or divided doses; administration of doses in excess of 20 mg daily for more than a few days is associated with an increased risk of gastrointestinal adverse effects. In acute musculoskeletal conditions an initial dose of 40 mg daily may be given for 2 days followed by 20 mg daily for a total of 1 to 2 weeks. Piroxicam is also used in acute gout, the usual dose being 40 mg daily for 5 to 7 days. Piroxicam is given in similar doses as a rectal suppository or on a short-term basis by intramuscular injection.

Piroxicam may also be used in children aged 6 years or over with juvenile idiopathic arthritis. The usual dose by mouth is 5 mg daily in those weighing less than 15 kg, 10 mg daily in those weighing 16 to 25 kg, 15 mg daily in those weighing 26 to 45 kg, and 20 mg daily in those weighing 46 kg or over.

Doses of piroxicam betadex are expressed in terms of the equivalent amount of piroxicam. In rheumatic and acute musculoskeletal disorders piroxicam betadex is given in a dose equivalent to 20 mg piroxicam daily as a single dose. This dose may be reduced to 10 mg daily in elderly patients.

Piroxicam is also used in the local treatment of a variety of painful or inflammatory conditions as a topical gel in a concentration of 0.5% applied three or four times daily; treatment should be reviewed after 4 weeks. Piroxicam has been used in some countries as a 1% cream and as eye drops in a concentration of 0.5%.

Other piroxicam salts or compounds that have also been used include piroxicam cinnamate (cinnoxicam), piroxicam choline, and piroxicam pivalate.

◊ Reviews.
1. Lee CR, Balfour JA. Piroxicam-β-cyclodextrin: a review of its pharmacodynamic and pharmacokinetic properties and therapeutic potential in rheumatic diseases and pain states. *Drugs* 1994; **48**: 907–29.
2. Edwards JE. Single dose piroxicam for acute postoperative pain (updated 30 August 2001). Available in The Cochrane Library; Issue 4. Oxford: Update Software; 2001.

Preparations

BP 2001: Piroxicam Capsules; Piroxicam Gel;
USP 25: Piroxicam Capsules.

Proprietary Preparations (details are given in Part 3)
Aust.: Brexin; Felden; Pirocam; Pirorheum; Piroxistad; Piroxityrol; **Austral.:** Candyl; Feldene; Fensaid†; Mobilis; Pirohexal-D; Pirox; Rosig; **Belg.:** Brexine; Feldene; Solicam; **Braz.:** Anartrit; Brexin; Cicladol; Feldene; Feldexican; Feldox; Felnan; Flamadene; Flamarene; Flamostat; Flogene; Flogoxen; Inflamene; Inflanan; Inflaxox; Inflax; Lisedema; Piroxene; Piroxifen; Piroxiflam; Piroxil; Piroxiplus; **Canad.:** Brexidol; Feldene; Fexicam; Novo-Pirocam; Nu-Pirox; **Denm.:** Brexidol; Felden; Pirkam; Pirom; Pironet†; **Fin.:** Brexidol; Felden; Piroxal; Piroxin; **Fr.:** Brexin; Cycladol; Feldene; Flexirox; Geldene; Inflaced; Olcam; Proxalyoc; Zofora; **Ger.:** Brexidol; durapirox; Fasax; Felden; Flexase; Jenapirox; Piro; Piro KD; Piro-Phlogont; Piro-Puren; Pirobeta; Piroflam; Pirorheum; PirorheumA; Pirox; Pirox-Spondyril; Piroximerck†; Pra-Brexidol; ratioMobil; Rheumitin; **Hong Kong:** Brexin; Feldene; Flamatrol; Hotemin; Piroxy; Sotilen; Syn-

oxicam; *Irl.:* Feldene; Geroxicam; Pericam; *Israel:* Exipan; Feldene; *Ital.:* Antiflog; Artroxicam; Brexin; Brexivel; Bruxicam; Cicladol; Ciclafast; Clevian; Dexicam; Euroxi; Feldene; Flodol; Flogobene; Lampoflex; Nirox†; Oxicam; Piroftal; Pivaloxicam†; Polipirox; Reucam; Reudene; Reumagil; Riacen; Roxene; Roxenil; Roxiden; Sinartrol; Zacam†; Zelis; Zen†; Zunden†; *Jpn:* Baxo; *Mex.:* Androxicam; Apopiran; Arlexicam; Artinor; Artyflam; Bioximil; Brexicam; Citoken; Dixonal; Dolzycam; Facicam; Farmicam; Feldene; Flogosan; Glandicin; Osteral; Oxicanol; Perfarin; Pirodax; Piromav; Piroxan; Piroxen; Reucam; Reufel; Reutricam; Rogal; Vatrem; *Neth.:* Brexine; Feldene; *Norw.:* Brexidol; Felden; Pirox; Tetram; *NZ:* Candyl-D; Feldene; Piram-D; *Port.:* Brexin; Feldene; Flexar; Flogocan; Reumoxican; Roxazin; *S.Afr.:* Brexecam; Feldene; Pixicam; Pyrocaps; Rheugesic; Roxacam; Xycam; *Singapore:* Brexin; Feldene; Mobilis; Rosiden; Sotilen; Vitaxicam; *Spain:* Artragil; Brexinil; Cycladol; Dekamega; Doblexan; Feldene; Improntal; Salcacam; Salvacam; Sasulen; Vitaxicam; *Swed.:* Brexidol; Felden; *Switz.:* Brexidol; Felden; Pirocam; Pirosol; pirox-basan; *Thai.:* Bicam; Brexin; Candyl; Felcam; Feldene; Felrox; Finfo; Flamic; Ifemed; Maswin; Neogel; Neotica; Piram; Pirax; Piroxam; Piroxcin; Piroxen; Piroxsil; Polyxicam; Posedene; Pyroxy; Roccaxin; Roxifen; Roxycam; Rumadene; Sotilen; Xicam; *UK:* Brexidol; Feldene; Flamatrol; Larapam; Piroflam; Pirozip; *USA:* Feldene.

Pranoprofen (3847-c)

Pranoprofen (rINN).

α-Methyl-5*H*-[1]-benzopyrano[2,3-*b*]pyridine-7-acetic acid.
$C_{15}H_{13}NO_3 = 255.3$.
CAS — 52549-17-4.
Pharmacopoeias. In Jpn.

Profile

Pranoprofen, a propionic acid derivative, is an NSAID (p.63). It has been given by mouth for the treatment of pain, inflammation, and fever. Pranoprofen has also been used as eye drops in a concentration of 0.1% for ocular inflammation.

◊ References.
1. Notivol R, *et al.* Treatment of chronic nonbacterial conjunctivitis with a cyclo-oxygenase inhibitor or a corticosteroid. *Am J Ophthalmol* 1994; **117:** 651–6.

Preparations

Proprietary Preparations (details are given in Part 3)
Belg.: Pranox; *Braz.:* Difen; *Jpn:* Niflan†; *Spain:* Oftalar.

Proglumetacin Maleate (13174-q)

Proglumetacin Maleate (BANM, rINNM).

CR-604; Protacine Maleate. 3-{4-[2-(1-*p*-Chlorobenzoyl-5-methoxy-2-methylindol-3-ylacetoxy)ethyl]piperazin-1-yl}propyl 4-benzamido-N,N-dipropylglutaramate dimaleate.
$C_{46}H_{58}ClN_5O_8.2C_4H_4O_4 = 1076.6$.
CAS — 57132-53-3 (proglumetacin); 59209-40-4 (proglumetacin maleate).

Profile

Proglumetacin maleate, an indoleacetic acid derivative related to indometacin (p.44), is an NSAID (p.63). It has been used in musculoskeletal and joint disorders in doses of up to 600 mg daily, in divided doses, by mouth.

◊ References.
1. Appelboom T, Franchimont P. Proglumetacin versus indometacin in rheumatoid arthritis: a double-blind multicenter study. *Adv Therapy* 1994; **11:** 228–34.
2. Martens M. Double-blind randomized comparison of proglumetacin and naproxen sodium in the treatment of patients with ankle sprains. *Curr Ther Res* 1995; **56:** 639–48.

Preparations

Proprietary Preparations (details are given in Part 3)
Aust.: Protaxon; *Belg.:* Tolindol; *Ger.:* Protaxon; *Hong Kong:* Afloxan; *Ital.:* Afloxan, Proxil; *Port.:* Protaxil; *Spain:* Prodamox; Protaxil; *Thai.:* Afloxan.

Propacetamol Hydrochloride (13537-a)

Propacetamol Hydrochloride (BANM, rINNM).

Propacetamoli Hydrochloridum. The hydrochloride of N,N-diethylglycine ester with paracetamol; 4-Acetamidophenyl diethylaminoacetate hydrochloride.
$C_{14}H_{20}N_2O_3,HCl = 300.8$.
CAS — 66532-85-2 (propacetamol).
Pharmacopoeias. In Eur. (see p.vi).

Pharmacopoeial description

Ph. Eur.: A white or almost white crystalline powder. Freely soluble in water; slightly soluble in dehydrated alcohol; practically insoluble in acetone. Protect from moisture.

Profile

Propacetamol hydrochloride, a para-aminophenol derivative, is hydrolysed to paracetamol (p.71) in the plasma. It has been given intramuscularly or intravenously in usual doses of 1 to 2 g for the treatment of pain (p.2) and fever (p.8).

◊ A report[1] of occupational contact dermatitis in 3 nurses arising from the preparation of injections of propacetamol.
1. Barbaud A, *et al.* Occupational allergy to propacetamol. *Lancet* 1995; **346:** 902.

Preparations

Proprietary Preparations (details are given in Part 3)
Belg.: Pro-Dafalgan; *Fin.:* Pro-Dafalgan; *Fr.:* Pro-Dafalgan; *Ital.:* Pro-Efferalgan; *Mex.:* Tempra; *Port.:* Pro-Dafalgan; *Spain:* Pro-Efferalgan; *Switz.:* Pro-Dafalgan.

Propiram Fumarate (2695-p)

Propiram Fumarate (BANM, USAN, rINNM).

Bay-4503; FBA-4503. N-(1-Methyl-2-piperidinoethyl)-N-(2-pyridyl)propionamide hydrogen fumarate.
$C_{16}H_{25}N_3O,C_4H_4O_4 = 391.5$.
CAS — 15686-91-6 (propiram); 13717-04-9 (propiram fumarate).

Profile

Propiram fumarate is an opioid analgesic (p.66) with agonist and antagonist properties; it is classified as a partial agonist at μ opioid receptors. It has been given by mouth for the relief of moderate to severe pain.

◊ References.
1. Goa KL, Brogden RN. Propiram: a review of its pharmacodynamic and pharmacokinetic properties, and clinical use as an analgesic. *Drugs* 1993; **46:** 428–45.

Propyl Nicotinate (19727-m)

$C_9H_{11}NO_2 = 165.2$.

Profile

Propyl nicotinate is used in topical preparations as a rubefacient.

Preparations

Proprietary Preparations (details are given in Part 3)
Ger.: Elacur; Nicodan; Nicodan N.

Propyphenazone (2696-s)

Propyphenazone (BAN, rINN).

Isopropylantipyrine; Isopropylantipyrinum; Isopropylphenazone; Propifenazona; Propyphenazonum. 4-Isopropyl-2,3-dimethyl-1-phenyl-3-pyrazolin-5-one.
$C_{14}H_{18}N_2O = 230.3$.
CAS — 479-92-5.
ATC — N02BB04.
Pharmacopoeias. In Eur. (see p.vi) and Jpn.

Pharmacopoeial description

Ph. Eur.: A white or slightly yellowish crystalline powder. Slightly soluble in water; freely soluble in alcohol and in dichloromethane; soluble in ether. Protect from light.

Profile

Propyphenazone, a pyrazolone derivative related to phenazone (p.77), has analgesic and antipyretic properties. It has been given by mouth and as a rectal suppository in the treatment of pain and fever. There have been some reports of severe hypersensitivity reactions in patients receiving propyphenazone.

Porphyria. Propyphenazone has been associated with acute attacks of porphyria and is considered unsafe in porphyric patients.

Preparations

Proprietary Preparations (details are given in Part 3)
Aust.: Dim-Antos; *Ger.:* Demex; Eufibron; Isoprochin P; *Ital.:* Cibalgina†; Pireuma; *Spain:* Cibalgina†.
Multi-ingredient: *Aust.:* Adolorin; Adoluron CC; APA; Asthma; Asticol; Avamigran; Cedanon†; Coldagrippin; Contraforte; Contraloren; Eu-Med; Gewadal; Influvidon; Melabon; Migradon; Montamed; Neokratin; Nervan; Neuro-Europan†; Normensan; Rapidol; Saridon; Spasmoplus; Tonopan; Toximer; Vivimed; *Belg.:* Migraine-Kranit Nova; Neuridon Forte; Optalidon; Saridon; Spasmo-Cibalgine†; Spasmoplus; *Braz.:* Optalidon; Saridon; Tonopan; *Denm.:* Kodamid; *Ger.:* Avamigran N; Copyrkal N; Ergo-Kranit; Eudorlin; Fomagrippin N; Gewodin; Ichtho-Bellol compositum S; Migrane-Kranit Kombi; Migrane-Kranit N; Migratan S; Milneuron Plus; Norgesic N; Novo Petrin; Optalidon N; Optalidon special NOC; RubieNex spezial; Saridon; Spasmo-Cibalgin compositum S; Spasmo-Cibalgin S; Tispol S†; Titretta; *Hong Kong:* APA; Epizon; Saridon; Tonterin; *Ital.:* Alfazina; Azerodol†; Caffalgina; Cistalgan; Flexidone†; Influrem; Influvit; Micranet; Mindol-Merck; Neo-Optalidon; Odontalgico Dr. Knapp con Vit. B1; Omniadol; Optalidon; Ribelfan; Saridon; Sedol; Spasmo-Cibalgina; Spasmoplus; Uniplus; Upsa Plus; Veramon; Vitialgin†; *Mex.:* Espasmo Cibalgina; Tonopan; *Neth.:* Daro Hoofdpijnpoeders†; Sanalgin; Saridon; *Port.:* Avamigran; Optalidon; Saridon N; *S.Afr.:* Ilvico; *Spain:* Abdominol; Bronquimar†; Calmoplex; Cibalgina Compuesta†; Dolodens; Fenalgin†; Flexagil; Hubergrip; Melabon; Meloka; Optalidon†; Quimpedor; Saridon; Sedalmerck; Sulmetin Papaver; Sulmetin Papaverina; Tabletas Quimpe; Tonopan; *Switz.:* Angifebrine†; Barbamin†; Caposan; Cerebrol; Comprimes analgesiques "S"; Dialgine forte; Dolopyrine†; Dolostop; Escalgin sans codeine†; Escogripp sans codeine; Febracyl; Gewodine; Gubamine†; Kafa; Nicaphlogyl; Novidol; Sanalgin; Saridon; Seranex sans codeine; Sinedal; Siniphen†; Sonotryl†; Spasmo-Barbamin†; Spasmo-Barbamine compositum†; Spasmo-Cibalgin, Spasmo-Cibalgin comp.; Spedralgin sans codeine; Tonopan.

Proquazone (13180-v)

Proquazone (BAN, USAN, rINN).

43-715; RU-43-715-n. 1-Isopropyl-7-methyl-4-phenylquinazolin-2(1H)-one.
$C_{18}H_{18}N_2O = 278.3$.
CAS — 22760-18-5.
ATC — M01AX13.

Profile

Proquazone is an NSAID (p.63). It was given by mouth in musculoskeletal and joint disorders. It has also been given by rectal suppository.

Preparations

Proprietary Preparations (details are given in Part 3)
Aust.: Biarison†.

Ramifenazone (2660-x)

Ramifenazone (rINN).

Isopropylaminophenazone; Isopyrin. 4-Isopropylamino-2,3-dimethyl-1-phenyl-3-pyrazolin-5-one.
$C_{14}H_{19}N_3O = 245.3$.
CAS — 3615-24-5.
NOTE. The name Isopyrin has also been applied to isoniazid.

Profile

Ramifenazone is an NSAID (p.63) that has been used in preparations for painful and inflammatory conditions. The hydrochloride salt was given by mouth and the salicylate applied topically.

Preparations

Proprietary Preparations (details are given in Part 3)
Multi-ingredient: *Aust.:* Delta-Tomanol†.

Remifentanil Hydrochloride (13662-d)

Remifentanil Hydrochloride (BANM, USAN, rINNM).

GI-87084B. 4-Carboxyl-4-(N-phenylpropionamido)-1-piperidine propionic acid dimethyl ester monohydrate.
$C_{20}H_{28}N_2O_5,HCl = 412.9$.
CAS — 132539-07-2.

Remifentanil hydrochloride 1.1 mg is approximately equivalent to 1 mg of remifentanil.

Incompatibility. Remifentanil hydrochloride should not be mixed in the same solution for intravenous administration as blood products. The UK manufacturer states that it should not be mixed with lactated Ringer's injection with or without 5% glucose; however, in the USA the manufacturer's literature states that remifentanil hydrochloride is stable for 4 hours at room temperature following reconstitution and dilution to 20 to 250 μg per mL with lactated Ringer's injection and for 24 hours if lactated Ringer's with 5% glucose is used. Incompatibilities have been reported between chlorpromazine hydrochloride 2 mg per mL and remifentanil 25 μg per mL (as the hydrochloride) in 5% glucose and cefoperazone sodium 40 mg per mL or amphotericin B 0.6 mg/mL and remifentanil 250 μg per mL (as the hydrochloride) in 5% glucose.[1]
1. Trissel LA, *et al.* Compatibility of remifentanil hydrochloride with selected drugs during simulated Y-site administration. *Am J Health-Syst Pharm* 1997; **54:** 2192–6.

Dependence and Withdrawal

As for Opioid Analgesics, p.66.

Adverse Effects and Treatment

As for Opioid Analgesics in general, p.67 and for Fentanyl, p.37.

Precautions

As for Opioid Analgesics in general, p.68.

Administration. Remifentanil hydrochloride injections containing glycine should not be given by the epidural or intrathecal routes.

Hepatic impairment. Although the pharmacokinetics of remifentanil are not changed in patients with severe hepatic impairment, such patients may be more sensitive to the respiratory depressant effects and should be monitored with doses titrated to individual requirements.

Renal impairment. The pharmacokinetics of remifentanil are not changed in patients with severe renal impairment (a creatinine clearance of less than 10 mL per minute) and the manufacturers have stated that the carboxylic acid metabolite is unlikely to accumulate to clinically active concentrations in such patients following remifentanil infusions of up to 2 μg per kg body-weight per minute for up to 12 hours. Dosage adjustment is considered to be unnecessary.

Interactions

For interactions associated with opioid analgesics, see p.68.

Pharmacokinetics

Following parenteral administration remifentanil hydrochloride has a rapid onset and short duration of action. Its effective biological half-life is about 3 to 10 minutes and is independent of dose. Remifentanil is about 70% bound to plasma proteins, principally to α_1-acid glycoprotein. It is hydrolysed by non-specific esterases in blood and tissues to an essentially inactive carboxylic acid metabolite. Approximately 95% of a dose of remifentanil is excreted in the urine as the metabolite.

◊ The manufacturers of remifentanil have given values for a three-compartment pharmacokinetic model with a rapid distribution half-life of 1 minute, a slower distribution half-life of 6 minutes, and a terminal elimination half-life of 10 to 20 minutes.

References.
1. Egan TD. Remifentanil pharmacokinetics and pharmacodynamics: a preliminary appraisal. *Clin Pharmacokinet* 1995; **29:** 80–94.

Uses and Administration

Remifentanil, an anilidopiperidine derivative, is an opioid analgesic (p.68) related to fentanyl (p.38). It is a short-acting μ-receptor opioid agonist used for analgesia during induction and/or maintenance of general anaesthesia. It is also used to provide analgesia into the immediate postoperative period, and may be used as the analgesic component of local or regional anaesthesia with or without benzodiazepine sedation.

Remifentanil is administered intravenously as the hydrochloride, usually by infusion. Its onset of action is within 1 minute and the duration of action is 5 to 10 minutes. Doses are expressed in terms of remifentanil base. Initial doses in elderly patients should be half the recommended adult doses and then titrated to individual requirements.

When used to provide **analgesia** during *induction* of anaesthesia an intravenous infusion is given in doses of 0.5 to 1 μg per kg body-weight per minute. An additional initial intravenous bolus of 1 μg per kg may be administered over 30 to 60 seconds if the patient is to be intubated less than 8 minutes after the start of the infusion.

For provision of analgesia during *maintenance* of anaesthesia in ventilated patients, usual infusion doses range from 0.05 to 2 μg per kg per minute depending on the anaesthetic drug employed and adjusted according to patient response. Supplemental intravenous boluses of 0.5 to 1 μg per kg may be given every 2 to 5 minutes in response to light anaesthesia or intense surgical stress. The infusion dosage in spontaneous respiration is initially 0.04 μg per kg per minute adjusted according to response within a usual range of 0.025 to 0.1 μg per kg per minute. Bolus doses are not recommended during spontaneous ventilation.

For continuation of analgesia into the immediate *postoperative* period typical doses by intravenous infusion range from 0.025 to 0.2 μg per kg per minute; supplemental intravenous bolus doses are not recommended during the postoperative period.

Remifentanil has a very rapid offset of action and no residual opioid action remains 5 to 10 minutes after discontinuation of an infusion. Consideration should therefore be given to provision of alternative analgesics administered in sufficient time before discontinuation of remifentanil to provide continuous and more prolonged postoperative pain relief when appropriate.

◊ References and reviews.
1. Bacon R, *et al.* Early extubation after open-heart surgery with total intravenous anaesthetic technique. *Lancet* 1995; **345:** 133–4.
2. Duthie DJR, *et al.* Remifentanil and coronary artery surgery. *Lancet* 1995; **345:** 649–50.
3. Patel SS, Spencer CM. Remifentanil. *Drugs* 1996; **52:** 417–27.
4. Duthie DJR. Remifentanil and tramadol. *Br J Anaesth* 1998; **81:** 51–7.

Preparations

Proprietary Preparations (details are given in Part 3)
Aust.: Ultiva; *Austral.:* Ultiva; *Belg.:* Ultiva; *Canad.:* Ultiva; *Denm.:* Ultiva; *Fin.:* Ultiva; *Fr.:* Ultiva; *Ger.:* Ultiva; *Israel:* Ultiva; *Ital.:* Ultiva; *Mex.:* Ultiva; *Neth.:* Ultiva; *Norw.:* Ultiva; *NZ:* Ultiva; *Port.:* Ultiva; *S.Afr.:* Ultiva; *Singapore:* Ultiva; *Spain:* Ultiva; *Swed.:* Ultiva; *Switz.:* Ultiva; *UK:* Ultiva; *USA:* Ultiva.

Rofecoxib (4728-k)

Rofecoxib (*BAN, USAN, rINN*).
MK-0966. 4-[p-(Methylsulfonyl)phenyl]-3-phenyl-2(5H)-furanone.
$C_{17}H_{14}O_4S = 314.4$.
CAS — 162011-90-7.

Adverse Effects and Precautions

As for NSAIDs in general, p.63. Mouth ulcers, chest pain, weight gain, atopic eczema, and muscle cramps have also been reported. Rofecoxib should not be used in patients with moderate to severe hepatic impairment. Therapy should be discontinued in patients if persistently abnormal liver function tests are detected. Rofecoxib is also contra-indicated in patients with severe heart failure, inflammatory bowel disease, and renal impairment associated with a creatinine clearance of less than 30 mL per minute.

Effects on the cardiovascular system. As of February 2001, the UK Committee on Safety of Medicines has received a small number of reports of myocardial infarction or ischaemia in association with the selective cyclo-oxygenase-2 (COX-2) inhibitors.[1] COX-2 inhibitors such as celecoxib do not possess the intrinsic antiplatelet activity associated with aspirin and possibly other non-selective NSAIDs and consequently do not provide protection against ischaemic cardiac events. Data from a large, randomised trial also showed the incidence of myocardial infarction to be greater in patients taking rofecoxib than in those taking naproxen.[2]

A randomised trial in elderly, hypertensive patients with osteoarthritis has suggested that the risk of developing increased systolic blood pressure is greater in those patients receiving rofecoxib than in those receiving celecoxib.[3] However, the manufacturers of rofecoxib have pointed out that the trial used doses of rofecoxib greater than those recommended for elderly or hypertensive patients.

1. Committee on Safety of Medicines/Medicines Control Agency. COX-2 selective NSAIDs lack antiplatelet activity. *Current Problems* 2001; **27:** 7.
2. Bombardier C, *et al.* Comparison of upper gastrointestinal toxicity of rofecoxib and naproxen in patients with rheumatoid arthritis. *N Engl J Med* 2000; **343:** 1520–8.
3. Whelton A, *et al.* Cyclooxygenase-2-specific inhibitors and cardiorenal function: a randomized, controlled trial of celecoxib and rofecoxib in older hypertensive osteoarthritis patients. *Am J Ther* 2001; **8:** 85–95.

Effects on the gastrointestinal tract. It is generally accepted that the inhibition of cyclo-oxygenase-1 (COX-1) results in the adverse gastrointestinal effects of the NSAIDs, and that the selective inhibition of the other isoform, COX-2, by NSAIDs such as rofecoxib may cause less gastrotoxicity than that seen with the non-selective inhibition of the traditional NSAIDs.

Results from controlled trials confirm that NSAIDs selective for COX-2 are associated with a lower incidence of serious gastrointestinal effects. A combined analysis of 8 pre-licensing trials concluded that the risk of upper gastrointestinal perforation, symptomatic gastroduodenal ulcers, or upper gastrointestinal bleeding with rofecoxib was significantly less than that with ibuprofen, diclofenac, or nabumetone.[1] In a comparative study,[2] rofecoxib given in doses of 50 mg daily (twice the maximum recommended dose for osteoarthritis) was associated with a significantly lower incidence of endoscopically-detected gastroduodenal ulceration than maximum recommended doses of ibuprofen (2.4 g daily). Another comparative study[3] in patients with rheumatoid arthritis also found rofecoxib, in doses of 50 mg daily, to be associated with significantly fewer incidences of clinically serious upper gastrointestinal events than naproxen, given in doses of 1 g daily.

There have been individual case reports of gastrotoxicity with rofecoxib.[4]

1. Langman MJ, *et al.* Adverse upper gastrointestinal effects of rofecoxib compared with NSAIDs. *JAMA* 1999; **282:** 1929–33.
2. Hawkey C, *et al.* Comparison of the effect of rofecoxib (a cyclooxygenase 2 inhibitor), ibuprofen, and placebo on the gastroduodenal mucosa of patients with osteoarthritis: a randomized, double-blind, placebo-controlled trial. *Arthritis Rheum* 2000; **43:** 370–7.
3. Bombardier C, *et al.* Comparison of upper gastrointestinal toxicity of rofecoxib and naproxen in patients with rheumatoid arthritis. *N Engl J Med* 2000; **343:** 1520–8.
4. Committee on Safety of Medicines/Medicines Control Agency. Rofecoxib (Vioxx). *Current Problems* 2000; **26:** 13.

Effects on the kidneys. Limited evidence of the renal toxicity of the selective cyclo-oxygenase-2 (COX-2) inhibitors such as rofecoxib suggests that such NSAIDs appear to have effects on renal function similar to those of the non-selective NSAIDs (see p.64).

Some references to the adverse renal effects of rofecoxib.
1. Swan SK, *et al.* Effect of cyclooxygenase-2 inhibition on renal function in elderly persons receiving a low-salt diet: a randomized controlled trial. *Ann Intern Med* 2000; **133:** 1–9.
2. Wolf G, *et al.* Acute renal failure associated with rofecoxib. *Ann Intern Med* 2000; **133:** 394.
3. Perazella MA, Tray K. Selective cyclooxygenase-2 inhibitors: a pattern of nephrotoxicity similar to traditional nonsteroidal anti-inflammatory drugs. *Am J Med* 2001; **111:** 64–7.
4. Rocha JL, Fernández-Alonso J. Acute tubulointerstitial nephritis associated with the selective COX-2 enzyme inhibitor, rofecoxib. *Lancet* 2001; **357:** 1946–7.

Interactions

For interactions associated with NSAIDs, see p.65.

Rifampicin. Co-administration of rifampicin and rofecoxib has resulted in a 50% decrease in rofecoxib plasma concentrations; the manufacturers recommend that the maximum dose (see below) be used when rofecoxib is administered with potent inducers of hepatic metabolism.

Pharmacokinetics

Rofecoxib is well absorbed from the gastrointestinal tract after oral administration. Peak plasma concentrations are reached in approximately 2 hours. Plasma protein binding is about 85%. Rofecoxib is extensively metabolised in the liver, mainly by reduction to *cis*- and *trans*-dihydrorofecoxib (as hydroxyl acids), which together account for 56% of a dose recovered in the urine. The 5-hydroxy glucuronide metabolite is also present. Excretion is mainly via the urine (72%) with only 14% of a dose appearing in the faeces. The elimination half-life is about 17 hours at steady state.

Uses and Administration

Rofecoxib is an NSAID (p.65) reported to be a selective inhibitor of cyclo-oxygenase-2 (COX-2). It is given by mouth for symptomatic relief in the treatment of osteoarthritis and rheumatoid arthritis, and is used in the management of acute pain and dysmenorrhoea.

In osteoarthritis, the usual starting dose is 12.5 mg once daily, which may be increased to a maximum of 25 mg once daily. Patients with rheumatoid arthritis should receive 25 mg daily. In patients with mild hepatic impairment the dose should not exceed 12.5 mg once daily.

An initial dose of 50 mg once daily is permitted for the short-term treatment of acute symptomatic pain; thereafter daily doses are 25 or 50 mg. In the USA, treatment is limited to 5 days.

◊ References.
1. Ehrich EW, *et al.* Characterization of rofecoxib as a cyclooxygenase-2 isoform inhibitor and demonstration of analgesia in the dental pain model. *Clin Pharmacol Ther* 1999; **65:** 336–47.
2. Scott LJ, Lamb HM. Rofecoxib. *Drugs* 1999; **58:** 499–505.
3. Matheson AJ, Figgitt DP. Rofecoxib: a review of its use in the management of osteoarthritis, acute pain and rheumatoid arthritis. *Drugs* 2001; **61:** 833–65.

Musculoskeletal and joint disorders. Rofecoxib is used in the treatment of the musculoskeletal disorders osteoarthritis and rheumatoid arthritis (see p.9 and p.9, respectively). However, in the UK, it is recommended that the use of rofecoxib and other selective cyclo-oxygenase-2 (COX-2) inhibitors is limited to those patients considered to be at high risk of developing serious gastrointestinal problems if given a non-selective NSAID (see p.63).

References.
1. Schnitzer TJ, *et al.* The safety profile, tolerability, and effective dose range of rofecoxib in the treatment of rheumatoid arthritis. *Clin Ther* 1999; **21:** 1688–1702.
2. Saag K, *et al.* Rofecoxib, a new cyclooxygenase 2 inhibitor, shows sustained efficacy, compared with other nonsteroidal anti-inflammatory drugs: a 6-week and a 1-year trial in patients with osteoarthritis. *Arch Fam Med* 2000; **9:** 1124–34.

Preparations

Proprietary Preparations (details are given in Part 3)
Austral.: Vioxx; *Canad.:* Vioxx; *Denm.:* Vioxx; *Fin.:* Vioxx; *Fr.:* Vioxx; *Ger.:* Vioxx; *Irl.:* Vioxx; *NZ:* Vioxx; *Port.:* Vioxx; *S.Afr.:* Vioxx; *Singapore:* Vioxx; *Spain:* Vioxx; *Swed.:* Vioxx; *Switz.:* Vioxx; *Thai.:* Vioxx; *UK:* Vioxx; *USA:* Vioxx.

Salamidacetic Acid (2622-j)

Carbamoylphenoxyacetic acid; Salicylamide O-acetic acid. (2-Carbamoylphenoxy)acetic acid.
$C_9H_9NO_4 = 195.2$.
CAS — 25395-22-6 (salamidacetic acid); 3785-32-8 (sodium salamidacetate).

Profile

Salamidacetic acid is a salicylic acid derivative (see Aspirin, p.14) that has also been used as the sodium and diethylamine salts for the treatment of musculoskeletal and joint disorders.

Preparations

Proprietary Preparations (details are given in Part 3)
Aust.: Akistin; **Ger.:** Clinit N; Hewedolor forte.

Multi-ingredient: Aust.: Ambene; Rheumesser; **Ger.:** Caye Balsam; Flexurat†; **Thai.:** Trabit.

Salicylamide (2700-l)

Salicylamide (BAN, rINN).
2-Hydroxybenzamide.
$C_7H_7NO_2 = 137.1$.
CAS — 65-45-2.
ATC — N02BA05.
Pharmacopoeias. In Aust., Pol., and US.

Pharmacopoeial description
USP 25: A white practically odourless crystalline powder. Slightly soluble in water and in chloroform; soluble in alcohol and in propylene glycol; freely soluble in ether and in solutions of alkalis.

Profile
Salicylamide is a salicylic acid derivative (see Aspirin, p.14) but is not hydrolysed to salicylate; it is almost completely metabolised to inactive metabolites during absorption and on first pass through the liver. It is given in doses of 325 to 650 mg or more by mouth, usually with other analgesics, three or four times daily for pain and fever. Salicylamide is also applied topically in rubefacient preparations in concentrations of about 5% for the relief of muscular and rheumatic pain.

Preparations

Proprietary Preparations (details are given in Part 3)
Aust.: Isosal.

Multi-ingredient: Aust.: Influvidon; Isosal; Rubriment; Sigmalin B₆; Sigmalin B₆ forte; Sigmalin B₆ ohne Coffein; Spalt; **Belg.:** Myalgesic; Percutalgine; **Braz.:** Benegrip; Coristina Reforcada; Gripin C; Neo Sativan; Resfry; Termigripe C; **Denm.:** Kodamid; Koffisal; **Fr.:** Percutalgine; **Ger.:** Coffalon; Glutisal; Salistoperm; **Hong Kong:** Antiflu Forte; Antiflu-N-Forte; Coryaid; Neosed; Neozep; **Israel:** Novocalm; **Ital.:** Anticorizza; Azerodol†; **S.Afr.:** Ascold†; Colcaps; Flutex; Histamed Compound; Ilvico; Intralgin†; **Spain:** Coricidin; Doloana†; Hubergrip; Percutalin†; Pridio; Rinomicine; Rinomicine Activada; Yendol; **Switz.:** Comba-Gripp†; Escalgin sans codeine†; Escogripp sans codeine; Grippalgine N; No Grip†; Novidol; Osa†; Siniphen†; **Thai.:** Fecol; Percutalgine; UAE: Adol Compound; Flukit; UK: Intralgin; USA: Anabar; Anodynos†; BC; Lobac; Presalin†; Rhinogesic†; Rid-a-Pain with Codeine†; S-A-C†; Saleto; Saleto-D†; Salocol†; Salphenyl†; Tri-Pain†; Trim-Elim.

Salix (11536-n)

Salicis Cortex; Willow Bark.
Pharmacopoeias. In Eur. (see p.vi).

Pharmacopoeial description
Ph. Eur.: The whole or fragmented dried bark of young branches or whole dried pieces of current year twigs of various species of the genus *Salix*, including *Salix purpurea, S. daphnoides*, and *S. fragilis*. It contains not less than 1.5% of total salicylic derivatives, expressed as salicin ($C_{13}H_{18}O_7 = 286.3$), calculated with reference to the dried drug. Protect from light.

Profile
Salix contains variable amounts of tannin and also of salicin which has antipyretic and analgesic actions similar to those of aspirin. Salix has been used in a variety of herbal remedies for painful and inflammatory conditions and for fever. It was once used as a bitter.

◊ References.
1. Chrubasik S, *et al.* Treatment of low back pain exacerbations with willow bark extract: a randomized double-blind study. *Am J Med* 2000; **109:** 9–14.

Preparations

Proprietary Preparations (details are given in Part 3)
Aust.: Biogelat Erkaltungs & Grippe†; **Canad.:** Saliton†; **Ger.:** Assalix; Assplant; Rheumakaps; Rheumatab Salicis; Tamanybonsan†.

Multi-ingredient: Aust.: Digestodoron; Grippefloran; Kneipp Grippe-Tee; Naturland Rheuma-Tee; **Austral.:** Arthritic Pain Herbal Formula 1; Bioglan Arthri Plus; Extralife Migrai-Care; Extralife PMS-Care; Harpagophytum Complex; Lifesystem Herbal Formula 1 Arthritic Aid; Lifesystem Herbal Formula 12 Willowbark†; Prost-1; Salagesic; Willowbark Plus Herbal Formula 11†; **Braz.:** Calman; Pasalix; Passicarbone; Passiflorine; **Canad.:** Arthrisan†; **Fr.:** Arkophytum; Mediflor Tisane Circulation du Sang No 12†; Santane A₄; **Ger.:** Dr Wiemanns Rheumatonikum; Hevert-Erkaltungs-Tee†; Hevert-Gicht-Rheuma-Tee comp†; Kneipp Rheuma Tee N†; Nephrubin†; **Ital.:** Bodyguard; Depurativo; Donalg; Fluend†; Passiflorine; Tauma; **Port.:** Bio-Strath No 5†; Neurocardol; **Spain:** Passiflorine; **Switz.:** Dragees antirhumatismales; Dragees contre les maux de tete; Phytomed Rhino†; Tisane antirhumatismale; UK: Bio-Strath Willow Formula; Digestodoron; Gerard House Ligvites; Gerard House Reumalex; Herbal Pain Relief; Hofels White Willow and Burdock; St Johnswort Compound.

Salol (9315-y)

Phenyl salicylate.
$C_{13}H_{10}O_3 = 214.2$.
CAS — 118-55-8.
Pharmacopoeias. In Aust. and Pol.

Profile
Salol is a salicylic acid derivative (see Aspirin, p.14). It was formerly used as an intestinal antiseptic, but effective doses were toxic owing to the liberation of phenol. It is used in oral preparations containing methenamine for the treatment of lower urinary-tract infections.
Salol has been used topically as a sunscreen.

Preparations

Proprietary Preparations (details are given in Part 3)
Austral.: Aussie Tan Sunstick.

Multi-ingredient: Aust.: Carl Baders Divinal; **Braz.:** Malvosulfam; **Canad.:** Franzbranns; **Fr.:** Borostyrol; Dermophil Indien; **Ger.:** Parodontal F5 med; **Swed.:** Munvatten†; **Switz.:** Borostyrol N; Dermophil Indien; USA: Atrosept; Dolsed; Prosed/DS; Trac Tabs 2X; UAA; Uridon Modified; Urimar-T; Urimax; Urised; Urogesic Blue.

Salsalate (2702-j)

Salsalate (BAN, USAN, rINN).
NSC-49171; Salicyl Salicylate; Salicylosalicylic Acid; Salicylsalicylic Acid; Salysal; Sasapyrine. O-(2-Hydroxybenzoyl)salicylic acid.
$C_{14}H_{10}O_5 = 258.2$.
CAS — 552-94-3.
Pharmacopoeias. In US.

Pharmacopoeial description
USP 25: Store in airtight containers.

Adverse Effects, Treatment, and Precautions
As for Aspirin, p.14.
The use of aspirin and other acetylated salicylates is generally not recommended for children under the age of 12 years because of the risk of Reye's syndrome, unless specifically indicated. Some authorities also extend this precaution to non-acetylated salicylates such as salsalate.

Effects on the gastrointestinal tract. Salsalate is associated with less faecal blood loss than aspirin and has been reported to cause fewer gastric lesions than piroxicam.[1] However, small-bowel ulcerations were reported in a patient when salsalate was added to a regimen of ranitidine and metoclopramide which had been prescribed for duodenal ulcer.[2]
1. Porro GB, *et al.* Salsalate in the treatment of rheumatoid arthritis: a double-blind clinical and gastroscopic trial versus piroxicam: II—endoscopic evaluation. *J Int Med Res* 1989; **17:** 320–3.
2. Souza Lima MA. Ulcers of the small bowel associated with stomach-bypassing salicylates. *Arch Intern Med* 1985; **145:** 1139.

Effects on the kidneys. A report of a case of minimal-change nephrotic syndrome associated with salsalate.[1]
1. Vallès M, Tovar JL. Salsalate and minimal-change nephrotic syndrome. *Ann Intern Med* 1987; **107:** 116.

Effects on the mouth. Ulcerated lesions on the tongue of a 77-year-old man were found to be due to incorrect administration of salsalate tablets.[1] The patient had placed the tablets under his tongue rather than swallowing them whole resulting in prolonged, direct contact with the tongue.
1. Ruscin JM, Astroth JD. Lingual lesions secondary to prolonged contact with salsalate tablets. *Ann Pharmacother* 1998; **32:** 1248.

Interactions
For interactions associated with salicylates, see Aspirin, p.16.

Pharmacokinetics
Salsalate is insoluble in acidic gastric fluids but is soluble in the small intestine. One molecule of salsalate is hydrolysed to 2 molecules of salicylic acid; hydrolysis occurs both in the small intestine and following absorption of the parent compound. Additional details on the pharmacokinetics of salicylic acid are provided in aspirin (see p.16). Not all of the absorbed salsalate is hydrolysed and about 13% of salsalate is excreted as glucuronide conjugates in the urine; thus, the amount of salicylic acid available from salsalate is less than that from aspirin when the two drugs are given in equimolar equivalents of salicylic acid.

Uses and Administration
Salsalate is a salicylic acid derivative that has analgesic, anti-inflammatory, and antipyretic actions similar to those of aspirin (see p.16). It is used for pain and fever and also in inflammatory disorders such as osteoarthritis and rheumatoid arthritis. A usual dose is up to 3 g daily given by mouth in divided doses with food.

Preparations

USP 25: Salsalate Capsules; Salsalate Tablets.

Proprietary Preparations (details are given in Part 3)
Canad.: Disalcid; **Spain:** Umbradol; **USA:** Amigesic; Argesic-SA; Artha-G; Disalcid; Marthritic; Mono-Gesic; Salflex; Salsitab.

Sarracenia Purpurea (18472-e)

Pitcher Plant.

Profile
The roots and leaves of *Sarracenia purpurea* (Sarraceniaceae) have been used in the form of an aqueous distillate, administered by local injection, for neuromuscular or neuralgic pain.

Preparations

Proprietary Preparations (details are given in Part 3)
USA: Sarapin.

Sodium Aurothiomalate (5296-k)

Sodium Aurothiomalate (rINN).
Gold Sodium Thiomalate; Sodium Aurothiosuccinate.
CAS — 12244-57-4 (anhydrous xNa); 39377-38-3 (2Na monohydrate).
ATC — M01CB01.
Pharmacopoeias. In Br., Jpn, and US.

Pharmacopoeial description
BP 2001: Fine, pale yellow, hygroscopic powder with a slight odour. It consists mainly of the disodium salt of (aurothio)succinic acid ($C_4H_3AuNa_2O_4S = 390.1$) and has a gold content of 44.5 to 46.0% calculated on the dried material. Very soluble in water. A 10% solution in water has a pH of 6.0 to 7.0. Protect from light.

USP 25: A mixture of the monosodium and disodium salts of gold thiomalic acid [(aurothio)succinic acid] ($C_4H_4AuNaO_4S = 368.1$ and $C_4H_3AuNa_2O_4S = 390.1$) that has a gold content of 44.8 to 49.6%, and 49.0 to 52.5% calculated on the dried alcohol-free and glycerol-free material. pH of a 10% solution in water is between 5.8 and 6.5. Store in airtight containers. Protect from light.

Adverse Effects
Reports show a wide range for the incidence of adverse effects of sodium aurothiomalate. However, authorities consider that with careful treatment about one-third of patients will experience adverse effects. It is also considered that about 5% of patients will experience severe adverse effects and that some of the effects will be fatal. The most common effects involve the skin and mucous membranes with pruritus (an early sign of intolerance) and stomatitis (often with a metallic taste) being the most prominent. Rashes with pruritus often occur after 2 to 6 months of intramuscular treatment and may necessitate discontinuation of therapy. Other reactions affecting the skin and mucous membranes include erythema, maculopapular eruptions, erythema multiforme, urticaria, eczema, seborrhoeic dermatitis, lichenoid eruptions, alopecia, exfoliative dermatitis, glossitis, pharyngitis, vaginitis, photosensitivity reactions, and irreversible pigmentation (chrysiasis).

Toxic effects on the blood include eosinophilia, thrombocytopenia, leucopenia, agranulocytosis, and aplastic anaemia.

Effects on the kidneys include mild transient proteinuria which may lead to heavy proteinuria, haematuria, and nephrosis.

Other effects reported include pulmonary fibrosis, toxic hepatitis, cholestatic jaundice, peripheral neuritis, encephalitis, psychoses, fever, and gastrointestinal disorders including enterocolitis. Gold deposits may occur in the eyes. Vasomotor or nitritoid reactions, with weakness, flushing, palpitations, and dyspnoea, may occur following injection of sodium aurothiomalate. Local irritation may also follow injection.

Sometimes there is an initial exacerbation of the arthritic condition.

A number of the adverse effects of gold have an immunogenic component.

◊ Reviews.
1. Tozman ECS, Gottlieb NL. Adverse reactions with oral and parenteral gold preparations. *Med Toxicol* 1987; **2:** 177–89.

Effects on the blood. Blood disorders such as leucopenia, granulocytopenia, and thrombocytopenia have occurred in patients receiving gold therapy. Eosinophilia has been reported to be the most frequent haematological abnormality.[1] It is estimated that thrombocytopenia develops in 1 to 3% of patients receiving gold salts.[2]

Fatal consumption coagulopathy occurred in 4 children follow-ing the second injection of sodium aurothioglucose or sodium aurothiomalate.[3]

1. Foster RT. Eosinophilia—a marker of gold toxicity. *Can J Hosp Pharm* 1985; **85**: 150–1.
2. Coblyn JS, *et al.* Gold-induced thrombocytopenia: a clinical and immunogenetic study of twenty-three patients. *Ann Intern Med* 1981; **95**: 178–81.
3. Jacobs JC, *et al.* Consumption coagulopathy after gold therapy for JRA. *J Pediatr* 1984; **105**: 674–5.

Effects on the cardiovascular system. Vasomotor or nitri-toid reactions associated with gold compounds are usually tran-sient and self-limiting and although they may be mild there have been isolated reports of associated complications such as myocardial infarction, stroke, transient ischaemic attack, and transient monocular visual loss.[1] Most reactions have been as-sociated with sodium aurothiomalate (a reported incidence of 4.7%) but they have also occurred with auranofin and sodium aurothioglucose. Tachyphylaxis usually occurs to the reactions and most patients are able to continue treatment but paradoxi-cally in some the severity increases with repeated doses; 2.8% of patients receiving sodium aurothiomalate may require a change of treatment due to recurrent reactions. Transfer to so-dium aurothioglucose may be an option in patients who derive significant benefit from gold injections but it is important firstly to distinguish such reactions from true anaphylactic reactions to gold.

1. Ho M, Pullar T. Vasomotor reactions with gold. *Br J Rheumatol* 1997; **36**: 154–6.

Effects on the gastrointestinal tract. A case report of en-terocolitis due to sodium aurothiomalate has been published[1] and 27 other cases associated with gold therapy reviewed.

1. Jackson CW, *et al.* Gold induced enterocolitis. *Gut* 1986; **27**: 452–56.

Effects on the immune system. Details of a patient who developed an immune deficiency syndrome that was attributed to gold therapy with sodium aurothiomalate.[1]

1. Haskard DO, Macfarlane D. Adult acquired combined immune deficiency in a patient with rheumatoid arthritis on gold. *J R Soc Med* 1988; **81**: 548–9.

Effects on the kidneys. Proteinuria developed in 21 patients while receiving a standard regimen of sodium aurothiomalate.[1] The severity of the proteinuria varied greatly and in 11 it in-creased for 4 months after treatment was stopped. Eight pa-tients were considered to have developed the nephrotic syn-drome. The median duration of proteinuria was 11 months, resolving in all 21 patients when treatment was withdrawn; at 24 months 3 patients were still experiencing proteinuria and it was not until 39 months that all were free of the condition. Re-nal biopsy indicated several types of kidney damage.

See under Auranofin (p.18) for a comparative incidence of pro-teinuria in patients receiving sodium aurothiomalate or auran-ofin.

1. Hall CL, *et al.* The natural course of gold nephropathy: long term study of 21 patients. *BMJ* 1987; **295**: 745–8.

Effects on the liver. Some reports of hepatotoxicity with so-dium aurothiomalate.[1,2]

1. Favreau M, *et al.* Hepatic toxicity associated with gold therapy. *Ann Intern Med* 1977; **87**: 717–19.
2. Edelman J, *et al.* Liver dysfunction associated with gold therapy for rheumatoid arthritis. *J Rheumatol* 1983; **10**: 510–11.

Effects on the lungs. 'Gold lung' is the term used to describe symptoms of dyspnoea on exertion, weakness, dry cough, and malaise developing some weeks or months after starting gold treatment. Pulmonary insufficiency may eventually develop. The pulmonary lesions usually subside on withdrawal of gold therapy, although persistent symptoms have been reported. Nonbacterial thrombotic endocarditis associated with gold-in-duced pulmonary disease has also been reported.[1] This was considered to be a manifestation of gold-induced immune com-plex deposition.

1. Kollef MH, *et al.* Nonbacterial thrombotic endocarditis associat-ed with gold induced pulmonary disease. *Ann Intern Med* 1988; **108**: 903–4.

Effects on the nervous system. Reports of sodium auro-thiomalate adversely affecting the nervous system.[1-5]

1. Dick DJ, Raman D. The Guillain-Barre syndrome following gold therapy. *Scand J Rheumatol* 1982; **11**: 119–20.
2. Schlumpf U, *et al.* Neurologic complications induced by gold treatment. *Arthritis Rheum* 1983; **26**: 825–31 (Guillain-Barré syndrome and neuropathy with myokymia).
3. Cerinic MM, *et al.* Gold polyneuropathy in juvenile rheumatoid arthritis. *BMJ* 1985; **290**: 1042.
4. Cohen M, *et al.* Acute disseminated encephalomyelitis as a com-plication of treatment with gold. *BMJ* 1985; **290**: 1179–80.
5. Dubowitz MN, *et al.* Gold-induced neuroencephalopathy re-sponding to dimercaprol. *Lancet* 1991; **337**: 850–1.

Effects on the skin. Chrysiasis is a distinctive pigmentation that develops in light-exposed skin of patients receiving parenteral gold salts. In a study[1] of 31 patients with chrysiasis who were receiving intramuscular sodium aurothiomalate for rheumatoid arthritis, it was noted that visible changes devel-oped above a threshold equivalent to 20 mg per kg body-weight gold content. The severity of the pigmentation depended upon cumulative dose. Focal aggregates of gold are deposited in the reticular and papillary dermis with no obvious increase in mel-anin. The pigmentation is permanent but benign, although the

cosmetic effects may cause some patients distress. Prevention of chrysiasis is difficult but avoidance of exposure to sunlight may be helpful.

1. Smith RW, *et al.* Chrysiasis revisited: a clinical and pathological study. *Br J Dermatol* 1995; **133**: 671–8.

Hypersensitivity. Many adverse effects associated with gold treatment have an immunological basis. Small amounts of nickel have been detected in sodium aurothiomalate injection[1] and in sodium aurothioglucose injection[2] and it has been sug-gested that gold therapy may exacerbate or induce hypersensi-tivity to nickel.[1-3]

Anaphylaxis may occur occasionally[4] but vasomotor or 'nitri-toid' reactions (see Effects on the Cardiovascular System above) may produce similar symptoms.

1. Choy EHS, *et al.* Nickel contamination of gold salts: link with gold-induced skin rash. *Br J Rheumatol* 1997; **36**: 1054–8.
2. Wijnands MJH, *et al.* Chrysotherapy provoking exacerbation of contact hypersensitivity to nickel. *Lancet* 1990; **335**: 867–8.
3. Fulton RA, *et al.* Another hazard of gold therapy? *Ann Rheum Dis* 1982; **41**: 100–1.
4. Neustadt DH. Another anaphylactic reaction after gold (auro-thiomalate) injection. *J Rheumatol* 1995; **22**: 190.

Pancreatitis. It was suggested that pancreatitis reported in a woman receiving gold injections and in a woman on oral gold therapy may have been due to a hypersensitivity reaction.[1]

1. Eisemann AD, *et al.* Pancreatitis and gold treatment of rheuma-toid arthritis. *Ann Intern Med* 1989; **111**: 860–1.

Treatment of Adverse Effects
The treatment of the adverse effects of gold is usually symptomatic and most effects resolve when gold therapy is withdrawn. In severe cases a chelator such as dimercaprol (p.1007) may be employed.

Precautions
Gold therapy is contra-indicated in exfoliative derma-titis, systemic lupus erythematosus, necrotising ente-rocolitis, and pulmonary fibrosis. It should be used with caution in patients with renal or hepatic impair-ment and in the elderly but is contra-indicated in se-vere renal or hepatic disorders. Patients with a history of haematological disorders or who have previously shown toxicity to heavy metals should not be given gold salts, nor should any severely debilitated patient.

It is recommended that diabetes mellitus and heart failure should be adequately controlled in any patient before gold is given. Patients with a history of urticar-ia, eczema, or colitis should be treated with caution. Patients with a poor sulfoxidation status may be more susceptible to adverse effects of sodium aurothioma-late.

It is generally recommended that gold salts should not be given to pregnant patients or to patients who are breast feeding.

Concurrent administration of gold salts with other therapy capable of inducing blood disorders should be undertaken with caution, if at all.

Due to the possibility of vasomotor reactions, patients should remain recumbent for about 10 minutes after each injection.

The urine should be tested for albumin before each injection and the blood should be examined for signs of depressed haematopoiesis. Patients receiving gold salts either orally or parenterally should be warned to report the appearance of sore throat or tongue, metal-lic taste, pruritus, rash, buccal ulceration, easy bruis-ing, purpura, epistaxis, bleeding gums, unexplained bleeding, menorrhagia, pyrexia, indigestion, diar-rhoea, or unexplained malaise. The development of breathlessness or cough should also be reported. Ef-fects such as eosinophilia, proteinuria, pruritus, and rash arising during gold treatment should be allowed to resolve before therapy is continued.

The manufacturer recommends that annual chest X-rays should be carried out.

Breast feeding. Gold has been detected in breast milk[1,2] and found bound to the red blood cells of breast-fed babies.[2] In a report[1] of one breast-fed infant it was calculated that the weight-adjusted dose of gold received by the infant exceeded that received by the mother although the infant exhibited no ill-effects during 100 days of breast feeding and developed nor-mally thereafter. Nonetheless, because of the relatively high ex-

posure it was recommended that breast-fed infants should be closely monitored.

1. Bennett PN, *et al.* Use of sodium aurothiomalate during lacta-tion. *Br J Clin Pharmacol* 1990; **29**: 777–9.
2. Needs CJ, Brooks PM. Antirheumatic medication during lacta-tion. *Br J Rheumatol* 1985; **24**: 291–7.

Porphyria. Sodium aurothiomalate has been associated with acute attacks of porphyria and is considered unsafe in porphy-ric patients.

Pregnancy. Although there have been a number of healthy neonates born after *in-utero* exposure to gold compounds,[1,2] *animal* studies and one report[1] of malformation in a child born to a woman treated with sodium aurothiomalate led to a sug-gestion that gold might possibly have teratogenic effects.

1. Rogers JG, *et al.* Possible teratogenic effects of gold. *Aust Pae-diatr J* 1980; **16**: 194–5.
2. Bennett PN, *et al.* Use of sodium aurothiomalate during lacta-tion. *Br J Clin Pharmacol* 1990; **29**: 777–9.

Interactions
There is an increased risk of toxicity when gold com-pounds are administered concurrently with other ne-phrotoxic, hepatotoxic, or myelosuppressive drugs. Concurrent use of gold compounds with penicilla-mine may increase the risk of haematologic or renal adverse reactions.

◊ For a discussion on the effects of previous therapy with gold salts affecting penicillamine toxicity, see p.1018.

Pharmacokinetics
Sodium aurothiomalate is absorbed readily after in-tramuscular injection and 85 to 95% becomes bound to plasma proteins. With doses of 50 mg weekly a steady-state serum concentration of gold of about 3 to 5 µg per mL is reached in 5 to 8 weeks. It is widely distributed to body tissues and fluids, including syno-vial fluid, and accumulates in the body.

The serum half-life of gold is about 5 to 6 days but this increases after successive doses and after a course of treatment, gold may be found in the urine for up to 1 year or more owing to its presence in deep body compartments. Sodium aurothiomalate is mainly ex-creted in the urine, with smaller amounts in the fae-ces.

Gold has been detected in the fetus following admin-istration of sodium aurothiomalate to the mother. Gold is distributed into breast milk.

◊ Reviews.

1. Blocka KLN, *et al.* Clinical pharmacokinetics of oral and inject-able gold compounds. *Clin Pharmacokinet* 1986; **11**: 133–43.
2. Tett SE. Clinical pharmacokinetics of slow-acting antirheumatic drugs. *Clin Pharmacokinet* 1993; **25**: 392–407.

Uses and Administration
Sodium aurothiomalate and other gold salts are used mainly for their anti-inflammatory effect in active progressive rheumatoid arthritis and progressive ju-venile idiopathic arthritis; they may also be beneficial in psoriatic arthritis. They are generally used as dis-ease-modifying antirheumatic drugs in patients whose symptoms are unresponsive to or inadequately controlled by NSAIDs alone.

Sodium aurothiomalate therapy should only be un-dertaken where facilities are available to carry out the tests specified under Precautions, above.

Sodium aurothiomalate is given by deep intramuscu-lar injection; the area should be gently massaged and, due to the possibility of vasomotor reactions, the pa-tient should remain recumbent for 10 minutes and kept under close observation for 30 minutes after each injection. In the UK, 10 mg is given in the first week to test the patient's tolerance. If satisfactory, this is followed by doses of 25 to 50 mg at weekly intervals until signs of remission occur, when the dosage inter-val is increased to 2 weeks until full remission occurs; the dosage interval is then further increased gradually to every 4 to 6 weeks and treatment may be continued for up to 5 years after remission. Improvement may not be seen until a total dose of 300 to 500 mg has been administered. If no major improvement has been observed after a total of 1 g has been given (excluding the test dose) therapy should be discontinued; alterna-tively in the absence of toxicity, 100 mg may be given weekly for a further 6 weeks; should there be no re-sponse at this dose other forms of therapy should be

The symbol † denotes a preparation no longer actively marketed

tried. In patients who relapse while receiving maintenance therapy, the interval between doses should be
reduced to one week and should not be increased
again until control has been obtained but if no response is obtained within 2 months, alternative treatment should be used. It is important to avoid complete
relapse since a second course of gold therapy is not
usually effective.

For children with progressive juvenile idiopathic arthritis the suggested initial weekly dose is 1 mg per
kg body-weight to a maximum of 50 mg weekly (one-
tenth to one-fifth of the calculated initial weekly dose
may be given for 2 to 3 weeks to test the patient's tolerance). With full remission, the dosage interval may
be increased to 4 weeks. If no improvement has occurred after 20 weeks, the dose could be raised slightly or another antirheumatic drug tried.

NSAIDs may be continued when sodium aurothiomalate therapy is initiated.

Other gold compounds that have been used include
auranofin (p.18), aurothioglucose (p.18), aurotioprol
(p.19), gold keratinate, and sodium aurotiosulfate
(p.84).

Pemphigus and pemphigoid. Corticosteroids are the main
treatment for blistering in pemphigus and pemphigoid
(p.1106). Systemic gold therapy has been used in combination
with corticosteroids to permit a reduction in corticosteroid dosage. However, it has been suggested that evidence for the steroid-sparing effect is lacking and that gold therapy should be
reserved for patients who cannot tolerate corticosteroids or in
whom they are contra-indicated.[1]
1. Bystryn J-C, Steinman NM. The adjuvant therapy of pemphigus:
an update. *Arch Dermatol* 1996; **132:** 203–12.

Rheumatic disorders. Gold compounds are among the disease-modifying antirheumatic drugs (DMARDs) that may be
used in the treatment of rheumatoid arthritis (p.9) and juvenile
idiopathic arthritis (p.9). There is little agreement on which of
the various DMARDs should be tried first and their selection is
largely based on individual experience and preference. Despite
its toxicity intramuscular gold has long been used for the treatment of rheumatoid arthritis and is often the standard against
which the efficacy of other treatments is measured. Oral gold is
less toxic but is also much less effective. Gold compounds may
also be of benefit in psoriatic arthritis (see under Spondyloarthropathies, p.10).
References.
1. Epstein WV, *et al.* Effect of parenterally administered gold therapy on the course of adult rheumatoid arthritis. *Ann Intern Med*
1991; **114:** 437–44.
2. Anonymous. Gold therapy in rheumatoid arthritis. *Lancet* 1991;
338: 19–20.
3. Klinkhoff AV, Teufel A. How low can you go? Use of very low
dosage of gold in patients with mucocutaneous reactions. *J
Rheumatol* 1995; **22:** 1657–9.
4. Clark P, *et al.* Injectable gold for rheumatoid arthritis (updated
22 March 2001). Available in The Cochrane Library; Issue 4. Oxford: Update Software; 2001.

Preparations
BP 2001: Sodium Aurothiomalate Injection;
USP 25: Gold Sodium Thiomalate Injection.

Proprietary Preparations (details are given in Part 3)
Aust.: Tauredon; **Austral.:** Myocrisin; **Braz.:** Myochrysine; **Canad.:** Myochrysine; **Denm.:** Myocrisin; **Fin.:** Myocrisin; **Ger.:**
Tauredon; **Hong Kong:** Myocrisin; **Irl.:** Myocrisin; **Norw.:** Myo-
crisin; **NZ:** Myocrisin; **Port.:** Tauredon; **S.Afr.:** Myocrisin; **Singapore:** Miocrin; **Spain:** Miocrin; **Swed.:** Myocrisin; **Switz.:** Tauredon; **Thai.:** Myocrisin; **UK:** Myocrisin; **USA:** Aurolate;
Myochrysine.

Sodium Aurotiosulfate   (5297-a)

Sodium Aurotiosulfate (rINN).

Gold Sodium Thiosulphate; Sodium Aurothiosulphate; Sodium
Dithiosulfatoaurate.

$Na_3Au(S_2O_3)_2, 2H_2O = 526.2.$
CAS — 10233-88-2 (anhydrous sodium aurotiosulfate);
10210-36-3 (sodium aurotiosulfate dihydrate).
ATC — M01CB02.

Sodium aurotiosulfate has a gold content of about 37%.

Profile
Sodium aurotiosulfate has similar actions and uses to those of
sodium aurothiomalate (p.82). It has been given by intramuscular injection.

Preparations
Proprietary Preparations (details are given in Part 3)
Ital.: Fosfocrisolo.

Sodium Gentisate   (2704-c)

Sodium Gentisate (rINN).

Gentisato Sodico; Natrii Gentisas. Sodium 2,5-dihydroxybenz-
oate dihydrate.

$C_7H_5NaO_4, 2H_2O = 212.1.$
CAS — 490-79-9 (gentisic acid); 4955-90-2 (anhydrous so-
dium gentisate).
Pharmacopoeias. In Fr.

Profile
Sodium gentisate was used in the treatment of musculoskeletal
and joint disorders.

Sodium Salicylate   (2705-k)

Natrii Salicylas. Sodium 2-hydroxybenzoate.
$C_7H_5NaO_3 = 160.1.$
CAS — 54-21-7.
ATC — N02BA04.
Pharmacopoeias. In Eur. (see p.vi), Int., Jpn, Pol., and US.

Sodium salicylate 1 g is approximately equivalent to 1.1 g of
aspirin.

Pharmacopoeial description

Ph. Eur.: Colourless small crystals or shiny flakes, or white
crystalline powder. Freely soluble in water; sparingly soluble in
alcohol. Store in airtight containers. Protect from light.

USP 25: Amorphous or microcrystalline powder or scales. It is
colourless or has not more than a faint pink tinge. It is odourless
or has a faint characteristic odour. A freshly made 10% solution
in water is neutral or acid to litmus. Freely (and slowly) soluble
in water and in glycerol; very soluble in boiling water and in
boiling alcohol; slowly soluble in alcohol. Protect from light.

Adverse Effects, Treatment, and Precautions
As for Aspirin, p.14.

When sodium salicylate is used in the treatment of rheumatic
fever its high sodium content may cause problems in patients
with cardiac complications.

The use of aspirin and other acetylated salicylates is generally
not recommended for children under the age of 12 years because of the risk of Reye's syndrome, unless specifically indicated. Some authorities also extend this precaution to non-acetylated salicylates such as sodium salicylate.

Effects on the eyes. Retinal haemorrhages were reported in
a 60-year-old woman taking sodium salicylate 6 g daily by
mouth for 2 months and in a 10-year-old girl taking sodium
salicylate, 4 g daily by mouth, for 40 days.[1] In both cases the
haemorrhages gradually resolved after the treatment was
stopped.
1. Mortada A, Abboud I. Retinal haemorrhages after prolonged use
of salicylates. *Br J Ophthalmol* 1973; **57:** 199–200.

Interactions
For interactions associated with salicylates, see Aspirin, p.16.

Uses and Administration
Sodium salicylate is a salicylic acid derivative that has analgesic, anti-inflammatory, and antipyretic actions similar to those
of aspirin (p.16). It is used in the treatment of pain, fever, and
in rheumatic disorders such as osteoarthritis and rheumatoid
arthritis. The usual oral dose of sodium salicylate for pain or
fever is 325 to 650 mg every four hours as required. The oral
dose for rheumatic disorders is 3.6 to 5.4 g daily in divided doses. Sodium salicylate has also been used in the symptomatic
treatment of rheumatic fever but its high sodium content may
cause problems in patients with cardiac complications.

Sodium salicylate has also been given by intravenous infusion.

◊ References.
1. Seymour RA, *et al.* The efficacy and pharmacokinetics of sodium
salicylate in post-operative dental pain. *Br J Clin Pharmacol*
1984; **17:** 161–3.

Preparations
USP 25: Sodium Salicylate Tablets.

Proprietary Preparations (details are given in Part 3)
Canad.: Dodds; **UK:** Jackson's Febrifuge.

Multi-ingredient: Belg.: Baseler Haussalbe†; **Braz.:** Abacatei-
rol; Pilulas De Witt's; **Canad.:** Plax; Thunas Tab for Menstrual
Pain; **Fr.:** Aromabyl†; Brulex; Buccawalter; Glyco-Thymoline;
Ger.: Gelonida NA; Salimar-Bad L; **S.Afr.:** Colphen; Ilvico; **UK:**
Doans Backache Pills; TCP; **USA:** Cystex; Pabalate†; Scot-Tussin
Original 5-Action; Tussirex.

Sodium Thiosalicylate   (16988-d)

$C_7H_5O_2NaS = 176.2.$

Profile
Sodium thiosalicylate is a salicylic acid derivative (see Aspirin,
p.14) used in the treatment of musculoskeletal disorders, osteoarthritis, rheumatic fever, and acute gout.

Preparations
Proprietary Preparations (details are given in Part 3)
USA: Pirosal†; Rexolate; Thiocyl†.

Sufentanil Citrate   (13274-e)

Sufentanil Citrate (BANM, USAN, rINNM).

R-33800; R-30730 (sufentanil); Sufentanili Citras. N-{4-(Methoxymethyl)-1-[2-(2-thienyl)ethyl]-4-piperidyl}propionanilide citrate.

$C_{22}H_{30}N_2O_2S, C_6H_8O_7 = 578.7.$
CAS — 56030-54-7 (sufentanil); 60561-17-3 (sufentanil
citrate).
Pharmacopoeias. In Eur. (see p.vi) and US. Eur. also includes sufentanil.

Sufentanil citrate 15 μg is approximately equivalent to 10 μg of
sufentanil.

Pharmacopoeial description

Ph. Eur.: A white or almost white powder. Soluble in water
and in alcohol; freely soluble in methyl alcohol. Protect from
light.

USP 25: A white powder. Soluble in water; sparingly soluble
in alcohol, in acetone, and in chloroform; freely soluble in
methyl alcohol.

◊ CAUTION. *Avoid contact with skin and the inhalation of particles of sufentanil citrate.*

Dependence and Withdrawal
As for Opioid Analgesics, p.66.

Adverse Effects, Treatment, and Precau-
tions
As for Opioid Analgesics in general, p.67 and Fentanyl, p.37.

Breast feeding. Concentrations of sufentanil were similar in
colostrum and serum in 7 women given sufentanil by continuous epidural infusion during the first postoperative day following caesarean section. In the light of its poor oral availability
such an amount was not considered to be a hazard to the breast-
feeding infant, and a maternal dose of 5 μg per hour epidurally
was considered to be safe for such infants.[1]
1. Ausseur A, *et al.* Continuous epidural infusion of sufentanil after
caesarean section: concentration in breast milk. *Br J Anaesth*
1994; **72** (suppl 1): 106.

Effects on the cardiovascular system. For a reference to
the effects of sufentanil on histamine release compared with
some other opioids, see under Pethidine, p.75.

Effects on the nervous system. There have been reports of
tonic-clonic movements or seizures in a few patients receiving
sufentanil.[1] There was no evidence of cortical seizure activity
in one patient whose EEG was recorded,[2] suggesting that the
observed myoclonus was not a convulsion or seizure.
1. Zaccara G, *et al.* Clinical features, pathogenesis and management of drug-induced seizures. *Drug Safety* 1990; **5:** 109–51.
2. Bowdle TA. Myoclonus following sufentanil without EEG seizure activity. *Anesthesiology* 1987; **67:** 593–5.

Effects on the respiratory system. Sufentanil, like other
opioid agonists, causes dose-related respiratory depression.
There have been reports of significant respiratory depression
associated with chest wall rigidity in the early postoperative period after anaesthesia with sufentanil.[1,2]
1. Goldberg M, *et al.* Postoperative rigidity following sufentanil administration. *Anesthesiology* 1985; **63:** 199–201.
2. Chang J, Fish KJ. Acute respiratory arrest and rigidity after anesthesia with sufentanil: a case report. *Anesthesiology* 1985; **63:**
710–11.

The elderly. The pharmacokinetics of sufentanil in elderly
patients have been variable in different studies, but a review[1]
considered that there had been no evidence overall for differences between the elderly and younger adults. Nevertheless, as
with fentanyl, the manufacturer advises reduced initial doses in
the elderly.
1. Monk JP, *et al.* Sufentanil: a review of its pharmacological properties and therapeutic use. *Drugs* 1988; **36:** 286–313.

Obesity. The elimination half-life and volume of distribution
of sufentanil were increased in obese subjects.[1] The manufacturers recommend that for obese patients more than 20% above
ideal body-weight the dosage of sufentanil should be determined on the basis of the patients' lean body-weight.
1. Schwartz AE, *et al.* Pharmacokinetics of sufentanil in the obese.
Anesthesiology 1986; **65** (suppl 3A): A562.

Interactions
For interactions associated with opioid analgesics,
see p.68.

Benzodiazepines. For the effects of concomitant use of opioids such as sufentanil with benzodiazepines, see under Analgesics in the Interactions of Diazepam, p.677.

Pharmacokinetics
Following parenteral administration sufentanil citrate
has a rapid onset and short duration of action. The terminal elimination half-life of sufentanil is about 2.5
hours. It is extensively bound to plasma proteins
(about 90%). It is metabolised in the liver and small

intestine by *N*-dealkylation and *O*-demethylation and the metabolites are excreted in the urine.

◊ **Reviews.**
1. Monk JP, *et al.* Sufentanil: a review of its pharmacological properties and therapeutic use. *Drugs* 1988; **36**: 286–313.
2. Scholz J, *et al.* Clinical pharmacokinetics of alfentanil, fentanyl and sufentanil: an update. *Clin Pharmacokinet* 1996; **31**: 275–92.

◊ Sufentanil is very lipid-soluble. Like alfentanil it is highly bound to plasma protein, principally to α_1-acid glycoprotein. The elimination half-life lies between that of alfentanil and fentanyl. The manufacturers of sufentanil have given values for a three-compartment pharmacokinetic model with a distribution half-life of 1.4 minutes, a redistribution half-life of 17.1 minutes, and an elimination half-life of 164 minutes. Accumulation may be relatively limited when compared with fentanyl. In practice the pharmacokinetics of sufentanil may vary according to the age and condition of the patient and the procedures undertaken. For example, the elimination half-life of sufentanil has been reported to be longer in patients undergoing cardiac surgery (595 minutes),[1] in hyperventilated patients (232 minutes),[2] and in those undergoing abdominal aortic surgery (more than 12 hours).[3]

1. Howie MB, *et al.* Serum concentrations of sufentanil and fentanyl in the post-operative course in cardiac surgery patients. *Anesthesiology* 1984; **61**: A131.
2. Schwartz AE, *et al.* Pharmacokinetics of sufentanil in neurosurgical patients undergoing hyperventilation. *Br J Anaesth* 1989; **63**: 385–8.
3. Hudson RJ, *et al.* Pharmacokinetics of sufentanil in patients undergoing abdominal aortic surgery. *Anesthesiology* 1989; **70**: 426–31.

Administration. References to the pharmacokinetics of sufentanil administered epidurally,[1] intrathecally,[1] and transdermally.[2]

1. Ionescu TI, *et al.* Pharmacokinetic study of extradural and intrathecal sufentanil anaesthesia for major surgery. *Br J Anaesth* 1991; **66**: 458–64.
2. Sebel PS, *et al.* Transdermal absorption of fentanyl and sufentanil in man. *Eur J Clin Pharmacol* 1987; **32**: 529–31.

Children. Neonates (up to 1 month old) had a significantly lower plasma clearance rate and greater elimination half-life than infants (1 month to 2 years), children, and adolescents.[1] Others[2] have found that infants and small children (1 month to 3 years) with cardiac disease had higher clearance rates and shorter elimination half-lives than reported for adults.

1. Greeley WJ, *et al.* Sufentanil pharmacokinetics in pediatric cardiovascular patients. *Anesth Analg* 1987; **66**: 1067–72.
2. Davis PJ, *et al.* Pharmacodynamics and pharmacokinetics of high-dose sufentanil in infants and children undergoing cardiac surgery. *Anesth Analg* 1987; **66**: 203–8.

Hepatic impairment. Because of the efficient hepatic extraction and clearance of sufentanil[1] liver dysfunction might be expected to affect its pharmacokinetics.

1. Schedewie H, *et al.* Sufentanil and fentanyl hepatic extraction rate and clearance in obese patients undergoing gastroplasty. *Clin Pharmacol Ther* 1988; **43**: 132.

Renal impairment. The pharmacokinetics of sufentanil were reported[1] to be unaffected in patients with chronic renal failure, although elevated plasma concentrations of sufentanil have been noted[2] in one such patient.

1. Sear JW. Sufentanil disposition in patients undergoing renal transplantation: influence of choice of kinetic model. *Br J Anaesth* 1989; **63**: 60–7.
2. Wiggum DC, *et al.* Postoperative respiratory depression and elevated sufentanil levels in a patient with chronic renal failure. *Anesthesiology* 1985; **63**: 708–10.

Uses and Administration

Sufentanil, a phenylpiperidine derivative, is an opioid analgesic (p.68) related to fentanyl (p.38). It is highly lipid-soluble and more potent than fentanyl. Sufentanil is used as an analgesic adjunct in anaesthesia and as a primary anaesthetic drug in procedures requiring assisted ventilation. It has a rapid onset and recovery is considered to be more rapid than with fentanyl.

Sufentanil is administered intravenously as the citrate either by slow injection or as an infusion. Lower initial doses are advised in the elderly and debilitated patients. For obese patients more than 20% above ideal body-weight the dosage of sufentanil should be determined on the basis of the patients' lean body-weight. In all patients supplementary maintenance doses should be according to individual response and length of procedure. Doses are expressed in terms of sufentanil base. Doses of up to 8 µg of sufentanil per kg body-weight produce profound analgesia. Doses of 8 µg or more per kg produce a deep level of anaesthesia but are associated with prolonged respiratory depression and assisted ventilation may be required in the postoperative period.

When used as an analgesic **adjunct to anaesthesia** with nitrous oxide and oxygen for surgical procedures

lasting up to 8 hours, the total dosage should not exceed 1 µg per kg per hour. It is customary to give up to 75% of the dose before intubation followed as necessary during surgery by additional injections of 10 to 50 µg or by a suitable continuous or intermittent infusion administered so that the total hourly dose is not exceeded. Thus, for an operation lasting 1 to 2 hours the total dose would be 1 to 2 µg per kg with 0.75 to 1.5 µg per kg being given before intubation.

When used as the **primary anaesthetic** drug in major surgery doses of 8 to 30 µg per kg are employed with 100% oxygen; doses of 25 to 30 µg per kg block sympathetic response including catecholamine release and are indicated in procedures such as cardiovascular surgery or neurosurgery. Anaesthesia may be maintained by additional injections of 0.5 to 10 µg per kg or by a suitable continuous or intermittent infusion administered so that the total dosage for the procedure does not exceed 30 µg per kg.

All the above doses relate to the use of sufentanil in adults; experience of paediatric use is more limited. **Children** undergoing cardiovascular surgery may be given sufentanil, with 100% oxygen, in an initial dose of 10 to 25 µg per kg with maintenance doses of up to 25 to 50 µg.

Sufentanil has also been given **epidurally** for the relief of pain (see below). Recommended doses for labour and delivery are 10 to 15 µg administered epidurally with 10 mL bupivacaine 0.125% with or without adrenaline [epinephrine]; the dose may be repeated twice at not less than one-hour intervals until delivery.

◊ **General reviews of sufentanil.**
1. Monk JP, *et al.* Sufentanil: a review of its pharmacological properties and therapeutic use. *Drugs* 1988; **36**: 286–313.
2. Clotz MA, Nahata MC. Clinical uses of fentanyl, sufentanil, and alfentanil. *Clin Pharm* 1991; **10**: 581–93.

Administration. Sufentanil is usually administered intravenously, but the epidural route is also used (see below). Intranasal administration (see under Anaesthesia and under Sedation, below) or intrathecal administration (see below) have also been tried.

EPIDURAL. In a laboratory assessment of epidural sufentanil in healthy subjects,[1] a dose of 50 µg produced analgesia for 2 to 3 hours; analgesia was intensified and prolonged and respiratory and other side-effects, especially drowsiness, were reduced by the addition of adrenaline [epinephrine]. Epidural sufentanil or fentanyl provided effective postoperative analgesia following caesarean section with comparable adverse effect profiles.[2] Sufentanil doses of 20 and 30 µg showed equivalent efficacy and provided greater analgesia for a longer duration than a dose of 10 µg; addition of sufentanil to the local anaesthetic bupivacaine has improved the quality of epidural analgesia.[3] Effective analgesia has been achieved in children with epidural sufentanil.[4]

Epidural administration of sufentanil has been tried for patient-controlled analgesia but appeared to have little advantage over patient-controlled analgesia using morphine given intravenously.[5]

1. Klepper ID, *et al.* Analgesic and respiratory effects of extradural sufentanil in volunteers and the influence of adrenaline as an adjuvant. *Br J Anaesth* 1987; **59**: 1147–56.
2. Grass JA, *et al.* A randomized, double-blind, dose-response comparison of epidural fentanyl versus sufentanil analgesia after cesarean section. *Anesth Analg* 1997; **85**: 365–71.
3. Reynolds F. Extradural opioids in labour. *Br J Anaesth* 1989; **63**: 251–3.
4. Benlabed M, *et al.* Analgesia and ventilatory response to CO$_2$ following epidural sufentanil in children. *Anesthesiology* 1987; **67**: 948–51.
5. Grass JA, *et al.* Patient-controlled analgesia after cesarean delivery: epidural sufentanil versus intravenous morphine. *Reg Anesth* 1994; **19**: 90–7.

INTRATHECAL. Sufentanil has been given by the intrathecal route for labour pain. There was no significant difference in terms of effects on fetal heart rate when intrathecal sufentanil was compared with epidural bupivacaine,[1] although the authors suggested that fetal heart rate should be monitored carefully when either drug is used. A combination of sufentanil, bupivacaine, and adrenaline [epinephrine] administered intrathecally provided excellent analgesia during labour and had a more rapid onset, a longer duration of action, and reduced local anaesthetic requirements compared with epidural administration.[2] Intrathecal sufentanil and bupivacaine provided shorter duration of analgesia when administered during the advanced stages of labour compared with early labour.[3]

1. Nielsen PE, *et al.* Fetal heart rate changes after intrathecal sufentanil or epidural bupivacaine for labor analgesia: incidence and clinical significance. *Anesth Analg* 1996; **83**: 742–6.

2. Kartawiadi SL, *et al.* Spinal analgesia during labor with low-dose bupivacaine, sufentanil, and epinephrine: a comparison with epidural analgesia. *Reg Anesth* 1996; **21**: 191–6.
3. Viscomi CM, *et al.* Duration of intrathecal labor analgesia: early versus advanced labor. *Anesth Analg* 1997; **84**: 1108–12.

Anaesthesia. Sufentanil, like fentanyl (p.39), appears to produce fewer circulatory changes than morphine and may be preferred for anaesthetic use, especially in cardiovascular surgery. In a comparative study fentanyl and sufentanil were equally preferable to morphine or pethidine as adjuncts to nitrous oxide anaesthesia in terms of haemodynamic changes to stress and rates of recovery.[1] A comparison[2] of these same 4 drugs found sufentanil to be the most satisfactory, especially in terms of the haemodynamic and autonomic stability achieved. Sufentanil also compared favourably with fentanyl when used for the induction and maintenance of anaesthesia for coronary artery bypass surgery[3] and when given in lower doses by continuous infusion for outpatient anaesthesia.[4]

Sufentanil anaesthesia for major surgery has been assessed in a multicentre study;[5] to prevent the majority of adverse reactions pre-operative assessment of the patient's circulatory volume, concomitant administration of muscle relaxants, ready availability of vagolytic agents, and a cumulative dose of no more than 1 µg per kg body-weight per hour, were recommended.

Premedication with sufentanil administered intranasally has been tried in children[6,7] and in adults.[8]

Neuroleptanalgesia. Sufentanil is one of the opioids that have been used with a neuroleptic to produce neuroleptanalgesia.

1. Ghoneim MM, *et al.* Comparison of four opioid analgesics as supplements to nitrous oxide anesthesia. *Anesth Analg* 1984; **63**: 405–12.
2. Flacke JW, *et al.* Comparison of morphine, meperidine, fentanyl, and sufentanil in balanced anesthesia: a double-blind study. *Anesth Analg* 1985; **64**: 897–910.
3. Mathews HML, *et al.* Comparison of fentanyl and sufentanil anaesthesia for patients undergoing coronary artery bypass grafting. *Br J Anaesth* 1987; **59**: 939–40P.
4. Phitayakorn P, *et al.* Comparison of continuous sufentanil and fentanyl infusions for outpatient anaesthesia. *Can J Anaesth* 1987; **34**: 242–5.
5. Murkin JM. Sufentanil anaesthesia for major surgery: the multicentre Canadian clinical trial. *Can J Anaesth* 1989; **36**: 343–9.
6. Henderson JM, *et al.* Pre-induction of anesthesia in pediatric patients with nasally administered sufentanil. *Anesthesiology* 1988; **68**: 671–5.
7. Zedie N, *et al.* Comparison of intranasal midazolam and sufentanil premedication in pediatric outpatients. *Clin Pharmacol Ther* 1996; **59**: 341–8.
8. Helmers JHJH, *et al.* Comparison of intravenous and intranasal sufentanil absorption and sedation. *Can J Anaesth* 1989; **36**: 494–7.

Pain. For the use of sufentanil in the management of pain, see under Epidural and Intrathecal Administration, above.

Sedation. Some references to the use of sufentanil for sedation are given below. See also under Anaesthesia, above.

1. Bates BA, *et al.* A comparison of intranasal sufentanil and midazolam to intramuscular meperidine, promethazine, and chlorpromazine for conscious sedation in children. *Ann Emerg Med* 1994; **24**: 646–51.
2. Lefrant JY, *et al.* Sufentanil short duration infusion for postoperative sedation in critically ill patients. *Br J Anaesth* 1995; **74** (suppl 1): 114.

Preparations

USP 25: Sufentanil Citrate Injection.

Proprietary Preparations (details are given in Part 3)
Aust.: Sufenta; *Belg.:* Sufenta; *Canad.:* Sufenta; *Denm.:* Sufenta; *Fin.:* Sufenta; *Fr.:* Sufenta; *Ger.:* Sufenta; *Ital.:* Fentatienil; *Neth.:* Sufenta; *Norw.:* Sufenta; *S.Afr.:* Sufenta; *Swed.:* Sufenta; *Switz.:* Sufenta; *USA:* Sufenta.

Sulindac   (2706-a)

Sulindac *(BAN, USAN, rINN).*
MK-231; Sulindacum. *(Z)*-[5-Fluoro-2-methyl-1-(4-methylsulphinylbenzylidene)inden-3-yl]acetic acid.
$C_{20}H_{17}FO_3S = 356.4.$
CAS — 38194-50-2.
ATC — M01AB02.
Pharmacopoeias. In *Eur.* (see p.vi) and *US.*

Pharmacopoeial description

Ph. Eur.: A yellow, polymorphic, crystalline powder. Very slightly soluble in water and in ether; sparingly soluble in alcohol; soluble in dichloromethane; dissolves in dilute solutions of alkali hydroxides. Protect from light.

USP 25: A yellow, odourless or practically odourless, crystalline powder. Practically insoluble in water and in hexane; slightly soluble in alcohol, in acetone, in chloroform, and in methyl alcohol; very slightly soluble in ethyl acetate and in isopropyl alcohol.

Adverse Effects and Precautions

As for NSAIDs in general, p.63. Urine discoloration has occasionally been reported with sulindac.

Sulindac metabolites have been reported as major or minor components in renal stones. It should therefore be used with caution in patients with a history of renal stones and such patients should be kept well hydrated while receiving sulindac.

The dose of sulindac may need to be reduced in patients with liver or renal function impairment.

◊ A report of 4 patients and a short review of 8 previously reported cases of serious adverse reactions to sulindac;[1] reactions included fever and skin, liver, CNS, lymph node, bone-marrow, and lung involvement.

1. Park GD, et al. Serious adverse reactions associated with sulindac. Arch Intern Med 1982; 142: 1292–4.

Effects on the blood. Agranulocytosis,[1] thrombocytopenia,[2] haemolytic anaemia,[3] and aplastic anaemia[4] have been reported in patients taking sulindac.

1. Romeril KR, et al. Sulindac induced agranulocytosis and bone marrow culture. Lancet 1981; ii: 523.
2. Karachalios GN, Parigorakis JG. Thrombocytopenia and sulindac. Ann Intern Med 1986; 104: 128.
3. Johnson FP, et al. Immune hemolytic anemia associated with sulindac. JAMA 1985; 145: 1515–16.
4. Andrews R, Russell N. Aplastic anaemia associated with a non-steroidal anti-inflammatory drug: relapse after exposure to another such drug. BMJ 1990; 301: 38.

Effects on the CNS. Acute deterioration of parkinsonism occurred in a patient following the introduction of sulindac therapy.[1]

See also under Hypersensitivity, below.

1. Sandyk R, Gillman MA. Acute exacerbation of Parkinson's disease with sulindac. Ann Neurol 1985; 17: 104–5.

Effects on the endocrine system. A case of reversible gynaecomastia associated with sulindac therapy has been reported.[1] There has also been a report[2] of reversible hypothyroidism in an elderly patient taking sulindac.

1. Kapoor A. Reversible gynecomastia associated with sulindac therapy. JAMA 1983; 250: 2294–5.
2. Iyer RP, Duckett GK. Reversible secondary hypothyroidism induced by sulindac. BMJ 1985; 290: 1788.

Effects on the gallbladder. A "sludge" composed of crystalline metabolites of sulindac has been found in the common bile duct during surgery for biliary obstruction in patients who had been taking sulindac.[1]

1. Anonymous. Rare complication with sulindac. FDA Drug Bull 1989; 19: 4.

Effects on the kidneys. Sulindac-induced renal impairment, interstitial nephritis, and nephrotic syndrome have been reported.[1] It has been suggested that sulindac, as a prodrug, may not inhibit renal prostaglandin synthesis in therapeutic doses. However, this potentially important therapeutic advantage has not been uniformly observed in short-term studies in patients with renal dysfunction.[2-4]

There have been reports of renal stones consisting of between 10 and 90% of sulindac metabolites developing in patients treated with sulindac.[5]

1. Whelton A, et al. Sulindac and renal impairment. JAMA 1983; 249: 2892.
2. Klassen DK, et al. Sulindac kinetics and effects on renal function and prostaglandin excretion in renal insufficiency. J Clin Pharmacol 1989; 29: 1037–42.
3. Eriksson L-O, et al. Effects of sulindac and naproxen on prostaglandin excretion in patients with impaired renal function and rheumatoid arthritis. Am J Med 1990; 89: 313–21.
4. Whelton A, et al. Renal effects of ibuprofen, piroxicam, and sulindac in patients with asymptomatic renal failure. Ann Intern Med 1990; 112: 568–76.
5. Anonymous. Rare complication with sulindac. FDA Drug Bull 1989; 19: 4.

Effects on the liver. Hepatotoxicity reported in patients receiving sulindac includes hepatocellular injury and cholestatic jaundice.[1,2] Symptoms of hypersensitivity including rash, fever, or eosinophilia have been reported in 35 to 55% of patients with sulindac-induced liver damage;[2] in these patients the liver damage occurred usually within 4 to 8 weeks of beginning sulindac therapy. For reference to a report citing the strongest evidence for an association of sulindac with liver disease compared with other NSAIDs, see under NSAIDs, p.64.

See also under Effects on the Skin, below.

1. Gallanosa AG, Spyker DA. Sulindac hepatotoxicity: a case report and review. Clin Toxicol 1985; 23: 205–38.
2. Tarazi EM, et al. Sulindac-associated hepatic injury: analysis of 91 cases reported to the Food and Drug Administration. Gastroenterology 1993; 104: 569–74.

Effects on the lungs. For reference to pneumonitis associated with sulindac therapy, see under Hypersensitivity, below.

Effects on the skin. Toxic epidermal necrolysis has occurred in patients taking sulindac.[1] In one patient toxic hepatitis and the Stevens-Johnson/toxic epidermal necrolysis syndrome resulted in death.[2]

An unusual pernio-like reaction affecting the toes and confirmed by rechallenge has also been reported.[3]

Sulindac has also been reported to cause photosensitivity reactions.[4]

1. Small RE, Garnett WR. Sulindac-induced toxic epidermal necrolysis. Clin Pharm 1988; 7: 766–71.
2. Klein SM, Khan MA. Hepatitis, toxic epidermal necrolysis and pancreatitis in association with sulindac therapy. J Rheumatol 1983; 10: 512–13.

3. Reinertsen JL. Unusual pernio-like reaction to sulindac. Arthritis Rheum 1981; 24: 1215.
4. Anonymous. Drugs that cause photosensitivity. Med Lett Drugs Ther 1986; 28: 51–2.

Hypersensitivity. Hypersensitivity reactions to sulindac include pneumonitis,[1,2] generalised lymphadenopathy,[3] aseptic meningitis,[4] and anaphylactoid reaction.[5]

See also under Effects on the Liver and under Effects on the Skin, above.

1. Smith FE, Lindberg PJ. Life-threatening hypersensitivity to sulindac. JAMA 1980; 244: 269–70.
2. Fein M. Sulindac and pneumonitis. Ann Intern Med 1981; 95: 245.
3. Sprung DJ. Sulindac causing a hypersensitivity reaction with peripheral and mediastinal lymphadenopathy. Ann Intern Med 1982; 97: 564.
4. Fordham von Reyn C. Recurrent aseptic meningitis due to sulindac. Ann Intern Med 1983; 99: 343–4.
5. Hyson CP, Kazakoff MA. A severe multisystem reaction to sulindac. Arch Intern Med 1991; 151: 387–8.

Pancreatitis. Reports[1-4] of pancreatitis associated with sulindac therapy.

1. Goldstein J, et al. Sulindac associated with pancreatitis. Ann Intern Med 1980; 93: 151.
2. Siefkin AD. Sulindac and pancreatitis. Ann Intern Med 1980; 93: 932–3.
3. Lilly EL. Pancreatitis after administration of sulindac. JAMA 1981; 246: 2680.
4. Memon AN. Pancreatitis and sulindac. Ann Intern Med 1982; 97: 139.

Interactions

For interactions associated with NSAIDs, see p.65.

Dimethyl sulfoxide reduces plasma concentrations of the active metabolite of sulindac and concomitant administration of the two drugs has also resulted in peripheral neuropathy. Diflunisal and aspirin are reported to reduce the plasma concentration of the active metabolite of sulindac. Unlike other NSAIDs, sulindac is reported not to reduce the antihypertensive effects of drugs such as thiazide diuretics, but nevertheless the manufacturers recommend that blood pressure be closely monitored in patients taking antihypertensives and sulindac together.

Pharmacokinetics

Sulindac is absorbed from the gastrointestinal tract. It is metabolised by reversible reduction to the sulfide metabolite, which appears to be the biologically active form, and by irreversible oxidation to the sulfone metabolite. Peak plasma concentrations of the sulfide metabolite are achieved in about 2 hours. The mean elimination half-life of sulindac is about 7 to 8 hours and of the sulfide metabolite about 16 to 18 hours. Sulindac and its metabolites are highly bound to plasma protein. About 50% is excreted in the urine mainly as the sulfone metabolite and its glucuronide conjugate, with smaller amounts of sulindac and its glucuronide conjugate. Sulindac and its metabolites are also excreted in bile and undergo extensive enterohepatic circulation.

◊ References.

1. Davies NM, Watson MS. Clinical pharmacokinetics of sulindac: a dynamic old drug. Clin Pharmacokinet 1997; 32: 437–59.

Uses and Administration

Sulindac is an NSAID (p.65) structurally related to indometacin (p.46); its biological activity appears to be due to its sulfide metabolite. Sulindac is used in musculoskeletal and joint disorders such as ankylosing spondylitis, osteoarthritis, and rheumatoid arthritis, and also in the short-term management of acute gout and peri-articular conditions such as bursitis and tendinitis. It is also used to reduce fever.

A usual dose of sulindac by mouth is initially 150 or 200 mg twice daily reduced according to response. The maximum recommended daily dose is 400 mg. The UK manufacturers recommend that the treatment of peri-articular disorders should be limited to 7 to 10 days; for acute gout, 7 days of therapy is usually adequate. The dose may need to be reduced in patients with liver or renal function impairment.

Sulindac sodium has been given by rectal suppository in doses of 200 to 400 mg daily.

Gastrointestinal disorders. In placebo-controlled studies[1,2] sulindac 150 to 200 mg twice daily for 6 to 9 months has reduced the number and size of polyps in patients with familial adenomatous polyposis but the effect may be incomplete and in

one study[2] only polyps less than 2 mm in size regressed. The size and number of polyps has been reported[1] to increase on discontinuation of treatment and long-term therapy is therefore being studied. However, some workers[3] have observed diminution of sulindac's effectiveness with long-term treatment although others[4] have reported that they have managed recurrences by adjustment of the maintenance dosage used; it appeared that there were individual variations in sensitivity to sulindac with respect to prevention of polyp recurrence although 200 mg daily appeared to be an average maintenance dose needed.[4] There is evidence[5] that sulindac alters the ratio of apoptosis of surface cells relative to those lying deeper in the crypt of rectal mucosa, thus altering epithelial homoeostasis. Whether sulindac prevents malignant degeneration is unknown but there has been a report[6] of a patient who developed rectal cancer during long-term therapy for familial adenomatous polyposis. Some[1] consider that sulindac is unlikely to replace surgery as primary therapy for familial adenomatous polyposis. Sulindac has also been reported to have produced beneficial effects in a patient with duodenal polyps associated with Gardner's syndrome[7] but a placebo-controlled study has suggested that it may not be effective against sporadic type colonic polyps.[8]

For a discussion of evidence suggesting that regular use of NSAIDs may protect against various types of malignant neoplasms of the gastrointestinal tract, see under Malignant Neoplasms in NSAIDs, p.66.

1. Giardiello FM, et al. Treatment of colonic and rectal adenomas with sulindac in familial adenomatous polyposis. N Engl J Med 1993; 328: 1313–16.
2. Debinski HS, et al. Effect of sulindac on small polyps in familial adenomatous polyposis. Lancet 1995; 345: 855–6.
3. Tonelli F, Valanzano R. Sulindac in familial adenomatous polyposis. Lancet 1993; 342: 1120.
4. Labayle D, et al. Sulindac in familial adenomatous polyposis. Lancet 1994; 343: 417–18.
5. Keller JJ, et al. Rectal epithelial apoptosis in familial adenomatous polyposis patients treated with sulindac. Gut 1999; 45: 822–8.
6. Thorson AG, et al. Rectal cancer in FAP patient after sulindac. Lancet 1994; 343: 180.
7. Parker AL, et al. Disappearance of duodenal polyps in Gardner's syndrome with sulindac therapy. Am J Gastroenterol 1993; 88: 93–4.
8. Ladenheim J, et al. Effect of sulindac on sporadic colonic polyps. Gastroenterology 1995; 108: 1083–7.

Premature labour. The most common approach to postponing premature labour (p.773) is with drugs is with a selective beta₂ agonist. However, as prostaglandins have a role in uterine contraction and cervical ripening and dilatation, prostaglandin synthetase inhibitors such as indometacin have also been used. Sulindac has also been tried[1,2] as an alternative to indometacin as it appears to have little placental transfer and may therefore have fewer fetal side-effects.[1] However, the authors of a more recent study suggested that sulindac has many of the same adverse fetal effects as indometacin and its use can only be described as investigational.[3]

1. Carlan SJ, et al. Randomized comparative trial of indomethacin and sulindac for the treatment of refractory preterm labor. Obstet Gynecol 1992; 79: 223–8.
2. Carlan SJ, et al. Outpatient oral sulindac to prevent recurrence of preterm labor. Obstet Gynecol 1995; 85: 769–74.
3. Kramer WB, et al. A randomized double-blind study comparing the fetal effects of sulindac to terbutaline during the management of preterm labor. Am J Obstet Gynecol 1999; 180: 396–401.

Preparations

BP 2001: Sulindac Tablets.
USP 25: Sulindac Tablets.

Proprietary Preparations (details are given in Part 3)
Aust.: Clinoril; *Austral.:* Aclin; Clinoril; Clusinol†; Saldac†; *Belg.:* Clinoril; *Canad.:* Apo-Sulin; Clinoril†; Novo-Sundac; *Denm.:* Clinoril; *Fr.:* Arthrocine; *Hong Kong:* Aclin; Clinoril; *Irl.:* Clinoril; *Ital.:* Aflodac†; Algocetil†; Citireuma; Clinoril; Lyndak; Sulartrene; Sulen; Sulic†; Sulinol†; *Mex.:* Clinoril; Copal; Kenalin; *Neth.:* Clinoril; *Norw.:* Clinoril; *NZ:* Clinoril; Daclin; Saldac; *Port.:* Artribid; *S.Afr.:* Clinoril; R-Flex†; *Spain:* Sulindal; *Swed.:* Clinoril; *Switz.:* Clinoril; *Thai.:* Cenlidac; Clinoril; *UK:* Clinoril; *USA:* Clinoril.

Superoxide Dismutase (992-n)

SOD.

A group of water-soluble protein congeners widely distributed in nature which catalyse the conversion of superoxide radicals to peroxide. Several different forms exist, which vary in their metal content; forms containing copper or copper and zinc are common.

Orgotein (13043-t)

Orgotein (BAN, USAN, rINN).

Bovine Superoxide Dismutase; Ormetein.

CAS — 9016-01-7.
ATC — M01AX14.

A superoxide dismutase produced from beef liver as Cu-Zn mixed chelate. Mol. wt about 33 000 with a compact conformation maintained by about 4 gram-atoms of chelated divalent metal.

Pegorgotein (17849-x)

Pegorgotein (USAN, rINN).

PEG-SOD; Win-22118.

CAS — 155773-57-2.

A superoxide dismutase conjugated with polyethylene glycol to prolong its duration of action.

Sudismase (5782-p)

Sudismase (rINN).

CAS — 110294-55-8.

A human N-acetylsuperoxide dismutase produced by recombinant DNA technology and containing a copper and zinc prosthetic group.

Adverse Effects

Anaphylaxis and other hypersensitivity reactions, sometimes fatal, have been reported with orgotein. Local reactions and pain may occur at the site of injection of orgotein.

Pharmacokinetics

◊ References.

1. Tsao D, et al. Pharmacokinetics of recombinant human superoxide dismutase in healthy volunteers. Clin Pharmacol Ther 1991; **50:** 713–20.
2. Uematsu T, et al. Pharmacokinetics and safety of intravenous recombinant human superoxide dismutase (NK341) in healthy subjects. Int J Clin Pharmacol Ther 1994; **32:** 638–41.
3. Jadot G, et al. Clinical pharmacokinetics and delivery of bovine superoxide dismutase. Clin Pharmacokinet 1995; **28:** 17–25.
4. Rosenfeld WN, et al. Safety and pharmacokinetics of recombinant human superoxide dismutase administered intrathecally to premature neonates with respiratory distress syndrome. Pediatrics 1996; **97:** 811–17.
5. Davis JM, et al. Safety and pharmacokinetics of multiple doses of recombinant human CuZn superoxide dismutase administered intrathecally to premature neonates with respiratory distress syndrome. Pediatrics 1997; **100:** 24–30.

Uses and Administration

Superoxide dismutases have anti-inflammatory properties. Orgotein, a bovine derived superoxide dismutase, has been given by local injection, into the joints for degenerative joint disorders, but hypersensitivity reactions have limited its use. It has also been tried for the amelioration of side-effects from radiotherapy. Forms of human superoxide dismutase derived by recombinant DNA technology have been developed.

Superoxide dismutases are also under investigation for their free-radical scavenging properties in a variety of conditions including the prevention of bronchopulmonary dysplasia in neonates.

Head injury. Pegorgotein was found[1] to be little more effective than placebo in improving neurological outcome or reducing mortality in patients with severe head injury.

1. Young B, et al. Effects of pegorgotein on neurologic outcome of patients with severe head injury: a multicenter, randomized controlled trial. JAMA 1996; **276:** 538–43.

Motor neurone disease. A small percentage of patients with familial amyotrophic lateral sclerosis (see Motor Neurone Disease, p.1658) have been shown to have a mutation in the gene encoding for the enzyme copper-zinc superoxide dismutase but there has been no consensus as to whether patients with this mutation should be given superoxide dismutase supplements.[1]

1. Orrell RW, deBelleroche JS. Superoxide dismutase and ALS. Lancet 1994; **344:** 1651–2.

Radiotherapy. Although some studies[1,2] indicate that orgotein can ameliorate the side-effects of radiotherapy for bladder tumours, one study[3] was terminated prematurely because of unacceptable hypersensitivity reactions and apparent inefficacy.

1. Edsmyr F, et al. Orgotein efficacy in ameliorating side effects due to radiation therapy I: double-blind, placebo-controlled trial in patients with bladder tumors. Curr Ther Res 1976; **19:** 198–211.
2. Sanchiz F, et al. Prevention of radioinduced cystitis by orgotein: a randomized study. Anticancer Res 1996; **16:** 2025–8.
3. Nielsen OS, et al. Orgotein in radiation treatment of bladder cancer: a report on allergic reactions and lack of radioprotective effect. Acta Oncol 1987; **26:** 101–4.

Preparations

Proprietary Preparations (details are given in Part 3)

Spain: Ontosein.

Suprofen (13292-y)

Suprofen (BAN, USAN, rINN).

R-25061; Sutoprofen. 2-[4-(2-Thenoyl)phenyl]propionic acid.

$C_{14}H_{12}O_3S = 260.3$.

CAS — 40828-46-4.

ATC — M01AE07.

Pharmacopoeias. In US.

Pharmacopoeial description

USP 25: A white to off-white powder, odourless or having a slight odour. Sparingly soluble in water.

Adverse Effects and Precautions

Ocular administration of suprofen may cause local reactions including discomfort, itching, redness, iritis, pain, chemosis,

photophobia, and rarely punctate epithelial staining. Hypersensitivity may occur. Suprofen eye drops should not be used in patients with active herpes simplex keratitis.

Adverse renal reactions following oral administration have ended its use as an oral NSAID.

Effects on the kidneys. A clinical syndrome of flank pain and acute renal failure associated with oral suprofen has been reported;[1] the syndrome is unlike other nephrotoxic syndromes related to NSAIDs.

1. Hart D, et al. Suprofen-related nephrotoxicity: a distinct clinical syndrome. Ann Intern Med 1987; **106:** 235–8.

Interactions

◊ The manufacturer of acetylcholine chloride ophthalmic preparations has stated that there have been reports that acetylcholine and carbachol have been ineffective when used in patients treated with topical (ophthalmic) NSAIDs.

Uses and Administration

Suprofen is an NSAID (p.65). Suprofen is used to inhibit the miosis that may occur during ocular surgery and is administered as 1% eye drops. On the day of surgery, 2 drops are instilled into the conjunctival sac 3 hours, 2 hours, and then 1 hour before surgery. Two drops may be instilled into the conjunctival sac every 4 hours during the day before surgery. It was formerly given by mouth in mild to moderate pain and in osteoarthritis and rheumatoid arthritis but, following reports of adverse renal reactions, marketing of the oral dose form was suspended worldwide.

Preparations

USP 25: Suprofen Ophthalmic Solution.

Proprietary Preparations (details are given in Part 3)

USA: Profenal.

Suxibuzone (2707-t)

Suxibuzone (BAN, rINN).

Suxibuzonum. 4-Butyl-4-hydroxymethyl-1,2-diphenylpyrazolidine-3,5-dione hydrogen succinate (ester).

$C_{24}H_{26}N_2O_6 = 438.5$.

CAS — 27470-51-5.

ATC — M02AA22.

Pharmacopoeias. In Eur. (see p.vi).

Pharmacopoeial description

Ph. Eur.: A white crystalline powder. Practically insoluble in water; soluble in alcohol; freely soluble in acetone; practically insoluble in cyclohexane.

Profile

Suxibuzone, a derivative of phenylbutazone (p.78), is an NSAID (p.63) that has been applied topically at a concentration of about 7% in musculoskeletal and joint disorders. Concern over safety and toxicity has led to its withdrawal from the market in many countries.

Preparations

Proprietary Preparations (details are given in Part 3)

Spain: Danilon; *Switz.:* Flamilon†.

Tenidap Sodium (4865-m)

Tenidap Sodium (BANM, USAN, rINNM).

CP-66248 (tenidap); CP-66248-2 (tenidap sodium); CP-66248-02 (tenidap sodium). (Z)-5-Chloro-3-(α-hydroxy-2-thenylidene)-2-oxoindoline-1-carboxamide sodium.

$C_{14}H_8ClN_2NaO_3S = 342.7$.

CAS — 120210-48-2 (tenidap); 119784-94-0 (tenidap sodium).

Profile

Tenidap is an NSAID (p.63) that also acts as a cytokine modulator. It has been studied in the treatment of rheumatoid arthritis and osteoarthritis but because of concern over its potential effect on bone mineral density its development for these indications was abandoned.

Tenoxicam (13305-h)

Tenoxicam (BAN, USAN, rINN).

Ro-12-0068; Ro-12-0068/000; Tenoxicamum. 4-Hydroxy-2-methyl-N-(2-pyridyl)-2H-thieno[2,3-e][1,2]thiazine-3-carboxamide 1,1-dioxide.

$C_{13}H_{11}N_3O_4S_2 = 337.4$.

CAS — 59804-37-4.

ATC — M01AC02.

Pharmacopoeias. In Eur. (see p.vi).

Pharmacopoeial description

Ph. Eur.: A yellow, polymorphic, crystalline powder. Practically insoluble in water; very slightly soluble in dehydrated alcohol; sparingly soluble in dichloromethane; it dissolves in solutions of acids and alkalis. Protect from light.

Adverse Effects and Precautions

As for NSAIDs in general, p.63.

◊ Adverse effects associated with tenoxicam have been reviewed.[1] The majority of adverse effects relate to the gastrointestinal tract (11.4%), nervous system (2.8%), or skin (2.5%).

1. Todd PA, Clissold SP. Tenoxicam: an update of its pharmacology and therapeutic efficacy in rheumatic diseases. Drugs 1991; **41:** 625–46.

Effects on the kidneys. A review[1] of the effects of tenoxicam on renal function concluded that tenoxicam could be given at normal recommended doses to elderly patients or those with mild to moderate renal impairment who were not at high risk of renal failure or receiving potentially nephrotoxic therapy. Data from the manufacturer's database[1] on 67 063 patients, including 17 005 over 65 years of age, who had received tenoxicam indicated that there had been 45 adverse events relating to urinary system function. The prevalence of adverse events was similar in elderly and non-elderly patients, the most common effects being dysuria and renal pain. Seven of the events had been described as severe.

1. Heintz RCA. Tenoxicam and renal function. Drug Safety 1995; **12:** 110–19.

Effects on the liver. A report[1] of acute hepatitis associated with the use of tenoxicam.

1. Sungur C, et al. Acute hepatitis caused by tenoxicam. Ann Pharmacother 1994; **28:** 1309.

Effects on the skin. A report of 3 cases of toxic epidermal necrolysis (Lyell's syndrome) associated with tenoxicam.[1] For the general incidence of dermatological effects see above.

1. Chosidow O, et al. Toxidermies sévères au ténoxicam (Tilcotil®). Ann Dermatol Venereol 1991; **118:** 903–4.

Interactions

For interactions associated with NSAIDs, see p.65.

Pharmacokinetics

Tenoxicam is well absorbed following oral administration; peak plasma concentrations occur within about 2 hours in fasting subjects; this may be delayed to about 6 hours when tenoxicam is given with food but the extent of absorption is not affected. Tenoxicam is over 98.5% protein bound and penetrates synovial fluid. The plasma elimination half-life is about 60 to 75 hours; with daily administration, steady-state concentrations are reached within 10 to 15 days. Tenoxicam is completely metabolised to inactive metabolites which are excreted mainly in the urine; there is some biliary excretion of glucuronide conjugates of the metabolites.

◊ References.

1. Nilsen OG. Clinical pharmacokinetics of tenoxicam. Clin Pharmacokinet 1994; **26:** 16–43.
2. Guentert TW, et al. Relative bioavailability of oral dosage forms of tenoxicam. Arzneimittelforschung 1994; **44:** 1051–4.

Uses and Administration

Tenoxicam, a piroxicam (p.79) analogue, is an NSAID (p.65). It is used in the symptomatic management of musculoskeletal and joint disorders such as osteoarthritis and rheumatoid arthritis, and also in the short-term management of soft-tissue injury. Tenoxicam is given by mouth as a single daily dose usually of 20 mg. In acute musculoskeletal disorders treatment for up to 7 days is usually sufficient but in severe cases it may be given for up to a maximum of 14 days. Doses similar to those given by mouth have been given by intramuscular or intravenous injection for initial treatment for 1 to 2 days. Tenoxicam has also been given by rectal suppository.

◊ References.

1. Todd PA, Clissold SP. Tenoxicam: an update of its pharmacology and therapeutic efficacy in rheumatic diseases. Drugs 1991; **41:** 625–46.

Preparations

BP 2001: Tenoxicam Injection; Tenoxicam Tablets.

Proprietary Preparations (details are given in Part 3)

Aust.: Liman; Tilcotil; *Austral.:* Tilcotil; *Belg.:* Tilcotil; *Braz.:* Legil; Tenoxen; Tilatil; *Canad.:* Mobiflex; *Denm.:* Tilcotil; *Fin.:* Tilcotil; *Fr.:* Tilcotil; *Ger.:* Liman†; Tilcotil†; *Hong Kong:* Nadamen; Tilcotil; *Irl.:* Mobiflex; *Ital.:* Dolmen; Rexalgan; Tilcotil; *Mex.:* Tilcotil; *Neth.:* Tilcotil; *NZ:* Tilcotil; *Port.:* Bioreucam; Calibral†; Doxican; Tilcotil; *S.Afr.:* Tilcotil; Tobitil; *Singapore:* Nadamen; Tilcotil; *Spain:* Artriunic; Reutenox; Tilcotil; *Swed.:* Alganex; *Switz.:* Tilcotil; *Thai.:* Menzotil; Nadamen; Seftil; Sinoral; Teconam; Tenax; Tenocam; Tenox; Tenoxil; Tilcotil; *UK:* Mobiflex.

Tetridamine (3915-l)

Tetridamine (rINN).

POLI-67; Tetrydamine (USAN). 4,5,6,7-Tetrahydro-2-methyl-3-(methylamino)-2H-indazole.

$C_9H_{15}N_3 = 165.2$.

CAS — 17289-49-5.

Profile

Tetridamine is an NSAID (p.63) that has been used as the maleate as a douche in the treatment of vaginitis.

Preparations

Proprietary Preparations (details are given in Part 3)

Ital.: Deb; *Spain:* Fomene; Tesos.

The symbol † denotes a preparation no longer actively marketed

Thurfyl Salicylate (2708-x)

Tetrahydrofurfuryl salicylate.
$C_{12}H_{14}O_4 = 222.2$.
$CAS — 2217-35-8$.

Profile

Thurfyl salicylate is a salicylic acid derivative that has been used similarly to methyl salicylate (p.55) in topical rubefacient preparations at concentrations of up to 14% for musculoskeletal, joint, peri-articular, and soft-tissue disorders.

Preparations

Proprietary Preparations (details are given in Part 3)
Multi-ingredient: *Belg.:* Transvane†; *Irl.:* Transvasin; *NZ:* Transvasin; *Swed.:* Transvasin†; *UK:* Transvasin Heat Rub.

Tiaprofenic Acid (2709-r)

Tiaprofenic Acid (BAN, rINN).
Acidum Tiaprofenicum; FC-3001; RU-15060. 2-(5-Benzoyl-2-thienyl)propionic acid.
$C_{14}H_{12}O_3S = 260.3$.
$CAS — 33005-95-7$.
$ATC — M01AE11$.
Pharmacopoeias. In Eur. (see p.vi).

Pharmacopoeial description

Ph. Eur.: A white or almost white, crystalline powder. Practically insoluble in water; freely soluble in alcohol, in acetone, and in dichloromethane. Protect from light.

Adverse Effects and Precautions

As for NSAIDs in general, p.63.
Tiaprofenic acid may cause cystitis, bladder irritation, and other urinary-tract symptoms (see below). It should not be given to patients with active urinary-tract disorders or prostatic disease or a history of recurrent urinary-tract disorders. It should be stopped immediately if urinary-tract symptoms occur and urinalysis and urine culture performed.

Breast feeding. See under Pharmacokinetics, below.

Effects on the urinary tract. Cystitis and bladder irritation have been associated with the use of tiaprofenic acid.[1-6] In August 1994 the UK Committee on Safety of Medicines (CSM) stated[4] that since the introduction of tiaprofenic acid in the UK in 1982 they had received 69 reports of cystitis and 32 other reports of urinary-tract symptoms associated with tiaprofenic acid including frequency, dysuria, and haematuria whereas only 8 cases of cystitis had been reported for all other NSAIDs combined. Analysis of spontaneous reports received by WHO[7] confirmed that cystitis was more commonly associated with tiaprofenic acid than with other NSAIDs. The Australian Adverse Drug Reaction Advisory Committee had received similar reports.[3] Since the 1994 warning, the CSM[8] had received reports of a further 74 cases of cystitis, but the majority of these had occurred before the warning was issued. The duration of treatment in patients affected had varied considerably. Most patients recovered when tiaprofenic acid was withdrawn.

The CSM recommended that tiaprofenic acid should not be given to patients with pre-existing urinary-tract disorders and that it should be stopped in patients who develop urinary-tract symptoms. Patients should be advised that if they develop symptoms such as urinary frequency, nocturia, urgency, or pain on urination, or have blood in their urine they should stop taking tiaprofenic acid and consult their doctor.

1. Ahmed M, Davison OW. Severe cystitis associated with tiaprofenic acid. *BMJ* 1991; **303:** 1376.
2. O'Neill GFA. Tiaprofenic acid as a cause of non-bacterial cystitis. *Med J Aust* 1994; **160:** 123–5.
3. Australian Adverse Drug Reactions Advisory Committee. Update on tiaprofenic acid and urinary symptoms. *Aust Adverse Drug React Bull* 1994; **13:** 6.
4. Committee on Safety of Medicines/Medicines Control Agency. Severe cystitis with tiaprofenic acid (Surgam). *Current Problems* 1994; **20:** 11.
5. Harrison WJ, *et al.* Adverse reactions to tiaprofenic acid mimicking interstitial cystitis. *BMJ* 1994; **309:** 574.
6. Mayall FG, *et al.* Cystitis and ureteric obstruction in patients taking tiaprofenic acid. *BMJ* 1994; **309:** 599.
7. The ADR Signals Analysis Project (ASAP) Team. How does cystitis affect a comparative risk profile of tiaprofenic acid with other non-steroidal antiinflammatory drugs? An international study based on spontaneous reports and drug usage data. *Pharmacol Toxicol* 1997; **80:** 211–17.
8. Crawford MLA, *et al.* Severe cystitis associated with tiaprofenic acid. *Br J Urol* 1997; **79:** 578–84.

Interactions

For interactions associated with NSAIDs, see p.65.

Pharmacokinetics

Tiaprofenic acid is absorbed from the gastrointestinal tract with peak plasma concentrations being reached within about 1.5 hours after oral administration. It has a short elimination half-life of about 2 hours and is highly bound to plasma proteins (about 98%). Excretion of tiaprofenic acid and its metabolites is mainly in the urine in the form of acyl glucuronides; some is excreted in the bile. Tiaprofenic acid is distributed into breast milk in amounts considered to be too small to be harmful to a breast-fed infant.

◊ References.
1. Davies NM. Clinical pharmacokinetics of tiaprofenic acid and its enantiomers. *Clin Pharmacokinet* 1996; **31:** 331–47.

Uses and Administration

Tiaprofenic acid, a propionic acid derivative, is an NSAID (p.65). It is used for the relief of pain and inflammation in musculoskeletal and joint disorders such as ankylosing spondylitis, osteoarthritis, and rheumatoid arthritis, in peri-articular disorders such as fibrositis and capsulitis, and in soft-tissue disorders such as sprains and strains. The usual dose by mouth is 600 mg daily given in 2 or 3 divided doses or once daily as a modified-release preparation. Tiaprofenic acid has also been given rectally. It has been given intramuscularly as the trometamol salt in acute conditions.

◊ References.
1. Plosker GL, Wagstaff AJ. Tiaprofenic acid: a reappraisal of its pharmacological properties and use in the management of rheumatic diseases. *Drugs* 1995; **50:** 1050–75.

Preparations

Proprietary Preparations (details are given in Part 3)
Austral.: Surgam; **Belg.:** Artiflam; Surgam; **Canad.:** Albert Tiafen; Surgam; **Denm.:** Surgamyl; **Fin.:** Surgamyl; **Fr.:** Flamirex; Flanid; Surgam; **Ger.:** Lindotabt†; Surgam; **Irl.:** Surgam; **Ital.:** Artroreuma; Suralgan; Surgamyl; Tiaprofen; Tiaprorex†; **Mex.:** Surdolin; Surgam; **Neth.:** Surgam; **NZ:** Surgam; **Port.:** Surgam; **S.Afr.:** Surgam; **Spain:** Derilate†; Surgamic; **Switz.:** Surgam†; **Thai.:** Anafen; Fengam; Gasam; Surgam; **UK:** Surgam.

Tiaramide Hydrochloride (2710-j)

Tiaramide Hydrochloride (BANM, USAN, rINNM).
NTA-194; Tiaperamide Hydrochloride. 5-Chloro-3-{2-[4-(2-hydroxyethyl)piperazin-1-yl]-2-oxoethyl}benzothiazolin-2-one hydrochloride.
$C_{15}H_{18}CIN_3O_3S,HCl = 392.3$.
$CAS — 32527-55-2$ (tiaramide); $35941-71-0$ (tiaramide hydrochloride).
Pharmacopoeias. In Jpn.

Tiaramide hydrochloride 110.3 mg is approximately equivalent to 100 mg of tiaramide.

Profile

Tiaramide hydrochloride is an NSAID (p.63) that has been given by mouth in usual doses equivalent to 100 mg of tiaramide up to three times daily for the relief of pain and inflammation.

Preparations

Proprietary Preparations (details are given in Part 3)
Jpn: Solantal.

Tilidate Hydrochloride (6262-z)

Tilidate Hydrochloride (BANM).
Tilidine Hydrochloride (USAN, pINNM); Gö 1261-C; W-5759A. (±)-Ethyl *trans*-2-dimethylamino-1-phenylcyclohex-3-ene-1-carboxylate hydrochloride hemihydrate.
$C_{17}H_{23}NO_2,HCl,\frac{1}{2}H_2O = 318.8$.
$CAS — 20380-58-9$ (tilidate); $27107-79-5$ (anhydrous tilidate hydrochloride); $24357-97-9$ (anhydrous +-trans-tilidate hydrochloride).

Dependence and Withdrawal

As for Opioid Analgesics in general, p.66.

Adverse Effects, Treatment, and Precautions

As for Opioid Analgesics in general, p.67.

Overdosage. Cyanosis, respiratory depression, and seizures developed in a 28-year-old woman after an overdose of a combination preparation of tilidate and naloxone.[1] The authors commented that the amount of naloxone in the preparation was insufficient to prevent respiratory depression after severe overdose, its intended role in such preparations being to prevent abuse.

1. Regenthal R, *et al.* Poisoning with tilidine and naloxone: toxicokinetic and clinical observations. *Hum Exp Toxicol* 1998; **17:** 593–7.

Porphyria. Tilidate has been associated with acute attacks of porphyria and is considered unsafe in porphyric patients.

Interactions

For interactions associated with opioid analgesics, see p.68.

Pharmacokinetics

Tilidate is absorbed from the gastrointestinal tract. It is metabolised and excreted in the urine mainly as metabolites nortilidate (nortilidine) and bisnortilidate (bisnortilidine). Nortilidate is responsible for the analgesic activity of tilidate.

◊ References.
1. Vollmer K-O, *et al.* Pharmacokinetics of tilidine and metabolites in man. *Arzneimittelforschung* 1989; **39:** 1283–8.

Uses and Administration

Tilidate hydrochloride is an opioid analgesic (p.68). It is used in the control of moderate to severe pain.
Tilidate hydrochloride may be given by intravenous, intramuscular, or subcutaneous injection in doses of up to 400 mg daily; usual doses as a suppository are 75 mg three or four times daily, or by mouth 50 mg four times daily. As a deterrent to abuse a

combined oral preparation of tilidate hydrochloride with naloxone hydrochloride is available in some countries.

Preparations

Proprietary Preparations (details are given in Part 3)
Belg.: Valoron; Valtran; **Ger.:** Findol N; Gruntin Tropfen; Tili; Tili-Puren; Tilicomp; Tilidalor; Tilidin comp; Tilidin N; Tilidin plus; Tilidin-saar; Tiligetic; Tilimerck; tilnalox; Valoron N; **S.Afr.:** Valoron; **Spain:** Tilitratet†; **Switz.:** Valoron.
Multi-ingredient: *Ger.:* Andolor; Nalidin.

Tinoridine Hydrochloride (2711-z)

Tinoridine Hydrochloride (rINNM).
Tienoridine Hydrochloride; Y-3642 (tinoridine). Ethyl 2-amino-6-benzyl-4,5,6,7-tetrahydrothieno[2,3-c]pyridine-3-carboxylate hydrochloride.
$C_{17}H_{20}N_2O_2S,HCl = 352.9$.
$CAS — 24237-54-5$ (tinoridine); $25913-34-2$ (tinoridine hydrochloride).

Profile

Tinoridine hydrochloride is an NSAID (p.63) that has been given for pain and inflammation.

Preparations

Proprietary Preparations (details are given in Part 3)
Jpn: Nonflamin†.

Tolfenamic Acid (2712-c)

Tolfenamic Acid (BAN, rINN).
Acidum Tolfenamicum. N-(3-Chloro-o-tolyl)anthranilic acid.
$C_{14}H_{12}CINO_2 = 261.7$.
$CAS — 13710-19-5$.
$ATC — M01AG02$.
Pharmacopoeias. In Eur. (see p.vi).

Pharmacopoeial description

Ph. Eur.: A white or slightly yellow crystalline powder. Practically insoluble in water; sparingly soluble in dehydrated alcohol and in dichloromethane; soluble in dimethylformamide. It dissolves in dilute solutions of alkali hydroxides. Protect from light.

Adverse Effects and Precautions

As for NSAIDs in general, p.63. Dysuria, most commonly in males and probably due to local irritation of the urethra by a metabolite, has been reported. Tremor, euphoria, and fatigue have also occurred.

Effects on the lungs. Pulmonary infiltration has been associated with tolfenamic acid treatment in 6 patients.[1]

1. Strömberg C, *et al.* Pulmonary infiltrations induced by tolfenamic acid. *Lancet* 1987; **ii:** 685.

Interactions

For interactions associated with NSAIDs, see p.65.

Pharmacokinetics

Tolfenamic acid is readily absorbed from the gastrointestinal tract. Peak plasma concentrations are reached about 60 to 90 minutes after administration of the tablets. Tolfenamic acid is about 99% bound to plasma proteins. The plasma half-life is about 2 hours. Tolfenamic acid is metabolised in the liver; the metabolites and unchanged drug are conjugated with glucuronic acid. About 90% of an ingested dose is excreted in the urine and the remainder in the faeces.

Uses and Administration

Tolfenamic acid, an anthranilic acid derivative related to mefenamic acid (p.51), is an NSAID (p.65). In the treatment of acute attacks of migraine tolfenamic acid is given in a usual dose of 200 mg by mouth when the first symptoms appear; if a satisfactory response is not obtained this dose may be repeated once after 1 to 2 hours. Tolfenamic acid has also been given for the relief of mild to moderate pain in disorders such as dysmenorrhoea, rheumatoid arthritis, or osteoarthritis in doses of 100 to 200 mg three times daily.

Preparations

Proprietary Preparations (details are given in Part 3)
Aust.: Clotam; **Braz.:** Clotam; **Denm.:** Clotam; Migea; **Fin.:** Clotam; Migea; **Mex.:** Bifenac; Flocur; **Neth.:** Rociclyn; **Switz.:** Clotam; **UK:** Clotam.

Tolmetin Sodium (2713-k)

Tolmetin Sodium (BANM, USAN, rINNM).
McN-2559-21-98; McN-2559 (tolmetin). Sodium (1-methyl-5-p-toluoylpyrrol-2-yl)acetate dihydrate.
$C_{15}H_{14}NNaO_3,2H_2O = 315.3$.
$CAS — 26171-23-3$ (tolmetin); $35711-34-3$ (anhydrous tolmetin sodium); $64490-92-2$ (tolmetin sodium dihydrate).
Pharmacopoeias. In US.

Pharmacopoeial description

USP 25: A light yellow to light orange crystalline powder. Freely soluble in water and in methyl alcohol; slightly soluble in alcohol; very slightly soluble in chloroform.

Adverse Effects and Precautions

As for NSAIDs in general, p.63.

Effects on the blood. Case reports of agranulocytosis[1] and thrombocytopenia[2] associated with tolmetin.

1. Sakai J, Joseph MW. Tolmetin and agranulocytosis. *N Engl J Med* 1978; **298:** 1203.
2. Lockhart JM. Tolmetin-induced thrombocytopenia. *Arthritis Rheum* 1982; **25:** 1144–5.

Effects on the CNS. See under Hypersensitivity, below.

Effects on the gastrointestinal tract. Erosive oesophagitis has been reported[1] in an 11-year-old child following ingestion of a dose of tolmetin while lying down and without drinking any water.

1. Palop V, *et al.* Tolmetin-induced esophageal ulceration. *Ann Pharmacother* 1997; **31:** 929.

Effects on the kidneys. Interstitial nephritis[1] and nephrotic syndrome[2,3] have been reported in patients given tolmetin.

1. Katz SM, *et al.* Tolmetin: association with reversible renal failure and acute interstitial nephritis. *JAMA* 1981; **246:** 243–5.
2. Chatterjee GP. Nephrotic syndrome induced by tolmetin. *JAMA* 1981; **246:** 1589.
3. Tietjen DP. Recurrence and specificity of nephrotic syndrome due to tolmetin. *Am J Med* 1989; **87:** 354–5.

Hypersensitivity. Anaphylactic shock,[1] urticaria and angioedema,[2] and aseptic meningitis[3] are among the hypersensitivity reactions reported in patients taking tolmetin.

1. Rossi AC, Knapp DE. Tolmetin-induced anaphylactoid reactions. *N Engl J Med* 1982; **307:** 499–500.
2. Ponte CD, Wisman R. Tolmetin-induced urticaria/angioedema. *Drug Intell Clin Pharm* 1985; **19:** 479–80.
3. Ruppert GB, Barth WF. Tolmetin-induced aseptic meningitis. *JAMA* 1981; **245:** 67–8.

Interactions

For interactions associated with NSAIDs, see p.65.

Pharmacokinetics

Tolmetin is almost completely absorbed from the gastrointestinal tract and peak plasma concentrations are attained about 30 to 60 minutes after ingestion. It is extensively bound to plasma proteins (over 99%) and has a biphasic plasma half-life of about 1 to 2 hours and 5 hours respectively. Tolmetin penetrates synovial fluid and very small amounts are distributed into breast milk. It is excreted in the urine as an inactive dicarboxylic acid metabolite and its glucuronide and as tolmetin glucuronide with small amounts of unchanged drug.

Uses and Administration

Tolmetin sodium is an NSAID (p.65). It is used in musculoskeletal and joint disorders such as osteoarthritis and rheumatoid arthritis, including juvenile idiopathic arthritis. For the treatment of rheumatoid arthritis and osteoarthritis, the usual initial dose in adults is the equivalent of 400 mg of tolmetin three times daily by mouth; maintenance doses of 600 mg to a maximum of 1800 mg daily in divided doses have been used. For the treatment of juvenile idiopathic arthritis in children aged 2 years and over it is given in usual initial doses equivalent to 20 mg of tolmetin per kg body-weight daily in divided doses; maintenance doses of 15 mg to a maximum of 30 mg per kg daily have been used.

Tolmetin has been used as the free acid in similar doses rectally, and has been applied as a 5% topical gel.

Preparations

USP 25: Tolmetin Sodium Capsules; Tolmetin Sodium Tablets.

Proprietary Preparations (details are given in Part 3)
Aust.: Tolectin; *Belg.:* Tolectin; *Canad.:* Tolectin; *Denm.:* Tolectin; *Irl.:* Tolectin†; *Ital.:* Tolectin†; *Mex.:* Tolectin; *Neth.:* Tolectin; *S.Afr.:* Tolectin†; *Spain:* Artrocaptin; *Switz.:* Tolectin; *UK:* Tolectin†; *USA:* Tolectin.

Tramadol Hydrochloride (6263-c)

Tramadol Hydrochloride (BANM, USAN, rINNM).
CG-315; CG-315E; U-26225A. (±)-*trans*-2-Dimethylaminomethyl-1-(3-methoxyphenyl)cyclohexanol hydrochloride.
$C_{16}H_{25}NO_2,HCl = 299.8$.
CAS — 27203-92-5 (tramadol); 22204-88-2 (tramadol hydrochloride); 36282-47-0 (tramadol hydrochloride).

Incompatibilities. An injection of tramadol hydrochloride 50 mg per mL is reported to be incompatible with injections of diazepam, diclofenac sodium, indometacin, midazolam, and piroxicam if mixed in the same syringe.

Dependence and Withdrawal

As for Opioid Analgesics, p.66. Tramadol may have lower potential for producing dependence than morphine.

◊ The UK Committee on Safety of Medicines[1] commented in October 1996 that since June 1994 they had received reports of drug dependence in 5 patients and withdrawal symptoms associated with tramadol in 28 patients, which corresponded to a reporting rate of about 1 in 6000. Doses in excess of the recommended maximum of 400 mg daily had been taken by 5 of the patients. The duration of treatment before onset of these effects ranged from 10 to 409 days (average 3 months). Withdrawal symptoms reported were typically those of opioid withdrawal in general.

1. Committee on Safety of Medicines/Medicines Control Agency. Tramadol—(Zydol, Tramake and Zamadol). *Current Problems* 1996; **22:** 11.

Adverse Effects and Treatment

As for Opioid Analgesics in general, p.67. Tramadol may produce fewer typical opioid adverse effects such as respiratory depression and constipation.

In addition to hypotension, hypertension has occasionally occurred. Anaphylaxis, hallucinations, and confusion have also been reported.

Effects on the CNS. The UK Committee on Safety of Medicines (CSM)[1] commented in February 1995 that since June 1994 they had received reports of 15 patients who had experienced confusion and/or hallucinations while taking tramadol. The majority of the reactions developed 1 to 7 days after starting treatment and in most patients resolved rapidly on withdrawal. It was noted that psychiatric reactions comprised about 10% of all reactions reported with tramadol. In a later comment[2] in October 1996, the CSM noted that 27 reports of convulsions and one of worsening epilepsy had been received, which corresponded to a reporting rate of about 1 in 7000. Of the 5 patients receiving intravenous tramadol, 2 had been given doses well in excess of those recommended (equivalent to 1.45 and 4 g daily). Of the patients receiving oral tramadol, the majority were taking other drugs, including tricyclic antidepressants and SSRIs. A similar pattern was reported by the FDA[3] in the USA: of 124 cases of seizures reported from March 1995 to July 1996, 30 suggested doses taken in excess of the recommended 400 mg or at shorter time intervals than those recommended, and in 72 cases drugs with the potential to lower the seizure threshold, including SSRIs and tricyclic antidepressants, had been taken.

A debilitating CNS-mediated reaction to an initial dose of tramadol has been described in a patient.[4] Symptoms, which lasted approximately 4 hours, included ataxia, dilatation of the pupils, numbness in all limbs, tremulousness, and dysphoria. Although the exact mechanism of the reaction is not known, it was suggested that since the patient was an extensive metaboliser with very high activity of the cytochrome P450 isoenzyme CYP2D6, high concentrations of the active *O*-desmethyl metabolite were the cause. The patient recovered with no sequelae.

1. Committee on Safety of Medicines/Medicines Control Agency. Tramadol (Zydol)—psychiatric reactions. *Current Problems* 1995; **21:** 2.
2. Committee on Safety of Medicines/Medicines Control Agency. Tramadol—(Zydol, Tramake and Zamadol). *Current Problems* 1996; **22:** 11.
3. Kahn LH, *et al.* Seizures reported with tramadol. *JAMA* 1997; **278:** 1661.
4. Gleason PP, *et al.* Debilitating reaction following the initial dose of tramadol. *Ann Pharmacother* 1997; **31:** 1150–2.

Effects on the respiratory system. Respiratory depression has been reported after tramadol infusion anaesthesia,[1] although in a postoperative study[2] tramadol had no significant respiratory depressant effect when equianalgesic doses of morphine, pentazocine, pethidine, piritramide, and tramadol were compared.

1. Paravicini D, *et al.* Tramadol-infusionsanaesthesie mit Substitution von Enfluran und differenten Lachgaskonzentrationen. *Anaesthesist* 1985; **34:** 20–7.
2. Fechner R, *et al.* Clinical investigations on the effect of morphine, pentazocine, pethidine, piritramide and tramadol on respiration. *Anasth Intensivmed* 1985; **26:** 126–32.

Precautions

As for Opioid Analgesics in general, p.68.

Tramadol should be used with caution in patients with renal or liver impairment and should be avoided if renal impairment is severe. Removal by haemodialysis is reported to be very slow.

Tramadol should be used with care in patients with a history of epilepsy or those susceptible to seizures. See also Effects on the CNS under Adverse Effects, above.

Anaesthesia. The manufacturers warn against using tramadol during very light planes of general anaesthesia because of possible intra-operative awareness, although it may be used intra-operatively provided anaesthesia is maintained by the continuous administration of a potent volatile or intravenous anaesthetic. Intra-operative awareness was reported in 65% of a group of 20 patients when used to provide analgesia during light general anaesthesia with nitrous oxide and intermittent enflurane.[1] However, in a study[2] of 51 patients given tramadol during stable light continuous isoflurane-nitrous oxide anaesthesia there was no clinically significant lightening of anaesthesia. Budd[3] had commented that during extensive use of tramadol intra-operatively over several years, there had not been any incidence of recall in any patient treated at their clinic.

1. Lehmann KA, *et al.* Zur Bedeutung von Tramadol als intraoperativem Analgetikum: eine randomisierte Doppelblindstudie im Vergleich zu Placebo. *Der Anaesthetist* 1985; **34:** 11–19.
2. Coetzee JF, *et al.* Effect of tramadol on depth of anaesthesia. *Br J Anaesth* 1996; **76:** 415–18.
3. Budd K. Tramadol. *Br J Anaesth* 1995; **75:** 500.

Interactions

For interactions associated with opioid analgesics, see p.68.

Carbamazepine is reported to diminish the analgesic activity of tramadol by reducing serum concentrations.

The risk of seizures is increased if tramadol is administered concomitantly with other drugs that have the potential to lower the seizure threshold. See also under Effects on the CNS under Adverse Effects, above.

Tramadol inhibits reuptake of noradrenaline and serotonin and enhances serotonin release and there is the possibility that it may interact with other drugs that enhance monoaminergic neurotransmission including lithium, tricyclic antidepressants, and selective serotonin reuptake inhibitors; it should not be given to patients receiving MAOIs or within 14 days of their discontinuation.

◊ Metabolism of tramadol is mediated by the cytochrome P450 isoenzyme CYP2D6. Concomitant administration with specific inhibitors of this enzyme, such as *quinidine*, may increase concentrations of tramadol and lower concentrations of its active metabolite but the clinical consequences of this effect are unclear.

Anticoagulants. Tramadol is reported to have potentiated the anticoagulant effect of *phenprocoumon* and of *warfarin*.[1,2] However, a randomised, double-blind, placebo-controlled study[3] in 19 patients failed to find evidence of an interaction between phenprocoumon and tramadol.

1. Scher ML, *et al.* Potential interaction between tramadol and warfarin. *Ann Pharmacother* 1997; **31:** 646–7.
2. Jensen K. Interaktion mellem tramadol og orale antikoagulantia. *Ugeskr Laeger* 1997; **159:** 785–6.
3. Boeijinga JK, *et al.* Lack of interaction between tramadol and coumarins. *J Clin Pharmacol* 1998; **38:** 966–70.

Antidepressants. For reference to a possible case of serotonin syndrome associated with concomitant administration of tramadol and *sertraline*, see under Fluoxetine, p.287.

Pharmacokinetics

Tramadol is readily absorbed following oral administration but is subject to first-pass metabolism. Tramadol is metabolised by *N*- and *O*-demethylation and glucuronidation or sulfation in the liver. The metabolite *O*-desmethyltramadol is pharmacologically active. Tramadol is excreted mainly in the urine predominantly as metabolites. Tramadol is widely distributed, crosses the placenta, and appears in small amounts in breast milk. The elimination half-life following oral administration is about 6 hours.

Metabolism. Production of the active metabolite *O*-desmethyltramadol is dependent on the cytochrome P450 isoenzyme CYP2D6, which exhibits genetic polymorphism.[1] For a reference to a debilitating CNS-mediated reaction in a patient who was an extensive metaboliser with high CYP2D6 activity, see under Effects on the CNS in Adverse Effects, above.

1. Poulsen L, *et al.* The hypoalgesic effect of tramadol in relation to CYP2D6. *Clin Pharmacol Ther* 1996; **60:** 636–44.

Uses and Administration

Tramadol hydrochloride is an opioid analgesic (p.68). It also has noradrenergic and serotonergic properties that may contribute to its analgesic activity. Tramadol is used for moderate to severe pain.

Tramadol hydrochloride is given by mouth, intravenously, or rectally as a suppository. The intramuscular route has also been used. It may also be given by infusion or as part of a patient-controlled analgesia system. Usual doses by mouth are 50 to 100 mg every 4 to 6 hours. Tramadol hydrochloride may also be given orally as a modified-release preparation once or twice daily. The total daily dosage by mouth should not exceed 400 mg.

A dose of 50 to 100 mg may be given every 4 to 6 hours by intravenous injection over 2 to 3 minutes, or by intravenous infusion. For the treatment of postoperative pain, the initial dose is 100 mg followed by 50 mg every 10 to 20 minutes if necessary to a total maximum (including the initial dose) of 250 mg in the first hour. Thereafter, doses are 50 to 100 mg every 4 to 6 hours up to a total daily dose of 600 mg.

Rectal doses by suppository are 100 mg up to 4 times daily.

The dosage interval should be increased to 12 hours in patients with a creatinine clearance less than 30 mL per minute; in the USA the manufacturers suggest that the maximum dose by mouth should not exceed 200 mg daily in these patients. Tramadol should not be given to patients with severe renal impairment (creatinine clearance less than 10 mL per minute). A dosage interval of 12 hours is also recommended in severe hepatic impairment.

◊ References.

1. Anonymous. Tramadol—a new analgesic. *Drug Ther Bull* 1994; **32:** 85–6. Correction. *ibid.:* 96.
2. Radbruch L, *et al.* A risk-benefit assessment of tramadol in the management of pain. *Drug Safety* 1996; **15:** 8–29.
3. Lewis KS, Han NH. Tramadol: a new centrally acting analgesic. *Am J Health-Syst Pharm* 1997; **54:** 643–52.
4. Duthie DJR. Remifentanil and tramadol. *Br J Anaesth* 1998; **81:** 51–7.
5. Budd K, Langford R. Tramadol revisited. *Br J Anaesth* 1999; **82:** 493–5.
6. Scott LJ, Perry CM. Tramadol: a review of its use in perioperative pain. *Drugs* 2000; **60:** 139–76.

Preparations

Proprietary Preparations (details are given in Part 3)
Aust.: Nobligan†; Nycodol; Tradolan; Tramabene; Tramal; Tramundal; *Austral.:* Tramal; *Belg.:* Contramal; Dolzam; Tradonal; *Braz.:* Sylador; Tramal; *Denm.:* Dolol; Mandolgin; Nobligan; Tradolan; *Fin.:* Tramadin; Tramol; *Fr.:* Biodalgic; Contramal; Predalgic; Topalgic; Tradol; Zamudol; Zumalgic; *Ger.:* Amadol; Tradol; Trama; Trama-Dorsch; Tramabeta; Tramadol-Dolgit; Tramadolor; Tramadura; Tramagetic; Tramagit; Tramal; Tramamerck; Tramedphano†; Tramundin; *Hong Kong:* Mabron; Tramal; Tramo; *Irl.:* Tradol; Tramake; Tramex; Zydol; *Israel:* Trabar; Tra-

madex; *Ital.*: Contramal; Fortradol; Fraxidol; Prontalgin; Tradonal; *Mex.*: Nobligan; Prontofort; Tradol; *Neth.*: Theradol; Tramagetic; Tramal; *Norw.*: Nobligan; *NZ*: Tramal; *Port.*: Paxilfar; Tramal; Travex; *S.Afr.*: Tramal; *Singapore*: Mabron; Pengesic; Sefmal; Tradol; Tramal; *Spain*: Adolonta; Tioner; Tradonal; Tralgiol; *Swed.*: Nobligan; Tiparol; Tradolan; *Switz.*: Tramadolor†; Tramal; *Thai.*: Anadol; Mabron; Madol; Madola; Sefmal; Tradonal; Tramal; Tramalan; Tramamed; Tramoda; Trosic; Volcidol-S; *UK*: Dromadol; Tramake; Zamadol; Zydol; *USA*: Ultram.

Multi-ingredient: *USA*: Ultracet.

Trolamine Salicylate   (9593-l)

Trolamine Salicylate (*pINNM*).

Triethanolamine Salicylate.

$C_{13}H_{21}NO_6 = 287.3$.
CAS — 2174-16-5.
Pharmacopoeias. In US.

Pharmacopoeial description

USP 25: A compounded mixture of trolamine and salicylic acid in propylene glycol. pH of a 5% solution in water is between 6.5 and 7.5. Store in airtight containers in a cool place.

Profile

Trolamine salicylate is a salicylic acid derivative used similarly to methyl salicylate (p.55) in topical rubefacient preparations in a concentration of 10 to 20% for the relief of muscular and rheumatic pain. It has also been used as a sunscreen.

◊ In contrast to methyl salicylate, which undergoes considerable absorption and produces high subcutaneous and dermal concentrations of salicylic acid after application to intact skin, concentrations of salicylic acid after topical application of trolamine salicylate were substantially lower in tissue[1] and undetectable in serum.[2]

1. Cross SE, *et al.* Is there tissue penetration after application of topical salicylate formulations? *Lancet* 1997; **350**: 636.
2. Morra P, *et al.* Serum concentrations of salicylic acid following topically applied salicylate derivatives. *Ann Pharmacother* 1996; **30**: 935–40.

Preparations

Proprietary Preparations (details are given in Part 3)
Austral.: Dencorub Arthritis; Goanna Arthritis Cream; Metsal AR Analgesic; *Canad.*: Antiphlogistine Rub A-535 No Odour; Aspercreme; Ben-Gay No Odor; Miosal; Myoflex; Royflex; *Mex.*: Myoflex; *Spain*: Bexidermil; Topicrem; *USA*: Analgesia Creme; Aspercreme; Coppertone Tan Magnifier; Mobisyl; Myoflex; Progesic†; Sportscreme; Tropical Blend Tan Magnifier.

Multi-ingredient: *Austral.*: Metsal Analgesic; *Canad.*: Ease Pain Away†; Myoflex Ice Plus.

Ufenamate   (3654-q)

Ufenamate (*rINN*).

Butyl Flufenamate. Butyl *N*-(α,α,α-trifluoro-*m*-tolyl)anthranilate.

$C_{18}H_{18}F_3NO_2 = 337.3$.
CAS — 67330-25-0.

Profile

Ufenamate is an NSAID (p.63) that has been used topically in inflammatory skin disorders.

Preparations

Proprietary Preparations (details are given in Part 3)
Jpn: Fenazol†.

Valdecoxib   (20242-a)

Valdecoxib (*USAN, rINN*).

SC-65872.   *p*-(5-Methyl-3-phenyl-4-isoxazolyl)benzenesulfonamide.

$C_{16}H_{14}N_2O_3S = 314.4$.
CAS — 181695-72-7.

Profile

Valdecoxib is an NSAID (p.63) reported to be a selective inhibitor of cyclo-oxygenase-2 (COX-2). It is given by mouth in the treatment of osteoarthritis and rheumatoid arthritis in doses of 10 mg daily, and for the pain of dysmenorrhoea in doses of 20 mg twice daily.

Preparations

Proprietary Preparations (details are given in Part 3)
USA: Bextra.

Vedaprofen   (17861-c)

Vedaprofen (*BAN, USAN, rINN*).

CERM-10202; PM-150. (±)-4-Cyclohexyl-α-methyl-1-naphthaleneacetic acid.

$C_{19}H_{22}O_2 = 282.4$.
CAS — 71109-09-6.

Profile

Vedaprofen, a propionic acid derivative, is an NSAID used in veterinary medicine for the treatment of inflammation and pain.

Viminol Hydroxybenzoate   (2715-t)

Viminol Hydroxybenzoate (*rINNM*).

Diviminol Hydroxybenzoate; Z-424 (viminol). 1-[1-(2-Chlorobenzyl)pyrrol-2-yl]-2-(di-*sec*-butyl)aminoethanol 4-hydroxybenzoate.

$C_{21}H_{31}ClN_2O,C_7H_6O_3 = 501.1$.
CAS — 21363-18-8 (viminol); 21466-60-4; 23784-10-3 (both viminol hydroxybenzoate).

Profile

Viminol hydroxybenzoate has analgesic and antipyretic properties. The equivalent of 400 mg of viminol has been given daily in divided doses by mouth.

Preparations

Proprietary Preparations (details are given in Part 3)
Ital.: Dividol.

Zaltoprofen   (3052-b)

Zaltoprofen (*rINN*).

CN-100. (±)-10,11-Dihydro-α-methyl-10-oxodibenzo[*b,f*]thiepin-2-acetic acid.

$C_{17}H_{14}O_3S = 298.4$.
CAS — 89482-00-8.

Profile

Zaltoprofen is an NSAID (p.63) which has been given by mouth for musculoskeletal and joint disorders.

◊ **References.**

1. Ishizaki T, *et al.* Pharmacokinetic profile of a new nonsteroidal anti-inflammatory agent, CN-100, in humans. *Drug Invest* 1991; **3**: 1–7.
2. Hatori M, Kokubun S. The long-term efficacy and tolerability of the new anti-inflammatory agent zaltoprofen in rheumatoid arthritis. *Curr Med Res Opin* 1998; **14**: 79–87.

Ziconotide   (20097-h)

Ziconotide (*USAN, rINN*).

SNX-111.   L-Cysteinyl-L-lysylglycyl-L-lysylglycl-L-alanyl-L-lysyl-L-cysteinyl-L-seryl-L-arginyl-L-leucyl-L-methionyl-L-tyrosyl-L-α-aspartyl-L-cysteinyl-L-cysteinyl-L-threonylglycyl-L-seryl-L-cysteinyl-L-arginyl-L-serylglycyl-L-lysyl-L-cysteinamide   cyclic(1→16),(8→20),(15→25)-tris(disulfide).

$C_{102}H_{172}N_{36}O_{32}S_7 = 2639.1$.
CAS — 107452-89-1.

Profile

Ziconotide is a peptide derived from sea snails. It is reported to be a neurone-specific calcium antagonist and is being studied in the management of various types of pain, including neuropathic pain, and in other conditions such as head trauma.

Anthelmintics

This chapter describes the important helminth or worm infections that occur in man (see Table, p.92) and the anthelmintics used to treat them.

Choice of Anthelmintic

Helminth infections are among the most common infections in man, affecting a large proportion of the world's population, mainly in tropical regions. In developing countries they pose a large threat to public health, and contribute to the prevalence of malnutrition, anaemia, eosinophilia, and pneumonia. Helminth infections causing severe morbidity include lymphatic filariasis (a cause of elephantiasis), onchocerciasis (river blindness), and schistosomiasis. These infections can affect the majority of populations in endemic areas with major economic and social consequences. WHO is making strenuous efforts to control a number of these infections in endemic areas. Control of these infections in both individuals and populations depends not only on the use of chemotherapeutic agents but also on preventing transmission by advice on food preparation and hygiene, the provision of adequate sanitation and sewage treatment (especially where sewage is used as fertiliser), the provision of safe potable water supplies, and effective vector control.

The worms that cause infection in man generally fall either into the phylum Platyhelminthes, which includes the cestodes or tapeworms and the trematodes or flukes, or into the phylum Nematoda which includes the nematodes or roundworms.

The **cestodes** (flatworms, segmented worms, or tapeworms) cause infection in man in most parts of the world. Man may be the definitive host and harbour the adult worm in the intestine or an intermediate host carrying the larval form. With the exception of *Hymenolepis nana* the adult worms do not usually multiply within the same host. However, larval forms may be produced and, as with infection or ingestion of these forms, systemic infection may develop.

Cestode infections include:

• cysticercosis
• diphyllobothriasis
• echinococcosis
• hymenolepiasis
• taeniasis.

The **nematodes** (or roundworms) represent a large group of worms, some of which are capable of producing infections in man. In many cases man is the primary (definitive) host but human infections caused by parasites for which animals are the primary hosts also occur. Nematodes do not generally multiply in man; strongyloidiasis is an exception as re-infection can occur without environmental re-exposure. Nematode infections are most common in warm, moist climates but some species of nematode can tolerate cool or arid conditions and infective forms can persist in the environment for long periods. An understanding of the life cycle of the infective species is necessary for diagnostic tests to be made at appropriate times, usually to coincide with the infective stage of the cycle, and for the choice of appropriate control measures.

The nematode infections can be divided into filarial infections, intestinal infections, and tissue infections. *Filarial nematodes* are endemic in large areas of the tropics and produce considerable morbidity. The adult worms may live for several years releasing large numbers of motile embryos known as microfilariae into the blood or skin, depending on the species. Transmission is usually by biting insects which form the intermediate host. In some endemic areas multiple infections with filarial nematodes are common.

Filarial nematode infections include:

• loiasis
• lymphatic filariasis
• mansonella infections
• onchocerciasis.

Intestinal nematode infections (roundworms) are very common especially in developing countries in the tropics and subtropics. Children are particularly at risk and these infections contribute to morbidity through malnutrition, vitamin deficiencies, diarrhoea, anaemia, and pneumonia. Poor sanitation and sewage disposal perpetuate infections with soil-borne nematodes. Several different worm infections may often be endemic in the same part of the world, resulting in mixed infections. When that occurs broad-spectrum anthelmintics may be used to reduce the overall infection burden in the population (see under Ascariasis, below).

Intestinal nematode infections include:

• angiostrongyliasis
• ascariasis
• capillariasis
• enterobiasis
• hookworm infections
• strongyloidiasis
• trichostrongyliasis
• trichuriasis.

The *tissue nematodes* represent a miscellaneous group causing a variety of pathological conditions in man. In cutaneous larva migrans and toxocariasis the nematodes have a primary animal host and the human disease is caused by infection with infective larvae which do not subsequently mature in man. Trichinosis and gnathostomiasis affect a number of carnivorous animals and man is an incidental host. Syngamosis is primarily an infection of domestic fowl and wild birds although infection in man has been reported rarely. In dracunculiasis man is the primary (definitive) host. Although these diseases are not generally fatal they cause a considerable degree of morbidity and treatment is complicated by the lack of effective, non-toxic systemic anthelmintics.

Tissue nematode infections include:

• angiostrongyliasis
• cutaneous larva migrans
• dracunculiasis
• gnathostomiasis
• syngamosis
• toxocariasis
• trichinosis.

Trematode (or fluke) infections are caused by parasitic worms of the class Trematoda. There are 4 categories of fluke which are pathogenic in man; the blood flukes *Schistosoma* spp., the intestinal flukes *Fasciolopsis, Heterophyes, Metagonimus,* and *Nanophyetus* spp., the liver flukes *Clonorchis, Fasciola,* and *Opisthorchis* spp., and the lung flukes *Paragonimus* spp. Symptoms are usually only seen in heavy infections and commonly include fever, pain, and eosinophilia.

Trematode infections include:

• intestinal fluke infections
• liver fluke infections
• lung fluke infections
• schistosomiasis.

Ancylostomiasis

See under Hookworm Infections, below. Larvae of *Ancylostoma* spp. are also a cause of cutaneous larva migrans (see below).

Angiostrongyliasis

Two forms of angiostrongyliasis are recognised and both are due to accidental infection with species of the animal nematode *Angiostrongylus*.

Infection with the larvae of the rat lungworm *A. cantonensis* causes an eosinophilic meningoencephalitis. Transmission follows ingestion of raw or undercooked snails or crustaceans or contaminated vegetables. The disease is generally self-limiting. Treatment with mebendazole has been suggested but severe host reaction to the dying larvae may result.

Intestinal infection with *A. costaricensis* can cause eosinophilic gastro-enteritis. It most commonly occurs in children following ingestion of vegetables contaminated by infected slugs. Surgical resection of the affected bowel may be necessary but treatment with mebendazole or tiabendazole has been suggested.

Ascariasis

Ascariasis is an infection caused by *Ascaris lumbricoides*, the common roundworm or giant roundworm. The term roundworm is also applied to nematodes in general. It is usually an infection of the small intestine but on rare occasions there may be severe ectopic infections. It is commonly found in the tropics and especially in rural areas. Eggs are excreted in the faeces and can remain viable in moist soil for several years. On ingestion of mature eggs the larvae hatch and penetrate the intestinal wall. They migrate in the blood stream via the liver to the lungs where they enter the alveoli. The larvae then move up the bronchial tree and are swallowed. The mature adult develops in the intestines, and it has been estimated that a gravid female is produced about 2 months after infection. The life span of the adult worm is 1 to 2 years. Ascariasis may be asymptomatic. When symptoms of intestinal infection do occur they include anorexia, abdominal pain, and diarrhoea; nutritional deficiency may result. The pulmonary stage may cause pneumonitis and bronchospasm often accompanied by eosinophilia. Heavy infections can cause intestinal or biliary obstruction. Migration of the worm from the small intestine can produce ectopic infection of the genito-urinary tract, lungs, liver, or heart. Such infections are rare but serious.

Children are at greatest risk of *Ascaris* infection and a study[1] has suggested that child-targeted treatment can be more cost effective in reducing disease cases than programmes of mass chemotherapy in areas where infection is endemic.

Treatment is with a benzimidazole carbamate derivative such as albendazole or mebendazole with both drugs being equally highly effective. Pyrantel embonate is an al-

Table 1. Helminths: classification and diseases.

Group	Helminth	Common Name	Clinical infection
Cestodes (tapeworms)	*Diphyllobothrium latum*	broad fish tapeworm	diphyllobothriasis
	Echinococcus spp.		echinococcosis (hydatid disease)
	Hymenolepis nana	dwarf tapeworm	hymenolepiasis
	*Taenia saginata**	beef tapeworm	taeniasis
	*Taenia solium**	pork tapeworm	cysticercosis (larval form), taeniasis (adult worm)
Nematodes (filarial)	*Brugia malayi*		lymphatic filariasis (Malayan, brugian)
	Brugia timori		lymphatic filariasis (Timorian, brugian)
	Loa loa	eye-worm	loiasis
	Mansonella spp.		Mansonella infections
	Onchocerca volvulus		onchocerciasis (river blindness)
	Wuchereria bancrofti		lymphatic filariasis (bancroftian)
Nematodes (intestinal)	*Ancylostoma duodenale*	Old World hookworm	ancylostomiasis
	Angiostrongylus costaricensis		angiostrongyliasis
	*Ascaris lumbricoides**	common roundworm, giant roundworm	ascariasis
	Capillaria philippinensis		capillariasis
	*Enterobius vermicularis**	threadworm, pinworm	enterobiasis
	Necator americanus	New World hookworm	necatoriasis
	Strongyloides stercoralis	sometimes called threadworm in USA	strongyloidiasis
	Trichostrongylus spp.		trichostrongyliasis
	*Trichuris trichiura**	whipworm	trichuriasis
Nematodes (tissue)	*Ancylostoma* spp.	dog/cat hookworm	cutaneous larva migrans (creeping eruption)
	Angiostrongylus cantonensis		angiostrongyliasis
	Dracunculus medinensis	guinea-worm	dracunculiasis (dracontiasis)
	Gnathostoma spinigerum		gnathostomiasis
	Syngamus spp.	gapeworm	syngamosis
	Toxocara spp.*		toxocariasis (visceral larva migrans, ocular larva migrans)
	*Trichinella spiralis**		trichinosis (trichinellosis)
Trematodes (flukes)	*Clonorchis sinensis*	Chinese liver fluke	clonorchiasis
	Fasciola hepatica	liver fluke	fascioliasis
	Fasciolopsis buski	intestinal fluke	fasciolopsiasis
	Heterophyes heterophyes	intestinal fluke	heterophyiasis
	Metagonimus yokogawi	intestinal fluke	metagonimiasis
	Nanophyetus salmincola	intestinal fluke	nanophyetiasis
	Opisthorchis spp.	liver fluke	opisthorchiasis
	Paragonimus spp.	oriental lung fluke	paragonimiasis
	Schistosoma spp.	blood fluke	schistosomiasis

NOTE: Infections due to worms marked with an asterisk may occur in temperate climates. Infections due to other worms are generally limited to tropical or localised areas, but may occur in travellers who have visited those areas.

ternative. Such broad-spectrum therapy can be useful if the patient is suffering from a mixed intestinal nematode infection. Drugs such as tiabendazole with little or no activity against *Ascaris* should be avoided for the initial treatment of mixed infections since they may stimulate the worm to migrate to a different body site. Other anthelmintics effective in ascariasis include levamisole and piperazine salts.

1. Guyatt HL, *et al.* Control of Ascaris infection by chemotherapy: which is the most cost-effective option? *Trans R Soc Trop Med Hyg* 1995; **89:** 16–20.

Capillariasis
Capillariasis is caused by infection with *Capillaria philippinensis*, a nematode endemic in the Philippines and southern Thailand. Infection in man is through eating raw or undercooked freshwater fish containing infective larvae. The larvae mature in the intestines and the adults produce both eggs and infective larvae so that auto-infection occurs and heavy infections can result. Symptoms are mostly gastrointestinal, with abdominal pain, vomiting, and severe prolonged diarrhoea leading to cachexia and muscle wasting. The infection has a mortality rate of between 20 and 30% if untreated. Prolonged treatment with mebendazole or, alternatively, albendazole, is necessary.

Clonorchiasis
See under Liver Fluke Infections, below.

Cutaneous larva migrans
Cutaneous larva migrans (creeping eruption) occurs when man becomes infected with the larvae of animal hookworms, usually *Ancylostoma braziliense* or *A. caninum*, hookworms of cats and dogs. Other hookworms may also be involved or may cause other infections (see Hookworm Infections, below). The larvae penetrate the skin and then migrate causing characteristic trails in the skin. This migration can persist for several months and can be a source of intense pruritus. Occasionally larvae migrate to the lungs causing eosinophilia and pulmonary symptoms. Tiabendazole given by mouth or applied topically is the standard treatment although albendazole and ivermectin are possible alternatives.

Infection with *Gnathostoma spinigerum* or *Strongyloides stercoralis* can also cause cutaneous larva migrans (see Gnathostomiasis and Strongyloidiasis, below). Ocular and visceral larva migrans are features of toxocariasis (see below).

References.

1. Rodilla F, *et al.* Current treatment recommendations for cutaneous larva migrans. *Ann Pharmacother* 1994; **28:** 672–3.

Cysticercosis
Cysticercosis is a systemic infection caused by the larval form (cysticercus) of *Taenia solium*. Infection is acquired through ingestion of eggs in contaminated food or water, or directly from individuals harbouring the adult worm. The eggs hatch in the intestine and the larvae spread systemically to almost any body tissue. Invasion of the brain is known as neurocysticercosis and is a common cause of epilepsy in endemic areas. The most effective treatment for neurocysticercosis has been debated.[1] In the absence of large randomised studies, opinion have been divided over whether cysticidal drugs should be given routinely in neurocysticercosis or reserved for selected patients.[1] Some have suggested that they might be associated with long-term sequelae,[2] and have reiterated that the ideal solution is prevention by ensuring adequate sanitation and sewage treatment and thorough cooking of meat that may be contaminated. A systematic review[3] has concluded that there is insufficient evidence to assess the benefit of cysticidal therapy in neurocysticercosis. When anthelmintics are considered necessary, praziquantel is used to treat neurocysticercosis and is usually given with a corticosteroid to prevent an inflammatory response to dead and dying larvae. Albendazole is an alternative treatment that some consider to be preferable; a corticosteroid or antihistamine is also administered to counter any inflammatory reaction. In some cases surgical removal of cysts may be the preferred treatment.

Infection with the adult worm of *T. solium* is discussed under Taeniasis, below.

1. Anonymous. Cerebral cysticercosis: what can be expected of cysticidal drugs? *WHO Drug Inf* 1995; **9:** 135–8.
2. Carpio A, *et al.* Is the course of neurocysticercosis modified by treatment with antihelminthic agents? *Arch Intern Med* 1995; **155:** 1982–8.
3. Salinas R, Prasad K. Drugs for treating neurocysticercosis (tapeworm infection of the brain) (updated 20 February 2001). Available in The Cochrane Library; Issue 3. Oxford: Update Software; 2001.

Diphyllobothriasis
Diphyllobothriasis is an intestinal infection with the fish tapeworm *Diphyllobothrium latum* and other *Diphyllobothrium* spp. and is acquired in man through ingestion of raw, infected, freshwater fish. The infection is rarely symptomatic. However, because the adult worm competes for vitamin B_{12}, some patients may develop megaloblastic anaemia with its associated neurological symptoms. Concentrations of other vitamins may also be reduced. Treatment is with a single dose of praziquantel. Niclosamide is an alternative. Vitamin supplements should also be given to correct any deficiencies.

Dracunculiasis
Dracunculiasis (dracontiasis, guinea-worm infection) is caused by infection with the nematode *Dracunculus medinensis*. It has been endemic in parts of Africa and Asia but is increasingly coming under control and the hope is that it will soon be eradicated. The disease is transmitted through drinking water containing larvae that develop in freshwater crustaceans. The larvae penetrate the intestinal mucosa and mature in connective tissue. The adult female migrates to the subcutaneous tissues normally of the legs after about 1 year. Ulceration of the overlying skin releases larvae which are ingested by the crustacean host to complete the life cycle. The first symptom is the lesion caused by the emerging worm, although a generalised hypersensitivity reaction may also occur. Secondary infection is a common complication.

The most effective method of controlling dracunculiasis is by provision of safe drinking water. The WHO eradication campaign is based on health education, and the provision of safe water by measures including water treatment with pesticides such as temefos and encouraging the use of domestic filters.

There is no effective direct drug therapy against any stage in man. The traditional treatment is removal of the adult worm by gentle traction sometimes over several weeks. Metronidazole or tiabendazole may provide symptomatic benefit in the management of dracunculiasis although they have no direct anthelmintic effect. They are thought to act by weakening the anchorage of the worms within the subcutaneous tissues, thus allowing them to be removed more quickly.

Echinococcosis
Echinococcosis, or hydatid disease, in man is infection with the larval stage of *Echinococcus granulosus* or *E. multilocularis*. These two species cause distinct forms of

the disease known as cystic echinococcosis and alveolar echinococcosis respectively. Various animals are involved in the transmission of the disease, man becoming infected through ingestion of eggs from contaminated faeces. The eggs hatch in the intestine and the embryos penetrate the intestinal wall and invade body organs, usually the liver. The embryo develops into a cyst which slowly increases in size and may remain intact for many years. Symptomatic infection usually only occurs when the cyst is large enough to cause obstruction or to compress adjacent structures, or if rupture occurs. Where possible, surgical removal of the intact cyst is the first line of treatment.

In **cystic echinococcosis**, drugs may be given locally or systemically before surgery to kill infective larvae within the cyst and reduce the risk of further infection. They are also given postoperatively if a cyst ruptures during surgery. Local injection of a larvicidal agent such as alcohol, cetrimide, or hypertonic saline has been used. Chemotherapy is also used as an adjunct or when surgery is not possible. The preferred drug for associated systemic treatment is albendazole. Mebendazole may be used, although some have suggested it is not as effective as albendazole. Praziquantel has also been reported to be effective. Albendazole may be a suitable alternative to surgery as initial treatment in uncomplicated cases; administration with cimetidine (to inhibit its metabolism) may increase its effectiveness.

A further option when surgery is not possible is the PAIR (puncture/aspiration/injection/re-aspiration) procedure which consists of ultrasound-guided cyst puncture followed by aspiration of the cyst fluid, local injection of alcohol or hypertonic saline into the cyst, and re-aspiration of the cyst contents. Concomitant chemotherapy is recommended.

E. multilocularis infection (**alveolar echinococcosis**) is more invasive and is characterised by a tumour-like infiltrative growth; it usually requires both surgery and long-term treatment with a benzimidazole such as albendazole although some patients have improved on albendazole alone.

References.

1. Kumar A, Chattopadhyay TK. Management of hydatid disease of the liver. *Postgrad Med J* 1992; **68:** 853–6.
2. Wen H, *et al.* Diagnosis and treatment of human hydatidosis. *Br J Clin Pharmacol* 1993; **35:** 565–74.
3. WHO Informal Working Group on Echinococcosis. Guidelines for treatment of cystic and alveolar echinococcosis in humans. *Bull WHO* 1996; **74:** 231–42.

Enterobiasis

Enterobiasis is an infection with *Enterobius vermicularis* (pinworm, threadworm). It is one of the few intestinal nematodes which is common in temperate climates and is particularly common in young children. Like trichuriasis (below) it is an infection of the large intestine and transmission follows ingestion or inhalation of mature eggs. The larvae mature in the gut in about 2 months. The eggs are not released into the gut contents but the mature female migrates to the anus at night and lays its eggs on the perianal and perineal skin. The eggs become infective within 6 hours. Diagnosis is based on detecting eggs around the anus. The most common symptom is perianal itching but many infections are asymptomatic. Rarely ectopic disease such as appendicitis or salpingitis may occur. The adult worm has a life span of about 6 weeks and, if re-infection can be prevented, the infection is self-limiting. While additional hygiene measures can prevent re-infection, treatment of the whole family with an anthelmintic should remain the main therapeutic response; more than one course may be required.

Treatment is with a benzimidazole carbamate derivative such as albendazole or mebendazole or with pyrantel embonate. Such broad-spectrum therapy can be useful if the patient is suffering from a mixed intestinal nematode infection. Other anthelmintics used in enterobiasis include piperazine or pyrvinium embonate.

Fascioliasis

See under Liver Fluke Infections, below.

Fasciolopsiasis

See under Intestinal Fluke Infections, below.

Gnathostomiasis

Gnathostomiasis is an infection with, in most cases, the larval form of the nematode *Gnathostoma spinigerum*, although other *Gnathostoma* spp. have been identified.

G. spinigerum inhabits the stomach of cats and dogs. Eggs shed in their faeces are ingested by freshwater crustaceans and hatch into larvae which are ingested by fish or other animals; man acquires the infection by consumption of the raw or undercooked flesh of these secondary hosts. Once ingested the larva penetrates the gut wall and migrates via the liver to a wide variety of other tissues including skin, eyes, and CNS. Rarely, dermal infiltration may result in cutaneous larva migrans (above).

The preferred treatment of gnathostomiasis is surgical removal of the gnathostome but this is rarely possible. Albendazole has been reported to be effective.

Heterophyiasis

See under Intestinal Fluke Infections, below.

Hookworm infections

Infections with the hookworms *Ancylostoma duodenale* (ancylostomiasis) and *Necator americanus* (necatoriasis) are a major cause of iron-deficiency anaemia in large areas of the tropics and sub-tropics, especially in rural communities. Eggs deposited in warm moist soil hatch into larvae which develop further into the infective form. Infection is normally by penetration through the skin although it may be by ingestion. The larvae migrate to the lungs from where they are swallowed and mature to the adult form in the small intestine. Eggs appear in the faeces about 6 to 8 weeks after infection and the adult worm may live for several years. *A. duodenale* larvae are capable of remaining dormant in the tissues, only maturing to the adult when climatic conditions are favourable. Symptoms correspond to the stage of infection. Visitors to endemic areas may develop intense pruritus, erythema, and a papulovesicular eruption at the site of infection known as ground itch. Migration through the lungs during the first infection may cause pneumonitis and bronchospasm with accompanying eosinophilia. The main symptoms of intestinal infection are iron-deficiency anaemia and severe hypoalbuminaemia. In addition, abdominal pain, diarrhoea, and weight loss may occur.

Treatment is usually with a benzimidazole carbamate derivative such as mebendazole or albendazole, and such broad-spectrum therapy can also be useful if the patient has a mixed intestinal nematode infection. Other anthelmintics used in hookworm include levamisole or pyrantel embonate, but these may be less effective against *N. americanus* than against *A. duodenale*. Iron-deficiency anaemia caused by hookworm infections responds rapidly to oral iron therapy; folic acid supplements may be necessary in some patients. Mass treatment programmes may be necessary in endemic areas to reduce the overall burden of infection.[1-3]

There is some evidence to suggest[4] that human infection with animal hookworms, some of which were previously thought to cause only cutaneous larva migrans (above), may also occasionally cause enteric infections characterised by eosinophilia.

1. Nahmias J, *et al.* Evaluation of albendazole, pyrantel, bephenium, pyrantel-praziquantel, and pyrantel-bephenium for single-dose mass treatment of necatoriasis. *Ann Trop Med Parasitol* 1989; **83:** 625–9.
2. Bradley M, *et al.* The epidemiology and control of hookworm infection in the Burma Valley area of Zimbabwe. *Trans R Soc Trop Med Hyg* 1993; **87:** 145–7.
3. Krepel HP, *et al.* Treatment of mixed Oesophagostomum and hookworm infection: effect of albendazole, pyrantel pamoate, levamisole and thiabendazole. *Trans R Soc Trop Med Hyg* 1993; **87:** 87–9.
4. Schad GA. Hookworms: pets to humans. *Ann Intern Med* 1994; **120:** 434–5.

Hymenolepiasis

Hymenolepiasis is an infection of the intestine with *Hymenolepis nana*, or dwarf tapeworm. Infection is acquired through ingestion of eggs in contaminated food or water or on hands and can be passed directly from person to person. It is more common in children. Clinical symptoms occur in heavy infections and include diarrhoea and abdominal pain. Treatment is with a single dose of praziquantel or a 7-day course of niclosamide.

Intestinal fluke infections

The intestinal fluke infections **fasciolopsiasis**, **heterophyiasis**, **metagonimiasis**, and **nanophyetiasis** are caused by *Fasciolopsis buski*, *Heterophyes heterophyes* and some other *Heterophyes* spp., *Metagonimus yokogawai*, and *Nanophyetus salmincola* respectively. Fasciolopsiasis, heterophyiasis, and metagonimiasis are endemic in the Far East and Southeast Asia, with hetero-

phyiasis also being common in the Middle East. Nanophyetiasis has occurred increasingly in the Pacific northwest of the USA. Fasciolopsiasis is caused by the ingestion of infected plants, while undercooked or raw infected fish are the sources of *H. heterophyes*, *M. yokogawai*, and *N. salmincola* infections.

Fasciolopsiasis is usually asymptomatic, but heavy infections can cause diarrhoea, abdominal pain, and, rarely, intestinal obstruction and an allergic oedematous reaction. Metagonimiasis is also generally asymptomatic but may cause mild diarrhoea, while pain and mucous diarrhoea are common in heterophyiasis. Similar gastrointestinal symptoms occur with eosinophilia in nanophyetiasis. Eggs of *M. yokogawai* and *H. heterophyes* may rarely penetrate the bowel wall and enter the blood stream to be deposited in various organs, leading to serious complications such as cardiac failure or fatal embolism in the heart or brain.

Treatment of intestinal fluke infections is with praziquantel.[1]

1. WHO. Control of foodborne trematode infections. *WHO Tech Rep Ser 849* 1995.

Liver fluke infections

Fasciola hepatica, *Opisthorchis viverrini*, *O. felineus*, and *Clonorchis sinensis* are liver flukes transmitted by the ingestion of infected aquatic plants, grasses or water (*F. hepatica*), or raw or undercooked fish (*Opisthorchis* spp., *C. sinensis*). **Fascioliasis** is primarily a disease of sheep and cattle and human infections occur where these animals are raised, whereas **clonorchiasis** and **opisthorchiasis** are seen mainly in Southeast Asia and eastern Europe.

Fascioliasis in the acute phase is usually characterised by fever, gastrointestinal symptoms, pain due to liver enlargement, and marked eosinophilia, but these symptoms decline as the worms enter their final habitat in the bile ducts. Acute symptoms occur rarely with clonorchiasis and opisthorchiasis and infections tend to be asymptomatic for many years. Adult flukes live in the bile ducts and symptoms of biliary-tract obstruction appear after repeated or heavy infections with liver flukes. Cholangiocarcinoma (bile duct cancer) is now generally accepted to be associated with liver fluke infection although its exact pathogenesis is unclear.

Praziquantel is used for the treatment of most liver fluke infections.[1] Bithionol is more effective than praziquantel in fascioliasis and is the preferred treatment, although triclabendazole may become the treatment of choice;[1] dehydroemetine has also been used.

Praziquantel remains the treatment of choice for clonorchiasis and opisthorchiasis.[1]

1. WHO. Control of foodborne trematode infections. *WHO Tech Rep Ser 849* 1995.

Loiasis

Loiasis is an infection with the filarial nematode *Loa loa* which occurs in areas of Central and West Africa. It is transmitted by the biting tabanid fly *Chrysops*. The infective larvae mature to adult worms which migrate through subcutaneous tissues and occasionally the subconjunctiva. Symptoms include pruritus, swelling, and pain, with occasional subcutaneous swellings, often on the arms or legs, that are characteristic of the disease. Passage of a worm through the subconjunctiva produces intense conjunctivitis. Eosinophilia may be severe, especially in visitors from non-endemic areas. Other complications include renal disease, endomyocardial fibrosis, encephalopathy, and peripheral neuropathy.

Treatment is with diethylcarbamazine which is effective against the microfilariae, larval forms, and a proportion of adult worms. In some cases, treatment has been associated with acute encephalitis, particularly in patients with heavy microfilaraemia. It has been assumed that this may be related to blockage of capillaries in the brain and meninges and for this reason small doses of diethylcarbamazine are given initially in combination with a corticosteroid and antihistamine, gradually increasing to full therapeutic doses over several days. However this does not eliminate the risk of encephalitis entirely and the role of the microfilariae in this syndrome has been questioned. Some consider that ivermectin could be useful but, as with diethylcarbamazine, there is concern over its potential neurotoxic effects in patients with heavy microfilaraemia.

Diethylcarbamazine is also used for prophylaxis but it has been suggested that it should be reserved for subjects at high risk of exposure. Vector control is regarded as impractical and methods aimed at reducing contact with the vector such as window screens and protective clothing are recommended.

Lung fluke infections

The lung fluke infection **paragonimiasis** is caused by *Paragonimus* spp., commonly *P. westermani*, with human infections occurring in Asia, Africa, and Central or South America. The disease is transmitted by the ingestion of raw infected freshwater crabs or crayfish, or from infected drinking water.

The flukes mature in the lungs where they cause local necrosis, haemorrhage, inflammation, and fibrosis. Symptoms of paragonimiasis include fever, pain, and chest complaints, but the majority of light to moderate infections are asymptomatic. The worms may also develop at other sites, particularly the brain where they can cause epilepsy, symptoms of cerebral tumours, or cerebral embolism, which may be fatal.

Treatment is with praziquantel or bithionol. Triclabendazole has been studied.

Lymphatic filariasis

Lymphatic filariasis arises from infection with *Wuchereria bancrofti* (bancroftian filariasis), *Brugia malayi*, or *B. timori* (both known as brugian filariasis and as Malayan and Timorian filariasis respectively). It occurs in tropical and subtropical regions. Larval forms are transmitted by mosquitoes. The larvae penetrate the lymphatic system where they mature to adult worms that may live for many years. Infective microfilariae are produced within 3 to 6 months and enter the peripheral blood stream, from where they are ingested by further mosquito vectors in which new larvae develop.

Lymphatic filariasis may be asymptomatic but both acute and chronic symptoms also occur. Inflammatory reactions to immature and adult worms in the lymphatic system produce episodic adenolymphangitis with fever. In men bancroftian filariasis characteristically presents as epididymo-orchitis. Abscesses may occasionally occur, particularly with brugian filariasis. Chronic lymphadenopathy is frequently seen. The main clinical features in chronic bancroftian filariasis are hydrocele, lymphoedema, elephantiasis, and chyluria. Chronic brugian filariasis typically causes lymphoedema and elephantiasis in the limb below the knee or elbow. Tropical pulmonary eosinophilia is a clinical variant of filarial disease, particularly of *W. bancrofti* infection. The symptoms include cough, wheezing, and eosinophilia. If untreated the condition can progress to chronic interstitial fibrosis.

There is no entirely satisfactory treatment of lymphatic filariasis. Diethylcarbamazine kills microfilariae and a proportion of immature and adult worms and is widely used for both treatment and prophylaxis. Treatment can precipitate severe immunological reactions to the dead and dying worms. Large hydroceles and elephantiasis are generally not reversible and usually require surgical intervention.[1] However, treatment with coumarins may reduce the lymphoedema and so lead to improvement.[2,3] There has also been a suggestion that elephantiasis may be linked to local secondary bacterial or fungal infections, and that simple measures such as regular washing could also produce improvement.[4] Tropical pulmonary eosinophilia responds to diethylcarbamazine but about 20% of patients may relapse and require re-treatment.[1] Diethylcarbamazine (p.99) is also used in the mass control of filariasis in all subjects in endemic areas. Ivermectin (p.100), which is also effective against microfilariae, has produced promising results in several studies. Albendazole, combined with diethylcarbamazine or ivermectin, has also shown promise. Indeed these drugs (with albendazole and ivermectin being donated by *SmithKline Beecham* and *Merck* respectively) are to be used in a global elimination campaign launched by WHO together with other international agencies. In areas where loiasis or onchocerciasis are co-endemic with bancroftian filariasis, albendazole and ivermectin are used together and where there is no loiasis or onchocerciasis then albendazole is given with diethylcarbamazine.

Control measures aimed at reducing the intensity of transmission include educating local communities on the use of insecticidal sprays and impregnated bed nets, and the use of mass chemotherapy treatment. Effective vector control is considered to be too expensive in most endemic areas.

1. WHO. Lymphatic filariasis: the disease and its control: fifth report of the WHO expert committee on filariasis. *WHO Tech Rep Ser* 821 1992.

2. Casley-Smith JR, *et al.* Treatment of filarial lymphoedema and elephantiasis with 5,6-benzo-α-pyrone (coumarin). *BMJ* 1993; **307:** 1037–41.
3. Anonymous. Coumarins: symptomatic relief of filarial lymphoedema. *WHO Drug Inf* 1993; **7:** 177–8.
4. McGregor A. Washing off elephantiasis. *Lancet* 1994; **344:** 121.

Mansonella infections

Infections with the filarial nematodes *Mansonella perstans*, *M. ozzardi*, and *M. streptocerca* are generally asymptomatic but a variety of symptoms including malaise, fever, joint pain, and meningeal symptoms have been described. Infection is transmitted by biting midges and flies. Treatment with diethylcarbamazine may be effective depending on the infecting species. Mebendazole may be effective alone or in combination with levamisole in *M. perstans*. Ivermectin has been suggested for *M. ozzardi* infections and may be the drug of choice for *M. streptocerca*.

Metagonimiasis

See under Intestinal Fluke Infections, above.

Nanophyetiasis

See under Intestinal Fluke Infections, above.

Necatoriasis

See under Hookworm Infections, above.

Onchocerciasis

Onchocerciasis (river blindness) is caused by infection with the filarial nematode *Onchocerca volvulus*. It is endemic in large areas of Africa and areas of Central or South America. It is particularly prevalent near fast flowing rivers, the breeding ground of the blackfly which is the vector of the parasite. Following infection, the larvae mature into adults in fibrous nodules, usually in the subcutaneous tissue. The adults release large numbers of microfilariae which are responsible for the major symptoms of the disease in the skin and the eye. Symptoms of skin involvement range from an intensely pruritic erythematous rash to chronic skin changes and severe pendulous lymphoedema. Microfilariae in the eye are a major cause of blindness in endemic areas.

Onchocerciasis is controlled with ivermectin.[1-3] Ivermectin rapidly eliminates microfilariae from the skin and more gradually from the eye.[3] It does not eliminate the adult worms although it suppresses release of microfilariae for several cycles. Ivermectin is donated without charge by *Merck* through the Mectizan Expert Committee (MEC) for human use in community-wide mass treatment programmes in all countries in which onchocerciasis is endemic, where it is given once a year to all but pregnant women, breast-feeding mothers of recently born babies, children weighing less than 15 kg, and those unable to walk or otherwise seriously ill.[4] Control of the disease in endemic areas thus relies upon the administration of ivermectin once or twice a year and this should be combined with vector control.[2] For further details, see under Ivermectin, p.100.

Before the introduction of ivermectin, diethylcarbamazine citrate was the usual treatment for onchocerciasis, but it is no longer recommended by WHO.[2,3] The major limitations to its use are the severe allergic reaction (the Mazzotti reaction) associated with its microfilaricidal action, aggravation of existing ocular lesions or precipitation of new ones, and the need to give repeated courses of treatment for continued suppression of the disease.[3] Suramin has also been used in the treatment of onchocerciasis and is effective against adult worms.[2,3] However, its use is restricted because of its toxicity. Amocarzine has also been evaluated in onchocerciasis.[3]

1. Van Laethen Y, Lopes C. Treatment of onchocerciasis. *Drugs* 1996; **52:** 861–9.
2. *WHO model prescribing information: drugs used in parasitic diseases.* 2nd ed. Geneva: WHO, 1995.
3. WHO. Onchocerciasis and its control: report of a WHO expert committee on onchocerciasis control. *WHO Tech Rep Ser* 852 1995.
4. Pond B. Distribution of ivermectin by health workers. *Lancet* 1990; **335:** 1539.

Opisthorchiasis

See under Liver Fluke Infections, above.

Paragonimiasis

See under Lung Fluke Infections, above.

Schistosomiasis

Schistosomiasis is a parasitic infection caused by *Schistosoma* spp., largely *S. mansoni*, *S. japonicum*, and *S. haematobium*, and to a lesser extent *S. intercalatum* and *S. mekongi*. The disease is seen mainly in Africa, Asia, South America, and the Caribbean, where it is a hazard to individuals exposed to fresh water containing the intermediate host, infected freshwater snails.

Free-swimming cercariae are released from the snail and penetrate human skin causing a pruritic papular rash in sensitised individuals (swimmer's itch). Parasites mature in the lungs and liver within about 6 weeks, then migrate to the blood vessels, the bladder, or intestines. Mature female worms produce eggs which are excreted in urine or stools, or become lodged in tissues, and immunological reaction to these eggs results in disease. The acute reaction to egg deposition has been termed Katayama fever, a self-limiting but sometimes fatal illness resembling serum sickness and most frequently seen in *S. japonicum* infection. The chronic phase of infection is often asymptomatic for many years but usually results in granuloma formation and fibrosis in tissues where eggs are deposited, such as the liver, lungs, intestines, or urinary tract, the site depending on the infecting species.

Praziquantel is used for the treatment of chronic schistosomiasis and is effective against all species of schistosomes. Metrifonate and oxamniquine are alternatives that may be used against *S. haematobium* and *S. mansoni* respectively.

Niclosamide is used as a molluscicide for the treatment of water in schistosomiasis control programmes. Copper sulfate or sodium pentachlorophenate have also been used but to a lesser extent.

Schistosomiasis vaccines are in development.

References.

1. WHO. The control of schistosomiasis: second report of the WHO expert committee. *WHO Tech Rep Ser* 830 1993.
2. Squires N. Interventions for treating schistosomiasis haematobium (updated 29 November 2000). Available in The Cochrane Library; Issue 1. Oxford: Update Software; 2001.
3. Saconato H, Atallah A. Interventions for treating schistosomiasis mansoni (updated 7 December 2000). Available in The Cochrane Library; Issue 3. Oxford: Update Software; 2001.

Strongyloidiasis

Strongyloidiasis is an infection of the small intestine caused by *Strongyloides stercoralis*, known as threadworm in the USA. It generally occurs in the tropics and subtropics and can also occur in some areas of South and East Europe, Japan, and the USA. In contrast with other intestinal nematodes, the eggs of *S. stercoralis* hatch before leaving the gastrointestinal tract, and can cause autoinfection, particularly in immunocompromised patients. Larvae reaching the soil can either mature into free-living adults or remain in an infective larval stage. Infective larvae cause infection by penetrating the skin. The larvae migrate to the lungs, move up the bronchial tree to be swallowed, and finally penetrate the mucosa of the small intestine where they mature. Eggs are deposited about 28 days after initial infection.

Infection may be asymptomatic, but commonly patients have symptoms relating to the stages of infection. Penetration of larvae through the skin causes intense pruritus and an erythematous rash. The rash may follow the course of migration and is one of the causes of cutaneous larva migrans (above). An inflammatory response to migration through the lungs may be seen and this may include pneumonitis and bronchospasm. In heavy infections, which are most common in immunocompromised patients as a result of autoinfection, massive pulmonary invasion may occur resulting in fatal alveolar haemorrhage. Abdominal symptoms include colicky pain, diarrhoea, and vomiting, leading to nutritional deficiencies and weight loss. Eosinophilia may also be present. Disseminated disease may occur in immunocompromised patients and may result in severe pulmonary and abdominal symptoms, shock, encephalopathy, meningitis, and Gram-negative septicaemia. Since strongyloidiasis is commonly fatal in these patients, vulnerable patients from endemic areas should be screened regularly and treated promptly at the first sign of infection.

Ivermectin is effective for the treatment of strongyloidiasis and is considered by some authorities to be the drug of choice. Tiabendazole was widely used and still is in some countries. Albendazole is more effective and better tolerated than tiabendazole. Mebendazole has also been suggested but it must be administered for longer periods than albendazole since it has only a limited effect on migrating larvae. These broad-spectrum anthelmintics (tiabendazole excepted) are also useful if the patient is suffering from a mixed intestinal nematode infection.

Syngamosis

Syngamosis, or gapeworm infection, is caused by *Syngamus* spp. and is primarily an infection of domestic fowl and wild birds and mammals, although infection in man has been reported rarely. Man may become infected by eating foods contaminated with infective larvae which penetrate the intestinal wall and migrate to the lungs where they mature into adult worms. The major symptom is cough, due to irritation of the bronchi and increased mucus production. The infection may be confused with asthma. Tiabendazole and mebendazole have been used successfully to treat the infection in man.

Taeniasis

Taeniasis is an infection of the intestine with beef tapeworm, *Taenia saginata*, or pork tapeworm, *T. solium*, acquired through ingestion of contaminated raw or undercooked meat. The larval form of *T. solium* can cause the systemic infection cysticercosis (see above).

Infection with the adult worm usually produces symptoms only when the worm reaches a size that can cause obstruction or related problems. Segments of the worm containing eggs may be excreted in the faeces so maintaining the cycle of reproduction. Treatment is with a single dose of praziquantel, which has the advantage of also being active, in higher doses, against the larval form of *T. solium*. Niclosamide is also effective but is only active against adult worms.

Toxocariasis

Toxocariasis is infection with the larval form of *Toxocara canis* and less commonly *T. cati*. The adult worms live in the intestines of dogs and cats respectively and man becomes infected when eggs excreted in animal faeces are ingested. Once ingested the eggs hatch and the larvae migrate from the intestine to other organs most commonly the liver, lung, and eye. Most infections are asymptomatic but two clinical syndromes, ocular larva migrans and visceral larva migrans, can occur, usually in children.

Ocular larva migrans occurs when larvae invade the eye causing a granuloma which may impair vision and can cause blindness. There is no specific treatment.[1] Anthelmintics such as albendazole or tiabendazole, corticosteroids, ocular surgery, and laser photocoagulation have been employed but assessment of their efficacy is difficult because of the variable natural course of the disease.

The clinical symptoms of visceral larva migrans depend upon the organs involved but commonly include cough, wheezing, fever, and hepatomegaly. Encephalitis and seizures may occur and there is usually eosinophilia. Acute infection normally resolves without treatment.[2] However, severe or prolonged infections may be treated with diethylcarbamazine citrate. Albendazole, mebendazole, and tiabendazole have also been used.

1. Shields JA. Ocular toxocariasis: a review. *Surv Ophthalmol* 1984; **28**: 361–81.
2. Gillespie SH. Human toxocariasis. *Commun Dis Rep* 1993; **3**: R140–R143.

Trichinosis

Trichinosis (trichinellosis) is an infection caused by *Trichinella spiralis*. Man becomes infected through ingestion of raw or undercooked meat, usually pork, containing infective larvae. The larvae mature into adult worms in the small intestine and the mature females deposit larvae which migrate in the blood to skeletal muscle and sometimes to the myocardium. Symptoms usually occur only in heavy infections. Invasion of the intestines by the maturing adult worms can cause diarrhoea, abdominal pain, and vomiting followed about a week later by hypersensitivity reactions to the migrating larvae. These may include eosinophilia, fever, muscle pain, periorbital oedema and more rarely encephalitis, myocarditis, or pneumonia which may be fatal.

All patients with confirmed or suspected infection should be treated to prevent the continued production of larvae. Mebendazole is considered to be the anthelmintic of choice in some countries. Albendazole, flubendazole, tiabendazole, or pyrantel embonate may also be effective. A corticosteroid should be given for severe hypersensitivity reactions.

Trichostrongyliasis

Trichostrongyliasis is an infection of the small intestine caused by *Trichostrongylus* spp. including *T. colubriformis*. It is normally a parasite of herbivores but infections in man have been found. *Trichostrongylus* spp. have a similar life cycle to *Ancylostoma duodenale* (see Hookworm Infections, above). Pyrantel embonate, albendazole, or mebendazole are recommended for the treatment of trichostrongyliasis.

Trichuriasis

Trichuriasis is an infection of the large intestine with *Trichuris trichiura*, sometimes known as whipworm. Distribution is worldwide but most infections occur in the tropics and subtropics. Eggs are excreted in the faeces and can remain viable in the soil for extended periods. Under optimum conditions the eggs become infective in about 2 to 4 weeks. Following ingestion, larvae are released from the eggs and develop within the wall of the small intestine for about 3 to 10 days before migrating to the lumen of the large intestine where they remain attached to the mucosal lining. Eggs are detectable in the faeces about 1 to 3 months after infection. Trichuriasis is often asymptomatic but heavy infection can result in anaemia, diarrhoea, and rectal prolapse.

Treatment is with a benzimidazole carbamate derivative such as albendazole or mebendazole and such broadspectrum therapy can be useful if the patient is suffering from a mixed intestinal nematode infection.

Abamectin (2774-q)

Abamectin (USAN, rINN).

MK-0936. A mixture of abamectin component B$_{1a}$ and abamectin component B$_{1b}$.

CAS — 65195-55-3 (component B$_{1a}$); 65195-56-4 (component B$_{1b}$).

Profile

Abamectin is an avermectin anthelmintic used in veterinary medicine for nematode infections. It is also used as a systemic veterinary ectoparasiticide.

Albendazole (752-p)

Albendazole (BAN, USAN, rINN).

Albendazolum; SKF-62979. Methyl 5-propylthio-1H-benzimidazol-2-ylcarbamate.

$C_{12}H_{15}N_3O_2S = 265.3$.

CAS — 54965-21-8.

ATC — P02CA03.

Pharmacopoeias. In *Chin.*, *Eur.* (see p.vi), and *US*.

Pharmacopoeial description

Ph. Eur.: A white to faintly yellowish powder. Practically insoluble in water and in alcohol; very slightly soluble in dichloromethane; freely soluble in anhydrous formic acid. Protect from light.

USP 25: A white to faintly yellowish powder. Practically insoluble in water and in alcohol; very slightly soluble in ether and in dichloromethane; freely soluble in anhydrous formic acid.

Adverse Effects and Precautions

As for Mebendazole, p.102.

Albendazole is teratogenic in *animals* (see Pregnancy and Breast Feeding, below).

◊ Although generally well-tolerated, the following adverse reactions were reported in the first phase of WHO-coordinated studies[1] involving 30 patients given *high-dose* therapy with albendazole for the treatment of cystic echinococcosis (hydatid disease): raised serum-transaminase levels (2 patients), reduced leucocyte counts (1), gastrointestinal symptoms (1), allergic conditions (1), and loss of hair (1). Treatment was stopped in a further patient with alveolar echinococcosis because of depressed bone-marrow activity. In the second phase of these studies[2] 109 patients were given albendazole and 20 experienced adverse effects; similar findings were reported with mebendazole. The range of effects with albendazole was: elevation of transaminases (5 patients), abdominal pain and other gastrointestinal symptoms (7), severe headache (4), loss of hair (2), leucopenia (2), fever and fatigue (1), thrombocytopenia (1), and urticaria and itching (1). Albendazole had to be withdrawn in 5 patients because of adverse effects, although in 3 the withdrawal was only temporary.

Albendazole should only be used in the treatment of echinococcosis if there is constant medical supervision with regular monitoring of serum-transaminase concentrations and of leucocyte and platelet counts. Patients with liver damage should

be treated with reduced doses of benzimidazole carbamates, if at all.[2]

1. Davis A, *et al.* Multicentre clinical trials of benzimidazolecarbamates in human echinococcosis. *Bull WHO* 1986; **64**: 383–8.
2. Davis A, *et al.* Multicentre clinical trials of benzimidazolecarbamates in human cystic echinococcosis (phase 2). *Bull WHO* 1989; **67**: 503–8.

Effects on growth. A multiple-dose regimen of albendazole in children with asymptomatic trichuriasis has been reported to be associated with impaired growth in those with low levels of infection.[1] However it was considered that this should not deter the use of single doses in mass treatment programmes.[2]

1. Forrester JE, *et al.* Randomised trial of albendazole and pyrantel in symptomless trichuriasis in children. *Lancet* 1998; **352**: 1103–4.
2. Winstanley P. Albendazole for mass treatment of asymptomatic trichuris infections. *Lancet* 1998; **352**: 1080–1.

Effects on the liver. In a series of 40 patients given albendazole for echinococcosis, 7 developed abnormalities in liver function tests during therapy.[1] Six had a hepatocellular type of abnormality attributable to albendazole; the seventh had cholestatic jaundice which was probably not due to albendazole.

1. Morris DL, Smith PG. Albendazole in hydatid disease—hepatocellular toxicity. *Trans R Soc Trop Med Hyg* 1987; **81**: 343–4.

Pregnancy and breast feeding. Albendazole is teratogenic in some *animal* species and the UK manufacturers have stated that it is contra-indicated in pregnant women or in women thought to be pregnant. They also advise that women of child-bearing age should take effective precautions, with non-hormonal contraceptive measures, against conception during and within one month of completing treatment with albendazole. In the USA the manufacturers, while not recommending albendazole for pregnant patients, have stated that if it is used in pregnancy, then such use should only be where the potential benefit justifies the risk to the fetus; this is in accordance with albendazole being classified in FDA pregnancy category C.

It is not known whether albendazole or its metabolites are distributed into breast milk.

Interactions

◊ Plasma concentrations of the active metabolite of albendazole (albendazole sulfoxide) were reported to be raised by approximately 50% in a study in 8 patients receiving concomitant *dexamethasone*.[1]

The plasma concentration of albendazole sulfoxide has also been increased by concomitant administration of *praziquantel*,[2] although the practical consequences of this were considered uncertain. Concentrations of albendazole sulfoxide have also been found to be raised in bile and hydatid cyst fluid by administration of albendazole with *cimetidine*, which may increase effectiveness in the treatment of echinococcosis.[3]

1. Jung H, *et al.* Dexamethasone increases plasma levels of albendazole. *J Neurol* 1990; **237**: 279–80.
2. Homeida M, *et al.* Pharmacokinetic interaction between praziquantel and albendazole in Sudanese men. *Ann Trop Med Parasitol* 1994; **88**: 551–9.
3. Wen H, *et al.* Initial observation on albendazole in combination with cimetidine for the treatment of human cystic echinococcosis. *Ann Trop Med Parasitol* 1994; **88**: 49–52.

Pharmacokinetics

Albendazole is poorly absorbed from the gastrointestinal tract, but rapidly undergoes extensive first-pass metabolism. The principal metabolite albendazole sulfoxide has anthelmintic activity and a plasma half-life of about 8.5 hours. Albendazole sulfoxide is widely distributed throughout the body including into the bile and the CSF. It is approximately 70% bound to plasma protein. Albendazole sulfoxide is eliminated in the bile; only a small amount appears to be excreted in the urine.

◊ References.

1. Marriner SE, *et al.* Pharmacokinetics of albendazole in man. *Eur J Clin Pharmacol* 1986; **30**: 705–8.
2. Morris DL, *et al.* Penetration of albendazole sulphoxide into hydatid cysts. *Gut* 1987; **28**: 75–80.
3. Steiger U, *et al.* Albendazole treatment of echinococcosis in humans: effects on microsomal metabolism and drug tolerance. *Clin Pharmacol Ther* 1990; **47**: 347–53.
4. Jung H, *et al.* Clinical pharmacokinetics of albendazole in patients with brain cysticercosis. *J Clin Pharmacol* 1992; **32**: 28–31.

Uses and Administration

Albendazole is a benzimidazole carbamate anthelmintic structurally related to mebendazole (p.102) and with similar activity. Albendazole is used in the treatment of the cestode infections cysticercosis and echinococcosis (hydatid disease) in relatively high doses. In some countries it is used in the treatment of single and mixed intestinal nematode infections including ascariasis, enterobiasis, hookworm, strongyloidiasis, and trichuriasis. It may also be used in the treatment of capillariasis, gnathostomiasis, and trichostrongyliasis. Albendazole may be effective in the treatment of the tissue nematode infections cutaneous larva migrans, toxocariasis, and trichinosis and in combination with other anthelmintics in the management of the filarial nematode infection lymphatic filariasis. For discussions of these infections and their treatment, see under Choice of Anthelmintic (p.91). See also below.

In the treatment of **echinococcosis**, albendazole is given by mouth with meals in a dose of 400 mg twice daily for 28 days for patients weighing over 60 kg. A dose of 15 mg per kg body-weight daily in two divided doses (to a maximum total daily dose of 800 mg) is used for patients weighing less than 60 kg. For cystic echinococcosis the 28-day course may be repeated after 14 days without treatment to a total of 3 treatment cycles. For alveolar echinococcosis, cycles of 28 days of treatment followed by 14 days without treatment may need to continue for months or years.

In the treatment of **neurocysticercosis**, albendazole 400 mg twice daily for patients weighing over 60 kg (or 15 mg per kg daily in two divided doses to a maximum total daily dose of 800 mg in those weighing less than 60 kg) is given by mouth for 8 to 30 days.

Albendazole is given by mouth, usually as a single dose, in the treatment of single or mixed **intestinal nematode infections**. The usual dose for adults and children aged 2 years or over with ascariasis, enterobiasis, hookworm infections, or trichuriasis is 400 mg as a single dose. In enterobiasis the dose may be repeated in 1 to 2 weeks. Some consider that children of 1 to 2 years of age may be given 200 mg for enterobiasis. In strongyloidiasis, 400 mg is given once or twice daily for 3 consecutive days; this may be repeated after 3 weeks if necessary.

Albendazole has also been used to treat children with **giardiasis** (p.583); suggested doses are 400 mg daily by mouth for 5 days.

Ascariasis. Albendazole is used as an alternative to mebendazole in the treatment of ascariasis (p.91). Both drugs are equally highly effective with a cure rate greater than 98% reported for albendazole in one study.[1]

1. Albonico M, et al. A randomized controlled trial comparing mebendazole and albendazole against Ascaris, Trichuris and hookworm infections. Trans R Soc Trop Med Hyg 1994; **88:** 585–9.

Capillariasis. Albendazole in a dose of 400 mg daily for 10 days has been suggested[1] as an alternative to mebendazole for the treatment of capillariasis (p.92).

1. Anonymous. Drugs for parasitic infections. Med Lett Drugs Ther 1998; **40:** 1–12.

Cutaneous larva migrans. Albendazole has been reported to be effective in the treatment of cutaneous larva migrans[1-3] and may be an alternative to standard treatment with tiabendazole (p.92). Albendazole, generally in a dose of 400 mg daily for three[1] or five[2] days, has alleviated the discomfort of cutaneous larva migrans. A single dose of 400 mg also appears to be effective.[3]

1. Jones SK, et al. Oral albendazole for the treatment of cutaneous larva migrans. Br J Dermatol 1990; **122:** 99–101.
2. Sanguigni S, et al. Albendazole in the therapy of cutaneous larva migrans. Trans R Soc Trop Med Hyg 1990; **84:** 831.
3. Orihuela AR, Torres JR. Single dose of albendazole in the treatment of cutaneous larva migrans. Arch Dermatol 1990; **126:** 398–9.

Cysticercosis. Albendazole is used in the treatment of neurocysticercosis (p.92) as an alternative to praziquantel;[1,2] some consider albendazole to be preferable.[3-5] Albendazole has also been reported to be effective in extra-ocular cysticercosis.[6]

1. Sotelo J, et al. Short course of albendazole therapy for neurocysticercosis. Arch Neurol 1988; **45:** 1130–3.
2. Botero D, et al. Short course albendazole treatment for neurocysticercosis in Columbia. Trans R Soc Trop Med Hyg 1993; **87:** 576–7.
3. Cruz M, et al. Albendazole versus praziquantel in the treatment of cerebral cysticercosis: clinical evaluation. Trans R Soc Trop Med Hyg 1991; **85:** 244–7.
4. Takayanagui OM, Jardim E. Therapy for neurocysticercosis: comparison between albendazole and praziquantel. Arch Neurol 1992; **49:** 290–4.
5. Mehta SS, et al. Albendazole versus praziquantel for neurocysticercosis. Am J Health-Syst Pharm 1998; **55:** 598–600.
6. Sihota R, Honavar SG. Oral albendazole in the management of extraocular cysticercosis. Br J Ophthalmol 1994; **78:** 621–3.

Echinococcosis. Albendazole is used in the treatment of echinococcosis (p.92) as an adjunct to, or instead of, surgery. It is generally preferred to mebendazole.

References.
1. Horton RJ. Chemotherapy of Echinococcus infection in man with albendazole. Trans R Soc Trop Med Hyg 1989; **83:** 97–102.

2. Davis A, et al. Multicentre clinical trials of benzimidazolecarbamates in human cystic echinococcosis (phase 2). Bull WHO 1989; **67:** 503–8.
3. Todorov T, et al. Factors influencing the response to chemotherapy in human cystic echinococcosis. Bull WHO 1992; **70:** 347–58.
4. Teggi A, et al. Therapy of human hydatid disease with mebendazole and albendazole. Antimicrob Agents Chemother 1993; **37:** 1679–84.
5. Gil-Grande LA, et al. Randomised controlled trial of efficacy of albendazole in intra-abdominal hydatid disease. Lancet 1993; **342:** 1269–72.
6. Liu Y-H, et al. Computer tomography of liver in alveolar echinococcosis treated with albendazole. Trans R Soc Trop Med Hyg 1993; **87:** 319–21.
7. Wen H, et al. Initial observation on albendazole in combination with cimetidine for the treatment of human cystic echinococcosis. Ann Trop Med Parasitol 1994; **88:** 49–52.

Gnathostomiasis. Albendazole has been reported to be effective in the treatment of gnathostomiasis (p.93). Doses of 400 mg once or twice daily have been given for 2 or 3 weeks.[1-3]

1. Kraivichian P, et al. Albendazole for the treatment of human gnathostomiasis. Trans R Soc Trop Med Hyg 1992; **86:** 418–21.
2. Suntharasamai P, et al. Albendazole stimulates outward migration of Gnathostoma spinigerum to the dermis in man. Southeast Asian J Trop Med Public Health 1992; **23:** 716–22.
3. Anonymous. Drugs for parasitic infections. Med Lett Drugs Ther 1998; **40:** 1–12.

Hookworm infections. Hookworm infections (p.93) are commonly treated with benzimidazole carbamates such as albendazole. In 77 patients with light necatoriasis (Necator americanus infection) albendazole, in a single 400-mg dose, produced an 84% cure rate and an 82% reduction in egg count in those patients not cured.[1] In another study,[2] although the cure rate was only 56.8% following a single 400-mg dose of albendazole this was superior to treatment with mebendazole which had a cure rate of 22.4%. A further study[3] comparing albendazole with mebendazole and pyrantel in the treatment of necatoriasis also found albendazole to be the most effective.

1. Nahmias J, et al. Evaluation of albendazole, pyrantel, bephenium, pyrantel-praziquantel and pyrantel-bephenium for single-dose mass treatment of necatoriasis. Ann Trop Med Parasitol 1989; **83:** 625–9.
2. Albonico M, et al. A randomized controlled trial comparing mebendazole and albendazole against Ascaris, Trichuris and hookworm infections. Trans R Soc Trop Med Hyg 1994; **88:** 585–9.
3. Sacko M, et al. Comparison of the efficacy of mebendazole, albendazole and pyrantel in treatment of human hookworm infections in the southern region of Mali, West Africa. Trans R Soc Trop Med Hyg 1999; **93:** 195–203.

Lymphatic filariasis. Albendazole is used in the management of lymphatic filariasis (p.94). In endemic areas where more than 5% of the population is infected, mass treatment of the entire population (excluding neonates, pregnant women, and debilitated individuals) can reduce the intensity of transmission and the incidence of disease. A global elimination campaign launched by WHO together with other international agencies advocates a single dose of albendazole 400 mg together with either a single dose of ivermectin 200 μg per kg body-weight (for bancroftian filariasis if there is co-endemic loiasis or onchocerciasis) or with a single dose of diethylcarbamazine 6 mg per kg (if there is no co-endemic loiasis or onchocerciasis); these doses are given once each year for 4 to 6 years.

Microsporidiosis. Albendazole has been tried[1-5] in the treatment of microsporidiosis (p.585), a protozoal infection increasingly seen in patients with AIDS. Albendazole has also been employed empirically in the treatment of HIV-associated diarrhoea (p.610).

1. Blanshard C, et al. Treatment of intestinal microsporidiosis with albendazole in patients with AIDS. AIDS 1992; **6:** 311–13.
2. Dieterich DT, et al. Treatment with albendazole for intestinal disease due to Enterocytozoon bieneusi in patients with AIDS. J Infect Dis 1994; **169:** 178–82.
3. Franzen C, et al. Intestinal microsporidiosis with Septata intestinalis in a patient with AIDS—response to albendazole. J Infect 1995; **31:** 237–9.
4. Dore GJ, et al. Disseminated microsporidiosis due to Septata intestinalis in nine patients infected with the human immunodeficiency virus: response to therapy with albendazole. Clin Infect Dis 1995; **21:** 70–6.
5. Molina J-M, et al. Albendazole for treatment and prophylaxis of microsporidiosis due to Encephalitozoon intestinalis in patients with AIDS: a randomized double-blind controlled trial. J Infect Dis 1998; **177:** 1373–7.

Strongyloidiasis. Albendazole is generally preferred to tiabendazole or mebendazole in the treatment of strongyloidiasis (p.94) although some authorities now consider ivermectin to be the drug of choice.

References.
1. Rossignol JF, Maisonneuve H. Albendazole: placebo-controlled study in 870 patients with intestinal helminthiasis. Trans R Soc Trop Med Hyg 1983; **77:** 707–11.
2. Chanthavanich P, et al. Repeated doses of albendazole against strongyloidiasis in Thai children. Southeast Asian J Trop Med Public Health 1989; **20:** 221–6.
3. Mojon M, Nielsen PB. Treatment of Strongyloides stercoralis with albendazole: a cure rate of 86 per cent. Zentralbl Bakteriol Mikrobiol Hyg [A] 1987; **263:** 619–24.
4. Archibald LK, et al. Albendazole is effective treatment for chronic strongyloidiasis. Q J Med 1993; **86:** 191–5.

Toxocariasis. Albendazole is one of the drugs that might be used for the treatment of toxocariasis (p.95) and in a small study[1] albendazole produced improvement similar to that achieved with tiabendazole but with fewer problems.

1. Stürchler D, et al. Thiabendazole vs albendazole in treatment of toxocariasis: a clinical trial. Ann Trop Med Parasitol 1989; **83:** 473–8.

Trichinosis. Albendazole may be effective in the treatment of trichinosis (p.95). A retrospective study in 44 patients with trichinosis comparing albendazole treatment with tiabendazole found that, while the two drugs were of comparable efficacy, albendazole was the better tolerated.[1] Albendazole has been used to treat a patient infected with Trichinella pseudospiralis, an organism related to T.spiralis, the usual cause of trichinosis.[2]

1. Cabié A, et al. Albendazole versus thiabendazole as therapy for trichinosis: a retrospective study. Clin Infect Dis 1996; **22:** 1033–5.
2. Andrews JRH, et al. Trichinella pseudospiralis in humans: description of a case and its treatment. Trans R Soc Trop Med Hyg 1994; **88:** 200–3.

Trichostrongyliasis. Albendazole in a single dose of 400 mg has been suggested[1] as an alternative to pyrantel embonate or mebendazole in the treatment of trichostrongyliasis (p.95).

1. Anonymous. Drugs for parasitic infections. Med Lett Drugs Ther 1998; **40:** 1–12.

Trichuriasis. Albendazole is used in the treatment of trichuriasis (p.95). It is normally given in a single dose and is often used in mixed intestinal nematode infections.[1] However, it has been reported[1-3] that in children with mixed intestinal worm infections single doses of albendazole are ineffective in eliminating Trichuris trichiura and multiple doses are required to produce worthwhile reductions in egg production. Treatment for 3 days has been suggested for heavy infection[4] (for a suggestion that such regimens may be associated with impaired growth in less heavily infected children, see Effects on Growth under Adverse Effects, above).

1. Hall A, Anwar KS. Albendazole and infections with Trichuris trichiura and Giardia intestinalis. Southeast Asian J Trop Med Public Health 1991; **22:** 84–7.
2. Hall A, Nahar Q. Albendazole and infections with Ascaris lumbricoides and Trichuris trichiura in children in Bangladesh. Trans R Soc Trop Med Hyg 1994; **88:** 110–12.
3. Albonico M, et al. A randomized controlled trial comparing mebendazole and albendazole against Ascaris, Trichuris and hookworm infections. Trans R Soc Trop Med Hyg 1994; **88:** 585–9.
4. Anonymous. Drugs for parasitic infections. Med Lett Drugs Ther 1998; **40:** 1–12.

Preparations

USP 25: Albendazole Tablets.

Proprietary Preparations (details are given in Part 3)

Aust.: Eskazole; *Austral.:* Eskazole; Zentel; *Braz.:* Alba-3; Alben; Alin; Amplozol; Bentiamin; Dazol; Helmintal; Mebenix; Parasin; Vermital; Zentel; Zolben; *Fr.:* Eskazole; Zentel; *Ger.:* Eskazole; *Israel:* Eskazole; *Ital.:* Zentel; *Mex.:* Albensil; Bendapar; Bradelmin; Dabenzol; Dazocan; Digezanol; Entoplus; Eskazole; Euralben; Gascop; Helmisons; Loveral; Lurdex; Tenibex; Vermilan; Vermin-Plus; Vermisen; Zelfin; Zenaxin; Zentel; *Neth.:* Eskazole; *Port.:* Zentel; *S.Afr.:* Bendex; Paranthil†; Zentel; *Singapore:* Alzental; Zentel; *Spain:* Eskazole; *Switz.:* Zentel; *Thai.:* Abentel; Albatel; Alben; Albenda; Alda; Alzol; Anthel; Gendazel; Leo-400; Masaworm; Mesin; Vermixide; Zeben; Zentel; *UAE:* Albenda; *UK:* Eskazole†; *USA:* Albenza.

Amocarzine (18938-g)

Amocarzine (rINN).

CGP-6140.   4-Methyl-4'-(p-nitroanilino)thio-1-piperazinecarboxanilide.

$C_{18}H_{21}N_5O_2S = 371.5$.

CAS — 36590-19-9.

NOTE. Amocarzine has sometimes been referred to as thiocarbamazine.

Profile

Amocarzine is an antifilarial anthelmintic, derived from amoscanate, that is active against the adult worms of Onchocerca volvulus. It is under investigation for the oral treatment of onchocerciasis (p.94).

◊ References.
1. Soula G, et al. Activity of thiocarbamazine in patients dually infected with schistosoma and onchocerca volvulus. Lancet 1989; **i:** 726.
2. Lecaillon JB, et al. Pharmacokinetics of CGP 6140 (amocarzine) after oral administration of single 100-1600 mg doses to patients with onchocerciasis. Br J Clin Pharmacol 1990; **30:** 625–8.
3. Lecaillon JB, et al. The influence of food on the pharmacokinetics of CGP 6140 (amocarzine) after oral administration of a 1200 mg single dose to patients with onchocerciasis. Br J Clin Pharmacol 1990; **30:** 629–33.
4. Poltera AA, et al. Onchocercacidal effects of amocarzine (CGP 6140) in Latin America. Lancet 1991; **337:** 583–4.
5. Cooper PJ, et al. Onchocerciasis in Ecuador: evolution of chorioretinopathy after amocarzine treatment. Br J Ophthalmol 1996; **80:** 337–42.

Amoscanate (12371-b)

Amoscanate (rINN).

C-9333-Go/CGP-4540; GO-9333; Nithiocyamine. 4-p-Nitro-anilinophenyl isothiocyanate.

$C_{13}H_9N_3O_2S = 271.3$.

CAS — 26328-53-0.

Profile

Amoscanate is an isothiocyanate anthelmintic that has been tried in the treatment of hookworm infections. In China it has been used against schistosomiasis due to *Schistosoma japonicum*.

Trivalent Antimony Compounds (14110-f)

Antimony Potassium Tartrate (755-e)

Antim. Pot. Tart.; Brechweinstein; Kalii Stibyli Tartras; Potassium Antimonyltartrate; Stibii et Kalii Tartras; Tartar Emetic; Tartarus Stibiatus. Dipotassium bis{μ-[2,3-dihydroxybutanedioato(4-)-$O^1,O^2:O^3,O^4$]}diantimonate(2-) trihydrate; Dipotassium bis[μ-tartrato(4-)]diantimonate(2-) trihydrate.

$C_8H_4K_2O_{12}Sb_2,3H_2O = 667.9$.

CAS — 11071-15-1 (anhydrous antimony potassium tartrate); 28300-74-5 (antimony potassium tartrate trihydrate).

Pharmacopoeias. In Fr., It., and US. In some pharmacopoeias the monograph substance is described as $C_4H_4KO_7Sb,\frac{1}{2}H_2O$ (= 333.9).

Pharmacopoeial description

USP 25: Odourless, colourless, transparent crystals or white powder. The crystals effloresce on exposure to air and do not readily rehydrate even on exposure to high humidity. Soluble 1 in 12 of water, 1 in 3 of boiling water, and 1 in 15 of glycerol; insoluble in alcohol. Its solutions are acid to litmus.

Antimony Sodium Tartrate (756-l)

Antim. Sod. Tart.; Sodium Antimonyltartrate; Stibium Natrium Tartaricum. Disodium bis{μ-[2,3-dihydroxybutanedioato(4-)-$O^1,O^2:O^3,O^4$]}diantimonate(2-); Disodium bis{μ-[L-(+)-tartrato(4-)]}diantimonate(2-).

$C_8H_4Na_2O_{12}Sb_2 = 581.6$.

CAS — 34521-09-0.

Pharmacopoeias. In Int. (as $C_4H_4NaO_7Sb$ = 308.8) and US.

Pharmacopoeial description

USP 25: Odourless, colourless, transparent crystals or white powder. The crystals effloresce on exposure to air. Freely soluble in water; insoluble in alcohol.

Sodium Stibocaptate (810-h)

Sodium Stibocaptate (BAN, rINN).

Antimony Sodium Dimercaptosuccinate; Ro-4-1544/6; Sb-58; Stibocaptate; TWSb/6. Antimony sodium meso-2,3-dimercaptosuccinate. The formula varies from:

$C_{12}H_{11}NaO_{12}S_6Sb_2 = 806.1$ to $C_{12}H_6Na_6O_{12}S_6Sb_2 = 916.0$.

CAS — 3064-61-7 ($C_{12}H_6Na_6O_{12}S_6Sb_2$).

Stibophen (811-m)

Estibofeno; Fouadin; Stibophenum. Bis[4,5-dihydroxybenzene-1,3-disulphonato(4−)-O^4,O^5]antimonate(5−) pentasodium heptahydrate.

$C_{12}H_4N_{a5}O_{16}S_4Sb,7H_2O = 895.2$.

CAS — 15489-16-4 (stibophen heptahydrate).

ATC — P02BX03.

Pharmacopoeias. In It.

Adverse Effects and Treatment

Trivalent antimony compounds are more toxic than pentavalent antimonials such as sodium stibogluconate, possibly because they are excreted much more slowly. The most serious adverse effects are on the heart and liver. There are invariably ECG changes during treatment, but hypotension, bradycardia, and cardiac arrhythmias are more serious. Sudden death or cardiovascular collapse may occur at any time. Elevated liver enzyme values are common; liver damage with hepatic failure and death is more likely in patients with pre-existing hepatic disease.

Adverse effects immediately after intravenous administration of trivalent antimonials, in particular the tartrates, have included coughing, chest pain, pain in the arms, vomiting, abdominal pain, fainting, and collapse, especially after rapid injection. Extravasation during injection is extremely painful because of tissue damage. An anaphylactoid reaction characterised by an urticarial rash, husky voice, and collapse has been reported after the sixth or seventh intravenous injection of a course of treatment.

Numerous less immediate adverse effects have occurred including gastrointestinal disturbances, muscular and joint pains, arthritis, pneumonia, dyspnoea, headache, dizziness, weak-

The symbol † denotes a preparation no longer actively marketed

ness, pruritus, skin rashes, facial oedema, fever, haemolytic anaemia, and kidney damage.

Large doses of antimony compounds taken by mouth have an emetic action. Continuous treatment with small doses of antimony may give rise to symptoms of subacute poisoning similar to those of chronic arsenical poisoning.

Treatment of severe poisoning with antimony compounds is similar to that for arsenic poisoning (p.1582); dimercaprol may be of benefit.

◊ References.
1. Stemmer KL. Pharmacology and toxicology of heavy metals: antimony. *Pharmacol Ther* 1976; 1: 157–60.

Precautions

Trivalent antimony therapy has generally been superseded by less toxic treatment. It is contra-indicated in the presence of lung, heart, liver, and kidney disease. Intravenous injections should be administered very slowly and stopped if coughing, vomiting, or substernal pain occurs; extravasation should be avoided.

Some antimony compounds such as the tartrates cause severe pain and tissue necrosis and should not be given by intramuscular or subcutaneous injection.

◊ In the event of trivalent antimony compounds being used then patients with glucose-6-phosphate dehydrogenase deficiency should be excluded. WHO lists stibophen[1] among the anthelmintics to be avoided in patients with this deficiency.
1. WHO. Glucose-6-phosphate dehydrogenase deficiency. *Bull WHO* 1989; 67: 601–11.

Pharmacokinetics

Antimony compounds are poorly absorbed from the gastrointestinal tract.

They are slowly excreted, mainly in the urine, following parenteral administration. Antimony accumulates in the body during treatment and persists for several months afterwards. Trivalent antimony has a greater affinity for cell proteins than for plasma proteins.

Uses and Administration

Trivalent antimony compounds were used in the treatment of the protozoal infection leishmaniasis until the advent of the less toxic pentavalent compounds. They continued to be used in the treatment of schistosomiasis, but have now been superseded by less toxic and more easily administered drugs such as praziquantel.

Antimony sodium tartrate was formerly used as an emetic and expectorant.

Preparations

Proprietary Preparations (details are given in Part 3)
Multi-ingredient: *Fr.:* Montavon†; *Hong Kong:* Cocillana Compound; *Thai.:* Brown Mixture.

Ascaridole (761-s)

Ascaridol. 1-Isopropyl-4-methyl-2,3-dioxabicyclo[2.2.2]oct-5-ene.

$C_{10}H_{16}O_2 = 168.2$.

CAS — 512-85-6.

The active principle of chenopodium oil. It is an unstable liquid which is liable to explode when heated or when treated with organic acids.

Profile

Ascaridole has the same actions as chenopodium oil (below).

Bephenium Hydroxynaphthoate (762-w)

Bephenium Hydroxynaphthoate (BAN, rINN).

Naphthammonum. Benzyldimethyl(2-phenoxyethyl)ammonium 3-hydroxy-2-naphthoate.

$C_{28}H_{29}NO_4 = 443.5$.

CAS — 7181-73-9 (bephenium); 3818-50-6 (bephenium hydroxynaphthoate).

Pharmacopoeias. In Int.

Profile

Bephenium hydroxynaphthoate is an anthelmintic formerly used in the treatment of hookworm infections due to *Ancylostoma duodenale*.

Preparations

Proprietary Preparations (details are given in Part 3)
Braz.: Debefenium.

Betanaphthol (763-e)

β-Naftol; Naphthol. Naphth-2-ol.

$C_{10}H_8O = 144.2$.

CAS — 135-19-3.

Pharmacopoeias. In Aust., Pol., and Swiss.

Profile

Betanaphthol was formerly used as an anthelmintic in hookworm and tapeworm infections, but it has been superseded by less toxic and more efficient drugs.

Betanaphthol has a potent parasiticidal effect and was used as an ointment in the treatment of scabies, ringworm, and other skin diseases.

Betanaphthyl benzoate was used similarly.

Preparations

Proprietary Preparations (details are given in Part 3)
Multi-ingredient: *Aust.:* Salvyl; *Spain:* Salva Infantes.

Bithionol (2210-k)

Bithionol (BAN, rINN).

Bitionol. 2,2′-Thiobis(4,6-dichlorophenol).

$C_{12}H_6Cl_4O_2S = 356.1$.

CAS — 97-18-7.

ATC — D10AB01; P02BX01.

Pharmacopoeias. Fr. includes bithionol oxide for veterinary use.

Adverse Effects

Adverse effects in patients taking bithionol by mouth include anorexia, nausea, vomiting, abdominal discomfort, diarrhoea, salivation, dizziness, headache, and skin rashes.

Photosensitivity reactions have occurred in persons using soap containing bithionol. Cross-sensitisation with other halogenated disinfectants has also occurred.

Uses and Administration

Bithionol is a chlorinated bis-phenol with bactericidal and anthelmintic properties. It is active against most trematodes (flukes). Bithionol is used in preference to praziquantel in fascioliasis (p.93) and is also used in paragonimiasis (p.94) as an alternative to praziquantel. It has been given in a dose of 30 to 50 mg per kg body-weight by mouth on alternate days for 10 to 15 doses. WHO recommends a regimen of 30 mg per kg body-weight daily for 5 days to treat fascioliasis.

Bithionol is no longer used topically as a bactericide because of photosensitivity reactions.

Bromofenofos (20577-a)

Bromofenofos (rINN).

Bromfenofos; Bromophenophos; Bromphenphos. 3,3′,5,5′-Tetrabromo-2,2′-biphenyldiolmono(dihydrogen phosphate).

$C_{12}H_7Br_4O_5P = 581.8$.

CAS — 21466-07-9.

Profile

Bromofenofos is an organophosphorus compound used as an anthelmintic in veterinary medicine for the treatment of fluke infections.

For a description of the toxic effects of organophosphorus compounds and the treatment of acute poisoning, see Organophosphorus Insecticides, p.1435.

Chenopodium Oil (768-c)

Aetheroleum Chenopodii; Esencia de Quenopodio Vermifuga; Oil of American Wormseed; Wurmsamenöl.

CAS — 8006-99-3.

Pharmacopoeias. In It.

Distilled with steam from the fresh flowering and fruiting plants, excluding roots, of *Chenopodium ambrosioides* var. *anthelminticum*. It contains ascaridole.

CAUTION. Chenopodium oil may explode when heated.

Profile

Chenopodium oil was formerly used as an anthelmintic for the expulsion of roundworms (*Ascaris*) and hookworms. It is toxic and has caused numerous fatalities.

Clorsulon (18980-p)

Clorsulon (BAN, USAN, rINN).

MK-401. 4-Amino-6-(trichlorovinyl)benzene-1,3-disulphonamide.

$C_8H_8Cl_3N_3O_4S_2 = 380.7$.

CAS — 60200-06-8.

Pharmacopoeias. In US for veterinary use only.

Pharmacopoeial description

USP 25: A white to off-white powder. Slightly soluble in water; freely soluble in acetonitrile and in methyl alcohol; very slightly soluble in dichloromethane.

Profile

Clorsulon is a veterinary anthelmintic used in the treatment of liver fluke infections.

Closantel (1984-s)

Closantel (BAN, USAN, rINN).

R-31520 (closantel); R-34828 (closantel sodium). 5′-Chloro-4′-(4-chloro-α-cyanobenzyl)-3,5-di-iodosalicyl-o-toluidide.

$C_{22}H_{14}Cl_2I_2N_2O_2 = 663.1$.

CAS — 57808-65-8 (closantel); 61438-64-0 (closantel sodium).

Profile

Closantel is a veterinary anthelmintic used in the treatment of liver fluke infections.

◊ Loss of eyesight was reported in 11 women who received closantel (Flukiver) in mistake for a gynaecological product.[1] Sight was restored after closantel administration was stopped but incapacitating eye pain remained.

1. 't Hoen E, et al. Harmful human use of donated veterinary drug. Lancet 1993; 342: 308–9.

Diamfenetide (12639-c)

Diamfenetide (BAN, rINN).

Diamfenetidum; Diamphenethide. β,β′-Oxybis(aceto-p-phenetidide).

$C_{20}H_{24}N_2O_5 = 372.4$.

CAS — 36141-82-9.

Profile

Diamfenetide is a veterinary anthelmintic that has been used for the control of fascioliasis in sheep.

Dichlorophen (771-e)

Dichlorophen (BAN, rINN).

Di-phenthane-70; G-4. 2,2′-Methylenebis(4-chlorophenol).

$C_{13}H_{10}Cl_2O_2 = 269.1$.

CAS — 97-23-4.

ATC — P02DX02.

Pharmacopoeias. In Aust., Br., and Fr.

Pharmacopoeial description

BP 2001: A white or slightly cream-coloured powder with a not more than slightly phenolic odour. Practically insoluble in water; freely soluble in alcohol; very soluble in ether.

Profile

Dichlorophen is an anthelmintic that was used in the treatment of infection by tapeworms but has been superseded by praziquantel or niclosamide.

Dichlorophen also has antifungal and antibacterial activity and has been used topically in the treatment of fungal infections and as a germicide in soaps and cosmetics.

Preparations

BP 2001: Dichlorophen Tablets.

Proprietary Preparations (details are given in Part 3)
Multi-ingredient: S.Afr.: Mycota; UK: Germolene; Mycota.

Diethylcarbamazine Citrate (772-I)

Diethylcarbamazine Citrate (BANM, rINNM).

Diethylcarbam. Cit.; Diethylcarbamazine Acid Citrate; Diethylcarbamazini Citras; Ditrazini Citras; RP-3799. NN-Diethyl-4-methylpiperazine-1-carboxamide dihydrogen citrate.

$C_{10}H_{21}N_3O,C_6H_8O_7 = 391.4$.

CAS — 90-89-1 (diethylcarbamazine); 1642-54-2 (diethylcarbamazine citrate).

Pharmacopoeias. In Chin., Eur. (see p.vi), Int., Jpn, and US.

Pharmacopoeial description

Ph. Eur.: A white, crystalline, slightly hygroscopic powder. M.p. about 138° with decomposition. Very soluble in water; soluble in alcohol; practically insoluble in acetone and in ether. Store in airtight containers.

USP 25: A white, crystalline, slightly hygroscopic powder, odourless or has a slight odour. M.p. about 136° with decomposition. Very soluble in water; sparingly soluble in alcohol; practically insoluble in acetone, in chloroform, and in ether. Store in airtight containers.

Adverse Effects

Adverse effects directly attributable to diethylcarbamazine include nausea and vomiting. Headache, dizziness, and drowsiness may occur.

Hypersensitivity reactions arise from the death of the microfilariae. These can be serious, especially in onchocerciasis where there may also be sight-threatening ocular toxicity; fatalities have been reported. Encephalitis may be exacerbated in patients with loiasis and fatalities have occurred.

◊ Reactions occurring during diethylcarbamazine treatment of lymphatic filariasis are basically of 2 types: pharmacological dose-dependent responses and a response of the infected host

to the destruction and death of parasites.[1] Reactions of the first type include weakness, dizziness, lethargy, anorexia, and nausea. They begin within 1 to 2 hours of taking diethylcarbamazine, and persist for a few hours. Reactions of the second type are less likely to occur and are less severe in bancroftian than in brugian filariasis. They may be systemic or local, both with and without fever. Systemic reactions may occur a few hours after the first oral dose of diethylcarbamazine and generally do not last for more than 3 days. They include headache, aches in other parts of the body, joint pain, dizziness, anorexia, malaise, transient haematuria, allergic reactions, vomiting, and sometimes attacks of bronchial asthma in asthmatic patients. Fever and systemic reactions are positively associated with microfilaraemia. Systemic reactions are reduced if diethylcarbamazine is given in spaced doses or in repeated small doses. They eventually cease spontaneously and interruption of treatment is rarely necessary; symptomatic treatment with antipyretics or analgesics may be helpful. Local reactions tend to occur later in the course of treatment and last longer; they also disappear spontaneously and interruption of treatment is not necessary. Local reactions include lymphadenitis, abscess, ulceration, and transient lymphoedema; funiculitis and epididymitis may also occur in bancroftian filariasis.

In most patients with onchocerciasis the microfilaricidal activity of diethylcarbamazine leads to a series of events with dermal, ocular, and systemic components, known as the Mazzotti reaction, within minutes to hours after its administration.[2] Clinical manifestations can be severe, dangerous, and debilitating and WHO no longer recommends the use of diethylcarbamazine in onchocerciasis. Systemic reactions include increased itching, rash, headache, aching muscles, joint pain, painful swollen and tender lymph nodes, fever, tachycardia and hypotension, and vertigo. Most patients experience eye discomfort in the first few hours after diethylcarbamazine treatment. Punctate keratitis can develop as can optic neuritis and visual field loss.

It has been suggested that the release of interleukin-6 may be implicated in diethylcarbamazine's adverse effects in patients with lymphatic filariasis.[3]

1. WHO. Lymphatic filariasis: the disease and its control: fifth report of the WHO expert committee on filariasis. WHO Tech Rep Ser 821 1992.
2. WHO. WHO expert committee on onchocerciasis: third report. WHO Tech Rep Ser 752 1987.
3. Yazdanbakhsh M, et al. Serum interleukin-6 levels and adverse reactions to diethylcarbamazine in lymphatic filariasis. J Infect Dis 1992; 166: 453–4.

Precautions

Treatment with diethylcarbamazine should be closely supervised since hypersensitivity reactions are common and may be severe, especially in patients with onchocerciasis or loiasis. Patients with onchocerciasis should be monitored for eye changes. (The use of diethylcarbamazine to treat onchocerciasis is no longer recommended.) In patients with heavy Loa loa infection there is a small risk of encephalopathy and diethylcarbamazine should be discontinued at the first sign of cerebral involvement.

Infants, pregnant women, the elderly, and the debilitated, especially those with cardiac or renal disease, are normally excluded when diethylcarbamazine is used in mass treatment schedules.

◊ The use of diethylcarbamazine 2 mg per kg body-weight as a provocative day test for the detection of microfilariae of nocturnally periodic Wuchereria bancrofti in the blood, was not suitable in the presence of onchocerciasis or loiasis.[1]

1. McMahon JE, et al. Tanzania filariasis project: a provocative day test with diethylcarbamazine for the detection of microfilariae of nocturnally periodic Wuchereria bancrofti in the blood. Bull WHO 1979; 57: 759–65.

Pregnancy. Animal studies[1] suggest that the uterine hypermotility induced by diethylcarbamazine is mediated via prostaglandin synthesis; this might explain the mechanism of the abortifacient action previously reported.[2]

1. Joseph CA, Dixon PAF. Possible prostaglandin-mediated effect of diethylcarbamazine on rat uterine contractility. J Pharm Pharmacol 1984; 36: 281–2.
2. Subbu VSV, Biswas AR. Ecbolic effect of diethyl carbamazine. Indian J Med Res 1971; 59: 646–7.

Renal impairment. For a study on the effects of renal impairment on the pharmacokinetics of diethylcarbamazine, see under Pharmacokinetics, below.

Pharmacokinetics

Diethylcarbamazine citrate is readily absorbed from the gastrointestinal tract and also through the skin and conjunctiva. It is widely distributed in tissues and is excreted in the urine unchanged and as the N-oxide metabolite. Urinary excretion and hence plasma half-life is dependent on urinary pH.

◊ A pharmacokinetic study in 6 patients with onchocerciasis[1] indicated that diethylcarbamazine is absorbed quickly and al-

most completely from the gastrointestinal tract and is eliminated largely as unchanged drug in urine with relatively small amounts being excreted as the N-oxide metabolite. Following a single radioactively labelled dose of diethylcarbamazine citrate 0.5 mg per kg body-weight, administered by mouth as an aqueous solution, peak plasma concentrations of 100 to 150 nanograms per mL were achieved in 1 to 2 hours, followed by a sharp decline, then a marked secondary rise 3 to 6 hours after dosing followed by a steady decline. The half-life ranged from 9 to 13 hours. Urinary excretion of diethylcarbamazine and diethylcarbamazine N-oxide was complete within 96 hours; between 4 and 5% of the dose was recovered in the faeces. Disposition kinetics were similar in 5 healthy subjects given a single 50-mg tablet of diethylcarbamazine citrate. Peak plasma concentrations were initially 80 to 200 nanograms per mL, with a secondary rise 3 to 9 hours after dosing, the terminal half-life ranged from 5 to 13 hours, and urinary excretion of unchanged diethylcarbamazine and the N-oxide was complete within 48 hours.

When an alkaline urinary pH was maintained the elimination half-life of diethylcarbamazine and the area under the plasma concentration versus time curve were significantly increased compared with values when an acidic urinary pH was maintained.[2] However, alkalinisation of the urine in an attempt to decrease the dose of diethylcarbamazine in onchocerciasis was unlikely to be of practical value.[3]

1. Edwards G, et al. Diethylcarbamazine disposition in patients with onchocerciasis. Clin Pharmacol Ther 1981; 30: 551–7.
2. Edwards G, et al. The effect of variations in urinary pH on the pharmacokinetics of diethylcarbamazine. Br J Clin Pharmacol 1981; 12: 807–12.
3. Awadzi K, et al. The effect of moderate urine alkalinisation on low dose diethylcarbamazine therapy in patients with onchocerciasis. Br J Clin Pharmacol 1986; 21: 669–76.

Renal impairment. Results in patients with chronic renal impairment and healthy subjects, given a single 50-mg dose of diethylcarbamazine citrate by mouth, indicated that the plasma half-life of diethylcarbamazine is prolonged and its 24-hour urinary excretion considerably reduced in those with moderate and severe degrees of renal impairment.[1] Mean plasma half-lives in 7 patients with severe renal impairment (creatinine clearance less than 25 mL per minute), 5 patients with moderate renal impairment (creatinine clearance between 25 and 60 mL per minute), and 4 healthy subjects were 15.1, 7.7, and 2.7 hours, respectively. The patient with the longest plasma half-life of 32 hours did not have the poorest renal function, but it was considered likely that the abnormally slow elimination of diethylcarbamazine was due to the high urine pH (7) resulting from sodium bicarbonate therapy. A further patient with a half-life longer than expected also had a less acidic urine.

1. Adjepon-Yamoah KK, et al. The effect of renal disease on the pharmacokinetics of diethylcarbamazine in man. Br J Clin Pharmacol 1982; 13: 829–34.

Uses and Administration

Diethylcarbamazine citrate is an anthelmintic used in the treatment of lymphatic filariasis due to Wuchereria bancrofti (bancroftian filariasis), Brugia malayi, or B. timori (both known as brugian filariasis and as Malayan and Timorian filariasis respectively). It is also used in loiasis due to Loa loa. It was used in onchocerciasis due to Onchocerca volvulus before ivermectin became available. Diethylcarbamazine is active against both the microfilariae and adult worms of W. bancrofti, B. malayi, and Loa loa, but only against the microfilariae of O. volvulus. It has been tried in Mansonella infections and may be most effective against M. streptocerca. Diethylcarbamazine is also used in the treatment of toxocariasis (visceral larva migrans). For discussions of these infections and their treatment, see under Choice of Anthelmintic, p.91. See also below.

Diethylcarbamazine citrate is usually administered by mouth as tablets.

In the treatment of filarial infections due to W. bancrofti, B. malayi, B. timori, and Loa loa the manufacturer recommends 6 mg per kg body-weight daily in 3 divided doses for 3 weeks, given in an initial dosage of 1 mg per kg daily, gradually increased to 6 mg per kg daily over 3 days then maintained for 3 weeks, to reduce the incidence and severity of hypersensitivity reactions due to the destruction of microfilariae. However, in bancroftian filariasis WHO recommends 6 mg per kg daily for 12 days, and in brugian filariasis a dose of 3 to 6 mg per kg daily for 6 to 12 days. In the treatment of loiasis, WHO recommends a dose of 1 mg per kg as a single dose initially, doubled on two successive days and then adjusted to 2 to 3 mg per kg three times daily for a further 18 days. A corticosteroid may be given concurrently in the treatment of filarial infections. Similar doses are given for 3 weeks in the treatment of toxocariasis.

In the prophylaxis of loiasis a dose of 300 mg weekly has been recommended.

In areas where lymphatic filariasis is endemic, mass treatment campaigns can reduce the intensity of transmission and incidence of disease. Diethylcarbamazine may also be used in the form of medicated salt to control lymphatic filariasis. For further details, see below.

Administration. Diethylcarbamazine was first used as the chloride, but is now produced as the dihydrogen citrate which contains only half its weight as base. In reporting doses it is therefore important to indicate whether they refer to a specific salt or to the base; unless otherwise stated, it can generally be assumed that the dose refers to the citrate.[1]

1. WHO. Lymphatic filariasis: fourth report of the WHO expert committee on filariasis. *WHO Tech Rep Ser 702* 1984.

Loiasis. Diethylcarbamazine citrate is the main drug used in the management of loiasis (p.93).

References.
1. Nutman TB, *et al.* Loa loa infection in temporary residents of endemic regions: recognition of a hyperresponsive syndrome with characteristic clinical manifestations. *J Infect Dis* 1986; **154:** 10–18.
2. Nutman TB, *et al.* Diethylcarbamazine prophylaxis for human loiasis: results of a double-blind study. *N Engl J Med* 1988; **319:** 752–6.
3. Nutman TB, Ottesen EA. Diethylcarbamazine and human loiasis. *N Engl J Med* 1989; **320:** 320.

Lymphatic filariasis. Diethylcarbamazine citrate is used in the management of lymphatic filariasis (p.94). In endemic areas where more than 5% of the population is infected, mass treatment of the entire population (excluding neonates, pregnant women, and debilitated individuals) can reduce the intensity of transmission and the incidence of disease. In countries where there is no co-endemic loiasis or onchocerciasis, a global elimination campaign launched by WHO together with other international agencies advocates a single dose of diethylcarbamazine 6 mg per kg body-weight together with a single dose of albendazole 400 mg, given once each year for 4 to 6 years. If diethylcarbamazine-medicated salt is to be employed then intake of salt needs to be on a daily basis for 6 to 12 months.

Diethylcarbamazine has also been used diagnostically. Detecting microfilariae in lymphatic filariasis can be difficult because of their nocturnal periodicity. Small doses of diethylcarbamazine can stimulate the microfilariae thus aiding their detection in the daytime in blood specimens.[1] For cautions against using such a test in patients with loiasis or onchocerciasis, see Precautions, above. Also it has been suggested that tests on finger-prick blood samples may not be as accurate as those carried out on samples of venous blood.[2]

1. Sabry M. A quantitative analysis of the diagnostic value of diethylcarbamazine provocation in endemic Wuchereria bancrofti infection. *Trans R Soc Trop Med Hyg* 1988; **82:** 117–21.
2. Eberhard ML, *et al.* Persistence of microfilaremia in bancroftian filariasis after diethylcarbamazine citrate therapy. *Trop Med Parasitol* 1988; **39:** 128–30.

Preparations

USP 25: Diethylcarbamazine Citrate Tablets.

Proprietary Preparations (details are given in Part 3)
Austral.: Hetrazan†; *Canad.:* Hetrazan†; *Fr.:* Notezine; *UK:* Hetrazan.

Disophenol (19115-r)

2,6-Diiodo-4-nitrophenol.
$C_6H_3I_2NO_3 = 390.9$.
CAS — 305-85-1.

Profile
Disophenol is an anthelmintic used in veterinary medicine.

Doramectin (14635-v)

Doramectin (*BAN, USAN, rINN*).
UK-67994.
CAS — 117704-25-3.

Profile
Doramectin is an avermectin anthelmintic used in veterinary medicine for nematode infections. It is also used as a systemic veterinary ectoparasiticide.

Embelia (777-k)

Vidang.
CAS — 550-24-3 (embelic acid).

The dried fruits of *Embelia ribes* and *E. robusta* (= *E. tsjeriamcottam*) (Myrsinaceae), containing about 2.5% of embelic acid (embelin).

Profile
Embelia has been used in India and other eastern countries for the expulsion of tapeworms.

Eprinomectin (19088-e)

Eprinomectin (*USAN, rINN*).
Eprinomectina; Eprinomectine; MK-397. A mixture of eprinomectin component B$_{1a}$ and eprinomectin component B$_{1b}$.
CAS — 159628-36-1 (eprinomectin); 123997-26-2 (eprinomectin); 133305-88-1 (component B$_{1a}$); 133305-89-2 (component B$_{1b}$).

Profile
Eprinomectin is an avermectin anthelmintic used in veterinary medicine for nematode infections. It is also used as a systemic veterinary ectoparasiticide.

Epsiprantel (2490-a)

Epsiprantel (*BAN, rINN*).
BRL-38705. 2-Cyclohexylcarbonyl-1,2,3,4,6,7,8,12b-octahydropyrazino[2,1-*a*][2]benzazepin-4-one.
$C_{20}H_{26}N_2O_2 = 326.4$.
CAS — 98123-83-2.

Profile
Epsiprantel is an anthelmintic closely related to praziquantel. It is used in veterinary medicine.

Febantel (12729-a)

Febantel (*BAN, USAN, rINN*).
Bay-h-5757; Bay-Vh-5757. 2′-[2,3-Bis(methoxycarbonyl)guanidino]-5′-phenylthio-2-methoxyacetanilide; Dimethyl {2-[2-(2-methoxyacetamido)-4-(phenylthio)phenyl]imidocarbonyl}dicarbamate.
$C_{20}H_{22}N_4O_6S = 446.5$.
CAS — 58306-30-2.

Profile
Febantel is a veterinary anthelmintic used in the treatment of nematode infections of the gastrointestinal tract and lungs and in tapeworm infections.

Fenbendazole (778-a)

Fenbendazole (*BAN, USAN, rINN*).
Hoe-881V. Methyl 5-phenylthio-1*H*-benzimidazol-2-ylcarbamate.
$C_{15}H_{13}N_3O_2S = 299.3$.
CAS — 43210-67-9.
ATC — P02CA06.
Pharmacopoeias. In *Eur.* (see p.vi) for veterinary use only.

Pharmacopoeial description
Ph. Eur.: A white or almost white powder. Practically insoluble in water; sparingly soluble in dimethylformamide; very slightly soluble in methyl alcohol. Protect from light.

Profile
Fenbendazole is a benzimidazole carbamate anthelmintic structurally related to mebendazole (p.102). It is used in veterinary practice.

Flubendazole (12756-r)

Flubendazole (*BAN, USAN, rINN*).
Fluoromebendazole; R-17889. Methyl 5-(4-fluorobenzoyl)-1*H*-benzimidazol-2-ylcarbamate.
$C_{16}H_{12}FN_3O_3 = 313.3$.
CAS — 31430-15-6.
ATC — P02CA05.

Profile
Flubendazole, a benzimidazole carbamate anthelmintic, is an analogue of mebendazole (p.102) and has similar actions and uses.

For the treatment of enterobiasis in adults and children, flubendazole 100 mg is given by mouth as a single dose, repeated if necessary after 2 to 3 weeks. For ascariasis, hookworm infections, and trichuriasis 100 mg is given twice daily for 3 days. For discussions of these infections and their treatment, see under Choice of Anthelmintic, p.91.

Preparations

Proprietary Preparations (details are given in Part 3)
Fr.: Fluvermal; *Port.:* Fluvermal; Teniverme; *Spain:* Flicum.

Haloxon (12815-c)

Haloxon (*BAN, rINN*).
Bis(2-chloroethyl) 3-chloro-4-methylcoumarin-7-yl phosphate.
$C_{14}H_{14}Cl_3O_6P = 415.6$.
CAS — 321-55-1.
Pharmacopoeias. In BP(Vet).

Pharmacopoeial description
BP(Vet) 2001: A white or almost white, odourless or almost odourless powder. M.p. 88° to 93°. Practically insoluble in water; freely soluble in alcohol, in acetone, and in chloroform.

Profile
Haloxon is an organophosphorus compound used as an anthelmintic in veterinary medicine.

For a description of the toxic effects of organophosphorus compounds and the treatment of acute poisoning, see Organophosphorus Insecticides, p.1435.

Hexachloroparaxylene (781-γ)

Chloxyle; Hetol; Hexachloroparaxylol. 1,4-Bis(trichloromethyl)benzene.
$C_8H_4Cl_6 = 312.8$.
CAS — 68-36-0.

Profile
Hexachloroparaxylene has been used in China and the former USSR as an anthelmintic, principally to treat the liver fluke infections clonorchiasis and opisthorchiasis, but other treatment is preferred.

Adverse effects reported with hexachloroparaxylene have included gastrointestinal disturbances, cardiac arrhythmias, nephrotoxicity, and haemolysis.

Hycanthone Mesilate (783-z)

Hycanthone Mesilate (*rINNM*).
Hycanthone Mesylate; Hydroxylucanthone Methanesulphonate; NSC-134434 (hycanthone); Win-24933 (hycanthone). 1-(2-Diethylaminoethylamino)-4-hydroxymethylthioxanthen-9-one methanesulphonate.
$C_{20}H_{24}N_2O_2S,CH_3SO_3H = 452.6$.
CAS — 3105-97-3 (hycanthone); 23255-93-8 (hycanthone mesilate).

NOTE. Hycanthone is *USAN*.

Profile
Hycanthone has been used as a schistosomicide in the individual or mass treatment of infection with *Schistosoma haematobium* and *S. mansoni*.

Owing to its toxicity and concern about possible carcinogenicity, mutagenicity, and teratogenicity, hycanthone has been replaced by other drugs such as praziquantel.

Hygromycin B (19322-v)

O-6-Amino-6-deoxy-L-glycero-D-galacto-heptopyranosylidene-(1→2-3)-O-β-D-talopyranosyl-(1→5)-2-deoxy-N³-methyl-D-streptamine.
$C_{20}H_{37}N_3O_{13} = 527.5$.

Profile
Hygromycin B is an anthelmintic used in veterinary practice.

Ivermectin (12874-b)

Ivermectin (*BAN, USAN, rINN*).
CAS — 70288-86-7 (ivermectin); 70161-11-4 (component B$_{1a}$); 70209-81-3 (component B$_{1b}$).
ATC — P02CF01.
Pharmacopoeias. In *Eur.* (see p.vi).

Pharmacopoeial description
Ph. Eur.: A mixture of ivermectin component H$_2$B$_{1a}$ (5-*O*-demethyl-22,23-dihydroavermectin A$_{1a}$; $C_{48}H_{74}O_{14} = 875.1$) and ivermectin component H$_2$B$_{1b}$ (5-*O*-demethyl-25-de(1-methylpropyl)-25-(1-methylethyl)-22,23-dihydroavermectin A$_{1a}$; $C_{47}H_{72}O_{14} = 861.1$).

A white or yellowish-white, slightly hygroscopic, crystalline powder. Practically insoluble in water; soluble in alcohol; freely soluble in dichloromethane. Store in airtight containers.

Adverse Effects and Precautions

The adverse effects reported with ivermectin are generally consistent with a mild Mazzotti reaction arising from its effect on the microfilariae. They include fever, pruritus, arthralgia, myalgia, asthenia, postural hypotension, tachycardia, oedema, lymphadenopathy, gastrointestinal symptoms, sore throat, cough, and headache. The effects tend to be transient and if

The symbol † denotes a preparation no longer actively marketed

treatment is required they respond to analgesics and antihistamines.

Ivermectin may cause mild ocular irritation. Somnolence, transient eosinophilia, and raised liver enzyme values have also been reported.

There is some distribution into breast milk (see Breast Feeding, below). Administration of ivermectin is not recommended during pregnancy. Mass treatment is generally withheld from pregnant women (see Pregnancy, below), children under 15 kg body-weight, and the seriously ill.

◊ Some studies have shown quite a high incidence of adverse effects with ivermectin and have associated the effects with the severity of infection.[1-3] However, in none of these studies were the reactions considered to be life-threatening and only symptomatic treatment was required. The severity, incidence, and duration of adverse reactions was reported to be reduced after repeated annual administration.[4] When larger groups of patients were considered in the Onchocerciasis Control Programme (OCP) in West Africa a much lower incidence of adverse reactions was observed in patients given ivermectin for the first time[5] and when treatment was repeated a year later that incidence was reduced even further. The results from several trials in this programme[6] showed 93 severe reactions in 50 929 patients (1.83%), most of the reactions being postural hypotension or dizziness (53). A more recent study[7] found 22 severe reactions in 17 877 patients treated for onchocerciasis in an area also endemic for *Loa loa* infection, and demonstrated a relationship to heavy *L. loa* microfilaraemia. It was suggested that ivermectin should be used with caution for mass onchocerciasis treatment programmes in areas where loiasis and onchocerciasis co-exist.

Some supervision is considered necessary after administration of ivermectin;[2,6] the OCP recommendation[6] is for resident nurses to monitor patients for a period of 36 hours after treatment, whatever the level of endemicity. However, the incidence of adverse reactions reported after repeated doses appears to be lower than after the first dose and the need for supervision on re-treatment has been questioned.[8]

Neurotoxicity observed in some breeds of *dogs* has not been seen in *cattle* or *horses*[9] nor was it reported in man in the above studies. Another potential concern was the prolongation of prothrombin times observed in 28 patients given ivermectin,[10] but others have not confirmed this effect[11] or observed any bleeding disorders.[12]

There has been some concern over the use of ivermectin to treat scabies in elderly patients following a report suggesting a possible link to an increased incidence of death among a cohort of 47 patients.[13] It has, however, been argued that no such association has been seen in other populations of elderly patients and that the statistical methods used by the original authors were deficient.[14-16] There was no evidence of an increase in death rate associated with ivermectin in a community-based trial in Papua New Guinea of diethylcarbamazine with or without ivermectin for lymphatic filariasis.[17]

1. Kumaraswami V, *et al.* Ivermectin for the treatment of Wuchereria bancrofti filariasis: efficacy and adverse reactions. *JAMA* 1988; **259**: 3150–3.
2. Rothova A, *et al.* Side-effects of ivermectin in treatment of onchocerciasis. *Lancet* 1989; **i**: 1439–41.
3. Zea-Flores R, *et al.* Adverse reactions after community treatment of onchocerciasis with ivermectin in Guatemala. *Trans R Soc Trop Med Hyg* 1992; **86**: 663–6.
4. Burnham GM. Adverse reactions to ivermectin treatment for onchocerciasis: results of a placebo-controlled, double-blind trial in Malawi. *Trans R Soc Trop Med Hyg* 1993; **87**: 313–17.
5. De Sole G, *et al.* Lack of adverse reactions in ivermectin treatment of onchocerciasis. *Lancet* 1990; **335**: 1106–7.
6. De Sole G, *et al.* Adverse reactions after large-scale treatment of onchocerciasis with ivermectin: combined results from eight community trials. *Bull WHO* 1989; **67**: 707–19.
7. Gardon J, *et al.* Serious reactions after mass treatment of onchocerciasis with ivermectin in an area endemic for Loa loa infection. *Lancet* 1997; **350**: 18–22.
8. Whitworth JAG, *et al.* A community trial of ivermectin for onchocerciasis in Sierra Leone: adverse reactions after the five treatment rounds. *Trans R Soc Trop Med Hyg* 1991; **85**: 501–5.
9. WHO. WHO expert committee on onchocerciasis: third report. *WHO Tech Rep Ser* 752 1987.
10. Homeida MMA, *et al.* Prolongation of prothrombin time with ivermectin. *Lancet* 1988; **i**: 1346–7.
11. Richards FO, *et al.* Ivermectin and prothrombin time. *Lancet* 1989; **i**; 1139–40.
12. Pacque MC, *et al.* Ivermectin and prothrombin time. *Lancet* 1989; **i**: 1140.
13. Barkwell R, Shields S. Deaths associated with ivermectin treatment of scabies. *Lancet* 1997; **349**: 1144–5.
14. Diazgranados JA, Costa JL. Deaths after ivermectin treatment. *Lancet* 1997; **349**: 1698.
15. Reintjes R, Hoek C. Deaths associated with ivermectin for scabies. *Lancet* 1997; **350**: 215.
16. Coyne PE, Addiss DG. Deaths associated with ivermectin for scabies. *Lancet* 1997; **350**: 215–16.
17. Alexander NDE, *et al.* Absence of ivermectin-associated excess deaths. *Trans R Soc Trop Med Hyg* 1998; **92**: 342.

Breast feeding. The distribution of ivermectin into breast milk has limited its use in breast-feeding mothers. Ivermectin concentrations measured in the milk of 4 healthy lactating women who had been given a standard dose of ivermectin found the mean concentration in breast milk to be 14.13 nanograms per mL.[1] It was felt that in view of this low

concentration the precaution of excluding lactating mothers from ivermectin mass treatment programmes should be reconsidered. Some authorities have recommended that ivermectin should not be given to mothers who are breast feeding until the infant is at least one week old.

1. Ogbuokiri JE, *et al.* Ivermectin levels in human breast milk. *Eur J Clin Pharmacol* 1994; **46**: 89–90.

Pregnancy. It is recommended that pregnant women should be excluded from mass treatment schedules with ivermectin. However, it is recognised that women not yet diagnosed as pregnant or unwilling to admit their pregnancy have been treated. An assessment[1] of 203 pregnancy outcomes to women who had received ivermectin during pregnancy mostly during the first 12 weeks found that the rates of major congenital malformation, miscarriage, and still-birth associated with ivermectin were similar to those in untreated mothers. In another study,[2] 110 women also inadvertently given ivermectin during pregnancy experienced a similar lack of adverse effect on pregnancy outcome; it was considered that the precaution of avoiding the use of ivermectin in women notifying a pregnancy should be adequate.

1. Pacqué M, *et al.* Pregnancy outcome after inadvertent ivermectin treatment during community-based distribution. *Lancet* 1990; **336**: 1486–9.
2. Chippaux J-P, *et al.* Absence of any adverse effect of inadvertent ivermectin treatment during pregnancy. *Trans R Soc Trop Med Hyg* 1993; **87**: 318.

Pharmacokinetics

Ivermectin is absorbed from the gastrointestinal tract following oral administration with peak plasma concentrations being obtained after about 4 hours. Ivermectin is reported to be approximately 93% bound to plasma proteins and has a plasma elimination half-life of about 12 hours. It undergoes metabolism and is excreted largely as metabolites over a period of about 2 weeks, chiefly in the faeces, with less than 1% appearing in the urine and less than 2% in breast milk (see also Breast Feeding, above).

Uses and Administration

Ivermectin is a semisynthetic derivative of one of the avermectins, a group of macrocyclic lactones produced by *Streptomyces avermitilis*.

It has a microfilaricidal action in onchocerciasis and reduces the microfilarial load without the toxicity seen with diethylcarbamazine. Ivermectin also has a microfilaricidal action in lymphatic filariasis and is used in its management. Ivermectin is also active in some other worm infections. It is used in the treatment of strongyloidiasis and has been tried in some *Mansonella* infections. For details of these infections and their treatment, see under Choice of Anthelmintic, p.91. See also below.

A single dose of 3 to 12 mg based roughly on 150 µg per kg body-weight by mouth for patients weighing more than 15 kg and over 5 years of age is given annually or every 6 months in the treatment of onchocerciasis. This schedule has been adopted in the mass treatment of subjects in infected areas. No food should be taken for 2 hours before or after the dose.

Ivermectin 200 µg per kg as a single dose, or daily on two consecutive days, is used for the treatment of strongyloidiasis.

◊ Reviews.
1. Ottesen EA, Campbell WC. Ivermectin in human medicine. *J Antimicrob Chemother* 1994; **34**: 195–203.

Cutaneous larva migrans. There are some reports[1,2] of ivermectin being effective in the treatment of cutaneous larva migrans (p.92).
1. Caumes E, *et al.* Efficacy of ivermectin in the therapy of cutaneous larva migrans. *Arch Dermatol* 1992; **128**: 994–5.
2. Caumes E, *et al.* A randomized trial of ivermectin versus albendazole for the treatment of cutaneous larva migrans. *Am J Trop Med Hyg* 1993; **49**: 641–4.

Intestinal nematode infections. Ivermectin activity has been observed in man against *Ascaris lumbricoides*, *Strongyloides stercoralis*, and *Trichuris trichiura*[1] although some have failed to detect activity against *Trichuris*.[2] Roundworm expulsion has been reported as a 'side-effect' of ivermectin when used in community-based treatment of onchocerciasis.[3] In a controlled study[4] single doses of 150 or 200 µg of ivermectin per kg body-weight produced cure rates of 94% in strongyloidiasis (see below) and above 67% in ascariasis, trichuriasis, and enterobiasis. Although some activity has been observed against *Necator americanus*,[1] cure rates for hookworm were considered unsatisfactory.[4]

1. Freedman DO, *et al.* The efficacy of ivermectin in the chemotherapy of gastrointestinal helminthiasis in humans. *J Infect Dis* 1989; **159**: 1151–3.

2. Whitworth JAG, *et al.* A field study of the effect of ivermectin on intestinal helminths in man. *Trans R Soc Trop Med Hyg* 1991; **85**: 232–4.
3. Whitworth JAG, *et al.* Community-based treatment with ivermectin. *Lancet* 1988; **ii**: 97–8.
4. Naquira C, *et al.* Ivermectin for human strongyloidiasis and other intestinal helminths. *Am J Trop Med Hyg* 1989; **40**: 304–9.

Loiasis. There is evidence of reduced microfilaraemia following ivermectin treatment[1-5] in patients with loiasis (p.93), but concern over its potential for neurotoxicity in patients with a high microfilarial burden.[6,7]

1. Martin-Prevel Y, *et al.* Reduction of microfilaraemia with single high-dose of ivermectin in loiasis. *Lancet* 1993; 342: 442.
2. Ranque S, *et al.* Decreased prevalence and intensity of Loa loa infection in a community treated with ivermectin every three months for two years. *Trans R Soc Trop Med Hyg* 1996; **90**: 429–30.
3. Duong TH, *et al.* Reduced Loa loa microfilaria count ten to twelve months after a single dose of ivermectin. *Trans R Soc Trop Med Hyg* 1997; **91**: 592–3.
4. Gardon J, *et al.* Marked decrease in Loa loa microfilaraemia six and twelve months after a single dose of ivermectin. *Trans R Soc Trop Med Hyg* 1997; **91**: 593–4.
5. Chippaux J-P, *et al.* Impact of repeated large scale ivermectin treatments on the transmission of Loa loa. *Trans R Soc Trop Med Hyg* 1998; **92**: 454–8.
6. Anonymous. Encephalitis following treatment of loiasis. *WHO Drug Inf* 1991; **5**: 113–14.
7. Gardon J, *et al.* Serious reactions after mass treatment of onchocerciasis with ivermectin in an area endemic for Loa loa infection. *Lancet* 1997; **350**: 18–22.

Lymphatic filariasis. Ivermectin is used in the management of lymphatic filariasis (p.94). In endemic areas where more than 5% of the population is infected, mass treatment of the entire population (excluding neonates, pregnant women, and debilitated individuals) can reduce the intensity of transmission and the incidence of disease. For bancroftian filariasis in countries where there is co-endemic loiasis or onchocerciasis, a global elimination campaign launched by WHO together with other international agencies advocates a single dose of ivermectin 200 µg per kg body-weight together with a single dose of albendazole 400 mg given once each year for 4 to 6 years.

Mansonella infections. The response of *Mansonella* infections (p.94) to ivermectin depends on the species. It may be effective against *Mansonella ozzardi*, but studies in *M. perstans* infection have not shown ivermectin to produce a substantial reduction in microfilaraemia.[1,2] A good response to ivermectin has been reported in infections with *M. streptocerca*.[3]

1. Schulz-Key H, *et al.* Efficacy of ivermectin in the treatment of concomitant Mansonella perstans infections in onchocerciasis patients. *Trans R Soc Trop Med Hyg* 1993; **87**: 227–9.
2. Van den Enden E, *et al.* Treatment failure of a single high dose of ivermectin for Mansonella perstans filariasis. *Trans R Soc Trop Med Hyg* 1993; **87**: 90.
3. Fischer P, *et al.* Treatment of human Mansonella streptocerca infection with ivermectin. *Trop Med Int Hlth* 1997; **2**: 191–9.

Onchocerciasis. Ivermectin has a microfilaricidal action against *Onchocerca volvulus* and is the main drug used in the control of onchocerciasis (p.94). A single dose rapidly eliminates microfilariae from the skin and gradually eliminates them from the cornea and anterior chamber of the eye.[1] Ivermectin does not eliminate the adult worms but does suppress the release of microfilariae from the adult worm for several cycles which accounts for its prolonged activity. Its action against *O. volvulus* has been attributed to a GABA-agonist effect. Studies have also indicated that ivermectin inhibits the transmission of microfilariae by reducing their uptake from man by the insect vector.[2-5]

Ivermectin is donated without charge by *Merck* through the Mectizan Expert Committee (MEC) for human use in community-wide mass treatment programmes in all countries in which onchocerciasis is endemic, where it is given once a year to all but pregnant women, breast-feeding mothers of recently born babies, children weighing less than 15 kg, and those unable to walk or otherwise seriously ill.[6] Several studies have confirmed the long-term safety and efficacy of such programmes.[7-11]

The ocular microfilarial load can be safely reduced by ivermectin[1,12] and early lesions of the anterior segment of the eye have improved.[12] A reduction in the incidence[13] and progression[14] of optic nerve damage has also been reported but the effect on posterior segment disease is less certain.[15] Improvements in skin lesions have been reported.[16] Administration every 6 months produces a more rapid reduction of microfilariae than administration every year,[17] but it is difficult to tell whether any long-term advantages outweigh the disadvantages of more frequent administration. In non-endemic areas, repeated doses may be necessary to reduce recurrence; a study in the UK found that patients given three doses at monthly intervals had fewer relapses at 6 months than patients who received a single dose, but relapses were nevertheless seen in 50% of patients at 12 months.[18] Others have suggested that treatment may need to be repeated every 4 to 6 months.[19]

1. Newland HS, *et al.* Effect of single-dose ivermectin therapy on human Onchocerca volvulus infection with onchocercal ocular involvement. *Br J Ophthalmol* 1988; **72**: 561–9.
2. Taylor HR, *et al.* Impact of mass treatment of onchocerciasis with ivermectin on the transmission of infection. *Science* 1990; **250**: 116–18.
3. Trpis M, *et al.* Effect of mass treatment of a human population with ivermectin on transmission of Onchocerca volvulus by Simulium yahense in Liberia, West Africa. *Am J Trop Med Hyg* 1990; **42**: 148–56.

4. Chavasse DC, *et al.* Low level ivermectin coverage and the transmission of onchocerciasis. *Trans R Soc Trop Med Hyg* 1995; **89:** 534–7.

5. Boussinesq M, *et al.* Onchocerca volvulus: striking decrease in transmission in the Vina valley (Cameroon) after eight annual large scale ivermectin treatments. *Trans R Soc Trop Med Hyg* 1997; **91:** 82–6.

6. Pond B. Distribution of ivermectin by health workers. *Lancet* 1990; **335:** 1539.

7. De Sole G, *et al.* Adverse reactions after large-scale treatment of onchocerciasis with ivermectin: combined results from eight community trials. *Bull WHO* 1989; **67:** 707–19.

8. Pacqué M, *et al.* Safety of and compliance with community-based ivermectin therapy. *Lancet* 1990; **335:** 1377–80.

9. Pacqué M, *et al.* Community-based treatment of onchocerciasis with ivermectin: safety, efficacy, and acceptability of yearly treatment. *J Infect Dis* 1991; **163:** 381–5.

10. Steel C, *et al.* Immunologic responses to repeated ivermectin treatment in patients with onchocerciasis. *J Infect Dis* 1991; **164:** 581–7.

11. Whitworth JAG, *et al.* A community trial of ivermectin for onchocerciasis in Sierra Leone: clinical and parasitological responses to four doses given at six-monthly interval. *Trans R Soc Trop Med Hyg* 1992; **86:** 277–80.

12. Dadzie KY, *et al.* Changes in ocular onchocerciasis after two rounds of community-based ivermectin treatment in a holo-endemic onchocerciasis focus. *Trans R Soc Trop Med Hyg* 1991; **85:** 267–71.

13. Abiose A, *et al.* Reduction in incidence of optic nerve disease with annual ivermectin to control onchocerciasis. *Lancet* 1993; **341:** 130–4.

14. Cousens SN, *et al.* Impact of annual dosing with ivermectin on progression of onchocercal visual field loss. *Bull WHO* 1997; **75:** 229–36.

15. Whitworth JAG, *et al.* Effects of repeated doses of ivermectin on ocular onchocerciasis: community-based trial in Sierra Lione. *Lancet* 1991; **338:** 1100–1103.

16. Pacqué M, *et al.* Improvements in severe onchocercal skin disease after a single dose of ivermectin. *Am J Med* 1991; **90:** 590–4.

17. Greene BM, *et al.* A comparison of 6-, 12-, and 24-monthly dosing with ivermectin for treatment of onchocerciasis. *J Infect Dis* 1991; **163:** 376–80.

18. Churchill DR, *et al.* A trial of a three-dose regimen of ivermectin for the treatment of patients with onchocerciasis in the UK. *Trans R Soc Trop Med Hyg* 1994; **88:** 242.

19. Greene BM. Modern medicine versus an ancient scourge: progress toward control of onchocerciasis. *J Infect Dis* 1992; **166:** 15–21.

Scabies and pediculosis. Scabies (p.1427) is usually treated with a topically applied acaricide. However, a single oral dose of ivermectin has been reported to be effective.[1,2] In a study of 11 patients with uncomplicated scabies, a single oral dose of ivermectin 200 μg per kg body-weight was effective in curing infection after 4 weeks. In a group of 11 patients, also infected with HIV, scabies was cured in 8 after 2 weeks.[1] Two of the remaining 3 patients received a second dose of ivermectin which cured the scabies infection by the fourth week. A single oral dose of ivermectin 150 μg per kg was partially effective in an outbreak of scabies in 1153 Tanzanian patients.[3] Crusted (Norwegian) scabies has also been reported to be effectively treated by a single oral dose of 12 mg of ivermectin in addition to topical application of 3% salicylic acid ointment in 2 patients; the treatment was effective in under one week.[2] A single oral dose of ivermectin 200 μg per kg was effective for crusted scabies in a 2-year-old infant who had contracted the disease following long-term corticosteroid use.[4]

Ivermectin has also been investigated as a possible treatment for pediculosis (p.1427), although again, topically applied insecticides are the usual method of control. A study *in vitro* and in *animals* showed that ivermectin killed nymphs and females of the human body louse (*Pediculus humanus humanus*). Ivermectin was known to be effective against other louse species that infect a range of *animals*.[5]

1. Meinking TL, *et al.* The treatment of scabies with ivermectin. *N Engl J Med* 1995; **333:** 26–30.

2. Aubin F, Humbert P. Ivermectin for crusted (Norwegian) scabies. *N Engl J Med* 1995; **332:** 612.

3. Leppard B, Naburi AE. The use of ivermectin in controlling an outbreak of scabies in a prison. *Br J Dermatol* 2000; **143:** 520–3.

4. Marlière V, *et al.* Crusted (Norwegian) scabies induced by use of topical corticosteroids and treated successfully with ivermectin. *J Pediatr* 1999; **135:** 122–4.

5. Mumcuoglu KY, *et al.* Systemic activity of ivermectin on the human body louse (Anoplura: Pediculidae) *J Med Entomol* 1990; **27:** 72–5.

Strongyloidiasis. Ivermectin is effective in the treatment of strongyloidiasis (p.94) and is considered by some authorities to be the drug of choice.
References.

1. Naquira C, *et al.* Ivermectin for human strongyloidiasis and other intestinal helminths. *Am J Trop Med Hyg* 1989; **40:** 304–9.

2. Wijesundera M de S, Sanmuganathan PS. Ivermectin therapy in chronic strongyloidiasis. *Trans R Soc Trop Med Hyg* 1992; **86:** 291.

3. Lyagoubi M, *et al.* Chronic persistent strongyloidiasis cured by ivermectin. *Trans R Soc Trop Med Hyg* 1992; **86:** 541.

4. Datry A, *et al.* Treatment of Strongyloides stercoralis infection with ivermectin compared with albendazole: results of an open study of 60 cases. *Trans R Soc Trop Med Hyg* 1994; **88:** 344–5.

5. Gann PH, *et al.* A randomized trial of single- and two-dose ivermectin versus thiabendazole for treatment of strongyloidiasis. *J Infect Dis* 1994; **169:** 1076–9.

Preparations

Proprietary Preparations (details are given in Part 3)
Austral.: Stromectol; *Fr.:* Mectizan; Stromectol; *USA:* Mectizan; Stromectol.

Levamisole Hydrochloride (788-x)

Levamisole Hydrochloride (*BANM, USAN, rINNM*).

Cloridrato de Levamizol; ICI-59623; Levamisoli Hydrochloridum; NSC-177023; R-12564; RP-20605; *l*-Tetramisole Hydrochloride; *l*-Tetramisole Hydrochloride. (−)-(S)-2,3,5,6-Tetrahydro-6-phenylimidazo[2,1-*b*]thiazole hydrochloride.

$C_{11}H_{12}N_2S,HCl = 240.8$.

CAS — 14769-73-4 (levamisole); 16595-80-5 (levamisole hydrochloride).

Pharmacopoeias. In Chin., Eur. (see p.vi), and US.

Levamisole hydrochloride 1.18 g is approximately equivalent to 1 g of levamisole.

Pharmacopoeial description

Ph. Eur.: A white to almost white crystalline powder. Freely soluble in water; soluble in alcohol; slightly soluble in dichloromethane; practically insoluble in ether. A 5% solution in water has a pH of 3.0 to 4.5. Protect from light.

USP 25: A white or almost white crystalline powder. Freely soluble in water; soluble in alcohol; slightly soluble in dichloromethane; practically insoluble in ether. pH of a 5% solution in water is between 3.0 and 4.5. Protect from light.

Adverse Effects

When given in single doses for the treatment of ascariasis or other worm infections, levamisole is generally well tolerated and side-effects are usually limited to nausea, vomiting, diarrhoea, abdominal pain, dizziness, and headache.

When levamisole is used as an immunostimulant and given for longer periods, adverse effects are more frequent and diverse and, in common with other immunomodulators, may sometimes result from exacerbation of the primary underlying disease. Adverse effects associated especially with the more prolonged administration of levamisole have included: hypersensitivity reactions such as fever, an influenza-like syndrome, arthralgia, muscle pain, skin rashes, and cutaneous vasculitis; CNS effects including headache, insomnia, dizziness, and convulsions; haematological abnormalities such as agranulocytosis, leucopenia, and thrombocytopenia; and gastrointestinal disturbances, including an abnormal taste in the mouth.

◊ A review from the manufacturers of 46 controlled studies in which 2635 cancer patients received adjuvant levamisole treatment.[1] Most patients received levamisole on 3 consecutive days every 2 weeks (1102 patients) or on 2 consecutive days every week (1156 patients), usually in a daily dose of 150 mg. Levamisole can cause several side-effects, such as skin rash, nausea, vomiting, and a metallic or bitter taste in the mouth, which although troublesome are relatively trivial and may regress during therapy or disappear on cessation of therapy. A total of 38 patients developed agranulocytosis and of these 36 had received weekly treatment. Several contracted possible life-threatening infections and 2 died of septic shock.

1. Amery WK, Butterworth BS. Review/commentary: the dosage regimen of levamisole in cancer: is it related to efficacy and safety? *Int J Immunopharmacol* 1983; **5:** 1–9.

Effects on the endocrine system. Rechallenge confirmed that levamisole was responsible for inappropriate antidiuretic hormone syndrome in a patient receiving levamisole with fluorouracil.[1]

1. Tweedy CR, *et al.* Levamisole-induced syndrome of inappropriate antidiuretic hormone. *N Engl J Med* 1992; **326:** 1164.

Effects on the liver. Elevated aspartate aminotransferase concentrations in 2 of 11 patients given levamisole for recurrent pyoderma suggested liver toxicity, a very rarely occurring side-effect.[1] More recently, liver enzyme concentrations were reported to be raised in a 14-year-old boy treated with levamisole for minimal change nephrotic syndrome.[2]

1. Papageorgiou P, *et al.* Levamisole in chronic pyoderma. *J Clin Lab Immunol* 1982; **8:** 121–7.

2. Bulugahapitiya DTD. Liver toxicity in a nephrotic patient treated with levamisole. *Arch Dis Child* 1997; **76:** 289.

Effects on the nervous system. Reports[1,2] of inflammatory leucoencephalopathy were associated with the use of fluorouracil and levamisole in 4 patients being treated for adenocarcinoma of the colon. Active demyelination was demonstrated in 2 patients.[1] Clinical improvement occurred when chemotherapy was stopped; 3 patients were treated with corticosteroids.[1] A similar syndrome has been reported in a patient with a history of hepatitis C who received levamisole alone.[3]

1. Hook CC, *et al.* Multifocal inflammatory leukoencephalopathy with 5-fluorouracil and levamisole. *Ann Neurol* 1992; **31:** 262–7.

2. Kimmel DW, Schutt AJ. Multifocal leukoencephalopathy: occurrence during 5-fluorouracil and levamisole therapy and resolution after discontinuation of chemotherapy. *Mayo Clin Proc* 1993; **68:** 363–5.

3. Lucia P, *et al.* Multifocal leucoencephalopathy induced by levamisole. *Lancet* 1996; **348:** 1450.

Precautions

The use of levamisole should be avoided in patients with pre-existing blood disorders. Patients receiving levamisole in combination with fluorouracil should undergo appropriate monitoring of haematological and hepatic function.

Rheumatoid arthritis. The presence of HLA B27 in seropositive rheumatoid arthritis is an important predisposing factor to the development of agranulocytosis during treatment with levamisole; it is recommended that the use of levamisole in this group should be avoided.[1]

1. Mielants H, Veys EM. A study of the hematological side effects of levamisole in rheumatoid arthritis with recommendations. *J Rheumatol* 1978; **5** (suppl 4): 77–83.

Sjögren's syndrome. The appearance of side-effects in 9 of 10 patients with rheumatoid arthritis and Sjögren's syndrome while being treated with levamisole led to abandonment of the study.[1] Levamisole should be given with caution, if at all, to patients with Sjögren's syndrome.

1. Balint G, *et al.* Sjögren's syndrome: a contraindication to levamisole treatment? *BMJ* 1977; **2:** 1386–7.

Interactions

◊ The US manufacturer reports that levamisole can produce a disulfiram-like reaction with *alcohol*.

Increased plasma-phenytoin concentrations have been observed in patients taking *phenytoin* with levamisole and fluorouracil (see Interactions, Antineoplastics, under Phenytoin, p.360).

For an increase in the activity of *warfarin* when given with levamisole and fluorouracil, see p.997.

Pharmacokinetics

Levamisole is rapidly absorbed from the gastrointestinal tract. Maximum plasma concentrations are attained within 1.5 to 4 hours. It is extensively metabolised in the liver. The plasma half-life for levamisole is 3 to 4 hours and for the metabolites is 16 hours. It is excreted mainly in the urine as metabolites and a small proportion in the faeces. About 70% of the administered dose is excreted in the urine over 3 days, with about 5% as unchanged levamisole.

◊ References.

1. Kouassi E, *et al.* Novel assay and pharmacokinetics of levamisole and p-hydroxylevamisole in human plasma and urine. *Biopharm Drug Dispos* 1986; **7:** 71–89.

2. Luyckx M, *et al.* Pharmacokinetics of levamisole in healthy subjects and cancer patients. *Eur J Drug Metab Pharmacokinet* 1982; **7:** 247–54.

Uses and Administration

Levamisole hydrochloride is the active laevo-isomer of tetramisole hydrochloride. It is used as an anthelmintic and as an adjuvant in malignant disease. It has also been tried in several conditions where its stimulant effect on the depressed immune response might be useful.

Levamisole is active against intestinal nematode worms and appears to act by paralysing susceptible worms which are subsequently eliminated from the intestines. In particular, levamisole is effective in the treatment of ascariasis (p.91). It is also used in hookworm infections (p.93).

Doses of levamisole hydrochloride are expressed in terms of the equivalent amount of levamisole. The usual adult dose in ascariasis is 150 mg of levamisole by mouth as a single dose; children have been given 3 mg per kg body-weight as a single dose. For the hookworm infection ancylostomiasis or for mixed ascariasis-hookworm infections, 300 mg is given over 1 or 2 days for adults; children have been given 6 mg per kg over 1 to 2 days. Another dose schedule widely used for ascariasis and hookworm infections in both adults and children is 2.5 mg per kg as a single dose, repeated after 7 days in cases of severe hookworm infection.

Levamisole affects the immune response. The term 'immunostimulant' has often been used; it is appropriate only in so far as restoration of a depressed response is concerned; stimulation above normal levels does not seem to occur. Levamisole influences host defences by modulating cell-mediated immune responses; it restores depressed T-cell functions. Levamisole has been tried in a wide variety of disorders involving the immune response, including bacterial

---

The symbol † denotes a preparation no longer actively marketed

and viral infections and rheumatic disorders, although in these conditions results have not been encouraging.

It is also used as an adjunct in patients with malignant disease, although it is not clear that any response is due to levamisole's action on the immune system. Recurrences of adenocarcinoma of the colon are inhibited by adjuvant treatment with levamisole and fluorouracil following resection of tumours with regional lymph node involvement. The dose is levamisole 50 mg by mouth every 8 hours for 3 days starting 7 to 30 days after surgery and this course is repeated every 14 days. Fluorouracil is given concurrently, but is not started until 21 to 34 days after surgery (i.e. if the first course of levamisole is given within 20 days of surgery, fluorouracil therapy is started with the second course of levamisole).

◊ Reviews.
1. Janssen PAJ. The levamisole story. *Prog Drug Res* 1976; **20:** 347–83.
2. Renoux G. The general immunopharmacology of levamisole. *Drugs* 1980; **20:** 89–99.
3. Amery WKP, Bruynseels JPJM. Levamisole, the story and the lessons. *Int J Immunopharmacol* 1992; **14:** 481–6.

Malignant neoplasms. Levamisole has been tried in the adjuvant treatment of various malignant neoplasms[1,2] with conflicting results. Based on the results of early adjuvant trials,[3-5] levamisole was used as standard therapy to modulate fluorouracil in patients with colorectal cancer (p.493), particularly in the USA. However, whether levamisole actually added to the beneficial effect of adjuvant fluorouracil was unclear. Adjuvant levamisole alone was no more effective than placebo in 1 study,[6] and more recent trials have indicated that levamisole is no more effective than placebo when added to fluorouracil,[7] or to fluorouracil plus folinic acid.[8]
1. Spreafico F. Use of levamisole in cancer patients. *Drugs* 1980; **20:** 105–16.
2. Amery WK, Butterworth BS. Review/commentary: the dosage regimen of levamisole in cancer: is it related to efficacy and safety? *Int J Immunopharmacol* 1983; **5:** 1–9.
3. Laurie JA, *et al.* Surgical adjuvant therapy of large-bowel carcinoma: an evaluation of levamisole and the combination of levamisole and fluorouracil: the North Central Cancer Treatment Group and the Mayo Clinic. *J Clin Oncol* 1989; **7:** 1447–56.
4. Moertel CG, *et al.* Levamisole and fluorouracil for adjuvant therapy of resected colon carcinoma. *N Engl J Med* 1990; **322:** 352–8.
5. Moertel CG, *et al.* Fluorouracil plus levamisole as effective adjuvant therapy after resection of stage III colon carcinoma: a final report. *Ann Intern Med* 1995; **122:** 321–6.
6. Chlebowski RT, *et al.* Long-term survival following levamisole or placebo adjuvant treatment of colorectal cancer: a Western Cancer Study Group trial. *Oncology* 1988; **45:** 141–3.
7. QUASAR Collaborative Group. Comparison of fluorouracil with additional levamisole, higher-dose folinic acid, or both, as adjuvant chemotherapy for colorectal cancer: a randomised trial. *Lancet* 2000; **355:** 1588–96.
8. Wolmark N, *et al.* Clinical trial to assess the relative efficacy of fluorouracil and leucovorin, fluorouracil and levamisole, and fluorouracil, leucovorin, and levamisole in patients with Dukes' B and C carcinoma of the colon: results from National Surgical Adjuvant Breast and Bowel Project C-04. *J Clin Oncol* 1999; **17:** 3553–9.

Mansonella infections. Levamisole is one of the drugs that has been suggested for the treatment of *Mansonella* infections (p.94). There have been reports[1,2] of response when given with mebendazole.
1. Maertens K, Wery M. Effect of mebendazole and levamisole on Onchocerca volvulus and Dipetalonema perstans. *Trans R Soc Trop Med Hyg* 1975; **69:** 359–60.
2. Bernberg HC, *et al.* The combined treatment with levamisole and mebendazole for a perstans-like filarial infection in Rhodesia. *Trans R Soc Trop Med Hyg* 1979; **73:** 233–4.

Mouth ulceration. Levamisole might be beneficial in severe mouth ulceration (p.1206) but is limited by its adverse effects. A review of its use indicated that beneficial results have been reported with levamisole in open studies, but results of double-blind studies have been conflicting. Nevertheless, there have been patients with severe recurrent aphthous stomatitis refractory to all other modes of treatment who have responded to levamisole. Dosage has been with 150 mg daily in divided doses given for 3 days at the first sign of ulceration, followed by 11 days without treatment, repeated as necessary.
1. Miller MF. Use of levamisole in recurrent aphthous stomatitis. *Drugs* 1980; **20:** 131–6.

Renal disorders. In a randomised double-blind study, children with frequently relapsing corticosteroid-sensitive and corticosteroid-dependent nephrotic syndrome were given placebo or levamisole 2.5 mg per kg body-weight on alternate days and steroid therapy was gradually withdrawn. Of 31 children being treated with levamisole 14 were still in remission 112 days after the start of the study compared with 4 of 30 receiving placebo. For a discussion of the treatment of glomerular kidney disorders, including the nephrotic syndrome, see p.1051.
1. British Association for Paediatric Nephrology. Levamisole for corticosteroid-dependent nephrotic syndrome in childhood. *Lancet* 1991; **337:** 1555–7.

Vitiligo. In a study[1] involving 36 patients with limited slow-spreading vitiligo response to levamisole treatment occurred in 34 within 2 to 4 months. Patients received 150 mg of oral levamisole daily on 2 consecutive days each week. Patients who were additionally treated with topical fluocinolone or clobetasol had higher rates of repigmentation.

The usual treatment of vitiligo is discussed under Pigmentation Disorders, p.1106.
1. Pasricha JS, Khera V. Effect of prolonged treatment with levamisole on vitiligo with limited and slow-spreading disease. *Int J Dermatol* 1994; **33:** 584–7.

Preparations

USP 25: Levamisole Hydrochloride Tablets.

Proprietary Preparations (details are given in Part 3)
Austral.: Ergamisol; *Belg.:* Ergamisol; *Braz.:* Ascaridil; *Canad.:* Ergamisol; *Fr.:* Solaskil†; *Ger.:* Ergamisol; *Hong Kong:* Decaris; *Irl.:* Ketrax; *Israel:* Ergamisol; *Ital.:* Ergamisol†; *Mex.:* Decaris; *Neth.:* Ergamisol; *S.Afr.:* Ergamisol; *UK:* Ketrax; *USA:* Ergamisol.

Male Fern (790-j)

Aspidium; Farnwurzel; Felce Maschio; Feto Macho; Filix Mas; Fougère Mâle; Helecho Macho; Rhizoma Filicis Maris.

The rhizome, frond-bases, and apical bud of *Dryopteris filix-mas* agg. (Polypodiaceae), collected late in the autumn, divested of the roots and dead portions and carefully dried, retaining the internal green colour. It contains not less than 1.5% of filicin. During storage the green colour of the interior gradually disappears, often after a lapse of 6 months, and such material is unfit for medicinal use.

Filicin is the mixture of ether-soluble substances obtained from male fern. Its activity is chiefly due to flavaspidic acid, a phloroglucinol derivative.

Profile

Male fern has anthelmintic properties and was formerly administered as male fern extract (aspidium oleoresin) for the expulsion of tapeworms. However, male fern is highly toxic and has been superseded by other drugs.

Adverse effects include headache, nausea and vomiting, severe abdominal cramp, diarrhoea, dyspnoea, albuminuria, hyperbilirubinaemia, dizziness, tremors, convulsions, visual disturbances including blindness (possibly permanent), stimulation of uterine muscle, coma, respiratory failure, bradycardia, and cardiac failure. Fatalities have occurred.

Preparations

Proprietary Preparations (details are given in Part 3)
Multi-ingredient: *Aust.:* Digestodoron; *Ger.:* Discmigon; *UK:* Digestodoron.

Mebendazole (791-z)

Mebendazole (BAN, USAN, rINN).
Mebendazolum; R-17635. Methyl 5-benzoyl-1H-benzimidazol-2-ylcarbamate.
$C_{16}H_{13}N_3O_3 = 295.3$.
CAS — 31431-39-7.
ATC — P02CA01.

Pharmacopoeias. In Chin., Eur. (see p.vi), Int., Pol., and US.

Pharmacopoeial description

Ph. Eur.: A white to faintly yellowish powder. It shows polymorphism. Practically insoluble in water, in alcohol, in dichloromethane, and in ether. Protect from light.

USP 25: A white to slightly yellow, almost odourless, powder. Practically insoluble in water, in alcohol, in chloroform, in ether, and in dilute mineral acids; freely soluble in formic acid.

Adverse Effects

Since mebendazole is poorly absorbed from the gastrointestinal tract at the usual therapeutic doses, side-effects have generally been restricted to gastrointestinal disturbances, such as transient abdominal pain and diarrhoea, and have tended to occur in patients being treated for heavy intestinal infection. Headache and dizziness have been reported. Adverse effects have been reported more frequently with the high doses tried in echinococcosis and have included allergic reactions, raised liver enzyme values, alopecia, and bone marrow depression.

◊ In the first phase[1] of WHO-coordinated multicentre studies on the treatment of echinococcosis (hydatid disease) involving *Echinococcus granulosus* or *E. multilocularis*, the most frequent adverse effects in the 139 patients given *high-dose* mebendazole, generally for 3 months, were reduced leucocyte count (25 patients), gastrointestinal symptoms (22), and raised serum-transaminase values (22). Other adverse effects were allergic conditions such as fever and skin reactions (4), CNS symptoms including headache (6), and loss of hair (7). Seven patients stopped treatment because of side-effects.

The second phase of studies[2] compared albendazole with mebendazole in more prolonged high-dosage schedules for cystic *E. granulosus* infection. Adverse effects were similar to those reported with the first phase. However, in the first phase the allergic consequences of the 14 ruptured lung cysts and the 4 ruptured liver cysts that occurred with mebendazole were not reported. In the second phase 2 patients suffered anaphylactic shock as a result of rupture of a lung cyst and a cyst in the abdominal cavity. These 2 patients were withdrawn from mebendazole treatment as were another 4 patients as a consequence of their adverse reactions, although in 3 the withdrawal was only temporary.

Although albendazole is preferred to mebendazole in the treatment of echinococcosis, if either drug is used, then there should be constant medical supervision with regular monitoring of serum-transaminase concentrations and of leucocyte and platelet counts. Patients with liver damage should be treated with reduced doses of benzimidazole carbamates, if at all.[2]
1. Davis A, *et al.* Multicentre clinical trials of benzimidazolecarbamates in human echinococcosis. *Bull WHO* 1986; **64:** 383–8.
2. Davis A, *et al.* Multicentre clinical trials of benzimidazolecarbamates in human cystic echinococcosis (phase 2). *Bull WHO* 1989; **67:** 503–8.

Overdosage. Respiratory arrest and tachyarrhythmia associated with continuous convulsions were reported[1] in an 8-week-old infant following accidental poisoning with mebendazole. Treatment by exchange transfusion and anticonvulsants was successful.
1. el Kalla S, Menon NS. Mebendazole poisoning in infancy. *Ann Trop Paediatr* 1990; **10:** 313–14.

Precautions

Mebendazole is teratogenic in *rats* (see Pregnancy and Breast Feeding, below).

Patients receiving high doses of mebendazole, such as those with echinococcosis, should be supervised closely with blood counts and liver function being monitored.

Monitoring drug concentrations. In a retrospective analysis of patients who had received high doses of mebendazole for echinococcosis,[1] no relationship was found between dose and plasma concentration of mebendazole and considerable intra- and interindividual variation in plasma concentrations was observed, emphasising the need for repeated monitoring. Several patients appeared to have what were considered to be subtherapeutic plasma concentrations.
1. Luder PJ, *et al.* Treatment of hydatid disease with high oral doses of mebendazole: long-term follow-up of plasma mebendazole levels and drug interactions. *Eur J Clin Pharmacol* 1986; **31:** 443–8.

Pregnancy and breast feeding. Mebendazole is teratogenic in *rats* and the manufacturers in the UK have stated that it is contra-indicated in pregnant women, including those who are thought to be, or may be, pregnant. In the USA the manufacturers have stated that mebendazole is not recommended in pregnant women and that patients should be informed of the potential risk to the fetus especially if it is taken during the first trimester; this is in accordance with mebendazole being classified in FDA pregnancy category C. However, they noted that in a survey of a limited number of pregnant women who had inadvertently taken mebendazole during the first trimester, the incidence of malformations and spontaneous abortions was no greater than that observed in the general population.

It is not known whether distribution into breast milk occurs.

Interactions

◊ The concomitant administration of *phenytoin* or *carbamazepine* has been reported to lower plasma-mebendazole concentrations in patients receiving high doses for echinococcosis, presumably as a result of enzyme induction; *valproate* had no such effect.[1] Plasma concentrations of mebendazole have been raised when the enzyme inhibitor *cimetidine* has been given concomitantly, and there has been a report of this effect resulting in the resolution of previously unresponsive hepatic hydatid cysts.[2]
1. Luder PJ, *et al.* Treatment of hydatid disease with high oral doses of mebendazole: long-term follow-up of plasma mebendazole levels and drug interactions. *Eur J Clin Pharmacol* 1986; **31:** 443–8.
2. Bekhti A, Pirotte J. Cimetidine increases serum mebendazole concentrations: implications for treatment of hepatic hydatid cysts. *Br J Clin Pharmacol* 1987; **24:** 390–2.

Pharmacokinetics

Mebendazole is poorly absorbed from the gastrointestinal tract and undergoes extensive first-pass elimination, being metabolised in the liver, eliminated in the bile as unchanged drug and metabolites, and excreted in the faeces. Only about 2% of a dose is excreted unchanged or as metabolites in the urine.

Mebendazole is highly protein bound.

Uses and Administration

Mebendazole, a benzimidazole carbamate derivative, is an anthelmintic with activity against most nematodes and some other worms; activity against some larval stages and ova has also been demonstrated. Mebendazole's anthelmintic activity is considered to be dependent on the inhibition or destruction of cytoplasmic microtubules in the worm's intestinal or absorptive cells. Inhibition of glucose uptake and depletion of glycogen stores follow as do other inhibitory effects leading to death of the worm within several days.

Mebendazole, being poorly absorbed from the gastrointestinal tract, is used principally in the treatment of the intestinal nematode infections ascariasis (roundworm infection), enterobiasis (pinworm or threadworm infections), hookworm infections (ancylostomiasis and necatoriasis), and trichuriasis (whipworm infection); it is useful in mixed infections. During treatment with mebendazole, migration of worms with expulsion through the mouth and nose has occurred in some patients heavily infected with *Ascaris*. Mebendazole is also used in the treatment of capillariasis and trichostrongyliasis and has been used in strongyloidiasis. Other nematode infections which may respond to mebendazole are infection with the filarial nematode *Mansonella perstans*, the tissue infections toxocariasis and trichinosis, and infections with the primary animal parasites *Angiostrongylus spp*. Mebendazole has also been tried in high doses in the treatment of echinococcosis (hydatid disease). For discussions of these infections and their treatment, see under Choice of Anthelmintic, p.91. See also below.

Mebendazole is given by mouth. The usual dose for adults and children aged over 2 years with enterobiasis is 100 mg as a single dose, repeated if necessary after 2 to 3 weeks; for ascariasis, hookworm infections, and trichuriasis the usual dose is 100 mg twice daily for 3 days, although a single dose of 500 mg may be effective.

Angiostrongyliasis. Mebendazole has been used for the treatment of angiostrongyliasis (p.91). A dose for infections with *Angiostrongylus cantonensis* is 100 mg twice daily for 5 days. For those due to *A. costaricensis* a higher dose of 200 to 400 mg three times daily for 10 days has been used.[1]

1. Anonymous. Drugs for parasitic infections. *Med Lett Drugs Ther* 1998; **40:** 1–12.

Capillariasis. Mebendazole in a dose of 200 mg twice daily for 20 days has been used[1] for the treatment of capillariasis (p.92).

1. Anonymous. Drugs for parasitic infections. *Med Lett Drugs Ther* 1998; **40:** 1–12.

Echinococcosis. Mebendazole has been used[1-6] in echinococcosis (p.92), but albendazole is generally preferred. The usual dose of mebendazole in cystic echinococcosis is 40 to 50 mg per kg body-weight daily for at least 3 to 6 months.[7] A similar dose is used as an adjuvant to surgery. For alveolar echinococcosis, the dose is adjusted after 4 weeks to produce a plasma concentration of at least 250 nanomoles per litre (74 nanograms per mL), although adults should not receive more than 6 g daily. Treatment is continued for at least 2 years following radical surgery, or indefinitely in inoperable cases.

1. Ammann RW, *et al.* Recurrence rate after discontinuation of long-term mebendazole therapy in alveolar echinococcosis (preliminary results). *Am J Trop Med Hyg* 1990; **43:** 506–15.
2. Messaritakis J, *et al.* High mebendazole doses in pulmonary and hepatic hydatid disease. *Arch Dis Child* 1991; **66:** 532–3.
3. Teggi A, *et al.* Therapy of human hydatid disease with mebendazole and albendazole. *Antimicrob Agents Chemother* 1993; **37:** 1679–84.
4. Göçmen A, *et al.* Treatment of hydatid disease in childhood with mebendazole. *Eur Respir J* 1993; **6:** 253–7.
5. Ammann RW, *et al.* Effect of chemotherapy on the larval mass and the long-term course of alveolar echinococcosis. *Hepatology* 1994; **19:** 735–42.
6. Erdinçler P, *et al.* The role of mebendazole in the surgical treatment of central nervous system hydatid disease. *Br J Neurosurg* 1997; **11:** 116–20.
7. WHO Informal Working Group on Echinococcosis. Guidelines for treatment of cystic and alveolar echinococcosis in humans. *Bull WHO* 1996; **74:** 231–42.

Mansonella infections. Mebendazole is one of the drugs that has been suggested for the treatment of infections with *Mansonella perstans* (p.94). Some patients have responded to mebendazole with levamisole[1,2] or to mebendazole alone.[3]

1. Maertens K, Wery M. Effect of mebendazole and levamisole on Onchocerca volvulus and Dipetalonema perstans. *Trans R Soc Trop Med Hyg* 1975; **69:** 359–60.

---

2. Bernberg HC, *et al.* The combined treatment with levamisole and mebendazole for a perstans-like filarial infection in Rhodesia. *Trans R Soc Trop Med Hyg* 1979; **73:** 233–4.
3. Wahlgren M, Frolov I. Treatment of Dipetalonema perstans infections with mebendazole. *Trans R Soc Trop Med Hyg* 1983; **77:** 422–3.

Strongyloidiasis. Mebendazole has been used for the treatment of strongyloidiasis (p.94), but needs to be given for longer periods than albendazole to control auto-infection, so that of the two benzimidazole carbamates albendazole is preferred.[1-3]

1. Wilson KH, Kauffman CA. Persistent Strongyloides stercoralis in a blind loop of the bowel: successful treatment with mebendazole. *Arch Intern Med* 1983; **143:** 357–8.
2. Mravak S, *et al.* Treatment of strongyloidiasis with mebendazole. *Acta Trop (Basel)* 1983; **40:** 93–4.
3. Pelletier LL, Baker CB. Treatment failures following mebendazole therapy for chronic strongyloidiasis. *J Infect Dis* 1987; **156:** 532–3.

Syngamosis. Mebendazole has been used successfully[1] to treat syngamosis (p.95).

1. Timmons RF, *et al.* Infection of the respiratory tract with Mammomanogamus (Syngamus) laryngeus: a new case in Largo, Florida, and a summary of previously reported cases. *Am Rev Respir Dis* 1983; **128:** 566–9.

Toxocariasis. Mebendazole has been used in the treatment of toxocariasis (p.95). In one study[1] mebendazole was reported to produce similar improvement to that obtained with tiabendazole but with a lower incidence of adverse effects.

1. Magnaval JF, Charlet JP. Efficacité comparée du thiabendazole et du mébendazole dans le traitement de la toxocarose. *Therapie* 1987; **42:** 541–4.

Trichinosis. Mebendazole is used for the treatment of trichinosis (p.95) and is considered the anthelmintic of choice in some countries.

References.

1. Levin ML. Treatment of trichinosis with mebendazole. *Am J Trop Med Hyg* 1983; **32:** 980–3.

Preparations

USP 25: Mebendazole Tablets.

Proprietary Preparations (details are given in Part 3)
Aust.: Pantelmin; *Austral.:* Chemists Own De Worm; Combantrin-1 with Mebendazole; Sqworm†; Vermox; *Belg.:* Vermox; *Braz.:* Ascariobel; Ascaritor; Ascarobex; Athelmin; Averpan; Bendrax; Bivalem; Certovermil; Cessaverm; Eraverm; Feller; Geophagol; Gran-Verm; Helmizil; Kindelmin; Meben; Mebendazotil; Mebendil; Moben; Necamin; Novelmin; Panfugan; Pantelmin; Parelmin; Pentazole; Pluriverm; Politelmin; Quintelmin; Sirben; Tetrahelmin; Vermepen; Vermirax; Vermonon; Vermoplex; Vermoral; Zol-Triq; *Canad.:* Vermox; *Denm.:* Vermox; *Ger.:* Surfont; Vermox; *Hong Kong:* Vermox; *Irl.:* Vermox; *Israel:* Vermox; *Ital.:* Vermox; *Mex.:* Amycil; Benedaxol; Bensolmin; Carbatil; Daben; Diazolen; Exaverm; Exbenzol; Exteny; Fanciadazol; Hedazol; Helminzole; Marben; Meban; Mebandozer; Mebelmin; Mebentiasis; Mebentine; Mizolmex; Nemapres; Oxizole; Prodazol; Profenzol; Revapol; Soltric; Vermicol; Vermidil; Vermin-Dazol; Vermox; Vertex; Vertizole; *Neth.:* Madicure; Vermox; *Norw.:* Vermox; *NZ:* Mindol; Vermox; *Port.:* Pantelmin; Toloxim; *S.Afr.:* Anthex; Cipex; D-Worm; Vermox; Wormgo; Wormstop; *Spain:* Bantenol; Lomper; Mebendan; Oxitover; Sufil; *Swed.:* Vermox; *Switz.:* Vermox; *Thai.:* Benda; Drivermide; Elmetin; Fugacar; Masaworm-1; Meba; Meben; Mebenda-P; Mebenlax; Medazole; Vagaka; Warca; *UAE:* Mebzol; *UK:* Ovex; Pripsen; Vermox; *USA:* Vermox.

Multi-ingredient: *Braz.:* Exelmin; Flenverme; Forverm; Helmi-Ped; Helmiben; Helmidrax; Neovermim; Poliben; Profium; Vermol; Zoles; *Mex.:* Mebeciclol.

Metrifonate (3594-e)

Metrifonate (BAN, rINN).

Bayer-L-1359; DETF; Metrifonatum; Metriphonate; Trichlorfon (USAN); Trichlorphon. Dimethyl 2,2,2-trichloro-1-hydroxyethylphosphonate.

$C_4H_8Cl_3O_4P = 257.4$.

CAS — 52-68-6.
ATC — P02BB01.

Pharmacopoeias. In *Eur.* (see p.vi), *Int.*, and *US*.

Pharmacopoeial description

Ph. Eur.: A white crystalline powder. M.p. is between 76° and 81°. Freely soluble in water, in alcohol, and in acetone; very soluble in dichloromethane. Protect from light.

USP 25: A white crystalline powder. M.p. about 78° with decomposition. Freely soluble in water, in alcohol, in acetone, in chloroform, in ether, and in benzene; very soluble in dichloromethane; very slightly soluble in hexane and in pentane. Decomposed by alkali. Store at a temperature not exceeding 25°.

◊ CAUTION. *Metrifonate is very toxic when inhaled, swallowed, or spilled on the skin. It can be removed from the skin by washing with soap and water. Contaminated material should be immersed in a 2% aqueous solution of sodium hydroxide for several hours.*

Adverse Effects, Treatment, and Precautions

Metrifonate is generally well tolerated, but may cause nausea, vomiting, abdominal pain, diarrhoea, headache, dizziness, and weakness.

It is an organophosphorus compound and because of its anticholinesterase properties depresses plasma-cholinesterase concentrations. Atropine has been used to relieve cholinergic side-effects without affecting metrifonate's activity against *Schistosoma haematobium*. Patients treated with metrifonate should not be given depolarising muscle relaxants such as suxamethonium for at least 48 hours. The administration of metrifonate should be avoided in those recently exposed to insecticides or other agricultural chemicals with anticholinesterase activity.

For a description of the toxic effects of organophosphorus compounds and the treatment of acute poisoning, see Organophosphorus Insecticides, p.1435.

◊ Metrifonate depresses cholinesterase activity and there has been the occasional report of severe cholinergic adverse effects.[1] However, it does not usually give rise to troublesome effects at doses normally employed, even though there may temporarily be almost complete inhibition of plasma cholinesterase and considerable inhibition of erythrocyte cholinesterase[2] (but see also under Alzheimer's Disease, below).

The environmental aspects of metrifonate usage have been considered by WHO.[3]

1. Jamnadas VP, Thomas JEP. Metriphonate and organophosphate poisoning. *Cent Afr J Med* 1979; **25:** 130.
2. Pleština R, *et al.* Effect of metrifonate on blood cholinesterases in children during the treatment of schistosomiasis. *Bull WHO* 1972; **46:** 747–59.
3. Trichlorfon. *Environmental Health Criteria 132*. Geneva: WHO, 1992.

Pregnancy. WHO reported[1] that metrifonate had not shown embryotoxicity or teratogenicity. Despite these negative findings WHO did not recommend the administration of metrifonate to pregnant patients unless immediate intervention was essential. There has been a report of an infant born with massive hydrocephalus and a large meningomyelocele whose mother had been treated twice during the second month of her pregnancy with metrifonate.[2] A possible link between congenital abnormalities and the use of metrifonate to eradicate fish parasites has also been postulated.[3]

1. WHO. The control of schistosomiasis: second report of the WHO expert committee. *WHO Tech Rep Ser 830* 1993.
2. Monson MH, Alexander K. Metrifonate in pregnancy. *Trans R Soc Trop Med Hyg* 1984; **78:** 565.
3. Czeizel AE, *et al.* Environmental trichlorfon and cluster of congenital abnormalities. *Lancet* 1993; **341:** 539–42.

Pharmacokinetics

Metrifonate is absorbed following oral administration and some is converted to dichlorvos which is considered to be the active moiety. Plasma concentrations of dichlorvos are about 1% of those of metrifonate with peak concentrations of both substances occurring within 2 hours. Excretion is via the kidney, mainly as glucuronides.

◊ References.

1. Nordgren I, *et al.* Plasma levels of metrifonate and dichlorvos during treatment of schistosomiasis with Bilarcil. *Am J Trop Med Hyg* 1980; **29:** 426–30.
2. Nordgren I, *et al.* Levels of metrifonate and dichlorvos in plasma and erythrocytes during treatment of schistosomiasis with Bilarcil. *Acta Pharmacol Toxicol* 1981; **49** (suppl V): 79–86.
3. Pettigrew LC, *et al.* Pharmacokinetics, pharmacodynamics, and safety of metrifonate in patients with Alzheimer's disease. *J Clin Pharmacol* 1998; **38:** 236–45.

Uses and Administration

Metrifonate is an organophosphorus compound and is converted in the body to the active metabolite dichlorvos (p.1431), an anticholinesterase.

Metrifonate has anthelmintic activity against *Schistosoma haematobium* and is given by mouth as an alternative to praziquantel in the treatment of schistosomiasis due to *S. haematobium*. It is usually given in three doses of 7.5 to 10 mg of metrifonate per kg body-weight at intervals of 2 weeks.

Metrifonate has also been used as an insecticide and as a parasiticide in fish and domestic animals.

Alzheimer's disease. Metrifonate, like a number of other cholinesterase inhibitors, has been tried in the treatment of Alzheimer's disease (see Dementia, p.1412). Studies[1,2] have indicated that it can produce modest benefits. However, clinical studies are reported to have been halted following reports of muscle weakness, sometimes requiring respiratory support.

1. Becker RE, *et al.* Effects of metrifonate on cognitive decline in Alzheimer disease: a double-blind, placebo-controlled, 6-month study. *Alzheimer Dis Assoc Disord* 1998; **12:** 54–7.
2. Morris JC, *et al.* Metrifonate benefits cognitive, behavioral, and global function in patients with Alzheimer's disease. *Neurology* 1998; **50:** 1222–30.

The symbol † denotes a preparation no longer actively marketed

Schistosomiasis. While praziquantel is now the main treatment for schistosomiasis (p.94), metrifonate is an alternative for infection due to *Schistosoma haematobium.*

Metrifonate owes its activity against *S. haematobium* to its metabolite dichlorvos which is a cholinesterase inhibitor; it is not active against other *Schistosoma* spp. The standard dose in the treatment of *S. haematobium* infection is 7.5 to 10 mg per kg body-weight given on 3 occasions at intervals of 2 weeks.[1] Cure rates with this schedule in schistosomiasis control programmes range from 40 to more than 80%, with a reduction of more than 80% in egg counts among those not cured. A comparison with praziquantel has shown praziquantel to be the more effective drug.[2] In addition, metrifonate's dosage schedule of 3 doses at intervals of 2 weeks has caused problems of patient compliance.[3] Other dosage schedules have been tried. In one group of trials, the cure rate at 6 months following treatment with 1, 2, or 3 doses was 28, 65, and 84% respectively. Another study showed that 5 mg per kg given three times in one day produced similar results to a standard dosage schedule.[4]

1. WHO. WHO model prescribing information: drugs used in parasitic diseases. Geneva: WHO, 1995.
2. Squires N. Interventions for treating schistosomiasis haematobium (updated 29 November 2000). Available in The Cochrane Library; Issue 3. Oxford: Update Software; 2001.
3. Aden Abdi Y, Gustafsson LL. Poor patient compliance reduces the efficacy of metrifonate treatment of Schistosoma haematobium in Somalia. *Eur J Clin Pharmacol* 1989; **36:** 161–4.
4. Aden Abdi Y, Gustafsson LL. Field trial of the efficacy of a simplified and standard metrifonate treatments of Schistosoma haematobium. *Eur J Clin Pharmacol* 1989; **37:** 371–4.

Milbemycin Oxime   (20588-r)

CGA-179246. A mixture of milbemycin A$_4$ 5-oxime and milbemycin A$_3$ 5-oxime.

CAS — 129496-10-2.

Profile
Milbemycin oxime is an anthelmintic used in veterinary medicine.

Morantel Citrate   (20912-k)

Morantel Citrate *(BANM, pINNM).*

(E)-1,4,5,6-Tetrahydro-1-methyl-2-[2-(3-methyl-2-thienyl)vinyl]pyrimidine citrate monohydrate.

$C_{12}H_{16}N_2S, C_6H_8O_7, H_2O = 430.5.$

CAS — 20574-50-9 (morantel); 69525-81-1 (morantel citrate).

Morantel Tartrate   (12977-e)

Morantel Tartrate *(BANM, USAN, pINNM).*

CP-12009-18; Moranteli Hydrogenotartras; UK-2964-18.

$C_{12}H_{16}N_2S, C_4H_6O_6 = 370.4.$

CAS — 20574-50-9 (morantel); 26155-31-7 (morantel tartrate).

Pharmacopoeias. In *Eur.* (see p.vi) for veterinary use only.

Pharmacopoeial description
Ph. Eur.: A white or pale yellow, crystalline powder. Very soluble in water and in alcohol; practically insoluble in ethyl acetate. A 1% solution in water has a pH of 2.8 to 3.2. Protect from light.

Profile
Morantel is an analogue of pyrantel. The citrate and the tartrate are used as veterinary anthelmintics in the treatment of gastrointestinal roundworms.

Moxidectin   (11024-d)

Moxidectin *(BAN, USAN, rINN).*

CL-301423.   (6R,15S)-5-O-Demethyl-28-deoxy-25-[(E)-1,3-dimethylbut-1-enyl]-6,28-epoxy-23-oxomilbemycin B (E)-23-O-methyloxime.

$C_{37}H_{53}NO_8 = 639.8.$

CAS — 113507-06-5.

Profile
Moxidectin is an anthelmintic used in veterinary medicine. It is also used as a systemic veterinary ectoparasiticide.

Naftalofos   (13000-p)

Naftalofos *(BAN, USAN, rINN).*

Bay-9002; E-9002; ENT-25567; Naphthalophos; Phthalophos; S-940. Diethyl naphthalimido-oxyphosphonate.

$C_{16}H_{16}NO_4P = 349.3.$

CAS — 1491-41-4.

Profile
Naftalofos is an organophosphorus compound used as an anthelmintic in veterinary medicine.

For a description of the toxic effects of organophosphorus compounds and the treatment of acute poisoning, see Organophosphorus Insecticides, p.1435.

Netobimin   (2190-g)

Netobimin *(BAN, USAN, rINN).*

Sch-32481. 2-{3-Methoxycarbonyl-2-[2-nitro-5-(propylthio)phenyl]guanidino}ethanesulphonic acid.

$C_{14}H_{20}N_4O_7S_2 = 420.5.$

CAS — 88255-01-0.

Profile
Netobimin is an anthelmintic used in veterinary medicine.

Niclosamide   (793-k)

Niclosamide *(BAN, USAN, rINN).*

Anhydrous Niclosamide; Bay-2353; Niclosamida Anidra; Niclosamidum Anhydricum; Phenasale. 2′,5-Dichloro-4′-nitrosalicylanilide; 5-Chloro-N-(2-chloro-4-nitrophenyl)-2-hydroxybenzamide.

$C_{13}H_8Cl_2N_2O_4 = 327.1.$

CAS — 50-65-7.

ATC — P02DA01.

Pharmacopoeias. In *Chin., Eur.* (see p.vi), *Int.,* and *Pol.*
Int. permits the anhydrous substance or the monohydrate.

Pharmacopoeial description
Ph. Eur.: Yellowish-white to yellowish, fine crystals. Practically insoluble in water; slightly soluble in dehydrated alcohol; sparingly soluble in acetone. Store in airtight containers. Protect from light.

Niclosamide Monohydrate   (15873-b)

Niclosamide Monohydrate *(BANM).*

Niclosamida Mono-hidratada; Niclosamidum Monohydricum.

$C_{13}H_8Cl_2N_2O_4, H_2O = 345.1.$

Pharmacopoeias. In *Eur.* (see p.vi).
Int. permits the monohydrate or the anhydrous substance under the title Niclosamide.

Pharmacopoeial description
Ph. Eur.: Yellowish, fine crystals. Practically insoluble in water; slightly soluble in dehydrated alcohol; sparingly soluble in acetone. Protect from light.

Adverse Effects
Gastrointestinal disturbances may occur occasionally with niclosamide. Lightheadedness and pruritus have been reported less frequently.

Pharmacokinetics
Niclosamide is not significantly absorbed from the gastrointestinal tract.

Uses and Administration
Niclosamide is an anthelmintic which is active against most tapeworms, including the beef tapeworm (*Taenia saginata*), the pork tapeworm (*T. solium*), the fish tapeworm (*Diphyllobothrium latum*), the dwarf tapeworm (*Hymenolepis nana*), and the dog tapeworm (*Dipylidium caninum*). For discussions of the treatment of tapeworm infections, see Diphyllobothriasis, p.92, Hymenolepiasis, p.93, and Taeniasis, p.95. The activity of niclosamide against these worms appears to be due to inhibition of mitochondrial oxidative phosphorylation; anaerobic ATP production is also affected.

Niclosamide is administered in tablets, which must be chewed thoroughly before swallowing and washed down with water.

For infections with pork tapeworm a single 2-g dose is given after a light breakfast. Niclosamide is not active against the larval form (cysticerci) and although the risk of inducing cysticercosis appears to be theoretical, a laxative is given about 2 hours after the dose to expel the killed worms and minimise the possibility of the migration of ova of *T. solium* into the stomach; also an antiemetic may be given before treatment.

For infections with beef or fish tapeworms the 2-g dose of niclosamide may be divided, with 1 g taken after breakfast and 1 g an hour later.

In dwarf-tapeworm infections an initial dose of 2 g is given on the first day followed by 1 g daily for 6 days. Children aged 2 to 6 years are given half the above doses and those under 2 years of age are given one-quarter the above doses.

Unless expulsion of the worm is aided by a laxative, portions are voided in a partially digested form after treatment with niclosamide; the scolex is rarely identifiable.

Niclosamide is used as a molluscicide for the treatment of water in schistosomiasis control programmes (p.94).

Preparations
BP 2001: Niclosamide Tablets.

Proprietary Preparations (details are given in Part 3)
Austral.: Yomesan†; *Belg.:* Yomesan; *Braz.:* Atenase; *Denm.:* Yomesan; *Fin.:* Kontal; *Fr.:* Tredemine; *Ger.:* Yomesan; *Israel:* Yomesan; *Ital.:* Yomesan; *Neth.:* Yomesan; *S.Afr.:* Yomesan; *Swed.:* Yomesan; *Thai.:* Niclosan; Telmitin; Unicide; Yomesan; *UK:* Yomesan.

Multi-ingredient: *Thai.:* Zenda.

Niridazole   (794-a)

Niridazole *(BAN, USAN, rINN).*

Ba-32644; NSC-136947. 1-(5-Nitrothiazol-2-yl)imidazolidin-2-one.

$C_6H_6N_4O_3S = 214.2.$

CAS — 61-57-4.

ATC — P02BX02.

Pharmacopoeias. In *Fr., Int.,* and *It.*

Adverse Effects
Common side-effects with niridazole include anorexia, nausea, vomiting, diarrhoea, abdominal pain, abnormal taste, dizziness, and headache.

Less frequent, but more serious, are effects on the CNS including insomnia, anxiety, agitation, confusion, hallucinations, and convulsions; they have occurred especially in patients with impaired liver function such as those with severe hepato-intestinal schistosomiasis.

Hypersensitivity reactions have been reported and may be associated with destruction of parasites; they have included skin rashes, fever, and peripheral eosinophilia.

Other adverse effects reported occasionally with niridazole include ECG abnormalities. Impaired spermatogenesis has been reported and niridazole has been shown in *animal* and *in-vitro* studies to have carcinogenic, mutagenic, and embryotoxic effects.

Haemolysis may occur in persons with a deficiency of glucose-6-phosphate dehydrogenase. The urine may be coloured a deep brown because of the presence of niridazole metabolites.

◊ References.
1. Urman HK, *et al.* Carcinogenic effects of niridazole. *Cancer Lett* 1975; **i:** 69–74.
2. El-Beheiry AH, *et al.* Niridazole and fertility in bilharzial men. *Arch Androl* 1982; **8:** 297–300.
3. Abdu-Aguye I, Sambo-Donga L. Influence of dosing interval and in-patient versus out-patient status on incidence of side-effects of niridazole. *Hum Toxicol* 1986; **5:** 275–8.

Uses and Administration
Niridazole is a nitrothiazole derivative that was formerly given in the treatment of schistosomiasis, but it has been superseded by less toxic drugs.

Nitroscanate   (13027-t)

Nitroscanate *(BAN, USAN, rINN).*

CGA-23654. 4-(4-Nitrophenoxy)phenyl isothiocyanate.

$C_{13}H_8N_2O_3S = 272.3.$

CAS — 19881-18-6.

Profile
Nitroscanate is an isothiocyanate anthelmintic used in veterinary practice.

Nitroxinil   (13029-r)

Nitroxinil *(BAN, rINN).*

Nitroxynil. 4-Hydroxy-3-iodo-5-nitrobenzonitrile.

$C_7H_3IN_2O_3 = 290.0.$

CAS — 1689-89-0 (nitroxinil); 27917-82-4 (nitroxinil eglumine).

Pharmacopoeias. In *BP(Vet).* Also in *Fr.* for veterinary use only.

Pharmacopoeial description
BP(Vet) 2001: A yellow to yellowish brown powder. Practically insoluble in water; slightly soluble in alcohol; sparingly sol-

uble in ether; it dissolves in solutions of alkali hydroxides. Protect from light.

Profile
Nitroxinil is a veterinary anthelmintic used in the treatment of fascioliasis and some gastrointestinal roundworms in cattle and sheep. It is also used to treat gapeworm infection (syngamosis) in game birds.

Oxamniquine (795-t)

Oxamniquine (BAN, USAN, rINN).

UK-4271. 1,2,3,4-Tetrahydro-2-isopropylaminomethyl-7-nitro-6-quinolylmethanol.
$C_{14}H_{21}N_3O_3 = 279.3$.
CAS — 21738-42-1.
ATC — P02BA02.

Pharmacopoeias. In Fr. and Int.

Adverse Effects
Oxamniquine caused severe pain at the injection site when administered intramuscularly and is no longer given by this route.

It is generally well tolerated following administration by mouth, although dizziness with or without drowsiness occurs in at least a third of patients, beginning up to 3 hours after a dose and usually lasting for up to 6 hours. Other common side-effects include headache and gastrointestinal effects such as nausea, vomiting, and diarrhoea.

Allergic-type reactions including urticaria, pruritic skin rashes, and fever may occur. Liver enzyme values have been raised transiently in some patients. Epileptiform convulsions have been reported, especially in patients with a history of convulsive disorders. Hallucinations and excitement have occurred rarely.

A reddish discoloration of urine, probably due to a metabolite of oxamniquine, has been reported.

Effects on body temperature. Although a modest post-treatment rise in temperature has been reported occasionally, fever is not a common side-effect of oxamniquine, except in Egypt where it appears to be characteristic. The cause is not known. Increased immune complexes and excretion of antigens occur in only half the cases, there is no evidence that Egyptian patients metabolise the drug differently to produce a pyrogenic metabolite, and the effect has not been seen in other areas where a similar high-dose regimen is used.[1]

1. Foster R. A review of clinical experience with oxamniquine. Trans R Soc Trop Med Hyg 1987; 81: 55–9.

Effects on the nervous system. In 37 patients with Schistosoma mansoni infection treated successfully with oxamniquine,[1] dizziness and drowsiness were most common but the only significant adverse effect was the development of EEG abnormalities in 6 of 34 patients whose pre-treatment EEG was normal. Of the 3 patients with pre-existing EEG abnormalities one suffered a tonic-clonic seizure during therapy as previously reported,[2] one did not suffer seizures, and the third received phenytoin prophylaxis during oxamniquine therapy. It was considered prudent to administer anticonvulsant drugs before starting oxamniquine therapy in patients with a history of seizure disorder. Since completion of this study a patient with no history of seizures suffered a tonic-clonic seizure 2 hours after each of the second and third doses of oxamniquine.

The main neuropsychiatric side-effects seen in 180 Brazilian patients with Schistosoma mansoni infection treated with single oral doses of oxamniquine were: drowsiness (50.6%), dizziness (41.1%), headache (16.1%), temporary amnesia (2.2%), behavioural disturbances (1.7%), chills (1.1%), and seizures (1.1%).[3] An EEG was performed before and after treatment in 20 patients; there were alterations in 3 but they were not associated with neuropsychiatric changes.

1. Krajden S, et al. Safety and toxicity of oxamniquine in the treatment of Schistosoma mansoni infections, with particular reference to electroencephalographic abnormalities. Am J Trop Med Hyg 1983; 32: 1344–6.
2. Keystone JS. Seizures and electroencephalograph changes associated with oxamniquine therapy. Am J Trop Med Hyg 1978; 27: 360–2.
3. de Carvalho SA, et al. Neurotoxicidade do oxamniquine no tratamento da infeção humana pelo Schistosoma mansoni. Rev Inst Med Trop S Paulo 1985; 27: 132–42.

Precautions
Oxamniquine should be used with caution in epileptics or patients with a history of epilepsy. Patients

should be warned that oxamniquine can cause dizziness or drowsiness and if affected they should not drive or operate machinery.

Pharmacokinetics
Oxamniquine is readily absorbed following administration by mouth. Peak plasma concentrations are achieved 1 to 3 hours after a dose and the plasma half-life is 1 to 2.5 hours.

It is extensively metabolised to inactive metabolites, principally the 6-carboxy derivative, which are excreted in the urine. About 70% of a dose of oxamniquine is excreted as the 6-carboxy metabolite within 12 hours of administration; traces of the 2-carboxy metabolite have also been detected in the urine.

◊ The pharmacokinetics of oxamniquine were studied[1] in Sudanese subjects, including 9 patients with advanced hepatosplenic schistosomiasis and 5 controls, following a single 1-g oral dose. In the 9 patients, peak plasma concentrations ranged from 300 to 2252 nanograms per mL (mean, 1267 nanograms per mL) 1 to 3 hours after the dose, compared with 1205 to 2619 nanograms per mL (mean, 1983 nanograms per mL) after 1 to 2 hours in the 5 healthy subjects. Mean plasma half-lives for patients and controls were 151.2 and 111.0 minutes respectively. There were no significant differences in time to reach peak concentration or plasma half-lives. It seemed that elimination of oxamniquine may be non-linear and, although the mean peak plasma concentration was 36% lower in patients than in controls, the higher dosage requirements noted in Sudanese patients were unlikely to be due to lower plasma concentrations. There was no correlation between severity of the disease and pharmacokinetic values.

1. Daneshmend TK, Homeida MA. Oxamniquine pharmacokinetics in hepatosplenic schistosomiasis in the Sudan. J Antimicrob Chemother 1987; 19: 87–93.

Uses and Administration
Oxamniquine is an anthelmintic used in the treatment of schistosomiasis caused by Schistosoma mansoni, but not by other Schistosoma spp. It causes worms to shift from the mesenteric veins to the liver where the male worms are retained; the female worms return to the mesentery, but can no longer release eggs. Resistance may occur.

Oxamniquine is given by mouth, preferably after food. Dosage depends on the geographical origin of the infection and total doses range from 15 mg per kg body-weight given as a single dose to 60 mg per kg given over 2 to 3 days. A single dose should not exceed 20 mg per kg.

Schistosomiasis. Oxamniquine is an alternative to praziquantel for the treatment of schistosomiasis (p.94) due to Schistosoma mansoni,[1] although resistance has occurred, particularly in South America.[2]

The dose ranges between a single dose of 15 mg per kg body-weight and 60 mg per kg given over 2 or 3 days.[1,2] Doses in the low range have been used effectively in South America, the Caribbean, and West Africa while patients in Egypt, South Africa, and Zimbabwe require doses at the top end of the range; intermediate doses may be effective in other parts of Africa.[2]

After the appropriate therapeutic dose of oxamniquine, cure rates of at least 60%, and often more than 90%, can be expected. Egg excretion in those not cured will be reduced by over 80%, and usually by over 90%, one year after treatment.[2]

1. WHO. The control of schistosomiasis: second report of the WHO expert committee. WHO Tech Rep Ser 830 1993.
2. WHO. The control of schistosomiasis: report of a WHO expert committee. WHO Tech Rep Ser 728 1985.

Preparations
Proprietary Preparations (details are given in Part 3)
Braz.: Mansil; USA: Vansil†.

Oxantel Embonate (796-x)

Oxantel Embonate (BANM, rINNM).

CP-14445-16; Oxantel Pamoate (USAN). (E)-3-[2-(1,4,5,6-Tetrahydro-1-methylpyrimidin-2-yl)vinyl]phenol 4,4'-methylenebis(3-hydroxy-2-naphthoate).
$C_{13}H_{16}N_2O, C_{23}H_{16}O_6 = 604.6$.
CAS — 36531-26-7 (oxantel); 68813-55-8 (oxantel embonate); 42408-84-4 (oxantel embonate).

Profile
Oxantel is an analogue of pyrantel that was formerly used as the embonate in the treatment of trichuriasis.

Oxfendazole (13060-x)

Oxfendazole (BAN, USAN, rINN).

Oxfendazolum; RS-8858. Methyl 5-phenylsulphinyl-1H-benzimidazol-2-ylcarbamate.
$C_{15}H_{13}N_3O_3S = 315.3$.
CAS — 53716-50-0.

Pharmacopoeias. In Eur. (see p.vi) and US for veterinary use only.

Pharmacopoeial description
Ph. Eur.: A white or almost white powder. It shows polymorphism. Practically insoluble in water; slightly soluble in alcohol and in dichloromethane. Protect from light.

USP 25: A white or almost white powder. Practically insoluble in water; slightly soluble in alcohol and in dichloromethane. Protect from light.

Profile
Oxfendazole is a benzimidazole carbamate anthelmintic structurally related to mebendazole (p.102). It is used in veterinary practice.

Oxibendazole (13062-f)

Oxibendazole (BAN, USAN, rINN).

SKF-30310. Methyl 5-propoxy-1H-benzimidazol-2-ylcarbamate.
$C_{12}H_{15}N_3O_3 = 249.3$.
CAS — 20559-55-1.

Profile
Oxibendazole is a benzimidazole carbamate anthelmintic structurally related to mebendazole (p.102). It is used in veterinary practice.

Oxyclozanide (13071-d)

Oxyclozanide (BAN, rINN).

ICI-46683. 3,3',5,5',6-Pentachloro-2'-hydroxysalicylanilide.
$C_{13}H_6Cl_5NO_3 = 401.5$.
CAS — 2277-92-1.

Pharmacopoeias. In BP(Vet).

Pharmacopoeial description
BP(Vet) 2001: A pale cream or cream-coloured, odourless or almost odourless powder. Very slightly soluble in water; soluble in alcohol; freely soluble in acetone; slightly soluble in chloroform.

Profile
Oxyclozanide is a veterinary anthelmintic used in the control of fascioliasis in cattle and sheep.

Piperazine (13973-z)

$C_4H_{10}N_2 = 86.14$.
CAS — 110-85-0.
ATC — P02CB01.

Pharmacopoeias. In US.

Piperazine 44.4 mg is approximately equivalent to 100 mg of piperazine hydrate.

Pharmacopoeial description
USP 25: White to off-white lumps or flakes having an ammoniacal odour. M.p. 109° to 113°. Soluble in water and in alcohol; insoluble in ether. Store in airtight containers. Protect from light.

Piperazine Adipate (799-d)

Piperaz. Adip.; Piperazini Adipas; Piperazinum Adipicum.
$C_4H_{10}N_2, C_6H_{10}O_4 = 232.3$.
CAS — 142-88-1.

Pharmacopoeias. In Eur. (see p.vi), Int., and Jpn.

Piperazine adipate 120 mg is approximately equivalent to 100 mg of piperazine hydrate.

Pharmacopoeial description
Ph. Eur.: A white crystalline powder. Soluble in water; practically insoluble in alcohol.

Piperazine Citrate (801-n)

Hydrous Triperazine Dicitrate; Piperazini Citras.
$(C_4H_{10}N_2)_3, 2C_6H_8O_7, xH_2O = 642.7$ (anhydrous substance).
CAS — 144-29-6 (anhydrous piperazine citrate); 41372-10-5 (piperazine citrate hydrate).

Pharmacopoeias. In Chin., Eur. (see p.vi), Int., and US.

Piperazine citrate 125 mg is approximately equivalent to 100 mg of piperazine hydrate; if calculations are based on anhydrous piperazine citrate, then 110 mg is approximately equivalent to 100 mg of piperazine hydrate.

The symbol † denotes a preparation no longer actively marketed

Pharmacopoeial description
Ph. Eur.: A white granular powder. It contains a variable amount of water. Freely soluble in water; practically insoluble in alcohol and in ether.
USP 25: A white, crystalline powder having not more than a slight odour. Soluble in water; insoluble in alcohol and in ether. pH of a 10% solution in water is about 5.

Stability. A decrease in the content of piperazine [as citrate] in syrups on storage was attributed to interaction with fructose and glucose formed by hydrolysis of sucrose.[1] A syrup prepared with sorbitol lost no potency when stored at 25° for 14 months.
1. Nielsen A, Reimer P. The stability of piperazine in syrup. *Arch Pharm Chemi (Sci)* 1975; **3:** 73–8.

Piperazine Hydrate (802-h)

Piperazini Hydras; Piperazinum Hydricum. Piperazine hexahydrate.
$C_4H_{10}N_2,6H_2O = 194.2$.
CAS — 142-63-2.
Pharmacopoeias. In Eur. (see p.vi).

The dosage of the salts of piperazine is usually expressed in terms of piperazine hydrate; 100 mg of piperazine hydrate is approximately equivalent to 44.4 mg of piperazine, to 120 mg of piperazine adipate, to 125 mg of piperazine citrate (110 mg of anhydrous piperazine citrate), and to 104 mg of piperazine phosphate.

Pharmacopoeial description
Ph. Eur.: Colourless deliquescent crystals. M.p. about 43°. Freely soluble in water and in alcohol; very slightly soluble in ether. A 5% solution in water has a pH of 10.5 to 12.0. Store in airtight containers. Protect from light.

Piperazine Phosphate (803-m)

Piperazini Phosphas.
$C_4H_{10}N_2,H_3PO_4,H_2O = 202.1$.
CAS — 14538-56-8 (anhydrous piperazine phosphate); 18534-18-4 (piperazine phosphate monohydrate).
Pharmacopoeias. In Br., Chin., and Jpn.

Piperazine phosphate 104 mg is approximately equivalent to 100 mg of piperazine hydrate.

Pharmacopoeial description
BP 2001: A white odourless or almost odourless crystalline powder. Sparingly soluble in water; practically insoluble in alcohol. A 1% solution in water has a pH of 6.0 to 6.5.

Adverse Effects

Serious adverse effects are rare with piperazine and generally indicate overdosage or impaired excretion. Nausea, vomiting, diarrhoea, abdominal pain, headache, skin rashes, and urticaria occasionally occur. Severe neurotoxicity and EEG abnormalities have been reported with symptoms including somnolence, dizziness, nystagmus, muscular incoordination and weakness, ataxia, paraesthesia, myoclonic contractions, choreiform movements, tremor, convulsions, and loss of reflexes.

Transient visual disturbances such as blurred vision have occurred occasionally and there were reports of cataract formation after treatment with piperazine although they do not appear to have been substantiated.

Hypersensitivity reactions such as bronchospasm, Stevens-Johnson syndrome, and angioedema have occurred in some individuals.

◊ Piperazine has been taken off the market in some European countries because of general concern about its safety.[1] A study carried out in Sweden on 2 subjects had indicated that mononitrosation of piperazine can occur in the stomach to produce the potential carcinogen *N*-mononitrosopiperazine; the more potent *N,N*-dinitrosopiperazine was not found.[2] However, the disease risk to man from such *N*-nitroso compounds has been questioned[3] and certainly reports of tumours associated with the use of piperazine have not been traced. Also in the UK the Committee on Review of Medicines concluded on reviewing piperazine that the incidence of serious adverse effects was low and that, with appropriate pack warnings, piperazine products could remain as medicines available to the public through pharmacies.[1]
1. Anonymous. Data sheet changes for piperazine in pregnancy. *Pharm J* 1988; **240:** 367.
2. Bellander BTD, *et al.* Nitrosation of piperazine in the stomach. *Lancet* 1981; **ii:** 372.
3. Tannenbaum SR. N-nitroso compounds: a perspective on human exposure. *Lancet* 1983; **i:** 629–32.

Effects on the blood. A 4-year-old African boy with glucose-6-phosphate dehydrogenase deficiency developed haemolytic anaemia.[1] No cause for the haemolysis was found except that 2 days previously he had taken Pripsen (piperazine and senna). Severe thrombocytopenia with epistaxis and haemoptysis which developed in a 61-year-old man after piperazine

self-medication was probably the result of sensitisation to piperazine 15 years earlier.[2]
1. Buchanan N, *et al.* G-6-PD deficiency and piperazine. *BMJ* 1971; **2:** 110.
2. Cork MJ, *et al.* Pruritus ani, piperazine, and thrombocytopenia. *BMJ* 1990; **301:** 1398.

Effects on the liver. A reaction resembling viral hepatitis occurred on 2 occasions in a 25-year-old woman after the administration of piperazine; it appeared to be a hypersensitivity reaction.[1]
1. Hamlyn AN, *et al.* Piperazine hepatitis. *Gastroenterology* 1976; **70:** 1144–7.

Hypersensitivity. There has been a report[1] of a patient experiencing a serum-sickness-like illness associated with piperazine and this was followed by a delayed hypersensitivity vasculitis.
See also Effects on the Blood and Effects on the Liver, above.
1. Balzan M, Cacciottolo JM. Hypersensitivity vasculitis associated with piperazine therapy. *Br J Dermatol* 1994; **131:** 133–4.

Precautions

Piperazine is contra-indicated in patients with epilepsy or severe renal impairment and should be given with care to patients with neurological disturbances or impaired renal function. It should also be avoided or given with extreme caution in patients with hepatic impairment.

Breast feeding. The UK manufacturers of Pripsen (piperazine and senna) report that piperazine is distributed into breast milk. Mothers should be advised to take a dose after breast feeding then not to breast feed for 8 hours during which period milk should be expressed and discarded at the regular feeding times.

Pregnancy. It has been reported that piperazine is teratogenic in *rabbits* and that there have been isolated reports of fetal malformations following clinical use, though no causal relationship has been established. Two infants with malformations have been described briefly:[1] one had bilateral hare lip, cleft palate, and anophthalmia; the other had an abnormality of one foot. Both mothers had taken Pripsen (piperazine with senna). The UK manufacturers of Pripsen advise against use in pregnancy, especially during the first trimester, unless immediate treatment with piperazine is essential.
1. Leach FN. Management of threadworm infestation during pregnancy. *Arch Dis Child* 1990; **65:** 399–400.

Interactions

The anthelmintic effects of piperazine and pyrantel may be antagonised when the two compounds are used together. The possibility that piperazine may enhance the adverse effects of phenothiazines such as chlorpromazine is discussed on p.665.

Pharmacokinetics

Piperazine is readily absorbed from the gastrointestinal tract and is almost completely excreted in the urine within 24 hours, partly as metabolites. The rate at which different individuals excrete piperazine has been reported to vary widely.

◊ References.
1. Hanna S, Tang A. Human urinary excretion of piperazine citrate from syrup formulations. *J Pharm Sci* 1973; **62:** 2024–5.
2. Bellander BTD, *et al.* Nitrosation of piperazine in the stomach. *Lancet* 1981; **ii:** 372.
3. Fletcher KA, *et al.* Urinary piperazine excretion in healthy Caucasians. *Ann Trop Med Parasitol* 1982; **76:** 77–82.

Uses and Administration

Piperazine is an anthelmintic effective against the intestinal nematodes *Ascaris lumbricoides* (roundworm) and *Enterobius vermicularis* (pinworm, threadworm), though other anthelmintics are usually preferred (see the discussions on the treatment of ascariasis and enterobiasis on p.91 and p.93). In roundworms piperazine produces a neuromuscular block leading to a flaccid muscle paralysis in susceptible worms which are then easily dislodged from their position by the movement of the gut and are expelled in the faeces.

Piperazine is usually administered as the citrate or phosphate, but the adipate may also be used. Dosage is generally stated in terms of the hexahydrate, piperazine hydrate.

For the treatment of roundworm infection a single dose, repeated once after 14 days, is used. In adults and children over 12 years of age, a dose equivalent to 4.5 g of piperazine hydrate is given by mouth. Chil-

dren aged 9 to 12 years may be given the equivalent of 3.75 g, those aged 6 to 8 years the equivalent of 3 g, those aged 4 to 5 years the equivalent of 2.25 g, and those aged 1 to 3 years the equivalent of 1.5 g. Children under 1 year should receive piperazine on medical advice only; a dose of 120 mg per kg bodyweight has been suggested.

For elimination of threadworms, treatment is generally given for 7 days. A second course after a 7-day interval may be required. Adults and children over 12 years of age are given the equivalent of 2.25 g of the hydrate once daily, children aged 7 to 12 years the equivalent of 1.5 g daily, those aged 4 to 6 years the equivalent of 1.125 g daily, and those aged 1 to 3 years the equivalent of 750 mg daily. Children under 1 year should receive piperazine on medical advice only; a dose of 45 to 75 mg per kg has been suggested.

Another schedule that is employed for a preparation of piperazine with senna is a single dose of 4 g of the phosphate for adults and children over 6 years of age, repeated after 14 days for threadworm infections, or repeated monthly if necessary for up to 3 months to treat and prevent re-infection with roundworms.

Preparations

BP 2001: Piperazine Citrate Elixir; Piperazine Phosphate Tablets; **USP 25:** Piperazine Citrate Syrup; Piperazine Citrate Tablets.

Proprietary Preparations (details are given in Part 3)
Aust.: Tasnon†; **Braz.:** Ascarin; Ortovermim; Oxiurazina; Pipercream; Pipervermin; Trivermon; Vermifran; Vermilen; **Canad.:** Entacyl; Veriga†; Verimex; Versol†; **Fr.:** Antelmina†; Solucamphre†; Vermifuge; **Irl.:** Citrazine†; **Ital.:** Citropiperazina; **Mex.:** Desparasil; Helmifar; Lu-Peracina; Overpon; Pipemed; Piperazil; Pipermed; Pirzinol; Verfid; Vermin; **Port.:** Lombrimade†; Pipermel; Pipertox; **S.Afr.:** Ascarient†; Pipralen†; Piprine; Wormelix†; **Spain:** Mimedran; Vermi; **Thai.:** Antepar; Vermex; **UK:** Ectodyne; Pripsen; Worm; Wormex.

Multi-ingredient: *Belg.:* Solucamphre†; *Braz.:* Licor de Cacau; Lumbriquil; *Irl.:* Pripsen; *Port.:* Urocrasina; *Switz.:* Carudol†; *UK:* Pripsen.

Pomegranate Bark (804-b)

Granado; Granati Cortex; Granatrinde; Granatum; Grenadier; Melograno; Pomegranate; Pomegranate Root Bark; Romeira.

The dried bark of the stem and root of *Punica granatum* (Punicaceae) containing about 0.4 to 0.9% of alkaloids.

Profile
Pomegranate bark has been used for the expulsion of tapeworms.

Praziquantel (13161-h)

Praziquantel (BAN, USAN, rINN).

EMBAY-8440; Praziquantelum. 2-Cyclohexylcarbonyl-1,2,3,6,7,11b-hexahydropyrazino[2,1-a]isoquinolin-4-one.
$C_{19}H_{24}N_2O_2 = 312.4$.
CAS — 55268-74-1.
ATC — P02BA01.
Pharmacopoeias. In Chin., Eur. (see p.vi), Int., and US.

Pharmacopoeial description
Ph. Eur.: White or almost white crystalline powder. Very slightly soluble in water; freely soluble in alcohol and in dichloromethane. Protect from light.
USP 25: A white or practically white crystalline powder; odourless or with a faint characteristic odour. Very slightly soluble in water; freely soluble in alcohol and in chloroform. Protect from light.

Adverse Effects

Side-effects with praziquantel may be common but they are usually mild and transient. Headache, diarrhoea, dizziness, drowsiness, malaise, abdominal discomfort, nausea, and vomiting have been reported most frequently. Hypersensitivity reactions such as fever, urticaria, pruritic skin rashes, and eosinophilia may occur; they may be due to death of the infecting parasites. Raised liver enzyme values have been reported rarely.

Most patients with neurocysticercosis who are given praziquantel suffer adverse nervous system effects, including headache, hyperthermia, seizures, and intracranial hypertension, which are thought to result from an inflammatory response to dead and dying parasites in the CNS. The concomitant administration of corticosteroids is advised in such patients.

Effects on the gastrointestinal tract. Colicky abdominal pain and bloody diarrhoea occurred in a small community in Zaire shortly after treatment for *Schistosoma mansoni* infection with single doses of praziquantel 40 mg per kg body-weight by mouth.[1] A similar syndrome has been reported in some patients with *Schistosoma japonicum* infection given praziquantel.[2] The abdominal pain occurring in these patients was very different from the mild abdominal discomfort much more commonly reported with praziquantel therapy.

1. Polderman AM, *et al.* Side effects of praziquantel in the treatment of Schistosoma mansoni in Maniema, Zaire. *Trans R Soc Trop Med Hyg* 1984; **78:** 752–4.
2. Watt G, *et al.* Bloody diarrhoea after praziquantel therapy. *Trans R Soc Trop Med Hyg* 1986; **80:** 345–6.

Effects on the nervous system. Adverse nervous system effects are common in patients with neurocysticercosis given praziquantel. Neurological symptoms have also been reported[1] with the much lower doses of praziquantel used in the treatment of taeniasis in a patient with undiagnosed neurocysticercosis.

1. Flisser A, *et al.* Neurological symptoms in occult neurocysticercosis after single taenicidal dose of praziquantel. *Lancet* 1993; **342:** 748.

Precautions

Praziquantel should not be used in patients with ocular cysticercosis because of the risk of severe eye damage resulting from destruction of the parasite.

Patients should be warned that praziquantel may cause dizziness or drowsiness and if affected they should not drive or operate machinery during or for 24 hours after treatment.

Praziquantel is distributed into breast milk and mothers should not breast feed during or for 72 hours after treatment.

Interactions

◊ Some workers have proposed the use of *dexamethasone* to prevent the inflammatory response due to destroyed cysticerci in praziquantel treatment of cysticercosis.[1] However, since dexamethasone has been reported to approximately halve plasma concentrations of praziquantel,[2] it has been suggested that it be reserved for the short-term treatment of praziquantel-induced intracranial hypertension.[1]

Carbamazepine,[3] *phenytoin,*[3] and *chloroquine*[4] have also been reported to reduce the bioavailability of praziquantel while *cimetidine* has been reported to increase praziquantel bioavailability.[5,6]

For reference to plasma concentrations of the active metabolite of *albendazole* being increased by concomitant administration of praziquantel, see p.95.

1. Del Brutto OH, Sotelo J. Neurocysticercosis: an update. *Rev Infect Dis* 1988; **10:** 1075–87.
2. Vazquez ML, *et al.* Plasma levels of praziquantel decrease when dexamethasone is given simultaneously. *Neurology* 1987; **37:** 1561–2.
3. Quinn DI, Day RO. Drug interactions of clinical importance: an updated guide. *Drug Safety* 1995; **12:** 393–452.
4. Masimirembwa CM, *et al.* The effect of chloroquine on the pharmacokinetics and metabolism of praziquantel in rats and in humans. *Biopharm Drug Dispos* 1994; **15:** 33–43.
5. Metwally A, *et al.* Effect of cimetidine, bicarbonate and glucose on the bioavailability of different formulations of praziquantel. *Arzneimittelforschung* 1995; **45:** 516–18.
6. Jung H, *et al.* Pharmacokinetic study of praziquantel administered alone and in combination with cimetidine in a single-day therapeutic regimen. *Antimicrob Agents Chemother* 1997; **41:** 1256–9.

Pharmacokinetics

Praziquantel is rapidly absorbed after administration by mouth, even when taken with a meal; more than 80% of a dose is reported to be absorbed. Peak plasma concentrations are achieved 1 to 3 hours after a dose, but there is a pronounced first-pass effect and praziquantel undergoes rapid and extensive metabolism in the liver, being hydroxylated to metabolites that are thought to be inactive. It is distributed into the CSF. The plasma elimination half-life of praziquantel is 1 to 1.5 hours and that of the metabolites about 4 hours.

It is excreted in the urine, mainly as metabolites, about 80% of the dose being eliminated within 4 days and more than 90% of this in the first 24 hours.

Praziquantel is distributed into breast milk.

◊ References to the pharmacokinetics of praziquantel.

1. Leopold G, *et al.* Clinical pharmacology in normal volunteers of praziquantel, a new drug against schistosomes and cestodes: an example of a complex study covering both tolerance and pharmacokinetics. *Eur J Clin Pharmacol* 1978; **14:** 281–91.

The symbol † denotes a preparation no longer actively marketed

---

2. Bühring KU, *et al.* Metabolism of praziquantel in man. *Eur J Drug Metab Pharmacokinet* 1978; **3:** 179–90.
3. Patzschke K, *et al.* Serum concentrations and renal excretion in humans after oral administration of praziquantel—results of three determination methods. *Eur J Drug Metab Pharmacokinet* 1979; **3:** 149–56.
4. Mandour M El M, *et al.* Pharmacokinetics of praziquantel in healthy volunteers and patients with schistosomiasis. *Trans R Soc Trop Med Hyg* 1990; **84:** 389–93.

Uses and Administration

Praziquantel is an anthelmintic with a broad spectrum of activity against trematodes (flukes) including all species of *Schistosoma* pathogenic to man, and against cestodes (tapeworms). It is used in the treatment of cysticercosis, diphyllobothriasis, hymenolepiasis, schistosomiasis, taeniasis, and intestinal, liver, and lung fluke infections. For discussions of these infections and their treatment, see under Choice of Anthelmintic, p.91. See also below.

Praziquantel is administered by mouth with food.

In the treatment of schistosomiasis in adults and children it is given on one day as three doses of 20 mg per kg body-weight at intervals of 4 to 6 hours or it is given as a single dose of 40 mg per kg (but see below).

Doses in adults and children in the liver fluke infections clonorchiasis and opisthorchiasis are 25 mg per kg three times daily for one or two days or a single dose of 40 mg per kg. Similar doses may be used in lung fluke and intestinal fluke infections (see below).

Single doses of 5 to 25 mg per kg are used in adults and children in tapeworm infections.

Praziquantel is used in the treatment of neurocysticercosis in a dose of 50 mg per kg daily in 3 divided doses for 15 days. A corticosteroid should be given concomitantly to reduce the severity of adverse effects.

◊ Reviews.
1. Pearson RD, Guerrant RL. Praziquantel: a major advance in anthelmintic therapy. *Ann Intern Med* 1983; **99:** 195–8. Correction. *ibid.;* 574.
2. King CH, Mahmoud AAF. Drugs five years later: praziquantel. *Ann Intern Med* 1989; **110:** 290–6.

Cysticercosis. Praziquantel is used in the treatment of neurocysticercosis (p.92) although albendazole may be more effective.

References.
1. Sotelo J, *et al.* Therapy of parenchymal brain cysticercosis with praziquantel. *N Engl J Med* 1984; **310:** 1001–7.
2. Sotelo J, *et al.* Praziquantel for cysticercosis of the brain parenchyma. *N Engl J Med* 1984; **311:** 1075–87.
3. Del Brutto OH, Sotelo J. Neurocysticercosis: an update. *Rev Infect Dis* 1988; **10:** 1075–87.
4. Ciferri F. Delayed CSF reaction to praziquantel. *Lancet* 1988; **i:** 642–3.
5. Moodley M, Moosa A. Treatment of neurocysticercosis: is praziquantel the new hope? *Lancet* 1989; **i:** 262–3.
6. Sotelo J. Praziquantel for neurocysticercosis. *Lancet* 1989; **i:** 897.
7. Crimmins D, *et al.* Neurocysticercosis: an under-recognized cause of neurological problems. *Med J Aust* 1990; **152:** 434–8.
8. Takayanagui JM, Jardim E. Therapy for neurocysticercosis: comparison between albendazole and praziquantel. *Arch Neurol* 1992; **49:** 290–4.
9. Mehta SS, *et al.* Albendazole versus praziquantel for neurocysticercosis. *Am J Health-Syst Pharm* 1998; **55:** 598–600.

Echinococcosis. Praziquantel may be used as an adjunct to surgery in echinococcosis (p.92). Praziquantel has been reported to possess a scolicidal effect *in vitro* against *Echinococcus granulosus*[1] and there has been a report of the successful treatment of disseminated peritoneal hydatid disease with praziquantel and surgery.[2] In this case praziquantel was effective against the small cysts; 2 large cysts were removed surgically, one before praziquantel was started. However, activity in 9 other patients given praziquantel was disappointing.[3]

1. Morris DL, *et al.* Protoscolicidal effect of praziquantel— in vitro and electron microscopical studies on Echinococcus granulosus. *J Antimicrob Chemother* 1986; **18:** 687–91.
2. Henriksen T-H, *et al.* Treatment of disseminated peritoneal hydatid disease with praziquantel. *Lancet* 1989; **i:** 272.
3. Piens MA, *et al.* Praziquantel dans l'hydatidose humaine: évaluation par traitement médical pré-opératoire. *Bull Soc Pathol Exot Filiales* 1989; **82:** 503–12.

Intestinal fluke infections. Praziquantel is used in the treatment of the intestinal fluke infections fasciolopsiasis, heterophyiasis, metagonimiasis, and nanophyetiasis (see p.93). It has been given in a usual recommended dose of 25 mg per kg body-weight three times daily for one day.[1] However, a single dose of 25 mg per kg has also been recommended.[2] In one study single doses of 15 mg per kg, 25 mg per kg, or 40 mg per kg all yielded a cure rate of 100% in a study in 72 primary-school children in Thailand who were harbouring *Fasciolopsis buski* suggesting that a single dose of 15 mg per kg at bedtime might

---

be tried.[3] In another study nine patients infected with the trematode *Nanophyetus salmincola* were treated with praziquantel 20 mg per kg body-weight three times daily for one day and were negative for eggs in their stools 2 to 12 weeks later.[4]

1. Anonymous. Drugs for parasitic infections. *Med Lett Drugs Ther* 1998; **40:** 1–12.
2. WHO. *WHO model prescribing information: drugs used in parasitic diseases.* Geneva: WHO, 1995.
3. Harinasuta T, *et al.* Efficacy of praziquantel on fasciolopsiasis. *Arzneimittelforschung* 1984; **34:** 1214–15.
4. Fritsche TR, *et al.* Praziquantel for treatment of human Nanophyetus salmincola (Troglotrema salmincola) infection. *J Infect Dis* 1989; **160:** 896–9.

Liver fluke infections. Praziquantel is used in the treatment of clonorchiasis and opisthorchiasis, and has also been used in the treatment of fascioliasis (p.93) although in this latter infection bithionol or triclabendazole are preferred.

Various studies have shown praziquantel to be effective in clonorchiasis[1-4] and opisthorchiasis,[5,6] although one study in opisthorchiasis[7] showed that re-infection was common despite praziquantel therapy, particularly in those with heavy initial infection. A study in Thailand[8] confirmed that mass treatment for opisthorchiasis with a single dose of praziquantel was beneficial, although it was suggested that ideally treatment should be given twice a year.

While praziquantel is not the drug of choice for fascioliasis, there has been a report[9] of successful treatment of a patient with severe fascioliasis. Subsequent studies[10-12] have, however, shown praziquantel to be of little benefit.

1. Soh C-J. Clonorchis sinensis: experimental and clinical studies with praziquantel in Korea. *Arzneimittelforschung* 1984; **34:** 1156–9.
2. Chen C-Y, Hsieh W-C. Clonorchis sinensis: epidemiology in Taiwan and clinical experience with praziquantel. *Arzneimittelforschung* 1984; **34:** 1160–2.
3. Kuang Q-H, *et al.* Clonorchiasis: treatment with praziquantel in 50 cases. *Arzneimittelforschung* 1984; **34:** 1162–3.
4. Lee S-H. Large scale treatment of clonorchis sinensis infections with praziquantel under field conditions. *Arzneimittelforschung* 1984; **34:** 1227–8.
5. Bunnag D, *et al.* Opisthorchis viverrini: clinical experience with praziquantel in hospital for tropical diseases. *Arzneimittelforschung* 1984; **34:** 1173–4.
6. Ambroise-Thomas P, *et al.* Therapeutic results in opisthorchiasis with praziquantel in a reinfection-free environment in France. *Arzneimittelforschung* 1984; **34:** 1177–9.
7. Upatham ES, *et al.* Rate of re-infection by Opisthorchis viverrini in an endemic northeast Thai community after chemotherapy. *Int J Parasitol* 1988; **18:** 643–9.
8. Pungpak S, *et al.* Opisthorchis viverrini infection in Thailand: studies on the morbidity of the infection and resolution following praziquantel treatment. *Am J Trop Med Hyg* 1997; **56:** 311–14.
9. Schiappacasse RH, *et al.* Successful treatment of severe infection with Fasciola hepatica with praziquantel. *J Infect Dis* 1985; **152:** 1339–40.
10. Farag HF, *et al.* A short note on praziquantel in human fascioliasis. *J Trop Med Hyg* 1986; **89:** 79–80.
11. Farid Z, *et al.* Unsuccessful use of praziquantel to treat acute fascioliasis in children. *J Infect Dis* 1986; **154:** 920–1.
12. Farid Z, *et al.* Treatment of acute toxaemic fascioliasis. *Trans R Soc Trop Med Hyg* 1988; **82:** 299.

Lung fluke infections. Praziquantel is used in the treatment of the lung fluke infection paragonimiasis (p.94).

References.
1. Vanijanonta S, *et al.* Paragonimus heterotremus and other Paragonimus spp. in Thailand: pathogenesis clinic and treatment. *Arzneimittelforschung* 1984; **34:** 1186–8.
2. Pachucki CT, *et al.* American paragonimiasis treated with praziquantel. *N Engl J Med* 1984; **311:** 582–3.

Schistosomiasis. Praziquantel is the main drug that is used in the treatment of schistosomiasis (p.94). It is effective against all species of schistosomes.[1] The manufacturers recommend a dose of 20 mg per kg body-weight given three times in one day for all schistosomal infections. WHO[1] recommends a single dose of 40 mg per kg. WHO considers[1] that in the field such treatment will produce a cure rate of 60 to 90% with a reduction in egg count in those not cured of 90 to 95%. Good as such results are, a single dose or one day's sole treatment should not be considered to be all that is required to achieve a permanent cure or prevent re-infection, and any treatment plan should be reassessed after 6 or 12 months.[2,3] Such an approach with annual screening and targeted chemotherapy is now accepted as providing, at least in some endemic areas, successful protection for children against intense infection and consequent hepatic disease.[3]

Several studies indicate that doses lower than those recommended above might be effective and in some control programmes 20 mg per kg might be enough for *S. haematobium*[4-6] or 30 mg per kg for *S. mansoni.*[4] It remains to be seen if such low doses lead to resistance as has been suggested with oxamniquine.[7] However, refractory infections have been reported. A 4-day treatment course was needed to produce a complete cure in a patient who relapsed twice following standard one-day treatment regimen.[8] Hepatic impairment, specifically hepatic fibrosis, is a feature of some schistosomal infections and patients with such liver involvement have benefited from treatment with praziquantel.[3,9]

1. WHO. The control of schistosomiasis: second report of the WHO expert committee. *WHO Tech Rep Ser 830* 1993.
2. Anonymous. The chemotherapy of schistosomiasis control. *Bull WHO* 1986; **64:** 23–5.
3. Anonymous. Mass treatment of schistosomiasis with praziquantel. *WHO Drug Inf* 1988; **2:** 184–5.

4. Taylor P, *et al.* Efficacy of low doses of praziquantel for Schistosoma mansoni and S. haematobium. *J Trop Med Hyg* 1988; **91**: 13–17.
5. King CH, *et al.* Dose-finding study for praziquantel therapy of Schistosoma haematobium in Coast Province, Kenya. *Am J Trop Med Hyg* 1989; **40**: 507–13.
6. Hatz C, *et al.* Ultrasound scanning for detecting morbidity due to Schistosoma haematobium and its resolution following treatment with different doses of praziquantel. *Trans R Soc Trop Med Hyg* 1990; **84**: 84–8.
7. Coles GC, *et al.* Tolerance of Kenyan Schistosoma mansoni to oxamniquine. *Trans R Soc Trop Med Hyg* 1987; **81**: 782–5.
8. Murray-Smith SQ, *et al.* A case of refractory schistosomiasis. *Med J Aust* 1996; **165**: 458.
9. Zwingenberger K, *et al.* Praziquantel in the treatment of hepatosplenic schistosomiasis: biochemical disease markers indicate deceleration of fibrogenesis and diminution of portal flow obstruction. *Trans R Soc Trop Med Hyg* 1990; **84**: 252–6.

Taeniasis. Praziquantel is used in the treatment of taeniasis (p.95). It has been studied in the mass control of taeniasis when a single dose of 5 mg per kg body-weight was used.[1]

Praziquantel is also effective against the larval form of *Taenia solium* and is used to treat neurocysticercosis (see above).

1. Cruz M, *et al.* Operational studies on the control of Taenia solium taeniasis/cysticercosis in Ecuador. *Bull WHO* 1989; **67**: 401–7.

Preparations

USP 25: Praziquantel Tablets.

Proprietary Preparations (details are given in Part 3)
Austral.: Biltricide; *Braz.:* Cestox; Cisticid; *Canad.:* Biltricide; *Fr.:* Biltricide; *Ger.:* Biltricide; Cesol; Cysticide; *Hong Kong:* Biltricide; *Israel:* Biltricide; *Mex.:* Cercon; Cesol; Cisticid; Ehliten; Extiser Q; Prozitel; Sincerck; Teniken; Waycital; Zifartel; *Neth.:* Biltricide; *S.Afr.:* Biltricide; Cysticide; *Thai.:* Biltricide; Opticide; Praquantel; Prasikon; Prazite; *USA:* Biltricide.

Pyrantel Embonate (805-v)

Pyrantel Embonate (BANM, rINNM).

CP-10423-16; Pirantel Pamoate; Pyrantel Pamoate (USAN). 1,4,5,6-Tetrahydro-1-methyl-2-[(E)-2-(2-thienyl)vinyl]pyrimidine 4,4'-methylenebis(3-hydroxy-2-naphthoate).

$C_{11}H_{14}N_2S,C_{23}H_{16}O_6 = 594.7$.

CAS — 15686-83-6 (pyrantel); 22204-24-6 (pyrantel embonate).

Pharmacopoeias. In Chin., Int., Jpn, Pol., and US.

Pyrantel embonate 2.9 g is approximately equivalent to 1 g of pyrantel.

Pharmacopoeial description

USP 25: A yellow to tan solid. Practically insoluble in water and in methyl alcohol; soluble in dimethyl sulfoxide; slightly soluble in dimethylformamide. Protect from light.

Adverse Effects and Precautions

The adverse effects of pyrantel embonate are generally mild and transient. The most frequent are gastrointestinal effects such as nausea and vomiting, anorexia, abdominal pain, and diarrhoea. Other adverse effects reported include headache, dizziness, drowsiness, insomnia, skin rashes, and elevated liver enzyme values.

Pyrantel embonate should be used with caution in patients with impaired liver function.

Interactions

The anthelmintic effects of both pyrantel and piperazine may be antagonised when the two drugs are used together.

Pharmacokinetics

Only a small proportion of a dose of pyrantel embonate is absorbed from the gastrointestinal tract. Up to about 7% is excreted as unchanged drug and metabolites in the urine but over half of the dose is excreted unchanged in the faeces.

Uses and Administration

Pyrantel embonate is an anthelmintic effective against intestinal nematodes including roundworms (*Ascaris lumbricoides*), threadworms (*Enterobius vermicularis*), and *Trichostrongylus* spp., the tissue nematode *Trichinella spiralis*, and hookworms, although it is possibly less effective against *Necator americanus* hookworms than against *Ancylostoma duodenale*. Pyrantel is not effective against whipworm (*Trichuris trichiura*). Pyrantel embonate is one of the anthelmintics that may be used in the treatment

---

of infections with these worms, as discussed under Choice of Anthelmintic, p.91. It appears to act by paralysing susceptible worms which are then dislodged by peristaltic activity.

Single or mixed infections due to susceptible worms in adults and children may be treated with a single oral dose equivalent to 10 mg of pyrantel per kg body-weight. Ascariasis occurring alone may only require 5 mg per kg; a single dose of 2.5 mg per kg given three or four times a year has been used in mass treatment programmes. In necatoriasis, 10 mg per kg daily for 3 days or 20 mg per kg daily for 2 days may be necessary. The response in enterobiasis may be improved by repeating the 10 mg per kg dose after 2 to 4 weeks. In trichinosis a dose of 10 mg per kg daily for 5 days has been used.

Preparations

USP 25: Pyrantel Pamoate Oral Suspension.

Proprietary Preparations (details are given in Part 3)
Aust.: Combantrin; *Austral.:* Anthel; Combantrin; Early Bird; *Braz.:* Ascarical; *Canad.:* Combantrin; Jaa Pyral; *Fr.:* Combantrin†; Helmintox; *Ger.:* Helmex; *Hong Kong:* Combantrin; Pyrantrin; *Israel:* Combantrin; *Ital.:* Combantrin; *Mex.:* Combantrin; Pirantrin; *NZ:* Combantrin; *Port.:* Combantrin; Vertel; *S.Afr.:* Combantrin; *Spain:* Lombriareu; Trilombrin; *Switz.:* Cobantril; *Thai.:* Bantel; Combantrin; Pyrapam; *USA:* Antiminth; Pin-Rid; Pin-X; Reese's Pinworm.

Pyrvinium Embonate (819-e)

Pyrvinium Embonate (rINNM).

Pyrvinium Pamoate (BAN); Viprynium Embonate; Viprynium Pamoate. Bis{6-dimethylamino-2-[2-(2,5-dimethyl-1-phenylpyrrol-3-yl)vinyl]-1-methylquinolinium} 4,4'-methylenebis(3-hydroxy-2-naphthoate).

$C_{52}H_{56}N_6,C_{23}H_{14}O_6 = 1151.4$.
CAS — 3546-41-6.

NOTE. Pyrvinium Chloride is rINN.

Pharmacopoeias. In US.

Pyrvinium embonate 7.5 mg is approximately equivalent to 5 mg of pyrvinium.

Pharmacopoeial description

USP 25: A bright orange or orange-red to practically black crystalline powder. Practically insoluble in water and in ether; slightly soluble in chloroform and in methoxyethanol; freely soluble in glacial acetic acid; very slightly soluble in methyl alcohol. Store in airtight containers. Protect from light.

Adverse Effects

Pyrvinium occasionally causes nausea, vomiting, and diarrhoea. Hypersensitivity reactions and photosensitivity have been reported.

Pyrvinium stains the stools bright red and may stain clothing if vomiting occurs.

Pharmacokinetics

Pyrvinium embonate is not significantly absorbed from the gastrointestinal tract.

Uses and Administration

Pyrvinium embonate is an effective anthelmintic in the treatment of enterobiasis (p.93), but has generally been superseded by other drugs.

It has been administered by mouth in a single dose equivalent to 5 mg of pyrvinium per kg body-weight, repeated after 2 to 3 weeks if necessary.

Preparations

USP 25: Pyrvinium Pamoate Oral Suspension; Pyrvinium Pamoate Tablets.

Proprietary Preparations (details are given in Part 3)
Aust.: Molevac; *Braz.:* Pyr-Pam; *Canad.:* Vanquin; *Denm.:* Vanquin; *Fin.:* Pyrvin; *Fr.:* Povanyl; *Ger.:* Molevac; *Ital.:* Vanquin†; *Norw.:* Vanquin; *Spain:* Pamoxan; *Swed.:* Vanquin; *Switz.:* Molevac†.

Multi-ingredient: *Braz.:* Contrelmin; Vermizol.

Rafoxanide (13206-f)

Rafoxanide (BAN, USAN, rINN).

MK-990. 3'-Chloro-4'-(4-chlorophenoxy)-3,5-di-iodosalicylanilide.

$C_{19}H_{11}Cl_2I_2NO_3 = 626.0$.
CAS — 22662-39-1.

Profile

Rafoxanide is an anthelmintic used for the treatment of fascioliasis in sheep and cattle.

Santonin (807-q)

Santoninum. (3S,3aS,5aS,9bS)-3a,5,5a,9b-Tetrahydro-3,5a,9-trimethylnaphtho[1,2-b]furan-2,8(3H,4H)-dione.

$C_{15}H_{18}O_3 = 246.3$.
CAS — 481-06-1.

Pharmacopoeias. In Jpn.

A crystalline lactone obtained from the dried unexpanded flowerheads of *Artemisia cina* (santonica, wormwood) and other species of *Artemisia* (Compositae).

Profile

Santonin was formerly used as an anthelmintic in the treatment of roundworm (*Ascaris*) infection, but has been superseded by other less toxic anthelmintics.

It is used as a flavour in food.

Selamectin (20389-j)

Selamectin (USAN, rINN).

UK-124114. (2aE,4E,5'S,6S,6'S,7S,8E,11R,13R,15S,17aR,20aR,20bS)-6'-Cyclohexyl-7-[(2,6-dideoxy-3-O-methyl-α-L-*arabino*-hexopyranosyl)oxy]-3',4',5',6,6',7,10,11,14,15,20a,20b-dodecahydro-20b-hydroxy-5',6,8,19-tetramethylspiro(11,15-methano-2H,13H,17H-furo[4,3,2-p,q][2,6]benzodioxacyclooctadecin-13,2'-[2H]pyran)-17,20(17aH)-dione 20-oxime.

$C_{43}H_{63}NO_{11} = 770.0$.
CAS — 165108-07-6.

Profile

Selamectin is an avermectin anthelmintic and ectoparasiticide used in veterinary medicine.

Tetramisole Hydrochloride (814-g)

Tetramisole Hydrochloride (BANM, USAN, rINNM).

ICI-50627; McN-JR-8299-11; R-8299. (±)-2,3,5,6-Tetrahydro-6-phenylimidazo[2,1-b]thiazole hydrochloride.

$C_{11}H_{12}N_2S,HCl = 240.8$.
CAS — 5036-02-2 (tetramisole); 5086-74-8 (tetramisole hydrochloride).

Pharmacopoeias. In Fr. for veterinary use only.

Profile

Tetramisole hydrochloride is an anthelmintic used in veterinary practice for the control of nematode infections. It is a racemic mixture and the laevo-isomer, levamisole hydrochloride (p.101), accounts for most of its activity.

Preparations

Proprietary Preparations (details are given in Part 3)
Braz.: Ascarotrat; Ascaverm; Cofasol; Tetramizotil.

Multi-ingredient: *Braz.:* Tetramizol Composto; Vermizol.

Thiacetarsamide (19922-g)

p-[Bis(carboxymethylmercapto)arsino]benzamide; 4-Carbamylphenyl bis[carboxymethylthio]arsenite.

$C_{11}H_{12}AsNO_5S_2 = 377.3$.
CAS — 531-72-6.

Pharmacopoeias. In US for veterinary use only.

Pharmacopoeial description

USP 25: A white to yellowish crystalline powder. Sparingly soluble in cold water but more soluble in water above 90°; sparingly soluble in cold dehydrated alcohol but soluble in warm dehydrated alcohol; insoluble in warm isopropyl alcohol; sparingly soluble in cold methyl alcohol but soluble in warm methyl alcohol.

Profile

Thiacetarsamide is an anthelmintic used in veterinary medicine.

Thiophanate (13328-s)

Thiophanate (BAN).

4,4'-o-Phenylenebis(ethyl 3-thioallophanate).

$C_{14}H_{18}N_4O_4S_2 = 370.4$.
CAS — 23564-06-9.

Profile

Thiophanate is an anthelmintic used in veterinary practice for the control of nematode infections.

Tiabendazole (816-p)

Tiabendazole (BAN, rINN).

E233; MK-360; Thiabendazole (USAN); Tiabendazolum. 2-(Thiazol-4-yl)-1H-benzimidazole.

$C_{10}H_7N_3S = 201.2$.

CAS — 148-79-8.

ATC — D01AC06; P02CA02.

Pharmacopoeias. In Chin., Eur. (see p.vi), Int., and US.

Pharmacopoeial description

Ph. Eur.: A white or almost white crystalline powder. Practically insoluble in water; slightly soluble in alcohol, in dichloromethane, and in ether; it dissolves in dilute mineral acids. Protect from light.

USP 25: A white to practically white, odourless or practically odourless, powder. Practically insoluble in water; slightly soluble in alcohol and in acetone; very slightly soluble in chloroform and in ether.

Adverse Effects

Dizziness and gastrointestinal disturbances, especially anorexia, nausea, and vomiting, are common during treatment with tiabendazole. Other adverse effects occurring occasionally include pruritus, skin rashes, headache, fatigue, drowsiness, drying of mucous membranes, hyperglycaemia, disturbance of vision including colour vision, leucopenia, tinnitus, effects on the liver including cholestasis and parenchymal damage (in some cases severe and irreversible), enuresis, crystalluria, and bradycardia and hypotension. There have also been reports of erythema multiforme, fatal Stevens-Johnson syndrome, toxic epidermal necrolysis, convulsions, and effects on mental state.

Fever, chills, angioedema, and lymphadenopathy have been reported, but may represent allergic response to dead parasites rather than to tiabendazole.

The urine of some patients taking tiabendazole may have a characteristic odour similar to that following the ingestion of asparagus; it is attributed to the presence of a tiabendazole metabolite.

Effects on the salivary glands. Dry mouth with swollen parotid and salivary glands suggestive of the sicca complex preceded the development of cholestatic jaundice in a 17-year-old boy given tiabendazole.[1]

1. Davidson RN, et al. Intrahepatic cholestasis after thiabendazole. Trans R Soc Trop Med Hyg 1988; **82:** 620.

Hypersensitivity. Severe erythema multiforme developed in a patient 16 days after a course of tiabendazole.[1] Many of the lesions encircled pre-existing melanocytic naevi.

1. Humphreys F, Cox NH. Thiabendazole-induced erythema multiforme with lesions around melanocytic naevi. Br J Dermatol 1988; **118:** 855–6.

Precautions

Tiabendazole is teratogenic in mice. It should be used with caution in patients with hepatic or renal impairment. Tiabendazole causes drowsiness in some patients and those affected should not drive or operate machinery.

Tiabendazole should not be used in mixed worm infections involving Ascaris lumbricoides as it can cause these roundworms to migrate; live roundworms have emerged through the mouth or nose.

Renal impairment. Tiabendazole and its 5-hydroxy metabolite did not accumulate in an anephric patient on haemodialysis and haemoperfusion and receiving treatment for severe strongyloidiasis.[1] However, the potentially toxic conjugated glucuronide and sulfate metabolites did accumulate. The clearance of all 3 metabolites was poor by haemodialysis; haemoperfusion was much more efficient, although for rapid removal the haemoperfusion columns should be changed every hour.

1. Bauer L, et al. The pharmacokinetics of thiabendazole and its metabolites in an anephric patient undergoing hemodialysis and hemoperfusion. J Clin Pharmacol 1982; **22:** 276–80.

Interactions

Theophylline. For the effect of tiabendazole on serum concentrations of theophylline, see p.782.

Pharmacokinetics

Tiabendazole is readily absorbed from the gastrointestinal tract and reaches peak concentrations in the plasma after 1 to 2 hours. It is metabolised to 5-hydroxythiabendazole and excreted principally in the urine as glucuronide or sulfate conjugates; about 90% is recovered in the urine within 48 hours of ingestion, but only 5% in the faeces. Absorption may occur from preparations applied to the skin or eyes.

◊ References.

1. Tocco DJ, et al. Absorption, metabolism, and excretion of thiabendazole in man and laboratory animals. Toxicol Appl Pharmacol 1966; **9:** 31–9.

Uses and Administration

Tiabendazole, a benzimidazole derivative, is an anthelmintic with activity against most nematode worms; activity against some larval stages and ova has also been demonstrated. The mode of action is not certain, but tiabendazole may inhibit the fumarate-reductase system of worms thereby interfering with their source of energy.

Tiabendazole is used in the treatment of cutaneous larva migrans, dracunculiasis (guinea worm infection), and toxocariasis. It may also be used in the treatment of strongyloidiasis, and can provide symptomatic relief during the larval invasion stage of trichinosis. Tiabendazole is also active against some intestinal nematodes, but should not be used as primary therapy; the treatment of mixed infections including ascariasis is not recommended since tiabendazole may cause the worms to migrate to other body organs causing serious complications. For discussions of the treatment of the above infections see under Choice of Anthelmintic, p.91. See also below.

Tiabendazole is given by mouth, with meals, usually in a dose of 25 mg per kg body-weight twice daily for 2 or more days, the duration depending on the type of infection; the daily dose should not exceed 3 g. For those unable to tolerate 2 doses daily, 25 mg per kg may be given after the largest meal on day 1 and repeated 24 hours later after a similar meal on day 2. For mass treatment, a single dose of 50 mg per kg after the evening meal is suggested although the incidence of adverse effects may be higher than with 2 doses of 25 mg per kg.

In cutaneous larva migrans, 25 mg per kg may be given twice daily for 2 days, repeated after 2 days if necessary; topical treatment with a 10 to 15% suspension intended for oral use has also been advocated as an alternative or adjunct to oral treatment.

In dracunculiasis, 25 to 50 mg per kg may be given twice daily for one day; in massive infection a further 50 mg per kg may be given after 5 to 8 days.

In strongyloidiasis, 25 mg per kg may be given twice daily for 2 or 3 days or 50 mg per kg as a single dose; when the infection is disseminated treatment for at least 5 days may be necessary.

In trichinosis, 25 mg per kg may be given twice daily for 2 to 4 successive days.

In toxocariasis, 25 mg per kg may be given twice daily for 7 days.

Tiabendazole also has some antifungal activity. It is used as a fungicidal preservative for certain foods.

Angiostrongyliasis. Tiabendazole has been suggested as an alternative to mebendazole for the treatment of infections with Angiostrongylus costaricensis (see p.91), although the high dose of 25 mg per kg body-weight three times daily for 3 days considered necessary is likely to be toxic and may have to be decreased.[1]

1. Anonymous. Drugs for parasitic infections. Med Lett Drugs Ther 1998; **40:** 1–12.

Dracunculiasis. Tiabendazole[1,2] may be used for symptomatic treatment of dracunculiasis (p.92), although it has no direct anthelmintic effect. It is used to facilitate removal of the worm from subcutaneous tissues.

1. Muller R. Guinea worm disease: epidemiology, control, and treatment. Bull WHO 1979; **57:** 683–9.
2. Kale OO, et al. Controlled comparative trial of thiabendazole and metronidazole in the treatment of dracontiasis. Ann Trop Med Parasitol 1983; **77:** 151–7.

Strongyloidiasis. Tiabendazole may be used in the treatment of strongyloidiasis (p.94), but albendazole or ivermectin are generally preferred.

References.

1. Grove DI. Treatment of strongyloidiasis with thiabendazole: an analysis of toxicity and effectiveness. Trans R Soc Trop Med Hyg 1982; **76:** 114–18.
2. Barnish G, Barker J. An intervention study using thiabendazole suspension against strongyloides fuelleborni-like infections in Papua New Guinea. Trans R Soc Trop Med Hyg 1987; **81:** 60–3.

Syngamosis. Tiabendazole has been used successfully[1,2] to treat syngamosis (p.95) when it has occurred in man.

1. Grell GAC, et al. Syngamus in a West Indian. BMJ 1978; **2:** 1464.
2. Leers W-D, et al. Syngamosis, an unusual case of asthma: the first reported case in Canada. Can Med Assoc J 1985; **132:** 269–70.

Preparations

BP 2001: Tiabendazole Tablets;
USP 25: Thiabendazole Oral Suspension; Thiabendazole Tablets.

Proprietary Preparations (details are given in Part 3)
Austral.: Mintezol; **Braz.:** Foldan; Folderm; Thiaben; Tiabiose; Tutiverm; **Canad.:** Mintezol; **Irl.:** Mintezol†; **Mex.:** Eprofil; **Spain:** Triasox; **UK:** Mintezol†; **USA:** Mintezol.

Multi-ingredient: Braz.: Contrelmin; Derms; Flenverme; Forverm; Helmi-Ped; Helmiben; Helmidrax; Micoplex; Neovermim; Poliben; Profium; Tetramizol Composto; Thiabena; Vermol; Zoles.

Triclabendazole (3230-g)

Triclabendazole (BAN, rINN).

5-Chloro-6-(2,3-dichlorophenoxy)-2-(methylthio)benzimidazole.

$C_{14}H_9Cl_3N_2OS = 359.7$.

CAS — 68786-66-3.

Profile

Triclabendazole is a benzimidazole anthelmintic used in veterinary practice and with a potential role in the treatment of human fascioliasis. Triclabendazole is also under investigation for the treatment of human paragonimiasis.

Liver fluke infections. Although bithionol or praziquantel are currently used to treat fascioliasis (p.93), WHO[1] anticipated that triclabendazole would become the drug of choice. A possible dosage schedule was two doses of 5 mg per kg body-weight given after meals, with an interval of 6 to 8 hours between the two doses.[1] In a study from Chile, 19 of 24 patients with chronic hepatic fascioliasis were treated successfully with a single dose of triclabendazole 10 mg per kg after an overnight fast.[2]

1. WHO. Control of foodborne trematode infections. WHO Tech Rep Ser 849 1995.
2. Apt W, et al. Treatment of human chronic fascioliasis with triclabendazole: drug efficacy and serologic response. Am J Trop Med Hyg 1995; **52:** 532–5.

Lung fluke infections. Encouraging results were reported from a pilot study of triclabendazole[1] in the treatment of paragonimiasis (p.94). In an open comparative study[2] in 62 patients, a more rapid parasitological response was obtained with triclabendazole in doses of 5 mg per kg body-weight once daily for 3 days, 10 mg per kg twice on one day, or 10 mg per kg as a single dose, than with praziquantel. Clinical symptoms resolved at a comparable rate in all groups.

1. Ripert C, et al. Therapeutic effect of triclabendazole in patients with paragonimiasis in Cameroon: a pilot study. Trans R Soc Trop Med Hyg 1992; **86:** 417.
2. Calvopiña M, et al. Treatment of human pulmonary paragonimiasis with triclabendazole: clinical tolerance and drug efficacy. Trans R Soc Trop Med Hyg 1998; **92:** 566–9.

The symbol † denotes a preparation no longer actively marketed

Antibacterials

In this chapter are antimicrobial drugs used principally in the treatment and prophylaxis of bacterial infections. In practice the term 'antibiotics' is often, and in some instances erroneously, used to encompass all of these agents. The various groups into which these drugs may be categorised are described below. Antibacterials described elsewhere in *Martindale* include metronidazole (p.594) which, as well as being an antiprotozoal, is used in the treatment of anaerobic bacterial infections. Immunological approaches to the treatment and prophylaxis of bacterial infections are discussed under Vaccines Immunoglobulins and Antisera, p.1529.

In addition, disinfectants and preservatives (p.1129) are used to kill or inhibit the growth of micro-organisms.

Drug Groups

Although antibiotics and other antibacterials are a very diverse class of compounds they are often classified and discussed in groups. They may be classified according to their mode of action or spectrum of antimicrobial activity, but generally those with similar chemical structures are grouped together.

Aminoglycosides

The aminoglycosides are a closely-related group of bactericidal antibiotics derived from bacteria of the order Actinomycetales or, more specifically, the genus *Streptomyces* (framycetin, kanamycin, neomycin, paromomycin (p.599), streptomycin, and tobramycin) and the genus *Micromonospora* (gentamicin and sisomicin). They are polycationic compounds that contain an aminocyclitol, usually 2-deoxystreptamine, or streptidine in streptomycin and related compounds, with cyclic amino-sugars at-

tached by glycosidic linkages. Therefore, they have also been termed aminoglycosidic aminocyclitols. The sulfate salts are generally used.

The aminoglycosides have broadly similar toxicological features. Ototoxicity is a major limitation to their use; streptomycin and gentamicin are generally considered to be more toxic to the vestibular branch of the eighth cranial nerve and neomycin and kanamycin to be more toxic to the auditory branch. Other adverse effects common to the group include nephrotoxicity, neuromuscular blocking activity, and allergy, including cross-reactivity.

The pharmacokinetics of the aminoglycosides are very similar. Little is absorbed from the gastrointestinal tract but they are generally well-distributed in the body after parenteral administration although penetration into the CSF is poor. They are excreted unchanged in the urine by glomerular filtration.

The aminoglycosides have a similar antimicrobial spectrum and appear to act by interfering with bacterial protein synthesis, possibly by binding irreversibly to the 30S and to some extent the 50S portions of the bacterial ribosome. The manner in which they bring about cell death is not fully understood. They are most active against Gram-negative rods. *Staphylococcus aureus* is susceptible to the aminoglycosides but otherwise most Gram-positive bacteria, and also anaerobic bacteria, are naturally resistant. They show enhanced activity with penicillins against some enterococci and streptococci. Bacterial resistance to streptomycin may occur by mutation, whereas with the other aminoglycosides it is usually associated with the plasmid-mediated production of inactivating enzymes which are capable of phosphorylation, acetylation, or adenylation. The aminoglycosides have a postantibiotic effect, that is antibacterial activity persisting after concentrations have dropped below minimum inhibitory concentrations.

Streptomycin was the first aminoglycoside to become available commercially and was isolated from a strain of *Streptomyces griseus* in 1944. Its use is now restricted mainly to the treatment of tuberculosis when it is always administered in association with other antituberculous drugs because of the rapid development of resistance. *Dihydrostreptomycin*, a reduction product of streptomycin, is only rarely used because of its toxicity. The *neomycin* complex of antibiotics were the next to be isolated; neomycin itself is mainly a mixture of the B and C isomers and neomycin B is considered to be identical with *framycetin*. Because of their toxicity they are not given systemically. The related compound *paromomycin* (p.599) also has antiprotozoal and anthelmintic properties and may be used in the treatment of intestinal amoebiasis, cestode infections, cryptosporidiosis, and leishmaniasis. *Kanamycin* is less toxic than neomycin and can be used systemically. Although it has been used in penicillin-resistant gonorrhoea, it is not active against *Pseudomonas aeruginosa* and has generally been replaced by gentamicin and other newer aminoglycosides.

Gentamicin was isolated from *Micromonospora purpurea* in 1963 and, being active against *Ps. aeruginosa* and *Serratia marcescens*, is widely used in the treatment of life-threatening infections. *Tobramycin* is one of several components of the nebramycin complex of aminoglycosides produced by *Streptomyces tenebrarius*. It has an antimicrobial spectrum very similar to that of gentamicin and is reported to be more active against *Ps. aeruginosa*. *Amikacin*, a semisynthetic derivative of kanamycin, has a side-chain rendering it less susceptible to inactivating enzymes. It has a spectrum of activity like that of gentamicin but Gram-negative bacteria resistant to gentamicin, tobramycin, and kanamycin are often sensitive. *Sisomicin* is closely related structurally to gentamicin, and *netilmicin* is the N-ethyl derivative of sisomicin. Netilmicin may be active against some gentamicin-resistant strains of bacteria although not to the same extent as amikacin. Other aminoglycosides include *isepamicin and micronomicin*.

Aminoglycosides should in general only be used for the treatment of serious infections because of their potential toxicity and antimicrobial spectrum. Doses must be carefully regulated to maintain plasma concentrations within the therapeutic range but avoiding accumulation, especially in patients with renal impairment. Neomycin and framycetin, which are considered too toxic to be given parenterally, have been given by mouth to suppress the intestinal flora. The topical use of neomycin and gentamicin has been associated with allergic reactions and the emergence of resistant bacteria. Gentamicin or tobramycin are the drugs of choice in the treatment of life-threatening infections due to aminoglycoside-sensitive organisms and are often used in association with other antibacterials. With the continuing emergence of resistant strains, amikacin and netilmicin should be reserved for severe infections resistant to gentamicin and the other aminoglycosides.

Described in this chapter are

Antimycobacterials

The antimycobacterials are a miscellaneous group of antibacterials whose spectrum of activity includes *Mycobacterium* spp. and which are used in the treatment of tuberculosis, leprosy, and other mycobacterial infections. They include the rifamycins, also known as ansamycins or rifomycins, a group of antibiotics isolated from a strain of *Amycolatopsis mediterranei* (*Nocardia mediterranei*; *Streptomyces mediterranei*). The main antibiotic in this group, *rifampicin*, is a mainstay of regimens for the treatment of tuberculosis and leprosy, and is increasingly being used for other infections. The related drug *rifabutin* is also used in mycobacterial disease, especially opportunistic mycobacterial infections due to *Mycobacterium avium* complex (MAC). Other rifamycins described in this chapter include *rifapentine*, *rifaximin* which is poorly absorbed and is mainly used for a local effect on the gastrointestinal tract, and *rifamycin sodium*, a rifamycin rarely used as it has been superseded by more effective drugs.

Another drug widely used for tuberculosis is *isoniazid*, a derivative of isonicotinic acid; it is invariably used in combination with other drugs to avoid or delay emergence of resistance. *Pyrazinamide*, a nicotinamide derivative, is also an important component of combination regimens for tuberculosis, while *ethambutol* and the aminoglycoside *streptomycin* are added unless resistance to first-line drugs is unlikely. The thiosemicarbazone derivative *thioacetazone* is now less widely used in tuberculosis because of its toxicity and because more effective drugs are available, but is sometimes employed in developing countries. Other drugs that have been used to treat tuberculosis including *aminosalicylic acid* and its salts, *capreomycin, cycloserine, ethionamide, protionamide*, and *kanamycin* are regarded as secondary drugs and are reserved for patients in whom resistance or toxicity to first-line drugs is a problem.

The sulfones have been employed since the 1940s in the treatment of leprosy, but the only one widely used now is *dapsone*, an important component of multidrug regimens. Its action is thought to involve inhibition of folate metabolism, similarly to the sulfonamides, and dapsone is also used for the prophylaxis of malaria and for prophylaxis and treatment of *Pneumocystis carinii* pneumonia. Also important in the treatment of leprosy is the phenazine dye *clofazimine*. Additionally, it has a role in the treatment of type 2 lepra reactions and has been used in other mycobacterial infections. The thioamides *ethionamide* and *protionamide* have been used in the treatment of leprosy and tuberculosis, but have generally been replaced by less toxic drugs, for example *clarithromycin, ofloxacin, minocycline*, or *pefloxacin*, in alternative antileprotic regimens.

Described in this chapter are

Cephalosporins and related Beta Lactams

The cephalosporins or cephem antibiotics are semisynthetic antibacterials derived from cephalosporin C a natural antibiotic produced by the mould *Cephalosporium acremonium*. The active nucleus, 7-aminocephalosporanic acid, is very closely related to the penicillin nucleus, 6-aminopenicillanic acid, and consists of a beta-lactam ring fused with a 6-membered dihydrothiazine ring and having an acetoxymethyl group at position 3. Cephalosporin C has a side-chain at position 7 derived from D-α-aminoadipic acid. Chemical modification of positions 3 and 7 has resulted in a series of drugs with different characteristics. Substitution at the 7-amino group tends to affect antibacterial action whereas at position 3 it may have more of an effect on pharmacokinetic properties.

The cephalosporins are bactericidal and, similarly to the penicillins, they act by inhibiting synthesis of the bacterial cell wall. The most widely used system of classification of cephalosporins is by generations and is based on the general features of their antibacterial activity, but may depend to some extent on when they were introduced. Succeeding generations generally have increasing activity against Gram-negative bacteria. *Cefalotin* was one of the first cephalosporins to become available and is representative of the **first-generation** cephalosporins. It has good activity against a wide spectrum of Gram-positive bacteria including penicillinase-producing, but not meticillin-resistant, staphylococci; enterococci are, however, resistant. Its activity against Gram-negative bacteria is modest. Cefalotin is not absorbed from the gastrointestinal tract and must be administered parenterally although intramuscular administration is painful. Cefalotin has generally been replaced by *cefazolin* or *cefradine*. *Cefaloridine* is now rarely used because of its nephrotoxicity. Cefradine is absorbed from the gastrointestinal tract and can be administered both by mouth and by injection. *Cefadroxil, cefatrizine*, and *cefalexin* are all administered by mouth. All of these drugs have a very similar spectrum of antimicrobial activity to cefalotin. *Cefaclor* is also given by mouth. It has similar activity to cefalotin against Gram-positive cocci, but because of its greater activity against Gram-negative bacteria, particularly *Haemophilus influenzae*, it is often classified as a second-generation drug. *Cefprozil* is an oral cephalosporin with a longer half-life than cefaclor.

Cefamandole was the first available **second-generation** cephalosporin. It has similar or slightly less activity than cefalotin against Gram-positive bacteria, but greater stability to hydrolysis by beta lactamases produced by Gram-negative bacteria and enhanced activity against many of the Enterobacteriaceae and *Haemophilus influenzae*. *Cefuroxime* has a similar spectrum of activity to cefamandole although it is even more resistant to hydrolysis by beta lactamases. *Cefuroxime axetil*, the acetoxyethyl ester of cefuroxime, is administered by mouth. Other drugs classified as second-generation cephalosporins and administered parenterally include *cefonicid, cefforanide*, and *cefotiam*; these all have spectra of activity similar to cefamandole. Cephamycins (see below) are also classified with second-generation cephalosporins.

The **third-generation** cephalosporins, sometimes referred to as **extended-spectrum** cephalosporins are even more stable to hydrolysis by beta lactamases than cefamandole and cefuroxime. Compared with the earlier generations of cephalosporins they have a wider spectrum and greater potency of activity against Gram-negative organisms including most clinically important Enterobacteriaceae. Their activity against Gram-positive organisms is said to be less than that of the first-generation drugs, but they are very active against streptococci. *Cefotaxime* was the first of this group to become available and it has relatively modest activity against *Pseudomonas aeruginosa*. *Cefmenoxime, cefodizime, ceftizoxime*, and *ceftriaxone* are all very similar to cefotaxime in their antimicrobial activity. These drugs are all administered parenterally and differ mainly in their pharmacokinetic characteristics. *Cefixime* is a third-generation cephalosporin given by mouth; others include *cefdinir, cefetamet pivoxil, cefpodoxime proxetil*, and *ceftibuten*. *Latamoxef* is an **oxacephalosporin** which differs from the true cephalosporins in that the sulfur atom of the 7-ami-

nocephalosporanic acid nucleus is replaced by an oxygen atom. It differs from cefotaxime mainly in its enhanced activity against *Bacteroides fragilis*. *Ceftazidime* is typical of a group of parenteral third-generation cephalosporins with enhanced activity against *Ps. aeruginosa*. *Cefoperazone* is similar in its activity to ceftazidime. *Cefpiramide* is structurally related to cefoperazone and has comparable activity. Although *cefsulodin* is classified as a third-generation cephalosporin its activity against Gram-negative bacteria is confined to *Ps. aeruginosa*.

The newer cephalosporins *cefepime* and *cefpirome* are generally considered to be **fourth-generation** because of their broad spectrum of activity.

The semisynthetic **cephamycins** are chemical modifications of cephamycin C, a beta-lactam antibiotic produced naturally by *Streptomyces* spp. They differ from the cephalosporins by the addition of a 7-α-methoxy group to the 7-aminocephalosporanic acid nucleus. Steric hindrance by this methoxy group is considered to be responsible for their greater stability to beta lactamases. For practical purposes they are generally classified with the second-generation cephalosporins, but are more active against anaerobic bacteria, especially *Bacteroides fragilis*. *Cefoxitin* was one of the first cephamycins available; *cefmetazole* and *cefotetan* have been introduced more recently. Another is *cefminox*. All these cephamycins must be administered by the parenteral route.

Imipenem was the first of the **carbapenem** group of antibiotics to become available; it is the *N*-formimidoyl derivative of thienamycin which is produced by *Streptomyces cattleya*. It is bactericidal, and, similarly to the cephalosporins, acts by inhibiting synthesis of the bacterial cell wall. It has a very broad spectrum of antimicrobial activity including Gram-positive and Gram-negative aerobic and anaerobic organisms; it has good activity against both *Ps. aeruginosa* and *B. fragilis*. Imipenem is administered parenterally in association with cilastatin, a dehydropeptidase I inhibitor which inhibits the renal metabolism of imipenem. Similarly, the carbapenem panipenem is given with the renal protectant betamipron. Another carbapenem, *meropenem*, is relatively stable to renal dehydropeptidase and can be administered without such an inhibitor.

The **monobactams** were first identified as monocyclic beta lactams isolated from bacteria; they are now produced synthetically. *Aztreonam* was the first commercially available monobactam. It too is bactericidal with a similar action on bacterial cell-wall synthesis to the cephalosporins. Its antimicrobial activity, however, differs from imipenem and the newer cephalosporins in that it is restricted to Gram-negative aerobic organisms. It has good activity against *Ps. aeruginosa*. Aztreonam is administered by the parenteral route. Other monobactams include *carumonam*.

Carbacephems are structurally related to the cephalosporins, but the sulfur atom of the 7-aminocephalosporanic acid nucleus is replaced by a methylene group. *Loracarbef* is an oral carbacephem.

Described in this chapter are

Chloramphenicols

Chloramphenicol is an antibiotic which was first isolated from cultures of *Streptomyces venezuelae* in 1947 but is now produced synthetically. It has a relatively simple structure and is a derivative of dichloroacetic acid with a nitrobenzene moiety. Chloramphenicol was the first broad-spectrum antibiotic to be discovered; it acts by interfering with bacterial protein synthesis and is mainly bacteriostatic. Its range of activity is similar to that of tetracycline and includes Gram-positive and Gram-negative bacteria, rickettsias, and chlamydias. The sensitivity of *Salmonella typhi*, *Haemophilus influenzae*, and *Bacteroides fragilis* to chloramphenicol have provided the principal indications for its use.

Shortly after its introduction chloramphenicol was found to have a serious and sometimes fatal depressant effect on the bone marrow. The 'grey syndrome', another potentially fatal adverse effect, was reported later in newborn infants. As a result of this toxicity the use of chloramphenicol has been restricted in many countries; it should only be given when there is no suitable alternative and never for minor infections.

Chloramphenicol is active when given by mouth and, unlike most other antibacterials, it diffuses into the CSF even when the meninges are not inflamed. The majority of a dose is inactivated in the liver, only a small proportion appearing unchanged in the urine.

Chloramphenicol is used for typhoid fever in many countries although resistance is a problem in some countries. For *Haemophilus influenzae* infections, especially meningitis, the emergence of ampicillin-resistant strains led to a reappraisal of the use of chloramphenicol. Some workers have considered that ampicillin and chloramphenicol should both be given empirically to patients with meningitis until the sensitivity of the infecting organisms is known, but the newer third-generation cephalosporins are increasingly preferred because of resistance. For proven *H. influenzae* meningitis chloramphenicol is used as an alternative to the third-generation cephalosporins, which are now regarded as treatment of choice. Chloramphenicol is also effective against many anaerobic bacteria and may be valuable in such conditions as cerebral abscess where anaerobes such as *Bacteroides fragilis* are often involved, although metronidazole may be preferred.

Chloramphenicol sodium succinate is used parenterally and the palmitate is given orally. Ophthalmic and other topical preparations of chloramphenicol are used widely in some countries for a variety of infections.

Thiamphenicol is a semisynthetic derivative of chloramphenicol in which the nitro group on the benzene ring has been replaced by a methylsulfonyl group, resulting, in general, in a loss of activity *in vitro*. It has been claimed that thiamphenicol is less toxic than chloramphenicol and there have been fewer reports of aplastic anaemia but reversible bone-marrow depression may occur more frequently. Unlike chloramphenicol, thiamphenicol is not metabolised in the liver to any extent and is excreted largely unchanged in the urine. It has been used similarly to chloramphenicol in some countries.

Azidamfenicol is another analogue of chloramphenicol that has been used topically in the treatment of eye infections.

Described in this chapter are
Azidamfenicol, p.152   Florfenicol, p.207
Chloramphenicol, p.179   Thiamphenicol, p.261

Glycopeptides

Vancomycin has a glycopeptide structure; it acts by interfering with bacterial cell wall synthesis and is very active against Gram-positive cocci. Intravenous vancomycin is reserved for the treatment of severe staphylococcal infections and for the treatment and prophylaxis of endocarditis when other antibacterials cannot be used, either because of patient sensitivity or bacterial resistance. It is the treatment of choice for infections caused by meticillin-resistant staphylococci. Vancomycin hydrochloride is poorly absorbed when taken by mouth; it is used in the treatment of pseudomembranous colitis. *Teicoplanin* is a glycopeptide with similar properties to vancomycin, but a longer duration of action. It can be given intramuscularly as well as intravenously. *Ramoplanin* is under investigation, especially for topical use in skin infections.

Described in this chapter are
Avoparcin, p.152   Teicoplanin, p.257
Ramoplanin, p.242   Vancomycin, p.267

Lincosamides

Lincomycin is an antibiotic produced by a strain of *Streptomyces lincolnensis* and was first described in 1962; *clindamycin* is the 7-chloro-7-deoxy derivative of lincomycin.

Although not related structurally to erythromycin and the other macrolide antibiotics, the lincosamides have similar antimicrobial activity and act at the same site on the bacterial ribosome to suppress protein synthesis.

The lincosamides are bacteriostatic or bactericidal depending on the concentration and are active mainly against Gram-positive bacteria, and against *Bacteroides* spp. They also appear to have some antiprotozoal activity. Clindamycin and lincomycin have qualitatively similar activity but clindamycin is more active than lincomycin *in vitro*. Cross-resistance occurs between the lincosamides, macrolides, and streptogramins.

The lincosamides have been used, like erythromycin, as an alternative to penicillin but reports of the occurrence of severe and sometimes fatal pseudomembranous colitis in association with lincomycin and clindamycin have led to the recommendation that they should only be used when there is no suitable alternative.

Both lincomycin and clindamycin can be given orally and parenterally but clindamycin is much better absorbed from the gastrointestinal tract and less affected by the presence of food in the stomach. They both penetrate well into bone and have been used successfully in osteomyelitis. They have also been used topically in the treatment of acne vulgaris.

The main indication for the use of lincosamides is now in the treatment of severe anaerobic infections although metronidazole (p.596) or some beta lactams may be a more suitable choice in such infections; clindamycin also has a role in the prophylaxis of endocarditis in penicillin-allergic patients. It has been used, usually with other antiprotozoals, in babesiosis, chloroquine-resistant malaria, toxoplasmosis, and *Pneumocystis carinii* pneumonia.

Described in this chapter are
Clindamycin, p.188   Pirlimycin, p.237
Lincomycin, p.219

Macrolides

The macrolides are a large group of antibiotics mainly derived from *Streptomyces* spp. and having a common macrocyclic lactone ring to which one or more sugars are attached. They are all weak bases and only slightly soluble in water. Their properties are very similar and in general they have low toxicity and a similar spectrum of antimicrobial activity with cross-resistance between individual members of the group. The macrolides are bacteriostatic or bactericidal, depending on the concentration and the type of micro-organism, and are thought to interfere with bacterial protein synthesis. Their antimicrobial spectrum is similar to that of benzylpenicillin but they are also active against such organisms as *Legionella pneumophila*, *Mycoplasma pneumoniae*, and some rickettsias and chlamydias. Macrolides and related drugs have a postantibiotic effect: that is, antibacterial activity persists after concentrations have dropped below the minimum inhibitory concentration.

Erythromycin was discovered in 1952 and is the macrolide used most widely. It is destroyed by gastric acid and must therefore be given as enteric-coated formulations or as one of its more stable salts or esters such as the stearate or ethyl succinate. Hepatotoxicity has been reported after the administration of erythromycin, most commonly as the estolate. Erythromycin lactobionate or gluceptate may be given intravenously. Cardiac arrhythmias have been reported occasionally after intravenous administration. Erythromycin is used as an alternative to penicillin in many infections, especially in patients who are allergic to penicillin. It has similar uses to tetracycline in the treatment of infections due to *Mycoplasma pneumoniae* and *Chlamydia trachomatis*, and in acne vulgaris. It is also used in the treatment of infections caused by *Legionella pneumophila*.

The other macrolides include *spiramycin* which has been used extensively in Europe and which has also been used in the treatment and prophylaxis of toxoplasmosis and may be useful in the treatment of cryptosporidiosis.

Oleandomycin has been used orally and parenterally as the phosphate. Its ester, *troleandomycin*, is better absorbed from the gastrointestinal tract but, like erythromycin estolate, has proved hepatotoxic. *Josamycin*, *kitasamycin*, *midecamycin*, and *rokitamycin* have been used in Europe and/or Japan.

More recent macrolides include *azithromycin*, *clarithromycin*, *dirithromycin*, and *roxithromycin*. These drugs all appear to have essentially similar properties to erythromycin although they may differ in their pharmacokinetics. Clarithromycin and, to a lesser extent, azithromycin are more active than erythromycin against opportunistic mycobacteria such as *Mycobacterium avium* complex. Clarithromycin is also used in the treatment of leprosy and in regimens for the eradication of *Helicobacter pylori* in peptic ulcer disease. Both azithromycin and clarithromycin have activity against protozoa including *Toxoplasma gondii*.

Flurithromycin is among other macrolides investigated.

The **streptogramin** group of antibiotics are also derived from *Streptomyces* spp. and include *pristinamycin* and *virginiamycin*. They consist of two components, which act synergistically and they are therefore also known as synergistins. One of the components is structurally related to the macrolides, and they have a similar spectrum of antimicrobial activity to erythromycin. Semisynthetic derivatives such as *quinupristin/dalfopristin* may be useful in the treatment of infections with multidrug-resistant organisms including meticillin-resistant *Staphylococcus aureus* and vancomycin-resistant enterococci.

Cross-resistance is often observed between the macrolides, lincosamides, and streptogramins.

Described in this chapter are
Azithromycin, p.153   Quinupristin/Dalfopristin,
Clarithromycin, p.186   p.241
Dirithromycin, p.199   Rokitamycin, p.247
Erythromycin, p.201   Roxithromycin, p.247
Flurithromycin, p.207   Spiramycin, p.248
Josamycin, p.217   Tilmicosin, p.263
Kitasamycin, p.218   Troleandomycin, p.266
Midecamycin, p.224   Tylosin, p.267
Oleandomycin, p.233   Virginiamycin, p.269
Pristinamycin, p.239

Penicillins

Penicillin was the first antibiotic to be used therapeutically and was originally obtained, as a mixture of penicillins known as F, G, X, and K, from the mould *Penicillium notatum*. Better yields were achieved using *P. chrysogenum* and benzylpenicillin (penicillin G) was selectively produced by adding the precursor phenylacetic acid to the fermentation medium. The term 'penicillin' is now used generically for the entire group of natural and semisynthetic penicillins. Penicillins are still widely used; they are generally well tolerated, apart from hypersensitivity reactions, and are usually bactericidal by virtue of their inhibitory action on the synthesis of the bacterial cell wall.

Penicillins all have the same ring structure and are monobasic acids which readily form salts and esters; 6-aminopenicillanic acid, the penicillin nucleus, consists of a fused thiazolidine ring and a beta-lactam ring with an amino group at the 6-position.

The earlier or so-called 'natural' penicillins were produced by adding different side-chain precursors to fermentations of the *Penicillium* mould; *benzylpenicillin*, with a phenylacetamido side-chain at the 6-position, and *phenoxymethylpenicillin* (penicillin V), with a phenoxyacetamido side-chain, were 2 of the first and are still widely used. Benzylpenicillin can be considered the parent compound of the penicillins and is active mainly against Gram-positive bacteria and *Neisseria* spp. It is inactivated by penicillinase-producing bacteria and because of its instability in gastric acid it is usually injected. Long-acting preparations include *procaine penicillin* [procaine benzylpenicillin] and *benzathine benzylpenicillin* which slowly release benzylpenicillin after injection. Phenoxymethylpenicillin is acid-stable and therefore given by mouth but it is also inactivated by penicillinase. It is generally used for relatively mild infections.

When no side-chain precursor is added to the fermentation medium, 6-aminopenicillanic acid itself is obtained. A range of penicillins has been synthesised from 6-aminopenicillanic acid by substitution at the 6-amino position in an effort to improve on the instability of benzylpenicillin to gastric acid and penicillinases, to widen its antimicrobial spectrum, and to reduce its rapid rate of renal excretion. Two phenoxypenicillins in which the side-chain is α-phenoxypropionamido (*pheneticillin*) or α-phenoxybutyramido (*propicillin*) are more stable to acid than benzylpenicillin but offer no advantage over phenoxymethylpenicillin.

Meticillin has a 2,6-dimethoxybenzamido group at the 6-position and was the first penicillin found to be resistant to destruction by staphylococcal penicillinase. However, it is not acid-resistant and has to be injected. The isoxazolyl penicillins, *cloxacillin, dicloxacillin, flucloxacillin,* and *oxacillin,* are resistant to penicillinase and gastric acid. They have very similar chemical structures and differ mainly in their absorption characteristics. *Nafcillin* is a similar penicillinase-resistant antibiotic but is irregularly absorbed when taken by mouth.

Ampicillin has a D(−)-α-aminophenylacetamido side-chain and a broader spectrum of activity than benzylpenicillin; although generally less active against Gram-positive bacteria, some Gram-negative organisms including *Escherichia coli, Haemophilus influenzae,* and *Salmonella* spp. are sensitive although resistance is being reported increasingly. *Pseudomonas* spp. are not sensitive. Ampicillin is acid-stable and can be given by mouth but is destroyed by penicillinase. A number of prodrugs including *bacampicillin, metampicillin,* and *pivampicillin* are also said to be better absorbed and are hydrolysed to ampicillin *in vivo. Amoxicillin,* with a D(−)-α-aminohydroxyphenylacetamido side-chain, only differs from ampicillin by the addition of a hydroxyl group, but is better absorbed from the gastrointestinal tract.

Carbenicillin, with an α-carboxyphenylacetamido side-chain, has marked activity against *Pseudomonas aeruginosa* and some *Proteus* spp. but otherwise is generally less active than ampicillin. It has to be given by injection and large doses are required. *Carfecillin* and *carindacillin* are the phenyl and indanyl esters of carbenicillin respectively and are hydrolysed to carbenicillin *in vivo* when taken by mouth. *Sulbenicillin* has an α-phenylsulfoacetamido side-chain and *ticarcillin* an α-carboxythienylacetamido side-chain and both have similar activity to carbenicillin; ticarcillin is more active against *Ps. aeruginosa.* The ureidopenicillins *azlocillin* and *mezlocillin,* and the closely related drug *piperacillin* are more active than carbenicillin against *Ps. aeruginosa* and have a wider range of activity against Gram-negative bacteria.

Temocillin, a 6-α-methoxy derivative of ticarcillin, is resistant to many beta lactamases and is active against most Gram-negative aerobic bacteria, but not *Ps. aeruginosa.*

Mecillinam is a penicillanic acid derivative with a substituted amidino group in the 6-position. Unlike the 6-aminopenicillanic acid derivatives it is active mainly against Gram-negative bacteria, although *Ps. aeruginosa,* and *Bacteroides* spp. are considered resistant. Mecillinam is not active orally and is given by mouth as *pivmecillinam* which is hydrolysed to mecillinam on absorption.

The beta-lactamase inhibitors *clavulanic acid, sulbactam,* and *tazobactam* are used to extend the antimicrobial range of certain beta-lactam antibiotics.

Quinolones

The quinolonecarboxylic acids, carboxyquinolones, or 4-quinolones are a group of synthetic antibacterials structurally related to nalidixic acid. The term 4-quinolone has been used as a generic name for the common 4-oxo-1,4-dihydroquinoline skeleton. Under this system nalidixic acid, a naphthyridine derivative, is an 8-aza-4-quinolone, cinoxacin, a cinnoline derivative, is a 2-aza-4-quinolone, and pipemidic and piromidic acids, pyridopyrimidine derivatives, are 6,8-diaza-4-quinolones.

Nalidixic acid is active against Gram-negative bacteria but has little activity against *Pseudomonas* and Gram-positive organisms. Because bactericidal concentrations

can only be achieved in urine its use has generally been limited to the treatment of urinary-tract infections.

Modification of the structure of nalidixic acid has produced related antibacterials such as *oxolinic acid, cinoxacin,* and *acrosoxacin [rosoxacin].* Although some of these have a greater activity *in vitro* against Gram-negative organisms and activity against some Gram-positive organisms, none has been considered to represent a significant clinical advance over nalidixic acid; acrosoxacin [rosoxacin] is only used in the treatment of gonorrhoea. Addition of a piperazinyl radical at position 7, as in *pipemidic acid,* appears to confer some activity against *Pseudomonas. Flumequine* was the first fluorinated 4-quinolone to be synthesised, but has no piperazinyl group. Addition of the 7-piperazinyl group and a fluorine atom at position 6 has produced a group of fluorinated piperazinyl quinolones or fluoroquinolones with a broader spectrum of activity than nalidixic acid and pharmacokinetic properties more suitable for the treatment of systemic infections. They include *ciprofloxacin, enoxacin, fleroxacin, gatifloxacin, gemifloxacin, levofloxacin, lomefloxacin, moxifloxacin, nadifloxacin, norfloxacin, ofloxacin, pefloxacin, rufloxacin, sparfloxacin,* and *trovafloxacin.* Marketing of trovafloxacin and its prodrug, alatrofloxacin, has been suspended in some countries following reports of unpredictable hepatotoxicity, including some fatalities. *Danofloxacin, enrofloxacin, marbofloxacin, orbifloxacin,* and *sarafloxacin* are used in veterinary practice. Development of *difloxacin* for human use was suspended because of the high incidence of adverse effects, but it is used in veterinary practice. *Temafloxacin* and, more recently, *grepafloxacin* were withdrawn worldwide because of toxicity.

The fluoroquinolones are very active against aerobic Gram-negative bacilli and cocci including the Enterobacteriaceae, *Haemophilus influenzae, Moraxella catarrhalis (Branhamella catarrhalis),* and *Neisseria gonorrhoeae* and are also active against *Pseudomonas aeruginosa.* They are generally less active against Gram-positive organisms such as staphylococci and much less active against streptococci such as *Streptococcus pneumoniae,* although some fluoroquinolones now developed have increased activity against these organisms. They also have activity against mycobacteria, mycoplasmas, rickettsias, and *Plasmodium falciparum.* Some, for example ofloxacin, have useful activity against *Chlamydia trachomatis.* Activity against anaerobic bacteria is generally poor. There is concern that the emergence of resistant strains of organisms may limit the usefulness of fluoroquinolones in future.

One disadvantage of the quinolone antibacterials is that they are generally not recommended for use in children, adolescents, and pregnant and breast feeding women because of their propensity to cause joint erosions in immature *animals.*

Sulfonamides and Diaminopyrimidines

The sulfonamides are analogues of *p*-aminobenzoic acid. The first sulfonamide of clinical importance was *Prontosil,* an azo dye which is metabolised *in vivo* to *sulfanilamide.* It was synthesised in Germany in 1932. Many sulfonamides have since been synthesised; they differ only slightly in their antimicrobial activity, but vary in their pharmacokinetic properties. The sulfonamides have been classified according to their rate of excretion as short-, medium- or intermediate-, long-, and ultra-long-acting. The **short-acting** sulfonamides are excreted in the urine in high concentrations and have therefore been of particular use in the treatment of urinary-tract infections. The solubility in urine of earlier short-acting sulfonamides, such as *sulfapyridine,* and their acetyl metabolites is low and hence crystalluria has been reported

frequently. Of the short-acting sulfonamides most commonly used, *sulfadiazine* also has low solubility in urine whereas *sulfadimidine* and *sulfafurazole* and their acetyl conjugates are very soluble. Three short-acting sulfonamides (triple sulfonamides) have been given together to reduce the risk of crystalluria, as the constituent sulfonamides can co-exist in solution in urine without affecting each other's solubility. Preparations of mixed sulfonamides have, however, generally been replaced by the more soluble sulfonamides. The **medium-acting** sulfonamides such as *sulfamethoxazole,* the **long-acting** sulfonamides such as *sulfadimethoxine, sulfamethoxypyridazine,* and *sulfametoxydiazine,* and the **ultra-long-acting** sulfonamides such as *sulfadoxine* and *sulfametopyrazine* do not attain such high concentrations in the urine and rarely cause crystalluria. Sulfonamides which are slowly excreted from the body do appear, however, to have been more commonly implicated in the development of reactions such as the Stevens-Johnson syndrome.

The sulfonamides are usually bacteriostatic, and interfere with folic acid synthesis of susceptible organisms; their broad spectrum of antimicrobial activity has, however, been limited by the development of resistance. The clinical use of sulfonamides has therefore been greatly reduced; in general they are indicated only in the treatment of urinary-tract infections and a few other disorders such as nocardiosis. Sulfonamides such as *sulfaguanidine, succinylsulfathiazole,* and *phthalylsulfathiazole* are poorly absorbed from the gastrointestinal tract and have been used for the treatment of gastrointestinal infections although they are now rarely indicated. *Sulfadiazine silver* and *mafenide* are applied topically for their antibacterial action in patients with burns. *Sulfasalazine* (p.1251), a conjugate of 5-aminosalicylic acid (mesalazine) and sulfapyridine, is used in the treatment of inflammatory bowel diseases and in rheumatoid arthritis.

Trimethoprim is a diaminopyrimidine which also inhibits folic acid synthesis but at a different stage in the metabolic pathway to that inhibited by the sulfonamides. It has a similar spectrum of antimicrobial activity to sulfonamides and often demonstrates synergy *in vitro* with these drugs. Trimethoprim was initially available only in combination with sulfonamides, most commonly with sulfamethoxazole as co-trimoxazole. It is now used alone particularly in the treatment of infections of the urinary and respiratory tracts. Analogues of trimethoprim include *baquiloprim, brodimoprim, ormetoprim,* and *tetroxoprim.*

Co-trimoxazole generally replaced sulfonamides alone in the treatment of systemic infections, although its use has also been restricted in some countries and trimethoprim may be preferred. Co-trimoxazole is however indicated for *Pneumocystis carinii* pneumonia and nocardiosis and may be useful in protozoal infections such as toxoplasmosis. Other sulfonamides which have been used in combination with trimethoprim include sulfadiazine (see *co-trimazine*), sulfamethoxypyridazine, sulfametopyrazine, sulfametrole, and sulfamoxole (see *co-trifamole*). Sulfadiazine has been used in combination with tetroxoprim (see *co-tetroxazine*).

Sulfonamides have also been used in association with the diaminopyrimidine, pyrimethamine (p.442) in the treatment or prophylaxis of some protozoal infections. Commonly used combinations are sulfadoxine and pyrimethamine for malaria, and sulfadiazine and pyrimethamine for the treatment of toxoplasmosis.

Tetracyclines

The tetracyclines are a group of antibacterials, originally derived from certain *Streptomyces* spp., having the same tetracyclic nucleus, naphthacene, and similar properties. Unlike the penicillins and aminoglycosides they are usually bacteriostatic at the concentrations achieved in the body but act similarly to the aminoglycosides by interfering with protein synthesis in susceptible organisms.

Tetracyclines all have a broad spectrum of activity which includes Gram-positive and Gram-negative bacteria, chlamydias, rickettsias, mycoplasmas, spirochaetes, some mycobacteria, and some protozoa, but the emergence of resistant strains and the development of other antimicrobials has often reduced their value. Adverse effects have also restricted their usefulness. Gastrointestinal disturbances are common and other important toxic effects include deposition in bones and teeth, precluding their use in pregnancy and young children; anti-anabolic effects, especially in patients with renal impairment; fatty changes in the liver; and photosensitivity, especially with demeclocycline. Allergic reactions are relatively uncommon. Because of these adverse effects tetracyclines should be avoided in pregnant women, children, and, apart from doxycycline and minocycline, patients with renal impairment.

The first tetracycline to be introduced was *chlortetracycline* in 1948 and, like chloramphenicol which was discovered at about the same time, it was found to have a broad spectrum of activity and to be active by mouth unlike benzylpenicillin or streptomycin, the only other antibiotics then in use. The discovery of chlortetracycline was followed closely by that of *oxytetracycline* and then *tetracycline*, a reduction product of chlortetracycline which may be produced semisynthetically. All three have very similar properties although chlortetracycline is less well absorbed, and oxytetracycline may cause less staining of teeth. *Demeclocycline*, demethylated chlortetracycline, has a longer half-life than tetracycline. However, phototoxic reactions have been reported most frequently with demeclocycline. It has been used with some success in patients with the syndrome of inappropriate secretion of antidiuretic hormone.

These four tetracyclines are all natural products that have been isolated from *Streptomyces* spp. The more recent tetracyclines, methacycline, doxycycline, and minocycline are semisynthetic derivatives. *Methacycline*, like demeclocycline, has a longer half-life than tetracycline and has been given twice daily. *Doxycycline* and *minocycline* are both more active *in vitro* than tetracycline against many species. More importantly, minocycline is active against some tetracycline-resistant bacteria including strains of staphylococci. Both are well absorbed and, unlike the other tetracyclines, absorption is not significantly affected by the presence of food. They can be given in lower doses than the older members of the group and, having long half-lives, doxycycline is usually given once daily and minocycline twice daily. Also, they do not accumulate significantly in patients with renal impairment and can, therefore, be given to such patients. Both doxycycline and minocycline are more lipid-soluble than the other tetracyclines and they penetrate well into tissues. The use of minocycline may, however, be limited by its vestibular side-effects.

Tetracyclines are not generally the antibacterials of choice in Gram-positive or Gram-negative infections because of the emergence of resistant organisms and the discovery of drugs with narrower antimicrobial spectra. However, they have a place in the treatment of chlamydial infections, rickettsial infections such as typhus and the spotted fevers, mycoplasmal infections such as atypical pneumonia, pelvic inflammatory disease, Lyme disease, brucellosis, tularaemia, plague, cholera, periodontal disease, and acne. The tetracyclines have also been useful in the treatment of penicillin-allergic patients suffering from venereal diseases, anthrax, actinomycosis, bronchitis, and leptospirosis. Minocycline may sometimes be used in multidrug regimens for leprosy.

Described in this chapter are

Miscellaneous Antibacterials

Spectinomycin is an aminocyclitol antibacterial with some similarities to streptomycin although it is not an aminoglycoside. Spectinomycin is active against a wide range of bacteria but its clinical use is restricted to the treatment of chancroid and gonorrhoea. Trospectomycin, a water-soluble derivative, has been investigated.

Mupirocin is an antibacterial produced by *Pseudomonas fluorescens* with activity against most strains of staphylococci and streptococci and also some Gram-negative bacteria. It is applied topically.

Fosfomycin is a derivative of phosphonic acid; it is active against a range of Gram-positive and Gram-negative bacteria and is administered by mouth or parenterally.

The fusidane antibacterial *fusidic acid* is derived from *Fusidium coccineum* and has narrow spectrum of antibacterial activity, but it is very active against *Staphylococcus aureus* and has been used both topically and systemically in the treatment of staphylococcal infections. Resistance develops readily and it is often given in conjunction with other antibacterials.

The polymyxins are basic antibacterials produced by the growth of different strains of *Bacillus polymyxa* (*B. aerosporus*). *Polymyxin B* and *colistin* have been used clinically, but their systemic use has been more or less abandoned because of their toxicity, notably to the kidneys and nervous system. They are not absorbed when taken by mouth and have therefore been given in gastrointestinal infections for their bactericidal activity against Gram-negative bacteria. They continue to be widely used as components of topical preparations.

Bacitracin, gramicidin, and *tyrothricin* are polypeptide antibacterials also produced by certain strains of *Bacillus* spp. but they are active against Gram-positive bacteria. Like the polymyxins, they are toxic when used systemically and are therefore mainly used topically.

The halogenated hydroxyquinoline *clioquinol* has antibacterial, antifungal, and antiprotozoal activity. It was formerly used in gastrointestinal infections including amoebiasis but is of little value and can produce severe neurotoxicity. It is now mainly used locally for superficial infections of the skin and external ear. Topical application to extensive areas of skin can result in significant systemic absorption, especially if an occlusive dressing is used. *Chlorquinaldol* and *halquinol* are used similarly.

Urinary antimicrobials such as *nitrofurantoin*, and also *methenamine* which has generally been given as the hippurate or mandelate, may be used in the treatment and prophylaxis of infections of the lower urinary tract. They are concentrated in the urine, but do not usually achieve antimicrobial concentrations in the blood.

The oxazolidinone *linezolid* has activity against Gram-positive organisms including vancomycin-resistant enterococci and meticillin-resistant *Staphylococcus aureus*. It is used in infections of the skin and respiratory tract due to these organisms.

Described in this chapter are

Choice of Antibacterial

Ideally, antibacterial treatment of infections should be chosen after the infecting organisms have been identified and the results of sensitivity tests are known. In practice, empirical treatment is often necessary initially, bearing in mind local patterns of infection and resistance. Other factors such as site of infection and tissue penetration are also important in deciding which antibacterial to give.

The prophylactic use of antibacterials is restricted mainly to patients undergoing some types of surgery. Other groups requiring infection prophylaxis include patients at special risk of developing endocarditis and those who have had rheumatic fever, who are splenectomised, or who are immunocompromised.

Abscess, abdominal

See under Abscess, Liver and under Peritonitis below.

Abscess, brain

Brain abscesses can result from otitis media, sinusitis, trauma, or dental sepsis, or they may be metastatic secondary to, for example, lung abscesses. Treatment entails removal of pus and administration of high doses of antibacterials. Ideally the choice of antibacterial depends on the infecting organisms and penetration by the antibacterial into brain tissue and abscess pus. Until organisms can be cultured empirical treatment should be given.

The site and origin of the brain abscess is a guide to the likely organisms; infections are often mixed and usually involve anaerobes. A report[1] from the UK noted that benzylpenicillin with metronidazole is appropriate against the *Streptococcus milleri* and anaerobes commonly found in frontal abscesses secondary to paranasal sinusitis; chloramphenicol or ampicillin or, more often, a third-generation cephalosporin with metronidazole and an aminoglycoside are used for temporal lobe and cerebellar abscesses which are often otogenic and may contain enterobacteria (usually *Proteus* spp.) with mixtures of anaerobes; and high-dose flucloxacillin with fusidic acid or rifampicin can be given for abscesses secondary to trauma, in which *Staphylococcus aureus* should be suspected (vancomycin is an alternative if allergy or bacterial resistance is a problem). Maximum doses of beta lactams are advocated to ensure adequate penetration into the brain abscess.

Opportunistic infections in immunocompromised patients may present as brain abscesses.

1. Donald FE. Treatment of brain abscess. *J Antimicrob Chemother* 1990; **25**: 310–12.

Abscess, liver

Bacteria commonly responsible for pyogenic liver abscesses include Enterobacteriaceae, especially *Escherichia coli*; anaerobes, especially *Bacteroides fragilis*; and *Streptococcus milleri* (these can be microaerophilic). As elsewhere in the abdomen (see under Peritonitis, below), infections are often mixed. Treatment involves removal of pus and the administration of high doses of antibacterials. Broad-spectrum empirical therapy should be started immediately; more specific therapy may be possible when the results of cultures following diagnostic percutaneous aspiration of the abscess are known. Antibacterial therapy has been successful without surgical intervention. Gentamicin with clindamycin has been commonly used[1,2] but various combinations of other antibacterials, including cefoxitin, chloramphenicol, carboxypenicillins, third-generation cephalosporins, and metronidazole, might be appropriate.[2] However, intravenous antibacterial treatment without surgical intervention was not consistently successful,[3] although this might have been due to inadequate treatment against enteric anaerobes, especially *B. fragilis*.[2]

For the treatment of amoebic liver abscess, see under Amoebiasis in Antiprotozoals, p.582.

1. Herbert DA, *et al.* Pyogenic liver abscesses: successful non-surgical therapy. *Lancet* 1982; **i**: 134–6.
2. Herbert DA, *et al.* Medical management of pyogenic liver abscesses. *Lancet* 1985; **i**: 1384.
3. McCorkell SJ, Niles NL. Pyogenic liver abscesses: another look at medical management. *Lancet* 1985; **i**: 803–6.

Abscess, lung

Lung abscesses are often secondary to aspiration pneumonia and are discussed under Pneumonia, below. The organisms involved are commonly anaerobic bacteria.

Actinomycosis

Actinomycosis is mainly caused by the oral commensal *Actinomyces israelii*, a Gram-positive anaerobic or microaerophilic bacterium. Other species sometimes responsible include *A. meyeri*, *A. naeslundii*, and *A. viscosus*. One of the commonest forms has been cervicofacial actinomycosis, generally associated with poor oral hygiene and dental procedures.[1] Other forms include abdominal,[2] pulmonary, and disseminated actinomycosis; pelvic actinomycosis is associated with the use of intra-uterine contraceptive devices.

The antibacterial of choice is benzylpenicillin intravenously in high doses for several weeks, followed by oral penicillin (e.g. phenoxymethylpenicillin) for several months.[1,2] Strains relatively resistant to benzylpenicillin have proved sensitive to amoxicillin.[3] Tetracycline is an alternative in patients allergic to penicillin. Other alternatives include erythromycin or clindamycin. In one patient, actinomyces resistant to conventional treatment responded to a prolonged course of ciprofloxacin.[4]

1. Anonymous. Essential drugs: systemic mycoses. *WHO Drug Inf* 1991; **5:** 129–36.
2. Stringer MD, Cameron AEP. Abdominal actinomycosis: a forgotten disease? *Br J Hosp Med* 1987; **38:** 125–7.
3. Martin MV. The use of oral amoxycillin for the treatment of actinomycosis: a clinical and in vitro study. *Br Dent J* 1984; **156:** 252–4.
4. Macfarlane DJ, *et al.* Treatment of recalcitrant actinomycosis with ciprofloxacin. *J Infect* 1993; **27:** 177–80.

Anaerobic bacterial infections

Anaerobic bacteria predominate in the normal microbial flora of man and are a common cause of infections, especially those arising from the gastrointestinal tract, upper respiratory tract, skin, or vagina. Common anaerobic pathogens are *Bacteroides, Prevotella* (formerly non-fragilis *Bacteroides*), *Fusobacterium, Clostridium, Peptostreptococcus,* and *Actinomyces* spp. Apart from single species infections such as tetanus, gas gangrene, pseudomembranous colitis, and actinomycosis, most anaerobic infections are of mixed aetiology. Abscesses are often a feature. Infections include: brain abscess; acute necrotising gingivitis and other periodontal infections; chronic otitis media and chronic sinusitis; aspiration pneumonia and lung abscess; peritonitis and intra-abdominal abscess; bacterial vaginosis and pelvic inflammatory disease; cellulitis, ulcers, bite and other wound infections.[1]

Sensitivity testing *in vitro* is often impractical and treatment for non-species-specific infections is usually empirical.[1-4] Benzylpenicillin was traditionally considered the antibacterial of choice when *B. fragilis* was unlikely (infections above the diaphragm) although resistance is increasingly a problem. Antibacterials with activity against the *B. fragilis* group and other anaerobic pathogens include metronidazole and other 5-nitroimidazole derivatives, chloramphenicol, clindamycin, cefoxitin, antipseudomonal penicillins, imipenem-cilastatin, and combinations of a beta lactam and a beta-lactamase inhibitor.[2]

Surveys of susceptibility patterns in clinical isolates of anaerobic bacteria in the USA[5] and France[6] have shown increasing resistance of the *B. fragilis* group (including *B. distasonis, B. fragilis, B. ovatus, B. thetaiotaomicron,* and *B. vulgatus*) to clindamycin, continuing penicillin resistance in non-fragilis *Bacteroides* spp. (now reclassified as *Prevotella* spp. and including the type species *P. melaninogenica*), and rare beta-lactamase-mediated resistance of *Fusobacterium* to penicillin. Resistance of some *Clostridium* spp. to penicillin and clindamycin had declined, but no changes were noted for *Cl. perfringens*.

The *B. fragilis* group are the most frequently isolated anaerobic bacteria in clinical infections and all members of the group may be pathogenic.[7] Most strains produce beta lactamase and thus are resistant to penicillins and cephalosporins although there is varied susceptibility within the group.[8] In an ongoing USA survey of susceptibility patterns[9] the most active drugs *in vitro* against *B. fragilis* group strains were imipenem, metronidazole, and chloramphenicol; resistance to cefoxitin, clindamycin, and piperacillin was not widespread and combinations of beta-lactamase inhibitors with penicillins or cephalosporins (e.g. ampicillin or cefoperazone with sulbactam; ticarcillin with clavulanate) were also very active. Others have reported similar results.[8] On the basis of activity *in vitro* in another study[10] metronidazole, imipenem, ticarcillin with clavulanate, cefoxitin, and amoxicillin with clavulanate were considered suitable for the treatment of *B. fragilis* group infections. A clinical isolate of *B. fragilis*, simultaneously resistant to metronidazole, amoxicillin with clavulanate, and imipenem, was reported in the UK;[11] treatment with clindamycin was successful on this occasion.

1. Styrt B, Gorbach SL. Recent developments in the understanding of the pathogenesis and treatment of anaerobic infections (first of two parts). *N Engl J Med* 1989; **321:** 240–6.
2. Styrt B, Gorbach SL. Recent developments in the understanding of the pathogenesis and treatment of anaerobic infections (second of two parts). *N Engl J Med* 1989; **321:** 298–302.
3. Finegold SM, Wexler HM. Present status of therapy for anaerobic infections. *Clin Infect Dis* 1996; **23** (suppl 1): S9–S14.
4. Brook I. Anaerobic infections. *Rev Med Microbiol* 1999; **10:** 137–53.

5. Musial CE, Rosenblatt JE. Antimicrobial susceptibilities of anaerobic bacteria isolated at the Mayo Clinic during 1982 through 1987: comparison with results from 1977 through 1981. *Mayo Clin Proc* 1989; **64:** 392–9.
6. Mory F, *et al.* Survey of anaerobic susceptibility patterns: a French multicentre study. *Int J Antimicrob Agents* 1998; **10:** 229–36.
7. Brook I. The clinical importance of all members of the Bacteroides fragilis group. *J Antimicrob Chemother* 1990; **25:** 473–4.
8. Cuchural GJ, *et al.* Comparative activities of newer β-lactam agents against members of the Bacteroides fragilis group. *Antimicrob Agents Chemother* 1990; **34:** 479–80.
9. Cornick NA, *et al.* The antimicrobial susceptibility patterns of the Bacteroides fragilis group in the United States, 1987. *J Antimicrob Chemother* 1990; **25:** 1011–19.
10. Jacobs MR, *et al.* β-Lactamase production, β-lactam sensitivity and resistance to synergy with clavulanate of 737 Bacteroides fragilis group organisms from thirty-three US centres. *J Antimicrob Chemother* 1990; **26:** 361–70.
11. Turner P, *et al.* Simultaneous resistance to metronidazole, co-amoxiclav, and imipenem in clinical isolate of Bacteroides fragilis. *Lancet* 1995; **345:** 1275–7.

Anthrax

Anthrax is a zoonotic disease caused by *Bacillus anthracis*, a spore-forming Gram-positive aerobe.[1] It is rare in western countries. The commonest type is cutaneous anthrax; pulmonary, gastrointestinal, and meningeal anthrax can also occur and in these types the prognosis is poor.

Benzylpenicillin is the antibacterial of choice[2,3] although some resistant strains of *B. anthracis* have been reported. The following treatment regimens have been cited:[2]

- mild uncomplicated cutaneous anthrax: phenoxymethylpenicillin potassium 7.5 mg per kg body-weight by mouth every 6 hours for 5 to 7 days
- more extensive cutaneous disease: procaine penicillin [procaine benzylpenicillin] 10 mg per kg intramuscularly every 12 hours for 5 to 7 days
- pulmonary, gastrointestinal, and meningeal anthrax: immediate treatment with benzylpenicillin by continuous intravenous infusion, 50 mg per kg in the first hour followed by 200 mg per kg every 24 hours.

Once septicaemia has developed a fatal outcome is likely due to toxin release and the use of anthrax antitoxin, if available, in conjunction with antibacterials has been advised.[2] Benzylpenicillin 10 mg per kg intramuscularly every 12 hours for 5 to 7 days has been used prophylactically if contaminated meat has been ingested or if *B. anthracis* has been inadvertently injected beneath the skin. Vaccine is available for active immunisation against anthrax. Combined penicillin and vaccine prophylaxis has been used for pulmonary anthrax prophylaxis.[2]

A tetracycline or erythromycin may be used in patients unable to take penicillin.[3,4] Ciprofloxacin is a further alternative,[3] and may be used[5,6] for initial treatment of clinically evident infection following the use of *B. anthracis* as an agent of biological warfare.

1. Dixon TC, *et al.* Anthrax. *N Engl J Med* 1999; **341:** 815–26.
2. Knudson GB. Treatment of anthrax in man: history and current concepts. *Milit Med* 1986; **151:** 71–7.
3. Anonymous. The choice of antibacterial drugs. *Med Lett Drugs Ther* 1999; **41:** 95–104.
4. Anonymous. Anthrax: memorandum from a WHO meeting. *Bull WHO* 1996; **74:** 465–70.
5. Inglesby TV, *et al.* Anthrax as a biological weapon: medical and public health management. *JAMA* 1999; **281:** 1735–45.
6. PHLS. *Anthrax: provisional PHLS guidelines for action in the event of a deliberate release.* Issue 1/version 2; issued 12/10/01. Available at: http://www.phls.co.uk/advice/anthrax_guidelines.pdf (accessed 16/10/01).

Antibiotic-associated colitis
See under Gastro-enteritis, below.

Arthritis, bacterial
See under Bone and Joint Infections, below.

Bacillary angiomatosis
See under Cat Scratch Disease, below.

Bacterial vaginosis

Bacterial vaginosis (anaerobic vaginosis; non-specific vaginitis) is a common and often distressing vaginal condition associated with a fishy-smelling vaginal discharge and an abnormal vaginal flora. The abnormal flora comprises *Gardnerella vaginalis* and *Bacteroides* and *Mobiluncus* spp.[1] It is not generally considered to be exclusively a sexually transmitted disease. An association has been reported between bacterial vaginosis and premature births of low-weight infants, and some have advised treatment early in the second trimester of pregnancy.[2,3] A systematic review[4] of randomised studies has concluded, however, that the current evidence does not

support screening and treatment of all pregnant women for bacterial vaginosis to prevent premature birth and its consequences, although it may be effective in preventing premature birth in women with a history of a previous premature birth.

Usual treatment is with metronidazole or clindamycin either by mouth or intravaginally;[3,5-7] the duration is usually 5 or 7 days depending on the drug and preparation used although single oral doses of metronidazole have been employed. However, relapse is common after any of these treatment regimens.[2]

1. Blackwell A. Anaerobic vaginosis: therapeutic and epidemiological aspects. *J Antimicrob Chemother* 1984; **14:** 445–8.
2. Hay PE. Therapy of bacterial vaginosis. *J Antimicrob Chemother* 1998; **41:** 6–9.
3. Anonymous. Management of bacterial vaginosis. *Drug Ther Bull* 1998; **36:** 33–5.
4. Brocklehurst P, *et al.* Interventions for treating bacterial vaginosis in pregnancy (updated 27 October 1999). Available in The Cochrane Library; Issue 4. Oxford: Update Software; 2001.
5. WHO. Guidelines for the management of sexually transmitted infections. Geneva: WHO, 2001.
6. Centers for Disease Control. 1998 Guidelines for treatment of sexually transmitted diseases. *MMWR* 1998; **47** (RR-1): 70–4.
7. Clinical Effectiveness Group (Association of Genitourinary Medicine and the Medical Society for the Study of Venereal Diseases). National guideline for the management of bacterial vaginosis. *Sex Transm Infect* 1999; **75** (suppl 1): S16–S18.

Biliary-tract infections

Infections of the biliary tract are usually associated with obstructive and inflammatory conditions such as cholecystitis and cholangitis. Complications can include gangrene, hepatic or intraperitoneal abscesses, peritonitis, and septicaemia. The organisms involved are typically gut flora including Gram-negative aerobes such as *Escherichia coli* and *Klebsiella* spp. and anaerobes including *Bacteroides fragilis*.

Treatment of uncomplicated acute cholecystitis is usually conservative. Antibacterials including cephalosporins, tetracyclines, or broad-spectrum penicillins are commonly given, although some have questioned that use.[1] For more severe infections including suppurative cholangitis, prompt treatment with appropriate antibacterial drugs is necessary. Since biliary obstruction prevents adequate concentrations of many antibacterials being achieved in the bile, the main aim of treatment is to control bacteraemia. Antibacterials used, often in combination, include cephalosporins, aminoglycosides, ampicillin (or amoxicillin), piperacillin, fluoroquinolones, metronidazole, clindamycin, and imipenem.[2-4] In most cases of obstruction, definitive treatment depends on restoring drainage of bile by surgical or medical treatment of gallstones (p.1678).

Antibacterial prophylaxis is commonly employed in biliary surgery (see Surgical Infection, below) to prevent acute cholangitis and wound infections. Cephalosporins are often used for this purpose.[2]

Antibacterials may also have a role as maintenance therapy in recurrent cholangitis.

1. Bouchier IAD. Gallstones. *BMJ* 1990; **300:** 592–7.
2. van den Hazel SJ, *et al.* Role of antibiotics in the treatment and prevention of acute and recurrent cholangitis. *Clin Infect Dis* 1994; **19:** 279–86.
3. Peña C, Gudiol F. Cholecystitis and cholangitis: spectrum of bacteria and role of antibiotics. *Dig Surg* 1996; **13:** 317–20.
4. Westphal J-F, Brogard J-M. Biliary tract infections: a guide to drug treatment. *Drugs* 1999; **57:** 81–91.

Bites and stings

Wound infections following cat or dog bites may be due to a mixture of organisms,[1] often including the Gram-negative aerobe *Pasteurella multocida*. The treatment of choice for *P. multocida* is benzylpenicillin[2] and it should be given for infections evident within 24 hours of a bite;[3] alternatives are amoxicillin-clavulanic acid, ampicillin-sulbactam, or a cephalosporin.[2] Tetracycline is a further alternative in patients allergic to penicillin. The fluoroquinolone ciprofloxacin has been used successfully to treat *P. multocida* cellulitis associated with a cat bite.[4]

In addition to *P. multocida*, other bacteria involved in cat or dog bite wound infections include *Staphylococcus, Streptococcus, Bacteroides,* and *Fusobacterium* spp. and their presence will influence the choice of treatment. For example, a penicillinase-resistant penicillin may be necessary if *Staph. aureus* is present. Also, combinations of antibacterials may be necessary in patients allergic to penicillin since tetracycline, the alternative suggested against *P. multocida* infection, has only limited activity against aerobic Gram-positive cocci.

More unusual organisms include *Capnocytophaga canimorsus* (formerly called dysgonic fermenter type 2 or DF-2) which has been associated in particular with dog bites,[5] but also with cat bites. It is an opportunistic pathogen especially hazardous to immunocompromised patients including splenectomised patients; the best treatment is benzylpenicillin,[6] amoxicillin-clavulanic acid, or erythromycin.[7] Infection with *C. canimorsus* following dog bites may be severe and has led to fatal septicaemia, disseminated intravascular coagulation, meningitis, or endocarditis,[5] highlighting the importance of early antibacterial treatment and debridement.

See also under Cat Scratch Disease (below).

A systematic review[8] has concluded that there is no evidence that the use of prophylactic antibacterials is effective for cat or dog bites, though, if necessary, prophylaxis or treatment for rabies (p.1561) should be instituted.

Among the more unusual infections acquired from animals is seal finger, caused by an as yet unidentified organism and treated with tetracycline.[9] The Gram-negative bacilli *Spirillum minus* (or *minor*) and *Streptobacillus moniliformis* are both causes of rat-bite fever. In each case the treatment of choice is benzylpenicillin;[2] a tetracycline or streptomycin are alternatives.

Envenomation following bites and stings by snakes, scorpions, spiders, and some marine animals is usually treated symptomatically and with specific antivenoms and antisera (see for example Box Jellyfish Sting, p.1546, Scorpion Stings, p.1563, Snake Bites, p.1564, Spider Bites, p.1564, and Stone Fish Venom Antisera, p.1565).

1. Talan DA, *et al.* Bacteriologic analysis of infected dog and cat bites. *N Engl J Med* 1999; **340:** 85–92.
2. Anonymous. The choice of antibacterial drugs. *Med Lett Drugs Ther* 1999; **41:** 95–104.
3. Elliot DL, *et al.* Pet-associated illness. *N Engl J Med* 1985; **313:** 985–95.
4. Richards CAL, Emmanuel FXS. Treatment of Pasteurella multocida cellulitis with ciprofloxacin. *J Infect* 1992; **24:** 216–17.
5. Pers C, *et al.* Capnocytophaga canimorsus septicemia in Denmark, 1982-1995: review of 39 cases. *Clin Infect Dis* 1996; **23:** 71–5.
6. McCarthy M, Zumla A. DF-2 infection. *BMJ* 1988; **297:** 1355–6.
7. Morgan MS, Cruickshank JG. Prevention of postsplenectomy sepsis. *Lancet* 1993; **341:** 700–1.
8. Medeiros I, Saconato H. Antibiotic prophylaxis for mammalian bites (updated 1 March 2001). Available in The Cochrane Library; Issue 4. Oxford: Update Software; 2001.
9. Beck B, Smith TG. Seal finger: an unsolved medical problem in Canada. *Can Med Assoc J* 1976; **115:** 105–9.

Bone and joint infections

In *bacterial arthritis* (septic arthritis) joints may be infected via the blood with a variety of organisms including staphylococci, streptococci, enterococci, Enterobacteriaceae, *Pseudomonas aeruginosa*, and anaerobes although the commonest is probably *Staphylococcus aureus*. *Haemophilus influenzae* is a common cause in young children as is *Neisseria gonorrhoeae* in sexually active young adults. In addition to gonococcal arthritis other specific types of bacterial arthritis include Lyme disease, and meningococcal, salmonellal, and tuberculous arthritis (see under the appropriate disease for further details).

With the exception of *N. gonorrhoeae*, infecting organisms in *osteomyelitis* (infection of bone) are similar to those in bacterial arthritis.[1-11]

In *reactive arthritis* (aseptic arthritis) joint inflammation follows infection elsewhere in the body. It is generally secondary to sexually transmitted infections, especially chlamydial infections, or to enteric infections. Reactive arthritis in association with urethritis or cervicitis, or both, is termed Reiter's syndrome.

Empirical treatment regimens for bacterial arthritis or osteomyelitis usually include antistaphylococcal antibacterials such as flucloxacillin, nafcillin, clindamycin, and fusidic acid; children under 5 years may be given amoxicillin or cefuroxime because of the likelihood of *H. influenzae* infection. Treatment is generally initiated with high doses given intravenously and may need to continue for 6 weeks in acute bacterial arthritis or osteomyelitis. Chronic disease may require longer term treatment although the oral route may be used after initial parenteral therapy.

Oral ciprofloxacin[12,13] or other fluoroquinolones[14,15] have been used successfully in the treatment of osteomyelitis due to susceptible organisms, but the value of fluoroquinolones against Gram-positive bacteria has been questioned and there is increasing resistance to them among meticillin-resistant *Staph. aureus* and coagulase-negative staphylococci.[16]

For reference to infection prophylaxis in orthopaedic patients, see under Surgical Infection, below.

Reactive arthritis is treated with anti-inflammatories; the role of antibacterials is less certain.[17] Results in arthritis associated with chlamydial infections have been more

promising than in that triggered by enteric infections.[18] Long-term treatment with a tetracycline in addition to an NSAID has been reported to shorten the duration of reactive arthritis resulting from *Chlamydia trachomatis* infection.[19]

For mention of the use of tetracyclines, usually minocycline, in the treatment of *rheumatoid arthritis*, see under Rheumatic Disorders, p.261.

1. Goldenberg DL, Reed JI. Bacterial arthritis. *N Engl J Med* 1985; **312:** 764–71.
2. Dickie AS. Current concepts in the management of infections in bones and joints. *Drugs* 1986; **32:** 458–75.
3. Anonymous. Bacterial arthritis. *Lancet* 1986; **ii:** 721–2.
4. Sexton DJ, McDonald M. Osteomyelitis: approaching the 1990s. *Med J Aust* 1990; **153:** 91–6.
5. Dirschl DR, Almekinders LC. Osteomyelitis: common causes and treatment recommendations. *Drugs* 1993; **45:** 29–43.
6. Haas DW, McAndrew MP. Bacterial osteomyelitis in adults: evolving considerations in diagnosis and treatment. *Am J Med* 1996; **101:** 550–61.
7. Hamed KA, *et al.* Pharmacokinetic optimisation of the treatment of septic arthritis. *Clin Pharmacokinet* 1996; **31:** 156–63.
8. Cimmino MA. Recognition and management of bacterial arthritis. *Drugs* 1997; **54:** 50–60.
9. Lew DP, Waldvogel FA. Osteomyelitis. *N Engl J Med* 1997; **336:** 999–1007.
10. Mader JT, *et al.* A practical guide to the diagnosis and management of bone and joint infections. *Drugs* 1997; **54:** 253–64.
11. Goldenberg DL. Septic arthritis. *Lancet* 1998; **351:** 197–202.
12. Gentry LO, Rodriguez GG. Oral ciprofloxacin compared with parenteral antibiotics in the treatment of osteomyelitis. *Antimicrob Agents Chemother* 1990; **34:** 40–3.
13. Dan M, *et al.* Oral ciprofloxacin treatment of Pseudomonas aeruginosa osteomyelitis. *Antimicrob Agents Chemother* 1990; **34:** 849–52.
14. Gentry LO, Rodriguez-Gomez G. Ofloxacin versus parenteral therapy for chronic osteomyelitis. *Antimicrob Agents Chemother* 1991; **35:** 538–41.
15. Greenberg RN, *et al.* Ciprofloxacin, lomefloxacin, or levofloxacin as treatment for chronic osteomyelitis. *Antimicrob Agents Chemother* 2000; **44:** 164–6.
16. Cruciani M, Bassetti D. The fluoroquinolones as treatment for infections caused by Gram-positive bacteria. *J Antimicrob Chemother* 1994; **33:** 403–17.
17. Toivanen A. Bacteria-triggered reactive arthritis: implications for antibacterial treatment. *Drugs* 2001; **61:** 343–51.
18. Svenungsson B. Reactive arthritis. *BMJ* 1994; **308:** 671–2.
19. Lauhio A. Reactive arthritis: consider combination treatment. *BMJ* 1994; **308:** 1302–3.

Botulism

For a discussion of botulism and its management, see p.1534.

Bronchitis

Bronchitis may be defined as inflammation of the bronchi and is associated with excessive sputum production and cough. The bronchi of healthy people are said to be nearly always sterile whereas the upper respiratory tract is often colonised with commensal bacteria including *Streptococcus pneumoniae* and *Haemophilus influenzae*.

Acute bronchitis in previously healthy subjects is commonly associated with viral respiratory infections such as colds and influenza. There may sometimes be secondary bacterial infection that responds to antibacterial therapy as for acute exacerbations of chronic bronchitis (see below). *Acute bronchiolitis* occurs in infants as a result mainly of viral infection and antibacterials are not given routinely (see Respiratory Syncytial Virus Infection, p.612).

Chronic bronchitis and emphysema often occur together and have been termed chronic obstructive pulmonary disease (chronic obstructive airways disease—p.759). Acute exacerbations of chronic bronchitis may be viral in origin, but bacteria are often present in purulent sputum, the commonest being *Str. pneumoniae* and *H. influenzae*; *Moraxella catarrhalis* (*Branhamella catarrhalis*) is increasingly reported.

The value of antibacterial treatment in both acute bronchitis and acute exacerbation of chronic disease has been controversial and difficult to assess.[1-5] Following a comparison of broad-spectrum antibacterial (amoxicillin, co-trimoxazole, or doxycycline) with placebo,[6] it was considered that antibacterials were justified in exacerbations of chronic obstructive pulmonary disease characterised by increased dyspnoea, sputum production, and sputum purulence. Also, a meta-analysis of randomised studies indicated a small improvement due to therapy in patients with exacerbations of disease.[7] However, a further meta-analysis[8] assessing the use of antibacterials for acute bronchitis concluded that, although there was some benefit to be obtained this did not outweigh the risks of adverse effects and increased resistance and that the use of antibacterials could therefore not be advocated in otherwise healthy patients with no evidence of chronic disease. A systematic review[9] also concluded that the modest benefit associated with antibacterial use in acute disease was of similar magnitude to the detriment from

potential adverse effects. If antibacterials are given it is common practice to give a 7- to 10-day oral course of a broad-spectrum drug such as amoxicillin with or without clavulanic acid, ampicillin, an oral cephalosporin such as cefaclor or cefuroxime axetil, co-trimoxazole, erythromycin or a newer macrolide such as azithromycin or clarithromycin, tetracycline, or trimethoprim (preferred to co-trimoxazole in the UK), the choice depending on local patterns of resistance. Long-term prophylaxis in patients with frequent exacerbations is controversial.

Bronchitis associated with *Chlamydia pneumoniae* (formerly TWAR strain of *C. psittaci*) and responding to tetracycline or erythromycin has also been reported.[10]

1. Gonzales R, Sande M. What will it take to stop physicians from prescribing antibiotics in acute bronchitis? *Lancet* 1995; **345:** 665–6.
2. Hahn DL. Antibiotics in acute bronchitis. *Lancet* 1995; **345:** 1244–5.
3. Anonymous. Antibiotics for exacerbations of chronic bronchitis? *Lancet* 1987; **ii:** 23–4.
4. Staley H, *et al.* Is an objective assessment of antibiotic therapy in exacerbations of chronic bronchitis possible? *J Antimicrob Chemother* 1993; **31:** 193–7.
5. O'Brien KL, *et al.* Cough illness/bronchitis—principles of judicious use of antimicrobial agents. *Pediatrics* 1998; **101** (suppl): 178–81.
6. Anthonisen NR, *et al.* Antibiotic therapy in exacerbations of chronic obstructive pulmonary disease. *Ann Intern Med* 1987; **106:** 196–204.
7. Saint S, *et al.* Antibiotics in chronic obstructive pulmonary disease exacerbations: a meta-analysis. *JAMA* 1995; **273:** 957–60.
8. Bent S, *et al.* Antibiotics in acute bronchitis: a meta-analysis. *Am J Med* 1999; **107:** 62–7.
9. Smucny J, *et al.* Antibiotics for acute bronchitis (updated 18 July 2001). Available in The Cochrane Library; Issue 4. Oxford: Update Software; 2001.
10. Grayston JT, *et al.* A new respiratory tract pathogen: Chlamydia pneumoniae strain TWAR. *J Infect Dis* 1990; **161:** 618–25.

Brucellosis

Brucellosis (formerly known as undulant fever) is caused by *Brucella* spp., aerobic Gram-negative bacteria found primarily in animals and transmitted to humans. The principal species affecting man are *Brucella abortus*, from cattle; *B. melitensis*, from sheep, goats, camels, and sometimes cattle; and *B. suis* from pigs. Brucellosis has often been associated with consumption of unpasteurised milk or its products and although rare or controlled in countries such as the UK it remains a problem in many areas, including the Mediterranean region and Middle East. Rarely, human infection can result from exposure to live veterinary vaccines.[1]

Treatment of brucellosis has been with rifampicin plus doxycycline, but some now prefer doxycycline plus streptomycin. The regimen recommended by WHO is rifampicin 600 to 900 mg with doxycycline 200 mg, both given daily in the morning as a single dose for at least 6 weeks.[2] Administration of doxycycline and rifampicin for 30 days was found by some workers[3] to result in higher relapse rates than those for the regimen of tetracycline and streptomycin previously recommended by WHO. However, in a multinational comparative study of 143 patients with acute brucellosis,[4] a 45-day regimen of rifampicin and doxycycline was comparable with a regimen of doxycycline 200 mg daily with a meal for 45 days and streptomycin 1 g intramuscularly daily for 21 days; a third regimen of tetracycline 500 mg 4 times daily for 21 days and streptomycin 1 g intramuscularly daily for 14 days was associated with a 41% failure rate and could not be recommended. Doxycycline for 6 weeks and streptomycin for the first 2 weeks also proved effective in a Spanish study,[5] and was considered preferable to doxycycline and rifampicin. An overview of studies also indicated that doxycycline plus streptomycin was associated with lower relapse rates than rifampicin plus doxycycline, and the former was recommended as the preferred combination.[6] An interaction between rifampicin and doxycycline, in which concentrations of doxycycline were reduced when the two were given together,[7] might explain the reduced efficacy of this combination. A suggested regimen in non-pregnant adults is thus doxycycline 200 mg daily for 6 weeks together with streptomycin 1 g daily for 2 to 3 weeks.[8]

Resistance to rifampicin has emerged following therapy despite administration with doxycycline.[9]

Thus, although treatment usually uses combinations of drugs, co-trimoxazole has been used alone but relapse was common.[2]

Rifampicin with co-trimoxazole was effective in the treatment of **children**,[10] although the authors of a multicentre study in Kuwaiti children[11] considered that rifampicin should be reserved for complicated brucellosis because of the risk of serious adverse effects and development of resistance in areas endemic for tuberculosis.

They recommended oxytetracycline or doxycycline for 3 weeks with gentamicin intramuscularly for the first 5 days in children over 8 years old, co-trimoxazole being given instead of a tetracycline in younger children.

For the treatment of brucellosis during **pregnancy**, WHO recommends rifampicin as the drug of choice and that co-trimoxazole or tetracycline should only be given if rifampicin is unavailable; streptomycin is contra-indicated.[2]

In the treatment of **neurobrucellosis**, the length of therapy appears to be of critical importance; relapses may occur after treatment lasting only 2 to 3 weeks and a regimen of tetracycline 2 g daily and rifampicin 600 to 900 mg daily given for 8 to 12 weeks supplemented with streptomycin 1 g daily for 6 weeks has consequently been recommended by some.[12] There have also been reports of the successful use of similar triple therapy in the treatment of endocarditis due to *Brucella melitensis*.[13]

A vaccine is available in some countries for active immunisation of individuals at high risk of contracting brucellosis.

1. Blasco JM, Díaz R. Brucella melitensis Rev-1 vaccine as a cause of human brucellosis. *Lancet* 1993; **342**: 805.
2. FAO/WHO. Joint FAO/WHO expert committee on brucellosis: sixth report. *WHO Tech Rep Ser 740* 1986.
3. Ariza J, *et al.* Comparative trial of rifampin-doxycycline versus tetracycline-streptomycin in the therapy of human brucellosis. *Antimicrob Agents Chemother* 1985; **28**: 548–51.
4. Acocella G, *et al.* Comparison of three different regimens in the treatment of acute brucellosis: a multicenter multinational study. *J Antimicrob Chemother* 1989; **23**: 433–9. Correction *ibid.*; **24**: 629.
5. Cisneros JM, *et al.* Multicenter prospective study of treatment of Brucella melitensis brucellosis with doxycycline for 6 weeks plus streptomycin for 2 weeks. *Antimicrob Agents Chemother* 1990; **34**: 881–3.
6. Solera J, *et al.* Recognition and optimum treatment of brucellosis. *Drugs* 1997; **53**: 245–56.
7. Colmenero JD, *et al.* Possible implications of doxycycline-rifampin interaction for treatment of brucellosis. *Antimicrob Agents Chemother* 1994; **38**: 2798–2802.
8. Friedland JS. Brucellosis. *Prescribers' J* 1993; **33**: 24–8.
9. De Rautlin de la Roy YM, *et al.* Rifampicin resistance in a strain of Brucella melitensis after treatment with doxycycline and rifampicin. *J Antimicrob Chemother* 1986; **18**: 648–9.
10. Llorens-Terol J, Busquets RM. Brucellosis treated with rifampicin. *Arch Dis Child* 1980; **55**: 486–8.
11. Lubani MM, *et al.* A multicenter therapeutic study of 1100 children with brucellosis. *Pediatr Infect Dis* 1989; **8**: 75–8.
12. Shakir RA. Neurobrucellosis. *Postgrad Med J* 1986; **62**: 1077–9.
13. Farid Z, Trabolsi B. Successful treatment of two cases of brucella endocarditis with rifampicin. *BMJ* 1985; **291**: 110.

Campylobacter enteritis
See under Gastro-enteritis, below.

Cat scratch disease
Cat scratch disease usually occurs after a cat scratch or bite. The condition is characterised by regional lymphadenopathy and is often self-limiting, but may be disseminated in immunocompromised patients.

In the 1980s a Gram-negative bacillus presumed to be responsible for cat scratch disease was isolated[1,2] and subsequently named *Afipia felis*.[3] However, it now appears that *Bartonella henselae* (formerly *Rochalimaea henselae*) is the main cause of cat scratch disease[3-5] and that *A. felis* causes few, if any, cases, although there is some evidence that both organisms might have a joint role.[6] With uncertainty over aetiology there has been no specific antibacterial therapy, but there are reports of successful treatment with gentamicin[7] or co-trimoxazole[8] in children and with ciprofloxacin[9] in adults. Bacillary angiomatosis, in which both *B. henselae* and *B. quintana*[10] (the causative organism of trench fever) have been implicated, may represent a disseminated form of cat scratch disease occurring predominantly in HIV-infected patients. However, in contrast to the response seen in cat scratch disease, the disseminated disease in immunocompromised patients has not responded to ciprofloxacin,[11,12] but has responded to treatment with doxycycline[11-14] or erythromycin.[11] Care is required in patients with AIDS since the lesions of bacillary angiomatosis closely resemble those of Kaposi's sarcoma, and if the diagnosis is missed life-saving antibacterial therapy may not be given.[15]

1. Wear DJ, *et al.* Cat scratch disease: a bacterial infection. *Science* 1983; **221**: 1403–5.
2. English CK, *et al.* Cat-scratch disease: isolation and culture of the bacterial agent. *JAMA* 1988; **259**: 1347–52.
3. Birtles RJ, *et al.* Cat scratch disease and bacillary angiomatosis: aetiological agents and the link with AIDS. *Commun Dis Rep* 1993; **3**: R107–R110.
4. Relman DA, *et al.* The agent of bacillary angiomatosis: an approach to the identification of uncultured pathogens. *N Engl J Med* 1990; **323**: 1573–80.
5. Flexman JP, *et al.* Bartonella henselae is a causative agent of cat scratch disease in Australia. *J Infect* 1995; **31**: 241–5.
6. Alkan S, *et al.* Dual role for Afipia felis and Rochalimaea henselae in cat-scratch disease. *Lancet* 1995; **345**: 385.
7. Bogue CW, *et al.* Antibiotic therapy for cat-scratch disease? *JAMA* 1989; **262**: 813–16.
8. Collipp PJ. Cat-scratch disease therapy. *Am J Dis Child* 1989; **143**: 1261.
9. Holley HP. Successful treatment of cat-scratch disease with ciprofloxacin. *JAMA* 1991; **265**: 1563–5.
10. Koehler JE, *et al.* Isolation of Rochalimaea species from cutaneous and osseous lesions of bacillary angiomatosis. *N Engl J Med* 1992; **327**: 1625–31.
11. Tappero JW, Koehler JE. Cat-scratch disease and bacillary angiomatosis. *JAMA* 1991; **266**: 1938–9.
12. Tucker RM, *et al.* Cat-scratch disease and bacillary angiomatosis. *JAMA* 1991; **266**: 1939.
13. Kemper CA, *et al.* Visceral bacillary epithelioid angiomatosis: possible manifestations of disseminated cat scratch disease in the immunocompromised host: a report of two cases. *Am J Med* 1990; **89**: 216–22.
14. Mui BSK, *et al.* Response of HIV-associated disseminated cat scratch disease to treatment with doxycycline. *Am J Med* 1990; **89**: 229–31.
15. Taylor AG, *et al.* Cat-scratch, Kaposi's sarcoma, and bacillary angiomatosis. *Lancet* 1993; **342**: 686.

Cellulitis
See under Skin Infections, below.

Cervicitis
Gonorrhoea in women occurs predominantly as cervicitis, but mucopurulent cervicitis is frequently caused by sexually transmitted *Chlamydia trachomatis*. The two infections often occur together and should be treated concurrently. Guidelines for treatment are given under Gonorrhoea, and Chlamydial Infections, below.

Chancroid
Chancroid is a sexually transmitted disease caused by the Gram-negative bacterium *Haemophilus ducreyi*. It occurs worldwide, but is endemic in parts of Africa and South East Asia where it is a frequent cause of genital ulceration and a risk factor in the transmission of HIV. Chancroid has also become an important sexually transmitted disease in the USA.[1]

The treatment of choice for chancroid in most endemic areas has been a multidose course of erythromycin or co-trimoxazole[2] although single-dose treatment regimens might be preferable if compliance is a problem. Treatment failure may be more common in patients also infected with HIV, especially with single-dose regimens.[1] Specific regimens have been provided in the UK,[3] the USA,[1] and by WHO.[4] Recommendations in both the UK and the USA are for either erythromycin 500 mg four times daily by mouth for 7 days; or a single intramuscular injection of ceftriaxone 250 mg; or a single oral dose of azithromycin 1 g; or ciprofloxacin 500 mg twice daily by mouth for 3 days. Alternatives listed in the UK guideline[3] are single oral doses of other fluoroquinolones such as fleroxacin 400 mg or norfloxacin 800 mg or a single intramuscular injection of spectinomycin 2 g. WHO has recommended[4] ciprofloxacin 500 mg twice daily by mouth for 3 days, or erythromycin 500 mg four times daily by mouth for 7 days, or azithromycin 1 g as a single oral dose; an alternative is a single intramuscular injection of ceftriaxone 250 mg. Co-trimoxazole 960 mg twice daily by mouth for 7 days has also been used in some countries. High failure rates with ceftriaxone[5] may limit its usefulness.

Sexual partners of patients with chancroid should also be treated.

1. Centers for Disease Control. 1998 Guidelines for treatment of sexually transmitted diseases. *MMWR* 1998; **47** (RR-1): 18–20.
2. Dangor Y, *et al.* Treatment of chancroid. *Antimicrob Agents Chemother* 1990; **34**: 1308–11.
3. Clinical Effectiveness Group (Association of Genitourinary Medicine and the Medical Society for the Study of Venereal Diseases). National guideline for the management of chancroid. *Sex Transm Infect* 1999; **75** (suppl 1): S43–S45.
4. WHO. Guidelines for the management of sexually transmitted infections. Geneva: WHO, 2001.
5. Tyndall M, *et al.* Ceftriaxone no longer predictably cures chancroid in Kenya. *J Infect Dis* 1993; **167**: 469–71.

Chlamydial infections
The species *Chlamydia pneumoniae*, *C. psittaci*, and *C. trachomatis* are all pathogens in man and are generally sensitive to tetracyclines or erythromycin. *C. pneumoniae* (formerly TWAR strain of *C. psittaci*) is a respiratory pathogen. It was first described as a cause of community-acquired pneumonia (see Pneumonia, below), but has since been associated with a wide variety of clinical presentations including pharyngitis (see below) and has been implicated in the pathogenesis of ischaemic heart disease (see Atherosclerosis, p.793). *C. psittaci* is transmitted to man from birds and causes psittacosis which also affects the lungs (see Psittacosis, below).

C. trachomatis causes a wide range of diseases. Many are sexually transmitted and the spectrum is similar to that with *Neisseria gonorrhoeae* (see Gonorrhoea, below); infections with the two organisms often occur concurrently. Pregnant women infected with *C. trachomatis* may be at risk of premature rupture of membranes and preterm labour (see Premature Labour, below). They may also infect their offspring to cause ophthalmia neonatorum (see Neonatal Conjunctivitis, below) or pneumonia (below).

Guidelines for the treatment of uncomplicated urethral, endocervical, or rectal infections with *C. trachomatis* from WHO[1] recommend a 7-day oral course of doxycycline or a single dose of azithromycin; alternatives are amoxicillin, erythromycin, ofloxacin, or tetracycline. UK guidelines[2] recommend a 7-day course of doxycycline or a single dose of azithromycin; alternatives include erythromycin, other tetracyclines, or ofloxacin. The Centers for Disease Control in the USA[3] also recommend either doxycycline for 7 days or a single oral dose of azithromycin; alternatives are ofloxacin or erythromycin. Sexual partners of those infected with *C. trachomatis* should be tested and treated.[1-3] Pregnant women should be given erythromycin or amoxicillin[1-3] to eradicate *C. trachomatis* infection and prevent perinatal transmission. Azithromycin[3] or clindamycin[4] are further alternatives.

For further reference to sexually transmitted *C. trachomatis* infections, see under Epididymitis, Pelvic Inflammatory Disease, and Urethritis, below.

Specific serotypes of *C. trachomatis* are responsible for another sexually transmitted disease, lymphogranuloma venereum (see Lymphogranuloma Venereum, below).

Reactive arthritis (see Bone and Joint Infections, above) may be secondary to chlamydial infections.

Other *C. trachomatis* infections that are not sexually transmitted include trachoma and inclusion conjunctivitis in adults (see Trachoma, below).

1. WHO. Guidelines for the management of sexually transmitted infections. Geneva: WHO, 2001.
2. Clinical Effectiveness Group (Association of Genitourinary Medicine and the Medical Society for the Study of Venereal Diseases). National guideline for the management of Chlamydia trachomatis genital tract infection. *Sex Transm Infect* 1999; **75** (suppl 1): S4–S8.
3. Centers for Disease Control. 1998 Guidelines for treatment of sexually transmitted diseases. *MMWR* 1998; **47** (RR-1): 53–9.
4. Brocklehurst P, Rooney G. Interventions for treating genital chlamydia trachomatis infection in pregnancy (updated 25 October 1999). Available in The Cochrane Library; Issue 4. Oxford: Update Software; 2001.

Cholera and other vibrio infections
See under Gastro-enteritis, below.

Cystic fibrosis
Cystic fibrosis is a genetic disorder associated with the production of abnormally viscous mucus. The underlying defect is mutation in the gene which codes for cystic fibrosis transmembrane conductance regulator (CFTR), a protein which functions as a chloride channel. Mutations result in defective ion transport with reduced chloride ion secretion and accelerated sodium ion absorption, and related changes in the composition and properties of mucin secreted. Now that patients with cystic fibrosis usually survive into adulthood, it is increasingly seen to be a multisystem disease. However, the main clinical manifestations are still pulmonary disease, with recurrent bacterial infections and the production of copious viscous sputum, and malabsorption due to pancreatic insufficiency. Other complications include male infertility and hepatobiliary disease. There is increased salt loss in sweat.

Various diagnostic methods are available[1-3] and clinical diagnosis of cystic fibrosis may be confirmed by establishing that chloride concentrations in sweat are raised, using the pilocarpine sweat test (see Pilocarpine, p.1423, and for further details, see *Martindale*, 29th ed. p.1335). Nowadays identification of gene mutation is possible and may be used for further confirmation of the diagnosis and identification of carrier status.[4]

The reduced morbidity in patients with cystic fibrosis and improved survival are largely due to the management of pulmonary disease with antibacterials and physiotherapy and to nutritional management. Several reviews have discussed both established and experimental therapy.[5-7]

Pulmonary disease is the major cause of mortality. Cystic fibrosis is an underlying cause of bronchiectasis (chronic dilatation of the bronchi) as a result of excessive secretion of mucus and recurrent infections. Cough and excessive production of sputum are characteristic of cystic fibrosis and the lungs are generally colonised with bacterial pathogens, especially mucoid strains of *Pseudomonas aeruginosa*. Pseudomonal pulmonary infection is the major cause of morbidity and mortality in cystic fibrosis. Monitoring of bacterial pathogens in the sputum, including their sensitivity, is necessary for rational treatment. Apart from *Ps. aeruginosa*, *Staphylococcus aureus* is often present and may be the predominant pathogen in infants. *Burkholderia cepacia* (formerly *Pseudomonas cepacia*) has been recognised as a cause of serious lung infection in cystic fibrosis. In a proportion who acquire it, *B. cepacia* has been associated with rapid deterioration and death.[8] Other bacteria isolated include *Haemophilus influenzae* and atypical *Mycobacteria* spp.

The approach to managing lung infections varies and the development of a consensus view has been hampered by the lack of clinical trials of sufficient power. Staphylococcal infections commonly develop during the first decade of life, and some clinicians start antistaphylococcal antibacterials on diagnosis of cystic fibrosis. Others wait until the first clinical infection occurs before starting treatment. Once started, antistaphylococcal therapy is continued indefinitely in some centres, while others only treat when symptomatic exacerbations or positive sputum cultures occur. Systematic reviews confirmed that antistaphylococcal treatment is effective and also concluded that prophylaxis is likely to be beneficial in young children with cystic fibrosis.[9,10] There was, however, insufficient evidence to determine whether intermittent or continuous therapy produces the best clinical outcome. In an accompanying editorial, concerns were expressed about the basis for even these conclusions.[11] Other potential disadvantages to prophylaxis are the possible early acquisition of *P. aeruginosa* infection and an increased incidence of drug-resistant staphylococci with continuous therapy.[11]

Once present, eradication of *Ps. aeruginosa* is difficult and not permanent. Acute exacerbations of pulmonary infection are treated with antipseudomonal antibacterials administered intravenously, usually an aminoglycoside (e.g. tobramycin) with a penicillin (e.g. ticarcillin) or a third-generation cephalosporin (e.g. ceftazidime); monotherapy, usually with ceftazidime, has also been given, but has been implicated in the emergence of resistant organisms.[12] High doses are necessary because of the poor penetration of these antipseudomonal antibacterials into the site of infection and their increased renal clearance in patients with cystic fibrosis.[13,14]

There is no consensus over the best strategy for managing chronic infection.[12] Some treat acute exacerbations as they occur whereas others give regular intermittent courses of intravenous antipseudomonal antibacterials. In one study,[15] chronic colonisation was prevented by giving ciprofloxacin and inhalations of colistin for 3 weeks whenever *Ps. aeruginosa* was isolated from routine sputum cultures. Intermittent elective intravenous therapy has become more practical with the development of regimens that enable patients to be treated at home.[12,16] Inhaled antibacterials including gentamicin with carbenicillin,[17] tobramycin alone[18] and with ticarcillin,[19] or colistin[20] have become increasingly popular.[21,22] In particular, studies have shown that nebulised tobramycin administered twice daily every alternate month produces clinical benefits[23] and is not associated with increased resistance or bacterial superinfections.[24] Active immunisation with a *Pseudomonas aeruginosa* vaccine or passive immunisation with antibodies against *Ps. aeruginosa* are under investigation.

Infection with *B. cepacia* is difficult to treat because the majority of antipseudomonal antibacterials are not effective. Co-trimoxazole has been suggested for *B. cepacia* infections[25] and temocillin has shown promise.[26] Results of a pilot study indicating that nebulised taurolidine could be beneficial have not been supported by a double-blind placebo-controlled crossover clinical trial.[27] Transmission of *B. cepacia* in cystic fibrosis patients appears to be mainly by social contact,[28,29] although some have reported otherwise.[30]

The effects of cystic fibrosis in the lungs are complex and treatment of infections may not halt the progression of lung destruction. Many other interventions have been tried.[31,32] Dornase alfa[33] is administered by aerosol inhalation and reduces the viscosity of the sputum by breaking down the large quantities of DNA released by degenerating inflammatory cells. The use of dornase alfa has been associated with some improvement in lung function and it might be a useful adjunct to bronchial drainage, although it is unclear whether it prevents the development of progressive lung damage (see p.1089). Mucolyt-

ics such as acetylcysteine are generally not considered to be effective in cystic fibrosis.[34,35]

Bronchodilators including both beta agonists and antimuscarinics may be useful in selected patients although there are few meaningful clinical trial results.[31,32] A therapeutic trial is often justified in individual patients since it is difficult to predict which patients will respond.[31] While administration by nebuliser is regarded as most effective, inhalers may be more practical but compatibility with other nebulised drugs could be a problem.[32]

Other interventions tried with some evidence of benefit include management of the inflammatory response in the lungs with corticosteroids[36] (by mouth[37] or more usually by inhalation,[31] although a systematic review[38] of randomised studies concluded that there was insufficient evidence to establish whether there was a beneficial or harmful effect of inhaled corticosteroids in cystic fibrosis patients), or with the NSAID ibuprofen.[39] Alpha$_1$-proteinase inhibitor, the main inhibitor of neutrophil elastase in the lung has also been investigated[40] as has oxpentifylline [pentoxifylline],[41] a drug with anticytokine activity.

Experimental treatment aimed at modifying the pulmonary disease process includes ion transport therapy involving the administration of aerosolised drugs which either inhibit sodium ion absorption across airway epithelia, for example the sodium channel blocker amiloride,[42] or induce chloride ion secretion, for example the triphosphate nucleotides adenosine triphosphate (ATP) and uridine triphosphate (UTP). However, nebulised amiloride was not found to be a useful adjunct in patients on optimal treatment.[43,44]

In patients with severe lung disease, oxygen therapy may give some relief of symptoms but its effect on mortality and morbidity is uncertain.[45,46] At present the only available treatment for patients with end stage pulmonary disease is lung transplantation.

Nutritional management of cystic fibrosis should ensure adequate calorie intake from a balanced diet in order to counteract malabsorption due to pancreatic insufficiency and the increased metabolic requirements of patients with cystic fibrosis.[47,48] Supplements of the fat-soluble vitamins A, D, and E, and sometimes vitamin K may be necessary. Investigation of bone mineral density[49] and direct assessment of vitamin status[50] suggest that current supplements may be inadequate. Pancreatic enzymes, as pancreatin or pancrelipase, are taken before or with each meal or snack.

Beneficial responses to ranitidine have been reported in some children with cystic fibrosis.

Somatic **gene therapy** represents the nearest approach to a cure for cystic fibrosis.[51] It aims to introduce the normal CFTR gene sequence into cells of affected tissue. Most effort has been directed at gene delivery to the lungs using adenovirus vectors or liposomes, but results have been variable.[52-54] Difficulties encountered include inefficient gene transfer, immunity to viral vectors, and a systemic inflammatory reaction provoked by plasmid DNA.[4] For a discussion of the general principles of gene therapy, see p.1614.

1. Stern RC. The diagnosis of cystic fibrosis. *N Engl J Med* 1997; **336:** 487–91.
2. Wallis C. Diagnosing cystic fibrosis: blood, sweat, and tears. *Arch Dis Child* 1997; **76:** 85–91.
3. Rosenstein BJ, *et al.* The diagnosis of cystic fibrosis: a consensus statement. *J Pediatr* 1998; **132:** 589–95.
4. Geddes DM, Alton EWFW. The CF gene: 10 years on. *Thorax* 1999; **54:** 1052–3.
5. Ramsey BW. Management of pulmonary disease in patients with cystic fibrosis. *N Engl J Med* 1996; **335:** 179–88.
6. Rosenstein BJ, Zeitlin PL. Cystic fibrosis. *Lancet* 1998; **351:** 277–82.
7. Bilton D, Mahadeva R. New treatments in adult cystic fibrosis. *J R Soc Med* 1997; **90** (suppl 31): 2–5.
8. Walters S, Smith EG. Pseudomonas cepacia in cystic fibrosis: transmissibility and its implications. *Lancet* 1993; **342:** 3–4.
9. McCaffery K, *et al.* Systematic review of antistaphylococcal antibiotic therapy in cystic fibrosis. *Thorax* 1999; **54:** 380–3.
10. Smyth A, Walters S. Prophylactic antibiotics for cystic fibrosis (updated 30 May 2001). Available in The Cochrane Library; Issue 4. Oxford: Update Software; 2001.
11. Elborn JS. Treatment of Staphylococcus aureus in cystic fibrosis. *Thorax* 1999; **54:** 377–8.
12. Denton M, Wilcox MH. Antimicrobial treatment of pulmonary colonization and infection by Pseudomonas aeruginosa in cystic fibrosis patients. *J Antimicrob Chemother* 1997; **40:** 468–74.
13. Rey E, *et al.* Drug disposition in cystic fibrosis. *Clin Pharmacokinet* 1998; **35:** 313–29.
14. Touw DJ, *et al.* Pharmacokinetic optimisation of antibacterial treatment in patients with cystic fibrosis: current practice and suggestions for future directions. *Clin Pharmacokinet* 1998; **35:** 437–59.
15. Valerius NH, *et al.* Prevention of chronic Pseudomonas aeruginosa colonisation in cystic fibrosis by early treatment. *Lancet* 1991; **338:** 725–6.
16. Gilbert J, *et al.* Home intravenous antibiotic treatment in cystic fibrosis. *Arch Dis Child* 1988; **63:** 512–17.
17. Hodson ME, *et al.* Aerosol carbenicillin and gentamicin treatment of Pseudomonas aeruginosa infection in patients with cystic fibrosis. *Lancet* 1981; **ii:** 1137–9.
18. Ramsey BW, *et al.* Efficacy of aerosolized tobramycin in patients with cystic fibrosis. *N Engl J Med* 1993; **328:** 1740–6.
19. Wall MA, *et al.* Inhaled antibiotics in cystic fibrosis. *Lancet* 1983; **i:** 1325.
20. Jensen T, *et al.* Colistin inhalation therapy in cystic fibrosis patients with chronic Pseudomonas aeruginosa lung infection. *J Antimicrob Chemother* 1987; **19:** 831–8.
21. Conway SP. Evidence for using nebulised antibiotics in cystic fibrosis. *Arch Dis Child* 1999; **80:** 307–9.
22. Campbell PW, Saiman L. Use of aerosolized antibiotics in patients with cystic fibrosis. *Chest* 1999; **116:** 775–88.
23. Ramsey BW, *et al.* Intermittent administration of inhaled tobramycin in patients with cystic fibrosis. *N Engl J Med* 1999; **340:** 23–30.
24. Burns JL, *et al.* Effect of chronic intermittent administration of inhaled tobramycin on respiratory microbial flora in patients with cystic fibrosis. *J Infect Dis* 1999; **179:** 1190–6.
25. Anonymous. The choice of antibacterial drugs. *Med Lett Drugs Ther* 1999; **41:** 95–104.
26. Taylor RFH, *et al.* Temocillin and cystic fibrosis: outcome of intravenous administration in patients infected with Pseudomonas cepacia. *J Antimicrob Chemother* 1992; **29:** 341–4.
27. Ledson MJ, *et al.* Nebulised taurolidine and B cepacia bronchiectasis. *Thorax* 2000; **55:** 91–2.
28. Govan JRW, *et al.* Evidence for transmission of Pseudomonas cepacia by social contact in cystic fibrosis. *Lancet* 1993; **342:** 15–19.
29. Mahenthiralingam E, *et al.* Burkholderia cepacia in cystic fibrosis. *N Engl J Med* 1995; **332:** 819.
30. Steinbach S, *et al.* Transmissibility of Pseudomonas cepacia infection in clinic patients and lung-transplant recipients with cystic fibrosis. *N Engl J Med* 1994; **331:** 981–7.
31. Conway SP, Watson A. Nebulised bronchodilators, corticosteroids, and rhDNase in adult patients with cystic fibrosis. *Thorax* 1997; **52** (suppl 2): S64–8.
32. Spencer DA. Nebulised bronchodilators, antibiotics and rhDNase for children with cystic fibrosis. *Thorax* 1997; **52** (suppl 2): S89–S91.
33. Kearney CE, Wallis CE. Deoxyribonuclease for cystic fibrosis (updated 22 August 2001). Available in The Cochrane Library; Issue 4. Oxford: Update Software; 2001.
34. Stafanger G, *et al.* The clinical effect and the effect on the ciliary motility of oral N-acetylcysteine in patients with cystic fibrosis and primary ciliary dyskinesia. *Eur Respir J* 1988; **1:** 161–7.
35. Ratjen F, *et al.* A double-blind placebo controlled trial with oral ambroxol and N-acetylcysteine for mucolytic treatment in cystic fibrosis. *Eur J Pediatr* 1985; **144:** 374–8.
36. Konstan MW. Therapies aimed at airway inflammation in cystic fibrosis. *Clin Chest Med* 1998; **19:** 505–13.
37. Cheng K, *et al.* Oral steroids for cystic fibrosis (updated 28 August 2001). Available in The Cochrane Library; Issue 4. Oxford: Update Software; 2001.
38. Dezateux C, *et al.* Inhaled corticosteroids for cystic fibrosis (updated 28 August 2001). Available in The Cochrane Library; Issue 4. Oxford: Update Software; 2001.
39. Konstan MW, *et al.* Effect of high-dose ibuprofen in patients with cystic fibrosis. *N Engl J Med* 1995; **332:** 848–54.
40. McElvaney NG, *et al.* Aerosol α-1-antitrypsin treatment for cystic fibrosis. *Lancet* 1991; **337:** 392–4.
41. Aronoff SC, *et al.* Effects of pentoxifylline on sputum neutrophil elastase and pulmonary function in patients with cystic fibrosis: preliminary observations. *J Pediatr* 1994; **125:** 992–7.
42. Knowles MR, *et al.* A pilot study of aerosolized amiloride for the treatment of lung disease in cystic fibrosis. *N Engl J Med* 1990; **322:** 1189–94.
43. Bowler IM, *et al.* Nebulised amiloride in respiratory exacerbations of cystic fibrosis: a randomised controlled trial. *Arch Dis Child* 1995; **73:** 427–30.
44. Graham A, *et al.* No added benefit from nebulized amiloride in patients with cystic fibrosis. *Eur Respir J* 1993; **6:** 1243–8.
45. Zinman R, *et al.* Nocturnal home oxygen in the treatment of hypoxemic cystic fibrosis patients. *J Pediatr* 1989; **114:** 368–77.
46. Dinwiddie R, *et al.* Oxygen therapy for cystic fibrosis. *J R Soc Med* 1999; **92** (suppl 37): 19–22.
47. Bowler IM, *et al.* Resting energy expenditure and substrate oxidation rates in cystic fibrosis. *Arch Dis Child* 1993; **68:** 754–9.
48. Green MR, *et al.* Nutritional management of the infant with cystic fibrosis. *Arch Dis Child* 1995; **72:** 452–6.
49. Haworth CS, *et al.* Low bone mineral density in adults with cystic fibrosis. *Thorax* 1999; **54:** 961–7.
50. Feranchak AP, *et al.* Prospective, long-term study of fat-soluble vitamin status in children with cystic fibrosis identified by newborn screen. *J Pediatr* 1999; **135:** 601–10.
51. Jaffé A, *et al.* Prospects for gene therapy in cystic fibrosis. *Arch Dis Child* 1999; **80:** 286–9.
52. Colledge WH, Evans MJ. Cystic fibrosis gene therapy. *Br Med Bull* 1995; **51:** 82–90.
53. Coutelle C. Gene therapy approaches for cystic fibrosis. *Biologicals* 1995; **23:** 21–5.
54. Southern KW. Gene therapy for cystic fibrosis: current issues. *Br J Hosp Med* 1996; **55:** 495–9.

Diarrhoea, infective

See under Gastro-enteritis, below.

Diphtheria

Diphtheria is caused by infection, usually of the upper respiratory tract or the skin, with the Gram-positive aerobe *Corynebacterium diphtheriae*. It is distributed worldwide and, despite the effectiveness of immunisation (see Diphtheria Vaccines, p.1536), is still common in parts of the world, including the tropics. Although the risk to travellers is said to be low, diphtheria should be considered in patients returning from tropical countries with a sore throat.[1] Russia and other republics of the former USSR have experienced an epidemic.[2]

The most serious manifestations of infection are due to exotoxin produced by toxigenic strains and thus treatment is primarily with diphtheria antitoxin. Erythromycin or benzylpenicillin are also given to eliminate C.

diphtheriae, thereby terminating toxin production and preventing the spread of infection to contacts. Close contacts of primary cases of diphtheria may be given a 7-day prophylactic course of erythromycin by mouth or a single intramuscular dose of benzylpenicillin,[3] in addition to boosters or primary immunisation with diphtheria vaccine. Non-toxigenic *C. diphtheriae* is the most common isolate in clinical cases in the UK[3,4] and generally causes a less severe form of the disease; it does, however, have the potential to cause invasive disease in some patients.[5] Asymptomatic carriers may harbour non-toxigenic strains of *C. diphtheriae* that can be converted to toxigenic strains. A single intramuscular injection of benzathine benzylpenicillin has been less effective than oral erythromycin, but may be used if compliance is uncertain;[6] clindamycin for 7 days by mouth has also eliminated the carrier state,[6] but erythromycin remains the drug of choice. Bacteriological follow-up should be carried out 2 weeks after completing treatment to be certain *C. diphtheriae* has been eradicated from carriers.[7]

1. Anonymous. Toxigenic Corynebacterium diphtheriae associated with the Haj. *Commun Dis Rep* 1991; **1:** 143.
2. Hardy IRB, *et al.* Current situation and control strategies for resurgence of diphtheria in newly independent states of the former Soviet Union. *Lancet* 1996; **347:** 1739–44.
3. Bonnet JM, Begg NT. Control of diphtheria: guidance for consultants in communicable disease control. *Commun Dis Public Health* 1999; **2:** 242–9.
4. Begg N, Balraj V. Diphtheria: are we ready for it? *Arch Dis Child* 1995; **73:** 568–72.
5. Efstratiou A, *et al.* Non-toxigenic Corynebacterium diphtheriae var gravis in England. *Lancet* 1993; **341:** 1592–3.
6. McCloskey RV, *et al.* Treatment of diphtheria carriers: benzathine penicillin, erythromycin, and clindamycin. *Ann Intern Med* 1974; **81:** 788–91.
7. Miller LW, *et al.* Diphtheria carriers and the effect of erythromycin therapy. *Antimicrob Agents Chemother* 1974; **6:** 166–9.

Ear infections
See under Otitis Externa, and Otitis Media, below.

Ehrlichiosis
Infections with rickettsia-like bacteria of the *Ehrlichia* genus are rare and at one time the only species isolated from humans was *E. sennetsu*, the cause of Sennetsu fever in Japan. *E. canis* is responsible for a tick-borne disease in *dogs* and a closely related species, *E. chaffeensis*, causes human monocytic ehrlichiosis.[1] A granulocytic *Ehrlichia* species closely related to *E. phagocytophila* and *E. equi* appears to be responsible for cases of human granulocytic ehrlichiosis in parts of the USA[1-3] and probably in Europe.[4] *E. ewingii* has recently been identified as a human pathogen[5] and there are likely to be others. A large proportion of infections occur after a tick bite. As with other rickettsial infections, treatment is with a tetracycline, commonly doxycycline;[1,2,6] chloramphenicol has been used as an alternative.[6] Antibiotic susceptibility testing has suggested that rifamycins and fluoroquinolones are promising alternatives in the granulocytic form of infections.[7] Successful treatment with rifampicin has been reported in 2 patients.[8]

1. Dumler JS, Bakken JS. Ehrlichial diseases of humans: emerging tick-borne infections. *Clin Infect Dis* 1995; **20:** 1102–10.
2. Bakken JS, *et al.* Clinical and laboratory characteristics of human granulocytic ehrlichiosis. *JAMA* 1996; **275:** 199–205.
3. IJdo JW, *et al.* The emergence of another tickborne infection in the 12-town area around Lyme, Connecticut: human granulocytic ehrlichiosis. *J Infect Dis* 2000; **181:** 1388–93.
4. Brouqui P, *et al.* Human granulocytic ehrlichiosis in Europe. *Lancet* 1995; **346:** 782–3.
5. Buller RS, *et al.* Ehrlichia ewingii, a newly recognized agent of human ehrlichiosis. *N Engl J Med* 1999; **341:** 148–55.
6. Schaffner W, Standaert SM. Ehrlichiosis—in pursuit of an emerging infection. *N Engl J Med* 1996; **334:** 262–3.
7. Klein MB, *et al.* Antibiotic susceptibility of the newly cultivated agent of human granulocytic ehrlichiosis: promising activity of quinolones and rifamycins. *Antimicrob Agents Chemother* 1997; **41:** 76–9.
8. Buitrago MI, *et al.* Human granulocytic ehrlichiosis during pregnancy treated successfully with rifampin. *Clin Infect Dis* 1998; **27:** 213–15.

Endocarditis
Infective endocarditis is caused by infection of the endocardium following invasion of the blood stream by bacteria or fungi and particularly affects the heart valves. Infection may follow an acute or subacute course depending in part on the organisms responsible. Virtually any organism can cause endocarditis but streptococci, enterococci, and staphylococci continue to be major culprits. The commonest bacteria responsible are the alpha-haemolytic streptococci originating mainly from the mouth and throat; they have been called viridans streptococci or even '*Streptococcus viridans*' (although this is not a true species) and include *Str. mitis*, *Str. mutans*, *Str. oralis*, *Str. salivarius*, and *Str. sanguis*. Other streptococci originate in the gut and include *Str. bovis*. Enterococci

(faecal streptococci) also originate in the gut and include *Enterococcus faecalis* and to a lesser extent *E. faecium*. Endocarditis due to all these bacteria is commonly subacute or insidious. Acute endocarditis is often due to *Staphylococcus aureus*, a common cause in intravenous drug abusers, but may also be caused by coagulase-negative staphylococci, particularly *Staph. lugdunensis*. *Staph. epidermidis* is often responsible for prosthetic valve infection. Less common causes of endocarditis are: Gram-negative bacteria such as the Enterobacteriaceae, *Pseudomonas* spp., and the HACEK group of slow-growing organisms (*Haemophilus*, *Actinobacillus*, *Cardiobacterium*, *Eikenella*, *Kingella*); the rickettsia *Coxiella burnetii* (the cause of Q fever, below); and fungi such as *Candida* and *Aspergillus*.

There are consensus recommendations for the treatment and prophylaxis of endocarditis.

Endocarditis treatment. Guidelines for the treatment of streptococcal, enterococcal, and staphylococcal endocarditis were produced by the British Society for Antimicrobial Chemotherapy in 1998[1] and, with the addition of HACEK endocarditis, by the American Heart Association in 1995.[2] Although these guidelines are broadly accepted there may be differing views on detail including choice of antibacterial, route of administration, and duration of treatment. Treatment depends on identification of the infecting organisms and their sensitivity to antibacterials. Blood should therefore be taken for culture before treatment is started; MICs should be measured. *Empirical treatment* with benzylpenicillin plus gentamicin may then be given until the laboratory results are known; vancomycin should be given instead of benzylpenicillin if staphylococcal infection is likely.[1] There is synergy between penicillin and aminoglycosides against streptococci. Viridans streptococci are generally much more sensitive to penicillin than enterococci and gentamicin may sometimes be stopped once the laboratory results are known.

Briefly, the 1998 **UK** guidelines[1] are as follows.

• STREPTOCOCCAL ENDOCARDITIS.

For *penicillin-sensitive streptococci* (viridans streptococci and *Str. bovis* with a benzylpenicillin MIC of 0.1 µg or less per mL): intravenous bolus injections of benzylpenicillin 1.2 g every 4 hours and gentamicin 80 mg twice daily both given for 2 weeks.

For *streptococci less sensitive to penicillin* (viridans streptococci and *Str. bovis* with a benzylpenicillin MIC of more than 0.1 µg per mL): benzylpenicillin and gentamicin as above, but both given for 4 weeks.

For *streptococci in penicillin-allergic patients*: initially either vancomycin 1 g intravenously twice daily or teicoplanin 400 mg intravenously every 12 hours for three doses and then a maintenance dose of 400 mg daily; either drug should be given for 4 weeks, together with gentamicin as above for the first 2 weeks.

• ENTEROCOCCAL ENDOCARDITIS.

For *gentamicin-sensitive or low-level resistant enterococci* (MIC less than 100 µg per mL): intravenous bolus injections of ampicillin or amoxicillin 2 g every 4 hours and gentamicin 80 mg twice daily, both given for 4 weeks.

For *gentamicin highly-resistant enterococci* (MIC at least 2000 µg per mL): ampicillin or amoxicillin as above, but for a minimum of 6 weeks; streptomycin may also be given if sensitivity can be demonstrated.

For *enterococci in penicillin-allergic patients*: as for streptococci in penicillin-allergic patients above, except that gentamicin should be given for all 4 weeks of treatment.

• STAPHYLOCOCCAL ENDOCARDITIS.

For *penicillin-sensitive staphylococci*: intravenous bolus injections of benzylpenicillin 1.2 g every 4 hours for four weeks plus gentamicin 80 to 120 mg every 8 hours for the first week.

For *staphylococci resistant to penicillins generally but sensitive to meticillin/flucloxacillin*: intravenous bolus injections of flucloxacillin 2 g every 4 hours for 4 weeks plus gentamicin as for penicillin-sensitive staphylococci.

For *staphylococci resistant to meticillin/flucloxacillin* and in *penicillin-allergic patients*: vancomycin 1 g intravenously twice daily for 4 weeks plus gentamicin as for penicillin-sensitive staphylococci.

In difficult cases of endocarditis due to coagulase-negative staphylococci or *Staph. aureus*, rifampicin may occasionally be added to therapy, usually with vancomycin.

The 1995 **USA** guidelines[2] are as follows.

• STREPTOCOCCAL AND ENTEROCOCCAL ENDOCARDITIS.

For *penicillin-sensitive streptococci* (viridans streptococci and *Str. bovis* with a benzylpenicillin MIC of 0.1 µg or less per mL): there are three alternative regimens, namely benzylpenicillin alone for 4 weeks; ceftriaxone alone for 4 weeks; or benzylpenicillin with gentamicin, each for 2 weeks only. Streptomycin has been used as an alternative to gentamicin but gentamicin is now preferred. Doses are: intravenous benzylpenicillin 7.2 to 10.8 g daily by continuous infusion or in 6 divided doses; intravenous or intramuscular ceftriaxone 2 g once daily; intramuscular or intravenous gentamicin 1 mg per kg body-weight every 8 hours.

For *relatively resistant streptococci* (viridans streptococci and *Str. bovis* with a benzylpenicillin MIC greater than 0.1 µg per mL but less than 0.5 µg per mL): intravenous benzylpenicillin 10.8 g daily by continuous infusion or in 6 divided doses for 4 weeks with gentamicin as above for 2 weeks.

For *more resistant bacteria* (enterococci or viridans streptococci with a benzylpenicillin MIC of 0.5 µg or more per mL): there are three alternative regimens, namely intravenous benzylpenicillin 10.8 to 18 g daily by continuous infusion or in 6 divided doses with gentamicin as above; or intravenous ampicillin 12 g daily by continuous infusion or in 6 divided doses again with gentamicin as above; or intravenous vancomycin 30 mg per kg daily in two divided doses, the total daily dose not exceeding 2 g, again with gentamicin as above. Both drugs in each regimen should be given for 4 to 6 weeks. Streptomycin has again been used as an alternative to gentamicin but gentamicin is now preferred. Resistance is, however, emerging among enterococcal strains to vancomycin and to gentamicin and streptomycin as well as to the penicillins. Where resistance to vancomycin is modest, teicoplanin is suggested as an alternative. Some patients with multiply-resistant enterococcal infection whose treatment fails may need to be considered for surgical intervention.

For *streptococci and enterococci in penicillin-allergic patients or those allergic to other beta lactams*: intravenous vancomycin 30 mg per kg daily in two divided doses for 4 weeks, the total daily dose not exceeding 2 g. For more resistant bacteria vancomycin should be given with gentamicin as above, both for 4 to 6 weeks.

• STAPHYLOCOCCAL ENDOCARDITIS.

For *meticillin-susceptible staphylococci in the absence of prosthetic material*: intravenous nafcillin or oxacillin 2 g every 4 hours for 4 to 6 weeks with or without gentamicin 1 mg per kg intramuscularly or intravenously every 8 hours for 3 to 5 days.

For *meticillin-resistant staphylococci in the absence of prosthetic material*, intravenous vancomycin 30 mg per kg daily in 2 divided doses is given for 4 to 6 weeks, the total daily dose not exceeding 2 g.

For *meticillin-susceptible staphylococci in the presence of prosthetic material*: intravenous nafcillin or oxacillin 2 g every 4 hours with oral rifampicin 300 mg every 8 hours for 6 weeks or more and gentamicin as above for the initial 2 weeks.

For *meticillin-resistant staphylococci in the presence of prosthetic material*, nafcillin or oxacillin are replaced by intravenous vancomycin 30 mg per kg daily in 2 or 4 divided doses for 6 weeks or more, the total daily dose not exceeding 2 g.

For *meticillin-susceptible staphylococci in penicillin-allergic patients or those allergic to other beta lactams in the absence of prosthetic material*, intravenous cefazolin 2 g every 8 hours for 4 to 6 weeks or other first-generation cephalosporin (except in immediate-type hypersensitivity) with or without gentamicin as above for 3 to 5 days. Alternatively intravenous vancomycin 30 mg per kg daily in 2 divided doses is given for 4 to 6 weeks, the total daily dose not exceeding 2 g.

For *meticillin-susceptible staphylococci in penicillin-allergic patients or those allergic to other beta lactams in the presence of prosthetic material*, as above but with nafcillin or oxacillin replaced by vancomycin or a first-generation cephalosporin.

• HACEK ENDOCARDITIS.

Traditionally the HACEK group of organisms have been susceptible to ampicillin, but recently resistant strains have been identified and monotherapy with ampicillin is no longer recommended. Preferred treatment is therefore with intramuscular or intravenous ceftriaxone 2 g once daily for 4 weeks, although cefotaxime or other third-generation cephalosporin may be substituted. Alternatively, intravenous ampicillin 12 g daily by continuous infusion or in 6 divided doses with intramuscular or intravenous gentamicin 1 mg per kg every 8 hours may be given, both for 4 weeks. Therapy should be extended to 6 weeks for prosthetic valve endocarditis.

Endocarditis prophylaxis. Patients at risk of developing endocarditis, including those with valvular heart disease, prosthetic valves, or other cardiac abnormalities and those with a history of endocarditis or rheumatic fever, should be given antibacterials prophylactically when about to undergo dental operations, tonsillectomy, or other procedures liable to lead to bacteraemia. Antibacterials should be administered so that adequate blood and tissue concentrations are achieved throughout the procedure. They are generally given as a single dose before the procedure, sometimes repeated about 6 hours later; the oral route is used if possible. A penicillin such as amoxicillin, with or without an aminoglycoside such as gentamicin, is used, reflecting the bacteria usually responsible (see above). Clindamycin, vancomycin, or teicoplanin are used in penicillin-allergic patients. UK and USA guidelines for prophylaxis are similar. Recommendations from the British Society for Antimicrobial Chemotherapy were published in 1982[3] and amended in 1986,[4] 1990,[5] 1992,[6] and 1997.[7] Updated recommendations from the American Heart Association were also published in 1997.[8]

UK guidelines are as follows.

• DENTAL PROCEDURES.

Prior application of chlorhexidine or other suitable antiseptic to the gingival margins may reduce the severity of any bacteraemia.

Under local or no anaesthesia (including patients with a prosthetic valve, but not in those who have had endocarditis): amoxicillin or clindamycin by mouth. Amoxicillin is preferred provided that patients are not penicillin-allergic and have not received penicillin more than once in the previous month. Doses are: amoxicillin 3 g or clindamycin 600 mg as a single oral dose 1 hour before the procedure.

Under general anaesthesia: amoxicillin in one of 3 regimens, namely: amoxicillin 1 g intravenously just before induction then 0.5 g by mouth 6 hours later; or 3 g by mouth 4 hours before anaesthesia and repeated once as soon as possible after the procedure; or amoxicillin 3 g with probenecid 1 g both by mouth 4 hours before the procedure. Those who are allergic to penicillin or have received it more than once in the previous month should be referred to hospital.

In special-risk patients referred to hospital (i.e. those who are to have a general anaesthetic and have prosthetic heart valves or are unable to receive penicillin because of allergy or receipt of penicillin more than once in the previous month; those who have previously had endocarditis): amoxicillin plus gentamicin or vancomycin plus gentamicin. When penicillin *can* be given: amoxicillin 1 g and gentamicin 120 mg both intravenously just before induction and amoxicillin 0.5 g by mouth 6 hours later. When penicillin *cannot* be used: vancomycin 1 g by slow intravenous infusion over at least 100 minutes followed by gentamicin 120 mg intravenously just before induction or 15 minutes before the surgical procedure. Intravenous teicoplanin 400 mg just before induction or 15 minutes before the procedure may be substituted for vancomycin. A second alternative is clindamycin 300 mg intravenously over at least 10 minutes just before induction or 15 minutes before the surgical procedure followed 6 hours later by 150 mg by mouth or by intravenous infusion over at least 10 minutes.

• UPPER RESPIRATORY-TRACT PROCEDURES.

As for dental procedures (above), but the postoperative antibacterial may need to be given parenterally if swallowing is painful.

• GENITO-URINARY PROCEDURES.

As for dental procedures in special-risk patients (above), but not clindamycin. If there is urinary infection prophylaxis should also be effective against these infecting organisms.

• GASTROINTESTINAL, OBSTETRIC, AND GYNAECOLOGICAL PROCEDURES.

Prophylaxis is only necessary in patients with prosthetic valves or those who have previously had endo-

carditis and then as for dental procedures in special-risk patients (above), but not clindamycin.

USA guidelines[8] are as follows.

• DENTAL, ORAL, RESPIRATORY-TRACT, OR OESOPHAGEAL PROCEDURES.

Standard oral regimen: amoxicillin 2 g an hour beforehand.

Patients unable to take oral antibacterials: ampicillin 2 g intravenously or intramuscularly up to 30 minutes before the procedure.

Penicillin-allergic patients: clindamycin 600 mg by mouth an hour beforehand, or cefalexin or cefadroxil 2 g by mouth an hour beforehand, or azithromycin or clarithromycin 500 mg by mouth an hour beforehand.

Penicillin-allergic patients unable to take oral antibacterials: clindamycin 600 mg intravenously or cefazolin 1 g intravenously or intramuscularly up to 30 minutes before the procedure.

• GENITO-URINARY AND GASTROINTESTINAL (EXCLUDING OESOPHAGEAL) PROCEDURES.

Moderate-risk patients: amoxicillin 2 g by mouth an hour beforehand, or ampicillin 2 g intravenously or intramuscularly up to 30 minutes before the procedure.

Moderate-risk patients who are penicillin-allergic: vancomycin 1 g intravenously over 1 to 2 hours, with completion of the infusion up to 30 minutes before the procedure.

High-risk patients: ampicillin 2 g plus gentamicin 1.5 mg per kg (up to a maximum total of 120 mg) intravenously or intramuscularly up to 30 minutes before the procedure, followed 6 hours later by ampicillin 1 g intravenously or intramuscularly or by amoxicillin 1 g by mouth.

High-risk patients who are penicillin-allergic: vancomycin 1 g intravenously over 1 to 2 hours plus gentamicin 1.5 mg per kg (up to 120 mg) intravenously or intramuscularly, with completion of the infusion and injection up to 30 minutes before the procedure.

1. Working Party of the British Society for Antimicrobial Chemotherapy. Antibiotic treatment of streptococcal, enterococcal, and staphylococcal endocarditis. *Heart* 1998; **79**: 207–10.
2. Wilson WR, *et al.* Antibiotic treatment of adults with infective endocarditis due to viridans streptococci, enterococci, staphylococci, and HACEK microorganisms. *JAMA* 1995; **274**: 1706–13.
3. Working Party of the British Society for Antimicrobial Chemotherapy. The antibiotic prophylaxis of infective endocarditis. *Lancet* 1982; **ii**: 1323–6.
4. Simmons NA, *et al.* Prophylaxis of infective endocarditis. *Lancet* 1986; **i**: 1267.
5. Endocarditis Working Party of the British Society for Antimicrobial Chemotherapy. Antibiotic prophylaxis of infective endocarditis. *Lancet* 1990; **335**: 88–9.
6. Simmons NA, *et al.* Antibiotic prophylaxis and infective endocarditis. *Lancet* 1992; **339**: 1292–3.
7. Littler WA, *et al.* Changes in recommendations about amoxycillin prophylaxis for prevention of endocarditis. *Lancet* 1997; **350**: 1100.
8. Dajani AS, *et al.* Prevention of bacterial endocarditis: recommendations by the American Heart Association. *JAMA* 1997; **277**: 1794–1801.

Endometritis

Endometritis (or endomyometritis) is a uterine infection that may be a part of pelvic inflammatory disease (below) or may be a postoperative complication of caesarean section.

Antibacterial prophylaxis may be given at caesarean section after cord clamping to prevent postpartum endometritis as well as wound infection. While the use of antimicrobial prophylaxis in patients at high risk of infection is well established, prophylaxis in low-risk patients remains controversial. A systematic literature review[1] has shown that prophylaxis was beneficial following both elective and non-elective caesarean section, but USA surgical guidelines do not recommend routine prophylaxis in low-risk patients.[2] A penicillin or first-generation cephalosporin such as cefazolin is commonly used.[2,3]

Early postpartum endometritis has a polymicrobial aetiology. In one study the most common organisms isolated included *Gardnerella vaginalis*, *Peptococcus* spp., *Bacteroides* spp., *Staphylococcus epidermidis*, group B streptococci, and *Ureaplasma urealyticum*.[4] *Chlamydia trachomatis* has been implicated more often in late postpartum endometritis, but a wide variety of micro-organisms may also be responsible including genital mycoplasmas and, to a lesser extent, facultative and anaerobic bacteria.[5]

In the USA, standard empirical therapy for postpartum endometritis has been a short course of intravenous antibacterials, often clindamycin with gentamicin, given until the patient has been afebrile and asymptomatic for 24

to 48 hours and may be followed by a course of oral treatment, often with amoxicillin. A systematic review[6] has confirmed the suitability of clindamycin with gentamicin and indicated that oral therapy is not necessary after successful intravenous therapy, although it may be recommended in patients with staphylococcal bacteraemia.[2]

1. Smaill F, Hofmeyr GJ. Antibiotic prophylaxis for cesarean section (updated 29 May 2001). Available in The Cochrane Library; Issue 4. Oxford: Update Software; 2001.
2. ACOG. Antimicrobial therapy for obstetric patients. *Int J Gynecol Obstet* 1998; **61**: 299–308.
3. Hopkins L, Smaill F. Antibiotic prophylaxis regimens and drugs for cesarean section (updated 27 February 2001). Available in The Cochrane Library; Issue 4. Oxford: Update Software; 2001.
4. Rosene K, *et al.* Polymicrobial early postpartum endometritis with facultative and anaerobic bacteria, genital mycoplasmas, and Chlamydia trachomatis: treatment with piperacillin or cefoxitin. *J Infect Dis* 1986; **153**: 1028–37.
5. Hoyme UB, *et al.* Microbiology and treatment of late postpartum endometritis. *Obstet Gynecol* 1986; **68**: 226–32.
6. French LM, Smaill FM. Antibiotic regimens for endometritis after delivery (updated 18 January 2001). Available in The Cochrane Library; Issue 4. Oxford: Update Software; 2001.

Enterococcal infections

Enterococcal infections are causing increasing concern, particularly with the emergence of drug-resistant strains.[1-6] Enterococci, principally *Enterococcus faecalis* (formerly *Streptococcus faecalis*) but also *E. faecium* and *E. avium*, can cause a variety of infections including those of the biliary tract and urinary tract, endocarditis, and peritonitis. Since they are frequently present in the gut flora they are a common cause of nosocomial infections. Enterococci are resistant to cephalosporins, tetracyclines, macrolides, and chloramphenicol. The emergence of resistance to gentamicin, penicillins, and the glycopeptide antimicrobials vancomycin and teicoplanin has compromised the previously standard treatment for enterococcal infections of a penicillin or glycopeptide with gentamicin. There can be no general recommendations for treatment at present and the choice of antibacterial should be made according to local patterns of resistance and antibacterial sensitivity tests. Because of the lack of effective antibacterials emphasis has been placed on measures to prevent the spread of vancomycin-resistant enterococci. Guidelines were published in 1995 by the USA Hospital Infection Control Practices Advisory Committee,[7] and it has been suggested that they could be adapted for use in other countries.[8]

1. Landman D, Quale JM. Management of infections due to resistant enterococci: a review of therapeutic options. *J Antimicrob Chemother* 1997; **40**: 161–70.
2. Murray BE. Vancomycin-resistant enterococci. *Am J Med* 1997; **102**: 284–93.
3. Antony SJ. Multidrug-resistant enterococci: the dawn of a new era in resistant pathogens. *J Natl Med Assoc* 1998; **90**: 537–40.
4. Moellering RC. Vancomycin-resistant enterococci. *Clin Infect Dis* 1998; **26**: 1196–9.
5. Linden PK, Miller CB. Vancomycin-resistant enterococci: the clinical effect of a common nosocomial pathogen. *Diagn Microbiol Infect Dis* 1999; **33**: 113–20.
6. Murray BE. Vancomycin-resistant enterococcal infections. *N Engl J Med* 2000; **342**: 710–21.
7. Hospital Infection Control Practices Advisory Committee (HICPAC). Recommendations for preventing the spread of vancomycin resistance. *MMWR* 1995; **44** (RR-12): 1–13.
8. Fraise AP. The treatment and control of vancomycin resistant enterococci. *J Antimicrob Chemother* 1996; **38**: 753–6.

Epididymitis

Epididymitis is often associated with urethritis and in young men occurs most commonly as a complication of sexually transmitted infection with *Neisseria gonorrhoeae* and especially *Chlamydia trachomatis*, but may occur in homosexual males as a result of infection with enteric organisms, particularly *Escherichia coli*.

In men over 35 years and in children epididymitis is usually secondary to urinary-tract infection with *Pseudomonas aeruginosa* and other Gram-negative bacilli and is not sexually transmitted.

For chlamydial epididymitis WHO[1] recommends a 7-day oral course of doxycycline 100 mg twice daily or azithromycin 1 g as a single dose. Alternatives include 7-day courses of amoxicillin 500 mg three times daily, erythromycin 500 mg four times daily, ofloxacin 300 mg twice daily, or tetracycline hydrochloride 500 mg four times daily. Unless it can be excluded, patients should also be treated concurrently for gonorrhoea (below).

In the UK, the recommended treatment[2] for disease most probably due to gonococcal infection is a single intramuscular dose of ceftriaxone 250 mg or a single oral dose of ciprofloxacin 500 mg plus doxycycline 100 mg by mouth twice daily for 10 to 14 days. For probable chlamydial infections or infections with other non-gonococcal, non-enteric organisms, doxycycline 100 mg by mouth twice daily for 10 to 14 days is recommended, and for infections with enteric organisms, ofloxacin 200 mg twice daily for 14 days is recommended. In patients allergic to cephalosporins and/or tetracyclines ofloxacin 200 mg by mouth twice daily for 14 days may be employed for infections of all causes.

In the USA, the Centers for Disease Control[3] recommends empirical treatment for epididymitis likely to have been caused by gonococcal or chlamydial infection with a single intramuscular dose of ceftriaxone 250 mg together with doxycycline 100 mg twice daily by mouth for 10 days; if the cause is thought to be an enteric organism ofloxacin 300 mg twice daily by mouth for 10 days is recommended.

1. WHO. Guidelines for the management of sexually transmitted infections. Geneva: WHO, 2001.
2. Clinical Effectiveness Group (Association of Genitourinary Medicine and the Medical Society for the Study of Venereal Diseases). National guideline for the management of epididymo-orchitis. *Sex Transm Infect* 1999; **75** (suppl 1): S51–S53.
3. Centers for Disease Control. 1998 Guidelines for treatment of sexually transmitted diseases. *MMWR* 1998; **47** (RR-1): 86–8.

Epiglottitis
In acute epiglottitis rapid swelling of the epiglottis and surrounding soft tissues results in sudden airway obstruction which can be fatal. It is often due to bacteraemic infection with *Haemophilus influenzae* type b (see below) and has occurred primarily in young children. However, the incidence has decreased in this age group since the introduction of haemophilus influenzae vaccine.[1] Acute epiglottitis also occurs in adults.[1]

Treatment and prophylaxis is similar to that for Haemophilus influenzae meningitis (see under Meningitis, below). Immediate management includes the maintenance of an adequate airway and the intravenous administration of antibacterials active against *H. influenzae* type b. Chloramphenicol has been the drug of choice, but third-generation cephalosporins such as cefotaxime and ceftriaxone are increasingly used.[2] Prophylaxis with rifampicin may be given to index cases and contacts.

1. Frantz TD, *et al.* Acute epiglottitis in adults: analysis of 129 cases. *JAMA* 1994; **272**: 1358–60.
2. Sawyer SM, *et al.* Successful treatment of epiglottitis with two doses of ceftriaxone. *Arch Dis Child* 1994; **70**: 129–32.

Escherichia coli enteritis
See under Gastro-enteritis, below.

Eye infections
Conjunctivitis is a common superficial eye disorder and may be caused by infection with a wide range of bacteria, viruses, and, less frequently, fungi. Acute bacterial conjunctivitis is commonly caused by staphylococci or streptococci in adults, and *Haemophilus influenzae* and *Moraxella catarrhalis* (*Branhamella catarrhalis*) particularly in children. Other causes of bacterial conjunctivitis include gonococci (see Gonorrhoea, below) and *Chlamydia trachomatis* (see Trachoma, below). Neonatal chlamydial and gonococcal conjunctivitis are discussed under Neonatal Conjunctivitis, below. Uncomplicated bacterial conjunctivitis may be self-limiting but empirical treatment with topical antibacterials is often given. In the UK, topical chloramphenicol remains the treatment of choice despite concerns over the potential risk of aplastic anaemia (see Ocular Use under Precautions of Chloramphenicol, p.180). Alternatives include gentamicin, tobramycin, erythromycin (especially when infection with Gram-positive organisms is suspected), fluoroquinolones including ciprofloxacin and ofloxacin, framycetin, fusidic acid (especially for staphylococcal infections), and polymyxin B in combination with bacitracin, trimethoprim, or neomycin.

Blepharitis is an infection of the lid margins. It usually presents as a chronic condition and may require prolonged treatment, typically involving local hygiene to remove encrustations and topical application of a broad-spectrum antibacterial ointment.

Keratitis may be caused by infection of the cornea by bacteria, fungi, viruses, or protozoa usually following trauma to the surface of the eye, including that due to contact lens wear (see Contact Lens Care, p.1129). Common bacterial pathogens include staphylococci, streptococci, *Pseudomonas* spp., and Enterobacteriaceae. Bacterial keratitis is potentially sight-threatening and requires prompt aggressive treatment with broad-spectrum antibacterials. It is customary to obtain material for sensitivity testing, but increasingly, empirical treatment is then instituted without delay. Frequent or continuous topical application of drops or the use of local drug delivery devices have been used to ensure prolonged elevated drug concentrations. Subconjunctival or systemic therapy may occasionally be necessary. Topical treatment with cefazolin and either gentamicin or tobramycin has traditionally been used when *Pseudomonas* is not suspected. More recently, fluoroquinolones or ceftazidime have been used, and semisynthetic penicillins or vancomycin are other alternatives. For the treatment of Acanthamoeba keratitis, see p.582.

Endophthalmitis is a devastating ocular disease resulting from infection of the ocular cavity, usually following penetrating trauma or surgery. Depending on the route of infection, causative organisms include staphylococci, streptococci, *H. influenzae*, *Bacillus cereus*, and *Propionibacterium acnes*. Fungal infections occur less commonly. Bacterial endophthalmitis requires immediate aggressive treatment with antibacterials, usually given intravitreally. The value of concurrent parenteral antibacterials is unclear. The choice of antibacterial for intravitreal use depends on the most likely pathogen. Third-generation cephalosporins or vancomycin are used, but aminoglycosides may produce retinal toxicity. Clindamycin may be effective if *B. cereus* is suspected. Adjunctive treatment includes vitrectomy, surgical removal of infected lens structures, and corticosteroids to control inflammatory and immune responses.

For a discussion of fungal infections of the eye, see p.374; for ocular herpes simplex infections, see under Herpes Simplex Infections, p.607.

Some general references are given below.

1. Baum J. Infections of the eye. *Clin Infect Dis* 1995; **21**: 479–88.
2. Leeming JP. Treatment of ocular infections with topical antibacterials. *Clin Pharmacokinet* 1999; **37**: 351–60.

Gas gangrene
Clostridium spp. are anaerobic Gram-positive bacteria some of which cause gas gangrene with muscle necrosis and systemic toxicity as a result of toxin formation. *Cl. perfringens* is the species most frequently responsible. Gas gangrene is usually associated with traumatic or surgical wounds. Treatment is primarily by surgical debridement of all necrotic muscle and the administration of large doses of benzylpenicillin. Alternative antibacterials have included clindamycin, metronidazole, imipenem, a tetracycline, or chloramphenicol. Hyperbaric oxygen is used as an adjunct to surgical debridement. Gas-gangrene antitoxins are rarely used nowadays.

Benzylpenicillin is also recommended as prophylaxis against gas gangrene in patients undergoing high amputations of lower limbs or following major trauma; metronidazole is an alternative in patients allergic to penicillin.

Gastro-enteritis
Diarrhoea is a symptom of simple gastro-enteritis and of most intestinal infections. It is a major problem in developing countries, but is common worldwide. Although viruses are often responsible, the severest forms of infectious diarrhoea are generally those due to bacteria. Common bacterial pathogens include *Campylobacter jejuni*, *Escherichia coli*, *Salmonella enteritidis*, *Shigella* spp., *Vibrio cholerae*, and *Yersinia enterocolitica*. Intestinal protozoa also cause diarrhoea and are of increasing importance in AIDS-associated diarrhoea. For discussions of viral and protozoal gastro-enteritis and their treatment, see p.605 and p.583 respectively. In acute diarrhoea of any aetiology the priority is to maintain hydration by prevention or treatment of fluid and electrolyte depletion, especially in infants and the elderly. Rehydration therapy is discussed under Diarrhoea on p.1203.

Acute, watery diarrhoea caused by non-invasive pathogens is usually self-limiting and may be treated conservatively. Inflammatory diarrhoea, predominantly caused by invasive pathogens and affecting the colon, often requires treatment with antibacterials. Guidelines published in the UK[1] recommended that empirical treatment of acute diarrhoea with antibacterials should be reserved for patients with symptoms suggesting infection with invasive pathogens and those at high risk of complications. Similarly antibacterial treatment was considered appropriate in tropical regions for diarrhoea due to invasive but not non-invasive organisms.[2] Nevertheless, some clinicians consider such an approach to be unnecessarily conservative in adults with severe acute diarrhoea in developed countries[3] in whom empirical treatment with fluoroquinolones can relieve symptoms and shorten the illness without significant adverse effects. In the USA, empirical therapy is considered for any patients in whom a bacterial cause is suspected.[4]

In **infants and children** oral rehydration therapy is universally recognised as initial treatment of acute diarrhoea, but has been underutilised in both developed and developing countries.[2,5,6] Nutritional support and management of secondary complications including systemic infections is also particularly important in this age-group.[2] Antibacterials have little place in management in most cases and their inappropriate use has contributed to a high prevalence of resistance in commensal bacteria.[5] WHO[6,7] has stipulated that antibacterials should only be used in children with acute diarrhoea when there is dysentery or suspected cholera; *Shigella* is the most important cause of dysentery in young children. Giardiasis and amoebiasis should also be treated. WHO emphasised[6] that oral preparations containing streptomycin or dihydrostreptomycin, neomycin, halogenated hydroxyquinolines, or nonabsorbable sulfonamides (sulfaguanidine, succinylsulfathiazole, phthalylsulfathiazole) should not be used.

Persistent or prolonged diarrhoea may not have an infective cause and antibacterial treatment should not be started unless a pathogen can be identified. **Tropical sprue**, a syndrome characterised by malabsorption often presenting as chronic diarrhoea, is believed to have an infective component and may respond to tetracycline, although this may be less effective in indigenous populations than in expatriates.[2]

HIV-associated diarrhoea. As discussed on p.610, diarrhoea is common in HIV infection and AIDS and causative organisms may be bacterial, protozoal, or viral.[8,9] The most common bacterial cause is the *Mycobacterium avium* complex (see Opportunistic Mycobacterial Infections, below); others include *Campylobacter*, *Salmonella*, and *Shigella* spp. Supportive care and appropriate conventional antibacterial therapy may be adequate, as described under the specific infections, below.

'Food poisoning' is generally a self-limiting form of gastro-enteritis although serious outbreaks of foodborne illness have been associated with bacteria such as *Salmonella enteritidis*. Other common food-poisoning organisms include *Listeria monocytogenes*, *Campylobacter* spp., *Yersinia enterocolitica*, *Vibrio parahaemolyticus*, and *E. coli*. An enterotoxin is responsible for food poisoning associated with *Staphylococcus aureus*, *Clostridium* spp., and *Bacillus* spp.[10,11]

Travellers' diarrhoea. Acute diarrhoea associated with travel occurs worldwide. The most common bacterial pathogen is enterotoxigenic *E. coli*, although enteroadherent *E. coli* is also sometimes involved. Other bacteria include *Campylobacter jejuni*, *Salmonella* and *Shigella* spp., *Vibrio cholerae*, and non-cholera vibrios such as *V. parahaemolyticus*. Viruses and the protozoa *Giardia intestinalis*, *Entamoeba histolytica*, and *Cryptosporidium* may also be responsible. Recommendations for the management of travellers' diarrhoea are published by national and international bodies including WHO, the Department of Health in the UK, and the Centers for Disease Control in the USA. Clinical features depend on the pathogen responsible and treatment varies according to severity and duration of diarrhoea. Onset of diarrhoea is generally delayed with *Giardia* and *Entamoeba* because of the incubation period. Diarrhoea is often mild and self-limiting and increased fluid intake or oral rehydration therapy is all that will be required. Symptomatic treatment with antimotility drugs such as loperamide may be of benefit in mild to moderate diarrhoea. Bismuth salicylate may be used to reduce the frequency of diarrhoea and is recommended for prophylaxis and treatment by US sources. Although antimicrobial therapy is not indicated in most cases of infective diarrhoea, empirical treatment with a fluoroquinolone has been effective for moderate to severe attacks. Co-trimoxazole has also been used, but there is a risk of severe skin reactions and bone-marrow depression and increasingly widespread bacterial resistance is causing concern. When the infecting bacteria are known, for example, *Campylobacter*, *Salmonella*, or *Shigella* spp., the specific therapy described below may be necessary.

The risk of developing travellers' diarrhoea can be reduced by avoiding possibly contaminated foods as embodied in the advice to 'cook it, boil it, peel it, or forget it'. A number of prophylactic drug regimens have been suggested, including various antibacterials, usually a fluoroquinolone or co-trimoxazole, in addition to bismuth salicylate as noted above. However, routine antimicrobial prophylaxis is not generally recommended because of the danger of drug reactions, supra-infections, and increasing bacterial resistance and should be reserved for those at special risk. Many authorities prefer early treatment, including self-medication, with clear instructions on when medical help should be sought.

1. Farthing M, et al. The management of infective gastroenteritis in adults: a consensus statement by an expert panel convened by the British Society for the Study of Infection. J Infect 1996; 33: 143–52.
2. Mathan VI. Diarrhoeal diseases. Br Med Bull 1998; 54: 407–19.
3. Gorbach SL. Treating diarrhoea. BMJ 1997; 314: 1776–7.
4. DuPont HL, The Practice Parameters Committee of the American College of Gastroenterology. Guidelines on acute infectious diarrhea in adults. Am J Gastroenterol 1997; 92: 1962–75.
5. Walker-Smith JA. Underutilisation of oral rehydration in the treatment of gastroenteritis. Drugs 1988; 36 (suppl 4): 61–4.
6. WHO. The rational use of drugs in the management of acute diarrhoea in children. Geneva: WHO, 1990.
7. WHO. The management and prevention of diarrhoea: practical guidelines. Geneva: WHO, 1993.
8. Dupont HL, Marshall GD. HIV-associated diarrhoea and wasting. Lancet 1995; 346: 352–6.
9. Sharpstone D, Gazzard B. Gastrointestinal manifestations of HIV infection. Lancet 1996; 348: 379–83.
10. Waites WM, Arbuthnott JP. Foodborne illness: an overview. Lancet 1990; 336: 722–5.
11. Roberts D. Sources of infection: food. Lancet 1990; 336: 859–61.

Antibiotic-associated colitis. Although other organisms, including Candida spp.,[1] have been implicated in antibiotic-associated diarrhoea, colonisation of the colon with Clostridium difficile, a toxin-producing Gram-positive anaerobe, is the most common identifiable cause of antibiotic-associated colitis and pseudomembranous colitis. Restrictive antibiotic policies have decreased the incidence of Cl. difficile-associated diarrhoea in some hospitals[2] but it remains a major hazard of antibacterial use. Antibiotic-associated colitis has been associated with the use of most antibacterials, but particularly with clindamycin, lincomycin, ampicillin, amoxicillin, and cephalosporins and less frequently with fluoroquinolones, tetracycline, carbapenems, and trimethoprim. The diarrhoea may be mild and self-limiting or debilitating and persistent and can be life-threatening. Although the diarrhoea generally resolves within a few days of discontinuation of the offending drug, together with fluid and electrolyte replacement, early specific antibacterial therapy should be given to patients with severe illness characterised by high fever, marked abdominal pain, and marked leucocytosis and to elderly, toxic, or debilitated patients, or those unresponsive to supportive therapy.[3,4] Antidiarrhoeal drugs should be avoided since they may aggravate the condition and may occasionally increase the possibility of toxic megacolon.[3]

Vancomycin or metronidazole are widely used when antibacterial treatment is necessary.[3-5] Metronidazole tends to be the drug of first choice and vancomycin is reserved for those who do not respond to, or who cannot tolerate, metronidazole, for those who are severely immunocompromised, and for those with severe illness.[3-6] This view is also endorsed by expert bodies in the USA whose aim is to provide guidelines for preventing the spread of vancomycin resistance.[7] Metronidazole can be given orally or intravenously as appropriate. Vancomycin is only given orally; it should not be given intravenously since it does not give rise to adequate concentrations of the drug in the bowel lumen.[3] The severity of the diarrhoea often decreases within 48 to 72 hours, but cessation may take a week or more. Treatment is usually continued for 10 days.[5] Relapses are quite common,[6] but usually respond to re-treatment with vancomycin or metronidazole.[3,6]

Other drugs that have been investigated in the treatment of antibiotic-associated colitis include teicoplanin,[8-10] fusidic acid,[10,11] and bacitracin,[12] although experience with their use remains limited.

The anion-exchange resins colestyramine and colestipol hydrochloride have been shown to bind the Cl. difficile toxin in vitro, and colestyramine has been used to treat pseudomembranous colitis.[13] The use of vancomycin together with colestyramine has been suggested,[14] but the value of the combination is uncertain. In general, the use of colestyramine is not recommended.[5]

Oral immunoglobulin A, used with vancomycin, was effective in controlling severe diarrhoea in a child who had not responded to other therapies.[15] Normal immunoglobulin given intravenously was also effective when added to vancomycin and metronidazole therapy in 2 elderly patients unresponsive to antibacterials alone.[16]

Treatment aimed at recolonising the gut with non-pathogenic organisms has included use of lactic-acid-producing organisms such as Lactobacillus,[17,18] and the yeasts Saccharomyces boulardii,[19,20] and S. cerevisiae.[21]

1. Danna PL, et al. Role of candida in pathogenesis of antibiotic-associated diarrhoea in elderly inpatients. Lancet 1991; 337: 511–14.
2. Gorbach SL. Antibiotics and Clostridium difficile. N Engl J Med 1999; 341: 1690–1.

3. Tabaqchali S, Jumaa P. Diagnosis and management of Clostridium difficile infection. BMJ 1995; 310: 1375–80.
4. Fekety R, Shah AB. Diagnosis and treatment of Clostridium difficile colitis. JAMA 1993; 269: 71–5.
5. ASHP. ASHP therapeutic position statement on the preferential use of metronidazole for the treatment of Clostridium difficile-associated disease. Am J Health-Syst Pharm 1998; 55: 1407–11.
6. Fekety R. Guidelines for the diagnosis and management of Clostridium difficile-associated diarrhea and colitis. Am J Gastroenterol 1997; 92: 739–50.
7. Hospital Infection Control Practices Advisory Committee (HICPAC). Recommendations for preventing the spread of vancomycin resistance. MMWR 1995; 44 (RR-12): 1–13.
8. de Lalla F, et al. Treatment of Clostridium difficile-associated disease with teicoplanin. Antimicrob Agents Chemother 1989; 33: 1125–7.
9. de Lalla F, et al. Prospective study of oral teicoplanin versus oral vancomycin for therapy of pseudomembranous colitis and Clostridium difficile-associated diarrhea. Antimicrob Agents Chemother 1992; 36: 2192–6.
10. Wenisch C, et al. Comparison of vancomycin, teicoplanin, metronidazole, and fusidic acid for the treatment of Clostridium difficile-associated diarrhea. Clin Infect Dis 1996; 22: 813–18.
11. Cronberg S, et al. Fusidic acid for the treatment of antibiotic-associated colitis induced by Clostridium difficile. Infection 1984; 12: 276–9.
12. Dudley MN, et al. Oral bacitracin vs vancomycin therapy for Clostridium difficile-induced diarrhea: a randomized double-blind trial. Arch Intern Med 1986; 146: 1101–4.
13. Pruksananonda P, Powell KR. Multiple relapses of Clostridium difficile-associated diarrhea responding to an extended course of cholestyramine. Pediatr Infect Dis J 1989; 8: 175–8.
14. Shwed JA, Rodvold KA. Anion-exchange resins and oral vancomycin in pseudomembranous colitis. DICP Ann Pharmacother 1989; 23: 70–1.
15. Tjellström B, et al. Oral immunoglobulin A supplement in treatment of Clostridium difficile enteritis. Lancet 1993; 341: 701–2.
16. Salcedo J, et al. Intravenous immunoglobulin therapy for severe Clostridium difficile colitis. Gut 1997; 41: 366–70.
17. Gorbach SL, et al. Successful treatment of relapsing Clostridium difficile colitis with Lactobacillus GG. Lancet 1987; ii: 1519.
18. Vanderhoof JA, et al. Lactobacillus GG in the prevention of antibiotic-associated diarrhea in children. J Pediatr 1999; 135: 564–8.
19. Surawicz CM, et al. Prevention of antibiotic-associated diarrhea by Saccharomyces boulardii: a prospective study. Gastroenterology 1989; 96: 981–8.
20. McFarland LV, et al. A randomized placebo-controlled trial of Saccharomyces boulardii in combination with standard antibiotics for Clostridium difficile disease. JAMA 1994; 271: 1913–18.
21. Schellenberg D, et al. Treatment of Clostridium difficile diarrhoea with brewer's yeast. Lancet 1994; 343: 171–2.

Campylobacter enteritis. Campylobacter jejuni is a major cause of acute diarrhoea. C. coli is less common and C. upsaliensis has been identified only recently as a probable enteropathogen.[1] Food is a common source of infection.[2] In the UK, several sources are responsible[3] including contaminated food and water and one important source is from doorstep deliveries of foil-topped bottled milk that have been pecked by birds.[3-5]

The macrolides erythromycin or azithromycin, or a fluoroquinolone are of benefit[6] in severely affected patients, but the infection is usually self-limiting and fluid and electrolyte replacement is generally sufficient. A tetracycline or gentamicin may be alternative antimicrobials.[6] Treatment with erythromycin can eradicate the organism from the faeces,[7-9] but may not reduce the duration of symptoms unless treatment is started early in the course of the disease.[7-9] Some strains of Campylobacter are resistant to erythromycin,[10] and resistance is also an increasing problem with ciprofloxacin.[11] Multiple drug resistance has been reported.[12]

Severe systemic infections with C. fetus require parenteral therapy with a carbapenem or gentamicin,[6] depending on susceptibility.

There is some evidence of an association between C. jejuni infection and the Guillain-Barré syndrome.[13]

1. Goossens H, et al. Is "Campylobacter upsaliensis" an unrecognised cause of human diarrhoea? Lancet 1990; 335: 584–6.
2. Skirrow MB. Foodborne illness: Campylobacter. Lancet 1990; 336: 921–3.
3. Pebody RG, et al. Outbreaks of campylobacter infection: rare events for a common pathogen. Commun Dis Rep 1997; 7: R33–R37.
4. Phillips CA. Bird attacks on milk bottles and campylobacter infection. Lancet 1995; 346: 386.
5. Stuart J, et al. Outbreak of campylobacter enteritis in a residential school associated with bird pecked bottle tops. Commun Dis Rep 1997; 7: R38–R40.
6. Anonymous. The choice of antibacterial drugs. Med Lett Drugs Ther 1999; 41: 95–104.
7. Anders BJ, et al. Double-blind placebo controlled trial of erythromycin for treatment of campylobacter enteritis. Lancet 1982; i: 131–2.
8. Mandal BK, et al. Double-blind placebo-controlled trial of erythromycin in the treatment of clinical campylobacter infection. J Antimicrob Chemother 1984; 13: 619–23.
9. Williams D, et al. Early treatment of Campylobacter jejuni enteritis. Antimicrob Agents Chemother 1989; 33: 248–50.
10. Taylor DN, et al. Erythromycin-resistant campylobacter infections in Thailand. Antimicrob Agents Chemother 1987; 31: 438–42.
11. Piddock LJV. Quinolone resistance and Campylobacter spp. J Antimicrob Chemother 1995; 36: 891–8.
12. Winstanley TG, et al. Multiple antibiotic resistance in a strain of Campylobacter jejuni acquired in Jordan. J Antimicrob Chemother 1993; 31: 178–9.
13. Rees JH, et al. Campylobacter jejuni infection and Guillain-Barré syndrome. N Engl J Med 1995; 333: 1374–9.

Cholera and other vibrio infections. Cholera results from infection with the enterotoxin-producing Gram-negative bacillus Vibrio cholerae which causes acute secretory diarrhoea. It can be associated with two serogroups of V. cholerae, O1 and O139. Serogroup O1 can then be divided into two biotypes (classical and El Tor) and each of these has three serotypes (Inaba, Ogawa, and Hikojima). The seventh pandemic began in 1961 in South East Asia, reached South America in January 1991,[1-6] and still shows no sign of abating. This pandemic is caused by V. cholerae O1 biotype El Tor. In late 1992 and 1993 epidemic cholera caused by V. cholerae O139 was reported in India and Bangladesh and subsequently identified in Thailand and other Asian countries. V. cholerae O139 became the dominant strain in India in less than 2 months and some workers declared it responsible for the eighth cholera pandemic.[2] However, there was some evidence that by 1994 it was abating and that by 1996 O1 was again the prevalent type in India and Bangladesh. There appears to be no cross-immunity between O1 and the O139 serogroup.

Individuals can reduce the risk of contracting cholera by avoiding possibly contaminated foodstuffs, good personal hygiene, and boiling or otherwise disinfecting drinking water. Methods of preventing or containing cholera epidemics include ensuring a safe water supply, providing good sanitation, and promoting safe handling and preparation of foods; mass chemoprophylaxis, vaccination, and travel and trade restrictions are not effective[7] although newer vaccines are showing more promise.

The majority of cases of vibrio gastro-enteritis are mild to moderate and generally require no therapy other than fluid and electrolyte replacement with an appropriate oral rehydration solution (see Diarrhoea, p.1203). Patients with severe gastro-enteritis, dehydration, and shock should receive vigorous fluid replacement, preferably intravenously.[8] Antimicrobial therapy has been shown to decrease the duration and volume of diarrhoea in cholera and may also decrease the duration of other vibrio diarrhoeas.[9] WHO[7] recommends a single dose of doxycycline as the treatment of choice for adults except pregnant women. Tetracycline, co-trimoxazole, furazolidone, erythromycin, and chloramphenicol are alternatives, with furazolidone being preferred for pregnant women and co-trimoxazole for children. Recommendations from the USA for adults specify a tetracycline as the first choice with co-trimoxazole or a fluoroquinolone such as ciprofloxacin as alternatives.[10] One study has suggested that single-dose ciprofloxacin might be preferred to doxycycline, particularly in areas of tetracycline resistance,[11] and in Bangladesh, ampicillin has been found to be as effective as either erythromycin or tetracycline[12] and may be a useful alternative in children. The O139 strain is reported to be sensitive to ciprofloxacin,[13] erythromycin,[13] and tetracyclines,[13] but resistant to co-trimoxazole.[2] There has also been some resistance to furazolidone.[2] Multiple drug resistance may be a problem; differing sensitivity and resistance patterns have been reported for the 2 biotypes classical and El Tor V. cholerae.[14] The outbreak strain in Rwandan refugees was resistant to tetracycline, doxycycline, co-trimoxazole, chloramphenicol, and ampicillin.[2]

Mass chemoprophylaxis is not recommended but may be justified for household contacts,[1,15] especially those at high risk because of age or pregnancy.[1] The type of cholera vaccines traditionally available are not very effective although some promising results have been reported with the use of oral vaccines in areas where cholera is endemic.

Marine or halophilic Vibrio spp. known to cause gastro-enteritis include V. parahaemolyticus which is responsible for food poisoning from raw or undercooked seafood especially in Japan.[16,17] Another halophilic sp., V. vulnificus, is increasingly associated with wound infection and septicaemia.[16] On the basis of in-vitro sensitivity testing[18] and anecdotal clinical experience, empirical therapy with aminoglycosides, ceftazidime, imipenem, or ciprofloxacin should all be effective.[19]

1. Anonymous. Cholera. Commun Dis Rep 1991; 1: R48–50.
2. Crowcroft NS. Cholera: current epidemiology. Commun Dis Rep 1994; 4: R157–64.
3. Swerdlow SL, Ries AA. Vibrio cholerae non-O1—the eighth pandemic? Lancet 1993; 342: 382–3.
4. Mahon BE, et al. Reported cholera in the United States, 1992–1994: a reflection of global changes in cholera epidemiology. JAMA 1996; 276: 307–12.
5. Seas C, Gotuzzo E. Cholera: overview of epidemiologic, therapeutic, and preventive issues learned from recent epidemics. Int J Infect Dis 1996; 1: 37–46.
6. Sánchez JL, Taylor DN. Cholera. Lancet 1997; 349: 1825–30.
7. WHO. Guidelines for cholera control. Geneva: WHO, 1993.

8. Morris JG, Black RE. Cholera and other vibrioses in the United States. *N Engl J Med* 1985; **312:** 343–50.
9. Blake PA. Vibrios on the half shell: what the walrus and the carpenter didn't know. *Ann Intern Med* 1983; **99:** 558–9.
10. Anonymous. The choice of antibacterial drugs. *Med Lett Drugs Ther* 1999; **41:** 95–104.
11. Khan WA, *et al.* Randomised controlled comparison of single-dose ciprofloxacin and doxycycline for cholera caused by Vibrio cholerae O1 or O139. *Lancet* 1996; **348:** 296–300.
12. Roy SK, *et al.* A randomized clinical trial to compare the efficacy of erythromycin, ampicillin and tetracycline for the treatment of cholera in children. *Trans R Soc Trop Med Hyg* 1998; **92:** 460–2.
13. Dhar U, *et al.* Clinical features, antimicrobial susceptibility and toxin production in Vibrio cholerae O139 infection: comparison with V. cholerae O1 infection. *Trans R Soc Trop Med Hyg* 1996; **90:** 402–5.
14. Siddique AK, *et al.* Simultaneous outbreaks of contrasting drug resistant classic and El Tor Vibrio cholerae O1 in Bangladesh. *Lancet* 1989; **ii:** 396.
15. WHO. WHO expert committee on cholera: second report. *WHO Tech Rep Ser 352* 1967.
16. Anonymous. Shuck your oysters with care. *Lancet* 1990; **336:** 215–16.
17. Doyle MP. Foodborne illness: pathogenic Escherichia coli, Yersinia enterocolitica, and Vibrio parahaemolyticus. *Lancet* 1990; **336:** 111–15.
18. French GL, *et al.* Antimicrobial susceptibilities of halophilic vibrios. *J Antimicrob Chemother* 1989; **24:** 183–94.
19. French GL. Antibiotics for marine vibrios. *Lancet* 1990; **336:** 568–9.

Escherichia coli enteritis. *Escherichia coli* is a normal intestinal commensal and member of the Gram-negative family of bacteria the Enterobacteriaceae. Pathogenic strains causing distinct syndromes of diarrhoeal disease and also associated with foodborne illness include: enteropathogenic *E. coli* (EPEC)—an important cause of infantile diarrhoea in many developing countries; enteroinvasive *E. coli* (EIEC)—producing an invasive type of diarrhoea resembling that of *Shigella* dysentery; enterotoxigenic *E. coli* (ETEC)—an important cause of travellers' diarrhoea (see Gastro-enteritis, above); and enterohaemorrhagic *E. coli* (EHEC)—associated with haemorrhagic colitis, haemolytic uraemic syndrome, and thrombotic thrombocytopenic purpura.[1] Enteroadherent *E. coli* (EAEC) is a cause of chronic diarrhoea in young children.[2]

Although these organisms are generally sensitive to a wide range of antibacterials only special categories of *E. coli* diarrhoea should be treated.[2]

Neonates with severe EPEC diarrhoea have been given oral non-absorbable antibacterials such as neomycin or gentamicin although in older children or adults this diarrhoea is said by some to be self-limiting.[2] Evidence for the efficacy of neomycin is largely limited to uncontrolled studies.[3] However, improvement with antibacterials has been noted beyond the neonatal period;[4] EPEC infection has been reported to be a common treatable cause of life-threatening *chronic* diarrhoea in infancy, possibly associated with travel to a developing country.[5] Symptoms could become persistent and life-threatening in previously healthy infants, requiring intravenous rehydration and parenteral antibacterials such as gentamicin and penicillin.[5]

Vero cytotoxin-producing strains of EHEC (VTEC; Shiga toxin producing *E. coli*), in particular serotype O157, have been associated with bloody diarrhoea, haemorrhagic colitis, and haemolytic uraemic syndrome.[6,7] Children and the elderly are regarded to be at high risk of severe disease,[6] but the illness is usually self-limiting.[7] Cases have generally been linked with the consumption of foods derived from cattle especially undercooked beef and raw milk, although there have been outbreaks associated with the consumption of fresh vegetables and unpasteurised juices, probably as a result of faecal contamination. Person-to-person spread is also common, and direct spread from infected animals may occur. *E. coli* O157 has also been reported as a cause of epidemic haemorrhagic colitis in Africa, where it may be difficult to distinguish from shigellosis.[8,9] Treatment is generally supportive, including correcting and maintaining the fluid and electrolyte balance.[7] Antibacterial treatment is controversial and there is uncertainty as to whether it influences the course of enterohaemorrhagic *E. coli* infection and the development of haemolytic-uraemic syndrome or thrombotic thrombocytopenic purpura;[6,7,10] the non-antibacterial treatment of these two latter complications is discussed in Plasma, under Thrombotic Microangiopathies, p.740. Oral preparations of Vero cytotoxin-binding resins are under investigation.

1. Doyle MP. Pathogenic Escherichia coli, Yersinia enterocolitica, and Vibrio parahaemolyticus. *Lancet* 1990; **336:** 1111–15.
2. Gorbach SL. Bacterial diarrhoea and its treatment. *Lancet* 1987; **ii:** 1378–82.
3. WHO. *The rational use of drugs in the management of acute diarrhoea in children.* Geneva: WHO, 1990.
4. Hill SM, *et al.* Antibiotics for Escherichia coli gastroenteritis. *Lancet* 1988; **i:** 771–2.
5. Hill SM, *et al.* Enteropathogenic Escherichia coli and life threatening chronic diarrhoea. *Gut* 1991; **32:** 154–8.
6. Mead PS, Griffin PM. Escherichia coli O157:H7. *Lancet* 1998; **352:** 1207–12.
7. Subcommittee of the PHLS Advisory Committee on Gastrointestinal Infections. Guidelines for the control of infection with Vero cytotoxin producing Escherichia coli (VTEC). *Commun Dis Public Health* 2000; **3:** 14–23.
8. Isaäcson M, *et al.* Haemorrhagic colitis epidemic in Africa. *Lancet* 1993; **341:** 961.
9. Paquet C, *et al.* Aetiology of haemorrhagic colitis epidemic in Africa. *Lancet* 1993; **342:** 175.
10. Farthing M, *et al.* The management of infective gastroenteritis in adults: a consensus statement by an expert panel convened by the British Society for the Study of Infection. *J Infect* 1996; **33:** 143–52.

Necrotising enterocolitis. Necrotising enterocolitis in the newborn is thought to result from hypoxia or ischaemic injury to the intestinal mucosa with subsequent infection. Bacteria implicated in the disease include *Pseudomonas, Escherichia coli, Klebsiella, Salmonella* spp., and *Clostridium* spp. Treatment involves suspension of oral feeding, intravenous fluid therapy, and surgical excision of the affected gut. References to the use of oral vancomycin for the treatment[1] of neonatal necrotising enterocolitis indicate that it may be of benefit. In a comparison of intravenous regimens to treat the condition it was reported that ampicillin with gentamicin appeared as effective as vancomycin with cefotaxime in neonates over 2200 g birth-weight, but in smaller neonates results were better with vancomycin and cefotaxime.[2] A systematic review has concluded that prophylactic oral antibacterials might well reduce the incidence of necrotising enterocolitis in very low birth-weight preterm infants in a high-risk environment,[3] but there are concerns about adverse outcomes, and prophylactic use (particularly of vancomycin) is not generally recommended because of the risk of inducing resistance.

Necrotising enteritis in older children and adults, known as pigbel, has been attributed to toxins produced by *Clostridium perfringens.* Both sporadic and epidemic forms are predominantly seen in the highlands of Papua New Guinea, but sporadic cases have been reported elsewhere. Treatment is supportive with surgical intervention where necessary. A vaccine is available for prophylaxis.

1. Han VKM. An outbreak of Clostridium difficile necrotizing enterocolitis: a case for oral vancomycin therapy? *Pediatrics* 1983; **71:** 935–41.
2. Scheifele DW, *et al.* Comparison of two antibiotic regimens for neonatal necrotizing enterocolitis. *J Antimicrob Chemother* 1987; **20:** 421–9.
3. Bury RG, Tudehope D. Enteral antibiotics for preventing necrotizing enterocolitis in low birthweight or preterm infants (updated 16 August 2001). Available in The Cochrane Library; Issue 4. Oxford: Update Software; 2001.

Salmonella enteritis. *Salmonella* spp. are Gram-negative bacteria belonging to the Enterobacteriaceae family. They can be divided into those causing enteric fever, namely *S. typhi* and *S. paratyphi*, where infection is systemic although affecting the gastrointestinal tract (see under Typhoid and Paratyphoid Fever, below) and non-typhoid *Salmonella*, including *S. enteritidis* and *S. typhimurium* which cause acute gastro-enteritis usually through food poisoning. There are numerous *Salmonella* serotypes identified with food poisoning and they have often been named according to the place where they were first isolated. The increase in salmonellosis in Great Britain has been almost entirely due to *S. enteritidis*[1] and this reflects an increase internationally.[2] Non-typhoid *Salmonella* spp. can cause invasive salmonellosis which may be manifest as septicaemia or localised infections such as meningitis or osteomyelitis.

Uncomplicated non-typhoid *Salmonella* enteritis is usually managed by fluid and electrolyte replacement. Antibacterial therapy produces no clinical benefit in uncomplicated *Salmonella* enteritis[3] and may prolong *Salmonella* detection in stools.[3] Attempts to eradicate the carrier state with antibacterial therapy (for example fluoroquinolones) appear to have been unsuccessful so far[4] and routine use is not recommended.[5] Patients with underlying debility or evidence of invasive salmonellosis should be given antibacterial therapy. Amoxicillin, ampicillin, or co-trimoxazole have been suggested[6,7] as have trimethoprim, cefotaxime,[7] ceftriaxone,[7] a fluoroquinolone[7] such as ciprofloxacin,[8] or chloramphenicol.[7] However, there is concern over the emergence of resistant strains, particularly to the fluoroquinolones.[9,10] Resistance to cephalosporins has also been recognised.[11] Multiresistant R-type strains of *S. typhimurium* DT 104 (another common cause of *Salmonella* enteritis in the UK) have severely limited the treatment options for infections with this organism.[12-15]

1. Baird-Parker AC. Foodborne salmonellosis. *Lancet* 1990; **336:** 1231–5.
2. Rodrigue DC, *et al.* International increase in Salmonella enteritidis: a new pandemic? *Epidemiol Infect* 1990; **105:** 21–7.
3. Sirinavin S, Garner P. Antibiotics for treating salmonella gut infections (updated 29 November 2000). Available in The Cochrane Library; Issue 4. Oxford: Update Software; 2001.
4. Nagler JM, *et al.* Salmonella gastroenteritis: longterm follow-up of an outbreak after treatment with norfloxacin or co-trimoxazole. *J Antimicrob Chemother* 1994; **34:** 291–4.
5. Farthing M. The management of infective gastroenteritis in adults: a consensus statement by an expert panel convened by the British Society for the Study of Infection. *J Infect* 1996; **33:** 143–52.
6. Gorbach SL. Bacterial diarrhoea and its treatment. *Lancet* 1987; **ii:** 1378–82.
7. Anonymous. The choice of antibacterial drugs. *Med Lett Drugs Ther* 1999; **41:** 95–104.
8. Leigh DA. The treatment of a large outbreak of acute bacterial gastroenteritis with ciprofloxacin. *J Antimicrob Chemother* 1992; **30:** 733–5.
9. Wilcox MH, Spencer RC. Quinolones and salmonella gastroenteritis. *J Antimicrob Chemother* 1992; **30:** 221–8.
10. Frost JA, *et al.* Increasing ciprofloxacin resistance in salmonellas in England and Wales 1991-1994. *J Antimicrob Chemother* 1996; **37:** 85–91.
11. Tzouvelekis LS, *et al.* Emergence of resistance to third-generation cephalosporins amongst Salmonella typhimurium isolates in Greece: report of the first three cases. *J Antimicrob Chemother* 1998; **42:** 273–5.
12. Threlfall EJ, *et al.* Increasing spectrum of resistance in multiresistant Salmonella typhimurium. *Lancet* 1996; **347:** 1053–4.
13. Anonymous. Multidrug-resistant Salmonella serotype typhimurium—United States, 1996. *JAMA* 1996; **277:** 1513.
14. Anonymous. Emergence of multidrug-resistant salmonella. *WHO Drug Inf* 1997; **11:** 21.
15. Trelfall EJ, *et al.* Multiresistant Salmonella typhimurium DT 104 and salmonella bacteraemia. *Lancet* 1998; **352:** 287–8.

Shigellosis. Shigellosis (bacillary dysentery) is an enteric infection caused by the *Shigella* spp. *S. dysenteriae, S. flexneri, S. boydii,* or *S. sonnei.* They are Gram-negative bacteria belonging to the Enterobacteriaceae and are able to invade the colon. Depending on the species involved, the disease ranges from mild self-limiting secretory diarrhoea to severe colitis and dysentery with blood and mucus in the stools. *S. dysenteriae* is the most common in the developing world and causes the most severe disease. In developed countries *S. flexneri* and *S. sonnei* are more common. Some *S. flexneri* can cause severe colitis and toxic dilatation of the colon has been reported in travellers.[1] *S. sonnei* is the least pathogenic of the species.

As with any form of diarrhoea rehydration is the key to treatment. Antibacterial therapy may be with ampicillin (amoxicillin appears to be less effective), co-trimoxazole (or trimethoprim), nalidixic acid, or fluoroquinolones such as ciprofloxacin, but will depend on the prevailing resistance patterns (see below) and the severity of the disease. Bacterial resistance is common and some consider that antibacterials should be restricted to the most severe cases, particularly those due to *S. dysenteriae;*[2] in the UK, the Public Health Laboratory Services (PHLS) Working Group has concluded that therapy is seldom indicated for *S. sonnei* infections.[3] WHO[4] has advised that children with *Shigella* dysentery should be given antimicrobial therapy and recommended co-trimoxazole as treatment of choice with nalidixic acid or ampicillin as alternatives; it was noted that resistance to ampicillin is frequent.[5]

The rapid development of resistance and the emergence of multiresistant strains of *Shigella*, particularly in developing countries, has led to some changes in treatment recommendations.[5] In 1992, nalidixic acid had become the preferred drug in developing countries unless ampicillin or co-trimoxazole were known to be effective in the region.[6] For *S. dysenteriae* it might be necessary to use pivmecillinam. It was concluded that the fluoroquinolones should continue to be reserved for infections resistant to nalidixic acid or pivmecillinam.[6] Reduced susceptibility to fluoroquinolones of some strains of *S. sonnei* has been reported from Japan.[7] Fluoroquinolones are generally not used in children although a study[8] in Bangladesh has used ciprofloxacin in children with shigellosis and found it to be of similar efficacy to pivmecillinam. In studies from Israel, the third-generation cephalosporins ceftriaxone[9] or cefixime[10] were more effective than ampicillin or co-trimoxazole, respectively, in children with shigellosis. Other studies in adults in Bangladesh found cefixime to be ineffective compared with pivmecillinam[11] and azithromycin to be effective, although slightly less so, than ciprofloxacin.[12]

Vitamin A may be a useful adjunct to treatment especially in children in developing countries (see Vitamin A, p.1383).

Oral shigella vaccines are being studied for prophylaxis.

1. Wilson APR, *et al.* Toxic dilatation of the colon in shigellosis. *BMJ* 1990; **301:** 1325–6.
2. Kaya IS, *et al.* Danger of antibiotic resistance in shigellosis. *Lancet* 1990; **336:** 186.

3. PHLS Working Group on the control of Shigella sonnei infection. Revised guidelines for the control of Shigella sonnei infection and other infective diarrhoeas. *Commun Dis Rep* 1993; **3**: R69–70.
4. WHO. *The rational use of drugs in the management of acute diarrhoea in children.* Geneva: WHO, 1990.
5. WHO. *The management and prevention of diarrhoea: practical guidelines.* 3rd ed. Geneva: WHO, 1993.
6. Bennish ML, Salam MA. Rethinking options for the treatment of shigellosis. *J Antimicrob Chemother* 1992; **30**: 243–7.
7. Horiuchi S, *et al.* Reduced susceptibilities of Shigella sonnei strains isolated from patients with dysentery to fluoroquinolones. *Antimicrob Agents Chemother* 1993; **37**: 2486–9.
8. Salam MA, *et al.* Randomised comparison of ciprofloxacin suspension and pivmecillinam for childhood shigellosis. *Lancet* 1998; **352**: 522–7.
9. Varsano I, *et al.* Comparative efficacy of ceftriaxone and ampicillin for treatment of severe shigellosis in children. *J Pediatr* 1991; **118**: 627–32.
10. Ashkenazi S, *et al.* A randomized, double-blind study comparing cefixime and trimethoprim-sulfamethoxazole in the treatment of childhood shigellosis. *J Pediatr* 1993; **123**: 817–21.
11. Salam MA, *et al.* Treatment of shigellosis: IV. Cefixime is ineffective in shigellosis in adults. *Ann Intern Med* 1995; **123**: 505–8.
12. Khan WA, *et al.* Treatment of shigellosis: V. Comparison of azithromycin and ciprofloxacin. *Ann Intern Med* 1997; **126**: 697–703.

Yersinia enteritis. *Yersinia enterocolitica* is a Gram-negative bacteria of the Enterobacteriaceae family and the species most commonly responsible for yersiniosis. The predominant form of infection is an enteric illness with or without mesenteric adenitis[1] although clinical manifestations can range from self-limited enterocolitis to potentially fatal systemic infection and post-infection complications can include erythema nodosum and reactive arthritis.[2] *Y. enterocolitica* is a recognised foodborne pathogen[3] and in some temperate countries rivals *Salmonella* and exceeds *Shigella* as a cause of acute gastro-enteritis; pigs are a major reservoir. Increased susceptibility to *Yersinia* infection has occurred in patients with iron overload treated with desferrioxamine and this is discussed further on p.1004.

Isolates of *Y. enterocolitica* are reported to be susceptible to co-trimoxazole, aminoglycosides, chloramphenicol, tetracycline, third-generation cephalosporins, and quinolones *in vitro*.[1,2] As with any form of diarrhoea rehydration is the key to treatment and most forms of mild uncomplicated enteritis do not require antibacterial treatment. There has been no general consensus concerning the antibacterial of choice when treatment becomes necessary: as with other enteric infections there is a lack of good clinical evidence. Drugs with good intracellular activity such as trimethoprim, co-trimoxazole, tetracycline, chloramphenicol, or fluoroquinolones may be preferred.[1] Doxycycline or co-trimoxazole have been recommended for complicated gastrointestinal and focal extra-intestinal infections or doxycycline and an aminoglycoside empirically in bacteraemia. Co-trimoxazole as first choice or alternatively a fluoroquinolone, an aminoglycoside, cefotaxime, or ceftizoxime have also been recommended.[4] A patient with chronic *Yersinia* infection who responded well to tetracycline or co-trimoxazole, but relapsed on withdrawal, has been treated successfully with ciprofloxacin.[5]

1. Hoogkamp-Korstanje JAA. Antibiotics in Yersinia enterocolitica infection. *J Antimicrob Chemother* 1987; **20**: 123–31.
2. Cover TL, Aber RC. Yersinia enterocolitica. *N Engl J Med* 1989; **321**: 16–24.
3. Doyle MP. Pathogenic Escherichia coli, Yersinia enterocolitica, and Vibrio parahaemolyticus. *Lancet* 1990; **336**: 1111–15.
4. Anonymous. The choice of antibacterial drugs. *Med Lett Drugs Ther* 1999; **41**: 95–104.
5. Reid RC, Barry RE. Relapsing yersinia infection. *BMJ* 1990; **300**: 164.

Gonorrhoea

Gonorrhoea is a sexually transmitted disease caused by infection of mucosa with *Neisseria gonorrhoeae* (gonococcus) a Gram-negative bacterium. It occurs predominantly as urethritis in men and cervicitis in women and also as pharyngitis, proctitis, or conjunctivitis. Complications of gonococcal infections include pelvic inflammatory disease (see below) in women and epididymitis (above) in men. Disseminated gonococcal infection results from gonococcal bacteraemia and may lead to septic arthritis, an arthritis-dermatitis syndrome (not to be confused with Reiter's disease which has been associated with non-gonococcal or non-specific urethritis), and more rarely with conditions such as endocarditis or meningitis. Gonorrhoea in pregnant women may cause neonatal conjunctivitis (ophthalmia neonatorum).

Infection with *Chlamydia trachomatis* (see under Chlamydial Infections, above) often occurs along with gonorrhoea and should be tested for or treated presumptively.

N. gonorrhoeae used to be sensitive to penicillins and tetracyclines but in some areas, including the USA, this is no longer the case. Gonococcal resistance includes plasmid-mediated penicillin resistance, due to penicillinase-producing *N. gonorrhoeae* (PPNG); high-level plasmid-mediated tetracycline resistance (TRNG); and chromosomally mediated resistance (CMRNG), not due to beta-lactamase production, including resistance to penicillin, tetracycline, cefoxitin, or spectinomycin.[1,2]

Although resistant strains of *N. gonorrhoeae* have generally been slower to emerge in the UK than in some other parts of the world, increasing world travel and population mixing means that clinicians in the UK have to be aware of the possibility of antibacterial resistant infections. Single doses of ciprofloxacin or ofloxacin are recommended for uncomplicated infections unless the organism can be demonstrated to be fully sensitive to penicillins, in which case ampicillin plus probenecid may be used.[3] Infections acquired outside the UK are presumed to be resistant to penicillins.

In the USA the wide distribution of antimicrobial-resistant *N. gonorrhoeae*, as documented by the Gonococcal Isolate Surveillance Project,[2] has necessitated revised treatment guidelines. In 1998 the Centers for Disease Control (CDC)[4] recommended single-dose cephalosporins or fluoroquinolones as the treatment of choice for uncomplicated gonorrhoea, rather than penicillin or tetracycline, plus treatment for chlamydial infection that commonly co-exists with gonorrhoea (see below for details).

Of concern are the increasing number of reports of resistance to newer antigonococcal drugs such as the fluoroquinolones from the UK,[5,6] the western Pacific region,[7,8] the Indian sub-continent,[9] Canada,[10] and the USA.[11,12] Recommended *treatment regimens* from WHO[13] in 2001 and CDC[4] in 1998 are as follows. Where appropriate, sexual partners should be tested and treated.

• UNCOMPLICATED GONOCOCCAL INFECTIONS IN ADULTS.

WHO (for anogenital infections): a single oral dose of ciprofloxacin 500 mg, azithromycin 2 g, or cefixime 400 mg, or a single intramuscular dose of ceftriaxone 125 mg or spectinomycin 2 g.

Alternatives that may be useful in some countries, depending on the prevalence of resistance, are kanamycin 2 g intramuscularly as a single dose or co-trimoxazole 4.8 g once daily by mouth for three days.

CDC (for uncomplicated infections in general): a single intramuscular dose of ceftriaxone 125 mg or single oral doses of cefixime 400 mg, ciprofloxacin 500 mg, or ofloxacin 400 mg. Other cephalosporins or fluoroquinolones may be substituted. Spectinomycin 2 g as a single intramuscular dose is an alternative in patients who cannot tolerate cephalosporins or fluoroquinolones. For pharyngeal infections ceftriaxone, ciprofloxacin, or ofloxacin are recommended (as they are also in the UK[3]). In each case CDC advocates concomitant treatment for presumptive chlamydial infections with either azithromycin 1 g orally as a single dose or doxycycline 100 mg twice daily for 7 days.

CDC recommends a cephalosporin or spectinomycin for pregnant women with gonorrhoea, and erythromycin or amoxicillin for chlamydial infection.

• GONOCOCCAL EYE INFECTIONS IN ADULTS.

WHO[13] recommends a single dose of ceftriaxone 125 mg intramuscularly, or spectinomycin 2 g intramuscularly, or ciprofloxacin 500 mg by mouth together with frequent irrigation of the infected eye with saline. Kanamycin 2 g intramuscularly is another alternative.

CDC[4] recommends a single dose of ceftriaxone 1 g intramuscularly together with irrigation of the infected eye with saline.

• DISSEMINATED GONOCOCCAL INFECTIONS IN ADULTS.

WHO[13] recommends ceftriaxone 1 g intramuscularly or intravenously once daily or spectinomycin 2 g intramuscularly twice daily for 7 days. Another third-generation cephalosporin may be substituted if neither of these drugs is available.

CDC[4] recommends the following regimens: initially ceftriaxone 1 g intramuscularly or intravenously every 24 hours, ceftizoxime 1 g intravenously every 8 hours, or cefotaxime 1 g intravenously every 8 hours. Ciprofloxacin 500 mg intravenously every 12 hours, ofloxacin 400 mg intravenously every 12 hours, or spectinomycin 2 g intramuscularly every 12 hours may be substituted in patients allergic to beta lactams. Once improvement has been established for 24 to 48

hours oral therapy with cefixime 400 mg, ciprofloxacin 500 mg, or ofloxacin 400 mg, all twice daily may be substituted for the remainder of the 1-week treatment period. For gonococcal *meningitis* and *endocarditis* CDC advises ceftriaxone 1 to 2 g intravenously every 12 hours initially. Treatment for meningitis should continue for 10 to 14 days and for endocarditis for at least 4 weeks.

• GONOCOCCAL INFECTIONS IN INFANTS AND CHILDREN.

Infants born to mothers with gonorrhoea are at high risk of infection and require prophylactic treatment.

WHO[13] recommends a single intramuscular injection of ceftriaxone 50 mg per kg body-weight (maximum 125 mg), or spectinomycin 25 mg per kg (maximum 75 mg), or kanamycin 25 mg per kg (maximum 75 mg) if ceftriaxone is not available.

CDC[4] suggests a single injection of ceftriaxone 25 to 50 mg per kg (maximum 125 mg). For those infants with disseminated gonococcal infection (sepsis, arthritis, meningitis) a 7-day course of ceftriaxone or cefotaxime is recommended, extended to 10 to 14 days if meningitis is present. The prevention and treatment of neonatal gonococcal conjunctivitis is discussed under Neonatal Conjunctivitis, below.

The treatment recommended by CDC[4] for *children* with gonococcal infections, most commonly due to sexual abuse in pre-adolescents, is as for adults in those weighing 45 kg or more. For those weighing less than 45 kg CDC recommends a single intramuscular dose of ceftriaxone 125 mg or spectinomycin 40 mg per kg (maximum 2 g) for those with uncomplicated infections; for disseminated infection they recommend an intramuscular or intravenous dose of ceftriaxone 50 mg per kg (maximum 1 g) once daily for 7 days, extended to 10 to 14 days and a maximum dose of 2 g in those weighing more than 45 kg.

1. Judson FN. Management of antibiotic-resistant Neisseria gonorrhoeae. *Ann Intern Med* 1989; **110**: 5–7.
2. Schwarcz SK, *et al.* National surveillance of antimicrobial resistance in Neisseria gonorrhoeae. *JAMA* 1990; **264**: 1413–17.
3. Clinical Effectiveness Group (Association of Genitourinary Medicine and the Medical Society for the Study of Venereal Diseases). National guideline for the management of gonorrhoea in adults. *Sex Transm Infect* 1999; **75** (suppl 1): S13–S15.
4. Centers for Disease Control. 1998 Guidelines for treatment of sexually transmitted diseases. *MMWR* 1998; **47** (RR-1): 59–69.
5. Gransden WR, *et al.* Decreased susceptibility of Neisseria gonorrhoeae to ciprofloxacin. *Lancet* 1990; **335**: 51. Correction. *ibid.*; 302.
6. Ison CA, *et al.* Drift in susceptibility of Neisseria gonorrhoeae to ciprofloxacin and emergence of therapeutic failure. *Antimicrob Agents Chemother* 1998; **42**: 2919–22.
7. Tapsall JW. Surveillance of antibiotic resistance in Neisseria gonorrhoeae and implications for the therapy of gonorrhoea. *Int J STD AIDS* 1995; **6**: 233–6.
8. Tanaka M, *et al.* Antimicrobial susceptibility of Neisseria gonorrhoeae in Fukuoka City, Japan, in the early 1980s and 1997-1998: emergence of high-level fluoroquinolone resistance. *Antimicrob Agents Chemother* 1999; **43**: 722–3.
9. Bhuiyan BU, *et al.* High prevalence of ciprofloxacin resistance amongst strains of Neisseria gonorrhoeae isolated from commercial sex workers in Bangladesh. *J Antimicrob Chemother* 1998; **48**: 675–6.
10. Yeung KH, Dillon JR. Norfloxacin resistant Neisseria gonorrhoeae in North America. *Lancet* 1990; **336**: 759.
11. Gordon SM, *et al.* The emergence of Neisseria gonorrhoeae with decreased susceptibility to ciprofloxacin in Cleveland, Ohio: epidemiology and risk factors. *Ann Intern Med* 1996; **125**: 465–70.
12. Knapp JS, *et al.* Emerging in vitro resistance to quinolones in penicillinase-producing Neisseria gonorrhoeae strains in Hawaii. *Antimicrob Agents Chemother* 1994; **38**: 2200–3.
13. WHO. Guidelines for the management of sexually transmitted infections. Geneva: WHO, 2001.

Granuloma inguinale

Granuloma inguinale or donovanosis is caused by the Gram-negative bacterium *Calymmatobacterium granulomatis* and occurs most commonly in the tropics and subtropics, especially Papua New Guinea and India. It is characterised by genital ulcers and is generally considered to be a sexually transmitted disease.

WHO[1] recommends azithromycin 1 g by mouth on the first day then 500 mg by mouth once daily, or doxycycline 100 mg orally twice daily. Alternative drugs include erythromycin, tetracycline, or co-trimoxazole. The addition of parenteral gentamicin should be considered for HIV-infected patients. All treatment should be continued until all lesions have completely resolved. Streptomycin is no longer recommended because of its toxicity and the need to reserve it for tuberculosis.

In the USA the Centers for Disease Control[2] recommend treatment with co-trimoxazole 960 mg twice daily or doxycycline 100 mg twice daily, both for a minimum of 3 weeks, with ciprofloxacin 750 mg twice daily or erythromycin 500 mg four times daily also for 3 weeks as alternatives. The addition of an aminoglycoside may be considered if lesions do not respond during the first few days of treatment.

Other drugs shown to be effective include azithromycin, ceftriaxone, and norfloxacin.[3]

1. WHO. Guidelines for the management of sexually transmitted infections. Geneva: WHO, 2001.
2. Centers for Disease Control. 1998 Guidelines for treatment of sexually transmitted diseases. *MMWR* 1998; **47** (RR-1): 26–7.
3. Clinical Effectiveness Group (Association of Genitourinary Medicine and the Medical Society for the Study of Venereal Diseases). National guideline for the management of donovanosis (granuloma inguinale). *Sex Transm Infect* 1999; **75** (suppl 1): S38–S39.

Haemophilus influenzae infections

Haemophilus influenzae is a Gram-negative bacterium that colonises the upper respiratory tract in the majority of healthy people. Most are carriers of non-encapsulated strains, but a small proportion carry *H. influenzae* type b, the commonest encapsulated strain. Serious invasive infections have usually been caused by type b strains and have occurred mainly in young children. They include the bacteraemic diseases meningitis, pneumonia, epiglottitis, cellulitis, and arthritis. Non-encapsulated strains commonly cause otitis media, sinusitis, and conjunctivitis and infect patients with chronic bronchitis. However, they too can cause invasive infections such as pneumonia, septicaemia, and meningitis[1] and, with the introduction of *H. influenzae* type b vaccines, non-encapsulated strains may be responsible for a greater proportion of invasive *H. influenzae* disease.

For further details of these infections and their management, see under the specific disease side-headings.

Ampicillin and chloramphenicol have been the antibacterials of choice against *H. influenzae*, but increasing resistance, especially to ampicillin, should be borne in mind; there have been several reports of multiresistant strains.[2-5] Injectable cephalosporins are popular alternatives for multiresistant type b organisms although there is controversy over their effectiveness against fully sensitive strains when compared with ampicillin or chloramphenicol or both; experience has been favourable with cefotaxime and ceftriaxone, but there have been treatment failures in *H. influenzae* meningitis with cefuroxime and there is argument over its efficacy.[6]

For serious *H. influenzae* infections cefotaxime, ceftriaxone, or chloramphenicol are currently preferred. For less serious infections, ampicillin, amoxicillin (with or without clavulanic acid), oral second- or third-generation cephalosporins, co-trimoxazole (or trimethoprim in the UK), tetracyclines, or the macrolides azithromycin and clarithromycin are suggested alternatives.[7]

In the UK, secondary prophylaxis with rifampicin is given following *H. influenzae* type b meningitis (see below). A vaccine against *H. influenzae* type b is available and vaccination is included in the infant immunisation schedules in some countries including the UK and USA.

1. Falla TJ, *et al.* Population-based study of non-typable Haemophilus influenzae invasive disease in children and neonates. *Lancet* 1993; **341**: 851–4.
2. Sturm AW, *et al.* Outbreak of multiresistant non-encapsulated Haemophilus influenzae infections in a pulmonary rehabilitation centre. *Lancet* 1990; **335**: 214–16.
3. Brightman CAJ, *et al.* Family outbreak of chloramphenicol-ampicillin resistant Haemophilus influenzae type b disease. *Lancet* 1990; **335**: 351–2.
4. Barclay K, *et al.* Multiresistant Haemophilus influenzae. *Lancet* 1990; **335**: 549.
5. Scott GM, *et al.* Outbreaks of multiresistant Haemophilus influenzae infection. *Lancet* 1990; **335**: 925.
6. Powell M. Chemotherapy for infections caused by Haemophilus influenzae: current problems and future prospects. *J Antimicrob Chemother* 1991; **27**: 3–7.
7. Anonymous. The choice of antibacterial drugs. *Med Lett Drugs Ther* 1999; **41**: 95–104.

Helicobacter pylori infections

Antibacterial therapy is used to eradicate *Helicobacter pylori* infection in peptic ulcer disease (p.1208) and MALT lymphoma of the stomach (p.488). The role of *H. pylori* and the value of its eradication in dyspepsia (p.1204) and gastro-oesophageal reflux disease (p.1204) is less clear.

Infections in immunocompromised patients

Patients with a defective immune system are at special risk of infection. Primary immune deficiency is rare, whereas secondary deficiency is more common: immunosuppressive therapy, cancer and its treatment, HIV infection, and splenectomy may all cause neutropenia and impaired humoral and cellular immunity in varying degrees. The risk and severity of infections depends upon the duration of compromised immunity, the degree to

which immune function is compromised, whether cellular or humoral functions are affected, and upon breaches in physical barriers, for example by severe mucositis or prolonged vascular access. Thus patients with profound neutropenia or a history of splenectomy are prone to rapidly progressive and potentially life-threatening infections; those with neutropenia induced by cytotoxic chemotherapy or by preparation for transplantation are particularly vulnerable to acute infections whereas those in whom immunosuppression results from viral infections or congenital defects are at lower risk of acute infections.[1] Patients in whom neutropenia persists for more than 10 days are not only at risk of opportunistic bacterial infections but also susceptible to viral, fungal, and parasitic infections.

Infectious diseases are a major cause of morbidity and mortality in patients with AIDS (see HIV-associated Infections, p.610). Some are due to common pathogens, and others are opportunistic and are caused by normally avirulent commensals. Children with HIV infection appear to be at special risk of serious bacterial infections with common encapsulated bacteria. For further reference to some bacterial infections associated with AIDS, see under Gastro-enteritis (above), Opportunistic Mycobacterial Infections (below), and Tuberculosis (below). Fungal, protozoal, and viral infections which can affect immunocompromised patients are discussed in the relevant chapters under Infections in Immunocompromised Patients, p.374, p.584, and p.611, respectively.

Common causative organisms of unexplained fever in neutropenic patients include the Gram-negative bacteria *Pseudomonas aeruginosa*, *Escherichia coli*, and *Klebsiella* spp. and Gram-positive organisms particularly staphylococci, streptococci, enterococci, and *Corynebacterium* spp. Gram-negative organisms have historically been responsible for most immediate life-threatening infections, but Gram-positive infections are increasing in importance and now predominate in many areas.[1,2] Factors influencing this change include the wider use of selective gut decontamination and of central venous catheters,[3] and possibly the prophylactic use of quinolones.

TREATMENT. Onset of fever in neutropenic patients is indicative of serious infection which may progress to septicaemia and death and empirical antibacterial therapy, usually parenterally, should be started immediately.

The severity of infections depends on a number of factors (see above) and it is consequently difficult to produce a standard drug regimen. In addition the choice of empirical therapy needs to be adapted depending on the prevailing infecting organisms and the emergence of drug resistant pathogens.[2,4,5]

While a combination of an aminoglycoside and an antipseudomonal cephalosporin or penicillin has been commonly used and remains the treatment of choice in many centres, monotherapy is becoming increasingly popular. Monotherapy with ceftazidime has been shown to be as effective as combination therapy, even in severely neutropenic patients,[6,7] although activity against Gram-positive infections may be inadequate. Carbapenems (imipenem/cilastatin or meropenem) have activity against both Gram-positive and Gram-negative organisms and provide an alternative monotherapy. However, imipenem has not been adopted for routine use because of its toxicity, and carbapenems have generally poor activity against meticillin-resistant *Staphylococcus aureus* and vancomycin-resistant enterococci.[2] The monobactams, which have little activity against Gram-positive organisms, are a less suitable choice. The fluoroquinolones have been studied but results are conflicting.[8-10]

There is some evidence[11,12] that oral empirical therapy may be practical.

Antibacterial combinations studied in an attempt to avoid aminoglycoside-related toxicity and the need for monitoring blood concentrations include combinations of two or more beta lactams[13] and the monobactam aztreonam with flucloxacillin.[14] However, there are concerns over both the activity and possible selection of resistant organisms with some of these regimens.[15] Withdrawal of the aminoglycoside when the patient stabilises or improves is less effective than continuing with the complete regimen.[16] Vancomycin or teicoplanin have been used in the initial regimen in centres with a high incidence of meticillin-resistant *Staphylococcus* spp.,[17] but have not been shown to produce additional benefits elsewhere.[18] They are more often used as adjuncts if there is evidence of Gram-positive infection.[2] The emergence of vancomycin-resistant strains of *Enterococcus* spp. and *Staphylo-*

coccus spp. means that empirical use of vancomycin should probably be discouraged.[19]

The optimum duration of therapy depends on the clinical situation. Antibacterial treatment can be discontinued after 5 to 7 days in patients in whom both the infection and the neutropenia resolve.[15] In those in whom the fever resolves but neutropenia persists treatment can probably be stopped after 10 days[2,15] or alternatively 5 to 7 days after the fever resolves[20] provided that patients are subsequently closely monitored and suitable prophylaxis is continued. In patients with continuing neutropenia, prolonged antibacterial use once the fever has resolved can predispose to fungal superinfections, but re-infection is a potential hazard if the drugs are stopped. In patients with persistent fever, it is sometimes possible to identify the pathogen and adjust the treatment accordingly. If no infecting organism can be identified and non-infective causes of fever can be ruled out, several options remain.[20] If the patient's condition does not deteriorate, the initial regimen can be continued unchanged, especially if neutropenia is expected to resolve within a few days. If there is clinical deterioration, vancomycin or teicoplanin can be added to improve cover against Gram-positive pathogens,[2,20] alternative broad spectrum antibacterials may be substituted for the original therapy,[2] or an antifungal[20] could be considered.

An ongoing series of studies by the International Antimicrobial Therapy Cooperative Group of the European Organisation for Research and Treatment of Cancer has attempted to assess the efficacy of a range of therapeutic and prophylactic strategies[5] and the Infectious Diseases Society of America is publishing a series of guidelines.[20]

The routine use of colony-stimulating factors as an adjunct to antibacterial treatment is not generally recommended[20] but may be indicated in neutropenic patients at high risk of serious infections or infection-related complications; examples include some patients with malignant neoplasms[21] and those with persistent severe neutropenia and infections that are not responsive to antibacterials alone.[20]

PROPHYLAXIS. Most infections in immunosuppressed patients are caused by organisms from their own alimentary tract and in cancer patients, for example, may follow chemotherapy-induced mucosal damage to the tract. Although antibacterial prophylaxis may be effective in non-febrile patients likely to be neutropenic, the efficacy of empirical treatment means that prophylaxis is less widely used[22] and the Infectious Diseases Society of America[20] discourages routine use; reasons include toxicity of the antibacterial, potential fungal overgrowth, and problems of bacterial resistance (see below). Most experience with prophylaxis has been in patients with leukaemia. Possible prophylactic regimens have included selective decontamination of the alimentary tract using oral nonabsorbable antibacterials (see also under Intensive Care, below). Co-trimoxazole has also been widely used.[22] More recently, prophylaxis with fluoroquinolones has been commonly used although, generally, prophylaxis with these drugs has resulted in reduction in Gram-negative but not in Gram-positive infections in immunocompromised patients,[23] and improved morbidity and mortality has not been observed.[24] Combination prophylaxis with fluoroquinolones and phenoxymethylpenicillin[25] or rifampicin[26] has been tried to improve cover against Gram-positive organisms. Nevertheless, concern about the emergence of resistant organisms has led to the recommendation that routine prophylaxis should be avoided.[20]

Immunocompromised patients may benefit from appropriate immunisation against common infections, although precautions relating to the administration of live vaccines in such patients should be observed (p.1530).

The duration and severity of neutropenia can be reduced by the use granulocyte or granulocyte-macrophage colony-stimulating factors, and this may be a useful adjunct in infection control in selected patients.[21] Bone marrow protective agents such as amifostine are also being studied.

For further reference to prophylaxis in high-risk patients, see under Intensive Care, below.

1. Pizzo PA. Fever in immunocompromised patients. *N Engl J Med* 1999; **341**: 893–900.
2. Plunkett T, *et al.* Complications of chemotherapy 1: the management of neutropenia and febrile neutropenia. *CME Oncol* 1998; **1**: 40–4.
3. Oppenheim BA. The changing pattern of infection in neutropenic patients. *J Antimicrob Chemother* 1998; **41** (suppl D): 7–11.
4. Klastersky J. Science and pragmatism in the treatment and prevention of neutropenic infection. *J Antimicrob Chemother* 1998; **41** (suppl D): 13–24.

5. Viscoli C. The evolution of the empirical management of fever and neutropenia in cancer patients. *J Antimicrob Chemother* 1998; **41** (suppl B): 65–80.
6. Pizzo PA, *et al.* A randomized trial comparing ceftazidime alone with combination antibiotic therapy in cancer patients with fever and neutropenia. *N Engl J Med* 1986; **315**: 552–8.
7. De Pauw BE, *et al.* Ceftazidime compared with piperacillin and tobramycin for the empiric treatment of fever in neutropenic patients with cancer: a multicenter randomized trial. *Ann Intern Med* 1994; **120**: 834–44.
8. Meunier F, *et al.* Prospective randomized evaluation of ciprofloxacin versus piperacillin plus amikacin for empiric antibiotic therapy of febrile granulocytopenic cancer patients with lymphomas and solid tumours. *Antimicrob Agents Chemother* 1991; **35**: 873–8.
9. Johnson PRE, *et al.* A randomized trial of high-dose ciprofloxacin versus azlocillin and netilmicin in the empirical therapy of febrile neutropenic patients. *J Antimicrob Chemother* 1992; **30**: 203–14.
10. Malik IA, *et al.* Randomised comparison of oral ofloxacin alone with combination of parenteral antibiotics in neutropenic febrile patients. *Lancet* 1992; **339**: 1092–6. [N.B. Correction to ofloxacin dosage (it should be 400 mg twice daily) in *Lancet* 1992; **340**: 128].
11. Freifeld A, *et al.* A double-blind comparison of empirical oral and intravenous antibiotic therapy for low-risk febrile patients with neutropenia during cancer chemotherapy. *N Engl J Med* 1999; **341**: 305–11.
12. Kern WV, *et al.* Oral versus intravenous empirical antimicrobial therapy for fever in patients with granulocytopenia who are receiving cancer chemotherapy. *N Engl J Med* 1999; **341**: 312–18.
13. Winston DJ, *et al.* Beta-lactam antibiotic therapy in febrile granulocytopenic patients: a randomized trial comparing cefoperazone plus piperacillin, ceftazidime plus piperacillin, and imipenem alone. *Ann Intern Med* 1991; **115**: 849–59.
14. Heney D, *et al.* Aztreonam therapy in children with febrile neutropenia: a randomized trial of aztreonam plus flucloxacillin versus piperacillin plus gentamicin. *J Antimicrob Chemother* 1991; **28**: 117–29.
15. Boogaerts MA. Anti-infective strategies in neutropenia. *J Antimicrob Chemother* 1995; **36** (suppl A): 167–78.
16. EORTC International Antimicrobial Therapy Cooperative Group. Ceftazidime combined with a short or long course of amikacin for empirical therapy of gram-negative bacteremia in cancer patients with granulocytopenia. *N Engl J Med* 1987; **317**: 1692–8.
17. Menichetti F, *et al.* Effects of teicoplanin and those of vancomycin in initial empirical antibiotic regimen for febrile, neutropenic patients with hematological malignancies. *Antimicrob Agents Chemother* 1994; **38**: 2041–6.
18. European Organization for Research and Treatment of Cancer (EORTC) International Antimicrobial Therapy Cooperative Group and the National Cancer Institute of Canada—Clinical Trials Group. Vancomycin added to empirical combination antibiotic therapy for fever in granulocytopenic cancer patients. *J Infect Dis* 1991; **163**: 951–8.
19. Centers for Disease Control. Hospital Infection Control Practices Advisory Committee (HICPAC). Recommendations for preventing the spread of vancomycin resistance. *MMWR* 1995; **44** (RR-12): 1–13.
20. Infectious Diseases Society of America. 1997 Guidelines for the use of antimicrobial agents in neutropenic patients with unexplained fever. *Clin Infect Dis* 1997; **25**: 551–73.
21. American Society of Clinical Oncology. 2000 Update of recommendations for the use of hematopoietic colony-stimulating factors: evidence-based, clinical practice guidelines. *J Clin Oncol* 2000; **18**: 3558–85.
22. Kerr KG. The prophylaxis of bacterial infections in neutropenic patients. *J Antimicrob Chemother* 1999; **44**: 587–91.
23. Engels EA, *et al.* Efficacy of quinolone prophylaxis in neutropenic cancer patients: a meta-analysis. *J Clin Oncol* 1998; **16**: 1179–87.
24. Cruciani M, *et al.* Prophylaxis with fluoroquinolones for bacterial infections in neutropenic patients: a meta-analysis. *Clin Infect Dis* 1996; **23**: 795–805.
25. International Antimicrobial Therapy Cooperative Group of the European Organization for Research and Treatment of Cancer (EORTC). Reduction of fever and streptococcal bacteremia in granulocytopenic patients with cancer: a trial of oral penicillin V or placebo combined with pefloxacin. *JAMA* 1994; **272**: 1183–9.
26. Bow EJ, *et al.* Quinolone-based antibacterial chemoprophylaxis in neutropenic patients: effect of augmented gram-positive activity on infectious morbidity. *Ann Intern Med* 1996; **125**: 183–90.

Intensive care

Similarly to immunocompromised patients (above), those in intensive care units are often very susceptible to endogenous infections, especially respiratory and urinary-tract infections, arising from gastrointestinal colonisation by aerobic Gram-negative bacilli acquired in hospital. Selective digestive tract decontamination (SDD), using oral non-absorbable antibacterial regimens, and selective parenteral and enteral antisepsis regimens (SPEAR), incorporating selective decontamination together with systemic antibacterial prophylaxis, have been used in an attempt to prevent colonisation and infection in these high-risk patients, although their effectiveness is debated. SDD has generally not been widely adopted in the USA[1] particularly in relation to prevention of nosocomial pneumonia.[2,3] It may be more effective in surgical patients.[4]

Selective decontamination is achieved by elimination of aerobic, potentially pathogenic, organisms from throat and intestines while preserving the indigenous, mostly anaerobic, flora.[5] Regimens commonly include two or three non-absorbable or poorly absorbed antibacterial drugs, for example colistin, neomycin, norfloxacin, or polymyxin, in combination with an antifungal, usually amphotericin B. The drugs are usually applied topically to the oropharyngeal mucosa in addition to oral or intragastric administration, although local application to the oropharynx alone is also reported to be effective.[6,7] A parenteral third-generation cephalosporin, usually cefotaxime, may be given for a few days until oral medication takes effect.[8,9] Strict adherence to the protocol is reported to be necessary for maximum efficacy[10] and constant monitoring for the emergence of antimicrobial resistance is considered essential[9,10] although so far this has rarely been seen in practice.[10,11] However, most regimens have little or no activity against potential Gram-positive pathogens such as *Enterococcus* spp., and so their use may increase the risk for colonisation and infection with these organisms.[12] There is particular concern over the emergence of vancomycin-resistant strains.

Despite numerous clinical studies, many of which have shown a reduction in potential Gram-negative pathogens[8,9,13] and in the incidence of respiratory-tract infections,[6,7] it has been difficult to demonstrate that SDD or SPEAR reduces mortality.[14-17] Although meta-analyses[18,19] of randomised controlled trials concluded that a combination of a systemic and topical antibacterial could be beneficial it has been argued that the effect was largely due to the systemic component of the treatment.[20] It has been suggested[21] that equivalent infection control could be achieved more economically by emphasis on high standards of hygiene and avoidance of histamine H_2-receptor antagonists, which could allow overgrowth of potentially pathogenic bacteria as a result of the change in gastric pH.

Another potential source of infection in intensive care is from the use of **intravascular catheters**. The organisms implicated most frequently have been coagulase-negative staphylococci.[22] Prevention and control of infection depend on good aseptic technique and care of the insertion site, and also catheter design.[22,23] Catheters should be removed as soon as possible (often after 48 to 72 hours for peripheral lines) and any infections treated promptly with antibacterials; vancomycin or teicoplanin are appropriate for empirical treatment so long as resistance is not a problem.[22] The effectiveness of antibacterial prophylaxis has not been fully tested, although there are some favourable studies.[24] Topical antiseptics and antibacterials have produced promising results.[22] Antibacterials could also prove useful in reducing or eliminating colonisation of the catheter lumen[25] and catheters coated with antibacterials[26] or heparin[27] are under investigation. Randomised clinical studies have shown that the use of catheters coated with minocycline and rifampicin[28] or with antiseptics (p.1130) can reduce the risk of systemic infections.

The importance of maintaining high standards of infection control, including handwashing, in intensive care units has been reinforced by the increasing incidence of nosocomial infections that are difficult to treat such as those due to vancomycin-resistant enterococci and *Acinetobacter*. In one such outbreak due to *A. baumannii* some strains were resistant to imipenem and all other antibacterials except polymyxin B and sulbactam.[29] Intensive infection control measures and irrigation of all open wounds with polymyxin B solution were used to eliminate infection and colonisation.

1. Kollef MH. The prevention of ventilator-associated pneumonia. *N Engl J Med* 1999; **340**: 627–34. Correction. *ibid.*; **341**: 294.
2. American Thoracic Society. Hospital-acquired pneumonia in adults: diagnosis, assessment of severity, initial antimicrobial therapy, and preventative strategies: a consensus statement. *Am J Respir Crit Care Med* 1995; **153**: 1711–25.
3. Centers for Disease Control. Guidelines for prevention of nosocomial pneumonia. *MMWR* 1997; **46** (RR-1): 1–79.
4. Nathens AB, Marshall JC. Selective decontamination of the digestive tract in surgical patients: a systematic review of the evidence. *Arch Surg* 1999; **134**: 170–6.
5. van Saene HKF, Stoutenbeek CP. Selective decontamination. *J Antimicrob Chemother* 1987; **20**: 462–5.
6. Rodriguez-Roldan JM, *et al.* Prevention of nosocomial lung infection in ventilated patients: use of an antimicrobial pharyngeal nonabsorbable paste. *Crit Care Med* 1990; **18**: 1239–42.
7. Pugin J, *et al.* Oropharyngeal decontamination decreases incidence of ventilator-associated pneumonia: a randomized, placebo-controlled, double-blind clinical trial. *JAMA* 1991; **265**: 2704–10.
8. Ledingham IM, *et al.* Triple regimen of selective decontamination of the digestive tract, systemic cefotaxime, and microbiological surveillance for prevention of acquired infection in intensive care. *Lancet* 1988; **i**: 785–90.
9. Tetteroo GWM, *et al.* Selective decontamination to reduce gram-negative colonisation and infections after oesophageal resection. *Lancet* 1990; **335**: 704–7.
10. Tetteroo GWM, *et al.* Bacteriology of selective decontamination: efficacy and rebound colonisation. *J Antimicrob Chemother* 1994; **34**: 139–48.
11. van Saene HKF, *et al.* Cefotaxime combined with selective decontamination in long term intensive care unit patients: virtual absence of emergence of resistance. *Drugs* 1988; **35** (suppl 2): 29–34.
12. Bonten MJM, *et al.* Colonization and infection with Enterococcus faecalis in intensive care units: the role of antimicrobial agents. *Antimicrob Agents Chemother* 1995; **39**: 2783–6.
13. Aerdts SJA, *et al.* Prevention of bacterial colonization of the respiratory tract and stomach of mechanically ventilated patients by a novel regimen of selective decontamination in combination with initial systemic cefotaxime. *J Antimicrob Chemother* 1990; **26** (suppl A): 59–76.
14. Loirat P, *et al.* Selective digestive decontamination in intensive care unit patients. *Intensive Care Med* 1992; **18**: 182–8.
15. Vandenbroucke-Grauls CMJE, Vandenbroucke JP. Effect of selective decontamination of the digestive tract on respiratory tract infections and mortality in the intensive care unit. *Lancet* 1991; **338**: 859–62.
16. van Saene HKF, *et al.* Selective decontamination of the digestive tract in the intensive care unit: current status and future prospects. *Crit Care Med* 1992; **20**: 691–703.
17. Selective Decontamination of the Digestive Tract Trialists' Collaborative Group. Meta-analysis of randomised controlled trials of selective decontamination of the digestive tract. *BMJ* 1993; **307**: 525–32.
18. Liberati A, *et al.* Antibiotics for preventing respiratory tract infections in adults receiving intensive care (updated 21 November 2000). Available in The Cochrane Library; Issue 2. Oxford: Update Software; 2001.
19. D'Amico R, *et al.* Effectiveness of antibiotic prophylaxis in critically ill adult patients: systematic review of randomised controlled trials. *BMJ* 1998; **316**: 1275–85.
20. Kollef MH. The prevention of ventilator-associated pneumonia. *N Engl J Med* 1999; **341**: 294.
21. Atkinson SW, Bihari DJ. Selective decontamination of the gut. *BMJ* 1993; **306**: 286–7.
22. Elliott TSJ. Line-associated bacteraemias. *Commun Dis Rep* 1993; **3**: R91–R96.
23. Raad I. Intravascular-catheter-related infections. *Lancet* 1998; **351**: 893–8.
24. Spafford PS, *et al.* Prevention of central venous catheter-related coagulase-negative staphylococcal sepsis in neonates. *J Pediatr* 1994; **125**: 259–63.
25. Yassien M, *et al.* Modulation of biofilms of Pseudomonas aeruginosa by quinolones. *Antimicrob Agents Chemother* 1995; **39**: 2262–8.
26. Raad I, *et al.* Antibiotics and prevention of microbial colonization of catheters. *Antimicrob Agents Chemother* 1995; **39**: 2397–2400.
27. Appelgren P, *et al.* Does surface heparinisation reduce bacterial colonization of central venous catheters? *Lancet* 1995; **345**: 130.
28. Raad I, *et al.* Central venous catheters coated with minocycline and rifampin for the prevention of catheter-related colonization and bloodstream infections: a randomized, double-blind trial. *Ann Intern Med* 1997; **127**: 267–74.
29. Go ES, *et al.* Clinical and molecular epidemiology of acinetobacter infections sensitive only to polymyxin B and sulbactam. *Lancet* 1994; **344**: 1329–32.

Legionnaires' disease

Legionnaires' disease is a legionella pneumonia caused by the Gram-negative bacterium *Legionella pneumophila*. Serious outbreaks have been associated with infected air-conditioning systems or water supplies. Pontiac fever is a milder, usually self-limiting, influenza-like illness also caused by *L. pneumophila* as well as by other *Legionella* spp. Legionellosis has been suggested as a broad term to cover pneumonic and non-pneumonic clinical syndromes caused by any *Legionella* spp., which may include *L. bozemanii*, *L. micdadei* (Pittsburgh pneumonia agent), and *L. wadsworthii*.

Erythromycin has been the usual treatment for *Legionella* infections but azithromycin is increasingly used in preference;[1,2] clarithromycin may be a further acceptable alternative macrolide.[3,4] Fluoroquinolones are also increasingly recommended as alternatives to the macrolides.[1,2,4] Rifampicin has been given in addition especially in severe or deteriorating illness or in immunocompromised patients,[3,4] although some consider this to be of little further benefit.[1]

1. Edelstein PH. Antimicrobial chemotherapy for Legionnaires disease: time for a change. *Ann Intern Med* 1998; **129**: 328–30.
2. Dedicoat M, Venkatesan P. The treatment of Legionnaires' disease. *J Antimicrob Chemother* 1999; **43**: 747–52.
3. Roig J, *et al.* Treatment of legionnaires' disease: current recommendations. *Drugs* 1993; **46**: 63–79.
4. Stout JE, Yu VL. Legionellosis. *N Engl J Med* 1997; **337**: 682–7.

Leprosy

Leprosy (Hansen's disease) is a chronic disease caused by *Mycobacterium leprae*; it affects the peripheral nervous system, the skin, and some other tissues. It is transmitted from person-to-person when bacilli are shed from the nose and skin lesions of infected patients, but most individuals are naturally immune, and symptoms are suppressed. Clinical leprosy may be regarded as a consequence of deficient cell-mediated immunity in susceptible individuals. For the purpose of grouping patients for chemotherapy, leprosy may be classified as multibacillary or paucibacillary.

Multibacillary leprosy occurs when cellular immunity is largely deficient, and includes the sub-groups lepromatous (LL), borderline lepromatous (BL), and midborderline leprosy (BB) as well as any other types giving a positive skin smear for acid-fast bacilli. Generally the lepromin test (p.1628) is negative. Paucibacillary leprosy results when cellular immunity is only partially deficient, and includes the sub-groups borderline tuberculoid (BT), tuberculoid (TT), and indeterminate leprosy (I) when the skin smear is negative. Generally the lepromin test is positive. For the purpose of treatment, WHO now classifies patients with more than 5 skin lesions as multibacillary, and those with 1 to 5 skin lesions as paucibacillary. It further classifies patients with only one skin lesion as having paucibacillary single-lesion leprosy. The use of this clinical classification avoids the necessity to provide facilities for bacteriological examination of skin smears.

Reactive episodes may be seen in leprosy patients undergoing treatment; they are known as *lepra reactions* and unless treated may lead to deformity and disability. Most reactions belong to one of two main types. *Type 1* lepra reactions or reversal reactions are delayed hypersensitivity reactions (type IV hypersensitivity). Prompt treatment with corticosteroids is necessary to prevent permanent nerve damage.[1-3] *Type 2* lepra reactions, also known as erythema nodosum leprosum (ENL), represent a humoral antibody response (type III hypersensitivity) to dead bacteria. Mild type 2 reactions may be treated with anti-inflammatories but moderate or severe reactions should be treated with corticosteroids or thalidomide.[1-4] The incidence of neuritis has decreased since the inclusion of clofazimine in multidrug regimens and is probably due to the drug's anti-inflammatory action; a further reduction in high-risk patients has been achieved by the use of an initial loading dose.[5] Clofazimine does not act as rapidly as either corticosteroids or thalidomide, nor is it as effective, but it may be used in chronic type 2 reactions in doses of up to 300 mg daily.[1,2,4,6] Antileprotic drug therapy is generally continued during lepra reactions.

Dapsone given on its own was for a long time the mainstay of leprosy treatment. However, the emergence of resistance to dapsone and to other antileprotics led to the use of multidrug therapy regimens consisting of 2 or 3 drugs with dapsone, rifampicin, and clofazimine being the standard ones. Newer alternatives include clarithromycin, minocycline, and fluoroquinolones such as ofloxacin. Ethionamide or protionamide have been used in place of clofazimine in light-skinned patients, but are no longer recommended because of their severe hepatotoxicity.

The most widely used multidrug regimens are those recommended by WHO[1] and in these the choice of drugs and length of treatment are based on the clinical classification outlined above.

MULTIBACILLARY LEPROSY.

The standard regimen recommended by WHO for multibacillary leprosy[1,3] is rifampicin 600 mg and clofazimine 300 mg both given once a month together with clofazimine 50 mg and dapsone 100 mg both daily. Treatment is continued for 12 months.[3] When multidrug therapy was introduced patient compliance was considered essential for successful treatment. Ideally, the monthly rifampicin and clofazimine doses were given under supervision and dapsone ingestion could be verified by a urine spot test. Subsequent demonstration of the high efficacy of the regimen has allowed WHO to take a pragmatic approach, recommending flexible delivery systems to ensure that patients have access to treatment even when supervision of the monthly dose is impractical.[1,3] A 2-year treatment duration was chosen originally because it is highly effective in the majority of cases and avoids the need to assess response with skin smears. However, such a long treatment duration is an obstacle to implementing treatment programmes in areas where healthcare is inaccessible or infrastructure poor. Ongoing clinical studies and experience with patients defaulting from treatment have encouraged WHO to now recommend that treatment for 12 months is adequate.[1,3] Nevertheless, there has been concern that prolonged treatment (beyond 2 years) may be necessary in patients with high pretreatment bacterial loads.[7-10] Early hopes that reducing duration of treatment to as little as one month would be possible have not been supported by a study using daily rifampicin and ofloxacin.[11]

In patients for whom rifampicin is unsuitable because of resistance or intolerance WHO recommends[1] daily treatment with clofazimine 50 mg, ofloxacin 400 mg, and minocycline 100 mg for the first 6 months; treatment is then continued for a further 18 months with clofazimine together with either minocycline or ofloxacin. When clofazimine cannot be given because of unacceptable skin pigmentation ofloxacin 400 mg daily or minocycline 100 mg daily may be substituted in the standard regimen.[12] Alternatively, rifampicin 600 mg, ofloxacin 400 mg, and minocycline 100 mg could be administered once a month for 24 months.[1]

PAUCIBACILLARY LEPROSY.

The WHO recommended regimen[1,3] for paucibacillary leprosy is rifampicin 600 mg once monthly and dapsone 100 mg daily. Treatment is continued for 6 months. If there are severe toxic effects with dapsone it should be stopped and clofazimine substituted.[12] On the basis of a clinical study[13] showing that a single dose of rifampicin 600 mg, ofloxacin 400 mg, and minocycline 100 mg given in combination is only slightly less effective than standard multidrug treatment, WHO has suggested that this is a suitable alternative for patients with single lesion paucibacillary leprosy.[1] However, reservations have been expressed about the study including concerns regarding the short follow-up[14] and poor microbiological rationale.[15]

RELAPSE.

Relapse following a recommended course of multidrug therapy for multibacillary or paucibacillary leprosy can occur and WHO recommends re-treatment with the appropriate regimen.[1,3] Although the relapse rate following multidrug therapy for multibacillary leprosy generally appears to be low,[1,16] there is concern that further reduction of treatment duration could be detrimental (see above).

PREGNANCY.

Pregnant and breast feeding leprosy patients experience clinical deterioration and in general antileprotic therapy is continued in such patients.

PROPHYLAXIS.

Leprosy is spread from person to person, so household contacts may be at risk. Administration of dapsone prophylaxis to some household contacts[17,18] may prevent disease in this high-risk group. WHO[1] suggests that contacts of newly diagnosed cases should be examined for evidence of leprosy and then advised how to watch for early signs of the disease; prophylaxis with rifampicin or other antileprotics is not recommended in leprosy control programmes. BCG vaccine appears to be protective. Vaccines specifically against leprosy are under investigation.

ELIMINATION.

The multidrug therapy regimens recommended by WHO have been widely implemented in recent years. Their success has led to the World Health Assembly setting a goal in 1991 of elimination of leprosy as a public health problem by the year 2000: that is, reducing the prevalence to less than 1 case per 10 000 population in endemic areas. This did not occur in 2000, although it was announced one year later, in May 2001, that the goal had been achieved. Full control of leprosy in all countries, however, had still not been attained and continued efforts were necessary for leprosy programmes.

1. WHO. WHO expert committee on leprosy. *WHO Tech Rep Ser* 874 1998.
2. Britton WJ, Lockwood DNJ. Leprosy reactions: current and future approaches to management. *Baillieres Clin Infect Dis* 1997; 4: 1–23.
3. WHO. *Guide to eliminate leprosy as a public health problem.* 1st ed. Geneva: WHO, 2000.
4. Lockwood DNJ. The management of erythema nodosum leprosum: current and future options. *Lepr Rev* 1996; 67: 253–9.
5. Arunthathi S, Satheesh KK. Does clofazimine have a prophylactic role against neuritis? *Lepr Rev* 1997; 68: 233–41.
6. Jacobson RR, Krahenbuhl JL. Leprosy. *Lancet* 1999; 353: 655–60.
7. Jakeman P. Risk of relapse in multibacillary leprosy. *Lancet* 1995; 345: 4–5.
8. Waters MFR. Relapse following various types of multidrug therapy in multibacillary leprosy. *Lepr Rev* 1995; 66: 1–9. Correction. *ibid.*; 192.
9. Jamet P, et al. Relapse after long-term follow-up of multibacillary patients treated by WHO multidrug regimen. *Int J Lepr* 1995; 63: 195–201.
10. Waters MFR. Is it safe to shorten multidrug therapy for lepromatous (LL and BL) leprosy to 12 months? *Lepr Rev* 1998; 69: 110–11.
11. Ji B, et al. High relapse rate among lepromatous leprosy patients treated with rifampin plus ofloxacin daily for 4 weeks. *Antimicrob Agents Chemother* 1997; 41: 1953–6.
12. WHO. Chemotherapy of leprosy. *WHO Tech Rep Ser* 847 1994.
13. Single-lesion Multicentre Trial Group. Efficacy of single-dose multidrug therapy for the treatment of single-lesion paucibacillary leprosy. *Indian J Lepr* 1997; 68: 341–9.
14. Lockwood DNJ. Rifampicin/minocycline and ofloxacin (ROM) for single lesions—what is the evidence? *Lepr Rev.* 1997; 68: 299–300.
15. Katoch VM. Is there a microbiological rationale for single-dose treatment of leprosy? *Lepr Rev* 1998; 69: 2–5.
16. World Health Organisation Leprosy Unit. Risk of relapse in leprosy. *Indian J Lepr* 1995; 67: 13–26.
17. Filice GA, Fraser DW. Management of household contacts of leprosy patients. *Ann Intern Med* 1978; 88: 538–42.
18. Dayal R, Bharadwaj VP. Prevention and early detection of leprosy in children. *J Trop Pediatr* 1995; 41: 132–8.

Leptospirosis

Leptospirosis is an infectious disease caused by serovars of the spirochaete *Leptospira interrogans*, the commonest in the UK being *L. hardjo* and *L. icterohaemorrhagiae*.[1] *Leptospira* are widely distributed in wild and domestic animals, including cattle. Rats are a common source of infection in man and transmission is often by contact with water or soil contaminated with infected urine. In England and Wales there were 299 confirmed cases of leptospirosis during 1985 to 1989;[1] the main occupational group at risk was farmers and agricultural workers. The data were insufficient to confirm whether recreational water users such as canoeists were at increased risk, but outbreaks among such groups have been reported elsewhere.[2] The majority of symptomatic patients have no more than a mild influenza-like illness, although a small proportion develop Weil's disease with haemorrhagic complications and severe liver and kidney failure.

The use of antibacterials is controversial since many recover without treatment. However, when leptospirosis is suspected treatment within 4 to 7 days has been recommended to prevent complications.[3,4] The intravenous administration of either benzylpenicillin 900 mg, ampicillin 1 g, or erythromycin 500 mg every 6 hours, or the oral administration of amoxicillin 500 mg every 8 hours or doxycycline 100 mg twice daily has been suggested;[4] treatment is continued for 7 days. Benzylpenicillin has been given intravenously in higher doses for severe leptospirosis; 7.2 to 9.6 g daily for 5 days followed by 1.44 g daily for a further 5 days has been advocated.[5] However, intravenous doses of 900 mg every 6 hours for 7 days have proved successful even when given late in the course of illness.[6] In severe infections, supportive therapy with analgesics and antiemetics may be required. Renal function should be monitored and dialysis instigated if necessary, and blood products may be necessary to control haemorrhagic complications.[3]

Doxycycline has reduced the incidence of leptospirosis when given prophylactically to USA soldiers in Panama.[7] Leptospirosis vaccines are available in some countries.

1. Ferguson IR. Leptospirosis update. *BMJ* 1991; 302 128–9.
2. Centers for Disease Control. Outbreak of leptospirosis among white-water rafters—Costa Rica, 1996. *MMWR* 1997; 46: 577–9.
3. Ferguson I. Uncommon infections I: leptospirosis. *Prescribers' J* 1991; 31: 185–9.
4. Ferguson IR. Leptospirosis surveillance: 1990-1992. *Commun Dis Rep* 1993; 3: R47–R48.
5. Anonymous. Leptospira outbreak in cattle and man. *J R Coll Gen Pract* 1985; 35: 36.
6. Watt G, et al. Placebo-controlled trial of intravenous penicillin for severe and late leptospirosis. *Lancet* 1988; i: 433–5.
7. Takafuji ET, et al. An efficacy trial of doxycycline chemoprophylaxis against leptospirosis. *N Engl J Med* 1984; 310: 497–500.

Listeriosis

Listeriosis is caused by *Listeria monocytogenes*, a Gram-positive bacterium widespread in the environment and capable of growing at low temperatures. Increased awareness of *L. monocytogenes* as a human pathogen has followed epidemics of listeriosis associated with the consumption of contaminated food products including soft cheeses, coleslaw, and milk. *L. monocytogenes* has since been detected in many types of food, especially uncooked hot dogs, undercooked chicken, and pâté.[1] A comprehensive review[2] acknowledged that it is a relatively rare infection and that despite epidemics associated with identified food products it typically occurs sporadically and the source is usually not certain. Infection occurs primarily in pregnant women, neonates, the elderly, and immunocompromised patients. Clinical manifestations vary. Pregnant women may have relatively mild flu-like symptoms, but infection may result in spontaneous abortion, fetal death, or perinatal sepsis or meningitis in the neonate. Non-perinatal listeriosis may cause sepsis but commonly presents as meningitis. Endocarditis has occurred in patients with cardiac lesions. Focal infections following initial bacteraemia occur mainly in immunocompromised patients.

The treatment of choice is generally ampicillin with gentamicin,[2-4] although some have advocated ampicillin alone;[5] synergy has been reported *in vitro*. Ampicillin or amoxicillin alone may be used in pregnant women.[6] In penicillin-allergic patients co-trimoxazole, erythromycin, and tetracycline are alternatives,[2] but the choice of treatment in these patients is more difficult. Gentamicin with chloramphenicol or with vancomycin has been used[3] as has erythromycin plus gentamicin.[7] According to some,[3] tetracycline should not be used to treat listeriosis in the UK because of bacterial resistance.

Further details specifically concerning neonatal listerial meningitis and its treatment can be found under Meningitis, below.

1. Jones D. Foodborne listeriosis. *Lancet* 1990; **336:** 1171–4.
2. Gellin BG, Broome CV. Listeriosis. *JAMA* 1989; **261:** 1313–20.
3. MacGowan AP. Listeriosis—the therapeutic options. *J Antimicrob Chemother* 1990; **26:** 721–2.
4. Temple ME, Nahata MC. Treatment of listeriosis. *Ann Pharmacother* 2000; **34:** 656–61.
5. Kessler SL, Dajani AS. Listeria meningitis in infants and children. *Pediatr Infect Dis J* 1990; **9:** 61–3.
6. Wilkinson P. Uncommon infections 2: listeriosis. *Prescribers' J* 1992; **32:** 26–31.
7. MacGowan AP, *et al.* Maternal listeriosis in pregnancy without fetal or neonatal infection. *J Infect* 1991; **22:** 53–7.

Lyme disease

Lyme disease is a seasonal infectious disease caused by the spirochaete *Borrelia burgdorferi* and transmitted primarily by *Ixodes* ticks. It was first recognised in the 1970s in Lyme, Connecticut, but when the spirochaete responsible was later identified, Lyme disease was found to occur worldwide with regional variations. Lyme disease is a multisystem disease that principally affects the skin, nervous system, heart, and joints, and can be divided into 3 stages. In the early stage a characteristic skin lesion, erythema migrans, may be accompanied by flu-like or meningitis-like symptoms. This may be followed weeks or months later by signs of disseminated infection including neurological and cardiac abnormalities and even years later by chronic arthritis and the late skin manifestation acrodermatitis chronica atrophicans, both signs of persistent infection.

Appropriate treatment should prove curative, especially in the early stages. Current recommendations for treatment[1,2] give oral doxycycline (or tetracycline) or amoxicillin as the antibacterials of choice for **early stage** Lyme disease and mild neurological and cardiac symptoms. Alternatives include oral cephalosporins such as cefuroxime or the macrolides azithromycin or clarithromycin. In pregnant women or young children amoxicillin (or phenoxymethylpenicillin) may be used or erythromycin in those allergic to penicillin, although erythromycin has been associated with a high failure rate. In general duration of treatment ranges from 14 to 21 days, but depends on individual response.

Intravenous ceftriaxone, cefotaxime, or benzylpenicillin are recommended for early stage Lyme disease with acute neurological symptoms of meningitis or radiculopathy, or for **late stage** Lyme disease including meningitis, serious cardiac symptoms, and arthritis; doxycycline or amoxicillin by mouth for 28 days may also be used in Lyme arthritis without clinically evident neurological disease.

Preventive measures against Lyme disease include the use of tick repellents and physical protection.[2,3] After tick bites empirical treatment with doxycycline may be warranted in endemic areas where the probability of infection is high,[4] but generally the risk of infection is low,[5] particularly if the tick is removed promptly. The risk of infection may be greater if the tick has fed to repletion.[6] Most guidelines[2,3] do not support the use of empirical antibacterial therapy following tick bites, and the cost effectiveness of parenteral therapy in those with positive serological test results and non-specific symptoms has been questioned.[7,8] Lyme disease vaccines are available in some countries.

1. Loewen PS, *et al.* Systematic review of the treatment of early Lyme disease. *Drugs* 1999; **57:** 157–73.
2. Infectious Diseases Society of America. Practice guidelines for the treatment of Lyme disease. *Clin Infect Dis* 2000; **31:** 1–14.
3. American Academy of Pediatrics Committee on Infectious Diseases. Prevention of Lyme disease. *Pediatrics* 2000; **105:** 142–7.
4. Magid D, *et al.* Prevention of Lyme disease after tick bites: a cost-effectiveness analysis. *N Engl J Med* 1992; **327:** 534–41.
5. Shapiro ED, *et al.* A controlled trial of antimicrobial prophylaxis for Lyme disease after deer-tick bites. *N Engl J Med* 1992; **327:** 1769–73.
6. Matuschka F-R, Spielman A. Risk of infection from and treatment of tick bite. *Lancet* 1993; **342:** 529–30.
7. Lightfoot RW, *et al.* Empiric parenteral antibiotic treatment of patients with fibromyalgia and fatigue and a positive serologic result for lyme disease: a cost-effectiveness analysis. *Ann Intern Med* 1993; **119:** 503–9.
8. Luft BJ, *et al.* Appropriateness of parenteral antibiotic treatment for patients with presumed Lyme disease: a joint statement of the American College of Rheumatology and the Council of the Infectious Diseases Society of America. *Ann Intern Med* 1993; **119:** 518.

Lymphogranuloma venereum

Lymphogranuloma venereum or chlamydial lymphogranuloma is caused by infection with certain serotypes of *Chlamydia trachomatis* and is endemic in tropical areas, but may also occur in the developed world. It is

a sexually transmitted disease and in the early phase may cause genital ulceration although the commonest clinical manifestation is inguinal lymphadenopathy. There is multisystem involvement and late complications, including those related to fibrosis and abnormal lymphatic drainage, may require surgery.

WHO[1] recommends treatment with doxycycline, erythromycin, or tetracycline, given by mouth for 2 weeks. UK[2] and US[3] guidelines recommend treatment for 3 weeks with doxycycline or alternatively with erythromycin.

1. WHO. Guidelines for the management of sexually transmitted infections. Geneva: WHO, 2001.
2. Clinical Effectiveness Group (Association of Genitourinary Medicine and the Medical Society for the Study of Venereal Diseases). National guideline for the management of lymphogranuloma venereum. *Sex Transm Infect* 1999; **75** (suppl 1): S40–S42.
3. Centers for Disease Control. 1998 Guidelines for treatment of sexually transmitted diseases. *MMWR* 1998; **47** (RR-1): 27–8.

Melioidosis

Melioidosis is caused by the Gram-negative aerobic bacterium *Burkholderia pseudomallei* (*Pseudomonas pseudomallei*), and has been found mainly in south-east Asia and northern Australia. Its true incidence and distribution may be much wider than originally thought;[1] diagnosis is difficult because of the broad spectrum of clinical manifestations. Pulmonary melioidosis is probably the commonest form and has been treated with doxycycline for 3 to 6 months.[2] Chronic or subacute non-bacteraemic melioidosis has also been treated long term with tetracycline or co-trimoxazole.[2]

Septicaemic melioidosis is an important cause of death in Thailand. Because *B. pseudomallei* is intrinsically resistant to many antibacterials, including aminoglycosides and the early beta lactams, it has been unresponsive to many empirical regimens for septicaemia.[1] Until recently, treatment has been based on anecdotal regimens, but in a study from Thailand[3] intravenous ceftazidime halved the mortality of severe melioidosis when compared with conventional parenteral treatment with high doses of chloramphenicol intravenously, doxycycline, and co-trimoxazole. As a result ceftazidime came to be considered the treatment of choice for septicaemic melioidosis.[1] A systematic review[4] of treatment of acute melioidosis has also concluded that regimens should contain ceftazidime or imipenem parenterally. Parenteral treatment for a minimum of 7 days is followed by oral maintenance therapy with amoxicillin-clavulanic acid or the conventional regimen (chloramphenicol, doxycycline, and co-trimoxazole);[3] amoxicillin-clavulanic acid has shown promise[3] and appears to be a safe alternative to the conventional regimen for the oral treatment of melioidosis.[5] However, resistance to ceftazidime and amoxicillin-clavulanic acid has been reported,[6] emphasising the importance of careful monitoring for the emergence of resistance during treatment. Ceftazidime plus co-trimoxazole, both given intravenously, has been advocated by some for severe melioidosis, especially in patients with septicaemia.[7]

B. pseudomallei has the potential for prolonged latency as demonstrated by a Vietnam war veteran who presented with melioidosis of the bone 18 years after exposure to the organism.[8] He was treated with ceftriaxone intravenously for 8 weeks followed by oral ciprofloxacin.

1. Dance DAB. Pseudomonas pseudomallei: danger in the paddy fields. *Trans R Soc Trop Med Hyg* 1991; **85:** 1–3.
2. Guard RW, *et al.* Melioidosis in far north Queensland: a clinical and epidemiological review of twenty cases. *Am J Trop Med Hyg* 1984; **33:** 467–73.
3. White NJ, *et al.* Halving of mortality of severe melioidosis by ceftazidime. *Lancet* 1989; **ii:** 697–701.
4. Samuel M, Ti TY. Interventions for treating melioidosis (updated 28 February 2001). Available in The Cochrane Library; Issue 4. Oxford: Update Software; 2001.
5. Rajchanuvong A, *et al.* A prospective comparison of co-amoxiclav and the combination of chloramphenicol, doxycycline, and co-trimoxazole for the oral maintenance treatment of melioidosis. *Trans R Soc Trop Med Hyg* 1995; **89:** 546–9.
6. Dance DAB, *et al.* Development of resistance to ceftazidime and co-amoxiclav in Pseudomonas pseudomallei. *J Antimicrob Chemother* 1991; **28:** 321–4.
7. Sookpranee M, *et al.* Multicenter prospective randomized trial comparing ceftazidime plus co-trimoxazole with chloramphenicol plus doxycycline and co-trimoxazole for treatment of severe melioidosis. *Antimicrob Agents Chemother* 1992; **36:** 158–62.
8. Koponen MA, *et al.* Melioidosis: forgotten but not gone. *Arch Intern Med* 1991; **151:** 605–8.

Meningitis

Initiation of bacterial meningitis involves colonisation of the nasopharynx by the bacterial pathogen, invasion into the blood stream (bacteraemia), survival in the blood stream (enhanced in encapsulated bacteria), invasion of the meninges, bacterial replication, and subarachnoid space inflammation.[1,2] The bacteria most often responsible for meningitis are *Streptococcus pneumoniae* (pneumococci), *Haemophilus influenzae*, and *Neisseria meningitidis* (meningococci). Other causes include *Listeria monocytogenes*, *Pseudomonas aeruginosa*, and Gram-negative enteric bacilli. *H. influenzae* is more common in infants and young children whereas in neonates *Escherichia coli* and group B streptococci are the most frequent causes. Overall *H. influenzae* meningitis has appeared to be more common in the USA than in the UK but, as elsewhere, its incidence has decreased following the introduction of immunisation with *H. influenzae* type b vaccine.

Choice of treatment. Doctors in the UK are advised[3] to give emergency treatment with parenteral benzylpenicillin to all suspected cases of meningitis before transfer to hospital (see also under Meningococcal Meningitis, below). Subsequent treatment depends on identification of the infecting organism and its susceptibility to antibacterials. Other factors affecting choice of antibacterial include penetration into the CSF and bactericidal activity once there. Once in hospital, penicillin and chloramphenicol have been the mainstays of treatment in adults and children and may be given **empirically** until the results of culture and susceptibility tests are known, but third-generation cephalosporins are increasingly preferred because of resistance. Authors working in the USA,[2,4] have advised the following empirical treatments: cefotaxime or ceftriaxone, with the addition of ampicillin in patients less than 3 months of age or over 50 years, in whom Listeria meningitis is more prevalent. They have also recommended addition of vancomycin to any empirical regimen when highly penicillin-resistant or cephalosporin-resistant pneumococcal meningitis is suspected. Vancomycin with ceftazidime is recommended in patients with recent head trauma, neurosurgery or CSF shunts.[4] Immunocompromised patients should receive ampicillin with ceftazidime.[4] Penicillin-allergic patients can be given chloramphenicol but it may not be effective against Gram-negative enteric bacilli or resistant pneumococci. There have been treatment failures with cefuroxime in *H. influenzae* meningitis[5] and, in comparative studies,[6,7] ceftriaxone has generally been superior to cefuroxime in children with bacterial meningitis; ceftriaxone and cefotaxime appear to have comparable efficacy.[8] Encouraging preliminary results have been obtained with meropenem as an alternative to cephalosporins for empirical treatment.[9,10]

The chosen antibacterials are generally given intravenously in relatively high doses. Treatment regimens should be reconsidered as soon as microbiological information is available. Management of the commonest forms of bacterial meningitis is discussed below.

Neonatal meningitis is uncommon but remains a life-threatening emergency often associated with bacteraemia and shock. Group B streptococci and *E. coli* are the commonest pathogens, *L. monocytogenes* is the third most common cause in the UK, and *Staphylococcus epidermidis* may be responsible for meningitis after invasive neurosurgery.[11] Empirical treatment with ampicillin or chloramphenicol together with gentamicin has been widely used, but extended-spectrum cephalosporins such as cefotaxime or ceftazidime are often preferred, plus ampicillin if *L. monocytogenes* is suspected.[12] USA authors[2] have advised that for neonates up to 4 weeks of age, ampicillin plus cefotaxime or ampicillin plus an aminoglycoside should be given; vancomycin should also be added when highly penicillin-resistant or cephalosporin-resistant pneumococcal meningitis is suspected. In preterm, low-birth-weight neonates, vancomycin should be given with ceftazidime because of the higher risk of nosocomial infection with staphylococci or Gram-negative bacilli.[4] A committee of the American Academy of Pediatrics[13] has recommended that, once the infecting organism is known, benzylpenicillin or ampicillin be given for group B streptococci and ampicillin for *L. monocytogenes*, both for 14 days; treatment of Gram-negative enteric infection should be based on susceptibility tests and continued for at least 3 weeks. A later update[14] suggested that vancomycin should be considered as additional therapy for suspected pneumococcal meningitis.

In the UK[11] an aggressive approach to the treatment of neonatal meningitis has been advocated with cefotaxime, penicillin, and gentamicin initially then, once the organisms were known, cefotaxime for *E. coli* and ceftazidime for *Pseudomonas*. Gentamicin was continued mainly to treat the associated septicaemia. The use of intraventricular gentamicin was supported but intrathecal administration via the lumbar route was considered to be ineffective. However, the necessity for gentamicin and its intraventricular administration were both severely criticised[15,16] and others[17] considered that, since the only studies to date had demonstrated a poorer outcome with intraventricular aminoglycosides, they should not be advocated. For other organisms the original report suggested[11] penicillin plus gentamicin for 3 weeks for group B streptococci, ampicillin with either cefotaxime or penicillin with gentamicin for *L. monocytogenes*, and systemic antibacterials with intraventricular vancomycin for *Staph. epidermidis* infection of ventriculoperitoneal shunts.

In **infants** immediately beyond the neonatal period (1 to 3 months of age) infecting organisms may be as for neonates or children older than 3 months (*N. meningitidis*, *Str. pneumoniae*, or *H. influenzae*) and initial treatment with ampicillin together with cefotaxime has been recommended in the UK.[18] Authors from the USA,[2,4] have advised ampicillin with either cefotaxime or ceftriaxone for infants aged 4 to 12 weeks; vancomycin should also be added when highly penicillin-resistant or cephalosporin-resistant pneumococcal meningitis is suspected.[2] A committee of the American Academy of Pediatrics has recommended[14] vancomycin plus cefotaxime or ceftriaxone for the initial treatment of all children older than 1 month with definite or probable meningitis. For **older infants and children** the UK authors[18] have recommended cefotaxime or ceftriaxone in preference to benzylpenicillin or ampicillin together with chloramphenicol. Opinion in the USA[2] is that ampicillin may or may not be given with the cephalosporin.

Adjunctive treatment. Mortality and morbidity, including deafness in children, remain high in meningitis despite increasingly effective antibacterials. As well as microbial virulence the host response to infection is important. Endotoxins and other microbial products, resulting from bacterial lysis following antibacterial treatment, are able to provoke an inflammatory response by triggering the release of cytokines including interleukin-1 and tumour necrosis factor. There is thus a possible role for anti-inflammatory drugs in the treatment of bacterial meningitis.[19,20] The role of corticosteroids has been the subject of considerable debate.[2,4,21-26] Some have suggested they may have a role in certain circumstances. There has been support for the use of dexamethasone in preventing deafness in children associated with *H. influenzae* type b meningitis[2,23-25] although the decreasing incidence of this type of meningitis since the introduction of immunisation casts further doubt on the value of such treatment. Additionally, some authors[2,4] have advocated dexamethasone use in bacterial meningitis in high-risk patients or in those with severe mental impairment, cerebral oedema, or very high intracranial pressure. However, the general view does appear to be against[2,4,21-26] *routine* adjunctive use, whether in children or adults.

GRAM-NEGATIVE ENTERIC AND PSEUDOMONAL MENINGITIS. Meningitis due to Gram-negative enteric bacteria occurs especially in neonates (see above), the elderly, and the immunocompromised and as a complication of neurosurgery. Treatment is generally with a third-generation cephalosporin such as cefotaxime; gentamicin or another suitable aminoglycoside may sometimes be given as well. For meningitis caused by *Pseudomonas aeruginosa* ceftazidime plus an aminoglycoside is used.[2,4,12] Intraventricular administration of an aminoglycoside has sometimes been judged necessary, but see under Neonatal Meningitis, above.

HAEMOPHILUS INFLUENZAE MENINGITIS. This is mainly a disease of pre-school children and was nearly always caused by encapsulated type b strains of *H. influenzae* acquired from close contact, but the incidence has decreased as a result of immunisation. A third-generation cephalosporin such as cefotaxime or ceftriaxone is the treatment of choice;[2,4,12] there have been treatment failures with cefuroxime.[5] Chloramphenicol is an alternative. Ampicillin is less useful now because of resistance, but can be given for beta-lactamase-negative strains. Treatment for a minimum of 7 to 10 days after fever has subsided may be necessary.[12,27] For a discussion of the treatment of *H. influenzae* infections in general, see above.

Prophylaxis. Since treatment does not eliminate nasopharyngeal carriage of *H. influenzae* type b, rifampicin should be given to index cases in the usual prophylactic dose for 4 days before discharge from hospital. Secondary cases should be prevented by giving rifampicin for 4 days to household and classroom contacts.[28]

For active immunisation of children against *H. influenzae* type b, see under Haemophilus Influenzae Vaccines, p.1540.

LISTERIA MENINGITIS. See above under Neonatal Meningitis. See also under Listeriosis, above.

MENINGOCOCCAL MENINGITIS. Benzylpenicillin is the treatment of choice for meningitis caused by *N. meningitidis*,[2,4,12] probably the commonest form of meningococcal infection (see under Meningococcal Infections, below), although reduced sensitivity has been reported in some strains[29-31] and has resulted in treatment failure;[32] high doses of benzylpenicillin are recommended. Alternatives are third-generation cephalosporins such as cefotaxime or ceftriaxone.[1,2,4,12,33] Parenteral benzylpenicillin is given, preferably intravenously, before transfer to hospital if meningococcal infection seems likely.[3,34-38] Duration of treatment is empirical but since *N. meningitidis* is rapidly cleared from the CSF and relapse is uncommon, treatment is generally continued for 5 days after resolution of fever and signs of meningitis;[12] a 7-day course is generally effective.[35] A single intramuscular dose of oily chloramphenicol may be a possibility in developing countries.[39]

Prophylaxis. Penicillin may not eliminate the carrier state and therefore rifampicin should be given for 2 days prior to hospital discharge, in the usual prophylactic dose. Secondary cases of meningococcal infection should be prevented by giving prophylactic treatment to close contacts of the index case, especially members of the same household who have had close prolonged contact with the case.[3,40] Rifampicin given for 2 days is the prophylactic of choice for the prevention of secondary cases.[3,40] Alternatives to rifampicin include a single oral dose of ciprofloxacin or an intramuscular dose of ceftriaxone.[3,40]

Where possible, vaccination should be performed in those contacts who have received prophylaxis.[3,40] Vaccines are available against group A and C meningococci or against groups A, C, Y, and W135 meningococci, and are under investigation against group B.

PNEUMOCOCCAL MENINGITIS. Meningitis due to *Str. pneumoniae* is most common in adults and infants, but can occur at any age. It is said to be the most serious form of meningitis with mortality exceeding 20%.[12] Benzylpenicillin or phenoxymethylpenicillin have been treatments of choice although strains with reduced sensitivity to penicillins are increasingly reported (see under Pneumonia, below) and a third-generation cephalosporin such as cefotaxime or ceftriaxone is often the initial treatment of choice; benzylpenicillin may be substituted if the organism is subsequently shown to be sensitive to it. Treatment should generally continue for 7 to 10 days after fever subsides,[12] with some clinicians preferring a minimum of 10 days.[27] Pneumococcal strains resistant to cephalosporins have recently emerged and vancomycin is recommended with or without rifampicin in addition to cefotaxime or ceftriaxone where such pneumococci are prevalent.[2,4] However, one difficulty is that third-generation cephalosporins may not be available in developing countries; chloramphenicol may still prove useful in those countries with a high incidence of bacterial meningitis,[41,42] but treatment failures have been reported with chloramphenicol in penicillin-resistant pneumococcal meningitis.[43]

Prophylaxis. A pneumococcal vaccine is available, but its effectiveness in preventing meningitis has not been established.

1. Tunkel AR, *et al.* Bacterial meningitis: recent advances in pathophysiology and treatment. *Ann Intern Med* 1990; **112**: 610–23.
2. Tunkel AR, Scheld WM. Acute bacterial meningitis. *Lancet* 1995; **346**: 1675–80.
3. PHLS Meningococcal Infections Working Group and Public Health Medicine Environmental Group. Control of meningococcal disease: guidance for consultants in communicable disease control. *Commun Dis Rep* 1995; **5**: R189–R195.
4. Quagliarello VJ, Scheld WM. Treatment of bacterial meningitis. *N Engl J Med* 1997; **336**: 708–16.
5. Arditi M, *et al.* Cefuroxime treatment failure and Haemophilus influenzae meningitis: case report and review of literature. *Pediatrics* 1989; **84**: 132–5.
6. Lebel MH, *et al.* Comparative efficacy of ceftriaxone and cefuroxime for treatment of bacterial meningitis. *J Pediatr* 1989; **114**: 1049–54.
7. Schaad UB, *et al.* A comparison of ceftriaxone and cefuroxime for the treatment of bacterial meningitis in children. *N Engl J Med* 1990; **322**: 141–7.
8. Scholz H, *et al.* Prospective comparison of ceftriaxone and cefotaxime for the short-term treatment of bacterial meningitis in children. *Chemotherapy* 1998; **44**: 142–7.
9. Schmutzhard E, *et al.* A randomised comparison of meropenem with cefotaxime or ceftriaxone for the treatment of bacterial meningitis in adults. *J Antimicrob Chemother* 1995; **36** (suppl A): 85–97.
10. Klugman KP, *et al.* Randomized comparison of meropenem with cefotaxime for treatment of bacterial meningitis. *Antimicrob Agents Chemother* 1995; **39**: 1140–6.
11. Gandy G, Rennie J. Antibiotic treatment of suspected neonatal meningitis. *Arch Dis Child* 1990; **65**: 1–2.
12. Finch R. Bacterial meningitis. *Prescribers' J* 1989; **29**: 2–11.
13. American Academy of Pediatrics Committee on Infectious Diseases. Treatment of bacterial meningitis. *Pediatrics* 1988; **81**: 904–7. [See also Savarino SJ, *et al. Pediatrics* 1989; **83**: 632–3 and McCracken GH, *ibid.*, 633 (correction; cefotaxime should *not* be used for pseudomonal meningitis).]
14. American Academy of Pediatrics. Therapy for children with invasive pneumococcal infections. *Pediatrics* 1997; **99**: 289–99.
15. Short A. Antibiotic treatment of suspected neonatal meningitis. *Arch Dis Child* 1990; **65**: 810.
16. Tarlow MJ. Antibiotic treatment of suspected neonatal meningitis. *Arch Dis Child* 1990; **65**: 810.
17. Heyderman RS, Levin M. Antibiotic treatment of suspected neonatal meningitis. *Arch Dis Child* 1990; **66**: 170.
18. Klein NJ, *et al.* Antibiotic choices for meningitis beyond the neonatal period. *Arch Dis Child* 1992; **67**: 157–9.
19. Anonymous. Steroids and meningitis. *Lancet* 1989; **ii**: 1307–8.
20. Finch RG, Mandragos C. Corticosteroids in bacterial meningitis. *BMJ* 1991; **302**: 607–8.
21. Harvey DR, Stevens JP. What is the role of corticosteroids in meningitis? *Drugs* 1995; **50**: 945–50.
22. Townsend GC, Scheld WM. The use of corticosteroids in the management of bacterial meningitis in adults. *J Antimicrob Chemother* 1996; **37**: 1051–61.
23. McIntyre PB, *et al.* Dexamethasone as adjunctive therapy in bacterial meningitis: a meta-analysis of randomized clinical trials since 1988. *JAMA* 1997; **278**: 925–31.
24. American Academy of Pediatrics Committee on Infectious Diseases. Dexamethasone therapy for bacterial meningitis in infants and children. *Pediatrics* 1990; **86**: 130–3.
25. The Meningitis Working Party of the British Paediatric Immunology and Infectious Diseases Group. Should we use dexamethasone in meningitis? *Arch Dis Child* 1992; **67**: 1398–1401.
26. Prasad K, Haines T. Dexamethasone treatment for acute bacterial meningitis: how strong is the evidence for routine use? *J Neurol Neurosurg Psychiatry* 1995; **59**: 31–7.
27. O'Neill P. Meningitis: how long to treat bacterial meningitis. *Lancet* 1993; **341**: 530. Correction. *ibid.*: 642.
28. Cartwright KAV, *et al.* Chemoprophylaxis for Haemophilus influenzae type b. *BMJ* 1991; **302**: 546–7.
29. Jones DM, Sutcliffe EM. Meningococci with reduced susceptibility to penicillin. *Lancet* 1990; **335**: 863–4.
30. Saez Nieto JA, *et al.* Meningococci moderately resistant to penicillin. *Lancet* 1990; **336**: 54.
31. Riley G, *et al.* Penicillin resistance in Neisseria meningitidis. *N Engl J Med* 1991; **324**: 997.
32. Turner PC, *et al.* Treatment failure in meningococcal meningitis. *Lancet* 1990; **335**: 732–3.
33. Klein NJ, *et al.* Management of meningococcal infections. *Br J Hosp Med* 1993; **50**: 42–9.
34. Welsby PD, Golledge CL. Meningococcal disease. *BMJ* 1990; **300**: 1150–1.
35. Begg N. Reducing mortality from meningococcal disease. *BMJ* 1992; **305**: 133–4.
36. Strang JR, Pugh EJ. Meningococcal infections: reducing the case fatality rate by giving penicillin before admission to hospital. *BMJ* 1992; **305**: 141–3.
37. Cartwright K, *et al.* Early treatment with parenteral penicillin in meningococcal disease. *BMJ* 1992; **305**: 143–7.
38. Cartwright K, *et al.* Initial management of suspected meningococcal infection: parenteral benzylpenicillin is vital. *BMJ* 1994; **309**: 1660–1.
39. Lewis RF, *et al.* Long-acting oily chloramphenicol for meningococcal meningitis. *Lancet* 1998; **352**: 823.
40. American Academy of Pediatrics, Canadian Paediatric Society. Meningococcal disease prevention and control strategies for practice-based physicians. *Pediatrics* 1996; **97**: 404–11.
41. Pécoul B, *et al.* Long-acting chloramphenicol versus intravenous ampicillin for treatment of bacterial meningitis. *Lancet* 1991; **338**: 862–6.
42. Kumar P, Verma IC. Antibiotic therapy for bacterial meningitis in children in developing countries. *Bull WHO* 1993; **71**: 183–8.
43. Friedland IR, Klugman KP. Failure of chloramphenicol therapy in penicillin-resistant pneumococcal meningitis. *Lancet* 1992; **339**: 405–8.

Meningococcal infections

The meningococcus *Neisseria meningitidis* is a Gram-negative bacterium classified into several serotypes including groups A, B, and C. It occurs worldwide and can cause endemic and epidemic infection. Group A is mainly responsible for epidemics in the developing world. In the USA most infections have been caused by group B or group C meningococci; the relative importance of group C has been increasing in North America. Group B has been the most prevalent in the UK and Europe although there has been some increase in group C infections. Infections have occurred predominantly in young children under 5 years, but there has been an increased incidence in teenagers and young adults in recent UK outbreaks. Meningococcal disease has traditionally been associated with poverty and overcrowding; the only established risk factor is close contact with an index case, hence the importance of prophylaxis. Clinical infection is preceded by asymptomatic nasopharyngeal carriage of meningococci and spread of infection is usually via respiratory droplets from asymptomatic carriers. Bacteraemia is probably the primary event in all forms of meningococcal disease; clinical manifestations range from mild sore throat or transient fever to fulminant disease. A vasculitic rash (petechiae or purpura) is often associated with meningococcal infection. Meningococcal infection most commonly manifests as septicaemia, which can be rapidly fatal, particularly if fulminating, with mortality ranging from 15% up to 80% in severe forms, or as meningococcal meningitis, in which the infection is confined to the CNS and is associated with mortality rates of 5% or less. Meningococcal meningitis may also occur in conjunction with meningococcal septicaemia. Less usual forms of metastatic meningococcal infection include polyarthritis, pericarditis, pneumonitis, and genito-urinary-tract infections.

Despite some uncertainty as to whether patients with suspected meningococcal septicaemia rather than meningitis would benefit from early penicillin treatment, it is still generally recommended for all patients with suspected meningococcal disease. Thus, when meningococcal infection seems likely benzylpenicillin should be given parenterally, preferably intravenously, before transfer to hospital. For details of the treatment and prophylaxis of meningococcal infections, see Meningococcal Meningitis, under Meningitis, above.

References.

1. Peltola H. Early meningococcal disease: advising the public and the profession. *Lancet* 1993; **342:** 509–10.
2. Klein NJ, *et al.* Management of meningococcal infections. *Br J Hosp Med* 1993; **50:** 42–9.
3. PHLS Meningococcal Infections Working Group and Public Health Medicine Environmental Group. Control of meningococcal disease: guidance for consultants in communicable disease control. *Commun Dis Rep* 1995; **5:** R189–R195. Updated: http://www.phls.co.uk/publications/CDR%20Weekly/archive/news0701.html (accessed 02.08.01).
4. American Academy of Pediatrics and Canadian Paediatric Society. Meningococcal disease prevention and control strategies for practice-based physicians. *Pediatrics* 1996; **97:** 404–11.

Mouth infections

Infections of the mouth include those of dental origin such as dental caries, abscesses, gingivitis, and periodontal infections, and those without a dental origin. Infections arising in the nasal cavity, middle ear, oropharynx, and paranasal sinuses can also affect the oral cavity. This discussion deals mainly with infections of dental origin.

The organisms most often encountered in oral infections are viridans streptococci, a variety of anaerobes, and facultative streptococci.[1] Over the years the emphasis has shifted from treatment to prevention of oral diseases.[2]

Dental caries is caused by the erosion of tooth enamel due to acid produced by bacteria (usually *Streptococcus mutans*) in plaque. Fluoride in various forms is used in dental caries prophylaxis, where it may promote remineralisation or reduce acid production by plaque bacteria.[2] Sugar-free chewing gum can help prevent caries by stimulating the production of saliva.[3] Dental caries vaccines have also been investigated.

The term periodontal disease encompasses specific conditions affecting the gingiva and the supporting connective tissue and alveolar bone.[4] Gingivitis is thought to be caused by a non-specific bacterial plaque flora that gradually changes from predominantly Gram-positive to more Gram-negative. Gingivitis may or may not develop into periodontitis, but periodontitis is always preceded by gingivitis. Periodontitis is associated with a Gram-negative anaerobic microflora. Most gingivitis and periodontitis can be prevented and treated by adequate oral hygiene and plaque removal using mechanical means such as toothbrushing. Mechanical removal of calculus is necessary where the build up is significant. Antiseptics may also help to reduce plaque accumulation and several, but most notably chlorhexidine, have been used.[5]

Penicillin has continued to be an effective drug in combating oral pathogens, and erythromycin or metronidazole can be alternatives. Fusiform bacteria and spirochaetes have been linked with acute necrotising ulcerative gingivitis (also called Vincent's infection or trench mouth);[6] systemic metronidazole is often the treatment of choice. Tinidazole has also been used. Tetracyclines or metronidazole have been used for chronic periodontal disease.[7] Antibacterials and antiseptics delivered locally to the periodontal pocket may be of value.

1. Guralnick W. Odontogenic infections. *Br Dent J* 1984; **156:** 440–7.
2. WHO. Recent advances in oral health: report of a WHO expert committee. *WHO Tech Rep Ser 826* 1992.
3. Edgar WM. Sugar substitutes, chewing gum and dental caries—a review. *Br Dent J* 1998; **184:** 29–32.
4. Williams RC. Periodontal disease. *N Engl J Med* 1990; **322:** 373–82.
5. Eley BM. Antibacterial agents in the control of supragingival plaque—a review. *Br Dent J* 1999; **186:** 286–96.
6. Johnson BD, Engel D. Acute necrotizing ulcerative gingivitis: a review of diagnosis, etiology and treatment. *J Periodontol* 1986; **57:** 141–50.
7. Watts TLP. Periodontitis for medical practitioners. *BMJ* 1998; **316:** 993–6.

Mycetoma

Mycetoma is a localised chronic infection seen especially in the tropics and subtropics and involving subcutaneous tissue, bone, and skin. It has been termed Madura foot when affecting the sole of the foot. Mycetomas caused by fungi (p.374) such as *Madurella mycetomatis* are called eumycetomas and those caused by the filamentous bacteria, actinomycetes, are called actinomycetomas. *Nocardia brasiliensis* is the commonest actinomycete responsible; others include *Actinomadura madurae*, *A. pelletieri*, and *Streptomyces somaliensis*. For details of systemic infections caused by *Nocardia* spp., see under Nocardiosis, below.

Various treatment regimens for actinomycetomas have been tried. Co-trimoxazole with streptomycin or dapsone with streptomycin have been found[1] to be the most effective although *Streptomyces somaliensis* infection did not always respond. Two further regimens, sulfadoxine with pyrimethamine and streptomycin or rifampicin with streptomycin, were suitable for second-line therapy.[1] Cures were achieved after treatment for 4 to 24 months.[1] In a study of antibacterial activity *in vitro* against strains of *Streptomyces somaliensis* isolated from mycetoma patients, rifampicin was the most effective followed by erythromycin, tobramycin, fusidic acid, and streptomycin in decreasing order of activity; all strains were resistant to trimethoprim.[2] The successful use of hyperbaric oxygen in addition to co-trimoxazole[3] or of amoxicillin-clavulanic acid[4] in the treatment of *N. brasiliensis* actinomycetoma previously resistant to conventional therapy has been described.

1. Mahgoub ES. Medical management of mycetoma. *Bull WHO* 1976; **54:** 303–10.
2. Nasher MA, *et al.* In vitro studies of antibiotic sensitivities of Streptomyces somaliensis—a cause of human actinomycetoma. *Trans R Soc Trop Med Hyg* 1989; **83:** 265–8.
3. Walker RM, *et al.* Beneficial effects of hyperbaric oxygen therapy in Nocardia brasiliensis soft-tissue infection. *Med J Aust* 1991; **155:** 122–3.
4. Gomez A, *et al.* Amoxicillin and clavulanic acid in the treatment of actinomycetoma. *Int J Dermatol* 1993; **32:** 218–20.

Necrotising enterocolitis

See under Gastro-enteritis, above.

Necrotising fasciitis

Necrotising fasciitis is a severe soft-tissue infection resulting in necrosis of the subcutaneous tissue and adjacent fascia together with severe systemic illness. It may be caused by a mixture of aerobic and anaerobic organisms, but can be due to group A streptococci or staphylococci alone and may be associated with a toxic shock syndrome (below).

Treatment involving radical surgical excision of the affected tissues may be avoided in some patients treated with large doses of appropriate antibacterials.[1] For streptococcal necrotising fasciitis high-dose benzylpenicillin should be used; clindamycin may be added in severe cases.[2] Erythromycin should be avoided because of the risk of resistance.[2] Staphylococcal infections are treated with a penicillinase-resistant penicillin, cefazolin, or vancomycin (for resistant strains).[1] Since diagnosis can be difficult, it may be advisable to treat as for a mixed infection with antibacterials active against anaerobes (e.g. clindamycin) and also an aminoglycoside or third-generation cephalosporin against Gram-negative rods initially, in addition to benzylpenicillin.[3] A broad-spectrum penicillin-beta-lactamase-inhibitor combination or imipenem-cilastatin may also be used.[1] Hyperbaric oxygen therapy has also been beneficial although prospective controlled studies are lacking.[4]

1. Gorbach SL. IDCP guidelines: necrotizing skin and soft tissue infections. Part I: necrotizing fasciitis. *Infect Dis Clin Pract* 1996; **5:** 406–11.
2. Anonymous. Invasive group A streptococcal infections in Gloucestershire. *Commun Dis Rep* 1994; **4:** 97.
3. Chelsom J, *et al.* Necrotising fasciitis due to group A streptococci in western Norway: incidence and clinical features. *Lancet* 1994; **344:** 1111–15.
4. Leach RM, *et al.* Hyperbaric oxygen therapy. *BMJ* 1998; **317:** 1140–3.

Neonatal conjunctivitis

Conjunctivitis of the newborn, also known as ophthalmia neonatorum, is defined as any conjunctivitis with discharge occurring during the first 28 days of life.[1] That due to *Neisseria gonorrhoeae* is the most serious; it usually appears by the third day after birth, can rapidly result in blindness, and systemic infections, especially severe septicaemia, may occur. *Chlamydia trachomatis* is another major cause of neonatal conjunctivitis; it charac-

teristically occurs 5 to 14 days after birth and is less threatening to sight than gonococcal infection, but may also infect the nasopharynx and may cause pneumonia. Chlamydial conjunctivitis is more common than gonococcal conjunctivitis in developed countries. Both these organisms are sexually transmitted and the infants of mothers with such genital-tract infections are infected during their passage through the birth canal. Other less serious bacterial causes of neonatal conjunctivitis include *Staphylococcus aureus*, *Streptococcus pneumoniae*, *Haemophilus* spp., and *Pseudomonas* spp.; they are often hospital-acquired.[1]

The management of gonococcal and chlamydial neonatal conjunctivitis varies from country to country depending on the prevalence of gonorrhoea and *C. trachomatis* infection and on bacterial resistance.

PROPHYLAXIS. The ideal method of prophylaxis is to treat the infected mother during pregnancy, but this is not always possible. Where the risk of *gonococcal infection* is high, ocular prophylaxis at birth is particularly important because of the rapid onset of conjunctivitis and its potential seriousness and is preferable to early diagnosis and treatment of the neonate.[2] Cleansing of the neonate's eyes immediately after birth followed by the topical application of either tetracycline 1% eye ointment, erythromycin 0.5% or 1% eye ointment, or silver nitrate 1% eye drops is advised[3,4] and is sometimes required by law.[3] Silver nitrate[1] is active against all strains of *N. gonorrhoeae* regardless of their susceptibility to antibacterials; it is inexpensive and widely available, but may cause chemical conjunctivitis and has been ineffective in preventing chlamydial conjunctivitis (see below). Tetracycline has been reported to be as effective as silver nitrate in protecting against gonococcal conjunctivitis caused by multiresistant strains[5] and WHO now lists it as the drug of choice.[4]

The value of prophylaxis against *chlamydial neonatal conjunctivitis* is less certain. Tetracycline ointment has been reported to be less effective in preventing chlamydial infection than gonococcal infection[5] and erythromycin ointment has also been unreliable.[6] Silver nitrate is generally considered ineffective,[1] despite an unexpected reduction in the incidence of chlamydial conjunctivitis in one study.[5] Screening and treatment of pregnant women for *C. trachomatis* infection may be a more effective method of control than ocular prophylaxis.[5,7] This approach also tackles the more serious problem of chlamydial pneumonia.[8]

Neonatal conjunctivitis continues to cause blindness, especially in developing countries. Povidone-iodine is less expensive and perhaps more readily available in such countries than silver nitrate or erythromycin. In a study in Kenya involving more than 3000 infants[9] a 2.5% ophthalmic solution of povidone-iodine appeared to be a more effective prophylactic than either a 1% ophthalmic solution of silver nitrate or erythromycin 0.5% eye ointment. In particular there were fewer cases of chlamydial conjunctivitis with povidone-iodine.

TREATMENT. *Gonococcal neonatal conjunctivitis* must be treated systemically. WHO[4] recommends ceftriaxone 50 mg per kg body-weight by intramuscular injection as a single dose (to a maximum of 125 mg) or, if ceftriaxone is not available, spectinomycin 25 mg per kg (to a maximum of 75 mg) or kanamycin 25 mg per kg (to a maximum of 75 mg) by intramuscular injection as a single dose. When systemic treatment is not available tetracycline 1% eye ointment should be applied to both eyes every hour until the infant can be transferred to a facility offering systemic treatment. Where the prevalence of penicillin-resistant gonococci is less than 1%, benzylpenicillin 60 mg per kg daily intravenously or intramuscularly in divided doses for 7 days might be given.[10] WHO formerly advised that systemic therapy should be accompanied by hourly conjunctival irrigation and by application of a topical antibacterial preparation such as tetracycline or erythromycin eye ointment until the discharge was eliminated.[1,10]

The CDC[3] recommends a single intravenous or intramuscular injection of ceftriaxone 25 to 50 mg per kg (up to 125 mg) when there is no evidence of disseminated infection.

See also under Gonorrhoea (above) for the treatment of infants exposed to gonorrhoea at birth or with established gonococcal infection at any site.

For *nongonococcal neonatal conjunctivitis* WHO[4] and CDC[3] recommend erythromycin 50 mg per kg daily in divided doses by mouth for 10 to 14 days. There is no indication that topical therapy is of additional benefit.[3,10]

1. WHO. *Conjunctivitis of the newborn: prevention and treatment at the primary health care level.* Geneva: WHO, 1986.
2. Laga M, *et al.* Epidemiology and control of gonococcal ophthalmia neonatorum. *Bull WHO* 1989; **67:** 471–8.
3. Centers for Disease Control. 1998 Guidelines for treatment of sexually transmitted diseases. *MMWR* 1998; **47** (RR-1): 56–7, 65–6, 69.
4. WHO. *Guidelines for the management of sexually transmitted infections.* Geneva: WHO, 2001.
5. Laga M, *et al.* Prophylaxis of gonococcal and chlamydial ophthalmia neonatorum: a comparison of silver nitrate and tetracycline. *N Engl J Med* 1988; **318:** 653–7.
6. Black-Payne C, *et al.* Failure of erythromycin ointment for post natal ocular prophylaxis of chlamydial conjunctivitis. *Pediatr Infect Dis J* 1989; **8:** 491–5.
7. Hammerschlag MR, *et al.* Efficacy of neonatal ocular prophylaxis for the prevention of chlamydial and gonococcal conjunctivitis. *N Engl J Med* 1989; **320:** 769–72.
8. Schachter J. Why we need a program for the control of Chlamydia trachomatis. *N Engl J Med* 1989; **320:** 802–4.
9. Isenberg SJ, *et al.* A controlled trial of povidone-iodine as prophylaxis against ophthalmia neonatorum. *N Engl J Med* 1995; **332:** 562–6.
10. WHO. WHO expert committee on venereal diseases and treponematoses: sixth report. *WHO Tech Rep Ser 736* 1986; 125.

Nocardiosis

Nocardia spp. are Gram-positive aerobic branching bacteria that cause systemic or localised infection. The principal pathogenic species in man is *N. asteroides*; others include *N. brasiliensis, N. pseudobrasiliensis,* and *N. caviae.* Localised chronic infection or actinomycetoma is described under Mycetoma (above). Systemic nocardiosis is primarily a lung infection and often involves abscess formation; it occurs especially in immunocompromised patients and may be disseminated with abscesses in the brain and subcutaneous tissues.

The treatment of choice has been a sulfonamide such as sulfadiazine or, more recently, co-trimoxazole,[1-4] although a study *in vitro* indicated that the fixed ratio of trimethoprim:sulfamethoxazole in co-trimoxazole might contain too little trimethoprim for optimal activity.[5] Sulfafurazole[6] has been used successfully. There have been reports of the effective treatment of nocardiosis with amikacin,[7,8] minocycline,[9,10] or ciprofloxacin with doxycycline.[11] Other suggested alternatives include imipenem or meropenem.[12] Treatment needs to be prolonged and may continue for 6 to 12 months.

1. Abdi EA, *et al.* Nocardia infection in splenectomized patients: case reports and a review of the literature. *Postgrad Med J* 1987; **63:** 455–8.
2. Smego RA, *et al.* Treatment of systemic nocardiosis. *Lancet* 1987; **i:** 456.
3. Filice GA. Treatment of nocardiosis. *Lancet* 1987; **i:** 1261–2.
4. Varghese GK, *et al.* Nocardia brasiliensis meningitis. *Postgrad Med J* 1992; **68:** 986.
5. Bennett JE, Jennings AE. Factors influencing susceptibility of Nocardia species to trimethoprim-sulfamethoxazole. *Antimicrob Agents Chemother* 1978; **13:** 624–7.
6. Poland GA, *et al.* Nocardia asteroides pericarditis: report of a case and review of the literature. *Mayo Clin Proc* 1990; **65:** 819–24.
7. Goldstein FW, *et al.* Amikacin-containing regimens for treatment of nocardiosis in immunocompromised patients. *Eur J Clin Microbiol* 1987; **6:** 198–200.
8. Meier B, *et al.* Successful treatment of a pancreatic Nocardia asteroides abscess with amikacin and surgical drainage. *Antimicrob Agents Chemother* 1986; **29:** 150–1.
9. Petersen EA, *et al.* Minocycline treatment of pulmonary nocardiosis. *JAMA* 1983; **250:** 930–2.
10. Naka W, *et al.* Unusually located lymphocutaneous nocardiosis caused by Nocardia brasiliensis. *Br J Dermatol* 1995; **132:** 609–13.
11. Bath PMW, *et al.* Treatment of multiple subcutaneous Nocardia asteroides abscesses with ciprofloxacin and doxycycline. *Postgrad Med J* 1989; **65:** 190–1.
12. Anonymous. The choice of antibacterial drugs. *Med Lett Drugs Ther* 1999; **41:** 95–104.

Obstetric disorders

See under: Endometritis (the prophylaxis and treatment of postpartum endometritis), above; Premature Labour, below; and Urinary-Tract Infections in Pregnancy, below. See also Neonatal Conjunctivitis, above, and Perinatal Streptococcal Infections, below.

Opportunistic mycobacterial infections

Environmental mycobacteria are widespread, and a number of species other than those responsible for leprosy and tuberculosis are facultative parasites capable of producing disease in man. These organisms, which have been referred to as atypical, nontuberculous, tuberculoid, opportunistic, or MOTT mycobacteria (mycobacteria other than tuberculous), are rarely, if ever, transmitted from person to person but are acquired from the environment. The diseases produced include localised skin and soft tissue lesions, pulmonary infections, and lymphadenitis, but disseminated infections may develop rapidly in immunocompromised patients such as those with AIDS and now represent one of the most common opportunistic bacterial infections in patients with advanced AIDS.

Localised lesions, invariably following inoculation, are most commonly due to the slow-growing species *Mycobacterium marinum* ('swimming pool' or 'fish-tank' granuloma), *M. ulcerans* (Buruli ulcer), and the fast-growing species *M. chelonae* (*M. chelonei*), *M. abscessus* (formerly *M. chelonae* subspecies), and *M. fortuitum.* Ulcerated lesions due to *M. haemophilum* have been described mainly in immunocompromised patients.

Pulmonary disease, which is clinically indistinguishable from pulmonary tuberculosis, has most frequently been attributed to the *M. avium* complex (MAC; *M. avium-intracellulare* complex; MAIC), *M. kansasii,* and to a lesser extent *M. xenopi;* less common causes include *M. abscessus, M. asiaticum, M. celatum, M. chelonae, M. fortuitum, M. malmoense, M. scrofulaceum, M. simiae,* and *M. szulgai.*

Lymphadenitis, which is usually self-limiting and occurs particularly in children under 5 years of age, may be caused by many species but the great majority of cases are due to the related *M. avium* complex, *M. genavense, M. malmoense,* and *M. scrofulaceum* (sometimes collectively known as the MAIS complex).

Dissemination of opportunistic mycobacterial infections may occur rapidly in patients with depressed cellular immunity. The majority of cases have been attributed to the *M. avium* complex; species implicated more recently include *M. abscessus, M. celatum, M. chelonae, M. genavense, M. haemophilum, M. kansasii, M. malmoense, M. scrofulaceum,* and *M. simiae.*

The course of treatment depends on the site and nature of infection. Response to chemotherapy is often difficult to predict as *in-vitro* sensitivity of the organisms may not reflect the response obtained *in vivo.*

Both HIV-negative and HIV-positive patients may be affected and the British Thoracic Society has published guidelines[1] on the management of opportunistic mycobacterial infections. It is noted that, on the whole, the evidence is not derived from controlled clinical trials as very few have been reported. In patients receiving antiretroviral therapy, the possibility of drug interactions should be borne in mind.

MYCOBACTERIUM AVIUM COMPLEX (MAC).

In HIV-negative patients with MAC pulmonary disease, treatment should be with rifampicin and ethambutol for 24 months; isoniazid may also be given if necessary. In extrapulmonary disease affecting lymph nodes, surgical excision of the nodes should be undertaken; chemotherapy with rifampicin, ethambutol, and clarithromycin for up to 2 years should be considered if disease recurs or where the excision is incomplete or impossible. In sites other than lymph nodes, chemotherapy should be given for 18 to 24 months.[1]

Treatment for HIV-positive patients with MAC pulmonary disease should consist of rifampicin (or rifabutin), ethambutol, and clarithromycin (or azithromycin). A quinolone such as ciprofloxacin, or even amikacin, may be added for patients who are intolerant of these drugs or who fail to respond. Treatment should be lifelong. In disseminated disease, the same treatment should be given and continued indefinitely.[1]

Chemoprophylaxis is used to reduce the incidence of disseminated MAC disease in patients with advanced HIV infection. There appears to be a tendency to delay starting prophylaxis until later in the disease process; in 1993 the National Institutes of Health (NIH) in the USA recommended[2] starting at a blood CD4+ count of less than 100 per mm³ whereas the 1999 guidelines[3] from the US Public Health Service and the Infectious Diseases Society of America (USPHS/IDSA) recommend starting prophylaxis at a CD4+ count of 50 per mm³.

In the UK, the British Thoracic Society note there is no general agreement about when prophylaxis should be used. If prophylaxis is to be given to patients with a CD4+ count below 50 per mm³ the first drug of choice would be azithromycin; clarithromycin is an alternative and azithromycin with rifabutin would be a third choice. Treatment should be continued indefinitely.[1] Two multicentre, double-blind, randomised studies[4,5] have concluded that prophylaxis (with azithromycin) may be safely discontinued in HIV-infected patients whose CD4+ count has increased from below 50 per mm³ to over 100 per mm³ in response to antiretroviral therapy.

MYCOBACTERIUM KANSASII INFECTION.

Infections with *M. kansasii* may be treated with rifampicin (or rifabutin) and ethambutol. For pulmonary disease, HIV-negative patients usually need only 9 months of therapy whereas HIV-positive patients should receive therapy for 2 years or until the sputum has been negative for 12 months. For disseminated infection in HIV-positive patients, clarithromycin should be added and possibly also isoniazid. The place of macrolides and fluoroquinolones in pulmonary or disseminated *M. kansasii* infection remain to be established. In extrapulmonary disease in HIV-negative patients, chemotherapy with rifampicin and ethambutol may be used prior to aspiration of an infected lymph node. In other extrapulmonary disease the data is rather insufficient to make recommendations, but rifampicin and ethambutol for 9 months appears sensible with the addition of protionamide and streptomycin and/or a macrolide if the condition is not responding.[1]

OTHER OPPORTUNISTIC MYCOBACTERIA.

In *M. malmoense* and *M. xenopi* pulmonary disease, rifampicin and ethambutol should be given for 24 months in HIV-negative states. Extrapulmonary *M. malmoense* infections should be treated in the same manner as extrapulmonary MAC or *M. kansasii* infections. *M. malmoense* infection rarely occurs in AIDS patients, but if necessary, treatment with rifampicin, ethambutol, and clarithromycin, and possibly isoniazid should be used. For *M. xenopi* in HIV-positive patients there is no evidence on which to base recommendations.[1]

For pulmonary disease due to rapidly growing bacteria (*M. abcessus, M. chelonae, M. fortuitum,* and *M. gordonae*) and other species (*M. genavense, M. haemophilum, M. simiae, M. szulgai,* and *M. ulcerans*) surgery should be employed if possible. Drug therapy should probably include rifampicin, ethambutol, and clarithromycin. Amikacin, cefoxitin, imipenem, quinolones, and sulfonamides may have a place in treatment. For extrapulmonary disease due to these organisms, there have been several anecdotal reports outlining treatment but there is no evidence from controlled clinical trials.[1] For *M. marinum* infections (swimming-pool granuloma or fish-tank granuloma) rifampicin with ethambutol[6] or isoniazid, rifabutin with ciprofloxacin,[7] minocycline with co-trimoxazole,[8] clarithromycin with rifabutin[9] or ciprofloxacin[7] or ethambutol,[7] and monotherapy with clarithromycin, minocycline, doxycycline, or co-trimoxazole[10] have been used, mainly in small series of patients. Surgical treatment and intensive antibacterial regimens have been used for *M. scrofulaceum* infections,[11] while Buruli ulcer, due to *M. ulcerans,* is difficult to treat, requires surgery, often major; responses to antimycobacterials have been disappointing.[12,13] Phenytoin, applied locally, was reported to induce healing in 3 patients with Buruli ulcer.[14] *M. haemophilum* infection in a patient with rheumatoid arthritis and ulcerated nodules on his legs responded to treatment with rifampicin, ciprofloxacin, and clarithromycin.[15] Symptomatic improvement was achieved in an AIDS patient with *M. celatum* infection with a regimen of isoniazid, rifampicin, and ethambutol.[16] Successful treatment of *M. simiae* infection in patients with AIDS was reported with clarithromycin, ethambutol, and ciprofloxacin.[17]

1. Subcommittee of the Joint Tuberculosis Committee of the British Thoracic Society. Management of opportunist mycobacterial infections: Joint Tuberculosis Committee guidelines 1999. *Thorax* 2000; **55:** 210–18.
2. Masur H, and the Public Health Service Task Force on Prophylaxis and Therapy for Mycobacterium avium Complex. Recommendations on prophylaxis and therapy for disseminated Mycobacterium avium complex disease in patients infected with the human immunodeficiency virus. *N Engl J Med* 1993; **329:** 898–904.
3. Centers for Disease Control. 1999 USPHS/IDSA guidelines for the prevention of opportunistic infections in persons infected with human immunodeficiency virus. *MMWR* 1999; **48** (RR-10): 1–59.
4. El-Sadr WM, *et al.* Discontinuation of prophylaxis against Mycobacterium avium complex disease in HIV-infected patients who have a response to antiretroviral therapy. *N Engl J Med* 2000; **342:** 1085–92.
5. Currier JS, *et al.* Discontinuation of Mycobacterium avium complex prophylaxis in patients with antiretroviral therapy-induced increases in CD4+ cell count: a randomised, double-blind, placebo-controlled trial. *Ann Intern Med* 2000; **133:** 493–503.
6. Donta ST, *et al.* Therapy of Mycobacterium marinum infections: use of tetracyclines vs rifampin. *Arch Intern Med* 1986; **146:** 902–4.
7. Laing RBS, *et al.* Antimicrobial treatment of fish tank granuloma. *J Hand Surg* 1997; **22B:** 135–7.
8. Gray SF, *et al.* Fish tank granuloma. *BMJ* 1990; **300:** 1069–70.
9. Laing RBS, *et al.* New antimicrobials against Mycobacterium marinum infection. *Br J Dermatol* 1994; **131:** 914.
10. American Thoracic Society. Diagnosis and treatment of disease caused by nontuberculous mycobacteria. *Am J Respir Crit Care Med* 1997; **156:** S1–S25.
11. Bailey WC. Treatment of atypical mycobacterial disease. *Chest* 1983; **84:** 625–8.
12. van der Werf TS, *et al.* Mycobacterium ulcerans infection. *Lancet* 1999; **354:** 1013–18.
13. Thangaraj HS, *et al.* Mycobacterium ulcerans disease; Buruli ulcer. *Trans R Soc Trop Med Hyg* 1999; **93:** 337–40.

14. Adjei O, et al. Phenytoin in the treatment of Buruli ulcer. Trans R Soc Trop Med Hyg 1998; 92: 108–9.
15. Darling TN, et al. Treatment of Mycobacterium haemophilum infection with an antibiotic regimen including clarithromycin. Br J Dermatol 1994; 131: 376–9.
16. Piersimoni C, et al. Disseminated infection due to Mycobacterium celatum in patient with AIDS. Lancet 1994; 344: 332.
17. Barzilai A, et al. Successful treatment of disseminated Mycobacterium simiae infection in AIDS patients. Scand J Infect Dis 1998; 30: 143–6.

Osteomyelitis

See under Bone and Joint Infections, above.

Otitis externa

Otitis externa or inflammation of the skin of the external auditory canal may be due to infection with bacteria, viruses, or fungi or secondary to skin disorders such as eczema, although more than one factor is often responsible for chronic disease. Treatment includes thorough cleansing and the use of appropriate antibacterial ear drops, often containing a corticosteroid as well, even though some have doubted the value of topical antibacterials. (Note that the UK Committee on Safety of Medicines has warned that ear drops containing aminoglycosides, such as gentamicin, neomycin, or framycetin, or polymyxins should not be used when the ear drum is perforated because of the risk of ototoxicity.[1]) Systemic antibacterials may be necessary in severe cases of otitis externa.

The various types of otitis externa and their management have been described.[2] Briefly, for a *boil or furuncle* in the ear canal a ribbon gauze wick soaked in ichthammol in glycerol ear drops or magnesium sulfate paste may be inserted to reduce the swelling; alternatively, dexamethasone, framycetin, and gramicidin ear drops may be used. Systemic treatment with flucloxacillin should be given if staphylococcal infection is likely.[2] In *acute diffuse otitis externa* (swimmer's ear) *Staphylococcus aureus* and *Pseudomonas* spp. are often present. Treatment includes instillation of ear drops such as dexamethasone, framycetin, and gramicidin or gentamicin and hydrocortisone, using a wick if it proves difficult.[2] Topical gentamicin has generally been successful and oral fluoroquinolones effective in most cases not responding to topical treatment.[3] 'Malignant' otitis externa, due to fulminating infection especially with *Pseudomonas*, is uncommon but can occur in, for example, elderly diabetics. Topical antibacterials are not effective and systemic treatment with antipseudomonal drugs such as gentamicin or ceftazidime, together with metronidazole if anaerobes are present, is essential.[2] Oral ciprofloxacin given for 6 or more weeks has been used successfully in infection due predominantly to *Ps. aeruginosa*[4,5] and some consider that fluoroquinolones, in particular ciprofloxacin, are the antibacterials of choice in malignant otitis externa.[6] However, resistance to ciprofloxacin has been reported.[7] In *eczematous otitis externa* gentamicin with hydrocortisone ear drops can be used if infection is suspected.[2]

1. Committee on Safety of Medicines. Preparations used in the topical treatment of otitis externa. Current Problems 5 1981.
2. Keene M. Otitis externa. Prescribers' J 1990; 30: 229–35.
3. Elies W. Local chemotherapy of selected bacterial infections of the ear. J Antimicrob Chemother 1990; 26: 303–5.
4. Hickey SA, et al. Treating malignant otitis with oral ciprofloxacin. BMJ 1989; 299: 550–1.
5. Lang R, et al. Successful treatment of malignant external otitis with oral ciprofloxacin: report of experience with 23 patients. J Infect Dis 1990; 161: 537–40.
6. Giamarellou H. Malignant otitis externa: the therapeutic evolution of a lethal infection. J Antimicrob Chemother 1992; 30: 745–51.
7. Cooper MA, et al. Ciprofloxacin resistance developing during treatment of malignant otitis externa. J Antimicrob Chemother 1993; 32: 163–4.

Otitis media

Otitis media or inflammation of the middle ear can be acute or chronic, serous (with effusion; secretory) or suppurative. Reviews[1,2] illustrate the continuing confusion over terminology and differences in management, despite the fact that otitis media is one of the most frequent childhood illnesses seen in general practice. Diagnosis can be difficult[3] and some consider that it can only be achieved by viewing the tympanic membrane (ear drum) or by the presence of a discharge.[1] The following classification has been applied[1] to otitis media:

- *acute serous otitis media*, secondary to Eustachian tube dysfunction and characterised by discomfort

- *acute suppurative otitis media*, due to bacterial or viral infection, with pain ranging from mild earache to severe pain and a red ear drum bulging from an acute purulent effusion that may rupture with purulent discharge

- *chronic serous otitis media*, or the 'glue ear' syndrome, characterised by deafness

- *chronic suppurative otitis media*, associated with perforation and/or cholesteatoma and characterised by discharge and deafness.

There may be some overlap in the use of these terms. It has been stated[4] that *serous otitis media* (also termed secretory or non-suppurative otitis media, otitis media with effusion, and 'glue ear') is the commonest middle ear disorder in children; the fluid present may be serous, mucoid, mucopurulent, or of mixed variety; there are no acute symptoms and signs of inflammation; and the fluid is often sterile. Some[5] consider terms such as 'acute suppurative' or 'acute serous' otitis media to be unhelpful since the diagnosis cannot be made in practice, and prefer the use of acute otitis media.

ACUTE OTITIS MEDIA is seen especially in young children and is often due to bacterial or viral infection (frequently both), although infecting organisms are not always identified. It is sometimes associated with upper respiratory-tract infection. The commonest bacterial pathogens are *Streptococcus pneumoniae*, followed by *Haemophilus influenzae*, with *Moraxella catarrhalis (Branhamella catarrhalis)*[6] an increasingly important cause. Treatment aims to relieve symptoms, avoid complications, and prevent relapse, recurrence, and progression to the chronic state.[1] Sometimes an analgesic such as paracetamol may be all that is required as long as frequent inspection is possible. However, it is common practice to prescribe a systemic antibacterial as well as an analgesic,[7] although the need for routine antibacterial treatment is questionable.[3,5,8–10] Ear drops containing antibacterials, corticosteroids, or local anaesthetics are not effective, neither are topical and systemic decongestants, antihistamines, and mucolytics.[1,11] Systemic antibacterial treatment aims to speed resolution and prevent complications. However, while clinical studies have shown only modest benefits from routine administration of antibacterials[12–14] and experience from countries where antibacterials are not given routinely for acute otitis media suggests that there is no consequent increase in complications,[9,14] some clinicians argue that the routine use of antibacterials is clinically justifiable[15–18] and a systematic review[19] has concluded that it does provide a small benefit in children. Amoxicillin is often the drug of choice; alternatives include erythromycin with or without a sulfonamide such as sulfafurazole, or an oral cephalosporin such as cefaclor, cefixime, or cefuroxime axetil. Co-trimoxazole is used in some countries but it is only recommended in the UK when there is good reason to prefer it. Amoxicillin with clavulanic acid may be given when beta-lactamase-resistant strains of *H. influenzae* or *M. catarrhalis* are prevalent. Penicillin-resistant strains of *Str. pneumoniae* have been reported in children with otitis media[20] and are reported to be increasingly prevalent.[21] However, many penicillin-resistant strains remain sensitive to amoxicillin, although the situation will need continued evaluation.[21,22] The Centers for Disease Control in the USA have produced guidelines[23] for the management and surveillance of acute otitis media, in which high-dose amoxicillin for those cases suspected to be caused by penicillin-resistant strains of *Str. pneumoniae* is still recommended. Alternatives in patients not responding after 3 days are amoxicillin with clavulanic acid, oral cefuroxime axetil, or intramuscular ceftriaxone.[23] A review[24] from the USA has suggested that co-trimoxazole or amoxicillin with clavulanic acid be given in cases refractory to high-dose amoxicillin alone, with ceftriaxone reserved for third-line treatment. Duration of therapy has varied from 5 to 10 or more days; some have claimed that the shorter courses of 5 days are as effective as 7 days or more[25,26] and in one study[27] amoxicillin for 3 days appeared to be as effective as for 10 days. However, a further study[28] has found a 10-day course of amoxicillin with clavulanic acid to be more effective than a 5-day course in children aged up to 30 months who were assessed 12 to 14 days after initiation of treatment, and it is considered by some that short courses should probably not be used in children under 2 years of age[18,25] or in others at high risk of treatment failure.[25] Longer treatment for 20 days has not been found to be more efficacious than 10 days.[29]

Antibacterial prophylaxis has been tried in children at high risk including those with *recurrent acute otitis media*,[30] but it remains controversial.[1] In the UK, it is suggested that prophylaxis with trimethoprim or erythromycin may be tried during the winter. In the USA amoxicillin or sulfafurazole has been recommended for

prophylaxis.[31] The use of xylitol chewing gum, which inhibits the growth of *Str. pneumoniae*, has been reported to reduce the incidence of acute otitis media.[32] There is also the prospect of vaccination against acute otitis media with pneumococcal vaccines, and one study has found such a vaccine to be safe and efficacious;[33] the results of this study were, however, questioned.

SEROUS OTITIS MEDIA (otitis media with effusion) is common in children and may be associated with recurrent upper respiratory-tract infection. Many are asymptomatic, the fluid is usually sterile, and the condition can resolve spontaneously.[4] Optimal treatment is controversial.[2] Careful assessment and follow-up without medication is the conservative approach, but some have advocated[4] a broad-spectrum antibacterial such as amoxicillin for 5 to 10 days in young children with serous otitis media following an infection. Those at special risk such as children with cleft palate should be referred to a specialist. In the USA, amoxicillin has been recommended as first-line therapy.[31] However, a meta-analysis of controlled studies has suggested that, although a short course of antibacterials might clear the effusion in the short term, the effect is not sustained.[34] Recent US guidelines for managing otitis media with effusion in young children[35] state that most cases resolve spontaneously, although it was noted that in the meta-analysis[34] there was a 14% increase in the resolution rate with antibacterial treatment; a typical course lasted for 10 days. Management options for uncomplicated otitis media with effusion in an otherwise healthy child of 1 to 3 years were considered to be either observation or antibacterial therapy; adverse effects and the possible development of bacterial resistance should be borne in mind.[35] Corticosteroids, antihistamines, and decongestants were not recommended.[35] Nevertheless, others[36] have stated that the use of corticosteroids in combination with antibacterials should still be considered a treatment option.

CHRONIC OTITIS MEDIA can include recurrent episodes of acute infection, chronic suppurative otitis media, and prolonged serous otitis media. There have been various definitions of *chronic suppurative otitis media*. One classification[1] has divided it into 2 types associated with deafness and/or discharge. In one (tubo-tympanic disease) there is typically perforation of the ear drum, deafness, and a profuse mucoid discharge associated with upper respiratory-tract infection, the commonest infecting organisms being *Str. pneumoniae*, *Staph. aureus*, and *H. influenzae*. In the other (attico-antral disease) there may be cholesteatoma with bone involvement and the commonest infecting organisms are *Pseudomonas aeruginosa* and *Proteus* spp. Treatment of chronic suppurative otitis media is controversial. Although the value of systemic antibacterials has been debated,[1] in the UK they are recommended for use during acute exacerbations. The mainstay of treatment is thorough cleansing. Local treatment with corticosteroids or astringents as in otitis externa (above) may be beneficial, particularly with infections of mastoid cavities. Antibacterial ear drops are suggested when perforation of the ear drum is present. The UK Committee on Safety of Medicines has warned of the dangers of ototoxicity when ear drops containing aminoglycosides or polymyxins are used in the presence of a perforated ear drum in patients with otitis externa, but specialists consider that untreated chronic suppurative otitis media is more likely to result in deafness than is the use of these ear drops.[1] In *Pseudomonas* infection ear drops containing gentamicin and hydrocortisone are frequently used.[1] Local application of the fluoroquinolones ciprofloxacin or ofloxacin[16] has shown promise and may prove a safer alternative than these ear drops.[37] A systematic review[38] has concluded that aural toilet procedures and topical antibacterials, particularly quinolones, are effective in resolving otorrhoea and eradicating bacteria from the middle ear.

In the USA initial oral therapy with amoxicillin-clavulanic acid, cefaclor, or erythromycin-sulfafurazole has been advocated for chronic suppurative otitis media,[39] but despite this ear drops continue to be popular.[2] In a study from Israel[40] intravenous mezlocillin or ceftazidime together with daily suction and debridement, but no topical antibacterial therapy, was reported to be successful in treating children with chronic suppurative otitis media without cholesteatoma. *Ps. aeruginosa* had been present in most cultures and other organisms included Gram-negative enteric bacilli, *Staph. aureus*, and *H. influenzae*. Anaerobic organisms have also been implicated frequently.[41] A community-based study in Kenya found that oral amoxicillin and topical antibacterial and corticosteroid drops given in addition to regular cleansing was more effective than either cleansing alone or no treatment.[42]

1. Glover GW. Otitis media. *Prescribers' J* 1990; **30:** 218–24.
2. Lisby-Sutch SM, *et al.* Therapy of otitis media. *Clin Pharm* 1990; **9:** 15–34.
3. Froom J, *et al.* Diagnosis and antibiotic treatment of acute otitis media: report from International Primary Care Network. *BMJ* 1990; **300:** 582–6.
4. Shah NS. Serous otitis media. *Prescribers' J* 1990; **30:** 225–8.
5. Bollag U, Bollag-Albrecht E. Recommendations derived from practice audit for the treatment of acute otitis media. *Lancet* 1991; **338:** 96–9.
6. Marchant CD. Spectrum of disease due to Branhamella catarrhalis in children with particular reference to acute otitis media. *Am J Med* 1990; **88** (suppl 5A): 15S–19S.
7. Anonymous. Management of acute otitis media and glue ear. *Drug Ther Bull* 1995; **33:** 12–15.
8. Browning GG. Childhood otalgia: acute otitis media 1. *BMJ* 1990; **300:** 1005–6.
9. Majeed A, Harris T. Acute otitis media in children. *BMJ* 1997; **315:** 321–2.
10. Damoiseaux RAMJ, *et al.* Primary care based randomised, double blind trial of amoxicillin versus placebo for acute otitis media in children aged under 2 years. *BMJ* 2000; **320:** 350–4.
11. Flynn CA, *et al.* Decongestants and antihistamines for acute otitis media in children (updated 18 July 2001). Available in The Cochrane Library; Issue 4. Oxford: Update Software; 2001.
12. Rosenfeld RM, *et al.* Clinical efficacy of antimicrobial drugs for acute otitis media: metaanalysis of 5400 children from thirty-three randomized trials. *J Pediatr* 1994; **124:** 355–67.
13. Del Mar C, *et al.* Are antibiotics indicated as initial treatment for children with acute otitis media? A meta-analysis. *BMJ* 1997; **314:** 1526–9.
14. Froom J, *et al.* Antimicrobials for acute otitis media? A review from the International Primary Care Network. *BMJ* 1997; **315:** 98–102.
15. Carlin SA, *et al.* Host factors and the early therapeutic response in acute otitis media. *J Pediatr* 1991; **118:** 178–83.
16. Burke P, *et al.* Acute red ear in children: controlled trial of non-antibiotic treatment in general practice. *BMJ* 1991; **303:** 558–62.
17. Dowell SF, *et al.* Otitis media—principles of judicious use of antimicrobial agents. *Pediatrics* 1998; **101** (suppl): 165–71.
18. Paradise JL. Short-course antimicrobial treatment for acute otitis media: not best for infants and young children. *JAMA* 1997; **278:** 1640–2.
19. Glasziou PP, *et al.* Antibiotics for acute otitis media in children (updated 29 August 2001). In The Cochrane Library; Issue 4. Oxford: Update Software; 2001.
20. Klugman KP. Management of antibiotic-resistant pneumococcal infections. *J Antimicrob Chemother* 1994; **34:** 191–3.
21. Klugman KP. Epidemiology, control and treatment of multiresistant pneumococci. *Drugs* 1996; **52** (suppl 2): 42–6.
22. Pelton SI. New concepts in the pathophysiology and management of middle ear disease in childhood. *Drugs* 1996; **52** (suppl 2): 62–7.
23. Dowell SF, *et al.* Acute otitis media: management and surveillance in an era of pneumococcal resistance—a report from the Drug-Resistant Streptococcus pneumoniae Therapeutic Working Group. *Pediatr Infect Dis J* 1999; **18:** 1–9.
24. Erramouspe J, Heyneman CA. Treatment and prevention of otitis media. *Ann Pharmacother* 2000; **34:** 1452–68.
25. Pichichero ME. Changing the treatment paradigm for acute otitis media in children. *JAMA* 1998; **279:** 1748–50.
26. Kozyrskyj AL, *et al.* Short course antibiotics for acute otitis media (updated 18 July 2001). In The Cochrane Library; Issue 4. Oxford: Update Software; 2001.
27. Chaput de Saintonge DM, *et al.* Trial of three-day and ten-day courses of amoxycillin in otitis media. *BMJ* 1982; **284:** 1078–81.
28. Cohen R, *et al.* A multicenter, randomized, double-blind trial of 5 versus 10 days of antibiotic therapy for acute otitis media in young children. *J Pediatr* 1998; **133:** 634–9.
29. Mandel EM, *et al.* Efficacy of 20- versus 10-day antimicrobial treatment for acute otitis media. *Pediatrics* 1995; **96:** 5–13.
30. Paradise JL. Antimicrobial drugs and surgical procedures in the prevention of otitis media. *Pediatr Infect Dis J* 1989; **8** (suppl 1): S35–7.
31. Bluestone CD. Management of otitis media in infants and children: current role of old and new antimicrobial agents. *Pediatr Infect Dis J* 1988; **7:** S129–36.
32. Uhari M, *et al.* Xylitol chewing gum in prevention of acute otitis media: double blind randomised trial. *BMJ* 1996; **313:** 1180–4.
33. Eskola J, *et al.* Efficacy of a pneumococcal conjugate vaccine against acute otitis media. *N Engl J Med* 2001; **344:** 403–9.
34. Williams RL, *et al.* Use of antibiotics in preventing recurrent acute otitis media and in treating otitis media with effusion: a meta-analytic attempt to resolve the brouhaha. *JAMA* 1993; **270:** 1344–51.
35. American Academy of Pediatrics Otitis Media Guideline Panel. Managing otitis media with effusion in young children. *Pediatrics* 1994; **94:** 766–73.
36. Berman S. Otitis media in children. *N Engl J Med* 1995; **332:** 1560–5.
37. Elies W. Local chemotherapy of selected bacterial infections of the ear. *J Antimicrob Chemother* 1987; **26:** 303–5.
38. Acuin J, *et al.* Interventions for chronic suppurative otitis media (updated 24 May 2001). In The Cochrane Library; Issue 4. Oxford: Update Software; 2001.
39. Nelson JD. Chronic suppurative otitis media. *Pediatr Infect Dis J* 1988; **7:** 446–8.
40. Fliss DM, *et al.* Medical management of chronic suppurative otitis media without cholesteatoma in children. *J Pediatr* 1990; **116:** 991–6.
41. Wintermeyer SM, Nahata MC. Chronic suppurative otitis media. *Ann Pharmacother* 1994; **28:** 1089–99.
42. Smith AW, *et al.* Randomised controlled trial of treatment of chronic suppurative otitis media Kenyan schoolchildren *Lancet* 1996; **348:** 1128–33.

Pancreatitis

The overall management of pancreatitis is discussed on p.1646. Although there has been some uncertainty about the value of prophylactic antibacterials in acute pancreatitis, early treatment with cefuroxime markedly reduced mortality in a study of patients with acute necrotising pancreatitis[1] and a retrospective study[2] reported a reduction in the incidence, but not in the time of onset, of infection in those receiving prophylactic therapy. A meta-analysis[3] of 8 studies showed a positive benefit for prophylactic antibiotics in reducing mortality in patients with acute pancreatitis. The advantage was limited to patients with severe pancreatitis who received broad-spectrum antibiotics that achieved therapeutic levels in pancreatic tissue.

1. Sainio V, *et al.* Early antibiotic treatment in acute necrotising pancreatitis. *Lancet* 1995; **346:** 663–7.
2. Ho HS, Frey CF. The role of antibiotic prophylaxis in severe acute pancreatitis. *Arch Surg* 1997; **132:** 487–93.
3. Golub R, *et al.* Role of antibiotics in acute pancreatitis: a meta-analysis. *J Gastrointest Surg* 1998; **2:** 496–503.

Pelvic inflammatory disease

Pelvic inflammatory disease is a broad term for infectious disorders of the upper genital tract in women and may include endometritis, salpingitis, tubo-ovarian abscess, and pelvic peritonitis. It is generally due to ascending infection through the cervix and uterus to the fallopian tubes, resulting in salpingitis, and from there may extend to the ovaries and peritoneum. Long-term complications include infertility and ectopic pregnancy. Pelvic inflammatory disease has become more common and has been the subject of several reviews.[1-3] The use of intrauterine contraceptive devices might increase the likelihood of pelvic inflammatory disease although the risk may have been overstated;[1] it appears to be greatest during the first 20 days after insertion of the device.[4]

The majority of these infections are probably sexually transmitted and at one time were mainly due to *Neisseria gonorrhoeae*, but *Chlamydia trachomatis* is increasingly responsible and may be the commonest cause of pelvic inflammatory disease in some areas. Other organisms that have been isolated include *Mycoplasma hominis*; *Ureaplasma urealyticum*; anaerobes such as *Bacteroides*, *Peptococcus*, and *Peptostreptococcus* spp.; Gram-negative enteric aerobes such as *Escherichia coli*; and Gram-positive aerobes such as group B streptococci. Some of these organisms occur in the abnormal vaginal flora associated with bacterial vaginosis (above). Thus, the aetiology of pelvic inflammatory disease appears to be polymicrobial; some think that primary infection with *N. gonorrhoeae* or *C. trachomatis*, or both, allows opportunistic infection with aerobic and anaerobic bacteria.[1]

Treatment regimens are of necessity broad spectrum and empirical and should include antibacterials active against the major pathogens. Many consider that treatment should be started in hospital so that drugs can be given parenterally.

WHO recommends three possible treatment regimens for inpatients:[5] intramuscular ceftriaxone, plus oral or intravenous doxycycline or oral tetracycline, plus oral or intravenous metronidazole or chloramphenicol; or intravenous clindamycin plus intravenous gentamicin; or oral ciprofloxacin or intramuscular spectinomycin, plus oral or intravenous doxycycline or oral tetracycline, plus oral or intravenous metronidazole or chloramphenicol. Therapy should be continued for at least 48 hours after clinical improvement, and followed by doxycycline or tetracycline orally for 14 days. For outpatients a single-dose treatment for uncomplicated gonorrhoea such as ceftriaxone intramuscularly is recommended[5] (see Gonorrhoea, above) together with metronidazole and either doxycycline or tetracycline by mouth for 14 days.

In the UK, recommended regimens[6] are: cefoxitin intravenously plus doxycycline intravenously (or by mouth if tolerated) then doxycycline plus metronidazole by mouth for a total of 14 days; clindamycin plus gentamicin both intravenously followed by either clindamycin by mouth or doxycycline plus metronidazole both by mouth for a total of 14 days; ofloxacin plus metronidazole both by mouth for 14 days; or single intramuscular doses of ceftriaxone or cefoxitin with probenecid by mouth followed by doxycycline plus metronidazole both by mouth for 14 days. Intravenous therapies should be continued until 24 hours after clinical improvement is noted and then oral therapy should be substituted. Alternative regimens are: ofloxacin plus metronidazole both intravenously; or ciprofloxacin plus metronidazole both intravenously, plus doxycycline intravenously or by mouth.

Further examples of suitable treatment regimens have been provided by the Centers for Disease Control in the USA.[7] For parenteral administration cefoxitin or cefotetan may be given intravenously together with doxycycline orally or intravenously (regimen A) or clindamycin intravenously together with gentamicin intramuscularly or intravenously (regimen B), in each case continued for 24 hours after substantial clinical improvement has occurred and then followed by doxycycline by mouth to complete a total of 14 days' treatment. In regimen A, clindamycin or metronidazole may be added to doxycycline for continued therapy in patients with tubo-ovarian abscesses. In regimen B continuation may be with oral clindamycin rather than doxycycline. For oral treatment ofloxacin plus metronidazole by mouth for 14 days may be employed. Alternatively, a single intramuscular dose of cefoxitin plus probenecid by mouth, or of ceftriaxone or equivalent cephalosporin, together with doxycycline by mouth for 14 days may be used.

1. Pearce JM. Pelvic inflammatory disease. *BMJ* 1990; **300:** 1090–1.
2. Dodson MG. Optimum therapy for acute pelvic inflammatory disease. *Drugs* 1990; **39:** 511–22.
3. McCormack WM. Pelvic inflammatory disease. *N Engl J Med* 1994; **330:** 115–19.
4. Farley TMM, *et al.* Intrauterine devices and pelvic inflammatory disease: an international perspective. *Lancet* 1992; **339:** 785–8.
5. WHO. Guidelines for the management of sexually transmitted infections. Geneva: WHO, 2001.
6. Clinical Effectiveness Group (Association of Genitourinary Medicine and the Medical Society for the Study of Venereal Diseases). National guideline for the management of pelvic infections and perihepatitis. *Sex Transm Infect* 1999; **75** (suppl 1): S54–S56.
7. Centers for Disease Control. 1998 Guidelines for treatment of sexually transmitted diseases. *MMWR* 1998; **47** (RR-1): 79–86.

Peptic ulcer disease

The Gram-negative bacterium *Helicobacter pylori* is involved in the aetiology of gastritis and peptic ulceration, and treatment regimens to eradicate the organism are recommended in peptic ulcer disease (p.1208).

Perinatal streptococcal infections

Group B streptococci are a major cause of perinatal infections, often leading to neonatal pneumonia or septicaemia, sometimes with meningitis, although the incidence varies in different parts of the world. Infections are acquired through maternal genital carriage during pregnancy. *Prevention* of group B streptococcal infection in infants may be achieved by giving appropriate antibacterials to the mother during labour.[1,2] Ideally maternal carriers of group B streptococci would be identified during pregnancy, but this may not be practical. Factors that increase the risk of acquiring neonatal infection include premature labour, prolonged rupture of membranes, maternal fever, a previous child with neonatal group B streptococcal infection, and multiple pregnancy and they will influence the decision of whether or not to give intrapartum antibacterial prophylaxis to the mother. A penicillin is the preferred drug.

Guidelines in the USA[1,3] allow prophylactic strategies based either on prenatal screening or on risk factor analysis. They have recommended ampicillin or benzylpenicillin given intravenously during labour, or alternatively clindamycin or erythromycin in women allergic to penicillin. However, these policies have their critics.[4,5] In other parts of the world, including Europe, the incidence of neonatal streptococcal infections is much lower and the US model for prophylaxis may not be appropriate.[6,7]

Another strategy suggested for areas with a high incidence of neonatal group B streptococcal disease (above 1.5 per 1000 live births) is administration of a single dose of penicillin to all neonates at birth.[8]

As mentioned under Premature Labour, below, the elimination of group B streptococci in pregnant women might also reduce the risk of premature labour.

Streptococcus group B vaccines are under investigation for administration to pregnant women to prevent neonatal infection.

1. Centers for Disease Control. Prevention of prenatal group B streptococcal disease: a public health perspective. *MMWR* 1996; **45** (RR-7): 1–24.
2. van Oppen C, Feldman R. Antibiotic prophylaxis of neonatal group B streptococcal infections. *BMJ* 1993; **301:** 411–12.
3. American Academy of Pediatrics, Committee on Infectious Diseases and Committee on Fetus and Newborn. Revised guidelines for prevention of early-onset group B streptococcal (GBS) infection. *Pediatrics* 1997; **99:** 489–96.
4. Benitz WE. The neonatal group B streptococcal debate. *Pediatrics* 1998; **101:** 494–5.
5. Ledger WJ. CDC guidelines for the prevention of perinatal group B streptococcal disease: are they appropriate? *Infect Dis Clin Pract* 1998; **7:** 188–93.
6. Simpson AJA, Heard SR. Group B Streptococcus. *Lancet* 1995; **346:** 700.
7. Jakobi P, *et al.* New CDC guidelines for prevention of perinatal group B streptococcal disease. *Lancet* 1996; **348:** 969.
8. Siegel JD, Cushion NB. Prevention of early-onset group B streptococcal disease: another look at single-dose penicillin at birth. *Obstet Gynecol* 1996; **87:** 692–8.

Peritonitis

Intra-abdominal infections include peritonitis, which may be complicated by intraperitoneal abscesses, and abscesses of the intra-abdominal viscera such as those of the liver (see under Abscess, Liver, above), pancreas, and spleen. Infective peritonitis may be primary or secondary or may be a complication of continuous ambulatory peritoneal dialysis (CAPD).

Primary peritonitis. In primary or spontaneous bacterial peritonitis there is no specific focus of infection and it occurs most often as a complication of ascites. Infecting bacteria include *Escherichia coli*, other Enterobacteriaceae, and streptococci. Initial empirical treatment has been with broad-spectrum chemotherapy such as ampicillin plus an aminoglycoside, but third-generation cephalosporins such as cefotaxime are considered by some to be the treatment of choice.[1-3] Other alternatives include other broad-spectrum penicillins, carbapenems, and combinations of penicillins with beta-lactamase inhibitors.[2,3] Ofloxacin by mouth has been reported to be as effective as intravenous cefotaxime in uncomplicated infections.[4] If infection with anaerobic organisms is suspected metronidazole or clindamycin may be added to the chosen regimen.[2] In cirrhotic patients with low levels of ascitic fluid protein[5] the administration of oral norfloxacin for selective intestinal decontamination appeared to prevent spontaneous bacterial peritonitis and prophylaxis with norfloxacin has been recommended to decrease the recurrence of spontaneous bacterial peritonitis.[1] However, prophylaxis with norfloxacin will not prevent infection by Gram-positive bacteria including *Staphylococcus aureus* and quinolone-resistant Gram-negative bacteria.[2] Co-trimoxazole has also been reported to be an effective prophylactic.[6]

Secondary peritonitis. Secondary peritonitis is associated with perforation of the gastrointestinal tract, conditions such as appendicitis and diverticulitis, and contamination at surgery. Infections are generally mixed and originate from the gastrointestinal tract. Bacteria responsible include *E. coli* and other Enterobacteriaceae; anaerobes, especially *Bacteroides fragilis*; enterococci; and sometimes *Pseudomonas aeruginosa*. Broad-spectrum antibacterial therapy is therefore usually employed, at least until the infecting organisms are known, and a combination of 2 or 3 drugs is often given. The intravenous route is generally preferred. Nevertheless, it is difficult to assess the relative merits of surgical therapy against medical management that includes antibacterial therapy.[2] An aminoglycoside such as gentamicin or a cephalosporin plus metronidazole or clindamycin has often been used, but many other regimens have been tried. Patterns of resistance further complicate the choice of antibacterial: resistance to beta lactams may emerge among some Gram-negative organisms which are most likely to infect patients with prolonged hospital stays, previous antibacterial treatment, postoperative peritonitis, or recurrent peritonitis. Such patients are best treated with a regimen that includes a carbapenem, cefepime, a fluoroquinolone, or an aminoglycoside.[2] Resistant isolates of *B. fragilis* and *Clostridium difficile* (with associated diarrhoea) are more common after clindamycin than after metronidazole.[2] Microaerophilic Gram-positive cocci are resistant to metronidazole but not to clindamycin,[2] so metronidazole should be used in combination with a beta lactam other than aztreonam.[2]

For reference to the prevention of postoperative infection, see under Surgical Infection, below.

CAPD peritonitis. Peritonitis is the main complication of CAPD, a technique widely used in end-stage renal failure. Unlike secondary peritonitis, above, a single infecting organism is often responsible. The most common infections have usually been due to Gram-positive organisms, especially staphylococci, but infections with Gram-negative bacteria (typically Enterobacteriaceae) are becoming more common,[7] and fungi are an increasingly important cause of peritonitis in CAPD.[2] The empirical treatment of CAPD peritonitis has changed in recent years because of the emergence of vancomycin-resistant organisms. While vancomycin in combination with an aminoglycoside has been recommended,[8] in order to avoid unnecessary exposure to vancomycin the International Society for Peritoneal Dialysis now recommends the use of a first-generation cephalosporin with an aminoglycoside, given intraperitoneally by mixing the antibacterials with the dialysate.[7] Alternatives to cephalosporins in this regimen are nafcillin, clindamycin, vancomycin, and ciprofloxacin in that order. Once-daily dosing regimens for aminoglycosides are considered

appropriate for CAPD patients.[7] Once the infecting organism is identified, an appropriate narrow-spectrum antibacterial can be substituted, although some physicians prefer to continue treatment with cephalosporins.[7] Treatment is generally continued for 14 days in patients who have a clinical response.[7] Treatment should be extended to 21 days in patients with *Staph. aureus* infections, and possibly also in those with pseudomonal infections.[7]

Exit-site infections can be treated with an oral penicillinase-resistant penicillin, cefalexin, or co-trimoxazole for Gram-positive infections, or an oral fluoroquinolone such as ciprofloxacin for Gram-negative infections.[7]

Long-term antibacterial prophylaxis is not generally effective, although intranasal mupirocin or oral rifampicin have been used to reduce nasal carriage of *Staph. aureus* in patients with exit-site infections.[7] Dramatic reductions in peritonitis rates have been achieved with programmes based on stringent aseptic wound care and on minimising contact of the CAPD system with domestic water.[9]

1. Gilbert JA, Kamath PS. Spontaneous bacterial peritonitis: an update. *Mayo Clin Proc* 1995; **70:** 365–70.
2. Johnson CC, et al. Peritonitis: update on pathophysiology, clinical manifestations, and management. *Clin Infect Dis* 1997; **24:** 1035–47.
3. Rimola A, et al. Diagnosis, treatment and prophylaxis of spontaneous bacterial peritonitis: a consensus document. *J Hepatol* 2000; **32:** 142–53.
4. Navasa M et al. Randomized comparative study of oral ofloxacin versus intravenous cefotaxime in spontaneous bacterial peritonitis. *Gastroenterology* 1996; **111:** 1011–17.
5. Soriano G, et al. Selective intestinal decontamination prevents spontaneous bacterial peritonitis. *Gastroenterology* 1991; **100:** 477–81.
6. Singh N, et al. Trimethoprim–sulfamethoxazole for the prevention of spontaneous bacterial peritonitis in cirrhosis: a randomized trial. *Ann Intern Med* 1995; **122:** 595–8.
7. Keane WF, et al. Peritoneal dialysis-related peritonitis treatment recommendations: 1996 update. *Perit Dial Int* 1996; **16:** 557–73.
8. Working Party of the British Society for Antimicrobial Chemotherapy. Diagnosis and management of peritonitis in continuous ambulatory peritoneal dialysis. *Lancet* 1987; **i:** 845–9.
9. Ludlam H, et al. Prevention of peritonitis in continuous ambulatory peritoneal dialysis. *Lancet* 1990; **335:** 1161.

Pertussis

Pertussis or whooping cough is caused by infection with the respiratory pathogen *Bordetella pertussis*, a Gram-negative aerobic bacterium. The related species *B. parapertussis* causes a similar but generally milder illness. Pertussis is very infectious and occurs most frequently in children, but may be more common in adults than once thought.[1-3] The incidence of pertussis has been greatly reduced by the active immunisation of infants (see under Pertussis Vaccines, p.1556) and effective prevention by the adequate uptake of vaccine remains the ultimate objective. In addition to an accelerated schedule of vaccination, prompt use of erythromycin for treatment and prophylaxis may help to contain epidemics.[4]

Erythromycin is the antibacterial of choice at any stage of the disease. Once infection has occurred erythromycin is thought to render the patient non-infectious by eliminating nasopharyngeal carriage of *B. pertussis*. Such treatment is unlikely to affect the clinical course of pertussis because diagnosis is difficult until the paroxysmal stage, by which time the bacteria have already damaged the respiratory tract and released their toxins.[5] Erythromycin is also given prophylactically to close contacts. Erythromycin 50 mg per kg body-weight daily for 14 days, whether for treatment or prophylaxis, has been recommended,[6] and the estolate ester was favoured in order to achieve maximum blood concentrations. However, a 7-day course of erythromycin was reported to be as effective as a 14-day course for treatment.[7] Courses of azithromycin for 5 days or clarithromycin for 7 days were also effective.[8] Decreased transmission and severity of the disease has been seen in adults and adolescents in a confined setting, when erythromycin was used for treatment, and prophylaxis in those exposed, and especially when started within 14 days of the first case being identified.[9] Erythromycin prophylaxis was also effective in a family setting, especially if started before the occurrence of the first secondary case.[10]

Strains of *B. pertussis* resistant to erythromycin have been reported in the USA, but do not appear to be widespread.[11] Co-trimoxazole has been suggested as an alternative to erythromycin for both treatment and prophylaxis.[11]

1. Mortimer EA. Pertussis and its prevention: a family affair. *J Infect Dis* 1990; **161:** 473–9.
2. Wright SW, et al. Pertussis infection in adults with persistent cough. *JAMA* 1995; **273:** 1044–6.
3. Cherry JD. Pertussis in adults. *Ann Intern Med* 1998; **128:** 64–6.
4. Christie CDC, et al. The 1993 epidemic of pertussis in Cincinnati: resurgence of disease in a highly immunized population of children. *N Engl J Med* 1994; **331:** 16–21.

5. Moxon ER, Rappuoli R. Modern vaccines: Haemophilus influenzae infections and whooping cough. *Lancet* 1990; **335:** 1324–9.
6. Bass JW. Pertussis: current status of prevention and treatment. *Pediatr Infect Dis* 1985; **4:** 614–19.
7. Halperin SA, et al. Seven days of erythromycin estolate is as effective as fourteen days for the treatment of Bordetella pertussis infections. *Pediatrics* 1997; **100:** 65–71.
8. Aoyama T, et al. Efficacy of short-term treatment of pertussis with clarithromycin and azithromycin. *J Pediatr* 1996; **129:** 761–4.
9. Steketee RW, et al. Evidence for a high attack rate and efficacy of erythromycin prophylaxis in a pertussis outbreak in a facility for the developmentally disabled. *J Infect Dis* 1988; **157:** 434–40.
10. De Serres G, et al. Field effectiveness of erythromycin prophylaxis to prevent pertussis within families. *Pediatr Infect Dis J* 1995; **14:** 969–75.
11. Centers for Disease Control. Erythromycin-resistant Bordetella pertussis—Yuma County, Arizona, May-October 1994. *MMWR* 1994; **43:** 807–10.

Pharyngitis

Pharyngitis and tonsillitis are upper respiratory-tract infections with similar causes and occur especially in children. Acute pharyngitis is an inflammatory syndrome of the oropharynx that may include the tonsils whereas tonsillitis is strictly speaking a more localised infection. The commonest causes are viral and 'sore throat' is often a symptom of the common cold as well as influenza and infectious mononucleosis. For further details of these viral infections, see under Choice of Antiviral, p.605.

The most important bacterial cause of acute pharyngitis and tonsillitis is the group A beta-haemolytic streptococcus, *Streptococcus pyogenes*. An erythrogenic toxin-producing strain causes pharyngitis and tonsillitis in scarlet fever.

In view of the prevalence of a viral cause, opinions have differed over whether and when to treat pharyngitis with antimicrobial drugs. Some have advocated waiting until a definite diagnosis of *Str. pyogenes* infection is made, but others treat immediately if streptococcal pharyngitis is suspected because of the risk of longer term complications such as rheumatic fever and the need to eradicate *Str. pyogenes* from the throat.[1-3] The incidence of rheumatic fever has been low for many years in developed countries, but there was evidence of a resurgence in parts of the USA in the mid-1980s. Thus, in addition to shortening the illness and interrupting transmission, the antibacterial treatment of streptococcal pharyngitis also serves as primary prevention of rheumatic fever (see below). However, in countries in which the incidence of rheumatic fever remains low the routine administration of antibacterials for the management of sore throats is discouraged.[4,5]

Penicillin is the standard treatment for streptococcal pharyngitis or tonsillitis,[6,7] generally as phenoxymethylpenicillin by mouth for 10 days; benzylpenicillin may be given by injection initially. A single intramuscular injection of benzathine benzylpenicillin is perhaps the treatment of choice, especially if compliance with a 10-day course of oral penicillin is unlikely, and is advocated by WHO and the American Heart Association for the primary prevention of rheumatic fever (see under Rheumatic Fever, below), but the injection may not be available in some countries. Ampicillin should probably be avoided because of the risk of maculopapular rash if the patient proves to have infectious mononucleosis.[8] Erythromycin or another macrolide may be given to penicillin-allergic patients, except where there is evidence of significant resistance, as in some parts of Europe,[7] Japan,[9] and Finland;[10] it may also be a better choice than penicillin if there is a likelihood of infection with *Arcanobacterium haemolyticum* (*Corynebacterium haemolyticum*) (see below). Oral cephalosporins are another alternative.

Despite the general effectiveness of penicillin a trend of increasing numbers of relapses and recurrent infections has been noted.[11] Some treatment failures have been attributed to poor patient compliance with a 10-day course of penicillin and attempts to overcome this have included giving fewer daily doses or shortening the length of treatment. Meta-analysis of studies supports the use of twice-daily dosing of phenoxymethylpenicillin which appears to be as effective as doses three or four times daily,[12] but a single daily dose is less effective. Courses of phenoxymethylpenicillin shorter than 10 days have not proved effective.[13,14] There is some evidence that shorter courses may be possible with some alternative antibacterials. Studies have shown that courses of 5 days or less of erythromycin,[15] cefotiam hexetil,[16] azithromycin,[17,18] or cefuroxime axetil[19,20] may be as effective as a 10-day course of phenoxymethylpenicillin. However, definitive studies have not been done, and the broader spectrum and higher cost of these regimens are drawbacks.[6,7]

Penicillin resistance in *Str. pyogenes* remains rare. In addition to poor compliance, treatment failures with penicillin, leading to recurrent infection, might be explained by the presence of beta-lactamase-producing oropharyngeal bacteria that are able to protect *Str. pyogenes* against penicillin,[21] although this theory was not supported by a study in 462 children.[22] Antibacterials less susceptible to beta lactamase have been effective, sometimes more so than phenoxymethylpenicillin. They include the oral cephalosporins cefaclor,[23] cefuroxime axetil,[24] cefixime,[25] cefprozil,[26] and cefadroxil[27] and the combined preparation amoxicillin with clavulanic acid[28,29] (like ampicillin, amoxicillin should perhaps be avoided because of the risk of maculopapular rash if the patient turns out to have infectious mononucleosis). Clindamycin has eradicated *Str. pyogenes* and beta-lactamase-producing bacteria in children of 12 years and under with recurrent tonsillitis, but might be less effective in older children.[30] It was also effective where penicillin and erythromycin had failed in an outbreak of streptococcal pharyngitis.[31]

Pharyngeal carriage of *Str. pyogenes* is common, especially in primary-school children and thus its presence does not necessarily reflect acute infection. Eradication may be beneficial in selected cases and has been achieved by a single intramuscular injection of benzathine benzylpenicillin together with a 4-day course of oral rifampicin;[32] a 10-day course of oral clindamycin has also been effective.[33] In order to ensure that outbreaks of *Str. pyogenes* are prevented in closely confined populations, some have recommended prophylactic antibacterials for *all* members of these populations, without exception.[34]

Other bacterial causes of pharyngitis include *Arcanobacterium haemolyticum* (*Corynebacterium haemolyticum*), *Chlamydia pneumoniae*, *Corynebacterium diphtheriae* (see under Diphtheria, above), *Neisseria gonorrhoeae* (see under Gonorrhoea, above), group C beta-haemolytic streptococci, and anaerobic bacteria.

A. haemolyticum is thought to be an important cause of pharyngitis in adolescents and young adults; there is often an accompanying scarlatiniform rash. It has been reported to respond to a single injection of benzathine benzylpenicillin or a 10-day course of erythromycin by mouth, but not to phenoxymethylpenicillin.[6]

Pharyngitis is often associated with infection with *Chlamydia pneumoniae* (formerly known as the TWAR strain of *C. psittaci*). Tetracycline or erythromycin are effective antibacterials.[35]

1. Anonymous. Bacterial pharyngitis. *Lancet* 1987; **i**: 1241–2.
2. Marcovitch H. Sore throats. *Arch Dis Child* 1990; **65**: 249–50.
3. Lang SDR, Singh K. The sore throat: when to investigate and when to prescribe. *Drugs* 1990; **40**: 854–62.
4. Little P, *et al.* Reattendance and complications in a randomised trial of prescribing strategies for sore throat: the medicalising effect of prescribing antibiotics. *BMJ* 1997; **315**: 350–2.
5. Del Mar CB, *et al.* Antibiotics for sore throat (updated 19 February 2001). Available in The Cochrane Library; Issue 2. Oxford: Update Software; 2001.
6. Bisno AL. Acute pharyngitis. *N Engl J Med* 2001; **344**: 205–11.
7. WHO. *WHO model prescribing information: drugs used in the treatment of streptococcal pharyngitis and prevention of rheumatic fever.* Geneva: WHO, 1999.
8. Green AD. Treatment of choice for childhood tonsillitis. *BMJ* 1986; **293**: 1030.
9. Maruyama S, *et al.* Sensitivity of group A streptococci to antibiotics: prevalence of resistance to erythromycin in Japan. *Am J Dis Child* 1979; **133**: 1143–5.
10. Seppälä H, *et al.* Resistance to erythromycin in group A streptococci. *N Engl J Med* 1992; **326**: 292–7.
11. Dillon HC. Streptococcal pharyngitis in the 1980s. *Pediatr Infect Dis J* 1987; **6**: 123–30.
12. Lan AJ, *et al.* The impact of dosing frequency on the efficacy of 10-day penicillin or amoxicillin therapy for streptococcal tonsillopharyngitis: a meta-analysis. Abstract: *Pediatrics* 2000; **105**: 414. Full version: http://www.pediatrics.org/cgi/content/full/105/2/e19
13. Gerber MA, *et al.* Five vs ten days of penicillin V therapy for streptococcal pharyngitis. *Am J Dis Child* 1987; **141**: 224–7.
14. Strömberg A, *et al.* Five versus ten days treatment of group A streptococcal pharyngotonsillitis: a randomized controlled clinical trial with phenoxymethylpenicillin and cefadroxil. *Scand J Infect Dis* 1988; **20**: 37–46.
15. Adam D, *et al.* Five days of erythromycin estolate versus ten days of penicillin V in the treatment of group A streptococcal tonsillopharyngitis in children. *Eur J Clin Microbiol Infect Dis* 1996; **15**: 712–17.
16. Carbon C, *et al.* A double-blind randomized trial comparing the efficacy and safety of a 5-day course of cefotiam hexetil with that of a 10-day course of penicillin V in adult patients with pharyngitis caused by group A β-haemolytic streptococci. *J Antimicrob Chemother* 1995; **35**: 843–54.
17. O'Doherty B, *et al.* Azithromycin versus penicillin V in the treatment of paediatric patients with acute streptococcal pharyngitis/tonsillitis. *Eur J Clin Microbiol Infect Dis* 1996; **15**: 718–24.
18. Hooton TM. A comparison of azithromycin and penicillin V for the treatment of streptococcal pharyngitis. *Am J Med* 1991; **91**(3A): 23S–26S.
19. Aujard Y, *et al.* Comparative efficacy and safety of four-day cefuroxime axetil and ten-day penicillin treatment of group A beta-hemolytic streptococcal pharyngitis in children. *Pediatr Infect Dis J* 1995; **14**: 295–300.
20. Adam D, *et al.* Comparison of short-course (5 day) cefuroxime axetil with a standard 10 day oral penicillin V regimen in the treatment of tonsillopharyngitis. *J Antimicrob Chemother* 2000; **45** (suppl): 23–30.
21. Brook I. The role of β-lactamase-producing bacteria in the persistence of streptococcal tonsillar infection. *Rev Infect Dis* 1984; **6**: 601–7.
22. Gerber MA, *et al.* Potential mechanisms for failure to eradicate group A streptococci from the pharynx. *Pediatrics* 1999; **104**: 911–17.
23. Stillerman M. Comparison of oral cephalosporins with penicillin therapy for group A streptococcal pharyngitis. *Pediatr Infect Dis* 1986; **5**: 649–54.
24. Gooch WM, *et al.* Efficacy of cefuroxime axetil suspension compared with that of penicillin V suspension in children with group A streptococcal pharyngitis. *Antimicrob Agents Chemother* 1993; **37**: 159–63.
25. Kiani R, *et al.* Comparative, multicenter studies of cefixime and amoxicillin in the treatment of respiratory tract infections. *Am J Med* 1988; **85** (suppl 3A): 6–13.
26. Milatovic D, *et al.* Cefprozil versus penicillin V in treatment of streptococcal tonsillopharyngitis. *Antimicrob Agents Chemother* 1993; **37**: 1620–3.
27. Milatovic D, Knauer J. Cefadroxil versus penicillin V in the treatment of streptococcal tonsillopharyngitis. *Eur J Clin Microbiol Infect Dis* 1989; **8**: 282–8.
28. Brook I. Treatment of patients with acute recurrent tonsillitis due to group A β-haemolytic streptococci: a prospective randomized study comparing penicillin and amoxycillin/clavulanate potassium. *J Antimicrob Chemother* 1989; **24**: 227–33.
29. Dykhuizen RS, *et al.* Phenoxymethyl penicillin versus co-amoxiclav in the treatment of acute streptococcal pharyngitis, and the role of β-lactamase activity in saliva. *J Antimicrob Chemother* 1996; **37**: 133–8.
30. Foote PA, Brook I. Penicillin and clindamycin therapy in recurrent tonsillitis: effect of microbial flora. *Arch Otolaryngol Head Neck Surg* 1989; **115**: 856–9.
31. Raz R, *et al.* Penicillin in the treatment of an outbreak of streptococcal pharyngitis in a kibbutz due to beta-lactamase producing organisms. *J Chemother* 1990; **2**: 182–4.
32. Tanz RR, *et al.* Penicillin plus rifampin eradicates pharyngeal carriage of group A streptococcus. *J Pediatr* 1985; **106**: 876–80.
33. Tanz RR, *et al.* Clindamycin treatment of chronic pharyngeal carriage of group A streptococcus. *J Pediatr* 1991; **119**: 123–8.
34. Gray GC, *et al.* Hyperendemic Streptococcus pyogenes infection despite prophylaxis with penicillin G benzathine. *N Engl J Med* 1991; **325**: 92–7.
35. Grayston JT, *et al.* A new respiratory tract pathogen: Chlamydia pneumoniae strain TWAR. *J Infect Dis* 1990; **161**: 618–25.

Pinta

See under Syphilis, below.

Plague

Plague is caused by the Gram-negative bacillus *Yersinia pestis* (*Yersinia pseudotuberculosis* subsp. *pestis*) and is usually transmitted to man via rodents and their infected fleas. It has occurred as worldwide pandemics, for example, the Black Death in Europe in the Middle Ages. In the 1980s the largest numbers of cases reported were in Tanzania, Vietnam, Brazil, and Peru.[1] More recently there has been a re-emergence in Madagascar.[2] Plague may take several forms of which bubonic plague is the most common; others include pneumonic, septicaemic, and meningitic plague. Treatment with streptomycin, tetracycline, or chloramphenicol is highly effective in all forms if recognised early.[3] Many consider streptomycin to be the antibacterial of choice,[1] but the possibility of a Jarisch-Herxheimer reaction resulting from the bactericidal effect of streptomycin has prompted some to prefer tetracycline or to use lower doses of streptomycin together with tetracycline. Chloramphenicol has been preferred in meningitic plague because it crosses the blood-brain barrier.

Commenting on the plague epidemic that occurred in India in 1994, workers from the US Centers for Disease Control[4] also noted that streptomycin continues to be the drug of choice for treating plague, that tetracycline and gentamicin are alternatives, and that chloramphenicol is preferred for plague meningitis. They considered that prophylaxis should be given to those who have had face-to-face contact or who have occupied a closed space with someone who has pneumonic plague. For prophylaxis, tetracycline can be given to adults and older children or sulfonamides to children of 8 years and less; chloramphenicol is also effective.[4]

Infection with a strain of *Y. pestis* resistant to all the drugs usually effective against plague identified in a patient from Madagascar[5] responded to treatment with co-trimoxazole and streptomycin.

A vaccine is available for active immunisation.

1. Butler T. The black death past and present 1: plague in the 1980s. *Trans R Soc Trop Med Hyg* 1989; **83**: 458–60.
2. Chanteau S, *et al.* Plague, a reemerging disease in Madagascar. *Emerg Infect Dis* 1998; **4**: 101–4.
3. Public Health Laboratory Service Communicable Disease Surveillance Centre. Plague. *BMJ* 1983; **287**: 118–19.
4. Campbell GL, Hughes JM. Plague in India: a new warning from an old nemesis. *Ann Intern Med* 1995; **122**: 151–3.
5. Galimand M, *et al.* Multidrug resistance in Yersinia pestis mediated by a transferable plasmid. *N Engl J Med* 1997; **337**: 677–80.

Pneumonia

Pneumonia, or inflammation of the lungs with consolidation, is mostly due to bacterial or viral infection, but may be caused by fungi in immunocompromised patients or by the aspiration of chemical irritants. Interstitial pneumonitis is a common complication in cancer patients and has also been associated with certain drugs, for example amiodarone, bleomycin, and nitrofurantoin; sometimes a hypersensitivity reaction has been suspected.

The aetiology of infective pneumonia, and therefore the choice of treatment, differs according to whether it is community-acquired or hospital-acquired (nosocomial) and whether the patient was previously healthy, has chronic lung disease or other debilitating condition, is very young or very old, is immunocompromised, or has pneumonia as a result of aspiration.

Community-acquired pneumonia. In community-acquired pneumonia[1-5] the commonest pathogen in previously healthy subjects is *Streptococcus pneumoniae* (pneumococcus). Onset of pneumococcal pneumonia can be very rapid and treatment should be started promptly. *Str. pneumoniae* has usually been considered sensitive to the penicillins benzylpenicillin, amoxicillin, or ampicillin; to cephalosporins; to erythromycin; or to co-trimoxazole, but a 1991 review of resistance patterns in Europe[6] concluded that *Str. pneumoniae* no longer had predictable antibacterial susceptibility. The problem of resistant pneumococci on a worldwide basis was noted in a further review[7] and such resistance is a major concern in the USA,[8,9] highlighting the need for a more effective pneumococcal vaccine. Penicillin-resistant strains, some with high levels of resistance, have been reported in various countries, notably Spain[10-13] and Australia.[14] In a survey between 1986 and 1989 of 61 centres in the UK all strains of *Str. pneumoniae* tested were sensitive to penicillin,[15] but localised pockets of resistance have been reported[16] and there has been a general trend in the UK toward an increased incidence of pneumococci resistant to, or with reduced susceptibility to, penicillin and other antibacterials commonly used for treatment.[17] However, the routine use of penicillin for community-acquired pneumonia may still be reasonable in many countries; indeed, the latest of the studies in Spain[13] noted that, although there were increased levels of resistance to penicillins and to cephalosporins, this had not been associated with increased mortality so that these antibacterials remained the drugs of choice. Erythromycin or macrolide resistance has also been reported in some countries,[18-20] especially in France where macrolide consumption is relatively high.[6] In the 1986–89 UK survey[15] 99% of strains were susceptible to erythromycin, although there was increased reporting of resistant strains in the 1992 review.[17] Resistance to co-trimoxazole and chloramphenicol has been noted in Pakistan.[21,22]

Mycoplasma pneumoniae is also an important cause of community-acquired pneumonia. Epidemics occur about every 4 years and the one underway in Europe in 1991 would probably have been responsible for up to 20% of all community-acquired pneumonia during 1992.[23] Erythromycin or tetracycline are the antibacterials of choice against *M. pneumoniae*; erythromycin is usually recommended when mycoplasmal pneumonia is suspected.[23,24] The wisdom of giving erythromycin alone for initial treatment of community-acquired pneumonia has been questioned[25] since even during *M. pneumoniae* epidemics pneumococci remain the commonest cause and, although they are usually sensitive to erythromycin, resistance has increasingly, albeit rarely,[15] been reported.[18-20] Giving erythromycin with a penicillin has therefore been suggested,[23] although as noted above penicillin-resistant pneumococci have also been reported.

Other bacteria that may be responsible for community-acquired pneumonia include *Staphylococcus aureus*, which usually occurs as a secondary bacterial infection following influenza and is associated with high mortality; *Haemophilus influenzae* and *Moraxella catarrhalis* (*Branhamella catarrhalis*),[26] especially in patients with chronic lung disease; *Legionella pneumophila* (see Legionnaires' Disease, above); *Chlamydia psittaci* (see Psittacosis, below); *Chlamydia pneumoniae* (formerly known as the TWAR strain of *Chlamydia psittaci*);[27] and *Coxiella burnetii* (see Q fever, below). Gram-negative bacilli rarely cause pneumonia in the community, especially in previously healthy patients. Anaerobic bacteria are associated with aspiration pneumonia. Viruses are the commonest pathogens in young children.

Guidelines for the management of community-acquired pneumonia in the UK[24] and in the USA[28] have been published by the British and the American Thoracic Societies respectively. In the UK,[24] initial *empirical* treatment is usually with benzylpenicillin, ampicillin, or amoxicillin. Erythromycin is an alternative in penicillin-allergic patients and should also be given during epidemics of mycoplasmal pneumonia and when *Legionella* is suspected. Second- or third-generation cephalosporins such as cefuroxime or cefotaxime are other alternatives to penicillin treatment.[24] An antistaphylococcal penicillin such as flucloxacillin should be added to treatment during influenza epidemics. Severe pneumonia of unknown aetiology may be treated by a combination of erythromycin and a second- or third-generation cephalosporin; an alternative regimen is ampicillin with flucloxacillin and erythromycin.[24] In the USA,[28] the preferred treatment in outpatients with uncomplicated disease is azithromycin or clarithromycin, or doxycycline if the patients are intolerant to macrolides. Outpatients who have co-existing cardiopulmonary disease and/or other complicating factors should be given a beta lactam such as oral cefpodoxime, cefuroxime, amoxicillin with or without clavulanic acid, or parenteral ceftriaxone followed by oral cefpodoxime, in addition to a macrolide or doxycycline. Alternatively, they may be given monotherapy with an antipneumococcal fluoroquinolone.[28] In hospitalised patients who are not in intensive care and have uncomplicated disease, intravenous azithromycin alone is recommended or, if there is macrolide intolerance, doxycycline with a beta lactam; alternatively such patients may be given monotherapy with an antipneumococcal fluoroquinolone. Inpatients not in intensive care, but who have co-existing cardiopulmonary disease and/or other complicating factors, should receive an intravenous beta lactam (cefotaxime, ceftriaxone, or ampicillin with or without sulbactam) together with an intravenous or oral macrolide or doxycycline; alternatively they may be given an intravenous antipneumococcal fluoroquinolone alone.[28] Inpatients who are in intensive care but in whom there is no risk of *Pseudomonas aeruginosa* infection, should receive an intravenous beta lactam such as cefotaxime or ceftriaxone together with either intravenous azithromycin or an intravenous fluoroquinolone. Where there is a risk of *Ps. aeruginosa*, an intravenous antipseudomonal beta lactam (such as cefepime, imipenem, meropenem, or piperacillin with tazobactam) should be given with either an intravenous antipseudomonal quinolone such as ciprofloxacin, or an intravenous aminoglycoside and either intravenous azithromycin or an intravenous fluoroquinolone; in patients who are allergic to beta lactams, aztreonam may be given in their place.[28]

Local patterns of resistance should be borne in mind (see, e.g. pneumococci, above). Definitive treatment recommendations for pneumonia due to penicillin-resistant pneumococci are lacking;[17] high-dose penicillin therapy may be adequate for strains with intermediate resistance.[13,29] Penicillin-resistant *H. influenzae* may be a problem in some areas. Many isolates of *Moraxella catarrhalis* (*Branhamella catarrhalis*) produce beta lactamase and are resistant to penicillins, but patients have responded to amoxicillin with clavulanic acid, cefotaxime, or co-trimoxazole.[26] An aminoglycoside has been added to initial therapy in patients at special risk of Gram-negative bacillary pneumonia, including those with chronic lung disease, alcoholism, diabetes, heart failure, or chronic debility.[30] Atypical pneumonias such as those caused by *Chlamydia* or *Coxiella burnetii* may be treated with erythromycin or tetracycline; azithromycin and clarithromycin are possible alternatives for *C. pneumoniae* infections.[31]

In *children* pneumonia is caused by a wider spectrum of organisms than in adults.[32] Pneumonia in neonates is usually due to organisms acquired from the mother's genital tract, especially group B streptococci, *Escherichia coli*, and *Klebsiella pneumoniae*; initial treatment with gentamicin and benzylpenicillin or ampicillin has been suggested. For prophylaxis against group B streptococci in neonates, see under Perinatal Streptococcal Infections, above. In the USA, *Chlamydia trachomatis* is said to be the commonest cause in infants up to 3 months of age;[32] erythromycin is the treatment of choice or, alternatively, sulfafurazole.[33] Viruses, especially respiratory syncytial virus, are the commonest pathogens in infants and children up to 4 years of age and, as in adults,

pneumococci are the commonest bacterial pathogens.[32] Although the pathogens are often not identified all children with pneumonia should be given antibacterials because of the possibility of bacterial infection.[32] Benzylpenicillin or ampicillin is effective, but severely ill infants should be given flucloxacillin and an aminoglycoside as well; erythromycin is used to treat chlamydial and mycoplasmal infection.[32] In developing countries acute lower respiratory-tract infection is a major cause of childhood mortality, especially in children under 5 years. Most die from pneumonia due to *Str. pneumoniae* or *H. influenzae*. In guidance from WHO[34] for the management of these infections in small hospitals, both organisms were considered to be sensitive usually to benzylpenicillin, ampicillin, amoxicillin, co-trimoxazole, and chloramphenicol and these drugs were included in protocols for the treatment of pneumonia, according to severity. However, in a study from Pakistan[21] the majority of isolates of *Str. pneumoniae* were resistant or had decreased susceptibility to at least one antibacterial, especially co-trimoxazole (62%) (recommended by WHO[34] as an alternative to procaine penicillin [procaine benzylpenicillin], amoxicillin, or ampicillin) and chloramphenicol (39%) (recommended by WHO[34] for very severe pneumonia). Even so, community-based treatment of pneumonia with a standard course of oral co-trimoxazole was of benefit in Nepalese[35] and Indian[36] infants. For children with only mild acute respiratory infections the WHO recommendation to provide supportive care without antibacterials[34] has been endorsed by an Indonesian study in which ampicillin was of no benefit.[37]

Hospital-acquired pneumonia. Most reports on hospital-acquired or nosocomial pneumonia have been from the USA.[1] Aerobic Gram-negative bacilli such as *Pseudomonas* and *Klebsiella* are the dominant cause and two or more pathogens are often found. *Staph. aureus* and *Legionella* spp. may also cause a substantial amount of nosocomial pneumonia.[1] Broad-spectrum antibacterial therapy is essential, initially with, for example, a third-generation cephalosporin such as cefotaxime or ceftazidime or an antipseudomonal penicillin together with an aminoglycoside. Monotherapy with monobactams, cephalosporins, or imipenem has also been used.[38] In one study,[39] intravenous ciprofloxacin was as effective as ceftazidime, but treatment failures with ciprofloxacin included persisting *Staph. aureus* and streptococcal infections. Nosocomial pneumonia is especially likely in immunocompromised or neutropenic patients. Prophylactic measures in ventilated patients are those mentioned under Intensive Care, above.

Immunocompromised patients. Immunosuppressed patients are at special risk of pneumonia. In addition to the bacteria mentioned above they are susceptible to opportunistic infections with *Mycobacterium tuberculosis* (see under Tuberculosis, below); viruses such as *Cytomegalovirus*; and fungi, in particular *Pneumocystis carinii* (see p.375), are also causes of pneumonia in these patients.

Interstitial pneumonitis is a common complication in cancer patients. It may sometimes be drug-related, but diagnosis of the cause is difficult. Early empirical treatment with erythromycin and co-trimoxazole, active against *Legionella*, *Mycoplasma*, and *Pneumocystis carinii*, has been advocated,[40] although individualised patient-directed care may be preferable.[41]

Aspiration pneumonia. Aspiration of organisms present in the upper respiratory tract into the lungs, often as a result of loss of consciousness or difficulty in swallowing, can cause aspiration pneumonia.[42] When community-acquired the organisms responsible are predominantly anaerobes, but in hospital-acquired aspiration pneumonia Gram-negative bacilli and *Staph. aureus* are also found.[1] Anaerobic pulmonary infections have been reviewed.[43] Confusion has arisen over the term 'aspiration pneumonia' because it has also been applied more generally to aspiration, for example, of gastric acid (Mendelson's syndrome), resulting in chemical pneumonitis and not associated with bacterial infection. *Lung abscess* generally characterises late-stage aspiration pneumonia involving anaerobic bacteria. The aetiology is rarely established, but specific anaerobic bacteria involved include *Peptostreptococcus*, *Prevotella melaninogenica* (*Bacteroides melaninogenicus*), and *Fusobacterium nucleatum*. Nearly all patients with anaerobic pulmonary infections are treated empirically. Benzylpenicillin used to be considered the treatment of choice, but this is less certain now because of increasing resistance

in anaerobes, often due to beta-lactamase production, and because of a study demonstrating the superiority of clindamycin.[44] Some, however,[42] have expressed the view that penicillin and clindamycin are inadequate and that antibacterials with activity against Gram-negative organisms, such as third-generation cephalosporins, fluoroquinolones, and piperacillin are usually required even in community-acquired aspiration pneumonia. However, one study demonstrated the value of clindamycin in the presence of penicillin-resistant *Prevotella melaninogenica*.[45] Responses to metronidazole alone have been poor. Antibacterial regimens advocated have included benzylpenicillin intravenously (despite its apparent inferiority to clindamycin); clindamycin orally or intravenously; or an aminopenicillin such as amoxicillin or ampicillin with metronidazole, each given intravenously or by mouth.[24,43] Most patients with lung abscess receive parenteral therapy until they become afebrile and show clinical improvement; oral therapy may then continue for weeks or months if necessary.

1. Macfarlane JT. Treatment of lower respiratory infections. *Lancet* 1987; **ii:** 1446–9.
2. Innes JA. Community acquired pneumonia. *BMJ* 1987; **295:** 1083–4.
3. Anonymous. Antibiotics for community-acquired pneumonia in adults. *Drug Ther Bull* 1988; **26:** 13–16.
4. Bartlett JG, Mundy LM. Community-acquired pneumonia. *N Engl J Med* 1995; **333:** 1618–24.
5. Brown PD, Lerner SA. Community-acquired pneumonia. *Lancet* 1998; **352:** 1295–1302.
6. Baquero F, *et al.* A review of antimicrobial resistance patterns of Streptococcus pneumoniae in Europe. *J Antimicrob Chemother* 1991; **28** (suppl C): 31–8.
7. Friedland IR, McCracken GH. Management of infections caused by antibiotic-resistant Streptococcus pneumoniae. *N Engl J Med* 1994; **331:** 377–82.
8. Breiman RF, *et al.* Emergence of drug-resistant pneumococcal infections in the United States. *JAMA* 1994; **271:** 1831–5.
9. Hofmann J, *et al.* The prevalence of drug-resistant Streptococcus pneumoniae in Atlanta. *N Engl J Med* 1995; **333:** 481–6.
10. Anonymous. Penicillin-resistant pneumococci. *Lancet* 1988; **i:** 1142–3.
11. Casal J, *et al.* Increase in resistance to penicillin in pneumococci in Spain. *Lancet* 1989; **i:** 735.
12. Klugman KP, Koornhof HJ. Worldwide increase in pneumococcal antibiotic resistance. *Lancet* 1989; **ii:** 444.
13. Pallares R, *et al.* Resistance to penicillin and cephalosporin and mortality from severe pneumococcal pneumonia in Barcelona, Spain. *N Engl J Med* 1995; **333:** 474–80. Correction. *ibid.*; 1655.
14. Collignon PJ, Bell JM. Drug-resistant Streptococcus pneumoniae: the beginning of the end for many antibiotics? *Med J Aust* 1996: **164:** 64–7.
15. Spencer RC, *et al.* A three year survey of clinical isolates in the United Kingdom and their antimicrobial susceptibility. *J Antimicrob Chemother* 1990; **26:** 435–46.
16. Ridgway EJ, Allen KD. Penicillin resistance in pneumococci. *J Antimicrob Chemother* 1991; **27:** 251–2.
17. George RC, *et al.* Antibiotic-resistant pneumococci in the United Kingdom. *Commun Dis Rep* 1992; **2:** R37–R43.
18. Eykyn SJ. Pneumococcaemia caused by erythromycin-resistant Streptococcus pneumoniae type 14. *Lancet* 1988; **ii:** 1086.
19. Verhaegen J, *et al.* Erythromycin-resistant Streptococcus pneumoniae. *Lancet* 1988; **ii:** 1432–3.
20. Warren RE, *et al.* Erythromycin-resistant Streptococcus pneumoniae. *Lancet* 1988; **ii:** 1433. Correction. *ibid.* 1989; **i:** 58.
21. Mastro TD, *et al.* Antimicrobial resistance of pneumococci in children with acute lower respiratory tract infection in Pakistan. *Lancet* 1991; **337:** 156–9.
22. Straus WL, *et al.* Antimicrobial resistance and clinical effectiveness of co-trimoxazole versus amoxycillin for pneumonia among children in Pakistan: randomised controlled trial. *Lancet* 1998; **352:** 270–4.
23. Anonymous. Mycoplasma pneumoniae. *Lancet* 1991; **337:** 651–2.
24. The British Thoracic Society. Guidelines for the management of community-acquired pneumonia in adults admitted to hospital. *Br J Hosp Med* 1993; **49:** 346–50.
25. Davies AJ, Jolley A. Community-acquired pneumonia. *Lancet* 1991; **337:** 1101.
26. Wright PW, *et al.* A descriptive study of 42 cases of Branhamella catarrhalis pneumonia. *Am J Med* 1990; **88** (suppl 5A): 2S–8S.
27. Grayston JT, *et al.* A new respiratory tract pathogen: Chlamydia pneumoniae strain TWAR. *J Infect Dis* 1990; **161:** 618–25.
28. American Thoracic Society. Guidelines for the management of adults with community-acquired pneumonia: diagnosis, assessment of severity, antimicrobial therapy, and prevention. *Am J Respir Crit Care Med* 2001; **163:** 1730–54.
29. Klugman KP. Pneumococcal resistance to antibiotics. *Clin Microbiol Rev* 1990; **3:** 171–96.
30. McGehee JL, *et al.* Treatment of pneumonia in patients at risk of infection with Gram-negative bacilli. *Am J Med* 1988; **84:** 597–602.
31. Hammerschlag MR. Antimicrobial susceptibility and therapy of infections caused by Chlamydia pneumoniae. *Antimicrob Agents Chemother* 1994; **38:** 1873–8.
32. Anonymous. Pneumonia in childhood. *Lancet* 1988; **i:** 741–3.
33. Anonymous. Drugs for sexually transmitted diseases. *Med Lett Drugs Ther* 1995; **37:** 117–22.
34. WHO. *Respiratory infections in children: management in small hospitals.* Geneva: WHO, 1988.
35. Pandey MR, *et al.* Reduction in total under-five mortality in western Nepal through community-based antimicrobial treatment of pneumonia. *Lancet* 1991; **338:** 993–7.
36. Bang AT, *et al.* Pneumonia in neonates: can it be managed in the community? *Arch Dis Child* 1993; **68:** 550–6.
37. Sutrisna B, *et al.* Randomised, controlled trial of effectiveness of ampicillin in mild acute respiratory infections in Indonesian children. *Lancet* 1991; **338:** 471–4.
38. LaForce FM. Systemic antimicrobial therapy of nosocomial pneumonia: monotherapy versus combination therapy. *Eur J Clin Microbiol Infect Dis* 1989; **8:** 61–8.

39. Rapp RP, *et al*. Intravenous ciprofloxacin versus ceftazidime for treatment of nosocomial pneumonia and urinary tract infection. *Clin Pharm* 1991; **10:** 49–55.
40. Browne MJ, *et al*. A randomized trial of open lung biopsy versus empiric antimicrobial therapy in cancer patients with diffuse pulmonary infiltrates. *J Clin Oncol* 1990; **8:** 222–9.
41. Bustamante CI, Wade JC. Treatment of interstitial pneumonia in cancer patients: is empiric antibiotic therapy the answer? *J Clin Oncol* 1990; **8:** 200–2.
42. Marik PE. Aspiration pneumonitis and aspiration pneumonia. *N Engl J Med* 2001; **344:** 665–71.
43. Bartlett JG. Treatment of anaerobic pulmonary infections. *J Antimicrob Chemother* 1989; **24:** 836–40.
44. Levison ME, *et al*. Clindamycin compared with penicillin for the treatment of anaerobic lung abscess. *Ann Intern Med* 1983; **98:** 466–71.
45. Gudiol F, *et al*. Clindamycin vs penicillin for anaerobic lung infections: high rate of penicillin failures associated with penicillin-resistant Bacteroides melaninogenicus. *Arch Intern Med* 1990; **150:** 2525–9.

Pregnancy and the neonate

For infections associated specifically with pregnancy, see under Endometritis (above), Perinatal Streptococcal Infections (above), and Premature Labour (below).

Premature labour

There is evidence of an association between premature rupture of membranes, maternal genito-urinary infection, and preterm labour. Various bacteria have been implicated, including group B streptococci, *Chlamydia trachomatis*, and those associated with bacterial vaginosis, and adjunctive antibacterial treatment is under evaluation. However, concerns have been expressed that delaying delivery in the presence of a subclinical infection may not produce the best outcome for the neonate.[1]

Meta-analysis[2] of studies of the routine use of antibacterials as adjuncts in the management of premature labour in women with intact membranes has failed to demonstrate an overall improvement in neonatal morbidity; indeed, an increase in neonatal mortality was actually noted.

In women with preterm premature rupture of membranes, meta-analyses[3,4] have shown that antibacterials could delay delivery, and reduce both maternal morbidity (chorioamnionitis and postpartum infections) and some aspects of neonatal morbidity (sepsis, pneumonia, and intraventricular haemorrhage). No effects on neonatal mortality or gestational age-related morbidity were noted.[4]

Clinical infections of the genito-urinary tract during pregnancy are a cause of significant morbidity in the neonate and intrapartum antimicrobial treatment is necessary (see Bacterial Vaginosis, p.115, Chlamydial Infections, p.117, and Perinatal Streptococcal Infections, above).

1. Brocklehurst P. Infection and preterm delivery. *BMJ* 1999; **318:** 548–9.
2. Egarter C, *et al*. Adjunctive antibiotic treatment in preterm labor and neonatal morbidity: a meta-analysis. *Obstet Gynecol* 1996; **88:** 303–9.
3. Mercer BM, Arheart KL. Antimicrobial therapy in expectant management of preterm premature rupture of the membranes. *Lancet* 1995; **346:** 1271–9. Correction. *ibid*. 1996; **347:** 410.
4. Egarter C, *et al*. Antibiotic treatment in preterm premature rupture of membranes and neonatal morbidity: a metaanalysis. *Am J Obstet Gynecol* 1996; **174:** 589–97.

Proctitis

The treatment of rectal infections caused by *Chlamydia trachomatis* and *Neisseria gonorrhoeae* is discussed under Chlamydial Infections and Gonorrhoea, above.

Ceftriaxone 125 mg intramuscularly together with doxycycline 100 mg twice daily by mouth for 7 days is recommended by the Centers for Disease Control in the USA[1] for empirical treatment of sexually transmitted proctitis and should be effective against *C. trachomatis* and *N. gonorrhoeae*.

Proctitis may also be associated with herpes simplex infections (p.607).

1. Centers for Disease Control. 1998 Guidelines for treatment of sexually transmitted diseases. *MMWR* 1998; **47** (RR-1): 104–5.

Prostatitis

See under Urinary-tract Infections, below.

Psittacosis

The causative organism of psittacosis is *Chlamydia psittaci*. It is usually transmitted to humans by direct or indirect contact with infected birds and the primary site of infection is the lung.[1] Transmission between humans is common with *C. pneumoniae* (formerly TWAR strain of *C. psittaci*)[2] that also causes pneumonia. The clinical presentation of psittacosis can vary widely from a mild 'flu-like' illness to a fulminating toxic state with multiple organ involvement.[1] Most patients will have a cough, although this is not always prominent. Tetracyclines are the treatment of choice[1,3] and early therapy may be life-saving; a 21-day course has been recommended since relapses have occurred after shorter periods.[1] An alternative is chloramphenicol.[3] Erythromycin or a similar macrolide have also been used successfully.[4,5]

1. Macfarlane JT, Macrae AD. Psittacosis. *Br Med Bull* 1983; **39:** 163–7.
2. Grayston JT, *et al*. A new respiratory tract pathogen: Chlamydia pneumoniae strain TWAR. *J Infect Dis* 1990; **161:** 618–25.
3. Anonymous. The choice of antibacterial drugs. *Med Lett Drugs Ther* 1999; **41:** 95–104.
4. Morrison WM, *et al*. An outbreak of psittacosis. *J Infect* 1991; **22:** 71–5.
5. Chang KP, Veitch PC. Fever, haematuria, proteinuria, and a parrot. *Lancet* 1997; **350:** 1674.

Q fever

Q fever (or query fever) is a rickettsial infection (below) caused by *Coxiella burnetii*. It is a zoonosis occurring worldwide and is transmitted to humans from domestic animals such as cattle and sheep, mainly by inhalation of infected dust. Acute infection generally presents as a febrile influenza-like illness that may progress to pneumonia. Endocarditis is the most frequent manifestation of chronic infection and the most serious form of Q fever; infection may be difficult to eradicate and prolonged treatment is generally required. There is also evidence of long-term sequelae including lethargy and fatigue in patients who have not experienced cardiac involvement.

A tetracycline such as doxycycline has been the treatment of choice for Q fever; alternatively chloramphenicol has been used. Erythromycin may be adequate for Q fever pneumonia,[1] at least in mild cases;[2] results with erythromycin were favourable in a retrospective review.[3] However, Q fever pneumonia may often resolve without treatment and the role of antibacterial therapy is not clear.[4]

Q fever endocarditis is more difficult to treat. Tetracycline has been described as the mainstay of treatment,[5] although it fails to eradicate *C. burnetii* when used alone and various combinations of antibacterials have been tried. A study *in vitro*[6] showed that isolates of *C. burnetii* associated with chronic infection were less sensitive to antibacterials than those from acute Q fever, but that fluoroquinolones alone or with rifampicin might be of value. Long-term treatment with doxycycline plus rifampicin[7] or with ciprofloxacin alone[8] has been successful in individual patients with endocarditis, whereas pefloxacin alone[9] was not. Following a retrospective comparison of doxycycline alone or with rifampicin, fluoroquinolones (ofloxacin or pefloxacin), or co-trimoxazole, treatment for at least 3 years with doxycycline plus a fluoroquinolone was recommended;[10] doxycycline plus rifampicin also appeared effective, but in most cases rifampicin had been stopped after a few months because of interactions with anticoagulants often prescribed at the same time. Different authors have also concluded[5] that no current treatment eradicated Q fever endocarditis within 2 years and similarly recommended[5] that it be treated with doxycycline together with a fluoroquinolone for a minimum of 3 years. Other regimens that have been investigated have included doxycycline with chloroquine[5] or with hydroxychloroquine.[11]

A vaccine is available in some countries for use in occupational groups who regularly handle potentially infected animal tissues.

1. D'Angelo LJ, Hetherington R. Q fever treated with erythromycin. *BMJ* 1979; **2:** 305–6.
2. Marrie TJ, *et al*. Q fever pneumonia associated with exposure to wild rabbits. *Lancet* 1986; **i:** 427–9.
3. Pérez-del-Molino A, *et al*. Erythromycin and the treatment of Coxiella burnetii pneumonia. *J Antimicrob Chemother* 1991; **28:** 455–9.
4. Lieberman D, *et al*. Q-fever pneumonia in the Negev region of Israel: a review of 20 patients hospitalised over a period of one year. *J Infect* 1995; **30:** 135–40.
5. Raoult D. Treatment of Q fever. *Antimicrob Agents Chemother* 1993; **37:** 1733–6.
6. Yeaman MR, *et al*. Antibiotic susceptibilities of two Coxiella burnetii isolates implicated in distinct clinical syndromes. *Antimicrob Agents Chemother* 1989; **33:** 1052–7.
7. Brecker SJD, Eykyn SJ. Q-fever endocarditis twenty-five years on. *Lancet* 1989; **ii:** 684–5.
8. Yebra M, *et al*. Ciprofloxacin in a case of Q fever endocarditis. *N Engl J Med* 1990; **323:** 614.
9. Cacoub P, *et al*. Q-fever endocarditis and treatment with the fluoroquinolones. *Arch Intern Med* 1991; **151:** 816, 818.
10. Levy PY, *et al*. Comparison of different antibiotic regimens for therapy of 32 cases of Q fever endocarditis. *Antimicrob Agents Chemother* 1991; **35:** 533–7.
11. Raoult D, *et al*. Treatment of Q fever endocarditis: comparison of 2 regimens containing doxycycline and ofloxacin or hydroxychloroquine. *Arch Intern Med* 1999; **159:** 167–73.

Relapsing fever

Relapsing fever is caused by spirochaetes of the *Borrelia* genus that are transmitted to humans by body lice or *Ornithodoros* ticks. *B. recurrentis* causes louse-borne relapsing fever and can occur widely, but is endemic especially in Ethiopia. Many species of *Borrelia* may cause tick-borne relapsing fever.

The treatment of choice for infection due to *B. recurrentis* is a tetracycline; benzylpenicillin is an alternative.[1] Therapy with single oral doses of tetracycline,[2,3] erythromycin,[2,3] or chloramphenicol[3] has been effective. Antibacterial treatment often causes a Jarisch-Herxheimer reaction characterised by rigor, fever and hypotension which may be fatal.[2,4] Therapies used in an attempt to prevent this reaction include paracetamol and corticosteroids;[2,4] the use of antibodies against tumour necrosis factor α has shown promise.[5]

Tick-borne relapsing fever is milder than the louse-borne variety, but has been treated similarly.

1. Anonymous. The choice of antibacterial drugs. *Med Lett Drugs Ther* 1999; **41:** 95–104.
2. Butler T, *et al*. Borrelia recurrentis infection: single-dose antibiotic regimens and management of the Jarisch-Herxheimer reaction. *J Infect Dis* 1978; **137:** 573–7.
3. Perine PL, Teklu B. Antibiotic treatment of louse-borne relapsing fever in Ethiopia: a report of 377 cases. *Am J Trop Med Hyg* 1983; **32:** 1096–1100.
4. Butler T. Relapsing fever: new lessons about antibiotic action. *Ann Intern Med* 1985; **102:** 397–9.
5. Fekade D, *et al*. Prevention of Jarisch-Herxheimer reactions by treatment with antibodies against tumor necrosis factor α. *N Engl J Med* 1996; **335:** 311–15.

Respiratory-tract infections

Principal community-acquired bacterial pathogens in the respiratory tract continue to be *Streptococcus pneumoniae* and *Haemophilus influenzae*,[1] although *Moraxella catarrhalis* (*Branhamella catarrhalis*)[2-4] is increasingly important in some areas. Other respiratory pathogens include *Chlamydia pneumoniae* (formerly TWAR strain of *C. psittaci*), *Legionella pneumophila*, and *Mycoplasma pneumoniae*. *Streptococcus pyogenes* is the predominant cause of pharyngitis. *Staphylococcus aureus* and aerobic Gram-negative bacilli such as *Pseudomonas aeruginosa* and *Klebsiella* spp. may be responsible for hospital-acquired (nosocomial) infections.

Community-acquired lower respiratory-tract infections are very common and are traditionally considered to be viral in origin, but bacterial pathogens similar to those causing pneumonia are commonly isolated from patients with these milder respiratory infections;[5] even so about one quarter of patients fail to respond satisfactorily to empirical antibacterial treatment.

Broad-spectrum antibacterials such as a penicillin or erythromycin may be necessary in some cases of uncomplicated upper or lower respiratory-tract infection. First line empirical treatment with a fluoroquinolone should be avoided because of poor activity against streptococci.[6,7] In respiratory-tract infections complicating chronic obstructive pulmonary disease, amoxicillin has been recommended for first-line treatment.[8] If a further course is necessary, drugs with activity against penicillin-resistant *H. influenzae* and *M. catarrhalis* should probably be given, such as amoxicillin with clavulanic acid, a fluoroquinolone (bearing in mind that they are not very active against *Str. pneumoniae*), or a second-generation cephalosporin.

For details on infections of the upper respiratory tract, see under Epiglottitis (p.121), Pharyngitis (p.134), and Sinusitis (p.139); see also Otitis Media (p.132). For infections of the lower respiratory tract, see under Bronchitis (p.116), Cystic Fibrosis (p.117), and Pneumonia (p.135); those with a specific cause include Legionnaires' Disease (p.126), Nocardiosis (p.131), Pertussis (p.134), and Tuberculosis (p.143).

1. Finch RG. Epidemiological features and chemotherapy of community-acquired respiratory tract infections. *J Antimicrob Chemother* 1990; **26** (suppl E): 53–61.
2. Davies BI, Maesen FPV. Treatment of Branhamella catarrhalis infections. *J Antimicrob Chemother* 1990; **25:** 1–4.
3. Wallace RJ, *et al*. Antibiotic susceptibilities and drug resistance in Moraxella (Branhamella) catarrhalis. *Am J Med* 1990; **88** (suppl 5A): 46S–50S.
4. Murphy TF. Branhamella catarrhalis: epidemiological and clinical aspects of a human respiratory tract pathogen. *Thorax* 1998; **53:** 124–8.
5. Macfarlane JT, *et al*. Prospective study of aetiology and outcome of adult lower-respiratory-tract infections in the community. *Lancet* 1993; **341:** 511–14.
6. Körner RJ, *et al*. Dangers of oral fluoroquinolone treatment in community acquired upper respiratory tract infections. *BMJ* 1994; **308:** 191–2.

7. Hosker HSR, *et al.* Management of community acquired lower respiratory tract infection. *BMJ* 1994; **308:** 701–5.

8. Hosker H, *et al.* Antibiotics in chronic obstructive pulmonary disease. *BMJ* 1994; **308:** 871–2.

Rheumatic fever

Acute rheumatic fever occurs especially in children aged 6 to 15 years as a consequence of upper respiratory-tract infections, such as pharyngitis or tonsillitis, with rheumatogenic strains of the group A beta-haemolytic streptococcus, *Streptococcus pyogenes*. The pathogenesis of rheumatic fever is not known, but an immune mechanism may be involved. There may be a latent period of 1 to 5 weeks after the initial infection, before clinical manifestations of rheumatic fever appear. The major ones are arthritis, carditis, chorea, erythema marginatum, and subcutaneous nodules. Those affecting the heart are the most serious and are a major cause of cardiovascular death in children and young adults in developing countries. Rheumatic fever has been associated with poverty and overcrowding and has declined dramatically in developed countries, but is still a major problem in the developing world. However, in the 1980s there was evidence of a resurgence in the USA with outbreaks of rheumatic fever reported in middle-class children[1] and military recruits.[2] Increased pathogenicity of *Str. pyogenes* serotypes might have contributed to this resurgence.[3]

Similar guidelines for the primary and secondary prevention of rheumatic fever have been published by WHO[4] and the American Heart Association (AHA).[5] Rheumatic fever can usually be prevented by *primary prophylaxis*, that is, by the prompt treatment of streptococcal upper respiratory-tract infection with penicillin of group A streptococci from the throat. Penicillin is the drug of choice, either as a single intramuscular injection of benzathine benzylpenicillin or as a course of phenoxymethylpenicillin by mouth for 10 days. An injection containing benzathine benzylpenicillin and procaine penicillin [procaine benzylpenicillin] has been used in children.[5] Erythromycin may be given to patients allergic to penicillin. Other macrolides or oral cephalosporins may also be used. For further details on the treatment of streptococcal sore throat, see under Pharyngitis, above. Treatment failure is more common after oral antibacterials and in the USA most of these patients are streptococcal carriers.[5] Treatment of chronic carriers is not usually necessary, but eradication of pharyngeal carriage has been achieved by an injection of benzathine benzylpenicillin plus rifampin by mouth for 4 days;[6] a 10-day course of oral clindamycin has also been effective.[7] Broad-based primary prophylaxis in communities rather than individuals is controversial and requires careful planning, but, for example, penicillin prophylaxis did control an epidemic of acute tonsillitis associated with *Str. pyogenes* in a junior detention centre.[8] However, a study in military recruits demonstrated that *Str. pyogenes* infection could not be prevented in closely confined communities unless all individuals in the population received prophylaxis.[9]

If acute rheumatic fever occurs, a full therapeutic course of penicillin should be given initially, as for primary prevention, to eradicate group A streptococci.[5] Treatment then comprises bed rest and anti-inflammatory drugs, usually corticosteroids or salicylates, in an attempt to prevent valvular scarring. However, it is unclear whether anti-inflammatory treatment has any influence on such long-term sequelae.[10] *Secondary prevention* is then continued with prolonged antibacterial prophylaxis because of the high risk of recurrent attacks of rheumatic fever following subsequent streptococcal upper respiratory-tract infections. Again, penicillin is the preferred antibacterial, the usual recommendation being an intramuscular injection of benzathine benzylpenicillin every 4 weeks, although injections every 3 weeks may be warranted where the risk of recurrence is high.[4,5] This advice has been influenced by reports of high recurrence rates with the monthly regimen in such situations.[11] A 12-year study in Taiwan[12] confirmed that prophylaxis with benzathine benzylpenicillin injections every 3 weeks is more effective than injections every 4 weeks and it was recommended that the 3-week regimen should be used in adults and children with a recent episode of rheumatic fever, especially in developing countries where exposure to streptococci is still intense. In addition, pharmacokinetic studies have indicated relatively low serum concentrations of penicillin in the fourth week after an intramuscular injection of benzathine benzylpenicillin,[13,14] despite the successful use of monthly injections in most patients. Alternatively, oral prophylaxis with phenoxymethylpenicillin

or sulfadiazine may be given; erythromycin is suggested for the rare patient who is allergic to penicillin and sulfonamides. Sulfonamides should *not* be used for primary prevention because they do not eradicate the streptococci. The duration of secondary prophylaxis depends on the individual patient, but in those who have not had rheumatic carditis it should generally continue for a minimum of 5 years after the last attack of rheumatic fever,[4,5] and at least until the age of 18 or early 20s. A study from Chile supported this view.[15] Those who have had rheumatic carditis but without residual valvular disease should perhaps receive prophylaxis for 10 years[5] or at least until the age of 25 years.[4] For those with carditis and persistent valvular disease, prophylaxis should continue at least until the age of 40 years, or sometimes for life.[5] Fears of serious allergic reactions associated with long-term benzathine benzylpenicillin prophylaxis appear to be unfounded.[16]

Household contacts of rheumatic fever patients who themselves have positive streptococcal cultures should be treated.[5]

Patients with rheumatic valvular heart disease as a result of rheumatic fever are at risk of developing infective endocarditis and should receive additional appropriate short-term antibacterial prophylaxis when undergoing dental and some surgical procedures (see Endocarditis, above).

1. Veasy LG, *et al.* Resurgence of acute rheumatic fever in the intermountain area of the United States. *N Engl J Med* 1987; **316:** 421–7.
2. Wallace MR, *et al.* The return of acute rheumatic fever in young adults. *JAMA* 1989; **262:** 2557–61.
3. Schwartz B, *et al.* Changing epidemiology of group A streptococcal infection in the USA. *Lancet* 1990; **336:** 1167–71.
4. WHO. *WHO model prescribing information: drugs used in the treatment of streptococcal pharyngitis and prevention of rheumatic fever.* Geneva: WHO, 1999.
5. Dajani A, *et al.* Treatment of acute streptococcal pharyngitis and prevention of rheumatic fever: a statement for health professionals. *Pediatrics* 1995; **96:** 758–64.
6. Tanz RR, *et al.* Penicillin plus rifampin eradicates pharyngeal carriage of group A streptococci. *J Pediatr* 1985; **106:** 876–80.
7. Tanz RR, *et al.* Clindamycin treatment of chronic pharyngeal carriage of group A streptococci. *J Pediatr* 1991; **119:** 123–8.
8. Colling A, *et al.* Minimum amount of penicillin prophylaxis required to control Streptococcus pyogenes epidemic in closed community. *BMJ* 1982; **285:** 95–6.
9. Gray GC, *et al.* Hyperendemic Streptococcus pyogenes infection despite prophylaxis with penicillin G benzathine. *N Engl J Med* 1991; **325:** 92–7.
10. Stollerman GH. Rheumatic fever. *Lancet* 1997; **349:** 935–42.
11. Ayoub EM. Prophylaxis in patients with rheumatic fever: every three or every four weeks? *J Pediatr* 1989; **115:** 89–91.
12. Lue H-C, *et al.* Long-term outcome of patients with rheumatic fever receiving benzathine penicillin G prophylaxis every three weeks versus every four weeks. *J Pediatr* 1994; **125:** 812–16.
13. Kaplan EL, *et al.* Pharmacokinetics of benzathine penicillin G: serum levels during the 28 days after intramuscular injection of 1,200,000 units. *J Pediatr* 1989; **115:** 146–50.
14. Meira ZMA, *et al.* Evaluation of secondary prophylactic schemes, based on benzathine penicillin G, for rheumatic fever in children. *J Pediatr* 1993; **123:** 156–8.
15. Berrios X, *et al.* Discontinuing rheumatic fever prophylaxis in selected adolescents and young adults: a prospective study. *Ann Intern Med* 1993; **118:** 401–6. Correction. *ibid.*; **119:** 173.
16. International Rheumatic Fever Study Group. Allergic reactions to long-term benzathine penicillin prophylaxis for rheumatic fever. *Lancet* 1991; **337:** 1308–10.

Rickettsial infections

Bacteria of the Rickettsiaceae family that infect man include *Rickettsia* spp. (see under Spotted Fevers and under Typhus, below) and *Coxiella burnetii* (see under Q fever, above). *Ehrlichia* spp. (see under Ehrlichiosis, above), are rickettsia-like bacteria. *Bartonella quintana* (*Rochalimaea quintana*) (see under Trench Fever, below) is no longer classified as a rickettsia. The treatment of choice for rickettsial infections is usually a tetracycline or chloramphenicol;[1,2] a fluoroquinolone such as ciprofloxacin has also been used.[2]

1. WHO Working Group on Rickettsial Diseases. Rickettsioses: a continuing disease problem. *Bull WHO* 1982; **60:** 157–64.
2. Raoult D, Drancourt M. Antimicrobial therapy of rickettsial diseases. *Antimicrob Agents Chemother* 1991; **35:** 2457–62.

Salmonella enteritis

See under Gastro-enteritis, above.

Salpingitis

See under Pelvic Inflammatory Disease, above.

Septicaemia

Traditionally, transient bacteraemia (the presence of bacteria in the blood) has been regarded as a fairly common condition which does not usually cause complications, whereas uncontrolled bacteraemia leads to septicaemia with serious symptoms such as fever and shock. This dis-

tinction has not always been adhered to in published sources and the terms have sometimes been used interchangeably. Added to this, the identification of the cascade of inflammatory mediators involved and the realisation that what had been called 'sepsis' could arise in the absence of infection have prompted reassessment of the terminology used both in the UK and in the USA.[1] In the UK, some authorities[2] considered that the term 'septicaemia' should no longer be used since it does not distinguish between mild and severe disease. The term 'sepsis syndrome' was preferred for patients with a generalised systemic response together with evidence of organ dysfunction and 'septic shock' to describe patients who also have hypotension not due to hypovolaemia or cardiac causes. The American College of Chest Physicians and Society of Critical Care Medicine proposed the following series of definitions to cover the spectrum of syndromes resulting from this inflammatory response:[1,3]

- **systemic inflammatory response syndrome** (SIRS), the systemic inflammatory response to infection or various other severe clinical insults including pancreatitis, ischaemia, trauma, and haemorrhagic shock

- **sepsis**, the SIRS caused specifically by infection

- **severe sepsis**, sepsis associated with organ dysfunction, perfusion abnormalities (such as lactic acidosis, oliguria, or an acute alteration in mental status), or hypotension

- **septic shock**, sepsis with hypotension, despite adequate fluid resuscitation, together with perfusion abnormalities

- **multiple organ dysfunction syndrome** (MODS), the presence of altered organ function in an acutely ill patient such that homoeostasis cannot be maintained without intervention; it may be a cause as well as a consequence of SIRS.

Septicaemia can be caused by a wide range of bacteria.[4] **Community-acquired** primary septicaemia is often associated with a specific infectious disease, such as meningococcal septicaemia with meningococcal meningitis (above) or streptococcal septicaemia with pneumonia (above). *Streptococcus pneumoniae* and *Haemophilus influenzae* are common causes of primary septicaemia in children (although this pattern is changing in countries where immunisation against *H. influenzae* type b is routine); Gram-negative rods and group B streptococci are commonest in neonates. **Hospital-acquired** septicaemia is often iatrogenic and may occur as a complication of surgery or indwelling catheters[5,6] or may be associated with neutropenia in immunosuppressed patients (see under Infections in Immunocompromised Patients, above). It is often associated with acute respiratory distress syndrome (p.1046).

Whatever the cause, septicaemia requires prompt treatment without waiting for the results of laboratory tests. Choice of antibacterial depends on the probable source of infection. For example, urinary-tract infection is likely to be associated with Gram-negative septicaemia due to *Escherichia coli*; abdominal sepsis with Gram-negative septicaemia due to mixed infection with *E. coli*, enterococci, and anaerobic bacteria; and skin sepsis, bacterial arthritis, acute osteomyelitis, and cardiovascular shunts with Gram-positive septicaemia due to staphylococci. The antibacterials used should also reflect current patterns of bacterial resistance in the community or hospital. *Empirical treatment* has often been initiated with a penicillin and an aminoglycoside, metronidazole being added if anaerobic infection is suspected. In the UK recommended initial empirical treatment for community-acquired septicaemia is with either a broad-spectrum penicillin plus an aminoglycoside, or a third-generation cephalosporin such as cefotaxime alone; for hospital-acquired septicaemia an aminoglycoside plus either a broad-spectrum antipseudomonal penicillin or ceftazidime is recommended, or meropenem alone, or imipenem-cilastatin alone. Metronidazole may be added if anaerobic organisms are suspected, and flucloxacillin or vancomycin if Gram-positive organisms are suspected. USA guidelines[7] recommend a third- or fourth-generation cephalosporin (cefotaxime, ceftizoxime, ceftriaxone, or cefepime), or ticarcillin-clavulanic acid, or piperacillin-tazobactam, or imipenem-cilastatin, or meropenem, each with an aminoglycoside (gentamicin, tobramycin, or amikacin) for the initial treatment of life-threatening sepsis in adults. When there is some information on which to base choice of treatment, but before the infecting organisms are definitely known, the following treatment is suggested:

- suspected bacterial endocarditis—gentamicin with vancomycin
- suspected meticillin-resistant staphylococci—vancomycin, with or without gentamicin and/or rifampicin
- intra-abdominal or pelvic infections likely to involve anaerobes—ticarcillin-clavulanic acid, ampicillin-sulbactam, piperacillin-tazobactam, imipenem-cilastatin, meropenem, cefoxitin, or cefotetan, each with or without an aminoglycoside
- suspected biliary-tract infection—piperacillin or mezlocillin plus metronidazole, piperacillin-tazobactam, or ampicillin-sulbactam, each with or without an aminoglycoside.

Once the infecting organisms have been identified, choice of treatment will again depend on their sensitivity and current patterns of resistance in the community or hospital. Specific types of septicaemia studied and reviewed in the literature include that due to Gram-negative bacteria in general,[8,9] *Pseudomonas aeruginosa*,[10] *Serratia* spp.,[11] staphylococci,[12] *Streptococcus pyogenes*,[13] *Str. pneumoniae*,[14] and enterococci.[15] For comments on the consequences of emerging multidrug-resistant strains of enterococci and staphylococci, see Enterococcal Infections, above, and Staphylococcal Infections, below.

In addition to antimicrobial therapy, patients with sepsis or septic shock[16-19] require rigorous supportive measures (p.813).

Septicaemia is generally most lethal in the very old and the very young.

Neonatal septicaemia may be divided into **early-onset**, which is acquired from the mother's genital tract and manifests itself during the first few days after birth, and **late-onset** which may be nosocomially acquired. Bacteria commonly causing early-onset sepsis include enterococci, *E. coli*, *H. influenzae*, *Listeria monocytogenes*, and streptococci. Some of these organisms may also produce meningitis in the neonate (above). Empirical treatment for both early- and late-onset sepsis is based on similar principles to those in other patients, giving consideration to local patterns of infection and resistance and to the suitability of individual antibacterials for this age group. However, early-onset sepsis is usually best controlled by prenatal treatment of the mother or by perinatal prophylaxis. Prophylaxis for group B streptococcal infections is discussed under Perinatal Streptococcal Infections, above. While vancomycin has been shown to prevent infections with coagulase-negative staphylococci, widespread prophylactic use of this drug is not recommended.[20] Intravenous administration of normal immunoglobulin has been tried for the prevention of septicaemia in preterm neonates with variable results (p.1554).

Treatment failure in sepsis or septic shock occurring in all patients, despite apparently adequate anti-infective therapy, might be due in part to a continuing inflammatory process and attempts to modify these are under investigation.[19,21] Endotoxin, a lipopolysaccharide associated with the cell membrane of Gram-negative bacteria, is an important mediator in the septic syndrome. Endotoxin release may occur spontaneously or during antibacterial therapy.[22] When in the circulation it stimulates the release of endogenous mediators such as interleukin-1, interleukin-6, tumour necrosis factor alpha, and other cytokines.[23] These in turn induce a cascade of secondary inflammatory mediators resulting eventually in endothelial damage and severe haemodynamic and metabolic derangements. It is now understood that a similar inflammatory response also occurs following non-infective insults. However, adjunctive therapy with endotoxin antibodies, anticytokines such as anakinra and tumour necrosis factor antibodies, soluble tumour necrosis factor receptor, bactericidal permeability increasing protein, nitric oxide synthase inhibitors, guanylate cyclase inhibitors such as methylene blue [methylthioninium chloride], and platelet-activating factor antagonists have generally produced disappointing results.[21,24,25] A systematic review[26] of the use of intravenous polyclonal immunoglobulin has concluded that it has a promising role as adjuvant therapy in sepsis and septic shock. Specific monoclonal immunoglobulins were not effective.[26] Recent theories suggest that a more complex interplay of pro- and anti-inflammatory responses may be involved in the pathophysiology of SIRS and MODS and this may explain the failure of many of these predominantly anti-inflammatory treatment modalities.[27]

1. Bone RC. Why new definitions of sepsis and organ failure are needed. *Am J Med* 1993; **95**: 348–50.
2. Lynn WA, Cohen J. Management of septic shock. *J Infect* 1995; **30**: 207–12.
3. American College of Chest Physicians/Society of Critical Care Medicine Consensus Conference Committee. Definitions for sepsis and organ failure and guidelines for the use of innovative therapies in sepsis. *Crit Care Med* 1992; **20**: 864–74.
4. Eykyn SJ, *et al.* The causative organisms of septicaemia and their epidemiology. *J Antimicrob Chemother* 1990; **25** (suppl C): 41–58.
5. Dickinson GM, Bisno AL. Infections associated with indwelling devices: concepts of pathogenesis; infections associated with intravascular devices. *Antimicrob Agents Chemother* 1989; **33**: 597–601.
6. Dickinson GM, Bisno AL. Infections associated with indwelling devices: infections related to extravascular devices. *Antimicrob Agents Chemother* 1989; **33**: 602–7.
7. Anonymous. The choice of antibacterial drugs. *Med Lett Drugs Ther* 1999; **41**: 95–104.
8. Dudley MN. Overview of gram-negative sepsis. *Am J Hosp Pharm* 1990; **47** (suppl 3): S3–S6.
9. DiPiro JT. Pathophysiology and treatment of gram-negative sepsis. *Am J Hosp Pharm* 1990; **47** (suppl 3): S6–S10.
10. Hilf M, *et al.* Antibiotic therapy for Pseudomonas aeruginosa bacteremia: outcome correlations in a prospective study of 200 patients. *Am J Med* 1989; **87**: 540–6.
11. Saito H, *et al.* Serratia bacteremia: review of 118 cases. *Rev Infect Dis* 1999; **11**: 912–20.
12. Eykyn SJ. Staphylococcal sepsis: the changing pattern of disease and therapy. *Lancet* 1988; **i**: 100–4.
13. Anonymous. Invasive streptococci. *Lancet* 1989; **ii**: 1255.
14. Davies AJ, Kumaratne DS. The continuing problem of pneumococcal infection. *J Antimicrob Chemother* 1988; **21**: 387–91.
15. Montecalvo MA, *et al.* Outbreak of vancomycin-, ampicillin-, and aminoglycoside-resistant Enterococcus faecium bacteremia in an adult oncology unit. *Antimicrob Agents Chemother* 1994; **38**: 1363–7.
16. Glauser MP, *et al.* Septic shock: pathogenesis. *Lancet* 1991; **338**: 732–6.
17. Cohen J, Glauser MP. Septic shock: treatment. *Lancet* 1991; **338**: 736–9.
18. Astiz ME, Rackow EC. Septic shock. *Lancet* 1998; **351**: 1501–5.
19. Wheeler AP, Bernard GR. Treating patients with severe sepsis. *N Engl J Med* 1999; **340**: 207–14.
20. Craft AP, *et al.* Vancomycin for prophylaxis against sepsis in preterm neonates (updated 27 February 2001). Available in The Cochrane Library; Issue 4. Oxford: Update Software; 2001.
21. Baumgartner J-D, Calandra T. Treatment of sepsis: past and future avenues. *Drugs* 1999; **57**: 127–32.
22. Prins JM. Clinical relevance of antibiotic-induced endotoxin release. *Antimicrob Agents Chemother* 1994; **38**: 1211–18.
23. Blackwell TS, Christman JW. Sepsis and cytokines: current status. *Br J Anaesth* 1996; **77**: 110–17.
24. Verhoef J, *et al.* Issues in the adjuvant therapy of severe sepsis. *J Antimicrob Chemother* 1996; **38**: 167–82.
25. Opal SM, Yu RL. Antiendotoxin strategies for the prevention and treatment of septic shock: new approaches and future directions. *Drugs* 1998; **55**: 497–508.
26. Alejandria MM, *et al.* Intravenous immunoglobulin for treating sepsis and septic shock (updated 29 May 2001). Available in The Cochrane Library; Issue 4. Oxford: Update Software; 2001.
27. Bone RC. Immunologic dissonance: a continuing evolution in our understanding of the systemic inflammatory response syndrome (SIRS) and the multiple organ dysfunction syndrome (MODS). *Ann Intern Med* 1996; **125**: 680–7.

Sexually transmitted diseases

The sexually transmitted diseases, formerly termed venereal diseases, are defined as a group of communicable diseases that are transferred mainly by sexual contact. More than 20 pathogens are known to be transmitted sexually. They include the bacteria *Haemophilus ducreyi* (see Chancroid, p.117), *Neisseria gonorrhoeae* (see Gonorrhoea, p.124), *Treponema pallidum* (see Syphilis, p.141), *Calymmatobacterium granulomatis* (see Granuloma Inguinale, p.124), *Chlamydia trachomatis* (see Lymphogranuloma Venereum, p.128 and Chlamydial Infections, p.117), and mycoplasmas including *Ureaplasma urealyticum*.

Clinical syndromes associated with sexually transmitted diseases include urethritis (p.146) and epididymitis (p.120) in men; cervicitis (p.117), pelvic inflammatory disease (p.133), and bacterial vaginosis (p.115) in women; and proctitis (p.137). Perinatal transmission of sexually transmitted pathogens from the mother can result in neonatal conjunctivitis (p.130) or pneumonia (p.135).

For discussions of some viral sexually transmitted diseases, see under HIV Infection and AIDS (p.608), Hepatitis (p.605), and Herpesvirus Infections (p.606) in Antivirals. Trichomoniasis is discussed in Antiprotozoals, p.586.

General guidelines for the management of sexually transmitted diseases are published,[1-3] and the epidemiology of sexually transmitted diseases and implications for travellers has been reviewed.[4]

The suggestion that spermicidal contraceptives may provide some protection against sexually transmitted diseases is discussed under Nonoxinols, p.1346.

1. Centers for Disease Control. 1998 Guidelines for treatment of sexually transmitted diseases. *MMWR* 1998 **47** (RR-1): 1–116.
2. Clinical Effectiveness Group (Association of Genitourinary Medicine and the Medical Society for the Study of Venereal Diseases). UK national guidelines on sexually transmitted infections and closely related conditions. *Sex Transm Infect* 1999; **75** (suppl 1): S1–S88.

3. WHO. Guidelines for the management of sexually transmitted infections. Geneva: WHO, 2001.
4. Mulhall BP. Sexually transmissible diseases and travel. *Br Med Bull* 1993; **49**: 394–411.

Shigellosis

See under Gastro-enteritis, above.

Sickle-cell disease

For prophylaxis against pneumococcal infection in sickle-cell disease, see under Spleen Disorders, below.

Sinusitis

Sinusitis or inflammation of the paranasal sinuses is more common in adults than children. It can be caused by viral, bacterial, or fungal infection or may be secondary to other disorders such as allergy. Serious complications include bacterial meningitis and brain abscess.

Acute sinusitis often results from viral upper respiratory-tract infections. Similarly to acute otitis media the most frequent bacterial pathogens are *Streptococcus pneumoniae* and unencapsulated *Haemophilus influenzae*, with *Moraxella catarrhalis* (*Branhamella catarrhalis*) increasingly important in children. Other bacterial causes, especially in adults, include mixed anaerobic bacteria (usually associated with dental disease and more frequent in chronic sinusitis), *Staphylococcus aureus*, *Streptococcus pyogenes*, and Gram-negative bacteria including Enterobacteriaceae and *Pseudomonas aeruginosa* (in nosocomial sinusitis). About 5% of primary sinusitis in young adults has been associated with *Chlamydia pneumoniae*.

Acute sinusitis may resolve spontaneously. In an evidence-based report on the diagnosis and treatment of rhinosinusitis,[1] the Agency for Health Care Policy and Research in the USA has stated that most patients with the acute condition will recover without recourse to antibacterial therapy, although they will recover faster if antibacterials are given. It was considered that the use of new antibacterials for treating uncomplicated community-acquired acute bacterial rhinosinusitis was not justified and that amoxicillin or folate inhibitors were sufficiently effective.[1] This view was supported by a meta-analysis.[2] A systematic review[3] has also supported the use of amoxicillin in confirmed acute sinusitis. If antibacterials are considered necessary treatment should be given for an adequate length of time, usually 2 weeks.[4,5] Topical decongestants may also be used to promote drainage and ventilation.[4,5] The choice of antibacterial is similar to that for acute otitis media (above). Effective antibacterials include amoxicillin with or without clavulanic acid, co-trimoxazole, cefuroxime, erythromycin, and azithromycin;[4] the emergence of penicillin-resistant strains of *H. influenzae*, *M. catarrhalis*, and *Str. pneumoniae* is causing concern.[6] Patients with evidence of severe infections may require intravenous therapy with vancomycin and ceftriaxone or cefotaxime initially.[6] Tetracycline or erythromycin are the most effective antibacterials against *Chlamydia pneumoniae*.[7]

Failure to treat acute sinusitis which does not resolve spontaneously can result in chronic sinusitis or occasionally in complications such as brain abscess or meningitis. Exacerbations of chronic sinusitis are treated as for acute infection. Management of chronic sinusitis is based on reducing obstruction of the sinus cavity using antihistamines, decongestants, anti-inflammatory drugs (including corticosteroids), and saline washes as appropriate.[4,8,9] The usefulness of antibacterials is more contentious,[8] although some clinicians advocate prolonged courses as part of initial treatment.[4,9] Surgical intervention may be necessary if medical treatment fails.

1. Agency for Health Care Policy and Research. *Diagnosis and treatment of acute bacterial rhinosinusitis*. Evidence Report/Technology Assessment: Number 9, March 1999. http://www.ahcpr.gov/clinic/sinussum.htm
2. de Ferranti SD, *et al.* Are amoxycillin and folate inhibitors as effective as other antibiotics for acute sinusitis? A meta-analysis. *BMJ* 1998; **317**: 632–7.
3. Williams JW, *et al.* Antibiotics for acute maxillary sinusitis (updated 29 August 2001). Available in The Cochrane Library; Issue 4. Oxford: Update Software; 2001.
4. Evans KL. Diagnosis and management of sinusitis. *BMJ* 1994; **309**: 1415–22.
5. Evans KL. Recognition and management of sinusitis. *Drugs* 1998. **56**: 59–71.
6. Gwaltney JM. Acute community-acquired sinusitis. *Clin Infect Dis* 1996; **23**: 1209–25.
7. Grayston JT, *et al.* A new respiratory tract pathogen: Chlamydia pneumoniae strain TWAR. *J Infect Dis* 1990; **161**: 618–25.
8. Rowe-Jones J, Mackay I. Management of sinusitis: sinusitis and rhinitis, or rhinosinusitis? *BMJ* 1995; **310**: 670.
9. Wald ER. Chronic sinusitis in children. *J Pediatr* 1995; **127**: 339–47.

Skin infections

Bacterial infections of the skin may result from invasion of skin structures by endogenous skin flora or by exogenous pathogenic organisms. They include the primary pyodermas (for example, impetigo, folliculitis, furunculosis, erysipelas, cellulitis, and ecthyma) and secondary infections complicating pre-existing skin lesions, for example diabetic or other chronic superficial skin ulcers, burns, bites and stings (p.115), eczema, and as opportunistic infections following skin trauma in immunocompromised patients.

The pyodermas are commonly caused by *Staphylococcus aureus* or, less commonly, by beta-haemolytic streptococci. Skin ulcers and burns may typically be colonised by *Staph. aureus* or *Pseudomonas aeruginosa*; chronic ulcers and fungating tumours may also be colonised by anaerobes which can cause an offensive odour.

Skin disorders of uncertain or mixed aetiology that are treated with antibacterials include acne (p.1103) and rosacea (p.1107). Systemic infections with cutaneous involvement include anthrax (p.115), diphtheria (p.118), and mycetoma (p.130).

Topical antibacterials and antiseptics may be useful for superficial skin infections, but antibacterials should only be used short term because of the risks of inducing bacterial resistance and contact allergy. Antibacterials of value systemically such as gentamicin are best avoided, although fusidic acid is used topically in the UK. Application of topical antibacterials to extensive areas of damaged skin can result in systemic toxicity.

Serious infections are treated systemically. Treatment of skin infections is increasingly based on knowledge of the likely infecting organisms and patterns of resistance; empirical treatment with broad-spectrum antibacterials is now discouraged in an attempt to minimise the emergence of resistant organisms.[1] For burns, however, control of infection is important to reduce the risk of sepsis. Topical application of sulfadiazine silver or mafenide acetate has been used in addition to aggressive systemic antibacterial therapy.

Gram-positive pathogens, especially staphylococci and beta-haemolytic streptococci, are commonly associated with primary pyodermas. *Staphylococcus aureus* is implicated in impetigo, cellulitis, folliculitis, furunculosis, and occasionally erysipelas and necrotising fasciitis (p.130), and may colonise burns. Staphylococcal scalded skin syndrome is a severe manifestation of bullous impetigo caused by infection with strains of *Staph. aureus* producing exfoliative exotoxins. The term toxic epidermal necrolysis is used to cover both this syndrome and a morphologically identical syndrome due to various aetiologies. A syndrome resembling scarlet fever may also occur. Staphylococcal infections are usually treated systemically with a penicillinase-resistant penicillin. Erythromycin is an alternative for patients unable to tolerate penicillin. Multidrug-resistant staphylococci are becoming increasingly common, particularly in hospitals, and treatment alternatives for infections with these organisms are discussed under Staphylococcal Infections, below. Less severe infections in folliculitis or furunculosis may respond to the application of moist heat without the need for antibacterials. In patients at risk of recurrent staphylococcal infections, nasal application of chlorhexidine plus neomycin or mupirocin alone is used to eliminate nasal carriage of staphylococci.

Beta-haemolytic streptococci are also implicated in pyodermas including impetigo, erysipelas, and cellulitis. Necrotising fasciitis (p.130) may be caused by group A streptococci. Streptococcal infections continue to respond to phenoxymethylpenicillin or benzylpenicillin. Erythromycin is an alternative in patients unable to tolerate penicillins, but increasing resistance may be a problem;[1] clindamycin may be effective in patients with aggressive infections not responding to penicillin.[2]

Resistance is also emerging in *Propionibacterium acnes*; strains resistant to erythromycin, clindamycin, and tetracycline are reported to be common in patients following treatment for acne.[1]

Gram-negative bacteria are less frequently implicated in skin infections, but *Pseudomonas aeruginosa* and *Proteus* spp. can cause infections especially if the skin is subjected to damp conditions. These organisms produce proteolytic enzymes that cause the resulting skin damage. *Ps. aeruginosa* may colonise burns and skin ulcers. Pseudomonal infections are treated with aminoglycosides and the antipseudomonal penicillins.

Anaerobic organisms may colonise wounds, particularly chronic ulcers and fungating tumours. Topical metronidazole has been used to control the offensive odour caused by these infections.

1. Espersen F. Resistance to antibiotics used in dermatological practice. *Br J Dermatol* 1998; **139** (suppl 53): 4–8.
2. Bisno AL, Stevens DL. Streptococcal infections of skin and soft tissues. *N Engl J Med* 1996; **334**: 240–5.

Spleen disorders

Splenectomised patients and those with hyposplenism associated with, for example, sickle-cell disease have impaired immunity and like other immunocompromised patients (above) are at increased risk of infection. Children are at special risk. *Streptococcus pneumoniae* is the commonest infecting bacterium and may cause severe overwhelming infection that is rapid in onset and sometimes fatal. Hence, prophylaxis with an oral penicillin such as phenoxymethylpenicillin is advocated. Pneumococcal vaccine is also used; the newer ones may be more effective than earlier vaccines. Other organisms implicated include *Neisseria meningitidis*, *Haemophilus influenzae*, and *Escherichia coli* in splenectomised patients and *Salmonella* in children with sickle-cell disease. More unusual organisms include *Capnocytophaga canimorsus* (formerly called DF-2) which may cause opportunistic infections in splenectomised patients following animal bites. There may also be an increased risk of falciparum malaria and babesiosis.

SPLENECTOMISED PATIENTS. Guidelines for prophylaxis based on published evidence and expert opinion have been published in the UK.[1] Immunisation with polyvalent pneumococcal vaccine is recommended for all asplenic patients and those with functional hyposplenism. *Haemophilus influenzae* (Hib) vaccine is recommended for all patients who have not previously received this vaccine. Meningococcal immunisation is not routinely recommended since the vaccine currently available does not protect against the group B strain of *N. meningitidis* causing most infections in the UK. However, it is recommended for patients travelling to destinations where group A and C strains are more prevalent. Influenza vaccination may be beneficial. Lifelong prophylaxis with a suitable antibacterial should be offered. Phenoxymethylpenicillin is usually given, but amoxicillin may be preferred, particularly in adults, as it is better absorbed following oral administration and has a broader spectrum of activity. Erythromycin is a suitable alternative in those unable to tolerate penicillins. On a practical level, compliance with lifelong prophylaxis is difficult, but is particularly important in patients with underlying immunodeficiency, in children up to the age of 16 years, and for the first two years after splenectomy. Patients should keep a supply of a suitable antibacterial for immediate administration should symptoms of infection occur, and be instructed to seek medical advice urgently.

SICKLE-CELL DISEASE. Children with sickle-cell disease are particularly susceptible to severe pneumococcal infection which may present as septicaemia, meningitis, or pneumonia.

Penicillin prophylaxis is usually combined with early administration of a polyvalent pneumococcal vaccine. However, despite the introduction of the 23-valent vaccine, there is little evidence that it produces substantial protection in children under 2 years of age. Phenoxymethylpenicillin 125 mg twice daily is effective in young children but amoxicillin may be preferred in adults since it is better absorbed and has a broader spectrum.[1] There is evidence to suggest that, in children who have received pneumococcal immunisation, there is no benefit in continuing penicillin prophylaxis beyond the age of 5 years[2] although indefinite prophylaxis has been recommended for those who have had a previous pneumococcal septic event.[3] Fears that prolonged prophylaxis could encourage the emergence of resistant pneumococci have not been substantiated,[4] although the prevalence of beta-lactam-resistant pneumococci continues to increase. Neonatal screening for sickle-cell disease is advocated, but compliance with regular penicillin prophylaxis may be poor and effective follow-up is necessary if the full benefit of such screening is to be achieved.[5,6] Nevertheless, availability of penicillin in the home, even if not taken regularly, means that it can be readily used if febrile illness occurs.[5] If children with sickle-cell disease develop a febrile illness they are generally treated in hospital with intravenous antibacterials, although outpatient management may often be possible.[7]

1. Working Party of the British Committee for Standards in Haematology Clinical Haematology Task Force. Guidelines for the prevention and treatment of infection in patients with an absent or dysfunctional spleen. *BMJ* 1996; **312**: 430–4.
2. Falletta JM, *et al.* Discontinuing penicillin prophylaxis in children with sickle cell anemia. *J Pediatr* 1995; **127**: 685–90.
3. Hongeng S, *et al.* Recurrent Streptococcus pneumoniae sepsis in children with sickle cell disease. *J Pediatr* 1997; **130**: 814–16. Correction. *ibid.*; **131**: 232.
4. Norris CF, *et al.* Pneumococcal colonization in children with sickle cell disease. *J Pediatr* 1996; **129**: 821–7.
5. Milne RIG. Assessment of care of children with sickle cell disease: implications for neonatal screening programmes. *BMJ* 1990; **300**: 371–4.
6. Cummins D, *et al.* Penicillin prophylaxis in children with sickle cell disease in Brent. *BMJ* 1991; **302**: 989–90.
7. Wilimas JA, *et al.* A randomized study of outpatient treatment with ceftriaxone for selected febrile children with sickle cell disease. *N Engl J Med* 1993; **329**: 472–6.

Spotted fevers

Rickettsial infections of the spotted fever group are transmitted to man by ticks and have also been called tick typhus. They include Rocky Mountain spotted fever, due to *Rickettsia rickettsii* and occurring especially in the USA; boutonneuse or Mediterranean spotted fever, due to *R. conorii* and occurring in Mediterranean countries including the Middle East, Africa, and India; Queensland tick typhus, due to *R. australis* and occurring in Australia; north Asian tick typhus, due to *R. sibirica* and occurring in Siberia and Mongolia; and oriental spotted fever, due to *R. japonica* and occurring in Japan. Rickettsialpox, due to *R. akari*, is transmitted from mice by mites and occurs in the USA, Russia, and Africa.

Spotted fevers are recognised increasingly as a cause of febrile illness associated usually, but not always, with a purpuric rash and are becoming an important cause of imported fevers in non-endemic areas.[1] Rocky Mountain spotted fever may be one of the most severe of these fevers, but others are potentially serious. A tetracycline, often doxycycline, or chloramphenicol is the treatment of choice for all the spotted fevers. In Rocky Mountain spotted fever tetracycline 25 to 50 mg per kg bodyweight daily or chloramphenicol 50 to 75 mg per kg daily for 7 to 10 days markedly reduced mortality.[1] Because tetracyclines are generally contra-indicated in young children, chloramphenicol has been recommended in the USA for children with Rocky Mountain spotted fever under the age of 9, but some still prefer to use a tetracycline;[2] as demonstrated in Mediterranean spotted fever, shorter courses of tetracycline might be effective.[3] Relapses have occurred in patients with Mediterranean spotted fever treated with chloramphenicol.[4] Other alternatives to tetracycline used in Mediterranean spotted fever have included erythromycin[5] and ciprofloxacin.[6] Erythromycin was effective, but less so than tetracycline, in children with Mediterranean spotted fever.[5] Short 2-day courses of ciprofloxacin or doxycycline were curative in adults whose disease was not severe, although there was a more rapid response to doxycycline.[6] A 5-day course of ciprofloxacin has also been used successfully to treat infection with *R. australis*.[7]

Rickettsialpox can be mistaken for chickenpox. However, it will respond to tetracycline although patients have generally recovered without treatment.[8]

1. Anonymous. Bitten, hot, and mostly spotty. *Lancet* 1991; **337**: 143–4.
2. Abramson JS, Givner LB. Should tetracycline be contraindicated for therapy of presumed Rocky Mountain spotted fever in children less than 9 years of age? *Pediatrics* 1990; **86**: 123–4.
3. Yagupsky P. Tetracycline for Rocky Mountain spotted fever. *Pediatrics* 1991; **87**: 124.
4. Shaked Y, *et al.* Relapse of rickettsial Mediterranean spotted fever and murine typhus after treatment with chloramphenicol. *J Infect* 1989; **18**: 35–7.
5. Muñoz-Espin T, *et al.* Erythromycin versus tetracycline for treatment of Mediterranean spotted fever. *Arch Dis Child* 1986; **61**: 1027–9.
6. Gudiol F, *et al.* Randomized double-blind evaluation of ciprofloxacin and doxycycline for Mediterranean spotted fever. *Antimicrob Agents Chemother* 1989; **33**: 987–8.
7. Hudson BJ, *et al.* Ciprofloxacin treatment for Australian spotted fever. *Med J Aust* 1996; **165**: 588.
8. Kass EM, *et al.* Rickettsialpox in a New York City hospital, 1980 to 1989. *N Engl J Med* 1994; **331**: 1612–17.

Staphylococcal infections

Staphylococci are Gram-positive bacteria pathogenic to man. Species may be differentiated by various methods including the coagulase test. Those species of clinical importance are *Staphylococcus aureus*, which is usually coagulase-positive, and *Staph. epidermidis* and *Staph. saprophyticus*, which are coagulase-negative.

Staph. aureus colonises the skin and mucous membranes naturally and many people, including neonates, may be staphylococcal carriers from time to time. Localised *Staph. aureus* infections may follow surgery or trauma and commonly result in abscess formation. Staphylococcal skin infections include impetigo and furunculosis. Conditions associated with staphylococcal extracellular toxin production include staphylococcal scalded skin syndrome, toxic shock syndrome, and staphylococcal food poisoning. Staphylococcal septicaemia is usually a consequence of local infection and may sometimes be associated with intravascular or intraperitoneal catheters or with intravenous drug abuse. Septicaemia often results in staphylococcal endocarditis. Other possible complications of septicaemia are pneumonia and bone and joint infections, although in these cases aspiration or local trauma, respectively, may be the cause.

Staph. epidermidis is also a natural inhabitant of skin and mucous membranes and an increasingly important nosocomial pathogen. Many infections are hospital-acquired and are often associated with indwelling catheters. There has been an increased incidence of bacteraemia due to *Staph. epidermidis* in neonatal units.

Staph. saprophyticus is a common cause of urinary-tract infections in young women.

Staphylococci were sensitive to benzylpenicillin when it was first introduced, but the majority of strains are now resistant as a result of penicillinase production. Meticillin and other penicillinase-resistant penicillins such as flucloxacillin were developed because of their activity against these resistant staphylococci. However, meticillin-resistant staphylococci soon emerged. Both coagulase-negative staphylococci and *Staph. aureus* resistant to meticillin are generally resistant to all beta lactams and often exhibit multiple resistance to other antibacterials (see Meticillin, p.223). More studies have been published on meticillin-resistant *Staph. aureus* (MRSA) than meticillin-resistant coagulase-negative staphylococci, but both types are a serious problem in hospitals around the world. Resistant strains may be endemic to a single hospital or may be epidemic causing outbreaks of infection at more than one hospital. Colonisation of hospital staff and patients with meticillin-resistant staphylococci is an important factor in the spread of these infections. Current trends are towards health care at home rather than in hospital and there are reports suggesting that MRSA is becoming more prevalent in the community.[1-4]

Revised guidelines[5] for the control of MRSA in hospital were produced by a combined working party of the British Society for Antimicrobial Chemotherapy, the Hospital Infection Society, and the Infection Control Nurses Association in 1998. They advise prompt isolation of infected or colonised patients, screening of patients and staff in contact with such patients, the use of protective clothing and handwashing with an antiseptic detergent or alcoholic rub; and the use by all patients of an antiseptic detergent for washing and bathing. For eradication of nasal carriage they recommend mupirocin nasal ointment or, if the strain is mupirocin-resistant, chlorhexidine and neomycin cream. Eradication at other colonised sites is more difficult: antiseptic detergents may be used for skin and hair washing; mupirocin in a macrogol basis for small infected skin lesions, but not for burns or large raw areas; hexachlorophene dusting powder for axillae and groins; and systemic rifampicin with fusidic acid or ciprofloxacin for throat or sputum colonisation if absolutely necessary.[5] For the treatment of severe infections due to MRSA they recommend vancomycin or teicoplanin, possibly combined with rifampicin, as the treatment of choice.[5] Similarly recommendations have been made in a consensus review published in the USA.[6]

Although ciprofloxacin may be used the emergence of widespread resistance in meticillin-sensitive and meticillin-resistant *Staph. aureus* limits its usefulness (see p.184). Combination therapy may be helpful. Rifampicin is highly active against MRSA, but it must always be used in combination with another drug to prevent the emergence of resistance. Combinations of rifampicin with gentamicin, vancomycin, co-trimoxazole, fusidic acid, quinolones, or novobiocin have been tried.

There has been concern over isolated reports from around the world of resistance or reduced susceptibility to vancomycin,[7,8] and in response the Centers for Disease Control in the USA produced interim guidelines.[9]

Staphylococcal vaccines have been used for the prophylaxis and treatment of staphylococcal infections.

For the management of staphylococcal infections in general, see under the specific disease headings.

1. Rosenberg J. Methicillin-resistant Staphylococcus aureus (MRSA) in the community: who's watching? *Lancet* 1995; **346:** 132–3.
2. Herold BC, et al. Community-acquired methicillin-resistant Staphylococcus aureus in children with no identified predisposing risk. *JAMA* 1998; **279:** 593–8.
3. Collignon P, et al. Community-acquired methicillin-resistant Staphylococcus aureus in Australia. *Lancet* 1998; **352:** 145–6.
4. Lowy FD. Staphylococcus aureus infections. *N Engl J Med* 1998; **339:** 520–32.
5. Combined Working Party of the British Society for Antimicrobial Chemotherapy, the Hospital Infection Society and the Infection Control Nurses Association. Revised guidelines for the control of methicillin-resistant Staphylococcus aureus infection in hospitals. *J Hosp Infect* 1998; **39:** 253–90.
6. Mulligan ME, et al. Methicillin-resistant Staphylococcus aureus: a consensus review of the microbiology, pathogenesis, and epidemiology with implications for prevention and management. *Am J Med* 1993; **94:** 313–28.
7. CDC. Update: Staphylococcus aureus with reduced susceptibility to vancomycin—United States, 1997. *MMWR* 1997; **46:** 813–15.
8. Smith TL, et al. Emergence of vancomycin resistance in Staphylococcus aureus. *N Engl J Med* 1999; **340:** 493–501.
9. CDC. Interim guidelines for prevention and control of staphylococcal infection associated with reduced susceptibility to vancomycin. *MMWR* 1997; **46:** 626–8, 635.

Surgical infection

Infection is an important cause of postoperative surgical morbidity and mortality and *antimicrobial prophylaxis* is one of several strategies used to reduce the risk of infection. The value of infection prophylaxis is well established in certain types of surgery, especially abdominal surgery and where prostheses are implanted, although recommendations as to the choice of antibacterial, the route, timing, and duration of administration may vary. Surgical wounds are classified as clean, clean-contaminated (potentially contaminated), contaminated, and those following dirty operations. Clean operations exclude those involving the gastrointestinal, genital, urinary, or respiratory tracts. Clean-contaminated operations include those where the gastrointestinal, genital, urinary, or respiratory tracts are opened, but without unusual contamination. Contaminated operations include those where there is acute inflammation or spillage from a hollow viscus. Dirty operations include those where there is pus, gangrene, or perforated viscera. In addition, surgery to repair compound fractures and lacerations due to animal or human bites is considered 'dirty'. The use of antibacterials for the management of contaminated or dirty surgery is considered to be therapeutic rather than prophylactic[1,2] and should continue for several days postoperatively.[3]

Guidelines for the *treatment* of intra-abdominal infections have been produced in the USA by the Surgical Infection Society.[4]

ANTIMICROBIAL PROPHYLAXIS. Strictly speaking the term 'prophylaxis' should be confined to elective procedures with no evidence of sepsis at the time of operation. If possible any pre-existing infections should be treated before admission for surgery. For prophylaxis it is customary to give antibacterials systemically as a single pre-operative dose whereas more prolonged administration is necessary when they are given therapeutically. Antimicrobial prophylaxis is used in clean-contaminated operations and in clean operations that involve the insertion of prosthetic materials or when an infection, however unlikely, would be catastrophic.[1]

Contaminating organisms. The choice of prophylactic antibacterial will be influenced by the likely contaminants for a particular surgical procedure. The most frequently isolated pathogens include *Staphylococcus aureus*, coagulase-negative staphylococci, *Enterococcus* spp., and *Escherichia coli*. Infections with antimicrobial-resistant pathogens including meticillin-resistant *Staph. aureus* (MRSA) and *Candida albicans* are increasing in some hospitals.[1] The most common source of infection is the endogenous flora of the patient's skin, mucous membranes, or viscera. Thus, aerobic Gram-positive organisms (for example staphylococci) are common infecting organisms when the source is the skin and mucous membranes, while infections with enterococci, Gram-negative aerobes (for example *E. coli*), and anaerobic bacteria (for example *Bacteroides fragilis*) can arise from the gastrointestinal tract.

Route of administration. Systemic administration, usually by the intravenous route, is generally preferred. The chosen antibacterial is usually given as a single dose intravenously just before operation at the induction of anaesthesia. The pharmacokinetic properties should be such that adequate serum concentrations are maintained throughout the surgical procedure.[1] Additional doses may be necessary when surgery is prolonged, when there is massive blood loss, or when an antibacterial with a short half-life is used.[3] More controversial routes have included topical or intra-incisional administration and peritoneal lavage. Oral administration of non-absorbable antibacterials to suppress the intestinal flora was traditionally used before large bowel surgery and neomycin

with erythromycin is still given for this purpose in the USA. For reference to selective digestive tract decontamination (SDD), see under Intensive Care, above. Other means of administration include bone cement and chains of beads for implantation, both containing gentamicin and used prophylactically in orthopaedic surgery,[5,6] and topical antibacterials for ophthalmic surgery.[5]

Choice of antibacterial. The most commonly used antibacterials are cephalosporins, aminoglycosides, and metronidazole. In the UK, gentamicin or a cephalosporin are given before abdominal surgery; metronidazole is given in addition before colorectal surgery and a cephalosporin with metronidazole is used before hysterectomy. In the USA, cefazolin is commonly given before surgery, except that involving the lower gastrointestinal tract, for which cefoxitin or cefotetan are used to provide activity against anaerobes.[1-3,7] Alternatively, cefazolin may be given with metronidazole in colorectal surgery.[3] The choice of prophylaxis for patients unable to tolerate cephalosporins is less well established. Aztreonam has been suggested as an alternative to cefazolin with the addition of clindamycin or metronidazole if activity against anaerobes is necessary.[1] However, the use of aztreonam plus metronidazole may provide inadequate activity against Gram-positive cocci.[7] Another suggested alternative to cefazolin is vancomycin,[3] but the routine use of vancomycin should be avoided because of the risk of inducing resistance.[8] Vancomycin may be indicated for high-risk procedures if MRSA infections are prevalent,[8] and combination with aztreonam or an aminoglycoside has been suggested to provide activity against Gram-negative organisms.[7] If vancomycin is used for prophylaxis, no more than two doses should be given.[8] Other alternatives for colorectal procedures include an aminoglycoside with either clindamycin or metronidazole.[7]

The necessity for antibacterial prophylaxis in minimally invasive procedures such as laparoscopy and endoscopy is often not clear.[9] Current US guidelines[1,7] suggest that standard prophylaxis should be used pending further evidence.

Certain categories of patient continue to be at long-term risk of infection after surgery and include splenectomised patients who have impaired immunity and are at risk of pneumococcal and other infections (see under Spleen Disorders, above). Patients at special risk of endocarditis require prophylaxis when undergoing dental and some surgical procedures (see Endocarditis, above). Some have advocated similar prophylaxis in patients with joint prostheses undergoing dental treatment,[10] but a working party for the British Society for Antimicrobial Chemotherapy considers such prophylaxis to be unjustified.[11]

1. Mangram AJ, et al. Guideline for prevention of surgical site infection, 1999. *Infect Control Hosp Epidemiol* 1999; **20:** 250–78.
2. ASHP. ASHP therapeutic guidelines on antimicrobial prophylaxis in surgery. *Am J Health-Syst Pharm* 1999; **56:** 1839–88.
3. Anonymous. Antimicrobial prophylaxis in surgery. *Med Lett Drugs Ther* 1999; **41:** 75–80.
4. Bohnen JMA, et al. Guidelines for clinical care: anti-infective agents for intra-abdominal infection: a Surgical Infection Society policy statement. *Arch Surg* 1992; **127:** 83–9.
5. Henry SL, Galloway KP. Local antibacterial therapy for the management of orthopaedic infections: pharmacokinetic considerations. *Clin Pharmacokinet* 1995; **29:** 36–45.
6. Wininger DA, Fass RJ. Antibiotic-impregnated cement and beads for orthopedic infections. *Antimicrob Agents Chemother* 1996; **40:** 2675–9.
7. Dellinger EP, et al. Quality standard for antimicrobial prophylaxis in surgical procedures. *Clin Infect Dis* 1994; **18:** 422–7.
8. CDC. Recommendations for preventing the spread of vancomycin resistance: recommendations of the Hospital Infection Control Practices Advisory Committee (HICPAC). *MMWR* 1995; **44** (RR-12): 1–13.
9. Wilson APR. Antibiotic prophylaxis and antibiotic control measures in minimally invasive surgery. *J Antimicrob Chemother* 1995; **36:** 1–5.
10. Grant A, Hoddinott C. Joint replacement, dental surgery, and antibiotic prophylaxis. *BMJ* 1992; **304:** 959.
11. Simmons NA, et al. Case against antibiotic prophylaxis for dental treatment of patients with joint prostheses. *Lancet* 1992; **339:** 301.

Syphilis

Syphilis is a sexually transmitted disease caused by the spirochaete *Treponema pallidum* and occurs worldwide. Non-venereal treponematoses occurring principally in the tropics include endemic syphilis or bejel, also caused by *T. pallidum*; pinta, caused by *T. carateum*; and yaws, caused by *T. pertenue*.

Syphilis may be acquired or congenital (see below) and in each case has early and late stages. In acquired sexually transmitted disease the *early* stage includes primary and secondary syphilis and early latent infection; early latent infection is defined as of not more than 2 years' duration in the UK[1] and by WHO,[2,3] or of less than

1 year's duration by the Centers for Disease Control (CDC) in the USA.[4] (Latent infection is when serological tests are positive, but the patient is asymptomatic.) *Late* stage disease includes late latent infection and all late clinical stages. Some term all these late clinical stages tertiary syphilis whereas others use tertiary for benign gummatous syphilis and quaternary for the more serious complications of cardiovascular syphilis and neurosyphilis.[5] The term *neurosyphilis* has generally been applied to late-stage symptomatic neurological disease, although it is recognised that CNS invasion by *T. pallidum* is common in early syphilis and that CNS involvement may occur at any stage.

The incidence of syphilis fell dramatically after the introduction of penicillin and *T. pallidum* remains sensitive to it. There has, however, been a resurgence of syphilis,[6] linked in part with HIV infection.[7] In HIV-infected patients syphilis appears more virulent and neurosyphilis occurs more quickly. Like other diseases causing genital ulcers, syphilis is a risk factor for HIV infection.

The **treatment** of choice for both early and late syphilis is still penicillin and long-acting injections are generally used. WHO guidelines[3] recommend either benzathine benzylpenicillin or procaine penicillin [procaine benzylpenicillin]. The preferred penicillin in the UK is procaine penicillin [procaine benzylpenicillin][1,8] although it is no longer commercially available. Benzathine benzylpenicillin is preferred in the USA.[4] Treatment for late syphilis is less well-established than that for early disease and is usually for longer. Benzylpenicillin may be preferred for neurosyphilis and congenital syphilis. For a summary of WHO, UK, and US treatment guidelines, see below.

CSF involvement is common in early syphilis and in the USA *neurosyphilis* has become more common especially among HIV-infected patients.[7] In the UK, CSF abnormalities are uncommon after treatment for early syphilis and the prevalence of late syphilis including neurosyphilis remains low.[1] The lower incidence of neurosyphilis throughout Europe may be attributable to the use of more intensive treatment courses for early syphilis than is customary in the USA,[9,10] and to the choice of penicillin.[1] In addition, since neither benzathine benzylpenicillin nor procaine penicillin [procaine benzylpenicillin] achieve treponemicidal concentrations in the CNS during standard regimens, host immune responses may play an essential part.[1] The use of multidose or augmented treatment regimens in the USA have not generally been associated with improved clinical responses.[11-13] In the UK, treatment of all cases of syphilis in HIV-infected patients as for neurosyphilis is advised; in the USA, standard treatment is considered sufficient (see below for details).[4]

Patients *allergic to penicillin* have been given a tetracycline or erythromycin although their efficacy is less well established.

A Jarisch-Herxheimer reaction may occur after the first dose of antibacterial, especially in patients with early syphilis, and some advocate corticosteroid cover.[5]

Congenital syphilis may result from transplacental infection at any stage of pregnancy and any stage of maternal syphilis. There has been a dramatic increase in its incidence in the USA and renewed concern about the efficacy of treatment with benzathine benzylpenicillin.[14] Benzylpenicillin or procaine penicillin [procaine benzylpenicillin] are preferred to benzathine benzylpenicillin for infants with congenital syphilis.[1-4]

Recommended **treatment regimens** from WHO,[3] UK,[1,8] and USA[4] for acquired and congenital syphilis are as follows. Sexual partners should be examined and treated.

• EARLY SYPHILIS

1. WHO: benzathine benzylpenicillin 1.8 g (2.4 million units) intramuscularly in a single session, usually given as 2 injections at separate sites, or procaine penicillin [procaine benzylpenicillin] 1.2 g (1.2 million units) intramuscularly daily for 10 days. Alternatives for non-pregnant penicillin-allergic patients: doxycycline 100 mg by mouth twice daily for 15 days or tetracycline hydrochloride 500 mg by mouth 4 times daily for 15 days. Pregnant women allergic to penicillin may be given erythromycin 500 mg by mouth 4 times daily for 15 days (but see below).

2. UK: procaine penicillin [procaine benzylpenicillin] 600 mg (600 000 units) intramuscularly daily for 10 to 14 days. Procaine penicillin [procaine benzylpenicillin] is given as a multi-ingredient preparation also containing benzylpenicillin. Alternatives for penicillin-allergic patients: doxycycline 200 mg daily for 14 days, or tetracycline 500 mg four times daily for

14 days, or erythromycin 500 mg four times daily for 14 days [all by mouth]. Additional alternative if parenteral therapy is refused: amoxicillin 500 mg plus probenecid 500 mg each four times daily for 14 days. Alternative for suspected non-compliance: benzathine benzylpenicillin 1.8 g (2.4 million units) intramuscularly weekly for 2 weeks.

3. USA: benzathine benzylpenicillin 1.8 g intramuscularly in a single dose. Alternatives for penicillin-allergic patients: doxycycline 100 mg twice daily, or tetracycline 500 mg four times daily, each by mouth for 2 weeks. A further though less effective alternative is erythromycin 500 mg four times daily, by mouth for 2 weeks; ceftriaxone may also be considered.

• LATE SYPHILIS

1. WHO: benzathine benzylpenicillin 1.8 g (2.4 million units) intramuscularly once weekly for 3 consecutive weeks or procaine penicillin [procaine benzylpenicillin] 1.2 g (1.2 million units) intramuscularly daily for 20 days. Alternatives for non-pregnant penicillin-allergic patients are doxycycline 100 mg twice daily, or tetracycline 500 mg four times daily, each by mouth for 30 days. For those with neurosyphilis: benzylpenicillin 1.2 to 2.4 g (2 to 4 million units) intravenously every 4 hours for 14 days, or, if compliance can be ensured, procaine penicillin [procaine benzylpenicillin] 1.2 g intramuscularly daily plus probenecid 500 mg orally 4 times daily for 10 to 14 days; non-pregnant penicillin-allergic patients may be given doxycycline 200 mg twice daily, or tetracycline 500 mg four times daily, each by mouth for 30 days.

2. UK: first-line therapy: procaine penicillin [procaine benzylpenicillin] 600 mg (600 000 units) intramuscularly daily for 17 to 21 days. Procaine penicillin [procaine benzylpenicillin] is given as a multi-ingredient preparation also containing benzylpenicillin. Alternative: benzathine benzylpenicillin 1.8 g (2.4 million units) intramuscularly weekly for 3 doses. Second-line therapy for patients allergic to penicillin and those declining parenteral therapy: doxycycline 200 mg by mouth twice daily for 28 days. For neurosyphilis: procaine penicillin [procaine benzylpenicillin] 1.8 to 2.4 g (1.8 to 2.4 million units) intramuscularly once daily plus probenecid 500 mg by mouth four times daily for 17 to 21 days. Alternative: benzylpenicillin 1.8 to 2.4 g (3 to 4 million units) intravenously every four hours for 17 to 21 days. Second-line therapies for neurosyphilis: doxycycline 200 mg by mouth four times daily for 28 days or amoxicillin 2 g three times daily plus probenecid 500 mg four times daily, both by mouth, for 28 days.

3. USA: benzathine benzylpenicillin 1.8 g intramuscularly weekly for 3 consecutive weeks. Alternatives: doxycycline or tetracycline by mouth for 4 weeks. For those with neurosyphilis: benzylpenicillin 1.8 to 2.4 g (3 to 4 million units) intravenously every 4 hours for 10 to 14 days or, if outpatient compliance can be ensured, procaine penicillin [procaine benzylpenicillin] 2.4 g (2.4 million units) intramuscularly daily together with probenecid 500 mg by mouth 4 times daily, both for 10 to 14 days.

• SYPHILIS IN PREGNANCY

Penicillin as under early and late syphilis together with close surveillance. In the USA CDC[4] note that some recommend a second dose of benzathine benzylpenicillin a week after the initial dose for patients with early syphilis. According to CDC[4] pregnant patients who are allergic to penicillin should be given penicillin, after desensitisation if necessary, since the alternatives, tetracyclines, are contra-indicated during pregnancy and erythromycin cannot be relied on to cure an infected fetus. WHO, on the other hand, advise against desensitisation in a primary care setting and suggest that erythromycin, although inferior, should be given in these circumstances. The mother should be re-treated with tetracyclines after delivery, and the infant assessed and treated. Similar advice to that of WHO is given in the UK.

• CONGENITAL SYPHILIS

1. WHO: for early congenital syphilis in infants up to 2 years of age and having abnormal CSF: benzylpenicillin 30 mg per kg body-weight (50 000 units per kg) intravenously twice daily for the first 7 days of life and three times daily thereafter for a total of 10 days, or procaine penicillin [procaine benzylpenicillin] 50 mg per kg (50 000 units per kg) intramuscularly daily in a single dose for 10 days. For infants with normal CSF: benzathine benzylpenicillin 37.5 mg per kg

(50 000 units per kg) intramuscularly as a single-session treatment (although some treat all as if the CSF were abnormal). Children older than 2 years: benzylpenicillin 120 to 180 mg per kg (200 000 to 300 000 units per kg) intramuscularly or intravenously daily in 4 or 6 divided doses for 10 to 14 days. An alternative regimen for penicillin-allergic infants aged over 1 month is erythromycin 7.5 to 12.5 mg per kg by mouth four times daily for 30 days.

2. UK: procaine penicillin [procaine benzylpenicillin] 50 mg per kg (50 000 units per kg) intramuscularly daily for 10 to 14 days. Procaine penicillin [procaine benzylpenicillin] is given as a multi-ingredient preparation also containing benzylpenicillin.

3. USA: benzylpenicillin 30 mg per kg intravenously every 12 hours for the first 7 days of life and every 8 hours thereafter for a total of 10 days or procaine penicillin [procaine benzylpenicillin] 50 mg per kg intramuscularly daily for 10 days. Infants at risk of congenital syphilis but without clinical evidence of infection may be given a single intramuscular injection of benzathine benzylpenicillin 37.5 mg per kg. Older infants and children thought to have congenital syphilis or neurological involvement should be given benzylpenicillin 30 mg per kg every 4 to 6 hours for 10 days.

• NON-VENEREAL TREPONEMATOSES

When the prevalence of endemic syphilis (bejel), pinta, or yaws is 10% or more WHO[2] recommend mass treatment of the entire population with a single intramuscular injection of benzathine benzylpenicillin 900 mg (1.2 million units) or half this dose in children under 10 years.

1. Clinical Effectiveness Group (Association of Genitourinary Medicine and the Medical Society for the Study of Venereal Diseases). National guideline for the management of early syphilis. *Sex Transm Infect* 1999; **75** (suppl 1): S29–S33.
2. WHO. WHO expert committee on venereal diseases and treponematoses: sixth report. *WHO Tech Rep Ser 736* 1986: 126–39.
3. WHO. Guidelines for the management of sexually transmitted infections. Geneva: WHO, 2001.
4. Centers for Disease Control. 1998 Guidelines for treatment of sexually transmitted diseases. *MMWR* 1998; **47** (RR-1): 28–46.
5. Thin RN. Treatment of venereal syphilis. *J Antimicrob Chemother* 1989; **24**: 481–3.
6. Rolfs RT, Nakashima AK. Epidemiology of primary and secondary syphilis in the United States, 1981 through 1989. *JAMA* 1990; **264**: 1432–7.
7. Flood JM, *et al.* Neurosyphilis during the AIDS epidemic, San Francisco, 1985–1992. *J Infect Dis* 1998; **177**: 931–40.
8. Clinical Effectiveness Group (Association of Genitourinary Medicine and the Medical Society for the Study of Venereal Diseases). National guideline for the management of late syphilis. *Sex Transm Infect* 1999; **75** (suppl 1): S34–S37.
9. Esselink R, *et al.* Low frequency of neurosyphilis in HIV-infected individuals. *Lancet* 1993; **341**: 571.
10. O'Farrell N, Thin RN. Neurosyphilis and HIV. *Lancet* 1993; **341**: 1224.
11. Malone JL, *et al.* Syphilis and neurosyphilis in a human immunodeficiency virus type-1 seropositive population: evidence for frequent serologic relapse after therapy. *Am J Med* 1995; **99**: 55–63.
12. Gordon SM, *et al.* The response of symptomatic neurosyphilis to high-dose intravenous penicillin G in patients with human immunodeficiency virus infection. *N Engl J Med* 1994; **331**: 1469–73.
13. Rolfs RT, *et al.* A randomized trial of enhanced therapy for early syphilis in patients with and without human immunodeficiency virus infection. *N Engl J Med* 1997; **337**: 307–14.
14. Ikeda MK, Janson HB. Evaluation and treatment of congenital syphilis. *J Pediatr* 1990; **117**: 843–52.

Tetanus

Clostridium tetani is a Gram-positive anaerobic spore-forming bacillus present in soil and faeces. The toxin it produces, tetanospasmin, causes tetanus or lockjaw, with uncontrolled muscle spasm. Tetanus can be prevented by active immunisation with tetanus vaccine or passive immunisation with tetanus immunoglobulin. Nowadays it occurs predominantly in developing countries and especially in neonates. In developed countries immunity may be relatively low in the elderly.

In addition to the control of muscle spasm with drugs such as diazepam (see p.1332 for the symptomatic treatment of tetanus), treatment includes the use of tetanus immunoglobulin to neutralise any circulating toxin and the administration of benzylpenicillin. A tetracycline[1] or metronidazole[2] have been suggested as possible alternatives to benzylpenicillin and some now consider metronidazole to be preferable to benzylpenicillin.[3]

In rural developing countries where tetanus is common and active immunisation little practised, pre-operative metronidazole or penicillin might be used for patients undergoing emergency operations who have not been immunised against tetanus; the duration of antibacterial cover depends on the contamination risk.[4]

1. Anonymous. The choice of antibacterial drugs. *Med Lett Drugs Ther* 1999; **41**: 95–104.

2. Ahmadsyah I, Salim A. Treatment of tetanus: an open study to compare the efficacy of procaine penicillin and metronidazole. *BMJ* 1985; **291:** 648–50.
3. Sanford JP. Tetanus—forgotten but not gone. *N Engl J Med* 1995; **332:** 812–13.
4. Anonymous. Postoperative tetanus. *Lancet* 1984; **ii:** 964–5.

Tonsillitis
See under Pharyngitis, above.

Toxic shock syndrome

Toxic shock syndrome is an acute febrile illness associated with multisystem failure and caused by a toxin, usually toxic shock syndrome toxin-1 (TSST-1), produced by *Staphylococcus aureus*.[1,2] Bacteraemia has been reported to be absent in most cases.[3] In the early 1980s toxic shock syndrome was reported predominantly in menstruating women using high-absorbency tampons, but it is now appreciated that foci of staphylococcal infection such as surgical wounds, burns, abscesses, and sinuses are often responsible.[1,2] Treatment of the acute phase requires prevention of further production or absorption of toxin by local measures such as removal of tampons or packing, wound debridement, or drainage of abscesses; elimination of the toxin-producing bacteria by antistaphylococcal antibacterials given intravenously initially; fluid replacement; and sometimes corticosteroids.[1,2] Continuing antibacterial treatment for 10 days during the convalescent phase to reduce the risk of recurrence has been recommended.[1]

More recently group A beta-haemolytic streptococci (*Streptococcus pyogenes*) have been associated with a similar toxin-related syndrome.[4,5] Benzylpenicillin is the treatment of choice[6] but, since it may be difficult to exclude staphylococcal toxic shock syndrome, an antistaphylococcal drug such as flucloxacillin should also be given.[6] Clinical improvement has been reported after administration of intravenous normal immunoglobulins.[7,8]

Toxic shock syndromes may be associated with necrotising fasciitis (see above).

1. Todd JK. Therapy of toxic shock syndrome. *Drugs* 1990; **39:** 856–61.
2. Williams GR. The toxic shock syndrome. *BMJ* 1990; **300:** 960.
3. Eykyn SJ. Staphylococcal sepsis: the changing pattern of disease and therapy. *Lancet* 1988; **i:** 100–4.
4. Cone LA, *et al.* Clinical and bacteriologic observations of a toxic shock-like syndrome due to Streptococcus pyogenes. *N Engl J Med* 1987; **317:** 146–9.
5. Stevens DL, *et al.* Severe group A streptococcal infections associated with a toxic shock-like syndrome and scarlet fever toxin A. *N Engl J Med* 1989; **321:** 1–7.
6. Sanderson P. Do streptococci cause toxic shock? *BMJ* 1990; **301:** 1006–7.
7. Barry W, *et al.* Intravenous immunoglobulin therapy for toxic shock syndrome. *JAMA* 1992; **267:** 3315–16.
8. Kaul R, *et al.* Intravenous immunoglobulin therapy for streptococcal toxic shock syndrome—a comparative observational study. *Clin Infect Dis* 1999; **28:** 800–7.

Trachoma

Trachoma results from chronic eye infection with certain *Chlamydia trachomatis* serotypes and is endemic in parts of Africa, the Middle East, and India where it is an important cause of blindness. It is not a sexually transmitted disease, but is associated with poverty, poor sanitation, and poor personal hygiene. The reservoir is chronic eye infection and transmission may be via fingers, fomites, and flies. Inclusion conjunctivitis in infants (see under Neonatal Conjunctivitis, above) and in adults is associated with sexually transmitted genital *C. trachomatis* infection and can progress to trachoma when there is persistent or recurrent eye infection.

Guidelines for trachoma control published by WHO in 1981 outlined topical or oral treatment with a tetracycline or alternatively with erythromycin or a sulfonamide.[1] Topical chemotherapy for trachoma must be intensive and prolonged, 6 weeks being the minimum recommended duration for continuous intensive treatment with tetracycline 1% ophthalmic ointment. With less frequent applications, the duration of treatment must be prolonged and may need to be extended to months or even years. The recommended intermittent treatment schedule consists of applications of tetracycline twice daily for 5 consecutive days or once daily for 10 days, each month and for 6 months each year, to be repeated as necessary. Short courses with topical tetracyclines can be used for the control of bacterial infections during seasonal epidemics of conjunctivitis and may have to be repeated annually. Oral therapy with tetracycline or doxycycline for 3 to 4 weeks has also been effective for selective treatment in well monitored programmes. Erythromycin and related macrolides administered by mouth or topically to the eye have been of benefit in trachoma, but have been less

widely used. Topical therapy with sulfonamides appears only partially effective; adequate treatment with oral sulfonamides requires full therapeutic doses for about 2 to 3 weeks and may be associated with adverse reactions.

A single oral dose of azithromycin has been reported to produce a similar rate of resolution to conventional treatment with topical tetracycline for 6 weeks.[2] In a more recent study,[3] mass treatment of African village communities with oral azithromycin once weekly for 3 weeks resulted in a lower incidence of trachoma at follow-up after one year than a standard course of topical tetracycline. Many[4] now recommend azithromycin as the treatment of choice for trachoma, with combined oral and topical treatment with either a tetracycline or a sulfonamide as an alternative.

The view has been expressed that in endemic areas the provision of clean water, regular face washing, and the use of tetracycline eye ointment by those infected might eradicate trachoma.[5] A programme[6] involving the use of azithromycin, surgery, facial cleanliness, and environmental improvements has been launched by WHO with the aim of eliminating trachoma by 2020.

A vaccine against *C. trachomatis* is also under investigation.[7]

1. Dawson CR, *et al.* Guide to trachoma control. Geneva: WHO, 1981.
2. Bailey RL, *et al.* Randomised controlled trial of single-dose azithromycin in treatment of trachoma. *Lancet* 1993; **342:** 453–6.
3. Schachter J, *et al.* Azithromycin in control of trachoma. *Lancet* 1999; **354:** 630–5.
4. Anonymous. The choice of antibacterial drugs. *Med Lett Drugs Ther* 1999; **41:** 95–104.
5. Potter AR. Avoidable blindness. *BMJ* 1991; **302:** 922–3.
6. Bailey R, Lietman T. The SAFE strategy for the elimination of trachoma by 2020: will it work? *Bull WHO* 2001; **79:** 233–6.
7. Coghlan A. Shapely vaccine targets chlamydia. *New Scientist* 1996; **152:** 18.

Trench fever

Trench fever is a louse-borne bacterial infection so named because of its prevalence among soldiers in the First World War. It is caused by *Bartonella quintana* (formerly *Rochalimaea quintana*) which was until recently classified as a rickettsia. *B. quintana* and *B. henselae* have also been implicated in bacillary angiomatosis, especially in immunocompromised patients, and *B. henselae* is considered to be a cause of cat scratch disease (above).

Reports from France[1,2] and the USA[3] of *B. quintana* bacteraemia, sometimes with endocarditis, in the urban poor prompted the suggestion that trench fever has returned.[4] Cases of trench fever in Marseilles have been reported[2] and might herald an increasing incidence as a result of migration from endemic areas, poverty, and louse infestation.

Treatment of trench fever has usually been with a tetracycline such as doxycycline or with erythromycin. Other antibacterials, for example ceftriaxone, were also used in cases of bacteraemia,[3] but there was limited follow-up and clear recommendations could not be given. Similarly, optimal therapy for *Bartonella* endocarditis has not been identified; however, it has been suggested that the usual treatment for blood culture-negative endocarditis (a penicillin plus an aminoglycoside) should be effective.[5]

1. Drancourt M, *et al.* Bartonella (Rochalimaea) quintana endocarditis in three homeless men. *N Engl J Med* 1995; **332:** 419–23.
2. Brouqui P, *et al.* Chronic Bartonella quintana bacteremia in homeless patients. *N Engl J Med* 1999; **340:** 184–9.
3. Spach DH, *et al.* Bartonella (Rochalimaea) quintana bacteremia in inner-city patients with chronic alcoholism. *N Engl J Med* 1995; **332:** 424–8.
4. Relman DA. Has trench fever returned? *N Engl J Med* 1995; **332:** 463–4.
5. Raoult D, *et al.* Diagnosis of 22 new cases of Bartonella endocarditis. *Ann Intern Med* 1996; **125:** 646–52. Correction. *ibid.* 1997; **127:** 249.

Tuberculosis

Tuberculosis is a chronic infectious disease caused primarily by *Mycobacterium tuberculosis* or sometimes *M. bovis*; the closely related form *M. africanum* has occasionally been implicated as a cause of human tuberculosis. Infection is usually due to inhalation of infected droplet nuclei and the lung is generally the first organ affected. The primary infection is usually asymptomatic.

In the majority of subjects infection and concomitant inflammatory reactions resolve once acquired immunity develops and any surviving organisms become dormant, but in a few patients, particularly in young children or immunocompromised patients, there may be a progression to active primary disease. Dormant organisms may also become reactivated in some patients to produce dis-

ease, particularly following changes in immune status. Hypersensitivity reactions to mycobacterial proteins may cause extensive tissue damage, and virtually any organ of the body can be involved.

During recent years there has been an increase in the incidence of tuberculosis, particularly among the urban poor, and also in association with the spread of HIV infection. WHO declared tuberculosis a global emergency in 1993. Particularly worrying is the increase in multidrug-resistant strains (see below) and poor compliance with drug treatment is seen as a contributory factor. In the USA, there has been emphasis on improving compliance with drug therapy and monitoring responses to limit the further spread of multidrug-resistant disease.[1,2] Direct supervision of treatment has been shown to be effective in both urban and rural settings,[3-6] and generally a higher proportion of patients complete treatment under direct observation than with unsupervised treatment.[7] However, directly observed treatment has not been successful in all settings,[8] and cultural and social attitudes are influential. Attempts have been made to simplify drug regimens including the use of intermittent therapy and combination preparations,[9] and fixed dose combination tablets are recommended by WHO to aid compliance.[10] The feasibility of implantable dosage forms has also been investigated.[11] A decrease in reported cases of tuberculosis in New York City from 1992 through 1994 was attributed mainly to better rates of treatment completion and expanded use of directly observed therapy.[12]

WHO applies the term DOTS to its tuberculosis control strategy which includes standards for diagnosis, ensuring secure drug supplies, and evaluating implementation in addition to the use of directly observed short course treatment regimens; it has also been used as an acronym for directly observed treatment, short-course. A survey has shown that countries adopting the WHO strategy achieved higher cure rates than those that did not.[13]

Treatment. The introduction of rifampicin, with its rapid bactericidal activity, in the 1970s allowed the development of short-course therapy for tuberculosis. Treatment regimens formerly relied on oral daily isoniazid and thioacetazone for periods of 12 to 18 months supplemented by parenteral streptomycin for the first 2 months. Reasons for the high failure rate commonly encountered with such regimens included poor compliance, failure of streptomycin to suppress active disease during the initial treatment phase, and toxicity of the drugs used. Modern short-course therapy involves an initial phase (2 months) using a combination of drugs to produce rapid killing of the bacilli, and a continuation phase of 4 to 6 months using fewer drugs with the aim of eliminating any remaining organisms and thus preventing recurrence. The majority of patients have no organisms detectable in sputum after 2 months with this regimen.

FIRST-LINE DRUGS. First-choice **antituberculous drugs**, often referred to as primary or 'first-line' drugs include isoniazid, rifampicin, pyrazinamide, ethambutol, and streptomycin. Thioacetazone has also been regarded as a first-line drug in developing countries but WHO recommends that ethambutol be substituted in patients with HIV infection whenever possible since this patient group is at high risk of severe and sometimes fatal skin reactions with thioacetazone. In fact, current WHO recommended treatment regimens do not include thioacetazone. However, the suggestion that thioacetazone should be dropped for routine treatment[14,15] in general has proved controversial.[16,17]

The short-course regimens recommended by WHO[18] combine drugs to ensure elimination of both metabolically active and dormant organisms: rifampicin and isoniazid are potent bactericides and one or both are used throughout the treatment course; pyrazinamide is bactericidal against intracellular organisms; and streptomycin and ethambutol are used to prevent the emergence of resistant strains. All first-line drugs except thioacetazone can be administered intermittently as an alternative to daily administration.

WHO categorises patients according to the site and severity of the disease, results of the sputum smear, and whether or not the patient has received treatment previously; treatment is then recommended accordingly.[18,19] To ensure compliance, WHO considers direct observation of therapy to be essential during the initial phase and desirable in patients receiving rifampicin during the continuation phase.[18,19]

For **newly diagnosed patients** with active pulmonary tuberculosis and patients with severe tuberculosis at any site the following regimens are recommended: for the initial phase, isoniazid, rifampicin, and pyrazinamide plus either streptomycin or ethambutol daily for 2 months; then for the continuation phase either isoniazid plus rifampicin daily (or 3 times each week for both drugs for intermittent therapy) for a further 4 months or isoniazid plus ethambutol daily for a further 6 months. (Ethambutol and streptomycin are omitted from the initial phase in some national guidelines for patient groups in whom the risk of drug resistance is small.)

For **re-treatment after relapse**, treatment failure, or default patients should receive isoniazid, rifampicin, pyrazinamide, and ethambutol daily for 3 months, supplemented with streptomycin daily for the first 2 months as directly observed therapy (initial phase) then, if the sputum is smear-negative, isoniazid, rifampicin, and ethambutol daily (or 3 times each week for all drugs) for a further 5 months (continuation phase).

For patients with smear-negative pulmonary tuberculosis and patients with **less severe infections** at other sites the preferred regimen is isoniazid, rifampicin, and pyrazinamide daily for 2 months (initial phase) then either isoniazid and ethambutol daily for 6 months or isoniazid and rifampicin daily (or 3 times each week for both drugs) for 4 months (continuation phase).

Short-course therapy is unsuitable for patients who **remain smear-positive** despite supervised re-treatment. These patients usually require treatment with second-line drugs (see below).

The choice of regimen depends on local patterns of drug resistance and the availability of drugs and medical supervision, and are embodied in national and regional treatment protocols in many countries including Europe,[20] the UK,[21] and USA.[22,23] Recently there has been increased awareness of the potential hepatotoxicity of first-line drugs such as isoniazid, rifampicin, and pyrazinamide. Pyrazinamide is generally regarded as being the most hepatotoxic of the three, and further details covering this and special precautions for its use in patients with liver disorders are given in the drug monograph (p.240). WHO and UK guidelines recommend interrupting drug therapy if liver dysfunction occurs, and cautiously re-introducing the same drugs (including pyrazinamide) on resolution.[18,24] Patients in whom complete cessation of therapy is hazardous may be given streptomycin and ethambutol until hepatic function recovers.

SECOND-LINE DRUGS. Other drugs used in the treatment of tuberculosis, such as the aminosalicylates, capreomycin, cycloserine, ethionamide, protionamide, and kanamycin are considered to be secondary drugs and have been used if resistance or toxicity to the 'first-line' drugs develops during therapy, and are generally less effective and/or more toxic. The increasing problem of tuberculosis resistant to conventional first-line drugs has also led to increased interest in the development of new agents, and in various drugs such as the fluoroquinolones, amoxicillin-clavulanic acid, and the rifampicin derivative rifabutin.

RESISTANCE. The incidence of drug-resistant strains of *Mycobacterium tuberculosis* has increased steadily over recent years in many countries, including the USA.[25-27] Isoniazid resistance is most common but multidrug-resistant strains have also occurred, often in HIV-infected individuals, resulting in disease which is very difficult to treat and often fatal. Such resistance is considered to result from poor management of tuberculosis control[28] and administration of tuberculosis treatment under direct observation has reduced the rates of primary drug resistance, acquired drug resistance, and relapse in the USA.[3,12] In the UK[29,30] rates of multidrug-resistant tuberculosis remain lower than those in the USA, but are rising. The first reported outbreak of hospital-acquired multidrug-resistant tuberculosis in England and Wales has occurred on an HIV unit.[31]

The key to controlling the development of multidrug-resistant tuberculosis is the adoption of the WHO DOTS programme,[32] but different strategies are necessary in areas where multidrug-resistance is established. In areas with a high rate of initial drug resistance, ethambutol or streptomycin is added during the initial phase;[18,19] drug selection may be re-evaluated once sensitivity results are available. As discussed above, patients who relapse after an initial treatment course are generally given a second prolonged and directly observed treatment course with first-line drugs. Patients who relapse following the WHO standard re-treatment regimen or who are otherwise suspected of having multidrug-resistant tuberculosis should receive at least three drugs which they have not already received and which do not share cross-resistance to drugs received previously; these should be given under direct

observation for at least 3 months followed by a continuation phase of at least 18 months with at least 2 of the drugs. WHO recommends inclusion of an injectable aminoglycoside (amikacin, capreomycin, or kanamycin) and pyrazinamide, even if the patient has previously received it, in the initial phase.[33] Cross-resistance exists between fluoroquinolones, between cycloserine and terizidone, and between thioacetazone and protionamide or ethionamide.[33] Cross-resistance between rifampicin and rifabutin is also commonly observed. There appears to be no cross-resistance between fluoroquinolones and other antituberculous drugs, but fluoroquinolone-resistant tuberculosis can emerge rapidly as a result of inadequate or inappropriate treatment.[34] Cross-resistance patterns among aminoglycosides are complex.[33]

CHILDREN. Children and infants can be treated with similar regimens to adults.[21-23] Ethambutol is not usually given to young children because of the perceived difficulty in detecting ocular toxicity in this age group although some clinicians have not found this to be a problem.[35]

PREGNANCY AND THE NEONATE. Tuberculosis during pregnancy poses a serious risk to the fetus and neonate if not detected early and treated properly in the mother.[36] Pregnant patients with clinical tuberculosis are treated similarly to non-pregnant patients, although streptomycin, other aminoglycosides, and capreomycin should be avoided because they can cause ototoxicity in the fetus. Ethionamide and protionamide are also best avoided.[21] The American Thoracic Society and the Centers for Disease Control (CDC)[23] have also advised against the routine use of pyrazinamide because the risk of teratogenicity had not been determined. Consequently, since the standard 6-month regimen includes pyrazinamide, they recommend a minimum of 9 months of therapy preferably with isoniazid, rifampicin, and ethambutol initially. However, others have used pyrazinamide in pregnancy.[36] Also in the USA, pregnant women who react positively to a tuberculin skin test, but who have a normal chest X-ray, may be offered immediate prophylaxis with isoniazid (see Preventive Therapy, below) if they have risk factors for tuberculosis; those without risk factors are referred for prophylaxis after delivery.[36] Following two reports of isoniazid-related hepatitis deaths in the postpartum period, some delay prophylaxis with isoniazid until 3 to 6 months post partum.[36]

The neonate of a mother with current tuberculosis should receive isoniazid for 6 weeks (UK)[37] or 6 months (USA)[23] after which time the infant should be re-evaluated. BCG vaccination is recommended by some authorities when isoniazid is stopped.[18,37]

HIV INFECTION. Patients with HIV infection are particularly prone to active tubercular disease, both pulmonary and extrapulmonary, and mortality is higher than in HIV-negative patients.[18,38] Studies suggest that such patients respond well to conventional regimens.[39,40] However, low drug concentrations can occur[41] possibly due to malabsorption of antimycobacterials[42,43] (although it has not invariably been found[44]); malabsorption has been associated with acquired drug resistance.[45] Paradoxical worsening of symptoms has been reported in patients receiving concurrent treatment with antimycobacterials and antiretrovirals.[46] Also, there may be an increased incidence of adverse reactions to antimycobacterials in HIV-positive individuals,[39] particularly to thioacetazone.[47] WHO recommend that ethambutol should be used in place of both thioacetazone and streptomycin in patients with HIV infection.[18] Most regimens suggested for treating tuberculosis in patients with HIV infection are versions of standard short-course therapy with rifampicin, isoniazid, ethambutol, and pyrazinamide (see above), and most commentators emphasise the importance of directly observed therapy to ensure compliance.[48] It has been suggested that regimens omitting thioacetazone should be adopted for treatment of all patients regardless of HIV status thus avoiding the necessity to test for HIV before starting treatment,[14,15] but this may not be practical in some developing countries.[16,17]

Drug interactions between rifamycins and antiretrovirals can complicate the choice of treatment.[49,50] In particular, rifamycins can reduce plasma concentrations of HIV-protease inhibitors to potentially subtherapeutic levels, and conversely, rifabutin concentrations may be increased to toxic levels (rifampicin is metabolised by a different mechanism and is not affected). Further details concerning the individual drugs affected, together with recommendations by the CDC for dosage adjustments where applicable, are given in Rifabutin under Interac-

tions, Antiretroviral Drugs, p.242 and Uses, Tuberculosis, p.243, respectively.

In patients who have not yet started antiretroviral therapy, it may be possible to delay it until treatment of tuberculosis is complete, but antiretroviral therapy, once started, should not be interrupted.[50] Alternatively, a regimen that does not contain a rifamycin may be used, although it is recommended that such regimens should continue for at least 9 months.[51] In addition, they typically include streptomycin and thus commit the patient to regular injections for 9 months which may jeopardize compliance. The non-rifamycin regimen recommended by the CDC consists of an initial phase of isoniazid, ethambutol, streptomycin, and pyrazinamide daily or daily then intermittently for 2 months, and a continuation phase of isoniazid, streptomycin, and pyrazinamide administered 2 or 3 times weekly for 7 months.

CDC recommends that the duration of therapy (regardless of the regimen used) should be increased by a further 3 months in patients with a delayed response to treatment during the primary phase.[50]

Drug-resistant tuberculosis is a problem,[52,53] with up to 90% of cases of drug-resistant disease in the USA occurring in HIV-infected persons:[52] regimens must be modified as in non-HIV-infected patients. Multiple drug-resistant tuberculosis can be rapidly fatal in patients with HIV infection and early, effective treatment is essential, and should continue for 18-24 months after smears become negative.[54]

Prolonged or lifetime prophylaxis with isoniazid has been given to patients with HIV infection following the completion of tuberculosis treatment in the UK,[55] and has been shown to reduce the rate of recurrence in other countries.[56] Preventive therapy is also used in some countries to prevent first episodes of active disease (see below).

ADJUNCTIVE THERAPY. Injection of suspensions of killed *Mycobacterium vaccae* has been shown to improve immune responsiveness in patients with pulmonary tuberculosis,[57-59] but not all studies have shown beneficial responses.[60] Several other forms of **immunotherapy** have also been tried as adjuncts to conventional chemotherapy.[61-64]

The use of **corticosteroids** in uncomplicated pulmonary tuberculosis should be avoided but they have a role in selected patients with severe pulmonary and severe extrapulmonary disease, and for patients with severe hypersensitivity reactions to antituberculous drugs.[18,65,66] They should never be given to patients with active disease without protective chemotherapy cover and they must be used with caution in patients with dormant disease in whom they may reactivate disease. For further details on the possible role of corticosteroids as an adjunct to antituberculous therapy, see p.1060.

Interferons have also been tried (see p.634).

Preventive therapy or chemoprophylaxis is intended to prevent the occurrence of acute tuberculosis in patients with asymptomatic tuberculous infection (that is, those with a positive tuberculin skin test but no evidence of active disease), and in susceptible contacts, and to curb its spread through the community.

Chemoprophylaxis is not recommended routinely in developing countries and the primary objective as elsewhere should be to treat active tuberculosis.[18] Chemoprophylaxis is more widely used in the USA than in the UK and other countries where vaccination with BCG vaccine (p.1534) is routinely employed.

The American Thoracic Society and the Centers for Disease Control[67] have issued detailed recommendations for chemoprophylaxis (treatment of latent tuberculosis infection). Administration of isoniazid for 9 months is the preferred regimen although treatment for 6 months may be adequate. Rifampicin, alone or in combination with pyrazinamide, is an alternative, but reports of severe and fatal liver damage associated with rifampicin and pyrazinamide administration have led to revised recommendations for the use of this combination.[68] Prophylaxis is generally recommended for patients at high risk of developing tuberculosis and who exhibit a positive tuberculin skin test, including:

• Household members and other close associates of newly diagnosed potentially infectious tuberculosis patients.

• Persons with an abnormal chest X-ray consistent with prior tuberculosis.

• Recent immigrants from countries with a high prevalence of tuberculosis.

• Patients in special clinical situations such as those with diabetes mellitus, lymphomas, leukaemia, carcinoma of the head or neck and lung, end-stage renal failure, or those receiving prolonged corticosteroid or immunosuppressive therapy, or intravenous drug abusers, or those with substantial rapid weight loss or chronic undernutrition.

In addition, chemoprophylaxis may be offered to persons with negative skin tests in certain high-risk situations.

Prophylaxis is also recommended for persons infected with HIV who react positively to tuberculin but have no evidence of disease. HIV-positive patients should not receive BCG vaccine because of the risk of disseminated infection.[69]

For reference to prophylaxis in pregnant women and the neonate, see above.

The British Thoracic Society's Joint Tuberculosis Committee advises that chemoprophylaxis may be given to some contacts with strongly positive tuberculin Heaf test reactions, but without clinical or radiological evidence of tuberculous disease.[37] They recommend that chemoprophylaxis should be given to contacts under 16 years old who have not had BCG vaccination and have positive tuberculin reactions and should be considered in children who have received BCG vaccination and who have a strongly positive tuberculin reaction. Also, children under 2 years old who are close contacts of cases with positive sputum smears and who have not had BCG vaccination should be given chemoprophylaxis whatever their tuberculin status.[21,37] Chemoprophylaxis is also recommended for patients in whom recent tuberculin conversion has been documented.[37]

The resurgence of tuberculosis has increased the risk of nosocomial infection in patients and health care workers and has prompted guidance on preventing its transmission in health care settings.[37,70] Guidance is also given on the management of bovine tuberculosis, and the risks of tuberculosis transmission during air travel and in schools.[37,71]

HIV INFECTION. Since HIV infection increases both the individual's susceptibility to primary infection with *M. tuberculosis* and to progression to active tuberculosis in individuals with existing *M. tuberculosis* infection, effective tuberculosis control is particularly important in this population. BCG immunisation is not recommended in individuals with HIV infection since there is a risk of disseminated infection. Chemoprophylaxis has been shown to reduce the incidence of tuberculosis when given to persons with HIV infection, particularly in those with a positive tuberculin reaction.[72] Current practice is to give chemoprophylaxis to individuals identified as being at greatest risk of tuberculosis, including close contacts of patients with infectious disease. In 1994, IUAT and WHO[73] supported prophylaxis with isoniazid for 6 to 12 months in HIV-infected individuals with a positive tuberculin test, once active tuberculosis had been excluded. Further research was necessary before, for example, the merits of life-long or extended preventive therapy in areas of high tuberculosis transmission or the role of prophylaxis in anergic individuals could be assessed. In the USA, chemoprophylaxis is also offered to HIV-infected persons who are considered to be at high risk of contracting the infection regardless of tuberculin test results.[50] Chemoprophylaxis with rifampicin or rifabutin with pyrazinamide for 2 months has also been used,[50,74,75] although, as mentioned above, rifamycins may interact with antiretroviral drugs.

In developing countries with a high prevalence of tuberculosis, the difficulties in providing preventive chemotherapy to all HIV-infected individuals at risk may be overwhelming.[76] WHO has suggested that preventive chemotherapy may be restricted to selected at-risk groups such as health-care workers and selected individuals.[18]

Inactivated *Mycobacterium vaccae* is under investigation.[77]

1. Bellin E. Failure of tuberculosis control: a prescription for change. *JAMA* 1994; **271**: 708–9.
2. Bloch AB, *et al.* Nationwide survey of drug-resistant tuberculosis in the United States. *JAMA* 1994; **271**: 665–71.
3. Weis SE, *et al.* The effect of directly observed therapy on the rates of drug resistance and relapse in tuberculosis. *N Engl J Med* 1994; **330**: 1179–84.
4. Wilkinson D. High-compliance tuberculosis treatment programme in a rural community. *Lancet* 1994; **343**: 647–8.
5. Bayer R, Wilkinson D. Directly observed therapy for tuberculosis: history of an idea. *Lancet* 1995; **345**: 1545–8. Correction. *ibid.*; **346**: 322.
6. China Tuberculosis Control Collaboration. Results of directly observed-therapy in 112 842 Chinese patients with smear-positive tuberculosis. *Lancet* 1996; **347**: 358–62.
7. Chaulk CP, *et al.* Directly observed therapy for treatment completion of pulmonary tuberculosis: consensus statement of the Public Health Tuberculosis Guidelines Panel. *JAMA* 1998; **279**: 943–8. Correction. *ibid.*; **280**: 134.
8. Zwarenstein M, *et al.* Randomised controlled trial of self-supervised and directly observed treatment of tuberculosis. *Lancet* 1998; **352**: 1340–3.
9. Moulding T, *et al.* Fixed-dose combinations of antituberculosis medications to prevent drug resistance. *Ann Intern Med* 1995; **122**: 951–4.
10. Blomberg B, *et al.* The rationale for recommending fixed-dose combination tablets for treatment of tuberculosis. *Bull WHO* 2001; **79**: 61–8.
11. Gangadharam PRJ, *et al.* Experimental chemotherapy of tuberculosis using single dose treatment with isoniazid in biodegradable polymers. *J Antimicrob Chemother* 1994; **33**: 265–71.
12. Frieden TR, *et al.* Tuberculosis in New York City—turning the tide. *N Engl J Med* 1995; **333**: 229–33.
13. Raviglione MC, *et al.* Assessment of worldwide tuberculosis control. *Lancet* 1997; **350**: 624–9.
14. Nunn P. Thiacetazone should not be used routinely—or primum non nocere. *Tubercle Lung Dis* 1995; **76** (suppl 2): 3.
15. Elliott AM, Foster SD. Thiacetazone: time to call a halt? *Tubercle Lung Dis* 1996; **77**: 27–9.
16. Rieder HL. Controversies in tuberculosis control: thioacetazone may be used routinely—pro. *Tubercle Lung Dis* 1995; **76** (suppl 2): 3.
17. van Gorkom J, Kibuga DK. Cost-effectiveness and total costs of three alternative strategies for the prevention and management of severe skin reactions attributable to thiacetazone in the treatment of human immunodeficiency virus positive patients with tuberculosis in Kenya. *Tubercle Lung Dis* 1996; **77**: 30–6.
18. WHO. *TB/HIV: A clinical manual.* Geneva: WHO, 1996.
19. WHO. *Treatment of tuberculosis: guidelines for national programmes.* Geneva: WHO, 1997.
20. Task Force of ERS, WHO and the Europe Region of IUATLD. Tuberculosis management in Europe: recommendations of a task force of the European Respiratory Society (ERS), the World Health Organisation (WHO) and the International Union Against Tuberculosis and Lung Disease (IUATLD) Europe region. *Eur Respir J* 1999; **14**: 978–92.
21. Joint Tuberculosis Committee of the British Thoracic Society. Chemotherapy and management of tuberculosis in the United Kingdom: recommendations 1998. *Thorax* 1998; **53**: 536–48.
22. Centers for Disease Control. Initial therapy for tuberculosis in the era of multidrug resistance: recommendations of the Advisory Council for the Elimination of Tuberculosis. *MMWR* 1993; **42**: 1–8.
23. American Thoracic Society and the Centers for Disease Control. Treatment of tuberculosis and tuberculosis infection in adults and children. *Am J Respir Crit Care Med* 1994; **149**: 1359–74.
24. Ormerod LP, *et al.* Hepatotoxicity of antituberculosis drugs. *Thorax* 1996; **51**: 111–13.
25. Iseman MD. Treatment of multidrug-resistant tuberculosis. *N Engl J Med* 1993; **329**: 784–91.
26. Pablos-Mendez A, *et al.* Global surveillance for antituberculosis-drug resistance, 1994-1997. *N Engl J Med* 1998; **338**: 1641–9. Correction. *ibid.*; **339**: 139.
27. Espinal MA, *et al.* Global trends in resistance to antituberculosis drugs. *N Engl J Med* 2001; **344**: 1294–1303.
28. Nunn P, Felten M. Surveillance of resistance to antituberculosis drugs in developing countries. *Tubercle Lung Dis* 1994; **75**: 163–7.
29. Bennett DE, *et al.* Drug resistant tuberculosis in England and Wales, 1993-1995. *Thorax* 1996; **51** (suppl 3): A8.
30. Irish C, *et al.* Database study of antibiotic resistant tuberculosis in the United Kingdom, 1994-6. *BMJ* 1999; **318**: 497–8.
31. Anonymous. Outbreak of hospital acquired multidrug resistant tuberculosis. *Commun Dis Rep* 1995; **5**: 161.
32. Farmer P, Kim JY. Community based approaches to the control of multidrug resistant tuberculosis: introducing "DOTS-plus". *BMJ* 1998; **317**: 671–4.
33. WHO. *Guidelines for the management of drug-resistant tuberculosis.* Geneva: WHO, 1997.
34. Sullivan EA, *et al.* Emergence of fluoroquinolone-resistant tuberculosis in New York City. *Lancet* 1995; **345**: 1148–50.
35. Trébucq A. Should ethambutol be recommended for routine treatment of tuberculosis in children? A review of the literature. *Int J Tuberc Lung Dis* 1997; **1**: 12–15.
36. Davidson PT. Managing tuberculosis during pregnancy. *Lancet* 1995; **346**: 199–200.
37. Joint Tuberculosis Committee of the British Thoracic Society. Control and prevention of tuberculosis in the United Kingdom: code of practice 2000. *Thorax* 2000; **55**: 887–901.
38. Havlir DV, Barnes PF. Tuberculosis in patients with human immunodeficiency virus infection. *N Engl J Med* 1999; **340**: 367–73.
39. Small PM, *et al.* Treatment of tuberculosis in patients with advanced human immunodeficiency virus infection. *N Engl J Med* 1991; **324**: 289–94.
40. Sterling TR, *et al.* Relapse rates after short-course (6-month) treatment of tuberculosis in HIV-infected and uninfected persons. *AIDS* 1999; **13**: 1899–1904.
41. Peloquin CA, *et al.* Low antituberculosis drug concentrations in patients with AIDS. *Ann Pharmacother* 1996; **30**: 919–25.
42. Peloquin CA, *et al.* Malabsorption of antimycobacterial medications. *N Engl J Med* 1993; **329**: 1122–3.
43. Sahai J, *et al.* Reduced plasma concentrations of antituberculosis drugs in patients with HIV infection. *Ann Intern Med* 1997; **127**: 289–93.
44. Choudhri SH, *et al.* Pharmacokinetics of antimycobacterial drugs in patients with tuberculosis, AIDS, and diarrhea. *Clin Infect Dis* 1997; **25**: 104–11.
45. Patel KB, *et al.* Drug malabsorption and resistant tuberculosis in HIV-infected patients. *N Engl J Med* 1995; **332**: 336–7.
46. Narita M, *et al.* Paradoxical worsening of tuberculosis following antiretroviral therapy in patients with AIDS. *Am J Respir Crit Care Med* 1998; **158**: 157–61.
47. Nunn P, *et al.* Cutaneous hypersensitivity reactions due to thiacetazone in HIV-1 seropositive patients treated for tuberculosis. *Lancet* 1991; **337**: 627–30.
48. De Cock KM, Wilkinson D. Tuberculosis control in resource-poor countries: alternative approaches in the era of HIV. *Lancet* 1995; **346**: 675–7.
49. Burman WJ, *et al.* Therapeutic implications of drug interactions in the treatment of human immunodeficiency virus-related tuberculosis. *Clin Infect Dis* 1999; **28**: 419–30.
50. Centers for Disease Control. Prevention and treatment of tuberculosis among patients infected with human immunodeficiency virus: principles of therapy and revised recommendations. *MMWR* 1998; **47** (RR-20): 1–51. Appendix—recommended treatment options for persons with human immunodeficiency virus-related tuberculosis infection and disease. *ibid.*: 53–8.
51. Schluger NW. Issues in the treatment of active tuberculosis in human immunodeficiency virus-infected patients. *Clin Infect Dis* 1999; **28**: 130–5.
52. Snider DE, Roper WL. The new tuberculosis. *N Engl J Med* 1992; **326**: 703–5.
53. Edlin BR, *et al.* An outbreak of multidrug-resistant tuberculosis among hospitalized patients with the acquired immunodeficiency syndrome. *N Engl J Med* 1992; **326**: 1514–21.
54. Drobniewski F. Is death inevitable with multiresistant TB plus HIV infection? *Lancet* 1997; **349**: 71–2.
55. Subcommittee of the Joint Tuberculosis Committee of the British Thoracic Society. Guidelines on the management of tuberculosis and HIV infection in the United Kingdom. *BMJ* 1992; **304**: 1231–3.
56. Fitzgerald DW, *et al.* Effect of post-treatment isoniazid on prevention of recurrent tuberculosis in HIV-1-infected individuals: a randomised trial. *Lancet* 2000; **356**: 1470–4.
57. Bahr GM, *et al.* Improved immunotherapy for pulmonary tuberculosis with Mycobacterium vaccae. *Tubercle* 1990; **71**: 259–66.
58. Corlan E, *et al.* Immunotherapy with Mycobacterium vaccae in the treatment of tuberculosis in Romania: 1, newly-diagnosed pulmonary disease. *Respir Med* 1997; **91**: 13–19.
59. Corlan E, *et al.* Immunotherapy with Mycobacterium vaccae in the treatment of tuberculosis in Romania: 2, chronic or relapsed disease. *Respir Med* 1997; **91**: 21–9.
60. Durban Immunotherapy Trial Group. Immunotherapy with Mycobacterium vaccae in patients with newly diagnosed pulmonary tuberculosis: a randomised controlled trial. *Lancet* 1999; **354**: 116–19.
61. Etemadi A, *et al.* Immunotherapy for drug-resistant tuberculosis. *Lancet* 1992; **340**: 1360–1.
62. Stanford JL, Grange JM. New concepts for the control of tuberculosis in the twenty first century. *J R Coll Physicians Lond* 1993; **27**: 218–23.
63. Prior JG, *et al.* Immunotherapy with Mycobacterium vaccae combined with second line chemotherapy in drug-resistant abdominal tuberculosis. *J Infect* 1995; **31**: 59–61.
64. Rook GAW, *et al.* Protection and immunopathology in tuberculosis: the role of immunotherapy. *J Pharm Pharmacol* 1997; **49** (suppl 1): 47–51.
65. Horne NW, ed. *Modern drug treatment of tuberculosis.* 7th ed. London: The Chest, Heart and Stroke Association, 1990.
66. Alzeer AH, FitzGerald JM. Corticosteroids and tuberculosis: risks and use as adjunct therapy. *Tubercle Lung Dis* 1993; **74**: 6–11.
67. American Thoracic Society and the Centers for Disease Control. Targeted tuberculin testing and treatment of latent tuberculosis infection. *Am J Respir Crit Care Med* 2000; **161** (suppl): S221–S247.
68. Centers for Disease Control. Update: fatal and severe liver injuries associated with rifampin and pyrazinamide for latent tuberculosis infection, and revisions in American Thoracic Society/CDC recommendations—United States, 2001. *MMWR* 2001; **50**: 733–5.
69. Centers for Disease Control. 1999 USPHS/IDSA guidelines for the prevention of opportunistic infections in persons infected with human immunodeficiency virus. *MMWR* 1999; **48** (RR-10): 1–59.
70. ACOEM. ACOEM guidelines for protecting health care workers against tuberculosis. *J Occup Environ Med* 1998; **40**: 765–7.
71. WHO. *International travel and health: vaccination requirements and health advice.* Geneva: WHO, 2001.
72. Wilkinson D, *et al.* Effect of preventive treatment for tuberculosis in adults infected with HIV: systematic review of randomised placebo controlled trials. *BMJ* 1998; **317**: 625–9.
73. International Union Against Tuberculosis and Lung Disease (IUATLD) and the Global Programme on AIDS and the Tuberculosis Programme of the World Health Organization (WHO). Tuberculosis preventive therapy in HIV-infected individuals: a joint statement. *Tubercle Lung Dis* 1994; **75**: 96–8.
74. Halsey NA, *et al.* Randomised trial of isoniazid versus rifampicin and pyrazinamide for prevention of tuberculosis in HIV-1 infection. *Lancet* 1998; **351**: 786–92.
75. Rose DN. Short-course prophylaxis against tuberculosis in HIV-infected persons. *Ann Intern Med* 1998; **129**: 779–86.
76. De Cock KM, *et al.* Preventive therapy for tuberculosis in HIV-infected persons: international recommendations, research, and practice. *Lancet* 1995; **345**: 833–6.
77. Fordham von Reyn C, *et al.* Cellular immune responses to mycobacteria in healthy and human immunodeficiency virus-positive subjects in the United States after a five-dose schedule of Mycobacterium vaccae vaccine. *Clin Infect Dis* 1998; **27**: 1517–20.

Tularaemia

Tularaemia is caused by the Gram-negative bacillus *Francisella tularensis* which primarily affects rodents and rabbits but may be transmitted to man, usually by handling infected animals or carcasses, or by the bites of insect vectors. It may take several forms, the most common of which is the ulceroglandular form, characterised by rash and ulceration at the site of inoculation accompanied by fever and lymphadenopathy; other forms include the typhoidal and pneumonic forms, which have a higher mortality rate.

Streptomycin is considered the antibacterial of choice in severe disease,[1,2] although gentamicin may be an alternative in patients who cannot tolerate streptomycin.[2] Tetracycline or chloramphenicol may be given by mouth; clinical relapses are more frequent than with the aminoglycosides,[2,3] although relapsed disease will respond to a further course. Some patients have also responded to high-dose intravenous erythromycin.[4]

Streptomycin is difficult to obtain in the USA but a review[5] of alternative drugs for the treatment of tularaemia concluded that:

- gentamicin is an acceptable alternative to streptomycin and should be considered the alternative antibacterial of choice for serious cases of nonmeningitic tularaemia
- tetracycline might be a reasonable alternative to gentamicin and could be given by mouth in less severely ill patients, but there is a relatively high relapse rate with tetracycline
- chloramphenicol should be considered when tularaemic meningitis is suspected—like tetracycline it is associated with a relatively high relapse rate, but has the advantage over both aminoglycosides and tetracycline of good penetration of the CNS
- imipenem-cilastatin (1 case) and the fluoroquinolones ciprofloxacin and norfloxacin (6 cases) have shown promise, but further studies are needed before they can be recommended.

A tularaemia vaccine is available in some countries for active immunisation against the disease.

1. Corwin WC, Stubbs SP. Further studies on tularemia in the Ozarks: review of forty-four cases during a three-year period. *JAMA* 1952; **149**: 343–5.
2. Evans ME, *et al.* Tularemia: a 30-year experience with 88 cases. *Medicine (Baltimore)* 1985; **64**: 251–69.
3. Ford-Jones L, *et al.* "Muskrat fever": two outbreaks of tularemia near Montreal. *Can Med Assoc J* 1982; **127**: 298–9.
4. Westerman EL, McDonald J. Tularemia pneumonia mimicking Legionnaires' disease: isolation of organism on CYE agar and successful treatment with erythromycin. *South Med J* 1983; **76**: 1169–70.
5. Enderlin G, *et al.* Streptomycin and alternative agents for the treatment of tularemia: review of the literature. *Clin Infect Dis* 1994; **19**: 42–7.

Typhoid and paratyphoid fever

Typhoid and paratyphoid fever are systemic infections caused respectively by *Salmonella typhi* and *S. paratyphi* A, B, or C, Gram-negative bacteria belonging to the Enterobacteriaceae family. They are sometimes termed collectively 'enteric fever' but, although infection follows invasion of the intestinal mucosa and re-infection of the intestines subsequently occurs, dissemination in the blood leads to more widespread systemic effects. Typhoid and paratyphoid are endemic in many countries and, in most, typhoid is more common. In the UK most cases are contracted abroad; in the period 1981-90 the majority of those in England and Wales with typhoid and paratyphoid A fever had been infected in the Indian subcontinent whereas the majority of paratyphoid B fever had been acquired in Mediterranean and Middle East countries.[1]

Treatment of typhoid fever has generally been with chloramphenicol or alternatively amoxicillin, ampicillin, or co-trimoxazole. However, there has been a spread of strains of *S. typhi* resistant to chloramphenicol, ampicillin, amoxicillin, trimethoprim, and co-trimoxazole,[2] especially in the Indian subcontinent, in the Middle East, and possibly in South and South-East Asia. Fluoroquinolones such as ciprofloxacin or third-generation cephalosporins such as cefotaxime, ceftriaxone, and cefoperazone are effective for typhoid fever due to multiresistant strains. Fluoroquinolones have been the preferred alternative to chloramphenicol for patients returning to the UK from the Indian subcontinent or other regions where multidrug-resistant strains are endemic[3,4] However, the increasing incidence of ciprofloxacin resistance in multiresistant *S. typhi* has been noted, mainly in cases originating in the Indian subcontinent,[5,6] and strains with decreased susceptibility to fluoroquinolones may now be endemic in this region.[7] Ciprofloxacin-resistant strains isolated in the UK have generally retained their sensitivity to cephalosporins.[7] Other alternative antimicrobials under investigation include the oral cephalosporin cefixime[8] and azithromycin.[9,10]

Fluoroquinolones are generally contra-indicated in children and in pregnant women because of potential toxicity, but there is evidence of the successful use of ciprofloxacin or ofloxacin in multiresistant infection in children.[11-13] Similarly, ciprofloxacin was effective in the second and third trimester of pregnancy[14,15] and some have suggested that it could be used in pregnancy if the organism was resistant to amoxicillin or ampicillin.[14]

On recovery, typhoid patients may continue to excrete *S. typhi* in the faeces or urine for several weeks. Unlike these convalescent carriers, chronic carriers may excrete *S. typhi* for years without any symptoms; eradication is difficult and prolonged treatment is necessary. An increased risk of biliary-tract and bile-related cancers has been associated with chronic carriage of *S. typhi*, and the importance of eradication has been emphasised.[16]

Typhoid vaccines are used for the prevention of typhoid fever.

Paratyphoid fever is less common and generally milder than typhoid fever. Treatment is similar.

1. Anonymous. Enteric fever England and Wales 1981-90. *Commun Dis Rep* 1991; **1**: 72.
2. Rowe B, *et al.* Multidrug-resistant Salmonella typhi: a worldwide epidemic. *Clin Infect Dis* 1997; **24** (suppl 1): S106–S109.
3. Rowe B, *et al.* Spread of multiresistant Salmonella typhi. *Lancet* 1990; **336**: 1065.
4. Rowe B, *et al.* Treatment of multiresistant typhoid fever. *Lancet* 1991; **337**: 1422.
5. Rowe B, *et al.* Ciprofloxacin-resistant Salmonella typhi in the UK. *Lancet* 1995; **346**: 1302.
6. Mitchell DH. Ciprofloxacin-resistant Salmonella typhi: an emerging problem. *Med J Aust* 1997; **167**: 172.
7. Threlfall EJ, *et al.* Ciprofloxacin-resistant Salmonella typhi and treatment failure. *Lancet* 1999; **353**: 1590–1.
8. Memon IA, *et al.* Cefixime: an oral option for the treatment of multidrug-resistant enteric fever in children. *South Med J* 1997; **90**: 1204–7.
9. Girgis NI, *et al.* Azithromycin versus ciprofloxacin for treatment of uncomplicated typhoid fever in a randomized trial in Egypt that included patients with multidrug resistance. *Antimicrob Agents Chemother* 1999; **43**: 1441–4.
10. Butler T, *et al.* Treatment of typhoid fever with azithromycin versus chloramphenicol in a randomized multicentre trial in India. *J Antimicrob Chemother* 1999; **44**: 243–50.
11. Cheesbrough JS, *et al.* Quinolones in children with invasive salmonellosis. *Lancet* 1991; **338**: 127.
12. Dutta P, *et al.* Ciprofloxacin for treatment of severe typhoid fever in children. *Antimicrob Agents Chemother* 1993; **37**: 1197–9.
13. Vinh H, *et al.* Two or three days of ofloxacin treatment for uncomplicated multidrug-resistant typhoid fever in children. *Antimicrob Agents Chemother* 1996; **40**: 958–61.
14. Leung D, *et al.* Treatment of typhoid in pregnancy. *Lancet* 1995; **346**: 648.
15. Koul PA, *et al.* Ciprofloxacin for multiresistant enteric fever in pregnancy. *Lancet* 1995; **346**: 307–8.
16. Caygill CPJ, *et al.* Cancer mortality in chronic typhoid and paratyphoid carriers. *Lancet* 1994; **343**: 83–4.

Typhus

Rickettsial infections or fevers of the typhus group are transmitted to man by various insect vectors. Louseborne or epidemic typhus, due to *Rickettsia prowazekii*, and flea-borne or murine typhus, due to the closely related *R. typhi* (formerly called *R. mooseri*), have occurred worldwide. Scrub typhus is due to *Orientia tsutsugamushi* (formerly *R. tsutsugamushi*) transmitted by mites and occurs mainly in Asia, Australia, and the Pacific Islands.

Tetracycline, often doxycycline, or chloramphenicol is the treatment of choice for these infections although strains of *O. tsutsugamushi* resistant to doxycycline and chloramphenicol have been reported in Thailand.[1,2] There is some evidence that ciprofloxacin may prove effective,[3] and rifampicin has been shown to be more effective against scrub typhus than doxycycline.[4] Prophylaxis for scrub typhus with doxycycline has shown promise when started before exposure to infection.[5] Typhus vaccines are available for active immunisation against louseborne typhus.

1. Watt G, *et al.* Scrub typhus infections poorly responsive to antibiotics in northern Thailand. *Lancet* 1996; **348**: 86–9.
2. Panpanich R, Garner P. Antibiotics for treating scrub typhus (updated 24 February 2001). Available in The Cochrane Library; Issue 2. Oxford: Update Software; 2001.
3. Eaton M, *et al.* Ciprofloxacin treatment of typhus. *JAMA* 1989; **262**: 772–3.
4. Watt G, *et al.* Doxycycline and rifampicin for mild scrub-typhus infections in northern Thailand: a randomised trial. *Lancet* 2000; **356**: 1057–61.
5. Twartz JC, *et al.* Doxycycline prophylaxis for human scrub typhus. *J Infect Dis* 1982; **146**: 811–18.

Urethritis

Infective urethritis is a sexually transmitted disease seen most frequently in men. One of the commonest causes is *Neisseria gonorrhoeae*. Nongonococcal urethritis or non-specific urethritis may be due to *Chlamydia trachomatis* in up to 50% of cases and *Ureaplasma urealyticum* (formerly T-strain mycoplasma) in up to 40%, but often the cause is unknown. Other organisms implicated have included *Mycoplasma genitalium*. Gonococcal and chlamydial infections frequently occur together and, since specific therapy for gonorrhoea is often not effective against *C. trachomatis*, treatment for the two infections should be given concomitantly otherwise postgonococcal urethritis due to *C. trachomatis* may follow the cure of gonorrhoea. The treatment of chlamydial urethritis is discussed under Chlamydial Infections (above) and that for gonococcal urethritis under Gonorrhoea (above).

For nongonococcal urethritis the UK guidelines[1] recommend a single 1-g dose of azithromycin by mouth or a 7-day course of doxycycline 100 mg twice daily. Alternative regimens are erythromycin 500 mg four times daily for 7 days or twice daily for 14 days, or a compound preparation of tetracycline, chlortetracycline, and demeclocycline (Detclo) twice daily for 7 days, or ofloxacin 400 mg daily in one single or two divided doses for 7 days, or tetracycline 500 mg four times daily for 7 days. In the USA,[2] the recommended first-choice therapy is the same as that in the UK. Alternative regimens listed in the USA are erythromycin 500 mg four times daily or ofloxacin 300 mg twice daily, in each case for 7 days.[2] Persistent or recurrent nongonococcal urethritis should be treated with a single oral 2-g dose of metronidazole plus oral erythromycin 500 mg four times daily for 7 days.[2]

1. Clinical Effectiveness Group (Association of Genitourinary Medicine and the Medical Society for the Study of Venereal Diseases). National guideline for the management of non-gonococcal urethritis. *Sex Transm Infect* 1999; **75** (suppl 1): S9–S12.
2. Centers for Disease Control. 1998 Guidelines for treatment of sexually transmitted diseases. *MMWR* 1998; **47** (RR-1): 49–52.

Urinary-tract infections

Infections of the urinary tract are especially common in women. They are frequently due to enteric bacteria, in particular *Escherichia coli*, although a common cause in young women is *Staphylococcus saprophyticus*, a coagulase-negative staphylococcus. Other urinary pathogens include *Staph. epidermidis*, enterococci, and *Pseudomonas* spp. An arbitrary definition of urinary-tract infection has been significant bacteriuria with 10^5 or more colony forming units per mL of a midstream urine specimen; some also consider lower counts to be indicative of infection. Most urinary-tract infections are isolated uncomplicated infections of the lower urinary tract. Recurrent infections may be due to relapse, or more often, re-infection, and are more serious. Patients with complicated urinary-tract infections associated with urinary-tract abnormalities or diseases such as diabetes mellitus may be at risk of kidney damage.

Infections of the lower urinary tract in *women* generally present as cystitis (inflammation of the bladder) and symptoms include dysuria, frequency, and urgency together with pyuria and significant bacteriuria; the urethral syndrome is similar, but there is no significant bacteriuria. In the upper urinary tract, acute pyelonephritis may occur as a complication of cystitis or, more rarely, may result from septicaemia. Asymptomatic bacteriuria may progress to acute pyelonephritis in *pregnant women* and should therefore be treated.

Urinary-tract infections in *men* are less common and are often associated with abnormalities of the genito-urinary tract such as prostatic hyperplasia. Acute bacterial prostatitis is usually caused by organisms similar to those responsible for cystitis in women. Chronic bacterial prostatitis is difficult to treat; the antibacterials used must be able to penetrate into the prostatic fluid. For other genito-urinary infections in men, see under Epididymitis and under Urethritis, above.

In preschool *children*, especially girls, asymptomatic bacteriuria together with vesicoureteric reflux can result in renal scarring and should be treated; the use of prophylactic antibacterials is complex and controversial. Long-term follow-up of girls who have had asymptomatic bacteriuria suggests that new kidney damage does not occur after 4 years of age, but highlights the importance of diagnosis and treatment in younger children.

The significance of asymptomatic bacteriuria in *old age* is disputed, but most consider treatment to be unnecessary.

Infections associated with *indwelling bladder catheters* occur in both men and women and probably account for the majority of hospital-acquired urinary-tract infections.

Treatment. Antibacterials used to treat urinary-tract infections need to be excreted in adequate concentrations in the urine. For *acute uncomplicated infections* oral amoxicillin, ampicillin, co-trimoxazole, nalidixic acid, nitrofurantoin, or trimethoprim (preferred to co-trimoxazole in the UK) have been given although the choice will depend on local patterns of bacterial resistance; *E. coli* resistant to ampicillin and amoxicillin is widespread. Alternatives when resistance is prevalent include amoxicillin with clavulanic acid, oral cephalosporins, fluoroquinolones such as ciprofloxacin or fosfomycin. In pregnant women, nitrofurantoin or a beta lactam can be used. Standard treatment schedules have been for 5 to 7 days; 3-day or single-dose regimens can also be effective and may be preferred in women. Urinary alkalinising agents such as potassium citrate and sodium citrate have been given by mouth to relieve the pain of cystitis caused by lower urinary-tract infections. Recurrent infections may require long-term low-dose antibacterial prophylaxis.

Acute pyelonephritis may require broad-spectrum parenteral treatment initially with, for example, aztreonam, ceftazidime, cefuroxime, ciprofloxacin, or gentamicin.

Chronic bacterial prostatitis may require treatment for several weeks with trimethoprim, erythromycin, or a fluoroquinolone.

Catheter-related bladder infections may sometimes respond to localised treatment with bladder washouts containing chlorhexidine.

References.
1. Brumfitt W. Progress in understanding urinary infections. *J Antimicrob Chemother* 1991; **27**: 9–22.
2. Wilkie ME, *et al.* Diagnosis and management of urinary tract infection in adults. *BMJ* 1992; **305**: 1137–41.
3. Stamm WE, Hooton TM. Management of urinary tract infections in adults. *N Engl J Med* 1993; **329**: 1328–34.
4. Grüneberg RN. Changes in urinary pathogens and their antibiotic sensitivities, 1971–1992. *J Antimicrob Chemother* 1994; **33** (suppl A): 1–8.
5. Thomson KS, *et al.* USA resistance patterns among UTI pathogens. *J Antimicrob Chemother* 1994; **33** (suppl A): 9–15.
6. Kunin CM. Chemoprophylaxis and suppressive therapy in the management of urinary tract infections. *J Antimicrob Chemother* 1994; **33** (suppl A): 51–62.
7. Reeves DS. A perspective on the safety of antibacterials used to treat urinary tract infections. *J Antimicrob Chemother* 1994; **33** (suppl A): 111–20.
8. Brumfitt W, Hamilton-Miller JMT. Consensus viewpoint on management of urinary infections. *J Antimicrob Chemother* 1994; **33** (suppl A): 147–53.
9. Maskell R. Management of recurrent urinary tract infections in adults. *Prescribers' J* 1995; **35**: 1–11.
10. Ronald A, Sanche SE. Antimicrobial management of urinary tract infections. *Curr Opin Infect Dis* 1995; **8**: 420–3.
11. Nicolle LE. A practical guide to the management of complicated urinary tract infection. *Drugs* 1997; **53**: 583–92.
12. Preston SL, *et al.* Empiric treatment of uncomplicated urinary tract infections. *Ann Pharmacother* 1998; **32**: 1231–3.

CATHETER-RELATED. References.
1. Anonymous. Catheter-acquired urinary tract infection. *Lancet* 1991; **338**: 857–8.
2. Harding GKM, *et al.* How long should catheter-acquired urinary tract infection in women be treated: a randomized controlled study. *Ann Intern Med* 1991; **114**: 713–19.
3. van der Wall E, *et al.* Prophylactic ciprofloxacin for catheter-associated urinary-tract infection. *Lancet* 1992; **339**: 946–51.

THE ELDERLY. References.
1. Morgan MG, *et al.* Treatment of urinary infection in the elderly. *Infection* 1990; **18**: 326–31.
2. Abrutyn E, *et al.* Does asymptomatic bacteriuria predict mortality and does antimicrobial treatment reduce mortality in elderly ambulatory women? *Ann Intern Med* 1994; **120**: 827–33. Correction. *ibid.*; **121**: 901.
3. Nicolle LE. Urinary tract infection in the elderly. *J Antimicrob Chemother* 1994; **33** (suppl A): 99–109.
4. Ouslander JG, *et al.* Does eradicating bacteriuria affect the severity of chronic urinary incontinence in nursing home residents? *Ann Intern Med* 1995; **122**: 749–54.
5. Abrutyn E, *et al.* Does treatment of asymptomatic bacteriuria in older ambulatory women reduce subsequent symptoms of urinary tract infection? *J Am Geriatr Soc* 1996; **44**: 293–5.

INFANTS AND CHILDREN. References.
1. Verrier Jones K. Antimicrobial treatment for urinary tract infections. *Arch Dis Child* 1990; **65**: 327–30.
2. White RHR. Management of urinary tract infection and vesicoureteric reflux in children: 1. *BMJ* 1990; **300**: 1391–2.
3. Working Group of the Research Unit, Royal College of Physicians. Guidelines for the management of acute urinary tract infection in childhood. *J R Coll Physicians Lond* 1991; **25**: 36–42.
4. Smellie JM, *et al.* Retrospective study of children with renal scarring associated with reflux and urinary infection. *BMJ* 1994; **308**: 1193–6.
5. Ansari BM, *et al.* Urinary tract infection in children: part 1: epidemiology, natural history, diagnosis and management. *J Infect* 1995; **30**: 3–6.
6. Watson AR. Urinary tract infection in early childhood. *J Antimicrob Chemother* 1994; **34** (suppl A): 53–60. Correction. *ibid.* 1995; **35**: 561.
7. Gordon I. Vesico-ureteric reflux, urinary-tract infection, and renal damage in children. *Lancet* 1995; **346**: 489–90.
8. Anonymous. The management of urinary tract infection in children. *Drug Ther Bull* 1997; **35**: 65–9.
9. American Academy of Pediatrics Committee on Quality Improvement, Subcommittee on Urinary Tract Infection. Practice parameter: the diagnosis, treatment, and evaluation of the initial urinary tract infection in febrile infants and young children. *Pediatrics* 1999; **103**: 843–52. Corrections. *ibid.*: 1052; *ibid.* 2000; **105**: 141.
10. Williams G, *et al.* Antibiotics for the prevention of urinary tract infection in children: a systematic review of randomized controlled trials. *J Pediatr* 2001; **138**: 868–74.
11. Tran D, *et al.* Short-course versus conventional length antimicrobial therapy for uncomplicated lower urinary tract infections in children: a meta-analysis of 1279 patients. *J Pediatr* 2001; **139**: 93–9.

MEN. References.
1. Lipsky BA. Urinary tract infections in men: epidemiology, pathophysiology, diagnosis, and treatment. *Ann Intern Med* 1989; **110**: 138–50.
2. Leigh DA. Prostatitis—an increasing clinical problem for diagnosis and management. *J Antimicrob Chemother* 1993; **32** (suppl A): 1–9.

3. Lipsky BA. Prostatitis and urinary tract infection in men: what's new; what's true? *Am J Med* 1999; **106**: 327–34.
4. Joly-Guillou M-L, Lasry S. Practical recommendations for the drug treatment of bacterial infections of the male genital tract including urethritis, epididymitis and prostatitis. *Drugs* 1999; **57**: 743–50.

PREGNANCY. References.
1. Tan JS, File TM. Treatment of bacteriuria in pregnancy. *Drugs* 1992; **44**: 972–80.
2. Vercaigne LM, Zhanel GG. Recommended treatment for urinary tract infection in pregnancy. *Ann Pharmacother* 1994; **28**: 248–51.
3. Bint AJ, Hill D. Bacteriuria of pregnancy—an update on significance, diagnosis and management. *J Antimicrob Chemother* 1994; **33** (suppl A): 93–7.
4. Maclean AB. Urinary tract infection in pregnancy. *Int J Antimicrob Agents* 2001; **17**: 273–6.
5. Krcmery S, *et al.* Treatment of lower urinary tract infection in pregnancy. *Int J Antimicrob Agents* 2001; **17**: 279–82.
6. Smaill F. Antibiotics for asymptomatic bacteriuria in pregnancy (updated 25 February 2001). Available in The Cochrane Library; Issue 2. Oxford: Update Software; 2001.

WOMEN. References.
1. Johnson JR, Stamm WE. Urinary tract infections in women: diagnosis and treatment. *Ann Intern Med* 1989; **111**: 906–17.
2. Brumfitt W, Hamilton-Miller JMT. Prophylactic antibiotics for recurrent urinary tract infections. *J Antimicrob Chemother* 1990; **25**: 505–12.
3. Hamilton-Miller JMT. The urethral syndrome and its management. *J Antimicrob Chemother* 1994; **33** (suppl A): 63–73.
4. Kunin CM. Urinary tract infections in females. *Clin Infect Dis* 1994; **18**: 1–12.
5. Anonymous. Managing urinary tract infection in women. *Drug Ther Bull* 1998; **36**: 30–2.
6. Warren JW, *et al.* Guidelines for antimicrobial treatment of uncomplicated acute bacterial cystitis and acute pyelonephritis in women. *Clin Infect Dis* 1999; **29**: 745–58.
7. Hooton TM. Recurrent urinary tract infection in women. *Int J Antimicrob Agents* 2001; **17**: 259–68.

Whipple's disease

Whipple's disease is a rare chronic systemic condition associated with infection with *Tropheryma whippelii*.[1] It was once considered to be a disease predominantly involving the small intestine and resulting in malabsorption, but may affect virtually all organs. There is probably CNS involvement in all patients with Whipple's disease, although it may only be evident in 10 to 20%.[2] Before the use of antibacterial therapy the disease was invariably fatal. The treatment generally recommended is benzylpenicillin (sometimes given as procaine penicillin [procaine benzylpenicillin]) and streptomycin parenterally for two weeks, followed by co-trimoxazole orally for one year.[2-5] Such long-term treatment with co-trimoxazole, a drug that crosses the blood-brain barrier, is advisable because of the relatively high frequency and seriousness of CNS relapse. These relapses respond less well to antibacterial treatment;[3] chloramphenicol has been used in those not responding to the above regimen and a patient with CNS relapse improved on ceftriaxone given intravenously.[6] A further alternative may be a tetracycline.[7] A patient intolerant of co-trimoxazole was given phenoxymethylpenicillin and probenecid after the initial 14-day course of benzylpenicillin and streptomycin.[8] There has also been a report of benefit in a penicillin-allergic patient treated with erythromycin.[9]

1. Relman DA, *et al.* Identification of the uncultured bacillus of Whipple's disease. *N Engl J Med* 1992; **327**: 293–301.
2. Dobbins WO. Whipple's disease. *Mayo Clin Proc* 1988; **63**: 623–4.
3. Keinath RD, *et al.* Antibiotic treatment and relapse in Whipple's disease: long-term follow-up of 88 patients. *Gastroenterology* 1985; **88**: 1867–73.
4. Fleming JL, *et al.* Whipple's disease: clinical, biochemical, and histopathologic features and assessment of treatment in 29 patients. *Mayo Clin Proc* 1988; **63**: 539–51.
5. Singer R. Diagnosis and treatment of Whipple's disease. *Drugs* 1998; **55**: 699–704.
6. Adler CH, Galetta SL. Oculo-facial-skeletal myorhythmia in Whipple disease: treatment with ceftriaxone. *Ann Intern Med* 1990; **112**: 467–9.
7. Anonymous. The choice of antibacterial drugs. *Med Lett Drugs Ther* 1999; **41**: 95–104.
8. Rickman LS, *et al.* Brief report: uveitis caused by Tropheryma whippelii (Whipple's bacillus). *N Engl J Med* 1995; **332**: 363–6.
9. Bowles KM, *et al.* A 35-year-old with swollen knees who had recurrent fever and pericarditis, then diarrhoea before getting better. *Lancet* 1996; **348**: 1356.

Yaws

See under Syphilis, above.

Yersinia enteritis

See under Gastro-enteritis, above.

Acediasulfone Sodium   (8231-n)

Acediasulfone Sodium *(rINN)*.

Sodium Diaphenylsulphonacetate. *N-p*-Sulphanilylphenylglycine sodium.

$C_{14}H_{13}N_2NaO_4S = 328.3$.
CAS — 127-60-6.

Profile
Acediasulfone sodium is reported to have antibacterial properties and is used topically in the treatment of local infections of the ear.

Preparations
Proprietary Preparations (details are given in Part 3)
Multi-ingredient: *Aust.:* Ciloprin cum Anaesthetico; *Denm.:* Ciloprin†; *Fin.:* Ciloprin cum Anaesthetico; *Swed.:* Ciloprin†; *Switz.:* Ciloprine ca.

Acrosoxacin   (12323-t)

Acrosoxacin *(BAN)*.

Rosoxacin *(BAN, USAN, rINN)*; Win-35213. 1-Ethyl-1,4-dihydro-4-oxo-7-(4-pyridyl)quinoline-3-carboxylic acid.

$C_{17}H_{14}N_2O_3 = 294.3$.
CAS — 40034-42-2.
ATC — J01MB01.

Adverse Effects and Precautions
As for Nalidixic Acid, p.227.

Dizziness, drowsiness, and visual disturbances may occur relatively frequently and patients should be advised not to drive or operate machinery if affected.

Uses and Administration
Acrosoxacin [rosoxacin] is a 4-quinolone antibacterial with actions similar to those of nalidixic acid (p.227). It is active against *Neisseria gonorrhoeae* and is given by mouth in the treatment of gonorrhoea (p.124) as a single dose of 300 mg, preferably on an empty stomach.

Preparations
Proprietary Preparations (details are given in Part 3)
Braz.: Eradacil; *Fr.:* Eracine; *Port.:* Eradacil.

Alatrofloxacin Mesilate   (5383-c)

Alatrofloxacin Mesilate *(rINNM)*.

Alatrofloxacin Mesylate *(USAN)*; CP-116517-27. 7-{(1R,5S,6s)-6-[(S)-2-((S)-2-Aminopropionamido)propionamido]-3-azabicyclo[3.1.0]hex-3-yl}-1-(2,4-difluorophenyl)-6-fluoro-1,4-dihydro-4-oxo-1,8-naphthyridine-3-carboxylic acid monomethanesulphonate.

$C_{26}H_{25}F_3N_6O_5,CH_3SO_3H = 654.6$.
CAS — 157182-32-6 (alatrofloxacin); 157605-25-9 (alatrofloxacin mesilate).

Profile
Alatrofloxacin is a prodrug of the fluoroquinolone antibacterial trovafloxacin (p.266) and is used intravenously as the mesilate in the treatment of susceptible infections. Details of doses are given under trovafloxacin.

Alatrofloxacin and trovafloxacin preparations have been withdrawn in many European countries following reports of unpredictable severe hepatic adverse effects, including some fatalities.

Preparations
Proprietary Preparations (details are given in Part 3)
Aust.: Trovan†; *Austral.:* Trovan; *Canad.:* Trovan; *Israel:* Trova; *Swed.:* Trovan†; *USA:* Trovan.

Amikacin   (184-z)

Amikacin *(BAN, rINN)*.

Amicacina; Amikacinum. 6-*O*-(3-Amino-3-deoxy-α-D-glucopyranosyl)-4-*O*-(6-amino-6-deoxy-α-D-glucopyranosyl)-*N*¹-[(2S)-4-amino-2-hydroxybutyryl]-2-deoxystreptamine.

$C_{22}H_{43}N_5O_{13} = 585.6$.
CAS — 37517-28-5.
ATC — D06AX12; J01GB06; S01AA21.

Pharmacopoeias. In *Eur.* (see p.vi), *Int., Pol.,* and *US.*

Pharmacopoeial description
Ph. Eur.: An antimicrobial substance obtained from kanamycin A. A white or almost white powder. Sparingly soluble in water; practically insoluble in alcohol and in acetone; slightly soluble in methyl alcohol. A 1% solution in water has a pH of 9.5 to 11.5.

USP 25: A white crystalline powder. Sparingly soluble in water. pH of a 1% solution in water is between 9.5 and 11.5. Store in airtight containers.

The symbol † denotes a preparation no longer actively marketed

Amikacin Sulfate (3-k)

Amikacin Sulfate (USAN, rINNM).
Amikacin Sulphate (BANM); Amikacini Sulfas; BB-K8.
$C_{22}H_{43}N_5O_{13},2H_2SO_4 = 781.8$.
CAS — 39831-55-5.
Pharmacopoeias. In Chin., Eur. (see p.vi), Int., Jpn, Pol., and US.

1.3 g of monograph substance is approximately equivalent to 1 g of amikacin. Solutions may darken from colourless to pale yellow but this does not indicate a loss of potency.
Incompatibilities. For discussion of the incompatibility of aminoglycosides, including amikacin, with beta lactams, see under Gentamicin Sulfate, p.210. Amikacin is also reported to be incompatible with various other drugs. However, reports are contradictory in many cases, and other factors, such as the strength and composition of the vehicles used, may play a role.

Pharmacopoeial description
Ph. Eur.: A white or almost white powder. It loses not more than 13.0% of its weight on drying. Freely soluble in water; practically insoluble in alcohol and in acetone. The pH of a 1% solution in water is between 2.0 and 4.0. Store in airtight containers.

USP 25: Amikacin sulfate having a molar ratio of amikacin to H_2SO_4 of 1:2 contains the equivalent of not less than 674 µg and not more than 786 µg of amikacin per mg, calculated on the dried basis. Amikacin sulfate having a molar ratio of amikacin to H_2SO_4 of 1:1.8 contains the equivalent of not less than 691 µg and not more than 806 µg of amikacin per mg, calculated on the dried basis.

A white crystalline powder. Freely soluble in water. pH of a 1% solution in water is between 2.0 and 4.0 (1:2 salt) and 6.0 to 7.3 (1:1.8 salt). Store in airtight containers.

Adverse Effects, Treatment, and Precautions
As for Gentamicin Sulfate, p.210. Peak plasma concentrations of amikacin greater than 30 to 35 µg per mL or trough concentrations greater than 5 to 10 µg per mL should be avoided. Amikacin affects auditory (cochlear) function to a greater extent than gentamicin.

Effects on the eyes. A report of retinal damage following intravitreal injection of amikacin.[1]
1. Jackson TL, Williamson TH. Amikacin retinal toxicity. Br J Ophthalmol 1999; 83: 1199–1200.

Interactions
As for Gentamicin Sulfate, p.211.

Antimicrobial Action
As for Gentamicin Sulfate, p.211. Amikacin is active against a similar range of organisms although it is also reported to have some activity against Nocardia asteroides, Mycobacterium tuberculosis, and some atypical mycobacterial strains. MICs of amikacin for the most sensitive organisms range from about 0.1 to 8 µg per mL or more, which are generally higher than those for gentamicin; however, higher doses than for gentamicin can be tolerated, permitting peak plasma concentrations up to about 30 to 35 µg per mL. Amikacin is not degraded by many of the common enzymes often responsible for acquired aminoglycoside resistance. In consequence, cross-resistance with gentamicin and other aminoglycosides is infrequent and amikacin may be effective against strains resistant to other aminoglycosides. However, resistant strains of Gram-negative bacteria and staphylococci have been reported, and some authorities feel that its use should be restricted to infections resistant to other aminoglycosides, although reports differ as to the extent and speed of the development of amikacin resistance where it has been widely used.

◊ References.
1. Ho YII, et al. In-vitro activities of aminoglycoside-aminocyclitols against mycobacteria. J Antimicrob Chemother 1997; 40: 27–32.

Pharmacokinetics
As for Gentamicin Sulfate, p.211.
After intramuscular injection of amikacin sulfate, peak plasma concentrations equivalent to about 20 µg of amikacin per mL are achieved one hour after a 500-mg dose, reducing to about 2 µg per mL 10 hours after injection. A plasma concentration of 38 µg per mL has been reported after the intravenous infusion of 500 mg over 30 minutes, reduced to 18 µg per mL one hour later. Amikacin has been detected in body tis-

sues and fluids after injection; it crosses the placenta but does not readily penetrate into the CSF, although substantial penetration of the blood-brain barrier has been reported in children with meningitis.
A plasma half-life of about 2 to 3 hours has been reported in patients with normal renal function. Most of a dose is excreted by glomerular filtration in the urine within 24 hours.

◊ References.
1. Vanhaeverbeek M, et al. Pharmacokinetics of once-daily amikacin in elderly patients. J Antimicrob Chemother 1993; 31: 185–7.
2. Gaillard J-L, et al. Cerebrospinal fluid penetration of amikacin in children with community-acquired bacterial meningitis. Antimicrob Agents Chemother 1995; 39: 253–5.
3. Bressolle F, et al. Population pharmacokinetics of amikacin in critically ill patients. Antimicrob Agents Chemother 1996; 40: 1682–9.
4. Canis F, et al. Pharmacokinetics and bronchial diffusion of single daily dose amikacin in cystic fibrosis patients. J Antimicrob Chemother 1997; 39: 431–3.
5. Tod M, et al. Population pharmacokinetic study of amikacin administered once or twice daily to febrile, severely neutropenic adults. Antimicrob Agents Chemother 1998; 42: 849–56.

Uses and Administration
Amikacin is a semisynthetic aminoglycoside antibiotic derived from kanamycin and is used similarly to gentamicin (p.212) in the treatment of severe Gram-negative and other infections. It is given as the sulfate, and is generally reserved for the treatment of severe infections caused by susceptible bacteria that are resistant to gentamicin and tobramycin. Amikacin has also been given with antimycobacterials in the treatment of opportunistic mycobacterial infections (p.131). As with gentamicin, amikacin may be used with penicillins and with cephalosporins; the injections should be given at separate sites.

Doses of amikacin sulfate are expressed in terms of amikacin base. Adults and children may be given the equivalent of 15 mg of amikacin per kg body-weight daily in equally divided doses every 8 or 12 hours by intramuscular injection. In life-threatening infections, the dose may be increased in adults up to a maximum of 500 mg every 8 hours. A dose of 7.5 mg per kg daily in two divided doses (equivalent to 250 mg twice daily in adults) may be given for the treatment of uncomplicated urinary-tract infections. The same doses may be given by slow intravenous injection over 2 to 3 minutes or by intravenous infusion. In adults, 500 mg in 100 to 200 mL of diluent has been infused over 30 to 60 minutes; proportionately less fluid should be given to children.

Neonates may be given the equivalent of 10 mg of amikacin per kg as a loading dose, followed by 15 mg per kg daily in two divided doses. If given by intravenous infusion an infusion period of 1 to 2 hours is recommended. It has been suggested that doses may need to be adjusted in preterm neonates.

Treatment should preferably not continue for longer than 7 to 10 days, and in consequence the total dose given to adults should not exceed 15 g. Peak plasma concentrations greater than 30 to 35 µg per mL or trough plasma concentrations greater than 5 to 10 µg per mL should be avoided. Dosage should be adjusted in all patients according to plasma-amikacin concentrations, and this is particularly important where factors such as age, renal impairment, or prolonged therapy may predispose to toxicity, or where there is a risk of subtherapeutic concentrations. For discussion of the methods of calculating aminoglycoside dosage requirements, see p.212. As with some other aminoglycosides, there are preliminary results suggesting that equivalent efficacy can be obtained from once-daily dosage with amikacin without increasing toxicity, but such dosage regimens are not yet established.

A 0.25% solution has been instilled into body cavities in adults.

A liposomal formulation of amikacin is under investigation.

Opportunistic mycobacterial infections. Amikacin has been included in multidrug regimens for the treatment of Mycobacterium avium complex infections (p.131). Treatment

with amikacin in combination with parenteral ethambutol and ciprofloxacin together with an oral macrolide produced negative blood cultures in 13 of 15 patients,[1] but the addition of amikacin to oral treatment with rifampicin, ciprofloxacin, clofazimine, and ethambutol did not influence the clinical response in an open study of 74 patients.[2]
1. Roger P-M, et al. Efficacy and safety of an intravenous induction therapy for treatment of disseminated Mycobacterium avium complex infection in AIDS patients: a pilot study. J Antimicrob Chemother 1999; 44: 129–31.
2. Parenti DM, et al. A phase II/III trial of antimicrobial therapy with or without amikacin in the treatment of disseminated Mycobacterium avium infection in HIV-infected individuals. AIDS 1998; 12: 2439–46.

Preparations
USP 25: Amikacin Sulfate Injection.

Proprietary Preparations (details are given in Part 3)
Aust.: Biklin; *Austral.:* Amikin; *Belg.:* Amukin; *Braz.:* Amikin; Novamin; *Canad.:* Amikin; *Denm.:* Biklin†; *Fin.:* Biklin; *Fr.:* Amiklin; *Ger.:* Biklin; *Hong Kong:* Amikin; *Irl.:* Amikin; *Israel:* Amikin; Likacin; *Ital.:* Amicasil; Amikan; BB-K8; Chemacin; Dramigel; Likacin; Lukadin; Migracin; Mikan; Mikavir; Nekacin; Pierami; Sifamic†; *Mex.:* Akacin; Amikafur; Amikalem; Amikason's; Amikavi; Amikayect; Amikin; AMK; Beramikin; Biclin; Cramigen; Gamikal; Georkacina; Mikazul; Oprad; Yectamid; *Neth.:* Amukin; *NZ:* Amikin; *Port.:* Biclin; *S.Afr.:* Amikin; Kacinth; *Singapore:* Amikin; Selemycin; *Spain:* Biclin; Kanbine; *Swed.:* Biklin; *Switz.:* Amikine; *Thai.:* Akacin; Akicin; Amikasol; Amikin; Anbikin; Siamik; Tipkin; Tybikin; *UAE:* Mikacin; *UK:* Amikin; *USA:* Amikin.

Aminosalicylic Acid (7551-s)

4-Aminosalicylic Acid; Aminosalylum; Para-aminosalicylic Acid; PAS; Pasalicylum. 4-Amino-2-hydroxybenzoic acid.
$C_7H_7NO_3 = 153.1$.
CAS — 65-49-6.
ATC — J04AA01.

NOTE. Distinguish from 5-aminosalicylic acid (Mesalazine, p.1234).
Pharmacopoeias. In Aust. and US.

Aqueous solutions are unstable.

Pharmacopoeial description
USP 25: A white or practically white, bulky powder that darkens on exposure to light and air; it is odourless or has a slight acetous odour. Slightly soluble in water and in ether; soluble in alcohol; practically insoluble in benzene. Under no circumstances use a solution if its colour is darker than that of a freshly prepared solution. pH of a saturated solution in water is between 3.0 to 3.7. Store in airtight containers at a temperature not exceeding 30°. Protect from light.

Calcium Aminosalicylate (7552-w)

Aminosalicylate calcium; Calcii Para-aminosalicylas; Calcium PAS. Calcium 4-amino-2-hydroxybenzoate trihydrate.
$(C_7H_6NO_3)_2Ca,3H_2O = 398.4$.
CAS — 133-15-3 (anhydrous calcium aminosalicylate).
ATC — J04AA03.
Pharmacopoeias. In Aust. Jpn includes the heptahydrate ($7H_2O$).

Calcium aminosalicylate 1.3 g is approximately equivalent to 1 g of aminosalicylic acid.

Sodium Aminosalicylate (7571-y)

Aminosalicylate Sodium; Aminosalylnatrium; Natrii Aminosalicylas; Natrii Para-aminosalicylas; Pasalicylum Solubile; Sodium Para-aminosalicylate; Sodium PAS. Sodium 4-amino-2-hydroxybenzoate dihydrate.
$C_7H_6NNaO_3,2H_2O = 211.1$.
CAS — 133-10-8 (anhydrous sodium aminosalicylate); 6018-19-5 (sodium aminosalicylate dihydrate).
ATC — J04AA02.
Pharmacopoeias. In Aust., Chin., It., Pol., Swiss, and US.

Sodium aminosalicylate 1.38 g is approximately equivalent to 1 g of aminosalicylic acid.
Aqueous solutions are unstable and should be freshly prepared.

Pharmacopoeial description
USP 25: A white to cream-coloured, practically odourless crystalline powder. Soluble 1 in 2 of water; sparingly soluble in alcohol; very slightly soluble in chloroform and in ether. Its solutions decompose slowly and darken in colour. Prepare solutions within 24 hours of administration. Under no circumstances use a solution if its colour is darker than that of a freshly prepared solution. pH of a 2% solution in water is between 6.5 and 8.5. Store in airtight containers at a temperature not exceeding 40°. Protect from light.

Stability. Solutions of sodium aminosalicylate in sorbitol or syrup degraded more quickly to m-aminophenol than those in glycerol or propylene glycol.[1] Colour developed in all solutions but was not found to be an accurate indicator of decomposition of sodium aminosalicylate as it reflected only oxidation of m-aminophenol.
1. Blake MI, et al. Effect of vehicle on the stability of sodium aminosalicylate in liquid dosage forms. Am J Hosp Pharm 1973; 30: 441–3.

Adverse Effects and Treatment

Aminosalicylic acid and its salts may cause the side-effects of salicylates (see Aspirin, p.14).

Gastrointestinal side-effects are common and include nausea, vomiting, and diarrhoea; they may be reduced by giving doses with food or in association with an antacid but occasionally may be severe enough that therapy has to be withdrawn. Alteration of gastrointestinal function may lead to malabsorption of vitamin B_{12}, folate, and lipids. Salts of aminosalicylic acid may be better tolerated than the acid. Tolerance in children is better than in adults.

Hypersensitivity reactions have been reported in 5 to 10% of adults, usually during the first few weeks of treatment, and include fever, skin rashes; less commonly, arthralgia, lymphadenopathy, and hepatosplenomegaly may occur and, rarely, a syndrome resembling infectious mononucleosis. Other adverse effects which have been attributed to a hypersensitivity reaction to aminosalicylate include jaundice and encephalitis. Blood disorders reported include haemolytic anaemia in patients with glucose-6-phosphate dehydrogenase deficiency, agranulocytosis, eosinophilia, leucopenia, and thrombocytopenia. Psychosis may occasionally occur. Prolonged treatment may induce goitre and hypothyroidism. Crystalluria may occur.

Effects on the liver. Drug-induced hepatitis occurred in 0.32% of 7492 patients receiving antituberculous drugs; aminosalicylic acid was the most common cause.[1]

1. Rossouw JE, Saunders SJ. Hepatic complications of antituberculous therapy. *Q J Med* 1975; **44:** 1–16.

Precautions

Aminosalicylic acid and its salts should be administered with great care to patients with impaired renal or hepatic function and in patients with gastric ulcer. They should be used with caution in patients with glucose-6-dehydrogenase deficiency. The sodium salt should be administered with caution to patients with heart failure.

Aminosalicylates interfere with tests for glycosuria using copper reagents and for urobilinogen using Erhlich's reagent.

Pregnancy and breast feeding. The use of aminosalicylic acid or its salts is not recommended in pregnant patients due to gastrointestinal intolerance.[1] In addition, the literature suggests that first-trimester exposure may be associated with congenital defects.[2]

Small amounts of aminosalicylic acid are present in breast milk. A maximum concentration of 1.1 µg per mL has been reported in a lactating woman 3 hours after administration of a 4 g dose of aminosalicylic acid.[3]

1. Snider D. Pregnancy and tuberculosis. *Chest* 1984; **86:** 10S–13S.
2. Briggs GG, *et al. Drugs in pregnancy and lactation.* 4th ed. Baltimore: Williams and Wilkins, 1994: 33a.
3. Holdiness MR. Antituberculosis drugs and breast feeding. *Arch Intern Med* 1984; **144:** 1888.

Interactions

The adverse effects of aminosalicylates and salicylates may be additive. Probenecid may also increase toxicity by delaying renal excretion and enhancing plasma concentrations of aminosalicylate. The activity of aminosalicylic acid may be antagonised by ester-type local anaesthetics such as procaine.

Antimicrobial Action

Aminosalicylic acid is bacteriostatic and is active only against mycobacteria. It has a relatively weak action compared with other antituberculous drugs but most strains of *Mycobacterium tuberculosis* have been reported to be inhibited by 1 µg per mL. Resistance develops quickly if aminosalicylic acid is used alone.

Pharmacokinetics

When given by mouth, aminosalicylic acid and its salts are readily absorbed, and peak plasma concentrations occur after about 1 to 4 hours.

Aminosalicylic acid diffuses widely through body tissues and fluids, although diffusion into the CSF occurs only if the meninges are inflamed. Some aminosalicylate is bound to plasma proteins.

Aminosalicylate is metabolised in the intestine and liver primarily by acetylation. Urinary excretion is rapid, and 80% or more of a dose is excreted within 24 hours; 50% or more of the dose is excreted as the acetylated metabolite. The half-life of aminosalicylic acid is approximately 1 hour.

Aminosalicylate is distributed into breast milk (see under Precautions above, for more details).

Uses and Administration

Aminosalicylic acid and its salts are second-line antimycobacterials given by mouth in the treatment of tuberculosis (p.143) when other more potent drugs cannot be used. They should always be given with other antituberculous drugs.

Aminosalicylic acid may be given, often as the sodium salt, in a daily dose of 10 to 12 g in 2 or 3 divided doses for adults and 150 to 300 mg per kg body-weight in 3 or 4 divided doses for children.

A wide range of dosage forms has been used in an attempt to overcome the bulk and exceedingly unpleasant taste of the aminosalicylates. The salts appear to be better tolerated than the free acid and solutions in iced water prepared immediately before use may be less unpleasant to take.

The symbol † denotes a preparation no longer actively marketed

---

Administration in renal impairment. Most clinicians recommend that aminosalicylic acid should be avoided in patients with renal impairment.[1] An increase in plasma clearance of aminosalicylic acid (attributed to increased hepatic metabolism) has been noted in patients with renal impairment, so attempting to give aminosalicylate in reduced doses to such patients may lead to subtherapeutic serum concentrations.[2]

1. Appel GB, Neu HC. The nephrotoxicity of antimicrobial agents (first of three parts). *N Engl J Med* 1977; **296:** 663–70.
2. Holdiness MR. Clinical pharmacokinetics of the antituberculosis drugs. *Clin Pharmacokinet* 1984; **9:** 511–44.

Diagnosis and testing. Aminosalicylic acid has been used in a test for pancreatic function.[1,2]

1. Hoek FJ, *et al.* Improved specificity of the PABA test with p-aminosalicylic acid (PAS). *Gut* 1987; **28:** 468–73.
2. Puntis JWL, *et al.* Simplified oral pancreatic function test. *Arch Dis Child* 1988; **63:** 780–4.

Inflammatory bowel disease. Together with corticosteroids, derivatives of 5-aminosalicylic acid are one of the mainstays of the treatment of inflammatory bowel disease (p.1205). However, aminosalicylic acid (4-aminosalicylic acid) has also been investigated, and promising results have been reported with enemas in ulcerative colitis.[1-4]

1. Campieri M, *et al.* 4-Aminosalicylic acid (4-ASA) and 5-aminosalicylic acid (5-ASA) in topical treatment of ulcerative colitis patients. *Gastroenterology* 1984; **86:** 1039.
2. Ginsberg AL, *et al.* Treatment of left-sided ulcerative colitis with 4-aminosalicylic acid enemas: a double-blind, placebo-controlled trial. *Ann Intern Med* 1988; **108:** 195–9.
3. Sharma MP, Duphare HV. 4-Aminosalicylic acid enemas for ulcerative colitis. *Lancet* 1989; **i:** 450.
4. O'Donnell LJD, *et al.* Double blind, controlled trial of 4-aminosalicylic acid and prednisolone enemas in distal ulcerative colitis. *Gut* 1992; **33:** 947–9.

Preparations

USP 25: Aminosalicylate Sodium Tablets; Aminosalicylic Acid Tablets.

Proprietary Preparations (details are given in Part 3)
Canad.: Nemasol; *Fr.:* Quadrasa; *Ger.:* Pas-Fatol N; *Ital.:* Quadrasa; Salf-Pas; *Switz.:* Perfusion de PAS; *USA:* Paser.

Amoxicillin   (4-a)

Amoxicillin *(BAN, rINN).*

Amoxycillin. (6R)-6-[α-D-(4-Hydroxyphenyl)glycylamino]penicillanic acid.
$C_{16}H_{19}N_3O_5S = 365.4$.
CAS — 26787-78-0.
ATC — J01CA04.

Amoxicillin Sodium   (5-t)

Amoxicillin Sodium *(BANM, USAN, rINNM).*

Amoxicilina Sódica; Amoxicillinum Natricum; Amoxycillin Sodium; BRL-2333AB-B.
$C_{16}H_{18}N_3NaO_5S = 387.4$.
CAS — 34642-77-8.
Pharmacopoeias. In *Eur.* (see p.vi) and *Pol.*

1.06 g of monograph substance is approximately equivalent to 1 g of amoxicillin. Each g of monograph substance represents about 2.6 mmol of sodium.

Pharmacopoeial description

Ph. Eur.: A white or almost white, very hygroscopic powder. Very soluble in water; sparingly soluble in dehydrated alcohol; very slightly soluble in acetone. A 10% solution in water has a pH of 8.0 to 10.0. Store in airtight containers.

Amoxicillin Trihydrate   (6-x)

Amoxicillin Trihydrate *(BANM, rINNM).*

Amoxicillin *(USAN);* Amoxicillinum Trihydricum; Amoxycillin Trihydrate; BRL-2333.
$C_{16}H_{19}N_3O_5S,3H_2O = 419.4$.
CAS — 61336-70-7.

NOTE. Compounded preparations of amoxicillin may be represented by the following names:

• Co-amoxiclav *x/y (BAN)*—amoxicillin (as the trihydrate or the sodium salt) and potassium clavulanate; *x* and *y* are the strengths in milligrams of amoxicillin and clavulanic acid respectively

• Co-amoxiclav *(USP 25)*—amoxicillin trihydrate and potassium clavulanate.

Pharmacopoeias. In *Chin., Eur.* (see p.vi), *Jpn, Pol.,* and *US.*

1.15 g of monograph substance is approximately equivalent to 1 g of amoxicillin.

Pharmacopoeial description

Ph. Eur.: A white or almost white, crystalline powder. Slightly soluble in water and in alcohol; practically insoluble in ether and in fatty oils. It dissolves in dilute acids and in dilute solu-

---

tions of alkali hydroxides. A 0.2% solution in water has a pH of 3.5 to 5.5. Store in airtight containers.

USP 25: A white, practically odourless crystalline powder. Slightly soluble in water and in methyl alcohol; insoluble in carbon tetrachloride, in chloroform, and in benzene. pH of a 0.2% solution in water is between 3.5 and 6.0. Store in airtight containers.

Adverse Effects and Precautions

As for Ampicillin, p.151.

The incidence of diarrhoea is less with amoxicillin than ampicillin.

Hepatitis and cholestatic jaundice have been reported with the combination amoxicillin with clavulanic acid; the clavulanic acid component has been implicated. Erythema multiforme, Stevens-Johnson syndrome, toxic epidermal necrolysis, and exfoliative dermatitis have also been attributed occasionally to amoxicillin with clavulanic acid.

Effects on the liver. Hepatitis and cholestatic jaundice associated with the combination amoxicillin with clavulanic acid (co-amoxiclav) have been reported[1-4] and by 1993 the UK Committee on Safety of Medicines (CSM) had received 138 reports of hepatobiliary disorders, 3 of which were fatal.[5] It warned that, although usually reversible, the reaction often occurred after stopping therapy with a delay of up to 6 weeks. It appeared that the clavulanic acid was probably responsible. Retrospective analysis of cases reported in Australia[6] and a cohort study in the UK[7] found increasing age and prolonged treatment to be major risk factors for jaundice following co-amoxiclav; male sex is also a risk factor. By 1997 the CSM considered that cholestatic jaundice occurred with a frequency of about 1 in 6000 adult patients and that the risk of acute liver injury was about six times greater with co-amoxiclav than with amoxicillin alone. Therefore it now recommends that co-amoxiclav should be reserved for bacterial infections likely to be caused by amoxicillin-resistant strains, and that treatment should not usually exceed 14 days.[8]

1. Stricker BHC, *et al.* Cholestatic hepatitis due to antibacterial combination of amoxicillin and clavulanic acid (Augmentin). *Dig Dis Sci* 1989; **34:** 1576–80.
2. Wong FS, *et al.* Augmentin-induced jaundice. *Med J Aust* 1991; **154:** 698–701.
3. Larrey D, *et al.* Hepatitis associated with amoxycillin-clavulanic acid combination report of 15 cases. *Gut* 1992; **33:** 368–71.
4. Hebbard GS, *et al.* Augmentin-induced jaundice with a fatal outcome. *Med J Aust* 1992; **156:** 285–6.
5. Committee on Safety of Medicines/Medicines Control Agency. Cholestatic jaundice with co-amoxiclav. *Current Problems* 1993; **19:** 2.
6. Thomson JA, *et al.* Risk factors for the development of amoxycillin-clavulanic acid associated jaundice. *Med J Aust* 1995; **162:** 638–40.
7. Rodríguez LAG, *et al.* Risk of acute liver injury associated with the combination of amoxicillin and clavulanic acid. *Arch Intern Med* 1996; **156:** 1327–32.
8. Committee on Safety of Medicines/Medicines Control Agency. Revised indications for co-amoxiclav (Augmentin). *Current Problems* 1997; **23:** 8.

Interactions

As for Ampicillin, p.151.

Antimicrobial Action

As for Ampicillin, p.151.

Amoxicillin has been reported to be more active *in vitro* than ampicillin against *Enterococcus faecalis, Helicobacter pylori,* and *Salmonella* spp., but less active against *Shigella* spp.

It is inactivated by beta lactamases and complete cross-resistance has been reported between amoxicillin and ampicillin. The spectrum of activity of amoxicillin may be extended by the concomitant use of a beta-lactamase inhibitor such as clavulanic acid (p.187). As well as reversing resistance to amoxicillin in beta-lactamase-producing strains of species otherwise sensitive, clavulanic acid has also been reported to enhance the activity of amoxicillin against several species not generally considered sensitive. These have included *Bacteroides, Legionella,* and *Nocardia* spp. and *Burkholderia pseudomallei (Pseudomonas pseudomallei).* However, *Ps. aeruginosa, Serratia marcescens,* and many other Gram-negative bacteria remain resistant. Transferable resistance has been reported in *H. pylori.*

Pharmacokinetics

Amoxicillin is resistant to inactivation by gastric acid. It is more rapidly and more completely absorbed than ampicillin when given by mouth. Peak plasma-amoxicillin concentrations of about 5 µg per mL have been observed 1 to 2 hours after a dose of 250 mg, with detectable amounts present for up to 8 hours. Doubling the dose can double the concentration. The presence of food in the stomach does not appear to diminish the total amount absorbed.

Amoxicillin is given by injection as the sodium salt and, in general, similar concentrations are achieved with intramuscular as with oral administration.

About 20% is bound to plasma proteins in the circulation and plasma half-lives of 1 to 1.5 hours have been reported. The half-life may be longer in neonates and the elderly; in renal failure the half-life may be 7 to 20 hours. Amoxicillin is widely distributed at varying concentrations in body tissues and fluids. It crosses the placenta; small amounts are distributed into breast milk. Little amoxicillin passes into the CSF unless the meninges are inflamed.

Amoxicillin is metabolised to a limited extent to penicilloic acid which is excreted in the urine. About 60% of an oral dose of amoxicillin is excreted unchanged in the urine in 6 hours by glomerular filtration and tubular secretion. Urinary concentrations above 300 µg per mL have been reported after a dose of 250 mg. Probenecid retards renal excretion. Amoxicillin is removed by haemodialysis. High concentrations have been reported in bile; some may be excreted in the faeces.

Amoxicillin with clavulanic acid. The pharmacokinetics of amoxicillin and clavulanic acid are broadly similar and neither appears to affect the other to any great extent.

Uses and Administration

Amoxicillin is the 4-hydroxy analogue of ampicillin (p.151) and is used in a similar variety of susceptible infections. These include actinomycosis, biliary-tract infections, bronchitis, endocarditis (particularly for prophylaxis), gastro-enteritis (including salmonella enteritis, but not shigellosis), gonorrhoea, Lyme disease, mouth infections, otitis media, pneumonia, spleen disorders (pneumococcal infection prophylaxis), typhoid and paratyphoid fever, and urinary-tract infections. The beta-lactamase inhibitor clavulanic acid (p.187) widens amoxicillin's antimicrobial spectrum and a combined preparation (co-amoxiclav) can be used when resistance to amoxicillin is prevalent, for example in respiratory-tract infections due to *Haemophilus influenzae* or *Moraxella catarrhalis* (*Branhamella catarrhalis*), in the empirical treatment of animal bites, or in infections such as chancroid and melioidosis. For details of these infections and their treatment, see under Choice of Antibacterial, p.114.

Amoxicillin is also given as part of treatment regimens to eradicate *Helicobacter pylori* infection in patients with peptic ulcer disease (p.1208).

Administration and dosage. Amoxicillin is given by mouth as the trihydrate and by injection as the sodium salt. Doses are expressed in terms of the equivalent amount of amoxicillin.

The usual oral dose is amoxicillin 250 to 500 mg every 8 hours. Children up to 10 years of age may be given 125 to 250 mg every 8 hours; under 20 kg body-weight, a dose of 20 to 40 mg per kg daily in divided doses every 8 hours may be employed; in infants less than 3 months of age, the maximum dose should be 30 mg per kg daily in divided doses every 12 hours.

Higher oral doses of amoxicillin, either as a single dose or in short courses, are used in some conditions. For example, amoxicillin is given as a single dose of 3 g, with probenecid 1 g, in the treatment of uncomplicated gonorrhoea in areas where gonococci remain sensitive. A dose of 3 g repeated once after 8 hours may be used for dental abscesses. A 3-g dose may be given for uncomplicated acute urinary-tract infections, and repeated once after 10 to 12 hours. For the prophylaxis of endocarditis in patients at risk, amoxicillin 2 or 3 g is given about 1 hour before dental procedures under local or no anaesthesia. A high-dose regimen of amoxicillin 3 g twice daily may be used in

patients with severe or recurrent infections of the respiratory tract. If necessary, children aged 3 to 10 years with otitis media may be given 750 mg twice daily for 2 days. For the eradication of *H. pylori*, amoxicillin is given in combination with either metronidazole or clarithromycin and a bismuth compound or an antisecretory drug; usual doses of amoxicillin are 0.75 or 1 g twice daily or 500 mg three times daily.

Amoxicillin is administered by intramuscular or slow intravenous injection in doses of 500 mg every 8 hours. In severe infections, 1 g of amoxicillin may be given every 6 hours by slow intravenous injection over 3 to 4 minutes or by infusion over 30 to 60 minutes. Children up to 10 years of age may be given 50 to 100 mg per kg body-weight daily by injection in divided doses.

Doses should be reduced in severe renal impairment.

Amoxicillin with clavulanic acid. Amoxicillin in combination with clavulanic acid (co-amoxiclav) is administered by mouth in a ratio of amoxicillin (as the trihydrate) 2, 4, or 7 parts to 1 part of clavulanic acid (as the potassium salt), or intravenously in a ratio of 5 parts of amoxicillin (as the sodium salt) to 1 part of clavulanic acid (as the potassium salt). Doses of the combination, calculated on amoxicillin content, are similar to those for amoxicillin alone.

◊ References.
1. Speller DCE, *et al.*, eds. Clavulanate/β-lactam antibiotics: further experience. *J Antimicrob Chemother* 1989; **24** (suppl B): 1–226.
2. Todd PA, Benfield P. Amoxicillin/clavulanic acid: an update of its antibacterial activity, pharmacokinetic properties and therapeutic use. *Drugs* 1990; **39**: 264–307.

Preparations

BP 2001: Amoxicillin Capsules; Amoxicillin Injection; Amoxicillin Oral Suspension; Co-amoxiclav Tablets;
USP 25: Amoxicillin and Clavulanate Potassium for Oral Suspension; Amoxicillin and Clavulanate Potassium Tablets; Amoxicillin Capsules; Amoxicillin for Oral Suspension; Amoxicillin Tablets.

Proprietary Preparations (details are given in Part 3)
Aust.: Amoxid; Amoxihexal; Amoxilan; Amoxistad; Clamoxyl; Eramox; Gonoform; Ospamox; Supramox; *Austral.:* Alphamox; Amohexal; Amoxil; Ampexin†; Bgramin; Cilamox; Fisamox; Ibiamox†; Moxacin; *Belg.:* Amoxi; Clamoxyl; Clavucid; Flemoxin; Hiconcil; Moxaline; Novabritine; *Braz.:* Amoxifar; Amoxil; Hiconcil; Novocilin; Novoxil; Penvicilin; Polimoxil; *Canad.:* Amoxil; Apo-Amoxi; Novamoxin; Nu-Amoxi; *Denm.:* Flemoxin; Imacillin; Imadrax; Spektramox; *Fin.:* Amorion; Amoxin; Clamox; Flemoxin; Penalta; *Fr.:* A-Gram; Amodex; Amophar; Bactox; Bristamox; Clamoxyl; Flemoxine; Gramidil; Hiconcil; Zamocilline†; *Ger.:* Amagesan; Amc-Puren; Amoxi; Amoxi-Diolan; Amoxi-Hefa; Amoxi-Puren; Amoxi-Tablinen; Amoxi-Wolff; Amoxibeta; Amoxibiocin; Amoxihexal; Amoxillat; Amoximerck; Amoxypen; Clamoxyl; Cuxacillin†; dura AX†; espa-moxin; Flui-Amoxicillin; InfectoMox; Jephoxin; Sigamopen; Ulcolind Amoxi†; *Hong Kong:* Amoxa; Amoxapen; Amoxil; Apo-Amoxi; Aroxin; Betamox; Moxlin; Ospamox; *Irl.:* Almodan†; Amoxil; Clonamox; Galenamox; Geramox; Oramox; Pinamox; Roxillin†; *Israel:* Amoxi; Apomoxyn; Hiconcil; Moxypen; Moxyvit; *Ital.:* Alfamox; Amoflux; Amoxi; Amoxillin; Amoxina; Amoxipen; Bradimox; Dodemox; Erremox; Neibmixt†; Hydramox; Ibiamox; Isimoxin; Majorpen; Mopen; Moxiren; Neo-Ampiplus; Neotetranase; Oralmox; Pamocil; Simoxil; Sintopen; Velamox; Zimox; *Mex.:* Acimox; Acroxil; Amoxifur; Amoxil; Amoxinovag; Amoxisol; Amoxivet; Ampliron; AMX; Ardine; Axcil; Brenoxil; Deniren; Flemoxon; Gimalxina; Grunicina; Hidramox; Limoxin; Moxicel; Moxlin; Penamox; Penticlox; Polymox; Servamox; Servamox-F; Solciclina; Xalyn-Or; Xiprocan; *Neth.:* Clamoxyl; Flemoxin; *Norw.:* Amimox†; Amoxillin; Imacillin; *NZ:* Amoxil; Apo-Amoxi; Ibiamox; Moxlin; Penamox; *Port.:* Amplamox; Bodisan†; Cipamox; Clamoxyl; Flemoxin; Moxadent; Moxipen; Oraminax; Ospamox; Penamox; *S.Afr.:* Acucil†; Amoxillin; Amoxil; Amoxyfizz†; AMX†; Arcanacillin†; Betamox; C-Mox†; Ipcamox; Maxcil; Moxan; Moxymax†; Moxypen; Norimox†; Penmox; Pharmoxin†; Promoxil; Ranmoxy; Rocillin; Saltermox; Spectramox; Ultramox†; Unimox†; Xeracil†; Xillin†; Zoxil; *Singapore:* Amoxa; Amoxapen; Amoxicap; Amoxigran; Amoxil; Amoxitab; Apo-Amoxi; Aroxin; Moxilen; Moxipen; Ospamox; Ranoxyl; *Spain:* Actimoxi; Agerpen; Amitron; Amoflamisan; Amox†; Amoxaren; Amoxi Gobens; Amoxibacter; Amoxidel; Amoximedical; Apamox; Ardine; Bioxidona†; Blenox; Bolchipen; Borbalan; Brondix; Clamoxyl; Co Amoxin; Combitora; Damoxicil; Dobriciclin; Edoxil; Eupen; Flubiotic NF; Halitol; Hosboral; Inexbron; Metifarma; Morgenxil; Novagcilina†; Precopen; Raudopen; Reloxyl; Remisan; Riotapen†; Salvapen; Suamoxil; Superpeni†; Tolodina; *Swed.:* Amimox; Amoxiferm†; Bristamox†; Flemoxin†; Imacillin; *Switz.:* amoxi-basan; Amoxi-Cophar; Amoxi-Mepha; Amoximex; Antiotic; Azilline; Clamoxyl; Flemoxin; Helvamox; Penamox; Rivoxicillin†; Servamox†; Spectroxyl; Supramox; *Thai.:* Acticillin; Amacin; Amox; Amoxa; Amoxil; Amoxylin; Asiamox; Biomox; Ibiamox; Kamoxin; Kenya-Mox; Meixil; Milamox; Moxapen; Moxcil; Moxcin; Moxilcap; Moxilen; Moxlin; Moximed; Moxipan; Pondnoxcill; Posmox; Rancil; Servamox; Sia-Mox; Sil-A-Mox; Unimox; *UAE:* Julphamox; *UK:* Almodan; Amix; Amopen; Amoram; Amoxil; Amrit†; Galenamox; Rimoxallin; *USA:* Amoxil; Biomox†; Polymox†; Trimox; Wymox.

Multi-ingredient: *Aust.:* Amoclan; Augmentin; Clavamox; Helicocin†; *Austral.:* Augmentin; Ausclav; Clamoxyl; Clavulin; Klac-

id HP 7; Losec Helicopak; Losec Hp 7; Pylorid-KA; *Belg.:* Augmentin; *Braz.:* Amoxifar Balsamico; Augmentin; Bronco Cilimox; Bronco-Amoxil; Bronco-Polimoxil; Clavoxil; Clavulin; Novamox; Novocilin Balsamico; Respicilin; *Canad.:* Clavulin; Hp-Pac; Losec 1-2-3 A; *Fin.:* Amoxin Comp; Augmentin; Helipak A; Helipak K; Losec Heliara; Spektramox; *Fr.:* Augmentin; Ciblor; *Ger.:* Amoclav; Amoxi-Clavulan; Amoxidura; Amoxiillat-Clav; Augmentan; Flanamox; *Hong Kong:* Amoksiklav; Augmentin; Curam; Moxiclav; *Irl.:* Augmentin; Clavamel; Germentin; *Israel:* Augmentin; *Ital.:* Augmentin; Clavulin; Neoduplamox; *Mex.:* Acimox-Ex; Amoxibron; Amoxiclav; Augmentin; Clavulin; Esteclin Bac; Eumetinex; Hidramox-M; Penamox M; Pentibroxil; Sekretovit Amoxi; Septacin Amoxi; Servamox CLV; *Neth.:* Augmentin; PantoPAC; *Norw.:* Bremide; *NZ:* Alpha-Amoxyclav; Augmentin; Helicosec; Klacid HP7; Losec Hp7; Synermox; *Port.:* Amoclavam; Augmentin; Betamox; Clavamox; Clavepen; Penilan; *S.Afr.:* Augmaxil; Augmentin; Clamentin; Flumox; Hiconcil-NS†; Losec 20 Triple; Macropen; Megapen; Ranclav; Suprapen; *Singapore:* Augmentin; Clamonex; Curam; Enhancin; Moxiclav; *Spain:* Agerpen Mucolitico; Amo Basan; Amoclave; Amoxi Gobens Mucol; Amoxidel Bronquial; Amoxtiol; Amoxyplus; Ardine Bronquial; Augmentine; Bigpen; Bisolvon Amoxycilina; Bronco Tonic; Bronconovag; Bronquium Amoxicilina†; Burmicin; Clamoxyl Mucolitico; Clavepen; Clavucid; Clavumox; Combitorax†; Damoxicil Mucolitico†; Duonasa; Edoxil Mucolitico; Eupeclanic; Eupen Bronquial; Halitol Mucolitico; Hosboral Bronquial; Inexbron Mucolitico; Inmupen; Kelsopen†; Metifarma Mucolit; Pangamox; Precopen Mucolitico; Pulmo Borbalan; Reloxyl Mucolitico; Remisan Mucolitico; Salvapen Mucolitico; Superpeni Mucolitico†; *Swed.:* Spektramox; *Switz.:* Augmentin; Aziclav; *Thai.:* Amoksiklav; Augmentin; Cavumox; Curam; *UAE:* Julmentin; *UK:* Amiclav; Augmentin; Augmentin-Duo; Heliclear; *USA:* Augmentin; Prevpac.

Ampicillin (8-f)

Ampicillin (BAN, USAN, rINN).

Aminobenzylpenicillin; Ampicillinum; Ampicillinum Anhydricum; Anhydrous Ampicillin; AY-6108; BRL-1341; NSC-528986; P-50. (6*R*)-6-(α-D-Phenylglycylamino)penicillanic acid.
$C_{16}H_{19}N_3O_4S = 349.4$.
CAS — 69-53-4.
ATC — J01CA01; S01AA19.

NOTE. Compounded preparations of ampicillin may be represented by the following names:
• Co-fluampicil (*BAN*)—flucloxacillin 1 part and ampicillin 1 part (w/w).
Pharmacopoeias. In *Eur.* (see p.vi), *Jpn*, and *Pol.*
Int. and *US* permit anhydrous or the trihydrate.

Pharmacopoeial description
Ph. Eur.: A white, crystalline powder. It exhibits polymorphism. Sparingly soluble in water; practically insoluble in alcohol, in acetone, in ether, and in fatty oils. It dissolves in dilute solutions of acids and of alkali hydroxides. A 0.25% solution in water has a pH of 3.5 to 5.5. Store at a temperature not exceeding 30° in airtight containers.
USP 25: Ampicillin is anhydrous or contains three molecules of water of hydration. A white, practically odourless crystalline powder. Slightly soluble in water and in methyl alcohol; insoluble in carbon tetrachloride, in chloroform, and in benzene. pH of a 1% solution in water is between 3.5 and 6.0. Store in airtight containers.

Ampicillin Sodium (9-d)

Ampicillin Sodium (BANM, USAN, rINNM).

Aminobenzylpenicillin Sodium; Ampicillinnatrium; Ampicillinum Natricum.
$C_{16}H_{18}N_3NaO_4S = 371.4$.
CAS — 69-52-3.
Pharmacopoeias. In *Chin.*, *Eur.* (see p.vi), *Int.*, *Jpn*, *Pol.*, and *US*.

1.06 g of monograph substance is approximately equivalent to 1 g of ampicillin. Each g of monograph substance represents about 2.7 mmol of sodium.

The stability of solutions of ampicillin sodium is dependent on many factors including concentration, pH, temperature, and the nature of the vehicle. Stability decreases in the presence of glucose, fructose, invert sugar, dextrans, hetastarch, sodium bicarbonate, and lactate. It is recommended that reconstituted solutions of ampicillin sodium for injection should be administered within 24 hours of preparation, and should be stored at 2° to 8° but should not be frozen. Solutions for infusion are stable for varying periods and details are given in the manufacturers' literature.

Incompatibility. The incompatibility of ampicillin sodium and aminoglycosides is well established. Incompatibilities have also been reported with a wide range of other drugs, including other antibacterials, and appear to be more pronounced at higher concentrations and in solutions also containing glucose.

Pharmacopoeial description
Ph. Eur.: A white hygroscopic powder. Freely soluble in water; sparingly soluble in acetone; practically insoluble in ether, in liquid paraffin, and in fatty oils. A 10% solution in water has a pH of 8.0 to 10.0. Store in airtight containers.
USP 25: A white to off-white, odourless or practically odourless, hygroscopic, crystalline powder. Very soluble in water and in isotonic sodium chloride and glucose solutions. pH of a

solution in water containing the equivalent of ampicillin 1% is between 8.0 and 10.0. Store in airtight containers.

◊ References.
1. Lynn B. The stability and administration of intravenous penicillins. *Br J Intraven Ther* 1981; **2**(Mar): 22–39.

Ampicillin Trihydrate   (10-c)

Ampicillin Trihydrate (BANM, rINNM).

Ampicillin; Ampicillinum Trihydricum.

$C_{16}H_{19}N_3O_4S,3H_2O = 403.5$.

CAS — 7177-48-2.

Pharmacopoeias. In Eur. (see p.vi) and *Pol.* In *Jpn* under the title Ampicillin. *Int.* and *US* permit anhydrous or the trihydrate under the title Ampicillin.

1.15 g of monograph substance is approximately equivalent to 1 g of ampicillin.

Pharmacopoeial description

Ph. Eur.: A white crystalline powder. Slightly soluble in water; practically insoluble in alcohol, in ether, and in fatty oils. It dissolves in dilute solutions of acids and of alkali hydroxides. A 0.25% solution in water has a pH of 3.5 to 5.5. Store at a temperature not exceeding 30° in airtight containers.

USP 25: Ampicillin is anhydrous or contains three molecules of water of hydration. A white, practically odourless crystalline powder. Slightly soluble in water and in methyl alcohol; insoluble in carbon tetrachloride, in chloroform, and in benzene. pH of a 1% solution in water is between 3.5 and 6.0. Store in airtight containers.

Adverse Effects

As for Benzylpenicillin p.157.

Skin rashes are among the most common side-effects and are generally either urticarial or maculopapular; the urticarial reactions are typical of penicillin hypersensitivity, while the erythematous maculopapular eruptions are characteristic of ampicillin and amoxicillin and often appear more than 7 days after commencing treatment. Such rashes may be due to hypersensitivity to the beta-lactam moiety or to the amino group in the side-chain, or to a toxic reaction. The occurrence of a maculopapular rash during ampicillin administration does not necessarily preclude the subsequent administration of other penicillins. Since it may be difficult in practice to distinguish between hypersensitive and toxic responses, skin testing for hypersensitivity may be advisable before another penicillin is used in patients who have had ampicillin rashes. Most patients with infectious mononucleosis develop a maculopapular rash when treated with ampicillin, and patients with other lymphoid disorders such as lymphatic leukaemia and possibly HIV infection also appear to be at higher risk. More serious skin reactions may occur and erythema multiforme associated with ampicillin has occasionally been reported.

Gastrointestinal adverse effects, particularly diarrhoea and nausea and vomiting, occur quite frequently, usually following administration by mouth. Pseudomembranous colitis has also been reported.

Precautions

As for Benzylpenicillin p.158.

Ampicillin should be discontinued if a skin rash occurs. It should preferably not be given to patients with infectious mononucleosis since they are especially susceptible to ampicillin-induced skin rashes; patients with lymphatic leukaemia or possibly HIV infection may also be at increased risk of developing skin rashes.

Myasthenia gravis. The symptoms of a woman with myasthenia gravis were exacerbated when she was given ampicillin.[1]

1. Argov Z, *et al.* Ampicillin may aggravate clinical and experimental myasthenia gravis. *Arch Neurol* 1986; **43**: 255–6.

Interactions

As for Benzylpenicillin, p.158.

Allopurinol. An increased frequency of skin rashes has been reported in patients receiving ampicillin or amoxicillin together with allopurinol, compared with those receiving antibacter-

ial alone,[1] but this could not be confirmed in a subsequent study.[2]

1. Jick H, Porter JB. Potentiation of ampicillin skin reactions by allopurinol or hyperuricemia. *J Clin Pharmacol* 1981; **21**: 456–8.
2. Hoigné R, *et al.* Occurrence of exanthems in relation to aminopenicillin preparations and allopurinol. *N Engl J Med* 1987; **316**: 1217.

Chloroquine. The absorption of ampicillin has been reduced in healthy subjects by chloroquine taken concomitantly.[1]

1. Ali HM. Reduced ampicillin bioavailability following oral coadministration with chloroquine. *J Antimicrob Chemother* 1985; **15**: 781–4.

Antimicrobial Action

Ampicillin is a beta-lactam antibiotic. It is bactericidal and has a similar mode of action to that of benzylpenicillin (p.158), but as an aminopenicillin with an amino group side-chain attached to the basic penicillin structure, ampicillin is better able to penetrate the outer membrane of some Gram-negative bacteria and has a broader spectrum of activity.

Spectrum of activity. Ampicillin resembles benzylpenicillin in its action against Gram-positive organisms, including *Streptococcus pneumoniae* and other streptococci, but, with the possible exception of activity against *Enterococcus faecalis,* it is slightly less potent than benzylpenicillin. *Listeria monocytogenes* is highly sensitive. The Gram-negative cocci *Moraxella catarrhalis* (*Branhamella catarrhalis*), *Neisseria gonorrhoeae,* and *N. meningitidis* are sensitive. Ampicillin is more active than benzylpenicillin against some Gram-negative bacilli, including *Haemophilus influenzae* and Enterobacteriaceae such as *Escherichia coli, Proteus mirabilis, Salmonella* and *Shigella* spp. It is inactive against *Pseudomonas aeruginosa.* Ampicillin also has activity similar to benzylpenicillin against other organisms including many anaerobes and *Actinomyces* spp.

Minimum inhibitory concentrations for sensitive Gram-positive organisms have been reported to range from 0.02 to 1.5 µg per mL and for Gram-negative organisms from 0.03 to 3 µg per mL.

Activity with other antimicrobials. There is synergy against some beta-lactamase-producing organisms between ampicillin and beta-lactamase inhibitors such as clavulanic acid or sulbactam, and also penicillinase-stable drugs such as cloxacillin or flucloxacillin. Synergy has also been demonstrated between ampicillin and aminoglycosides against a range of organisms, including enterococci. Variable effects ranging from synergy to antagonism have been reported between ampicillin and other beta-lactams, bacteriostatic drugs such as chloramphenicol, and rifampicin.

Resistance. Like benzylpenicillin, ampicillin is inactivated by beta lactamases, although other mechanisms may be responsible for resistance in some species. There are geographical variations in the incidence of resistance, but most staphylococci and many strains of *E. coli, H. influenzae, M. catarrhalis, N. gonorrhoeae,* and *Salmonella* and *Shigella* spp. are resistant.

Pharmacokinetics

Ampicillin is relatively resistant to inactivation by gastric acid and is moderately well absorbed from the gastrointestinal tract after oral administration. Food can interfere with the absorption of ampicillin so doses should preferably be taken at least 30 minutes before meals. Peak concentrations in plasma are attained in about 1 to 2 hours and following a dose of 500 mg by mouth are reported to range from 2 to 6 µg per mL.

Ampicillin is given by injection as the sodium salt and, following the intramuscular administration of 500 mg, peak plasma concentrations occur within about 1 hour and are reported to range from 7 to 14 µg per mL.

Ampicillin is widely distributed and therapeutic concentrations can be achieved in ascitic, pleural, and joint fluids. It crosses the placenta into the fetal circulation and small amounts are distributed into breast

milk. There is little diffusion into the CSF except when the meninges are inflamed. About 20% is bound to plasma proteins and the plasma half-life is about 1 to 1.5 hours, but this may be increased in neonates and the elderly; in renal impairment half-lives of 7 to 20 hours have been reported.

Ampicillin is metabolised to some extent to penicilloic acid which is excreted in the urine.

Renal clearance of ampicillin occurs partly by glomerular filtration and partly by tubular secretion; it is retarded by the concomitant administration of probenecid. About 20 to 40% of an orally administered dose may be excreted unchanged in the urine in 6 hours; urinary concentrations have ranged from 0.25 to 1 mg per mL following a dose of 500 mg. Following parenteral administration about 60 to 80% is excreted in the urine within 6 hours. Ampicillin is removed by haemodialysis. High concentrations are reached in bile; it undergoes enterohepatic recycling and some is excreted in the faeces.

Ampicillin with sulbactam. The pharmacokinetics of ampicillin and sulbactam are broadly similar and neither appears to affect the other to any great extent.

Uses and Administration

Ampicillin is used in the treatment of a variety of infections due to susceptible organisms (see Antimicrobial Action, above). They include biliary-tract infections, bronchitis, endocarditis, gastro-enteritis (including salmonella enteritis and shigellosis), gonorrhoea, listeriosis, meningitis, otitis media, perinatal streptococcal infections (intrapartum prophylaxis against group B streptococci), peritonitis, pneumonia, septicaemia, typhoid and paratyphoid fever, and urinary-tract infections. Resistance to ampicillin is increasingly a problem in some infections, for example, gonorrhoea, pneumococcal infections, respiratory-tract infections due to *Haemophilus influenzae* or *Moraxella catarrhalis* (*Branhamella catarrhalis*), salmonella infections, shigellosis, and infections due to *Escherichia coli.* For details of these infections and their treatment, see under Choice of Antibacterial, p.114. If beta-lactamase-producing organisms are present, ampicillin can be administered with a beta-lactamase inhibitor such as sulbactam (see below) or a penicillinase-resistant drug such as cloxacillin, dicloxacillin, or flucloxacillin (known as co-fluampicil). It may also be administered in association with an aminoglycoside to increase the spectrum of organisms covered; it is advisable to administer the injections separately.

Administration and dosage. The dosage of ampicillin will depend on the severity of the disease, the age of the patient, and renal function; the dose should be reduced, or the dose interval increased, in severe renal impairment (creatinine clearance less than 10 mL per minute). Ampicillin is usually administered by mouth as the trihydrate and by injection as the sodium salt. Doses are expressed in terms of the equivalent amount of ampicillin. The usual adult dose by mouth is 0.25 to 1 g every 6 hours taken at least 30 minutes before or 2 hours after food. Children may be given half the adult dose.

For urinary-tract infections, ampicillin 500 mg is given every 8 hours.

For typhoid and paratyphoid where *Salmonella typhi* strains remain sensitive to ampicillin, a dose of 1 to 2 g may be given every 6 hours for two weeks for acute infections, and for 4 to 12 weeks in carriers.

Ampicillin 2 g administered, in association with probenecid 1 g, as a single dose by mouth, has been used in the treatment of uncomplicated gonorrhoea, in areas where gonococci remain sensitive; repeated doses are recommended in females.

Ampicillin is administered by injection in usual adult doses of 500 mg every 4 to 6 hours intramuscularly or by slow intravenous injection over 3 to 5 minutes or by infusion. Higher parenteral doses of 2 g given intravenously every 6 hours have been suggested for meningitis. Children may be given half the adult dose.

The symbol † denotes a preparation no longer actively marketed

For infants and children with meningitis, a dose of 150 mg per kg daily in divided doses has been suggested. A suggested dose, given to the mother, for intrapartum prophylaxis against group B streptococcal infection in the neonate is 2 g by intravenous injection initially then 1 g every 4 hours until delivery.

Ampicillin may also be administered by other routes usually as a supplement to systemic therapy. Intraperitoneal or intrapleural injections are given in a dose of 500 mg daily dissolved in 5 to 10 mL of water. For intra-articular injection, ampicillin 500 mg daily is given dissolved in up to 5 mL of water or a solution of procaine hydrochloride 0.5%.

Ampicillin benzathine has also been administered by intramuscular injection.

Ampicillin with sulbactam. The sodium salts of ampicillin and sulbactam (p.250) may be given intramuscularly or intravenously in the treatment of infections due to beta-lactamase-producing organisms. Doses are expressed in terms of the equivalent amounts of ampicillin and sulbactam; available injections contain ampicillin and sulbactam in the ratio 2:1, respectively. The usual dose is ampicillin 1 g with sulbactam 0.5 g every 6 hours; doses may be doubled in severe infections.

For oral administration sultamicillin (p.257), a mutual prodrug of ampicillin and sulbactam, may be used.

Preparations

BP 2001: Ampicillin Capsules; Ampicillin Injection; Ampicillin Oral Suspension; Co-fluampicil Capsules; Co-fluampicil Oral Suspension;
USP 25: Ampicillin and Probenecid for Oral Suspension; Ampicillin and Sulbactam for Injection; Ampicillin Capsules; Ampicillin for Injectable Suspension; Ampicillin for Injection; Ampicillin for Oral Suspension; Ampicillin Tablets.

Proprietary Preparations (details are given in Part 3)
Aust.: Binotal†; Doktacillin†; Standacillin; *Austral.:* Alphacin; Ampicyn; Austrapen; *Belg.:* Penbritin†; Pentrexyl; *Braz.:* Ampicil; Ampicilase; Ampicler; Ampicler com Probenecide; Ampicrom; Ampifar; Ampispectrin; Ampitotal; Amplacilina; Amplimed; Amplitor; Amplofen; Bacterinil; Bacterion; Binopen; Binotal; Binotine; Cilipen; Degona; Gonocilin; Gonol; Gonorrels; Gramcilina; Makrocilin; Natuscilin; Probenzima; Tandrexin; Totapen; *Canad.:* Ampicin; Apo-Ampi; Nu-Ampi; Penbritin†; *Denm.:* Anhypen†; Doktacillin; Pentrexyl; *Fin.:* A-Pen; *Fr.:* Totapen; *Ger.:* Ampi; Binotal; duraampicillin†; Jenampin†; *Hong Kong:* Ampilin; Dhacillin; Pamecil; Penbritin; Pentrexyl; *Irl.:* Amfipen; Clonamp; Novapen; Penbritin; Vidopen†; *Israel:* Penibrin; Pentrexyl; Vitapen; *Ital.:* Ampilisa; Ampilux; Ampiplus Simplex†; Amplital; Amplizer; Citicil†; Ibimicyn; Lampocillina; Pentrexyl; Platocillina†; *Jpn:* Herpen†; *Mex.:* Acimpil; Ambiosol; Ampi-Quim; Ampi-Tecno; Ampimex; Ampisuspen; Amsapen; Anglopen; Bacticil; Binotal; Dibacilina; Diferin; Expicin; Fenipencil; Flamicina; Ifecin; Iqfacilina; Lampicin; Linapen; Marovilina; Meprizina; Omnipen; Penbritin; Pentiver; Pentrexyl; Prodifer; Promecilina; Rayepen; Riganpil; Sinaplin; Totipen; Tronex; Unicilin; Yapamicin; *Neth.:* Pentrexyl; *Norw.:* Doktacillin; Pentrexyl; *Port.:* Amplifar; Britacil; Hiperbiotico; Hiperbiotico Retard; *S.Afr.:* Ampi-Rol; Ampimax; Ampipen; Ampisalt†; Be-Ampicil; Co-Cillin†; Dyna-Ampcil; Excillin; Hexacillin†; M-P-Cil†; Penbritin; Penrite†; Petercillin; Ranamp; Spectracil; Statcillin†; *Singapore:* Ampicap; Ampilin; Ampitab; Dhacillin; Pamecil; Penbritin; Pricillin; Standacillin; *Spain:* Ampiplus; Antibiopen; Britapen; Ciarbiot†; Electopen†; Gobemicina; Nuvapen; *Swed.:* Doktacillin; Pentrexyl; *Thai.:* Amcillin; Amilin; Ampat; Ampexin; Ampicyn; Ampilin; Ampillin; Ampra; Amprexyl; Ampro; Eracillin; Penbritin; Pencotrex; Pentrexyl; Servicillin; Siampicil; Sumapen; Vacillin; Viccillin; *UK:* Amfipen; Flu-Amp; Magnapen; Penbritin; Rimacillin; Vidopen†; *USA:* D-Amp†; Marcillin; Omnipen; Omnipen-N; Polycillin-N†; Polycillin-PRB†; Polycillin†; Principen; Totacillin; Totacillin-N†.

Multi-ingredient: *Aust.:* Unasyn; *Braz.:* Ambezetal; Ampifar Balsamico; Ampizan; Amplotal; Benzotal; Benzotal Balsamico; Binotine Balsamico; Dibendril; Durapen; Durapen Balsamico; Expectocilin Balsamico; Genitopen; Labfcilina; Optacilin; Optacilin Balsamico; Parenzyme Ampicilina; Penbritin Balsamico; Soma; Soma Balsamico; Urobiotic; Uropielon; *Fr.:* Unacim; *Ger.:* Unacid; *Hong Kong:* Ampiclox; Pamedox; Unasyn; *Irl.:* Ampiclox; *Ital.:* Ampiplus†; Amplium; Bethacil; Diamplicil; Duplexcillina; Duplexil; Infectin†; Loricin; Unasyn; *Mex.:* Ampiclox-D; Pentibrom; Pentrexyl Expec; Unasyn; *S.Afr.:* Ampiclox; Apen; Cloxam; Megamox; *Singapore:* Unasyn; *Spain:* Alongamicina Balsa; Bacimex; Bactosone Retard; Bio Espectrum; Bronco Pensusan†; Electopen Balsam Retard; Electopen Retard†; Espectral; Espectral Balsamico; Espectrosira; Etro; Etro Balsamico; Galotam†; Gobemicina Retard; Hispamicina Retard; Maxicilina; Miliken Mucol Med Retard; Miliken Mucol Retard; Miliken Mucolitico; Mucorex Ampicilina; Pectosan Ampicilina; Pectox Ampicilina†; Penisintex Bronquial; Pulminflamatoria; Pulmospin; Pulmosterin Retard; Resan Mucolitico; Resan Retard; Resisten Retard; Retarpen; Retarpen Balsamico; Retarpen Mucolitico; Sulquibron; Ultrabion; Ultrabion Balsamico; Ultrapenil; Unasyn; *Thai.:* Ampiclox; Polyclox; Unasyn; Viccillin-S; *UK:* Ampiclox†; Flu-Amp; Magnapen; *USA:* Unasyn.

Apramycin Sulfate   (15966-s)

Apramycin Sulfate *(rINNM)*.

47657 (apramycin); Apramycin Sulphate *(BANM)*; EL-857 (apramycin); EL-857/820 (apramycin); Nebramycin Factor 2 (apramycin).   4-O-[(2R,3R,4aS,6R,7S,8R,8aR)-3-Amino-6-(4-amino-4-deoxy-α-D-glucopyranosyloxy)-8-hydroxy-7-methyl-aminoperhydropyrano[3,2-b]pyran-2-yl]-2-deoxystreptamine sulphate.
$C_{21}H_{41}N_5O_{11},2\frac{1}{2}H_2SO_4 = 784.8$.
CAS — 37321-09-8 (apramycin); 41194-16-5 (apramycin sulfate).

NOTE. Apramycin is *USAN*.
Pharmacopoeias. In *BP(Vet)*.

Pharmacopoeial description

BP(Vet) 2001: The sulfate of an antibiotic produced by certain strains of *Streptomyces tenebrarius* or by other means. A light brown hygroscopic powder or granules. Freely soluble in water; practically insoluble in alcohol, in acetone, in ether, and in methyl alcohol. Store at a temperature not exceeding 25°.

Profile

Apramycin is an aminoglycoside antibiotic used as the sulfate in veterinary practice.

Arbekacin Sulfate   (19281-l)

Arbekacin Sulfate *(rINNM)*.

ABK (arbekacin); AHB-DBK (arbekacin); Arbekacin Sulphate; HABA-Dibekacin (arbekacin). O-3-Amino-3-deoxy-α-D-glucopyranosyl-(1→4)-O-[2,6-diamino-2,3,4,6-tetradeoxy-α-D-erythro-hexopyranosyl-(1→6)]-N′-[(2S)-4-amino-2-hydroxybutyryl]-2-deoxy-L-streptamine sulphate.
$C_{22}H_{44}N_6O_{10},xH_2SO_4$.
CAS — 51025-85-5 (arbekacin).
Pharmacopoeias. In *Jpn*.

Profile

Arbekacin is an aminoglycoside derived from dibekacin and has general properties similar to those of gentamicin (p.210). It has been used as the sulfate in the treatment of serious infections due to meticillin-resistant *Staphylococcus aureus*.

Preparations

Proprietary Preparations (details are given in Part 3)
Jpn: Habekacin†.

Arsanilic Acid   (12394-e)

Arsanilic Acid *(BAN, rINN)*.

Aminarsonic Acid; AS-101. p-Aminobenzenearsonic acid; 4-Aminophenylarsonic acid.
$C_6H_8AsNO_3 = 217.1$.
CAS — 98-50-0.

NOTE. The code AS-101 has been used for an immunomodulator that was investigated in the treatment of AIDS.
Pharmacopoeias. In *US* for veterinary use only.

Pharmacopoeial description

USP 25: A white to off-white crystalline powder. Soluble in hot water, in amyl alcohol, and in solutions of alkali carbonates; slightly soluble in cold water, in alcohol, and in acetic acid; insoluble in acetone, in chloroform, in ether, in benzene, and in dilute mineral acids; sparingly soluble in concentrated mineral acids.

Sodium Arsanilate   (13241-h)

Sodium Arsanilate *(BANM, rINNM)*.

Sodium Aminarsonate; Sodium Anilarsonate. Sodium 4-aminophenylarsonate.
$C_6H_7AsNNaO_3 = 239.0$.
CAS — 127-85-5.
Pharmacopoeias. Fr. includes the anhydrous substance and the trihydrate.

Profile

Arsanilic acid and sodium arsanilate are used in veterinary medicine for the prophylaxis and treatment of enteric infections in pigs and also as growth-promoting agents.

Aspoxicillin   (1960-n)

Aspoxicillin *(rINN)*.

TA-058.   (2S,5R,6R)-6-{(2R)-2-[(2R)-2-Amino-3-(methylcarbamoyl)propionamido]-2-(p-hydroxyphenyl)acetamido}-3,3-dimethyl-7-oxo-4-thia-1-azabicyclo[3.2.0]heptane-2-carboxylic acid.
$C_{21}H_{27}N_5O_7S = 493.5$.
CAS — 63358-49-6.
Pharmacopoeias. Jpn includes the trihydrate.

Profile

Aspoxicillin is a ureidopenicillin that has been given intravenously in the treatment of susceptible infections.

Preparations

Proprietary Preparations (details are given in Part 3)
Jpn: Doyle†.

Astromicin Sulfate   (12404-x)

Astromicin Sulfate *(USAN, pINNM)*.

Abbott-44747; Astromicin Sulphate; Fortimicin A Sulphate; KW-1070.   4-Amino-1-(2-amino-N-methylacetamido)-1,4-dideoxy-3-O-(2,6-diamino-2,3,4,6,7-pentadeoxy-β-L-lyxo-heptopyranosyl)-6-O-methyl-L-chiro-inositol sulphate.
$C_{17}H_{35}N_5O_6,2H_2SO_4 = 601.6$.
CAS — 55779-06-1 (astromicin); 72275-67-3 (astromicin sulfate); 66768-12-5 (xH_2SO_4).
Pharmacopoeias. In *Jpn*.

An antibiotic produced by *Micromonospora* spp.

Profile

Astromicin is an aminoglycoside with actions and uses similar to those of gentamicin (p.210). It is used as the sulfate but doses are expressed in terms of the base. It is administered intramuscularly or by intravenous infusion over 0.5 to 1 hour in a usual dosage equivalent to 400 mg of astromicin daily in 2 divided doses. Dosage should be adjusted based on serum-astromicin concentration monitoring.

Preparations

Proprietary Preparations (details are given in Part 3)
Jpn: Fortimicin.

Avilamycin   (3342-j)

Avilamycin *(BAN, USAN)*.

LY-048740 (avilamycin or avilamycin A).
$C_{61}H_{88}Cl_2O_{32}$ (avilamycin A) = 1404.2.
CAS — 11051-71-1 (avilamycin); 69787-79-7 (avilamycin A); 69787-80-0 (avilamycin C).

Profile

Avilamycin is an antibacterial used in veterinary medicine as a growth promotor.

Avoparcin   (11-k)

Avoparcin *(BAN, USAN, rINN)*.

Compound 254.
CAS — 37332-99-3.

A glycopeptide antibiotic produced by *Amycolatopsis coloradensis* (*Streptomyces candidus*) or by any other means.

Profile

Avoparcin is a glycopeptide antibiotic that has been incorporated into animal feedstuffs to promote growth.

◊ There is evidence of cross-resistance between avoparcin and vancomycin.[1] Suggestions that vancomycin-resistant organisms could enter the human population from the food chain as a result of the use of avoparcin as a growth promotor in animals[2,3] have been disputed by the manufacturers of avoparcin.[4,5] Following a ban in the European Union on the use of avoparcin as a growth promotor in animals there has been some evidence[6] of a decrease in the occurrence of vancomycin-resistant enterococci in poultry meat.

1. Klare I, *et al.* vanA-mediated high-level glycopeptide resistance in Enterococcus faecium from animal husbandry. *FEMS Microbiol Lett* 1995; **125:** 165–72.
2. Howarth F, Poulter D. Vancomycin resistance: time to ban avoparcin? *Lancet* 1996; **347:** 1047.
3. Wise R. Avoparcin and animal feedstuff. *Lancet* 1996; **347:** 1835.
4. Mudd A. Vancomycin resistance and avoparcin. *Lancet* 1996; **347:** 1412.
5. Mudd AJ. Is it time to ban all antibiotics as animal growth-promoting agents? *Lancet* 1996; **348:** 1454–5.
6. Pantosti A, *et al.* Decrease of vancomycin-resistant enterococci in poultry meat after avoparcin ban. *Lancet* 1999; **354:** 741–2.

Azidamfenicol   (12-a)

Azidamfenicol *(BAN, rINN)*.

Azidamphenicol; Azidoamphenicol; Bayer 52910. 2-Azido-N-[(αR,βR)-β-hydroxy-α-hydroxymethyl-4-nitrophenethyl]acetamide.
$C_{11}H_{13}N_5O_5 = 295.3$.
CAS — 13838-08-9.
ATC — S01AA25.

Profile

Azidamfenicol is an antibiotic that is related structurally to chloramphenicol (p.179). It is used as 1% eye drops or eye ointment in the treatment of bacterial eye infections.

Preparations

Proprietary Preparations (details are given in Part 3)
Ger.: Berlicetin; Posifenicol; Thilocanfol.

Azidocillin (13-t)

Azidocillin (BAN, rINN).

Azidobenzylpenicillin; BRL-2534; SPC-297D. (6R)-6-(D-2-Azido-2-phenylacetamido)penicillanic acid.

$C_{16}H_{17}N_5O_4S = 375.4$.

CAS — 17243-38-8.

ATC — J01CE04.

Profile

Azidocillin is a semisynthetic penicillin with actions and uses similar to those of phenoxymethylpenicillin (p.235). It is given by mouth as the sodium salt in doses of 750 mg twice daily in the treatment of susceptible infections. The potassium salt has also been used.

Preparations

Proprietary Preparations (details are given in Part 3)
Aust.: Longatren; *Ger.:* InfectoBicillin H; Syncillin.

Azithromycin (3467-b)

Azithromycin (BAN, USAN, rINN).

CP-62993; XZ-450. (2R,3S,4R,5R,8R,10R,11R,12S,13S,14R)-13-(2,6-Dideoxy-3-C-3-O-dimethyl-α-L-ribo-hexopyranosyloxy)-2-ethyl-3,4,10-trihydroxy-3,5,6,8,10,12,14-heptamethyl-11-(3,4,6-trideoxy-3-dimethylamino-β-D-xylo-hexopyranosyloxy)-1-oxa-6-azacyclopentadecan-15-one dihydrate; 9-Deoxo-9a-aza-9a-methyl-9a-homoerythromycin A dihydrate.

$C_{38}H_{72}N_2O_{12},2H_2O = 785.0$.

CAS — 83905-01-5 (anhydrous azithromycin); 117772-70-0 (azithromycin dihydrate).

ATC — J01FA10.

Pharmacopoeias. In US.

Pharmacopoeial description

USP 25: pH of a 0.2% solution in a mixture of methyl alcohol and water (1:1) is between 9.0 and 11.0. Store in airtight containers.

Adverse Effects and Precautions

As for Erythromycin, p.201. Gastrointestinal disturbances are the most frequent adverse effect but are usually mild and less frequent than with erythromycin. Transient elevations of liver enzyme values have been reported and, rarely, cholestatic jaundice. Rashes, headache, and dizziness may occur. Severe hypersensitivity reactions occur rarely but may be prolonged. Transient alterations in neutrophil counts have been seen in patients receiving azithromycin. Pain and inflammation may occur at the site of intravenous infusions. The manufacturers suggest that azithromycin should not be used in patients with hepatic impairment.

◊ In patients receiving long-term daily administration of azithromycin for mycobacterial infections,[1] gastrointestinal disorders occurred in 32 of 39 patients (82%), hearing impairment in 10 patients (26%), tinnitus in 18 patients (46%), and poor balance or dizziness in 11 patients (28%). In general, adverse effects were associated with higher serum-azithromycin concentrations.
1. Brown BA, *et al.* Relationship of adverse events to serum drug levels in patients receiving high-dose azithromycin for mycobacterial lung disease. *Clin Infect Dis* 1997; **24:** 958–64.

Effects on the ears. Reversible sensorineural hearing loss was reported in 3 patients who received azithromycin 500 mg daily together with clofazimine and ethambutol for the treatment of disseminated *Mycobacterium avium* complex infection.[1]
See also above.
1. Wallace MR, *et al.* Ototoxicity with azithromycin. *Lancet* 1994; **343:** 241.

Effects on fluid and electrolyte homoeostasis. The syndrome of inappropriate antidiuretic hormone secretion was associated with azithromycin treatment in a patient.[1,2]
1. Cadle RM, *et al.* Symptomatic syndrome of inappropriate antidiuretic hormone secretion associated with azithromycin. *Ann Pharmacother* 1997; **31:** 1308–10.
2. Kintzel PE. Correction: symptomatic syndrome of inappropriate antidiuretic hormone secretion associated with azithromycin. *Ann Pharmacother* 1998; **32:** 388.

Effects on the kidneys. Acute interstitial nephritis leading to irreversible renal failure has been reported in a patient who received azithromycin for 9 days.[1]
1. Mansoor GA, *et al.* Azithromycin-induced acute interstitial nephritis. *Ann Intern Med* 1993; **119:** 636–7.

Eosinophilia. A syndrome characterised by eosinophilia, arthralgia, fever, and rash was associated with administration of azithromycin or roxithromycin to a patient on separate occasions.[1] The original authors believed the condition represented the Churg-Strauss syndrome, although this was disputed in

The symbol † denotes a preparation no longer actively marketed

correspondence[2] and attributed to the eosinophilia-myalgia syndrome.
1. Hübner C, *et al.* Macrolide-induced Churg-Strauss syndrome in a patient with atopy. *Lancet* 1997; **350:** 563.
2. Kränke B, Aberer W. Macrolide-induced Churg-Strauss syndrome in patient with atopy. *Lancet* 1997; **350:** 1551–2.

Interactions

For a discussion of drug interactions of macrolide antibacterials, see Erythromycin, p.202. Concurrent administration of antacids containing aluminium or magnesium salts can reduce the rate, but not the extent, of absorption of azithromycin.

Increased rifabutin toxicity has been reported in patients receiving azithromycin and rifabutin.

Antimicrobial Action

As for Erythromycin, p.203. Azithromycin is less active than erythromycin against streptococci and staphylococci, but has greater activity than erythromycin *in vitro* against some Gram-negative pathogens such as *Haemophilus influenzae* and *Moraxella catarrhalis* (*Branhamella catarrhalis*), as well as having activity against some of the Enterobacteriaceae such as *Escherichia coli* and *Salmonella* and *Shigella* spp. Azithromycin is also more active than erythromycin against *Chlamydia trachomatis* and some opportunistic mycobacteria, including *Mycobacterium avium* complex. It has activity against the protozoa *Toxoplasma gondii* and *Plasmodium falciparum*.

◊ References.
1. Hamilton-Miller JMT. In-vitro activities of 14-, 15- and 16-membered macrolides against Gram-positive cocci. *J Antimicrob Chemother* 1992; **29:** 141–7.
2. Gordillo ME, *et al.* In vitro activity of azithromycin against bacterial enteric pathogens. *Antimicrob Agents Chemother* 1993; **37:** 1203–5.
3. Agacfidan A, *et al.* In vitro activity of azithromycin (CP-62, 993) against Chlamydia trachomatis and Chlamydia pneumoniae. *Antimicrob Agents Chemother* 1993; **37:** 1746–8.
4. Odenholt I, *et al.* Studies of the killing kinetics of benzylpenicillin, cefuroxime, azithromycin, and sparfloxacin on bacteria in the postantibiotic phase. *Antimicrob Agents Chemother* 1997; **41:** 2522–6.
5. Fuentes F, *et al.* Postantibiotic and sub-MIC effects of azithromycin and isepamicin against Staphylococcus aureus and Escherichia coli. *Antimicrob Agents Chemother* 1998; **42:** 414–18.
6. Watt G, *et al.* Azithromycin activities against Orientia tsutsugamushi strains isolated in cases of scrub typhus in Northern Thailand. *Antimicrob Agents Chemother* 1999; **43:** 2817–18.

Resistance. The pattern of resistance to azithromycin is similar to that seen with clarithromycin (p.186).

Pharmacokinetics

Following oral administration about 40% of a dose of azithromycin is bioavailable. Absorption from the capsule formulation, but not the tablet formulation, is reduced by food. Peak plasma concentrations are achieved 2 to 3 hours after a dose, but azithromycin is extensively distributed to the tissues, and tissue concentrations subsequently remain much higher than those in the blood; in contrast to most other antibacterials, plasma concentrations are therefore of little value as a guide to efficacy. High concentrations are taken up into white blood cells. There is little diffusion into the CSF when the meninges are not inflamed. Small amounts of azithromycin are demethylated in the liver, and it is excreted in bile as unchanged drug and metabolites. About 6% of an oral dose (representing about 20% of the amount in the systemic circulation) is excreted in the urine. The terminal elimination half-life is probably in excess of 40 hours.

◊ Reviews and references.
1. Lalak NJ, Morris DL. Azithromycin clinical pharmacokinetics. *Clin Pharmacokinet* 1993; **25:** 370–4.
2. Nahata MC, *et al.* Pharmacokinetics of azithromycin in pediatric patients after oral administration of multiple doses of suspension. *Antimicrob Agents Chemother* 1993; **37:** 314–16.
3. Luke DR, *et al.* Safety, toleration, and pharmacokinetics of intravenous azithromycin. *Antimicrob Agents Chemother* 1996; **40:** 2577–81.
4. Rapp RP. Pharmacokinetics and pharmacodynamics of intravenous and oral azithromycin: enhanced tissue activity and minimal drug interactions. *Ann Pharmacother* 1998; **32:** 785–93.
5. Amsden GW, *et al.* Pharmacokinetics in serum and leukocyte exposures of oral azithromycin, 1,500 milligrams, given over a 3- or 5-day period in healthy subjects. *Antimicrob Agents Chemother* 1999; **43:** 163–5.

Uses and Administration

Azithromycin is a nitrogen-containing macrolide or azalide with actions and uses similar to those of erythromycin (p.203).

Azithromycin may also be used as a component of regimens in the treatment of *Mycobacterium avium* complex (MAC) infections (see under Opportunistic Mycobacterial Infections, p.131) and may be used for prophylaxis. It is used in some countries for the prophylaxis of endocarditis in at-risk patients unable to take penicillin. It has been tried in protozoal infections including toxoplasmosis (p.585).

It is given by mouth as the dihydrate; doses are calculated in terms of the base. The capsule formulation should be given at least an hour before, or 2 hours after, meals.

The usual adult dose of azithromycin is 500 mg as a single dose daily for 3 days. Alternatively, an initial dose of 500 mg may be followed by 250 mg daily for a further 4 days. For uncomplicated genital infections due to *Chlamydia trachomatis*, the equivalent of 1 g of azithromycin is given as a single dose. A single dose of 2 g may be given for uncomplicated gonorrhoea. For prophylaxis of disseminated MAC infections, azithromycin 1.2 g may be given once weekly. In children over 6 months of age, the dose in the UK is 10 mg per kg body-weight once daily for 3 days. In the USA, the dose for children over 6 months of age for pneumonia or otitis media is 10 mg per kg on the first day, then 5 mg per kg daily for a further 4 days, and the dose for pharyngitis or tonsillitis in children aged over 2 years is 12 mg per kg once daily for 5 days.

Azithromycin dihydrate may also be given initially by intravenous infusion in doses equivalent to 500 mg of azithromycin as a single daily dose in the treatment of community-acquired pneumonia and pelvic inflammatory disease. It may be administered either in a solution containing 1 mg per mL over 3 hours or in a solution containing 2 mg per mL over 1 hour.

◊ Reviews.
1. Peters DH, *et al.* Azithromycin: a review of its antimicrobial activity, pharmacokinetic properties and clinical efficacy. *Drugs* 1992; **44:** 750–99.
2. Langtry HD, Balfour JA. Azithromycin: a review of its use in paediatric infectious disease. *Drugs* 1998; **56:** 273–97.
3. Alvarez-Elcoro S, Enzler MJ. The macrolides: erythromycin, clarithromycin, and azithromycin. *Mayo Clin Proc* 1999; **74:** 613–34.
4. Garey KW, Amsden GW. Intravenous azithromycin. *Ann Pharmacother* 1999; **33:** 218–28.

Ischaemic heart disease. Azithromycin is being investigated in the prevention of ischaemic heart disease, based on a suggested link between atherosclerosis and *Chlamydia pneumoniae* infection (see p.117). Pilot studies[1,2] and preliminary results of prospective studies[3] have demonstrated that treatment with azithromycin is tolerable but large-scale long-term studies are needed to assess outcome.
1. Gupta S, *et al.* Elevated Chlamydia pneumoniae antibodies, cardiovascular events, and azithromycin in male survivors of myocardial infarction. *Circulation* 1997; **96:** 404–7.
2. Jackson LA, *et al.* Safety and effect on anti-Chlamydia pneumoniae antibody titres of a 1 month course of daily azithromycin in adults with coronary artery disease. *J Antimicrob Chemother* 1999; **44:** 411–14.
3. Anderson JL, *et al.* Randomized secondary prevention trial of azithromycin in patients with coronary artery disease and serological evidence for Chlamydia pneumoniae infection. *Circulation* 1999; **99:** 1540–7.

Preparations

USP 25: Azithromycin Capsules.

Proprietary Preparations (details are given in Part 3)

Aust.: Zithromax; *Austral.:* Zithromax; *Belg.:* Zitromax; *Braz.:* Azitromin; Zitromax; *Canad.:* Zithromax; *Denm.:* Zitromax; *Fin.:* Zithromax; *Fr.:* Azadose; Zithromax; *Ger.:* Ultreon; Zithromax; *Hong Kong:* Zithromax; *Irl.:* Zithromax; *Israel:* Azenil; Zeto; *Ital.:* Azitrocin; Ribotrex; Trozocina; Zitromax; *Mex.:* Azitrocin; *Neth.:* Zithromax; *Norw.:* Azitromax; *NZ:* Zithromax; *Port.:* Zithromax; *S.Afr.:* Zithromax; *Singapore:* Zithromax; *Spain:* Goxil; Toraseptol; Vinzam; Zentavion; Zitromax; *Swed.:* Azitromax; *Switz.:* Zithromax; *Thai.:* Zithromax; *UAE:* Azomycin; *UK:* Zithromax; *USA:* Zithromax.

Azlocillin Sodium (14-x)

Azlocillin Sodium (BANM, rINNM).

Bay-e-6905. Sodium (6R)-6-[D-2-(2-oxoimidazolidine-1-carboxamido)-2-phenylacetamido]penicillanate.

$C_{20}H_{22}N_5NaO_6S = 483.5$.

CAS — 37091-66-0 (azlocillin); 37091-65-9 (azlocillin sodium).

NOTE. Azlocillin is USAN.

Pharmacopoeias. In Pol.

1.05 g of monograph substance is approximately equivalent to 1 g of azlocillin. Each g of monograph substance represents about 2.1 mmol of sodium.

Incompatibility has been reported with aminoglycosides, ciprofloxacin, metronidazole, and tetracyclines.

Adverse Effects and Precautions

As for Carbenicillin Sodium, p.160.

As azlocillin sodium has a lower sodium content than carbenicillin sodium, hypernatraemia and hypokalaemia are less likely to occur. Prolongation of bleeding time has been less frequent and less severe than with carbenicillin.

Hypouricaemia. Reports of transient asymptomatic decreases in serum-uric acid concentrations during treatment with azlocillin.[1,2]

1. Faris HM, Potts DW. Azlocillin and serum uric acid. Ann Intern Med 1983; 98: 414.
2. Ernst JA, Sy ER. Effect of azlocillin on uric acid levels in serum. Antimicrob Agents Chemother 1983; 24: 609–10.

Interactions

As for Benzylpenicillin, p.158.

◊ For the effect of azlocillin on the clearance of cefotaxime, and a report of neurotoxicity, see p.169. For reference to azlocillin affecting the disposition of ciprofloxacin, see p.184.

See also above for incompatibilities.

Antimicrobial Action

Azlocillin has an antimicrobial action similar to that of piperacillin (p.236). Its activity in vitro against Enterobacteriaceae is generally less than that of mezlocillin or piperacillin, but it has comparable activity to piperacillin against Pseudomonas aeruginosa.

Pharmacokinetics

Azlocillin is not absorbed from the gastrointestinal tract to any significant extent. It has nonlinear dose-dependent pharmacokinetics. Doubling of an intravenous dose results in more than double the plasma concentration. Between 20 and 46% of azlocillin in the circulation is bound to plasma proteins. The plasma half-life is usually about 1 hour, but longer in neonates; in patients with renal impairment half-lives of 2 to 6 hours have been reported.

Azlocillin is widely distributed in body tissues and fluids. It crosses the placenta into the fetal circulation and small amounts are distributed into breast milk. There is little diffusion into the CSF except when the meninges are inflamed.

Azlocillin is metabolised to a limited extent. About 50 to 70% of a dose is excreted unchanged in the urine by glomerular filtration and tubular secretion within 24 hours of administration, so that high urinary concentrations are achieved. Azlocillin is partly excreted in the bile where it is also found in high concentrations.

Plasma concentrations are enhanced if probenecid is administered concomitantly.

Azlocillin is removed by haemodialysis.

Uses and Administration

Azlocillin is a ureidopenicillin and, like piperacillin (p.236), is used primarily for the treatment of infections caused by Pseudomonas aeruginosa. It has been used particularly for septicaemia, and infections of the respiratory and urinary tracts, and also for peritonitis; for details of these infections, see under Choice of Antibacterial, p.114.

Azlocillin is commonly administered in association with an aminoglycoside; however they should be administered separately as they have been shown to be incompatible.

Administration and dosage. Azlocillin is administered intravenously as the sodium salt. Doses are expressed in terms of the equivalent amount of azlocillin. A 10% solution in a suitable diluent is given by slow injection for doses of 2 g or less; higher doses should be infused over 20 to 30 minutes.

The usual adult dose is 5 g every 8 hours for life-threatening infections, or 2 g every 8 hours for less severe infections and urinary-tract infections.

The following doses may be used for children: premature infants, 50 mg per kg body-weight twice daily; neonates less than 7 days old, 100 mg per kg twice daily; infants between 7 days and 1 year, 100 mg per kg three times daily; children up to 14 years, 75 mg per kg three times daily.

The interval between doses may need to be increased to every 12 hours in moderate to severe renal impairment; additional dosage reductions may be needed in patients with both renal and hepatic impairment.

Preparations

Proprietary Preparations (details are given in Part 3)
Aust.: Securopen; **Ger.:** Securopen; **Irl.:** Securopen; **Ital.:** Securopen†; **Norw.:** Securopen†; **UK:** Securopen†.

Aztreonam (13266-e)

Aztreonam (BAN, USAN, rINN).

Azthreonam; SQ-26776. (Z)-2-{2-Aminothiazol-4-yl-[(2S,3S)-2-methyl-4-oxo-1-sulphoazetidin-3-ylcarbamoyl]methyleneamino-oxy}-2-methylpropionic acid.

$C_{13}H_{17}N_5O_8S_2 = 435.4$.

CAS — 78110-38-0.

ATC — J01DF01.

Pharmacopoeias. In Jpn and US.

Aztreonam has been reported to be **incompatible** with metronidazole, nafcillin, and vancomycin.

Pharmacopoeial description

USP 25: A white, odourless crystalline powder. Very slightly soluble in dehydrated alcohol; practically insoluble in chloroform, in ethyl acetate, and in toluene; soluble in dimethylformamide and in dimethyl sulfoxide; slightly soluble in methyl alcohol. Store in airtight containers.

Incompatibility and stability. References.

1. Bell RG, et al. Stability of intravenous admixtures of aztreonam and cefoxitin, gentamicin, metronidazole, or tobramycin. Am J Hosp Pharm 1986; 43: 1444–53.
2. Riley CM, Lipford LC. Interaction of aztreonam with nafcillin in intravenous admixtures. Am J Hosp Pharm 1986; 43: 2221–4.
3. Belliveau PP, et al. Stability of aztreonam and ampicillin sodium-sulbactam sodium in 0.9% sodium chloride injection. Am J Hosp Pharm 1994; 51: 901–4.
4. Trissel LA, Martinez JF. Compatibility of aztreonam with selected drugs during simulated Y-site administration. Am J Health-Syst Pharm 1995; 52: 1086–90.
5. Trissel LA, et al. Compatibility and stability of aztreonam and vancomycin hydrochloride. Am J Health-Syst Pharm 1995; 52: 2560–4.

Adverse Effects

The adverse effects of aztreonam are similar to those of other beta lactams (see Benzylpenicillin, p.157, and Cefalotin, p.162). Hypersensitivity reactions, including skin rashes, urticaria, eosinophilia, and rarely anaphylaxis, may occur in patients receiving aztreonam, although it has been reported to be only weakly immunogenic (see also under Precautions, below). Gastrointestinal effects include diarrhoea, nausea, vomiting, and an abnormal taste.

Phlebitis or thrombophlebitis has been reported after the intravenous administration of aztreonam, and pain or swelling after intramuscular injection.

Administration of aztreonam may result in the overgrowth of non-susceptible organisms, including Gram-positive cocci. Pseudomembranous colitis may develop.

Other adverse effects that have been reported with aztreonam include jaundice and hepatitis, increases in liver enzymes, and prolongation of prothrombin and partial thromboplastin times.

Effects on the skin. References.

1. McDonald BJ, et al. Toxic epidermal necrolysis possibly linked to aztreonam in bone marrow transplant patients. Ann Pharmacother 1992; 26: 34–5.

Precautions

Aztreonam should not be given to patients who are hypersensitive to it and should be administered with caution to those known to be hypersensitive to other beta-lactams, although the incidence of cross-sensitivity appears to be low (but see below).

It should be used with caution in patients with renal or hepatic impairment.

Hypersensitivity. Aztreonam is said to show little cross-reactivity with other beta-lactams,[1,2] but there have been isolated reports of immediate hypersensitivity to aztreonam in patients with a history of hypersensitivity to penicillin.[3,4]

1. Saxon A, et al. Lack of cross-reactivity between aztreonam, a monobactam antibiotic, and penicillin in penicillin-allergic subjects. J Infect Dis 1984; 149: 16–22.
2. Adkinson NF. Immunogenicity and cross-allergenicity of aztreonam. Am J Med 1990; 88 (suppl 3C): 12S–15S.
3. Alvarez JS, et al. Immediate hypersensitivity to aztreonam. Lancet 1990; 335: 1094.
4. Hantson P, et al. Immediate hypersensitivity to aztreonam and imipenem. BMJ 1991; 302: 294–5.

Interactions

Caution is recommended in patients receiving aztreonam and oral anticoagulant therapy because of the possibility of increased prothrombin time.

Antimicrobial Action

Aztreonam is bactericidal and acts similarly to the penicillins by inhibiting synthesis of the bacterial cell wall; it has a high affinity for the penicillin-binding protein 3 (PBP-3) of Gram-negative bacteria. The activity of aztreonam is restricted to Gram-negative aerobic organisms, including beta-lactamase-producing strains, with poor or no activity against Gram-positive aerobes or anaerobic organisms. It is active against most Enterobacteriaceae including Escherichia coli, Klebsiella, Proteus, Providencia, Salmonella, Serratia, Shigella, and Yersinia spp. Most of these organisms are inhibited in vitro by a concentration of aztreonam of 4 µg or less per mL. Some strains of Enterobacter and Citrobacter spp. are resistant. Aztreonam is active against Pseudomonas aeruginosa with MICs of 16 µg or less per mL. Most strains of other Pseudomonas spp. are insensitive. Aztreonam has good activity against Haemophilus influenzae and Neisseria spp.; most strains are inhibited by concentrations of 0.5 µg or less per mL.

Synergy has been reported in vitro between aztreonam and aminoglycosides against Ps. aeruginosa and some Enterobacteriaceae.

Aztreonam is stable to hydrolysis by many beta-lactamases and appears to be a poor inducer of beta-lactamase production. Acquired resistance has occasionally been reported.

Pharmacokinetics

Aztreonam is poorly absorbed from the gastrointestinal tract and is therefore administered parenterally. Absorption after intramuscular injection is good; peak plasma concentrations of about 46 µg per mL have been achieved within one hour of a 1-g dose. Aztreonam has a plasma half-life of approximately 1.7 hours. The half-life may be prolonged in neonates, in renal impairment, and to some extent in patients with hepatic impairment. About 56% in the circulation is bound to plasma proteins. It is widely distributed in body tissues and fluids, including bile. Diffusion into the CSF is poor unless the meninges are inflamed. It crosses the placenta and enters the fetal circulation; small amounts are distributed into breast milk.

Aztreonam is not extensively metabolised. The principal metabolite, SQ-26992, is inactive and is formed by opening of the beta-lactam ring; it has a much longer half-life than the parent compound. Aztreonam is excreted predominantly in the urine, by renal tubular secretion and glomerular filtration; about 60 to 70% of a dose appears within 8 hours as unchanged drug with only small quantities of metabolites. Only small amounts of unchanged drug and metabolites are excreted in the faeces.

Aztreonam is removed by haemodialysis and to a lesser extent by peritoneal dialysis.

◊ Reviews.

1. Mattie H. Clinical pharmacokinetics of aztreonam: an update. Clin Pharmacokinet 1994; 26: 99–106.

Uses and Administration

Aztreonam is a monobactam or monocyclic beta-lactam antibiotic used parenterally as an alternative to aminoglycosides or third-generation cephalosporins for the treatment of infections caused by susceptible Gram-negative aerobic organisms. These have included bone and joint infections, gonorrhoea, intra-abdominal and pelvic infections, lower respiratory-tract infections including pseudomonal infections in patients with cystic fibrosis, meningitis, septicaemia, skin and soft tissue infections, and urinary-tract infections. For details of these infections and their treatment, see under Choice of Antibacterial, p.114. To broaden the spectrum of activity for empirical treatment of infections, aztreonam should be used with other antibacterials. Concurrent use of an aminoglycoside may be of benefit in serious *Pseudomonas aeruginosa* infections.

Aztreonam is usually administered parenterally by deep intramuscular injection, by slow intravenous injection over 3 to 5 minutes, or by intravenous infusion over 20 to 60 minutes. It is given to adults in doses ranging from 1 to 8 g daily, administered in divided doses every 6 to 12 hours, according to the severity of the infection. Single doses over 1 g should be administered by the intravenous route.

Infants older than one week and children may be given aztreonam 30 mg per kg body-weight every 6 or 8 hours. For severe infections, children of 2 years or older may be given 50 mg per kg every 6 or 8 hours up to a maximum total daily dose of 8 g.

Dosage should be reduced in moderate to severe renal impairment. Patients with renal impairment may be given a usual initial dose followed by a maintenance dose adjusted according to their creatinine clearance: those with a clearance of 10 to 30 mL per minute, half the initial dose; less than 10 mL per minute, one-quarter of the initial dose. A supplementary dose of one-eighth of the initial dose may be given to patients undergoing haemodialysis after each dialysis session.

A single intramuscular dose of 1 g has been recommended for the treatment of gonorrhoea or cystitis.

◊ General references.
1. Brogden RN, Heel RC. Aztreonam: a review of its antibacterial activity, pharmacokinetic properties and therapeutic use. *Drugs* 1986; **31:** 96–130.
2. Neu HC. ed. Aztreonam's role in the treatment of Gram-negative infections. *Am J Med* 1990; **88** (suppl 3C): 1S–43S.
3. Hellinger WC, Brewer NS. Carbapenems and monobactams: imipenem, meropenem, and aztreonam. *Mayo Clin Proc* 1999; **74:** 420–34.

Preparations
USP 25: Aztreonam for Injection; Aztreonam Injection.

Proprietary Preparations (details are given in Part 3)
Aust.: Azactam; *Austral.:* Azactam; *Belg.:* Azactam; *Braz.:* Azactam; *Denm.:* Azactam; *Fin.:* Azactam; *Fr.:* Azactam; *Ger.:* Azactam; *Hong Kong:* Azactam; *Irl.:* Azactam; *Israel:* Azactam; *Ital.:* Azactam; Primbactam; *Jpn:* Azactam†; *Mex.:* Monobac; *Neth.:* Azactam; *Norw.:* Azactam; *NZ:* Azactam; *Port.:* Azactam; *S.Afr.:* Azactam; *Singapore:* Azactam; *Spain:* Azactam; Urobactam; *Swed.:* Azactam; *Switz.:* Azactam; *Thai.:* Azactam; *UK:* Azactam; *USA:* Azactam.

Bacampicillin Hydrochloride (15-r)
Bacampicillin Hydrochloride *(BANM, USAN, rINNM)*.
Ampicillin Ethoxycarbonyloxyethyl Hydrochloride; Bacampicillini Hydrochloridum; Carampicillin; EPC-272. 1-(Ethoxycarbonyloxy)ethyl *(6R)*-6-(α-D-phenylglycylamino)penicillanate hydrochloride.
$C_{21}H_{27}N_3O_7S,HCl = 502.0$.
CAS — 50972-17-3 (bacampicillin); 37661-08-8 (bacampicillin hydrochloride).
Pharmacopoeias. In *Eur.* (see p.vi), *Jpn,* and *US.*

1.44 g of monograph substance is approximately equivalent to 1 g of ampicillin.

Pharmacopoeial description
Ph. Eur.: A white or almost white hygroscopic powder or granules. Soluble in water and in dichloromethane; freely soluble in alcohol. A 2% solution in water has a pH of 3.0 to 4.5. Store in airtight containers.
USP 25: A white or practically white, hygroscopic, powder. Soluble in water and in dichloromethane; freely soluble in alcohol and in chloroform; very slightly soluble in ether. pH of a 2% solution in water is between 3.0 and 4.5. Store in airtight containers.

Adverse Effects and Precautions
As for Ampicillin, p.151. Diarrhoea has been reported to occur less frequently with bacampicillin.

Interactions
As for Benzylpenicillin, p.158.

Antimicrobial Action
Bacampicillin has the antimicrobial action of ampicillin *in vivo* (p.151). It possesses no intrinsic activity and needs to be hydrolysed to ampicillin.

Pharmacokinetics
Bacampicillin is more rapidly and completely absorbed from the gastrointestinal tract than ampicillin, to which it is hydrolysed in the intestinal wall and plasma. Peak plasma-ampicillin concentrations occur about 30 to 60 minutes after administration by mouth, and are approximately two to three times those after an equivalent dose of ampicillin. The absorption of bacampicillin from tablets does not appear to be affected by the presence of food in the stomach. About 75% of a dose is excreted in the urine as ampicillin within 8 hours.

The symbol † denotes a preparation no longer actively marketed

Uses and Administration
Bacampicillin has actions and uses similar to those of ampicillin (p.151) to which it is rapidly hydrolysed after administration. It is given as the hydrochloride in adult doses of 400 to 800 mg two or three times daily by mouth; children over 5 years of age have been given 25 to 50 mg per kg body-weight daily in two or three divided doses.
In uncomplicated gonorrhoea a single dose of bacampicillin hydrochloride 1.6 g together with probenecid 1 g may be given in areas where gonococci remain sensitive.

Preparations
USP 25: Bacampicillin Hydrochloride for Oral Suspension; Bacampicillin Hydrochloride Tablets.
Proprietary Preparations (details are given in Part 3)
Aust.: Penglobe; *Belg.:* Bacampicin; Bacocil; Penglobe†; *Canad.:* Penglobe; *Denm.:* Penglobe†; *Fr.:* Bacampicine; Penglobe; *Ger.:* Ambacamp; Penglobe; *Hong Kong:* Penglobe; *Ital.:* Bacacil; Bacagen; Bacasint; Bacillin; Penglobe; Rebacil; *Mex.:* Penglobe; *Port.:* Bacampicin; *Singapore:* Penglobe; *Spain:* Ambaxino; Penglobe; Velbacil; *Swed.:* Penglobe; *Switz.:* Bacampicin; *Thai.:* Penglobe; *UK:* Ambaxin†; *USA:* Spectrobid†.

Bacitracin (17-d)
Bacitracin *(BAN, rINN)*.
Bacitracinum.
CAS — 1405-87-4.
ATC — D06AX05; R02AB04.
Pharmacopoeias. In *Chin., Eur.* (see p.vi), *Int., Pol.,* and *US.*

Pharmacopoeial description
Ph. Eur.: It consists of one or more of the antimicrobial polypeptides produced by certain strains of *Bacillus licheniformis* and by *B. subtilis* var. *Tracy.* The potency is not less than 60 units per mg, calculated with reference to the dried substance. A white or almost white hygroscopic powder. Freely soluble in water and in alcohol; practically insoluble in ether. A 1% solution in water has a pH of 6.0 to 7.0. Store at a temperature of 8° to 15° in airtight containers.
USP 25: A polypeptide produced by the growth of an organism of the *licheniformis* group of *Bacillus subtilis* (Bacillaceae). It has a potency of not less than 40 units per mg. It is a white to pale buff, hygroscopic, powder, odourless or having a slight odour. Freely soluble in water; soluble in alcohol, in glacial acetic acid, and in methyl alcohol, the solution in the organic solvents usually showing some insoluble residue; insoluble in acetone, in chloroform, and in ether. Its solutions deteriorate rapidly at room temperature. It is precipitated from its solutions and is inactivated by salts of many of the heavy metals. pH of a solution in water containing 10 000 units per mL is between 5.5 and 7.5. Store in airtight containers at a temperature of 8° to 15°.

Bacitracin Zinc (16-f)
Bacitracin Zinc *(BANM, rINNM)*.
Bacitracins Zinc Complex; Bacitracinum Zincum; Zinc Bacitracin.
CAS — 1405-89-6.
Pharmacopoeias. In *Eur.* (see p.vi), *Int., Pol.,* and *US.*

Pharmacopoeial description
Ph. Eur.: The zinc complex of bacitracin. The potency is not less than 60 units per mg, calculated with reference to the dried substance. A white or light-yellowish-grey hygroscopic powder. Slightly soluble in water and in alcohol; very slightly soluble in ether. The filtrate of a saturated solution has a pH of 6.0 to 7.5. Store in airtight containers.
USP 25: The zinc salt of a kind of bacitracin or a mixture of two or more such salts. It has a potency of not less than 40 units per mg. A white or pale tan, hygroscopic powder, odourless or having a slight odour. Sparingly soluble in water. pH of a saturated solution in water is between 6.0 and 7.5. Store in airtight containers at a temperature of 8° to 15°.

Incompatibility. Bacitracin was slowly inactivated in bases containing stearyl alcohol, cholesterol, polyoxyethylene derivatives, and sodium laurilsulfate, and was rapidly inactivated in bases containing water, macrogols, propylene glycol, glycerol, cetylpyridinium chloride, benzalkonium chloride, ichthammol, phenol, and tannic acid.[1]
1. Plaxco JM, Husa WJ. The effect of various substances on the antibacterial activity of bacitracin in ointments. *J Am Pharm Assoc (Sci)* 1956; **45:** 141–5.

Stability. Bacitracin zinc was more stable than bacitracin and could be stored for 18 months at temperatures up to 40° without appreciable loss. Lozenges of bacitracin zinc and ointments and tablets containing bacitracin zinc with neomycin were more stable than the corresponding bacitracin preparations. Bacitracin zinc was less bitter than bacitracin and the taste was more readily disguised.[1]
1. Gross HM, *et al.* Zinc bacitracin in pharmaceutical preparations. *Drug Cosmet Ind* 1954; **75:** 612–13.

Units
The second International Standard Preparation (1964) of bacitracin zinc contains 74 units per mg.

Adverse Effects
When administered systemically bacitracin may produce severe nephrotoxicity. Nausea and vomiting may occur, as well as pain at the site of injection. Hypersensitivity reactions, including rashes and anaphylaxis, have occurred with both systemic, and more rarely with topical, administration.

Interactions
Additive nephrotoxicity would be anticipated if bacitracin is given systemically with other nephrotoxic drugs. Bacitracin is reported to enhance the neuromuscular blocking action of other drugs.

Antimicrobial Action
Bacitracin interferes with bacterial cell wall synthesis by blocking the function of the lipid carrier molecule that transfers cell wall subunits across the cell membrane. It is active against many Gram-positive bacteria including staphylococci, streptococci (particularly group A streptococci), and clostridia. It is also active against *Actinomyces, Treponema pallidum,* and some Gram-negative species such as *Neisseria* and *Haemophilus influenzae,* although most Gram-negative organisms are resistant.

Acquired bacterial resistance to bacitracin rarely occurs, but resistant strains of staphylococci have been detected.

Pharmacokinetics
Bacitracin is not appreciably absorbed from the gastrointestinal tract. When administered by intramuscular injection it is rapidly absorbed. About 10 to 40% of a single injected dose is excreted in the urine within 24 hours. Bacitracin readily diffuses into the pleural and ascitic fluids but little passes into the CSF. Absorption is reported to be negligible following topical application but may occur after peritoneal lavage.

Uses and Administration
Bacitracin and bacitracin zinc are applied topically, often in conjunction with other antibacterials such as neomycin and polymyxin B, and sometimes with corticosteroids, in the treatment of local infections due to susceptible organisms. Absorption from open wounds and from the bladder or peritoneal cavity may lead to adverse effects, although the dose-limiting toxicity of combined preparations is considered to be due to neomycin.

Bacitracin has been given by mouth in the treatment of antibiotic-associated colitis due to *Clostridium difficile.* Parenteral administration is usually avoided because of toxicity but bacitracin has been given intramuscularly.

Preparations
BP 2001: Polymyxin and Bacitracin Eye Ointment;
USP 25: Bacitracin and Polymyxin B Sulfate Topical Aerosol; Bacitracin for Injection; Bacitracin Ointment; Bacitracin Ophthalmic Ointment; Bacitracin Zinc and Polymyxin B Sulfate Ointment; Bacitracin Zinc and Polymyxin B Sulfate Ophthalmic Ointment; Bacitracin Zinc Ointment; Neomycin and Polymyxin B Sulfates and Bacitracin Ointment; Neomycin and Polymyxin B Sulfates and Bacitracin Ophthalmic Ointment; Neomycin and Polymyxin B Sulfates and Bacitracin Zinc Ointment; Neomycin and Polymyxin B Sulfates and Bacitracin Zinc Ophthalmic Ointment; Neomycin and Polymyxin B Sulfates, Bacitracin Zinc, and Hydrocortisone Acetate Ophthalmic Ointment; Neomycin and Polymyxin B Sulfates, Bacitracin Zinc, and Hydrocortisone Ointment; Neomycin and Polymyxin B Sulfates, Bacitracin Zinc, Hydrocortisone Ophthalmic Ointment; Neomycin and Polymyxin B Sulfates, Bacitracin Zinc, and Lidocaine Ointment; Neomycin and Polymyxin B Sulfates, Bacitracin, and Hydrocortisone Acetate Ointment; Neomycin and Polymyxin B Sulfates, Bacitracin, and Hydrocortisone Acetate Ophthalmic Ointment; Neomycin and Polymyxin B Sulfates, Bacitracin, and Lidocaine Ointment; Neomycin Sulfate and Bacitracin Ointment; Neomycin Sulfate and Bacitracin Zinc Ointment; Polymyxin B Sulfate and Bacitracin Zinc Topical Aerosol; Polymyxin B Sulfate and Bacitracin Zinc Topical Powder.

Proprietary Preparations (details are given in Part 3)
Aust.: Rhinocillin B; *Canad.:* Baciguent; Bacitin; *Hong Kong:* Bacitin; *Port.:* Dermimade Bacitracina†; *USA:* Ak-Tracin; Baci-IM; Baciguent.

Multi-ingredient: *Aust.:* Baneocin; Cicatrex; Eucillin; Nebacetin; Polybactrin†; Riker Antibiotic-Spray†; *Austral.:* Cicatrin; Nemdyn; Neosporin; Spersin†; *Belg.:* Neobacitracine; *Braz.:* Bacigem; Cicatrene; Cicatrizan; Dermase; Duplocitrin; Infectacina; Nebacetin; Neotricin; *Canad.:* Antibiotic Ointment; Antibiotique Onguent; Baciguent Plus Pain Reliever†; Bacimyxin;

Band-Aid Antibiotic; Bioderm; Cicatrin; Cortisporin; Emercreme No 4; Lanabiotic†; Lid-Pack; Neo Bace; Neosporin; Neotopic; Optimyxin; Ozonol Antibiotic Plus; Polycidin; Polyderm; Polysporin; Polysporin Triple Antibiotic; Polytopic; Polytracin†; *Fin.:* Bacibact; *Fr.:* Bacicoline; Collunovar; Lysopaine; Maxilase-Bacitracine; Oropivalone Bacitracine; *Ger.:* Anginomycin; Batrax; Bivacyn; Cicatrex; Nebacetin; Neobac; Neotracin; Polyspectran; Polyspectran HC; Prednitracin; *Hong Kong:* Bacimycin; Bivacyn; Nebacetin; Neosporin; Neotopic; Polyfax; Polyspectran; Prednitracin; *Irl.:* Cicatrin; Polybactrin†; Polyfax; *Israel:* Bamyxin; *Ital.:* Bimixin; Cicatrene; Enterostop; Orobicin; *Mex.:* Nebacetina; Neosporin; Polixin; Tribiot; Tribiot†; *Neth.:* Bacicoline-B†; Polyspectran B†; *Norw.:* Bacimycin; *Port.:* Baciderma; Bacitracina-Neo; Cicatrin; Davimicina; Dermobiotico; Dimicina; Oralbiotico; Polisulfade; Tri-Sinerge; *S.Afr.:* Cicatrin; Nebacetin†; Neosporin; Polysporin; *Singapore:* Baneocin; Batramycin; Fast Powder; Polybamycin; *Spain:* Alantomicina Complex†; Alantomicina†; Bacisporin; Banedif; Bio Hubber Fuerte†; Dermisone Tri Antibiotic; Dermo Hubber; Edifaringen; Linitul Antibiotico; Lizipaina; Neo Bacitrin; Neo Bacitrin Hidrocortis; Oxidermiol Enzima; Phonal; Pomada Antibiotica; Rinobanedif; Tulgrasum Antibiotico; Tyroneomicin†; *Swed.:* Nebacetin†; *Switz.:* Bacimycine; Baneopol; Batramycine; Cicatrex; Lysopaine; Nebacetin; Neotracin; Oro-Pivalone; Prednitracin; *Thai.:* Banocin; Genquin; Lobacin; Mybacin; Mybacin Dermic; *UK:* Cicatrin; Polyfax; *USA:* Ak-Poly-Bac; Ak-Spore; Alba-3†; Aquaphor Antibiotic†; Bactine First Aid Antibiotic Plus Anesthetic†; Betadine First Aid Antibiotics + Moisturizer†; Betadine Plus First Aid Antibiotics & Pain Reliever; Campho-Phenique Antibiotic Plus Pain Reliever Ointment†; Clomycin†; Coracin†; Cortimycin; Cortisporin; Lanabiotic; Mycitracin; Mycitracin Plus†; Neocin; Neomixin†; Neosporin; Neosporin + Pain Relief; Neosporin Plus†; Neotal†; Neotricin HC; Ocu-Spor-B; Ocutricin; Polycin-B; Polymycin; Polysporin; Polytracin; Septa†; Spectrocin Plus; Tri-Biozene; Tribiotic Plus†; Triple Antibiotic†.

Balofloxacin (17613-d)

Balofloxacin (rINN).

Q-35. (±)-1-Cyclopropyl-6-fluoro-1,4-dihydro-8-methoxy-7-[3-(methylamino)piperidino]-4-oxo-3-quinolinecarboxylic acid.
$C_{20}H_{24}FN_3O_4 = 389.4$.
CAS — 127294-70-6.

Profile
Balofloxacin is a fluoroquinolone antibacterial.

Bambermycin (12416-n)

Bambermycin (BAN, pINN).
Bambermycins (USAN); Flavophospholipol.
CAS — 11015-37-5.

An antibiotic complex containing mainly moenomycin A and moenomycin C and which may be obtained from cultures of *Streptomyces bambergiensis* or by other means.

Profile
Bambermycin is used as a growth promotor in veterinary practice.

Baquiloprim (2485-r)

Baquiloprim (BAN, rINN).

138OU. 5-(8-Dimethylamino-7-methyl-5-quinolylmethyl)pyrimidin-2,4-diyldiamine.
$C_{17}H_{20}N_6 = 308.4$.
CAS — 102280-35-3.

Profile
Baquiloprim is a diaminopyrimidine antibacterial used in veterinary medicine in combination with sulfadimethoxine or sulfadimidine.

Bekanamycin Sulfate (18-n)

Bekanamycin Sulfate (rINNM).
Aminodeoxykanamycin Sulphate; Bekanamycin Sulphate; Bekanamycini Sulfas; Kanamycin B Sulphate; KDM; NK-1006. 6-*O*-(3-Amino-3-deoxy-α-D-glucopyranosyl)-2-deoxy-4-*O*-(2,6-diamino-2,6-dideoxy-α-D-glucopyranosyl)-D-streptamine sulphate.
$C_{18}H_{37}N_5O_{10}, 2\frac{1}{2}H_2SO_4 = 728.7$.
CAS — 4696-76-8 (bekanamycin); 70550-99-1 (bekanamycin sulfate).
Pharmacopoeias. In Jpn.

1.5 g of monograph substance is approximately equivalent to 1 g of bekanamycin.

Profile
Bekanamycin is an aminoglycoside and is a congener of kanamycin. It has properties similar to those of gentamicin (p.210). It is given topically as the sulfate for the treatment of eye infections. It has also been given intramuscularly and by mouth. It is reported to be more toxic than kanamycin.

Preparations

Proprietary Preparations (details are given in Part 3)
Ital.: Kanendos†; *Jpn:* Kanendomycin†; *Port.:* Kanacyl.
Multi-ingredient: *Ital.:* Situalin Antibiotico†; Visucloben Antibiotico; Visumetazone Antibiotico; Visumicina.

Benethamine Penicillin (19-h)

Benethamine Penicillin (BAN, rINN).
Benzyl(phenethyl)ammonium (6R)-6-(2-phenylacetamido)penicillanate.
$C_{15}H_{17}N, C_{16}H_{18}N_2O_4S = 545.7$.
CAS — 751-84-8.
Pharmacopoeias. In Br.

Benethamine penicillin 950 mg is approximately equivalent to 600 mg of benzylpenicillin (1 million units).

Pharmacopoeial description
BP 2001: A white crystalline powder. Very slightly soluble in water; slightly soluble in alcohol; sparingly soluble in acetone and in chloroform. Store at a temperature not exceeding 30° in airtight containers.

Profile
Benethamine penicillin is a poorly soluble derivative of benzylpenicillin (p.157) with similar actions and uses, although it is not recommended for chronic, severe, or deep-seated infections. After deep intramuscular injection it forms a depot from which it is slowly absorbed and hydrolysed to benzylpenicillin. Benethamine penicillin is usually given in conjunction with benzylpenicillin sodium and also sometimes procaine penicillin [procaine benzylpenicillin] to produce both an immediate and a prolonged effect; overall, the effect lasts for 2 to 3 days.

Preparations
Proprietary Preparations (details are given in Part 3)
Port.: Atralmicina.
Multi-ingredient: *Fr.:* Biclinocilline.

Benzathine Benzylpenicillin (20-a)

Benzathine Benzylpenicillin (BAN, rINN).
Benzathine Penicillin; Benzathini Benzylpenicillinum; Benzethacil; Benzilpenicillina Benzatinica; Benzylpenicillinum Benzathinum; Penicillin G Benzathine; Penzaethinum G. NN'-Dibenzylethylenediammonium bis[(6R)-6-(2-phenylacetamido)penicillanate].
$C_{16}H_{20}N_2(C_{16}H_{18}N_2O_4S)_2 = 909.1$.
CAS — 1538-09-6 (anhydrous benzathine benzylpenicillin); 5928-83-6 (benzathine benzylpenicillin monohydrate); 41372-02-5 (benzathine benzylpenicillin tetrahydrate).
ATC — J01CE08.
Pharmacopoeias. In Chin., Eur. (see p.vi), Int., Pol., and US (as the tetrahydrate).

Benzathine benzylpenicillin 900 mg is approximately equivalent to 720 mg of benzylpenicillin (1.2 million units).

Pharmacopoeial description
Ph. Eur.: A white powder. Very slightly soluble in water; slightly soluble in alcohol; freely soluble in dimethylformamide and in formamide. Store in airtight containers.
USP 25: The tetrahydrate is a white, odourless, crystalline powder. Soluble 1 in 5000 of water and 1 in 65 of alcohol. pH in a solution prepared by dissolving 50 mg in 50 mL of dehydrated alcohol, and adding 50 mL of water is between 4.0 and 6.5. Store in airtight containers.

Adverse Effects and Precautions
As for Benzylpenicillin, p.157.

Non-allergic (embolic-toxic) reactions similar to those reported after administration of procaine penicillin [procaine benzylpenicillin], p.239, have been reported rarely with benzathine benzylpenicillin.

Benzathine benzylpenicillin should not be injected intravascularly since ischaemic reactions may occur.

Interactions
As for Benzylpenicillin, p.158.

Pharmacokinetics
When benzathine benzylpenicillin is given by intramuscular injection, it forms a depot from which it is slowly released and hydrolysed to benzylpenicillin. Peak plasma concentrations are produced in about 24 hours and are lower than those following an equivalent dose of benzylpenicillin potassium or sodium. However, depending on the dose, benzylpenicillin is usually detectable in plasma for up to 4 weeks (but see below).
Distribution into the CSF is reported to be poor.

Due to the slow absorption from the site of injection, benzylpenicillin has been detected in the urine for up to 12 weeks after a single dose.

Benzathine benzylpenicillin is relatively stable in the presence of gastric juice, but absorption from the gastrointestinal tract is variable. Plasma concentrations of benzylpenicillin achieved following an oral dose are lower than those from the same dose of a soluble penicillin; peak concentrations are also produced less rapidly, but may persist for longer.

Plasma concentrations. Benzathine benzylpenicillin has been given every 4 weeks for secondary prophylaxis against rheumatic fever, although some advocate administration every 3 weeks to ensure adequate plasma concentrations of benzylpenicillin. Typical concentrations achieved after a single intramuscular injection of benzathine benzylpenicillin 900 mg have been cited as about 0.1, 0.02, and 0.002 μg per mL on days 1, 14, and 32 respectively. In one study[1] adequate concentrations (defined as 0.02 μg or more per mL) were seen in more than 80% of serum samples at 3 weeks, but in only 36% at 4 weeks. In a further study,[2] in which single doses of 900 mg, 1.35 g and 1.8 g were compared, it appeared that doses higher than the 900-mg dose of benzathine benzylpenicillin usually recommended might prolong the duration of protective plasma concentrations of benzylpenicillin (defined as above 0.025 μg per mL) and improve the efficacy of dosing every 4 weeks for prophylaxis against rheumatic fever.
1. Kaplan EL, *et al.* Pharmacokinetics of benzathine penicillin G: serum levels during the 28 days after intramuscular injection of 1 200 000 units. *J Pediatr* 1989; **115:** 146–50.
2. Currie BJ, *et al.* Penicillin concentrations after increased doses of benzathine penicillin G for prevention of secondary rheumatic fever. *Antimicrob Agents Chemother* 1994; **38:** 1203–4.

Pregnancy. The pharmacokinetics of benzathine benzylpenicillin appear to be altered in late pregnancy. Of 10 healthy pregnant women given benzathine benzylpenicillin 1.8 g intramuscularly before caesarean section, only 4 achieved adequate serum concentrations of benzylpenicillin (for syphilis, at least 0.018 μg per mL) for 7 days.[1]
1. Nathan L, *et al.* Penicillin levels following the administration of benzathine penicillin G in pregnancy. *Obstet Gynecol* 1993; **82:** 338–42.

Uses and Administration
Benzathine benzylpenicillin has the same antimicrobial action as benzylpenicillin (p.158), to which it is hydrolysed gradually following deep intramuscular injection. This results in a prolonged effect, but because of the relatively low blood concentrations of benzylpenicillin produced, its use should be restricted to micro-organisms that are highly susceptible to benzylpenicillin. In acute infections, and when bacteraemia is present, the initial treatment should be with benzylpenicillin by injection.

Infections treated with benzathine benzylpenicillin include diphtheria (asymptomatic carriers), pharyngitis (*Streptococcus pyogenes; Arcanobacterium haemolyticum (Corynebacterium haemolyticum)*), and syphilis (including non-venereal treponematoses). It is also used for primary and secondary prophylaxis of rheumatic fever. For details of these infections and their treatment, see under Choice of Antibacterial, p.114.

Administration and dosage. Benzathine benzylpenicillin is administered by deep intramuscular injection, sometimes in association with procaine penicillin [procaine benzylpenicillin] and benzylpenicillin itself. It has been given by mouth for mild infections, although phenoxymethylpenicillin is usually preferred.

For early syphilis, a single dose of benzathine benzylpenicillin 1.8 g by deep intramuscular injection is given, usually as 2 injections at separate sites. In late syphilis, 1.8 g is given at weekly intervals for 3 consecutive weeks. Benzathine benzylpenicillin is not usually recommended for the treatment of neurosyphilis because of reports of inadequate penetration into the CSF. Infants up to 2 years of age may be given a single intramuscular dose of 37.5 mg per kg bodyweight for the treatment of congenital syphilis, provided there is no evidence of infection in the CSF.

For the treatment of other treponemal infections, such as yaws, pinta, and endemic syphilis (bejel), a single intramuscular dose of benzathine benzylpenicillin 900 mg is given; a dose of 450 mg may be used in children.

For streptococcal pharyngitis and the primary prevention of rheumatic fever, the adult dose is a single intramuscular injection of 900 mg; children under 30 kg body-weight may be given 450 to 675 mg. To prevent recurrences of acute rheumatic fever, 900 mg is given intramuscularly every 3 or 4 weeks to adults; a dose of 450 mg has been used for children under 30 kg body-weight.

Preparations

USP 25: Penicillin G Benzathine and Penicillin G Procaine Injectable Suspension; Penicillin G Benzathine Injectable Suspension; Penicillin G Benzathine Oral Suspension; Penicillin G Benzathine Tablets.

Proprietary Preparations (details are given in Part 3)
Aust.: Retarpen; *Austral.:* Bicillin L-A; *Belg.:* Penadur; *Braz.:* Ampiretard; Benzetacil; Longacilin; Normabenzil; *Canad.:* Bicillin L-A; Megacillin†; *Fr.:* Extencilline; *Ger.:* Pendysin; *Israel:* Durabiotic; *Ital.:* Diaminocillina; Wycillina; *Mex.:* Bencelin; Benzanil Simple; Benzetacil; Lentopenil; *Neth.:* Penidural; *NZ:* Bicillin L-A; *Port.:* Lentocilin-S; Penadur; *S.Afr.:* Bicillin L-A†; Penilente LA; *Singapore:* Penadur; Retarpen; *Spain:* Benzetacil; Cepacilina; *Thai.:* Penadur; *USA:* Bicillin L-A; Permapen.

Multi-ingredient: *Aust.:* Retarpen compositum; *Austral.:* Bicillin All Purpose†; *Braz.:* Kitapen; *Canad.:* Bicillin A-P†; *Ger.:* Retacillin; Tardocillin; *Ital.:* Tri-Wycillina; *Mex.:* Bencelin Combinado; Benzanil Compuesto; Benzetacil Combinado; Pendiben Compuesto; *Neth.:* Penidural D/F; *Port.:* Penadur 6.3.3; *S.Afr.:* Penilente Forte; Ultracillin; *Spain:* Benzetacil Compuesta; Cepacilina 321, 621, or 633†; Neocepacilina†; Penilevel Retard; *USA:* Bicillin C-R.

Benzathine Phenoxymethylpenicillin   (21-t)

Penicillin V Benzathine (*USAN*); Phenoxymethylpenicillini Dibenzylaethylendiaminum.   *N,N′*-Dibenzylethylenediammonium bis[(6R)-6-(2-phenoxyacetamido)penicillanate].
(C$_{16}$H$_{18}$N$_2$O$_5$S)$_2$,C$_{16}$H$_{20}$N$_2$ = 941.1.
CAS — 5928-84-7 (*anhydrous benzathine phenoxymethylpenicillin*); 63690-57-3 (*benzathine phenoxymethylpenicillin tetrahydrate*).
ATC — J01CE10.
Pharmacopoeias. In Aust. and US.

Benzathine phenoxymethylpenicillin 1.3 g is approximately equivalent to 1 g of phenoxymethylpenicillin.

Pharmacopoeial description

USP 25: A practically white powder having a characteristic odour. Soluble 1 in 3200 of water, 1 in 330 of alcohol, 1 in 37 of acetone, 1 in 42 of chloroform, and 1 in 910 of ether. pH of a 3% suspension in water is between 4.0 and 6.5. Store in airtight containers.

Profile

Benzathine phenoxymethylpenicillin has actions and uses similar to those of phenoxymethylpenicillin (p.235) and is administered by mouth in the treatment of susceptible mild to moderate infections. Doses are expressed in terms of phenoxymethylpenicillin.

Preparations

USP 25: Penicillin V Benzathine Oral Suspension.

Proprietary Preparations (details are given in Part 3)
Aust.: Ospen; Pen-Os†; Star-Pen; *Austral.:* Abbocillin-V; Cilicaine V; *Belg.:* Oracilline; *Canad.:* Pen-Vee; PVF†; *Fr.:* Oracilline; *Ger.:* InfectoBicillin; *Spain:* Benoral; *Switz.:* Ospen; Phenocillin.

Benzylpenicillin   (181-I)

Benzylpenicillin (*BAN, rINN*).
Crystalline Penicillin G; Penicillin; Penicillin G. (2S,5R,6R)-3,3-Dimethyl-7-oxo-6-(2-phenylacetamido)-4-thia-1-azabicyclo[3.2.0]heptane-2-carboxylic acid; (6R)-6-(2-Phenylacetamido)penicillanic acid.
C$_{16}$H$_{18}$N$_2$O$_4$S = 334.4.
CAS — 61-33-6.
ATC — J01CE01; S01AA14.

The name benzylpenicillin is commonly used to describe either benzylpenicillin potassium or benzylpenicillin sodium as these are the forms in which benzylpenicillin is used.
In *Martindale*, benzylpenicillin means either the potassium or sodium salt.

Benzylpenicillin Potassium   (182-y)

Benzylpenicillin Potassium (*BANM, rINNM*).
Benzylpenicillinum Kalicum; Penicillin G Potassium.
C$_{16}$H$_{17}$KN$_2$O$_4$S = 372.5.
CAS — 113-98-4.
Pharmacopoeias. In Chin., Eur. (see p.vi), Int., Jpn, Pol., and US.

The potassium salt of 6-phenylacetamidopenicillanic acid.
Each g of monograph substance represents about 2.7 mmol of potassium.
Stability and incompatibility, as for Benzylpenicillin Sodium, below.

The symbol † denotes a preparation no longer actively marketed

---

Pharmacopoeial description

Ph. Eur.: The potassium salt of a substance produced by growing certain strains of *Penicillium notatum* or related organisms or obtained by any other means. A white or almost white crystalline powder. Very soluble in water; practically insoluble in fatty oils and in liquid paraffin. A 10% solution in water has a pH of 5.5 to 7.5. Store in airtight containers.

USP 25: Colourless or white crystals, or white crystalline powder. It is odourless or practically so, and is moderately hygroscopic. Very soluble in water, in sodium chloride 0.9%, and in glucose solutions; sparingly soluble in alcohol. Its solutions retain substantially full potency for several days at temperatures below 15°, but are rapidly inactivated by acids, by alkali hydroxides, by glycerol, and by oxidising agents. pH of a 6% solution in water is between 5.0 and 7.5. Store in airtight containers.

Benzylpenicillin Sodium   (22-x)

Benzylpenicillin Sodium (*BANM, rINNM*).
Benzylpenicillinum Natricum; Penicillin G Sodium.
C$_{16}$H$_{17}$N$_2$NaO$_4$S = 356.4.
CAS — 69-57-8.
Pharmacopoeias. In Chin., Eur. (see p.vi), Int., Pol., and US.

The sodium salt of 6-phenylacetamidopenicillanic acid.
Each g of monograph substance represents about 2.8 mmol of sodium.

Stability. Benzylpenicillin sodium or potassium is hydrolysed in aqueous solutions by degradation of the β-lactam ring and hydrolysis is accelerated by increased temperature and alkaline conditions; inactivation also occurs under acid conditions. Degradation products include penillic, penicillenic, and penicilloic acids which lower the pH and cause a progressive increase in the rate of deterioration; *N*-formylpenicillamine and very small amounts of penicillamine have also been detected. Degradation is minimal at about pH 6.8 and deterioration of benzylpenicillin in solution may be retarded by using a citrate buffer. Dilute solutions are more stable than concentrated ones.

Incompatibility. Benzylpenicillin has been reported to be incompatible with metal ions and some rubber products. Its stability may be affected by ionic and nonionic surfactants, oxidising and reducing agents, alcohols, glycerol, glycols, macrogols and other hydroxy compounds, some paraffins and bases, some preservatives for example chlorocresol or thiomersal, carbohydrate solutions in an alkaline pH, fat emulsions, blood and blood products, and viscosity modifiers. Benzylpenicillin is incompatible with a wide range of acidic and basic drugs (see Stability, above) and with a number of other antimicrobials, including amphotericin B, some cephalosporins, and vancomycin. Benzylpenicillin and aminoglycosides are mutually incompatible and injections should be administered at separate sites.

Pharmacopoeial description

Ph. Eur.: The sodium salt of a substance produced by growing certain strains of *Penicillium notatum* or related organisms or obtained by any other means. A white or almost white crystalline powder. Very soluble in water; practically insoluble in fatty oils and in liquid paraffin. A 10% solution in water has a pH of 5.5 to 7.5. Store in airtight containers.

USP 25: Colourless or white crystals, or white to slightly yellow crystalline powder. It is odourless or practically so, and is moderately hygroscopic. Its solutions lose potency fairly rapidly at room temperature, but retain substantially full potency for several days at temperatures below 15°. Its solutions are rapidly inactivated by acids, by alkali hydroxides, by oxidising agents, and by penicillinase. pH of a 6% solution in water is between 5.0 and 7.5. Store in airtight containers.

◊ **References.**
1. Lynn B. The stability and administration of intravenous penicillins. *Br J Intraven Ther* 1981; **2** (Mar): 22–39.
2. Bird AE, *et al.* N-Formylpenicillamine and penicillamine as degradation products of penicillins in solution. *J Pharm Pharmacol* 1986; **38:** 913–17.

Units

The second International Standard Preparation (1952) of benzylpenicillin sodium contained 1670 units of penicillin per mg but was discontinued in 1968 since penicillin can now be characterised completely by chemical tests. Despite this, doses of benzylpenicillin are still expressed in units in some countries.

Benzylpenicillin potassium 600 mg or benzylpenicillin sodium 600 mg have generally been considered to be approximately equivalent to 1 million units (1 mega unit).

Adverse Effects

The most common adverse effects of benzylpenicillin are hypersensitivity reactions, especially skin rashes; anaphylaxis occasionally occurs and has sometimes been fatal. Other adverse effects have generally been associated with large intravenous doses of benzylpen-

---

icillin; patients with impaired renal function are also at increased risk. These adverse effects include haemolytic anaemia and neutropenia, both of which might have some immunological basis; prolongation of bleeding time and defective platelet function; convulsions and other signs of CNS toxicity (encephalopathy has followed intrathecal administration and can be fatal); and electrolyte disturbances because of the administration of large amounts of potassium or sodium when benzylpenicillin potassium or sodium, respectively, are administered.

Hepatitis and cholestatic jaundice have been reported rarely with some penicillins, notably penicillinase-resistant penicillins such as flucloxacillin and oxacillin, and also combinations of amoxicillin or ticarcillin with clavulanic acid.

Nephropathy and interstitial nephritis, which may have some immunological basis, have been especially associated with meticillin, but may be produced by other penicillins.

Some patients with syphilis and other spirochaete infections may experience a Jarisch-Herxheimer reaction shortly after starting treatment with penicillin, which is probably due to the release of endotoxins from the killed treponemes and should not be mistaken for a hypersensitivity reaction. Symptoms include fever, chills, headache, and reactions at the site of the lesions. The reaction can be dangerous in cardiovascular syphilis, or where there is a serious risk of increased local damage, such as with optic atrophy.

Gastrointestinal effects such as diarrhoea and nausea are the most common adverse effects following oral administration of benzylpenicillin; a sore mouth or tongue or a black hairy tongue have occasionally been reported. Pseudomembranous colitis has been associated with the use of most antibiotics; of the penicillins, ampicillin or amoxicillin have been implicated most frequently (see Antibiotic-associated Colitis, p.122).

Hypersensitivity. The overall incidence of allergic reactions to penicillin has been reported to vary from about 1 to 10% although some patients may have been incorrectly labelled 'allergic to penicillin'. Anaphylactic reactions occur in about 0.05% of patients, usually after parenteral administration but they have also been reported after taking penicillin by mouth.

Hypersensitivity to penicillin gives rise to a wide variety of clinical syndromes. Immediate reactions include anaphylaxis, angioedema, urticaria, and some maculopapular rashes. Late reactions may include serum sickness-like reactions and haemolytic anaemia. Reactions are considered to be due mainly to breakdown products (produced *in vitro* before administration) or metabolites of penicillin, and possibly penicillin itself, acting as haptens which when combined with proteins and other macromolecules produce potential antigens. As the hypersensitivity is related to the basic penicillin structure, patients who are genuinely allergic to benzylpenicillin must be assumed to be allergic to all penicillins; sensitised patients may also react to the cephalosporins and other beta-lactam antibiotics. For comment on crossreactivity with penicillamine, see under Penicillamine, Precautions, p.1018.

Tests for hypersensitivity may be used to determine those patients most likely to develop serious allergic reactions to penicillins. Skin tests are used to evaluate the current risk of immediate or accelerated IgE-mediated reactions, the most serious being anaphylaxis. Both the major and minor determinants of penicillin hypersensitivity should be used; the major determinant is available as penicilloyl-polylysine (p.1649) and a minor-determinant mixture consisting of benzylpenicillin and its derivatives, including penicilloic acid and benzylpenicilloylamine can be used, although if this is not available a solution of benzylpenicillin may be substituted. Adrenaline [epinephrine] should be available in case an anaphylactic reaction develops. The results of skin tests are unreliable if a significant time has elapsed before beginning therapy. A number of *in-vitro* tests including the radi-oallergosorbent test (RAST) have been developed.

Desensitisation may be attempted in patients allergic to penicillin when treatment with penicillin is considered essential. It involves the administration of very small doses of penicillin given at relatively short intervals of 15 minutes or more, and gradually increased to therapeutic concentrations. However, desensitisation may be hazardous and should only be carried out if the patient can be monitored continuously and adrenaline [epinephrine] and resuscitation equipment are immediately available. Desensitisation should be regarded as temporary, and allergic reactions may recur during the next exposure to penicillin.

Neutropenia. Neutropenia has been widely reported in patients receiving high doses of beta-lactams and an incidence of from 5 to more than 15% has been reported in patients treated for 10 days or more. Warning signs include fever, rash, and eosinophilia. Monitoring of the leucocyte count is recommended during long-term treatment with high doses. Some have proposed a direct toxic effect whereas others have postulated an immune mechanism.

◊ References to hypersensitivity reactions associated with penicillins.
1. Sullivan TJ, et al. Skin testing to detect penicillin allergy. *J Allergy Clin Immunol* 1981; **68:** 171–80.
2. Beeley L. Allergy to penicillin. *BMJ* 1984; **288:** 511–12.
3. Holgate ST. Penicillin allergy: how to diagnose and when to treat. *BMJ* 1988; **296:** 1213–14.
4. Anonymous. Penicillin allergy in childhood. *Lancet* 1989; **i:** 420.
5. Surtees SJ, et al. Allergy to penicillin: fable or fact? *BMJ* 1991; **302:** 1051–2. [With comments from several authors— *BMJ* 1991; **302:** 1462–3.]
6. Lin RY. A perspective on penicillin allergy. *Arch Intern Med* 1992; **152:** 930–7.
7. Anonymous. Penicillin allergy. *Drug Ther Bull* 1996; **34:** 87–8.

◊ References to neutropenia associated with penicillins.
1. Anonymous. Antibiotic-induced neutropenia. *Lancet* 1985; **ii:** 814.
2. Neftel KA, et al. Inhibition of granulopoiesis in vivo and in vitro by β-lactam antibiotics. *J Infect Dis* 1985; **152:** 90–8.
3. Olaison L, Alestig K. A prospective study of neutropenia induced by high doses of β-lactam antibiotics. *J Antimicrob Chemother* 1990; **25:** 449–53.

◊ References to CNS effects associated with penicillins.
1. Schliamser SE, et al. Neurotoxicity of β-lactam antibiotics: predisposing factors and pathogenesis. *J Antimicrob Chemother* 1991; **27:** 405–25.

Precautions
Patients known to be hypersensitive to penicillins should be given an antibacterial of another class. However, sensitised patients may also react to the cephalosporins and other beta-lactams. Desensitisation may be attempted if treatment with a penicillin is considered essential (see Adverse Effects, above). Penicillins should be given with caution to patients with a history of allergy, especially to drugs.

Care is necessary if very high doses of penicillins are given, especially if renal function is poor, because of the risk of neurotoxicity. The intrathecal route should be avoided. Care is also necessary if large doses of the potassium or sodium salts are given to patients with impaired renal function or heart failure, and high doses of benzylpenicillin potassium should be used with caution in patients receiving potassium-containing drugs or potassium-sparing diuretics. Renal and haematological status should be monitored during prolonged and high-dose therapy. Because of the Jarisch-Herxheimer reaction, care is also necessary when treating patients with spirochaete infections, particularly syphilis.

Contact with penicillin should be avoided since skin sensitisation may occur.

Penicillin therapy changes the normal bacterial flora and can lead to supra-infection with penicillin-resistant organisms including *Pseudomonas* or *Candida*, particularly with prolonged use.

Penicillins may interfere with some diagnostic tests such as those for urinary glucose using copper sulfate, direct antiglobulin (Coombs') tests, and some tests for urinary or serum proteins. Penicillins may interfere with tests that use bacteria, for example the Guthrie test for phenylketonuria using *Bacillus subtilis* organisms.

Interactions
Probenecid prolongs the half-life of benzylpenicillin by competing with it for renal tubular secretion and may be used therapeutically for this purpose. Benzylpenicillin may also interact with bacteriostatic antibacterials such as chloramphenicol and tetracyclines (see Antimicrobial Action, below), and may be incompatible *in vitro* with other drugs, including a number of other antibacterials (see above).

The possibility of a prolonged bleeding time following oral treatment with a broad-spectrum drug like ampicillin should be borne in mind in patients receiving anticoagulants.

◊ For the effect of penicillins on *methotrexate*, see p.555 and for the effect on *oral contraceptives*, see p.1458.

Antimicrobial Action
Benzylpenicillin is a beta lactam antibiotic and has a bactericidal action against Gram-positive bacteria, Gram-negative cocci, some other Gram-negative bacteria, spirochaetes, and actinomycetes.

Mechanism of action. It exerts its killing action on growing and dividing bacteria by inhibiting bacterial cell-wall synthesis, although the mechanisms involved are still not precisely understood. Bacterial cell walls are held rigid and protected against osmotic rupture by peptidoglycan. Benzylpenicillin inhibits the final cross-linking stage of peptidoglycan production by binding to and inactivating transpeptidases, penicillin-binding proteins on the inner surface of the bacterial cell membrane. However, it is now realised that other earlier stages in cell-wall synthesis can also be inhibited. Other mechanisms involved include bacterial lysis by the inactivation of endogenous inhibitors of bacterial autolysins.

Its action is inhibited by penicillinase and other beta-lactamases that are produced during the growth of certain micro-organisms.

Many Gram-negative organisms are intrinsically resistant by virtue of the inability of benzylpenicillin to penetrate their outer membranes. Intrinsic resistance can also be due to structural differences in the target penicillin-binding proteins. See under Resistance, below, for reference to acquired resistance.

Spectrum of activity. The following pathogenic organisms are usually sensitive to benzylpenicillin:

Gram-positive aerobes and anaerobes including *Bacillus anthracis, Clostridium perfringens, Cl. tetani, Corynebacterium diphtheriae, Erysipelothrix rhusiopathiae, Listeria monocytogenes, Peptostreptococcus* spp., non-beta-lactamase-producing staphylococci, and streptococci including *Streptococcus agalactiae* (group B), *Str. pneumoniae* (pneumococci), *Str. pyogenes* (group A), and some viridans streptococci; enterococci are relatively insensitive.

Gram-negative cocci including *Neisseria meningitidis* (meningococci) and *Neisseria gonorrhoeae* (gonococci).

Gram-negative bacilli including *Pasteurella multocida, Streptobacillus moniliformis,* and *Spirillum minus* (or *minor*); most Gram-negative bacilli, including *Pseudomonas* spp. and Enterobacteriaceae, are insensitive although some strains of *Proteus mirabilis* and *Escherichia coli* may be inhibited by high concentrations of benzylpenicillin.

Gram-negative anaerobes including *Prevotella* (non-fragilis *Bacteroides*) and *Fusobacterium* spp.

Other organisms including *Actinomyces* and the spirochaetes, *Borrelia, Leptospira,* and *Treponema* spp.

Mycobacteria, fungi, mycoplasmas, and rickettsias are not sensitive.

Minimum inhibitory concentrations (MICs) of benzylpenicillin for the most sensitive organisms (gonococci, meningococci, non-beta-lactamase-producing staphylococci, and streptococci) have been reported to range from 0.005 to 0.05 μg per mL; the maximum bactericidal effect is at concentrations about 4 times the MIC.

Activity with other antimicrobials. Benzylpenicillin may exhibit synergy with other antimicrobials particularly the aminoglycosides and such combinations have been used against enterococci and other relatively insensitive bacteria. Its activity may be enhanced by clavulanic acid and other beta-lactamase inhibitors, and both enhancement and antagonism have been demonstrated for beta-lactam combinations. Antagonism has been reported to occur with some bacteriostatic drugs, such as chloramphenicol, that interfere with active bacterial growth necessary for benzylpenicillin to achieve its effect.

Resistance. Susceptible Gram-positive bacteria acquire resistance to beta lactams mainly through the induction of beta-lactamases, including penicillinases. These enzymes are liberated extracellularly and hydrolyse the beta-lactam ring. This resistance is usually plasmid-mediated and can be transferred from one bacterium to another. Gram-negative bacteria produce beta-lactamases within their cell membranes which may be chromosomally or plasmid-mediated; all Gram-negative species probably contain small amounts of beta-lactamases. Resistance in Gram-negative species may also be due to changes in their outer membrane resulting in the failure of beta lactams to reach their target penicillin-binding proteins. Changes in the binding characteristics of penicillin-binding proteins may also result in resistance in Gram-positive and Gram-negative bacteria.

Most strains of *Staphylococcus aureus* are now resistant to benzylpenicillin. *Streptococcus pneumoniae* with reduced susceptibility or complete resistance to benzylpenicillin have increasingly been reported. Strains of *Neisseria meningitidis* with reduced sensitivity to benzylpenicillin have been reported. Penicillinase-producing *Neisseria gonorrhoeae* are widespread; reduced sensitivity of gonococci to benzylpenicillin may also result from alterations in penicillin-binding proteins. Resistant strains of other species usually sensitive to benzylpenicillin have emerged among *Bacillus anthracis* and *Corynebacterium diphtheriae*. Most strains of *Haemophilus influenzae* and *Moraxella catarrhalis* (*Branhamella catarrhalis*) are now resistant.

Some organisms, usually Gram-positive cocci such as staphylococci or streptococci, may develop tolerance and are inhibited but not killed by benzylpenicillin; in such cases the minimum bactericidal concentration is much greater than the minimum inhibitory concentration.

Pharmacokinetics
Benzylpenicillin rapidly appears in the blood following intramuscular injection of water-soluble salts, and maximum concentrations are usually reached in 15 to 30 minutes; peak plasma concentrations of about 12 μg per mL have been reported after single doses of 600 mg.

When given by mouth, benzylpenicillin is inactivated fairly rapidly by gastric acid and only up to about 30% is absorbed, mainly from the duodenum; maximum plasma-penicillin concentrations usually occur in about 1 hour. In order to attain plasma-penicillin concentrations after oral administration similar to those following intramuscular injection, up to 5 times as much benzylpenicillin may be necessary. Absorption varies greatly in different individuals and is better in patients with reduced gastric acid production, including neonates and the elderly. Food decreases the absorption of benzylpenicillin and oral doses are best given at least half an hour before or 2 to 3 hours after a meal.

Benzylpenicillin is widely distributed at varying concentrations in body tissues and fluids. It appears in pleural, pericardial, peritoneal, and synovial fluids, but in the absence of inflammation diffuses only to a small extent into abscess cavities, avascular areas, the eye, the middle ear, and the CSF. Inflamed tissue is, however, more readily penetrated and, for example, in meningitis higher concentrations of benzylpenicillin are achieved in the CSF. Active transport out of the CSF is reduced by probenecid. In patients with uraemia, other organic acids may accumulate in the CSF and compete with benzylpenicillin for active transport; toxic concentrations of benzylpenicillin sufficient to cause convulsions can result.

Benzylpenicillin diffuses across the placenta into the fetal circulation, and small amounts appear in breast milk.

The plasma half-life is about 30 minutes although it may be longer in neonates and the elderly because of incomplete renal function. In renal impairment the half-life may be increased to about 10 hours. Approximately 60% is reported to be bound to plasma protein.

Benzylpenicillin is metabolised to a limited extent and the penicilloic acid derivative has been recovered in the urine. Benzylpenicillin is rapidly excreted in the urine, principally by tubular secretion and about 20% of a dose given by mouth appears unchanged in the urine; about 60 to 90% of a dose of aqueous benzylpenicillin given intramuscularly appears in the urine, mainly within the first hour. Significant concentrations are achieved in bile, but in patients with normal renal function only small amounts are excreted via the bile. Benzylpenicillin is removed by haemodialysis.

Renal tubular secretion is inhibited by probenecid (p.402), which is sometimes given to increase plasma-penicillin concentrations.

Uses and Administration

Benzylpenicillin is used in the treatment of a variety of infections due to susceptible organisms (see Antimicrobial Action, above). They include abscess, actinomycosis, anthrax, bites and stings, diphtheria, endocarditis, gas gangrene, leptospirosis, Lyme disease, meningitis, meningococcal infections, necrotising enterocolitis, necrotising fasciitis, neonatal conjunctivitis (if gonococci are sensitive), perinatal streptococcal infections (intrapartum prophylaxis against group B streptococci), pharyngitis (or tonsillitis), pneumonia, skin infections, syphilis (neurosyphilis and congenital syphilis), tetanus, toxic shock syndrome, and Whipple's disease. It is also used for surgical infection prophylaxis in first trimester abortion in women at high risk of pelvic infection. For details of these infections and their treatment, see under Choice of Antibacterial, p.114.

Administration and dosage. Benzylpenicillin is usually administered intramuscularly or intravenously. For some indications benzathine benzylpenicillin (p.156) or procaine penicillin [procaine benzylpenicillin] (p.239), which provide a prolonged effect, are preferred; they are given intramuscularly. Benzylpenicillin is sometimes given by mouth for infections of moderate severity, but one of the acid-resistant penicillins such as phenoxymethylpenicillin (p.235) is preferable.

Benzylpenicillin is available as the potassium or sodium salt. The dose of benzylpenicillin should be sufficient to achieve an optimum bactericidal concentration in the blood as rapidly as possible; concentrations may be increased by concurrent administration of probenecid (p.402). In some countries, doses are still expressed in units (see above).

For some infections, adult doses of 0.6 to 2.4 g of benzylpenicillin daily in 2 to 4 divided doses by intramuscular or slow intravenous injection or intravenous infusion may be adequate, but higher doses given intravenously, often by infusion, are more usual for severe infections. For example, in endocarditis, benzylpenicillin 7.2 g daily (1.2 g every 4 hours) intravenously, usually with an aminoglycoside, is recommended; doses of 18 g or more daily are not unusual for less sensitive streptococci and enterococci. In meningococcal and pneumococcal meningitis, benzylpenicillin 9.6 to 14.4 g daily (2.4 g every 4 to 6 hours) intravenously is recommended; up to 18 g daily has been recommended for meningococcal menin-

gitis. High doses should be administered slowly to avoid irritation of the CNS and electrolyte imbalance, and a rate of not more than 300 mg per minute is recommended for intravenous doses above 1.2 g. High doses may need to be reduced in patients with renal impairment.

Infants and children from 1 month to 12 years may be given 100 mg per kg body-weight daily in 4 divided doses; infants aged 1 to 4 weeks, 75 mg per kg daily in 3 divided doses; and neonates 50 mg per kg daily in 2 divided doses.

As in adults, higher paediatric doses may be necessary in severe infections. A dose of 180 to 300 mg per kg daily given intravenously in 4 to 6 divided doses is recommended for meningococcal meningitis in infants and children from 1 month to 12 years of age; infants aged 1 to 4 weeks may be given 150 mg per kg daily in 3 divided doses; neonates up to 7 days old may be given 100 mg per kg daily in 2 divided doses.

In patients with suspected meningococcal infection, an intravenous or intramuscular injection of benzylpenicillin should be given before transfer to hospital. Doses are: adults and children aged 10 years or more, 1.2 g; children aged 1 to 9 years, 600 mg; children under 1 year, 300 mg.

A dose for intrapartum prophylaxis against group B streptococcal infection is benzylpenicillin 3 g initially then 1.5 g every 4 hours until delivery.

Other routes. For subconjunctival injection, 300 or 600 mg of benzylpenicillin may be dissolved in 0.5 to 1.0 mL of water, or another suitable solvent such as lignocaine [lidocaine] 2% with or without adrenaline [epinephrine] 1 in 100 000.

Benzylpenicillin is sometimes given by mouth in adult doses of 125 to 312 mg every 4 to 6 hours administered on an empty stomach.

Intrathecal injections are no longer recommended.

Preparations

BP 2001: Benzylpenicillin Injection; Fortified Procaine Benzylpenicillin Injection;
USP 25: Penicillin G Potassium Capsules; Penicillin G Potassium for Injection; Penicillin G Potassium for Oral Solution; Penicillin G Potassium Injection; Penicillin G Potassium Tablets; Penicillin G Sodium for Injection.

Proprietary Preparations (details are given in Part 3)

Austral.: Benpen; *Braz.:* Isacilin; Megapen; *Canad.:* Crystapen; Megacillin†; Novo-Pen-G†; *Fin.:* Geepenil; *Irl.:* Crystapen; *Mex.:* Hidrociclina; Pengesod; Sodipen; *NZ:* Benpen; *Port.:* Atralcilina; Atralmicina; *S.Afr.:* Benzatec; Novopen; *Spain:* Coliriocilina; Pekamin; Penibiot; Penibiot Lidocaina†; Penilevel; Peniroger†; Sodiopen; Unicilina; *UK:* Crystapen; *USA:* Pfizerpen.

Multi-ingredient: *Aust.:* Antipen†; Fortepen†; Ophcillin N; Retarpen compositum; *Austral.:* Bicillin All Purpose†; *Braz.:* Benapen; Climacilin; Despacilina; Drenovac; Expectovac; Ginurovac; Linfocilin; Odontovac; Ortocilin; Pulmocilin; Wycillin R; *Canad.:* Bicillin A-P†; *Fr.:* Biclinocilline; Gomenol-Syner-Penicilline†; *Ger.:* Bipensaar; Hydracillin†; Jenacillin A; Retacillin; *Israel:* Duplo-Penicillin; Penicillin Fortified; *Ital.:* Tri-Wycillina; *Mex.:* Anapenil; Bencelin Combinado; Benzanil Compuesto; Benzetacil Combinado; Megapenil Forte; Pendiben Compuesto; Penicil; Penipot; Penisodina; Penprocilina; *Neth.:* Bicilline†; Penidural D/F; *Port.:* Penadur 6.3.3; Prevecilina; *S.Afr.:* Penilente Forte; Ultracillin; *Spain:* Anapen†; Aqucilina D A; Benzetacil Compuesta; Cepacilina 321, 621, or 633†; Neocepacilina†; Neopenyl; Neumobiot†; Penilevel Retard; *UK:* Bicillin†.

Betamipron   (15257-m)

Betamipron *(rINN)*.

N-Benzoyl-β-alanine; CS-443. 3-Benzamidopropionic acid.
$C_{10}H_{11}NO_3 = 193.2$.
CAS — 3440-28-6.

Profile

Betamipron is a renal protectant used in combination with the carbapenem antibiotic panipenem to reduce its adverse renal effects.

Preparations

Proprietary Preparations (details are given in Part 3)

Multi-ingredient: *Jpn:* Carbenin.

Biapenem   (13919-s)

Biapenem *(USAN, rINN)*.

CL-186815; L-627; LJC-10627. 6-{[(4R,5S,6S)-2-Carboxy-6-[(1R)-1-hydroxyethyl]-4-methyl-7-oxo-1-azabicyclo[3.2.0]hept-2-en-3-yl]thio}-6,7-dihydro-5H-pyrazolo[1,2-a]s-triazol-4-ium hydroxide, inner salt.
$C_{15}H_{18}N_4O_4S = 350.4$.
CAS — 120410-24-4.

Profile

Biapenem is a carbapenem beta-lactam antibiotic similar to imipenem (p.214). Like meropenem (p.222) it is reported to be more stable to renal dehydropeptidase I than imipenem.

◊ References.

1. Malanoski GJ, et al. In vitro activity of biapenem against clinical isolates of Gram-positive and Gram-negative bacteria. *Antimicrob Agents Chemother* 1993; **37:** 2009–16.
2. Aldridge KE, et al. In vitro activity of biapenem (L-627), a new carbapenem, against anaerobes. *Antimicrob Agents Chemother* 1994; **38:** 889–93.
3. Yeo S-F, Livermore DM. Comparative in-vitro activity of biapenem and other carbapenems against Haemophilus influenzae isolates with known resistance mechanisms to ampicillin. *J Antimicrob Chemother* 1994; **33:** 861–5.
4. Chen HY, Livermore DM. In-vitro activity of biapenem, compared with imipenem and meropenem, against Pseudomonas aeruginosa strains and mutants with known resistance mechanisms. *J Antimicrob Chemother* 1994; **33:** 949–58.
5. Piddock LJV, Jin YF. Activity of biapenem (LJC 10627) against 51 imipenem-resistant bacteria and selection and characterisation of biapenem-resistant mutants. *J Antimicrob Chemother* 1995; **36:** 845–50.
6. Koeppe P, et al. Biapenem pharmacokinetics in healthy volunteers and in patients with impaired renal function. *Arzneimittelforschung* 1997; **47:** 1250–6.
7. Kozawa O, et al. Pharmacokinetics and safety of a new parenteral carbapenem antibiotic, biapenem (L-627), in elderly subjects. *Antimicrob Agents Chemother* 1998; **42:** 1433–6.

Brodimoprim   (16546-x)

Brodimoprim *(rINN)*.

2,4-Diamino-5-(4-bromo-3,5-dimethoxybenzyl)pyrimidine.
$C_{13}H_{15}BrN_4O_2 = 339.2$.
CAS — 56518-41-3.
ATC — J01EA02.

Profile

Brodimoprim is closely related structurally to trimethoprim (p.264) and is used in the treatment of infections of the respiratory tract and ear.

◊ References.

1. Braunsteiner AR, Finsinger F. Brodimoprim: therapeutic efficacy and safety in the treatment of bacterial infections. *J Chemother* 1993; **5:** 507–11.

Preparations

Proprietary Preparations (details are given in Part 3)
Ital.: Hyprim†; Unitrim†; *Mex.:* Novatrim.

Calcium Sulfaloxate   (4901-j)

Calcium Sulfaloxate *(BANM, rINNM)*.

Calcium Sulphaloxate. Calcium 4'-[(hydroxymethylcarbamoyl)sulphamoyl]phthalanilate pentahydrate.
$(C_{16}H_{14}N_3O_7S)_2Ca,5H_2O = 914.9$.
CAS — 14376-16-0 (sulfaloxic acid); 59672-20-7 (calcium sulfaloxate).

Profile

Calcium sulfaloxate is a sulfonamide with properties similar to those of sulfamethoxazole (p.254). It is poorly absorbed, about 95% remaining in the intestine, and has been given for its antibacterial action in the gastrointestinal tract.

Capreomycin Sulfate   (7554-l)

Capreomycin Sulfate *(USAN, rINN)*.

34977; Capreomycin Sulphate *(BANM)*; Capreomycin Sulphate.
CAS — 11003-38-6 (capreomycin); 1405-37-4 (capreomycin sulfate).
Pharmacopoeias. In Br., Chin., and US.

Capreomycin I consists of capreomycin IA ($C_{25}H_{44}N_{14}O_8 = 668.7$) and capreomycin IB ($C_{25}H_{44}N_{14}O_7 = 652.7$) which predominates. Capreomycin II which makes up about 10% of the mixture consists of capreomycin IIA and capreomycin IIB.

Pharmacopoeial description

BP 2001: A mixture of the sulfates of antimicrobial substances produced by certain strains of *Streptomyces capreolus*. The potency is not less than 700 units per mg. A white or almost white solid. Very soluble in water; practically insoluble in alcohol, in chloroform, and in ether. A 3% solution has a pH of 4.5 to 7.5. Store at a temperature not exceeding 25°.

USP 25: The disulfate of capreomycin, a polypeptide mixture produced by the growth of *Streptomyces capreolus*. It contains not less than 90% of capreomycin I. A white to practically white amorphous powder. Freely soluble in water; practically insoluble in most organic solvents. pH of a 3% solution in water is between 4.5 and 7.5. Store in airtight containers.

Adverse Effects and Treatment

The effects of capreomycin on the kidney and eighth cranial nerve are similar to those of aminoglycosides such as gentamicin (p.210). Nitrogen retention, renal tubular dysfunction, and progressive renal damage may occur. Hypokalaemia and other electrolyte abnormalities have been reported. Vertigo, tinnitus, and hearing loss may also occur and are sometimes irreversible. Abnormalities in liver function have been reported when capreomycin has been administered with other antituberculous drugs. Hypersensitivity reactions including urticaria, maculopapular rashes, and sometimes fever have been reported. Leucocytosis and leucopenia have also been observed. Thrombocytopenia has been reported rarely. Eosinophilia commonly occurs with capreomycin. Capreomycin also has a neuromuscular blocking action. There may be pain, induration, and excessive bleeding at the site of intramuscular injection; sterile abscesses may also form.

Teratogenicity has been observed following high doses in *rodents*.

Treatment of overdose is generally supportive. Patients with normal renal function should be hydrated to maintain adequate urine output. Capreomycin is removed by haemodialysis.

Precautions

Capreomycin should be given with care and in reduced dosage to patients with impaired renal function. Care is also essential in patients with signs of eighth cranial nerve damage. It is advisable to monitor renal and auditory function and serum-potassium concentrations in patients before and during therapy. Periodic assessment of hepatic function is also recommended.

Interactions

Care should be taken when capreomycin is used with other drugs that have neuromuscular blocking activity. It should not be administered with other drugs that are ototoxic or nephrotoxic.

Antimicrobial Action

Capreomycin is bacteriostatic against various mycobacteria. An MIC of 10 µg per mL has been reported for *Mycobacterium tuberculosis*, though this varies greatly with the media used. Resistance develops readily if capreomycin is used alone. It shows cross-resistance with kanamycin and neomycin.

◊ References.
1. Ho YII, *et al.* In-vitro activities of aminoglycoside-aminocyclitols against mycobacteria. *J Antimicrob Chemother* 1997; **40**: 27–32.

Pharmacokinetics

Capreomycin is poorly absorbed from the gastrointestinal tract. A dose of 1 g administered intramuscularly has been reported to give a peak serum concentration of about 30 µg per mL after 1 or 2 hours. About 50% of a dose is excreted unchanged in the urine by glomerular filtration within 12 hours. Capreomycin is removed by haemodialysis.

Uses and Administration

Capreomycin is a second-line antimycobacterial that may be used in the treatment of tuberculosis (p.143) as part of a multidrug regimen when resistance to or toxicity from primary drugs has developed.

Capreomycin is administered as the sulfate by deep intramuscular injection or by intravenous infusion. The usual adult dose is the equivalent of 1 g of capreomycin base (maximum 20 mg per kg body-weight) given daily for 2 to 4 months, then two or three times weekly for the remainder of therapy. Experience in children is limited.

As with aminoglycosides, the dose of capreomycin in patients with reduced renal function must be adjusted based on creatinine clearance; the desired steady-state serum capreomycin level is 10 µg per mL.

Preparations

BP 2001: Capreomycin Injection;
USP 25: Capreomycin for Injection.

Proprietary Preparations (details are given in Part 3)
Aust.: Capastat; **Austral.:** Capastat; **Canad.:** Capastat†; **Spain:** Capastat; **UK:** Capastat; **USA:** Capastat.

Carbadox (12522-m)

Carbadox (BAN, USAN, pINN).
GS-6244. Methyl 3-quinoxalin-2-ylmethylenecarbazate 1,4-dioxide.
$C_{11}H_{10}N_4O_4 = 262.2$.
CAS — 6804-07-5.

Profile

Carbadox is an antibacterial that has been used in veterinary practice for treating swine dysentery and enteritis and for promoting growth. However, its use has been prohibited in the UK following reports of carcinogenicity.

Carbenicillin Sodium (24-f)

Carbenicillin Sodium (BANM, rINNM).
BRL-2064; Carbenicillin Disodium (USAN); Carbenicillinum Natricum; α-Carboxybenzylpenicillin Sodium; CP-15-639-2; GS-3159 (carbenicillin potassium); NSC-111071. The disodium salt of (6R)-6-(2-carboxy-2-phenylacetamido)penicillanic acid .
$C_{17}H_{16}N_2Na_2O_6S = 422.4$.
CAS — 4697-36-3 (carbenicillin); 4800-94-6 (carbenicillin disodium); 17230-86-3 (carbenicillin potassium).
Pharmacopoeias. In Eur. (see p.vi), Pol., and US.

1.1 g of monograph substance is approximately equivalent to 1 g of carbenicillin. Each g of monograph substance represents about 4.7 mmol of sodium.

Carbenicillin sodium has been reported to be incompatible with aminoglycosides, tetracyclines, and a number of other drugs including other antimicrobials.

Pharmacopoeial description

Ph. Eur.: A white or slightly yellowish, hygroscopic powder. Freely soluble in water; soluble in alcohol and in methyl alcohol. A 5% solution in water has a pH of 5.5 to 7.5. Store at a temperature between 2° and 8° in airtight containers. Protect from light.

USP 25: A white to off-white crystalline powder. Freely soluble in water; soluble in alcohol; practically insoluble in chloroform and in ether. pH of a solution in water containing the equivalent of carbenicillin 1% is between 6.5 and 8.0. Store in airtight containers.

Adverse Effects

As for Benzylpenicillin, p.157.

Pain at the injection site and phlebitis may occur. Electrolyte disturbances, particularly hypokalaemia or hypernatraemia, may follow the administration of large doses of carbenicillin sodium.

A dose-dependent coagulation defect has been reported, especially in patients with renal failure. Carbenicillin appears to interfere with platelet function thereby prolonging bleeding time; purpura and haemorrhage from mucous membranes and elsewhere may result.

Precautions

As for Benzylpenicillin, p.158.

Carbenicillin sodium should be given with caution to patients on a restricted sodium diet.

Carbenicillin sodium and other antipseudomonal penicillins have been shown to be incompatible with gentamicin and some other aminoglycosides *in vitro* and they should therefore be administered separately.

Interactions

As for Benzylpenicillin, p.158.

Antimicrobial Action

Carbenicillin has a bactericidal mode of action similar to that of benzylpenicillin, but with an extended spectrum of activity against Gram-negative bacteria. The most important feature of carbenicillin is its activity against *Pseudomonas aeruginosa*, although high concentrations are generally necessary. Activity against *Ps. aeruginosa* and some other organisms can be enhanced by gentamicin and other aminoglycosides. Carbenicillin is also active against *Proteus*, including indole-positive spp. such as *Pr. vulgaris*. It is comparable with ampicillin against other Gram-negative bacteria. Sensitive organisms include some Enterobacteriaceae, for example *Escherichia coli* and *Enterobacter* spp.; *Haemophilus influenzae*; and *Neisseria* spp. *Klebsiella* spp. are usually insensitive. Its activity against Gram-positive bacteria is less than that of benzylpenicillin. Anaerobic organisms are generally susceptible to carbenicillin, but for *Bacteroides fragilis* high concentrations are required.

Minimum inhibitory concentrations (MICs) of carbenicillin against bacteria considered susceptible range from about 0.1 to 32 µg per mL. Against *Ps. aeruginosa* an MIC of 16 to 32 µg per mL has been cited, but much higher concentrations may be necessary; isolates have been considered by some to be resistant when the MIC exceeds 128 µg per mL.

Resistance. Carbenicillin is inactivated by penicillinases and some other beta-lactamases, although it is more stable to the chromosomally mediated beta-lactamases produced by some Gram-negative organisms, including *Ps. aeruginosa* and some *Proteus* spp. Resistance to carbenicillin may develop in *Ps. aeruginosa* during treatment with carbenicillin or other beta-lactams. This resistance may be intrinsic where there are changes in cell wall permeability or penicillin-binding proteins, or it may be due to plasmid-mediated beta-lactamase production that may be transferred to and from certain strains of Enterobacteriaceae.

There may be cross-resistance between carbenicillin and other antipseudomonal penicillins.

Outbreaks of pseudomonal resistance to carbenicillin have been associated with extensive use in, for example, hospital burns units.

Pharmacokinetics

Carbenicillin is not absorbed from the gastrointestinal tract and

has therefore been given either intramuscularly or intravenously.

The half-life of carbenicillin is reported to be about 1 to 1.5 hours; it is increased in patients with renal impairment, especially if there is hepatic impairment, and also in neonates. Half-lives of 10 to 20 hours have been reported in severe renal impairment. Clearance is enhanced in patients with cystic fibrosis. Carbenicillin is approximately 50% bound to plasma proteins. Distribution of carbenicillin in the body is similar to that of other penicillins. Small amounts have been detected in breast milk. There is little diffusion into the CSF except when the meninges are inflamed.

Relatively high concentrations have been reported in bile, but carbenicillin is excreted principally by renal tubular secretion and glomerular filtration.

Administration of probenecid increases and prolongs the plasma concentrations of carbenicillin.

Carbenicillin is removed by haemodialysis and, to some extent, by peritoneal dialysis.

Uses and Administration

Carbenicillin is a carboxypenicillin that has been given by injection as the disodium salt, often in association with gentamicin, in the treatment of infections due to *Pseudomonas aeruginosa*; however, other antipseudomonal penicillins such as ticarcillin (p.262) or piperacillin (p.236) are now preferred. It has also been given to treat serious infections due to non-penicillinase-producing strains of *Proteus* spp.

Esters of carbenicillin, such as carfecillin (p.160) and carindacillin (p.160), have been given by mouth in the treatment of urinary-tract infections.

Preparations

USP 25: Carbenicillin for Injection.

Proprietary Preparations (details are given in Part 3)
Ital.: Geopen†; **Mex.:** Carbecin; Myciclid; **Spain:** Geopen†.

Carfecillin Sodium (25-d)

Carfecillin Sodium (BANM, pINNM).
BRL-3475; Carbenicillin Phenyl Sodium (USAN). Sodium (6R)-6-(2-phenoxycarbonyl-2-phenylacetamido)penicillanate.
$C_{23}H_{21}N_2NaO_6S = 476.5$.
CAS — 27025-49-6 (carfecillin); 21649-57-0 (carfecillin sodium).

Profile

Carfecillin is the phenyl ester of carbenicillin (p.160) to which it is hydrolysed following absorption from the gastrointestinal tract. Its use has been restricted to the treatment of urinary-tract infections due to *Pseudomonas* spp. and other sensitive bacteria including *Proteus* spp.

Preparations

Proprietary Preparations (details are given in Part 3)
Ital.: Urocarf†.

Carindacillin Sodium (26-n)

Carindacillin Sodium (BANM, pINNM).
Carbenicillin Indanyl Sodium (USAN); CP-15464-2. Sodium (6R)-6-[2-(indan-5-yloxycarbonyl)-2-phenylacetamido]penicillanate.
$C_{26}H_{25}N_2NaO_6S = 516.5$.
CAS — 35531-88-5 (carindacillin); 26605-69-6 (carindacillin sodium).
Pharmacopoeias. In US.

1.4 g of monograph substance is approximately equivalent to 1 g of carbenicillin. Each g of monograph substance represents about 1.9 mmol of sodium.

Pharmacopoeial description

USP 25: A white to off-white powder. Soluble in water and in alcohol. pH of a 10% solution in water is between 5.0 and 8.0. Store in airtight containers.

Profile

Carindacillin is the indanyl ester of carbenicillin (p.160) to which it is hydrolysed following absorption from the gastrointestinal tract. Its use is restricted to the treatment of urinary-tract infections due to *Pseudomonas* spp. and other sensitive bacteria including *Proteus* spp.

It is given by mouth as carindacillin sodium. Usual doses, expressed in terms of carbenicillin, are 382 to 764 mg four times daily.

Preparations

USP 25: Carbenicillin Indanyl Sodium Tablets.

Proprietary Preparations (details are given in Part 3)
Hong Kong: Geopen; **USA:** Geocillin.

Carumonam Sodium (18916-d)

Carumonam Sodium (BANM, USAN, rINNM).

AMA-1080 (carumonam); Ro-17-2301 (carumonam); Ro-17-2301/006 (carumonam sodium). (Z)-(2S,3S)-2-carbamoyloxymethyl-4-oxo-1-sulphoazetidin-3-yl]carbamoyl}methyleneamino-oxyacetic acid, disodium salt.

$C_{12}H_{12}N_6Na_2O_{10}S_2 = 510.4$.

CAS — 87638-04-8 (carumonam); 86832-68-0 (carumonam sodium).

Pharmacopoeias. In Jpn.

Profile

Carumonam sodium is a monobactam antibiotic with a spectrum of antimicrobial action in vitro similar to that of aztreonam (p.154). It is given by intramuscular or intravenous injection in a usual dose of 1 to 2 g daily in two divided doses.

Preparations

Proprietary Preparations (details are given in Part 3)
Jpn: Amasulin.

Cefaclor (27-h)

Cefaclor (BAN, USAN, pINN).

Cefaclorum; Compound 99638. (7R)-3-Chloro-7-(α-D-phenylglycylamino)-3-cephem-4-carboxylic acid monohydrate.

$C_{15}H_{14}ClN_3O_4S,H_2O = 385.8$.

CAS — 53994-73-3 (anhydrous cefaclor); 70356-03-5 (cefaclor monohydrate).

ATC — J01DA08.

Pharmacopoeias. In Eur. (see p.vi) and US. Jpn includes the anhydrous substance.

1.05 g of monograph substance is approximately equivalent to 1 g of anhydrous cefaclor.

Pharmacopoeial description

Ph. Eur.: A white or slightly yellow powder. Slightly soluble in water; practically insoluble in dichloromethane and in methyl alcohol. A 2.5% suspension in water has a pH of 3.0 to 4.5.
USP 25: A white to off-white crystalline powder. Slightly soluble in water; practically insoluble in chloroform, in methyl alcohol, and in benzene. pH of a 2.5% suspension in water is between 3.0 and 4.5. Store in airtight containers.

Adverse Effects and Precautions

As for Cefalexin, p.162.

Hypersensitivity. Serum-sickness-like reactions may be more common with cefaclor than several other oral antibacterials[1] especially in young children who have received a number of courses of cefaclor;[2] typical features include skin reactions and arthralgia. A relatively high incidence of anaphylactic reactions has been reported from Japan.[3]

There has been a report of myocarditis that developed as a hypersensitivity reaction to cefaclor in a 12-year-old child.[4]

1. McCue JD. Delayed detection of serum sickness caused by oral antimicrobials. Adv Therapy 1990; 7: 22–7.
2. Vial T, et al. Cefaclor-associated serum sickness-like disease: eight cases and review of the literature. Ann Pharmacother 1992; 26: 910–14.
3. Hama R, Mori K. High incidence of anaphylactic reactions to cefaclor. Lancet 1988; i: 1331.
4. Beghetti M, et al. Hypersensitivity myocarditis caused by an allergic reaction to cefaclor. J Pediatr 1998; 132: 172–3.

Interactions

As for Cefalexin, p.162.

Anticoagulants. The UK manufacturer recommends that monitoring of prothrombin time should be considered in patients receiving cefaclor and warfarin following rare reports of increased prothrombin times. It is not known whether this interaction is related to the vitamin K-related hypoprothrombinaemia observed with some cephalosporins (see Cefamandole, p.163), but cefaclor does not contain the side-chain usually implicated in this reaction.

Antimicrobial Action

Cefaclor is bactericidal and has antimicrobial activity similar to that of cefalexin (p.162) but is reported to be more active against Gram-negative bacteria including Escherichia coli, Klebsiella pneumoniae, Neisseria gonorrhoeae, and Proteus mirabilis, and especially against Haemophilus influenzae. It is active against some beta-lactamase-producing strains of H. influenzae. It may be less resistant to staphylococcal penicillinase than cefalexin or cefradine and a marked inoculum effect has been reported in vitro.

Pharmacokinetics

Cefaclor is well absorbed from the gastrointestinal tract but plasma concentrations are slightly lower than those achieved with cefalexin or cefradine. Doses of 250 mg, 500 mg, and 1 g by mouth produce peak plasma concentrations of about 7, 13, and 23 µg per mL respectively after 0.5 to 1 hour. The presence of food may delay the absorption of cefaclor, but the total amount absorbed is unchanged. A plasma half-life of 0.5 to 1 hour has been reported; it may be slightly prolonged in patients with renal impairment. About 25% is bound to plasma proteins.

Cefaclor appears to be widely distributed in the body; it crosses the placenta and low concentrations have been detected in breast milk. It is rapidly excreted by the kidneys; up to 85% of a dose appears unchanged in the urine within 8 hours, the greater part within 2 hours. High concentrations of cefaclor are achieved in the urine within 8 hours of a dose; peak concentrations of 600, 900, and 1900 µg per mL have been reported after doses of 250 mg, 500 mg, and 1 g respectively. Probenecid delays excretion. Some cefaclor is removed by haemodialysis.

◊ References.
1. Wise R. The pharmacokinetics of the oral cephalosporins—a review. J Antimicrob Chemother 1990; 26 (suppl E): 13–20.

Uses and Administration

Cefaclor is a cephalosporin antibiotic given by mouth similarly to cefalexin in the treatment of susceptible infections including upper and lower respiratory-tract infections, skin infections, and urinary-tract infections. Some classify cefaclor as a second-generation cephalosporin and its greater activity against Haemophilus influenzae makes it more suitable than cefalexin for the treatment of infections such as otitis media. For details of these infections and their treatment, see under Choice of Antibacterial, p.114.

Cefaclor is given as the monohydrate. Doses are expressed in terms of the equivalent amount of anhydrous cefaclor. The usual adult dose is 250 to 500 mg every 8 hours; up to 4 g daily has been given. A suggested dose for children over 1 month of age is 20 mg per kg body-weight daily in three divided doses, increased if necessary to 40 mg per kg daily, but not exceeding a total daily dose of 1 g. A common dosage regimen is: children over 5 years, 250 mg three times daily; 1 to 5 years, 125 mg three times daily; under 1 year, 62.5 mg three times daily.

Preparations

BP 2001: Cefaclor Capsules; Cefaclor Oral Suspension; Slow Cefaclor Tablets;
USP 25: Cefaclor Capsules; Cefaclor Extended-Release Tablets; Cefaclor for Oral Suspension.

Proprietary Preparations (details are given in Part 3)
Aust.: Cec; Ceclor; Austral.: Ceclor; Cefkor; Keflor; Vercef; Belg.: Ceclor; Braz.: Ceclor; Canad.: Ceclor; Fin.: Kefolor; Fr.: Alfatil; Alphexine; Ger.: Cec; Ceclorbeta; Cef-Diolan; Cefa-Wolff; Cefallone; Ceph-Biocin; InfectoCef; Kefspor; Panoral; Sigacefal; Hong Kong: Ceclor; Irl.: Distaclor; Keftid; Israel: Ceclor; Cefalor; Ital.: Citiclor; Clorad; Fuclode; Kliacef; Panacef; Mex.: Ceclor; Neth.: Ceclor; N.Z.: Ceclor; Port.: Ceclor; S.Afr.: Cec; Ceclor; CloraCEF; Kloclor†; Vercef; Singapore: Cleancef; Distaclor; Vercef; Spain: Ceclor; Swed.: Kefolor†; Switz.: Ceclor; Thai.: Distaclor; Kefaclor; Sifaclor; Tefaclor; Vercef; UAE: Recocef; UK: Distaclor; Keftid; USA: Ceclor.

Multi-ingredient: Ger.: Muco Panoral.

Cefadroxil (28-m)

Cefadroxil (BAN, USAN, pINN).

BL-S578; Cefadroxilum; Cephadroxil; MJF-11567-3. (7R)-7-(α-D-4-Hydroxyphenylglycylamino)-3-methyl-3-cephem-4-carboxylic acid monohydrate.

$C_{16}H_{17}N_3O_5S,H_2O = 381.4$.

CAS — 50370-12-2 (anhydrous cefadroxil); 119922-85-9 (cefadroxil hemihydrate); 66592-87-8 (cefadroxil monohydrate).

ATC — J01DA09.

Pharmacopoeias. In Chin., Eur. (see p.vi), and US. Jpn includes the anhydrous substance.

Pharmacopoeial description

Ph. Eur.: A white or almost white powder. Slightly soluble in water; very slightly soluble in alcohol; practically insoluble in ether. A 5% suspension in water has a pH of 4.0 to 6.0. Store at a temperature not exceeding 30°. Protect from light.
USP 25: A white to off-white crystalline powder. Slightly soluble in water; practically insoluble in alcohol, in chloroform, and in ether. pH of a 5% suspension in water is between 4.0 and 6.0. Store in airtight containers.

Adverse Effects and Precautions

As for Cefalexin, p.162.

Interactions

As for Cefalexin, p.162.

Antimicrobial Action

As for Cefalexin, p.162.

Pharmacokinetics

Cefadroxil is well absorbed from the gastrointestinal tract. After doses of 500 mg and 1 g by mouth, peak plasma concentrations of about 16 and 30 µg per mL respectively are obtained after 1.5 to 2 hours. Although peak concentrations are similar to those of cefalexin, plasma concentrations are more sustained. Administration with food does not appear to affect the absorption of cefadroxil. About 20% of cefadroxil in the circulation is reported to be bound to plasma proteins. The plasma half-life of cefadroxil is about 1.5 hours and is prolonged in patients with impaired renal function.

Cefadroxil is widely distributed to body tissues and fluids. It crosses the placenta and appears in breast milk.

More than 90% of a dose of cefadroxil may be excreted unchanged in the urine within 24 hours by glomerular filtration and tubular secretion; peak urinary concentrations of greater than 1 mg per mL have been reported after a dose of 500 mg. Cefadroxil is removed by haemodialysis.

◊ References.
1. Tanrisever B, Santella PJ. Cefadroxil: a review of its antibacterial, pharmacokinetic and therapeutic properties in comparison with cephradine and cephalexin. Drugs 1986; 32 (suppl 3): 1–16.
2. Wise R. The pharmacokinetics of the oral cephalosporins—a review. J Antimicrob Chemother 1990; 26 (suppl E): 13–20.
3. Garrigues TM, et al. Dose-dependent absorption and elimination of cefadroxil in man. Eur J Clin Pharmacol 1991; 41: 179–83.

Uses and Administration

Cefadroxil is a first-generation cephalosporin antibiotic that is the para-hydroxy derivative of cefalexin (p.162), and is used similarly in the treatment of mild to moderate susceptible infections. It is administered by mouth, and doses are expressed in terms of the anhydrous substance. Usually, 1 to 2 g is given daily as a single dose or in 2 divided doses to adults. The following doses are used in children: 500 mg twice daily for those over 6 years of age, 250 mg twice daily for children aged 1 to 6 years, and 25 mg per kg body-weight daily in divided doses for infants under 1 year.

Doses should be reduced in patients with impaired renal function.

Preparations

BP 2001: Cefadroxil Capsules; Cefadroxil Oral Suspension;
USP 25: Cefadroxil Capsules; Cefadroxil for Oral Suspension; Cefadroxil Tablets.

Proprietary Preparations (details are given in Part 3)
Aust.: Biodroxil†; Duracef; Belg.: Duracef; Moxacef; Braz.: Cefamox; Drocef; Canad.: Duricef; Fin.: Duracef; Fr.: Oracefal; Ger.: Bidocef†; Cedrox; Gruncef; Hong Kong: Amben; Androxyl; Biodroxil; Duracef; Irl.: Ultracef; Israel: Duracef; Ital.: Cefadril; Ceoxil; Cephos; Crenodyn; Foxil; Oradroxil; Jpn: Sedral†; Mex.: Cefamox; Duracef; Port.: Biofaxil; Cefacile; Ceforal; Cefra†; S.Afr.: Cedrox; Cipadur; Dacef; Duracef†; Singapore: Biodroxil; Duricef; Spain: Duracef; Swed.: Cefamox; Switz.: Duracef; Thai.: Cefadril; Duricef; UK: Baxan; USA: Duricef.

Cefalexin (37-b)

Cefalexin (BAN, pINN).

66873; Cefalexinum; Cephalexin (USAN). (7R)-3-Methyl-7-(α-D-phenylglycylamino)-3-cephem-4-carboxylic acid monohydrate.

$C_{16}H_{17}N_3O_4S,H_2O = 365.4$.

CAS — 15686-71-2 (anhydrous cefalexin); 23325-78-2 (cefalexin monohydrate).

ATC — J01DA01.

Pharmacopoeias. In Chin., Eur. (see p.vi), Jpn, Pol., and US. It. also includes Cephalexin Sodium.

1.05 g of monograph substance is approximately equivalent to 1 g of anhydrous cefalexin.

The symbol † denotes a preparation no longer actively marketed

Pharmacopoeial description

Ph. Eur.: A white or almost white crystalline powder. Soluble 1 in about 100 of water; practically insoluble in alcohol and in ether. A 0.5% solution in water has a pH of 4.0 to 5.5. Store at a temperature not exceeding 30°. Protect from light.

USP 25: A white to off-white crystalline powder. Slightly soluble in water; practically insoluble in alcohol, in chloroform, and in ether. pH of a 5% suspension in water is between 3.0 and 5.5. Store in airtight containers.

Cefalexin Hydrochloride (9391-h)

Cefalexin Hydrochloride (BANM, pINNM).
Cephalexin Hydrochloride (USAN); LY-061188.
$C_{16}H_{17}N_3O_4S,HCl,H_2O = 401.9$.
CAS — 105879-42-3.
Pharmacopoeias. In US.

1.16 g of monograph substance is approximately equivalent to 1 g of anhydrous cefalexin.

Pharmacopoeial description

USP 25: A white to off-white crystalline powder. Soluble 1 in 100 in water, in acetone, in acetonitrile, in alcohol, in dimethylformamide, and in methyl alcohol; practically insoluble in chloroform, in ether, in ethyl acetate, and in isopropyl alcohol. pH of a 1% solution in water is between 1.5 and 3.0. Store in airtight containers.

Adverse Effects and Precautions

As for Cefalotin Sodium, p.162.

The most common adverse effects of cefalexin and other oral cephalosporins are generally gastrointestinal disturbances and hypersensitivity reactions. Pseudomembranous colitis has been reported.

◊ References.
1. Dave J, et al. Cephalexin induced toxic epidermal necrolysis. J Antimicrob Chemother 1991; **28:** 477–8.
2. Baran R, Perrin C. Fixed-drug eruption presenting as an acute paronychia. Br J Dermatol 1991; **125:** 592–5.
3. Clark RF. Crystalluria following cephalexin overdose. Pediatrics 1992; **89:** 672–4.
4. Murray KM, Camp MS. Cephalexin-induced Stevens-Johnson syndrome. Ann Pharmacother 1992; **26:** 1230–3.

Porphyria. Cefalexin is considered to be unsafe in patients with porphyria although there is conflicting experimental evidence of porphyrinogenicity.

Interactions

The renal excretion of cefalexin, and many other cephalosporins, is delayed by probenecid.

Hormonal contraceptives. There have been isolated reports of cefalexin decreasing the efficacy of oestrogen-containing oral contraceptives.[1] For a discussion of decreased efficacy of oral contraceptives and the need for additional contraceptive methods in patients taking broad-spectrum antibacterials, see under Hormonal Contraceptives, p.1458.
1. Friedman M, et al. Cephalexin and Microgynon-30 do not go well together. J Obstet Gynaecol 1982; **2:** 195–6.

Antimicrobial Action

As for Cefalotin Sodium, p.163, although cefalexin is generally less potent. Some strains of Gram-negative bacteria may be inhibited only by the high concentrations achievable in the urinary tract. Haemophilus influenzae shows varying sensitivity to cefalexin.

Pharmacokinetics

Cefalexin is almost completely absorbed from the gastrointestinal tract and produces a peak plasma concentration of about 18 µg per mL one hour after a 500-mg oral dose; doubling the dose doubles the peak concentration. If cefalexin is taken with food, absorption may be delayed, but the total amount absorbed is not appreciably altered. Up to 15% of a dose is bound to plasma proteins. The plasma half-life is about 1 hour; it increases with reduced renal function.

Cefalexin is widely distributed in the body but does not enter the CSF in significant quantities. It crosses the placenta and small quantities are found in breast milk. Cefalexin is not metabolised. About 80% or more of a dose is excreted unchanged in the urine in the first 6 hours by glomerular filtration and tubular secretion; urinary concentrations greater than 1 mg per mL have been achieved after a dose of 500 mg. Probenecid delays urinary excretion. Therapeutically effective concentrations may be found in the bile and some may be excreted by this route.

Cefalexin is removed by haemodialysis and peritoneal dialysis.

◊ References.
1. Wise R. The pharmacokinetics of the oral cephalosporins—a review. J Antimicrob Chemother 1990; **26** (suppl E): 13–20.

Uses and Administration

Cefalexin is a first-generation cephalosporin antibacterial. It is administered by mouth for the treatment of susceptible infections including those of the respiratory and urinary tracts and of the skin (see under Choice of Antibacterial, p.114). For severe infections treatment with parenteral cephalosporins is to be preferred.

Cefalexin is usually given as the monohydrate although the hydrochloride is sometimes used. Doses are expressed in terms of the equivalent amount of anhydrous cefalexin.

The usual dose for adults is 1 to 2 g daily given in divided doses at 6-, 8-, or 12-hourly intervals; in severe or deep-seated infections the dose can be increased to up to 6 g daily but when high doses are required the use of a parenteral cephalosporin should be considered. Children may be given 25 to 100 mg per kg body-weight daily in divided doses to a maximum of 4 g daily.

For the prophylaxis of recurrent urinary-tract infection, cefalexin may be given in a dose of 125 mg at night.

Doses may need to be reduced in severe renal impairment.

Cefalexin sodium or cefalexin lysine have been used parenterally.

Preparations

BP 2001: Cefalexin Capsules; Cefalexin Oral Suspension; Cefalexin Tablets;
USP 25: Cephalexin Capsules; Cephalexin for Oral Suspension; Cephalexin Tablets.

Proprietary Preparations (details are given in Part 3)
Aust.: Cepexin; Cephalobene; Keflex; Ospexin; Sanaxin; *Austral.:* Ceflin; Cilex; Ibilex; Keflex; *Belg.:* Ceporex; Keforal; *Braz.:* Cefalen; Cefaporex; Ceporexin; Keflex; *Canad.:* Apo-Cephalex; Keflex; Novo-Lexin; Nu-Cephalex; *Denm.:* Keflex; *Fin.:* Kefalex; Kefexin; Orakef; *Fr.:* Cefacet; Ceporexine; Keforal; *Ger.:* Cephalex; Ceporexin; Oracef; *Hong Kong:* Apo-Cepalex; Ceporex; Felexin; Keflex; Medolexin; Ospexin; Solulexin; *Irl.:* Ceporex; Kefexin; Keflex; *Israel:* Cefalin; Ceforal; Cefovit; Keflex; *Ital.:* Ceporex; Keforal; Lafarin; *Mex.:* Cefalver; Ceporex; Falexol; Keflex; Meta-K; Quimosporina; Servicef; *Neth.:* Keforal; *Norw.:* Keflex; *NZ:* Keflex; *Port.:* Ceflax†; Ceporex; Keflex; *S.Afr.:* Betacef; Cerexin†; Fexin; Keflex; Lenocef; Ranceph; *Singapore:* Celexin; Ceporex; Felexin; Ospexin; Sofilex; Sporidex; *Spain:* Bioscefal; Cefalexgobens; Cefamiso; Defaxina; Efemida†; Karilexina; Kefloridina; Lexibiotico; Lexincef; Sulquipen; Torlasporin; *Swed.:* Keflex; *Switz.:* Keflex†; Servispor†; *Thai.:* Anxer; Cefexin; Celex; Celexin; Cephin; Ceporex; Felexin; Ibilex; Keflex; Servispor; Sialexin; Sporicef; Toflex; Zeplex; *UAE:* Cefrin; *UK:* Ceporex; Keflex; Kiflone†; *USA:* Biocef; Cefanex; Keflex; Keftab.

Multi-ingredient: *Mex.:* Mucocef; Rombox; *Spain:* Kefloridina Mucolitico.

Cefalonium (39-g)

Cefalonium (BAN, pINN).
41071; Carbamoylcefaloridine; Cephalonium. (7R)-3-(4-Carbamoyl-1-pyridiniomethyl)-7-[2-(2-thienyl)acetamido]-3-cephem-4-carboxylate.
$C_{20}H_{18}N_4O_5S_2 = 458.5$.
CAS — 5575-21-3.
Pharmacopoeias. BP(Vet) includes the dihydrate.

Pharmacopoeial description

BP(Vet) 2001: The dihydrate is a white or almost white crystalline powder. Very slightly soluble in water and in methyl alcohol; insoluble in alcohol, in dichloromethane, and in ether; soluble in dimethyl sulfoxide. It dissolves in dilute acids and in alkaline solutions. Store at temperature not exceeding 30°. Protect from light.

Profile

Cefalonium is a cephalosporin antibacterial used in veterinary practice.

Cefaloridine (40-f)

Cefaloridine (BAN, pINN).
40602; Cefaloridinum; Cephaloridine (USAN). (7R)-3-(1-Pyridiniomethyl)-7-[2-(2-thienyl)acetamido]-3-cephem-4-carboxylate.
$C_{19}H_{17}N_3O_4S_2 = 415.5$.
CAS — 50-59-9.
ATC — J01DA02.
Pharmacopoeias. In Aust., Belg., Fr., It., Jpn, Neth., and Port.

Profile

Cefaloridine was one of the first cephalosporin antibacterials to be available clinically. It has properties similar to those of cefalotin (below), but is more nephrotoxic and is seldom used now.

Preparations

Proprietary Preparations (details are given in Part 3)
Mex.: Ceporan.

Cefalotin Sodium (41-d)

Cefalotin Sodium (BANM, pINNM).
38253; Cefalotinum Natricum; Cephalothin Sodium (USAN); Sodium Cephalothin. Sodium (7R)-7-[2-(2-thienyl)acetamido]cephalosporanate; Sodium (7R)-3-acetoxymethyl-7-[2-(2-thienyl)acetamido]-3-cephem-4-carboxylate.
$C_{16}H_{15}N_2NaO_6S_2 = 418.4$.
CAS — 153-61-7 (cefalotin); 58-71-9 (cefalotin sodium).
Pharmacopoeias. In Chin., Eur. (see p.vi), Jpn, Pol., and US.

1.06 g of monograph substance is approximately equivalent to 1 g of cefalotin. Each g of monograph substance represents 2.39 mmol of sodium.

Cefalotin sodium has been reported to be incompatible with aminoglycosides and with many other drugs. Precipitation may occur in solutions with a pH of less than 5.

Pharmacopoeial description

Ph. Eur.: A white or almost white powder. Freely soluble in water; slightly soluble in dehydrated alcohol. A 10% solution in water has a pH of 4.5 to 7.0. Store in airtight containers. Protect from light.

USP 25: A white to off-white, practically odourless, crystalline powder. Freely soluble in water, in sodium chloride 0.9%, and in glucose solutions; insoluble in most organic solvents. pH of a 25% solution in water is between 4.5 and 7.0. Store in airtight containers.

Adverse Effects

The adverse effects associated with cefalotin and other cephalosporins are broadly similar to those described for penicillins (see Benzylpenicillin, p.157). The most common are hypersensitivity reactions, including skin rashes, urticaria, eosinophilia, fever, reactions resembling serum sickness, and anaphylaxis.

There may be a positive response to the Coombs' test although haemolytic anaemia rarely occurs. Neutropenia and thrombocytopenia have occasionally been reported. Agranulocytosis has been associated rarely with some cephalosporins. Bleeding complications related to hypoprothrombinaemia and/or platelet dysfunction have occurred especially with cephalosporins and cephamycins having a methylthiotetrazole side-chain, including cefamandole, cefbuperazone, cefmenoxime, cefmetazole, cefonicid, cefoperazone, ceforanide, cefotetan, cefpiramide, and latamoxef. The presence of a methylthiadiazolethiol side-chain, as in cefazolin, or a methylthiotriazine ring, as in ceftriaxone, might also be associated with such bleeding disorders.

Nephrotoxicity has been reported with cefalotin although it is less toxic than cefaloridine. Acute renal tubular necrosis has followed excessive dosage and has also been associated with its use in older patients or those with pre-existing renal impairment, or with the concomitant administration of nephrotoxic drugs such as aminoglycosides. Acute interstitial nephritis is also a possibility as a manifestation of hypersensitivity.

Transient increases in liver enzyme values have been reported. Hepatitis and cholestatic jaundice have occurred rarely with some cephalosporins.

Convulsions and other signs of CNS toxicity have been associated with high doses, especially in patients with severe renal impairment.

Gastrointestinal adverse effects such as nausea, vomiting, and diarrhoea have been reported rarely. Prolonged use may result in overgrowth of non-susceptible organisms and, as with other broad-spectrum antibiotics, pseudomembranous colitis may develop (see also below).

There may be pain at the injection site following intramuscular administration, and thrombophlebitis has occurred following intravenous infusion of cephalosporins. Cefalotin appears to be more likely to cause such local reactions than other cephalosporins.

Antibiotic-associated colitis. Pseudomembranous colitis has occurred with most antibiotics, including the cephalosporins. The newer broad-spectrum cephalosporins have also been implicated[1-3] and the UK Committee on Safety of Medicines (CSM) has warned[4] of the dangers of pseudomembranous colitis with the newer, as well as the older, oral cephalosporins. In addition to 33 reports of pseudomembranous colitis associated with cefalexin, cefradine, cefadroxil, and cefaclor, 6 of which proved fatal, they had received 12 reports of probable or confirmed cases with cefuroxime axetil and 15 with cefixime, one of them fatal. In clinical trials of cefuroxime axetil and cefixime, diarrhoea and pseudomembranous colitis appeared to be dose-related and therefore the CSM recommended that higher doses should be reserved for severe infections. In any event they advised that treatment should be discontinued if symptoms suggestive of pseudomembranous colitis arise.
For further discussion of the management of this condition, see p.122.

1. de Lalla F, et al. Third generation cephalosporins as a risk factor for Clostridium difficile-associated disease: a four-year survey in a general hospital. *J Antimicrob Chemother* 1989; **23:** 623–31.
2. Golledge CL, et al. Extended spectrum cephalosporins and Clostridium difficile. *J Antimicrob Chemother* 1989; **23:** 929–31.
3. Freiman JP, et al. Pseudomembranous colitis associated with single-dose cephalosporin prophylaxis. *JAMA* 1989; **262:** 902.
4. Committee on Safety of Medicines. Pseudomembranous (antibiotic-associated) colitis and diarrhoea with cephalosporins. *Current Problems 32* 1991.

Effects on the kidneys. References.
1. Zhanel GG. Cephalosporin-induced nephrotoxicity: does it exist? *DICP Ann Pharmacother* 1990; **24:** 262–5.

Precautions
Cefalotin should not be given to patients who are hypersensitive to it or to other cephalosporins. About 10% of penicillin-sensitive patients may also be allergic to cephalosporins although the true incidence is uncertain; great care should be taken if cefalotin is to be given to such patients. Care is also necessary in patients with a history of allergy.

Cefalotin should be given with caution to patients with renal impairment; a dosage reduction may be necessary. Renal and haematological status should be monitored especially during prolonged and high-dose therapy. Cefalotin and some other cephalosporins and cephamycins (ceforanide, cefotetan, cefoxitin, and cefpirome) may interfere with the Jaffé method of measuring creatinine concentrations and may produce falsely high values; this should be borne in mind when measuring renal function. Positive results to the direct Coombs' test have been found during treatment with cefalotin and these can interfere with blood cross-matching. The urine of patients being treated with cefalotin may give false-positive reactions for glucose using copper-reduction reactions.

Porphyria. Cephalosporins are considered to be unsafe in patients with porphyria although there is conflicting experimental evidence of porphyrinogenicity.

Interactions
The concomitant use of a nephrotoxic drug such as the aminoglycoside gentamicin may increase the risk of kidney damage with cefalotin. There is also some evidence for enhanced nephrotoxicity with a loop diuretic like frusemide [furosemide], but this is less certain than with frusemide [furosemide] and cefaloridine. Similarly to the penicillins, the renal excretion of cefalotin and many other cephalosporins is inhibited by probenecid. There may be antagonism between cefalotin and bacteriostatic antibacterials.

Antimicrobial Action
Cefalotin is a beta-lactam antibiotic. It is bactericidal and acts similarly to benzylpenicillin (p.158) by inhibiting synthesis of the bacterial cell wall. It is most active against Gram-positive cocci, and has moderate activity against some Gram-negative bacilli.

Sensitive Gram-positive cocci include both penicillinase- and non-penicillinase-producing staphylococci, although meticillin-resistant staphylococci are usually resistant; most streptococci are also sensitive, but not penicillin-resistant *Streptococcus pneumoniae;* enterococci are usually resistant. Some Gram-positive anaerobes are also sensitive. Cefalotin is usually inactive against *Listeria monocytogenes*.

The symbol † denotes a preparation no longer actively marketed

Among Gram-negative bacteria cefalotin has activity against some Enterobacteriaceae including strains of *Escherichia coli, Klebsiella pneumoniae, Proteus mirabilis, Salmonella,* and *Shigella* spp., but not against *Enterobacter,* indole-positive *Proteus,* or *Serratia* spp. It is also active against *Haemophilus influenzae, Moraxella catarrhalis (Branhamella catarrhalis),* and *Neisseria* spp. *Bacteroides fragilis* and *Pseudomonas aeruginosa* are not sensitive, neither are mycobacteria, mycoplasma, and fungi.

The minimum inhibitory concentrations of cefalotin for susceptible Gram-positive cocci range from about 0.1 to 1 μg per mL; for the majority of susceptible Gram-negative bacteria concentrations of 1 to 16 μg or more per mL are usually required.

Resistance of bacteria to cefalotin may be due to several mechanisms: the drug may be prevented from reaching its site of action, for example in some Gram-negative organisms the cell wall may be a potential barrier; the target penicillin-binding proteins may be altered so that cefalotin cannot bind with these proteins; or, most importantly, the organism may produce beta-lactamases (cephalosporinases). Cefalotin is relatively resistant to hydrolysis by staphylococcal beta-lactamase, but is inactivated by a variety of beta-lactamases produced by Gram-negative organisms; resistance of Gram-negative organisms often depends on more than one factor. Resistance can be chromosomally or plasmid-mediated and may sometimes be inducible by cephalosporins.

Certain strains of bacteria may be inhibited but not killed by cephalosporins or penicillins and in such cases the minimum bactericidal concentration is much greater than the minimum inhibitory concentration; this is known as tolerance.

As well as with other cephalosporins, some cross-resistance may occur between cefalotin and the penicillinase-resistant penicillins.

Pharmacokinetics
Cefalotin is poorly absorbed from the gastrointestinal tract. After intramuscular injection peak plasma concentrations of about 10 and 20 μg per mL are achieved within 30 minutes of doses of 0.5 and 1 g, respectively. A concentration of 30 μg per mL has been reported 15 minutes after the intravenous injection of a 1-g dose; a range of 14 to 20 μg per mL has been achieved by the continuous intravenous infusion of 500 mg per hour.

Cefalotin is widely distributed in body tissues and fluids except the brain and CSF where the concentrations achieved are low and unpredictable. It crosses the placenta into the fetal circulation and low concentrations have been detected in breast milk. The plasma half-life varies from about 30 to 50 minutes, but may be longer in patients with renal impairment, especially that of the metabolite. About 70% of cefalotin in the circulation is bound to plasma proteins.

Approximately 20 to 30% of cefalotin is rapidly deacetylated in the liver and about 60 to 70% of a dose is excreted in the urine by the renal tubules within 6 hours as cefalotin and the relatively inactive metabolite, desacetylcefalotin. High urine concentrations of 0.8 and 2.5 mg per mL have been observed following intramuscular doses of 0.5 and 1 g, respectively. Probenecid blocks the renal excretion of cefalotin. A very small amount is excreted in bile.

Uses and Administration
Cefalotin is a first-generation cephalosporin antibiotic that has been used in the treatment of infections due to susceptible bacteria, particularly staphylococci, but has generally been replaced by cefazolin or cefradine; these in turn are being replaced by newer cephalosporins.

Cefalotin is given as the sodium salt by slow intravenous injection over 3 to 5 minutes or by intermittent or continuous infusion. It may be given intramuscularly but this route is painful. Doses are expressed in terms of the equivalent amount of cefalotin. The usual

dose has been 0.5 to 1 g of cefalotin every 4 to 6 hours; up to 12 g daily has been given in severe infections.

Reduced doses are recommended if cefalotin has to be given to patients with impaired renal function.

Preparations
USP 25: Cephalothin for Injection; Cephalothin Injection.

Proprietary Preparations (details are given in Part 3)
Aust.: Keflin; *Austral.:* Keflin Neutral; *Braz.:* Keflin; *Canad.:* Ceporacin; Keflin; *Denm.:* Keflin; *Fin.:* Keflin†; *Fr.:* Keflin†; *Israel:* Keflin; *Ital.:* Keflin; *Mex.:* Ceftina; Keflin; *Neth.:* Keflin; *Norw.:* Keflin; *NZ:* Keflin; *S.Afr.:* Keflin; *Spain:* Keflin; *Swed.:* Keflin†; *Thai.:* Cefadin; Keflin.

Cefamandole (42-n)

Cefamandole (BAN, USAN, rINN).

83405; Cephamandole; Compound 83405. (7R)-7-D-Mandelamido-3-(1-methyl-1H-tetrazol-5-ylthiomethyl)-3-cephem-4-carboxylic acid; {6R-[6α,7β(R')]}-7-[(hydroxyphenylacetyl)amino]-3-{[(1-methyl-1H-tetrazol-5-yl)thio]methyl}-8-oxo-5-thia-1-azabicyclo[4.2.0]oct-2-ene-2-carboxylic acid.
$C_{18}H_{18}N_6O_5S_2 = 462.5$.
CAS — 34444-01-4.
ATC — J01DA07.

Cefamandole Nafate (18358-s)

Cefamandole Nafate (BAN, USAN, rINNM).

106223; Cefmandoli Nafas; Cephamandole Nafate. Sodium (7R)-7-[(2R)-2-formyloxy-2-phenylacetamido]-3-(1-methyl-1H-tetrazol-5-ylthiomethyl)-3-cephem-4-carboxylate.
$C_{19}H_{17}N_6NaO_6S_2 = 512.5$.
CAS — 42540-40-9.
Pharmacopoeias. In *Eur.* (see p.vi), *Pol.,* and *US.*

1.11 g of monograph substance is approximately equivalent to 1 g of cefamandole activity and represents 2.2 mmol of sodium.

Cefamandole nafate has been reported to be **incompatible** with aminoglycosides and with metronidazole. Formulations of cefamandole nafate available for injection contain sodium carbonate and are incompatible with solutions containing calcium or magnesium salts. When reconstituted with water the sodium carbonate rapidly hydrolyses about 30% of the ester to cefamandole sodium; during storage of the reconstituted solution at room temperature carbon dioxide is produced.

Pharmacopoeial description
Ph. Eur.: A white, or almost white powder. Freely soluble in water; sparingly soluble in methyl alcohol. A 10% solution in water has a pH, measured after 30 minutes, of 6.0 to 8.0. Store in airtight containers. Protect from light.

USP 25: A white, odourless, crystalline solid. Soluble in water and in methyl alcohol; practically insoluble in chloroform, in cyclohexane, in ether, and in benzene. pH of a 10% solution in water is between 3.5 and 7.0. Store in airtight containers.

Incompatibility and stability. References.
1. Frable RA, et al. Stability of cefamandole nafate injection with parenteral solutions and additives. *Am J Hosp Pharm* 1982; **39:** 622–7. Correction. *ibid.;* 1479.

Cefamandole Sodium (43-h)

Cefamandole Sodium (BANM, rINNM).
Cephamandole Sodium.
$C_{18}H_{17}N_6NaO_5S_2 = 484.5$.
CAS — 30034-03-8.
Pharmacopoeias. In *Jpn.*

1.05 g of monograph substance is approximately equivalent to 1 g of cefamandole and represents 2.2 mmol of sodium.

Adverse Effects and Precautions
As for Cefalotin Sodium, p.162.

Cefamandole has an *N*-methylthiotetrazole side-chain and may cause bleeding as a result of hypoprothrombinaemia which is usually reversible with administration of vitamin K. An alteration in intestinal flora was once thought responsible for this vitamin K-associated hypoprothrombinaemia, but interference with prothrombin synthesis now seems more likely.

Effects on the blood. References.
1. Lipsky JJ. Antibiotic-associated hypoprothrombinaemia. *J Antimicrob Chemother* 1988; **21:** 281–300.
2. Shearer MJ, et al. Mechanism of cephalosporin-induced hypoprothrombinemia: relation to cephalosporin side chain, vitamin K metabolism, and vitamin K status. *J Clin Pharmacol* 1988; **28:** 88–95.
3. Welage LS, et al. Comparative evaluation of the pharmacokinetics of N-methylthiotetrazole following administration of cefoperazone, cefotetan, and cefmetazole. *Antimicrob Agents Chemother* 1990; **34:** 2369–74.

Interactions

A disulfiram-like interaction with alcohol may occur and has been attributed to the *N*-methylthiotetrazole side-chain of cefamandole. Patients receiving cefamandole should therefore avoid alcohol during, and for at least several days after, treatment. Interactions are also possible with preparations containing significant amounts of alcohol.

Cefamandole, and other cephalosporins containing an *N*-methylthiotetrazole side-chain, may enhance the hypoprothrombinaemic response to anticoagulants as discussed under Warfarin (p.994).

Probenecid reduces the renal clearance of cefamandole and many other cephalosporins.

◊ References.
1. Portier H, *et al.* Interaction between cephalosporins and alcohol. *Lancet* 1980; **ii:** 263.
2. Drummer S, *et al.* Antabuse-like effect of β-lactam antibiotics. *N Engl J Med* 1980; **303:** 1417–18.

Antimicrobial Action

Cefamandole is bactericidal and acts similarly to cefalotin, but has a broader spectrum of activity. It generally has similar or less activity against Gram-positive staphylococci and streptococci, but is resistant to some beta-lactamases produced by Gram-negative bacteria. It is more active than cefalotin against many of the Enterobacteriaceae including some strains of *Enterobacter, Escherichia coli, Klebsiella, Salmonella,* and indole-positive *Proteus* spp. However, resistance to cefamandole and other beta lactams has emerged in some species, notably *Enterobacter,* during treatment with cefamandole. Cefamandole is very active *in vitro* against *Haemophilus influenzae* although an inoculum effect has been reported for beta-lactamase-producing strains. Like cefalotin, most strains of *Bacteroides fragilis* are resistant to cefamandole, as are *Pseudomonas* spp.

The minimum inhibitory concentrations of cefamandole for susceptible Gram-positive bacteria have been reported to range from about 0.1 to 2.0 μg per mL; for most susceptible Gram-negative bacteria concentrations of 0.5 to 8.0 μg per mL are usually required.

◊ References.
1. Sabath LD. Reappraisal of the antistaphylococcal activities of first-generation (narrow-spectrum) and second-generation (expanded-spectrum) cephalosporins. *Antimicrob Agents Chemother* 1989; **33:** 407–11.

Pharmacokinetics

Cefamandole is poorly absorbed from the gastrointestinal tract. It is given intramuscularly or intravenously, usually as the nafate which is rapidly hydrolysed to release cefamandole *in vivo*. Peak plasma concentrations for cefamandole of about 13 and 25 μg per mL have been achieved 0.5 to 2 hours after intramuscular doses of 0.5 and 1 g respectively; concentrations are very low after 6 hours. About 70% is bound to plasma proteins. The plasma half-life varies from about 0.5 to 1.2 hours depending on the route of injection; it is prolonged in patients with renal impairment.

Cefamandole is widely distributed in body tissues and fluids including bone, joint fluid, and pleural fluid; it diffuses into the CSF when the meninges are inflamed, but concentrations are unpredictable. Cefamandole has also been detected in breast milk. It is rapidly excreted unchanged by glomerular filtration and renal tubular secretion; about 80% of a dose is excreted within 6 hours and high urinary concentrations are achieved. Probenecid competes for renal tubular secretion with cefamandole resulting in higher and prolonged plasma concentrations of cefamandole. Therapeutic concentrations of cefamandole are achieved in bile.

It is removed by haemodialysis to some extent.

Uses and Administration

Cefamandole is a second-generation cephalosporin antibiotic used in the treatment of infections due to susceptible bacteria (see Antimicrobial Action, above) and for surgical infection prophylaxis.

It is given principally as cefamandole nafate (the sodium salt of cefamandole formyl ester). Doses are expressed in terms of the equivalent amount of cefamandole. It is administered by deep intramuscular injection, by slow intravenous injection over 3 to 5 minutes, or by intermittent or continuous infusion in doses of 0.5 to 2 g every 4 to 8 hours for adults depending on the severity of the infection. Children over 1 month of age may be given 50 to 100 mg per kg body-weight daily in divided doses; 150 mg per kg daily may be given in severe infections, but this dose should not be exceeded.

Doses should be reduced for patients with impaired renal function. After an initial dose of 1 to 2 g the following maintenance doses have been recommended: for patients with a creatinine clearance of 50 to 80 mL per minute, 0.75 to 2 g every 6 hours; 25 to 50 mL per minute, 0.75 to 2 g every 8 hours; 10 to 25 mL per minute, 0.5 to 1.25 g every 8 hours; 2 to 10 mL per minute, 0.5 to 1 g every 12 hours; and less than 2 mL per minute, 0.25 to 0.75 g every 12 hours.

If the addition of an aminoglycoside to cefamandole therapy is necessary, then they should be administered separately.

For surgical infection prophylaxis, a dose of 1 or 2 g intravenously or intramuscularly one-half to one hour before surgical incision, followed by 1 or 2 g every 6 hours for 24 to 48 hours, is recommended. For patients undergoing procedures involving implantation of prosthetic devices, cefamandole should be continued for up to 72 hours.

Preparations

USP 25: Cefamandole Nafate for Injection.

Proprietary Preparations (details are given in Part 3)
Aust.: Mandokef; *Austral.:* Mandol; *Belg.:* Mandol; *Canad.:* Mandol†; *Ger.:* Mandokef; *Hong Kong:* Mandol; *Irl.:* Kefadol; *Ital.:* Cedol; Cefam; Cefiran†; Cemado; Lampomandol; Mancef; Mandokef; Mandolsan; Neocefal; Septomandolo; *Neth.:* Mandol; *NZ:* Mandokef; *Port.:* Mandokef; *S.Afr.:* Mandokef; *Spain:* Mandokef; *Switz.:* Mandokef; *Thai.:* Cefadol; Cefmandol; Mandol; *UK:* Kefadol; *USA:* Mandol.

Cefapirin Sodium   (29-b)

Cefapirin Sodium *(BANM, pINNM).*

BL-P-1322; Cephapirin Sodium *(USAN).* Sodium (7R)-7-[2-(4-pyridylthio)acetamido]cephalosporanate; Sodium (7R)-3-acetoxymethyl-7-[2-(4-pyridylthio)acetamido]-3-cephem-4-carboxylate.

$C_{17}H_{16}N_3NaO_6S_2 = 445.4.$
CAS — 21593-23-7 (cefapirin); 24356-60-3 (cefapirin sodium).

Pharmacopoeias. In It., Jpn, and US.
US also includes Cephapirin Benzathine for veterinary use.

1.05 g of monograph substance is approximately equivalent to 1 g of cefapirin. Each g of monograph substance represents about 2.2 mmol of sodium.

Pharmacopoeial description

USP 25: A white to off-white crystalline powder, odourless or having a slight odour. Very soluble in water; insoluble in most organic solvents. pH of a solution in water containing the equivalent of cefapirin 1% is between 6.5 and 8.5. Store in airtight containers.

Profile

Cefapirin is a first-generation cephalosporin antibiotic with actions and uses very similar to those of cefalotin (p.162).

It is used as the sodium salt and the usual adult dose is the equivalent of 0.5 to 1 g of cefapirin every 4 to 6 hours by intramuscular injection or intravenously. In severe infections up to 12 g daily may be given, preferably intravenously.

Reduced doses may be necessary in patients with impaired renal function.

Preparations

USP 25: Cephapirin for Injection.

Proprietary Preparations (details are given in Part 3)
Fr.: Cefaloject; *Hong Kong:* Lopitrex; *Spain:* Brisfirina; *USA:* Cefadyl†.

Multi-ingredient: *Spain:* Brisfirina Balsamica†.

Cefatrizine   (30-x)

Cefatrizine *(BAN, USAN, pINN).*

BL-S640; SKF-60771; S-640P. (7R)-7-(α-D-4-Hydroxyphenylglycylamino)-3-(1H-1,2,3-triazol-4-ylthiomethyl)-3-cephem-4-carboxylic acid.

$C_{18}H_{18}N_6O_5S_2 = 462.5.$
CAS — 51627-14-6.
ATC — J01DA21.

Pharmacopoeias. Eur. (see p.vi) *and Jpn* include Propylene Glycol Cefatrizine.

Profile

Cefatrizine is a cephalosporin antibiotic with actions and uses similar to those of cefalexin (p.161), although it might be more active *in vitro.* It is given by mouth, as a compound with propylene glycol, in usual doses equivalent to 500 mg twice daily of cefatrizine.

Preparations

Proprietary Preparations (details are given in Part 3)
Belg.: Cefaperos; *Fr.:* Cefaperos; *Ital.:* Biotrixina; Cefatrix; Cefotrizin; Cetrazil; Cetrinox; Faretrizin; Ipatrizina; Kefoxina; Ketrizin; Latocef†; Miracef; Novacef; Tamyl; Tricef; Trixidine†; Trixilan; Trizina; Zinaf; Zitrix; *Jpn:* Cepticol†; *Port.:* Macropen.

Cefazolin   (18366-s)

Cefazolin *(BAN, pINN).*

Cephazolin. 3-[(5-Methyl-1,3,4-thiadiazol-2-yl)thiomethyl]-7-(tetrazol-1-ylacetamido)-3-cephem-4-carboxylic acid.

$C_{14}H_{14}N_8O_4S_3 = 454.5.$
CAS — 25953-19-9.
ATC — J01DA04.
Pharmacopoeias. In US.

Pharmacopoeial description

USP 25: A white to slightly off-white, odourless crystalline powder. Slightly soluble in water, in alcohol, and in methyl alcohol; sparingly soluble in acetone; practically insoluble in chloroform, in dichloromethane, in ether, and in benzene; soluble in dimethylformamide and in pyridine; very slightly soluble in ethyl acetate, in isopropyl alcohol, and in methyl isobutyl ketone. Store in airtight containers.

Cefazolin Sodium   (44-m)

Cefazolin Sodium *(BANM, USAN, pINNM).*

46083; Cefazolinum Natricum; Cephazolin Sodium; SKF-41558.
$C_{14}H_{13}N_8NaO_4S_3 = 476.5.$
CAS — 27164-46-1.
Pharmacopoeias. In Chin., Eur. (see p.vi), *Jpn, and US.*

1.05 g of monograph substance is approximately equivalent to 1 g of cefazolin. Each g of monograph substance represents about 2.1 mmol of sodium.

Cefazolin sodium has been reported to be incompatible with aminoglycosides and many other drugs. When the pH of a solution exceeds 8.5 there may be hydrolysis and when it is below 4.5 insoluble cefazolin may be precipitated.

Pharmacopoeial description

Ph. Eur.: A white or almost white, very hygroscopic powder. Freely soluble in water; very slightly soluble in alcohol; practically insoluble in ether. A 10% solution in water has a pH of 4.0 to 6.0. Store at a temperature not exceeding 30° in airtight containers. Protect from light.

USP 25: A white to off-white, practically odourless, crystalline powder, or a white to off-white solid. Freely soluble in water, in sodium chloride 0.9%, and in glucose solutions; very slightly soluble in alcohol; practically insoluble in chloroform and in ether. pH of a solution in water containing the equivalent of cefazolin 10% is between 4.0 and 6.0. Store in airtight containers.

Stability. References.
1. Nahata MC, Ahalt PA. Stability of cefazolin sodium in peritoneal dialysis solutions. *Am J Hosp Pharm* 1991; **48:** 291–2.

Adverse Effects and Precautions

As for Cefalotin Sodium, p.162.

Similarly to cephalosporins with a *N*-methylthiotetrazole side-chain, cefazolin has been associated with hypoprothrombinaemia (see Cefamandole, p.163).

Effects on the nervous system. References.
1. Manzella JP, *et al.* CNS toxicity associated with intraventricular injection of cefazolin: report of three cases. *J Neurosurg* 1988; **68:** 970–1.
2. Martin ES, *et al.* Seizures after intraventricular cefazolin administration. *Clin Pharm* 1992; **11:** 104–5.

Interactions

Cefazolin contains a methylthiadiazolethiol side-chain and, similarly to cephalosporins containing the related *N*-methyltetrazole side-chain (see Cefamandole, p.164), may cause a disulfiram-like reaction with alcohol, and possibly enhance the effects of warfarin.

The renal excretion of cefazolin and many other cephalosporins is delayed by probenecid.

Antimicrobial Action
As for Cefalotin Sodium, p.163, although cefazolin is more sensitive to staphylococcal beta-lactamase.

The minimum inhibitory concentrations of cefazolin for susceptible Gram-positive cocci range from about 0.1 to 1 µg per mL; for the majority of susceptible Gram-negative bacteria concentrations of greater than 1 µg per mL are required.

Pharmacokinetics
Cefazolin is poorly absorbed from the gastrointestinal tract and is given by intramuscular or intravenous injection. Following a dose of 500 mg given intramuscularly, peak plasma concentrations of 30 µg or more per mL are obtained after 1 to 2 hours. About 85% of cefazolin in the circulation is bound to plasma proteins. The plasma half-life of cefazolin is about 1.8 hours, and is increased in patients with renal impairment. Cefazolin diffuses into bone and into ascitic, pleural, and synovial fluid but not appreciably into the CSF. It crosses the placenta into the fetal circulation; only low concentrations are detected in breast milk.

Cefazolin is excreted unchanged in the urine, mainly by glomerular filtration with some renal tubular secretion, at least 80% of a dose given intramuscularly being excreted within 24 hours. Peak urine concentrations of more than 1 and 4 mg per mL have been reported after intramuscular doses of 0.5 and 1 g respectively. Probenecid delays excretion. Cefazolin is removed to some extent by haemodialysis.

High biliary concentrations have been reported, although the amount excreted by this route is small.

Uses and Administration
Cefazolin is a first-generation cephalosporin antibiotic used in the treatment of a variety of infections due to susceptible organisms, including biliary-tract infections, endocarditis (staphylococcal), and peritonitis (associated with continuous ambulatory peritoneal dialysis). It is also used for surgical infection prophylaxis, including prophylaxis of endometritis at caesarean section. For details of these infections, and their treatment, see under Choice of Antibacterial, p.114.

Administration and dosage. Cefazolin is given as the sodium salt by deep intramuscular injection, by slow intravenous injection over 3 to 5 minutes, or by intravenous infusion. Doses are expressed in terms of the equivalent amount of cefazolin. The usual adult dose is 0.5 to 1 g every 6 to 12 hours. The usual maximum daily dose is 6 g, although up to 12 g has been used in severe life-threatening infections. Children over 1 month may be given 25 to 50 mg per kg body-weight daily in three or four divided doses, increased in severe infections to a maximum of 100 mg per kg daily.

For the prophylaxis of infection during surgery, a 1-g dose is given half to one hour before the operation, followed by 0.5 to 1 g during surgery for lengthy procedures. A dose of 0.5 to 1 g is given every 6 to 8 hours postoperatively for 24 hours, or up to 5 days in certain cases.

Dosage should be reduced in patients with renal impairment and various modifications have been recommended. The manufacturers suggest the following for adults following a loading dose: creatinine clearance 55 mL or more per minute, usual doses; 35 to 54 mL per minute, usual doses but at intervals of at least 8 hours; 11 to 34 mL per minute, half the usual dose every 12 hours; 10 mL or less per minute, half the usual dose every 18 to 24 hours.

Other routes of administration used for cefazolin sodium include intraperitoneal administration in peritoneal dialysis solutions and intra-ocular injections.

In some countries a modified-release intramuscular formulation of cefazolin sodium together with the less soluble dibenzylamine salt of cefazolin, in the ratio of 1:4, has been used.

Preparations
BP 2001: Cefazolin Injection;
USP 25: Cefazolin for Injection; Cefazolin Injection; Cefazolin Ophthalmic Solution.
Proprietary Preparations (details are given in Part 3)
Aust.: Gramaxin; Kefzol; Zolicef; *Austral.:* Cefamezin; Kefzol; *Belg.:* Cefacidal; Kefzol; *Braz.:* Cefamezin; Kefzol; *Canad.:* Ancef; Kefzol; *Fr.:* Cefacidal; Kefzol†; *Ger.:* Basocef; Elzogram; Gramaxin†; *Hong Kong:* Cefamezin; Kefzol; *Israel:* Cefamezin; Kefazin; Kefzol; Totacef; *Ital.:* Acef; Biazolina†; Cefabiozim; Cefamezin; Cefazil; Cromezin; Firmacef; Recef; Sicef; Silzolin; Totacef; Zolin; Zolisint†; *Jpn:* Cefamezin; *Mex.:* Cefacidal; *Neth.:* Cefacidal; Kefzol; *NZ:* Kefzol; *Port.:* Cefamezin†; Kurgan; *S.Afr.:* Cefacidal; Izacef; Kefzol; Ranzol; *Spain:* Areuzolin; Brizolina; Caricef; Cefa Resan; Cefacene; Cefadrex; Cefakes; Cefamezin; Cefamusel†; Fazoplex; Filoklin; Gencefal; Intrazolina; Karidina; Kefol; Kurgan; Neofazol; Tasep; Tecfazolina; Zolival; *Switz.:* Kefzol; Servicef†; *Thai.:* Cefacidal; Cefalin; Cefamezin; Cefazillin; Cefzol; Fazolin; Kefzol; Zefa; Zepilen; *UK:* Kefzol; *USA:* Ancef; Kefzol; Zolicef.

Cefcapene (17075-y)
Cefcapene (rINN).

(6R,7R)-7-[(Z)-2-(2-Amino-4-thiazolyl)-2-pentenamido]-3-(hydroxymethyl)-8-oxo-5-thia-1-azabicyclo[4.2.0]oct-2-ene-2-carboxylic acid carbamate.
$C_{17}H_{19}N_5O_6S_2 = 453.5$.
CAS — 135889-00-8.

Profile
Cefcapene is an oral cephalosporin antibacterial given by mouth as the pivaloyloxymethyl ester, cefcapene pivoxil hydrochloride in usual doses of 100 mg three times daily.

For reference to carnitine deficiency occurring after the administration of some pivaloyloxymethyl esters, see Pivampicillin, p.237.

Preparations
Proprietary Preparations (details are given in Part 3)
Jpn: Flomox.

Cefdinir (10948-y)
Cefdinir (BAN, USAN, rINN).

CI-983; FK-482. (−)-(6R,7R)-7-[2-(2-Amino-4-thiazolyl)glyoxylamido]-8-oxo-3-vinyl-5-thia-1-azabicyclo[4.2.0]oct-2-ene-2-carboxylic acid, 7^2-(Z)-oxime; 7-{(2-Amino-1,3-thiazol-4-yl)-2-[(Z)-hydroxyimino]acetamido}-3-vinylcephem-4-carboxylic acid.
$C_{14}H_{13}N_5O_5S_2 = 395.4$.
CAS — 91832-40-5.
ATC — J01DA42.

Adverse Effects and Precautions
As for Cefalotin Sodium, p.162. There have been reports of reddish stools in patients who have received cefdinir with iron supplements (see also Interactions, below).

Interactions
Absorption of cefdinir is decreased by concurrent ingestion of antacids or of iron supplements; thus, an interval of at least 2 hours should elapse between taking cefdinir and either an antacid or an iron supplement. Probenecid reduces the renal excretion of cefdinir.

Antimicrobial Action
As for Cefixime, p.166. However, cefdinir is reported to be much more active *in vitro* than cefixime against *Staphylococcus aureus* and *Enterococcus faecalis*, but is less active against some Enterobacteriaceae.

◊ References.
1. Neu HC, *et al.* Comparative in vitro activity and β-lactamase stability of FK-482, a new oral cephalosporin. *Antimicrob Agents Chemother* 1989; **33:** 1795–1800.
2. Wise R, *et al.* The in-vitro activity of cefdinir (FK-482), a new oral cephalosporin. *J Antimicrob Chemother* 1991; **28:** 239–48.
3. Perea EJ, Iglesias MCG. Comparative in-vitro activity of cefdinir against multiresistant Haemophilus influenzae. *J Antimicrob Chemother* 1994; **34:** 161–4.
4. Marchese A, *et al.* Antistaphylococcal activity of cefdinir, a new oral third-generation cephalosporin, alone and in combination with other antibiotics, at supra- and sub-MIC levels. *J Antimicrob Chemother* 1995; **35:** 53–66.

Pharmacokinetics
Cefdinir is absorbed from the gastrointestinal tract following oral administration, peak plasma concentrations occurring 2 to 4 hours after a dose. Bioavailability following administration by mouth has been estimated to range from 16 to 25%. It is widely distributed into tissues and is 60 to 70% bound to plasma proteins. Cefdinir is not appreciably metabolised and is excreted in the urine with an elimination half-life of 1.7 hours.

Cefdinir is removed by dialysis.

◊ References.
1. Cook PJ, *et al.* Distribution of cefdinir, a third generation cephalosporin antibiotic, in serum and pulmonary compartments. *J Antimicrob Chemother* 1996; **37:** 331–9.

Uses and Administration
Cefdinir is a third-generation oral cephalosporin antibiotic with actions and uses similar to those of cefixime (p.166). It is given by mouth in a usual adult dose of 600 mg daily as a single dose or in two divided doses. Children may be given 14 mg per kg body-weight daily up to a maximum of 600 mg. Doses should be reduced in patients with renal impairment (with a creatinine clearance of less than 30 mL per minute) to 300 mg once daily.

◊ Reviews.
1. Guay DRP. Cefdinir: an expanded-spectrum oral cephalosporin. *Ann Pharmacother* 2000; **34:** 1469–77.

Preparations
Proprietary Preparations (details are given in Part 3)
Jpn: Cefzon; *Thai.:* Omnicef; *USA:* Omnicef.

Cefditoren (15883-g)
Cefditoren (rINN).

(+)-(6R,7R)-7-[2-(2-Amino-4-thiazolyl)glyoxylamido]-3-[(Z)-2-(4-methyl-5-thiazolyl)vinyl]-8-oxo-5-thia-1-azabicyclo[4.2.0]oct-2-ene-2-carboxylic acid 7^2-(Z)-(O-methyloxime).
$C_{19}H_{18}N_6O_5S_3 = 506.6$.
CAS — 104145-95-1.

Profile
Cefditoren is a cephalosporin antibiotic with a broad spectrum of activity. It is given by mouth as the pivaloyloxymethyl ester, cefditoren pivoxil in usual doses equivalent to 100 to 200 mg of cefditoren three times daily.

For reference to carnitine deficiency occurring after the administration of some pivaloyloxymethyl esters, see Pivampicillin, p.237.

Preparations
Proprietary Preparations (details are given in Part 3)
Jpn: Meiact; *USA:* Spectracef.

Cefepime Hydrochloride (17329-t)
Cefepime Hydrochloride (BANM, USAN, rINNM).

BMY-28142 (cefepime). {6R-[6α,7β(Z)]}-1-[(7-{[(2-Amino-4-thiazolyl)-(methoxyimino)acetyl]amino}-2-carboxy-8-oxo-5-thia-1-azabicyclo[4.2.0]oct-2-en-3-yl)methyl]-1-methylpyrrolidinium chloride monohydrochloride monohydrate; 7-{(2-Amino-1,3-thiazol-4-yl)-2-[(Z)-methoxyimino]acetamido}-3-(1-methylpyrrolidiniomethyl)-3-cephem-4-carboxylate hydrochloride.
$C_{19}H_{25}ClN_6O_5S_2,HCl,H_2O = 571.5$.
CAS — 88040-23-7 (cefepime); 123171-59-5 (cefepime hydrochloride monohydrate).

Stability. References.
1. Stewart JT, *et al.* Stability of cefepime hydrochloride injection in polypropylene syringes at −20°C, 4°C, and 22-24°C. *Am J Health-Syst Pharm* 1999; **56:** 457–9.
2. Stewart JT, *et al.* Stability of cefepime hydrochloride in polypropylene syringes. *Am J Health-Syst Pharm* 1999; **56:** 1134.
3. Williamson JC, *et al.* Stability of cefepime in peritoneal dialysis solution. *Ann Pharmacother* 1999; **33:** 906–9.

Adverse Effects and Precautions
As for Cefalotin Sodium, p.162.

◊ References.
1. Neu HC. Safety of cefepime: a new extended-spectrum parenteral cephalosporin. *Am J Med* 1996; **100** (suppl 6A): 68S–75S.

Antimicrobial Action
Cefepime is a fourth-generation cephalosporin antibiotic and is active against a wide range of Gram-positive and Gram-negative aerobic organisms. Against Gram-positive cocci, its activity is similar to that of cefotaxime (p.169) and includes staphylococci (but not meticillin-resistant *Staphylococcus aureus*) and streptococci. Against Enterobacteriaceae, it has a broader spectrum of activity than other cephalosporins, including activity against organisms producing chromosomally mediated beta-lactamases such as *Enterobacter* spp. and *Proteus vulgaris*. Against *Pseudomonas aeruginosa*, it has similar or slightly less activity than ceftazidime (p.175), although it may be active against some strains resistant to ceftazidime.

◊ References.
1. Neu HC, *et al.* The activity of BMY 28142, a new broad spectrum β-lactamase stable cephalosporin. *J Antimicrob Chemother* 1986; **17:** 441–52.
2. Watanabe N, *et al.* Comparative in-vitro activities of newer cephalosporins cefclidin, cefepime, and cefpirome against ceftazidime- or imipenem-resistant Pseudomonas aeruginosa. *J Antimicrob Chemother* 1992; **30:** 633–41.

The symbol † denotes a preparation no longer actively marketed

3. Thornsberry C, et al. In-vitro activity of cefepime and other antimicrobials: survey of European isolates. J Antimicrob Chemother 1993; 32 (suppl B): 31–53.
4. Kessler RE, Fung-Tomc J. Susceptibility of bacterial isolates to β-lactam antibiotics from US clinical trials over a 5-year period. Am J Med 1996; 100 (suppl 6A): 13S–19S.
5. Palmer SM, et al. Bactericidal killing activities of cefepime, ceftazidime, cefotaxime, and ceftriaxone against Staphylococcus aureus and β-lactamase-producing strains of Enterobacter aerogenes and Klebsiella pneumoniae in an in vitro infection model. Antimicrob Agents Chemother 1995; 39: 1764–71.

Pharmacokinetics

Cefepime is administered by injection as the hydrochloride. It is rapidly and almost completely absorbed following intramuscular injection and mean peak plasma concentrations of about 14 and 30 μg per mL have been reported about 1.5 hours after doses of 0.5 and 1 g respectively. Within 30 minutes of intravenous administration of similar doses, peak plasma concentrations of about 40 and 80 μg per mL are achieved. The plasma half-life of cefepime is approximately 2 hours and is prolonged in patients with renal impairment. About 20% of cefepime is bound to plasma proteins.

Cefepime is widely distributed in body tissues and fluids. High concentrations are achieved in bile. Low concentrations have been detected in breast milk.

Cefepime is eliminated principally by the kidneys and about 85% of a dose is recovered unchanged in the urine. Cefepime is substantially removed by haemodialysis.

◊ References.
1. Okamoto MP, et al. Cefepime clinical pharmacokinetics. Clin Pharmacokinet 1993; 25: 88–102.
2. Rybak M. The pharmacokinetic profile of a new generation of parenteral cephalosporin. Am J Med 1996; 100 (suppl 6A): 39S–44S.
3. Reed MD, et al. Pharmacokinetics of intravenously and intramuscularly administered cefepime in infants and children. Antimicrob Agents Chemother 1997; 41: 1783–7.
4. Allaouchiche B, et al. Pharmacokinetics of cefepime during continuous venovenous hemodiafiltration. Antimicrob Agents Chemother 1997; 41: 2424–7.

Uses and Administration

Cefepime is a fourth-generation cephalosporin antibiotic used in the treatment of infections due to susceptible organisms. They include infections of the urinary tract, respiratory tract, and skin. For details of these infections and their treatment, see under Choice of Antibacterial, p.114.

Cefepime is given as the hydrochloride by deep intramuscular injection, or intravenously by slow injection over 3 to 5 minutes or by infusion over at least 30 minutes. Doses are expressed in terms of the equivalent amount of cefepime. The usual dose is 1 to 2 g daily in two divided doses for mild to moderate infections, increased to 4 g daily in severe infections, although up to 6 g daily in three divided doses has been given. Children aged over 2 months and weighing up to 40 kg may be given 50 mg per kg body-weight twice daily; this dose may be given three times daily for febrile neutropenia.

Dosage should be modified in renal impairment; after a normal initial loading dose the maintenance dosage should be adjusted according to the patient's creatinine clearance and the severity of the infection: creatinine clearance 30 to 60 mL per minute, 0.5 to 2 g every 24 hours; 11 to 29 mL per minute, 0.5 to 1 g every 24 hours; and 10 mL per minute or less, 0.25 to 0.5 g every 24 hours. Patients undergoing haemodialysis should be given a repeat dose after each dialysis session, while those undergoing continuous ambulatory peritoneal dialysis should receive normal recommended doses at intervals of 48 hours.

◊ Reviews.
1. Various. Cefepime: a β-lactamase-stable extended-spectrum cephalosporin. J Antimicrob Chemother 1993; 32 (suppl B): 1–214.
2. Barradell LB, Bryson HM. Cefepime: a review of its antibacterial activity, pharmacokinetic properties and therapeutic use. Drugs 1994; 47: 471–505.
3. Okamoto MP, et al. Cefepime: a new fourth-generation cephalosporin. Am J Hosp Pharm 1994; 51: 463–77.
4. Wynd MA, Paladino JA. Cefepime: a fourth-generation parenteral cephalosporin. Ann Pharmacother 1996; 30: 1414–24.

Preparations

Proprietary Preparations (details are given in Part 3)
Aust.: Maxipime; *Austral.:* Maxipime; *Belg.:* Maxipime; *Canad.:* Maxipime; *Denm.:* Maxipime; *Fin.:* Maxipime; *Fr.:* Axepim; *Ger.:* Maxipime; *Hong Kong:* Maxipime; *Irl.:* Maxipime; *Israel:* Maxcef; *Ital.:* Cepim; Cepimex; Maxipime; *Mex.:* Maxipime; *Neth.:* Maxipime; *NZ:* Maxipime; *Port.:* Maxipime; *S.Afr.:* Maxipime; *Singapore:* Maxipime; *Spain:* Maxipime; *Swed.:* Maxipime; *Switz.:* Maxipime; *Thai.:* Maxipime; *USA:* Maxipime.

Cefetamet (3412-I)

Cefetamet (USAN, rINN).

LY-097964; Ro-15-8074; Ro-15-8075 (cefetamet pivoxil). (Z)-7-[2-(2-Aminothiazol-4-yl)-2-methoxyiminoacetamido]-3-methyl-3-cephem-4-carboxylic acid.
$C_{14}H_{15}N_5O_5S_2 = 397.4.$
CAS — 65052-63-3 (cefetamet); 65243-33-6 (cefetamet pivoxil).
ATC — J01DA26.

Profile
Cefetamet is a third-generation cephalosporin antibiotic similar to cefixime (below). It is given by mouth as the hydrochloride of the pivaloyloxymethyl ester, cefetamet pivoxil hydrochloride, which is hydrolysed to cefetamet in vivo. The usual dose is 500 mg twice daily.

For reference to carnitine deficiency occurring after the administration of some pivaloyloxymethyl esters, see Pivampicillin, p.237.

◊ Reviews.
1. Bryson HM, Brogden RN. Cefetamet pivoxil: a review of its antibacterial activity, pharmacokinetic properties and therapeutic use. Drugs 1993; 45: 589–621.
2. Blouin RA, Stoeckel K. Cefetamet pivoxil clinical pharmacokinetics. Clin Pharmacokinet 1993; 25: 172–88.

Preparations

Proprietary Preparations (details are given in Part 3)
Aust.: Globocef†; *Braz.:* Globocef; *Ger.:* Globocef; *Hong Kong:* Globocef; *Ital.:* Globocef; *Mex.:* Globocef; *Port.:* Cefec; Globocef; *Switz.:* Globocef.

Cefixime (12006-g)

Cefixime (BAN, USAN, rINN).

Cefiximum; CL-284635; FK-027; FR-17027. (Z)-7-[2-(2-Aminothiazol-4-yl)-2-(carboxymethoxyimino)acetamido]-3-vinyl-3-cephem-4-carboxylic acid trihydrate.
$C_{16}H_{15}N_5O_7S_2,3H_2O = 507.5.$
CAS — 79350-37-1.
ATC — J01DA23.

Pharmacopoeias. In Eur. (see p.vi) and US. Jpn includes the anhydrous substance.

1.12 g of monograph substance is approximately equivalent to 1 g of anhydrous cefixime.

Pharmacopoeial description
Ph. Eur.: A white or almost white, slightly hygroscopic, powder. Slightly soluble in water; sparingly soluble in dehydrated alcohol; practically insoluble in ethyl acetate; freely soluble in methyl alcohol. A 5% suspension in water has a pH of 2.6 to 4.1. Store in airtight containers. Protect from light.

USP 25: A white to light yellow crystalline powder. Practically insoluble in water, in ether, in ethyl acetate, and in hexane; slightly soluble in alcohol, in acetone, and in glycerol; freely soluble in methyl alcohol; soluble in propylene glycol; very slightly soluble in 70% sorbitol and in octanol; pH of a solution in water containing the equivalent of cefixime 0.07% is between 2.6 and 4.1. Store in airtight containers.

Adverse Effects and Precautions
As for Cefalotin Sodium, p.162.

The most frequently reported adverse effects of cefixime are gastrointestinal disturbances, especially diarrhoea. Cefixime should be discontinued if diarrhoea is severe.

Although cefixime does not have the N-methylthiotetrazole side-chain usually associated with hypoprothrombinaemia (see Cefamandole, p.163), increases in prothrombin times have occurred in a few patients.

Antibiotic-associated colitis. For reports of diarrhoea and pseudomembranous colitis associated with cefixime, see Cefalotin, p.163.

Interactions
Care should be exercised in patients receiving anticoagulants and cefixime concomitantly due to the possibility that cefixime may increase prothrombin times (see above).

Antimicrobial Action
Cefixime is a bactericidal antibiotic and is stable to hydrolysis by many beta-lactamases. It has a mode of action and spectrum of activity similar to those of the third-generation cephalosporin cefotaxime (p.169), but some Enterobacteriaceae are less susceptible to cefixime. *Haemophilus influenzae, Moraxella catarrhalis (Branhamella catarrhalis),* and *Neisseria gonorrhoeae* are sensitive, including penicillinase-producing strains. Of the Gram-positive bacteria, streptococci are sensitive to cefixime but most strains of staphylococci, enterococci, and *Listeria* spp. are not.

Enterobacter spp., *Pseudomonas aeruginosa,* and *Bacteroides* spp. are resistant to cefixime.

◊ References.
1. Barry AL, Jones RN. Cefixime: spectrum of antibacterial activity against 16 016 clinical isolates. Pediatr Infect Dis J 1987; 6: 954–7.
2. Neu HC. In vitro activity of a new broad spectrum, beta-lactamase-stable oral cephalosporin, cefixime. Pediatr Infect Dis J 1987; 6: 958–62.
3. Stone JW, et al. Cefixime, in-vitro activity, pharmacokinetics and tissue penetration. J Antimicrob Chemother 1989; 23: 221–8.

Pharmacokinetics
Only 40 to 50% of an oral dose of cefixime is absorbed from the gastrointestinal tract, whether taken before or after meals, although the rate of absorption may be decreased in the presence of food. Cefixime is better absorbed from oral suspension than from tablets. Absorption is fairly slow. Peak plasma concentrations of 2 to 3 μg per mL and 3.7 to 4.6 μg per mL have been reported between 2 and 6 hours after single doses of 200 and 400 mg, respectively. The plasma half-life is usually about 3 to 4 hours and may be prolonged when there is renal impairment. About 65% of cefixime in the circulation is bound to plasma proteins.

Information on the distribution of cefixime in body tissues and fluids is limited. It crosses the placenta. Relatively high concentrations may be achieved in bile and urine. About 20% of an oral dose (or 50% of an absorbed dose) is excreted unchanged in the urine within 24 hours. Up to 60% may be eliminated by nonrenal mechanisms; there is no evidence of metabolism but some is probably excreted into the faeces from bile. It is not substantially removed by dialysis.

◊ References.
1. Brittain DC, et al. The pharmacokinetic and bactericidal characteristics of oral cefixime. Clin Pharmacol Ther 1985; 38: 590–4.
2. Guay DRP, et al. Pharmacokinetics of cefixime (CL-284,635; FK027) in healthy subjects and patients with renal insufficiency. Antimicrob Agents Chemother 1986; 30: 485–90.
3. Faulkner RD, et al. Pharmacokinetics of cefixime in the young and elderly. J Antimicrob Chemother 1988; 21: 787–94.
4. Stone JW, et al. Cefixime, in-vitro activity, pharmacokinetics and tissue penetration. J Antimicrob Chemother 1989; 23: 221–8.
5. Westphal JF, et al. Biliary excretion of cefixime: assessment in patients provided with T-tube drainage. Antimicrob Agents Chemother 1993; 37: 1488–91.
6. Somekh E, et al. Penetration and bactericidal activity of cefixime in synovial fluid. Antimicrob Agents Chemother 1996; 40: 1198–1200.

Uses and Administration
Cefixime is generally classified as a third-generation cephalosporin antibiotic and is given by mouth in the treatment of susceptible infections (see Antimicrobial Action, above), including gonorrhoea, otitis media, pharyngitis, lower respiratory-tract infections such as bronchitis, and urinary-tract infections. For details of these infections and their treatment, see under Choice of Antibacterial, p.114.

Cefixime is available as the trihydrate and doses are expressed in terms of anhydrous cefixime. It is given by mouth in adult doses of 200 to 400 mg daily as a single dose or in two divided doses. Children under 50 kg body-weight may be given 8 mg per kg daily as an oral suspension, again as a single dose or in two divided doses.

Doses should be reduced in patients with moderate to severe renal impairment. A dose of 200 mg daily should not be exceeded in patients with a creatinine clearance of less than 20 mL per minute.

For uncomplicated gonorrhoea, a single oral dose of 400 mg is given.

◊ General references.

1. Brogden RN, Campoli-Richards DM. Cefixime: a review of its antibacterial activity, pharmacokinetic properties and therapeutic potential. *Drugs* 1989; **38**: 524–50.
2. Leggett NJ, *et al.* Cefixime. *DICP Ann Pharmacother* 1990; **24**: 489–95.
3. Adam D, Wallace RJ, eds. Symposium on cefixime. *Drugs* 1991; **42** (suppl 4): 1–32.
4. Markham A, Brogden RN. Cefixime: a review of its therapeutic efficacy in lower respiratory tract infections. *Drugs* 1995; **49**: 1007–22.

Preparations

USP 25: Cefixime for Oral Suspension; Cefixime Tablets.

Proprietary Preparations (details are given in Part 3)
Aust.: Aerocef; Tricef; **Braz.:** Plenax; **Canad.:** Suprax; **Fin.:** Supracef; **Fr.:** Oroken; **Ger.:** Cephoral; Suprax; Uro-Cephoral; **Irl.:** Suprax; **Israel:** Supran; **Ital.:** Cefixoral; Suprax; Unixime; **Jpn:** Cefspan; **Mex.:** Denvar; Novacef; **Neth.:** Fixim; **Port.:** Neocef; Tricef; **S.Afr.:** Fixime; **Spain:** Denvar; Necopen; **Swed.:** Tricef; **Switz.:** Cephoral; **Thai.:** Cefspan; **UK:** Suprax; **USA:** Suprax.

Cefluprenam (17616-m)

Cefluprenam (*rINN*).

(−)-{(*E*)-3-[(6*R*,7*R*)-7-[2-(5-Amino-1,2,4-thiadiazol-3-yl)glyoxylamido]-2-carboxy-8-oxo-5-thia-1-azabicyclo[4.2.0]oct-2-en-3-yl]allyl}(carbamoylmethyl)ethylmethylammonium hydroxide, inner salt, 7²-(*Z*)-[*O*-(fluoromethyl)oxime].
$C_{20}H_{25}FN_8O_6S_2 = 556.6$.
$CAS — 116853-25-9$.

Profile

Cefluprenam is a cephalosporin antibacterial. It has been investigated in the treatment of susceptible infections.

Cefmenoxime Hydrochloride (15312-k)

Cefmenoxime Hydrochloride (*USAN, rINNM*).

Abbott-50192; Cefmenoxime Hemihydrochloride; SCE-1365 (cefmenoxime). (*Z*)-(7*R*)-7-[2-(2-Aminothiazol-4-yl)-2-methoxyiminoacetamido]-3-[(1-methyl-1*H*-tetrazol-5-yl)thiomethyl]-3-cephem-4-carboxylic acid hydrochloride.
$(C_{16}H_{17}N_9O_5S_3)_2,HCl = 1059.6$.
$CAS — 65085-01-0 (cefmenoxime); 75738-58-8 (cefmenoxime hydrochloride)$.

Pharmacopoeias. In *Jpn* and *US*.

Pharmacopoeial description

USP 25: White to light orange-yellow crystals or crystalline powder. Very slightly soluble in water; practically insoluble in dehydrated alcohol and in ether; freely soluble in formamide; slightly soluble in methyl alcohol. Store in airtight containers.

Profile

Cefmenoxime is a third-generation cephalosporin antibiotic with actions and uses similar to those of cefotaxime (p.169). It is administered as the hydrochloride by intramuscular injection, or intravenously by injection or infusion in the treatment of susceptible infections. Doses are expressed in terms of the equivalent amount of cefmenoxime. The usual adult dose is 1 to 4 g daily in 2 to 4 divided doses, although up to 9 g daily has been given in severe infections. Children have been given 40 to 80 mg per kg body-weight daily in 2 to 4 divided doses; higher doses have been used in severe infections. Neonates have been given 40 to 60 mg per kg in 2 or 3 divided doses.

Like cefamandole (p.163), cefmenoxime has an *N*-methylthiotetrazole side-chain and coagulopathy and a disulfiram-like interaction with alcohol have been reported rarely.

◊ Reviews.

1. Campoli-Richards DM, Todd PA. Cefmenoxime: a review of its antibacterial activity, pharmacokinetic properties and therapeutic use. *Drugs* 1987; **34**: 188–221.

Preparations

USP 25: Cefmenoxime for Injection.

Proprietary Preparations (details are given in Part 3)
Aust.: Tacef; **Ger.:** Tacef†; **Jpn:** Bestcall; Bestron.

Cefmetazole (17134-p)

Cefmetazole (*USAN, rINN*).

U-72791. (6*R*,7*S*)-7-{2-[(Cyanomethyl)thio]acetamido}-7-methoxy-3-{[(1-methyl-1*H*-tetrazol-5-yl)thio]methyl}-8-oxo-5-thia-1-azabicyclo-[4.2.0]oct-2-ene-2-carboxylic acid.
$C_{15}H_{17}N_7O_5S_3 = 471.5$.
$CAS — 56796-20-4$.
$ATC — J01DA40$.

Pharmacopoeias. In *US*.

Pharmacopoeial description

USP 25: Store in airtight containers.

Cefmetazole Sodium (12540-v)

Cefmetazole Sodium (*USAN, rINNM*).

CS-1170; SKF-83088; U-72791A.
$C_{15}H_{16}N_7NaO_5S_3 = 493.5$.
$CAS — 56796-39-5$.

Pharmacopoeias. In *Jpn* and *US*.

1.05 g of cefmetazole sodium is approximately equivalent to 1 g of cefmetazole. Each g of monograph substance represents about 2 mmol of sodium.

Pharmacopoeial description

USP 25: A white solid. Very soluble in water and in methyl alcohol; soluble in acetone; practically insoluble in chloroform. pH of a 10% solution in water is between 4.2 and 6.2. Store in airtight containers.

Adverse Effects and Precautions

As for Cefalotin Sodium, p.162.
Cefmetazole contains an *N*-methylthiotetrazole side-chain and like cefamandole (p.163) has the potential to cause hypoprothrombinaemia and bleeding.

Effects on the blood. References.

1. Breen GA, St Peter WL. Hypoprothrombinemia associated with cefmetazole. *Ann Pharmacother* 1997; **31**: 180–3.

Interactions

As for Cefamandole, p.164.

Antimicrobial Action

Cefmetazole is a cephamycin antibiotic with a similar spectrum of antibacterial activity to that of cefoxitin (p.171), including the anaerobe *Bacteroides fragilis*.

◊ References.

1. Cornick NA, *et al.* Activity of cefmetazole against anaerobic bacteria. *Antimicrob Agents Chemother* 1987; **31**: 2010–12.

Pharmacokinetics

Following administration of cefmetazole 2 g intravenously every 6 hours, as the sodium salt, peak and trough plasma concentrations of 138 and 6 μg per mL have been achieved. Cefmetazole is 65 to 85% bound to plasma proteins, depending on the plasma concentration. A plasma half-life of about 1.1 to 1.5 hours has been reported; it is prolonged in patients with renal impairment. Small amounts have been detected in breast milk. Relatively high concentrations have been achieved in bile. The majority of a dose is excreted unchanged in the urine resulting in high concentrations; up to 85% of a dose has been recovered within 12 hours. Cefmetazole is partly excreted by renal tubular secretion and probenecid prolongs elimination. Cefmetazole is removed to some extent by haemodialysis.

◊ References.

1. Ito MK, *et al.* Intraoperative serum, bile, and gallbladder-wall concentrations of cefmetazole in patients undergoing cholecystectomy. *Clin Pharm* 1988; **7**: 447–51.
2. Ko H, *et al.* Pharmacokinetics of intravenously administered cefmetazole and cefoxitin and effects of probenecid on cefmetazole elimination. *Antimicrob Agents Chemother* 1989; **33**: 356–61.
3. Ko H, *et al.* Pharmacokinetics of single-dose cefmetazole following intramuscular administration of cefmetazole sodium to healthy male volunteers. *Antimicrob Agents Chemother* 1989; **33**: 508–12.
4. Tan JS, *et al.* Pharmacokinetics of intravenous cefmetazole with emphasis on comparison between predicted theoretical levels in tissue and actual skin window fluid levels. *Antimicrob Agents Chemother* 1989; **33**: 924–7.
5. Halstenson CE, *et al.* Disposition of cefmetazole in healthy volunteers and patients with impaired renal function. *Antimicrob Agents Chemother* 1990; **34**: 519–23.
6. Borin MT, *et al.* Pharmacokinetics and dose proportionality of cefmetazole in healthy young and elderly volunteers. *Antimicrob Agents Chemother* 1990; **34**: 1944–8.

Uses and Administration

Cefmetazole is a cephamycin antibiotic generally classified with the second-generation cephalosporins and used similarly to cefoxitin (p.171) in the treatment and prophylaxis of anaerobic and mixed bacterial infections, especially intra-abdominal and pelvic infections. It may also be used in the treatment of gonorrhoea. For details of these infections and their treatment, see under Choice of Antibacterial, p.114.

It is administered intravenously as the sodium salt by infusion over 10 to 60 minutes or by slow injection over 3 to 5 minutes. Cefmetazole sodium is also administered intramuscularly in some countries. Doses are expressed in terms of the equivalent amount of cefmetazole.

The usual adult dose is 2 g intravenously every 6 to 12 hours. The interval between doses should be 12, 16, or 24 hours in patients with mild, moderate, or severe renal impairment, respectively; patients with virtually no renal function may be given cefmetazole every 48 hours, after haemodialysis.

For uncomplicated gonorrhoea the usual dose is 1 g as a single intramuscular injection, together with probenecid 1 g by mouth.

For surgical infection prophylaxis, a single dose of 1 or 2 g may be given intravenously 30 to 90 minutes before surgery and repeated if necessary after 8 and 16 hours. At caesarean section a single 2-g dose may be given intravenously to the mother after the umbilical cord is clamped; alternatively a 1-g dose may be given and repeated after 8 and 16 hours.

◊ References.

1. Finch R, *et al.* eds. Cefmetazole: a clinical appraisal. *J Antimicrob Chemother* 1989; **23** (suppl D): 1–142.

Preparations

USP 25: Cefmetazole for Injection; Cefmetazole Injection.

Proprietary Preparations (details are given in Part 3)
Hong Kong: Cefmetazon; **Ital.:** Cefadel; Decacef†; Metacaf; Metafar; Metasal; Metazol; **Jpn:** Cefmetazon; **Spain:** Cemetol†; **Thai.:** Cefmetazon; **USA:** Zefazone.

Cefminox Sodium (18922-r)

Cefminox Sodium (*pINN*).

MT-141. Sodium 7-{2-[((*S*)-2-amino-2-carboxyethyl]thioacetamido}-7-methoxy-3-(1-methyl-1*H*-tetrazol-5-ylthiomethyl)-3-cephem-4-carboxylate.
$C_{16}H_{20}N_7NaO_7S_3 = 541.6$.
$CAS — 75481-73-1 (cefminox)$.

Pharmacopoeias. Jpn includes the heptahydrate.

Profile

Cefminox sodium is a cephamycin antibiotic with properties similar to those of cefoxitin sodium (p.171). It is given intravenously.

Cefminox has an *N*-methylthiotetrazole side-chain. For adverse effects and drug interactions associated with this side-chain, see under Cefamandole, p.163.

◊ References.

1. Watanabe S, Omoto S. Pharmacology of cefminox, a new bactericidal cephamycin. *Drugs Exp Clin Res* 1990; **16**: 461–7.
2. Soriano F, *et al.* Comparative susceptibility of cefminox and cefoxitin to β-lactamases of Bacteroides spp. *J Antimicrob Chemother* 1991; **28**: 55–60.
3. Aguilar L, *et al.* Cefminox: correlation between in-vitro susceptibility and pharmacokinetics and serum bactericidal activity in healthy volunteers. *J Antimicrob Chemother* 1994; **33**: 91–101.
4. Mayama T, *et al.* Postmarketing surveillance on side-effects of cefminox sodium (Meicelin). *Int J Clin Pharmacol Ther* 1995; **33**: 149–55.
5. Hoellman DB, *et al.* In vitro activities of cefminox against anaerobic bacteria compared with those of nine other compounds. *Antimicrob Agents Chemother* 1998; **42**: 495–501.

Preparations

Proprietary Preparations (details are given in Part 3)
Jpn: Meicelin; **Spain:** Alteporina; Tencef.

Cefodizime Sodium (18923-f)

Cefodizime Sodium (*BANM, rINNM*).

HR-221; S-771221B; THR-221; TRH-221. (*Z*)-7-[2-(2-Aminothiazol-4-yl)-2-methoxyiminoacetamido]-3-(5-carboxymethyl-4-methylthiazol-2-ylthiomethyl)-3-cephem-4-carboxylic acid, disodium salt.
$C_{20}H_{18}N_6Na_2O_7S_4 = 628.6$.
$CAS — 69739-16-8 (cefodizime); 86329-79-5 (cefodizime sodium)$.

1.08 g of monograph substance is approximately equivalent to 1 g of cefodizime. Each g of monograph substance represents about 3.2 mmol of sodium.

Adverse Effects and Precautions

As for Cefotaxime Sodium, p.169.

Interactions

Probenecid reduces the renal clearance of cefodizime.

Antimicrobial Action

Cefodizime has similar antimicrobial activity to that of cefotaxime (p.169) although cefodizime has no active metabolite. It has variable activity against *Citrobacter* spp., and *Pseudomonas aeruginosa* and *Bacteroides fragilis* are generally resistant.

Pharmacokinetics

Cefodizime is administered by injection as the sodium salt. Intramuscular administration of 1 g cefodizime produces peak plasma concentrations of about 60 to 75 μg per mL at about 1 to 1.5 hours. Immediately after intravenous administration of 1 or 2 g cefodizime mean peak plasma concentrations of 215 and 394 μg per mL, respectively, have been achieved. Cefodizime is about 80% bound to plasma proteins and is widely distributed into body tissues and fluids. It crosses the placenta and small amounts have been detected in breast milk. Plasma elimination is reported to be triphasic with a terminal elimination half-life of about 4 hours. The half-life is prolonged by renal impairment.

The majority of a dose is excreted unchanged in the urine; up to 80% of a dose has been recovered within 24 hours. Cefodizime is mainly excreted by glomerular filtration with some tubular secretion. Probenecid delays excretion. Cefodizime is removed by dialysis.

◊ References.

1. Conte JE. Pharmacokinetics of cefodizime in volunteers with normal or impaired renal function. *J Clin Pharmacol* 1994; **34**: 1066–70.
2. Lenfant B, *et al.* Pharmacokinetics of cefodizime following single doses of 0.5, 1.0, 2.0, and 3.0 grams administered intravenously to healthy volunteers. *Antimicrob Agents Chemother* 1995; **39**: 2037–41.
3. Scaglione F, *et al.* Pharmacokinetic study of cefodizime and ceftriaxone in sera and bones of patients undergoing hip arthroplasty. *Antimicrob Agents Chemother* 1997; **41**: 2292–4.

The symbol † denotes a preparation no longer actively marketed

Uses and Administration

Cefodizime is a third-generation cephalosporin antibiotic with uses similar to those of cefotaxime (p.170).

Cefodizime is administered as the disodium salt by intramuscular injection or intravenously by injection or infusion in the treatment of susceptible infections. Doses are expressed in terms of the equivalent amount of cefodizime. Adults have usually been given 1 g every 12 hours for urinary-tract infections and lower respiratory-tract infections; alternatively, a single daily dose of 2 g has been given in urinary-tract infections. Single doses over 1 g should be given intravenously. Doses should be reduced to one-half the usual dose in renal impairment when the creatinine clearance is less than 30 mL per minute.

◊ References.
1. Finch RG, et al., eds. Cefodizime: a third generation cephalosporin with immunomodulating properties. J Antimicrob Chemother 1990; 26 (suppl C): 1–134.
2. Barradell LB, Brogden RN. Cefodizime: a review of its antibacterial activity, pharmacokinetic properties and therapeutic use. Drugs 1992; 44: 800–834.

Preparations

Proprietary Preparations (details are given in Part 3)
Aust.: Timecef; *Braz.:* Timecef; *Ger.:* Opticef; *Irl.:* Modivid; *Ital.:* Diezime; Modivid; Timecef; *Mex.:* Modivid; *Port.:* Modivid; *Thai.:* Modivid; *UK:* Timecef†.

Cefonicid Sodium (16566-n)

Cefonicid Sodium (BANM, USAN, rINNM).
SKF-D-75073-Z₂; SKF-D-75073-Z (cefonicid monosodium). 7-[(R)-Mandelamido]-3-(1-sulphomethyl-1H-tetrazol-5-ylthiomethyl)-3-cephem-4-carboxylic acid, disodium salt.
C₁₈H₁₆N₆Na₂O₈S₃ = 586.5.
CAS — 61270-58-4 (cefonicid); 61270-78-8 (cefonicid disodium); 71420-79-6 (cefonicid monosodium).
Pharmacopoeias. In US.

1.08 g of monograph substance is approximately equivalent to 1 g of cefonicid. Each g of monograph substance represents about 3.4 mmol of sodium.

Pharmacopoeial description

USP 25: A white to off-white solid. Freely soluble in water, in sodium chloride 0.9%, and in glucose 5%; very slightly soluble in dehydrated alcohol; soluble in methyl alcohol. pH of a 5% solution in water is between 3.5 and 6.5. Store in airtight containers.

Adverse Effects and Precautions

As for Cefalotin Sodium, p.162.

Cefonicid contains a substituted N-methylthiotetrazole side-chain, a structure associated with hypoprothrombinaemia (see Cefamandole, p.163).

Effects on the blood. References.
1. Riancho JA, et al. Life-threatening bleeding in a patient treated with cefonicid. Ann Intern Med 1995; 123: 472–3.

Interactions

As for Cefamandole, p.164.

Antimicrobial Action

Cefonicid sodium has an antimicrobial action and pattern of resistance similar to those of cefamandole (p.164), although it is generally less active against Gram-positive cocci.

Pharmacokinetics

Cefonicid is administered parenterally as the sodium salt. After intramuscular administration of a dose of 1 g peak plasma concentrations ranging from 67 to 126 µg per mL have been achieved after 1 to 2 hours. More than 90% of cefonicid in the circulation is bound to plasma proteins. Cefonicid has a plasma half-life of approximately 4.5 hours, which is prolonged in patients with renal impairment.

Therapeutic concentrations of cefonicid have been reported in a wide range of body tissues and fluids.

Up to 99% of a dose of cefonicid is excreted unchanged in the urine within 24 hours. The excretion of cefonicid is decreased by the concomitant administration of probenecid.

◊ References.
1. Trang JM, et al. Effect of age and renal function on cefonicid pharmacokinetics. Antimicrob Agents Chemother 1989; 33: 142–6.
2. Furlanut M, et al. Pharmacokinetics of cefonicid in children. Eur J Clin Pharmacol 1989; 36: 79–82.
3. Benson JM, et al. In vitro protein binding of cefonicid and cefuroxime in adult and neonatal sera. Antimicrob Agents Chemother 1993; 37: 1343–7.

Uses and Administration

Cefonicid is a second-generation cephalosporin antibiotic used similarly to cefamandole in the treatment of susceptible infections and for surgical infection prophylaxis.

It is given as the sodium salt by deep intramuscular injection, or intravenously by slow injection over 3 to 5 minutes or by infusion. Doses are expressed in terms of the equivalent amount of cefonicid. The usual dose is cefonicid 1 g once daily. For uncomplicated urinary-tract infections a dose of 0.5 g once daily is recommended; up to 2 g once daily has been given in severe infections. More than 1 g should not be injected intramuscularly into a single site.

For patients with renal impairment a loading dose of 7.5 mg per kg body-weight is recommended followed by reduced maintenance doses according to the creatinine clearance and the severity of the infection. A dose supplement is not required after dialysis.

For surgical infection prophylaxis, a single dose of 1 g given one hour before surgical incision is usually sufficient, but may be given daily for a further 2 days in prosthetic arthroplasty or open-heart surgery.

◊ References.
1. Saltiel E, Brogden RN. Cefonicid: a review of its antibacterial activity, pharmacological properties and therapeutic use. Drugs 1986; 32: 222–59.

Preparations

USP 25: Cefonicid for Injection.

Proprietary Preparations (details are given in Part 3)
Belg.: Monocid; *Hong Kong:* Monocid; *Israel:* Monocef; *Ital.:* Abiocef; Bacid; Biocil; Cefobacter; Cefodie; Cefoger; Cefok; Cefoplus; Cefosporin; Cefovis; Chefir; Daycef; Delsacid; Diespor; Emidoxin; Epicef; Fonicef; Fonisal; Framecef; Ipacid; Krucef; Lampocef; Lisa; Maxid; Modicef; Modiem; Monobios; Monocid; Necid; Nokid; Pantacid; Parecid; Praticef; Rocid; Silvercef; Sintocef; Unicef†; Unicid; Valecid; *Port.:* Monocid; *Spain:* Monocid; Unidie; *USA:* Monocid.

Cefoperazone Sodium (187-a)

Cefoperazone Sodium (BANM, USAN, rINNM).
Cefoperazonum Natricum; CP-52640-2; CP-52640 (anhydrous cefoperazone); CP-52640-3 (cefoperazone dihydrate); T-1551 (cefoperazone or sodium salt). Sodium (7R)-7-[(R)-2-(4-ethyl-2,3-dioxopiperazin-1-ylcarboxamido)-2-(4-hydroxyphenyl)acetamido]-3-[(1-methyl-1H-tetrazol-5-yl)thiomethyl]-3-cephem-4-carboxylate.
C₂₅H₂₆N₉NaO₈S₂ = 667.6.
CAS — 62893-19-0 (cefoperazone); 62893-20-3 (cefoperazone sodium).
Pharmacopoeias. In Chin., Eur. (see p.vi), Jpn, Pol., and US.

1.03 g of monograph substance is approximately equivalent to 1 g of cefoperazone. Each g of monograph substance represents about 1.5 mmol of sodium.

Pharmacopoeial description

Ph. Eur.: A white or slightly yellow, hygroscopic, powder. If crystalline it exhibits polymorphism. Freely soluble in water; slightly soluble in alcohol; soluble in methyl alcohol. A 25% solution in water has a pH of 4.5 to 6.5. Store in airtight containers at a temperature of 2° to 8°. Protect from light.

USP 25: A white to pale buff crystalline powder. Freely soluble in water and in methyl alcohol; slightly soluble in dehydrated alcohol; insoluble in acetone, in ether, and in ethyl acetate. pH of a 25% solution in water is between 4.5 and 6.5. Store in airtight containers.

Incompatibility. As with most beta-lactams, admixture of cefoperazone sodium with aminoglycosides is not recommended because of the potential for inactivation of either drug.

There have been reports of incompatibility with other drugs including diltiazem,[1] doxorubicin,[2] pentamidine,[3] perphenazine,[4] pethidine,[5] promethazine,[6] and remifentanil.[7]

1. Gayed AA, et al. Visual compatibility of diltiazem injection with various diluents and medications during simulated Y-site injection. Am J Health-Syst Pharm 1995; 52: 516–20.
2. Trissel LA, et al. Compatibility of doxorubicin hydrochloride liposome injection with selected other drugs during simulated Y-site administration. Am J Health-Syst Pharm 1997; 54: 2708–13.
3. Lewis JD, El-Gendy A. Cephalosporin-pentamidine isethionate incompatibilities. Am J Health-Syst Pharm 1996; 53: 1461–2.
4. Gasca M, et al. Visual compatibility of perphenazine with various antimicrobials during simulated Y-site injection. Am J Hosp Pharm 1987; 44: 574–5.
5. Nieves-Cordero AL, et al. Compatibility of narcotic analgesic solutions with various antibiotics during simulated Y-site injection. Am J Hosp Pharm 1985; 42: 1108–9.
6. Scott SM. Incompatibility of cefoperazone and promethazine. Am J Hosp Pharm 1990; 47: 519.
7. Trissel LA, et al. Compatibility of remifentanil hydrochloride with selected drugs during simulated Y-site administration. Am J Health-Syst Pharm 1997; 54: 2192–6.

Adverse Effects and Precautions

As for Cefalotin Sodium, p.162.

Like cefotaxime (p.169), cefoperazone has the potential for colonisation and superinfection with resistant organisms. Changes in bowel flora may be more marked than with cefotaxime because of the greater biliary excretion of cefoperazone; diarrhoea may occur more often.

Cefoperazone contains an N-methylthiotetrazole side-chain, a structure associated with hypoprothrombinaemia (see Cefamandole, p.163). Hypoprothrombinaemia has been reported in patients treated with cefoperazone and has rarely been associated with bleeding episodes. Prothrombin time should be monitored in patients at risk of hypoprothrombinaemia and vitamin K administered if necessary.

Interactions

As for Cefamandole, p.164.

Antimicrobial Action

Cefoperazone has antimicrobial activity similar to that of ceftazidime (p.175), although it is slightly less active against some Enterobacteriaceae. It has good activity against Pseudomonas aeruginosa, but is less active than ceftazidime.

Cefoperazone is more susceptible than cefotaxime to hydrolysis by certain beta-lactamases.

Activity, particularly against Enterobacteriaceae and Bacteroides spp. has been enhanced in the presence of the beta-lactamase inhibitor sulbactam; resistant Ps. aeruginosa are not sensitive to the combination.

◊ References.
1. Fass RJ, et al. In vitro activities of cefoperazone and sulbactam singly and in combination against cefoperazone-resistant members of the family Enterobacteriaceae and nonfermenters. Antimicrob Agents Chemother 1990; 34: 2256–9.
2. Clark RB, et al. Multicentre study on antibiotic susceptibilities of anaerobic bacteria to cefoperazone-sulbactam and other antimicrobial agents. J Antimicrob Chemother 1992; 29: 57–67.

Pharmacokinetics

Cefoperazone is administered parenterally as the sodium salt. After intramuscular administration of doses equivalent to cefoperazone 1 or 2 g, peak plasma concentrations of 65 and 97 µg per mL have been reported after 1 to 2 hours. The plasma half-life of cefoperazone is about 2 hours, but may be prolonged in neonates and in patients with hepatic or biliary-tract disease. Cefoperazone is 82 to 93% bound to plasma proteins, depending on the concentration.

Cefoperazone is widely distributed in body tissues and fluids, although penetration into the CSF is generally poor. It crosses the placenta, and low concentrations have been detected in breast milk.

Cefoperazone is excreted mainly in the bile where it rapidly achieves high concentrations. Urinary excretion is primarily by glomerular filtration. Up to 30% of a dose is excreted unchanged in the urine within 12 to 24 hours; this proportion may be increased in patients with hepatic or biliary disease. Cefoperazone A, a degradation product less active than cefoperazone, has been found only rarely in vivo.

Uses and Administration

Cefoperazone is a third-generation cephalosporin antibiotic used similarly to ceftazidime (p.175) in the treatment of susceptible infections, especially those due to Pseudomonas spp. It is not recommended for the treatment of meningitis because of poor penetration into the CSF.

Cefoperazone is given as the sodium salt by deep intramuscular injection or intravenously by intermittent or continuous infusion. Doses are expressed in terms of the equivalent amount of cefoperazone. The usual dose for adults is 2 to 4 g daily in two divided doses. In severe infections, up to 12 g daily in two to four divided doses may be given. In general, the dose should not exceed 4 g daily in patients with liver disease or biliary obstruction or 1 to 2 g daily in those with both liver and kidney impairment; if higher doses are used plasma concentrations of cefoperazone should be monitored. If cefoperazone is given in association with an aminoglycoside, the drugs should be administered separately.

Cefoperazone has also been given with the beta-lactamase inhibitor sulbactam.

Preparations

USP 25: Cefoperazone for Injection; Cefoperazone Injection.

Proprietary Preparations (details are given in Part 3)
Aust.: Cefobid; **Braz.:** Cefobid; **Fr.:** Cefobis†; **Ger.:** Cefobis†; **Hong Kong:** Cefobid; Cefozone; **Ital.:** Bioperazone; Cefazone†; Cefogram; Cefoneg; Cefoper; Cefosint†; Dardum; Farecef; Ipazone; Kefazon; Novobiocyl; Perocef†; Prontokef†; Tomabef; Zoncef; **Singapore:** Cefobid; Cefozone; Dardum; Medocef; **Spain:** Cefobid; **Thai.:** Cefobid; Cefozone; Medocef; **USA:** Cefobid.

Multi-ingredient: Thai.: Sulperazon.

Ceforanide (12541-g)

Ceforanide (BAN, USAN, rINN).
BL-S786. 7-[2-(α-Amino-o-tolyl)acetamido]-3-(1-carboxymethyl-1H-tetrazol-5-ylthiomethyl)-3-cephem-4-carboxylic acid.
$C_{20}H_{21}N_7O_6S_2 = 519.6$.
CAS — 60925-61-3.
Pharmacopoeias. In US.

Pharmacopoeial description
USP 25: A white to off-white powder. Practically insoluble in water, in chloroform, in ether, and in methyl alcohol; very soluble in 1N sodium hydroxide. pH of a 5% suspension in water is between 2.5 and 4.5. Store in airtight containers.

Profile
Ceforanide is a second-generation cephalosporin antibiotic with actions and uses similar to those of cefamandole (p.163), although it is reported to be less active in vitro against some bacteria, including staphylococci and Haemophilus influenzae. It is used in the treatment of susceptible infections and for surgical infection prophylaxis.

It is given as the lysine salt but doses are expressed in terms of the equivalent amount of ceforanide. It has been administered by deep intramuscular injection, or intravenously by slow injection over 3 to 5 minutes or by infusion, in doses of 1 to 2 g every 12 hours to adults. Children have been given 20 mg per kg body-weight daily in two divided doses. For surgical infection prophylaxis a dose of 1 to 2 g intravenously one hour before surgical incision has been used in adults.

Ceforanide contains a substituted N-methylthiotetrazole side-chain, a structure associated with hypoprothrombinaemia and alcohol intolerance (see Cefamandole, p.163). Probenecid does not affect the renal excretion of ceforanide.

◊ References.
1. Campoli-Richards DM, et al. Ceforanide: a review of its antibacterial activity, pharmacokinetic properties and clinical efficacy. Drugs 1987; **34:** 411–37.

Preparations
USP 25: Ceforanide for Injection.

Proprietary Preparations (details are given in Part 3)
Belg.: Precef.

Cefoselis (17617-b)

Cefoselis (rINN).
(−)-5-Amino-2-({(6R,7R)-7-[2-(2-amino-4-thiazolyl)glyoxylamido]-2-carboxy-8-oxo-5-thia-1-azabicyclo[4.2.0]oct-2-en-3-yl}methyl)-1-(2-hydroxyethyl)pyrazolium hydroxide, inner salt, 7²-(Z)-(O-methyloxime).
$C_{19}H_{22}N_8O_6S_2 = 522.6$.
CAS — 122841-10-5.

Profile
Cefoselis is a cephalosporin antibacterial used in the treatment of susceptible bacterial infections. It is given as the sulfate by intravenous infusion in a usual dose of 1 to 2 g daily in two divided doses. For severe infections, up to 4 g daily may be given.

Preparations
Proprietary Preparations (details are given in Part 3)
Jpn: Wincef.

Cefotaxime Sodium (32-f)

Cefotaxime Sodium (BANM, USAN, rINNM).
Cefotaximum Natricum; CTX; HR-756; RU-24756. Sodium (7R)-7-[(Z)-2-(2-aminothiazol-4-yl)-2-(methoxyimino)acetamido]cephalosporanate; Sodium (7R)-3-acetoxymethyl-7-[(Z)-2-(2-aminothiazol-4-yl)-2-(methoxyimino)acetamido]-3-cephem-4-carboxylate.
$C_{16}H_{16}N_5NaO_7S_2 = 477.4$.
CAS — 63527-52-6 (cefotaxime); 64485-93-4 (cefotaxime sodium).
Pharmacopoeias. In Chin., Eur. (see p.vi), Jpn, Pol., and US.

The symbol † denotes a preparation no longer actively marketed

---

1.05 g of monograph substance is approximately equivalent to 1 g of cefotaxime. Each g of monograph substance represents about 2.09 mmol of sodium.

Pharmacopoeial description
Ph. Eur.: A white or slightly yellow, hygroscopic, powder. Very soluble in water; practically insoluble in ether; sparingly soluble in methyl alcohol. A 10% solution in water has a pH of between 4.5 and 6.5. Store in airtight containers at a temperature not exceeding 30°. Protect from light.

USP 25: An off-white to pale yellow crystalline powder. Freely soluble in water; practically insoluble in organic solvents. pH of a 10% solution in water is between 4.5 and 6.5. Store in airtight containers.

Incompatibility. Cefotaxime sodium has been reported to be incompatible with alkaline solutions such as sodium bicarbonate. The manufacturers recommend that it should be administered separately from aminoglycosides.

Adverse Effects and Precautions
As for Cefalotin Sodium, p.162. Arrhythmias have been associated with rapid bolus infusion through a central venous catheter in a few cases.

The broad-spectrum third-generation cephalosporins have the potential for colonisation and superinfection with resistant organisms such as Pseudomonas aeruginosa, Enterobacter spp., Candida, and enterococci, at various sites in the body, although the incidence has generally been low with cefotaxime. Changes in bowel flora are a predisposing factor and have been more marked with cefoperazone and ceftriaxone, possibly because of their greater biliary excretion. Pseudomembranous colitis, associated with Clostridium difficile infection, may occasionally be seen with any of the third-generation cephalosporins.

◊ Reviews on adverse effects associated with third-generation cephalosporins.
1. Neu HC. Third generation cephalosporins: safety profiles after 10 years of clinical use. J Clin Pharmacol 1990; **30:** 396–403.
2. Fekety FR. Safety of parenteral third-generation cephalosporins. Am J Med 1990; **88** (suppl 4A): 38S–44S.

Antibiotic-associated colitis. It has been suggested[1] that cefotaxime is associated with an increased risk of Clostridium difficile diarrhoea in elderly patients; however, the manufacturer[2] has disputed this, arguing that cefotaxime compares favourably with alternative third-generation cephalosporins.
1. Impallomeni M, et al. Increased risk of diarrhoea caused by Clostridium difficile in elderly patients receiving cefotaxime. BMJ 1995; **311:** 1345–6.
2. Rothschild E, et al. Risk of diarrhoea due to Clostridium difficile during cefotaxime treatment. BMJ 1996; **312:** 778.

Interactions
As for many cephalosporins, probenecid reduces the renal clearance of cefotaxime, resulting in higher and prolonged plasma concentrations of cefotaxime and its desacetyl metabolite.

Antibacterials. The total body clearance of cefotaxime has been reduced in patients with normal and reduced renal function by the concomitant administration of the ureidopenicillins azlocillin[1] or mezlocillin.[2] Doses of cefotaxime may need to be reduced if either of these penicillins is being given. Encephalopathy with focal motor status and generalised convulsions have been reported in a patient with renal failure given cefotaxime and high doses of azlocillin.[3]
1. Kampf D, et al. Kinetic interactions between azlocillin, cefotaxime, and cefotaxime metabolites in normal and impaired renal function. Clin Pharmacol Ther 1984; **35:** 214–20.
2. Rodondi LC, et al. Influence of coadministration on the pharmacokinetics of mezlocillin and cefotaxime in healthy volunteers and in patients with renal failure. Clin Pharmacol Ther 1989; **45:** 527–34.
3. Wroe SJ, et al. Focal motor status epilepticus following treatment with azlocillin and cefotaxime. Med Toxicol 1987; **2:** 233–4.

Antimicrobial Action
Cefotaxime is a third-generation cephalosporin antibiotic. It has a bactericidal action similar to cefamandole, but a broader spectrum of activity. It is highly stable to hydrolysis by most beta-lactamases and has greater activity than first- or second-generation cephalosporins against Gram-negative bacteria. Although cefotaxime is generally considered to have slightly less activity than first-generation cephalosporins against Gram-positive bacteria, many streptococci are very sensitive to it.

Desacetylcefotaxime is an active metabolite of cefotaxime and there may be additive or synergistic effects against some species.

Minimum inhibitory concentrations (MICs) of cefotaxime for susceptible organisms have been reported to range from about 0.03 to 16 μg per mL. An MIC of 8 μg or less per mL has been taken to indicate susceptibility, and 64 μg or more per mL resistance. Many studies express activity in terms of MIC_{90}, the concentration at which 90% of organisms are inhibited. MICs are generally close to minimum bactericidal concentrations although tolerance has been reported.

Spectrum of activity. Among Gram-negative bacteria cefotaxime is active in vitro against many Enterobacteriaceae including Citrobacter and Enterobacter spp., Escherichia coli, Klebsiella spp., both indole-positive and indole-negative Proteus, Providencia, Salmonella, Serratia, Shigella, and Yersinia spp. Other Gram-negative bacteria, including penicillin-resistant strains, are Haemophilus influenzae, Moraxella catarrhalis, (Branhamella catarrhalis), Neisseria gonorrhoeae, and N. meningitidis. Brucella melitensis is also reported to be sensitive. For many of these Gram-negative bacteria the MIC is under 1 μg per mL and often much less. Some strains of Pseudomonas spp. are moderately susceptible to cefotaxime, but most are resistant. Desacetylcefotaxime is active against many of these Gram-negative bacteria, but not against Pseudomonas spp.

Among Gram-positive bacteria cefotaxime is active against staphylococci and streptococci. Staphylococcus aureus, including penicillinase-producing strains but not methicillin-resistant Staph. aureus, is sensitive with an MIC_{90} of about 2 to 4 μg per mL, reduced in the presence of desacetylcefotaxime. Staph. epidermidis is sensitive with an MIC_{90} of about 8 μg per mL, but penicillinase-producing strains are resistant. Streptococcus agalactiae (group B streptococci), Str. pneumoniae, and Str. pyogenes (group A streptococci) are all very sensitive (MIC_{90} 0.1 μg or less per mL) although truly penicillin-resistant pneumococci are apparently not sensitive. Enterococci and Listeria monocytogenes are resistant.

Cefotaxime is active against some anaerobic bacteria. Bacteroides fragilis may be moderately sensitive, but many strains are resistant; synergy has been demonstrated with desacetylcefotaxime in vitro. Clostridium perfringens is sensitive, but most Cl. difficile are resistant.

Other organisms sensitive to cefotaxime include the spirochaete Borrelia burgdorferi and the causative organism of chancroid, Haemophilus ducreyi.

Activity with other antimicrobials. In addition to possible synergy or additive effects with desacetylcefotaxime, the activity of cefotaxime may be enhanced by aminoglycosides such as gentamicin; synergy has been demonstrated in vitro against Gram-negative bacteria including Pseudomonas aeruginosa. There have also been reports of enhanced activity in vitro with other antibacterials including fosfomycin and ciprofloxacin and variable results with penicillins.

Resistance may develop during treatment with cefotaxime due to derepression of chromosomally mediated beta-lactamases, and has been reported particularly in Enterobacter spp., with multiresistant strains emerging during treatment. This type of resistance has also developed in other bacteria including Citrobacter, Serratia, and Pseudomonas spp. Another mechanism of cefotaxime resistance is the development of plasma-mediated, extended-spectrum beta-lactamases, and this has occurred in Klebsiella spp. and also other Enterobacteriaceae. Resistance in Str. pneumoniae is due to the production of altered penicillin-binding proteins.

◊ References to the antimicrobial activity of cefotaxime and other third-generation cephalosporins, including the problem of bacterial resistance.
1. Neu HC. Pathophysiologic basis for the use of third-generation cephalosporins. Am J Med 1991; **115:** 585–90.
2. Chow JW, et al. Enterobacter bacteremia: clinical features and emergence of antibiotic resistance during therapy. Ann Intern Med 1991; **115:** 585–90.
3. Sanders CC. New β-lactams: new problems for the internist. Ann Intern Med 1991; **115:** 650–1.

4. Thomson KS, *et al.* High-level resistance to cefotaxime and ceftazidime in Klebsiella pneumoniae isolates from Cleveland, Ohio. *Antimicrob Agents Chemother* 1991; **35**: 1001–3.
5. Piddock LJV, *et al.* Prevalence and mechanism of resistance to 'third-generation' cephalosporins in clinically relevant isolates of Enterobacteriaceae from 43 hospitals in the UK, 1990-1991. *J Antimicrob Chemother* 1997; **39**: 177–87.

Pharmacokinetics

Cefotaxime is administered by injection as the sodium salt. It is rapidly absorbed after intramuscular injection and mean peak plasma concentrations of about 12 and 20 µg per mL have been reported 30 minutes after 0.5 and 1 g of cefotaxime, respectively. Immediately after the intravenous injection of 0.5, 1, or 2 g of cefotaxime mean peak plasma concentrations of 38, 102, and 215 µg per mL, respectively, have been achieved with concentrations ranging from about 1 to 3 µg per mL after 4 hours. The plasma half-life of cefotaxime is about one hour and that of the active metabolite desacetylcefotaxime is about 1.5 hours; half-lives are increased in neonates and in patients with severe renal impairment, especially those of the metabolite, and a reduction in dosage may be necessary. The effects of liver disease on clearance of cefotaxime and its metabolite have been variable, but in general dosage adjustment has not been considered necessary. About 40% of cefotaxime in the circulation is reported to be bound to plasma proteins.

Cefotaxime and desacetylcefotaxime are widely distributed in body tissues and fluids; therapeutic concentrations are achieved in the CSF particularly when the meninges are inflamed. It crosses the placenta and low concentrations have been detected in breast milk.

Following partial metabolism in the liver to desacetylcefotaxime and inactive metabolites, elimination is mainly by the kidneys and about 40 to 60% of a dose has been recovered unchanged in the urine within 24 hours; a further 20% is excreted as the desacetyl metabolite. Relatively high concentrations of cefotaxime and desacetylcefotaxime are achieved in bile and about 20% of a dose has been recovered in the faeces.

Probenecid competes for renal tubular secretion with cefotaxime resulting in higher and prolonged plasma concentrations of cefotaxime and its desacetyl metabolite. Cefotaxime and its metabolites are removed by haemodialysis.

When microbiological assays have been used, reported pharmacokinetic values may relate to cefotaxime plus its active metabolite, desacetylcefotaxime.

◊ Studies of the pharmacokinetics of cefotaxime.

a. General.
1. Asmar BI, *et al.* Cefotaxime diffusion into the cerebrospinal fluid of children with meningitis. *Antimicrob Agents Chemother* 1985; **28**: 138–40.
2. Fick RB, *et al.* Penetration of cefotaxime into respiratory secretions. *Antimicrob Agents Chemother* 1987; **31**: 815–17.
3. Kearns GL, *et al.* Cefotaxime and desacetylcefotaxime pharmacokinetics in very low birth weight neonates. *J Pediatr* 1989; **114**: 461–7.
4. Sjölin J, *et al.* Penetration of cefotaxime and desacetylcefotaxime into brain abscesses in humans. *Antimicrob Agents Chemother* 1991; **35**: 2606–10.
5. Nau R, *et al.* Passage of cefotaxime and ceftriaxone into cerebrospinal fluid of patients with uninflamed meninges. *Antimicrob Agents Chemother* 1993; **37**: 1518–24.

◊ b. Pharmacokinetics in liver disease.
1. Höffken G, *et al.* Pharmacokinetics of cefotaxime and desacetylcefotaxime in cirrhosis of the liver. *Chemotherapy* 1984; **30**: 7–17.
2. Graninger W, *et al.* Cefotaxime and desacetyl-cefotaxime blood levels in hepatic dysfunction. *J Antimicrob Chemother* 1984; **14** (suppl B): 143–6.
3. Hary L, *et al.* The pharmacokinetics of ceftriaxone and cefotaxime in cirrhotic patients with ascites. *Eur J Clin Pharmacol* 1989; **36**: 613–16.
4. Ko RJ, *et al.* Pharmacokinetics of cefotaxime and desacetylcefotaxime in patients with liver disease. *Antimicrob Agents Chemother* 1991; **35**: 1376–80.

◊ c. Pharmacokinetics in renal impairment.
1. Matzke GR, *et al.* Cefotaxime and desacetyl cefotaxime kinetics in renal impairment. *Clin Pharmacol Ther* 1985; **38**: 31–6.
2. Paap CM, *et al.* Pharmacokinetics of cefotaxime and its active metabolite in children with renal dysfunction. *Antimicrob Agents Chemother* 1991; **35**: 1879–83.
3. Paap CM, *et al.* Cefotaxime and metabolite disposition in two pediatric continuous ambulatory peritoneal dialysis patients. *Ann Pharmacother* 1992; **26**: 341–3.
4. Paap CM, Nahata MC. The relation between type of renal disease and renal drug clearance in children. *Eur J Clin Pharmacol* 1993; **44**: 195–7.

Uses and Administration

Cefotaxime is a third-generation cephalosporin antibiotic used in the treatment of infections due to susceptible organisms (see Antimicrobial Action, above), especially serious and life-threatening infections. They include brain abscess, endocarditis, gonorrhoea, intensive care (selective parenteral and enteral antisepsis regimens), Lyme disease, meningitis, peritonitis (primary or spontaneous), pneumonia, septicaemia, and typhoid fever. It is also used for surgical infection prophylaxis. For details of these infections and their treatment, see under Choice of Antibacterial, p.114.

Administration and dosage. Cefotaxime is given as the sodium salt by deep intramuscular injection or intravenously by slow injection over 3 to 5 minutes or by infusion over 20 to 60 minutes. Doses are expressed in terms of the equivalent amount of cefotaxime. It is usually given in doses of 2 to 6 g daily in 2 to 4 divided doses to adults. In severe infections up to 12 g may be given daily by the intravenous route in up to 6 divided doses; pseudomonal infections usually require more than 6 g daily, but a cephalosporin with greater antipseudomonal activity, such as ceftazidime, is preferable. Children may be given 100 to 150 mg per kg body-weight (50 mg per kg for neonates) daily in 2 to 4 divided doses, increased in severe infections to 200 mg per kg (150 to 200 mg per kg for neonates) daily if necessary. Doses of cefotaxime should be reduced in severe renal impairment; after an initial loading dose of 1 g for adults, halving the dose while maintaining the usual frequency of dosing has been suggested.

In the treatment of gonorrhoea a single 1-g dose of cefotaxime is given.

For surgical infection prophylaxis, 1 g is administered 30 to 90 minutes before surgery. At caesarean section 1 g is given intravenously to the mother as soon as the umbilical cord is clamped and two further doses intramuscularly or intravenously 6 and 12 hours later.

Cefotaxime may be administered in association with an aminoglycoside as synergy may occur against some Gram-negative organisms, but the drugs should be administered separately. It has sometimes been used with another beta-lactam to broaden the spectrum of activity. Cefotaxime has also been used in association with metronidazole in the treatment of mixed aerobic-anaerobic infections.

◊ General references to third-generation cephalosporins.
1. Neu HC, *et al.*, eds. Third-generation cephalosporins: a decade of progress in the treatment of severe infections. *Am J Med* 1990; **88** (suppl 4A): 1S–54S.

◊ General references to cefotaxime.
1. Todd PA, Brogden RN. Cefotaxime: an update of its pharmacology and therapeutic use. *Drugs* 1990; **40**: 608–51.
2. Gentry LO. Cefotaxime and prophylaxis: new approaches with a proven agent. *Am J Med* 1990; **88** (suppl 4A): 32S–37S.
3. Davies A, Speller DCE, eds. Cefotaxime—recent clinical investigations. *J Antimicrob Chemother* 1990; **26** (suppl A): 1–83.
4. Brogden RN, Spencer CM. Cefotaxime: a reappraisal of its antibacterial activity and pharmacokinetic properties, and a review of its therapeutic efficacy when administered twice daily for the treatment of mild to moderate infections. *Drugs* 1997; **53**: 483–510.

Preparations

BP 2001: Cefotaxime Injection;
USP 25: Cefotaxime for Injection; Cefotaxime Injection.

Proprietary Preparations (details are given in Part 3)

Aust.: Claforan; *Austral.:* Claforan; *Belg.:* Claforan; *Braz.:* Claforan; *Canad.:* Claforan; *Denm.:* Claforan; *Fin.:* Claforan; *Fr.:* Claforan; *Ger.:* Claforan; *Hong Kong:* Claforan; Valoran; *Irl.:* Claforan; *Israel:* Claforan; *Ital.:* Claforan; Zarivíz; *Mex.:* Benaxima; Biosint; Cefradil; Claforan; Fotexina; Taporin; Viken; *Neth.:* Claforan; *Norw.:* Claforan; *NZ:* Claforan; *Port.:* Ralopar; *S.Afr.:* Claforan; Oritaxim; *Singapore:* Claforan; *Spain:* Cefacron†; Claforan; Primafen; *Swed.:* Claforan; *Switz.:* Claforan; *Thai.:* Cefomic; Ceforan; Cefotax; Ceftaran; Claforan; Claraxim; Fotax; Valoran; *UAE:* Primocef; *UK:* Claforan; *USA:* Claforan.

Cefotetan Disodium (15313-a)

Cefotetan Disodium (BANM, USAN, rINNM).

ICI-156834; YM-09330 (both cefotetan or disodium salt). (7S)-7-[(4-Carbamoylcarboxymethylene-1,3-dithietan-2-yl)carboxamido]-7-methoxy-3-[(1-methyl-1H-tetrazol-5-yl)thiomethyl]-3-cephem-4-carboxylic acid, disodium salt.
$C_{17}H_{15}N_7Na_2O_8S_4 = 619.6$.

CAS — 69712-56-7 (cefotetan); 74356-00-6 (cefotetan disodium).

Pharmacopoeias. US includes Cefotetan and Cefotetan Disodium. Jpn includes Cefotetan.

1.08 g of cefotetan disodium is approximately equivalent to 1 g of cefotetan. A 10% solution in water has a pH of 4.0 to 6.5. Each g of monograph substance represents about 3.2 mmol of sodium.

There may be incompatibility with aminoglycosides. Precipitation has been reported with promethazine hydrochloride.

Pharmacopoeial description

USP 25: pH of a 10% solution in water is between 4.0 and 6.5. Store in airtight containers.

Incompatibility and stability. References.
1. Das Gupta V, *et al.* Chemical stability of cefotetan disodium in 5% dextrose and 0.9% sodium chloride injections. *J Clin Pharm Ther* 1990; **15**: 109–14.
2. Erickson SH, Ulici D. Incompatibility of cefotetan disodium and promethazine hydrochloride. *Am J Health-Syst Pharm* 1995; **52**: 1347.

Adverse Effects and Precautions

As for Cefalotin Sodium, p.162.

Cefotetan contains an *N*-methylthiotetrazole side-chain and like cefamandole (p.163) has the potential to cause hypoprothrombinaemia and bleeding.

Cefotetan, especially at high doses, may interfere with the Jaffé method of measuring creatinine concentrations to produce falsely elevated values; this should be borne in mind when measuring renal function.

Effects on the blood. Haemolytic anaemia occurred following cefotetan treatment in a patient on two occasions.[1] On the second occasion, haemolysis was accompanied by acute renal failure. The mechanism of the reaction was thought to be due to immune complex formation.
1. Wagner BKJ, *et al.* Cefotetan disodium-induced hemolytic anemia. *Ann Pharmacother* 1992; **26**: 199–200.

Interactions

As for Cefamandole, p.164.

Antimicrobial Action

Cefotetan is a cephamycin antibiotic with a mode of action and spectrum of activity similar to those of cefoxitin (p.171). It is generally much more active *in vitro* than cefoxitin against the Gram-negative Enterobacteriaceae, but has similar activity against *Bacteroides fragilis* and may be less active against some other *Bacteroides* spp.

◊ References.
1. Wexler HM, Finegold SM. In vitro activity of cefotetan compared with that of other antimicrobial agents against anaerobic bacteria. *Antimicrob Agents Chemother* 1988; **32**: 601–4.

Pharmacokinetics

After intramuscular injection of cefotetan, peak plasma concentrations of about 70 µg per mL at 1 hour and 90 µg per mL at 3 hours have been reported after doses of 1 and 2 g, respectively. The plasma half-life of cefotetan is usually in the range of 3.0 to 4.6 hours and is prolonged in patients with renal impairment. About 88% of cefotetan in the circulation may be bound to plasma proteins, depending on the plasma concentration.

Cefotetan is widely distributed in body tissues and fluids. It crosses the placenta and low concentrations have been detected in breast milk. High concentrations are achieved in bile.

Cefotetan is excreted in the urine, primarily by glomerular filtration, as unchanged drug; 50 to 80% of a dose has been recovered in the urine in 24 hours and high concentrations are achieved. Small amounts of the tautomeric form of cefotetan have been detected in both plasma and urine.

Biliary excretion of cefotetan probably accounts for nonrenal clearance.

Some cefotetan is removed by dialysis.

◊ References.

1. Owen AWMC, *et al*. The pharmacokinetics of cefotetan excretion in the unobstructed biliary tree. *J Antimicrob Chemother* 1983; **11** (suppl A): 217–21.
2. Smith BR, *et al*. Cefotetan pharmacokinetics in volunteers with various degrees of renal function. *Antimicrob Agents Chemother* 1986; **29**: 887–93.
3. Browning MJ, *et al*. Pharmacokinetics of cefotetan in patients with end-stage renal failure on maintenance dialysis. *J Antimicrob Chemother* 1986; **18**: 103–6.
4. Carver PL, *et al*. Pharmacokinetics and pharmacodynamics of total and unbound cefoxitin and cefotetan in healthy volunteers. *J Antimicrob Chemother* 1989; **23**: 99–106.
5. Zimmerman J, *et al*. Absolute bioavailability and noncompartmental analysis of intravenous and intramuscular Cefotan (cefotetan) in normal volunteers. *J Clin Pharmacol* 1989; **29**: 151–7.
6. Martin C, *et al*. Clinical pharmacokinetics of cefotetan. *Clin Pharmacokinet* 1994; **26**: 248–58.

Uses and Administration

Cefotetan is a cephamycin antibiotic generally classified with the second-generation cephalosporins and used similarly to cefoxitin (p.171) in the treatment and prophylaxis of anaerobic and mixed bacterial infections, especially intra-abdominal and pelvic infections.

It is administered as the disodium salt by deep intramuscular injection or intravenously by slow injection over 3 to 5 minutes or by infusion. Doses are expressed in terms of the equivalent amount of cefotetan. The usual dose for adults is 1 or 2 g every 12 hours. For the treatment of life-threatening infections, 3 g every 12 hours may be given intravenously. Dosage should be reduced in patients with severely impaired renal function. Those with a creatinine clearance of 10 to 30 mL per minute may be given the usual dose every 24 hours or one-half the usual dose every 12 hours, and those with a creatinine clearance of less than 10 mL per minute the usual dose every 48 hours or one-quarter the usual dose every 12 hours. In patients undergoing haemodialysis, one-quarter the usual dose may be given every 24 hours on days between dialysis and one-half the usual dose on the day of dialysis.

For infection prophylaxis during surgical procedures, an intravenous dose of 1 or 2 g is administered 30 to 60 minutes before surgery or, in caesarean section, as soon as the umbilical cord is clamped.

Preparations

USP 25: Cefotetan for Injection; Cefotetan Injection.

Proprietary Preparations (details are given in Part 3)

Aust.: Ceftenon†; *Austral.:* Apatef; *Belg.:* Apacef; *Canad.:* Cefotan; *Fr.:* Apacef; *Ital.:* Apatef; *Jpn:* Yamatetan; *NZ:* Apatef; *Port.:* Apatef; *USA:* Cefotan.

Cefotiam Hydrochloride   (12542-q)

Cefotiam Hydrochloride *(BANM, USAN, rINNM)*.

Abbott-48999; CGP-14221E (cefotiam or hydrochloride); SCE-963. 7-[2-(2-Amino-1,3-thiazol-4-yl)acetamido]-3-[1-(2-dimethylaminoethyl)-1*H*-tetrazol-5-ylthiomethyl]-3-cephem-4-carboxylic acid dihydrochloride.

$C_{18}H_{23}N_9O_4S_3,2HCl = 598.6$.

CAS — 61622-34-2 *(cefotiam)*; 66309-69-1 *(cefotiam hydrochloride)*.

Pharmacopoeias. In Jpn and US. Jpn also includes cefotiam hexetil hydrochloride.

1.14 g of monograph substance is approximately equivalent to 1 g of cefotiam.

Pharmacopoeial description

USP 25: Store in airtight containers.

Profile

Cefotiam is a third-generation cephalosporin antibiotic with actions and uses similar to those of cefamandole (p.163). It is administered intravenously or intramuscularly as the hydrochloride in doses equivalent to up to 6 g of cefotiam daily in divided doses, according to the severity of the infection.

Cefotiam hexetil hydrochloride, a prodrug of cefotiam, is given by mouth in doses equivalent to 200 to 400 mg of cefotiam twice daily.

◊ References.

1. Brogard JM, *et al*. Clinical pharmacokinetics of cefotiam. *Clin Pharmacokinet* 1989; **17**: 163–74.

The symbol † denotes a preparation no longer actively marketed

Preparations

USP 25: Cefotiam for Injection.

Proprietary Preparations (details are given in Part 3)

Aust.: Spizef; *Fr.:* Taketiam; Texodil; *Ger.:* Spizef; *Hong Kong:* Ceradolan; *Jpn:* Pansporin; *Singapore:* Ceradolan; *Thai.:* Ceradolan.

Cefoxitin Sodium   (33-d)

Cefoxitin Sodium *(BANM, USAN, rINNM)*.

Cefoxitinum Natricum; L-620388; MK-306. Sodium 3-carbamoyloxymethyl-7-methoxy-7-(2-thienylacetamido)-3-cephem-4-carboxylate.

$C_{16}H_{16}N_3NaO_7S_2 = 449.4$.

CAS — 35607-66-0 *(cefoxitin)*; 33564-30-6 *(cefoxitin sodium)*.

Pharmacopoeias. In Eur. (see p.vi), Jpn, Pol., and US.

1.05 g of cefoxitin sodium is approximately equivalent to 1 g of cefoxitin. Each g of monograph substance represents about 2.2 mmol of sodium.

Pharmacopoeial description

Ph. Eur.: A white or almost white, very hygroscopic, powder. Very soluble in water; sparingly soluble in alcohol; practically insoluble in ether. A 1% solution in water has a pH between 4.2 and 7.0. Store in airtight containers at a temperature not exceeding 30°.

USP 25: White to off-white, somewhat hygroscopic, granules or powder, having a slight characteristic odour. Very soluble in water; slightly soluble in acetone; insoluble in chloroform and in ether; sparingly soluble in dimethylformamide; soluble in methyl alcohol. pH of a 10% solution in water is between 4.2 and 7.0. Store in airtight containers at a temperature not exceeding 8°.

Adverse Effects and Precautions

As for Cefalotin Sodium, p.162.

Cefoxitin may interfere with the Jaffé method of measuring creatinine concentrations to produce falsely high values; this should be borne in mind when measuring renal function.

Effects on the gastrointestinal tract. Marked changes in anaerobic, facultative, and aerobic faecal flora have been noted with cefoxitin.[1]

1. Mulligan ME, *et al*. Alterations in human fecal flora, including ingrowth of Clostridium difficile, related to cefoxitin therapy. *Antimicrob Agents Chemother* 1984; **26**: 343–6.

Interactions

Probenecid reduces the renal clearance of cefoxitin.

Antimicrobial Action

Cefoxitin is a cephamycin antibiotic which, like the other beta lactams, is bactericidal and is considered to act through the inhibition of bacterial cell wall synthesis.

It has a similar spectrum of activity to cefamandole (p.164) but is more active against anaerobic bacteria, especially *Bacteroides fragilis*.

Cefoxitin can induce the production of beta-lactamases by some bacteria, and combinations of cefoxitin with other beta lactams have been shown to be antagonistic *in vitro*.

Cefoxitin itself is considered to be resistant to a wide range of beta-lactamases, including those produced by *Bacteroides* spp. However, acquired resistance to cefoxitin has been reported in *B. fragilis* (see Anaerobic Bacterial Infections, p.115) and has been attributed to beta-lactamase as well as to alterations in penicillin-binding proteins or to outer membrane proteins; there may be cross-resistance to other antibacterials.

◊ References.

1. Cuchural GJ, *et al*. Transfer of β-lactamase-associated cefoxitin resistance in Bacteroides fragilis. *Antimicrob Agents Chemother* 1986; **29**: 918–20.
2. Piddock LJV, Wise R. Cefoxitin resistance in Bacteroides species: evidence indicating two mechanisms causing decreased susceptibility. *J Antimicrob Chemother* 1987; **19**: 161–70.
3. Brogan O, *et al*. Bacteroides fragilis resistant to metronidazole, clindamycin and cefoxitin. *J Antimicrob Chemother* 1989; **23**: 660–2.
4. Wexler HM, Halebian S. Alterations to the penicillin-binding proteins in the Bacteroides fragilis group: a mechanism for non-β-lactamase mediated cefoxitin resistance. *J Antimicrob Chemother* 1990; **26**: 7–20.
5. Cherubin CE, Appleman MD. Susceptibility of cefoxitin-resistant isolates of bacteroides to other agents including β-lactamase inhibitor/β-lactam combinations. *J Antimicrob Chemother* 1993; **32**: 168–70.

Pharmacokinetics

Cefoxitin is not absorbed from the gastrointestinal tract; it is given parenterally as the sodium salt. After 1 g by intramuscular injection a peak plasma concentration of up to 30 µg per mL at 20 to 30 minutes has been reported whereas concentrations of 125, 72, and 25 µg per mL have been achieved after the intravenous injection of 1 g over 3, 30, and 120 minutes respectively. Cefoxitin is about 70% bound to plasma proteins. It has a plasma half-life of 45 to 60 minutes which is prolonged in renal impairment. Cefoxitin is widely distributed in the body but there is normally little penetration into the CSF, even when the meninges are inflamed. It crosses the placenta and has been detected in breast milk. Relatively high concentrations are achieved in bile.

The majority of a dose is excreted unchanged by the kidneys, up to about 2% being metabolised to descarbamylcefoxitin which is virtually inactive. Cefoxitin is excreted in the urine by glomerular filtration and tubular secretion and about 85% of a dose is recovered within 6 hours; probenecid slows this excretion. After an intramuscular dose of 1 g, peak concentrations in the urine are usually greater than 3 mg per mL.

Cefoxitin is removed by haemodialysis.

◊ References.

1. Feldman WE, *et al*. Penetration of cefoxitin into cerebrospinal fluid of infants and children with bacterial meningitis. *Antimicrob Agents Chemother* 1982; **21**: 468–71.
2. Hansbrough JF, Clark JE. Concentrations of cefoxitin in gallbladder bile of cholecystectomy patients. *Antimicrob Agents Chemother* 1982; **22**: 709–10.

Uses and Administration

Cefoxitin is a cephamycin antibiotic which differs structurally from the cephalosporins by the addition of a 7-α-methoxy group to the 7-β-aminocephalosporanic acid nucleus.

It is generally classified with the second-generation cephalosporins and can be used similarly to cefamandole for the treatment of susceptible infections. However, because of its activity against *Bacteroides fragilis* and other anaerobic bacteria, it is used principally in the treatment and prophylaxis of anaerobic and mixed bacterial infections, especially intra-abdominal and pelvic infections. Indications include endometritis (prophylaxis at caesarean section), pelvic inflammatory disease, and surgical infection (prophylaxis). It may also be used in the treatment of gonorrhoea and urinary-tract infections. For details of these infections and their treatment, see under Choice of Antibacterial, p.114.

Administration and dosage. Cefoxitin is administered as the sodium salt by deep intramuscular injection, by slow intravenous injection over 3 to 5 minutes, or by intermittent or continuous intravenous infusion.

Doses are expressed in terms of the equivalent amount of cefoxitin. The usual adult dose is 1 or 2 g every 8 hours although it may be given more frequently (every 4 or 6 hours). In severe infections up to 12 g daily has been recommended. Children and neonates may be given 20 to 40 mg per kg bodyweight every 12 hours for neonates up to 1 week old, every 8 hours for those aged 1 to 4 weeks, and every 6 to 8 hours for older infants and children; in severe infections, up to 200 mg per kg daily may be given, to a maximum of 12 g daily.

For the treatment of uncomplicated urinary-tract infections, cefoxitin 1 g twice daily has been given intramuscularly.

In renal impairment, dosage should be reduced according to the creatinine-clearance rate. In adults, after an initial loading dose of 1 to 2 g, maintenance doses are: creatinine clearance of 30 to 50 mL per minute, 1 to 2 g every 8 to 12 hours; 10 to 29 mL per minute, 1 to 2 g every 12 to 24 hours; 5 to 9 mL per minute, 0.5 to 1 g every 12 to 24 hours; and below 5 mL per minute, 0.5 to 1 g every 24 to 48 hours. In patients undergoing haemodialysis, the loading dose should be repeated after each dialysis session.

For the treatment of uncomplicated gonorrhoea, a single dose of 2 g intramuscularly has been given in association with probenecid 1 g by mouth.

For surgical infection prophylaxis, the usual adult dose is cefoxitin 2 g intramuscularly or intravenously 30 to 60 minutes prior to the procedure and then every 6 hours, not usually for more than 24 hours. Infants and children undergoing surgical procedures can be given doses of 30 to 40 mg per kg, at the same time intervals as adults; neonates may also be given 30 to 40 mg per kg, but at intervals of 8 to 12 hours.

At caesarean section a single 2-g dose may be given intravenously to the mother as soon as the umbilical cord is clamped. If necessary, a 3-dose regimen, with further 2-g doses 4 and 8 hours after the initial dose, may be employed.

◊ Reviews.
1. DiPiro JT, May JR. Use of cephalosporins with enhanced antianaerobic activity for treatment and prevention of anaerobic and mixed infections. *Clin Pharm* 1988; **7:** 285–302.
2. Goodwin CS. Cefoxitin 20 years on: is it still useful? *Rev Med Microbiol* 1995; **6:** 146–53.

Preparations

BP 2001: Cefoxitin Injection;
USP 25: Cefoxitin for Injection; Cefoxitin Injection.

Proprietary Preparations (details are given in Part 3)
Aust.: Mefoxin; *Austral.:* Mefoxin; *Belg.:* Mefoxin; *Braz.:* Mefoxin; *Canad.:* Mefoxin; *Fin.:* Mefoxin; *Fr.:* Mefoxin; *Ger.:* Mefoxitin; *Hong Kong:* Mefoxin; *Irl.:* Mefoxin; *Ital.:* Betacef; Cefociclin; Mefoxin; Tifox; *Neth.:* Mefoxin; *Norw.:* Mefoxitin; *NZ:* Mefoxin; *Port.:* Mefoxin; *S.Afr.:* Mefoxin; *Spain:* Cefaxicina†; Mefoxitin; *Swed.:* Mefoxitin; *Switz.:* Mefoxitin; *Thai.:* Cefoxin; Cefxitin; *UK:* Mefoxin; *USA:* Mefoxin.

Cefozopran (15884-q)

Cefozopran (rINN).

SCE-2787. (−)-1-{[(6R,7R)-7-[2-(5-Amino-1,2,4-thiadiazol-3-yl)glyoxylamido]-2-carboxy-8-oxo-5-thia-1-azabicyclo[4.2.0]oct-2-en-3-yl]methyl}-1H-imidazo[1,2-b]pyridazin-4-ium hydroxide inner salt, 7²-(Z)-(O-methyloxime).
$C_{19}H_{17}N_9O_5S_2 = 515.5.$
$CAS — 113359-04-9.$

Profile

Cefozopran is a cephalosporin antibiotic used parenterally as the hydrochloride.

◊ References.
1. Iwahi T, *et al.* In vitro and in vivo activities of SCE-2787, a new parenteral cephalosporin with a broad antibacterial spectrum. *Antimicrob Agents Chemother* 1992; **36:** 1358–66.
2. Paulfeuerborn W, *et al.* Comparative pharmacokinetics and serum bactericidal activities of SCE-2787 and ceftazidime. *Antimicrob Agents Chemother* 1993; **37:** 1835–41.

Cefpiramide (14940-j)

Cefpiramide (USAN, rINN).

SM-1652; Wy-44635. (7R)-7-[(R)-2-(4-Hydroxy-6-methylnicotinamido)-2-(4-hydroxyphenyl)acetamido]-3-(1-methyl-1H-tetrazol-5-ylthiomethyl)-3-cephem-4-carboxylic acid.
$C_{25}H_{24}N_8O_7S_2 = 612.6.$
$CAS — 70797-11-4.$
$ATC — J01DA27.$
Pharmacopoeias. In US.

Pharmacopoeial description

USP 25: Store in airtight containers. pH of a 0.5% suspension in water is between 3.0 and 5.0.

Cefpiramide Sodium (16569-b)

Cefpiramide Sodium (USAN, rINN).
$C_{25}H_{23}N_8NaO_7S_2 = 634.6.$
$CAS — 74849-93-7.$
Pharmacopoeias. In Jpn.

1.04 g of monograph substance is approximately equivalent to 1 g of cefpiramide. Each g of monograph substance represents about 1.6 mmol of sodium.

Profile

Cefpiramide is a third-generation cephalosporin antibiotic related to cefoperazone (p.168) and with similar activity against *Pseudomonas aeruginosa*, but possibly less active against Enterobacteriaceae. Cefpiramide is also active against staphylococci and streptococci and marginal activity against enterococci *in vitro* has been reported. Cefpiramide contains an N-methylthiotetrazole side-chain, a structure associated with hypoprothrombinaemia (see Cefamandole, p.163), alcohol intolerance, and potentiation of anticoagulants.

It is given by intravenous injection or infusion as the sodium salt in the treatment of susceptible infections. A usual adult dose is 1 to 2 g daily in two divided doses.

◊ References to the antibacterial activity of cefpiramide.
1. Barry AL, *et al.* Cefpiramide: comparative in-vitro activity and β-lactamase stability. *J Antimicrob Chemother* 1985; **16:** 315–25.
2. Quentin C, *et al.* Comparative in vitro activity of cefpiramide, a new parenteral cephalosporin. *Eur J Clin Microbiol Infect Dis* 1988; **7:** 544–9.

◊ References to the pharmacokinetics of cefpiramide.
1. Nakagawa K, *et al.* Pharmacokinetics of cefpiramide (SM-1652) in humans. *Antimicrob Agents Chemother* 1984; **25:** 221–5.
2. Conte JE. Pharmacokinetics of cefpiramide in volunteers with normal or impaired renal function. *Antimicrob Agents Chemother* 1987; **31:** 1585–8.
3. Brogard JM, *et al.* High hepatic excretion in humans of cefpiramide, a new cephalosporin. *Antimicrob Agents Chemother* 1988; **32:** 1360–4.
4. Demotes-Mainard F, *et al.* Pharmacokinetics and protein binding of cefpiramide in patients with alcoholic cirrhosis. *Clin Pharmacol Ther* 1991; **49:** 263–9.
5. Demotes-Mainard F, *et al.* Cefpiramide kinetics and plasma protein binding in cholestasis. *Br J Clin Pharmacol* 1994; **37:** 295–7.

Preparations

USP 25: Cefpiramide for Injection.

Proprietary Preparations (details are given in Part 3)
Jpn: Sepatren.

Cefpirome Sulfate (18924-d)

Cefpirome Sulfate (USAN, rINN).

Cefpirome Sulphate (BANM); HR-810 (cefpirome or cefpirome sulfate). (Z)-7-[2-(2-Aminothiazol-4-yl)-2-methoxyiminoacetamido]-3-(1-pyrindiniomethyl)-3-cephem-4-carboxylate sulphate.
$C_{22}H_{22}N_6O_5S_2,H_2SO_4 = 612.7.$
$CAS — 84957-29-9 (cefpirome); 98753-19-6 (cefpirome sulfate).$

Adverse Effects and Precautions

As for Cefalotin, p.162.

Cefpirome is reported to interfere with the Jaffé method of measuring creatinine concentrations to determine renal function.

◊ References.
1. Rubinstein E, *et al.* A review of the adverse events profile of cefpirome. *Drug Safety* 1993; **9:** 340–5.

Interactions

Probenecid reduces the renal clearance of cefpirome.

Antimicrobial Action

Cefpirome is a fourth-generation cephalosporin antibiotic that is stable to a wide range of beta-lactamases. It has a spectrum of activity similar to that of the third-generation cephalosporin cefotaxime (p.169), but it appears to be more active *in vitro* against staphylococci, some enterococci, some Enterobacteriaceae, and *Pseudomonas aeruginosa*. Cefpirome may be less active than ceftazidime (p.175) against *Ps. aeruginosa*.

◊ References to the antibacterial action of cefpirome *in vitro*.
1. Wise R, *et al.* The antimicrobial activity of cefpirome, a new cephalosporin. *J Antimicrob Chemother* 1985; **15:** 449–56.
2. Jones RN, Fuchs PC. Activity of cefepime (BMY-28142) and cefpirome (HR-810) against Gram-negative bacilli resistant to cefotaxime or ceftazidime. *J Antimicrob Chemother* 1989; **23:** 163–5.
3. Eng RHK, *et al.* In-vitro and in-vivo activity of cefpirome (HR-810) against methicillin-susceptible and -resistant Staphylococcus aureus and Streptococcus faecalis. *J Antimicrob Chemother* 1989; **23:** 373–81.
4. Schäfer V, *et al.* In-vitro activity of cefpirome against isolates from patients with urinary tract, lower respiratory tract and wound infections. *J Antimicrob Chemother* 1992; **29** (suppl A): 7–12.
5. Cheng AFB, *et al.* The antimicrobial activity and β-lactamase stability of cefpirome, a new fourth-generation cephalosporin in comparison with other agents. *J Antimicrob Chemother* 1993; **31:** 699–709.
6. Piérard D, *et al.* Comparative in-vitro activity of cefpirome against isolates from intensive care and haematology/oncology units. *J Antimicrob Chemother* 1998; **41:** 443–50.

Pharmacokinetics

Cefpirome is administered by injection as the sulfate. Mean peak serum concentrations of 80 to 90 μg per mL are attained after a single intravenous 1-g dose. The elimination half-life is about 2 hours and is prolonged in patients with renal impairment. Cefpirome is less than 10% bound to plasma proteins.

Cefpirome is widely distributed into body tissues and fluids and appears in breast milk. It is mainly excreted by the kidneys and 80 to 90% of a dose is recovered unchanged in the urine. Significant amounts are removed by haemodialysis.

◊ References.
1. Kavi J, *et al.* Pharmacokinetics and tissue penetration of cefpirome, a new cephalosporin. *J Antimicrob Chemother* 1988; **22:** 911–16.
2. Saxby MF, *et al.* Penetration of cefpirome in prostatic tissue. *J Antimicrob Chemother* 1990; **25:** 488–90.
3. Baldwin DR, *et al.* The penetration of cefpirome into the potential sites of pulmonary infection. *J Antimicrob Chemother* 1991; **28:** 79–86.
4. Wilcox MH, *et al.* Relationship between cefpirome clearance, serum creatinine, weight and age in patients treated for infection. *J Antimicrob Chemother* 1991; **28:** 291–9.
5. Nakayama I, *et al.* Single- and multiple-dose pharmacokinetics of intravenous cefpirome (HR-810) to healthy volunteers. *J Clin Pharmacol* 1992; **32:** 256–66.
6. Veys N, *et al.* Single-dose pharmacokinetics of cefpirome in patients receiving hemodialysis and in patients treated by continuous ambulatory peritoneal dialysis. *Clin Pharmacol Ther* 1993; **54:** 459–401.
7. Strenkoski LC, Nix DE. Cefpirome clinical pharmacokinetics. *Clin Pharmacokinet* 1993; **25:** 263–73.
8. Nahata MC, *et al.* Pharmacokinetics of cefpirome in pediatric patients. *Antimicrob Agents Chemother* 1995; **39:** 2348–9.
9. Friedland IR, *et al.* Concentrations of cefpirome in cerebrospinal fluid of children with bacterial meningitis after a single intravenous dose. *Antimicrob Agents Chemother* 1998; **42:** 199–201.

Uses and Administration

Cefpirome is a fourth-generation cephalosporin antibiotic used in the treatment of infections due to susceptible organisms. They include infections of the urinary tract, respiratory tract, and skin, and also septicaemia and infections in immunocompromised patients. For details of these infections and their treatment, see under Choice of Antibacterial, p.114.

Cefpirome is given by intravenous injection over 3 to 5 minutes or infusion over 20 to 30 minutes as the sulfate in doses of 1 or 2 g every 12 hours.

Dosage should be modified in renal impairment; after a loading dose of 1 or 2 g depending on the severity of infection the maintenance dosage should be adjusted according to the patient's creatinine clearance and the severity of infection: creatinine clearance 20 to 50 mL per minute, 0.5 or 1 g twice daily; 5 to 20 mL per minute, 0.5 or 1 g once daily; 5 mL per minute or less (in haemodialysis patients), 0.5 or 1 g once daily plus a half-dose after each dialysis session.

◊ References.
1. Brown EM, *et al.* eds. Cefpirome: a novel extended spectrum cephalosporin. *J Antimicrob Chemother* 1992; **29** (suppl A): 1–104.
2. Wiseman LR, Lamb HM. Cefpirome: a review of its antibacterial activity, pharmacokinetic properties and clinical efficacy in the treatment of severe nosocomial infections and febrile neutropenia. *Drugs* 1997; **54:** 117–40.

Preparations

Proprietary Preparations (details are given in Part 3)
Aust.: Cedixen; Cefrom; *Austral.:* Cefrom; *Belg.:* Cefrom; *Braz.:* Cefrom; *Denm.:* Cefrom†; *Fin.:* Cefrom; *Fr.:* Cefrom; *Hong Kong:* Cefrom; *Irl.:* Cefrom; *Mex.:* Cefrom; *Neth.:* Cefrom; *NZ:* Cefrom; *S.Afr.:* Cefrom; *Singapore:* Cefrom; *Spain:* Metran; *Swed.:* Cefrom; *Switz.:* Cefrom†; *Thai.:* Cefrom; *UK:* Cefrom.

Cefpodoxime Proxetil (1990-q)

Cefpodoxime Proxetil (BANM, USAN, rINN).

CS-807; U-76252. The 1-[(isopropoxycarbonyl)oxy]ethyl ester of (Z)-7-[2-(2-amino-1,3-thiazol-4-yl)-2-methoxyiminoacetamido]-3-methoxymethyl-3-cephem-4-carboxylic acid.
$C_{21}H_{27}N_5O_9S_2 = 557.6.$
$CAS — 80210-62-4 (cefpodoxime); 87239-81-4 (cefpodoxime proxetil).$

1.3 g of cefpodoxime proxetil is approximately equivalent to 1 g of cefpodoxime.

Adverse Effects and Precautions

As for Cefalotin Sodium, p.162.

The most frequently reported adverse effects of cefpodoxime are gastrointestinal disturbances, especially diarrhoea.

Interactions

Absorption of cefpodoxime is decreased by concurrent ingestion of antacids or histamine H_2-receptor antagonists. Probenecid reduces the renal excretion of cefpodoxime.

Antimicrobial Action

As for Cefixime, p.166. Cefpodoxime also has some activity against *Staphylococcus aureus*, and may be more active than cefixime against penicillin-resistant strains of *Streptococcus pneumoniae*.

◊ References.
1. Valentini S, *et al.* In-vitro evaluation of cefpodoxime. *J Antimicrob Chemother* 1994; **33**: 495–508.

Pharmacokinetics

Cefpodoxime proxetil is de-esterified in the intestinal epithelium following oral administration, to release active cefpodoxime in the blood stream. Bioavailability is about 50% in fasting subjects and may be increased in the presence of food. Absorption is decreased in conditions of low gastric acidity. Plasma concentrations of about 1.5, 2.5, and 4.0 μg per mL have been achieved 2 to 3 hours after oral doses of 100, 200, and 400 mg cefpodoxime respectively. About 20 to 30% of cefpodoxime is bound to plasma proteins. The plasma half-life is about 2 to 3 hours and is prolonged in patients with impaired renal function.

Cefpodoxime reaches therapeutic concentrations in the respiratory and genito-urinary tracts and bile. It has been detected in low concentrations in breast milk.

Cefpodoxime is excreted unchanged in the urine. It is removed by dialysis.

◊ Pharmacokinetics of cefpodoxime.
1. Hughes GS, *et al.* Effects of gastric pH and food on the pharmacokinetics of a new oral cephalosporin, cefpodoxime proxetil. *Clin Pharmacol Ther* 1989; **46**: 674–85.
2. O'Neill P, *et al.* Pharmacokinetics and inflammatory fluid penetration of cefpodoxime proxetil in volunteers. *Antimicrob Agents Chemother* 1990; **34**: 232–4.
3. Borin MT, *et al.* Pharmacokinetics of cefpodoxime in plasma and skin blister fluid following oral dosing of cefpodoxime proxetil. *Antimicrob Agents Chemother* 1990; **34**: 1094–9.
4. Borin MT, *et al.* Pharmacokinetic and tolerance studies of cefpodoxime after single- and multiple-dose oral administration of cefpodoxime proxetil. *J Clin Pharmacol* 1991; **31**: 1137–45.
5. Peter JVS, *et al.* Disposition of cefpodoxime proxetil in healthy volunteers and patients with impaired renal function. *Antimicrob Agents Chemother* 1992; **36**: 126–31.
6. Muller-Serieys C, *et al.* Penetration of cefpodoxime proxetil in lung parenchyma and epithelial lining fluid of non-infected patients. *Antimicrob Agents Chemother* 1992; **36**: 2099–2103.
7. Borin MT, *et al.* Disposition of cefpodoxime proxetil in hemodialysis patients. *J Clin Pharmacol* 1992; **32**: 1038–44.
8. Johnson CA, *et al.* Pharmacokinetics and ex vivo susceptibility of cefpodoxime proxetil in patients receiving continuous ambulatory peritoneal dialysis. *Antimicrob Agents Chemother* 1993; **37**: 2650–5.
9. Borin MT, *et al.* Pharmacokinetics of cefpodoxime proxetil in healthy young and elderly volunteers. *J Clin Pharmacol* 1994; **34**: 774–81.
10. Borin MT, Forbes KK. Effect of food on absorption of cefpodoxime proxetil oral suspension in adults. *Antimicrob Agents Chemother* 1995; **39**: 273–5.
11. Takasugi N, *et al.* Penetration of cefpodoxime into uterine and vaginal secretions from postpartum women after a single oral dose of cefpodoxime proxetil. *Antimicrob Agents Chemother* 1996; **40**: 1832–4.

Uses and Administration

Cefpodoxime is a third-generation cephalosporin antibiotic used similarly to cefixime (p.166) in the treatment of susceptible infections. It is given by mouth as the proxetil ester which is hydrolysed on absorption to cefpodoxime. Doses are expressed in terms of the equivalent amount of cefpodoxime. Absorption may be enhanced if cefpodoxime proxetil is administered with food. The usual adult dose is 100 to 200 mg every 12 hours for respiratory-tract and urinary-tract infections. A dose of 200 or 400 mg every 12 hours may be given for skin infections. In children doses of 8 to 10 mg per kg body-weight daily may be given in two divided doses, up to a maximum of 200 mg daily for respiratory-tract infections or 400 mg daily for otitis media.

The interval between doses should be extended in patients with severe renal impairment (creatinine clearance of less than about 40 mL per minute).

For uncomplicated gonorrhoea, a single dose of 200 mg may be given.

◊ References.
1. Moore EP, *et al.*, eds. Cefpodoxime proxetil: a third-generation oral cephalosporin. *J Antimicrob Chemother* 1990; **26** (suppl E): 1–101.
2. Adam D, *et al.*, eds. Cefpodoxime proxetil: a new third generation oral cephalosporin. *Drugs* 1991; **42** (suppl 3): 1–66.
3. Frampton JE, *et al.* Cefpodoxime proxetil: a review of its antibacterial activity, pharmacokinetic properties and therapeutic potential. *Drugs* 1992; **44**: 889–917.

4. Chocas EC, *et al.* Cefpodoxime proxetil: a new, broad-spectrum, oral cephalosporin. *Ann Pharmacother* 1993; **27**: 1369–77.
5. Fulton B, Perry CM. Cefpodoxime proxetil: a review of its use in the management of bacterial infections in paediatric patients. *Paediatr Drugs* 2001; **3**: 137–58.

Preparations

Proprietary Preparations (details are given in Part 3)
Aust.: Biocef; Otreon; ***Austral.:*** Orelox; ***Denm.:*** Orelox†; ***Fr.:*** Orelox; ***Ger.:*** Orelox; Podomexef; ***Hong Kong:*** Banan; ***Irl.:*** Cefodox; ***Ital.:*** Cefodox; Orelox; Otreon; ***Jpn:*** Banan; ***Mex.:*** Orelox; ***Neth.:*** Orelox; ***S.Afr.:*** Orelox; ***Spain:*** Kelbium; Orelox; Otreon; ***Swed.:*** Orelox; ***Switz.:*** Orelox; Podomexef; ***Thai.:*** Banan; ***UK:*** Orelox; ***USA:*** Vantin.

Cefprozil   (9390-n)

Cefprozil (BAN, USAN, rINN).

BMY-28100-03-800; BMY-28100 (*cis*-isomer); BMY-28167 (*trans*-isomer);   (6R,7R)-7-[(R)-2-Amino-2-(p-hydroxyphenyl)acetamido]-8-oxo-3-(1-propenyl)-5-thia-1-azabicyclo[4.2.0]oct-2-ene-2-carboxylic acid monohydrate; 7-(D-4-Hydroxyphenylglycylamino)-3-[(E)prop-1-enyl]cephem-4-carboxylic acid monohydrate.
$C_{18}H_{19}N_3O_5S,H_2O = 407.4$.
CAS — 92665-29-7 (anhydrous cefprozil); 121123-17-9 (cefprozil monohydrate).
ATC — J01DA41.

Pharmacopoeias. In US.

1.05 g of monograph substance is approximately equivalent to 1 g of anhydrous cefprozil.

Pharmacopoeial description
USP 25: pH of a 0.5% solution in water is between 3.5 and 6.5. Store in airtight containers.

Adverse Effects and Precautions

As for Cefalexin, p.162.

Hypersensitivity. Serum sickness-like reactions were reported in 4 patients, 3 of them children, given cefprozil.[1] Such reactions have been associated with cefaclor (p.161), but whether they represent a class-related hypersensitivity reaction is not yet clear.
1. Lowery N, *et al.* Serum sickness-like reactions associated with cefprozil therapy. *J Pediatr* 1994; **125**: 325–8.

Interactions

As for Cefalexin, p.162.

Antimicrobial Action

Cefprozil is bactericidal and has antimicrobial activity similar to that of cefaclor (p.161).

◊ References.
1. Leitner F, *et al.* BMY-28100, a new oral cephalosporin. *Antimicrob Agents Chemother* 1987; **31**: 238–43.
2. Chin N-X, Neu HC. Comparative antibacterial activity of a new oral cephalosporin, BMY-28100. *Antimicrob Agents Chemother* 1987; **31**: 480–3.
3. Scribner RK, *et al.* In vitro activity of BMY-28100 against common isolates from pediatric infections. *Antimicrob Agents Chemother* 1987; **31**: 630–1.
4. Eliopoulos GM, *et al.* In vitro activity of BMY-28100, a new oral cephalosporin. *Antimicrob Agents Chemother* 1987; **31**: 653–6.
5. Arguedas AG, *et al.* In-vitro activity of cefprozil (BMY-28100) and loracarbef (LY-163892) against pathogens obtained from middle ear fluid. *J Antimicrob Chemother* 1991; **27**: 311–18.

Pharmacokinetics

Cefprozil is well absorbed from the gastrointestinal tract with a reported bioavailability of 90 to 95%. Doses of 250 mg, 500 mg, and 1 g by mouth produce peak plasma concentrations of 6, 10, and 18 μg per mL respectively at 1 to 2 hours. The presence of food is reported to have little or no effect on the absorption of cefprozil. A plasma half-life of 1 to 1.4 hours has been reported; it is increased in patients with impaired renal function, up to about 6 hours in those with end-stage renal failure. Approximately 35 to 45% of cefprozil is bound to plasma proteins.

Cefprozil is widely distributed in the body tissues. Concentrations of cefprozil in tonsillar and adenoidal tissue are reported to be about 40 to 50% of those in plasma, and less than 0.3% of a 1-g dose has been recovered in breast milk in 24 hours. About 60% of a dose is excreted unchanged in the urine in the first 8 hours by glomerular filtration and tubular secretion. High concentrations of cefprozil are achieved in the urine; concentrations of 700, 1000, and 2900 μg per mL have been reported within 4 hours of doses of 250 mg, 500 mg, and 1 g respectively. Some cefprozil is removed by haemodialysis.

◊ References.
1. Nye K, *et al.* Pharmacokinetics and tissue penetration of cefprozil. *J Antimicrob Chemother* 1990; **25**: 831–5.
2. Barbhaiya RH, *et al.* Comparison of cefprozil and cefaclor pharmacokinetics and tissue penetration. *Antimicrob Agents Chemother* 1990; **34**: 1204–9.
3. Barbhaiya RH, *et al.* Comparison of the effects of food on the pharmacokinetics of cefprozil and cefaclor. *Antimicrob Agents Chemother* 1990; **34**: 1210–13.
4. Sáez-Llorens X, *et al.* Pharmacokinetics of cefprozil in infants and children. *Antimicrob Agents Chemother* 1990; **34**: 2152–5.
5. Shyu WC, *et al.* Pharmacokinetics of cefprozil in healthy subjects and patients with renal impairment. *J Clin Pharmacol* 1991; **31**: 362–71.
6. Shyu WC, *et al.* Pharmacokinetics of cefprozil in healthy subjects and patients with hepatic impairment. *J Clin Pharmacol* 1991; **31**: 372–6.
7. Lode H, *et al.* Multiple-dose pharmacokinetics of cefprozil and its impact on intestinal flora of volunteers. *Antimicrob Agents Chemother* 1992; **36**: 144–9.
8. Shyu WC, *et al.* Oral absolute bioavailability and intravenous dose-proportionality of cefprozil in humans. *J Clin Pharmacol* 1992; **32**: 798–803.
9. Shyu WC, *et al.* Penetration of cefprozil into tonsillar and adenoidal tissues. *Antimicrob Agents Chemother* 1993; **37**: 1080–3.
10. Shyu WC, *et al.* Penetration of cefprozil into middle ear fluid of patients with otitis media. *Antimicrob Agents Chemother* 1994; **38**: 2210–12.

Uses and Administration

Cefprozil is an oral cephalosporin antibiotic consisting of *cis*- and *trans*- isomers in a ratio of about 90:10. It is used similarly to cefaclor (p.161) in the treatment of susceptible infections, including upper and lower respiratory-tract infections and skin and soft tissue infections, and should probably be classified as a second-generation cephalosporin.

Cefprozil is given as the monohydrate. Doses are expressed in terms of the equivalent amount of anhydrous cefprozil. The usual adult dose is 500 mg daily (as a single dose or in two divided doses), increased to 500 mg twice daily if necessary. Children may be given up to 20 mg per kg once or twice daily (to a maximum of 500 mg once daily, or twice daily if necessary for otitis media).

Doses should be reduced in patients with impaired renal function; half the standard dose may be given to patients with a creatinine clearance of less than 30 mL per minute.

◊ Reviews.
1. Wiseman LR, Benfield P. Cefprozil: a review of its antibacterial activity, pharmacokinetic properties, and therapeutic potential. *Drugs* 1993; **45**: 295–317.
2. Barriere SL. Review of in vitro activity, pharmacokinetic characteristics, safety, and clinical efficacy of cefprozil, a new oral cephalosporin. *Ann Pharmacother* 1993; **27**: 1082–9.

Preparations

USP 25: Cefprozil for Oral Suspension; Cefprozil Tablets.

Proprietary Preparations (details are given in Part 3)
Canad.: Cefzil; ***Fin.:*** Procef; ***Hong Kong:*** Procef; ***Ital.:*** Cronocef; Procef; Rozicel; ***Mex.:*** Procef; ***Port.:*** Procef; ***S.Afr.:*** Procef; ***Singapore:*** Procef; ***Spain:*** Arzimol; Brisoral; ***Switz.:*** Procef; ***Thai.:*** Procef; ***UK:*** Cefzil; ***USA:*** Cefzil.

Cefquinome   (6466-b)

Cefquinome (BAN, rINN).

HR111V.   (Z)-7-[2-(2-Amino-1,3-thiazol-4-yl)-2-(methoxyimino)acetamido]-3-(5,6,7,8-tetrahydroquinoliniomethyl)-3-cephem-4-carboxylate.
$C_{23}H_{24}N_6O_5S_2 = 528.6$.
CAS — 84957-30-2 (cefquinome); 123766-80-3 (cefquinome sulfate).

NOTE. Cefquinome Sulfate is *USAN*.

Profile

Cefquinome is a fourth-generation cephalosporin antibacterial used in veterinary medicine.

Cefradine   (45-b)

Cefradine (BAN, rINN).

Cefradinum; Cephradine (USAN); SKF-D-39304; SQ-11436; SQ-22022 (cefradine dihydrate). (7R)-7-(α-D-Cyclohexa-1,4-dienylglycylamino)-3-methyl-3-cephem-4-carboxylic acid.
$C_{16}H_{19}N_3O_4S = 349.4$.
CAS — 38821-53-3 (anhydrous cefradine); 31828-50-9 (non-stoichiometric cefradine hydrate); 58456-86-3 (cefradine dihydrate).
ATC — J01DA31.

Pharmacopoeias. In Eur. (see p.vi), Jpn, Pol., and US (which allows the anhydrous form, the monohydrate, or the dihydrate).

Commercially available injections contain sodium carbonate or arginine as neutralisers. Injections containing sodium carbonate are incompatible with solutions such as compound sodium lactate injection which contain calcium salts.

Pharmacopoeial description

Ph. Eur.: A white to slightly yellow, hygroscopic powder. Sparingly soluble in water; practically insoluble in alcohol and in ether. A 1% solution in water has a pH of 3.5 to 6.0. Store at a temperature not exceeding 30° in airtight containers. Protect from light.

USP 25: A white to off-white crystalline powder. Sparingly soluble in water; very slightly soluble in alcohol and in chloroform; practically insoluble in ether. pH of a 1% solution in water is between 3.5 and 6.0. Store in airtight containers.

Incompatibility and stability. References.
1. Wang Y-C J, Monkhouse DC. Solution stability of cephradine neutralized with arginine or sodium bicarbonate. *Am J Hosp Pharm* 1983; **40:** 432.
2. Mehta AC, *et al.* Chemical stability of cephradine injection solutions. *Intensive Therapy Clin Monit* 1988; **9:** 195–6.

Adverse Effects and Precautions

As for Cefalexin, p.162. Intramuscular injections of cefradine can be painful and thrombophlebitis has occurred following intravenous injection.

Porphyria. Cefradine is considered to be unsafe in patients with porphyria although there is conflicting experimental evidence of porphyrinogenicity.

Interactions

As for Cefalexin, p.162.

Antimicrobial Action

As for Cefalexin, p.162.

Pharmacokinetics

Cefradine is rapidly and almost completely absorbed from the gastrointestinal tract. Doses of 250 mg, 500 mg, and 1 g given by mouth have produced peak plasma concentrations of about 9, 17, and 24 μg per mL respectively at 1 hour and are similar to those achieved with cefalexin. Absorption is delayed by the presence of food although the total amount absorbed is not appreciably altered. Following intramuscular injection peak plasma concentrations of about 6 and 14 μg per mL have been obtained within 1 to 2 hours of doses of 500 mg and 1 g respectively.

Only about 6 to 20% is reported to be bound to plasma proteins. A plasma half-life of about 1 hour has been reported; this is prolonged in patients with renal impairment. Cefradine is widely distributed to body tissues and fluids, but does not enter the CSF in significant quantities. Therapeutic concentrations may be found in the bile. It crosses the placenta into the fetal circulation and is distributed in small amounts into breast milk.

Cefradine is excreted unchanged in the urine by glomerular filtration and tubular secretion, over 90% of an oral dose or 60 to 80% of an intramuscular dose being recovered within 6 hours. Peak urinary concentrations of about 3 mg per mL have been achieved after a 500-mg dose by mouth. Probenecid delays excretion.

Cefradine is removed by haemodialysis and peritoneal dialysis.

◊ References.
1. Wise R. The pharmacokinetics of the oral cephalosporins—a review. *J Antimicrob Chemother* 1990; **26** (suppl E): 13–20.
2. Schwinghammer TL, *et al.* Pharmacokinetics of cephradine administered intravenously and orally to young and elderly subjects. *J Clin Pharmacol* 1990; **30:** 893–9.

Uses and Administration

Cefradine is a first-generation cephalosporin antibiotic administered by mouth similarly to cefalexin (p.162) and by the parenteral route similarly to cefazolin (p.165) in the treatment of susceptible infections and in the prophylaxis of infections during surgical procedures.

Cefradine is given by mouth in doses of 1 to 2 g daily in two to four divided doses to adults; up to 4 g daily may be given by this route. In severe infections it should be given parenterally, by deep intramuscular injection or intravenously by slow injection over 3 to 5 minutes or by infusion, in doses of 2 to 4 g daily in four divided doses; up to 8 g daily may be given by

the parenteral route. The usual daily dose by mouth for children is 25 to 50 mg per kg body-weight although 75 to 100 mg per kg daily may be given for otitis media. By injection 50 to 100 mg per kg daily may be given, increasing to 300 mg per kg daily if necessary.

For surgical infection prophylaxis, 1 to 2 g may be given pre-operatively by intramuscular or intravenous injection; subsequent parenteral or oral doses are given as appropriate.

Dosage should be reduced in patients with severe renal impairment.

Preparations

BP 2001: Cefradine Capsules;
USP 25: Cephradine Capsules; Cephradine for Injection; Cephradine for Oral Suspension; Cephradine Tablets.

Proprietary Preparations (details are given in Part 3)
Aust.: Sefril†; *Belg.:* Velosef; *Fr.:* Cefirex; Dexef; Doncef; Kelsef; Zadyl†; Zeefra; *Hong Kong:* Velosef; *Irl.:* Velosef; *Israel:* Velosef; *Ital.:* Cefrabiotic; Citicef; Ecosporina; Lisacef; *Mex.:* Veracef; *Neth.:* Maxisporin; Velosef; *NZ:* Velosef; *Port.:* Cefradur; Novacefrex; Velosef; *S.Afr.:* Bactocef; Cefril; *Spain:* Septacef; Velocef; *UAE:* Eskacef; *UK:* Nicef; Velosef; *USA:* Velosef.

Cefsulodin Sodium (12544-s)

Cefsulodin Sodium *(BANM, USAN, rINNM).*

Abbott-46811; CGP-7174E; SCE-129; Sulcephalosporin Sodium. Sodium 3-(4-carbamoylpyridiniomethyl)-7-[(2R)-2-phenyl-2-sulphoacetamido]-3-cephem-4-carboxylate.

$C_{22}H_{19}N_4NaO_8S_2$ = 554.5.

CAS — 62587-73-9 *(cefsulodin);* 52152-93-9 *(cefsulodin sodium).*

Pharmacopoeias. In *Jpn.*

1.04 g of monograph substance is approximately equivalent to 1 g of cefsulodin. Each g of monograph substance represents about 1.8 mmol of sodium.

Adverse Effects and Precautions

As for Cefalotin Sodium, p.162.

Antimicrobial Action

Cefsulodin is a bactericidal antibiotic with activity against *Pseudomonas aeruginosa* as great as that of ceftazidime (p.175), but no significant activity against other Gram-negative bacteria. Gram-positive bacteria and anaerobes are not very susceptible. Its activity against *Ps. aeruginosa* may be enhanced by aminoglycosides.

Cefsulodin is stable to hydrolysis by many beta-lactamases, but emergence of resistant *Ps. aeruginosa* has been reported.

Pharmacokinetics

Cefsulodin is given parenterally as the sodium salt. It has a plasma half-life of approximately 1.6 hours, which is prolonged in renal impairment. Up to 30% of cefsulodin in the circulation is bound to plasma proteins. Therapeutic concentrations have been reported in a wide range of body tissues and fluids. The major route of excretion of cefsulodin is via the urine, mainly by glomerular filtration. Clearance may be enhanced in cystic fibrosis, although there have been conflicting reports.

◊ References.
1. Granneman GR, *et al.* Cefsulodin kinetics in healthy subjects after intramuscular and intravenous injection. *Clin Pharmacol Ther* 1982; **31:** 95–103.
2. Reed MD, *et al.* Single-dose pharmacokinetics of cefsulodin in patients with cystic fibrosis. *Antimicrob Agents Chemother* 1984; **25:** 579–81.
3. Hedman A, *et al.* Increased renal clearance of cefsulodin due to higher glomerular filtration rate in cystic fibrosis. *Clin Pharmacokinet* 1990; **18:** 168–75.

Uses and Administration

Cefsulodin is a third-generation cephalosporin antibiotic with a narrow spectrum of activity that has been used similarly to ceftazidime (below) for the treatment of infections caused by susceptible strains of *Pseudomonas aeruginosa.*

It is given as the sodium salt by intramuscular injection, or intravenously by slow injection or by infusion. Doses are expressed in terms of the equivalent amount of cefsulodin. The usual dose for adults is 1 to 4 g daily in two to four divided doses; in severe infections daily doses of 6 g or more may be required. Children may be given doses of 20 to 50 mg per kg body-weight daily; up to 100 mg per kg daily has been given in severe infections.

Patients with renal impairment should be given cefsulodin sodium in a usual loading dose; subsequent doses should be reduced or the dosage interval prolonged.

◊ References.
1. Smith BR. Cefsulodin and ceftazidime, two antipseudomonal cephalosporins. *Clin Pharm* 1984; **3:** 373–85.
2. Wright DB. Cefsulodin. *Drug Intell Clin Pharm* 1986; **20:** 845–9.

Preparations

Proprietary Preparations (details are given in Part 3)
Aust.: Monaspor; Pseudocef; *Fr.:* Pyocefal; *Ger.:* Pseudocef; *Jpn:* Takesulin.

Ceftazidime (12545-w)

Ceftazidime *(BAN, USAN, rINN).*

Ceftazidimum; GR-20263; LY-139381. (Z)-(7R)-7-[2-(2-Aminothiazol-4-yl)-2-(1-carboxy-1-methylethoxyimino)acetamido]-3-(1-pyridiniomethyl)-3-cephem-4-carboxylate pentahydrate.

$C_{22}H_{22}N_6O_7S_2,5H_2O$ = 636.7.

CAS — 72558-82-8 *(anhydrous ceftazidime);* 78439-06-2 *(ceftazidime pentahydrate).*
ATC — J01DA11.

Pharmacopoeias. In *Eur.* (see p.vi), *Jpn, Pol.,* and *US.*

Ceftazidime pentahydrate 1.16 g is approximately equivalent to 1 g of anhydrous ceftazidime.

Pharmacopoeial description

Ph. Eur.: A white or almost white crystalline powder. Slightly soluble in water and in methyl alcohol; practically insoluble in alcohol and in acetone; it dissolves in acid and alkali solutions. A 0.5% solution in water has a pH of 3.0 to 4.0. Store in airtight containers.

USP 25: A white to cream-coloured crystalline powder. Slightly soluble in water, in dimethylformamide, and in methyl alcohol; insoluble in alcohol, in acetone, in chloroform, in dioxan, in ether, in ethyl acetate, and in toluene; soluble in alkali and in dimethyl sulfoxide. pH of a 0.5% solution in water is between 3.0 and 4.0. Store in airtight containers.

◊ Ceftazidime for injection is available as a dry powder containing ceftazidime together with sodium carbonate. When reconstituted ceftazidime sodium is formed with the evolution of carbon dioxide. An alternative formulation, ceftazidime with arginine, appears to overcome the problems associated with effervescence.[1] In some countries a frozen injection containing ceftazidime sodium is also used.
1. Stiles ML, *et al.* Gas production of three brands of ceftazidime. *Am J Hosp Pharm* 1991; **48:** 1727–9.

Incompatibility. It has been reported that ceftazidime does not cause decreased activity when incubated in solution with *gentamicin*[1] or *tobramycin*[2] at 37°, or when mixed with tobramycin in serum.[3] Ceftazidime and tobramycin[4] were also stable for up to 16 hours at room temperature when combined in a glucose-containing dialysis solution, and for a further 8 hours at 37°. However the manufacturers recommend that ceftazidime, like most other beta lactams, should not be mixed with an aminoglycoside in the same giving set or syringe because of the potential for inactivation of either drug.

Ceftazidime is generally considered to be compatible with *metronidazole*, but degradation of ceftazidime has been reported.[5] Precipitation has occurred with *vancomycin*[6] and therefore the manufacturers consider it prudent to flush giving sets and intravenous lines between administration of the two drugs. However, in one study[7] ceftazidime and/or vancomycin were stable in a glucose-containing peritoneal dialysis solution when kept for 6 days in a refrigerator or 48 to 72 hours at room temperature, and in a further study[8] the two drugs were stable when combined in similar solutions containing 1.5% or 4.25% glucose for up to 12 hours when stored at 37° and for 24 hours when stored at 4° and 24°. Ceftazidime and *teicoplanin*[9] were stable in combination in a peritoneal dialysis solution at 37° for 8 hours when it had been previously stored at 4°, but not when previously stored at 25°. Ceftazidime was not stable when mixed in solution with *aminophylline*.[10] There was some evidence of possible incompatibility with *pentamidine*.[11]

1. Elliott TSJ, *et al.* Stability of gentamicin in combination with selected new β-lactam antibiotics. *J Antimicrob Chemother* 1984; **14:** 668–9.
2. Elliott TSJ, *et al.* Stability of tobramycin in combination with selected new β-lactam antibiotics. *J Antimicrob Chemother* 1986; **17:** 680–1.
3. Pennell AT, *et al.* Effect of ceftazidime, cefotaxime, and cefoperazone on serum tobramycin concentrations. *Am J Hosp Pharm* 1991; **48:** 520–2.
4. Mason NA, *et al.* Stability of ceftazidime and tobramycin sulfate in peritoneal dialysis solution. *Am J Hosp Pharm* 1992; **49:** 1139–42.
5. Messerschmidt W. Pharmazeutische kompatibilität von ceftazidim und metronidazol. *Pharm Ztg* 1990; **135:** 36–8.
6. Cairns CJ, Robertson J. Incompatibility of ceftazidime and vancomycin. *Pharm J* 1987; **238:** 577.
7. Vaughan LM, Poon CY. Stability of ceftazidime and vancomycin alone and in combination in heparinized and nonheparinized peritoneal dialysis solution. *Ann Pharmacother* 1994; **28:** 572–6.
8. Stamatakis MK, *et al.* Stability of high-dose vancomycin and ceftazidime in peritoneal dialysis solutions. *Am J Health-Syst Pharm* 1996; **56:** 246–8.
9. Manduru M, *et al.* Stability of ceftazidime sodium and teicoplanin sodium in a peritoneal dialysis solution. *Am J Health-Syst Pharm* 1996; **53:** 2731–4.
10. Pleasants RA, *et al.* Compatibility of ceftazidime and aminophylline admixtures for different methods of intravenous infusion. *Ann Pharmacother* 1992; **26:** 1221–6.
11. Lewis JD. El-Gendy A. Cephalosporin-pentamidine isethionate incompatibilities. *Am J Health-Syst Pharm* 1996; **53:** 1462–3.

Stability. References.

1. Richardson BL, *et al.* The pharmacy of ceftazidime. *J Antimicrob Chemother* 1981; **8** (suppl B): 233–6.
2. Brown AF, *et al.* Freeze thaw stability of ceftazidime. *Br J Parenter Ther* 1985; **6**: 43, 45, 50.
3. Walker SE, Dranitsaris G. Ceftazidime stability in normal saline and dextrose in water. *Can J Hosp Pharm* 1988; **41**: 65–6, 69–71.
4. Wade CS, *et al.* Stability of ceftazidime and amino acids in parenteral nutrient solutions. *Am J Hosp Pharm* 1991; **48**: 1515–19.
5. Stiles ML, *et al.* Stability of ceftazidime (with arginine) and of cefuroxime sodium in infusion-pump reservoirs. *Am J Hosp Pharm* 1992; **49**: 2761–4.
6. Stewart JT, *et al.* Stability of ceftazidime in plastic syringes and glass vials under various storage conditions. *Am J Hosp Pharm* 1992; **49**: 2765–8.
7. Nahata MC, *et al.* Stability of ceftazidime (with arginine) stored in plastic syringes at three temperatures. *Am J Hosp Pharm* 1992; **49**: 2954–6.
8. Bednar DA, *et al.* Stability of ceftazidime (with arginine) in an elastomeric infusion device. *Am J Health-Syst Pharm* 1995; **52**: 1912–14.
9. van Doorne H, *et al.* Ceftazidime degradation rates for predicting stability in a portable infusion-pump reservoir. *Am J Health-Syst Pharm* 1996; **53**: 1302–5.
10. Stendal TL, *et al.* Drug stability and pyridine generation in ceftazidime injection stored in an elastomeric infusion device. *Am J Health-Syst Pharm* 1998; **55**: 683–5.

Adverse Effects and Precautions

As for Cefalotin Sodium, p.162.

Like cefotaxime (p.169), ceftazidime has the potential for colonisation and superinfection with resistant organisms. The risk of superinfection with, for example, *Staphylococcus aureus* may be higher than with cefotaxime, since ceftazidime is less active against staphylococci.

Effects on the blood. References.

1. Hui CH, Chan LC. Agranulocytosis associated with cephalosporin. *BMJ* 1993; **307**: 484.

Effects on the nervous system. References.

1. Al-Zahawi MF, *et al.* Hallucinations in association with ceftazidime. *BMJ* 1988; **297**: 858.
2. Jackson GD, Berkovic SF. Ceftazidime encephalopathy: absence status and toxic hallucinations. *J Neurol Neurosurg Psychiatry* 1992; **55**: 333–4.

Effects on the skin. References.

1. Vinks SATMM, *et al.* Photosensitivity due to ambulatory intravenous ceftazidime in cystic fibrosis patient. *Lancet* 1993; **341**: 1221–2.

Interactions

Unlike many other cephalosporins, probenecid has little effect on the renal clearance of ceftazidime.

◊ References.

1. Verhagen CA, *et al.* The renal clearance of cefuroxime and ceftazidime and the effect of probenecid on their tubular excretion. *Br J Clin Pharmacol* 1994; **37**: 193–7.

Antimicrobial Action

Ceftazidime has a bactericidal action and broad spectrum of activity similar to that of cefotaxime (p.169), but increased activity against *Pseudomonas* spp.; it is less active against staphylococci and streptococci. Unlike cefotaxime it has no active metabolite.

Ceftazidime is highly stable to hydrolysis by most beta-lactamases. It is active *in vitro* against many Gram-negative bacteria including *Pseudomonas aeruginosa*, *Burkholderia pseudomallei* (*Pseudomonas pseudomallei*), and Enterobacteriaceae including *Citrobacter* and *Enterobacter* spp., *Escherichia coli*, *Klebsiella* spp., both indole-positive and indole-negative *Proteus*, *Providencia*, *Salmonella*, *Serratia*, and *Shigella* spp. and *Yersinia enterocolitica*. Other susceptible Gram-negative bacteria include *Haemophilus influenzae*, *Moraxella catarrhalis* (*Branhamella catarrhalis*), and *Neisseria* spp. Among Gram-positive bacteria it is active against some staphylococci and streptococci, but meticillin-resistant staphylococci, enterococci, and *Listeria monocytogenes* are generally resistant. Ceftazidime is active against some anaerobes, although most strains of *Bacteroides fragilis* and *Clostridium difficile* are resistant.

Minimum inhibitory concentrations (MICs) of 8 µg or less per mL have been taken to indicate susceptibility to ceftazidime and MICs of 32 µg or more per mL, resistance. An MIC of about 4 µg per mL has been reported for *Ps. aeruginosa*.

The activity of ceftazidime against *Pseudomonas aeruginosa* and some Enterobacteriaceae may be enhanced by aminoglycosides. Antagonism has been re-

ported *in vitro* between ceftazidime and chloramphenicol.

Resistance. As with cefotaxime, resistance may develop during treatment due to the derepression of chromosomally mediated beta-lactamases. It has been noted particularly in *Pseudomonas* spp. and in Enterobacteriaceae including *Citrobacter*, *Enterobacter* spp. and *Proteus vulgaris*. Resistance may also occur due to the production of plasmid-mediated extended-spectrum beta-lactamases, particularly in *Klebsiella* spp. and *E. coli*.

Pharmacokinetics

Ceftazidime is administered by injection as the sodium salt or in solution with arginine. Mean peak plasma concentrations of 17 and 39 µg per mL have been reported approximately one hour after intramuscular administration of 0.5 and 1 g of ceftazidime, respectively. Five minutes after intravenous bolus injections of 0.5, 1, and 2 g of ceftazidime, mean plasma concentrations of 45, 90, and 170 µg per mL, respectively, have been reported. The plasma half-life of ceftazidime is about 2 hours, but this is prolonged in patients with renal impairment and in neonates. Clearance may be enhanced in patients with cystic fibrosis. It is about 10% bound to plasma proteins.

Ceftazidime is widely distributed in body tissues and fluids; therapeutic concentrations are achieved in the CSF when the meninges are inflamed. It crosses the placenta and is distributed into breast milk.

Ceftazidime is passively excreted in bile, although only a small proportion is eliminated by this route. It is mainly excreted by the kidneys, almost exclusively by glomerular filtration; probenecid has little effect on the excretion. About 80 to 90% of a dose appears unchanged in the urine within 24 hours. It is removed by haemodialysis and peritoneal dialysis.

◊ Studies of the pharmacokinetics of ceftazidime.

a. General.

1. Mouton JW, *et al.* Pharmacokinetics of ceftazidime in serum and suction blister fluid during continuous and intermittent infusions in healthy volunteers. *Antimicrob Agents Chemother* 1990; **34**: 2307–11.
2. Bressolle F, *et al.* Endotracheal and aerosol administrations of ceftazidime in patients with nosocomial pneumonia: pharmacokinetics and absolute bioavailability. *Antimicrob Agents Chemother* 1992; **36**: 1404–11.

◊ b. Biliary excretion.

1. Bouza E, *et al.* Comparison of ceftazidime concentrations in bile and serum. *Antimicrob Agents Chemother* 1983; **24**: 104–6.
2. Leung JWC, *et al.* The effect of obstruction on the biliary excretion of cefoperazone and ceftazidime. *J Antimicrob Chemother* 1990; **25**: 399–406.

◊ c. CNS distribution.

1. Modai J, *et al.* Penetration of ceftazidime into cerebrospinal fluid of patients with bacterial meningitis. *Antimicrob Agents Chemother* 1983; **24**: 126–8.
2. Fong IW, Tomkins KB. Penetration of ceftazidime into the cerebrospinal fluid of patients with and without evidence of meningeal inflammation. *Antimicrob Agents Chemother* 1984; **26**: 115–16.
3. Green HT, *et al.* Penetration of ceftazidime into intracranial abscess. *J Antimicrob Chemother* 1989; **24**: 431–6.
4. Nau R, *et al.* Cerebrospinal fluid ceftazidime kinetics in patients with external ventriculostomies. *Antimicrob Agents Chemother* 1996; **40**: 763–6.

◊ d. Other distribution.

1. O'Donoghue MAT, *et al.* Ceftazidime in middle ear fluid. *J Antimicrob Chemother* 1989; **23**: 664–6.
2. Langer M, *et al.* Penetration of ceftazidime into bronchial secretions in critically ill patients. *J Antimicrob Chemother* 1991; **28**: 925–32.

◊ e. Pharmacokinetics in cystic fibrosis.

1. Leeder JS, *et al.* Ceftazidime disposition in acute and stable cystic fibrosis. *Clin Pharmacol Ther* 1984; **36**: 355–62.
2. Hedman A, *et al.* Influence of the glomerular filtration rate on renal clearance of ceftazidime in cystic fibrosis. *Clin Pharmacokinet* 1988; **15**: 57–65.
3. Vinks AATMM, *et al.* Continuous infusion of ceftazidime in cystic fibrosis patients during home treatment: clinical outcome, microbiology and pharmacokinetics. *J Antimicrob Chemother* 1997; **40**: 125–33.

◊ f. Pharmacokinetics in the elderly.

1. LeBel M, *et al.* Pharmacokinetics of ceftazidime in elderly volunteers. *Antimicrob Agents Chemother* 1985; **28**: 713–15.
2. Higbee MD, *et al.* Pharmacokinetics of ceftazidime in elderly patients. *Clin Pharm* 1989; **8**: 59–62.
3. Sirgo MA, Norris S. Ceftazidime in the elderly: appropriateness of twice-daily dosing. *DICP Ann Pharmacother* 1991; **25**: 284–8.

◊ g. Pharmacokinetics in hepatic impairment.

1. El Touny M, *et al.* Pharmacokinetics of ceftazidime in patients with liver cirrhosis and ascites. *J Antimicrob Chemother* 1991; **28**: 95–100.

◊ h. Pharmacokinetics in premature neonates.

1. van den Anker JN, *et al.* Ceftazidime pharmacokinetics in preterm infants: effects of renal function and gestational age. *Clin Pharmacol Ther* 1995; **58**: 650–9.
2. van den Anker JN, *et al.* Ceftazidime pharmacokinetics in preterm infants: effect of postnatal age and postnatal exposure to indomethacin. *Br J Clin Pharmacol* 1995; **40**: 439–43.
3. van den Anker JN, *et al.* Once-daily versus twice-daily administration of ceftazidime in the preterm infant. *Antimicrob Agents Chemother* 1995; **39**: 2048–50.

◊ i. Pharmacokinetics in renal impairment.

1. Welage LS, *et al.* Pharmacokinetics of ceftazidime in patients with renal insufficiency. *Antimicrob Agents Chemother* 1984; **25**: 201–4.
2. Leroy A, *et al.* Pharmacokinetics of ceftazidime in normal and uremic subjects. *Antimicrob Agents Chemother* 1984; **25**: 638–42.
3. Ackerman BH, *et al.* Effect of decreased renal function on the pharmacokinetics of ceftazidime. *Antimicrob Agents Chemother* 1984; **25**: 785–6.
4. Lin N-S, *et al.* Single- and multiple-dose pharmacokinetics of ceftazidime in infected patients with varying degrees of renal function. *J Clin Pharmacol* 1989; **29**: 331–7.
5. Kinowski J-M, *et al.* Multiple-dose pharmacokinetics of amikacin and ceftazidime in critically ill patients with septic multiple-organ failure during intermittent hemofiltration. *Antimicrob Agents Chemother* 1993; **37**: 464–73.
6. Demotes-Mainard F, *et al.* Pharmacokinetics of intravenous and intraperitoneal ceftazidime in chronic ambulatory peritoneal dialysis. *J Clin Pharmacol* 1993; **33**: 475–9.

Uses and Administration

Ceftazidime is a third-generation cephalosporin antibiotic with enhanced activity against *Pseudomonas aeruginosa*. It is used in the treatment of susceptible infections (see Antimicrobial Action, above), especially those due to *Pseudomonas* spp. They include biliary-tract infections, bone and joint infections, cystic fibrosis (respiratory-tract infections), endophthalmitis, infections in immunocompromised patients (neutropenic patients), melioidosis, meningitis, peritonitis, pneumonia, upper respiratory-tract infections, septicaemia, skin infections (including burns, ecthyma gangrenosum, and ulceration), and urinary-tract infections. It is also used for surgical infection prophylaxis. For details of these infections and their treatment, see under Choice of Antibacterial, p.114.

Administration and dosage. Ceftazidime is available as the pentahydrate but it is formulated with sodium carbonate, to form the sodium salt in solution, or with arginine. Doses are expressed in terms of anhydrous ceftazidime. It is given by deep intramuscular injection, slow intravenous injection over 3 to 5 minutes, or intravenous infusion over up to 30 minutes. The usual dose for adults ranges from 1 to 6 g daily in divided doses every 8 or 12 hours. The higher doses are used in severe infections especially in immunocompromised patients. In adults with cystic fibrosis who have pseudomonal lung infections, high doses of 90 to 150 mg per kg body-weight daily in 3 divided doses are used; up to 9 g daily has been given to adults with normal renal function. Single doses of more than 1 g should be given intravenously.

Children are usually given ceftazidime 30 to 100 mg per kg daily in 2 or 3 divided doses, but in severely ill children up to 150 mg per kg daily to a maximum of 6 g daily may be given in 3 divided doses. Neonates and infants up to 2 months old have been given 25 to 60 mg per kg daily in 2 divided doses.

In the elderly the dose should generally not exceed 3 g daily.

In patients with renal impairment the dosage of ceftazidime may need to be reduced. Following a loading dose of 1 g, maintenance doses are based on the creatinine clearance. Maintenance doses are: creatinine clearance 31 to 50 mL per minute, 1 g every 12 hours; 16 to 30 mL per minute, 1 g every 24 hours; 6 to 15 mL per minute, 0.5 g every 24 hours; and less than 5 mL per minute, 0.5 g every 48 hours. In severe infections these doses may need to be increased by 50%. In these patients ceftazidime trough serum concentrations should not exceed 40 µg per mL. In patients undergoing peritoneal dialysis a loading dose of 1 g may be given followed by 500 mg every 24 hours; ceftazidime sodium may also be added to the dialysis fluid, usually 125 to 250 mg of ceftazidime for 2 litres of dialysis fluid. In patients undergoing haemodialysis a loading dose of 1 g is given and should be repeated after each dialysis period.

For surgical infection prophylaxis in patients undergoing prostatic surgery, a dose of 1 g may be given at induction of anaesthesia and repeated if necessary when the catheter is removed.

Ceftazidime can be used in association with an aminoglycoside, another beta lactam such as piperacillin, or vancomycin in patients with severe neutropenia, or, if infection with *Bacteroides fragilis* is suspected, in association with an antimicrobial such as clindamycin or metronidazole. The drugs should generally be administered separately (see also Incompatibility, above).

◊ References.
1. Rains CP, *et al*. Ceftazidime: an update of its antibacterial activity, pharmacokinetic properties and therapeutic efficacy. *Drugs* 1995; **49:** 577–617.

Preparations

USP 25: Ceftazidime for Injection; Ceftazidime Injection.

Proprietary Preparations (details are given in Part 3)
Aust.: Fortum; Kefazim; *Austral.:* Fortum; *Belg.:* Glazidim; Kefadim; *Braz.:* Fortaz; Kefadim; Tazidem; *Canad.:* Ceptaz; Fortaz; Tazidime; *Denm.:* Fortum; *Fin.:* Glazidim; *Fr.:* Fortum; Fortumset; *Ger.:* Fortum; *Hong Kong:* Fortum; *Irl.:* Fortum; *Israel:* Fortum; *Ital.:* Ceftim; Glazidim; Panzid; Spectrum; Starcef; *Mex.:* Bac-Zidim; Fortum; Izadima; Lezidim; Tagal; Taxifur; Waytrax; Zidicef; *Neth.:* Fortum; *Norw.:* Fortum; *NZ:* Fortum; *S.Afr.:* Fortum; Kefzim; *Singapore:* Fortum; *Spain:* Fortam; Kefamin; Potendal; *Swed.:* Fortum; *Switz.:* Fortam; *Thai.:* CEF-4; Cefodime; Fortum; Forzid; Kefadim; Zeftam; *UAE:* Negacef; *UK:* Fortum; Kefadim; *USA:* Ceptaz; Fortaz; Tazicef; Tazidime.

Cefteram (2899-x)

Cefteram (rINN).

Ro-19-5247; T-2525. (Z)-7-[2-(2-Aminothiazol-4-yl)-2-methoxyiminoacetamido]-3-(5-methyl-2H-tetrazol-2-ylmethyl)-3-cephem-4-carboxylic acid.
$C_{16}H_{17}N_9O_5S_2 = 479.5.$
CAS — 82547-58-8.
Pharmacopoeias. Jpn includes Cefteram Pivoxil.

Profile
Cefteram is a cephalosporin antibacterial used for the treatment of susceptible infections. It is given by mouth as the pivaloyloxymethyl ester, cefteram pivoxil, in a usual adult dose of 150 to 300 mg daily in three divided doses after meals.

Ceftezole Sodium (34-n)

Ceftezole Sodium (rINNM).

Sodium (7R)-7-[2-(1H-tetrazol-1-yl)acetamido]-3-(1,3,4-thiadiazol-2-ylthiomethyl)-3-cephem-4-carboxylate.
$C_{13}H_{11}N_8NaO_4S_3 = 462.5.$
CAS — 26973-24-0 (ceftezole); 41136-22-5 (ceftezole sodium).

Profile
Ceftezole is a cephalosporin antibiotic with properties similar to those of cefalotin (p.162). It may be administered as the sodium salt by the intramuscular route in usual adult doses of 2 to 4 g daily in two or three divided doses.

Preparations

Proprietary Preparations (details are given in Part 3)
Ital.: Alomen.

Ceftibuten (1793-h)

Ceftibuten (BAN, USAN, rINN).

7432-S; Sch-39720. 7-[2-(2-Amino-1,3-thiazol-4-yl)-4-carboxyisocrotonamide]-3-cephem-4-carboxylic acid.
$C_{15}H_{14}N_4O_6S_2 = 410.4.$
CAS — 97519-39-6.
ATC — J01DA39.

Adverse Effects and Precautions
As for Cefalotin Sodium, p.162.

The most frequently reported adverse effects of ceftibuten are gastrointestinal disturbances, especially diarrhoea, and headache.

Antimicrobial Action
As for Cefixime, p.166. It is less active *in vitro* against *Streptococcus pneumoniae*.

◊ References.
1. Shawar R, *et al*. Comparative in vitro activity of ceftibuten (Sch-39720) against bacterial enteropathogens. *Antimicrob Agents Chemother* 1989; **33:** 781–4.
2. Bragman SGL, Casewell MW. The in-vitro activity of ceftibuten against 475 clinical isolates of Gram-negative bacilli, compared with cefuroxime and cefadroxil. *J Antimicrob Chemother* 1990; **25:** 221–6.
3. Wise R, *et al*. Ceftibuten—in-vitro activity against respiratory pathogens, β-lactamase stability and mechanism of action. *J Antimicrob Chemother* 1990; **26:** 209–13.

Pharmacokinetics
Ceftibuten is rapidly absorbed from the gastrointestinal tract following oral administration, although the rate and extent of absorption are somewhat decreased by the presence of food. Peak plasma concentrations of about 17 µg per mL are attained about 2 hours after a 400-mg dose. The plasma half-life of ceftibuten is about 2.0 to 2.3 hours and is prolonged in patients with renal impairment. Ceftibuten is 60 to 77% bound to plasma proteins.

Ceftibuten distributes into middle-ear fluid and bronchial secretions. About 10% of a dose is converted to the *trans*-isomer, which has about one-eighth of the activity of the *cis*-isomer. Ceftibuten is excreted mainly in the urine and also in the faeces. Significant amounts are removed by haemodialysis.

◊ References.
1. Wise R, *et al*. Pharmacokinetics and tissue penetration of ceftibuten. *Antimicrob Agents Chemother* 1990; **34:** 1053–5.
2. Kearns GL, *et al*. Single-dose pharmacokinetics of ceftibuten (SCH-39720) in infants and children. *Antimicrob Agents Chemother* 1991; **35:** 2078–84.
3. Kelloway JS, *et al*. Pharmacokinetics of ceftibuten-cis and its trans metabolite in healthy volunteers and in patients with chronic renal insufficiency. *Antimicrob Agents Chemother* 1991; **35:** 2267–74.
4. Kearns GL, Young RA. Ceftibuten pharmacokinetics and pharmacodynamics: focus on paediatric use. *Clin Pharmacokinet* 1994; **26:** 169–89.
5. Lin C, *et al*. Multiple-dose pharmacokinetics of ceftibuten in healthy volunteers. *Antimicrob Agents Chemother* 1995; **39:** 356–8.
6. Lin C, *et al*. Pharmacokinetics and dose proportionality of ceftibuten in men. *Antimicrob Agents Chemother* 1995; **39:** 359–61.
7. Lin C, *et al*. Penetration of ceftibuten into middle ear fluid. *Antimicrob Agents Chemother* 1996; **40:** 1394–6.

Uses and Administration
Ceftibuten is an oral third-generation cephalosporin antibiotic used similarly to cefixime (p.166) in the treatment of urinary-tract and respiratory-tract infections. It is given by mouth as the dihydrate, but doses are expressed in terms of anhydrous ceftibuten. The usual adult dose is 400 mg once daily. Children over 6 months of age and weighing 45 kg or less may be given 9 mg per kg body-weight daily as a single dose.

Doses should be reduced in patients with moderate to severe renal impairment. The following doses based on creatinine clearance may be used: 30 to 49 mL per minute, 200 mg once daily and 5 to 29 mL per minute, 100 mg once daily.

◊ Reviews.
1. Wiseman LR, Balfour JA. Ceftibuten: review of its antibacterial activity, pharmacokinetic properties and clinical efficacy. *Drugs* 1994; **47:** 784–808.
2. Nelson JD, McCracken GH (eds). Ceftibuten: a new orally active cephalosporin for pediatric infections. *Pediatr Infect Dis J* 1995; **14** (suppl): S76–S133.
3. Guay DRP. Ceftibuten: a new expanded-spectrum oral cephalosporin. *Ann Pharmacother* 1997; **31:** 1022–33.

Preparations

Proprietary Preparations (details are given in Part 3)
Aust.: Caedax; *Fin.:* Cedax; *Ger.:* Keimax; *Hong Kong:* Cedax; *Irl.:* Cedax; *Israel:* Cedax; *Ital.:* Cedax; *Isocef*; *Jpn:* Seftem; *Mex.:* Cedax; *Neth.:* Cedax; *Port.:* Caedax; *S.Afr.:* Cedax; Sepexin; *Singapore:* Cedax; *Spain:* Biocef; Cedax; Cepifran; *Swed.:* Cedax; *Switz.:* Cedax; *Thai.:* Cedax; *UK:* Cedax†; *USA:* Cedax.

Ceftiofur Sodium (3853-j)

Ceftiofur Sodium (BANM, USAN).

CM-31-916; CM-31916 (ceftiofur); U-64279A (ceftiofur hydrochloride); U-64279E. Sodium (6R,7R)-7-[2-(2-Amino-4-thiazolyl)-glyoxylamido]-3-mercaptomethyl-8-oxo-5-thia-1-azabicyclo[4.2.0]oct-2-ene-2-carboxylate, 7²-(Z)-(O-methyloxime), 2-furoate (ester).
$C_{19}H_{16}N_5NaO_7S_3 = 545.5.$
CAS — 80370-57-6 (ceftiofur); 103980-44-5 (ceftiofur hydrochloride); 104010-37-9 (ceftiofur sodium).

Profile
Ceftiofur is a cephalosporin antibiotic used as the sodium salt in veterinary practice.

Ceftizoxime Sodium (12546-e)

Ceftizoxime Sodium (BANM, USAN, rINNM).

FK-749; FR-13749; SKF-88373-Z. Sodium (Z)-7-[2-(2-aminothiazol-4-yl)-2-methoxyiminoacetamido]-3-cephem-4-carboxylate.
$C_{13}H_{12}N_5NaO_5S_2 = 405.4.$
CAS — 68401-81-0 (ceftizoxime); 68401-82-1 (ceftizoxime sodium).
Pharmacopoeias. In Jpn and US.

1.06 g of monograph substance is approximately equivalent to 1 g of ceftizoxime. Each g of monograph substance represents about 2.5 mmol of sodium.

Pharmacopoeial description
USP 25: A white to pale yellow crystalline powder. Freely soluble in water. pH of a 10% solution in water is between 6.0 and 8.0. Store in airtight containers.

Stability. References.
1. Lesko AB, *et al*. Ceftizoxime stability in iv solutions. *DICP Ann Pharmacother* 1989; **23:** 615–18.

Adverse Effects and Precautions
As for Cefotaxime Sodium, p.169.

Interactions
Probenecid reduces the renal clearance of ceftizoxime.

Antimicrobial Action
As for Cefotaxime Sodium, p.169, although ceftizoxime has no active metabolite.

Pharmacokinetics
After intramuscular injection of 0.5 and 1 g of ceftizoxime, mean peak plasma concentrations of about 14 and 39 µg per mL respectively have been reported after 1 hour. The plasma half-life of ceftizoxime is about 1.7 hours and is prolonged in neonates and in renal impairment. Only 30% of ceftizoxime in the circulation is bound to plasma proteins.

Ceftizoxime is widely distributed in body tissues and fluids; therapeutic concentrations are achieved in the CSF when the meninges are inflamed. It crosses the placenta and low concentrations have been detected in breast milk.

Nearly all of a dose is excreted unchanged in the urine within 24 hours of administration, thus achieving high urinary concentrations. Ceftizoxime is excreted by tubular secretion as well as glomerular filtration and the concomitant administration of probenecid results in higher and more prolonged plasma concentrations. Some ceftizoxime is removed by dialysis.

◊ References.
1. Jordan NS, *et al*. Comparative pharmacokinetics of ceftizoxime and cefotaxime in healthy volunteers. *Curr Ther Res* 1986; **40:** 133–40.
2. Vallée F, LeBel M. Comparative study of pharmacokinetics and serum bactericidal activity of ceftizoxime and cefotaxime. *Antimicrob Agents Chemother* 1991; **35:** 2057–64.
3. Fujii R. Investigation of half-life and clinical effects of ceftizoxime in premature and newborn infants. *Drug Invest* 1990; **2:** 143–9.
4. Reed MD, *et al*. Ceftizoxime disposition in neonates and infants during the first six months of life. *DICP Ann Pharmacother* 1991; **25:** 344–7.
5. Guglielmo BJ, *et al*. Pharmacokinetics and pharmacodynamics of ceftizoxime in abscess fluid. *J Antimicrob Chemother* 1997; **39:** 437–8.

Uses and Administration
Ceftizoxime is a third-generation cephalosporin antibiotic used similarly to cefotaxime (p.170) for the treatment of susceptible infections.

It is administered as the sodium salt by deep intramuscular injection, or intravenously as a slow injection over 3 to 5 minutes or as a continuous or intermittent infusion. If 2 g of ceftizoxime is injected intramuscularly the dose should be divided between sites.

Doses are expressed in terms of the equivalent amount of ceftizoxime. It is usually given in an adult dose of 1 to 2 g every 8 to 12 hours. In severe or life-threatening infections 2 to 4 g may be given intravenously every 8 hours.

Children over 6 months of age may be given 50 mg per kg body-weight every 6 to 8 hours.

For the treatment of uncomplicated urinary-tract infections, a dose of 0.5 g every 12 hours is used.

Doses should be modified in renal impairment; after a loading dose of 0.5 to 1 g the maintenance dosage should be adjusted according to the patient's creatinine clearance and the severity of the infection: creatinine clearance 50 to 79 mL per minute, 0.5 to 1.5 g every 8 hours; 5 to 49 mL per minute, 0.25 to 1 g every 12 hours; less than 5 mL per minute, 0.25 to 0.5 g every 24 hours or 0.5 to 1 g every 48 hours, after dialysis.

A single intramuscular dose of 1 g has been given in uncomplicated gonorrhoea.

◊ References.
1. Richards DM, Heel RC. Ceftizoxime: a review of its antibacterial activity, pharmacokinetic properties and therapeutic use. *Drugs* 1985; **29:** 281–329.

Preparations

USP 25: Ceftizoxime for Injection; Ceftizoxime Injection.

Proprietary Preparations (details are given in Part 3)
Aust.: Cefizox; **Canad.:** Cefizox; **Fin.:** Epocelin; **Fr.:** Cefizox; **Ger.:** Ceftix†; **Irl.:** Cefizox; **Israel:** Tefizox; **Ital.:** Eposerin; **Jpn:** Epocelin; **Mex.:** Cefizox; Ultracef; **Neth.:** Cefizox; **Port.:** Cefizox†; **Spain:** Cefizox; Epocelin†; **Thai.:** Epocelin; **USA:** Cefizox.

Ceftriaxone Sodium (12547-I)

Ceftriaxone Sodium (BANM, USAN, rINNM).

Ceftriaxonum Natricum; Ro-13-9904; Ro-13-9904/000 (ceftriaxone). (Z)-7-[2-(2-Aminothiazol-4-yl)-2-methoxyiminoacetamido]-3-[(2,5-dihydro-6-hydroxy-2-methyl-5-oxo-1,2,4-triazin-3-yl)thiomethyl]-3-cephem-4-carboxylic acid, disodium salt, sesquaterhydrate.
$C_{18}H_{16}N_8Na_2O_7S_3,3\frac{1}{2}H_2O = 661.6$.
CAS — 73384-59-5 (ceftriaxone); 74578-69-1 (anhydrous ceftriaxone sodium); 104376-79-6 (ceftriaxone sodium sesquaterhydrate).

Pharmacopoeias. In *Eur.* (see p.vi), *Jpn, Pol.,* and *US.*

1.19 g of monograph substance is approximately equivalent to 1 g of ceftriaxone. Each g of monograph substance represents about 3.0 mmol of sodium.

Pharmacopoeial description

Ph. Eur.: An almost white to yellowish, slightly hygroscopic, crystalline powder. Freely soluble in water; very slightly soluble in dehydrated alcohol; sparingly soluble in methyl alcohol. A 12% solution in water has a pH of 6.0 to 8.0. Store in airtight containers. Protect from light.

USP 25: A white to yellowish-orange crystalline powder. Freely soluble in water; very slightly soluble in alcohol; sparingly soluble in methyl alcohol. pH of a 10% solution in water is between 6.0 and 8.0. Store in airtight containers.

Incompatibility. The UK manufacturer warns of incompatibility if ceftriaxone sodium is mixed with calcium-containing solutions or with aminoglycosides, fluconazole, labetalol, vancomycin, or amsacrine. Published reports of incompatibility have included that between ceftriaxone and vancomycin[1] or pentamidine.[2]
1. Pritts D, Hancock D. Incompatibility of ceftriaxone with vancomycin. *Am J Hosp Pharm* 1991; **48:** 77.
2. Lewis JD, El-Gendy A. Cephalosporin-pentamidine isethionate incompatibilities. *Am J Health-Syst Pharm* 1996; **53:** 1461–2.

Stability. References.
1. Nahata MC. Stability of ceftriaxone sodium in peritoneal dialysis solutions. *DICP Ann Pharmacother* 1991; **25:** 741–2.
2. Canton E, Esteban MJ. Stability of ceftriaxone solution. *J Antimicrob Chemother* 1992; **30:** 397–8.
3. Bailey LC, et al. Stability of ceftriaxone sodium in injectable solutions stored frozen in syringes. *Am J Hosp Pharm* 1994; **51:** 2159–61.
4. Plumridge RJ et al. Stability of ceftriaxone sodium in polypropylene syringes at −20, 4, and 20°C. *Am J Health-Syst Pharm* 1996; **53:** 2320–3.

Adverse Effects and Precautions

As for Cefotaxime Sodium, p.169.

Changes in bowel flora may be more marked than with cefotaxime because of the greater biliary excretion of ceftriaxone; diarrhoea may occur more often, especially in children. Biliary sludge or pseudolithiasis due to a precipitate of calcium ceftriaxone has been seen occasionally in patients receiving ceftriaxone. Similarly, deposition of the calcium salt has occurred rarely in the urine. Ceftriaxone is highly protein-bound and is able to displace bilirubin from

albumin binding sites, causing hyperbilirubinaemia; its use should be avoided in jaundiced neonates.

Neutropenia has been reported with most cephalosporins; a complex mechanism has been attributed to that associated with ceftriaxone. There have been rare reports of fatal haemolysis associated with ceftriaxone.

Although ceftriaxone has an *N*-methylthiotriazine ring rather than the *N*-methylthiotetrazole side-chain seen in cephalosporins such as cefamandole (p.163), it might still have the potential to cause hypoprothrombinaemia.

Effects on the biliary tract. Using abdominal ultrasonography, biliary sludge or pseudolithiasis was found in about 40% of severely ill children being treated with high doses of ceftriaxone[1] and was later reported in adults.[2,3] The sludge has been identified as a calcium salt of ceftriaxone.[4] Patients are often asymptomatic and the sludge usually dissolves once ceftriaxone is discontinued. Gallstones with ceftriaxone as a major component have been identified in a patient given long-term high-dose treatment.[5] Similarly, a bile-duct stone composed of ceftriaxone occurred with high-dose ceftriaxone in a child.[6] In another report, intractable hiccups were associated with ceftriaxone-related pseudolithiasis in a 10-year-old boy.[7]
1. Schaad UB, et al. Reversible ceftriaxone-associated biliary pseudolithiasis in children. *Lancet* 1988; **ii:** 1411–13.
2. Pigrau C, et al. Ceftriaxone-associated biliary pseudolithiasis in adults. *Lancet* 1989; **ii:** 165.
3. Heim-Duthoy KL, et al. Apparent biliary pseudolithiasis during ceftriaxone therapy. *Antimicrob Agents Chemother* 1990; **34:** 1146–9.
4. Park HZ, et al. Ceftriaxone-associated gallbladder sludge: identification of calcium-ceftriaxone salt as a major component of gallbladder precipitate. *Gastroenterology* 1991; **100:** 1665–70.
5. Lopez AJ, et al. Ceftriaxone-induced cholelithiasis. *Ann Intern Med* 1991; **115:** 712–14.
6. Robertson FM, et al. Ceftriaxone choledocholithiasis. *Pediatrics* 1996; **98:** 133–5.
7. Bonioli E, et al. Pseudolithiasis and intractable hiccups in a boy receiving ceftriaxone. *N Engl J Med* 1994; **331:** 1532.

Effects on the blood. References.
1. Haubenstock A, et al. Hypoprothrombinaemic bleeding associated with ceftriaxone. *Lancet* 1983; **i:** 1215–16.
2. Rey D, et al. Ceftriaxone-induced granulopenia related to a peculiar mechanism of granulopoiesis inhibition. *Am J Med* 1989; **87:** 591–2.
3. Bernini JC, et al. Fatal hemolysis induced by ceftriaxone in a child with sickle cell anemia. *J Pediatr* 1995; **126:** 813–15.
4. Lascari AD, Amyot K. Fatal hemolysis caused by ceftriaxone. *J Pediatr* 1995; **126:** 816–17.
5. Scimeca PG, et al. Hemolysis after treatment with ceftriaxone. *J Pediatr* 1996; **128:** 163.
6. Moallem HJ, et al. Ceftriaxone-related fatal hemolysis in an adolescent with perinatally acquired human immunodeficiency virus infection. *J Pediatr* 1998; **133:** 279–81.

Effects on the gastrointestinal tract. References.
1. Nahata MC, Miller MA. Diarrhoea associated with ceftriaxone and its implications in paediatric patients. *J Clin Pharm Ther* 1989; **14:** 305–7.
2. Samonis G, et al. Prospective evaluation of effects of broad-spectrum antibiotics on gastrointestinal yeast colonization of humans. *Antimicrob Agents Chemother* 1993; **37:** 51–3.

Effects on the pancreas. References.
1. Zimmermann AE, et al. Ceftriaxone-induced acute pancreatitis. *Ann Pharmacother* 1993; **27:** 36–7.

Use in neonates. References to the displacement of bilirubin by ceftriaxone in neonates.
1. Gulian J-M, et al. Bilirubin displacement by ceftriaxone in neonates: evaluation by determination of 'free' bilirubin and erythrocyte-bound bilirubin. *J Antimicrob Chemother* 1987; **19:** 823–9.
2. Fink S, et al. Ceftriaxone effect on bilirubin-albumin binding. *Pediatrics* 1987; **80:** 873–5.

Interactions

Ceftriaxone has an *N*-methylthiotriazine side-chain and may have the potential to increase the effects of anticoagulants and to cause a disulfiram-like reaction with alcohol.

Unlike many cephalosporins, probenecid does not affect the renal excretion of ceftriaxone.

Antimicrobial Action

As for Cefotaxime Sodium, p.169, although ceftriaxone has no active metabolite.

◊ References.
1. Goldstein FW, et al. Resistance to ceftriaxone and other β-lactams in bacteria isolated in the community. *Antimicrob Agents Chemother* 1995; **39:** 2516–19.

Pharmacokinetics

Ceftriaxone demonstrates nonlinear dose-dependent pharmacokinetics because of its protein binding; about 85 to 95% is bound to plasma protein depending on the plasma concentration of ceftriaxone.

Mean peak plasma concentrations of about 40 and 80 µg per mL have been reported 2 hours after intramuscular injection of 0.5 and 1 g of ceftriaxone respectively. The plasma half-life of ceftriaxone is not dependent on the dose and varies between 6 and 9 hours; it may be prolonged in neonates. The half-life does not change appreciably in patients with moderate renal impairment, but it may be prolonged in severe renal impairment especially when there is also hepatic impairment.

Ceftriaxone is widely distributed in body tissues and fluids. It crosses both inflamed and non-inflamed meninges, generally achieving therapeutic concentrations in the CSF. It crosses the placenta and low concentrations have been detected in breast milk. High concentrations are achieved in bile.

About 40 to 65% of a dose of ceftriaxone is excreted unchanged in the urine, principally by glomerular filtration; the remainder is excreted in the bile and is ultimately found in the faeces as unchanged drug and microbiologically inactive compounds.

◊ Reviews.
1. Hayton WL, Stoeckel K. Age-associated changes in ceftriaxone pharmacokinetics. *Clin Pharmacokinet* 1986; **11:** 76–86.
2. Yuk JH, et al. Clinical pharmacokinetics of ceftriaxone. *Clin Pharmacokinet* 1989; **17:** 223–35.

◊ Some studies of the pharmacokinetics of ceftriaxone.
a. Distribution into the CNS.
1. Latif R, Dajani AS. Ceftriaxone diffusion into cerebrospinal fluid of children with meningitis. *Antimicrob Agents Chemother* 1983; **23:** 46–8.
2. Chandrasekar PH, et al. Diffusion of ceftriaxone into the cerebrospinal fluid of adults. *J Antimicrob Chemother* 1984; **14:** 427–30.
3. Lucht F, et al. The penetration of ceftriaxone into human brain tissue. *J Antimicrob Chemother* 1990; **26:** 81–6.
4. Nau R, et al. Passage of cefotaxime and ceftriaxone into cerebrospinal fluid of patients with uninflamed meninges. *Antimicrob Agents Chemother* 1993; **37:** 1518–24.
5. Gaillard J-L, et al. Concentrations of ceftriaxone in cerebrospinal fluid of children with meningitis receiving dexamethasone therapy. *Antimicrob Agents Chemother* 1994; **38:** 1209–10.

◊ b. Pharmacokinetics in hepatobiliary disease.
1. Stoeckel K, et al. Single-dose ceftriaxone kinetics in liver insufficiency. *Clin Pharmacol Ther* 1984; **36:** 500–9.
2. Hary L, et al. The pharmacokinetics of ceftriaxone and cefotaxime in cirrhotic patients with ascites. *Eur J Clin Pharmacol* 1989; **36:** 613–16.
3. Toth A, et al. Pharmacokinetics of ceftriaxone in liver-transplant recipients. *J Clin Pharmacol* 1991; **31:** 722–8.
4. Van Delden OM, et al. Biliary excretion of ceftriaxone into non-stagnant and stagnant bile. *J Antimicrob Chemother* 1994; **33:** 193–4.

◊ c. Pharmacokinetics in pregnancy and lactation.
1. Bourget P, et al. Pharmacokinetics and protein binding of ceftriaxone during pregnancy. *Antimicrob Agents Chemother* 1993; **37:** 54–9.
2. Bourget P, et al. Ceftriaxone distribution and protein binding between maternal blood and milk postpartum. *Ann Pharmacother* 1993; **27:** 294–7.

◊ d. Pharmacokinetics in renal impairment.
The pharmacokinetics of ceftriaxone are not markedly altered in mild to moderate renal impairment,[1] but the half-life can be prolonged in severe or end-stage renal disease.[1-4] Ceftriaxone is generally not removed by peritoneal dialysis[4] or by haemodialysis[1-3] although a decrease in half-life has been reported during haemodialysis.[5] In many patients no alteration in dosage is necessary, but some individuals have reduced non-renal clearance despite apparently normal hepatic function.[2,3] It is advisable to monitor plasma ceftriaxone in patients with severe renal impairment and unknown non-renal clearance.
1. Patel IH, et al. Ceftriaxone pharmacokinetics in patients with various degrees of renal impairment. *Antimicrob Agents Chemother* 1984; **25:** 438–42.
2. Stoeckel K, et al. Single-dose ceftriaxone kinetics in functionally anephric patients. *Clin Pharmacol Ther* 1983; **33:** 633–41.
3. Cohen D, et al. Pharmacokinetics of ceftriaxone in patients with renal failure and in those undergoing hemodialysis. *Antimicrob Agents Chemother* 1983; **24:** 529–32.
4. Ti T-Y, et al. Kinetic disposition of intravenous ceftriaxone in normal subjects and patients with renal failure on hemodialysis or peritoneal dialysis. *Antimicrob Agents Chemother* 1984; **25:** 83–7.
5. Garcia RL, et al. Single-dose pharmacokinetics of ceftriaxone in patients with end-stage renal disease and hemodialysis. *Chemotherapy* 1988; **34:** 261–6.

◊ e. Pharmacokinetics in surgery.
1. Jungbluth GL, et al. Ceftriaxone disposition in open-heart surgery patients. *Antimicrob Agents Chemother* 1989; **33:** 850–6.
2. Martin C, et al. Pharmacokinetics and tissue penetration of a single dose of ceftriaxone (1,000 milligrams intravenously) for antibiotic prophylaxis in thoracic surgery. *Antimicrob Agents Chemother* 1992; **36:** 2804–7.
3. Martin C, et al. Concentrations of prophylactic ceftriaxone in abdominal tissues during pancreatic surgery. *J Antimicrob Chemother* 1997; **40:** 445–8.
4. Scaglione F, et al. Pharmacokinetic study of cefodizime and ceftriaxone in sera and bones of patients undergoing hip arthroplasty. *Antimicrob Agents Chemother* 1997; **41:** 2292–4.

The symbol † denotes a preparation no longer actively marketed

Uses and Administration

Ceftriaxone is a third-generation cephalosporin antibiotic used similarly to cefotaxime for the treatment of susceptible infections. They include chancroid, endocarditis, gastro-enteritis (invasive salmonellosis; shigellosis), gonorrhoea, Lyme disease, meningitis (including meningococcal meningitis prophylaxis), septicaemia, syphilis, typhoid fever, and Whipple's disease. It is also used for surgical infection prophylaxis. For details of these infections and their treatment, see under Choice of Antibacterial, p.114.

Administration and dosage. Ceftriaxone is given as the sodium salt by slow intravenous injection over at least 2 to 4 minutes, by intermittent intravenous infusion over at least 30 minutes, or by deep intramuscular injection. If more than 1 g is to be injected intramuscularly then the dose should be divided between more than one site. Doses are expressed in terms of the equivalent amount of ceftriaxone. It is usually given to adults in a dose of 1 to 2 g daily as a single dose or in two divided doses; in severe infections up to 4 g daily may be given. Doses for infants and children are 20 to 50 mg per kg body-weight once daily; for severe infections up to 80 mg per kg daily may be given. In neonates, the maximum dose should not exceed 50 mg per kg daily; intravenous doses in neonates should be given over 60 minutes. Doses above 50 mg per kg should be given by intravenous infusion only.

A reduction in dosage may be necessary in patients with severe renal impairment and in those with both impaired renal and hepatic function; plasma concentrations should be monitored in such patients.

A single intramuscular dose of 250 mg is recommended for the treatment of uncomplicated gonorrhoea in adults.

For surgical infection prophylaxis in adults, a single dose of 1 g may be administered 0.5 to 2 hours before surgery; a 2-g dose is suggested before colorectal surgery.

For the prevention of secondary cases of meningococcal meningitis, a single intramuscular dose of 250 mg may be used for adults and 125 mg for children.

◊ References.
1. Brogden RN, Ward A. Ceftriaxone: a reappraisal of its antibacterial activity and pharmacokinetic properties, and an update on its therapeutic use with particular reference to once-daily administration. *Drugs* 1988; **35:** 604–45.

Preparations

BP 2001: Ceftriaxone Injection;
USP 25: Ceftriaxone for Injection; Ceftriaxone Injection.

Proprietary Preparations (details are given in Part 3)
Aust.: Rocephin; *Austral.:* Rocephin; *Belg.:* Rocephine; *Braz.:* Rocefin; *Canad.:* Rocephin; *Denm.:* Rocephalin; *Fin.:* Rocephalin; *Fr.:* Rocephine; *Ger.:* Rocephin; *Hong Kong:* Rocephin; *Irl.:* Rocephin; *Israel:* Rocephin; *Ital.:* Rocefin; *Mex.:* Benaxona; Cefaxona; Cefraden; Ceftrex; Rocephin; Tacex; Terbac; Triaken; *Neth.:* Rocephin; *Norw.:* Rocephin; *NZ:* Rocephin; *Port.:* Mesporin; Rocephin; *S.Afr.:* Rocephin; *Singapore:* Cefaxone; Cefin; Rocephin; Trexofin; *Spain:* Rocefalin; *Swed.:* Rocephalin; *Switz.:* Rocephine; *Thai.:* CEF-3; Cefine; Ceftrex; Ceftriphin; Oframax; Rocephin; Sedalin; Tricephin; Trixone; Zefaxone; *UAE:* Triaxone; *UK:* Rocephin; *USA:* Rocephin.

Cefuroxime (15872-m)

Cefuroxime *(BAN, USAN, rINN).*
640/359. (Z)-3-Carbamoyloxymethyl-7-[2-(2-furyl)-2-methoxyiminoacetamido]-3-cephem-4-carboxylic acid.
$C_{16}H_{16}N_4O_8S = 424.4.$
CAS — 55268-75-2.
ATC — J01DA06.

Cefuroxime Axetil (16570-x)

Cefuroxime Axetil *(BANM, USAN, rINNM).*
CCI-15641.
$C_{20}H_{22}N_4O_{10}S = 510.5.$
CAS — 64544-07-6.
Pharmacopoeias. In Eur. (see p.vi), Jpn, Pol., and US.

1.20 g of cefuroxime axetil is approximately equivalent to 1 g of cefuroxime.

Pharmacopoeial description

Ph. Eur.: A white or almost white amorphous powder. Slightly soluble in water and in alcohol; soluble in acetone, in ethyl ac-

etate, and in methyl alcohol. Store in airtight containers. Protect from light.

USP 25: A white or almost white powder. The amorphous form is insoluble in water and in ether; slightly soluble in dehydrated alcohol; freely soluble in acetone; soluble in chloroform, in ethyl acetate, and in methyl alcohol. The crystalline form is insoluble in water and in ether; slightly soluble in dehydrated alcohol; freely soluble in acetone; sparingly soluble in chloroform, in ethyl acetate, and in methyl alcohol. Store in airtight containers.

Cefuroxime Sodium (35-h)

Cefuroxime Sodium *(BANM, rINNM).*
Cefuroximum Natricum.
$C_{16}H_{15}N_4NaO_8S = 446.4.$
CAS — 56238-63-2.
Pharmacopoeias. In Eur. (see p.vi), Jpn, Pol., and US.

1.05 g of cefuroxime sodium is approximately equivalent to 1 g of cefuroxime. Each g of monograph substance represents about 2.2 mmol of sodium.

Cefuroxime sodium may be incompatible with aminoglycosides.

Pharmacopoeial description

Ph. Eur.: A white or almost white slightly hygroscopic powder. Freely soluble in water; very slightly soluble in alcohol. A 1% solution in water has a pH of 5.5 to 8.5. Store in airtight containers.

USP 25: A white or faintly yellow powder. Freely soluble in water; very slightly soluble in alcohol, in chloroform, in ether, and in ethyl acetate; soluble in methyl alcohol. pH of a 10% solution in water is between 6.0 and 8.5. Store in airtight containers.

Stability. References.
1. Barnes AR. Chemical stabilities of cefuroxime sodium and metronidazole in an admixture for intravenous infusion. *J Clin Pharm Ther* 1990; **15:** 187–96.
2. Stiles ML, *et al.* Stability of ceftazidime (with arginine) and of cefuroxime sodium in infusion-pump reservoirs. *Am J Hosp Pharm* 1992; **49:** 2761–4.
3. Hebron B, Scott H. Shelf life of cefuroxime eye-drops when dispensed in artificial tear preparations. *Int J Pharm Pract* 1993; **2:** 163–7.

Adverse Effects and Precautions

As for Cefalotin Sodium, p.162.

Gastrointestinal disturbances, including diarrhoea, nausea, and vomiting, have occurred in some patients receiving cefuroxime axetil. There have been rare reports of erythema multiforme, Stevens-Johnson syndrome, and toxic epidermal necrolysis.

Antibiotic-associated colitis. For reports of pseudomembranous colitis associated with cefuroxime axetil, see Cefalotin, p.163.

Porphyria. Cefuroxime is considered to be unsafe in patients with porphyria although there is conflicting experimental evidence of porphyrinogenicity.

Interactions

Probenecid reduces the renal clearance of cefuroxime.

Antimicrobial Action

Cefuroxime is bactericidal and has a similar spectrum of antimicrobial action and pattern of resistance to those of cefamandole (p.164). It is more resistant to hydrolysis by beta-lactamases than cefamandole, and therefore may be more active against beta-lactamase-producing strains of, for example, *Haemophilus influenzae* and *Neisseria gonorrhoeae.* However, treatment failures have occurred in patients with *H. influenzae* meningitis given cefuroxime and might be associated with a relatively high minimum bactericidal concentration when compared with the minimum inhibitory concentration or with a significant inoculum effect. Reduced affinity of penicillin-binding proteins for cefuroxime has also been reported to be responsible for resistance in a beta-lactamase-negative strain of *H. influenzae.*

◊ References.
1. Arditi M, *et al.* Cefuroxime treatment failure and Haemophilus influenzae meningitis: case report and review of literature. *Pediatrics* 1989; **84:** 132–5.
2. Mendelman PM, *et al.* Cefuroxime treatment failure of nontypable Haemophilus influenzae meningitis associated with alteration of penicillin-binding proteins. *J Infect Dis* 1990; **162:** 1118–23.
3. Brown NM, *et al.* Cefuroxime resistance in Haemophilus influenzae. *Lancet* 1992; **340:** 552.

Pharmacokinetics

Cefuroxime axetil is absorbed from the gastrointestinal tract and is rapidly hydrolysed in the intestinal mucosa and blood to cefuroxime; absorption is enhanced in the presence of food. Peak plasma concentrations are reported about 2 to 3 hours after an oral dose. The sodium salt is given by intramuscular or intravenous injection. Peak plasma concentrations of about 27 µg per mL have been achieved 45 minutes after an intramuscular dose of 750 mg with measurable amounts present 8 hours after a dose. Up to 50% of cefuroxime in the circulation is bound to plasma proteins. The plasma half-life is about 70 minutes and is prolonged in patients with renal impairment and in neonates.

Cefuroxime is widely distributed in the body including pleural fluid, sputum, bone, synovial fluid, and aqueous humour, but only achieves therapeutic concentrations in the CSF when the meninges are inflamed. It crosses the placenta and has been detected in breast milk.

Cefuroxime is excreted unchanged, by glomerular filtration and renal tubular secretion, and high concentrations are achieved in the urine. Following injection, most of a dose of cefuroxime is excreted within 24 hours, the majority within 6 hours. Probenecid competes for renal tubular secretion with cefuroxime resulting in higher and more prolonged plasma concentrations of cefuroxime. Small amounts of cefuroxime are excreted in bile.

Plasma concentrations are reduced by dialysis.

◊ References to the pharmacokinetics of cefuroxime.
1. Winter J, Dhillon P. Penetration of cefuroxime into bronchial mucosa following oral administration of cefuroxime axetil. *J Antimicrob Chemother* 1991; **27:** 556–8.
2. Ridgway E, *et al.* The pharmacokinetics of cefuroxime axetil in the sick elderly patient. *J Antimicrob Chemother* 1991; **27:** 663–8.
3. Powell DA, *et al.* Pharmacokinetics of cefuroxime axetil suspension in infants and children. *Antimicrob Agents Chemother* 1991; **35:** 2042–5.
4. Konishi K, *et al.* Pharmacokinetics of cefuroxime axetil in patients with normal and impaired renal function. *J Antimicrob Chemother* 1993; **31:** 413–20.
5. Kossmann T, *et al.* Penetration of cefuroxime into the cerebrospinal fluid of patients with traumatic brain injury. *J Antimicrob Chemother* 1996; **37:** 161–7.
6. Jenkins CDG, *et al.* Comparative intraocular penetration of topical and injected cefuroxime. *Br J Ophthalmol* 1996; **80:** 685–8.
7. Stoeckel K, *et al.* Penetration of cefetamet pivoxil and cefuroxime axetil into the maxillary sinus mucosa at steady state. *Antimicrob Agents Chemother* 1996; **40:** 780–3.

Uses and Administration

Cefuroxime is a second-generation cephalosporin antibiotic used in the treatment of susceptible infections (see Antimicrobial Action, above). These have included bone and joint infections, bronchitis (and other lower respiratory-tract infections), gonorrhoea, meningitis (although treatment failures have been reported in *H. influenzae* meningitis, see p.128), otitis media, peritonitis, pharyngitis, sinusitis, skin infections (including soft-tissue infections), and urinary-tract infections. It is also used for surgical infection prophylaxis. For details of all these infections and their treatment, see under Choice of Antibacterial, p.114.

Administration and dosage. Cefuroxime is given by mouth as the acetoxyethyl ester, cefuroxime axetil, in the form of tablets or suspension with or after food, or by injection as the sodium salt. Cefuroxime sodium may be given by deep intramuscular injection, by slow intravenous injection over 3 to 5 minutes, or by intravenous infusion. Doses of cefuroxime axetil and cefuroxime sodium are expressed in terms of the equivalent amount of cefuroxime.

Usual oral doses for adults are 125 mg twice daily for uncomplicated urinary-tract infections and 250 to 500 mg twice daily for respiratory-tract infections. A dose for children more than 3 months of age is 125 mg twice daily or 10 mg per kg body-weight twice daily to a maximum of 250 mg daily. Children over 2 years of age with otitis media may be given 250 mg twice daily or 15 mg per kg twice daily to a maximum of 500 mg daily.

By injection the usual adult dose is 750 mg of cefuroxime every 8 hours but in more severe infections 1.5 g may be given intravenously every 8, or in some cases every 6, hours. Infants and children can be given 30 to 60 mg per kg body-weight daily, increased to 100 mg per kg daily if necessary, given in 3 or 4 divided doses. Neonates may be given similar total daily doses but administered in 2 or 3 divided doses.

Parenteral doses may need to be reduced in renal impairment. The manufacturers suggest that the usual adult dose of 750 mg should only be given twice daily when the creatinine clearance is between 10 and 20 mL per minute and once daily when it is below 10 mL per minute. Patients undergoing haemodialysis should receive an additional 750-mg dose following each dialysis; those undergoing continuous peritoneal dialysis may be given 750 mg twice daily.

For the treatment of meningitis due to sensitive strains of bacteria, cefuroxime is administered intravenously in doses of 3 g every 8 hours for adults. Infants and children are given 200 to 240 mg per kg daily intravenously in 3 or 4 divided doses, which may be decreased to 100 mg per kg daily after 3 days or when there is clinical improvement. For neonates, a dose of 100 mg per kg daily, decreased to 50 mg per kg daily when indicated, has been used.

In the treatment of gonorrhoea, a single dose of 1.5 g by intramuscular injection, divided between 2 injection sites, has been used. A single 1-g oral dose of cefuroxime has been given for uncomplicated gonorrhoea. In each case an oral dose of probenecid 1 g may be given with cefuroxime.

For surgical infection prophylaxis, the usual dose is 1.5 g of cefuroxime intravenously before the procedure; this may be supplemented by 750 mg intravenously or intramuscularly every 8 hours for up to 24 to 48 hours depending upon the procedure. For total joint replacement, 1.5 g of cefuroxime powder may be mixed with the methylmethacrylate cement.

◊ References.
1. Perry CM, Brogden RN. Cefuroxime axetil: a review of its antibacterial activity, pharmacokinetic properties and therapeutic efficacy. *Drugs* 1996; **52:** 125–58.
2. Scott LJ, *et al.* Cefuroxime axetil: an updated review of its use in the management of bacterial infections. *Drugs* 2001; **61:** 1455–1500.

Preparations

BP 2001: Cefuroxime Axetil Tablets; Cefuroxime Injection;
USP 25: Cefuroxime Axetil Tablets; Cefuroxime for Injection; Cefuroxime Injection.

Proprietary Preparations (details are given in Part 3)
Aust.: Curocef; Zinnat; *Austral.:* Zinnat; *Belg.:* Kefurox; Zinacef; Zinnat; *Braz.:* Zinacef; Zinnat; *Canad.:* Ceftin; Kefurox; Zinacef; *Denm.:* Axacef; Lifurox†; Zinacef; Zinnat; *Fin.:* Kefurion; Lifurox; Zinacef; Zinnat; *Fr.:* Cepazine; Zinnat; *Ger.:* Cefurox-Reu; Elobact; Zinacef; Zinnat; *Hong Kong:* Zinacef; Zinnat; *Irl.:* Zinacef; Zinnat; *Israel:* Kefurim; Zinacef; Zinnat; *Ital.:* Biociclin; Biofurex; Bioxima†; Cefamar; Cefoprim; Cefumax; Cefur; Cefurex; Cefurin; Colifossim; Curoxim; Deltacef; Duxima; Gibicef; Ipacef; Itorex; Kefox; Kesint; Lafurex; Medoxim; Oraxim; Poliximat†; Supero; Tileximt†; Zinnat; Zoref; *Mex.:* Cefuracet; Cetoxil; Froxal; Zinnat; *Neth.:* Zinacef; Zinnat; *Norw.:* Lifurox; Zinacef; *NZ:* Zinacef; Zinnat; *Port.:* Curoxime; Zipos; Zoref; *S.Afr.:* Intracef; Lifurom; Zinacef; Zinnat; *Singapore:* Zinacef; Zinnat; *Spain:* Curoxima; Lifurox; Nivador; Selan; Zinnat; *Swed.:* Axacef; Lifurox†; Zinacef; Zinnat; *Switz.:* Zinacef; Zinnat; *Thai.:* Axetine; Cefamar; Cefurim; Furoxime; Zinacef; Zinnat; *UAE:* Cefuzime; *UK:* Zinacef; Zinnat; *USA:* Ceftin; Kefurox; Zinacef.

Chloramphenicol (49-p)

Chloramphenicol (BAN, rINN).

Chloramphenicolum; Chloranfenicol; Cloranfenicol; Kloramfenikol; Laevomycetinum. 2,2-Dichloro-N-[(αR,βR)-β-hydroxy-α-hydroxymethyl-4-nitrophenethyl]acetamide.
$C_{11}H_{12}Cl_2N_2O_5 = 323.1$.
CAS — 56-75-7.
ATC — D06AX02; D10AF03; G01AA05; J01BA01; S01AA01; S02AA01; S03AA08.

NOTE. CPL is a code approved by the BP 2001 for use on single unit doses of eye drops containing chloramphenicol where the individual container may be too small to bear all the appropriate labelling information.

Pharmacopoeias. In *Chin., Eur.* (see p.vi), *Int., Jpn, Pol.,* and *US.*

Pharmacopoeial description

Ph. Eur.: A substance produced by the growth of certain strains of *Streptomyces venezuelae,* but now mainly prepared synthetically. A white, greyish-white or yellowish-white, fine crystalline powder or fine crystals, needles, or elongated plates. Slightly soluble in water and in ether; freely soluble in alcohol and in propylene glycol. Protect from light.
USP 25: Fine, white to greyish-white or yellowish-white, needle-like crystals or elongated plates. Soluble 1 in 400 of water; freely soluble in alcohol, in acetone, in ethyl acetate, and in propylene glycol. pH of a 2.5% suspension in water is between 4.5 and 7.5. Its solutions are practically neutral to litmus. It is reasonably stable in neutral or moderately acid solutions. Store in airtight containers.

Chloramphenicol Palmitate (48-q)

Chloramphenicol Palmitate (BANM, rINNM).
Chloramphenicol α-Palmitate; Chloramphenicoli Palmitas; Palmitylchloramphenicol.
$C_{27}H_{42}Cl_2N_2O_6 = 561.5$.
CAS — 530-43-8.
Pharmacopoeias. In *Chin., Eur.* (see p.vi), *Int.,* and *US.*

1.7 g of monograph substance is approximately equivalent to 1 g of chloramphenicol.

Pharmacopoeial description

Ph. Eur.: A fine, white or almost white, unctuous, powder. M.p. 87° to 95°. Chloramphenicol palmitate shows polymorphism and the thermodynamically stable form has low bioavailability following oral administration. Practically insoluble in water; sparingly soluble in alcohol; freely soluble in acetone; soluble in ether; very slightly soluble in hexane. Protect from light.
USP 25: A fine, white, unctuous, crystalline powder, having a faint odour. M.p. 87° to 95°. Insoluble in water; sparingly soluble in alcohol; freely soluble in acetone and in chloroform; soluble in ether; very slightly soluble in hexane. Store in airtight containers.

Chloramphenicol Sodium Succinate (46-v)

Chloramphenicol Sodium Succinate (BANM, rINNM).
Chloramphenicol α-Sodium Succinate; Chloramphenicoli Natrii Succinas.
$C_{15}H_{15}Cl_2N_2NaO_8 = 445.2$.
CAS — 982-57-0.
Pharmacopoeias. In *Eur.* (see p.vi) and *US. Chin.* includes Chloramphenicol Hydrogen Succinate.

1.4 g of monograph substance is approximately equivalent to 1 g of chloramphenicol. Each g of monograph substance represents about 2.2 mmol of sodium.

Incompatibilities. Incompatibility or loss of activity has been reported between chloramphenicol and a wide variety of other substances. Other factors, especially, drug concentration, may play a part and many interactions are chiefly seen with concentrated solutions.

Pharmacopoeial description

Ph. Eur.: A white or yellowish-white hygroscopic powder. Very soluble in water; freely soluble in alcohol; practically insoluble in ether. A 25% solution in water has a pH of 6.4 to 7.0. Store in airtight containers. Protect from light.
USP 25: A light yellow powder. Freely soluble in water and in alcohol. pH of a solution in water containing the equivalent of chloramphenicol 25% is between 6.4 and 7.0. Store in airtight containers.

Adverse Effects

Chloramphenicol may cause serious and sometimes fatal adverse effects. Some of its toxicity is thought to be due to effects on mitochondrial protein synthesis. The most serious adverse effect of chloramphenicol is its depression of the bone marrow, which can take 2 different forms. The first is a fairly common dose-related reversible depression occurring usually when plasma-chloramphenicol concentrations exceed 25 µg per mL and is characterised by morphological changes in the bone marrow, decreased iron utilisation, reticulocytopenia, anaemia, leucopenia, and thrombocytopenia. This effect may be due to inhibition of protein synthesis in the mitochondria of bone marrow cells.

The second and apparently unrelated form of bone-marrow toxicity is severe irreversible aplastic anaemia. This is fairly rare, with a suggested incidence of about 1:20 000 to 1:50 000, although the incidence varies throughout the world, and is not considered to be dose-related. The aplasia usually develops after a latent period of weeks or even months and has been suggested to be the result of a nitrated benzene radical produced *in vivo.* It is considered that there may be some genetic or biochemical predisposition, but there is no way of identifying susceptible patients. Although the majority of cases have followed oral administration, aplasia has also occurred after intravenous and topical (eye drops) use of chloramphenicol. Survival is most likely in those with early onset aplasia, but they may subsequently develop acute myeloid leukaemia.

A toxic manifestation—the 'grey syndrome'—characterised by abdominal distension, vomiting, ashen colour, hypothermia, progressive pallid cyanosis, irregular respiration, and circulatory collapse followed by death in a few hours or days, has occurred in premature and other newborn infants receiving large doses of chloramphenicol. The syndrome is associated with high plasma concentrations of chloramphenicol, due to reduced capacity for glucuronidation and decreased glomerular filtration in children of this age, leading to drug accumulation. Recovery is usually complete if the drug is withdrawn early enough after onset, but up to 40% of infants with the full-blown syndrome may die. The syndrome has also been reported in infants born to mothers given chloramphenicol in late pregnancy. A similar syndrome has been reported in adults and older children given very high doses.

Prolonged oral administration of chloramphenicol may induce bleeding, either by bone-marrow depression or by reducing the intestinal flora with consequent inhibition of vitamin K synthesis. Haemolytic anaemia has occurred in some patients with the Mediterranean form of glucose 6-phosphate dehydrogenase deficiency, but is rare in patients with milder forms of the deficiency.

Peripheral as well as optic neuritis has been reported in patients receiving chloramphenicol, usually over prolonged periods. Although ocular symptoms are often reversible if treatment is withdrawn early, permanent visual impairment or blindness has occurred.

Other neurological symptoms have included encephalopathy with confusion and delirium, mental depression, and headache. Ototoxicity has also occurred, especially after the use of ear drops.

Hypersensitivity reactions including rashes, fever, and angioedema may occur especially after topical use; anaphylaxis has occurred but is rare. Jarisch-Herxheimer reactions may also occur. Gastrointestinal symptoms including nausea, vomiting, and diarrhoea can follow oral administration. Disturbances of the oral and intestinal flora may cause stomatitis, glossitis, and rectal irritation. Patients may experience an intensely bitter taste following rapid intravenous administration of chloramphenicol sodium succinate.

◊ A review[1] of the toxicity of chloramphenicol and related drugs, including the potential role of the *p*-nitro group in producing aplastic anaemia, indicated that derivatives such as thiamphenicol, which lack this grouping, are not associated with increased incidence of aplastic anaemia.

1. Yunis AA. Chloramphenicol: relation of structure to activity and toxicity. *Ann Rev Pharmacol Toxicol* 1988; **28:** 83–100.

Overdosage. Charcoal haemoperfusion was found to be far superior to exchange transfusion in the removal of chloramphenicol from blood, although it did not prevent death in a 7-week-old infant with the 'grey syndrome' following a dosage error.[1]

1. Freundlich M, *et al.* Management of chloramphenicol intoxication in infancy by charcoal hemoperfusion. *J Pediatr* 1983; **103:** 485–7.

Precautions

Chloramphenicol is contra-indicated in patients with a history of hypersensitivity or toxic reaction to the drug. It should never be given systemically for minor infections or for prophylaxis. Repeated courses and prolonged treatment should be avoided and it should not be used in patients with pre-existing bone-marrow depression or blood dyscrasias. Routine periodic blood examinations are advisable in all patients, but will not warn of aplastic anaemia.

Concomitant administration of chloramphenicol with other drugs liable to depress bone-marrow function should be avoided.

Reduced doses should be given to patients with impaired liver function. Excessive blood concentrations

---

The symbol † denotes a preparation no longer actively marketed

may also occur following administration of usual doses to patients with severe renal impairment and in premature and full-term neonates who have immature metabolic processes. Monitoring of plasma-chloramphenicol concentrations may be desirable in patients with risk factors. A suggested range for peak plasma concentrations is 10 to 25 μg per mL and 5 to 15 μg per mL for trough concentrations.

Because of the risk of the 'grey syndrome' neonates should never be given chloramphenicol systemically, unless it may be life-saving and there is no alternative treatment. The use of chloramphenicol is probably best avoided during pregnancy, particularly in the last trimester, and in nursing mothers since chloramphenicol is distributed into breast milk.

Chloramphenicol may interfere with the development of immunity and it should not be given during active immunisation.

Ocular use. Ocular chloramphenicol is widely used in Britain for the treatment of superficial eye infections. In view of the potential for serious toxicity, such as aplastic anaemia, following systemic absorption some, particularly in the USA, have advised that its ocular use should be restricted to situations where there is no alternative treatment.[1] However, apart from patients with a personal or family history of blood dyscrasias, the use, particularly of short courses, was defended by several specialists in the UK,[2-4] and the arguments have been the subject of several reviews.[5-7] Prospective case-control studies should help to clarify the risk.[8] One such study,[9] involving 145 patients with aplastic anaemia and 1226 controls, found that only 3 of the patients had been exposed to ocular chloramphenicol, and calculated that the absolute risk was no more than 0.5 cases per million treatment courses. Similarly, data[10] from 2 other studies revealed that none of 426 patients with aplastic anaemia and 7 of 3118 controls had used chloramphenicol eye drops. In a survey[11] of patients who received prescriptions for chloramphenicol eye drops the risk of serious haematological toxicity was 3 per 442 543 patients or 3 per 674 148 prescriptions.

1. Doona M, Walsh JB. Use of chloramphenicol as topical eye medication: time to cry halt? *BMJ* 1995; **310:** 1217–18.
2. Mulla RJ, *et al.* Is it time to stop using chloramphenicol on the eye: fears are based on only six cases. *BMJ* 1995; **311:** 450.
3. Buckley RJK, *et al.* Is it time to stop using chloramphenicol on the eye: safe in patients with no history of blood dyscrasia. *BMJ* 1995; **311:** 450.
4. Hall AV, *et al.* Is it time to stop using chloramphenicol on the eye: risk is low in short courses. *BMJ* 1995; **311:** 450–1.
5. McGhee CNJ, Anastas CN. Widespread ocular use of topical chloramphenicol: is there justifiable concern regarding idiosyncratic aplastic anaemia? *Br J Ophthalmol* 1996; **80:** 182–4.
6. Rayner SA, Buckley RJ. Ocular chloramphenicol and aplastic anaemia: is there a link? *Drug Safety* 1996; **14:** 273–6.
7. Titcomb L. Ophthalmic chloramphenicol and blood dyscrasias: a review. *Pharm J* 1997; **258:** 28–35.
8. Gordon-Smith EC, *et al.* Is it time to stop using chloramphenicol on the eye: prospective study of aplastic anaemia should give definitive answer. *BMJ* 1995; **311:** 451.
9. Laporte J-R, *et al.* Possible association between ocular chloramphenicol and aplastic anaemia—the absolute risk is very low. *Br J Clin Pharmacol* 1998; **46:** 181–4.
10. Wiholm B-E, *et al.* Relation of aplastic anaemia to use of chloramphenicol eye drops in two international case-control studies. *BMJ* 1998; **316:** 666.
11. Lancaster T, *et al.* Risk of serious haematological toxicity with use of chloramphenicol eye drops in a British general practice database. *BMJ* 1998; **316:** 667.

Porphyria. Chloramphenicol has been associated with acute attacks of porphyria and is considered unsafe in porphyric patients.

Interactions

Chloramphenicol is inactivated in the liver and may, therefore, interact with drugs that are metabolised by hepatic microsomal enzymes. For example, chloramphenicol enhances the effects of coumarin anticoagulants such as dicoumarol and warfarin sodium, some hypoglycaemics such as chlorpropamide and tolbutamide, and antiepileptics such as phenytoin, and may reduce the metabolism of tacrolimus and of cyclophosphamide to its active form. Conversely the metabolism of chloramphenicol may be increased by inducers of hepatic enzymes such as phenobarbital or rifampicin. Some other interactions affecting the activity of chloramphenicol are discussed below.

Chloramphenicol may decrease the effects of iron and vitamin B_{12} in anaemic patients and impair the action of oral contraceptives.

For the effects of chloramphenicol on the activity of other antibacterials, see under Antimicrobial Action, below.

Antiepileptics. Serum concentrations of chloramphenicol are usually reduced by the hepatic enzyme induction that occurs

with *phenobarbital*,[1,2] and similar reductions have been reported in a case study during *phenytoin* administration.[3] Conversely, elevated and potentially toxic serum-chloramphenicol concentrations have resulted during concurrent phenytoin administration,[2] apparently due to competition for binding sites, although increased metabolism may alternatively lead to decreased serum-chloramphenicol concentrations.
For reference to the effects of chloramphenicol on phenobarbital and phenytoin, see p.355 and p.359, respectively.

1. Bloxham RA, *et al.* Chloramphenicol and phenobarbitone—a drug interaction. *Arch Dis Child* 1979; **54:** 76–7.
2. Krasinski K, *et al.* Pharmacologic interactions among chloramphenicol, phenytoin and phenobarbital. *Pediatr Infect Dis* 1982; **1:** 232–5.
3. Powell DA, *et al.* Interactions among chloramphenicol, phenytoin, and phenobarbital in a pediatric patient. *J Pediatr* 1981; **98:** 1001–3.

Ciclosporin. For the effect of chloramphenicol on ciclosporin, see p.520.

Cimetidine. Fatal aplastic anaemia of rapid onset has occurred in 2 patients who received intravenous chloramphenicol and cimetidine concomitantly.[1,2] As there is usually a latent period of 2 weeks to 12 months before aplastic anaemia develops following chloramphenicol therapy it is plausible that an additive or synergistic effect may have occurred between the 2 drugs to cause bone-marrow toxicity.

1. Farber BF, Brody JP. Rapid development of aplastic anemia after intravenous chloramphenicol and cimetidine therapy. *South Med J* 1981; **74:** 1257–8.
2. West BC, *et al.* Aplastic anemia associated with parenteral chloramphenicol: review of 10 cases, including the second case of possible increased risk with cimetidine. *Rev Infect Dis* 1988; **10:** 1048–51.

Cyclophosphamide. For the effect of chloramphenicol on cyclophosphamide, see p.528.

Oral contraceptives. For the suggestion that chloramphenicol may reduce the efficacy of oral contraceptives, see Hormonal Contraceptives, p.1458.

Paracetamol. A report of an increase in chloramphenicol half-life from 3.25 to 15 hours when intravenous paracetamol was given to 6 patients in intensive care 2 hours after intravenous chloramphenicol[1] has not been confirmed by subsequent studies in patients receiving oral paracetamol. A study in 5 children found that the half-life of intravenous chloramphenicol was reduced from 3 to 1.2 hours, concomitant with an increase in clearance, when oral paracetamol was given 30 minutes beforehand.[2] Furthermore, a study in 26 children found no evidence of altered disposition when oral paracetamol was given to patients receiving intravenous chloramphenicol,[3] and no significant change in chloramphenicol pharmacokinetics was found in 5 patients given oral chloramphenicol and paracetamol.[4]

1. Buchanan N, Moodley GP. Interaction between chloramphenicol and paracetamol. *BMJ* 1979; **2:** 307–8.
2. Spika JS, *et al.* Interaction between chloramphenicol and acetaminophen. *Arch Dis Child* 1986; **61:** 1121–4.
3. Kearns GL, *et al.* Absence of a pharmacokinetic interaction between chloramphenicol and acetaminophen in children. *J Pediatr* 1985; **107:** 134–9.
4. Stein CM, *et al.* Lack of effect of paracetamol on the pharmacokinetics of chloramphenicol. *Br J Clin Pharmacol* 1989; **27:** 262–4.

Tacrolimus. For the effect of chloramphenicol on tacrolimus, see p.570.

Antimicrobial Action

Chloramphenicol is a bacteriostatic antibiotic with a broad spectrum of action against both Gram-positive and Gram-negative bacteria, as well as some other organisms.

Mechanism of action. Chloramphenicol is thought to enter sensitive cells by an active transport process. Within the cell it binds to the 50S subunit of the bacterial ribosome at a site adjacent to the site of action of the macrolides and clindamycin, and inhibits bacterial protein synthesis by preventing attachment of aminoacyl transfer RNA to its acceptor site on the ribosome, thus preventing peptide bond formation by peptidyl transferase. The block in protein synthesis results in a primarily bacteriostatic action, although it may be bactericidal to some organisms, including *Haemophilus influenzae*, *Neisseria meningitidis*, and *Streptococcus pneumoniae*, at concentrations about 2 to 4 times the inhibitory concentration.

Spectrum of activity. Chloramphenicol has activity against many types of bacteria, although in most cases there are less toxic alternatives available. The following pathogens are usually susceptible (but see also Resistance, below).

Gram-positive cocci including staphylococci such as *Staph. epidermidis* and some strains of *Staph. aureus*, and streptococci such as *Str., pneumoniae*, *Str. pyo-*

genes, and the viridans streptococci. Meticillin-resistant staphylococci and *Enterococcus faecalis* are considered to be resistant.

Other Gram-positive species including *Bacillus anthracis*, *Corynebacterium diphtheriae*, and anaerobes such as *Peptococcus* and *Peptostreptococcus* spp.

Gram-negative cocci such as *Neisseria meningitidis* and *N. gonorrhoeae* are usually highly sensitive, as are *Haemophilus influenzae* and a variety of other Gram-negative bacteria including *Brucella abortus*, *Campylobacter* spp., *Legionella pneumophila*, *Pasteurella*, and *Vibrio* spp. The Enterobacteriaceae vary in their susceptibility, and many strains have shown acquired resistance, but *Escherichia coli*, and strains of *Klebsiella* spp., *Proteus mirabilis*, *Salmonella*, *Shigella*, and *Yersinia* spp. have been reported to be susceptible. Many strains of *Enterobacter*, indole positive *Proteus*, and *Serratia* spp. are resistant, or at best moderately susceptible. *Pseudomonas aeruginosa* is invariably resistant, although *Burkholderia* (formerly *Pseudomonas*) spp. may be susceptible.

Some Gram-negative anaerobes are susceptible, or moderately so, including *Bacteroides fragilis*, *Veillonella*, and *Fusobacterium* spp.

Other susceptible organisms include *Actinomyces* spp., *Leptospira* spp., spirochaetes such as *Treponema pallidum*, chlamydias, mycoplasmas, and rickettsias. *Nocardia* spp. are resistant. Chloramphenicol is ineffective against fungi, protozoa, and viruses.

Minimum inhibitory concentrations (MICs) for the most sensitive organisms such as *Haemophilus influenzae* or *Neisseria* spp. range from about 0.25 to 2 μg per mL, but organisms with MICs of up to about 12 μg per mL are generally considered susceptible.

Activity with other antimicrobials. As with other bacteriostatic antimicrobials, the possibility exists of an antagonistic effect if chloramphenicol is given with a bactericidal drug, and some antagonism has been demonstrated *in vitro* between chloramphenicol and various beta lactams and aminoglycosides, but the clinical significance of most of these interactions is usually held to be doubtful. Because of the adjacency of their binding sites on the ribosome, chloramphenicol may competitively inhibit the effects of macrolides or lincosamides such as clindamycin.

Resistance. Acquired resistance has been widely reported, although the prevalence of resistance has tended to decline where use of the drug has become less frequent. The most commonly seen form of resistance has been the production of an acetyltransferase that inactivates the drug. Such resistance is usually plasmid-mediated and may be associated with resistance to other drugs such as the tetracyclines. Other mechanisms that may reduce sensitivity to chloramphenicol include reduced permeability or uptake, and ribosomal mutation.

The actual incidence of resistance varies considerably in different countries and different centres. Epidemics of chloramphenicol-resistant *Salmonella* and *Shigella* spp. have occurred in the past, and although the prevalence of resistance in *Salmonella* spp. has been reported to be negligible except in parts of South or South-east Asia, resistant salmonellal infections acquired in these regions are increasingly being seen elsewhere. Resistance among *Haemophilus* and *Neisseria* spp. occurs, and the latter may be problematic in developing countries, although it does not yet seem to be widespread. However, resistant strains of enterococci and pneumococci are reported to be relatively common in some areas, and over 50% of staphylococcal strains have been reported to show resistance in some hospitals.

◊ In India, 91.6% of strains of *Salmonella typhi* were sensitive to chloramphenicol compared with 71.9% in 1994.[1] The re-emergence of chloramphenicol-sensitive strains may be attributable to restricted use of the drug in the community for the treatment of typhoid.

1. Sood S, *et al.* Re-emergence of chloramphenicol-sensitive Salmonella typhi. *Lancet* 1999; **353:** 1241–2.

◊ Chloramphenicol has been reported to be effective against vancomycin-resistant *Enterococcus faecium*.[1-3] However, no significant effect of chloramphenicol on mortality was found in one small study.[4]

1. Norris AH, *et al.* Chloramphenicol for the treatment of vancomycin-resistant enterococcal infections. *Clin Infect Dis* 1995; **20:** 1137–44.
2. Papanicolaou GA, *et al.* Nosocomial infections with vancomycin-resistant Enterococcus faecium in liver transplant recipients: risk factors for acquisition and mortality. *Clin Infect Dis* 1996; **23:** 760–6.
3. Mato SP, *et al.* Vancomycin-resistant Enterococcus faecium meningitis successfully treated with chloramphenicol. *Pediatr Infect Dis J* 1999; **18:** 483–4.
4. Lautenbach E, *et al.* The role of chloramphenicol in the treatment of bloodstream infection due to vancomycin-resistant Enterococcus. *Clin Infect Dis* 1998; **27:** 1259–65.

Pharmacokinetics

Chloramphenicol is readily absorbed when given by mouth. Blood concentrations of 10 μg per mL or more may be reached about 1 or 2 hours after a single dose of 1 g by mouth, and blood concentrations of about 18.5 μg per mL have been reported after multiple 1-g doses. Chloramphenicol palmitate is hydrolysed to chloramphenicol in the gastrointestinal tract prior to absorption, and the sodium succinate, which is given parenterally, is probably hydrolysed to free drug mainly in the liver, lungs, and kidneys; such hydrolysis may be incomplete in infants and neonates, contributing to the variable pharmacokinetics in this age group. Chloramphenicol sodium succinate is, even in adults, only partially and variably hydrolysed, so that blood concentrations of chloramphenicol obtained after parenteral administration of the sodium succinate are often lower than those obtained after administration of chloramphenicol by mouth, with up to 30% of a dose excreted unchanged in the urine before hydrolysis can take place (but see under Administration, below).

Chloramphenicol is widely distributed in body tissues and fluids; it enters the CSF, giving concentrations of about 50% of those existing in the blood even in the absence of inflamed meninges; it diffuses across the placenta into the fetal circulation, into breast milk, and into the aqueous and vitreous humours of the eye. It also enters the aqueous humour following topical application. Up to about 60% in the circulation is bound to plasma protein. The half-life of chloramphenicol has been reported to range from 1.5 to 4 hours; the half-life is prolonged in patients with severe hepatic impairment and is also much longer in neonates. Renal impairment has relatively little effect on the half-life of the active drug, due to its extensive metabolism, but may lead to accumulation of the inactive metabolites.

Chloramphenicol is excreted mainly in the urine but only 5 to 10% of an oral dose appears unchanged; the remainder is inactivated in the liver, mostly by conjugation with glucuronic acid. About 3% is excreted in the bile. However, most is reabsorbed and only about 1%, mainly in the inactive form, is excreted in the faeces.

The absorption, metabolism, and excretion of chloramphenicol are subject to considerable interindividual variation, especially in infants and children, making monitoring of plasma concentrations necessary to determine pharmacokinetics in a given patient.

Uses and Administration

The liability of chloramphenicol to provoke life-threatening adverse effects, particularly bone-marrow aplasia, has severely limited its clinical usefulness, although it is still widely used in some countries. It should never be given systemically for minor infections and regular blood counts are usually advisable during treatment. The third-generation cephalosporins are now favoured for many of the former indications of chloramphenicol. There are consequently few unambiguous indications for the use of chloramphenicol. It has been used in severe typhoid and other salmonellal infections, although it does not eliminate the carrier state. Chloramphenicol is an alternative to a third-generation cephalosporin in the treatment of bacterial meningitis, both empirically and against sensitive organisms such as *Haemophilus influenzae*. It has been used in the treatment of severe anaerobic infections, particularly in brain abscesses, and in infections below the diaphragm where *Bacteroides fragilis* is often implicated; however, other drugs are usually preferred. Although the tetracyclines remain the treatment of choice in rickettsial infections such as typhus and the spotted fevers, chloramphenicol is also used as an alternative where the tetracyclines cannot be given.

Other bacterial infections in which chloramphenicol may be used as an alternative to other drugs include anthrax, severe systemic infections with *Campylobacter fetus*, ehrlichiosis, severe gastro-enteritis (including *Salmonella* enteritis, cholera, and *Yersinia* enteritis), gas gangrene, granuloma inguinale, severe *Haemophilus influenzae* infections other than meningitis (for example in epiglottitis), listeriosis, severe melioidosis, plague (especially if meningitis develops), pneumonia, psittacosis, Q fever, tularaemia (especially when meningitis is suspected), and Whipple's disease. For details of these infections and their treatment, see under Choice of Antibacterial, p.114.

Chloramphenicol is extensively used in the topical treatment of ear and, in particular, eye infections, despite the fact that many of these are mild and self-limiting. It is also used topically in the treatment of skin infections.

When given by mouth, chloramphenicol is usually administered in capsules or as a suspension of chloramphenicol palmitate. When oral administration is not feasible, water-soluble chloramphenicol sodium succinate may be given intravenously, but oral therapy should be substituted as soon as possible; an intravenous dose should be injected over at least one minute. Administration by intramuscular injection is controversial because of doubts whether absorption is adequate. In some countries chloramphenicol has been given rectally as suppositories.

Doses are expressed in terms of chloramphenicol base and are similar whether administered by mouth or intravenously. For adults and children the usual dose is 50 mg per kg body-weight daily in divided doses every 6 hours; up to 100 mg per kg daily may be given in meningitis or severe infections due to moderately resistant organisms, although these higher doses should be reduced as soon as possible. To minimise the risk of relapse it has been recommended that treatment should be continued after the patient's temperature has returned to normal for a further 4 days in rickettsial diseases and for 8 to 10 days in typhoid fever.

Where there is no alternative to the use of chloramphenicol, premature and full-term neonates may be given daily doses of 25 mg per kg, in 4 divided doses, and full-term infants over the age of 2 weeks may be given up to 50 mg per kg daily, in 4 divided doses. Monitoring of plasma concentrations is essential to avoid toxicity.

In patients with impaired hepatic function or severe renal impairment, the dose of chloramphenicol may need to be reduced because of decreased metabolism or excretion.

In the treatment of eye infections, chloramphenicol is usually applied as a 0.5% solution or as a 1% ointment.

Chloramphenicol has also been used in the form of various other derivatives including the arginine succinate, the cinnamate, the glycinate, the glycinate sulfate, the palmitoylglycolate, the pantothenate, the steaglate, the stearate, and the hydrogen succinate.

Administration. INTRAMUSCULAR ADMINISTRATION. When parenteral administration of chloramphenicol is necessary the intravenous route is generally preferred, although the intramuscular route has been advocated. Adequate serum concentrations after intramuscular injection have been reported,[1,2] although this is contrary to the widely held belief that chloramphenicol sodium succinate is poorly absorbed by this route. Pain on injection was also claimed to be minimal.[1] Following a study in children with bacterial meningitis,[3] treatment with intramuscular chloramphenicol for 2 or 3 days followed by oral therapy has been suggested, although a later study[2] found that the intramuscular route produced therapeutic concentrations when the oral route did not. However, it has been said[4] that children describe intramuscular chloramphenicol as amongst the worst treatments they ever receive, and certainly much worse than the insertion of intravenous cannulae.

1. Shann F, *et al.* Absorption of chloramphenicol sodium succinate after intramuscular administration in children. *N Engl J Med* 1985; **313:** 410–14.
2. Weber MW, *et al.* Chloramphenicol pharmacokinetics in infants less than three months of age in the Philippines and The Gambia. *Pediatr Infect Dis J* 1999; **18:** 896–901.
3. Shann F, *et al.* Chloramphenicol alone versus chloramphenicol plus penicillin for bacterial meningitis in children. *Lancet* 1985; **ii** 681–3.
4. Coulthard MG, Lamb WH. Antibiotics: intramuscular or intravenous? *Lancet* 1985; **ii:** 1015.

Preparations

BP 2001: Chloramphenicol Capsules; Chloramphenicol Ear Drops; Chloramphenicol Eye Drops; Chloramphenicol Eye Ointment; Chloramphenicol Sodium Succinate Injection;
USP 25: Chloramphenicol and Hydrocortisone Acetate for Ophthalmic Suspension; Chloramphenicol and Polymyxin B Sulfate Ophthalmic Ointment; Chloramphenicol and Prednisolone Ophthalmic Ointment; Chloramphenicol Capsules; Chloramphenicol Cream; Chloramphenicol for Ophthalmic Solution; Chloramphenicol Ophthalmic Ointment; Chloramphenicol Ophthalmic Solution; Chloramphenicol Otic Solution; Chloramphenicol Palmitate Oral Suspension; Chloramphenicol Sodium Succinate for Injection; Chloramphenicol, Polymyxin B Sulfate, and Hydrocortisone Acetate Ophthalmic Ointment.

Proprietary Preparations (details are given in Part 3)
Aust.: Biophenicol†; Halomycetin; Kemicetin; Oleomycetin; *Austral.:* Chloromycetin; Chlorsig; *Belg.:* Kemicetina; *Braz.:* Clorfenil; Farmicetina P7; Quemicetina; Sintomicetina; Vixmicina; *Canad.:* Chloromycetin; Chloroptic†; Diochloram; Novo-Chlorocap†; Ophtho-Chloram; Pentamycetin; *Fin.:* Chloromycetin; Oftan Akvakol; Oftan Chlora; *Fr.:* Cebenicol; *Ger.:* Aquamycetin-N; Berlicetin†; Chloramsaar N; Oleomycetin; Paraxin; Posifenicol C; Thilocanfol C; *Hong Kong:* Chloment; Chlorsig; Isopto Fenicol; Kemicetine; Spersanicol; Vanafen-S; Vista-Phenicol; Xepanicol; *Irl.:* Chloromycetin; Chloroptic; Israel: Chloroptic; Phenicol; Synthomycin; Synthomycine; Tarophenicol; *Ital.:* Chemicetina; Chloromycetin; Cloramfen; Mycetin; Optafen; Sificetina; Vitamfenicolo; *Mex.:* Alcan; Brocil; Cetina; Chloromycetin; Clorafen; Cloramed; Cloramfeni; Cloramfenil; Cloran; Clorazin; Clordil; Clorfenil; Dilclor; Domicetina; Fenisol; Fenizzard; Furocloran; Italmicin; K-Biofen; Lebrocetin; Leclor A; Naxo; Oftadil; Palcol; Palmiclor; Palmiffer; Palmisol; Procloril; Pronicol; Quemicetina; Solufen; Spersanicol; Uniclor; Vixin; Wilyfenicol; *Neth.:* Globenicol; *NZ:* Chloromycetin; Chloroptic; Chlorsig; Isopto Fenicol; *Port.:* Clorocil; Dermimade Cloranfenicol; Fenoptic; Micetinoftalmina; *S.Afr.:* Chloramex; Chlorcol; Chlornicol; Chloromycetin; Chloroptic; Chlorphen; Fenicol; Lennacol†; Spersanicol; Troymycetin†; *Singapore:* Beaphenicol; Isopto Fenicol; Kemicetine; Spersanicol; Vanafen-S; Xepanicol; *Spain:* Chemicetina; Chloromycetin; Cloranfe†; Cloranfenic; Isopto Fenicol; Normofenicol; *Swed.:* Chloromycetin; Isopto Fenicol; *Switz.:* Chloromycetin†; Septicol; Spersanicol; *Thai.:* Antibi-Otic; Archifen; Chloracil; Chloram-D; Chloroph; Chlorosin; Cogenate; Cogetine; Fenicol; Genercin; Kemicetine; Koro; Levomycetin; Mycochlorin; Nicolmycetin; Opsaram; Pharmacetin; Servicol; Silmycetin; Succi Pharmacetin; Syncholim; Unison Ointment; Vanafen; *UK:* Chloromycetin; Kemicetine; Sno Phenicol; *USA:* Ak-Chlor; Chloromycetin; Chloroptic.

Multi-ingredient: *Aust.:* Cortison Kemicetin; Oleomycetin-Prednison; *Austral.:* Chlorocort†; *Belg.:* De Icol; Viscocort†; *Braz.:* Adermycin-C; Dexacloran; Dexafenicol; Epitezan; Fenidex; Fibrase com Clorafenicol; Fluo-Fenicol; Gino-Cauterex; Gino-Fibrase; Gyno Iruxol; Hipoglos Oftalmico; Iruxol; Lisofenicol; Naxogin Composto; Oto-Biotic; Otofenicol-D; Otoflogin; Otomicina; Otopen; Ouvidonal; Sulnil; *Canad.:* Actinac; Elase-Chloromycetin†; Ophthocort†; Pentamycetin-HC; *Denm.:* Spersadex Comp; *Fin.:* Iruxol; Oftan C-C; Oftan Dexa-Chlora; *Fr.:* Cebedexacol; *Ger.:* Aquapred; Berlicetin-Ohrentropfen; Corti-Flexiole†; Ichthoseptal; Iruxol; Oleomycetin-Prednison; Spersadex Comp; Spersadexolin; *Hong Kong:* Chlomy-P; Cortiphenol H; Cortison-Kemicetine; Ginetris; Neo-Dex (Improved); Oftalmolosa Cusi de Icol; Spersacet C; Spersadex Comp; Spersadexoline; *Irl.:* Actinac; *Israel:* Phenimixin; Tarocidin; Tarocidin D; Threolone; *Ital.:* Antibioptal; Betabioptal; Colbiocin; Cortison Chemicetina; Cosmiciclina; Dexoline; Eubetal Antibiotico; Fluorobioptal; Idracemi; Iruxol; Otomicetina†; Vasofen; Vitecaf; Xantervit Antibiotico; *Mex.:* Cloran Otico; Fibrase; Levodexan; Levofenil; Pre Clor; Soldrin; Solfranicol; Sulfa Cloran; Ulcoderma; *Norw.:* Spersadex med kloramfenikol; *Port.:* Blefarida†; Cloranpectina; Clorcorticil; Medrivas Antibiotico; Predniftalmina; *S.Afr.:* Chloramex H†; Corti-Flexiole†; Covomycin; Covomycin-D; Covotop; Spersacet C; Spersadex Comp; Spersadexoline; *Singapore:* Neo-Dex (Improved); Spersadex Comp; Spersadexoline; *Spain:* Blefarida; Clo Zinc†; Cloranfe Hemidex; Cloranfenic Zinc; Cortison Chemicet Topica; Cortivel†; Dexa Fenic†; Dexafenicol; Dexam Constric; Epitelizante; Fluo Fenic; Hidroc Cloranf; Icol; Icolamida; Medricol; Medrivas Antib; Otosedol Biotico; Parkelase Chloromycetin†; Predni Azuleno; *Swed.:* Chloromycetin Hydrocortison†; Spersacet C; *Switz.:* Septicortin†; Spersacet C; Spersadex Comp; Spersadexoline; *Thai.:* Archifen; Chlorotracin; Dermasol; Levoptin; Otosil; Spersacet C; Spersadexoline; Vagicin; *UK:* Actinac; Chloromycetin Hydrocortisone†; *USA:* Chloromycetin Hydrocortisone†; Elase-Chloromycetin†.

The symbol † denotes a preparation no longer actively marketed

Chlorquinaldol (1601-n)

Chlorquinaldol (BAN, rINN).

5,7-Dichloro-2-methylquinolin-8-ol.

$C_{10}H_7Cl_2NO = 228.1$.

CAS — 72-80-0.

ATC — D08AH02; G01AC03; P01AA04; R02AA11.

Pharmacopoeias. In Pol.

Profile
Chlorquinaldol is a halogenated hydroxyquinoline with properties similar to those of clioquinol (p.190). It is mainly applied topically in infected skin conditions and in vaginal infections.

Preparations
Proprietary Preparations (details are given in Part 3)

Multi-ingredient: *Aust.*: Neriquinol; Ultraquinol†; *Braz.*: Bi-Nerisona; *Denm.*: Locoidol; *Fin.*: Locoidol; *Fr.*: Nerisone C; *Ger.*: Nerisona C; Proctospre; *Hong Kong:* Colposeptine; Nerisone C; *Irl.*: Locoid C; *Israel:* Multiderm; *Ital.*: Impetex; Nerisona C; *Mex.*: Bi-Nerisona; *Mon.*: Colposeptine; *Norw.*: Locoidol; *NZ:* Locoid C; Nerisona C; *Port.*: Locoid C; Nerisona C; Trophoseptine; *S.Afr.*: Locoid C†; *Singapore:* Nerisone C; *Spain:* Amplidermis; Claral Plus; Quinortar; *Swed.*: Sterosan-Hydrocortisone†; *Switz.*: Proctospre; *UK:* Locoid C.

Chlortetracycline (50-n)

Chlortetracycline (BAN, rINN).

(4S,4aS,5aS,6S,12aS)-7-Chloro-4-dimethylamino-1,4,4a,5,5a,6,11,12a-octahydro-3,6,10,12,12a-pentahydroxy-6-methyl-1,11-dioxonaphthacene-2-carboxamide; 7-Chlorotetracycline.

$C_{22}H_{23}ClN_2O_8 = 478.9$.

CAS — 57-62-5.

ATC — A01AB21; D06AA02; J01AA03; S01AA02.

Chlortetracycline Hydrochloride (52-m)

Chlortetracycline Hydrochloride (BANM, rINNM).

Chlortetracyclini Hydrochloridum.

$C_{22}H_{23}ClN_2O_8,HCl = 515.3$.

CAS — 64-72-2.

Pharmacopoeias. In *Chin.*, *Eur.* (see p.vi), *Int.*, *Pol.*, and *US*.

US also includes Chlortetracycline Bisulfate for veterinary use.

Incompatibilities. Preparations of chlortetracycline have an acid pH and incompatibility may reasonably be expected with alkaline preparations or drugs unstable at low pH.

Pharmacopoeial description
Ph. Eur.: The hydrochloride of a substance produced by the growth of certain strains of *Streptomyces aureofaciens* or by any other means. A yellow powder. Slightly soluble in water and in alcohol; it dissolves in solutions of alkali hydroxides and carbonates. A 1% solution in water has a pH of 2.3 to 3.3. Protect from light.

USP 25: A yellow, odourless crystalline powder. Soluble 1 in 75 of water and 1 in 560 of alcohol; practically insoluble in acetone, in chloroform, in dioxan, and in ether; soluble in solutions of alkali hydroxides and carbonates. pH of a 1% solution in water is between 2.3 and 3.3. Store in airtight containers. Protect from light.

Adverse Effects and Precautions
As for Tetracycline Hydrochloride, p.259.

Interactions
As for Tetracycline Hydrochloride, p.259.

Antimicrobial Action
As for Tetracycline Hydrochloride, p.259. It is somewhat less active against many Gram-negative organisms.

Pharmacokinetics
As for Tetracycline Hydrochloride, p.260.

Chlortetracycline is poorly absorbed from the gastrointestinal tract compared with other tetracyclines. It is reported to be rapidly inactivated in the body with a half-life of about 6 hours, and is largely eliminated by biliary excretion. About 45% of a dose is protein bound. Only a small amount is excreted in the urine and, although it is not recommended in patients with renal impairment, accumulation would not be likely despite an increase in half-life to 7 to 11 hours.

Uses and Administration
Chlortetracycline is a tetracycline derivative with uses similar to those of tetracycline (p.260). It is used as the hydrochloride and is administered as a 1% ophthalmic ointment and as a 3% ointment for application to the skin. It is also sometimes given by mouth as the hydrochloride in combination with other tetracycline derivatives.

Preparations
BP 2001: Chlortetracycline Eye Ointment; Chlortetracycline Ointment;

USP 25: Chlortetracycline Hydrochloride Ointment; Chlortetracycline Hydrochloride Ophthalmic Ointment.

Proprietary Preparations (details are given in Part 3)

Aust.: Aureomycin; *Austral.*: Aureomycin; *Belg.*: Aureomycine; *Canad.*: Aureomycin; *Denm.*: Aureomycin†; *Fin.*: Aureomycin; Chlortralim; *Irl.*: Aureomycin; *Israel:* Aureomycin; *Ital.*: Aureomicina; *Mex.*: Aureomycin; *Neth.*: Aureomycin;

Norw.: Aureomycin; *NZ:* Aureomycin; *Port.*: Aurecil; Aureodermil; Aureomicina†; *S.Afr.*: Aureomycin; *Singapore:* Chlortralim; *Spain:* Aureomicina; Dermosa Aureomicina; *Swed.*: Aureomycin; *Switz.*: Aureomycine; *Thai.*: Aureomycin; Chlortralim; *UK:* Aureomycin.

Multi-ingredient: *Aust.*: Aureocort; *Braz.*: Corciclen; *Fin.*: Aureocort; *Ger.*: Auredelf; Aureomycin N; *Irl.*: Aureocort; Deteclo; *Ital.*: Aureocort; Aureomix; *S.Afr.*: Tritet†; *Spain:* Antiblefarica; Poliantib; *UK:* Aureocort; Deteclo.

Ciclacillin (63-g)

Ciclacillin (BAN, rINN).

Cyclacillin (USAN); Wy-4508. (6R)-6-(1-Aminocyclohexanecarboxamido)penicillanic acid.

$C_{15}H_{23}N_3O_4S = 341.4$.

CAS — 3485-14-1.

Pharmacopoeias. In *Jpn.*

Profile
Ciclacillin is an aminopenicillin with properties similar to those of ampicillin (p.150), although it is generally less active *in vitro*.

Preparations
Proprietary Preparations (details are given in Part 3)

Braz.: Cilinase.

Cilastatin Sodium (16578-v)

Cilastatin Sodium (BANM, USAN, rINNM).

Cilastatinum Natricum; MK-791. (Z)-(S)-6-Carboxy-6-[(S)-2,2-dimethylcyclopropanecarboxamido]hex-5-enyl-L-cysteine, monosodium salt.

$C_{16}H_{25}N_2NaO_5S = 380.4$.

CAS — 82009-34-5 (cilastatin); 81129-83-1 (cilastatin sodium).

Pharmacopoeias. In *Eur.* (see p.vi) and *US*.

Pharmacopoeial description
Ph. Eur.: A white or light yellow, hygroscopic, amorphous powder. Very soluble in water and in methyl alcohol; slightly soluble in dehydrated alcohol; practically insoluble in acetone and in dichloromethane; soluble in dimethyl sulfoxide. A 1% solution in water has a pH of 6.5 to 7.5. Store at a temperature not exceeding 8° in airtight containers.

USP 25: A white to tan-coloured powder. Soluble in water and in methyl alcohol. pH of a 1% solution in water is between 6.5 and 7.5. Store at a temperature less than 8°.

Profile
Cilastatin sodium is an inhibitor of dehydropeptidase I, an enzyme found in the brush border of the renal tubules. It is administered concurrently with the antibiotic imipenem (p.214) to prevent its renal metabolism to microbiologically inactive and potentially nephrotoxic products. This increases the concentrations of imipenem achieved in the urine and protects against any nephrotoxic effects, which were seen with high doses of imipenem given experimentally to *animals*.

Cilastatin has no antibacterial activity itself, and does not affect the antibacterial activity of imipenem.

Preparations
USP 25: Imipenem and Cilastatin for Injectable Suspension; Imipenem and Cilastatin for Injection.

Proprietary Preparations (details are given in Part 3)

Multi-ingredient: *Aust.*: Zienam; *Austral.*: Primaxin; *Belg.*: Tienam; *Braz.*: Tienam; *Canad.*: Primaxin; *Denm.*: Tienam; *Fin.*: Tienam; *Fr.*: Tienam; *Ger.*: Zienam; *Hong Kong:* Tienam; *Israel:* Tienam; *Ital.*: Imipem; Tenacid; Tienam; *Mex.*: Tienam; *Neth.*: Tienam; *Norw.*: Tienam; *NZ:* Primaxin; *Port.*: Tienam; *S.Afr.*: Tienam; *Singapore:* Tienam; *Spain:* Tienam; *Swed.*: Tienam; *Switz.*: Tienam; *Thai.*: Tienam; *UK:* Primaxin; *USA:* Primaxin.

Cinoxacin (5655-n)

Cinoxacin (BAN, USAN, rINN).

64716; Azolinic Acid; Compound 64716. 1-Ethyl-1,4-dihydro-4-oxo-1,3-dioxolo[4,5-g]cinnoline-3-carboxylic acid.

$C_{12}H_{10}N_2O_5 = 262.2$.

CAS — 28657-80-9.

ATC — G04AB05.

Pharmacopoeias. In *US*.

Pharmacopoeial description
USP 25: A white to yellowish-white, odourless crystalline solid. Insoluble in water and in most common organic solvents; soluble in alkaline solution. Store in airtight containers.

Adverse Effects and Precautions
As for Nalidixic Acid, p.227.

Cinoxacin is not recommended in patients with severe renal impairment, and the dosage should be reduced in those with mild to moderate renal impairment.

◊ References.
1. Stricker BHC, *et al.* Anaphylactic reactions to cinoxacin. *BMJ* 1988; **297:** 1434–5.

Interactions
As for Nalidixic Acid, p.227.

Antimicrobial Action
As for Nalidixic Acid, p.227. Cross-resistance with nalidixic acid has been shown.

Pharmacokinetics
Cinoxacin is rapidly and almost completely absorbed following administration by mouth. Peak serum concentrations of about 15 µg per mL have been obtained 1 to 3 hours after a 500-mg dose. The plasma half-life is about 1 to 1.5 hours. Cinoxacin has been reported to be more than 60% bound to plasma proteins.

Cinoxacin appears to be metabolised in the liver and is excreted via the kidney. Over 95% of a dose appears in the urine within 24 hours, over half as unaltered drug and the remainder as inactive metabolites. Mean urinary concentrations of about 300 µg per mL have been achieved during the first 4 hours after administration of a 500-mg dose by mouth. Urinary excretion is reduced by probenecid and in patients with renal impairment.

Uses and Administration
Cinoxacin is a 4-quinolone antibacterial with actions and uses similar to those of nalidixic acid (p.227). In the treatment of urinary-tract infections the usual adult dose is 500 mg twice daily by mouth; for prophylaxis a single dose of 500 mg daily at bedtime is given. Dosage should be reduced in mild to moderate renal impairment; cinoxacin is not recommended in patients with severe renal impairment.

◊ References.
1. Sisca TS, *et al.* Cinoxacin: a review of its pharmacological properties and therapeutic efficacy in the treatment of urinary tract infections. *Drugs* 1983; **25:** 544–69.

Preparations
USP 25: Cinoxacin Capsules.

Proprietary Preparations (details are given in Part 3)

Aust.: Cinobac†; *Belg.*: Cinobac†; *Ger.*: Cinobactin†; *Ital.*: Cinobac; Cinoxen; Nossacin; Noxigram; Uroc; Uronorm; Uroxacin; *Mex.*: Gugecin; *S.Afr.*: Cinobactin; *Swed.*: Cinobactin†; *UK:* Cinobac†; *USA:* Cinobac.

Ciprofloxacin (16850-v)

Ciprofloxacin (BAN, USAN, rINN).

Bay-q-3939; Ciprofloxacinum. 1-Cyclopropyl-6-fluoro-1,4-dihydro-4-oxo-7-piperazin-1-ylquinoline-3-carboxylic acid.

$C_{17}H_{18}FN_3O_3 = 331.3$.

CAS — 85721-33-1.

ATC — J01MA02; S01AX13; S03AA07.

Pharmacopoeias. In *Eur.* (see p.vi) and *US*.

Pharmacopoeial description
Ph. Eur.: A pale yellow, crystalline powder. Practically insoluble in water; very slightly soluble in dehydrated alcohol and in dichloromethane; soluble in dilute acetic acid. Protect from light.

USP 25: Store in airtight containers. Protect from light.

Ciprofloxacin Hydrochloride (11305-s)

Ciprofloxacin Hydrochloride (BANM, USAN, rINNM).

Bay-q-9867; Ciprofloxacini Hydrochloridum. Ciprofloxacin hydrochloride monohydrate.

$C_{17}H_{18}FN_3O_3,HCl,H_2O = 385.8$.

CAS — 86483-48-9 (anhydrous ciprofloxacin hydrochloride); 86393-32-0 (ciprofloxacin hydrochloride monohydrate).

Pharmacopoeias. In *Eur.* (see p.vi), *Pol.*, and *US*.

291.1 mg of monograph substance is approximately equivalent to 250 mg of ciprofloxacin.

Pharmacopoeial description
Ph. Eur.: A pale yellow, crystalline powder. Soluble in water; very slightly soluble in dehydrated alcohol; practically insoluble in acetone, in dichloromethane, and in ethyl acetate; slightly soluble in methyl alcohol. A 2.5% solution in water has a pH of 3.0 to 4.5. Store in airtight containers. Protect from light.

USP 25: Faintly yellowish to light yellow crystals. Sparingly soluble in water; very slightly soluble in dehydrated alcohol; slightly soluble in acetic acid and in methyl alcohol; practically insoluble in acetone, in acetonitrile, in dichloromethane, in ethyl acetate, and in hexane. pH of a 2.5% solution in water is between 3.0 and 4.5. Store in airtight containers. Protect from light.

Ciprofloxacin Lactate (11306-w)

Ciprofloxacin Lactate (BANM, rINNM).

$C_{17}H_{18}FN_3O_3,C_3H_6O_3 = 421.4$.

CAS — 97867-33-9.

127 mg of monograph substance is approximately equivalent to 100 mg of ciprofloxacin.

Incompatibility. Ciprofloxacin infusion is stated by the manufacturers to have a pH of 3.9 to 4.5 and to be incompatible with injections chemically or physically unstable at this pH range. Incompatibility has been reported between ciprofloxacin and a range of drugs including some other antibacterials.[1-4]

1. Lyall A, Blythe J. Ciprofloxacin lactate infusion. *Pharm J* 1987; **238:** 290.
2. Jankegt R, *et al.* Quinolones and penicillins incompatibility. *DICP Ann Pharmacother* 1989; **23:** 91-2.
3. Goodwin SD, *et al.* Compatibility of ciprofloxacin injection with selected drugs and solutions. *Am J Hosp Pharm* 1991; **48:** 2166-71.
4. Jim LK. Physical and chemical compatibility of intravenous ciprofloxacin with other drugs. *Ann Pharmacother* 1993; **27:** 704-7.

Adverse Effects

Ciprofloxacin is generally well tolerated. The range of adverse effects associated with ciprofloxacin and the other fluoroquinolone antibacterials is broadly similar to that with earlier quinolones such as nalidixic acid (p.227). They most often involve the gastrointestinal tract, CNS, or skin.

Gastrointestinal disturbances include nausea, vomiting, diarrhoea, abdominal pain, and dyspepsia and are the most frequent adverse effects. Pseudomembranous colitis has been reported rarely.

Headache, dizziness, and restlessness are among the commonest effects on the CNS. Others include tremor, drowsiness, insomnia, nightmares, and visual and other sensory disturbances, depression, and convulsions. Paraesthesia and peripheral neuropathy have occurred occasionally.

In addition to rash and pruritus, hypersensitivity-type reactions affecting the skin have included, rarely, vasculitis, erythema multiforme, Stevens-Johnson syndrome, and toxic epidermal necrolysis. Photosensitivity has occurred, although it may be more frequent with some newer fluoroquinolones such as lomefloxacin and sparfloxacin. Anaphylaxis has been associated with some quinolone antibacterials. As with other quinolone antibacterials, reversible arthralgia has sometimes occurred and joint erosions have been documented in immature *animals*. Tendon damage has been reported.

Other adverse effects reported with ciprofloxacin include transient increases in serum creatinine or blood urea nitrogen and, occasionally, acute renal failure secondary to interstitial nephritis; crystalluria; elevated liver enzyme values, jaundice, and hepatitis; haematological disturbances including eosinophilia, leucopenia, thrombocytopenia and, very rarely, haemolytic anaemia or agranulocytosis; myalgia; gynaecomastia; and cardiovascular effects including tachycardia.

As with other antibacterials, superinfection with organisms not very susceptible to ciprofloxacin is possible. Such organisms include *Candida*, *Clostridium difficile*, and *Streptococcus pneumoniae*. There is some evidence that ciprofloxacin use may be associated with an increased risk of colonisation by meticillin-resistant *Staphylococcus aureus* and vancomycin-resistant enterococci.

Pain and irritation may occur at the site of injection accompanied rarely by phlebitis or thrombophlebitis.

◊ General reviews of the adverse effects of antibacterials.
1. Stahlmann R. Safety profile of the quinolones. *J Antimicrob Chemother* 1990; **26** (suppl D): 31-44.
2. Paton JH, Reeves DS. Adverse reactions to the fluoroquinolones. *Adverse Drug React Bull* 1992; (April): 575-8.
3. Domagala JM. Structure-activity and structure-side-effect relationships for the quinolone antibacterials. *J Antimicrob Chemother* 1994; **33:** 685-706.
4. Rubinstein E, *et al.* The use of fluoroquinolones in neutropenic patients—analysis of adverse effects. *J Antimicrob Chemother* 1994; **34:** 7-19.
5. Ball P, Tillotson G. Tolerability of fluoroquinolone antibiotics: past, present and future. *Drug Safety* 1995; **13:** 343-58.
6. Lipsky BA, Baker CA. Fluoroquinolone toxicity profiles: a review focusing on newer agents. *Clin Infect Dis* 1999; **28:** 352-64.
7. Ball P, *et al.* Comparative tolerability of the newer fluoroquinolone antibacterials. *Drug Safety* 1999; **21:** 407-21.

◊ Reviews and surveys of the adverse effects of ciprofloxacin and the antibacterials.
1. Arcieri GM, *et al.* Safety of intravenous ciprofloxacin: a review. *Am J Med* 1989; **87** (suppl 5A): 92S-97S.
2. Schacht P, *et al.* Safety of oral ciprofloxacin: an update based on clinical trial results. *Am J Med* 1989; **87** (suppl 5A): 98S-102S.

Effects on the blood. Haematological disturbances including eosinophilia, leucopenia, thrombocytopenia, and, very rarely, haemolytic anaemia have been reported with ciprofloxacin; in addition, transient reductions in factor VIII and von Willebrand's factor leading to bleeding in 2 patients receiving ciprofloxacin has been reported.[1]
1. Kennedy N, *et al.* Safety profile of ciprofloxacin during long-term therapy for pulmonary tuberculosis. *J Antimicrob Chemother* 1993; **32:** 897-902.
2. Segev S, *et al.* Safety of long-term ciprofloxacin therapy: data analysis of controlled clinical trials and review. *Clin Infect Dis* 1999; **28:** 299-308.
3. Castaman G, Rodeghiero F. Acquired transitory von Willebrand syndrome with ciprofloxacin. *Lancet* 1994; **343:** 492.

Effects on the gastrointestinal tract. Reports of pseudomembranous colitis or superinfection with *Clostridium difficile* associated with ciprofloxacin and other fluoroquinolones.
1. Dan M, Samra Z. Clostridium difficile colitis associated with ciprofloxacin therapy. *Am J Med* 1989; **87:** 479.
2. Cain DB, O'Connor ME. Pseudomembranous colitis associated with ciprofloxacin. *Lancet* 1990; **336:** 946.
3. Bates CJ, *et al.* Clostridium difficile and Clostridium difficile-associated diarrhoea. *Lancet* 1990; **336:** 1193.
4. Low N, Harries AD. Ciprofloxacin and pseudomembranous colitis. *Lancet* 1990; **336:** 1510.
5. Hillman RJ, *et al.* Ciprofloxacin as a cause of Clostridium difficile-associated diarrhoea in an HIV antibody-positive patient. *Lancet* 1990; **336:** 1510.
6. Golledge CL, *et al.* Ciprofloxacin and Clostridium difficile-associated diarrhoea. *J Antimicrob Chemother* 1992; **30:** 141-7.
7. McFarland LV, *et al.* Ciprofloxacin-associated Clostridium difficile disease. *Lancet* 1995; **346:** 977-8.

Effects on the kidneys. References to renal toxicity associated with ciprofloxacin and other fluoroquinolones.
1. Rippelmeyer DJ, Synhavsky A. Ciprofloxacin and allergic interstitial nephritis. *Ann Intern Med* 1988; **109:** 170.
2. Ying LS, Johnson CA. Ciprofloxacin-induced interstitial nephritis. *Clin Pharm* 1989; **8:** 518-21.
3. Rastogi S, *et al.* Allergic nephropathy associated with ciprofloxacin. *Mayo Clin Proc* 1990; **65:** 987-9.
4. Allon M, *et al.* Acute renal failure due to ciprofloxacin. *Arch Intern Med* 1990; **150:** 2187-9.
5. George M, *et al.* Acute renal failure after an overdose of ciprofloxacin. *Arch Intern Med* 1991; **151:** 620.
6. Simpson J, *et al.* Typhoid fever, ciprofloxacin, and renal failure. *Arch Dis Child* 1991; **66:** 1083-4.
7. Yew WW, *et al.* Ciprofloxacin-induced renal dysfunction in patients with mycobacterial lung infections. *Tubercle Lung Dis* 1995; **76:** 173-5.
8. Hesin BM, *et al.* Norfloxacin-induced nephrotic syndrome. *Lancet* 1995; **345:** 732-3.
9. Lomaestro BM. Fluoroquinolone-induced renal failure. *Drug Safety* 2000; **22:** 479-85.

Effects on the liver. References to hepatotoxicity associated with ciprofloxacin and other fluoroquinolones.
1. Grassmick BK, *et al.* Fulminant hepatic failure possibly related to ciprofloxacin. *Ann Pharmacother* 1992; **26:** 636-9.
2. Sherman O, Beizer JL. Possible ciprofloxacin-induced acute cholestatic jaundice. *Ann Pharmacother* 1994; **28:** 1162-4.
3. Villeneuve J-P, *et al.* Suspected ciprofloxacin-induced hepatotoxicity. *Ann Pharmacother* 1995; **29:** 257-9.
4. Jones SE, Smith RH. Quinolones may induce hepatitis. *BMJ* 1997; **314:** 869.

Effects on the musculoskeletal system. Reversible arthralgia has sometimes occurred with the fluoroquinolone antibacterials; joint erosions have been documented in immature *animals*. In one report, treatment with pefloxacin might have contributed to the destructive arthropathy that occurred in a 17-year-old youth.[2]
More recently there have been reports of tendinitis and tendon rupture associated with fluoroquinolones.[3-6] By July 1995, the UK Committee on Safety of Medicines (CSM) had received 21 reports of tendon damage, often of the Achilles tendon, associated with these antibacterials—11 with ciprofloxacin and 10 with ofloxacin.[5] The risk of tendon damage might be increased by the concomitant use of corticosteroids and appeared more common with increasing age.[5] The CSM warned that at the first sign of pain or inflammation the quinolone should be discontinued and the affected limb rested until the tendon symptoms had resolved.[5] Similar warnings have been issued in other countries.
1. Alfaham M, *et al.* Arthropathy in a patient with cystic fibrosis taking ciprofloxacin. *BMJ* 1987; **295:** 699.
2. Chevalier X, *et al.* A case of destructive polyarthropathy in a 17-year-old youth following pefloxacin treatment. *Drug Safety* 1992; **7:** 310-14.
3. Huston KA. Achilles tendinitis and tendon rupture due to fluoroquinolone antibiotics. *N Engl J Med* 1994; **331:** 748.
4. Szarfman A, *et al.* More on fluoroquinolone antibiotics and tendon rupture. *N Engl J Med* 1995; **332:** 193.
5. Committee on Safety of Medicines/Medicines Control Agency. Tendon damage associated with quinolone antibiotics. *Current Problems* 1995; **21:** 8.
6. Carrasco JM, *et al.* Tendinitis associated with ciprofloxacin. *Ann Pharmacother* 1997; **31:** 120.

Effects on the nervous system. By 1991 the UK Committee on Safety of Medicines had received 26 reports of convulsions associated with ciprofloxacin, 1 with norfloxacin, and 1 with ofloxacin.[1] It was noted that convulsions could occur both in patients with epilepsy and in those with no previous history of convulsions.
Other recent reports of CNS toxicity associated with ciprofloxacin have included eosinophilic meningitis,[2] delirium,[3] and acute psychoses.[4,5] Peripheral neuropathy,[6] dysaesthesia,[7] catatonia,[8] sleep disturbances,[9] hemiparesis,[10] and tinnitus[11] have also been reported. There has also been a report of a Tourette-like syndrome associated with ofloxacin.[12]
1. Committee on Safety of Medicines. Convulsions due to quinolone antimicrobial agents. *Current Problems* 32 1991.
2. Asperilla MO, *et al.* Eosinophilic meningitis associated with ciprofloxacin. *Am J Med* 1989; **87:** 589-90.
3. Jay GT, Fitzgerald JM. Ciprofloxacin-induced delirium. *Ann Pharmacother* 1997; **31:** 252.
4. McCue JD, Zandt JR. Acute psychoses associated with the use of ciprofloxacin and trimethoprim-sulfamethoxazole. *Am J Med* 1991; **90:** 528-9.
5. Reeves RR. Ciprofloxacin-induced psychosis. *Ann Pharmacother* 1992; **26:** 930-1.
6. Aoun M, *et al.* Peripheral neuropathy associated with fluoroquinolones. *Lancet* 1992; **340:** 127.
7. Zehnder D, *et al.* Painful dysaesthesia with ciprofloxacin. *BMJ* 1995; **311:** 1204.
8. Akhtar S, Ahmad H. Ciprofloxacin-induced catatonia. *J Clin Psychiatry* 1993; **54:** 115-16.
9. Upton C. Sleep disturbance in children treated with ofloxacin. *BMJ* 1994; **309:** 1411.
10. Rosolen A, *et al.* Acute hemiparesis associated with ciprofloxacin. *BMJ* 1994; **309:** 1411.
11. Paul J, Brown NM. Tinnitus and ciprofloxacin. *BMJ* 1995; **311:** 232.
12. Thomas RJ, Reagan DR. Association of a Tourette-like syndrome with ofloxacin. *Ann Pharmacother* 1996; **30:** 138-41.

Hypersensitivity. Hypersensitivity and skin reactions have been associated with ciprofloxacin and other fluoroquinolones. Reports have included anaphylaxis (which has been fatal),[1-4] serum sickness,[5] toxic epidermal necrolysis,[6-8] laryngeal oedema,[9] and vasculitis.[10-12] Fatal vasculitis has been reported with ofloxacin.[13]
1. Davis H, *et al.* Anaphylactoid reactions reported after treatment with ciprofloxacin. *Ann Intern Med* 1989; **111:** 1041-3.
2. Peters B, Pinching AJ. Fatal anaphylaxis associated with ciprofloxacin in a patient with AIDS related complex. *BMJ* 1989; **298:** 605.
3. Wurtz RM, *et al.* Anaphylactoid drug reactions to ciprofloxacin and rifampicin in HIV-infected patients. *Lancet* 1989; **i:** 955-6.
4. Assoaud M, *et al.* Anaphylactoid reactions to ciprofloxacin. *Ann Intern Med* 1995; **122:** 396-7.
5. Slama TG. Serum sickness-like illness associated with ciprofloxacin. *Antimicrob Agents Chemother* 1990; **34:** 904-5.
6. Tham TCK, *et al.* Possible association between toxic epidermal necrolysis and ciprofloxacin. *Lancet* 1991; **338:** 522.
7. Moshfeghi M, Mandler HD. Ciprofloxacin-induced toxic epidermal necrolysis. *Ann Pharmacother* 1993; **27:** 1467-9.
8. Yerasi AB, Oertel MD. Ciprofloxacin-induced toxic epidermal necrolysis. *Ann Pharmacother* 1996; **30:** 297.
9. Baciewicz AM, *et al.* Laryngeal edema related to ciprofloxacin therapy. *Ann Pharmacother* 1992; **26:** 1456.
10. Choe U, *et al.* Ciprofloxacin-induced vasculitis. *N Engl J Med* 1989; **320:** 257-8.
11. Stubbings J, *et al.* Cutaneous vasculitis due to ciprofloxacin. *BMJ* 1992; **305:** 29.
12. Drago F, *et al.* Henoch-Schönlein purpura induced by fluoroquinolones. *Br J Dermatol* 1994; **131:** 448.
13. Pace JL, Gatt P. Fatal vasculitis associated with ofloxacin. *BMJ* 1989; **299:** 658.

Superinfection. Reports of superinfection with *Streptococcus pneumoniae*.[1-3] For references to superinfection with *Clostridium difficile* see under Effects on the Gastrointestinal Tract, above.
1. Righter J. Pneumococcal meningitis during intravenous ciprofloxacin therapy. *Am J Med* 1990; **88:** 548.
2. Gordon JJ, Kaufman CA. Superinfection with Streptococcus pneumoniae during therapy with ciprofloxacin. *Am J Med* 1990; **89:** 383-4.
3. Lee BL, *et al.* Infectious complications with respiratory pathogens despite ciprofloxacin therapy. *N Engl J Med* 1991; **325:** 520-1.

Precautions

Ciprofloxacin should be used with caution in patients with epilepsy or a history of CNS disorders. Since ciprofloxacin and related fluoroquinolones have, like nalidixic acid, been shown to cause degenerative changes in weight-bearing joints of young *animals*, it has been suggested that these compounds should not be used in children, adolescents, pregnant women, or breast-feeding mothers. Tendon damage may occur rarely with fluoroquinolones (see Effects on the Musculoskeletal System, above) and treatment should be discontinued if patients experience tendon pain, inflammation, or rupture.

Care is necessary in patients with impaired hepatic or renal function, glucose-6-phosphate dehydrogenase deficiency, or myasthenia gravis. An adequate fluid intake should be maintained during treatment with ciprofloxacin and excessive alkalinity of the urine avoided because of the risk of crystalluria. Exposure to strong sunlight or sunlamps should also be avoided. The ability to drive or operate machinery may be impaired by ciprofloxacin, especially when alcohol is also taken.

Ciprofloxacin should be avoided in meticillin-resistant *Staphylococcus aureus* infections because of the high level of resistance.

Administration in children. Since ciprofloxacin and other fluoroquinolones can cause degenerative changes in weight-bearing joints of young animals they should only be used in children and adolescents where their use may be justified if the benefits outweigh the risks.[1,2]

1. Schaad UB, et al. Use of fluoroquinolones in pediatrics: consensus report of an International Society of Chemotherapy commission. Pediatr Infect Dis J 1995; 14: 1–9.
2. Green SDR. Indications and restrictions fluoroquinolone use in children. Br J Hosp Med 1996; 56: 420–3.

Exposure to ultraviolet light. Loss of antibacterial activity has been reported following irradiation of ciprofloxacin solutions by ultraviolet light.[1] In addition to the possible hazard of photosensitivity reactions, a reduction in both cutaneous and circulating levels of ciprofloxacin was predicted in patients exposed to sunlight through window glass or longer wavelength ultraviolet (UVA) radiation from sunbeds.[1]

1. Phillips G, et al. The loss of antibiotic activity of ciprofloxacin by photodegradation. J Antimicrob Chemother 1990; 26: 783–9.

Interference with diagnostic tests. Ciprofloxacin did not interfere with determination of urinary-glucose concentrations carried out with Clinitest, Diastix, or Tes-Tape,[1] but pseudoglycosuria, a false-positive reaction for glucose in urine, has been reported with BM-Test-7 in elderly patients given ciprofloxacin for urinary-tract infections.[2]

1. Tartaglione TA, Flint NB. Effect of imipenem-cilastatin and ciprofloxacin on tests for glycosuria. Am J Hosp Pharm 1985; 42: 602–5.
2. Drysdale L, et al. Pseudoglycosuria and ciprofloxacin. Lancet 1988; ii: 961.

Myasthenia gravis. Caution is advised in patients with myasthenia gravis given fluoroquinolones following reports of the possible exacerbation of symptoms in a patient,[1] and unmasking of subclinical myasthenia gravis in another,[2] by ciprofloxacin. Exacerbation of myasthenia gravis has also been reported with norfloxacin.[3]

1. Moore B, et al. Possible exacerbation of myasthenia gravis by ciprofloxacin. Lancet 1988; i: 882.
2. Mumford CJ, Ginsberg L. Ciprofloxacin and myasthenia gravis. BMJ 1990; 301: 818.
3. Rauser EH, et al. Exacerbation of myasthenia gravis by norfloxacin. DICP Ann Pharmacother 1990; 24: 207–8.

Interactions

Fluoroquinolones are known to inhibit hepatic drug metabolism and may interfere with the clearance of drugs, such as theophylline, that are metabolised by the liver. Cations like aluminium, magnesium, or iron reduce the absorption of ciprofloxacin and related drugs when given concomitantly.

For physical or chemical incompatibilities with ciprofloxacin, see above.

Analgesics. Concurrent administration of fenbufen with quinolones may increase the incidence of quinolone CNS adverse effects. Reviews[1,2] have noted that 7 cases of convulsions associated with the use of fenbufen and enoxacin have been reported to the Japanese regulatory authorities. The UK Committee on Safety of Medicines has recognised that convulsions may occur due to an interaction between the quinolones and NSAIDs; by 1991, 3 such interactions had been reported to them.[3] Adverse neurological effects have also been reported in a patient receiving naproxen and chloroquine when ciprofloxacin was administered, which abated when the antirheumatic drugs were withdrawn.[4]

Ciprofloxacin also interacts with opioid analgesics; peak serum concentrations of ciprofloxacin given by mouth pre-operatively were significantly reduced when intramuscular papaveretum was injected concomitantly.[5] The manufacturers recommend that opioids should not be administered perioperatively to patients receiving ciprofloxacin.

1. Janknegt R. Drug interactions with quinolones. J Antimicrob Chemother 1990; 26 (suppl D): 7–29.
2. Christ W. Central nervous system toxicity of quinolones: human and animal findings. J Antimicrob Chemother 1990; 26 (suppl B): 219–25.
3. Committee on Safety of Medicines. Convulsions due to quinolone antibiotics. Current Problems 32 1991.
4. Rollof J, Vinge E. Neurologic adverse effects during concomitant treatment with ciprofloxacin, NSAIDs, and chloroquine. Ann Pharmacother 1993; 27: 1058–9.
5. Morran C, et al. Brief report: pharmacokinetics of orally administered ciprofloxacin in abdominal surgery. Am J Med 1989; 87 (suppl 5A): 86S–88S.

Antacids and metal ions. The absorption of ciprofloxacin and other fluoroquinolones is reduced by antacids containing aluminium or magnesium and also by calcium, iron, and zinc salts.[1] Sucralfate releases aluminium ions in the stomach and thereby reduces the absorption of ciprofloxacin[2,3] and other fluoroquinolones, including norfloxacin[4] and ofloxacin.[5] In addition, concomitant administration of antacids or oral iron preparations might antagonise the antibacterial activity of fluoroquinolones within the gut lumen.[5] Dairy products with a high calcium content might also interfere with the absorption of some fluoroquinolones.[6-8] Enteral feeds, which contain cations, have also been found to reduce absorption of ciprofloxacin.[9] A reduction in ciprofloxacin bioavailability has also been reported following concomitant administration of chewable tablets of didanosine which contain aluminium and magnesium ion buffering agents.[10]

1. Lomaestro BM, Bailie GR. Absorption interactions with fluoroquinolones: 1995 update. Drug Safety 1995; 12: 314–33.
2. Garrelts JC, et al. Sucralfate significantly reduces ciprofloxacin concentrations in serum. Antimicrob Agents Chemother 1990; 34: 931–3.
3. Van Slooten AD, et al. Combined use of ciprofloxacin and sucralfate. DICP Ann Pharmacother 1991; 25: 578–82.
4. Parpia SH, et al. Sucralfate reduces the gastrointestinal absorption of norfloxacin. Antimicrob Agents Chemother 1989; 33: 99–102.
5. Lewin CS, Smith JT. 4-Quinolones and multivalent ions. J Antimicrob Chemother 1990; 26: 149.
6. Neuvonen PJ, et al. Interference of dairy products with the absorption of ciprofloxacin. Clin Pharmacol Ther 1991; 50: 498–502.
7. Kivistö KT, et al. Inhibition of norfloxacin absorption by dairy products. Antimicrob Agents Chemother 1992; 36: 489–91.
8. Neuvonen PJ, Kivistö KT. Milk and yoghurt do not impair the absorption of ofloxacin. Br J Clin Pharmacol 1992; 33: 346–8.
9. Healy DP, et al. Ciprofloxacin absorption is impaired in patients given enteral feedings orally and via gastrostomy and jejunostomy tubes. Antimicrob Agents Chemother 1996; 40: 6–10.
10. Sahai J, et al. Cations in the didanosine tablet reduce ciprofloxacin bioavailability. Clin Pharmacol Ther 1993; 53: 292–7.

Antibacterials. The simultaneous administration of parenteral ciprofloxacin and azlocillin has resulted in higher and more prolonged serum concentrations of ciprofloxacin.[1]

1. Barriere SL, et al. Alteration in the pharmacokinetic disposition of ciprofloxacin by simultaneous administration of azlocillin. Antimicrob Agents Chemother 1990; 34: 823–6.

Anticoagulants. For reports of ciprofloxacin and other quinolones enhancing the effect of oral anticoagulants, see under Warfarin, p.994.

Antiepileptics. For conflicting reports of the effect of ciprofloxacin on serum-phenytoin concentrations, see p.359.

Antimigraine drugs. For a recommendation to reduce the dosage of zolmitriptan when given concurrently with ciprofloxacin, see p.458.

Antineoplastics and immunosuppressants. Absorption of oral ciprofloxacin appears to be reduced after cytotoxic chemotherapy.[1] There has been a report of enhanced nephrotoxicity in a patient who received ciprofloxacin and ciclosporin,[2] although a review[3] found no correlation between concurrent treatment and alterations in pharmacokinetics or pharmacodynamics.

1. Johnson EJ, et al. Reduced absorption of oral ciprofloxacin after administration for haematological malignancy. J Antimicrob Chemother 1990; 25: 837–42.
2. Elston RA, Taylor J. Possible interaction of ciprofloxacin with cyclosporin A. J Antimicrob Chemother 1988; 21: 679–80.
3. Hoey LL, Lake KD. Does ciprofloxacin interact with cyclosporine? Ann Pharmacother 1994; 28: 93–6.

Antivirals. Both ciprofloxacin and foscarnet can cause convulsions and 2 patients developed generalised tonic-clonic seizures while receiving the drugs concurrently.[1]

1. Fan-Havard P, et al. Concurrent use of foscarnet and ciprofloxacin may increase the propensity for seizures. Ann Pharmacother 1994; 28: 869–72.

Anxiolytics. For an isolated report of increased blood concentrations of midazolam associated with the concomitant administration of ciprofloxacin, see under Diazepam, p.677.

Histamine H₂-antagonists. Cimetidine has been reported to reduce the clearance of pefloxacin,[1] and ranitidine given intravenously has reduced the bioavailability of oral enoxacin.[2]

1. Sörgel F, et al. Effects of cimetidine on the pharmacokinetics of pefloxacin in healthy volunteers. Rev Infect Dis 1988; 10 (suppl 1): S137.
2. Grasela TH, et al. Inhibition of enoxacin absorption by antacids or ranitidine. Antimicrob Agents Chemother 1989; 33: 615–17.

Probenecid. The urinary excretion of ciprofloxacin and some other fluoroquinolones is reduced by the concomitant administration of probenecid; plasma concentrations are not necessarily increased.

Xanthines. Ciprofloxacin and other fluoroquinolones (to a greater or lesser extent) decrease the clearance of theophylline (p.780) and caffeine (p.762) from the body. Seizures have occurred in patients given ciprofloxacin and theophylline concomitantly and in one such report[1] serum-theophylline concentrations were normal. Fluoroquinolones can be neurotoxic in their own right (see Effects on the Nervous System, above).

1. Bader MB. Role of fluoroquinolones in fatal seizures. Chest 1992; 101: 883–4.

Antimicrobial Action

Ciprofloxacin is bactericidal and acts by inhibiting the A subunit of DNA gyrase (topoisomerase) which is essential in the reproduction of bacterial DNA. It has a broader spectrum of activity and is more potent in vitro than the non-fluorinated quinolone nalidixic acid. Activity may be reduced in acid media.

Spectrum of activity (see also Resistance, below). Among Gram-negative aerobic bacteria, ciprofloxacin is active in vitro against Enterobacteriaceae, including Escherichia coli and Citrobacter, Enterobacter, Klebsiella, Proteus, Providencia, Salmonella, Serratia, Shigella, and Yersinia spp; the MIC_{90} for most of these is reported to be 1 μg or less per mL. It is also active against Pseudomonas aeruginosa (MIC_{90} about 2 μg per mL), but less so against other Pseudomonas spp. Haemophilus ducreyi, H. influenzae, Moraxella catarrhalis (Branhamella catarrhalis), Neisseria gonorrhoeae, and N. meningitidis are all very sensitive, including beta-lactamase-producing strains of H. influenzae, M. catarrhalis, and N. gonorrhoeae. Other Gram-negative aerobic bacteria reported to be sensitive to ciprofloxacin have included Acinetobacter spp., Campylobacter spp. Gardnerella vaginalis, Helicobacter pylori, Legionella spp., Pasteurella multocida, and Vibrio spp. Variable activity has been reported against Brucella melitensis.

Among Gram-positive aerobic bacteria, ciprofloxacin is active against staphylococci, including penicillinase-producing and penicillinase-nonproducing strains (MIC_{90} 1 μg or less per mL), and against some meticillin-resistant strains. Streptococci, in particular Streptococcus pneumoniae and enterococci, are less susceptible. Other Gram-positive bacteria sensitive to ciprofloxacin in vitro are Corynebacterium spp. and Listeria monocytogenes.

Most anaerobic bacteria, including Bacteroides fragilis and Clostridium difficile, are resistant to ciprofloxacin, although some other Bacteroides and Clostridium spp. may be susceptible.

Ciprofloxacin has some activity against mycobacteria, mycoplasmas, rickettsias, and the protozoan Plasmodium falciparum. Chlamydia trachomatis is not very susceptible and Nocardia asteroides and Ureaplasma urealyticum are usually considered to be resistant. The spirochaete Treponema pallidum and fungi are also resistant.

Activity with other antimicrobial agents. There have been some reports of enhanced activity in vitro when ciprofloxacin has been used with other antimicrobials, such as azlocillin against Staphylococcus aureus and Pseudomonas aeruginosa, imipenem against Ps. aeruginosa, and cefotaxime or clindamycin against anaerobic bacteria.

Acquired resistance. Resistant strains, particularly of Staph. aureus (including meticillin-resistant strains) and Ps. aeruginosa have emerged during treatment with ciprofloxacin (see below for reports of other resistant bacteria). There is complete cross-resistance between ciprofloxacin and the other fluoroquinolones, but not between ciprofloxacin and nalidixic acid. Like nalidixic acid, resistance to ciprofloxacin appears, so far, to be chromosomally rather than plasmid-mediated.

Resistance. Acquired resistance to ciprofloxacin and other fluoroquinolones has occurred most frequently in staphylococci[1-3] and Pseudomonas aeruginosa;[4] cross-resistance to unrelated antibacterials has been described in Ps. aeruginosa.[5] Resistance has also been reported in Campylobacter spp. initially linked with the widespread veterinary use of quinolones[6,7] and subsequently becoming more clinically important[8,9] including isolated reports of possible resistance in C. fetus infections in immunocompromised patients.[10] Similarly there have been reports of increasing quinolone resistance in both non-typhoid Salmonella spp.[11] as well as S. typhi[12-15] and S. paratyphi.[16] Resistance to fluoroquinolones has also been reported in other Enterobacteriaceae including Escherichia coli,[17,18] Serratia marcescens,[19] Shigella sonnei,[20] and Haemophilus influenzae.[21,22] Decreased susceptibility of Neisseria gonorrhoeae has been reported.[23,24] and resistant strains have now been reported.[25,26] Mutational resistance has developed in mycobacteria following monotherapy with ciprofloxacin.[27] Fluoroquinolone-resistant strains of Mycobacterium tuberculosis have been isolated from patients with tuberculosis.[28]

Excretion of ciprofloxacin in sweat has been suggested to be a contributory factor in the development of resistance to Staphylococcus epidermidis and possibly other skin-dwelling bacteria.[29]

1. Oppenheim BA, et al. Outbreak of coagulase negative staphylococcus highly resistant to ciprofloxacin in a leukaemia unit. BMJ 1989; 299: 294–7.
2. Blumberg HM, et al. Rapid development of ciprofloxacin resistance in meticillin-susceptible and resistant Staphylococcus aureus. J Infect Dis 1991; 163: 1279–85.
3. Trucksis M, et al. Emerging resistance to fluoroquinolones in staphylococci: an alert. Ann Intern Med 1991; 114: 424–6.
4. Acar JF, Francoual S. The clinical problems of bacterial resistance to the new quinolones. J Antimicrob Chemother 1990; 26 (suppl B): 207–13.

Pharmacokinetics

Ciprofloxacin is rapidly and well absorbed from the gastrointestinal tract. Oral bioavailability is approximately 70% and a peak plasma concentration of about 2.5 μg per mL is achieved 1 to 2 hours after a dose of 500 mg by mouth. Absorption may be delayed by the presence of food, but is not substantially affected overall. The plasma half-life is about 3.5 to 4.5 hours and there is evidence of modest accumulation. Half-life may be prolonged in severe renal disease—a value of 8 hours has been reported in end-stage renal disease—and to some extent in the elderly. There is limited information on the effect of liver dysfunction; in one study the half-life of ciprofloxacin was slightly prolonged in patients with severe cirrhosis of the liver. With one or two exceptions, most studies have shown the pharmacokinetics of ciprofloxacin to be not markedly affected by cystic fibrosis.

Plasma protein binding ranges from 20 to 40%. Ciprofloxacin is widely distributed in the body and tissue penetration is generally good. It appears in the CSF, but concentrations are only about 10% of those in plasma when the meninges are not inflamed. Ciprofloxacin crosses the placenta and is distributed into breast milk. High concentrations are achieved in bile.

Ciprofloxacin is eliminated principally by urinary excretion, but non-renal clearance may account for about a third of elimination and includes hepatic metabolism, biliary excretion, and possibly transluminal secretion across the intestinal mucosa. At least 4 active metabolites have been identified. Oxociprofloxacin appears to be the major urinary metabolite and sulfociprofloxacin the primary faecal metabolite. Urinary excretion is by active tubular secretion as well as glomerular filtration and is reduced by probenecid; it is virtually complete within 24 hours. About 40 to 50% of an oral dose is excreted unchanged in the urine and about 15% as metabolites. Up to 70% of a parenteral dose may be excreted unchanged within 24 hours and 10% as metabolites. Faecal excretion over 5 days has accounted for 20 to 35% of an oral dose and 15% of an intravenous dose.

Only small amounts of ciprofloxacin are removed by haemodialysis or peritoneal dialysis.

◊ Comparative pharmacokinetics of the fluoroquinolones.

1. Aminimanzani A, *et al.* Comparative pharmacokinetics and pharmacodynamics of the newer fluoroquinolone antibacterials. *Clin Pharmacokinet* 2001; 40: 169–187.

◊ Reviews of the pharmacokinetics of ciprofloxacin.

1. Vance-Bryan K, *et al.* Clinical pharmacokinetics of ciprofloxacin. *Clin Pharmacokinet* 1990; 19: 434–61.

◊ Studies on the distribution of ciprofloxacin.

1. Sweeney G, *et al.* Penetration of ciprofloxacin into the aqueous humour of the uninflamed human eye after oral administration. *J Antimicrob Chemother* 1990; 26: 99–105.
2. Cover DL, Mueller BA. Ciprofloxacin penetration into human breast milk: a case report. *DICP Ann Pharmacother* 1990; 24: 703–4.
3. Nau R, *et al.* Penetration of ciprofloxacin into the cerebrospinal fluid of patients with uninflamed meninges. *J Antimicrob Chemother* 1990; 25: 965–73.
4. Trautmann M, *et al.* Penetration of ciprofloxacin into the spinal fluid in patients with viral and bacterial meningitis. *Arzneimittelforschung* 1990; 40: 611–13.
5. Mertes PM, *et al.* Penetration of ciprofloxacin into heart valves, myocardium, mediastinal fat, and sternal bone marrow in humans. *Antimicrob Agents Chemother* 1990; 34: 398–401.
6. Darouiche R, *et al.* Levels of rifampin and ciprofloxacin in nasal secretions: correlation with MIC_{90} and eradication of nasopharyngeal carriage of bacteria. *J Infect Dis* 1990; 162: 1124–7.
7. Jacobs F, *et al.* Penetration of ciprofloxacin into human pleural fluid. *Antimicrob Agents Chemother* 1990; 34: 934–6.
8. Fabre D, *et al.* Steady-state pharmacokinetics of ciprofloxacin in plasma from patients with nosocomial pneumonia: penetration of the bronchial mucosa. *Antimicrob Agents Chemother* 1991; 35: 2521–5.
9. Dan M, *et al.* Distribution of ciprofloxacin in ascitic fluid following administration of a single oral dose of 750 milligrams. *Antimicrob Agents Chemother* 1992; 36: 677–8.
10. Dan M, *et al.* The penetration of ciprofloxacin into bronchial mucosa, lung parenchyma, and pleural tissue after intravenous administration. *Eur J Clin Pharmacol* 1993; 44: 101–2.
11. Decré D, Bergogne-Bérézin E. Pharmacokinetics of quinolones with special reference to the respiratory tree. *J Antimicrob Chemother* 1993; 31: 331–43.
12. Catchpole C, *et al.* The comparative pharmacokinetics and tissue penetration of single-dose ciprofloxacin 400 mg iv and 750 mg po. *J Antimicrob Chemother* 1994; 33: 103–10.
13. Leeming JP, *et al.* Ocular penetration of topical ciprofloxacin and norfloxacin drugs and their effect upon eyelid flora. *Br J Ophthalmol* 1994; 78: 546–8.
14. Edmiston CE, *et al.* Penetration of ciprofloxacin and fleroxacin into biliary tract. *Antimicrob Agents Chemother* 1996; 40: 787–8.

◊ b. Pharmacokinetics in patients with cystic fibrosis.

1. LeBel M, *et al.* Pharmacokinetics of ciprofloxacin in cystic fibrosis patients. *Antimicrob Agents Chemother* 1986; 30: 260–6.
2. Davis RL, *et al.* Pharmacokinetics of ciprofloxacin in cystic fibrosis. *Antimicrob Agents Chemother* 1987; 31: 915–19.
3. Steen HJ, *et al.* Clinical and pharmacokinetic aspects of ciprofloxacin in the treatment of acute exacerbations of pseudomonas infection in cystic fibrosis patients. *J Antimicrob Chemother* 1989; 24: 787–95.
4. Christensson BA, *et al.* Increased oral bioavailability of ciprofloxacin in cystic fibrosis patients. *Antimicrob Agents Chemother* 1992; 36: 2512–17.
5. Schaefer HG, *et al.* Penetration of ciprofloxacin into paediatric cystic fibrosis patients. *Antimicrob Agents Chemother* 1996; 40: 29–34.

◊ c. Pharmacokinetics in the elderly.

1. LeBel M, *et al.* Pharmacokinetics of ciprofloxacin in elderly subjects. *Pharmacotherapy* 1986; 6: 87–91.
2. Kees F, *et al.* Pharmacokinetics of ciprofloxacin in elderly patients. *Arzneimittelforschung* 1989; 39: 524–7.
3. Ljungberg B, Nilsson-Ehle I. Pharmacokinetics of ciprofloxacin in the elderly: increased oral bioavailability and reduced renal clearance. *Eur J Clin Microbiol Infect Dis* 1989; 8: 515–20.
4. Shah A, *et al.* Pharmacokinetics of high-dose intravenous ciprofloxacin in young and elderly and in male and female subjects. *Antimicrob Agents Chemother* 1995; 39: 1003–6.

◊ d. Pharmacokinetics in hepatic impairment.

1. Esposito S, *et al.* Pharmacokinetics of ciprofloxacin in impaired liver function. *Int J Clin Pharmacol Res* 1989; 9: 37–41.

◊ e. Pharmacokinetics in renal impairment.

1. Roberts DE, Williams JD. Ciprofloxacin in renal failure. *J Antimicrob Chemother* 1989; 23: 820–3.
2. Dharmasena R, *et al.* Pharmacokinetics of ciprofloxacin in patients on CAPD. *J Antimicrob Chemother* 1989; 23: 253–9.
3. Plaisance KI, *et al.* Pharmacokinetics of intraperitoneal ciprofloxacin in patients on CAPD. *J Antimicrob Chemother* 1989; 23: 1031–4.
4. MacGowan AP, *et al.* Serum ciprofloxacin concentrations in patients with severe sepsis being treated with ciprofloxacin 200 mg iv bd irrespective of renal function. *J Antimicrob Chemother* 1994; 33: 1051–4.
5. Shah A, *et al.* Pharmacokinetics of intravenous ciprofloxacin in normal and renally impaired subjects. *J Antimicrob Chemother* 1996; 38: 103–16.

◊ f. Pharmacokinetics in seriously ill patients.

1. Forrest A, *et al.* Development of a population pharmacokinetic model and optimal sampling strategies for intravenous ciprofloxacin. *Antimicrob Agents Chemother* 1993; 37: 1065–72.
2. Forrest A, *et al.* Pharmacodynamics of intravenous ciprofloxacin in seriously ill patients. *Antimicrob Agents Chemother* 1993; 37: 1073–81.
3. Cohn SM, *et al.* Enteric absorption of ciprofloxacin during the immediate postoperative period. *J Antimicrob Chemother* 1995; 36: 717–21.
4. Garrelts JC, *et al.* Ciprofloxacin pharmacokinetics in burn patients. *Antimicrob Agents Chemother* 1996; 40: 1153–6.
5. Owens RC, *et al.* Oral bioavailability and pharmacokinetics of ciprofloxacin in patients with AIDS. *Antimicrob Agents Chemother* 1997; 41: 1508–11.
6. Lipman J, *et al.* Pharmacokinetic profiles of high-dose intravenous ciprofloxacin in severe sepsis. *Antimicrob Agents Chemother* 1998; 42: 2235–9.

Uses and Administration

Ciprofloxacin is a fluorinated 4-quinolone or fluoroquinolone antibacterial with a wider spectrum of activity than nalidixic acid (see Antimicrobial Action, above) and more favourable pharmacokinetics for use in systemic infections. It has been used in the treatment of a wide range of infections including anthrax, biliary-tract infections, infected bites and stings, bone and joint infections, brucellosis, cat scratch disease, chancroid, exacerbations of cystic fibrosis, gastro-enteritis (including travellers' diarrhoea and campylobacter enteritis, cholera, salmonella enteritis, and shigellosis), gonorrhoea, infections in immunocompromised patients (neutropenia), legionnaires' disease, otitis externa, otitis media, peritonitis, Q fever, lower respiratory-tract infections (including pneumococcal pneumonia such as *Streptococcus pneumoniae* pneumococcal pneumonia), septicaemia, skin infections (including soft-tissue infections), spotted fevers, typhoid and paratyphoid fever, typhus, and urinary-tract infections. Ciprofloxacin is used for meningococcal meningitis prophylaxis. It is also used for surgical infection prophylaxis. Fluoroquinolones such as ciprofloxacin and ofloxacin have been tried in the treatment of opportunistic mycobacterial infections and tuberculosis; ofloxacin may be used in the treatment of leprosy. Fluoroquinolones such as ciprofloxacin and ofloxacin are used topically in the treatment of eye infections. For details of all these infections and their treatment, see under Choice of Antibacterial, p.114.

Administration and dosage. Ciprofloxacin is given by mouth as the hydrochloride or base or by intravenous infusion over 30 to 60 minutes as a solution of ciprofloxacin lactate in a concentration of 1 to 2 mg per mL. Eye drops containing ciprofloxacin hydrochloride equivalent to 0.3% of the base are also available.

The usual adult oral dose of ciprofloxacin ranges from 250 to 750 mg twice daily depending on the severity and nature of the infection. The usual intravenous dose is 100 to 400 mg twice daily. A dose of 100 mg twice daily by mouth is suitable in women with acute uncomplicated cystitis.

For acute exacerbations of cystic fibrosis associated with *Pseudomonas aeruginosa* infection, ciprofloxacin may be given to adolescents and children aged 5 years or more in a dose of 20 mg per kg body-weight by mouth twice daily, up to a maximum of 750 mg twice daily. Alternatively a dose of 10 mg per kg may be given by intravenous infusion over 60 minutes three times daily, to a maximum of 400 mg three times daily.

Ciprofloxacin is not generally recommended for other uses in children and adolescents (see Precautions, above) but, if considered essential, doses of 5 to 15 mg per kg twice daily by mouth or 4 to 8 mg per kg twice daily intravenously have been suggested.

Doses should be reduced in patients with severe renal impairment. Halving the dose has been suggested when the creatinine clearance is less than 20 mL per minute or alternatively the dosage interval may be increased; ideally plasma concentrations of ciprofloxacin should be monitored.

Single oral doses of 250 or 500 mg are used for the treatment of gonorrhoea, depending upon patterns of resistance. A single oral dose of 500 mg is suggested for meningococcal meningitis prophylaxis. A single oral dose of 750 mg is suggested for surgical infec...

5. Aubert G, *et al.* Emergence of quinolone-imipenem cross-resistance in Pseudomonas aeruginosa after fluoroquinolone therapy. *J Antimicrob Chemother* 1992; 29: 307–12.
6. Endtz HP, *et al.* Quinolone resistance in campylobacter isolated from man and poultry following the introduction of fluoroquinolones in veterinary medicine. *J Antimicrob Chemother* 1991; 27: 199–208.
7. Bowler I, Day D. Emerging quinolone resistance in campylobacters. *Lancet* 1992; 340: 245.
8. Segreti J, *et al.* High-level quinolone resistance in clinical isolates of Campylobacter jejuni. *J Infect Dis* 1992; 165: 667–70.
9. McIntyre M, Lyons M. Resistance to ciprofloxacin in Campylobacter spp. *Lancet* 1993; 341: 188.
10. Meier PA, *et al.* Development of quinolone-resistant Campylobacter fetus bacteraemia in human immunodeficiency virus-infected patients. *J Infect Dis* 1998; 177: 951–4.
11. Frost JA, *et al.* Increasing ciprofloxacin resistance in salmonellas in England and Wales 1991–1994. *J Infect* 1996; 37: 85–91.
12. Rowe B, *et al.* Ciprofloxacin-resistant Salmonella typhi in the UK. *Lancet* 1995; 346: 1302.
13. Mitchell DH. Ciprofloxacin-resistant Salmonella typhi: an emerging problem. *Med J Aust* 1997; 167: 172.
14. Murdoch DA, *et al.* Epidemic ciprofloxacin-resistant Salmonella typhi in Tajikistan. *Lancet* 1998; 351: 339.
15. Threlfall EJ, *et al.* Ciprofloxacin-resistant Salmonella typhi and treatment failure. *Lancet* 1999; 353: 1590–1.
16. Bhutta ZA. Quinolone-resistant Salmonella paratyphi B meningitis in a newborn: a case report. *J Infect* 1997; 35: 308–10.
17. Aguiar JM, *et al.* The emergence of highly fluoroquinolone-resistant Escherichia coli in community-acquired urinary tract infections. *J Antimicrob Chemother* 1992; 29: 349–50.
18. Threlfall EJ, *et al.* High-level resistance to ciprofloxacin in Escherichia coli. *Lancet* 1997; 349: 403.
19. Fujimaki K, *et al.* Quinolone resistance in clinical isolate of Serratia marcescens. *Antimicrob Agents Chemother* 1989; 33: 785–7.
20. Horiuchi S, *et al.* Reduced susceptibilities of Shigella sonnei strains isolated from patients with dysentery to fluoroquinolones. *Antimicrob Agents Chemother* 1993; 37: 2486–9.
21. Barriere SL, Hindler JA. Ciprofloxacin-resistant Haemophilus influenzae infection in a patient with chronic lung disease. *Ann Pharmacother* 1993; 27: 309–10.
22. Gould IM, *et al.* Quinolone resistant Haemophilus influenzae. *J Antimicrob Chemother* 1994; 33: 187–8.
23. Jephcott AE, Turner A. Ciprofloxacin resistance in gonococci. *Lancet* 1990; 335: 165.
24. Gordon SM, *et al.* The emergence of Neisseria gonorrhoeae with decreased susceptibility to ciprofloxacin in Cleveland, Ohio: epidemiology and risk factors. *Ann Intern Med* 1996; 125: 465–70.
25. Kam K, *et al.* Quinolone-resistant Neisseria gonorrhoeae in Hong Kong. *Sex Transm Dis* 1996; 23: 103–8.
26. Ison CA, *et al.* Drift in susceptibility of Neisseria gonorrhoeae to ciprofloxacin and emergence of therapeutic failure. *Antimicrob Agents Chemother* 1998; 42: 2919–22.
27. Wallace RJ, *et al.* Activities of ciprofloxacin and ofloxacin against rapidly growing mycobacterial with demonstration of acquired resistance following single-drug therapy. *Antimicrob Agents Chemother* 1990; 34: 65–70.
28. Sullivan EA, *et al.* Emergence of fluoroquinolone-resistant tuberculosis in New York City. *Lancet* 1995; 345: 1148–50.
29. Holby N, *et al.* Excretion of ciprofloxacin in sweat and multiresistant Staphylococcus epidermidis. *Lancet* 1997; 349: 167–9.

tion prophylaxis, given 60 to 90 minutes before the procedure.

◊ General references to fluoroquinolone antibacterials.

1. Hooper DC, Wolfson JS. Fluoroquinolone antimicrobial agents. *N Engl J Med* 1991; **324:** 384–94.
2. von Rosensteil N, Adam D. Quinolone antibacterials: an update of their pharmacology and therapeutic use. *Drugs* 1994; **47:** 872–901.
3. Balfour JA, Goa KL, eds. Proceedings of the 5th International symposium on new quinolones. *Drugs* 1995; **49** (suppl 2): 1–505.
4. Walker RC. The fluoroquinolones. *Mayo Clin Proc* 1999; **74:** 1030–7.
5. Smith A, *et al.* Fluoroquinolones: place in ocular therapy. *Drugs* 2001; **61:** 747–61.

◊ General references to ciprofloxacin.

1. Campoli-Richards DM, *et al.* Ciprofloxacin: a review of its antibacterial activity, pharmacokinetic properties and therapeutic use. *Drugs* 1988; **35:** 373–447.
2. Neu HC, ed. Ciprofloxacin: major advances in intravenous and oral quinolone therapy. *Am J Med* 1989; **87** (suppl 5A): 1S–287S.
3. Brown EM, *et al.* eds. Ciprofloxacin—defining its role today. *J Antimicrob Chemother* 1990; **26** (suppl F): 1–193.
4. Davis R, *et al.* Ciprofloxacin: an updated review of its pharmacology, therapeutic efficacy and tolerability. *Drugs* 1996; **51:** 1019–74.
5. Gould FK, *et al.*, eds. Ten years of ciprofloxacin: the past, present and future. *J Antimicrob Chemother* 1999; **43** (suppl A): 1–134.

Administration. Although the usual maximum doses of ciprofloxacin are 750 mg orally or 400 mg intravenously twice daily, higher doses have been used. Notably, the US manufacturer recommends an intravenous dose of 400 mg three times daily in severe infections other than those of the urinary tract.

In a study in patients with suspected shigellosis,[1] a single oral dose of ciprofloxacin 1 g or 1 g daily for 2 days was as effective as the conventional dose of 500 mg twice daily for 5 days except in patients infected with *Shigella dysenteriae* type 1. A single oral dose of ciprofloxacin 500 mg appeared to be effective when given early for the empirical treatment of travellers' diarrhoea.[2] A patient with a renal cyst infection unresponsive to conventional antibacterial therapy improved on ciprofloxacin 600 mg intravenously twice daily for 7 days followed by oral therapy without evidence of toxicity.[3] Long-term therapy with a single 1-g daily dose was also found to be probably more effective than 500 mg twice daily in a study in patients with pulmonary tuberculosis.[4]

1. Bennish ML, *et al.* Treatment of shigellosis III: comparison of one- or two-dose ciprofloxacin with standard 5-day therapy: a randomized, blinded trial. *Ann Intern Med* 1992; **117:** 727–34.
2. Salam I, *et al.* Randomised trial of single-dose ciprofloxacin for travellers' diarrhoea. *Lancet* 1994; **344:** 1537–9.
3. Rossi SJ, *et al.* High-dose ciprofloxacin in the treatment of a renal cyst infection. *Ann Pharmacother* 1993; **27:** 38–9.
4. Bergstermann H, Richardt A. Ciprofloxacin once daily versus twice daily for the treatment of pulmonary tuberculosis. *Infection* 1997; **25:** 227–32.

Inflammatory bowel disease. Ciprofloxacin has been given in combination with metronidazole to treat active Crohn's disease[1] (see Inflammatory Bowel Disease, p.1205).

1. Prantera C, *et al.* An antibiotic regimen for the treatment of active Crohn's disease: a randomized, controlled clinical trial of metronidazole plus ciprofloxacin. *Am J Gastroenterol* 1996; **91:** 328–32.

Preparations

BP 2001: Ciprofloxacin Intravenous Infusion; Ciprofloxacin Tablets;
USP 25: Ciprofloxacin Injection; Ciprofloxacin Ophthalmic Solution; Ciprofloxacin Tablets.

Proprietary Preparations (details are given in Part 3)

Aust.: Ciloxan; Ciproxin; *Austral.:* Ciloquin; Ciloxan; Ciproxin; *Belg.:* Ciloxan; Ciproxine; *Braz.:* Biamotil; Cifox; Ciloxan; Ciprex; Cipro; Procin; Quinoflox; *Canad.:* Ciloxan; Cipro; *Denm.:* Ciloxan; Ciproxin; *Fin.:* Ciloxan; Ciproxin; *Fr.:* Ciflox; Ciloxan; Uniflox; *Ger.:* Ciloxan; Ciprobay; *Hong Kong:* Ciloxan; *Ital.:* Ciproxin; *Irl.:* Ciproxin; Oftacilox; *Mex.:* Arfloxina; Bioflox; Cloxan; Cimogal; Ciprain; Ciprobiotic; Ciprofur; Ciproser; Ciproxina; Ehlikaxin; Eni; Floxakin; Infoxa; Italnik; Kenzoflex; Lemyflox; Lifenxina; Microrgan; Mitroken; Nivoflox; Novoquin; Opthaflox; Proxitec; Quifloxona; Quinoflox; Sophixen; Suiflox; Zipra; *Neth.:* Ciproxin; *Norw.:* Cilox; Ciproxin; *NZ:* Ciloxan; Ciproxin; *Port.:* Carmicina; Ciflan; Ciplox; Ciproquinol; Ciproxina; Estecina; Floxacipron; Giroflox; Keefloxin; Megaflox; Nivoflox; Nixin; Quinox; Xorpic; *S.Afr.:* Ciproxin; Baycip; *Singapore:* Ciloxan; Ciprobay; Uroxin; *Spain:* Aceoto; Baycip; Belmacina; Catex; Ceprimax; Cetraxal; Cipobacter; Ciprenil Otico; Ciprok; Cunesin; Estecina; Felixene; Globuce; Huberdoxina; Inkamil; Oftacilox; Piprol; Plenolyt; Quipro; Rigoran; Sepcen; Septocipro; Tam; Ultramicina; Velmonit; *Swed.:* Ciloxan; Ciproxin; *Switz.:* Ciloxan; Ciproxine; *Thai.:* Cifloxin; Ciprobid; Ciprofrin; Cilab; Ciloxan; Cipflocin; Ciprobay; Ciprobid; Ciprofin; Ciprogen; Ciprolet; Ciprom-H; Ciprosun; Forexin; Medociprin; Policiflox; Proflox; Serviflox; Uroxin; *UAE:* Sarf; *UK:* Ciloxan; Ciproxin; *USA:* Ciloxan; Cipro.

Multi-ingredient: *Austral.:* Ciproxin HC; *Braz.:* Biamctil-D; *Canad.:* Cipro HC; *Denm.:* Ciflox; *Fin.:* Ciproxin-Hydrcorti-son; *USA:* Cipro HC.

Clarithromycin (191-b)

Clarithromycin (BAN, USAN, rINN).

A-56268; Abbott-56268; TE-031. (2R,3S,4S,5R,6R,8R,10R,11R, 12S,13R)-3-(2,6-Dideoxy-3-C,3O-dimethyl-α-L-*ribo*-hexopyranosyloxy)-11,12-dihydroxy-6-methoxy-2,4,6,8,10,12-hexamethyl-9-oxo-5-(3,4,6-trideoxy-3-dimethylamino-β-D-*xylo*-hexopyranosyloxy)pentadecan-13-olide; 6-O-Methylerythromycin.

$C_{38}H_{69}NO_{13} = 748.0$.

CAS — 81103-11-9.

ATC — J01FA09.

Pharmacopoeias. In US.

USP 25: A white to off-white crystalline powder. Practically insoluble in water; slightly soluble in dehydrated alcohol, in methyl alcohol, and in acetonitrile; soluble in acetone; slightly soluble in phosphate buffer at pH values of 2 to 5. pH of a 0.2% suspension in a mixture of water and methyl alcohol (19:1) is between 7.5 and 10.0. Store in airtight containers.

Adverse Effects and Precautions

As for Erythromycin, p.201. Gastrointestinal disturbances are the most frequent adverse effect but are usually mild and less frequent than with erythromycin. Taste disturbances, stomatitis, glossitis, and tooth discoloration have occurred. Transient elevations of liver enzyme values, cholestatic jaundice, and hepatitis have been reported. Headache and rashes from mild skin eruptions to, rarely, Stevens-Johnson syndrome have occurred. There have also been reports of transient CNS effects such as anxiety, dizziness, insomnia, hallucinations, and confusion. Hearing loss has been reported occasionally and is usually reversible. Other adverse effects include hypoglycaemia and thrombocytopenia. Interstitial nephritis and renal failure have been reported rarely.

Intravenous administration may cause phlebitis and pain at the injection site.

Caution is required in patients with impaired renal or hepatic function and doses should be reduced in those with severe renal impairment. It should not be used during pregnancy if possible: high doses have been associated with embryotoxicity in *animal* studies.

Effects on the blood. Single cases of thrombocytopenia[1] and thrombocytopenic purpura[2] associated with clarithromycin administration have been reported.

1. Price TA, Tuazon CU. Clarithromycin-induced thrombocytopenia. *Clin Infect Dis* 1992; **15:** 563–4.
2. Oteo JA, *et al.* Clarithromycin-induced thrombocytopenic purpura. *Clin Infect Dis* 1994; **19:** 1170–1.

Effects on the eyes. Corneal opacities, reversible on discontinuation of treatment, were reported in a patient receiving clarithromycin as part of a regimen for disseminated *Mycobacterium avium* complex infection.[1]

1. Dorrell L, *et al.* Toxicity of clarithromycin in the treatment of *Mycobacterium avium* complex infection in a patient with AIDS. *J Antimicrob Chemother* 1994; **34:** 605–6.

Effects on the gastrointestinal tract. Pseudomembranous colitis associated with *Clostridium difficile* developed in a child receiving clarithromycin.[1]

1. Braeger CP, Nadal D. Clarithromycin and pseudomembranous enterocolitis. *Lancet* 1994; **343:** 241–2.

Effects on the heart. QT prolongation and torsade de pointes was associated with clarithromycin administration in 2 patients.[1] Impaired renal function in 1 patient and impaired hepatic function and organic heart disease in both could have increased their susceptibility to these adverse effects.

1. Lee KL, *et al.* QT prolongation and torsades de pointes associated with clarithromycin. *Am J Med* 1998; **104:** 395–6.

Effects on mental state. Acute psychoses occurred in 2 patients receiving clarithromycin as part of prophylactic treatment for *Helicobacter pylori* infection and were similar to 3 previously reported cases in either AIDS patients or elderly subjects.[1]

1. Gómez-Gil E, *et al.* Clarithromycin-induced acute psychoses in peptic ulcer disease. *Eur J Clin Microbiol Infect Dis* 1999; **18:** 70–1.

Effects on the pancreas. A case of pancreatitis was reported in a patient receiving clarithromycin.[1]

1. Liviu L, *et al.* Pancreatitis induced by clarithromycin. *Ann Intern Med* 1996; **125:** 701.

Effects on the skin. In addition to skin rashes and other hypersensitivity reactions which occasionally occur in patients receiving macrolides, leukocytoclastic vasculitis has been reported in a patient receiving clarithromycin.[1]

1. Gavura SR, Nusinowitz S. Leukocytoclastic vasculitis associated with clarithromycin. *Ann Pharmacother* 1998; **32:** 543–5.

Fever. Fever associated with clarithromycin has been reported in a patient.[1]

1. Kadayifci A, *et al.* Clarithromycin-induced fever in a patient with Helicobacter pylori gastritis. *Ann Pharmacother* 1997; **31:** 788.

Interactions

For a discussion of drug interactions of macrolide antibacterials, see Erythromycin, p.202.

Increased rifabutin toxicity has been reported in patients receiving clarithromycin and rifabutin (p.242) and there has been a report of delirium following concurrent use with fluoxetine (p.287).

Antiretroviral drugs. In studies in healthy subjects[1,2] concurrent administration of the HIV-protease inhibitor *ritonavir* inhibited the metabolism of clarithromycin, producing elevated plasma concentrations and a prolonged half-life. The metabolism of ritonavir was not affected significantly. The manufacturer recommends that the dose of clarithromycin should be reduced in patients with impaired renal function receiving ritonavir and it should be noted that this is an extra reduction over and above that which may be needed for the impaired renal function alone. It has been suggested that other HIV-protease inhibitors and non-nucleoside reverse transcriptase inhibitors may have a similar effect on clarithromycin. Administration of *efavirenz* with clarithromycin has resulted in decreases in the plasma concentration of clarithromycin and increases in its hydroxy metabolite. The combination has been associated with a high incidence of skin rashes.

Decreased concentrations of *zidovudine* (p.646) have been reported in patients also taking clarithromycin and the manufacturer recommends that doses of the two drugs should be separated by 1 to 2 hours.

1. Ouellet D, *et al.* Assessment of the pharmacokinetic interaction between ritonavir and clarithromycin. *Clin Pharmacol Ther* 1996; **59:** 143.
2. Ouellet D, *et al.* Pharmacokinetic interaction between ritonavir and clarithromycin. *Clin Pharmacol Ther* 1998; **64:** 355–62.

Cimetidine. Although a study in healthy subjects suggested that some pharmacokinetic parameters of clarithromycin are altered by concurrent cimetidine administration,[1] the clinical significance of such changes are unknown.

1. Amsden GW, *et al.* Oral cimetidine prolongs clarithromycin absorption. *Antimicrob Agents Chemother* 1998; **42:** 1578–80.

Omeprazole. In a study in healthy subjects, increased concentrations of clarithromycin and its active metabolite were observed in gastric tissue and mucus and, to a lesser extent, in plasma during concomitant administration of omeprazole.[1] In addition, administration of clarithromycin with omeprazole resulted in higher and more prolonged plasma concentrations of omeprazole. The investigators suggest that this interaction could account for the synergistic action observed with this combination when used for eradication of *Helicobacter pylori*. However, the manufacturers of clarithromycin have noted that no dosage alteration to either drug is necessary.

1. Gustavson LE, *et al.* Effect of omeprazole on concentrations of clarithromycin in plasma and gastric tissue at steady state. *Antimicrob Agents Chemother* 1995; **39:** 2078–83.

Antimicrobial Action

As for Erythromycin, p.203. Clarithromycin is reported to be more active than erythromycin against susceptible streptococci and staphylococci *in vitro*, as well as against some other species including *Moraxella catarrhalis* (*Branhamella catarrhalis*), *Legionella* spp., *Chlamydia trachomatis*, and *Ureaplasma urealyticum*. MICs are usually two- to fourfold lower than for erythromycin. Clarithromycin is reported to be more active than erythromycin or azithromycin against some mycobacteria, including *Mycobacterium avium* complex, and against *M. leprae*. It is reported to have some *in-vitro* activity against the protozoan *Toxoplasma gondii*, and may have some activity against cryptosporidia. The major metabolite, 14-hydroxyclarithromycin, is also active, and may enhance the activity of clarithromycin *in vivo*, notably against *Haemophilus influenzae*.

Activity with other antimicrobials. Clarithromycin has been reported to enhance the activity of a number of antimycobacterials including ethambutol, isoniazid, pyrazinamide, and rifampicin against *Mycobacterium tuberculosis*.[1,2]

1. Cavalieri SJ, *et al.* Synergistic activities of clarithromycin and antituberculous drugs against multi-drug-resistant Mycobacterium tuberculosis. *Antimicrob Agents Chemother* 1995; **39:** 1542–5.
2. Mor N, Esfandiari A. Synergistic activities of clarithromycin and pyrazinamide against Mycobacterium tuberculosis in human macrophages. *Antimicrob Agents Chemother* 1997; **41:** 2035–6.

Resistance. Erythromycin-resistant isolates of *Streptococcus pneumoniae* are commonly cross-resistant to clarithromycin.[1] The incidence of resistance to clarithromycin and other macrolides is higher among penicillin-resistant strains than among penicillin-sensitive strains.[2] Clarithromycin-resistant isolates of *Helicobacter pylori* are also emerging.[3,4] Genetic mutations responsible for clarithromycin resistance have been identified in *H. pylori*[5] and in *Mycobacterium* spp.[6,7] Since resistance develops rapidly in *Mycobacterium avium* during clarithromycin monotherapy, combination therapy is usually recommended. However, resistance to clarithromycin in an AIDS patient with systemic *Mycobacterium avium* complex infection, despite combined treatment with clofazimine, has been described.[8]

1. Lonks JR, Medeiros AA. High rate of erythromycin and clarithromycin resistance among Streptococcus pneumoniae isolates from blood cultures from Providence, RI. *Antimicrob Agents Chemother* 1993; **37:** 1742–5.
2. Barry AL, *et al.* Macrolide resistance among Streptococcus pneumoniae and Streptococcus pyogenes isolates from out-patients in the USA. *J Antimicrob Chemother* 1997; **40:** 139–40.
3. López-Brea M, *et al.* Evolution of resistance to metronidazole and clarithromycin in Helicobacter pylori clinical isolates from Spain. *J Antimicrob Chemother* 1997; **40:** 279–81.
4. Hultén K, *et al.* Macrolide resistance in Helicobacter pylori: mechanism and stability in strains from clarithromycin-treated patients. *Antimicrob Agents Chemother* 1997; **41:** 2550–3.
5. Versalovic J, *et al.* Mutations in 23S rRNA are associated with clarithromycin resistance in Helicobacter pylori. *Antimicrob Agents Chemother* 1996; **40:** 477–80.
6. Nash KA, Inderlied CB. Genetic basis of macrolide resistance in Mycobacterium avium isolated from patients with disseminated disease. *Antimicrob Agents Chemother* 1995; **39:** 2625–30.
7. Wallace RJ, *et al.* Genetic basis for clarithromycin resistance among isolates of Mycobacterium chelonae and Mycobacterium abscessus. *Antimicrob Agents Chemother* 1996; **40:** 1676–81.
8. De Wit S, *et al.* Acquired resistance to clarithromycin as combined therapy in Mycobacterium avium intracellulare infection. *Lancet* 1993; **341:** 53–4.

Pharmacokinetics

Clarithromycin is rapidly absorbed from the gastrointestinal tract following oral administration, and undergoes first-pass metabolism; the bioavailability of the parent drug is about 55%. The extent of absorption is relatively unaffected by the presence of food. Peak concentrations of clarithromycin and its principal active metabolite 14-hydroxyclarithromycin are reported to be about 0.6 and 0.7 µg per mL respectively following a single 250-mg dose by mouth; at steady state the same dose given every 12 hours as tablets produces peak concentrations of clarithromycin of about 1 µg per mL. The same dose given as a suspension produces a steady-state plasma concentration of about 2 µg per mL.

The pharmacokinetics of clarithromycin are non-linear and dose dependent; high doses may produce disproportionate increases in peak concentration of the parent drug, due to saturation of the metabolic pathways.

The drug and its principal metabolite are widely distributed, and tissue concentrations exceed those in serum, in part because of intracellular uptake. Clarithromycin has been detected in breast milk. It is extensively metabolised in the liver, and excreted in faeces via the bile. Substantial amounts are excreted in urine; at steady state about 20% and 30% of a 250-mg or 500-mg dose, respectively, is excreted in this way, as unchanged drug. 14-Hydroxyclarithromycin as well as other metabolites are also excreted in the urine accounting for 10 to 15% of the dose. The terminal half-life of clarithromycin is reportedly about 3 to 4 hours in patients receiving 250-mg doses twice daily, and about 5 to 7 hours in those receiving 500 mg twice daily. The half-life is prolonged in renal impairment.

◊ Reviews.
1. Rodvold KA. Clinical pharmacokinetics of clarithromycin. *Clin Pharmacokinet* 1999; **37:** 385–98.

Uses and Administration

Clarithromycin is a macrolide derived from erythromycin with similar actions and uses (p.203). It is given in the treatment of respiratory-tract infections (including otitis media) and in skin and soft-tissue infections. Clarithromycin is also used in the treatment of leprosy and for prophylaxis and treatment of opportunistic mycobacterial infections. It is used in some countries as an alternative to penicillins for prophylaxis of endocarditis. For details of all these infections and their treatment, see under Choice of Antibacterial, p.114.

Clarithromycin may be given to eradicate *Helicobacter pylori* in treatment regimens for peptic ulcer disease (p.1208). It has been tried in protozoal infections, including toxoplasmosis (p.585).

Clarithromycin is given by mouth or by intravenous infusion. Usual doses in adults are 250 mg twice daily by mouth, increased to 500 mg twice daily if necessary in severe infection. Modified-release tablets allowing once-daily administration are available in some countries. A course is usually for 7 to 14 days. Children may be given 7.5 mg per kg body-weight twice daily for 5 to 10 days.

The usual intravenous dose is 500 mg twice daily, given as an intravenous infusion over 60 minutes using a solution containing about 0.2% of clarithromycin. Intravenous treatment may continue for 2 to 5 days, but should be changed to clarithromycin by mouth when possible.

For disseminated infection due to *Mycobacterium avium* complex, clarithromycin may be given in a dose of 500 mg twice daily by mouth, with other antimycobacterials. For leprosy, clarithromycin 500 mg daily by mouth has been given as part of an alternative multidrug therapy regimen (p.126).

For the eradication of *H. pylori* associated with peptic ulcer disease, clarithromycin, usually in a dose of 500 mg twice daily, is given with another antibacterial and either a proton pump inhibitor or a histamine H_2-receptor antagonist, for 7 to 14 days.

In patients with severe renal impairment (creatinine clearance of less than 30 mL per minute) dosage may need to be halved.

◊ Reviews.
1. Peters DH, Clissold SP. Clarithromycin: a review of its antimicrobial activity, pharmacokinetic properties and therapeutic potential. *Drugs* 1992; **44:** 117–64.
2. Barradell LB, *et al.* Clarithromycin: a review of its pharmacological properties and therapeutic use in Mycobacterium avium-intracellulare complex infection in patients with acquired immune deficiency syndrome. *Drugs* 1993; **46:** 289–312.
3. Williams JD, Sefton AM. Comparison of macrolide antibiotics *J Antimicrob Chemother* 1993; **31** (suppl C): 11–26.
4. Markham A, McTavish D. Clarithromycin and omeprazole: as Helicobacter pylori eradication therapy in patients with H. pylori-associated gastric disorders. *Drugs* 1996; **51:** 161–78.
5. Alvarez-Elcoro S, Enzler MJ. The macrolides: erythromycin, clarithromycin, and azithromycin. *Mayo Clin Proc* 1999; **74:** 613–34.

Preparations

USP 25: Clarithromycin for Oral Suspension; Clarithromycin Tablets.

Proprietary Preparations (details are given in Part 3)
Aust.: Klacid; Maclar; *Austral.:* Klacid; *Belg.:* Biclar; Heliclar; Maclar; Monaxin; *Braz.:* Klaricid; *Canad.:* Biaxin; *Denm.:* Klacid; *Fin.:* Klacid; Zeclar; *Fr.:* Naxy; Zeclar; *Ger.:* Biaxin; Cyllind; Klacid; Mavid; *Hong Kong:* Klacid; *Irl.:* Klacid; *Israel:* Karin; Klacid; *Ital.:* Klacid; Macladin; Veclam; *Mex.:* Adel; Klaricid; Mabicrol; *Neth.:* Klacid; *Norw.:* Klacid; *NZ:* Klacid; *Port.:* Klacid; Maclar; *S.Afr.:* Klacid; *Singapore:* Klacid; *Spain:* Bremon; Klacid; Kofron; *Swed.:* Klacid; *Switz.:* Klacid; Klaciped; *Thai.:* Klacid; *UAE:* Clamycin; *UK:* Klaricid; *USA:* Biaxin.

Multi-ingredient: *Austral.:* Klacid HP 7; Losec Hp 7; PyloridKA; *Canad.:* Hp-Pac; Losec 1-2-3 A; Losec 1-2-3 M; *Fin.:* Helipak K; *Neth.:* PantoPAC; *NZ:* Klacid HP7; Losec Hp7; *S.Afr.:* Losec 20 Triple; *UK:* Heliclear; HeliMet; *USA:* Prevpac.

Clavulanic Acid (18258-v)

Clavulanic Acid (BAN, rINN).
BRL-14151; MM-14151. (Z)-(2R,5R)-3-(2-Hydroxyethylidene)-7-oxo-4-oxa-1-azabicyclo[3.2.0]heptane-2-carboxylic acid.
$C_8H_9NO_5 = 199.2$.
CAS — 58001-44-8 (clavulanic acid); 57943-81-4 (sodium clavulanate).

Potassium Clavulanate (153-p)

Potassium Clavulanate (BANM, rINNM).
BRL-14151K; Clavulanate Potassium (USAN); Kalii Clavulanas.
$C_8H_8KNO_5 = 237.3$.
CAS — 61177-45-5.

NOTE. Compounded preparations of potassium clavulanate may be represented by the following names:

- Co-amoxiclav *x/y* (*BAN*)—amoxicillin (as the trihydrate or the sodium salt) and potassium clavulanate; *x* and *y* are the strengths in milligrams of amoxicillin and clavulanic acid respectively
- Co-amoxiclav (*USP 25*)—amoxicillin trihydrate and potassium clavulanate.

Pharmacopoeias. In Eur. (see p.vi), Jpn, Pol., and US.

1.19 g of potassium clavulanate is approximately equivalent to 1 g of clavulanic acid.

Pharmacopoeial description

Ph. Eur.: The potassium salt of a substance produced by the growth of certain strains of *Streptomyces clavuligerus* or by any other means. A white or almost white, hygroscopic, crystalline powder. Freely soluble in water; slightly soluble in alcohol; very slightly soluble in acetone. A 1% solution in water has a pH of 5.5 to 7.5. Store in airtight containers.

USP 25: A white to off-white powder. Freely soluble in water; soluble in methyl alcohol with decomposition. Stability in aqueous solutions is not good, optimum stability at a pH of 6.0 to 6.3. pH of a 1% solution in water is between 5.5 and 8.0. Store in airtight containers.

Profile

Clavulanic acid is produced by cultures of *Streptomyces clavuligerus*. It has a beta-lactam structure resembling that of the penicillin nucleus, except that the fused thiazolidine ring of the penicillins is replaced by an oxazolidine ring. In general, clavulanic acid has only weak antibacterial activity. It is a potent progressive inhibitor of plasmid-mediated and some chromosomal beta-lactamases produced by Gram-negative bacteria including *Haemophilus ducreyi*, *H. influenzae*, *Neisseria gonorrhoeae*, *Moraxella catarrhalis* (*Branhamella catarrhalis*), *Bacteroides fragilis*, and some Enterobacteriaceae. It is also an inhibitor of the beta-lactamases produced by *Staphylococcus aureus*. Clavulanic acid can permeate bacterial cell walls and can therefore inactivate both extracellular enzymes and those that are bound to the cell. Its mode of action depends on the particular enzyme inhibited, but it generally acts as a competitive, and often irreversible, inhibitor. Clavulanic acid consequently enhances the activity of penicillin and cephalosporin antibacterials against many resistant strains of bacteria. However, it is generally less effective against chromosomally mediated type 1 beta-lactamases; therefore, many *Citrobacter*, *Enterobacter*, *Morganella*, and *Serratia* spp., and *Pseudomonas aeruginosa* remain resistant. Some plasmid-mediated extended-spectrum beta-lactamases in *Klebsiella pneumoniae*, some other Enterobacteriaceae, and *Ps. aeruginosa* are also not inhibited by beta-lactamase inhibitors.

It is given as potassium clavulanate by mouth and injection in combination with amoxicillin (co-amoxiclav) (p.149), and by injection in combination with ticarcillin (p.262).

Administration of clavulanate with penicillins has been associated with the development of cholestatic jaundice and hepatitis (see Amoxicillin, Adverse Effects, p.149) and therefore the use of co-amoxiclav has declined (see below).

◊ Because of the risk of cholestatic jaundice co-amoxiclav is not a treatment of choice for common bacterial infections. The UK Committee on Safety of Medicines[1] recommends that it should be reserved for bacterial infections likely to be caused by amoxicillin-resistant beta-lactamase producing strains and that treatment should not usually exceed 14 days. It may be considered for the following main indications:

- sinusitis, otitis media, recurrent tonsillitis
- acute exacerbations of chronic bronchitis
- bronchopneumonia
- urinary-tract infections, especially when recurrent or complicated, but not prostatitis
- septic abortion, pelvic or puerperal sepsis, and intra-abdominal sepsis
- cellulitis, animal bites, and severe dental abscess with spreading cellulitis.

1. Committee on Safety of Medicines/Medicines Control Agency. Revised indications for co-amoxiclav (Augmentin). *Current Problems* 1997; **23:** 8.

◊ References.
1. Watson ID, *et al.* Clinical pharmacokinetics of enzyme inhibitors in antimicrobial chemotherapy. *Clin Pharmacokinet* 1988; **15:** 133–64.

Preparations

BP 2001: Co-amoxiclav Tablets;
USP 25: Amoxicillin and Clavulanate Potassium for Oral Suspension; Amoxicillin and Clavulanate Potassium Tablets; Ticarcillin and Clavulanic Acid for Injection; Ticarcillin and Clavulanic Acid Injection.

Proprietary Preparations (details are given in Part 3)
Belg.: Clavucid; *Denm.:* Spektramox.

Multi-ingredient: *Aust.:* Amoclan; Augmentin; Clavamox; Timenten†; *Austral.:* Augmentin; Ausclav; Clamoxyl; Clavulin; Timentin; *Belg.:* Augmentin; Timentin; *Braz.:* Augmentin; Clavoxil; Clavulin; Novamox; Timentin; *Canad.:* Clavulin; Timentin; *Fin.:* Amoxin Comp; Augmentin; Spektramox; *Fr.:* Augmentin; Ciblor; Claventin; *Ger.:* Amoclav; Amoxi-Clavulan; Amoxidura; Amoxillat-Clav; Augmentan; Betabactyl†; *Hong Kong:* Amoksiklav; Augmentin; Curam; Moxiclav; Timentin; *Irl.:* Augmentin; Clavamel; Germentin; Timentin; *Israel:* Augmentin; Timentin; *Ital.:* Augmentin; Clavucar; Clavulin; Neoduplamox; Timentin; *Mex.:* Amoxiclav; Augmentin; Clavulin; Eumetinex; Servamox CLV; Timentin; *Neth.:* Augmentin; Timentin; *Norw.:* Bremide; *NZ:* Alpha-Amoxyclav; Augmentin; Synermox; Timentin; *Port.:* Amoclavam; Augmentin; Betamox; Clavamox; Clavepen; Penilan; *S.Afr.:* Augmaxil; Augmentin; Clamentin; Ranclav; Servamox CLV; Timentin; *Singapore:* Augmentin; Clamonex; Curam; Enhancin; Moxiclav; *Spain:* Amoclave; Amoxyplus; Augmentine; Bigpen; Burmicin; Clavepen; Clavucid; Clavumox; Duonasa; Eupeclanic; Inmupen;

Kelsopen†; Pangamox; **Swed.:** Spektramox; **Switz.:** Augmentin; Aziclav; Timenten; **Thai.:** Amoksiklav; Augmentin; Cavumox; Curam; **UAE:** Julmentin; **UK:** Amiclav; Augmentin; Augmentin-Duo; Timentin; **USA:** Augmentin; Timentin.

Clemizole Penicillin (53-b)

Clemizole Penicillin (BAN, rINN).

Clemizole Benzylpenicillin; Penicillin G Clemizole. 1-[1-(4-Chlorobenzyl)benzimidazol-2-ylmethyl]pyrrolidinium (6R)-6-(2-phenylacetamido)penicillanate.

$C_{16}H_{18}N_2O_4S,C_{19}H_{20}ClN_3 = 660.2$.

CAS — 6011-39-8.

Profile

Clemizole penicillin is a long-acting preparation of benzylpenicillin (p.157) with similar properties and uses.

Preparations

Proprietary Preparations (details are given in Part 3)

Aust.: Clemipen†; **Mex.:** Megapenil; **Switz.:** Megacilline.

Multi-ingredient: Aust.: Antipen†; **Mex.:** Anapenil; Megapenil Forte; **Port.:** Previcilina; **Spain:** Anapen†; Neopenyl.

Clinafloxacin Hydrochloride (15475-y)

Clinafloxacin Hydrochloride (USAN, rINN).

CI-960 (clinafloxacin); PD-127391. (±)-7-(3-Amino-1-pyrrolidinyl)-8-chloro-1-cyclopropyl-6-fluoro-1,4-dihydro-4-oxo-3-quinolinecarboxylic acid hydrochloride.

$C_{17}H_{17}ClFN_3O_3,HCl = 402.2$.

CAS — 105956-97-6 (clinafloxacin); 105956-99-8 (clinafloxacin hydrochloride).

Profile

Clinafloxacin is a fluoroquinolone antibacterial.

◊ References.

1. Humphrey GH, et al. Pharmacokinetics of clinafloxacin enantiomers in humans. J Clin Pharmacol 1999; **39:** 1143–50.

Clindamycin Hydrochloride (55-g)

Clindamycin Hydrochloride (BANM, rINN).

Chlorodeoxylincomycin Hydrochloride; (7S)-Chloro-7-deoxylincomycin Hydrochloride; Clindamycini Hydrochloridum; U-21251 (clindamycin). Methyl 6-amino-7-chloro-6,7,8-trideoxy-N-[(2S,4R)-1-methyl-4-propylprolyl]-1-thio-L-threo-D-galacto-octopyranoside hydrochloride.

$C_{18}H_{33}ClN_2O_5S,HCl = 461.4$.

CAS — 18323-44-9 (clindamycin); 21462-39-5 (anhydrous clindamycin hydrochloride); 58207-19-5 (clindamycin hydrochloride monohydrate).

NOTE. Clindamycin is USAN.

The name Clinimycin, which was formerly used for clindamycin, has also been used for a preparation of oxytetracycline.

Pharmacopoeias. In Chin., Eur. (see p.vi), Pol., and US.

1.13 g of monograph substance is approximately equivalent to 1 g of clindamycin.

Pharmacopoeial description

Ph. Eur.: A white or almost white, crystalline powder. It contains a variable quantity of water. Very soluble in water; slightly soluble in alcohol. A 10% solution in water has a pH of 3.0 to 5.0. Store at a temperature not exceeding 30° in airtight containers.

USP 25: A white or practically white crystalline powder, odourless or has a faint mercaptan-like odour. Freely soluble in water, in dimethylformamide, and in methyl alcohol; soluble in alcohol; practically insoluble in acetone. pH of a 10% solution in water is between 3.0 and 5.5. Store in airtight containers.

Clindamycin Palmitate Hydrochloride (54-v)

Clindamycin Palmitate Hydrochloride (BANM, USAN, rINN).

U-25179E. Clindamycin 2-palmitate hydrochloride.

$C_{34}H_{63}ClN_2O_6S,HCl = 699.9$.

CAS — 36688-78-5 (clindamycin palmitate); 25507-04-4 (clindamycin palmitate hydrochloride).

Pharmacopoeias. In US.

1.6 g of monograph substance is approximately equivalent to 1 g of clindamycin.

Pharmacopoeial description

USP 25: A white to off-white amorphous powder having a characteristic odour. Freely soluble in water, in chloroform, in ether, and in benzene; soluble 1 in 3 of alcohol and 1 in 9 of ethyl acetate; very soluble in dimethylformamide. pH of a 1% solution in water is between 2.8 and 3.8. Store in airtight containers.

Clindamycin Phosphate (56-q)

Clindamycin Phosphate (BANM, USAN, rINN).

Clindamycini Phosphas; U-28508. Clindamycin 2-(dihydrogen phosphate).

$C_{18}H_{34}ClN_2O_8PS = 505.0$.

CAS — 24729-96-2.

Pharmacopoeias. In Eur. (see p.vi), Jpn, and US.

1.2 g of monograph substance is approximately equivalent to 1 g of clindamycin.

Incompatibilities. Solutions of clindamycin salts have an acid pH and incompatibility may reasonably be expected with alkaline preparations, or with drugs unstable at low pH. Clindamycin phosphate is incompatible with natural rubber closures.

Pharmacopoeial description

Ph. Eur.: A white or almost white, slightly hygroscopic powder. It exhibits polymorphism. Freely soluble in water; very slightly soluble in alcohol; practically insoluble in dichloromethane and in ether. A 1% solution in water has a pH of 3.5 to 4.5. Store at a temperature not exceeding 30° in airtight containers.

USP 25: A white to off-white, odourless or practically odourless, hygroscopic, crystalline powder. Soluble 1 in 2.5 of water; slightly soluble in dehydrated alcohol; very slightly soluble in acetone; practically insoluble in chloroform, in ether, and in benzene. pH of a 1% solution in water is between 3.5 and 4.5. Store in airtight containers.

Adverse Effects

Clindamycin is reported to produce diarrhoea in about 2 to 20% of patients after systemic administration; in some patients severe antibiotic-associated or pseudomembranous colitis may develop, and has proved fatal. The syndrome, which may develop during therapy or several weeks later, appears to be due to toxins produced by Clostridium spp., most notably C. difficile. It has been reported to be more frequent in women and in elderly patients, and may also occur rarely after topical administration. Other gastrointestinal effects reported with clindamycin include nausea, vomiting, abdominal pain or cramps, and unpleasant or metallic taste after high intravenous doses.

Hypersensitivity reactions, including skin rashes in up to 10% of patents, urticaria, and very rarely anaphylaxis, have occurred. Other adverse effects include transient leucopenia or occasionally agranulocytosis, eosinophilia, thrombocytopenia, erythema multiforme, exfoliative and vesiculobullous dermatitis, polyarthritis, and abnormalities of liver function tests; in some cases overt jaundice and hepatic damage have been reported. Although local irritation is stated to be rare, intramuscular injection has led to sterile abscess, and thrombophlebitis may occur after intravenous administration. Some parenteral formulations contain benzyl alcohol which may cause fatal 'gasping syndrome' in neonates.

Topical application may be associated with local irritation and contact dermatitis; sufficient clindamycin may be absorbed to produce systemic effects. Cervicitis, vaginitis, or vulvovaginal irritation has been reported with intravaginal use; a small amount of systemic absorption also occurs.

Effects on the cardiovascular system. Cardiac arrest occurred in a 50-year-old woman after rapid injection of 600 mg of undiluted clindamycin phosphate into a central intravenous line. Further injections were given over 30 minutes without cardiovascular complications.[1]

1. Aucoin P, et al. Clindamycin-induced cardiac arrest. South Med J 1982; **75:** 768.

Effects on the gastrointestinal tract. References to antibiotic-associated colitis and the role of clindamycin.

1. Tedesco FJ, et al. Clindamycin-associated colitis: a prospective study. Ann Intern Med 1974; **81:** 429–33.
2. Robertson MB, et al. Incidence of antibiotic-related diarrhoea and pseudomembranous colitis: a prospective study of lincomycin, clindamycin and ampicillin. Med J Aust 1977; **1:** 243–6.
3. Committee on Safety of Medicines. Antibiotic induced colitis. Adverse Reactions Series 17 1979.
4. Borriello SP, Larson HE. Antibiotic and pseudomembranous colitis. J Antimicrob Chemother 1981; **7** (suppl A): 53–62.
5. Milstone EB, et al. Pseudomembranous colitis after topical application of clindamycin. Arch Dermatol 1981; **117:** 154–5.
6. Parry MF, Rha C-K. Pseudomembranous colitis caused by topical clindamycin phosphate. Arch Dermatol 1986; **122:** 583–4.
7. Young GP, et al. Antibiotic-associated colitis caused by Clostridium difficile: relapse and risk factors. Med J Aust 1986; **144:** 303–6.

Effects on the lymphatic system. Lymphadenitis was associated with clindamycin administration in a patient.[1]

1. Southern PM. Lymphadenitis associated with the administration of clindamycin. Am J Med 1997; **103:** 164–5.

Effects on the skin. A report of toxic epidermal necrolysis associated with clindamycin.[1]

1. Paquet P, et al. Toxic epidermal necrolysis following clindamycin treatment. Br J Dermatol 1995; **132:** 665–6.

Treatment of Adverse Effects

Clindamycin should be withdrawn immediately if significant diarrhoea or colitis occurs. Metronidazole or vancomycin may be used to treat antibiotic-associated pseudomembranous colitis. For further details, see under Gastro-enteritis, p.122.

Precautions

Clindamycin should not be given to patients hypersensitive to it or to the closely-related drug lincomycin. It should be used with caution in patients with gastrointestinal disease, particularly those with a history of colitis. Clindamycin should be withdrawn immediately if significant diarrhoea or colitis occurs. Elderly and female patients may be more likely to experience severe diarrhoea or pseudomembranous colitis. Caution has also been advised in atopic patients. Patients with hepatic or renal impairment may require dosage adjustment. Periodic tests of liver and kidney function and blood counts have been recommended in patients receiving prolonged therapy, and in infants. Clindamycin is distributed into breast milk and it should be given with caution during breast feeding.

AIDS. Clindamycin was poorly tolerated by patients with AIDS in a study of its use for prophylaxis of toxoplasmic encephalitis. Despite the use of relatively low doses of clindamycin (300 mg twice daily) 23 of 52 patients reported adverse effects that necessitated temporary or permanent withdrawal of the drug, the most frequent adverse reactions being diarrhoea and skin rash. The clindamycin arm of the study had to be terminated prematurely.[1] Nevertheless, clindamycin has been used successfully in patients with AIDS for the treatment of both toxoplasmic encephalitis (below) and Pneumocystis carinii pneumonia (below).

1. Jacobson MA, et al. Toxicity of clindamycin as prophylaxis for AIDS-associated toxoplasmic encephalitis. Lancet 1992; **339:** 333–4.

Interactions

Clindamycin has neuromuscular blocking activity in high doses and may enhance the effect of other drugs with this action (p.1334), with a potential danger of respiratory depression. Clindamycin may antagonise the activity of parasympathomimetics. For reports of synergistic and antagonistic antimicrobial activity with other antibacterials, see Antimicrobial Action, below.

Adsorbents. In 16 healthy subjects given clindamycin alone and with a kaolin-pectin suspension it was found that the suspension had no effect on the extent of clindamycin absorption but did markedly reduce the absorption rate.[1]

1. Albert KS, et al. Pharmacokinetic evaluation of a drug interaction between kaolin-pectin and clindamycin. J Pharm Sci 1978; **67:** 1579–82.

Antimicrobial Action

Clindamycin is a lincosamide antibiotic with a primarily bacteriostatic action against Gram-positive aerobes and a wide range of anaerobic bacteria.

Mechanism of action. Lincosamides such as clindamycin bind to the 50S subunit of the bacterial ribosome, similarly to macrolides such as erythromycin (p.203), and inhibit the early stages of protein synthesis. The action of clindamycin is predominantly bacteriostatic, although high concentrations may be slowly bactericidal against sensitive strains.

Spectrum of activity. Clindamycin is active against most aerobic Gram-positive bacteria including streptococci, staphylococci, Bacillus anthracis, and Corynebacterium diphtheriae; enterococci, however, are generally resistant.

Clindamycin has good activity against a wide range of anaerobic bacteria. Susceptible Gram-positive anaerobes include Eubacterium, Propionibacterium, Peptococcus, and Peptostreptococcus spp., and many strains of Clostridium perfringens and Cl. tetani. Among Gram-negative anaerobes susceptible to clindamycin are Fusobacterium spp. (although F. varium is usually resistant), Veillonella, and Bacteroides spp., including the B. fragilis group.

Apart from *Mycoplasma hominis,* clindamycin is generally less active than erythromycin against *Mycoplasma* spp. Several *Actinomyces* spp. and *Nocardia asteroides* are reported to be susceptible.

Most Gram-negative aerobic bacteria, including the Enterobacteriaceae, are resistant to clindamycin; unlike erythromycin, *Neisseria gonorrhoeae, N. meningitidis,* and *Haemophilus influenzae* are generally resistant to clindamycin.

Fungi, yeasts, and viruses are also resistant; however, clindamycin has been reported to have some antiprotozoal activity against *Toxoplasma gondii* and *Plasmodium* spp.

Minimum inhibitory concentrations (MICs) of clindamycin have been reported to be as low as 0.002 µg per mL for the most sensitive strains of *Streptococcus pneumoniae* but MICs for sensitive streptococci, staphylococci, and anaerobes such as *Bacteroides fragilis* or *Fusobacterium* spp. are usually in the range 0.01 to 0.5 µg per mL. Organisms with MICs up to about 1.6 µg per mL are considered sensitive, and those with MICs between about 1.6 and 4.8 µg per mL of moderate sensitivity.

Activity with other antimicrobials. Synergistic activity has been reported between clindamycin and ceftazidime or metronidazole, and also with ciprofloxacin against some anaerobes. However, there is some evidence that clindamycin inhibits the bactericidal activity of the aminoglycosides, although conflicting reports have suggested variable degrees of synergy against anaerobic organisms. Because of the adjacency of their binding sites on the ribosome, clindamycin may competitively inhibit the effects of macrolides or chloramphenicol. Clindamycin has been reported to diminish the activity of ampicillin *in vitro* against *Staph. aureus.* It is reported to enhance the activity of primaquine against *Pneumocystis carinii.*

Resistance. Most Gram-negative aerobes, such as the Enterobacteriaceae, are intrinsically resistant to clindamycin, but acquired resistance also occurs in normally sensitive strains. The mechanisms of resistance are the same as those for erythromycin, namely methylation of the ribosomal binding site, chromosomal mutation of the ribosomal protein, and in a few staphylococcal isolates enzymic inactivation by a plasmid-mediated adenyltransferase. Methylation of the ribosome leads to cross-resistance between the lincosamides and macrolides and streptogramins (the MLS$_B$ phenotype); this type of resistance is usually plasmid-mediated and inducible. Complete cross-resistance exists between clindamycin and lincomycin.

The incidence of resistance varies with the organism and the geographical location; it is more frequent in organisms that are also erythromycin resistant, and many strains of meticillin-resistant *Staphylococcus aureus* are also resistant to clindamycin. In some countries and institutions there is evidence of an increase in resistance amongst the *Bacteroides fragilis* group to 25% of strains or more.

Action. References suggesting that clindamycin may reduce microbial adherence and enhance phagocytosis by its effects on bacterial slime (glycocalyx)[1-3] and that its antibacterial effects may be independent of plasma concentrations.[4,5]

1. Veringa EM, *et al.* Enhancement of opsonophagocytosis of Bacteroides spp by clindamycin in subinhibitory concentrations. *J Antimicrob Chemother* 1981; **23**: 577–87.
2. Veringa EM, *et al.* The role of glycocalyx in surface phagocytosis of Bacteroides spp, in the presence and absence of clindamycin. *J Antimicrob Chemother* 1989; **23**: 711–20.
3. Khardori N, *et al.* Effect of subinhibitory concentrations of clindamycin and trospectomycin on the adherence of Staphylococcus epidermidis in an in vitro model of vascular catheter colonization. *J Infect Dis* 1991; **164**: 108–13.
4. Xue IB, *et al.* Variation in postantibiotic effect of clindamycin against clinical isolates of Staphylococcus aureus and implications for dosing of patients with osteomyelitis. *Antimicrob Agents Chemother* 1996; **40**: 1403–7.
5. Klepser ME, *et al.* Bactericidal activity of low-dose clindamycin administered at 8- and 12-hour intervals against Staphylococcus aureus, Streptococcus pneumoniae, and Bacteroides fragilis. *Antimicrob Agents Chemother* 1997; **41**: 630–5.

Activity against protozoa and fungi. References.

1. Lewis C. Antiplasmodial activity of 7-halogenated lincomycins. *J Parasitol* 1968; **54**: 169–70.

2. Araujo FG, Remington JS. Effect of clindamycin on acute and chronic toxoplasmosis in mice. *Antimicrob Agents Chemother* 1874; **5**: 647–51.
3. Mack DG, McLeod R. New micromethod to study the effect of antimicrobial agents on Toxoplasma gondii: comparison of sulfadoxine and sulfadiazine individually and in combination with pyrimethamine and study of clindamycin, metronidazole, and cyclosporin A. *Antimicrob Agents Chemother* 1984; **26**: 26–30.
4. Queener SF, *et al.* Activity of clindamycin with primaquine against Pneumocystis carinii in vitro and in vivo. *Antimicrob Agents Chemother* 1988; **32**: 807–13.
5. Blais J, *et al.* Effect of clindamycin on intracellular replication, protein synthesis, and infectivity of Toxoplasma gondii. *Antimicrob Agents Chemother* 1993; **37**: 2571–7.
6. Fichera ME, *et al.* In vitro assays elucidate peculiar kinetics of clindamycin action against Toxoplasma gondii. *Antimicrob Agents Chemother* 1995; **39**: 1530–7.

Activity with other antimicrobials. References to antimicrobial synergy or antagonism between clindamycin and other antimicrobials.

1. Meers PD. Bacteroides infections. *Lancet* 1973; **ii**: 573.
2. Busch DF, *et al.* Activity of combinations of antimicrobial agents against Bacteroides fragilis. *J Infect Dis* 1976; **133**: 321–8.
3. Sanders CC, *et al.* Effects of clindamycin on derepression of β-lactamases in Gram-negative bacteria. *J Antimicrob Chemother* 1983; **12** (suppl C): 97–104.
4. Brook I, *et al.* Synergism between penicillin, clindamycin, or metronidazole and gentamicin against species of the Bacteroides melaninogenicus and Bacteroides fragilis groups. *Antimicrob Agents Chemother* 1984; **25**: 71–7.
5. George WL. In vitro antibacterial activity of the combination of clindamycin and ceftazidime. *Antimicrob Agents Chemother* 1984; **25**: 657–8.
6. Brook I, Walker RI. Interaction between penicillin, clindamycin or metronidazole and gentamicin against species of clostridia and anaerobic and facultatively anaerobic Gram-positive cocci. *J Antimicrob Chemother* 1984; **15**: 31–7.
7. Whiting JL, *et al.* Interactions of ciprofloxacin with clindamycin, metronidazole, cefoxitin, cefotaxime, and mezlocillin against Gram-positive and Gram-negative anaerobic bacteria. *Antimicrob Agents Chemother* 1987; **31**: 1379–82.
8. Arditi M, Yogev R. In vitro interaction between rifampin and clindamycin against pathogenic coagulase-negative staphylococci. *Antimicrob Agents Chemother* 1989; **33**: 245–7.

Resistance. Although there is usually cross-resistance between clindamycin and macrolides (above), a resistance pattern has recently been identified that results in streptococcal resistance to macrolides while retaining susceptibility to clindamycin.[1]

1. Sutcliffe J, *et al.* Streptococcus pneumoniae and Streptococcus pyogenes resistant to macrolides but sensitive to clindamycin: a common resistance pattern mediated by an efflux system. *Antimicrob Agents Chemother* 1996; **40**: 1817–24.

Pharmacokinetics

About 90% of a dose of clindamycin hydrochloride is absorbed from the gastrointestinal tract following administration by mouth; concentrations of 2 to 3 µg per mL occur within 1 hour after a 150-mg dose of clindamycin, with average concentrations of about 0.7 µg per mL after 6 hours. After doses of 300 and 600 mg peak plasma concentrations of 4 and 8 µg per mL, respectively, have been reported. Absorption is not significantly diminished by food in the stomach but the rate of absorption may be reduced. Clindamycin palmitate hydrochloride is rapidly hydrolysed following oral administration to provide free clindamycin.

Following parenteral administration, the biologically inactive clindamycin phosphate is also hydrolysed to clindamycin. When the equivalent of 300 mg of clindamycin is injected intramuscularly, a mean peak plasma concentration of 6 µg per mL is achieved within 3 hours; 600 mg gives a peak concentration of 9 µg per mL. In children, peak concentrations may be reached within 1 hour. When the same doses are infused intravenously, peak concentrations of 7 and 10 µg per mL are achieved by the end of infusion.

Small amounts of clindamycin may be absorbed after topical application to the skin; bioavailability from topical preparations of the hydrochloride and phosphate (the former in an extemporaneous formulation) has been reported to be about 7.5% and 2% respectively.

About 5% of an intravaginal dose may be absorbed systemically.

Clindamycin is widely distributed in body fluids and tissues including bone, but it does not reach the CSF in significant concentrations. It diffuses across the placenta into the fetal circulation and has been reported to appear in breast milk. High concentrations occur in bile. It accumulates in leucocytes and macrophages. Over 90% of clindamycin in the circulation is bound to plasma proteins. The half-life is 2 to 3 hours,

although this may be prolonged in preterm neonates and in patients with severe renal impairment.

Clindamycin undergoes metabolism, presumably in the liver, to the active *N*-demethyl and sulfoxide metabolites, and also to some inactive metabolites. About 10% of a dose is excreted in the urine as active drug or metabolites and about 4% in the faeces; the remainder is excreted as inactive metabolites. Excretion is slow, and takes place over several days. It is not effectively removed from the blood by dialysis.

AIDS patients. Clindamycin was reported to have higher bioavailability, lower plasma clearance, and a lower volume of distribution in patients with AIDS than in healthy volunteers.[1] This may partly be explained by increased binding to plasma proteins.[2]

Although it is generally considered that penetration of clindamycin into the CSF is insignificant, parasiticidal CSF concentrations against *Toxoplasma gondii* were achieved following intravenous administration of clindamycin to patients with AIDS.[3]

1. Gatti G, *et al.* Comparative study of bioavailabilities and pharmacokinetics of clindamycin in healthy volunteers and patients with AIDS. *Antimicrob Agents Chemother* 1993; **37**: 1137–43.
2. Flaherty JF, *et al.* Protein binding of clindamycin in sera of patients with AIDS. *Antimicrob Agents Chemother* 1996; **40**: 1134–8.
3. Gatti G, *et al.* Penetration of clindamycin and its metabolite N-demethylclindamycin into cerebrospinal fluid following intravenous infusion of clindamycin phosphate in patients with AIDS. *Antimicrob Agents Chemother* 1998; **42**: 3014–17.

Uses and Administration

Clindamycin is a lincosamide antibiotic which is a chlorinated derivative of lincomycin. It is a primarily bacteriostatic antibacterial used chiefly in the treatment of serious anaerobic infections, notably due to *Bacteroides fragilis,* and in some staphylococcal and streptococcal infections. However, because of its potential for causing pseudomembranous colitis (see Adverse Effects, above) it is usually used only when alternative drugs are unsuitable. Amongst the conditions that it may be used to treat are liver abscess, actinomycosis, biliary-tract infections, staphylococcal bone and joint infections, the carrier state of diphtheria, gas gangrene, various gynaecological infections including bacterial vaginosis, endometritis, and pelvic inflammatory disease (the latter two in combination with an aminoglycoside), necrotising fasciitis, secondary peritonitis, streptococcal pharyngitis (usually to treat the carrier state), pneumonia (especially lung abscess), septicaemia, and skin infections involving heavy colonisation with streptococci or anaerobes. It is used in the prophylaxis of endocarditis in penicillin-allergic patients, in the prevention of perinatal streptococcal infections, and in combination with other drugs for the prophylaxis of surgical infection. For details of these bacterial infections and their treatment, see under Choice of Antibacterial, p.114.

Clindamycin is also applied topically in the treatment of acne (p.1103).

Clindamycin also has some antiprotozoal actions, and has been used, usually in combination with other antiprotozoals, in various infections (see below) including babesiosis, malaria, and toxoplasmosis; it may also be used in combination with primaquine in the treatment of *Pneumocystis carinii* pneumonia (below).

Clindamycin is given by mouth as capsules containing the hydrochloride or as oral liquid preparations containing the palmitate hydrochloride. The capsules should be taken with a glass of water. Doses are expressed in terms of the equivalent amount of clindamycin.

The usual adult dose by mouth is the equivalent of 150 to 300 mg of clindamycin every 6 hours; in severe infections the dose may be increased to 450 mg every 6 hours. Children may be given 3 to 6 mg per kg body-weight every 6 hours; those under one-year-old or weighing 10 kg or less should receive at least 37.5 mg every 8 hours.

For prophylaxis in patients at risk of developing endocarditis and who cannot be given a penicillin, an oral dose of clindamycin 600 mg given one hour before procedures such as dental extractions under local

The symbol † denotes a preparation no longer actively marketed

or no anaesthesia has been suggested. For patients at special risk undergoing dental procedures involving general anaesthesia, a suggested regimen is clindamycin 300 mg given intravenously over at least 10 minutes, at induction or 15 minutes before the procedure, followed 6 hours later by oral or intravenous clindamycin 150 mg.

Clindamycin is given parenterally as the phosphate by intramuscular injection or by intermittent or continuous intravenous infusion. For intravenous use a solution containing the equivalent of 6 mg of clindamycin per mL is employed in the UK, although solutions containing up to 18 mg per mL are allowed in the USA; the rate of infusion should be not more than 30 mg per minute. Not more than 1.2 g should be administered as a single one-hour infusion, and not more than 600 mg should be given as a single intramuscular injection.

The usual parenteral dose is the equivalent of 0.6 to 2.7 g of clindamycin daily in divided doses; up to 4.8 g daily has been given intravenously in very severe infections. Children over the age of 1 month may be given the equivalent of 15 to 40 mg per kg bodyweight daily in divided doses; in severe infections they should receive a total dose of not less than 300 mg of clindamycin daily. Neonates have been given 15 to 20 mg per kg daily.

Topical formulations containing 1% of clindamycin phosphate are used for the treatment of acne. The hydrochloride may be applied similarly, but systemic absorption may be greater (see Pharmacokinetics, above).

A 2% cream containing clindamycin phosphate is used for the treatment of bacterial vaginosis, the equivalent of about 100 mg clindamycin being given intravaginally at night for 3 to 7 days.

Administration. A number of studies have suggested that a parenteral regimen of clindamycin 600 mg three times daily is as effective as giving the same dose four times daily,[1] or as giving 900 mg three times daily.[2,3]

1. Buchwald D, et al. Effect of hospitalwide change in clindamycin dosing schedule on clinical outcome. Rev Infect Dis 1989; 11: 619–24.
2. Chin A, et al. Cost analysis of two clindamycin dosing regimens. DICP Ann Pharmacother 1989; 23: 980–3.
3. Chatwani A, et al. Clindamycin dosage scheduling for acute pelvic infection. Am J Obstet Gynecol 1990; 163: 240.

Babesiosis. Clindamycin 1.2 g twice daily intravenously or 600 mg three times daily by mouth, in association with quinine 650 mg three times daily by mouth, has been recommended in the USA for the treatment of babesiosis (p.583) caused by Babesia microti.[1] Children could be given clindamycin 20 to 40 mg per kg body-weight daily and quinine 25 mg per kg daily, both by mouth in 3 divided doses.[1] Treatment is continued for 7 days. However, WHO, while noting that the combination was reported to be successful in the few patients requiring specific treatment, stated that further confirmation of its effectiveness was required.[2]

1. Anonymous. Drugs for parasitic infections. Med Lett Drugs Ther 1998; 40: 1–12.
2. WHO. WHO model prescribing information—drugs used in parasitic diseases. Geneva: WHO, 1995.

Malaria. Clindamycin 900 mg three times daily for 5 days in a regimen with quinine sulfate 650 mg three times daily for 3 to 7 days, both given by mouth, is one of the suggested treatments[1] for chloroquine-resistant falciparum malaria (p.428). Parenteral clindamycin plus quinine has also been tried in severe falciparum malaria.[2]

1. Anonymous. Drugs for parasitic infections. Med Lett Drugs Ther 1998; 40: 1–12.
2. Kremsner PG, et al. Quinine plus clindamycin improves chemotherapy of severe malaria in children. Antimicrob Agents Chemother 1995; 39: 1603–5.

Pneumocystis carinii pneumonia. Clindamycin may be used with primaquine as an alternative to co-trimoxazole for the treatment of Pneumocystis carinii pneumonia in patients with AIDS (p.375). A suggested dose[1] is clindamycin 600 mg intravenously, or 300 to 450 mg by mouth, every 6 hours with primaquine 30 mg by mouth daily, for 21 days.
A randomised multicentre study[2] compared the use of a combination of primaquine (30 mg daily) and clindamycin (600 mg three times daily) with co-trimoxazole and with a combination of dapsone and trimethoprim in 181 AIDS patients who had confirmed mild to moderate Pneumocystis carinii pneumonia. Primaquine/clindamycin was as effective as the other two regimens, although the authors suggested that the combination might be best avoided in patients with severe myelosuppression.
Clindamycin with primaquine is not normally recommended for prophylaxis although there are reports of it being tried.[3]

1. Anonymous. Drugs for parasitic infections. Med Lett Drugs Ther 1998; 40: 1–12.
2. Safrin S, et al. Comparison of three regimens for treatment of mild to moderate Pneumocystis carinii pneumonia in patients with AIDS: a double-blind, randomized trial of oral trimethoprim-sulfamethoxazole, dapsone-trimethoprim, and clindamycin-primaquine. Ann Intern Med 1996; 124: 792–802.
3. Kay R, DuBois RE. Clindamycin/primaquine therapy and secondary prophylaxis against Pneumocystis carinii pneumonia in patients with AIDS. South Med J 1990; 83: 403–4.

Rosacea. Topical clindamycin[1] has improved the inflammatory episodes of rosacea (p.1107), although other features of the skin disorder may not respond.

1. Wilkin JK, DeWitt S. Treatment of rosacea: topical clindamycin versus oral tetracycline. Int J Dermatol 1993; 32: 65–7.

Toxoplasmosis. Primaquine with clindamycin has been used for the treatment of toxoplasmosis (p.585) instead of the more usual treatment with pyrimethamine plus sulfadiazine, in patients unable to tolerate sulfonamides. In patients with AIDS and toxoplasmic encephalitis, a suggested dose has been clindamycin 600 mg by mouth every 6 hours for at least 3 weeks, then maintenance therapy with at least 1200 mg daily;[1] patients also received pyrimethamine. Another schedule[2] has been oral clindamycin 600 mg four times daily together with pyrimethamine 75 mg daily for 6 weeks. Other studies found acute therapy with pyrimethamine and clindamycin, 600 mg four times daily by mouth[3] or 1200 mg every 6 hours intravenously,[4] to be as effective as pyrimethamine and sulfadiazine, but maintenance therapy with pyrimethamine and clindamycin 300 mg four times daily by mouth was less effective than pyrimethamine and sulfadiazine at preventing relapses in a population followed for 3 years or more.[3] Clindamycin with fluorouracil produced beneficial responses in a study involving 16 patients.[5]
In contrast, another study, comparing clindamycin alone (in lower doses—300 mg twice daily by mouth) with pyrimethamine alone for prophylaxis of toxoplasmic encephalitis, reported an unacceptably high incidence of adverse effects with clindamycin, which forced premature termination of the clindamycin arm—see under Precautions, above.

1. Remington JS, Vildé JL. Clindamycin for toxoplasma encephalitis in AIDS. Lancet 1991; 338: 1142–3.
2. Luft BJ, et al. Toxoplasmic encephalitis in patients with the acquired immunodeficiency syndrome. N Engl J Med 1993; 329: 995–1000.
3. Katlama C, et al. Pyrimethamine-clindamycin vs pyrimethamine-sulphadiazine as acute and long-term therapy for toxoplasmic encephalitis in patients with AIDS. Clin Infect Dis 1996; 22: 268–75.
4. Dannemann B, et al. Treatment of toxoplasmic encephalitis in patients with AIDS: a randomized trial comparing pyrimethamine plus clindamycin to pyrimethamine plus sulfadiazine. Ann Intern Med 1992; 116: 33–43.
5. Dhiver C, et al. 5-Fluoro-uracil-clindamycin for treatment of cerebral toxoplasmosis. AIDS 1993; 7: 143–4.

Preparations

BP 2001: Clindamycin Capsules; Clindamycin Injection;
USP 25: Clindamycin for Injection; Clindamycin Hydrochloride Capsules; Clindamycin Hydrochloride Oral Solution; Clindamycin Injection; Clindamycin Palmitate Hydrochloride for Oral Solution; Clindamycin Phosphate Gel; Clindamycin Phosphate Topical Solution; Clindamycin Phosphate Topical Suspension; Clindamycin Phosphate Vaginal Cream.

Proprietary Preparations (details are given in Part 3)
Aust.: Cleocin; Clindac; Dalacin; Lanacine; Austral.: Cleocin; Clindatech; Dalacin C; Dalacin T; Dalacin V; Belg.: Dalacin C; Dalacin Topical; Dalacin Vaginal; Braz.: Dalacin C; Dalacin T; Canad.: Dalacin C; Dalacin T; Dalacin Vaginal; Denm.: Dalacin; Fin.: Dalacin; Fr.: Dalacine; Dalacine T; Ger.: Aclinda; Basocin; Clin-Sanorania; Clinda; Clinda-saar; Clindabeta; Clindahexal; Clindastad; Sobelin; Turimycin; Hong Kong: Clinac; Dalacin C; Dalacin T; Dalacin V; Irl.: Dalacin; Dalacin C; Dalacin T; Israel: Dalacin C; Dalacin Vaginal; Dalagis T; Ital.: Cleocin; Dalacin C; Dalacin T; Mex.: Clindazyn; Cutaclin; Dalacin C; Dalacin T; Dalacin V; Galecin; Klyndaken; Neth.: Dalacin C; Dalacin T; Norw.: Dalacin; NZ: Clinac; Dalacin; Dalacin T; Dalacin V; Topicil; Port.: Dalacin C; Dalacin T; Dalacin V; S.Afr.: Clindac; Clindahexal; Dalacin C; Dalacin T; Dalacin VC; Singapore: Dalacin; Spain: Clinwas; Dalacin; Swed.: Dalacin; Switz.: Dalacin C; Dalacin T; Dalacin V; Thai.: Dalacin; Klimicin; Klinna; Lacin; UK: Dalacin; Dalacin C; Dalacin T; USA: C/T/S; Cleocin; Cleocin T; Clinda-Derm; Clindagel; Clindets.

Multi-ingredient: USA: BenzaClin.

Clioquinol (4770-t)

Clioquinol (BAN, rINN).
Chinoform; Chloroiodoquine; Cliochinolum; Iodochlorhydroxyquin; Iodochlorhydroxyquinoline; Quiniodochlor. 5-Chloro-7-iodoquinolin-8-ol.
$C_9H_5ClINO = 305.5$.
CAS — 130-26-7.
ATC — D08AH30; D09AA10; G01AC02; P01AA02; S02AA05.
Pharmacopoeias. In Aust., Br., It., Swiss, and US.

Pharmacopoeial description
BP 2001: A yellowish-white to brownish-yellow, voluminous powder with a faint characteristic odour. Practically insoluble in water and in alcohol; freely soluble in dimethylformamide and in pyridine; Protect from light.
USP 25: A voluminous, spongy, yellowish-white to brownish-yellow powder having a slight characteristic odour. It darkens

on exposure to light. Practically insoluble in water; soluble 1 in 3500 of alcohol, 1 in 120 of chloroform, and 1 in 4500 of ether; soluble in hot ethyl acetate and in hot glacial acetic acid. Store in airtight containers. Protect from light.

Adverse Effects and Precautions
Clioquinol may rarely cause iodism in sensitive patients. Local application of clioquinol in ointments or creams may occasionally cause severe irritation or hypersensitivity and there may be cross-sensitivity with other halogenated hydroxyquinolines.
Clioquinol stains clothing and linen yellow on contact and may stain the skin and discolour fair hair.
Clioquinol given by mouth has been associated with severe neurotoxicity. In Japan, the epidemic development of subacute myelo-opticoneuropathy (SMON) in the 1960s was associated with the ingestion of normal or high doses of clioquinol for prolonged periods, and the sale of clioquinol and related hydroxyquinolines were subsequently banned in Japan. Symptoms of subacute myelo-opticoneuropathy are principally those of peripheral neuropathy, including optic atrophy, and myelopathy. Abdominal pain and diarrhoea often precede neurological symptoms, such as paraesthesias in the legs progressing to paraplegia in some patients, and loss of visual acuity sometimes leading to blindness. A characteristic green pigment, a chelate of clioquinol with iron, is often seen on the tongue and in the urine and faeces. Cerebral disturbances, including confusion and retrograde amnesia, have also been reported. Although many patients improved when clioquinol was withdrawn, others had residual disablement.
It was suggested that the Japanese epidemic might be due to genetic susceptibility, but a few similar cases of subacute myelo-opticoneuropathy associated with clioquinol or related hydroxyquinoline derivatives, such as broxyquinoline or diiodohydroxyquinoline have been reported from several other countries. Oral preparations of clioquinol have now been banned in most countries.

◊ Absorption of clioquinol through the skin has been noted following topical application.[1,2] Significant toxicity has been found in dogs treated with 5 g of a 3% clioquinol topical preparation for 28 days.[3] The Committee on Drugs of the American Academy of Pediatrics[4] considered that there was a potential risk of toxicity to infants and children from clioquinol and diiodohydroxyquinoline applied topically. Since alternative effective preparations are available for dermatitis the Committee recommended that products containing either of these compounds should not be used.

1. Fischer T, Hartvig P. Skin absorption of 8-hydroxyquinolines. Lancet 1977; i: 603.
2. Stohs SJ, et al. Percutaneous absorption of iodochlorhydroxyquin in humans. J Invest Dermatol 1984; 82: 195–8.
3. Ezzedeen FW, et al. Percutaneous absorption and disposition of iodochlorhydroxyquin in dogs. J Pharm Sci 1984; 73: 1369–72.
4. Kauffman RE, et al. Clioquinol (iodochlorhydroxyquin, Vioform) and iodoquinol (diiodohydroxyquin): blindness and neuropathy. Pediatrics 1990; 86: 797–8.

Hypersensitivity. Clioquinol is classified as a contact allergen which can commonly cause sensitisation, especially when applied to eczematous skin; chlorquinaldol can also cause sensitisation, but less frequently.[1] It is important to include clioquinol and chlorquinaldol in routine patch testing since the clinical reaction may be relatively mild and sensitivity easily missed, particularly in the presence of a corticosteroid which suppresses or attenuates the reaction.

1. Anonymous. Skin sensitisers in topical corticosteroids Drug Ther Bull 1986; 24: 57–9.

Uses and Administration
Clioquinol is a halogenated hydroxyquinoline with antibacterial and antifungal activity and is used in creams and ointments, usually containing 3%, in the treatment of skin infections. It is applied together with a corticosteroid in inflammatory skin conditions complicated by bacterial or fungal infections. It is also used in ear drops for otitis externa. The treatment of bacterial and fungal skin infections is described on p.140 and p.376 respectively.
For a discussion of the risks from topical application of clioquinol, see Adverse Effects and Precautions, above.
Clioquinol was formerly given by mouth in the treatment of intestinal amoebiasis. It was also formerly used for the prophylaxis and treatment of traveller's diarrhoea and similar infections but was of doubtful value. Oral preparations have now been withdrawn because of neurotoxicity (see Adverse Effects and Precautions, above).

Preparations
BP 2001: Betamethasone and Clioquinol Cream; Betamethasone and Clioquinol Ointment; Hydrocortisone and Clioquinol Cream; Hydrocortisone and Clioquinol Ointment;
USP 25: Clioquinol and Hydrocortisone Cream; Clioquinol and Hydrocortisone Ointment; Clioquinol Cream; Clioquinol Ointment; Compound Clioquinol Topical Powder.

Proprietary Preparations (details are given in Part 3)
Canad.: Vioform†; Ger.: Linola-sept; Irl.: Oralcer; Mex.: Lasalar-Y Simple; Quindoleina; Vioformo; Yoquin; Port.: Quinodermil; S.Afr.: Bioform; Switz.: Vioform; USA: Vioform†.

Multi-ingredient: Aust.: Betnovate-C; Locacorten Vioform; Austral.: Hydroform; Locacorten Vioform; Quinaband; Belg.: Betnelan-VC; Locacortene Vioforme; Braz.: Atacoly; Betnovate-Q; Dreniformio; Hidrocorete; Locorten Vioformio; Quadriderm; Quadrilon; Vioformio-Hidrocortisona; Canad.: Locacorten Vioform; Phenoris; Vioform-Hydrocortisone; Denm.: Betnovat med

Chinoform; Celeston med Chinoform; Diproform; Locacorten Vioform; Synalar med Chinoform; **Fin.:** Betnovat-C; Celestoderm cum Chinoform; Locacorten Vioform; **Fr.:** Diprosept; **Ger.:** Locacorten Vioform; Millicorten-Vioform; **Hong Kong:** Betnovate-C; Quadriderm; Triaforma; **Irl.:** Betnovate-C; Synalar C; Vioform-Hydrocortisone; **Israel:** Betnovate-C; Topicorten V; **Ital.:** Diproform; Locorten; Locorten Vioformio; Viobeta; **Mex.:** Cetoquina Y; Clio-Betnovate; Dealan; Diprosone-Y; Ditayod; Lasalar-Y; Sebryl; Sebryl Plus; Solfurol; Sultroquin; Synalar C; Topsyn-V; Vioformo-Cort; **Neth.:** Betnelan Clioquinol†; Celestoform; Locacorten Vioform; **Norw.:** Betnovat med Chinoform; Locacorten Vioform; Synalar med Chinoform; **NZ:** Betnovate-C; Locorten Vioform; **Port.:** Betnovate-N; Dexaval V; Locorten Vioformio; **S.Afr.:** Betnovate-C; Locacorten Vioform; Manoderm†; Propaderm-C†; Quadriderm; **Singapore:** Betnovate-C; Quadriderm; Synalar C; **Spain:** Antiblef Eczem; Cuatroderm; Locortene Vioformo; Menaderm Clio; Menaderm Otologico; Recto Menaderm†; Synobel; **Swed.:** Betnovat med Chinoform; Celeston valerat med chinoform; Locacorten Vioform; **Switz.:** Betnovate-C; Quadriderm; **Thai.:** Banocin; Beta-C; Betnovate-C; Betosone-CE; Chlorotracin; Genquin; Quadriderm; **UK:** Betnovate-C; Locorten Vioform; Oralcer; Quinaband; Synalar C; Vioform-Hydrocortisone; **USA:** 1 + 1-F; Ala-Quin†; Albaform HC†; Corque; Hysone; Pedi-Cort V†.

Clofazimine (6553-m)

Clofazimine (BAN, USAN, rINN).

B-663; G-30320; NSC-141046. 3-(4-Chloroanilino)-10-(4-chlorophenyl)-2,10-dihydro-2-phenazin-2-ylideneisopropylamine.

$C_{27}H_{22}Cl_2N_4 = 473.4$.

CAS — 2030-63-9.

ATC — J04BA01.

Pharmacopoeias. In Br., Fr., Int. and US.

Pharmacopoeial description

BP 2001: A fine reddish-brown, odourless or almost odourless powder. It exhibits polymorphism. Practically insoluble in water; slightly soluble in alcohol; soluble in chloroform; very slightly soluble in ether.

USP 25: Dark red crystals. Practically insoluble in water; sparingly soluble in alcohol, in acetone, and in ethyl acetate; soluble in chloroform and in benzene; Store in airtight containers. Protect from light.

Adverse Effects

Adverse effects to clofazimine are dose-related, the most common being red to brown discoloration of the skin especially on areas exposed to sunlight; leprotic lesions may become mauve to black. These changes are more noticeable in light-skinned people and may limit its acceptance. The conjunctiva and cornea may also show some signs of red to brown pigmentation. The generalised discoloration may take months to years to disappear after stopping therapy with clofazimine. Discoloration of hair, tears, sweat, sputum, breast milk, urine, and faeces may occur.

Gastrointestinal effects are uncommon for doses of clofazimine less than 100 mg daily and usually are not severe. Symptoms of nausea, vomiting, and abdominal pain experienced shortly after the start of treatment may be due to direct irritation of the gastrointestinal tract and such symptoms usually disappear on dose reduction. Administration of doses of 300 mg daily or more for several months sometimes produces abdominal pain, diarrhoea, weight loss, gastrointestinal bleeding, and in severe cases the small bowel may become oedematous and symptoms of bowel obstruction may develop. This may be due to deposition of crystals of clofazimine in the wall of the small bowel and in the mesenteric lymph nodes. Crystal deposition may also occur in other organs including the liver and spleen and cause adverse effects. Symptoms usually regress on withdrawal of treatment.

Clofazimine may produce a dryness of the skin and ichthyosis as well as decreased sweat production and rashes. Pruritus and photosensitivity reactions have also been reported.

Eye irritation and decreased tear production may occur.

Headache, drowsiness, dizziness, and taste disorders have been reported rarely.

◊ The incidence of adverse effects experienced with clofazimine was reviewed in 65 patients who were receiving or had received clofazimine in doses of either 700 mg per week or less as antimycobacterial therapy, or more than 700 mg per week as anti-inflammatory therapy.[1] Length of treatment ranged from 1

---

to 83 months. Adverse effects on the skin included discoloration (20% of patients), pigmentation (64.6%), dry skin (35.4%), and pruritus (5%). Ocular adverse effects experienced were conjunctival pigmentation (49.2% of patients), subjective dimness of vision (12.3%), and dry eyes, burning and other ocular irritation (24.6%). Gastrointestinal adverse effects included abdominal pain (33.8% of patients), nausea (9.2%), diarrhoea (9.2%), and weight loss, vomiting, or loss of appetite (13.8%). The different dose regimens for antimycobacterial therapy or anti-inflammatory effect had similar incidences of adverse effects. Skin pigmentation in 8 patients disappeared on average 8.5 months after stopping therapy with clofazimine, the maximum time required being one year. Adverse effects of clofazimine were considered to be well tolerated.

In another report covering 540 patients receiving clofazimine 100 mg on alternate days or 300 mg daily, the most common adverse effect was skin pigmentation which occurred in 77.8% of the patients. Ichthyotic changes were reported in 66.7% and pruritus in 20.2%. Gastrointestinal symptoms occurred in 20 patients (about 4%); other effects such as discoloration of sweat, urine, and tears were minor.[2]

1. Moore VJ. A review of side-effects experienced by patients taking clofazimine. *Lepr Rev* 1983; **54:** 327–35.
2. Kumar B, *et al.* More about clofazimine—3 years experience and review of the literature. *Indian J Lepr* 1987; **59:** 63–74.

Effects on the eyes. Accumulation of clofazimine crystals in the eye can lead to pigmentation of the cornea and conjunctiva. Degeneration of the retinal pigment epithelium has also been attributed to clofazimine therapy in a patient.[1] Slight repigmentation was observed following withdrawal of clofazimine.

1. Forster DJ, *et al.* Bull's eye retinopathy and clofazimine. *Ann Intern Med* 1992; **116:** 876–7.

Effects on the heart. Ventricular tachycardia, thought to be probably torsade de pointes, was reported to be associated with clofazimine in a patient.[1]

1. Choudhri SH, *et al.* Clofazimine induced cardiotoxicity—a case report. *Lepr Rev* 1995; **66:** 63–8.

Splenic infarction. A case report[1] of splenic infarction associated with clofazimine.

1. McDougall AC, *et al.* Splenic infarction and tissue accumulation of crystals associated with the use of clofazimine (Lamprene; B663) in the treatment of pyoderma gangrenosum. *Br J Dermatol* 1980; **102:** 227–30.

Precautions

Clofazimine should be used with caution in patients with gastrointestinal symptoms such as abdominal pain and diarrhoea. If gastrointestinal symptoms develop during treatment with clofazimine, the dose should be reduced and, if necessary, the interval between doses increased, or the drug should be discontinued. Daily doses of more than 100 mg of clofazimine should not be administered for more than 3 months because of dose-related adverse effects on the gastrointestinal tract; patients receiving doses greater than 100 mg daily should be under medical supervision.

Patients should be warned that clofazimine may cause a reddish-brown discoloration of skin, conjunctiva, tears, sputum, sweat, urine, and faeces.

As clofazimine crosses the placental barrier and is distributed into breast milk, neonates of women receiving clofazimine may have skin discoloration at birth or from breast feeding.

Pregnancy. Two successful pregnancies in women who received clofazimine throughout pregnancy have been reported[1] but a literature review revealed 28 neonatal deaths in 13 pregnancies, although the deaths could not be directly attributed to clofazimine. However, WHO[2] now states that its recommended multiple drug therapy regimens, which may include clofazimine, are safe during pregnancy.

1. Farb H, *et al.* Clofazimine in pregnancy complicated by leprosy. *Obstet Gynecol* 1982; **59:** 122–3.
2. WHO. *Guide to eliminate leprosy as a public health problem.* 1st ed. Geneva: WHO, 2000.

Interactions

Some preliminary data has suggested that the anti-inflammatory action of clofazimine in Type 2 lepra reactions may be reduced by dapsone, although the manufacturers have stated that these findings have not been confirmed; the antimycobacterial effect was not affected.

In patients receiving high doses of clofazimine and also receiving isoniazid, elevated plasma and urine concentrations of clofazimine have been detected, although skin concentrations were found to be lower.

For a report of the effect of clofazimine on rifampicin absorption, see p.244.

Antimicrobial Action

Clofazimine is bacteriostatic and weakly bactericidal against *Mycobacterium leprae*. The minimum inhibitory concentration for *Mycobacterium leprae* in mouse tissue has been estimated to lie between 0.1 and 1 μg per gram; uneven tissue distribution precludes a more accurate estimate. Tissue antimicrobial activity in humans cannot be demonstrated until after about 50 days of therapy.

Clofazimine is active *in vitro* against various other species of *Mycobacterium*.

Resistance has been reported rarely.

Pharmacokinetics

Clofazimine is absorbed from the gastrointestinal tract in amounts varying from 45 to 70%. Absorption is greatest when clofazimine is given in microcrystalline formulations and when it is taken immediately after food. The time to steady-state plasma concentrations has not been determined but exceeds 30 days.

Average plasma concentrations in leprosy patients receiving 100 or 300 mg daily are reported as 0.7 μg per mL and 1.0 μg per mL, respectively.

Because of its lipophilic nature, clofazimine is mainly distributed to fatty tissue and reticuloendothelial cells, including macrophages. Clofazimine is distributed to most organs and tissues and into breast milk; it crosses the placenta but not the blood-brain barrier.

The tissue half-life following a single dose has been reported to be about 10 days; that following multiple oral doses has been variously estimated to be between 25 and 90 days. Clofazimine accumulates in the body and is largely excreted unchanged in the faeces, both as unabsorbed drug and via biliary excretion. About 1% of the dose is excreted in 24 hours in the urine as unchanged clofazimine and metabolites. A small amount of clofazimine is also excreted through sebaceous and sweat glands.

◊ References to the pharmacokinetics of clofazimine.

1. Holdiness MR. Clinical pharmacokinetics of clofazimine: a review. *Clin Pharmacokinet* 1989; **16:** 74–85.

Uses and Administration

Clofazimine is an antimycobacterial and is one of the main drugs used in regimens for the treatment of multibacillary leprosy (p.126), although because of its adverse effect on skin colour it may be replaced by other drugs in light-skinned patients. It has anti-inflammatory properties and has been given in chronic Type 2 lepra reactions and in a variety of skin disorders. It may also be used as a component of regimens for the treatment of opportunistic mycobacterial infections (p.131) due to *Mycobacterium avium* complex.

Clofazimine is administered orally with, or immediately after, food or milk for optimum absorption.

For multibacillary leprosy the most common regimen is that recommended by WHO, in which rifampicin 600 mg and clofazimine 300 mg are both given once a month together with clofazimine 50 mg daily [or 100 mg every other day depending on what preparations are available] and dapsone 100 mg daily; this treatment continues for 12 months. Children aged 10 to 14 years may be given clofazimine 150 mg once a month and 50 mg on alternate days.

Clofazimine 50 mg daily is given in combination with ofloxacin and minocycline in patients unable to take rifampicin. Clofazimine is not usually given in paucibacillary leprosy. However, it may be used in association with rifampicin instead of dapsone when the latter has caused severe toxicity.

Clofazimine has been used in the treatment of chronic Type 2 lepra reactions, although the effect may not be evident for 4 to 6 weeks. A dose of up to 300 mg daily has been suggested but it should not be given for longer than 3 months. Corticosteroids may be given in conjunction with clofazimine, and standard antileprosy treatment should be continued. Clofazimine is not used in Type 1 lepra reactions.

The symbol † denotes a preparation no longer actively marketed

In the treatment of opportunistic mycobacterial infections, doses of 100 to 200 mg daily have been given, and have been increased up to 300 mg daily in patients with AIDS and disseminated *M. avium* complex infection; again, the increased risk of gastrointestinal toxicity may preclude the use of daily doses above 100 mg for more than 3 months.

Preparations

BP 2001: Clofazimine Capsules;
USP 25: Clofazimine Capsules.

Proprietary Preparations (details are given in Part 3)
Austral.: Lamprene; *Fr.:* Lamprene; *Hong Kong:* Lamprene; *Irl.:* Lamprene†; *Jpn:* Lampren; *Neth.:* Lampren; *NZ:* Lamprene; *S.Afr.:* Lamprene; *Spain:* Lampren; *Switz.:* Lamprene; *UK:* Lamprene; *USA:* Lamprene.

Multi-ingredient: *S.Afr.:* MB-Combi†.

Clofoctol (12586-t)

Clofoctol *(rINN)*.

2-(2,4-Dichlorobenzyl)-4-(1,1,3,3-tetramethylbutyl)phenol.
$C_{21}H_{26}Cl_2O = 365.3$.
CAS — 37693-01-9.
ATC — J01XX03.

Profile

Clofoctol is an antimicrobial compound with bacteriostatic or bactericidal activity against Gram-positive organisms such as staphylococci and streptococci. It is given in doses of 20 to 40 mg per kg daily by the rectal route in the treatment of respiratory-tract infections.

Preparations

Proprietary Preparations (details are given in Part 3)
Fr.: Octofene; *Ital.:* Gramplus; Octofene; *Port.:* Octofene.

Clometocillin Potassium (57-p)

Clometocillin Potassium *(rINNM)*.

3,4-Dichloro-α-methoxybenzylpenicillin Potassium; Penicillin 356 (clometocillin). Potassium (6R)-6-[2-(3,4-dichlorophenyl)-2-methoxyacetamido]penicillanate.
$C_{17}H_{17}Cl_2KN_2O_5S = 471.4$.
CAS — 1926-49-4 (clometocillin); 15433-28-0 (clometocillin potassium).

Profile

Clometocillin is a penicillin given by mouth as the potassium salt in the treatment of susceptible bacterial infections. Doses are expressed in terms of the base. The usual adult dose is 500 mg two or three times daily.

Preparations

Proprietary Preparations (details are given in Part 3)
Belg.: Rixapen.

Cloxacillin (14777-t)

Cloxacillin *(BAN, rINN)*.

(6R)-6-[3-(2-Chlorophenyl)-5-methylisoxazole-4-carboxamido]penicillanic acid.
$C_{19}H_{18}ClN_3O_5S = 435.9$.
CAS — 61-72-3.
ATC — J01CF02.

Cloxacillin Benzathine (12594-t)

Cloxacillin Benzathine *(BANM)*.

The *N,N'*-dibenzylethylenediamine salt of cloxacillin.
$C_{16}H_{20}N_2,(C_{19}H_{18}ClN_3O_5S)_2 = 1112.1$.
CAS — 23736-58-5; 32222-55-2.
Pharmacopoeias. In US for veterinary use only. Also in BP(Vet).

Pharmacopoeial description

BP(Vet) 2001: A white or almost white powder. Slightly soluble in water, in alcohol, and in isopropyl alcohol; soluble in chloroform; freely soluble in methyl alcohol. Store at a temperature not exceeding 25° in airtight containers.
USP 25: White or almost white, almost odourless, crystals or crystalline powder. Slightly soluble in water, in alcohol, and in isopropyl alcohol; sparingly soluble in acetone; soluble in chloroform and in methyl alcohol. pH of a 1% suspension in water is between 3.0 and 6.5. Store in airtight containers.

Cloxacillin Sodium (60-m)

Cloxacillin Sodium *(BANM, USAN, rINNM)*.

BRL-1621; Cloxacilina Sódica; Cloxacillinum Natricum; P-25.
$C_{19}H_{17}ClN_3NaO_5S,H_2O = 475.9$.
CAS — 642-78-4 (anhydrous cloxacillin sodium); 7081-44-9 (cloxacillin sodium monohydrate).
Pharmacopoeias. In Eur. (see p.vi), Int., Jpn, Pol., and US. Chin. includes anhydrous cloxacillin sodium.

1.09 g of monograph substance is approximately equivalent to 1 g of anhydrous cloxacillin. Each g of monograph substance represents about 2.1 mmol of sodium.

Cloxacillin sodium has been reported to be incompatible with aminoglycosides and a number of other antimicrobials.

Pharmacopoeial description

Ph. Eur.: A white or almost white, hygroscopic, crystalline powder. Freely soluble in water and in methyl alcohol; soluble in alcohol. A 10% solution in water has a pH of 5.0 to 7.0. Store at a temperature not exceeding 25° in airtight containers.
USP 25: A white, odourless, crystalline powder. Freely soluble in water; soluble in alcohol; slightly soluble in chloroform. pH of a 1% solution in water is between 4.5 and 7.5. Store in airtight containers at a temperature not exceeding 25°.

Adverse Effects and Precautions

As for Flucloxacillin, p.207.

Effects on the kidneys. References.
1. García-Ortiz R, *et al.* Cloxacillin-induced acute tubulo interstitial nephritis. *Ann Pharmacother* 1992; **26:** 1241–2.

Effects on the liver. References.
1. Enat R, *et al.* Cholestatic jaundice caused by cloxacillin: macrophage inhibition factor test in preventing rechallenge with hepatotoxic drugs. *BMJ* 1980; **280:** 982–3.
2. Konikoff F, *et al.* Cloxacillin-induced cholestatic jaundice. *Am J Gastroenterol* 1986; **81:** 1082–3.

Interactions

As for Benzylpenicillin, p.158.

Antimicrobial Action

As for Flucloxacillin, p.207.

Pharmacokinetics

Cloxacillin is incompletely absorbed from the gastrointestinal tract after oral administration, and absorption is further reduced by the presence of food in the stomach. After an oral dose of 500 mg, a peak plasma concentration of 7 to 14 µg per mL is attained in fasting subjects in 1 to 2 hours. Absorption is more complete when given by intramuscular injection and peak plasma concentrations of about 15 µg per mL have been observed 30 minutes after a dose of 500 mg. Doubling the dose can double the plasma concentration. About 94% of cloxacillin in the circulation is bound to plasma proteins. Cloxacillin has been reported to have a plasma half-life of 0.5 to 1 hour. The half-life is prolonged in neonates.

Cloxacillin crosses the placenta and is distributed into breast milk. There is little diffusion into the CSF except when the meninges are inflamed. Therapeutic concentrations can be achieved in pleural and synovial fluids and in bone.

Cloxacillin is metabolised to a limited extent, and the unchanged drug and metabolites are excreted in the urine by glomerular filtration and renal tubular secretion. About 35% of an oral dose is excreted in the urine and up to 10% in the bile. Cloxacillin is not removed by haemodialysis.

Plasma concentrations are enhanced if probenecid is given concomitantly. Reduced concentrations in patients with cystic fibrosis have been attributed to enhanced nonrenal clearance of cloxacillin.

Uses and Administration

Cloxacillin is an isoxazolyl penicillin used similarly to flucloxacillin (p.207) in the treatment of infections due to staphylococci resistant to benzylpenicillin.

It is administered by mouth as the sodium salt. It should be given at least 30 minutes before meals as the presence of food in the stomach reduces absorption. All doses are expressed in terms of the equivalent amount of cloxacillin.

Usual oral doses are 250 to 500 mg four times daily. Children may be given 50 to 100 mg per kg bodyweight daily in divided doses every 6 hours.

Cloxacillin sodium has also been administered by intramuscular or slow intravenous injection or infusion. Other routes of administration have included intra-articular or intrapleural injection, and inhalation.

Cloxacillin may be administered in combination with other antibacterials, including ampicillin, to produce a wider spectrum of activity.

Cloxacillin benzathine is used in veterinary medicine.

Preparations

BP 2001: Cloxacillin Capsules; Cloxacillin Injection; Cloxacillin Oral Solution;
USP 25: Cloxacillin Sodium Capsules; Cloxacillin Sodium for Oral Solution.

Proprietary Preparations (details are given in Part 3)
Austral.: Alclox†; *Belg.:* Orbenin†; Penstaphon; *Canad.:* Apo-Cloxi; Novo-Cloxin; Nu-Cloxi; Tegopen; *Denm.:* Ekvacillin; *Fin.:* Ekvacillin; Staflocil; *Fr.:* Orbenine; *Hong Kong:* Apo-Cloxi; Cloxil; Monoclox; Orbenin; *Irl.:* Orbenin; *Israel:* Loxavit; Orbenil; Prostaphlin-A; *Neth.:* Orbenin; *Norw.:* Ekvacillin; *S.Afr.:* Clocillin; Cloxin; Orbenin; *Singapore:* Axocillin; Cloxacap; Monoclox; Orbenin; *Spain:* Anaclosil; Orbenin; *Swed.:* Ekvacillin; *Thai.:* Cloxa; Cloxalin; Cloxanbin; Cloxapan; Cloxasian; Cloxgen; Cloxil; Corbin; Greater-Gloxa; K-Cil; Lidoxin; Meiclox; Monoclox; Orbenin; Serviclox; Socloxin; Syntoclox; Theraclox; Vaclox; *UK:* Orbenin†; *USA:* Cloxapen; Tegopen†.

Multi-ingredient: *Hong Kong:* Ampiclox; Pamedox; *Irl.:* Ampiclox; *Ital.:* Amplium; *S.Afr.:* Ampiclox; Apen; Cloxam; Megamox; *Thai.:* Ampiclox; Polyclox; Viccillin-S; *UK:* Ampiclox†.

Colistin Sulfate (61-b)

Colistin Sulfate *(pINNM)*.

Colistin Sulphate *(BANM)*; Colistini Sulfas; Polymyxin E Sulphate.
CAS — 1066-17-7 (colistin); 1264-72-8 (colistin sulfate).
Pharmacopoeias. In Chin., Eur. (see p.vi), Pol., and US.

The base is precipitated from aqueous solution above pH 7.5.

Pharmacopoeial description

Ph. Eur.: A mixture of the sulfates of polypeptides produced by certain strains of *Bacillus polymyxa* var. *colistinus* or obtained by other means. The potency is not less than 19 000 units per mg, calculated with reference to the dried substance. A white or almost white, hygroscopic powder. Freely soluble in water; slightly soluble in alcohol; practically insoluble in acetone and in ether. A 1% solution in water has a pH of 4.0 to 6.0. Store in airtight containers. Protect from light.
USP 25: The sulfate salt of an antibacterial substance produced by the growth of *Bacillus polymyxa* var. *colistinus*. It has a potency of not less than 500 µg of colistin per mg. A white to slightly yellow, odourless, fine powder. Freely soluble in water; insoluble in acetone and in ether; slightly soluble in methyl alcohol. pH of a 1% solution in water is between 4.0 and 7.0. Store in airtight containers.

Colistimethate Sodium (62-v)

Colistimethate Sodium *(BANM, USAN, rINN)*.

Colistimetato de Sódio; Colistimethatum Natrium; Colistin Sulphomethate Sodium; Colistineméthanesulfonate Sodique; Pentasodium Colistinmethanesulfonate; Sodium Colistimethate; Sodium Colistinmethanesulphonate; W-1929.
CAS — 30387-39-4 (colistimethate); 8068-28-8 (colistimethate sodium).
Pharmacopoeias. In Eur. (see p.vi), Jpn, Pol., and US.

Incompatibilities. Lack of compatibility has been reported with various drugs including other antibacterials.

Pharmacopoeial description

Ph. Eur.: It is prepared from colistin by the action of formaldehyde and sodium bisulfite. The potency is not less than 11 500 units per mg, calculated with reference to the dried substance. A white or almost white, hygroscopic powder. Very soluble in water; slightly soluble in alcohol; practically insoluble in acetone. A 1% solution in water has a pH of 6.5 to 8.5. Store in airtight containers. Protect from light.
USP 25: A white to slightly yellow, odourless, fine powder. It has a potency equivalent to not less than 390 µg of colistin per mg. Freely soluble in water; insoluble in acetone and in ether; soluble in methyl alcohol. pH of a 1% solution in water is between 6.5 and 8.5.

Units

The first International Standard Preparation (1968) for colistin contains 20 500 units per mg of colistin sulfate and the first International Reference Preparation (1966) for colistimethate contains 12 700 units per mg of colistimethate.

Adverse Effects, Treatment, and Precautions

As for Polymyxin B Sulfate, p.238.

Colistin sulfate is poorly absorbed from the gastrointestinal tract and adverse effects do not normally follow its administration in the usual oral doses. Bronchospasm may occur during inhalation. Overgrowth of non-susceptible organisms, particularly *Proteus* spp., may occur after prolonged administration. Pain and local irritation are reported to be less troublesome following intramuscular injection of colistimethate sodium than with polymyxin B.

Cystic fibrosis. Colistin sulfate was reported to be associated with a lower rate of severe nephrotoxicity among 19 patients with cystic fibrosis than has been previously reported in other patient populations.[1]

1. Bosso JA, *et al.* Toxicity of colistin in cystic fibrosis patients. *DICP Ann Pharmacother* 1991; **25:** 1168–70.

Porphyria. Colistin has been associated with acute attacks of porphyria and is considered unsafe in porphyric patients.

Interactions
As for Polymyxin B Sulfate, p.238.

Antimicrobial Action
The antimicrobial spectrum and mode of action of colistin is similar to that of polymyxin B (p.238) but colistin sulfate is slightly, and colistimethate significantly, less active. MICs for most sensitive species range from about 0.01 to 4 µg per mL; susceptible strains of *Pseudomonas aeruginosa* generally respond to concentrations below 8 µg per mL.

Pharmacokinetics
Colistin sulfate and colistimethate sodium are poorly absorbed from the gastrointestinal tract. They are not absorbed through intact skin. Peak plasma activity usually occurs 2 to 3 hours after an intramuscular injection of colistimethate sodium. Some colistimethate sodium may be hydrolysed to colistin *in vivo*. The serum half-life of colistimethate sodium is 2 to 3 hours. Colistin is reversibly bound to body tissues, but binding does not occur with colistimethate.

Colistimethate is mainly excreted by glomerular filtration as changed and unchanged drug and up to 80% of a parenteral dose may be recovered in the urine within 8 hours. Excretion is more rapid in children than in adults; it is diminished in patients with impaired kidney function. Colistin diffuses across the placenta but diffusion into the CSF is negligible except occasionally in infants. It is distributed into breast milk.

Neonates. The biological half-life of colistimethate sodium was variously reported as 9 hours in newborn infants falling to 2.6 hours 3 or 4 days later and 2.3 to 2.6 hours (according to age) in premature infants.[1]

1. Sereni F, Principi N. Developmental pharmacology. *Annu Rev Pharmacol* 1968; **8:** 453–66.

Renal impairment. Colistimethate was administered intramuscularly in a dose equivalent to 75 mg of colistin base to 10 healthy persons and 8 patients with renal impairment. The serum half-life was 4.5 hours in normal persons, 12.75 hours in patients with severe renal impairment (creatinine clearance 5 to 20 mL per minute), and 10.25 hours in those with negligible renal function (creatinine clearance less than 5 mL per minute).[1]

1. Goodwin NJ, Friedman EA. The effects of renal impairment, peritoneal dialysis and hemodialysis on serum sodium colistimethate levels. *Ann Intern Med* 1968; **68:** 984–94.

Uses and Administration
Colistin is a polymyxin antibiotic that has been used in the treatment of severe Gram-negative infections, especially those due to *Pseudomonas aeruginosa*, although other drugs are usually preferred. It has been used by mouth as the sulfate for the treatment of gastrointestinal infections and in combination with other drugs for the selective decontamination of the gastrointestinal tract in patients at high risk of endogenous infections (see under Intensive Care, p.126). Colistimethate sodium has been used by inhalation in the management of respiratory infections, especially in patients with cystic fibrosis (p.117).

The usual dose of colistin sulfate by mouth is 1.5 to 3 million units three times daily; children weighing up to 15 kg body-weight may be given 0.25 to 0.5 million units three times daily, and those weighing 15 to 30 kg may be given 0.75 to 1.5 million units three times daily.

Colistin is given parenterally, as colistimethate sodium, by intramuscular injection or slow intravenous injection or infusion. In the UK usual doses are 6 million units daily in three divided doses for adults weighing more than 60 kg; children weighing up to

60 kg may be given 50 000 units per kg body-weight daily in three divided doses. In the USA, the usual dose is equivalent to colistin base 2.5 to 5 mg per kg daily in two to four divided doses. Dosage must be adjusted in renal impairment; both reduction in dose and decreased frequency of dosing may be required.

Colistimethate sodium may be given by inhalation in respiratory infections as an adjunct to parenteral administration. The UK manufacturers recommend 6 million units daily in three divided doses by inhalation but lower doses have been recommended by some UK authorities; patients over 40 kg may be given 1 million units every 12 hours, those weighing less than 40 kg may be given 0.5 million units every 12 hours.

Colistimethate sodium has also been given by subconjunctival injection and as a bladder instillation. Both colistin sulfate and colistimethate sodium have been applied topically, often with other antibacterials, in the management of ear, eye, and skin infections.

Preparations
BP 2001: Colistimethate Injection; Colistin Tablets;
USP 25: Colistimethate for Injection; Colistin and Neomycin Sulfates and Hydrocortisone Acetate Otic Suspension; Colistin Sulfate for Oral Suspension.

Proprietary Preparations (details are given in Part 3)
Austral.: Coly-Mycin M; *Belg.:* Colimycine; *Canad.:* Coly-Mycin M; *Denm.:* Colimycin; *Fr.:* Colimycine; *Ger.:* Diaront mono; *Irl.:* Colomycin; *Israel:* Coliracin; *Ital.:* Colimicina; *Neth.:* Belcomycine; Colimycine; *Norw.:* Colimycin; *NZ:* Coly-Mycin M; *Spain:* Colimicina; *UK:* Colomycin; *USA:* Coly-Mycin M.

Multi-ingredient: *Aust.:* AZK; *Denm.:* Antibiotic Simplex†; *Fr.:* Bacicoline; Colicort; *Ger.:* Ecolicin; *Ital.:* Colbiocin; Eubetal Antibiotico; Iducol; *Mex.:* Colfur; *Neth.:* Bacicoline-B†; *NZ:* Coly-Mycin S Otic; *Switz.:* AZK†; *USA:* Coly-Mycin S Otic; Cortisporin-TC.

Co-tetroxazine (12612-v)

Co-tetroxazine (BAN).
CAS — 73173-12-3.

A mixture of tetroxoprim and sulfadiazine in the proportion of 2:5.

Profile
Co-tetroxazine has properties similar to those of co-trimoxazole (below) and is used similarly, mainly in the treatment of infections of the urinary and respiratory tracts, including *Pneumocystis carinii* pneumonia. It is given by mouth in an initial dose of 700 mg (tetroxoprim 200 mg or its equivalent as the embonate and sulfadiazine 500 mg), followed by 350 mg twice daily.

Preparations
Proprietary Preparations (details are given in Part 3)
Ger.: Sterinor; *Ital.:* Oxosint; Sterinor†.

Co-trifamole (4902-z)

Co-trifamole (BAN).
CN-3123.

A mixture of 5 parts of sulfamoxole and 1 part of trimethoprim.

Profile
Co-trifamole has properties similar to those of co-trimoxazole (below) and has been used similarly.

Preparations
Proprietary Preparations (details are given in Part 3)
S.Afr.: Supristol†.

Co-trimazine (4903-c)

Co-trimazine (BAN).
CAS — 39474-58-3.

A mixture of 5 parts of sulfadiazine and 1 part of trimethoprim.

Profile
Co-trimazine has properties similar to those of co-trimoxazole (below) and has been used similarly.
Preparations are available in some countries which contain trimethoprim and sulfadiazine in proportions different to co-trimazine.

Preparations
Proprietary Preparations (details are given in Part 3)
Fr.: Trimadiaz Antrima†.

Co-trimoxazole (4904-k)

Co-trimoxazole (BAN).
CAS — 8064-90-2.

A mixture of 5 parts of sulfamethoxazole and 1 part of trimethoprim.

Diluted infusion solutions of co-trimoxazole have a limited stability and eventually form a precipitate: this happens more rapidly at higher concentrations. The manufacturers recommend a dilution of 480 mg in 130 mL, which is usually stable for up to 6 hours, but more concentrated solutions should be used within shorter periods of time, and a dilution of 480 mg in 80 mL should be used within one hour. The usual diluent is glucose 5%, although other solutions, including sodium chloride 0.9%, have been stated to be compatible for adequate periods.

Adverse Effects and Treatment
The adverse effects of co-trimoxazole are those of its components (see Sulfamethoxazole, p.254, and Trimethoprim, p.264). Gastrointestinal disturbances (mainly nausea and vomiting) and skin reactions are the most common adverse effects. There have been occasional deaths, especially in elderly patients, mainly due to blood disorders or severe skin reactions.

A high incidence of adverse effects has been reported in AIDS patients; desensitisation may sometimes be considered (see Immunocompromised Patients under Precautions, below).

◊ There has been concern over the safety of co-trimoxazole. In 1985, reporting on 85 deaths associated with the use of co-trimoxazole,[1] predominantly due to blood dyscrasias (50 reports) and skin reactions (14 reports), the UK Committee on Safety of Medicines (CSM) found that fatalities showed a marked increase with age: below 40 years, there were 0.25 reported deaths per million prescriptions, but for patients over 65 years of age the number of reported deaths per million prescriptions was more than 15-fold greater. However, at that time the CSM felt that it would be unwise to assume that trimethoprim was substantially less liable than co-trimoxazole to cause fatal adverse reactions.[1] Others suggested[2] that most of the deaths associated with the use of co-trimoxazole were typical of sulfonamide toxicity and that the indications for the use of co-trimoxazole should be reduced; this included the suggestion that it should be contra-indicated in the elderly. The CSM stated that their main message was that the risks of treatment of co-trimoxazole were more apparent in the elderly, but that there was no significant difference between the numbers of reports received for serious adverse reactions to trimethoprim and co-trimoxazole when corrected for prescription volumes.[3] In practice, despite further occasional reports of fatalities in elderly patients,[4] there did not appear to have been a marked reduction in the prescribing of this drug in the UK.[5] A similar warning of increased risk from co-trimoxazole in elderly patients was issued by the Adverse Drug Reactions Advisory Committee in Australia.[6]

More recently, a large population-based follow-up study in the UK[7] indicated that the risks of serious liver, blood, skin, and kidney disorders with either co-trimoxazole, trimethoprim, or cefalexin were small and were similar to those with many other antibacterials. Although in 1995 the CSM did restrict the use of co-trimoxazole on the grounds that its place in therapy had changed[8] (see under Uses and Administration, below), they also noted that co-trimoxazole continued to show a similar pattern of serious suspected adverse reactions to that reported 10 years earlier and that adverse drug reactions with trimethoprim were similar; blood dyscrasias and generalised skin disorders were the most serious reactions in each case and remained predominantly in elderly patients.

1. Committee on Safety of Medicines. Deaths associated with co-trimoxazole, ampicillin and trimethoprim. *Current Problems* 15 1985.
2. Lacey RW, *et al.* Co-trimoxazole toxicity. *BMJ* 1985; **291:** 481.
3. Goldberg A. Co-trimoxazole toxicity. *BMJ* 1985; **291:** 673.
4. Whittington RM. Toxic epidermal necrolysis and co-trimoxazole. *Lancet* 1989; **ii:** 574.
5. Carmichael AJ, Tan CY. Fatal toxic epidermal necrolysis associated with co-trimoxazole. *Lancet* 1989; **ii:** 808–9.
6. Adverse Drug Reactions Advisory Committee. Trimethoprim-sulphamethoxazole warning on elderly. *Aust Adverse Drug React Bull* February 1990.
7. Jick H, Derby LE. Is co-trimoxazole safe? *Lancet* 1995; **345:** 1118–19.
8. Committee on Safety of Medicines. Revised indications for co-trimoxazole (Septrin, Bactrim, various generic preparations). *Current Problems* 1995; **21:** 6.

Precautions
As for Sulfamethoxazole, p.254 and Trimethoprim, p.264.

Co-trimoxazole should not be given to patients with a history of hypersensitivity to it or to the sulfonamides or trimethoprim. It is contra-indicated in patients with severe hepatic failure and should be used with caution

---

The symbol † denotes a preparation no longer actively marketed

in patients with lesser degrees of hepatic impairment. Like its components, co-trimoxazole should be used with caution in impaired renal function, and dosage adjustment may be necessary; it should not be used in severe renal impairment without monitoring of plasma drug concentrations. An adequate fluid intake should be maintained to reduce the risk of crystalluria, but alkalinisation of the urine, although it increases urinary excretion of the sulfamethoxazole component, decreases urinary trimethoprim excretion. Regular blood counts and urinalyses and renal-function tests should be carried out in patients receiving prolonged treatment with co-trimoxazole. Elderly patients may be more susceptible to adverse effects (see above). Folate supplementation may be necessary in patients predisposed to folate deficiency, such as elderly patients and when high doses of co-trimoxazole are given for a prolonged period.

Glucose 6-phosphate dehydrogenase deficiency. Some have expressed the opinion that co-trimoxazole should be avoided by people with glucose 6-phosphate dehydrogenase deficiency.[1]

1. WHO. Glucose-6-phosphate dehydrogenase deficiency. *Bull WHO* 1989; **67**: 601–11.

Immunocompromised patients. An extraordinarily high frequency of adverse reactions to co-trimoxazole has been reported in patients with AIDS being treated for *Pneumocystis carinii* pneumonia. The comment has been made that, when therapeutic doses of co-trimoxazole are used, hypersensitivity rashes and leucopenia each develop in 30% of patients, compared with less than 5% for each complication in patients without AIDS.[1] Other studies have reported an even higher incidence of toxicity, and the overall incidence of adverse effects, including fever, malaise, and hepatitis, may be 80% or more.[2-4] Adverse reactions also appear to be unusually frequent when prophylactic doses are used.[4]

The occurrence of high serum concentrations of trimethoprim and sulfamethoxazole in patients has been proposed as a contributing factor to the high incidence of adverse effects,[5,6] and it was noted[5] that adverse effects, and in particular myelosuppression, were kept to tolerable levels in a group of patients in whom the dose of co-trimoxazole was adjusted to maintain serum-trimethoprim concentrations at 5 to 8 µg per mL. However, others[7] demonstrated no difference in the frequency of side-effects when the sulfamethoxazole dose was modified. A lower frequency of cutaneous reactions has been reported among African, Haitian, and American black AIDS patients compared with white AIDS patients, suggesting a genetic susceptibility to such reactions.[8]

It was suggested[9] that it was the reactive hydroxylamine metabolites of sulfamethoxazole which produced the adverse effects in HIV-infected individuals, but later work by the same authors[10] cast some doubt on this hypothesis.

Some workers have used diphenhydramine alone or with adrenaline [epinephrine] to manage hypersensitivity reactions associated with co-trimoxazole therapy, thus allowing continuation of treatment,[11,12] while other workers have tried desensitisation to co-trimoxazole in patients with AIDS.[13-18] For mention of desensitisation to sulfonamides in patients with AIDS, see under Sulfamethoxazole, p.254.

An increased incidence of myelosuppression, although not, apparently, of other adverse effects, has been reported in patients with leukaemia receiving maintenance chemotherapy.[19,20]

1. Masur H. Treatment of infections and immune defects. In: Fauci AS, moderator. Acquired immunodeficiency syndrome: epidemiologic, clinical, immunologic, and therapeutic considerations. *Ann Intern Med* 1984; **100**: 92–106.
2. Gordin FM, et al. Adverse reactions to trimethoprim-sulfamethoxazole in patients with the acquired immunodeficiency syndrome. *Ann Intern Med* 1984; **100**: 495–9.
3. Jaffe HS, et al. Complications of co-trimoxazole in treatment of AIDS-associated Pneumocystis carinii pneumonia in homosexual men. *Lancet* 1983; **ii**: 1109–11.
4. Mitsuyasu R, et al. Cutaneous reaction to trimethoprim-sulfamethoxazole in patients with AIDS and Kaposi's sarcoma. *N Engl J Med* 1983; **308**: 1535.
5. Sattler FR, et al. Trimethoprim-sulfamethoxazole compared with pentamidine for treatment of Pneumocystis carinii pneumonia in the acquired immunodeficiency syndrome. *Ann Intern Med* 1988; **109**: 280–7.
6. Stevens RC, et al. Pharmacokinetics and adverse effects of 20-mg/kg/day trimethoprim and 100-mg/kg/day sulfamethoxazole in healthy adult subjects. *Antimicrob Agents Chemother* 1991; **35**: 1884–90.
7. McLean I, et al. Modified trimethoprim-sulfamethoxazole doses in Pneumocystis carinii pneumonia. *Lancet* 1987; **ii**: 857–8.
8. Colebunders R, et al. Cutaneous reactions to trimethoprim-sulfamethoxazole in African patients with the acquired immunodeficiency syndrome. *Ann Intern Med* 1987; **107**: 599–600.
9. van der Ven AJAM, et al. Adverse reactions to co-trimoxazole in HIV infection. *Lancet* 1991; **338**: 431–3.
10. ter Hofstede HJM, et al. Drug reactions to cotrimoxazole in HIV infection: possibly not due to the hydroxylamine metabolites of sulphamethoxazole. *Br J Clin Pharmacol* 1999; **47**: 571–3.
11. Gibbons RB, Fraimow HA. Successful treatment of Pneumocystis carinii pneumonia with trimethoprim-sulfamethoxazole in hypersensitive AIDS patients. *JAMA* 1985; **253**: 1259–60.
12. Toma E, Fournier S. Adverse reactions to co-trimoxazole in HIV infection. *Lancet* 1991; **338**: 954.
13. Kreuz W, et al. "Treating through" hypersensitivity to co-trimoxazole in children with HIV infection. *Lancet* 1990; **336**: 508–9.
14. Carr A, et al. Efficacy and safety of rechallenge with low-dose trimethoprim-sulfamethoxazole in previously hypersensitive HIV-infected patients. *AIDS* 1993; **7**: 65–71.
15. Absar N, et al. Desensitization to trimethoprim/sulfamethoxazole in HIV-infected patients. *J Allergy Clin Immunol* 1994; **93**: 1001–5.
16. Cortese LM, et al. Trimethoprim/sulfamethoxazole desensitization. *Ann Pharmacother* 1996; **30**: 184–6.
17. Caumes E, et al. Efficacy and safety of desensitization with sulfamethoxazole and trimethoprim in 48 previously hypersensitive patients infected with human immunodeficiency virus. *Arch Dermatol* 1997; **133**: 465–9.
18. Demoly P, et al. Six-hour trimethoprim-sulfamethoxazole-graded challenge in HIV-infected patients. *J Allergy Clin Immunol* 1998; **102**: 1033–6.
19. Woods WG, et al. Myelosuppression associated with co-trimoxazole as a prophylactic antibiotic in the maintenance phase of childhood acute lymphocytic leukemia. *J Pediatr* 1984; **105**: 639–44.
20. Drysdale HC, Jones LF. Co-trimoxazole prophylaxis in leukaemia. *Lancet* 1982; **i**: 448.

Interference with diagnostic tests. Co-trimoxazole has been reported[1,2] to cause a small reduction in serum-thyroxine and tri-iodothyronine concentrations, probably due to the sulfonamide component.[2] It is suggested that, although co-trimoxazole cannot be concluded to be a cause of hypothyroidism (as all concentrations remained within the normal range), tests of thyroid function should be interpreted with care in patients on such treatment.

1. Cohen HN, et al. Effects on human thyroid function of sulphonamide and trimethoprim combination drugs. *BMJ* 1980; **281**: 646–7.
2. Cohen HN, et al. Trimethoprim and thyroid function. *Lancet* 1981; **i**: 676–7.

Porphyria. See under Sulfamethoxazole, p.254, and Trimethoprim, p.265.

Interactions

Any of the drug interactions reported with sulfamethoxazole (p.255) or trimethoprim (p.265) may occur with co-trimoxazole.

Antimicrobial Action

The actions and spectrum of activity of co-trimoxazole are essentially those of its components, sulfamethoxazole (p.255) and trimethoprim (p.265).

Because they act at different points of the folate metabolic pathway a potent synergy exists between its components in vitro with an increase of up to about 10-fold in antibacterial activity, and a frequently bactericidal action where the components individually are generally bacteriostatic. The optimum effect against most organisms is seen at a ratio of 1 part trimethoprim to 20 of sulfamethoxazole: although co-trimoxazole is formulated as a 1 to 5 ratio, differences in the pharmacokinetics of the two drugs mean that the ratio of the peak concentrations is approximately 1:20. However, it is not clear that the optimum ratio is achieved at all sites and, given that both drugs are present in therapeutic concentrations, the contribution of synergy to the effects of co-trimoxazole in vivo is uncertain.

Resistance to co-trimoxazole develops more slowly in vitro than to either component alone. Resistance has increased, and although initially slow, a more rapid increase was seen in many countries during the 1980s, occurring in both Gram-positive and Gram-negative organisms. Resistance has occurred notably among Enterobacteriaceae. Resistant strains of *Haemophilus influenzae*, streptococci, and *Vibrio cholerae* have been reported rarely. Although resistant organisms are usually resistant to both components of the mixture, strains resistant to either the sulfonamide or trimethoprim, and with a reduced sensitivity to co-trimoxazole, have been reported.

Pharmacokinetics

As for sulfamethoxazole (p.255) and trimethoprim (p.265). When co-trimoxazole is administered by mouth, plasma concentrations of trimethoprim and sulfamethoxazole are generally around the optimal ratio of 1:20, although they may vary from 1:2 to 1:30 or more. The ratio of the two drugs is usually much lower in the tissues (often around 1:2 to 1:5) since trimethoprim, the more lipophilic drug, penetrates many tissues better than sulfamethoxazole and has a much larger volume of distribution. In urine the ratio may vary from 1:1 to 1:5 depending on the pH.

Uses and Administration

Co-trimoxazole is a mixture of the sulfonamide, sulfamethoxazole, and the diaminopyrimidine, trimethoprim, and has been used in a wide variety of infections due to susceptible organisms, particularly those of the urinary, respiratory, and gastrointestinal tracts, although the indications for its use are restricted in the UK (see below). Its main uses now are in *Pneumocystis carinii* pneumonia, toxoplasmosis, and nocardiosis.

Its other uses have included the treatment of: acne; biliary-tract infections; brucellosis (generally in combination with other drugs); cat scratch disease; chancroid; *Burkholderia cepacia* (*Pseudomonas cepacia*) infections in cystic fibrosis; some forms of AIDS-associated diarrhoea such as the protozoal infection isosporiasis; gonorrhoea; granuloma inguinale; listeriosis; melioidosis; mycetoma; otitis media; pertussis; typhoid and paratyphoid fever; and Whipple's disease. It has also been used for the prophylaxis of infections in immunocompromised patients and for selective decontamination for patients in intensive care. For details of the bacterial infections listed above and their treatment, see under Choice of Antibacterial, p.114.

Co-trimoxazole is usually given by mouth in a dose of 960 mg (trimethoprim 160 mg and sulfamethoxazole 800 mg) twice daily; in severe infections 2.88 g daily in 2 divided doses has been given. Lower doses are given for long-term treatment and in patients with renal impairment: half the usual dosage for patients with a creatinine clearance between 15 and 30 mL per minute; co-trimoxazole is generally not employed when the creatinine clearance is less than 15 mL per minute unless facilities for haemodialysis are available.

Doses of co-trimoxazole to be given twice daily to children are: from 6 weeks to 5 months of age, 120 mg; 6 months to 5 years, 240 mg; 6 to 12 years, 480 mg. Co-trimoxazole should not generally be given to infants below 6 weeks of age because of the risk of kernicterus from the sulfonamide component (see Pregnancy and Breast Feeding, under Precautions of Sulfamethoxazole, p.254), although it may be used in infants from 4 weeks of age for the treatment or prophylaxis of *Pneumocystis carinii* pneumonia.

Higher doses of co-trimoxazole of up to 120 mg per kg body-weight daily given in two to four divided doses for 14 to 21 days are used in the treatment of *Pneumocystis carinii* pneumonia; serum concentrations should be monitored and folate supplementation possibly considered (but see Pneumocystis carinii Pneumonia, below). For prophylaxis in patients with AIDS, the standard dose of co-trimoxazole (960 mg twice daily) may be given, but has been associated with a high incidence of adverse effects (see under Precautions, above). Alternatively the following dose regimens may be used: 960 mg daily (7 days each week); 960 mg daily on alternate days (3 days each week); or 960 mg twice daily on alternate days (3 days each week).

For serious infections, if oral administration is not possible, co-trimoxazole may be given initially by intravenous infusion diluted immediately before use in a suitable diluent. The contents of each ampoule containing 480 mg of co-trimoxazole in 5 mL are added to 125 mL of diluent and infused over 60 to 90 minutes, unless fluid restriction is required, in which case only 75 mL of diluent may be used. Dosage is similar to that by mouth.

◊ The current place of co-trimoxazole in therapy was reviewed by the UK Committee on Safety of Medicines in 1995 (see also under Adverse Effects and Treatment, above).[1] As a result they recommended that its use should be limited to: *Pneumocystis carinii* pneumonia, toxoplasmosis, and nocardiosis; urinary-tract infections and acute exacerbations of chronic bronchitis, but only when there is bacteriological evidence of sensitivity to co-trimoxazole and good reason to prefer it to a single antibac-

has variable activity against Gram-positive and Gram-negative bacteria including *Escherichia coli* and *Staphylococcus aureus*. Cycloserine is active against *Mycobacterium tuberculosis* and some other mycobacteria. Minimum inhibitory concentrations *in vitro* for *M. tuberculosis* range from 5 to 20 µg per mL. Resistance develops if cycloserine is used alone.

Pharmacokinetics

Cycloserine is readily and almost completely absorbed from the gastrointestinal tract. Peak plasma concentrations of 10 µg per mL have been obtained in 3 to 4 hours after a dose of 250 mg, rising to 20 to 30 µg per mL on repeating the dose every 12 hours. The plasma half-life is about 10 hours and is prolonged in patients with renal impairment.

Cycloserine is widely distributed into body tissues and fluids, including the CSF and breast milk. It crosses the placenta producing fetal blood concentrations approaching those in maternal serum.

Cycloserine is excreted largely unchanged by glomerular filtration. About 50% of a single 250-mg dose is excreted unchanged in the urine within 12 hours and about 70% is excreted within 72 hours. As negligible amounts of cycloserine appear in the faeces, it is assumed that the remainder of a dose is metabolised to unidentified metabolites. It is removed by haemodialysis.

Pregnancy and breast feeding. Cycloserine has been shown to pass to the fetus, amniotic fluid,[1] and into breast milk.[2] Concentrations in breast milk after 250 mg four times daily have been reported to range from 6 to 19 µg per mL.[2]

1. Holdiness MR. Transplacental pharmacokinetics of the antituberculosis drugs. *Clin Pharmacokinet* 1987; **13:** 125–9.
2. Snider DE, Powell KE. Should women taking antituberculosis drugs breast-feed? *Arch Intern Med* 1984; **144:** 589–90.

Uses and Administration

Cycloserine is a second-line antimycobacterial that may be used in the treatment of tuberculosis (p.143) as part of a multi-drug regimen when resistance to or toxicity from primary drugs has developed. It has been used in urinary-tract infections although less toxic drugs are preferred.

The usual adult dose in tuberculosis is 0.5 to 1 g daily by mouth in divided doses. The maximum daily dose is 1 g. Some recommend an initial dose of 250 mg twice daily for 2 weeks. Experience in children is limited; an initial paediatric dose of 10 mg per kg body-weight daily has been suggested. Dosage in patients with renal impairment should be reduced and doses for all patients should be adjusted by monitoring plasma concentrations (see Precautions, above).

L-Cycloserine (levcycloserine) has been investigated for the treatment of Gaucher disease (p.1575).

Preparations

USP 25: Cycloserine Capsules.

Proprietary Preparations (details are given in Part 3)
Austral.: Closina; *Canad.:* Seromycin†; *Hong Kong:* Seromycin; *UK:* Cycloserine; *USA:* Seromycin.

Danofloxacin Mesilate (10962-e)

Danofloxacin Mesilate *(BANM, rINNM)*.

CP-76136 (danofloxacin); CP-76136-27 (danofloxacin mesilate); Danofloxacin Mesylate *(USAN)*. 1-Cyclopropyl-6-fluoro-1,4-dihydro-7- [(1S,4S)-5-methyl-2,5-diazabicyclo[2.2.1]hept-2-yl]-4-oxo-3-quinolinecarboxylic acid monomethanesulphonate.

$C_{19}H_{20}FN_3O_3,CH_4O_3S = 453.5$.
CAS — 112398-08-0 (danofloxacin); 119478-55-6 (danofloxacin mesilate).

Profile

Danofloxacin is a fluoroquinolone antibacterial used as the mesilate in veterinary medicine.

Dapsone (6554-b)

Dapsone *(BAN, USAN, rINN)*.

DADPS; Dapsonum; DDS; Diaminodiphenylsulfone; Diaphenylsulfone; Disulone; NSC-6091; Sulphonyldianiline. Bis(4-aminophenyl) sulphone.

$C_{12}H_{12}N_2O_2S = 248.3$.
CAS — 80-08-0.
ATC — J04BA02.
Pharmacopoeias. In *Chin., Eur.* (see p.vi), *Int.,* and *US*.

Pharmacopoeial description

Ph. Eur.: A white or slightly yellowish-white, crystalline powder. Very slightly soluble in water; sparingly soluble in alcohol; freely soluble in acetone. It dissolves freely in dilute mineral acids. Protect from light.

USP 25: A white or creamy-white, odourless crystalline powder. Very slightly soluble in water, freely soluble in alcohol; soluble in acetone and in dilute mineral acids. Protect from light.

Adverse Effects

Varying degrees of dose-related haemolysis and

methaemoglobinaemia are the most frequently reported adverse effects of dapsone, and occur in most subjects given more than 200 mg daily; doses of up to 100 mg daily do not cause significant haemolysis, but subjects deficient in glucose-6-phosphate dehydrogenase are affected by doses above about 50 mg daily. Although agranulocytosis has been reported rarely with dapsone when used alone, reports have been more common when dapsone has been used with other drugs in the prophylaxis of malaria.

Rash and pruritus may develop. Serious cutaneous hypersensitivity reactions occur rarely and include maculopapular rash, exfoliative dermatitis, toxic epidermal necrolysis, and Stevens-Johnson syndrome. Fixed drug eruptions have occurred.

A 'dapsone syndrome' may occur and resembles mononucleosis in its presentation (see below).

Peripheral neuropathy with motor loss has been reported in patients on dapsone for dermatological conditions. Peripheral neuropathy may occur as part of leprosy reaction states and is not an indication to discontinue dapsone.

Other adverse effects occur infrequently and include nausea, vomiting, anorexia, headache, hepatitis, psychosis, and tachycardia.

Carcinogenicity. A survey of 1678 leprosy patients admitted for treatment to the National Hansen's Disease Center in Carville between 1939 and 1977 indicated that, although dapsone has been implicated as a carcinogen in *animals*, the use of dapsone did not appear to affect significantly the risk of any cancer in these patients.[1]

1. Brinton LA, *et al.* Cancer mortality among patients with Hansen's disease. *J Natl Cancer Inst* 1984; **72:** 109–14.

Effects on the blood. *Haemolysis* is the most frequent serious adverse effect of dapsone and may occur at doses of 200 mg or higher daily.[1] Red blood cells may contain Heinz bodies and there is a reduction in their life span. Well-known risk factors include glucose-6-phosphate deficiency, methaemoglobin reductase deficiency, and haemoglobin M trait; haemoglobin E trait may also increase susceptibility to haemolytic reactions.[2] Haemolytic anaemia has been reported in a neonate following ingestion of dapsone in breast milk.[3]

Methaemoglobinaemia, though common, is rarely symptomatic.[1] However, severe cyanosis was associated with methaemoglobinaemia in an HIV-positive patient with suspected *Pneumocystis carinii* pneumonia following inadvertent overdosing with dapsone.[4]

Agranulocytosis has occurred rarely following dapsone use in leprosy and skin disease. More cases have been observed when used for malaria prophylaxis[5] (see also under Pyrimethamine, p.442) and dermatitis herpetiformis.[6] The reaction is usually self-limiting once the drug is withdrawn, but fatalities have occurred.[6,7]

Aplastic anaemia has been reported.[8,9] Of 11 fatalities attributed to dapsone reported to the British and Swedish adverse reaction registers[10] between 1968 and 1988, 7 were due to white blood cell dyscrasias; none were attributed to red cell dyscrasias, although such reactions formed almost half of all serious reactions reported for dapsone.

Thrombocytosis was reported in a patient with AIDS receiving dapsone prophylactically.[11]

See also Hypoalbuminaemia, below.

1. Jopling WH. Side-effects of antileprosy drugs in common use. *Lepr Rev* 1983; **54:** 261–70.
2. Lachant NA, Tanaka KR. Case report: dapsone-associated Heinz body hemolytic anemia in a Cambodian woman with hemoglobin E trait. *Am J Med Sci* 1987; **294:** 364–8.
3. Sanders SW, *et al.* Hemolytic anemia induced by dapsone transmitted through breast milk. *Ann Intern Med* 1982; **96:** 465–6.
4. Seaton RA, *et al.* Blue and breathless. *Hosp Med* 1999; **60:** 530.
5. Firkin FC, Mariani AF. Agranulocytosis due to dapsone. *Med J Aust* 1977; **2:** 247–51.
6. Cockburn EM, *et al.* Dapsone-induced agranulocytosis: spontaneous reporting data. *Br J Dermatol* 1993; **128:** 702–3.
7. Barss P. Fatal dapsone agranulocytosis in a Melanesian. *Lepr Rev* 1986; **57:** 63–6.
8. Foucauld J, *et al.* Dapsone and aplastic anemia. *Ann Intern Med* 1985; **102:** 139.
9. Meyerson MA, Cohen PR. Dapsone-induced aplastic anaemia in a woman with bullous systemic lupus erythematosus. *Mayo Clin Proc* 1994; **69:** 1159–62.
10. Björkman A, Phillips-Howard PA. Adverse reactions to sulfa drugs: implications for malaria chemotherapy. *Bull WHO* 1991; **69:** 297–304.
11. Wynn RF, *et al.* Case report of dapsone-related thrombocytosis in an AIDS patient. *Am J Med* 1995; **98:** 602.

Effects on the eyes. References to eye damage associated with acute or subacute dapsone poisoning.[1,2]

1. Daneshmend TK. The neurotoxicity of dapsone. *Adverse Drug React Acute Poisoning Rev* 1984; **3:** 43–58.
2. Alexander TA, *et al.* Presumed DDS ocular toxicity. *Indian J Ophthalmol* 1989; **37:** 150–1.

Effects on the liver. Toxic hepatitis and cholestatic jaundice have been reported by the manufacturer to occur early in dapsone therapy. Jaundice may also form part of the dapsone reac-

tion (see Hypersensitivity Reactions, below). Deterioration in liver function tests during dapsone treatment has been noted in a patient with dermatitis herpetiformis and primary sclerosing cholangitis.[1]

1. Kirby B, *et al.* Abnormal liver function tests induced by dapsone in a patient with dermatitis herpetiformis and primary sclerosing cholangitis. *Br J Dermatol* 1999; **141:** 172–3.

Effects on the lungs. Pulmonary eosinophilia occurred on 2 occasions in a woman receiving dapsone for urticaria.[1] On each occasion symptoms resolved when dapsone was stopped.

1. Jaffuel D, *et al.* Eosinophilic pneumonia induced by dapsone. *BMJ* 1998; **317:** 181.

Effects on mental state. Psychosis has been reported in leprosy patients receiving dapsone, but the role of dapsone in this effect is poorly defined.[1] Manic-depressive reactions have been reported in 2 patients with skin disorders.[2] These reactions appeared to be idiosyncratic reactions to dapsone.[2,3]

1. Daneshmend T. Idiosyncratic dapsone induced manic depression. *BMJ* 1989; **299:** 324.
2. Carmichael AJ, Paul CJ. Idiosyncratic dapsone induced manic depression. *BMJ* 1989; **298:** 1524. Correction. *ibid.*; **299:** 56.
3. Gawkrodger D. Manic depression induced by dapsone in patient with dermatitis herpetiformis. *BMJ* 1989; **299:** 860.

Effects on the nervous system. Clinical details of 13 patients who experienced dapsone-induced neuropathy. Patients received a mean dose of 115 g (range 6 to 380 g) over 19 months for various dermatological conditions.[1] All patients had motor weakness and some experienced sensory impairment. Most recovered within several months of discontinuing dapsone.

1. Daneshmend TK. The neurotoxicity of dapsone. *Adverse Drug React Acute Poisoning Rev* 1984; **3:** 43–58.

Effects on taste. A persistent sweet taste and tingling of the face and lips was described in a patient receiving dapsone for ocular cicatricial pemphigoid.[1] The symptoms resolved when dapsone was stopped.

1. Stafanous SN, Morgan SJ. A previously unrecognised side effect of dapsone. *Br J Ophthalmol* 1997; **81:** 1113–14.

Hyperpigmentation. Hyperpigmented macules were reported in 32 of about 800 children who received dapsone with pyrimethamine for 3 months or more for malaria prophylaxis.[1] The reaction was attributed to dapsone.

1. David KP, *et al.* Hyperpigmented dermal macules in children following the administration of Maloprim for malaria chemoprophylaxis. *Trans R Soc Trop Med Hyg* 1997; **91:** 204–8.

Hypersensitivity reactions. Dapsone syndrome is a rare hypersensitivity reaction although it has been suggested[1,2] that the incidence has increased since the introduction of multidrug therapy for leprosy. It occurs in the first 6 weeks of therapy and symptoms include rash, which is always present, fever, jaundice, and eosinophilia. The syndrome has occurred in leprosy patients,[3-5] in patients with skin disorders,[6,7] and in patients taking weekly dapsone (in association with pyrimethamine) for malaria prophylaxis.[8] Fatalities have occurred.[4,9] Desensitisation has been successfully carried out in several patients with AIDS who exhibited hypersensitivity to dapsone.[10,11]

1. Richardus JH, Smith TC. Increased incidence in leprosy of hypersensitivity reactions to dapsone after introduction of multidrug therapy. *Lepr Rev* 1989; **60:** 267–73.
2. Kumar RH, *et al.* Dapsone syndrome—a five year retrospective analysis. *Indian J Lepr* 1998; **70:** 271–6.
3. Joseph MS. Hypersensitivity reaction to dapsone. *Lepr Rev* 1985; **56:** 315–20.
4. Jamrozik K. Dapsone syndrome occurring in two brothers. *Lepr Rev* 1986; **57:** 57–62.
5. Hortaleza AR, *et al.* Dapsone syndrome in a Filipino man. *Lepr Rev* 1995; **66:** 307–13.
6. Tomecki KJ, Catalano CJ. Dapsone hypersensitivity: the sulfone syndrome revisited. *Arch Dermatol* 1981; **117:** 38–9.
7. Kromann NP, *et al.* The dapsone syndrome. *Arch Dermatol* 1982; **118:** 531–2.
8. Grayson ML, *et al.* Severe dapsone syndrome due to weekly Maloprim. *Lancet* 1988; **i:** 531.
9. Frey HM, *et al.* Fatal reaction to dapsone during treatment of leprosy. *Ann Intern Med* 1981; **94:** 777–9.
10. Metroka CE, *et al.* Desensitization to dapsone in HIV-positive patients. *JAMA* 1992; **267:** 512.
11. Cook DE, Kossey JL. Successful desensitization to dapsone for Pneumocystis carinii prophylaxis in an HIV-positive patient. *Ann Pharmacother* 1998; **32:** 1302–5.

Hypoalbuminaemia. Severe and often life-threatening hypoalbuminaemia has been reported rarely in patients taking dapsone for extended periods for dermatitis herpetiformis.[1-3] Hypoalbuminaemia usually resolves rapidly once dapsone is withdrawn.

1. Kingham JGC, *et al.* Dapsone and severe hypoalbuminaemia. *Lancet* 1979; **ii:** 662–4 and 1018.
2. Foster PN, Swan CHJ. Dapsone and fatal hypoalbuminaemia. *Lancet* 1981; **ii:** 806–7.
3. Sinclair SA, *et al.* Life threatening hypoalbuminaemia associated with dapsone therapy. *Br J Dermatol* 1996; **135** (suppl 47): 45.

Photosensitivity. A report of photosensitivity in 6 patients who had taken dapsone.[1]

1. Dhanapaul S. DDS-induced photosensitivity with reference to six case reports. *Lepr Rev* 1989; **60:** 147–50.

Treatment of Adverse Effects

In severe overdosage the stomach should be emptied by lavage. Repeated doses of activated charcoal should be given by mouth with the aim of preventing absorption of dapsone but also to aid the elimination of dapsone and its monoacetyl metabolite. Methaem-oglobinaemia has been treated with slow intravenous injections of methylene blue [methylthioninium chloride] 1 to 2 mg per kg body-weight repeated after one hour if necessary. Methylene blue [methylthioninium chloride] should not be administered to patients with glucose-6-phosphate dehydrogenase deficiency since it will not be effective. Haemolysis has been treated by infusion of concentrated human red blood cells to replace the damaged cells. Supportive therapy includes administration of oxygen and fluids.

◊ References to the treatment of dapsone overdosage.
1. Dawson AH, Whyte IM. Management of dapsone poisoning complicated by methaemoglobinaemia. *Med Toxicol Adverse Drug Exp* 1989; **4:** 387–92.
2. Endre ZH, et al. Successful treatment of acute dapsone intoxication using charcoal hemoperfusion. *Aust N Z J Med* 1983; **13:** 509–12.
3. Hoetelmans RMW, et al. Combined dapsone and clofazimine intoxication. *Hum Exp Toxicol* 1996; **15:** 625–8.
4. Ferguson JY, Lavery GG. Deliberate self-poisoning with dapsone: a case report and summary of relevant pharmacology and treatment. *Anaesthesia* 1997; **52:** 359–63.

Prevention of haemotoxicity. Administration of cimetidine with dapsone may reduce the incidence or severity of dapsone-induced methaemoglobinaemia and haemolysis, probably by reducing N-hydroxylation.[1,2] Other strategies, such as the use of the antioxidant alpha tocopherol, were considered less successful.[3]
1. Coleman MD, et al. The use of cimetidine as a selective inhibitor of dapsone N-hydroxylation in man. *Br J Clin Pharmacol* 1990; **30:** 761–7.
2. Rhodes LE, et al. Cimetidine improves the therapeutic/toxic ratio of dapsone in patients on chronic dapsone therapy. *Br J Dermatol* 1995; **132:** 257–62.
3. Coleman MD, Coleman NA. Drug-induced methaemoglobinaemia: treatment issues. *Drug Safety* 1996; **14:** 394–405.

Precautions

Dapsone should not be used in patients with severe anaemia. It is recommended that regular blood counts be performed during treatment. Patients deficient in glucose-6-phosphate dehydrogenase, or methaemoglobin reductase, or with haemoglobin M are more susceptible to the haemolytic effects of dapsone.

Where possible, liver function should be monitored during treatment.

It is now generally considered that the benefits of dapsone in the treatment of leprosy during pregnancy outweigh any potential risk to the pregnant patient. Some leprologists recommend folic acid 5 mg daily for leprosy patients receiving dapsone during pregnancy. Dapsone is distributed into breast milk and there has been a report of haemolytic anaemia in a breast-fed infant (see Effects on the Blood, under Adverse Effects, above). While some authorities feel that dapsone should not be used in mothers who are breast feeding, in general treatment for leprosy is continued in such patients.

Porphyria. Dapsone has been associated with acute attacks of porphyria and is considered unsafe in porphyric patients.

Interactions

Serum concentrations of dapsone are increased, with a consequent increased risk of adverse effects, during concurrent administration of probenecid, probably as a result of reduced renal excretion of dapsone. Increased dapsone concentrations have also been reported in patients receiving trimethoprim, and patients receiving this combination may be at increased risk of dapsone toxicity. Rifampicin reduces serum concentrations of dapsone to a level that may compromise efficacy in infections other than leprosy. Rifampicin concentrations are generally unaffected. Dapsone may antagonise the anti-inflammatory properties of clofazimine (p.191).

Pyrimethamine. Although some manufacturers warn that dapsone-induced haematotoxicity could be potentiated by folic acid antagonists such as pyrimethamine, the tolerability of dapsone plus pyrimethamine was similar to dapsone alone when each treatment was given on a once-weekly basis to patients with HIV infection.[1] Dapsone concentrations were not significantly higher in patients receiving dapsone plus pyrimethamine than in those receiving dapsone alone.
1. Falloon J, et al. Pharmacokinetics and safety of weekly dapsone and dapsone plus pyrimethamine for prevention of pneumocystis pneumonia. *Antimicrob Agents Chemother* 1994; **38:** 1580–7.

Trimethoprim. In a study of AIDS patients with *Pneumocystis carinii* pneumonia, the mean peak serum concentrations

of dapsone were 1.5 µg per mL following 100 mg daily for 7 days and 2.1 µg per mL following dapsone in combination with trimethoprim 20 mg per kg body-weight daily; concentrations of trimethoprim were also increased.[1] Elevated dapsone concentrations may contribute to the toxicity and the efficacy of this combination.
1. Lee BL, et al. Dapsone, trimethoprim, and sulfamethoxazole plasma levels during treatment of pneumocystis pneumonia in patients with the acquired immuno deficiency syndrome (AIDS). *Ann Intern Med* 1989; **110:** 606–11.

Antimicrobial Action

Dapsone is a sulfone active against a wide range of bacteria, but it is mainly employed for its action against *Mycobacterium leprae*. Its mechanism of action is probably similar to that of the sulfonamides, which involves inhibition of folic acid synthesis in susceptible organisms. It is usually considered to be bacteriostatic against *M. leprae*, although it may also possess weak bactericidal activity. It is also active against *Plasmodium* and *Pneumocystis carinii*. As with the sulfonamides, antibacterial activity is inhibited by *p*-aminobenzoic acid.

Using the mouse foot-pad technique the minimum inhibitory concentration for *M. leprae* has been reported to be less than 10 nanograms per mL.

Secondary (acquired) dapsone resistance of *Mycobacterium leprae* is mainly associated with dapsone being used on its own. Primary dapsone resistance has also been reported with increasing frequency in areas with secondary resistance. Resistance of *M. leprae* to dapsone should be suspected whenever a patient relapses clinically and bacteriologically.

◊ Combinations of dapsone with the folate antagonists sulfadimidine,[1] cycloguanil,[1] or pyrimethamine[2] showed synergistic activity against *Mycobacterium avium* complex *in vitro*.
1. Gonzalez AH, et al. In-vitro activity of dapsone and two potentiators against Mycobacterium avium complex. *J Antimicrob Chemother* 1989; **24:** 19–22.
2. Shah LM, et al. Enhanced in vitro activity of pyrimethamine in combination with dapsone against Mycobacterium avium complex. *Antimicrob Agents Chemother* 1996; **40:** 2426–7.

Multidrug resistance. Strains of *Mycobacterium leprae* with multiple resistance to rifampicin, ofloxacin, and dapsone have been isolated from patients who have previously received dapsone monotherapy followed by treatment with rifampicin in combination with ofloxacin.[1]
1. Cambau E, et al. Multidrug-resistance to dapsone, rifampicin, and ofloxacin in Mycobacterium leprae. *Lancet* 1997; **349:** 103–4.

Pharmacokinetics

Dapsone is almost completely absorbed from the gastrointestinal tract with peak plasma concentrations occurring from 2 to 8 hours after a dose. Steady-state concentrations are not attained until after at least 8 days of daily administration; doses of 100 mg daily provide trough concentrations of 0.5 µg per mL, which are well in excess of the MIC for *M. leprae*. About 50 to 80% of dapsone in the circulation is bound to plasma proteins and nearly 100% of its monoacetylated metabolite is bound.

Dapsone undergoes enterohepatic recycling. It is widely distributed; it is present in saliva and breast milk and crosses the placenta. The half-life ranges from 10 to 50 hours.

Dapsone is acetylated to monoacetyldapsone, the major metabolite, and other mono and diacetyl derivatives. Acetylation exhibits genetic polymorphism. Hydroxylation is the other major metabolic pathway resulting in hydroxylamine dapsone, which may be responsible for dapsone-associated methaemoglobinaemia and haemolysis.

Dapsone is mainly excreted in the urine, only 20% of a dose as unchanged drug.

◊ References.
1. Zuidema J, et al. Clinical pharmacokinetics of dapsone. *Clin Pharmacokinet* 1986; **11:** 299–315.
2. Pieters FAJM, Zuidema J. The pharmacokinetics of dapsone after oral administration to healthy volunteers. *Br J Clin Pharmacol* 1986; **22:** 491–4.
3. May DG, et al. The disposition of dapsone in cirrhosis. *Clin Pharmacol Ther* 1992; **51:** 689–700.
4. Mirochnick M, et al. Pharmacokinetics of dapsone in children. *J Pediatr* 1993; **122:** 806–9.
5. Opravil M, et al. Levels of dapsone and pyrimethamine in serum during once-weekly dosing for prophylaxis of Pneumocystis carinii pneumonia and toxoplasmic encephalitis. *Antimicrob Agents Chemother* 1994; **38:** 1197–9.

6. Gatti G, et al. Pharmacokinetics of dapsone in human immunodeficiency virus-infected children. *Antimicrob Agents Chemother* 1995; **39:** 1101–6.
7. Gatti G, et al. Population pharmacokinetics of dapsone administered biweekly to human immunodeficiency virus-infected patients. *Antimicrob Agents Chemother* 1996; **40:** 2743–8.
8. Gatti G, et al. Penetration of dapsone into cerebrospinal fluid of patients with AIDS. *J Antimicrob Chemother* 1997; **40:** 113–15.
9. Mirochnick M, et al. Pharmacokinetics of dapsone administered daily and weekly in human immunodeficiency virus-infected children. *Antimicrob Agents Chemother* 1999; **43:** 2586–91.

Metabolism. Measurement of the relative activity of the two main routes of dapsone metabolism (acetylation and hydroxylation) suggests that the risk of adverse effects is greater in individuals in whom the N-hydroxylation route predominates.[1] This is consistent with the hypothesis that the toxicity of dapsone is related to production of an active metabolite.
1. Bluhm RE, et al. Development of dapsone toxicity in patients with inflammatory dermatoses: activity of acetylation and hydroxylation of dapsone as risk factors. *Clin Pharmacol Ther* 1999; **65:** 598–605.

Uses and Administration

Dapsone is used as part of multi-drug regimens in the treatment of all forms of leprosy (p.126). It has also been used in the prophylaxis of leprosy and in the management of household contacts of leprosy patients. Dapsone is used as an alternative to co-trimoxazole or pentamidine for the treatment and prophylaxis of *Pneumocystis carinii* pneumonia (below), and in combination with pyrimethamine for the prophylaxis of malaria (see under Pyrimethamine, p.444). It is also used in dermatitis herpetiformis and other dermatoses (see Skin Disorders, below). It has been tried for the prophylaxis of toxoplasmosis (p.585) and for the treatment of cutaneous leishmaniasis (p.584) and actinomycetoma (p.130).

Dapsone is usually given by mouth. There are some reports of it being given by intramuscular injection, but such injections can be painful and cause abscess formation.

The most common regimens for leprosy are those recommended by WHO. For multibacillary leprosy, rifampicin 600 mg and clofazimine 300 mg are both given once a month together with dapsone 100 mg and clofazimine 50 mg both daily for 12 months. Doses of all 3 drugs are reduced in children and in those aged 10 to 14 years daily doses of dapsone 50 mg, or 1 to 2 mg per kg if their body-weight is low, are given. Adults weighing less than 35 kg also receive reduced doses of rifampicin and dapsone and in such patients the dapsone dose is 50 mg or 1 to 2 mg per kg daily.

The WHO regimen for paucibacillary leprosy consists of rifampicin 600 mg once a month and dapsone 100 mg daily; both are given for 6 months. Doses are reduced in children and low-weight patients as for multibacillary leprosy.

The doses of dapsone used for the prophylaxis of *Pneumocystis carinii* pneumonia are discussed in more detail under Pneumocystis carinii Pneumonia, below. Dapsone has also been given with trimethoprim for treatment.

The adult dose of dapsone for malaria prophylaxis is 100 mg weekly with pyrimethamine 12.5 mg weekly.

The dose required for the treatment of dermatitis herpetiformis has to be titrated for individual patients, but it is usual to start with 50 mg daily by mouth, gradually increased to 300 mg daily or more if required. This dose should be reduced to a minimum as soon as possible. Maintenance dosage can often be reduced in patients receiving a gluten-free diet.

Connective tissue disorders. Dapsone has been used in a number of inflammatory disorders. Relapsing polychondritis (p.1056) has responded to dapsone, as has Behçet's syndrome (p.1047) and systemic lupus erythematosus (p.1059). Vasculitic syndromes such as hypersensitivity vasculitis (p.1052) have also improved following dapsone.

Kaposi's sarcoma. For a report of the control of non-epidemic (not HIV-related) Kaposi's sarcoma by the use of dapsone, see p.501.

Pneumocystis carinii pneumonia. Dapsone is used alone and in combination with pyrimethamine[1] for primary prophylaxis of *Pneumocystis carinii* pneumonia in patients unable to tolerate co-trimoxazole (see p.375). A dose of dapsone 100 mg daily in one or two doses is commonly used and has been reported to have similar efficacy to co-trimoxazole.[2] Dapsone has

The symbol † denotes a preparation no longer actively marketed

also been given in combination with pyrimethamine in various regimens including dapsone 50 mg daily with pyrimethamine 50 mg once weekly,[3] dapsone 100 mg plus pyrimethamine 50 mg both given twice weekly,[4] and dapsone 200 mg plus pyrimethamine 75 mg both given once weekly.[5]

For treatment, dapsone 100 mg daily with trimethoprim 20 mg per kg body-weight daily for 21 days has been suggested.

1. Centers for Disease Control. USPHS/IDSA guidelines for the prevention of opportunistic infections in persons infected with human immunodeficiency virus. *MMWR* 1999; **48** (RR-10): 1–59.
2. Bozzette SA, *et al.* A randomized trial of three antipneumocystis agents in patients with advanced human immunodeficiency virus infection. *N Engl J Med* 1995; **332:** 693–9.
3. Girard P-M, *et al.* Dapsone-pyrimethamine compared with aerosolized pentamidine as primary prophylaxis against Pneumocystis carinii pneumonia and toxoplasmosis in HIV infection. *N Engl J Med* 1993; **328:** 1514–20.
4. Podzamczer D, *et al.* Intermittent trimethoprim-sulfamethoxazole compared with dapsone-pyrimethamine for the simultaneous primary prophylaxis of pneumocystis pneumonia and toxoplasmosis in patients infected with HIV. *Ann Intern Med* 1995; **122:** 755–61.
5. Opravil M, *et al.* Once-weekly administration of dapsone/pyrimethamine vs. aerosolized pentamidine as combined prophylaxis for Pneumocystis carinii pneumonia and toxoplasmic encephalitis in human immunodeficiency virus-infected patients. *Clin Infect Dis* 1995; **20:** 531–41.

Skin disorders. Dapsone is used in a variety of skin disorders including the suppression of skin lesions in dermatitis herpetiformis (p.1104). The mechanism of action is unknown but unrelated to its antimicrobial activity. Reports, generally involving small numbers of patients, suggest that dapsone may also be beneficial for bullous or cicatricial pemphigoid (p.1106), pyoderma gangrenosum (p.1107), recurrent erythema multiforme (p.1105), and urticaria (p.1107).

Spider bites. As discussed on p.1564, necrotic araneism resulting from the bite of spiders of the genus *Loxosceles* is usually treated conservatively with surgical repair of any persistent defect. A prospective clinical study of 31 patients with brown recluse spider bites indicated[1] that treatment with dapsone 100 mg daily for 14 days followed by delayed surgical intervention if necessary reduced the incidence of wound complications and residual scarring compared with treatment by immediate surgical excision. A dose of 100 mg twice daily has also been given for 14 days.[2]

1. Rees RS, *et al.* Brown recluse spider bites: a comparison of early surgical excision versus dapsone and delayed surgical excision. *Ann Surg* 1985; **202:** 659–63.
2. King LE, Rees RS. Dapsone treatment of a brown recluse bite. *JAMA* 1983; **250:** 648.

Preparations

BP 2001: Dapsone Tablets;
USP 25: Dapsone Tablets.

Proprietary Preparations (details are given in Part 3)
Canad.: Avlosulfon; *Israel:* Avlosulfon; *Mex.:* Dapsoderm-X; Novasulfon; *Port.:* Sulfona; *Spain:* Sulfona; *Thai.:* Servidapsone.

Multi-ingredient: *Aust.:* Isoprodian; *Austral.:* Maloprim†; *Fr.:* Disulone; *Ger.:* Isoprodian; *Irl.:* Maloprim; *S.Afr.:* Maloprim; MB-Combi†; *UK:* Maloprim.

Daptomycin (3854-z)

Daptomycin (*BAN, USAN, rINN*).

Ly-146032. *N*-Decanoyl-L-tryptophyl-L-asparaginyl-L-aspartyl-L-threonylglycyl-L-ornithyl-L-aspartyl-D-alanyl-L-aspartylglycyl-D-seryl-*threo*-3-methyl-L-glutamyl-3-anthraniloyl-L-alanine   1.13-3.4-lactone.

$C_{72}H_{101}N_{17}O_{26} = 1620.7$.
CAS — 103060-53-3.

Profile
Daptomycin is a lipopeptide antibacterial that is reported to have a spectrum of antibacterial activity similar to that of vancomycin (p.268) and greater potency against many bacterial strains *in vitro*. It is reported to show antimicrobial synergy *in vitro* with the aminoglycosides against enterococci and *Staphylococcus aureus*. It is under investigation for the intravenous treatment of complicated Gram-positive infections of the skin and soft tissues.

◊ References.

1. Pryka RD, *et al.* Clinical pharmacokinetics of daptomycin. *DICP Ann Pharmacother* 1990; **24:** 255–6.
2. Kreft B, *et al.* Experimental studies on nephrotoxicity and pharmacokinetics of LY 146032 (daptomycin) in rats. *J Antimicrob Chemother* 1990; **25:** 635–43.
3. Woodworth JR, *et al.* Single-dose pharmacokinetics and antibacterial activity of daptomycin, a new lipopeptide antibiotic, in healthy volunteers. *Antimicrob Agents Chemother* 1992; **36:** 318–25.
4. Woodworth JR, *et al.* Tobramycin and daptomycin disposition when co-administered to healthy volunteers. *J Antimicrob Chemother* 1994; **33:** 655–9.
5. Tally FP, DeBruin MF. Development of daptomycin for gram-positive infections. *J Antimicrob Chemother* 2000; **46:** 523–6.
6. Snydman DR, *et al.* Comparative in vitro activities of daptomycin and vancomycin against resistant Gram-positive pathogens. *Antimicrob Agents Chemother* 2000; **44:** 3447–50.

Demeclocycline (65-p)

Demeclocycline (*BAN, rINN*).

Demethylchlortetracycline. (4S,4aS,5aS,6S,12aS)-7-Chloro-4-dimethylamino-1,4,4a,5,5a,6,11,12a-octahydro-3,6,10,12,12a-pentahydroxy-1,11-dioxonaphthacene-2-carboxamide; 7-Chloro-6-demethyltetracycline.

$C_{21}H_{21}ClN_2O_8 = 464.9$.

CAS — 127-33-3 (demeclocycline); 13215-10-6 (demeclocycline sesquihydrate).
ATC — D06AA01; J01AA01.
Pharmacopoeias. In US.

Pharmacopoeial description

USP 25: A yellow, odourless crystalline powder. Sparingly soluble in water; soluble 1 in 200 of alcohol and 1 in 40 of methyl alcohol; dissolves readily in 3N hydrochloric acid and in alkaline solutions. pH of a 1% solution in water is between 4.0 and 5.5. Store in airtight containers. Protect from light.

Demeclocycline Hydrochloride (66-s)

Demeclocycline Hydrochloride (*BANM, rINNM*).
Demeclocyclini Hydrochloridum.
$C_{21}H_{21}ClN_2O_8,HCl = 501.3$.
CAS — 64-73-3.
Pharmacopoeias. In Eur. (see p.vi) and US.

Pharmacopoeial description

Ph. Eur.: The hydrochloride of a substance produced by certain strains of *Streptomyces aureofaciens* or by any other means. A yellow powder. Soluble or sparingly soluble in water; slightly soluble in alcohol; very slightly soluble in acetone; practically insoluble in ether. It dissolves in solutions of alkali hydroxides and carbonates. A 1% solution in water has a pH of 2.0 to 3.0. Protect from light.

USP 25: A yellow, odourless, crystalline powder. Soluble 1 in 60 of water and 1 in 50 of methyl alcohol; slightly soluble in alcohol; practically insoluble in acetone and in chloroform; sparingly soluble in solutions of alkali hydroxides and carbonates. pH of a 1% solution in water is between 2.0 and 3.0. Store in airtight containers. Protect from light.

Adverse Effects and Precautions
As for Tetracycline Hydrochloride, p.259.

Phototoxic reactions occur more frequently with demeclocycline than with other tetracyclines and patients should avoid exposure to direct sunlight.

Reversible nephrogenic diabetes insipidus with polyuria, polydipsia, and weakness may occur in patients treated with demeclocycline. Plasma creatinine should be monitored in patients receiving demeclocycline for long periods for the treatment of inappropriate secretion of antidiuretic hormone, since tetracycline-induced renal impairment may not otherwise be apparent in the absence of oliguria. For a comment that the usefulness of demeclocycline for this indication may be limited by nephrotoxicity in patients with cardiac or hepatic disease, see Syndrome of Inappropriate ADH Secretion under Uses and Administration, below.

Interactions
As for Tetracycline Hydrochloride, p.259.

Antimicrobial Action
As for Tetracycline Hydrochloride, p.259. Demeclocycline is stated to be somewhat more active against certain strains of some organisms including *Neisseria gonorrhoeae* and *Haemophilus influenzae*, as well as to being the most active of the tetracyclines *in vitro* against *Brucella* spp.

Pharmacokinetics
As for Tetracycline Hydrochloride, p.260.
Peak plasma concentrations of about 1.5 to 1.7 µg per mL have been reported 3 to 4 hours after a single oral dose of 300 mg of demeclocycline, but higher plasma concentrations may be achieved with repeated dosage. Its biological half-life is about 12 hours. The renal clearance of demeclocycline is about half that of tetracycline.

Uses and Administration
Demeclocycline is a tetracycline derivative with uses similar to those of tetracycline (p.260). It is excreted more slowly and effective blood concentrations are maintained for a longer period.

It is given by mouth as the hydrochloride in a usual adult dosage of 0.6 g daily in 2 or 4 divided doses, preferably 1 hour before or 2 hours after meals; 0.9 g daily in 3 divided doses may be given for atypical pneumonia. Older children (over 8 years) have been given approximately 6 to 12 mg per kg body-weight daily in divided doses, but the effect of tetracyclines on teeth and bones should be considered.

Demeclocycline may be given to adults in the treatment of chronic hyponatraemia associated with the inappropriate secretion of antidiuretic hormone, when water restriction has proved ineffective. Initially demeclocycline hydrochloride 0.9 to 1.2 g is given daily in divided doses, reduced to maintenance doses of 0.6 to 0.9 g daily.

Like other tetracyclines, demeclocycline should be avoided in patients with renal impairment and doses reduced if it has to be given. Patients with liver disease should not receive more than 1 g daily.

The calcium and magnesium salts of demeclocycline have also been used.

Syndrome of inappropriate ADH secretion. Demeclocycline may be given in the treatment of the syndrome of inappropriate ADH (antidiuretic hormone) secretion (SIADH—p.1277) to antagonise the effect of ADH on the renal tubules; lithium has been given as an alternative. Both lithium and demeclocycline act by interfering with the cellular action of ADH to produce nephrogenic diabetes insipidus. Demeclocycline was reported to be superior to lithium[1] and became the preferred treatment for chronic SIADH if water restriction was unsuccessful,[2] although fluid restriction is probably still the treatment of choice. However, since nephrotoxicity has been reported in patients with cardiac or hepatic disease, the usefulness of demeclocycline in the treatment of hyponatraemic states might be limited; this view was supported by studies in patients with heart failure[3] and cirrhosis.[4]

1. Forrest JN, *et al.* Superiority of demeclocycline over lithium in the treatment of chronic syndrome of inappropriate secretion of antidiuretic hormone. *N Engl J Med* 1978; **298:** 173–7.
2. Schrier RW. Treatment of hyponatremia. *N Engl J Med* 1985; **312:** 1121–2.
3. Zegers de Beyl D, *et al.* Demeclocycline treatment of water retention in congestive heart failure. *BMJ* 1978; **1:** 760.
4. Miller PD, *et al.* Plasma demeclocycline levels and nephrotoxicity: correlation in hyponatremic cirrhotic patients. *JAMA* 1980; **243:** 2513–15.

Preparations

BP 2001: Demeclocycline Capsules;
USP 25: Demeclocycline Hydrochloride Capsules; Demeclocycline Hydrochloride Tablets; Demeclocycline Oral Suspension.

Proprietary Preparations (details are given in Part 3)
Aust.: Ledermycin; *Austral.:* Ledermycin; *Belg.:* Ledermycin†; *Canad.:* Declomycin; *Irl.:* Ledermycin; *Ital.:* Ledermicina†; *Neth.:* Ledermycin; *NZ:* Ledermycin; *S.Afr.:* Ledermycin†; *UK:* Ledermycin; *USA:* Declomycin.

Multi-ingredient: *Aust.:* Ledermix; *Denm.:* Ledermix; *Irl.:* Deteclo; Ledermix; *Israel:* Ledermix; *Ital.:* Rubrociclina; *S.Afr.:* Ledermix; Tritet†; *Spain:* Varibiotic; *Switz.:* Ledermix; *UK:* Deteclo; Ledermix.

Dibekacin Sulfate (67-w)

Dibekacin Sulfate (*rINNM*).

Dibekacin Sulphate (*BANM*); 3′,4′-Dideoxykanamycin B. 6-*O*-(3-Amino-3-deoxy-α-D-glucopyranosyl)-2-deoxy-4-*O*-(2,6-diamino-2,3,4,6-tetradeoxy-α-D-*erythro*-hexopyranosyl)-streptamine sulphate.

$C_{18}H_{37}N_5O_8,xH_2SO_4$.

CAS — 34493-98-6 (dibekacin); 58580-55-5 (dibekacin sulfate).
Pharmacopoeias. In Jpn.

Profile
Dibekacin is an aminoglycoside derived from kanamycin with actions and uses similar to those of gentamicin (p.210). It is given as the sulfate, intramuscularly in doses equivalent to 1 to 3 mg of dibekacin per kg body-weight daily in divided doses; doses in the upper half of this range are mostly recommended in Europe while those in the lower half have been preferred in the Far East. It may be given in similar doses by intravenous infusion and has also been given subcutaneously. Dosage should be adjusted based on serum-dibekacin concentration monitoring. It has also been used topically for eye infections.

Preparations

Proprietary Preparations (details are given in Part 3)
Belg.: Dikacine; *Fr.:* Debekacyl†; *Jpn:* Panimycin.

Dicloxacillin (14178-t)

Dicloxacillin (BAN, USAN, rINN).

BRL-1702; R-13423. (6R)-6-[3-(2,6-Dichlorophenyl)-5-methyl-isoxazole-4-carboxamido]penicillanic acid.

$C_{19}H_{17}Cl_2N_3O_5S = 470.3$.

CAS — 3116-76-5.

ATC — J01CF01.

Dicloxacillin Sodium (68-e)

Dicloxacillin Sodium (BANM, USAN, rINNM).

Dicloxacilina Sódica; Dicloxacillinum Natricum; P-1011. Sodium dicloxacillin monohydrate.

$C_{19}H_{16}Cl_2N_3NaO_5S,H_2O = 510.3$.

CAS — 343-55-5 (anhydrous dicloxacillin sodium); 13412-64-1 (dicloxacillin sodium, monohydrate).

Pharmacopoeias. In Eur. (see p.vi), Int., Jpn, and US.

1.09 g of monograph substance is approximately equivalent to 1 g of anhydrous dicloxacillin. Each g of monograph substance represents approximately 2 mmol of sodium.

Pharmacopoeial description

Ph. Eur.: A white or almost white, hygroscopic, crystalline powder. Freely soluble in water; soluble in alcohol and in methyl alcohol. A 10% solution in water has a pH of 5.0 to 7.0. Store at a temperature not exceeding 25° in airtight containers.

USP 25: A white to off-white crystalline powder. Freely soluble in water. pH of a 1% solution in water is between 4.5 and 7.5. Store in airtight containers.

Adverse Effects and Precautions

As for Flucloxacillin, p.207.

Effects on the liver. References.

1. Kleinman MS, Presberg JE. Cholestatic hepatitis after dicloxacillin-sodium therapy. J Clin Gastroenterol 1986; **8:** 77–8.

Interactions

As for Benzylpenicillin, p.158.

Antimicrobial Action

As for Flucloxacillin, p.207.

Pharmacokinetics

Dicloxacillin, like flucloxacillin, is about twice as well absorbed from the gastrointestinal tract as cloxacillin but absorption is also reduced by the presence of food in the stomach. After an oral dose of 500 mg, peak plasma concentrations of 10 to 18 µg per mL in about 1 hour have been reported in fasting subjects. Doubling the dose can double the plasma concentration. About 97% of dicloxacillin in the circulation is bound to plasma proteins. Dicloxacillin has been reported to have a plasma half-life of 0.5 to 1 hour. The half-life is prolonged in neonates.

The distribution of dicloxacillin in body tissues and fluids is similar to that of cloxacillin (p.192).

Dicloxacillin is metabolised to a limited extent and the unchanged drug and metabolites are excreted in the urine by glomerular filtration and renal tubular secretion. About 60% of a dose given by mouth is excreted in the urine. Only small amounts are excreted in the bile. Dicloxacillin is not removed by haemodialysis.

Plasma concentrations are enhanced if probenecid is given concomitantly. Reduced concentrations have been reported in patients with cystic fibrosis.

Uses and Administration

Dicloxacillin is an isoxazolyl penicillin used similarly to flucloxacillin (p.207) in the treatment of infections due to staphylococci resistant to benzylpenicillin.

It is administered by mouth, as the sodium salt, at least 1 hour before, or 2 hours after, meals since the presence of food in the stomach reduces absorption. Doses are expressed in terms of the equivalent amount of dicloxacillin. The usual adult dose is 125 to 250 mg of dicloxacillin every 6 hours. Children may be given 12.5 to 25 mg per kg body-weight daily in four divided doses. Doses may be increased in severe infections. Dicloxacillin sodium has also been given parenterally.

The symbol † denotes a preparation no longer actively marketed

Preparations

USP 25: Dicloxacillin Sodium Capsules; Dicloxacillin Sodium for Oral Suspension.

Proprietary Preparations (details are given in Part 3)

Austral.: Diclocil; Dicloxsig; Distaph; *Denm.:* Dicillin; Diclocil; *Fin.:* Diclocil; *Ger.:* Dichlor-Stapenor; *Hong Kong:* Diclocil; *Ital.:* Diclo; *Mex.:* Brispen; Cilpen; Cloxil; Cloxipen; Diclo-Tecno; Dipxapen; Ditterolina; Dixen; Penclox; Posipen; *Norw.:* Diclocil; *NZ:* Diclocil; *Port.:* Diclocil; *Swed.:* Diclocil; *Thai.:* Diclex; Diclocil; Diclocillin; Dicloson; Diclox; Dicloxia; Ditum; Dixocillin; Dorox; Servidiclox; *USA:* Dycill; Dynapen; Pathocil.

Multi-ingredient: *Ital.:* Ampiplus†; Diamplicil; Duplexcillina; Duplexil; *Mex.:* Ampiclox-D.

Difloxacin Hydrochloride (20535-p)

Difloxacin Hydrochloride (USAN, rINNM).

A-56619; Abbott-56619. 6-Fluoro-1-(p-fluorophenyl)-1,4-dihydro-7-(4-methyl-1-piperazinyl)-4-oxo-3-quinolinecarboxylic acid hydrochloride.

$C_{21}H_{19}F_2N_3O_3,HCl = 435.9$.

CAS — 98106-17-3 (difloxacin); 91296-86-5 (difloxacin hydrochloride).

Profile

Difloxacin is a fluoroquinolone antibacterial used as the hydrochloride in veterinary medicine. It was formerly used in humans but was associated with an unacceptably high incidence of adverse CNS effects.

Dihydrostreptomycin Sulfate (71-g)

Dihydrostreptomycin Sulfate (rINNM).

Dihydrostreptomycin Sulphate (BANM); Dihydrostreptomycini Sulfas. O-2-Deoxy-2-methylamino-α-L-glucopyranosyl-(1→2)-O-5-deoxy-3-C-hydroxymethyl-α-L-lyxofuranosyl-(1→4)-N^1,N^3-diamidino-D-streptamine sulphate.

$(C_{21}H_{41}N_7O_{12})_2,3H_2SO_4 = 1461.4$.

CAS — 128-46-1 (dihydrostreptomycin); 5490-27-7 (dihydrostreptomycin sulfate).

Pharmacopoeias. In Eur. (see p.vi) and US for veterinary use only.

1.25 g of monograph substance is approximately equivalent to 1 g of dihydrostreptomycin.

Pharmacopoeial description

Ph. Eur.: The sulfate of a substance obtained by catalytic hydrogenation of streptomycin or by any other means. Stabilisers may be added. The potency is not less than 730 units per mg, calculated with reference to the dried substance. A white or almost white powder; it may be hygroscopic. Freely soluble in water; practically insoluble in alcohol, in acetone, and in methyl alcohol. A 25% solution in water has a pH of 5.0 to 7.0. Store in airtight containers. Protect from light.

USP 25: A white or almost white amorphous or crystalline powder; the amorphous form is hygroscopic. Freely soluble in water; practically insoluble in acetone, in chloroform, and in methyl alcohol. pH of a solution in water containing the equivalent of dihydrostreptomycin 20% is between 4.5 and 7.0, except that if it is labelled as being solely for oral use, the pH is between 3.0 and 7.0. Store in airtight containers.

Profile

Dihydrostreptomycin is an aminoglycoside antibacterial with actions similar to those of streptomycin (p.249). As it is not absorbed following oral administration it has been given by this route for gastrointestinal infections. Since it is more likely than streptomycin to cause partial or complete loss of hearing it is not used parenterally in humans, although it is used as the sulfate in veterinary medicine.

Preparations

Proprietary Preparations (details are given in Part 3)

Multi-ingredient: *Braz.:* Fluocal com Pectina; *Mex.:* Estrefen; *Spain:* Cilinafosal DHD Estrep; Citrocil; Estreptoenterol; Salitanol Estreptomicina; Sulfintestin Neomicina.

Dirithromycin (18782-h)

Dirithromycin (BAN, USAN, rINN).

ASE-136BS; Dirithromycinum; LY-237216. (1R,2R,3R,6R,7S,8S,9R,10R,12R,13S,15R,17S)-7-(2,6-Dideoxy-3-C,3-O-dimethyl-α-L-ribo-hexopyranosyloxy)-3-ethyl-2,10-dihydroxy-15-(2-methoxyethoxymethyl)-2,6,8,10,12,17-hexamethyl-9-(3,4,6-trideoxy-3-dimethylamino-β-L-xylo-hexopyranosyloxy)-4,16-dioxa-14-azabicyclo[11.3.1]heptadecan-5-one; (9S)-9-Deoxo-11-deoxy-9,11-{imino[(1R)-2-(2-methoxyethoxy)-ethylidene]oxy}erythromycin.

$C_{42}H_{78}N_2O_{14} = 835.1$.

CAS — 62013-04-1.

ATC — J01FA13.

Pharmacopoeias. In Eur. (see p.vi) and US.

Pharmacopoeial description

Ph. Eur.: A white or almost white powder. It exhibits polymorphism. Very slightly soluble in water; very soluble in dichloromethane and in methyl alcohol.

USP 25: A white or practically white powder. Very slightly soluble in water; very soluble in dichloromethane and in methyl alcohol.

Adverse Effects and Precautions

As for Erythromycin, p.201. Dirithromycin should be used with caution in patients with moderate to severe hepatic impairment since its metabolite erythromycylamine is primarily eliminated in the bile.

Interactions

For a discussion of drug interactions of macrolide antibacterials, see Erythromycin, p.202.

Antimicrobial Action

As for Erythromycin, p.203.

◊ Dirithromycin and its isomer epidirithromycin form an equilibrium mixture in aqueous solution and both are rapidly hydrolysed to 9(S)-erythromycylamine in vitro and in vivo.[1] Consequently, the antibacterial activity of these compounds is difficult to distinguish. Dirithromycin has a spectrum of activity and pattern of resistance similar to those of erythromycin. It is generally less active than erythromycin in vitro,[2,3] and in particular some strains of Bacteroides fragilis[2,3] and other anaerobes,[3,4] Haemophilus influenzae,[2-5] Listeria spp.,[4] and Neisseria gonorrhoeae[3,4] are less susceptible. It is more effective than erythromycin against Campylobacter jejuni.[2,4] However, activity was generally improved by the addition of human serum to the nutrient medium,[2] and results with H. influenzae in particular could be adversely influenced by test conditions.[5] Dirithromycin may show greater activity in vivo than is indicated by in-vitro studies,[6] and may have beneficial effects due to a postantibiotic effect.[7]

1. Kirst HA, et al. Antimicrobial characterization and interrelationships of dirithromycin and epidirithromycin. Antimicrob Agents Chemother 1995; **39:** 1436–41.
2. Hardy DJ, et al. Comparative in vitro activities of new 14-, 15-, and 16-membered macrolides. Antimicrob Agents Chemother 1988; **32:** 1710–19.
3. Yu K-W, Neu HC. In vitro activity of dirithromycin (LY 237216) compared with activities of other macrolide antibiotics. Antimicrob Agents Chemother 1990; **34:** 1839–42.
4. Bauernfeind A. In-vitro activity of dirithromycin in comparison with other new and established macrolides. J Antimicrob Chemother 1993; **31** (suppl C): 39–49.
5. Biedenbach DJ, et al. Comparative in vitro evaluation of dirithromycin tested against recent clinical isolates of Haemophilus influenzae, Moraxella catarrhalis, and Streptococcus pneumoniae, including effects of medium supplements and test conditions on MIC results. Diagn Microbiol Infect Dis 1999; **33:** 275–82.
6. Counter FT, et al. Synthesis and antimicrobial evaluation of dirithromycin (AS-E 136; LY237216), a new macrolide antibiotic derived from erythromycin. Antimicrob Agents Chemother 1991; **35:** 1116–26.
7. Fuursted K, et al. Comparative study of bactericidal activities, postantibiotic effects, and effects on bacterial virulence of penicillin G and six macrolides against Streptococcus pneumoniae. Antimicrob Agents Chemother 1997; **41:** 781–4.

Pharmacokinetics

Dirithromycin is readily absorbed following oral administration and undergoes rapid non-enzymatic hydrolysis to erythromycylamine. Absorption is enhanced by food. Bioavailability is about 10%. Daily administration of dirithromycin 500 mg produces peak plasma concentrations of erythromycylamine of about 0.4 µg per mL.

Erythromycylamine is widely distributed and tissue concentrations exceed those in plasma. Protein binding is 15 to 30%. Erythromycylamine is mainly excreted unchanged in the bile with only about 2% in the urine. The mean plasma half-life is about 8 hours and the mean urinary terminal elimination half-life is about 44 hours.

◊ References.

1. Sides GD, et al. Pharmacokinetics of dirithromycin. J Antimicrob Chemother 1993; **31** (suppl C): 65–75.
2. LaBreque D, et al. Pharmacokinetics of dirithromycin in patients with impaired hepatic function. J Antimicrob Chemother 1993; **32:** 741–50.
3. Mazzei T, et al. Pharmacokinetics of dirithromycin in patients with mild or moderate cirrhosis. Antimicrob Agents Chemother 1999; **43:** 1556–9.

Uses and Administration

Dirithromycin is a prodrug of the macrolide antibiotic erythromycylamine, which has similar properties to those of erythromycin (p.201) and is used in pulmonary, skin, and soft tissue infections caused by susceptible organisms.

Dirithromycin is given by mouth as enteric-coated tablets in a usual dose of 500 mg once daily.

◊ General references.

1. Various. Dirithromycin: a new once-daily macrolide. J Antimicrob Chemother 1993; **31** (suppl C): 1–185.
2. Brogden RN, Peters DH. Dirithromycin: a review of its antimicrobial activity, pharmacokinetic properties and therapeutic efficacy. Drugs 1994; **48:** 599–616.

Preparations

USP 25: Dirithromycin Delayed-Release Tablets.

Proprietary Preparations (details are given in Part 3)
Aust.: Dimac; **Belg.:** Unibac; **Braz.:** Dynabac; **Fr.:** Dynabac; **Hong Kong:** Dynabac; **Ital.:** Dinabac†; **Spain:** Balodin; Noriclan; Nortron; **USA:** Dynabac.

Doxycycline (72-q)

Doxycycline (BAN, USAN, rINN).
Doxycycline Monohydrate; Doxycyclinum; GS-3065. (4S,4aR,5S,5aR,6S,12aS)-4-Dimethylamino-1,4,4a,5,5a,6,11,12a-octahydro-3,5,10,12,12a-pentahydroxy-6-methyl-1,11-dioxonaphthacene-2-carboxamide monohydrate; 6-Deoxy-5β-hydroxytetracycline monohydrate.
$C_{22}H_{24}N_2O_8,H_2O = 462.4$.
CAS — 564-25-0 (anhydrous doxycycline); 17086-28-1 (doxycycline monohydrate).
ATC — J01AA02.
Pharmacopoeias. In *Eur.* (see p.vi) and *US*.

Pharmacopoeial description

Ph. Eur.: A yellow crystalline powder. Very slightly soluble in water and in alcohol; practically insoluble in ether. It dissolves in dilute solutions of mineral acids and in solutions of alkali hydroxides and carbonates. A 1% suspension in water has a pH of 5.0 to 6.5. Store in airtight containers. Protect from light.
USP 25: A yellow crystalline powder. Very slightly soluble in water; sparingly soluble in alcohol; practically insoluble in chloroform and in ether; freely soluble in dilute acid and in alkali hydroxide solutions. pH of a 1% suspension in water is between 5.0 and 6.5. Store in airtight containers. Protect from light.

Doxycycline Calcium (73-p)

Doxycycline Calcium (BANM, rINNM).

Doxycycline Fosfatex (18633-l)

Doxycycline Fosfatex (BAN, USAN).
AB-08; DMSC. 6-Deoxy-5β-hydroxytetracycline—metaphosphoric acid—sodium metaphosphate in the ratio 3:3:1.
$(C_{22}H_{24}N_2O_8)_3(HPO_3)_3NaPO_3 = 1675.2$.
CAS — 83038-87-3.

Doxycycline Hyclate (74-s)

Doxycycline Hyclate (BANM, rINNM).
Dossiciclina Iclato; Doxycycline Hydrochloride; Doxycyclini Hyclas. Doxycycline hydrochloride hemiethanolate hemihydrate.
$C_{22}H_{24}N_2O_8,HCl,\frac{1}{2}C_2H_5OH,\frac{1}{2}H_2O = 512.9$.
CAS — 10592-13-9 (doxycycline hydrochloride); 24390-14-5 (doxycycline hyclate).
Pharmacopoeias. In *Chin., Eur.* (see p.vi), *Int., Jpn, Pol.,* and *US*.

Doxycycline hyclate 115 mg is approximately equivalent to 100 mg of anhydrous doxycycline.

Incompatibilities. Preparations of doxycycline hyclate have an acid pH and incompatibility may reasonably be expected with alkaline preparations or with drugs unstable at low pH. Reduced antimicrobial activity has been reported *in vitro* when doxycycline hyclate was mixed with riboflavin.

Pharmacopoeial description

Ph. Eur.: A yellow hygroscopic crystalline powder. Freely soluble in water and in methyl alcohol; sparingly soluble in alcohol; practically insoluble in ether; dissolves in solutions of alkali hydroxides and of carbonates. A 1% solution in water has a pH of 2.0 to 3.0. Store in airtight containers. Protect from light.
USP 25: A yellow crystalline powder. Soluble in water; slightly soluble in alcohol; practically insoluble in chloroform and in ether; soluble in solutions of alkali hydroxides and carbonates. pH of a solution in water containing the equivalent of doxycycline 1% is between 2.0 and 3.0. Store in airtight containers. Protect from light.

Adverse Effects and Precautions

As for Tetracycline Hydrochloride, p.259.

Gastrointestinal disturbances with doxycycline are reported to be less frequent than with tetracycline and doxycycline may also cause less tooth discoloration.

Oesophageal ulceration may be a particular problem if capsules or tablets are taken with insufficient fluid or in a recumbent posture: doxycycline should be taken with at least half a glass of water, in an upright position, and well before retiring to bed. There is some evidence from studies in *animals* that preparations of the base, which have a higher pH, cause less oesophageal damage than those of the more acid hyclate. Dispersible tablets or liquid formulations

should be used in elderly patients, who may be at greater risk of oesophageal injury.

Unlike many tetracyclines, doxycycline does not appear to accumulate in patients with impaired renal function, and aggravation of renal impairment may be less likely.

Anosmia. Anosmia or dysosmia (absent or impaired sense of smell) have occasionally been reported in patients receiving doxycycline, although the association has not been definitely established.[1]
1. Bleasel AF, *et al.* Anosmia after doxycycline use. *Med J Aust* 1990; **152:** 440.

Porphyria. Doxycycline has been associated with acute attacks of porphyria and is considered unsafe in porphyric patients.

Interactions

As for Tetracycline Hydrochloride, p.259.

Doxycycline has a lower affinity for binding with calcium than many tetracyclines. In consequence its absorption is less likely to be affected by milk or food, although it is still affected by antacids and iron preparations.

The metabolism of doxycycline may be accelerated by drugs that induce hepatic enzymes such as alcohol (chronic use), rifampicin, and antiepileptics including carbamazepine, phenobarbital, phenytoin, and primidone. It has been suggested that doxycycline could increase ciclosporin concentrations, but evidence for this seems to be scant.

Antimicrobial Action

As for Tetracycline Hydrochloride, p.259. Doxycycline is more active than tetracycline against many bacterial species including the enterococci and various anaerobes. Cross-resistance is common although some tetracycline-resistant *Staphylococcus aureus* respond to doxycycline. Doxycycline is also more active against protozoa, particularly *Plasmodium* spp.

Pharmacokinetics

For the general pharmacokinetics of the tetracyclines, see Tetracycline Hydrochloride, p.260.

Doxycycline is readily and almost completely absorbed from the gastrointestinal tract and absorption is not significantly affected by the presence of food in the stomach or duodenum. Mean peak plasma concentrations of 2.6 µg per mL have been reported 2 hours after a 200-mg dose by mouth, falling to 1.45 µg per mL at 24 hours. After intravenous infusion of the same dose peak plasma concentrations are briefly somewhat higher, but become very similar to those after oral administration following equilibration into the tissues.

From 80 to 95% of doxycycline in the circulation is reported to be bound to plasma proteins. Its biological half-life varies from about 12 to 24 hours. Doxycycline is more lipid-soluble than tetracycline. It is widely distributed in body tissues and fluids.

In patients with normal renal function about 40% of a dose is slowly excreted in the urine, although more is excreted by this route if the urine is made alkaline. However, the majority of a dose of doxycycline is excreted in the faeces following chelation in the intestines. Although doxycycline has been reported to undergo some inactivation in the liver, some sources consider this doubtful; however, the kinetics of doxycycline have been reportedly altered in patients receiving drugs which induce hepatic metabolism.

Doxycycline is stated not to accumulate significantly in patients with renal impairment, although excretion in the urine is reduced; increased amounts of doxycycline are excreted in the faeces in these patients. Nevertheless, there have been reports of some accumulation in renal failure. Removal of doxycycline by haemodialysis is insignificant.

◊ Reviews.
1. Saivin S, Houin G. Clinical pharmacokinetics of doxycycline and minocycline. *Clin Pharmacokinet* 1988; **15:** 355–66.

Distribution. Concentrations of doxycycline in CSF of patients with neurological manifestations of Lyme disease receiving doxycycline 200 mg daily by mouth ranged from 0.4 to

2.5 µg per mL at 4 hours after a dose.[1] This represented 3 to 36% of the serum concentration at that time and was reported to be adequate for the treatment of the infection.
1. Karlsson M, *et al.* Concentrations of doxycycline and penicillin G in sera and cerebrospinal fluid of patients treated for neuroborreliosis. *Antimicrob Agents Chemother* 1996; **40:** 1104–7.

Uses and Administration

Doxycycline is a tetracycline derivative with uses similar to those of tetracycline (p.260). It may sometimes be preferred to other tetracyclines in the treatment of sensitive infections because of its fairly reliable absorption and its long half-life which permits less frequent (often once daily) dosage. It also has the advantage that it can be given (with care) to patients with renal insufficiency. However, relatively high doses may need to be given for urinary-tract infections because of its low renal excretion. Doxycycline has antiprotozoal actions and may be given in conjunction with quinine in the management of falciparum malaria resistant to chloroquine (below).

Doxycycline is normally administered by mouth as doxycycline or its various derivatives. Doses are expressed in terms of doxycycline. The usual dose is 200 mg of doxycycline on the first day (as a single dose or in divided doses), followed by 100 mg daily. Older children (over 8 years) weighing 45 kg or less have been given approximately 4 mg per kg bodyweight in two divided doses initially and thereafter 2 mg per kg daily but the effect of tetracyclines on teeth and bones should be considered. In severe infections the initial dosage is maintained throughout the course of treatment. In patients with sensitive gonococcal infections, doxycycline 100 mg twice daily for 7 days is given, although it has occasionally been given in a single dose of 300 mg, alone or followed by a second similar dose one hour later. For syphilis, doxycycline 200 or 300 mg is given daily in divided doses for at least 15 or 10 days, respectively. In the treatment of acne, a dose of 50 mg daily may be adequate. For relapsing fever and louse-borne typhus, doxycycline 100 or 200 mg may be given as a single dose. For prophylaxis of scrub typhus, 200 mg may be taken as a single dose.

Doxycycline capsules and tablets should be given with plenty of fluid, with the patient in an upright position, and well before retiring for the night. It may be given with food or milk if gastric irritation occurs. Dispersible tablets or liquid formulations are advisable in elderly patients.

In patients in whom oral therapy is not feasible, doxycycline may be given as the hyclate by slow intravenous infusion of a solution containing 0.1 to 1 mg per mL, in doses equivalent to those by mouth. Infusions should be given over 1 to 4 hours.

Solutions of doxycycline are also used for malignant effusions (p.489).

Doxycycline is also administered as a subgingival gel for the treatment of periodontal disease.

Malaria. Doxycycline is used in some areas for the treatment of chloroquine-resistant falciparum malaria (p.428) in a dose of 200 mg daily for at least 7 days following treatment with quinine. Doxycycline 100 mg daily has been used for prophylaxis in areas of high risk where other drugs are likely to be ineffective, but it is not suitable for extended prophylactic use.

Preparations

BP 2001: Dispersible Doxycycline Tablets; Doxycycline Capsules;
USP 25: Doxycycline Calcium Oral Suspension; Doxycycline Capsules; Doxycycline for Injection; Doxycycline for Oral Suspension; Doxycycline Hyclate Capsules; Doxycycline Hyclate Delayed-release Capsules; Doxycycline Hyclate Tablets.

Proprietary Preparations (details are given in Part 3)
Aust.: Biocyclin†; Dotur; Doxybene; Doxyderm; Doxydyn; Doxyhexal; Doxylan; Doxystad; Gewacyclin; Mundicycline†; Sigadoxin; Supracyclin; Vibramycin; Vibravenos; **Austral.:** Doryx; Doxsig; Doxy; Doxyhexal; Doxylin; Vibra-Tabs; Vibramycin; Vizam†; **Belg.:** Clifordin; Dagramycine†; Doxyfim; Doxylets; Unidox; Vibracare†; Vibramycine; Vibratab; **Braz.:** Vibramicina; **Canad.:** Apo-Doxy; Doryx†; Doxycin; Doxytec; Novo-Doxylin; Vibra-Tabs; Vibramycin†; **Denm.:** Dumoxin†; Vibradox; Vibramycin; **Fin.:** Apodoxin; Dosyklin; Doximed; Doximycin; Doxitin; **Fr.:** Doxy; Doxygram†; Doxylets†; Granudoxy; Monocline; Spanor; Tolexine; Vibramycine N; Vibraveineuse; **Ger.:** Azudoxat; Doxakne; Clinofug D; Doxakne; Doxy; Doxy Komb; Doxy M; Doxy S+K; Doxy-Diolan; Doxy-HP; Doxy-N-Tablinen; Doxy-P†; Doxy-Puren; Doxy-Tablinen†; Doxy-Wolff; Doxybioc-

in; Doxyderma; Doxydoc; Doxyhexal; Doxymerck; Doxymono; Doxytem†; duradoxal†; Jenacyclin; Mespafin; Neodox; Sigadoxin; Supracyclin; Vibramycin; Vibravenos; **Hong Kong:** Medomycin; Servidoxyne; Tolexine; Vibramycin; Wanmycin; Zadorin; **Irl.:** By-Mycin; Vibramycin; **Israel:** Apodoxy; Doxibiotic; Doxy; Doxylin; Doxytrim; Vibramycin; Vibravenos; **Ital.:** Bassado; Doxina; Gram-Val; Miraclin; Monodoxin†; Ribociclina; Unacil; **Mex.:** Apociclina; Bioximicina; Kenciclen; Vibramicina; Vivradoxil; **Neth.:** Dagracycline, Doxy; Doxymycin†; Neo-Dagracycline; Unidox; Vibra-S; Vibramycin; **Norw.:** Doryx; Doxylin; Doxysol; Dumoxin; Vibramycin; **NZ:** Doryx; Doxine; Doxy; **Port.:** Actidox; Biocin; Doxytrex; Pluridoxina; Sigadoxin; Vibramicina; **S.Afr.:** Acne-Cy-Clean†; Bok-C-Lin†; Cyclidox; Doryx; Doxitab; Doxyclin†; Doxycyl; Doxylets†; Doxymycin†; Dumoxin; Noritet; Thedox†; Viacin; Vibramycin; **Singapore:** Apo-Doxy; Bronmycin; Doryx; Doxilin; Doxine; Doxycap; Doxymycin; Medomycin; Remycin; Servidoxyne; Tetradox; Vibramycin; **Spain:** Cildox; Cliseminat†; Docostyl; Dosil; Doxi Crisol; Doxi Sergo; Doxiclat; Doxinate; Doxiten Bio; Doxiten†; Novelciclina; Peledox; Retens; Rexilen; Solupen; Tetrasan†; Vibracina; Vibravenosa; **Swed.:** Doryx; Doxyferm; Idocyklin†; Vibramycin; **Switz.:** Diocimex; Doxy-basan; Doxyclin; Doxysol; Helvedoclyn; Rudocycline; Sigadoxin; Supracycline; Vibramycine; Vibraveineuse; Zadorin; **Thai.:** Amermycin; Bronmycin; Docline; Doxin; Doxy; Doxy-100; Doxy-P; Doxycline; Doxylin; Doxymycin; Dumoxin; Ibimycin; Medomycin; Medoxin; Poli-Cycline; Servidoxyne; Siadocin; Tetradox; Torymycin; Vibramycin; **UAE:** Duradox; **UK:** Atridox; Cyclodox; Demix; Doxylar; Periostat; Ramysis; Vibramycin; Vibramycin D; **USA:** Adoxa; Bio-Tab; Doryx; Doxy; Doxychel; Monodox; Periostat; Vibra-Tabs; Vibramycin.

Multi-ingredient: **Aust.:** Mucotectan; Vibrabron†; **Ger.:** Ambrodoxy; Ambroxol AL comp; Ambroxol comp; Amdox-Puren; Azudoxat comp; Doxam; Doximucol; Doxy Comp; Doxy Lindoxyl; Doxy Plus; Doxy-duramucal; Doxy-Wolff Mucolyt; Doxysolvat; Jenabroxol comp; Mucotectan; Sagittamuc; Sigamuc; Terelit; **Spain:** Dosil Enzimatico; Doxiten Enzimatico; Duo Gobens; Pulmotropic; Solupen Enzimatico; Sorciclina.

Enoxacin (16623-k)

Enoxacin (BAN, USAN, rINN).

AT-2266; CI-919; PD-107779. 1-Ethyl-6-fluoro-1,4-dihydro-4-oxo-7-(1-piperazinyl)-1,8-naphthyridine-3-carboxylic acid.

$C_{15}H_{17}FN_4O_3 = 320.3$.

CAS — 74011-58-8.

ATC — J01MA04.

Pharmacopoeias. In Jpn.

Adverse Effects and Precautions

As for Ciprofloxacin, p.183.

Interactions

As for Ciprofloxacin, p.184.

Of the fluoroquinolones, enoxacin has been reported to cause the strongest interaction with theophylline (p.780) and with caffeine (p.762).

Antimicrobial Action

As for Ciprofloxacin, p.184, although enoxacin is less potent *in vitro*.

Pharmacokinetics

Peak plasma concentrations of 2 to 3 µg per mL are achieved 1 to 2 hours after a 400-mg dose of enoxacin by mouth. A plasma half-life of about 4 to 6 hours has been reported. Plasma protein binding has ranged from 18 to 57%. Enoxacin appears to be widely distributed in the body and concentrations higher than those in plasma have been reported in tissues such as lung, kidney, and prostate. High concentrations are achieved in bile, but the extent of biliary excretion is not completely clear.

Enoxacin is eliminated from the body mainly by urinary excretion, but also by metabolism. The major metabolite, 3-oxo-enoxacin, has some antibacterial activity. Urinary excretion of enoxacin is by both tubular secretion and glomerular filtration and may be reduced by probenecid. High concentrations are achieved in the urine since about 60% of an oral dose of enoxacin appears unchanged in the urine within 24 hours; about 10% is recovered as 3-oxo-enoxacin. In renal impairment the half-life of enoxacin may be prolonged and the oxometabolite may accumulate.

Uses and Administration

Enoxacin is a fluoroquinolone antibacterial with properties similar to those of ciprofloxacin (p.182) but it is generally less potent *in vitro*. It is used mainly in the treatment of urinary-tract infections (p.146) and gonorrhoea (p.124).

For urinary-tract infections enoxacin is given by mouth in doses of 200 to 400 mg twice daily. A single 400-mg dose is given for uncomplicated gonorrhoea.

Half the usual dose is recommended in renal impairment when the creatinine clearance is 30 mL or less per minute.

◊ References.
1. Henwood JM, Monk JP. Enoxacin: a review of its antibacterial activity, pharmacokinetic properties and therapeutic use. *Drugs* 1988; **36:** 32–66.
2. Jaber LA, *et al.* Enoxacin: a new fluoroquinolone. *Clin Pharm* 1989; **8:** 97–107.
3. Patel SS, Spencer CM. Enoxacin: a reappraisal of its clinical efficacy in the treatment of genitourinary tract infections. *Drugs* 1996; **51:** 137–60.

The symbol † denotes a preparation no longer actively marketed

Preparations

Proprietary Preparations (details are given in Part 3)
Aust.: Gyramid†; **Austral.:** Enoxin; **Fr.:** Enoxor; **Ger.:** Enoxor; **Ital.:** Bactidan; Enoxen; **Jpn:** Flumark; **Mex.:** Comprecin; **Port.:** Vinone†; **S.Afr.:** Bactidron; **Spain:** Almitil; **USA:** Penetrex.

Enrofloxacin (2489-h)

Enrofloxacin (BAN, USAN, rINN).

Bay-Vp-2674. 1-Cyclopropyl-7-(4-ethylpiperazin-1-yl)-6-fluoro-1,4-dihydro-4-oxoquinoline-3-carboxylic acid.

$C_{19}H_{22}FN_3O_3 = 359.4$.

CAS — 93106-60-6.

Profile

Enrofloxacin is a fluoroquinolone antibacterial that is used in veterinary practice.

Erythromycin (77-l)

Erythromycin (BAN, rINN).

Eritromicina; Erythromycinum. Erythromycin A is (2R,3S,4S,5R,6R,8R,10R,11R,12S,13R)-5-(3-amino-3,4,6-trideoxy-N,N-dimethyl-β-D-xylo-hexopyranosyloxy)-3-(2,6-dideoxy-3-C,3-O-dimethyl-α-L-ribo-hexopyranosyloxy)-13-ethyl-6,11,12-trihydroxy-2,4,6,8,10,12-hexamethyl-9-oxotridecan-13-olide.

$C_{37}H_{67}NO_{13} = 733.9$.

CAS — 114-07-8.

ATC — D10AF02; J01FA01; S01AA17.

Pharmacopoeias. In Chin., Eur. (see p.vi), Int., Jpn, Pol., and US.

Pharmacopoeial description

Ph. Eur.: Erythromycin is produced by the growth of a strain of *Streptomyces erythreus* and is a mixture of macrolide antibiotics consisting largely of erythromycin A. It occurs as a white or slightly yellow powder or colourless or slightly yellow crystals; slightly hygroscopic. Slightly soluble in water but less soluble at higher temperatures; freely soluble in alcohol; soluble in methyl alcohol. It dissolves in dilute hydrochloric acid. A 0.067% solution in water has a pH of 8.0 to 10.5. Store at a temperature not exceeding 30°. Protect from light.

USP 25: Erythromycin consists primarily of erythromycin A. A white or slightly yellow, odourless or practically odourless, crystalline powder. Soluble 1 in 1000 of water; soluble in alcohol, in chloroform, and in ether. Store in airtight containers.

Erythromycin Acistrate (2798-z)

Erythromycin Acistrate (USAN, rINN).

Acetylerythromycin Stearate. Erythromycin 2′-acetate stearate.

$C_{39}H_{69}NO_{14},C_{18}H_{36}O_2 = 1060.4$.

CAS — 96128-89-1.

Erythromycin Estolate (78-y)

Erythromycin Estolate (BAN, USAN, rINNM).

Erythromycin Propionate Lauryl Sulfate; Erythromycin Propionate Lauryl Sulphate; Erythromycini Estolas; Propionylerythromycin Lauryl Sulphate. Erythromycin 2′-propionate dodecyl sulphate.

$C_{40}H_{71}NO_{14},C_{12}H_{26}O_4S = 1056.4$.

CAS — 3521-62-8.

Pharmacopoeias. In Chin., Eur. (see p.vi), Pol., and US.

1.44 g of monograph substance is approximately equivalent to 1 g of erythromycin.

Pharmacopoeial description

Ph. Eur.: A white, crystalline powder. The potency is not less than 610 units per mg calculated on the anhydrous basis. Practically insoluble in water; freely soluble in alcohol; soluble in acetone; practically insoluble in dilute hydrochloric acid. A saturated solution in water has a pH of 5.5 to 7.0. Store in airtight containers at a temperature not exceeding 30°. Protect from light.

USP 25: A white, odourless or practically odourless, crystalline powder. It has a potency equivalent to not less than 600 µg of erythromycin per mg, calculated on the anhydrous basis. Practically insoluble in water; soluble 1 in 20 of alcohol, 1 in 15 of acetone, and 1 in 10 of chloroform. Store in airtight containers.

Erythromycin Ethyl Succinate (80-q)

Erythromycin Ethyl Succinate (BANM).

Erythromycin Ethylsuccinate; Erythromycini Ethylsuccinas. Erythromycin 2′-(ethylsuccinate).

$C_{43}H_{75}NO_{16} = 862.1$.

CAS — 41342-53-4.

NOTE. Compounded preparations of erythromycin ethyl succinate may be represented by the following names:

• Co-erynsulfisox (USP 25)—erythromycin ethyl succinate and acetyl sulfafurazole.

Pharmacopoeias. In Chin., Eur. (see p.vi), Int., Jpn, Pol., and US.

1.17 g of monograph substance is approximately equivalent to 1 g of erythromycin.

Pharmacopoeial description

Ph. Eur.: A white hygroscopic crystalline powder. The potency is not less than 780 units per mg calculated on the anhydrous basis. Practically insoluble in water; freely soluble in dehydrated alcohol, in acetone, and in methyl alcohol. A 1% suspension in water has a pH of 6.0 to 8.5. Store in airtight containers at a temperature not exceeding 30°. Protect from light.

USP 25: A white or slightly yellow, odourless or practically odourless, crystalline powder. It has a potency equivalent to not less than 765 µg of erythromycin per mg, calculated on the anhydrous basis. Very slightly soluble in water; freely soluble in alcohol, in chloroform, and in macrogol 400. Store in airtight containers.

Erythromycin Gluceptate (81-p)

Erythromycin Gluceptate (BANM, rINNM).

Erythromycin glucoheptonate.

$C_{37}H_{67}NO_{13},C_7H_{14}O_8 = 960.1$.

CAS — 304-63-2; 23067-13-2.

Pharmacopoeias. US includes Sterile Erythromycin Gluceptate.

1.3 g of monograph substance is approximately equivalent to 1 g of erythromycin.

Pharmacopoeial description

USP 25: pH of a 2.5% solution in water of Sterile Erythromycin Gluceptate is between 6.0 and 8.0.

Erythromycin Lactobionate (82-s)

Erythromycin Lactobionate (BANM, rINNM).

Erythromycini Lactobionas. Erythromycin mono(4-O-β-D-galactopyranosyl-D-gluconate).

$C_{37}H_{67}NO_{13},C_{12}H_{22}O_{12} = 1092.2$.

CAS — 3847-29-8.

Pharmacopoeias. In Chin., Eur. (see p.vi), and Pol. US includes Sterile Erythromycin Lactobionate.

1.5 g of monograph substance is approximately equivalent to 1 g of erythromycin.

Pharmacopoeial description

Ph. Eur.: White or slightly yellow, hygroscopic powder. Soluble in water; freely soluble in dehydrated alcohol and in methyl alcohol; very slightly soluble in acetone and in dichloromethane; practically insoluble in ether. A 2% solution in water has a pH of 6.5 to 7.5. Store in airtight containers at a temperature not exceeding 25°.

USP 25: Sterile Erythromycin Lactobionate has a potency equivalent to not less than 525 µg of erythromycin per mg, calculated on the anhydrous basis. pH of a solution in water containing the equivalent of erythromycin 5% is between 6.5 and 7.5.

Erythromycin Propionate (83-w)

Erythromycin Propionate (BANM, USAN, rINNM).

Erythromycin Propanoate; Propionylerythromycin. Erythromycin 2′-propionate.

$C_{40}H_{71}NO_{14} = 790.0$.

CAS — 134-36-1.

Pharmacopoeias. In Fr.

1.08 g of monograph substance is approximately equivalent to 1 g of erythromycin.

Erythromycin Stearate (84-e)

Erythromycin Stearate (BANM, rINNM).

Erythromycini Stearas. Erythromycin octadecanoate.

$C_{37}H_{67}NO_{13},C_{18}H_{36}O_2 = 1018.4$.

CAS — 643-22-1.

Pharmacopoeias. In Eur. (see p.vi), Int., Jpn, Pol., and US.

1.39 g of monograph substance is approximately equivalent to 1 g of erythromycin.

Incompatibilities. The stability of erythromycin derivatives is dependent upon pH, with particularly rapid degradation occurring at a pH greater than 10 or less than 5.5. Incompatibility might reasonably be expected, therefore, when erythromycin preparations are mixed with drugs or preparations that have a highly acidic or alkaline pH. In practice, reports of incompatibility are not always consistent, and other factors such as the temperature and concentration of solutions, and the diluents used, may play a role.

Pharmacopoeial description

Ph. Eur.: A white crystalline powder. Practically insoluble in water; soluble in acetone and in methyl alcohol. Solutions may be opalescent.

USP 25: the stearic acid salt of erythromycin with an excess of stearic acid. White or slightly yellow crystals or powder, odourless or may have a slight, earthy odour. Practically insoluble in water; soluble in alcohol, in chloroform, in ether, and in methyl alcohol. Store in airtight containers.

Adverse Effects

Erythromycin and its salts and esters are generally well tolerated and serious adverse effects are rare.

Gastrointestinal disturbances such as abdominal discomfort and cramp, nausea, vomiting, and diarrhoea are fairly common after both oral and parenteral administration, probably because of the stimulant activity of erythromycin on the gut. Gastrointestinal effects are dose-related and appear to be more common in young than in older subjects. Supra-infection with resistant organisms may occur and pseudomembranous colitis has been reported.

Hypersensitivity reactions appear to be uncommon, having been reported in about 0.5% of patients, and include pruritus, urticaria and skin rash as well as occasional cases of anaphylaxis. Hypersensitivity or irritation may occur following topical application of erythromycin.

A hypersensitivity reaction may also be responsible for the hepatotoxicity sometimes reported in patients receiving erythromycin or its derivatives. Symptoms indicative of cholestasis, including upper abdominal pain (sometimes very severe), nausea and vomiting, abnormal liver function values, raised serum bilirubin and usually jaundice, may be accompanied by rash, fever, and eosinophilia. Symptoms usually occur initially in patients who have been receiving the drug for more than 10 days, although they may develop more quickly in patients given the drug in a previous course of treatment. Erythromycin may interfere with tests for serum aspartate aminotransferase, which might make diagnosis of hepatotoxicity more difficult.

The majority of reports of liver dysfunction have been in patients receiving the estolate, and it has been suggested that the propionyl ester linkage is particularly associated with hepatotoxicity, but symptoms have been reported in patients receiving the base and most of the other derivatives, both by mouth and parenterally. Hepatic dysfunction seems to be rare in children. The effects of erythromycin on the liver are generally reversible on discontinuing treatment.

A generally reversible sensorineural deafness, sometimes with tinnitus, has been reported in patients receiving erythromycin and appears to be related to serum concentration, with an increased likelihood of such effects in patients given doses of 4 g or more daily of base or its equivalent, in those given intravenous therapy, and in those with renal or hepatic impairment.

Other adverse effects that have been reported in patients receiving erythromycin include agranulocytosis, arrhythmias, central neurotoxicity including psychotic reactions and nightmares, a myasthenia-like syndrome, and pancreatitis. Parenteral formulations of erythromycin are irritant and intravenous administration may produce thrombophlebitis, particularly at high doses. Intramuscular injection is generally avoided as it may produce severe pain.

◊ General reviews.
1. Periti P, et al. Adverse effects of macrolide antibacterials. Drug Safety 1993; 9: 346–64.
2. Principi N, Esposito S. Comparative tolerability of erythromycin and newer macrolide antibacterials in paediatric patients. Drug Safety 1999; 20: 25–41.

Effects on body temperature. A report of 2 cases of hypothermia associated with oral erythromycin in children.[1] Symptoms resolved on withdrawal of the medication. The children were cousins, perhaps indicating a genetic predisposition to the effect.
1. Hassel B. Hypothermia from erythromycin. Ann Intern Med 1991; 115: 69–70.

Effects on the gastrointestinal tract. Comparison in patients with upper respiratory-tract infections has suggested that erythromycin ethyl succinate was associated with less abdominal pain than an equivalent dosage of erythromycin base; the ethyl succinate and acistrate did not differ in their gastrointestinal tolerability.[1] Another study has indicated that there was no significant difference in gastrointestinal symptoms between plain and enteric-coated formulations of erythromycin base.[2] Severe nausea and vomiting following rapid intravenous infusion of erythromycin lactobionate ceased in 2 patients who were converted to erythromycin base or ethyl succinate by mouth.[3] However, the adverse effects with the lactobionate may have been due to the rate of administration, since in 2 further patients symptoms resolved when the lactobionate was given more slowly as a more dilute solution.[3]

A retrospective cohort study[4] of 7 cases of infantile hypertrophic pyloric stenosis, occurring in a group of about 200 neonates given erythromycin for postexposure prophylaxis of pertussis, suggested that the drug may have had a causal role.

For reference to the stimulant effects of erythromycin on the gastrointestinal tract, see Decreased Gastrointestinal Motility under Uses and Administration, below.

1. Saloranta P, et al. Erythromycin ethylsuccinate, base and acistrate in the treatment of upper respiratory tract infection: two comparative studies of tolerability. J Antimicrob Chemother 1989; 24: 455–62.
2. Ellsworth AJ, et al. Prospective comparison of patient tolerance to enteric-coated vs non-enteric-coated erythromycin. J Fam Pract 1990; 31: 265–70.
3. Seifert CF, et al. Intravenous erythromycin lactobionate-induced severe nausea and vomiting. DICP Ann Pharmacother 1989; 23: 40–4.
4. Honein MA, et al. Infantile hypertrophic pyloric stenosis after pertussis prophylaxis with erythromycin: a case review and cohort study. Lancet 1999; 354: 2101–5. Correction. ibid. 2000; 355: 758.

Effects on the heart. References to prolongation of the QT interval and associated arrhythmias in patients receiving erythromycin intravenously.
1. McComb JM, et al. Recurrent ventricular tachycardia associated with QT prolongation after mitral valve replacement and its association with intravenous administration of erythromycin. Am J Cardiol 1984; 54: 922–3.
2. Schoenenberger RA, et al. Association of intravenous erythromycin and potentially fatal ventricular tachycardia with Q-T prolongation (torsades de pointes). BMJ 1990; 330: 1375–6.
3. Nattel S, et al. Erythromycin-induced long QT syndrome: concordance with quinidine and underlying cellular electrophysiologic mechanism. Am J Med 1990; 89: 235–8.
4. Gitler B, et al. Torsades de pointes induced by erythromycin. Chest 1994; 105: 368–72.
5. Gouyon JB, et al. Cardiac toxicity of intravenous erythromycin lactobionate in preterm infants. Pediatr Infect Dis J 1994; 13: 840–1.
6. Drici M-D, et al. Cardiac actions of erythromycin: influence of female sex. JAMA 1998; 280: 1774–6.

Effects on the neonate. For a suggestion that erythromycin might be associated with an increased risk of infantile hypertrophic pyloric stenosis in neonates, see under Effects on the Gastrointestinal Tract, above.

Effects on the skin. Skin reactions ranging from mild eruptions to erythema multiforme, Stevens-Johnson syndrome, and toxic epidermal necrolysis have rarely been reported with macrolides.
References.
1. Lestico MR, Smith AD. Stevens-Johnson syndrome following erythromycin administration. Am J Health-Syst Pharm 1995; 52: 1805–7.

Overdosage. Acute pancreatitis was reported in a 12-year-old girl after ingestion of about 5 g of erythromycin base.[1]
1. Berger TM, et al. Acute pancreatitis in a 12-year-old girl after an erythromycin overdose. Pediatrics 1992; 90: 624–6.

Precautions

Erythromycin and its derivatives should be avoided in those known to be hypersensitive to it, or in those who have previously developed liver disorders while receiving it. All forms of erythromycin should be used with care in patients with existing liver disease or hepatic impairment, and the estolate is best avoided in such patients. Repeated courses of the estolate or administration for longer than 10 days increase the risk of hepatotoxicity. Erythromycin may aggravate muscle weakness in patients with myasthenia gravis. It has been suggested that erythromycin should be used with care in patients with a history of arrhythmias or a prolonged QT interval.

Erythromycin may interfere with some diagnostic tests including measurements of urinary catecholamines and 17-hydroxycorticosteroids. The estolate has been associated with falsely-elevated serum aspartate aminotransferase values when measured colorimetrically, although genuine elevations of this enzyme, due to hepatotoxicity, also occur.

Erythromycin is irritant; solutions for parenteral administration should be suitably diluted and administered by intravenous infusion over up to 60 minutes to reduce the incidence of thrombophlebitis.

Porphyria. Erythromycin has been associated with acute attacks of porphyria and is considered unsafe in porphyric patients.

Pregnancy. Of 298 pregnant women who took erythromycin estolate, clindamycin, or placebo for 3 weeks or longer, about 14, 4, and 3% respectively had abnormally high serum aspartate aminotransferase values.[1] Erythromycin estolate should probably not be given to pregnant women.
1. McCormack WM, et al. Hepatotoxicity of erythromycin estolate during pregnancy. Antimicrob Agents Chemother 1977; 12: 630–5.

Interactions

Erythromycin and other macrolides have the potential to interact with a large number of drugs through their action on hepatic cytochrome P450 isoenzymes, particularly CYP1A2 and CYP3A4. Macrolides inhibit drug metabolism by microsomal cytochromes by competitive inhibition and by the formation of inactive complexes. Such interactions can result in severe adverse effects, including ventricular arrhythmias with the non-sedative antihistamines astemizole and terfenadine and with the prokinetic drug cisapride. Enzyme inhibition is reported to be particularly pronounced with macrolides such as erythromycin and troleandomycin. Clarithromycin is less likely to inhibit the hepatic metabolism of other drugs, although those undergoing first-pass metabolism may still be affected. Other macrolides such as azithromycin and dirithromycin are reported to have little or no effect on hepatic cytochromes, and consequently may produce fewer interactions.

Macrolides themselves have been reported rarely to prolong the QT interval and should be used with care with other drugs known to also have this effect.

Other mechanisms by which macrolides cause interactions include suppression of the gastrointestinal flora responsible for the intraluminal metabolism of digoxin and possibly oral contraceptives, and the stimulant effect of macrolides on gastrointestinal motility which is believed to be responsible for the interaction between spiramycin and levodopa.

Cimetidine is one of the few drugs reported to affect erythromycin (see below).

The effect on antimicrobial action when erythromycin is given with other antimicrobials is discussed under Antimicrobial Action, below.

◊ General references to interactions associated with macrolide antibacterials.
1. Westphal JF. Macrolide-induced clinically relevant drug interactions with cytochrome P-450A (CYP) 3A4: an update focused on clarithromycin, azithromycin and dirithromycin. Br J Clin Pharmacol 2000; 50: 285–95.
2. Pai MP, et al. Macrolide drug interactions: an update. Ann Pharmacother 2000; 34: 495–513.

◊ For reference to the effects of erythromycin and other macrolides on other drugs, see alfentanil (p.12), bromocriptine (p.1166), carbamazepine (p.344), ciclosporin (p.520), clozapine (p.672), colchicine (p.400), digoxin (p.871), dihydroergotamine and ergotamine (p.452), disopyramide (p.879), levodopa (p.1171), lovastatin (p.923), midazolam and triazolam (p.677), phenytoin (p.359), pimozide (p.664), quinidine (p.965), rifabutin (p.242), sildenafil (p.1663), tacrolimus (p.570), terfenadine (p.425), theophylline (p.780), valproate (p.368), vinblastine (p.578), warfarin (p.994), and zopiclone (p.713).

In the case of astemizole, cisapride, and terfenadine the UK Committee on Safety of Medicines (CSM) has warned that there is a risk of inducing ventricular arrhythmias if erythromycin, or possibly other macrolides, are given concomitantly,[1,2] and that, in particular, cisapride should not be administered with macrolides.[3]
1. Committee on Safety of Medicines. Ventricular arrhythmias due to terfenadine and astemizole. Current Problems 35 1992.
2. Committee on Safety of Medicines/Medicines Control Agency. Cisapride (Prepulsid, Alimax): interactions with antifungals and antibiotics can lead to ventricular arrhythmias. Current Problems 1996; 22: 1.
3. Committee on Safety of Medicines/Medicines Control Agency. Cisapride (Prepulsid): risk of arrhythmias. Current Problems 1998; 24: 11.

Cimetidine. The concomitant administration of cimetidine may increase plasma concentrations of erythromycin and was associated with deafness in a patient.[1]
1. Mogford N, et al. Erythromycin deafness and cimetidine treatment. BMJ 1994; 309: 1620.

Mechanism. In rats and humans, troleandomycin, and erythromycin and some of its derivatives, induce microsomal enzymes; the nitrosoalkane metabolites so formed produce stable inactive complexes with the iron of cytochrome P450. Eventually the oxidative metabolism of other drugs may be decreased. These effects are marked after administration of troleandomycin, moderate after erythromycin, small after oleandomycin, and absent or negligible after josamycin, midecamycin, or spiramycin.[1,2]
1. Pessayre D, et al. Drug interactions and hepatitis produced by some macrolide antibiotics. J Antimicrob Chemother 1985; 16 (suppl A): 181–94.
2. Periti P, et al. Pharmacokinetic drug interactions of macrolides. Clin Pharmacokinet 1992; 23: 106–31.

Antimicrobial Action

Erythromycin is a macrolide antibiotic with a broad and essentially bacteriostatic action against many Gram-positive and to a lesser extent some Gram-negative bacteria, as well as other organisms including mycoplasmas, spirochaetes, chlamydias, and rickettsias.

Mechanism of action. Erythromycin and other macrolides bind reversibly to the 50S subunit of the ribosome, resulting in blockage of the transpeptidation or translocation reactions, inhibition of protein synthesis, and hence inhibition of cell growth. Its action is predominantly bacteriostatic, but high concentrations are slowly bactericidal against the more sensitive strains. Because of the ready penetration of macrolides into white blood cells and macrophages there has been some interest in their potential synergy with host defence mechanisms *in vivo*. The actions of erythromycin are increased at moderately alkaline pH (up to about 8.5), particularly in Gram-negative species, probably because of the improved cellular penetration of the nonionised form of the drug.

Spectrum of activity. Erythromycin has a broad spectrum of activity. The following pathogenic organisms are usually sensitive to erythromycin (but see also Resistance, below).

Gram-positive cocci, particularly streptococci such as *Streptococcus pneumoniae* and *Str. pyogenes* are sensitive. Most strains of *Staphylococcus aureus* remain susceptible, although resistance can emerge rapidly, and some enterococcal strains are also susceptible.

Many other Gram-positive organisms respond to erythromycin, including *Bacillus anthracis*, *Corynebacterium diphtheriae*, *Erysipelothrix rhusiopathiae*, and *Listeria monocytogenes*. Anaerobic *Clostridium* spp. are also usually susceptible, as is *Propionibacterium acnes*. *Nocardia* spp. vary in their susceptibility.

Gram-negative cocci including *Neisseria meningitidis* and *N. gonorrhoeae*, and *Moraxella catarrhalis* (*Branhamella catarrhalis*) are usually sensitive.

Other Gram-negative organisms vary in their susceptibility, but *Bordetella* spp., some *Brucella* strains, *Flavobacterium*, and *Legionella* spp. are usually susceptible. *Haemophilus ducreyi* is reportedly susceptible, but *H. influenzae* is somewhat less so. The Enterobacteriaceae are not susceptible in general, although some strains may respond at alkaline pH. *Helicobacter pylori* and most strains of *Campylobacter jejuni* are sensitive (about 10% of the latter are reported to be resistant).

Among the Gram-negative anaerobes more than half of all strains of *Bacteroides fragilis* and many *Fusobacterium* strains are resistant.

Other organisms usually sensitive to erythromycin include *Actinomyces*, *Chlamydia*, rickettsias, spirochaetes such as *Treponema pallidum* and *Borrelia burgdorferi*, some mycoplasmas (notably *Mycoplasma pneumoniae*) and some of the opportunistic mycobacteria: *Mycobacterium scrofulaceum* and *M. kansasii* are usually susceptible, but *M. intracellulare* is often resistant and *M. fortuitum* usually so.

Fungi, yeasts, and viruses are resistant to erythromycin.

Minimum inhibitory concentrations (MICs) of erythromycin may be as little as 0.001 µg per mL for the most sensitive strains of *Str. pneumoniae* and *Mycoplasma pneumoniae*, but MICs for these and other organisms most sensitive to erythromycin (such as *Str. pyogenes*, *Listeria*, the more sensitive strains of *Neisseria gonorrhoeae* and *Corynebacterium diphtheriae*, *Moraxella catarrhalis*, and *Bordetella pertussis*) range from about 0.01 to 0.25 µg per mL. Organisms with MICs up to about 0.5 µg per mL are considered sensitive, and those with MICs between about 0.5 and 2 µg per mL of moderate sensitivity.

Activity with other antimicrobials. As with other bacteriostatic antimicrobials, the possibility of an antagonistic effect if erythromycin is given with a bacteri-

cide exists, and some antagonism has been shown *in vitro* between erythromycin and various penicillins and cephalosporins or gentamicin. However, in practice the results of such concurrent use are complex, and depend on the organism; in some cases synergy has been seen. Because of the adjacency of their binding sites on the ribosome, erythromycin may competitively inhibit the effects of chloramphenicol or lincosamides such as clindamycin. A synergistic effect has been seen when erythromycin was combined with a sulfonamide, notably against *Haemophilus influenzae*. Erythromycin has also been reported to enhance the antiplasmodial actions of chloroquine.

Resistance. Several mechanisms of acquired resistance to erythromycin have been reported of which the most common is a plasmid-mediated ability to methylate ribosomal RNA, resulting in decreased binding of the antimicrobial drug. This can result in cross-resistance between erythromycin, other macrolides, lincosamides, and streptogramin B, because they share a common binding site on the ribosome and this pattern of resistance is referred to as the MLS_B phenotype. It is seen in staphylococci, and to a somewhat lesser extent in streptococci, as well as in a variety of other species including *Bacteroides fragilis*, *Clostridium perfringens*, *Corynebacterium diphtheriae*, *Listeria*, and *Legionella* spp.

Decreased binding of antimicrobial to the ribosome may also occur as a result of a chromosomal mutation, resulting in an alteration of the ribosomal proteins in the 50S subunit, which conveys one-step high-level erythromycin resistance. This form of resistance has been demonstrated in *Escherichia coli* and some strains of *Str. pyogenes*, and probably occurs in *Staphylococcus aureus*.

Other forms of erythromycin resistance may be due to the elaboration of a plasmid-determined erythromycin esterase which can inactivate the drug, or to decreased drug penetration. The latter may be partly responsible for the intrinsic resistance of Gram-negative bacteria like the Enterobacteriaceae, but has also been shown to be acquired as a plasmid-mediated determinant in some organisms; production of a protein which increases drug efflux from the cell is thought to explain the MS form of resistance, in which organisms are resistant to 14-carbon ring macrolides and streptogramins, but retain sensitivity to 16-carbon ring macrolides and lincosamides.

The incidence of resistance varies greatly with the area and the organism concerned and, although the emergence of resistance is rarely a problem in the short-term treatment of infection, it is quite common in conditions requiring prolonged treatment such as endocarditis due to *Staph. aureus*. The incidence of resistance in *Staph. aureus* has been reported to be about 30 to 40% among hospital isolates and 5 to 10% in general practice. The incidence of resistance in streptococci is generally lower but shows geographical variation and may be increasing in some countries including the UK. In addition, localised outbreaks of resistant strains may occur and produce a much higher incidence of resistance.

◊ Although macrolides have limited direct antibacterial activity against *Pseudomonas aeruginosa*, prolonged exposure has produced antipseudomonal effects *in vitro*[1,2] and synergy has been demonstrated with other antipseudomonals.[3] Erythromycin and clarithromycin appear to have the greatest activity. This action has been attributed to the ability of macrolides to reduce the protective biofilm produced by some strains of *P. aeruginosa*.[4]

1. Tateda K, *et al.* Effects of sub-MICs of erythromycin and other macrolide antibiotics on serum sensitivity of Pseudomonas aeruginosa. *Antimicrob Agents Chemother* 1993; **37**: 675–80.
2. Tateda K, *et al.* Direct evidence of antipseudomonal activity of macrolides: exposure-dependent bactericidal activity and inhibition of protein synthesis by erythromycin, clarithromycin, and azithromycin. *Antimicrob Agents Chemother* 1996; **40**: 2271–5.
3. Bui KQ, *et al.* In vitro and in vivo influence of adjunct clarithromycin on the treatment of mucoid Pseudomonas aeruginosa. *J Antimicrob Chemother* 2000; **45**: 57–62.
4. Yasuda H, *et al.* Interaction between biofilms formed by Pseudomonas aeruginosa and clarithromycin. *Antimicrob Agents Chemother* 1993; **37**: 1749–55.

◊ References to erythromycin resistance.
1. Eady EA, *et al.* Multiple mechanisms of erythromycin resistance. *J Antimicrob Chemother* 1990; **26**: 461–5.
2. Seppälä H, *et al.* Resistance to erythromycin in group A streptococci. *N Engl J Med* 1992; **326**: 292–7.
3. Eady EA, *et al.* Antibiotic resistant propionibacteria in acne: need for policies to modify antibiotic usage. *BMJ* 1993; **306**: 555–6.
4. Lonks JR, Medeiros AA. High rate of erythromycin and clarithromycin resistance among Streptococcus pneumoniae isolates from blood cultures from Providence, RI. *Antimicrob Agents Chemother* 1993; **37**: 1742–5.
5. Soriano F, Fernández-Roblas R. High rates of erythromycin-resistant Streptococcus pneumoniae among penicillin-resistant strains. *J Antimicrob Chemother* 1993; **31**: 440.
6. Sutcliffe J, *et al.* Streptococcus pneumoniae and Streptococcus pyogenes resistant to macrolides but sensitive to clindamycin: a common resistance pattern mediated by an efflux system. *Antimicrob Agents Chemother* 1996; **40**: 1817–24.
7. Barry AL, *et al.* Macrolide resistance among Streptococcus pneumoniae and Streptococcus pyogenes isolated from out-patients in the USA. *J Antimicrob Chemother* 1997; **40**: 139–40.
8. Amsden GW. Pneumococcal macrolide resistance—myth or reality? *J Antimicrob Chemother* 1999; **44**: 1–6.
9. Shortridge VD, *et al.* Prevalence of macrolide resistance mechanisms in Streptococcus pneumoniae isolates from a multicenter antibiotic resistance surveillance study conducted in the United States in 1994–1995. *Clin Infect Dis* 1999; **29**: 1186–8.
10. Bingen E, *et al.* Resistance to macrolides in Streptococcus pyogenes in France in pediatric patients. *Antimicrob Agents Chemother* 2000; **44**: 1453–7.

Pharmacokinetics

Erythromycin base is unstable in gastric acid, and absorption is therefore variable and unreliable. In consequence, the base is usually administered in film- or enteric-coated preparations, or one of the more acid-stable salts or esters is employed. Food may reduce the absorption of the base or the stearate, although this depends to some extent on the formulation, but the esters are generally more reliably and quickly absorbed and their absorption is little affected by food, obviating any need to take them before food.

Peak plasma concentrations generally occur between 1 and 4 hours after administration, and have been reported to range between about 0.3 and 0.5 µg per mL after 250 mg of erythromycin base, and from 0.3 to 1.9 µg per mL after 500 mg. Similar concentrations have been seen after equivalent doses of the stearate. Somewhat higher peak concentrations may be achieved on repeated administration four times daily. Higher total concentrations are achieved after oral administration of the acistrate, estolate, or ethyl succinate, but only about 20 to 35% of acistrate or estolate or 55% of ethyl succinate is present as the active base, the rest being present as the ester (in the case of the estolate as the propionate). Peak concentrations of about 0.5 µg per mL of erythromycin base have been reported following 250 mg of the acistrate or estolate, or 500 mg of the ethyl succinate. A peak of 3 to 4 µg per mL can be achieved after intravenous administration of 200 mg of gluceptate or lactobionate.

Erythromycin is widely distributed throughout body tissues and fluids, although it does not cross the blood-brain barrier well and concentrations in CSF are low. Relatively high concentrations are found in the liver and spleen, and some is taken up into polymorphonuclear lymphocytes and macrophages. Around 70 to 75% of the base is protein bound, but after administration as the estolate the propionate ester is stated to be about 95% protein bound. Erythromycin crosses the placenta: fetal plasma concentrations are variously stated to be 5 to 20% of those in the mother. It is distributed into breast milk.

Erythromycin is excreted in high concentrations in the bile and 2 to 5% of an oral dose is excreted in the urine. As much as 12 to 15% of an intravenous dose may be excreted by the urinary route. Some erythromycin is demethylated in the liver but its metabolic fate has not been completely determined. The half-life of erythromycin is usually reported to be roughly in the range 1.5 to 2.5 hours, although this may be somewhat longer in patients with renal impairment.

Uses and Administration

Erythromycin is a macrolide antibiotic with a wide spectrum of activity, that has been used in the treatment of a wide variety of infections caused by susceptible organisms (see Antimicrobial Action, above).

Its uses have included bronchitis, severe campylobacter enteritis, chancroid, diphtheria, legionnaires' disease and other *Legionella* infections, neonatal conjunctivitis, pertussis, pneumonia (mycoplasmal and other atypical pneumonias as well as streptococcal), sinusitis, and trench fever, and, combined with neomycin, for the prophylaxis of surgical infection in patients undergoing bowel surgery.

Erythromycin is used as an alternative to penicillin in penicillin-allergic patients with various conditions including anthrax, actinomycosis, leptospirosis, listeriosis, mouth infections, otitis media (usually with a sulfonamide such as sulfafurazole), pharyngitis, the prevention of perinatal streptococcal infections, rheumatic fever, and infections in splenectomised patients, and staphylococcal and streptococcal skin infections. It has also been used in the treatment of penicillin-allergic patients with syphilis, but there are doubts about its efficacy. In penicillin-allergic patients in the early stages of Lyme disease, erythromycin may be employed as an alternative to a tetracycline. The use is generally restricted to pregnant women and young children, since it is less effective than other drugs. It is also used as an alternative to the tetracyclines in patients with chlamydial infections (such as epididymitis, lymphogranuloma venereum, nongonococcal urethritis, chlamydial pneumonia, pelvic inflammatory disease, psittacosis, and trachoma), in Q fever, and in spotted fevers.

For details of all these infections and their treatment, see under Choice of Antibacterial, p.114.

Both oral and topical erythromycin may be employed in acne (see Skin Disorders, below).

Administration and dosage. Erythromycin may be given as the base or its salts or esters; doses are expressed in terms of the base. The usual oral adult dose is the equivalent of erythromycin 1 to 2 g daily in 2 to 4 divided doses; for severe infections this may be increased to up to 4 g daily in divided doses. Daily doses higher than 1 g should be given in more than two divided doses. A maximum of 1.5 g daily has been suggested for patients with severe renal impairment. For children the dose is usually about 30 to 50 mg per kg body-weight daily although it may be doubled in severe infections; based on age, children of 2 to 8 years may be given 1 g daily in divided doses and infants and children up to 2 years of age may be given 500 mg daily in divided doses.

For the management of acne, maintenance doses as low as 250 mg daily have been used in adults, but resistant strains of propionibacteria are widespread.

In the patient who is unable to take erythromycin by mouth and in severely ill patients in whom it is necessary to attain an immediate high blood concentration, erythromycin may be given intravenously in the form of one of its more soluble salts such as the gluceptate or the lactobionate, in doses equivalent to those by mouth.

To reduce the risk of venous irritation it should be administered only by continuous or intermittent intravenous infusion of a solution containing not more than 0.5% of erythromycin. Intermittent infusions should be given every 6 hours over 20 to 60 minutes.

For the preparation of solutions of erythromycin gluceptate or lactobionate for infusion, a primary solution containing not more than 5% of erythromycin should be prepared with water. Sodium chloride or other inorganic salt solution should not be used in preparing the primary solution. It should be further diluted before intravenous administration with sodium chloride 0.9% or other suitable intravenous fluid. Acidic solutions, such as glucose, should only be used if neutralised with sodium bicarbonate.

Other routes. Erythromycin was formerly given by intramuscular injection, but such injections are painful and are no longer generally recommended. Erythromycin is used as a 0.5 to 1% ophthalmic ointment for the treatment and prophylaxis of infections of the eye, particularly of neonatal conjunctivitis. It may also be applied topically as a 2 to 4% solution for the treatment of acne vulgaris.

Propionyl erythromycin mercaptosuccinate is also used. Erythromycin salnacedin, a prodrug of erythromycin, acetylcysteine, and salicylic acid, is under investigation for the treatment of acne. Erythromycin thiocyanate and erythromycin phosphate are used in veterinary medicine.

◊ Reviews.
1. Zhanel GG, *et al.* Review of macrolides and ketolides: focus on respiratory tract infections. *Drugs* 2001; **61**: 443–98.

Administration. A discussion of the significance of different formulations and salts used for oral preparations of erythromycin concluded that there was no clear evidence that any was superior in terms of clinical effect.[1]
1. Anonymous. Giving erythromycin by mouth. *Drug Ther Bull* 1995; **33**: 77–9.

Decreased gastrointestinal motility. Erythromycin stimulates gut motility, apparently by acting as a motilin receptor agonist although it has been suggested that it may have other actions as well.[1] It has been tried, with some success, for its prokinetic action in a small number of patients with decreased gastrointestinal motility (p.1202) including those with gastroparesis,[2-5] reflux ileus,[6] acute colonic pseudo-obstruction (Ogilvie's syndrome),[6,7] delayed gastric emptying following pancreatic-duodenal surgery,[8] and neonatal postoperative intestinal dysmotility.[9] However, side-effects associated with the long-term use of erythromycin necessary in, for example, diabetic gastroparesis, may be problematic.[10]
1. Catnach SM, Fairclough PD. Erythromycin and the gut. *Gut* 1992; **33**: 397–401.
2. Janssens J, *et al.* Improvement of gastric emptying in diabetic gastroparesis by erythromycin: preliminary studies. *N Engl J Med* 1990; **322**: 1028–31.
3. Dull JS, *et al.* Successful treatment of gastroparesis with erythromycin in a patient with progressive systemic sclerosis. *Am J Med* 1990; **89**: 528–30.
4. Wadhwa NK, *et al.* Intraperitoneal erythromycin for gastroparesis. *Ann Intern Med* 1991; **114**: 912.
5. Richards RD, *et al.* The treatment of idiopathic and diabetic gastroparesis with acute intravenous and chronic oral erythromycin. *Am J Gastroenterol* 1993; **88**: 203–7.
6. Armstrong DN, *et al.* Erythromycin for reflux ileus in Ogilvie's syndrome. *Lancet* 1991; **337**: 378.
7. Bonacini M, *et al.* Erythromycin as therapy for acute colonic pseudo-obstruction (Ogilvie's syndrome). *J Clin Gastroenterol* 1991; **13**: 475–6.
8. Yeo CJ, *et al.* Erythromycin accelerates gastric emptying after pancreaticoduodenectomy: a prospective, randomized, placebo-controlled trial. *Ann Surg* 1993; **218**: 229–38.
9. Simkiss DE, *et al.* Erythromycin in neonatal postoperative intestinal dysmotility. *Arch Dis Child* 1994; **71**: F128–9.
10. Tanis AA, *et al.* Side-effects of oral erythromycin for treatment of diabetic gastroparesis. *Lancet* 1993; **342**: 1431.

Skin disorders. ACNE. Erythromycin may be used topically or orally in the treatment of acne (p.1103). Topical erythromycin may be used for mild inflammatory acne if benzoyl peroxide is ineffective or poorly tolerated. It is also used as adjunctive treatment in more severe acne. Erythromycin is also available as a complex with zinc (as the acetate) that has been reported to be more effective than topical erythromycin alone[1] or oral minocycline.[2] However, development of antibiotic resistance by the skin flora is an increasing problem. Combination therapy with benzoyl peroxide and erythromycin has been reported to be helpful in preventing the selection of antibiotic-resistant mutants[3,4] and to be more effective than topical clindamycin alone.[5] Alternatively, short intervening courses of benzoyl peroxide during antibacterial therapy may help to eliminate any resistant bacteria that have been selected.[6] It has also been recommended that courses of topical antibiotics be continued for no longer than necessary (although treatment should be used for at least 6 months), that the same drug be used if further treatment is required, and that concomitant treatment with different oral and topical antibiotics or antibiotic rotation be avoided.[6]

Oral erythromycin may be used as an alternative to a tetracycline in moderate acne. However, resistance to erythromycin is increasing so it is usually reserved for those patients in whom other antibacterials are unsuitable.
1. Habbema L, *et al.* A 4% erythromycin and zinc combination (Zineryt®) versus 2% erythromycin (Eryderm®) in acne vulgaris: a randomized, double-blind comparative study. *Br J Dermatol* 1989; **121**: 497–502.
2. Stainforth J, *et al.* A single-blind comparison of topical erythromycin/zinc lotion and oral minocycline in the treatment of acne vulgaris. *J Dermatol Treat* 1993; **4**: 119–22.
3. Eady EA, *et al.* Effects of benzoyl peroxide and erythromycin alone and in combination against antibiotic-sensitive and -resistant skin bacteria from acne patients. *Br J Dermatol* 1994; **131**: 331–6.
4. Eady EA, *et al.* The effects of acne treatment with a combination of benzoyl peroxide and erythromycin on skin carriage of erythromycin-resistant propionibacteria. *Br J Dermatol* 1996; **134**: 107–13.
5. Packman AM, *et al.* Treatment of acne vulgaris: combination of 3% erythromycin and 5% benzoyl peroxide in a gel compared to clindamycin phosphate lotion. *Int J Dermatol* 1996; **35**: 209–11.
6. Eady EA, *et al.* Antibiotic resistant propionibacteria in acne: need for policies to modify antibiotic usage. *BMJ* 1993; **306**: 555–6.

Preparations

BP 2001: Erythromycin Estolate Capsules; Erythromycin Ethyl Succinate Oral Suspension; Erythromycin Ethyl Succinate Tablets; Erythromycin Lactobionate Intravenous Infusion; Erythromycin Stearate Tablets; Erythromycin Tablets;
USP 25: Erythromycin and Benzoyl Peroxide Topical Gel; Erythromycin Delayed-release Capsules; Erythromycin Delayed-release Tablets; Erythromycin Estolate and Sulfisoxazole Acetyl Oral Suspension; Erythromycin Estolate Capsules; Erythromycin Estolate for Oral Suspension; Erythromycin Estolate Oral Suspension; Erythromycin Estolate Tablets; Erythromycin Ethylsuccinate and Sulfisoxazole Acetyl for Oral Suspension; Erythromycin Ethylsuccinate for Oral Suspension; Erythromycin Ethylsuccinate Injection; Erythromycin Ethylsuccinate Oral Suspension; Erythromycin Ethylsuccinate Tablets; Erythromycin Lactobionate for Injection; Erythromycin Ointment; Erythromycin Ophthalmic Ointment; Erythromycin Pledgets; Erythromycin Stearate Tablets; Erythromycin Tablets; Erythromycin Topical Gel; Erythromycin Topical Solution; Sterile Erythromycin Ethylsuccinate; Sterile Erythromycin Gluceptate; Sterile Erythromycin Lactobionate.

Proprietary Preparations (details are given in Part 3)

Aust.: Akne; Aknemycin; Emuvin†; Ery-Maxin†; Eryaknen; Erybesan†; Erycinum†; Eryhexal; Erysolvan; Erythrocin; Ilosone; Meromycin; Monomycin; Stiemycine; **Austral.:** E-Mycin; EES; Emu-V; Eryace; Eryc; Eryhexal; Erythrocin; Ilosone; **Belg.:** Acneryne; Aknemycin; Eryderm; Erythrocine; Erythroforte; Inderm; **Braz.:** Eribiotic; Eriflogin; Eritrex; Eritrofar; Eryacnen; Ilocin; Ilosone; Ilotrex; Infectoso; Kanazima; Lisotrex; Ortociclina; Pantomicina; Plenomicina; Stiemycin; **Canad.:** Apo-Erythro; Diomycin; E-Mycin†; EES; Erybid; Eryc; Erysol; Erythrocin; Erythromid; Ilosone; Ilotycin†; Novo-Rythro; PCE; Staticin; T-Stat; **Denm.:** Abboticin; Erycin; Erystrat; Escumycin; Hexabotin; **Fin.:** Abboticin; Erasis; Erymysin; **Fr.:** Abboticine; Egery; Ery; Eryacne; Erycocci†; Eryfluid; Erythrocine; Erythrogel; Erythrogram; Logecine; Propiocine†; Stimycine; **Ger.:** Akne Cordes; Aknederm Ery; Aknefug-EL; aknemago; Aknemycin; Aknin; Bisolvonat Mono†; Clinofug Gel†; duraerythromycin; durapaediat; Ery-Diolan; Ery-Reu†; Eryaknen; Erybeta; Erycinum; Erydermec; Eryhexal; Erysec; Erythro; Erythro-Hefa; Erythrocin; Erythrocin Neo; Erythrogenat; Erytop; Eupragin; Hydrodermed; Inderm; InfectoMyn; Karex; Lederpaediat†; Medismon; Monomycin; Paediathrocin; Sanasepton; Semibiocin; Skid E†; Stiemycine; Udima Ery†; **Hong Kong:** Aknemycin; Apo-Erythro; E-Mycin; EES; Eryacne; Eryc; Eryped; Erysol; Erythro Ethyl; Erythrocin; Ilosone; PCE; Porphyrocin; Servitrocin; Stiemycin; **Irl.:** Erymax; Erythrocin; Erythromid†; Erythroped; Ilosone; Primacine; Stiemycin; Tiprocin; **Israel:** Acnetrim; E-Mycin; Eryc; Eryderm; Erytab; Erythro-Teva; Erythrocin; Erythroderm; Erythrol; Erythroped; **Ital.:** Eritrocina; Eritrocast; Eryacne; Erytrociclin; Ilosone†; Lauromicina; Stellamicina†; Zalig†; **Mex.:** Biotril; Eriber; Eribus; Erimicina; Erisuspen; Eritolat; Eriterba; Eritrofarmin; Eritrolat; Eritroquim; Eritrosol; Eritrovier; Eritrowel; Eryacnen; Eryderm; Erylar; Esteromicin; Examicyn; Galentromicina; Ilosone; Latotryd; Lauricin; Laurimicina; Laurithran; Lederpax; Mexcyn; Optomicin; Pantomicina; Procephal; Quimolauril; Sansacne; Stiemycin; T-Stat; Totatrom; Tromigal; Verytracin; Witromin; **Neth.:** Aknemycin; Eryacne; Eryc; Eryderm; Erythrocine; Inderm; Stiemycin; **Norw.:** Abboticin; Ery-Max; **NZ:** E-Mycin; EES; Era; Eromycin; Eryacne; Eryc; Stiemycin; **Port.:** Akne-Mycin; Clinac; Eritina; Eritrocina; Eritromicina; Eryc; Eryfluid; ESE; **S.Afr.:** Acu-Erylate S†; Arcanamycin†; Betamycin; E-Mycin†; Emsyn; Emu-K†; Emu-V†; Eromel; Eromel-S†; Erycette; Eryderm; Erymax†; Erymin S†; Erymycin; Erystat†; Erythrocin; Erythromid†; Erythroped; Estomycin†; Ethimycin†; Ilosone; Ilotycin; Macrolate†; Purmycin; Rubimycin†; Ryped; Spectrasone; Stiemycin; Succilate; Succin; Xeramel; **Singapore:** Acnetrim; Akne-Mycin; E-Mycin; EES; Ermycin; Erotab; Eryacne; Eryderm; Eryped; Erysol; Eryson; Erytab-S; Erythrocin; Erotin; Ranthrocin; Servitrocin; Stiemycin; T Stat; **Spain:** Bio Exazol†; Bronsema; Deripil; Eridosis; Eritrogobens; Eritroveinte; Ery-Max; Euskin; Lagarmicin; Lederpax; Loderm; Neo Iloticina; Pantodrin; Pantomicina; **Swed.:** Abboticin; Ery-Max; **Switz.:** Aknemycin; Aknilox; Cimetrin†; Ericosol; Erios; Ery†; Eryaknen; Eryderm; Erythrocine; Erytran; Helvemycin†; Ilotycin†; Inderm; Monomycine; Servitrocin†; Staticine; Stiemycine; **Thai.:** Elocin; Erathrom; Ericin; Erimit; Erimycin; Ery-Tab; Eryacne; Eryc; Erymin; Erysil; Erythrocin; Ilosone; Malocin; Pocin; Redrocin; Rythocin; Servitrocin; Stiemycin; Tomcin; **UAE:** Eromycin; **UK:** Arpimycin; Eryacne; Erycen†; Erymax; Erymin†; Erythrocin; Erythromid; Erythroped; Ilosone†; Retcin; Rommix; Ronmix†; Stiemycin; Tiloryth; **USA:** Ak-Mycin†; Akne-Mycin; ATS; Del-Mycin; E-Base; E-Mycin; E/Gel†; EES; Emgel; Eramycin; Ery-Ped; Ery-Tab; Eryc; Erycette; Eryderm; Erygel; Erymax; Erythra-Derm; Erythrocin; Ilosone; Ilotycin; PCE; Robimycin Robitabs; Staticin; T-Stat; Theramycin Z.

Multi-ingredient: Aust.: Aknemycin compositum; AKZ; **Belg.:** Benzamycin; Zineryt; **Braz.:** Baknyl; Cifrantil; Eritrex A; Eritrosima; **Canad.:** Benzamycin; Pediazole; Sans-Acne; Stievamycin; **Denm.:** Antibiotic Simplex†; **Fr.:** Antibio-Aberel; Antibiotrex; Erylik; Pediazole; **Ger.:** Aknemycin; Aknemycin Plus; Bisolvonat; Clinesfar; Ecolicin; Isotrexin; Synergomycin; Zineryt; **Hong Kong:** Benzamycin; Dermabaz; Pediazole; **Irl.:** Benzamycin; Isotrexin; Zineryt; **Israel:** Aknemycin; Benzamycin; Pediazole; **Ital.:** Isotrexin; Lauromicina; Rubrociclina; Zineryt; **Mex.:** Benzamycin; Pantobron; Pediazole; Quimobrom; **Neth.:** Zineryt; **Port.:** Isotrexin; Zineryt; **S.Afr.:** Benzamycine; Pediazole†; **Singapore:** Benzamycin; Zineryt; **Spain:** Bronsema Expectorante; Erifoscin; Isotrex Eritromicina; Tosdiazina; Zineryt; **Switz.:** Aknemycin; AKZ†; Pediazole†; **UK:** Aknemycin Plus; Benzamycin; Isotrexin; Zineryt; **USA:** Benzamycin; Eryzole; Pediazole.

Ethambutol Hydrochloride (7556-j)

Ethambutol Hydrochloride (BANM, USAN, rINNM).

CL-40881; Ethambutoli Hydrochloridum. (S,S)-N,N'-Ethyleneb-is(2-aminobutan-1-ol) dihydrochloride.

$C_{10}H_{24}N_2O_2,2HCl = 277.2$.

CAS — 74-55-5 (ethambutol); 1070-11-7 (ethambutol hydrochloride).

Pharmacopoeias. In Chin., Eur. (see p.vi), Int., Jpn, Pol., and US.

Pharmacopoeial description

Ph. Eur.: A white, crystalline powder. Freely soluble in water; soluble in alcohol; very slightly soluble in ether. A 2% solution in water has a pH of 3.7 to 4.0. Store in airtight containers.

USP 25: A white crystalline powder. Freely soluble in water; soluble in alcohol and in methyl alcohol; slightly soluble in chloroform and in ether.

Adverse Effects and Treatment

The most important adverse effect of ethambutol is retrobulbar neuritis with a reduction in visual acuity, constriction of visual field, central or peripheral scotoma, and green-red colour blindness. One or both eyes may be affected. The degree of visual impairment appears to depend on the dose and duration of therapy; toxicity is observed most frequently at daily doses of 25 mg per kg body-weight and after 2 months of therapy. Recovery of vision usually takes place over a period of a few weeks or months, but in rare cases it may take up to one year or more or the effect may be permanent. Retinal haemorrhage has occurred rarely.

Renal clearance of urate may be reduced and acute gout has been precipitated rarely.

Hypersensitivity reactions including skin rashes, pruritus, leucopenia, fever, and joint pains have occurred but appear to be rare with ethambutol. Other adverse effects which have been reported include confusion, disorientation, hallucinations, headache, dizziness, malaise, jaundice or transient liver dysfunction, peripheral neuritis, thrombocytopenia, pulmonary infiltrates, eosinophilia, and gastrointestinal disturbances such as nausea, vomiting, anorexia, and abdominal pain.

Teratogenicity has been observed in *animals*.

Blood concentrations of ethambutol following overdosage may be reduced by haemodialysis or peritoneal dialysis.

Effects on the blood. Neutropenia has been reported in a patient on ethambutol, isoniazid, and rifampicin.[1] Each drug induced neutropenia individually on rechallenge. Thrombocytopenia attributable to ethambutol has been reported in 2 patients.[2,3]

1. Jenkins PF, et al. Neutropenia with each standard antituberculosis drug in the same patients. *BMJ* 1980; **280:** 1069–70.
2. Rabinovitz M, et al. Ethambutol-induced thrombocytopenia. *Chest* 1982; **81:** 765–6.
3. Prasad R, Mukerji PK. Ethambutol-induced thrombocytopaenia. *Tubercle* 1989; **70:** 211–12.

Effects on the eyes. Ophthalmic effects have been found in 10 of 2184 patients receiving ethambutol in doses of 25 mg or less per kg body-weight daily, although few of the 10 patients complained of symptoms.[1] In 9 of the 10 patients, ocular changes occurred after the second month of treatment. In the 928 patients who only received 2 months of ethambutol therapy, ocular toxicity was not reported. While short-term use of ethambutol is usually safe, deterioration of vision leading to long-term blindness has been reported after only a few doses of ethambutol;[2] it was suspected that this was an idiosyncratic reaction. Rapid onset reversible ocular toxicity has also occurred.[3] Visual defects occurring with ethambutol generally resolve when the drug is discontinued; for long-term visual loss hydroxocobalamin or cyanocobalamin[2,4,5] have been used with varying success.

1. Citron KM, Thomas GO. Ocular toxicity from ethambutol. *Thorax* 1986; **41:** 737–9.
2. Karnik AM, et al. A case of ocular toxicity to ethambutol—an idiosyncratic reaction? *Postgrad Med J* 1985; **61:** 811–13.
3. Schild HS, Fox BC. Rapid-onset reversible ocular toxicity from ethambutol therapy. *Am J Med* 1991; **90:** 404–6.
4. Harada T, et al. Ocular toxicity of ethambutol. *Jpn J Clin Ophthalmol* 1979; **33:** 1345–55.
5. Guerra R, Casu L. Hydroxycobalamin for ethambutol-induced optic neuropathy. *Lancet* 1981; **ii:** 1176.

Effects on the kidneys. Interstitial nephritis has been reported[1,2] in 5 patients receiving ethambutol and isoniazid; 3 were also receiving additional antimycobacterials.

1. Collier J, et al. Two cases of ethambutol nephrotoxicity. *BMJ* 1976; **2:** 1105–6.
2. Stone WJ, et al. Acute diffuse interstitial nephritis related to chemotherapy of tuberculosis. *Antimicrob Agents Chemother* 1976; **10:** 164–72.

The symbol † denotes a preparation no longer actively marketed

Effects on the liver. Although transient abnormalities in liver function commonly occur during the early stages of antituberculosis treatment, drugs other than ethambutol are generally considered responsible. Ethambutol has generated fewer reports of hepatotoxicity to the UK Committee on Safety of Medicines than rifampicin, isoniazid, or pyrazinamide,[1] and the use of regimens containing ethambutol has been recommended for patients unable to tolerate standard regimens due to hepatotoxicity.[1-3]

1. Ormerod LP, et al. Hepatotoxicity of antituberculosis drugs. *Thorax* 1996; **51:** 111–13.
2. Ormerod LP. Chemotherapy and management of tuberculosis in the United Kingdom: recommendations of the Joint Tuberculosis Committee of the British Thoracic Society. *Thorax* 1990; **45:** 403–8.
3. WHO. *TB/HIV: a clinical manual.* Geneva: WHO, 1996.

Effects on the skin. Details of a patient in whom toxic epidermal necrolysis was associated with the use of ethambutol.[1] The manufacturer noted that isolated cases of photosensitive lichenoid eruptions, Stevens-Johnson syndrome, and bullous dermatitis had also occurred.

1. Pegram PS, et al. Ethambutol-induced toxic epidermal necrolysis. *Arch Intern Med* 1981; **141:** 1677–8.

Hyperuricaemia. In a controlled study of 71 patients receiving ethambutol 20 mg per kg body-weight daily by mouth with other antimycobacterials, serum-uric acid concentrations increased in 66, mainly in the first 2 weeks of treatment.[1] One patient experienced arthralgia and another acute gouty arthritis. Serum-uric acid concentrations did not change in 60 control patients receiving other antimycobacterials.

1. Khanna BK, Gupta VP. Ethambutol-induced hyperuricaemia. *Tubercle* 1984; **65:** 195–9.

Precautions

Ethambutol is generally contra-indicated in patients with optic neuritis. It should be used with great care in patients with visual defects, the elderly, and in children in whom evaluation of changes in visual acuity may be difficult; it should generally not be used in children under 6 years of age and some consider that it should not be used in children under 13 years of age nor in patients with visual defects. Ocular examination is recommended before treatment with ethambutol and some consider that regular examinations are necessary during treatment especially in children. Patients should be advised to report visual disturbances immediately and to discontinue ethambutol pending visual evaluation.

Ethambutol should be given in reduced dosage to patients with impaired kidney function and dosage adjustments may need to be made according to serum concentrations.

Ethambutol may precipitate attacks of gout.

Although ethambutol crosses the placenta and may be teratogenic in *animals*, problems in humans have not been documented. It is generally considered that the benefits of ethambutol in the treatment of tuberculosis outweigh any potential risks in pregnancy.

Children. A review of experience of using ethambutol in children suggests that visual toxicity is not a particular problem except perhaps when CNS infection is involved.[1]

1. Graham SM, et al. Ethambutol in tuberculosis: time to reconsider? *Arch Dis Child* 1998; **78:** 274–8.

Antimicrobial Action

Ethambutol is bacteriostatic against *Mycobacterium tuberculosis* with an MIC of 0.5 to 8 μg per mL; it is bactericidal at higher concentrations. It possesses little sterilising activity. Resistant strains of *M. tuberculosis* are readily produced if ethambutol is used alone.

Mycobacterium avium complex. Strains of *Mycobacterium avium* complex have been reported to be resistant *in-vitro* to ethambutol[1] but appear to be susceptible to a combination of ethambutol and rifampicin[2] or ethambutol and ciprofloxacin.[3]

Studies have suggested that ethambutol increases the effectiveness of other antibacterial drugs by increasing cell-wall permeability.[4] Other investigators have proposed inhibition of synthesis of the outermost layer of the cell envelope by ethambutol as a mechanism for the increased drug susceptibility of *M. avium* complex.[5]

1. Kiehn TE, et al. Infections caused by Mycobacterium avium complex in immunocompromised patients: diagnosis by blood culture and fecal examination, antimicrobial susceptibility tests, and morphological and seroagglutination characteristics. *J Clin Microbiol* 1985; **21:** 168–73.
2. Zimmer BL, et al. In vitro synergistic activity of ethambutol, isoniazid, kanamycin, rifampin, and streptomycin against Mycobacterium avium-intracellulare complex. *Antimicrob Agents Chemother* 1982; **22:** 148–50.

3. Hoffner SE, et al. In-vitro synergistic activity between ethambutol and fluorinated quinolones against Mycobacterium avium complex. *J Antimicrob Chemother* 1989; **24:** 317–24.
4. Hoffner SE, et al. Microcalorimetric studies of the initial interaction between antimycobacterial drugs and Mycobacterium avium. *J Antimicrob Chemother* 1990; **25:** 353–9.
5. Rastogi N, et al. Enhancement of drug susceptibility of Mycobacterium avium by inhibitors of cell envelope synthesis. *Antimicrob Agents Chemother* 1990; **34:** 759–64.

Pharmacokinetics

About 80% of an oral dose of ethambutol is absorbed from the gastrointestinal tract, and the remainder appears in the faeces unchanged. Absorption is not significantly impaired by food (but see also Bioavailability, below). After a single dose of 25 mg per kg body-weight, peak plasma concentrations of up to 5 μg per mL appear within 4 hours, and are less than 1 μg per mL by 24 hours.

Ethambutol is distributed to most tissues, including the lungs, kidneys, and erythrocytes. It diffuses into the CSF when the meninges are inflamed. It has been reported to cross the placenta and is distributed into breast milk. The elimination half-life following oral administration is about 3 to 4 hours.

Ethambutol is partially metabolised in the liver to the aldehyde and dicarboxylic acid derivatives which are inactive and then excreted in the urine. Most of a dose appears in the urine within 24 hours as unchanged drug and 8 to 15% as the inactive metabolites. About 20% of the dose is excreted unchanged in the faeces.

Bioavailability. Although the absorption of ethambutol is not generally regarded as being impaired by food, a study in 14 healthy subjects[1] suggested that administration with a high fat meal or an antacid could delay absorption and reduce the maximum plasma concentration.

1. Peloquin CA, et al. Pharmacokinetics of ethambutol under fasting conditions, with food, and with antacids. *Antimicrob Agents Chemother* 1999; **43:** 568–72.

Distribution. In a study of the absorption of ethambutol[1] given in a dose of 25 mg per kg body-weight to 13 healthy subjects and to 21 patients with tuberculous meningitis, mean serum concentrations measured at 3 hours were 4.1 μg per mL (range 2.6 to 6.6) and 4.9 μg per mL (range 3.4 to 8) respectively. A CSF concentration of 0.07 μg per mL was measured at 3 hours in 2 of 5 healthy subjects, no ethambutol being detected in the other 3. The mean CSF concentration at 3 hours was 0.48 μg per mL (0.05 to 1.6) in 4 of 5 patients, no ethambutol being detected in the fifth.

1. Pilheu JA, et al. Concentrations of ethambutol in the cerebrospinal fluid after oral administration. *Tubercle* 1971; **52:** 117–22.

HIV-infected patients. In patients with HIV infections receiving standard multidrug therapy for tuberculosis, serum concentrations of ethambutol were low or very low compared with those expected.[1]

1. Peloquin CA, et al. Low antituberculosis drug concentrations in patients with AIDS. *Ann Pharmacother* 1996; **30:** 919–25.

Pregnancy and breast feeding. Ethambutol crosses the placenta and is present in fetal tissue in amounts of at least 74.5% of the maternal serum concentration.[1] Use of ethambutol during pregnancy has not been associated with fetal abnormalities.[2]

Ethambutol diffuses into breast milk to produce concentrations similar to those in plasma.[3]

1. Holdiness MR. Transplacental pharmacokinetics of the antituberculosis drugs. *Clin Pharmacokinet* 1987; **13:** 125–9.
2. Snider DE, et al. Treatment of tuberculosis during pregnancy. *Am Rev Respir Dis* 1980; **122:** 65–79.
3. Snider DE, Powell KE. Should women taking antituberculosis drugs breast-feed? *Arch Intern Med* 1984; **144:** 589–90.

Uses and Administration

Ethambutol is used with other antituberculous drugs in the primary treatment of pulmonary and extrapulmonary tuberculosis (p.143) to suppress emergence of resistance to the other drugs used in the regimens. It is also used as a component of regimens for the treatment of opportunistic mycobacterial infections (p.131).

In the treatment of tuberculosis, ethambutol is given, as the hydrochloride, usually with isoniazid, rifampicin, and pyrazinamide in the initial 8-week phase and sometimes in combinations with isoniazid and rifampicin in the continuation phase. It is given by mouth in a single daily dose of 15 mg per kg body-weight, or 30 mg per kg three times weekly, or 45 mg per kg twice weekly. Initial doses of ethambutol 25 mg per kg daily for 60 days may be given to patients who have previously received antimycobacterial therapy, reduced to 15 mg per kg daily thereafter.

Ethambutol has also been used occasionally with other drugs for prophylaxis if the likelihood of resistance to isoniazid is high, when daily doses of 15 mg per kg have been employed, for 6 months or more. If it is used in patients with renal impairment (see Precautions, above), then doses should be adjusted according to serum concentrations.

Preparations

BP 2001: Ethambutol Tablets;
USP 25: Ethambutol Hydrochloride Tablets; Rifampin, Isoniazid, Pyrazinamide, and Ethambutol Hydrochloride Tablets.

Proprietary Preparations (details are given in Part 3)
Aust.: Etibi; Myambutol; *Austral.:* Myambutol; *Belg.:* Myambutol; *Canad.:* Etibi; Myambutol; *Denm.:* Myambutol; *Fin.:* Oributol; *Fr.:* Dexambutol; Myambutol; *Ger.:* EMB; Myambutol; *Hong Kong:* Etibi; Lambutol; Myambutol; *Irl.:* Myambutol; *Israel:* Myambutol; *Ital.:* Etapiam; Etibi†; Myambutol; *Mex.:* Myambutol; Tambutec; Tubetam; *Neth.:* Myambutol; *NZ:* Myambutol; *Port.:* Turresis; *S.Afr.:* Myambutol; Mycrol†; *Spain:* Myambutol; *Swed.:* Myambutol; *Switz.:* Myambutol; *Thai.:* Ethbutol; Lambutol; Myambutol; Myrin; Myrin-P; Servambutol; Tobutol; *UK:* Myambutol†; *USA:* Myambutol.

Multi-ingredient: *Aust.:* Myambutol-INH; *Fr.:* Dexambutol-INH; *Ger.:* EMB-INH; Myambutol-INH; *Ital.:* Etanicozid B6; Etibi-INH†; Miazide B6; Miazide†; *S.Afr.:* Mynah†; Myrin; Myrin Plus; Rifafour; Tuberol†; *Spain:* Isoetam†; *Switz.:* Myambutol-INH.

Ethionamide (7557-z)

Ethionamide *(BAN, USAN, rINN)*.
Ethionamidum; Etionamide; 1314-TH. 2-Ethylpyridine-4-carbothioamide.
$C_8H_{10}N_2S = 166.2$.
CAS — 536-33-4.
ATC — J04AD03.
Pharmacopoeias. In Eur. (see p.vi), Int., Jpn, Pol., and US.

Pharmacopoeial description
Ph. Eur.: Small yellow crystals or a yellow crystalline powder. Practically insoluble in water; sparingly soluble in alcohol; slightly soluble in ether; soluble in methyl alcohol.
USP 25: A bright yellow powder having a faint to moderate sulfide-like odour. Slightly soluble in water, in chloroform, and in ether; sparingly soluble in alcohol and in propylene glycol; soluble in methyl alcohol. pH of a 1% slurry in water is between 6.0 and 7.0. Store in airtight containers.

Adverse Effects and Treatment

Many patients cannot tolerate therapeutic doses of ethionamide and have to discontinue treatment. The most common adverse effects are dose-related gastrointestinal disturbances, including anorexia, excessive salivation, a metallic taste, nausea, vomiting, abdominal pain, and diarrhoea. Tolerance may be improved by reducing the dose, adjusting the timing of administration, or administering an antiemetic.

Mental disturbances including depression, anxiety, and psychosis have been provoked. Dizziness, drowsiness, headache, postural hypotension, and asthenia may also occur occasionally. Peripheral and optic neuropathy and a pellagra-like syndrome have occurred. Pyridoxine or nicotinamide have been suggested for the treatment or prevention of neurotoxic effects. Although rare, hepatitis may occur with or without jaundice. The incidence of hepatotoxicity is increased when ethionamide is given in association with rifampicin.

Other side-effects reported include hypersensitivity reactions, thrombocytopenia and purpura, alopecia, dermatitis (including photodermatitis); endocrine disturbances, hypoglycaemia, and hypothyroidism with or without goitre.

Teratogenic effects have been reported in *animals.*

Effects on the liver. Use of ethionamide or protionamide with rifampicin for the treatment of multibacillary leprosy has been associated with a high incidence of hepatotoxicity. A hepatitis incidence of 4.5 to 5% has been reported for patients on ethionamide or protionamide, rifampicin, and either dapsone or clofazimine.[1,2] In these studies, diagnosis of hepatitis was based on clinical assessment. When laboratory monitoring was used, an incidence of 13% was reported with a regimen of ethionamide or protionamide with rifampicin and dapsone.[3] A regimen of protionamide, dapsone, rifampicin, and clofazimine has been associated with a 22% incidence based on laboratory monitoring.[4] Administration of ethionamide in association with pyrazinamide has also resulted in a high incidence of abnormal liver function tests.[5]

In the above studies rifampicin was administered daily during part or all of the regimens. The incidence of hepatotoxicity when ethionamide or protionamide is administered in association with once-monthly rifampicin may be lower; hepatotoxicity was not reported in patients receiving monthly rifampicin and daily protionamide, isoniazid, and dapsone.[6]

1. Pattyn SR, *et al.* Hepatotoxicity of the combination of rifampin-ethionamide in the treatment of multibacillary leprosy. *Int J Lepr* 1984; **52:** 1–6.

2. Pattyn SR, *et al.* Combined regimens of one year duration in the treatment of multibacillary leprosy—II: combined regimens with rifampicin administered during 6 months. *Lepr Rev* 1989; **60:** 118–23.
3. Cartel J-L, *et al.* Hepatitis in leprosy patients treated by a daily combination of dapsone, rifampin, and a thioamide. *Int J Lepr* 1983; **51:** 461–5.
4. Ji B, *et al.* Hepatotoxicity of combined therapy with rifampicin and daily prothionamide for leprosy. *Lepr Rev* 1984; **55:** 283–9.
5. Schless JM, *et al.* The use of ethionamide in combined drug regimens in the re-treatment of isoniazid-resistant pulmonary tuberculosis. *Am Rev Respir Dis* 1965; **91:** 728–37.
6. Ellard GA, *et al.* Long-term prothionamide compliance: a study carried out in India using a combined formulation containing prothionamide, dapsone and isoniazid. *Lepr Rev* 1988; **59:** 163–75.

Precautions

Ethionamide should not be given to patients with severe liver disease. Liver function tests should be carried out before and during treatment with ethionamide.

Caution is necessary in administering ethionamide to patients with depression or other psychiatric illness. Difficulty may be experienced in the management of diabetes mellitus. Periodic monitoring of blood glucose, thyroid function, and visual function is desirable.

Ethionamide is best avoided during pregnancy.

Porphyria. Ethionamide is considered to be unsafe in patients with porphyria because it has been shown to be porphyrinogenic in *animals* or *in-vitro* systems.

Interactions

The side-effects of other antimycobacterials may be increased when ethionamide is administered concomitantly (see Effects on the Liver, above, and under Cycloserine, p.195).

Alcohol. Psychotic reactions have been reported in patients receiving ethionamide following excessive intake of alcohol.

Antimicrobial Action

Ethionamide is active only against mycobacteria including *Mycobacterium tuberculosis, M. kansasii, M. leprae,* and some strains of *M. avium* complex. Most susceptible organisms are inhibited by 10 μg or less per mL. It is considered to be bactericidal against *M. leprae* and an MIC of 0.05 μg per mL has been reported.

Resistance develops rapidly if used alone and there is complete cross-resistance between ethionamide and protionamide. Cross-resistance has been reported *in vitro* and in *animals* with isoniazid or with thioacetazone.

Pharmacokinetics

Ethionamide is readily absorbed from the gastrointestinal tract, and peak plasma concentrations of about 2 μg per mL occur 2 hours after an oral dose of 250 mg. It is widely distributed throughout body tissues and fluids. It crosses the placenta and penetrates the uninflamed meninges, appearing in the CSF in concentrations equivalent to those in serum. It is about 30% bound to plasma proteins. The half-life is reported to be 2 to 3 hours. Ethionamide is extensively metabolised, probably in the liver, to the active sulfoxide and other inactive metabolites and less than 1% of a dose appears in the urine as unchanged drug.

Distribution. Following single oral doses of ethionamide 15 or 20 mg per kg body-weight in children with tuberculous meningitis, the peak spinal fluid concentration was reached in 1½ to 2½ hours.[1] A wide range of concentrations was reported but doses of 20 mg per kg were more likely to produce spinal fluid concentrations above 2.5 μg per mL, the concentration considered by the authors to be essential for therapeutic success.

1. Donald PR, Seifart HI. Cerebrospinal fluid concentrations of ethionamide in children with tuberculous meningitis. *J Pediatr* 1989; **115:** 483–6.

Uses and Administration

Ethionamide is a thioamide derivative considered to be interchangeable with protionamide. It has been used in combination with other antituberculous drugs for the treatment of tuberculosis (p.143) when resistance to, or toxicity from, primary drugs has developed. It has also been used, as a substitute for clofazimine, in regimens for the treatment of leprosy (p.126) but less toxic alternatives are now preferred.

In the treatment of resistant tuberculosis, adults may be given 15 to 20 mg per kg body-weight daily (maximum 1 g daily) by mouth. Children have been given 10 to 20 mg per kg daily (maximum 750 mg daily). Ethionamide may be given in divided doses with meals, or as a single daily dose after the evening meal, or at bedtime, to minimise gastrointestinal adverse effects. Similar doses were used for the treatment of leprosy.

Ethionamide has also been administered as rectal suppositories; the hydrochloride has been given intravenously.

Preparations

USP 25: Ethionamide Tablets.

Proprietary Preparations (details are given in Part 3)
S.Afr.: Ethatyl; *USA:* Trecator.

Evernimicin (3266-a)

Evernimicin *(USAN, rINN)*.
Sch-27899. O-(1R)-2,3-O-Methylene-4-O-(6-methyl-β-resorcyloyl)-D-xylopyranosylidene-(1→3-4)-α-L-lyxopyranosyl   O-2,3,6-trideoxy-3-C-methyl   4-O-methyl-3-nitro-α-L-arabino-hexopyranosyl-(1→3)-O-2,6-dideoxy-4-O-(3,5-dichloro-6-methoxy-4,2-cresotoyl)-β-D-arabino-hexopyranosyl-(1→4)-O-(1R)-2,6-dideoxy-D-arabino-hexopyranosylidene-(1→3-4)-O-6-deoxy-3-C-methyl-β-D-mannopyranosyl-(1→3)-O-6-deoxy-4-O-methyl-β-D-galactopyranosyl-(1→4)-2,6-di-O-methyl-β-D-mannopyranoside.
$C_{70}H_{97}Cl_2NO_{38} = 1631.4$.
CAS — 109545-84-8.

Profile

Evernimicin is an everninomicin antibacterial with activity against Gram-positive bacteria. It has been investigated for the treatment of infections due to penicillin-resistant pneumococci. Development has been discontinued because of disappointing efficacy.

Faropenem Sodium (17297-b)

Faropenem Sodium *(rINNM)*.
Fropenem Sodium. Sodium (+)-(5R,6S)-6-[(1R)-1-hydroxyethyl]-7-oxo-3-[(2R)-tetrahydro-2-furyl]-4-thia-1-azabicyclo[3.2.0]hept-2-ene-2-carboxylate.
$C_{12}H_{15}NaNO_5S = 308.3$.
CAS — 106560-14-9 (faropenem); 122547-49-3 (faropenem sodium).

Profile

Faropenem is a penem antibacterial that is given by mouth as the sodium salt for the treatment of susceptible infections.

◊ References.
1. Woodcock JM, *et al.* The in-vitro activity of faropenem, a novel oral penem. *J Antimicrob Chemother* 1997; **39:** 35–43.

Preparations

Proprietary Preparations (details are given in Part 3)
Jpn: Farom.

Fleroxacin (2953-w)

Fleroxacin *(BAN, USAN, rINN)*.
AM-833; Ro-23-6240; Ro-23-6240/000. 6,8-Difluoro-1-(2-fluoroethyl)-1,4-dihydro-7-(4-methyl-1-piperazinyl)-4-oxo-3-quinolinecarboxylic acid.
$C_{17}H_{18}F_3N_3O_3 = 369.3$.
CAS — 79660-72-3.
ATC — J01MA08.

Profile

Fleroxacin is a fluoroquinolone antibacterial with actions and uses similar to those of ciprofloxacin (p.182), but is reported to have greater systemic bioavailability and a longer half-life. It is given by mouth or by intravenous infusion for the treatment of susceptible infections in usual doses of 200 or 400 mg once daily.

The incidence of adverse effects associated with fleroxacin has been relatively high.

◊ General references.
1. Leigh D, *et al.* eds. Fleroxacin, a long acting fluoroquinolone with broad spectrum activity. *J Antimicrob Chemother* 1988; **22** (suppl D): 1–234.
2. Balfour JA, *et al.* Fleroxacin: a review of its pharmacology and therapeutic efficacy in various infections. *Drugs* 1995; **49:** 794–850.

◊ References to adverse effects associated with fleroxacin.
1. Bowie WR, *et al.* Adverse reactions in a dose-ranging study with a new long-acting fluoroquinolone, fleroxacin. *Antimicrob Agents Chemother* 1989; **33:** 1778–82.

Preparations

Proprietary Preparations (details are given in Part 3)
Aust.: Quinodis; *Belg.:* Quinodis†; *Denm.:* Quinodis; *Ger.:* Quinodis; *Jpn:* Megalocin; *Switz.:* Quinodis.

Flomoxef (1792-n)

Flomoxef *(rINN)*.
6315-S. 7R-7-[2-(Difluoromethylthio)acetamido]-3-[1-(2-hydroxyethyl)-1H-tetrazol-5-ylthiomethyl]-7-methoxy-1-oxa-3-cephem-4-carboxylic acid.
$C_{15}H_{18}F_2N_6O_7S_2 = 496.5$.
CAS — 99665-00-6.
Pharmacopoeias. Jpn includes flomoxef sodium.

Profile

Flomoxef is an oxacephalosporin or oxacephem antibiotic with properties similar to latamoxef (p.218). It is given as the sodium salt in doses equivalent to 1 to 2 g daily of flomoxef by intravenous injection or infusion.

Preparations

Proprietary Preparations (details are given in Part 3)
Jpn: Flumarin.

Florfenicol (824-p)

Florfenicol *(BAN, USAN, rINN)*.
Sch-25298. 2,2-Dichloro-N-[(αS,βR)-α-(fluoromethyl)-β-hydroxy-4-methanesulfonylphenethyl]acetamide.
$C_{12}H_{14}Cl_2FNO_4S = 358.2$.
CAS — 76639-94-6.

Profile

Florfenicol, a fluorinated analogue of chloramphenicol, is an antibacterial used in veterinary medicine.

Flucloxacillin (12125-y)

Flucloxacillin *(BAN, rINN)*.
BRL-2039; Floxacillin *(USAN)*. (6R)-6-[3-(2-Chloro-6-fluorophenyl)-5-methylisoxazole-4-carboxamido]penicillanic acid.
$C_{19}H_{17}ClFN_3O_5S = 453.9$.
CAS — 5250-39-5.
ATC — J01CF05.

NOTE. Compounded preparations of flucloxacillin may be represented by the following names:
• Co-fluampicil *(BAN)*—flucloxacillin 1 part and ampicillin 1 part (w/w).

Flucloxacillin Magnesium (3868-r)

Flucloxacillin Magnesium *(BANM, rINNM)*.
$(C_{19}H_{16}ClFN_3O_5S)_2Mg,8H_2O = 1074.2$.
CAS — 58486-36-5.
Pharmacopoeias. In *Br.*

2.4 g of monograph substance is approximately equivalent to 1 g of anhydrous flucloxacillin. Each g of monograph substance represents about 0.9 mmol of magnesium.

Pharmacopoeial description

BP 2001: A white or almost white powder. Slightly soluble in water and in chloroform; freely soluble in methyl alcohol. A 0.5% solution in water has a pH of 4.5 to 6.5. Store at a temperature not exceeding 25°. Protect from moisture.

Flucloxacillin Sodium (85-l)

Flucloxacillin Sodium *(BANM, rINNM)*.
Flucloxacilina Sódica; Flucloxacillinum Natricum.
$C_{19}H_{16}ClFN_3NaO_5S,H_2O = 493.9$.
CAS — 1847-24-1.
Pharmacopoeias. In *Eur.* (see p.vi).

1.09 g of monograph substance is approximately equivalent to 1 g of anhydrous flucloxacillin. Each g of monograph substance represents about 2 mmol of sodium.
As with other penicillins, flucloxacillin sodium is incompatible with aminoglycosides.

Pharmacopoeial description

Ph. Eur.: A white or almost white, crystalline hygroscopic, powder. Freely soluble in water and in methyl alcohol; soluble in alcohol. A 10% solution in water has a pH of 5.0 to 7.0. Store at a temperature not exceeding 25° in airtight containers.

Adverse Effects and Precautions

As for Benzylpenicillin p.157.

Hepatitis and cholestatic jaundice have been reported occasionally with flucloxacillin and may be delayed in onset for up to several weeks after treatment has been stopped; older patients and those receiving flucloxacillin for more than two weeks are at greater risk. Agranulocytosis and neutropenia have been associated rarely with isoxazolyl penicillins such as flucloxacillin. Phlebitis has followed intravenous infusion.

Effects on the liver. References.
1. Bengtsson F, *et al.* Flucloxacillin-induced cholestatic liver damage. *Scand J Infect Dis* 1985; **17:** 125–8.
2. Turner IB, *et al.* Prolonged hepatic cholestasis after flucloxacillin therapy. *Med J Aust* 1989; **151:** 701–5.
3. Fairley CK, *et al.* Flucloxacillin jaundice. *Lancet* 1992; **339:** 679.
4. Committee on Safety of Medicines. Flucloxacillin-induced cholestatic jaundice. *Current Problems 35* 1992.
5. Fairley CK, *et al.* Risk factors for development of flucloxacillin associated jaundice. *BMJ* 1993; **306:** 233–5. Correction. *ibid.*; **307:** 1179.

Porphyria. Flucloxacillin has been associated with acute attacks of porphyria and is considered unsafe in porphyric patients.

Interactions

As for Benzylpenicillin, p.158.

The symbol † denotes a preparation no longer actively marketed

Antimicrobial Action

Flucloxacillin is bactericidal with a mode of action similar to that of benzylpenicillin, but is resistant to staphylococcal penicillinase. It is active therefore against penicillinase-producing and non-penicillinase-producing staphylococci, with minimum inhibitory concentrations in the range of 0.25 to 0.5 μg per mL. Its activity against streptococci such as *Streptococcus pneumoniae* and *Str. pyogenes* is less than that of benzylpenicillin, but sufficient to be useful when these organisms are present with penicillin-resistant staphylococci. Flucloxacillin is virtually ineffective against *Enterococcus faecalis*.

Resistance. The resistance of staphylococci to flucloxacillin and other penicillinase-resistant penicillins is described under meticillin (p.223).

Pharmacokinetics

Flucloxacillin, like dicloxacillin, is about twice as well absorbed from the gastrointestinal tract as cloxacillin, but absorption is also reduced by the presence of food in the stomach. After an oral dose of 250 mg to 1 g, in fasting subjects, peak plasma concentrations in about 1 hour are usually in the range of 5 to 15 μg per mL. Plasma concentrations following the intramuscular injection of flucloxacillin sodium are similar, but peak concentrations are achieved in about 30 minutes. Doubling the dose can double the plasma concentration. About 95% of flucloxacillin in the circulation is bound to plasma proteins. Flucloxacillin has been reported to have a plasma half-life of approximately 1 hour. The half-life is prolonged in neonates.

The distribution of flucloxacillin into body tissues and fluids is similar to that of cloxacillin (p.192).
Flucloxacillin is metabolised to a limited extent and the unchanged drug and metabolites are excreted in the urine by glomerular filtration and renal tubular secretion. About 50% of a dose by mouth and up to 90% of an intramuscular dose is excreted in the urine within 6 hours. Only small amounts are excreted in the bile. Flucloxacillin is not removed by haemodialysis. Plasma concentrations are enhanced if probenecid is given concomitantly.

Uses and Administration

Flucloxacillin is an isoxazolyl penicillin used primarily for the treatment of infections due to staphylococci resistant to benzylpenicillin. These include bone and joint infections, endocarditis, peritonitis (associated with continuous ambulatory peritoneal dialysis), pneumonia, skin infections (including soft-tissue infections), and toxic shock syndrome. For discussions of these infections and their treatment, see under Choice of Antibacterial, p.114.

Administration and dosage. Flucloxacillin is administered by mouth as the sodium or magnesium salt. It should be taken at least 30 minutes before meals as the presence of food in the stomach reduces absorption. It is administered parenterally as the sodium salt. All doses are expressed as flucloxacillin. In severe renal impairment a reduction in dosage may be necessary.
The usual adult dose by mouth or by intramuscular injection is 250 mg four times daily. It is administered intravenously in a dose of 250 mg to 1 g four times daily by slow injection over 3 to 4 minutes or by intravenous infusion. All systemic doses may be doubled in severe infections; up to 8 g daily in three or four divided doses may be given for endocarditis or osteomyelitis.
Flucloxacillin has been administered by other routes in conjunction with systemic therapy. It has been administered in a dose of 250 to 500 mg daily by intra-articular injection, dissolved if necessary in a 0.5% solution of lignocaine [lidocaine] hydrochloride, or by intrapleural injection in a dose of 250 mg daily. Using powder for injection, 125 to 250 mg has been dissolved in 3 mL of sterile water and inhaled by nebuliser 4 times daily.

Children up to 2 years of age may be given one-quarter the adult dose and those aged 2 to 10 years one-half the adult dose.
Flucloxacillin may be administered in combination with other antibacterials, including ampicillin (known as co-fluampicil), to produce a wider spectrum of activity. If flucloxacillin is used concurrently with an aminoglycoside the two drugs should not be mixed.

Preparations

BP 2001: Co-fluampicil Capsules; Co-fluampicil Oral Suspension; Flucloxacillin Capsules; Flucloxacillin Injection; Flucloxacillin Oral Solution; Flucloxacillin Oral Suspension.

Proprietary Preparations (details are given in Part 3)
Aust.: Floxapen; *Austral.:* Flopen; Floxapen; Flucil; Staphylex; *Belg.:* Floxapen; Staphycid; *Denm.:* Heracillin; *Ger.:* Fluclox-Reu; Staphylex; *Hong Kong:* Flucloxil; *Irl.:* Floxapen; Flucillin; Fluclon†; Geriflox; Ladropen†; Stafoxil†; *Ital.:* Betabiotic; Cloxillin; Evercid; Flucinal; *Mex.:* Floxapen; *Neth.:* Floxapen; Stafoxil; *NZ:* Floxapen; Flucloxin; Staphlex; *Port.:* Floxapen; Floxil; *S.Afr.:* Floxapen; Flucillin; *Singapore:* Fluoclox; Staphlex; *Swed.:* Heracillin; *Switz.:* Floxapen; Flucloxin†; *UK:* Floxapen; Fluclomix; Galfloxin; Ladropen†; Stafoxil†; Zoxin†.

Multi-ingredient: *Aust.:* Fluxapril; *Ger.:* Flanamox; Fluxapril†; *Ital.:* Infectrin†; *S.Afr.:* Flumox; Macropen; Megapen; Suprapen; *UK:* Flu-Amp; Magnapen.

Flumequine (12757-f)

Flumequine *(BAN, USAN, rINN)*.
Flumequinum; R-802. 9-Fluoro-6,7-dihydro-5-methyl-1-oxo-1H,5H-pyrido[3,2,1-ij]quinoline-2-carboxylic acid.
$C_{14}H_{12}FNO_3 = 261.2$.
CAS — 42835-25-6.
ATC — G04AB06.
Pharmacopoeias. In *Eur.* (see p.vi).

Pharmacopoeial description

Ph. Eur.: A microcrystalline white powder. Practically insoluble in water; sparingly soluble in dichloromethane; very slightly soluble in methyl alcohol; freely soluble in dilute solutions of alkali hydroxides.

Profile

Flumequine is a 4-quinolone antibacterial with actions and uses similar to those of nalidixic acid (p.227). It may be more active *in vitro* against some Enterobacteriaceae. In the treatment of urinary-tract infections doses of 400 mg are given three times daily by mouth.

Porphyria. Flumequine is considered to be unsafe in patients with porphyria because it has been shown to be porphyrinogenic in *in-vitro* systems.

Preparations

Proprietary Preparations (details are given in Part 3)
Belg.: Apurone†; *Fr.:* Apurone; *Ital.:* Flumural†.

Flurithromycin (3075-e)

Flurithromycin *(rINN)*.
CI-932; P-0501A. (8S)-8-Fluoroerythromycin.
$C_{37}H_{66}FNO_{13} = 751.9$.
CAS — 82664-20-8.
ATC — J01FA14.

Profile

Flurithromycin is a fluorinated macrolide antibacterial derived from erythromycin (p.201). It is given by mouth as the ethyl succinate in the treatment of susceptible infections.

◊ References.
1. Saverino D, *et al.* Antibacterial profile of flurithromycin, a new macrolide. *J Antimicrob Chemother* 1992; **30:** 261–72.

Preparations

Proprietary Preparations (details are given in Part 3)
Ital.: Flurizic; Mizar; Ritro.

Formosulfathiazole (4905-a)

Formaldehyde-sulphathiazole; Formosulphathiazole; Methylenesulfathiazole.
CAS — 13968-86-0.

A condensation product of sulfathiazole with formaldehyde.

Profile

Formosulfathiazole is a sulfonamide with properties similar to those of sulfamethoxazole (p.254). It is poorly absorbed and has been given for its antibacterial action in the gastrointestinal tract, often in combination with other antibacterials.

Preparations

Proprietary Preparations (details are given in Part 3)
Multi-ingredient: *Spain:* Sulfintestin Neom†; Sulfintestin Neomicina.

Fosfomycin (179-a)

Fosfomycin (BAN, USAN, rINN).
MK-955; Phosphomycin; Phosphonomycin. (1R,2S)-1,2-Epoxy-propylphosphonic acid.
$C_3H_7O_4P = 138.1$.
CAS — 23155-02-4 (fosfomycin); 26016-98-8 (fosfomycin calcium); 26016-99-9 (fosfomycin disodium); 78964-85-9 (fosfomycin trometamol).
ATC — J01XX01.
Pharmacopoeias. Eur. (see p.vi) and Jpn include the calcium and disodium salts. Eur. also includes Fosfomycin Trometamol.

An antibiotic isolated from Streptomyces fradiae and other Streptomyces spp. or produced synthetically.

Pharmacopoeial description

Ph. Eur.: Fosfomycin Calcium is a white or almost white powder. Slightly soluble in water; practically insoluble in acetone, in dichloromethane, and in methyl alcohol. A 0.1% solution in water has a pH of 8.1 to 9.6. Store in airtight containers. Protect from light.
Fosfomycin Sodium is a white or almost white, very hygroscopic powder. Very soluble in water; practically insoluble in dehydrated alcohol and in dichloromethane; sparingly soluble in methyl alcohol. A 5% solution in water has a pH of 9.0 to 10.5. Store in airtight containers. Protect from light.
Fosfomycin Trometamol is a white or almost white, hygroscopic powder. Very soluble in water; slightly soluble in alcohol and in methyl alcohol; practically insoluble in acetone. A 5% solution in water has a pH of 3.5 to 5.5. Store in airtight containers.

Adverse Effects and Precautions

Gastrointestinal disturbances including nausea and diarrhoea, transient increases in serum concentrations of aminotransferases, headache, visual disturbances, and skin rashes have been reported following the use of fosfomycin. Eosinophilia and, rarely, angioedema, aplastic anaemia, exacerbation of asthma, cholestatic jaundice, hepatic necrosis, and toxic megacolon, have also occurred.

Antimicrobial Action

Fosfomycin is a bactericidal antibacterial. Following active uptake into the cell it is reported to interfere with the first step in the synthesis of bacterial cell walls. It is active in vitro against a range of Gram-positive and Gram-negative bacteria including Staphylococcus aureus, some streptococci, most Enterobacteriaceae, Haemophilus influenzae, Neisseria spp., and some strains of Pseudomonas aeruginosa although some are resistant. Bacteroides spp. are not sensitive. MICs are very variable and depend on the type of test medium used as well as inoculum size: glucose 6-phosphate potentiates its activity in vitro but MICs determined in the presence of glucose 6-phosphate correlate better with activity in vivo. MICs for the most sensitive strains have been reported to range from about 1 to 4 μg per mL, but organisms with MICs up to about 16 μg per mL have been considered sensitive and those with MICs between about 16 and 64 μg per mL of moderate sensitivity. Bacterial resistance to fosfomycin has been reported and can be chromosomal or, in some organisms, transferred by plasmids encoding multiple resistance (for example in Serratia marcescens). However, there appears to be little cross-resistance with other antibacterials.

Fosfomycin has been reported to demonstrate antimicrobial synergy with a wide range of antibacterials against organisms such as enterococci, meticillin-resistant Staph. aureus, and the enterobacteria. Such synergistic effects have been reported particularly with the beta lactams, but also with aminoglycosides, macrolides, tetracyclines, chloramphenicol, rifamycin, and lincomycin. Antimicrobial antagonism with a beta lactam has also been reported.

There is some suggestion that co-administration of fosfomycin with an aminoglycoside may also reduce the nephrotoxicity of the latter in vivo.

◊ References.
1. Barry AL, Brown SD. Antibacterial spectrum of fosfomycin trometamol. J Antimicrob Chemother 1995; 35: 228–30.

Pharmacokinetics

Fosfomycin or fosfomycin calcium are poorly absorbed from the gastrointestinal tract. Peak plasma concentrations about 4 hours after a 1-g dose of fosfomycin are around 7 μg per mL, and bioavailability has been calculated at about 30 to 40%. Similar bioavailability has been reported for the trometamol salt, and plasma concentrations of about 22 to 32 μg per mL have been reported 2 hours after a dose of 50 mg per kg bodyweight (about 3 g fosfomycin). Fosfomycin disodium is administered by the intramuscular or intravenous routes: intravenous infusion of a 3-g dose results in peak serum concentrations of around 220 μg per mL. The plasma half-life is about 2 hours. Fosfomycin does not appear to be bound to plasma proteins. It diffuses across the placenta and is widely distributed in body fluids including the CSF; small amounts have been found in breast milk and bile. The majority of a parenteral dose is excreted unchanged in the urine, by glomerular filtration, within 24 hours.

Following oral administration of fosfomycin trometamol, urinary concentrations of 3 mg per mL have been reported within 2 to 4 hours of a 3-g dose; therapeutic concentrations are maintained for about 36 hours following a single oral dose.

◊ References.
1. Bergan T, et al. Pharmacokinetic profile of fosfomycin trometamol. Chemotherapy 1993; 39: 297–301.

Uses and Administration

Fosfomycin is a phosphonic acid antibacterial administered by mouth as the trometamol salt in the treatment of acute uncomplicated infections of the urinary tract (p.146). It is given to adults as a single dose equivalent to 3 g of fosfomycin; children over 5 years have been given 2 g.

Fosfomycin trometamol has also been used for the prophylaxis of infection in transurethral surgical procedures; the equivalent of 3 g of fosfomycin has been given by mouth 3 hours before and repeated 24 hours after the procedure. For a discussion of surgical infections and their prophylaxis and treatment, see p.141.

Fosfomycin has also been given by mouth as the calcium salt and intramuscularly or intravenously as the disodium salt in the treatment of a variety of bacterial infections due to susceptible organisms. Doses are calculated in terms of the base. The usual adult dose by mouth is 1 g of fosfomycin every 6 to 8 hours. Higher doses have been given parenterally, with up to 20 g daily having been given intravenously in severe infection.

Fosfomycin has been administered as an ingredient of combination preparations also containing a beta lactam.

◊ References.
1. Reeves DS. Fosfomycin trometamol. J Antimicrob Chemother 1994; 34: 853–8.
2. Patel SS, et al. Fosfomycin tromethamine: a review of its antibacterial activity, pharmacokinetic properties and therapeutic efficacy as a single-dose oral treatment for acute uncomplicated lower urinary tract infections. Drugs 1997; 53: 637–56.

Preparations

Proprietary Preparations (details are given in Part 3)
Aust.: Monuril; **Belg.:** Monuril; **Braz.:** Monuril; **Fin.:** Monurol; **Fr.:** Fosfocine; Monuril; Uridoz; **Ger.:** Fosfocin; InfectoFos; Monuril; **Hong Kong:** Monurol; **Irl.:** Monuril; **Israel:** Monuril; **Ital.:** Afos; Biocin; Faremicin; Fonofos†; Fosfocin; Fosforal†; Foximin; Francital; Ipamicina; Lofoxin†; Monuril; Ultramicina; **Jpn:** Fosmicin-S; **Mex.:** Fosfocil; Monurol; **Neth.:** Monuril; **Port.:** Monuril; **S.Afr.:** Urizone; **Spain:** Fosfocina; Monofoscin; Monurol; Solufos; **Swed.:** Monuril; **Switz.:** Fosfocin†; Monuril; **Thai.:** Fosmicin; **UK:** Monuril†; **USA:** Monurol.
Multi-ingredient: Spain: Erifoscin.

Framycetin Sulfate (86-y)

Framycetin Sulfate (rINNM).
Framycetin Sulphate (BANM); Framycetini Sulfas; Neomycin B Sulphate. 2-Deoxy-4-O-(2,6-diamino-2,6-dideoxy-α-D-glucopyranosyl)-5-O-[3-O-(2,6-diamino-2,6-dideoxy-β-L-idopyranosyl)-β-D-ribofuranosyl]streptamine sulphate.
$C_{23}H_{46}N_6O_{13}.xH_2SO_4$.
CAS — 119-04-0 (framycetin); 4146-30-9 (framycetin sulfate).
Pharmacopoeias. In Eur. (see p.vi).

Pharmacopoeial description

Ph. Eur.: A substance produced by growth of selected strains of Streptomyces fradiae or S. decaris or obtained by any other means. It contains not more than 3% of neomycin C (p.228) and loses not more than 8% of its weight on drying. A white or yellowish-white, hygroscopic powder. The potency is not less than 630 units of neomycin B per mg, calculated with reference to the dried substance. Freely soluble in water; very slightly soluble in alcohol; practically insoluble in acetone and in ether. A 1% solution in water has a pH of 6 to 7. Store in airtight containers. Protect from light.

Profile

Framycetin is an aminoglycoside antibiotic which forms the major component of neomycin (p.228) and has similar actions and uses. It is used as the sulfate and is administered topically in usual concentrations of 1% for the treatment of infections of the skin, and in concentrations of 0.5% for infections of the eye and ear. It is often used in combination with other antibacterials and corticosteroids in topical preparations.

Framycetin sulfate is poorly absorbed from the gastrointestinal tract and has been given by mouth for the treatment of gastrointestinal infections and pre-operatively for bowel preparation. It has sometimes been given prophylactically as part of regimens for the selective decontamination of the digestive tract in patients in intensive care.

Preparations

Proprietary Preparations (details are given in Part 3)
Aust.: Sofra-Tull; **Austral.:** Sofra-Tulle; **Soframycin; Belg.:** Soframcyne; **Canad.:** Sofra-Tulle; Soframycin; **Denm.:** Sofra-Tulle†; **Fin.:** Sofra-Tulle; **Fr.:** Framybiotal†; Isofra; Rhinalene a la framycetine†; Rhinobiotal; Soframycine; **Ger.:** Leukase N; Sofra-Tull; **Hong Kong:** Sofra-Tulle; **Irl.:** Sofra-Tulle; Soframycin; **Israel:** Sofra-Tulle; **Neth.:** Sofra-Tulle; Soframycin; **Norw.:** Sofra-Tulle; **NZ:** Sofra-Tulle; Soframycin; **S.Afr.:** Sofra-Tulle; Soframycin†; **Singapore:** Sofra-Tulle; Soframycin; **Swed.:** Sofra-Tulle; **Switz.:** Frakitacine; Sofra-Tulle; Soframycine; **Thai.:** Sofra-Tulle; **UK:** Sofra-Tulle; Soframycin.
Multi-ingredient: Aust.: Leukase; Leukase-Kegel; **Austral.:** Otodex; Sofradex; **Braz.:** Sofraline; Sofrasolone; **Braz.:** Fonergin; Oftcor; Oftrim; **Canad.:** Proctosedyl; Proctosone; Sofracort; Soframycin; **Denm.:** Proctosedyl; Sofradex; **Fin.:**

Proctosedyl; Sofradex; **Fr.:** Cortibiotique; Corticetine; Dermocalm†; Frakidex; Framyxone; Frazoline; Neoparyl Framycetine†; Polyfra; Rhinotrophyl; Rhinyl; Soframycine Hydrocortisone; Soframycine Naphazoline; Topifram†; **Ger.:** Leukase N; **Hong Kong:** Proctosedyl; Sofradex; **Irl.:** Proctosedyl; Sofradex; Soframycin; **Neth.:** Proctosedyl; Sofradex; **Norw.:** Proctosedyl; Sofradex; **NZ:** Sofradex; Soframycin; **Port.:** Frakidex; Sofradex; **S.Afr.:** Proctosedyl; Sofradex; **Singapore:** Proctosedyl; Sofradex; Topifram; **Spain:** Abrasone; Aldo Otico; Aldoderma; Nesfare Antibiotico; Otomidrin; **Swed.:** Proctosedyl; Sofradex; **Switz.:** Corticetine; Dexalocal-F; Frakidex; Pulpomixine; Septomixine; Sofradex; **Thai.:** Proctosedyl; Sofradex; Topifram; **UK:** Sofradex; Soframycin†.

Furaltadone Hydrochloride (14192-k)

Furaltadone Hydrochloride (BANM, rINNM).
(±)-5-Morpholinomethyl-3-(5-nitrofurfurylideneamino)oxazolidin-2-one hydrochloride.
$C_{13}H_{16}N_4O_6,HCl = 360.8$.
CAS — 139-91-3 (furaltadone); 59302-14-6 (±-furaltadone).
Pharmacopoeias. Fr. includes Furaltadone for veterinary use.

Profile

Furaltadone was formerly administered by mouth as an antibacterial but was later withdrawn owing to its toxic effects. Furaltadone hydrochloride is still used topically in preparations for ear disorders.
Furaltadone has been used in veterinary medicine.

Preparations

Proprietary Preparations (details are given in Part 3)
Multi-ingredient: Spain: Panotile.

Fusafungine (87-j)

Fusafungine (BAN, rINN).
CAS — 1393-87-9.
ATC — R02AB03.

A depsipeptide antibiotic produced by Fusarium lateritium strain 437.

Profile

Fusafungine is a depsipeptide antibiotic active against some Gram-positive and Gram-negative organisms and Candida albicans. It has also been stated to possess anti-inflammatory activity.

It is used in the form of an aerosol spray in the treatment of infections of the upper respiratory tract, inhaled in usual adult doses of 500 μg every 4 hours into each nostril or via the mouth.

Preparations

Proprietary Preparations (details are given in Part 3)
Aust.: Locabiosol; **Belg.:** Locabiotal; **Braz.:** Locabiotal; **Fr.:** Locabiotal; **Ger.:** Locabiosol; **Hong Kong:** Locabiotal; **Irl.:** Locabiotal; **Ital.:** Locabiotal; **Mex.:** Locabiotal; **Port.:** Locabiosol; **S.Afr.:** Locabiotal; **Spain:** Fusaloyos; **Switz.:** Locabiotal; **UK:** Locabiotal.

Fusidic Acid (88-z)

Fusidic Acid (BAN, USAN, rINN).
Acidum Fusidicum; SQ-16603. ent-16α-Acetoxy-3β-dihydroxy-4β,8β,14-trimethyl-18-nor-5β,10α-cholesta-(17Z)-17(20),24-dien-21-oic acid hemihydrate.
$C_{31}H_{48}O_6,\frac{1}{2}H_2O = 525.7$.
CAS — 6990-06-3 (anhydrous fusidic acid).
ATC — D06AX01; D09AA02; J01XC01; S01AA13.
Pharmacopoeias. In Eur. (see p.vi).

Pharmacopoeial description

Ph. Eur.: An antimicrobial substance produced by the growth of certain strains of Fusidium coccineum or by any other means. A white or almost white crystalline powder. Practically insoluble in water; freely soluble in alcohol. Store at a temperature of 2° to 8°. Protect from light.

Sodium Fusidate (154-s)

Sodium Fusidate (BANM, rINNM).
Fusidate Sodium (USAN); Natrii Fusidas; SQ-16360.
$C_{31}H_{47}NaO_6 = 538.7$.
CAS — 751-94-0.
Pharmacopoeias. In Eur. (see p.vi).

1 g of monograph substance is approximately equivalent to 0.98 g of fusidic acid.

Pharmacopoeial description

Ph. Eur.: A white or almost white, slightly hygroscopic, crystalline powder. Freely soluble in water and in alcohol. A 1.25% solution in water has a pH of 7.5 to 9.0. Store in airtight containers at a temperature of 2° to 8°. Protect from light.

Incompatibility. The UK manufacturers state that the reconstituted sodium fusidate injection is incompatible with infusion solutions containing glucose 20% or more, and that precipitation may occur in solutions with a pH of less than 7.4.

Adverse Effects and Precautions

Apart from mild gastrointestinal upsets fusidic acid or sodium fusidate appear to be well tolerated when given by mouth. Treatment with fusidates, by mouth or especially by the intravenous route, has been associated with jaundice and changes in liver function; normal liver function is usually restored when treatment is discontinued. Therefore fusidates should be given with caution to patients with impaired liver function, and periodic monitoring of hepatic function is recommended in these patients and in those receiving high or prolonged oral doses.

Venospasm, thrombophlebitis, and haemolysis have occurred in patients given fusidates intravenously. To reduce this it is recommended that solutions be buffered and that the solution should be given as a slow infusion into a large vein where there is a good blood flow. Hypocalcaemia has occurred after intravenous administration of doses above those recommended, and has been attributed to the phosphate-citrate buffer in the preparation. Intramuscular or subcutaneous administration may lead to tissue necrosis and is contra-indicated.

Hypersensitivity reactions in the form of rashes and irritation may occur after the topical administration of fusidates; rash is rare after systemic administration. Fusidic acid or its derivatives should be avoided in patients known to be hypersensitive to fusidates.

Fusidic acid competes with bilirubin for binding to albumin *in vitro* and caution has been advised if it is given to premature, jaundiced, acidotic or seriously-ill neonates because of the possible risk of kernicterus.

Effects on the blood. There have been occasional reports of granulocytopenia[1-3] and one case of thrombocytopenia[3] following the use of fusidic acid systemically.

1. Revell P, *et al.* Granulocytopenia due to fusidic acid. *Lancet* 1988; **ii:** 454–5.
2. Evans DIK. Granulocytopenia due to fusidic acid. *Lancet* 1988; **ii:** 851.
3. Leibowitz G, *et al.* Leukopenia and thrombocytopenia due to fusidic acid. *Postgrad Med J* 1991; **67:** 591–2.

Antimicrobial Action

Fusidic acid is a steroidal antibiotic with a bacteriostatic or bactericidal activity, mainly against Gram-positive bacteria.

Mechanism of action. Fusidic acid inhibits bacterial protein synthesis although, in contrast to drugs such as the macrolides or tetracyclines, it does not bind to the bacterial ribosome, but inhibits a factor necessary for translocation of peptide subunits and elongation of the peptide chain. It is capable of inhibiting protein synthesis in mammalian cells but exerts a selective action against susceptible infecting organisms because of poor penetration into the host cell.

Spectrum of activity. Fusidic acid is very active against staphylococci, notably *Staph. aureus* and *Staph. epidermidis* (including meticillin-resistant strains). *Nocardia asteroides* and many clostridial strains are also highly susceptible. The streptococci and enterococci are less susceptible.

Most Gram-negative bacteria are intrinsically resistant but fusidic acid is active against *Neisseria* spp. and *Bacteroides fragilis*. It has some activity against strains of *Mycobacterium tuberculosis* and *M. leprae*. Fungi are resistant, but fusidic acid has some activity against a range of protozoa including *Giardia lamblia* and *Plasmodium falciparum*. High concentrations of fusidate are reported to inhibit viral growth *in vitro*, including that of HIV, although it is unclear whether this represents a surfactant effect, a general cytotoxic effect, or a genuine antiviral action.

Minimum inhibitory concentrations (MICs) for susceptible *Staph. aureus* isolates are reported to range from about 0.03 to 0.1 µg per mL; up to 16 µg per mL may be required to inhibit streptococci. The activity is reduced in the presence of protein. Fusidic acid is bactericidal for many strains at concentrations close to the MIC, but in most meticillin-resistant *Staph. aureus* the ratio of the bactericidal to the inhibitory concentration is much greater.

The symbol † denotes a preparation no longer actively marketed

Activity with other antimicrobials. No synergy has been demonstrated *in vitro* in most studies between fusidic acid and rifampicin or vancomycin, and antagonism of the effects of ciprofloxacin has been reported. Interactions with the penicillins are complex, with either antagonism of the effect of one or both drugs, or no interaction. However, the combination of an antistaphylococcal penicillin with fusidic acid may prevent the emergence of fusidic acid-resistant staphylococcal mutants, and such combinations may be clinically effective.

Resistance. Resistant strains of staphylococci are readily selected *in vitro*, and occasionally during therapy, but the number of clinical isolates that are initially resistant remains relatively low at about 1 to 2% overall, despite widespread topical use. Resistance may be chromosomally mediated, representing altered protein synthesis, or plasmid-mediated, which appears to be due to reduced penetration of active drug into the cell.

Pharmacokinetics

Sodium fusidate is well absorbed from the gastrointestinal tract, and a single 500-mg dose is reported to produce mean plasma concentrations of about 30 µg per mL 2 to 4 hours after administration, although there is considerable interindividual variation. Oral suspensions of fusidic acid are less well absorbed, and a 500-mg dose of such a suspension is reported to produce peak plasma concentrations of about 23 µg per mL. Absorption may be delayed by food, but may be more rapid in children than adults. Some accumulation occurs with repeated administration and plasma concentrations of 100 µg per mL or more have been reported following 500 mg of sodium fusidate three times daily for 4 days.

Fusidate is widely distributed into tissues and body fluids, including bone, pus, and synovial fluid; it penetrates cerebral abscesses but does not enter CSF in appreciable amounts. It has been found in the fetal circulation and in breast milk. About 95% or more of fusidate in the circulation is bound to plasma protein. Fusidate has a plasma half-life that has been variously reported as 5 to 6 and 10 to 15 hours. It is excreted in the bile, almost entirely as metabolites some of which have weak antimicrobial activity. About 2% appears unchanged in the faeces. Little is excreted in the urine or removed by haemodialysis.

◊ References.
1. Reeves DS. The pharmacokinetics of fusidic acid. *J Antimicrob Chemother* 1987; **20:** 467–76.
2. Peter J-D, *et al.* Pharmacokinetics of intravenous fusidic acid in patients with cholestasis. *Antimicrob Agents Chemother* 1993; **37:** 501–6.
3. Brown NM, *et al.* The pharmacokinetics and protein-binding of fusidic acid in patients with severe renal failure requiring either haemodialysis or continuous ambulatory peritoneal dialysis. *J Antimicrob Chemother* 1997; **39:** 803–9.

Uses and Administration

Fusidic acid and its salts are antibiotics used mainly in the treatment of staphylococcal infections, often in conjunction with other drugs. They have been used in the treatment of abscess, including brain abscess, in bone and joint infections, in staphylococcal infections in patients with cystic fibrosis, in the treatment of staphylococcal endocarditis, and topically in eye infections and infections of the skin. For details of these infections and their treatment, see under Choice of Antibacterial, p.114.

Administration and dosage. The fusidates are given by mouth or topically as fusidic acid or sodium fusidate, or intravenously as sodium fusidate. The diolamine salt was formerly used intravenously. Sodium fusidate is administered as tablets in a usual adult dose of 500 mg by mouth every 8 hours, although this dose may be doubled in severe infection. For cutaneous staphylococcal infections, a dose of 250 mg twice daily is suitable. Because of differences in absorption (see Pharmacokinetics, above) 250 mg of fusidic acid is therapeutically equivalent to only 175 mg of the sodium salt, so doses of fusidic acid suspension (commonly employed in children) appear relatively higher.

Doses are: up to 1 year, 50 mg per kg body-weight daily in 3 divided doses; 1 to 5 years, 250 mg three times daily; 5 to 12 years, 500 mg three times daily; over 12 years and adults, 750 mg three times daily.

In severe infections in adults weighing over 50 kg, sodium fusidate 500 mg is given three times daily by slow intravenous infusion. Each 500-mg dose is usually administered as a buffered solution (pH 7.4 to 7.6) diluted to 500 mL with sodium chloride or other suitable intravenous solution. For children and adults weighing less than 50 kg, a dose of 6 to 7 mg per kg three times daily is used.

Sodium fusidate as an ointment (2%) or medicated dressing, or fusidic acid as a cream or gel (2%), are used in the local treatment of skin infections. Eye drops containing fusidic acid 1% are used in eye infections. Topical use may lead to problems of resistance.

Preparations

BP 2001: Fusidic Acid Cream; Fusidic Acid Eye Drops; Fusidic Acid Oral Suspension; Sodium Fusidate Ointment.

Proprietary Preparations (details are given in Part 3)
Aust.: Fucidin; Fucithalmic; *Austral.:* Fucidin; *Belg.:* Fucidin; Fucithalmic; *Braz.:* Verutex; *Canad.:* Fucidin; *Denm.:* Fucidin; Fucithalmic; *Fin.:* Fucidin; Fucithalmic; *Fr.:* Fucidine; Fucithalmic; *Ger.:* Fucidine; Fucithalmic; *Hong Kong:* Fucidin; Fucithalmic; *Irl.:* Fucidin; Fucithalmic; *Israel:* Fucidin; Fucithalmic; *Ital.:* Dermomycin; Fucithalmic; *Mex.:* Fucidin; *Neth.:* Fucidin; Fucithalmic; *Norw.:* Fucidin; Fucithalmic; *NZ:* Fucidin; Fucithalmic; *Port.:* Fucidine; Fucithalmic; *S.Afr.:* Fucidin; Fucithalmic; *Singapore:* Balad; Foban; Fucidin; Fucithalmic; *Spain:* Fucidine; Fucithalmic; *Swed.:* Fucidin; Fucithalmic; *Switz.:* Fucidine; Fucithalmic; *Thai.:* Fucidin; Fucithalmic; Fusid; *UAE:* Futasole; *UK:* Fucidin; Fucithalmic.

Multi-ingredient: *Belg.:* Fucicort; Fucidin Hydrocortisone; *Canad.:* Fucidin H; *Denm.:* Fucicort; Fucidin-Hydrocortison; *Fin.:* Fucicort; Fucidin-Hydrocortison; *Ger.:* Fucicort; Fucidine plus; *Hong Kong:* Fucicort; *Irl.:* Fucibet; Fucidin H; *Israel:* Fucicort; Fucidin H; *Ital.:* Piodermina; *Mex.:* Fucicort; *Norw.:* Fucidin-hydrocortison; *NZ:* Fucicort; *Port.:* Fucicort; Fucidine H; *S.Afr.:* Fucidin H; *Singapore:* Fucicort; Fucidin H; *Spain:* Fucibet; Fucidine H; *Swed.:* Fucidin-Hydrocortison; *Switz.:* Fucicort; Fucidin H; *Thai.:* Fucicort; *UAE:* Futasone; *UK:* Fucibet; Fucidin H.

Gatifloxacin (3078-j)

Gatifloxacin (USAN, rINN).
AM-1155; BMS-206584-01; CG-5501. (±)-1-Cyclopropyl-6-fluoro-1,4-dihydro-8-methoxy-7-(3-methyl-1-piperazinyl)-4-oxo-3-quinolinecarboxylic acid sesquihydrate.
$C_{19}H_{22}FN_3O_4,1\frac{1}{2}H_2O = 402.4$.
CAS — 160738-57-8 (anhydrous gatifloxacin); 180200-66-2 (gatifloxacin sesquihydrate).

Adverse Effects and Precautions

As for Ciprofloxacin, p.183.

Gatifloxacin may have the potential to prolong the QT interval and should be avoided in patients with existing QT prolongation.

Interactions

As for Ciprofloxacin, p.184.

As gatifloxacin may have the potential to prolong the QT interval, it should not be given to patients receiving class Ia antiarrhythmic drugs (such as quinidine and procainamide) or class III antiarrhythmics (such as amiodarone and sotalol). In addition, caution should be exercised when gatifloxacin is used with other drugs known to have this effect (such as the antihistamines astemizole and terfenadine, cisapride, erythromycin, pentamidine, phenothiazines, or tricyclic antidepressants).

Antimicrobial Action

As for Ciprofloxacin, p.184.

◊ References.
1. Hoellman DB, *et al.* Anti-pneumococcal activity of gatifloxacin compared with other quinolone and non-quinolone agents. *J Antimicrob Chemother* 1999; **43:** 645–9.
2. Odland BA, *et al.* Antimicrobial activity of gatifloxacin (AM-1155, CG5501), and four other fluoroquinolones tested against 2,284 recent clinical strains of Streptococcus pneumoniae from Europe, Latin America, Canada, and the United States. *Diagn Microbiol Infect Dis* 1999; **34:** 315–20.

Pharmacokinetics

Gatifloxacin is readily absorbed from the gastrointestinal tract following oral administration with an absolute bioavailability of 96%. Peak plasma concentrations are achieved within 1 to 2 hours of a dose. Gatifloxacin is widely distributed into body tissues and is approximately 20% bound to plasma proteins. It undergoes limited metabolism and has an elimination half-life of 7 to 14 hours. It is excreted primarily unchanged in the urine with less than 1% as metabolites. A small amount (5%) is also excreted unchanged in the faeces.

Uses and Administration

Gatifloxacin is a fluoroquinolone antibacterial with actions and uses similar to those of ciprofloxacin (p.185).

It is given by mouth, or by intravenous infusion as a 2 mg per mL solution over 60 minutes, for the treatment of susceptible infections, including respiratory- and urinary-tract infections. The usual adult dose is 400 mg once daily. A single dose of 400 mg or a dose of 200 mg daily for 3 days may be adequate for uncomplicated urinary-tract infections. A single dose of 400 mg may also be given for the treatment of uncomplicated gonorrhoea.

Dosage should be reduced in patients with renal impairment; the initial dose of 400 mg should be followed by maintenance doses of 200 mg daily in those with a creatinine clearance less than 40 mL per minute.

◊ Reviews.
1. Perry CM, et al. Gatifloxacin. Drugs 1999; 58: 683–96.

Preparations

Proprietary Preparations (details are given in Part 3)
Austral.: Tequin; *USA:* Tequin.

Gemifloxacin Mesilate (5217-h)

Gemifloxacin Mesilate (rINNM).
Gemifloxacin Mesylate (USAN); LB-20304 (gemifloxacin); LB-20304a; SB-265805 (gemifloxacin); SB-265805S. (±)-7-[3-(Aminomethyl)-4-oxo-1-pyrrolidinyl]-1-cyclopropyl-6-fluoro-1,4-dihydro-4-oxo-1,8-naphthyridine-3-carboxylic acid 7⁴-(Z)-(O-methyloxime) methanesulfonate.
$C_{18}H_{20}FN_5O_4,CH_4O_3S = 485.5$.
CAS — 204519-64-2 (gemifloxacin); 204519-65-3 (gemifloxacin mesilate).

Profile

Gemifloxacin is a fluoroquinolone antibacterial under investigation as the mesilate for the treatment of susceptible respiratory- and urinary-tract infections.

◊ Reviews.
1. Lowe MN, Lamb HM. Gemifloxacin. Drugs 2000; 59: 1137–47.

Gentamicin Sulfate (89-c)

Gentamicin Sulfate (USAN, pINNM).
Gentamicin Sulphate (BANM); Gentamicini Sulfas; NSC-82261; Sch-9724.
CAS — 1403-66-3 (gentamicin); 1405-41-0 (gentamicin sulfate).

NOTE. GNT is a code approved by the BP 2001 for use on single unit doses of eye drops containing gentamicin sulfate where the individual container may be too small to bear all the appropriate labelling information.
Pharmacopoeias. In *Chin., Eur.* (see p.vi), *Int., Jpn, Pol.,* and *US.*

The sulfates of a mixture of antimicrobial substances produced by *Micromonospora purpurea.* Gentamicin sulfate is a complex mixture of the sulfates of gentamicin C_1, gentamicin C_{1A}, and gentamicin C_2. Some commercial samples may contain significant quantities of the minor components gentamicin C_{2A} and gentamicin C_{2B}.
Incompatibilities. The aminoglycosides are inactivated *in vitro* by various penicillins and cephalosporins via an interaction with the beta-lactam ring, the extent of inactivation depending on temperature, concentration, and duration of contact. The different aminoglycosides vary in their stability, with amikacin apparently the most resistant and tobramycin the most susceptible to inactivation; gentamicin and netilmicin are of intermediate stability. The beta lactams also vary in their ability to produce inactivation, with ampicillin, benzylpenicillin, and antipseudomonal penicillins such as carbenicillin and ticarcillin producing marked inactivation. Inactivation has also been reported with clavulanic acid.

Gentamicin is also incompatible with frusemide [furosemide], heparin, sodium bicarbonate (the acid pH of gentamicin solutions may liberate carbon dioxide) and some solutions for parenteral nutrition. Interactions with preparations having an

alkaline pH (for example sulfadiazine sodium), or drugs unstable at acid pH (for example erythromycin salts), might reasonably be expected.

Given their potential for incompatibility, gentamicin and other aminoglycosides should not generally be mixed with other drugs in syringes or infusion solutions nor given through the same intravenous line. When aminoglycosides are given with a beta lactam administration should generally be at separate sites.

Pharmacopoeial description

Ph. Eur.: A mixture of the sulfates of antimicrobial substances produced by *Micromonospora purpurea.* The potency is not less than 590 units per mg, calculated with reference to the anhydrous substance. A white or almost white powder. Freely soluble in water; practically insoluble in alcohol and in ether. A 4% solution in water has a pH of 3.5 to 5.5.

USP 25: The sulfate salt, or a mixture of such salts, of antibiotic substances produced by the growth of *Micromonospora purpurea.* It has a potency equivalent to not less than 590 µg of gentamicin per mg, calculated on the dried basis. A white to buff powder. Freely soluble in water; insoluble in alcohol, in acetone, in chloroform, in ether, and in benzene. pH of a 4% solution in water is between 3.5 and 5.5. Store in airtight containers.

Incompatibility. References to the incompatibility of aminoglycosides with beta lactams (see also above).
1. Henderson JL, et al. In vitro inactivation of gentamicin, tobramycin, and netilmicin by carbenicillin, azlocillin, or mezlocillin. Am J Hosp Pharm 1981; 38: 1167–70.
2. Tindula RJ, et al. Aminoglycoside inactivation by penicillins and cephalosporins and its impact on drug-level monitoring. Drug Intell Clin Pharm 1983; 17: 906–8.
3. Wright DN, et al. In vitro inactivation of aminoglycosides by apalcillin. Antimicrob Agents Chemother 1986; 29: 353–4.
4. Navarro AS, et al. In-vitro interaction between dibekacin and penicillins. J Antimicrob Chemother 1986; 17: 83–9.
5. Courcol RJ, Martin GR. Comparative aminoglycoside inactivation by potassium clavulanate. J Antimicrob Chemother 1986; 17: 682–4.

Stability. There was an average 16% potency loss of gentamicin sulfate from solutions containing 10 and 40 mg per mL when stored at 4° or 25° in plastic disposable syringes for 30 days, and a brown precipitate formed in several. Storage in glass disposable syringes for 30 days produced an average 7% potency loss, which was considered acceptable, but storage for longer resulted in precipitate formation in some cases and was not recommended.[1]
1. Weiner B, et al. Stability of gentamicin sulfate injection following unit dose repackaging. Am J Hosp Pharm 1976; 33: 1254–9.

Adverse Effects

The aminoglycosides can produce irreversible, cumulative ototoxicity affecting both the cochlea (manifest as hearing loss, initially of higher tones, and which, because speech recognition relies greatly on lower frequencies, may not be at first apparent) and the vestibular system (manifest as dizziness or vertigo). The incidence and relative toxicity with different aminoglycosides is a matter of some dispute, but netilmicin is probably less cochleotoxic than gentamicin or tobramycin, and amikacin more so. Netilmicin also exhibits less vestibular toxicity than gentamicin, tobramycin, or amikacin, while streptomycin produces a high incidence of vestibular damage. Vestibular damage is more common than hearing loss in patients receiving gentamicin.

Reversible nephrotoxicity may occur and acute renal failure has been reported, often in association with the concurrent administration of other nephrotoxic drugs. Renal impairment is usually mild, although acute tubular necrosis and interstitial nephritis have occurred. Decreased glomerular filtration rate is usually seen only after several days, and may even occur after therapy has been discontinued. Electrolyte disturbances (notably hypomagnesaemia, but also hypocalcaemia and hypokalaemia) have occurred. The nephrotoxicity of gentamicin is reported to be largely due to the gentamicin C_2 component.

Although particularly associated with high plasma concentrations, many risk factors have been suggested for ototoxicity and nephrotoxicity in patients receiving aminoglycosides—see Precautions below.

Aminoglycosides possess a neuromuscular-blocking action and respiratory depression and muscular paralysis have been reported, notably after absorption from serous surfaces. Neomycin has the most potent action and several deaths have been associated with its use.

Hypersensitivity reactions have occurred, especially after local use, and cross-sensitivity between

aminoglycosides may occur. Very rarely, anaphylactic reactions to gentamicin have occurred. Some hypersensitivity reactions have been attributed to the presence of sulfites in parenteral formulations, and endotoxic shock has also been reported.

Infrequent effects reported for gentamicin include blood dyscrasias, purpura, nausea and vomiting, stomatitis, and signs of liver dysfunction such as increased serum-aminotransferase values and increased serum-bilirubin concentrations. Neurotoxicity has occurred, with both peripheral neuropathies and central symptoms being reported including encephalopathy, confusion, lethargy, hallucinations, convulsions, and mental depression.

Atrophy or fat necrosis has been reported at injection sites. There have been isolated reports of meningeal irritation, arachnoiditis, polyradiculitis, and ventriculitis following the intrathecal, intracisternal, or intraventricular administration of aminoglycosides. Subconjunctival injection of gentamicin may lead to pain, hyperaemia, and conjunctival oedema, while severe retinal ischaemia has followed intra-ocular injection.

Effects on the ears. Reviews and references to aminoglycoside-induced ototoxicity.
1. Cone LA. A survey of prospective, controlled clinical trials of gentamicin, tobramycin, amikacin, and netilmicin. Clin Ther 1982; 5: 155–62.
2. Kahlmeter G, Dahlager JI. Aminoglycoside toxicity—a review of clinical studies published between 1975 and 1982. J Antimicrob Chemother 1984; 13 (suppl A): 9–22.
3. Brummett RE, Fox KE. Aminoglycoside-induced hearing loss in humans. Antimicrob Agents Chemother 1989; 33: 797–800.
4. Mattie H, et al. Determinants of efficacy and toxicity of aminoglycosides. J Antimicrob Chemother 1989; 24: 281–93.

Effects on the kidneys. Some references and reviews on aminoglycoside-induced nephrotoxicity.
1. Cone LA. A survey of prospective, controlled clinical trials of gentamicin, tobramycin, amikacin, and netilmicin. Clin Ther 1982; 5: 155–62.
2. Lietman PS, Smith CR. Aminoglycoside nephrotoxicity in humans. Rev Infect Dis 1983; 5 (suppl 2): S284–93.
3. Kahlmeter G, Dahlager JI. Aminoglycoside toxicity—a review of clinical studies published between 1975 and 1982. J Antimicrob Chemother 1984; 13 (suppl A): 9–22.
4. Kohlhepp SJ, et al. Nephrotoxicity of the constituents of the gentamicin complex. J Infect Dis 1984; 149: 605–14.
5. Mattie H, et al. Determinants of efficacy and toxicity of aminoglycosides. J Antimicrob Chemother 1989; 24: 281–93.
6. Appel GB. Aminoglycoside nephrotoxicity. Am J Med 1990; 88 (suppl 3C): 16S–20S.
7. Bertino JS, et al. Incidence of and significant risk factors for aminoglycoside-associated nephrotoxicity in patients dosed by using individualized pharmacokinetic monitoring. J Infect Dis 1993; 167: 173–9.

Endotoxin reactions. Reports of endotoxin reactions associated with intravenous gentamicin have been received by the Centers for Disease Control and the FDA in the USA.[1] Although endotoxin concentrations in the injections used were within USP limits, administration as a single daily dose rather than in divided doses was thought to have resulted in toxic serum concentrations of endotoxins.[1,2]
1. Centers for Disease Control. Endotoxin-like reactions associated with intravenous gentamicin—California, 1998. MMWR 1998; 47: 877–80.
2. Krieger JA, Duncan L. Gentamicin contaminated with endotoxin. N Engl J Med 1999; 340: 1122.

Treatment of Adverse Effects

Aminoglycosides may be removed by haemodialysis or to a much lesser extent by peritoneal dialysis. Calcium salts given intravenously have been used to counter neuromuscular blockade; the effectiveness of neostigmine has been variable.

◊ For the suggestion that calcium-channel blockers may reduce aminoglycoside-related nephrotoxicity, see Kidney Disorders, under Uses of Verapamil, p.991.

Precautions

Gentamicin is contra-indicated in patients with a known history of allergy to it, and probably in those allergic to other aminoglycosides. Great care is required in patients with myasthenia gravis, parkinsonism, and other conditions characterised by muscular weakness.

Because the risk of ototoxicity and nephrotoxicity is increased at high plasma concentrations, it is generally desirable to determine dosage requirements of the aminoglycosides by individual monitoring. In patients receiving standard multiple-dose regimens of gentamicin, dosage should be adjusted to avoid peak plasma concentrations above 10 to 12 µg per mL, or trough concentrations (immediately before next dose) exceeding 2 μg per mL. Monitoring is particularly important in patients receiving high doses or prolonged courses, in infants and the elderly, and in patients with impaired renal function, who generally require reduced doses. Some authorities consider that monitoring is also important in obese patients and those with cystic fibrosis. See Pharmacokinetics below for other patient groups in whom pharmacokinetics may be altered. Impaired hepatic function or auditory function, bacteraemia, fever, and perhaps exposure to loud noises have also been reported to increase the risk of ototoxicity, while volume depletion or hypotension, liver disease, or female sex have been reported as additional risk factors for nephrotoxicity. Regular assessment of auditory and renal function is particularly necessary in patients with additional risk factors.

Topical application of gentamicin into the ear is contra-indicated in patients with known or suspected perforation of the ear drum.

Use of aminoglycosides during pregnancy may damage the eighth cranial nerve of the fetus.

Interference with assay procedures. The implications of drug interference with assays for aminoglycosides have been reviewed.[1] A number of other antimicrobials and antineoplastics may alter the results of microbiological assays but this might be overcome by selection of an appropriate assay organism.

Microbiological assays for aminoglycosides in samples also containing *imipenem* could be accomplished by using cysteine hydrochloride to inactivate imipenem, since it is stable to most beta-lactamases and resistant strains are extremely rare.[2] Because aminoglycosides may be inactivated by *penicillins* and *cephalosporins*, it has been recommended that aminoglycoside sampling times should be chosen to coincide with a trough plasma concentration for the beta lactam. Samples should be frozen if there is to be a delay before they are assayed[3] or a penicillinase added. However, one group of workers reported loss of gentamicin activity after storage at −60° before assay.[4] Furthermore, there have been reports that concentrations of aminoglycosides in patients also receiving beta lactams have been overestimated using a homogeneous enzyme immunoassay, probably because of an inability to differentiate between active drug and inactivated products.[5,6]

The radionuclide *gallium-67* interferes with radio-enzymatic assays, and it has been suggested that an agar diffusion method should be used in patients who have received a gallium scan.[7,8]

Heparin has been shown to produce underestimation of aminoglycoside concentrations when using microbiological, enzymatic, or immunoassays.[9-11] It has been recommended that either serum should be used or that blood samples should not be collected in heparinised tubes or from indwelling catheter lines. Some consider that concentrations of heparin reached in the blood of patients receiving heparin are too low to affect gentamicin.[12]

Falsely low concentrations have also been reported in microbiological assays in the presence of *zinc* salts.[13]

Heat treatment of whole *blood* to inactivate human immunodeficiency virus leads to an increase in the concentration of gentamicin subsequently found on assay.[14]

1. Yosselson-Superstine S. Drug interferences with plasma assays in therapeutic drug monitoring. *Clin Pharmacokinet* 1984; **9:** 67–87.
2. McLeod KM, *et al.* Gentamicin assay in the presence of imipenem, *J Antimicrob Chemother* 1986; **17:** 828–9.
3. Tindula RJ, *et al.* Aminoglycoside inactivation by penicillins and cephalosporins and its impact on drug-level monitoring. *Drug Intell Clin Pharm* 1983; **17:** 906–8.
4. Carlson LG, *et al.* Potential liabilities of gentamicin homogeneous enzyme immunoassay. *Antimicrob Agents Chemother* 1982; **21:** 192–4.
5. Ebert SC, Clementi WA. In vitro inactivation of gentamicin by carbenicillin, compared by Emit and microbiological assays. *Drug Intell Clin Pharm* 1983; **17:** 451.
6. Dalmady-Israel C, *et al.* Ticarcillin and assay of tobramycin. *Ann Intern Med* 1984; **100:** 460.
7. Bhattacharya I, *et al.* Effects of radiopharmaceuticals on radioenzymatic assays of aminoglycoside antibiotics: interference by gallium-67 and its elimination. *Antimicrob Agents Chemother* 1978; **14:** 448–53.
8. Shannon K, *et al.* Interference with gentamicin assays by gallium-67. *J Antimicrob Chemother* 1980; **6:** 285–300.
9. Nilsson L. Factors affecting gentamicin assay. *Antimicrob Agents Chemother* 1980; **17:** 918–21. Correction. *ibid.*; **18:** 839.
10. Nilsson L, *et al.* Inhibition of aminoglycoside activity by heparin. *Antimicrob Agents Chemother* 1981; **20:** 155–8.
11. O'Connell MB, *et al.* Heparin interference with tobramycin, netilmicin, and gentamicin concentrations determined by Emit. *Drug Intell Clin Pharm* 1984; **18:** 503–4.
12. Regamey C, *et al.* Inhibitory effect of heparin on gentamicin concentrations in blood. *Antimicrob Agents Chemother* 1972; **1:** 329–32.
13. George RH, Healing DE. The effect of zinc on aminoglycoside assay. *J Antimicrob Chemother* 1978; **4:** 186.
14. Eley A, *et al.* Effect of heat on gentamicin assays. *Lancet* 1987; **ii:** 335–6.

Interactions

Concurrent use of other nephrotoxic drugs, including other aminoglycosides, vancomycin, some of the cephalosporins, ciclosporin, cisplatin, and fludarabine, or potentially ototoxic drugs such as etacrynic acid and perhaps frusemide [furosemide], may increase the risk of aminoglycoside toxicity. It has been suggested that concurrent use of an antiemetic such as dimenhydrinate may mask the early symptoms of vestibular ototoxicity. Care is also required if other drugs with a neuromuscular-blocking action are given concomitantly (p.1334). The neuromuscular-blocking properties of aminoglycosides may be sufficient to provoke severe respiratory depression in patients receiving general anaesthetics or opioids.

There is a theoretical possibility that the antibacterial effects of aminoglycosides could be reduced by use with a bacteriostatic antibacterial, but such combinations have been used successfully in practice.

Since aminoglycosides have been shown to be incompatible with some beta lactams *in vitro* (see Incompatibility, above), these antibacterials should be administered separately if both are required; antagonism *in vivo* has been reported only in a few patients with severe renal impairment, in whom aminoglycoside activity was diminished. Aminoglycosides exhibit synergistic activity with a number of beta lactams *in vivo* (see Antimicrobial Action, below).

Renal excretion of zalcitabine (p.644) may be reduced by concurrent administration of aminoglycosides.

For a report of severe hypocalcaemia in a patient receiving aminoglycosides and bisphosphonates, see p.749.

Antimicrobial Action

Gentamicin is an aminoglycoside antibiotic and has a bactericidal action against many Gram-negative aerobes and against some strains of staphylococci.

Mechanism of action. Aminoglycosides are taken up into sensitive bacterial cells by an active transport process which is inhibited in anaerobic, acidic, or hyperosmolar environments. Within the cell they bind to the 30S, and to some extent to the 50S subunits of the bacterial ribosome, inhibiting protein synthesis and generating errors in the transcription of the genetic code. The manner in which cell death is brought about is imperfectly understood, and other mechanisms may contribute, including effects on membrane permeability.

Spectrum of activity. The following pathogenic organisms are usually sensitive to gentamicin (but see also Resistance, below).

Many strains of Gram-negative bacteria including species of *Brucella, Calymmatobacterium, Campylobacter, Citrobacter, Escherichia, Enterobacter, Klebsiella, Proteus, Providencia, Pseudomonas, Serratia, Vibrio,* and *Yersinia.* Some activity has been reported against isolates of *Neisseria* although aminoglycosides are rarely used clinically in neisserial infections.

Among the Gram-positive organisms many strains of *Staphylococcus aureus* are highly sensitive to gentamicin. *Listeria monocytogenes* and some strains of *Staph. epidermidis* may also be sensitive to gentamicin, but enterococci and streptococci are insensitive to gentamicin.

Some actinomycetes and mycoplasmas have been reported to be sensitive to gentamicin but mycobacteria are insensitive at clinically achievable concentrations; anaerobic organisms, yeasts, and fungi are resistant.

Minimum inhibitory concentrations (MICs) of gentamicin for the most sensitive organisms (some staphylococci, enterobacteria, sensitive *Pseudomonas aeruginosa* strains) are 0.03 to 2 μg per mL; the aminoglycosides are usually bactericidal at concentrations not far above the MIC. Organisms with MICs up to about 8 μg per mL are generally considered sensitive to gentamicin. Bacterial regrowth does not resume immediately when the concentration of gen-

tamicin falls below the MIC, and this prolonged postantibiotic effect is the basis for once-daily dosing (see below).

Activity with other antimicrobials. Gentamicin exhibits synergy with beta lactams, probably because the effects of the latter on bacterial cell walls enhance aminoglycoside penetration. Enhanced activity has been demonstrated with a penicillin (such as ampicillin or benzylpenicillin) and gentamicin against the enterococci, and gentamicin has been combined with an antipseudomonal penicillin such as ticarcillin for enhanced activity against *Pseudomonas* spp., and with vancomycin for enhanced activity against staphylococci and streptococci.

Resistance to the aminoglycosides may be acquired by three main mechanisms. The first is by mutation of ribosomal target sites leading to reduced affinity for binding; this type of resistance is generally only relevant for streptomycin and, even then, it appears to be rare in Gram-negative bacteria. Secondly, penetration of aminoglycosides into bacterial cells is by an oxygen-dependent active transport process and resistance may occur because of elimination or reduction of this uptake; when it occurs this generally results in cross-resistance to all aminoglycosides. Thirdly, and by far the most important cause of resistance to the aminoglycosides, is inactivation by enzymatic modification. Three main classes of enzyme conferring resistance have been found, operating by phosphorylation, acetylation, or addition of a nucleotide group, usually adenyl. Enzyme production is usually plasmid-determined and resistance can therefore be transferred between bacteria, even of different species. Resistance to other antibacterials may be transferred at the same time. In *Staph. aureus* such transfer of resistance is reportedly facilitated when these drugs are used topically. Each type of enzyme produces characteristic patterns of resistance, but their overlapping and variable affinities for their substrates result in a wide range of permutations of cross-resistance to the different aminoglycosides.

The different enzymes vary in their distribution and prevalence in different locations, and at different times, presumably with variations in antibacterial usage, but relationships to the use of specific aminoglycosides are difficult to establish. These variations in drug sensitivity require local testing to determine resistance and establish susceptibility of bacteria to the aminoglycoside being used.

Because of such local variations, estimates of the incidence of resistance are of limited value. In general, the occurrence of resistant pathogens seems to be greater in southern than in northern Europe, and perhaps greater in the USA than in Europe. There has been particular concern over the increasing incidence of high-level gentamicin resistance among enterococci (in up to 50% of isolates from some centres) since they already possess inherent or acquired resistance to many drugs, including vancomycin in some cases; a similar problem exists with gentamicin resistance in meticillin-resistant strains of *Staph. aureus.* Such multiply-resistant strains pose a major therapeutic problem in those centres where they occur, since the usual synergistic combinations with other antibacterials are ineffective. However, results from some centres indicate that rational use of a wider range of aminoglycosides (including amikacin which is not affected by most of the aminoglycoside degrading enzymes) has resulted in a modest decline in overall aminoglycoside resistance.

◊ References.

1. Mingeot-Leclercq M-P, *et al.* Aminoglycosides: activity and resistance. *Antimicrob Agents Chemother* 1999; **43:** 727–37.

Pharmacokinetics

Gentamicin and other aminoglycosides are poorly absorbed from the gastrointestinal tract but are rapidly absorbed after intramuscular injection. Average peak plasma concentrations of about 4 μg per mL have been attained in patients with normal renal function

30 to 60 minutes after intramuscular administration of a dose equivalent to 1 mg of gentamicin per kg body-weight, which is similar to concentrations achieved after intravenous infusion. There may be considerable individual variation. Several doses are required before plasma equilibrium concentrations occur and this may represent the saturation of binding sites in body tissues such as the kidney. Binding of gentamicin to plasma proteins is usually low.

Following parenteral administration gentamicin and other aminoglycosides diffuse mainly into extracellular fluids. However, there is little diffusion into the CSF and even when the meninges are inflamed effective concentrations may not be achieved; diffusion into the eye is also poor. Aminoglycosides diffuse readily into the perilymph of the inner ear. They cross the placenta but only small amounts have been reported in breast milk.

Systemic absorption of gentamicin and other aminoglycosides has been reported after topical use on denuded skin and burns and following instillation into, and irrigation of, wounds, body-cavities (except the urinary bladder), and joints.

The plasma elimination half-life for gentamicin has been reported to be 2 to 3 hours though it may be considerably longer in neonates and patients with renal impairment. Gentamicin and other aminoglycosides do not appear to be metabolised and are excreted virtually unchanged in the urine by glomerular filtration. At steady state at least 70% of a dose may be recovered in the urine in 24 hours and urine concentrations in excess of 100 µg per mL may be achieved. However, gentamicin and the other aminoglycosides appear to accumulate in body tissues to some extent, mainly in the kidney, although the relative degree to which this occurs may vary with different aminoglycosides. Release from these sites is slow and small amounts of aminoglycosides may be detected in the urine for up to 20 days or more after administration ceases. Small amounts of gentamicin appear in the bile.

The pharmacokinetics of the aminoglycosides are affected by many factors, which may become significant because of the relatively small difference between therapeutic and toxic concentrations, reinforcing the need for monitoring. Absorption from intramuscular sites may be reduced in critically-ill patients, especially in conditions that reduce perfusion such as shock. Plasma concentrations may also be reduced in patients with conditions which expand extracellular fluid volume or increase renal clearance including ascites, cirrhosis, heart failure, malnutrition, spinal cord injury, burns, cystic fibrosis, and possibly leukaemia. Clearance is also reportedly increased in intravenous drug abusers, and in patients who are febrile. In contrast, renal impairment or reduced renal clearance for any reason (for example in neonates with immature renal function, or in the elderly in whom glomerular function tends to decline with age) can result in markedly increased plasma concentrations and/or prolonged half-lives. However, in neonates initial plasma concentrations may actually be reduced, due to a larger volume of distribution. Plasma concentrations may also be higher than expected for a given dose in obese patients (in whom extracellular volume is low relative to weight), and in patients with anaemia.

Renal clearance, and hence plasma concentrations, of aminoglycosides may vary according to a circadian cycle, and it has been suggested that this should be taken into account when determining and comparing plasma aminoglycoside concentrations.

Uses and Administration

Gentamicin is an aminoglycoside antibiotic used, usually in combination, to treat severe systemic infections due to sensitive Gram-negative and other organisms (see Antimicrobial Action above). They include biliary-tract infections (acute cholecystitis or cholangitis), brucellosis, cat scratch disease, cystic fibrosis, endocarditis (in the treatment and prophylaxis of en-

docarditis due to streptococci, enterococci, or staphylococci), endometritis, gastro-enteritis, granuloma inguinale, listeriosis, meningitis, otitis externa, otitis media, pelvic inflammatory disease, peritonitis, plague, pneumonia, septicaemia, skin infections such as in burns or ulcers (given systemically for pseudomonal and other Gram-negative infections), and urinary-tract infections (acute pyelonephritis), as well as in the prophylaxis of surgical infection and the treatment of immunocompromised patients and those in intensive care. Gentamicin is also applied topically for localised infections. For details of these infections and their treatment, see under Choice of Antibacterial, p.114.

Gentamicin is often used concomitantly with other antibacterials to extend its spectrum of efficacy or increase its effectiveness, e.g. with a penicillin for enterococcal and streptococcal infections, or an antipseudomonal beta lactam for pseudomonal infections, or with metronidazole or clindamycin for mixed aerobic-anaerobic infections.

Administration and dosage. Gentamicin is used as the sulfate but doses are expressed in terms of gentamicin base. In the management of many of the infections above it is commonly given intramuscularly every 8 hours to provide a total daily dose of 3 to 5 mg of gentamicin per kg body-weight. Slightly lower doses have been suggested in the prophylaxis and treatment of streptococcal and enterococcal endocarditis: in the UK a dose of 80 mg of gentamicin, given twice daily in association with penicillin or vancomycin has been suggested for treatment, and 120 mg before induction of anaesthesia, with a penicillin or vancomycin or teicoplanin, for prophylaxis in high-risk patients. For urinary-tract infections, if renal function is not impaired, 160 mg once daily may be used.

Gentamicin sulfate may also be given intravenously in similar doses to those used intramuscularly, but there is some disagreement as to the appropriate method. In the USA, intravenous infusion over 30 minutes to 2 hours is favoured, but sources in the UK differ, with some manufacturers recommending infusion over no more than 20 minutes, in a limited fluid volume, while others suggest that it should not be given by infusion, recommending bolus injection over 2 to 3 minutes, and yet others recommend administration in a similar way to the USA. Both methods present problems: intravenous infusion has been associated with both subtherapeutic and excessive trough concentrations of gentamicin, while bolus injection may increase the risk of neuromuscular blockade.

The course of treatment should generally be limited to 7 to 10 days. As gentamicin is poorly distributed into fatty tissue some authorities suggest that dosage calculations should be based on an estimate of lean body-weight.

Doses in infants and children are usually somewhat higher than those in adults but exact dosage recommendations vary. One suggested dose is 3 mg of gentamicin per kg every 12 hours in premature infants and those up to 2 weeks of age, with older neonates and children receiving 2 mg per kg every 8 hours. Alternatively, 2.5 mg per kg every 12 hours in the first week of life, 2.5 mg per kg every 8 hours in infants and neonates, and 2.0 to 2.5 mg per kg every 8 hours in children has been suggested.

Dose adjustment and monitoring. Dosage should be adjusted in all patients according to plasma-gentamicin concentrations, and this is particularly important where factors such as age, renal impairment, or high dose may predispose to toxicity, or where there is a risk of subtherapeutic concentrations (see Pharmacokinetics, above, for factors that may affect plasma concentrations). Although there has been some dispute about the relationship between plasma concentrations and toxicity it is generally recommended that trough plasma concentrations (measured just before the next dose) should be less than 2 µg per mL, and peak concentrations should reach at least 4 µg per mL but not exceed 10 to 12 µg per mL. In the UK

peak concentrations are generally measured one hour after intramuscular and intravenous administration, but the latter has varied between centres and countries and may lead to difficulties in comparing figures.

Various methods, none universally accepted, have been proposed for calculating aminoglycoside dosage requirements. Predictive nomograms, although possibly valuable in determining an initial dose, for example in renal impairment, are considered to be unsuitable for further dose determination, and methods based on the use of individualised pharmacokinetic parameters are recommended. Good results have been reported with the method of Sawchuk and Zaske, or with methods using Bayesian statistics which may be somewhat simpler to implement (for references see Dosage Calculation, below).

Once-daily dosage. Some sources consider, in contrast to what has been the accepted view, that there may be advantages to administering the total daily requirement as a single dose (see Once-daily Dosage, below). However, it is not yet clear whether once-daily dosage is as effective as conventional dosage regimens in all cases, particularly in children, or in patients with endocarditis or renal impairment. With once-daily dosage, traditional methods of monitoring peak and trough plasma concentrations may not be applicable and advice on dosage and plasma concentrations should be sought.

Other routes. Gentamicin has sometimes been given by mouth for enteric infections and to suppress intestinal flora and has occasionally been given by inhalation in cystic fibrosis. In meningitis it has been administered intrathecally or intraventricularly usually in doses of 1 to 5 mg daily in conjunction with intramuscular therapy. Gentamicin has also been given by subconjunctival injection.

A bone cement impregnated with gentamicin is used in orthopaedic surgery. Acrylic beads containing gentamicin and threaded on to surgical wire are implanted in the management of bone infections.

Gentamicin is also used topically for skin infections in concentrations of 0.1%, but as topical use may lead to the emergence of resistance it is considered inadvisable. Concentrations of 0.3% are used in preparations for topical application to the eyes and ears.

A liposomal formulation of gentamicin is under investigation.

◊ Reviews.
1. Edson RS. Terrell CL. The aminoglycosides. *Mayo Clin Proc* 1999; **74:** 519–28.

Administration and dosage. CONCENTRATION MONITORING. References to the problems of drug concentration monitoring of the aminoglycosides, and the difficulty in correlating concentrations with toxicity.
1. Scott DK, *et al.* Aminoglycoside trough levels: a source of error. *Lancet* 1982; **ii:** 441–2.
2. Wenk M, *et al.* Serum level monitoring of antibacterial drugs: a review. *Clin Pharmacokinet* 1984; **9:** 475–92.
3. Rodvold KA, *et al.* Aminoglycoside pharmacokinetic monitoring: an integral part of patient care? *Clin Pharm* 1988; **7:** 608–13.
4. Banks BEC. Monitoring of aminoglycosides. *J Antimicrob Chemother* 1990; **26:** 145–8.
5. McCormack JP, *et al.* A critical reevaluation of the therapeutic range of aminoglycosides. *Clin Infect Dis* 1992; **14:** 320–39.
6. Aronson JK, Reynolds DJM. Aminoglycoside antibiotics. *BMJ* 1992; **305;** 1421–4.

DOSAGE CALCULATION. References to methods of dosage calculation for aminoglycosides including nomograms[1-6] and pharmacokinetic methods,[7-16] such as those of Sawchuk and Zaske,[7,8] and Bayesian analysis.[9-11,17,18]
1. Hull JH, Sarubbi FA. Gentamicin serum concentrations: pharmacokinetic predictions. *Ann Intern Med* 1976; **85:** 183–9.
2. Sarubbi FA, Hull JH. Amikacin serum concentrations: prediction of levels and dosage guidelines. *Ann Intern Med* 1978; **89:** 612–18.
3. Chan RA, *et al.* Gentamicin therapy in renal failure: a nomogram for dosage. *Ann Intern Med* 1972; **76:** 773–8.
4. Lesar TS, *et al.* Gentamicin dosing errors with four commonly used nomograms. *JAMA* 1982; **248:** 1190–3.
5. Platt DR, *et al.* Comparison of four methods of predicting serum gentamicin concentrations in adult patients with impaired renal function. *Clin Pharm* 1982; **1:** 361–5.
6. Watling SM, Kisor DF. Population pharmacokinetics: development of a medical intensive care unit-specific gentamicin dosing nomogram. *J Pharmacokinet Biopharm* 1993; **27:** 151–4.
7. Sawchuk RJ, Zaske DE. Pharmacokinetics of dosing regimens which utilize multiple intravenous infusions: gentamicin in burn patients. *J Pharmacokinet Biopharm* 1976; **4:** 183–95.
8. Sawchuk RJ, *et al.* Kinetic model for gentamicin dosing with the use of individual patient parameters. *Clin Pharmacol Ther* 1977; **21:** 362–9.

9. Burton ME, *et al.* A Bayesian feedback method of aminoglycoside dosing. *Clin Pharmacol Ther* 1985; **37**: 349–57.
10. Koup JR, *et al.* Multiple-dose non-linear regression analysis program: aminoglycoside dose prediction. *Clin Pharmacokinet* 1983; **8**: 456–62.
11. Chrystyn H. Validation of the use of Bayesian analysis in the optimization of gentamicin therapy from the commencement of dosing. *Drug Intell Clin Pharm* 1988; **22**: 49–53.
12. Lackner TE, *et al.* A nonexponential, nonlogarithmic pharmacokinetic dosing method for gentamicin. *Clin Pharm* 1991; **10**: 706–10.
13. Burton ME, *et al.* Accuracy of Bayesian and Sawchuk-Zaske dosing methods for gentamicin. *Clin Pharm* 1986; **5**: 143–9.
14. Rodvold KA, *et al.* Aminoglycoside pharmacokinetics monitoring: an integral part of patient care? *Clin Pharm* 1988; **7**: 608–13.
15. Erdman SM, *et al.* An updated comparison of drug dosing methods part III: aminoglycoside antibiotics. *Clin Pharmacokinet* 1991; **20**: 374–88.
16. Watling SM, Dasta JF. Aminoglycoside dosing considerations in intensive care unit patients. *Ann Pharmacother* 1993; **27**: 351–7.
17. Radomski KM, *et al.* General versus subpopulation values in Bayesian prediction of aminoglycoside pharmacokinetics in hematology-oncology patients. *Am J Health-Syst Pharm* 1997; **54**: 541–4.
18. Duffull SB, *et al.* Comparison of two Bayesian approaches to dose-individualization for once-daily aminoglycoside regimens. *Br J Clin Pharmacol* 1997; **43**: 125–35.

IN NEONATES AND INFANTS. References.

1. Gennrich JL, Nitake M. Devising an aminoglycoside dosage regimen for neonates seven to ninety days chronological age. *Neonatal Pharmacol Q* 1992; **1**: 45–50.
2. Sidhu JS, *et al.* Assessment of bioelectrical impedance for individualising gentamicin therapy in neonates. *Eur J Clin Pharmacol* 1993; **44**: 253–8.
3. Weber W, *et al.* Population kinetics of gentamicin in neonates. *Eur J Clin Pharmacol* 1993; **44** (suppl 1): S23–S25.
4. Isemann BT, *et al.* Optimal gentamicin therapy in preterm neonates including loading doses and early monitoring. *Ther Drug Monit* 1996; **18**: 549–55.
5. Logsdon BA, Phelps SJ. Routine monitoring of gentamicin serum concentrations in pediatric patients with normal renal function is unnecessary. *Ann Pharmacother* 1997; **31**: 1514–18.

IN PATIENTS WITH NON-IDEAL BODY-WEIGHT. References.

1. Traynor AM, *et al.* Aminoglycoside dosing weight correction factors for patients of various body sizes. *Antimicrob Agents Chemother* 1995; **39**: 545–8.

IN RENAL IMPAIRMENT. Although a number of nomograms, schedules, and rules have been devised for the calculation of aminoglycoside dosage in renal impairment, where possible dosage modification should be based on the monitoring of individual pharmacokinetic parameters. Standard dosage calculation methods should not be used for patients undergoing dialysis as they may require supplementary post-dialysis doses.

ONCE-DAILY DOSAGE. The concept of administering aminoglycosides once daily rather than in divided doses is attractive on the grounds of convenience and economy. The rationale cited by proponents of single daily doses for preferring high intermittent plasma concentrations includes the prolonged postantibiotic effect of aminoglycosides (persistent antibacterial activity after plasma concentrations have fallen below the MIC), potentially higher antibacterial concentrations at the site of infection, and theoretical reductions in the incidence of adaptive resistance, with no apparent increase in nephrotoxicity. There have been numerous clinical and *animal* studies but clinical studies have generally included small numbers of patients with uncomplicated infections and have excluded patients with altered pharmacokinetic profiles. Despite the deficiencies of these studies, several meta-analyses have been published which have concluded that once-daily administration appears to be at least as effective as, and no more toxic than, multiple daily dosing in such patient populations.[1-7] Some have questioned the validity of these conclusions[8] while others take a more optimistic view.[9] Despite the reports of good tolerability, an increase in endotoxin reactions has recently been associated with the administration of single daily doses (see under Adverse Effects, above).

Several methods for calculating doses and monitoring treatment have been proposed[10-12] but consensus is still needed on appropriate treatment regimens and suitable target serum concentrations.[12-14] There is currently insufficient information for pregnant or breast-feeding women, or patients with burns or impaired renal or hepatic function.[12-14] However, preliminary reports suggest that once-daily administration may be practical in trauma patients,[15] neonates and children,[16-18] including those with neutropenia,[19] and patients with cystic fibrosis.[20,21] Once daily dosage may, though, be inappropriate for elderly patients[22] due to an increased incidence of nephrotoxicity, patients in whom the volume of drug distribution or clearance is difficult to predict or markedly abnormal,[23] and in the treatment of enterococcal endocarditis.[12]

1. Barza M, *et al.* Single or multiple daily doses of aminoglycosides: a meta-analysis. *BMJ* 1996; **312**: 338–45.
2. Hatala R, *et al.* Once-daily aminoglycoside dosing in immunocompetent adults: a meta-analysis. *Ann Intern Med* 1996; **124**: 717–25.
3. Ferriols-Lisart R, Alos-Almiñana M. Effectiveness and safety of once-daily aminoglycosides: a meta-analysis. *Am J Health-Syst Pharm* 1996; **53**: 1141–50.
4. Munckhof WJ, *et al.* A meta-analysis of studies on the safety and efficacy of aminoglycosides given either once daily or as divided doses. *J Antimicrob Chemother* 1996; **37**: 645–63.
5. Bailey TC, *et al.* A meta-analysis of extended-interval dosing versus multiple daily dosing of aminoglycosides. *Clin Infect Dis* 1997; **24**: 786–95.
6. Ali MZ, Goetz MB. A meta-analysis of the relative efficacy and toxicity of single daily dosing versus multiple daily dosing of aminoglycosides. *Clin Infect Dis* 1997; **24**: 796–809.
7. Hatala R, *et al.* Single daily dosing of aminoglycosides in immunocompromised adults: a systematic review. *Clin Infect Dis* 1997; **24**: 810–15.
8. Bertino JS, *et al.* Single daily dosing of aminoglycosides—a concept whose time has not yet come. *Clin Infect Dis* 1997; **24**: 820–3.
9. Gilbert DN. Meta-analyses are no longer required for determining the efficacy of single daily dosing of aminoglycosides. *Clin Infect Dis* 1997; **24**: 816–19.
10. Begg EJ, *et al.* A suggested approach to once-daily aminoglycoside dosing. *Br J Clin Pharmacol* 1995; **39**: 605–9.
11. Prins JM, *et al.* Validation and nephrotoxicity of a simplified once-daily aminoglycoside dosing schedule and guidelines for monitoring therapy. *Antimicrob Agents Chemother* 1996; **40**: 2494–9.
12. Freeman CD, *et al.* Once-daily dosing of aminoglycosides: review and recommendations for clinical practice. *J Antimicrob Chemother* 1997; **39**: 677–86.
13. Rodvold KA, *et al.* Single daily doses of aminoglycosides. *Lancet* 1997; **350**: 1412.
14. Anonymous. Aminoglycosides once daily? *Drug Ther Bull* 1997; **35**: 36–7.
15. Finnell DL, *et al.* Validation of the Hartford nomogram in trauma surgery patients. *Am J Health-Syst Pharm* 1998; **32**: 417–21.
16. Langlass TM, Mickle TR. Standard gentamicin dosage regimen in neonates. *Am J Health-Syst Pharm* 1999; **56**: 440–3.
17. Thureen PJ, *et al.* Once- versus twice-daily gentamicin dosing in neonates ≥34 weeks' gestation: cost-effectiveness analyses. *Pediatrics* 1999; **103**: 594–8.
18. Lundergan FS, *et al.* Once-daily gentamicin dosing in newborn infants. *Pediatrics* 1999; **103**: 1228–34.
19. Tomlinson RJ, *et al.* Once daily ceftriaxone and gentamicin for the treatment of febrile neutropenia. *Arch Dis Child* 1999; **80**: 125–31.
20. Bragonier R, Brown NM. The pharmacokinetics and toxicity of once-daily tobramycin therapy in children with cystic fibrosis. *J Antimicrob Chemother* 1998; **42**: 103–6.
21. Vic P, *et al.* Efficacy, tolerance, and pharmacokinetics of once daily tobramycin for pseudomonas exacerbations in cystic fibrosis. *Arch Dis Child* 1998; **78**: 536–9.
22. Koo J, *et al.* Comparison of once-daily versus pharmacokinetic dosing of aminoglycosides in elderly patients. *Am J Med* 1996; **101**: 177–83.
23. Gerberding JL. Aminoglycoside dosing: timing is of the essence. *Am J Med* 1998; **105**: 256–8.

Ménière's disease. Gentamicin and streptomycin have been used for medical ablation in advanced Ménière's disease (p.407). Although gentamicin given systemically is considered to be more ototoxic than streptomycin evidence from *animal* studies suggests that intratympanic administration may be less ototoxic. This, and a higher incidence of side-effects with streptomycin, has meant that intratympanic gentamicin is now preferred. Intratympanic gentamicin has been reported to control vertigo symptoms in 91% of patients, though 19% experienced a worsening of their hearing loss immediately after treatment.[1] Other workers using similar methods have also had successful outcomes.[2,3] However, the ideal regimen for intratympanic gentamicin has yet to be defined.

1. Beck C. Intratympanic application of gentamicin for treatment of Ménière's disease. *Keio J Med* 1986; **35**: 36–41.
2. Nedzelski JM, *et al.* Chemical labyrinthectomy: local application of gentamicin for the treatment of unilateral Meniere's disease. *Am J Otol* 1992; **13**: 18–22.
3. Pyykkö I, *et al.* Intratympanic gentamicin in bilateral Meniere's disease. *Otolaryngol Head Neck Surg* 1994; **110**: 162–7.

Preparations

BP 2001: Gentamicin Cream; Gentamicin Eye Drops; Gentamicin Injection; Gentamicin Ointment;
USP 25: Gentamicin and Prednisolone Acetate Ophthalmic Ointment; Gentamicin Injection; Gentamicin Sulfate Cream; Gentamicin Sulfate Ointment; Gentamicin Sulfate Ophthalmic Ointment; Gentamicin Sulfate Ophthalmic Solution.

Proprietary Preparations (details are given in Part 3)
Aust.: Gentax; Refobacin; Sulmycin; *Austral.:* Garamycin†; Genoptic; *Belg.:* Gentamytrex; Geomycine; *Braz.:* Ampligen; Amplomicina; Garamicina; Gentaplus; Gentaxil; *Canad.:* Alcomicin; Cidomycin; Diogent; Garamycin; Garatec; Gentacidin†; Ocugram†; *Denm.:* Garamycin; Gensumycin; Gentacoll; Hexamycin; *Fin.:* Gensumycin; Gentacoll; *Fr.:* Gentabilles†; Gentalline; Ophtagram†; *Ger.:* Dispagent; duragentamicin; Gencin; Gent-Ophtal; Genta; Gentamytrex; Ophtagram; Refobacin; Sulmycin; *Hong Kong:* Garamycin; Genoptic; Miramycin; Optigen; *Irl.:* Cidomycin; Genticin; *Israel:* Cidomycin; Garamycin; Gentatrim; Lacromycin; Opti-Genta; *Ital.:* Gentalyn; Gentamen; Gentibioptal; Genticol; Gentomil; Ribomicin; *Mex.:* Barmicil; Beramicina; Fustermicina; Garacoll; Garalen; Garamicina; Genemicin; Genexal; Genkova; Genrex; Genta; Gentabac; Gentacarnot; Gentacin; Gentanacin; Gentapat; Gentarim; Gentavivant; Gentazaf Z; Gentialoquin; Geracin; GI; Gy-Sol; Ikatin; Migent; Nozolon; Oftagen; Quilagen; Servigenta; Tamigen; Tondex; Yectamicina; *Neth.:* Garacol; Garamycin; Gentamytrex; *Norw.:* Garamycin; Gensumycin; *NZ:* Genoptic; Ophtagram; *Port.:* Cronocol; Garalone; GentaGobens; Gentocil; Ophtagram; *S.Afr.:* Cidomycin; Fermentmycin; Garamycin; Gencin; Servigenta; Sabax Gentamix; *Singapore:* Garamycin; Genoptic; Gentamytrex; Miramycin; Ophtagram; *Spain:* Colirocilina Gentam; Genta Gobens; Gentalodina†; Gentamedical; Gentamival; Genticina; Gentralay†; Gevramycin; Gevramycin Topica; Lantogent; Rexgenta; *Swed.:* Garamycin; Gensumycin; *Switz.:* Garamycin; Ophtagram; Servigenta†; Yedoc†; *Thai.:* Garamycin; Genta; Genta-Oph; Gentac; Gentacin; Gental; Gramicin; Grammixin; Miramycin; Servigenta; Versigen; *UAE:* Gental; *UK:* Cidomycin; Garamycin; Genticin; *USA:* G-Myticin; Garamycin; Genoptic; Gentacidin; Gentak; Gentasol; Jenamicin†; Ocu-Mycin.

Multi-ingredient: *Aust.:* Decoderm compositum; Decoderm trivalent; Dexagenta; Diprogenta; Refobacin-Palacos R; Septopal; Terra-Cortril mit Gentamicin†; *Austral.:* Celestone VG; Palacos E with Garamycin; Palacos R with Garamycin; Septopal; *Belg.:* De-coderm Comp; Duracoll; Garasone; Palacos R avec Gentamicine; Septopal; *Braz.:* Cauterex com Gentamicina; Diprogenta; Emecort; Garasone; Gentacort; Ginometrim; Otigent; Pan-Emecort; Quadriderm; Quadrilon; Septopal; *Canad.:* Diprogen; Garasone; Valisone-G; *Denm.:* Palacos cum Gentamicin; Septopal; *Fin.:* Celestoderm cum Garamycin; Palacos R cum Gentamicin; Septopal; *Fr.:* Gentasone; Indobiotic; Palacos LV avec Gentamicine; Palacos R avec Gentamicine; Voltamicine; *Ger.:* Betagentam; Cibaflam; Decoderm Comp; Dexa-Gentamicin; Dexamytrex; Diprogenta; Inflanegent; Refobacin-Palacos R; Septopal; Sulmycin mit Celestan-V; *Hong Kong:* Celestoderm-V with Garamycin; Colircusi Gentadexa; Diprogenta; Garasone; Infectoflam; Novoter Gentamicin; Quadriderm; Septopal; Triderm; Triditol-G; *Irl.:* Gentisone HC; Palacos R with Gentamicin; Septopal; *Israel:* Aflumycin; Betacorten-G; Celestoderm-V with Garamycin; Cicloderm-C; Diprogenta; Triderm; *Ital.:* Citrizan Antibiotico; Diprogenta†; Formomicin; Genalfa; Genatrop; Gentacort; Gentalyn Beta; Vasosterone Oto; Voltamicin; *Mex.:* Diprosone G; Garamicina V; Garasone; Genrex-B; Quadriderm NF; *Neth.:* Dexagenta-POS†; Dexamytrex; Palacos met gentamicine; Septopal; *Norw.:* Palacos cum Gentamicin†; Septopal; *NZ:* Palacos with Garamycin; *Port.:* Dexamytrex; Diprogenta; Epione; Gentadexa; Palacos R com Gentamicina†; Quadriderme; *S.Afr.:* Celestoderm-V with Garamycin; Diprogenta; Garasone; Palacos R with Garamycin; Pred G; Quadriderm; Septopal; *Singapore:* B-Tasone-G; Beprogent; Betnovate-GM; Celestoderm-V with Garamycin; Combiderm; Conazole; Dexamytrex; Diprogenta; Garasone; Gentrisone; Infectoflam; Neoderm; Quadriderm; Refobacin-Palacos R; Septopal; Tri-Micon; Triderm; *Spain:* Celestoderm Gentamicina; Cuatroderm; Diprogenta; Flugen; Flutenal Gentamicina; Gentadexa; Gentavasor; Interderm; Novoter Gentamicina; *Swed.:* Celeston valerat med gentamicin; Palacos cum gentamicin†; Septopal; *Switz.:* Diprogenta; Infectoflam; Ophtasone; Palacos avec Garamycin†; Pred G†; Quadriderm; Septopal; Triderm; Voltamicin; *Thai.:* Beprogenta; Dexamytrex; Diprogenta; Genquin; Gental-F; Infectoflam; Pred Oph; Quadriderm; Refobacin-Palacos R; Septopal; *UK:* Gentisone HC; Palacos LV with Gentamicin; Palacos R with Gentamicin; Septopal; Vipsogal; *USA:* Pred G.

Gramicidin   (90-s)

Gramicidin (BAN, rINN).

Gramicidin D; Gramicidin (Dubos); Gramicidinum.
CAS — 1405-97-6 (gramicidin); 113-73-5 (gramicidin S).
ATC — R02AB30.

NOTE. The name gramicidin was formerly applied to tyrothricin. *Pharmacopoeias.* In *Eur.* (see p.vi) and US.

Pharmacopoeial description

Ph. Eur.: A mixture consisting mainly of three pairs of linear polypeptides usually obtained by extraction from tyrothricin, the complex isolated from the fermentation broth of *Bacillus brevis*. The potency is not less than 900 units per mg calculated with reference to the dried substance. A white or almost white, slightly hygroscopic, crystalline powder. Practically insoluble in water; sparingly soluble in alcohol; practically insoluble in cyclohexane. Store in airtight containers.

USP 25: An antibacterial substance produced by the growth of *Bacillus brevis* (Bacillaceae); it may be obtained from tyrothricin. It has a potency of not less than 900 μg of gramicidin per mg, calculated on the dried basis. A white or practically white, odourless, crystalline, powder. Insoluble in water; soluble in alcohol. Store in airtight containers.

Profile

Gramicidin has properties similar to those of tyrothricin (p.267) and is too toxic to be administered systemically. It has been used for the local treatment of susceptible infections usually with other antibacterials such as neomycin and polymyxin B, and frequently with a corticosteroid as well.

Gramicidin sulfate has also been used. Gramicidin S or 'Soviet gramicidin' ($C_{60}H_{92}N_{12}O_{10} = 1141.4$) has been used.

Porphyria. Gramicidin is considered to be unsafe in patients with porphyria because it has been shown to be porphyrinogenic in *animals* or *in-vitro* systems.

Preparations

USP 25: Neomycin and Polymyxin B Sulfates and Gramicidin Cream; Neomycin and Polymyxin B Sulfates and Gramicidin Ophthalmic Solution; Neomycin and Polymyxin B Sulfates, Gramicidin, and Hydrocortisone Acetate Cream; Neomycin Sulfate and Gramicidin Ointment; Nystatin, Neomycin Sulfate, Gramicidin, and Triamcinolone Acetonide Cream; Nystatin, Neomycin Sulfate, Gramicidin, and Triamcinolone Acetonide Ointment.

Proprietary Preparations (details are given in Part 3)
Fr.: Argicilline†; Pharmaciline†.

Multi-ingredient: *Aust.:* Mycostatin V; Topsym polyvalent; Volon A antibiotikahaltig; *Austral.:* Aristocomb†; Kenacomb; Neosporin; Otocomb Otic; Otodex; Sofradex; Soframycin; *Belg.:* Graneodine†; Mycolog; *Braz.:* Fonergin; Oftrim; Omcilon AM; *Canad.:* Antibiotic Cream; Diosporin†; Kenacomb; Lidosporin; Neosporin; Optimyxin; Optimyxin Plus; Polycidin; Polysporin; Polysporin Plus Pain Relief; Polysporin Triple Antibiotic; Polytopic; Sofracort; Soframycin; Trisomcin; Viaderm-KC; *Denm.:* Kenalog Comp; Kenalog Comp med Mycostatin; Sofradex; *Fin.:* Bafucin; Polysporin; Sofradex; *Fr.:* Topifram†; *Ger.:* Kombi-Stulln; Polyspectran; Ultexiv; *Hong Kong:* Dexa-Polyspectran; Kenacomb; Neosporin; Polyspectran; Sofradex; Triacomb; *Irl.:* Graneodin; Kenacomb; Neosporin; Sofradex; Soframycin; *Israel:* Dermacombin; Kenacomb; *Ital.:* Eta Biocortilen VC; Neogram; Vasosterone Antibiotico; *Mex.:* Kenacomb; Neosporin; Polixin; Septilisin; *Neth.:* Mycolog; Polyspectran G†; Sofradex; *Norw.:* Sofradex; *NZ:* Kenacomb; Sofradex; Soframycin; *Port.:* Dropcina; Gramixina; Kenacomb; Polysporina†; *S.Afr.:* Kenacomb; Sofradex; *Singapore:* Kenacomb; Neosporin; Sofradex; Topifram; *Spain:* Deltasiton†; Flodermol; Fludronef; Intradermo Cort Ant Fung; Midacina; Oftalmowell; Poxider†; Spectrocin; Tivitis; Trigon Topico; *Swed.:* Bafucin; Kenacombin†; Sofradex; *Switz.:* Angidine; Korticoid polyvalent; Mycolog; Neosporin; Sofradex; Topsym polyvalent; Tyrothricine + Gramicidine; *Thai.:* Dermacombin; Kenacomb; Neosporin; Opsacin; Polyoph; Sofradex; Topifram; Xanalin; *UAE:* Panderm; *UK:* Adcortyl with Graneodin†; Graneodin; Neosporin; Sofradex; Soframycin†; Tri-Adcortyl; *USA:* Ak-Spore; Alba-3†; Neosporin; Ocu-Spor-G; Ocutricin; Polymycin.

Grepafloxacin Hydrochloride (17086-c)

Grepafloxacin Hydrochloride (BANM, USAN, rINNM).
OPC-17116. (±)-1-Cyclopropyl-6-fluoro-1,4-dihydro-5-methyl-7-(3-methyl-1-piperazinyl)-4-oxo-3-quinolinecarboxylic acid monohydrochloride.
$C_{19}H_{22}FN_3O_3,HCl$ = 395.9.
CAS — 119914-60-2 (grepafloxacin); 161967-81-3 (grepafloxacin hydrochloride).

Profile
Grepafloxacin is a fluoroquinolone antibacterial with properties similar to those of ciprofloxacin (p.182). It was formerly used as the hydrochloride but was withdrawn worldwide in October 1999 following reports of cardiovascular toxicity; prolongation of the QT interval was associated with the drug.

Preparations
Proprietary Preparations (details are given in Part 3)
Aust.: Raxar†; *Austral.:* Raxar†; *Canad.:* Raxar†; *Denm.:* Raxar†; *Ger.:* Vaxar†; *Israel:* Raxar†; *Mex.:* Raxar†; *Neth.:* Raxar†; *Switz.:* Raxar†; *UK:* Raxar†; *USA:* Raxar†.

Halquinol (4785-m)

Halquinol (BAN).
Chlorhydroxyquinoline; Chlorquinol; Halquinols (USAN); SQ-16401. A mixture of the chlorinated products of quinolin-8-ol containing 57 to 74% of 5,7-dichloroquinolin-8-ol (chloroxine), 23 to 40% of 5-chloroquinolin-8-ol (cloxyquin), and not more than 4% of 7-chloroquinolin-8-ol.
CAS — 8067-69-4 (halquinol); 773-76-2 (5,7-dichloroquinolin-8-ol).

Profile
Halquinol is a halogenated hydroxyquinoline with properties similar to those of clioquinol (p.190). It is used topically in infected skin conditions and one of its constituents, 5,7-dichloroquinolin-8-ol (chloroxine), has been applied as a 2% shampoo in the treatment of dandruff and seborrhoeic dermatitis of the scalp.

Preparations
Proprietary Preparations (details are given in Part 3)
UK: Valpeda; *USA:* Capitrol.

Multi-ingredient: *Aust.:* Decoderm trivalent; *Denm.:* Kenacutan; *Israel:* Antiseptic Foot Balm; *Ital.:* Beben Clorossina; *Norw.:* Kenacutan; *Spain:* Decoderm Trivalente; Deltasiton†; *Swed.:* Kenacutan; *UK:* Antiseptic Foot Balm.

Imipenem (16849-l)

Imipenem (BAN, USAN, rINN).
N-Formimidoyl Thienamycin; Imipemide; MK-787; MK-0787. (5R,6S)-6-[(R)-1-Hydroxyethyl]-3-(2-iminomethylaminoethylthio)-7-oxo-1-azabicyclo[3.2.0]hept-2-ene-2-carboxylic acid monohydrate.
$C_{12}H_{17}N_3O_4S,H_2O$ = 317.4.
CAS — 64221-86-9 (anhydrous imipenem); 74431-23-5 (imipenem monohydrate).
Pharmacopoeias. In Eur. (see p.vi), *Jpn*, and *US*.

The *N*-formimidoyl derivative of thienamycin, an antibiotic produced by *Streptomyces cattleya*. Imipenem is unstable at alkaline or acidic pH and the commercially available injection of imipenem with cilastatin sodium for intravenous use, is buffered to provide, when reconstituted, a solution with pH 6.5 to 7.5. The manufacturers advise against mixing with other antibacterials.

Pharmacopoeial description
Ph. Eur.: A white, almost white, or pale yellow powder. Sparingly soluble in water; slightly soluble in methyl alcohol. A 0.5% solution in water has a pH of 4.5 to 7.0. Store in airtight containers at a temperature of 2° to 8°.
USP 25: A white to tan-coloured crystalline powder. Sparingly soluble in water; slightly soluble in methyl alcohol. Store at a temperature not exceeding 8°.

◊ References.
1. Bigley FP, *et al.* Compatibility of imipenem-cilastatin sodium with commonly used intravenous solutions. *Am J Hosp Pharm* 1986; **43:** 2803–9.
2. Smith GB, *et al.* Stability and kinetics of degradation of imipenem in aqueous solution. *J Pharm Sci* 1990; **79:** 732–40.

Adverse Effects

Imipenem is only given in association with the enzyme inhibitor cilastatin and thus clinical experience relates to the combination.

Adverse effects with imipenem-cilastatin are similar in general to those with other beta lactams (see Benzylpenicillin, p.157, and Cefalotin, p.162). They include hypersensitivity reactions such as skin rashes, urticaria, eosinophilia, fever, and rarely, anaphylaxis; gastrointestinal effects such as nausea, vomiting, diarrhoea, tooth or tongue discoloration, and altered taste; and superinfection with non-susceptible organisms such as *Enterococcus faecium*, strains of *Pseudomonas aeruginosa* with acquired resistance, and *Candida*. Pseudomembranous colitis may develop. Toxic epidermal necrolysis has been reported rarely. Increases in liver enzymes and abnormalities in haematological parameters, including a positive Coombs' test, have been noted.

Local reactions such as pain or thrombophlebitis may occur following injection.

Seizures or convulsions have been reported with imipenem-cilastatin, particularly in patients with a history of CNS lesions and/or poor renal function, but sometimes in those without predisposing factors for seizures given recommended doses. Mental disturbances and confusion have also been reported.

Cilastatin has protected against the nephrotoxicity seen with high doses of imipenem given experimentally to *animals*. A harmless reddish coloration of urine has been observed in children.

Effects on the nervous system. References.
1. Eng RH, *et al.* Seizure propensity with imipenem. *Arch Intern Med* 1989; **149:** 1881–3.
2. Brown RB, *et al.* Seizure propensity with imipenem. *Arch Intern Med* 1990; **150:** 1551.
3. Job ML, Dretler RH. Seizure activity with imipenem therapy: incidence and risk factors. *DICP Ann Pharmacother* 1990; **24:** 467–9.
4. Leo RJ, Ballow CH. Seizure activity associated with imipenem use: clinical case reports and review of the literature. *DICP Ann Pharmacother* 1991; **25:** 351–4.
5. Duque A, *et al.* Vertigo caused by intravenous imipenem/cilastatin. *DICP Ann Pharmacother* 1991; **25:** 1009.
6. Lucena M, *et al.* Imipenem/cilastatin-associated hiccups. *Ann Pharmacother* 1992; **26:** 1459.
7. Norrby SR. Neurotoxicity of carbapenem antibacterials. *Drug Safety* 1996; **15:** 87–90.

Superinfection. References.
1. Gray JW, *et al.* Enterococcal superinfection in paediatric oncology patients treated with imipenem. *Lancet* 1992; **339:** 1487–8.

Precautions

Imipenem-cilastatin should not be given to patients known to be hypersensitive to it, and should be given with caution to patients known to be hypersensitive to penicillins, cephalosporins, or other beta lactams because of the possibility of cross-sensitivity.

It should be given with caution to patients with renal impairment, and the dose reduced appropriately. Particular care is necessary in patients with CNS disorders such as epilepsy.

Interactions

Seizures have been reported in patients given ganciclovir with imipenem-cilastatin.

Antimicrobial Action

Imipenem is bactericidal and acts similarly to the penicillins by inhibiting synthesis of the bacterial cell wall. It has a very broad spectrum of activity *in vitro*, including activity against Gram-positive and Gram-negative aerobic and anaerobic organisms, and is stable to hydrolysis by beta-lactamases produced by most bacterial species. Cilastatin, the enzyme inhibitor given in association with imipenem, appears to have no antibacterial activity.

Most Gram-positive cocci are sensitive to imipenem (MIC$_{90}$ ranging from 0.01 to 0.1 μg per mL) including most streptococci, and both penicillinase- and non-penicillinase-producing staphylococci, although its activity against meticillin-resistant *Staphylococcus aureus* is variable. Imipenem has good to moderate activity against *Enterococcus faecalis*, but most *E.*

faecium are resistant. *Nocardia, Rhodococcus,* and *Listeria* spp. are also sensitive.

Among Gram-negative bacteria, imipenem is active against many of the Enterobacteriaceae (MIC$_{90}$ ranging from 0.1 to 8 μg per mL) including *Citrobacter* and *Enterobacter* spp., *Escherichia coli, Klebsiella, Proteus, Providencia, Salmonella, Serratia, Shigella,* and *Yersinia* spp. Its activity against *Pseudomonas aeruginosa* is similar to that of ceftazidime and the MIC$_{90}$ has ranged from 2 to 8 μg per mL. Imipenem is also active against *Acinetobacter* spp. and *Campylobacter jejuni,* and also against *Haemophilus influenzae* and *Neisseria* spp., including beta-lactamase-producing strains.

Many anaerobic bacteria, including *Bacteroides* spp., are sensitive to imipenem, but *Clostridium difficile* is only moderately susceptible.

Imipenem is not active against *Chlamydia trachomatis, Mycoplasma* spp., fungi, or viruses.

There have been reports of antagonism between imipenem and other beta lactams *in vitro*. Imipenem and aminoglycosides often act synergistically.

Imipenem is a potent inducer of beta-lactamases of some Gram-negative bacteria, but generally remains stable to them. Acquired resistance has been reported in *Ps. aeruginosa* during therapy with imipenem.

Resistance. References.
1. King A, *et al.* Resistance to imipenem in Pseudomonas aeruginosa. *J Antimicrob Chemother* 1995; **36:** 1037–41.
2. Ballestero S, *et al.* Carbapenem resistance in Pseudomonas aeruginosa from cystic fibrosis patients. *J Antimicrob Chemother* 1996; **38:** 39–45.
3. Rasmussen BA, Bush K. Carbapenem-hydrolyzing β-lactamases. *Antimicrob Agents Chemother* 1997; **41:** 223–32.
4. Livermore DM. Acquired carbapenemases. *J Antimicrob Chemother* 1997; **39:** 673–6.
5. MacKenzie FM, *et al.* Emergence of a carbapenem-resistant Klebsiella pneumoniae. *Lancet* 1997; **350:** 783.
6. Pikis A, *et al.* Decreased susceptibility to imipenem among penicillin-resistant Streptococcus pneumoniae. *J Antimicrob Chemother* 1997; **40:** 105–8.
7. Mainardi J-L, *et al.* Carbapenem resistance in a clinical isolate of Citrobacter freundii. *Antimicrob Agents Chemother* 1997; **41:** 2352–4.

Pharmacokinetics

Imipenem is not appreciably absorbed from the gastrointestinal tract and is administered parenterally.

It is excreted primarily in the urine by glomerular filtration and tubular secretion and undergoes partial metabolism in the kidneys by dehydropeptidase I, an enzyme in the brush border of the renal tubules, to inactive, nephrotoxic metabolites, with only 5 to 45% of a dose excreted in the urine as unchanged active drug. Imipenem is administered in conjunction with cilastatin sodium (p.182), a dehydropeptidase inhibitor, resulting in increased urinary-imipenem concentrations. Cilastatin does not affect serum concentrations of imipenem.

The pharmacokinetics of imipenem and cilastatin are similar and both have plasma half-lives of approximately one hour; half-lives, especially those of cilastatin, may be prolonged in neonates and in patients with renal impairment. Following intramuscular administration of imipenem with cilastatin peak plasma concentrations of 10 to 12 μg per mL are achieved at about 2 hours and prolonged absorption results in plasma concentrations of above 2 μg per mL for 6 to 8 hours. The bioavailability of imipenem following intramuscular injection is about 75%. Up to 20% of imipenem and 40% of cilastatin in the circulation is bound to plasma proteins. Imipenem is widely distributed in body tissues and fluids and crosses the placenta. Information on penetration into the CSF is limited, but concentrations appear to be relatively low.

When given with cilastatin about 70% of an intravenous dose of imipenem is recovered unchanged in the urine within 10 hours. A total of 50% of an intramuscular dose is recovered in the urine and concentrations above 10 μg per mL are maintained for 12 hours following a dose of 500 or 750 mg. Cilastatin is also excreted mainly in the urine, the majority as unchanged drug and about 12% as *N*-acetyl cilastatin. Both imipenem and cilastatin are removed by haemodialysis.

About 1% of imipenem is excreted via the bile in the faeces.

◊ **Reviews.**
1. Drusano GL. An overview of the pharmacology of imipenem/cilastatin. *J Antimicrob Chemother* 1986; **18** (suppl E): 79–92.
2. Watson ID, *et al.* Clinical pharmacokinetics of enzyme inhibitors in antimicrobial chemotherapy. *Clin Pharmacokinet* 1988; **15**: 133–64.
3. Mouton JW, *et al.* Comparative pharmacokinetics of the carbapenems: clinical implications. *Clin Pharmacokinet* 2000; **39**: 185–201.

◊ **Studies of the pharmacokinetics of imipenem.**
a. In the elderly.
1. Finch RG, *et al.* Pharmacokinetic studies of imipenem/cilastatin in elderly patients. *J Antimicrob Chemother* 1986; **18** (suppl E): 103–7.

◊ b. In liver disease.
1. Rolando N, *et al.* The penetration of imipenem/cilastatin into ascitic fluid in patients with chronic liver disease. *J Antimicrob Chemother* 1994; **33**: 163–7.

◊ c. In pregnancy and the neonate.
1. Reed MD, *et al.* Clinical pharmacology of imipenem and cilastatin in premature infants during the first week of life. *Antimicrob Agents Chemother* 1990; **34**: 1172–7.
2. Heikkilä A, *et al.* Pharmacokinetics and transplacental passage of imipenem during pregnancy. *Antimicrob Agents Chemother* 1992; **36**: 2652–5.

◊ d. In renal impairment.
1. Verbist L, *et al.* Pharmacokinetics and tolerance after repeated doses of imipenem/cilastatin in patients with severe renal failure. *J Antimicrob Chemother* 1986; **18** (suppl E): 115–20.
2. Alarabi AA, *et al.* Pharmacokinetics of intravenous imipenem/cilastatin during intermittent haemofiltration. *J Antimicrob Chemother* 1990; **26**: 91–8.
3. Pietroski NA, *et al.* Steady-state pharmacokinetics of intramuscular imipenem-cilastatin in elderly patients with various degrees of renal function. *Antimicrob Agents Chemother* 1991; **35**: 972–5.
4. Konishi K, *et al.* Removal of imipenem and cilastatin by hemodialysis in patients with end-stage renal failure. *Antimicrob Agents Chemother* 1991; **35**: 1616–20.
5. Chan CY, *et al.* Pharmacokinetics of parenteral imipenem/cilastatin in patients on continuous ambulatory peritoneal dialysis. *J Antimicrob Chemother* 1991; **27**: 225–32.
6. Tegeder I, *et al.* Pharmacokinetics of imipenem-cilastatin in critically ill patients undergoing continuous venovenous hemofiltration. *Antimicrob Agents Chemother* 1997; **41**: 2640–5.

Uses and Administration

Imipenem is a carbapenem beta-lactam antibiotic, differing from the penicillins in that the 5-membered ring is unsaturated and contains a carbon rather than a sulfur atom. Since imipenem is metabolised in the kidney by the enzyme dehydropeptidase I it is administered only in association with cilastatin (p.182), an inhibitor of the enzyme; this enhances urinary concentrations of active drug and was found to protect against the nephrotoxicity of high doses of imipenem in *animals*.

Imipenem is used for the treatment of infections caused by susceptible organisms (see Antimicrobial Action, above). They include infections in immunocompromised patients (with neutropenia), intra-abdominal infections, bone and joint infections, skin and soft-tissue infections, urinary-tract infections, biliary-tract infections, hospital-acquired pneumonia, and septicaemia. It may also be used for the treatment of gonorrhoea and for surgical infection prophylaxis. For details of these infections and their treatment, see under Choice of Antibacterial, p.114. It is not indicated for CNS infections.

Administration and dosage. Commercial preparations contain imipenem and cilastatin, as the sodium salt, in a ratio of 1 to 1. Doses of the combination are expressed in terms of the amount of anhydrous imipenem. Imipenem is administered by intravenous infusion or deep intramuscular injection. When administered intravenously, doses of 250 or 500 mg are infused over 20 to 30 minutes, and doses of 750 mg or 1 g over 40 to 60 minutes. The usual intravenous dose in adults and children weighing more than 40 kg is 1 to 2 g daily in divided doses every 6 or 8 hours, depending on the severity of the infection. A maximum daily dose of 4 g or 50 mg per kg body-weight is advised.

Children of 3 months or more and weighing less than 40 kg may be given 15 mg per kg every 6 hours by intravenous infusion; the total daily dose should not exceed 2 g.

The symbol † denotes a preparation no longer actively marketed

For surgical infection prophylaxis in adults, imipenem 1 g may be given intravenously on induction of anaesthesia, followed by a further 1 g three hours later, with additional doses of 500 mg at 8 and 16 hours if necessary.

Imipenem may be administered intramuscularly in adults with mild to moderate infections in doses of 500 or 750 mg every 12 hours. A single 500-mg intramuscular dose may be given in uncomplicated gonorrhoea.

Doses should be reduced in patients with renal impairment; in the UK the following are the recommended maximum *intravenous* doses in patients with a creatinine clearance of 70 mL per minute or less: creatinine clearance 31 to 70 mL per minute, 500 mg every 6 to 8 hours; 21 to 30 mL per minute, 500 mg every 8 to 12 hours; 6 to 20 mL per minute, 250 mg (or 3.5 mg per kg, whichever is the lower) every 12 hours or occasionally 500 mg every 12 hours. Patients with a creatinine clearance of 5 mL per minute or less should only be given imipenem if haemodialysis is started within 48 hours. Imipenem and cilastatin are cleared from the body by haemodialysis and doses should be given after a dialysis session and then every 12 hours. Information is lacking on the safety or effectiveness of the intramuscular route in patients with renal impairment.

◊ **General reviews.**
1. Buckley MM, *et al.* Imipenem/cilastatin: a reappraisal of its antibacterial activity, pharmacokinetic properties and therapeutic efficacy. *Drugs* 1992; **44**: 408–44. Correction. *ibid.*; 1012.
2. Balfour JA, *et al.* Imipenem/cilastatin: an update of its antibacterial activity, pharmacokinetics and therapeutic efficacy in the treatment of serious infections. *Drugs* 1996; **51**: 99–136.
3. Hellinger WC, Brewer NS. Carbapenems and monobactams: imipenem, meropenem, and aztreonam. *Mayo Clin Proc* 1999; **74**: 420–34.
4. Norrby SR. Carbapenems in serious infections: a risk-benefit assessment. *Drug Safety* 2000; **22**: 191–4.

Preparations

USP 25: Imipenem and Cilastatin for Injectable Suspension; Imipenem and Cilastatin for Injection.

Proprietary Preparations (details are given in Part 3)

Multi-ingredient: *Aust.:* Zienam; *Austral.:* Primaxin; *Belg.:* Tienam; *Braz.:* Tienam; *Canad.:* Primaxin; *Denm.:* Tienam; *Fin.:* Tienam; *Fr.:* Tienam; *Ger.:* Zienam; *Hong Kong:* Tienam; *Israel:* Tienam; *Ital.:* Impem; Tenacid; Tienam; *Mex.:* Tienam; *Neth.:* Tienam; *Norw.:* Tienam; *NZ:* Primaxin; *Port.:* Tienam; *S.Afr.:* Tienam; *Singapore:* Tienam; *Spain:* Tienam; *Swed.:* Tienam; *Switz.:* Tienam; *Thai.:* Tienam; *UK:* Primaxin; *USA:* Primaxin.

Isepamicin (2173-v)

Isepamicin (BAN, USAN, rINN).

HAPA-B; Sch-21420; Sch-21420. 4-O-(6-Amino-6-deoxy-α-D-glucopyranosyl)-1-N-(3-amino-L-lactoyl)-2-deoxy-6-O-(3-deoxy-4-C-methyl-3-methylamino-β-L-arabinopyranosyl)streptamine;   1N-(S-3-Amino-2-hydroxypropionyl)-gentamicin B.

$C_{22}H_{43}N_5O_{12} = 569.6$.
$CAS — 58152-03-7; 67479-40-7$.
$ATC — J01GB11$.

Isepamicin Sulfate (19892-c)

Isepamicin Sulfate (rINNM).
Isepamicin Sulphate (BANM).

$C_{22}H_{43}N_5O_{12}, 2H_2SO_4 = 765.8$.
$CAS — 68000-78-2$.

Pharmacopoeias. In *Jpn*, which specifies a variable amount of H_2SO_4.

Profile

Isepamicin is a semisynthetic aminoglycoside with actions and uses similar to those of gentamicin (p.210). It is reported not to be degraded by many of the enzymes responsible for aminoglycoside resistance. It is given by intramuscular injection or intravenous infusion as the sulfate in a dose of up to 15 mg per kg body-weight daily in 2 divided doses. Once-daily dosage may be possible in selected patients. Dosage should be adjusted based on serum-isepamicin concentration monitoring. In adults, the total daily dose should not exceed 1.5 g.

◊ **References.**
1. Tod M, *et al.* Clinical pharmacokinetics and pharmacodynamics of isepamicin. *Clin Pharmacokinet* 2000; **38**: 205–23.

Preparations

Proprietary Preparations (details are given in Part 3)
Belg.: Isepacine; *Fr.:* Isepalline; *Ital.:* Isepacin; Vizax†; *Mex.:* Isepacin; *Port.:* Isepacin.

Isoniazid (7559-k)

Isoniazid (BAN, pINN).

INAH; INH; Isoniazidum; Isonicotinic Acid Hydrazide; Isonicotinylhydrazide; Isonicotinylhydrazine; Tubazid. Isonicotinohydrazide.

$C_6H_7N_3O = 137.1$.
$CAS — 54-85-3$.
$ATC — J04AC01$.

NOTE. The name Isopyrin, which has been applied to isoniazid, has also been applied to isopropylaminophenazone.

Pharmacopoeias. In *Chin., Eur.* (see p.vi), *Int., Jpn, Pol.,* and *US*.

Solutions are sterilised by autoclaving.
Incompatible with sugars.

Pharmacopoeial description

Ph. Eur.: A white, crystalline powder or colourless crystals. Freely soluble in water; sparingly soluble in alcohol; very slightly soluble in ether. A 5% solution in water has a pH of 6.0 to 8.0.

USP 25: Colourless, or white, odourless crystals, or white crystalline powder. Soluble 1 in 8 of water and 1 in 50 of alcohol; slightly soluble in chloroform; very slightly soluble in ether. pH of a 10% solution in water is between 6.0 and 7.5. Store in airtight containers. Protect from light.

Adverse Effects

Isoniazid is generally well tolerated at currently recommended doses. However, patients who are slow acetylators of isoniazid appear to have a higher incidence of some adverse effects. Also patients whose nutrition is poor are at risk of peripheral neuritis which is one of the commonest adverse effects of isoniazid. Other neurological adverse effects include psychotic reactions and convulsions. Pyridoxine may be given to prevent or treat these adverse effects. Optic neuritis has also been reported.

Transient increases in liver enzymes occur in 10 to 20% of patients during the first few months and usually return to normal despite continued treatment. Elevated liver enzymes associated with clinical signs of hepatitis such as nausea and vomiting, or fatigue may indicate hepatic damage; in these circumstances, isoniazid should be stopped pending evaluation and should only be reintroduced cautiously once hepatic function has recovered. The incidence of liver damage is highest in patients over 35 years of age. The influence of acetylator status is uncertain. Fatalities have occurred following liver necrosis.

Haematological effects reported following use of isoniazid include various anaemias, agranulocytosis, thrombocytopenia, and eosinophilia.

Hypersensitivity reactions occur infrequently and include skin eruptions (including erythema multiforme), fever, and vasculitis.

Other adverse effects include nausea, vomiting, pellagra, purpura, hyperglycaemia, lupus-like syndrome, urinary retention, and gynaecomastia.

Symptoms of overdosage include slurred speech, metabolic acidosis, hyperglycaemia, convulsions, and coma; fatalities can occur.

Carcinogenicity. Concern about the carcinogenicity of isoniazid arose in the 1970s when an increased risk of bladder cancer in patients treated with isoniazid was reported.[1-3] However, no evidence to support a carcinogenic effect of isoniazid was found in more than 25 000 patients followed up for 9 to 14 years in studies organised by the USA Public Health Service[4] and in 3842 patients followed up for 16 to 24 years in the UK.[5]
1. Miller CT. Isoniazid and cancer risks. *JAMA* 1974; **230**: 1254.
2. Kerr WK, Chipman ML. The incidence of cancer of bladder and other sites after INH therapy. *Am J Epidemiol* 1976; **104**: 335–6.
3. Miller CT, *et al.* Relative importance of risk factors in bladder carcinogenesis. *J Chron Dis* 1978; **31**: 51–6.
4. Glassroth JL, *et al.* An assessment of the possible association of isoniazid with human cancer deaths. *Am Rev Respir Dis* 1977; **116**: 1065–74.
5. Stott H, *et al.* An assessment of the carcinogenicity of isoniazid in patients with pulmonary tuberculosis. *Tubercle* 1976; **57**: 1–15.

Effects on the blood. In addition to the effects mentioned above, rare reports of adverse effects of isoniazid on the blood include bleeding associated with acquired inhibition of fibrin stabilisation[1] or of factor XIII[2] and red cell aplasia.[3-5]

For a reference to neutropenia, see Effects on the Blood under Ethambutol Hydrochloride, p.205.
1. Otis PT, *et al.* An acquired inhibitor of fibrin stabilization associated with isoniazid therapy: clinical and biochemical observations. *Blood* 1974; **44**: 771–81.

2. Krumdieck R, *et al.* Hemorrhagic disorder due to an isoniazid-associated acquired factor XIII inhibitor in a patient with Waldenström's macroglobulinemia. *Am J Med* 1991; **90:** 639–45.
3. Claiborne RA, Dutt AK. Isoniazid-induced pure red cell aplasia. *Am Rev Respir Dis* 1985; **131:** 947–9.
4. Lewis CR, Manoharan A. Pure red cell hypoplasia secondary to isoniazid. *Postgrad Med J* 1987; **63:** 309–10.
5. Veale KS, *et al.* Pure red cell aplasia and hepatitis in a child receiving isoniazid therapy. *J Pediatr* 1992; **120:** 146–8.

Effects on the CNS. References.

1. Blumberg EA, Gil RA. Cerebellar syndrome caused by isoniazid. *DICP Ann Pharmacother* 1990; **24:** 829–31.
2. Pallone KA, *et al.* Isoniazid-associated psychosis: case report and review of the literature. *Ann Pharmacother* 1993; **27:** 167–70.
3. Cheung WC, *et al.* Isoniazid induced encephalopathy in dialysis patients. *Tubercle Lung Dis* 1993; **74:** 136–9.
4. Shah BR, *et al.* Acute isoniazid neurotoxicity in an urban hospital. *Pediatrics* 1995; **95:** 700–4.
5. Alao AO, Yolles JC. Isoniazid-induced psychosis. *Ann Pharmacother* 1998; **32:** 889–91.

Effects on the liver. In a review[1] of hepatotoxicity of antituberculous regimens containing isoniazid, it was stressed that hepatitis occurring during chemotherapy may be due to the disease itself, alcoholism, cirrhosis, or other infections. When treatment is implicated, it may not be possible to identify which drug or drugs are responsible.

A multicentre study[2] considered the incidence of hepatotoxicity in a short-term regimen of daily isoniazid, rifampicin, and pyrazinamide for 8 weeks in the initial phase followed by daily isoniazid and rifampicin for 16 weeks in the continuing phase. Analysis from 617 patients showed an incidence of hepatotoxic reactions of 1.6%; the incidence of elevated aspartate aminotransferase was 23.2%. In the same study, 445 patients on a nine-month regimen of daily isoniazid and rifampicin had a 1.2% incidence of hepatotoxicity and 27.1% incidence of elevated liver enzymes. A similar incidence of hepatitis of 1.4% among 350 patients on a 9-month regimen of rifampicin and isoniazid has also been reported.[3] A retrospective analysis[4] of 430 children on isoniazid and rifampicin revealed hepatotoxic reactions in 3.3%, the highest incidence being in children with severe disease. The incidence of hepatotoxicity is lower in patients receiving isoniazid for prophylaxis than in those receiving treatment for active disease. During a 7-year period[5] an incidence of 0.15% was recorded in 11 141 patients who started prophylactic therapy, whereas it was 1.25% amongst 1427 patients receiving treatment.

While increasing age,[6-9] high isoniazid doses, and pre-existing hepatic disease appear to increase the risk of isoniazid-induced hepatotoxicity, the influence of other factors is less certain. Speculation that fast acetylators of isoniazid could be at increased risk of hepatotoxicity due to production of a hepatotoxic hydrazine metabolite have not been supported;[10] in fact, slow acetylators have generally been found to have a higher risk than fast.[7,11] This could reflect a reduced rate of subsequent metabolism to non-toxic compounds. In addition, concentrations of hydrazine in the blood have not been found to correlate with acetylator status.[12,13]

The Joint Tuberculosis Committee of the British Thoracic Society is anxious that fears over the safety of treatment regimens do not compromise adequate therapy of the disease itself. They make recommendations[14] for initial measurement of liver function in all patients and regular monitoring in patients with known chronic liver disease. Tests should be repeated if symptoms of liver dysfunction occur, and details are given concerning the response to deteriorating liver function depending on the clinical situation, and include guidelines for prompt re-introduction of appropriate antituberculosis therapy once normal liver function is restored.

1. Girling DJ. The hepatic toxicity of antituberculosis regimens containing isoniazid, rifampicin and pyrazinamide. *Tubercle* 1978; **59:** 13–32.
2. Combs DL, *et al.* USPHS tuberculosis short-course chemotherapy trial 21: effectiveness, toxicity, and acceptability: the report of final results. *Ann Intern Med* 1990; **112:** 397–406.
3. Dutt AK, *et al.* Short-course chemotherapy for extrapulmonary tuberculosis: nine years' experience. *Ann Intern Med* 1986; **104:** 7–12.
4. O'Brien RJ, *et al.* Hepatotoxicity from isoniazid and rifampin among children treated for tuberculosis. *Pediatrics* 1983; **72:** 491–9.
5. Nolan CM, *et al.* Hepatotoxicity associated with isoniazid preventive therapy: a 7-year survey from a public health tuberculosis clinic. *JAMA* 1999; **281:** 1014–18.
6. Black M, *et al.* Isoniazid-associated hepatitis in 114 patients. *Gastroenterology* 1975; **69:** 289–302.
7. Dickinson DS, *et al.* Risk factors for isoniazid (INH)-induced liver dysfunction. *J Clin Gastroenterol* 1981; **3:** 271–9.
8. Stead WW, *et al.* Benefit-risk considerations in preventive treatment for tuberculosis in elderly persons. *Ann Intern Med* 1987; **107:** 843–5.
9. Døssing M, *et al.* Liver injury during antituberculosis treatment: an 11-year study. *Tubercle Lung Dis* 1996; **77:** 335–40.
10. Gurumurthy P, *et al.* Lack of relationship between hepatic toxicity and acetylator phenotype in three thousand South Indian patients during treatment with isoniazid for tuberculosis. *Am Rev Respir Dis* 1984; **129:** 58–61.
11. Pande JN, *et al.* Risk factors for hepatotoxicity from antituberculosis drugs: a case-control study. *Thorax* 1996; **51:** 132–6.
12. Gent WL, *et al.* Factors in hydrazine formation from isoniazid by paediatric and adult tuberculosis patients. *Eur J Clin Pharmacol* 1992; **43:** 131–6.
13. Donald PR, *et al.* Hydrazine production in children receiving isoniazid for the treatment of tuberculous meningitis. *Ann Pharmacother* 1994; **28:** 1340–3.
14. Ormerod LP, *et al.* Hepatotoxicity of antituberculosis drugs. *Thorax* 1996; **51:** 111–13.

Effects on the pancreas. Pancreatitis was associated with isoniazid therapy in 2 patients.[1,2] Chronic pancreatic insufficiency was reported in a patient following administration of isoniazid, rifampicin, ethambutol, and pyrazinamide.[3]

1. Chan KL, *et al.* Recurrent acute pancreatitis induced by isoniazid. *Tubercle Lung Dis* 1994; **75:** 383–5.
2. Rabassa AA, *et al.* Isoniazid-induced acute pancreatitis. *Ann Intern Med* 1994; **121:** 433–4.
3. Liu BA, *et al.* Pancreatic insufficiency due to antituberculosis therapy. *Ann Pharmacother* 1997; **31:** 724–6.

Effects on the skin and hair. Isoniazid causes cutaneous drug reactions in less than 1% of patients.[1,2] These reactions include urticaria, purpura, acneform syndrome,[3] a lupus erythematosus-like syndrome (see below),[4] and exfoliative dermatitis.[5] Pellagra is also associated with isoniazid.[6] Isoniazid was considered the most likely cause of alopecia in 5 patients receiving antituberculosis regimens which also included rifampicin, ethambutol, and pyrazinamide.[7]

1. Arndt KA, Jick H. Rates of cutaneous reactions to drugs: a report from the Boston Collaborative Drug Surveillance Program. *JAMA* 1976; **235:** 918–23.
2. Bigby M, *et al.* Drug-induced cutaneous reactions: a report from the Boston Collaborative Drug Surveillance Program on 15 438 consecutive inpatients, 1975 to 1982. *JAMA* 1986; **256:** 3358–63.
3. Thorne N. Skin reactions to systemic drug therapy. *Practitioner* 1973; **211:** 606–13.
4. Smith AG. Drug-induced photosensitivity. *Adverse Drug React Bull* 1989; **136:** 508–11.
5. Rosin MA, King LE. Isoniazid-induced exfoliative dermatitis. *South Med J* 1982; **75:** 81.
6. Ishii N, Nishihara Y. Pellagra encephalopathy among tuberculous patients: its relation to isoniazid therapy. *J Neurol Neurosurg Psychiatry* 1985; **48:** 628–34.
7. FitzGerald JM, *et al.* Alopecia side-effect of antituberculosis drugs. *Lancet* 1996; **347:** 472–3.

Lupus. Antinuclear antibodies have been reported to occur in up to 22% of patients receiving isoniazid; however, patients are usually asymptomatic and overt lupoid syndrome is rare.[1] The incidence of antibody induction has been reported to be higher in slow acetylators than in fast acetylators[2] but the difference was not statistically significant and acetylator phenotype is not considered an important determinant of the risk of isoniazid-induced lupus.[1,3] The syndrome appeared to be due to isoniazid itself rather than its metabolite acetylisoniazid.[4]

1. Hughes GRV. Recent developments in drug-associated systemic lupus erythematosus. *Adverse Drug React Bull* 1987; **123:** 460–3.
2. Alarcon-Segovia D, *et al.* Isoniazid acetylation rate and development of antinuclear antibodies upon isoniazid treatment. *Arthritis Rheum* 1971; **14:** 748–52.
3. Clark DWJ. Genetically determined variability in acetylation and oxidation: therapeutic implications. *Drugs* 1985; **29:** 342–75.
4. Sim E, *et al.* Drugs that induce systemic lupus erythematosus inhibit complement component C4. *Lancet* 1984; **ii:** 422–4.

Treatment of Adverse Effects

Pyridoxine hydrochloride 10 mg daily has been recommended in the UK for prophylaxis of peripheral neuritis associated with isoniazid although some have suggested using up to 50 mg daily.

Nicotinamide has been given, usually in association with pyridoxine, in patients who develop pellagra.

Treatment of overdosage is symptomatic and supportive and consists of gastric lavage, administration of activated charcoal, control of convulsions, and correction of metabolic acidosis. Large doses of pyridoxine may be needed intravenously for control of convulsions and may be given in conjunction with diazepam. Isoniazid is removed by haemodialysis.

◊ Pyridoxine deficiency associated with isoniazid in doses of 5 mg per kg body-weight daily is uncommon. Patients at risk of developing pyridoxine deficiency include those with diabetes, uraemia, alcoholism, HIV infection, and malnutrition.[1,2] Supplementation with pyridoxine should be considered for this at-risk group as well as for pregnant women and patients with seizure disorders.[1] For the prophylaxis of peripheral neuritis it is common practice to give a dose of 10 mg daily, although a dose of 6 mg daily might be sufficient.[3] However, in one patient a dose of pyridoxine 10 mg daily failed to prevent psychosis, the symptoms of which only resolved after stopping isoniazid and increasing the pyridoxine dosage to 100 mg daily.[4] Doses of 100 to 200 mg of pyridoxine daily have been suggested for the treatment of peripheral neuritis.[3]

1. American Thoracic Society and the Centers for Disease Control. Treatment of tuberculosis and tuberculosis infection in adults and children. *Am J Respir Crit Care Med* 1994; **149:** 1359–74.
2. Joint Tuberculosis Committee of the British Thoracic Society. Chemotherapy and management of tuberculosis in the United Kingdom: recommendations 1998. *Thorax* 1998; **53:** 536–48.
3. Snider DE. Pyridoxine supplementation during isoniazid therapy. *Tubercle* 1980; **61:** 191–6.
4. Chan TYK. Pyridoxine ineffective in isoniazid-induced psychosis. *Ann Pharmacother* 1999; **33:** 1123–4.

Overdosage. Isoniazid doses of 6 g or more are associated with severe toxicity and doses above 15 g may be fatal without appropriate treatment. Symptoms may not occur until 2 hours after ingestion. Treatment includes early removal of the drug from the stomach, supportive treatment, and intravenous administration of pyridoxine in a dose at least equal to the amount of isoniazid ingested. Diazepam may be given intravenously to assist seizure control and sodium bicarbonate for metabolic acidosis. Dialysis has been used but may not be necessary.[1] An initial dose of pyridoxine hydrochloride 5 g (even if the amount of isoniazid ingested is unknown), given intravenously over 3 to 5 minutes, has been recommended. This dose is repeated at 5 to 20 minute intervals until the dose greatly exceeds that of ingested isoniazid, seizures cease, or consciousness is regained. Other methods of pyridoxine administration have been proposed, including administration of the total amount of pyridoxine as a single intravenous infusion in glucose 5% over 30 to 60 minutes.[2] A maximum dose of pyridoxine has not been set; doses in the range of 70 to 357 mg per kg body-weight over 1 hour[2] and 52 g intravenously[3] have been used in isoniazid overdosage without pyridoxine toxicity.

1. Cameron WM. Isoniazid overdose. *Can Med Assoc J* 1978; **118:** 1413–15.
2. Wason S, *et al.* Single high-dose pyridoxine treatment for isoniazid overdose. *JAMA* 1981; **246:** 1102–4.
3. Sievers ML, Herrier RN. Treatment of acute isoniazid toxicity. *Am J Hosp Pharm* 1975; **32:** 202–6.

Precautions

Isoniazid should be administered with caution to patients with convulsive disorders, a history of psychosis, or hepatic or renal dysfunction. Patients who are at risk of neuropathy or pyridoxine deficiency, including those who are diabetic, alcoholic, malnourished, uraemic, pregnant, or infected with HIV, should receive pyridoxine usually in a dose of 10 mg daily, although some have suggested using up to 50 mg daily. If symptoms of hepatitis such as malaise, fatigue, anorexia, and nausea develop isoniazid should be discontinued pending evaluation.

Liver function should be checked before treatment with isoniazid and special care should be taken in alcoholic patients or those with pre-existing liver disease. Regular monitoring of liver function is recommended in patients with pre-existing liver disease, and isoniazid treatment should be suspended if serum aspartate aminotransferase concentrations are elevated to 3 to 5 times the normal upper limit or the bilirubin concentration rises. Careful monitoring should be considered for black and Hispanic women, in whom there may be an increased risk of fatal hepatitis.

Periodic eye examinations during isoniazid treatment have also been suggested.

Breast feeding. Isoniazid is distributed into breast milk. Peak concentrations of 6 μg per mL of milk following isoniazid doses of 5 mg per kg body-weight and 16.6 μg per mL of milk following a 300-mg dose have been reported.[1] Adverse effects on infants during breast feeding have not been reported,[2] although such infants should be monitored for toxic reactions.[1]

1. Snider D, Powell KE. Should women taking antituberculosis drugs breast-feed? *Arch Intern Med* 1984; **144:** 589–90.
2. American Academy of Pediatrics, Committee on Drugs. The transfer of drugs and other chemicals into human milk. *Pediatrics* 2001; **108:** 776 89.

Porphyria. Isoniazid is considered to be unsafe in patients with porphyria although there is conflicting experimental evidence of porphyrinogenicity.

Pregnancy and the neonate. In a review[1] of antituberculous treatment in pregnant patients it was reported that over 95% of 1480 pregnancies in which isoniazid had been given resulted in a normal term infant. Slightly more than 1% of the infants/fetuses were abnormal and many of these abnormalities were CNS related. Isoniazid is therefore recognised as being suitable for use in regimens for the **treatment** of tuberculosis in **pregnant** patients.[2,3] Pyridoxine supplementation is recommended[2] (see Treatment of Adverse Effects, above). **Preventive therapy** with isoniazid is generally delayed until after delivery unless other risk factors are present.[2]

Isoniazid crosses the placenta and average fetal concentrations of 61.5 and 72.8% of maternal serum or plasma concentration have been reported.[4] The half-life of isoniazid may be prolonged in neonates.[4]

Isoniazid is also suitable for use in the **neonate**.[2]

1. Snider DE, *et al.* Treatment of tuberculosis during pregnancy. *Am Rev Respir Dis* 1980; **122:** 65–79.
2. American Thoracic Society and the Centers for Disease Control. Treatment of tuberculosis and tuberculosis infection in adults and children. *Am J Respir Crit Care Med* 1994; **149:** 1359–74.
3. Joint Tuberculosis Committee of the British Thoracic Society. Chemotherapy and management of tuberculosis in the United Kingdom: recommendations 1998. *Thorax* 1998; **53:** 536–48.
4. Holdiness MR. Transplacental pharmacokinetics of the antituberculosis drugs. *Clin Pharmacokinet* 1987; **13:** 125–9.

Interactions

The risk of hepatotoxicity may be increased in patients receiving isoniazid in combination with rifampicin or other potentially hepatotoxic drugs.

Isoniazid can inhibit the hepatic metabolism of a number of drugs, in some cases leading to increased toxicity. These include the antiepileptics carbamazepine (p.344), ethosuximide (p.348), and phenytoin (p.359), the benzodiazepines diazepam and triazolam (p.677), chlorzoxazone (p.1327), and theophylline (p.780). The metabolism of enflurane (p.1258) may be increased in patients receiving isoniazid, resulting in potentially nephrotoxic levels of fluoride. Isoniazid has been associated with increased concentrations or toxicity of clofazimine (p.191), cycloserine (p.195), and warfarin (p.994).

For interactions affecting isoniazid, see below.

Alcohol. The metabolism of isoniazid may be increased in chronic alcoholics: this may lead to reduced isoniazid effectiveness.[1] These patients may also be at increased risk of developing isoniazid-induced peripheral neuropathies and hepatic damage (see Precautions, above).
1. Anonymous. Interaction of drugs with alcohol. *Med Lett Drugs Ther* 1981; **23**: 33–4.

Antacids. Oral absorption of isoniazid is reduced by aluminium-containing antacids; isoniazid should be given one hour before the antacid.[1]
1. Hurwitz A, Schluzman DL. Effects of antacids on gastrointestinal absorption of isoniazid in rat and man. *Am Rev Respir Dis* 1974; **109**: 41–7.

Corticosteroids. Administration of prednisolone 20 mg to 13 slow acetylators and 13 fast acetylators receiving isoniazid 10 mg per kg body-weight reduced plasma concentrations of isoniazid by 25 and 40% respectively.[1] Renal clearance of isoniazid was also enhanced in both acetylator phenotypes and the rate of acetylation increased in slow acetylators only.[1] The clinical significance of this effect is not established.
1. Sarma GR, *et al.* Effect of prednisolone and rifampin on isoniazid metabolism in slow and rapid inactivators of isoniazid. *Antimicrob Agents Chemother* 1980; **18**: 661–6.

Food. Palpitations, headache, conjunctival irritation, severe flushing, tachycardia, tachypnoea, and sweating have been reported in patients taking isoniazid following ingestion of cheese, red wine,[1] and some fish.[2,3] Accumulation of tyramine[1] or histamine[2] has been proposed as the cause of these food-related reactions, and they could be mistaken for anaphylaxis.[3]
1. Toutoungi M, *et al.* Cheese, wine, and isoniazid. *Lancet* 1985; **ii**: 671.
2. Kottegoda SR. Cheese, wine, and isoniazid. *Lancet* 1985; **ii**: 1074.
3. O'Sullivan TL. Drug-food interaction with isoniazid resembling anaphylaxis. *Ann Pharmacother* 1997; **31**: 928.

Ketoconazole. Serum concentrations of isoniazid were below the limits of detection in a patient also receiving rifampicin and ketoconazole.[1] For the effect of isoniazid on ketoconazole, see p.389.
1. Abadie-Kemmerly S, *et al.* Failure of ketoconazole treatment of Blastomyces dermatitidis due to interaction of isoniazid and rifampin. *Ann Intern Med* 1988; **109**: 844–5. Correction. *ibid.* 1989; **111**: 96.

Zalcitabine. The clearance of isoniazid was approximately doubled when zalcitabine was given to 12 HIV-positive patients.[1] In addition, care is needed since zalcitabine also causes peripheral neuropathy.
1. Lee BL, *et al.* The effect of zalcitabine on the pharmacokinetics of isoniazid in HIV-infected patients. *Intersci Conf Antimicrob Agents Chemother* 1994; **34**: 3(A4).

Antimicrobial Action

Isoniazid is highly active against *Mycobacterium tuberculosis* which it inhibits *in vitro* at concentrations of 0.02 to 0.2 μg per mL. Isoniazid may have activity against some strains of other mycobacteria including *M. kansasii*.

Although it is rapidly bactericidal against actively dividing *M. tuberculosis*, it is considered to be only bacteriostatic against semi-dormant organisms and has less sterilising activity than rifampicin or pyrazinamide.

Resistance to isoniazid develops rapidly if it is used alone in the treatment of clinical infection, and may be due in some strains to loss of the gene for catalase production. Resistance is delayed or prevented by combination with other antimycobacterials and it appears to be highly effective in preventing emergence of resistance to other antituberculous drugs. Resistance does not appear to be a problem when isoniazid is used alone in prophylaxis, probably because the bacillary load is low.

The symbol † denotes a preparation no longer actively marketed

Mycobacterium avium complex. Synergistic activity of isoniazid plus streptomycin and, to a lesser degree, isoniazid plus clofazimine against *Mycobacterium avium* complex (MAC) has been demonstrated *in vitro* and *in vivo*.[1]
1. Reddy MV, *et al.* In vitro and in vivo synergistic effect of isoniazid with streptomycin and clofazimine against Mycobacterium avium complex (MAC). *Tubercle Lung Dis* 1994; **75**: 208–12.

Pharmacokinetics

Isoniazid is readily absorbed from the gastrointestinal tract and following intramuscular injection. Peak concentrations of about 3 to 8 μg per mL appear in blood 1 to 2 hours after a fasting dose of 300 mg by mouth. The rate and extent of absorption of isoniazid is reduced by food. Isoniazid is not considered to be bound appreciably to plasma proteins and diffuses into all body tissues and fluids, including the CSF. It appears in fetal blood if given during pregnancy, and is distributed into breast milk (see above).

The plasma half-life for isoniazid ranges from about 1 to 6 hours, those who are fast acetylators having shorter half-lives. The primary metabolic route is the acetylation of isoniazid to acetylisoniazid by *N*-acetyltransferase found in the liver and small intestine. Acetylisoniazid is then hydrolysed to isonicotinic acid and monoacetylhydrazine; isonicotinic acid is conjugated with glycine to isonicotinyl glycine (isonicotinuric acid) and monoacetylhydrazine is further acetylated to diacetylhydrazine. Some unmetabolised isoniazid is conjugated to hydrazones. The metabolites of isoniazid have no tuberculostatic activity and, apart from possibly monoacetylhydrazine, they are also less toxic. The rate of acetylation of isoniazid and monoacetylhydrazine is genetically determined and there is a bimodal distribution of persons who acetylate them either slowly or rapidly. Various ethnic groups contain differing proportions of genetic phenotypes. When isoniazid is administered daily or 2 or 3 times weekly, clinical effectiveness is not influenced by acetylator status.

In patients with normal renal function, over 75% of a dose appears in the urine in 24 hours, mainly as metabolites. Small amounts of drug are also excreted in the faeces. Isoniazid is removed by dialysis.

Distribution. Therapeutic concentrations of isoniazid have been detected in CSF[1,2] and synovial fluid[3] several hours after oral administration. Diffusion into saliva is good and it has been suggested that salivary concentrations could be used in place of serum concentrations in pharmacokinetic studies.[4]
1. Forgan-Smith R, *et al.* Pyrazinamide and other drugs in tuberculous meningitis. *Lancet* 1973; **ii**: 374.
2. Miceli JN, *et al.* Isoniazid (INH) kinetics in children. *Fedn Proc* 1983; **42**: 1140.
3. Mouries D, *et al.* Passage articulaire de l'isoniazide et de l'éthambutol: deux observations de synovite tuberculeuse du genou. *Nouv Presse Med* 1975; **4**: 2734.
4. Gurumurthy P, *et al.* Salivary levels of isoniazid and rifampicin in tuberculous patients. *Tubercle* 1990; **71**: 29–33.

HIV-infected patients. Malabsorption of isoniazid may occur in patients with HIV infection. However, it is not clear whether this is related to the infection itself or associated diarrhoea. In a report of treatment failure during observed antituberculosis therapy in 2 patients with HIV infection, serum concentrations of isoniazid in 1 patient were low or undetectable for up to 12 hours after a dose.[1] However, serum concentrations of isoniazid in 26 HIV-positive patients undergoing intermittent antituberculosis treatment were generally regarded as adequate in a single sample taken 2 hours after a dose.[2] A pharmacokinetic study in volunteers without tuberculosis indicated that the presence of diarrhoea had a greater influence on absorption than either the presence or severity of HIV infection.[3]
1. Patel KB, *et al.* Drug malabsorption and resistant tuberculosis in HIV-infected patients. *N Engl J Med* 1995; **332**: 336–7.
2. Peloquin CA, *et al.* Low antituberculosis drug concentrations in patients with AIDS. *Ann Pharmacother* 1996; **30**: 919–25.
3. Sahai J, *et al.* Reduced plasma concentrations of antituberculosis drugs in patients with HIV infection. *Ann Intern Med* 1997; **127**: 289–93.

Uses and Administration

Isoniazid is a hydrazide derivative that is the mainstay of the primary treatment of pulmonary and extrapulmonary tuberculosis (p.143). It is administered with other antituberculous drugs usually including rifampicin and pyrazinamide. Isoniazid is also used in high risk subjects for the prophylaxis of tuberculosis.

Isoniazid is given in the initial and continuation phases of short-course tuberculosis regimens. The usual adult dose is 300 mg daily by mouth on an empty stomach. Children's doses vary between 5 mg per kg body-weight daily (WHO and UK) and 10 to 20 mg per kg daily (USA), all with a maximum of 300 mg daily. For intermittent therapy, WHO recommend 10 mg per kg three times a week or 15 mg per kg twice a week, while the recommended dose in the UK is 15 mg per kg three times a week. In the USA 15 mg per kg two or three times a week is recommended for adults and 20 to 40 mg per kg two or three times a week for children (maximum 900 mg). Doses may need to be reduced in patients with hepatic impairment or moderate to severe renal impairment.

Similar doses to those used orally may be given by intramuscular injection when isoniazid cannot be taken by mouth; it may also be given by intravenous injection. Isoniazid has also been given intrathecally and intrapleurally.

In tuberculosis prophylaxis, daily doses of 300 mg are given for at least 6 months and sometimes for up to 1 year. Alternatively it may be given with rifampicin for 3 months. Doses of 5 to 10 mg per kg isoniazid daily to a maximum of 300 mg daily have been suggested for prophylaxis in children in the UK.

Isoniazid aminosalicylate (pasiniazid) and isoniazid sodium glucuronate have also been used in the treatment of tuberculosis.

Preparations

BP 2001: Isoniazid Injection; Isoniazid Tablets;
USP 25: Isoniazid Injection; Isoniazid Syrup; Isoniazid Tablets; Rifampin and Isoniazid Capsules; Rifampin, Isoniazid, and Pyrazinamide Tablets; Rifampin, Isoniazid, Pyrazinamide, and Ethambutol Hydrochloride Tablets.

Proprietary Preparations (details are given in Part 3)
Belg.: Nicotibine; **Canad.:** Isotamine; **Fin.:** Tubilysin; **Fr.:** Rimifon; **Ger.:** Isozid; Isozid comp N; tebesium; tebesium-s; **Hong Kong:** Trisofort; **Ital.:** Nicizina; Nicozid; **Mex.:** Dipasic; Erbazid; Hidrasix; Pas Hain; **Port.:** Hidrazida; **Spain:** Cemidon; Cemidon B6; Pyreazid†; Rimifon; **Swed.:** Tibinide; **Switz.:** Isoamin; **Thai.:** Myrin; Myrin-P; **UK:** Rimifon; **USA:** Laniazid; Nydrazid.

Multi-ingredient: Aust.: Isoprodian; Myambutol-INH; Rifater; Rifoldin INH; Rimactan + INH; **Braz.:** Fluodrazin F; **Canad.:** Rifater; **Fr.:** Dexambutol-INH; Rifater; Rifinah; **Ger.:** EMB-INH; Iso-Eremfat; Isoprodian; Myambutol-INH; Rifater; Rifinah; **Hong Kong:** Ricinis; Rifater; Rifinah; **Irl.:** Rifater; Rifinah; Rimactazid; **Ital.:** Etanicozid B6; Etibi-INH†; Miazide B6; Miazide†; Rifanicozid†; Rifater; Rifinah; **Mex.:** Rifater; Rifinah; **Neth.:** Rifinah; **NZ:** Rifinah; **Port.:** Rifater; Rifinah; Tuberen; **S.Afr.:** Mynah†; Myrin; Myrin Plus; Pyrifin†; Rifafour; Rifater; Rifinah; Rimactazid; Rimcure; Tuberol†; **Singapore:** Rifater; Rifinah; Rimactazid; **Spain:** Amiopia; Duplicalcio 150; Duplicalcio B12; Duplicalcio Hidraz; Duplicalcio†; Isoetam†; Rifater; Rifinah; Rimactazid; Victogon†; **Switz.:** Myambutol-INH; Rifater; Rifinah; Rimactazide; Rimactazide + Z†; **Thai.:** Ricinis; Rifamiso; Rifater; Rifinah; Rimactazid; **UK:** Rifater; Rifinah; Rimactazid; **USA:** Rifamate; Rifater.

Josamycin (94-y)

Josamycin (BAN, USAN, rINN).

EN-141; Josamycinum; Leucomycin A₃. A stereoisomer of 7-(formylmethyl)-4,10-dihydroxy-5-methoxy-9,16-dimethyl-2-oxo-oxacyclohexadeca-11,13-dien-6-yl 3,6-dideoxy-4-O-(2,6-dideoxy-3-C-methyl-α-L-ribo-hexopyranosyl)-3-(dimethylamino)-β-D-glucopyranoside 4'-acetate 4''-isovalerate.
$C_{42}H_{69}NO_{15}$ = 828.0.
CAS — 16846-24-5; 56689-45-3.
ATC — J01FA07.
Pharmacopoeias. In Eur. (see p.vi) and Jpn.

Pharmacopoeial description
Ph. Eur.: A macrolide antibiotic produced by certain strains of *Streptomyces narbonensis* var. *josamyceticus* var. *nova*, or obtained by any other means. A white or slightly yellowish, slightly hygroscopic powder. It contains a minimum of 900 Ph. Eur. units per mg calculated with reference to the dried substance. Very slightly soluble in water; soluble in acetone; freely soluble in dichloromethane and in methyl alcohol. Store in airtight containers.

Josamycin Propionate (18281-b)

Josamycin Propionate (BANM, rINNM).

Josamicini Propionas; YS-20P. Josamycin 10-propionate.
$C_{45}H_{73}NO_{16}$ = 884.1.
CAS — 56111-35-4; 40922-77-8.
Pharmacopoeias. In Eur. (see p.vi) and Jpn.

1.07 mg of josamycin propionate is approximately equivalent to 1 mg of josamycin base.

Pharmacopoeial description
Ph. Eur.: Josamycin propionate is derived from a macrolide antibiotic produced by certain strains of *Streptomyces narbonensis* var. *josamyceticus* var. *nova*, or obtained by any other means. A white or slightly yellowish, slightly hygroscopic,

crystalline powder. It contains a minimum of 843 Ph. Eur. units per mg, calculated with reference to the dried substance. Practically insoluble in water; soluble in acetone; freely soluble in dichloromethane and in methyl alcohol. Store in airtight containers.

Adverse Effects and Precautions

As for Erythromycin, p.201. Josamycin is reported to produce less gastrointestinal disturbance than erythromycin.

◊ A report of josamycin-induced pedal oedema.[1]

1. Bosch X, *et al.* Josamycin-induced pedal oedema. *BMJ* 1993; **307:** 26.

Interactions

For a discussion of drug interactions of macrolide antibacterials, see Erythromycin, p.202.

◊ As discussed under Interactions of Erythromycin (Mechanism, p.202), josamycin is reported to have little or no effect on hepatic cytochrome P450 and may therefore interact less than erythromycin with other drugs metabolised by this enzyme system. The lack of interaction between josamycin and theophylline (p.780) would appear to support this.

Antimicrobial Action

As for Erythromycin, p.203. Some reports suggest that josamycin may be more active against some strains of anaerobic species such as *Bacteroides fragilis*.

Uses and Administration

Josamycin is a macrolide antibiotic with actions and uses similar to those of erythromycin (p.203). It is given by mouth as the base or the propionate but doses are calculated in terms of the base. Usual doses are 1 to 2 g daily in two or more divided doses.

Preparations

Proprietary Preparations (details are given in Part 3)
Aust.: Josalid; *Fr.:* Josacine; *Ger.:* Wilprafen; *Ital.:* Iosalide; Josaxin; *Jpn:* Josamy; *Spain:* Josamina; Josaxin; *Switz.:* Josacine.
Multi-ingredient: *Ital.:* Corti-Fluoral.

Kanamycin Acid Sulfate (95-j)

Kanamycin Acid Sulphate *(BANM)*; Kanamycini Sulfas Acidus.
Pharmacopoeias. In *Eur.* (see p.vi).

1.34 g of monograph substance is approximately equivalent to 1 g of kanamycin.

Pharmacopoeial description

Ph. Eur.: A form of kanamycin sulfate prepared by adding sulfuric acid to a solution of kanamycin sulfate and drying by a suitable method. A white or almost white, hygroscopic powder containing not less than 670 units per mg and 23 to 26% of sulfate, calculated with reference to the dried material. Soluble 1 in about 1 of water; practically insoluble in alcohol, in acetone, and in ether. A 1% solution in water has a pH of 5.5 to 7.5.

Kanamycin Sulfate (96-z)

Kanamycin Sulfate *(rINNM)*.
Kanamycin A Sulphate; Kanamycin Monosulphate; Kanamycin Sulphate *(BANM)*; Kanamycini Monosulfas. 6-*O*-(3-Amino-3-deoxy-α-D-glucopyranosyl)-4-*O*-(6-amino-6-deoxy-α-D-glucopyranosyl)-2-deoxystreptamine sulphate monohydrate.
$C_{18}H_{36}N_4O_{11},H_2SO_4,H_2O = 600.6$.
CAS — 59-01-8 (kanamycin); 25389-94-0 (anhydrous kanamycin sulfate).
Pharmacopoeias. In *Chin., Eur.* (see p.vi), *Jpn, Pol.,* and *US*.

Incompatibilities. For discussion of the incompatibility of aminoglycosides such as kanamycin with beta lactams, see under Gentamicin Sulfate, p.210. Kanamycin is also reported to be incompatible with various other drugs including some other antimicrobials as well as with some electrolytes. 1.2 g of monograph substance is approximately equivalent to 1 g of kanamycin.

Pharmacopoeial description

Ph. Eur.: The sulfate of an antimicrobial substance produced by the growth of certain strains of *Streptomyces kanamyceticus*. A white or almost white, crystalline powder containing not less than 750 units per mg and 15.0 to 17.0% of sulfate, calculated with reference to the dried material. Soluble 1 in about 8 of water; practically insoluble in alcohol, in acetone, and in ether. A 1% solution in water has a pH of 6.5 to 8.5.

USP 25: A white, odourless crystalline powder. It has a potency equivalent to not less than 750 µg of kanamycin per mg, calculated on the dried basis. Freely soluble in water; insoluble in acetone, in ethyl acetate, and in benzene. pH of a 1% solution in water is between 6.5 and 8.5. Store in airtight containers.

Adverse Effects, Treatment, and Precautions

As for Gentamicin Sulfate, p.210.

Peak plasma concentrations of kanamycin greater than 30 µg per mL, and trough concentrations greater than 10 µg per mL, should be avoided. Auditory (co-

chlear) toxicity is more frequent than vestibular toxicity.

Local pain and inflammation, as well as bruising and haematoma, have been reported at the site of intramuscular injections.

Gastrointestinal disturbances and a malabsorption syndrome, similar to that seen with oral neomycin (p.228), have occurred following administration of kanamycin by mouth. Oral kanamycin (local therapy) should be avoided in patients with gastrointestinal ulceration.

Interactions

As for Gentamicin Sulfate, p.211.

Antimicrobial Action

As for Gentamicin Sulfate, p.211. It is active against a similar range of organisms although it is not active against *Pseudomonas* spp. Some strains of *Mycobacterium tuberculosis* are sensitive. MICs of kanamycin for the most sensitive organisms range from about 0.5 to 4 µg per mL but organisms with MICs less than about 8 µg per mL are considered sensitive.

Resistance has been reported in strains of many of the organisms normally sensitive to kanamycin, and at one time was widespread, but a decline in the use of kanamycin has meant that resistance has become somewhat less prevalent. Cross-resistance occurs between kanamycin and neomycin, framycetin, and paromomycin, and partial cross-resistance has been reported between kanamycin and streptomycin.

◊ References.
1. Ho YII, *et al.* In-vitro activities of aminoglycoside-aminocyclitols against mycobacteria. *J Antimicrob Chemother* 1997; **40:** 27–32.

Pharmacokinetics

As for Gentamicin Sulfate, p.211.

Less than 1% of an oral dose is absorbed, although this may be significantly increased if the gastrointestinal mucosa is inflamed or ulcerated.

After intramuscular injection peak plasma concentrations of kanamycin of about 20 and 30 µg per mL are attained in about 1 hour following doses of 0.5 and 1 g respectively. A plasma half-life of about 3 hours has been reported. Absorption after intraperitoneal instillation is similar to that from intramuscular administration.

Kanamycin is rapidly excreted by glomerular filtration and most of a parenteral dose appears in the urine within 24 hours. It has been detected in cord blood and in breast milk.

Uses and Administration

Kanamycin is an aminoglycoside antibacterial with actions similar to those of gentamicin (p.212). It has been used in the treatment of susceptible Gram-negative and staphylococcal infections, including gonorrhoea (p.124) and neonatal gonococcal eye infections (p.130), although its use has declined in many centres because of the development of resistance. As with gentamicin it may be used with penicillins and with cephalosporins; the injections should be given at separate sites. Kanamycin has also been used as a second-line drug in tuberculosis (p.143), but other, safer drugs are usually preferred.

The sulfate or acid sulfate salts are often used: in the USA, preparations containing the bisulfate $(C_{18}H_{36}N_4O_{11},2H_2SO_4)$, but referred to as the sulfate, are available. Doses are expressed in terms of kanamycin base. It is usually administered by intramuscular injection, and in acute infections adults may be given 15 mg per kg body-weight daily, to a maximum of 1.5 g daily, in two to four divided doses. The same doses may be given by intravenous infusion of a 0.25 to 0.5% solution over 30 to 60 minutes; in the UK the manufacturers suggest that up to 30 mg per kg daily may be given by this route in overwhelming infection. Similar doses are used in children. Treatment should preferably not continue for longer than 7 to 10 days or exceed a cumulative dose of 10 g kanamycin. A sin-

gle intramuscular dose of 2 g has been used in the treatment of penicillin-resistant gonorrhoea. A dose of 3 to 4 g weekly has been suggested by the UK manufacturers for patients with chronic bacterial infections, up to a cumulative dose not to exceed 50 g, but prolonged administration increases the risk of nephrotoxicity and is not generally recommended.

In the treatment and prophylaxis of neonatal gonococcal infections in infants born to mothers with gonorrhoea, the equivalent of kanamycin 25 mg per kg, up to a maximum of 75 mg, may be given as a single intramuscular dose.

Peak plasma concentrations of greater than 30 µg per mL and trough concentrations greater than 10 µg per mL should be avoided. It is recommended that dosage should be adjusted in all patients according to plasma-kanamycin concentrations, and this is particularly important where factors such as age, renal impairment, or prolonged therapy may predispose to toxicity, or where there is a risk of subtherapeutic concentrations. For discussion of the methods of calculating aminoglycoside dosage requirements, see p.212.

Kanamycin has been used by mouth similarly to neomycin (p.228), for the suppression of intestinal flora. For pre-operative use, the equivalent of 1 g of kanamycin may be given every hour for 4 hours, then 1 g every 6 hours for 36 to 72 hours. In the management of hepatic encephalopathy, 8 to 12 g daily in divided doses may be given.

Kanamycin has also been administered in doses equivalent to 250 mg as a nebulised inhalation, two to four times daily. Solutions of kanamycin 0.25% have been used for the irrigation of body cavities.

Kanamycin tannate has also been used.

Preparations

USP 25: Kanamycin Injection; Kanamycin Sulfate Capsules.

Proprietary Preparations (details are given in Part 3)
Fr.: Kamycine†; *Ger.:* Kan-Ophtal; Kana-Stulln; Kanamytrex; *Irl.:* Kannasyn†; *Ital.:* Keimicina†; *Mex.:* Kanapat; Kanibel; Reukamicin; Solkan; Sulmyn; *Singapore:* Kancin-L; *Spain:* Kanacolirio; Kanescin; Kantrex; *Thai.:* Anbikan; Kan-Mycin; Kancin; Kangen; KMH; *UK:* Kannasyn†; *USA:* Kantrex.

Multi-ingredient: *Fr.:* Sterimycine; *Ital.:* Dermaflogil; Fluomicetina†; Kanazone; *S.Afr.:* Kantrexil; *Spain:* Kanafosal; Kanafosal Predni; Kanapomada; Lysokana†; Naso Pekamin; *Thai.:* KA-Cilone.

Kitasamycin (97-c)

Kitasamycin *(BAN, USAN, rINN)*.
Leucomycin.
CAS — 1392-21-8.
Pharmacopoeias. In *Jpn* which also includes Acetylkitasamycin.

An antimicrobial substance produced by *Streptomyces kitasatoensis*, consisting mainly of kitasamycins A_4 and A_5.

Profile

Kitasamycin is a macrolide antibiotic with actions and uses similar to those of erythromycin (p.201). It has been administered by mouth as kitasamycin base or intravenously as the tartrate. Acetylkitasamycin has also been administered by mouth.

Latamoxef Disodium (186-k)

Latamoxef Disodium *(BANM, rINNM)*.
LY-127935; Moxalactam Disodium *(USAN)*; 6059-S. (7R)-7-[2-Carboxy-2-(4-hydroxyphenyl)acetamido]-7-methoxy-3-(1-methyl-1*H*-tetrazol-5-ylthiomethyl)-1-oxa-3-cephem-4-carboxylic acid, disodium salt.
$C_{20}H_{18}N_6Na_2O_9S = 564.4$.
CAS — 64952-97-2 (latamoxef); 64953-12-4 (latamoxef disodium).
Pharmacopoeias. In *Jpn*.

Profile

Latamoxef is an oxacephalosporin antibiotic that has been given intramuscularly or intravenously as the disodium salt in the treatment of susceptible infections. It differs from the cephalosporins in that the sulfur atom of the 7-aminocephalosporanic acid nucleus is replaced by oxygen. Like cefamandole, it has a methylthiotetrazole side-chain and may cause hypoprothrombinaemia. Serious bleeding episodes have been reported with latamoxef and prophylaxis with vitamin K and monitoring of bleeding time have been recommended during treatment. In addition to hypoprothrombinaemia, inhibition of platelet function and more rarely immune-mediated thrombocytopenia may be responsible for interference with haemostasis. As with the methylthiotetrazole-containing cephalosporins, a disulfiram-like reaction with alcohol may occur.

Latamoxef has antimicrobial activity similar to that of the third-generation cephalosporin cefotaxime (p.169), although it is generally less active against Gram-positive bacteria and more active against *Bacteroides fragilis*.

Preparations

Proprietary Preparations (details are given in Part 3)
Ital.: Mactam†; Sectam†; *Jpn:* Shiomarin.

Levofloxacin (15283-v)

Levofloxacin (BAN, USAN, rINN).
DR-3355; HR-355; *S*-(–)-Ofloxacin; RWJ-25213. (–)-(S)-9-Fluoro-2,3-dihydro-3-methyl-10-(4-methyl-1-piperazinyl)-7-oxo-7H-pyrido[1,2,3-de]-1,4-benzoxazine-6-carboxylic acid.
$C_{18}H_{20}FN_3O_4 = 361.4$.
CAS — 100986-85-4 (levofloxacin); 138199-71-0 (levofloxacin hemihydrate).
ATC — J01MA12.

Adverse Effects and Precautions

As for Ciprofloxacin, p.183.

Interactions

As for Ciprofloxacin, p.184.

◊ References.
1. Liao S, *et al.* Absence of an effect of levofloxacin on warfarin pharmacokinetics and anticoagulation in male volunteers. *J Clin Pharmacol* 1996; **36:** 1072–7.
2. Gisclon LG, *et al.* Absence of a pharmacokinetic interaction between intravenous theophylline and orally administered levofloxacin. *J Clin Pharmacol* 1997; **37:** 744–50.
3. Doose DR, *et al.* Levofloxacin does not alter cyclosporine disposition. *J Clin Pharmacol* 1998; **38:** 90–3.

Antimicrobial Action

As for Ciprofloxacin, p.184.

Levofloxacin is generally considered to be about twice as active as its isomer, ofloxacin (p.232). It has a broad spectrum of activity which includes Gram-positive bacteria.

◊ References.
1. George J, Morrissey I. The bactericidal activity of levofloxacin compared with ofloxacin, D-ofloxacin, ciprofloxacin, sparfloxacin and cefotaxime against Streptococcus pneumoniae. *J Antimicrob Chemother* 1997; **39:** 719–23.
2. Licata L, *et al.* Comparison of the postantibiotic and postantibiotic sub-MIC effects of levofloxacin and ciprofloxacin on Staphylococcus aureus and Streptococcus pneumoniae. *Antimicrob Agents Chemother* 1997; **41:** 950–5.
3. Entenza JM, *et al.* Levofloxacin versus ciprofloxacin, flucloxacillin, or vancomycin for treatment of experimental endocarditis due to methicillin-susceptible or -resistant Staphylococcus aureus. *Antimicrob Agents Chemother* 1997; **41:** 1662–7.
4. Spangler SK, *et al.* Postantibiotic effect and postantibiotic sub-MIC effect of levofloxacin compared to those of ofloxacin, ciprofloxacin, erythromycin, azithromycin, and clarithromycin against 20 pneumococci. *Antimicrob Agents Chemother* 1998; **42:** 1253–5.

Pharmacokinetics

Levofloxacin is rapidly and almost completely absorbed following oral administration with peak plasma concentrations achieved within an hour of a dose. It is distributed into body tissues including the bronchial mucosa and lungs, but penetration into CSF is relatively poor. Levofloxacin is approximately 30 to 40% bound to plasma proteins. It is only metabolised to a small degree to inactive metabolites. The elimination half-life of levofloxacin is 6 to 8 hours, although this may be prolonged in patients with renal impairment. Levofloxacin is excreted largely unchanged, primarily in the urine. It is not removed by haemodialysis or peritoneal dialysis.

◊ References.
1. Fish DN, Chow AT. The clinical pharmacokinetics of levofloxacin. *Clin Pharmacokinet* 1997; **32:** 101–19.
2. Chien S-C, *et al.* Pharmacokinetic profile of levofloxacin following once-daily 500-milligram oral or intravenous doses. *Antimicrob Agents Chemother* 1997; **41:** 2256–60.
3. Preston SL, *et al.* Pharmacodynamics of levofloxacin: a new paradigm for early clinical trials. *JAMA* 1998; **279:** 125–9.
4. Chien S-C, *et al.* Double-blind evaluation of the safety and pharmacokinetics of multiple oral once-daily 750-milligram and 1-gram doses of levofloxacin in healthy volunteers. *Antimicrob Agents Chemother* 1998; **42:** 885–8.
5. Piscitelli SC, *et al.* Pharmacokinetics and safety of high-dose and extended-interval regimens of levofloxacin in human immunodeficiency virus-infected patients. *Antimicrob Agents Chemother* 1999; **43:** 2323–7.

Uses and Administration

Levofloxacin is the *S*-(–)-isomer of the fluoroquinolone antibacterial ofloxacin (p.232). It is given by mouth or intravenously for the treatment of susceptible infections in a usual dose of 250 or 500 mg once or twice daily. Doses should be reduced in patients with renal impairment.

Levofloxacin is also administered topically as 0.5% eye drops for the treatment of bacterial conjunctivitis.

◊ Reviews.
1. Davis R, Bryson HM. Levofloxacin: a review of its antibacterial activity, pharmacokinetics and therapeutic efficacy. *Drugs* 1994; **4:** 677–700.
2. Martin SJ, *et al.* Levofloxacin and sparfloxacin: new quinolone antibiotics. *Ann Pharmacother* 1998; **32:** 320–36.
3. Langtry HD, Lamb HM. Levofloxacin: its use in infections of the respiratory tract, skin, soft tissues and urinary tract. *Drugs* 1998; **56:** 487–515.
4. Martin SJ, *et al.* A risk-benefit assessment of levofloxacin in respiratory, skin and skin structure, and urinary tract infections. *Drugs* 2001; **24:** 199–222.

Preparations

Proprietary Preparations (details are given in Part 3)
Aust.: Tavanic; *Belg.:* Tavanic; *Canad.:* Levaquin; *Fin.:* Tavanic; *Fr.:* Tavanic; *Ger.:* Tavanic; *Hong Kong:* Cravit; *Irl.:* Tavanic; *Ital.:* Levoxacin; Tavanic; *Jpn:* Cravit; *Mex.:* Elequine; Tavanic; *Neth.:* Tavanic; *Port.:* Tavanic; *S.Afr.:* Tavanic; *Singapore:* Cravit; *Spain:* Tavanic; *Swed.:* Tavanic; *Switz.:* Tavanic; *Thai.:* Cravit; *UK:* Tavanic; *USA:* Levaquin; Quixin.

Lincomycin Hydrochloride (98-k)

Lincomycin Hydrochloride (BANM, rINNM).
Lincomycini Hydrochloridum; NSC-70731; U-10149 (lincomycin). Methyl 6-amino-6,8-dideoxy-N-[(2S,4R)-1-methyl-4-propylprolyl]-1-thio-α-D-*erythro*-D-*galacto*-octopyranoside hydrochloride monohydrate.
$C_{18}H_{34}N_2O_6S,HCl,H_2O = 461.0$.
CAS — 154-21-2 (lincomycin); 859-18-7 (anhydrous lincomycin hydrochloride); 7179-49-9 (lincomycin hydrochloride, monohydrate).
NOTE. Lincomycin is *USAN*.
Pharmacopoeias. In *Chin., Eur.* (see p.vi), *Jpn, Pol.,* and *US*.

1.13 g of monograph substance is approximately equivalent to 1 g of lincomycin.

Incompatibilities. Solutions of lincomycin hydrochloride have an acid pH and incompatibility may be expected with alkaline preparations, or with drugs unstable at low pH.

Pharmacopoeial description

Ph. Eur.: An antimicrobial substance produced by *Streptomyces lincolnensis* var. *lincolnensis* or by any other means. A white or almost white crystalline powder. It contains not more than 5% of lincomycin B. Very soluble in water; slightly soluble in alcohol; very slightly soluble in acetone; practically insoluble in ether. A 10% solution in water has a pH of 3.5 to 5.5. Store at a temperature not exceeding 30° in airtight containers.

USP 25: A white or practically white crystalline powder, odourless or with a faint odour. Freely soluble in water; very slightly soluble in acetone; soluble in dimethylformamide. pH of a 10% solution in water is between 3.0 and 5.5. Store in airtight containers.

Adverse Effects, Treatment, and Precautions

As for Clindamycin, p.188.

Hypotension, ECG changes, and on rare occasions cardiac arrest, have followed rapid intravenous injections. Other adverse reactions reported rarely with lincomycin include aplastic anaemia, pancytopenia, and tinnitus.

Interactions

As for Clindamycin, p.188.

Absorption of lincomycin is reduced by adsorbent antidiarrhoeals and cyclamate sweeteners.

Antimicrobial Action

As for Clindamycin (p.188) but it is less potent. The minimum inhibitory concentrations of lincomycin have been reported to range from 0.05 to 2 μg per mL for the most sensitive organisms. There is complete cross-resistance between clindamycin and lincomycin.

Pharmacokinetics

About 20 to 30% of a dose of lincomycin given by mouth is absorbed from the gastrointestinal tract and following a 500-mg dose, peak plasma concentrations of 2 to 7 μg per mL are reached within 2 to 4 hours. Food markedly reduces the rate and extent of absorption. The intramuscular injection of 600 mg produces peak plasma concentrations of 8 to 18 μg per mL usually within 30 minutes.

The biological half-life of lincomycin is about 5 hours. Lincomycin is widely distributed in the tissues including bone and body fluids but diffusion into the CSF is poor, although it may be slightly better when the meninges are inflamed. It diffuses across the placenta and is distributed into breast milk. Lincomycin is partially inactivated in the liver; unchanged drug and metabolites are excreted in the urine, bile, and faeces. Lincomycin is not effectively removed from the blood by dialysis.

Uses and Administration

Lincomycin is a lincosamide antibiotic with actions and uses similar to those of its chlorinated derivative, clindamycin (p.189). Clindamycin is usually preferred to lincomycin because of its greater activity and better absorption. However, the usefulness of both drugs is limited by their potential to cause pseudomembranous colitis.

Lincomycin hydrochloride is administered by mouth in adult doses equivalent to 500 mg of lincomycin 3 or 4 times daily, taken at least 1 hour before food. It is also given parenterally by intramuscular injection in a dose of 600 mg once or twice daily, or by slow intravenous infusion in a dose of 600 mg to 1 g two or three times daily. Higher doses have been given in very severe infections, up to a total daily dose of about 8 g. Children over the age of 1 month may be given 20 to 60 mg per kg body-weight daily in divided doses by mouth, or 10 to 20 mg per kg daily in divided doses by intramuscular injection or intravenous infusion. Doses may need to be reduced in patients with severe renal impairment; a reduction down to 25 to 30% of the usual dose may be appropriate.

Lincomycin hydrochloride may be administered into the eye by subconjunctival injection in a dose equivalent to 75 mg of lincomycin.

Preparations

BP 2001: Lincomycin Capsules; Lincomycin Injection;
USP 25: Lincomycin Hydrochloride Capsules; Lincomycin Hydrochloride Syrup; Lincomycin Injection.

Proprietary Preparations (details are given in Part 3)
Austral.: Lincocin; *Belg.:* Lincocin; *Braz.:* Frademicina; Fredcina; Linco-Plus; Macrolin; *Canad.:* Lincocin; *Fr.:* Lincocine; *Ger.:* Albiotic; *Hong Kong:* Lincocin; *Ital.:* Lincocin; *Mex.:* Lincocin; Princol; Rimsalin; *Neth.:* Lincocin; *Port.:* Lincocina; *S.Afr.:* Lincocin; *Singapore:* Lincocin; *Spain:* Cillimicina; Lincocin; *Swed.:* Lincocin†; *Switz.:* Lincocin; *Thai.:* Anbycin; Linco; Lincocin; Lincogin; Lincolan; Lincomy; Lingo; Linmycin; *USA:* Lincocin; Lincorex.

Linezolid (9770-y)

Linezolid (BAN, USAN, rINN).
U-100766. N-{[(S)-3-(3-Fluoro-4-morpholinophenyl)-2-oxo-5-oxazolidinyl]methyl}acetamide.
$C_{16}H_{20}FN_3O_4 = 337.3$.
CAS — 165800-03-3.

Adverse Effects and Precautions

The adverse effects most frequently reported in patients receiving linezolid include diarrhoea, nausea and vomiting, metallic taste, headache, insomnia, constipation, rashes, dizziness, and abnormal liver function tests. Reversible myelosuppression including anaemia, leucopenia, pancytopenia and, in particular, thrombocytopenia has been reported and blood counts should be monitored weekly in patients receiving linezolid. Patients particularly at risk are those who have received linezolid for more than 10 to 14 days or who have pre-existing myelosuppression or severe renal impairment.

Effects on the blood. Reversible myelosuppression with red cell hypoplasia occurred in 3 patients treated with linezolid.[1] Features of the myelosuppression were considered to be similar to those associated with chloramphenicol.

During the initial 8 months of licensed use in the UK 12 reports of haematopoietic disorders (including thrombocytopenia,

---

The symbol † denotes a preparation no longer actively marketed

anaemia, leucopenia, and pancytopenia) were received by the UK Committee on Safety of Medicines.[2]

1. Green SL, et al. Linezolid and reversible myelosuppression. JAMA 2001; 285: 1291.
2. Committee on Safety of Medicines/Medicines Control Agency. Reminder: linezolid (Zyvox) and myelosuppression. Current Problems 2001; 27: 14.

Interactions

Linezolid is a reversible, nonselective MAOI and therefore has the potential to interact with adrenergic and serotonergic drugs. Enhanced pressor activity has been reported in patients receiving linezolid in combination with phenylpropanolamine or pseudoephedrine. The interactions of conventional MAOIs, both with other drugs and with foods, are described under Phenelzine, p.305.

Antimicrobial Action

Linezolid is a oxazolidinone antibacterial with activity against a range of aerobic Gram-positive bacteria including vancomycin-resistant enterococci and meticillin-resistant *Staphylococcus aureus*. It is less active against Gram-negative bacteria, but has some *in vitro* activity against *Haemophilus influenzae*, *Legionella* spp., *Moraxella catarrhalis* (*Branhamella catarrhalis*), *Neisseria gonorrhoeae*, and *Pasteurella* spp. It is not active against *Acinetobacter* spp., Enterobacteriaceae, or *Pseudomonas* spp.

Oxazolidinone antibacterials are bacteriostatic and act by inhibition of ribosomal protein synthesis. Cross-resistance between oxazolidinones and other classes of antibacterial is considered unlikely.

Resistant strains of *Enterococcus faecium* have been reported.

Pharmacokinetics

Linezolid is rapidly and completely absorbed following oral administration. Maximum plasma concentrations are achieved 1 to 2 hours after dosing. It is about 31% bound to plasma proteins. It is metabolized mainly by oxidation and is excreted in the urine as unchanged drug and inactive metabolites. The elimination half-life is 4.8 hours following intravenous administration and 4.6 to 5.4 hours following oral administration.

Uses and Administration

Linezolid is an oxazolidinone antibacterial used for the treatment of Gram-positive infections of the skin and respiratory tract, including those due to vancomycin-resistant enterococci and meticillin-resistant *Staphylococcus aureus*. It is given in a dose of 600 mg by mouth or by intravenous infusion every 12 hours for 10 to 28 days. In uncomplicated skin and skin structure infections the dose is 400 mg by mouth every 12 hours for 10 to 14 days.

◊ Reviews.
1. Diekema DJ, Jones RN. Oxazolidinones: a review. Drugs 2000; 59: 7–16.
2. Plouffe JF. Emerging therapies for serious gram-positive bacterial infections: a focus on linezolid. Clin Infect Dis 2000; 31(suppl 4): S144–S149.
3. French G. Linezolid. Int J Clin Pract 2001; 55: 59–63.
4. Fung HB, et al. Linezolid: an oxazolidinone antimicrobial agent. Clin Ther 2001; 23: 356–91.
5. Perry CM, Jarvis B. Linezolid: a review of its use in the management of serious gram-positive infections. Drugs 2001; 61: 525–51.
6. Bain KT, Wittbrodt ET. Linezolid for the treatment of resistant gram-positive cocci. Ann Pharmacother 2001; 35: 566–75.

Preparations

Proprietary Preparations (details are given in Part 3)
UK: Zyvox; *USA:* Zyvox.

Lomefloxacin Hydrochloride (5472-k)

Lomefloxacin Hydrochloride (BANM, USAN, rINNM).
NY-198; SC-47111; SC-47111A (lomefloxacin); SC-47111B (lomefloxacin mesilate). (RS)-1-Ethyl-6,8-difluoro-1,4-dihydro-7-(3-methylpiperazin-1-yl)-4-oxoquinoline-3-carboxylic acid hydrochloride.
$C_{17}H_{19}F_2N_3O_3$,HCl = 387.8.
CAS — 98079-51-7 (lomefloxacin); 98079-52-8 (lomefloxacin hydrochloride); 114394-67-1 (lomefloxacin mesilate).

NOTE. Lomefloxacin Mesilate is also USAN.

Adverse Effects and Precautions

As for Ciprofloxacin, p.183.

Concern has been expressed over the relatively high incidence of phototoxicity reactions in patients receiving lomefloxacin. Patients should be advised to avoid exposure to sunlight during, and for a few days after, lomefloxacin therapy, and to discontinue the drug immediately if phototoxicity occurs.

◊ References.
1. Arata J, et al. Photosensitivity reactions caused by lomefloxacin hydrochloride: a multicenter survey. Antimicrob Agents Chemother 1998; 42: 3141–5.

Interactions

As for Ciprofloxacin, p.184. Lomefloxacin does not appear to interact significantly with theophylline or caffeine.

Antimicrobial Action

As for Ciprofloxacin, p.184. Most streptococci, including *Streptococcus pneumoniae*, are relatively resistant to lomefloxacin. Cross-resistance between lomefloxacin and other quinolones has been reported.

◊ References.
1. Van der Auwera P, et al. In-vitro activity of lomefloxacin in comparison with pefloxacin and ofloxacin. J Antimicrob Chemother 1989; 23: 209–19.
2. Chambers ST, et al. Antimicrobial effects of lomefloxacin in vitro. J Antimicrob Chemother 1991; 27: 481–9.
3. Leigh DA, et al. Antibacterial activity of lomefloxacin. J Antimicrob Chemother 1991; 27: 589–98.
4. Banerjee DK, et al. In-vitro activity of lomefloxacin against pathogenic and environmental mycobacteria. J Antimicrob Chemother 1992; 30: 236–8.

Pharmacokinetics

Lomefloxacin is rapidly and almost completely absorbed following oral administration, peak plasma concentrations of about 3 µg per mL being attained about 1 to 1.5 hours after a 400-mg dose. Lomefloxacin is approximately 10% bound to plasma proteins. It is widely distributed into body tissues including the lungs and prostate.

The elimination half-life of lomefloxacin is about 7 to 8 hours, and is prolonged in patients with renal impairment. Lomefloxacin is excreted in the urine, mainly as unchanged drug but also in small amounts as the glucuronide and other metabolites. Small amounts are also eliminated unchanged in the faeces. Lomefloxacin is only removed in negligible amounts by haemodialysis.

◊ References.
1. Freeman CD, et al. Lomefloxacin clinical pharmacokinetics. Clin Pharmacokinet 1993; 25: 6–19.

Uses and Administration

Lomefloxacin is a fluoroquinolone antibacterial with actions and uses similar to those of ciprofloxacin (p.185).

It is given by mouth, as the hydrochloride, for the treatment of susceptible infections, including bronchitis due to *Haemophilus influenzae* or *Moraxella catarrhalis*, and urinary-tract infections. The usual dose is the equivalent of 400 mg of lomefloxacin base once daily. Evening administration may minimise the risk of phototoxicity reactions.

Dosage should be reduced in patients with moderate to severe renal impairment; the initial dose of 400 mg should be followed by maintenance doses of 200 mg daily in those with a creatinine clearance less than 40 mL per minute.

It is also administered topically as the hydrochloride as 0.3% eye drops for the treatment of bacterial conjunctivitis.

◊ General references.
1. Wadworth AN, Goa KL. Lomefloxacin: a review of its antibacterial activity, pharmacokinetic properties and therapeutic use. Drugs 1991; 42: 1018–60.
2. Neu HC, ed. Lomefloxacin: development of a once-a-day quinolone. Am J Med 1992; 92 (suppl 4A): 1S–137S.

Preparations

Proprietary Preparations (details are given in Part 3)
Aust.: Uniquin; *Braz.:* Maxaquin; *Denm.:* Okacin; *Fin.:* Okacin; *Fr.:* Decalogiflox; Logiflox; *Hong Kong:* Maxaquin; Okacin; *Israel:* Maxaquin; *Ital.:* Chimono; Maxaquin; Okacin; Uniquin; *Jpn:* Bareon†; Lomeflon†; *Mex.:* Lomacin; Maxaquin; *Port.:* Loxina; Maxaquin; Monoquin; Okacin; Uniquin; *S.Afr.:* Maxaquin; Okacyn; Uniquin; *Switz.:* Maxaquin; Okacin; *Thai.:* Maxaquin; Okacin; *UAE:* Lomax; *UK:* Okacyn; *USA:* Maxaquin.

Loracarbef (5477-f)

Loracarbef (BAN, USAN, rINN).
LY-163892. (6R,7S)-3-Chloro-8-oxo-7-D-phenylglycylamino-1-azabicyclo[4.2.0]oct-2-ene-2-carboxylic acid monohydrate.
$C_{16}H_{16}ClN_3O_4$,H_2O = 367.8.
CAS — 76470-66-1 (anhydrous loracarbef); 121961-22-6 (loracarbef monohydrate).
ATC — J01DA38.
Pharmacopoeias. In US.

Approximately 105 mg of loracarbef monohydrate is equivalent to 100 mg of anhydrous loracarbef.

Pharmacopoeial description
USP 25: pH of a 10% suspension in water is between 3.0 and 5.5. Store in airtight containers.

Adverse Effects and Precautions

Adverse effects of loracarbef are generally similar to those of other beta lactams (see Benzylpenicillin, p.157, and Cefalotin, p.162). They include gastrointestinal disturbances, particularly diarrhoea, and hypersensitivity reactions such as skin rashes. Increases in liver enzymes and abnormalities in haematological parameters have been reported.

Loracarbef should not be given to patients known to be hypersensitive to it or to other beta lactams because of the possibility of cross-sensitivity. It should be given with caution, with appropriate dosage reduction, in patients with impaired renal function.

Effects on the kidneys. References.
1. Thieme RE, et al. Acute interstitial nephritis associated with loracarbef therapy. J Pediatr 1995; 127: 997–1000.

Interactions

Probenecid decreases the renal excretion of loracarbef thereby increasing its plasma concentrations.

Antimicrobial Action

Loracarbef is bactericidal with antibacterial activity similar to that of cefaclor (p.161).

◊ References.
1. Knapp CC, Washington JA. In vitro activities of LY-163892, cefaclor, and cefuroxime. Antimicrob Agents Chemother 1988; 32: 131–3.
2. Cao C, et al. In-vitro activity and β-lactamase stability of LY-163892. J Antimicrob Chemother 1988; 22: 155–65.
3. Jones RN, Barry AL. Antimicrobial activity of LY-163892, an orally administered 1-carbacephem. J Antimicrob Chemother 1988; 22: 315–20.
4. Howard AJ, Dunkin KT. Comparative in-vitro activity of a new oral carbacephem, LY-163892. J Antimicrob Chemother 1988; 22: 445–56.
5. Shelton S, Nelson JD. In vitro susceptibilities of common pediatric pathogens to LY-163892. Antimicrob Agents Chemother 1988; 32: 268–70.
6. Doern GV, et al. In vitro activity of loracarbef (LY-163892), a new oral carbacephem antimicrobial agent, against respiratory isolates of Haemophilus influenzae and Moraxella catarrhalis. Antimicrob Agents Chemother 1991; 35: 1504–7.
7. Arguedas AG, et al. In-vitro activity of cefprozil (BMY-28100) and loracarbef (LY-163892) against pathogens obtained from middle ear fluid. J Antimicrob Chemother 1991; 27: 311–18.

Pharmacokinetics

Loracarbef is well absorbed from the gastrointestinal tract with a bioavailability of 90%. Peak plasma concentrations following 200- and 400-mg doses as capsules are about 8 and 14 µg per mL respectively at 1.2 hours. Peak concentrations are achieved more rapidly following administration as oral suspension and a paediatric dose of 15 mg per kg body-weight produces a concentration of approximately 19 µg per mL within 40 to 60 minutes. Absorption is delayed by the presence of food. A plasma half-life of about 1 hour has been reported which may be prolonged in renal impairment. About 25% is bound to plasma proteins.

Loracarbef is excreted largely unchanged in the urine, and therapeutic concentrations are maintained in the urine for up to 12 hours. Probenecid delays excretion. Loracarbef is removed by haemodialysis.

◊ References.
1. Nelson JD, et al. Pharmacokinetics of LY-163892 in infants and children. Antimicrob Agents Chemother 1988; 32: 1738–9.
2. Kusmiesz H, et al. Loracarbef concentrations in middle ear fluid. Antimicrob Agents Chemother 1990; 34: 2030–1.

3. Therasse DG, *et al.* Effects of renal dysfunction on the pharmacokinetics of loracarbef. *Clin Pharmacol Ther* 1993; **54:** 311–16.
4. Lees AS, *et al.* The pharmacokinetics, tissue penetration and in-vitro activity of loracarbef, a β-lactam antibiotic of the carbacephem class. *J Antimicrob Chemother* 1993; **32:** 853–9.
5. Hill SL, *et al.* Sputum and serum pharmacokinetics of loracarbef (LY163892) in patients with chronic bronchial sepsis. *J Antimicrob Chemother* 1994; **33:** 129–36.
6. Sitar DS, *et al.* Pharmacokinetic disposition of loracarbef in healthy young men and women at steady state. *J Clin Pharmacol* 1994; **34:** 924–9.

Uses and Administration

Loracarbef is an oral carbacephem antibiotic. The carbacephems are closely related to the cephalosporins, but replacement of the sulfur atom in the 7-aminocephalosporanic acid nucleus by a methylene group is said to enhance stability. It is used similarly to cefaclor in the treatment of susceptible infections of the respiratory and urinary tracts and of skin and soft tissue. For details of these infections and their treatment, see under Choice of Antibacterial, p.114.

Loracarbef is given as the monohydrate. Doses are expressed in terms of the equivalent amount of anhydrous loracarbef. The usual adult dose is 200 to 400 mg every 12 hours. In uncomplicated urinary-tract infections, a dose of 200 mg daily may be adequate. A dose for children is 7.5 mg per kg body-weight every 12 hours for uncomplicated infections or 15 mg per kg every 12 hours for acute otitis media or acute maxillary sinusitis. Loracarbef should be given an hour before food or on an empty stomach. Doses should be reduced in patients with renal function impairment; patients with a creatinine clearance of 10 to 49 mL per minute may be given half the usual dose at the usual dosage interval or the full usual dose at twice the usual interval; patients with a creatinine clearance of less than 10 mL per minute may be treated with the usual dose given every 3 to 5 days. Patients on haemodialysis should receive another dose following dialysis.

◊ General references.
1. Moellering RC, Jacobs NF. Advances in outpatient antimicrobial therapy: loracarbef. *Am J Med* 1992; **92** (suppl 6A): 1S–10S.
2. Brogden RN, McTavish D. Loracarbef: a review of its antimicrobial activity, pharmacokinetic properties and therapeutic efficacy. *Drugs* 1993; **45:** 716–36.

Preparations

USP 25: Loracarbef Capsules; Loracarbef for Oral Suspension.

Proprietary Preparations (details are given in Part 3)
Aust.: Lorabid; Lorax; *Ger.:* Lorafem; *Hong Kong:* Lorabid; *Ital.:* Carbem†; *Mex.:* Carbac; Lorabid; *Neth.:* Lorax; *S.Afr.:* Lorabid; *Swed.:* Lorabid; *USA:* Lorabid.

Lymecycline   (100-a)

Lymecycline *(BAN, rINN)*.
Limeciclina; Tetracyclinemethylene lysine.
$C_{29}H_{38}N_4O_{10} = 602.6$.
CAS — 992-21-2.
ATC — J01AA04.
Pharmacopoeias. In *Br.*

Lymecycline 407 mg is approximately equivalent to 300 mg of tetracycline and to 325 mg of tetracycline hydrochloride.

Pharmacopoeial description

BP 2001: A water-soluble combination of tetracycline, lysine, and formaldehyde. A yellow, very hygroscopic, powder. Very soluble in water; slightly soluble in alcohol; practically insoluble in acetone, in chloroform, and in ether. It contains not more than 5% by weight of water. A 1% solution in water has a pH of 7.8 to 8.1. Store at a temperature not exceeding 25°. Protect from light.

Profile

Lymecycline is a tetracycline derivative with general properties similar to those of tetracycline (p.259).

Doses are expressed in terms of the equivalent amount of tetracycline base. The usual adult dose is the equivalent of 300 mg of tetracycline administered twice daily by mouth; in severe infections total daily doses of up to the equivalent of 1.2 g may be given. In the treatment of acne, the equivalent of 300 mg of tetracycline is given daily.

Preparations

BP 2001: Lymecycline Capsules.

Proprietary Preparations (details are given in Part 3)
Aust.: Tetralysal; *Belg.:* Tetralysal; *Denm.:* Tetralysal; *Fin.:* Tetralysal; *Fr.:* Tetralysal; *Irl.:* Tetralysal; *Norw.:* Tetralysal; *S.Afr.:* Tetralysal; *Swed.:* Tetralysal; *UK:* Tetralysal.

Mafenide Acetate   (4908-r)

Mafenide Acetate *(BANM, rINNM)*.
NSC-34632 (mafenide). α-Aminotoluene-*p*-sulphonamide acetate.
$C_7H_{10}N_2O_2S,C_2H_4O_2 = 246.3$.
CAS — 138-39-6 (mafenide); 13009-99-9 (mafenide acetate).

NOTE. Mafenide is *USAN*.
Pharmacopoeias. In *Chin.* and *US.* .

11.2 g of monograph substance is approximately equivalent to 8.5 g of mafenide.

Pharmacopoeial description

USP 25: A white to pale yellow crystalline powder. Freely soluble in water. pH of a 10% solution in water is between 6.4 and 6.8. Store in airtight containers. Protect from light.

Adverse Effects, Treatment, and Precautions

Mafenide is absorbed to some extent following topical application and may produce systemic effects similar to those of other sulfonamides (see Sulfamethoxazole, p.254). Fatal haemolytic anaemia with disseminated intravascular coagulation, related to glucose-6-phosphate dehydrogenase deficiency, has been reported.

Mafenide acetate cream may cause pain or a burning sensation on application to the burnt area, with occasional bleeding or excoriation. The separation of the eschar may be delayed and fungal invasion of the wound has been reported. By its action in inhibiting carbonic anhydrase, mafenide may cause metabolic acidosis and hyperventilation; acid-base balance should therefore be monitored, particularly in patients with extensive burns, or with pulmonary or renal impairment, and treatment should be temporarily suspended and continuous fluid therapy given if persistent acidosis occurs.

Pharmacokinetics

Mafenide is absorbed from wounds into the circulation and is metabolised to *p*-carboxybenzenesulfonamide which is excreted in the urine. The metabolite has no antibacterial action but retains the ability to inhibit carbonic anhydrase.

Uses and Administration

Mafenide is a sulfonamide that is not inactivated by *p*-aminobenzoic acid or by pus and serum. The acetate is used as a cream, containing the equivalent of mafenide 8.5%, in conjunction with debridement, for the prevention and treatment of infection, including *Pseudomonas aeruginosa*, in second- and third-degree burns (p.1104). A solution containing mafenide acetate 5% is also available for use under moist dressings in burns. Mafenide hydrochloride and mafenide propionate have also been used.

Preparations

USP 25: Mafenide Acetate Cream; Mafenide Acetate for Topical Solution.

Proprietary Preparations (details are given in Part 3)
USA: Sulfamylon.
Multi-ingredient: *Braz.:* Otosulf; *Ger.:* Combiamid†; *Spain:* Pental Forte; Pentalmicina†.

Magainins   (5484-r)

Profile

The magainins are a group of antimicrobial peptides derived from amphibians. A number of semisynthetic derivatives including MSI-78 (pexiganan acetate), MSI-93, and MSI-94 are under development as topical anti-infectives.

◊ References.
1. Chopra I. The magainins: antimicrobial peptides with potential for topical application. *J Antimicrob Chemother* 1993; **32:** 351–3.
2. Levison ME, *et al.* The bactericidal activity of magainins against Pseudomonas aeruginosa and Enterococcus faecium. *J Antimicrob Chemother* 1993; **32:** 577–85.
3. Fuchs PC, *et al.* In vitro antimicrobial activity of MSI-78, a magainin analog. *Antimicrob Agents Chemother* 1998; **42:** 1213–16.
4. Lamb HM, Wiseman LR. Pexiganan acetate. *Drugs* 1998; **56:** 1047–52.

Mandelic Acid   (5662-d)

Amygdalic Acid; Phenylglycolic Acid; Racemic Mandelic Acid. 2-Hydroxy-2-phenylacetic acid.
$C_8H_8O_3 = 152.1$.
CAS — 90-64-2; 17199-29-0 ((+)-mandelic acid); 611-72-3 ((±)-mandelic acid); 611-71-2 ((−)-mandelic acid).
ATC — B05CA06; G04AG05.
Pharmacopoeias. In *Neth.*

Profile

Mandelic acid has bacteriostatic properties and has been given by mouth in the treatment of urinary-tract infections, usually as the ammonium or calcium salt. It is excreted unchanged in the urine and has been effective against uncomplicated infections due to Gram-negative and a few Gram-positive species, provided that the pH is maintained below 5.5. Mandelic acid has also

been used as a 1% flushing solution for the maintenance of indwelling urinary catheters. Mandelic acid and acetyl mandelic acid have been used topically in preparations for the treatment of acne.

Gastrointestinal disturbances, dizziness and tinnitus, and dysuria or haematuria have been reported occasionally following ingestion of mandelic acid or its salts. It is contra-indicated in patients with impaired renal function.

Mandelic acid is a component of methenamine mandelate (p.223).

Preparations

Proprietary Preparations (details are given in Part 3)
Multi-ingredient: *Fr.:* Zeniac LP Fort; *Ital.:* NeoCeuticals Clear Skin; NeoCeuticals Spot Treatment; *Port.:* Mandelip.

Marbofloxacin   (15416-h)

Marbofloxacin *(BAN, rINN)*.
9-Fluoro-2,3-dihydro-3-methyl-10-(4-methyl-1-piperazinyl)-7-oxo-7*H*-pyrido[3,2,1-*ij*][4,1,2]benzoxadiazine-6-carboxylic acid.
$C_{17}H_{19}FN_4O_4 = 362.4$.
CAS — 115550-35-1.

Profile

Marbofloxacin is a fluoroquinolone antibacterial used in veterinary medicine.

Mecillinam   (102-x)

Mecillinam *(BAN, rINN)*.
Amdinocillin *(USAN)*; FL-1060; Ro-10-9070. (6*R*)-6-(Perhydroazepin-1-ylmethyleneamino)penicillanic acid.
$C_{15}H_{23}N_3O_3S = 325.4$.
CAS — 32887-01-7.
ATC — J01CA11.

Adverse Effects and Precautions

As for Benzylpenicillin, p.157.

Porphyria. Mecillinam has been associated with acute attacks of porphyria and is considered unsafe in porphyric patients.

Interactions

As for Benzylpenicillin, p.158.

Antimicrobial Action

Mecillinam is a derivative of amidinopenicillanic acid. Unlike benzylpenicillin and related antibiotics, it is active against many Gram-negative bacteria, in particular Enterobacteriaceae including *Escherichia coli*, *Enterobacter*, *Klebsiella*, *Salmonella*, and *Shigella* spp.; indole-positive *Proteus* and *Serratia marcescens* are generally resistant. It is less active against *Neisseria* spp. and *Haemophilus influenzae*. *Pseudomonas aeruginosa* and *Bacteroides* spp. are considered to be resistant. It is much less active against Gram-positive bacteria; enterococci including *Enterococcus faecalis* are resistant.

Mecillinam interferes with the synthesis of the bacterial cell wall by binding with a different penicillin-binding protein from benzylpenicillin. This difference in mode of action may explain the synergism against many Gram-negative organisms that has been reported *in vitro* between mecillinam and various penicillins or cephalosporins.

Mecillinam is inactivated by beta-lactamases, but is more stable than ampicillin.

Pharmacokinetics

Mecillinam is poorly absorbed from the gastrointestinal tract. Peak plasma concentrations of about 6 and 12 μg per mL have been achieved half an hour after intramuscular doses of 200 and 400 mg, respectively. The usual plasma half-life of about 1 hour has been reported to be prolonged to 3 or 4 hours in severe renal failure. Between 5 and 10% of mecillinam is bound to plasma proteins. Mecillinam is widely distributed into body tissues and fluids; little passes into the CSF unless the meninges are inflamed. It crosses the placenta into the fetal circulation; little appears to be distributed into breast milk.

Mecillinam is metabolised to only a limited extent. From 50 to 70% of a parenteral dose may be excreted in the urine within 6 hours by glomerular filtration and tubular secretion. Renal tubular secretion can be reduced by the concomitant use of probenecid. Some mecillinam is excreted in bile where high concentrations are achieved.

Mecillinam is removed by haemodialysis.

Uses and Administration

Mecillinam is a semisynthetic penicillin with a substituted amidino group at the 6-position of the penicillanic acid nucleus. It is given by slow intravenous injection, by intravenous infusion, or intramuscularly in the treatment of susceptible Gram-negative infections (see under Antimicrobial Action, above).

For urinary-tract infections a dose of 800 mg is given every 6 to 8 hours. A total dose of up to 60 mg per kg daily may be used in very severe infections.

Mecillinam has been administered in combination with other beta-lactams, particularly ampicillin (p.150), to extend the spectrum of antimicrobial activity to Gram-positive organisms and because of reported synergism against Gram-negative bacteria *in vitro*.

The pivaloyloxymethyl ester of mecillinam, pivmecillinam, is used orally (see p.237).

Preparations

Proprietary Preparations (details are given in Part 3)
Denm.: Selexid; *Norw.*: Selexid; *Swed.*: Selexid.

Meclocycline Sulfosalicylate (103-r)

Meclocycline Sulfosalicylate (USAN).

GS-2989 (meclocycline); Meclocycline Sulphosalicylate; NSC-78502 (meclocycline). (4S,4aR,5S,5aR,6S,12aS)-7-Chloro-4-dimethylamino-1,4,4a,5,5a,6,11,12a-octahydro-3,5,10,12,12a-pentahydroxy-6-methylene-1,11-dioxonaphthacene-2-carboxamide 5-sulphosalicylate; 7-Chloro-6-demethyl-6-deoxy-5β-hydroxy-6-methylenetetracycline 5-sulphosalicylate.

$C_{22}H_{21}ClN_2O_8,C_7H_6O_6S = 695.0$.
$CAS — 2013-58-3$ (meclocycline); 73816-42-9 (meclocycline sulfosalicylate).

NOTE. Meclocycline is *BAN*, *USAN*, and *rINN*.
Pharmacopoeias. In US.

Pharmacopoeial description

USP 25: pH of a 1% solution in water is between 2.5 and 3.5. Store in airtight containers. Protect from light.

Profile

Meclocycline is a tetracycline antibiotic derived from oxytetracycline (p.234). It is applied topically as the sulfosalicylate for the treatment of acne vulgaris and superficial skin infections. Potency is expressed in terms of meclocycline. Preparations containing the equivalent of 1 or 2% are available. Meclocycline sulfosalicylate has also been given as a pessary in the treatment of vulvovaginal infections.

Preparations

USP 25: Meclocycline Sulfosalicylate Cream.

Proprietary Preparations (details are given in Part 3)
Ger.: Meclosorb; *Ital.*: Mecloderm; Mecloderm Antiacne; Mecloderm Ovuli; Mecloderm Polvere Aspersoria; Meclutin Semplice; Novacnyl; Traumatociclina; *Spain*: Quoderm; *USA*: Meclan.

Multi-ingredient: *Ital.*: Anti-Acne; Mecloderm F; Meclutin.

Meropenem (5491-x)

Meropenem (BAN, USAN, rINN).

ICI-194660; SM-7338. (4R,5S,6S)-3-[(3S,5S)-5-Dimethylcarbamoylpyrrolidin-3-ylthio]-6-[(R)-1-hydroxyethyl]-4-methyl-7-oxo-1-azabicyclo[3.2.0]hept-2-ene-2-carboxylic acid trihydrate.

$C_{17}H_{25}N_3O_5S,3H_2O = 437.5$.
$CAS — 96036-03-2$ (meropenem); 119478-56-7 (meropenem trihydrate).
$ATC — J01DH02$.

Pharmacopoeias. In US.

Pharmacopoeial description

USP 25: Colourless to white crystals. Sparingly soluble in water; very slightly soluble in alcohol; practically insoluble in acetone and in ether; soluble in dimethylformamide and in 5% monobasic potassium phosphate solution. pH of a 1% solution in water is between 4.0 and 6.0. Store in airtight containers.

Adverse Effects and Precautions

As for Imipenem, p.214.

Meropenem is more stable to renal dehydropeptidase I than imipenem and administration with cilastatin, which inhibits this enzyme, is not required. Meropenem may have less potential to induce seizures than imipenem (see also below).

Effects on the nervous system. *Animal* studies have indicated that meropenem induces fewer seizures than imipenem-cilastatin and clinical data from the manufacturer have substantiated this.[1] Comparison of data from 3125 patients with a variety of infections (sometimes including meningitis) treated with meropenem with that from 2886 patients who received other antibacterials, principally cephalosporin-based regimens or imipenem-cilastatin, showed that meropenem was not associated with any greater risk of seizures than the other antibacterials and was likely to have less neurotoxic potential than imipenem-cilastatin, making it a suitable drug to use in the treatment of meningitis.

1. Norrby SR, *et al.* Safety profile of meropenem: international clinical experience based on the first 3125 patients treated with meropenem. *J Antimicrob Chemother* 1995; **36** (suppl A): 207–23.

Interactions

Probenecid inhibits the renal excretion of meropenem thereby increasing its plasma concentrations and prolonging its elimination half-life.

Antiepileptics. For a report of decreased plasma-*valproate* concentrations associated with antibacterial therapy containing meropenem, see p.368.

Antimicrobial Action

As for Imipenem, p.214.

Meropenem is slightly more active than imipenem against Enterobacteriaceae and slightly less active against Gram-positive organisms.

Pharmacokinetics

Following intravenous injection of meropenem 0.5 and 1.0 g over 5 minutes, peak plasma concentrations of about 50 and 112 μg per mL respectively are attained. The same doses infused over 30 minutes produce peak plasma concentrations of 23 and 49 μg per mL, respectively.

Meropenem has a plasma elimination half-life of about one hour; this may be prolonged in patients with renal impairment and is also slightly prolonged in children. Meropenem is widely distributed into body tissues and fluids including the CSF and bile. It is more stable to renal dehydropeptidase I than imipenem and is mainly excreted in the urine by tubular secretion and glomerular filtration. About 70% of a dose is recovered unchanged in the urine over a 12-hour period and urinary concentrations above 10 μg per mL are maintained for up to 5 hours after a 500-mg dose. Meropenem has one inactive metabolite which is excreted in the urine.

Meropenem is removed by haemodialysis.

◊ References.

1. Hextall A, *et al.* Intraperitoneal penetration of meropenem. *J Antimicrob Chemother* 1991; **28**: 314–16.
2. Leroy A, *et al.* Pharmacokinetics of meropenem (ICI 194,660) and its metabolite (ICI 213,689) in healthy subjects and in patients with renal impairment. *Antimicrob Agents Chemother* 1992; **36**: 2794–8.
3. Chimata M, *et al.* Pharmacokinetics of meropenem in patients with various degrees of renal function, including patients with end-stage renal disease. *Antimicrob Agents Chemother* 1993; **37**: 229–33.
4. Bergogne-Bérézin E, *et al.* Concentration of meropenem in serum and in bronchial secretions in patients undergoing fibreoptic bronchoscopy. *Eur J Clin Pharmacol* 1994; **46**: 87–8. Correction. *ibid.*; 282.
5. Dagan R, *et al.* Penetration of meropenem into the cerebrospinal fluid of patients with inflamed meninges. *J Antimicrob Chemother* 1994; **34**: 175–9.
6. Mouton JW, Van den Anker JN. Meropenem clinical pharmacokinetics. *Clin Pharmacokinet* 1995; **28**: 275–86.
7. Blumer JL, *et al.* Sequential, single-dose pharmacokinetic evaluation of meropenem in hospitalized infants and children. *Antimicrob Agents Chemother* 1995; **39**: 1721–5.
8. Novelli A, *et al.* Clinical pharmacokinetics of meropenem after the first and tenth intramuscular administration. *J Antimicrob Chemother* 1996; **37**: 775–81.
9. Krueger WA, *et al.* Pharmacokinetics of meropenem in critically ill patients with acute renal failure treated by continuous hemodiafiltration. *Antimicrob Agents Chemother* 1998; **42**: 2421–4.
10. Tegeder I, *et al.* Pharmacokinetics of meropenem in critically ill patients with acute renal failure undergoing continuous venovenous hemofiltration. *Clin Pharmacol Ther* 1999; **65**: 50–7.
11. Thalhammer F, *et al.* Continuous infusion versus intermittent administration of meropenem in critically ill patients. *J Antimicrob Chemother* 1999; **43**: 523–7.

Uses and Administration

Meropenem is a carbapenem beta-lactam antibiotic with actions and uses similar to those of imipenem (p.215). It is more stable to renal dehydropeptidase I than imipenem and need not be given in association with an enzyme inhibitor such as cilastatin. It is used in the treatment of susceptible infections including intra-abdominal infections, meningitis, respiratory-tract infections (including in cystic fibrosis patients), septicaemia, skin infections, urinary-tract infections, and infections in immunocompromised patients. For details of these infections and their treatment, see under Choice of Antibacterial, p.114.

Meropenem is administered intravenously as the trihydrate, but doses are expressed in terms of the amount of anhydrous meropenem. It is given by slow injection over 3 to 5 minutes or by infusion over 15 to 30 minutes in a usual adult dose of 0.5 to 1 g every 8 hours, increased to 2 g every 8 hours for meningitis; doses of up to 2 g every 8 hours have also been used in cystic fibrosis. Doses should be reduced in patients

with renal impairment. The following doses may be given based on creatinine clearance: creatinine clearance 26 to 50 mL per minute, the usual dose given every 12 hours; 10 to 25 mL per minute, one-half the usual dose every 12 hours; less than 10 mL per minute, one-half the usual dose every 24 hours.

Children over 3 months of age and weighing less than 50 kg may be given 10 to 20 mg per kg body-weight every 8 hours, increased to 40 mg per kg every 8 hours for meningitis. Doses of 25 to 40 mg per kg every 8 hours have been used in children with cystic fibrosis.

◊ Reviews.

1. Pryka RD, Haig GM. Meropenem: a new carbapenem antimicrobial. *Ann Pharmacother* 1994; **28**: 1045–54.
2. Wiseman LR, *et al.* Meropenem: a review of its antibacterial activity, pharmacokinetic properties and clinical efficacy. *Drugs* 1995; **50**: 73–101.
3. Finch RG, *et al.* eds. Meropenem: focus on clinical performance. *J Antimicrob Chemother* 1995; **36** (suppl A): 1–223.
4. Hellinger WC, Brewer NS. Carbapenems and monobactams: imipenem, meropenem, and aztreonam. *Mayo Clin Proc* 1999; **74**: 420–34.
5. Hurst M, Lamb HM. Meropenem: a review of its use in patients in intensive care. *Drugs* 2000; **59**: 653–80.
6. Lowe MN, Lamb HM. Meropenem: an updated review of its use in the management of intra-abdominal infections. *Drugs* 2000; **60**: 619–46.

Preparations

USP 25: Meropenem for Injection.

Proprietary Preparations (details are given in Part 3)
Aust.: Optinem; *Austral.*: Merrem; *Belg.*: Meronem; *Canad.*: Merrem; *Denm.*: Meronem; *Fin.*: Meronem; *Ger.*: Meronem; *Hong Kong*: Meronem; *Irl.*: Meronem; *Israel*: Meronem; *Ital.*: Merrem; *Jpn*: Meropen; *Mex.*: Merrem; *Neth.*: Meronem; *Norw.*: Meronem; *NZ*: Merrem; *Port.*: Meronem; *S.Afr.*: Meronem; *Singapore*: Meronem; *Spain*: Meronem; *Swed.*: Meronem; *Switz.*: Meronem; *Thai.*: Meronem; *UK*: Meronem; *USA*: Merrem.

Metampicillin (185-c)

Metampicillin (rINN).

(6R)-6-(D-2-Methyleneamino-2-phenylacetamido)penicillanic acid.

$C_{17}H_{19}N_3O_4S = 361.4$.
$CAS — 6489-97-0$.
$ATC — J01CA14$.

Metampicillin Sodium (104-f)

Metampicillin Sodium (rINNM).
$C_{17}H_{18}N_3NaO_4S = 383.4$.
$CAS — 6489-61-8$.

Profile

Metampicillin has actions and uses similar to those of ampicillin (p.150).

After oral administration it is almost completely hydrolysed to ampicillin. When given parenterally, however, a proportion of the administered dose exists in the circulation as unchanged metampicillin which has some antibacterial activity of its own. Metampicillin has been given by mouth or by intramuscular or intravenous injection in usual doses of 1 to 2 g daily in four divided doses, as metampicillin or as the sodium salt.

Preparations

Proprietary Preparations (details are given in Part 3)
Braz.: Pravacilin; *Fr.*: Suvipen†; *Spain*: Dompil; Meta Framan; Metakes; Serfabiotic.

Multi-ingredient: *Spain*: Pulmosterin Meta†.

Methacycline Hydrochloride (105-d)

Methacycline Hydrochloride (BANM).

Metacycline Hydrochloride (pINNM); GS-2876 (methacycline); Metacyclini Chloridum; Méthylènecycline Chlorhydrate; 6-Methyleneoxytetracycline Hydrochloride. (4S,4aR,5S,5aR,6S,12aS)-4-Dimethylamino-1,4,4a,5,5a,6,11,12a-octahydro-3,5,10,12,12a-pentahydroxy-6-methylene-1,11-dioxonaphthacene-2-carboxamide hydrochloride; 6-Demethyl-6-deoxy-5β-hydroxy-6-methylenetetracycline hydrochloride.

$C_{22}H_{22}N_2O_8,HCl = 478.9$.
$CAS — 914-00-1$ (methacycline); 3963-95-9 (methacycline hydrochloride).

NOTE. Methacycline is *USAN*.
Pharmacopoeias. In Pol. and US.

Methacycline 92 mg is approximately equivalent to 100 mg of methacycline hydrochloride.

Pharmacopoeial description

USP 25: A yellow to dark yellow crystalline powder. Soluble 1 in 100 of water, 1 in 300 of alcohol, and 1 in 25 of 0.1N sodium hydroxide; very slightly soluble in chloroform and in ether. pH of a solution in water containing the equivalent of methacycline 1% is between 2.0 and 3.0. Store in airtight containers. Protect from light.

Adverse Effects and Precautions
As for Tetracycline Hydrochloride, p.259.

Interactions
As for Tetracycline Hydrochloride, p.259.

Antimicrobial Action
As for Tetracycline Hydrochloride, p.259.

Pharmacokinetics
As for Tetracycline Hydrochloride, p.260.

Around 60% of a dose by mouth is absorbed. About 80 to 95% of methacycline in the circulation is bound to plasma proteins. Plasma concentrations of up to 2.6 µg per mL have been reported 4 hours after a 300-mg dose of methacycline. Its biological half-life is about 14 to 15 hours. About 60% of a dose is slowly excreted unchanged in the urine.

Uses and Administration
Methacycline is a tetracycline derivative with uses similar to those of tetracycline (p.260). Like demeclocycline, it is excreted more slowly than tetracycline and effective blood concentrations are maintained for longer periods.

Methacycline hydrochloride is administered by mouth in a usual dose of 600 mg daily in two divided doses, preferably 1 hour before or 2 hours after meals.

Preparations
USP 25: Methacycline Hydrochloride Capsules; Methacycline Hydrochloride Oral Suspension.

Proprietary Preparations (details are given in Part 3)
Aust.: Optimycin†; *Austral.:* Rondomycin†; *Fr.:* Lysocline; Physiomycine; *Ital.:* Esarondil; Rotilen; Stafilon; *Swed.:* Rondomycin†.

Multi-ingredient: *Aust.:* Optimycin S†.

Methaniazide (7562-I)
Methaniazide *(rINN)*.

Isoniazid Mesylate; Isoniazid Methanesulfonate. 2-Isonicotinoylhydrazinomethanesulphonic acid.
$C_7H_9N_3O_4S = 231.2.$
CAS — 13447-95-5 (methaniazide); 6059-26-3 (calcium methaniazide); 3804-89-5 (sodium methaniazide).

Profile
Methaniazide is a derivative of isoniazid (p.215). It has been administered as the calcium salt in the treatment of tuberculosis. The sodium salt has also been used.

Preparations
Proprietary Preparations (details are given in Part 3)
Aust.: Neo-Tizide†.

Methenamine (5657-m)
Methenamine *(rINN)*.

Aminoform; E239; Esametilentetrammina; Esammina; Formine; Hexamethylenamine; Hexamine; Metenammina; Urotropine. Hexamethylenetetramine; 1,3,5,7-Tetraazatricyclo[3.3.1.1³,⁷]decane.
$C_6H_{12}N_4 = 140.2.$
CAS — 100-97-0.
ATC — G04AA01.
Pharmacopoeias. In Chin., Eur. (see p.vi), Pol., and US.

Pharmacopoeial description
Ph. Eur.: A white crystalline powder or colourless crystals. Freely soluble in water; soluble in alcohol and in dichloromethane. Protect from light.
USP 25: Colourless, practically odourless, lustrous crystals or white crystalline powder. Soluble 1 in 1.5 of water, 1 in 12.5 of alcohol, 1 in 10 of chloroform, and 1 in 320 of ether. Its solutions are alkaline to litmus.

Methenamine Hippurate (5660-r)
Methenamine Hippurate *(BAN, USAN, rINNM)*.

Hexamine Hippurate. Hexamethylenetetramine hippurate.
$C_6H_{12}N_4,C_9H_9NO_3 = 319.4.$
CAS — 5714-73-8.
Pharmacopoeias. In US.

Methenamine Mandelate (5661-f)
Methenamine Mandelate *(rINNM)*.

Hexamine Amygdalate; Hexamine Mandelate; Mandelato de Metenamina. Hexamethylenetetramine mandelate.
$C_6H_{12}N_4,C_8H_8O_3 = 292.3.$
CAS — 587-23-5.
Pharmacopoeias. In US.

Pharmacopoeial description
USP 25: A white, practically odourless crystalline powder. Very soluble in water; soluble 1 in 10 of alcohol, 1 in 20 of chloroform, and 1 in 350 of ether. Its solutions have a pH of about 4.

The symbol † denotes a preparation no longer actively marketed

---

Adverse Effects and Precautions
Methenamine and its salts are generally well tolerated but may cause gastrointestinal disturbances such as nausea, vomiting, and diarrhoea. Skin rashes, and occasionally other hypersensitivity reactions, may occur.

Comparatively large amounts of the active moiety formaldehyde may be formed during prolonged administration or when large doses are used, and may give rise to irritation and inflammation of the urinary tract especially the bladder, painful and frequent micturition, haematuria, and proteinuria. The effect of the formaldehyde may be diluted by administering alkalinising drugs such as sodium bicarbonate or large quantities of water but it is then less effective.

Methenamine and its salts are contra-indicated in patients with hepatic insufficiency because of the liberation of ammonia in the gastrointestinal tract. Although methenamine itself is not contra-indicated in renal insufficiency, the salts should be avoided, at any rate in severe insufficiency, because of the risk of mandelate or hippurate crystalluria. They should also be avoided in patients with severe dehydration, metabolic acidosis, or gout.

Interference with laboratory estimations for catecholamines, 17-hydroxycorticosteroids, and oestrogens in the urine has been reported.

Interactions
The concomitant use of drugs that alkalinise the urine, including some antacids, potassium citrate, and diuretics such as acetazolamide or the thiazides should be avoided because the activation of methenamine to formaldehyde may be inhibited.

The concomitant administration of methenamine and sulfonamides may increase the risk of crystalluria since methenamine requires low urinary pH for its effect, at which sulfonamides and their metabolites are poorly soluble; methenamine may also form poorly soluble compounds with some sulfonamides.

Antimicrobial Action
Methenamine owes its antibacterial properties to formaldehyde, a non-specific bactericide, which is slowly liberated by hydrolysis at acid pH. Most Gram-positive and Gram-negative organisms and fungi are susceptible, usually at MICs of around 20 µg per mL. Hippuric and mandelic acids have some antibacterial activity *in vitro*, but their contribution to the antibacterial action of the salts *in vivo*, beyond assisting the maintenance of low urinary pH, is uncertain. Urea-splitting organisms such as *Proteus* and some *Pseudomonas* spp. tend to increase urinary pH and inhibit the release of formaldehyde, thereby decreasing the effectiveness of methenamine. The concomitant use of acetohydroxamic acid, a potent inhibitor of bacterial urease, has been suggested for urinary infections due to these organisms. True resistance to formaldehyde does not appear to be a problem in clinical use.

Pharmacokinetics
Methenamine is readily absorbed from the gastrointestinal tract and widely distributed in the body. Under acid conditions methenamine is slowly hydrolysed to formaldehyde and ammonia: about 10 to 30% of a dose may be converted in the stomach unless it is given as an enteric-coated preparation. Almost no hydrolysis of methenamine takes place at physiological pH, and it is therefore virtually inactive in the body. The half-life is reported to be approximately 4 hours. Methenamine is rapidly and almost completely eliminated in the urine, and provided this is acid (preferably below pH 5.5) bactericidal concentrations of formaldehyde are achieved; because of the time taken for hydrolysis, however, these are not achieved until the urine reaches the bladder, with peak concentrations up to 2 hours after administration. Absorption, and hence excretion, may be somewhat delayed in patients given enteric-coated formulations.

Small amounts of methenamine may be distributed into breast milk.

The mandelate and hippurate moieties are also rapidly absorbed and are excreted in urine by tubular secretion as well as glomerular filtration.

Uses and Administration
Methenamine is used, usually as the hippurate or mandelate, in the prophylaxis and treatment of chronic or recurrent, uncomplicated, lower urinary-tract infections and asymptomatic bacteriuria. It has been considered suitable for long-term use because acquired resistance does not appear to develop.

Methenamine and its salts should not be used in upper urinary-tract infections because it is eliminated too rapidly to exert an effect, nor in acute urinary infections. It is only active in acid urine, when formaldehyde is released, and although hippuric or mandelic acid helps to acidify the urine, administration of ammonium chloride or ascorbic acid may be tried. If urea-splitting bacteria such as *Proteus* or some *Pseudomonas* spp. are present they may produce so much ammonia that the urine cannot be acidified (see also Antimicrobial Action, above).

The usual adult dose of methenamine or methenamine mandelate is 1 g by mouth four times daily; a dose of about 15 mg per kg body-weight four times daily has been suggested in children up to 6 years of age and 0.5 g four times daily in those aged 6 to 12 years. Methenamine hippurate is given in a usual adult dose of 1 g twice daily, or 0.5 g twice daily in children 6 to 12 years of age.

Topically, methenamine has been used in deodorant preparations, since in the presence of acid sweat it liberates formaldehyde. Methenamine calcium thiocyanate has been used in combination with other ingredients in preparations for upper respiratory-tract disorders.

Preparations
USP 25: Methenamine Elixir; Methenamine Hippurate Tablets; Methenamine Mandelate Delayed-release Tablets; Methenamine Mandelate for Oral Solution; Methenamine Mandelate Oral Suspension; Methenamine Mandelate Tablets; Methenamine Tablets.

Proprietary Preparations (details are given in Part 3)
Aust.: Antihydral; Hiprex; *Austral.:* Hiprex; *Belg.:* Hiprex; *Braz.:* Neohexal; *Canad.:* Dehydral; Hiprex†; Mandelamine; Urasal; *Denm.:* Geasalol; Haiprex; *Fin.:* Hipeksal; Hiprex; *Ger.:* Antihydral; Mandelamine†; Urotractan; *Irl.:* Hiprex; *Israel:* Hiprex; *Mex.:* Mandelan; Mandepiril; *Neth.:* Reflux†; *Norw.:* Hiprex; *NZ:* Hiprex; *S.Afr.:* Hippramine; Mandelamine; *Swed.:* Hippuran†; Hiprex; *Switz.:* Antihydral; Mandelamine†; *UK:* Hiprex; *USA:* Hiprex; Mandelamine; Urex.

Multi-ingredient: *Aust.:* Antihydral M; *Belg.:* Carbobel; Mictasol; *Braz.:* Abacaterol; Acridin; Cezane; Colagolen; Cystex; Pyelodion; Sepurin; Urodonal; Uropirite; Urosalin; Uroseptin; *Fr.:* Aromalgyl†; Mictasol; *Ger.:* Antihydral M; *Hong Kong:* Antihydral M; *Mex.:* Furanton; *Port.:* Urocrasina; *S.Afr.:* Azo-Mandelamine†; *Switz.:* Antihydral M; *USA:* Atrosept; Cystex; Dolsed; Prosed/DS; Trac Tabs 2X; UAA; Uridon Modified; Urimar-T; Urimax; Urised; Urisedamine; Uro-Phosphate; Urogesic Blue; Uroqid-Acid.

Meticillin Sodium (106-n)
Meticillin Sodium *(rINNM)*.

BRL-1241; Dimethoxyphenecillin Sodium; Dimethoxyphenyl Penicillin Sodium; Methicillin Sodium *(BANM, USAN)*; Meticillinum Natricum; SQ-16123; X-1497. Sodium (6R)-6-(2,6-dimethoxybenzamido)penicillanate monohydrate.
$C_{17}H_{19}N_2NaO_6S,H_2O = 420.4.$
CAS — 61-32-5 (meticillin); 132-92-3 (anhydrous meticillin sodium); 7246-14-2 (meticillin sodium monohydrate).
Pharmacopoeias. In It.

1.11 g of monograph substance is approximately equivalent to 1 g of anhydrous meticillin. Each g of monograph substance represents about 2.4 mmol of sodium.

Meticillin sodium has been reported to be incompatible with aminoglycosides and a number of other antimicrobials. It has also been reported to be incompatible with acidic and alkaline drugs.

Adverse Effects and Precautions
As for Benzylpenicillin, p.157.

Meticillin is the penicillin most commonly associated with acute interstitial nephritis.

Effects on the kidneys. References.
1. Sanjad SA, *et al.* Nephropathy, an underestimated complication of methicillin therapy. *J Pediatr* 1974; **84:** 873–7.
2. Galpin JE, *et al.* Acute interstitial nephritis due to methicillin. *Am J Med* 1978; **65:** 756–65.

Interactions
As for Benzylpenicillin, p.158.

Antimicrobial Action
Meticillin has a mode of action similar to that of benzylpenicillin (p.158) but it is resistant to staphylococcal penicillinase. There is evidence that meticillin is more stable to staphylococcal penicillinase than the other penicillinase-resistant penicillins.

Meticillin is active against both penicillinase-producing and non-penicillinase-producing staphylococci, and also against *Streptococcus pyogenes* (group A beta-haemolytic streptococci), *Str. pneumoniae*, and some viridans streptococci. It is virtually ineffective against *Enterococcus faecalis*.

The minimum inhibitory concentration against susceptible penicillinase-producing and non-penicillinase-producing staphylococci, is usually within the range of 1 to 4 µg per mL. Its activity against penicillin-sensitive staphylococci and streptococci is less than that of benzylpenicillin.

Resistance of staphylococci to meticillin is due to the expression of an altered penicillin-binding protein and is not dependent on penicillinase production. There is cross-resistance with other penicillins, including the penicillinase-resistant penicillins cloxacillin, dicloxacillin, flucloxacillin, nafcillin, and oxacillin, and with the cephalosporins. Meticillin-resistant staphylococci are also frequently resistant to other antibacterials including aminoglycosides, chloramphenicol, ciprofloxacin, clindamycin, erythromycin, and tetracycline. The incidence of such resistance has varied considerably. However, both endemic (restricted to one hospital) and epidemic (affecting more than one hospital) strains of meticillin-resistant *Staphylococcus aureus* (MRSA) are now recognised and infections are a problem in many hospitals. There have been fewer studies on coagulase-negative staphylococci, but patterns of meticillin resistance in *Staph. epidermidis* are similar to those for MRSA and the frequency of resistance may be higher.

For further details on meticillin-resistant staphylococci and the management of infections, see under Staphylococcal Infections, p.140.

◊ References to meticillin-resistant staphylococci.
1. Hackbarth CJ, Chambers HF. Methicillin-resistant staphylococci: genetics and mechanisms of resistance. *Antimicrob Agents Chemother* 1989; **33**: 991–4.
2. Maple PAC, *et al.* World-wide antibiotic resistance in methicillin-resistant Staphylococcus aureus. *Lancet* 1989; **i**: 537–40.
3. Mouton RP, *et al.* Correlations between consumption of antibiotics and methicillin resistance in coagulase negative staphylococci. *J Antimicrob Chemother* 1990; **26**: 573–83.
4. Marples RR, Reith S. Methicillin-resistant Staphylococcus aureus in England and Wales. *Commun Dis Rep* 1992; **2**: R25–R29.
5. de Lencastre H, *et al.* Molecular aspects of methicillin resistance in Staphylococcus aureus. *J Antimicrob Chemother* 1994; **33**: 7–24.
6. Fluckiger U, Widmer AF. Epidemiology of methicillin-resistant Staphylococcus aureus. *Chemotherapy* 1999; **45**: 121–34.

Pharmacokinetics
Meticillin is inactivated by gastric acid and must be given by injection. Peak plasma concentrations are attained within 0.5 to 1 hour of an intramuscular injection; concentrations of up to 18 µg per mL have been achieved after a dose of 1 g. A half-life of 0.5 to 1 hour has been reported, although this may be increased to 3 to 6 hours in renal impairment. About 40% of the meticillin in the circulation is bound to plasma proteins. It is widely distributed in body fluids and in tissues, but there is little diffusion into the CSF unless the meninges are inflamed. Meticillin also crosses the placenta and appears in breast milk. Relatively high concentrations are achieved in bile compared with plasma, although only small amounts are excreted in bile. The majority is rapidly excreted by tubular secretion and glomerular filtration; up to 80% of an injected dose has been detected unchanged in the urine.

Plasma concentrations are enhanced if probenecid is given concomitantly. They may be reduced in patients with cystic fibrosis.

Uses and Administration
Meticillin is a penicillinase-resistant penicillin and has been used similarly to flucloxacillin (p.207) in the treatment of staphylococcal infections resistant to benzylpenicillin.

It is not active by mouth and is given by injection as the sodium salt. In severe renal impairment a reduction in dosage may be necessary.

The usual dosage of meticillin sodium is 1 g every 4 to 6 hours intramuscularly, or intravenously by slow injection over 3 to 4 minutes or by intravenous infusion. In severe infections up to 12 g daily may be given intravenously in divided doses.

Preparations
Proprietary Preparations (details are given in Part 3)
Denm.: Lucopenin†; **Ital.:** Staficyn; **USA:** Staphcillin†.

Mezlocillin Sodium (107-h)

Mezlocillin Sodium (BANM, rINNM).
Bay-f-1353. Sodium (6R)-6-[D-2-(3-mesyl-2-oxoimidazolidine-1-carboxamido)-2-phenylacetamido]penicillanate monohydrate.
$C_{21}H_{24}N_5NaO_8S_2,H_2O = 579.6$.
CAS — 51481-65-3 (mezlocillin); 42057-22-7 (anhydrous mezlocillin sodium); 59798-30-0 (anhydrous mezlocillin sodium).

NOTE. Mezlocillin is *USAN*.
Pharmacopoeias. In US.

1.07 g of monograph substance is approximately equivalent to 1 g of anhydrous mezlocillin. Each g of monograph substance represents about 1.7 mmol of sodium.

Incompatibility has been reported with aminoglycosides, ciprofloxacin, metronidazole, and tetracyclines.

Pharmacopoeial description
USP 25: A white to pale yellow crystalline powder. Freely soluble in water. pH of a 10% solution in water is between 4.5 and 8.0. Store in airtight containers.

Adverse Effects and Precautions
As for Carbenicillin Sodium, p.160.

As mezlocillin sodium has a lower sodium content than carbenicillin sodium, hypernatraemia and hypokalaemia are less likely to occur. Prolongation of bleeding time has been less frequent and less severe than with carbenicillin.

Interactions
As for Benzylpenicillin, p.158.

◊ For the effect of mezlocillin on the clearance of *cefotaxime*, see p.169.
See also above for incompatibilities.

Antimicrobial Action
Mezlocillin has a similar antimicrobial action to piperacillin (p.236). Its activity against *Pseudomonas aeruginosa* is less than that of azlocillin or piperacillin.

Pharmacokinetics
Mezlocillin is not absorbed from the gastrointestinal tract to any significant extent. It is well absorbed after intramuscular administration, peak plasma concentrations of 15 to 25 µg per mL having been observed 45 to 90 minutes after a single dose of 1 g. It is reported to have nonlinear dose-dependent pharmacokinetics. Between 16 and 42% of mezlocillin in the circulation is bound to plasma proteins. Mezlocillin is reported to have a plasma half-life of about one hour, but longer in neonates; in patients with renal impairment half-lives of up to about 6 hours have been reported.

Mezlocillin is widely distributed in body tissues and fluids. It crosses the placenta into the fetal circulation and small amounts are distributed into breast milk. There is little diffusion into CSF except when the meninges are inflamed.

Mezlocillin is reported to be metabolised to a limited extent. About 55% of a dose is excreted unchanged in the urine by glomerular filtration and tubular secretion within 6 hours of administration, hence achieving high urinary concentrations. High concentrations are also found in the bile; up to 30% of a dose has been reported to be excreted by this route.

Plasma concentrations are enhanced if probenecid is administered concomitantly.

Mezlocillin is removed by haemodialysis, and to some extent by peritoneal dialysis.

Uses and Administration
Mezlocillin is a ureidopenicillin with uses similar to those of piperacillin (p.236). It is commonly administered in association with an aminoglycoside; however they should be administered separately as they have been shown to be incompatible.

Administration and dosage. Mezlocillin is given by injection as the sodium salt. Doses are expressed in terms of the equivalent amount of mezlocillin. Dosage may need to be reduced in renal impairment. It may be administered by slow intravenous injection over 3 to 5 minutes, by intravenous infusion over 30 minutes, or by deep intramuscular injection. Single intramuscular doses should not exceed 2 g.

For the treatment of serious infections, 200 to 300 mg per kg body-weight daily in divided doses may be administered intravenously; usual doses are 4 g every 6 hours or 3 g every 4 hours. For life-threatening infections, up to 350 mg per kg daily may be given, but the total daily dose should not normally exceed 24 g. For uncomplicated urinary-tract infections, a dose of 1.5

to 2 g may be given intramuscularly or intravenously every 6 hours.

Uncomplicated gonorrhoea may be treated by a single intramuscular or intravenous dose of mezlocillin 1 to 2 g. Probenecid 1 g by mouth may be given at the same time or up to half-an-hour before the injection.

For the prophylaxis of infection during surgery, an intravenous pre-operative dose of mezlocillin 4 g, followed by 2 postoperative doses at 6-hourly intervals, may be given.

Preparations
USP 25: Mezlocillin for Injection.
Proprietary Preparations (details are given in Part 3)
Aust.: Baypen; **Fr.:** Baypen; **Ger.:** Baypen; Melocin†; **Israel:** Baypen; **Ital.:** Baypen; **Spain:** Baypen; **USA:** Mezlin.
Multi-ingredient: Aust.: Optocillin; **Ger.:** Optocillin.

Micronomicin Sulfate (736-p)

Micronomicin Sulfate (pINNM).
Gentamicin C_{2B} Sulphate; KW-1062 (micronomicin); 6′-N-Methylgentamicin C_{1A} Sulphate; Micronomicin Sulphate; Sagamicin Sulphate. O-2-Amino-2,3,4,6-tetradeoxy-6-(methylamino)-α-D-erythro-hexopyranosyl-(1→4)-O-[3-deoxy-4-C-methyl-3-(methylamino)-β-L-arabinopyranosyl-(1→6)]-2-deoxy-D-streptamine hemipentasulphate.
$(C_{20}H_{41}N_5O_7)_2,5H_2SO_4 = 1417.5$.
CAS — 52093-21-7 (micronomicin).
Pharmacopoeias. In Jpn.

Profile
Micronomicin is an aminoglycoside with general properties similar to those of gentamicin (p.210). It may be given as the sulfate by intramuscular injection or by intravenous infusion over 0.5 to 1 hour in doses of 120 to 240 mg daily in 2 or 3 divided doses. Dosage should be adjusted based on serum-micronomicin concentration monitoring. It is also used topically as eye drops or ointment in a concentration of 0.3% for infections of the eye.

Preparations
Proprietary Preparations (details are given in Part 3)
Ital.: Luxomicina; Sagamicina; **Jpn:** Sagamicin; **Mon.:** Micro-phta.

Midecamycin (108-m)

Midecamycin (rINN).
Midecamycin A_1; Mydecamycin. 7-(Formylmethyl)-4,10-dihydroxy-5-methoxy-9,16,-dimethyl-2-oxo-oxacyclohexadeca-11,13-dien-6-yl 3,6-dideoxy-4-O-(2,6-dideoxy-3-C-methyl-α-L-ribo-hexopyranosyl)-3-(dimethylamino)-β-D-glucopyranoside 4′,4″-dipropionate.
$C_{41}H_{67}NO_{15} = 814.0$.
CAS — 35457-80-8 (midecamycin); 55881-07-7 (midecamycin acetate).
ATC — J01FA03.
Pharmacopoeias. In Jpn which also includes Midecamycin Acetate.

Profile
Midecamycin is a macrolide antibiotic produced by the growth of *Streptomyces mycarofaciens* and with actions and uses similar to those of erythromycin (p.201) but somewhat less active. It is given by mouth as the base or as the acetate.

Preparations
Proprietary Preparations (details are given in Part 3)
Belg.: Merced; **Braz.:** Mosil; **Fr.:** Mosil; **Ital.:** Macroral; Midecin; Miocamen; Miokacin; **Jpn:** Medemycin; Miocamycin; **Mex.:** Midecamin; **Port.:** Miocacin; **Spain:** Momicine; Myoxam; Normicina; **Thai.:** Miotin.

Minocycline Hydrochloride (109-b)

Minocycline Hydrochloride (BANM, rINNM).
Minocyclini Hydrochloridim. (4S,4aR,5aR,6S,12aS)-4,7-Bis(dimethylamino)-1,4,4a,5,5a,6,11,12a-octahydro-3,10,12,12a-tetrahydroxy-6-methyl-1,11-dioxonaphthacene-2-carboxamide hydrochloride; 6-Demethyl-6-deoxy-7-dimethylaminotetracycline hydrochloride.
$C_{23}H_{27}N_3O_7,HCl = 493.9$.
CAS — 10118-90-8 (minocycline); 13614-98-5 (minocycline hydrochloride).

NOTE. Minocycline is *USAN*.
Pharmacopoeias. In Eur. (see p.vi), Jpn, and US.

Minocycline hydrochloride 108 mg is approximately equivalent to 100 mg of minocycline.

Incompatibilities. Preparations of minocycline hydrochloride have an acid pH and incompatibility may reasonably be expected with alkaline preparations or with drugs unstable at low pH.

Pharmacopoeial description

Ph. Eur.: A yellow, hygroscopic, crystalline powder. Sparingly soluble in water; slightly soluble in alcohol; practically insoluble in ether. It dissolves in solutions of alkali hydroxides and carbonates. A 1% solution in water has a pH of 3.5 to 4.5. Store in airtight containers. Protect from light.

USP 25: A yellow crystalline powder. Sparingly soluble in water; slightly soluble in alcohol; practically insoluble in chloroform and in ether; soluble in solutions of alkali hydroxides and carbonates. pH of a solution in water containing the equivalent of minocycline 1% is between 3.5 and 4.5. Store in airtight containers. Protect from light.

Adverse Effects and Precautions

As for Tetracycline Hydrochloride, p.259.

Vestibular side-effects including dizziness or vertigo may occur with minocycline, particularly in women. Patients should be advised not to drive or operate machinery if affected.

Severe adverse effects including erythema nodosum, hepatitis, and systemic lupus erythematosus have been reported, often in patients taking the drug long-term for acne. Hypersensitivity reactions may include arthralgia, myalgia, pulmonary infiltration, and anaphylaxis. Other adverse effects include alopecia, myocarditis, and vasculitis.

Minocycline has also been associated with pigmentation of the skin and other tissues. Three patterns of skin pigmentation have been described: blue-black macules occurring in areas of inflammation and scarring and possibly due to an iron chelate of minocycline within macrophages; blue-grey macules or hyperpigmentation affecting normal skin and which may be due to a breakdown product of minocycline; or a greyish-brown discoloration occurring particularly in sun-exposed areas of skin ('muddy skin syndrome'), apparently due to melanin deposition. Skin pigmentation appears to resolve slowly on discontinuing the drug although recovery may be incomplete.

Unlike many tetracyclines, minocycline does not appear to accumulate in patients with impaired renal function, and aggravation of renal impairment may be less likely.

◊ There have been several reports of severe complications in patients receiving minocycline for acne including serum-sickness-like disease,[1,2] lupus erythematosus,[3] and hepatitis.[3,4] The number of cases reported probably reflects the widespread use of this drug and the true incidence of such adverse effects is difficult to assess.[5] A study of 700 patients receiving minocycline for acne revealed adverse effects in 13.6%, mostly benign.[6] Gastrointestinal disturbances and vestibular disturbances were the most common, each occurring in about 2% of patients, and pigmentation in up to 4% of patients. Another problem is that of assessing the incidence of severe adverse effects relative to other antibacterials commonly used in acne such as tetracycline and erythromycin. Nevertheless, minocycline should probably be regarded as a second-line oral antibacterial for the treatment of acne until further evidence is available.[3,5]

1. Knowles SR, et al. Serious adverse reactions induced by minocycline: report of 13 patients and review of the literature. Arch Dermatol 1996; **132:** 934–9.
2. Harel L, et al. Serum-sickness-like reaction associated with minocycline therapy in adolescents. Ann Pharmacother 1996; **30:** 481–3.
3. Gough A, et al. Minocycline induced autoimmune hepatitis and systemic lupus erythematosus-like syndrome. BMJ 1996; **312:** 169–72.
4. Australian Adverse Drug Reactions Advisory Committee. Minocycline and the liver, the CNS, the skin. Aust Adverse Drug React Bull 1996; **15:** 14.
5. Seukeran DC, et al. Benefit-risk assessment of acne therapies. Lancet 1997; **349:** 1251–2.
6. Goulden V, et al. Safety of long-term high-dose minocycline in the treatment of acne. Br J Dermatol 1996; **134:** 693–5.

Effects on the liver. References.

1. Lawrenson RA, et al. Liver damage associated with minocycline use in acne: a systematic review of the published literature and pharmacovigilance data. Drug Safety 2000; **23:** 333–49.

Effects on the lungs. References to minocycline-induced pneumonitis.

1. Guillon J-M, et al. Minocycline-induced cell-mediated hypersensitivity pneumonitis. Ann Intern Med 1992; **117:** 476–81.
2. Bridges AJ. Minocycline-induced pneumonia. Ann Intern Med 1993; **118:** 749–50.
3. Sigmann P. Minocycline-induced pneumonia. Ann Intern Med 1993; **118:** 750.
4. Sitbon O, et al. Minocycline pneumonitis and eosinophilia: a report on 8 patients. Arch Intern Med 1994; **154:** 1633–40.
5. Dykhuizen RS, et al. Minocycline and pulmonary eosinophilia. BMJ 1995; **310:** 1520–1.

The symbol † denotes a preparation no longer actively marketed

Effects on the nervous system. Some references to the vestibular adverse effects of minocycline.

1. Williams DN, et al. Minocycline: possible vestibular side-effects. Lancet 1974; **ii:** 744–6.
2. Nicol CS, Oriel JD. Minocycline: possible vestibular side-effects. Lancet 1974; **ii:** 1260.
3. Yeadon A. Chemoprophylaxis of meningococcal infection. Lancet 1975; **i:** 109.
4. Fanning WL, et al. Side effects of minocycline: a double-blind study. Antimicrob Agents Chemother 1977; **11:** 712–17.
5. Gump DW, et al. Side effects of minocycline: different dosage regimens. Antimicrob Agents Chemother 1977; **12:** 642–6.
6. Greco TP, et al. Minocycline toxicity: experience with an altered dosage regimen. Curr Ther Res 1979; **25:** 193–201.

Hyperpigmentation. References to skin and tissue pigmentation in patients receiving minocycline.

1. Attwood HD, Dennett X. A black thyroid and minocycline treatment. BMJ 1976; **2:** 1109–10.
2. Fenske NA, et al. Minocycline-induced pigmentation at sites of cutaneous inflammation. JAMA 1980; **244:** 1103–6.
3. Ridgway HA, et al. Hyperpigmentation associated with oral minocycline. Br J Dermatol 1982; **107:** 95–102.
4. Zijdenbos AM, Balmus KJ. Pigmentation secondary to minocycline therapy. Br J Dermatol 1984; **110:** 117–18.
5. Basler RSW. Minocycline-related hyperpigmentation. Arch Dermatol 1985; **121:** 606–8.
6. Noble JG, et al. The black thyroid: an unusual finding during neck exploration. Postgrad Med J 1989; **65:** 34–5.
7. Dwyer CM, et al. Skin pigmentation due to minocycline treatment of facial dermatoses. Br J Dermatol 1993; **129:** 158–62.
8. Okada N, et al. Characterization of pigmented granules in minocycline-induced cutaneous pigmentation: observations using fluorescence microscopy and high-performance liquid chromatography. Br J Dermatol 1993; **129:** 403–7.

Interactions

As for Tetracycline Hydrochloride, p.259.

Minocycline has a lower affinity for binding with calcium than tetracycline. In a consequence its absorption is less affected by milk and food, although it is still affected by iron salts and antacids.

Antimicrobial Action

Minocycline has a spectrum of activity and mode of action similar to that of tetracycline (p.259) but it is more active against many species including *Staphylococcus aureus*, streptococci, *Neisseria meningitidis*, various enterobacteria, *Acinetobacter*, *Bacteroides*, *Haemophilus*, *Nocardia*, and some mycobacteria, including *M. leprae*.

Partial cross-resistance exists between minocycline and other tetracyclines but some strains resistant to other drugs of the group remain sensitive to minocycline, perhaps because of better cell-wall penetration.

Pharmacokinetics

For the general pharmacokinetics of the tetracyclines, see Tetracycline Hydrochloride, p.260.

Minocycline is readily absorbed from the gastrointestinal tract and is not significantly affected by the presence of food or moderate amounts of milk. Oral doses of 200 mg followed by 100 mg every 12 hours are reported to produce plasma concentrations within the range of 2 to 4 μg per mL. It is more lipid-soluble than doxycycline and the other tetracyclines and is widely distributed in body tissues and fluids with high concentrations being achieved in the hepatobiliary tract, lungs, sinuses and tonsils, as well as in tears, saliva, and sputum. Penetration into the CSF is relatively poor, although a higher ratio of CSF to blood concentrations has been reported with minocycline than with doxycycline. It crosses the placenta and is distributed into breast milk. About 75% of minocycline in the circulation is bound to plasma proteins. It has a low renal clearance: only about 5 to 10% of a dose is excreted in the urine and up to about 34% is excreted in the faeces. However, in contrast to most tetracyclines it appears to undergo some metabolism in the liver, mainly to 9-hydroxyminocycline. Sources differ as to whether the normal plasma half-life of 11 to 26 hours is prolonged, with a consequent risk of accumulation, in patients with renal impairment, but hepatic impairment does not appear to lead to accumulation. Little minocycline is removed by dialysis.

◊ Reviews.

1. Saivin S, Houin G. Clinical pharmacokinetics of doxycycline and minocycline. Clin Pharmacokinet 1988; **15:** 355–66.

Uses and Administration

Minocycline is a tetracycline derivative with uses similar to those of tetracycline (p.260). It is also a component of multidrug regimens for the treatment of leprosy (p.126) and has been used in the prophylaxis of meningococcal infection to eliminate the carrier state, but the high incidence of vestibular disturbances means that it is not the drug of choice for the latter. Despite some conflicting pharmacokinetic data, patients with impaired renal function do not usually require adjustment of minocycline dosage, although this may be considered if renal impairment is severe.

Minocycline is normally given by mouth as the hydrochloride. Doses are expressed in terms of minocycline base. The usual adult dose is 200 mg of minocycline daily in divided doses, usually every 12 hours. An initial loading dose of 200 mg may be given. A dose of 50 mg twice daily or 100 mg once daily by mouth is used for the treatment of acne. For leprosy, minocycline 100 mg daily or intermittently has been recommended (by WHO) as part of alternative multidrug regimens. In asymptomatic meningococcal carriers, 100 mg may be given twice daily for 5 days, usually followed by a course of rifampicin.

Older children (over 8 years) have been given 4 mg per kg body-weight initially followed by 2 mg per kg every 12 hours, but the effect of tetracyclines on teeth and bones should be considered.

In patients in whom oral therapy is not feasible minocycline may be given as the hydrochloride, by slow intravenous infusion, in doses equivalent to those by mouth. In some countries it has also been given by intramuscular injection.

Minocycline is applied as a 2% gel for periodontal infections.

Rheumatic disorders. For reference to the use of minocycline in the treatment of rheumatoid arthritis, see under Tetracycline Hydrochloride, p.261.

Preparations

BP 2001: Minocycline Tablets;
USP 25: Minocycline for Injection; Minocycline Hydrochloride Capsules; Minocycline Hydrochloride Oral Suspension; Minocycline Hydrochloride Tablets.

Proprietary Preparations (details are given in Part 3)
Aust.: Auramin; Klinoc; Minocin; Minostad; Oracyclin; *Austral.:* Akamin; Minomycin; *Belg.:* Klinotab; Mino-50; Minocin; Minotab; *Braz.:* Minomax; *Canad.:* Minocin; *Fr.:* Dermirex; Logryx; Mestacine; Minolis; Mynocine; Spicline†; Zacnan; *Ger.:* Akne-Puren; Aknereduct†; Aknin-Mino; Aknosan; durakne; Icht-Oral†; Klinomycin; Lederderm; Minakne; Mino-Wolff; Minoclir; Minogalen; Minoplus; Skid; Udima; *Hong Kong:* Minocin; *Irl.:* Dentomycin; Minocin; Minox; *Israel:* Apominocin; Minocin; Minoclir; *Ital.:* Minocin; *Jpn:* Periocline; *Mex.:* Minocin; *Neth.:* Aknemin†; Minocin; Minotab†; *NZ:* Minomycin; Minotabs; *Port.:* Minocin; Minotrext†; *S.Afr.:* Cyclimycin; Mino T†; Minomycin; Minotabs; Romin; Triomin; *Singapore:* Minocin; *Spain:* Minocin; *Switz.:* Aknin-N; Aknoral; Dentomycine†; Minac 50; Minocin; *Thai.:* Minocin; *UK:* Aknemin; Blemix; Cyclomin†; Dentomycin; Minocin; Minogal; *USA:* Arestin; Dynacin; Minocin; Vectrin.

Morinamide (7563-y)

Morinamide (pINN)

Morphazinamide. *N*-Morpholinomethylpyrazine-2-carboxamide.

$C_{10}H_{14}N_4O_2 = 222.2.$
CAS — 952-54-5.
ATC — J04AK04.

Profile

Morinamide is an antimycobacterial that is given by mouth as the hydrochloride in the treatment of tuberculosis.

Preparations

Proprietary Preparations (details are given in Part 3)
Ital.: Piazofolina.

Moxifloxacin Hydrochloride (20404-x)

Moxifloxacin Hydrochloride (BANM, USAN, rINNM).

Bay-12-8039. 1-Cyclopropyl-6-fluoro-1,4-dihydro-8-methoxy-7-[(4aS,7aS)-octahydro-6H-pyrrolo[3,4-b]pyridin-6-yl]-4-oxo-3-quinolinecarboxylic acid hydrochloride.

$C_{21}H_{24}FN_3O_4,HCl = 437.9.$
CAS — 151096-09-2 (moxifloxacin); 186826-86-8 (moxifloxacin hydrochloride).

Adverse Effects and Precautions
As for Ciprofloxacin, p.183.
Moxifloxacin has been shown to prolong the QT interval and should be avoided in patients with existing QT prolongation.

Interactions
As for Ciprofloxacin, p.184.
As moxifloxacin has been shown to prolong the QT interval, it should not be given to patients receiving class Ia antiarrhythmic drugs (such as quinidine and procainamide) or class III antiarrhythmics (such as amiodarone and sotalol). In addition, caution should be exercised when moxifloxacin is used with other drugs known to have this effect (such as the antihistamines astemizole and terfenadine, cisapride, erythromycin, pentamidine, phenothiazines, or tricyclic antidepressants).

Antimicrobial Action
As for Ciprofloxacin, p.184.
Moxifloxacin is reported to have greater activity against Gram-positive bacteria, including pneumococci, than ciprofloxacin.

Pharmacokinetics
Moxifloxacin is readily absorbed from the gastrointestinal tract following oral administration with an absolute bioavailability of about 90%. Moxifloxacin has an elimination half-life of approximately 12 hours, allowing once-daily dosing. It is metabolised principally via sulfate and glucuronide conjugation.

Uses and Administration
Moxifloxacin is a fluoroquinolone antibacterial given by mouth as the hydrochloride in the treatment of susceptible infections. Doses are expressed in terms of the base; the usual adult dose is 400 mg daily.

◊ Reviews.
1. Barman Balfour JA, Wiseman LR. Moxifloxacin. *Drugs* 1999; **57**: 363–73.
2. Barman Balfour JA, Lamb HM. Moxifloxacin: a review of its clinical potential in the management of community-acquired respiratory tract infections. *Drugs* 2000; **59**: 115–39.
3. Anonymous. Gatifloxacin and moxifloxacin: two new fluoroquinolones. *Med Lett Drugs Ther* 2000; **42**: 15–17.
4. Culley CM, *et al.* Moxifloxacin: clinical efficacy and safety. *Am J Health-Syst Pharm* 2001; **58**: 379–88.

Preparations
Proprietary Preparations (details are given in Part 3)
Austral.: Avelox; *Fin.:* Avelox; *Ger.:* Avalox; *Irl.:* Avelox; *Swed.:* Avelox; *USA:* Avelox.

Mupirocin   (16906-v)

Mupirocin (BAN, USAN, rINN).
BRL-4910A; Mupirocinum; Pseudomonic Acid. 9-[(2E)-4-[(2S,3R,4R,5S)-5-[(2S,3S,4S,5S)-2,3-Epoxy-5-hydroxy-4-methylhexyl]tetrahydro-3,4-dihydroxypyran-2-yl]-3-methylbut-2-enoyloxy]nonanoic acid.
$C_{26}H_{44}O_9 = 500.6$.
CAS — 12650-69-0.
ATC — D06AX09; R01AX06.

Pharmacopoeias. In Eur. (see p.vi) and US. Eur. also includes the calcium salt.

An antibiotic produced by *Pseudomonas fluorescens.*

Pharmacopoeial description
Ph. Eur.: Mupirocin is a white or almost white powder. It shows polymorphism. Slightly soluble in water; freely soluble in dehydrated alcohol, in acetone, and in dichloromethane. It shows polymorphism. The pH of a freshly prepared saturated solution in water is 3.5 to 4.0. Protect from light.
Mupirocin Calcium is a white or almost white powder. Very slightly soluble in water; sparingly soluble in dehydrated alcohol and in dichloromethane.

USP 25: A white to off-white crystalline solid. Very slightly soluble in water; freely soluble in dehydrated alcohol, in acetone, in chloroform, and in methyl alcohol; slightly soluble in ether. pH of a saturated solution in water is between 3.5 and 4.5. Store in airtight containers.

Adverse Effects and Precautions
Mupirocin is usually well tolerated but local reactions such as burning, stinging, and itching may occur after the application of mupirocin to the skin.

Some mupirocin products are formulated in a macrogol base: such formulations are not suitable for application to mucous membranes and should be used with caution in patients with extensive burns or wounds because of the possibility of macrogol toxicity. Care is also required in patients with renal impairment.

Antimicrobial Action
Mupirocin is an antibiotic which inhibits bacterial protein synthesis by binding to isoleucyl transfer RNA synthetase. It is primarily bacteriostatic at low concentrations, although it is usually bactericidal in the high concentrations achieved on the skin. At these concentrations it may have some activity against organisms reported to be relatively resistant to mupirocin *in vitro.*

It is mainly active against Gram-positive aerobes. Most strains of staphylococci (including meticillin-resistant and multiply-resistant *Staph. aureus*) and streptococci are susceptible *in vitro*, although the enterococci are relatively resistant. Mupirocin is also active against *Listeria monocytogenes* and *Erysipelothrix rhusiopathiae.* The Gram-negative organisms are generally insensitive, but *Haemophilus influenzae, Neisseria* spp. and a few others are sensitive. Anaerobic organisms, both Gram-positive and Gram-negative, are generally resistant, and activity against fungi is low.

MICs for the most sensitive strains of staphylococci range between about 0.01 to 0.25 µg per mL and those for sensitive streptococcal strains from around 0.06 to 0.5 µg per mL; *Listeria* is inhibited by 8 µg per mL. Mupirocin is more active *in vitro* at acid pH than in alkaline conditions.

Naturally resistant strains of *Staph. aureus* occur rarely but resistance, including high-level plasmid-mediated transferable resistance, has emerged, particularly during long-term treatment. With as many as 8% of staphylococcal strains from some centres proving resistant there has been some concern that inappropriate prescribing of mupirocin has led to steadily increasing resistance.

Activity against fungi. Activity of mupirocin 2% *in vitro* against *Candida albicans* was comparable to that of other commonly used topical antifungals. Although MICs were considerably in excess of those reported for susceptible bacteria, clinical responses in 10 patients suggested that adequate concentrations of mupirocin were achieved following topical application.[1]
1. Rode H, *et al.* Efficacy of mupirocin in cutaneous candidiasis. *Lancet* 1991; **338**: 578.

Resistance. Reports and discussions of mupirocin resistance.
1. Rahman M, *et al.* Transmissible mupirocin resistance in Staphylococcus aureus. *Epidemiol Infect* 1989; **102**: 261–70.
2. Cookson BD. Mupirocin resistance in staphylococci. *J Antimicrob Chemother* 1990; **25**: 497–503.
3. Wise R, Johnson J. Mupirocin resistance. *Lancet* 1991; **338**: 578.
4. Cookson B, *et al.* Mupirocin-resistant Staphylococcus aureus. *Lancet* 1992; **339**: 625.
5. Gilbart J, *et al.* High-level mupirocin resistance in Staphylococcus aureus: evidence for two distinct isoleucyl-tRNA synthetases. *Antimicrob Agents Chemother* 1993; **37**: 32–8.
6. Janssen DA, *et al.* Detection and characterization of mupirocin resistance in staphylococcus aureus. *Antimicrob Agents Chemother* 1993; **37**: 2003–6.
7. Cookson BD. The emergence of mupirocin resistance: a challenge to infection control and antibiotic prescribing practice. *J Antimicrob Chemother* 1998; **41**: 11–18.
8. Schmitz F-J, *et al.* The prevalence of low- and high-level mupirocin resistance in staphylococci from 19 European hospitals. *J Antimicrob Chemother* 1998; **42**: 489–95.

Pharmacokinetics
Only very small amounts of topically applied mupirocin are absorbed into the systemic circulation where it is rapidly metabolised to monic acid.

Uses and Administration
Mupirocin is an antibiotic which is applied topically as a 2% ointment in a macrogol basis in the treatment of various bacterial skin infections. It should be applied up to three times daily for up to 10 days. This ointment is not suitable for application to mucous membranes, and mupirocin 2%, as the calcium salt, in a paraffin basis is used for eradication of the nasal carriage of *Staphylococcus aureus*, particularly epidemic meticillin-resistant strains.

For further details of skin infections and staphylococcal infections and their treatment, see under Choice of Antibacterial, p.140.

Preparations
USP 25: Mupirocin Ointment.

Proprietary Preparations (details are given in Part 3)
Aust.: Bactroban; *Austral.:* Bactroban; *Belg.:* Bactroban; *Braz.:* Bactroban; *Canad.:* Bactroban; *Denm.:* Bactroban; *Fin.:* Bactroban; *Fr.:* Bactroban; Mupiderm; *Ger.:* Turixin; *Hong Kong:* Bactroban; *Irl.:* Bactroban; *Israel:* Bactoderm; Bactroban; *Ital.:* Bactroban; *Jpn:* Bactroban; *Mex.:* Bactroban; *Neth.:* Bactroban; *NZ:* Bactroban; *S.Afr.:* Bactroban; *Singapore:* Bactroban; *Spain:* Bactroban; Plasimine; *Swed.:* Bactroban; *Switz.:* Bactroban; *Thai.:* Bactroban; *UK:* Bactroban; *USA:* Bactroban.

Nadifloxacin   (15296-w)

Nadifloxacin (BAN, rINN).
Jinofloxacin; OPC-7251. (±)-9-Fluoro-6,7-dihydro-8-(4-hydroxypiperidino)-5-methyl-1-oxo-1H,5H-benzo[ij]quinolizine-2-carboxylic acid.
$C_{19}H_{21}FN_2O_4 = 360.4$.
CAS — 124858-35-1.

Profile
Nadifloxacin is a fluoroquinolone antibacterial. It is applied topically in the treatment of acne.

Preparations
Proprietary Preparations (details are given in Part 3)
Jpn: Acuatim.

Nafcillin Sodium   (110-x)

Nafcillin Sodium (BANM, USAN, rINNM).
Nafcillinum Natricum; Wy-3277. Sodium (6R)-6-(2-ethoxy-1-naphthamido)penicillanate monohydrate.
$C_{21}H_{21}N_2NaO_5S,H_2O = 454.5$.
CAS — 147-52-4 (nafcillin); 985-16-0 (anhydrous nafcillin sodium); 7177-50-6 (nafcillin sodium, monohydrate).

Pharmacopoeias. In US.

1.1 g of monograph substance is approximately equivalent to 1 g of anhydrous nafcillin. Each g of monograph substance represents 2.2 mmol of sodium.

Nafcillin sodium has been reported to be incompatible with aminoglycosides and a number of other antibacterials. It has also been reported to be incompatible with acidic and alkaline drugs.

Pharmacopoeial description
USP 25: A white to yellowish-white powder having not more than a slight characteristic odour. Freely soluble in water and in chloroform; soluble in alcohol. pH of a 3% solution in water is between 5.0 and 7.0. Store in airtight containers.

Adverse Effects and Precautions
As for Benzylpenicillin, p.157.

Thrombophlebitis may occur when nafcillin is given by intravenous injection, and tissue damage has been reported on extravasation.

Effects on the kidneys. References.
1. Lestico MR, *et al.* Hepatic and renal dysfunction following nafcillin administration. *Ann Pharmacother* 1992; **26**: 985–90.
2. Guharoy SR, *et al.* Suspected nafcillin-induced interstitial nephritis. *Ann Pharmacother* 1993; **27**: 170–3.

Effects on the liver. References.
1. Lestico MR, *et al.* Hepatic and renal dysfunction following nafcillin administration. *Ann Pharmacother* 1992; **26**: 985–90.

Interactions
As for Benzylpenicillin, p.158.

◊ For the effect of nafcillin on *ciclosporin*, see p.520, and on *warfarin*, see p.994.

Antimicrobial Action
As for Flucloxacillin, p.207.

Pharmacokinetics
Nafcillin is incompletely and irregularly absorbed from the gastrointestinal tract, especially when administered after a meal. After intramuscular injection it is absorbed more reliably, an injection of 0.5 to 1 g producing peak plasma concentrations of 5 to 8 µg per mL within about 0.5 to 2 hours. Up to 90% of nafcillin in the circulation is bound to plasma proteins. Nafcillin has been reported to have a plasma half-life of about 0.5 to 1 hour. The half-life is prolonged in neonates.

Nafcillin crosses the placenta into the fetal circulation and is distributed into breast milk. There is little diffusion into the CSF except when the meninges are inflamed. Therapeutic concentrations can be achieved in pleural and synovial fluids and in bone.

Nafcillin differs from most other penicillins in that it is largely inactivated by hepatic metabolism. It is excreted via the bile although some reabsorption takes place in the small intestine. Only about 10% of a dose given by mouth before food, and about 30% of a dose given intramuscularly, is excreted in the urine.

Plasma concentrations are enhanced if probenecid is given concomitantly.

Uses and Administration

Nafcillin is a penicillinase-resistant penicillin used similarly to flucloxacillin (p.207) in the treatment of infections due to staphylococci resistant to benzyl-penicillin.

It is administered by mouth or by injection as the sodium salt. Doses are expressed in terms of the equivalent amount of nafcillin. By intramuscular injection the usual adult dose is 500 mg of nafcillin every 4 to 6 hours. Children may be given 25 mg per kg body-weight twice daily, and neonates 10 mg per kg twice daily. Nafcillin sodium may also be given intravenously by slow injection over 5 to 10 minutes or by slow infusion; adult doses are 0.5 to 1.5 g of nafcillin every 4 hours, although it is usually recommended that it be used for not more than 24 to 48 hours because of the risk of thrombophlebitis.

The dose by mouth for adults is 0.25 to 1 g of nafcillin every 4 to 6 hours; for children it is 6.25 to 12.5 mg per kg four times daily; and for neonates it is 10 mg per kg three or four times daily. It should preferably be given at least one hour before, or 2 hours after, meals.

Preparations

USP 25: Nafcillin for Injection; Nafcillin Injection; Nafcillin Sodium Capsules; Nafcillin Sodium for Oral Solution; Nafcillin Sodium Tablets.

Proprietary Preparations (details are given in Part 3)
USA: Nafcil†; Nallpen†; Unipen†.

Nalidixic Acid (5663-n)

Nalidixic Acid *(BAN, USAN, rINN).*

Acidum Nalidixicum; Nalidixinic Acid; NSC-82174; Win-18320. 1-Ethyl-1,4-dihydro-7-methyl-4-oxo-1,8-naphthyridine-3-carboxylic acid.

$C_{12}H_{12}N_2O_3 = 232.2$.

CAS — 389-08-2.
ATC — G04AB01.

Pharmacopoeias. In *Chin., Eur.* (see p.vi), *Jpn, Pol.,* and *US.*

Pharmacopoeial description

Ph. Eur.: An almost white or pale yellow, crystalline powder. Practically insoluble in water; slightly soluble in alcohol and in acetone; soluble in dichloromethane. It dissolves in dilute solutions of alkali hydroxides. Store in airtight containers. Protect from light.

USP 25: A white to very pale yellow, odourless crystalline powder. Very slightly soluble in water and in ether; soluble 1 in 910 of alcohol and 1 in 29 of chloroform; slightly soluble in acetone, in methyl alcohol, and in toluene; soluble in dichloromethane and in solutions of fixed alkali hydroxides and carbonates. Store in airtight containers.

Adverse Effects

The most frequent adverse reactions to nalidixic acid involve the gastrointestinal tract, skin, and CNS. Gastrointestinal effects have been reported in about 8% of patients and include nausea, vomiting, diarrhoea, and abdominal pain.

Neurological side-effects include visual disturbances, headache, dizziness or vertigo, drowsiness, and sometimes confusion, depression, excitement, and hallucinations. Toxic psychoses or convulsions have occurred, especially after large doses; convulsions are most likely in patients with predisposing factors such as cerebrovascular insufficiency, parkinsonism, or epilepsy. There have been reports of intracranial hypertension, especially in infants and young children, and also of metabolic acidosis. Peripheral neuropathies, muscular weakness, and myalgia are occasional side-effects.

Adverse effects on the skin include photosensitivity reactions with erythema and bullous eruptions, allergic rashes, urticaria, and pruritus. Eosinophilia, fever, angioedema, and, rarely, anaphylactoid reactions have occurred. Arthralgia has been reported (degen-

The symbol † denotes a preparation no longer actively marketed

erative changes in weight-bearing joints of young *animals* are documented). Tendon damage has occasionally been associated with related compounds, the fluoroquinolones (see under Ciprofloxacin: Effects on the Musculoskeletal System, p.183).

Cholestatic jaundice, thrombocytopenia, and leucopenia have occurred rarely, as has haemolytic anaemia in patients who may or may not be deficient in glucose-6-phosphate dehydrogenase. There have been isolated reports of fatal auto-immune haemolytic anaemia in elderly patients.

Precautions

Nalidixic acid should be avoided in patients subject to convulsions. It should be given with care to patients with impaired renal or hepatic function or with glucose-6-phosphate dehydrogenase deficiency. Blood counts and renal and hepatic function should be monitored if treatment continues for more than 2 weeks.

It should be avoided in babies less than 3 months old. Since nalidixic acid and related antimicrobials have been shown to cause degenerative changes in weight-bearing joints of young *animals*, it has been suggested that these compounds should not be used in children, adolescents, pregnant women, or during breast feeding. Treatment should be discontinued if symptoms of arthralgia occur.

Exposure to strong sunlight or sunlamps should be avoided during treatment with nalidixic acid.

Nalidixic acid may cause false-positive reactions in urine tests for glucose using copper reduction methods.

Porphyria. Nalidixic acid has been associated with acute attacks of porphyria and is considered unsafe in porphyric patients.

Interactions

The excretion of nalidixic acid is reduced and plasma concentrations increased by the concomitant administration of probenecid. Nitrofurantoin and nalidixic acid are antagonistic *in vitro* and should not be used together. Fatal haemorrhagic enterocolitis has been associated with the concomitant use of nalidixic acid and high-dose intravenous melphalan in children. There is a possible risk of increased nephrotoxicity when nalidixic acid is administered with ciclosporin.

Nalidixic acid is reported to enhance the effect of oral anticoagulants such as warfarin (p.994); this may be due in part to displacement of anticoagulant from its plasma binding sites. The dose of anticoagulant may need to be reduced.

For the effect of some quinolone antibacterials on xanthines, see under Caffeine, p.762, and Theophylline, p.780.

Convulsions may be precipitated by the administration of some quinolones with NSAIDs (see Analgesics, under Interactions of Ciprofloxacin, p.184), although this has not been reported with nalidixic acid.

Antimicrobial Action

Nalidixic acid is considered to act by interfering with the replication of bacterial DNA, probably by inhibiting DNA gyrase (topoisomerase) activity. It is active against Gram-negative bacteria including *Escherichia coli, Klebsiella* spp., *Proteus* spp., *Enterobacter* spp., *Salmonella* spp., and *Shigella* spp., and is usually bactericidal. Most susceptible organisms are inhibited by 16 µg or less per mL. *Pseudomonas aeruginosa,* Gram-positive bacteria, and anaerobes are not generally susceptible.

Bacterial resistance may develop rapidly, sometimes within a few days of commencing treatment, but it does not appear to be transferable or R-plasmid mediated (see also below). Cross-resistance occurs with oxolinic acid and cinoxacin.

The antibacterial activity of nalidixic acid is not significantly affected by differences in urinary pH. Antagonism between nitrofurantoin and nalidixic acid has been demonstrated *in vitro.*

◊ Bacterial plasmid-mediated resistance to quinolones had not been seen by the late 1980s.[1] A report of such resistance to nalidixic acid in *Shigella dysenteriae* responsible for an epidemic of shigellosis in Bangladesh in 1987,[2] was questioned at the time.[3] On reinspection of the data, chromosomal mutation rather than plasmid-mediated resistance was confirmed as the mechanism responsible so far for resistance to quinolones.[1] More recent data[4] in an isolate of *Klebsiella pneumoniae* has, however, suggested that plasma-mediated resistance to quinolones may be possible.

1. Courvalin P. Plasmid-mediated 4-quinolone resistance: a real or apparent absence? *Antimicrob Agents Chemother* 1990; **34:** 681–4.
2. Munshi MH, *et al.* Plasmid-mediated resistance to nalidixic acid in Shigella dysenteriae type 1. *Lancet* 1987; **ii:** 419–21.
3. Crumplin GC. Plasmid-mediated resistance to nalidixic acid and new 4-quinolones? *Lancet* 1987; **ii:** 854–5.
4. Martínez-Martínez L, *et al.* Quinolone resistance from a transferable plasmid. *Lancet* 1998; **351:** 797–9.

Pharmacokinetics

Nalidixic acid is rapidly and almost completely absorbed from the gastrointestinal tract, and peak plasma concentrations of 20 to 50 µg per mL have been reported 2 hours after the administration of 1 g by mouth. Plasma half-lives of about 1 to 2.5 hours have been reported (but see below).

Nalidixic acid is partially metabolised to hydroxynalidixic acid, which has antibacterial activity similar to that of nalidixic acid and accounts for about 30% of active drug in the blood. About 93% of nalidixic acid and 63% of hydroxynalidixic acid are bound to plasma proteins. Both nalidixic acid and hydroxynalidixic acid are rapidly metabolised to inactive glucuronide and dicarboxylic acid derivatives; the major inactive metabolite carboxynalidixic acid is usually only detected in urine.

Nalidixic acid and its metabolites are excreted rapidly in the urine, nearly all of a dose being eliminated within 24 hours. About 80 to 90% of the drug excreted in the urine is as inactive metabolites, but urinary concentrations of unchanged drug and active metabolite ranging from 25 to 250 µg per mL are achieved after a single 1-g dose. Hydroxynalidixic acid accounts for about 80 to 85% of activity in the urine. Urinary excretion is reduced by probenecid.

Traces of nalidixic acid are distributed into breast milk and appear to cross the placenta. About 4% of a dose is excreted in the faeces.

◊ Although a plasma half-life of 1 to 2.5 hours is generally cited for nalidixic acid, values of 6 to 7 hours have been reported for active drug (nalidixic acid and hydroxynalidixic acid) after using more specific and sensitive assay techniques and longer sampling periods than previously.[1]

The elimination rate of nalidixic acid appears to be not markedly altered by renal impairment, but the elimination of hydroxynalidixic acid is significantly reduced. 7-Carboxynalidixic acid has appeared in the plasma of patients with renal impairment.[2] Plasma concentrations of active drug were higher and the half-life prolonged in elderly subjects.[3]

1. Ferry N, *et al.* Nalidixic acid kinetics after single and repeated oral doses. *Clin Pharmacol Ther* 1981; **29:** 695–8.
2. Cuisinaud G, *et al.* Nalidixic acid kinetics in renal insufficiency. *Br J Clin Pharmacol* 1982; **14:** 489–93.
3. Barbeau G, Belanger P-M. Pharmacokinetics of nalidixic acid in old and young volunteers. *J Clin Pharmacol* 1982; **22:** 490–6.

Uses and Administration

Nalidixic acid is a 4-quinolone antibacterial used in the treatment of uncomplicated lower urinary-tract infections due to Gram-negative bacteria other than *Pseudomonas* spp. (p.146). It has also been used to treat shigellosis (bacillary dysentery) (p.123).

The usual adult dose is 4 g daily by mouth in 4 divided doses for at least 7 days in acute infections. Since bacterial resistance may develop rapidly it has been suggested that if treatment with nalidixic acid has not resulted in a negative urine culture within 48 hours another antimicrobial should be used. If therapy continues for longer than 2 weeks the dose should usually be halved. Children over 3 months have been given 50 to 55 mg per kg body-weight daily in 4 divided doses reduced to 30 to 33 mg per kg daily for prolonged treatment (but see Precautions, above).

Although the antibacterial activity of nalidixic acid does not appear to be influenced by urinary pH, the concomitant administration of sodium bicarbonate or sodium citrate does increase the concentration of active drug in the urine. The adult dose of nalidixic acid, in conjunction with sodium citrate, is 660 mg three times daily for 3 days.

Preparations

BP 2001: Nalidixic Acid Oral Suspension; Nalidixic Acid Tablets; *USP 25:* Nalidixic Acid Oral Suspension; Nalidixic Acid Tablets.

Proprietary Preparations (details are given in Part 3)
Austral.: Negram†; *Braz.:* Wintomylon; *Canad.:* NegGram; *Denm.:* Negram†; *Fr.:* Negram; *Hong Kong:* Wintomylon; *Irl.:* Negram; *Israel:* NegGram; Urigram; *Ital.:* Betaxina; Nalidixin; Naligram; Nalissina; NegGram; Uralgin; Uri-Flor; Urogram; *Mex.:* Acidix; Acinal; Fardixon; Labydon; Lidinal; Lidixin; Nadiwil; Nalidixan; Nalidoid; Nalix; Neo-Uridixico; Seltomylon; Unidixina; Urlix; Uronalin; Wintomylon; *Norw.:* Negram; *NZ:* Negram; *Port.:* Wintomilon; *S.Afr.:* Puromylon; Winlomylon; *Swed.:* Negram†; *UK:* Negram; Uriben; *USA:* NegGram.

Multi-ingredient: *Braz.:* Azo-Wintomylon; *Irl.:* Mictral; *Mex.:* Azo-Wintomylon; Nalixone; Naxilan-Plus; Pirifur; *UK:* Mictral.

Neomycin (III-r)

Neomycin *(BAN, rINN).*
CAS — 1404-04-2 (neomycin); 3947-65-7 (neomycin A); 119-04-0 (neomycin B); 66-86-4 (neomycin C).
ATC — A01AB08; A07AA01; B05CA09; D06AX04; J01GB05; R02AB01; S01AA03; S02AA07; S03AA01.

A mixture of 2 isomers, neomycin B ($C_{23}H_{46}N_6O_{13}$ = 614.6) and neomycin C ($C_{23}H_{46}N_6O_{13}$ = 614.6) with neomycin A (neamine, $C_{12}H_{26}N_4O_6$ = 322.4); neomycins B and C are glycoside esters of neamine and neobiosamines B and C. Framycetin (p.208) consists of neomycin B.

Pharmacopoeial description
The BP 2001 states that when Neomycin is prescribed or demanded, Neomycin Sulfate must be dispensed or supplied.

Neomycin Sulfate (112-f)

Neomycin Sulfate *(rINNM).*
Fradiomycin Sulfate; Neomycin Sulphate *(BANM);* Neomycini Sulfas.
CAS — 1405-10-3.

NOTE. NEO is a code approved by the BP 2001 for use on single unit doses of eye drops containing neomycin sulfate where the individual container may be too small to bear all the appropriate labelling information.
Pharmacopoeias. In *Chin., Eur.* (see p.vi), *Int., Jpn, Pol.,* and *US.*

Pharmacopoeial description
Ph. Eur.: A mixture of the sulfates of substances produced by the growth of certain selected strains of *Streptomyces fradiae.* The potency is not less than 680 units per mg, calculated with reference to the dried substance. A white or yellowish-white, hygroscopic powder. Very soluble in water; very slightly soluble in alcohol; practically insoluble in acetone. A 1% solution in water has a pH of 5.0 to 7.5. Store in airtight containers. Protect from light.

USP 25: The sulfate salt of a kind of neomycin, an antibacterial substance produced by the growth of *Streptomyces fradiae* (Streptomycetaceae), or a mixture of two or more such salts. It has a potency equivalent to not less than 600 μg of neomycin per mg, calculated on the dried basis. A white to slightly yellow powder, or cryodesiccated solid. It is odourless or practically so, and is hygroscopic. Soluble 1 in 1 of water; very slightly soluble in alcohol; insoluble in acetone, in chloroform, and in ether. pH of a solution in water containing the equivalent of neomycin 3.3% is between 5.0 and 7.5. Store in airtight containers. Protect from light.

Neomycin Undecenoate (113-d)

Neomycin Undecenoate *(BANM, rINNM).*
Neomycin Undecylenate *(USAN).* The 10-undecenoate salt of neomycin.
CAS — 1406-04-8.

Adverse Effects and Treatment
As for Gentamicin Sulfate, p.210.
Neomycin has particularly potent nephrotoxic and ototoxic properties which have led to the general abandonment of parenteral administration. However, sufficient may be absorbed by other routes, e.g. following oral administration, instillation into cavities or open wounds, or topical administration to damaged skin, to produce irreversible partial or total deafness. The effect is dose-related and is enhanced by renal impairment. Nephrotoxic effects may also occur.

When given by mouth in large doses, neomycin causes nausea, vomiting, and diarrhoea. Prolonged oral therapy may cause a malabsorption syndrome with steatorrhoea and diarrhoea which can be very severe.

Supra-infection may occur, especially with prolonged oral treatment.

Neomycin has a neuromuscular blocking action similar to, but stronger than, that of other aminoglycosides, and respiratory depression and arrest has followed the intraperitoneal instillation of neomycin. Fatalities have occurred.

Hypersensitivity reactions, such as rashes, pruritus, and sometimes drug fever or even anaphylaxis, occur frequently during local treatment with neomycin and may be masked by the combined use of a corticosteroid. Cross-sensitivity with other aminoglycoside antibiotics may occur.

Precautions
As for Gentamicin Sulfate, p.210. Parenteral administration of neomycin, or its use for irrigation of wounds or serous cavities such as the peritoneum, is no longer recommended.

Neomycin is contra-indicated for intestinal disinfection when an obstruction is present and in patients with a known history of allergy to aminoglycosides. It should be used with great care in patients with kidney or liver disease or neuromuscular disorders and in those with impaired hearing. The topical use of neomycin in patients with extensive skin damage or perforated tympanic membranes may result in deafness. Neomycin sulfate should not be used topically or for urological purposes in doses greater than 1 g daily; it should not be used urologically for longer than 10 days.

Prolonged local use should be avoided as it may lead to skin sensitisation and possible cross-sensitivity to other aminoglycosides.

Hypersensitivity and vaccination. Neomycin was thought to be responsible for a hypersensitivity reaction[1] in a child given measles mumps and rubella vaccine containing neomycin 25 μg. However, there is also a report of successful vaccination with measles mumps and rubella vaccine in a neomycin-sensitive child.[2] Although the vaccine may contain small amounts of neomycin or kanamycin, and sensitivity to either is considered a contra-indication to its use, it is only rarely necessary to withold it once appropriate expert advice has been taken. There is little logic to intradermal testing since test solutions contain 4 to 40 times as much neomycin as the vaccine.[2]

1. Kwittken PL, *et al.* MMR vaccine and neomycin allergy. *Am J Dis Child* 1993; **147:** 128–9.
2. Elliman D, Dhanraj B. Safe MMR vaccination despite neomycin allergy. *Lancet* 1991; **337:** 365.

Interactions
As for Gentamicin Sulfate, p.211. Absorption following oral or local administration may be sufficient to produce interactions with other drugs administered systemically.

Neomycin, taken by mouth, has been reported to impair the absorption of other drugs including phenoxymethylpenicillin, digoxin, methotrexate, and some vitamins; the efficacy of oral contraceptives might be reduced. The effects of acarbose may be enhanced by oral neomycin.

Antimicrobial Action
Neomycin has a mode of action and spectrum of activity similar to that of gentamicin (p.211) but it lacks activity against *Pseudomonas aeruginosa.* It is reported to be active against *Mycobacterium tuberculosis.*

Because of its extensive topical use resistance has been reported to be relatively widespread, notably among staphylococci, and some *Salmonella, Shigella,* and *Escherichia coli* strains. Cross-resistance with kanamycin, framycetin, and paromomycin occurs.

Pharmacokinetics
Neomycin is poorly absorbed from the gastrointestinal tract, about 97% of an orally administered dose being excreted unchanged in the faeces. Doses of 3 g by mouth produce peak plasma concentrations of up to 4 μg per mL and absorption is similar after administration by enema. Absorption may be increased in

conditions which damage or inflame the mucosa. Absorption has also been reported to occur from the peritoneum, respiratory tract, bladder, wounds, and inflamed skin.

Once neomycin is absorbed it is rapidly excreted by the kidneys in active form. It has been reported to have a half-life of 2 to 3 hours.

Uses and Administration
Neomycin is an aminoglycoside antibiotic used topically in the treatment of infections of the skin, ear, and eye due to susceptible staphylococci and other organisms. Most preparations contain the sulfate, but neomycin undecenoate is also used. Neomycin is often used in combination with another antibacterial such as bacitracin, colistin, gramicidin, or polymyxin B. Such combinations have been used topically in the eye before ophthalmic surgery for infection prophylaxis (p.141) and, in conjunction with propamidine isetionate, in the treatment of acanthamoeba keratitis (p.582). A cream containing neomycin sulfate and chlorhexidine hydrochloride has been used for application to the nostrils in the treatment of staphylococcal nasal carriers (p.140) but, as with other topical antibacterial preparations, development of resistance may be a problem. Neomycin is often combined with topical corticosteroid preparations, but such combinations should be used with caution because of the risk that signs of resistant infection may be suppressed. Care must also be taken where there is skin trauma because of the risk of increased absorption and toxicity (see Adverse Effects, above). For details of bacterial skin infections and their treatment, see p.140.

Because neomycin sulfate is poorly absorbed from the gastrointestinal tract, it has been given by mouth for bowel preparation before abdominal surgery, often in combination with erythromycin (p.141). Neomycin sulfate is also used in combination with other antibacterials and antifungals in the selective decontamination of the digestive tract in patients in intensive care (p.126).

Neomycin is rarely used in the treatment of existing gastrointestinal infections. Although it has been used in the treatment of diarrhoea due to infection with enteropathogenic *Escherichia coli* (EPEC) (p.123), the use of neomycin in children with acute diarrhoea is generally not recommended.

Neomycin sulfate may be given by mouth to patients with incipient hepatic encephalopathy (p.1205) to reduce the flora of the gastrointestinal tract.

Neomycin has lipid regulating properties and has occasionally been given by mouth in the treatment of hyperlipidaemias (see below). It has also been used for the irrigation of wounds and body cavities but such use is no longer recommended because of the risk of toxicity.

Administration and dosage. For pre-operative use, 1 g of neomycin sulfate has been given hourly for 4 hours and then every 4 hours for a day or more before surgery, up to a maximum of 3 days; suggested doses in children, given every 4 hours, are 1 g in those aged over 12 years and 250 to 500 mg in those aged 6 to 12 years.

As an adjunct in the management of hepatic encephalopathy, 4 to 12 g may be given daily in divided doses, usually for 5 to 7 days; children may be given 50 to 100 mg per kg body-weight daily in divided doses. Prolonged administration may cause malabsorption.

Topical preparations typically contain the equivalent of 0.35% neomycin base.

Neomycin hydrochloride has also been used.

Hyperlipidaemias. Neomycin has been given in doses of up to 2 g daily by mouth in the treatment of hypercholesterolaemia (p.800). It is thought to reduce intestinal absorption of cholesterol through its action on microbial flora, resulting in greater catabolism of low-density lipoproteins in the body.[1] However, more effective and safer drugs are preferred.

1. Illingworth DR. Lipid-lowering drugs: an overview of indications and optimum use. *Drugs* 1987; **33:** 259–79.

Preparations

BP 2001: Hydrocortisone Acetate and Neomycin Ear Drops; Hydrocortisone Acetate and Neomycin Eye Drops; Hydrocortisone Acetate and Neomycin Eye Ointment; Hydrocortisone and Neomycin Cream; Neomycin Eye Drops; Neomycin Eye Ointment; Neomycin Oral Solution; Neomycin Tablets;

USP 25: Colistin and Neomycin Sulfates and Hydrocortisone Acetate Otic Suspension; Neomycin and Polymyxin B Sulfates and Bacitracin Ointment; Neomycin and Polymyxin B Sulfates and Bacitracin Ophthalmic Ointment; Neomycin and Polymyxin B Sulfates and Bacitracin Zinc Ophthalmic Ointment; Neomycin and Polymyxin B Sulfates and Bacitracin Zinc Ointment; Neomycin and Polymyxin B Sulfates and Dexamethasone Ophthalmic Ointment; Neomycin and Polymyxin B Sulfates and Dexamethasone Ophthalmic Suspension; Neomycin and Polymyxin B Sulfates and Gramicidin Ointment; Neomycin and Polymyxin B Sulfates and Gramicidin Ophthalmic Solution; Neomycin and Polymyxin B Sulfates and Hydrocortisone Acetate Cream; Neomycin and Polymyxin B Sulfates and Hydrocortisone Acetate Ophthalmic Suspension; Neomycin and Polymyxin B Sulfates and Hydrocortisone Ophthalmic Suspension; Neomycin and Polymyxin B Sulfates and Hydrocortisone Otic Solution; Neomycin and Polymyxin B Sulfates and Hydrocortisone Otic Suspension; Neomycin and Polymyxin B Sulfates and Lidocaine Cream; Neomycin and Polymyxin B Sulfates and Pramoxine Hydrochloride Cream; Neomycin and Polymyxin B Sulfates and Prednisolone Acetate Ophthalmic Suspension; Neomycin and Polymyxin B Sulfates Cream; Neomycin and Polymyxin B Sulfates Ophthalmic Ointment; Neomycin and Polymyxin B Sulfates Ophthalmic Solution; Neomycin and Polymyxin B Sulfates Solution for Irrigation; Neomycin and Polymyxin B Sulfates, Bacitracin Zinc, and Hydrocortisone Acetate Ophthalmic Ointment; Neomycin and Polymyxin B Sulfates, Bacitracin Zinc, and Hydrocortisone Ointment; Neomycin and Polymyxin B Sulfates, Bacitracin Zinc, and Hydrocortisone Ophthalmic Ointment; Neomycin and Polymyxin B Sulfates, Bacitracin Zinc, and Lidocaine Ointment; Neomycin and Polymyxin B Sulfates, Bacitracin, and Hydrocortisone Acetate Ointment; Neomycin and Polymyxin B Sulfates, Bacitracin, and Hydrocortisone Acetate Ophthalmic Ointment; Neomycin and Polymyxin B Sulfates, Bacitracin, and Hydrocortisone Ointment; Neomycin and Polymyxin B Sulfates, Bacitracin, and Lidocaine Ointment; Neomycin and Polymyxin B Sulfates, Gramicidin, and Hydrocortisone Acetate Cream; Neomycin for Injection; Neomycin Sulfate and Bacitracin Ointment; Neomycin Sulfate and Bacitracin Zinc Ointment; Neomycin Sulfate and Dexamethasone Sodium Phosphate Cream; Neomycin Sulfate and Dexamethasone Sodium Phosphate Ophthalmic Ointment; Neomycin Sulfate and Dexamethasone Sodium Phosphate Ophthalmic Solution; Neomycin Sulfate and Fluocinolone Acetonide Cream; Neomycin Sulfate and Fluorometholone Ointment; Neomycin Sulfate and Flurandrenolide Cream; Neomycin Sulfate and Flurandrenolide Lotion; Neomycin Sulfate and Flurandrenolide Ointment; Neomycin Sulfate and Gramicidin Ointment; Neomycin Sulfate and Hydrocortisone Acetate Cream; Neomycin Sulfate and Hydrocortisone Acetate Lotion; Neomycin Sulfate and Hydrocortisone Acetate Ointment; Neomycin Sulfate and Hydrocortisone Acetate Ophthalmic Ointment; Neomycin Sulfate and Hydrocortisone Acetate Ophthalmic Suspension; Neomycin Sulfate and Hydrocortisone Acetate Cream; Neomycin Sulfate and Hydrocortisone Ointment; Neomycin Sulfate and Hydrocortisone Otic Suspension; Neomycin Sulfate and Methylprednisolone Acetate Cream; Neomycin Sulfate and Prednisolone Acetate Ointment; Neomycin Sulfate and Prednisolone Acetate Ophthalmic Ointment; Neomycin Sulfate and Prednisolone Acetate Ophthalmic Suspension; Neomycin Sulfate and Prednisolone Sodium Phosphate Ophthalmic Ointment; Neomycin Sulfate and Triamcinolone Acetonide Cream; Neomycin Sulfate and Triamcinolone Acetonide Ophthalmic Ointment; Neomycin Sulfate Cream; Neomycin Sulfate Ointment; Neomycin Sulfate Ophthalmic Ointment; Neomycin Sulfate Oral Solution; Neomycin Sulfate Tablets; Neomycin Sulfate, Sulfacetamide Sodium, and Prednisolone Acetate Ophthalmic Ointment; Nystatin, Neomycin Sulfate, Gramicidin, and Triamcinolone Acetonide Cream; Nystatin, Neomycin Sulfate, Gramicidin, and Triamcinolone Acetonide Ointment.

Proprietary Preparations (details are given in Part 3)

Aust.: Bykomycin; **Austral.:** Neosulf; Siguent Neomycin; **Braz.:** Dermazon; **Canad.:** Mycifradin; Myciguent†; **Fr.:** Bacteomycine; **Ger.:** Bykomycin; Cysto-Myacyne N; Myacyne; Nebacetin N; Uro-Nebacetin N; Vagicillin; **Hong Kong:** Mycifradin; **Irl.:** Mycifradin; **Israel:** Neocin; **Mex.:** Gemicina; Neomixen; **NZ:** Neosulf; **Port.:** Dermimade Bacitracina†; Enteromicina; **S.Afr.:** Mycifradin†; **Switz.:** Uro-Beniktol N†; **UK:** Mycifradin†; Nivemycin; **USA:** Mycifradin; Myciguent; Neo-fradin; Neo-Tabs†.

Multi-ingredient: Aust.: Banecin; Betnesol-N; Betnovate-N; Cicatrex; Dexa-Rhinospray†; Dolothricin†; Dorithricin; Ecomytrin-Hydrocortison†; Ecomytrin†; Hydoftal; Hydrocortimycin; Locacorten mit Neomycin; Mycostatin V; Nebacetin; Neo-Delphicort; Neocones; Otosporin; Polybactrin†; Riker Antibiotic-Spray†; Synalar N; Topsym polyvalent; Tropoderm; Tyrothricin comp; Ulcurilen; Volon A antibiotikahaltig; **Austral.:** Aristocomb†; Cicatrin; Kenacomb; Nemdyn; Neo-Medrol; Neosporin; Otocomb Otic; Spersin†; **Belg.:** Betnelan-VN†; De Icin; Decadron avec Neomycine; Flogocid; Graneodine†; Maxitrol; Mycolog; Neobactracine; Neodexon†; Otosporin; Panotile; Pimafucort; Polydexa; Polygynax; Predmycin; Pulvo Neomycine; Rhinovalon Neomycine; Spitalen; Statrol; Synalar Bi-Otic; **Braz.:** Amigdagen; Amigdamicin; Anaseptil; Anfomicin; Angino Tricin; Atacoly; Bacigem; Betnovate-N; Bismu-Jet; Cicatrene; Cicatrizan; Colpagex N; Colpolase; Colutoide; Conjuntin; Decadron Nasal; Decadron Oftalmico; Dermase; Dermogen; Dermoxin; Derms; Dexacort; Dexavison; Dimicin; Drenison N; Duplocitrin; Elotin; Enterocler; Enterodina; Enteroftal; Enterozol; Esperson N; Flumex-N; Fluo-Vaso; Fluocal com Pectina; Gargosedans; Gingilone; Gotas Ototilan; Gynax-N; Hidrocin; Hipodex; Histalergi; Infectracina; Larintil; Locorten Neomicina; Maxitrol; Micoplex; Nazobel; Nebacetin; Neocinolon; Neocortin; Neomicina Composta; Neotricin; Novacort; Omcilon AM; Oto Xilodase; Otocort; Otodol; Otolin; Otolone; Otomixyn; Otosporin; Otosynalar; Panotil; Parenterin; Penetran; Poliginax; Polipred; Prenefrin; Providex; Rhinosept; Rinosite; Testinfex; Thiabena; Trivagel N; Trofodermin; Vagitrin-N; Xilodase; **Canad.:** Cicatrin; Cortisporin; Dioptrol; Diospor HC†; Diosporin†; Kenacomb;

The symbol † denotes a preparation no longer actively marketed

Maxitrol; Neo-Cortef; Neo-Medrol Acne; Neo-Medrol Veriderm; NeoDecadron†; Neosporin; Neotopic; Optimyxin Plus; Triacomb; Viaderm-KC; **Denm.:** Decadron med Neomycin; Kenalog Comp; Kenalog Comp med Mycostatin; **Fin.:** Bacibact; Maxitrol; Neo-Medrol comp; Otomize; Pimafucort; Polysporin; **Fr.:** Antibio-Synalar†; Antibiotulle Lumiere; Atebemyxine; Betneval-Neomycine; Cebemyxine; Chibro-Cadron; Cidermex; Corticotulle Lumiere; Dexagrane; Diprosone Neomycine; Halog Neomycine†; Locoide N; Madecassol Neomycine Hydrocortisone; Maxidrol; Myco-Ultralan; Mycolog; Panotile; Penticort Neomycine†; Pivalone Neomycine; Plastenan Neomycine†; Polydexa; Polydexa a la Phenylephrine; Polygynax; Polygynax Virgo; Pulvo 47 Neomycine; Synalar Neomycine†; Tergynan†; Topsyne Neomycine†; Trofoseptine; **Ger.:** Antibiotulle Lumiere; Batrax; Bivacyn; Chibro-Cadron†; Cicatrex; Corticotulle Lumiere; Cortidexason comp; Dexa Polyspectran N; Dispadex comp; Efflumycin; Farco-Uromycin; Halog Tri; Isopto Max; Jellin polyvalent; Jellin-Neomycin; Jellisoft-Neomycin; Kombi-Stulln; Linola-H-compositum N; Lokalison-antimikrobiell Creme N; Myacyne†; Nebacetin; Neobac; Neotracin; Otosporin; Pimafucort; Polygynax; Polyspectran; Prednitracin; Pulvo Neomycin; Topoderm N; Topsym polyvalent; Ulcurilen N; Ultexiv; Volon A antibiotikahaltig N; **Hong Kong:** Bacimycin; Betnovate-N; Bivacyn; Celestoderm-V with Neomycin; Chlomy-P; Decadron with Neomycin; Dexa-Polyspectran; Dextracin; Drenison N; Flunolone; Kenacomb; Maxitrol; Nebacetin; Neo-Medrol Acne; Neosporin; Neotopic; Otosporin; Polygynax; Polyspectran; Prednitracin; Proctosone; Protozone; Spersapolymyxin; Synco-CFN; Triacomb; **Irl.:** Audicort; Betnesol-N; Betnovate-N; Cicatrin; Dexa-Rhinaspray; Graneodin; Kenacomb; Maxitrol; Naseptin; Neo-Cortef; Neo-Medrone†; Neosporin; Otomize; Otosporin; Polybactrin†; Synalar N; Vista-Methasone N; **Israel:** Bamyxin; Betnesol-N; Betnovate-N; Dermacombin; Desoren; Dethamycin; Dethaprine; Dex-Otic; Dexamycin; Dexefrin; FML Neo; Hycocin; Hycomycin; Kenacomb; Locacorten; Maxitrol; Nazodin; Neo-Medrol; Nodryl; Otomize; Otomycin; Otosporin; Polycutan; **Ital.:** Abiostil; Anauran; Antibioptal; Bimixin; Bio-Delta Cortilen; Cicatrene; Desalfa; Desamix-Neomicina; Doricum; Ecoval con Neomicina; Enterostop; Eta Biocortilen; Eta Biocortilen VC; Halcidermo Combi; Idracemi; Idrocet; Idroneomicil; Idustatin†; Kataval; Localyn; Localyn-Neomicina; Locorten; Menaderm; Mixotone; Nefluan; Neo-Audiocort; Neo-Cortofen; Neo-Medrol Veriderm; Neogram; Nevacort; Orobicin; Otomicetina†; Otosporin; Rinojet SF; Solprene; Streptosil con Neomicina-Fher; Trofodermin; Vasosterone Antibiotico; Vasosterone Collirio; **Mex.:** Alin Nasal; Alin Oftalmico; Baycuten N; Biodexan; Cortisporin; Decadron Con Neomicina; Dermalog-C; Dexamicin; Dexsul; Fluo Grin; Hidropolicin; Kaomycin; Kenacomb; Maxitrol; Nebacetina; Neobacigrin; Neosporin; Polixin; Recoveron N; Scheriderm; Septilisin; Soldrin; Synalar N; Synalar Neo; Synalar O; Synalar Oftalmico; Tapzol Con Neomicina; Treda; Tribiot; **Neth.:** Betnelan Neomycine†; Celestoderm met Neomycine; Decadron met neomycine; Maxitrol†; Mycolog; Otosporin; Panotile; Pimafucort†; Polyspectran B†; Polyspectran G†; Predmycin-P Liquifilm†; Synalar Bi-Otic; **Norw.:** Maxitrol; **NZ:** Betnesol-N; Coly-Mycin S Otic; Kenacomb; Maxitrol; Pimafucort; Ultrazon N; **Port.:** Baciderma; Bacitracina-Neo; Betnovate-N; Bienterico; Cicatrin; Conjunctilone; Conjunctilone-S; Davimicina; Decadron; Dermobiotico; Dermovate-NN; Dexaval N; Dexaval O; Dimicina; FML Neo; Kenacomb; Leuco Hubber†; Meocil; Neo-Davisolona; Neo-Preocil; Otolys†; Otosporin; Pimafucort; Plastenan Neomicina; Polydexa; Polygynax; Polysporina†; Predniderma; Tri-Sinerge; **S.Afr.:** Betnesol-N; Betnovate-N; Cicatrin; Covomycin; Covomycin-D; FML Neo; Kaoneo†; Kenacomb; Maxitrol; Naseptin; Nasomixin; Nebacetin†; Neo-Medrol; Neoderm; Neopan; Neopec†; Neosporin; Otoseptil†; Otosporin; Synalar N; Trialone; Vibrocil; **Singapore:** Banecin; Batramycin; Besone-N; Betnovate-N; Celestoderm-V with Neomycin; Dextracin; Fast Powder; Flunolone; Kenacomb; Maxitrol; Neo-Daca; Neo-Medrol; Neosporin; Otosporin; Pivalone Neomycin; Polybamycin; Polydexa; Polygynax; Predmycin-P; Synalar N; Uniflex-N; **Spain:** Alantomicina Complex†; Alantomicina†; Anasilpiel; Antihemorroidal; Bacisporin; Banedif; Betamatil con Neomicina; Bexicortil; Bio Hubber Fuerte†; Bio Hubber†; Blastoestimulina; Cilinafosal Hidrocort; Cilinafosal Neomicina; Cilinavagin Neomicina; Coliriocilina Espectro; Coliriocilina Prednisona; Creanolona; Decadran Neomicina; Decoderm Trivalente; Deltacina; Deltasiton†; Derbitan Antibiotico†; Dermisone Tri Antibiotic; Dermo Hubber; Dermomycose Talco; Drenison Neomicina†; Edifaringen; Flodermol; Fludronef; Fluo Vaso; FML Neo; Gingilone; Grietalgen Hidrocort; Hidroc Neomic; Intradermo Cort Ant Fung; Iruxol Neo; Leuco Hubber; Linitul Antibiotico; Liquipom Dexa Antib; Maxitrol; Menaderm Neomicina; Midacina; Mirantal†; Nasotic Oto; Neo Analsona; Neo Bacitrin; Neo Bacitrin Hidrocortis; Neo Hubber; Neo Moderin; Neo-Synalar†; Neocones; Neodexa; Oftalmo; Oftalmowell; Oto Difusor; Oto Nemoicin Calm†; Otonina; Otosporin; Oxidermiol Enzima; Panotile; Pentalmicina†; Phonal; Plaskine Neomicina; Poly Pred; Pomada Antibiotica; Positon; Poxider†; Prednis Neomic; Rino Dexa; Rinobanedif; Rinoblanco Dexa Antib; Rinovel; Spectrocin; Statrol; Sulfintestin Neom†; Sulfintestin Neomicina; Synalar Nasal; Synalar Neomicina; Synalar Otico; Tisuderma; Tivitis; Trigon Topico; Tulgrasum Antibiotico; Tyroneomicin†; Vasocon Ant; Vinciseptil Otico; **Swed.:** Betnovat med Neomycin; Celeston valerat comp; Decadron cum neomycin; Ecomytrin-Hydrocortison†; Ecomytrin†; Isopto Biotic; Kenacombin†; Nebacetin†; **Switz.:** Bacimycine; Baneopol; Batramycine; Betnovate-N; Cicatrex; Cloptison-N†; Cortifluid N; Cortimycine; Dermovate-NN; Flogocid NN†; FML Neo; Korticoid polyvalent; Maxitrol; Mycinopred; Mycolog; Nebacetin; Neo-Hydro; Neocones; Neosporin; Neotracin; Otosporin; Otospray; Panotile; Pivalone compositum; Polydexa; Prednitracin; Riccomycine†; Spersapolymyxin; Synalar N; Topsym polyvalent; Tyrocombine; **Thai.:** Archidex; Banocin; Benn; Besone-N; Beta-N; Betama-EN; Bethasone-N; Betnovate-N; Cadexcin-N; Celestoderm-V with Neomycin; Coccila; Decadron with Neomycin; Dermacombin; Dex-Otic; Dexacin; Dexasil; Dexoph; Dexylin; Disento; Eyedex; Farakil; Fluciderm-N; Fluonid-N; Fluonolone; FML Neo; Kaopectal-N; Kenacomb; Lobacin; Maxitrol; Mybacin; Mybacin Dermic; Mysolone-N; Neo-Hytisone; Neo-Medrol; Neo-Optal; Neopred; Neosporin; Neozolone; Opsacin; Opsardex; Otosporin; Polyoph; Predex; Predmycin; Prednisil; Prednisil-N; Spersapolymyxin; Statrol; Supra-

lan-N; Synalar N; Trilosil N; Trofodermin; Valbet-N; Xanalin; **UAE:** Panderm; **UK:** Adcortyl with Graneodin†; Audicort; Betnesol-N; Betnovate-N; Cicatrin; Cloburate-N†; Dermovate-NN; Dexa-Rhinaspray†; FML Neo Liquifilm†; Graneodin; Gregoderm; Maxitrol; Naseptin; Neo-Cortef; Neosporin; Otomize; Otosporin; Predsol-N; Synalar N; Tri-Adcortyl; Uniroid†; Vista-Methasone N; **USA:** Ak-Neo-Dex; Ak-Spore; Ak-Spore HC; Ak-Trol; Alba-3†; AntibiOtic; Bacticort†; Bactine First Aid Antibiotic Plus Anesthetic†; Campho-Phenique Antibiotic Plus Pain Reliever Ointment†; Clomycin†; Coly-Mycin S Otic; Coracin†; Cortatrigen; Cortimycin; Cortisporin; Cortisporin-TC; Dexacidin; Dexacine; Dexasporin; Ear-Eze; Lanabiotic; LazerSporin-C; Maxitrol; Mycitracin; Mycitracin Plus†; Neo-Cortef†; Neo-Dexair†; Neo-Dexameth; Neocin; NeoDecadron; Neodexasone; Neomixin†; Neopolydex; Neosporin; Neosporin + Pain Relief; Neosporin GU; Neosporin Plus†; Neotal†; Neotricin HC; Octicair; Ocu-Spor-B; Ocu-Spor-G; Ocu-Trol; Ocutricin; Otic-Care; Oticin HC†; OtiTricin; Otocort; Otomycin-HPN; Otosporin; Pediotic; Poly-Dex; Poly-Pred; Polymycin; Septa†; Spectrocin Plus; Storz-N-D†; Storz-N-P-D†; Tri-Biozene; Tribiotic Plus†; Triple Antibiotic†; UAD-Otic.

Netilmicin Sulfate (114-n)

Netilmicin Sulfate (USAN, rINNM).

N¹-Ethylsissomicin; Netilmicin Sulphate (BANM); Netilmicini Sulfas; Sch-20569. 4-O-[(2R,3R)-cis-3-Amino-6-aminomethyl-3,4-dihydro-2H-pyran-2-yl]-2-deoxy-6-O-(3-deoxy-4-C-methyl-3-methylamino-β-L-arabinopyranosyl)-1-N-ethyl-streptamine sulphate.

$(C_{21}H_{41}N_5O_7)_2,5H_2SO_4 = 1441.6.$

CAS — 56391-56-1 (netilmicin); 56391-57-2 (netilmicin sulfate).

Pharmacopoeias. In Eur. (see p.vi), Jpn, Pol., and US.

1.5 g of monograph substance is approximately equivalent to 1 g of netilmicin.

Incompatibilities. For discussion of the incompatibility of aminoglycosides, including netilmicin, with beta lactams, see under Gentamicin Sulfate, p.210. Netilmicin is also reported to be incompatible with frusemide [furosemide], heparin, and vitamin B complex.

Pharmacopoeial description

Ph. Eur.: A substance obtained by synthesis from sisomicin. The potency is not less than 650 units per mg, calculated with reference to the dried substance. A white or yellowish-white, very hygroscopic, powder. Very soluble in water; practically insoluble in alcohol and in acetone. A 4% solution in water has a pH of 3.5 to 5.5. Store in airtight containers. Protect from light.

USP 25: A white to pale yellowish-white powder. Freely soluble in water; practically insoluble in dehydrated alcohol and in ether. pH of a solution in water containing the equivalent of netilmicin 4% is between 3.5 and 5.5. Store in airtight containers.

Adverse Effects, Treatment, and Precautions

As for Gentamicin Sulfate, p.210. Some studies suggest that netilmicin is less nephrotoxic and ototoxic than gentamicin or tobramycin, although others have not found any significant differences in their toxicity.

Prolonged peak plasma concentrations of netilmicin greater than 16 µg per mL, and trough concentrations greater than 4 µg per mL, should be avoided, and some suggest that peaks below 12 µg per mL and troughs below 2 µg per mL are preferable.

Effects on the cardiovascular system. Severe hypotension was associated with administration of netilmicin in a patient undergoing artificial ventilation.[1] Hypotensive episodes were of short duration and coincided with netilmicin injection. They almost disappeared when sedation was stopped.

1. Rygnestad T. Severe hypotension associated with netilmicin treatment. *BMJ* 1997; **315:** 31.

Interactions

As for Gentamicin Sulfate, p.211.

Antimicrobial Action

As for Gentamicin Sulfate, p.211. It is active against a similar range of organisms although it is also reported to have some activity against *Nocardia*. It may be somewhat less effective against *Pseudomonas aeruginosa*. MICs of netilmicin for the most sensitive organisms range from about 0.25 to 2 µg per mL, but organisms with MICs less than about 8 µg per mL are considered sensitive. It is not degraded by all of the enzymes responsible for aminoglycoside resistance, and may be active against some strains resistant to gentamicin or tobramycin, but this is less marked than with amikacin: for example, gentamicin-resistant *Proteus*, *Providencia*, *Pseudomonas*, and *Serratia* are usually also netilmicin-resistant. Between about 5 and 20% of Gram-negative isolates are reported to be resistant to netilmicin.

Pharmacokinetics
As for Gentamicin Sulfate, p.211.

Following intramuscular injection of netilmicin, peak plasma concentrations are achieved within half to 1 hour, and concentrations of about 7 µg per mL have been reported following doses of 2 mg per kg body-weight; similar concentrations are obtained after intravenous infusion of the same dose over 1 hour. Peak concentrations following rapid intravenous injection may transiently be 2 or 3 times higher than those following infusion. Administration of standard, once-daily doses may produce transient peak concentrations of 20 to 30 µg per mL. In multiple dosing studies, administration of netilmicin in usual doses every 12 hours produced steady-state concentrations on the second day which were less than 20% higher than those seen after the first dose.

The half-life of netilmicin is usually 2.0 to 2.5 hours. About 80% of a dose is excreted in the urine within 24 hours.

Uses and Administration
Netilmicin is a semisynthetic aminoglycoside antibiotic with actions and uses similar to those of gentamicin (p.212). It may be used as an alternative to amikacin (p.148) in the treatment of infections caused by susceptible bacteria that are resistant to gentamicin and tobramycin. As with gentamicin, netilmicin may be used with penicillins and with cephalosporins; the injections should be given separately.

Netilmicin is given as the sulfate but doses are expressed in terms of the equivalent amount of base. It is usually given intramuscularly in doses equivalent to netilmicin 4 to 6 mg per kg body-weight daily as a single dose; alternatively, it may be given in equally divided doses every 8 or 12 hours; for the control of life-threatening infections, up to 7.5 mg per kg may be given daily in divided doses every 8 hours for short periods. In the management of urinary-tract infections, regimens consisting of either a single daily dose of 150 mg for 5 days or of 3 to 4 mg per kg daily in divided doses every 12 hours have been suggested. A single dose of 300 mg has been suggested for gonorrhoea (p.124) although it is not recommended in current treatment guidelines.

The same doses may be given by slow intravenous injection over 3 to 5 minutes or infused intravenously over half to 2 hours in 50 to 200 mL of infusion fluid; proportionately less fluid should be given to children.

Treatment with netilmicin is usually given for 7 to 14 days. Prolonged peak plasma concentrations greater than 16 µg per mL and trough plasma concentrations greater than 4 µg per mL should be avoided. Some sources suggest peaks below 12 µg per mL and troughs below 2 µg per mL for divided daily dose regimens.

Dosage recommendations in infants and children vary somewhat. One regimen is the equivalent of 7.5 to 9 mg of netilmicin per kg daily in infants and neonates older than 1 week, and 6 to 7.5 mg per kg daily in older children, both given in divided doses every 8 hours. Premature infants, and neonates less than 1 week old, would be given 6 mg per kg daily in divided doses of 3 mg per kg every 12 hours. An alternative regimen is 4 to 6.5 mg per kg daily in neonates less than 6 weeks of age, in divided doses every 12 hours, and 5.5 to 8 mg per kg daily in divided doses every 8 or 12 hours in older infants and children.

Dosage should be adjusted in all patients according to plasma-netilmicin concentrations, and this is particularly important where factors such as age, renal impairment, or prolonged therapy may predispose to toxicity, or where there is a risk of subtherapeutic concentrations. For discussion of the methods of calculating aminoglycoside dosage requirements, see p.212.

Preparations
USP 25: Netilmicin Sulfate Injection.

Proprietary Preparations (details are given in Part 3)
Aust.: Certomycin; *Austral.:* Netromycin; *Belg.:* Netromycine; *Braz.:* Netromicina; *Canad.:* Netromycin; *Denm.:* Netilyn; *Fin.:* Netilyn; *Fr.:* Netromicine; *Ger.:* Certomycin; *Hong Kong:* Netromycin; *Irl.:* Netillin; *Ital.:* Nettacin; *Mex.:* Netromicina; *Neth.:* Netromycine; *Norw.:* Netilyn; *NZ:* Netromycin; *Port.:* Netromicina; *S.Afr.:* Netromycin; *Spain:* Dalinar; Netrocin; *Swed.:* Netilyn; *Switz.:* Netromycine; *Thai.:* Netromycin; *UK:* Netillin; *USA:* Netromycin.

Nifuroxazide (13014-j)
Nifuroxazide (rINN).
2′-(5-Nitrofurfurylidene)-4-hydroxybenzohydrazide.
$C_{12}H_9N_3O_5 = 275.2$.
CAS — 965-52-6.
ATC — A07AX03.
Pharmacopoeias. In *Fr.*

Profile
Nifuroxazide is an antibacterial that is poorly absorbed from the gastrointestinal tract. It has been given by mouth in a dose of 800 mg daily in divided doses in the treatment of colitis and diarrhoea.

Preparations
Proprietary Preparations (details are given in Part 3)
Belg.: Bacifurane; Ercefuryl; *Braz.:* Passifuril; *Fr.:* Ambatrol†; Antinal†; Bifix; Ercefuryl; Erceryl; Lumifurex; Nifur; Panfurex; Septidiaryl; *Hong Kong:* Antidia; Ercefuryl; *Ital.:* Diarret; ErceFuryl†; *Mex.:* Akabar; Diarim; Eskapar; Topron; *Singapore:* ErceFuryl; Niraben; *Thai.:* ErceFuryl.

Nifurtoinol (13016-c)
Nifurtoinol (rINN).
Hydroxymethylnitrofurantoin. 3-Hydroxymethyl-1-(5-nitrofurfurylideneamino)hydantoin.
$C_9H_8N_4O_6 = 268.2$.
CAS — 1088-92-2.
ATC — G04AC02.

Profile
Nifurtoinol is a nitrofuran antibacterial with properties similar to those of nitrofurantoin (p.230) and is used in the treatment of urinary-tract infections. It is given by mouth in doses of up to 300 mg daily in divided doses.

Preparations
Proprietary Preparations (details are given in Part 3)
Belg.: Urfadyn PL; *Switz.:* Urfadyne†.

Nifurzide (19569-v)
Nifurzide (rINN).
5-Nitro-2-thiophenecarboxylic acid [3-(5-nitro-2-furyl)allylidene]hydrazide.
$C_{12}H_8N_4O_6S = 336.3$.
CAS — 39978-42-2.
ATC — A07AX04.

Profile
Nifurzide is an antibacterial that is poorly absorbed from the gastrointestinal tract. It has been given by mouth in a dose of 450 mg daily in divided doses in the treatment of diarrhoea.

Preparations
Proprietary Preparations (details are given in Part 3)
Fr.: Ricridene; *Mex.:* Normodiar.

Nisin (13021-y)
E234.
CAS — 1414-45-5.

Profile
Nisin is a polypeptide antibiotic produced by *Streptococcus lactis*. It is used as a preservative for foods.
It is under investigation for treating various infections including those caused by *Helicobacter pylori* and *Clostridium difficile*.

Nitrofurantoin (5651-x)
Nitrofurantoin (BAN, rINN).
Furadoninum; Nitrofurantoinum. 1-(5-Nitrofurfurylideneamino)hydantoin; 1-(5-Nitrofurfurylideneamino)imidazolidine-2,4-dione.
$C_8H_6N_4O_5 = 238.2$.
CAS — 67-20-9 (anhydrous nitrofurantoin); 17140-81-7 (nitrofurantoin monohydrate).
ATC — G04AC01.

Pharmacopoeias. In *Chin.* and *Eur.* (see p.vi).
Int. and *US* specify anhydrous or monohydrate.

Pharmacopoeial description
Ph. Eur.: A yellow, odourless or almost odourless, crystalline powder or crystals. Very slightly soluble in water and in alcohol; soluble in dimethylformamide. Store at a temperature not exceeding 25°. Protect from light.

USP 25: It is anhydrous or contains one molecule of water of hydration. Lemon-yellow, odourless crystals or fine powder. Nitrofurantoin and its solutions are discoloured by alkalis and by exposure to light, and are decomposed on contact with metals other than stainless steel or aluminium. Very slightly soluble in water and in alcohol; soluble in dimethylformamide. Store in airtight containers. Protect from light.

Nitrofurantoin Sodium (5652-r)
Nitrofurantoin Sodium (BANM, rINNM).
$C_8H_5N_4NaO_5 = 260.1$.
CAS — 54-87-5.

Adverse Effects
The estimated incidence of adverse effects with nitrofurantoin has varied enormously, but may be around 10% overall; an incidence of serious reactions of about 0.001% for pulmonary, and 0.0007% for neurological reactions has been suggested. The most common adverse effects encountered with nitrofurantoin involve the gastrointestinal tract. They are dose-related and generally include nausea, vomiting, and anorexia; abdominal pain and diarrhoea occur less frequently. It has been reported that adverse effects on the gastrointestinal tract are less common when nitrofurantoin is administered in a macrocrystalline form or with food.

Neurological adverse effects include headache, drowsiness, vertigo, dizziness, nystagmus, and intracranial hypertension. Severe and sometimes irreversible peripheral polyneuropathy has developed, particularly in patients with impaired renal function and in those given prolonged therapy.

Hypersensitivity reactions such as skin rashes, urticaria, pruritus, fever, and angioedema may occur. Anaphylaxis, erythema multiforme, Stevens-Johnson syndrome, exfoliative dermatitis, pancreatitis, a lupus-like syndrome, myalgia, and arthralgia have also been reported. Patients with a history of asthma may experience acute asthmatic attacks.

Acute pulmonary sensitivity reactions characterised by sudden onset of fever, chills, eosinophilia, cough, chest pain, dyspnoea, pulmonary infiltration or consolidation, and pleural effusion may occur within hours to a few days of beginning therapy, but they usually resolve on discontinuation.

Subacute or chronic pulmonary symptoms including interstitial pneumonitis and pulmonary fibrosis may develop more insidiously in patients on long-term therapy and the latter are not always reversible, particularly if therapy is continued after onset of symptoms.

Hepatotoxicity including cholestatic jaundice and hepatitis may develop rarely, particularly in women, and probably represents a hypersensitivity reaction. Other adverse effects include megaloblastic anaemia, leucopenia, granulocytopenia or agranulocytosis, thrombocytopenia, aplastic anaemia, and haemolytic anaemia in persons with a genetic deficiency of glucose-6-phosphate dehydrogenase. Transient alopecia has been reported.

There is limited evidence from *animal* studies that nitrofurantoin may be carcinogenic, although this has not been demonstrated conclusively in humans.

◊ References.
1. Koch-Weser J, *et al.* Adverse reactions to sulfisoxazole, sulfamethoxazole, and nitrofurantoin: manifestations and specific reaction rates during 2118 courses of therapy. *Arch Intern Med* 1971; **128:** 399–404.
2. Holmberg L, *et al.* Adverse reactions to nitrofurantoin: analysis of 921 reports. *Am J Med* 1980; **69:** 733–8.
3. Penn RG, Griffin JP. Adverse reactions to nitrofurantoin in the United Kingdom, Sweden, and Holland. *BMJ* 1982; **284:** 1440–2.
4. D'Arcy PF. Nitrofurantoin. *Drug Intell Clin Pharm* 1985; **19:** 540–7.

Precautions

Nitrofurantoin should not be given to patients with impaired renal function since antibacterial concentrations in the urine may not be attained and toxic concentrations in the plasma can occur. Nitrofurantoin is also contra-indicated in patients known to be hypersensitive to nitrofurans, in those with a deficiency of glucose-6-phosphate dehydrogenase, and in infants less than three months old. It has been suggested that nitrofurantoin should not be used in pregnant patients at term because of the possibility of producing haemolytic anaemia in the neonate, and that it should be avoided, or used with caution, in mothers who are breast feeding infants who have a deficiency of glucose-6-phosphate dehydrogenase since traces are found in breast milk.

Nitrofurantoin should be used with care in the elderly, who may be at increased risk of toxicity, particularly acute pulmonary reactions. All patients undergoing prolonged therapy should be monitored for changes in pulmonary function, and the drug withdrawn at the first signs of pulmonary damage. Care is required in patients with pre-existing pulmonary, hepatic, neurological or allergic disorders, and in those with conditions (such as anaemia, diabetes mellitus, electrolyte imbalance, debility, or vitamin B deficiency) which may predispose to peripheral neuropathy. Nitrofurantoin should be withdrawn if signs of peripheral neuropathy develop.

Nitrofurantoin may cause false positive reactions in urine tests for glucose using copper reduction methods.

Nitrofurantoin may cause a brownish discoloration of the urine.

Porphyria. Nitrofurantoin has been associated with acute attacks of porphyria and is considered to be unsafe in porphyric patients.

Interactions

Nitrofurantoin and the quinolone antibacterials are antagonistic *in vitro* and their concomitant use is not recommended. The antibacterial activity of nitrofurantoin may be decreased in the presence of carbonic anhydrase inhibitors and other drugs that alkalinise the urine.

Probenecid or sulfinpyrazone may reduce the excretion of nitrofurantoin and should not be given with it. Magnesium trisilicate may reduce the absorption of nitrofurantoin but it is not clear whether this applies to other antacids.

◊ For reference to the effect of nitrofurantoin on *phenytoin,* see p.359. For mention of a possible decrease in contraceptive efficacy when nitrofurantoin was given concomitantly with *oral contraceptives,* see under Hormonal Contraceptives, p.1458.

Antimicrobial Action

Nitrofurantoin is bactericidal *in vitro* to most Gram-positive and Gram-negative urinary-tract pathogens. The mode of action is uncertain but appears to depend on the formation of reactive intermediates by reduction; this process occurs more efficiently in bacterial than in mammalian cells.

It is effective against the enterococci *in vitro,* as well as various other Gram-positive species including staphylococci, streptococci, and corynebacteria, although this is of little clinical significance. Most strains of *Escherichia coli* are particularly sensitive to nitrofurantoin but *Enterobacter* and *Klebsiella* spp. are less susceptible and some may be resistant. *Pseudomonas aeruginosa* is resistant as are most strains of *Proteus* spp.

The symbol † denotes a preparation no longer actively marketed

---

Organisms with MICs below 32 μg per mL are usually considered susceptible, as such concentrations are readily achievable in urine, while strains with MICs above about 128 μg per mL are considered resistant. Nitrofurantoin is generally bactericidal at concentrations not much above the MIC. It is most active in acid urine, and if the pH exceeds 8 most of the antibacterial activity is lost. Resistance rarely develops during nitrofurantoin treatment but may occur during prolonged treatment. Plasmid-encoded resistance has been reported in *E. coli.* Resistance may be due to the loss of nitrofuran reductases which generate the active intermediates.

Pharmacokinetics

Nitrofurantoin is readily absorbed from the gastrointestinal tract. The absorption rate is dependent on crystal size. The macrocrystalline form has slower dissolution and absorption rates, produces lower serum concentrations than the microcrystalline form, and takes longer to achieve peak concentrations in the urine. The presence of food in the gastrointestinal tract may increase the bioavailability of nitrofurantoin and prolong the duration of therapeutic urinary concentrations. Preparations of nitrofurantoin from different sources may not be bioequivalent, and care may be necessary if changing from one brand to another.

Following absorption, concentrations in blood and body tissues are low because of rapid elimination, and antibacterial concentrations are not achieved. Nitrofurantoin crosses the placenta and the blood-brain barrier and traces have been detected in breast milk. There is some disagreement about the degree of protein binding, and although figures of up to about 60% are quoted by some sources, others suggest that the figure should be as much as 90 to 95%. The plasma half-life is reported to range from 0.3 to 1 hour.

Nitrofurantoin is metabolised in the liver and most body tissues while about 30 to 40% of a dose is excreted rapidly in the urine as unchanged nitrofurantoin. Some tubular reabsorption may occur in acid urine. Average doses give a concentration of 50 to 200 μg per mL in the urine in patients with normal renal function.

Uses and Administration

Nitrofurantoin is a nitrofuran derivative which is used in the treatment of uncomplicated lower urinary-tract infections (p.146), including for prophylaxis or long-term suppressive therapy in recurrent infection.

It is given by mouth usually in a dose of 50 to 100 mg four times daily, with food or milk. In uncomplicated infection 100 mg twice daily may be adequate. Treatment is usually continued for 7 days. A usual long-term prophylactic dose is 50 to 100 mg at bedtime.

Infants over 3 months of age and older children may be given 3 mg per kg body-weight daily in 4 divided doses by mouth. For long-term prophylactic therapy 1 mg per kg once daily may be adequate.

Preparations

BP 2001: Nitrofurantoin Oral Suspension; Nitrofurantoin Tablets; **USP 25:** Nitrofurantoin Capsules; Nitrofurantoin Oral Suspension; Nitrofurantoin Tablets.

Proprietary Preparations (details are given in Part 3)
Aust.: Furadantin; Urolong†; **Austral.:** Furadantin; Macrodantin; Ralodantin; **Belg.:** Furadantine; **Braz.:** Macrodantina; Uro Furan Urogen; **Canad.:** Macrobid; Macrodantin; Novo-Furantoin; **Fin.:** Nitrofur-C; **Fr.:** Furadantine; Furadoine; Microdoine; **Ger.:** Cystit; Furadantin; Nifurantin; Nifuretten; Uro-Tablinen; **Irl.:** Furadantin; Macrobid; Macrodantin; **Israel:** Macrodantin; Urantoin; Uvamin; **Ital.:** Cistofuran†; Furadantin; Furedan; Furil; Macrodantin; Neo-Furadantin; **Mex.:** Biofurin; Furadantina; Futroken; Macrodantina; Macrofurin; Promac; Teguran; Urobac; **Neth.:** Furabid; Furadantine MC; **Norw.:** Furadantin; **NZ:** Furadantin; Nifuran; **Port.:** Furadantina†; **S.Afr.:** Furadantin; Macrodantin; Urantin†; **Spain:** Chemiofurin†; Furantoina; Furobactina; **Swed.:** Furadantin; **Switz.:** Furadantine; Urodin; Uvamine retard; **UK:** Furadantin; Macrobid; Macrodantin; Urantoin; **USA:** Furadantin; Macrobid; Macrodantin.

Multi-ingredient: Aust.: Spasmo-Urolong†; Urospasmon sine phenazopyridino†; **Braz.:** Nipactrin; Urofen; Uropac; **Ger.:** Nifurantin B 6; Urospasmon; Urospasmon sine; **Mex.:** Furanton; **Spain:** Urogobens Antiespasmo†.

Nitrofurazone (1626-w)

Nitrofurazone *(BAN).*

Nitrofural *(pINN);* Furacilinum; Nitrofuralum. 5-Nitro-2-furaldehyde semicarbazone.
$C_6H_6N_4O_4 = 198.1.$
CAS — 59-87-0.
ATC — B05CA03; D08AF01; D09AA03; P01CC02; S01AX04; S02AA02.
Pharmacopoeias. In *Eur.* (see p.vi), *Pol.,* and *US.*

It discolours on contact with alkalis.

Pharmacopoeial description
Ph. Eur.: A yellow or brownish-yellow, crystalline powder. Very slightly soluble in water; slightly soluble in alcohol; practically insoluble in ether. The filtrate from a 1% suspension in water has a pH of 5.0 to 7.0. Protect from light.

USP 25: A lemon-yellow, odourless crystalline powder. It darkens slowly on exposure to light. Soluble 1 in 4200 of water, 1 in 590 of alcohol, and 1 in 350 of propylene glycol; practically insoluble in chloroform and in ether; soluble in dimethylformamide; slightly soluble in polyethylene glycol mixtures. The filtrate from a 1% suspension in water has a pH of 5.0 to 7.5. Store in airtight containers at a temperature not exceeding 40°. Protect from light.

Sterilisation. Autoclaving gauze dressings impregnated with nitrofurazone, as recommended by the US manufacturer of the preparation, resulted in a greater than 10% loss of the drug.[1] Since the spectroscopic assay used may not distinguish between nitrofurazone and some of its degradation products, the degree of degradation may have been greater than this.
1. Phillips C, Fisher E. Effect of autoclaving on stability of nitrofurazone soluble dressing. *Am J Health-Syst Pharm* 1996; **53:** 1169–71.

Adverse Effects
Sensitisation and generalised allergic skin reactions may be produced by the topical application of nitrofurazone.

Nitrofurazone is a toxic drug when given by mouth and serious adverse effects include severe peripheral neuropathy; haemolysis may occur in patients with a deficiency of glucose-6-phosphate dehydrogenase. Nitrofurazone in high oral doses is carcinogenic in *rats.*

Precautions
Topical preparations of nitrofurazone are contra-indicated in patients with known hypersensitivity. Those preparations containing macrogols should be used with caution in patients with renal dysfunction since macrogols can be absorbed and their accumulation in such patients may result in symptoms of progressive renal impairment.

Because of the risk of haemolysis nitrofurazone by mouth should be used with caution in patients with glucose-6-phosphate dehydrogenase deficiency.

Antimicrobial Action
Nitrofurazone is a nitrofuran derivative with a broad spectrum of antibacterial activity, but with little activity against *Pseudomonas* spp. It also has antitrypanosomal activity.

Uses and Administration
Nitrofurazone is a nitrofuran derivative which is used as a local application for wounds, burns, ulcers, and skin infections, and for the preparation of surfaces before skin grafting. It is usually applied in a concentration of 0.2% in a water-soluble or water-miscible basis. A solution of nitrofurazone is used for bladder irrigation.

Preparations
USP 25: Nitrofurazone Ointment; Nitrofurazone Topical Solution.
Proprietary Preparations (details are given in Part 3)
Belg.: Furacine; **Braz.:** Alivioderm; Caziderm; Furacin; **Ger.:** Furacin-Sol; Nifucin†; **Israel:** Rafuzone; **Ital.:** Furacin†; **Mex.:** Furacin; Nifurol; **Neth.:** Furacine; **S.Afr.:** Furacin; Furasept; Furex; Germex†; **Spain:** Furacin; **Thai.:** Polycin; **USA:** Furacin.

Multi-ingredient: Braz.: Colpacid; Dermilan; Elocort; Furazolon; Infladerm; Nitrileno; Nitronasal; Otodol; Otolin; Panotil; Rinocron; Solucao Nasal de Nafazolina; **Ger.:** Nifucin†; **Ital.:** Furanvit; Furotricina; **Mex.:** Madecassol C; **Spain:** Dertrase; **Thai.:** Denson.

Nitroxoline (5664-h)

Nitroxoline *(BAN, pINN).*
5-Nitroquinolin-8-ol.
$C_9H_6N_2O_3 = 190.2.$
CAS — 4008-48-4.
ATC — G04AG06.

Profile
Nitroxoline has antibacterial and antifungal properties and is used in the treatment of urinary-tract infections in usual doses of 600 mg daily by mouth in divided doses before food. It has also been given in combination with sulfamethizole.

Preparations
Proprietary Preparations (details are given in Part 3)
Fr.: Nibiol; *Mex.:* Noxigur; *S.Afr.:* Nicene N.
Multi-ingredient: Braz.: Urotril; **S.Afr.:** Nicene†.

Norfloxacin (12349-g)

Norfloxacin *(BAN, USAN, rINN)*.

AM-715; MK-366; Norfloxacinum. 1-Ethyl-6-fluoro-1,4-dihydro-4-oxo-7-(piperazin-1-yl)quinoline-3-carboxylic acid.
$C_{16}H_{18}FN_3O_3 = 319.3$.
CAS — 70458-96-7.
ATC — J01MA06; S01AX12.
Pharmacopoeias. In Chin., Eur. (see p.vi), Pol., and US.

Pharmacopoeial description
Ph. Eur.: A white or pale yellow, hygroscopic, photosensitive, crystalline powder. Very slightly soluble in water; slightly soluble in alcohol and in acetone. Store in airtight containers. Protect from light.

USP 25: A white to pale yellow crystalline powder. Slightly soluble in water, in alcohol, and in acetone; freely soluble in acetic acid; sparingly soluble in chloroform; practically insoluble in ether; very slightly soluble in ethyl acetate and in methyl alcohol. Store in airtight containers. Protect from light.

Adverse Effects and Precautions
As for Ciprofloxacin, p.183.

Effects on the kidneys. References.
1. Hestin D, *et al.* Norfloxacin-induced nephrotic syndrome. *Lancet* 1995; **345:** 732–3.

Interactions
As for Ciprofloxacin, p.184.

Antimicrobial Action
As for Ciprofloxacin, p.184, although norfloxacin is less potent *in vitro*. Norfloxacin is not active against *Chlamydia* spp., mycoplasmas, or mycobacteria.

Pharmacokinetics
About 30 to 40% of an oral dose of norfloxacin is absorbed. Peak plasma concentrations of about 1.5 µg per mL have been achieved 1 to 2 hours after the administration of a 400-mg dose by mouth; the presence of food can delay absorption. The plasma half-life is about 4 hours and may be prolonged in renal impairment; a value of 6.5 hours or more has been reported when creatinine clearance is below 30 mL per minute. Norfloxacin has been reported to be 14% bound to plasma proteins. It is probably widely distributed, but information is limited. Norfloxacin penetrates well into tissues of the genito-urinary tract. It crosses the placenta. Relatively high concentrations are achieved in bile.

About 30% of a dose is excreted unchanged in the urine within 24 hours, producing high urinary concentrations; norfloxacin is least soluble at a urinary pH of 7.5. Urinary excretion is by tubular secretion and glomerular filtration and is reduced by probenecid, although plasma concentrations of norfloxacin are not generally affected. Some metabolism occurs, possibly in the liver, and several metabolites have been identified in urine, some with antibacterial activity. About 30% of an oral dose is recovered from the faeces.

◊ References.
1. Norrby SR. Pharmacokinetics of norfloxacin: clinical implications. *Eur J Chemother Antibiot* 1983; **3:** 19–25.
2. Swanson BN, *et al.* Norfloxacin disposition after sequentially increasing oral doses. *Antimicrob Agents Chemother* 1983; **23:** 284–8.
3. Fillastre JP, *et al.* Pharmacokinetics of norfloxacin in renal failure. *J Antimicrob Chemother* 1984; **14:** 439.
4. Arrigo G, *et al.* Pharmacokinetics of norfloxacin in chronic renal failure. *Int J Clin Pharmacol Ther Toxicol* 1985; **23:** 491–6.
5. MacGowan AP, *et al.* The pharmacokinetics of norfloxacin in the aged. *J Antimicrob Chemother* 1988; **22:** 721–7.
6. Kelly JG, *et al.* Chronic dose urinary and serum pharmacokinetics of norfloxacin in the elderly. *Br J Clin Pharmacol* 1988; **26:** 787–90.

Uses and Administration
Norfloxacin is a fluoroquinolone antibacterial with properties similar to those of ciprofloxacin, but it is generally less potent *in vitro*.

Norfloxacin is used mainly in the treatment of urinary-tract infections (p.146). It is also used for the treatment of gonorrhoea (p.124).

Norfloxacin is administered by mouth. In urinary-tract infections the usual dose is 400 mg twice daily for 3 to 10 days. Treatment may need to be continued for up to 12 weeks in chronic relapsing urinary-tract

infections; it may be possible to reduce the dose to 400 mg once daily if there is an adequate response within the first 4 weeks.

Doses may need to be reduced in renal impairment; 400 mg once daily may be given to patients with a creatinine clearance of 30 mL or less per minute.

A single oral dose of 800 mg is given in the treatment of uncomplicated gonorrhoea.

Eye drops containing 0.3% of norfloxacin are used to treat eye infections.

◊ Reviews.
1. Holmes B, *et al.* Norfloxacin: a review of its antibacterial activity, pharmacokinetic properties and therapeutic use. *Drugs* 1985; **30:** 482–513.
2. Wolfson JS, Hooper DC. Norfloxacin: a new targeted fluoroquinolone antimicrobial agent. *Ann Intern Med* 1988; **108:** 238–51.

Preparations
BP 2001: Norfloxacin Eye Drops; Norfloxacin Tablets;
USP 25: Norfloxacin Ophthalmic Solution; Norfloxacin Tablets.

Proprietary Preparations (details are given in Part 3)
Aust.: Urobacid; Zoroxin; **Austral.:** Insensye; Norflohexal; Noroxin; **Belg.:** Chibroxol; Zoroxin; **Braz.:** Chibroxin; Floxacin; Floxinol; Noracin; Quinoform; Respexil; Uritrat NF; Uroflox; Uroplex; **Canad.:** Apo-Norflox; Noroxin; **Denm.:** Zoroxin; **Fin.:** Lexinor; Noroxin; **Fr.:** Chibroxine; Noroxine; **Ger.:** Bactracid; Barazan; Chibroxin; Firin; Norflosal; Norflox-Azu; **Hong Kong:** Chibroxin; Lexiflox; Lexinor; **Israel:** Apirol; Chibroxin; **Ital.:** Flossac; Fulgram; Norflox; Noroxin; Sebercim; Utinor; **Jpn:** Baccidal; **Mex.:** Difoxacil; Floxacin; Microxen; Noroxin; Oranor; **Neth.:** Chibroxol; Noroxin; **NZ:** Noroxin; **Port.:** Chibroxol; Noroxin; Quinoflex; Taflox; Uroflox; **S.Afr.:** Noroxin; Utin; **Singapore:** Bexinor; Chibroxin; Effectsal; Gyrablock; Lexinor; Norbactin; Trizolin; Urobacid; **Spain:** Amicrobin; Baccidal; Chibroxin; Esclebin; Espeden; Nalion; Noroxin; Senro; Uroctal; Vicnas; **Swed.:** Lexinor; **Switz.:** Chibroxol; Norflocin; Noroxin; Norsol; **Thai.:** Floxenor; Foxin; Foxinon; Gonorcin; Gyrablock; Janacin; Lexfor; Lexinor; Noracin; Noraxin; Norbactin; Norcin; Norfcin; Norflo; Norflocin; Norfloxin; Norsa; Noraxacin; Norxia; Noxine; Noxinor; Rexacin; Trizolin; Urinox; Xacin; **UAE:** Uroxin; **UK:** Utinor; **USA:** Chibroxin; Noroxin.

Novobiocin (115-h)

Novobiocin *(BAN, rINN)*.

Crystallinic Acid; PA-93; Streptonivicin; U-6591. 4-Hydroxy-3-[4-hydroxy-3-(3-methylbut-2-enyl)benzamido]-8-methylcoumarin-7-yl 3-O-carbamoyl-5,5-di-C-methyl-α-L-lyxofuranoside.
$C_{31}H_{36}N_2O_{11} = 612.6$.
CAS — 303-81-1.

An antimicrobial substance produced by the growth of *Streptomyces niveus* and *S. spheroides* or related organisms.

Novobiocin Calcium (116-m)

Novobiocin Calcium *(BANM, rINNM)*.

Calcium Novobiocin; Novobiocinum Calcium.
$(C_{31}H_{35}N_2O_{11})_2Ca = 1263.3$.
CAS — 4309-70-0.

Novobiocin Sodium (117-b)

Novobiocin Sodium *(BANM, rINNM)*.

Novobiocinum Natricum; Sodium Novobiocin.
$C_{31}H_{35}N_2NaO_{11} = 634.6$.
CAS — 1476-53-5.
Pharmacopoeias. In Fr., Int., and US.

1.04 g of monograph substance is approximately equivalent to 1 g of novobiocin. Each g of monograph substance represents about 1.6 mmol of sodium.

Pharmacopoeial description
USP 25: A white or yellowish-white, odourless, hygroscopic crystalline powder. Freely soluble in water, in alcohol, in methyl alcohol, in glycerol, and in propylene glycol; practically insoluble in acetone, in chloroform, and in ether; slightly soluble in butyl acetate. pH of a 2.5% solution in water is between 6.5 and 8.5. Store in airtight containers.

Profile
Novobiocin is an antimicrobial which is structurally related to coumarin. It is active against Gram-positive bacteria such as *Staphylococcus aureus* (including meticillin-resistant strains) and other staphylococci; the enterococci are usually resistant. Some Gram-negative organisms including *Haemophilus influenzae* and *Neisseria* spp. are also susceptible, as are some strains of *Proteus*, but most of the Enterobacteriaceae are resistant. Its action is primarily bacteriostatic, although it may be bactericidal against more sensitive species at high concentrations. It is an inhibitor of DNA gyrase and is effective in eliminating plasmids, but resistance to novobiocin develops readily *in vitro* and during therapy.

Although novobiocin has been used alone or with other drugs such as rifampicin or tetracycline in the treatment of infections due to staphylococci and other susceptible organisms, it has been largely superseded by other drugs because of the problems of resistance and toxicity.

Novobiocin is a potent sensitiser and hypersensitivity reactions are relatively common; they include rashes, fever, and pruritus, and more serious reactions such as Stevens-Johnson syndrome and pneumonitis. Jaundice and liver damage have occurred, although apparent jaundice may be due to a yellow metabolite of the drug rather than hyperbilirubinaemia. Other adverse effects include eosinophilia, leucopenia, thrombocytopenia, agranulocytosis, and haemolytic anaemia; gastrointestinal disturbances are common.

Porphyria. Novobiocin has been associated with acute attacks of porphyria and is considered unsafe in porphyric patients.

Preparations
Proprietary Preparations (details are given in Part 3)
USA: Albamycin†.
Multi-ingredient: *Spain:* Tetra Tripsin.

Ofloxacin (16935-w)

Ofloxacin *(BAN, USAN, rINN)*.

DL-8280; Hoe-280; Ofloxacinum. (±)-9-Fluoro-2,3-dihydro-3-methyl-10-(4-methyl-1-piperazinyl)-7-oxo-7H-pyrido[1,2,3-de]-1,4-benzoxazine-6-carboxylic acid.
$C_{18}H_{20}FN_3O_4 = 361.4$.
CAS — 82419-36-1; 83380-47-6.
ATC — J01MA01; S01AX11.
Pharmacopoeias. In Eur. (see p.vi) and US.

Pharmacopoeial description
Ph. Eur.: A pale yellow or bright yellow crystalline powder. Slightly soluble in water and in methyl alcohol; slightly soluble to soluble in dichloromethane; soluble in glacial acetic acid. Store in airtight containers. Protect from light.

USP 25: Pale yellowish-white to light yellowish-white crystals or crystalline powder. Slightly soluble in water, in alcohol, and in methyl alcohol; sparingly soluble in chloroform. Protect from light.

Adverse Effects and Precautions
As for Ciprofloxacin, p.183.

Interactions
As for Ciprofloxacin, p.184.

Antimicrobial Action
As for Ciprofloxacin, p.184.

Ofloxacin is more active than ciprofloxacin against *Chlamydia trachomatis*. It is also active against *Mycobacterium leprae* as well as *M. tuberculosis* and some other *Mycobacterium* spp. Synergistic activity against *M. leprae* has been reported between ofloxacin and rifabutin.

The optically active *S*-(−)-isomer levofloxacin (p.219) has twice the activity of the racemate ofloxacin.

Resistance has been reported in some strains of *Neisseria gonorrhoeae*.

◊ References.
1. Dhople AM, *et al.* In vitro synergistic activity between ofloxacin and ansamycins against *Mycobacterium leprae*. *Arzneimittelforschung* 1993; **43:** 384–6.
2. Kam K-M, *et al.* Ofloxacin susceptibilities of 5667 *Neisseria gonorrhoea* strains isolated in Hong Kong. *Antimicrob Agents Chemother* 1993; **37:** 2007–8.
3. Kam KM, *et al.* Quinolone-resistant *Neisseria gonorrhoeae* in Hong Kong. *Sex Transm Dis* 1996; **23:** 103–8.
4. Cambau E, *et al.* Multidrug-resistance to dapsone, rifampicin, and ofloxacin in *Mycobacterium leprae*. *Lancet* 1997; **349:** 103–4.

Pharmacokinetics
Ofloxacin is rapidly and well absorbed from the gastrointestinal tract. Oral bioavailability is almost 100% and a peak plasma concentration of 3 to 4 µg per mL is achieved 1 to 2 hours after a dose of 400 mg by mouth. Absorption may be delayed by the presence of food, but the extent of absorption is not substantially affected. The plasma half-life ranges from 5 to 8 hours; in renal impairment values of 15 to 60 hours have been reported.

About 25% is bound to plasma proteins. Ofloxacin is widely distributed in body fluids, including the CSF, and tissue penetration is good. It crosses the placenta and is distributed into breast milk. Relatively high concentrations are achieved in bile.

There is limited metabolism to desmethyl and *N*-oxide metabolites; desmethylofloxacin has moderate antibacterial activity. Ofloxacin is eliminated mainly by the kidneys. Excretion is by tubular secretion and glomerular filtration and 75 to 80% of a dose is excreted unchanged in the urine over 24 to 48 hours, resulting in high urinary concentrations. Less than 5% is excreted in the urine as metabolites. From 4 to 8% of a dose may be excreted in the faeces.

Only small amounts of ofloxacin are removed by haemodialysis.

◊ References.

1. Lamp KC, et al. Ofloxacin clinical pharmacokinetics. Clin Pharmacokinet 1992; 22: 32–46.
2. Flor SC, et al. Bioequivalence of oral and intravenous ofloxacin after multiple-dose administration to healthy male volunteers. Antimicrob Agents Chemother 1993; 37: 1468–72.
3. Nau R, et al. Kinetics of ofloxacin and its metabolites in cerebrospinal fluid after a single intravenous infusion of 400 milligrams of ofloxacin. Antimicrob Agents Chemother 1994; 38: 1849–53.
4. Tang-Liu DD-S, et al. Comparative tear concentrations over time of ofloxacin and tobramycin in human eyes. Clin Pharmacol Ther 1994; 55: 284–92.
5. Bethell DB, et al. Pharmacokinetics of oral and intravenous ofloxacin in children with multidrug-resistant typhoid fever. Antimicrob Agents Chemother 1996; 40: 2167–72.
6. Durmaz B, et al. Aqueous humor penetration of topically applied ciprofloxacin, ofloxacin and tobramycin. Arzneimittelforschung 1997; 47: 413–15.
7. McMullin CM, et al. The pharmacokinetics of once-daily oral 400 mg ofloxacin in patients with peritonitis complicating continuous ambulatory peritoneal dialysis. J Antimicrob Chemother 1997; 39: 829–31.

Uses and Administration

Ofloxacin is a fluoroquinolone antibacterial used similarly to ciprofloxacin (p.185). It is also used in chlamydial infections including nongonococcal urethritis (p.117 and p.146) and in the treatment of mycobacterial infections such as leprosy (p.126).

Ofloxacin is given by mouth as the base or intravenously as the hydrochloride. All doses are expressed in terms of the base.

The adult oral or intravenous dose ranges from 200 mg daily to 400 mg twice daily depending on the severity and the nature of the infection. Oral doses up to 400 mg may be given as a single dose, preferably in the morning. For intravenous use a 0.2% solution is infused over 30 minutes or a 0.4% solution over 60 minutes. A dose of 400 mg daily or intermittently by mouth has been recommended (by WHO) as part of alternative multidrug therapy regimens for leprosy.

Lower doses may be necessary in patients with impaired renal function. Following a normal initial dose, subsequent doses are halved to 100 to 200 mg daily or the usual dose is given every 24 hours in patients with a creatinine clearance of 20 to 50 mL per minute; the dose should be reduced to 100 mg every 24 hours when the creatinine clearance is less than 20 mL per minute. Patients on dialysis may be given 100 mg every 24 hours.

A single 400-mg dose of ofloxacin may be given by mouth for uncomplicated gonorrhoea.

Ofloxacin is also employed as 0.3% eye drops and 0.3% ear drops.

◊ Reviews.

1. Todd PA, Faulds D. Ofloxacin: a reappraisal of its antimicrobial activity, pharmacology and therapeutic use. Drugs 1991; 42: 825–76.
2. Onrust SV, et al. Ofloxacin: a reappraisal of its use in the management of genitourinary tract infections. Drugs 1998; 56: 895–928.
3. Simpson KL, Markham A. Ofloxacin otic solution: a review of its use in the management of ear infections. Drugs 1999; 58: 509–31.

Preparations

USP 25: Ofloxacin Ophthalmic Solution.

Proprietary Preparations (details are given in Part 3)
Aust.: Floxal; Tarivid; *Austral.:* Ocuflox; Oflocet; *Belg.:* Tarivid; Trafloxal; *Braz.:* Floxstat; Oflox; Ofloxan; *Canad.:* Apo-Oflox; Floxin; Ocuflox; *Denm.:* Exocin; Tarivid; *Fin.:* Exocin; Tarivid; *Fr.:* Exocine; Monoflocet; Oflocet; *Ger.:* Tarivid; Uro-Tarivid; *Hong Kong:* Tarivid; *Irl.:* Exocin; Tarivid; *Israel:* Oflox; Tarivid; *Ital.:* Exocin; Flobacin; Oflocin; *Jpn:* Tarivid; *Mex.:* Bactocin; Floxil; Floxstat; Ocuflox; *Neth.:* Tarivid; Trafloxal; *Norw.:* Tarivid; *NZ:* Oflocet; *Port.:* Bactoflox; Bioquil; Exocin; Floxedol; Megacina†; Megasin; Oflocet; Tarivid; *S.Afr.:* Exocin; Tarivid; *Singapore:* Inoflox; Tarivid; *Spain:* Exocin; Oflovir; Surnox; Tarivid; *Swed.:* Tarivid; *Switz.:* Floxal; Tarivid; *Thai.:* Konovid; O-Flox; Occidal; Ofloxa; Ofloxcin; Qinolon; Seracin; Tarivid; *UK:* Exocin; Tarivid; *USA:* Floxin; Ocuflox.

Oleandomycin Phosphate (118-v)

Oleandomycin Phosphate (BANM, rINNM).

PA-105 (oleandomycin). (2R,3S,4R,5S,6S,8R,10R,11S,12R,13R)-3-(2,6-Dideoxy-3-O-methyl-α-L-arabino-hexopyranosyloxy)-8,8-epoxymethano-11-hydroxy-2,4,6,10,12,13-hexamethyl-9-oxo-5-(3,4,6-trideoxy-3-dimethylamino-β-D-xylo-hexopyranosyloxy)tridecan-13-olide phosphate.

$C_{35}H_{61}NO_{12},H_3PO_4$ = 785.9.

CAS — 3922-90-5 (oleandomycin); 7060-74-4 (oleandomycin phosphate).

Profile

Oleandomycin is a macrolide antibiotic produced by the growth of certain strains of *Streptomyces antibioticus* with actions and uses similar to those of erythromycin (p.201). It has antimicrobial activity weaker than that of erythromycin. It has been given by mouth or intravenously as the phosphate.

The triacetyl ester, troleandomycin (p.266), has also been used.

Orbifloxacin (17102-d)

Orbifloxacin (rINN).

1-Cyclopropyl-7-(cis-3,5-dimethyl-1-piperazinyl)-5,6,8-trifluoro-1,4-dihydro-4-oxo-3-quinolinecarboxylic acid.

$C_{19}H_{20}F_3N_3O_3$ = 395.4.

CAS — 113617-63-3.

Profile

Orbifloxacin is a fluoroquinolone antibacterial used in veterinary medicine.

Ormetoprim (6350-z)

Ormetoprim (USAN, rINN).

NSC-95072; Ro-5-9754. 5-(4,5-Dimethoxy-2-methylphenyl)methyl-2,4-pyrimidinediamine.

$C_{14}H_{18}N_4O_2$ = 274.3.

CAS — 6981-18-6.

Profile

Ormetoprim is a diaminopyrimidine antibacterial used in veterinary medicine in combination with sulfadimethoxine.

Oxacillin Sodium (119-g)

Oxacillin Sodium (BANM, USAN, rINNM).

(5-Methyl-3-phenyl-4-isoxazolyl)penicillin Sodium; Oxacillinum Natricum; Oxacillinum Natrium; P-12; SQ-16423. Sodium (6R)-6-(5-methyl-3-phenylisoxazole-4-carboxamido)penicillanate monohydrate.

$C_{19}H_{18}N_3NaO_5S,H_2O$ = 441.4.

CAS — 66-79-5 (oxacillin); 1173-88-2 (anhydrous oxacillin sodium); 7240-38-2 (oxacillin sodium, monohydrate).

Pharmacopoeias. In Chin. and US.

1.1 g of monograph substance is approximately equivalent to 1 g of anhydrous oxacillin. Each g of monograph substance represents about 2.3 mmol of sodium.

Oxacillin sodium has been reported to be incompatible with aminoglycosides and tetracyclines.

Pharmacopoeial description

USP 25: A fine white crystalline powder, odourless or having a slight odour. Freely soluble in water, in dimethyl sulfoxide, and in methyl alcohol; slightly soluble in dehydrated alcohol, in chloroform, in methyl acetate, and in pyridine; insoluble in ether, in ethyl acetate, in ethylene chloride, and in benzene. pH of a 3% solution in water is between 4.5 and 7.5. Store in airtight containers at a mean temperature not exceeding 25°.

Adverse Effects and Precautions

As for Flucloxacillin, p.207.

Effects on the liver. References.

1. Onorato IM, Axelrod JL. Hepatitis from intravenous high-dose oxacillin therapy: findings in an adult inpatient population. Ann Intern Med 1978; 89: 497–500.
2. Saliba B, Herbert PN. Oxacillin hepatotoxicity in HIV-infected patients. Ann Intern Med 1994; 120: 1048.

Interactions

As for Benzylpenicillin, p.158.

Antimicrobial Action

As for Flucloxacillin, p.207.

◊ The isolation of pneumococci resistant to oxacillin but sensitive to benzylpenicillin has been reported.[1,2] The resistance was due to acquisition of a low-affinity penicillin-binding protein and conferred cross-resistance to meticillin and cloxacillin, and, to a lesser degree, to cefotaxime.

1. Johnson AP, et al. Oxacillin-resistant pneumococci sensitive to penicillin. Lancet 1993; 341: 1222.
2. Dowson CG, et al. Genetics of oxacillin resistance in clinical isolates of Streptococcus pneumoniae that are oxacillin resistant and penicillin susceptible. Antimicrob Agents Chemother 1994; 38: 49–53.

Pharmacokinetics

Oxacillin is incompletely absorbed from the gastrointestinal tract. Absorption is reduced by the presence of food in the stomach and is less than with cloxacillin. Peak plasma concentrations of 3 to 6 µg per mL have been achieved 1 hour after a dose of 500 mg given by mouth to fasting subjects. Following the intramuscular injection of 500 mg, peak plasma concentrations of up to 15 µg per mL have been achieved after 30 minutes. Doubling the dose can double the plasma concentration. About 93% of the oxacillin in the circulation is bound to plasma proteins. Oxacillin has been reported to have a plasma half-life of 0.5 to 1 hour. The half-life is prolonged in neonates.

The distribution of oxacillin into body tissues and fluids is similar to that of cloxacillin (p.192).

Oxacillin undergoes some metabolism, and the unchanged drug and metabolites are excreted in the urine by glomerular filtration and renal tubular secretion.

About 20 to 30% of an oral dose, and more than 40% of an intramuscular dose, is rapidly excreted in the urine. Oxacillin is also excreted in the bile.

Plasma concentrations are enhanced if probenecid is given.

Uses and Administration

Oxacillin is an isoxazolyl penicillin used similarly to flucloxacillin (p.207) in the treatment of infections due to staphylococci resistant to benzylpenicillin.

Oxacillin is administered as the sodium salt, by mouth, preferably at least 1 hour before, or 2 hours after, meals, or by injection. Doses are expressed in terms of the equivalent amount of oxacillin. Usual adult oral doses are 500 mg to 1 g of oxacillin every 4 to 6 hours. Similar doses may be given by intramuscular injection, by slow intravenous injection over about 10 minutes, or by intravenous infusion.

Children weighing less than 40 kg may be given 50 to 100 mg per kg body-weight daily in divided doses by mouth or parenterally.

Doses may be increased in severe infections.

Preparations

USP 25: Oxacillin for Injection; Oxacillin Injection; Oxacillin Sodium Capsules; Oxacillin Sodium for Oral Solution.

Proprietary Preparations (details are given in Part 3)
Aust.: Stapenor; *Belg.:* Penstapho; *Braz.:* Staficilin N; *Fr.:* Bristopen; *Ger.:* Stapenor; *Ital.:* Penstapho; *USA:* Bactocill; Prostaphlin†.

Multi-ingredient: *Aust.:* Optocillin; *Ger.:* Optocillin.

Oxolinic Acid (5665-m)

Oxolinic Acid (BAN, USAN, rINN).

Acidum Oxolinicum; NSC-110364; W-4565. 5-Ethyl-5,8-dihydro-8-oxo-1,3-dioxolo[4,5-g]quinoline-7-carboxylic acid.

$C_{13}H_{11}NO_5$ = 261.2.

CAS — 14698-29-4.

ATC — G04AB04.

Pharmacopoeias. In Eur. (see p.vi).

Pharmacopoeial description

Ph. Eur.: An almost white or pale yellow crystalline powder. Practically insoluble in water and in alcohol; very slightly soluble in dichloromethane; dissolves in dilute solutions of alkali hydroxides. Protect from light.

Profile

Oxolinic acid is a 4-quinolone antibacterial with properties similar to those of nalidixic acid (p.227), although adverse effects on the CNS may be more frequent. It is given in the treatment of urinary-tract infections in a usual dose of 750 mg by mouth every 12 hours, preferably after food.

Preparations

Proprietary Preparations (details are given in Part 3)
Belg.: Uritrate; *Braz.:* Urilin; *Fr.:* Urotrate†; *Port.:* Cistopax†; *Spain:* Oribiox; Oxinex.

Oxytetracycline (121-d)

Oxytetracycline (BAN, rINN).

Glomycin; Hydroxytetracycline; Oxytetracyclinum; Riomitsin; Terrafungine. 4S,4aR,5S,5aR,6S,12aS-4-Dimethylamino-1,4,4a,5,5a,6,11,12a-octahydro-3,5,6,10,12,12a-hexahydroxy-6-methylene-1,11-dioxonaphthacene-2-carboxamide; 5β-Hydroxytetracycline.

$C_{22}H_{24}N_2O_9 = 460.4$.

CAS — 79-57-2 (anhydrous oxytetracycline); 6153-64-6 (oxytetracycline dihydrate).

ATC — D06AA03; G01AA07; J01AA06; S01AA04.

Pharmacopoeias. In Eur. (see p.vi), which specifies a variable amount of water; Pol. and US allow the anhydrous substance or the dihydrate ($C_{22}H_{24}N_2O_9,2H_2O = 496.5$); Int. includes the dihydrate.

Oxytetracycline dihydrate 1.08 g is approximately equivalent to 1 g of oxytetracycline.

Pharmacopoeial description

Ph. Eur.: A substance produced by the growth of certain strains of Streptomyces rimosus or obtained by any other means. It contains a variable amount of water. A yellow, crystalline powder. Very slightly soluble in water; dissolves in dilute acid and alkaline solutions. A 1% suspension in water has a pH of 4.5 to 7.5. Store in airtight containers. Protect from light.

USP 25: A pale yellow to tan, odourless crystalline powder, that darkens on exposure to strong sunlight. Soluble 1 in 4150 of water, 1 in 66 of dehydrated alcohol, and 1 in 6250 of ether; sparingly soluble in alcohol; practically insoluble in chloroform; freely soluble in 3N hydrochloric acid and in alkaline solutions. pH of a 1% suspension in water is between 4.5 and 7.0. It loses potency in solutions of pH below 2 and is rapidly destroyed by alkali hydroxide solutions. Store in airtight containers. Protect from light.

Oxytetracycline Calcium (120-f)

Oxytetracycline Calcium (BANM, rINNM).

$C_{44}H_{46}CaN_4O_{18} = 958.9$.

CAS — 15251-48-6 (xCa).

Pharmacopoeias. In Br. and US.

Oxytetracycline calcium 1.04 g is approximately equivalent to 1 g of oxytetracycline.

Pharmacopoeial description

BP 2001: A pale yellow to greenish-fawn, crystalline powder. Practically insoluble in water; soluble in dilute acids; dissolves slowly in dilute ammonia solution. A 2.5% suspension in water has a pH of 6.0 to 7.5. Store at a temperature of 2° to 8°. Protect from light.

USP 25: A yellow to light brown crystalline powder. Insoluble in water; soluble 1 in more than 1000 of alcohol, of chloroform, and of ether, and 1 in 15 of 0.1N sodium hydroxide. pH of a 2.5% suspension in water is between 6.0 and 8.0. Store in airtight containers at a temperature between 8° and 15°. Protect from light.

Oxytetracycline Hydrochloride (122-n)

Oxytetracycline Hydrochloride (BANM, rINNM).

Oxytetracyclini Hydrochloridum.

$C_{22}H_{24}N_2O_9,HCl = 496.9$.

CAS — 2058-46-0.

Pharmacopoeias. In Chin., Eur. (see p.vi), Int., Jpn, Pol., and US.

Oxytetracycline hydrochloride 1.08 g is approximately equivalent to 1 g of oxytetracycline.

Incompatibilities. Oxytetracycline injections have an acid pH and incompatibility may reasonably be expected with alkaline preparations, or with drugs unstable at low pH. Tetracyclines can chelate metal cations to produce insoluble complexes, and incompatibility has been reported with solutions containing metallic salts.

Reports of incompatibility are not always consistent, and other factors, such as the strength and composition of the vehicles used, may play a role.

Pharmacopoeial description

Ph. Eur.: A yellow, hygroscopic, crystalline powder. Freely soluble in water; sparingly soluble in alcohol. Solutions in water become turbid on standing owing to the precipitation of oxytetracycline. A 1% solution in water has a pH of 2.3 to 2.9. Store in airtight containers. Protect from light.

USP 25: A yellow, odourless, hygroscopic, crystalline powder. It decomposes at temperatures exceeding 180° and exposure to strong sunlight or temperatures exceeding 90° in moist air causes it to darken. Its potency is diminished in solutions having a pH below 2, and it is rapidly destroyed by alkali hydroxide solutions. Freely soluble in water, but crystals of oxytetracycline separate as a result of partial hydrolysis of the hydrochloride; sparingly soluble in alcohol and in methyl alcohol, and even less soluble in dehydrated alcohol; insoluble in chloroform and in ether. pH of a 1% solution in water is between 2.0 and 3.0. Store in airtight containers. Protect from light.

Adverse Effects and Precautions

As for Tetracycline Hydrochloride, p.259.

Oxytetracycline may produce less tooth discoloration than some other tetracyclines but gastrointestinal symptoms tend to be more severe.

Porphyria. For the suggestion that oxytetracycline might be porphyrinogenic, see under Tetracycline Hydrochloride, p.259.

Interactions

As for Tetracycline Hydrochloride, p.259.

Antimicrobial Action

As for Tetracycline Hydrochloride, p.259. It is somewhat less active against many organisms.

Pharmacokinetics

As for Tetracycline Hydrochloride, p.260. A dose of 500 mg every 6 hours by mouth is reported to produce steady-state plasma concentrations of 3 to 4 μg per mL. Plasma protein binding is reported to be about 20 to 40% and the half-life to be 9 hours.

Uses and Administration

Oxytetracycline is a tetracycline derivative with actions and uses similar to those of tetracycline (p.260).

Oxytetracycline dihydrate or hydrochloride are usually used in tablets and capsules, and for injections, and the calcium salt in aqueous oral suspensions; all three are also used in topical preparations. Doses have been expressed as anhydrous oxytetracycline, the dihydrate, or the hydrochloride but in practice this appears to make little difference.

Oxytetracycline is usually given in adult doses of 250 to 500 mg four times daily by mouth, usually one hour before food or 2 hours after food. Older children (over 8 years) have been given 25 to 50 mg per kg body-weight daily by mouth, in 4 divided doses, but the effect of tetracyclines on teeth and bones should be considered.

Doses of oxytetracycline 250 to 500 mg daily have been used in acne.

Oxytetracycline is sometimes given intramuscularly, in doses of 250 to 300 mg daily, but this route may be painful and produces lower blood concentrations than oral administration in the recommended doses. It has also been given by intravenous infusion, in usual adult doses of 250 to 500 mg every 12 hours, although up to 2 g daily in divided doses may be given.

Oxytetracycline and its salts have been applied topically, often in combination with other agents, as a variety of eye and ear drops, ointments, creams, and sprays.

Preparations

BP 2001: Oxytetracycline Capsules; Oxytetracycline Tablets;
USP 25: Oxytetracycline and Nystatin Capsules; Oxytetracycline and Nystatin for Oral Suspension; Oxytetracycline Calcium Oral Suspension; Oxytetracycline for Injection; Oxytetracycline Hydrochloride and Hydrocortisone Acetate Ophthalmic Suspension; Oxytetracycline Hydrochloride and Hydrocortisone Ointment; Oxytetracycline Hydrochloride and Polymyxin B Sulfate Ointment; Oxytetracycline Hydrochloride and Polymyxin B Sulfate Ophthalmic Ointment; Oxytetracycline Hydrochloride and Polymyxin B Sulfate Topical Powder; Oxytetracycline Hydrochloride and Polymyxin B Sulfate Vaginal Tablets; Oxytetracycline Hydrochloride Capsules; Oxytetracycline Injection; Oxytetracycline Tablets.

Proprietary Preparations (details are given in Part 3)
Aust.: Tetra-Tablinen†; **Braz.:** Terramicina; **Denm.:** Oxytetral; **Fr.:** Posicycline; Terramycine Solu-Retard†; Tetranase; **Ger.:** Tetra-Tablinen†; **Hong Kong:** Oxylim; Terramycin; **Irl.:** Berkmycen†; Clinimycin; **Mex.:** Metrecina; Oxitraklin; Terrados; Terramicina; Tracin; **Norw.:** Oxytetral; **Port.:** Geomicina; Terricil; **S.Afr.:** Acu-Oxytet†; Be-Oxytet; Cotet; Dynoxytet; O-4 Cycline; O-Tet†; Oxy†; Oxymycin†; Oxypan; Rocap†; Roxy; Spectratet; Terramycin†; Tetracem; Tetramel; **Spain:** Terramicina; **Swed.:** Oxytetral; **Thai.:** Oxycline; Oxylim; Servicyclin; Terramycin; **UK:** Berkmycen†; Oxymycin; Oxytetramix; Terramycin; **USA:** Terramycin; Uri-Tet†.

Multi-ingredient: Aust.: Bisolvomycin†; Terra-Cortril mit Gentamicin†; Terra-Cortril mit Polymyxin B-Sulfat†; Terra-Cortril†; Terramycin mit Polymyxin-B-Sulfat†; Tetra-Gelomyrtol; **Belg.:** Eoline; Terra-Cortril; Terramycine; **Braz.:** Asseptobron; Terra-Cortril; Terra-Cortril com Polimixina B; Terramicina Polimixina B; **Denm.:** Terramycin-Polymyxin B; **Fin.:** Terra-Cortril; Terra-Cortril P; **Fr.:** Auriculaum; Pyrmycine; Ster-Dex; **Ger.:** Bisolvomycin; Corti Biciron N; Farco-Tril; Oxy Biciron; Terracortril; Terramycin; Tetra-Gelomyrtol; **Hong Kong:** Terramycin with Poly-

myxin B; **Irl.:** Terra-Cortril; Terra-Cortril Nystatin; **Israel:** Auricularum; Tarocyn; Terramycin; **Ital.:** Cosmiciclina; **Mex.:** Andociclina Balsamica; Terramicina; **Neth.:** Terra-Cortril Gel Steraject met polymyxine-B; Terra-Cortril met polymyxine-B; Terra-Cortril†; Terramycin met polymyxine-B†; **Norw.:** Terra-Cortril; Terra-Cortril Polymyxin B; Terramycin Polymyxin B; **Port.:** Corticil T; **S.Afr.:** Bisolvomycin; Terra-Cortril; Terramycin; Vernacycline-V†; **Singapore:** Terramycin; **Spain:** Coliriociclina Espectro; Pulmonilo Synergium†; Terra-Cortril; Terramicina; **Swed.:** Terracortril; Terracortril med polymyxin B; Terramycin Polymyxin B; **Switz.:** Terracortril; Terramycine†; **Thai.:** Terramycin; Terrasil; **UK:** Terra-Cortril; Terra-Cortril Nystatin; Trimovate; **USA:** Terak; Terra-Cortril; Terramycin with Polymyxin B; Urobiotic-250.

Panipenem (15342-d)

Panipenem (rINN).

(+)-(5R,6S)-3{[(S)-1-Acetimidoyl-3-pyrrolidinyl]thio}-6-[(R)-1-hydroxyethyl]-7-oxo-1-azabicyclo[3.2.0]hept-2-ene-2-carboxylic acid.

$C_{15}H_{21}N_3O_4S = 339.4$.

CAS — 87726-17-8.

Profile

Panipenem is a carbapenem beta-lactam antibiotic similar to imipenem (p.214). It is given in combination with betamipron (p.159) to reduce adverse renal effects, by intravenous infusion in a usual adult dose of 500 mg twice daily.

Preparations

Proprietary Preparations (details are given in Part 3)
Multi-ingredient: Jpn: Carbenin.

Pefloxacin Mesilate (10363-e)

Pefloxacin Mesilate (BANM, rINNM).

EU-5306 (pefloxacin); Pefloxacin Mesylate (USAN); Pefloxacini Mesilas Dihydricus; 1589-RB (pefloxacin); 41982-RP. 1-Ethyl-6-fluoro-1,4-dihydro-7-(4-methyl-1-piperazinyl)-4-oxo-3-quinolinecarboxylic acid methanesulphonate dihydrate.

$C_{17}H_{20}FN_3O_3,CH_4O_3S,2H_2O = 465.5$.

CAS — 70458-92-3 (pefloxacin); 70458-95-6 (pefloxacin mesilate).

Pharmacopoeias. In Eur. (see p.vi) and Pol.

Pharmacopoeial description

Ph. Eur.: A fine, white or almost white powder. Freely soluble in water; slightly soluble in alcohol; very slightly soluble in dichloromethane. A 1% solution in water has a pH of 3.5 to 4.5. Store in airtight containers. Protect from light.

Profile

Pefloxacin is a fluoroquinolone antibacterial with actions and uses similar to those of ciprofloxacin (p.182). It also has bactericidal activity against Mycobacterium leprae and has been tried in the treatment of leprosy (p.126).

Pefloxacin has a longer plasma half-life than ciprofloxacin (about 8 to 13 hours) and is also extensively metabolised, the principal metabolite being N-desmethylpefloxacin which is otherwise known as norfloxacin (p.232).

Pefloxacin is given by mouth or by intravenous infusion as the mesilate in the treatment of susceptible infections. Doses are expressed in terms of the equivalent amount of pefloxacin and are usually 400 mg twice daily by mouth or by intravenous infusion.

Fluoroquinolones have caused adverse effects on the musculoskeletal system (see under Ciprofloxacin, p.183) and in the case of pefloxacin this has led to certain restrictions in some countries.

◊ General references.
1. Gonzalez JP, Henwood JM. Pefloxacin: a review of its antibacterial activity, pharmacokinetic properties and therapeutic use. Drugs 1989; 37: 628–68.
2. Bint AJ, et al. eds. Pefloxacin in clinical practice. J Antimicrob Chemother 1990; 26(suppl B): 1–229.

◊ Adverse effects.
1. Chevalier X, et al. A case of destructive polyarthropathy in a 17-year-old youth following pefloxacin treatment. Drug Safety 1992; 7: 310–14.
2. Al-Hedaithy MA, Noreddin AM. Hypersensitivity anaphylactoid reaction to pefloxacin in a patient with AIDS. Ann Pharmacother 1996; 30: 612–14.

◊ Pharmacokinetics.
1. Bressolle F, et al. Pefloxacin clinical pharmacokinetics. Clin Pharmacokinet 1994; 27: 418–46.

Preparations

Proprietary Preparations (details are given in Part 3)
Aust.: Peflacine; **Belg.:** Peflacine; **Braz.:** Peflacin; **Fr.:** Peflacine; **Ger.:** Peflacin; **Hong Kong:** Abaktal; Peflacine; **Israel:** Peflacine; **Ital.:** Peflacine; **Mex.:** Nopriken; Peflacine; **Neth.:** Peflacin†; **Port.:** Peflacine; **Spain:** Azuben; Peflacine; **Thai.:** Abaktal; Peflacine.

Penethamate Hydriodide (125-b)

Penethamate Hydriodide (BAN).

Diethylaminoethyl Penicillin G Hydroiodide. 2-Diethylamino-ethyl (6R)-6-(2-phenylacetamido)penicillanate hydriodide.

$C_{22}H_{31}N_3O_4S$,HI = 561.5.

CAS — 3689-73-4 (penethamate); 808-71-9 (penethamate hydriodide).

Profile

Penethamate hydriodide is a penicillin antibacterial used in veterinary medicine.

Pheneticillin Potassium (129-p)

Pheneticillin Potassium (BANM, rINNM).

Penicillin B; Phenethicillin Potassium; Pheneticillinum Kalicum; Potassium α-Phenoxyethylpenicillin. A mixture of the D(+)- and L(−)-isomers of potassium (6R)-6-(2-phenoxypropionamido)penicillanate.

$C_{17}H_{19}KN_2O_5S$ = 402.5.

CAS — 147-55-7 (pheneticillin); 132-93-4 (pheneticillin potassium).

Profile

Pheneticillin is a phenoxypenicillin with actions and uses similar to those of phenoxymethylpenicillin (below). It is given by mouth, as the potassium salt, for the treatment of susceptible mild to moderate infections in a usual dose of 250 mg three times daily. Pheneticillin sodium has also been used.

Preparations

Proprietary Preparations (details are given in Part 3)
Neth.: Broxil.

Phenoxymethylpenicillin (130-n)

Phenoxymethylpenicillin (BAN, rINN).

Fenoximetilpenicilina; Penicillin, Phenoxymethyl; Penicillin V (USAN); Phénomycilline; Phenoxymethyl Penicillin; Phenoxymethylpenicillinum. (6R)-6-(2-Phenoxyacetamido)penicillanic acid.

$C_{16}H_{18}N_2O_5S$ = 350.4.

CAS — 87-08-1.
ATC — J01CE02.

Pharmacopoeias. In Eur. (see p.vi), Int., Pol., and US.

Pharmacopoeial description

Ph. Eur.: A substance produced by the growth of certain strains of *Penicillium notatum* or related organisms on a culture medium containing an appropriate precursor, or obtained by any other means. A white, slightly hygroscopic, crystalline powder. Very slightly soluble in water; soluble in alcohol. A 0.5% suspension in water has a pH of 2.4 to 4.0. Store protected from moisture.

USP 25: A white, odourless crystalline powder. Very slightly soluble in water; freely soluble in alcohol and in acetone; insoluble in fixed oils. pH of a 3% suspension in water is between 2.5 and 4.0. Store in airtight containers.

Phenoxymethylpenicillin Calcium (131-h)

Phenoxymethylpenicillin Calcium (BANM, rINNM).

Penicillin V Calcium; Phenoxymethylpenicillinum Calcicum.

$(C_{16}H_{17}N_2O_5S)_2Ca,2H_2O$ = 774.9.

CAS — 147-48-8 (anhydrous phenoxymethylpenicillin calcium); 73368-74-8 (phenoxymethylpenicillin calcium dihydrate).

Pharmacopoeias. In Int.

A white crystalline powder. 1.1 g of monograph substance is approximately equivalent to 1 g of phenoxymethylpenicillin. Each g of monograph substance represents about 1.3 mmol of calcium.

Phenoxymethylpenicillin Potassium (132-m)

Phenoxymethylpenicillin Potassium (BANM, rINNM).

Fenoximetilpenicilina Potássica; Penicillin V Potassium (USAN); Phenoxymethylpenicillinum Kalicum.

$C_{16}H_{17}KN_2O_5S$ = 388.5.

CAS — 132-98-9.

Pharmacopoeias. In Eur. (see p.vi), Int., Jpn, Pol., and US.

1.1 g of monograph substance is approximately equivalent to 1 g of phenoxymethylpenicillin. Each g of monograph substance represents about 2.6 mmol of potassium.

Pharmacopoeial description

Ph. Eur.: A white, crystalline powder. Freely soluble in water; practically insoluble in alcohol. A 0.5% solution in water has a pH of 5.5 to 7.5.

The symbol † denotes a preparation no longer actively marketed

---

USP 25: A white, odourless crystalline powder. Very soluble in water; soluble 1 in 150 of alcohol; insoluble in acetone. pH of a 3% solution in water is between 4.0 and 7.5. Store in airtight containers.

Units

The first International Standard Preparation (1957) of phenoxymethylpenicillin contained 1695 units per mg but was discontinued in 1968. Despite this, doses of phenoxymethylpenicillin are still expressed in units in some countries.

Phenoxymethylpenicillin 250 mg is approximately equivalent to 400 000 units.

Adverse Effects and Precautions

As for Benzylpenicillin, p.157.

Phenoxymethylpenicillin is usually well tolerated but may occasionally cause transient nausea and diarrhoea.

Interactions

As for Benzylpenicillin, p.158.

Antibacterials. Reduced absorption was reported when phenoxymethylpenicillin was given following a course of *neomycin* by mouth.[1]

1. Cheng SH, White A. Effect of orally administered neomycin on the absorption of penicillin V. *N Engl J Med* 1962; **267:** 1296–7.

Beta blockers. Beta blockers might have potentiated anaphylactic reactions in 2 patients on *nadolol* and *propranolol*, respectively, who died following a dose of phenoxymethylpenicillin.[1]

1. Berkelman RL, et al. Beta-adrenergic antagonists and fatal anaphylactic reactions to oral penicillin. *Ann Intern Med* 1986; **104:** 134.

Antimicrobial Action

Phenoxymethylpenicillin has a range of antimicrobial activity similar to that of benzylpenicillin (p.158) and a similar mode of action. It may be less active against some susceptible organisms, particularly Gram-negative bacteria.

The mechanisms and patterns of resistance to phenoxymethylpenicillin are similar to those of benzylpenicillin.

Pharmacokinetics

Phenoxymethylpenicillin is more resistant to inactivation by gastric acid and is more completely absorbed than benzylpenicillin from the gastrointestinal tract following administration by mouth. Absorption is usually rapid, although variable, with about 60% of an oral dose being absorbed. The calcium and potassium salts are better absorbed than the free acid. Peak plasma concentrations of 3 to 5 μg per mL have been observed 30 to 60 minutes after a dose of 500 mg. The effect of food on absorption appears to be slight. The plasma half-life of phenoxymethylpenicillin is about 30 to 60 minutes and may be increased to about 4 hours in severe renal impairment. About 80% is reported to be protein bound. The distribution and elimination of phenoxymethylpenicillin is similar to that of benzylpenicillin (p.158). It is metabolised in the liver to a greater extent than benzylpenicillin; several metabolites have been identified including penicilloic acid. The unchanged drug and metabolites are excreted rapidly in the urine. Only small amounts are excreted in the bile.

Uses and Administration

Phenoxymethylpenicillin is used similarly to benzylpenicillin (p.159) in the treatment or prophylaxis of infections caused by susceptible organisms, especially streptococci. It is used only for the treatment of mild to moderate infections, and not for chronic, severe, or deep-seated infections since absorption can be unpredictable. Patients treated initially with parenteral benzylpenicillin may continue treatment with phenoxymethylpenicillin by mouth once a satisfactory clinical response has been obtained. Specific indications for phenoxymethylpenicillin include anthrax (mild uncomplicated infections), Lyme disease

---

(early stage in pregnant women or young children), pharyngitis or tonsillitis, rheumatic fever (primary and secondary prophylaxis), streptococcal skin infections, and spleen disorders (pneumococcal infection prophylaxis). For details of these infections and their treatment, see under Choice of Antibacterial, p.114.

Administration and dosage. Phenoxymethylpenicillin is administered by mouth, usually as the potassium or calcium salt, preferably at least 30 minutes before, or 2 hours after, food. Benzathine phenoxymethylpenicillin (p.157) and hydrabamine phenoxymethylpenicillin have also been used.

Doses are expressed in terms of the equivalent amount of phenoxymethylpenicillin.

Usual adult doses have been 250 to 500 mg every 6 hours, but authorities in the UK now recommend 500 to 750 mg every 6 hours. Children may be given the following doses every 6 hours: up to 1 year, 62.5 mg; 1 to 5 years, 125 mg; and 6 to 12 years, 250 mg. Dosage may need to be modified in severe renal impairment.

To prevent recurrences of rheumatic fever, WHO and other authorities recommend 250 mg twice daily.

Preparations

BP 2001: Phenoxymethylpenicillin Oral Solution; Phenoxymethylpenicillin Tablets;
USP 25: Penicillin V for Oral Suspension; Penicillin V Potassium for Oral Solution; Penicillin V Potassium Tablets; Penicillin V Tablets.

Proprietary Preparations (details are given in Part 3)
Aust.: Cliacil; Mack Pen†; Megacillin; Ospen; Pen-V; Penbene; Penstad; Star-Pen; *Austral.:* Abbocillin-VK; Cilicaine VK; Cilopen VK; LPV; Penhexal VK; PVK; *Belg.:* Peni-Oral; *Braz.:* Meracilina; Oracilin; Pen-Ve-Oral; *Canad.:* Apo-Pen-VK; Ledercillin VK†; Nadopen-V; Novo-Pen-VK; Nu-Pen-VK; Pen-Vee; PVFK; V-Cillin K†; *Denm.:* Calcipen; Fenoxcillin†; Pancillin; Primcillin; Rocilin; Vepicombin; *Fin.:* Medicillin; Milcopen; V-Pen; *Fr.:* Oracilline; Ospen; *Ger.:* Antibiocin†; Arcasin; durapenicillin; InfectoCillin; Isocillin; Ispenoral; Jenacillin V; Megacillin oral; P-Mega-Tablinen; Pen; Pen-BASF; Pen-V-Merck; Penbeta; Penhexal; Penicillat; V-Tablopen; *Hong Kong:* Ospen; Pen-V; *Irl.:* Calvepen; Kopen; *Israel:* Rafapen Mega; Rafapen V-K; V-Pen; *Ital.:* Fenospen; *Mex.:* Anapenil; Kavipen; Megapenil; Pen-Vi-K; Pota-Vi-Kin; *Neth.:* Acipen; Acipen-V; Norw.: Apocillin; Calcipen; Femepen; Kavepenin; Rocilin; Weifapenin; *NZ:* Cilicaine VK; Compocillin; *S.Afr.:* Betapen; Copent†; Daroradillin†; Deltacillin†; Dynapen†; Len V.K.; Novo V-K; V-Cil-K†; Veekay†; *Singapore:* Ospen; *Spain:* Penilevel; *Swed.:* Abbopen†; Calciopen†; Kavepenin; Penferm†; Tikacillin; Vepenicillin†; *Switz.:* Arcasin†; Brunocillin; Fenoxypen†; Megacilline; Monocilline†; Ospen; Penisol; Phenocillin; Rivopen-V†; Stabicilline; *Thai.:* Pen-V; Pener; Servipen-V; *UK:* Apsin VK†; Distaquaine V-K; Rimapen†; *USA:* Beepen-VK; Betapen-VK†; Ledercillin VK†; Pen-V†; Pen-Vee K; Robicillin VK†; V-Cillin K†; Veetids.

Multi-ingredient: *Spain:* Penilevel Retard.

Phthalylsulfathiazole (4912-k)

Phthalylsulfathiazole (BAN, rINN).

Ftalilsulfatiazol; Phthalazolum; Phthalylsulfathiazolum; Phthalylsulphathiazole; Sulfaphtalylthiazol. 4′-(1,3-Thiazol-2-ylsulphamoyl)phthalanilic acid.

$C_{17}H_{13}N_3O_5S_2$ = 403.4.

CAS — 85-73-4.
ATC — A07AB02.

Pharmacopoeias. In Eur. (see p.vi).

Pharmacopoeial description

Ph. Eur.: A white or yellowish-white crystalline powder. Practically insoluble in water and in ether; slightly soluble in alcohol and in acetone; freely soluble in dimethylformamide. Protect from light.

Profile

Phthalylsulfathiazole is a sulfonamide with properties similar to those of sulfamethoxazole (p.254). It is poorly absorbed, about 95% remaining in the intestine and only about 5% being slowly hydrolysed to sulfathiazole and absorbed.

It is given for its antibacterial action in the gastrointestinal tract, in combination with other antibacterials, for the treatment of infections and for bowel decontamination before surgery.

Preparations

Proprietary Preparations (details are given in Part 3)
Mex.: Kaotalil.

Multi-ingredient: *Aust.:* Hylakombun; *Braz.:* Enterodina; Enteroftal; Enteromicina; Furazolin; Parenterin; Tratocoli; *Mex.:* Ditayod; Sultroquin; *Port.:* Cloranpectina; *S.Afr.:* Diastat†; *Spain:* Derbitan Antibiotico†; Estreptoenterol; *Thai.:* Chlorotracin; Coccila; Disento; Mediocin.

Pipemidic Acid (5666-b)

Pipemidic Acid (BAN, rINN).

Acidum Pipemidicum; Piperamic Acid; 1489-RB. 8-Ethyl-5,8-di-hydro-5-oxo-2-(piperazin-1-yl)pyrido[2,3-d]pyrimidine-6-carb-oxylic acid.

$C_{14}H_{17}N_5O_3 = 303.3$.
CAS — 51940-44-4 (anhydrous pipemidic acid); 72571-82-5 (pipemidic acid trihydrate).
ATC — G04AB03.

Pharmacopoeias. In Chin., Eur. (see p.vi), and Jpn (all as the trihydrate).

Pharmacopoeial description

Ph. Eur.: Pipemidic acid trihydrate is a pale yellow or yellow crystalline powder. Very slightly soluble in water. It dissolves in dilute solutions of acids and of alkali hydroxides. Protect from light.

Profile

Pipemidic acid is a 4-quinolone antibacterial with properties similar to those of nalidixic acid (p.227), but is more active in vitro against some bacteria, including Pseudomonas aeruginosa. It is used (as the trihydrate) in the treatment of urinary-tract infections in doses equivalent to 400 mg of the anhydrous substance twice daily by mouth.

Interactions. For the effect of pipemidic acid on the clearance of xanthines, see under Caffeine, p.762, and Theophylline, p.780.

Porphyria. Pipemidic acid is considered to be unsafe in patients with porphyria because it has been shown to be porphyrinogenic in in-vitro systems.

Preparations

Proprietary Preparations (details are given in Part 3)
Aust.: Deblaston; Belg.: Pipram†; Braz.: Balurol; Pipram; Pipurol; Uroxina; Fr.: Pipram; Ger.: Deblaston; Hong Kong: Urotractin; Ital.: Acipem; Biopim†; Cistomid; Diperpen; Faremid; Filtrax; Pipeacid; Pipedac; Pipefort; Pipemid; Pipram; Pipurin; Pro-Uro†; Tractur; Urodene; Uropimid; Urosan; Urosetic; Urotractin; Uroval; Jpn: Dolcol; Mex.: Anurin; Dicofarm; Fustermid; Pipemidol; Uribac; Uriken; Uripiser; Urmidin; Urogal; Uronovag; Uropipemid; Urotal; Neth.: Pipram; S.Afr.: Deblaston; Septidron; Singapore: Urotractin; Spain: Galusan; Nuril; Urisan; Uropipedil†; Switz.: Deblaston; Thai.: Pipedic; Urotractin.

Piperacillin (14850-l)

Piperacillin (BAN, rINN).

Piperacillinum. (6R)-6-[R-2-(4-Ethyl-2,3-dioxopiperazine-1-carboxamido)-2-phenylacetamido]penicillanic acid monohydrate; 3-Dimethyl-7-oxo-4-thia-1-azabicyclo[3.2.0]heptane-2-carboxylic acid monohydrate.

$C_{23}H_{27}N_5O_7S,H_2O = 535.6$.
CAS — 61477-96-1 (anhydrous piperacillin); 66258-76-2 (piperacillin monohydrate).
ATC — J01CA12.

Pharmacopoeias. In Chin., Eur. (see p.vi), and US.

Pharmacopoeial description

Ph. Eur.: A white or almost white powder. Slightly soluble in water and in ethyl acetate; freely soluble in methyl alcohol.
USP 25: A white to off-white crystalline powder. Very slightly soluble in water; slightly soluble in ethyl acetate; sparingly soluble in isopropyl alcohol; very soluble in methyl alcohol.

Piperacillin Sodium (133-b)

Piperacillin Sodium (BANM, USAN, rINNM).
CL-227193; Piperacillinum Natricum; T-1220.
$C_{23}H_{26}N_5NaO_7S = 539.5$.
CAS — 59703-84-3.

Pharmacopoeias. In Eur. (see p.vi), Jpn, Pol., and US.

1.04 g of monograph substance is approximately equivalent to 1 g of piperacillin. Each g of monograph substance represents 1.85 mmol of sodium.

Incompatibility has been reported with aminoglycosides and sodium bicarbonate.

Pharmacopoeial description

Ph. Eur.: A white or almost white, hygroscopic powder. Freely soluble in water and in methyl alcohol; practically insoluble in ethyl acetate. A 10% solution in water has a pH of 5.0 to 7.0. Store in airtight containers.
USP 25: A white to off-white solid. Freely soluble in water and in alcohol. pH of a 40% solution in water is between 5.5 and 7.5. Store in airtight containers.

Adverse Effects and Precautions

As for Carbenicillin Sodium, p.160.

As piperacillin sodium has a lower sodium content than carbenicillin sodium, hypernatraemia and hypokalaemia are less likely to occur. Prolongation of bleeding time has been less frequent and less severe than with carbenicillin.

Hypersensitivity. In the mid 1980s there were reports of a relatively high incidence of adverse reactions to piperacillin, especially fever, in patients with cystic fibrosis.[1-3] However, the manufacturers[4] considered such patients to be particularly prone to allergy and cited reactions with other semisynthetic penicillins including carbenicillin and azlocillin.

Similar apparent hypersensitivity reactions have been reported in patients taking high doses of piperacillin and other ureidopenicillins, over long periods for other indications,[5] and with other penicillins in patients with cystic fibrosis,[6] although piperacillin does appear to be most frequently implicated.[6]

1. Stead RJ, et al. Adverse reactions to piperacillin in cystic fibrosis. Lancet 1984; i: 857–8.
2. Strandvik B. Adverse reactions to piperacillin in patients with cystic fibrosis. Lancet 1984; i: 1362.
3. Stead RJ, et al. Adverse reactions to piperacillin in adults with cystic fibrosis. Thorax 1985; 40: 184–6.
4. Brock PG, Roach M. Adverse reactions to piperacillin in cystic fibrosis. Lancet 1984; i: 1070–1.
5. Lang R, et al. Adverse reactions to prolonged treatment with high doses of carbenicillin and ureidopenicillins. Rev Infect Dis 1991; 13: 68–72.
6. Pleasants RA, et al. Allergic reactions to parenteral beta-lactam antibiotics in patients with cystic fibrosis. Chest 1994; 106: 1124–8.

Interactions

As for Benzylpenicillin, p.158.

Neuromuscular blockers. Piperacillin and other ureidopenicillins are reported to prolong the action of competitive muscle relaxants such as vecuronium (see Atracurium, p.1334).

Antimicrobial Action

Piperacillin has a similar antimicrobial action to carbenicillin (p.160) and ticarcillin (p.263), but is active against a wider range of Gram-negative organisms, including Klebsiella pneumoniae. It is also generally more active in vitro, especially against Pseudomonas aeruginosa and the Enterobacteriaceae, against Gram-positive Enterococcus faecalis, and possibly against Bacteroides fragilis. There is, however, an inoculum effect, i.e. minimum inhibitory concentrations of piperacillin increase with the size of the inoculum.

Combinations of piperacillin and aminoglycosides have been shown to be synergistic in vitro against Ps. aeruginosa and Enterobacteriaceae. The effect of combining piperacillin with other beta lactams has been less predictable. The activity of piperacillin against some organisms, resistant because of the production of beta-lactamases, may be restored by tazobactam, a beta-lactamase inhibitor. Such organisms include beta-lactamase-producing strains of staphylococci, Escherichia coli, Haemophilus influenzae, and Bacteroides spp.; the activity of piperacillin against Ps. aeruginosa is not enhanced by tazobactam.

Resistance has developed in Ps. aeruginosa during treatment with piperacillin, especially when used alone. There may be some cross-resistance with other antipseudomonal penicillins.

◊ References.
1. Higashitani F, et al. Inhibition of β-lactamases by tazobactam and in-vitro antibacterial activity of tazobactam combined with piperacillin. J Antimicrob Chemother 1990; 25: 567–74.
2. Mehtar S, et al. The in-vitro activity of piperacillin/tazobactam, ciprofloxacin, ceftazidime and imipenem against multiple resistant Gram-negative bacteria. J Antimicrob Chemother 1990; 25: 915–19.
3. Kempers J, MacLaren DM. Piperacillin/tazobactam and ticarcillin/clavulanic acid against resistant Enterobacteriaceae. J Antimicrob Chemother 1990; 26: 598–9.
4. Kadima TA, Weiner JH. Mechanism of suppression of piperacillin resistance in enterobacteria by tazobactam. Antimicrob Agents Chemother 1997; 41: 2177–83.
5. Klepser ME, et al. Comparison of the bactericidal activities of piperacillin-tazobactam, ticarcillin-clavulanate, and ampicillin-sulbactam against clinical isolates of Bacteroides fragilis, Enterococcus faecalis, Escherichia coli, and Pseudomonas aeruginosa. Antimicrob Agents Chemother 1997; 41: 435–9.

Pharmacokinetics

Piperacillin is not absorbed from the gastrointestinal tract. It is well absorbed after intramuscular administration, peak plasma concentrations of 30 to 40 µg per mL being observed 30 to 50 minutes after a dose of 2 g. The pharmacokinetics of piperacillin are reported to be nonlinear and dose-dependent. The plasma half-life is about one hour, but is prolonged in neonates. In patients with severe renal insufficiency there may be a threefold increase in half-life; in those with end-stage renal failure half-lives of 4 to 6 hours have been reported, and in those with both renal and hepatic im-

pairment much longer half-lives may result. About 20% of piperacillin in the circulation is bound to plasma proteins.

Piperacillin is widely distributed in body tissues and fluids. It crosses the placenta into the fetal circulation and small amounts are distributed into breast milk. There is little diffusion into the CSF except when the meninges are inflamed.

About 60 to 80% of a dose is excreted unchanged in the urine by glomerular filtration and tubular secretion within 24 hours, achieving high concentrations. High concentrations are also found in the bile and about 20% of a dose may be excreted by this route. Plasma concentrations are enhanced if probenecid is administered concomitantly.

Piperacillin is removed by haemodialysis.

Piperacillin with tazobactam. The pharmacokinetics of piperacillin do not appear to be altered by the coadministration of tazobactam, but piperacillin reduces the renal clearance of tazobactam.

◊ References.
1. Heikkilä A, Erkkola R. Pharmacokinetics of piperacillin during pregnancy. J Antimicrob Chemother 1991; 28: 419–23.
2. Wise R, et al. Pharmacokinetics and tissue penetration of tazobactam administered alone and with piperacillin. Antimicrob Agents Chemother 1991; 35: 1081–4.
3. Johnson CA, et al. Single-dose pharmacokinetics of piperacillin and tazobactam in patients with renal disease. Clin Pharmacol Ther 1992; 51: 32–41.
4. Dupon M, et al. Plasma levels of piperacillin and vancomycin used as prophylaxis in liver transplant patients. Eur J Clin Pharmacol 1993; 45: 529–34.
5. Sörgel F, Kinzig M. The chemistry, pharmacokinetics and tissue distribution of piperacillin/tazobactam. J Antimicrob Chemother 1993; 31 (suppl A): 39–60.
6. Reed MD, et al. Single-dose pharmacokinetics of piperacillin and tazobactam in infants and children. Antimicrob Agents Chemother 1994; 38: 2817–26.
7. Bourget P, et al. Clinical pharmacokinetics of piperacillin-tazobactam combination in patients with major burns and signs of infection. Antimicrob Agents Chemother 1996; 40: 139–45.
8. Occhipinti DJ, et al. Pharmacokinetics and pharmacodynamics of two multiple-dose piperacillin-tazobactam regimens. Antimicrob Agents Chemother 1997; 41: 2511–17.

Uses and Administration

Piperacillin is a ureidopenicillin that is used similarly to ticarcillin (p.263) for the treatment of infections caused by Pseudomonas aeruginosa, and also infections due to other susceptible bacteria (see Antimicrobial Action, above). It has been used particularly in immunocompromised patients (neutropenic patients) and for biliary-tract infections (cholangitis). Other indications have included uncomplicated gonorrhoea due to penicillin-sensitive gonococci, and urinary-tract infections. It has also been used for surgical infection prophylaxis. For details of these infections and their treatment, see under Choice of Antibacterial, p.114. For the treatment of serious infections piperacillin is commonly given with an aminoglycoside, but they should be administered separately because of possible incompatibility.

Administration and dosage. Piperacillin is given by injection as the sodium salt. Doses are expressed in terms of the equivalent amount of piperacillin. Doses should generally be reduced in moderate to severe renal impairment.

Piperacillin may be administered by slow intravenous injection over 3 to 5 minutes, by intravenous infusion over 20 to 40 minutes, or by deep intramuscular injection. Single doses of more than 2 g for adults or 0.5 g for children should not be given by the intramuscular route.

For the treatment of serious or complicated infections, adults may be given piperacillin 200 to 300 mg per kg body-weight daily in divided doses intravenously; the usual dose is 4 g every 6 or 8 hours. In life-threatening infections, particularly those caused by Pseudomonas or Klebsiella spp., it should be given in a dose of not less than 16 g daily. The usual maximum daily dose is 24 g, although this has been exceeded.

For mild or uncomplicated infections, 100 to 150 mg per kg daily may be given to adults; usual doses are 2 g every 6 or 8 hours, or 4 g every 12 hours, by intravenous administration, or 2 g every 8 or 12 hours by intramuscular injection.

Uncomplicated gonorrhoea may be treated by a single intramuscular dose of 2 g. Probenecid 1 g by mouth may be given half an hour before the injection.

For the prophylaxis of infection during surgery, 2 g just before the procedure, or when the umbilical cord is clamped in caesarean section, followed by at least 2 doses of 2 g at intervals of 4 or 6 hours within 24 hours of the procedure, may be given.

The intravenous route is preferred for infants and children. Those aged 1 month to 12 years may be given 100 to 300 mg per kg daily in 3 or 4 divided doses. Neonates less than 7 days old or weighing less than 2 kg may be given 150 mg per kg daily in 3 divided doses. Those more than 7 days old and weighing more than 2 kg may be given 300 mg per kg daily in 3 or 4 divided doses.

Piperacillin with tazobactam. Piperacillin has also been administered in association with tazobactam (p.257), a beta-lactamase inhibitor, to widen its antibacterial spectrum to organisms usually resistant because of the production of beta-lactamases. It is given intravenously in a ratio of piperacillin (as the sodium salt) 8 parts to 1 part of tazobactam (as the sodium salt). Doses of the combination, calculated on piperacillin content, are similar to those of piperacillin alone.

◊ References.
1. Greenwood D, Finch RG, eds. Piperacillin/tazobactam: a new β-lactam/β-lactamase inhibitor combination. *J Antimicrob Chemother* 1993; **31** (suppl A): 1–124.
2. Schoonover LL, *et al.* Piperacillin/tazobactam: a new beta-lactam/beta-lactamase inhibitor combination. *Ann Pharmacother* 1995; **29:** 501–14.
3. Perry CM, Markham A. Piperacillin/tazobactam: an updated review of its use in the treatment of bacterial infections. *Drugs* 1999; **57:** 805–43.

Preparations
BP 2001: Piperacillin Intravenous Infusion;
USP 25: Piperacillin for Injection.

Proprietary Preparations (details are given in Part 3)
Aust.: Pripil; **Austral.:** Pripil; **Belg.:** Pipcil; **Canad.:** Pipracil; **Denm.:** Ivacin; **Fr.:** Piperilline†; **Ger.:** Pipril; **Hong Kong:** Pipracil; **Irl.:** Pripil; **Israel:** Picillin; Pipril; **Ital.:** Avocin; Eril; Peracil; Picillin; Piperital; Pipersal; Picardin; **Jpn:** Pentcillin; **Neth.:** Pipril; **NZ:** Pipril; **S.Afr.:** Pipril; **Spain:** Piperzam†; Pipril; **Swed.:** Ivacin; **Switz.:** Pipril; **Thai.:** Pipracil; **UK:** Pipril†; **USA:** Pipracil.

Multi-ingredient: Aust.: Fluxapril; Tazonam; **Austral.:** Tazocin; **Belg.:** Tazocin; **Canad.:** Tazocin; **Fin.:** Tazocin; **Fr.:** Tazocilline; **Ger.:** Fluxapril†; Tazobac; **Hong Kong:** Tazocin; **Irl.:** Tazocin; **Israel:** Tazocin; **Ital.:** Tazobact†; Tazocin; **Neth.:** Tazocin; **NZ:** Tazocin; **Port.:** Tazobac; **S.Afr.:** Tazocin; **Singapore:** Tazocin; **Spain:** Tazocel; **Swed.:** Tazocin; **Switz.:** Tazobac; **Thai.:** Tazocin; **UK:** Tazocin; **USA:** Zosyn.

Pirlimycin Hydrochloride (147-w)

Pirlimycin Hydrochloride (USAN, rINNM).
U-57930E.   Methyl   7-chloro-6,7,8-trideoxy-6-(cis-4-ethyl-L-pipecolamido)-1-thio-L-threo-α-D-galacto-octopyranoside monohydrochloride monohydrate.
$C_{17}H_{31}ClN_2O_5S,HCl,H_2O = 465.4.$
CAS — 79548-73-5 (pirlimycin); 77495-92-2 (pirlimycin hydrochloride).

Profile
Pirlimycin is a lincosamide antibacterial used in veterinary medicine.

Piromidic Acid (5667-v)

Piromidic Acid (rINN).
PD-93.   8-Ethyl-5,8-dihydro-5-oxo-2-(pyrrolidin-1-yl)pyrido[2,3-d]pyrimidine-6-carboxylic acid.
$C_{14}H_{16}N_4O_3 = 288.3.$
CAS — 19562-30-2.
ATC — G04AB02.

Profile
Piromidic acid is a 4-quinolone antibacterial with properties similar to those of nalidixic acid (p.227). It is used in the treatment of susceptible infections in doses of up to 3 g daily by mouth in divided doses.

Preparations
Proprietary Preparations (details are given in Part 3)
Ital.: Enteromix.

Pivampicillin (188-t)

Pivampicillin (BAN, rINN).
MK-191.   Pivaloyloxymethyl   (6R)-6-(α-D-phenylglycylamino)penicillanate.
$C_{22}H_{29}N_3O_6S = 463.5.$
CAS — 33817-20-8.
ATC — J01CA02.
Pharmacopoeias. In Eur. (see p.vi).

1.3 g of monograph substance is approximately equivalent to 1 g of ampicillin.

Pharmacopoeial description
Ph. Eur.: A white or almost white crystalline powder. Practically insoluble in water; soluble in dehydrated alcohol; freely soluble in methyl alcohol. It dissolves in dilute acids. Store in airtight containers.

Pivampicillin Hydrochloride (135-g)

Pivampicillin Hydrochloride (BANM, USAN, rINNM).
$C_{22}H_{29}N_3O_6S,HCl = 500.0.$
CAS — 26309-95-5.

1.43 g of monograph substance is approximately equivalent to 1 g of ampicillin.

Adverse Effects and Precautions
As for Ampicillin, p.151. Pivampicillin is reported to cause a lower incidence of diarrhoea than ampicillin, although upper gastrointestinal discomfort may be more frequent. These effects appear to be more common when pivampicillin is taken on an empty stomach.

Pivaloyloxymethyl esters such as pivampicillin have been associated with the induction of carnitine deficiency (see below).

Carnitine deficiency. Carnitine deficiency (see under Levocarnitine, p.1356) has been reported following the administration of pivampicillin and pivmecillinam.[1] It is thought that the pivalic acid liberated on hydrolysis of these pivaloyloxymethyl esters *in vivo* is excreted as pivaloyl-carnitine with a consequent depletion in plasma and muscle concentrations of carnitine.[2] Low plasma-carnitine concentrations persisted in a patient after discontinuing pivampicillin, despite 6 weeks of replacement therapy with carnitine 1g daily by mouth. She had originally presented with skeletal myopathy after receiving pivampicillin for 3 months. A more intensive carnitine replacement regimen might be necessary in such patients.[3]

1. Holme E, *et al.* Carnitine deficiency induced by pivampicillin and pivmecillinam therapy. *Lancet* 1989; **ii:** 469–73.
2. Anonymous. Carnitine deficiency. *Lancet* 1990; **335:** 631–3.
3. Rose SJ, *et al.* Carnitine deficiency associated with long-term pivampicillin treatment: the effect of a replacement therapy regime. *Postgrad Med J* 1992; **68:** 932–4.

Porphyria. Pivampicillin has been associated with acute attacks of porphyria and is considered unsafe in porphyric patients.

Interactions
As for Benzylpenicillin, p.158.
There is a theoretical possibility that carnitine deficiency may be increased in patients receiving pivampicillin and valproate.

Antimicrobial Action
Pivampicillin has the antimicrobial activity of ampicillin to which it is hydrolysed *in vivo* (p.151).

Pharmacokinetics
Pivampicillin is acid-stable and is readily absorbed from the gastrointestinal tract. On absorption it is rapidly and almost completely hydrolysed to ampicillin, pivalic acid, and formaldehyde. Plasma-ampicillin concentrations 1 hour after administration are 2 to 3 times those attained after an equivalent dose of ampicillin. The absorption of pivampicillin is generally not significantly affected by food. About 70% of a dose is excreted in the urine as ampicillin within 6 hours.

Uses and Administration
Pivampicillin is the pivaloyloxymethyl ester of ampicillin (p.151) and has similar uses. It is given by mouth to adults in doses of 0.5 g twice daily with food. Doses in children are: 3 months to 1 year of age, 40 to 60 mg per kg body-weight daily in two divided doses; 1 to 3 years, 350 mg daily in two divided doses; 4 to 6 years, 525 mg daily in two divided doses; 7 to 10 years, 700 mg daily in two divided doses. Doses may be doubled in severe infections. In gonorrhoea a single dose of 1.5 g is given, in association with probenecid 1 g, in areas where gonococci remain sensitive.

Pivampicillin hydrochloride is used in some countries.
Pivampicillin has also been administered in association with pivmecillinam hydrochloride (p.237).

Preparations
Proprietary Preparations (details are given in Part 3)
Aust.: Pondocillin†; **Canad.:** Pondocillin; **Denm.:** Pondocillin; **Fr.:** Proampi; **Irl.:** Pondocillin†; **Norw.:** Pondocillin; **S.Afr.:** Pondocillin†; **Spain:** Lervipan; Pivamiser; **Swed.:** Pondocillin; **UK:** Pondocillin†.

Multi-ingredient: Aust.: Miraxid; **Swed.:** Miraxid†.

Pivmecillinam (136-q)

Pivmecillinam (BAN, rINN).
Amdinocillin Pivoxil (USAN); FL-1039; Pivamdinocillin; Ro-10-9071. Pivaloyloxymethyl (6R)-6-(perhydroazepin-1-ylmethyleneamino)penicillanate.
$C_{21}H_{33}N_3O_5S = 439.6.$
CAS — 32886-97-8.
ATC — J01CA08.

Pivmecillinam Hydrochloride (137-p)

Pivmecillinam Hydrochloride (BANM, rINNM).
Pivmecillinami Hydrochloridum.
$C_{21}H_{33}N_3O_5S,HCl = 476.0.$
CAS — 32887-03-9.
Pharmacopoeias. In Eur. (see p.vi) and Jpn.

Pivmecillinam 1.35 g and pivmecillinam hydrochloride 1.46 g are each approximately equivalent to 1 g of mecillinam.

Pharmacopoeial description
Ph. Eur.: A white or almost white crystalline powder. Freely soluble in water, in dehydrated alcohol, and in methyl alcohol; slightly soluble in acetone. A 10% solution in water has a pH of 2.8 to 3.8. Store at a temperature of 2° to 8°. Protect from light.

Adverse Effects and Precautions
As for Benzylpenicillin, p.157.
Pivaloyloxymethyl esters such as pivmecillinam have been associated with the induction of carnitine deficiency (see Pivampicillin, p.237).

Administration. Oesophageal injury has been associated rarely with pivmecillinam tablets.[1,2] Patients are advised to take them during a meal, while sitting or standing, and with at least half a glass of water.[3]

1. Committee on Safety of Medicines. Pivmecillinam and oesophageal injury. *Current Problems 19* 1987.
2. Mortimer Ö, Wiholm B-E. Oesophageal injury associated with pivmecillinam tablets. *Eur J Clin Pharmacol* 1989; **37:** 605–7.
3. Anonymous. CSM warning on pivmecillinam. *Pharm J* 1987; **238:** 443.

Porphyria. Pivmecillinam has been associated with acute attacks of porphyria and is considered unsafe in porphyric patients.

Interactions
As for Benzylpenicillin, p.158.

Antimicrobial Action
Pivmecillinam has the antimicrobial activity of mecillinam (p.221) to which it is hydrolysed *in vivo*.

Pharmacokinetics
Pivmecillinam is well absorbed from the gastrointestinal tract and is rapidly hydrolysed to the active drug mecillinam (p.221), pivalic acid, and formaldehyde. The presence of food in the stomach does not appear to have a significant effect on absorption. Peak plasma concentrations of mecillinam of up to 5 μg per mL have been achieved 1 to 2 hours after a 400-mg dose of pivmecillinam.

About 45% of a dose may be excreted in the urine as mecillinam, mainly within the first 6 hours.

◊ References.
1. Heikkilä A, *et al.* The pharmacokinetics of mecillinam and pivmecillinam in pregnant and non-pregnant women. *Br J Clin Pharmacol* 1992; **33:** 629–33.

Uses and Administration
Pivmecillinam is the pivaloyloxymethyl ester of mecillinam (p.221), to which it is hydrolysed on oral administration. It is used in the treatment of urinary-tract infections (p.146) and in salmonellosis (p.123).

Doses of pivmecillinam have often been expressed in a confusing manner since no differentiation has been made between the hydrochloride, used in tablets, and the base, used in suspensions for oral use.

In acute uncomplicated cystitis, the initial adult dose is 400 mg by mouth followed by 200 mg three times daily for 8 doses. In chronic or recurrent bacteriuria, 400 mg may be given three or four times daily. The dose for children (body-weight less than 40 kg) with urinary-tract infections is 20 to 40 mg per kg daily in three or four divided doses.

In salmonellosis, a dose of 1.2 to 2.4 g daily for 14 days is used in adults with enteric fever; carriers may be treated with the same daily dose for 2 to 4 weeks.

The symbol † denotes a preparation no longer actively marketed

The dose for children is 30 to 60 mg per kg daily in three or four divided doses.

Pivmecillinam should preferably be taken with food (see also under Adverse Effects and Precautions, above).

Pivmecillinam has been administered in combination with other beta lactams, particularly pivampicillin (p.237), to extend the spectrum of antimicrobial activity to Gram-positive organisms and because of reported synergism against Gram-negative bacteria *in vitro*.

For parenteral administration, mecillinam is used.

Preparations
Proprietary Preparations (details are given in Part 3)
Aust.: Selexid; **Belg.:** Selexid; **Canad.:** Selexid; **Denm.:** Selexid; **Fin.:** Selexid; **Fr.:** Selexid; **Norw.:** Selexid; **Port.:** Selecid; **Swed.:** Selexid; **UK:** Selexid.

Multi-ingredient: Aust.: Miraxid; **Swed.:** Miraxid†.

Polymyxin B Sulfate (139-w)

Polymyxin B Sulfate (rINNM).
Polymyxin B Sulphate (BANM); Polymyxini B Sulfas.
CAS — 1404-26-8 (polymyxin B); 1405-20-5 (polymyxin B sulfate).
Pharmacopoeias. In Eur. (see p.vi), Jpn, Pol., and US.

Incompatibilities. Lack of compatibility has been reported with many other drugs including antimicrobials. Polymyxin B sulfate is rapidly inactivated by strong acids and alkalis.

Pharmacopoeial description
Ph. Eur.: A mixture of the sulfates of polypeptides produced by the growth of certain strains of *Bacillus polymyxa* or obtained by other means. The potency is not less than 6500 units per mg, calculated with reference to the dried substance. A white or almost white, hygroscopic powder. Soluble in water; slightly soluble in alcohol. A 2% solution in water has a pH of 5.0 to 7.0. Store in airtight containers. Protect from light.

USP 25: The sulfate salt of a kind of polymyxin, a substance produced by the growth of *Bacillus polymyxa* (Bacillaceae), or a mixture of two or more such salts. A white to buff-coloured, powder, odourless or has a faint odour. It has a potency of not less than 6000 Polymyxin B units per mg, calculated on the dried substance. Freely soluble in water; slightly soluble in alcohol. pH of a 0.5% solution in water is between 5.0 and 7.5. Store in airtight containers. Protect from light.

Units
The second International Standard Preparation (1969) of polymyxin B sulfate contains 8403 units per mg.

NOTE. The available forms of polymyxin B sulfate are generally less pure than the International Standard Preparation and doses are sometimes stated in terms of pure polymyxin base; 100 mg of pure polymyxin B is considered to be equivalent to 1 million units (1 mega unit).

Adverse Effects, Treatment, and Precautions
When given parenterally the major adverse effects of the polymyxins are dose-related neurotoxicity and nephrotoxicity. Hypersensitivity reactions are rare, although rashes and fever have been reported, and polymyxins cause histamine release which may lead to bronchoconstriction and other anaphylactoid symptoms.

Neurotoxic reactions include both peripheral effects such as circumoral and 'stocking-glove' pattern paraesthesias, visual disturbances, and dizziness, ataxia, confusion, drowsiness, and other central effects. The polymyxins are potent neuromuscular blockers, and respiratory paralysis and apnoea may result, especially in patients with impaired renal function or pre-existing disorders of neuromuscular transmission such as myasthenia gravis, in whom particular care is needed. Neostigmine or calcium salts are of little value in reversing neuromuscular blockade and artificial ventilation may be required if it develops.

Nephrotoxicity may occur in up to 20% of patients following parenteral use and may be marked by nitrogen retention, haematuria, proteinuria, and tubular necrosis. Electrolyte disturbances frequently occur. Patients with pre-existing renal impairment are at par-

ticular risk and require dosage reduction. Renal function should be monitored. Signs of increasing nitrogen retention are an indication for dosage reduction in all patients and the drugs should be withdrawn if oliguria occurs. Although polymyxin B is stated to be more nephrotoxic than colistin on a weight-for-weight basis their effects on the kidney seem to be similar at therapeutically equivalent doses.

Polymyxin B is irritant and pain following intramuscular injection may be severe. Meningeal irritation may follow the intrathecal administration of polymyxin B.

Polymyxins should be avoided in patients with a history of hypersensitivity to any of the group. Serum concentrations of polymyxins should be monitored in patients receiving parenteral therapy.

Ear drops containing polymyxins should not be used in patients with perforated ear drums, and topical application to large areas of broken skin should be avoided, because of the risk of systemic absorption.

Interactions
Polymyxins may enhance the action of neuromuscular blockers (p.1334). Additive nephrotoxicity may occur if polymyxins are given with other potentially nephrotoxic drugs including aminoglycosides and cefalotin.

Antimicrobial Action
Polymyxin B and the other polymyxin antibiotics act primarily by binding to membrane phospholipids and disrupting the bacterial cytoplasmic membrane. Polymyxin B has a bactericidal action on most Gram-negative bacilli except *Proteus* spp. It is particularly effective against *Pseudomonas aeruginosa*. Of the other Gram-negative organisms, *Acinetobacter* spp., *Escherichia coli, Enterobacter* and *Klebsiella* spp., *Haemophilus influenzae, Bordetella pertussis, Salmonella,* and *Shigella* spp. are sensitive. Classical *Vibrio cholerae* is sensitive but the El Tor and O139 biotypes are resistant. *Serratia marcescens, Providencia* spp., and *Bacteroides fragilis* are usually resistant. It is not active against *Neisseria* spp., obligate anaerobes, and Gram-positive bacteria. Some fungi such as *Coccidioides immitis* are susceptible but most are resistant.

Polymyxins have been reported to demonstrate antimicrobial synergy with a variety of other drugs, including chloramphenicol, tetracyclines, and the sulfonamides and trimethoprim.

MICs for the most sensitive species generally range from about 0.01 to 4 µg per mL. The action of polymyxin B is reduced by divalent cations such as calcium and magnesium, and so activity *in vivo* is less marked than *in vitro*.

Acquired resistance to polymyxin B is uncommon, although adaptive resistance may develop in enterobacteria exposed to sublethal concentrations. There is complete cross-resistance between polymyxin B and colistin.

Pharmacokinetics
Polymyxin B sulfate is not absorbed from the gastrointestinal tract, except in the newborn. It is not absorbed through the intact skin.

Peak plasma concentrations after intramuscular administration are usually obtained within 2 hours, but are variable and it is partially inactivated by serum. It is widely distributed and extensively bound to cell membranes in the tissues. Accumulation may occur after repeated doses. Polymyxin B is reported to have a half-life of about 6 hours. There is no diffusion into the CSF.

Polymyxin B sulfate is excreted mainly by the kidneys, up to 60% being recovered in the urine, but there is a time lag of 12 to 24 hours before polymyxin B is recovered in the urine.

Uses and Administration
Polymyxin B sulfate is used topically, often in combination with other drugs, in the treatment of skin, ear, and eye infections due to susceptible organisms. Eye drops of polymyxin B with neomycin and gramicidin have been used for the prophylaxis of infection in patients undergoing ocular surgery and, in combination with propamidine isetionate, for the treatment of acanthamoeba keratitis (p.582). Polymyxin B has been given orally for oropharyngeal decontamination or the suppression of intestinal flora in patients at high risk of endogenous infections (see under Intensive Care, p.126). Polymyxin B has also been used parenterally for the treatment of infections due to susceptible Gram-negative bacteria, especially *Pseudomonas aeruginosa,* but other drugs are generally preferred.

For topical application polymyxin B is usually available as a 0.1% solution or ointment. Parenteral doses have ranged from 15 000 to 25 000 units (about 1.5 to 2.5 mg) per kg body-weight daily, preferably by intravenous infusion, although the intramuscular route has been used despite the severe pain which may be associated with it. Higher doses have been given to neonates, but dosage must be reduced in patients with impaired renal function.

Polymyxin B has also been given intrathecally in meningeal infection, and by subconjunctival injection for eye infections.

Preparations
BP 2001: Polymyxin and Bacitracin Eye Ointment;
USP 25: Bacitracin and Polymyxin B Sulfate Topical Aerosol; Bacitracin Zinc and Polymyxin B Sulfate Ointment; Bacitracin Zinc and Polymyxin B Sulfate Ophthalmic Ointment; Chloramphenicol and Polymyxin B Sulfate Ophthalmic Ointment; Chloramphenicol, Polymyxin B Sulfate, and Hydrocortisone Acetate Ophthalmic Ointment; Neomycin and Polymyxin B Sulfates and Bacitracin Ointment; Neomycin and Polymyxin B Sulfates and Bacitracin Ophthalmic Ointment; Neomycin and Polymyxin B Sulfates and Bacitracin Zinc Ointment; Neomycin and Polymyxin B Sulfates and Bacitracin Zinc Ophthalmic Ointment; Neomycin and Polymyxin B Sulfates and Dexamethasone Ophthalmic Ointment; Neomycin and Polymyxin B Sulfates and Dexamethasone Ophthalmic Suspension; Neomycin and Polymyxin B Sulfates and Hydrocortisone Acetate Cream; Neomycin and Polymyxin B Sulfates and Hydrocortisone Acetate Ophthalmic Suspension; Neomycin and Polymyxin B Sulfates and Hydrocortisone Ophthalmic Suspension; Neomycin and Polymyxin B Sulfates and Hydrocortisone Otic Solution; Neomycin and Polymyxin B Sulfates and Hydrocortisone Otic Suspension; Neomycin and Polymyxin B Sulfates and Lidocaine Cream; Neomycin and Polymyxin B Sulfates and Pramoxine Hydrochloride Cream; Neomycin and Polymyxin B Sulfates and Prednisolone Acetate Ophthalmic Suspension; Neomycin and Polymyxin B Sulfates Cream; Neomycin and Polymyxin B Sulfates Ophthalmic Ointment; Neomycin and Polymyxin B Sulfates Ophthalmic Solution; Neomycin and Polymyxin B Sulfates Solution for Irrigation; Neomycin and Polymyxin B Sulfates, Bacitracin Zinc, and Hydrocortisone Acetate Ophthalmic Ointment; Neomycin and Polymyxin B Sulfates, Bacitracin Zinc, and Hydrocortisone Ointment; Neomycin and Polymyxin B Sulfates, Bacitracin Zinc, and Hydrocortisone Ophthalmic Ointment; Neomycin and Polymyxin B Sulfates, Bacitracin Zinc, and Lidocaine Ointment; Neomycin and Polymyxin B Sulfates, Bacitracin, and Hydrocortisone Acetate Ointment; Neomycin and Polymyxin B Sulfates, Bacitracin, and Hydrocortisone Acetate Ophthalmic Ointment; Neomycin and Polymyxin B Sulfates, Bacitracin, and Hydrocortisone Ointment; Neomycin and Polymyxin B Sulfates, Bacitracin, and Lidocaine Ointment; Neomycin and Polymyxin B Sulfates, Gramicidin, and Hydrocortisone Acetate Cream; Oxytetracycline Hydrochloride and Polymyxin B Sulfate Ointment; Oxytetracycline Hydrochloride and Polymyxin B Sulfate Ophthalmic Ointment; Oxytetracycline Hydrochloride and Polymyxin B Sulfate Topical Powder; Oxytetracycline Hydrochloride and Polymyxin B Sulfate Vaginal Tablets; Polymyxin B for Injection; Polymyxin B Sulfate and Bacitracin Zinc Topical Aerosol; Polymyxin B Sulfate and Bacitracin Zinc Topical Powder; Polymyxin B Sulfate and Hydrocortisone Otic Solution; Polymyxin B Sulfate and Trimethoprim Ophthalmic Solution.

Proprietary Preparations (details are given in Part 3)
Canad.: Aerosporin†; **USA:** Aerosporin†.

Multi-ingredient: Aust.: Neocones; Otosporin; Polybactrin†; Polytrim; Riker Antibiotic-Spray†; Terra-Cortril mit Polymyxin B-Sulfat†; Terramycin mit Polymyxin-B-Sulfat†; **Austral.:** Neosporin; Spersin†; **Belg.:** De Icin; Maxitrol; Ophtalmotrim; Otosporin; Panotile; Polydexa; Polygynax; Polytrim; Predmycin; Statrol; Synalar Bi-Otic; Terra-Cortril; Terramycine; **Braz.:** Anaseptil; Colpolase; Conjuntin; Dermicin; Lidosporin; Maxitrol; Oftcor; Oftrim; Otocort; Otolone; Otomixyn; Otosporin; Otosynalar; Panotil; Pertrim; Poliginax; Polipred; Predmicin; Terra-Cortril com Polimixina B; Terramicina Polimixina B; **Canad.:** Antibiotic Cold Sore Ointment; Antibiotic Cream; Antibiotic Ointment; Antibiotique Onguent; Bacimyxin; Band-Aid Antibiotic; Bioderm; Cortimyxin; Cortisporin; Dioptrol; Diospor HC†; Diosporin†; Lanabiotic†; Lid-Pack; Lidomyxin; Lidosporin; Maxitrol; Neo Bace; Neosporin; Neotopic; Ophthocort†; Optimyxin; Optimyxin Plus; Ozonol Antibiotic Plus; Polycidin; Polyderm; Polysporin; Polysporin Plus Pain Relief; Polysporin Triple

Antibiotic; Polytopic; Polytracin†; Polytrim; Webber Antibiotic Cold Sore Ointment†; **Denm.:** Terramycin-Polymyxin B; **Fin.:** Maxitrol; Polysporin; Terra-Cortil P; **Fr.:** Antibio-Synalar†; Antibiotulle Lumiere; Atebemyxine; Auriculanum; Cebemyxine; Corticotulle Lumiere; Framyxone; Maxidrol; Panotile; Polydexa; Polydexa a la Phenylephrine; Polyfra; Polygynax; Polygynax Virgo; Primyxine; Sterimycine; **Ger.:** Antibiotulle Lumiere; Corticotulle Lumiere; Dexa Polyspectran N; Farco-Tril; Isopto Max; Kombi-Stulln; Otosporin; Panotile N; Polygynax; Polyspectran; Polyspectran HC; Terracortril; Terramycin; **Hong Kong:** Dexa-Polyspectran; Maxitrol; Neosporin; Neotopic; Oftalmotrim; Otosporin; Polyfax; Polygynax; Polyspectran; Spersapolymyxin; Terramycin with Polymyxin B; **Irl.:** Maxitrol; Neosporin; Otosporin; Polyfax; Polyfax; **Israel:** Auriculanum; Bamyxin; Desoren; Dex-Otic; Maxitrol; Otosporin; Phenimixin; Tarocidin; Tarocidin D; Tarocyn; Terramycin; **Ital.:** Anauran; Cicatrene; Dermobios†; Mixotone; Otosporin; Rinojet SF; **Mex.:** Biodexan; Cortisporin; Dexsul; Hidropolicin; Maxitrol; Neobacigrin; Neosporin; Polixin; Septilisin; Synalar N; Synalar O; Synalar Oftalmico; Terramicina; Tribiot; **Neth.:** Maxitrol†; Otosporin; Panotile; Polyspectran B†; Polyspectran G†; Polytrim; Predmycin-P Liquifilm†; Synalar Bi-Otic; Terra-Cortril Gel Steraject met polymyxine-B; Terra-Cortril met polymyxine-B; Terramycin met polymyxine-B†; **Norw.:** Maxitrol; Terra-Cortril Polymyxin B; Terramycin Polymyxin B; **NZ:** Maxitrol; **Port.:** Conjunctilone; Conjunctilone-S; Gramixina; Oftalmotrim; Otolys†; Otosporin; Polisulfade; Polydexa; Polygynax; Polysporina†; **S.Afr.:** Maxitrol; Neosporin; Otosporin; Polysporin; Polytrim; Terra-Cortril; Terramycin; **Singapore:** Lignosporin; Maxitrol; Neosporin; Oftalmotrim; Otosporin; Polybamycin; Polydexa; Polygynax; Predmycin-P; Terramycin; **Spain:** Bacisporin; Blastoestimulina; Creanolona; Dermisone Tri Antibiotic; Linitul Antibiotico; Liquipom Dexa Antib; Maxitrol; Nasotic Oto; Neocones; Oftalmotrim; Oftalmotrim Dexa; Oftalmowell; Otix; Otosporin; Panotile; Phonal; Poliantib; Poly Pred; Pomada Antibiotica; Statrol; Synalar Nasal; Synalar Otico; Terra-Cortril; Terramicina; Tivitis; Tulgrasum Antibiotico; Vinciseptil Otico; **Swed.:** Isopto Biotic; Terracortril med polymyxin B; Terramycin Polymyxin B; **Switz.:** Baneopol; Maxitrol; Mycinopred; Neosporin; Otosporin; Panotile; Polydexa; Pulpomixine; Spersapolymyxin; Terracortril; Terramycine†; **Thai.:** Banocin; Dex-Otic; Maxitrol; Neosporin; Opsacin; Otosporin; Polyoph; Predmycin; Spersapolymyxin; Statrol; Terramycin; Terrasil; Xanalin; **UK:** Gregoderm; Maxitrol; Neosporin; Otosporin; Polyfax; Polytrim; Uniroid†; **USA:** Ak-Poly-Bac; Ak-Spore; Ak-Spore HC; Ak-Trol; Alba-3†; AntibiOtic; Aquaphor Antibiotic†; Bacticort†; Bactine First Aid Antibiotic Plus Anesthetic†; Betadine First Aid Antibiotics + Moisturizer†; Betadine Plus First Aid Antibiotics & Pain Reliever; Campho-Phenique Antibiotic Plus Pain Reliever Ointment†; Clomycin†; Coracin†; Cortatrigen; Cortimycin; Cortisporin; Dexacidin; Dexacine; Dexasporin; Ear-Eze; Lanabiotic; LazerSporin-C; Maxitrol; Mycitracin; Mycitracin Plus†; Neocin; Neomixin†; Neopolydex; Neosporin; Neosporin + Pain Relief; Neosporin GU; Neosporin Plus†; Neotal†; Neotricin HC; Octicair; Ocu-Spor-B; Ocu-Spor-G; Ocu-Trol; Ocutricin; Otic-Care; Oticin HC†; OtiTricin; Otobiotic; Otocort; Otomycin-HPN; Otosporin; Pediotic; Poly-Dex; Poly-Pred; Polycin-B; Polymycin; Polysporin; Polytracin; Polytrim; Septa†; Spectrocin Plus; Storz-N-P-D†; Terak; Terramycin with Polymyxin B; Tri-Biozene; Tribiotic Plus†; Triple Antibiotic†; UAD-Otic.

Pristinamycin (140-m)

Pristinamycin (BAN, rINN).
RP-7293.
CAS — 11006-76-1.
ATC — J01FA04.

Profile
Pristinamycin is a streptogramin antibiotic produced by the growth of *Streptomyces pristina spiralis*, with actions and uses similar to those of virginiamycin (p.269). It is administered by mouth in the treatment of susceptible infections (particularly staphylococcal infections) in a dose of 2 to 4 g daily in divided doses. Children have been given 50 to 100 mg per kg body-weight daily.

◊ Pristinamycin is a naturally occurring mixture of two synergistic components, pristinamycin I which is a macrolide, and pristinamycin II which is a depsipeptide.[1] It has been available for many years as an oral antistaphylococcal drug, and also acts against streptococci. It is effective against strains showing resistance to erythromycin; resistance to pristinamycin is currently rare, although resistance in staphylococci has been reported.[2,3] It is effective against meticillin-resistant *Staphylococcus aureus* (MRSA) but its usefulness in severe infection is limited by its poor solubility, which prevents development of an intravenous formulation. Mixtures of water-soluble derivatives of pristinamycins I and II, including quinupristin/dalfopristin (p.241), are in clinical use or under investigation.

1. Hamilton-Miller JMT. From foreign pharmacopoeias: 'new' antibiotics from old? *J Antimicrob Chemother* 1991; **27:** 702–5.
2. Loncle V, *et al.* Analysis of pristinamycin-resistant *Staphylococcus epidermidis* isolates responsible for an outbreak in a Parisian hospital. *Antimicrob Agents Chemother* 1993; **37:** 2159–65.
3. Allignet J, *et al.* Distribution of genes encoding resistance to streptogramin A related compounds among staphylococci resistant to these antibiotics. *Antimicrob Agents Chemother* 1996; **40:** 2523–8.

Preparations
Proprietary Preparations (details are given in Part 3)
Belg.: Pyostacine; **Fr.:** Pyostacine; **Israel:** Pyostacine.

Procaine Penicillin (141-b)

Procaine Penicillin (BAN).

Procaine Benzylpenicillin (BAN, rINNM); Benzylpenicillin Novocaine; Benzylpenicillinum Procainum; Penicillin G Procaine; Procaine Penicillin G; Procaini Benzylpenicillinum. 2-(4-Aminobenzoyloxy)ethyldiethylammonium (6R)-6-(2-phenylacetamido)penicillanate monohydrate.

$C_{13}H_{20}N_2O_2,C_{16}H_{18}N_2O_4S,H_2O = 588.7$.

CAS — 54-35-3 (anhydrous procaine penicillin [procaine benzylpenicillin]); 6130-64-9 (procaine penicillin [procaine benzylpenicillin] monohydrate).
ATC — J01CE09.

Pharmacopoeias. In Chin., Eur. (see p.vi), Int., Pol., and US.

Procaine penicillin [procaine benzylpenicillin] 600 mg is approximately equivalent to 360 mg of benzylpenicillin (600 000 units).

Pharmacopoeial description
Ph. Eur.: A white, crystalline powder. Slightly soluble in water; sparingly soluble in alcohol. A 0.33% solution in water has a pH of 5.0 to 7.5. Store in airtight containers.

USP 25: White crystals or white, very fine, microcrystalline powder, odourless or practically odourless. Slightly soluble in water; soluble in alcohol and in chloroform. It is rapidly inactivated by acids, by alkali hydroxides, and by oxidising agents. pH of a saturated solution in water is between 5.0 and 7.5.

Adverse Effects and Precautions
As for Benzylpenicillin, p.157.

Procaine penicillin [procaine benzylpenicillin] should not be given to patients known to be hypersensitive to either of its components.

Severe, usually transient, reactions with symptoms of severe anxiety and agitation, psychotic reactions, including visual and auditory hallucinations, seizures, tachycardia and hypertension, cyanosis, and a sensation of impending death have occasionally been reported with procaine penicillin [procaine benzylpenicillin] and may be due to accidental intravascular injection. Since similar reactions have also occurred with other depot penicillin preparations that do not contain procaine, its presence is unlikely to be the major cause of such reactions, but may be a contributory factor, especially after injection of high doses. These reactions have been termed non-allergic, pseudoallergic, pseudoanaphylactic, or Hoigné's syndrome and the term 'embolic-toxic reaction' has also been proposed.

Procaine penicillin [procaine benzylpenicillin] should not be injected intravascularly since ischaemic reactions may occur.

Interactions
As for Benzylpenicillin, p.158.

Pharmacokinetics
When procaine penicillin [procaine benzylpenicillin] is given by intramuscular injection, it forms a depot from which it is slowly released and hydrolysed to benzylpenicillin. Peak plasma concentrations are produced in 1 to 4 hours, and effective concentrations of benzylpenicillin are usually maintained for 12 to 24 hours. However, plasma concentrations are lower than those following an equivalent dose of benzylpenicillin potassium or sodium.

Distribution into the CSF is reported to be poor.

Uses and Administration
Procaine penicillin [procaine benzylpenicillin] has the same antimicrobial action as benzylpenicillin (p.158) to which it is hydrolysed gradually following deep intramuscular injection. This results in a prolonged effect, but because of the relatively low blood concentrations produced, its use should be restricted to infections caused by micro-organisms that are highly sensitive to penicillin. Procaine penicillin [procaine benzylpenicillin] should not be used as the sole treatment for severe acute infections, or when bacteraemia is present.

It is used mainly in the treatment of syphilis; other indications have included anthrax, pneumonia (in children in developing countries), and Whipple's disease. For details of these infections and their treatment, see under Choice of Antibacterial, p.114.

Administration and dosage. Procaine penicillin [procaine benzylpenicillin] is administered by deep intramuscular injection in usual doses of 0.6 to 1.2 g daily.

Patients with syphilis are given procaine penicillin [procaine benzylpenicillin] 1.2 g daily for 10 to 15 days; infants up to 2 years of age with congenital syphilis may be given 50 mg per kg body-weight daily. Treatment may be continued for 3 weeks in patients with late syphilis.

Procaine penicillin [procaine benzylpenicillin] is also administered in combined preparations with other penicillins, including benzylpenicillin and benzathine benzylpenicillin.

Preparations
BP 2001: Fortified Procaine Benzylpenicillin Injection; Procaine Benzylpenicillin Injection;
USP 25: Penicillin G Benzathine and Penicillin G Procaine Injectable Suspension; Penicillin G Procaine for Injectable Suspension; Penicillin G Procaine Injectable Suspension.

Proprietary Preparations (details are given in Part 3)
Austral.: Cilicaine Syringe; **Braz.:** Probecilin; **Canad.:** Ayercillin†; **Ger.:** Jenacillin O; **NZ:** Cilicaine Syringe; **Port.:** Atralcilina; **S.Afr.:** Novocillin; **Spain:** Aquilina; Farmaproina; Fradicilina†; **USA:** Crysticillin; Pfizerpen-AS†; Wycillin.

Multi-ingredient: Aust.: Fortepen†; Retarpen compositum; **Austral.:** Bicillin All Purpose†; **Braz.:** Benapen; Climacilin; Despacilina; Drenovac; Expectovac; Ginurovac; Linfocilin; Odontovac; Ortocilin; Pulmocilin; Wycillin R; **Canad.:** Bicillin A-P†; **Ger.:** Bipensaar; Hydracillin†; Jenacillin A; Retacillin; **Israel:** Duplo-Penicillin; Penicillin Fortified; **Ital.:** Tri-Wycillina; **Mex.:** Bencelin Combinado; Benzanil Compuesto; Benzetacil Combinado; Pendiben Compuesto; Penicil; Penipot; Penisodina; Penprocilina; **Neth.:** Bicilline†; Penidural D/F†; **Port.:** Penadur 6.3.3; **S.Afr.:** Penilente Forte; Ultracilin; **Spain:** Aquilina D A; Benzetacil Compuesta; Cepacilina 321, 621, or 633†; Neocepacilina†; **UK:** Bicillin†; **USA:** Bicillin C-R.

Propicillin Potassium (142-v)

Propicillin Potassium (BANM, pINNM).

Potassium α-Phenoxypropylpenicillin; Propicillinum Kalicum. A mixture of the D(+)- and L(−)-isomers of potassium (6R)-6-(2-phenoxybutyramido)penicillanate.
$C_{18}H_{21}KN_2O_5S = 416.5$.
CAS — 551-27-9 (propicillin); 1245-44-9 (propicillin potassium).

Profile
Propicillin is a phenoxypenicillin with actions and uses similar to those of phenoxymethylpenicillin (p.235). It is given by mouth, as the potassium salt, for the treatment of susceptible mild to moderate infections in a usual dose of 700 mg three times daily.

Preparations
Proprietary Preparations (details are given in Part 3)
Ger.: Baycillin; **Mex.:** Propibay.

Protionamide (7567-k)

Protionamide (BAN, rINN).

Prothionamide; RP-9778; TH-1321. 2-Propylpyridine-4-carbothioamide.
$C_9H_{12}N_2S = 180.3$.
CAS — 14222-60-7.
ATC — J04AD01.

Pharmacopoeias. In Chin., Int., and Jpn.

Adverse Effects, Precautions, and Antimicrobial Action
As for Ethionamide, p.206; it may be better tolerated than ethionamide.

Pharmacokinetics
Protionamide is readily absorbed from the gastrointestinal tract and produces peak plasma concentrations about 2 hours after a dose by mouth. It is widely distributed throughout body tissues and fluids, including the CSF. Protionamide is metabolised to the active sulfoxide and other inactive metabolites and less than 1% of a dose appears in the urine as unchanged drug.

Uses and Administration
Protionamide is a thioamide derivative considered to be interchangeable with ethionamide (p.206). Complete cross-resistance occurs between the two drugs. Protionamide has been administered by mouth in doses similar to those used for ethionamide. It has also been administered as rectal suppositories; protionamide hydrochloride has been given intravenously. Like ethionamide, it has generally been replaced by less toxic antimycobacterials.

The symbol † denotes a preparation no longer actively marketed

Preparations

Proprietary Preparations (details are given in Part 3)
Ger.: ektebin; Peteha.

Multi-ingredient: *Aust.:* Isoprodian; *Ger.:* Isoprodian; Peteha.

Prulifloxacin (15200-s)

Prulifloxacin *(rINN)*.

NM-441. (±)-7-{4-[(Z)-2,3-Dihydroxy-2-butenyl]-1-piperazinyl}-6-fluoro-1-methyl-4-oxo-1H,4H-[1,3]thiazeto[3,2-a]quinoline-3-carboxylic acid cyclic carbonate.
$C_{21}H_{20}FN_3O_6S = 461.5$.
CAS — 123447-62-1.

Profile

Prulifloxacin is a fluoroquinolone antibacterial.

Pyrazinamide (7568-a)

Pyrazinamide *(BAN, rINN)*.

Pyrazinamidum; Pyrazinoic Acid Amide. Pyrazine-2-carboxamide.
$C_5H_5N_3O = 123.1$.
CAS — 98-96-4.
ATC — J04AK01.

Pharmacopoeias. In *Chin.*, *Eur.* (see p.vi), *Int.*, *Jpn*, *Pol.*, and *US*.

Pharmacopoeial description

Ph. Eur.: A white, crystalline powder. Sparingly soluble in water, slightly soluble in alcohol and in dichloromethane; very slightly soluble in ether.

USP 25: A white to practically white, odourless or practically odourless, crystalline powder. Soluble 1 in 67 of water, 1 in 175 of dehydrated alcohol, 1 in 135 of chloroform, 1 in 1000 of ether, and 1 in 72 of methyl alcohol; slightly soluble in alcohol.

Adverse Effects and Treatment

Hepatotoxicity is the most serious side-effect of pyrazinamide therapy and its frequency appears to be dose-related. However, in currently recommended doses, when given with isoniazid and rifampicin, the incidence of hepatitis has been reported to be less than 3%. Patients may experience a transient increase in liver enzyme values; more seriously hepatomegaly, splenomegaly, and jaundice may develop and on rare occasions death has occurred.

Hyperuricaemia commonly occurs and may lead to attacks of gout.

Other side-effects are anorexia, nausea, vomiting, arthralgia, malaise, fever, sideroblastic anaemia, and dysuria. Photosensitivity and skin rashes have been reported on rare occasions.

Effects on blood pressure. Acute hypertension was associated with pyrazinamide administration in a previously normotensive woman.[1]

1. Goldberg J, *et al.* Acute hypertension as an adverse effect of pyrazinamide *JAMA* 1997; **277:** 1356.

Effects on the liver. The risk of hepatitis with antituberculous regimens containing pyrazinamide may be lower than suggested by early studies, in which large doses were used, often for long periods. The incidence of hepatitis in studies of short-course regimens containing pyrazinamide has ranged from 0.2% in Africa, to 0.6% in Hong Kong, to 2.8% in Singapore.[1] These and later studies[2-4] have shown that hepatotoxicity is not increased when pyrazinamide is added to the initial phase of short-term chemotherapy containing rifampicin and isoniazid. Nevertheless, a report[5] of 4 cases of fulminant hepatic failure in patients given triple therapy with the potentially hepatotoxic drugs rifampicin, isoniazid, and pyrazinamide (one patient also received ethambutol) highlighted the importance of strict liver function monitoring and this was reinforced by others. However, the Joint Tuberculosis Committee of the British Thoracic Society is anxious that fears over the safety of treatment regimens do not compromise adequate therapy of the disease itself. They recommend[6] initial measurement of liver function in all patients and regular monitoring in patients with known chronic liver disease. Tests should be repeated if symptoms of liver dysfunction occur, and details are given concerning the response to deteriorating liver function and include guidelines for prompt re-introduction of appropriate antituberculous therapy once normal liver function is restored.

1. Girling DJ. The role of pyrazinamide in primary chemotherapy for pulmonary tuberculosis. *Tubercle* 1984; **65:** 1–4.
2. Parthasarathy R, *et al.* Hepatic toxicity in South Indian patients during treatment of tuberculosis with short-course regimens containing isoniazid, rifampicin and pyrazinamide. *Tubercle* 1986; **67:** 99–108.
3. Combs DL, *et al.* USPHS tuberculosis short-course chemotherapy trial 21: effectiveness, toxicity, and acceptability: the report of final results. *Ann Intern Med* 1990; **112:** 397–406.

4. le Bourgeois M, *et al.* Good tolerance of pyrazinamide in children with pulmonary tuberculosis. *Arch Dis Child* 1989; **64:** 177–8.
5. Mitchell I, *et al.* Anti-tuberculous therapy and acute liver failure. *Lancet* 1995; **345:** 555–6.
6. Ormerod LP, *et al.* Hepatotoxicity of antituberculosis drugs. *Thorax* 1996; **51:** 111–13.

Effects on the nervous system. Convulsions which developed in a 2-year-old child receiving antituberculous therapy appeared to be due to pyrazinamide, administered in a dose of 250 mg daily.[1]

1. Herlevsen P, *et al.* Convulsions after treatment with pyrazinamide. *Tubercle* 1987; **68:** 145–6.

Hyperuricaemia. Hyperuricaemia during therapy with pyrazinamide may be due to inhibition of uric acid excretion by pyrazinoic acid, the main metabolite of pyrazinamide.[1]

In a large multicentre study,[2] the incidence of elevated serum concentrations of uric acid for patients receiving rifampicin, isoniazid, and pyrazinamide was 52.2% at 8 weeks while the incidence for patients receiving rifampicin and isoniazid was 5.4%. Arthralgia was reported in 6 of 617 patients receiving rifampicin, isoniazid, and pyrazinamide, but in none of 445 patients receiving rifampicin and isoniazid.

Slight increases in plasma concentrations of uric acid occurred in 9 of 43 children after one month's treatment with rifampicin, isoniazid, ethambutol, and pyrazinamide. Arthralgias and gout did not occur. Uric acid concentrations were normal on completion of treatment with pyrazinamide.[3] Some studies have suggested a relationship between elevated serum uric acid levels and arthralgia,[4] but this has not been confirmed.[5]

1. Ellard GA, Haslam RM. Observations on the reduction of the renal elimination of urate in man caused by the administration of pyrazinamide. *Tubercle* 1976; **57:** 97–103.
2. Combs DL, *et al.* USPHS tuberculosis short-course chemotherapy trial 21: effectiveness, toxicity, and acceptability: the report of final results. *Ann Intern Med* 1990; **112:** 397–406.
3. le Bourgeois M, *et al.* Good tolerance of pyrazinamide in children with pulmonary tuberculosis. *Arch Dis Child* 1989; **64:** 177–8.
4. Hong Kong Tuberculosis Treatment Services/British MRC. Adverse reactions to short-course regimens containing streptomycin, isoniazid, pyrazinamide and rifampicin in Hong Kong. *Tubercle* 1976; **57:** 81–95.
5. Jenner PJ, *et al.* Serum uric acid concentrations and arthralgia among patients treated with pyrazinamide-containing regimens in Hong Kong and Singapore. *Tubercle* 1981; **62:** 175–9.

Pellagra. Pellagra, probably due to pyrazinamide, developed in a 26-year-old woman receiving antituberculous therapy.[1] Symptoms regressed, without stopping therapy, on administration of nicotinamide.

1. Jørgensen J. Pellagra probably due to pyrazinamide: development during combined chemotherapy of tuberculosis. *Int J Dermatol* 1983; **22:** 44–5.

Precautions

Pyrazinamide is contra-indicated by the manufacturers in patients with liver damage, although some consider that it can be used with care when the liver damage is not severe. Liver function should be assessed before and regularly during treatment. The British Thoracic Society recommends that, in patients with chronic liver disease, pyrazinamide treatment should be suspended if serum aminotransferase concentrations are elevated to 5 times the normal upper limit or the bilirubin concentration rises. Although the manufacturer recommends that pyrazinamide should not be restarted in patients with evidence of hepatocellular damage, the UK guidelines allow cautious re-introduction of antimycobacterial drugs, including pyrazinamide, once liver function has returned to normal.

Pyrazinamide should not be given to patients with acute gout or hyperuricaemia and should be used with caution in patients with a history of gout. Caution should also be observed in patients with impaired renal function. Increased difficulty has been reported in controlling diabetes mellitus when diabetics are given pyrazinamide.

Porphyria. Pyrazinamide has been associated with acute attacks of porphyria and is considered unsafe in porphyric patients.

Pregnancy. Although the American Thoracic Society[1,2] considers that there is insufficient teratogenicity data to recommend the routine use of pyrazinamide during pregnancy, others, including the IUAT[3] and the British Thoracic Society,[4] do not contra-indicate pyrazinamide in pregnant patients.

For details on distribution into breast milk, see Pharmacokinetics, below.

1. American Thoracic Society. Treatment of tuberculosis and tuberculosis infection in adults and children. *Am Rev Respir Dis* 1986; **134:** 355–63.
2. American Thoracic Society and the Centers for Disease Control. Treatment of tuberculosis and tuberculosis infection in adults and children. *Am J Respir Crit Care Med* 1994; **149:** 1359–74.

3. Anonymous. Antituberculosis regimens of chemotherapy: recommendations from the Committee on Treatment of the International Union Against Tuberculosis and Lung Disease. *Bull Int Union Tuberc Lung Dis* 1988; **63:** 60–4.
4. Joint Tuberculosis Committee of the British Thoracic Society. Chemotherapy and management of tuberculosis in the United Kingdom: recommendations 1998. *Thorax* 1998; **53:** 536–48.

Interactions

Probenecid. A study of the complex interactions occurring when pyrazinamide and probenecid are given to patients with gout.[1] Urinary excretion of urate depends on the relative size and timing of doses of the two drugs. Probenecid is known to block the excretion of pyrazinamide.

1. Yü TF, *et al.* The effect of the interaction of pyrazinamide and probenecid on urinary uric acid excretion in man. *Am J Med* 1977; **63:** 723–8.

Zidovudine. Low or undetectable concentrations of pyrazinamide occurred in 4 patients also taking zidovudine.[1] In the same study, 6 of 7 patients with HIV infections taking pyrazinamide without zidovudine had normal serum pyrazinamide concentrations.

1. Peloquin CA, *et al.* Low antituberculosis drug concentrations in patients with AIDS. *Ann Pharmacother* 1996; **30:** 919–25.

Antimicrobial Action

Pyrazinamide has a bactericidal effect on *Mycobacterium tuberculosis* but appears to have no activity against other mycobacteria or micro-organisms *in vitro*. The MIC for *M. tuberculosis* is less than 20 µg per mL at pH 5.6; it is almost completely inactive at a neutral pH. Pyrazinamide is effective against persisting tubercle bacilli within the acidic intracellular environment of the macrophages. The initial inflammatory response to chemotherapy increases the number of organisms in the acidic environment. As inflammation subsides and pH increases, the sterilising activity of pyrazinamide decreases. This pH-dependent activity explains the clinical effectiveness of pyrazinamide as part of the initial 8-week phase in short-course treatment regimens.

Resistance to pyrazinamide rapidly develops when it is used alone.

◊ Although the antimicrobial activity of pyrazinamide has been recognised since the 1950s, the mode of action is still unclear. One proposal is that pyrazinoic acid is the active moiety. Pyrazinamidase produced by the tubercle bacilli is known to convert pyrazinamide to pyrazinoic acid. A further proposal[1] is that the pyrazinoic acid formed within the macrophage would be trapped, thereby lowering intracellular pH to levels toxic to tubercle bacilli.

1. Salfinger M, *et al.* Pyrazinamide and pyrazinoic acid activity against tubercle bacilli in cultured human macrophages and in the BACTEC system. *J Infect Dis* 1990; **162:** 201–7.

Activity with other antimicrobials. Pyrazinamide exhibited synergistic activity against *Mycobacterium tuberculosis* with clarithromycin.[1]

1. Mor N, Esfandiari A. Synergistic activities of clarithromycin and pyrazinamide against Mycobacterium tuberculosis in human macrophages. *Antimicrob Agents Chemother* 1997; **41:** 2035–6.

Pharmacokinetics

Pyrazinamide is readily absorbed from the gastrointestinal tract. Peak serum concentrations occur about 2 hours after a dose by mouth and have been reported to be about 35 µg per mL after 1.5 g, and 66 µg per mL after 3 g. Pyrazinamide is widely distributed in body fluids and tissues and diffuses into the CSF. The half-life has been reported to be about 9 to 10 hours. It is metabolised primarily in the liver by hydrolysis to the major active metabolite pyrazinoic acid which is subsequently hydroxylated to the major excretory product 5-hydroxypyrazinoic acid. It is excreted through the kidney mainly by glomerular filtration. About 70% of a dose appears in the urine within 24 hours mainly as metabolites and 4 to 14% as unchanged drug. Pyrazinamide is removed by dialysis. Pyrazinamide is distributed into breast milk.

◊ A short distribution phase and an elimination phase of 9.6 hours in healthy subjects following a single oral dose of pyrazinamide 27 mg per kg body-weight has been reported;[1] the half-life for the major metabolite pyrazinoic acid was 11.8 hours.

In the major metabolic pathway, pyrazinamide was deaminated to pyrazinoic acid which was hydroxylated to hydroxypyrazinoic acid; in the minor pathway, pyrazinamide was hydroxylated to hydroxypyrazinamide which was then deaminated to hydroxypyrazinoic acid. The limiting step was deamination; oxidation by xanthine oxidase occurred very quickly.

A similar study was carried out in 10 patients with cirrhosis of the liver.[2] Following a dose of 19.3 mg per kg, the elimination phase was about 15 hours for pyrazinamide and 24 hours for pyrazinoic acid.

1. Lacroix C, *et al.* Pharmacokinetics of pyrazinamide and its metabolites in healthy subjects. *Eur J Clin Pharmacol* 1989; **36:** 395–400.
2. Lacroix C, *et al.* Pharmacokinetics of pyrazinamide and its metabolites in patients with hepatic cirrhotic insufficiency. *Arzneimittelforschung* 1990; **40:** 76–9.

Bioavailability. The oral bioavailability of rifampicin and isoniazid, but not of pyrazinamide, was decreased by food in many patients.[1]

1. Zent C, Smith P. Study of the effect of concomitant food on the bioavailability of rifampicin, isoniazid and pyrazinamide. *Tubercle Lung Dis* 1995; **76:** 109–13.

Breast feeding. The peak concentration of pyrazinamide in breast milk of a 29-year-old woman was 1.5 µg per mL 3 hours after administration of a 1-g dose of pyrazinamide.[1] The peak plasma concentration was 42 µg per mL after 2 hours.

1. Holdiness MR. Antituberculosis drugs and breast-feeding. *Arch Intern Med* 1984; **144:** 1888.

Distribution. Pyrazinamide was given to 28 patients with suspected tuberculous meningitis in doses of 34 to 41 mg per kg body-weight. The mean concentration of pyrazinamide in the CSF 2 hours after administration was 38.6 µg per mL and represented about 75% of that in serum; concentrations at 5 and 8 hours were 44.5 and 31.0 µg per mL respectively and were about 10% higher than those in serum.[1] The use of corticosteroids appeared to have no influence on penetration of pyrazinamide into the CSF of patients with tuberculous meningitis.[2]

1. Ellard GA, *et al.* Penetration of pyrazinamide into the cerebrospinal fluid in tuberculous meningitis. *BMJ* 1987; **294:** 284–5.
2. Woo J, *et al.* Cerebrospinal fluid and serum levels of pyrazinamide and rifampicin in patients with tuberculous meningitis. *Curr Ther Res* 1987; **42:** 235–42.

Uses and Administration

Pyrazinamide is used as part of multidrug regimens for the treatment of tuberculosis (p.143), primarily in the initial 8-week phase of short-course treatment. Pyrazinamide is usually given daily or 2 or 3 times weekly. In the UK recommended doses by mouth for adults and children are up to 35 mg per kg body-weight daily (maximum daily dose is 3 g) or 50 mg per kg three times weekly, or up to 75 mg per kg twice weekly. To standardise administration, the usual dose for patients under 50 kg is 1.5 g daily, 2.0 g three times weekly, or 3.0 g twice weekly. For patients 50 kg or greater, the usual dose is 2.0 g daily, 2.5 g three times weekly, or 3.5 g twice weekly. The recommended doses in the USA are 15 to 30 mg per kg daily (maximum 2 g) or 50 to 70 mg per kg three times weekly (maximum 3 g each day) or twice weekly (maximum 4 g each day). WHO recommends 25 mg per kg daily or 35 mg per kg three times weekly or 50 mg per kg twice weekly.

Administration in hepatic impairment. See Precautions, above.

Administration in renal impairment. The manufacturer in the UK recommends dosage reduction in patients with impaired renal function.

In a study of 6 patients on haemodialysis,[1] the average amount of pyrazinamide and its metabolites removed during a dialysis session was 926 mg after an oral dose of 1700 mg. It was recommended that the usual pyrazinamide dose be given to patients on dialysis as the risk of accumulation was negligible, and that the dose on dialysis days be given after the procedure.

1. Lacroix C, *et al.* Haemodialysis of pyrazinamide in uraemic patients. *Eur J Clin Pharmacol* 1989; **37:** 309–11.

Preparations

BP 2001: Pyrazinamide Tablets;
USP 25: Pyrazinamide Tablets; Rifampin, Isoniazid, and Pyrazinamide Tablets; Rifampin, Isoniazid, Pyrazinamide, and Ethambutol Hydrochloride Tablets.

Proprietary Preparations (details are given in Part 3)

Aust.: Rifater; *Austral.:* Zinamide; *Belg.:* Tebrazid; *Canad.:* Tebrazid; *Fin.:* Tisamid; *Fr.:* Pirilene; *Ger.:* Pyrafat; PZA; *Hong Kong:* Pyrafat; *Irl.:* Zinamide; *Ital.:* Piraldina; *Mex.:* Braccopiral; Pirafoid; Pirazer; Premox; *NZ:* Zinamide; *Port.:* Piraside; Pramide; *S.Afr.:* Pyrazide; Rozide; Tebezide; *Singapore:* PZA; *Thai.:* Myrin-P; Pyratab; PZA; *UK:* Zinamide.

Multi-ingredient: *Aust.:* Rifater; *Canad.:* Rifater; *Fr.:* Rifater; *Ger.:* Rifater; *Hong Kong:* Rifater; *Irl.:* Rifater; *Ital.:* Rifater; *Mex.:* Rifater; *Port.:* Rifater; Tuberen; *S.Afr.:* Myrin Plus; Pyrifin†; Rifafour; Rifater; Rimcure; *Singapore:* Rifater; *Spain:* Rifater; *Switz.:* Rifater; Rimactazide + Z†; *Thai.:* Rifater; *UK:* Rifater; *USA:* Rifater.

Quinupristin/Dalfopristin   (12225-k)

RP-59500.
CAS — 126602-89-9; 176861-85-1.

Dalfopristin Mesilate   (20414-f)

Dalfopristin Mesilate (*BANM, rINNM*).
Dalfopristin Mesylate; RP-54476 (dalfopristin). (3R,4R,5E,10E,12E,14S,26R,26aS)-26-{[2-(Diethylamino)ethyl]sulfonyl}-8,9,14,15,24,25,26,26a-octahydro-14-hydroxy-3-isopropyl-4,12-dimethyl-3H-21,18-nitrilo-1H,22H-pyrrolo[2.1-c][1,8,4,19]dioxadiazacyclotetracosine-1,7,16,22(4H,17H)-tetrone methanesulphonate;   (26R,27S)-26-{[2-(Diethylamino)-ethyl]sulfonyl}-26,27-dihydrovirginiamycin M₁ methanesulphonate.
$C_{34}H_{50}N_4O_9S$,CH_4O_3S = 787.0.
CAS — 112362-50-2 (dalfopristin).

NOTE. Dalfopristin is *USAN*.

Quinupristin Mesilate   (20423-d)

Quinupristin Mesilate (*BANM, rINNM*).
Quinupristin Mesylate; RP-57669 (quinupristin). N-{(6R,9S,10R,13S,15aS,18R,22S,24aS)-22-[p-(Dimethylamino)benzyl]-6-ethyldocosahydro-10,23-dimethyl-5,8,12,15,17,21,24-heptaoxo-13-phenyl-18-{[(3S)-3-quinuclidinylthio)methyl}-12H-pyrido[2,1-f]pyrrolo[2,1-f][1,4,7,10,13,16]-oxapentaazacyclononadecin-9-yl}-3-hydroxy-picolinamide methanesulphonate; 4-[4-(Dimethylamino)-N-methyl-L-phenylalamine]-5-(cis-5-{[(S)-1-azabicyclo[2.2.2]oct-3-ylthio]methyl}-4-oxo-L-2-piperidinecarboxylic acid)-virginiamycin S₁ methanesulphonate.
$C_{53}H_{67}N_9O_{10}S$,CH_4O_3S = 1118.3.
CAS — 120138-50-3 (quinupristin).

NOTE. Quinupristin is *USAN*.

Adverse Effects and Treatment

The adverse effects most frequently reported in patients receiving quinupristin/dalfopristin include nausea and vomiting, diarrhoea, skin rash, pruritus, headache, and pain. Myalgia and arthralgia have occurred and may be severe; symptoms may be improved by decreasing the dose frequency. Pseudomembranous colitis has been reported. Hyperbilirubinaemia and raised liver enzyme values may occur. Individual cases of severe thrombocytopenia and pancytopenia have been reported.

Pain and inflammation at the injection site is common, and thrombophlebitis has occurred.

Quinupristin/dalfopristin is not removed by peritoneal dialysis, and removal by haemodialysis is considered unlikely.

Precautions

Quinupristin/dalfopristin should be used with caution in patients with impaired hepatic function and is contra-indicated in severe hepatic impairment, as elevated plasma concentrations of quinupristin and dalfopristin and their metabolites have been found in patients with hepatic dysfunction, and elevated concentrations of quinupristin metabolites have occurred in patients with hyperbilirubinaemia.

Interactions

Quinupristin/dalfopristin inhibits the cytochrome P450 isoenzyme CYP3A4 and it may therefore inhibit the metabolism of a number of drugs. In particular there is a theoretical possibility of serious ventricular arrhythmias with cisapride and the non-sedating antihistamines astemizole and terfenadine. Concomitant administration of quinupristin/dalfopristin has been shown to increase plasma concentrations of ciclosporin, midazolam, nifedipine, and tacrolimus.

Antimicrobial Action

Quinupristin/dalfopristin is a semisynthetic streptogramin antibacterial. Quinupristin and dalfopristin each have bacteriostatic activity and in combination usually act synergistically to produce bactericidal activity. The streptogramins act on the ribosome to block protein synthesis.

Quinupristin/dalfopristin is active against a range of Gram-positive bacteria including meticillin- and multidrug-resistant strains of *Staphylococcus aureus*, *S. epidermidis*, vancomycin-resistant *Enterococcus faecium* (but not *E. faecalis*), and penicillin- and mac-

rolide-resistant *Streptococcus pneumoniae*. It is also active against the anaerobe *Clostridium perfringens*, and Gram-negative bacteria *Legionella pneumophila*, *Moraxella catarrhalis* (*Branhamella catarrhalis*), *Mycoplasma pneumoniae*, and *Neisseria meningitidis*.

◊ References.

1. Schouten MA, Hoogkamp-Korstanje JAA. Comparative in-vitro activities of quinupristin-dalfopristin against Gram-positive bloodstream isolates. *J Antimicrob Chemother* 1997; **40:** 213–19.
2. Pankuch GA, *et al.* Postantibiotic effect and postantibiotic sub-MIC effect of quinupristin-dalfopristin against Gram-positive andnegative organisms. *Antimicrob Agents Chemother* 1998; **42:** 3028–31.
3. Johnson AP, *et al.* Susceptibility to quinupristin/dalfopristin and other antibiotics of vancomycin-resistant enterococci from the UK, 1997 to mid-1999. *J Antimicrob Chemother* 2000; **46:** 125–8.

Resistance. Although uncommon, isolated reports of *E. faecium* resistant to quinupristin/dalfopristin have emerged,[1-3] and have included a link to the use of the streptogramin virginiamycin as an animal food additive.[3]

1. Eliopoulos GM, *et al.* Characterization of vancomycin-resistant Enterococcus faecium isolates from the United States and their susceptibility in vitro to dalfopristin-quinupristin. *Antimicrob Agents Chemother* 1998; **42:** 1088–92.
2. Bozdogan B, *et al.* Plasmid-mediated coresistance to streptogramins and vancomycin in Enterococcus faecium HM1032. *Antimicrob Agents Chemother* 1999; **43:** 2097–8.
3. Werner G, *et al.* Association between quinupristin/dalfopristin resistance in glycopeptide-resistant Enterococcus faecium and the use of additives in animal feed. *Eur J Clin Microbiol Infect Dis* 1998; **17:** 401–2.

Pharmacokinetics

Following parenteral administration, quinupristin and dalfopristin are rapidly metabolised. At steady state, the half-life of quinupristin and its metabolites is about 3 hours and that of dalfopristin and its metabolites about 1 hour. Elimination half-lives of unchanged quinupristin and dalfopristin are 0.9 and 0.75 hours respectively. Protein binding of quinupristin is 55 to 78% and for dalfopristin, 11 to 26%. The main route of excretion is biliary, with 75 to 77% of a dose detectable in the faeces. Urinary excretion accounts for 15% of the quinupristin and 19% of the dalfopristin dose. Negligible amounts are removed by peritoneal dialysis and probably also by haemodialysis.

Uses and Administration

Quinupristin/dalfopristin is a streptogramin antibacterial related to pristinamycin. Quinupristin and dalfopristin are semisynthetic derivatives of pristinamycin I and pristinamycin IIA respectively, and are used in the ratio 3:7. Quinupristin/dalfopristin is active against a range of Gram-positive and some Gram-negative organisms, but it is reserved for the treatment of serious infections with multidrug-resistant Gram-positive bacteria, specifically multidrug-resistant *Staphylococcus aureus* and pneumococci and vancomycin-resistant *Enterococcus faecium*.

Quinupristin/dalfopristin is given by intravenous infusion in glucose 5% over 60 minutes through a central venous catheter. The vein should be flushed following each infusion to minimise venous irritation. The injection should not be diluted with saline solutions since it is incompatible with sodium chloride. Quinupristin/dalfopristin is given as the mesilate salts in a dose of 7.5 mg per kg body-weight (equivalent to quinupristin 2.25 mg per kg and dalfopristin 5.25 mg per kg) every 8 or 12 hours for 7 to 10 days.

◊ References.

1. Finch RG. Antibacterial activity of quinupristin/dalfopristin: rationale for clinical use. *Drugs* 1996; **51** (suppl 1): 31–7.
2. Bryson HM, Spencer CM. Quinupristin-dalfopristin. *Drugs* 1996; **52:** 406–15.
3. Bayston R, *et al.*, eds. Quinupristin/dalfopristin—update on the first injectable streptogramin. *J Antimicrob Chemother* 1997; **39** (suppl A): 1–151.
4. Wood MJ (ed). Quinupristin/dalfopristin–a novel approach for the treatment of serious Gram-positive infections. *J Antimicrob Chemother* 1999; **44** (suppl A): 1–46.
5. Lamb HM, *et al.* Quinupristin/dalfopristin: a review of its use in the management of serious Gram-positive infections. *Drugs* 1999; **58:** 1061–97.

The symbol † denotes a preparation no longer actively marketed

Preparations

Proprietary Preparations (details are given in Part 3)
Multi-ingredient: *Austral.:* Synercid; *Fin.:* Synercid; *Fr.:* Synercid; *UK:* Synercid; *USA:* Synercid.

Ramoplanin (3759-c)

Ramoplanin (USAN, rINN).
A-16686; MDL-62198.
CAS — 76168-82-6.

Profile

Ramoplanin is a glycopeptide antibiotic with a spectrum of activity *in vitro* similar to that of vancomycin (p.268) but considerably more potent. It is also active against *Bacteroides* spp. It is under investigation, notably in the topical treatment of acne and skin infections, the prevention of infection due to vancomycin-resistant enterococci, and the reduction of nasal carriage of staphylococci.

Rifabutin (16512-w)

Rifabutin (BAN, USAN, rINN).
Ansamicin; Ansamycin; LM-427; Rifabutine. (9S,12E,14S,15R,16S,17R,18R,19R,20S,21S,22E,24Z)-6,16,18,20-Tetrahydroxy-1'-isobutyl-14-methoxy-7,9,15,17,19,21,25-heptamethylspiro[9,4-(epoxypentadeca[1,11,13]trienimino)-2H-furo-[2',3':7,8]naphth[1,2-d]imidazole-2,4'-piperidine]-5,10,26-(3H,9H)-trione-16-acetate.
$C_{46}H_{62}N_4O_{11}$ = 847.0.
CAS — 72559-06-9.
ATC — J04AB04.
Pharmacopoeias. In US.

Pharmacopoeial description

USP 25: An amorphous red-violet powder. Very slightly soluble in water; sparingly soluble in alcohol; soluble in chloroform and in methyl alcohol. Store at a temperature not exceeding 40°. Protect from light.

Stability. Study of the stability of two extemporaneous oral liquid preparations of rifabutin.[1]

1. Haslam JL, et al. Stability of rifabutin in two extemporaneously compounded oral liquids. *Am J Health-Syst Pharm* 1999; **56:** 333–6.

Adverse Effects and Precautions

As for Rifampicin, p.243. It produces a syndrome of polyarthralgia-arthritis at doses greater than 1 g daily. Uveitis has been reported, especially in patients also receiving clarithromycin or fluconazole. Asymptomatic corneal opacities have been reported following long-term administration.

◊ A polyarthralgia-arthritis syndrome has been reported[1] in 9 of 10 patients receiving a daily dose of rifabutin greater than 1 g. The syndrome did not occur in patients receiving less than 1 g daily and disappeared on drug withdrawal. Two patients with polyarthralgia-arthritis symptoms developed uveitis (see also below under Effects on the Eyes) and aphthous stomatitis at doses of approximately 1.8 g per day.
An orange-tan skin pigmentation has been reported to occur in most patients receiving rifabutin.[1] Urine may be discoloured.[2] An influenza-like syndrome has been reported in 2 of 12 patients given 300 mg daily for Crohn's disease,[3] in 1 of 16 HIV-infected patients on continuous rifabutin,[1] and in 8 of 15 HIV-infected patients receiving increasing doses of rifabutin.[2]
Other reported adverse effects include hepatitis,[1] leucopenia[2] (including neutropenia[4]), epigastric pain,[3] rash,[3] erythema,[2] and ageusia.[5]
Rash, fever, and vomiting occurred in 1 of 2 children receiving 6.5 mg per kg body-weight per day.[6]

1. Siegal FP, et al. Dose-limiting toxicity of rifabutin in AIDS-related complex: syndrome of arthralgia/arthritis. *AIDS* 1990; **4:** 433–41.
2. Torseth J, et al. Evaluation of the antiviral effect of rifabutin in AIDS-related complex. *J Infect Dis* 1989; **159:** 1115–18.
3. Basilisco G, et al. Controlled trial of rifabutin in Crohn's disease. *Curr Ther Res* 1989; **46:** 245–50.
4. Apseloff G, et al. Severe neutropenia caused by recommended prophylactic doses of rifabutin. *Lancet* 1996; **348:** 685.
5. Morris JT, Kelly JW. Rifabutin-induced ageusia. *Ann Intern Med* 1993; **119:** 171–2.
6. Levin RH, Bolinger AM. Treatment of nontuberculous mycobacterial infections in pediatric patients. *Clin Pharm* 1988; **7:** 545–51.

Effects on the eyes. Uveitis may occur a few weeks or months after starting rifabutin, and generally necessitates withdrawal of the drug and treatment with topical or systemic corticosteroids and cycloplegics.[1] The UK Committee on Safety of Medicines was aware of 48 reports of uveitis in patients taking rifabutin.[2] Most patients were also receiving clarithromycin for treatment of AIDS-related *Mycobacterium avium* complex (MAC) infection and some were also receiving fluconazole (see Interactions, below). A dosage reduction to 300 mg rifabutin daily is now recommended in patients also receiving mac-

rolides or triazole antifungals[2,3] and is reported to produce a satisfactory response in MAC infections.[4]
Asymptomatic corneal opacities have been reported following long-term administration.

1. Tseng AL, Walmsley SL. Rifabutin-associated uveitis. *Ann Pharmacother* 1995; **29:** 1149–55.
2. Committee on Safety of Medicines. Rifabutin (Mycobutin)–uveitis. *Current Problems 20* 1994.
3. Committee on Safety of Medicines. Revised indications and drug interactions of rifabutin. *Current Problems* 1997; **23:** 14.
4. Shafran SD, et al. A comparison of two regimens for the treatment of Mycobacterium avium complex bacteremia in AIDS; rifabutin, ethambutol, and clarithromycin versus rifampin, ethambutol, clofazimine, and ciprofloxacin. *N Engl J Med* 1996; **335:** 377–83.

Interactions

As for Rifampicin, p.244. Rifabutin is reported to be a less potent inducer of microsomal enzymes than rifampicin, but similar interactions should nevertheless be anticipated.

Plasma concentrations of rifabutin are increased by concurrent administration of clarithromycin (and possibly other macrolides) and fluconazole resulting in increased rifabutin toxicity, in particular uveitis and neutropenia (see also above).

Antiretroviral drugs. Rifabutin interacts with *HIV-protease inhibitors*, resulting in reductions in plasma concentrations of the HIV-protease inhibitor and increases in rifabutin plasma concentrations, with a possible risk of uveitis. Most clinical experience appears to have been gained with rifabutin in combination with indinavir. The Centers for Disease Control in the USA suggest[1,2] that in patients with HIV infection who need treatment for tuberculosis, rifabutin could be used in those receiving amprenavir, indinavir, nelfinavir, or nevirapine and could probably be used in those receiving efavirenz, ritonavir, or saquinavir; however, dose modifications are required for some combinations and should be substantial (150 mg two or three times per week) for rifabutin when given with ritonavir in particular[2] (see Tuberculosis under Uses, below). Rifabutin should not be given with delavirdine.
Although rifabutin is reported to reduce the plasma concentrations of *zidovudine*, studies have shown that the effect is not marked (see p.646), and the manufacturer suggests that the reduction may not be clinically relevant.

1. Centers for Disease Control. Prevention and treatment of tuberculosis among patients infected with human immunodeficiency virus: principles of therapy and revised recommendations. *MMWR* 1998; **47** (RR-20): 1–51.
2. Centers for Disease Control. Notice to readers: updated guidelines for the use of rifabutin or rifampin for the treatment and prevention of tuberculosis among HIV-infected patients taking protease inhibitors or nonnucleoside reverse transcriptase inhibitors. *MMWR* 2000; **49:** 185–9.

Azole antifungals. As reported under Adverse Effects, above, many reports of rifabutin-associated uveitis have occurred in patients also receiving *fluconazole*. Increases in the area under the concentration-time curve for rifabutin and its active 25-deacetyl metabolite were increased by 82% and 216% respectively when fluconazole was given concurrently to 12 HIV-infected patients,[1] and elevated plasma-rifabutin concentrations were reported in a patient who developed uveitis while also receiving *itraconazole*.[2] The mechanism of the interaction remains uncertain but could involve microsomal cytochrome P450 isoenzyme CYP3A4 (see Metabolism under Pharmacokinetics, below).

1. Trapnell CB, et al. Increased plasma rifabutin levels with concomitant fluconazole therapy in HIV-infected patients. *Ann Intern Med* 1996; **124:** 573–6.
2. Lefort A, et al. Uveitis associated with rifabutin prophylaxis and itraconazole therapy. *Ann Intern Med* 1996; **125:** 939–40.

Macrolides. As discussed under Effects on the Eyes, above, most patients developing uveitis during rifabutin treatment are also receiving *clarithromycin*. In a study of the treatment of *Mycobacterium avium* complex infection in AIDS patients,[1] uveitis or pseudojaundice or both were noted in those receiving rifabutin, ethambutol, and clarithromycin, but not in those receiving rifabutin, ethambutol, ciprofloxacin, and clofazimine. A retrospective study following an outbreak of uveitis in a similar patient population[2] also found concurrent clarithromycin to be a risk factor, with a trend towards greater risk at higher rifabutin doses, although patient numbers were small. In 26 patients taking rifabutin with either clarithromycin or *azithromycin*,[3] the incidence and severity of adverse effects in general was similar, although the 2 patients who developed uveitis were both receiving clarithromycin.
Pharmacokinetic studies have demonstrated increased rifabutin concentrations when clarithromycin is taken concurrently. A study in healthy subjects[4] was terminated prematurely because of the high incidence of adverse effects, including neutropenia, fevers, and myalgia, particularly in subjects receiving rifabutin with azithromycin or clarithromycin. Mean serum concentrations of rifabutin and the 25-O-deacetyl metabolite in subjects also receiving clarithromycin were more than 400% and 3700% respectively of those in subjects receiving rifabutin alone. Plasma concentrations were unaffected by azithromycin. Similar effects on rifabutin concentrations were found in HIV-

infected subjects receiving clarithromycin[5] and reductions in clarithromycin concentrations were also noted.

1. Shafran SD, et al. Uveitis and pseudojaundice during a regimen of clarithromycin, rifabutin, and ethambutol. *N Engl J Med* 1994; **330:** 438–9.
2. Kelleher P, et al. Uveitis associated with rifabutin and macrolide therapy for Mycobacterium avium intracellulare infection in AIDS patients. *Genitourin Med* 1996; **72:** 419–21.
3. Griffith DE, et al. Adverse events associated with high-dose rifabutin in macrolide-containing regimens for the treatment of Mycobacterium avium complex lung disease. *Clin Infect Dis* 1995; **21:** 594–8.
4. Apseloff G, et al. Comparison of azithromycin and clarithromycin in their interactions with rifabutin in healthy volunteers. *J Clin Pharmacol* 1998; **38:** 830–5.
5. Hafner R, et al. Tolerance and pharmacokinetic interactions of rifabutin and clarithromycin in human immunodeficiency virus-infected volunteers. *Antimicrob Agents Chemother* 1998; **42:** 631–9.

Antimicrobial Action

Rifabutin possesses a spectrum of antibacterial activity similar to that of rifampicin (p.245). However, most investigations have concentrated on its action against mycobacteria. Cross-resistance is common with rifampicin.

Antibacterial action. Rifabutin is active against many Gram-positive and Gram-negative bacteria, including *Helicobacter pylori*.[1] Resistance can be induced *in vitro* in H. pylori but is currently rare in clinical isolates.[2]

1. Kunin CM. Antimicrobial activity of rifabutin. *Clin Infect Dis* 1996; **22** (suppl 1): S3–S14.
2. Heep M, et al. Rifampin and rifabutin resistance mechanism in Helicobacter pylori. *Antimicrob Agents Chemother* 1999; **43:** 1497–9.

Antimycobacterial action. Rifabutin possesses activity against most species of mycobacteria. One study[1] found the MIC of rifabutin against rifampicin-sensitive *Mycobacterium tuberculosis* strains to be 8 times lower than that of rifampicin. At a concentration of 0.6 µg per mL, 69% of *Mycobacterium avium* complex strains were sensitive to rifabutin while 35% were sensitive to this concentration of rifampicin.
Another study[2] has reported the MIC for rifabutin against clinical isolates of M. avium complex as 1.53 µg per mL for an agar dilution method and 1.25 µg per mL for a radiometric broth method.
Rifabutin may be more active *in vivo* than *in vitro* studies suggest, as a result of its favourable pharmacokinetic profile and prolonged postantibiotic effect.[3]
Rifabutin has been reported to be active in *animal* assays against *Mycobacterium leprae*,[4] including a rifampicin-resistant strain.[5] Synergistic activity against M. leprae has been reported[6] *in vitro* for rifabutin with clinafloxacin and rifabutin with sparfloxacin.

1. Dickinson JM, Mitchison DA. In vitro activity of new rifamycins against rifampicin-resistant M. tuberculosis and MAIS-complex mycobacteria. *Tubercle* 1987; **68:** 177–82.
2. Heifets LB, et al. Determination of ansamycin MICs for Mycobacterium avium complex in liquid medium by radiometric and conventional methods. *Antimicrob Agents Chemother* 1985; **28:** 570–5.
3. Kunin CM. Antimicrobial activity of rifabutin. *Clin Infect Dis* 1996; **22** (suppl 1): S3–S14.
4. Hastings RC, Jacobson RR. Activity of ansamycin against Mycobacterium leprae in mice. *Lancet* 1983; **ii:** 1079–80. Correction. *ibid.* 1210.
5. Hastings RC, et al. Ansamycin activity against rifampicin-resistant Mycobacterium leprae. *Lancet* 1984; **i:** 1130.
6. Dhople AM, Ibanez MA. In-vitro activity of three new fluoroquinolones and synergy with ansamycins against Mycobacterium leprae. *J Antimicrob Chemother* 1993; **32:** 445–51.

Antiprotozoal action. Rifabutin was shown to have activity *in vitro* and in *mice* against *Toxoplasma gondii*.[1] Synergistic activity was shown for rifabutin in combination with atovaquone.

1. Romand S, et al. In vitro and in vivo effects of rifabutin alone or combined with atovaquone against Toxoplasma gondii. *Antimicrob Agents Chemother* 1996; **40:** 2015–20.

Resistance. Rifampicin-resistant strains of *Mycobacterium tuberculosis* have been identified in 2 patients receiving rifabutin alone as prophylaxis against M. avium complex.[1,2] It is therefore important to exclude M. tuberculosis infection before beginning rifabutin prophylaxis.
Rifampicin-resistant M. kansasii has also been reported in a patient receiving rifabutin.[3]

1. Weltman AC, et al. Rifampicin-resistant Mycobacterium tuberculosis. *Lancet* 1995; **345:** 1513.
2. Bishai WR, et al. Brief report: rifampin-resistant tuberculosis in a patient receiving rifabutin prophylaxis. *N Engl J Med* 1996; **334:** 1573–6.
3. Meynard JL, et al. Rifampin-resistant Mycobacterium kansasii infection in a patient with AIDS who was receiving rifabutin. *Clin Infect Dis* 1997; **24:** 1262–3.

Pharmacokinetics

Rifabutin is poorly absorbed from the gastrointestinal tract, but is widely distributed. Approximately 70% is bound to plasma proteins. Both hepatic and renal clearance occurs. A terminal half-life of 36 hours has been reported.

HIV-infected patients. The pharmacokinetics of rifabutin were studied in HIV-infected patients with normal renal and hepatic function.[1] A two-compartment open pharmacokinetic model was proposed. Rifabutin was rapidly but incompletely absorbed from the gastrointestinal tract and bioavailability was poor, being 20% on day 1 of the study and 12% on day 28. Mean peak plasma concentrations occurred 2 to 3 hours following oral doses and were about 350, 500, and 900 nanograms per mL following oral doses of 300, 600, and 900 mg respectively. The peak and trough concentrations following 600 mg twice daily were about 900 and 200 nanograms per mL respectively. Rifabutin is approximately 70% bound to plasma proteins. The area under the curve showed a decrease on repeated dosage which might be explained by the induction of drug-metabolising liver enzymes. A large volume of distribution of 8 to 9 litres per kg body-weight, indicative of extensive tissue distribution, and a mean terminal half-life of 32 to 38 hours were reported. This study[1] also showed that the peak plasma concentration of the major metabolite, 25-deacetylrifabutin, was 10% of the parent compound. Only 4% of unchanged rifabutin was excreted in the urine following oral administration and between 6 to 14% following intravenous administration. Total urinary excretion of rifabutin and metabolite 72 hours after intravenous administration was 44%; total faecal excretion was between 30 and 49%.

Peak and trough concentrations at steady state were reported as 900 and 200 nanograms per mL respectively in a patient with tuberculosis given rifabutin 450 mg daily.[2] While these figures were the same as those previously reported with 600 mg twice daily,[1] that earlier study showed that there was considerable interpatient variability.

CSF concentrations in 5 patients with AIDS on rifabutin 450 mg daily ranged from 36 to 70% of serum concentrations.[3]

1. Skinner MH, et al. Pharmacokinetics of rifabutin. *Antimicrob Agents Chemother* 1989; **33:** 1237–41.
2. Gillespie SH, et al. The serum rifabutin concentrations in a patient successfully treated for multi-resistant mycobacterium tuberculosis infection. *J Antimicrob Chemother* 1990; **25:** 490–1. Correction. *ibid.* 1991; **27:** 877.
3. Siegal FP, et al. Dose-limiting toxicity of rifabutin in AIDS-related complex: syndrome of arthralgia/arthritis. *AIDS* 1990; **4:** 433–41.

Metabolism. Five metabolites of rifabutin were identified in an *in-vitro* study[1] using human hepatic and enterocyte microsomes. Cytochrome P450 isoenzyme CYP3A4 was involved in the formation of all metabolites except 25-*O*-deacetylrifabutin. Deacetylation of rifabutin was apparently mediated by microsomal cholinesterase,[1] although another study[2] showed that further metabolism of 25-*O*-deacetylrifabutin is dependent on CYP3A4. The results[1] also suggested that metabolism by intestinal CYP3A4 contributes significantly to presystemic metabolism of rifabutin (and consequently its low bioavailability) and to drug interactions with azole antifungals (see above) and macrolides.

1. Iatsimirskaia E, et al. Metabolism of rifabutin in human enterocyte and liver microsomes: kinetic parameters, identification of enzyme systems, and drug interactions with macrolides and antifungal agents. *Clin Pharmacol Ther* 1997; **61:** 554–62.
2. Trapnell CB, et al. Metabolism of rifabutin and its 25-desacetyl metabolite, LM565, by human liver microsomes and recombinant human cytochrome P-450 3A4: relevance to clinical interaction with fluconazole. *Antimicrob Agents Chemother* 1997; **41:** 924–6.

Uses and Administration

Rifabutin is a rifamycin antibiotic used for the *prophylaxis* of *Mycobacterium avium* complex (MAC) infection in immunocompromised patients and for the *treatment* of opportunistic mycobacterial infections (including those due to MAC) (p.131) and tuberculosis (p.143). When used for treatment rifabutin, like rifampicin, should be given in combination with other antibacterials to prevent the emergence of resistant organisms.

Rifabutin is given by mouth as a single daily dose. The dose for the prophylaxis of *M. avium* complex infection is 300 mg daily. For the treatment of opportunistic mycobacterial infections the dose is 450 to 600 mg daily and for pulmonary tuberculosis the dose is 150 to 450 mg daily, in each case as part of a multidrug regimen. Doses should be reduced to 300 mg daily in patients also receiving macrolides or azole antifungals (see under Adverse Effects, Effects on the Eyes, above). Dosage alterations may also be necessary in patients receiving HIV-protease inhibitors (see under Tuberculosis, below).

◊ Reviews.
1. Brogden RN, Fitton A. Rifabutin: a review of its antimicrobial activity, pharmacokinetic properties and therapeutic efficacy. *Drugs* 1994; **47:** 983–1009.

Cryptosporidiosis. Rifabutin may have a potential prophylactic effect against cryptosporidiosis (p.583).

Mycobacterium avium complex infections. Alterations in rifabutin dosage may be necessary in patients concurrently

The symbol † denotes a preparation no longer actively marketed

---

receiving antiretrovirals for the management of HIV infection, and further details are given under Tuberculosis, below.

Toxoplasmosis. A beneficial response to rifabutin in combination with pyrimethamine was reported in a patient with AIDS-related *Toxoplasma gondii* encephalitis.[1] The patient was allergic to sulfonamides and clindamycin, the drugs most commonly used (see p.585).

1. Schürmann D, et al. Rifabutin appears to be a promising agent for combination treatment of AIDS-related toxoplasma encephalitis. *J Infect* 1998; **36:** 352–3.

Tuberculosis. The Centers for Disease Control in the USA recommends that rifabutin should be used in place of rifampicin in short-course therapy for tuberculosis in patients receiving antiretroviral drugs for HIV infection.[1] However, dose modifications are often necessary;[1,2] additionally, some combinations, notably rifabutin with delavirdine, should not be employed.

In patients receiving ritonavir, the dose of rifabutin should be substantially reduced from 300 mg daily or twice weekly to 150 mg two or three times per week. In those receiving amprenavir, indinavir, or nelfinavir the daily dose of rifabutin should be decreased from 300 mg to 150 mg, although the dose for intermittent therapy remains unchanged at 300 mg two or three times weekly. The doses of indinavir and nelfinavir will need to be increased. In patients receiving efavirenz, the dose of rifabutin should be increased from 300 mg daily or twice weekly to 450 mg or 600 mg daily or 600 mg two or three times per week.

1. Centers for Disease Control. Prevention and treatment of tuberculosis among patients infected with human immunodeficiency virus: principles of therapy and revised recommendations. *MMWR* 1998; **47** (RR-20): 1–51.
2. Centers for Disease Control. Notice to readers: updated guidelines for the use of rifabutin or rifampin for the treatment and prevention of tuberculosis among HIV-infected patients taking protease inhibitors or nonnucleoside reverse transcriptase inhibitors. *MMWR* 2000; **49:** 185–9.

Preparations

USP 25: Rifabutin Capsules.

Proprietary Preparations (details are given in Part 3)
Aust.: Mycobutin; *Austral.:* Mycobutin; *Belg.:* Mycobutin; *Canad.:* Mycobutin; *Fin.:* Ansatipin; *Fr.:* Ansatipine; *Ger.:* Alfacid; Mycobutin; *Hong Kong:* Mycobutin; *Israel:* Mycobutin; *Ital.:* Mycobutin; *Neth.:* Mycobutin; *NZ:* Mycobutin; *Port.:* Mycobutin; *S.Afr.:* Mycobutin; *Spain:* Ansatipin; *Swed.:* Ansatipin; *Switz.:* Mycobutin; *UK:* Mycobutin; *USA:* Mycobutin.

Rifampicin (7569-t)

Rifampicin *(BAN, rINN)*.
Ba-41166/E; L-5103; NSC-113926; Rifaldazine; Rifampicinum; Rifampin *(USAN)*; Rifamycin AMP. 3-(4-Methylpiperazin-1-yliminomethyl)rifamycin SV; (12Z,14E,24E)-(2S,16S,17S,18R,19R, 20R,21S,22R,23S)-1,2-Dihydro-5,6,9,17,19-pentahydroxy-23-methoxy-2,4,12,16,18,20,22-heptamethyl-8-(4-methylpiperazin-1-yliminomethyl)-1,11-dioxo-2,7-(epoxypentadeca[1,11,13]trienimino)naphtho[2,1-*b*]furan-21-yl acetate.
$C_{43}H_{58}N_4O_{12} = 822.9$.
CAS — 13292-46-1.
ATC — J04AB02.

Pharmacopoeias. In *Chin., Eur.* (see p.vi), *Int., Jpn, Pol.,* and *US.*

Pharmacopoeial description

Ph. Eur.: A reddish-brown or brownish-red, crystalline powder. Slightly soluble in water, in alcohol, in acetone, and in ether; soluble in methyl alcohol. A 1% suspension has a pH of 4.5 to 6.5. Store at a temperature not exceeding 25° in an atmosphere of nitrogen in airtight containers. Protect from light.

USP 25: A red-brown crystalline powder. Very slightly soluble in water; freely soluble in chloroform; soluble in ethyl acetate and in methyl alcohol. A 1% suspension in water has a pH of 4.5 to 6.5. Store at a temperature not exceeding 40° in airtight containers. Protect from light.

Stability. The method employed when preparing an oral liquid from commercial rifampicin capsules influenced the dispersion of the powder and consequently the measured concentration of rifampicin in the final product.[1]

1. Nahata MC, et al. Effect of preparation method and storage on rifampin concentration in suspensions. *Ann Pharmacother* 1994; **28:** 182–5.

Adverse Effects

Rifampicin is usually well tolerated. Adverse effects are more common during intermittent therapy or after restarting interrupted treatment.

Some patients may experience a cutaneous syndrome which presents 2 to 3 hours after a daily or intermittent dose as facial flushing, itching, rash, or rarely eye irritation. A 12-hour 'flu' syndrome of fever, chills, bone pain, shortness of breath, and malaise has been associated with intermittent administration. It usually occurs after 3 to 6 months of intermittent treatment and has a higher incidence with doses of 20 mg or

---

more per kg body-weight given once weekly than with currently recommended regimens. Anaphylaxis or shock has occurred rarely.

Gastrointestinal adverse effects include nausea, vomiting, anorexia, diarrhoea, and epigastric distress. Administration on an empty stomach is recommended for maximal absorption, but this has to be balanced against administration after a meal to minimise gastrointestinal intolerance. Pseudomembranous colitis has been reported. Rifampicin produces transient abnormalities in liver function. Hepatitis occurs rarely. Fatalities due to hepatotoxicity have been reported occasionally (see Effects on the Liver, below).

Rifampicin can cause thrombocytopenia and purpura, usually when administered as an intermittent regimen, and if this occurs further administration of rifampicin is contra-indicated. Other haematological adverse effects include eosinophilia, leucopenia, and haemolytic anaemia.

Alterations in kidney function and renal failure have occurred, particularly during intermittent therapy. Menstrual disturbances have been reported.

Nervous system adverse effects include headache, drowsiness, ataxia, dizziness, and numbness.

Oedema, myopathy, and muscular weakness have been reported.

Thrombophlebitis has occurred following prolonged intravenous infusion. Extravasation during intravenous infusion may cause local irritation and inflammation.

Rifampicin causes a harmless orange-red discoloration of the urine and other body fluids.

Effects on the blood. Thrombocytopenia may occur in patients taking rifampicin, most commonly as intermittent therapy, and probably has an immunological basis. The platelet count may fall within 3 hours of a dose and return to normal within 36 hours, if additional doses are not given.[1] There may also be a risk of thrombocytopenia when re-introducing rifampicin to patients who have interrupted their treatment.[2] Thrombocytopenia has also been reported in a patient taking rifampicin for the first time for meningococcal prophylaxis.[3] Fatalities have occurred when rifampicin was not withdrawn once thrombocytopenic purpura had developed or when treatment with rifampicin was resumed in patients who had experienced purpura.[1] However, there is a report of the successful re-introduction of rifampicin in a patient who developed thrombocytopenia without rifampicin-dependent antibodies.[4]

Bleeding from the oral cavity not associated with thrombocytopenia has been reported in a patient taking rifampicin.[5] Leucopenia[6,7] and haemolysis or haemolytic anaemia[8] or red cell aplasia[9] have occurred. Disseminated intravascular coagulation has been reported in a patient receiving intermittent rifampicin therapy.[10] The incidence of deep-vein thrombosis increased in one group of hospitalised tuberculosis patients when rifampicin was introduced as standard therapy,[11] but data from others have not supported a causal relationship.[12]

1. Girling DJ. Adverse effects of antituberculosis drugs. *Drugs* 1982; **23:** 56–74.
2. Burnette PK, et al. Rifampin-associated thrombocytopenia secondary to poor compliance. *Drug Intell Clin Pharm* 1989; **23:** 382–4.
3. Hall AP, et al. New hazard of meningococcal chemoprophylaxis. *J Antimicrob Chemother* 1993; **31:** 451.
4. Bhasin DK, et al. Can rifampicin be restarted in patients with rifampicin-induced thrombocytopenia? *Tubercle* 1991; **72:** 306–7.
5. Sule RR. An unusual reaction to rifampicin in a once monthly dose. *Lepr Rev* 1996; **67:** 227–33.
6. Van Assendelft AHW. Leucopenia in rifampicin chemotherapy. *J Antimicrob Chemother* 1985; **16:** 407–8.
7. Vijayakumaran P, et al. Leucocytopenia after rifampicin and ofloxacin therapy in leprosy. *Lepr Rev* 1997; **68:** 10–15.
8. Lakshminarayan S, et al. Massive haemolysis caused by rifampicin. *BMJ* 1973; **2:** 282–3.
9. Mariette X, et al. Rifampicin-induced pure red cell aplasia. *Am J Med* 1989; **87:** 459–60.
10. Souza CS, et al. Disseminated intravascular coagulopathy as an adverse reaction to intermittent rifampin schedule in the treatment of leprosy. *Int J Lepr* 1997; **65:** 366–71.
11. White NW. Venous thrombosis and rifampicin. *Lancet* 1989; **ii:** 434–5.
12. Cowie RL, et al. Deep-vein thrombosis and pulmonary tuberculosis. *Lancet* 1989; **ii:** 1397.

Effects on the gastrointestinal tract. In addition to symptoms of gastrointestinal intolerance, gastrointestinal bleeding and erosive gastritis,[1] ulcerative colitis,[2] and eosinophilic colitis[3] have been reported in patients receiving rifampicin.

1. Zargar SA, et al. Rifampicin-induced upper gastrointestinal bleeding. *Postgrad Med J* 1990; **66:** 310–11.
2. Tajima A, et al. Rifampicin-associated ulcerative colitis. *Ann Intern Med* 1992; **116:** 778–9.
3. Lange P, et al. Eosinophilic colitis due to rifampicin. *Lancet* 1994; **344:** 1296–7.

Effects on the immune system. Symptoms including malaise, arthralgia, arthritis, and oedema of the extremities occurring in 4 patients taking rifampicin and 3 taking rifabutin were considered to be due to drug-induced lupus syndrome.[1] Cutaneous lupus erythematosus was reported in a patient receiving rifampicin with clarithromycin and ethambutol.[2] All patients had positive anti-nuclear antibody titres.[1,2]

1. Berning SE, Iseman MD. Rifamycin-induced lupus syndrome. *Lancet* 1997; **349:** 1521–2.
2. Patel GK, Anstey A. Rifampicin-induced cutaneous lupus erythematosus. *Br J Dermatol* 1999; **141** (suppl 55): 77.

Effects on the liver. Transient abnormalities in liver function are common during the early stages of antituberculous therapy with rifampicin and other drugs, but sometimes there is more serious hepatotoxicity that may require a change of treatment especially in patients with pre-existing liver disease.

The use of rifampicin daily with ethionamide or protionamide for the treatment of multibacillary leprosy has long been associated with a high incidence of hepatotoxicity (see under Adverse Effects of Ethionamide, p.206) and ethionamide and protionamide are no longer recommended for the treatment of leprosy because of their severe hepatotoxicity. However, hepatic reactions have also been reported with rifampicin, isoniazid, and pyrazinamide, the drugs most commonly used to treat tuberculosis, and have occasionally proved fatal. A report[1] of 4 cases of fulminant hepatic failure in patients given triple therapy with this potentially hepatotoxic combination regimen (one patient also received ethambutol) highlighted the importance of strict liver function monitoring and this was reinforced by others.

The Joint Tuberculosis Committee of the British Thoracic Society is nevertheless anxious that fears over the safety of treatment regimens do not compromise adequate therapy of the disease itself. They make recommendations[2] for initial measurement of liver function in all patients and regular monitoring in patients with pre-existing liver disease. Tests should be repeated if symptoms of liver dysfunction occur, and details are given concerning the response to deteriorating liver function and include guidelines for prompt re-introduction of appropriate antituberculosis therapy once normal liver function is restored.

1. Mitchell I, *et al.* Anti-tuberculous therapy and acute liver failure. *Lancet* 1995; **345:** 555–6.
2. Ormerod LP, *et al.* Hepatotoxicity of antituberculosis drugs. *Thorax* 1996; **51:** 111–13.

Effects on the lungs. Pulmonary fibrosis in an elderly man was attributed to rifampicin.[1]

1. Umeki S. Rifampicin and pulmonary fibrosis. *Arch Intern Med* 1988; **148:** 1663, 7.

Effects on the pancreas. Report of chronic pancreatic insufficiency in a patient following administration of rifampicin, isoniazid, ethambutol, and pyrazinamide.[1]

1. Liu BA, *et al.* Pancreatic insufficiency due to antituberculosis therapy. *Ann Pharmacother* 1997; **31:** 724–6.

Effects on the skin. Skin reactions to rifampicin are usually mild, irrespective of it being given daily or intermittently.[1] However, there have been a few isolated reports of severe reactions.[2-4] Contact dermatitis has been observed.[5]

1. Girling DJ. Adverse reactions to rifampicin in antituberculosis regimens. *J Antimicrob Chemother* 1977; **3:** 115–32.
2. Okano M, *et al.* Toxic epidermal necrolysis due to rifampicin. *J Am Acad Dermatol* 1987; **17:** 303–4.
3. Goldin HM, *et al.* Rifampin and exfoliative dermatitis. *Ann Intern Med* 1987; **107:** 789.
4. Mimouni A, *et al.* Fixed drug eruption following rifampin treatment. *DICP Ann Pharmacother* 1990; **24:** 947–8.
5. Anker N, Da Gunha Bang F. Long-term intravenous rifampicin treatment: advantages and disadvantages. *Eur J Respir Dis* 1981; **62:** 84–6.

Hypersensitivity. References.

1. Girling DJ. Adverse reactions to rifampicin in antituberculosis regimens. *J Antimicrob Chemother* 1977; **3:** 115–32.
2. Wurtz RM, *et al.* Anaphylactoid drug reactions to ciprofloxacin and rifampicin in HIV-infected patients. *Lancet* 1989; **i:** 955–6.
3. Harland RW, *et al.* Anaphylaxis from rifampin. *Am J Med* 1992; **92:** 581–2.
4. Cnudde F, Leynadier F. The diagnosis of allergy to rifampicin confirmed by skin test. *Am J Med* 1994; **97:** 403–4.
5. Sharma VK, *et al.* Rifampicin-induced urticaria in leprosy. *Lepr Rev* 1997; **68:** 331–2.

Overdosage. Cases of skin pigmentation induced by rifampicin overdose have been reviewed.[1] Reddish-orange discoloration of the skin appeared within a few hours of drug administration; urine, mucous membranes, and sclera were also discoloured. Periorbital or facial oedema, pruritus, and gastrointestinal intolerance occurred in most patients. Treatment was supportive and clinical symptoms resolved in most patients over 3 to 4 days, although fatalities occurred with doses over 14 g.

1. Holdiness MR. A review of the redman syndrome and rifampicin overdosage. *Med Toxicol Adverse Drug Exp* 1989; **4:** 444–51.

Precautions

Liver function should be checked before treatment with rifampicin and special care should be taken in alcoholic patients or those with pre-existing liver disease who require regular monitoring during therapy. Some manufacturers contra-indicate its use in pa-

tients with jaundice. A self-limiting hyperbilirubinaemia may occur in the first 2 or 3 weeks of treatment. Alkaline phosphatase values may be raised moderately due to rifampicin's enzyme-inducing capacity. When other liver function tests are within normal limits, hyperbilirubinaemia in the first few weeks or moderately elevated alkaline phosphatase are not indications to withdraw rifampicin. However, dose adjustment is necessary when there is other evidence of hepatic impairment and treatment should be suspended when there is evidence of more serious liver toxicity.

Blood counts should be monitored during prolonged treatment and in patients with hepatic disorders. Should thrombocytopenia or purpura occur then rifampicin should be withdrawn permanently. Some manufacturers also recommend such withdrawal in patients who develop haemolytic anaemia or renal failure.

Administration of rifampicin following interruption of treatment has been associated with increased risk of serious adverse effects.

Patients should be advised that rifampicin may colour faeces, saliva, sputum, sweat, tears, urine, and other body-fluids orange-red. Soft contact lenses worn by patients receiving rifampicin may become permanently stained.

Rifampicin should not be given by the intramuscular or subcutaneous route. When given by intravenous infusion care should be taken to avoid extravasation.

Adrenocortical insufficiency. Acute adrenal crisis has been precipitated by rifampicin in patients with adrenal insufficiency[1] and induction of microsomal enzymes may be enough to compromise even patients with mildly impaired cortisol production. Critical hypotension has also developed in non-Addisonian patients within a week to 10 days of starting rifampicin therapy. However, it has not been necessary to suspend the use of rifampicin if patients are treated with corticosteroids.[2] The effectiveness of corticosteroid therapy can be reduced by rifampicin (see Interactions, below).

1. Elansary EH, Earis JE. Rifampicin and adrenal crisis. *BMJ* 1983; **286:** 1861–2.
2. Boss G. Rifampicin and adrenal crisis. *BMJ* 1983; **287:** 62.

Porphyria. Rifampicin has been associated with acute attacks of porphyria and is considered unsafe in porphyric patients.

Pregnancy and breast feeding. The International Union Against Tuberculosis[1] and the WHO Expert Committee on Leprosy[2] recommend **treatment** of **pregnant** patients with the same rifampicin-containing multidrug regimens as would be used in nonpregnant patients. Of the standard drugs recommended for leprosy or tuberculosis, only streptomycin has proven teratogenicity.[3] While administration of rifampicin to pregnant patients is generally considered to be safe, the drug does cross into the fetus[4] and malformations and bleeding tendencies have been reported.[3] A literature review[3] revealed 386 normal term infants and 29 elective terminations out of 446 pregnancies in patients who took rifampicin in association with other antimycobacterial drugs. A variety of malformations were reported; there were 14 abnormal infants or fetuses, 2 premature births, 9 still-births and 7 spontaneous abortions. It was considered that rifampicin did not increase the overall risk of congenital malformations.

Rifampicin treatment can increase the metabolism of vitamin K resulting in clotting disorders associated with vitamin K deficiency. Bleeding disorders in 2 mothers shortly after delivery, and scalp haemorrhage, anaemia, and shock in one of the infants have been reported.[5] The authors recommended blood coagulation monitoring and prophylactic administration of vitamin K to mothers and neonates when the mother has received rifampicin during pregnancy.

Rifampicin is present in small amounts in breast milk; 1 to 3 μg per mL has been reported.[6] The American Academy of Pediatrics considers that mothers taking rifampicin may **breast feed**.[7]

1. Committee on Treatment of the International Union against Tuberculosis and Lung Disease. Antituberculosis regimens of chemotherapy. *Bull Int Union Tuberc Lung Dis* 1988; **63:** 60–4.
2. WHO. WHO expert committee on leprosy: sixth report. *WHO Tech Rep Ser* 768 1988.
3. Snider DE, *et al.* Treatment of tuberculosis during pregnancy. *Am Rev Respir Dis* 1980; **122:** 65–79.
4. Holdiness MR. Transplacental pharmacokinetics of the antituberculosis drugs. *Clin Pharmacokinet* 1987; **13:** 125–9.
5. Chouraqui JP, *et al.* Hémorragie par avitaminose K chez la femme enceinte et le nouveau-né: rôle éventuel de la rifampicine: a propos de 2 observations. *Therapie* 1982; **37:** 447–50.
6. Vorherr H. Drug excretion in breast milk. *Postgrad Med* 1974; **56:** 97–104.
7. American Academy of Pediatrics, Committee on Drugs. The transfer of drugs and other chemicals into human milk. *Pediatrics* 2001; **108:** 776–89.

Interactions

Rifampicin accelerates the metabolism of some drugs by inducing microsomal liver enzymes and possibly by interfering with hepatic uptake. A number of drugs have been reported to be affected but the clinical significance of some of these interactions remains to be determined. Although most drugs involved may require an increase in dosage to maintain effectiveness, women taking oral contraceptives should change to another form of contraception (see p.1459). Other drugs reported to be affected include atovaquone, azathioprine, chloramphenicol, ciclosporin, cimetidine, clofibrate, corticosteroids, coumarin anticoagulants, dapsone, diazepam and other benzodiazepines, doxycycline, fluconazole, haloperidol, hexobarbital, HIV-protease inhibitors, itraconazole, ketoconazole, lamotrigine, methadone, non-nucleoside reverse transcriptase inhibitor antiretrovirals, ondansetron, oral hypoglycaemics, phenytoin, quinine, rofecoxib, statins (HMG-CoA reductase inhibitors), sulfasalazine, tacrolimus, theophylline, thyroid hormones, zidovudine, and several cardiovascular drugs including beta blockers, digitalis alkaloids, and antiarrhythmics such as disopyramide, lorcainide, mexiletine, propafenone, quinidine, tocainide, and verapamil and other calcium-channel blockers.

The absorption of rifampicin may be reduced by administration with antacids, drugs that reduce gastric motility (anticholinergics and opioids), ketoconazole, or preparations containing bentonite (for example some aminosalicylic acid preparations). However, such interactions can be overcome by giving rifampicin a few hours before any of these drugs. Some other interactions affecting the activity of rifampicin are discussed below.

◊ Reviews.
1. Venkatesan K. Pharmacokinetic drug interactions with rifampicin. *Clin Pharmacokinet* 1992; **22:** 47–65.
2. Borcherding SM, *et al.* Update on rifampin drug interactions II. *Arch Intern Med* 1992; **152:** 711–16.
3. Grange JM, *et al.* Clinically significant drug interactions with antituberculosis agents. *Drug Safety* 1994; **11:** 242–51.

Antiretroviral drugs. Rifamycins can induce the metabolism of zidovudine, the non-nucleoside reverse transcriptase inhibitors delavirdine, efavirenz, and nevirapine, and HIV-protease inhibitors, resulting in potentially subtherapeutic plasma concentrations. In addition HIV-protease inhibitors inhibit the metabolism of rifamycins resulting in elevated plasma-rifamycin concentrations and an increased incidence of adverse effects.[1,2] In general, rifampicin and HIV-protease inhibitors should not be used concurrently. See also p.242 for comment on the interaction of HIV-protease inhibitors with rifabutin.

1. Anonymous. Clinical update: impact of HIV protease inhibitors on the treatment of HIV-infected tuberculosis patients with rifampin. *MMWR* 1996; **45:** 921–5.
2. Centers for Disease Control. Notice to readers: updated guidelines for the use of rifabutin or rifampin for the treatment and prevention of tuberculosis among HIV-infected patients taking protease inhibitors or nonnucleoside reverse transcriptase inhibitors. *MMWR* 2000; **49:** 185–9.

Clofazimine. Concomitant administration of clofazimine to leprosy patients receiving rifampicin with or without dapsone may decrease the rate of absorption of rifampicin and increase the time to peak plasma concentration.[1] In patients receiving clofazimine, rifampicin, and dapsone, the area under the curve for rifampicin was reduced.[1] However, a multiple dose study showed that the pharmacokinetics of rifampicin were similar after 7 days' treatment with rifampicin and dapsone or rifampicin, dapsone, and clofazimine.[2]

1. Mehta J, *et al.* Effect of clofazimine and dapsone on rifampicin (Lositril) pharmacokinetics in multibacillary and paucibacillary leprosy cases. *Lepr Rev* 1986; **57** (suppl 3): 67–76.
2. Venkatesan K, *et al.* The effect of clofazimine on the pharmacokinetics of rifampicin and dapsone in leprosy. *J Antimicrob Chemother* 1986; **18:** 715–18.

Co-trimoxazole. In 15 patients receiving combination therapy including rifampicin for tuberculosis, administration of a course of co-trimoxazole resulted in increases in maximum plasma concentrations and in the area under the concentration-time curve for rifampicin.[1] No adverse effects were observed and the clinical implications of this observation remain unclear.

1. Bhatia RS, *et al.* Drug interaction between rifampicin and cotrimoxazole in patients with tuberculosis. *Hum Exp Toxicol* 1991; **10:** 419–21.

Isoniazid. There is little significant pharmacokinetic interaction between rifampicin and isoniazid.[1] Although lower blood concentrations of rifampicin have been reported with concomitant isoniazid administration, the effect is not considered clinically significant.[2]

Since both drugs are hepatotoxic, concurrent administration could be associated with an increased incidence of hepatic damage, although the benefits of using this combination are considered to outweigh any potential risks.

1. Acocella G, et al. Kinetics of rifampicin and isoniazid administered alone and in combination to normal subjects and patients with liver disease. Gut 1972; 13: 47–53.
2. Mouton RP, et al. Blood levels of rifampicin, desacetylrifampicin and isoniazid during combined therapy. J Antimicrob Chemother 1979; 5: 447–54.

Ketoconazole. Concomitant administration of rifampicin, ketoconazole, and isoniazid have produced low serum concentrations of each drug resulting in failure of antifungal treatment.[1] Rifampicin serum concentrations are reduced when rifampicin is given concurrently with ketoconazole;[2] separation of the doses by 30 minutes[3] to 12 hours[2] may result in similar rifampicin concentrations to those attained when rifampicin is given alone, although serum concentrations of ketoconazole remain depressed regardless of the time of administration.

1. Abadie-Kemmerly S, et al. Failure of ketoconazole treatment of Blastomyces dermatitidis due to interaction of isoniazid and rifampin. Ann Intern Med 1988; 109: 844–5. Correction. ibid. 1989; 111: 96.
2. Engelhard D, et al. Interaction of ketoconazole with rifampin and isoniazid. N Engl J Med 1984; 311: 1681–3.
3. Doble N, et al. Pharmacokinetic study of the interaction between rifampicin and ketoconazole. J Antimicrob Chemother 1988; 21: 633–5.

Probenecid. Although one study[1] showed that concomitant administration of probenecid could increase serum-rifampicin concentrations, another[2] subsequently found that the effect was uncommon and inconsistent and concluded that probenecid had no place as an adjunct to routine rifampicin therapy.

1. Kenwright S, Levi AJ. Impairment of hepatic uptake of rifamycin antibiotics by probenecid and its therapeutic implications. Lancet 1973; ii: 1401–5.
2. Fallon RJ, et al. Probenecid and rifampicin serum levels. Lancet 1975; ii: 792–4.

Antimicrobial Action

Rifampicin is bactericidal against a wide range of micro-organisms and interferes with their synthesis of nucleic acids by inhibiting DNA-dependent RNA polymerase. It has the ability to kill intracellular organisms. It is active against mycobacteria, including *Mycobacterium tuberculosis* and *M. leprae* and, having high sterilising activity against these organisms, it possesses the ability to eliminate semi-dormant or persisting organisms. Rifampicin is active against Gram-positive bacteria, especially staphylococci, but less active against Gram-negative organisms. The most sensitive Gram-negative bacteria include *Neisseria meningitidis*, *N. gonorrhoeae*, *Haemophilus influenzae*, and *Legionella* spp. Rifampicin also has activity against *Chlamydia trachomatis* and some anaerobic bacteria. At high concentrations it is active against some viruses. Rifampicin has no effect on fungi but has been reported to enhance the antifungal activity of amphotericin B.

Minimum inhibitory concentrations tend to vary with the medium used; MICs for the most sensitive organisms (chlamydia, staphylococci) tend to range from about 0.01 to 0.02 µg per mL, while the MIC for most susceptible mycobacteria ranges from 0.1 to 2 µg per mL. The concomitant use of other antimicrobials may enhance or antagonise the bactericidal activity of rifampicin.

Strains of *Mycobacterium tuberculosis*, *M. leprae*, and other usually susceptible bacteria have demonstrated resistance, both initially and during treatment. Thus in tuberculosis and leprosy regimens, rifampicin is used in combination with other drugs to delay or prevent the development of rifampicin resistance. There does not appear to be cross-resistance apart from that between rifampicin and other rifamycins. However, there have been isolated reports of the emergence of multidrug-resistant strains of *M. leprae* (see below).

Multidrug resistance. Strains of *Mycobacterium leprae* with multiple resistance to rifampicin, ofloxacin, and dapsone have been isolated from patients who have previously received dapsone monotherapy followed by treatment with rifampicin in combination with ofloxacin.[1,2]

1. Cambau E, et al. Multidrug-resistance to dapsone, rifampicin, and ofloxacin in Mycobacterium leprae. Lancet 1997; 349: 103–4.
2. Ji B, et al. High relapse rate among lepromatous leprosy patients treated with rifampicin plus ofloxacin daily for 4 weeks. Antimicrob Agents Chemother 1997; 41: 1953–6.

Pharmacokinetics

Rifampicin is readily absorbed from the gastrointestinal tract and peak plasma concentrations of about 7 to 10 µg per mL have been reported 2 to 4 hours after a dose of 600 mg, although there may be considerable interindividual variation. Food may reduce and delay absorption. Rifampicin is approximately 80% bound to plasma proteins. It is widely distributed in body tissues and fluids and diffusion into the CSF is increased when the meninges are inflamed. Rifampicin crosses the placenta and is distributed into breast milk (see Pregnancy and Breast Feeding, under Precautions, above). Half-lives for rifampicin have been reported to range initially from 2 to 5 hours, the longest elimination times occurring after the largest doses. However, as rifampicin induces its own metabolism, elimination time may decrease by up to 40% during the first 2 weeks, resulting in half-lives of about 1 to 3 hours. The half-life is prolonged in patients with liver disease.

Rifampicin is rapidly metabolised in the liver mainly to active 25-*O*-deacetylrifampicin; rifampicin and deacetylrifampicin are excreted in the bile. Deacetylation diminishes intestinal reabsorption and increases faecal excretion, although significant enterohepatic circulation still takes place. About 60% of a dose eventually appears in the faeces. The amount excreted in the urine increases with increasing doses and up to 30% of a dose of 900 mg may be excreted in the urine, about half of it within 24 hours. The metabolite formylrifampicin is also excreted in the urine. In patients with impaired renal function the half-life of rifampicin is not prolonged at doses of 600 mg or less.

Distribution. Rifampicin is widely distributed in most body tissues and fluids following oral or intravenous administration.[1] Rifampicin is also able to penetrate into polymorphonuclear leucocytes to kill intracellular pathogens.[2] Rifampicin does not appear to diffuse well through the uninflamed meninges[3] but therapeutic concentrations have been attained in the CSF following daily doses of 600 and 900 mg when the meninges are inflamed;[4] concentrations in the CSF are about 10 to 20% of simultaneous serum concentrations, and approximately represent the fraction unbound to plasma proteins. Administration of corticosteroids does not appear to influence the penetration of rifampicin into the CSF of patients with tuberculous meningitis.[5]

1. Holdness MR. Clinical pharmacokinetics of the antituberculosis drugs. Clin Pharmacokinet 1984; 9: 511–44.
2. Prokesch RC, Hand WL. Antibiotic entry into human polymorphonuclear leukocytes. Antimicrob Agents Chemother 1982; 21: 373–80.
3. Sippel JE, et al. Rifampin concentrations in cerebrospinal fluid of patients with tuberculous meningitis. Am Rev Respir Dis 1974; 109: 579–80.
4. D'Oliveira JJG. Cerebrospinal fluid concentrations of rifampin in meningeal tuberculosis. Am Rev Respir Dis 1972; 106: 432–7.
5. Woo J, et al. Cerebrospinal fluid and serum levels of pyrazinamide and rifampicin in patients with tuberculous meningitis. Curr Ther Res 1987; 42: 235–42.

Intravenous administration. Mean peak plasma concentrations of 10 µg per mL have been reported following administration of 600 mg of rifampicin by intravenous infusion over 3 hours. Peak plasma concentrations declined with repeated administration but to a less marked extent than occurs with oral administration.[1] Mean peak plasma concentrations of 27 µg per mL have been attained in children following doses of 11.5 mg per kg body-weight infused over 30 minutes. Mean concentrations of 1.9 µg per mL were reported 8 hours after the dose.[2]

1. Acocella G, et al. Serum and urine concentrations of rifampicin administered by intravenous infusion in man. Arzneimittelforschung 1977; 27: 1221–6.
2. Koup JR, et al. Pharmacokinetics of rifampin in children I. Multiple dose intravenous infusion. Ther Drug Monit 1986; 8: 11–16.

Oral administration. Gastrointestinal absorption of rifampicin is considered good. However, analysis of serum-rifampicin concentrations in children indicated that only 50 ± 22% of a freshly prepared suspension was absorbed following oral administration.[1] Also varying oral bioavailability from capsule formulations has been reported and could result in ineffective therapy[2] or higher than needed serum concentrations.[3] The oral bioavailability of rifampicin and isoniazid, but not of pyrazinamide, was decreased by food in many patients.[4] Subtherapeutic plasma rifampicin concentrations have been reported in patients with HIV infection, possibly related to impaired absorption.[5-7]

1. Koup JR, et al. Pharmacokinetics of rifampin in children II. Oral bioavailability. Ther Drug Monit 1986; 8: 17–22.
2. Holdness MR. Clinical pharmacokinetics of the antituberculosis drugs. Clin Pharmacokinet 1984; 9: 511–44.
3. Ganiswarna SG, et al. Bioavailability of rifampicin caplets (600 mg and 450 mg) in healthy Indonesian subjects. Int J Clin Pharmacol Ther Toxicol 1986; 24: 60–4.
4. Zent C, Smith P. Study of the effect of concomitant food on the bioavailability of rifampicin, isoniazid and pyrazinamide. Tubercle Lung Dis 1995; 76: 109–13.
5. Patel KB, et al. Drug malabsorption and resistant tuberculosis in HIV-infected patients. N Engl J Med 1995; 332: 336–7.
6. Peloquin CA, et al. Low antituberculosis drug concentrations in patients with AIDS. Ann Pharmacother 1996; 30: 919–25.
7. Sahai J, et al. Reduced plasma concentrations of antituberculosis drugs in patients with HIV infection. Ann Intern Med 1997; 127: 289–93.

Uses and Administration

Rifampicin belongs to the rifamycin group of antimycobacterials (p.111) and is used in the treatment of various infections due to mycobacteria and other susceptible organisms (see Antimicrobial Action, above). It is usually given combined with other antibacterials to prevent the emergence of resistant organisms.

Rifampicin is used, notably in combination with isoniazid and pyrazinamide, as a component of multidrug regimens for the treatment of tuberculosis, and with dapsone and clofazimine in the treatment of leprosy. It is a component of various regimens for the treatment of opportunistic mycobacterial infections.

Other uses include brucellosis, chancroid, chlamydial infections, the treatment of staphylococcal endocarditis, penicillin-resistant pneumococcal meningitis, prophylaxis of epiglottitis due to *Haemophilus influenzae*, Legionnaires' disease, the prophylaxis of meningococcal and *H. influenzae* meningitis, mycetoma, the eradication of pharyngeal streptococcal carriage in pharyngitis, Q fever, and in various staphylococcal infections for treatment or prophylactically to reduce staphylococcal carriage. For discussions of all these infections and their treatment, see under Choice of Antibacterial, p.114.

The usual adult dose of rifampicin is 600 mg daily by mouth, preferably on an empty stomach, or by intravenous infusion as the base or the sodium salt; higher doses are sometimes employed (see below).

Rifampicin is used in the initial and continuation phases of short-course **tuberculosis** regimens (p.143) in combination with other antimycobacterials. Rifampicin is administered orally on an empty stomach in single daily doses of 10 mg per kg body-weight (maximum 600 mg) to children and adults or may be given intermittently two or three times weekly in doses of 10 or 15 mg per kg (maximum 900 mg) to children and adults. Alternatively doses may be expressed as follows: with daily administration, adults weighing less than 50 kg receive 450 mg and those over 50 kg receive 600 mg; with intermittent administration, adults receive 600 to 900 mg two or three times weekly. The maximum recommended dose is considered to be 900 mg because a greater incidence of adverse effects is associated with doses above 900 mg.

In **leprosy** regimens (p.126), rifampicin is usually given with dapsone for paucibacillary leprosy, and with dapsone and clofazimine for multibacillary leprosy. Rifampicin is given once monthly in a usual adult dose of 600 mg by mouth. Guidelines for monthly doses in low-body-weight adults and in children are rifampicin 450 mg for adults weighing less than 35 kg and children 10 to 14 years old. Low body-weight children may be given 12 to 15 mg per kg monthly. Single-dose treatment with rifampicin, ofloxacin, and minocycline may be an alternative in patients with single-lesion paucibacillary leprosy.

For **prophylaxis** against meningococcal meningitis and the treatment of meningococcal carriers, rifampicin is usually given in a dose of 600 mg twice daily by mouth for 2 days. Recommended doses for children in the UK are 10 mg per kg for children between 1 and 12 years of age and 5 mg per kg for children under 12 months each twice daily for 2 days; in the USA children aged 1 month or more are given 10 mg per kg and infants less then 1 month old are given 5 mg per kg, both twice daily for 2 days. For prophylaxis against meningitis due to *Haemophilus influenzae*, a dose of 600 mg daily by mouth for 4 days is given to adults. Recommended doses for children in the UK are 10 mg per kg once daily by mouth for 4 days for children aged 1 to 3 months, and 20 mg per kg once daily by mouth for 4 days for those aged over 3 months, with a maximum daily dose of 600 mg.

In the treatment of **brucellosis**, **Legionnaires' disease**, and serious **staphylococcal infections** a dose of 600 to 1200 mg daily in divided doses has been recommended in combination with other drugs.

Reduced doses are recommended for patients with impaired hepatic function and a maximum of 8 mg per kg daily has been suggested.

Administration in hepatic and renal impairment. See Precautions, above.

Ehrlichiosis. Beneficial responses to rifampicin have been reported[1] in 2 pregnant women with granulocytic ehrlichiosis (p.119), in whom the usual treatment with a tetracycline was contra-indicated.

1. Buitrago MI, et al. Human granulocytic ehrlichiosis during pregnancy treated successfully with rifampin. Clin Infect Dis 1998; 27: 213–15.

Meningitis prophylaxis. HAEMOPHILUS INFLUENZAE MENINGITIS PROPHYLAXIS. Meningeal infection with *Haemophilus influenzae* type b (Hib) in children is associated with substantial morbidity, but the incidence has decreased since the introduction of immunisation with *H. influenzae* type b vaccine. Although a world-wide problem, the disease and its prophylaxis has been studied mainly in the USA, where it has been shown that children under 4 years of age form the highest risk group for primary infection while children under 2 years of age form the highest risk group for secondary infection.[1] The goal of prophylaxis in close contacts is to eliminate carriage of the organism to prevent spread to young children. Risk of infection to young children with recent household contact to the primary case of infection with *Haemophilus influenzae* type b is increased 600- to 800-fold,[1,2] but only increased 20-fold[3] from day-care or school contact. The risk may be higher when more than 1 index patient is identified.

Rifampicin in doses of 20 mg per kg per day once daily for 4 days (maximum dose 600 mg) has been shown to eradicate Hib nasopharyngeal carriage in at least 95% of contacts of the primary case.[4] There is some evidence from a study involving 68 families of patients with Hib infection that rifampicin 20 mg per kg daily for 2 days may be as effective as a 4-day course in eradicating Hib pharyngeal colonisation.[5] Rifampicin prophylaxis appears to be successful in preventing infection in household contacts, but benefit in school settings where there has been a single index case has not been established.[3]

Various recommendations have been made for rifampicin prophylaxis. Administration of rifampicin to all persons, regardless of vaccine status, with close, recent (within 2 weeks) contact to the primary case and who are likely to be exposed to susceptible children has been endorsed by the American Academy of Pediatrics;[6] similar recommendations have been made in the UK.[2] Rifampicin should also be given to the primary case since treatment of the infection does not eradicate nasopharyngeal carriage.[2,6] Rifampicin prophylaxis following exposure through day-care or school contact may be given and has been endorsed by the American Centers for Disease Control.[7]

In the UK prophylaxis is recommended for all room contacts when 2 or more cases of *H. influenzae* disease have occurred in a playgroup or nursery within 120 days.[2]

Rifampicin prophylaxis is not recommended for pregnant women,[2,6] and in the UK prophylaxis is not recommended in breast-feeding mothers.[2]

Treatment of *H. influenzae* meningitis is discussed on p.128.

1. Casto DT, Edwards DL. Preventing Haemophilus influenzae type b disease. Clin Pharm 1985; 4: 637–48.
2. Cartwright KAV, et al. Chemoprophylaxis for Haemophilus influenzae type b: rifampicin should be given to close contacts. BMJ 1991; 302: 546–7.
3. ASHP Commission on Therapeutics. ASHP therapeutic guidelines on nonsurgical antimicrobial prophylaxis. Clin Pharm 1990; 9: 423–45.
4. Band JD, et al. Prevention of Hemophilus influenzae type b disease. JAMA 1984; 251: 2381–6.
5. Green M, et al. Duration of rifampin chemoprophylaxis for contacts of patients infected with Haemophilus influenzae type B. Antimicrob Agents Chemother 1992; 36: 545–7.
6. American Academy of Pediatrics. Revision of recommendation for use of rifampin prophylaxis of contacts of patients with Haemophilus influenzae infection. Pediatrics 1984; 74: 301–2.
7. Broome CV, et al. Use of chemoprophylaxis to prevent the spread of Hemophilus influenzae b in day-care facilities. N Engl J Med 1987; 36: 1226–8.

MENINGOCOCCAL MENINGITIS PROPHYLAXIS. *Neisseria meningitidis* is an important cause of bacterial meningitis; all age groups are at risk during epidemics but children are usually at highest risk during endemic outbreaks. Vaccines are available for meningococci groups A and C but not for group B, therefore antimicrobial prophylaxis remains important in preventing the spread of the disease. The aim of prophylaxis is to eliminate nasopharyngeal carriage of the organism. Sulfadiazine and minocycline are no longer used because of resistance and adverse effects. The current antibacterial of choice is rifampicin; rates of 70 to 90% have been reported for eradication of nasal carriage.[1] Alternative drugs are ceftriaxone and ciprofloxacin. Once a meningococcal infection occurs, the risk of infection in

household contacts increases 500- to 1200-fold.[2] Antibacterial prophylaxis should be given as soon as possible to household contacts and persons exposed to the patient's oral secretions (ideally within 24 hours of diagnosis of the index case). It is also recommended for child care or nursery school contacts in the USA,[1] but is not usually advised for this group in the UK following a single case.[2] The index patient should also receive rifampicin or other prophylaxis since treatment with penicillin does not necessarily eradicate nasopharyngeal carriage.

Treatment of meningococcal meningitis is discussed on p.128.

1. Committee on Infectious Diseases of the American Academy of Pediatrics, Infectious Diseases and Immunization Committee of the Canadian Pediatric Society. Meningococcal disease prevention and control strategies for practice-based physicians. Pediatrics 1996; 97: 404–11.
2. PHLS Meningococcal Infections Working Group and Public Health Medicine Environmental Group. Control of meningococcal disease: guidance for consultants in communicable disease control. Commun Dis Rep 1995; 5 (review 13): R189–R195.

Naegleria infections. For mention of the use of rifampicin in primary amoebic meningoencephalitis, see p.582.

Preparations

BP 2001: Rifampicin Capsules; Rifampicin Oral Suspension;
USP 25: Rifampin and Isoniazid Capsules; Rifampin Capsules; Rifampin for Injection; Rifampin Oral Suspension; Rifampin, Isoniazid, and Pyrazinamide Tablets; Rifampin, Isoniazid, Pyrazinamide, and Ethambutol Hydrochloride Tablets.

Proprietary Preparations (details are given in Part 3)
Aust.: Eremfat; Rifoldin; Rimactan; *Austral.:* Rifadin; Rimycin; *Belg.:* Rifadine; Rimactan†; *Braz.:* Rifaldin; *Canad.:* Rifadin; Rimactane†; Rofact; *Denm.:* Rimactan; *Fin.:* Rimapen; *Fr.:* Rifadine; Rimactan; *Ger.:* Eremfat; Rifa; Rimactan†; *Hong Kong:* Ricin; Rifadin; Rifasynt; Rimactane; *Irl.:* Rifadin; Rimactane; *Israel:* Rimactan; *Ital.:* Rifadin; Rifapiam; *Mex.:* Eurifam; Fampin; Finamicina; Pestarin; Ricilin; Rifadin; Rifamcilin; Rimactan; Simar; Turifarm; *Neth.:* Rifadin; Rimactan; *Norw.:* Rifadin†; Rimactan; *NZ:* Rifadin; *Port.:* Rifadin; Rifex; *S.Afr.:* Rifadin; Rifcin; Rimactane; *Singapore:* Rimactane; *Spain:* Rifagen; Rifaldin; Rifocina†; Rimactan; *Swed.:* Rifadin; Rimactan; *Switz.:* Rifoldine†; Rimactan; *Thai.:* Cinifa; Myrin; Myrin-P; Ramfin; Rampicin; Ricin; Rifadin; Rifagen; Rifam; Rifam-P; Rifano; Rifasynt; Rimactane; RP-Pose; Tibirim; *UK:* Rifadin; Rimactane; *USA:* Rimactane.

Multi-ingredient: *Aust.:* Rifater; Rifoldin INH; Rimactan + INH; *Canad.:* Rifater; *Fr.:* Rifater; Rifinah; *Ger.:* Iso-Eremfat; Rifater; Rifinah; Rifoga; Rimactazid; *Irl.:* Rifater; Rifinah; *Irl.:* Rifater; Rifinah; Rimactazid; *Ital.:* Rifanicozid†; Rifater; Rifinah; *Mex.:* Rifaprim; Rifater; Rifinah; *Neth.:* Rifinah; *NZ:* Rifinah; *Port.:* Rifater; Rifinah; Tuberen; *S.Afr.:* MB-Combi†; Myrin; Myrin Plus; Pyrifin†; Rifafour; Rifater; Rifinah; Rimactazid; Rimcure; *Singapore:* Rifater; Rifinah; Rimactazid; *Spain:* Rifater; Rifinah; Rimactazid; *Switz.:* Rifater; Rifinah; Rimactazide; Rimactazide + Z†; *Thai.:* Ricinis; Rifamiso; Rifater; Rifinah; Rimactazid; *UK:* Rifater; Rifinah; Rimactazid; *USA:* Rifamate; Rifater.

Rifamycin Sodium (146-s)

Rifamycin Sodium (BANM, rINNM).
M-14 (rifamycin); Rifamycin SV Sodium; Rifamycinum Natricum. Sodium (12Z,14E,24E)-(2S,16S,17S,18R,19R,20R,21S,22R, 23S)-21-acetoxy-1,2-dihydro-6,9,17,19-tetrahydroxy-23-methoxy-2,4,12,16,18,20,22-heptamethyl-1,11-dioxo-2,7-(epoxypentadeca-1,11,13-trienimino)-naphtho[2,1-b]furan-5-olate.
$C_{37}H_{46}NNaO_{12} = 719.8.$
$CAS — 6998-60-3$ (rifamycin); 14897-39-3; 15105-92-7 (both rifamycin sodium).
Pharmacopoeias. In Eur. (see p.vi) and Pol.

Pharmacopoeial description
Ph. Eur.: The monosodium salt of rifamycin SV, a substance obtained by chemical transformation of rifamycin B which is produced during growth of certain strains of *Amycolatopsis mediterranei*. Rifamycin SV may also be obtained directly from certain mutants of *A. mediterranei*. The potency is not less than 900 units per mg calculated with reference to the anhydrous substance. A red, fine or slightly granular powder. Soluble in water; freely soluble in dehydrated alcohol; practically insoluble in ether. A 5% solution in water has a pH of 6.5 to 8.0. Store in airtight containers at a temperature of 2° to 8°. Protect from light.

Adverse Effects and Precautions
Some gastrointestinal side-effects have occurred following injections of rifamycin. High doses may produce alterations in liver function. Hypersensitivity reactions including rashes, pruritus, and anaphylaxis have occurred rarely, but prolonged administration increases the risk of sensitisation. A reddish coloration of the urine has been reported. It should be used with care in patients with hepatic dysfunction.

Antimicrobial Action
Rifamycin has similar antimicrobial actions to those of rifampicin (p.245).

Pharmacokinetics
Rifamycin is not effectively absorbed from the gastrointestinal tract. Plasma concentrations of 2 μg per mL have been achieved 2 hours after a dose of 250 mg by intramuscular injection. The plasma half-life is reported to be about 1 hour.
It is excreted mainly in the bile and only small amounts appear in the urine.

Uses and Administration
Rifamycin is a rifamycin antibacterial that has been used in the treatment of infections caused by susceptible organisms such as staphylococci. It has been given as the sodium salt by intramuscular injection and by slow intravenous infusion and is also administered by local instillation and topical application.

Preparations
Proprietary Preparations (details are given in Part 3)
Aust.: Rifocin; *Belg.:* Rifocine; *Braz.:* Rifocina; *Fr.:* Otofa; Rifocine†; *Ital.:* Rifocin; *Mex.:* Rifocyna; *Port.:* Otofa; Rifocina; *Switz.:* Otofa.

Multi-ingredient: *Braz.:* Rifocort.

Rifapentine (16978-r)

Rifapentine (BAN, USAN, rINN).
DL-473; DL-473-IT; L-11473; MDL-473. 3-[N-(4-Cyclopentyl-1-piperazinyl)formimidoyl]rifamycin.
$C_{47}H_{64}N_4O_{12} = 877.0.$
$CAS — 61379-65-5.$

Adverse Effects
As for Rifampicin, p.243. A higher incidence of hyperuricaemia has been reported with rifapentine than with rifampicin.

Precautions
As for Rifampicin, p.244.
Rifapentine is teratogenic in *animals*.

Interactions
As for Rifampicin, p.244.

Antimicrobial Action
As for Rifampicin, p.245. Cross-resistance is common between rifapentine and rifampicin in *Mycobacterium tuberculosis*.

Antimycobacterial action. References.
1. Mor N, et al. Comparison of activities of rifapentine and rifampin against Mycobacterium tuberculosis residing in human macrophages. Antimicrob Agents Chemother 1995; 39: 2073–7.
2. Vernon A, et al. Acquired rifamycin monoresistance in patients with HIV-related tuberculosis treated with once-weekly rifapentine and isoniazid. Lancet 1999; 353: 1843–7.

Pharmacokinetics
Rifapentine is absorbed following oral administration. Absorption is enhanced when rifapentine is taken with food. Peak plasma concentrations are achieved 5 to 6 hours after a single dose of 600 mg and steady-state concentrations are achieved by day 10 during daily administration. A half-life of about 13 hours has been reported. Rifapentine does not appear to induce its own metabolism. Rifapentine and its active metabolite 25-deacetylrifapentine are 98% and 93% bound to plasma proteins, respectively.
Rifapentine and 25-deacetylrifapentine are excreted mainly in the faeces with a small amount appearing in the urine.

◊ References.
1. Keung ACF, et al. Pharmacokinetics of rifapentine in patients with varying degrees of hepatic dysfunction. J Clin Pharmacol 1998; 38: 517–24.
2. Keung AC-F, et al. Pharmacokinetics of rifapentine in subjects seropositive for the human immunodeficiency virus: a phase I study. Antimicrob Agents Chemother 1999; 43: 1230–3.
3. Conte JE, et al. Single-dose intrapulmonary pharmacokinetics of rifapentine in normal subjects. Antimicrob Agents Chemother 2000; 44: 985–90.

Uses and Administration
Rifapentine is a rifamycin antibacterial (see Rifampicin, p.243) that is used, in combination with other antimycobacterials, for the treatment of tuberculosis. It is under investigation for the prophylaxis of *Mycobacterium avium* complex infections in patients with AIDS.
Rifapentine is given by mouth in a dose of 600 mg twice weekly during the initial phase of short-course tuberculosis regimens, then once weekly during the continuation phase of treatment.

◊ Reviews.
1. Jarvis B, Lamb HM. Rifapentine. Drugs 1998; 56: 607–16.
2. Temple ME, Nahata MC. Rifapentine: its role in the treatment of tuberculosis. Ann Pharmacother 1999; 33: 1203–10.

Preparations
Proprietary Preparations (details are given in Part 3)
USA: Priftin.

Rifaximin (503-j)

Rifaximin (USAN, rINN).
L-105; Rifaxidin; Rifaximine. (2S,16Z,18E,20S,21S,22R,23R,24R, 25S,26S,27S,28E)-5,6,21,23,25-Pentahydroxy-27-methoxy-2,4,11,16,20,22,24,26-octamethyl-2,7-(epoxypentadeca[1,11,13]trienimino)benzofuro[4,5-e]pyrido[1,2-a]benzimidazole-1,15(2H)-dione 25-acetate.
$C_{43}H_{51}N_3O_{11} = 785.9.$
$CAS — 80621-81-4.$
$ATC — A07AA11; D06AX11.$
NOTE. The code L-105 has also been applied to the cephalosporin cefuzonam.

Profile
Rifaximin is a rifamycin antibacterial with antimicrobial actions similar to those of rifampicin (p.245), but which is poorly absorbed from the gastrointestinal tract. It has been given by mouth in the treatment of gastrointestinal infections, for surgical infection prophylaxis, and to reduce hyperammonaemia in hepatic encephalopathy (p.1205). Doses in adults have ranged from 10 to 15 mg per kg body-weight daily, or from 800 to 1200 mg daily, both in divided doses.

It has also been used topically as a 5% ointment.

◊ References.
1. Gillis JC, Brogden RN. Rifaximin: a review of its antibacterial activity, pharmacokinetic properties and therapeutic potential in conditions mediated by gastrointestinal bacteria. *Drugs* 1995; **49:** 467–84.

Preparations
Proprietary Preparations (details are given in Part 3)
Ital.: Dermodis†; Normix; Redactiv; Rifacol; *Mex.:* Redactiv.

Rokitamycin (2827-b)
Rokitamycin *(rINN)*.

M-19-Q; 3″-Propionyl-leucomycin A₅; Rikamycin; TMS-19Q. [(4R,5S,6S,7R,9R,10R,11E,13E,16R)-7-(Formylmethyl)-4,10-dihydroxy-5-methoxy-9,16-dimethyl-2-oxooxacyclohexadeca-11,13-dien-6-yl]-3,6-dideoxy-4-O-(2,6-dideoxy-3-C-methyl-α-L-ribo-hexopyranosyl)-3-(dimethylamino)-β-D-glucopyranoside 4″-butyrate 3″-propionate.
$C_{42}H_{69}NO_{15} = 828.0$.
CAS — 74014-51-0.
ATC — J01FA12.
Pharmacopoeias. In Jpn.

Profile
Rokitamycin is a macrolide antibiotic with actions and uses similar to those of erythromycin (p.201). It has been given by mouth in doses of 400 mg twice daily.

Preparations
Proprietary Preparations (details are given in Part 3)
Ital.: Paidocin; Rokital.

Rolitetracycline (149-I)
Rolitetracycline *(BAN, USAN, rINN)*.

PMT; Pyrrolidinomethyltetracycline; SQ-15659. N^2-(Pyrrolidin-1-ylmethyl)tetracycline.
$C_{27}H_{33}N_3O_8 = 527.6$.
CAS — 751-97-3.
ATC — J01AA09.
Pharmacopoeias. In It.

Rolitetracycline Nitrate (150-v)
Rolitetracycline Nitrate *(BANM, USAN, rINNM)*.

Pyrrolidinomethyltetracycline Nitrate Sesquihydrate.
$C_{27}H_{33}N_3O_8,HNO_3,1\frac{1}{2}H_2O = 617.6$.
CAS — 20685-78-3 (anhydrous rolitetracycline nitrate); 7681-32-5 (anhydrous rolitetracycline nitrate); 26657-13-6 (rolitetracycline nitrate sesquihydrate).

1.17 mg of rolitetracycline nitrate is approximately equivalent to 1 mg of rolitetracycline.

Stability. Rolitetracycline is unstable in the presence of water: aqueous solutions of the base or the nitrate are hydrolysed in solution to tetracycline,[1,2] more than 50% being so converted in 3 hours at 25° according to one report,[1] while 15% of a reconstituted injection of the base has been reported[2] to be lost in 21 to 25 hours when stored at 5°.
1. Hughes DW, *et al.* Stability of rolitetracycline in aqueous solution. *J Pharm Pharmacol* 1974; **26:** 79–80.
2. Wilson WL, *et al.* Chemical stability of reconstituted rolitetracycline formulations. *Can J Pharm Sci* 1976; **11:** 126–8.

Adverse Effects and Precautions
As for Tetracycline Hydrochloride, p.259.

Shivering, and more rarely rigor due to a Jarisch-Herxheimer reaction, may be associated with the first few injections of rolitetracycline in infections due to organisms highly sensitive to tetracyclines. Injections may be followed by a peculiar taste sensation, often similar to ether. Rapid intravenous injection may cause transient giddiness, hot flushes, reddening of the face and, occasionally, peripheral circulatory failure.

Symptoms of myasthenia gravis have been exacerbated by the intravenous administration of rolitetracycline, although it has been suggested that this may be due to magnesium ions in the formulation.

Interactions
As for Tetracycline Hydrochloride, p.259.

Antimicrobial Action
As for Tetracycline Hydrochloride, p.259.

Pharmacokinetics
As for Tetracycline Hydrochloride, p.260.

The symbol † denotes a preparation no longer actively marketed

---

Rolitetracycline is not absorbed from the gastrointestinal tract. When administered by injection about 50% of rolitetracycline in the circulation is bound to plasma proteins. Peak plasma concentrations have been reported about 0.5 to 1 hour after an intramuscular dose. The half-life has been reported to range from about 5 to 8 hours. About 50% of a dose is excreted in the urine.

Uses and Administration
Rolitetracycline is a tetracycline derivative with uses similar to those of tetracycline (p.260). It is included in some topical eye preparations. It has also been given by slow intravenous injection or by deep intramuscular injection.

Rolitetracycline citrate has also been used.

Preparations
Proprietary Preparations (details are given in Part 3)
Aust.: Reverin†; *Canad.:* Reverin†; *S.Afr.:* Reverin†.
Multi-ingredient: *Ital.:* Colbiocin; Eubetal Antibiotico; Iducol; Vitecaf.

Roxithromycin (680-p)
Roxithromycin *(USAN, rINN)*.

Roxithromycinum; RU-965; RU-28965. Erythromycin 9-{O-[(2-methoxyethoxy)methyl]oxime}.
$C_{41}H_{76}N_2O_{15} = 837.0$.
CAS — 80214-83-1.
ATC — J01FA06.
Pharmacopoeias. In Eur. (see p.vi) and Jpn.

Pharmacopoeial description
Ph. Eur.: A white crystalline powder. It exhibits polymorphism. Very slightly soluble in water; freely soluble in alcohol, in acetone, and in dichloromethane; slightly soluble in dilute hydrochloric acid. Store in airtight containers.

Adverse Effects and Precautions
As for Erythromycin, p.201. Gastrointestinal disturbances are the most frequent adverse effect, but are less frequent than with erythromycin. Increases in liver enzyme values and hepatitis have been reported. Rashes and other hypersensitivity reactions, headache, dizziness, weakness, and changes in blood cell counts have also occurred.

Effects on the pancreas. Acute pancreatitis, with duodenal inflammation, pain, pancreatic enlargement and raised serum-amylase developed within 24 hours of substitution of roxithromycin for erythromycin ethyl succinate in a patient being treated for respiratory-tract infection.[1] Symptoms resolved rapidly once roxithromycin was withdrawn.
1. Souweine B, *et al.* Acute pancreatitis associated with roxithromycin therapy. *DICP Ann Pharmacother* 1991; **25:** 1137.

Eosinophilia. For a report of an eosinophilic syndrome in a patient following treatment with azithromycin or roxithromycin, see Azithromycin, p.153.

Interactions
For a discussion of drug interactions of macrolide antibacterials, see Erythromycin, p.202.

Antimicrobial Action
As for Erythromycin, p.203. It is reported to be as active or slightly less active than erythromycin.

Pharmacokinetics
Following oral administration roxithromycin is absorbed, with a bioavailability of about 50%. Peak plasma concentrations of about 6 to 8 μg per mL occur around 2 hours after a single dose of 150 mg. The mean peak plasma concentration at steady state after a dose of 150 mg twice daily is 9.3 μg per mL. Absorption is reduced when taken after, but not before, a meal. It is widely distributed in tissues and body fluids. It is reported to be about 96% bound to plasma protein (mainly α₁-acid glycoprotein) at trough concentrations, but binding is saturable, and only about 86% is bound at usual peak concentrations. Small amounts of roxithromycin are metabolised in the liver, and the majority of a dose is excreted in the faeces as unchanged drug and metabolites; about 7 to 12% is excreted in urine, and up to 15% via the lungs. The elimination half-life is reported to range between about 8 and 13 hours, but may be more prolonged in patients with impaired hepatic or renal function and in children.

◊ References.
1. Puri SK, Lassman HB. Roxithromycin: a pharmacokinetic review of a macrolide. *J Antimicrob Chemother* 1987; **20** (suppl B): 89–100.
2. Periti P, *et al.* Clinical pharmacokinetic properties of the macrolide antibiotics: effects of age and various pathophysiological states (part I). *Clin Pharmacokinet* 1989; **16:** 261–82.

Uses and Administration
Roxithromycin is a macrolide antibiotic with actions and uses similar to those of erythromycin (p.203). It is given by mouth to adults in a dose of 150 mg twice daily or sometimes 300 mg once daily, before meals, in the treatment of susceptible infections. In children of up to 40 kg body-weight a dose of 5 to 8 mg per kg daily may be used.

◊ References.
1. Williams JD, Sefton AM. Comparison of macrolide antibiotics. *J Antimicrob Chemother* 1993; **31** (suppl C): 11–26.

---

2. Markham A, Faulds D. Roxithromycin: an update of its antimicrobial activity, pharmacokinetic properties and therapeutic use. *Drugs* 1994; **48:** 297–326.
3. Young LS, Lode H, eds. Roxithromycin: first of a new generation of macrolides: update and perspectives. *Infection* 1995; **23** (suppl 1): S1–S52.
4. Lovering AM, *et al.*, eds. Roxithromycin—additional therapeutic potential. *J Antimicrob Chemother* 1998; **41** (suppl B): 1–97.

Preparations
Proprietary Preparations (details are given in Part 3)
Aust.: Rulide; *Austral.:* Biaxin†; Biaxsig; Rulide; *Belg.:* Claramid; Rulid; *Braz.:* Rulid; *Denm.:* Forilin; Surlid; *Fin.:* Roxibion; Surlid; *Fr.:* Claramid; Rulid; *Ger.:* Rulid; *Hong Kong:* Rulid; *Israel:* Rulid; *Ital.:* Assoral; Overal; Rossitrol; Rulid; *Mex.:* Roxitrol; Rulid; Surlid; *Neth.:* Rulide; *NZ:* Rulide; *Port.:* Rulide; *S.Afr.:* Rulide; *Singapore:* Rulid; *Spain:* Macrosil; Rotesan; Rotramin; Rulide; *Swed.:* Surlid; Rulide; *Switz.:* Rulid; *Thai.:* Eroxade; Poliroxin; Rothricin; Roxcin; Roxicin; Roxilan; Roximin; Roxitin; Roxlecon; Roxomycin; Roxthomed; Roxthrin; Roxto; Roxtrocin; Rucin; Rulid; Uonin.

Rufloxacin (3763-I)
Rufloxacin *(BAN, rINN)*.

MF-934. 9-Fluoro-2,3-dihydro-10-[4-methylpiperazin-1-yl]-7-oxo-7H-pyrido[1,2,3-de]-1,4-benzothiazine-6-carboxylic acid.
$C_{17}H_{18}FN_3O_3S = 363.4$.
CAS — 101363-10-4.
ATC — J01MA10.

Profile
Rufloxacin is a fluoroquinolone antibacterial with properties similar to those of ciprofloxacin (p.182). It is given by mouth as the hydrochloride in the treatment of susceptible infections in an initial dose of 400 mg followed by 200 mg daily. A plasma half-life of 30 hours or more has been reported.

Preparations
Proprietary Preparations (details are given in Part 3)
Ital.: Monos; Qari; Tebraxin.

Sarafloxacin Hydrochloride (2999-n)
Sarafloxacin Hydrochloride *(BANM, USAN, rINN)*.

A-57135 (sarafloxacin); A-56620 (sarafloxacin or sarafloxacin hydrochloride); Abbott-56620 (sarafloxacin or sarafloxacin hydrochloride).
$C_{20}H_{17}F_2N_3O_3,HCl = 421.8$.
CAS — 98105-99-8 (sarafloxacin); 91296-87-6 (sarafloxacin hydrochloride).

Profile
Sarafloxacin is a fluoroquinolone antibacterial used as the hydrochloride in veterinary medicine.

Sisomicin Sulfate (152-q)
Sisomicin Sulfate *(USAN, rINN)*.

Antibiotic 6640 (sisomicin); Rickamicin Sulphate; Sch-13475 (sisomicin); Sisomicin Sulphate *(BANM)*; Sissomicin Sulphate. 4-O-[(2R,3R)-cis-3-Amino-6-aminomethyl-3,4-dihydro-2H-pyran-2-yl]-2-deoxy-6-O-(3-deoxy-4-C-methyl-3-methylamino-β-L-arabinopyranosyl)streptamine sulphate; 2-Deoxy-6-O-(3-deoxy-4-C-methyl-3-methylamino-β-L-arabinopyranosyl)-4-O-(2,6-diamino-2,3,4,6-tetradeoxy-D-glycero-hex-4-enopyranosyl)streptamine sulphate.
$(C_{19}H_{37}N_5O_7)_2,5H_2SO_4 = 1385.4$.
CAS — 32385-11-8 (sisomicin); 53179-09-2 (sisomicin sulfate).
Pharmacopoeias. In Jpn and US.

Sisomicin is an antibiotic produced by *Micromonospora inyoensis* and closely related to gentamicin C_{1A}. 1.5 g of monograph substance is approximately equivalent to 1 g of sisomicin.

Pharmacopoeial description
USP 25: It loses not more than 15% of its weight on drying. 1 mg of monograph substance has a potency equivalent to not less than 580 μg of sisomicin calculated on the dried basis. A 4% solution in water of sisomicin has a pH of 3.5 to 5.5. Store in airtight containers.

Profile
Sisomicin is an aminoglycoside with general properties similar to those of gentamicin (p.210). It is given as the sulfate and the usual dose for adults is the equivalent of 3 mg of sisomicin per kg body-weight daily given intramuscularly in 2 or 3 divided doses. Sisomicin may be given by intravenous infusion if necessary.

Preparations
USP 25: Sisomicin Sulfate Injection.

Proprietary Preparations (details are given in Part 3)
Ital.: Mensiso; *Spain:* Sisomina†.

Sparfloxacin (9355-r)

Sparfloxacin (BAN, USAN, rINN).

AT-4140; CI-978. 5-Amino-1-cyclopropyl-7-(cis-3,5-dimethyl-piperazin-1-yl)-6,8-difluoro-1,4-dihydro-4-oxoquinoline-3-car-boxylic acid.

$C_{19}H_{22}F_2N_4O_3 = 392.4$.

CAS — 110871-86-8.

ATC — J01MA09.

Adverse Effects and Precautions

As for Ciprofloxacin, p.183.

Concern over phototoxicity associated with sparfloxacin has led to restriction of its use in some countries; patients should be advised to avoid exposure to sunlight during, and for a few days after, sparfloxacin therapy, and to discontinue the drug immediately if phototoxicity occurs.

Sparfloxacin may prolong the QT interval and various cardiac arrhythmias have been reported.

Photosensitivity. In a survey[1] of the reporting rate for phototoxicity associated with sparfloxacin in France, there were 371 reports to either the manufacturer or to the French Pharmacovigilance System of severe phototoxic reactions during the first 9 months following marketing of the drug; this approximated to between 4 and 25 times the rate reported for other fluoroquinolones.

1. Pierfitte C, et al. The link between sunshine and phototoxicity of sparfloxacin. Br J Clin Pharmacol 2000; 49: 609–12.

Interactions

As for Ciprofloxacin, p.184.

As sparfloxacin may prolong the QT interval it should not be used with other drugs known to have this effect (such as the antihistamines astemizole and terfenadine, cisapride, erythromycin, pentamidine, phenothiazines, or tricyclic antidepressants).

Sparfloxacin does not appear to interact with theophylline or caffeine, nor with warfarin or cimetidine. Probenecid does not alter the pharmacokinetics of sparfloxacin.

Antimicrobial Action

As for Ciprofloxacin, p.184.

Sparfloxacin is reported to be more active in vitro than ciprofloxacin against mycobacteria and against Gram-positive bacteria, including Streptococcus pneumoniae and other streptococci and staphylococci.

◊ References.

1. Richard MP, et al. Sensitivity to sparfloxacin and other antibiotics, of Streptococcus pneumoniae, Haemophilus influenzae and Moraxella catarrhalis strains isolated from adult patients with community-acquired lower respiratory tract infections: a European multicentre study. J Antimicrob Chemother 1998; 41: 207–14.

Pharmacokinetics

Sparfloxacin is well absorbed from the gastrointestinal tract following oral administration with a reported bioavailability of about 90%. Peak plasma concentrations are achieved 3 to 6 hours after a dose. Sparfloxacin is widely distributed into body tissues and fluids, including respiratory tissues, but is only about 45% bound to plasma proteins. It is metabolised in the liver by glucuronidation and has an elimination half-life of about 20 hours. It is excreted in equal amounts in the faeces and urine as unchanged drug and as the glucuronide metabolite.

◊ References.

1. Shimada J, et al. Clinical pharmacokinetics of sparfloxacin. Clin Pharmacokinet 1993; 25: 358–69.
2. Fillastre JP, et al. Pharmacokinetics of sparfloxacin in patients with renal impairment. Antimicrob Agents Chemother 1994; 38: 733–7.
3. Trautmann M, et al. Pharmacokinetics of sparfloxacin and serum bactericidal activity against pneumococci. Antimicrob Agents Chemother 1996; 40: 776–9.

Uses and Administration

Sparfloxacin is a fluoroquinolone antibacterial with actions similar to those of ciprofloxacin (p.185). It is used for the treatment of community-acquired pneumonia and acute bacterial exacerbations of chronic bronchitis including those caused by pneumococci. The usual dose by mouth is 400 mg initially followed by 200 mg daily.

Doses should be reduced in patients with renal impairment; 200 mg may be given on alternate days for maintenance.

◊ General references.

1. Finch RG, et al., eds. Sparfloxacin: focus on clinical performance. J Antimicrob Chemother 1996; 37 (suppl A): 1–167.
2. Goa KL, et al. Sparfloxacin: a review of its antibacterial activity, pharmacokinetic properties, clinical efficacy and tolerability in lower respiratory tract infections. Drugs 1997; 53: 700–25.
3. Martin SJ, et al. Levofloxacin and sparfloxacin: new quinolone antibiotics. Ann Pharmacother 1998; 32: 320–36.

Preparations

Proprietary Preparations (details are given in Part 3)

Fr.: Zagam†; Ger.: Zagam; Hong Kong: Zagam; Jpn: Spara; NZ: Zagam; S.Afr.: Zagam; Switz.: Zagam†; Thai.: Zagam; USA: Zagam.

Spectinomycin (155-w)

Spectinomycin (BAN, rINN).

Actinospectacin. Perhydro-4a,7,9-trihydroxy-2-methyl-6,8-bis(methylamino)pyrano[2,3-b][1,4]benzodioxin-4-one.

$C_{14}H_{24}N_2O_7 = 332.3$.

CAS — 1695-77-8.

ATC — J01XX04.

An antimicrobial substance produced by the growth of Streptomyces spectabilis or by any other means.

Spectinomycin Hydrochloride (157-l)

Spectinomycin Hydrochloride (BANM, USAN, rINNM).

M-141; Spectinomycini Hydrochloridum; U-18409AE. Spectinomycin dihydrochloride pentahydrate.

$C_{14}H_{24}N_2O_7,2HCl,5H_2O = 495.3$.

CAS — 21736-83-4 (anhydrous spectinomycin hydrochloride); 22189-32-8 (spectinomycin hydrochloride pentahydrate).

Pharmacopoeias. In Eur. (see p.vi), Int., and US.

1.5 g of monograph substance is approximately equivalent to 1 g of spectinomycin.

Pharmacopoeial description

Ph. Eur.: A white or almost white, slightly hygroscopic, powder. Freely soluble in water; very slightly soluble in alcohol; practically insoluble in ether. A 10% solution in water has a pH of 3.8 to 5.6. Store at a temperature not exceeding 30° in airtight containers.

USP 25: A white to pale buff crystalline powder. 1 mg of monograph substance has a potency equivalent to not less than 603 µg of spectinomycin. Freely soluble in water; practically insoluble in alcohol, in chloroform, and in ether. A 1% solution in water has a pH of 3.8 to 5.6. Store in airtight containers.

Adverse Effects and Precautions

Nausea, headache, dizziness, fever and chills, insomnia, and urticaria have occasionally occurred with single doses of spectinomycin. Anaphylaxis has occurred rarely. Mild to moderate pain has been reported following intramuscular injections. Alterations in kidney and liver function and a decrease in haemoglobin and haematocrit have occasionally been observed with repeated doses. Although a reduction in urine output has occasionally been seen after single and multiple dose administration, spectinomycin has not been observed to produce functional changes indicative of nephrotoxicity.

Spectinomycin is ineffective in the treatment of syphilis and patients being treated for gonorrhoea should be observed for evidence of syphilis.

Interactions

Lithium. For the effect of spectinomycin on lithium, see Antimicrobials, under Interactions of Lithium, p.295.

Antimicrobial Action

Spectinomycin is an aminocyclitol antibiotic that acts by binding to the 30S subunit of the bacterial ribosome and inhibiting protein synthesis. Its activity is generally modest, particularly against Gram-positive organisms. Anaerobic organisms are mostly resistant. Various Gram-negative organisms are sensitive, including many enterobacteria and also Haemophilus ducreyi, and it is particularly effective against Neisseria gonorrhoeae. Although generally bacteriostatic, spectinomycin is bactericidal against susceptible gonococci at concentrations not much above the MIC. Most strains of N. gonorrhoeae are inhibited by concentrations in the range 2 to 20 µg per mL.

Resistance may develop by chromosomal mutation or may be plasmid-mediated in some organisms; resistant gonococci have been reported clinically, notably in the Far East, but in most parts of the world resistant neisserial strains have been uncommon to date.

Pharmacokinetics

Spectinomycin is poorly absorbed by mouth but is rapidly absorbed following the intramuscular injection of the hydrochloride. A 2-g dose produces peak plasma concentrations of about 100 µg per mL at 1 hour while a 4-g dose produces peak concentrations of about 160 µg per mL at 2 hours. Therapeutic plasma concentrations are maintained for up to 8 hours. Distribution into saliva is poor (which limits its value in pharyngeal gonorrhoea). It is poorly bound to plasma proteins. Spectinomycin is excreted in an active form in the urine and up to 100% of a dose has been recovered within 48 hours. A half-life of about 1 to 3 hours has been reported. The half-life is prolonged in patients with impaired renal function. Spectinomycin is partially removed by dialysis.

Uses and Administration

Spectinomycin is used as an alternative to cephalosporins or fluoroquinolones in the treatment of gonorrhoea (p.124) although poor distribution into saliva limits its usefulness in pharyngeal infections. It has also been used in the treatment of chancroid (p.117).

Spectinomycin is administered as the hydrochloride but doses are calculated in terms of the base. In the treatment of gonorrhoea it is given by deep intramuscular injection as a single dose equivalent to 2 g of spectinomycin, although a dose of 4 g may sometimes be required divided between two injection sites. Multiple-dose courses have been used for the treatment of disseminated infections.

Spectinomycin is not effective against syphilis or chlamydial infections and additional therapy for these infections may be given concomitantly.

Doses equivalent to spectinomycin 40 mg per kg body-weight have been administered to children.

Preparations

BP 2001: Spectinomycin Injection;

USP 25: Spectinomycin for Injectable Suspension.

Proprietary Preparations (details are given in Part 3)

Aust.: Trobicin; Austral.: Trobicin; Belg.: Trobicin; Braz.: Trobicin; Canad.: Trobicin†; Fr.: Trobicine; Ger.: Stanilo; Hong Kong: Kirin; Trobicin; Irl.: Trobicin†; Israel: Togamycin; Ital.: Trobicin; Mex.: Trobicin; Port.: Trobicin; S.Afr.: Trobicin; Singapore: Trobicin; Spain: Kempi; Swed.: Trobicin†; Switz.: Trobicin; Thai.: Trobicin; Vabicin; UK: Trobicin†; USA: Trobicin.

Spiramycin (158-y)

Spiramycin (BAN, USAN, rINN).

Espiramicina; IL-5902; NSC-55926; NSC-64393 (spiramycin hydrochloride); RP-5337; Spiramycinum. A mixture comprised principally of (4R,5S,6S,7R,9R,10R,16R)-(11E,13E)-6-[(O-2,6-dideoxy-3-C-methyl-α-L-ribo-hexopyranosyl)-(1→4)-(3,6-dideoxy-3-dimethylamino-β-D-glucopyranosyl)oxy]-7-formylmethyl-4-hydroxy-5-methoxy-9,16-dimethyl-10-[(2,3,4,6-tetradeoxy-4-dimethylamino-D-erythro-hexopyranosyl)oxy]oxacyclohexadeca-11,13-dien-2-one (Spiramycin I).

$C_{43}H_{74}N_2O_{14} = 843.1$.

CAS — 8025-81-8.

ATC — J01FA02.

Pharmacopoeias. In Eur. (see p.vi). Jpn includes Acetylspiramycin.

Pharmacopoeial description

Ph. Eur.: A macrolide antibiotic produced by the growth of certain strains of Streptomyces ambofaciens or obtained by any other means.

A white or slightly yellowish, slightly hygroscopic powder. The potency is not less than 3900 units per mg, calculated with reference to the dried substance. Slightly soluble in water; freely soluble in alcohol, in acetone, and in methyl alcohol; sparingly soluble in ether. A 0.5% solution in methyl alcohol and water has a pH of 8.5 to 10.5. Store in airtight containers.

Units

3200 units of spiramycin are contained in 1 mg of the first International Reference Preparation (1962).

Adverse Effects and Precautions

As for Erythromycin, p.201. The most frequent adverse effects are gastrointestinal disturbances. Skin hypersensitivity reactions have also occurred. Transient paraesthesia has been reported during parenteral administration.

Interactions

For a discussion of drug interactions of macrolide antibacterials, see Erythromycin, p.202.

◊ As discussed under Interactions of Erythromycin (Mechanism, p.202), spiramycin is reported to have little or no effect on hepatic cytochrome P450 isoenzymes and may therefore produce fewer interactions than erythromycin with other drugs metabolised by this enzyme system. The lack of interactions between spiramycin and theophylline (p.780) and ciclosporin (p.520) would appear to support this. Nevertheless, a report of torsade de pointes in a patient with a congenital long QT syndrome during treatment with spiramycin and *mequitazine*[1] suggests that caution is still needed.

Reduced plasma concentrations of *levodopa* have been reported during concurrent administration of spiramycin (see p.1171).

1. Verdun F, *et al.* Torsades de pointes sous traitement par spiramycine et méquitazine: à propos d'un cas. *Arch Mal Coeur Vaiss* 1997; **90:** 103–6.

Antimicrobial Action

As for Erythromycin, p.203, although it is somewhat less active *in vitro* against many species. It is active against *Toxoplasma gondii.*

Pharmacokinetics

Spiramycin is incompletely absorbed from the gastrointestinal tract and is widely distributed in the tissues. A dose of 6 million units produces peak blood concentrations of 3.3 µg per mL after 1.5 to 3 hours; concentrations fall with a half-life of about 8 hours. High tissue concentrations are achieved and persist long after the plasma concentration has fallen to low levels, but it does not diffuse into the CSF to an appreciable extent.

Spiramycin is metabolised in the liver to active metabolites; substantial amounts are excreted in the bile and about 10% in the urine. It is distributed into breast milk.

Uses and Administration

Spiramycin is a macrolide antibiotic that has been used similarly to erythromycin (p.203) in the treatment of susceptible bacterial infections. It has also been used in the protozoal infections cryptosporidiosis (p.583) and toxoplasmosis (p.585).

Spiramycin is given by mouth as the base or rectally or intravenously as the adipate. The usual adult dose is 6 to 9 million units by mouth daily, in 2 or 3 divided doses. Doses of up to 15 million units have been given daily in divided doses for severe infections. Doses of about 1.5 million units of spiramycin may be given by slow intravenous infusion every 8 hours; in severe infection the dose may be doubled. Children may be given 150 000 to 300 000 units per kg body-weight daily in divided doses by mouth.

Acetylspiramycin is also used.

◊ Reviews.
1. Rubinstein E, Keller N. Spiramycin renaissance. *J Antimicrob Chemother* 1998; **42:** 572–6.

Preparations

Proprietary Preparations (details are given in Part 3)
Aust.: Rovamycin; *Belg.:* Rovamycine; *Braz.:* Rovamicina; *Canad.:* Rovamycine; *Denm.:* Rovamycin; Spiravet†; *Fr.:* Rovamycine; *Ger.:* Rovamycine; Selectomycin; *Hong Kong:* Rovamycine; *Israel:* Rovamycine; *Ital.:* Rovamicina; *Mex.:* Provamicina; *Neth.:* Rovamycine; *Norw.:* Rovamycine; *Port.:* Rovamycine; *Singapore:* Rovamycine; *Spain:* Dicorvin; Rovamycine; *Swed.:* Rovamycin†; *Switz.:* Rovamycine; *Thai.:* Rovamycin.

Multi-ingredient: *Braz.:* Periodontil; *Fr.:* Birodogyl; Rodogyl; *Spain:* Rhodogil.

Streptomycin   (160-q)

Streptomycin (BAN, rINN).

Estreptomicina. *O*-2-Deoxy-2-methylamino-α-L-glucopyranosyl-(1→2)-*O*-5-deoxy-3-*C*-formyl-α-L-lyxofuranosyl-(1→4)-N^3,N^3-diamidino-D-streptamine.
$C_{21}H_{39}N_7O_{12} = 581.6$.
CAS — 57-92-1.
ATC — A07AA04; J01GA01.

An antimicrobial organic base produced by the growth of certain strains of *Streptomyces griseus,* or by any other means.

Streptomycin Hydrochloride   (162-s)

Streptomycin Hydrochloride (BANM, rINNM).
$C_{21}H_{39}N_7O_{12}$,3HCl = 691.0.
CAS — 6160-32-3.

1.19 g of monograph substance is approximately equivalent to 1 g of streptomycin.

Streptomycin Sulfate   (163-w)

Streptomycin Sulfate (rINNM).
Streptomycin Sesquisulphate; Streptomycin Sulphate (BANM); Streptomycini Sulfas.
$(C_{21}H_{39}N_7O_{12})_2$,3$H_2SO_4$ = 1457.4.
CAS — 3810-74-0.
Pharmacopoeias. In Chin., Eur. (see p.vi), *Int., Jpn, Pol.,* and *US.*

1.25 g of monograph substance is approximately equivalent to 1 g of streptomycin.

Incompatible with acids and alkalis.

Pharmacopoeial description

Ph. Eur.: A white or almost white, hygroscopic powder. The potency is not less than 720 units per mg, calculated with reference to the dried substance. Very soluble in water; practically insoluble in dehydrated alcohol and in ether. A 25% solution in water has a pH of 4.5 to 7.0. Store in airtight containers.

USP 25: A white or practically white, hygroscopic powder; odourless or with not more than a faint odour. It has a potency equivalent to not less than 650 µg and not more than 850 µg of streptomycin per mg. Freely soluble in water; very slightly soluble in alcohol; practically insoluble in chloroform. A solution in water containing the equivalent of streptomycin 20% has a pH of 4.5 to 7.0. Store in airtight containers.

◊ CAUTION. *Streptomycin may cause severe dermatitis in sensitised persons, and pharmacists, nurses, and others who handle the drug frequently should wear masks and rubber gloves.*

Adverse Effects, Treatment, and Precautions

As for Gentamicin Sulfate, p.210. Like gentamicin the ototoxic effects of streptomycin are manifested mainly on vestibular rather than auditory function. Ototoxicity has been observed in infants whose mothers had been given streptomycin during pregnancy. However, streptomycin is reported to be somewhat less nephrotoxic than the other aminoglycosides.

Paraesthesia in and around the mouth is not uncommon after intramuscular injection of streptomycin, and other neurological symptoms, including peripheral neuropathies, optic neuritis, and scotoma have occasionally occurred. Intrathecal administration has resulted in symptoms of meningeal inflammation including radiculitis, arachnoiditis, nerve root pain, and paraplegia, and some authorities recommend that such administration be avoided.

Hypersensitivity skin reactions are reported in about 5% of patients, and eosinophilia may occur. There have been reports of severe exfoliative dermatitis and anaphylaxis. Sensitisation is common among those who handle streptomycin occupationally. Topical and inhalational use of streptomycin should be avoided. If necessary, hypersensitivity can usually be overcome by desensitisation. Aplastic anaemia and agranulocytosis have been reported rarely.

Although sources differ, it is usually suggested that peak plasma concentrations greater than about 15 to 40 µg per mL, and trough concentrations greater than 3 to 5 µg per mL should be avoided; in the UK it has been suggested that trough concentrations in excess of 1 µg per mL should be avoided in elderly patients. A total cumulative dose in excess of 100 g may be associated with a higher incidence of adverse effects.

Interactions

As for Gentamicin Sulfate, p.211.

Antimicrobial Action

Streptomycin has a mode of action and antimicrobial spectrum similar to that of gentamicin (p.211), although most strains of *Pseudomonas aeruginosa* are resistant. It is effective against *Yersinia pestis, Francisella tularensis,* and *Brucella* spp. Streptomycin has particular activity against *Mycobacterium tuberculosis.*

The MIC of streptomycin for most susceptible organisms is in the range of 1 to 8 µg per mL. Resistance has commonly been reported in many of the species normally sensitive to streptomycin, and may develop in strains which are initially sensitive within a few days or weeks of beginning therapy. The widespread emergence of resistance has largely put paid to its use in infections due to the common Gram-negative aerobes. Primary resistance in *M. tuberculosis* is relatively uncommon in the UK and USA but may be seen in a third or more of cases in the Far East.

Both low-level and high-level resistance have been reported; the latter is thought to be due to mutation of the ribosomal binding site of the antibiotic and cannot be overcome by the synergistic use of another drug such as a beta lactam, whereas strains with moderate

resistance due to decreased uptake or permeability of streptomycin may respond to combined use.

Organisms resistant to framycetin, kanamycin, neomycin, and paromomycin usually show cross-resistance to streptomycin, although streptomycin-resistant strains sometimes respond to one of these drugs.

◊ References.
1. Cooksey RC, *et al.* Characterization of streptomycin resistance mechanisms among Mycobacterium tuberculosis isolates from patients in New York City. *Antimicrob Agents Chemother* 1996; **40:** 1186–8.
2. Ho YII, *et al.* In-vitro activities of aminoglycoside-aminocyclitols against mycobacteria. *J Antimicrob Chemother* 1997; **40:** 27–32.

Pharmacokinetics

As for Gentamicin Sulfate, p.211. After intramuscular injection of streptomycin, maximum concentration in the blood is reached in 0.5 to 2 hours but the time taken and the concentration attained, which may be as high as about 50 µg per mL after a dose of 1 g, vary considerably. The half-life of streptomycin is about 2.5 hours. About one-third of streptomycin in the circulation is bound to plasma proteins. It is rapidly excreted by glomerular filtration and the concentration of streptomycin in the urine is often very high, with about 30 to 90% of a dose usually being excreted within 24 hours.

Uses and Administration

Streptomycin is an aminoglycoside antibacterial mainly used as a first-line drug in the treatment of tuberculosis in conjunction with other antimycobacterials. It is given during the initial phase of treatment unless the risk of drug resistance is small. Streptomycin has been used as an alternative to gentamicin in combination with a penicillin in the treatment of bacterial endocarditis. Streptomycin is effective in the treatment of plague, tularaemia, and, in conjunction with a tetracycline, in brucellosis. It has also been used, in combination with other drugs, in various other infections including mycetoma and Whipple's disease. For details of these infections and their treatment, see under Choice of Antibacterial, p.114.

Streptomycin is mostly used as the sulfate but doses are expressed in terms of the base. It is given by intramuscular injection.

In the treatment of tuberculosis, streptomycin is given during the initial phase of short-course regimens in usual adult doses of 15 mg per kg body-weight daily, up to a maximum of 1 g daily. A reduction in the maximum dose to 500 to 750 mg in adults aged over 40 years, and in those weighing less than 50 kg, has been suggested. Streptomycin may also be given as part of an intermittent regimen 2 or 3 times weekly. It has been given by the intrathecal route, together with intramuscular administration, for tuberculous meningitis, but this is no longer recommended.

Children with tuberculosis may also be given streptomycin 15 to 20 mg per kg daily (to a maximum of 1 g daily).

In the treatment of non-tuberculous infections, streptomycin has been given in usual adult doses of 1 to 2 g daily in divided doses, depending on the susceptibility and severity of infection; children may be given up to 40 mg per kg daily (maximum 1 g daily), usually in divided doses.

The course of treatment (other than in tuberculosis) should usually be limited to 7 to 14 days, and peak plasma concentrations greater than 15 to 40 µg per mL and trough concentrations greater than 3 to 5 µg per mL should be avoided. In all patients dosage should preferably be adjusted according to plasma-streptomycin concentrations, and particularly where factors such as age, renal impairment, or prolonged therapy may predispose to toxicity. For discussion of the methods used to calculate aminoglycoside dosage requirements, see under Gentamicin Sulfate, p.212.

Streptomycin has also been used as the hydrochloride, the pantothenate, and as a complex with calcium chloride.

The symbol † denotes a preparation no longer actively marketed

Administration and dosage. A report of the successful use of streptomycin 7 to 15 mg per kg body-weight as an intravenous infusion over half to one hour in 4 patients with tuberculosis. Despite the view that streptomycin should be given intramuscularly because of the greater risk of toxicity with the intravenous route, this study was considered to indicate that intravenous administration was feasible in selected patients unable to tolerate the intramuscular route.[1]

1. Driver AG, Worden JP. Intravenous streptomycin. *DICP Ann Pharmacother* 1990; **24**: 826–8.

Ménière's disease. Streptomycin and gentamicin have been used for medical ablation in advanced Ménière's disease (p.407). Systemic treatment has generally been limited by the development of chronic ataxia and oscillopsia (oscillating vision). However, streptomycin sulfate 1 g twice daily by intramuscular injection on 5 days each week for 2 weeks, repeated as necessary to a total dose of up to 60 g, has produced improvements in vestibular symptoms without hearing loss in patients with bilateral Ménière's disease.[1,2] Local (intratympanic) injections have also been tried,[3] but gentamicin is considered to be less toxic and is now generally preferred.

1. Graham MD, *et al.* Titration streptomycin therapy for bilateral Meniere's disease: a preliminary report. *Otolaryngol Head Neck Surg* 1984; **92**: 440–7.
2. Shea JJ, *et al.* Long-term results of low dose intramuscular streptomycin for Ménière's disease. *Am J Otol* 1994; **15**: 540–4.
3. Beck C, Schmidt CL. 10 Years of experience with intratympanally applied streptomycin (gentamycin) in the therapy of Morbus Menière. *Arch Otorhinolaryngol* 1978; **221**: 149–52.

Preparations

BP 2001: Streptomycin Injection;
USP 25: Streptomycin for Injection; Streptomycin Injection.

Proprietary Preparations (details are given in Part 3)
Ger.: Strepto-Fatol; Strepto-Hefa; *Ital.:* Streptocol†; *Mex.:* Sulfestrep; *S.Afr.:* Novostrep; Solustrep; *Thai.:* Strepto.

Multi-ingredient: *Braz.:* Climacilin; Enteromicina; Ortocilin; *Port.:* Bienterico; Tri-Sinerge; *S.Afr.:* Diastat†; *Spain:* Bio Hubber Fuerte†; Bio Hubber†; Derbitan Antibiotico†; *Thai.:* Diolin.

Succinylsulfathiazole (4914-t)

Succinylsulfathiazole *(BAN, rINN).*

Succinilsolfatiazolo; Succinylsulfathiazolum; Succinylsulphathiazole. 4′-(1,3-Thiazol-2-ylsulphamoyl)succinanilic acid monohydrate.
$C_{13}H_{13}N_3O_5S_2,H_2O = 373.4.$
CAS — 116-43-8 *(anhydrous succinylsulfathiazole).*
ATC — A07AB04.
Pharmacopoeias. In *Eur.* (see p.vi).

Pharmacopoeial description

Ph. Eur.: A white or yellowish-white crystalline powder. Very slightly soluble in water; slightly soluble in acetone and in alcohol; practically insoluble in ether; dissolves in solutions of alkali hydroxides and carbonates. Protect from light.

Profile

Succinylsulfathiazole is a sulfonamide with properties similar to those of sulfamethoxazole (p.254). It is poorly absorbed and has been given for its antibacterial activity in the gastrointestinal tract.

Sulbactam (13275-l)

Sulbactam *(BAN, rINN).*

CP-45899. Penicillanic acid 1,1-dioxide; (2S,5R)-3,3-Dimethyl-7-oxo-4-thia-1-azabicyclo[3.2.0]heptane-2-carboxylic acid 4,4-dioxide.
$C_8H_{11}NO_5S = 233.2.$
CAS — 68373-14-8.
ATC — J01CG01.

Sulbactam Sodium (11563-b)

Sulbactam Sodium *(BANM, USAN, rINNM).*

CP-45899-2.
$C_8H_{10}NNaO_5S = 255.2.$
CAS — 69388-84-7.
Pharmacopoeias. In *Jpn* and *US.*

1.09 g of sulbactam sodium is approximately equivalent to 1 g of sulbactam.

Pharmacopoeial description

USP 25: A white to off-white crystalline powder. It contains not less than 886 μg and not more than 941 μg of sulbactam per mg, calculated on the anhydrous basis. Freely soluble in water and in dilute acid; sparingly soluble in acetone, in chloroform, and in ethyl acetate. Store in airtight containers.

Profile

Sulbactam is a penicillanic acid sulfone with beta-lactamase inhibitory properties. It generally has only weak antibacterial activity, except against Neisseriaceae, but it is an irreversible inhibitor of many plasmid-mediated and some chromosomal beta-lactamases and has a similar spectrum of beta-lactamase inhibition to clavulanic acid (p.187), although it is regarded as less potent. Sulbactam can therefore enhance the activity of

penicillins and cephalosporins against many resistant strains of bacteria.

It is given in association with ampicillin (p.150) in the treatment of various infections where beta-lactamase production is suspected. Sulbactam is poorly absorbed from the gastrointestinal tract and is given by injection as the sodium salt. The pharmacokinetics of parenteral sulbactam and ampicillin are similar. For oral administration the mutual prodrug sultamicillin (p.257) is available in some countries. Sulbactam has also been given with cefoperazone.

◊ General references.

1. Campoli-Richards DM, Brogden RN. Sulbactam/ampicillin: a review of its antibacterial activity, pharmacokinetic properties, and therapeutic use. *Drugs* 1987; **33**: 577–609.
2. Payne DJ, *et al.* Comparative activities of clavulanic acid, sulbactam, and tazobactam against clinically important β-lactamases. *Antimicrob Agents Chemother* 1994; **38**: 767–72.
3. Nicolas-Chanoine MH. Inhibitor-resistant β-lactamases. *J Antimicrob Chemother* 1997; **40**: 1–3.

Preparations

USP 25: Ampicillin and Sulbactam for Injection.

Proprietary Preparations (details are given in Part 3)
Aust.: Combactam; *Fr.:* Betamaze†; *Ger.:* Combactam.

Multi-ingredient: *Aust.:* Unasyn†; *Fr.:* Unacim; *Ger.:* Unacid; *Hong Kong:* Sulperazon; Unasyn; *Ital.:* Bethacil; Loricin; Unasyn; *Mex.:* Unasyna; *Singapore:* Unasyn; *Spain:* Bacimex; Galotam†; Unasyn; *Thai.:* Sulperazon; Unasyn; *USA:* Unasyn.

Sulbenicillin Sodium (164-e)

Sulbenicillin Sodium *(rINNM).*

α-Sulfobenzylpenicillin Sodium; Sulfocillin Sodium. The disodium salt of (6R)-6-(2-phenyl-2-sulphoacetamido)penicillanic acid.
$C_{16}H_{16}N_2Na_2O_7S_2 = 458.4.$
CAS — 34779-28-7; 41744-40-5 *(both sulbenicillin).*
Pharmacopoeias. In *Chin.* and *Jpn.*

Profile

Sulbenicillin sodium has actions and uses similar to those of carbenicillin sodium (p.160). It is given by intramuscular or intravenous injection or infusion, usually in doses equivalent to sulbenicillin 2 to 4 g daily in divided doses. Higher doses may be necessary for severe infections.

Preparations

Proprietary Preparations (details are given in Part 3)
Ital.: Kedacillina†; *Jpn:* Lilacillin; *Mex.:* Kedacillin.

Sulfabenzamide (4915-x)

Sulfabenzamide *(BAN, USAN, rINN).*

N-Sulphanilylbenzamide.
$C_{13}H_{12}N_2O_3S = 276.3.$
CAS — 127-71-9.
Pharmacopoeias. In *US.*

Pharmacopoeial description

USP 25: A fine, white, practically odourless powder. Insoluble in water and in ether; soluble in alcohol, in acetone, and in sodium hydroxide 4% solution. Protect from light.

Profile

Sulfabenzamide is a sulfonamide with properties similar to those of sulfamethoxazole (p.254). It is reported to exert an optimal bacteriostatic action at pH 4.6. It is used with sulfacetamide and sulfathiazole in pessaries or a vaginal cream for the treatment of bacterial vaginosis, although its value has been questioned. The vaginal cream is also used for the prevention of bacterial infection following cervical and vaginal surgery.

Preparations

USP 25: Triple Sulfa Vaginal Cream; Triple Sulfa Vaginal Tablets.

Proprietary Preparations (details are given in Part 3)
Multi-ingredient: *Austral.:* Sultrin; *Belg.:* Sultrin; *Canad.:* Sultrin; *Irl.:* Sultrin; *Port.:* Sultrin; *S.Afr.:* Sultrin; *UK:* Sultrin; *USA:* Alba Gyn†; Dayto Sulf†; Gyne-Sulf†; Sultrin; Triple Sulfa; Trysul†; VVS†.

Sulfacarbamide (4956-g)

Sulfacarbamide *(BAN, rINN).*

Sulfanilcarbamide; Sulfaurea; Sulphacarbamide; Sulphanilylurea; Sulphaurea; Urosulphanum. Sulphanilylurea monohydrate.
$C_7H_9N_3O_3S,H_2O = 233.2.$
CAS — 547-44-4 *(anhydrous sulfacarbamide);* 6101-35-5 *(sulfacarbamide monohydrate).*
Pharmacopoeias. In *Pol.*

Profile

Sulfacarbamide is a sulfonamide with properties similar to those of sulfamethoxazole (p.254). It has been used in the treatment of urinary-tract infections, sometimes in combination with other drugs.

Preparations

Proprietary Preparations (details are given in Part 3)
Multi-ingredient: *Norw.:* Trisulfamid†.

Sulfacetamide (4927-n)

Sulfacetamide *(BAN, rINN).*

Acetosulfaminum; Sulphacetamide. N-Sulphaniloylacetamide.
$C_8H_{10}N_2O_3S = 214.2.$
CAS — 144-80-9.
ATC — S01AB04.
Pharmacopoeias. In *Aust., Int., Neth.,* and *US.*

Pharmacopoeial description

USP 25: A white, odourless, crystalline powder. Slightly soluble in water and in ether; soluble in alcohol; very slightly soluble in chloroform; freely soluble in dilute mineral acids and in solutions of potassium and sodium hydroxides; practically insoluble in benzene. Solutions in water are acid to litmus and sensitive to light; they are unstable when acidic or strongly alkaline. Protect from light.

Sulfacetamide Sodium (4928-h)

Sulfacetamide Sodium *(BANM, rINNM).*

Soluble Sulphacetamide; Sulfacetamidum Natricum; Sulfacylum; Sulphacetamide Sodium; Sulphacetamidum Sodium.
$C_8H_9N_2NaO_3S,H_2O = 254.2.$
CAS — 127-56-0 *(anhydrous sulfacetamide sodium);* 6209-17-2 *(sulfacetamide sodium monohydrate).*
NOTE. SULF is a code approved by the BP 2001 for use on single unit doses of eye drops containing sulfacetamide sodium where the individual container may be too small to bear all the appropriate labelling information.
Pharmacopoeias. In *Chin., Eur.* (see p.vi), *Int., Pol.,* and *US.*

1.19 g of monograph substance is approximately equivalent to 1 g of sulfacetamide.

When solutions are heated, hydrolysis occurs forming sulfanilamide which may be deposited as crystals, especially from concentrated solutions and under cold storage conditions.

Pharmacopoeial description

Ph. Eur.: A white or yellowish-white, crystalline powder. Freely soluble in water; slightly soluble in dehydrated alcohol; practically insoluble in ether. A 5% solution in water has a pH of 8.0 to 9.5. Protect from light.

USP 25: A white odourless crystalline powder. Soluble 1 in 2.5 of water; sparingly soluble in alcohol; practically insoluble in chloroform and in ether. A 5% solution in water has a pH of 8.0 to 9.5. Store in airtight containers. Protect from light.

Adverse Effects, Treatment, and Precautions

As for Sulfamethoxazole, p.254.

Local application of sulfacetamide sodium to the eye may cause burning or stinging but this is rarely severe enough to necessitate discontinuation of treatment.

Antimicrobial Action

As for Sulfamethoxazole, p.255.

Pharmacokinetics

When sulfacetamide sodium is applied to the eye it penetrates into ocular tissues and fluids; sulfacetamide may be absorbed into the blood when the conjunctiva is inflamed.

Uses and Administration

Sulfacetamide is a sulfonamide antibacterial that is used with sulfabenzamide and sulfathiazole in preparations for vaginal use, and is applied, as the sodium salt, in infections or injuries of the eyes, although it is rarely of much value. Eye drops containing sulfacetamide sodium 10% to 30% and eye ointments containing up to 10% have been used. The sodium salt is also applied topically in the treatment of skin infections.

Preparations

USP 25: Neomycin Sulfate, Sulfacetamide Sodium, and Prednisolone Acetate Ophthalmic Ointment; Sulfacetamide Sodium and Prednisolone Acetate Ophthalmic Ointment; Sulfacetamide Sodium and Prednisolone Acetate Ophthalmic Suspension; Sulfacetamide Sodium Ophthalmic Ointment; Sulfacetamide Sodium Ophthalmic Solution; Sulfacetamide Sodium Topical Suspension; Triple Sulfa Vaginal Cream; Triple Sulfa Vaginal Tablets.

Proprietary Preparations (details are given in Part 3)
Aust.: Beocid Puroptal†; Cetazin; *Austral.:* Acetopt; Bleph-10; Optamide; *Belg.:* Anginamide; Antebor; Isopto Cetamide; Sulfa 10; Ultra; *Braz.:* Sulfanil; *Canad.:* Bleph-10 Liquifilm†; Cetamide; Diosulf; Ophtho-Sulf†; Sodium Sulamyd; Sulfex†; *Fr.:* Antebor; Vitaseptine†; *Ger.:* Albucid; *Hong Kong:* Bleph-10; Spersacet; Sulfex; Vista-Cetamide; *Israel:* Optisol; Sulfacid; Sulphamide; *Ital.:* Optamid; Prontamid†; *Mex.:* Blef-10; Ceta Sulfa; *NZ:* Acetopt; Bleph-10; *S.Afr.:* Albucid†; Bleph-10; Covosulf; Spersamide; *Spain:* Sulfacet†; Sulfacetam; *Switz.:* Keratosept; *Thai.:* Bleph-10; Cetasil; Opsar; Optal; *USA:* Ak-Sulf; Bleph-10; Cetamide; Isopto Cetamide; Klaron; Ocusulf-10; Sebizon; Sodium Sulamyd; Storz-Sulf†; Sulf-10; Sulfac; Vanocin.

Multi-ingredient: *Aust.:* Blephamide; *Austral.:* Blephamide; Sultrin; *Belg.:* Cetapred; Isopto Cetapred; *Braz.:* Isopto Cetapred; Oto-Biotic; Paraqueimol; Pyelodion; Sunil; Uromix; *Canad.:* Blephamide; Dioptimyd; Metimyd†; Sulfacet-R†; Sultrin; Vasocidin; Vasosulf†; *Fr.:* Antebor B₆†; *Ger.:* Blefcon; Blephamide; Combiamid†; *Hong Kong:* Blephamide; Spersacet C; *Irl.:* Sultrin; *Israel:* Blephamide; Prednistyle; *Ital.:* Antisettico Astringente Sedativo; Aureomix; Brumeton Colloidale S; Cosmiciclina; Visublefarite; *Mex.:* Blefamide SF; Deltamid; Metimyd; Premid; Sulfa Cloran; Sulfa Hidro; *NZ:* Blephamide; *Port.:* Blifamol; Meocil; Sultrin; *S.Afr.:* Blephamide; Covancaine; Covosan; Spersacet C; Sultrin; *Singapore:* Blephamide; *Spain:* Betamida; Celestone S; Icolamida; Liquipom Dexamida; Oto Neomicin Calm†; Visublefarite†; *Swed.:* Blefcon†; Metimyd; *Switz.:* Blephamide; Spersacet C; *Thai.:* Spersacet C; *UK:* Sultrin; *USA:* Ak-Cide; Alba Gyn†; Blephamide; Cetapred; Dayto Sulf†; FML-S; GyneSulf†; Isopto Cetapred; Metimyd; Novacet; Optimyd†; Sulfacet-R; Sulfamide; Sulster†; Sultrin; Triple Sulfa; Trysul†; Vasocidin; Vasocine; Vasosulf; VVS†.

Sulfachlorpyridazine (4929-m)

Sulfachlorpyridazine (BAN, rINN).
Sulphachlorpyridazine. N^1-(6-Chloropyridazin-3-yl)sulphanilamide.
$C_{10}H_9ClN_4O_2S$ = 284.7.
CAS — 80-32-0.
Pharmacopoeias. In US for veterinary use only.

Pharmacopoeial description
USP 25: Protect from light.

Profile
Sulfachlorpyridazine is a sulfonamide antibacterial used in veterinary medicine.

Preparations
Proprietary Preparations (details are given in Part 3)
Multi-ingredient: *Braz.:* Mictasol com Sulfa.

Sulfachrysoidine (20445-g)

Sulfachrysoidine (rINN).
Carboxysulfamidochrysoidine.   3,5-Diamino-2-(*p*-sulfamoylphenylazo) benzoic acid.
$C_{13}H_{13}N_5O_4S$ = 335.3.
CAS — 485-41-6.

Profile
Sulfachrysoidine is a sulfonamide antibacterial used topically for infections of the oral mucosa.

Preparations
Proprietary Preparations (details are given in Part 3)
Braz.: Colubiazol.

Sulfaclozine (8640-a)

Sulfaclozine (rINN).
N^1-(6-Chloropyrazinyl)sulfanilamide.
$C_{10}H_9ClN_4O_2S$ = 284.7.
CAS — 102-65-8; 27890-59-1.

Profile
Sulfaclozine is a sulfonamide antibacterial that has been used in veterinary medicine.

Sulfadiazine (4930-t)

Sulfadiazine (BAN, rINN).
Solfadiazina; Solfapirimidina; Sulfadiazinum; Sulphadiazine. N^1-(Pyrimidin-2-yl)sulphanilamide.
$C_{10}H_{10}N_4O_2S$ = 250.3.
CAS — 68-35-9.
ATC — J01EC02.

NOTE. Sulfadiazine may be given with tetroxoprim or trimethoprim; such combinations have been given approved names Cotetroxazine (p.193) and Co-trimazine (p.193) respectively.
Pharmacopoeias. In Chin., Eur. (see p.vi), and US.

Pharmacopoeial description
Ph. Eur.: White, yellowish-white, or pinkish-white, crystalline powder or crystals. Practically insoluble in water; very slightly soluble in alcohol; slightly soluble in acetone. It dissolves in solutions of alkali hydroxides and in dilute mineral acids. Protect from light.
USP 25: White or slightly yellow, odourless or nearly odourless, powder, slowly darkening on exposure to light. Soluble 1 in 13 000 of water; sparingly soluble in alcohol and in acetone; freely soluble in dilute mineral acids and in solutions of potassium and sodium hydroxides, and ammonia. Protect from light.

Sulfadiazine Sodium (4931-x)

Sulfadiazine Sodium (BANM, rINN).
Sodium Sulphadiazine; Soluble Sulphadiazine; Sulfadiazinum Natricum; Sulphadiazine Sodium.
$C_{10}H_9N_4NaO_2S$ = 272.3.
CAS — 547-32-0.
Pharmacopoeias. In Aust., Chin., and US.

1.09 g of monograph substance is approximately equivalent to 1 g of sulfadiazine.

The symbol † denotes a preparation no longer actively marketed

Incompatibilities. Solutions of sulfadiazine sodium are alkaline, and incompatibility may reasonably be expected with acidic drugs or with preparations unstable at high pH.

Pharmacopoeial description
USP 25: A white powder. Soluble 1 in 2 of water; slightly soluble in alcohol. On prolonged exposure to humid air it absorbs carbon dioxide with the liberation of sulfadiazine and becomes incompletely soluble in water. Store in airtight containers. Protect from light.

Adverse Effects, Treatment, and Precautions
As for Sulfamethoxazole, p.254.

Because of the low solubilities of sulfadiazine and its acetyl derivative in urine, crystalluria is more likely after administration of sulfadiazine than after sulfamethoxazole.

Sulfadiazine sodium solution is strongly alkaline; it should therefore be administered intravenously in a strength not exceeding 5% to reduce the risk of thrombosis of the vein; extravasation may cause sloughing and necrosis. For the same reason, intramuscular injections are painful and sulfadiazine sodium should not be given by intrathecal or subcutaneous injection.

Carnitine deficiency. A case of hyperammonaemia and carnitine deficiency in an immunosuppressed patient receiving sulfadiazine and pyrimethamine for the treatment of toxoplasmosis.[1]
1. Sekas G, Harbhajan SP. Hyperammonemia and carnitine deficiency in a patient receiving sulfadiazine and pyrimethamine. *Am J Med* 1993; **95:** 112–13.

Effects on the eyes. Numerous white stone-like concretions of sulfadiazine occurred in the conjunctiva of a woman who had used sulfadiazine eye drops for about one year.[1]
1. Boettner EA, *et al.* Conjunctival concretions of sulfadiazine. *Arch Ophthalmol* 1974; **92:** 446–8.

Effects on the kidneys. Reports of crystalluria and renal failure associated with the use of sulfadiazine in patients with AIDS,[1-4] including the suggestion that such patients may be particularly prone to sulfadiazine-induced renal toxicity.[3]
1. Goadsby PJ, *et al.* Acquired immunodeficiency syndrome (AIDS) and sulfadiazine-associated acute renal failure. *Ann Intern Med* 1987; **107:** 783–4.
2. Ventura MG, *et al.* Sulfadiazine revisited. *J Infect Dis* 1989; **160:** 556–7.
3. Simon DI, *et al.* Sulfadiazine crystalluria revisited: the treatment of Toxoplasma encephalitis in patients with acquired immunodeficiency syndrome. *Arch Intern Med* 1990; **150:** 2379–84.
4. Díaz F, *et al.* Sulfadiazine-induced multiple urolithiasis and acute renal failure in a patient with AIDS and Toxoplasma encephalitis. *Ann Pharmacother* 1996; **30:** 41–2.

Effects on the salivary glands. Enlargement of the salivary glands (sialadenitis) has been reported[1] in a patient who received a preparation containing sulfadiazine; complete recovery followed within 3 days of stopping therapy. Rechallenge confirmed that sulfadiazine was the causative agent.
1. Añíbarro B, Fontela JL. Sulfadiazine-induced sialadenitis. *Ann Pharmacother* 1997; **31:** 59–60.

Interactions
As for Sulfamethoxazole, p.255.

Antimicrobial Action
As for Sulfamethoxazole, p.255.

Pharmacokinetics
Sulfadiazine is readily absorbed from the gastrointestinal tract, peak blood concentrations being reached 3 to 6 hours after a single dose; 20 to 55% has been reported to be bound to plasma proteins. It penetrates into the CSF within 4 hours of oral administration to produce therapeutic concentrations which may be more than half those in the blood. Up to 40% of sulfadiazine in the blood is present as the acetyl derivative. The half-life of sulfadiazine is about 10 hours; it is prolonged in renal impairment.

About 50% of a single dose of sulfadiazine given by mouth is excreted in the urine in 24 hours; 15 to 40% is excreted as the acetyl derivative.

◊ The urinary excretion of sulfadiazine and the acetyl derivative is dependent on pH. About 30% is excreted unchanged in both fast and slow acetylators when the urine is acidic whereas about 75% is excreted unchanged by slow acetylators when the urine is alkaline. The half-life of sulfadiazine ranges from 7 to 12 hours and that of its metabolite from 8 to 12 hours.[1]
1. Vree TB, *et al.* Determination of the acetylator phenotype and pharmacokinetics of some sulphonamides in man. *Clin Pharmacokinet* 1980; **5:** 274–94.

Uses and Administration
Sulfadiazine is a short-acting sulfonamide that has been used similarly to sulfamethoxazole (p.255) in the treatment of infections due to susceptible organisms. It has been used in the treatment of nocardiosis and lymphogranuloma venereum, and has been given for the prophylaxis of rheumatic fever in penicillin-allergic patients. For details of these infections and their treatment, see Choice of Antibacterial, p.114. Sulfadiazine is also given with pyrimethamine for the treatment of toxoplasmosis (p.585) and has been tried in disseminated *Acanthamoeba* infection (p.582).

In the treatment of susceptible infections, sulfadiazine may be given by mouth in usual doses of 2 to 4 g, followed by up to 6 g daily in divided doses, although up to 8 g daily has been suggested for toxoplasmosis; a dose in children is 75 mg per kg bodyweight initially, then 150 mg per kg daily in divided doses to a maximum of 6 g daily. A concentration in the blood of 100 to 150 µg per mL is desirable. Sulfadiazine is used in infants less than 2 months of age for congenital toxoplasmosis. For the prophylaxis of rheumatic fever, patients weighing less than about 30 kg are given 500 mg once daily, while those over 30 kg may receive 1 g once daily.

Sulfadiazine is also given intravenously as the sodium salt. The usual dose is the equivalent of sulfadiazine 2 to 3 g initially, followed by 1 g four times daily for 2 days; subsequent treatment is given by mouth. Children and infants over 2 months of age may be given the equivalent of 50 mg per kg initially, followed by 25 mg per kg four times daily.

Intravenous doses of sulfadiazine sodium are given by infusion or by slow intravenous injection of a solution containing up to 5%. It may be diluted with sodium chloride 0.9%. Sulfadiazine sodium has been given by deep intramuscular injection, but great care must be taken to prevent damage to subcutaneous tissues; the intravenous route is preferred.

Sulfadiazine is used with trimethoprim as co-trimazine (p.193). Sulfadiazine has also been given in association with other sulfonamides, particularly sulfamerazine and sulfadimidine, to reduce the problems of low solubility in urine.

Preparations
BP 2001: Sulfadiazine Injection;
USP 25: Sulfadiazine Sodium Injection; Sulfadiazine Tablets; Trisulfapyrimidines Oral Suspension; Trisulfapyrimidines Tablets.
Proprietary Preparations (details are given in Part 3)
Fr.: Adiazine; *Port.:* Labdiazina; *Thai.:* Balin.

Multi-ingredient: *Aust.:* Bisolvonamid†; Ophcillin N; Rhinon; Triglobe; Urospasmon sine phenazopyridino†; *Braz.:* Anfomicin; Enterodina; Enterozol; Gargosedans; Testinfex; Triglobe; *Canad.:* Coptin; Trisulfaminic; *Fin.:* Ditrim; Trimetin Duplo; *Fr.:* Trimadiaz Antrima†; *Ger.:* Sterinor; Triglobe; Urospasmon; Urospasmon sine; *Ital.:* Kombinax; Oxosint; Sterinor†; *Mex.:* Estrefen; *Norw.:* Trisulfamid†; *Port.:* Broncodiazina; *Singapore:* Balin; Triglobe; *Spain:* Bio Hubber Fuerte†; Bio Hubber†; Bronco Aseptilex†; Broncomicin Bals†; Triglobe†; *Swed.:* Trimin sulfa; *Thai.:* Sulfatril.

Sulfadiazine Silver (4913-a)

Sulfadiazine Silver (BANM, rINNM).
Silver Sulfadiazine (USAN); Silver Sulphadiazine; Sulphadiazine Silver.
$C_{10}H_9AgN_4O_2S$ = 357.1.
CAS — 22199-08-2.
ATC — D06BA01.
Pharmacopoeias. In Chin., Jpn, and US.

Pharmacopoeial description
USP 25: A white to creamy-white, odourless or almost odourless crystalline powder. It becomes yellow on exposure to light. Practically insoluble in alcohol, in chloroform, and in ether; slightly soluble in acetone; freely soluble in 30% ammonia solution. It decomposes in moderately strong mineral acids. Protect from light.

Adverse Effects, Treatment, and Precautions
Sulfadiazine silver may be absorbed following topical application and produce systemic effects similar to those of other sulfonamides (see Sulfamethoxazole, p.254).

Local pain or irritation are uncommon; the separation of the eschar may be delayed and fungal invasion of the wound may occur.

Transient leucopenia does not usually require withdrawal of sulfadiazine silver, but blood counts should be monitored to ensure they return to normal within a few days. Systemic absorption of silver, resulting in argyria, can occur when sulfadiazine silver is applied to large area wounds or over prolonged periods.

Argyria. A report of argyria, with discoloration of the skin and sensorimotor neuropathy, caused by excessive application of sulfadiazine silver 1% cream to extensive leg ulcers.[1]

1. Payne CMER, et al. Argyria from excessive use of topical silver sulphadiazine. Lancet 1992; 340: 126.

Interactions
As for Sulfamethoxazole, p.255.

Sulfadiazine silver is not antagonised by p-aminobenzoic acid or related compounds. The silver content of sulfadiazine silver may inactivate enzymatic debriding agents.

Antimicrobial Action
Sulfadiazine silver has broad antimicrobial activity against Gram-positive and Gram-negative bacteria including *Pseudomonas aeruginosa*, and some yeasts and fungi. Sulfadiazine silver has a bactericidal action; in contrast to sulfadiazine, the silver salt acts primarily on the cell membrane and cell wall and its action is not antagonised by p-aminobenzoic acid. Resistance to sulfadiazine silver has been reported and may develop during therapy.

Pharmacokinetics
Sulfadiazine silver slowly releases sulfadiazine when in contact with wound exudates. Up to about 10% of the sulfadiazine may be absorbed; concentrations in blood of 10 to 20 µg per mL have been reported, although higher concentrations may be achieved when extensive areas of the body are treated. Some silver may also be absorbed.

Uses and Administration
Sulfadiazine silver is a sulfonamide that is used, in conjunction with debridement, as a 1% cream for the prevention and treatment of infection in severe burns (p.1104).

Sulfadiazine silver has also been used in other skin conditions, such as leg ulcers (p.1108), where infection may prevent healing and for the prophylaxis of infection in skin grafting. It has also been applied to the eyes in the treatment of superficial *Aspergillus* infections.

Preparations
USP 25: Silver Sulfadiazine Cream.

Proprietary Preparations (details are given in Part 3)
Aust.: Flammazine; *Belg.:* Flammazine; *Braz.:* Dermazine; *Canad.:* Dermazin; Flamazine; SSD; *Denm.:* Flamazine; *Fin.:* Flamazine; *Fr.:* Flammazine; Sicazine; *Ger.:* Brandiazin; Flammazine; *Hong Kong:* Dermazin; Flamazine; Silverol; *Irl.:* Flamazine; *Israel:* Silverol; *Ital.:* Bacternil; Sofargen; *Mex.:* Argental; Silvadene; *Neth.:* Flammazine; *Norw.:* Flamazine; *Port.:* Flamazine; Sicazine; *S.Afr.:* Argent-Eze†; Bactrazine; Flamazine; *Singapore:* Flamazine; *Spain:* Flammazine; Silvederma; *Switz.:* Flammazine; Silvadene†; Silvertone; *Thai.:* Dermazin; Flamazine; Silverol; *UK:* Flamazine; *USA:* Silvadene; SSD; Thermazine.

Multi-ingredient: *Austral.:* Silvazine; *Belg.:* Flammacerium; *Canad.:* Flamazine C; *Fr.:* Flammacerium; *Israel:* Flammacerium; *Ital.:* Connettivina Plus; *Neth.:* Flammacerium; *NZ:* Silvazine; *Singapore:* Silvazine; *Spain:* Unitul Complex; *Switz.:* Ialugen Plus; *UK:* Flammacerium.

Sulfadicramide   (13277-j)
Sulfadicramide (rINN).

N'-(3,3-Dimethylacroyl)sulphanilamide.
$C_{11}H_{14}N_2O_3S = 254.3$.
CAS — 115-68-4.
ATC — S01AB03.

Profile
Sulfadicramide is a sulfonamide with properties similar to those of sulfamethoxazole (p.254). It is applied as a 15% ointment for superficial infections of the eye.

Preparations
Proprietary Preparations (details are given in Part 3)
Denm.: Irgamid; *Fin.:* Irgamid; *Neth.:* Irgamid; *Switz.:* Irgamid.

Sulfadimethoxine   (4932-r)
Sulfadimethoxine (BAN, rINN).

Solfadimetossina; Solfadimetossipirimidina; Sulphadimethoxine. N'-(2,6-Dimethoxypyrimidin-4-yl)sulphanilamide.
$C_{12}H_{14}N_4O_4S = 310.3$.
CAS — 122-11-2.
ATC — J01ED01.
Pharmacopoeias. In Fr. and It. In US for veterinary use only.

Pharmacopoeial description
USP 25: Practically white, crystalline powder. Practically insoluble in water; slightly soluble in alcohol, in chloroform, in ether, and in hexane; soluble in 2N sodium hydroxide; sparingly soluble in 2N hydrochloric acid. Protect from light.

Profile
Sulfadimethoxine is a long-acting sulfonamide with properties similar to those of sulfamethoxazole (p.254). It is used in veterinary medicine, sometimes in combination with baquiloprim or ormetoprim. It was formerly used in humans for the treatment of urinary-tract infections.

Sulfadimidine   (4933-f)
Sulfadimidine (BAN, rINN).

Solfametazina; Sulfadimerazine; Sulfadimezinum; Sulfadimidinum; Sulfamethazine; Sulphadimethylpyrimidine; Sulphadimidine; Sulphamethazine. N'-(4,6-Dimethylpyrimidin-2-yl)sulphanilamide.
$C_{12}H_{14}N_4O_2S = 278.3$.
CAS — 57-68-1.
ATC — J01EB03.

NOTE. Sulfadimethylpyrimidine has been used as a synonym for sulfisomidine (p.257). Care should be taken to avoid confusion between the two compounds, which are isomeric.
Pharmacopoeias. In Chin., Eur. (see p.vi), Int., and US.

Pharmacopoeial description
Ph. Eur.: White or almost white powder or crystals. Very slightly soluble in water and in ether; slightly soluble in alcohol; soluble in acetone. It dissolves in solutions of alkali hydroxides and in dilute mineral acids. Protect from light.

USP 25: White to yellowish-white, practically odourless, powder. It may darken on exposure to light. Very slightly soluble in water and in ether; slightly soluble in alcohol; soluble in acetone. Protect from light.

Sulfadimidine Sodium   (4934-d)
Sulfadimidine Sodium (BANM, rINNM).

Soluble Sulphadimidine; Sulfamethazine Sodium; Sulphadimidine Sodium.
$C_{12}H_{13}N_4NaO_2S = 300.3$.
CAS — 1981-58-4.
Pharmacopoeias. In Aust., Br., and Int.

1.08 g of monograph substance is approximately equivalent to 1 g of sulfadimidine.

Pharmacopoeial description
BP 2001: White or creamy-white, odourless or almost odourless, hygroscopic crystals or powder. Freely soluble in water; sparingly soluble in alcohol. A 10% solution in water has a pH of 10.0 to 11.0. Protect from light.

Profile
Sulfadimidine is a short-acting sulfonamide with properties similar to those of sulfamethoxazole (p.254).

It is well absorbed from the gastrointestinal tract and about 80 to 90% has been stated to be bound to plasma protein. Reported half-lives have ranged from 1.5 to 4 hours in fast and 5.5 to 8.8 hours in slow acetylators. Because of the relatively high solubility of the drug and its acetyl metabolite, crystalluria may be less likely than with sulfamethoxazole.

In the treatment of susceptible infections, sulfadimidine is given by mouth in an initial dose of 2 g, followed by 0.5 to 1.0 g every 6 to 8 hours. It has also been given parenterally as the sodium salt.

Sulfadimidine has also been used in association with other sulfonamides, particularly sulfamerazine and sulfadiazine. It is also used in veterinary medicine, sometimes in combination with baquiloprim or trimethoprim.

Because its pharmacokinetics differ in fast and slow acetylators, sulfadimidine has been used to determine acetylator status.

Preparations
USP 25: Trisulfapyrimidines Oral Suspension; Trisulfapyrimidines Tablets.

Proprietary Preparations (details are given in Part 3)
Multi-ingredient: *Canad.:* Trisulfaminic; *Norw.:* Trisulfamid†; *Thai.:* Sulfatril.

Sulfadoxine   (4917-f)
Sulfadoxine (BAN, USAN, rINN).

Ro-4-4393; Sulfadoxinum; Sulformethoxine; Sulforthomidine; Sulphormethoxine; Sulphorthodimethoxine. N'-(5,6-Dimethoxypyrimidin-4-yl)sulphanilamide.
$C_{12}H_{14}N_4O_4S = 310.3$.
CAS — 2447-57-6.
Pharmacopoeias. In Eur. (see p.vi), Int., and US.

Pharmacopoeial description
Ph. Eur.: White or yellowish-white crystalline powder or crystals. Very slightly soluble in water; slightly soluble in alcohol and in methyl alcohol; practically insoluble in ether. It dissolves in solutions of alkali hydroxides and in dilute mineral acids. Protect from light.

USP 25: Protect from light.

Adverse Effects, Treatment, and Precautions
As for Sulfamethoxazole, p.254. For reference to the adverse effects of a combination of sulfadoxine and pyrimethamine, see Pyrimethamine, p.443.

If side-effects occur, sulfadoxine has the disadvantage that several days are required for elimination from the body.

Interactions
As for Sulfamethoxazole, p.255.

Antimicrobial Action
As for Sulfamethoxazole, p.255. Synergy exists between sulfadoxine and pyrimethamine, which act against folate metabolism at different points of the metabolic cycle.

Resistance to the combination of sulfadoxine and pyrimethamine in plasmodia, first noted in Thailand in the late 1970s, has become widespread in many malarious areas of the world. For further details of resistance to antimalarial drugs, see p.428.

Pharmacokinetics
Sulfadoxine is readily absorbed from the gastrointestinal tract. High concentrations in the blood are reached in about 4 hours; the half-life in the blood is about 4 to 9 days. About 90 to 95% is reported to be bound to plasma proteins.

Sulfadoxine is widely distributed to body tissues and fluids; it passes into the fetal circulation and has been detected in low concentrations in breast milk. Sulfadoxine is excreted very slowly in urine, primarily unchanged.

Uses and Administration
Sulfadoxine is a long-acting sulfonamide that has been used in the treatment of various infections but is now rarely used alone.

It is given as a fixed-dose combination of 20 parts sulfadoxine with 1 part pyrimethamine (Fansidar) in the treatment of falciparum malaria resistant to other therapies (p.428), usually following a course of quinine. Although formerly used in the prophylaxis of malaria, the risk of toxicity from the combination is now generally considered to outweigh its value.

In the treatment of malaria, the usual dose by mouth is 1.5 g of sulfadoxine with 75 mg of pyrimethamine as a single dose; this should not be repeated for at least 7 days. Oral doses for children are: 5 to 10 kg body-weight, 250 mg sulfadoxine with 12.5 mg pyrimethamine; 11 to 20 kg, 500 mg sulfadoxine with 25 mg pyrimethamine; 21 to 30 kg, 750 mg sulfadoxine with 37.5 mg pyrimethamine; 31 to 45 kg, 1 g sulfadoxine with 50 mg pyrimethamine.

The combination of sulfadoxine with pyrimethamine has also been administered intramuscularly.

Sulfadoxine with pyrimethamine has also been tried in the treatment of actinomycetomas (see Mycetoma p.130), and for prophylaxis of *Pneumocystis carinii* pneumonia in immunocompromised patients (see p.375 for the more usual prophylactic regimens).

A mixture of 5 parts of sulfadoxine with 1 part trimethoprim is used in veterinary medicine.

Preparations

USP 25: Sulfadoxine and Pyrimethamine Tablets.

Proprietary Preparations (details are given in Part 3)
Ital.: Fansil†.

Multi-ingredient: *Aust.:* Fansidar†; *Austral.:* Fansidar; *Belg.:* Fansidar†; *Braz.:* Fansidar; *Canad.:* Fansidar; *Denm.:* Fansidar; *Fr.:* Fansidar; *Irl.:* Fansidar; *Israel:* Fansidar; *Neth.:* Fansidar†; *S.Afr.:* Fansidar; *Singapore:* Madomine; *Swed.:* Fansidar†; *Switz.:* Fansidar; Fansimef; *Thai.:* Vivaxine; *UK:* Fansidar; *USA:* Fansidar.

Sulfafurazole (4936-h)

Sulfafurazole *(BAN, pINN)*.

Sulfafurazolum; Sulfisoxazole; Sulphafuraz; Sulphafurazole. N^1-(3,4-Dimethylisoxazol-5-yl)sulphanilamide.
$C_{11}H_{13}N_3O_3S = 267.3$.
CAS — 127-69-5.
ATC — J01EB05; S01AB02.
Pharmacopoeias. In Eur. (see p.vi), *Jpn, Pol.,* and *US.*

Pharmacopoeial description

Ph. Eur.: White or yellowish-white, crystalline powder or crystals. Practically insoluble in water; sparingly soluble in alcohol; slightly soluble in dichloromethane and in ether. It dissolves in solutions of alkali hydroxides and in dilute mineral acids. Protect from light.

USP 25: A white to slightly yellowish, odourless crystalline powder. Soluble 1 in 7700 of water and 1 in 10 of boiling alcohol; soluble in 3N hydrochloric acid. Store in airtight containers. Protect from light.

Acetyl Sulfafurazole (4937-m)

Acetyl Sulphafurazole; Sulfisoxazole Acetyl. N^1-Acetyl Sulphafurazole; N-(3,4-Dimethylisoxazol-5-yl)-N-sulphanilylacetamide.
$C_{13}H_{15}N_3O_4S = 309.3$.
CAS — 80-74-0.

NOTE. Acetyl sulfafurazole is to be distinguished from the N^4-acetyl derivative formed from sulfafurazole by conjugation in the body.
Compounded preparations of acetyl sulfafurazole may be represented by the following names:

• Co-erynsulfisox (*USP 25*)—acetyl sulfafurazole and erythromycin ethyl succinate.

Pharmacopoeias. In US.

1.16 g of monograph substance is approximately equivalent to 1 g of sulfafurazole.

Pharmacopoeial description

USP 25: A white or slightly yellow crystalline powder. Practically insoluble in water; soluble 1 in 176 of alcohol, 1 in 35 of chloroform, 1 in 1064 of ether, and 1 in 203 of methyl alcohol. Store in airtight containers. Protect from light.

Sulfafurazole Diolamine (4938-b)

Sulfafurazole Diolamine *(pINNM)*.

NU-445; Sulfisoxazole Diolamine *(USAN)*; Sulphafurazole Diethanolamine; Sulphafurazole Diolamine. The 2,2′-iminobisethanol salt of sulphafurazole .
$C_{11}H_{13}N_3O_3S,C_4H_{11}NO_2 = 372.4$.
CAS — 4299-60-9.

Adverse Effects, Treatment, and Precautions

As for Sulfamethoxazole, p.254.

Sulfafurazole and its acetyl derivative are relatively soluble in urine and the risk of crystalluria is generally slight, but nevertheless adequate fluid intake is recommended.

Interactions

As for Sulfamethoxazole, p.255.

Sulfafurazole has been reported to increase the anaesthetic effect of thiopental sodium.

Eye preparations of sulfafurazole diolamine should not be applied concomitantly with preparations of silver salts.

Antimicrobial Action

As for Sulfamethoxazole, p.255.

Pharmacokinetics

Sulfafurazole is readily absorbed from the gastrointestinal tract with peak plasma concentrations occurring 1 to 4 hours after a dose by mouth. Acetyl sulfafurazole (the N^1-acetyl derivative) is broken down to sulfafurazole in the gastrointestinal tract before absorption, resulting in delayed and somewhat lower peak concentrations. Following absorption about 85 to 90% is bound to plasma proteins. Sulfafurazole readily diffuses into extracellular fluid, but very little diffuses into cells. Concentrations in the CSF are about one-third of those in the blood. It crosses the placenta into the fetal circulation and is distributed into breast milk. About 30% of sulfafurazole in the blood and in the urine is in the form of the N^4-acetyl derivative.

Sulfafurazole is excreted rapidly, up to 95% of a single dose being eliminated in 24 hours. The half-life is reported to range from about 5 to 8 hours. Both sulfafurazole and its N^4-acetyl derivative are more soluble than many other sulfonamides in urine.

Uses and Administration

Sulfafurazole is a short-acting sulfonamide that is used similarly to sulfamethoxazole (p.255), notably in the treatment of chlamydial infections such as lymphogranuloma venereum, chlamydial pneumonia, urethritis, and trachoma. It is used, usually with erythromycin, in the treatment of otitis media. For details of these infections and their treatment see Choice of Antibacterial, p.114.

Sulfafurazole is usually administered by mouth. In the treatment of susceptible infections, it has been given in an initial dose of 2 to 4 g, followed by 4 to 8 g daily in divided doses every 4 to 6 hours. For children, the dose has been 75 mg per kg body-weight initially, followed by 150 mg per kg daily in divided doses to a maximum of 6 g daily. Dosage modification may be necessary in patients with renal impairment. Acetyl sulfafurazole is tasteless and is used in liquid oral preparations of the drug; doses are expressed in terms of sulfafurazole.

Sulfafurazole diolamine has been used, as an ophthalmic ointment or solution containing the equivalent of 4% of sulfafurazole, in the topical treatment of susceptible eye infections.

Sulfafurazole diolamine has also been given parenterally.

Preparations

USP 25: Erythromycin Estolate and Sulfisoxazole Acetyl Oral Suspension; Erythromycin Ethylsuccinate and Sulfisoxazole Acetyl for Oral Suspension; Sulfisoxazole Acetyl Oral Suspension; Sulfisoxazole Tablets.

Proprietary Preparations (details are given in Part 3)
Canad.: Novo-Soxazole†; *Mex.:* Sulfizax; *USA:* Gantrisin; SS-Tab†.

Multi-ingredient: *Canad.:* Pediazole; *Fr.:* Pediazole; *Hong Kong:* Pediazole; *Israel:* Pediazole; *Mex.:* Pediazole; *S.Afr.:* Pediazole†; *Switz.:* Pediazole†; *USA:* Eryzole; Pediazole.

Sulfaguanidine (4939-v)

Sulfaguanidine *(BAN, rINN)*.

Solfaguanidina; Sulfaguanidinum; Sulfamidinum; Sulginum; Sulphaguanidine. 1-Sulphanilylguanidine; N′-Amidinosulphanilamide.
$C_7H_{10}N_4O_2S = 214.2$.
CAS — 57-67-0 *(anhydrous sulfaguanidine)*; 6190-55-2 *(sulfaguanidine monohydrate)*.
ATC — A07AB03.
Pharmacopoeias. In Eur. (see p.vi).
Pol. includes the monohydrate.

Pharmacopoeial description

Ph. Eur.: A white or almost white, fine crystalline powder. Very slightly soluble in water and in alcohol; slightly soluble in acetone; practically insoluble in dichloromethane. It dissolves in dilute solutions of mineral acids. Protect from light.

Profile

Sulfaguanidine is a sulfonamide with properties similar to those of sulfamethoxazole (p.254). It is absorbed to a limited extent from the gastrointestinal tract and may therefore be more likely to cause systemic effects than less well absorbed drugs such as phthalylsulfathiazole and succinylsulfathiazole. It is used, usually in combination with other drugs, in the treatment of gastrointestinal infections, and has also been applied locally to the skin and throat.

Preparations

Proprietary Preparations (details are given in Part 3)
Fr.: Enteropathyl.

Multi-ingredient: *Braz.:* Enteroftal; Testinfex; *Fr.:* Litoxol; *Thai.:* Biodan.

Sulfamazone (3943-c)

Sulfamazone *(rINN)*.

Sulfenazone; Sulphenazone. α-{p-[(6-Methoxy-3-pyridazinyl)sulfamoyl]anilino}-2,3-dimethyl-5-oxo-1-phenyl-3-pyrazoline-4-methanesulphonic acid.
$C_{23}H_{24}N_6O_7S_2 = 560.6$.
CAS — 65761-24-2 *(sulfamazone)*; 13061-27-3 *(sulfamazone sodium)*.

Profile

Sulfamazone is an antibacterial with antipyretic activity that is given as the sodium salt, by mouth or rectally, in infections of the upper respiratory tract.

Preparations

Proprietary Preparations (details are given in Part 3)
Ital.: Marespin.

Sulfamerazine (4918-d)

Sulfamerazine *(BAN, rINN)*.

RP-2632; Solfamerazina; Sulfamerazinum; Sulfamethyldiazine; Sulfamethylpyrimidine; Sulphamerazine. N^1-(4-Methylpyrimidin-2-yl)sulphanilamide.
$C_{11}H_{12}N_4O_2S = 264.3$.
CAS — 127-79-7.
ATC — J01ED07.
Pharmacopoeias. In Eur. (see p.vi) and *Pol.*

Pharmacopoeial description

Ph. Eur.: White, yellowish-white, or pinkish-white, crystalline powder or crystals. Very slightly soluble in water and in dichloromethane; slightly soluble in alcohol; sparingly soluble in acetone. It dissolves in solutions of alkali hydroxides and in dilute mineral acids. Protect from light.

Sulfamerazine Sodium (4919-n)

Sulfamerazine Sodium *(BANM, rINN)*.

Soluble Sulphamerazine; Sulfamerazinum Natricum; Sulphamerazine Sodium.
$C_{11}H_{11}N_4NaO_2S = 286.3$.
CAS — 127-58-2.
Pharmacopoeias. In Aust. .

1.08 g of monograph substance is approximately equivalent to 1 g of sulfamerazine.

Profile

Sulfamerazine is a short-acting sulfonamide with properties similar to those of sulfamethoxazole (p.254). It has usually been administered in conjunction with other sulfonamides, or with trimethoprim.

Preparations

USP 25: Trisulfapyrimidines Oral Suspension; Trisulfapyrimidines Tablets.

Proprietary Preparations (details are given in Part 3)
Multi-ingredient: *Canad.:* Trisulfaminic; *Ger.:* Berlocombin; *Thai.:* Sulfatril.

Sulfamethizole (4941-f)

Sulfamethizole *(BAN, rINN)*.

Sulfamethizolum; Sulphamethizole. N^1-(5-Methyl-1,3,4-thiadiazol-2-yl)sulphanilamide.
$C_9H_{10}N_4O_2S_2 = 270.3$.
CAS — 144-82-1.
ATC — B05CA04; D06BA04; J01EB02; S01AB01.
Pharmacopoeias. In Eur. (see p.vi), *Jpn,* and *US.*

Pharmacopoeial description

Ph. Eur.: White or yellowish-white crystalline powder or crystals. Very slightly soluble in water and in ether; sparingly soluble in alcohol; soluble in acetone. It dissolves in dilute solutions of alkali hydroxides and in dilute mineral acids. Protect from light.

USP 25: Practically odourless, white crystals or powder. Soluble 1 in 2000 of water, 1 in 38 of alcohol, 1 in 13 of acetone, and 1 in 1900 of chloroform and of ether; freely soluble in solutions of ammonium, potassium, and sodium hydroxides; soluble in dilute mineral acids; practically insoluble in benzene. Protect from light.

Adverse Effects, Treatment, and Precautions

As for Sulfamethoxazole, p.254.

Sulfamethizole and its acetyl derivative are relatively soluble in urine, and the risk of crystalluria is quite low, but an adequate fluid intake should generally be maintained.

Interactions

As for Sulfamethoxazole, p.255.

The symbol † denotes a preparation no longer actively marketed

Antimicrobial Action
As for Sulfamethoxazole, p.255.

Pharmacokinetics
Sulfamethizole is readily absorbed from the gastrointestinal tract; about 90% has been reported to be bound to plasma proteins. Its half-life has been reported to range from about 1.5 to 3 hours. It is only slightly acetylated in the body and is rapidly excreted, about 60% of a dose being eliminated in the urine in 5 hours and around 90% within 10 hours. Sulfamethizole and its acetyl derivative are readily soluble in urine over a wide pH range. Only low concentrations are achieved in blood and tissues because of its rapid excretion.

Uses and Administration
Sulfamethizole is a short-acting sulfonamide that is given by mouth in the treatment of infections of the urinary tract, sometimes in combination with other antibacterials; it is unsuitable for the treatment of systemic infection since only relatively low concentrations of drug are achieved in the blood and tissues.

It is given in adult doses of 1.5 to 4 g daily in 3 or 4 divided doses. A usual dose for children is 30 to 45 mg per kg body-weight daily in 4 divided doses.

Sulfamethizole monoethanolamine has also been used.

Preparations
USP 25: Sulfamethizole Oral Suspension; Sulfamethizole Tablets.
Proprietary Preparations (details are given in Part 3)
Aust.: Lucosil†; Urolucosil†; **Denm.:** Lucosil; **Fr.:** Rufol; **Norw.:** Lucosil; **Thai.:** Luco-Oph; **USA:** Thiosulfil Forte†.
Multi-ingredient: Braz.: Uromix; **Ger.:** Harnosal†; **S.Afr.:** Nicene†; **Spain:** Micturol Sedante; **USA:** Urobiotic-250.

Sulfamethoxazole (4942-d)

Sulfamethoxazole (BAN, USAN, rINN).
Ro-4-2130; Sulfamethoxazolum; Sulfisomezole; Sulphamethoxazole. N^1-(5-Methylisoxazol-3-yl)sulphanilamide.
$C_{10}H_{11}N_3O_3S = 253.3$.
CAS — 723-46-6.
ATC — J01EC01.

NOTE. Sulfamethoxazole may be given with trimethoprim and a preparation of such a combination has been given the approved name Co-trimoxazole, p.193.
Pharmacopoeias. In Chin., Eur. (see p.vi), Int., Jpn, Pol., and US.

Pharmacopoeial description
Ph. Eur.: A white or almost white, crystalline powder. Practically insoluble in water; sparingly soluble in alcohol; freely soluble in acetone; slightly soluble in ether. It dissolves in dilute solutions of sodium hydroxide. Protect from light.

USP 25: A white to off-white, practically odourless, crystalline powder. Soluble 1 in 3400 of water, 1 in 50 of alcohol, and 1 in 1000 of chloroform and of ether; slowly and usually incompletely soluble 1 in 2 of carbon disulfide; freely soluble in acetone and in dilute solutions of sodium hydroxide. Protect from light.

Adverse Effects and Treatment
Nausea, vomiting, anorexia, and diarrhoea are relatively common following the administration of sulfamethoxazole and other sulfonamides.

Hypersensitivity reactions to sulfonamides have proved a problem. Fever is relatively common, and reactions involving the skin may include rashes, pruritus, photosensitivity reactions, exfoliative dermatitis, and erythema nodosum. Severe, potentially fatal, skin reactions including toxic epidermal necrolysis and the Stevens-Johnson syndrome have occurred in patients treated with sulfonamides. Dermatitis may also occur from contact of sulfonamides with the skin. Systemic lupus erythematosus, particularly exacerbation of pre-existing disease, has also been reported.

Nephrotoxic reactions including interstitial nephritis and tubular necrosis, which may result in renal failure, have been attributed to hypersensitivity to sulfamethoxazole. Lumbar pain, haematuria, oliguria, and anuria may also occur due to crystallisation in the urine of sulfamethoxazole or its less soluble acetylat-

ed metabolite. The risk of crystalluria can be reduced by the administration of fluids to maintain a high urine output. If necessary, alkalinisation of the urine by administration of sodium bicarbonate may increase solubility and aid the elimination of sulfonamides.

Blood disorders have occasionally occurred during treatment with the sulfonamides including sulfamethoxazole, and include agranulocytosis, aplastic anaemia, thrombocytopenia, leucopenia, hypoprothrombinaemia, and eosinophilia. Many of these effects on the blood may result from hypersensitivity reactions. Sulfonamides may rarely cause cyanosis due to methaemoglobinaemia. Acute haemolytic anaemia is a rare complication which may be associated with glucose-6-phosphate dehydrogenase deficiency.

Other adverse effects which may be manifestations of a generalised hypersensitivity reaction to sulfonamides include a syndrome resembling serum sickness, liver necrosis, hepatomegaly and jaundice, myocarditis, pulmonary eosinophilia and fibrosing alveolitis, and vasculitis including polyarteritis nodosa. Anaphylaxis has been reported only very rarely.

Other adverse reactions that have been reported after the administration of sulfamethoxazole or other sulfonamides include hypoglycaemia, hypothyroidism, neurological reactions including aseptic meningitis, ataxia, benign intracranial hypertension, convulsions, dizziness, drowsiness, fatigue, headache, insomnia, mental depression, peripheral or optic neuropathies, psychoses, tinnitus, vertigo, and pancreatitis.

Sulfonamides may displace serum-bound bilirubin, resulting in jaundice and kernicterus in premature neonates.

As with other antimicrobials, sulfamethoxazole may cause alterations of the bacterial flora in the gastrointestinal tract. There is, therefore, the possibility, although it appears to be small, that pseudomembranous colitis may occur.

Slow acetylators of sulfamethoxazole may be at greater risk of adverse reactions than fast acetylators.

Precautions
In patients receiving sulfamethoxazole, adequate fluid intake is necessary to reduce the risk of crystalluria; the daily urine output should be 1200 to 1500 mL or more. The administration of compounds which render the urine acidic may increase the risk of crystalluria; the risk may be reduced with alkaline urine.

Treatment with sulfonamides should be discontinued immediately a rash appears because of the danger of severe allergic reactions such as the Stevens-Johnson syndrome.

Sulfamethoxazole should be given with care to patients with renal or hepatic impairment and is contra-indicated in patients with severe renal or hepatic failure or with blood disorders. Dosage reduction may be necessary in renal impairment. Complete blood counts and urinalyses with microscopic examination should be carried out particularly during prolonged therapy. Sulfamethoxazole should not be given to patients with a history of hypersensitivity to sulfonamides as cross-sensitivity may occur between drugs of this group. Care is generally advisable in patients with a history of allergy or asthma. Caution is also needed in the elderly, who may be more likely to have other risk factors for reactions. Some authorities consider sulfamethoxazole to be contra-indicated in lupus erythematosus as it may exacerbate the condition. Patients with glucose 6-phosphate dehydrogenase deficiency may be at risk of haemolytic reactions.

Sulfamethoxazole and other sulfonamides are not usually given to infants within 1 to 2 months of birth because of the risk of producing kernicterus; for the same reason, they are generally contra-indicated in women prior to delivery, and in breast-feeding mothers.

Patients with AIDS may be particularly prone to adverse reactions, especially when sulfamethoxazole is

given in combination with trimethoprim as co-trimoxazole.

Sulfonamides have been reported to interfere with some diagnostic tests, including those for urea, creatinine, and urinary glucose and urobilinogen.

Immunocompromised patients. Sulfamethoxazole is mainly conjugated in the liver to the N^4-acetyl derivative, but is also oxidised, to a limited extent, to the hydroxylamine metabolite.[1-5] Although this metabolite was originally implicated[6] in the development of adverse reactions to sulfonamides, recent work[7] has cast some doubt on this hypothesis. The metabolite appears to be produced through cytochrome P450 oxidative metabolism, and it has been suggested that slow acetylators of sulfamethoxazole exhibit increased oxidation compared with other metabolic routes.[1] AIDS patients also exhibit increased oxidation, since they may be depleted of substrates such as acetylcoenzyme A or glutathione necessary for acetylation or detoxification, and this may explain their susceptibility to sulfamethoxazole toxicity.[2,3]

There have been attempts to inhibit the formation of the hydroxylamine metabolite by competitive inhibition of cytochrome P450 enzymes, notably with fluconazole and ketoconazole.[4,5] Encouraging results have been obtained with fluconazole in healthy volunteers, but the potential for clinical benefit in AIDS patients requires further study.[5]

However, one successful method of overcoming adverse effects in AIDS patients has been desensitisation. Desensitisation by administration of initial doses of 4 mg of sulfamethoxazole or 5 mg of sulfadiazine every 6 hours, doubled at 24-hour intervals until the desired dose was reached, was uneventful in 9 of 13 patients with AIDS requiring sulfonamide treatment for opportunistic infections.[8] The remaining 4 had cutaneous reactions with fever, but in 2 of these the reactions were successfully managed with an antihistamine. Although there is a risk of anaphylaxis, patients with AIDS can be successfully treated with sulfonamides if desensitisation is employed.

See also Immunocompromised Patients under Precautions of Co-trimoxazole, p.194.

1. Cribb AE, Spielberg SP. Sulfamethoxazole is metabolized to the hydroxylamine in humans. Clin Pharmacol Ther 1992; 51: 522–6.
2. Lee BL, et al. The hydroxylamine of sulfamethoxazole and adverse reactions in patients with acquired immunodeficiency syndrome. Clin Pharmacol Ther 1994; 56: 184–9.
3. van der Ven AJA, et al. Urinary recovery and kinetics of sulphamethoxazole and its metabolites in HIV-seropositive patients and healthy volunteers after a single oral dose of sulphamethoxazole. Br J Clin Pharmacol 1995; 39: 621–5.
4. Mitra AK, et al. Inhibition of sulfamethoxazole hydroxylamine formation by fluconazole in human liver microsomes and healthy volunteers. Clin Pharmacol Ther 1996; 59: 332–40.
5. Gill HJ, et al. The effect of fluconazole and ketoconazole on the metabolism of sulphamethoxazole. Br J Clin Pharmacol 1996; 42: 347–53.
6. van der Ven AJAM, et al. Adverse reactions to co-trimoxazole in HIV infection. Lancet 1991; 338: 431–3.
7. ter Hofstede HJM, et al. Drug reactions to cotrimoxazole in HIV infection: possibly not due to the hydroxylamine metabolites of sulphamethoxazole. Br J Clin Pharmacol 1999; 47: 571–3.
8. Torgovnick J, Arsura E. Desensitization in sulfonamide-sensitive patients with HIV infection. Am J Med 1990; 88: 548–9.

Porphyria. Sulfonamides have been associated with acute attacks of porphyria and are considered unsafe in porphyric patients.

Pregnancy and breast feeding. Some sulfonamides have been shown to cause fetal abnormalities including cleft palate in animals, but fears of teratogenic effects in humans do not appear to be substantiated. Sulfonamides are probably safe in the first trimester of pregnancy, although throughout pregnancy they should be used only in the absence of a suitable alternative drug.[1] Sulfonamides may displace serum-bound bilirubin and they should be avoided close to delivery because of the risk of kernicterus in the neonate. The risk of drug-induced bilirubin displacement has been reviewed.[2] The initial evidence suggesting a kernicterus-promoting effect of drugs in neonates was reported for sulfafurazole, and this drug now serves as a standard displacing agent against which other drugs are evaluated. Although all sulfonamides are highly protein bound, each has a different capacity to displace bilirubin. Sulfadiazine and sulfanilamide have been found to be the least displacing of the sulfonamides and the effects of sulfadiazine on bilirubin may not be clinically significant; an increased incidence of hyperbilirubinaemia and kernicterus has not been demonstrated following its use for prophylaxis of rheumatic fever during pregnancy. Sulfasalazine should theoretically cause significant bilirubin displacement, but studies suggest that the drug may be given to patients with Crohn's disease who are pregnant or breast feeding. Metabolites of sulfonamides have also been evaluated for kernicterus-promoting effects; glucuronide metabolites are expected to compete for binding sites less effectively than the parent compound, whereas acetylated metabolites of some sulfonamides appear to be more potent bilirubin displacers.

1. Wise R. Prescribing in pregnancy: antibiotics. BMJ 1987; 294: 42–4.
2. Walker PC. Neonatal bilirubin toxicity: a review of kernicterus and the implications of drug-induced bilirubin displacement. Clin Pharmacokinet 1987; 13: 26–50.

Interactions

The action of sulfonamides may be antagonised by *p*-aminobenzoic acid and compounds derived from it, particularly potassium aminobenzoate and the procaine group of local anaesthetics.

Sulfamethoxazole and other sulfonamides may potentiate the effects of some drugs, such as oral anticoagulants (p.994), methotrexate (p.555), and phenytoin (p.359); this may be due to displacement of the drug from plasma protein binding sites or to inhibition of metabolism. However, the clinical significance of these interactions appears to depend on the particular sulfonamide involved. The possibility of interactions with other highly protein-bound drugs, such as NSAIDs, should be considered.

High doses of sulfonamides have been reported to have a hypoglycaemic effect; the antidiabetic effect of the sulfonylurea compounds may be enhanced by the concomitant administration of sulfonamides (p.336). Some sulfonamides have been associated with a decrease in plasma-ciclosporin concentrations when used concomitantly (p.521). Isolated reports have described possible failures of hormonal contraceptives resulting in pregnancy in patients given sulfonamides (p.1458).

The administration of compounds which render the urine acidic may increase the risk of crystalluria.

Antimicrobial Action

Sulfamethoxazole and other sulfonamides have a similar structure to *p*-aminobenzoic acid and interfere with the synthesis of nucleic acids in sensitive microorganisms by blocking the conversion of *p*-aminobenzoic acid to the coenzyme dihydrofolic acid, a reduced form of folic acid; in man, dihydrofolic acid is obtained from dietary folic acid so sulfonamides do not affect human cells. Their action is primarily bacteriostatic, although they may be bactericidal where concentrations of thymine are low in the surrounding medium. The sulfonamides have a broad spectrum of action, but the development of widespread resistance (see below) has greatly reduced their usefulness, and susceptibility often varies widely even among nominally sensitive pathogens.

Gram-positive cocci, particularly the Group A streptococci and some strains of *Streptococcus pneumoniae*, are usually sensitive and staphylococci also demonstrate sensitivity but to a lesser extent. Enterococci and many of the clostridia are more or less resistant, although strains of *Clostridium perfringens* are moderately susceptible. Among other Gram-positive organisms that have been reported to be sensitive are *Bacillus anthracis* and many strains of Nocardia, especially *N. asteroides*.

The Gram-negative cocci *Neisseria meningitidis* and *N. gonorrhoeae* were formerly extremely susceptible to sulfonamides, but most strains are now resistant. Susceptibility is often seen in *Haemophilus influenzae* and *H. ducreyi* but varies widely among the Enterobacteriaceae: strains of *Escherichia coli*, *Klebsiella*, *Proteus*, *Salmonella*, and *Serratia* are sometimes sensitive, and few strains of *Shigella* are now susceptible. *Vibrio cholerae* may be sensitive.

Other organisms that have been reported to be sensitive include *Actinomyces* spp., *Brucella*, *Calymmatobacterium granulomatis*, *Legionella*, and *Yersinia pestis*. Chlamydia are sensitive, but not mycoplasmas, rickettsias, or spirochaetes, nor in general the mycobacteria. *Pseudomonas aeruginosa* is resistant, although sulfonamides may be effective against *Burkholderia pseudomallei* (*Pseudomonas pseudomallei*).

Sulfonamides have some activity against the protozoa *Plasmodium falciparum* and *Toxoplasma gondii*. They are also active against *Pneumocystis carinii*, but are ineffective against most fungi.

Sulfamethoxazole and other sulfonamides demonstrate synergy with the dihydrofolate reductase inhibitors pyrimethamine and trimethoprim which inhibit a later stage in folic acid synthesis. For reports of the

antimicrobial activity of sulfamethoxazole with trimethoprim, see Co-trimoxazole, p.194.

The *in-vitro* antimicrobial activity of sulfamethoxazole is very dependent on both the culture medium and size of inoculum used.

Resistance. Acquired resistance to sulfonamides is common and widespread among formerly susceptible organisms, particularly *Neisseria* spp., *Shigella* and some other enterobacteria, staphylococci, and streptococci.

There appear to be several mechanisms of resistance including alteration of dihydropteroate synthetase, the enzyme inhibited by sulfonamides, to a less sensitive form, or an alteration in folate biosynthesis to an alternative pathway; increased production of *p*-aminobenzoic acid; or decreased uptake or enhanced metabolism of sulfonamides.

Resistance may result from chromosomal alteration, or may be plasmid-mediated and transferable, as in many resistant strains of enterobacteria. High-level resistance is usually permanent and irreversible. There is complete cross-resistance between the different sulfonamides.

Pharmacokinetics

Sulfamethoxazole is readily absorbed from the gastrointestinal tract and peak plasma concentrations are reached after about 2 hours. Doses of 1 g twice daily should produce blood concentrations of unconjugated sulfamethoxazole in excess of 50 μg per mL. About 70% is bound to plasma proteins and the plasma half-life is about 6 to 12 hours; it is prolonged in patients with severe renal impairment.

Sulfamethoxazole, like most sulfonamides, diffuses freely throughout the body tissues and may be detected in the urine, saliva, sweat, and bile, in the cerebrospinal, peritoneal, ocular, and synovial fluids, and in pleural and other effusions. It crosses the placenta into the fetal circulation and low concentrations have been detected in breast milk.

Sulfamethoxazole undergoes conjugation mainly in the liver, chiefly to the inactive N^4-acetyl derivative; this metabolite represents about 15% of the total amount of sulfamethoxazole in the blood. Metabolism is increased in patients with renal impairment and decreased in those with hepatic impairment. Elimination in the urine is dependent on pH. About 80 to 100% of a dose is excreted in the urine, of which about 60% is in the form of the acetyl derivative, with the remainder as unchanged drug and glucuronide.

Sulfamethoxazole is also oxidised to the hydroxylamine, a metabolite that has been implicated in adverse reactions to sulfonamides (see also Immunocompromised Patients, under Precautions, above), although some doubt has been cast upon this hypothesis.

Uses and Administration

The use of sulfamethoxazole and other sulfonamides has been limited by the increasing incidence of resistant organisms. Their main use has been in the treatment of acute, uncomplicated urinary-tract infections, particularly those caused by *Escherichia coli*. They have also been used in nocardiosis, and in some other bacterial infections such as otitis media, chlamydial infections, and prophylaxis of meningococcal meningitis, but have largely been replaced by other drugs: even where pathogens retain some sensitivity to sulfonamides, a combination such as co-trimoxazole (sulfamethoxazole with trimethoprim) has often been preferred. The usual treatment of these infections is discussed under Choice of Antibacterial, p.114. Sulfonamides are also used, often in combination with pyrimethamine or trimethoprim, in the treatment of protozoal infections, particularly malaria (p.428) and toxoplasmosis (p.585). They are also used similarly in *Pneumocystis carinii* pneumonia (p.375).

Sulfamethoxazole is an intermediate-acting sulfonamide given by mouth in a usual dose of 2 g initially,

followed by 1 g twice daily. In severe infections 1 g three times daily may be given.

The dose for children is 50 to 60 mg per kg bodyweight initially, followed by 25 to 30 mg per kg twice daily. A total daily dose of 75 mg per kg should not be exceeded.

Reduction of dosage may be required in patients with renal impairment.

For the uses and dosage of sulfamethoxazole with trimethoprim, see Co-trimoxazole, p.194.

Sulfamethoxazole lysine has also been used.

Administration. The USA manufacturers of sulfamethoxazole have recommended that blood concentrations be measured in patients receiving sulfonamides for serious infections. The following concentrations of free sulfonamide in the blood were considered to be therapeutically effective: for most infections, 50 to 150 μg per mL, and for serious infections, 120 to 150 μg per mL. Concentrations of 200 μg per mL should not be exceeded since the incidence of adverse reactions may be increased.

Preparations

BP 2001: Co-trimoxazole Intravenous Infusion; Co-trimoxazole Oral Suspension; Co-trimoxazole Tablets; Dispersible Co-trimoxazole Tablets; Paediatric Co-trimoxazole Oral Suspension; Paediatric Co-trimoxazole Tablets;
USP 25: Sulfamethoxazole and Trimethoprim Injection; Sulfamethoxazole and Trimethoprim Oral Suspension; Sulfamethoxazole and Trimethoprim Tablets; Sulfamethoxazole Oral Suspension; Sulfamethoxazole Tablets.

Proprietary Preparations (details are given in Part 3)
USA: Gantanol†; Urobak†.

Multi-ingredient: *Aust.:* Bactrim; Cotribene; Eusaprim; Oecotrim; Supracombin; Trimetho comp; *Austral.:* Bactrim; Cosig; Resprim; Septrin; Trimoxazole; *Belg.:* Bactrim; Eusaprim; *Braz.:* Assepium; Assepium Balsamico; Bac Septin; Bacfar; Bacfar Balsamico; Bacgen; Bacgen Balsamico; Bacris; Bacteracin; Bacteracin Balsamico; Bactox; Bactox Balsamico; Bactren; Bactrex; Bactricin; Bactricin Balsamico; Bactrim; Bactrisan; Bactrisan Balsamico; Bactropin; Bactropin Balsamico; Balsandin; Balsiprin; Baxapril; Becaltrin; Benectrin; Benectrin Balsamico; Binoctrin; Diazol; Dientrin; Diteutrin; Duoctrin; Duoctrin Balsamico; Duoctrin Enterico; Ectrin; Ectrin Balsamico; Entercal; Entero Heractrin; Enterone; Espectrin; Gamactrin; Heractrin; Imuneprim; Infecteracin; Infectrin; Infectrin Balsamico; Katrim; Katrim Balsamico; Leotrim; Lupectrim; Lupectrim Balsamico; Metoprin; Metoprin Balsamico; Mictrex; Neotrin; Neotrin Balsamico; Qiftrim; Quimio-Ped; Quimio-Ped Balsamico; Roytrin; Sedactrim; Sedactrim Balsamico; Septiolan; Septiolan Balsamico; Septoprin; Silpin; Sulfatrex; Suss; Suss Balsamico; Teutrin; Teutrin Balsamico; Trimetoprim Balsamico; Trimexazol; Trimexazol Balsamico; Trizol Balsamico; Urizal; Uro Bac Septin; Uro Bactrim; Uro Batrox; Uro Duoctrim; Uro Heractrim; Uro Septoprin; Uro-Bacteracin; Uro-Baxapril; Uro-Leotrim; Uro-Septiolan; Uro-Teutrin; Urobactrex; Urobioctrin; Uroctrim; Urofar; Uroneotrim; Uropol; Uroxazol; Utrim; *Canad.:* Apo-Sulfatrim; Bactrim; Novo-Trimel; Nu-Cotrimox; Roubac†; Septra; *Denm.:* Bactrim; Sulfotrim; *Fin.:* Cotrim; *Fr.:* Bactrim; Cotrimazol†; Eusaprim; *Ger.:* Bactoreduct; Bactrim†; Berlocid; Co-trim-Tablinen†; Cotrim; Cotrim E; Cotrim K; Cotrim-Diolan; Cotrim-Hefa; Cotrim-Puren†; Cotrimhexal; Cotrimox-Wolff; Cotrimstada; Drylin; Eusaprim; Jenamoxazol†; Kepinol; Linaris†; Microtrim; Sigaprim; Supracombin; TMS; *Hong Kong:* Apo-Sulfatrim; Bacin; BS; Chemitrim; Chemoprim; Dhatrin; Septrin; *Irl.:* Antrimox†; Bactrim; Cotrimel; Duobact; Septrin; Tricomox†; *Israel:* Diseptyl; Resprim; Septrin; Sulfatrim; *Ital.:* Abacin; Bacterial†; Bactrim; Chemitrim; Eusaprim; Gantrim; Isotrim†; Medixin†; Strepto-Plus†; *Mex.:* Anitrim; Bacpiryl; Bactelan; Bactilen; Bactiver; Bactrim; Bactrim Compositum; Bactropin; Bateral; Batrizol; Bioprim; Dertrin; Dibaprim; Ectaprim; Enterobacticel; Esteprim; Fectri; Isobac; Lidaprim; Maxtrim; Metoxiprim; Microbactim; Octiban; Pisatrina; Polibatrim; Protaxol; Septrin; Servitrim; Sulfawal; Sulfoid Trimetho; Sulfort; Sulprim; Supristol; Syraprim; Thriazol; Tribakin; Trim-Vit; Trimesul; Trimesuxol; Trimetoger; Trimetox; Trimexazol; Trimexole; Trimexole Compositum; Trimzol; Trinelax; Trisufin; Zaprin; *Neth.:* Bactrimel; Eusaprim; Trimoxol; *Norw.:* Bactrim; *NZ:* Apo-Sulfatrim; Bactrim; Trimel; Trisul; *Port.:* Bactrim; Cotrim; Metomide; Septrin; *S.Afr.:* Acuco†; Arcanaprim†; Bactrim; Bencole; Briscotrim†; Cocydal; Cotrivant; Cozole; Doctrim†; Durobac; Dynazole; Fabubac; Mezenol†; Microbac†; Norisept†; Partrim†; Purbac; Septran; Spectrim; Thoxaprim†; Tri-Co; Trimethox; Trimoks†; Trimzol†; Troxazole†; Ultrasept; Ultrazole; Xerazole; Xeroprim; *Singapore:* Apo-Sulfatrim; Bacin; Bactrim; BS; Chemoprim; Dhatrin; Septrin; Suprim; Trimezole; *Spain:* Abactrim†; Bactifor†; Bactopumon; Balsoprim; Bridotrim; Bronco Aseptilex Fuerte; Bronco Bactifor; Bronco Sergo; Broncorema†; Broncovir; Brongenit; Bronquicisteina; Bronquidiazina CR; Bronquimar; Bronquimucil; Bronquium; Cotrazol; Eduprim; Eduprim Mucolitico; Gobens Trim; Lotusix†; Momentol; Mucorama TS; Neumopectolina; Pulmo Menal; Pulmosterin Duo; Salvatrim; Septrin; Soltrim; Toose†; Tosdetan†; Traquivan; Tresium†; *Swed.:* Bactrim; Eusaprim; Trimetoprim-Sulfa†; *Switz.:* Agoprim; Bactrim; Cotrim; Escoprim; Eusaprim†; Groprim; Helveprim; Imexim†; Lagatrim; Nopil; Sigaprim; Supracombin; *Thai.:* Actin; Bacin; Bacta; Bactrim; Baczole; Chemoprim; Co-Tasian; Co-Trimed; Conprim; Cotamox; Lastrim; Letus; Med-Sultrim; Mega-Prim; Metrim; Metxaprim; Mycosamthong; Po-Trim; Pulvicin; Septrin; Servitrim; Sulbacta; Sulfometh; Tampo; Toprim; Trimexazole; Trimox; Trimoxzol; Triprim; Trixzol; Zoleprim; *UAE:* Trimol; *UK:* Bactrim†; Chemotrim; Comixco†; Fectrim; Laratrim; Septrin; *USA:* Bactrim; Cotrim; Septra; SMZ-TMP; Sulfamethoprim†; Sulfatrim; Uroplus†.

Sulfamethoxypyridazine (4944-h)

Sulfamethoxypyridazine (BAN, rINN).

Solfametossipiridazina; Sulfamethoxypyridazinum; Sulphamethoxypyridazine. N^1-(6-Methoxypyridazin-3-yl)sulphanilamide.
$C_{11}H_{12}N_4O_3S = 280.3$.
CAS — 80-35-3.
ATC — J01ED05.

Pharmacopoeias. In Int. In Eur. (see p.vi) for veterinary use only.

Pharmacopoeial description

Ph. Eur.: A white or slightly yellowish crystalline powder which colours slowly on exposure to light. Practically insoluble in water; slightly soluble in alcohol; sparingly soluble in acetone; very slightly soluble in dichloromethane; dissolves in dilute mineral acids and solutions of alkali hydroxides. Protect from light.

Acetyl Sulfamethoxypyridazine (4945-m)

Acetyl Sulphamethoxypyridazine; Sulfamethoxypyridazine Acetyl. N-(6-Methoxypyridazin-3-yl)-N-sulphanilylacetamide.
$C_{13}H_{14}N_4O_4S = 322.3$.
CAS — 3568-43-2.

NOTE. Acetyl sulfamethoxypyridazine is to be distinguished from the N^4-acetyl derivative formed from sulfamethoxypyridazine by conjugation in the body.

1.15 g of monograph substance is approximately equivalent to 1 g of sulfamethoxypyridazine.

Profile

Sulfamethoxypyridazine is a long-acting sulfonamide with properties similar to those of sulfamethoxazole (p.254) and is used for the treatment of susceptible infections. It is rapidly absorbed from the gastrointestinal tract and excreted slowly in urine, partly as the N^4-acetyl metabolite; it remains detectable for up to 7 days after a dose. It has also been used with trimethoprim similarly to co-trimoxazole.

Acetyl sulfamethoxypyridazine, which is hydrolysed in the gastrointestinal tract forming sulfamethoxypyridazine, and sulfamethoxypyridazine sodium have also been used.

Preparations

Proprietary Preparations (details are given in Part 3)
Mex.: Dibasul; Exasul.
Multi-ingredient: Braz.: Nipactrin; Testinfex; Urofen; Uropac; Ital.: Velaten†.

Sulfamethylthiazole (14272-k)

Methylsulfathiazole. 4-Amino-N-(4-methyl-2-thiazolyl)benzenesulfonamide.
$C_{10}H_{11}N_3O_2S_2 = 269.3$.
CAS — 515-59-3.

Profile

Sulfamethylthiazole is a sulfonamide with properties similar to those of sulfamethoxazole (p.254). It is applied topically in combination with tetracycline in the treatment of eye infections.

Preparations

Proprietary Preparations (details are given in Part 3)
Multi-ingredient: Ital.: Pensulvit.

Sulfametopyrazine (4920-k)

Sulfametopyrazine (BAN).

Sulfalene (USAN, pINN); AS-18908; NSC-110433; Solfametopirazina; Solfametossipirazina; Sulfamethoxypyrazine; Sulfapirazinmetossina; Sulfapyrazin Methoxyne; Sulphalene. N^1-(3-Methoxypyrazin-2-yl)sulphanilamide.
$C_{11}H_{12}N_4O_3S = 280.3$.
CAS — 152-47-6.
ATC — J01ED02.

Pharmacopoeias. In It.

Adverse Effects, Treatment, and Precautions

As for Sulfamethoxazole, p.254.

If side-effects occur, sulfametopyrazine has the disadvantage that several days are required for its elimination from the body.

Interactions

As for Sulfamethoxazole, p.255.

Antimicrobial Action

As for Sulfamethoxazole, p.255.

Pharmacokinetics

Sulfametopyrazine is readily absorbed from the gastrointestinal tract; 60 to 80% is bound to plasma proteins. Only about 5% of a dose is metabolised to the acetyl derivative. It is slowly excreted in the urine. The biological half-life has been reported to be about 60 to 65 hours.

Uses and Administration

Sulfametopyrazine is a long-acting sulfonamide that has been used in the treatment of respiratory- and urinary-tract infections due to sensitive organisms. It is usually given by mouth in a single dose of 2 g once each week.

Sulfametopyrazine is given in the ratio 4 parts of sulfametopyrazine to 5 parts of trimethoprim as a combination with uses similar to those of co-trimoxazole (p.194). It is also given with pyrimethamine (p.444) in the treatment of malaria.

Preparations

Proprietary Preparations (details are given in Part 3)
Belg.: Kelfizina†; Longum; Ger.: Longum; Irl.: Kelfizine W; Ital.: Kelfizina; UK: Kelfizine W.
Multi-ingredient: Braz.: Periodine Anti-Malarico; Ital.: Kelfiprim; Metakelfin; Mex.: Kelfiprim; Thai.: Kelfiprim.

Sulfametrole (4921-a)

Sulfametrole (BAN, rINN).

N^1-(4-Methoxy-1,2,5-thiadiazol-3-yl)sulphanilamide.
$C_9H_{10}N_4O_3S_2 = 286.3$.
CAS — 32909-92-5.

Profile

Sulfametrole is a sulfonamide with properties similar to those of sulfamethoxazole (p.254). It is given in the ratio of 5 parts of sulfametrole to 1 part of trimethoprim as a combination with uses similar to those of co-trimoxazole (p.194). Usual doses are 960 mg (800 mg of sulfametrole and 160 mg of trimethoprim) twice daily by mouth. It has also been given by intravenous infusion.

Preparations

Proprietary Preparations (details are given in Part 3)
Multi-ingredient: Aust.: Lidaprim; Hong Kong: Lidaprim; Ital.: Lidaprim; Switz.: Maderan†; Thai.: Lidaprim.

Sulfamonomethoxine (4922-t)

Sulfamonomethoxine (BAN, USAN, rINN).

DJ-1550; DS-36; ICI-32525; Ro-4-3476. N^1-(6-Methoxypyrimidin-4-yl)sulphanilamide monohydrate.
$C_{11}H_{12}N_4O_3S,H_2O = 298.3$.
CAS — 1220-83-3 (anhydrous sulfamonomethoxine).

Pharmacopoeias. In Chin. and Jpn.

Profile

Sulfamonomethoxine is a sulfonamide antibacterial with properties similar to those of sulfamethoxazole (p.254). It is used in veterinary medicine.

Sulfamoxole (4946-b)

Sulfamoxole (BAN, USAN, rINN).

Sulphadimethyloxazole; Sulphamoxole. N^1-(4,5-Dimethyloxazol-2-yl)sulphanilamide.
$C_{11}H_{13}N_3O_3S = 267.3$.
CAS — 729-99-7.
ATC — J01EC03.

NOTE. Sulfamoxole may be given with trimethoprim and a preparation of such a combination has been given the approved name Co-trifamole, p.193.

Pharmacopoeias. In Fr.

Profile

Sulfamoxole is a sulfonamide antibacterial with properties similar to those of sulfamethoxazole (p.254). It has been used in combination with trimethoprim as co-trifamole (p.193).

Preparations

Proprietary Preparations (details are given in Part 3)
Multi-ingredient: S.Afr.: Supristol†.

Sulfanilamide (4947-v)

Sulfanilamide (rINN).

Solfamide; Streptocidum; Sulfaminum; Sulfanilamidum; Sulphanilamide. 4-Aminobenzenesulphonamide; p-Sulphamidoaniline.
$C_6H_8N_2O_2S = 172.2$.
CAS — 63-74-1.
ATC — J01EB06.

Pharmacopoeias. In Eur. (see p.vi).

Pharmacopoeial description

Ph. Eur.: White or yellow-white crystals or fine powder. Slightly soluble in water; sparingly soluble in alcohol; freely soluble in acetone; practically insoluble in dichloromethane; dissolves in solutions of alkali hydroxides and in dilute mineral acids. Protect from light.

Profile

Sulfanilamide is a short-acting sulfonamide with properties similar to those of sulfamethoxazole (p.254). Its antibacterial activity is less than that of sulfamethoxazole. It has been used topically, including as pessaries or as a vaginal cream, for the treatment of susceptible infections, often in combination with other drugs. The sodium, sodium mesilate, and camsilate salts have also been used.

Preparations

Proprietary Preparations (details are given in Part 3)
Belg.: Astreptine†; Canad.: AVC; Spain: Azol; USA: AVC†.
Multi-ingredient: Belg.: Mucorhinyl†; Polyseptol; Pyal†; Rhinamide; Sulfaryl†; Braz.: Malvosulfam; Yatropan; Port.: Otocalma; S.Afr.: Achromide; AMS; Daromide; Ung Vernleigh; Spain: Buco Regis; Cilinafosal; Cilinafosal DHD Estrep; Cilinafosal Hidrocort; Cilinavagin Neomicina; Kanafosal; Kanafosal Predni; Nasopomada; Odontocromil c Sulfamida; Oto Difusor; Otonasal; Pental Forte; Pentalmicina†; Polvos Wilfe; Pomada Heridas; Pomada Wilfe; Quimpe Amida; Vitavox Pastillas; USA: Alasulf; Deltavac; DIT1-2.

Sulfapyridine (4949-q)

Sulfapyridine (BAN, rINN).

Sulphapyridine. N^1-(2-Pyridyl)sulphanilamide.
$C_{11}H_{11}N_3O_2S = 249.3$.
CAS — 144-83-2.
ATC — J01EB04.

Pharmacopoeias. In Fr. and US.

Pharmacopoeial description

USP 25: White or faintly yellowish-white, odourless or practically odourless, crystals, granules, or powder. It slowly darkens on exposure to light. Soluble 1 in 3500 of water, 1 in 440 of alcohol, 1 in 65 of acetone; freely soluble in dilute mineral acids and in solutions of potassium and sodium hydroxides. Protect from light.

Profile

Sulfapyridine is a short- or intermediate-acting sulfonamide, with properties similar to those of sulfamethoxazole (p.254). It is slowly and incompletely absorbed from the gastrointestinal tract and excreted in urine; sulfapyridine and its acetyl metabolite are poorly soluble in urine and the risk of crystalluria is relatively high. Adverse effects are common, and gastrointestinal disturbances may preclude continued therapy. Because of its toxicity, sulfapyridine is now little used except occasionally for dermatitis herpetiformis and related skin disorders where alternative treatment cannot be used; doses of up to 1 g four times daily by mouth are given initially, reduced to the minimum effective maintenance dose once improvement occurs.

◊ Benefit has been seen with sulfapyridine in cicatricial pemphigoid.[1]

1. Elder MJ, et al. Sulphapyridine—a new agent for the treatment of ocular cicatricial pemphigoid. Br J Ophthalmol 1996; 80: 549–52.

Preparations

USP 25: Sulfapyridine Tablets.

Proprietary Preparations (details are given in Part 3)
Canad.: Dagenan.
Multi-ingredient: Fr.: Pommade Lelong†.

Sulfaquinoxaline (4924-r)

Sulfaquinoxaline (BAN, rINN).

Sulfabenzpyrazine; Sulphaquinoxalina; Sulphaquinoxaline. N^1-(Quinoxalin-2-yl)sulphanilamide.
$C_{14}H_{12}N_4O_2S = 300.3$.
CAS — 59-40-5 (sulfaquinoxaline); 967-80-6 (sulfaquinoxaline sodium).

Pharmacopoeias. In Fr. Also in BP(Vet) and in US for veterinary use only.
Fr. also includes Sulfaquinoxaline Sodium, $C_{14}H_{11}N_4NaO_2S = 322.3$.

Pharmacopoeial description

BP(Vet) 2001: A yellow, odourless or almost odourless, powder. Practically insoluble in water and in ether; very slightly soluble in alcohol. It dissolves in aqueous solutions of alkalis. Protect from light.
USP 25: Protect from light.

Profile

Sulfaquinoxaline is a sulfonamide antibacterial used in veterinary medicine, sometimes in combination with trimethoprim.

Sulfasuccinamide (13570-t)

Sulfasuccinamide (rINN).

4'-Sulphamoylsuccinanilic acid.
$C_{10}H_{12}N_2O_5S = 272.3$.
CAS — 3563-14-2.

Profile

Sulfasuccinamide is a sulfonamide antibacterial with properties similar to those of sulfamethoxazole (p.254). It is applied topically in the treatment of local infections of the ear, nose, and throat. It has also been given as the sodium salt.

Preparations

Proprietary Preparations (details are given in Part 3)
Multi-ingredient: Fr.: Otoralgyl sulfamide†; RhinATP; Switz.: Otoralgyl†.

Sulfathiazole (4953-m)

Sulfathiazole *(BAN, rINN)*.

M&B-760; Norsulfazole; RP-2090; Solfatiazolo; Sulfanilamidothiazolum; Sulfathiazolum; Sulfonazolum; Sulphathiazole. N^1-(1,3-Thiazol-2-yl)sulphanilamide.
$C_9H_9N_3O_2S_2 = 255.3$.
CAS — 72-14-0.
ATC — D06BA02; J01EB07.
Pharmacopoeias. In *Eur.* (see p.vi) and *US*.

Pharmacopoeial description

Ph. Eur.: A white or slightly yellowish, crystalline powder. Practically insoluble in water; slightly soluble in alcohol; practically insoluble in dichloromethane and in ether. It dissolves in dilute solutions of alkali hydroxides and in dilute mineral acids. Protect from light.

USP 25: A white or faintly yellowish-white, practically odourless, fine powder. Very slightly soluble in water; slightly soluble in alcohol; soluble in acetone, in dilute mineral acids, in solutions of alkali hydroxides, and in 6N ammonium hydroxide. Protect from light.

Sulfathiazole Sodium (4954-b)

Sulfathiazole Sodium *(BANM, rINNM)*.

Soluble Sulphathiazole; Sulfathiazolum Natricum; Sulphathiazole Sodium.
$C_9H_8N_3NaO_2S_2,5H_2O = 367.4$.
CAS — 144-74-1 (anhydrous sulfathiazole sodium); 6791-71-5 (sulfathiazole sodium pentahydrate).
Pharmacopoeias. In *Aust.* ($1\frac{1}{2}H_2O$). Also in *BP(Vet)* ($1\frac{1}{2}H_2O$ or $5H_2O$).

1.44 g of monograph substance is approximately equivalent to 1 g of sulfathiazole.

Pharmacopoeial description

BP(Vet) 2001: A white or yellowish-white, odourless or almost odourless, crystalline powder or granules. Freely soluble in water; soluble in alcohol. A solution in water containing the equivalent of 1% of the anhydrous substance has a pH of 9.0 to 10.0. Protect from light.

Profile

Sulfathiazole is a short-acting sulfonamide with properties similar to those of sulfamethoxazole (p.254). It is now rarely used systemically due to its toxicity.

Sulfathiazole is used with other sulfonamides, usually sulfabenzamide and sulfacetamide, in preparations for the topical treatment of vaginal infections and is also applied in combination with other drugs in the treatment of skin infections.

Sulfathiazole sodium has been applied topically with other drugs in the treatment of eye infections.

Preparations

USP 25: Triple Sulfa Vaginal Cream; Triple Sulfa Vaginal Tablets.
Proprietary Preparations (details are given in Part 3)
Mex.: Sulfagine; *Port.:* Stopex.
Multi-ingredient: *Aust.:* Linobion-Sulfonamid; *Austral.:* Sultrin; *Belg.:* Pyal†; Sultrin; *Braz.:* Otobel; *Canad.:* Sultrin; *Irl.:* Sultrin; *Port.:* Streptosil con Neomicina-Fher; *Port.:* Sultrin; *S.Afr.:* Sultrin; *Spain:* Cremsol; Polvos Wilfe; Pomada Wilfe; Sabanotropico; Salitanol Estreptomicina; *UK:* Sultrin; *USA:* Alba Gyn†; Dayto Sulf†; Gyne-Sulf†; Sultrin; Triple Sulfa; Trysul†; VVS†.

Sulfatroxazole (8641-t)

Sulfatroxazole *(BAN, rINN)*.

N^1-(4,5-Dimethyl-1,2-oxazol-3-yl)sulfanilamide.
$C_{11}H_{13}N_3O_3S = 267.3$.
CAS — 23256-23-7.

Profile

Sulfatroxazole is a sulfonamide antibacterial used in combination with trimethoprim in veterinary medicine.

Sulfisomidine (4952-h)

Sulfisomidine *(BAN, rINN)*.

Sulfa-isodimérazine; Sulfaisodimidine; Sulfasomidine; Sulfisomidinum; Sulphasomidine. N^1-(2,6-Dimethylpyrimidin-4-yl)sulphanilamide.
$C_{12}H_{14}N_4O_2S = 278.3$.
CAS — 515-64-0.
ATC — J01EB01.
NOTE. Sulfadimethylpyrimidine has been used as a synonym for sulfisomidine, and sulphadimethylpyrimidine is sometimes used as a synonym for sulfadimidine (p.252). Care should be taken to avoid confusion between the two compounds, which are isomeric.
Pharmacopoeias. In *Eur.* (see p.vi).

Pharmacopoeial description

Ph. Eur.: White or yellowish-white powder or crystals. Very slightly soluble in water; slightly soluble in alcohol and in acetone; dissolves in dilute solutions of alkali hydroxides and in dilute mineral acids. Protect from light.

The symbol † denotes a preparation no longer actively marketed

Profile

Sulfisomidine is a short-acting sulfonamide with properties similar to those of sulfamethoxazole (p.254). It has been applied topically for skin or vaginal infections and has also been administered by mouth. The sodium salt has also been used.

Preparations

Proprietary Preparations (details are given in Part 3)
Multi-ingredient: *S.Afr.:* Oestro-Gynedron†; Poly-Gynedron†.

Sultamicillin (17000-k)

Sultamicillin *(BAN, USAN, rINN)*.

CP-49952. Penicillanoyloxymethyl (6R)-6-(D-2-phenylglycylamino)penicillanate S',S'-dioxide.
$C_{25}H_{30}N_4O_9S_2 = 594.7$.
CAS — 76497-13-7.
ATC — J01CR04.
Pharmacopoeias. Jpn includes sultamicillin tosilate.

Profile

Sultamicillin is a prodrug of ampicillin (p.150) and the beta-lactamase inhibitor sulbactam (p.250); it consists of the two compounds linked chemically as a double ester. During absorption from the gastrointestinal tract it is hydrolysed, releasing equimolar quantities of ampicillin and sulbactam.

Sultamicillin is given by mouth as tablets containing sultamicillin tosilate or as oral suspension containing sultamicillin. It is used in the treatment of infections where beta-lactamase-producing organisms might occur, including uncomplicated gonorrhoea, otitis media, and respiratory-tract and urinary-tract infections. The usual dose is 375 to 750 mg of sultamicillin (equivalent to 147 to 294 mg of sulbactam and 220 to 440 mg of ampicillin) twice daily. A single dose of sultamicillin 2.25 g together with probenecid 1 g may be used for uncomplicated gonorrhoea.

When parenteral therapy is necessary a combined preparation of ampicillin with sulbactam is given.

◊ References.
1. Friedel HA, *et al.* Sultamicillin: a review of its antibacterial activity, pharmacokinetic properties and therapeutic use. *Drugs* 1989; **37:** 491–522.

Preparations

Proprietary Preparations (details are given in Part 3)
Aust.: Dynapen; Unasyn; *Fr.:* Unacim†; *Ger.:* Unacid PD; *Hong Kong:* Unasyn; *Ital.:* Bethacil†; Unasyn; *Mex.:* Unasyna; *Singapore:* Unasyn; *Spain:* Bacimex†; Unasyn; *Thai.:* Unasyn.

Taurolidine (17001-a)

Taurolidine *(BAN, rINN)*.

4,4'-Methylenebis(perhydro-1,2,4-thiadiazine 1,1-dioxide).
$C_7H_{16}N_4O_4S_2 = 284.4$.
CAS — 19388-87-5.
ATC — B05CA05.

Profile

Taurolidine is a broad-spectrum antimicrobial that is hydrolysed in aqueous solution to its monomeric form taurultam and other metabolites, with the release of what was originally thought to be formaldehyde but is now considered to be activated methylene glycol or methylol groups, from which it is believed to derive its activity. Its antibacterial activity *in vitro* is modest but is reported to be enhanced in the presence of serum or urine: it is active against a variety of pathogens including *Staphylococcus aureus*, *Escherichia coli*, and *Pseudomonas aeruginosa*. Taurolidine is also reported to inactivate bacterial endotoxin.

It is used in peritonitis; a solution containing 0.5% is used for irrigation and another containing 2% is available for instillation. Taurolidine has been given experimentally as an intravenous infusion in the treatment of severe sepsis or endotoxic shock and in pancreatitis.

Preparations

Proprietary Preparations (details are given in Part 3)
Aust.: Taurolin; *Ger.:* Taurolin; *Switz.:* Taurolin.

Tazobactam Sodium (10443-e)

Tazobactam Sodium *(BANM, USAN, rINNM)*.

CL-307579; CL-298741 (tazobactam); YTR-830; YTR-830H (tazobactam). Sodium (2S,3S,5R)-3-methyl-7-oxo-3-(1H-1,2,3-triazol-1-ylmethyl)-4-thia-1-azabicyclo[3.2.0]-heptane-2-carboxylate 4,4-dioxide.
$C_{10}H_{11}N_4NaO_5S = 322.3$.
CAS — 89786-04-9 (tazobactam); 89785-84-2 (tazobactam sodium).

Profile

Tazobactam is a penicillanic acid sulfone derivative with beta-lactamase inhibitory properties similar to those of sulbactam (p.250) although it is regarded as more potent. It has the potential to enhance the activity of beta-lactam antibacterials against beta-lactamase-producing bacteria.

The combination of piperacillin sodium (p.236) with tazobactam sodium is given intravenously for the treatment of bacterial infections. The pharmacokinetics of tazobactam and piperacillin are similar.

◊ References.
1. Bush K, *et al.* Kinetic interactions of tazobactam with β-lactamases from all major structural classes. *Antimicrob Agents Chemother* 1993; **37:** 851–8.
2. Payne DJ, *et al.* Comparative activities of clavulanic acid, sulbactam, and tazobactam against clinically important β-lactamases. *Antimicrob Agents Chemother* 1994; **38:** 767–72.

Preparations

Proprietary Preparations (details are given in Part 3)
Denm.: Tazocin.

Multi-ingredient: *Aust.:* Tazonam; *Austral.:* Tazocin; *Belg.:* Tazocin; *Canad.:* Tazocin; *Fin.:* Tazocin; *Fr.:* Tazocilline; *Ger.:* Tazobac; *Hong Kong:* Tazocin; *Irl.:* Tazocin; *Israel:* Tazocin; *Ital.:* Tazobac†; Tazocin; *Neth.:* Tazocin; *NZ:* Tazocin; *Port.:* Tazobac; *S.Afr.:* Tazocin; *Singapore:* Tazocin; *Spain:* Tazocel; *Swed.:* Tazocin; *Switz.:* Tazobac; *Thai.:* Tazocin; *UK:* Tazocin; *USA:* Zosyn.

Teicoplanin (18689-v)

Teicoplanin *(BAN, USAN, rINN)*.

A-8327; DL-507-IT; L-12507; MDL-507; Teichomycin A_2.
CAS — 61036-62-2 (teichomycin); 61036-64-4 (teichomycin A_2).
ATC — J01XA02.

A glycopeptide antibiotic obtained from cultures of *Actinoplanes teichomyceticus* or the same substance obtained by any other means.

Adverse Effects and Precautions

Fever and chills, skin rash and pruritus, and occasional bronchospasm and anaphylaxis have been reported in patients receiving teicoplanin, but, in comparison with vancomycin (p.267), it appears to be better tolerated when given by rapid intravenous injection and, although erythema and flushing of the upper body have occurred, the 'red-man syndrome' has been reported less often. In addition, unlike vancomycin, teicoplanin does not appear to cause tissue necrosis and can be administered by intramuscular injection. Other hypersensitivity reactions have included rigors, angioedema, and, rarely, severe skin reactions including exfoliative dermatitis, erythema multiforme, Stevens-Johnson syndrome, and toxic epidermal necrolysis.

Other reported reactions include gastrointestinal disturbances, dizziness, headache, thrombocytopenia (especially at high doses), leucopenia, neutropenia, eosinophilia, disturbances in liver enzyme values, and pain, erythema, and thrombophlebitis or abscess at the site of administration. Rare cases of agranulocytosis have occurred. Impairment of renal function, and ototoxicity, have been reported but both appear to be less frequent than with vancomycin.

Renal and auditory function should be monitored during prolonged therapy in patients with pre-existing renal insufficiency, and in those receiving other ototoxic or nephrotoxic drugs concurrently, although opinions conflict on whether increased risk of nephrotoxicity has been demonstrated from combined therapy with drugs such as the aminoglycosides. In general, periodic blood counts and liver- and renal-function tests are advised during treatment.

No relationship has yet been established between plasma concentration and toxicity, and plasma-concentration monitoring is not generally considered necessary. Dosage adjustment is required in renal impairment.

Hypersensitivity. Although there have been occasional reports of cross-sensitivity to teicoplanin in patients hypersensitive to vancomycin,[1,2] the majority of reports suggest that cross-sensitivity is very rare and teicoplanin can usually be used in patients intolerant of vancomycin.[3-5]

1. McElrath MJ, *et al.* Allergic cross-reactivity of teicoplanin and vancomycin. *Lancet* 1986; **i:** 47.
2. Grek V, *et al.* Allergic cross-reaction of teicoplanin and vancomycin. *J Antimicrob Chemother* 1991; **28:** 476–7.
3. Schlemmer B, *et al.* Teicoplanin for patients allergic to vancomycin. *N Engl J Med* 1988; **318:** 1127–8.
4. Smith SR, *et al.* Teicoplanin administration in patients experiencing reactions to vancomycin. *J Antimicrob Chemother* 1989; **23:** 810–12.
5. Wood G, Whitby M. Teicoplanin in patients who are allergic to vancomycin. *Med J Aust* 1989; **150:** 668.

Red-man syndrome. Although teicoplanin is believed[1,2] to be less likely than vancomycin to induce the red-man syndrome, symptoms consistent with the syndrome have nevertheless been reported following intravenous administration.[3]

1. Sahai J, *et al.* Comparison of vancomycin- and teicoplanin-induced histamine release and "red man syndrome". *Antimicrob Agents Chemother* 1990; **34:** 765–9.
2. Rybak MJ, *et al.* Absence of "red man syndrome" in patients being treated with vancomycin or high-dose teicoplanin. *Antimicrob Agents Chemother* 1992; **36:** 1204–7.
3. Dubettier S, *et al.* Red man syndrome with teicoplanin. *Rev Infect Dis* 1991; **13:** 770.

Antimicrobial Action

As for Vancomycin Hydrochloride, p.268. It may be more active *in vitro* against enterococci and some anaerobic organisms, including strains of *Clostridium,* but some coagulase-negative staphylococci are less sensitive to teicoplanin than to vancomycin. MICs for the most sensitive organisms, such as sensitive strains of *Staphylococcus aureus* or *Streptococcus pneumoniae,* range from about 0.03 to 0.25 µg per mL, but organisms with MICs below 8 µg per mL are generally considered sensitive, and those with MICs between about 8 and 16 µg per mL of intermediate sensitivity. There have been difficulties in the determination of the MIC for coagulase-negative staphylococci.

Acquired resistance to teicoplanin has developed in staphylococci during treatment with teicoplanin. Cross-resistance with vancomycin has occurred in staphylococci and enterococci.

Pharmacokinetics

Teicoplanin is poorly absorbed from the gastrointestinal tract. Following intravenous administration of a 400-mg dose peak plasma concentrations one hour later are reported to be in the range 20 to 50 µg per mL. It is well absorbed following intramuscular injection with a bioavailability of about 90%; following administration of 3 mg per kg body-weight intramuscularly, peak plasma concentrations of 7 µg per mL have been reported after 2 hours.

The pharmacokinetics of teicoplanin are triphasic, with a biphasic distribution and a prolonged elimination. Penetration into the CSF is poor. It is taken up into white blood cells, and about 90 to 95% of teicoplanin in plasma is protein bound. It is excreted almost entirely by glomerular filtration in the urine, as unchanged drug. The terminal half-life is prolonged, but reported half-lives have ranged from about 30 to over 160 hours, depending on the sampling time; an effective clinical half-life of about 60 hours has been suggested for use in calculating dosage regimens. Half-life is prolonged in patients with reduced or impaired renal function. Teicoplanin is not removed by haemodialysis.

Teicoplanin is a mixture of several components, the pharmacokinetics of which have been shown to vary slightly, depending on their lipophilicity.

◊ Reviews.
1. Wilson APR. Clinical pharmacokinetics of teicoplanin. *Clin Pharmacokinet* 2000; **39:** 167–83.

Uses and Administration

Teicoplanin is a glycopeptide antibiotic that may be used as an alternative to vancomycin (p.269) in the treatment of serious Gram-positive infections where other drugs cannot be used, including the treatment and prophylaxis of infective endocarditis, peritonitis associated with continuous ambulatory peritoneal dialysis, and suspected infection in neutropenic or otherwise immunocompromised patients. Teicoplanin, administered orally, has been suggested as a possible alternative to vancomycin or metronidazole in antibiotic-associated colitis. For details of these infections and their treatment, see under Choice of Antibacterial, p.114.

Teicoplanin is given intravenously, as a bolus dose or by infusion over 30 minutes, or else by intramuscular injection. The usual dose is 400 mg (or 6 mg per kg body-weight) intravenously or intramuscularly initially, followed by 200 mg (or 3 mg per kg) intrave-

nously or intramuscularly on each subsequent day of treatment. In more severe infections, 400 mg may be given intravenously every 12 hours for the first 3 doses, followed by intravenous or intramuscular maintenance doses of 400 mg daily. Higher doses of up to 12 mg per kg daily have been given intravenously occasionally.

For the prophylaxis of endocarditis in high-risk penicillin-allergic patients undergoing dental or other procedures, teicoplanin may be given in a single dose of 400 mg by intravenous injection together with gentamicin, before the procedure. A similar dose of teicoplanin is given for prophylaxis in orthopaedic surgery at induction of anaesthesia.

In children, loading doses of 10 mg per kg every 12 hours for 3 doses may be followed by 6 to 10 mg per kg daily, depending on the severity of infection. In neonates, a loading dose of 16 mg per kg on the first day may be followed by maintenance doses of 8 mg per kg daily given by intravenous infusion.

Dosage should be adjusted in patients with impaired renal function. One regimen is the administration of usual doses for the first 3 days of therapy, followed by half the normal daily dose in patients with mild renal insufficiency (creatinine clearance between 40 and 60 mL per minute) or one-third of the normal dose in those with more marked insufficiency (creatinine clearance below 40 mL per minute). Alternatively, dosage may be adjusted by giving the usual daily dose only every 2 or 3 days.

◊ Reviews.
1. Brogden RN, Peters DH. Teicoplanin: a reappraisal of its antimicrobial activity, pharmacokinetic properties and therapeutic efficacy. *Drugs* 1994; **47:** 823–54.
2. Murphy S, Pinney RJ. Teicoplanin or vancomycin in the treatment of Gram-positive infections? *J Clin Pharm Ther* 1995; **20:** 5–11.
3. de Lalla F, Tramarin A. A risk-benefit assessment of teicoplanin in the treatment of infections. *Drug Safety* 1995; **13:** 317–28.
4. Periti P, *et al.* Antimicrobial prophylaxis in orthopaedic surgery: the role of teicoplanin. *J Antimicrob Chemother* 1998; **41:** 329–40.

Preparations

Proprietary Preparations (details are given in Part 3)
Aust.: Targocid; *Austral.:* Targocid; *Belg.:* Targocid; *Braz.:* Targocid; *Denm.:* Targocid; *Fin.:* Targocid; *Fr.:* Targocid; *Ger.:* Targocid; *Hong Kong:* Targocid; *Irl.:* Targocid; *Israel:* Targocid; *Ital.:* Targosid; Teicomid†; *Jpn:* Targocid; *Mex.:* Targocid; *Neth.:* Targocid; *Norw.:* Targocid; *NZ:* Targocid; *Port.:* Targosid; *S.Afr.:* Targocid; *Singapore:* Targocid; *Spain:* Targocid; *Swed.:* Targocid; *Switz.:* Targocid; *Thai.:* Targocid; *UK:* Targocid.

Telithromycin   (20246-f)

Telithromycin (BAN, rINN).
HMR-3647. (3aS,4R,7R,9R,10R,11R,13R,15R,15aR)-4-Ethyloctahydro-11-methoxy-3a,7,9,11,13,15-hexamethyl-1-{4-[4-(3-pyridyl)imidazol-1-yl]butyl}-10-{[3,4,6-trideoxy-3-(dimethylamino)-β-D-*xylo*-hexopyranosyl]oxy}-2H-oxacyclotetradecino[4,3-d][1,3]oxazole-2,6,8,14(1H,7H,9H)-tetrone.
$C_{43}H_{65}N_5O_{10}$ = 812.0.
CAS — 173838-31-8.

Profile
Telithromycin is a ketolide antibacterial used for the treatment of susceptible respiratory-tract infections.

Preparations
Proprietary Preparations (details are given in Part 3)
UK: Ketek.

Temafloxacin   (5794-l)

Temafloxacin (BAN, rINN).
A-62254; Abbott-62254. (RS)-1-(2,4-Difluorophenyl)-6-fluoro-1,4-dihydro-7-(3-methylpiperazin-1-yl)-4-oxoquinoline-3-carboxylic acid.
$C_{21}H_{18}F_3N_3O_3$ = 417.4.
CAS — 108319-06-8 (temafloxacin); 105784-61-0 (temafloxacin hydrochloride).
ATC — J01MA05.
NOTE. Temafloxacin Hydrochloride is *USAN*.

Profile
Temafloxacin is a fluoroquinolone antibacterial with properties similar to those of ciprofloxacin (p.182). It was formerly given by mouth in the treatment of susceptible infections but was withdrawn worldwide in 1992 following reports of serious adverse events, mainly in the USA. These adverse effects included symptoms of severe hypoglycaemia, hepatic dysfunction,

haemolytic anaemia, renal dysfunction sometimes requiring dialysis, anaphylaxis, and death.

Temocillin Sodium   (17002-t)

Temocillin Sodium (BANM, rINNM).
BRL-17421; Temocillin Disodium. The disodium salt of (6S)-6-[2-carboxy-2-(3-thienyl)acetamido]-6-methoxypenicillanic acid.
$C_{16}H_{16}N_2Na_2O_7S_2$ = 458.4.
CAS — 66148-78-5 (temocillin); 61545-06-0 (temocillin disodium).
NOTE. Temocillin is *USAN*.

Profile
Temocillin is a semisynthetic penicillin that is highly resistant to a wide range of beta-lactamases and has been used for the treatment of infections caused by Gram-negative aerobic bacteria, including those resistant to third-generation cephalosporins.

It has been given, as the sodium salt, intramuscularly or intravenously.

Preparations
Proprietary Preparations (details are given in Part 3)
Belg.: Negaban†; *UK:* Temopen†.

Terizidone   (13309-g)

Terizidone (rINN).
B-2360. 4,4′-[p-Phenylenebis(methyleneamino)]bis(isoxazolidin-3-one).
$C_{14}H_{14}N_4O_4$ = 302.3.
CAS — 25683-71-0.
ATC — J04AK03.

Profile
Terizidone has been used in the treatment of infections of the urinary tract and of pulmonary and extrapulmonary tuberculosis.

Preparations
Proprietary Preparations (details are given in Part 3)
Aust.: Terivalidin; *S.Afr.:* Terivalidin†.

Tetracycline   (168-z)

Tetracycline (BAN, rINN).
Tetraciclina; Tetracyclinum. A variably hydrated form of (4S,4aS,5aS,6S,12aS)-4-Dimethylamino-1,4,4a,5,5a,6,11,12a-octahydro-3,6,10,12,12a-pentahydroxy-6-methyl-1,11-dioxonaphthacene-2-carboxamide.
$C_{22}H_{24}N_2O_8$ = 444.4.
CAS — 60-54-8 (anhydrous tetracycline); 6416-04-2 (tetracycline trihydrate).
ATC — A01AB13; D06AA04; J01AA07; S01AA09; S02AA08; S03AA02.
Pharmacopoeias. In *Eur.* (see p.vi), *Jpn,* and *US.*

Tetracycline (anhydrous) 1 g is approximately equivalent to 1.08 g of tetracycline hydrochloride.

Pharmacopoeial description
Ph. Eur.: A yellow crystalline powder. Very slightly soluble in water; soluble in alcohol and in methyl alcohol; sparingly soluble in acetone; practically insoluble in ether. It dissolves in dilute acid and alkaline solutions. A 1% suspension in water has a pH of 3.5 to 6.0. Protect from light.

USP 25: A yellow, odourless, crystalline powder. It darkens in strong sunlight. Soluble 1 in 2500 of water and 1 in 50 of alcohol; practically insoluble in chloroform and in ether; soluble in methyl alcohol; freely soluble in dilute acids and in alkali hydroxide solutions. It loses not more than 13% of its weight on drying. A 1% suspension in water has a pH of 3.0 to 7.0. The potency of tetracycline is reduced in solutions having a pH below 2 and it is rapidly destroyed in solutions of alkali hydroxides. Store in airtight containers. Protect from light.

Tetracycline Hydrochloride   (169-c)

Tetracycline Hydrochloride (BANM, rINNM).
Tetracyclini Hydrochloridum.
$C_{22}H_{24}N_2O_8,HCl$ = 480.9.
CAS — 64-75-5.
Pharmacopoeias. In *Chin., Eur.* (see p.vi), *Int., Jpn, Pol.,* and *US.*
US also includes Epitetracycline Hydrochloride.

Incompatibilities. Tetracycline injections have an acid pH and incompatibility may reasonably be expected with alkaline preparations, or with drugs unstable at low pH. Tetracyclines can chelate metal cations to produce insoluble complexes, and incompatibility has been reported with solutions containing metallic salts. Reports of incompatibility are not always consistent, and other factors, such as the strength and composition of the vehicles used, may play a role.

Pharmacopoeial description

Ph. Eur.: A yellow crystalline powder. Soluble in water; slightly soluble in alcohol; practically insoluble in acetone and in ether. It dissolves in solutions of alkali hydroxides and carbonates. Solutions in water become turbid on standing, owing to the precipitation of tetracycline. A 1% solution in water has a pH of 1.8 to 2.8. Store in airtight containers. Protect from light.

USP 25: A yellow, odourless, hygroscopic, crystalline, powder. Tetracycline hydrochloride darkens in moist air when exposed to strong sunlight. Soluble 1 in 10 of water and 1 in 100 of alcohol; practically insoluble in chloroform and in ether; soluble in solutions of alkali hydroxides and carbonates, although it is rapidly destroyed by alkali hydroxide solutions. A 1% solution in water has a pH of 1.8 to 2.8. The potency of tetracycline hydrochloride is reduced in solutions having a pH below 2. Store in airtight containers. Protect from light.

Tetracycline Phosphate Complex (170-s)

Tetracycline Phosphate Complex (BAN).
CAS — 1336-20-5.
Pharmacopoeias. Jpn includes Tetracycline Metaphosphate ($C_{22}H_{24}N_2O_8$, HPO_3, $\frac{1}{5}NaPO_3$ = 544.8).

A complex of sodium metaphosphate and tetracycline.

Stability. Tetracycline undergoes reversible epimerisation in solution to the less active 4-epitetracycline;[1,2] the degree of epimerisation is dependent on pH, and is greatest at a pH of about 3, with conversion of some 55% to the epimer at equilibrium.[1] The rate at which epimerisation occurs is affected by a variety of factors including temperature and the presence of phosphate or citrate ions.[1] Intravenous solutions of tetracycline hydrochloride with a pH between 3 and 5 have been reported to be stable for 6 hours, but to lose approximately 8 to 12% of their potency in 24 hours at room temperature.[3] Although epimerisation has been observed to be the dominant degradation reaction at pH 2.5 to 5, outside this pH range other reactions become important, with the pH-dependent formation of anhydrotetracycline at very low pH, and oxidation to isotetracycline at alkaline pH.[4]

In contrast to the case in solution, suspensions of tetracycline hydrochloride with a pH between 4 and 7 are stable for at least 3 months.[2] This is because epimerisation, which continues until an equilibrium is achieved between tetracycline and its epimer, depends only on the portion in solution, and the solubility of tetracycline at this pH range is low.

The stability of solid dosage forms and powder at various temperatures and humidities has also been studied; tetracycline hydrochloride was fairly stable when stored at 37° and 66% humidity for 2 months, with about a 10% loss of potency, but the phosphate was rather less stable, with potency losses of 25 to 40% and the formation of potentially toxic degradation products.[5] Comparison with other tetracyclines indicated that tetracycline was less stable than demeclocycline and more stable than rolitetracycline.[5] However, although this study, and an accelerated stability study carried out by WHO[6] indicate that there is a risk of deterioration of solid dose tetracycline, in practice a study of its stability during shipment to the tropics found that deterioration was not a problem.[7]

1. Remmers EG, *et al.* Some observations on the kinetics of the C4 epimerization of tetracycline. *J Pharm Sci* 1963; **52**: 752–6.
2. Grobben-Verpoorten A, *et al.* Determination of the stability of tetracycline suspensions by high performance liquid chromatography. *Pharm Weekbl (Sci)* 1985; **7**: 104–8.
3. Parker EA. Solution additive chemical incompatibility study. *Am J Hosp Pharm* 1967; **24**: 434–9.
4. Vej-Hansen B, Bundgaard H. Kinetic study of factors affecting the stability of tetracycline in aqueous solution. *Arch Pharm Chemi (Sci)* 1978; **6**: 201–14.
5. Walton VC, *et al.* Anhydrotetracycline and 4-epianhydrotetracycline in market tetracyclines and aged tetracycline products. *J Pharm Sci* 1970; **59**: 1160–4.
6. WHO. WHO expert committee on specifications for pharmaceutical preparations: thirty-first report. *WHO Tech Rep Ser 790* 1990.
7. Hogerzeil HV, *et al.* Stability of essential drugs during shipment to the tropics. *BMJ* 1992; **304**: 210–14.

Adverse Effects

The side-effects of tetracycline are common to all tetracyclines. Gastrointestinal effects including nausea, vomiting, and diarrhoea are common especially with high doses and most are attributed to irritation of the mucosa. Other effects that have been reported include dry mouth, glossitis and discoloration of the tongue, stomatitis, and dysphagia. Oesophageal ulceration has also been reported, particularly after ingestion of capsules or tablets with insufficient water at bedtime.

Oral candidiasis, vulvovaginitis, and pruritus ani occur, mainly due to overgrowth with *Candida albicans*, and there may be overgrowth of resistant coliform organisms, such as *Pseudomonas* spp. and *Proteus* spp., causing diarrhoea. More seriously, enterocolitis due to superinfection with resistant staphylococci and pseudomembranous colitis due to *Clostridium difficile* have occasionally been reported. It has been suggested that disturbances in the intestinal flora

are more common with tetracycline than with better absorbed analogues such as doxycycline.

Renal dysfunction has been reported with tetracyclines, and particularly exacerbation of dysfunction in those with pre-existing renal impairment. Usual therapeutic doses given to patients with renal disease increase the severity of uraemia with increased excretion of nitrogen and losses of sodium, accompanied by acidosis and hyperphosphataemia. These effects are related to the dose and the severity of renal impairment and are probably due to the anti-anabolic effects of the tetracycline. Acute renal failure and nephritis have occurred rarely.

Increases in liver enzyme values have been reported with tetracyclines, and in some cases severe and sometimes fatal hepatotoxicity, associated with fatty changes in the liver and pancreatitis, has occurred in pregnant women given tetracycline intravenously for pyelonephritis, and in patients with renal impairment or those given high doses.

Tetracyclines are deposited in deciduous and permanent teeth during their formation, causing discoloration and enamel hypoplasia. They are also deposited in calcifying areas in bone and the nails and interfere with bone growth when given in therapeutic doses to young infants or pregnant women. An increase in intracranial pressure with headache, visual disturbances, and papilloedema has been reported in patients given tetracyclines; the use of tetracyclines in infants has been associated with a bulging fontanelle. If raised intracranial pressure occurs tetracycline treatment should be stopped.

Hypersensitivity to the tetracyclines is much less common than to the beta-lactams, but hypersensitivity reactions, including rashes, fixed drug eruptions, exfoliative dermatitis, toxic epidermal necrolysis, drug fever, pericarditis, angioedema, urticaria, and asthma have been reported; anaphylaxis has occurred very rarely. Photosensitivity, which has been reported with most tetracyclines but particularly with demeclocycline and other long-acting analogues, appears to be phototoxic rather than photoallergic in nature. Paraesthesia may be an early sign of impending phototoxicity. Nail discoloration and onycholysis may occur. Abnormal pigmentation of the skin and eye has occurred rarely: permanent discoloration of the cornea has been reported in infants born to mothers given tetracycline in high doses during pregnancy. Myopia in patients taking tetracyclines may be due to transient hydration of the lens. Local pain and irritation can occur when tetracyclines are given parenterally and thrombophlebitis may follow intravenous injections. A Jarisch-Herxheimer reaction occurs commonly in patients with relapsing fever treated with tetracycline.

Although rare, agranulocytosis, aplastic anaemia, haemolytic anaemia, eosinophilia, neutropenia, and thrombocytopenia have been reported. Tetracyclines may produce hypoprothrombinaemia. They have also been associated with reductions in serum-vitamin B concentrations, including a case of folate deficiency and concomitant megaloblastic anaemia.

The use of out-of-date or deteriorated tetracyclines has been associated with the development of a reversible Fanconi-type syndrome characterised by polyuria and polydipsia with nausea, glycosuria, aminoaciduria, hypophosphataemia, hypokalaemia, and hyperuricaemia with acidosis and proteinuria; these effects have been attributed to the presence of degradation products, in particular anhydroepitetracycline.

Other adverse effects that have occasionally been reported with tetracyclines include increased muscle weakness in patients with myasthenia gravis and provocation of lupus erythematosus.

Precautions

The tetracyclines are contra-indicated in patients hypersensitive to any of this group of antibacterials, since cross-sensitivity may occur. They should be avoided in patients with systemic lupus erythematosus. In general the tetracyclines, with the exception of doxycycline and perhaps minocycline, are considered to be contra-indicated in renal impairment, particularly if severe: if they must be given, doses should be reduced.

Tetracyclines should not be used during pregnancy because of the risk of hepatotoxicity in the mother as well as the effects on the developing fetus. They should also be avoided during breast feeding and in children up to the age of 8, or some authorities say 12, years. Use in pregnancy, potentially during breast feeding, or in childhood, may result in impaired bone growth and permanent discoloration of the child's teeth.

Care should be taken if tetracyclines are given to patients with impaired liver function and high doses should be avoided. Patients who may be exposed to direct sunlight should be warned of the risk of photosensitivity. Care is advisable in patients with myasthenia gravis, who may be at risk of neuromuscular blockade. Serum-monitoring of tetracyclines may be helpful in patients with risk factors receiving parenteral therapy: it has been suggested that serum concentrations of tetracycline should not exceed 15 µg per mL. When administered by mouth, tetracyclines (notably doxycycline, see p.200) should be taken with plenty of fluid while sitting or standing to avoid the risk of oesophageal ulceration.

Tetracycline may interfere with some diagnostic tests including determination of urinary catecholamines or glucose.

Porphyria. Tetracyclines are considered to be probably safe in patients with porphyria, although there is conflicting experimental evidence of porphyrinogenicity. Doxycycline has been associated with acute attacks of porphyria and is considered unsafe in porphyric patients, and results from *animals* or *in-vitro* systems suggest that oxytetracycline might be porphyrinogenic.

Interactions

The absorption of the tetracyclines is reduced by divalent and trivalent cations such as aluminium, bismuth, calcium, iron, magnesium, and zinc, and therefore concomitant administration of tetracyclines with antacids, iron preparations, some foods such as milk and dairy products, or other preparations containing such cations, whether as active ingredients or excipients, may result in subtherapeutic serum concentrations of the antibacterial. Sodium bicarbonate, colestipol, and kaolin-pectin are also reported to reduce tetracycline absorption, but potential reductions due to cimetidine or sucralfate are probably of little clinical significance.

The nephrotoxic effects of the tetracyclines may be exacerbated by diuretics, methoxyflurane, or other potentially nephrotoxic drugs. Potentially hepatotoxic drugs should be used with caution in patients receiving tetracyclines. An increased incidence of benign intracranial hypertension has been reported when retinoids and tetracyclines are given together. Tetracyclines have been reported to produce increased concentrations of lithium, digoxin, and theophylline (although these interactions are not strongly established); the effects of oral anticoagulants may also be increased. There have been occasional reports of tetracyclines increasing the toxic effects of ergot alkaloids and methotrexate. Tetracyclines may decrease plasma-atovaquone concentrations. Ocular inflammation has occurred following the use of ocular preparations preserved with thiomersal in some patients receiving tetracyclines. Tetracyclines may decrease the effectiveness of oral contraceptives.

Because of possible antagonism of the action of the penicillins by predominantly bacteriostatic tetracyclines it has been recommended that the two types of drug should not be given concomitantly, especially when a rapid bactericidal action is necessary.

Antimicrobial Action

The group of tetracycline antibiotics is mainly bacteriostatic, with a broad spectrum of antimicrobial activity including chlamydias, mycoplasmas, rickettsias, and spirochaetes, many aerobic and anaerobic Gram-positive and Gram-negative pathogenic bacteria, and some protozoa.

Mechanism of action. Tetracyclines are taken up into sensitive bacterial cells by an active transport process. Once within the cell they bind reversibly to the 30S subunit of the ribosome, preventing the binding of aminoacyl transfer RNA and inhibiting protein synthesis and hence cell growth. Although tetracyclines also inhibit protein synthesis in mammalian cells they are not actively taken up, permitting selective activity against the infecting organism.

Spectrum of activity. The following pathogenic organisms are usually sensitive to tetracyclines.

Gram-positive cocci including some strains of *Staphylococcus aureus* and coagulase-negative staphylococci, and streptococci including *Str. pneumoniae, Str. pyogenes* (group A), some *Str. agalactiae* (group B), and some viridans streptococci. Enterococci are essentially resistant.

Other sensitive Gram-positive bacteria include strains of *Actinomyces israelii, Bacillus anthracis, Erysipelothrix rhusiopathiae, Listeria monocytogenes,* and among the anaerobes some *Clostridium* spp. *Nocardia* spp. are generally much less susceptible although some are sensitive to minocycline. *Propionibacterium acnes* is susceptible although the action of the tetracyclines in acne is complex and benefit may be seen even at subinhibitory concentrations.

Gram-negative cocci including *Neisseria meningitidis* (meningococci) and *N. gonorrhoeae* (gonococci), *Acinetobacter* spp., and *Moraxella catarrhalis* (*Branhamella catarrhalis*).

Other sensitive Gram-negative aerobes include *Bordetella pertussis, Brucella* spp., *Calymmatobacterium granulomatis, Campylobacter* spp., *Eikenella corrodens, Francisella tularensis, Haemophilus influenzae* and some strains of *Haemophilus ducreyi, Legionella* spp., *Pasteurella multocida, Streptobacillus moniliformis,* and various members of the Vibrionaceae including *Aeromonas hydrophila, Plesiomonas shigelloides, Vibrio cholerae* and *Vibrio parahaemolyticus.* Although many of the Enterobacteriaceae, including *Salmonella, Shigella,* and *Yersinia* spp., are susceptible, resistant strains are common; *Proteus* and *Providencia* spp. are not susceptible. *Pseudomonas aeruginosa* is not susceptible either, although some other species formerly classified as *Pseudomonas* respond, including *Burkholderia mallei, B. pseudomallei,* and *Stenotrophomonas maltophilia* (*Xanthomonas maltophilia*).

Among the Gram-negative anaerobes *Bacteroides fragilis* may sometimes be susceptible, although wild strains are often resistant, and *Fusobacterium* may also be sensitive.

Other organisms usually sensitive to tetracyclines include *Helicobacter pylori, Chlamydia* spp., *Rickettsia* and *Coxiella* spp., many spirochaetes including *Borrelia burgdorferi, Leptospira* spp., and *Treponema pallidum,* atypical mycobacteria such as *Mycobacterium marinum,* and mycoplasmas including *Mycoplasma pneumoniae* and *Ureaplasma urealyticum.* In addition the tetracyclines are active against some protozoa including *Plasmodium falciparum* and *Entamoeba histolytica.*

Fungi, yeasts, and viruses are generally resistant.

Minimum inhibitory concentrations (MICs) of tetracycline for the most sensitive organisms (*Streptococci, Neisseria,* sensitive *Shigella* and *Salmonella* spp., *Bacteroides fragilis*) range from about 0.25 to 2 µg per mL, but organisms with MICs up to about 4 µg per mL are considered sensitive. MICs for the other tetracyclines are generally similar, although minocycline, and to a lesser extent doxycycline, are somewhat more active *in vitro* against many susceptible organisms than the other tetracyclines.

Resistance. Resistance to the tetracyclines is usually plasmid-mediated and transferable. It is often inducible, and appears to be associated with the ability to prevent accumulation of the antibiotic within the bacterial cell, both by decreasing active transport of the drug into the cell and by increasing tetracycline efflux.

Unsurprisingly, given the widespread use of the tetracyclines (including as components of animal feeds, although this is now banned in some countries), resistant strains of the majority of sensitive species have now been reported. Resistance has increased particularly among Enterobacteriaceae such as *Escherichia coli, Enterobacter, Salmonella,* and *Shigella* spp., especially in hospital isolates, and multiple resistance is common. Staphylococci are commonly resistant, although doxycycline or minocycline are occasionally effective against tetracycline-resistant strains. Resistance is now also common among the streptococci, with reported resistance rates of 15 to 62% among group A, and even more among group B streptococci; resistance among pneumococci is reported to range from 3 to 23%, with multiple drug resistance becoming common. Emergence of high-level tetracycline-resistant strains of *Neisseria gonorrhoeae* is common in some areas. Frequent resistance is also seen in clostridia, and in *Bacteroides fragilis* (among more than 60% of isolates in some countries), while increasing resistance amongst *Haemophilus ducreyi* has limited the value of tetracyclines in chancroid.

Pharmacokinetics

Most tetracyclines are incompletely absorbed from the gastrointestinal tract, about 60 to 80% of a dose of tetracycline usually being available. The degree of absorption is diminished by the presence of divalent and trivalent metal ions, with which tetracyclines form stable insoluble complexes, and to a variable degree by milk or food. However, the more lipophilic analogues doxycycline and minocycline are almost completely absorbed (more than 90%), and they are little affected by food. Formulation with phosphate may enhance the absorption of tetracycline.

Administration of tetracycline 500 mg by mouth every 6 hours generally produces steady-state plasma concentrations of 4 to 5 µg per mL, whereas with doxycycline a dose of 200 mg is sufficient to produce peak concentrations of about 3 µg per mL. Peak plasma concentrations occur about 1 to 3 hours after ingestion. Higher concentrations can be achieved after intravenous administration; concentrations may be higher in women than in men.

In the circulation, tetracyclines are bound to plasma proteins in varying degrees, but reported values differ considerably ranging from about 20 to 40% for oxytetracycline, 20 to 65% for tetracycline, about 45% for chlortetracycline, 35 to 90% for demeclocycline, 75% for minocycline, and about 80 to 95% for methacycline and for doxycycline.

The tetracyclines are widely distributed throughout the body tissues and fluids. Concentrations in CSF are relatively low, but may be raised if the meninges are inflamed. Small amounts appear in saliva, and in the fluids of the eye and lung; higher concentrations are achieved with more lipid-soluble analogues such as minocycline and doxycycline. Tetracyclines appear in breast milk, where concentrations may be 60% or more of those in the plasma. They diffuse across the placenta and appear in the fetal circulation in concentrations of about 25 to 75% of those in the maternal blood. Tetracyclines are retained at sites of new bone formation and recent calcification and in developing teeth.

The tetracyclines have been classified in terms of their duration of action in the body, although the divisions appear to overlap somewhat. Of the 'short-acting' derivatives, chlortetracycline has a reported half-life of about 6 hours, oxytetracycline 9 hours, and tetracycline 8 hours, although reported values for the latter two range from about 6 to 12 hours. The 'intermediate-acting' tetracyclines, demeclocycline and methacycline, have reported half-lives of about 12 and 14 hours respectively, although various sources cite values of 7 to 17 hours, and the 'long-acting' minocycline and doxycycline have half-lives of about 16 to 18 hours, with reported values anywhere between 11 to 26 and 12 to 24 hours respectively.

The tetracyclines are excreted in the urine and in the faeces. Renal clearance is by glomerular filtration. Up to 60% of an intravenous dose of tetracycline, and up to 55% of a dose by mouth, is eliminated unchanged in the urine; tetracycline concentrations in the urine of up to 300 µg per mL may be reached 2 hours after a usual dose is taken and be maintained for up to 12 hours. For most tetracyclines between about 40 to 70% of a dose is excreted in the urine, but for chlortetracycline, doxycycline, and minocycline, rather less is eliminated by this route since chlortetracycline and minocycline undergo metabolism, and doxycycline is excreted mainly in the faeces. Urinary excretion is increased if urine is alkalinised.

The tetracyclines are excreted in the bile, where concentrations 5 to 25 times those in plasma can occur. Since there is some enterohepatic reabsorption complete elimination is slow. Considerable quantities occur in the faeces after administration by mouth and lesser amounts after administration by injection.

Uses and Administration

The tetracyclines are bacteriostatic antibiotics with a wide spectrum of activity and have been used in the treatment of a large number of infections caused by susceptible organisms (see Antimicrobial Action, above). With the emergence of bacterial resistance and the development of other antibacterials their use has become more restricted, but they remain the usual drugs of choice in rickettsial infections, including ehrlichiosis, typhus, spotted fevers, trench fever, and Q fever; chlamydial infections, including psittacosis, lymphogranuloma venereum, trachoma, non-gonococcal urethritis, chlamydial conjunctivitis, and pharyngitis, sinusitis, or pneumonia due to *Chlamydia pneumoniae*; and mycoplasmal infections, especially pneumonia caused by *Mycoplasma pneumoniae*. They are widely used as part of regimens for pelvic inflammatory disease. A tetracycline is often used in the treatment of cholera, in conjunction with fluid and electrolyte replacement, and is usually the treatment of choice in relapsing fever and in the early stages of Lyme disease. They are also used in the oral treatment of acne (below) and rosacea. Tetracyclines may be of benefit in the treatment of melioidosis. They may be used for mouth infections, especially in destructive forms of periodontal disease. Tetracyclines are used, often in association with streptomycin or rifampicin, in the treatment of brucellosis, and may be given with streptomycin in plague, and as an alternative to streptomycin in the treatment of tularaemia. Tetracyclines are used as an alternative to other drugs in the treatment of actinomycosis, infected animal bites, anthrax, bronchitis, gastro-enteritis (due to *Campylobacter* or *Yersinia enterocolitica*), granuloma inguinale, leptospirosis, and syphilis. Opinions differ as to their value in listeriosis. There are now relatively few areas where tetracycline-resistant gonococci are uncommon, which limits the value of tetracyclines in gonorrhoea, but they are often given with antigonorrhoeal therapy to treat concomitant chlamydial infections, and they retain some value in the prophylaxis and treatment of neonatal gonococcal conjunctivitis by topical application. For details of these infections and their treatment, see under Choice of Antibacterial, p.114.

Tetracyclines have antiprotozoal actions and tetracycline or doxycycline may be given in conjunction with quinine in the management of falciparum malaria resistant to chloroquine (below). Tetracyclines are the usual treatment for balantidiasis (p.583) and they have been used in amoebiasis in association with an amoebicide in the treatment of severe amoebic dysentery and in *Dientamoeba fragilis* infections (p.582).

Tetracycline has been used in the management of malabsorption syndromes such as tropical sprue.

Tetracycline has been instilled as a sclerosant solution for pleurodesis and in the management of malignant effusions (p.489).

Administration and dosage. In the treatment of systemic infections the tetracyclines are usually administered by mouth. They should be taken with plenty of fluid while sitting or standing to avoid the risk of oesophageal ulceration. In severe acute infections they may be given by slow intravenous infusion or, rarely, by intramuscular injection; parenteral therapy should be substituted by oral administration as soon as practicable. Doses of tetracycline base and tetracycline hydrochloride are expressed in terms of tetracycline hydrochloride.

The usual adult dosage of tetracycline hydrochloride is 250 or 500 mg every 6 hours by mouth, preferably one hour before or 2 hours after meals. Higher doses, up to 4 g daily have occasionally been given in severe infection, but increase the risk of adverse effects. Modified-release formulations are available in some countries.

In severe infections, tetracycline hydrochloride has been administered by slow intravenous infusion every 12 hours as a solution containing not more than 0.5% in a usual total dose of 0.5 to 1 g daily, although up to 2 g daily has been given. If the intramuscular route is to be used, tetracycline hydrochloride has been given in a dosage of 200 to 300 mg daily in divided doses. As intramuscular injections are painful, procaine hydrochloride is usually included in the solution.

In children, the effects on teeth should be considered and tetracyclines only used when absolutely essential. Tetracycline hydrochloride has been given to older children (over 8 years) in doses of 25 to 50 mg per kg body-weight daily by mouth in divided doses.

Care is required if tetracyclines are given to the elderly. They should be avoided if possible in renal impairment (with the exception of doxycycline and minocycline) and doses reduced if they must be used.

Other routes. Although topical application carries the risk of sensitisation and may contribute to the development of resistance tetracycline hydrochloride has been applied as a 3% ointment; a 0.2% solution has been used in acne but systemic treatment appears to produce better results. A 1% eye ointment or eye drops have been used in the treatment of ocular infections due to sensitive organisms. For the treatment of pleural effusions, 500 mg of tetracycline hydrochloride has been dissolved in 30 to 50 mL of sodium chloride 0.9% and instilled into the pleural space. For periodontal disease, fibres that release tetracycline are available in some countries; they are inserted into the periodontal pocket.

◊ Reviews.
1. Chopra I, *et al.* Tetracyclines, molecular and clinical aspects. *J Antimicrob Chemother* 1992; **29**: 245–77.

Malaria. Tetracyclines have been used when necessary in combination with quinine to treat malaria (p.428).[1] They are active against both blood and tissue forms of the parasite, and high cure rates have been obtained with such combinations. The action of tetracyclines is relatively slow and they should never be used alone to treat malaria.

The dose of tetracycline hydrochloride given by mouth with quinine on days 1 to 3 has varied; doses of 1 to 2 g daily have been given for 7 days or 1 g daily for 7 to 10 days. The total daily dose should be divided, and that usually recommended is 250 mg four times daily, although 500 mg twice daily may be more practical in the field. If the patient is too ill for oral medication quinine should be given parenterally until the oral therapy can be begun; tetracycline should not be administered parenterally. Although tetracycline therapy is normally contra-indicated in pregnant women and children, it may have to be given if the risk of withholding the drug is judged to outweigh the risk to developing teeth and bones.

The dose of doxycycline given by mouth following treatment with quinine is 200 mg daily for at least 7 days.

Tetracyclines are not considered suitable for extended prophylactic use, although doxycycline 100 mg daily has been used for short-term prophylaxis in areas of high risk where other drugs are likely to be ineffective.

1. WHO. *WHO model prescribing information: drugs used in parasitic diseases.* 2nd ed. Geneva: WHO, 1995.

Mouth ulceration. In recurrent aphthous stomatitis(p.1206) tetracyclines, used as mouthwashes, reportedly reduce ulcer pain and duration,[1] but their potential for adverse effects if swallowed must be borne in mind, and their acidity may damage tooth enamel if poorly formulated. Topical application of a tetracycline has been considered the treatment of choice for oral ulceration associated with Behçet's syndrome (p.1047).

The symbol † denotes a preparation no longer actively marketed

1. Henricsson V, Axéll T. Treatment of recurrent aphthous ulcers with Aureomycin mouth rinse or Zendium dentifrice. *Acta Odontol Scand* 1985; **43**: 47–52.

Peptic ulcer disease. Tetracycline has been used as part of triple therapy to eradicate *Helicobacter pylori* in patients with peptic ulcer disease (p.1208). The usual dose of tetracycline in these regimens has been 500 mg four times daily for 2 weeks.

Rheumatic disorders. Tetracyclines, usually minocycline, are among the wide range of drugs tried in rheumatoid arthritis (p.9). Studies[1,2] indicate that minocycline can produce modest beneficial effects in patients with advanced rheumatoid arthritis, but the clinical significance of these improvements has been questioned.[3] Greater symptomatic improvements have been obtained with minocycline when it is used in patients with early rheumatoid arthritis;[4] continued treatment with minocycline may also reduce the need for disease-modifying antirheumatic drugs.[5] Its mechanism of action, whether antibacterial or anti-inflammatory, remains to be determined.[6] There has been speculation over the role of infection as a cause of rheumatoid arthritis.[3,7]

The role of antibacterials is also uncertain in reactive arthritis (p.116), although long-term treatment with a tetracycline in addition to an NSAID has been reported to shorten the duration of reactive arthritis resulting from *Chlamydia trachomatis* infection.[8]

1. Kloppenburg M, *et al.* Minocycline in active rheumatoid arthritis. *Arthritis Rheum* 1994; **37**: 629–36.
2. Tilley BC, *et al.* Minocycline in rheumatoid arthritis: a 48-week, double-blind, placebo-controlled trial. *Ann Intern Med* 1995; **122**: 81–9.
3. McKendry RJR. Is rheumatoid arthritis caused by an infection? *Lancet* 1995; **345**: 1319–20.
4. O'Dell JR, *et al.* Treatment of early rheumatoid arthritis with minocycline or placebo: results of a randomized double-blind, placebo-controlled trial. *Arthritis Rheum* 1997; **40**: 842–8.
5. O'Dell JR, *et al.* Treatment of early seropositive rheumatoid arthritis with minocycline: four-year follow-up of a double-blind, placebo-controlled trial. *Arthritis Rheum* 1999; **42**: 1691–5.
6. Paulus HE. Minocycline treatment of rheumatoid arthritis. *Ann Intern Med* 1995; **122**: 147–8.
7. O'Dell JR. Is there a role for antibiotics in the treatment of patients with rheumatoid arthritis? *Drugs* 1999; **57**: 279–82.
8. Lauhio A. Reactive arthritis: consider combination treatment. *BMJ* 1994; **308**: 1302–3.

Skin disorders. ACNE. Tetracyclines may be used topically or orally in the treatment of acne (p.1103). In acne, antibacterials appear to act by suppressing the growth of *Propionibacterium acnes*, but also by suppressing inflammation. Topical tetracycline is used for mild inflammatory acne and as an adjunct to systemic treatment in more severe forms. Tetracyclines, given orally, are the drugs of choice for moderate acne and may be considered, in high doses, for severe acne. Licensed doses in the UK are: doxycycline 50 mg daily; minocycline 100 mg daily; oxytetracycline 250 to 500 mg daily; and tetracycline 1 g daily. Higher doses for doxycycline of 100 mg daily and for oxytetracycline of 1 g daily are advocated in the *British National Formulary*. Treatment should be changed to another antibacterial if there has been no improvement in the first 3 months. Maximum improvement is said to occur after 3 to 6 months, but treatment may need to continue for 2 or more years.

Minocycline has been reported to have superior antibacterial activity against *P. acnes*[1] and a reduced incidence of resistance,[1] and has also been more effective than erythromycin against oxytetracycline-resistant acne.[2] However, it can cause skin pigmentation and may be associated rarely with immunologically mediated reactions[3] and some dermatologists do not favour its use. Although the usual dose of minocycline is 100 mg daily in one or two divided doses some patients may need up to 200 mg daily.[4]

1. Eady EA, *et al.* Superior antibacterial action and reduced incidence of bacterial resistance in minocycline compared to tetracycline-treated acne patients. *Br J Dermatol* 1990; **122**: 233–44.
2. Knaggs HE, *et al.* The role of oral minocycline and erythromycin in tetracycline therapy-resistant acne—a retrospective study and a review. *J Dermatol Treat* 1993; **4**: 53–6.
3. Ferner RE, Moss C. Minocycline for acne. *BMJ* 1996; **312**: 138.
4. Goulden V, *et al.* Safety of long-term high-dose minocycline in the treatment of acne. *Br J Dermatol* 1996; **134**: 693–5.

PEMPHIGUS AND PEMPHIGOID. Corticosteroids are generally given to control the blistering in pemphigus and pemphigoid (p.1106), although there have been reports[1-3] suggesting that a tetracycline (often minocycline) may be of value in controlling the lesions associated with various types of pemphigus and pemphigoid.

1. Sawai T, *et al.* Pemphigus vegetans with oesophageal involvement: successful treatment with minocycline and nicotinamide. *Br J Dermatol* 1995; **132**: 668–70.
2. Poskitt L, Wojnarowska F. Minimizing cicatricial pemphigoid orodynia with minocycline. *Br J Dermatol* 1995; **132**: 784–9.
3. Kolbach DN, *et al.* Bullous pemphigoid successfully controlled by tetracycline and nicotinamide. *Br J Dermatol* 1995; **133**: 88–90.

ROSACEA. Tetracycline is the oral antibacterial of choice for the treatment of rosacea (p.1107). Long-term treatment is usually necessary. Tetracycline and doxycycline have also been shown to improve ocular manifestations of rosacea.[1]

1. Frucht-Pery J, *et al.* Efficacy of doxycycline and tetracycline in ocular rosacea. *Am J Ophthalmol* 1993; **116**: 88–92.

Preparations

BP 2001: Tetracycline Capsules; Tetracycline Tablets;
USP 25: Tetracycline Hydrochloride and Nystatin Capsules; Tet-

racycline Hydrochloride Capsules; Tetracycline Hydrochloride for Injection; Tetracycline Hydrochloride for Topical Solution; Tetracycline Hydrochloride Ointment; Tetracycline Hydrochloride Ophthalmic Ointment; Tetracycline Hydrochloride Ophthalmic Suspension; Tetracycline Hydrochloride Oral Suspension; Tetracycline Hydrochloride Tablets; Tetracycline Oral Suspension.

Proprietary Preparations (details are given in Part 3)
Aust.: Achromycin; Actisite; Hostacyclin; Latycin†; Steclin†; Tetrarco†; *Austral.:* Achromycin; Achromycin V; Latycin; Mysteclin; Tetrex; *Belg.:* Hostacycline†; *Braz.:* Ambra-Sinto T; Combitrex; Infex; Miociclin; Statinclyne; Tetrex; *Canad.:* Achromycin V†; Achromycin†; Apo-Tetra; Novo-Tetra; Nu-Tetra; Tetracyn†; *Denm.:* Achromycin†; Actisite†; Dumocyclin; *Fin.:* Apocyclin; Oricyclin; *Fr.:* Florocycline†; *Ger.:* Achromycin; Actisite; Dispatetrin†; Hostacyclin†; Imex; Sagittacin N†; Supramycin; Tefilin; Tetralution; *Hong Kong:* Achromycin V; Apo-Tetra; Medocycline; *Irl.:* Achromycin; Hostacycline†; Topicycline; Tetrex† Recycline; Tevacycline; *Ital.:* Acromicina†; Actisite; Ambramicina; Calociclina†; Spaciclina†; Tetrabioptal; Tetrafosammina; *Mex.:* Acromicina; Ambotetra; Berciclina Enzimatica; Biotricina; Dibaterr; Droclina; Forciclina; Imacol; Inacol; Istix; Laur; Macrocilin; Miciclin; Ofticlin; Parenciclina; Pavitron; Quimocyclar; Rayetetra; Senociclin; Solclin; Te-Br; Tecyn; Terranumonyl; Tetra; Tetranovax; Tetrapres; Tetraprocyn; Tetrazil; Tetrerba; Tetrex; Triclin; Tromicol; *NZ:* Panmycin; *Port.:* Ciclobiotico; Neociclina; *S.Afr.:* Achromycin†; Arcanacycline†; Gammatet†; Hostacycline; Rotet†; Tetrex†; *Singapore:* Latycin; *Spain:* Actisite; Ambramicina†; Bristaciclina†; Kinciclina; Quimpe Antibiotico; Tetra Hubber; *Swed.:* Achromycin†; *Switz.:* Achromycine†; Actisite; Tetraseptine†; Triphacycline; *Thai.:* Achromycin; Hydromycin; Lenocin; Pantocycline; Servitet; Tetralim; Tetrana; *UK:* Achromycin; Economycin; Sustamycin†; Tetrachel†; Topicycline; *USA:* Achromycin V; Actisite; Nor-Tet†; Panmycin; Robitet Robicaps†; Sumycin; Teline†; Tetracap; Tetralan†; Topicycline.

Multi-ingredient: *Aust.:* Eftapan Tetra†; Fluorex Plus; Mysteclin; *Austral.:* Helidac; Mysteclin-V; *Braz.:* Acobiotic; Monocetin; Parenzyme Tetraciclina; Talsutin; Tericin AT; Tricangine-A; Trinotrex; Velutrix; *Fin.:* Helipak T; *Fr.:* Amphocycline; Colicort; *Ger.:* Mysteclin; Polcortolon TC; *Hong Kong:* Talsutin; *Irl.:* Deteclo; *Ital.:* Alfaflor; Colbiocin; Dermobios†; Eubetal Antibiotico; Flumetol Antibiotico; Iducol; Mictasone; Pensulvit; Vitecaf; *Mex.:* Solfranicol; *Port.:* Ciclobiotico; Neociclina Vitaminada; *S.Afr.:* Mysteclin-V†; Riostatin; Tetrex-F†; Tritet†; Vagmycin; *Spain:* Bristaciclina Dental; Bronquinflamatoria†; Gine Heyden; Mucorex Ciclin; Nasopomada; Sanicel; Tantum Ciclina; Terranilo; Tetra Tripsin; *UK:* Deteclo; *USA:* Helidac.

Tetroxoprim (13315-b)

Tetroxoprim *(BAN, USAN, rINN)*.
5-[3,5-Dimethoxy-4-(2-methoxyethoxy)benzyl]pyrimidine-2,4-diyldiamine.
$C_{16}H_{22}N_4O_4 = 334.4.$
CAS — 53808-87-0.

NOTE. Tetroxoprim may be given with sulfadiazine and a preparation of such a combination has been given the approved name Co-tetroxazine, p.193.

Profile
Tetroxoprim is a dihydrofolate reductase inhibitor similar to, but less active than, trimethoprim (p.264). It is used, in conjunction with sulfadiazine, as co-tetroxazine (p.193).
Tetroxoprim embonate has been used similarly.

Preparations
Proprietary Preparations (details are given in Part 3)
Multi-ingredient: *Ger.:* Sterinor; *Ital.:* Oxosint; Sterinor†.

Thenoic Acid (13319-p)

Tenoic Acid; 2-Thiophenic Acid. Thiophene-2-carboxylic acid.
$C_5H_4O_2S = 128.1.$
CAS — 527-72-0.

Profile
Thenoic acid has been administered by mouth, rectally, or as nasal drops as the sodium salt, and by mouth as the lithium salt, in the treatment of respiratory-tract infections. The monoethanolamine salt has been used as a mucolytic.

Preparations
Proprietary Preparations (details are given in Part 3)
Fr.: Soufrane; *Spain:* Trophires†.

Multi-ingredient: *Fr.:* Glossithiase; Rhinotrophyl; Trophires; Trophires Compose; *Spain:* Trophires.

Thiamphenicol (171-w)

Thiamphenicol *(BAN, USAN, rINN)*.
CB-8053; Dextrosulphenidol; Thiamfenicol; Thiamphenicolum; Thiophenicol; Tiamfenicolo; Win-5063-2; Win-5063 (racephenicol). (αR,βR)-2,2-Dichloro-N-(β-hydroxy-α-hydroxymethyl-4-methylsulphonylphenethyl)acetamide.
$C_{12}H_{15}Cl_2NO_5S = 356.2.$
CAS — 15318-45-3 (thiamphenicol); 847-25-6 (racephenicol).
ATC — J01BA02.

NOTE. Racephenicol, the racemic form of thiamphenicol, is *USAN*.

Pharmacopoeias. In Eur. (see p.vi).

Pharmacopoeial description

Ph. Eur.: A fine, white or yellowish-white, crystalline powder or crystals. Slightly soluble in water, in ether, and in ethyl acetate; sparingly soluble in dehydrated alcohol and in acetone; freely soluble in acetonitrile and in dimethylformamide; very soluble in dimethylacetamide; soluble in methyl alcohol. Protect from light and moisture.

Thiamphenicol Glycinate Hydrochloride

(172-e)

Thiamphenicol Aminoacetate Hydrochloride; Tiamfenicolo Glicinato Cloridrato.
$C_{14}H_{18}Cl_2N_2O_6S,HCl = 449.7$.
CAS — 2393-92-2 (thiamphenicol glycinate); 2611-61-2 (thiamphenicol glycinate hydrochloride).
Pharmacopoeias. In It.

1.26 g of monograph substance is approximately equivalent to 1 g of thiamphenicol.

Adverse Effects and Precautions

As for Chloramphenicol, p.179.

Thiamphenicol is probably more liable to cause dose-dependent reversible depression of the bone marrow than chloramphenicol but it is not usually associated with aplastic anaemia. Thiamphenicol also appears to be less likely to cause the 'grey syndrome' in neonates.

Doses of thiamphenicol should be reduced in patients with renal impairment. It is probably not necessary to reduce doses in patients with impaired liver function.

Interactions

As for Chloramphenicol, p.180.

Although thiamphenicol is not metabolised in the liver and might not be expected to be affected by drugs which induce hepatic enzymes, it is reported to inhibit hepatic microsomal enzymes and may affect the metabolism of other drugs.

Antimicrobial Action

Thiamphenicol has a broad spectrum of activity resembling that of chloramphenicol (p.180). Although in general it is less active than chloramphenicol it is reported to be equally effective, and more actively bactericidal, against *Haemophilus* and *Neisseria* spp. MICs for the most sensitive strains range from about 0.1 to 2 μg per mL.

Cross-resistance has been reported between thiamphenicol and chloramphenicol. However, some strains resistant to chloramphenicol may be susceptible to thiamphenicol.

Pharmacokinetics

Thiamphenicol is absorbed from the gastrointestinal tract following oral administration and peak serum concentrations of 3 to 6 μg per mL have been achieved about 2 hours after a 500-mg dose.

Thiamphenicol has been reported to diffuse into the CSF, across the placenta, into breast milk, and to penetrate well into the lungs. About 10% is bound to plasma proteins. The half-life of thiamphenicol is around 2 to 3 hours but unlike chloramphenicol the half-life is increased in patients with renal impairment. It is excreted in the urine, about 70% of a dose being excreted in 24 hours as unchanged drug. It undergoes little or no conjugation with glucuronic acid in the liver. A small amount is excreted in the bile and the faeces.

Uses and Administration

Thiamphenicol has been used similarly to chloramphenicol (p.181) in the treatment of susceptible infections, including sexually transmitted diseases. The usual adult dose is 1.5 g daily by mouth in divided doses; up to 3 g daily has been given initially in severe infections. A daily dose of 30 to 100 mg per kg body-weight may be used in children. Equivalent doses may be administered by intramuscular or intravenous injection as the more water-soluble glycinate. Doses of thiamphenicol should be reduced in patients with renal insufficiency and may be 0.5 g twice daily for patients with a creatinine clearance of 30 to 60 mL per minute and 0.5 g once daily for patients with a creatinine clearance of 10 to 30 mL per minute.

For the treatment of gonorrhoea, oral doses have ranged from thiamphenicol 2.5 g daily for 1 or 2 days through to thiamphenicol 2.5 g on the first day followed by 2 g daily on each of 4 subsequent days. The single daily dose may be most appropriate for male patients with uncomplicated gonorrhoea and has also been recommended for the treatment of bacterial vaginitis.

Thiamphenicol glycinate may also be given by inhalation, or by endobronchial or intracavitary instillation.

Thiamphenicol has also been used as thiamphenicol glycine acetylcysteinate, thiamphenicol sodium glycinate isophthalolate, and thiamphenicol palmitate.

Preparations

Proprietary Preparations (details are given in Part 3)
Belg.: Fluimucil Antibiotic; Urfamycine; **Braz.:** Flogotisol; Glitisol; **Fr.:** Fluimucil Antibiotic; Thiophenicol; **Ital.:** Flogotisol; Fluimucil Antibiotico; Glitisol; **Mex.:** Tiofenicin; **Spain:** Fluimucil Antibiotico; Urfamycin; **Switz.:** Urfamycine; **Thai.:** Ervin; Thiamcin; Treomycin; Urfamycin.

Multi-ingredient: Braz.: Acobiotic; Fluimucil Biotic; **Thai.:** Fluimucil Antibiotic.

Thioacetazone (7572-j)

Thioacetazone *(BAN, rINN)*.

Amithiozone; TBI/698; Tebezonum; Thiacetazone. 4-Acetamidobenzaldehyde thiosemicarbazone.
$C_{10}H_{12}N_4OS = 236.3$.
CAS — 104-06-3.
Pharmacopoeias. In Int.

Adverse Effects

Gastrointestinal disorders, hypersensitivity reactions including skin rashes, conjunctivitis, and vertigo are the side-effects most frequently reported with thioacetazone although the incidence appears to vary from country to country. Toxic epidermal necrolysis, exfoliative dermatitis, which has sometimes been fatal, and the Stevens-Johnson syndrome have been reported; the incidence of severe skin reactions is especially high in patients with HIV infection (see below). Thioacetazone may cause bone-marrow depression with leucopenia, agranulocytosis, and thrombocytopenia. Acute haemolytic anaemia may occur and a large percentage of patients will have some minor degree of anaemia. Hepatotoxicity with jaundice may also develop and acute hepatic failure has been reported. Cerebral oedema has been reported. Dose-related ototoxicity may occur rarely.

◊ In a 10-year series of 1212 patients with tuberculosis who were treated with a regimen of streptomycin, isoniazid, and thioacetazone, 171 (14%) had adverse reactions associated with thioacetazone. The most common side-effects were giddiness (10%), occurring mainly in association with streptomycin, and skin rashes (3%) including exfoliation and the Stevens-Johnson syndrome.[1]

1. Pearson CA. Thiacetazone toxicity in the treatment of tuberculosis patients in Nigeria. *J Trop Med Hyg* 1978; **81:** 238–42.

Effects on the nervous system. Acute peripheral neuropathy which occurred in a 50-year-old man on 2 separate occasions within 15 minutes of administration of thioacetazone may have been due to an allergic reaction.[1]

1. Gupta PK, *et al.* Acute severe peripheral neuropathy due to thiacetazone. *Indian J Tuberc* 1984; **31:** 126–7.

Effects on the skin. A high incidence of severe and sometimes fatal cutaneous hypersensitivity reactions to thioacetazone has been reported in patients with HIV infection being treated for tuberculosis.[1,2] WHO advised that thioacetazone should be avoided in such patients.[3] Unfortunately, thioacetazone has been one of the mainstays of tuberculosis treatment in the developing world because of its relatively low cost.[4] Some have supported a change to rifampicin-based regimens in, for example, parts of Africa with a high incidence of HIV infection.[5] Others have found a lower frequency of fatalities from adverse cutaneous reactions to thioacetazone than reported previously and have suggested that improved management might allow retention of thioacetazone in tuberculosis programmes.[6] This was rejected by other workers who considered that better and more cost-effective regimens were available than those containing thioacetazone.[7] A pragmatic approach may be to adopt a strategy depending upon the prevailing incidence of HIV infection in the population.[8] Thus, where the incidence of HIV infection is high, ethambutol should be substituted for thioacetazone; where the incidence is moderate, routine HIV testing could be used to identify patients at risk; and where the incidence is low, education of patients on the risks of skin reaction would be adequate.

1. Nunn P, *et al.* Cutaneous hypersensitivity reactions due to thiacetazone in HIV-1 seropositive patients treated for tuberculosis. *Lancet* 1991; **337:** 627–30.
2. Chintu C, *et al.* Cutaneous hypersensitivity reactions due to thiacetazone in the treatment of tuberculosis in Zambian children infected with HIV-I. *Arch Dis Child* 1993; **68:** 665–8.
3. Raviglione MC, *et al.* HIV-associated tuberculosis in developing countries: clinical features, diagnosis, and treatment. *Bull WHO* 1992; **70:** 515–26.
4. Nunn P, *et al.* Thiacetazone—avoid like poison or use with care? *Trans R Soc Trop Med Hyg* 1993; **87:** 578–82.
5. Okwera A, *et al.* Randomised trial of thiacetazone and rifampicin-containing regimens for pulmonary tuberculosis in HIV-infected Ugandans. *Lancet* 1994; **344:** 1323–8.
6. Ipuge YAI, *et al.* Adverse cutaneous reactions to thiacetazone for tuberculosis treatment in Tanzania. *Lancet* 1995; **346:** 657–60.
7. Elliott AM, *et al.* Treatment of tuberculosis in developing countries. *Lancet* 1995; **346:** 1098–9.
8. van Gorkom J, Kibuga DK. Cost-effectiveness and total costs of three alternative strategies for the prevention and management of severe skin reactions attributable to thiacetazone in the treatment of human immunodeficiency virus positive patients with tuberculosis in Kenya. *Tubercle Lung Dis* 1996; **77:** 30–6.

Hypertrichosis. Hypertrichosis occurred in 2 children and was associated with the use of thioacetazone.[1]

1. Nair LV, Sugathan P. Thiacetazone induced hypertrichosis. *Indian J Dermatol Venereol* 1982; **48:** 161–3.

Precautions

The efficacy and toxicity of a regimen of treatment which includes thioacetazone should be determined in a community before it is used widely since there appear to be geographical differences.

Thioacetazone should not be given to patients with hepatic impairment. It has also been suggested that, because thioacetazone has a low therapeutic index and is excreted mainly in the urine, it should not be given to patients with renal impairment. It should probably be avoided in HIV-positive patients because

they are at increased risk of severe adverse effects (see Effects on the Skin, above).

Interactions

Thioacetazone may enhance the ototoxicity of streptomycin.

Antimicrobial Action

Thioacetazone is bacteriostatic. It is effective against most strains of *Mycobacterium tuberculosis*, although sensitivity varies in different parts of the world. The MIC for sensitive strains is 1 μg per mL.

Thioacetazone is also bacteriostatic against *Mycobacterium leprae*. Resistance to thioacetazone develops when used alone. Cross-resistance can develop between thioacetazone and ethionamide or protionamide.

Pharmacokinetics

Thioacetazone is absorbed from the gastrointestinal tract and peak plasma concentrations of 1 to 2 μg per mL have been obtained about 4 to 5 hours after a 150-mg dose. About 20% of a dose is excreted unchanged in the urine. A half-life of about 12 hours has been reported.

Uses and Administration

Thioacetazone has been used in association with other antimycobacterials in the initial and continuation treatment phases of tuberculosis (p.143). Thioacetazone-containing regimens are less effective than the short-course regimens recommended by WHO and are used in long-term regimens combined with isoniazid in some developing countries to reduce drug costs. However, thioacetazone is not generally recommended for use in HIV-positive patients because of the risk of severe adverse reactions (but see Effects on the Skin, above).

Thioacetazone has been used in the treatment of leprosy (p.126), but WHO now considers that such use is no longer justified.

In the treatment of tuberculosis, thioacetazone has been given orally in doses of 150 mg daily or 2.5 mg per kg body-weight daily. Thioacetazone may be used with isoniazid, usually in the continuation phase of some longer treatment regimens, to prevent emergence of isoniazid resistance. Thioacetazone has also been used in the initial phase in association with streptomycin and isoniazid. Daily administration is recommended as the drug is less effective when given intermittently.

Thiostrepton (8708-f)

$C_{72}H_{85}N_{19}O_{18}S_5 = 1664.9$.
CAS — 1393-48-2.
Pharmacopoeias. In US for veterinary use only.

Pharmacopoeial description

USP 25: An antibacterial substance produced by the growth of strains of *Streptomyces azureus*. A white to off-white crystalline solid. Practically insoluble in water, in the lower alcohols, in nonpolar organic solvents, and in dilute aqueous acids or alkalis; soluble in glacial acetic acid, in chloroform, in dimethylformamide, in dimethyl sulfoxide, in dioxan, and in pyridine. Store in airtight containers.

Profile

Thiostrepton is an antibacterial produced by strains of *Streptomyces azureus*. It is included in topical antibacterial preparations for veterinary use.

Tiamulin Fumarate (13337-w)

Tiamulin Fumarate *(BANM, USAN, rINNM)*.

81723-hfu; SQ-14055 (tiamulin); SQ-22947 (tiamulin fumarate). 11-Hydroxy-6,7,10,12-tetramethyl-1-oxo-10-vinylperhydro-3a,7-pentanoinden-8-yl (2-diethylaminoethylthio)acetate hydrogen fumarate.
$C_{28}H_{47}NO_4S,C_4H_4O_4 = 609.8$.
CAS — 55297-95-5 (tiamulin); 555297-96-6 (tiamulin fumarate).

Profile

Tiamulin fumarate is an antibacterial used in veterinary medicine.

Ticarcillin Sodium (173-l)

Ticarcillin Sodium *(BANM, rINNM)*.

BRL-2288; Ticarcillin Disodium *(USAN)*; Ticarcillinum Natricum. The disodium salt of (6R)-6-[2-carboxy-2-(3-thienyl)acetamido]penicillanic acid.
$C_{15}H_{14}N_2Na_2O_6S_2 = 428.4$.
CAS — 34787-01-4 (ticarcillin); 3973-04-4 (ticarcillin); 4697-14-7 (ticarcillin disodium); 29457-07-6 (ticarcillin disodium); 74682-62-5 (ticarcillin monosodium).
Pharmacopoeias. In Eur. (see p.vi), Jpn, and US.
US also includes Ticarcillin Monosodium.

1.1 g of monograph substance is approximately equivalent to 1 g of ticarcillin. Each g of monograph substance represents about 4.7 mmol of sodium.

Incompatibility has been reported with aminoglycosides.

Pharmacopoeial description

Ph. Eur.: A white or slightly yellow, hygroscopic powder. Freely soluble in water; practically insoluble in ether; soluble in methyl alcohol. A 5% solution in water has a pH of 5.5 to 7.5. Store in airtight containers at a temperature of 2° to 8°.

USP 25: A white to pale yellow powder or solid. 1 mg of monograph substance has a potency equivalent to not less than 800 µg of ticarcillin, calculated on the anhydrous basis. Freely soluble in water. A 1% solution in water has a pH of 6.0 to 8.0. Store in airtight containers.

◊ References.
1. Swenson E, *et al.* Compatibility of ticarcillin disodium clavulanate potassium with commonly used intravenous solutions. *Curr Ther Res* 1990; **48**: 385–94.

Adverse Effects and Precautions

As for Carbenicillin Sodium, p.160.

Cholestatic jaundice and hepatitis have been reported with the combination ticarcillin with clavulanic acid; the clavulanic acid component has been implicated.

Effects on the liver. Cholestatic jaundice and hepatitis have been associated with combined preparations of a penicillin and clavulanic acid (see Amoxicillin, p.149) and 2 cases had been reported to the UK Committee on Safety of Medicines in association with ticarcillin and clavulanic acid.[1] It appeared that the clavulanic acid was probably responsible.
1. Committee on Safety of Medicines/Medicines Control Agency. Cholestatic jaundice with co-amoxiclav. *Current Problems* 1993; **19**: 2.

Interactions

As for Benzylpenicillin, p.158.

Antimicrobial Action

Ticarcillin is bactericidal and has a mode of action and range of activity similar to that of carbenicillin (p.160), but is reported to be 2 to 4 times more active against *Pseudomonas aeruginosa*.

Combinations of ticarcillin and aminoglycosides have been shown to be synergistic *in vitro* against *Ps. aeruginosa* and Enterobacteriaceae.

The activity of ticarcillin against organisms usually resistant because of the production of certain beta-lactamases is enhanced by clavulanic acid, a beta-lactamase inhibitor. Such organisms have included staphylococci, many Enterobacteriaceae, *Haemophilus influenzae*, and *Bacteroides* spp.; the activity of ticarcillin against *Ps. aeruginosa* is not enhanced by clavulanic acid. Resistance to ticarcillin with clavulanic acid has been reported.

There is cross-resistance between carbenicillin and ticarcillin.

◊ References.
1. Pulverer G, *et al.* In-vitro activity of ticarcillin with and without clavulanic acid against clinical isolates of Gram-positive and Gram-negative bacteria. *J Antimicrob Chemother* 1986; **17** (suppl C): 1–5.
2. Masterton RG, *et al.* Timentin resistance. *Lancet* 1987; **ii**: 975–6.
3. Fass RJ, Prior RB. Comparative in vitro activities of piperacillin-tazobactam and ticarcillin-clavulanate. *Antimicrob Agents Chemother* 1989; **33**: 1268–74.
4. Kempers J, MacLaren DM. Piperacillin/tazobactam and ticarcillin/clavulanic acid against resistant Enterobacteriaceae. *J Antimicrob Chemother* 1990; **26**: 598–9.
5. Klepser ME, *et al.* Comparison of the bactericidal activities of piperacillin-tazobactam, ticarcillin-clavulanate, and ampicillin-sulbactam against clinical isolates of Bacteroides fragilis, Enterococcus faecalis, Escherichia coli, and Pseudomonas aeruginosa. *Antimicrob Agents Chemother* 1997; **41**: 435–9.

Pharmacokinetics

Ticarcillin is not absorbed from the gastrointestinal tract. After intramuscular injection of 1 g peak plasma concentrations in the range of 20 to 30 µg per mL are achieved after 0.5 to 1 hour. About 50% of ticarcillin in the circulation is bound to plasma proteins. A plasma half-life of 70 minutes has been reported. A shorter half-life in patients with cystic fibrosis (about 50 minutes in one study) has been attributed to increased renal and non-renal elimination. The half-life is prolonged in neonates and also in patients with renal impairment, especially if hepatic function is also impaired. A half-life of about 15 hours has been reported in severe renal impairment.

Distribution of ticarcillin in the body is similar to that of carbenicillin. Relatively high concentrations have been reported in bile, but ticarcillin is excreted principally by glomerular filtration and tubular secretion. Concentrations of 2 to 4 mg per mL are achieved in

the urine after the intramuscular injection of 1 or 2 g. Ticarcillin is metabolised to a limited extent. Up to 90% of a dose is excreted unchanged in the urine, mostly within 6 hours after administration. The concomitant administration of probenecid produces higher plasma-ticarcillin concentrations.

Ticarcillin is removed by haemodialysis and, to some extent, by peritoneal dialysis.

Ticarcillin with clavulanic acid. The pharmacokinetics of ticarcillin and clavulanic acid are broadly similar and neither appears to affect the other to any great extent.

◊ References.
1. Staniforth DH, *et al.* Pharmacokinetics of parenteral ticarcillin formulated with clavulanic acid: Timentin. *Int J Clin Pharmacol Ther Toxicol* 1986; **24**: 123–9.
2. Brogard JM, *et al.* Biliary elimination of ticarcillin plus clavulanic acid (Claventin®): experimental and clinical study. *Int J Clin Pharmacol Ther Toxicol* 1989; **27**: 135–44.
3. de Groot R, *et al.* Pharmacokinetics of ticarcillin in patients with cystic fibrosis: a controlled prospective study. *Clin Pharmacol Ther* 1990; **47**: 73–8.
4. Wang J-P, *et al.* Disposition of drugs in cystic fibrosis IV: mechanisms for enhanced renal clearance of ticarcillin. *Clin Pharmacol Ther* 1993; **54**: 293–302.
5. Burstein AH, *et al.* Ticarcillin-clavulanic acid pharmacokinetics in preterm neonates with presumed sepsis. *Antimicrob Agents Chemother* 1994; **38**: 2024–8.

Uses and Administration

Ticarcillin is a carboxypenicillin used in the treatment of severe Gram-negative infections, especially those due to *Pseudomonas aeruginosa*. Pseudomonal infections where ticarcillin is used include those in cystic fibrosis (respiratory-tract infections), immunocompromised patients (neutropenia), peritonitis, and septicaemia. Other infections that may be due to *Ps. aeruginosa* include bone and joint infections, meningitis, otitis media (chronic), skin infections (burns, ecthyma gangrenosum, ulceration), and urinary-tract infections. For details of these infections and their treatment, see under Choice of Antibacterial, p.114.

Administration and dosage. Ticarcillin is given by injection as the sodium salt. Doses are expressed in terms of the equivalent amount of ticarcillin. They may need to be reduced in renal impairment.

Ticarcillin is given to adults and children in a dose of 200 to 300 mg per kg body-weight daily by intravenous infusion in divided doses every 4 or 6 hours.

In adults the concomitant administration of probenecid 1 g three times daily by mouth may achieve higher and more prolonged plasma concentrations of ticarcillin, but caution is advised in patients with impaired renal function.

In the treatment of complicated urinary-tract infections, adults and children may be given a dose of ticarcillin 150 to 200 mg per kg daily by intravenous infusion in divided doses every 4 or 6 hours. In uncomplicated urinary-tract infections, the usual adult dose is ticarcillin 1 g every 6 hours intramuscularly or by slow intravenous injection. Children with uncomplicated urinary-tract infections may be given 50 to 100 mg per kg body-weight daily in divided doses. Not more than 2 g of ticarcillin should be injected intramuscularly into one site.

In patients with cystic fibrosis, ticarcillin has been administered by nebuliser in the management of respiratory-tract infections.

Ticarcillin is often used with an aminoglycoside but the injections must be administered separately because of possible incompatibility.

Ticarcillin with clavulanic acid. Ticarcillin may be administered in a combination preparation with clavulanic acid (p.187), a beta-lactamase inhibitor, to widen its antibacterial spectrum to organisms usually resistant because of the production of beta-lactamases. This combination is administered by intravenous infusion in a ratio of 15 or 30 parts of ticarcillin (as the sodium salt) to 1 part of clavulanic acid (as the potassium salt). Doses are according to the content of ticarcillin, similar to those specified above.

Preparations

USP 25: Ticarcillin and Clavulanic Acid for Injection; Ticarcillin and Clavulanic Acid Injection; Ticarcillin for Injection.

Proprietary Preparations (details are given in Part 3)
Austral.: Tarcil†; Ticillin†; *Belg.:* Triacilline†; *Canad.:* Ticar†; *Fr.:* Ticarpen; *Neth.:* Ticarpen; *Spain:* Ticarpen; *UK:* Ticar†; *USA:* Ticar.

Multi-ingredient: *Aust.:* Timentin†; *Austral.:* Timentin; *Belg.:* Timentin; *Braz.:* Timentin; *Canad.:* Timentin; *Fr.:* Claventin; *Ger.:* Betabactyl†; *Hong Kong:* Timentin; *Irl.:* Timentin; *Israel:* Timentin; *Ital.:* Clavucar; Timentin; *Mex.:* Timentin; *Neth.:* Timentin; *NZ:* Timentin; *Switz.:* Timenten; *UK:* Timentin; *USA:* Timentin.

Tilmicosin (3769-a)

Tilmicosin (BAN, USAN, rINN).

EL-870; LY-177370. 4^A-O-De(2,6-dideoxy-3-C-methyl-α-L-ribo-hexopyranosyl)-20-deoxo-20-(cis-3,5-dimethyl-piperidino)tylosin.

$C_{46}H_{80}N_2O_{13}$ = 869.1.
CAS — 108050-54-0.

NOTE. Tilmicosin Phosphate is *USAN*.
Pharmacopoeias. In US for veterinary use only.

Pharmacopoeial description

USP 25: White to off-white amorphous solid. Slightly soluble in water and in *n*-hexane. Store at a temperature not exceeding 40°. Protect from light.

◊ Contact with tilmicosin should be avoided. It is irritating to the eyes and may cause allergic reactions.

Profile

Tilmicosin is a macrolide antibacterial used in veterinary medicine.

◊ A report[1] of accidental self-injection of tilmicosin by a farm worker, resulting in asthenia and temporary pulmonary, gastrointestinal, and neuromuscular toxicity.
1. Crown LA, Smith RB. Accidental veterinary antibiotic injection into a farm worker. *Tenn Med* 1999; **92**: 339–40.

Tobramycin (18310-c)

Tobramycin (BAN, USAN, rINN).

47663; Nebramycin Factor 6; Tobramycinum. 6-O-(3-Amino-3-deoxy-α-D-glucopyranosyl)-2-deoxy-4-O-(2,6-diamino-2,3,6-trideoxy-α-D-ribo-hexopyranosyl)streptamine.
$C_{18}H_{37}N_5O_9$ = 467.5.
CAS — 32986-56-4.
ATC — J01GB01; S01AA12.
Pharmacopoeias. In Eur. (see p.vi), Jpn, Pol., and US.

Pharmacopoeial description

Ph. Eur.: An antimicrobial substance produced by *Streptomyces tenebrarius* or by any other means. A white or almost white powder. Freely soluble in water; very slightly soluble in alcohol; practically insoluble in ether. A 10% solution in water has a pH of 9.0 to 11.0. Store at a temperature not exceeding 25°.

USP 25: A white to off-white, hygroscopic powder. Freely soluble in water; very slightly soluble in alcohol; practically insoluble in chloroform and in ether. Contains not more than 8.0% w/w of water. A 10% solution in water has a pH of 9.0 to 11.0. Store in airtight containers.

Tobramycin Sulfate (174-y)

Tobramycin Sulfate (rINNM).
Tobramycin Sulphate (BANM).
$(C_{18}H_{37}N_5O_9)_2,5H_2SO_4$ = 1425.4.
CAS — 49842-07-1 ($C_{18}H_{37}N_5O_9,xH_2SO_4$); 79645-27-5 (($C_{18}H_{37}N_5O_9)_2,5H_2SO_4$).
Pharmacopoeias. In Pol. and US.

1.5 g of monograph substance is approximately equivalent to 1 g of tobramycin.

Incompatibilities. For discussion of the incompatibility of aminoglycosides, including tobramycin, with beta lactams, see under Gentamicin Sulfate, p.210. Tobramycin is also reported to be incompatible with various other drugs and, as injections have an acid pH, incompatibility with alkaline preparations or with drugs unstable at acid pH may reasonably be expected.

Pharmacopoeial description

USP 25: The monograph substance has a potency of not less than 634 µg and not more than 739 µg of tobramycin per mg. A 4% solution in water has a pH of 6.0 to 8.0. Store in airtight containers.

Adverse Effects, Treatment, and Precautions

As for Gentamicin Sulfate, p.210. Some studies suggest that tobramycin is slightly less nephrotoxic than gentamicin, but others have not found any significant difference in their effects on the kidneys.

Peak plasma-tobramycin concentrations greater than 12 µg per mL (some suggest 10 µg per mL) and trough concentrations greater than 2 µg per mL should be avoided.

Interactions
As for Gentamicin Sulfate, p.211.

Antimicrobial Action
As for Gentamicin Sulfate, p.211. Tobramycin is reported to be somewhat more effective *in vitro* than gentamicin against *Pseudomonas aeruginosa* and less effective against *Serratia*, staphylococci, and enterococci; however these differences do not necessarily translate into differences in clinical effectiveness. MICs are generally similar to those of gentamicin.

Cross-resistance between tobramycin and gentamicin is generally seen, but about 10% of strains resistant to gentamicin are susceptible to tobramycin.

◊ References to activity against *Pseudomonas aeruginosa*.
1. Barclay ML, *et al.* Adaptive resistance to tobramycin in Pseudomonas aeruginosa lung infection in cystic fibrosis. *J Antimicrob Chemother* 1996; **37:** 1155–64.
2. den Hollander JG, *et al.* Synergism between tobramycin and ceftazidime against a resistant Pseudomonas aeruginosa strain, tested in an in vitro pharmacokinetic model. *Antimicrob Agents Chemother* 1997; **41:** 95–100.
3. Wu YL, *et al.* Ability of azlocillin and tobramycin in combination to delay or prevent resistance development in Pseudomonas aeruginosa. *J Antimicrob Chemother* 1999; **44:** 389–92.
4. Shawar RM, *et al.* Activities of tobramycin and six other antibiotics against Pseudomonas aeruginosa isolates from patients with cystic fibrosis. *Antimicrob Agents Chemother* 1999; **43:** 2877–80.

Pharmacokinetics
As for Gentamicin Sulfate, p.211.

Following intramuscular administration of tobramycin, peak plasma concentrations are achieved within 30 to 90 minutes and concentrations of about 4 µg per mL have been reported following doses of 1 mg per kg body-weight. Administration of usual doses by slow intravenous injection may result in plasma concentrations which briefly exceed 12 µg per mL. A plasma half-life of 2 to 3 hours has been reported.

Inhalation. References.
1. Touw DJ, *et al.* Pharmacokinetics of aerosolized tobramycin in adult patients with cystic fibrosis. *Antimicrob Agents Chemother* 1997; **41:** 184–7.
2. Beringer PM, *et al.* Pharmacokinetics of tobramycin in adults with cystic fibrosis: implications for once-daily administration. *Antimicrob Agents Chemother* 2000; **44:** 809–13.

Uses and Administration
Tobramycin is an aminoglycoside antibiotic with actions and uses similar to those of gentamicin (p.212). It is used, usually as the sulfate, particularly in the treatment of pseudomonal infections.

As with gentamicin, tobramycin may be used with penicillins or cephalosporins; the injections should be administered separately.

Doses of tobramycin sulfate are expressed in terms of tobramycin base, and are similar to those of gentamicin, with the usual adult dose ranging from 3 to 5 mg of tobramycin per kg daily in 3 or 4 divided doses. In patients with cystic fibrosis, doses of 8 to 10 mg per kg daily in divided doses may be necessary to achieve therapeutic plasma concentrations.

For mild to moderate urinary-tract infections, a dose of 2 to 3 mg per kg once daily may be effective in adults.

The usual dose for children is 6 to 7.5 mg per kg daily in 3 or 4 divided doses. Premature and full-term neonates may be given 2 mg per kg every 12 hours.

See under Gentamicin Sulfate (p.213) for reference to once-daily dosage of aminoglycosides.

Tobramycin sulfate is given by intramuscular injection, or by intravenous infusion over 20 to 60 minutes in 50 to 100 mL of sodium chloride 0.9% or glucose 5% injection; proportionately less fluid should be given to children. It has also been given slowly by direct intravenous injection.

Treatment should generally be limited to 7 to 10 days, and peak plasma concentrations greater than 12 µg per mL (some suggest 10 µg per mL) or trough concentrations greater than 2 µg per mL should be avoid-ed. In all patients, dosage should be adjusted according to plasma-tobramycin concentrations and particularly where factors such as age, renal impairment, or prolonged therapy may predispose to toxicity (see Uses and Administration of Gentamicin Sulfate, p.212).

Tobramycin may be administered into the eye as a 0.3% ointment or drops in the treatment of eye infections. It is also given by inhalation in patients with cystic fibrosis to control *Pseudomonas aeruginosa* infections in a dose of 300 mg every 12 hours for 28 days using a suitable nebuliser. Treatment is then stopped for 28 days before being resumed for another treatment period. This cycle may be repeated indefinitely.

Preparations
BP 2001: Tobramycin Injection;
USP 25: Tobramycin and Dexamethasone Ophthalmic Ointment; Tobramycin and Dexamethasone Ophthalmic Suspension; Tobramycin and Fluorometholone Acetate Ophthalmic Suspension; Tobramycin for Injection; Tobramycin Injection; Tobramycin Ophthalmic Ointment; Tobramycin Ophthalmic Solution.

Proprietary Preparations (details are given in Part 3)
Aust.: Brulamycin; Tobrasix; Tobrex; *Austral.:* Nebcin; Tobi; Tobrex; *Belg.:* Obracin; Tobrex; *Braz.:* Tobramina; Tobrex; *Canad.:* Nebcin; Tobi; Tobrex; Tomycine; *Denm.:* Nebcina; Tobrex; *Fin.:* Nebcina; Tobrex; Tomycin; *Fr.:* Nebcine; Tobrex; *Ger.:* Brulamycin; Gernebcin; Tobra-cell; Tobramaxin; *Hong Kong:* Nebcin; Tobrex; *Irl.:* Nebcin; Tobralex; *Israel:* Nebcin; Tobrex; *Ital.:* Nebicina; Tobral; Tobrex; *Mex.:* Tobra; Tobrex; Trazil; *Neth.:* Obracin; Tobrex†; *Norw.:* Nebcina; *NZ:* Nebcin; Tobrex; *Port.:* Distobram; Tobra Gobens; Tobracil; Tobrex; Tobridavi; *S.Afr.:* Mytobrin; Nebcin; Tobrex; *Singapore:* Tobrex; *Spain:* Tobra Gobens; Tobradistin; Tobrex; *Swed.:* Nebcina; Tobrex; *Switz.:* Obracin; Tobrex; *Thai.:* Tobrex; *UK:* Nebcin; Tobi; Tobralex†; *USA:* AkTob; Defy†; Nebcin; Tobi; Tobrasol; Tobrex.

Multi-ingredient: *Belg.:* Tobradex; *Braz.:* Tobradex; *Canad.:* Tobradex; *Fr.:* Tobradex; *Hong Kong:* Tobradex; *Ital.:* Tobradex; *Mex.:* Trazidex; Trazinac; *Neth.:* Tobradex†; *NZ:* Tobradex; Tobrasone; *S.Afr.:* Tobradex; *Singapore:* Tobradex; *Spain:* Ocubrax; Tobradex; *Switz.:* Tobradex; Tobrafen; *Thai.:* Tobradex; *UK:* Tobradex; *USA:* Tobradex.

Tosufloxacin Tosilate (20339-b)
Tosufloxacin Tosilate *(rINNM)*.
Abbott-61827 (tosufloxacin); Tosufloxacin Tosylate. (±)-7-(3-Amino-1-pyrrolidinyl)-1-(2,4-difluorophenyl)-6-fluoro-1,4-dihydro-4-oxo-1,8-naphthyridine-3-carboxylic acid toluene-4-sulphonate monohydrate.
$C_{19}H_{15}F_3N_4O_3,C_7H_8O_3S,H_2O = 594.6$.
CAS — 108138-46-1 (anhydrous tosufloxacin); 107097-79-0 (tosufloxacin monohydrate); 115964-29-9 (tosufloxacin tosilate); 144742-63-2 (tosufloxacin tosilate).

NOTE. Tosufloxacin is USAN.

Profile
Tosufloxacin is a fluoroquinolone antibacterial with properties similar to those of ciprofloxacin (p.182). It is given by mouth as the tosilate in the treatment of susceptible infections in usual doses of 300 to 450 mg daily in two or three divided doses.

Preparations
Proprietary Preparations (details are given in Part 3)
Jpn: Ozex.

Trimethoprim (1401-c)
Trimethoprim *(BAN, USAN, rINN)*.
BW-56-72; NSC-106568; Trimethoprimum; Trimethoxyprim. 5-(3,4,5-Trimethoxybenzyl)pyrimidine-2,4-diamine.
$C_{14}H_{18}N_4O_3 = 290.3$.
CAS — 738-70-5 (trimethoprim); 56585-33-2 (trimethoprim sulfate).
ATC — J01EA01.

NOTE. Trimethoprim may be given with various sulfonamides and some preparations of such combinations have been given approved names: see Co-trifamole, p.193; Co-trimazine, p.193; and Co-trimoxazole, p.193.
Pharmacopoeias. In Chin., Eur. (see p.vi), Int., Pol., and US. US also includes Trimethoprim Sulfate.

Pharmacopoeial description
Ph. Eur.: A white or yellowish-white powder. Very slightly soluble in water; slightly soluble in alcohol.

USP 25: White to cream-coloured, odourless crystals or crystalline powder. Very slightly soluble in water; slightly soluble in alcohol and in acetone; soluble in benzyl alcohol; practically insoluble in carbon tetrachloride and in ether; sparingly soluble in chloroform and in methyl alcohol. Store in airtight containers. Protect from light.

Incompatibility. The UK manufacturers state that trimethoprim injections (containing the lactate) should not be mixed with solutions of sulfonamides because of incompatibility. Although a former such preparation stated that it should not be diluted in chloride-containing infusion solutions, because of the risk of precipitating trimethoprim hydrochloride, others are stated to be compatible with sodium chloride 0.9% and some other chloride-containing solutions including Ringer's solution. Injections are considered compatible with glucose 5% and with sodium lactate.

Adverse Effects and Treatment
Trimethoprim is reasonably well tolerated in general, and the most frequent adverse effects at usual doses are pruritus and skin rash (in about 3 to 7% of patients) and mild gastrointestinal disturbances including nausea, vomiting, and sore mouth.

Rarely, more severe effects have been reported. Sulfonamide-like skin reactions including exfoliative dermatitis, erythema multiforme, Stevens-Johnson syndrome, and toxic epidermal necrolysis have occurred. Disturbances of liver enzyme values and cholestatic jaundice have been associated with trimethoprim. Rises in serum creatinine and blood-urea nitrogen have been reported although it is unclear whether this represents genuine renal dysfunction or inhibition of tubular secretion of creatinine. Photosensitivity has been reported. Fever is not uncommon but occasionally hypersensitivity reactions may be severe and manifest as anaphylaxis. Cases of aseptic meningitis have also been reported.

Trimethoprim may cause a depression of haematopoiesis due to interference of the drug in the metabolism of folic acid, particularly when given over a prolonged period or in high doses. This may manifest as megaloblastic anaemia, or as thrombocytopenia and leucopenia; methaemoglobinaemia has also been seen. Calcium folinate 5 to 15 mg daily by mouth may be given to counter this effect. Trimethoprim is teratogenic in *animals*.

For reports of adverse effects of trimethoprim when used with sulfamethoxazole, see Co-trimoxazole, p.193.

Hyperkalaemia. Trimethoprim has been reported to induce hyperkalaemia,[1] particularly in HIV-infected patients being treated for *Pneumocystis carinii* pneumonia or in the elderly. The hyperkalaemia may be due to amiloride-like potassium-sparing properties of trimethoprim, and may be potentiated by ACE inhibitors.
1. Perazella MA. Trimethoprim-induced hyperkalaemia: clinical data, mechanism, prevention and management. *Drug Safety* 2000; **22:** 227–36.

Precautions
Trimethoprim should not be given to patients with a history of hypersensitivity to the drug, and it should be discontinued if a skin rash appears. Care is necessary in administering trimethoprim to patients with impaired renal function to avoid accumulation and toxicity: it should not be given in severe renal impairment unless blood concentrations can be monitored. It should be used with caution in patients with severe hepatic damage as changes may occur in the absorption and metabolism of trimethoprim.

It is suggested that regular haematological examination should be made during prolonged courses of treatment; trimethoprim should not usually be given to patients with serious haematological disorders and particularly not in megaloblastic anaemia secondary to folate depletion. Caution should be taken in patients with actual, or possible, folate deficiency and administration of folinic acid should be considered. Trimethoprim should be avoided during pregnancy. Trimethoprim appears in breast milk and care is required when it is used in breast-feeding mothers. Elderly patients may be more susceptible to adverse effects and a lower dosage may be advisable.

Trimethoprim may interfere with some diagnostic tests, including serum-methotrexate assay where dihydrofolate reductase is used and the Jaffé reaction for creatinine.

For reports dealing with precautions for trimethoprim given with sulfamethoxazole, see Co-trimoxazole, p.193.

Fragile X syndrome. A warning that trimethoprim and other folate antagonists should be avoided in children with the fragile X chromosome which is associated with mental retardation and is folate sensitive.[1]

1. Hecht F, Glover TW. Antibiotics containing trimethoprim and the fragile X chromosome. *N Engl J Med* 1983; **308**: 285–6.

Porphyria. Trimethoprim has been associated with acute attacks of porphyria and is considered unsafe in porphyric patients.

Interactions
Trimethoprim may increase serum concentrations and potentiate the effect of a number of drugs, including phenytoin, digoxin, and procainamide. The effect may be due to competitive inhibition of renal excretion, decreased metabolism, or both. It has been suggested that trimethoprim may potentiate the effects of warfarin. Trimethoprim has been reported to reduce the renal excretion and increase blood concentrations of zidovudine, zalcitabine, and lamivudine. Trimethoprim and dapsone increase each other's serum concentrations when given concomitantly, whereas rifampicin may decrease trimethoprim concentrations.

An increased risk of nephrotoxicity has been reported with the use of trimethoprim or co-trimoxazole and ciclosporin. Intravenous administration of trimethoprim and sulfonamides may reduce ciclosporin concentrations in blood. In patients given trimethoprim who were also receiving diuretics, hyponatraemia has been reported (an increased risk of thrombocytopenia has been seen in elderly patients given co-trimoxazole with diuretics, although it is unclear which component is responsible).

Administration of trimethoprim with other depressants of bone marrow function may increase the likelihood of myelosuppression, and there may be a particular risk of megaloblastic anaemia if it is given with other folate inhibitors, such as pyrimethamine or methotrexate.

Severe hyperkalaemia has been noted in patients given trimethoprim (or co-trimoxazole) together with an ACE inhibitor.

Antimicrobial Action
Trimethoprim is a dihydrofolate reductase inhibitor. It inhibits the conversion of bacterial dihydrofolic acid to tetrahydrofolic acid which is necessary for the synthesis of certain amino acids, purines, thymidine, and ultimately DNA. It acts in the same metabolic pathway as the sulfonamides. It exerts its selective action because of a far greater affinity for the bacterial than the mammalian enzyme. Trimethoprim may be bacteriostatic or bactericidal depending on growth conditions; pus, for example, may inhibit the action of trimethoprim because of the presence of thymine and thymidine.

Spectrum of activity. Trimethoprim is active against a wide range of Gram-negative and Gram-positive aerobes, as well as some protozoa. The following species are usually susceptible (but see also Resistance, below).

Many Gram-positive cocci are sensitive, including *Staphylococcus aureus*, streptococci including *Streptococcus pyogenes*, *Str. pneumoniae*, and the viridans streptococci, and to a variable extent enterococci, although their sensitivity is reduced in the presence of folate.

Other sensitive Gram-positive organisms include strains of *Listeria*, *Corynebacterium diphtheriae*, and the Gram-positive bacilli.

Among the Gram-negative organisms most of the Enterobacteriaceae are susceptible, or moderately so, including *Citrobacter*, *Enterobacter*, *Escherichia coli*, *Hafnia*, *Klebsiella*, *Proteus mirabilis*, *Providencia*, *Salmonella*, some *Serratia*, *Shigella*, and *Yersinia*. *Legionella* and *Vibrio* are also sensitive, and so are *Haemophilus influenzae* and *H. ducreyi*.

Anaerobic species are usually resistant, and so, to varying degrees are *Brucella*, *Neisseria*, and *Nocardia*. *Mycobacterium tuberculosis* is resistant although *M. marinum* may not be. *Pseudomonas aeruginosa* is re-

sistant, and so are the chlamydias, mycoplasmas, and rickettsias, as well as the spirochaetes.

Trimethoprim has some activity against *Pneumocystis carinii* and against some protozoa such as *Naegleria*, *Plasmodium*, and *Toxoplasma*.

Minimum inhibitory concentrations (MICs) vary considerably with the medium; in particular the media should contain minimal amounts of thymine or thymidine. MICs for the most sensitive strains range from about 0.01 to 0.5 μg per mL; in the treatment of urinary-tract infections organisms with MICs up to about 8 μg per mL are considered sensitive and those with MICs between 8 and 16 μg per mL of moderate sensitivity, but since concentrations in blood are lower than those in urine such MICs would not indicate sensitivity in systemic infections.

Activity with other antimicrobials. Because their modes of action are complementary, affecting different stages in folate metabolism, a potent synergistic effect exists between trimethoprim and sulfonamides against many organisms *in vitro*. The effect is most marked when the two drugs are present in the ratio of their MICs: i.e. an organism susceptible to 1 μg per mL of trimethoprim and 20 μg per mL of sulfonamide will be maximally inhibited by a 1:20 mixture.

Fixed-dose combinations of trimethoprim with various sulfonamides are available, of which co-trimoxazole (trimethoprim with sulfamethoxazole in a 1:5 mixture) is the most widely used. For further details on the antimicrobial action of co-trimoxazole, see p.194.

Synergy has also been reported with rifampicin, and with the polymyxins.

Resistance. Resistance to trimethoprim may be due to several mechanisms. Clinical resistance is often due to plasmid-mediated dihydrofolate reductases that are resistant to trimethoprim: such genes may become incorporated into the chromosome via transposons. Resistance may also be due to overproduction of dihydrofolate reductase, changes in cell permeability, or bacterial mutants which are intrinsically resistant to trimethoprim because they depend on exogenous thymine and thymidine for growth. Despite fears of a rapid increase in resistance if trimethoprim was used alone there is little evidence that this has been any worse than in areas where it has been used in combination with sulfonamides. Nonetheless, trimethoprim resistance has been reported in many species, and very high frequencies of resistance have been seen in some developing countries, particularly among the Enterobacteriaceae.

◊ References.
1. Huovinen P, *et al.* Trimethoprim and sulfonamide resistance. *Antimicrob Agents Chemother* 1995; **39**: 279–89.

Pharmacokinetics
Trimethoprim is rapidly and almost completely absorbed from the gastrointestinal tract and peak concentrations in the circulation occur about 1 to 4 hours after an oral dose; peak plasma concentrations of about 1 μg per mL have been reported after a single dose of 100 mg. About 45% is bound to plasma proteins. Trimethoprim is widely distributed to various tissues and fluids including kidneys, liver, lung and bronchial secretions, saliva, aqueous humour, prostatic tissue and fluid, and vaginal secretions; concentrations in many of these tissues are reported to be higher than serum concentrations but concentrations in the CSF are about one-quarter to one-half of those in serum. Trimethoprim readily crosses the placenta and it appears in breast milk. The half-life is about 8 to 11 hours in adults and somewhat less in children, but is prolonged in severe renal impairment and in neonates, whose renal function is immature.

Trimethoprim is excreted primarily by the kidneys through glomerular filtration and tubular secretion. About 10 to 20% of trimethoprim is metabolised in the liver and small amounts are excreted in the faeces via the bile, but most, about 40 to 60% of a dose, is excreted in urine, predominantly as unchanged drug,

within 24 hours. Trimethoprim is removed from the blood by haemodialysis to some extent.

Uses and Administration
Trimethoprim is a diaminopyrimidine antibacterial that is used for the treatment of infections due to sensitive organisms, including gastro-enteritis and respiratory-tract infections, and in particular for the treatment and prophylaxis of urinary-tract infections. For details of these infections and their treatment, see Choice of Antibacterial, p.114.

Trimethoprim is also used in conjunction with sulfonamides. The most common combination is co-trimoxazole (trimethoprim with sulfamethoxazole) (p.193). Other combinations are co-trimazine (with sulfadiazine) and co-trifamole (with sulfamoxole); trimethoprim is also used with sulfamerazine, sulfametopyrazine, sulfametrole, and sulfamethoxypyridazine, and, in veterinary practice, with sulfadoxine, sulfaquinoxaline, sulfatroxazole, sulfadimethoxine, sulfadimidine, or sulfafurazole.

The combination of trimethoprim with sulfamethoxazole (co-trimoxazole) or with dapsone is used in the management of *Pneumocystis carinii* pneumonia (p.375).

The usual adult dose of trimethoprim in acute infection is 200 mg twice daily by mouth; doses of 200 or 300 mg daily as a single dose are also used. For the dosage of trimethoprim when given with sulfamethoxazole, see under Co-trimoxazole, p.194. Up to 20 mg per kg body-weight daily may be given in combination with dapsone for the treatment of *Pneumocystis carinii* pneumonia.

Children may be given 6 to 8 mg per kg daily of trimethoprim in 2 divided doses: regimens for children are, 6 to 12 years, 100 mg twice daily; 6 months to 5 years, 50 mg twice daily; 6 weeks to 5 months, 25 mg twice daily.

For long-term prophylaxis the usual dose is 100 mg at night for adults; children aged 6 to 12 years may be given 50 mg at night and those aged 6 months to 5 years, 25 mg at night.

Trimethoprim is also administered intravenously by injection or infusion as the lactate although doses are in terms of the base. The usual dose is 200 mg every 12 hours in adults; children may be given 8 mg per kg daily in 2 or 3 divided doses. Initial doses may be higher or given more frequently in severely ill patients.

Care should be taken in patients with moderate to severe renal impairment and doses generally should be reduced. If the creatinine clearance is between 15 and 27 mL per minute, the normal dose may be given for 3 days but should then be reduced to one-half; if the creatinine clearance is below 15 mL per minute, half the normal dose should be employed from the start of the treatment period. Plasma concentrations should be monitored in patients with severe renal impairment.

Combinations of trimethoprim and polymyxin B have been used topically in the treatment and prophylaxis of eye infections. Trimethoprim sulfate and trimethoprim hydrochloride are also used.

Administration. SINGLE-DOSE THERAPY. Although there are obvious advantages to a single-dose regimen, one study[1] found that there was about a 1 in 4 risk of recurrence of urinary-tract infection within 10 days in 50 children given, according to age, a single dose of 75 to 450 mg of trimethoprim. The problems with a single-dose regimen were confirmed by others[2] in a study involving 344 evaluated cases of cystitis in 306 women. Only 122 of 173 cases treated with trimethoprim 320 mg as a single dose were evaluated as cured after 5 weeks, compared with 149 of 171 given 160 mg twice daily for 1 week (71 versus 87%). Again, these results suggest that about 1 patient in 4 would have to be re-treated.

1. Nolan T, *et al.* Single dose trimethoprim for urinary tract infection. *Arch Dis Child* 1989; **64**: 581–6.
2. Österberg E, *et al.* Efficacy of single-dose versus seven-day trimethoprim treatment of cystitis in women: a randomized double-blind study. *J Infect Dis* 1990; **161**: 942–7.

Preparations
BP 2001: Co-trimoxazole Intravenous Infusion; Co-trimoxazole Oral Suspension; Co-trimoxazole Tablets; Dispersible Co-trimox-

azole Tablets; Paediatric Co-trimoxazole Oral Suspension; Paediatric Co-trimoxazole Tablets; Trimethoprim Tablets;
USP 25: Polymyxin B Sulfate and Trimethoprim Ophthalmic Solution; Sulfamethoxazole and Trimethoprim Injection; Sulfamethoxazole and Trimethoprim Oral Suspension; Sulfamethoxazole and Trimethoprim Tablets; Trimethoprim Tablets.

Proprietary Preparations (details are given in Part 3)
Aust.: Monoprim; Motrim; Solotrim; Triprim; Wellcoprim; *Austral.:* Alprim; Triprim; *Belg.:* Wellcoprim; *Canad.:* Proloprim;
Denm.: Monotrim; Triprim; *Fin.:* Trimetin; Trimex; Trimopan;
Fr.: Wellcoprim; *Ger.:* InfectoTrimet; TMP-ratiopharm; Trimono†; Uretrim†; *Irl.:* Ipral; Monotrim; *Ital.:* Abaprim†; *Neth.:* Wellcoprim; *NZ:* TMP; Triprim; *S.Afr.:* Monotrim†; Triprim; *Singapore:* Alprim; *Spain:* Tediprima; *Swed.:* Idotrim; *Switz.:* Monotrim; Primosept†; *Thai.:* Balin; *UK:* Ipral†; Monotrim; Tiempe; Trimogal; Trimopan; Triprimix†; *USA:* Primsol; Proloprim; Trimpex.

Multi-ingredient: *Aust.:* Bactrim; Cotribene; Eusaprim; Lidaprim; Oecotrim; Polytrim; Supracombin; Triglobe; Trimethe comp; *Austral.:* Bactrim; Cosig; Resprim; Septrin; Trimoxazole; *Belg.:* Bactrim; Eusaprim; Ophtalmotrim; Polytrim; *Braz.:* Assepium; Assepium Balsamico; Bac Septin; Bacfar; Bacfar Balsamico; Bacgen; Bacgen Balsamico; Bacris; Bacteracin; Bacteracin Balsamico; Bactox; Bactox Balsamico; Bactren; Bactrex; Bactricin; Bactricin Balsamico; Bactrim; Bactrisan; Bactrisan Balsamico; Bactropin; Bactropin Balsamico; Balsamin; Balsiprin; Baxapril; Becaltrin; Benectrin; Benectrin Balsamico; Binoctrin; Diazol; Dientrin; Diteutrin; Duoctrin; Duoctrin Balsamico; Duoctrin Enterico; Ectrin; Ectrin Balsamico; Entercal; Entero Heractrin; Enterone; Espectrin; Gamactrin; Heractrin; Imuneprim; Infecteracin; Infectrin; Infectrin Balsamico; Katrim; Katrim Balsamico; Leotrim; Lupectrim; Lupectrim Balsamico; Metoprin; Metoprin Balsamico; Mictrex; Neotrin; Neotrin Balsamico; Pertrim; Qiftrim; Quimio-Ped; Quimio-Ped Balsamico; Roytrin; Sedactrim; Sedactrim Balsamico; Septiolan; Septiolan Balsamico; Septoprin; Silpin; Sulfatrex; Suss; Suss Balsamico; Teutrin; Teutrin Balsamico; Triglobe; Trimetoprim Balsamico; Trimexazol; Trimexazol Balsamico; Trizol Balsamico; Urizal; Uro Bac Septin; Uro Bactrim; Uro Batrox; Uro Duoctrim; Uro Heractrim; Uro Septoprin; Uro-Bacteracin; Uro-Baxapril; Uro-Leotrim; Uro-Septiolan; Uro-Teutrim; Urobactrex; Urobioctrin; Uroctrim; Urofar; Uroneotrim; Uropol; Uroxazol; Utrim; *Canad.:* Apo-Sulfatrim; Bactrim; Coptin; Novo-Trimel; Nu-Cotrimox; Polytrim; Roubac†; Septra; *Denm.:* Bactrim; Sulfotrim; *Fin.:* Cotrim; Ditrim; Trimetin Duplo; *Fr.:* Bactrim; Cotrimazol†; Eusaprim; Trimadiaz Antima†; *Ger.:* Bactoreduct; Bactrim†; Berlocid; Berlocombin; Co-trim-Tablinen†; Cotrim; Cotrim E; Cotrim K; Cotrim-Diolan; Cotrim-Hefa; Cotrim-Puren†; Cotrimhexal; Cotrimox-Wolff; Cotrimstada; Drylin; Eusaprim; Jenamoxazol†; Kepinol; Linaris†; Microtrim; Sigaprim; Supracombin; TMS; Triglobe; *Hong Kong:* Apo-Sulfatrim; Bacin; BS; Chemitrim; Chemoprim; Dhatrin; Lidaprim; Oftalmotrim; Septrin; *Irl.:* Antrimox†; Bactrim; Cotrimel; Duobact; Septrin; Tricomox†; *Israel:* Diseptyl; Resprim; Septrin; Sulfatrim; *Ital.:* Abacin; Bacterial†; Bactrim; Chemitrim; Eusaprim; Gantrim; Isotrim†; Kelfiprim; Kombinax; Lidaprim; Medixin†; Strepto-Plus†; Velaten†; *Mex.:* Anitrim; Bacpiryl; Bactelan; Bactilen; Bactiver; Bactrim; Bactrim Compositum; Bactropin; Bateral; Batrizol; Bioprim; Dertrin; Dibaprim; Ectaprim; Enterobacticel; Esteprim; Fectri; Isobac; Kelfiprim; Lidaprim; Maxtrim; Metoxiprim; Microbactrim; Octiban; Pisatrina; Polibatrin; Protaxol; Rifaprim; Septrin; Servitrim; Sulfawal; Sulfoid Trimetho; Sulfort; Sulprim; Supristol; Syraprim; Thriazol; Tribakin; Trim-Vit; Trimesul; Trimesuxol; Trimetoger; Trimetox; Trimexazol; Trimexole; Trimexole Compositum; Trimzol; Trinelax; Trisufin; Zaprin; *Neth.:* Bactrimel; Eusaprim; Polytrim; Trimoxol; *Norw.:* Bactrim; *NZ:* Apo-Sulfatrim; Bactrim; Trimel; Trisul; *Port.:* Bactrim; Cotrim; Metomide; Oftalmotrim; Septrin; *S.Afr.:* Acuco†; Arcanaprim†; Bactrim; Bencole; Briscotrim†; Cocydal; Cotrivan†; Cozole; Doctrim†; Durobac; Dynazole; Fabubac; Mezenol†; Microbac†; Norisep†; Partrim†; Polytrim; Purbac; Septran; Spectrim; Supristol†; Thoxaprim†; Tri-Co; Trimethox; Trimoks†; Trimzol†; Troxazole†; Ultrasept; Ultrazole; Xerazole; Xeroprim; *Singapore:* Apo-Sulfatrim; Bacin; Bactrim; Balin; BS; Chemoprim; Dhatrin; Oftalmotrim; Septrin; Suprim; Triglobe; Trimezole; *Spain:* Abactrim†; Bactifor†; Bactopumon; Balsoprim; Bridotrim; Bronco Aseptilex Fuerte; Bronco Bactifor; Bronco Sergo; Broncorema†; Broncovir; Bronquial; Bronquicisteina; Bronquidiazina CR; Bronquimar; Bronquimucil; Bronquium; Cotrazol; Eduprim; Eduprim Mucolitico; Gobens Trim; Lotusix†; Momentol; Mucorama TS; Neumopectolina; Oftalmotrim; Oftalmotrim Dexa; Otix; Pulmo Menal; Pulmosterin Duo; Salvatrim; Septrin; Soltrim; Toose†; Tosdetan†; Traquivan; Tresium†; Triglobe†; *Swed.:* Bactrim; Eusaprim; Trimetoprim-Sulfa†; Trimin sulfa; *Switz.:* Agoprim; Bactrim; Cotrim; Escoprim; Eusaprim†; Groprim; Helveprim; Imexim†; Lagatrim; Maderan†; Nopil; Sigaprim; Supracombin; *Thai.:* Actin; Bacin; Bacta; Bactrim; Baczole; Chemoprim; Co-Tasian; Co-Trimed; Conprim; Cotamox; Kelfiprim; Lastrim; Letus; Lidaprim; Med-Sultrim; Mega-Prim; Metrim; Metxaprim; Mycosamthong; Po-Trim; Pulvicin; Servitrim; Sulbacta; Sulfometh; Tampo; Triprim; Trimexazole; Trimox; Trimoxzol; Triprim; Trixzol; Zoleprim; *UAE:* Trimol; *UK:* Bactrim†; Chemotrim; Comixco†; Fectrim; Laratrim; Polytrim; Septrin; *USA:* Bactrim; Cotrim; Polytrim; Septra; SMZ-TMP; Sulfamethoprim†; Sulfatrim; Uroplus†.

Troleandomycin (175-j)

Troleandomycin (*BAN, USAN, rINN*).

NSC-108166; Triacetyloleandomycin. The triacetyl ester of oleandomycin .

$C_{41}H_{67}NO_{15} = 814.0$.

CAS — 2751-09-9.

ATC — J01FA08.

Pharmacopoeias. In *Fr.* and *US.*

1.18 g of monograph substance is approximately equivalent to 1 g of oleandomycin.

Pharmacopoeial description

USP 25: A white, odourless, crystalline powder. It contains the equivalent of not less than 750 μg of oleandomycin per mg. Slightly soluble in water and in ether; freely soluble in alcohol; soluble in chloroform. A 10% solution in alcohol and water (1:1) has a pH of 7.0 to 8.5. Store in airtight containers.

Adverse Effects and Precautions

As for Erythromycin, p.201. After administration of troleandomycin for 2 weeks or more, or in repeated courses, hepatotoxicity with transient disturbances of liver function and jaundice, as described for erythromycin, have occurred and liver function should be monitored in patients who receive the drug for more than 14 days or in repeated courses. It should be used with care in patients with hepatic impairment and avoided in those who have previously developed liver toxicity on receiving it.

Interactions

For a discussion of drug interactions of macrolide antibacterials, see Erythromycin, p.202.

◊ For the effect of troleandomycin on serum concentrations of *carbamazepine*, see p.344 and for its effect on *triazolam*, see under Diazepam, p.677. The concomitant administration of troleandomycin and *cisapride* can increase plasma concentrations of cisapride which may result in serious ventricular arrhythmias. Troleandomycin has a more potent effect on hepatic cytochrome P450 than erythromycin (see Interactions, Mechanism, p.202), and interactions reported between drugs such as *astemizole*, the ergot alkaloids, *terfenadine*, or *theophylline* and other macrolides are at least as likely if they are taken with troleandomycin.

For the effects of troleandomycin on *methylprednisolone*, see Administration in Asthma under Uses, below.

Antimicrobial Action

Troleandomycin is hydrolysed *in vivo* to oleandomycin (p.233) which has a range of activity similar to but, in general, less effective than that of erythromycin (p.203). It has a similar pattern of resistance to erythromycin.

Pharmacokinetics

Troleandomycin is more rapidly and completely absorbed from the gastrointestinal tract than is oleandomycin, to which it is hydrolysed *in vivo*. Peak plasma-oleandomycin concentrations of about 2 μg per mL are attained 2 hours after a single dose of 500 mg, and detectable amounts are present in plasma after 12 hours. It is excreted in the faeces via the bile; about 20% of the dose can be recovered in active form from the urine.

Uses and Administration

Troleandomycin is a macrolide antibiotic with actions similar to those of erythromycin (p.203). It has been given by mouth in the treatment of susceptible infections although more effective antibacterials are generally preferred. The usual adult dose is the equivalent of 1 to 2 g daily of oleandomycin in divided doses by mouth. Children have been given the equivalent of about 25 to 45 mg per kg body-weight daily.

Administration in asthma. Troleandomycin inhibits the elimination of methylprednisolone[1] and has been given to children with corticosteroid-dependent asthma (p.757), to permit a reduction in the oral dosage of methylprednisolone.[2-4] It is unclear whether troleandomycin has actions in asthma beyond its effect on methylprednisolone metabolism; there is some evidence that it may reduce airway hyperresponsiveness,[3] and there is a report of a patient who was successfully maintained on troleandomycin alone after her corticosteroid therapy was tapered to zero.[5] However, a systematic review[6] concluded that there is insufficient evidence to support its use in steroid-dependent asthma.

1. Szefler SJ, *et al.* Dose- and time-related effect of troleandomycin on methylprednisolone elimination. *Clin Pharmacol Ther* 1982; **32:** 166–71.
2. Eitches RW, *et al.* Methylprednisolone and troleandomycin in treatment of steroid-dependent asthmatic children. *Am J Dis Child* 1985; **139:** 264–8.
3. Ball BD, *et al.* Effect of low-dose troleandomycin on glucocorticoid pharmacokinetics and airway hyperresponsiveness in severely asthmatic children. *Ann Allergy* 1990; **65:** 37–45.
4. Kamada AK, *et al.* Efficacy and safety of low-dose troleandomycin therapy in children with severe, steroid-requiring asthma. *J Allergy Clin Immunol* 1993; **91:** 873–82.
5. Rosenberg SM, *et al.* Use of TAO without methylprednisolone in the treatment of severe asthma. *Chest* 1991; **100:** 849–50.
6. Evans DJ, *et al.* Troleandomycin as an oral corticosteroid sparing agent in stable asthma (updated 19 May 2001). Available in The Cochrane Library; Issue 3. Oxford: Update Software; 2001.

Preparations

USP 25: Troleandomycin Capsules.

Proprietary Preparations (details are given in Part 3)
Ital.: Triocetin; *USA:* TAO.

Trospectomycin Sulfate (1363-m)

Trospectomycin Sulfate (*USAN, rINN*).

Trospectomycin Sulphate (*BANM*); U-63366 (trospectomycin); U-63366F. (2R,4aR,5aR,6S,7S,8R,9S,9aR,10aS)-2-Butyl-4a,7,9-trihydroxy-6,8-bis(methylamino)perhydropyrano[2,3-b][1,4]benzodioxin-4-one sulphate pentahydrate.

$C_{17}H_{30}N_2O_7,H_2SO_4,5H_2O = 562.6$.

CAS — 88669-04-9 (trospectomycin); 88851-61-0 (trospectomycin sulfate).

Profile

Trospectomycin is a water-soluble derivative of spectinomycin (p.248) but is more active against Gram-positive organisms, *Haemophilus influenzae*, and *Chlamydia trachomatis* as well as *Neisseria*. It has been investigated in various infections and given as the sulfate intravenously or intramuscularly. Reported adverse effects include perioral paraesthesia, pain at the injection site, nausea, and dizziness.

◊ References.

1. Novak E, *et al.* Human safety and pharmacokinetics of a single intramuscular dose of a novel spectinomycin analog, trospectomycin (U-63366F). *Antimicrob Agents Chemother* 1990; **34:** 2342–7.
2. Nichols DJ, *et al.* Pharmacokinetics of trospectomycin sulphate in healthy subjects after single intravenous and intramuscular doses. *Br J Clin Pharmacol* 1991; **32:** 255–7.
3. Keefer MC, *et al.* Single-dose trospectomycin for chlamydial urethritis in men. *Antimicrob Agents Chemother* 1991; **35:** 986–7.
4. Beam TR, *et al.* In-vitro activity of trospectomycin [sic] against Gram-positive cocci. *J Antimicrob Chemother* 1995; **36:** 874–8.
5. Chisari G, *et al.* The in vitro activity of trospectomycin against anaerobic bacteria. *J Chemother* 1995; **7:** 515–18.
6. Chatwani A, *et al.* Trospectomycin in acute pelvic inflammatory disease: a preliminary report. *Infect Dis Obstet Gynecol* 1997; **5:** 215–18.
7. Chatwani A, *et al.* Double-blind, multicenter, prospective randomized study of trospectomycin vs clindamycin, both with aztreonam, in non-community acquired obstetric and gynecologic infections. *Infect Dis Obstet Gynecol* 1997; **5:** 280–5.

Trovafloxacin Mesilate (17529-b)

Trovafloxacin Mesilate (*rINNM*).

CP-99219-27; CP-99219 (trovafloxacin); Trovafloxacin Mesylate (*USAN*). 7-[(1R,5S,6S)-6-Amino-3-azabicyclo[3.1.0]hex-3-yl]-1-(2,4-difluorophenyl)-6-fluoro-1,4-dihydro-4-oxo-1,8-naphthyridine-3-carboxylic acid monomethanesulphonate.

$C_{20}H_{15}F_3N_4O_3,CH_4O_3S = 512.5$.

CAS — 147059-72-1 (trovafloxacin); 147059-75-4 (trovafloxacin mesilate).

Adverse Effects and Precautions

As for Ciprofloxacin, p.183.

Dizziness is the most common adverse effect reported with trovafloxacin.

Trovafloxacin preparations have been withdrawn in many European countries following reports of unpredictable severe hepatic adverse effects, including some fatalities. Symptomatic pancreatitis has also been reported. In those countries (such as the USA) where trovafloxacin is still available, it is recommended that liver function tests and pancreatic tests should be performed when symptoms develop and, if necessary, that the drug be discontinued.

Antimicrobial Action

As for Ciprofloxacin, p.184. It is more active against pneumococci.

Pharmacokinetics

Trovafloxacin is readily absorbed from the gastrointestinal tract following oral administration, peak plasma concentrations being achieved after about 1 to 2 hours. Following intravenous administration, alatrofloxacin is rapidly converted to trovafloxacin. Bioavailability following oral administration of trovafloxacin has been reported to be 88%. Trovafloxacin is widely distributed into body tissues and is about 76% bound to plasma proteins. It appears in breast milk.

The serum half-life of trovafloxacin ranges from about 9 to 12 hours. Trovafloxacin is metabolised by conjugation, 13% of a dose appearing in the urine as the glucuronide and 9% in the faeces as the N-acetyl metabolite; other metabolites appear in both the urine and faeces in minor amounts, but approximately 50% of an oral dose is excreted unchanged, mainly in the faeces but also in the urine.

Uses and Administration

Trovafloxacin is a fluoroquinolone antibacterial with actions and uses similar to those of ciprofloxacin (p.185). It is given as the mesilate by mouth for the treatment of susceptible infections. The prodrug alatrofloxacin (p.147) is used as the mesilate for intravenous infusion.

Trovafloxacin and alatrofloxacin preparations have been withdrawn in many European countries following reports of unpredictable severe hepatic adverse effects, including some fatalities; the use in some other countries such as the USA is restricted to specified serious conditions and usually for a treatment period of up to a maximum of 2 weeks. Doses of both trovafloxacin mesilate and alatrofloxacin mesilate are expressed in terms of trovafloxacin base. Usual daily doses are the equivalent of 200 mg of trovafloxacin by mouth or 200 to 300 mg intravenously.

◊ General references.

1. Haria M, Lamb HM. Trovafloxacin. *Drugs* 1997; **54:** 435–45.
2. Amyes SGN, *et al.* (eds.) Trovafloxacin: a novel extended spectrum quinolone. *J Antimicrob Chemother* 1997; **39** (suppl B): 1–97.
3. Alghasham AA, Nahata MC. Trovafloxacin: a new fluoroquinolone. *Ann Pharmacother* 1999; **33:** 48–60.

Preparations

Proprietary Preparations (details are given in Part 3)
Aust.: Trovan†; **Austral.:** Trovan; **Canad.:** Trovan; **Hong Kong:** Trovan; **Mex.:** Trovan; **Swed.:** Trovan†; **USA:** Trovan.

Tylosin (13388-r)

Tylosin (BAN, rINN).
$C_{46}H_{77}NO_{17} = 916.1$.
CAS — 1401-69-0.
Pharmacopoeias. In Eur. (see p.vi) and *US*, both for veterinary use.

Pharmacopoeial description

Ph. Eur.: A mixture of macrolide antibiotics produced by a strain of *Streptomyces fradiae* or by any other means. The main component of the mixture is tylosin A, but tylosin B (desmycosin), tylosin C (macrocin), and tylosin D (relomycin) may also be present. An almost white or slightly yellow powder. Slightly soluble in water; freely soluble in dehydrated alcohol and in dichloromethane. It dissolves in dilute solutions of mineral acids. A 2.5% suspension in water has a pH of 8.5 to 10.5. Protect from light.

USP 25: A macrolide antibiotic substance or mixture of such substances produced by the growth of *Streptomyces fradiae* or by any other means. A white to buff-coloured powder. Slightly soluble in water; soluble in alcohol, in amyl acetate, in chloroform and in dilute mineral acids; freely soluble in methyl alcohol. It loses not more than 5% of its weight on drying. Protect from light, moisture, and temperatures exceeding 40°.

Tylosin Tartrate (13389-f)

Tylosin Tartrate (BANM, rINNM).
$(C_{46}H_{77}NO_{17})_2,C_4H_6O_6 = 1982.3$.
CAS — 1405-54-5.
Pharmacopoeias. In Eur. (see p.vi) for veterinary use.

1.1 g of monograph substance is approximately equivalent to 1 g of tylosin.

Pharmacopoeial description

Ph. Eur.: An almost white or slightly yellow hygroscopic powder. Freely soluble in water and in dichloromethane; slightly soluble in dehydrated alcohol. It dissolves in dilute solutions of mineral acids. A 2.5% solution in water has a pH of 5.0 to 7.2. Store in airtight containers. Protect from light.

Profile

Tylosin is a macrolide antibiotic with actions similar to those of erythromycin (p.201). Tylosin and its phosphate and tartrate salts are used in veterinary medicine in the prophylaxis and treatment of various infections caused by susceptible organisms.

Tylosin and tylosin phosphate have been added to animal feeding stuffs as growth promotors for pigs.

Tyrothricin (176-z)

Tyrothricin (BAN, rINN).
Tirotricina.
CAS — 1404-88-2.
ATC — D06AX08; R02AB02; S01AA05.
Pharmacopoeias. In Fr., Swiss, and *US.*

Pharmacopoeial description

USP 25: An antibacterial substance produced by the growth of *Bacillus brevis.* It is a mixture consisting chiefly of gramicidin and tyrocidine, the latter being usually present as the hydrochloride. Store in airtight containers.

Adverse Effects and Precautions

Tyrothricin is too toxic to be administered systemically; effects that have been reported include liver and kidney damage as well as Stevens-Johnson syndrome. It damages the sensory epithelium of the nose and instances of prolonged loss of smell have occurred after its use as a nasal spray or instillation. Tyrothricin should not be instilled into the nasal cavities or into closed body cavities.

Uses and Administration

Tyrothricin is unsuitable for systemic treatment. It is active *in vitro* against many Gram-positive bacteria and has been used either alone or in conjunction with other antibacterials in the local treatment of infections mainly of the skin and mouth.

The symbol † denotes a preparation no longer actively marketed

Preparations

Proprietary Preparations (details are given in Part 3)
Fr.: Codetricine; **Ger.:** Tyrosur; **Hong Kong:** Tyrosur; **Israel:** Rafathricin; **Ital.:** Faringotricina; Hydrotricine; Rinotricina; **Port.:** Hydrotricine.

Multi-ingredient: Aust.: Dolothricin†; Dorithricin; Lemocin; Neocones; Recessan†; Sanoral; Tongill; Tonsicur; Tyrosolvin†; Tyrothricin comp; **Belg.:** Lemocin; Tricidine; Tyro-Drops; **Braz.:** Amidalin; Amigdagen; Amigdalol; Amigdamicin; Anapyon; Anfomicin; Angino Tricin; Anginozetes; Auritricin; Cloraseptic; Colpacid; Colpagex N; Colpolase; Dermosed; Eucament; Filogargan; Gargosedans; Gynax-N; Gyrol; Higienex; Lacto Vagin; Lacto-Gin; Laringex; Larintil; Malvatricin; Naso Instil; Neomicina Composta; Oturga; Rinocron; Sedauric; Trivagel N; Vagitrin-N; Varigerm; Vulgix; **Canad.:** Antibiotic Cold Sore Ointment; Emercreme No 4; Soropon; Webber Antibiotic Cold Sore Ointment†; **Fr.:** Broncorinol rhinites; Bronpax†; Codetricine vitamine C; Collunovar; Ergix; Pharyngine a la Vitamine C; Solutricine Tetracaine; Solutricine Vitamine C; Tyrcine; Tyrothricine Lafran†; Veybirol-Tyrothyricine; **Ger.:** Anginomycin; Dori; Dorithricin Limone; Dorithricin Original; Inspirol Halsschmerztabletten; Lemocin; Myacyne†; Nordathricin N; Pellit dermal Wund- und Heilsalbe; Trachisan; Tyrosur; **Hong Kong:** Deq; Tyrocaine; Tyrothricin Co; **Irl.:** Tyrozets; **Israel:** Acnex; Kalgaron; Rafathricin with Benzocaine; **Ital.:** Bio-Arscolloid; Deltavagin; Furotricina; Golamixin; Kinogen; Rinocidina; **Port.:** Afonina; Mebocaina; Medifon; Mentocaina R; Oralbiotico; Tyrozets†; **S.Afr.:** Otoseptil†; Tyrogel†; **Singapore:** Beathricin; Deq; Trachisan; **Spain:** Anginovag; Bucometasana; Cicatral; Cohortan; Cohortan Antibiotico†; Diformiltricina; Gradin Del D Andreu; Hemodren Compuesto; Miozets; Neocones; Otosedol Biotico; Oxidermiol Antihist; Pastillas Koki Ment Tiro; Piorlis; Roberfarin; Sedofarin; Viberol Tirotricina; **Switz.:** Lemocin; Mebucaine; Otothricinol; Rhinothricinol; Sangerol; Solmucaine; Solutricine†; Trachisan†; Tyrocombine; Tyroqualine; Tyrothricin; Tyrothricine + Gramicidine; **Thai.:** Deq; Iwazin; Trocacin; Troneo; **UAE:** B-Cool; **UK:** Tyrozets.

Valnemulin (3218-w)

Valnemulin (rINN).
Valnemulina; Valnémuline. ({2-[(R)-2-Amino-3-methylbutyramido]-1,1-dimethylethyl}thio)acetic acid 8-ester with (3aS,4R,5S,6S,8R,9R,9aR,10R)-octahydro-5,8-dihydroxy-4,6,9,10-tetramethyl-6-vinyl-3a,9-propano-3aH-cyclopentacycloocten-1(4H)-one.
$C_{31}H_{52}N_2O_5S = 564.8$.
CAS — 101312-92-9.

Profile

Valnemulin is an antibacterial used as the hydrochloride in veterinary medicine.

Vancomycin Hydrochloride (177-c)

Vancomycin Hydrochloride (BANM, rINNM).
Vancomycini Hydrochloridum. (S_a)-(3S,6R,7R,22R,23S,26S,36R,38aR)-44-{[2-O-(3-Amino-2,3,6-trideoxy-3-C-methyl-α-L-lyxo-hexopyranosyl)-β-D-glucopyranosyl]oxy}-3-(carbamoylmethyl)-10,19-dichloro-2,3,4,5,6,7,23,24,25,26,36,37,38,38a-tetradecahydro-7,22,28,30,32-pentahydroxy-6-[(2R)-4-methyl-2-(methylamino)valeramido]-2,5,24,38,39-pentaoxo-22H-8,11:18,21-dietheno-23,36-(iminomethano)-13,16:31,35-dimetheno-1H,16H-[1,6,9]oxadiazacyclohexadecino[4,5-m][10,2,16]-benzoxadiazacyclotetracosine-26-carboxylic acid, monohydrochloride.
$C_{66}H_{75}Cl_2N_9O_{24},HCl = 1485.7$.
CAS — 1404-90-6 (vancomycin); 1404-93-9 (vancomycin hydrochloride).
Pharmacopoeias. In Eur. (see p.vi), *Jpn, Pol.* and *US.*
US also includes vancomycin base.

A glycopeptide antimicrobial substance or mixture of glycopeptides produced by the growth of certain strains of *Amycolatopsis orientalis* (*Nocardia orientalis, Streptomyces orientalis*), or by any other means. 1.03 g of monograph substance is approximately equivalent to 1 g of vancomycin.

Incompatibilities. Solutions of vancomycin hydrochloride have an acid pH and incompatibility may reasonably be expected with alkaline preparations, or with drugs unstable at low pH. Reports of incompatibility are not always consistent, and other factors such as the strength of solution, and composition of the vehicles used, may play a part.

Pharmacopoeial description

Ph. Eur.: A mixture of related glycopeptides, consisting principally of vancomycin B, a substance produced by certain strains of *Amycolatopsis orientalis* or obtained by any other means. A white or almost white, hygroscopic powder. Freely soluble in water; slightly soluble in alcohol. A 5% solution in water has a pH of 2.5 to 4.5. Store in airtight containers. Protect from light.

USP 25: A substance or mixture of substances produced by the growth of *Streptomyces orientalis*. A tan to brown, odourless, free-flowing powder. Freely soluble in water; insoluble in chloroform and in ether. A 5% solution in water has a pH of 2.5 to 4.5. Store in airtight containers.

Stability. Although the manufacturers recommend storage at 2° to 8°, solutions of vancomycin hydrochloride in various diluents (sodium chloride 0.9%, glucose 5%, and peritoneal dialysis solution) have been found to be stable for at least 14 days at room temperature.[1-3]
The stability of vancomycin in ophthalmic solution has also been studied.[4]

1. Das Gupta V, *et al.* Stability of vancomycin hydrochloride in 5% dextrose and in 0.9% sodium chloride injections. *Am J Hosp Pharm* 1986; **43:** 1729–31.
2. Walker SE, Birkhans B. Stability of intravenous vancomycin. *Can J Hosp Pharm* 1988; **41:** 233–8.
3. Mauhinuey WM, *et al.* Stability of vancomycin hydrochloride in peritoneal dialysis solution. *Am J Hosp Pharm* 1992; **49:** 137–9.
4. Fuhrman LC, Stroman RT. Stability of vancomycin in an extemporaneously compounded ophthalmic solution. *Am J Health-Syst Pharm* 1998; **55:** 1386–8.

Adverse Effects

The intravenous administration of vancomycin may be associated with the so-called 'red-neck' or 'red-man' syndrome, characterised by erythema, flushing, or rash over the face and upper torso, and sometimes by hypotension and shock-like symptoms. The effect appears to be due in part to the release of histamine and is usually related to rapid infusion.

Hypersensitivity reactions may occur in about 5% of patients and include rashes, fever, chills, and rarely, anaphylactoid reactions, exfoliative dermatitis, Stevens-Johnson syndrome, toxic epidermal necrolysis, and vasculitis. Many reactions have become less frequent with the availability of more highly purified preparations. Reversible neutropenia, eosinophilia, and rarely thrombocytopenia and agranulocytosis have been reported; neutropenia is stated to be more common in patients who have received a total dose of 25 g or more. Nephrotoxicity may occur, particularly at high doses or in patients with predisposing factors, but has declined in frequency with greater awareness of the problem and appropriate monitoring of plasma concentrations and renal function.

Ototoxicity is also associated with vancomycin administration, and is more likely in patients with high plasma concentrations. It may progress after drug withdrawal, and may be irreversible. Hearing loss may be preceded by tinnitus, which must be regarded as a sign to discontinue treatment.

Vancomycin is irritant; intravenous administration may be associated with thrombophlebitis, although this can be minimised by the slow infusion of dilute solutions, and by using different infusion sites. Extravasation may cause tissue necrosis.

Because of its poor absorption, relatively few adverse effects have been reported after the oral administration of vancomycin, although mild gastrointestinal disturbances have occurred.

Effects on the ears. Reviews of ototoxicity associated with vancomycin therapy:[1,2] the actual number of cases is quite small, and close examination suggests that in most cases where hearing loss occurred patients had also received an aminoglycoside. The degree, and the reversibility, of ototoxicity associated with vancomycin alone is uncertain.

1. Bailie GR, Neal D. Vancomycin ototoxicity and nephrotoxicity: a review. *Med Toxicol* 1988; **3:** 376–86.
2. Brummett RE, Fox KE. Vancomycin- and erythromycin-induced hearing loss in humans. *Antimicrob Agents Chemother* 1989; **33:** 791–6.

Effects on the gastrointestinal tract. A 25-year-old woman developed *Clostridium difficile* colitis following a course of vancomycin and metronidazole, both by mouth, for pelvic inflammatory disease.[1] The condition resolved after treatment with vancomycin given alone.

1. Bingley PJ, Harding GM. Clostridium difficile colitis following treatment with metronidazole and vancomycin. *Postgrad Med J* 1987; **63:** 993–4.

Effects on the heart. A report[1] of cardiac arrest associated with inadvertent and rapid intravenous administration of vancomycin 150 mg to a neonate.

1. Boussemart T, *et al.* Cardiac arrest associated with vancomycin in a neonate. *Arch Dis Child* 1995; **73:** F123.

Effects on the kidneys. In a study,[1] nephrotoxicity was seen in 14 of 101 patients assigned to vancomycin 1 g before and after vascular surgery for infection prophylaxis compared with 2 of 99 assigned to saline placebo, suggesting that even short regimens of vancomycin can affect renal function. In another study involving 224 patients, nephrotoxicity was seen in 8 of 168 given vancomycin alone, 14 of 63 given vancomycin with an aminoglycoside, and 11 of 103 given an aminoglycoside without vancomycin.[2] This latter study found that concomitant aminoglycoside therapy, trough serum concentrations of vancomycin greater than 10 µg per mL, and prolonged vancomycin therapy (for more than 21 days) were associated with an increased risk of nephrotoxicity. In both studies nephrotoxicity was defined in terms of increased serum-creatinine.

1. Gudmundsson GH, Jensen LJ. Vancomycin and nephrotoxicity. *Lancet* 1989; i: 625.
2. Rybak MJ, *et al.* Nephrotoxicity of vancomycin, alone and with an aminoglycoside. *J Antimicrob Chemother* 1990; 25: 679–87.

Effects on the nervous system. Reports of encephalopathy[1] (associated with high CSF concentrations after oral administration) and peripheral neuropathy[2] associated with vancomycin.

1. Thompson CM, *et al.* Absorption of oral vancomycin—possible associated toxicity. *Int J Pediatr Nephrol* 1983; 4: 1–4.
2. Leibowitz AL, *et al.* Mononeuritis multiplex associated with prolonged vancomycin treatment. *BMJ* 1990; 300: 1344.

Effects on the skin. Skin reactions associated with vancomycin have commonly been rash, erythema, or pruritus but there have also been reports of linear IgA dermatosis,[1-4] Stevens-Johnson-like reaction,[5] bullous eruption,[6] and exfoliative dermatitis.[6] In an analysis, risk factors for adverse cutaneous reactions were suggested to be age under 40 years and duration of therapy greater than 7 days.[6]

1. Piketty C, *et al.* Linear IgA dermatosis related to vancomycin. *Br J Dermatol* 1994; 130: 130–1.
2. Nousari HC, *et al.* Vancomycin-associated linear IgA bullous dermatosis. *Ann Intern Med* 1998; 129: 507–8.
3. Bernstein EF, Schuster M. Linear IgA bullous dermatosis associated with vancomycin. *Ann Intern Med* 1998; 129: 508–9.
4. Danielson AG, Thomsen K. Vancomycin-induced linear IgA bullous disease. *Br J Dermatol* 1999; 141: 756–7.
5. Laurencin CT, *et al.* Stevens-Johnson-like reaction with vancomycin treatment. *Ann Pharmacother* 1992; 26: 1520–1.
6. Korman TM, *et al.* Risk factors for adverse cutaneous reactions associated with intravenous vancomycin. *J Antimicrob Chemother* 1997; 39: 371–81.

Local reactions. Despite the view that thrombophlebitis is less frequent with more highly purified preparations of vancomycin, it may still be common:[1] in 6 patients receiving vancomycin as solutions containing 4 or 5 mg per mL, phlebitis developed at 32 of 35 sites used. The intraperitoneal infusion of vancomycin has been associated with chemical peritonitis and, although it may be associated with less highly purified brands of the drug,[2] this has not been confirmed.[3]

1. Garrelts JC, *et al.* Phlebitis associated with vancomycin therapy. *Clin Pharm* 1988; 7: 720–1.
2. Smith TA, *et al.* Chemical peritonitis associated with intraperitoneal vancomycin. *DICP Ann Pharmacother* 1991; 25: 602–3.
3. Abel SR. Lack of chemical peritonitis after intraperitoneal use of two brands of vancomycin hydrochloride. *Clin Pharm* 1989; 8: 91–2.

Red-man syndrome. References[1-13] to the 'red-man syndrome', including the suggestion that pretreatment with an antihistamine can provide significant protection against it.[8,10] Similar reactions appear to be much less of a problem with teicoplanin and substitution of teicoplanin for vancomycin may be a viable alternative in patients at risk.[12-14] Skin tests are reported[15] to be of little value in predicting the severity of 'red-man syndrome'.

1. Pau AK, Khakoo R. "Red-neck" syndrome with slow infusion of vancomycin. *N Engl J Med* 1985; 313: 756–7.
2. Southorn PA, *et al.* Adverse effects of vancomycin administered in the perioperative period. *Mayo Clin Proc* 1986; 61: 721–4.
3. Davis RL, *et al.* The "red man's syndrome" and slow infusion of vancomycin. *Ann Intern Med* 1986; 104: 285–6.
4. Best CJ, *et al.* Perioperative complications following the use of vancomycin in children: a report of two cases. *Br J Anaesth* 1989; 62: 576–7.
5. Sahai J, *et al.* Influence of antihistamine pretreatment on vancomycin-induced red-man syndrome. *J Infect Dis* 1989; 160: 876–81.
6. Healy DP, *et al.* Vancomycin-induced histamine release and "red man syndrome": comparison of 1- and 2-hour infusions. *Antimicrob Agents Chemother* 1990; 34: 550–4.
7. Levy M, *et al.* Vancomycin-induced red man syndrome. *Pediatrics* 1990; 86: 572–80.
8. Bailie GR, *et al.* Red-neck syndrome associated with intraperitoneal vancomycin. *Clin Pharm* 1990; 9: 671–2.
9. Anonymous. Red men should go: vancomycin and histamine release. *Lancet* 1990; 335: 1006–7.
10. Sahai J, *et al.* Comparison of vancomycin- and teicoplanin-induced histamine release and "red man syndrome". *Antimicrob Agents Chemother* 1990; 34: 765–9.
11. Wallace MR, *et al.* Red man syndrome: incidence, etiology, and prophylaxis. *J Infect Dis* 1991; 164: 1180–5.
12. Polk RE. Anaphylactoid reactions to glycopeptide antibiotics. *J Antimicrob Chemother* 1991; 27 (suppl B): 17–29.
13. Rybak MJ, *et al.* Absence of "red man syndrome" in patients being treated with vancomycin or high-dose teicoplanin. *Antimicrob Agents Chemother* 1992; 36: 1204–7.
14. Smith SR. Vancomycin and histamine release. *Lancet* 1990; 335: 1341.
15. Polk RE, *et al.* Vancomycin skin tests and prediction of "red man syndrome" in healthy volunteers. *Antimicrob Agents Chemother* 1993; 37: 2139–43.

AFTER ORAL ADMINISTRATION. Reports of rash[1] and 'red-man syndrome'[2,3] following oral administration of vancomycin.

1. McCullough JM, *et al.* Oral vancomycin-induced rash: case report and review of the literature. *DICP Ann Pharmacother* 1991; 25: 1326–8.
2. Killian AD, *et al.* Red man syndrome after oral vancomycin. *Ann Intern Med* 1991; 115: 410–11.
3. Bergeron L, Boucher FD. Possible red-man syndrome associated with systemic absorption of oral vancomycin in a child with normal renal function. *Ann Pharmacother* 1994; 28: 581–4.

Precautions

Vancomycin should not be given to patients who have experienced a hypersensitivity reaction to it. It should not be given intramuscularly, and care should be taken when it is given intravenously to avoid extravasation, because of the risk of tissue necrosis. The adverse effects of infusion may be minimised by dilution of each 500 mg of vancomycin in at least 100 mL of fluid, and by infusion of doses over not less than 60 minutes.

Because the risk of ototoxicity and nephrotoxicity is thought to be increased at high plasma concentrations it may be desirable to adjust dosage requirements according to plasma-vancomycin concentrations. It has been suggested that dosage should be adjusted to avoid peak plasma concentrations above 30 to 40 µg per mL and trough concentrations exceeding 10 µg per mL, although uncertainty about the optimum methods and sampling times for monitoring, as well as some uncertainty about the degree of risk, means that there is less general agreement than for the aminoglycosides. It is agreed, however, that vancomycin should be generally avoided in patients with a history of impaired hearing and that particular care is necessary in patients with renal impairment, in neonates (especially if premature), and in the elderly, all of whom may be at increased risk of toxicity. Renal function and blood counts should be monitored regularly in all patients, and monitoring of auditory function is advisable, especially in patients with the risk factors mentioned. Vancomycin should be discontinued in patients who develop tinnitus.

Since vancomycin is poorly absorbed, toxicity is much less of a problem following oral administration than with the intravenous route but care is required in patients with inflammatory gastrointestinal disorders, including antibiotic-associated colitis, in whom absorption may be enhanced.

Interactions

Other ototoxic or nephrotoxic drugs, such as the aminoglycosides, polymyxins, and loop diuretics, markedly increase the risk of toxicity and should be given concomitantly with vancomycin only with great caution.

Some of the adverse effects of vancomycin may be enhanced by the concurrent use of general anaesthetics; it has been suggested that, where patients require both, vancomycin infusions should be completed before the induction of anaesthesia.

Vancomycin may increase neuromuscular blockade produced by drugs such as suxamethonium or vecuronium.

Antimicrobial Action

Vancomycin is a glycopeptide antibiotic with a primarily bactericidal action against a variety of Gram-positive bacteria.

Mechanism of action. It exerts its action by inhibiting the formation of the peptidoglycan polymers of the bacterial cell wall. Unlike penicillins which act primarily to prevent the cross-linking of peptidoglycans which gives the cell wall its strength, vancomycin prevents the transfer and addition of the muramylpentapeptide building blocks that make up the peptidoglycan molecule itself. Vancomycin may also exert some effects by damaging the cytoplasmic membrane of the protoplast, and by inhibiting bacterial RNA synthesis.

Spectrum of activity. Staphylococci, notably *Staph. aureus* and *Staph. epidermidis* (including meticillin-resistant strains), *Streptococcus pneumoniae*, *Str. pyogenes*, and some strains of Group B streptococci are reported to be susceptible to vancomycin. The viridans streptococci, and enterococci such as *Enterococcus faecalis*, are often 'tolerant', i.e. inhibition, but no bactericidal effect, can be achieved at usual plasma concentrations (but see Activity with other Antimicrobials and Resistance, below).

Clostridium difficile is usually highly susceptible but other clostridia vary somewhat in their susceptibility; *Actinomyces* spp., *Bacillus anthracis*, *Corynebacterium* spp., some lactobacilli, and *Listeria* are usually susceptible. Virtually all Gram-negative organisms, as well as mycobacteria and fungi, are intrinsically resistant.

Minimum inhibitory concentrations (MICs) of vancomycin for the most susceptible organisms range from about 0.1 to 2 µg per mL; for most organisms it is bactericidal at concentrations not far above the MIC. Organisms with MICs up to about 4 µg per mL are generally considered sensitive to vancomycin, and those with MICs between about 4 and 16 µg per mL of intermediate sensitivity.

Activity with other antimicrobials. Vancomycin exhibits synergy with the aminoglycosides against enterococci; such combinations are usually bactericidal, even against vancomycin-tolerant strains. The synergistic effect is reported to be greater with gentamicin than with streptomycin. Combinations with an aminoglycoside are also reported to demonstrate synergy against *Staph. aureus*; however, variable results, including antimicrobial antagonism, or lack of synergy, have been reported against strains of *Staph. aureus* when vancomycin was combined with rifampicin. Synergy has been reported with the third-generation cephalosporins against *Staph. aureus* and enterococci.

Resistance to vancomycin in normally susceptible organisms has until recently remained relatively uncommon, although high-level intrinsic resistance has been seen in some species of *Lactobacillus*, *Leuconostoc*, and *Erysipelothrix*. However, there are an increasing number of reports of high-level acquired resistance amongst enterococci, apparently plasmid-mediated and transferable to other Gram-positive organisms, notably *Staph. aureus*, which are causing considerable concern. Organisms exhibiting high-level vancomycin resistance demonstrate cross-resistance to teicoplanin. Low-level resistance has also been reported in enterococci, but these organisms remain sensitive to teicoplanin, and this form of resistance does not appear to be transferable. Low-level vancomycin resistance has also been seen rarely among some staphylococcal strains: in contrast to the enterococci, these are often cross-resistant to teicoplanin. The mechanism of acquired resistance is uncertain, although it appears to be associated with the development of novel cell-membrane proteins.

◊ Reference[1] to increasing resistance to vancomycin amongst enterococci, including its possible transferral to *Staphylococcus aureus*,[2-6] and guidelines to prevent its spread.[7,8]

1. Murray BE. Vancomycin-resistant enterococci. *Am J Med* 1997; 102: 284–93.
2. Hiramatsu K, *et al.* Methicillin-resistant Staphylococcus aureus clinical strain with reduced vancomycin susceptibility. *J Antimicrob Chemother* 1997; 40: 135–6.
3. Johnson AP. Intermediate vancomycin resistance in Staphylococcus aureus: a major threat or a minor inconvenience? *J Antimicrob Chemother* 1998; 42: 289–91.
4. Ploy MC, *et al.* First clinical isolate of vancomycin-intermediate Staphylococcus aureus in a French hospital. *Lancet* 1998; 351: 1212.
5. Smith TL, *et al.* Emergence of vancomycin resistance in Staphylococcus aureus. *N Engl J Med* 1999; 340: 493–501.
6. Sieradzki K, *et al.* The development of vancomycin resistance in a patient with methicillin-resistant Staphylococcus aureus infection. *N Engl J Med* 1999; 340: 517–23.
7. Hospital Infection Control Practices Advisory Committee (HICPAC). Recommendations for preventing the spread of vancomycin resistance. *Infect Control Hosp Epidemiol* 1995; 16: 105–13.
8. Edmond MB, *et al.* Vancomycin-resistant Staphylococcus aureus: perspectives on measures needed for control. *Ann Intern Med* 1996; 124: 329–34.

Pharmacokinetics

Vancomycin is only poorly absorbed from the gastrointestinal tract, although absorption may be somewhat greater when the gastrointestinal tract is inflamed. Intramuscular administration is associated with pain and tissue necrosis; systemic doses are therefore given intravenously. Infusion of a 1-g dose intravenously over 60 minutes has reportedly been associated with plasma concentrations of up to about 60 µg per mL immediately after completion of the infusion, and about 25 µg per mL 2 hours later, falling to under 10 µg per mL after 11 hours. However, there may be considerable interindividual variation in the pharmacokinetics of vancomycin: a range of half-lives between 3 and 13 hours has been reported, with an average of about 6 hours, in patients with normal renal function. Half-life may be prolonged in patients with renal impairment, to 7 days or more in anephric patients. About 55% is bound to plasma proteins, although large variations have been reported.

Vancomycin diffuses into extracellular fluid, including pleural, pericardial, ascitic, and synovial fluid. Small amounts are found in bile. However, there is little diffusion into the CSF and even when the meninges are inflamed effective concentrations may not be achieved. Vancomycin crosses the peritoneal cavity; about 60% of an intraperitoneal dose is reported to be absorbed in 6 hours. It is reported to cross the placenta. It is also distributed into breast milk.

Little or no metabolism of vancomycin is thought to take place. It is excreted unchanged by the kidneys, mostly by glomerular filtration. Some 80 to 90% of the dose is excreted in urine within 24 hours. There appears to be a small amount of non-renal clearance, although the mechanism for this has not been determined.

As for the aminoglycosides, the pharmacokinetics of vancomycin may be altered by conditions which affect renal clearance: clearance of vancomycin has been reported to be enhanced in burn patients, whereas in those with renal impairment, or reduced renal function (such as neonates or the elderly), clearance is reduced and plasma-concentrations and half-lives increased. Dosage adjustment is often necessary in patients with reduced or impaired renal function; ideally, this should be based on plasma-concentration monitoring. Although clearance is also altered in hepatic impairment, it has been suggested that dosage adjustment is not necessary in the absence of other factors.

Plasma concentrations of vancomycin are reported to be little affected by conventional haemodialysis, although the use of high-flux membranes may significantly reduce vancomycin concentrations. Peritoneal dialysis, although it may decrease concentrations, is also thought not to do so by significant amounts, but haemoperfusion or haemofiltration effectively removes vancomycin from the blood.

Uses and Administration

Vancomycin is a glycopeptide antibiotic that is used in the treatment of serious staphylococcal or other Gram-positive infections where other drugs such as the penicillins cannot be used because of resistance or patient intolerance. It is used particularly in the treatment of meticillin-resistant staphylococcal infections (p.140), in conditions such as brain abscess, staphylococcal meningitis, peritonitis associated with continuous ambulatory peritoneal dialysis, and septicaemia. It is used alone, or in combination with another drug such as an aminoglycoside, in the treatment and prophylaxis of endocarditis, for the prophylaxis of surgical infection, and in intensive care and the management of immunocompromised patients. It is also used (by mouth) in the treatment of antibiotic-associated colitis (see under Gastro-enteritis, p.122). For details of all these infections and their treatment, see under Choice of Antibacterial, p.114.

Vancomycin may be used concomitantly with other antibacterials to extend the spectrum of efficacy or increase effectiveness, notably with gentamicin or other aminoglycosides, or with rifampicin (but see Antimicrobial Action, above).

Administration and dosage. Vancomycin is given as the hydrochloride but doses are expressed in terms of the base. It is administered intravenously, preferably by intermittent infusion, although continuous infusion has been used. For intermittent infusion, a concentrated solution containing the equivalent of 500 mg of vancomycin in 10 mL of water is prepared

and then added to glucose 5% or sodium chloride 0.9% to produce a diluted solution containing not more than 5 mg per mL; this diluted solution is then infused over at least 60 minutes for a 500-mg dose or 100 minutes for a 1-g dose. Final concentrations of up to 10 mg per mL may be used for patients requiring fluid restriction, although there is an increased risk of adverse events. For continuous intravenous infusion, the equivalent of 1 to 2 g is added to a sufficiently large volume of glucose or sodium chloride to permit the daily dose to be given over a period of 24 hours.

The usual adult dose is the equivalent of 500 mg of vancomycin every 6 hours or 1 g every 12 hours. Response is generally seen within 48 to 72 hours in sensitive infections. In patients with staphylococcal endocarditis, treatment for at least 3 weeks has been recommended.

For the prophylaxis of endocarditis in high-risk penicillin-allergic patients undergoing dental or other procedures, vancomycin may be given before the procedure in a single dose of 1 g by intravenous infusion over at least 100 minutes followed by intravenous gentamicin.

Doses in infants and children. Children and infants over 4 weeks of age may be given 10 mg per kg bodyweight every 6 hours. Neonates and infants up to 4 weeks old may be given an initial dose of 15 mg per kg; this is followed by 10 mg per kg every 12 hours in the first week of life or by 10 mg per kg every 8 hours in those aged 1 to 4 weeks.

For the prophylaxis of endocarditis in children a single dose of 20 mg per kg may be used.

Dose adjustment and monitoring. It has been recommended that dosage should be adjusted if necessary according to plasma-vancomycin concentrations, and this is particularly important where factors such as age or renal impairment may predispose to toxicity, or where there is a risk of subtherapeutic concentrations. There has been some dispute about the relationship between plasma concentrations and toxicity, and this, complicated by differences in the sampling time after the end of infusion and by differences in the regimens administered and assay method used, has meant that suggested peak and trough concentrations have varied considerably. However in order to avoid toxic concentrations immediately after the end of infusion the consensus appears to be that concentrations of not more than 30 to 40 µg per mL should be aimed for 1 to 2 hours after completion of infusion. It is usually recommended that trough concentrations (measured just before the next dose) should be below 10 µg per mL.

Various methods, including predictive nomograms based on creatinine clearance and pharmacokinetic methods such as those using Bayesian statistics, have been suggested for calculating vancomycin dosage requirements in patients with reduced renal function (see also below). One suggested approach has been a loading dose of 15 mg per kg followed by a daily dose in mg equivalent to about 15 times the glomerular filtration rate in mL per minute; or in anuric patients a dose of 1 g every 7 to 10 days. However, individualised dosage based on plasma concentrations is generally to be preferred.

Other routes. Vancomycin hydrochloride is administered by mouth in the treatment of staphylococcal enterocolitis and antibiotic-associated colitis including pseudomembranous colitis associated with the overgrowth of *Clostridium difficile.* It is given in a dose of 0.5 to 2.0 g daily in 3 or 4 divided doses for 7 to 10 days; the lowest dose of 0.5 g daily is often considered adequate. A dose for children is 40 mg per kg daily in 3 or 4 divided doses; some authorities suggest that half this dose is adequate.

In meningitis or other CNS infections vancomycin has sometimes been given by the intrathecal or intraventricular route in order to ensure adequate CSF concentrations of antibiotic. Vancomycin has also been applied topically to the eye or given by subcon-

junctival or intravitreal injection; it has also been given by inhalation.

◊ Reviews.
1. Wilhelm MP, Estes L. Vancomycin. *Mayo Clin Proc* 1999; **74:** 928–35.

Administration. References to methods of determining vancomycin dosage and the necessity for monitoring plasma concentrations.
1. Nielsen HE, *et al.* Renal excretion of vancomycin in kidney disease. *Acta Med Scand* 1975; **197:** 261–4.
2. Moellering RC, *et al.* Vancomycin therapy in patients with impaired renal function: a nomogram for dosage. *Ann Intern Med* 1981; **94:** 343–6.
3. Rotschafer JC, *et al.* Pharmacokinetics of vancomycin; observations in 28 patients and dosage recommendations. *Antimicrob Agents Chemother* 1982; **22:** 391–4.
4. Matzke GR, *et al.* Pharmacokinetics of vancomycin in patients with various degrees of renal function. *Antimicrob Agents Chemother* 1984; **25:** 433–7.
5. Matzke GR, *et al.* Evaluation of the vancomycin-clearance: creatinine-clearance relationship for predicting vancomycin dosage. *Clin Pharm* 1985; **4:** 311–15.
6. Rybak MJ, Boike SC. Monitoring vancomycin therapy. *Drug Intell Clin Pharm* 1986; **20:** 757–61.
7. Healy DP, *et al.* Comparison of steady-state pharmacokinetics of two dosage regimens of vancomycin in normal volunteers. *Antimicrob Agents Chemother* 1987; **31:** 393–7.
8. Rodvold KA, *et al.* Evaluation of a two-compartment Bayesian forecasting program for predicting vancomycin concentrations. *Ther Drug Monit* 1989; **11:** 269–75.
9. Pryka RD, *et al.* Individualizing vancomycin dosage regimens: one- vs two-compartment Bayesian models. *Ther Drug Monit* 1989; **11:** 450–4.
10. Pryka RD, *et al.* An updated comparison of drug dosing methods part IV: vancomycin. *Clin Pharmacokinet* 1991; **20:** 463–76.
11. Gabriel MH, *et al.* Prospective evaluation of a vancomycin dosage guideline for neonates. *Clin Pharm* 1991; **10:** 129–32.
12. Ackerman BH, Vanmier AM. Necessity of a loading dose when using vancomycin in critically ill patients. *J Antimicrob Chemother* 1992; **29:** 460–1.
13. Freeman CD, *et al.* Vancomycin therapeutic drug monitoring: is it necessary? *Ann Pharmacother* 1993; **27:** 594–8.
14. Saunders NJ. Why monitor peak vancomycin concentrations? *Lancet* 1994; **344:** 1748–50. [Subsequent correspondence. *ibid.* 1995; **345:** 645–7.]
15. Leader WG, *et al.* Pharmacokinetic optimisation of vancomycin therapy. *Clin Pharmacokinet* 1995; **28:** 327–42.
16. Marra F, *et al.* Vancomycin serum concentration monitoring: the middle ground is best. *Clin Drug Invest* 1996; **12:** 105–18.
17. Shackley F, *et al.* Trough-only monitoring of serum vancomycin concentrations in neonates. *J Antimicrob Chemother* 1998; **41:** 141–2.

Preparations

BP 2001: Vancomycin Injection;
USP 25: Sterile Vancomycin Hydrochloride; Vancomycin Hydrochloride Capsules; Vancomycin Hydrochloride for Injection; Vancomycin Hydrochloride for Oral Solution; Vancomycin Injection.

Proprietary Preparations (details are given in Part 3)
Austral.: Vancocin; Vancoled; *Belg.:* Vancocin; *Braz.:* Vancocina; *Canad.:* Vancocin; *Denm.:* Vancocin; *Fin.:* Orivan; Vancocin; *Fr.:* Vancocine; *Ger.:* VANCO; Vanco-saar; *Hong Kong:* Lyphocin; Vanco-Teva; Vancocin; *Irl.:* Vancocin; *Israel:* Vanco-Teva; Vancocin; Vancoled; *Ital.:* Vancocin; *Mex.:* Balcoran; Vancocin; Vancox; Vanmicina; *Neth.:* Vancocin; *Norw.:* Vancocin; *NZ:* Vancocin; *Port.:* Glipep; Vancocina; *S.Afr.:* Vancocin; *Spain:* Diatracin; *Swed.:* Vancocin; Vancoscand; *Switz.:* Vancocin; Vancoled; *Thai.:* Edicin; Vancocin; *UAE:* Vancolin; *UK:* Vancocin; *USA:* Lyphocin; Vancocin; Vancoled.

Virginiamycin (178-k)

Virginiamycin *(BAN, USAN, rINN).*
Antibiotic 899; SKF-7988; Virgimycin.
CAS — 11006-76-1; 21411-53-0 *(virginiamycin M₁)*; 23152-29-6 *(virginiamycin S₁)*.
ATC — D06AX10.

A mixture consisting principally of 2 antimicrobial substances, virginiamycin M₁, and virginiamycin S₁, produced by the growth of *Streptomyces virginiae.*

Adverse Effects

Virginiamycin may cause gastrointestinal disturbances including diarrhoea and vomiting. A few instances of hypersensitivity have been observed.

Antimicrobial Action

Virginiamycin has a spectrum of antimicrobial activity similar to that of erythromycin (p.203). It is active against staphylococci and some streptococci; *Neisseria gonorrhoeae* and *Haemophilus influenzae* are reported to be sensitive.
Cross-resistance is often observed between streptogramins, macrolides, and lincosamides.

Pharmacokinetics

Virginiamycin is incompletely absorbed following a dose by mouth. It is widely distributed in tissues and body fluids but does not cross the blood-brain barrier. It is metabolised in the liver and excreted in the bile; about 13% of a dose is excreted in the urine. The half-life is reported to be about 5 hours.

Uses and Administration

Virginiamycin is a streptogramin antibiotic used for the treatment of infections due to sensitive organisms, particularly Gram-positive cocci. It has been given by mouth and applied locally.
Virginiamycin has been used in animal feeding stuffs as a growth promotor.

Preparations

Proprietary Preparations (details are given in Part 3)
Fr.: Staphylomycine†.
Multi-ingredient: *Belg.:* Spitalen.

Xibornol　(14022-f)

Xibornol *(BAN, rINN).*
CP3H; 1HP; 1BX. 6-(Isoborn-2-yl)-3,4-xylenol; 6-[(1*R,*2*S,*4*S*)-Born-2-yl]-3,4-xylenol.
$C_{18}H_{26}O = 258.4.$
CAS — 38237-68-2; 13741-18-9.
ATC — J01XX02.

Profile

Xibornol is an antimicrobial that is reported to have a bacteriostatic action on Gram-positive organisms such as staphylococci and streptococci, as well as activity against *Haemophilus influenzae.* It has been given by mouth in doses of 1 to 1.5 g daily; it has also been given rectally.

Preparations

Proprietary Preparations (details are given in Part 3)
Fr.: Nanbacine†; *Ital.:* Bornilene.
Multi-ingredient: *Spain:* Xibornol Prodes.

Antidepressants

This chapter describes drugs used principally in the treatment of affective disorders. Affective disorders are disorders of mood that may manifest as *depression* or *mania* or, in some cases, as *mixed affective states* in which depressive and manic episodes may coexist or alternate.

The core features of depressive disorders are low mood, anhedonia (the loss of interest in former pleasures or activities), pessimism, and lethargy. They were formerly classified either as *endogenous*, in which the symptoms were independent of external factors and considered to be a consequence of factors within the patient, or *reactive*, in which depressive symptoms were a result of external stressors (i.e. exogenous). It is now recognised that depressive disorders are composed of both endogenous and reactive factors. Similarly, the classification of *neurotic depression* is no longer considered useful because it encompasses several different syndromes. Depressive episodes are classified according to severity as mild, moderate, severe, or severe with psychosis. *Recurrent brief depression* is defined as depressive episodes of a few days' duration that recur regularly. Depression is often accompanied by characteristic *somatic* symptoms, including anorexia, weight loss, insomnia, early morning waking, and psychomotor retardation. Symptoms associated with *atypical depression* include overeating and oversleeping.

The main symptoms of *mania* are overactivity, mood changes ranging from elation to irritability, expansive ideas, and inflated self-importance. Manic episodes are classified according to severity in a similar manner to depressive disorders: namely, mild, moderate, severe, or severe with psychosis. *Hypomania* is differentiated from mania in terms of a reduction in intensity of symptoms and social incapacity.

Alternating episodes of mania and depression are termed *bipolar disorder*. Since it is very rare for repeated episodes of mania to occur without alternating episodes of depression, it is accepted practice to include mania without depression within the bipolar category. The term *unipolar disorder* (*unipolar depression*) is reserved for depressive disorders without mania.

States of persistent but mild disturbances of mood exist in which the symptoms are not severe enough to meet the criteria for classification as a major depressive or hypomanic disorder, but may nevertheless cause considerable suffering to the patient. *Dysthymia* is the term used to describe a chronic depressive state whereas *cyclothymia* has some similarity to bipolar disorder, the instability characterised by long periods of milder elation and milder depression.

The term *seasonal affective disorder* has been applied to depressive disorders repeatedly occurring seasonally, but not related to seasonal stressful life events; the depressive symptoms usually occur during the autumn and winter months. There have also been reports of patients developing seasonal bipolar disorder with hypomania or mania occurring in the summer months.

Anxiety is often associated with depressive disorders at all levels of severity and it may be difficult to distinguish between the two conditions, especially in the milder forms. *Mixed anxiety and depressive disorder* defines a state in which anxiety and depressive symptoms coexist but neither component is severe enough to merit classification as an anxiety disorder or a depressive disorder.

Classification of antidepressants. Antidepressants are classified into different groups either structurally or depending on which central neurotransmitters they act upon. The older tricyclic (e.g. amitriptyline) and related cyclic antidepressants and the monoamine oxidase inhibitors (MAOIs) (e.g. phenelzine) have now been joined by the selective serotonin reuptake inhibitors (SSRIs) (e.g. fluoxetine), the reversible inhibitors of monoamine oxidase type A (RIMAs) (e.g. moclobemide), and more recently by the serotonin and noradrenaline reuptake inhibitors (SNRIs) (e.g. venlafaxine). Other antidepressants that do not fit exactly into these groups include bupropion, the herbal preparation hypericum (St John's wort), mirtazapine, nefazodone, reboxetine, and trazodone.

Lithium salts provide a source of lithium ions that compete with sodium ions at various sites in the body and thus have an action and side-effects distinct and separate from those of other antidepressants.

Bipolar disorder

Bipolar disorder (manic depression) is a mixed affective disorder in which the patient experiences alternating episodes of hypomania or mania and depression. Although isolated episodes of mania may occur, they are more usually part of bipolar disorder; for the purposes of classification, mania without depression is therefore included in the bipolar category. Bipolar disorder is usually treated with mood-stabilising drugs, the most important of which is lithium. Electroconvulsive therapy (ECT) is also effective and is used for example in patients for whom lithium treatment is unsuitable or in patients refractory to lithium or other drugs.

Drug therapy of the manic phase is directed at controlling the acute attack, maintaining that response, and preventing further attacks. Lithium is effective in acute mania but it may take a few days before an antimanic effect is seen. Treatment in acutely manic patients with coexisting psychotic features, agitation, or disruptive behaviour is therefore usually initiated with an antipsychotic to produce a rapid tranquillising effect; typical drugs include the phenothiazine chlorpromazine and the butyrophenones droperidol and haloperidol although the atypical antipsychotics such as olanzapine are becoming more widely used. Clozapine may be useful in refractory mania although its use is restricted by adverse effects. The antipsychotic may be used in conjunction with lithium, and then gradually withdrawn once lithium becomes effective, but due consideration should be given to the risks from interactions between antipsychotics and lithium (see under Interactions of Lithium, p.295). Alternatively, initiation of lithium therapy may be postponed until the acute attack has been stabilised with the antipsychotic. Benzodiazepines are also used in manic patients with coexisting agitation or insomnia until lithium has achieved its full effect; they should not be used for long periods owing to the risk of dependence.

Once the acute phase has been brought under control drug treatment should continue until it is safe to expect that the patient will not suffer a relapse; this might entail maintaining treatment for several months. High doses of lithium are usually required to control the acute phase, but as the margin between the therapeutic and the toxic concentration of lithium is narrow, the dose should be reduced to maintenance levels as soon as practicable. Regular monitoring of serum concentrations of lithium is essential during the initial and maintenance phases of therapy to minimise the risks of lithium toxicity (see under Pharmacokinetics of Lithium, p.296).

The treatment of the subsequent depressive phase of bipolar disorder depends on the severity of the depression and whether psychotic symptoms are still present. In some milder cases optimal therapy with lithium may suffice, as lithium itself possesses antidepressant activity; however in more severe cases or in those receiving only an antipsychotic additional antidepressant therapy may be required. Treatment with antidepressants is essentially similar to that of unipolar depression (see below), but extra caution is warranted because antidepressants may precipitate hypomania or mania. Antidepressants have also been implicated in the induction of rapid cycling, in which there are four or more affective episodes in a year. Some authorities recommend that, if the use of an antidepressant is necessary, it should be given in the lowest effective dose and for the shortest time possible, or should not be given long term without the cover of a mood-stabilising drug. Tricyclic antidepressants should only be used with caution and data for the newer antidepressants such as nefazodone and venlafaxine are limited. Bupropion is the antidepressant of choice of many clinicians in the USA; SSRIs are also an alternative. MAOIs may be less likely to induce mania than other antidepressants, but troublesome side-effects and safety issues have limited their use to second-line. ECT is a valuable alternative and should be considered for bipolar depression.

Patients with recurrent episodes of bipolar disorder may require prophylactic therapy with lithium. Sometimes prophylaxis may be instituted following treatment of a first episode where there is an expectation of repeated attacks. Lithium prophylaxis usually entails extending the maintenance treatment and continuing to monitor serum concentrations as before; it may need to be continued for a prolonged period. Some authorities have also given antipsychotics, either alone or with lithium, for prophylaxis.

When lithium therapy is to be discontinued, withdrawal should be gradual over a period of weeks to allay any concerns about relapse.

Should the above treatments fail then mood-stabilising antiepileptics such as carbamazepine and valproate are alternatives to lithium. Carbamazepine and valproate are both effective in the treatment of acute mania and in the maintenance and prophylactic phases; they are also particularly effective for rapid cycling bipolar disorder. If patients fail to respond after several weeks of therapy with a mood stabiliser then a different one should be substituted, with gradual tapering of the first drug. If there is only a partial response after several weeks then a second mood stabiliser may be added. For example carbamazepine or valproate may be added to existing lithium therapy or alternatively lithium can be added to treatment with carbamazepine or valproate. Some of the newer antiepileptics such as gabapentin or lamotrigine are also being investigated.

References.

1. American Psychiatric Association. Practice guideline for the treatment of patients with bipolar disorder. *Am J Psychiatry* 1994; **151** (suppl): 1–36.
2. Silverstone T, Romans S. Long term treatment of bipolar disorder. *Drugs* 1996; **51**: 367–82.
3. The Expert Consensus Panel for Bipolar Disorder. Treatment of bipolar disorder. *J Clin Psychiatry* 1996; **57**: (suppl 12A): 1–89.
4. Daly I. Mania. *Lancet* 1997; **349**: 1157–60.
5. Bauer MS, *et al.* Clinical practice guidelines for bipolar disorder from the Department of Veterans Affairs. *J Clin Psychiatry* 1999; **60**: 9–21.
6. Sachs GS, *et al.* The expert consensus guideline series: medication treatment of bipolar disorder 2000. *Postgrad Med* 2000; **Apr** (spec no): 1–104. Also available at: http://www.psychguides.com/Bipolar_2000.pdf (accessed 13/06/01).

Depression

Clinical depression (unipolar depression) is a disturbance of mood that is distinguishable from the usual mood fluctuations of everyday life. A depressed mood is usually the major symptom, which may be accompanied by a variety of other mental or somatic symptoms representing several depressive syndromes.

The aetiology of depression is unknown but it may represent an interaction between psychological and biochemical mechanisms rather than any single factor. The symptoms appear to be mediated through alterations in levels of some central neurotransmitters, although it is not certain that this represents a cause of the disorder. However, it is at this level that the antidepressant drugs currently in clinical use exert their action.

There are several approaches to the treatment of depression depending on the severity of the condition and the risks to the patient, and these have been summarised in consensus statements and guidelines in the UK[1,2] and the USA.[3,4] Guidelines in the UK have recently been revised.[5] Although the most common form of treatment is with an antidepressant, other forms of treatment may also be of value in some situations. Psychosocial or psychotherapeutic management may be effective alone in mild depressive disorders or may be used in conjunction with antidepressants[1,3] or following ECT. ECT is used in severe depression or when the patient has not responded to drug therapy; it has been given in repeated courses without evidence of brain damage.[6] ECT is of particular value when a rapid improvement in symptoms is essential (e.g. patients at high risk of suicide), and for patients with depressive psychosis or psychomotor retardation.[3,6] Light therapy appears to be effective in patients with seasonal affective disorder.[7] Exposure to bright artificial light may take place at any time of the day,[3] and the therapy should continue until the natural seasonal remission of the disorder; antidepressant drugs may also be used.[3]

There has been much debate about the **choice of antidepressant** therapy. Tricyclic antidepressants have long been preferred over MAOIs because of the problem of drug interactions and the need for strict dietary precautions required for the latter group. Tricyclics with sedative properties may be more suitable for agitated and anxious patients, whereas those with less sedative properties may be preferred for withdrawn and apathetic patients. Unfortunately, the traditional tricyclics such as amitriptyline are associated to varying degrees with antimuscarinic and cardiotoxic adverse effects that can limit their use. Their cardiotoxicity also means that they are associated with a high risk of fatality in patients taking overdoses with suicidal intent (see toxicity in overdosage, below). The emergence of newer antidepressants has improved the treatment options for patients.[8,9] These have included lofepramine and drugs related to the tricyclic group such as mianserin that are less cardiotoxic than the earlier tricyclics.[2] The subsequent introduction of SSRIs such as fluoxetine has provided a group of drugs with still fewer antimuscarinic and cardiotoxic side-effects. However, the SSRIs themselves have characteristic side-effects; gastrointestinal symptoms such as nausea and vomiting may be a problem, and sleep disturbances and anxiety may be exacerbated at the start of treatment. Moreover, those in current clinical use interact to varying degrees with cytochrome P450 isoenzymes, which carries a potential for interaction with a wide range of compounds.[8]

There are arguments supporting both the first-choice use of SSRIs, because of fewer unpleasant side-effects,[10] and the tricyclics, because of wide experience with their use and familiarity with their pharmacological actions.[1,2,11] Meta-analyses[12-14] comparing the efficacy of SSRIs and tricyclics in general find no difference in efficacy although there is the suggestion of a greater efficacy for some tricyclics when given to inpatients. However, drop-out rates due to adverse effects have generally been higher in patients receiving tricyclics than in those taking SSRIs.

More recently serotonin and noradrenaline reuptake inhibitors (SNRIs) such as venlafaxine have been developed, as well as reversible inhibitors of monoamine oxidase type A (RIMAs) such as moclobemide. RIMAs offer a safer alternative to the MAOIs and fewer dietary restrictions are necessary.[15] Antidepressants such as nefazodone, mirtazapine, and reboxetine, which have slightly different biochemical profiles from the major groups, have also been recently introduced. Like the SSRIs, most of these newer drugs seem to be associated with fewer severe adverse effects; their efficacy is also comparable to that of the SSRIs.[16]

The improvement in treatment options offered by the newer antidepressants has meant that choice of therapy is increasingly being tailored to individual patient requirements.[4,5]

Other drugs used in the treatment of depression include flupentixol, the antidepressant dose of which is lower than that used for the treatment of psychoses. Ademetionine, the active derivative of methionine, has been tried in depressive disorders, and extracts of the plant hypericum (St John's Wort) are widely used in some countries for depression. Lithium may be used for the prophylaxis of recurrent unipolar depression as an alternative to standard antidepressants, although it is more commonly used in the management of bipolar disorder (see above); its role in unipolar depression is more usually to augment the effect of standard antidepressants in drug-resistant patients.

The sedative properties of some of the antidepressants may adversely affect the performance of potentially hazardous tasks such as driving and the operation of machinery. It would therefore be prudent to select one of the less sedative antidepressants where appropriate, although caution is warranted in this respect with all psychotropic drugs, especially at the start of treatment.

An area of particular concern with regard to initial choice of an antidepressant is the most appropriate drug for patients considered to be a high suicide risk.[17] Varying relative risks of **toxicity in overdosage** for different groups of antidepressant have been assessed:[18-20] older tricyclics and the tetracyclic maprotiline[21] appear to be more toxic in overdosage than the tetracyclic mianserin[22] and the SSRIs;[20] MAOIs have an intermediate risk.[23] Within the tricyclic group, desipramine[18,19] has been reported to be associated more frequently with fatal overdosage whereas lofepramine[24] may be one of the safer tricyclics. Although such analyses cannot determine to what extent the data reflect prescribing patterns and patient selection as opposed to drug toxicity[18,19,24] it is widely accepted that the older tricyclics are more toxic in overdosage, and that safer options are the SSRIs[25,26] and the newer tricyclic and related cyclic antidepressants.[26] In practice, it is often difficult to identify patients at high risk for suicide, and it has therefore been suggested that a routine strategy should be to initiate antidepressant therapy in all patients with drugs that have low toxicity in overdose.[17,26] However, whichever antidepressant is chosen, all patients should be closely monitored during early therapy until improvement in depression has been observed and limited quantities of antidepressants should be prescribed at any one time. It is important to remember that suicide is an inherent risk in depression; it is generally accepted that with all antidepressants therapies the risk of suicide may increase in the early stages of recovery.

When **starting antidepressant therapy** a low initial dose will minimise adverse effects; this is then increased until an adequate response is observed.[1] When this is done with the newer antidepressants, including the SSRIs, the dose can generally be increased after a few days; for the tricyclics the increase should be more gradual.[27] Gradual introduction of treatment is of particular importance in the elderly who may be more susceptible to adverse effects. Although some adverse effects of antidepressant drugs appear soon after treatment is initiated, there is a delay of about two weeks before any therapeutic benefit is observed, and at least six weeks before maximum improvement in depressive symptoms occurs.[8] Claims of a fast onset of action have been made for several antidepressants, but in a review[28] of data relating to onset of action with currently available antidepressants, none have been shown conclusively to work faster than any other. The delay in onset of antidepressant effect may relate to a combination of pharmacokinetic and neurochemical factors. Patients should not be considered resistant to the chosen drug until they have been maintained at an adequate dose for at least 4 weeks,[5] (the *British National Formulary* has recommended 6 weeks in the elderly). Patients with a partial response should continue for a further 2 weeks before being considered resistant.[5] Treatment failure is often due to subtherapeutic doses being used,[2] particularly with the older tricyclics whose adverse effects limit maximum tolerable doses in many patients.[29] Where lack of compliance leads to subtherapeutic doses therapeutic drug monitoring may be of value.[3]

In those who show little or no response to an adequate trial of the first-choice antidepressant two options exist: either switching to another antidepressant or adding another drug (augmentation). If switching therapies a drug with a different biochemical profile may be substituted;[5] alternatively, some patients may respond preferentially to another drug within the same group.[30,31] MAOIs can be tried in patients who are refractory to or intolerant of treatment with other antidepressants.

When **changing a patient from one type of antidepressant to another** due regard should be given to allowing the appropriate drug-free interval between the 2 drugs. An MAOI (including a RIMA) should not be started until at least one week after stopping a tricyclic antidepressant, an SSRI, or any related antidepressant; in the case of the SSRIs paroxetine and sertraline the drug-free interval is extended to two weeks, and for fluoxetine, to five weeks because of their longer half-lives. For the tricyclics clomipramine and imipramine a drug-free interval of 3 weeks should be allowed. Conversely, two weeks should elapse between discontinuing MAOI therapy and starting patients on a tricyclic antidepressant (3 weeks in the case of clomipramine or imipramine), an SSRI, or any related antidepressant. Although some manufacturers recommend a similar treatment-free period between stopping a reversible inhibitor of monoamine oxidase type A (RIMA) and starting an SSRI there does not seem to be any evidence to support such a requirement.

Drugs that have been used in **augmentation strategies** for resistant depression include thyroid hormones (liothyronine)[32] and central stimulants[3,32] such as methylphenidate. Pindolol has also been studied as an augmentation agent in combination with several SSRIs and other serotonergic antidepressants.[32] Another method is to combine different classes of antidepressants. Although this has been used successfully in the treatment of drug-resistant depression,[3,32] it may result in enhanced adverse reactions or interactions and is therefore considered unsuitable or controversial by some authorities; it should only ever be employed under expert supervision. For further details of the interactions between different antidepressants when coadministered, see under Interactions of Phenelzine, p.306.

If the response to treatment is good, the patient should continue with the same treatment for at least 4 to 6 months,[1-3] and perhaps 12 months in the elderly; symptoms are likely to recur if treatment is discontinued prematurely.[33] It is often recommended that doses should be reduced for **maintenance treatment** but this view has been challenged and the recommendation made that the dose closest to that which achieved clinical response should be used unless adverse effects are intolerable.[1-3] Continuation of antidepressant therapy beyond this phase[34] is a matter of clinical judgement. **Prophylactic maintenance therapy** should be considered for recurrent depressive disorders,[1-3,33,35] and may be necessary for several years in some cases. Again, full therapeutic doses are recommended for prophylaxis rather than reduced doses.[35]

When stopping treatment, the sudden **discontinuation of antidepressant therapy** after regular administration for 8 weeks or more may precipitate withdrawal symptoms.[36-38] Such symptoms can be minimised by a gradual reduction in dosage; most authorities recommend reducing the dose over a period of about 4 weeks although considerably longer periods may be required when withdrawing maintenance therapy.[38]

Depressive disorders may arise in **childhood and adolescence**, the prevalence increasing with age.[39] Treatment generally commences with psychosocial and psychotherapeutic methods, followed by antidepressant therapy if no improvement is seen after 4 to 6 weeks.[39,40] SSRIs[39-42] and lofepramine[39] are considered the optimum first choices in children and adolescents because they are less toxic in overdose. The older tricyclics are reserved for refractory cases in adolescents and may be augmented with lithium;[40] ECT may be used in severe depression.[39] Some authorities recommend avoiding desipramine because of reports of death due to cardiac toxicity in children.[41]

Depression in the **elderly** may be particularly severe and the suicide risk higher compared with younger adults.[43,44] SSRIs are often the first choice of treatment in the elderly because of their favourable adverse effect profile and low toxicity in overdose.[45] They may be especially appropriate in patients with an existing cardiovascular disease or in those concurrently taking other medications that may lower the blood pressure. Tricyclics such as amitriptyline and imipramine are probably best avoided in the elderly as their cardiotoxic, antimuscarinic, and sedative effects may be particularly troublesome. However, the tricyclics desipramine and nortriptyline are considered by some to be an alternative first-choice as they are less cardiotoxic and have fewer antimuscarinic and sedative actions compared with amitriptyline or imipramine. Other antidepressants may also be useful in specific situations. As in younger patients, MAOIs may be tried in those who have failed to respond to other therapies, and bupropion has the advantage of a relative lack of cardiotoxicity and drug interactions. Lower initial doses of antidepressant drugs are often recommended in the elderly to minimise adverse effects but individual differences in metabolism and excretion may mean that some patients are undertreated.[44] The elderly tend to respond more slowly to antidepressants than younger patients and therefore concomitant psychosocial or psychotherapeutic management may be warranted. ECT is a safe and effective treatment in the elderly, although temporary memory impairment after treatment in some patients may limit its use to those at high risk for suicide or who are refractory to or intolerant of antidepressant drugs. Depression late in life may require long-term antidepressant treatment beyond the recovery phase, even after first episodes of depression and should be a continuation of the treatment that was successful in the initial acute phase.[46]

Treatment of women with depressive disorders during and after **pregnancy** raises concerns about the risk of teratogenicity, fetal growth retardation, or perinatal problems; the ratio of risk to benefit must therefore be considered very carefully before antidepressants are given.[47,48] Maternal mood disorders in the immediate postpartum period are related to hormonal changes, particularly falling progesterone levels; the symptoms are mild and resolve spontaneously after several days, therefore no treatment is required.[49] Of greater concern are major depressive episodes that occur beyond this initial phase, which are clinically identical to depressive disorders in general and call for the same principles of management. These depressive episodes have been found to be related to the presence of immediate postpartum mood disorders, although no hormonal basis to this association has been identified.[50] Nevertheless, there is interest in the use of oestrogen as a treatment.

As with use of any medication in nursing mothers, the risks to the infant from drugs distributed into breast milk must be considered. The American Academy of Pediatrics[51] considers that all antidepressants are drugs whose effect on nursing infants could be of concern.

Symptoms of **anxiety and depression** often coexist, and although it may be difficult to distinguish which is the predominant disorder, especially in milder forms, patients usually require an antidepressant. Anxiolytics and antipsychotics can be useful adjuncts in agitated depression, but a sedative antidepressant might be preferable. Combination preparations of antidepressants with antipsychotics or anxiolytics should not be used because the dosage of the individual components should be adjusted separately. Also, anxiolytics should only be prescribed on a short-term basis whereas antidepressants are given for several months.

Although no randomised double-blind studies assessing the efficacy of antidepressants in **chronic fatigue syndrome** have been published it has been suggested that antidepressant therapy should be tried in patients with co-existing depression.[52] Cognitive therapy may also be useful. Controlled trials of antidepressants in non-depressed patients with chronic fatigue syndrome are particularly needed.[52]

1. Paykel ES, Priest RG. Recognition and management of depression in general practice: consensus statement. *BMJ* 1992; **305:** 1198–1202.
2. Montgomery SA, *et al.* Guidelines for treating depressive illness with antidepressants: a statement from the British Association for Psychopharmacology. *J Psychopharmacol* 1993; **7:** 19–23.
3. American Psychiatric Association. Practice guidelines for major depressive disorder in adults. *Am J Psychiatry* 1993; **150** (suppl): 1–26.
4. Snow V, *et al.* Clinical guidelines, part 1. Pharmacologic treatment of acute depression and dysthymia. *Ann Intern Med* 2000; **132:** 738–42.
5. Anderson IM, *et al.* Evidence-based guidelines for treating depressive disorders with antidepressants: a revision of the 1993 British Association for Psychopharmacology guidelines. *J Psychopharmacol* 2000; **14:** 3–30.
6. Scott AIF. Contemporary practice of electroconvulsive therapy. *Br J Hosp Med* 1994; **51:** 334–8.
7. Partonen T, Lönnqvist J. Seasonal affective disorder. *Lancet* 1998; **352:** 1369–74.
8. Richelson E. Pharmacology of antidepressants—characteristics of the ideal drug. *Mayo Clin Proc* 1994; **69:** 1069–81.
9. Möller H-J, Volz H-P. Drug treatment of depression in the 1990s: an overview of achievements and future possibilities. *Drugs* 1996; **52:** 625–38.
10. Harrison G. New or old antidepressants: new is better. *BMJ* 1994; **309:** 1280–1.
11. Owens D. New or old antidepressants: benefits of new drugs are exaggerated. *BMJ* 1994; **309:** 1281–2.
12. Trindade E, Menon D. *Selective serotonin reuptake inhibitors (SSRIs) for major depression. Part 1: evaluation of the clinical literature.* Ottawa: Canadian Coordinating Office for Health Technology Assessment, 1997.
13. Anderson IM. SSRIs versus tricyclic antidepressants in depressed inpatients: a meta-analysis of efficacy and tolerability. *Depress Anxiety* 1998; **7** (suppl 1): 11–17.
14. Geddes JR, *et al.* Selective serotonin reuptake inhibitors (SSRIs) for depression (updated 28 May 2001). Available in The Cochrane Library; Issue 3. Oxford: Update Software; 2001.
15. Lecrubier Y. Risk-benefit assessment of newer versus older monoamine oxidase (MAO) inhibitors. *Drug Safety* 1994; **10:** 292–300.
16. Kent JM. SNaRIs, NaSSAs, and NaRIs: new agents for the treatment of depression. *Lancet* 2000; **355:** 911–8. Correction. *ibid.;* 2000.
17. Henry JA. Epidemiology and relative toxicity of antidepressant drugs in overdose. *Drug Safety* 1997; **16:** 374–90.
18. Beaumont G. The toxicity of antidepressants. *Br J Psychiatry* 1989; **154:** 454–8.
19. Kapur S, *et al.* Antidepressant medications and the relative risk of suicide attempt and suicide. *JAMA* 1992; **268:** 3441–5.
20. de Jonghe F, Swinkels JA. The safety of antidepressants. *Drugs* 1992; **43** (suppl 2): 40–7.
21. Knudsen KAI, Heath A. Effects of self poisoning with maprotiline. *BMJ* 1984; **288:** 601–3.
22. Inman WHW. Blood disorders and suicide in patients taking mianserin or amitriptyline. *Lancet* 1988; **ii:** 90–2.
23. Cassidy S, Henry J. Fatal toxicity of antidepressant drugs in overdose. *BMJ* 1987; **295:** 1021–4.
24. Malmvik J, *et al.* Antidepressants in suicide: differences in fatality and drug utilisation. *Eur J Clin Pharmacol* 1994; **46:** 291–4.
25. Henry JA, *et al.* Relative mortality from overdose of antidepressants. *BMJ* 1995; **310:** 221–4. Correction. *ibid.;* 911.
26. Freemantle N, *et al.* Prescribing selective serotonin reuptake inhibitors as strategy for prevention of suicide. *BMJ* 1994; **309:** 249–53.
27. Spigset O, Mårtensson B. Drug treatment of depression. *BMJ* 1999; **318:** 1188–91.
28. Soares JC, Gershon S. Prospects for the development of new treatments with a rapid onset of action in affective disorders. *Drugs* 1996; **52:** 477–82.
29. Kendrick T. Prescribing antidepressants in general practice. *BMJ* 1996; **313:** 829–30.
30. Brown WA, Harrison W. Are patients who are intolerant to one serotonin selective reuptake inhibitor intolerant to another? *J Clin Psychiatry* 1995; **56:** 30–4.
31. Joffe RT, *et al.* Response to an open trial of a second SSRI in major depression. *J Clin Psychiatry* 1996; **57:** 114–15.
32. Schweitzer I, Tuckwell V. Risk of adverse events with the use of augmentation therapy for the treatment of resistant depression. *Drug Safety* 1998; **19:** 45–64.
33. Angst J. A regular review of the long term follow up of depression. *BMJ* 1997; **315:** 1143–6.
34. Edwards JG. Long term pharmacotherapy of depression. *BMJ* 1998; **316:** 1180–1.
35. Montgomery SA. Prophylactic treatment of depression. *Br J Hosp Med* 1994; **52:** 5–7.
36. Dilsaver SC. Withdrawal phenomena associated with antidepressant and antipsychotic agents. *Drug Safety* 1994; **10:** 103–114.
37. Haddad P, *et al.* Antidepressant discontinuation reactions. *BMJ* 1998; **316:** 1105–6.
38. Anonymous. Withdrawing patients from antidepressants. *Drug Ther Bull* 1999; **37:** 49–52.
39. Mirza KAH, Michael A. Major depression in children and adolescents. *Br J Hosp Med* 1996; **55:** 57–61.
40. Harrington R. Depressive disorder in adolescence. *Arch Dis Child* 1995; **72:** 193–5.
41. Carrey NJ, *et al.* Pharmacological treatment of psychiatric disorders in children and adolescents: focus on guidelines for the primary care practitioner. *Drugs* 1996; **51:** 750–9.
42. Renaud J, *et al.* A risk-benefit assessment of pharmacotherapies for clinical depression in children and adolescents. *Drug Safety* 1999; **20:** 59–75.
43. Wattis J. What an old age psychiatrist does. *BMJ* 1996; **313:** 101–4.
44. Waern M, *et al.* High rate of antidepressant treatment in elderly people who commit suicide. *BMJ* 1996; **313:** 1118.
45. The American Society of Health-System Pharmacists (ASHP). ASHP therapeutic position statement on the recognition and treatment of depression in older adults. *Am J Health-Syst Pharm* 1998; **55:** 2514–18.
46. Lebowitz BD, *et al.* Diagnosis and treatment of depression in late life: consensus statement update. *JAMA* 1997; **278:** 1186–90.
47. Robert E. Treating depression in pregnancy. *N Engl J Med* 1996; **335:** 1056–8.
48. Schou M. Treating recurrent affective disorders during and after pregnancy: what can be taken safely? *Drug Safety* 1998; **18:** 143–52.
49. Harris B, *et al.* Maternity blues and major endocrine changes: Cardiff puerperal mood and hormone study II. *BMJ* 1994; **308:** 949–53.
50. Cooper PJ, Murray L. Postnatal depression. *BMJ* 1998; **316:** 1884–6.
51. American Academy of Pediatrics Committee on Drugs. The transfer of drugs and other chemicals into human milk. *Pediatrics* 2001; **108:** 776–89.
52. The Royal Colleges of Physicians, Psychiatrists and General Practitioners. *Chronic Fatigue Syndrome.* London, 1997.

Mania

Although isolated episodes of mania may occur, mania is usually followed by depression when it is considered to be part of bipolar disorder. It is accepted practice to include mania without depression within the bipolar category. The treatment of acute attacks of mania and their prophylaxis are therefore described under Bipolar Disorder, above.

Amineptine Hydrochloride (12358-q)

Amineptine Hydrochloride (rINNM).

S-1694.   7-[(10,11-Dihydro-5H-dibenzo[a,d]cyclohepten-5-yl)amino]heptanoic acid hydrochloride.

$C_{22}H_{27}NO_2,HCl$ = 373.9.

CAS — 57574-09-1 (amineptine); 30272-08-3 (amineptine hydrochloride).

Profile

Amineptine hydrochloride is a tricyclic antidepressant (see Amitriptyline, below). It has been given by mouth in the treatment of depression.

Hepatic adverse effects seem to be more common than with most other tricyclic antidepressants (see Effects on the Liver, p.274). Also amineptine has been subject to abuse and withdrawal has been both prolonged and difficult; for these reasons, it is no longer marketed in a number of countries.

Adverse effects. In 5 patients very severe acne-type lesions were associated with the chronic self-increased administration of high doses of amineptine (200 to 1000 mg daily).[1] The presence of an unusual lactam form of metabolites was detected in all patients and in 2 these metabolites were still present, along with the lesions, 3 months after therapy had been withdrawn.

1. Vexiau P, *et al.* Severe acne-like lesions caused by amineptine overdose. *Lancet* 1988; **i:** 585.

Porphyria. Amineptine is considered to be unsafe in patients with porphyria because it has been shown to be porphyrinogenic in *in-vitro* systems.

Preparations

Proprietary Preparations (details are given in Part 3)
Braz.: Survector; *Fr.:* Survector†; *Ital.:* Maneon†; *Survector†;* *Port.:* Directim†; Survector†; *Spain:* Survector†.

Amitriptyline (12293-g)

Amitriptyline (BAN, rINN).

3-(10,11-Dihydro-5H-dibenzo[a,d]cyclohepten-5-ylidene)propyldimethylamine;   10,11-Dihydro-N,N-dimethyl-5H-dibenzo[a,d]cycloheptene-Δ$^{5,\gamma}$-propylamine.

$C_{20}H_{23}N$ = 277.4.

CAS — 50-48-6.

ATC — N06AA09.

Amitriptyline Embonate (2501-v)

Amitriptyline Embonate (BANM, rINNM).

$(C_{20}H_{23}N)_2,C_{23}H_{16}O_6$ = 943.2.

CAS — 17086-03-2.

Pharmacopoeias. In Br.

Amitriptyline embonate 1.5 g is approximately equivalent to 1 g of amitriptyline hydrochloride and 0.88 g of amitriptyline.

Pharmacopoeial description

BP 2001: A pale yellow to brownish-yellow, odourless or almost odourless powder. Practically insoluble in water; slightly soluble in alcohol; freely soluble in chloroform. Protect from light.

Amitriptyline Hydrochloride (2502-g)

Amitriptyline Hydrochloride (BANM, rINNM).

Amitriptylini Hydrochloridum.

$C_{20}H_{23}N,HCl$ = 313.9.

CAS — 549-18-8.

Pharmacopoeias. In Chin., Eur. (see p.vi), Int., Jpn, Pol., and US.

Pharmacopoeial description

Ph. Eur.: A white or almost white powder or colourless crystals. Freely soluble in water, in alcohol, and in dichloromethane. Protect from light.

USP 25: A white or practically white, odourless or practically odourless, crystalline powder or small crystals. Freely soluble in water, in alcohol, in chloroform, and in methyl alcohol; insoluble in ether. pH of a 1% solution in water is between 5.0 and 6.0.

Stability. Decomposition occurred when solutions of amitriptyline hydrochloride in water or phosphate buffers were autoclaved at 115° to 116° for 30 minutes in the presence of excess oxygen.[1] The decomposition of amitriptyline as the hydrochloride in buffered aqueous solution was accelerated by metal ions particularly from amber glass ampoules.[2] Disodium edetate 0.1% significantly reduced the decomposition rate of these amitriptyline solutions but propyl gallate and hydroquinone were less effective. Sodium metabisulfite produced an initial lowering of amitriptyline concentration and subsequently an acceleration of decomposition.

Solutions of amitriptyline hydrochloride in water are stable for at least 8 weeks at room temperature if protected from light either by storage in a cupboard or in amber containers.[3] Decomposition to ketone and, to a lesser extent, other unidentified products was found to occur on exposure to light.

1. Enever RP, *et al.* Decomposition of amitriptyline hydrochloride in aqueous solution: identification of decomposition products. *J Pharm Sci* 1975; **64:** 1497–9.
2. Enever RP, *et al.* Factors influencing decomposition rate of amitriptyline hydrochloride in aqueous solution. *J Pharm Sci* 1977; **66:** 1087–9.
3. Buckles J, Walters V. The stability of amitriptyline hydrochloride in aqueous solution. *J Clin Pharm* 1976; **1:** 107–12.

Adverse Effects

Many side-effects of amitriptyline and similar tricyclic antidepressants are caused by their antimuscarinic actions. The antimuscarinic side-effects are relatively common and occur before an antidepressant effect is obtained. Tolerance is often achieved if treatment is continued and side-effects may be less troublesome if treatment is initiated with small doses and then increased gradually, although this may delay the clinical response. Antimuscarinic effects include dry mouth, constipation occasionally leading to paralytic ileus, urinary retention, blurred vision and disturbances in accommodation, increased intra-ocular pressure, and hyperthermia.

Drowsiness may also be a common side-effect. Conversely, a few tricyclic antidepressants possess little or no sedative potential and nervousness and insomnia may occur.

Other neurological adverse effects include headache, peripheral neuropathy, tremor, ataxia, epileptiform seizures, tinnitus, and occasional extrapyramidal symptoms including speech difficulties (dysarthria). Confusion or delirium may occur, particularly in the elderly and mania or hypomania, and behavioural disturbances (particularly in children) have been reported. Gastrointestinal complaints include sour or metallic taste, stomatitis, and gastric irritation with nausea and vomiting.

Various effects on the cardiovascular system have been reported and are discussed in more detail under Effects on the Cardiovascular System, below. Orthostatic hypotension and tachycardia may occur in patients without a history of cardiovascular disease, and may be particularly troublesome in the elderly.

Hypersensitivity reactions, such as urticaria and angioedema, and photosensitisation have been reported and, rarely, cholestatic jaundice and blood disorders, including eosinophilia, bone-marrow depression, thrombocytopenia, leucopenia, and agranulocytosis.

Endocrine effects include testicular enlargement, gynaecomastia and breast enlargement, and galactorrhoea. Sexual dysfunction may also occur. Changes in blood sugar concentrations may also occur, and, very occasionally, hyponatraemia associated with inappropriate secretion of antidiuretic hormone.

Other side-effects that have been reported are increased appetite with weight gain (or occasionally anorexia with weight loss). Sweating may be a problem.

Symptoms of **overdosage** may include excitement and restlessness with marked antimuscarinic effects, including dryness of the mouth, dilated pupils, tachycardia, urinary retention, and intestinal stasis. Severe symptoms include unconsciousness, convulsions and myoclonus, hyperreflexia, hypotension, metabolic acidosis, and respiratory and cardiac depression, with life-threatening cardiac arrhythmias that may recur some days after apparent recovery. Delirium, with confusion, agitation and hallucinations, is common during recovery.

◊ Studies in vitro showed antidepressant affinities for human muscarinic acetylcholine receptors and therefore the likelihood of antimuscarinic effects to be, in descending order: amitriptyline, protriptyline, clomipramine, trimipramine, doxepin, imipramine, nortriptyline, desipramine, amoxapine, maprotiline, trazodone.[1] The effect of affinities for other receptor sites was less certain, although those antidepressants with high affinity for histamine H_1 receptors might be expected to be more sedating. Affinities for murine histamine H_1 receptors in descending order were: doxepin, trimipramine, amitriptyline, maprotiline, amoxapine, nortriptyline, imipramine, clomipramine, protriptyline, trazodone, desipramine.

1. Richelson E. Antimuscarinic and other receptor-blocking properties of antidepressants. *Mayo Clin Proc* 1983; **58:** 40–6.

Effects on the blood. Following a case report of agranulocytosis linked with imipramine, review of the literature suggested that agranulocytosis associated with tricyclic antidepressant use was a rare idiosyncratic condition, resulting from a direct toxic effect rather than an allergic mechanism, and particularly affected the elderly from 4 to 8 weeks after beginning treatment.[1]

Between 1963 and 1993 the UK Committee on Safety of Medicines (CSM) received 912 reports of drug-induced agranulocytosis of which 38 were due to tricyclic antidepressants (12 fatal) and 1499 cases of neutropenia of which 46 were due to tricyclics (none fatal).[2] In a report[3] on a patient who developed aplastic anaemia associated with concomitant therapy with remoxipride and dothiepin [dosulepin] it was noted that up to May 1993 the CSM had received 11 reports of aplastic anaemia secondary to use of dothiepin [dosulepin].

Neutropenia reported[4] in a patient after separate exposure to imipramine and nortriptyline, indicated that there might be cross-intolerance between the tricyclic antidepressants and if neutropenia developed with one member of the group the use of others on future occasions should be avoided.

1. Albertini RS, Penders TM. Agranulocytosis associated with tricyclics. *J Clin Psychiatry* 1978; **39:** 483–5.
2. Committee on Safety of Medicines/Medicines Control Agency. Drug-induced neutropenia and agranulocytosis. *Current Problems* 1993; **19:** 10–11.
3. Philpott NJ, et al. Aplastic anaemia and remoxipride. *Lancet* 1993; **342:** 1244–5.
4. Draper BM, Manoharan A. Neutropenia with cross-intolerance between two tricyclic antidepressant agents. *Med J Aust* 1987; **146:** 452–3.

Effects on the cardiovascular system. The cardiotoxic potential of tricyclic antidepressants after overdosage is widely acknowledged; symptoms include arrhythmias, conduction defects, and hypotension. This factor was, in part, responsible for the development of antidepressants with different chemical structures and pharmacological properties that are less cardiotoxic. It also led to some concern over whether tricyclic antidepressants had adverse effects on the heart or cardiovascular system when used in usual therapeutic doses.

Since the introduction of the tricyclic antidepressants, several reports, often anecdotal, have been published of adverse cardiovascular effects and have included malignant hypertension

with amitriptyline,[1] and cardiomyopathy in a patient who had received amitriptyline and imipramine.[2] QT prolongation, which is considered a risk factor for torsade de pointes, has also been associated with the use of some tricyclics.[3] Sudden cardiac death in patients with pre-existing cardiac disease has been linked with amitriptyline[4-6] or imipramine,[5] although the Boston Collaborative Drug Surveillance Program failed to substantiate these findings.[7] There have also been reports of sudden death in children given desipramine[8-10] or imipramine;[10] in at least some of these cases plasma concentrations were not elevated and the children had no cardiac abnormality. Again, however, evaluation of much of the evidence for the association suggests it is weak;[11] nonetheless, the American Heart Association recommends baseline ECG monitoring in children who are to be treated with tricyclic antidepressants, and a repeat ECG when steady-state dosage is achieved.[12]

Re-evaluations and reviews of this topic[13,14] concluded that the only significant or serious cardiovascular side-effects, seen in patients with no previous history of cardiovascular disease given therapeutic doses of tricyclic antidepressants, are orthostatic hypotension and tachycardia, and that these effects may be particularly troublesome in elderly patients. However, a more recent study[15] also considers that prolongation of the QT interval may occur with therapeutic doses of tricyclics in non-risk patients.

In patients with overt heart disease it was considered[13] that increased risk was likely in those with intraventricular conduction abnormalities; in patients with a history of myocardial infarction or angina, but free of conduction defects, the use of tricyclics appeared to be primarily limited by the degree to and frequency with which they developed orthostatic hypotension. In a re-evaluation of the risks/benefits of tricyclics in patients with ischaemic heart disease no consensus was reached.[16] In practice the authors used SSRIs or bupropion as first-choice therapy in patients with ischaemic heart disease who were mildly or moderately depressed; tricyclics were reserved for patients not responding and were also used as first-choice therapy for patients with more severe depression despite cardiac risks. Recently an increased risk of myocardial infarction has been found in patients receiving tricyclic antidepressants (but not SSRIs) and concomitant treatment for heart disease.[17] Results of a later case-control study[18] examining the risk of ischaemic heart disease for different types of antidepressants and individual antidepressants support these findings. After adjustment for confounders and use of other antidepressants the risk of ischaemic heart disease was significantly raised in patients who had ever taken tricyclics but not in those who had received other antidepressants. When the risk was calculated for the tricyclics amitriptyline, dothiepin [dosulepin], and lofepramine, and confounders had been adjusted for, an increased risk of ischaemic heart disease remained only for dothiepin [dosulepin] with evidence of a dose-response relationship.

1. Dunn FG. Malignant hypertension associated with use of amitriptyline hydrochloride. *South Med J* 1982; **75:** 1124–5.
2. Howland JS, et al. Cardiomyopathy associated with tricyclic antidepressants. *South Med J* 1983; **76:** 1455–6.
3. Baker B, et al. Electrocardiographic effects of fluoxetine and doxepin in patients with major depressive disorder. *J Clin Psychopharmacol* 1997; **17:** 15–21.
4. Coull DC, et al. Amitriptyline and cardiac disease. *Lancet* 1970; **ii:** 590–1.
5. Moir DC, et al. Cardiotoxicity of amitriptyline. *Lancet* 1972; **ii:** 561–4.
6. Moir DC, et al. Medicines evaluation and monitoring group: a follow-up study of cardiac patients receiving amitriptyline. *Eur J Clin Pharmacol* 1973; **6:** 98–101.
7. Boston Collaborative Drug Surveillance Program. Adverse reactions to the tricyclic-antidepressant drugs: report from Boston Collaborative Drug Surveillance Program. *Lancet* 1972; **i:** 529–31.
8. Anonymous. Sudden death in children treated with a tricyclic antidepressant. *Med Lett Drugs Ther* 1990; **32:** 53.
9. Riddle MA, et al. Another sudden death in a child treated with desipramine. *J Am Acad Child Adolesc Psychiatry* 1993; **32:** 792–7.
10. Varley CK, McClellan J. Case study: two additional sudden deaths with tricyclic antidepressants. *J Am Acad Child Adolesc Psychiatry* 1997; **36:** 390–4.
11. Biederman J, et al. Estimation of the association between desipramine and the risk for sudden death in 5- to 14-year-old children. *J Clin Psychiatry* 1995; **56:** 87–93.
12. Gutgesell H, et al. Cardiovascular monitoring of children and adolescents receiving psychotropic drugs: a statement for healthcare professionals from the Committee on Congenital Cardiac Defects, Council on Cardiovascular Disease in the Young, American Heart Association. *Circulation* 1999; **99:** 979–82.
13. Glassman AH. Cardiovascular effects of tricyclic antidepressants. *Annu Rev Med* 1984; **35:** 503–11.
14. Mortensen SA. Cyclic antidepressants and cardiotoxicity. *Practitioner* 1984; **228:** 1180–3.
15. Reilly JG, et al. QTc-interval abnormalities and psychotropic drug therapy in psychiatric patients. *Lancet* 2000; **355:** 1048–52.
16. Glassman AH, et al. The safety of tricyclic antidepressants in cardiac patients: risk-benefit reconsidered. *JAMA* 1993; **269:** 2673–5.
17. Cohen HW, et al. Excess risk of myocardial infarction in patients treated with antidepressant medications: association with use of tricyclic agents. *Am J Med* 2000; **108:** 2–8.
18. Hippisley-Cox J, et al. Antidepressants as risk factor for ischaemic heart disease: case-control study in primary care. *BMJ* 2001; **323:** 666–9.

EFFECTS ON THE PERIPHERAL CIRCULATION. Painful vasospastic episodes, characterised by cold and blue hands and feet, occurred in a woman each time she received imipramine 150 mg daily but with amitriptyline only when the dose was increased to

200 mg daily.[1] This suggested that the ability of tricyclic antidepressants to induce vasospasm was not limited to imipramine and that the effect might be partly dose-dependent. Additionally, acrocyanosis of the hands and feet has occurred in a child receiving imipramine for nocturnal enuresis.[2]

1. Appelbaum PS, Kapoor W. Imipramine-induced vasospasm: a case report. *Am J Psychiatry* 1983; **140:** 913–15.
2. Anderson RP, Morris BAP. Acrocyanosis due to imipramine. *Arch Dis Child* 1988; **63:** 204–5.

Effects on the endocrine system. The syndrome of inappropriate antidiuretic hormone secretion with hyponatraemia has been reported in patients receiving tricyclics and other antidepressants. The UK Committee on Safety of Medicines, commenting on reports it had received of hyponatraemia associated with antidepressants (fluoxetine, paroxetine, lofepramine, clomipramine, and imipramine), considered that it was likely to occur with any antidepressant and usually involved elderly patients.[1] Case reports of hyponatraemia in 24 patients treated with tricyclics and 20 patients treated with other antidepressants have been summarised.[2]

In a review covering the effects of drugs on prolactin secretion[3] it was stated that antidepressants could affect prolactin secretion by disturbing the balance of catecholaminergic inhibition and serotonergic stimulation of prolactin release, although any change is less than with antipsychotic therapy. Clomipramine and nortriptyline had been reported to stimulate prolactin release whereas amitriptyline, desipramine, and imipramine had been reported to be without effect. Such stimulation may account for symptoms of galactorrhoea or amenorrhoea reported with some tricyclics.

1. Committee on Safety of Medicines/Medicines Control Agency. Antidepressant-induced hyponatraemia. *Current Problems* 1994; **20:** 5–6.
2. Spigset O, Hedenmalm K. Hyponatraemia and the syndrome of inappropriate antidiuretic hormone secretion (SIADH) induced by psychotropic drugs. *Drug Safety* 1995; **12:** 209–25.
3. Hell K, Wernze H. Drug-induced changes in prolactin secretion: clinical implications. *Med Toxicol* 1988; **3:** 463–98.

Effects on the gastrointestinal tract. By 1978 the UK Committee on Safety of Medicines had been notified of cases of ileus, probably resulting from the antimuscarinic effects of tricyclic antidepressants.[1] Various tricyclics were taken by different patients, there being no suggestion that any one was especially liable to cause ileus. Fortunately the complication appeared to be rare.

1. Committee on Safety of Medicines. *Current Problems 3* 1978.

Effects on the kidneys and urine. Haematuria has been observed in a patient receiving amitriptyline and carbamazepine;[1] carbamazepine had previously been taken alone for an extensive period without producing this symptom.

Amitriptyline may have produced a blue-green colour in urine,[2] although it was considered to be a rare phenomenon.

1. Gillman MA, Sandyk R. Hematuria following tricyclic therapy. *Am J Psychiatry* 1984; **141:** 463–4.
2. Beeley L. *BMJ* 1986; **293:** 750.

Effects on the liver. Of 91 cases of hepatitis due to antidepressant therapy, 63 occurred in patients receiving the tricyclic antidepressant amineptine, sometimes with other psychotropic drugs; in approximately 50% of these amineptine cases, benzodiazepines had also been taken and it was postulated that the benzodiazepines may have increased the oxidation of amineptine to a toxic metabolite.[1] Most patients presented with abdominal pain and mixed liver damage with predominant cholestasis. One died after myocardial infarction, but all the others recovered. The mean amineptine dosage was 200 mg daily. In comparison, only a few cases were attributed to other tricyclic antidepressants—amitriptyline (4), clomipramine (3), and dibenzepin (1). Cross hepatotoxicity has also been reported in one patient between amineptine and clomipramine.[2]

Hepatotoxicity has also been noted with lofepramine. The UK Committee on Safety of Medicines had by the end of 1987 received 57 reports of abnormal liver function tests associated with lofepramine.[3] They included hepatic failure (1), jaundice (9), and hepatitis (5). All reactions occurred within the first 8 weeks of treatment and all were reversible on discontinuation of the drug.

1. Lefebure B, et al. Hépatites aux antidépresseurs. *Therapie* 1984; **39:** 509–16.
2. Larrey D, et al. Cross hepatotoxicity between tricyclic antidepressants. *Gut* 1986; **27:** 726–7.
3. Committee on Safety of Medicines. Lofepramine (Gamanil) and abnormal blood tests of liver function. *Current Problems 23* 1988.

Effects on the mouth. The inhibition of salivation caused by tricyclic antidepressants (in this case clomipramine) has been implicated in dental caries formation.[1]

1. deVries MW, Peeters F. Dental caries with longterm use of antidepressants. *Lancet* 1995; **346:** 1640.

Effects on the nervous system. A variety of effects on the nervous system have been attributed to tricyclic antidepressants, including drowsiness (especially with those with antihistaminic activity), peripheral neuropathy, tremor, ataxia, confusion, and delirium. Of particular concern is a reduction in the seizure threshold (see Epileptogenic Effect, below). Extrapyramidal effects and neuroleptic malignant syndrome (see below) may also occasionally occur.

Effects on sexual function. Loss of libido and impotence are common symptoms of depression, often making the role of drugs in producing sexual dysfunction difficult to assess.[1]

Sedation due to tricyclic antidepressants may lead to loss of libido and many of the tricyclics have been reported to cause impotence.[1,2] Amitriptyline, clomipramine, desipramine, doxepin, nortriptyline, and trimipramine have been stated to delay or inhibit ejaculation, and amoxapine, imipramine, and protriptyline, also to cause painful ejaculation. However, some tricyclics have been used for their effect on ejaculation to treat patients for premature ejaculation (see Clomipramine, p.282).

In women, anorgasmia or delayed orgasm has been reported with amitriptyline, amoxapine, clomipramine, and imipramine,[1-3] although spontaneous orgasm associated with yawning has been reported with clomipramine.[4]

1. Beeley L. Drug-induced sexual dysfunction and infertility. *Adverse Drug React Acute Poisoning Rev* 1984; **3:** 23–42.
2. Anonymous. Drugs that cause sexual dysfunction. *Med Lett Drugs Ther* 1987; **29:** 65–70.
3. Shen WW, Sata LS. Inhibited female orgasm resulting from psychotropic drugs: a clinical review. *J Reprod Med* 1983; **28:** 497–9.
4. McLean JD, *et al.* Unusual side effects of clomipramine associated with yawning. *Can J Psychiatry* 1983; **28:** 569–70.

Effects on the skin. Hypersensitivity reactions to tricyclic antidepressants are said to be uncommon.[1] Urticaria and angioedema have occurred, the urticaria occasionally clearing without drug withdrawal. Pruritus is also uncommon, but may be associated with transient erythema. Photosensitivity reactions are far less common than with phenothiazines; protriptyline has been the tricyclic most frequently implicated.[2,3] Rarely exfoliative dermatitis has developed, and purpura, pigmentation, and lichen planus have been noted in isolated reports. Toxic epidermal necrolysis has been reported in a patient 2 weeks after commencing therapy with amoxapine.[4] Hypersensitivity reactions to tricyclic antidepressants usually occur between 14 and 60 days after the start of treatment.[5]

Amitriptyline and fluoxetine have been implicated in the development of atypical cutaneous lymphoid hyperplasia in 8 patients, 7 of whom either had an underlying immunosuppressant systemic disease or were receiving concomitant therapy with immunomodulatory drugs.[6] The lesions improved or resolved on discontinuation of the antidepressant, although in some patients other factors may have contributed to lesional resolution.

1. Almeida J. Drug reactions XIII: cutaneous reactions to imipramine and chlordiazepoxide. *Br J Dermatol* 1971; **84:** 298–9.
2. Smith AG. Drug-induced photosensitivity. *Adverse Drug React Bull* 1989; **136** (June): 508–11.
3. Harth Y, Rapoport M. Photosensitivity associated with antipsychotics, antidepressants and anxiolytics. *Drug Safety* 1996; **14:** 252–9.
4. Camisa C, Grines C. Amoxapine: a cause of toxic epidermal necrolysis? *Arch Dermatol* 1983; **119:** 709–10.
5. Quitkin F. Cross-tolerance of tricyclic antidepressant drugs. *JAMA* 1979; **241:** 1625.
6. Crowson AN, Magro CM. Antidepressant therapy: a possible cause of atypical cutaneous lymphoid hyperplasia. *Arch Dermatol* 1995; **131:** 925–9.

Epileptogenic effect. Seizures have been reported after normal therapeutic doses of tricyclic antidepressants as well as after overdosage, although the mechanism by which the seizures are induced is unclear.[1] Seizures usually appear within a few days of starting the drug or changing to a higher dose but in patients with no previous history of epilepsy or no predisposing medical condition the frequency seems[1] to be very low with an incidence of approximately 1 in 1000. An incidence of 0.4 per 1000 was reported[2] based on 16 cases out of an estimated group of 42 000 patients receiving tricyclics and who had no predisposing factors, but in another review[3] a reasonable estimate of the incidence was considered to be 3 to 6 per 1000. However, it is widely agreed that tricyclics should be used very cautiously in patients with epilepsy or those with a low convulsive threshold.

In a retrospective analysis of 1313 cases[4] of overdosage involving cyclic antidepressants, seizures occurred more commonly with the tricyclics amoxapine (24.5%) and desipramine (17.9%), and the tetracyclic maprotiline (12.2%). In another analysis of 302 consecutive cases of tricyclic overdose a higher rate of seizures was seen with dothiepin [dosulepin] in overdosage (13%) than other tricyclics.[5]

1. Zaccara G, *et al.* Clinical features, pathogenesis and management of drug-induced seizures. *Drug Safety* 1990; **5:** 109–51.
2. Jick SS, *et al.* Antidepressants and convulsions. *J Clin Psychopharmacol* 1992; **12:** 241–5.
3. Rosenstein DL, *et al.* Seizures associated with antidepressants: a review. *J Clin Psychiatry* 1993; **54:** 289–99.
4. Wedin GP, *et al.* Relative toxicity of cyclic antidepressants. *Ann Emerg Med* 1986; **15:** 797–804.
5. Buckley NA, *et al.* Greater toxicity in overdose of dothiepin than of other tricyclic antidepressants. *Lancet* 1994; **343:** 159–62.

Extrapyramidal effects. Various extrapyramidal effects such as orofacial and choreoathetoid movements, and dyskinesias have been attributed to treatment with tricyclic antidepressants. Some patients with panic disorder may be sensitive to imipramine, developing symptoms of insomnia, jitteriness, and irritability.[1] These symptoms have also been observed in patients with panic disorder treated with low doses of desipramine although the symptoms usually subsided when the dose of the tricyclic was gradually increased. It has been suggested[2] that these symptoms may be related to akathisia and

are more likely to occur with those tricyclics that have a more potent effect on inhibition of noradrenaline reuptake.

Dysarthria has been reported[3] and was said to be not uncommon in those taking higher doses of tricyclic antidepressants, but unusual at lower doses.[4]

Reviews of adverse effects of drugs on the nervous system have also listed acute torsion dystonias and tremors[5] as being caused or exacerbated by tricyclic antidepressants.

1. Yeragani VK, *et al.* Tricyclic induced jitteriness—a form of akathisia? *BMJ* 1986; **292:** 1529.
2. Cole JO, Bodkin JA. Antidepressant drug side effects. *J Clin Psychiatry* 1990; **51** (suppl): 21–6.
3. Quader SE. Dysarthria: an unusual side effect of tricyclic antidepressants. *BMJ* 1977; **2:** 97.
4. Saunders M. Dysarthria with tricyclic antidepressants. *BMJ* 1977; **2:** 317.
5. Lane RJM, Routledge PA. Drug-induced neurological disorders. *Drugs* 1983; **26:** 124–47.

Hypersensitivity. See under Effects on the Skin, above.

Hyponatraemia. See Effects on the Endocrine System, above.

Neuroleptic malignant syndrome. Of 16 cases of neuroleptic malignant syndrome reported to the UK Committee on Safety of Medicines by July 1986, 3 cases occurred in patients receiving a tricyclic antidepressant; a combination of amitriptyline and perphenazine had been taken by one patient and dothiepin [dosulepin] or clomipramine alone by two other patients. The clomipramine case was fatal.[1] Other reports have been associated with amoxapine,[2] and the combined use of clomipramine and triazolam.[3]

1. Committee on Safety of Medicines. Neuroleptic malignant syndrome—an underdiagnosed condition? *Current Problems 18* 1986.
2. Madakasira S. Amoxapine-induced neuroleptic malignant syndrome. *DICP Ann Pharmacother* 1989; **23:** 50–1.
3. Domingo P, *et al.* Benign type of malignant syndrome. *Lancet* 1989; **i:** 50.

Overdosage. In a 1993 report[1] tricyclic antidepressants were associated with a higher risk of fatality following suicide attempts by drug overdose than were non-tricyclics available at the time. Some have considered desipramine to be associated more frequently than other tricyclic antidepressants with fatal overdosage.[2]

1. Anonymous. Antidepressant drugs and the risk of suicide. *WHO Drug Inf* 1993; **7:** 18–20.
2. Amitai Y, Frischer H. The toxicity and dose of desipramine hydrochloride. *JAMA* 1994; **272:** 1719–20.

Treatment of Adverse Effects

The basis of the management of tricyclic antidepressant poisoning is intensive supportive care and symptomatic therapy.

Since tricyclic antidepressants slow gastrointestinal transit time, absorption may be delayed in overdosage. Activated charcoal may be given by mouth or nasogastric tube if more than 4 mg per kg body-weight has been ingested within 1 hour; a second dose may be considered after 2 hours in patients with central features of toxicity. Gastric lavage has also been used, alone or in combination with charcoal. Multiple doses of charcoal may be appropriate in patients who have ingested modified-release preparations. The patient should be monitored for cardiac arrhythmias. UK authorities consider that although cardiac arrhythmias are of concern they are best treated by correction of hypoxia and acidosis and that the use of antiarrhythmic drugs is best avoided.

Convulsions can be managed by giving diazepam intravenously. Diazepam by mouth is usually adequate to sedate delirious patients, although large doses may be needed.

Physostigmine salicylate has been reported to be beneficial in some forms of cardiotoxicity, and in convulsions and coma, but its routine use cannot be recommended because of the serious adverse effects it may cause (see Antimuscarinic Poisoning in Uses of Physostigmine, p.1422). Peritoneal dialysis, haemodialysis, and measures to increase urine production are not of value in tricyclic antidepressant poisoning, and charcoal haemoperfusion is of doubtful benefit.

Precautions

The antimuscarinic effects of tricyclic antidepressants warrant their cautious use in patients with urinary retention, prostatic hyperplasia, or chronic constipation; caution has also been advised in untreated angle-closure glaucoma and in phaeochromocytoma.

The epileptogenic potential of tricyclic antidepressants leads to caution in administering them to pa-

tients with a history of epilepsy and their potential cardiotoxicity to caution in cardiovascular disease and avoidance in heart block, cardiac arrhythmias, or in the immediate recovery period after myocardial infarction.

Blood-sugar concentrations may be altered in diabetic patients.

Because tricyclic antidepressants are metabolised and inactivated in the liver they should be used with caution in patients with impaired liver function; they should be avoided in severe liver disease. Caution has also been recommended in patients with hyperthyroidism as administration of tricyclics may precipitate cardiac arrhythmias.

Patients should be closely monitored during early antidepressant therapy until improvement in depression is observed because suicide is an inherent risk in depressed patients. For further details, see under Depression, p.271.

If tricyclic antidepressants are used for the depressive component of bipolar disorder, mania may be precipitated; similarly, psychotic symptoms may be aggravated if tricyclics are used for a depressive component of schizophrenia.

Drowsiness is often experienced particularly at the start of therapy and patients, if affected, should not drive or operate machinery.

Regular dental check-ups are recommended for patients on long-term therapy with tricyclic antidepressants, particularly those with marked antimuscarinic actions.

Elderly patients can be particularly sensitive to the side-effects of tricyclic antidepressants and a reduced dose, especially initially, should be employed.

Tricyclic antidepressants are not recommended for depression in children. If they are used for nocturnal enuresis in children they should be limited to short courses with a full physical examination before subsequent courses.

Tricyclic antidepressants should be withdrawn gradually to reduce the risk of withdrawal symptoms (see below).

It has been recommended that, where possible, tricyclic antidepressants should be stopped some days before elective surgery, and that they should be used with caution in patients requiring concurrent electroconvulsive therapy, but see also under Anaesthesia, below.

Anaesthesia. Patients receiving tricyclic antidepressants are at an increased risk of developing hypotension or cardiac arrhythmias during anaesthesia. Tricyclics may also dangerously potentiate the cardiovascular effects of vasopressor drugs such as sympathomimetics that may be required during anaesthesia. Although some manufacturers recommend stopping tricyclics several days before elective surgery where possible, the *British National Formulary* advises that this is unnecessary as long as the anaesthetist is informed if they are not stopped.

Commenting on the anaesthetic considerations relevant to ECT,[1] it was considered that concurrent therapy with tricyclic antidepressants should not be a contra-indication to anaesthesia for ECT. A major consideration, though, was said to be the interaction of tricyclics with barbiturates resulting in increased sleep time and duration of anaesthesia. This meant that lower doses of barbiturate anaesthetics should be employed.

1. Gaines GY, Rees DI. Electroconvulsive therapy and anesthetic considerations. *Anesth Analg* 1986; **65:** 1345–56.

Breast feeding. In general, only small amounts of tricyclic antidepressants are distributed into breast milk. Nevertheless, most manufacturers advise that tricyclics should be avoided by the mother during breast feeding.

Case reports indicate that amitriptyline and its metabolite, nortriptyline,[1,2] desipramine and its metabolite, 2-hydroxydesipramine,[3] dothiepin [dosulepin] and its primary metabolites (nordothiepin, dothiepin-*S*-oxide, and nordothiepin-*S*-oxide),[4] doxepin and its metabolite, *N*-desmethyldoxepin,[5,6] imipramine and its metabolite, desipramine,[7] and maprotiline[8] are all present in breast milk in concentrations similar to those in maternal blood; amoxapine and its metabolite, 8-hydroxyamoxapine,[9] have also been detected in breast milk but in concentrations lower than in maternal blood. In the above cases all but one of the infants were breast fed without experiencing side-effects and tricyclics were undetectable in the infant's blood or present only in minute amounts. In the affected infant[6] adverse effects included sedation and shallow respiration. The infant's mother had received doxepin and, although doxepin was almost undetectable in the infant's serum, the desmethyl metabolite appeared to have accumulated. There were no data for the effects of amoxapine on breast-fed infants because the case reported[9] involved samples of milk taken from a woman experiencing galactorrhoea as an adverse effect of tricyclic administration. No adverse effects were seen during a 27-month follow-up of 14 breast-fed infants whose mothers had received imipramine 100 to 225 mg daily for 4 to 24 weeks.[10]

The American Academy of Pediatrics[11] considers that all antidepressants, including tricyclics, are drugs whose effect on nursing infants is unknown but may be of concern.

1. Bader TF, Newman K. Amitriptyline in human breast milk and the nursing infant's serum. *Am J Psychiatry* 1980; **137:** 855–6.
2. Brixen-Rasmussen L, *et al.* Amitriptyline and nortriptyline excretion in human breast milk. *Psychopharmacology (Berl)* 1982; **76:** 94–5.
3. Stancer HC, Reed KL. Desipramine and 2-hydroxydesipramine in human breast milk and the nursing infant's serum. *Am J Psychiatry* 1986; **143:** 1597–1600.
4. Ilett KF, *et al.* The excretion of dothiepin and its primary metabolites in breast milk. *Br J Clin Pharmacol* 1992; **33:** 635–9.
5. Kemp J, *et al.* Excretion of doxepin and N-desmethyldoxepin in human milk. *Br J Clin Pharmacol* 1985; **20:** 497–9.
6. Matheson I, *et al.* Respiratory depression caused by N-desmethyldoxepin in breast milk. *Lancet* 1985; **ii:** 1124.
7. Sovner R, Orsulak PJ. Excretion of imipramine and desipramine in human breast milk. *Am J Psychiatry* 1979; **136:** 451–2.
8. Lloyd AH. Practical considerations in the use of maprotiline (Ludiomil) in general practice. *J Int Med Res* 1977; **5** (suppl 4): 122–38.
9. Gelenberg AJ. Amoxapine, a new antidepressant, appears in human milk. *J Nerv Ment Dis* 1979; **167:** 635–6.
10. Misri S, Sivertz K. Tricyclic drugs in pregnancy and lactation: a preliminary report. *Int J Psychiatry Med* 1991; **21:** 157–71.
11. American Academy of Pediatrics Committee on Drugs. The transfer of drugs and other chemicals into human milk. *Pediatrics* 2001; **108:** 776–89.

Cardiovascular disease. For comments on the potential cardiotoxicity of tricyclic antidepressants and precautions to be observed in patients with pre-existing cardiovascular disorders, see under Effects on the Cardiovascular System in Adverse Effects, above.

Contact lenses. Based on reports involving amitriptyline[1] and maprotiline[2] it has been considered that the antimuscarinic action of tricyclic antidepressants may decrease tear flow enough to cause corneal drying and staining of contact lenses.[3]

1. Litovitz GL. Amitriptyline and contact lenses. *J Clin Psychiatry* 1984; **45:** 188.
2. Troiano G. Amitriptyline and contact lenses. *J Clin Psychiatry* 1985; **46:** 199.
3. Anonymous. Drugs interfering with contact lenses. *Aust J Hosp Pharm* 1987; **17:** 55–6.

Diabetes mellitus. The fact that tricyclic antidepressants may cause alterations in blood-glucose concentrations has led to the recommendation that these drugs be used with caution in diabetic patients. Additionally, amitriptyline has been reported[1] to cause hypoglycaemic unawareness; one patient did not experience her usual adrenergic symptoms that preceded or accompanied a hypoglycaemic episode.

1. Sherman KE, Bornemann M. Amitriptyline and asymptomatic hypoglycemia. *Ann Intern Med* 1988; **109:** 683–4.

Driving. While affective disorders probably adversely affect driving skill,[1,2] treatment with antidepressant drugs may also be hazardous,[1] although patients may be safer drivers with medication than without.[2] Impairment of performance is largely related to sedative and antimuscarinic effects both of which are more pronounced at the start of treatment; sedative tricyclics, such as amitriptyline and doxepin, are likely to cause greater psychomotor impairment than less sedative tricyclics such as imipramine and nortriptyline.[1] However, an epidemiological study[3] was unable to confirm any increased risk of road-traffic accidents in those drivers receiving tricyclic antidepressants or SSRIs. In healthy subjects fluoxetine (an SSRI) and dothiepin [dosulepin] appeared to have a similar but apparently small potential for impairing psychomotor and driving performance.[4]

In the UK, the Driver and Vehicle Licensing Authority (DVLA) considers that drugs with antimuscarinic adverse effects, such as tricyclic antidepressants, should be avoided in drivers, and that care is needed when taking antidepressants with antihistamine effects, because of the risk of drowsiness.[5] Patients with severe depressive illnesses complicated by significant memory or concentration problems, agitation, behavioural disturbances or suicidal thoughts should cease driving pending the outcome of medical enquiry. It has been mentioned[2] that the UK Medical Commission on Accident Prevention has recommended that patients on long-term psychotropic medication are unsuitable to be drivers of heavy goods or public service vehicles.

1. Ashton H. Drugs and driving. *Adverse Drug React Bull* 1983; **98:** 360–3.
2. Cremona A. Mad drivers: psychiatric illness and driving performance. *Br J Hosp Med* 1986; **35:** 193–5.
3. Barbone F, *et al.* Association of road-traffic accidents with benzodiazepine use. *Lancet* 1998; **352:** 1331–6.
4. Ramaekers JG, *et al.* A comparative study of acute and subchronic effects of dothiepin, fluoxetine and placebo on psychomotor and actual driving performance. *Br J Clin Pharmacol* 1995; **39:** 397–404.
5. Driver and Vehicle Licensing Agency. At a glance: a guide for medical practitioners. Available at: http://www.dvla.gov.uk/at_a_glance/ch4_psychiatric.htm (accessed 14/08/01).

Electroconvulsive therapy. For comments concerning the precautions to be observed in patients receiving electroconvulsive therapy, see under Anaesthesia, above.

Epilepsy. For comments on the epileptogenic effect of tricyclic antidepressants and the need for caution in patients with a history of epilepsy or other risk factors for development of seizures, see under Epileptogenic Effect in Adverse Effects, above.

Food. There has been a report of 3 patients in whom a high-fibre diet reduced or abolished the effectiveness of their tricyclic antidepressant therapy;[1] the tricyclics involved were doxepin in two patients and desipramine in one.

1. Stewart DE. High-fiber diet and serum tricyclic antidepressant levels. *J Clin Psychopharmacol* 1992; **12:** 438–40.

Gastro-oesophageal reflux disease. The antimuscarinic action of tricyclic antidepressants may cause relaxation of the lower oesophageal sphincter and could aggravate nocturnal symptoms of gastro-oesophageal reflux if given in the late evening.[1]

1. Atkinson M. Use and misuse of drugs in the treatment of gastro-oesophageal reflux. *Prescribers' J* 1982; **22:** 129–36.

Glaucoma. It has been considered by the manufacturers that tricyclic antidepressants, because of their antimuscarinic actions, should be used with caution in patients with angle-closure glaucoma or raised intra-ocular pressure. There have been few reports of glaucoma associated with tricyclics, although acute angle-closure glaucoma was reported in 4 patients with narrow angles while taking imipramine in usual doses,[1] and in another patient taking clomipramine.[2] In the latter case, the presenting sign was amaurosis fugax, caused by the combination of an abnormally large drop in blood pressure on standing and raised intra-ocular pressure.

1. Ritch R, *et al.* Oral imipramine and acute angle closure glaucoma. *Arch Ophthalmol* 1994; **112:** 67–8.
2. Schlingemann RO, *et al.* Amaurosis fugax on standing and angle-closure glaucoma with clomipramine. *Lancet* 1996; **347:** 465.

Phaeochromocytoma. Administration of imipramine[1,2] or desipramine[3] has caused adverse effects such as seizures and cardiovascular abnormalities (tachycardia and hypertension or hypotension) which have led to the recognition of a previously undiagnosed phaeochromocytoma. It has been suggested[3] that imipramine and its metabolite, desipramine, may be particularly effective in unmasking phaeochromocytoma and that this may be a reflection of their relative potency among the tricyclic antidepressants in inhibiting the noradrenaline reuptake mechanism.

1. Kaufmann JS. Phaeochromocytoma and tricyclic antidepressants. *JAMA* 1974; **229:** 1282.
2. Mok J, Swann I. Diagnosis of phaeochromocytoma after ingestion of imipramine. *Arch Dis Child* 1978; **53:** 676–7.
3. Achong MR, Keane PM. Pheochromocytoma unmasked by desipramine therapy. *Ann Intern Med* 1981; **94:** 358–9.

Porphyria. Amitriptyline has been associated with acute attacks of porphyria and is considered unsafe in porphyric patients.

Pregnancy. Although there have been isolated reports[1] attributing *congenital malformations* to the use of tricyclic antidepressants during pregnancy, large-scale studies and case-control data[2,3] have failed to substantiate any such association. Indeed, one report[4] on experience in 8 pregnant women being treated with a tricyclic antidepressant suggested that the antidepressant dose might need to be increased during the second half of pregnancy to achieve a response.

Fetal tachyarrhythmia detected at 37 weeks of gestation was attributed to maternal ingestion of dothiepin [dosulepin] during pregnancy. Following discontinuation of therapy by the mother no abnormalities in fetal heart rate were found and an uneventful labour followed with a healthy infant being delivered. However, the authors expressed concern that fetal tachycardias may result in *in-utero* cardiac failure and considered that tricyclic antidepressants should be used during pregnancy only if there were compelling reasons.[5]

Withdrawal syndromes manifesting as hypothermia and jitteriness,[6] convulsions,[7,8] or myoclonus[9] have been reported in neonates whose mothers took clomipramine during pregnancy. Management has been with phenobarbital or clomipramine. The manufacturers advise that if it is justifiable to do so, clomipramine should be withdrawn at least 7 weeks before the calculated date of delivery.

1. Barson AJ. Malformed infant. *BMJ* 1972; **2:** 45.
2. Greenberg G, *et al.* Maternal drug histories and congenital abnormalities. *BMJ* 1977; **2:** 853–6.
3. Winship KA, *et al.* Maternal drug histories and central nervous system anomalies. *Arch Dis Child* 1984; **59:** 1052–60.
4. Wisner KL, *et al.* Tricyclic dose requirements across pregnancy. *Am J Psychiatry* 1993; **150:** 1541–2.
5. Prentice A, Brown R. Fetal tachyarrhythmia and maternal antidepressant treatment. *BMJ* 1989; **298:** 190.
6. Musa AB, Smith CS. Neonatal effects of maternal clomipramine therapy. *Arch Dis Child* 1979; **54:** 405.
7. Cowe L, *et al.* Neonatal convulsions caused by withdrawal from maternal clomipramine. *BMJ* 1982; **284:** 1837–8.
8. Bromiker R, Kaplan M. Apparent intrauterine fetal withdrawal from clomipramine hydrochloride. *JAMA* 1994; **272:** 1722–3.
9. Bloem BR, *et al.* Clomipramine withdrawal in newborns. *Arch Dis Child Fetal Neonatal Ed* 1999; **81:** F77–F79.

Surgery. For comments regarding the precautions to be observed in patients undergoing surgery, see under Anaesthesia, above.

Withdrawal. Sudden discontinuation of antidepressant therapy after regular administration for 8 weeks or more may precipitate withdrawal symptoms. The symptoms associated with withdrawal of tricyclic antidepressants appear to form four distinct syndromes:[1] a range of gastrointestinal disturbances and generalised somatic symptoms such as malaise, chills, headache, and increased perspiration, which may also be accompanied by anxiety and agitation; sleep disturbances characterised by insomnia followed by excessive and vivid dreams; parkinsonism or akathisia; and hypomania or mania. Tricyclic withdrawal has also resulted in cardiac arrhythmias in some patients. Withdrawal symptoms seem to be more common and more severe in children.[2]

Many of the symptoms associated with discontinuation of tricyclic therapy may be produced by cholinergic rebound[1] and can be minimised by a gradual reduction in antidepressant dosage. The *British National Formulary* has recommended reduction over a period of at least 4 weeks, or as much as 6 months in patients who have been receiving long-term maintenance therapy. If withdrawal symptoms do occur, they may be managed by reinstitution of the tricyclic in a dose sufficient to eliminate them, followed by gradual discontinuation thereafter.[1,2] On the occasions that it may be necessary to stop a tricyclic abruptly, the withdrawal symptoms may be treated with a centrally active antimuscarinic such as atropine or benzatropine,[1] or alternatively, an antimuscarinic that does not cross the blood-brain barrier, such as propantheline, if the only withdrawal symptoms are gastrointestinal in nature.[1] Awareness of the possibility of withdrawal syndromes helps to avoid misinterpreting new symptoms after withdrawal as evidence of relapse.

Tricyclic antidepressants have been included in some classifications as drugs of dependence because of their potential to produce withdrawal syndromes, but this concept has been challenged by Lichtigfeld and Gillman[3] after reviewing several substance abuse studies and finding no evidence of abuse or dependence of the barbiturate type developing with the tricyclics.

For reports of withdrawal symptoms in neonates born to mothers who took tricyclic antidepressants during pregnancy, and their management, see under Pregnancy, above.

1. Dilsaver SC. Withdrawal phenomena associated with antidepressant and antipsychotic agents. *Drug Safety* 1994; **10:** 103–14.
2. Anonymous. Problems when withdrawing antidepressives. *Drug Ther Bull* 1986; **24:** 29–30.
3. Lichtigfeld FJ, Gillman MA. The possible abuse of and dependence on major tranquillisers and tricyclic antidepressants. *S Afr Med J* 1994; **84:** 5–6.

Interactions

Interactions involving tricyclic antidepressants often result from additive side-effects shared by each drug or from altered metabolism of one drug by the other. Drugs that inhibit the cytochrome P450 isoenzyme CYP2D6 may produce substantial decreases in tricyclic metabolism and marked increases in plasma concentrations.

Side-effects may be enhanced by the concurrent administration of antimuscarinic drugs or CNS depressants, including alcohol. Barbiturates and other enzyme inducers such as rifampicin and some antiepileptics can increase the metabolism of tricyclic antidepressants and may result in lowered plasma concentrations and reduced antidepressant response. Cimetidine, methylphenidate, antipsychotics, and calcium-channel blockers may reduce the metabolism of the tricyclics leading to the possibility of increased plasma concentrations and accompanying toxicity.

Patients taking thyroid preparations may show an accelerated response to tricyclic antidepressants and occasionally liothyronine has been employed to produce this effect in patients with refractory depression. However, concomitant administration of tricyclics with thyroid hormone therapy may precipitate cardiac arrhythmias.

The antihypertensive effects of betanidine, debrisoquine, guanethidine, and clonidine may be reduced by tricyclic antidepressants. The pressor effects of sympathomimetics, especially those of the direct-acting drugs adrenaline [epinephrine] and noradrenaline [norepinephrine], can be enhanced by tricyclic antidepressants; however, there is no clinical evidence of dangerous interactions between adrenaline [epinephrine]-containing local anaesthetics and tricyclic antidepressants. Great care should however be taken to avoid inadvertent intravenous administration of the local anaesthetic preparation.

Drugs which prolong the QT interval including antiarrhythmics such as quinidine, the antihistamines astemizole and terfenadine, some antipsychotics (notably pimozide and sertindole), cisapride, halofantrine, and sotalol, may increase the likelihood of ventricular arrhythmias when taken with tricyclic antidepressants. The problem may be exacerbated where the interacting drug (such as quinidine or some antipsychotics) also reduces tricyclic metabolism.

Although different antidepressants have been used together under expert supervision in refractory cases of depression, severe adverse reactions including the serotonin syndrome (see p.304) may occur. For this reason an appropriate drug-free interval should elapse between discontinuing some types of antidepressant and starting another. Tricyclic antidepressants should not generally be given to patients receiving MAOIs or for at least two weeks (3 weeks if starting clomipramine or imipramine) after their discontinuation. No treatment-free period is necessary after stopping a reversible inhibitor of monoamine oxidase type A (RIMA) and starting a tricyclic. At least 1 to 2 weeks (3 weeks in the case of clomipramine or imipramine) should elapse between withdrawing a tricyclic antidepressant and starting any drug liable to provoke a serious reaction (e.g. phenelzine).

Further details concerning some of the above interactions, and others, are given below.

Alcohol. For reference to the effect of alcohol on amitriptyline, see under CNS depressants, below.

Analgesics. Doubling of plasma-doxepin concentrations with associated lethargy has been reported in one patient following the addition of dextropropoxyphene to the tricyclic therapy.[1] This was consistent with previous studies indicating that dextropropoxyphene can impair the hepatic metabolism of other drugs.

For general reference to the effect of tricyclic antidepressants, notably amitriptyline and clomipramine, on opioid analgesics, see under Morphine, p.57.

1. Abernethy DR, et al. Impairment of hepatic drug oxidation by propoxyphene. *Ann Intern Med* 1982; **97:** 223–4.

Antiarrhythmics. Antiarrhythmics that prolong the QT interval may increase the likelihood of ventricular arrhythmias when given concomitantly with tricyclic antidepressants. There has been a report[1] of a patient receiving desipramine who had raised serum-desipramine concentrations and signs of toxicity after starting treatment with digoxin and propafenone for paroxysmal atrial fibrillation. It was considered that propafenone probably reduced the metabolism and clearance of desipramine.

1. Katz MR. Raised serum levels of desipramine with the antiarrhythmic propafenone. *J Clin Psychiatry* 1991; **52:** 432–3.

Anticoagulants. For the effect of tricyclic antidepressants on anticoagulants, see under Warfarin, p.995.

Antidepressants. Combination therapy with differing classes of antidepressants has been used successfully in the treatment of drug-resistant depression. It should be emphasised, however, that such combinations may result in enhanced adverse reactions or interactions, and should be employed only under expert supervision. This practice is considered unsuitable or controversial by some authorities. For further details of the interactions between different antidepressants when coadministered, see Phenelzine, p.306. For details of the serotonin syndrome that can arise when two serotonergic drugs with different mechanisms of action are administered, see under Adverse Effects of Phenelzine, p.304.

Antidiabetics. For the effect of tricyclic antidepressants on sulfonylurea antidiabetics, see Interactions, p.335.

Antiepileptics. Antidepressants may antagonise the activity of antiepileptics by lowering the convulsive threshold.

A review[1] of drug interactions with phenytoin noted that although there had been a number of reports of interactions between antiepileptics and tricyclic or related antidepressants, most involved enzyme-inducing antiepileptics other than phenytoin or phenytoin in combination with other drugs. In the only report where phenytoin could be identified as the sole antiepileptic used, 2 patients required high doses of desipramine to achieve an antidepressant effect and to maintain plasmadesipramine concentrations in the range usually associated with therapeutic efficacy.

Concomitant use of nortriptyline and carbamazepine in a patient led to a decrease in serum-nortriptyline concentration; an increase in nortriptyline dose was required.[2]

Valproate has been reported to increase plasma concentrations of amitriptyline and its metabolite nortriptyline.[3]

For the effects of tricyclic antidepressants on phenytoin, see p.360.

1. Nation RL, et al. Pharmacokinetic drug interactions with phenytoin (part II). *Clin Pharmacokinet* 1990; **18:** 131–50.
2. Brøsen K, Kragh-Sørensen P. Concomitant intake of nortriptyline and carbamazepine. *Ther Drug Monit* 1993; **15:** 258–60.
3. Wong SL, et al. Effects of divalproex sodium on amitriptyline and nortriptyline pharmacokinetics. *Clin Pharmacol Ther* 1996; **60:** 48–53.

Antifungals. Increased serum concentrations of nortriptyline[1] or amitriptyline[2,3] have been observed in patients also being given fluconazole. In some patients the combination of amitriptyline and fluconazole has led to syncope[3] or torsade de pointes.[4] Raised serum concentrations of nortriptyline and associated symptoms of intoxication occurred in a patient during concomitant treatment with terbinafine;[5] the interaction was confirmed on rechallenge.

1. Gannon RH. Fluconazole-nortriptyline drug interaction. *Ann Pharmacother* 1992; **26:** 1456.
2. Newberry DL, et al. A fluconazole/amitriptyline drug interaction in three male adults. *Clin Infect Dis* 1997; **24:** 270–1.
3. Robinson RF, et al. Syncope associated with concurrent amitriptyline and fluconazole therapy. *Ann Pharmacother* 2000; **34:** 1406–1409.
4. Dorsey ST, Biblo LA. Prolonged QT interval and torsades de pointes caused by the combination of fluconazole and amitriptyline. *Am J Emerg Med* 2000; **18:** 227–9.
5. van der Kuy P-HM, et al. Nortriptyline intoxication induced by terbinafine. *BMJ* 1998; **316:** 441.

Antihypertensives. In general, the hypotensive effect of antihypertensives is enhanced by tricyclic antidepressants, but there may be antagonism of the effect of adrenergic neurone blockers and of clonidine.

Antineoplastics. For the effect of tricyclic antidepressants on altretamine, see p.506.

Antiprotozoals. Furazolidone, an antiprotozoal with monoamine oxidase inhibiting activity, resulted in a toxic psychosis when given with amitriptyline to one patient.[1]

1. Aderhold RM, Muniz CE. Acute psychosis with amitriptyline and furazolidone. *JAMA* 1970; **213:** 2080.

Antipsychotics. For a discussion of interactions between antipsychotics and tricyclic antidepressants, see Chlorpromazine (p.664).

Antivirals. HIV-protease inhibitors may increase the plasma concentrations of tricyclic antidepressants whose metabolism is mediated through common cytochrome P450 isoenzymes. Ritonavir has produced moderate increases in the plasma concentrations of desipramine and the manufacturer has warned that a similar increase may occur for other tricyclics. Monitoring of drug concentrations and/or adverse effects is recommended when tricyclics are used with ritonavir.

Anxiolytics. For a suggestion that benzodiazepines may increase the oxidation of amineptine to a toxic metabolite, see under Effects on the Liver in Adverse Effects, above. For a possible interaction of desipramine and other antidepressants with zolpidem see p.712.

Barbiturates. For details of the interaction of tricyclic antidepressants with barbiturate anaesthetics, see under Anaesthesia in Precautions, above.

Beta blockers. Labetalol increased the bioavailability of imipramine in healthy subjects and inhibited its metabolism.[1]

The risk of ventricular arrhythmias may be increased when tricyclic antidepressants are taken with sotalol.

1. Hermann DJ, et al. Comparison of verapamil, diltiazem, and labetalol on the bioavailability and metabolism of imipramine. *J Clin Pharmacol* 1992; **32:** 176–83.

Calcium-channel blockers. Diltiazem and verapamil each increased the bioavailability of imipramine in healthy subjects; second-degree heart block developed in 2 subjects.[1] Diltiazem also increased the bioavailability of nortriptyline in one patient,[2] probably by reducing the first-pass metabolism of nortriptyline. Increased serum concentrations of trimipramine have been reported when taken concomitantly with diltiazem,[3] although there was no evidence of toxicity.

1. Hermann DJ, et al. Comparison of verapamil, diltiazem, and labetalol on the bioavailability and metabolism of imipramine. *J Clin Pharmacol* 1992; **32:** 176–83.
2. Krähenbühl S, et al. Pharmacokinetic interaction between diltiazem and nortriptyline. *Eur J Clin Pharmacol* 1996; **49:** 417–19.
3. Cotter PA, et al. Asymptomatic tricyclic toxicity associated with diltiazem. *Ir J Psychol Med* 1996; **13:** 168–9.

CNS depressants. Drugs with depressant actions on the CNS may be expected to enhance the drowsiness and related effects produced by the sedating type of tricyclic antidepressants. Such an interaction may occur between alcohol and tricyclic antidepressants and one study has shown that alcohol decreases the hepatic first-pass extraction of amitriptyline resulting in increased free plasma-amitriptyline concentrations, especially during the period of drug absorption.[1]

The problems that may be encountered with barbiturate anaesthetics are discussed under Anaesthesia in Precautions, above.

1. Dorian P, et al. Amitriptyline and ethanol: pharmacokinetic and pharmacodynamic interaction. *Eur J Clin Pharmacol* 1983; **25:** 325–31.

Disulfiram. Acute organic brain syndrome has been reported in 2 patients receiving disulfiram following the addition of amitriptyline to their treatment.[1] It was suspected that the syndrome was potentiated by the combined action of the two drugs and the synergistic elevation in dopamine concentration.

For a report of the enhancement of the disulfiram-alcohol reaction by amitriptyline, see p.1605.

1. Maany I, et al. Possible toxic interaction between disulfiram and amitriptyline. *Arch Gen Psychiatry* 1982; **39:** 743–4.

Dopaminergics. Serious adverse effects have been reported[1] when selegiline, an irreversible selective inhibitor of monoamine oxidase type B, and tricyclic antidepressants have been used concomitantly. In some instances results resembled the potentially fatal serotonin syndromes reported when tricyclics are administered together with non-selective MAOIs (see under Phenelzine, p.304).

Some authorities advise that tricyclic antidepressants should not generally be given to patients receiving selegiline, or for at least two weeks after it has been discontinued. Similarly, at least one week should elapse between withdrawing a tricyclic antidepressant and starting selegiline.

For reference to the effect of tricyclic antidepressants on levodopa, see p.1171.

1. Anonymous. Selegiline and antidepressants: risk of serious interactions. *WHO Drug Inf* 1995; **9:** 160–1.

General anaesthetics. For the effect of amitriptyline on enflurane, see p.1258. For the effects of concomitant use of tricyclic antidepressants and barbiturates see under Anaesthesia in Precautions, above.

Histamine H₂-antagonists. Cimetidine is a known inhibitor of hepatic metabolism of drugs and symptoms of tricyclic toxicity have been reported in patients receiving cimetidine concurrently with desipramine[1] and imipramine;[1] there has been a report of psychosis developing in a patient given imipramine in addition to cimetidine treatment.[2] Elevated tricyclic concentrations during combined therapy or reductions in tricyclic concentrations after withdrawal of cimetidine have been reported for imipramine[3] and nortriptyline.[4] Studies in healthy subjects have also indicated increased bioavailability and/or impaired hepatic metabolism of doxepin[5,6] and imipramine[7] during cimetidine therapy. This evidence points to the fact that adjustment of tricyclic antidepressant dosage may be required if cimetidine therapy is initiated or discontinued. Ranitidine has been reported not to alter the pharmacokinetics of amitriptyline,[8] doxepin,[6] or imipramine.[7]

1. Miller DD, Macklin M. Cimetidine-imipramine interaction: a case report. *Am J Psychiatry* 1983; **140:** 351–2.
2. Miller ME, et al. Psychosis in association with combined cimetidine and imipramine treatment. *Psychosomatics* 1987; **28:** 217–19.
3. Shapiro PA. Cimetidine-imipramine interaction: case report and comments. *Am J Psychiatry* 1984; **141:** 152.
4. Miller DD, et al. Cimetidine's effect on steady-state serum nortriptyline concentrations. *Drug Intell Clin Pharm* 1983; **17:** 904–5.
5. Abernethy DR, Todd EL. Doxepin-cimetidine interaction: increased doxepin bioavailability during cimetidine treatment. *J Clin Psychopharmacol* 1986; **6:** 8–12.
6. Sutherland DL, et al. The influence of cimetidine versus ranitidine on doxepin pharmacokinetics. *Eur J Clin Pharmacol* 1987; **32:** 159–64.
7. Wells BG, et al. The effect of ranitidine and cimetidine on imipramine disposition. *Eur J Clin Pharmacol* 1986; **31:** 285–90.
8. Curry SH, et al. Lack of interaction of ranitidine with amitriptyline. *Eur J Clin Pharmacol* 1987; **32:** 317–20.

Muscle relaxants. There has been an isolated report[1] of a patient taking baclofen for spasticity who experienced leg weakness and was unable to stand after starting treatment with nortriptyline. Symptoms improved on discontinuation of nortriptyline but recurred when imipramine was given.

1. Silverglat MJ. Baclofen and tricyclic antidepressants: possible interaction. *JAMA* 1981; **246:** 1659.

Sex hormones. There have been anecdotal reports of interactions between tricyclic antidepressants and oestrogens[1-3] resulting in either lack of antidepressant response or tricyclic toxicity; the significance of these interactions is not, however, established.

1. Prange AJ, et al. Estrogen may well affect response to antidepressant. *JAMA* 1972; **219:** 143–4.
2. Khurana RC. Estrogen-imipramine interaction. *JAMA* 1972; **222:** 702–3.
3. Somani SM, Khurana RC. Mechanism of estrogen-imipramine interaction. *JAMA* 1973; **223:** 560.

Smoking. Tobacco smoke has been reported to reduce the plasma levels of tricyclic antidepressants.[1-3] The clinical significance is not, however, fully established as the plasma concentration of unbound drug may not be affected.[3] The mechanism is probably by stimulation of hepatic drug metabolism by components present in cigarette smoke.

1. Perel JM, et al. Pharmacodynamics of imipramine in depressed patients. *Psychopharmacol Bull* 1975; **11:** 16–18.
2. John VA, et al. Effects of age, cigarette smoking and the oral contraceptive on the pharmacokinetics of clomipramine and its desmethyl metabolite during chronic dosing. *J Int Med Res* 1980; **8** (suppl 3): 88–95.
3. Perry PJ, et al. Effects of smoking on nortriptyline plasma concentrations in depressed patients. *Ther Drug Monit* 1986; **8:** 279–84.

Sympathomimetics. The pressor effects of sympathomimetics can be enhanced by tricyclic antidepressants.

For precautions to be observed in patients on tricyclic therapy who may require sympathomimetics during anaesthesia, see under Anaesthesia in Precautions, above.

Thyroid hormones. An increase in receptor sensitivity to catecholamines produced by thyroid hormones has been proposed as the reason for an increase in response to tricyclic antidepressants given concomitantly with *liothyronine*.[1,2]

1. Banki CM. Cerebrospinal fluid amine metabolites after combined amitriptyline-triiodothyronine treatment of depressed women. *Eur J Clin Pharmacol* 1977; **11:** 311–15.
2. Goodwin FK, *et al.* Potentiation of antidepressant effects by L-triiodothyronine in tricyclic nonresponders. *Am J Psychiatry* 1982; **139:** 34–8.

Pharmacokinetics

Amitriptyline is readily absorbed from the gastrointestinal tract, peak plasma concentrations occurring within a few hours of oral administration.

Amitriptyline undergoes extensive first-pass metabolism and is demethylated in the liver to its primary active metabolite, nortriptyline. Other paths of metabolism of amitriptyline include hydroxylation (possibly to active metabolites) and *N*-oxidation; nortriptyline follows similar paths. Amitriptyline is excreted in the urine, mainly in the form of its metabolites, either free or in conjugated form.

Amitriptyline and nortriptyline are widely distributed throughout the body and are extensively bound to plasma and tissue protein. Amitriptyline has been estimated to have an elimination half-life ranging from about 9 to 36 hours, which may be considerably extended in overdosage. Plasma concentrations of amitriptyline and nortriptyline vary very widely between individuals and no simple correlation with therapeutic response has been established.

Amitriptyline and nortriptyline cross the placenta and are distributed into breast milk (see Breast Feeding under Precautions, above).

◊ References.

1. Schulz P, *et al.* Discrepancies between pharmacokinetic studies of amitriptyline. *Clin Pharmacokinet* 1985; **10:** 257–68.
2. Task Force on the Use of Laboratory Tests in Psychiatry. Tricyclic antidepressants—blood level measurements and clinical outcome: an APA Task Force Report. *Am J Psychiatry* 1985; **142:** 155–62.
3. Brøsen K, Gram LF. Clinical significance of the sparteine/debrisoquine oxidation polymorphism. *Eur J Clin Pharmacol* 1989; **36:** 537–47.
4. Caccia S, Garattini S. Formation of active metabolites of psychotropic drugs: an updated review of their significance. *Clin Pharmacokinet* 1990; **18:** 434–59.
5. Wood AJJ, Zhou HH. Ethnic differences in drug disposition and responsiveness. *Clin Pharmacokinet* 1991; **20:** 350–73.
6. Llerena A, *et al.* Debrisoquin and mephenytoin hydroxylation phenotypes and CYP2D6 genotype in patients treated with neuroleptic and antidepressant agents. *Clin Pharmacol Ther* 1993; **54:** 606–11.

Uses and Administration

Tricyclic antidepressants such as amitriptyline were developed from phenothiazine compounds related to chlorpromazine and, as the name suggests, possess a 3-ring molecular structure. They inhibit the neuronal reuptake of noradrenaline in the CNS; some, in addition, inhibit the reuptake of serotonin (5-HT). Prevention of the reuptake of these monoamine neurotransmitters, which potentiates their action in the brain, appears to be associated with antidepressant activity. Tricyclic antidepressants also possess affinity for muscarinic and histamine H_1 receptors to varying degrees, see under Adverse Effects, above. Amitriptyline is one of the more sedating tricyclics. Antidepressants with one, two, or four rings have also been developed, and these share only some of the properties of the tricyclics.

While the sedative action and other adverse effects of amitriptyline and other tricyclics are soon apparent, it may be 2 to 4 weeks before the antidepressant effect is seen. After a response has been obtained, maintenance therapy should be continued at the optimum dose for at least 4 to 6 months (12 months in the elderly) to avoid relapse on discontinuation of therapy. It is important to use doses that are sufficiently high for

effective treatment, but not so high as to cause toxic effects.

Amitriptyline, a dibenzocycloheptadiene, is usually given by mouth as the hydrochloride; the hydrochloride may also be administered by intramuscular or intravenous injection.

In the treatment of **depression**, amitriptyline hydrochloride is given by mouth initially in a daily dose of 75 mg in divided doses (or as a single dose at night). Thereafter, the dose may be gradually increased, if necessary, to 150 mg daily, the additional doses being given in the late afternoon or evening. Therapy may also be initiated with a single dose of 50 to 100 mg at bedtime, increased by 25 or 50 mg as necessary to a total of 150 mg daily. Doses of up to 200 mg daily and, occasionally, up to 300 mg daily have been used in severely depressed patients in hospital.

Adolescent and elderly patients often have reduced tolerance to tricyclic antidepressants and initial doses of amitriptyline hydrochloride 30 to 75 mg daily may be adequate, given either as divided doses or as a single dose, preferably at bedtime.

Amitriptyline may also be given by mouth in liquid form as the hydrochloride or the embonate with doses expressed in terms of the base. Amitriptyline oxide (amitriptylinoxide) is also given by mouth.

In the initial stages of treatment, if administration by mouth is impracticable or inadvisable, the hydrochloride may be given by intravenous or intramuscular injection, but oral administration should be substituted as soon as possible. In some countries only the intramuscular route is used for parenteral administration in doses of 20 to 30 mg of the hydrochloride four times daily.

Amitriptyline is also used for the treatment of **nocturnal enuresis** in children in whom organic pathology has been excluded. However, drug therapy for nocturnal enuresis should be reserved for when other methods have failed and should preferably only be given to cover periods away from home; tricyclic antidepressants are not recommended in children under 6 years of age (the *British National Formulary* recommends that they should not be given until 7 years of age). Doses of amitriptyline hydrochloride that have been suggested are 10 to 20 mg at bedtime for children aged 6 to 10 years, and 25 to 50 mg at bedtime for children over 11 years of age. Treatment for enuresis, including the period of gradual withdrawal, should not continue for longer than 3 months. A full physical examination is recommended before a further course.

Tricyclic antidepressants including amitriptyline may be helpful in some disorders characterised by anxiety.

Amitriptyline should be withdrawn gradually to reduce the risk of withdrawal symptoms.

Anxiety disorders. See under Clomipramine, p.282.

Bulimia nervosa. A combination of counselling, support, psychotherapy, and antidepressants is the usual treatment for bulimia nervosa. Antidepressants can help to reduce the frequency of overeating and some other symptoms of bulimia but relapse tends to occur on discontinuation. A wide range of antidepressants has been tried, but the tricyclic desipramine and the SSRI fluoxetine have been the most commonly used and are considered to be well tolerated.

Ciguatera poisoning. Amitriptyline has relieved some of the neurological symptoms associated with ciguatera poisoning (see Mannitol, p.925).

Cocaine dependence. See under Desipramine, p.283.

Depression. As discussed on p.271, there is very little difference in efficacy between the different groups of antidepressant drugs, and choice is often made on the basis of adverse effect profile. Tricyclic antidepressants are often still chosen because of wide experience with their use and familiarity with their pharmacological actions. The more sedating tricyclics such as amitriptyline, clomipramine, dothiepin [dosulepin], doxepin, and trimipramine may be of value in depression with associated agitation or anxiety. The less sedating tricyclics such as desipramine, imipramine, lofepramine, nortriptyline, and protriptyline may be of value for withdrawn or apathetic depressed patients.

Combination therapy with differing classes of antidepressants, including the tricyclics, has been used in the treatment of refractory or drug-resistant depression. However, such therapy

may result in enhanced adverse reactions or interactions and requires expert supervision; it is considered unsuitable or controversial by some. For further details, see Antidepressants under Interactions of Phenelzine, p.306.

Headache. Tricyclic antidepressants can be effective in the management of some types of headache and, although they are especially useful when the headache is accompanied by depression, their beneficial effects appear to be independent of their antidepressant action. They are used for the prophylaxis of migraine (p.449) when drugs such as propranolol or pizotifen have proved ineffective. A suggested dosage for amitriptyline in the prophylaxis of migraine is 10 mg at night increased to a maintenance dose of 50 to 75 mg at night; the need for continuing prophylaxis should be reviewed at intervals of about 6 months. They are also used prophylactically in the control of chronic tension-type headache (p.450) although benefit is rarely complete. Improvement is generally seen with low doses, but full antidepressant doses are necessary in the presence of underlying depression. Amitriptyline is the tricyclic usually used but others have been tried.

References.

1. Mathew NT. Prophylaxis of migraine and mixed headache: a randomized controlled study. *Headache* 1981; **21:** 105–9.
2. Pfaffenrath V, *et al.* Combination headache: practical experience with a combination of a β-blocker and an antidepressive. *Cephalalgia* 1986; **6** (suppl 5): 25–32.
3. Wörz R, Scherhag R. Treatment of chronic tension headache with doxepin or amitriptyline—results of a double-blind study. *Headache Q* 1990; **1:** 216–23.
4. Ziegler DK, *et al.* Propranolol and amitriptyline in prophylaxis of migraine: pharmacokinetic and therapeutic effects. *Arch Neurol* 1993; **50:** 825–30.
5. Pfaffenrath V, *et al.* Efficacy and tolerability of amitriptylinoxide in the treatment of chronic tension-type headache: a multi-centre controlled study. *Cephalalgia* 1994; **14:** 149–55.
6. Holroyd KA, *et al.* Management of chronic tension-type headache with tricyclic antidepressant medication, stress management therapy, and their combination: a randomized controlled trial. *JAMA* 2001; **285:** 2208–15.

Hiccup. Amitriptyline is one of a wide range of drugs for which there are anecdotal reports[1] of success in the treatment of intractable hiccup. A protocol for the management of intractable hiccups may be found under Chlorpromazine, p.667.

1. Stalnikowicz R, *et al.* Amitriptyline for intractable hiccups. *N Engl J Med* 1986; **315:** 64–5.

Hyperactivity. When drug therapy is required for attention deficit hyperactivity disorder (p.1505), initial treatment is usually with a central stimulant. Tricyclic antidepressants such as imipramine or desipramine are reserved for patients who fail to respond to or who are intolerant of stimulants. They may also be of use for selected patients with certain co-existing disorders.

Interstitial cystitis. Tricyclic antidepressants such as amitriptyline or imipramine have been found to be of benefit in the treatment of interstitial cystitis (see Dimethyl Sulfoxide, p.1402) given at night in conjunction with methenamine hippurate during the day.[1]

1. Cardozo L. Postmenopausal cystitis. *BMJ* 1996; **313:** 129.

Irritable bowel syndrome. A tricyclic antidepressant may be tried in irritable bowel syndrome (p.1206), particularly where diarrhoea and abdominal pain are presenting symptoms.

Micturition disorders. Tricyclic antidepressants are among the drugs used as an alternative or adjunct to nonpharmacological methods for the treatment of **nocturnal enuresis** in children (p.459) in whom organic pathology has been excluded. However, because of their potentially fatal toxicity in overdosage, there has been concern over the safety of using tricyclics in households with children. Most experience in nocturnal enuresis has been with imipramine, but other tricyclics such as amitriptyline, nortriptyline, and clomipramine have also been used. Their mechanism of action in nocturnal enuresis is unclear. It may be the result of a combination of their antimuscarinic and antispasmodic actions as well as their effect on sleep patterns and possible stimulation of antidiuretic hormone secretion. Imipramine appears to be most effective in older children, but many patients develop tolerance and increasingly higher doses are required.

Tricyclic antidepressants are also sometimes used in the management of **urinary incontinence** (p.459).

References.

1. Glazener CMA, Evans JHC. Tricyclic and related drugs for nocturnal enuresis in children (updated 23 May 2001). Available in The Cochrane Library; Issue 3. Oxford: Update Software; 2001.

Narcoleptic syndrome. Tricyclic antidepressants are the primary treatment for cataplexy and sleep paralysis associated with narcolepsy (p.1505). Imipramine appears to be one of the most widely used for these symptoms. The onset of action is quicker than when used for depression and doses required appear to be lower. Doses should be titrated to provide maximal protection for the time of day when symptoms usually occur. Clomipramine and protriptyline are also commonly used.

Pain. Tricyclic antidepressants, usually amitriptyline, are useful in alleviating some types of pain when given in subantidepressant doses. This is discussed in Choice of Analgesic on p.2. Chronic neuropathic pain as seen in cancer (p.5), central post-stroke pain (p.5), diabetic neuropathy (p.5), phantom limb pain (p.7), and postherpetic neuralgia (p.7) responds to therapy with tricyclics. Tricyclics are also often of benefit in the treatment of idiopathic orofacial pain (p.7), and may be of value for patients with refractory reflex sympathetic dystrophy (p.8). Pain and sleep quality may be improved by tricyclics in patients with fibromyalgia (see Soft-tissue Rheumatism, p.10), a condition that responds poorly to analgesics and anti-inflammatory drugs. Patients with migraine or chronic tension-type headache may also benefit from tricyclics (see Headache, above). There is little evidence for an analgesic effect of tricyclics in acute pain.

References.
1. Onghena P, Van Houdenhove, B. Antidepressant-induced analgesia in chronic non-malignant pain: a meta-analysis of 39 placebo-controlled studies. *Pain* 1992; **49:** 205–19.
2. McQuay HJ, *et al.* A systematic review of antidepressants in neuropathic pain. *Pain* 1996; **68:** 217–27.
3. Godfrey RG. A guide to the understanding and use of tricyclic antidepressants in the overall management of fibromyalgia and other chronic pain syndromes. *Arch Intern Med* 1996; **156:** 1047–52.
4. McQuay HJ, Moore RA. Antidepressants and chronic pain. *BMJ* 1997; **314:** 763–4.
5. Joss JD. Tricyclic antidepressant use in diabetic neuropathy. *Ann Pharmacother* 1999; **33:** 996–1000.

Pathological crying or laughing. Pathological crying or laughing can result from lesions in certain areas of the brain. Attempts at treatment have mostly been with antidepressants and favourable results have been reported in double-blind studies with amitriptyline[1] and nortriptyline.[2]
1. Schiffer RB, *et al.* Treatment of pathologic laughing and weeping with amitriptyline. *N Engl J Med* 1985; **312:** 1480–2.
2. Robinson RG, *et al.* Pathological laughing and crying following stroke: validation of a measurement scale and a double-blind treatment study. *Am J Psychiatry* 1993; **150:** 286–93.

Premenstrual syndrome. See under Clomipramine, p.282.

Schizophrenia. Antidepressants such as the tricyclics are considered worth trying as an adjunct in the treatment of patients with schizophrenia (p.651) who develop depression during the recovery phase after an acute episode of psychosis. There is, however, no clear evidence that they are effective during acute psychotic episodes or for depression during periods of remission in patients with chronic schizophrenia.[1]
1. Anonymous. The drug treatment of patients with schizophrenia. *Drug Ther Bull* 1995; **33:** 81–6.

Sexual dysfunction. Impotence or ejaculatory problems have been reported as adverse effects of tricyclic antidepressants (see Effects on Sexual Function in Adverse Effects, above). Such properties have been studied as a potential form of treatment for men with premature ejaculation (see Clomipramine, p.282).

Skin disorders. See under Doxepin, p.284.

Smoking cessation. Tricyclic antidepressants are among the drugs that have been tried with varying degrees of success as alternatives to nicotine replacement therapy (NRT) to alleviate the withdrawal syndrome associated with smoking cessation (p.1642). Nortriptyline is recommended by some as a second-line treatment in those patients who cannot tolerate or relapse after NRT.

References.
1. Hughes JR, *et al.* Antidepressants for smoking cessation (updated 30 August 2000). Available in The Cochrane Library; Issue 4. Oxford: Update Software; 2000.

Stuttering. See under Clomipramine, p.282.

Preparations

BP 2001: Amitriptyline Tablets;
USP 25: Amitriptyline Hydrochloride Injection; Amitriptyline Hydrochloride Tablets; Chlordiazepoxide and Amitriptyline Hydrochloride Tablets; Perphenazine and Amitriptyline Hydrochloride Tablets.

Proprietary Preparations (details are given in Part 3)
Aust.: Saroten; Tryptizol; *Austral.:* Amitrol†; Endep; Tryptanol; Tryptine; *Belg.:* Redomex; Tryptizol; *Braz.:* Tryptil; *Canad.:* Elavil; Levate†; Novo-Triptyn†; *Denm.:* Saroten; Tryptizol; *Fin.:* Klotriptyl; Saroten; Triptyl; *Fr.:* Elavil; Laroxyl; *Ger.:* Amineurin; Amioxid; Equilibrin; Novoprotect; Saroten; Syneudon; *Hong Kong:* Domical; Tryptanol; *Irl.:* Domical†; Lentizol; Tryptizol; *Israel:* Elatrol; Tryptal; *Ital.:* Adepril; Amilit-IFI; Laroxyl; Triptizol; *Mex.:* Anapsique; Tryptanol; *Neth.:* Sarotex; Tryptizol; *Norw.:* Sarotex; Tryptizol; *NZ:* Amitrip; Tryptanol; *Port.:* ADT; Tryptizol; *S.Afr.:* Endep; Noriline†; Saroten; Trepiline; Tryptanol; *Singapore:* Tryptal; *Spain:* Deprelio; Tryptizol; Swed.: Saroten; Tryptizol; *Switz.:* Saroten; Tryptizol; *Thai.:* Polytanol; Tripta; Triptyline; Tryptanol; *UK:* Domical†; Elavil; Lentizol; Tryptizol†; *USA:* Elavil.

Multi-ingredient: *Aust.:* Limbitrol; Pantrop; *Austral.:* Mutabon D†; *Belg.:* Limbitrol†; *Braz.:* Limbitrol; Tryptanol; *Canad.:* Elavil Plus; Etrafon; PMS-Levazine†; Triavil; *Fin.:* Limbitrol; Pertriptyl; *Ger.:* Limbatril; *Irl.:* Triptafen†; *Ital.:* Diapatol; Limbitryl; Mutabon; Sedans; *Mex.:* Adepsique; *Neth.:* Limbitrol†; *Port.:* Mutabon; *S.Afr.:* Etrafon; Limbitrol; *Spain:* Mutabase; Nobritol; *Switz.:* Limbitrol; *Thai.:* Anxipress-D; Neuragon; *UK:* Triptafen; *USA:* Etrafon; Limbitrol; Triavil.

Amoxapine (2503-q)

Amoxapine (BAN, USAN, rINN).
CL-67772.   2-Chloro-11-(piperazin-1-yl)dibenz[b,f][1,4]oxazepine.
$C_{17}H_{16}ClN_3O = 313.8$.
CAS — 14028-44-5.
ATC — N06AA17.
Pharmacopoeias. In Jpn and US.

Pharmacopoeial description
USP 25: A white to yellowish crystalline powder. Practically insoluble in water; slightly soluble in acetone; freely soluble in chloroform; sparingly soluble in methyl alcohol and in toluene; soluble in tetrahydrofuran. Store in airtight containers.

Adverse Effects, Treatment, and Precautions
As for tricyclic antidepressants in general (see Amitriptyline, p.273).

Amoxapine has also been associated with tardive dyskinesias and the neuroleptic malignant syndrome has been reported.

Antidopaminergic effects. Amoxapine is a derivative of the antipsychotic loxapine (p.690) and possesses some neuroleptic activity. It also demonstrates dopamine-receptor blocking properties as do its hydroxylated metabolites. A variety of adverse effects that are symptoms of such blockade have been reported and reviewed[1,2] and include akinesia, akathisia, withdrawal dyskinesia, reversible tardive dyskinesia, persistent dyskinesia, elevated serum concentration of prolactin, and galactorrhoea. Chorea[3] and oculogyric crisis[4] have also been reported.
1. Tao GK, *et al.* Amoxapine-induced tardive dyskinesia. *Drug Intell Clin Pharm* 1985; **19:** 548–9.
2. Devarajan S. Safety of amoxapine. *Lancet* 1989; **ii:** 1455.
3. Patterson JF. Amoxapine-induced chorea. *South Med J* 1983; **76:** 1077.
4. Hunt-Fugate AK, *et al.* Adverse reactions due to dopamine blockade by amoxapine. *Pharmacotherapy* 1984; **4:** 35–9.

Antimuscarinic effects. While amoxapine has been reported to produce in depressed patients adverse effects associated with antimuscarinic activity (such as constipation, blurred vision, and dry mouth), Bourne *et al.*[1] considered that such reports did not reflect *in-vitro* findings that amoxapine had considerably less affinity for muscarinic binding sites than amitriptyline and this was supported by their results in healthy subjects. The adverse effects described as antimuscarinic could possibly be explained by amoxapine affecting noradrenergic mechanisms.
1. Bourne M, *et al.* A comparison of the effects of single doses of amoxapine and amitriptyline on autonomic functions in healthy volunteers. *Eur J Clin Pharmacol* 1993; **44:** 57–62.

Effects on the endocrine system. Reversible nonketotic hyperglycaemia developed in a 49-year-old woman with no history of diabetes mellitus within 5 days of therapy with amoxapine 50 mg three times daily by mouth.[1] She had previously experienced nonketotic hyperglycaemic coma after loxapine 150 mg daily. 7-Hydroxyamoxapine, a metabolite common to both amoxapine and loxapine, was implicated.
See also Antidopaminergic Effects, above, for mention of galactorrhoea and hyperprolactinaemia.
1. Tollefson G, Lesar T. Nonketotic hyperglycemia associated with loxapine and amoxapine: case report. *J Clin Psychiatry* 1983; **44:** 347–8.

Overdosage. In overdosage, amoxapine is reported to cause acute renal failure with rhabdomyolysis,[1,2] coma, and seizures.[3-5] Although there has been some debate as to whether the incidence of seizures and death is higher with overdosage of amoxapine than with other tricyclic antidepressants, some[6] consider that evidence does seem to favour increased neurological consequences.
It has been reported that amoxapine is not cardiotoxic in overdosage[3] but later evidence would suggest that there is cardiotoxic potential.[6,7]
1. Pumariega AJ, *et al.* Acute renal failure secondary to amoxapine overdose. *JAMA* 1982; **248:** 3141–2.
2. Jennings AE, *et al.* Amoxapine-associated acute renal failure. *Arch Intern Med* 1983; **143:** 1525–7.
3. Kulig K, *et al.* Amoxapine overdose: coma and seizures without cardiotoxic effects. *JAMA* 1982; **248:** 1092–4.
4. Litovitz TL, Troutman WG. Amoxapine overdose: seizures and fatalities. *JAMA* 1983; **250:** 1069–71.
5. Jefferson JW. Convulsions associated with amoxapine. *JAMA* 1984; **251:** 603–4.
6. Leonard BE. Safety of amoxapine. *Lancet* 1989; **ii:** 808.
7. Sørensen MR. Acute myocardial failure following amoxapine intoxication. *J Clin Psychopharmacol* 1988; **8:** 75.

Interactions
For interactions associated with tricyclic antidepressants, see Amitriptyline, p.276.

Pharmacokinetics
Amoxapine is readily absorbed from the gastrointestinal tract. It bears a close chemical relationship to loxapine (p.690) and is similarly metabolised by hydroxylation. It is excreted in the urine, mainly as its metabolites in conjugated form as glucuronides.

Amoxapine has been reported to have a plasma half-life of 8 hours and its major metabolite, 8-hydroxyamoxapine, has been reported to have a biological half-life of 30 hours; another metabolite, 7-hydroxyamoxapine, has a half-life of 6.5 hours. Both metabolites are pharmacologically active. Amoxapine is extensively bound to plasma proteins.

Amoxapine and its metabolite 8-hydroxyamoxapine are distributed into breast milk (see Breast Feeding under Precautions for Amitriptyline, p.275).

Uses and Administration
Amoxapine, the N-desmethyl derivative of loxapine (p.690), is a dibenzoxazepine tricyclic antidepressant with actions and uses similar to those of amitriptyline (p.278). Amoxapine is one of the less sedating tricyclics and its antimuscarinic effects are mild; it also inhibits the reuptake of dopamine.

In the treatment of depression (p.271) amoxapine is given in oral doses of 50 mg two or three times daily initially, gradually increased up to 100 mg three times daily as necessary. Higher doses of up to 600 mg daily may be required in severely depressed patients in hospital. A suggested dose for the elderly is 25 mg two or three times daily initially, increased after 5 to 7 days to up to 150 mg daily as necessary; some patients may require further increases to a maximum of 300 mg daily.

Once-daily dosage regimens, usually given at night, are suitable for amoxapine up to 300 mg daily; divided-dosage regimens are recommended for doses above 300 mg daily.

It has been claimed that, in the treatment of depression, amoxapine has a more rapid onset of action than amitriptyline or imipramine with a clinical effect possibly appearing 4 to 7 days after the initiation of therapy, although this has sometimes been disputed.

Amoxapine should be withdrawn gradually to reduce the risk of withdrawal symptoms.

◊ References.
1. Jue SG, *et al.* Amoxapine: a review of its pharmacology and efficacy in depressed states. *Drugs* 1982; **24:** 1–23.

Preparations
USP 25: Amoxapine Tablets.

Proprietary Preparations (details are given in Part 3)
Canad.: Asendin; *Denm.:* Demolox; *Fr.:* Defanyl; *Irl.:* Asendis; *NZ:* Asendin; *Spain:* Demolox; *UK:* Asendis; *USA:* Asendin.

Atomoxetine Hydrochloride (1270-r)

Atomoxetine Hydrochloride (BANM, USAN).
Tomoxetine Hydrochloride (pINNM); LY-135252; LY-139602; LY-139603.   (–)-N-Methyl-γ-(2-methylphenoxy)-benzenepropanamine hydrochloride.
$C_{17}H_{21}NO,HCl = 291.8$.
CAS — 83015-26-3 (atomoxetine); 82248-59-7 (atomoxetine hydrochloride).

Profile
Atomoxetine hydrochloride is a selective noradrenaline reuptake inhibitor under investigation in the treatment of attention deficit hyperactivity disorder in adults and children.

◊ References.
1. Spencer T, *et al.* Effectiveness and tolerability of tomoxetine in adults with attention deficit hyperactivity disorder. *Am J Psychiatry* 1998; **155:** 693–5.

Befloxatone (15879-w)

Befloxatone (rINN).
(R)-5-(Methoxymethyl)-3-{p-[(R)-4,4,4-trifluoro-3-hydroxybutoxy]phenyl}-2-oxazolidinone.
$C_{15}H_{18}F_3NO_5 = 349.3$.
CAS — 134564-82-2.

Profile
Befloxatone, an oxazolidinone derivative, is a reversible inhibitor of monoamine oxidase type A (RIMA) (see Moclobemide, p.299) under investigation for the treatment of depression.

◊ References.
1. Durrieu G, *et al.* Oral tyramine pressor effect after chronic treatment with befloxatone in healthy volunteers. *Br J Clin Pharmacol* 1995; **39:** 574P.

The symbol † denotes a preparation no longer actively marketed

2. Patat A, et al. Pharmacodynamics and pharmacokinetics of two dose regimens of befloxatone, a new reversible and selective monoamine oxidase inhibitor, at steady state in healthy volunteers. *J Clin Pharmacol* 1996; **36:** 216–29.
3. Warot D, et al. Effects of befloxatone, a reversible selective monoamine oxidase-A inhibitor, on psychomotor function and memory in healthy subjects. *J Clin Pharmacol* 1996; **36:** 942–50.
4. Rosenzweig P, et al. Clinical pharmacology of befloxatone: a brief review. *J Affect Disord* 1998; **51:** 305–12.

Benactyzine Hydrochloride (7005-g)

Benactyzine Hydrochloride (BANM, rINNM).
2-Diethylaminoethyl benzilate hydrochloride.
$C_{20}H_{25}NO_3,HCl = 363.9$.
CAS — 302-40-9 (benactyzine); 57-37-4 (benactyzine hydrochloride).

Profile
Benactyzine has antidepressant and antimuscarinic activity. It has been used as the hydrochloride in the management of depression and associated anxiety. It is also used as a pharmacological tool. Methylbenactyzium bromide (p.470), the methobromide of benactyzine, has been used for its antimuscarinic activity in the treatment of gastrointestinal spasm and nocturnal enuresis.

Brofaromine (2840-n)

Brofaromine (rINN).
CGP-11305A (brofaromine hydrochloride). 4-(7-Bromo-5-methoxy-2-benzofuranyl)piperidine.
$C_{14}H_{16}BrNO_2 = 310.2$.
CAS — 63638-91-5.

Profile
Brofaromine is a reversible inhibitor of monoamine oxidase type A (RIMA) (see Moclobemide, p.299). It has been studied in the treatment of depression and in anxiety disorders including social phobia.

◊ References.
1. Steiger A, et al. Results of an open clinical trial of brofaromine (CGP 11305 A), a competitive, selective, and short-acting inhibitor of MAO-A in major endogenous depression. *Pharmacopsychiatry* 1987; **20:** 262–9.
2. van Vliet IM, et al. MAO inhibitors in panic disorder: clinical effects of treatment with brofaromine: a double blind placebo controlled study. *Psychopharmacology (Berl)* 1993; **112:** 483–9.
3. Zeeh J, et al. Influence of age, frailty and liver function on the pharmacokinetics of brofaromine. *Eur J Clin Pharmacol* 1996; **49:** 387–91.
4. Volz H-P, et al. Brofaromine—a review of its pharmacological properties and therapeutic use. *J Neural Transm* 1996; **103:** 217–45.
5. Lott M, et al. Brofaromine for social phobia: a multicenter, placebo-controlled, double-blind study. *J Clin Psychopharmacol* 1997; **17:** 255–60.
6. Lotufo-Neto F, et al. Meta-analysis of the reversible inhibitors of monoamine oxidase type A moclobemide and brofaromine for the treatment of depression. *Neuropsychopharmacology* 1999; **20:** 226–47.

Bupropion Hydrochloride (12469-j)

Bupropion Hydrochloride (BANM, USAN, rINNM).
Amfebutamone Hydrochloride; BW-323. (±)-2-(tert-Butylamino)-3'-chloropropiophenone hydrochloride.
$C_{13}H_{18}ClNO,HCl = 276.2$.
CAS — 34911-55-2 (bupropion); 31677-93-7 (bupropion hydrochloride).

Adverse Effects and Treatment
Agitation, anxiety, and insomnia often occur during the initial stages of bupropion therapy. Other relatively common side-effects reported with bupropion include fever, dry mouth, headache or migraine, dizziness, nausea and vomiting, constipation, tremor, sweating, and skin rashes. Hypersensitivity reactions, ranging from pruritus and urticaria to, less commonly, angioedema, dyspnoea, and anaphylactoid reactions, have occurred, as have symptoms suggestive of serum sickness. There have been rare reports of Stevens-Johnson syndrome and erythema multiforme. Tachycardia, chest pain, and hypertension (sometimes severe), or occasionally vasodilatation, postural hypotension, and syncope have been reported. Psychotic episodes, confusion, loss of appetite, tinnitus and visual disturbances have also been reported.

Seizures, which appear to be partially dose-related, may occur with bupropion and have been particularly notable in patients with anorexia nervosa or bulimia nervosa; the risk is also increased in patients with a history of seizure disorders or other predisposing fac-

tor. The manufacturers state that the overall incidence of seizure in patients receiving bupropion at recommended doses is about 0.1 to 0.4%.

Symptoms of overdosage include hallucinations, nausea and vomiting, tachycardia, loss of consciousness, and death (following massive overdose); seizures have occurred in approximately one-third of all bupropion overdose cases. Gastric lavage or administration of activated charcoal within the first 12 hours of ingestion may decrease absorption. Treatment is supportive. Benzodiazepines may be tried for seizures. Diuresis, dialysis, and haemoperfusion are unlikely to be of benefit.

◊ Up to 24 September 2001 (the first 16 months of marketing), the UK Committee on Safety of Medicines (CSM) had received 6570 reports of suspected adverse reactions associated with the use of bupropion.[1] Of these reports, 51 were associated with a fatal outcome although the contribution of bupropion to these fatalities is unproven and in the majority of the cases underlying conditions may provide an alternative explanation. The CSM also commented that adverse reactions were mainly recognised ones and listed in the manufacturer's product information.
1. Committee on Safety of Medicines/Medicines Control Agency. Zyban (bupropion hydrochloride) - safety update. Available at: http://www.mca.gov.uk/ourwork/monitorsafequalmed/safetymessages/zyban260901.pdf (accessed 29/10/01).

Effect on the cerebrovascular system. A 67-year-old male experienced paraesthesia, dizziness, tinnitus, confusion, and gait impairment after taking bupropion for smoking cessation.[1] Although a transient ischaemic attack was suspected symptoms resolved on discontinuation of bupropion and recurred on rechallenge.
1. Humma LM, Swims MP. Bupropion mimics a transient ischemic attack. *Ann Pharmacother* 1999; **33:** 305–7.

Hypersensitivity. Eosinophilia has been reported[1] in a patient 12 days after bupropion was added to her existing treatment regimen of glibenclamide and tolmetin. The eosinophil count returned to normal after all medication was stopped. Bupropion appeared to be the causative drug. Serum sickness associated with bupropion exposure has also been reported.[2,3]
1. Malesker MA, et al. Eosinophilia associated with bupropion. *Ann Pharmacother* 1995; **29:** 867–8.
2. Yolles JC, et al. Serum sickness induced by bupropion. *Ann Pharmacother* 1999; **33:** 931–3.
3. McCollom RA, et al. Bupropion-induced serum sickness-like reaction. *Ann Pharmacother* 2000; **34:** 471–3.

Precautions
Bupropion may induce seizures and consequently its use is contra-indicated in patients with epilepsy. It is also contra-indicated in patients with a history of anorexia nervosa or bulimia nervosa as a higher incidence of seizures has been noted in such patients treated with bupropion. It should be used with extreme caution, if at all, in patients with a history of seizure disorders or other predisposing factors such as severe hepatic cirrhosis or a CNS tumour, and in those undergoing abrupt withdrawal from alcohol or benzodiazepines. The use of bupropion in patients with other risk factors for seizures (for example, alcohol abuse, a history of head trauma, diabetes, and drugs known to lower the seizure threshold) should only be undertaken when there are compelling clinical reasons.

Bupropion should be used with caution in patients with bipolar disorder or psychoses because of the risk of precipitating mania; use for smoking cessation in such patients may be contra-indicated. It should also be used cautiously in patients with a recent history of myocardial infarction or unstable heart disease, and in hepatic or renal impairment.

When bupropion is used for depression, patients should be closely monitored during early therapy until improvement is observed because suicide is an inherent risk in depressed patients. For further details, see under Depression, p.271.

As with other CNS-active drugs, the ability to perform tasks requiring motor or cognitive skills or judgement may be impaired by bupropion, and patients, if affected, should not drive or operate machinery.

Bupropion is distributed into breast milk and therefore has the potential for serious adverse effects in the infant.

Interactions
Bupropion should not be given concurrently with or within 14 days of stopping an MAOI.

The use of alcohol with bupropion should be minimised or avoided completely because it may alter the seizure threshold. Similarly, other drugs that lower the seizure threshold, such as other antidepressants, antimalarials, antipsychotics, sedating antihistamines, quinolones, tramadol, theophylline, or systemic corticosteroids, should be used with extreme caution together with bupropion.

Use of nicotine transdermal patches concurrently with bupropion has been associated with hypertension, and patients using this combination should therefore have their blood pressure monitored.

Caution has been advised in patients receiving levodopa because of reports of a higher incidence of adverse effects in patients receiving these two drugs concurrently.

Animal studies have indicated that bupropion may induce drug-metabolising enzymes and interactions with other drugs are therefore a possibility. It is itself metabolised by hepatic enzyme systems and drugs known to affect such systems may interact with bupropion. For example carbamazepine, phenobarbital, or phenytoin may induce the metabolism of bupropion while other drugs such as cimetidine or ritonavir may inhibit its metabolism. *In-vitro* studies have demonstrated that bupropion is metabolised by the cytochrome P450 isoenzyme CYP2B6. Consequently interactions may occur between bupropion and drugs that affect this isoenzyme, for example orphenadrine, cyclophosphamide, and ifosfamide.

In-vitro studies have also shown that bupropion is an inhibitor of another isoenzyme, CYP2D6, and, therefore, caution should be exercised when it is given with drugs metabolised by this enzyme and they should be initiated at the lower end of their dose range. Such drugs include some antidepressants, antipsychotics, beta blockers, and type Ic antiarrhythmics.

Antiepileptics. Plasma-bupropion concentrations became undetectable in 2 patients who were also receiving carbamazepine; plasma concentrations of hydroxybupropion, an active metabolite of bupropion, were high.[1]
1. Popli AP, et al. Bupropion and anticonvulsant drug interactions. *Ann Clin Psychiatry* 1995; **7:** 99–101.

Pharmacokinetics
Bupropion is well absorbed from the gastrointestinal tract but may undergo extensive first-pass metabolism. Several metabolites of bupropion are pharmacologically active and have longer half-lives, and achieve higher plasma concentrations, than the parent compound. Hydroxybupropion is the major metabolite, produced by the metabolism of bupropion by the cytochrome P450 isoenzyme CYP2B6; it is comparable in potency to bupropion. Threohydrobupropion and erythrohydrobupropion are produced by hydroxylation and/or reduction and are about one-half to one-tenth the potency of the parent compound. Bupropion is 80% or more bound to plasma proteins. The terminal plasma half-life of bupropion is about 14 hours. The metabolites of bupropion are excreted primarily in the urine; less than 1% of the parent drug is excreted unchanged. Bupropion and its metabolites cross the placenta and are distributed into breast milk.

◊ References.
1. Sweet RA, et al. Pharmacokinetics of single- and multiple-dose bupropion in elderly patients with depression. *J Clin Pharmacol* 1995; **35:** 876–84.

Distribution into breast milk. There has been a report of accumulation of bupropion in human breast milk in concentrations higher than those in maternal plasma.[1] However, neither bupropion nor its metabolites were detected in the plasma of the infant breast-fed twice daily by the affected mother and no adverse effects were noted in the infant (but see Precautions, above).
1. Briggs GC, et al. Excretion of bupropion in breast milk. *Ann Pharmacother* 1993; **27:** 431–3.

Smoking. No clinically significant differences were observed between the pharmacokinetics of bupropion or its metabolites in cigarette smokers and non-smokers.[1]

1. Hsyu P-H, *et al.* Pharmacokinetics of bupropion and its metabolites in cigarette smokers versus nonsmokers. *J Clin Pharmacol* 1997; **37:** 737–43.

Uses and Administration

Bupropion is a chlorpropiophenone antidepressant chemically unrelated to other classes of antidepressants but similar in structure to the central stimulant diethylpropion (p.1508). It is a weak blocker of neuronal reuptake of serotonin and noradrenaline compared with tricyclic antidepressants; it also inhibits the neuronal reuptake of dopamine. The antidepressant effect may not be evident until after 4 weeks of therapy. Bupropion is also used as an aid to smoking cessation.

Bupropion is given by mouth as the hydrochloride. To minimise agitation, anxiety, and insomnia often experienced at the start of therapy, and to reduce the risk of seizures, doses should be increased gradually; the total daily dose should be administered in equally divided doses and the maximum recommended single and total daily doses should not be exceeded. Insomnia at the start of therapy may be minimised by avoiding bedtime doses. Patients with renal or hepatic impairment should be given reduced doses and monitored for toxic effects.

In the treatment of **depression** bupropion hydrochloride is given in initial doses of 100 mg twice daily increased, if necessary, after at least 3 days to 100 mg three times daily. In severe cases, if no improvement has been observed after several weeks of therapy, the dose may be increased further to a maximum of 150 mg three times daily. Bupropion hydrochloride is also available as a modified-release preparation given in an initial dose of 150 mg once daily in the morning increased, if necessary, after at least 3 days to 150 mg twice daily; in severe cases, the dose of the modified-release preparation may be increased further after several weeks to 200 mg twice daily.

Bupropion hydrochloride is given as a modified-release preparation as an aid to **smoking cessation** in an initial dose of 150 mg once daily for 6 days, increasing to 150 mg twice daily on day 7. In the USA, the dose may be increased after 3 days. The maximum recommended dose for patients with predisposing risk factors for seizure (see Precautions, above) is 150 mg daily. Treatment should be started about 1 week before the patient attempts to stop smoking, to allow steady-state blood levels of bupropion to be reached, and normally continues for 7 to 12 weeks; if there is no significant progress towards smoking abstinence by the seventh week, then therapy should be stopped. Use with nicotine transdermal patches may be warranted in some patients, although there is a risk of hypertension with such therapy (see Interactions, above).

Depression. The management of depression is discussed on p.271. References to the use of bupropion in patients with depression are given below.

1. Anonymous. Bupropion for depression. *Med Lett Drugs Ther* 1989; **31:** 97–8.
2. Weisler RH, *et al.* Comparison of bupropion and trazodone for the treatment of major depression. *J Clin Psychopharmacol* 1994; **14:** 170–9.
3. Kavoussi RJ, *et al.* Double-blind comparison of bupropion sustained release and sertraline in depressed outpatients. *J Clin Psychiatry* 1997; **58:** 532–7.

Hyperactivity. When drug therapy is indicated for attention deficit hyperactivity disorder (p.1505) initial treatment is usually with a central stimulant. Antidepressants may be used for patients who fail to respond to, or who are intolerant of, central stimulants. Data from open and controlled studies involving small numbers of patients suggest that bupropion is effective in adults and children.[1,2]

1. Cantwell DP. ADHD through the life span: the role of bupropion in treatment. *J Clin Psychiatry* 1998; **59** (suppl 4): 92–4.
2. Wilens TE, *et al.* A controlled clinical trial of bupropion for attention deficit hyperactivity disorder in adults. *Am J Psychiatry* 2001; **158:** 282–8.

Smoking cessation. The management of smoking cessation is discussed on p.1642. References to the use of bupropion in smoking cessation are given below.

1. Anonymous. Bupropion (Zyban) for smoking cessation. *Med Lett Drugs Ther* 1997; **39:** 77–8.

The symbol † denotes a preparation no longer actively marketed

2. Benowitz NL. Treating tobacco addiction—nicotine or no nicotine? *N Engl J Med* 1997; **337:** 1230–1.
3. Hurt RD, *et al.* A comparison of sustained-release bupropion and placebo for smoking cessation. *N Engl J Med* 1997; **337:** 1195–1202.
4. Jorenby DE, *et al.* A controlled trial of sustained-release bupropion, a nicotine patch, or both for smoking cessation. *N Engl J Med* 1999; **340:** 685–91.
5. Holm KJ, Spencer CM. Bupropion: a review of its use in the management of smoking cessation. *Drugs* 2000; **59:** 1007–1024.
6. Hughes JR, *et al.* Antidepressants for smoking cessation (updated 29 August 2000). Available in The Cochrane Library; Issue 3. Oxford: Update Software; 2001.
7. Tashkin DP, *et al.* Smoking cessation in patients with chronic obstructive pulmonary disease: a double-blind, placebo-controlled, randomised trial. *Lancet* 2001; **357:** 1571–5.
8. Gonzales DH, *et al.* Bupropion SR as an aid to smoking cessation in smokers treated previously with bupropion: a randomized placebo-controlled study. *Clin Pharmacol Ther* 2001; **69:** 438–44.

Preparations

Proprietary Preparations (details are given in Part 3)
Austral.: Zyban; *Canad.:* Wellbutrin; Zyban; *Irl.:* Zyban; *Mex.:* Wellbutrin; *Port.:* Zyban; *UK:* Zyban; *USA:* Wellbutrin; Zyban.

Butriptyline Hydrochloride (2505-s)

Butriptyline Hydrochloride (*BANM, USAN, rINNM*).
AY-62014. (±)-3-(10,11-Dihydro-5*H*-dibenzo[*a,d*]cyclohepten-5-yl)-2-methylpropyldimethylamine hydrochloride.
$C_{21}H_{27}N,HCl = 329.9$.
CAS — 35941-65-2 (butriptyline); 5585-73-9 (butriptyline hydrochloride).

Butriptyline hydrochloride 28.1 mg is approximately equivalent to 25 mg of butriptyline.

Profile

Butriptyline hydrochloride is a tricyclic antidepressant with actions and uses similar to those of amitriptyline (p.273). It is one of the less sedating tricyclics.

In the treatment of depression (p.271) it has been given by mouth as the hydrochloride in doses equivalent to butriptyline 25 mg three times daily initially, gradually increased to a maximum of 150 mg daily as necessary.

Butriptyline should be withdrawn gradually to reduce the risk of withdrawal symptoms.

Preparations

Proprietary Preparations (details are given in Part 3)
Aust.: Evasidol; *Ital.:* Evadene.

Citalopram (20405-r)

Citalopram (*BAN, rINN*).
Lu-10-171. 1-(3-Dimethylaminopropyl)-1-(4-fluorophenyl)-1,3-dihydroisobenzofuran-5-carbonitrile.
$C_{20}H_{21}FN_2O = 324.4$.
CAS — 59729-33-8.
ATC — N06AB04.

Citalopram Hydrobromide (12575-c)

Citalopram Hydrobromide (*BANM, USAN, rINNM*).
Lu-10-171B; Nitalapram Hydrobromide.
$C_{20}H_{21}FN_2O,HBr = 405.3$.
CAS — 59729-32-7.

Citalopram hydrobromide 24.99 mg is equivalent to 20 mg of citalopram.

Citalopram Hydrochloride (17588-z)

Citalopram Hydrochloride (*BANM, rINNM*).
$C_{20}H_{21}FN_2O,HCl = 360.9$.

Citalopram hydrochloride 22.25 mg is equivalent to 20 mg of citalopram.

Adverse Effects, Treatment, and Precautions

As for SSRIs in general (see Fluoxetine, p.284) although increased appetite and weight gain have also been reported with citalopram.

Interactions

For interactions associated with SSRIs, see Fluoxetine, p.287.

Pharmacokinetics

Citalopram is readily absorbed from the gastrointestinal tract and maximum plasma concentrations are reached 2 to 4 hours after oral administration. Citalopram is widely distributed throughout the body; protein binding is low. Citalopram is metabolised by demethylation, deamination, and oxidation to active and inactive metabolites. The elimination half-life of citalopram is reported to be about 33 hours. It is excreted mainly via the liver (85%) with the remainder via the kidneys. About 12% of the daily dose is excreted in the urine as unchanged drug. Citalopram is distributed into breast milk in very low concentrations.

Uses and Administration

Citalopram, a phthalane derivative, is an SSRI with actions and uses similar to those of fluoxetine (p.288). Citalopram is given by mouth as the hydrobromide or hydrochloride, usually as a single daily dose. Doses are expressed in terms of citalopram.

In the treatment of **depression**, the initial dose of citalopram is 20 mg daily by mouth. After at least one week, the dose may be increased to 40 mg once daily; a dose of 60 mg daily may be necessary in some patients. Citalopram hydrochloride has also been given by intravenous infusion in similar doses when the oral route is impracticable.

In the treatment of **panic disorder** with or without agoraphobia, the initial dose of citalopram is 10 mg daily by mouth increasing to 20 mg daily after one week. The dose may be increased thereafter as required up to a maximum of 60 mg daily.

Doses at the lower end of the therapeutic range, up to a maximum of 40 mg, should be employed in elderly patients and those with hepatic impairment.

Citalopram should be withdrawn gradually to reduce the risk of withdrawal symptoms.

The *S*-enantiomer of citalopram, escitalopram (*S*-citalopram) is under investigation for the treatment of depression.

◊ Reviews.

1. Milne RJ, Goa KL. Citalopram: a review of its pharmacodynamic and pharmacokinetic properties, and therapeutic potential in depressive illness. *Drugs* 1991; **41:** 450–77.

Anxiety disorders. Citalopram has been given in a variety of anxiety disorders (p.649) including panic attacks (p.649), obsessive-compulsive disorder (p.649), and social phobia (see under Phobic Disorders, p.649).

References.

1. Koponen H, *et al.* Citalopram in the treatment of obsessive-compulsive disorder: an open pilot study. *Acta Psychiatr Scand* 1997; **96:** 343–6.
2. Bouwer C, Skin DJ. Use of the selective serotonin reuptake inhibitor citalopram in the treatment of generalized social phobia. *J Affect Disord* 1998; **49:** 79–82.
3. Lepola UM, *et al.* A controlled, prospective, 1-year trial of citalopram in the treatment of panic disorder. *J Clin Psychiatry* 1998; **59:** 528–34.

Depression. As discussed on p.271, there is very little difference in efficacy between the different groups of antidepressant drugs. SSRIs such as citalopram are widely used as an alternative to the older tricyclics as they have fewer side-effects and are safer in overdosage.

References.

1. Shaw DM, *et al.* A comparison of the antidepressant action of citalopram and amitriptyline. *Br J Psychiatry* 1986; **149:** 515–17.
2. Andersen G, *et al.* Effective treatment of poststroke depression with the selective serotonin reuptake inhibitor citalopram. *Stroke* 1994; **25:** 1099–1104.
3. Montgomery SA, *et al.* The optimal dosing regimen for citalopram—a meta-analysis of nine placebo-controlled studies. *Int Clin Psychopharmacol* 1994; **9** (suppl 1): 35–40.
4. Rosenberg C, *et al.* Citalopram and imipramine in the treatment of depressive patients in general practice: a Nordic Multicentre Clinical Study. *Int Clin Psychopharmacol* 1994; **9** (suppl 1): 41–8.
5. Patris M, *et al.* Citalopram versus fluoxetine: a double-blind, controlled, multicentre, phase III trial in patients with unipolar major depression treated in general practice. *Int Clin Psychopharmacol* 1996; **11:** 129–36.
6. Eleselius L, *et al.* A double-blind multicenter trial comparing sertraline and citalopram in patients with major depression treated in general practice. *Int Clin Psychopharmacol* 1997; **12:** 323–31.
7. Kyle CJ, *et al.* Comparison of the tolerability and efficacy of citalopram and amitriptyline in elderly depressed patients treated in general practice. *Depress Anxiety* 1998; **8:** 147–53.
8. Keller MB. Citalopram therapy for depression: a review of 10 years of European experience and data from US trials. *J Clin Psychiatry* 2000; **61:** 896–908.

Pathological crying or laughing. Inappropriate or uncontrolled crying or laughing can occur in patients with lesions in certain areas of the brain. Attempts at treatment have mostly been with antidepressant drugs, including SSRIs. Favourable results have been reported in a double-blind placebo-controlled study[1] with citalopram.

1. Andersen G, *et al.* Citalopram for post-stroke pathological crying. *Lancet* 1993; **342:** 837–9.

Schizophrenia. The treatment of schizophrenia consists mainly of a combination of social therapy and antipsychotic drugs (see p.651). In a preliminary placebo-controlled study[1] in

15 patients with chronic schizophrenia who exhibited signs of impulsive aggression, citalopram given in addition to existing antipsychotic therapy significantly reduced the frequency, but not the average severity, of aggressive incidents. In a subsequent study involving 90 patients, although citalopram appeared to improve subjective well-being the drug had no clear effect on psychopathological symptoms.[2]

1. Vartiainen H, et al. Citalopram, a selective serotonin reuptake inhibitor, in the treatment of aggression in schizophrenia. *Acta Psychiatr Scand* 1995; **91:** 348–51.
2. Salokangas RKR, et al. Citalopram as an adjuvant in chronic schizophrenia: a double-blind placebo-controlled study. *Acta Psychiatr Scand* 1996; **94:** 175–80.

Preparations

Proprietary Preparations (details are given in Part 3)
Aust.: Seralgan†; Seropram; *Austral.:* Cipramil; Talohexal; *Belg.:* Cipramil; *Braz.:* Cipramil; *Canad.:* Celexa; *Denm.:* Akarin; Cipramil; *Fin.:* Cipramil; *Fr.:* Seropram; *Ger.:* Cipramil; Sepram; *Hong Kong:* Cipram; *Irl.:* Cipramil; *Israel:* Cipramil; *Ital.:* Elopram; Seropram; *Mex.:* Seropram; *Neth.:* Cipramil; *Norw.:* Cipramil; *NZ:* Cipramil; *S.Afr.:* Cipramil; *Singapore:* Cipram; *Spain:* Prisdal; Seropram; *Swed.:* Cipramil; *Switz.:* Seropram; *Thai.:* Cipram; *UK:* Cipramil; *USA:* Celexa.

Clomipramine Hydrochloride

(2507-e)

Clomipramine Hydrochloride (BANM, USAN, rINNM).

Chlorimipramine Hydrochloride; Clomipramini Hydrochloridum; G-34586; Monochlorimipramine Hydrochloride. 3-(3-Chloro-10,11-dihydro-5H-dibenz[b,f]azepin-5-yl)propyldimethylamine hydrochloride.

$C_{19}H_{23}ClN_2,HCl = 351.3$.

CAS — 303-49-1 (clomipramine); 17321-77-6 (clomipramine hydrochloride).

Pharmacopoeias. In *Eur.* (see p.vi) and *Jpn.*

Pharmacopoeial description

Ph. Eur.: A white or slightly yellow, slightly hygroscopic, crystalline powder. Freely soluble in water and in dichloromethane; soluble in alcohol; practically insoluble in ether. A 10% solution in water has a pH of 3.5 to 5.0. Protect from light.

Adverse Effects, Treatment, and Precautions

As for tricyclic antidepressants in general (see Amitriptyline, p.273).

Porphyria. Clomipramine is considered to be unsafe in patients with porphyria because it has been shown to be porphyrinogenic in *in-vitro* systems, although there is conflicting evidence of porphyrinogenicity.

Interactions

For interactions associated with tricyclic antidepressants, see Amitriptyline, p.276.

MAOIs. In relation to interactions with other antidepressants, it should be noted that the combination of clomipramine and tranylcypromine is particularly hazardous, and that the serotonin syndrome (p.304) has occurred in patients receiving clomipramine and moclobemide (see under Interactions of Antidepressants in Phenelzine, p.306).

Pharmacokinetics

Clomipramine is readily absorbed from the gastrointestinal tract, and extensively demethylated during first-pass metabolism in the liver to its primary active metabolite, desmethylclomipramine.

Clomipramine and desmethylclomipramine are widely distributed throughout the body and are extensively bound to plasma and tissue protein. Clomipramine has been estimated to have a plasma elimination half-life of about 21 hours, which may be considerably extended in overdosage; that of desmethylclomipramine is longer (about 36 hours).

Paths of metabolism of both clomipramine and desmethylclomipramine include hydroxylation and N-oxidation. Approximately two-thirds of a single dose of clomipramine is excreted in the urine, mainly in the form of its metabolites, either free or in conjugated form; the remainder of the dose is excreted in the faeces. Clomipramine crosses the placenta and is distributed into breast milk.

◊ References.

1. Gex-Fabry M, et al. Clomipramine metabolism: model-based analysis of variability factors from drug monitoring data. *Clin Pharmacokinet* 1990; **19:** 241–55.

2. Balant-Gorgia AE, et al. Clinical pharmacokinetics of clomipramine. *Clin Pharmacokinet* 1991; **20:** 447–62.
3. Nielsen KK, et al. Single-dose kinetics of clomipramine: relationship to the sparteine and S-mephenytoin oxidation polymorphisms. *Clin Pharmacol Ther* 1994; **55:** 518–27.

Uses and Administration

Clomipramine is a dibenzazepine tricyclic antidepressant with actions and uses similar to those of amitriptyline (p.278). It has antimuscarinic properties and is also a potent serotonin reuptake inhibitor. Clomipramine is one of the more sedating tricyclics. It is used as the hydrochloride.

In the treatment of **depression**, clomipramine hydrochloride is given by mouth in doses of 10 mg daily initially, increasing gradually to 30 to 150 mg daily if required; up to 250 mg daily may be given in severe cases. A suggested initial dose for the elderly is 10 mg daily increasing gradually to 30 to 75 mg daily if required. Clomipramine may be given in divided doses throughout the day, but since it has a prolonged half-life, once-daily dosage regimens are also suitable, usually given at night.

In the treatment of **obsessive-compulsive disorders** and **phobias**, clomipramine hydrochloride may be given by mouth in an initial dose of 25 mg daily (or 10 mg daily for elderly patients) increased gradually over two weeks to 100 to 150 mg daily. In the USA, maximum doses of 250 mg daily have been used. In the USA clomipramine hydrochloride is also used for the treatment of obsessive-compulsive disorders in children and adolescents, in initial doses of 25 mg daily, increased gradually during the first 2 weeks to a maximum daily dose of 3 mg per kg body-weight or 100 mg, whichever is smaller. Further increases are permitted, over several weeks to a maximum of 3 mg per kg or 200 mg, whichever is smaller.

In the adjunctive treatment of **cataplexy associated with narcolepsy**, clomipramine hydrochloride is given by mouth in an initial dose of 10 mg daily and gradually increased until a satisfactory response occurs, usually within the range of 10 to 75 mg daily.

In the *initial stages of treatment* of depression or obsessional or phobic states only, if administration by mouth is impracticable or inadvisable clomipramine may be given by the intramuscular or intravenous routes. The daily dose of clomipramine hydrochloride by intramuscular injection is 25 to 50 mg, increasing by 25 mg a day up to a maximum of 100 to 150 mg daily; oral administration should be substituted as soon as possible. Clomipramine hydrochloride may also be given by intravenous infusion in initial doses of 25 to 50 mg diluted in 250 to 500 mL of sodium chloride 0.9% or glucose 5% and infused over 1.5 to 3 hours to assess tolerance; the dose may then be increased by 25 mg daily until an optimum therapeutic dose is achieved; this is usually about 100 mg daily, although more may be required. As the initial dose is gradually increased the volume of infusion fluid may be decreased to a minimum of 125 mL, and the duration of infusion decreased to a minimum of 45 minutes. When a satisfactory response to intravenous infusion has been obtained (usually after 7 to 10 days) oral therapy should be substituted, initially giving double the maximum intravenous dose by mouth and subsequently adjusting if necessary. Patients must be carefully supervised during intravenous infusion of clomipramine hydrochloride and the blood pressure carefully monitored owing to the risk of hypotension.

Clomipramine should be withdrawn gradually to reduce the risk of withdrawal symptoms.

Anxiety disorders. Tricyclic antidepressants that inhibit serotonin reuptake, such as clomipramine and imipramine, have been given in the management of anxiety disorders including obsessive-compulsive disorder (p.649), phobic disorders (p.649), panic attacks (p.649), and trichotillomania.

References.

1. Swedo SE, et al. A double-blind comparison of clomipramine and desipramine in the treatment of trichotillomania (hair pulling). *N Engl J Med* 1989; **321:** 497–501.

2. McTavish D, Benfield P. Clomipramine: an overview of its pharmacological properties and a review of its therapeutic use in obsessive compulsive disorder and panic disorder. *Drugs* 1990; **39:** 136–53.
3. Kelly MW, Myers CW. Clomipramine: a tricyclic antidepressant effective in obsessive compulsive disorder. *DICP Ann Pharmacother* 1990; **24:** 739–44.
4. Papp LA, et al. Clomipramine treatment of panic disorder: pros and cons. *J Clin Psychiatry* 1997; **58:** 423–5.

Autism. There is an anecdotal report that clomipramine alleviated adventitious movements when tried in 5 boys with autistic disorder.[1]

1. Brasic JR, et al. Clomipramine ameliorates adventitious movements and compulsions in prepubertal boys with autistic disorder and severe mental retardation. *Neurology* 1994; **44:** 1309–12.

Premenstrual syndrome. Clomipramine has been shown in a placebo-controlled trial[1] to be effective in reducing premenstrual irritability and depressed mood when administered during the luteal phase. Doses of clomipramine ranged from 25 to 75 mg daily. It was postulated that the efficacy of clomipramine in relieving premenstrual symptoms is related to its serotonin reuptake inhibitor activity. For the overall management of premenstrual syndrome, see p.1475.

1. Sundblad C, et al. Clomipramine administered during the luteal phase reduces the symptoms of premenstrual syndrome: a placebo-controlled trial. *Neuropsychopharmacology* 1993; **9:** 133–45.

Sexual dysfunction. Clomipramine has been used for its inhibitory effect on ejaculation to treat men for premature ejaculation.[1-4] Any benefits may relate to its effect as a serotonin reuptake inhibitor; other antidepressants with serotonin reuptake inhibiting actions, such as fluoxetine and sertraline, have also been tried in this condition.[4]

1. Hawton K. Erectile dysfunction and premature ejaculation. *Br J Hosp Med* 1988; **40:** 428–36.
2. Althof SE, et al. A double-blind crossover trial of clomipramine for rapid ejaculation in 15 couples. *J Clin Psychiatry* 1995; **56:** 402–7.
3. Haensel SM, et al. Clomipramine and sexual function in men with premature ejaculation and controls. *J Urol (Baltimore)* 1996; **156:** 1310–15.
4. Kim SC, Seo KK. Efficacy and safety of fluoxetine, sertraline and clomipramine in patients with premature ejaculation: a double-blind, placebo controlled study. *J Urol (Baltimore)* 1998; **159:** 425–7.

Stuttering. Clomipramine was of modest success in a controlled study[1] of 17 patients with developmental stuttering (p.687). It was suggested that its efficacy may be related to its serotonin reuptake inhibitor activity.

1. Gordon CT, et al. A double-blind comparison of clomipramine and desipramine in the treatment of developmental stuttering. *J Clin Psychiatry* 1995; **56:** 238–42.

Preparations

BP 2001: Clomipramine Capsules.

Proprietary Preparations (details are given in Part 3)
Aust.: Anafranil; *Austral.:* Anafranil; Placil; *Belg.:* Anafranil; *Braz.:* Anafranil; *Canad.:* Anafranil; Novo-Clopamine; *Denm.:* Anafranil; *Fin.:* Anafranil; *Fr.:* Anafranil; *Ger.:* Anafranil; Hydiphen; *Hong Kong:* Anafranil; *Irl.:* Anafranil; *Israel:* Anafranil; Maronil; *Ital.:* Anafranil; *Mex.:* Anafranil; *Neth.:* Anafranil; *Norw.:* Anafranil; *NZ:* Anafranil; Clopress; *Port.:* Anafranil; *S.Afr.:* Anafranil; Equinorm; *Singapore:* Anafranil; *Spain:* Anafranil; *Swed.:* Anafranil; *Switz.:* Anafranil; *Thai.:* Anafranil; Clofranil; *UK:* Anafranil; Tranquax†; *USA:* Anafranil.

Clorgiline Hydrochloride (2508-l)

Clorgiline Hydrochloride (BANM, rINNM).

Clorgyline Hydrochloride; M&B-9302. 3-(2,4-Dichlorophenoxy)propyl(methyl)prop-2-ynylamine hydrochloride.

$C_{13}H_{15}Cl_2NO,HCl = 308.6$.

CAS — 17780-72-2 (clorgiline); 17780-75-5 (clorgiline hydrochloride).

Profile

Clorgiline hydrochloride, a propylamine derivative, is an irreversible inhibitor of monoamine oxidase type A (see Phenelzine, p.303). Although research and development as an antidepressant appears to have been abandoned clorgiline is sometimes used as a pharmacological tool.

Desipramine Hydrochloride (2509-y)

Desipramine Hydrochloride (BANM, USAN, rINNM).

Desipramini Hydrochloridum; Desmethylimipramine Hydrochloride; DMI; EX-4355; G-35020; JB-8181; NSC-114901; RMI-9384A. 3-(10,11-Dihydro-5H-dibenz[b,f]azepin-5-yl)propyl(methyl)amine hydrochloride.

$C_{18}H_{22}N_2,HCl = 302.8$.

CAS — 50-47-5 (desipramine); 58-28-6 (desipramine hydrochloride).

Pharmacopoeias. In *Eur.* (see p.vi) and *US.*

Pharmacopoeial description

Ph. Eur.: A white or almost white crystalline powder. Soluble in water and in alcohol. Protect from light.

USP 25: A white to off-white crystalline powder. Soluble 1 in 12 of water, 1 in 14 of alcohol, and 1 in 3.5 of chloroform; insoluble in ether; freely soluble in methyl alcohol. Store in airtight containers.

Adverse Effects, Treatment, and Precautions

As for tricyclic antidepressants in general (see Amitriptyline, p.273).

Interactions

For interactions associated with tricyclic antidepressants, see Amitriptyline, p.276.

Pharmacokinetics

Desipramine is the principal active metabolite of imipramine (p.291).

Uses and Administration

Desipramine, the principal active metabolite of imipramine (p.291), is a dibenzazepine tricyclic antidepressant with actions and uses similar to those of amitriptyline (p.278). It is one of the less sedating tricyclics and its antimuscarinic effects are mild. Desipramine is used as the hydrochloride.

In the treatment of depression, desipramine hydrochloride is given by mouth in daily doses of 100 to 200 mg; higher doses of up to 300 mg daily may be required in severely depressed patients in hospital. Lower doses should be used in adolescents and the elderly and are usually 25 to 100 mg daily; higher doses of up to 150 mg daily may be required for severe depression. Initial doses should be at a lower level and gradually increased according to tolerance and clinical response. Therapy may initially be given as a single daily dose or in divided doses; maintenance therapy may be given as a single daily dose usually at night.

Desipramine should be withdrawn gradually to reduce the risk of withdrawal symptoms.

Cocaine dependence. Since dopamine depletion may be the cause of the depression often associated with cocaine craving and with relapse, drugs such as desipramine that interact with dopaminergic systems have been tried in managing cocaine withdrawal symptoms (p.1310). However, studies[1-7] have provided conflicting results on the use of desipramine for the management of persons who abuse cocaine, and the idea of giving desipramine to cocaine-dependent persons has been criticised[8] and defended.[9]

1. Giannini AJ, et al. Treatment of depression in chronic cocaine and phencyclidine abuse with desipramine. *J Clin Pharmacol* 1986; **26:** 211–14.
2. Weiss RD. Relapse to cocaine abuse after initiating desipramine treatment. *JAMA* 1988; **260:** 2545–6.
3. Gawin FH, et al. Desipramine facilitation of initial cocaine abstinence. *Arch Gen Psychiatry* 1989; **46:** 117–21.
4. Fischman MW, et al. Effects of desipramine maintenance on cocaine self-administration by humans. *J Pharmacol Exp Ther* 1990; **253:** 760–70.
5. Carroll KM, et al. Psychotherapy and pharmacotherapy for ambulatory cocaine abusers. *Arch Gen Psychiatry* 1994; **51:** 177–87.
6. Hall SM, et al. Continuity of care and desipramine in primary cocaine abusers. *J Nerv Ment Dis* 1994; **182:** 570–5.
7. Oliveto A, et al. Desipramine, amantadine, or fluoxetine in buprenorphine-maintained cocaine users. *J Subst Abuse Treat* 1995; **12:** 423–8.
8. Clark RJ. The treatment of chemical dependence. *JAMA* 1989; **261:** 3239.
9. Weiss RD. The treatment of chemical dependence. *JAMA* 1989; **261:** 3239.

Hyperactivity. When drug therapy is required for attention deficit hyperactivity disorder, initial treatment is usually with a central stimulant (see p.1505). Tricyclic antidepressants such as imipramine or desipramine[1-3] are also used but are reserved for patients who fail to respond to, or who are intolerant of, stimulants. They may also be of use for selected patients with co-existing disorders such as Tourette's syndrome, anxiety, and enuresis.

1. Rapport MD, et al. Methylphenidate and desipramine in hospitalized children: I. separate and combined effects on cognitive function. *J Am Acad Child Adolesc Psychiatry* 1993; **32:** 333–42.
2. Pataki CS, et al. Side effects of methylphenidate and desipramine alone and in combination in children. *J Am Acad Child Adolesc Psychiatry* 1993; **32:** 1065–72.
3. Singer HS, et al. The treatment of attention-deficit hyperactivity disorder in Tourette's syndrome: a double-blind placebo-controlled study with clonidine and desipramine. *Pediatrics* 1995; **95:** 74–81.

Pain. Antidepressants, usually amitriptyline or another tricyclic, are useful in alleviating some types of pain (p.2) when given in subantidepressant doses.

References to the use of desipramine.

1. Kishore-Kumar R, et al. Desipramine relieves postherpetic neuralgia. *Clin Pharmacol Ther* 1990; **47:** 305–12.
2. Max MB, et al. Effects of desipramine, amitriptyline, and fluoxetine on pain in diabetic neuropathy. *N Engl J Med* 1992; **326:** 1250–6.
3. Coquoz D, et al. Central analgesic effects of desipramine, fluvoxamine, and moclobemide after single oral dosing: a study in healthy volunteers. *Clin Pharmacol Ther* 1993; **54:** 339–44.
4. Gordon NC, et al. Temporal factors in the enhancement of morphine analgesia by desipramine. *Pain* 1993; **53:** 273–6.

Preparations

BP 2001: Desipramine Tablets;
USP 25: Desipramine Hydrochloride Tablets.

Proprietary Preparations (details are given in Part 3)
Aust.: Pertofran; *Austral.:* Pertofran; *Belg.:* Pertofran; *Canad.:* Norpramin; Pertofrane†; *Fr.:* Pertofran; *Ger.:* Pertofran; Petylyl; *Israel:* Deprexan; *Ital.:* Nortimil; *Neth.:* Pertofran; *NZ:* Pertofran; *S.Afr.:* Pertofran†; *UK:* Pertofran†; *USA:* Norpramin; Pertofrane†.

Dibenzepin Hydrochloride (2510-g)

Dibenzepin Hydrochloride (BANM, USAN, rINNM).
HF-1927. 10-(2-Dimethylaminoethyl)-5,10-dihydro-5-methyldibenzo[b,e][1,4]diazepin-11-one hydrochloride.
$C_{18}H_{21}N_3O,HCl = 331.8$.
CAS — 4498-32-2 (dibenzepin); 315-80-0 (dibenzepin hydrochloride).

Profile

Dibenzepin hydrochloride is a tricyclic antidepressant (see Amitriptyline, p.273).

In the treatment of depression dibenzepin hydrochloride is given by mouth in doses of 240 to 480 mg daily; higher doses of up to 720 mg daily may be required in some patients with severe depression.

Dibenzepin hydrochloride has also been given in doses of up to 360 mg daily by intravenous infusion.

Dibenzepin should be withdrawn gradually to reduce the risk of withdrawal symptoms.

◊ References.

1. Wirtheim E, Bloch Y. Dibenzepin overdose causing pulmonary edema. *Ann Pharmacother* 1996; **30:** 789–90.

Preparations

Proprietary Preparations (details are given in Part 3)
Aust.: Noveril; *Ger.:* Noveril; *Israel:* Victoril; *S.Afr.:* Noveril†; *Switz.:* Noveril.

Dothiepin Hydrochloride (2512-p)

Dothiepin Hydrochloride (BANM, USAN).
Dosulepin Hydrochloride (BANM, rINNM); Dosulepini Hydrochloridum. 3-(Dibenzo[b,e]thiepin-11-ylidene)propyldimethylamine hydrochloride.
$C_{19}H_{21}NS,HCl = 331.9$.
CAS — 113-53-1 (dothiepin [dosulepin]); 897-15-4 (dothiepin [dosulepin] hydrochloride).
Pharmacopoeias. In Eur. (see p.vi).

Pharmacopoeial description

Ph. Eur.: A white or faintly yellow crystalline powder. It consists chiefly of the *E*-isomer. Freely soluble in water, in alcohol, and in dichloromethane. A 10% solution in water has a pH of 4.2 to 5.2. Protect from light.

Adverse Effects, Treatment, and Precautions

As for tricyclic antidepressants in general (see Amitriptyline, p.273).

Effects on the cardiovascular system. For reference to an increased risk of ischaemic heart disease in patients treated with dothiepin [dosulepin], see under Amitriptyline, p.274.

Porphyria. Dothiepin [dosulepin] hydrochloride is considered to be unsafe in patients with porphyria because it has been shown to be porphyrinogenic in *animals*.

Interactions

For interactions associated with tricyclic antidepressants, see Amitriptyline, p.276.

Pharmacokinetics

Dothiepin [dosulepin] hydrochloride is readily absorbed from the gastrointestinal tract, and extensively demethylated by first-pass metabolism in the liver to its primary active metabolite, desmethyldothiepin (also termed northiaden). Paths of metabolism also include *S*-oxidation.

Dothiepin [dosulepin] is excreted in the urine, mainly in the form of its metabolites; small amounts are also excreted in the faeces. Elimination half-lives of about 14 to 24 and 23 to 46 hours have been reported for dothiepin [dosulepin] and its metabolites respectively.

Dothiepin [dosulepin] is distributed into breast milk (see Breast Feeding under Precautions in Amitriptyline, p.275).

◊ References.

1. Maguire KP, et al. Clinical pharmacokinetics of dothiepin: single-dose kinetics and prediction of steady-state concentrations. *Clin Pharmacokinet* 1983; **8:** 179–85.
2. Yu DK, et al. Pharmacokinetics of dothiepin in humans: a single dose dose-proportionality study. *J Pharm Sci* 1986; **75:** 582–5.
3. Ilett KF, et al. The excretion of dothiepin and its primary metabolites in breast milk. *Br J Clin Pharmacol* 1992; **33:** 635–9.

Uses and Administration

Dothiepin [dosulepin] hydrochloride is a tricyclic antidepressant with actions and uses similar to those of amitriptyline (p.278). It is one of the more sedating tricyclics.

In the treatment of depression, dothiepin [dosulepin] hydrochloride is given by mouth in doses of 25 mg three times daily initially, gradually increased to 50 mg three times daily if necessary; alternatively a single dose at night may be given. Higher doses of up to 225 mg daily have been given to severely depressed patients in hospital. The recommended initial dose for the elderly is 50 to 75 mg daily.

Dothiepin [dosulepin] should be withdrawn gradually to reduce the risk of withdrawal symptoms.

Preparations

BP 2001: Dosulepin Capsules; Dosulepin Tablets.

Proprietary Preparations (details are given in Part 3)
Aust.: Xerenal; *Austral.:* Dothep; Prothiaden; *Belg.:* Prothiaden; *Denm.:* Prothiaden; *Fr.:* Prothiaden; *Ger.:* Idom†; *Hong Kong:* Prothiaden; *Irl.:* Dothep; Prothiaden; *Ital.:* Protiaden; *Neth.:* Prothiaden; *NZ:* Dopress; Prothiaden; *Port.:* Protiadene; *S.Afr.:* Jardin; Prothiaden; Thaden; *Singapore:* Prothiaden; *Spain:* Prothiaden; *Switz.:* Protiaden; *Thai.:* Dopin; Prothiaden; *UK:* Dothapax; Prepadine; Prothiaden; Thaden.

Multi-ingredient: *Aust.:* Harmomed.

Doxepin Hydrochloride (2513-s)

Doxepin Hydrochloride (BANM, USAN, rINNM).
Doxepini Hydrochloridum; NSC-108160; P-3693A. (E)-3-(Dibenz[b,e]oxepin-11-ylidene)propyldimethylamine hydrochloride.
$C_{19}H_{21}NO,HCl = 315.8$.
CAS — 1668-19-5 (doxepin); 1229-29-4 (doxepin hydrochloride); 4698-39-9 (doxepin hydrochloride, E-isomer); 25127-31-5 (doxepin hydrochloride, Z-isomer).
Pharmacopoeias. In Eur. (see p.vi), Pol., and US.

Doxepin hydrochloride 113 mg is approximately equivalent to 100 mg of doxepin.

Pharmacopoeial description

Ph. Eur.: A white or almost white crystalline powder. Freely soluble in water, in alcohol, and in dichloromethane. Protect from light.

USP 25: It consists of a mixture of *Z*- and *E*-isomers.

Adverse Effects, Treatment, and Precautions

As for tricyclic antidepressants in general (see Amitriptyline, p.273). Drowsiness and other systemic effects can also occur following topical application.

Overdosage. An infant became difficult to arouse following the application of doxepin cream 5% to approximately 50% of her body-surface; an entire 30-g tube of the cream was used in only 2 applications.[1] The cream is not recommended for use in children.

1. Zell-Kanter M, et al. Doxepin toxicity in a child following topical application. *Ann Pharmacother* 2000; **34:** 328–9.

Interactions

For interactions associated with tricyclic antidepressants, see Amitriptyline, p.276.

Pharmacokinetics

Doxepin is readily absorbed from the gastrointestinal tract, and extensively demethylated by first-pass metabolism in the liver, to its primary active metabolite, desmethyldoxepin. Doxepin is also absorbed through the skin following topical application.

Paths of metabolism of both doxepin and desmethyldoxepin include hydroxylation and *N*-oxidation. Doxepin is excreted in the urine, mainly in the form of its metabolites, either free or in conjugated form.

Doxepin and desmethyldoxepin are widely distributed throughout the body and are extensively bound to plasma and tissue protein. Doxepin has been estimated to have a plasma elimination half-life ranging from 8 to 24 hours, which may be considerably extended in overdosage; that of desmethyldoxepin is longer.

Doxepin crosses the blood-brain barrier and the placenta. It is distributed into breast milk (see Breast Feeding under Precautions in Amitriptyline, p.275).

◊ References.

1. Faulkner RD, et al. Multiple-dose doxepin kinetics in depressed patients. *Clin Pharmacol Ther* 1983; **34:** 509–15.
2. Joyce PR, Sharman JR. Doxepin plasma concentrations in clinical practice: could there be a pharmacokinetic explanation for low concentrations? *Clin Pharmacokinet* 1985; **10:** 365–70.

Uses and Administration

Doxepin is a dibenzoxepine tricyclic antidepressant with actions and uses similar to those of amitriptyline (p.278). It has moderate antimuscarinic and marked sedative properties and has serotonin reuptake inhibitor activity.

In the treatment of depression doxepin is given by mouth as the hydrochloride in doses equivalent to doxepin 75 mg daily initially, gradually adjusted according to individual response. Doses of up to 300 mg daily may be required in severely depressed patients; mildly affected patients may respond to as little as 25 to 50 mg daily. Daily doses up to 100 mg may be given in divided doses or as a single dose at bedtime. If the total daily dose exceeds 100 mg, it should be given in divided doses, although the largest portion, up to a maximum of 100 mg, may be given at bedtime. In the USA, the maximum single dose is 150 mg. A suggested starting dose in the elderly is 10 to 50 mg daily.

Doxepin hydrochloride has also been given by intramuscular or intravenous injection.

Doxepin should be withdrawn gradually to reduce the risk of withdrawal symptoms.

Doxepin has histamine H_1- and H_2-antagonist activity and is used topically in a cream containing 5% of the hydrochloride for the short-term (up to 8 days) relief of moderately severe pruritus associated with various types of dermatitis (see below).

Headache. Tricyclic antidepressants can be effective in the management of some types of headache—see p.278.

References to the use of doxepin.
1. Wörz R, Scherhag R. Treatment of chronic tension headache with doxepin or amitriptyline—results of a double-blind study. *Headache Q* 1990; **1:** 216–23.

Skin disorders. Tricyclic antidepressants have a wide range of pharmacological activity and some members of the group have notable antihistaminic actions. Doxepin in particular has very potent antihistaminic activity. It has been shown to be an effective oral alternative to conventional antihistamines in the treatment of chronic urticaria,[1-3] and to be an effective oral treatment for idiopathic cold urticaria.[4,5] In the case of cold urticaria it was suggested that the action of doxepin was due to inhibition of platelet-activating factor-like lipid release.[5]

For an overview of the possible treatments for the various urticarias, including mention of the use of doxepin, see p.1107.

Like standard antihistamines (p.407) doxepin has also been used topically for the relief of pruritus (see also p.1106) associated with various types of allergic and inflammatory skin disorders[6,7] although some authorities remain to be convinced of its efficacy.[8,9] Topical application of doxepin can also produce contact dermatitis and drowsiness and other systemic effects.
1. Greene SL, *et al.* Double-blind crossover study comparing doxepin with diphenhydramine for the treatment of chronic urticaria. *J Am Acad Dermatol* 1985; **12:** 669–75.
2. Harto A, *et al.* Doxepin in the treatment of chronic urticaria. *Dermatologica* 1985; **170:** 90–3.
3. Goldsobel AB, *et al.* Efficacy of doxepin in the treatment of chronic idiopathic urticaria. *J Allergy Clin Immunol* 1986; **78:** 867–73.
4. Neittaanmäki H, *et al.* Comparison of cinnarizine, cyproheptadine, doxepin, and hydroxyzine in treatment of idiopathic cold urticaria: usefulness of doxepin. *J Am Acad Dermatol* 1984; **11:** 483–9.
5. Grandel KE, *et al.* Association of platelet-activating factor with primary acquired cold urticaria. *N Engl J Med* 1985; **313:** 405–9.
6. Drake LA, *et al.* Relief of pruritus in patients with atopic dermatitis after treatment with topical doxepin cream. *J Am Acad Dermatol* 1994; **31:** 613–16.
7. Smith PF, Corelli RL. Doxepin in the management of pruritus associated with allergic cutaneous reactions. *Ann Pharmacother* 1997; **31:** 633–5.
8. Anonymous. Doxepin cream for pruritus. *Med Lett Drugs Ther* 1994; **36:** 99–100.
9. Anonymous. Doxepin cream for eczema? *Drug Ther Bull* 2000; **38:** 31–2.

Preparations

BP 2001: Doxepin Capsules; **USP 25:** Doxepin Hydrochloride Capsules; Doxepin Hydrochloride Oral Solution.

Proprietary Preparations (details are given in Part 3)
Aust.: Sinequan; *Austral.:* Deptran; Sinequan; *Belg.:* Quitaxon; Sinequan; *Canad.:* Sinequan; Triadapin†; Zonalon; *Denm.:* Quitaxon†; Sinequan; *Fin.:* Doxal; *Fr.:* Quitaxon; Sinequan†; *Ger.:* Aponal; Desidoxepin; Doneurin; Mareen; Sinquan; *Hong Kong:* Sinequan; *Irl.:* Sinequan; Xepin; *Israel:* Gilex; *Mex.:* Sinequan; *Neth.:* Sinequan; *Norw.:* Sinequan; *NZ:* Anten; *Spain:* Sinequan; *Switz.:* Sinquane; *Thai.:* Sinequan; *UK:* Sinequan; Xepin; *USA:* Sinequan; Zonalon.

Duloxetine Hydrochloride (17135-s)

Duloxetine Hydrochloride *(BANM, USAN, rINNM)*.
LY-248686 (duloxetine). (+)-(S)-N-Methyl-γ-(1-naphthyloxy)-2-thiophenepropylamine hydrochloride.
$C_{18}H_{19}NOS,HCl = 333.9$.
CAS — 116539-59-4 (duloxetine); 136434-34-9 (duloxetine hydrochloride).

Profile

Duloxetine hydrochloride is a serotonin and noradrenaline reuptake inhibitor (SNRI) under investigation for the treatment of depression. It is also being studied in the management of urinary incontinence.

◊ **References.**
1. Mulcahy JJ, *et al.* Efficacy and safety of duloxetine in stress incontinence patients. *Neurourol Urodyn* 1996; **15:** 395–6.
2. Berk M, *et al.* An open-label study of duloxetine hydrochloride, a mixed serotonin and noradrenaline reuptake inhibitor, in patients with DSM-111-R major depressive disorder. *Int Clin Psychopharmacol* 1997; **12:** 137–40.
3. Sharma A, *et al.* Pharmacokinetics and safety of duloxetine, a dual-serotonin and norepinephrine reuptake inhibitor. *J Clin Pharmacol* 2000; **40:** 161–7.

Etoperidone Hydrochloride (12721-w)

Etoperidone Hydrochloride *(USAN, rINNM)*.
Clopradone Hydrochloride; McN-A-2673-11; ST-1191 (etoperidone). 2-{3-[4-(3-Chlorophenyl)piperazin-1-yl]propyl}-4,5-diethyl-2,4-dihydro-3H-1,2,4-triazol-3-one hydrochloride.
$C_{19}H_{28}ClN_5O,HCl = 414.4$.
CAS — 52942-31-1 (etoperidone); 57775-22-1 (etoperidone hydrochloride).

Profile

Etoperidone hydrochloride is a triazolopyridine antidepressant related structurally to trazodone (p.310). It has been used in the treatment of depression.

Preparations

Proprietary Preparations (details are given in Part 3)
Spain: Depraser†.

Fluoxetine Hydrochloride (12763-x)

Fluoxetine Hydrochloride *(BANM, USAN, rINNM)*.
Fluoxetini Hydrochloridum; LY-110140. (±)-N-Methyl-3-phenyl-3-(α,α,α-trifluoro-p-tolyloxy)propylamine hydrochloride.
$C_{17}H_{18}F_3NO,HCl = 345.8$.
CAS — 54910-89-3 (fluoxetine); 59333-67-4 (fluoxetine hydrochloride).
Pharmacopoeias. In *Eur.* (see p.vi) and *US*.

Fluoxetine hydrochloride 22.4 mg is approximately equivalent to 20 mg of fluoxetine.

Pharmacopoeial description

Ph. Eur.: A white or almost white crystalline powder. Sparingly soluble in water and in dichloromethane; freely soluble in methyl alcohol. A 1% solution in water has a pH of 4.5 to 6.5.

USP 25: A white to off-white crystalline powder. Sparingly soluble in water and in dichloromethane; freely soluble in alcohol and in methyl alcohol; practically insoluble in ether. Store in airtight containers.

Stability. References.
1. Peterson JA, *et al.* Stability of fluoxetine hydrochloride in fluoxetine solution diluted with common pharmaceutical diluents. *Am J Hosp Pharm* 1994; **51:** 1342–5.

Adverse Effects

SSRIs such as fluoxetine are less sedative than tricyclic antidepressants and have fewer antimuscarinic or cardiotoxic effects. Adverse effects reported with fluoxetine include dry mouth and gastrointestinal disturbances such as nausea, vomiting, dyspepsia, constipation, and diarrhoea. Anorexia and weight loss may also occur. Neurological side-effects have included either anxiety, restlessness, nervousness, and insomnia, or drowsiness and fatigue; headache, tremor, dizziness, convulsions, hallucinations, extrapyramidal effects, sexual dysfunction, and symptoms suggestive of a serotonin syndrome (p.304) have also occurred. The concern that some SSRIs may be associated with increased suicidal ideation is discussed under Effects on Mental State, below.

Excessive sweating, pruritus, skin rashes, and urticaria have also been reported. Angioedema and anaphylaxis have occurred. In some patients who have developed rashes while taking fluoxetine, systemic hypersensitivity reactions involving the lungs, kidneys, or liver, and possibly related to vasculitis, have

developed; it has therefore been advised that fluoxetine therapy should be discontinued in any patient who develops a skin rash. Dyspnoea and pulmonary fibrosis have been reported.

Hyponatraemia, possibly due to inappropriate secretion of antidiuretic hormone, has been associated with the use of antidepressants, particularly in the elderly. Hyperprolactinaemia and galactorrhoea have occurred, as have changes in blood sugar, in patients receiving SSRIs.

Arthralgia and myalgia have been reported. Abnormal liver function tests have been reported rarely. SSRIs have occasionally been associated with bleeding disorders and other effects on the blood.

In overdosage nausea, vomiting, and excitation of the CNS are considered to be prominent features; death has been reported.

◊ In June 1992 the UK Committee on Safety of Medicines (CSM) had received 1236 reports of adverse effects with fluvoxamine (from about 280 000 prescriptions) compared with 2422 for fluoxetine (from about 480 000 prescriptions).[1] The overall adverse reactions profiles were similar but dermatological reactions were more likely with fluoxetine and gastrointestinal reactions with fluvoxamine. Reports of attempted suicide increased after adverse publicity about SSRIs in 1990, and the number of reports per million prescriptions were similar for the 2 drugs (25 for fluoxetine and 20 for fluvoxamine); such figures were not considered disconcerting given that features of depression, including attempted suicide, can worsen after the introduction of any antidepressant. A more recent review[2] by the CSM of the 5 SSRIs available in the UK (citalopram, fluoxetine, fluvoxamine, paroxetine, and sertraline) found that the SSRIs were broadly similar with respect to their safety profile. A list of adverse reactions common to all SSRIs was provided.

A review[3] of 1861 adverse reactions to citalopram, fluoxetine, fluvoxamine, paroxetine, or sertraline reported to the Swedish Adverse Drug Reactions Advisory Committee found that the most commonly reported reactions were neurological (22.4% of all reports), psychiatric (19.5%), and gastrointestinal (18.0%). Compared with other SSRIs, gastrointestinal symptoms were more common with fluvoxamine, psychiatric symptoms were more common with sertraline, and dermatological symptoms were more common with fluoxetine.
1. Committee on Safety of Medicines. Safety of fluoxetine (Prozac): comparison with fluvoxamine (Faverin). *Current Problems* 34 1992.
2. Committee on Safety of Medicines/Medicines Control Agency. Selective serotonin reuptake inhibitors (SSRIs). *Current Problems* 2000; **26:** 11–12.
3. Spigset O. Adverse reactions of selective serotonin reuptake inhibitors: reports from a spontaneous reporting system. *Drug Safety* 1999; **20:** 277–87.

Effects on the blood. Abnormalities in platelet aggregation were associated with fluoxetine given to a severely underweight patient.[1] Platelet activity returned to normal when fluoxetine was discontinued. Fluoxetine was also suspected of being the cause of bruising in a patient whose blood clotting parameters were within normal limits.[2] Purpura and bruising have been reported to be the commonest adverse blood effects associated with fluoxetine, paroxetine, or sertraline although cases of thrombocytopenia have been recorded for all three antidepressants.[3] The suggested mechanism was inhibition of uptake of serotonin into platelets, thereby disrupting platelet aggregation; caution was recommended when treating patients with a history of bleeding disorders with SSRIs. However, a subsequent cohort study based on prescription event monitoring provided only weak evidence of a link between the use of SSRIs and the development of bleeding disorders.[4] A similar study[5] found no evidence of a major increased risk of intracranial haemorrhage with the use of SSRIs, although smaller increases in risk could not be ruled out.

For mention of a possibly increased risk of gastrointestinal bleeding, see Effects on the Gastrointestinal Tract, below.
1. Alderman CP, *et al.* Abnormal platelet aggregation associated with fluoxetine therapy. *Ann Pharmacother* 1992; **26:** 1517–19.
2. Pai VB, Kelly MW. Bruising associated with the use of fluoxetine. *Ann Pharmacother* 1996; **30:** 786–8.
3. Anonymous. Bruising and bleeding with SSRIs. *Aust Adverse Drug React Bull* 1998; **17:** 10.
4. Layton D, *et al.* Is there an association between selective serotonin reuptake inhibitors and risk of abnormal bleeding? Results from a cohort study based on prescription event monitoring in England. *Eur J Clin Pharmacol* 2001; **57:** 167–76.
5. de Abajo FJ, *et al.* Intracranial haemorrhage and use of selective serotonin reuptake inhibitors. *Br J Clin Pharmacol* 2000; **50:** 43–7.

Effects on the cardiovascular system. SSRIs are not associated with the same degree of cardiotoxicity as the tricyclic antidepressants (see p.274), although orthostatic hypotension has been reported in some patients. The manufacturers of fluvoxamine state that a decrease in heart rate with ECG changes has been noted. However, a study[1] on long-term fluvoxamine treatment in 311 patients followed for 1 year revealed no significant effect on ECG findings compared with patients given placebo.

Concern over the use of sertraline in patients with coronary heart disease was raised following a report[2] of a 53-year-old man with a history of coronary heart disease who experienced attacks of sudden precordial chest pain after starting treatment with sertraline. The pain responded to glyceryl trinitrate. The manufacturers[3] pointed out that there had been no ECG changes confirming an ischaemic origin of the disorder in this patient and that in studies sertraline had had no demonstrable clinical effects on intraventricular conduction or ECG intervals. Furthermore, no significant changes in cardiovascular indices had been recorded in patients who had taken overdoses of up to 6 g of sertraline. It was suggested that this might have been an effect on the gastrointestinal tract possibly at the oesophageal level.

1. Hochberg HM, et al. Electrocardiographic findings during extended clinical trials of fluvoxamine in depression: one years experience. Pharmacopsychiatry 1995; 28: 253–6.
2. Iruela LM. Sudden chest pain with sertraline. Lancet 1994; 343: 1106.
3. Berti CA, Doogan DP. Sudden chest pain with sertraline. Lancet 1994; 343: 1510–11.

Effects on the endocrine system. The *syndrome of inappropriate antidiuretic hormone secretion (SIADH)* with *hyponatraemia* has been reported in patients receiving antidepressants. The UK Committee on Safety of Medicines, commenting on reports it had received of hyponatraemia associated with antidepressants (fluoxetine, paroxetine, lofepramine, clomipramine, and imipramine), considered that it was likely to occur with any antidepressant, and usually involved elderly patients.[1] Case reports of hyponatraemia in 16 patients treated with SSRIs have been summarised.[2] A further review[3] of reports on 15 patients with hyponatraemia with SIADH induced by fluoxetine (12 cases), fluvoxamine (2 cases), and paroxetine (1 case) showed that the risk was greatest during the early treatment phase. This is borne out by single-case reports[4-9] of hyponatraemia with SIADH in elderly patients receiving either paroxetine or sertraline. A retrospective study[10] of hyponatraemia associated with either fluoxetine or paroxetine use also showed the early onset of the condition and identified low body-weight as being another risk factor for developing hyponatraemia.

SSRI-associated *hyperprolactinaemia* has been reported.[11] Lactation and raised prolactin levels occurred in a teenager 3 days after fluoxetine was added to her existing therapy which included pimozide. Stopping fluoxetine had no effect on lactation, which only ceased after withdrawing pimozide. In another report,[12] hyperprolactinaemia and galactorrhoea in an elderly woman receiving fluoxetine resolved on discontinuing the drug.

1. Committee on Safety of Medicines/Medicines Control Agency. Antidepressant-induced hyponatraemia. Current Problems 1994; 20: 5–6.
2. Spigset O, Hedenmalm K. Hyponatraemia and the syndrome of inappropriate antidiuretic hormone secretion (SIADH) induced by psychotropic drugs. Drug Safety 1995; 12: 209–25.
3. Canadian Medical Association. Hyponatraemia and selective serotonin reuptake inhibitors. Can Med Assoc J 1996; 154: 63.
4. Bluff DD. SIADH in a patient receiving sertraline. Ann Intern Med 1995; 123: 811.
5. Adverse Drug Reactions Advisory Committee. Selective serotonin reuptake inhibitors and SIADH. Med J Aust 1996; 164: 562.
6. Kessler J, Samuels SC. Sertraline and hyponatremia. N Engl J Med 1996; 335: 524.
7. Robinson D, et al. SIADH—compulsive drinking or SSRI influence? Ann Pharmacother 1996; 30: 885.
8. Monmany J, et al. Syndrome of inappropriate secretion of antidiuretic hormone induced by paroxetine. Arch Intern Med 1999; 159: 2089–90.
9. Odeh M, et al. Severe life-threatening hyponatremia during paroxetine therapy. J Clin Pharmacol 1999; 39: 1290–1.
10. Wilkinson TJ, et al. Incidence and risk factors for hyponatraemia following treatment with fluoxetine or paroxetine in elderly people. Br J Clin Pharmacol 1999; 47: 211–17.
11. Arya DK, et al. Lactation associated with fluoxetine treatment. Aust N Z J Psychiatry 1995; 29: 697.
12. Peterson MC. Reversible galactorrhea and prolactin elevation related to fluoxetine use. Mayo Clin Proc 2001; 76: 215–16.

Effects on the eyes. Symptoms of glaucoma developed in a patient receiving fluoxetine; the symptoms subsided within 2 days of drug withdrawal.[1] Similar symptoms have been reported[2] with paroxetine. Intra-ocular pressure following fluoxetine administration was recorded in 20 patients in a placebo-controlled crossover double-blind study.[3] Significant increases were demonstrated in all patients 2 hours after receiving fluoxetine by mouth; some patients still had raised intra-ocular pressure after 8 hours.

There has been a report[4] of anisocoria (uneven pupillary dilatation) in one patient taking paroxetine and in another taking sertraline. It was noted that the UK Committee on Safety of Medicines had received 21 reports of mydriasis associated with paroxetine but it appeared that noticeably asymmetrical mydriasis as seen in these 2 patients had not previously been reported.

1. Ahmad S. Fluoxetine and glaucoma. DICP Ann Pharmacother 1991; 25: 436.
2. Eke T, Carr S. Acute glaucoma, chronic glaucoma, and serotoninergic drugs. Br J Ophthalmol 1998; 82: 976–7.
3. Costagliola C, et al. Fluoxetine oral administration increases intraocular pressure. Br J Ophthalmol 1996; 80: 678.
4. Barrett J. Anisocoria associated with selective serotonin reuptake inhibitors. BMJ 1994; 309: 1620.

Effects on the gastrointestinal tract. A case-control study[1] has suggested that treatment with SSRIs produces a moderately increased risk of upper gastrointestinal bleeding (adjusted relative risk 3.0). The risk was greatly increased if SSRIs were given concomitantly with NSAIDs (relative risk 15.6). Treatment with SSRIs did not appear to increase the risk of ulcer perforation. The absolute risk of bleeding was estimated at one case per 8000 prescriptions, a risk similar to that of low dose ibuprofen. Others, however, have questioned whether such an association exists.[2] A subsequent retrospective cohort study[3] in elderly patients found that there was an increasing risk of upper gastrointestinal bleeding as the extent of inhibition of serotonin reuptake by the antidepressant used increased. The effect was considered to be clinically important for patients with a high risk of such bleeding, namely the very elderly and those with a history of previous upper gastrointestinal bleeding.

1. de Abajo FJ, et al. Association between selective serotonin reuptake inhibitors and upper gastrointestinal bleeding: population based case-control study. BMJ 1999; 319: 1106–9.
2. Dunn NR, et al. Association between SSRIs and upper gastrointestinal bleeding. BMJ 2000; 320: 1405–6.
3. van Walraven C, et al. Inhibition of serotonin reuptake by antidepressants and upper gastrointestinal bleeding in elderly patients: retrospective cohort study. BMJ 2001; 323: 655–8.

Effects on the hair. A report[1] on 2 patients who experienced hair loss associated with the use of fluoxetine noted 4 other published cases and stated that up to the end of 1991 the US manufacturers had received 498 reports of fluoxetine-associated alopecia.

1. Ogilvie AD. Hair loss during fluoxetine treatment. Lancet 1993; 342: 1423.

Effects on the liver. Acute hepatitis occurred in 2 patients after several months of fluoxetine treatment;[1] it was noted that 5 other cases of acute hepatitis with fluoxetine had been reported. Abnormal liver function tests were seen in a patient after a suicide attempt with sertraline and cefalexin.[2] The patient was then started on venlafaxine but, again abnormal liver function tests were noted. When these abnormal values had decreased, sertraline was restarted at therapeutic doses, with a subsequent increase in liver function tests. Values returned to normal once all medications were stopped.

1. Cai Q, et al. Acute hepatitis due to fluoxetine therapy. Mayo Clin Proc 1999; 74: 692–4.
2. Kim KY, et al. Acute liver damage possibly related to sertraline and venlafaxine ingestion. Ann Pharmacother 1999; 33: 381–2.

Effects on mental state. There has been concern that fluoxetine increases *suicidal ideation* and there have been suggestions that there may be a link with akathisia[1] or dosage.[2] However meta-analyses[3,4] (criticism of statistical power notwithstanding[5]) have not confirmed an increased risk and this appears to be supported by the results of prescription event monitoring,[6] and is the view of various regulatory authorities. However some reviewers consider that under certain conditions all antidepressants and antipsychotics can induce suicidal ideation in some individuals and comment that there does appear to be enough anecdotal evidence to indicate that fluoxetine may induce suicidal ideation on rare occasions.[7,8] It has been suggested that as suicidal ideation has been associated with induction of akathisia, agitation, or panic by fluoxetine, propranolol might be added to therapy to control these effects.[7,8] There has also been concern that fluvoxamine, like fluoxetine, may increase suicidal ideation and a suggestion that it might be dose-related.[9]

For a discussion of the choice of antidepressant with respect to safety in overdosage, see under Depression, p.271.

For further effects on mental function, see also under Withdrawal and under Mania in Precautions, below.

There have also been suggested links between the use of fluoxetine and *irritability, hostility, and aggression*.[10] However, one review[8] noted that an unpublished analysis by Heiligenstein et al. indicated that patients taking fluoxetine for a variety of disorders were not more likely to be aggressive than those taking placebo. Prescription event monitoring has also found no evidence to suggest that fluoxetine increases the frequency of aggression.[6]

Initiation of antidepressant therapy with paroxetine or sertraline has been associated with either worsening or a new onset of *flashback syndrome* in 2 patients with a history of lysergide abuse.[11]

1. Rothschild AJ, Locke CA. Reexposure to fluoxetine after serious suicide attempts by three patients: the role of akathisia. J Clin Psychiatry 1991; 52: 491–3.
2. Fichtner CG, et al. Does fluoxetine have a therapeutic window? Lancet 1991; 338: 520–1.
3. Beasley CM, et al. Fluoxetine and suicide: a meta-analysis of controlled trials of treatment for depression. BMJ 1991; 303: 685–92. Correction. ibid.: 968.
4. Goldstein DJ, et al. Analyses of suicidality in double-blind, placebo-controlled trials of fluoxetine for weight reduction. J Clin Psychiatry 1993; 54: 309–16.
5. Li Wan Po A. Fluoxetine and suicide: meta-analysis and Monte-Carlo simulations. Pharmacoepidemiol Drug Safety 1993; 2: 79–84.
6. Nakielny J. Fluoxetine and suicide. Lancet 1994; 343: 1359.
7. Healy D. The fluoxetine and suicide controversy: a review of the evidence. CNS Drugs 1994; 1: 223–31.
8. Power AC, Cowen PJ. Fluoxetine and suicidal behaviour; some clinical and theoretical aspects of a controversy. Br J Psychiatry 1992; 161: 735–41.
9. Pitchot W, et al. Therapeutic window for 5-HT reuptake inhibitors. Lancet 1992; 339: 689.

10. Anonymous. Fluoxetine, suicide and aggression. Drug Ther Bull 1992; 30: 5–6.
11. Markel H, et al. LSD flashback syndrome exacerbated by selective serotonin reuptake inhibitor antidepressants in adolescents. J Pediatr 1994; 125: 817–19.

Effects on sexual function. It has been considered that sexual dysfunction occurs in up to 1.9% of patients taking fluoxetine, with impotence or ejaculatory problems occurring in less than 1% of patients.[1] These figures were based on information supplied by the US manufacturer for the data sheet but have been disputed.[2,3] More recent studies and anecdotal reports quote rates of 7.8 to 75% for sexual dysfunction with fluoxetine but it appears that only small numbers of men were studied.[4] The reported frequency of sexual dysfunction is usually higher in men taking SSRIs than in women; complaints include a decrease in or loss of libido, delayed ejaculation, erectile difficulty, or anorgasmia.[5] However, loss of libido, delayed orgasm, or anorgasmia have also been reported in women.[5,6]

Suggested[5,7] strategies for managing SSRI-induced sexual dysfunction include reducing the dosage of the SSRI or altering the timing of its administration or changing to another antidepressant. Various drugs have also been tried but evidence of efficacy is mainly anecdotal. Cyproheptadine is the drug most commonly reported to have been used but the SSRI may become less effective (see under Interactions, below) and patients should be monitored for worsening symptoms of depression.

The effects of the SSRIs on sexual function have been studied as a potential form of treatment for men with premature ejaculation (see Sexual Dysfunction in Uses, below).

1. Hollander JB. Fluoxetine and sexual dysfunction. JAMA 1994; 272: 242.
2. Balon R. Fluoxetine and sexual dysfunction. JAMA 1995; 273: 1489.
3. Hopkins HS, Gelenberg AJ. Fluoxetine and sexual dysfunction. JAMA 1995; 273: 1489–90.
4. Hollander JB. Fluoxetine and sexual dysfunction. JAMA 1995; 273: 1490.
5. Frye CB, Berger JE. Treatment of sexual dysfunction induced by selective serotonin-reuptake inhibitors. Am J Health-Syst Pharm 1998; 55: 1167–9.
6. Feiger A, et al. Nefazodone versus sertraline in outpatients with major depression: focus on efficacy, tolerability, and effects on sexual function and satisfaction. J Clin Psychiatry 1996; 57 (suppl 2): 53–62.
7. Woodrum ST, Brown CS. Management of SSRI-induced sexual dysfunction. Ann Pharmacother 1998; 32: 1209–15.

Effects on the skin. *Toxic epidermal necrolysis* developed in a 16-year-old girl 8 days after beginning fluvoxamine therapy.[1] Other drugs, which included metoclopramide, clorazepate, and clomipramine were discounted as possible causes.

Amitriptyline and fluoxetine have been implicated in the development of *atypical cutaneous lymphoid hyperplasia* in 8 patients, 7 of whom either had an underlying immunosuppressant systemic disease or were receiving concomitant therapy with immunomodulatory drugs.[2] The lesions improved or resolved on discontinuation of the antidepressant, although in some patients other factors may have contributed to lesional resolution.

Bullous pemphigoid induced by fluoxetine has been reported in a 75-year-old woman.[3] Spontaneous resolution followed within 3 weeks of discontinuing the drug.

1. Wolkenstein P, et al. Toxic epidermal necrolysis after fluvoxamine. Lancet 1993; 342: 304–5.
2. Crowson AN, Magro CM. Antidepressant therapy: a possible cause of atypical cutaneous lymphoid hyperplasia. Arch Dermatol 1995; 131: 925–9.
3. Rault S, et al. Bullous pemphigoid induced by fluoxetine. Br J Dermatol 1999; 141: 755–6.

Epileptogenic effect. Generalised seizures have been reported in two patients with no previous history of seizures following initiation of fluoxetine therapy.[1,2] Although convulsions have been noted in patients receiving fluvoxamine (see p.289), a small clinical study involving 35 depressed epileptic patients[3] found no change in the number of seizures or in their nature when fluvoxamine was given in doses of up to 200 mg daily.

1. Weber JJ. Seizure activity associated with fluoxetine therapy. Clin Pharm 1989; 8: 296–8.
2. Ware MR, Stewart RB. Seizures associated with fluoxetine therapy. DICP Ann Pharmacother 1989; 23: 428.
3. Harmant J, et al. Fluvoxamine: an antidepressant with low (or no) epileptogenic effect. Lancet 1990; 336: 386.

Extrapyramidal effects. Extrapyramidal effects, such as tics[1] and akathisia,[2,3] have been reported with fluoxetine. By 1993, the UK Committee on Safety of Medicines had received 39 reports of extrapyramidal reactions with paroxetine including 15 of dystonia of the face and mouth.[4] It was noted that, although extrapyramidal effects may occur with other SSRIs, orofacial dystonias appeared to be more common with paroxetine. However, evidence from monitoring prescriptions within the UK has shown that the overall incidence of extrapyramidal effects is the same for paroxetine as for other SSRIs.[5] Orofacial dystonias (teeth clenching) or dyskinesias (teeth grinding), with resultant severe damage to teeth and gums in the majority of cases, have been reported[6] in 6 patients receiving fluoxetine, fluvoxamine, paroxetine, or sertraline. The authors concluded that these adverse effects were not specific for any particular SSRI.

Dyskinesia associated with withdrawal of citalopram and risperidone has been reported in a patient.[7]

1. Eisenhauer G, Jermain DM. Fluoxetine and tics in an adolescent. Ann Pharmacother 1993; 27: 725–6.

The symbol † denotes a preparation no longer actively marketed

2. Lipinski JF, et al. Fluoxetine-induced akathisia: clinical and the-oretical implications. J Clin Psychiatry 1989; 50: 339–42.
3. Rothschild AJ, Locke CA. Reexposure to fluoxetine after serious suicide attempts by three patients: the role of akathisia. J Clin Psychiatry 1991; 52: 491–3.
4. Committee on Safety of Medicines/Medicines Control Agency. Dystonia and withdrawal symptoms with paroxetine (Seroxat). Current Problems 1993; 19: 1.
5. Choo V. Paroxetine and extrapyramidal reactions. Lancet 1993; 341: 624.
6. Fitzgerald K, Healy D. Dystonias and dyskinesias of the jaw as-sociated with the use of SSRIs. Hum Psychopharmacol Clin Exp 1995; 10: 215–19.
7. Miller LJ. Withdrawal-emergent dyskinesia in a patient taking risperidone/citalopram. Ann Pharmacother 2000; 34: 269.

Hyponatraemia. See Effects on the Endocrine System, above.

Overdosage. SSRIs are generally regarded as being less toxic in overdosage than tricyclic antidepressants or MAOIs. A review[1] of SSRI overdosage, covering the period 1985 to 1997, noted that there had been remarkably few fatal overdoses when taken alone. Moderate overdoses (up to about 30 times the usu-al daily dose) were generally associated with minor symptoms at most; only at very high doses (more than 75 times the usual daily dose) did more serious effects such as seizures, ECG abnormalities, and decreased consciousness tend to occur. Tox-icity was greatly increased, however, when overdoses of SSRIs were taken in combination with alcohol or other drugs. There was no evidence of a difference in the various SSRIs with re-spect to safety in overdosage.

A report involving 87 cases in which fluoxetine was taken in overdosage without other drugs found that the main symptoms were tachycardia, drowsiness, tremor, and nausea and vomit-ing.[2] These were considered relatively minor, and were of short duration, and supportive care was considered to be the only in-tervention necessary. Of 41 cases of self-poisoning with flu-voxamine, only one patient died and even here fluvoxamine was not implicated.[3] Prolonged cerebral depression occurred in a patient following fluvoxamine overdose,[3] but this may have been due to an interaction with temazepam which the patient also took in overdose. One hour after taking 40 sertraline 50-mg tablets in a suicide attempt a 42-year-old woman was flushed, angry, emotionally labile, and easily distracted but not psychotic.[4] Apart from watery bowel movements recovery was mainly uneventful following treatment with gastric lavage, oral activated charcoal with sorbitol, and intravenous hydration. Abnormal liver function tests have also been noted after a sui-cide attempt with sertraline (see Effects on the Liver, above).

Fatal overdose has been reported with citalopram in 6 patients,[5] although the suggested cause of death as cardiac dysfunction rather than seizures was disputed.[6]

For a discussion of choice of antidepressant with respect to safety in overdosage, see under Depression, p.271.

1. Barbey JT, Roose SP. SSRI safety in overdose. J Clin Psychiatry 1998; 59 (suppl 15): 42–8.
2. Borys DJ, et al. Acute fluoxetine overdose: a report of 234 cases. Am J Emerg Med 1992; 10: 115–20.
3. Banerjee AK. Recovery from prolonged cerebral depression af-ter fluvoxamine overdose. BMJ 1988; 296: 1774.
4. Brown DF, Kerr HD. Sertraline overdose. Ann Pharmacother 1994; 28: 1307.
5. Öström M, et al. Fatal overdose with citalopram. Lancet 1996; 348: 339–40.
6. Brion F, et al. Fatal overdose with citalopram? Lancet 1996; 348: 1380.

Treatment of Adverse Effects

Treatment of overdosage with an SSRI involves ap-propriate symptomatic and supportive therapy. Acti-vated charcoal may be given by mouth if the amount ingested was large and treatment is within an hour of ingestion. Some consider that gastric lavage may be appropriate if the overdose is likely to be life-threat-ening (but see Overdosage, above). Dialysis, haemo-perfusion, exchange transfusion, and measures to in-crease urine production are considered unlikely to be of benefit.

Precautions

Fluoxetine and other SSRIs that undergo hepatic me-tabolism and renal excretion should be used with cau-tion and in reduced doses in patients with impaired hepatic or renal function; some authorities recom-mend that they should not be used in severe hepatic or renal failure. Because of their epileptogenic effect SSRIs should be used with caution in patients with epilepsy or a history of such disorders (and should be avoided if the epilepsy is poorly controlled); care is advised in patients receiving concomitant ECT. SS-RIs should also be used with caution in patients with cardiac disease or a history of bleeding disorders. Fluoxetine may alter glycaemic control and therefore caution is also warranted in diabetic subjects. Fluox-etine should be discontinued in patients who develop

a rash since systemic effects, possibly related to vas-culitis, have occurred in such patients.

Patients should be closely monitored during early therapy until improvement in depression is observed because suicide is an inherent risk in depressed pa-tients. For further details, see under Depression, p.271. For a discussion of the concern that SSRIs, particularly fluoxetine, may increase suicidal idea-tion, see Effects on Mental State in Adverse Effects, above.

If SSRIs are given for the depressive component of bipolar disorder, mania may be precipitated.

SSRIs may impair performance of skilled tasks and, if affected, patients should not drive or operate ma-chinery.

Some authorities recommend reduced or less frequent dosage of SSRIs for elderly patients.

Significant amounts of fluoxetine are distributed into breast milk and the manufacturers have reported that adverse effects have been observed in a breast-fed in-fant; consequently fluoxetine is not recommended for nursing mothers. Similarly, the manufacturers of some other SSRIs have recommended that they should be avoided during breast feeding (fluvoxamine and paroxetine) or used with caution (citalopram).

SSRIs should be withdrawn gradually to reduce the risk of withdrawal symptoms.

◊ For the opinion that the SSRIs may produce a clinically im-portant increase in the risk of upper gastrointestinal bleeding in patients with a high risk of such bleeding, see under Effects on the Gastrointestinal Tract, p.285.

Abuse. There have been occasional reports of individuals abusing fluoxetine.[1,2]

1. Tinsley JA, et al. Fluoxetine abuse. Mayo Clin Proc 1994; 69: 166–8.
2. Pagliaro LA, Pagliaro AM. Fluoxetine abuse by an intravenous drug user. Am J Psychiatry 1993; 150: 1898.

Blood disorders. For a reference recommending cautious use of fluoxetine in patients with thrombocytopenia or platelet dys-function, see Effects on the Blood in Adverse Effects, above.

Breast feeding. Symptoms of colic were reported[1] in a 6-week-old infant whose mother was taking fluoxetine 20 mg daily. The concentrations of fluoxetine and its active metabolite norfluoxetine were 69 nanograms per mL and 90 nanograms per mL respectively in breast milk, and 340 nanograms per mL and 208 nanograms per mL respectively in the infant's plasma. The infant's symptoms resolved when he was formula fed. Post-natal weight gain has been reduced in infants exposed to fluoxetine during breast feeding, although in all cases the re-duction was less than 2 standard deviations below the norm.[2] In a study[3] of 10 women taking fluoxetine while breast feeding 11 infants, breast milk concentrations of fluoxetine ranged from 17.4 to 293 nanograms per mL and of norfluoxetine from 23.4 to 379.1 nanograms per mL. No adverse effects were noted in the infants. Fluoxetine and norfluoxetine were detected in the milk of 14 nursing women.[4] Blood samples were taken from 9 of the infants in the study, and of these, fluoxetine was detected in the plasma of 5 and norfluoxetine in 7. Although it was felt that many infants would tolerate the mean combined dose of fluoxetine and norfluoxetine transmitted to infants via breast milk in this study, there was considerable interpatient variabil-ity in estimated infant dose and caution should be exercised; neonates in particular exhibited higher concentrations of nor-fluoxetine than older infants. Moreover, since both fluoxetine and norfluoxetine have long half-lives, neonates already ex-posed in utero may have an additional risk of adverse effects during breast feeding.

The excretion of fluvoxamine into breast milk was studied[5] in a woman who had been receiving fluvoxamine maleate 100 mg twice daily for 2 weeks. The concentration of fluvoxamine base 4.75 hours after a dose was 310 nanograms per mL in maternal plasma and 90 nanograms per mL in breast milk. It was esti-mated that an infant would ingest only 0.5% of the daily mater-nal intake. It was considered that these data supported the no-tion that administration of fluvoxamine to nursing mothers posed little risk to the infant. Although paroxetine was detected in measurable concentrations in the breast milk of a group of 10 nursing mothers receiving paroxetine no adverse effects were reported in any of their breast-fed infants.[6] Paroxetine could not be detected in the plasma of 7 of the 8 infants from whom samples were obtained and in the other infant concentra-tions were not quantifiable. Another study involving 7 women suggested that the dose of paroxetine to suckling infants would be 0.7 to 2.9% of the weight-adjusted maternal dose.[7]

Plasma concentrations of sertraline were undetectable in a breast-fed infant despite the presence of concentrations in the mother's breast milk ranging from 8.8 to 43 nanograms per mL over a 24-hour period.[8] However, the authors pointed out that metabolite levels were not measured and that sertraline may have been present in the infant at a concentration below the

level of sensitivity of the assay. Two further studies[9,10] detected desmethylsertraline in breast milk, which was also detected in the plasma of some of the infants in one of the studies[9] but not in any of the infants in the other study.[10]

Citalopram appears in breast milk in very low concentrations.

1. Lester BM, et al. Possible association between fluoxetine hydro-chloride and colic in an infant. J Am Acad Child Adolesc Psychi-atry 1993; 32: 1253–5.
2. Chambers CD, et al. Weight gain in infants breastfed by mothers who take fluoxetine. Pediatrics 1999; 104: 1120–1.
3. Taddio A, et al. Excretion of fluoxetine and its metabolite, nor-fluoxetine, in human breast milk. J Clin Pharmacol 1996; 36: 42–7.
4. Kristensen JH, et al. Distribution and excretion of fluoxetine and norfluoxetine in human milk. Br J Clin Pharmacol 1999; 48: 521–7.
5. Wright S, et al. Excretion of fluvoxamine in breast milk. Br J Clin Pharmacol 1991; 31: 209.
6. Begg EJ, et al. Paroxetine in human milk. Br J Clin Pharmacol 1999; 48: 142–7.
7. Öhman R, et al. Excretion of paroxetine into breast milk. J Clin Psychiatry 1999; 60: 519–23.
8. Altshuler LL, et al. Breastfeeding and sertraline: a 24-hour anal-ysis. J Clin Psychiatry 1995; 56: 243–5.
9. Stowe ZN, et al. Sertraline and desmethylsertraline in human breast milk and nursing infants. Am J Psychiatry 1997; 154: 1255–60.
10. Kristensen JH, et al. Distribution and excretion of sertraline and N-desmethylsertraline in human milk. Br J Clin Pharmacol 1998; 45: 453–7.

Diabetes mellitus. A report of the loss of hypoglycaemic awareness in a patient with type 1 diabetes mellitus following the start of treatment with fluoxetine.[1] Awareness returned fol-lowing reduction and discontinuation of fluoxetine dosage. Changes in blood sugar concentrations may occur in patients with diabetes treated for depression with SSRIs; however, these may represent an improvement in glycaemic control.[2]

1. Sawka AM, et al. Loss of hypoglycemia awareness in an adoles-cent with type 1 diabetes mellitus during treatment with fluoxet-ine hydrochloride. J Pediatr 2000; 136: 394–6.
2. Lustman PJ, et al. Fluoxetine for depression in diabetes: a rand-omized double-blind placebo-controlled trial. Diabetes Care 2000; 23: 618–23.

Driving. While affective disorders probably adversely affect driving skill,[1,2] treatment with antidepressants may also be haz-ardous,[1] although patients may be safer drivers with medication than without.[2] Impairment of performance is largely related to sedative and antimuscarinic effects, both of which are more pronounced with older antidepressants such as the tricyclic antidepressants than with the SSRIs, although a comparative study[3] of fluoxetine (an SSRI) and dothiepin [dosulepin] (a tri-cyclic) in healthy subjects demonstrated a similar but apparent-ly small potential for impairing psychomotor and driving per-formance. However, a recent epidemiological study[4] was unable to confirm any increased risk of road-traffic accidents in those drivers receiving tricyclic antidepressants or SSRIs.

In the UK, the Driver and Vehicle Licensing Authority (DVLA) considers that SSRIs, MAOIs, and noradrenaline reuptake in-hibitors have fewer adverse effects on drivers than antidepres-sants with antimuscarinic or antihistaminic adverse effects, such as tricyclic antidepressants. However some patients have idiosyncratic responses and should be advised accordingly.[5] Patients with severe depressive illnesses complicated by signif-icant memory or concentration problems, agitation, behaviour-al disturbances or suicidal thoughts should cease driving pend-ing the outcome of medical enquiry. It has been mentioned[2] that the UK Medical Commission on Accident Prevention has recommended that patients on long-term psychotropic medica-tion are unsuitable to be drivers of heavy goods or public serv-ice vehicles.

1. Ashton H. Drugs and driving. Adverse Drug React Bull 1983; 98: 360–3.
2. Cremona A. Mad drivers: psychiatric illness and driving per-formance. Br J Hosp Med 1986; 35: 193–5.
3. Ramaekers JG, et al. A comparative study of acute and subchron-ic effects of dothiepin, fluoxetine and placebo on psychomotor and actual driving performance. Br J Clin Pharmacol 1995; 39: 397–404.
4. Barbone F, et al. Association of road-traffic accidents with ben-zodiazepine use. Lancet 1998; 352: 1331–6.
5. Driver and Vehicle Licensing Agency. At a glance: a guide for medical practitioners. Available at: http://www.dvla.gov.uk/at_a_glance/ch4_psychiatric.htm (accessed 16/08/01).

Mania. Hypomania or mania have been reported with some of the SSRIs.

Fluvoxamine was associated with manic behaviour in 8 pa-tients who were being treated for major depression;[1] three also had concurrent obsessive-compulsive disorder. Daily doses of fluvoxamine ranged from 75 to 300 mg and duration of therapy to development of manic behaviour from 2 to 6 weeks. The au-thors were unable to determine whether fluvoxamine had in-duced mania or unmasked latent bipolar disorder in these pa-tients. However, they recommended that fluvoxamine-treated patients should be monitored for manic behaviour.

1. Dorevitch A, et al. Fluvoxamine-associated manic behavior: a case series. Ann Pharmacother 1993; 27: 1455–7.

Pregnancy. In an early prospective study[1] comparing 128 pregnant women exposed to a mean daily dose of about 26 mg of fluoxetine during their first trimester with control groups re-ceiving tricyclic antidepressants or non-teratogens, the inci-dence of neonatal malformations was similar in all groups and did not exceed that in the general population. However, there was a tendency for a higher incidence of miscarriages in the groups receiving fluoxetine or tricyclics. A more recent prospective study[2] comparing 228 pregnant women taking fluoxetine with a control group taking non-teratogens confirmed that there was no significant increased incidence in major fetal abnormalities in the fluoxetine group, but it did not reveal an increased risk of miscarriage. There was an increase in the incidence of minor fetal abnormalities in infants exposed to fluoxetine during the first trimester. Also, infants exposed to fluoxetine during the third trimester experienced more perinatal complications such as prematurity, low full-term birth-weight and length, and poor neonatal adaptation compared with infants exposed only during the first and second trimesters. However, the design of this study was criticised[3] because of several methodological problems such as unmatched controls and a higher maternal age in the fluoxetine group, which may partly explain the excess of poor perinatal outcomes. The manufacturer evaluated the outcome of 796 pregnancies in which the mother received fluoxetine during the first trimester and considered that it was unlikely that fluoxetine increased the risk of miscarriage or fetal malformation.[4] The effects of fluoxetine on fetal neurodevelopment were studied[5] in 55 pregnant women by later assessing global IQ of the children; no differences were seen in those exposed to fluoxetine in utero compared with those exposed to tricyclic antidepressants or non-teratogens. CNS toxicity and an increased heart rate were reported in a neonate whose mother had received 20 mg of fluoxetine daily throughout most of her pregnancy.[6] The neonate's symptoms resolved 96 hours after delivery.

A prospective controlled study[7] on pregnancy outcome in women exposed to fluvoxamine, paroxetine, or sertraline found that, when used in recommended doses, there appeared to be no increase in the risk of major congenital malformations, miscarriages, or still-births when compared with women exposed to non-teratogens.

1. Pastushak A, et al. Pregnancy outcome following first-trimester exposure to fluoxetine (Prozac). JAMA 1993; 269: 2246–8.
2. Chambers CD, et al. Birth outcomes in pregnant women taking fluoxetine. N Engl J Med 1996; 335: 1010–15.
3. Robert E. Treating depression in pregnancy. N Engl J Med 1996; 335: 1056–8.
4. Goldstein DJ, et al. Effects of first-trimester fluoxetine exposure on the newborn. Obstet Gynecol 1997; 89: 713–18.
5. Nulman I, et al. Neurodevelopment of children exposed in utero to antidepressant drugs. N Engl J Med 1997; 336: 258–62.
6. Spencer MJ. Fluoxetine hydrochloride (Prozac) toxicity in a neonate. Pediatrics 1993; 92: 721–2.
7. Kulin NA, et al. Pregnancy outcome following maternal use of the new selective serotonin reuptake inhibitors: a prospective controlled multicenter study. JAMA 1998; 279: 609–10.

Withdrawal. Withdrawal symptoms have been reported for SSRIs,[1-6] although the number of cases is greatest for paroxetine. The UK Committee on Safety of Medicines (CSM) has advised that normally paroxetine should not be discontinued abruptly.[1] Up to July 1994 the CSM had received 430 reports of symptoms occurring on withdrawal of paroxetine, including dizziness, sweating, nausea, insomnia, tremor, and confusion. The reactions, which had been reported more often with paroxetine than with other SSRIs, tended to start 1 to 4 days after stopping paroxetine and resolved in some patients on re-instating treatment. An update[6] by the CSM in September 2000 confirmed that in most cases the symptoms occurred within 3 days of stopping treatment with the most common symptoms being dizziness, headache, nausea, and paraesthesia. A retrospective analysis[5] has also found that withdrawal symptoms occur significantly more frequently in patients treated with the shorter half-life SSRIs, such as paroxetine, than in those receiving an SSRI with a longer half-life metabolite, such as fluoxetine. There has also been a report[2] of 2 patients without a history of major psychiatric disorder who developed severe behavioural symptoms when paroxetine was withdrawn. Discontinuation was abrupt in one patient and gradual, over a 12-day period, in the other. Symptoms were predominantly hypomanic over the first few days, followed by a period of escalated ego-dystonic aggression, behavioural dyscontrol, and suicidal intention.

Some authorities recommend that any antidepressant, including an SSRI, that has been administered regularly for 8 weeks or more should be discontinued gradually over a period of about 4 weeks.

The withdrawal syndrome of the SSRIs is not considered to be a consequence of dependence.[6]

See also Extrapyramidal Effects under Adverse Effects, above.

1. Price JS, et al. A comparison of the post-marketing safety of four selective serotonin re-uptake inhibitors including the investigation of symptoms occurring on withdrawal. Br J Clin Pharmacol 1996; 42: 757–63.
2. Bloch M, et al. Severe psychiatric symptoms associated with paroxetine withdrawal. Lancet 1995; 346: 57.
3. Szabadi E. Fluvoxamine withdrawal syndrome. Br J Psychiatry 1992; 160: 283–4.
4. Adverse Drug Reactions Advisory Committee (ADRAC). SSRI's and withdrawal syndrome. Aust Adverse Drug React Bull 1996; 15: 3.
5. Coupland NJ, et al. Serotonin reuptake inhibitor withdrawal. J Clin Psychopharmacol 1996; 16: 356–62.
6. Committee on Safety of Medicines/Medicines Control Agency. Selective serotonin reuptake inhibitors (SSRIs). Current Problems 2000; 26: 11–12.

Interactions

SSRIs interact with a range of other drugs mainly as a result of their inhibitory activity on hepatic cyto-

chrome P450 isoenzymes. Individual SSRIs do not all exhibit the same degree of inhibition nor do they react with the same isoenzymes. The range of drugs inhibited by specific SSRIs varies according to which isoenzyme is affected.

The effects of alcohol may possibly be enhanced by SSRIs.

Although different antidepressants have been used together under expert supervision in refractory cases of depression, severe adverse reactions including the serotonin syndrome (see p.304) may occur. Sequential prescribing of different types of antidepressant may also produce adverse reactions, and an appropriate drug-free interval should elapse between discontinuing one type of antidepressant and starting another. SSRIs should not generally be given to patients receiving MAOIs or for at least two weeks after their discontinuation. Although some manufacturers recommend a similar treatment-free period between stopping a reversible inhibitor of monoamine oxidase type A (RIMA) and starting an SSRI there does not seem to be any evidence to support such a requirement. At least one week should elapse between withdrawing an SSRI and starting any drug liable to provoke a serious reaction (e.g. phenelzine); in the case of the SSRIs paroxetine and sertraline the drug-free interval is extended to two weeks, and for fluoxetine five weeks, because of their longer half-lives. Adverse effects such as the serotonin syndrome may also occur when the SSRIs are given with other drugs known to act on the same neurotransmitter, a consequence of synergistic interaction.

Further details concerning some of these interactions, and others, are given below.

◊ References.
1. Mitchell PB. Drug interactions of clinical significance with selective serotonin reuptake inhibitors. Drug Safety 1997; 17: 390–406.
2. Sproule BA, et al. Selective serotonin reuptake inhibitors and CNS drug interactions: a critical review of the evidence. Clin Pharmacokinet 1997; 33: 454–71.

Antibacterials. Rapid development of delirium was reported[1] in a patient when clarithromycin was added to his existing regimen of fluoxetine and nitrazepam. It was suggested that his delirium was a result of increased plasma-fluoxetine concentrations produced by the inhibition of cytochrome P450 enzymes by clarithromycin. A report[2] of a serotonin syndrome in a patient given erythromycin in addition to sertraline was attributed to inhibition of CYP3A4 by the antibacterial, resulting in accumulation of the SSRI.

1. Pollak PT, et al. Delirium probably induced by clarithromycin in a patient receiving fluoxetine. Ann Pharmacother 1995; 29: 486–8.
2. Lee DO, Lee CD. Serotonin syndrome in a child associated with erythromycin and sertraline. Pharmacotherapy 1999; 19: 894–6.

Anticoagulants. SSRIs may increase the anticoagulant activity of warfarin (see p.995).

Antidepressants. Combination therapy with differing classes of antidepressants has been used successfully in the treatment of drug-resistant depression. It should be emphasised, however, that such combinations may result in enhanced adverse reactions or interactions, and should be employed only under expert supervision. This practice is considered unsuitable or controversial by some authorities. For further details of the interactions between different antidepressants when coadministered, see Phenelzine, p.306. For details of the serotonin syndrome that can arise when two serotonergic drugs with different mechanisms of action are administered, see under Adverse Effects of Phenelzine, p.304.

Antiepileptics. Antidepressants may antagonise the activity of antiepileptics by lowering the convulsive threshold.

There has been a report of the serotonin syndrome (see p.304) developing in a patient 14 days after fluoxetine had been added to carbamazepine therapy.[1]

Phenobarbital has been reported to reduce serum concentrations of paroxetine.[2] Steady-state serum concentrations of paroxetine were found to be lower in patients taking phenytoin than in those taking carbamazepine or valproate.[3]

Some SSRIs have been reported to increase plasma concentrations of carbamazepine (see p.344) and phenytoin (see p.360).

1. Dursun SM, et al. Toxic serotonin syndrome after fluoxetine plus carbamazepine. Lancet 1993; 342: 442–3.
2. Greb WH, et al. The effect of liver enzyme inhibition by cimetidine and enzyme induction by phenobarbitone on the pharmacokinetics of paroxetine. Acta Psychiatr Scand 1989; 80 (suppl 350): 95–8.
3. Andersen BB, et al. No influence of the antidepressant paroxetine on carbamazepine, valproate and phenytoin. Epilepsy Res 1991; 10: 201–4.

Antihistamines. Cyproheptadine given to male and female patients as treatment for sexual dysfunction induced by fluoxetine or paroxetine produced re-emergence of previously controlled depressive symptoms[1,2] or bulimia nervosa.[3] Citalopram, fluoxetine, and fluvoxamine may increase plasma concentrations of astemizole or terfenadine by inhibition of their hepatic cytochrome P450 metabolism, increasing the risk of ventricular arrhythmias; concomitant use should be avoided.

1. Feder R. Reversal of antidepressant activity of fluoxetine by cyproheptadine in three patients. J Clin Psychiatry 1991; 52: 163–4.
2. Christensen RC. Adverse interaction of paroxetine and cyproheptadine. J Clin Psychiatry 1995; 56: 433–4.
3. Goldbloom DS, Kennedy SH. Adverse interaction of fluoxetine and cyproheptadine in two patients with bulimia nervosa. J Clin Psychiatry 1991; 52: 261–2.

Antimalarials. For mention of the effect of the SSRI fluvoxamine on the metabolism of proguanil, see p.441.

Antimigraine drugs. There is a risk of CNS toxicity with SSRIs and sumatriptan (see p.457).

Antimuscarinics. For the effect of SSRIs on benzatropine, see p.463.

Antipsychotics. For reports of adverse effects in patients given concomitant treatment with SSRIs and antipsychotics, see under Chlorpromazine, p.664.

Antivirals. Plasma concentrations of fluoxetine and other SSRIs are possibly increased by HIV-protease inhibitors. For the effect of fluoxetine on delavirdine, see p.617.

Anxiolytics. Fluoxetine and fluvoxamine increase plasma concentrations of some benzodiazepines (see under Diazepam, p.678). There is a report of hyponatraemia and serotonin syndrome developing in a patient who received high doses of citalopram and buspirone.[1]

1. Spigset O, Adielsson G. Combined serotonin syndrome and hyponatraemia caused by a citalopram-buspirone interaction. Int Clin Psychopharmacol 1997; 12: 61–3.

Beta blockers. For the effect of fluoxetine and fluvoxamine on beta blockers, see p.846.

Ciclosporin. For the effect of fluoxetine on ciclosporin, see p.521.

Cough suppressants. For the effect of fluoxetine and paroxetine on dextromethorphan, see p.1088.

Dopaminergics. Selegiline is an irreversible selective inhibitor of monoamine oxidase type B. Serious adverse effects have been reported when selegiline and SSRIs have been used concomitantly (see p.1177). In some instances, these reactions resemble the potentially fatal serotonin syndromes reported when SSRIs are administered together with non-selective MAOIs (see p.304).

Some authorities advise that SSRIs should not generally be given to patients receiving selegiline, or for at least two weeks after it has been discontinued. Similarly, at least one week should elapse between withdrawing an SSRI and starting selegiline; this interval should be increased to two weeks for paroxetine and sertraline, and to five weeks for fluoxetine because of their longer half-lives.

Gastrointestinal drugs. Acute dystonia has been noted in a patient after the coadministration of fluvoxamine and metoclopramide.[1] Similar reports have been published for other SSRIs (fluoxetine[2] or sertraline[3]) and metoclopramide.

1. Palop V, et al. Acute dystonia associated with fluvoxamine-metoclopramide. Ann Pharmacother 1999; 33: 382.
2. Coulter DM, Pillans PI. Fluoxetine and extrapyramidal side effects. Am J Psychiatry 1995; 152: 122–5.
3. Christensen RC, Byerly MJ. Mandibular dystonia associated with the combination of sertraline and metoclopramide. J Clin Psychiatry 1996; 57: 596.

General anaesthetics. For a report of a generalised tonic-clonic seizure in a patient receiving paroxetine and methohexital sodium, see p.1263.

Hypnotics. For reference to visual hallucinations in patients receiving an SSRI concomitantly with zolpidem, see p.712.

NSAIDs. For reference to an increased risk of upper gastrointestinal bleeding in patients taking SSRIs and NSAIDs together, see under Effects on the Gastrointestinal Tract, above.

Opioid analgesics. A possible case of serotonin syndrome (p.304) has been reported with coadministration of tramadol and sertraline,[1] and another when sertraline was given with high doses of oxycodone.[2] There have also been occasional reports of the syndrome in patients given tramadol with paroxetine.[3,4] For reference to SSRIs enhancing the effects and toxicity of methadone, see p.53.

1. Mason BJ, Blackburn KH. Possible serotonin syndrome associated with tramadol and sertraline coadministration. Ann Pharmacother 1997; 31: 175–7.
2. Rosebraugh CJ, et al. Visual hallucination and tremor induced by sertraline and oxycodone in a bone marrow transplant patient. J Clin Pharmacol 2001; 41: 224–7.
3. Egberts ACG, et al. Serotonin syndrome attributed to tramadol addition to paroxetine therapy. Int Clin Psychopharmacol 1997; 12: 181–2.
4. Lantz MS, et al. Serotonin syndrome following the administration of tramadol with paroxetine. Int J Geriatr Psychiatry 1998; 13: 343–5.

Parasympathomimetics. For the effect of fluvoxamine on *tacrine*, see p.1425.

Sibutramine. There is a risk of CNS toxicity due to synergistic serotonergic actions when an SSRI is given with sibutramine.

Smoking. Serum concentrations of fluvoxamine were lower in smokers than non-smokers in a single-dose study.[1] It was proposed that the polycyclic hydrocarbons present in cigarette smoke stimulated hepatic metabolism of fluvoxamine by cytochrome P450 enzymes.

1. Spigset O, *et al.* Effect of cigarette smoking on fluvoxamine pharmacokinetics in humans. *Clin Pharmacol Ther* 1995; **58:** 399–403.

Theophylline. For the effect of fluvoxamine on theophylline, see p.780.

Thyroxine [levothyroxine]. For mention of a decreased effect of thyroxine [levothyroxine] in patients given sertraline concomitantly, see p.1527.

Pharmacokinetics

Fluoxetine is readily absorbed from the gastrointestinal tract with peak plasma concentrations appearing about 6 to 8 hours after administration. The systemic bioavailability does not appear to be affected by food. It is extensively metabolised, by demethylation, in the liver to its primary active metabolite norfluoxetine. Excretion is mainly via the urine. Protein binding is reported to be about 95%.

Fluoxetine used clinically is a racemic mixture consisting of *R* and *S* enantiomers in equal amounts. Both enantiomers are active according to *animal* studies, but *S*-fluoxetine is eliminated more slowly. Metabolism is believed to be mediated by cytochrome P450 isoenzyme CYP2D6 (but see below), and leads to *R* and *S* enantiomers of norfluoxetine, with the *S* enantiomer being considered as active as the parent drug; the *R* enantiomer is considered to be much less active. This metabolism is subject to genetic polymorphism. While the small proportion of the population known as slow metabolisers do show a different spectrum of parent drug and metabolite, the overall activity does not appear to be altered.

Fluoxetine is widely distributed throughout the body.

Fluoxetine has a relatively long elimination half-life of about 1 to 3 days; that of its metabolite, norfluoxetine, is even longer, being about 4 to 16 days. These long half-lives have clinical implications. Steady-state plasma concentrations will only be attained after several weeks. Additionally, after discontinuation fluoxetine and its metabolites may persist for a considerable time and this has led to precautions concerning the subsequent administration of other serotonergic antidepressants (see Interactions, above).

Fluoxetine and norfluoxetine are distributed into breast milk (see Breast Feeding under Precautions, above).

◊ References.
1. van Harten J. Clinical pharmacokinetics of selective serotonin reuptake inhibitors. *Clin Pharmacokinet* 1993; **24:** 203–20.
2. Altamura AC, *et al.* Clinical pharmacokinetics of fluoxetine. *Clin Pharmacokinet* 1994; **26:** 201–14.
3. Baumann P. Pharmacokinetic-pharmacodynamic relationship of the selective serotonin reuptake inhibitors. *Clin Pharmacokinet* 1996; **31:** 444–69.
4. Greenblatt DJ, *et al.* Inhibition of human cytochrome P450-3A isoforms by fluoxetine and norfluoxetine: in vitro and in vivo studies. *J Clin Pharmacol* 1996; **36:** 792–8.
5. Hamelin BA, *et al.* The disposition of fluoxetine but not sertraline is altered in poor metabolizers of debrisoquin. *Clin Pharmacol Ther* 1996; **60:** 512–21.
6. Preskorn SH. Clinically relevant pharmacology of selective serotonin reuptake inhibitors: an overview with emphasis on pharmacokinetics and effects on oxidative drug metabolism. *Clin Pharmacokinet* 1997; **32** (suppl 1): 1–21.

Metabolism. Although fluoxetine is stated by the manufacturers to be metabolised by the cytochrome P450 isoenzyme CYP2D6, which is supported by studies[1] indicating that its disposition is altered in poor metabolisers of debrisoquine (a substrate for this enzyme), others have suggested that CYP2C19, and perhaps CYP2C9, play an important role.[2]

1. Hamelin BA, *et al.* The disposition of fluoxetine but not sertraline is altered in poor metabolizers of debrisoquin. *Clin Pharmacol Ther* 1996; **60:** 512–21.
2. Liu Z-Q, *et al.* Effect of the CYP2C19 oxidation polymorphism on fluoxetine metabolism in Chinese healthy subjects. *Br J Clin Pharmacol* 2001; **52:** 96–9.

Uses and Administration

SSRIs such as fluoxetine preferentially inhibit the reuptake of serotonin compared with noradrenaline, and have limited direct action at other neurotransmitter sites, including muscarinic receptors. They therefore cause fewer antimuscarinic or sedative side-effects than the tricyclic antidepressants and are less cardiotoxic. Specific SSRIs differ in selectivity and potency for the reuptake of serotonin and the two parameters are not interdependent. Thus, citalopram is the most selective of the currently available serotonin reuptake inhibitors, whereas paroxetine is the most potent.

Prevention of the reuptake of monoamine transmitters such as serotonin, which potentiates their action in the brain, appears to be associated with antidepressant activity.

SSRIs provide an alternative to the tricyclics for the treatment of depression. As with the tricyclics, it may be several weeks before an antidepressant effect is seen. After a response has been obtained, maintenance therapy should be continued for 4 to 6 months after the depression has resolved to avoid relapse on discontinuation of therapy.

Some SSRIs are also used as part of the management of obsessive-compulsive disorder and panic disorders with or without agoraphobia, and as part of the management of bulimia nervosa. Fluoxetine is also used in the treatment of premenstrual dysphoric disorder.

Fluoxetine, a phenylpropylamine derivative, is given by mouth as the hydrochloride; doses are expressed in terms of fluoxetine.

In the treatment of **depression** the usual dose of fluoxetine is 20 mg daily and some authorities recommend giving this dose in the morning. In the USA, it is recommended that if no clinical response is seen after several weeks, the daily dose may be gradually increased, up to a maximum of 80 mg daily. Doses above 20 mg daily may be administered in 2 divided doses, for example in the morning and at noon, or as a once daily dose. A once-weekly, modified-release preparation equivalent to 90 mg of fluoxetine is available in the USA for use in patients whose depressive symptoms have stabilised, and who require long-term treatment.

Fluoxetine is used in doses of 60 mg daily in the management of **bulimia nervosa**.

In the management of **obsessive-compulsive disorder** the initial dose of fluoxetine is 20 mg daily increased after several weeks if there is no response to up to 60 mg daily. Up to 80 mg daily has been used in the USA where twice daily, as well as once daily, regimens may also be employed.

A dose of 20 mg once daily is used in the treatment of **premenstrual dysphoric disorder**. Treatment may be continued for 6 months; benefit should then be reassessed before continuing further.

Because fluoxetine is subject to hepatic metabolism, lower doses, such as alternate-day dosing, have been recommended in patients with significant hepatic impairment; some authorities recommend that SSRIs should be avoided if hepatic impairment is severe. Similar recommendations, because of renal excretion, have been made for patients with mild to moderate renal impairment; it should not, however, be used at all in patients with severe renal impairment. Some authorities recommend a lower or less frequent dosage in elderly patients.

It should be noted that the prolonged half-lives of fluoxetine and norfluoxetine will result in the need for several weeks of therapy to be employed before steady-state concentrations are attained; similarly after dosage adjustments a time lag will occur before steady-state concentrations are again achieved.

Fluoxetine should be withdrawn gradually to reduce the risk of withdrawal symptoms.

◊ References.
1. Gram LF. Fluoxetine. *N Engl J Med* 1994; **331:** 1354–61.

2. Finley PR. Selective serotonin reuptake inhibitors: pharmacologic profiles and potential therapeutic distinctions. *Ann Pharmacother* 1994; **28:** 1359–69.
3. Hyttel J. Pharmacological characterization of selective serotonin reuptake inhibitors (SSRIs). *Int Clin Psychopharmacol* 1994; **9** (suppl 1): 19–26.
4. Edwards JG, Anderson I. Systematic review and guide to selection of selective serotonin reuptake inhibitors. *Drugs* 1999; **57:** 507–33.

Anorexia nervosa. Counselling and psychotherapy form the major part of treatment of anorexia nervosa and there is little or no role for specific drug therapy. Antidepressants may be indicated when there is co-existing depression but malnourished anorexic patients may be more susceptible to adverse effects and less responsive than other patients with depression. Fluoxetine has been tried with some success, although the efficacy and safety of SSRIs has been questioned.
References.
1. Bergh C, *et al.* Selective serotonin reuptake inhibitors in anorexia. *Lancet* 1996; **348:** 1459–60.
2. Mayer LES, Walsh BT. The use of selective serotonin reuptake inhibitors in eating disorders. *J Clin Psychiatry* 1998; **59:** (suppl 15): 28–34.
3. Kaye WH, *et al.* Double-blind placebo-controlled administration of fluoxetine in restricting- and restricting-purging-type anorexia nervosa. *Biol Psychiatry* 2001; **49:** 644–52.

Anxiety disorders. SSRIs have been given in a variety of anxiety disorders but their role in these disorders is most well established in the treatment of *obsessive-compulsive disorder* (p.649). Efficacy in obsessive-compulsive disorder appears to have been best demonstrated for fluvoxamine and fluoxetine but other SSRIs are also effective and patients unresponsive to one SSRI may respond to another. SSRIs are also of use in the treatment of *panic attacks* (p.649) and *post-traumatic stress disorder* (p.650). Encouraging results have been obtained with various SSRIs in the treatment of *social phobia* (see under Phobic Disorders, p.649). Fluoxetine is one of the SSRIs that has been tried in the treatment of *trichotillomania*.
References.
1. Montgomery SA, *et al.* A double-blind, placebo-controlled study of fluoxetine in patients with DSM-III-R obsessive-compulsive disorder. *Eur Neuropsychopharmacol* 1993; **3:** 143–52.
2. Wood A, *et al.* Pharmacotherapy of obsessive compulsive disorder—experience with fluoxetine. *Int Clin Psychopharmacol* 1993; **8:** 301–6.
3. Van Ameringen M, *et al.* Fluoxetine efficacy in social phobia. *J Clin Psychiatry* 1993; **54:** 27–32.
4. Tollefson GD, *et al.* A multicenter investigation of fixed-dose fluoxetine in the treatment of obsessive-compulsive disorder. *Arch Gen Psychiatry* 1994; **51:** 559–67.
5. Yanchick JK, *et al.* Efficacy of fluoxetine in trichotillomania. *Ann Pharmacother* 1994; **28:** 1245–6.
6. Boyer W. Serotonin uptake inhibitors are superior to imipramine and alprazolam in alleviating panic attacks: a meta-analysis. *Int Clin Psychopharmacol* 1995; **10:** 45–9.
7. Michelson D, *et al.* Continuing treatment of panic disorder after acute response: randomised, placebo-controlled trial with fluoxetine. *Br J Psychiatry* 1999; **174:** 213–18.
8. Connor KM, *et al.* Fluoxetine in post-traumatic stress disorder: randomised, double-blind study. *Br J Psychiatry* 1999; **175:** 17–22.

Bipolar disorder. Treatment of the depressive phase of bipolar disorder (p.271) with antidepressants needs caution since these drugs may precipitate mania or hypomania. The SSRIs such as fluoxetine are one group of antidepressants that have been used in bipolar disorder with some success.
References.
1. Amsterdam JD, *et al.* Efficacy and safety of fluoxetine in treating bipolar II major depressive episode. *J Clin Psychopharmacol* 1998; **18:** 435–40.
2. Megna JL, Devitt PJ. Treatment of bipolar depression with twice-weekly fluoxetine: an antidepressant-induced mania. *Ann Pharmacother* 2001; **35:** 45–7.

Bulimia nervosa. A combination of counselling, support, psychotherapy, and antidepressants is the usual treatment for bulimia nervosa. Fluoxetine and the tricyclic desipramine have been suggested as the antidepressants of choice because they have been used extensively and are considered to be well tolerated. Other SSRIs that have been tried include sertraline, fluvoxamine, and paroxetine. Antidepressants in general do not appear to alter the patient's disturbed self-image, although disturbed attitudes might improve during short-term therapy with fluoxetine.
References.
1. Goldbloom DS, Olmsted MP. Pharmacotherapy of bulimia nervosa with fluoxetine: assessment of clinically significant attitudinal change. *Am J Psychiatry* 1993; **150:** 770–4.
2. Mayer LES, Walsh BT. The use of selective serotonin reuptake inhibitors in eating disorders. *J Clin Psychiatry* 1998; **59** (suppl 15): 28–34.

Depression. As discussed on p.271, there is very little difference in efficacy between the different groups of antidepressant drugs, and choice is often made on the basis of adverse effect profile. SSRIs such as fluoxetine are widely used as an alternative to the older tricyclics as they have fewer unpleasant side-effects and are safer in overdosage.

Combination therapy with differing classes of antidepressants, including the SSRIs, has been used in the treatment of drug-resistant depression. However, such therapy may result in enhanced adverse reactions or interactions and is considered unsuitable or controversial by some workers. For further details, see Antidepressants under Interactions of Phenelzine, p.306.

References to the use of SSRIs in general and to the use of fluoxetine are given below.

1. Song F, *et al.* Selective serotonin reuptake inhibitors: meta-analysis of efficacy and acceptability. *BMJ* 1993; **306**: 683–7.
2. Montgomery SA, *et al.* Selective serotonin reuptake inhibitors: meta-analysis of discontinuation rates. *Int Clin Psychopharmacol* 1994; **9**: 47–53.
3. Fava M, *et al.* Lithium and tricyclic augmentation of fluoxetine treatment for resistant major depression: a double blind, controlled study. *Am J Psychiatry* 1994; **151**: 1372–4.
4. Roose SP, *et al.* Comparative efficacy of selective serotonin reuptake inhibitors and tricyclics in the treatment of melancholia. *Am J Psychiatry* 1994; **151**: 1735–9.
5. Lam RW, *et al.* Multicenter, placebo-controlled study of fluoxetine in seasonal affective disorder. *Am J Psychiatry* 1995; **152**: 1765–70.
6. Anderson IM, Tomenson BM. Treatment discontinuation with selective serotonin reuptake inhibitors compared with tricyclic antidepressants: a meta-analysis. *BMJ* 1995; **310**: 1433–8.
7. Brown WA, Harrison W. Are patients who are intolerant to one serotonin selective reuptake inhibitor intolerant to another? *J Clin Psychiatry* 1995; **56**: 30–4.
8. Fava M, *et al.* Relapse in patients on long-term fluoxetine treatment: response to increased fluoxetine dose. *J Clin Psychiatry* 1995; **56**: 52–5.
9. Joffe RT, *et al.* Response to an open trial of a second SSRI in major depression. *J Clin Psychiatry* 1996; **57**: 114–15.
10. Nobler MS, *et al.* Fluoxetine treatment of dysthymia in the elderly. *J Clin Psychiatry* 1996; **57**: 254–6.
11. Burke WJ, *et al.* Fluoxetine and norfluoxetine serum concentrations and clinical response in weekly versus daily dosing. *Psychopharmacol Bull* 1996; **32**: 27–32.
12. Mourilhe P, Stokes PE. Risks and benefits of selective serotonin reuptake inhibitors in the treatment of depression. *Drug Safety* 1998; **18**: 57–82.
13. Trindade E, Menion D. *Selective serotonin reuptake inhibitors (SSRIs) for major depression. Part 1. Evaluation of the clinical literature.* Ottawa: Canadian Coordinating Office for Health Technology Assessment, 1997.
14. Anderson IM. SSRIs versus tricyclic antidepressants in depressed inpatients: a meta-analysis of efficacy and tolerability. *Depress Anxiety* 1998; **7** (suppl 1): 11–17.
15. Cheer SM, Goa KL. Fluoxetine: a review of its therapeutic potential in the treatment of depression associated with physical illness. *Drugs* 2001; **61**: 81–110.
16. Sampson SM. Treating depression with selective serotonin reuptake inhibitors: a practical approach. *Mayo Clin Proc* 2001; **76**: 739–44.
17. Geddes JR, *et al.* Selective serotonin reuptake inhibitors (SSRIs) for depression (updated 28 May 2001). Available in The Cochrane Library; Issue 3. Oxford: Update Software; 2001.

Disturbed behaviour. SSRIs appear to have been of some benefit in controlling symptoms such as impulsiveness and aggression[1-3] when tried in various disorders for the management of disturbed behaviour (see p.650). There have been several case reports of fluoxetine being used with some success in the control of fantasies associated with various paraphilias.[4]

1. Coccaro EF, Kavoussi RJ. Fluoxetine and impulsive aggressive behavior in personality-disordered subjects. *Arch Gen Psychiatry* 1997; **54**: 1081–8.
2. Cornelius JR, *et al.* Fluoxetine trial in borderline personality disorder. *Psychopharmacol Bull* 1990; **26**: 151–4.
3. Vartiainen H, *et al.* Citalopram, a selective serotonin reuptake inhibitor, in the treatment of aggression in schizophrenia. *Acta Psychiatr Scand* 1995; **91**: 348–51.
4. Richer M, Crismon ML. Pharmacotherapy of sexual offenders. *Ann Pharmacother* 1993; **27**: 316–19.

Headache. The results of several studies have suggested that SSRIs may be of benefit in the treatment of chronic tension-type headache (p.450); however, results in the prophylaxis of migraine (p.449) have been conflicting.

References.
1. Sosin D. Clinical efficacy of fluoxetine vs sertraline in a headache clinic population. *Headache* 1993; **33**: 284.
2. Solomon GD, Pearson E. Sertraline in the management of headache. *Clin Pharmacol Ther* 1994; **55**: 130.
3. Jung AC, *et al.* The efficacy of selective serotonin reuptake inhibitors for the management of chronic pain. *J Gen Intern Med* 1997; **12**: 384–9.

Hyperactivity. When drug therapy is indicated for attention deficit hyperactivity disorder (ADHD—p.1505) initial treatment is usually with a central stimulant. SSRIs such as fluoxetine have produced beneficial effects as an adjunct to central stimulants in small numbers of patients with comorbid disorders such as depression or obsessive-compulsive disorder;[1,2] although there is insufficient evidence to assess their efficacy in ADHD alone.

1. Gammon GD, Brown TE. Fluoxetine and methylphenidate in combination for treatment of attention deficit disorder and comorbid depressive disorder. *J Child Adolesc Psychopharmacol* 1993; **3**: 1–10.
2. Bussing R, Levin GM. Methamphetamine and fluoxetine treatment of a child with attention-deficit hyperactivity disorder and obsessive-compulsive disorder. *J Child Adolesc Psychopharmacol* 1993; **3**: 53–8.

Hypochondriasis. Fluoxetine in an initial dose of 20 mg daily gradually increased up to 80 mg daily produced some beneficial results in 10 of 14 patients with hypochondriasis (p.650) who completed 12 weeks of treatment.[1]

1. Fallon BA, *et al.* Fluoxetine for hypochondriacal patients without major depression. *J Clin Psychopharmacol* 1993; **13**: 438–41.

Hypotension. SSRIs have been suggested for patients with neurally mediated hypotension refractory to standard treatment (see p.805).

See also Orthostatic Hypotension, below.

Obesity. Fluoxetine has been tried with some success as part of the management of obesity (p.1505). Fluoxetine's mecha-

The symbol † denotes a preparation no longer actively marketed

nism of action in obesity is unknown. Serotonin is believed to be involved in the regulation of satiety[1] but fluoxetine has also been shown to increase resting energy expenditure and raise basal body temperature.[2] A common dose for fluoxetine in the management of obesity has been 60 mg daily; it appears that fluoxetine has a dose-related effect on weight loss.[3] Reviews[1,4,5] agree that fluoxetine can aid weight reduction in the short term but after 16 to 20 weeks some patients have started to regain weight and its long-term efficacy remains to be established. Troublesome adverse effects can occur.[1] Some patients treated with fluoxetine for depression have experienced an increase of appetite and some have gained weight. There has been a report[6] of a patient who lost weight during treatment with fluoxetine for depression despite an increased appetite and food intake.

1. Anonymous. Fluoxetine (Prozac) and other drugs for treatment of obesity. *Med Lett Drugs Ther* 1994; **36**: 107–8.
2. Bross R, Hoffer LJ. Fluoxetine increases resting energy expenditure and basal body temperature in humans. *Am J Clin Nutr* 1995; **61**: 1020–5.
3. Levine LR, *et al.* Use of fluoxetine, a selective serotonin-uptake inhibitor, in the treatment of obesity: a dose-response study. *Int J Obes* 1989; **13**: 635–45.
4. Bray GA. Use and abuse of appetite-suppressant drugs in the treatment of obesity. *Ann Intern Med* 1993; **119**: 707–13.
5. Mayer LE, Walsh BT. The use of selective serotonin reuptake inhibitors in eating disorders. *J Clin Psychiatry* 1998; **59** (suppl 15): 28–34.
6. Fichtner CG, Braun BG. Hyperphagia and weight loss during fluoxetine treatment. *Ann Pharmacother* 1994; **28**: 1350–2.

Orthostatic hypotension. Although orthostatic hypotension has been reported in some patients taking SSRIs there has been a report[1] that fluoxetine 20 mg daily for 6 to 8 weeks produced beneficial effects in 4 of 5 patients with chronic symptomatic orthostatic hypotension (p.1070) refractory to other treatment.

1. Grubb BP, *et al.* Fluoxetine hydrochloride for the treatment of severe refractory orthostatic hypotension. *Am J Med* 1994; **97**: 366–8.

Pain. SSRIs have been tried in the treatment of painful disorders including fibromyalgia and diabetic neuropathy.

See also Headache, above.

References.
1. Geller SA. Treatment of fibrositis with fluoxetine hydrochloride (Prozac). *Am J Med* 1989; **87**: 594–5.
2. Cantini F, *et al.* Fluoxetina associata a ciclobenzaprina nel trattamento della fibromialgia. *Minerva Med* 1994; **85**: 97–100.
3. Goldenberg D, *et al.* A randomized, double-blind crossover trial of fluoxetine and amitriptyline in the treatment of fibromyalgia. *Arthritis Rheum* 1996; **39**: 1852–9.
4. Jung AC, *et al.* The efficacy of selective serotonin reuptake inhibitors for the management of chronic pain. *J Gen Intern Med* 1997; **12**: 384–9.
5. Smith AJ. The analgesic effects of selective serotonin reuptake inhibitors. *J Psychopharmacol* 1998; **12**: 407–13.

Parkinsonism. It has been suggested that fluoxetine might be of use in the management of selected patients with Parkinson's disease (p.1160) who have levodopa-induced dyskinesias unresponsive to other measures.[1] However, although fluoxetine has been reported to have produced beneficial results in such patients[2] there has also been a report of increased disability in patients with Parkinson's disease given fluoxetine.[3] Extrapyramidal effects have also been reported in other patients taking fluoxetine (see under Adverse Effects, above).

1. Giron LT, Koller WC. Methods of managing levodopa-induced dyskinesias. *Drug Safety* 1996; **14**: 365–74.
2. Durif F, *et al.* Levodopa-induced dyskinesias are improved by fluoxetine. *Neurology* 1995; **45**: 1855–8.
3. Steur ENHJ. Increase of Parkinson disability after fluoxetine medication. *Neurology* 1993; **43**: 211–3.

Pathological crying or laughing. Inappropriate or uncontrolled crying or laughing can occur in patients with lesions in certain areas of the brain. Attempts at treatment have mostly been with antidepressant drugs, including SSRIs. Beneficial effects have been claimed for fluoxetine in a number of uncontrolled studies and reports.[1-4]

1. Seliger GM, *et al.* Fluoxetine improves emotional incontinence. *Brain Inj* 1992; **6**: 267–70.
2. Sloan RL, *et al.* Fluoxetine as a treatment for emotional lability after brain injury. *Brain Inj* 1992; **6**: 315–19.
3. Hanger HC. Emotionalism after stroke. *Lancet* 1993; **342**: 1235–6.
4. Tsai WC, *et al.* Treatment of emotionalism with fluoxetine during rehabilitation. *Scand J Rehabil Med* 1998; **30**: 145–9.

Peripheral vascular disease. There have been anecdotal reports[1,2] of fluoxetine in a daily dose of 20 to 60 mg producing favourable therapeutic responses in patients with Raynaud's syndrome (p.809).

1. Bolte MA, Avery D. Case of fluoxetine-induced remission of Raynaud's phenomenon—a case report. *Angiology* 1993; **44**: 161–3.
2. Jaffe IA. Serotonin reuptake inhibitors in Raynaud's phenomenon. *Lancet* 1995; **345**: 1378.

Premenstrual syndrome. Fluoxetine is used to control both the psychological and somatic symptoms of women with premenstrual syndrome (p.1475). Other SSRIs also appear to be useful, although evidence is so far more limited.

References.
1. Romano S, *et al.* The role of fluoxetine in the treatment of premenstrual dysphoric disorder. *Clin Ther* 1999; **21**: 615–33.
2. Dimmock PW, *et al.* Efficacy of selective serotonin-reuptake inhibitors in premenstrual syndrome: a systematic review. *Lancet* 2000; **356**: 1131–6.

Sexual dysfunction. Impotence or ejaculatory problems have been reported as adverse effects of SSRIs (see Effects on Sexual Function in Adverse Effects, above). Such properties of the SSRIs have been studied as a potential form of treatment for men with premature ejaculation (see Paroxetine, p.303 and Sertraline, p.309). Fluoxetine has been reported to be less effective in this condition than sertraline or clomipramine.[1]

1. Kim SC, Seo KK. Efficacy and safety of fluoxetine, sertraline and clomipramine in patients with premature ejaculation: a double-blind, placebo controlled study. *J Urol (Baltimore)* 1998; **159**: 425–7.

Preparations

BP 2001: Fluoxetine Capsules; Fluoxetine Oral Solution;
USP 25: Fluoxetine Capsules; Fluoxetine Oral Solution.

Proprietary Preparations (details are given in Part 3)
Aust.: Felicium; Fluctine; Fluoxibene; Flux; Mutan; Positivum; **Austral.:** Auscap; Erocap†; Fluohexal; Lovan; Prozac; Zactin; **Belg.:** Prozac; **Braz.:** Daforin; Deprax; Eufor; Fluxene; Prozac; Verotina; **Canad.:** Prozac; **Denm.:** Afeksin; Flutin; Fluxantin; Fondur; Fontex; Fonzac; Nycoflox; **Fin.:** Fluxantin; Fontex; Seromex; Seronil; **Fr.:** Prozac; **Ger.:** Fluctin; Fluneurin; Fluox-Puren; Fluoxemerck; Fluxet; Motivone; **Hong Kong:** Magrilan; Provatine; Prozac; **Irl.:** Affex; Gerozac; Norzac; Prozac; Prozamel; Prozatan; **Israel:** Affectine; Flutine; Prizma; Prozac; **Ital.:** Diesan; Fluoxeren; Prozac; **Mex.:** Fluoxac; Prozac; Siqual; **Neth.:** Prozac; **Norw.:** Fontex; Nycoflox; **NZ:** Fluox; Lovan; Plinzene; Prozac; **Port.:** Digassim; Nodepe; Prozac; Psipax; Salipax; Tuneluz; **S.Afr.:** Lorien; Nuzak; Prozac; Prozynt†; Sanzur; **Singapore:** Deprexin; Fluxetin; Magrilan; Prodep; Prozac; Zactin; **Spain:** Adofen; Astrin; Nodepe; Prozac; Reneuron; **Swed.:** Fontex; Seroscand; **Switz.:** Fluctine; Fluocim; Fluoxifar; Flusol; **Thai.:** Atd; Deproxin; Flumed; Fluoxine; Flutine; Fluxetil; Fluxetin; Fluzac; Magrilan; Oxetine; Oxsac; Prodep; Prozac; **UAE:** Flutin; **UK:** Felicium; Prozac; **USA:** Prozac; Sarafem.

Fluvoxamine Maleate (12768-h)

Fluvoxamine Maleate (*BANM, USAN, rINNM*).
DU-23000. (*E*)-5-Methoxy-4′-trifluoromethylvalerophenone O-2-aminoethyloxime maleate.
$C_{15}H_{21}F_3N_2O_2,C_4H_4O_4 = 434.4$.
CAS — 54739-18-3 (fluvoxamine); 61718-82-9 (fluvoxamine maleate).

Pharmacopoeias. In Br.

Pharmacopoeial description

BP 2001: A white to almost white crystalline powder. Sparingly soluble in water; freely soluble in alcohol and in methyl alcohol.

Adverse Effects, Treatment, and Precautions

As for SSRIs in general (see Fluoxetine, p.284).

Bradycardia with ECG changes has been noted with fluvoxamine (see also Effects on the Cardiovascular System in Adverse Effects of Fluoxetine, p.284).

It is recommended that fluvoxamine should be withdrawn in patients who have an increase in serum concentrations of liver enzymes.

Fluvoxamine should be given in low initial dosage to patients with hepatic impairment. US and UK manufacturers vary in that they recommend similar reductions in the elderly and those with renal impairment respectively.

◊ The UK Committee on Safety of Medicines has reported[1] that between 25 September 1986 and 23 March 1988 it had received 961 reports of adverse reactions associated with the use of fluvoxamine and that these included 5 deaths. The most frequently reported reactions were nausea (183) and vomiting (101). Other reactions included dizziness, somnolence, agitation, headache, tremor, and, during the first few days, worsening of anxiety. There were 13 reports of convulsions. Reports of appetite stimulation and antimuscarinic reactions were unusual. The effects sometimes resolved with time or dose reduction.
The safety profile of fluvoxamine has been reviewed.[2] For a comparison of the adverse reaction profile of fluoxetine with that of fluvoxamine, see under Adverse Effects of Fluoxetine, p.284.

1. Committee on Safety of Medicines. Fluvoxamine (Faverin): adverse reaction profile. *Current Problems* 22 1988.
2. Wagner W, *et al.* Fluvoxamine: a review of its safety profile in world-wide studies. *Int Clin Psychopharmacol* 1994; **9**: 223–7.

Interactions

For interactions associated with SSRIs, see Fluoxetine, p.287.

Fluvoxamine can greatly increase plasma concentrations of theophylline (see p.780), and it is recommended that concomitant use should be avoided or, if this is not possible, the dose of theophylline should be halved and plasma-theophylline concentrations monitored more closely.

◊ References.
1. Wagner W, Vause EW. Fluvoxamine: a review of global drug-drug interaction data. *Clin Pharmacokinet* 1995; **29** (suppl 1): 26–32.

Pharmacokinetics

Fluvoxamine is readily absorbed from the gastrointestinal tract with peak plasma concentrations occurring 2 to 8 hours after administration. Systemic bioavailability does not appear to be affected by food. It is extensively metabolised, by oxidative demethylation and deamination, in the liver to inactive metabolites. Excretion is mainly in the urine. Fluvoxamine is widely distributed throughout the body and protein binding is reported to be about 80%; it has a plasma-elimination half-life of about 15 hours. Fluvoxamine is distributed into breast milk (see Breast Feeding under Precautions in Fluoxetine, p.286).

◊ References.
1. De Bree H, *et al.* Fluvoxamine maleate: disposition in man. *Eur J Drug Metab Pharmacokinet* 1983; **8:** 175–9.
2. Overmars H, *et al.* Fluvoxamine maleate: metabolism in man. *Eur J Drug Metab Pharmacokinet* 1983; **8:** 269–80.
3. van Harten J, *et al.* Pharmacokinetics of fluvoxamine maleate in patients with liver cirrhosis after single-dose oral administration. *Clin Pharmacokinet* 1993; **24:** 177–82.
4. Perucca E, *et al.* Clinical pharmacokinetics of fluvoxamine. *Clin Pharmacokinet* 1994; **27:** 175–90.
5. van Harten J. Overview of the pharmacokinetics of fluvoxamine. *Clin Pharmacokinet* 1995; **29** (suppl 1): 1–9.
6. Xu Z-H, *et al.* In vivo inhibition of CYP2C19 but not CYP2D6 by fluvoxamine. *Br J Clin Pharmacol* 1996; **42:** 518–21.
7. Spigset O, *et al.* Non-linear fluvoxamine disposition. *Br J Clin Pharmacol* 1998; **45:** 257–63.

Uses and Administration

Fluvoxamine, an aralkylketone derivative, is an SSRI with actions and uses similar to those of fluoxetine (p.288). It is used as the maleate

In the treatment of **depression** fluvoxamine maleate is given by mouth in an initial dose of 100 mg daily; in some patients the dose may need to be gradually increased up to a maximum of 300 mg daily. It is recommended that daily dosages exceeding 100 mg should be given in divided doses.

Fluvoxamine is also used in the management of **obsessive-compulsive disorder**. In the UK, doses are similar to those used in the treatment of depression. The recommended starting dose in the USA is fluvoxamine maleate 50 mg once daily; this dose may be increased by increments of 50 mg every 4 to 7 days to a maximum of 300 mg daily. Doses above 100 mg daily should be given in two divided doses. In the USA, fluvoxamine may also be used in children of 8 years and over with obsessive-compulsive disorder. The recommended starting dose is fluvoxamine maleate 25 mg once daily, which may be increased in increments of 25 mg every 4 to 7 days to a maximum daily dose of 200 mg daily. Daily doses of more than 50 mg should be given as two divided doses. It is recommended that if no improvement of symptoms is observed within 10 weeks, treatment with fluvoxamine should be re-assessed.

Therapy should be begun with a low dose in patients with hepatic impairment, and the patient carefully monitored. Similar caution is recommended by US sources for elderly patients, and by UK sources for those with renal impairment.

Fluvoxamine should be withdrawn gradually to reduce the risk of withdrawal symptoms.

◊ Reviews.
1. Mendlewicz J. Efficacy of fluvoxamine in severe depression. *Drugs* 1992; **43** (suppl 2): 32–9.
2. Wilde ME, *et al.* Fluvoxamine: an updated review of its pharmacology, and therapeutic use in depressive illness. *Drugs* 1993; **46:** 895–924.
3. Palmer KJ, Benfield P. Fluvoxamine: an overview of its pharmacological properties and review of its therapeutic potential in non-depressive disorders. *CNS Drugs* 1994; **1:** 57–87.

Anxiety disorders. Fluvoxamine has been given in a variety of anxiety disorders including obsessive-compulsive disorder (p.649), panic attacks (p.649), and social phobia (see under Phobic Disorders, p.649).

References.
1. Jenike MA, *et al.* A controlled trial of fluvoxamine in obsessive-compulsive disorder: implications for a serotonergic theory. *Am J Psychiatry* 1990; **147:** 1209–15.
2. Mallya GK, *et al.* Short- and long-term treatment of obsessive-compulsive disorder with fluvoxamine. *Ann Clin Psychiatry* 1992; **4:** 77–80.

3. Black DW, *et al.* A comparison of fluvoxamine, cognitive therapy, and placebo in the treatment of panic disorder. *Arch Gen Psychiatry* 1993; **50:** 44–50.
4. Hoehn-Saric R, *et al.* Effect of fluvoxamine on panic disorder. *J Clin Psychopharmacol* 1993; **13:** 321–6.
5. van Vliet IM, *et al.* Psychopharmacological treatment of social phobia: a double blind placebo controlled study with fluvoxamine. *Psychopharmacology (Berl)* 1994; **115:** 128–34.
6. Freeman CPL, *et al.* Fluvoxamine versus clomipramine in the treatment of obsessive compulsive disorder: a multicenter, randomized, double-blind, parallel group comparison. *J Clin Psychiatry* 1994; **55:** 301–5.
7. Greist JH, *et al.* Efficacy of fluvoxamine in obsessive-compulsive disorder: results of a multicentre, double blind, placebo-controlled trial. *Eur J Clin Res* 1995; **7:** 195–204.
8. Stein MB, *et al.* Fluvoxamine treatment of social phobia (social anxiety disorder): a double-blind placebo-controlled study. *Am J Psychiatry* 1999; **156:** 756–60.
9. The Research Unit on Pediatric Psychopharmacology Anxiety Study Group. Fluvoxamine for the treatment of anxiety disorders in children and adolescents. *N Engl J Med* 2001; **344:** 1279–85.

Preparations

BP 2001: Fluvoxamine Tablets.

Proprietary Preparations (details are given in Part 3)
Aust.: Floxyfral; *Austral.:* Faverin; Luvox; *Belg.:* Floxyfral; *Canad.:* Luvox; *Denm.:* Fevarin; *Fin.:* Fevarin; *Fr.:* Floxyfral; *Ger.:* Desifluvoxamin; Fevarin; Fluvoxadura; *Hong Kong:* Faverin; *Irl.:* Faverin; *Israel:* Favoxil; *Ital.:* Dumirox; Fevarin; Maveral; *Mex.:* Luvox; *Neth.:* Fevarin; *Norw.:* Fevarin; *Port.:* Dumyrox; *S.Afr.:* Luvox; *Singapore:* Faverin; *Spain:* Dumirox; *Swed.:* Fevarin; *Switz.:* Floxyfral; *Thai.:* Faverin; *UK:* Faverin; *USA:* Luvox.

Hypericum (314-s)

Hyperici Herba; Johanniskraut; Millepertuis; St. John's Wort.
CAS — 548-04-9 (hypericin).

Pharmacopoeias. In Eur. (see p.vi) and Pol. Also in USNF. Swiss also includes monographs for hypericum (fresh flowering tops) and hypericum oil.

Pharmacopoeial description
Ph. Eur.: The whole or cut, dried flowering tops of *Hypericum perforatum* gathered during flowering. It contains not less than 0.08% of total hypericins, expressed as hypericin $(C_{30}H_{16}O_8 = 504.4)$ calculated with reference to the dried drug. Protect from light.
USNF 20: The dried flowering tops or aerial parts of *Hypericum perforatum* (Hypericaceae), gathered shortly before or during flowering. It contains not less than 0.04% of total hypericins, calculated as hypericin $(C_{30}H_{16}O_8)$. Store in airtight containers. Protect from light.

Adverse Effects and Precautions
Adverse effects reported with hypericum have included gastrointestinal symptoms, allergic reactions, and fatigue. Photosensitivity has also been reported; hypericin and pseudohypericin are the constituents of hypericum thought to be responsible for this reaction.

Effects on the nervous system. Subacute polyneuropathy following sun exposure developed in a woman who had taken hypericum for mild depression; she improved following drug withdrawal.[1]
1. Bove GM. Acute neuropathy after exposure to sun in a patient treated with St John's Wort. *Lancet* 1998; **352:** 1121–2.

Effects on the skin. In addition to photosensitivity reactions associated with hypericum use,[1] there has been a report of severe erythroderma in a patient who supplemented his regular antidepressant medication (dothiepin [dosulepin]) with hypericum.[2] The reaction was seen on both light-exposed and non-exposed areas, and was thought to be due to the hypericum although there remained a possibility that it was due to an interaction between the 2 drugs.
1. Lane-Brown MM. Photosensitivity associated with herbal preparations of St John's wort (Hypericum perforatum). *Med J Aust* 2000; **172:** 302.
2. Holme SA, Roberts DL. Erythroderma associated with St John's wort. *Br J Dermatol* 2000; **143:** 1127–8.

Interactions
Hypericum has been shown to induce several drug metabolising enzymes including some cytochrome P450 isoenzymes (in particular CYP3A4) and the transport protein P-glycoprotein. Clinically important interactions resulting in decreased plasma concentrations of the interacting drug have been reported with ciclosporin, digoxin, HIV-protease inhibitors such as indinavir, oral contraceptives, theophylline, and warfarin. There is also a theoretical possibility of an interaction between hypericum and antiepileptics such as carbamazepine (p.344), phenobarbital (p.355), and phenytoin (p.360). In addition, stopping hypericum may result in increased, and possibly toxic, concentrations of the interacting drug.

In many countries, including the UK, preparations of hypericum are not required to be licensed, and the amount of active ingredient may vary widely between preparations. Changing preparations may therefore alter the degree of enzyme induction.

Concomitant administration of hypericum with drugs known to act on the same neurotransmitters may result in synergistic interactions and an increased risk of adverse effects may also occur. Examples include the SSRIs (see p.306) and the selective serotonin (5-HT$_1$) agonists (see p.457) used to treat migraine.

◊ References.
1. Roby CA, *et al.* St John's Wort: effect on CYP3A4 activity. *Clin Pharmacol Ther* 2000; **67:** 451–7.
2. Committee on Safety of Medicines/Medicines Control Agency. Reminder: St John's Wort (Hypericum perforatum) interactions. *Current Problems* 2000; **26:** 6–7.
3. Dürr D, *et al.* St John's Wort induces intestinal p-glycoprotein/MDR1 and intestinal and hepatic CYP3A4. *Clin Pharmacol Ther* 2000; **68:** 598–604.

Anticoagulants. For mention of a possible interaction between hypericum and warfarin, see p.997.

Antivirals. For details of a possible interaction between hypericum and HIV-protease inhibitors such as indinavir, see p.626.

Cardiac glycosides. For details of a possible interaction between hypericum and digoxin, see p.872.

Ciclosporin. For details of possible interactions between hypericum and ciclosporin, see p.521.

Oral contraceptives. For a report of a possible interaction between hypericum and oral contraceptives, see p.1459.

Xanthines. For details of a possible interaction between hypericum and theophylline, see p.780.

Uses and Administration
Herbal preparations containing hypericum are used, frequently for self-medication, in the treatment of depression. Such preparations are also promoted for the treatment of other nervous disorders such as insomnia and anxiety, particularly if associated with the menopause. Hypericum oil has also been used as an astringent. Hypericin, a major constituent of hypericum, has been investigated as an antiviral in the treatment of HIV infection and AIDS (but see below).

The amount of active constituents can vary between different preparations and doses depend on the preparation being taken. Hypericum has been used in homoeopathic preparations.

◊ References.
1. McIntyre M. A review of the benefits, adverse events, drug interactions, and safety of St. John's Wort (Hypericum perforatum): the implications with regard to the regulation of herbal medicines. *J Altern Complement Med* 2000; **6:** 115–24.

Antiviral action. A study involving 30 HIV-infected patients suggested that hypericin, given intravenously or by mouth, produced significant phototoxicity and had no effect on virological markers or CD4 cell count.[1]
1. Gulick RM, *et al.* Phase I studies of hypericin, the active compound in St John's Wort, as an antiretroviral agent in HIV-infected adults. *Ann Intern Med* 1999; **130:** 510–14.

Depression. Hypericum extracts are widely used in some countries for the treatment of depression (p.271).

A meta-analysis[1] of randomised trials found hypericum extracts to be more effective than placebo in mild to moderately severe depressive disorders, and was supported by a subsequent systematic review.[2] However, there was insufficient evidence available to establish relative efficacy and tolerability compared with standard antidepressants,[1] although experience from those populations in whom hypericum extracts are widely used suggests that the herb may offer an advantage in terms of relative safety and tolerability.[3] Longer term studies are required before the herb can be recommended in major depression;[2,3] a multicentre randomised controlled trial found hypericum extract to be ineffective in patients with major depression.[4]

The mechanism of action of hypericum extracts in the treatment of depression remains unclear. Extracts contain at least 10 active principles. It was originally believed that hypericin, one of the major constituents of hypericum, was responsible for the antidepressant effect since it had an inhibitory action on monoamine oxidase *in vitro*. However it was subsequently demonstrated that this action was, at best, weak and it is now generally believed that monoamine oxidase inhibition is not responsible for the antidepressant effect of hypericum. More recent studies have suggested that hyperforin may be one of the major constituents responsible for the antidepressant effect.[5] Although the evidence is mainly from *in vitro* studies, hyperforin inhibits the reuptake of several major neurotransmitters including serotonin, dopamine, and noradrenaline.[6]

1. Linde K, Mulrow CD. St John's wort for depression (updated 20 September 1999). Available in the Cochrane Library; Issue 4. Oxford: Update Software; 2000.
2. Stevinson C, Ernst E. Hypericum for depression: an update of the clinical evidence. *Eur Neuropsychopharmacol* 1999; **9:** 501–5.
3. de Smet PAGM, Nolen WA. St John's wort as an antidepressant. *BMJ* 1996; **313:** 241–2.
4. Shelton RC, *et al.* Effectiveness of St John's Wort in major depression: a randomized controlled trial. *JAMA* 2001; **285:** 1978–86.
5. Laakmann G, *et al.* St. John's Wort in mild to moderate depression: the relevance of hyperforin for the clinical efficacy. *Pharmacopsychiatry* 1998; **31** (suppl.): 54–9.
6. Chatterjee SS, *et al.* Hyperforin as a possible antidepressant component of hypericum extracts. *Life Sci* 1998; **63:** 499–510.

Preparations

Proprietary Preparations (details are given in Part 3)
Aust.: Esbericum; Jarsin; Kira; Psychotonin; *Austral.:* Bioglan Stress-Relax; Hyperiforte; Remotiv; *Ger.:* Aristo; Aristoforat; Cesradyston; Cesran; Divinal Seda†; dysto-lux; Esbericum; Felis; Futuran; Helarium; Herbaneurin; Hyperforat; Hypericaps; Hyperimerck; Hyperpur; Jarsin; Jukunda Rotol; Kira; Kytta-Modal;

Laif; LomaHypericum; mct Psycho Dragees N†; Nervei; Neuroplant; Neurotisan†; Neurovegetalin; Psychotonin; Psychotonin M; Remotiv; Rephahyval†; Rotol†; Sedovegan; Spilan; Syxal; Texx; Tonizin; Turineurin; Viviplus; **Mex.:** Hiperikan; Remotiv; **Singapore:** Lomahypericum; **Spain:** Arkocapsulas Hiperico; Hiperico; Kajel; Quetzal; Tolecen; **Switz.:** Felis; Hyperiforce; HyperiMed; Hyperiplant; Hyperval; Jarsin; Lucilium; Mandal 425; Movina; ReBalance; Remotiv; Valverde Hyperval†; **UK:** Kira.

Multi-ingredient: Aust.: Eryval; Magentee EF-EM-ES; Nervetee; Species nervinae; Vulpuran; Wechseltee; **Austral.:** Anti-Flamme; Bioglan 3B Beer Belly Buster; Feminine Herbal Complex; Infant Tonic; Irontona; Joint & Muscle Relief Cream; Nappy Rash Relief Cream; Skin Healing Cream; Vitatona; **Fr.:** Cicaderma†; **Ger.:** anabol-loges; Anisan; Arthrodynat P; Befelka-Oel; Cefaktivon; Cefaktivon "novum"†; Cheiranthol; Discmigon; Dolo-cyl; Gastritol; Gastrol S; Gutnacht; Hewepsychon duo; Hocura-Spondylose novo; Hyperesa; Hyperforat-forte; JuCholan S†; JuDorm; JuNeuron S†; JuViton; Kneipp Herz- und Kreislauf-Tee; Kneipp Krauter Taschenkur Nerven und Schlaf N; Marianon; Neurapas; Oxacant N; Phytogran; Presselin Arterien K 5 P; Presselin Nerven K 1 N; Psychotonin-sed; Remifemin plus; Rhoival; Salus Nerven-Schlaf-Tee Nr.22†; Salusan†; Sedariston; Sedariston Konzentrat; Sinedyston†; Valena N; Venacton; Vollmers praprarierter gruner; **Ital.:** Elisir Depurativo Ambrosiano; Mithen; Neumoral; **Port.:** Cicaderma; **Switz.:** Alpina Gel a la consoude†; Cetona Plus; Gel a la consoude; Huile de millepertuis A. Vogel (huile de St. Jean); Hyperiforce comp; Keppur; Malvedrin; Phytoberidin; Pommade Po-Ho N A Vogel; Saltrates; Saltrates Rodell; Tai Ginseng N; Yakona N†; **UK:** Savlon Natural First Aid for Burns; Savlon Natural First Aid for Cuts & Sores; Savlon Natural First Aid for Insect Bites & Stings; St Johnswort Compound.

Imipramine   (2514-w)

Imipramine (BAN, rINN).

3-(10,11-Dihydro-5H-dibenz[b,f]azepin-5-yl)propyldimethylamine.

$C_{19}H_{24}N_2 = 280.4$.
CAS — 50-49-7.
ATC — N06AA02.

Imipramine 8.8 mg is approximately equivalent to 10 mg of imipramine hydrochloride.

Imipramine Embonate   (2515-e)

Imipramine Embonate (BANM, rINNM).
Imipramine Pamoate.
$(C_{19}H_{24}N_2)_2, C_{23}H_{16}O_6 = 949.2$.
CAS — 10075-24-8.

Imipramine embonate 15 mg is approximately equivalent to 10 mg of imipramine hydrochloride.

Imipramine Hydrochloride   (2516-l)

Imipramine Hydrochloride (BANM, rINNM).
Imipram. Hydrochlor.; Imipramini Chloridum; Imipramini Hydrochloridum; Imizine.
$C_{19}H_{24}N_2, HCl = 316.9$.
CAS — 113-52-0.
Pharmacopoeias. In Chin., Eur. (see p.vi), Int., Jpn, Pol., and US.

Pharmacopoeial description

Ph. Eur.: A white or slightly yellow crystalline powder. Freely soluble in water and in alcohol; practically insoluble in ether. A 10% solution in water has a pH of 3.6 to 5.0. Protect from light.

USP 25: A white to off-white, odourless or practically odourless, crystalline powder. Freely soluble in water and in alcohol; soluble in acetone; insoluble in ether and in benzene. Store in airtight containers.

Adverse Effects, Treatment, and Precautions

As for tricyclic antidepressants in general (see Amitriptyline, p.273).

Porphyria. Imipramine has been associated with acute attacks of porphyria and is considered unsafe in porphyric patients.

Interactions

For interactions associated with tricyclic antidepressants, see Amitriptyline, p.276.

Pharmacokinetics

Imipramine is readily absorbed from the gastrointestinal tract, and extensively demethylated by first-pass metabolism in the liver, to its primary active metabolite, desipramine.

Paths of metabolism of both imipramine and desipramine include hydroxylation and N-oxidation. Imipramine is excreted in the urine, mainly in the form of its metabolites, either free or in conjugated form; small amounts are excreted in the faeces via the bile.

Imipramine and desipramine are widely distributed throughout the body and are extensively bound to

plasma and tissue protein. Imipramine has been estimated to have an elimination half-life ranging from 9 to 28 hours, which may be considerably extended in overdosage. Plasma concentrations of imipramine and desipramine vary very widely between individuals but some correlation with therapeutic response has been established.

Imipramine and desipramine cross the blood-brain barrier and placenta and are distributed into breast milk (see Breast Feeding under Precautions in Amitriptyline, p.275).

◊ References.
1. Sallee FR, Pollock BG. Clinical pharmacokinetics of imipramine and desipramine. Clin Pharmacokinet 1990; 18: 346–64.

Uses and Administration

Imipramine is a dibenzazepine tricyclic antidepressant with actions and uses similar to those of amitriptyline (p.278). Imipramine is one of the less sedating tricyclics and has moderate antimuscarinic activity. Imipramine is usually given by mouth as the hydrochloride or embonate, with doses expressed in terms of the hydrochloride.

In the treatment of **depression**, the usual daily dose of imipramine hydrochloride is up to 75 mg in divided doses initially, gradually increased to 150 to 200 mg daily as necessary; higher doses of up to 300 mg daily may be required in severely depressed patients in hospital. A suggested initial dose for the elderly in the UK is 10 mg at night, gradually increasing to 30 to 50 mg daily. In the USA, daily doses of 25 to 50 mg are recommended for initial therapy in the elderly and adolescents increasing to a maximum of 100 mg daily as required. Since imipramine has a prolonged half-life, once-daily dosage regimens may also be suitable, usually given at night.

In the initial stages of treatment, if administration by mouth is impracticable or inadvisable, up to 100 mg of imipramine hydrochloride may be given daily in divided doses by intramuscular injection, but oral administration should be substituted as soon as possible.

Imipramine is also used for the treatment of **nocturnal enuresis** in children in whom organic pathology has been excluded. However, drug therapy for nocturnal enuresis should be reserved for those in whom other methods have failed and should preferably only be given to cover periods away from home; tricyclic antidepressants are not recommended in children under 6 years of age (some authorities recommend that they should not be given until 7 years of age). Suggested doses of imipramine hydrochloride are 25 mg for children aged 6 to 7 years (20 to 25 kg bodyweight), 25 to 50 mg for children aged 8 to 11 years (25 to 35 kg body-weight), and 50 to 75 mg for children aged over 11 years (35 to 54 kg body-weight). The dose should be taken just before bedtime and treatment, including the gradual period of withdrawal, should not continue for longer than 3 months. A full physical examination is recommended before a further course.

Imipramine oxide hydrochloride (imipraminoxide hydrochloride) is also used as an antidepressant and for nocturnal enuresis.

Imipramine should be withdrawn gradually to reduce the risk of withdrawal symptoms.

Anxiety disorders. See under Clomipramine, p.282.
Some references to the use of imipramine in anxiety disorders are given below.
1. Cross-National Collaborative Panic Study, Second Phase Investigators. Drug treatment of panic disorder: comparative efficacy of alprazolam, imipramine, and placebo. Br J Psychiatry 1992; 160: 191–202.
2. Lepola UM, et al. Three-year follow-up of patients with panic disorder after short-term treatment with alprazolam and imipramine. Int Clin Psychopharmacol 1993; 8: 115–18.
3. Rickels K, et al. Antidepressants for the treatment of generalised anxiety disorder: a placebo-controlled comparison of imipramine, trazodone, and diazepam. Arch Gen Psychiatry 1993; 50: 884–95.
4. Clark DM, et al. A comparison of cognitive therapy, applied relaxation and imipramine in the treatment of panic disorder. Br J Psychiatry 1994; 164: 759–69.
5. Barlow DH, et al. Cognitive-behavioral therapy, imipramine, or their combination for panic disorder: a randomized controlled trial. JAMA 2000; 283: 2529–36. Correction. ibid.; 284: 2597.

Hyperactivity. See under Desipramine, p.283.

Pain. Antidepressants, usually amitriptyline or another tricyclic, are useful in alleviating some types of pain (p.2) when given in subantidepressant doses.
Some references to the use of imipramine are given below.
1. Kvinesdal B, et al. Imipramine treatment of painful diabetic neuropathy. JAMA 1984; 251: 1727–30.
2. Walsh TD. Controlled study of imipramine and morphine in chronic pain due to advanced cancer. Proc Am Soc Clin Oncol 1986; 5: 237.
3. Hummel T, et al. A comparison of the antinociceptive effects of imipramine, tramadol and anpirtoline. Br J Clin Pharmacol 1994; 37: 325–33.
4. Cannon RO, et al. Imipramine in patients with chest pain despite normal coronary angiograms. N Engl J Med 1994; 330: 1411–17.
5. Godfrey RG. A guide to the understanding and use of tricyclic antidepressants in the overall management of fibromyalgia and other chronic pain syndromes. Arch Intern Med 1996; 156: 1047–52.

Preparations

BP 2001: Imipramine Tablets;
USP 25: Imipramine Hydrochloride Injection; Imipramine Hydrochloride Tablets.

Proprietary Preparations (details are given in Part 3)
Aust.: Tofranil; **Austral.:** Melipramine; Tofranil; **Belg.:** Tofranil; **Braz.:** Tofranil; **Canad.:** Impril†; Novo-Pramine†; Tofranil; **Fr.:** Tofranil; **Ger.:** Pryleugan; Tofranil; **Hong Kong:** Tofranil; **Irl.:** Tofranil; **Israel:** Primonil; Tofranil; **Ital.:** Tofranil; **Mex.:** Talpramin; Tofranil; **Neth.:** Tofranil; **Norw.:** Tofranil†; **Port.:** Tofranil; **S.Afr.:** Ethipramine; Medipramine†; Mipralin†; Tofranil; **Spain:** Tofranil; **Swed.:** Tofranil; **Switz.:** Tofranil; **Thai.:** Antidep; Celamine; Sermonil; Tofranil; Topramine; **UK:** Tofranil; **USA:** Imp-Tab†; Janimine†; Tofranil; Tofranil-PM.

Iprindole Hydrochloride   (2518-j)

Iprindole Hydrochloride (BANM, rINNM).
Pramindole Hydrochloride; Wy-3263 (iprindole). 5-(3-Dimethylaminopropyl)-6,7,8,9,10,11-hexahydrocyclo-oct[b]indole hydrochloride.
$C_{19}H_{28}N_2, HCl = 320.9$.
CAS — 5560-72-5 (iprindole); 20432-64-8 (iprindole hydrochloride).
NOTE. Iprindole is USAN.

Profile
Iprindole hydrochloride has actions and uses similar to those of amitriptyline (p.273), but it only has weak antimuscarinic and sedative effects. It has been used as an alternative to tricyclic antidepressants for the treatment of depression.

Iproniazid Phosphate   (2520-p)

Iproniazid Phosphate (BANM, rINNM).
2'-Isopropylisonicotinohydrazide phosphate.
$C_9H_{13}N_3O, H_3PO_4 = 277.2$.
CAS — 54-92-2 (iproniazid); 305-33-9 (iproniazid phosphate).

Iproniazid phosphate 155 mg is approximately equivalent to 100 mg of iproniazid.

Adverse Effects, Treatment, and Precautions
As for MAOIs in general (see Phenelzine, p.303).

Effects on the liver. Of 91 cases of hepatitis due to antidepressant therapy, cytolytic reactions occurred in 11 treated with iproniazid.[1] Five patients died, 3 of them after involuntary rechallenge. High levels of antimitochondrial antibody were found in 5 patients.
1. Lefebure B, et al. Hépatites aux antidépresseurs. Therapie 1984; 39: 509–16.

Porphyria. Iproniazid has been associated with acute attacks of porphyria and is considered unsafe in porphyric patients.

Interactions
For interactions associated with MAOIs, see Phenelzine, p.305.

Uses and Administration
Iproniazid, a hydrazine derivative, is an irreversible inhibitor of both monoamine oxidase types A and B with actions and uses similar to those of phenelzine (p.307).

Iproniazid is used in the treatment of depression, but as discussed on p.271 the risks associated with irreversible non-selective MAOIs usually mean that other antidepressants are preferred. It is given by mouth as the phosphate in initial doses equivalent to iproniazid 50 to 150 mg daily. Once a response has been obtained the dosage may be gradually reduced for maintenance therapy; some patients may respond to 25 to 50 mg daily or every other day.

Iproniazid should be withdrawn gradually to reduce the risk of withdrawal symptoms.

Iproniazid is the isopropyl derivative of isoniazid (see p.215) and was developed for use in tuberculosis, but owing to its toxicity is no longer used for this purpose.

Preparations
Proprietary Preparations (details are given in Part 3)
Fr.: Marsilid.

The symbol † denotes a preparation no longer actively marketed

Isocarboxazid (2521-s)

Isocarboxazid (BAN, rINN).

Ro-50831. 2'-Benzyl-5-methylisoxazole-3-carbohydrazide.

$C_{12}H_{13}N_3O_2 = 231.3$.

CAS — 59-63-2.

ATC — N06AF01.

Adverse Effects, Treatment, and Precautions
As for MAOIs in general (see Phenelzine, p.303).

Interactions
For interactions associated with MAOIs, see Phenelzine, p.305.

Pharmacokinetics
Isocarboxazid is readily absorbed from the gastrointestinal tract reaching peak plasma concentrations 3 to 5 hours after ingestion. It is metabolised by the liver, and is excreted in the urine mainly in the form of metabolites.

Uses and Administration
Isocarboxazid, a hydrazine derivative, is an irreversible inhibitor of both monoamine oxidase types A and B with actions and uses similar to those of phenelzine (p.307).

Isocarboxazid is used in the treatment of depression but as discussed on p.271 the risks associated with irreversible non-selective MAOIs usually mean that other antidepressants are preferred. It is given by mouth in an initial dose of 30 mg daily in single or divided doses. If no improvement occurs after 4 weeks, doses of up to 60 mg daily can be tried for up to 4 to 6 weeks. Once a response has been obtained the dosage may be gradually reduced to a maintenance dose of 10 to 20 mg daily, although doses of up to 40 mg daily may be needed in some patients. Half the normal maintenance dose may be adequate in the elderly.

Isocarboxazid should be withdrawn gradually to reduce the risk of withdrawal symptoms.

Preparations
Proprietary Preparations (details are given in Part 3)
Denm.: Marplan; *UK:* Marplan; *USA:* Marplan.

Lithium Carbonate (5057-h)

Lithium Carbonate (USAN).

CP-15467-61; Lithii Carbonas; Lithium Carb.; NSC-16895.

$Li_2CO_3 = 73.89$.

CAS — 554-13-2.

NOTE. Commercially available lithium materials have atomic weights ranging from 6.939 to 6.996. The molecular weight of lithium carbonate of 73.89 given above has been calculated using the lowest atomic weight; using the highest figure would give a molecular weight of 74.00. This difference does not affect the figure of 27 mmol of lithium being provided by 1 g of lithium carbonate. Nor should it affect the outcome of assays of serum-lithium concentrations given the limits of error of the assay methods. However, while it is doubtful that there would be any discernible effect on serum concentrations resulting from this atomic weight variance in a patient changing to a different lithium preparation, the different pharmacokinetic characteristics still have to be considered.

Pharmacopoeias. In Chin., Eur. (see p.vi), Int., Jpn, Pol., and US.

Each g represents 27 mmol of lithium.

Pharmacopoeial description

Ph. Eur.: A white powder. Slightly soluble in water; practically insoluble in alcohol.

USP 25: A white odourless granular powder. Sparingly soluble in water, very slightly soluble in alcohol; dissolves, with effervescence, in dilute mineral acids.

Lithium Citrate (7058-t)

Lithii Citras.

$C_6H_5Li_3O_7,4H_2O = 282.0$.

CAS — 919-16-4 (anhydrous lithium citrate); 6080-58-6 (lithium citrate tetrahydrate).

NOTE. Commercially available lithium materials have atomic weights ranging from 6.939 to 6.996. The molecular weight of lithium citrate of 282.0 given above has been calculated using the lowest atomic weight; using the highest figure would give a molecular weight of 282.1. This difference does not affect the figure of 10.6 mmol of lithium being provided by 1 g of lithium citrate. Nor should it affect the outcome of assays of serum-lithium concentrations given the limits of error of the assay methods. However, while it is doubtful that there would be any discernible effect on serum concentrations resulting from this atomic weight variance in a patient changing to a different lithium preparation, the different pharmacokinetic characteristics still have to be considered.

Pharmacopoeias. In Eur. (see p.vi) and US.

US also includes lithium hydroxide.

Each g represents 10.6 mmol of lithium.

Pharmacopoeial description

Ph. Eur.: A white or almost white fine crystalline powder. Freely soluble in water; slightly soluble in alcohol.

USP 25: A white odourless deliquescent powder or granules. Freely soluble in water; slightly soluble in alcohol. pH of a 5% solution in water is between 7.0 and 10.0. Store in airtight containers.

Adverse Effects

Many of the side-effects of lithium are dose-related and the margin between the therapeutic and toxic dose is narrow.

Initial adverse effects of lithium therapy include nausea, diarrhoea, vertigo, muscle weakness, and a dazed feeling; these effects often abate with continued therapy. Fine hand tremors, polyuria, and polydipsia may, however, persist. Other adverse effects that may occur at therapeutic serum-lithium concentrations include weight gain and oedema (which should not be treated with diuretics). Hypercalcaemia, hypermagnesaemia, and hyperparathyroidism have been reported. Skin disorders such as acne, psoriasis, and rashes may be exacerbated by lithium therapy. Leucocytosis is a relatively common adverse effect. Long-term adverse effects include hypothyroidism and/or goitre, rarely hyperthyroidism, and mild cognitive and memory impairment. Histological and functional changes in the kidney have been noted following long-term use of therapeutic concentrations of lithium (but see under Effects on the Kidneys, below).

Toxic effects may be expected at serum-lithium concentrations of about 1.5 mmol per litre, although they can appear at lower concentrations. They call for immediate withdrawal of treatment and should always be considered very seriously.

Signs of lithium toxicity include increasing diarrhoea, vomiting, anorexia, muscle weakness, lethargy, giddiness with ataxia, lack of coordination, tinnitus, blurred vision, coarse tremor of the extremities and lower jaw, muscle hyperirritability, choreoathetoid movements, dysarthria, and drowsiness. Symptoms of severe overdosage at serum-lithium concentrations above 2 mmol per litre include hyperreflexia and hyperextension of limbs, syncope, toxic psychosis, seizures, polyuria, renal failure, electrolyte imbalance, dehydration, circulatory failure, coma, and occasionally death. The hazards of lithium in pregnant patients are discussed under Pregnancy in Precautions, below.

Effects on the blood. There has been a report of a patient developing thrombocytopenia after restarting lithium therapy following a gap of some weeks.[1] Withdrawing the lithium led to an improvement in platelet count, but the count fell when lithium therapy was tried again. Leucocytosis is a recognised effect of lithium which this patient also experienced. Although concerns about leukaemia induction have not been verified, the author noted earlier reports of aplastic and megaloblastic anaemia and a case of fatal haemolytic anaemia reported to the UK Committee on Safety of Medicines.

1. Collins S. Thrombocytopenia associated with lithium carbonate. BMJ 1992; **305:** 159.

Effects on the cardiovascular system. Reports of adverse effects on the heart associated with lithium have included bradycardia due to sinus node dysfunction,[1] which has persisted after stopping lithium,[2] premature ventricular contractions,[3] atrioventricular block,[4] and T-wave depression.[5] For the adverse cardiac effects associated with lithium intoxication, see under Overdosage, below.

For mention of myocarditis associated with lithium therapy, see under Effects on the Musculoskeletal System, below.

1. Montalescot G, *et al.* Serious sinus node dysfunction caused by therapeutic doses of lithium. *Int J Cardiol* 1984; **5:** 94–6.
2. Palileo EV, *et al.* Persistent sinus node dysfunction secondary to lithium therapy. *Am Heart J* 1983; **106:** 1443–4.
3. Tangedahl TN, Gau GT. Myocardial irritability associated with lithium carbonate therapy. *N Engl J Med* 1972; **287:** 867–9.
4. Martin CA, Piascik MT. First degree A-V block in patients on lithium carbonate. *Can J Psychiatry* 1985; **30:** 114–16.
5. Demers RG, Heninger GR. Electrocardiographic T-wave changes during lithium carbonate treatment. *JAMA* 1971; **218:** 381–6.

Effects on the endocrine system. The effects of lithium on the endocrine system have been reviewed.[1] Although the published prevalence figures have varied widely there is a small, but definite, risk that patients taking lithium in therapeutic doses will develop clinical *goitre, hypothyroidism,* or, rarely, both; the risk appears to be greatest during the first 2 years of lithium therapy.[2] However some authors[3] suggest that the incidence of clinical hypothyroidism is not more frequent in patients taking lithium than in the general population. Auto-immune atrophic thyroiditis is now thought to be one important pre-disposing factor.[1] Early goitre and lithium-induced hypothyroidism are both reversible if lithium is discontinued; if continued treat-

ment with lithium is desirable the patient should be treated with thyroxine [levothyroxine].

There have been rare reports of *hyperthyroidism* in lithium-treated patients and the association may only be one of coincidence, although it is important to realise that hyperthyroidism can precipitate mania and can also be mistaken for an attack of mania.

Increases in serum concentrations of calcium and parathyroid hormone have been described in patients receiving lithium therapy. Although these are considered to be slight,[1] some patients have experienced *parathyroid hyperplasia.*[4,5]

Cases of *diabetes mellitus* developing in patients treated with lithium have been reported but reviewers did not consider this was attributable to lithium.[1,6]

1. Myers DH, West TET. Hormone systems. In: Johnson FN, ed. *Depression & mania: modern lithium therapy.* Oxford: IRL Press, 1987: 220–6.
2. Vincent A, *et al.* Lithium-associated hypothyroidism: a practical review. *Lithium* 1994; **5:** 73–4.
3. Bocchetta A, *et al.* Six-year follow-up of thyroid function during lithium treatment. *Acta Psychiatr Scand* 1996; **94:** 45–8.
4. Nordenström J, *et al.* Hyperparathyroidism associated with treatment of manic-depressive disorders by lithium. *Eur J Surg* 1992; **158:** 207–11.
5. Taylor JW, Bell AJ. Lithium-induced parathyroid dysfunction: a case report and review of the literature. *Ann Pharmacother* 1993; **27:** 1040–3.
6. Pandit MK, *et al.* Drug-induced disorders of glucose tolerance. *Ann Intern Med* 1993; **118:** 529–39.

Effects on the eyes. The adverse effects of lithium on the eyes have been reviewed by Fraunfelder *et al.*[1] Decrease in accommodation has been reported in up to 10% of patients taking lithium but mainly younger patients are affected. Blurred vision may also occur, most commonly early in therapy, but this may improve with time. Lithium can affect extra-ocular muscles and produce diplopia. A reduction in dosage or discontinuation of therapy may be required. Lithium reduces lachrymal secretions and is excreted in tears in increased concentrations. In rare cases this may result in ocular irritation but this usually causes few problems when artificial tears are used. Photophobia, which occurs rarely with lithium therapy, may also be associated with the excretion of lithium in tears. Lithium can reduce dark adaptation due to a direct neural effect but whether this can progress further to cause irreversible macular or retinal degeneration is not proven. There are some rare but poorly documented reports of deposits in the cornea or conjunctiva. Fraunfelder *et al.* considered that on the evidence available it was unlikely that lithium increased the risk of developing senile cataracts.

Lithium can cause various forms of nystagmus, many of which are reversible on reducing the dose or withdrawal of the drug. However, downbeat nystagmus is a serious adverse effect and is often irreversible. Irreversible oscillopsia can occur rarely secondary to nystagmus. Oculogyric crisis has been associated with lithium therapy and may be exacerbated by concomitant treatment with haloperidol.

Some ocular effects may occur secondary to the effects of lithium on other systems. Exophthalmos and other thyroid-related eye disorders may occur rarely as a secondary effect of lithium on the thyroid. Lithium can also cause pseudotumour cerebri with papilloedema (benign intracranial hypertension). Most cases have occurred a few years after starting therapy but there has been one report of this condition after only 7 months of treatment. Ptosis has been reported, mainly associated with unmasking of myasthenia gravis.

1. Fraunfelder FT, *et al.* The effects of lithium on the human visual system. *J Toxicol Cutan Ocul Toxicol* 1992; **11:** 97–169.

Effects on the kidneys. Lithium is primarily excreted by renal mechanisms. Polyuria, with associated polydipsia, is the most common symptom that results from the effects of lithium on the kidney; the incidence in studies has been stated[1] to range from 4 to 50%. The symptoms are associated with a decreased urinary concentrating ability and are believed to be due to a lithium-induced nephrogenic diabetes insipidus-like syndrome. The polyuria was originally assumed to be a reversible effect, but as a result of several studies showing persisting nephrogenic diabetes insipidus it was suggested that lithium may cause irreversible kidney damage. Patients were identified with renal histological changes that included tubular atrophy, focal interstitial nephropathy and focal fibrosis, and impairment of glomerular filtration rate. However, many of these patients had suffered acute lithium toxicity or severe polyuria and many of the non-specific histological lesions have also been identified in psychiatric patients who have never received lithium. Thus, although patients on long-term maintenance lithium therapy did appear to be susceptible to the development of progressive impairment of urinary concentrating ability it was most noticeable in patients with a history of acute lithium toxicity. The risk of renal damage and impaired glomerular filtration rate was thought to be extremely small in patients on stable maintenance lithium therapy without prior episodes of acute lithium intoxication.[1]

These conclusions were broadly similar to those published later by George[2] who considered that, although it was necessarily an oversimplified view, many, and perhaps all, of the renal side-effects of lithium are induced by excessive dosage. Others have also defended lithium with respect to its renal toxicity and stated that long-term therapy, if properly controlled, does not necessarily lead to chronic or irreversible renal damage.[3-5]

1. Walker RG, Kincaid-Smith P. Kidneys and the fluid regulatory system. In: Johnson FN, ed. *Depression & mania: modern lithium therapy.* Oxford: IRL Press, 1987: 206–13.
2. George CRP. Renal aspects of lithium toxicity. *Med J Aust* 1989; **150:** 291–2.
3. Schou M. Serum lithium monitoring of prophylactic treatment: critical review and updated recommendations. *Clin Pharmacokinet* 1988; **15:** 283–6.
4. Schou M. Lithium treatment of manic-depressive illness: past, present, and perspectives. *JAMA* 1988; **259:** 1834–6.
5. Gitlin M. Lithium and the kidney: an updated review. *Drug Safety* 1999; **20:** 231–43.

Effects on the musculoskeletal system. The effects of lithium on skeletal muscle are represented mainly by varying degrees of weakness and tremor (for further details see under Effects on the Nervous and Neuromuscular Systems, below). Aggravation of myasthenia gravis has been reported. Acute or subacute painful proximal myopathy causing myalgia, cramps, myokymia, or weakness has also been described. Lithium has also been listed as causing toxic myocarditis but a review in 1987 could only trace three cases possibly associated with lithium.[1]

1. Baandrup U, *et al.* Muscle. In: Johnson FN, ed. *Depression & mania: modern lithium therapy.* Oxford: IRL Press, 1987: 236–8.

Effects on the nervous and neuromuscular systems. Neurotoxicity has long been recognised as a potential adverse effect of lithium. The effects of lithium on the nervous system may be minor (which can be minimised by reduction of lithium dose during maintenance therapy) or severe (which warrant immediate and complete withdrawal of the drug).[1] Minor effects have been considered to include decreased concentration and comprehension, impaired short-term memory, restlessness and anxiety, depression, fine rapid tremors, and easy fatigue. Serious or severe effects might include declining cognition and mental status, gait disturbances, movement disorders such as choreoathetosis, myoclonus, and parkinsonism, seizures, cerebellar signs, pseudotumour cerebri (although this was rare), neuroleptic malignant syndrome, myopathy, axonal neuropathy, a myasthenic syndrome, and exacerbation of underlying neuromuscular disease.

In comments[2] on lithium-induced tremor it has been emphasised that there are 2 types. The first is a coarse tremor occurring with impending and actual lithium toxicity and appears to have both cerebellar and parkinsonian components. It is often associated with incoordination, facial spasms, twitching of muscles and limbs, hyperactive reflexes, and more general systemic signs of toxicity. With this type of tremor it was mandatory to stop or decrease the dose of lithium. The second type, which is more common, is a fine tremor, usually occurring within normal therapeutic concentrations, either transiently within a few days of starting treatment or later as a long-standing side-effect. With this type of fine tremor there was evidence to show that a slight decrease in dose may be beneficial.

In addition to the effects mentioned above impairment of taste perception (mainly involving butter and celery)[3] and speech disturbances with few other signs of toxicity[4-6] have been reported.

For further details of the effects of lithium on the nervous system, see under Effects on the Eyes above, Effects on the Musculoskeletal System, above, and under Epileptogenic Effect, below.

1. Sansone ME, Ziegler DK. Brain and nervous system. In: Johnson FN, ed. *Depression & mania: modern lithium therapy.* Oxford: IRL Press, 1987: 240–5.
2. Johns S, Harris B. Tremor. *BMJ* 1984; **288:** 1309.
3. Himmelhoch JM, Hanin I. Side effects of lithium carbonate. *BMJ* 1974; **4:** 233.
4. Solomon K, Vickers R. Dysarthria resulting from lithium carbonate: a case report. *JAMA* 1975; **231:** 280.
5. Worrall EP, Gillham RA. Lithium-induced constructional dyspraxia. *BMJ* 1983; **286:** 189.
6. McGovern GP. Lithium induced constructional dyspraxia. *BMJ* 1983; **286:** 646.

Effects on respiration. Lithium is not generally recognised as a respiratory depressant but an episode of reversible respiratory failure about 3 weeks after the start of lithium therapy has been described in a patient with stable chronic airways obstruction.[1] Recovery of consciousness and resolution of hypercapnia occurred within 24 to 36 hours of lithium discontinuation.

1. Weiner M, *et al.* Effect of lithium on the responses to added respiratory resistances. *N Engl J Med* 1983; **308:** 319–22.

Effects on sexual function and fertility. Lithium does not seem to interfere with sexual function in most patients, but there have been isolated reports of impotence and loss of libido attributed to lithium therapy.[1]

Studies *in vitro* have demonstrated that in concentrations comparable with those reported to be achieved in semen lithium can inhibit sperm motility,[2] but concentrations found in cervico-vaginal mucus were considered unlikely to affect motility.[3]

1. Beeley L. Drug-induced sexual dysfunction and infertility. *Adverse Drug React Acute Poisoning Rev* 1984; **3:** 23–42.
2. Raoof NT, *et al.* Lithium inhibits human sperm motility in vitro. *Br J Clin Pharmacol* 1989; **28:** 715–17.
3. Salas IG, *et al.* Lithium carbonate concentration in cervico-vaginal mucus and serum after repeated oral dose administration. *Br J Clin Pharmacol* 1989; **28:** 751P.

Effects on the skin and hair. Cutaneous side-effects associated with lithium therapy have been reviewed.[1] Approximately

1% of patients present with some kind of skin disorder though they are not necessarily serious or severe. Although the onset varies from 2 or 3 weeks to 7 or more years, a large number of reactions start to appear once optimal serum-lithium concentrations have been attained. Effects reported include psoriasis which may be severe and require lithium withdrawal. Seborrhoeic dermatitis and follicular keratosis are also encountered and can improve spontaneously or after discontinuation of lithium. Acneform eruptions are found in areas not usually affected by acne vulgaris; in general the face is less affected or not affected at all.

Hair loss, not always severe, is more frequent than cutaneous effects. About 6% of patients may be affected and all kinds of alopecias have been found. The onset occurs several weeks or months after the start of lithium therapy. The hair usually regrows despite continuing therapy but in some cases regrowth only occurs after withdrawal of lithium. Fraunfelder *et al.*,[2] in their review of the effects on the ocular system, stated that loss of eyebrows and eyelashes had been associated with lithium therapy but was a rare event. They advised that patients affected should have their thyroid function assessed as hair loss due to lithium-induced hypothyroidism could be corrected by medication.

For references to the association of lithium with lupus, see under Lupus, below.

1. Lambert D, Dalac S. Skin, hair and nails. In: Johnson FN, ed. *Depression & mania: modern lithium therapy.* Oxford: IRL Press, 1987: 232–4.
2. Fraunfelder FT, *et al.* The effects of lithium on the human visual system. *J Toxicol Cutan Ocul Toxicol* 1992; **11:** 97–169.

Epileptogenic effect. Seizures occurring during lithium therapy are usually indicative of toxicity or impending toxicity. There have, however, been a few isolated reports describing seizures in patients with serum-lithium concentrations within the normally accepted therapeutic range.[1,2]

1. Demers R, *et al.* Convulsion during lithium therapy. *Lancet* 1970; **ii:** 315–16.
2. Massey EW, Folger WN. Seizures activated by therapeutic levels of lithium carbonate. *South Med J* 1984; **77:** 1173–5.

Lupus. Studies have found that antinuclear antibodies were more common in patients taking lithium carbonate than in controls.[1,2] The absence of anti-DNA antibodies indicated that they did not have true systemic lupus erythematosus but it was considered that patients ingesting lithium might be at risk. Dermatological manifestations of lupus together with antinuclear antibodies have been reported in a patient taking lithium.[3]

1. Johnstone EC, Whaley K. Antinuclear antibodies in psychiatric illness: their relationship to diagnosis and drug treatment. *BMJ* 1975; **2:** 724–5.
2. Presley AP, *et al.* Antinuclear antibodies in patients on lithium carbonate. *BMJ* 1976; **2:** 280–1.
3. Shukla VR, Borison RL. Lithium and lupuslike syndrome. *JAMA* 1982; **248:** 921–2.

Overdosage. Nausea, vomiting, and diarrhoea are common early features of lithium toxicity, and are followed by coarse tremor, increased muscle tone, cogwheel rigidity, fasciculation, and myoclonus.[1] Coma and convulsions may occur in serious cases and cardiac effects (first-degree heart block and QRS and QT prolongation) have been described rarely. A patient may appear to be aware with open eyes but have an expressionless face and be unable to move or speak (coma vigil). Acute renal failure and nephrogenic diabetes insipidus may develop.

One reviewer considered that the great majority of lithium intoxications reported had occurred in patients with an intercurrent reduction of renal function or in patients who had been treated with dosages of lithium that were, in fact, too high.[2] The patient usually experiences a prodromal period of days to a few weeks with minor 'nervous' symptoms which are signs of a manifest slight intoxication. At an unpredictable point renal function starts to deteriorate and within hours or at the most within a few days, the patient will become severely intoxicated. By this point lithium should have been discontinued and efficient detoxification measures (see Treatment of Adverse Effects, below) instituted if the patient is to make a complete recovery.

Lithium therapy should be controlled by measuring serum concentrations to ensure that values for lithium do not rise to levels associated with toxicity. Some patients may have concentrations considered to be toxic without showing any symptoms; unfortunately other patients may develop signs of toxicity at therapeutic serum concentrations.[3]

In acute overdosage[2] vomiting often occurs within an hour of ingestion due to the high concentration of lithium in the stomach, but significant amounts of lithium can still reach the systemic circulation. The typical clinical symptoms often appear after a latency period and gastrointestinal symptoms can re-appear at a later time. The symptoms of overdosage are reported to be mainly related to the alimentary and nervous systems and include abdominal pain, anorexia, nausea, and vomiting, occasionally mild diarrhoea, giddiness, tremor, ataxia, slurring speech, myoclonus, twitching, asthenia, and depression; renal symptoms have also been noted by some investigators. Again efficient detoxification procedures (see Treatment of Adverse Effects, below) should be instituted as rapidly as possible.

In a series of 28 patients with lithium self-poisoning or therapeutic intoxication many of the features and symptoms mentioned above were noted.[4] Other workers[5] have also reported

cases which illustrate the differences between acute and chronic toxicity encountered clinically.

Other symptoms that have been noted in case reports of lithium intoxication in individual patients include photophobia,[6] acute polyarthritis involving several large joints,[7] severe hypertension,[8] deep venous thrombophlebitis,[9] reduction of central temperature,[10] and severe leucopenia.[11]

1. Proudfoot AT. Acute poisoning with antidepressants and lithium. *Prescribers' J* 1986; **26:** 97–106.
2. Amdisen A. Clinical features and management of lithium poisoning. *Med Toxicol* 1988; **3:** 18–32.
3. Stern R. Lithium in the treatment of mood disorders. *N Engl J Med* 1995; **332:** 127–8.
4. Dyson EH, *et al.* Self-poisoning and therapeutic intoxication with lithium. *Hum Toxicol* 1987; **6:** 325–9.
5. Ananth J, *et al.* Acute and chronic lithium toxicity: case reports and a review. *Lithium* 1992; **3:** 139–45.
6. Caplan RP, Fry AH. Photophobia in lithium intoxication. *BMJ* 1982; **285:** 1314–15.
7. Black DW, Waziri R. Arthritis associated with lithium toxicity: case report. *J Clin Psychiatry* 1984; **45:** 135–6.
8. Michaeli J, *et al.* Severe hypertension and lithium intoxication. *JAMA* 1984; **251:** 1680.
9. Lyles MR. Deep venous thrombophlebitis associated with lithium toxicity. *J Natl Med Assoc* 1984; **76:** 633–4.
10. Follézou J-Y, Bleibel J-M. Reduction of temperature and lithium poisoning. *N Engl J Med* 1985; **313:** 1609.
11. Green ST, Dunn FG. Severe leucopenia in fatal lithium poisoning. *BMJ* 1985; **290:** 517.

Treatment of Adverse Effects

In recent acute overdosage with lithium, consideration should be given to emptying the stomach, although gastric lavage may be of limited value following overdosage with modified-release preparations, which do not disintegrate in the stomach and may be too large to pass through a lavage tube. Activated charcoal is of no value. Whole bowel irrigation has been suggested although there do not appear to be clinical studies to confirm efficacy.

Further measures may involve procedures to enhance the renal clearance of lithium or its active removal. Adequate hydration should be ensured and any electrolyte imbalance corrected, but forced diuresis or diuretics are contra-indicated. Appropriate supportive care may include measures to control hypotension and convulsions. Maintenance of fluid and electrolyte balance is particularly important because of the risk of hypernatraemia. The ECG should be monitored in symptomatic patients.

In severe poisoning, haemodialysis is the treatment of choice (particularly if there is renal impairment). Although effective in reducing serum-lithium concentrations, substantial rebound increases can be expected when dialysis is stopped, and prolonged or repeated treatments may be required. Peritoneal dialysis is less effective and only appropriate if haemodialysis facilities are not available. Haemofiltration has been tried to good effect.

Serum lithium concentrations should be monitored regularly throughout treatment. Once the serum and dialysis fluid are free of lithium, it has been recommended that serum-lithium concentrations should be monitored for at least another week so that allowance can be made for delayed diffusion from body tissues.

As a result of the narrow margin between therapeutic and toxic serum concentrations lithium poisoning may also develop during the course of therapeutic lithium administration. In some instances temporary withdrawal of lithium therapy and administration of generous amounts of sodium and fluid may be all that is required while adverse effects abate. In any serious or severe case of intoxication active measures such as dialysis and supportive measures outlined above may need to be instituted.

◊ References.

1. Gomolin IH. Coping with excessive doses. In: Johnson FN, ed. *Depression & mania: modern lithium therapy.* Oxford: IRL Press, 1987: 154–7.
2. Amdisen A. Clinical features and management of lithium poisoning. *Med Toxicol* 1988; **3:** 18–32.
3. Smith SW, *et al.* Whole-bowel irrigation as a treatment for acute lithium overdose. *Ann Emerg Med* 1991; **20:** 536–9.
4. Okusa MD, *et al.* Clinical manifestations and management of acute lithium intoxication. *Am J Med* 1994; **97:** 383–9.
5. Swartz CM, Jones P. Hyperlithemia correction and persistent delirium. *J Clin Pharmacol* 1994; **34:** 865–70.
6. Wells BG. Amiloride in lithium-induced polyuria. *Ann Pharmacother* 1994; **28:** 888–9.
7. Tyrer SP. Lithium intoxication: appropriate treatment. *CNS Drugs* 1996; **6:** 426–39.

Precautions

The margin between the therapeutic and the toxic concentration of lithium is narrow so therapy usually requires specialist advice, and serum concentrations should be monitored regularly under controlled conditions. Patients receiving lithium therapy should be taught to recognise the symptoms of early toxicity (see under Adverse Effects, above) and, should these occur, to discontinue therapy and request medical aid at once. They should be warned not to compensate for an omitted dose by subsequently taking a double dose. Additionally, patients should not be switched between different formulations or preparations of lithium without therapeutic monitoring as bioavailability may be different.

Lithium should be avoided in patients with cardiac disease or renal impairment, and cardiac and renal function should be monitored regularly. It should also be avoided in Addison's disease or other conditions with a sodium imbalance and in severely debilitated or dehydrated patients.

Patients receiving lithium should be examined periodically for abnormal thyroid function, since goitre and hypothyroidism may develop. Lithium should be avoided in untreated hypothyroidism. Lithium should be used with caution in patients with myasthenia gravis because exacerbation of this disorder has been reported (see Effects on the Musculoskeletal System in Adverse Effects, above).

Lithium should be used with particular care in the elderly since this group may be particularly susceptible to toxicity due to decreasing renal function.

Impaired driving performance or machine operating skills may occur in patients receiving lithium (see Driving, below).

A temporary dose reduction or discontinuation of lithium therapy may be necessary in vomiting, diarrhoea, excessive sweating, or any other condition that causes excessive sodium loss, thereby increasing serum-lithium concentrations. Conversely, increased sodium levels are likely to reduce serum-lithium concentrations. Patients taking lithium should therefore maintain an adequate fluid intake and should avoid increasing or decreasing sodium intake through dietary changes or ingestion of sodium-containing medicaments. Significant changes in caffeine intake may affect serum-lithium concentrations (see Xanthines under Interactions, below).

Lithium therapy should, where possible, be withdrawn slowly over a period of weeks to allay any concerns about relapse (see below).

If lithium is used during pregnancy then dose adjustments will be required to compensate for the altered renal handling. The risks of using lithium in pregnant patients are described under Pregnancy, below.

Lithium should be temporarily discontinued 24 hours before major surgery to safeguard the patient from accumulation (see under Anaesthesia, below).

Anaesthesia. The *British National Formulary* states that lithium should be discontinued 24 hours before major surgery, but the normal dose can be continued for minor surgery if fluids and electrolytes are carefully monitored. There is no clinical evidence of interaction between lithium and anaesthetics, although lithium may prolong the action of neuromuscular blockers.[1] Lithium may accumulate due to reduced renal clearance associated with anaesthesia; lithium treatment should be resumed as soon as possible after surgery, when kidney function and fluid-electrolyte balance have become normal. Patients are often not allowed fluids or foods by mouth the night before surgery but patients with lithium-induced polyuria should be given fluids parenterally during the night before the operation, if they vomit copiously, or if they are unconscious for several hours.

1. Schou M, Hippus H. Guidelines for patients receiving lithium treatment who require major surgery. *Br J Anaesth* 1987; **59:** 809–10.

Breast feeding. Lithium is distributed into breast milk and most manufacturers in the UK suggest that mothers receiving lithium should bottle feed their babies. A review[1] of a few rare cases of adverse effects associated with lithium in breast-fed infants also concluded that it would be best to avoid breast feeding during lithium therapy. However others[2] had previously questioned whether the advantages of such a course would be outweighed by the losses when breast feeding is avoided. It

was recommended[1] that if a mother did want to breast feed this should be done at times to avoid peak blood concentrations of lithium and the infant carefully monitored. Medication should be withheld or breast feeding stopped if the infant developed an infection or dehydration as they would be more susceptible to the adverse effects of lithium.

1. Ananth J. Lithium during pregnancy and lactation. *Lithium* 1993; **4:** 231–7.
2. Schou M. Lithium treatment during pregnancy, delivery, and lactation: an update. *J Clin Psychiatry* 1990; **51:** 410–13.

Cystic fibrosis. Reduced renal excretion of lithium was demonstrated in eight patients with cystic fibrosis compared with healthy subjects.[1] The authors recommended caution when prescribing standard doses of lithium to patients with cystic fibrosis until more definitive data were available.

1. Brager NPD, *et al.* Reduced renal fractional excretion of lithium in cystic fibrosis. *Br J Clin Pharmacol* 1996; **41:** 157–9.

Driving. While affective disorders probably adversely affect driving skill,[1,2] treatment with antidepressant drugs, including lithium, may also be hazardous,[1] although patients may be safer drivers with medication than without.[2] Lithium has been reported[1] to adversely affect the choice reaction time (a test to assess the time taken to respond correctly to some signals but not others) to a level considered dangerous for driving.

It has been mentioned[2] that the UK Medical Commission on Accident Prevention has recommended that patients on long-term psychotropic medication are unsuitable to be drivers of heavy goods or public service vehicles.

1. Ashton H. Drugs and driving. *Adverse Drug React Bull* 1983; **98:** 360–3.
2. Cremona A. Mad drivers: psychiatric illness and driving performance. *Br J Hosp Med* 1986; **35:** 193–5.

Pregnancy. Case reports of mothers taking lithium during pregnancy pointed to an increased risk of congenital abnormalities with the heart being mainly affected.[1] Support for this increased risk came from a study[2] of the records of 59 children born to women who had taken lithium during pregnancy. However, a later study[3] prospectively followed 138 pregnant women being treated with lithium and did not identify any difference in pregnancy outcome between them and a control group. The authors considered that lithium was not a major teratogen and felt that women with major affective disorders could continue lithium treatment during pregnancy provided that adequate fetal screening tests were carried out. A subsequent review[4] considered that the teratogenic risk was lower than previously thought, but that it would still be wise for women who wished to become pregnant to discontinue lithium if at all possible, at least during the period of embryogenesis.

There is limited evidence that lithium treatment during pregnancy may increase the risk of fetal macrosomia, premature delivery, and perinatal mortality.[1,5]

The renal clearance of lithium by the mother is not constant during pregnancy; in the second half of the pregnancy clearance rises gradually by 30 to 50% but falls abruptly and significantly after delivery to pre-pregnancy values.[1,6] The increased doses of lithium that may be given during pregnancy to compensate for this increased clearance may result in lithium toxicity.[6] It is generally considered[1,7] advisable to discontinue lithium during the last few days of pregnancy to reduce the risk of maternal lithium toxicity due to accumulation of lithium but it should be started again a few days later after delivery at reduced dosage because of the increased postpartum risk of manic and depressive relapse.[1] *Polyhydramnios* (an excess of amniotic fluid) in the last trimester of pregnancy has been reported and has been attributed to fetal lithium toxicity (polyuria and diabetes insipidus).[8,9]

Reducing the dosage during the last few days of pregnancy also helps to reduce lithium concentrations in the neonate and avoid associated adverse effects.[1,7] Adverse effects that have been reported in neonates exposed *in utero* to lithium include cyanosis, lethargy, flaccidity, hypotonia, poor gag and sucking reflexes, feeding problems, bradycardia, tachycardia, goitre, hypothyroidism, nephrogenic diabetes, and jaundice;[7] withdrawal symptoms have also been observed.

1. Schou M. Lithium treatment during pregnancy, delivery, and lactation: an update. *J Clin Psychiatry* 1990; **51:** 410–13.
2. Källén B, Tandberg A. Lithium and pregnancy: a cohort study on manic-depressive women. *Acta Psychiatr Scand* 1983; **68:** 134–9.
3. Jacobson SJ, *et al.* Prospective multicentre study of pregnancy outcome after lithium exposure during first trimester. *Lancet* 1992; **339:** 530–3.
4. Cohen LS, *et al.* A reevaluation of risk of in utero exposure to lithium. *JAMA* 1994; **271:** 146–50.
5. Troyer WA, *et al.* Association of maternal lithium exposure and premature delivery. *J Perinatol* 1993; **XIII:** 123–7.
6. Lemoine J-M. Pregnancy, delivery and lactation. In: Johnson FN, ed. *Depression & mania: modern lithium therapy.* Oxford: IRL Press, 1987: 139–46.
7. Ananth J. Lithium during pregnancy and lactation. *Lithium* 1993; **4:** 231–7.
8. Krause S, *et al.* Polyhydramnios with maternal lithium treatment. *Obstet Gynecol* 1990; **75:** 504–6.
9. Ang MS, *et al.* Maternal lithium therapy and polyhydramnios. *Obstet Gynecol* 1990; **76:** 517–19.

Surgery. For comments regarding the precautions to be observed in patients undergoing Surgery, see under Anaesthesia, above.

Withdrawal. A withdrawal syndrome consisting of symptoms such as anxiety, tremor, fatigue, nausea, sweating, head-

ache, sleep disturbances, diarrhoea, or blurred vision, usually develops within days of sudden cessation of treatment with lithium.[1] These may simply be a recurrence of symptoms of mood change. Uncontrolled studies of withdrawal symptoms have raised the possibility of a lithium-withdrawal state but controlled studies have not been convincingly negative. It is, however, wise to reduce lithium dosage gradually rather than stop high-dosage treatment abruptly.

A frequent worry associated with the termination of lithium therapy is that of relapse. Most evidence has supported the view that any relapses occurring in the first weeks after lithium withdrawal are simply part of a pattern of recurrence of bipolar disorder in general and are not indicative of a higher rate of recurrence. Some,[2] however, have found the proportion of patients relapsing on sudden withdrawal of lithium therapy to be 50%, a figure they consider to be too high to be accounted for by the natural history of the disease process. They and others[3] advise that this risk should be considered when prescribing lithium for bipolar disorder. In patients who previously had been stable on lithium for at least 18 months, the risk of early recurrence of bipolar disorder was higher when therapy was withdrawn rapidly in less than 2 weeks than when it was withdrawn gradually over 2 to 4 weeks.[4]

1. Goodnick PJ. Terminating treatment. In: Johnson FN, ed. *Depression & mania: modern lithium therapy.* Oxford: IRL Press, 1987: 115–17.
2. Mander AJ, Loudon JB. Rapid recurrence of mania following abrupt discontinuation of lithium. *Lancet* 1988; **ii:** 15–17.
3. Goodwin GM. Recurrence of mania after lithium withdrawal. *Br J Psychiatry* 1994; **164:** 149–52.
4. Faedda GL, *et al.* Outcome after rapid vs gradual discontinuation of lithium treatment in bipolar disorders. *Arch Gen Psychiatry* 1993; **50:** 448–55.

Interactions

Concurrent administration of some diuretics with lithium reduces lithium excretion and may result in toxicity (see below for further details). Thiazide diuretics may also show a paradoxical antidiuretic effect. Consequently diuretics should be avoided or used with great caution in those receiving lithium. Further interactions reported with lithium are discussed below.

◊ Reviews of drug interactions with lithium.

1. Amdisen A. Lithium and drug interactions. *Drugs* 1982; **24:** 133–9.
2. Beeley L. Drug interactions with lithium. *Prescribers' J* 1986; **26:** 160–2.
3. Harvey NS, Merriman S. Review of clinically important drug interactions with lithium. *Drug Safety* 1994; **10:** 455–63.
4. Finley PR, *et al.* Clinical relevance of drug interactions with lithium. *Clin Pharmacokinet* 1995; **29:** 172–91.

ACE inhibitors. Concurrent administration of lithium with ACE inhibitors has been reported[1-5] to increase serum-lithium concentrations. ACE inhibitors such as *captopril*,[1] *enalapril*,[2-4] and *lisinopril*[4,5] have been implicated, although in a study[6] of enalapril and lithium in healthy volunteers, the lithium levels remained unchanged. The mechanism is unclear but it has been suggested[7] that suppression of the renin-angiotensin-aldosterone system by ACE inhibitors may be responsible. Lithium excretion by the kidney is dependent on both glomerular filtration and sodium concentration in the proximal tubule, both of which are reduced by ACE inhibitors. It has also been suggested[4] that inhibition of angiotensin II production may lead to reduced fluid intake through lack of activation of the thirst stimulus and this would enhance the tendency to volume depletion caused by natriuresis. Patients considered[7] to be at risk from this reaction would include those whose renal function is largely dependent on the effect of angiotensin II, those with congestive heart failure, and those with volume depletion.

1. Pulik M, Lida H. Interaction lithium-inhibiteurs de l'enzyme de conversion. *Presse Med* 1988; **17:** 755.
2. Douste-Blazy P, *et al.* Angiotensin converting enzyme inhibitors and lithium treatment. *Lancet* 1986; **i:** 1448.
3. Navis GJ, *et al.* Volume homeostasis, angiotensin converting enzyme inhibition, and lithium therapy. *Am J Med* 1989; **86:** 621.
4. Correa FJ, Eiser AR. Angiotensin-converting enzyme inhibitors and lithium toxicity. *Am J Med* 1992; **93:** 108–9.
5. Baldwin CM, Safferman AZ. A case of lisinopril-induced lithium toxicity. *DICP Ann Pharmacother* 1990; **24:** 946–7.
6. DasGupta K, *et al.* The effect of enalapril on serum lithium levels in healthy men. *J Clin Psychiatry* 1992; **53:** 398–400.
7. Mignat C, Unger T. Ace inhibitors: drug interactions of clinical significance. *Drug Safety* 1995; **12:** 334–47.

Analgesics. See NSAIDs, below.

Antidepressants. Lithium has been used to augment the effect of other antidepressants in refractory depression. However, there have been reports of adverse reactions with some of these combinations. For further details, see Antidepressants under Interactions of Phenelzine, p.306.

Antiepileptics. Severe CNS toxicity despite 'normal' serum-lithium concentrations has been described in a patient also taking *phenytoin* together with *phenobarbital*.[1] Symptoms indicative of lithium toxicity have also been reported in a patient receiving *phenytoin* concomitantly,[2] again where concentrations were not abnormal.

For reports of neurotoxicity in patients receiving *carbamazepine* and lithium, see p.344. Carbamazepine-induced renal failure has also resulted in toxic serum-lithium concentrations in 1 report.[3]

1. Speirs J, Hirsch SR. Severe lithium toxicity with "normal" serum concentrations. *BMJ* 1978; **1:** 815–16.
2. MacCallum WAG. Interaction of lithium and phenytoin. *BMJ* 1980; **280:** 610–11.
3. Mayan H, *et al.* Lithium intoxication due to carbamazepine-induced renal failure. *Ann Pharmacother* 2001; **35:** 560–2.

Antimicrobials. Lithium toxicity has been reported on isolated occasions in patients receiving *metronidazole*,[1] *spectinomycin*,[2] and *tetracycline*.[3]

However, it has been noted that lithium and tetracycline have been used concomitantly without serious problems in many patients and that additionally tetracycline has been used to treat the acneform skin eruptions induced by lithium.[4] These same authors investigating healthy subjects found that lithium concentrations were decreased, rather than increased, following the addition of tetracycline but considered this was probably of no clinical significance.

1. Teicher MH, *et al.* Possible nephrotoxic interaction of lithium and metronidazole. *JAMA* 1987; **257:** 3365–6.
2. Anonymous. Possible adverse drug-drug interaction report: lithium intoxication in a spectinomycin-treated patient. *Int Drug Ther Newslett* 1978; **13:** 15.
3. McGennis AJ. Lithium carbonate and tetracycline interaction. *BMJ* 1978; **1:** 1183.
4. Fankhauser MP, *et al.* Evaluation of lithium-tetracycline interaction. *Clin Pharm* 1988; **7:** 314–17.

Antimigraine drugs. For comment on the suggestion that there may be a risk of increased CNS toxicity when *sumatriptan* and lithium are given together, see p.457.

Antineoplastics. Transient decreases in serum-lithium concentration occurred in a patient after administration of *cisplatin*.[1] The relative contributions of cisplatin itself, or the fluid loading procedure involving intravenous fluids and mannitol, or their combined effects were unclear. The interaction, however, had no apparent clinical significance in this patient although a risk of undertreatment with lithium may occur in other patients.

1. Pietruszka LJ, *et al.* Evaluation of cisplatin-lithium interaction. *Drug Intell Clin Pharm* 1985; **19:** 31–2.

Antipsychotics and anxiolytics. In the control of acute mania lithium is often too slow in onset to be used alone and therefore additional therapy with an antipsychotic may be necessary. It should be noted, however, that such combinations should be used with care as interactions and adverse reactions have occurred.

The renal excretion of lithium is increased during concurrent *chlorpromazine* treatment,[1] which means that subsequent withdrawal of chlorpromazine can result in an abrupt rise in serum-lithium concentrations.[2] The serum concentration of chlorpromazine can also be reduced by the concurrent administration of lithium,[3] and chlorpromazine toxicity may be precipitated by the abrupt withdrawal of lithium in patients previously stabilised on the two drugs together. Ventricular fibrillation has been described following withdrawal of lithium in a patient concurrently taking chlorpromazine;[4] it was suggested that the chlorpromazine dose should be reduced if lithium is to be discontinued.

There have been isolated reports of neurotoxicity or brain damage, characterised by delirium, seizures, encephalopathy, or an increased incidence of extrapyramidal symptoms in patients receiving lithium concomitantly with *flupentixol decanoate*,[5] *fluphenazine decanoate*,[6] or high-dose *haloperidol*,[7-9] although two earlier retrospective studies of patients taking lithium with antipsychotics had failed to detect such adverse reactions.[10,11] Neurological reactions have continued to be reported in patients receiving lithium concomitantly with *thioridazine*,[12,13] *sulpiride*,[14] *clozapine*,[15] and *risperidone*.[16] Although a causal relationship between these events and concomitant use of lithium and antipsychotics has not been fully established, patients should be monitored for signs of neurotoxicity if receiving such combinations.

Ross and Coffey[17] in a discussion of the interactions between lithium and antipsychotics made the following comments. The neurotoxicity induced by lithium and antipsychotics is a rare entity, about 40 cases have been reported in the literature. There is controversy whether the combination produces any greater risk than either drug alone and also whether the neurotoxicity is a distinct diagnostic entity or simply represents atypical cases of lithium toxicity or the neuroleptic malignant syndrome. They mentioned suggestions that have been made that the interaction between lithium and haloperidol represents a form of neuroleptic malignant syndrome while that between lithium and the phenothiazines, especially thioridazine, represents a form of lithium toxicity. They concluded that the risk from combination therapy was very small but that the clinician should, nevertheless, be aware of it.

Although lithium has been reported to interact with *diazepam* resulting in hypothermic episodes,[18] Ross and Coffey[17] considered that this was more likely to be an idiosyncratic response rather than a true drug interaction; they stated that in general it was considered quite safe to use lithium and benzodiazepines in combination.

1. Sletten I, *et al.* The effect of chlorpromazine on lithium excretion in psychiatric subjects. *Curr Ther Res* 1966; **8:** 441–6.
2. Pakes GE. Lithium toxicity with phenothiazine withdrawal. *Lancet* 1979; **ii:** 701.

3. Rivera-Calimlim L, *et al.* Effect of lithium on plasma chlorpromazine levels. *Clin Pharmacol Ther* 1978; **23:** 451–5.
4. Stevenson RN, *et al.* Ventricular fibrillation due to lithium withdrawal—an interaction with chlorpromazine? *Postgrad Med J* 1989; **65:** 936–8.
5. West A. Adverse effects of lithium treatment. *BMJ* 1977; **2:** 642.
6. Singh SV. Lithium carbonate/fluphenazine decanoate producing irreversible brain damage. *Lancet* 1982; **ii:** 278.
7. Cohen WJ, Cohen NH. Lithium carbonate, haloperidol, and irreversible brain damage. *JAMA* 1974; **230:** 1283–7.
8. Loudon JB, Waring H. Toxic reactions to lithium and haloperidol. *Lancet* 1976; **ii:** 1088.
9. Thomas C, *et al.* Lithium/haloperidol combinations and brain damage. *Lancet* 1982; **i:** 626.
10. Baastrup PC, *et al.* Adverse reactions in treatment with lithium carbonate and haloperidol. *JAMA* 1976; **236:** 2645–6.
11. Prakash R. Lithium-haloperidol combination and brain damage. *Lancet* 1982; **i:** 1468–9.
12. Standish-Barry HMAS, Shelly MA. Toxic neurological reaction to lithium/thioridazine. *Lancet* 1983; **i:** 771.
13. Cantor CH. Encephalopathy with lithium and thioridazine in combination. *Med J Aust* 1986; **144:** 164–5.
14. Dinan TG, O'Keane V. Acute extrapyramidal reactions following lithium and sulpiride co-administration: two case reports. *Hum Psychopharmacol Clin Exp* 1991; **6:** 67–9.
15. Blake LM, *et al.* Reversible neurologic symptoms with clozapine and lithium. *J Clin Psychopharmacol* 1992; **12:** 297–9.
16. Swanson CL, *et al.* Effects of concomitant risperidone and lithium treatment. *Am J Psychiatry* 1995; **152:** 1096.
17. Ross DR, Coffey CE. Neuroleptics and anti-anxiety agents. In: Johnson FN, ed. *Depression & mania: modern lithium therapy.* Oxford: IRL Press, 1987: 167–71.
18. Naylor GJ, McHarg A. Profound hypothermia on combined lithium carbonate and diazepam treatment. *BMJ* 1977; **2:** 22.

Benzodiazepines. See Antipsychotics and Anxiolytics, above.

Calcium-channel blockers. Neurotoxicity has been reported in a patient receiving lithium following the addition of *verapamil*.[1] Serum-lithium concentrations were still inside the accepted therapeutic range and it was considered that the similar actions of lithium and verapamil on neurosecretory processes may have been responsible. Verapamil has also been reported to decrease serum-lithium concentrations.[2] Neurotoxicity has also been reported in a patient receiving lithium and *diltiazem*[3] as well as other drugs. Psychosis, possibly induced by the use of diltiazem and lithium together, has been reported in another patient.[4]

1. Price WA, Giannini AJ. Neurotoxicity caused by lithium-verapamil synergism. *J Clin Pharmacol* 1986; **26:** 717–19.
2. Weinrauch LA, *et al.* Decreased serum lithium during verapamil therapy. *Am Heart J* 1984; **108:** 1378–80.
3. Valdiserri EV. A possible interaction between lithium and diltiazem: case report. *J Clin Psychiatry* 1985; **46:** 540–1.
4. Binder EF, *et al.* Diltiazem-induced psychosis and a possible diltiazem-lithium interaction. *Arch Intern Med* 1991; **151:** 373–4.

Central stimulants. There is a report of a woman who had been stabilised on lithium treatment for 15 months developing lithium toxicity within a few days of being given *mazindol*.[1]

1. Hendy MS, *et al.* Mazindol-induced lithium toxicity. *BMJ* 1980; **280:** 684–5.

Diuretics. *Thiazide diuretics* produce sodium depletion by inhibiting distal tubular sodium reabsorption. The consequent increase in proximal tubular reabsorption frequently results in an increase in serum-lithium concentrations.[1] Patients who are stabilised on lithium therapy and begin taking thiazide diuretics are at significant risk of developing lithium toxicity. Toxic lithium concentrations may be seen within 3 to 5 days of diuretic initiation. *Loop diuretics* (frusemide [furosemide], bumetanide, and etacrynic acid) seem less likely to cause lithium retention, although caution is warranted, especially with patients in whom dietary sodium is restricted.[1] *Amiloride*, and probably other potassium-sparing diuretics, have no effect on lithium excretion, but *acetazolamide* increases lithium excretion. However, the diuretic action of acetazolamide is short-lived and the interaction may therefore be transient.[1]

It has therefore been suggested that if diuretic therapy is necessary in patients stabilised on lithium a reduction of 25 to 50% of the lithium dose should be initiated,[1] lithium concentrations measured twice weekly until re-stabilisation occurs, and that perhaps loop diuretics such as bumetanide or frusemide [furosemide] would be preferable.

The topic of lithium-diuretic interaction and precautions to be observed has also been discussed by Grau.[3]

1. Beeley L. Drug interactions with lithium. *Prescribers' J* 1986; **26:** 160–3.
2. Ramsay LE. Interactions that matter: diuretics and antihypertensive drugs. *Prescribers' J* 1984; **24:** 60–5.
3. Grau E. Diuretics. In: Johnson FN, ed. *Depression & mania: modern lithium therapy.* Oxford: IRL Press, 1987: 180–3.

Gastrointestinal drugs. Administration of *sodium bicarbonate* with lithium has led to reduced blood-lithium concentrations and has been attributed to increased renal excretion of the lithium cation in response to the extra load of bicarbonate anion to be excreted.[1] *Antacids* containing combinations of *aluminium and magnesium hydroxides* and *simeticone* had no effect on the dissolution and solubility of lithium carbonate *in vitro*[2] nor on its bioavailability *in vivo*.[3]

There has been a case report describing a possible interaction between lithium and *ispaghula* where the ispaghula may have inhibited intestinal absorption of lithium resulting in low serum concentrations.[4]

There is an increased risk of extrapyramidal effects and the possibility of neurotoxicity when drugs such as *metoclopramide* are given to patients receiving lithium.

Concomitant use of *cisapride* and lithium may increase the risk of ventricular arrhythmias.

1. McSwiggan C. A significant drug interaction. *Aust J Pharm* 1978; **59:** 6.
2. Schiessler DM, *et al.* Effect of antacids on lithium carbonate dissolution and solubility in vitro. *Am J Hosp Pharm* 1983; **40:** 825–8.
3. Goode DL, *et al.* Effect of antacid on the bioavailability of lithium carbonate. *Clin Pharm* 1984; **3:** 284–7.
4. Perlman BB. Interaction between lithium salts and ispaghula husk. *Lancet* 1990; **335:** 416.

Methyldopa. Lithium toxicity induced by concurrent administration of methyldopa has been described on a number of occasions.[1-3] Symptoms of toxicity may occur even though serum-lithium concentrations remain within the therapeutic range.

1. Byrd GJ. Methyldopa and lithium carbonate: suspected interaction. *JAMA* 1975; **233:** 320.
2. O'Regan JB. Adverse interaction of lithium carbonate and methyldopa. *Can Med Assoc J* 1976; **115:** 385–6.
3. Osanloo E, Deglin JH. Interaction of lithium and methyldopa. *Ann Intern Med* 1980; **92:** 433–4.

Muscle relaxants. For reports of hypothermic episodes occurring during the concomitant administration of lithium and *diazepam* see under Antipsychotics and Anxiolytics, above.

Severe aggravation of hyperkinetic symptoms occurred in 2 patients with Huntington's chorea when *baclofen* was added to their treatment with lithium and haloperidol.[1]

1. Andén N-E, *et al.* Baclofen and lithium in Huntington's chorea. *Lancet* 1973; **ii:** 93.

Neuromuscular blockers. For reports of prolongation of neuromuscular blockade by lithium see under Atracurium, p.1335. For further comments relating to surgery and anaesthesia, see under Anaesthesia in Precautions, above.

NSAIDs. Decreased clearance and increased serum concentrations of lithium, resulting in toxicity on some occasions, have been reported after the concomitant use of lithium with *diclofenac*,[1] *ibuprofen*,[2,3] *indometacin*,[4,5] *mefenamic acid*,[6,7] *naproxen*,[8] and *piroxicam*;[9,10] secondary sources have also implicated *azapropazone*, *ketoprofen*,[11] and *phenylbutazone*.[11] However, serum-lithium concentration is not increased by the concomitant use of *sulindac*.[8,12,13] Although serum-lithium concentrations were increased in one patient receiving *aspirin*[14] this has not been substantiated by others and an interaction is considered unlikely;[5,15] it has also been pointed out that control of sodium balance is necessary in such studies[15] and in the report purporting to demonstrate an interaction the diet had not been controlled.

In a discussion Furnell[11] has stated that for mild occasional aches, pains, and fever paracetamol is the preferred analgesic in patients receiving lithium, although occasional doses of aspirin are acceptable. Sulindac appeared to be the safest NSAID for long-term use. Diclofenac, ibuprofen, indometacin, ketoprofen, naproxen, phenylbutazone, and piroxicam should be avoided where possible but if it was necessary to use one of these drugs the maintenance dose of lithium should be reduced. He also considered that perhaps other NSAIDs, for which no information was available at that time, should be regarded as having the potential to cause a rise in serum-lithium concentrations. Subsequent to Furnell's discussion, decreased renal clearance and increased serum concentrations of lithium, sometimes resulting in toxicity, have been found when lithium was taken with *ketorolac*[16,17] or *tiaprofenic acid*.[18]

1. Reimann IW, Frölich JC. Effects of diclofenac on lithium kinetics. *Clin Pharmacol Ther* 1981; **30:** 348–52.
2. Kristoff CA, *et al.* Effect of ibuprofen on lithium plasma and red blood cell concentrations. *Clin Pharm* 1986; **5:** 51–5.
3. Ragheb M. Ibuprofen can increase serum lithium level in lithium-treated patients. *J Clin Psychiatry* 1987; **48:** 161–3.
4. Frölich JC, *et al.* Indomethacin increases plasma lithium. *BMJ* 1979; **1:** 1115–16.
5. Reimann IW, *et al.* Indomethacin but not aspirin increases plasma lithium ion levels. *Arch Gen Psychiatry* 1983; **40:** 283–6.
6. Shelley RK. Lithium toxicity and mefenamic acid: a possible interaction and the role of prostaglandin inhibition. *Br J Psychiatry* 1987; **151:** 847–8.
7. MacDonald J, Neale TJ. Toxic interaction of lithium carbonate and mefenamic acid. *BMJ* 1988; **297:** 1339.
8. Ragheb M, Powell AL. Lithium interaction with sulindac and naproxen. *J Clin Psychopharmacol* 1986; **6:** 150–4.
9. Kerry RJ, *et al.* Possible toxic interaction between lithium and piroxicam. *Lancet* 1983; **i:** 418–19.
10. Walbridge DG, Bazire SR. An interaction between lithium carbonate and piroxicam presenting as lithium toxicity. *Br J Psychiatry* 1985; **147:** 206–7.
11. Furnell MM. Non-steroidal anti-inflammatory drugs. In: Johnson FN, ed. *Depression & mania: modern lithium therapy.* Oxford: IRL Press, 1987: 183–6.
12. Furnell MM, Davies J. The effect of sulindac on lithium therapy. *Drug Intell Clin Pharm* 1985; **19:** 374–6.
13. Ragheb MA, Powell AL. Failure of sulindac to increase serum lithium levels. *J Clin Psychiatry* 1986; **47:** 33–4.
14. Bendz H, Feinberg M. Aspirin increases serum lithium ion levels. *Arch Gen Psychiatry* 1984; **41:** 310–11.
15. Reimann I. Aspirin increases serum lithium ion levels. *Arch Gen Psychiatry* 1984; **41:** 311.
16. Langlois R, Paquette D. Increased serum lithium levels due to ketorolac therapy. *Can Med Assoc J* 1994; **150:** 1455–6.
17. Iyer V. Ketorolac (Toradol®) induced lithium toxicity. *Headache* 1994; **34:** 442–4.
18. Alderman CP, Lindsay KSW. Increased serum lithium concentration secondary to treatment with tiaprofenic acid and fosinopril. *Ann Pharmacother* 1996; **30:** 1411–3.

Parasympathomimetics. For the effect of lithium on parasympathomimetics, see p.1420.

Xanthines. It has been reported[1] that *theophylline* enhances the renal clearance of lithium, thus tending to reduce serum-lithium concentrations. Lithium blood concentrations increased by 24% when *caffeine* was eliminated from the diet of 11 patients taking lithium.[2] No toxicity was observed but these patients had been maintained on low baseline lithium concentrations; toxicity might occur in patients maintained at higher concentrations.

1. Cook BL, *et al.* Theophylline-lithium interaction. *J Clin Psychiatry* 1985; **46:** 278–9.
2. Mester R, *et al.* Caffeine withdrawal increases lithium blood levels. *Biol Psychiatry* 1995; **37:** 348–50.

Pharmacokinetics

Lithium is readily and completely absorbed from the gastrointestinal tract when taken as one of its salts. Absorption can be affected by the formulation of the preparation taken. Peak serum concentrations are obtained between 0.5 and 3 hours after ingestion from conventional tablets or capsules; following modified-release formulations peak concentrations are delayed and may occur between 2 and 12 hours after administration. Lithium is distributed throughout the body and distribution is complete within about 6 to 10 hours; higher concentrations occur in the bones, the thyroid gland, and portions of the brain, than in the serum.

Lithium is excreted unchanged, predominantly in the urine; only a small amount can be detected in the faeces, saliva, and sweat. It is not bound to plasma proteins. It crosses the placenta and is distributed into breast milk. The elimination half-life in patients with normal renal function is about 20 to 24 hours, but increases with decreasing renal function; half-lives of up to 36 hours have been reported for elderly patients and 40 to 50 hours for patients with renal impairment. Steady-state concentrations may not, therefore, be attained until 4 to 7 days after the initiation of treatment.

Following administration of lithium salts there is wide intersubject variation between both the serum concentrations obtained following a given dose, and between those required for therapeutic effect. Concentrations also vary considerably according to factors such as the dosage regimen (whether given in single or divided daily doses), renal function, the dietary regimen of the patient, the patient's state of health, the time at which the blood sample is taken, and concomitant medication, such as sodium salts or diuretics, as well as by formulation and bioavailability. Moreover, there is only a narrow margin between the therapeutic and the toxic serum concentration of lithium. Therefore, not only is individual titration of lithium dosage essential to ensure constant appropriate concentrations for the patient, but the conditions under which the blood samples are taken for monitoring must be carefully controlled. In practice, a blood sample drawn 12 hours after the last dose of lithium following a consistent dosing schedule for 4 to 7 days is used for measurement of serum-lithium concentrations. Under these conditions the distribution of the last dose of lithium is complete and steady-state concentrations will have been attained. The usual maintenance therapeutic serum concentrations of lithium are 0.4 to 1.0 mmol per litre; toxic effects may be expected at concentrations exceeding 1.5 mmol per litre. For further details regarding monitoring of serum concentrations of lithium, see under Uses and Administration, below. Estimation of lithium concentrations in other body fluids such as saliva has been investigated as a less invasive method of monitoring. However, results have been equivocal and these methods have not replaced serum monitoring in general practice.

◊ References.
1. Ward ME, *et al.* Clinical pharmacokinetics of lithium. *J Clin Pharmacol* 1994; **34:** 280–5.
2. Reiss RA, *et al.* Lithium pharmacokinetics in the obese. *Clin Pharmacol Ther* 1994; **55:** 392–8.
3. Thomsen K, Schou M. Avoidance of lithium intoxication: advice based on knowledge about the renal lithium clearance under various circumstances. *Pharmacopsychiatry* 1999; **32:** 83–6.
4. Sproule BA, *et al.* Differential pharmacokinetics of lithium in elderly patients. *Drugs Aging* 2000; **16:** 165–77.

Administration. References concerning the pharmacokinetic methods of predicting lithium dosage requirements.
1. Marken PA, *et al.* Preliminary comparison of predictive and empiric lithium dosing: impact on patient outcome. *Ann Pharmacother* 1994; **28:** 1148–52.
2. Taright N, *et al.* Nonparametric estimation of population characteristics of the kinetics of lithium from observational and experimental data: individualization of chronic dosing regimen using a new Bayesian approach. *Ther Drug Monit* 1994 **16:** 258–69.
3. Sproule BA, *et al.* Fuzzy logic pharmacokinetic modeling: application to lithium concentration prediction. *Clin Pharmacol Ther* 1997; **62:** 29–40.

Cystic fibrosis. For a reference to reduced renal excretion of lithium in patients with cystic fibrosis, see Precautions, above.

Distribution into breast milk. For references to the distribution of lithium into breast milk, see Precautions, above.

Pregnancy. For references to changes in renal clearance of lithium during pregnancy, see Precautions, above.

Uses and Administration

Lithium, as one of its salts, provides a source of lithium ions, which compete with sodium ions at various sites in the body. It thus has an action and side-effects distinct and separate from those of other antidepressants. Its mode of action is not understood, but it is effective in the treatment and prophylaxis of **mania**, and prophylaxis of **bipolar disorder** and **recurrent unipolar depression**. Since the margin between therapeutic and toxic serum concentrations is narrow the decision to give lithium is usually based on specialist advice; lithium should not be prescribed unless facilities for monitoring serum concentrations are available.

As toxic effects are associated with concentrations above 1.5 mmol per litre, and may occur with concentrations as low as 1.0 mmol per litre in susceptible patients such as the elderly, it is recommended that doses are adjusted to provide a serum-lithium concentration of 0.4 to 1.0 mmol per litre (at the lower end of the range for maintenance therapy and elderly patients). Treatment with lithium thus needs to be monitored through measurement of serum concentrations. It should be emphasised that serum concentrations should be adjusted for each individual patient to those that give a clinical response without evidence of toxicity. Patients must be taught to recognise the symptoms of early lithium intoxication in order to omit further doses of lithium and seek medical care should it be impending.

The dose of lithium given depends on the preparation chosen since different preparations of lithium salts vary widely in bioavailability. Recommended doses for some UK preparations are as follows:

• *Camcolit* tablets (Norgine, UK) containing lithium carbonate; for treatment, initially 1 to 1.5 g daily; for prophylaxis, initially 0.3 to 0.4 g daily.

• *Li-Liquid* oral solution (Rosemont, UK) containing lithium citrate; for treatment and prophylaxis, initially 1.018 to 3.054 g daily in two divided doses (elderly or patients less than 50 kg body-weight, 0.509 g twice daily).

• *Liskonum* tablets (SmithKline Beecham, UK) containing lithium carbonate; for treatment, initially 450 to 675 mg twice daily (elderly, 225 mg twice daily); for prophylaxis, initially 450 mg twice daily (elderly, 225 mg twice daily).

• *Priadel* tablets (Sanofi Synthelabo, UK) containing lithium carbonate; for treatment and prophylaxis, initially 0.4 to 1.2 g daily as a single dose or in two divided doses (elderly or patients less than 50 kg body-weight, 0.4 g daily).

• *Priadel* syrup (Sanofi Synthelabo, UK) containing lithium citrate; for treatment and prophylaxis, initially 1.04 to 3.12 g daily in two divided doses (elderly or patients less than 50 kg body-weight, 0.52 g twice daily).

Lithium is not recommended for use in children.

The initial dose given is adjusted after 4 to 7 days according to the results of serum-lithium estimations obtained under controlled conditions (samples being taken 12 hours after the preceding dose). Serum-lithium concentrations are then checked once a week until the dosage has remained constant for 4 weeks. The frequency of estimations can then be reduced to about once every 3 months. Should the patient's circumstances change such that the lithium pharmacokinetics or requirements might be affected, close control of serum concentrations should be reinstated until the concentrations stabilise once more. Such circum

stances could involve a change of lithium preparation, an intercurrent illness (including a urinary-tract infection), a manic or depressive phase, a change in dietary regimen or body temperature, pregnancy, and concomitant administration of medication (in particular, sodium-containing preparations and diuretics). For further details see under Precautions and Interactions, above. Long-term use of lithium has been associated with thyroid disorders and mild cognitive and memory impairment. Therefore, long-term treatment should only be undertaken if it is definitely indicated. Patients need to be carefully reassessed after a period of 3 to 5 years and lithium continued only if the benefit persists.

Lithium is also used for the management of **aggressive or self-mutilating behaviour**. The doses are similar to those used in the prophylaxis of recurrent affective disorders described above.

Lithium therapy should, where possible, be withdrawn slowly over a period of weeks to allay any concerns about relapse. For further details, see Withdrawal under Precautions, above.

Other lithium salts have been used in the treatment of psychiatric disorders and these include the acetate, gluconate, glutamate, and sulfate.

Lithium carbonate is used in homoeopathic medicines.

Administration. A double-blind study in unipolar and bipolar patients on prophylactic lithium supported the trend towards using lithium in lower dosage.[1] It indicated that a plasma concentration as low as 0.45 mmol per litre was as effective as what had been the traditionally accepted concentration of 0.8 mmol per litre and above.
1. Abou-Saleh MT, Coppen A. The efficacy of low-dose lithium: clinical, psychological and biological correlates. *J Psychiatr Res* 1989; **23:** 157–62.

Bipolar disorder. The management of bipolar disorder is discussed on p.271 where the role of lithium is covered. Briefly, lithium's main role is in prophylaxis. It is sometimes used in the control of the acute manic stage, but, because of its slow onset of action, usually in conjunction with an antipsychotic drug.
References.
1. Aronson JK, Reynolds DJM. Lithium. *BMJ* 1992; **305:** 1273–6.
2. Birch NJ, *et al.* Lithium prophylaxis: proposed guidelines for good clinical practice. *Lithium* 1993; **4:** 225–30.
3. Peet M, Pratt JP. Lithium: current status in psychiatric disorders. *Drugs* 1993; **46:** 7–17.
4. Price LH, Heninger GR. Lithium in the treatment of mood disorders. *N Engl J Med* 1994; **331:** 591–8.
5. Jensen HV, *et al.* Lithium prophylaxis of manic-depressive disorder: daily lithium dosing schedule versus every second day. *Acta Psychiatr Scand* 1995; **92:** 69–74.
6. Moncrieff J. Lithium revisited: a re-examination of the placebo-controlled trials of lithium prophylaxis in manic-depressive disorder. *Br J Psychiatry* 1995; **167:** 569–74.
7. Jensen HV, *et al.* Twelve-hour brain lithium concentration in lithium maintenance treatment of manic-depressive disorder: daily versus alternate-day dosing schedule. *Psychopharmacology (Berl)* 1996; **124:** 275–8.
8. Maj M, *et al.* Late non-responders to lithium prophylaxis in bipolar patients: prevalence and predictors. *J Affect Disord* 1996; **39:** 39–42.
9. Anonymous. Using lithium safely. *Drug Ther Bull* 1999; **37:** 22–4.
10. Burgess S, *et al.* Lithium for maintenance treatment of mood disorders (updated 16 May 2001). Available in The Cochrane Library; Issue 3. Oxford: Update Software; 2001.

Depression. Lithium may be used in the treatment and prophylaxis of recurrent unipolar depression, usually when standard antidepressants have failed (p.271). Lithium is also used to augment the efficacy of other antidepressants in refractory cases.
References.
1. Heit S, Nemeroff CB. Lithium augmentation of antidepressants in treatment-refractory depression. *J Clin Psychiatry* 1998; **59** (suppl 6): 28–33.
2. Sackeim HA, *et al.* Continuation pharmacotherapy in the prevention of relapse following electroconvulsive therapy; a randomized controlled trial. *JAMA* 2001; **285:** 1299–1307.

Headache. Lithium is one of a number of drugs tried in cluster headache (p.449) to prevent headache attacks during cluster periods when ergotamine is ineffective or has had to be withdrawn. In a double-blind study[1] lithium and verapamil were found to be of similar efficacy for cluster headache prophylaxis although verapamil appeared to produce fewer adverse effects.
1. Bussone G, *et al.* Double blind comparison of lithium and verapamil in cluster headache prophylaxis. *Headache* 1990; **30:** 411–17.

Hyperthyroidism. Lithium has been tried in hyperthyroidism (p.1519), though its practical value is a matter of debate and, rarely, it may even cause hyperthyroidism (see Effects on the Endocrine System in Adverse Effects, above). Pretreatment with lithium has also been reported to prolong the expo sure of the thyroid to radioactive iodine in a patient with Graves' thyrotoxicosis resistance to previous iodine treatment.[1]

1. Hoogenberg K, et al. Lithium as an adjunct to radioactive iodine in treatment-resistant Graves thyrotoxicosis. *Ann Intern Med* 1998; **129:** 670.

Schizophrenia. The addition of lithium to antipsychotic treatment may be worthwhile in patients with schizophrenia (p.651) or schizoaffective disorders who fail to respond to an antipsychotic alone, but the danger of an interaction between the drugs should be borne in mind (see under Interactions, above). Although affective symptoms need not be present for patients with schizophrenia to respond to adjunctive lithium their presence does appear to predict a greater likelihood of response.[1]

1. Christison GW, et al. When symptoms persist: choosing among alternative somatic treatments for schizophrenia. *Schizophr Bull* 1991; **17:** 217–45.

Preparations

BP 2001: Lithium Carbonate Tablets; Lithium Citrate Oral Solution; Slow Lithium Carbonate Tablets;
USP 25: Lithium Carbonate Capsules; Lithium Carbonate Extended-release Tablets; Lithium Carbonate Tablets; Lithium Citrate Syrup.

Proprietary Preparations (details are given in Part 3)
Aust.: Neurolepsin; Quilonorm; *Austral.:* Lithicarb; Quilonum; *Belg.:* Camcolit; Maniprex; Priadel; *Braz.:* Carbolim; Carbolitium; Litiocar; *Canad.:* Carbolith; Duralith; Lithane; Lithizine†; *Denm.:* Litarex; *Fin.:* Lito; *Fr.:* Neurolithium; Teralithe; *Ger.:* Hypnorex; leukominerase; Li 450; Quilonum; *Hong Kong:* Camcolit; Lithicarb; Lithiofor; *Irl.:* Camcolit; Priadel; *Israel:* Licarbium; *Ital.:* Carbolithium; *Mex.:* Carbolit; Litheum; *Neth.:* Priadel; *Norw.:* Litarex†; Lithionit; *NZ:* Lithicarb; Priadel; *Port.:* Priadel; *S.Afr.:* Camcolit; Lentolith; Quilonum; *Singapore:* Camcolit; Lithosun; Priadel; *Spain:* Plenur; *Swed.:* Litarex†; Lithionit; *Switz.:* Litarex; Lithiofor; Neurolithium; Priadel; Quilonorm; *Thai.:* Licab; Licarb; Limed; Lit-300; Phanate; *UK:* Camcolit; Li-Liquid; Liskonum; Litarex†; Lithonate; Priadel; *USA:* Eskalith; Lithobid; Lithonate†; Lithotabs†.

Multi-ingredient: *Aust.:* Togal; *Austral.:* Caprilate; *Ger.:* Ney-Dop N (Revitorgan-Dilutionen N Nr 97); Togal; *Spain:* Citinoides.

Lofepramine Hydrochloride   (2522-w)

Lofepramine Hydrochloride *(BANM, USAN, rINNM).*
Leo-640; Lopramine Hydrochloride; WHR-2908A. 5-{3-[N-(Chlorophenacyl)-N-methylamino]propyl}-10,11-5H-dihydrodibenz[b,f]azepine hydrochloride.
$C_{26}H_{27}ClN_2O,HCl = 455.4.$
CAS — 23047-25-8 (lofepramine); 26786-32-3 (lofepramine hydrochloride).
Pharmacopoeias. In Br.

Pharmacopoeial description

BP 2001: A fine, yellowish-white to green-yellow powder with a faint characteristic odour. It exhibits polymorphism. Very slightly soluble in alcohol and in methyl alcohol; slightly soluble in acetone. Store in airtight containers. Protect from light.

Adverse Effects, Treatment, and Precautions

As for tricyclic antidepressants in general (see Amitriptyline, p.273). Lofepramine should be avoided in patients with severe hepatic or severe renal impairment.

Effects on the liver. See under Amitriptyline, p.274.

Overdosage. Lofepramine is a newer tricyclic antidepressant that may be less toxic in overdosage than earlier tricyclics.[1]

1. Reid F, Henry JA. Lofepramine overdosage. *Pharmacopsychiatry* 1990; **23:** 23–27.

Interactions

For interactions associated with tricyclic antidepressants, see Amitriptyline, p.276.

Pharmacokinetics

Lofepramine is readily absorbed from the gastrointestinal tract, and extensively demethylated by first-pass metabolism in the liver to its primary metabolite, desipramine (p.282). Since lofepramine slows gastrointestinal transit time absorption can, however, be delayed, particularly in overdosage. Paths of metabolism also include *N*-oxidation and hydroxylation. Lofepramine is mainly excreted in the urine, chiefly in the form of its metabolites. It is highly bound to plasma proteins. Lofepramine is distributed into breast milk.

Uses and Administration

Lofepramine is a dibenzazepine tricyclic antidepressant with actions and uses similar to those of amitriptyline (p.278). One of its metabolites is desipramine (p.282). Lofepramine is one of the less sedating tricyclics.

In the treatment of depression lofepramine is given by mouth as the hydrochloride in divided doses equivalent to lofepramine 140 to 210 mg daily.

Lofepramine should be withdrawn gradually to reduce the risk of withdrawal symptoms.

◊ References.

1. Lancaster SG, Gonzalez JP. Lofepramine: a review of its pharmacodynamic and pharmacokinetic properties, and therapeutic efficacy in depressive illness. *Drugs* 1989; **37:** 123–40.

Administration in the elderly. The UK manufacturer has suggested that some elderly patients may respond to lower than usual doses of lofepramine, but in a study[1] involving 46 elderly

patients with various grades of depression lofepramine 70 mg once daily was no more effective than placebo at the end of 28 days of treatment.

1. Tan RSH, et al. The effect of low dose lofepramine in depressed elderly patients in general medical wards. *Br J Clin Pharmacol* 1994; **37:** 321–4.

Preparations

BP 2001: Lofepramine Tablets.

Proprietary Preparations (details are given in Part 3)
Aust.: Tymelyt; *Belg.:* Tymelyt†; *Denm.:* Tymelyt; *Ger.:* Gamonil; *Irl.:* Gamanil; *Ital.:* Timelit; *Port.:* Deprimil; *S.Afr.:* Emdalen; *Spain:* Deftan; *Swed.:* Tymelyt; *Switz.:* Gamonil; *UK:* Feprapax; Gamanil; Lomont.

Maprotiline Hydrochloride   (2524-l)

Maprotiline Hydrochloride *(BANM, rINNM).*
Ba-34276; Maprotilini Hydrochloridum. 3-(9,10-Dihydro-9,10-ethanoanthracen-9-yl)propyl(methyl)amine hydrochloride.
$C_{20}H_{23}N,HCl = 313.9.$
CAS — 10262-69-8 (maprotiline); 10347-81-6 (maprotiline hydrochloride).

NOTE. Maprotiline is *USAN*.
Pharmacopoeias. In Eur. (see p.vi) and *US*.

Pharmacopoeial description

Ph. Eur.: A white or almost white crystalline powder. It shows polymorphism. Slightly soluble in water; soluble in alcohol; very slightly soluble in acetone; sparingly soluble in dichloromethane; freely soluble in methyl alcohol.

USP 25: A fine white or off-white, practically odourless, crystalline powder. Slightly soluble in water; freely soluble in chloroform and in methyl alcohol; practically insoluble in isooctane. Store in airtight containers.

Adverse Effects, Treatment, and Precautions

Adverse effects with maprotiline, a tetracyclic antidepressant, are broadly similar to those with tricyclic antidepressants (see Amitriptyline, p.273) but antimuscarinic effects are less frequent.

Skin rashes seem more common with maprotiline than with tricyclic antidepressants. Seizures have occurred in patients with no prior history of such disorders as well as in those with a history of epilepsy and the risk is increased if high doses of maprotiline are employed. It should not be used in patients with epilepsy or a lowered seizure threshold.

◊ By March 1985 the UK Committee on Safety of Medicines[1] had received reports of the following adverse reactions associated with maprotiline from a cumulative total of 2.5 million prescriptions: convulsions (124), hepatic reactions (4), and haematological reactions (8). There had also been 454 reports of skin rashes.

1. Committee on Safety of Medicines. Dangers of newer antidepressants. *Current Problems 15* 1985.

Effects on the skin. In addition to many recorded instances of skin rashes with maprotiline (see above) cutaneous vasculitis, which resolved on discontinuation of therapy, has also been observed.[1]

1. Oakley AMM, Hodge L. Cutaneous vasculitis from maprotiline. *Aust N Z J Med* 1985; **15:** 256–7.

Epileptogenic effect. In a retrospective review of 186 psychiatric patients with no history of prior seizures, 5 of 32 patients receiving maprotiline developed generalised tonic-clonic seizures, compared with 1 of 45 receiving a tricyclic antidepressant.[1] There were no seizures in the remaining patients who received other medications, or no drug treatment. Two of the 5 patients experiencing seizures with maprotiline were receiving doses of 75 to 150 mg daily, 2 were receiving daily doses of 200 to 300 mg, and one patient experienced partial complex seizures with a daily dose of 150 mg and generalised tonic-clonic seizures after increasing the daily dose to 300 mg.

1. Jabbari B, et al. Incidence of seizures with tricyclic and tetracyclic antidepressants. *Arch Neurol* 1985; **42:** 480–1.

Overdosage. Apart from seizures being more common with maprotiline, features of overdosage are similar to those experienced with tricyclic antidepressant poisonings (see under Adverse Effects of Amitriptyline, p.273).

For a discussion of choice of antidepressant with respect to safety in overdosage, see under Depression, p.271.

References.
1. Crome P, Newman B. Poisoning with maprotiline and mianserin. *BMJ* 1977; **2:** 260.
2. Curtis RA, et al. Fatal maprotiline intoxication. *Drug Intell Clin Pharm* 1984; **18:** 716–20.
3. Knudsen K, Heath A. Effects of self poisoning with maprotiline. *BMJ* 1984; **288:** 601–3.
4. Crome P, Ali C. Clinical features and management of self-poisoning with newer antidepressants. *Med Toxicol* 1986; **1:** 411–20.

Porphyria. Maprotiline hydrochloride is considered to be unsafe in patients with porphyria because it has been shown to be porphyrinogenic in *animals*.

Interactions

Interactions associated with maprotiline are similar to those associated with tricyclic antidepressants (see Amitriptyline, p.276).

Pharmacokinetics

Maprotiline is slowly but completely absorbed from the gastrointestinal tract.

Maprotiline is extensively demethylated in the liver to its principal active metabolite, desmethylmaprotiline; paths of metabolism of both maprotiline and desmethylmaprotiline include *N*-oxidation, aliphatic and aromatic hydroxylation, and the formation of aromatic methoxy derivatives. In addition to desmethylmaprotiline, maprotiline-*N*-oxide is also reported to be pharmacologically active. The average elimination half-life of maprotiline is reported to be about 51 hours and that of its active metabolite even longer (range 60 to 90 hours). Maprotiline is excreted in the urine, mainly in the form of its metabolites, either in free or in conjugated form; appreciable amounts are also excreted in the faeces.

Maprotiline is widely distributed throughout the body and is extensively bound to plasma protein. Maprotiline is distributed into breast milk (see Breast Feeding under Precautions of Amitriptyline, p.275).

◊ References.

1. Maguire KP, et al. An evaluation of maprotiline: intravenous kinetics and comparison of two oral doses. *Eur J Clin Pharmacol* 1980; **18:** 249–54.
2. Alkalay D, et al. Bioavailability and kinetics of maprotiline. *Clin Pharmacol Ther* 1980; **27:** 697–703.
3. Firkusny L, Gleiter H. Maprotiline metabolism appears to cosegregate with the genetically-determined CYP2D6 polymorphic hydroxylation of debrisoquine. *Br J Clin Pharmacol* 1994; **37:** 383–8.

Uses and Administration

Maprotiline is a tetracyclic antidepressant with actions and uses similar to those of tricyclic antidepressants (see Amitriptyline, p.278). It is one of the more sedating antidepressants but antimuscarinic effects are less marked. Like the tricyclics, maprotiline is an inhibitor of the reuptake of noradrenaline; it also has weak affinity for central adrenergic (α_1) receptors.

Maprotiline is usually given by mouth as the hydrochloride but it has also been given by injection as the mesilate and in oral drops as the resinate.

In the treatment of depression (p.271) maprotiline hydrochloride is given by mouth in doses of 25 to 75 mg daily in three divided doses, gradually increased to 150 mg daily if necessary; up to 225 mg daily may be required in severely depressed patients in hospital. The dosage should be adjusted after 1 or 2 weeks according to response. Because of the prolonged half-life of maprotiline the total daily dose may also be given as a single dose, usually at night. A suggested initial dose for elderly patients is 10 mg three times daily or 30 mg at night gradually increased according to response over a period of 1 to 2 weeks to 25 mg three times daily or 75 mg at night.

Maprotiline should be withdrawn gradually to reduce the risk of withdrawal symptoms.

Preparations

USP 25: Maprotiline Hydrochloride Tablets.

Proprietary Preparations (details are given in Part 3)
Aust.: Ludiomil; *Belg.:* Ludiomil; *Braz.:* Ludiomil; *Canad.:* Ludiomil; *Denm.:* Ludiomil; Maludil; *Fr.:* Ludiomil; *Ger.:* Aneural; Deprilept; Ludiomil; Mapro-GRY†; Maprolu; Mirpan; Psymion; *Hong Kong:* Ludiomil; *Israel:* Ludiomil; Melodil; *Ital.:* Ludiomil; *Mex.:* Ludiomil; *Neth.:* Ludiomil; *NZ:* Ludiomil; *Port.:* Ludiomil; *S.Afr.:* Ludiomil; *Singapore:* Ludiomil; *Spain:* Ludiomil; *Swed.:* Ludiomil; *Switz.:* Ludiomil; *Thai.:* Ludiomil; *UK:* Ludiomil; *USA:* Ludiomil†.

Medifoxamine   (12920-k)

Medifoxamine *(rINN).*
NN-Dimethyl-2,2-diphenoxyethylamine.
$C_{16}H_{19}NO_2 = 257.3.$
CAS — 32359-34-5.
ATC — N06AX13.

Profile

Medifoxamine is an antidepressant. It was withdrawn because of adverse hepatic effects.

Preparations

Proprietary Preparations (details are given in Part 3)
Fr.: Cledial†.

Melitracen Hydrochloride   (2526-j)

Melitracen Hydrochloride *(USAN, rINNM).*
N7001; U-24973A. 3-(9,10-Dihydro-10,10-dimethyl-9-anthrylidene)propyldimethylamine hydrochloride.
$C_{21}H_{25}N,HCl = 327.9.$
CAS — 5118-29-6 (melitracen); 10563-70-9 (melitracen hydrochloride).

Melitracen hydrochloride 28.1 mg is approximately equivalent to 25 mg of melitracen.

Profile

Melitracen is a tricyclic antidepressant (see Amitriptyline, p.273).

In the treatment of depression it is given by mouth as the hydrochloride in initial doses equivalent to melitracen 25 mg two or three times daily gradually increased to a total of 225 mg daily if necessary. Elderly patients should generally be given reduced doses equivalent to melitracen 25 mg daily initially.

Melitracen should be withdrawn gradually to reduce the risk of withdrawal symptoms.

Preparations

Proprietary Preparations (details are given in Part 3)
Aust.: Dixeran; *Belg.*: Dixeran; *Switz.*: Dixerant†.

Multi-ingredient: *Aust.*: Deanxit; *Belg.*: Deanxit; *Hong Kong:* Deanxit; *Ital.*: Deanxit; *Singapore:* Deanxit; *Spain:* Deanxit; *Switz.*: Deanxit; *Thai.*: Deanxit.

Mianserin Hydrochloride (2527-z)

Mianserin Hydrochloride (BANM, USAN, rINNM).

Mianserini Hydrochloridum; Org-GB-94. 1,2,3,4,10,14b-Hexahydro-2-methyldibenzo[c,f]pyrazino[1,2-a]azepine hydrochloride.

$C_{18}H_{20}N_2$,HCl = 300.8.

CAS — 24219-97-4 (mianserin); 21535-47-7 (mianserin hydrochloride).

Pharmacopoeias. In Eur. (see p.vi).

Pharmacopoeial description

Ph. Eur.: A white or almost white crystalline powder or crystals. Sparingly soluble in water; slightly soluble in alcohol; soluble in dichloromethane. A 1% solution in water has a pH of 4.0 to 5.5. Protect from light.

Adverse Effects

Antimuscarinic and cardiac side-effects are fewer and milder with mianserin, a tetracyclic antidepressant, than with tricyclic antidepressants but effects are otherwise broadly similar (see Amitriptyline, p.273); mianserin may be associated with a lower risk of cardiotoxicity in overdosage.

The most common adverse effect associated with mianserin is drowsiness. Mianserin also causes bone-marrow depression usually presenting as leucopenia, granulocytopenia, or agranulocytosis; aplastic anaemia has been reported. These adverse haematological reactions generally occur during the first few weeks of therapy and especially in the elderly.

Other side-effects reported include disturbances of liver function and jaundice, breast disorders (gynaecomastia, nipple tenderness, and non-puerperal lactation), and polyarthropathy.

Effects on the blood. Between 1976 and the end of 1988 the UK Committee on Safety of Medicines (CSM) had received 239 reports of adverse haematological reactions associated with mianserin.[1] The reports included 68 of agranulocytosis and 84 of granulocytopenia or leucopenia where mianserin was considered to be the probable or possible cause; there had been 17 fatalities. Allowing for the pattern of prescribing there was a greater number of reports of white blood cell disorders in patients over 65 years of age but there was no sex difference. The data also indicated that the adverse reactions were most likely to develop during the first three months of therapy. By the end of 1992 the number of reports of mianserin-induced agranulocytosis received by the CSM[2] had risen to 79 and the number of reports of mianserin-induced neutropenia was 105.

A case of fatal aplastic anaemia associated with mianserin has also been reported.[3]

Proposed mechanisms of mianserin haematotoxicity have included a direct toxicity[4] and an immunologically-mediated mechanism.[5] There is evidence from *in vitro* studies of a significant correlation between the desmethyl metabolite and cytotoxicity. Mianserin is administered as a racemic preparation and the formation of metabolites was greater with the R(−)-enantiomer than with the S(+)-enantiomer.[6]

1. Committee on Safety of Medicines. Mianserin and white blood cell disorders in the elderly. *Current Problems 25* 1989.
2. Committee on Safety of Medicines/Medicines Control Agency. Drug-induced neutropenia and agranulocytosis. *Current Problems* 1993; **19**: 10–11.
3. Durrant S, Read D. Fatal aplastic anaemia associated with mianserin. *BMJ* 1982; **285**: 437.
4. O'Donnell JL, et al. Possible mechanism for mianserin induced neutropenia associated with saturable elimination kinetics. *BMJ* 1985; **291**: 1375–6.
5. Stricker BHC, et al. Thrombocytopenia and leucopenia with mianserin-dependent antibodies. *Br J Clin Pharmacol* 1985; **19**: 102–4.
6. Riley RJ, et al. A stereochemical investigation of the cytotoxicity of mianserin metabolites in vitro. *Br J Clin Pharmacol* 1989; **27**: 823–30.

Effects on the cardiovascular system. Although mianserin is considered to be less cardiotoxic than the tricyclic antidepressants adverse effects have been noted in individual patients. Two elderly patients developed signs of disturbed cardiac function (cardiac failure, atrial and ventricular fibrillation, bradycardia, and frequent ventricular ectopic beats) which resolved after the drug was discontinued.[1] One of the patients also developed hypokalaemia which was possibly caused by mianserin. It was suggested that persons most likely to experience problems were the elderly with a past history of cardiovascular disorders. Further reports of mianserin-induced cardiac effects include recurrent ventricular fibrillation in a 61-year-old

man after an overdose of mianserin[2] and bradycardia in a 50-year-old woman following a therapeutic dose.[3]

1. Whiteford H, et al. Disturbed cardiac function possibly associated with mianserin therapy. *Med J Aust* 1984; **140**: 166–7.
2. Haefeli WE, et al. Recurrent ventricular fibrillation in mianserin intoxication. *BMJ* 1991; **302**: 415–16.
3. Carcone B, et al. Symptomatic bradycardia caused by mianserin at therapeutic doses. *Hum Exp Toxicol* 1991; **10**: 383–4.

Effects on the liver. By March 1985 the UK Committee on Safety of Medicines had received 57 reports of hepatic reactions associated with mianserin from a total of 5 million prescriptions. Reactions had included jaundice and other abnormalities of liver function, but no fatalities had been reported.[1] Case reports have also been published concerning jaundice;[2-5] the liver function returned to normal after discontinuation of mianserin or dose reduction.

1. Committee on Safety of Medicines. Dangers of newer antidepressants. *Current Problems 15* 1985.
2. Adverse Drug Reactions Advisory Committee. Mianserin: a possible cause of neutropenia and agranulocytosis. *Med J Aust* 1980; **2**: 673–4.
3. Goldstraw PW, et al. Mianserin and jaundice. *N Z Med J* 1983; **96**: 985.
4. Zarski J-P, et al. Toxicité hépatique des nouveaux anti-dépresseurs: à propos d'une observation. *Gastroenterol Clin Biol* 1983; **7**: 220–1.
5. Otani K, et al. Hepatic injury caused by mianserin. *BMJ* 1989; **299**: 519.

Effects on the musculoskeletal system. A patient developed an acute polyarthritis affecting the hands and feet 6 days after commencing therapy with mianserin;[1] the authors of the report also mentioned that the UK Committee on Safety of Medicines had received 19 reports of arthritis and arthralgia associated with mianserin.

1. Hughes A, Coote J. Arthropathy associated with treatment with mianserin. *BMJ* 1986; **292**: 1050.

Effects on the skin. Reports of adverse dermatological reactions in individual patients related to mianserin therapy have included toxic epidermal necrolysis[1] and erythema multiforme.[2,3]

1. Randell P. Tolvon and toxic epidermal necrolysis. *Med J Aust* 1979; **2**: 653.
2. Quraishy E. Erythema multiforme during treatment with mianserin—a case report. *Br J Dermatol* 1981; **104**: 481.
3. Cox NH. Erythema multiforme due to mianserin—a case against generic prescribing. *Br J Clin Pract* 1985; **39**: 293–4.

Effects on the tongue. Glossitis associated with mianserin therapy has been reported in 2 patients.[1] Additionally, glossitis accompanied by severe facial oedema has been noted in another patient.[2] In all cases symptoms resolved after withdrawal of mianserin.

1. de la Fuente JR, Berlanga C. Glossitis associated with mianserin. *Lancet* 1984; **i**: 233.
2. Leibovitch G, et al. Severe facial oedema and glossitis associated with mianserin. *Lancet* 1989; **ii**: 871–2.

Epileptogenic effect. By March 1985 the UK Committee on Safety of Medicines had received 64 reports of convulsions associated with mianserin from a total of 5 million prescriptions.[1] In a previous review[2] concerning 40 of these cases it was considered that a causal connection could be established only in a minority. It was suggested that mianserin is no more epileptogenic than tricyclic antidepressants, an opinion that was also shared by other reviewers.[3]

1. Committee on Safety of Medicines. Dangers of newer antidepressants. *Current Problems 15* 1985.
2. Edwards JG, Glen-Bott M. Mianserin and convulsive seizures. *Br J Clin Pharmacol* 1983; **15**: 299S–311S.
3. Richens A, et al. Antidepressant drugs, convulsions and epilepsy. *Br J Clin Pharmacol* 1983; **15**: 295S–298S.

Overdosage. Experience with 100 consecutive cases of intoxication with mianserin[1] revealed that when it was the only drug ingested symptoms were mild and neither deep coma nor convulsions occurred. More serious symptoms were seen in patients who had taken multiple drug overdoses and there were 2 fatalities. The results suggested that following an acute overdose mianserin is less toxic than the tricyclic antidepressants. This conclusion was also supported by a large follow-up study[2] comparing the outcome of suicide attempts among patients who had taken mianserin in overdose with those who had taken amitriptyline.

1. Chand S, et al. One hundred cases of acute intoxication with mianserin hydrochloride. *Pharmakopsychiatrie* 1981; **14**: 15–17.
2. Inman WHW. Blood disorders and suicide in patients taking mianserin or amitriptyline. *Lancet* 1988; **ii**: 90–2.

Precautions

As for tricyclic antidepressants in general (see Amitriptyline, p.275). Although mianserin does not have the cardiotoxicity of the tricyclic antidepressants, it should be used with caution in patients with cardiovascular disorders, such as heart block, or after recent myocardial infarction. Patients with angle-closure glaucoma or prostatic hyperplasia should be monitored even though antimuscarinic effects are rare. Mianserin should be used with caution in patients with diabetes mellitus, epilepsy, and hepatic or renal insufficiency.

Patients should be carefully monitored during early antidepressant therapy until improvement in depression is observed because suicide is an inherent risk in depressed patients. For further details, see under Depression, p.271.

A full blood count is recommended every 4 weeks during the first 3 months of treatment with mianserin, because of the risk

of bone-marrow depression. Similarly, if a patient receiving mianserin develops fever, sore throat, stomatitis, or other signs of infection, treatment should be stopped and a full blood count obtained. The elderly are considered to be at special risk of blood disorders from mianserin. For further details see Effects on the Blood under Adverse Effects, above.

The manufacturers recommend that mianserin should not be given during breast feeding, but some authorities consider the amount distributed into breast milk too small to be harmful.

Porphyria. Mianserin hydrochloride is considered to be unsafe in patients with porphyria because it has been shown to be porphyrinogenic in *animals*.

Interactions

It is recommended that mianserin should not be given to patients receiving MAOIs or for at least 14 days after their discontinuation. At least one week should elapse between withdrawing mianserin and starting any drug liable to provoke a serious reaction (e.g. phenelzine). Unlike the tricyclics (p.276), mianserin does not diminish the effects of the antihypertensives guanethidine, hydralazine, propranolol, clonidine, or betanidine. However, it is still recommended that blood pressure be monitored when mianserin is prescribed with antihypertensive therapy. Plasma-phenytoin concentrations should be monitored carefully in patients treated concurrently with mianserin; phenytoin has been reported to reduce concentrations of mianserin. There may be potentiation of effects when mianserin is given concomitantly with CNS depressants such as alcohol, anxiolytics, or antipsychotics.

Antiepileptics. Reduced plasma concentrations and half-lives of mianserin and desmethylmianserin were observed in 6 patients also receiving antiepileptic therapy consisting of phenytoin with either carbamazepine or phenobarbital.[1] Carbamazepine alone may also reduce the plasma concentration of mianserin.[2,3]

Mianserin may antagonise the action of antiepileptics by lowering the convulsive threshold.

1. Nawishy S, et al. Kinetic interaction of mianserin in epileptic patients on anticonvulsant drugs. *Br J Clin Pharmacol* 1982; **13**: 612P–13P.
2. Leinonen E, et al. Effects of carbamazepine on serum antidepressant concentrations in psychiatric patients. *J Clin Psychopharmacol* 1991; **11**: 313–18.
3. Eap CB, et al. Effects of carbamazepine coadministration on plasma concentrations of the enantiomers of mianserin and of its metabolites. *Ther Drug Monit* 1999; **21**: 166–70.

Pharmacokinetics

Mianserin is readily absorbed from the gastrointestinal tract, but its bioavailability is reduced by extensive first-pass metabolism in the liver.

Paths of metabolism of mianserin include aromatic hydroxylation, N-oxidation, and N-demethylation. Desmethylmianserin and 8-hydroxymianserin are pharmacologically active.

Mianserin is excreted in the urine, almost entirely as its metabolites, either free or in conjugated form; some is also found in the faeces.

Mianserin is widely distributed throughout the body and is extensively bound to plasma proteins. It has been found to have a biphasic plasma half-life with the duration of the terminal phase ranging from about 6 to 40 hours. Mianserin crosses the blood-brain barrier and the placenta. It is distributed into breast milk.

◊ References.

1. Hrdina PD, et al. Mianserin kinetics in depressed patients. *Clin Pharmacol Ther* 1983; **33**: 757–62.
2. Pinder RM, Van Delft AML. The potential therapeutic role of enantiomers and metabolites of mianserin. *Br J Clin Pharmacol* 1983; **15**: 269S–276S.
3. Timmer CJ, et al. Absolute bioavailability of mianserin tablets and solution in healthy humans. *Eur J Drug Metab Pharmacokinet* 1985; **10**: 315–23.
4. Begg EJ, et al. Variability in the elimination of mianserin in elderly patients. *Br J Clin Pharmacol* 1989; **27**: 445–51.
5. Buist A, et al. Mianserin in breast milk. *Br J Clin Pharmacol* 1993; **36**: 133–4.
6. Dahl M-L, et al. Stereoselective disposition of mianserin is related to debrisoquin hydroxylation polymorphism. *Clin Pharmacol Ther* 1994; **56**: 176–83.

Uses and Administration

Mianserin is a tetracyclic antidepressant. It does not appear to have significant antimuscarinic properties, but has a marked sedative action. Unlike the tricyclic antidepressants (see Amitriptyline, p.278), mianserin does not prevent the peripheral re-uptake of noradrenaline; it blocks presynaptic adrenergic (α_2) receptors and increases the turnover of brain noradrenaline. Mianserin is also an antagonist of serotonin receptors in some parts of the brain. It is used as the hydrochloride.

In the treatment of depression (p.271) mianserin hydrochloride is given by mouth in initial doses of 30 to 40 mg daily increased gradually thereafter as necessary. The effective daily dosage is usually between 30 and 90 mg. The daily dosage may be divided throughout the day or given as a single dose at night. Divided daily dosages of up to 200 mg have been given. The recommended initial daily dose in the elderly is not more than 30 mg, which may be slowly increased if necessary.

Mianserin should be withdrawn gradually to reduce the risk of withdrawal symptoms.

Preparations

BP 2001: Mianserin Tablets.

Proprietary Preparations (details are given in Part 3)
Aust.: Miabene; Tolvon; *Austral.:* Lerivon; Lumin; Tolvon; *Belg.:* Lerivon; *Braz.:* Tolvon; *Denm.:* Tolmin; Tolvon; *Fin.:* Miaxan; Tolvon; *Fr.:* Athymil; *Ger.:* Hopacem; Mianeurin; Prisma; Tolvin; *Hong Kong:* Tolvon; *Irl.:* Tolvon; *Israel:* Bolvidon; Bonserin; *Ital.:* Lantanon; *Mex.:* Tolvon; *Neth.:* Tolvon; *Norw.:* Tolvon; *NZ:* Tolvon; *Port.:* Tolvon; *S.Afr.:* Lantanon; *Singapore:* Tolvon; *Spain:* Lantanon; *Swed.:* Tolvon; *Switz.:* Tolvon; *Thai.:* Mealin; Servin; Tolimed; Tolvon.

Milnacipran Hydrochloride (5030-j)

Milnacipran Hydrochloride *(BANM, rINNM).*

F-2207 (milnacipran); Midalcipran Hydrochloride. (±)-*cis*-2-(Aminomethyl)-*N,N*-diethyl-1-phenylcyclopropanecarboxamide hydrochloride.

$C_{15}H_{22}N_2O,HCl = 282.8.$

CAS — 92623-85-3 (milnacipran); 101152-94-7 (milnacipran hydrochloride); 175131-61-0 (milnacipran hydrochloride).

Profile

Milnacipran hydrochloride is a serotonin and noradrenaline reuptake inhibitor (SNRI) used for the treatment of depression (p.271). It is given by mouth in doses of 100 mg daily.

◊ References.

1. Ansseau M, *et al.* Controlled comparison of milnacipran and fluoxetine in major depression. *Psychopharmacology (Berl)* 1994; **114:** 131–7.
2. Leinonen E, *et al.* Long-term efficacy and safety of milnacipran compared to clomipramine in patients with major depression. *Acta Psychiatr Scand* 1997; **96:** 497–504.
3. Tignol J, *et al.* Double-blind study of the efficacy and safety of milnacipran and imipramine in elderly patients with major depressive episode. *Acta Psychiatr Scand* 1998; **97:** 157–65.
4. Spencer CM, Wilde MI. Milnacipran: a review of its use in depression. *Drugs* 1998; **56:** 405–27.

Preparations

Proprietary Preparations (details are given in Part 3)
Aust.: Dalcipran; Ixel; *Fr.:* Ixel; *Israel:* Ixel; *Port.:* Ixel.

Mirtazapine (11022-r)

Mirtazapine *(BAN, USAN, rINN).*

Org-3770. (*RS*)-1,2,3,4,10,14b-Hexahydro-2-methylpyrazino[2,1-*a*]pyrido[2,3-*c*][2]benzazepine.

$C_{17}H_{19}N_3 = 265.4.$

CAS — 61337-67-5.

ATC — N06AX11.

Adverse Effects

Side-effects commonly reported with mirtazapine are an increase in appetite and weight; drowsiness or sedation generally occur during the first few weeks of treatment. Dizziness, headache, oedema, and increases in liver enzyme levels have been reported less commonly; jaundice may occur. Other rarely reported side-effects include postural hypotension, exanthema, nightmares, agitation, mania, hallucinations, paraesthesia, convulsions, tremor, myoclonus, restless legs syndrome, arthralgia, myalgia, and reversible agranulocytosis, leucopenia, and granulocytopenia.

Hyponatraemia, possibly due to inappropriate secretion of antidiuretic hormone, has been associated with the use of antidepressants, particularly in the elderly.

Precautions

Mirtazapine should be used with caution in patients with epilepsy, hepatic or renal impairment, and cardiac disorders such as conduction disturbances, angina pectoris, and recent myocardial infarction, and also in patients with hypotension, diabetes mellitus, psychoses, and in those with a history of bipolar disorder. Treatment should be stopped if jaundice develops. Although mirtazapine has only weak antimuscarinic activity, caution should nevertheless be exercised in patients with micturition disturbances, angle-closure glaucoma, and raised intra-ocular pressure.

Patients should be advised to report any of the following symptoms during treatment: fever, sore throat, stomatitis, or other signs of infection; treatment should be stopped and a blood count performed.

Drowsiness is often experienced at the start of therapy and patients, if affected, should not drive or operate machinery.

Patients should be closely monitored during early therapy until improvement in depression is observed because suicide is an inherent risk in depressed patients. For further details, see under Depression, p.271.

Mirtazapine should be withdrawn gradually to reduce the risk of withdrawal symptoms.

Interactions

Mirtazapine should not be used concomitantly with or within two weeks of discontinuing an MAOI; at least one week should elapse between discontinuation of mirtazapine and starting any drug liable to provoke a serious reaction (e.g. phenelzine). Use of mirtazapine with alcohol, anxiolytics, or hypnotics may potentiate sedative effects.

Pharmacokinetics

Mirtazapine is well absorbed from the gastrointestinal tract with peak plasma levels occurring after about 2 hours. Plasma protein binding is about 85%. Mirtazapine is extensively metabolised in the liver and the major biotransformation pathways are demethylation and oxidation followed by glucuronide conjugation; cytochrome P450 isoenzymes involved are CYP2D6, CYP1A2, and CYP3A4. The *N*-desmethyl metabolite is pharmacologically active. Elimination is via urine (75%) and faeces (15%). The mean plasma elimination half-life is 20 to 40 hours. Data from *animal* studies indicate that mirtazapine crosses the placenta and is distributed into breast milk.

◊ References.

1. Timmer CJ, *et al.* Clinical pharmacokinetics of mirtazapine. *Clin Pharmacokinet* 2000; **38:** 461–74.

Uses and Administration

Mirtazapine, a piperazinoazepine, is an analogue of mianserin (p.298); it is a noradrenergic and specific serotonergic antidepressant. It enhances the release of noradrenaline and, indirectly, serotonin through blockade of central presynaptic adrenergic (α_2) receptors. The effects of released serotonin are mediated via $5\text{-}HT_1$ receptors as mirtazapine blocks both $5\text{-}HT_2$ and $5\text{-}HT_3$ receptors. Mirtazapine is given as a racemic mixture: the S(+)-enantiomer blocks α_2 and $5\text{-}HT_2$ receptors whereas the R(−)-enantiomer blocks $5\text{-}HT_3$ receptors. Mirtazapine is also a potent antagonist at histamine (H_1) receptors which gives it sedative properties; it has very little antimuscarinic activity.

In the treatment of depression (p.271), mirtazapine is given by mouth in an initial daily dose of 15 mg, which may be increased gradually according to clinical response. Changes in dose should be made at intervals of at least 1 to 2 weeks because of the long half-life. The usual effective dose lies within the range of 15 to 45 mg. Daily doses may be given as a single dose, preferably at bedtime, or in 2 equally divided doses.

Mirtazapine should be withdrawn gradually to reduce the risk of withdrawal symptoms.

◊ References.

1. Sitsen JMA, Moors J. Mirtazapine, a novel antidepressant, in the treatment of anxiety symptoms: results from a placebo-controlled trial. *Drug Invest* 1994; **8:** 339–44.
2. Kasper S, *et al.* A risk-benefit assessment of mirtazapine in the treatment of depression. *Drug Safety* 1997; **17:** 251–64.
3. Puzantian T. Mirtazapine, an antidepressant. *Am J Health-Syst Pharm* 1998; **55:** 44–9.
4. Holm KJ, Markham A. Mirtazapine: a review of its use in major depression. *Drugs* 1999; **57:** 607–31.

Preparations

Proprietary Preparations (details are given in Part 3)
Aust.: Remeron; *Austral.:* Avanza; *Denm.:* Remeron; *Fin.:* Remeron; *Fr.:* Norset; *Ger.:* Remergil; *Hong Kong:* Remeron; *Irl.:* Zispin; *Israel:* Remeron; *Ital.:* Remeron; *Mex.:* Remeron; *Neth.:* Remeron; *Port.:* Remeron; *S.Afr.:* Remeron; *Singapore:* Remeron; *Spain:* Rexer; *Swed.:* Remeron; *Thai.:* Remeron; *UK:* Zispin; *USA:* Remeron.

Moclobemide (19529-x)

Moclobemide *(BAN, USAN, rINN).*

Ro-11-1163; Ro-11-1163/000. 4-Chloro-*N*-(2-morpholinoethyl)benzamide.

$C_{13}H_{17}ClN_2O_2 = 268.7.$

CAS — 71320-77-9.

ATC — N06AG02.

Pharmacopoeias. In *Swiss.*

Adverse Effects

Adverse effects reported to occur with moclobemide include sleep disturbances, dizziness, agitation, feelings of anxiety, restlessness, irritability, and headache. Gastrointestinal disturbances include dry mouth, diarrhoea, constipation, and nausea and vomiting. Paraesthesia, visual disturbances, and oedema have also been reported, and skin reactions include rash, pruritus, urticaria, and flushing. Confusional states that disappear rapidly on discontinuation of the drug have been observed. Raised liver enzymes have been reported.

Hyponatraemia, possibly due to inappropriate secretion of antidiuretic hormone, has been associated with the use of antidepressants, particularly in the elderly.

Effects on the cardiovascular system. Hypertension has been reported[1,2] rarely in patients taking moclobemide. Some of these patients were taking other drugs concomitantly although moclobemide was suspected to be the cause. Blood pressure usually returned to normal after discontinuation of moclobemide.

1. Coulter DM, Pillans PI. Hypertension with moclobemide. *Lancet* 1995; **346:** 1032.
2. Boyd IW. Hypertension with moclobemide. *Lancet* 1995; **346:** 1498.

Effects on the endocrine system. A prescription-event monitoring study demonstrated that galactorrhoea is significantly associated with the use of moclobemide.[1]

1. Dunn NR, *et al.* Galactorrhoea with moclobemide. *Lancet* 1998; **351:** 802.

Overdosage. Symptoms that have been reported with overdosage of moclobemide include agitation, aggression, behavioural disturbances, and gastrointestinal irritation.

References.

1. Hetzel W. Safety of moclobemide taken in overdose for attempted suicide. *Psychopharmacology (Berl)* 1992; **106:** S127–S129.
2. Hackett LP, *et al.* Disposition and clinical effects of moclobemide and three of its metabolites following overdose. *Drug Invest* 1993; **5:** 281–4.
3. Myrenfors PG, *et al.* Moclobemide overdose. *J Intern Med* 1993; **233:** 113–15.

Precautions

Moclobemide is contra-indicated in patients with acute confusional states and in those with phaeochromocytoma. It should be avoided in excited or agitated patients, unless given in combination with a sedative. Manic episodes may be provoked in patients with bipolar disorders. Care is also required in patients with thyrotoxicosis as moclobemide may theoretically precipitate a hypertensive reaction. Reduced doses should be used in patients with severe hepatic impairment.

Patients should be closely monitored during early antidepressant therapy until improvement in depression is observed because suicide is an inherent risk in depressed patients. For further details, see under Depression, p.271.

Although impairment of mental alertness is generally not expected with moclobemide, caution should be exercised with respect to driving or operating machinery until individual reactions have been assessed.

Antidepressants, particularly MAOIs, should be withdrawn gradually to reduce the risk of withdrawal symptoms.

Although the amounts of moclobemide distributed into breast milk are reported to be small (see under Pharmacokinetics, below), the manufacturers advise caution and consideration of the benefits of moclobemide therapy to the mother against possible risks to the infant.

Interactions

The dietary restrictions that need to be followed with selective reversible inhibitors of monoamine oxidase type A such as moclobemide are less stringent than

---

The symbol † denotes a preparation no longer actively marketed

those for non-selective inhibitors of monoamine oxidase types A and B (see under Interactions of Phenelzine, p.305). However, the manufacturers of moclobemide recommend that since some patients may be especially sensitive to tyramine, consumption of large amounts of tyramine-rich food should be avoided.

Medicines containing *sympathomimetics, dextromethorphan,* or *anorectics* should not be taken with moclobemide. Moclobemide should not be given with *other antidepressants* although, owing to its short duration of action, a treatment-free period is generally considered unnecessary following its cessation. For further details, see Antidepressants under Interactions of Phenelzine, p.306. Therapy with moclobemide should not be started until at least a week following cessation of a tricyclic or related antidepressant or a selective serotonin reuptake inhibitor or related antidepressant (2 weeks in the case of paroxetine and sertraline; at least 5 weeks in the case of fluoxetine) or for at least a week after stopping treatment with non-selective MAOIs. CNS excitation or depression may occur if moclobemide is taken concomitantly with *opioid analgesics,* and there is also a risk of CNS toxicity if taken with *serotonin (5-HT₁)* agonists. Moclobemide may enhance the effects of *ibuprofen* and possibly *other NSAIDs.* There has also been a warning that a hypertensive crisis may occur if moclobemide and *levodopa* are used together. The metabolism of moclobemide is inhibited by *cimetidine,* leading to increased plasma concentrations and a need for reduced dosage (see below).

Antimigraine drugs. For the effects of moclobemide on serotonin (5-HT₁) agonists, see under Sumatriptan, p.457.

Cimetidine. Administration of cimetidine 1 g daily for 2 weeks increased the mean maximum plasma concentration of moclobemide in 8 healthy subjects from 575 nanograms per mL to 787 nanograms per mL; several other parameters associated with moclobemide absorption and disposition were also affected.[1] It was suggested that a reduction in the dosage of moclobemide might be required. The manufacturers of moclobemide recommend reducing the dose by half in patients also receiving cimetidine.

1. Schoerlin M-P, *et al.* Cimetidine alters the disposition kinetics of the monoamine oxidase-A inhibitor moclobemide. *Clin Pharmacol Ther* 1991; **49:** 32–8.

Dopaminergics. Caution is required when *selegiline* and moclobemide are given together. Dietary restrictions with this combination (see under Phenelzine, p.305) are recommended by one manufacturer of selegiline, whereas another advises that this combination should be avoided (as does the manufacturer of moclobemide).

For the effects of moclobemide on *levodopa,* see p.1171, and on selegiline, see p.1177.

Omeprazole. Omeprazole, which is an inhibitor of cytochrome P450 isoenzyme CYP2C19, increased plasma concentrations and elimination half-life of moclobemide in extensive metabolisers of the drug towards values seen in poor metabolisers.[1] It had little effect on pharmacokinetic parameters in poor metabolisers. The clinical effects were uncertain but extra care might be warranted if the 2 drugs are given together.

1. Yu K-S, *et al.* Effect of omeprazole on the pharmacokinetics of moclobemide according to the genetic polymorphism of CYP2C19. *Clin Pharmacol Ther* 2001; **69:** 266–73.

Opioid analgesics. Symptoms suggestive of a mild serotonin syndrome (p.304) developed in a 73-year-old woman taking moclobemide, nortriptyline, and lithium after she was given *pethidine* intravenously.[1]

1. Gillman PK. Possible serotonin syndrome with moclobemide and pethidine. *Med J Aust* 1995; **162:** 554.

Sympathomimetics. Symptoms resembling phaeochromocytoma occurred in an elderly woman who was receiving treatment with the reversible MAOI toloxatone;[1] the woman had also been receiving a preparation containing *phenylephrine* without ill-effect but the symptoms occurred after addition of *terbutaline* therapy. It was noted that such an interaction is more typical of older, irreversible, less selective MAOIs.

1. Lefebvre H, *et al.* Life-threatening pseudo-phaeochromocytoma after toloxatone, terbutaline, and phenylephrine. *Lancet* 1993; **341:** 555–6.

Pharmacokinetics

Moclobemide is readily absorbed from the gastrointestinal tract, peak plasma concentrations occurring within 1 to 2 hours of ingestion. Absorption is virtually complete but first-pass metabolism reduces bioavailability of the drug. Moclobemide is widely distributed throughout the body and undergoes extensive

metabolism in the liver, in part by the cytochrome P450 isoenzymes CYP2C19 and CYP2D6. Metabolites of moclobemide and a small amount of unchanged drug are excreted in the urine. Moclobemide has a plasma elimination half-life of 1 to 4 hours. Moclobemide is distributed into breast milk.

◊ References.
1. Mayersohn M, Guentert TW. Clinical pharmacokinetics of the monoamide oxidase-A inhibitor moclobemide. *Clin Pharmacokinet* 1995; **29:** 292–332.
2. Gram LF, *et al.* Moclobemide: a substrate of CYP2C19 and an inhibitor of CYP2C19, CYP2D6, and CYP1A2: a panel study. *Clin Pharmacol Ther* 1995; **57:** 670–7.

Distribution into breast milk. In a study[1] of the distribution of moclobemide into the breast milk of 6 lactating mothers given a single 300-mg dose of moclobemide, a mean of 0.057% of the dose appeared in breast milk as moclobemide and 0.031% as its major metabolite Ro-12-8095 within 24 hours of administration. It was considered that this small amount of moclobemide was unlikely to be hazardous to suckling infants.

1. Pons G, *et al.* Moclobemide excretion in human breast milk. *Br J Clin Pharmacol* 1990; **29:** 27–31.

Uses and Administration

Moclobemide, a benzamide derivative, is a reversible inhibitor of monoamine oxidase type A (RIMA) (see under Phenelzine, p.307) used for the treatment of depression and of social phobia.

In the treatment of **depression** the usual initial daily dose of moclobemide is 300 mg by mouth in divided doses. This may be increased to up to 600 mg daily according to response. In some patients, a maintenance dose of 150 mg daily may be sufficient.

In the treatment of **social phobia,** the initial daily dose of moclobemide is 300 mg increased after 3 days to 600 mg given in 2 divided doses. Treatment should be continued for 8 to 12 weeks to assess efficacy; patients should be periodically re-evaluated thereafter to determine the need for further treatment. Moclobemide should be taken after food.

Doses in patients with severe hepatic impairment may need to be reduced by half to one-third.

Antidepressants, particularly MAOIs, should be withdrawn gradually to reduce the risk of withdrawal symptoms.

◊ Reviews.
1. Fulton B, Benfield P. Moclobemide: an update of its pharmacological properties and therapeutic use. *Drugs* 1996; **52:** 450–74.

Anxiety disorders. The use of MAOIs in general in the management of anxiety disorders is discussed under Phenelzine on p.307. For a discussion of the overall treatment of anxiety disorders, see p.649.

References.
1. Noyes R, *et al.* Moclobemide in social phobia: a controlled dose-response trial. *J Clin Psychopharmacol* 1997; **17:** 247–54.
2. Neal LA, *et al.* An open trial of moclobemide in the treatment of post-traumatic stress disorder. *Int Clin Psychopharmacol* 1997; **12:** 231–7.
3. Schneier FR, *et al.* Placebo-controlled trial of moclobemide in social phobia. *Br J Psychiatry* 1998; **172:** 70–7.
4. Tiller JW, *et al.* Moclobemide and fluoxetine for panic disorder. *Eur Arch Psychiatry Clin Neurosci* 1999; **249** (suppl 1): S7–S10.

Depression. As discussed on p.271 there is very little difference in efficacy between the different groups of antidepressant drugs, and choice is often made on the basis of adverse effects. The traditional MAOIs such as phenelzine are rarely used as first-choice antidepressants because of the dangers of dietary and drug interactions. Reversible inhibitors of monoamine oxidase type A (RIMAs) such as moclobemide offer a safer alternative to the irreversible non-selective MAOIs and fewer dietary restrictions are necessary.

References.
1. Fitton A, *et al.* Moclobemide: a review of its pharmacological properties and therapeutic use in depressive illness. *Drugs* 1992; **43:** 561–96.
2. Angst J, Stabl M. Efficacy of moclobemide in different patient groups: a meta-analysis of studies. *Psychopharmacology (Berl)* 1992; **106** (suppl): S109–S113.
3. Freeman H. Moclobemide. *Lancet* 1993; **342:** 1528–32.
4. Lonnqvist J, *et al.* Moclobemide and fluoxetine in atypical depression: a double-blind trial. *J Affect Disord* 1994; **32:** 169–77.
5. Anonymous. Moclobemide for depression. *Drug Ther Bull* 1994; **32:** 6–8.
6. Norman TR, Burrows GD. A risk-benefit assessment of moclobemide in the treatment of depressive disorders. *Drug Safety* 1995; **12:** 46–54.
7. Roth M, *et al.* Moclobemide in elderly patients with cognitive decline and depression: an international double-blind, placebo-controlled trial. *Br J Psychiatry* 1996; **168:** 149–57.
8. Lotufo-Neto F, *et al.* Meta-analysis of the reversible inhibitors of monoamine oxidase type A moclobemide and brofaromine for the treatment of depression. *Neuropsychopharmacology* 1999; **20:** 226–47.

Smoking cessation. In a preliminary double-blind, placebo-controlled parallel-group study in 88 smokers, moclobemide facilitated smoking cessation (p.1642) in highly dependent smokers.[1]

1. Berlin I, *et al.* A reversible monoamine oxidase A inhibitor (moclobemide) facilitates smoking cessation and abstinence in heavy, dependent smokers. *Clin Pharmacol Ther* 1995; **58:** 444–52.

Preparations

Proprietary Preparations (details are given in Part 3)
Aust.: Aurorix; **Austral.:** Arima; Aurorix; Mohexal; **Belg.:** Aurorix; **Braz.:** Aurorix; **Canad.:** Manerix; **Denm.:** Aurorix; **Fin.:** Aurorix; **Fr.:** Moclamine; **Ger.:** Aurorix; **Hong Kong:** Aurorix; **Irl.:** Manerix; **Israel:** Mobemide; **Ital.:** Aurorix; **Mex.:** Aurorex; Feraken; **Neth.:** Aurorix; **Norw.:** Aurorix; **NZ:** Aurorix; **Port.:** Aurorix; **S.Afr.:** Aurorix; **Singapore:** Aurorix; **Spain:** Manerix; **Swed.:** Aurorix; **Switz.:** Aurorix; **Thai.:** Aurorix; **UK:** Manerix.

Nefazodone Hydrochloride (6275-x)

Nefazodone Hydrochloride (BANM, USAN, rINNM).
BMY-13754; MJ-13754-1.
CAS — 83366-66-9 *(nefazodone);* 82752-99-6 *(nefazodone hydrochloride).*

Adverse Effects and Treatment

The most common adverse effects seen with nefazodone are weakness, dry mouth, nausea, constipation, somnolence, dizziness, and lightheadedness. Other effects which have occurred less frequently include chills, fever, orthostatic hypotension, incoordination, vasodilatation, arthralgia, paraesthesia, confusion, memory impairment, abnormal dreams, ataxia, and amblyopia and other visual disturbances. Syncope has occurred rarely and there have been reports of sinus bradycardia. Hepatotoxicity has occurred (see below).

Hyponatraemia, possibly due to inappropriate secretion of antidiuretic hormone, has been associated with the use of antidepressants, particularly in the elderly.

In overdosage, the symptoms that have been reported most frequently include hypotension, nausea, vomiting, and drowsiness. Treatment of overdosage involves gastric lavage followed by symptomatic and supportive therapy.

◊ Reviews.
1. Robinson DS, *et al.* The safety profile of nefazodone. *J Clin Psychiatry* 1996; **57** (suppl 2): 31–8.

Effects on the liver. Subfulminant hepatic failure developed in 3 women given nefazodone for depression.[1] Two patients required liver transplantation although this was unsuccessful in one case and the patient died. Hepatitis, positive on rechallenge, has also been reported with nefazodone.[2]

The manufacturers of nefazodone state that rare events of raised liver enzymes, hepatitis, liver failure and necrosis have been reported since marketing but no causal relationship has been established. The Canadian manufacturers have indicated[3] that as of June 2001 there had been 109 reports of serious hepatic adverse events associated with nefazodone from postmarketing surveillance worldwide. These included 23 cases of liver failure, of which 16 led to transplantation and/or death. Most cases occurred within 4 months of beginning treatment although a few were after continuous use for up to 2 years.

1. Aranda-Michel J, *et al.* Nefazodone-induced liver failure: report of three cases. *Ann Intern Med* 1999; **130:** 285–8.
2. Schrader GD, Roberts-Thompson IC. Adverse effect of nefazodone: hepatitis. *Med J Aust* 1999; **170:** 452.
3. Bristol-Myers Squibb Canada Inc/Linson Pharama Inc. Important safety information on nefazodone HCl: severe and serious hepatic events. Available at: http://www.hc-sc.gc.ca./hpb-dgps/therapeut/zfiles/english/advisory/industry/nefazodone_e.pdf (accessed 20/08/01).

Overdosage. A 27-year-old woman developed no serious toxicity after taking 3 g of nefazodone in a suicide attempt.[1] Somnolence was the most severe effect noted. In another case, a 31-year-old woman attempted suicide with 16.8 g of nefazodone and an unknown quantity of verapamil.[2] The patient was lethargic, and developed significant bradycardia and hypotension; she recovered after supportive therapy. The authors reported that among the 7 cases of overdose occurring during clinical trials, there were no fatalities or permanent sequelae.

1. Gaffney PW, *et al.* Nefazodone overdose. *Ann Pharmacother* 1998; **32:** 1249–50.
2. Catalano G, *et al.* Nefazodone overdose: a case report *Clin Neuropharmacol* 1999; **22:** 63–5.

Precautions

Nefazodone should be used with caution in patients with epilepsy, a history of hypomania or mania, or hepatic or severe renal impairment. It should also be used with caution in cardiovascular or cerebrovascular disease that could be exacerbated by hypotension (for example recent history of myocardial infarction, unstable heart disease, angina, or ischaemic stroke), and in any condition such as dehydration or hypovolaemia that may predispose patients to hypotension.

Since nefazodone is structurally related to trazodone which is known to have caused priapism (see p.310), the manufacturer recommends that any patient developing inappropriate or prolonged penile erections should discontinue nefazodone immediately.

Patients should be closely monitored during early antidepressant therapy until improvement in depression is observed because suicide is an inherent risk in depressed patients. For further details, see under Depression, p.271.

Nefazodone may impair performance of skilled tasks and, if affected, patients should not drive or operate machinery.

Antidepressants should be withdrawn gradually to reduce the risk of withdrawal symptoms.

Breast feeding. A study[1] in 2 nursing mothers receiving nefazodone for postpartum depression indicated that nefazodone, but not its major active metabolites, was distributed into breast milk in variable amounts; the quantity present did not seem to be dose related. The calculated exposure of the two women's offspring was 2.2% and 0.4% of the maternal dose respectively. Another report suggested that even such low exposures might result in clinically significant effects:[2] drowsiness, inability to maintain normal body temperature, and poor feeding were reported in the breast-fed infant of a woman receiving nefazodone. After breast feeding was discontinued the symptoms resolved, suggesting an association between the two despite a calculated exposure in the infant of only 0.45% of the maternal dose.

The manufacturers of nefazodone advise against breast feeding by women receiving the drug.

1. Dodd S, *et al.* Nefazodone in the breast milk of nursing mothers: a report of two patients. *J Clin Psychopharmacol* 2000; **20:** 717–18.
2. Yapp P, *et al.* Drowsiness and poor feeding in a breast-fed infant: association with nefazodone and its metabolites. *Ann Pharmacother* 2000; **34:** 1269–72.

Interactions

Nefazodone should not be given to patients receiving MAOIs or for at least 14 days after their discontinuation; it has also been recommended that any drug liable to provoke a serious reaction (e.g. phenelzine) should not be given within one week after discontinuation of nefazodone therapy. For further details on the coadministration of antidepressants, see Antidepressants under Interactions of Phenelzine, p.306.

Orthostatic hypotension can be a problem with nefazodone, and therefore a reduction in dose of antihypertensive drugs administered concomitantly may be required.

Nefazodone is an inhibitor of the cytochrome P450 isoenzyme CYP3A4 responsible for the metabolism of some benzodiazepines, and consequently concomitant administration may produce clinically important increases in their plasma concentrations. The potential also exists for increased plasma concentrations of astemizole, cisapride, pimozide, and terfenadine (which are metabolised by the same isoenzyme), and concomitant administration is best avoided because of the risk of inducing ventricular arrhythmias. Other substrates for this isoenzyme may also interact with nefazodone: lovastatin and simvastatin should be used with caution with nefazodone since there have been rare reports of rhabdomyolysis with such combinations. Increased serum levels of ciclosporin, another substrate, have been reported in patients receiving concomitant nefazodone. Monitoring of serum ciclosporin levels is recommended when these two drugs are given together.

Plasma concentrations of digoxin are increased by the concomitant administration of nefazodone and it is recommended that, because of digoxin's narrow therapeutic index, plasma concentrations of digoxin should be monitored if coadministration with nefazodone is necessary.

Caution should be exercised when haloperidol is given concomitantly with nefazodone as the clearance of haloperidol may be reduced. Plasma concentrations

of carbamazepine are also increased when given with nefazodone and concomitant administration should be avoided if possible, or carbamazepine levels monitored if coadministration is necessary. Conversely, nefazodone plasma concentrations may decrease with coadministration of carbamazepine.

The potential for interaction between nefazodone and general anaesthetics exists and the manufacturer recommends that nefazodone should be stopped before elective surgery for as long as clinically feasible.

Pharmacokinetics

Nefazodone is readily absorbed from the gastrointestinal tract and peak plasma concentrations have been obtained 1 to 3 hours after oral administration. Absorption is delayed and reduced by food but this is not considered to be clinically significant. Nefazodone undergoes extensive first-pass metabolism and is more than 99% bound to plasma proteins; it is widely distributed. It is extensively metabolised by N-dealkylation and hydroxylation in the liver to several metabolites, two of which, hydroxynefazodone and *m*-chlorophenylpiperazine, are known to be pharmacologically active. Excretion is predominantly as metabolites via the urine (approximately 55%) and the faeces (20 to 30%). The plasma elimination half-life is 2 to 4 hours. Pharmacokinetic parameters are reported to be non-linear with increasing doses. Nefazodone is distributed in small amounts into breast milk (see Precautions, above).

◊ Reviews.
1. Greene DS, Barbhaiya RH. Clinical pharmacokinetics of nefazodone. *Clin Pharmacokinet* 1997; **33:** 260–75.

Uses and Administration

Nefazodone is a phenylpiperazine antidepressant structurally related to trazodone (see p.310). It blocks the reuptake of serotonin at presynaptic neurones and is an antagonist at postsynaptic 5-HT$_2$ receptors. Unlike trazodone, nefazodone inhibits the reuptake of noradrenaline. It blocks α_1-adrenoceptors but has no apparent effect on dopamine receptors. Nefazodone does not appear to have very significant antimuscarinic properties compared with tricyclic antidepressants. It is used as the hydrochloride.

Nefazodone hydrochloride is given by mouth for the treatment of depression in a usual initial dose of 50 to 100 mg twice daily, increased after 5 to 7 days to 200 mg twice daily. The dose may be increased gradually, if necessary, to a maximum of 300 mg twice daily. Elderly patients, especially females, may have higher plasma concentrations than other patients and a maximal therapeutic effect is usually achieved at doses of 100 to 200 mg twice daily. Initial doses should be restricted to 50 mg twice daily. Doses should be restricted to the lower end of the range in patients with hepatic or severe renal impairment.

Antidepressants should be withdrawn gradually to reduce the risk of withdrawal symptoms.

◊ Reviews.
1. Ellingrod VL, Perry PJ. Nefazodone: a new antidepressant. *Am J Health-Syst Pharm* 1995; **52:** 2799–2812.

Anxiety disorders. Nefazodone has been tried in a variety of anxiety disorders including panic attacks (p.649) with or without associated depression and post-traumatic stress disorder (p.650).
References.
1. DeMartinis NA, *et al.* An open-label trial of nefazodone in high comorbidity panic disorder. *J Clin Psychiatry* 1996; **57:** 245–8.
2. Hidalgo R, *et al.* Nefazodone in post-traumatic stress disorder: results from six open-label trials. *Int Clin Psychopharmacol* 1999; **14:** 61–8.

Depression. As discussed on p.271, there is very little difference in efficacy between the different groups of antidepressant drugs, and choice is often made on the basis of adverse effect profile. Nefazodone has a different biochemical profile from both the tricyclics and the SSRIs.
References.
1. Rickels K, *et al.* Nefazodone and imipramine in major depression: a placebo-controlled trial. *Br J Psychiatry* 1994; **164:** 802–5.
2. Fontaine R, *et al.* A double-blind comparison of nefazodone, imipramine, and placebo in major depression. *J Clin Psychiatry* 1994; **55:** 234–41.

3. Ansseau M, *et al.* Controlled comparison of nefazodone and amitriptyline in major depressive inpatients. *Psychopharmacology (Berl)* 1994; **115:** 254–60.
4. Anonymous. Nefazodone for depression. *Med Lett Drugs Ther* 1995; **37:** 33–4.
5. Baldwin DS, *et al.* A multicenter double-blind comparison of nefazodone and paroxetine in the treatment of outpatients with moderate-to-severe depression. *J Clin Psychiatry* 1996; **57** (suppl 2): 46–52.
6. Feiger A, *et al.* Nefazodone versus sertraline, in outpatients with major depression: focus on efficacy, tolerability, and effects on sexual function and satisfaction. *J Clin Psychiatry* 1996; **57** (suppl 2): 53–62.
7. Anonymous. Three new antidepressants. *Drug Ther Bull* 1996; **34:** 65–8.
8. Cyr M, Brown CS. Nefazodone: its place among antidepressants. *Ann Pharmacother* 1996; **30:** 1006–12.
9. Davis R, *et al.* Nefazodone: a review of its pharmacology and clinical efficacy in the management of major depression. *Drugs* 1997; **53:** 608–36.

Preparations

Proprietary Preparations (details are given in Part 3)
Aust.: Dutonin; *Austral.:* Serzone; *Braz.:* Serzone; *Canad.:* Serzone; *Denm.:* Nefadar; *Fin.:* Nefadar; *Ger.:* Nefadar; *Hong Kong:* Serzone; *Irl.:* Dutonin; *Israel:* Serzonil; *Ital.:* Reseril; *Mex.:* Serzone; *Neth.:* Dutonin; *Norw.:* Nefadar; *NZ:* Serzone; *S.Afr.:* Serzone; *Singapore:* Serzone; *Spain:* Dutonin; Menfazona; Rulivan; *Swed.:* Nefadar; *Switz.:* Nefadar; *Thai.:* Serzone; *UK:* Dutonin; *USA:* Serzone.

Nialamide (2528-c)

Nialamide (BAN, rINN).
N′-(2-Benzylcarbamoylethyl)isonicotinohydrazide.
$C_{16}H_{18}N_4O_2 = 298.3$.
CAS — 51-12-7.
ATC — N06AF02.

Profile
Nialamide, a hydrazine derivative, is an irreversible inhibitor of monoamine oxidase types A and B (see Phenelzine, p.303). It has been used in the treatment of depression and is sometimes used as a pharmacological tool.

Preparations
Proprietary Preparations (details are given in Part 3)
Belg.: Niamid†.

Nortriptyline Hydrochloride (2530-w)

Nortriptyline Hydrochloride (BANM, USAN, rINNM).
38489; Nortriptylini Hydrochloridum. 3-(10,11-Dihydro-5H-dibenzo[*a,d*]cyclohepten-5-ylidene)propyl(methyl)amine hydrochloride.
$C_{19}H_{21}N,HCl = 299.8$.
CAS — 72-69-5 (nortriptyline); 894-71-3 (nortriptyline hydrochloride).
Pharmacopoeias. In Eur. (see p.vi), Jpn, and US.

Nortriptyline hydrochloride 22.8 mg is approximately equivalent to 20 mg of nortriptyline.

Pharmacopoeial description
Ph. Eur.: A white or almost white powder. Sparingly soluble in water; soluble in alcohol and in dichloromethane. Protect from light.
USP 25: A white to off-white powder having a slight characteristic odour. Soluble 1 in 90 of water, 1 in 30 of alcohol, 1 in 20 of chloroform, and 1 in 10 of methyl alcohol; practically insoluble in ether, in benzene, and in most other organic solvents. pH of a 1% solution in water is about 5. Store in airtight containers. Protect from light.

Adverse Effects, Treatment, and Precautions
As for tricyclic antidepressants in general (see Amitriptyline, p.273).

Effects on ventilation. Severe hyperventilation developed in a 61-year-old man with end-stage renal disease after receiving nortriptyline 125 mg daily;[1] mechanical ventilation was necessary to correct severe respiratory alkalosis.
1. Sunderrajan S, *et al.* Nortriptyline-induced severe hyperventilation. *Arch Intern Med* 1985; **145:** 746–7.

Porphyria. Nortriptyline is considered to be unsafe in patients with porphyria although there is conflicting experimental evidence of porphyrinogenicity.

Interactions
For interactions associated with tricyclic antidepressants, see Amitriptyline, p.276.

Pharmacokinetics
Nortriptyline is the principal active metabolite of amitriptyline (p.278). Nortriptyline has been reported to have a longer plasma half-life than amitriptyline.

Nortriptyline is subject to extensive first-pass metabolism in the liver to 10-hydroxynortriptyline, which is active.

Metabolism. There is evidence that individuals with a poor debrisoquine hydroxylation phenotype may be at greater risk of confusional states when taking nortriptyline.[1] This was thought to be because the polymorphic hydroxylation of debrisoquine and nortriptyline are mediated by similar enzymatic mechanisms, with poor oxidisers having higher plasma nortriptyline concentrations.[2,3] A nonlinear (dose-dependent) relationship between dose and plasma-nortriptyline concentrations has been observed during therapeutic drug monitoring[4] in subjects who were considered to be extensive metabolisers of debrisoquine; nonlinearity did not appear to occur in poor metabolisers. There was no significant correlation between hydroxylation phenotype and amitriptyline concentrations, suggesting that demethylation and hydroxylation of tricyclic antidepressants are mediated by different cytochrome P450 isoenzymes.[5]

The pharmacokinetics and pharmacological actions of 10-hydroxynortriptyline, the major active metabolite of nortriptyline, have been reviewed.[3]

1. Park BK, Kitteringham NR. Adverse reactions and drug metabolism. *Adverse Drug React Bull* 1987; **122:** 456–9.
2. Nordin C, *et al.* Plasma concentrations of nortriptyline and its 10-hydroxy metabolite in depressed patients—relationship to the debrisoquine hydroxylation metabolic ratio. *Br J Clin Pharmacol* 1985; **19:** 832–5.
3. Nordin C, Bertilsson L. Active hydroxymetabolites of antidepressants: emphasis on E-10-hydroxy-nortriptyline. *Clin Pharmacokinet* 1995; **28:** 26–40.
4. Jerling M, Alván G. Nonlinear kinetics of nortriptyline in relation to nortriptyline clearance as observed during therapeutic drug monitoring. *Eur J Clin Pharmacol* 1994; **46:** 67–70.
5. Bertilsson L, *et al.* Metabolism of various drugs in subjects with different debrisoquine and sparteine oxidation phenotypes. *Br J Clin Pharmacol* 1982; **14:** 602P.

Plasma concentrations. Nortriptyline appears to have an optimum antidepressant effect between 50 and 150 nanograms per mL. Above and below this specific plasma concentration range, there is a poor clinical response. Plasma concentration measurements are unequivocally useful in problem patients who do not respond to usual oral doses or in high-risk patients for whom, because of age or medical illness, it is especially important to use the lowest possible effective dose of the drug.[1]

It has been suggested[2] that within this window of total nortriptyline concentrations there is a probability of an antidepressant response of 68% or more with free concentrations of 7 to 10 nanograms per mL.

For reference to dose-dependent kinetics of nortriptyline observed in individuals with an extensive debrisoquine hydroxylation phenotype, see under Metabolism, above.

1. Task Force on the Use of Laboratory Tests in Psychiatry. Tricyclic antidepressants—blood level measurements and clinical outcome: an APA task force report. *Am J Psychiatry* 1985; **142:** 155–62.
2. Perry PJ, *et al.* The relationship of free nortriptyline levels to antidepressant response. *Drug Intell Clin Pharm* 1984; **18:** 510.

Uses and Administration

Nortriptyline is a dibenzocycloheptadiene tricyclic antidepressant with actions and uses similar to those of amitriptyline (p.278). It is the principal active metabolite of amitriptyline. Nortriptyline is one of the less sedating tricyclics and its antimuscarinic effects are mild.

In the treatment of **depression** nortriptyline is given by mouth as the hydrochloride starting with a low dose and gradually increasing to the equivalent of nortriptyline 75 to 100 mg daily in divided doses. Up to a maximum of 150 mg daily may be required in patients with severe depression. The manufacturers recommend that plasma concentrations of nortriptyline should be monitored when doses above 100 mg daily are given. Adolescents and the elderly may be given 30 to 50 mg daily in divided doses. Since nortriptyline has a prolonged half-life, once-daily dosage regimens are also suitable, usually given at night.

Nortriptyline is also used for the treatment of **nocturnal enuresis** in children in whom organic pathology has been excluded. However, drug therapy for nocturnal enuresis should be reserved for those in whom other methods have failed and should preferably only be given to cover periods away from home; tricyclic antidepressants are not recommended in children under 6 years of age (some authorities recommend that they should not be given until 7 years of age). Suggested doses are 10 mg for children aged 6 to 7 years, 10 to 20 mg for children aged 8 to 11 years, and 25 to 35 mg for children aged over 11 years. The dose should be given 30 minutes before bedtime and treat-

ment should not continue for longer than 3 months, which should include a period of gradual withdrawal. A full physical examination is recommended before a further course.

Nortriptyline should be withdrawn gradually to reduce the risk of withdrawal symptoms.

Smoking cessation. For reference to the use of nortriptyline in management of smoking cessation, see p.279.

Preparations

BP 2001: Nortriptyline Capsules; Nortriptyline Tablets;
USP 25: Nortriptyline Hydrochloride Capsules; Nortriptyline Hydrochloride Oral Solution.

Proprietary Preparations (details are given in Part 3)
Aust.: Nortrilen; **Austral.:** Allegron; **Belg.:** Nortrilen; **Braz.:** Pamelor; **Canad.:** Aventyl; **Denm.:** Noritren; **Fin.:** Noritren; **Ger.:** Nortrilen; **Hong Kong:** Nortrilen; **Irl.:** Aventyl; **Ital.:** Noritren; Vividyl†; **Neth.:** Nortrilen; **Norw.:** Noritren; **NZ:** Allegron; Norpress; **Port.:** Norterol; Nortrix†; **S.Afr.:** Aventyl; **Spain:** Martimil; Norfenazin; Paxtibi; **Swed.:** Sensaval; **Switz.:** Nortrilen; **Thai.:** Norline; Nortrilen; Nortyline; Ortrip; **UK:** Allegron; **USA:** Aventyl; Pamelor.

Multi-ingredient: **Fr.:** Motival†; **Hong Kong:** Motival; **Irl.:** Motipress†; Motival; **Ital.:** Dominans; **S.Afr.:** Motival; **Spain:** Tropargal; **Thai.:** Motival; **UK:** Motipress; Motival.

Opipramol Hydrochloride (2532-l)

Opipramol Hydrochloride (BANM, USAN, rINNM).
G-33040. 2-[4-(3-5*H*-Dibenz[*b,f*]azepin-5-ylpropyl)piperazin-1-yl]ethanol dihydrochloride.
$C_{23}H_{29}N_3O,2HCl = 436.4$.
CAS — 315-72-0 (opipramol); 909-39-7 (opipramol dihydrochloride).

Pharmacopoeias. In Pol.

Profile
Opipramol hydrochloride is a tricyclic antidepressant (see Amitriptyline, p.273) given by mouth in doses of 50 to 300 mg daily in the treatment of depression.

It should be withdrawn gradually to reduce the risk of withdrawal symptoms.

Preparations

Proprietary Preparations (details are given in Part 3)
Aust.: Insidon; **Belg.:** Insidon†; **Fr.:** Insidon†; **Ger.:** Insidon; **Irl.:** Insidon; **Israel:** Oprimol; **Ital.:** Insidon†; **Neth.:** Insidon†; **Switz.:** Insidon.

Oxaflozane Hydrochloride (2295-z)

Oxaflozane Hydrochloride (rINNM).
1766-Cerm (oxaflozane); CERM-1766 (oxaflozane). 4-Isopropyl-2-(α,α,α-trifluoro-*m*-tolyl)morpholine hydrochloride.
$C_{14}H_{18}F_3NO,HCl = 309.8$.
CAS — 26629-87-8 (oxaflozane); 26629-86-7 (oxaflozane hydrochloride).

Profile
Oxaflozane hydrochloride is an antidepressant.

Preparations

Proprietary Preparations (details are given in Part 3)
Fr.: Conflictan†.

Oxitriptan (12836-r)

Oxitriptan (rINN).
5-HTP; L-5-Hydroxytryptophan; Ro-0783/B. L-2-Amino-3-(5-hydroxy-1*H*-indol-3-yl)propionic acid.
$C_{11}H_{12}N_2O_3 = 220.2$.
CAS — 4350-09-8 (oxitriptan); 56-69-9 (DL-5-hydroxytryptophan).
ATC — N06AX01.

Profile
Oxitriptan is the L form of 5-hydroxytryptophan, a precursor of serotonin. Like tryptophan (p.311) it is used in the treatment of depression; it is given in doses of up to 600 mg daily by mouth.

Oxitriptan is also used in doses of up to 1 g daily in myoclonic disorders, especially posthypoxic myoclonus (p.342). It has also been employed in various neurological conditions including migraine, pain syndromes, and sleep disorders, and as an adjunct in epilepsy and parkinsonism.

DL-Oxitriptan has also been used as an antidepressant.

Preparations

Proprietary Preparations (details are given in Part 3)
Fr.: Levotonine; **Ger.:** Levothym; **Ital.:** Oxyfan†; Tript-OH; **Port.:** Cincofarm; **Spain:** Cincofarm; Telesol; **Switz.:** Tript-OH.

Paroxetine Hydrochloride (18670-k)

Paroxetine Hydrochloride (BANM, rINNM).
BRL-29060 (paroxetine); BRL-29060A (paroxetine hydrochloride); FG-7051 (paroxetine). (−)-*trans*-5-(4-*p*-Fluorophenyl-3-piperidylmethoxy)-1,3-benzodioxole hydrochloride.
$C_{19}H_{20}FNO_3,HCl = 365.8$.
CAS — 61869-08-7 (paroxetine); 78246-49-8 (paroxetine hydrochloride).

NOTE. Paroxetine is *USAN*.

Paroxetine hydrochloride 22.2 mg is approximately equivalent to 20 mg of paroxetine.

Adverse Effects, Treatment, and Precautions

As for SSRIs in general (see Fluoxetine, p.284).

Extrapyramidal reactions (including orofacial dystonias) and withdrawal symptoms associated with paroxetine have been reported to the UK Committee on Safety of Medicines more commonly than with other SSRIs. For further details, see Extrapyramidal Effects under Adverse Effects of Fluoxetine, p.285 and Withdrawal under Precautions, p.287.

There is a potential for worsening of panic symptoms during the initial treatment of panic disorder with paroxetine.

Interactions

For interactions associated with SSRIs, see Fluoxetine, p.287.

Pharmacokinetics

Paroxetine is readily absorbed from the gastrointestinal tract with peak plasma concentrations occurring within about 5 hours of ingestion. It undergoes extensive first-pass metabolism in the liver. The main metabolic pathway is oxidation followed by methylation and formation of glucuronide and sulfate conjugates. Paroxetine is widely distributed throughout body tissues and is about 95% bound to plasma proteins. The elimination half-life of paroxetine is reported to be about 21 hours. Excretion is via the urine (approximately 64%) and the faeces (approximately 36%), mainly as metabolites in both cases. Paroxetine is distributed into breast milk (see Breast Feeding under Precautions in Fluoxetine, p.286).

◊ References.
1. Dalhoff K, *et al.* Pharmacokinetics of paroxetine in patients with cirrhosis. *Eur J Clin Pharmacol* 1991; **41:** 351–4.

Uses and Administration

Paroxetine, a phenylpiperidine derivative, is an SSRI with actions and uses similar to those of fluoxetine (p.288). Paroxetine is given by mouth as paroxetine hydrochloride, usually in the morning as a single dose with food. Doses are expressed in terms of paroxetine.

In the treatment of **depression**, the usual dose of paroxetine is 20 mg daily, increased gradually, if necessary, by increments of 10 mg to a maximum of 50 mg daily.

In the treatment of **obsessive-compulsive disorder**, the initial dose is 20 mg daily increased weekly in 10-mg increments to a usual maintenance dose of 40 mg daily; some patients may require up to 60 mg daily.

In the treatment of **panic disorder** with or without agoraphobia, the initial dose is 10 mg daily increased weekly in 10-mg increments according to clinical response; the usual recommended maintenance dose is 40 mg daily, although some patients may benefit from 50 or 60 mg daily.

The initial dose for the treatment of **social phobia** is 20 mg daily increased after at least 2 weeks, if necessary, by increments of 10 mg at weekly intervals to a maximum of 50 or 60 mg daily.

In the treatment of **generalised anxiety disorder**, the initial dose is 20 mg daily increased in weekly increments of 10 mg to a maximum of 50 mg.

The recommended starting dose for the treatment of **post-traumatic stress disorder** is 20 mg daily. If necessary this may be increased in increments of 10 mg up to a maximum of 50 mg daily.

A suggested maximum daily dose in elderly or debilitated patients is 40 mg. A recommended dose for patients with severe renal or severe hepatic impairment is 10 mg daily in the USA, and 20 mg daily in the UK; incremental dosage if required should be restricted to the lower end of the range.

Paroxetine should be withdrawn gradually to reduce the risk of withdrawal symptoms. For further details, see Withdrawal under Precautions of Fluoxetine, p.287.

◊ Reviews.
1. Grimsley SR, Jann MW. Paroxetine, sertraline, and fluvoxamine: new selective serotonin reuptake inhibitors. *Clin Pharm* 1992; **11:** 930–57.
2. Anonymous. Paroxetine for treatment of depression. *Med Lett Drugs Ther* 1993; **35:** 24–5.
3. Caley CF, Weber SS. Paroxetine: a selective serotonin reuptake inhibiting antidepressant. *Ann Pharmacother* 1993; **27:** 1212–22.
4. Gunasekara NS, et al. Paroxetine: an update of its pharmacology and therapeutic use in depression and a review of its use in other disorders. *Drugs* 1998; **55:** 85–120.

Anxiety disorders. Paroxetine is used in a variety of anxiety disorders including generalised anxiety disorder (p.649), obsessive-compulsive disorder (p.649), panic attacks (p.649), post-traumatic stress disorder (p.650), and social phobia (see under Phobic Disorders, p.649). It has also been tried for adult night terrors (see under Parasomnias, p.653).

References.
1. Oehrberg S, et al. Paroxetine in the treatment of panic disorder: a randomised, double-blind, placebo-controlled study. *Br J Psychiatry* 1995; **167:** 374–9.
2. Stein MB, et al. Paroxetine in the treatment of generalized social phobia: open-label treatment and double-blind placebo-controlled discontinuation. *J Clin Psychopharmacol* 1996; **16:** 218–22.
3. Zohar J, et al. Paroxetine versus clomipramine in the treatment of obsessive-compulsive disorder. *Br J Psychiatry* 1996; **169:** 468–74.
4. Lecrubier Y, et al. Long-term evaluation of paroxetine, clomipramine and placebo in panic disorder. *Acta Psychiatr Scand* 1997; **95:** 153–60.
5. Wilson SJ, et al. Adult night terrors and paroxetine. *Lancet* 1997; **350:** 185.
6. Stein MB, et al. Paroxetine treatment of generalized social phobia (social anxiety disorder). *JAMA* 1998; **280:** 708–13.

Depression. As discussed on p.271, there is very little difference in efficacy between the different groups of antidepressant drugs, and choice is often made on the basis of adverse effect profile. SSRIs such as paroxetine are widely used as an alternative to the older tricyclics as they have fewer unpleasant side-effects and are safer in overdosage.

References.
1. De Wilde J, et al. A double-blind, comparative, multicentre study comparing paroxetine with fluoxetine in depressed patients. *Acta Psychiatr Scand* 1993; **87:** 141–5.
2. Arminen S-L, et al. A 12-week double-blind multi-centre study of paroxetine and imipramine in hospitalized depressed patients. *Acta Psychiatr Scand* 1994; **89:** 382–9.
3. Ansseau M, et al. Controlled comparison of paroxetine and fluvoxamine in major depression. *Hum Psychopharmacol Clin Exp* 1994; **9:** 329–36.
4. Montgomery SA, et al. Reduction of suicidal thoughts with paroxetine in comparison with reference antidepressants and placebo. *Eur Neuropsychopharmacol* 1995; **5:** 5–13.
5. Geretsegger C, et al. Multicenter double blind study of paroxetine and amitriptyline in elderly depressed inpatients. *Psychopharmacology (Berl)* 1995; **119:** 277–81.
6. Leyman S, et al. Paroxetine: post-marketing experience on 4024 depressed patients in Belgium. *Eur J Clin Res* 1995; **7:** 287–96.
7. Rodríguez-Ramos P, et al. Effects of paroxetine in depressed adolescents. *Eur J Clin Res* 1996; **8:** 49–61.
8. Schnyder U, Koller-Leiser A. A double-blind, multicentre study of paroxetine and maprotiline in major depression. *Can J Psychiatry* 1996; **41:** 239–44.
9. Moon C, Vince M. Treatment of major depression in general practice: a double-blind comparison of paroxetine and lofepramine. *Br J Clin Pract* 1996; **50:** 240–4.
10. Williams JW, et al. Treatment of dysthymia and minor depression in primary care: a randomized controlled trial in older adults. *JAMA* 2000; **284:** 1519–26.

Premenstrual syndrome. Paroxetine in doses ranging from 10 to 30 mg daily throughout the menstrual cycle has produced beneficial effects in controlling both the psychological and somatic symptoms of premenstrual syndrome;[1] it was more effective than the tetracyclic antidepressant maprotiline.

For a discussion of the overall management of premenstrual syndrome, see p.1475.
1. Eriksson E, et al. The serotonin reuptake inhibitor paroxetin is superior to the noradrenaline reuptake inhibitor maprotiline in the treatment of premenstrual syndrome. *Neuropsychopharmacology* 1995; **12:** 167–76.

Sexual dysfunction. Impotence or ejaculatory problems have been reported as adverse effects of SSRIs (see Effects on Sexual Function in Adverse Effects of Fluoxetine, p.285). Such properties of the SSRIs have been studied as a potential form of treatment for men with premature ejaculation. Paroxetine was found to be effective in delaying premature ejaculation in a

study involving 17 patients with primary (lifelong) or a history of at least 2 years' premature ejaculation.[1]
1. Waldinger MD, et al. Paroxetine treatment of premature ejaculation: a double-blind, randomized, placebo-controlled study. *Am J Psychiatry* 1994; **151:** 1377–9.

Preparations

Proprietary Preparations (details are given in Part 3)
Aust.: Seroxat; **Austral.:** Aropax; **Belg.:** Aropax; Seroxat; **Braz.:** Aropax; **Canad.:** Paxil; **Denm.:** Seroxat; **Fin.:** Seroxat; **Fr.:** Deroxat; **Ger.:** Seroxat; Tagonis; **Hong Kong:** Seroxat; **Irl.:** Seroxat; **Israel:** Seroxat; **Ital.:** Sereupin; Seroxat; **Mex.:** Aropax; Paxil; **Neth.:** Seroxat; **Norw.:** Seroxat; **NZ:** Aropax; **Port.:** Paxetil; Seroxat; **S.Afr.:** Aropax; **Singapore:** Seroxat; **Spain:** Casbol; Frosinor; Motivan; Seroxat; **Swed.:** Seroxat; **Switz.:** Deroxat; **Thai.:** Seroxat; **UK:** Seroxat; **USA:** Paxil.

Phenelzine Sulfate (2533-γ)

Phenelzine Sulfate *(pINNM)*.

Phenelzine Sulphate *(BANM)*. Phenethylhydrazine hydrogen sulphate.

$C_8H_{12}N_2,H_2SO_4 = 234.3$.

CAS — 51-71-8 (phenelzine); 156-51-4 (phenelzine sulfate).

Pharmacopoeias. In Br. and US.

Phenelzine sulfate 25.8 mg is approximately equivalent to 15 mg of phenelzine.

Pharmacopoeial description

BP 2001: A white powder or pearly platelets with a pungent odour. Freely soluble in water; practically insoluble in alcohol, in chloroform, and in ether. Protect from light.

USP 25: A white to yellowish-white powder having a characteristic odour. Freely soluble in water; practically insoluble in alcohol, in chloroform, and in ether. pH of a 1% solution in water is between 1.4 and 1.9. Store in airtight containers. Protect from heat and light.

Adverse Effects

Adverse effects commonly associated with phenelzine and other MAOIs include orthostatic hypotension and attacks of dizziness. Other common side-effects include headache, dryness of the mouth, constipation and other gastrointestinal disturbances (including nausea and vomiting), and oedema. Drowsiness, weakness, and fatigue are reported frequently although CNS stimulation may occur and symptoms include agitation, nervousness, euphoria, restlessness, insomnia, and convulsions. Psychotic episodes, with manic reactions, or toxic delirium, may be induced in susceptible persons.

Sweating and muscle tremors, twitching, or hyperreflexia may occur, which in overdosage may present as extreme hyperpyrexia and neuromuscular irritability. Other reported reactions include blurred vision, urinary retention or difficulty in micturition, skin rashes, leucopenia, sexual disturbances, and weight gain with inappropriate appetite. Jaundice has been reported with hydrazine MAOIs and, on rare occasions, fatal progressive hepatocellular necrosis. Peripheral neuropathies associated with the hydrazine derivatives may be caused by pyridoxine deficiency. Hyponatraemia, possibly due to inappropriate secretion of antidiuretic hormone, has been associated with the use of antidepressants, particularly in the elderly.

Symptoms of overdosage may be mild initially and progress over the ensuing 24 to 48 hours. Following mild overdosage and symptomatic and supportive therapy, recovery may occur in 3 to 4 days, but following massive overdosage symptoms may persist for up to 2 weeks. Symptoms of CNS depression including drowsiness have been observed with overdosage, but CNS stimulation is more common and is manifested by irritability, hyperactivity, agitation, hallucinations, or convulsions. Respiratory depression and coma may ultimately occur. Cardiovascular effects include hypertension, sometimes with severe headache, although hypotension is more frequently observed; cardiac arrhythmias and peripheral collapse can also develop. Profuse sweating, hyperpyrexia, and neuromuscular excitation with hyperreflexia are also prominent features of overdosage.

MAOIs have been the most commonly implicated drugs in the serotonin syndrome (see below). A severe hypertensive crisis, sometimes fatal, may occur

if an MAOI is given simultaneously with some other drugs or certain foods (see Interactions, below). These reactions are characterised by severe headache and a rapid and sometimes prolonged rise in blood pressure followed by intracranial haemorrhage or acute cardiac failure.

For the adverse effects of reversible inhibitors of monoamine oxidase type A (RIMAs), see Moclobemide, p.299.

◊ A suspicion that the reported side-effects of MAOIs were both exaggerated and overemphasised prompted a comparative study in patients receiving phenelzine or imipramine.[1] The report noted that the dosages of phenelzine used were at the upper end of the usual therapeutic range (mean 77 mg daily) while those of imipramine were in the middle of the usual therapeutic range (mean 139 mg daily). A very similar profile of side-effects in the two groups was observed. With the exception of significantly increased incidence of drowsiness in the phenelzine-treated group, the 2 groups did not differ in the frequency of autonomic, CNS, cardiovascular, or psychological side-effects. However, a significantly greater number of phenelzine-treated patients had to discontinue their treatment because of the severity of the side-effects. Nonetheless it was considered that phenelzine was reasonably well-tolerated when compared with imipramine.

Others have also studied the side-effect profile of phenelzine and made comparisons with tranylcypromine and imipramine.[2,3] A retrospective review involving 198 patients led them to believe that although phenelzine was more likely than the other two drugs to induce side-effects, drug discontinuation because of side-effects was less likely to occur. This was probably because phenelzine showed clear-cut clinical efficacy resulting in prescribers being reluctant to discontinue therapy.
1. Evans DL, et al. Early and late side effects of phenelzine. *J Clin Psychopharmacol* 1982; **2:** 208–10.
2. Rabkin J, et al. Adverse reactions to monoamine oxidase inhibitors. Part I: a comparative study. *J Clin Psychopharmacol* 1984; **4:** 270–8.
3. Rabkin JG, et al. Adverse reactions to monoamine oxidase inhibitors. Part II: treatment correlates and clinical management. *J Clin Psychopharmacol* 1985; **5:** 2–9.

Effects on the cardiovascular system. MAOIs are generally considered to be relatively free of adverse cardiovascular effects. The hypertensive reaction that may follow interactions of MAOIs with foods or other drugs is well known (see Interactions, below) but it should not be forgotten that orthostatic hypotension may be encountered as a side-effect when these drugs are used on their own.

In one study[1] involving 14 patients it was found that phenelzine produced both a significant decrease in lying systolic blood pressure and significant orthostatic hypotension; in 2 patients these effects on blood pressure necessitated modification of treatment regimens. Differences between the effects of phenelzine and those reported for the tricyclic antidepressants were noted. Tricyclics were not known to affect lying systolic blood pressure and although both tricyclics and phenelzine could cause orthostatic hypotension, that occurring with the tricyclics typically reaches a maximum within the first week of treatment whereas with phenelzine the maximum effect was noted after 4 weeks. Additionally, the study provided some indication that the blood pressure effects of phenelzine may attenuate with time, a phenomenon that is not known to occur with the tricyclics.
1. Kronig MH, et al. Blood pressure effects of phenelzine. *J Clin Psychopharmacol* 1983; **3:** 307–10.

Effects on the endocrine system. MAOIs may induce *hyperprolactinaemia*[1] and this has led to galactorrhoea in women.[2] Occasionally, MAOIs may cause *dilutional hyponatraemia* due to a reduction in the renal excretion of free water mediated by both enhanced vasopressin release and increased antidiuretic action on the renal tubule.[3] The UK Committee on Safety of Medicines, commenting on reports[4] it had received of hyponatraemia with antidepressants (fluoxetine, paroxetine, lofepramine, clomipramine, and imipramine), considered that it was likely to occur with any antidepressant and usually involved elderly patients.
1. Slater SL, et al. Elevation of plasma-prolactin by monoamine-oxidase inhibitors. *Lancet* 1977; **ii:** 275–6.
2. Segal M, Heys RF. Inappropriate lactation. *BMJ* 1969; **4:** 236.
3. Baylis PH. Drug-induced endocrine disorders. *Adverse Drug React Bull* 1986; No 116: 432–5.
4. Committee on Safety of Medicines/Medicines Control Agency. Antidepressant-induced hyponatraemia. *Current Problems* 1994; **20:** 5–6.

Effects on the liver. Published case reports of hepatotoxic reactions to MAOIs have included jaundice in 4 patients[1] and hepatic failure progressing to encephalopathy in 2 patients;[2] this latter reaction was attributed to a hypersensitivity reaction.

Of 91 cases of hepatitis associated with antidepressants reported to French pharmacovigilance centres during the years 1977 to 1983 an MAOI (iproniazid) was implicated in 11. These 11 cases were associated with cytolytic reactions and 5 patients died.[3]

Two cases of fulminant hepatic failure have been reported[4] following administration of phenelzine for 4 months; all other causes of acute liver damage were ruled out. Both patients recovered after emergency liver transplantation.

1. Holdsworth CD, *et al.* Hepatitis caused by the newer amine-oxidase-inhibiting drugs. *Lancet* 1961; **ii**: 621–3.
2. Wilkinson SP, *et al.* Frequency and type of renal and electrolyte disorders in fulminant hepatic failure. *BMJ* 1974; **1**: 186–9.
3. Lefebure B, *et al.* Hépatites aux antidépresseurs. *Therapie* 1984; **39**: 509–16.
4. Gómez-Gil E, *et al.* Phenelzine-induced fulminant hepatic failure. *Ann Intern Med* 1996; **124**: 692–3.

Effects on the nervous system. MAOIs produce a variety of effects on the nervous system. Drowsiness is frequently reported but symptoms of CNS stimulation, including agitation, nervousness, and euphoria may also occur; psychotic episodes may be induced in susceptible individuals. Further adverse neurological reactions are described under Epileptogenic Effect and Extrapyramidal Effects, below.

Peripheral neuropathies, sometimes associated with a documented pyridoxine deficiency, have been reported in patients receiving phenelzine.[1,2] In most of the patients the neuropathies developed 6 weeks to 4 months after the initiation of phenelzine,[2] although in one case symptoms did not occur for 11 years.[1] The symptoms also generally disappeared when pyridoxine was given together with continued phenelzine therapy.[2] The possibility that the dietary restrictions imposed on persons taking phenelzine might have contributed to a low pyridoxine intake was considered unlikely. The most probable mechanism for the induced pyridoxine deficiency was combination of the hydrazine moiety with the pyridoxal form of the vitamin to form an inactive compound.

Many drugs can inhibit transmission at the myoneural junction under experimental conditions and it has been said that phenelzine may cause postoperative respiratory depression, possibly through a combined action with neuromuscular blockers.[3] For further details, see Anaesthesia under Precautions, below.

1. Heller CA, Friedman PA. Pyridoxine deficiency and peripheral neuropathy associated with long-term phenelzine therapy. *Am J Med* 1983; **75**: 887–8.
2. Stewart JW, *et al.* Phenelzine-induced pyridoxine deficiency. *J Clin Psychopharmacol* 1984; **4**: 225–6.
3. Lane RJM, Routledge PA. Drug-induced neurological disorders. *Drugs* 1983; **26**: 124–47.

Effects on sexual function. MAOIs such as phenelzine and tranylcypromine have been implicated in producing both impotence and failure of ejaculation.[1,2] Priapism has been reported with phenelzine.[3] There have also been several reports of anorgasmia in women attributed to MAOIs, an effect which appears to be dose-related.[4] It should be remembered that loss of libido and impotence are common symptoms of depression, often making the role of drugs in producing sexual dysfunction difficult to assess.

1. Simpson GM, *et al.* Effects of anti-depressants on genito-urinary function. *Dis Nerv Syst* 1965; **26**: 787–9.
2. Wyatt RJ, *et al.* Treatment of intractable narcolepsy with a monoamine oxidase inhibitor. *N Engl J Med* 1971; **285**: 987–91.
3. Yeragani VK, Gershon S. Priapism related to phenelzine therapy. *N Engl J Med* 1987; **317**: 117–18.
4. Shen WW, Sata LS. Inhibited female orgasm resulting from psychotropic drugs: a clinical review. *J Reprod Med* 1983; **28**: 497–9.

Epileptogenic effect. Convulsions represent one of the less common adverse effects of MAOIs; they may be a feature of overdosage.

A typical grand-mal seizure with tonic-clonic convulsions has been reported in a patient with no history of epilepsy or predisposing factors shortly after the start of phenelzine therapy.[1] The point was made that phenelzine-induced seizures had rarely been observed.

1. Bhugra DK, Kaye N. Phenelzine induced grand mal seizure. *Br J Clin Pract* 1986; **40**: 173–4.

Extrapyramidal effects. A parkinsonian syndrome developed in a patient about 5 weeks after the start of therapy with phenelzine. Symptoms gradually resolved over 10 days following the withdrawal of phenelzine. The mechanisms by which phenelzine could have induced these effects were discussed.[1]

1. Gillman MA, Sandyk R. Parkinsonism induced by a monoamine oxidase inhibitor. *Postgrad Med J* 1986; **62**: 235–6.

Hyponatraemia. See Effects on the Endocrine System, above.

Lupus. A reversible lupus-like reaction has been reported in a patient who had been taking phenelzine sulfate for 8 months.[1]

1. Swartz C. Lupus-like reaction to phenelzine. *JAMA* 1978; **239**: 2693.

Overdosage. MAOIs in overdose rarely produce severe hypertension; the blood pressure may be high or low, or may alternate between the two. More commonly the patient gradually develops widespread muscle spasms, trismus, and opisthotonus with widely dilated pupils and a hot and sweating skin. About 16 to 24 hours after ingestion potentially fatal hyperthermia may develop; temperatures of 42.1 to 43.8° have been recorded immediately before death. Disseminated intravascular coagulation, rhabdomyolysis, and acute tubular necrosis can also occur. It is recommended that the temperature of a patient who has taken an overdose of an MAOI should be closely monitored, and, if the rectal temperature increases to more than 39°, the trachea should be intubated and the patient's lungs ventilat-

ed using pancuronium bromide as a neuromuscular blocker; this produces a dramatic decrease in temperature.[1]

1. Henry JA. Specific problems of drug intoxication. *Br J Anaesth* 1986; **58**: 223–33.

Serotonin syndrome. The serotonin syndrome most commonly results from an additive adverse effect between two or more drugs that enhance serotonergic activity at central receptors, usually by different mechanisms; the pathogenesis and management have been reviewed.[1-5] It is characterised by the development of at least three of the following clinical features after a recent change in a treatment regimen involving serotonergic drugs: agitation, ataxia, diaphoresis, diarrhoea, fever, hyperreflexia, myoclonus, shivering, and changes in mental status. The onset of the syndrome may occur within minutes of the change, or several weeks later.[3] The occurrence and severity of the syndrome do not appear to be dose-related,[3] and it is distinct from the hypertensive crises produced by the interaction between MAOIs and tyramine (see Interactions of MAOIs with Foods, below), and from the neuroleptic malignant syndrome (see p.662).[4]

The serotonin syndrome is relatively uncommon and, in the majority of cases, the symptoms are mild. However, severe complications, including disseminated intravascular coagulation, severe hyperthermia, respiratory failure, and seizures have been reported; there have also been fatalities, hence the need for great caution when giving serotonergic drugs together. The use of combination therapy with serotonergic antidepressant drugs for the treatment of refractory or drug-resistant depression is discussed under Interactions of MAOIs with other Drugs, below.

MAOIs have been the most commonly implicated drugs in this syndrome, and cases have been reported when MAOIs have been combined with other antidepressants such as the tricyclics, SSRIs, serotonin and noradrenaline reuptake inhibitors (SNRIs), trazodone, lithium, and tryptophan. MAOIs combined with the opioids dextromethorphan and pethidine have also produced the serotonin syndrome. The interaction can occur with both irreversible and reversible MAOIs, and with those selective for monoamine oxidase type A such as moclobemide as well as with non-selective MAOIs.[6] The selective inhibitor of monoamine oxidase type B, selegiline, may also pose problems at high doses when selectivity starts to diminish. As usage of the SSRIs has increased, so too has the number of reports of adverse reactions when these drugs have been combined with other serotonergic drugs including the herbal preparation hypericum.

Other drugs that may potentially cause serotonin syndrome in certain circumstances include buspirone, carbamazepine, and methylenedioxyamfetamine.[2] Rarely, a single serotonergic drug has produced the serotonin syndrome.[3]

Serotonergic potentiation may also occur if one serotonergic drug is used after another without allowing a sufficient drug-free interval after discontinuation of the first. This is a particular problem when the first drug is an irreversible MAOI or a drug with a long half-life such as the SSRI fluoxetine.

Most cases of serotonin syndrome resolve within 24 hours following withdrawal of the offending drugs and administration of supportive therapy.[1-5] The management of fever and hyperthermia is described on p.8. Benzodiazepines may be of value to control myoclonus and seizures. Serotonin antagonists have been tried as specific drug therapy for the serotonin syndrome. The non-specific antagonists cyproheptadine and methysergide have been tried with some success.[3,4] Other drugs that have been tried but with inconsistent results include propranolol, chlorpromazine, and dantrolene.[3,4]

1. Sternbach H. The serotonin syndrome. *Am J Psychiatry* 1991; **148**: 705–13.
2. Nierenberg DW, Semprebon M. The central nervous system serotonin syndrome. *Clin Pharmacol Ther* 1993; **53**: 84–8.
3. Sporer KA. The serotonin syndrome: implicated drugs, pathophysiology and management. *Drug Safety* 1995; **13**: 94–104.
4. Corkeron MA. Serotonin syndrome—a potentially fatal complication of antidepressant therapy. *Med J Aust* 1995; **163**: 481–2.
5. Brown TM, *et al.* Pathophysiology and management of the serotonin syndrome. *Ann Pharmacother* 1996; **30**: 527–33.
6. Livingston MG. Interactions with selective MAOIs. *Lancet* 1995; **345**: 533–4.

Treatment of Adverse Effects

In cases of overdosage with MAOIs activated charcoal may be given by mouth, or the stomach may be emptied by lavage. Management then largely involves intensive symptomatic and supportive therapy with particular attention being given to CNS effects, raised body temperature which may develop into malignant hyperthermia, and cardiovascular effects. It should not be forgotten that delayed effects, even in patients who are initially asymptomatic, may develop some time after the overdose and therefore prolonged monitoring is warranted. Other drugs taken with an overdose of MAOIs may complicate the features and result in the need for an even longer period of monitoring. Special care should be observed with any drug therapy used in the management of MAOI over-

dosage in view of the many known interactions which occur with this class of drugs.

Muscle spasm, agitation, and convulsions should be treated with diazepam. Severe neuromuscular irritability may call for the use of a competitive neuromuscular blocker such as pancuronium and intubation with assisted ventilation. Hyperthermia may be a particular problem; if simple antipyretics such as paracetamol and external cooling measures fail a competitive neuromuscular blocker has often been advocated; dantrolene has also been suggested.

Hypotension, which is a fairly common feature, should be managed by intravenous fluid therapy and volume expansion; vasopressors should be avoided. Conversely, a hypertensive crisis may occasionally occur following an overdose with MAOIs and can be managed with phentolamine given by slow intravenous injection. A short-acting beta blocker such as esmolol has also been advocated for persistent tachycardia and hypertension.

Precautions

Phenelzine and other MAOIs should not be given to patients with liver disease or, because of their effects on blood pressure, to patients with cerebrovascular disease or phaeochromocytoma. (Blood pressure should be monitored in all patients.) MAOIs should be avoided or only used with great caution in patients with blood disorders or cardiovascular disease. MAOIs should similarly be avoided or used with great caution in elderly or agitated patients who may be particularly susceptible to their adverse effects. They should be given with caution to epileptic patients. Caution has also been advised in diabetic patients because of conflicting evidence whether glucose metabolism is altered or requirements for hypoglycaemics changed. MAOIs should be used with caution, if at all, in patients with hyperthyroidism because of increased sensitivity to pressor amines.

Patients should be closely monitored during early antidepressant therapy until improvement in depression is observed because suicide is an inherent risk in depressed patients. For further details, see under Depression, p.271.

Mania may be precipitated if MAOIs are used for the depressive component of bipolar disorder, and they are not usually indicated; similarly psychotic symptoms may be aggravated if they are used for a depressive component of schizophrenia.

MAOIs have a prolonged action so patients should not take any of the foods or drugs known to cause reactions (see Interactions, below) for at least 14 days after stopping treatment. A similar drug-free period has been advised before any patient undergoes surgery since it may involve the use of drugs that can interact with MAOIs, although not all agree that this is necessary; caution has been advised in patients requiring MAOIs concurrently with ECT; for further details see under Anaesthesia, below. Patients should carry cards giving details of their MAOI therapy; they and their relatives should be fully conversant with the implications of food and drug interactions and the precautions to be taken.

Patients liable to take charge of vehicles or other machinery should be warned that MAOIs may modify behaviour and state of alertness. Patients affected by drowsiness should not drive or operate machinery.

MAOIs should be withdrawn gradually to reduce the risk of withdrawal symptoms (see below).

For the precautions to be observed with reversible inhibitors of monoamine oxidase A (RIMAs), see Moclobemide, p.299.

Anaesthesia. The considerations given to patients receiving tricyclic antidepressants before receiving anaesthesia for ECT or surgery (see Amitriptyline, p.275) are also generally applicable to patients being treated with MAOIs; the manufacturer of phenelzine also warns that cardiovascular depression following ECT has been reported. The interactions of other drugs with MAOIs may be more numerous or more severe than those with tricyclics and the interaction with pethidine should not be forgotten.

Reviewing the potential problems of anaesthesia in patients receiving MAOIs Stack et al.[1] considered that the advice that MAOIs should be stopped about 2 weeks before anaesthesia was unreasonable, as there was a wide range of safe and suitable anaesthetics available, but that the dangers of sympathetic overactivity must always be remembered. This view, that it is safe to continue MAOIs throughout the period of anaesthesia and surgery, has also been advocated by Hirshman and Lindeman[2,3] although others have registered disapproval.[4]

Regardless of any decision, the anaesthetist should be informed of all drugs that the patient is or has been taking; this is particularly important when emergency surgery is required in a patient receiving MAOI therapy.

- It has been stated[1] that the interaction between MAOIs and *opioid analgesics* has two distinct forms: an excitatory form, which may be due to central serotonergic overactivity, characterised by sudden agitation, unmanageable behaviour, headache, hypertension or hypotension, rigidity, hyperpyrexia, convulsions, and coma; and a depressive form consisting of respiratory depression, hypotension, and coma as a result of the inhibition of hepatic microsomal enzymes by the MAOI leading to accumulation of free opioid analgesic. *Pethidine* is the only commonly used opioid analgesic to have elicited the excitatory response which has frequently been severe and often fatal. For this reason, pethidine should never be administered to patients receiving MAOIs. *Morphine* does not block neuronal serotonin uptake but its narcotic effects may be potentiated in the presence of MAOIs and a single case report of the depressive type of reaction has been described. Thus, morphine is the opioid analgesic of choice but must be given in reduced dosage and the dosage carefully titrated against clinical response. *Phenoperidine* is probably best avoided as its metabolites are norpethidine and, to a lesser extent, pethidine. *Papaveretum* would appear to have no advantage over morphine. Although interactions of MAOIs with *pentazocine* have occurred in *animals*, it is not clear if this occurs in man. *Methadone* has been used in a patient without mishap and there is also anecdotal evidence to support the safety of *fentanyl*. A case report[5] described the successful use of *alfentanil* (together with propofol and atracurium) mentioning that this was the first report of such use in patients receiving MAOIs. A further case report[6] described a patient who underwent successful anaesthesia with *sufentanil* (together with thiopental, lignocaine [lidocaine], and vecuronium) while continuing to take an MAOI (tranylcypromine) as well as a tricyclic antidepressant (imipramine) and lorazepam.
- With regard to induction agents,[1] the use of *ketamine* in patients receiving MAOIs should be avoided on theoretical grounds, although no interactions have been reported. Potentiation of *barbiturates* may be expected.
- With neuromuscular blockers, phenelzine has been shown to decrease plasma cholinesterase concentrations and there have been case reports of a prolonged effect with *suxamethonium*; additionally this prolongation of the effect of suxamethonium may lead to apnoea and modification of the convulsion during ECT. There appeared to be a theoretical hazard with *pancuronium* since it releases stored adrenaline (although its use has been advocated in the treatment of symptoms of overdosage with MAOIs, see above), but *alcuronium*, *atracurium*, or *vecuronium* would all appear to be suitable alternatives.
- *Enflurane*, *halothane*, *isoflurane*, and *nitrous oxide* are all safe in the presence of MAOIs, although there is a theoretical possibility of an increased risk of hepatic damage with halothane.
- *Indirect-acting sympathomimetics* pose the risk of a serious and possibly lethal hypertensive interaction but *direct-acting sympathomimetics*, such as *adrenaline [epinephrine]*, *isoprenaline*, and *noradrenaline [norepinephrine]*, are reliable vasopressors in the presence of MAOIs although great care should be taken with their use because of enhanced receptor sensitivity.

1. Stack CG, et al. Monoamine oxidase inhibitors and anaesthesia: a review. *Br J Anaesth* 1988; 60: 222–7.
2. Hirshman CA, Lindeman K. MAO inhibitors: must they be discontinued before anesthesia? *JAMA* 1988; 260: 3507–8.
3. Hirshman CA, Lindeman KS. Anesthesia and monoamine oxidase inhibitors. *JAMA* 1989; 261: 3407–8.
4. Gevirtz C. Anesthesia and monoamine oxidase inhibitors. *JAMA* 1989; 261: 3407.
5. Powell H. Use of alfentanil in a patient receiving monoamine oxidase inhibitor therapy. *Br J Anaesth* 1990; 64: 528.
6. O'Hara JF, et al. Sufentanil-isoflurane-nitrous oxide anesthesia for a patient treated with monoamine oxidase inhibitor and tricyclic antidepressant. *J Clin Anesth* 1995; 7: 148–50.

Driving. While affective disorders probably adversely affect driving skill,[1,2] treatment with antidepressant drugs may also be hazardous,[1] although patients may be safer drivers with medication than without.[2] Impairment of performance is largely related to sedative properties and some MAOIs can adversely affect psychomotor performance.[1,2]

In the UK, the Driver and Vehicle Licensing Authority (DVLA) considers that SSRIs, MAOIs, and noradrenaline reuptake inhibitors have fewer adverse effects on drivers than antidepressants with antimuscarinic or antihistaminic adverse effects,

such as tricyclic antidepressants. However some patients have idiosyncratic responses and should be advised accordingly.[3] Patients with severe depressive illnesses complicated by significant memory or concentration problems, agitation, behavioural disturbances or suicidal thoughts should cease driving pending the outcome of medical enquiry. It has been mentioned[2] that the UK Medical Commission on Accident Prevention has recommended that patients on long-term psychotropic medication are unsuitable to be drivers of heavy goods or public service vehicles.

1. Ashton H. Drugs and driving. *Adverse Drug React Bull* 1983; 98: 360–3.
2. Cremona A. Mad drivers: psychiatric illness and driving performance. *Br J Hosp Med* 1986; 35: 193–5.
3. Driver and Vehicle Licensing Agency. At a glance: a guide for medical practitioners. Available at: http://www.dvla.gov.uk/at_a_glance/ch4_psychiatric.htm (accessed 21/08/01).

Electroconvulsive therapy. For comments concerning the precautions to be observed in patients receiving ECT, see under Anaesthesia, above.

Porphyria. Phenelzine is considered to be unsafe in patients with porphyria because it has been shown to be porphyrinogenic in *animals*.

Surgery. For comments regarding the precautions to be observed in patients undergoing surgery, see under Anaesthesia, above.

Withdrawal. Sudden discontinuation of antidepressant therapy after regular administration for 8 weeks or more may precipitate withdrawal symptoms which may be very severe.

Symptoms associated with withdrawal of MAOIs[1,2] include gastrointestinal disturbances and generalised somatic symptoms such as nausea and vomiting, anorexia, chills, headache, and giddiness; sleep disturbances characterised by insomnia, severe nightmares, and somnolence; and a range of CNS symptoms including panic, anxiety, restlessness, agitation, cognitive impairment, mood swings, depression and suicidal ideation, hypomania, delusions, and hallucinations. Some of the above may be ameliorated by reinstitution of the MAOI in low doses, but the best management is considered to be prevention by gradually discontinuing the drug.[2] Some authorities recommend reducing the dose over a period of 4 weeks.

The pathophysiology of the MAOI withdrawal syndrome has not been fully elucidated, although it has been hypothesised that some of the symptoms represent adrenergic hyperactivity[1] produced by the release of excessive amounts of dopamine and noradrenaline.[2]

With the exception of tranylcypromine, the withdrawal syndrome of MAOIs is not a consequence of drug dependence.[1] Tranylcypromine has been reported to produce dependence and tolerance in patients receiving high doses irrespective of whether or not they had a previous history of substance abuse. Tranylcypromine is similar in structure to amfetamine, which may be responsible for its addictive properties.[1]

1. Anonymous. Problems when withdrawing antidepressives. *Drug Ther Bull* 1986; 24: 29–30.
2. Dilsaver SC. Withdrawal phenomena associated with antidepressant and antipsychotic agents. *Drug Safety* 1994; 10: 103–14.

Interactions of MAOIs with Foods

A major disadvantage of MAOIs such as phenelzine is that by inhibiting monoamine oxidase they cause an accumulation of amine neurotransmitters. This means that the pressor effects of *tyramine*, which occurs in a number of common foods and is also metabolised by monoamine oxidase, can be dangerously enhanced. Reactions to foods rich in pressor amines such as tyramine can therefore occur in patients being treated with MAOIs producing hypertensive crises. Cheese, especially aged or matured cheeses, meat or yeast extracts, pickled herrings, smoked foods, and broad bean pods have caused such reactions. Patients should be warned not to eat any of these foods while being treated with an MAOI and for at least 14 days after its discontinuation. Some foods will only cause a reaction if large amounts are eaten, and foods may vary in tyramine content depending upon methods of manufacture and storage. Any protein-containing food such as meat, fish, or game subject to hydrolysis, fermentation, pickling, smoking, or spoilage could contain tyramine derived from tyrosine as a result of these processes or of deterioration. Patients taking MAOIs should therefore be advised to eat protein-containing foods only if fresh.

Alcoholic beverages, including wines, beers, and drinks that are de-alcoholised or are low in alcohol, contain variable amounts of tyramine and are best avoided.

The above dietary restrictions that need to be observed with MAOIs may be less stringent for reversible inhibitors of monoamine oxidase type A (RIMAs)

such as moclobemide (see p.299), although the manufacturers recommend that since some patients may be especially sensitive to tyramine, consumption of large amounts of tyramine-rich food should be avoided.

◊ MAOIs can, when taken with certain foodstuffs, cause a potentially fatal hypertensive reaction. This effect is accepted and well documented and has led to the publication of many lists of prohibited foods and drinks. Some workers have expressed the opinion that the dangers of the interaction may have been slightly overemphasised or exaggerated and that the published lists may have been overinclusive;[1-3] this may have led to reduced compliance in a number of patients.

A review and discussion[1] of the MAOI interaction with tyramine made the following observations and recommendations:

- the hyperadrenergic state resulting from this interaction consisted of three syndromes although significant overlap between them existed: paroxysmal headache of great severity; cardiovascular symptoms with paroxysmal hypertension; and intracerebral haemorrhage and death
- the most common offending drug reported had been tranylcypromine at doses of 20 to 50 mg daily although a few reports had involved phenelzine
- only 4 foodstuffs clearly warranted total prohibition: aged cheese, pickled herring or fish, concentrated yeast extracts, and broad bean pods
- the ingestion of cheese was said to have been associated with 80% of all case reports and with virtually all fatalities. It was agreed that aged cheese should not be permitted, although cottage and cream cheese required no restriction. There was less agreement concerning dairy products such as yogurt and sour cream and it was suggested that limited amounts were permissible
- pickled herring or smoked fish were to be avoided because of several well-documented cases of hypertensive crisis as well as detection of high levels of tyramine. Any meat may become dangerous unless consumed while fresh as tyramine is formed from bacterial protein degradation
- concentrated yeast extracts have a significant tyramine content and yeast vitamin supplements may also constitute a hazard; baker's yeast was considered to be safe
- broad bean pods contain dopamine although the beans were stated to have little pressor activity and carried no prohibition
- other foods which had been reported to have caused a hypertensive reaction but for which these authors considered that there was insufficient evidence to warrant dietary restriction were chocolate and caffeine-containing beverages, soy sauce, fresh fish, wild game, and fruits although caution was necessary with avocados and bananas.

Other reviews of foods[2,4] give broadly similar recommendations.

The consumption of alcoholic beverages, and in particular Chianti wine, has frequently been advised against. However, sources have differed with respect to whether particular types of drink (white wine, red wine, spirits, or beer) are safe or not. One study[5] demonstrated no significant differences in mean free tyramine concentration between white wine, red wine, Chianti, and beer although within each category of wine there could be up to a fiftyfold variation even if from the same grape stock. Mention has also been made[6,7] that alcohol-free or low-alcohol beers are likely to contain similar amounts of tyramine as alcoholic beers. The consumption of alcoholic drinks with MAOIs still appears to be controversial with some advocating total abstinence while others permit a modest intake.

1. Brown C, et al. The monoamine oxidase inhibitor-tyramine interaction. *J Clin Pharmacol* 1989; 29: 529–32.
2. Lippman SB, Nash K. Monoamine oxidase inhibitor update: potential adverse food and drug interactions. *Drug Safety* 1990; 5: 195–204.
3. Folks DG. Monoamine oxidase inhibitors: reappraisal of dietary considerations. *J Clin Psychopharmacol* 1983; 3: 249–52.
4. Anonymous. Foods interacting with MAO inhibitors. *Med Lett Drugs Ther* 1989; 31: 11–12.
5. Hannah P, et al. Tyramine in wine and beer. *Lancet* 1988; i: 879.
6. Sandler M. Monoamine oxidase inhibitors and low alcohol or alcohol free drinks. *BMJ* 1990; 300: 1527.
7. Beswick DT, Rogers ML. Monoamine oxidase inhibitors and low alcohol or alcohol free drinks. *BMJ* 1990; 301: 179–80.

Interactions of MAOIs with other Drugs

MAOIs inhibit the metabolism of some *amine drugs* (notably indirect-acting sympathomimetics), which can lead to dangerous enhancement of their pressor effects. MAOIs also inhibit other drug-metabolising enzymes and are therefore responsible for a large number of *other drug interactions*. Moreover, they have an additive effect with serotonergic drugs which may result in the *serotonin syndrome* (see under Adverse Effects, above). As in the case of foods, the danger of an interaction persists for at least 14 days after treatment with an MAOI has been discontinued.

Severe hypertensive reactions due to enhancement of pressor activity have followed the administration of sympathomimetics such as *amfetamines, dopamine, ephedrine, levodopa, phenylephrine, phenylpropanolamine,* and *pseudoephedrine*. Reactions may also follow the use of anorectics and stimulants with sympathomimetic activity such as *fenfluramine, methylphenidate, pemoline,* and *phentermine*. There have been case reports of fatalities in patients who took cough preparations containing *dextromethorphan*. There is no clinical evidence of dangerous interactions between *local anaesthetic preparations containing adrenaline [epinephrine]* and MAOIs but great care should be taken to avoid inadvertent intravenous administration of the local anaesthetic. Significant rises in blood pressure have been reported following the use of *buspirone* with MAOIs.

Inhibition of drug-metabolising enzymes by MAOIs may enhance the effects of *barbiturates* and possibly other *hypnotics, hypoglycaemics,* and possibly *antimuscarinics. Alcohol* metabolism may be altered and its effects enhanced; see also under Interactions of MAOIs with Foods, above. *Antihypertensives* including *guanethidine, reserpine,* and *methyldopa* should be given with caution; hypotensive and hypertensive reactions have been suggested; the hypotensive effects of *beta blockers* and *thiazide diuretics* may be enhanced.

The administration of *pethidine* and possibly other *opioid analgesics* to patients taking an MAOI has also been associated with very severe and sometimes fatal reactions. When it is considered essential to use an opioid analgesic a test dose of morphine should be given. It has been suggested that the test dose should be one-tenth to one-fifth of the normal dose and if this produces no untoward reaction, the dose of morphine can be gradually and carefully increased over a period of 2 to 3 hours. The use of opioid analgesics and other drugs employed during general anaesthesia in patients continuing to take MAOIs is discussed in Anaesthesia under Precautions, above.

Clozapine may enhance the CNS effects of MAOIs.

Although different antidepressants have been used together under expert supervision in refractory cases of depression, severe adverse reactions may occur. MAOIs should not generally be given to patients receiving *tricyclic antidepressants, SSRIs, serotonin and noradrenaline reuptake inhibitors (SNRIs),* or *nefazodone* or *trazodone*. An appropriate drug-free interval should elapse between discontinuing one type of antidepressant and starting another. An MAOI should not be started until at least 1 or 2 weeks after stopping a tricyclic antidepressant. For the tricyclic antidepressants clomipramine and imipramine a drug-free interval of 3 weeks should be allowed. For an SSRI, an SNRI, nefazodone, trazodone, or any related antidepressant the drug-free interval should be at least one week; in the case of the SSRIs paroxetine and sertraline, the interval is extended to two weeks, and for fluoxetine, five weeks because of their longer half-lives. Conversely, two weeks should elapse between discontinuing MAOI therapy and starting patients on a tricyclic antidepressant (3 weeks in the case of clomipramine or imipramine), an SSRI, an SNRI, or any related antidepressant. For further warnings on the coadministration of antidepressants, see below. Interactions can also occur between MAOIs themselves.

For details of the less severe interactions associated with reversible inhibitors of monoamine oxidase A (RIMAs), see Interactions of Moclobemide, p.299.

◊ References.
1. Lippman SB, Nash K. Monoamine oxidase inhibitor update: potential adverse food and drug interactions. *Drug Safety* 1990; **5:** 195–204.
2. Blackwell B. Monoamine oxidase inhibitor interactions with other drugs. *J Clin Psychopharmacol* 1991; **11:** 55–9.
3. Livingston MC, Livingston HM. Monoamine oxidase inhibitors: an update on drug interactions. *Drug Safety* 1996; **14:** 219–27.

Anticoagulants. For the effects of MAOIs on warfarin, see p.995.

Antidepressants. Combination therapy with differing classes of antidepressants has been used successfully in the treatment of drug-resistant depression. It should be emphasised, however, that such combination therapy may result in interactions or enhanced adverse reactions such as the serotonin syndrome (see under Adverse Effects, above), and is therefore considered unsuitable or controversial by some authorities. Because combination therapy poses increased risks it should be employed only under expert supervision. Despite these drawbacks certain combinations of drugs have been found to be beneficial, although others are considered unsuitable; it should be noted that absence of information documenting unsuitability or hazard does not necessarily imply that the two drugs may be used safely together but may merely reflect an untried combination.

MAOIs have been used fairly frequently under expert supervision with tricyclics in refractory depression and it has been stated[1] that the risk of serious problems in combining *tricyclic antidepressant and MAOI* antidepressant therapy is almost exclusively limited to sequential prescribing, in particular the addition of a tricyclic to established treatment with an MAOI. The recommended procedure was said to be to allow a drug-free interval of at least one week and then to start both drugs together at a low dosage. The dosage of both drugs is then gradually increased to around half that normally prescribed for the drugs when given on their own. The dietary restrictions for MAOIs alone apply equally to the combined antidepressant regimen. Amitriptyline and trimipramine were considered to be the tricyclics least likely to produce side-effects in combination with MAOIs, while phenelzine and isocarboxazid were the safest MAOIs.

Two tricyclic antidepressants that have been considered particularly unsuitable for combination therapy with MAOIs are clomipramine, a tricyclic with serotonin reuptake inhibiting activity, and imipramine. Reports of interactions have occurred with both these drugs.[2,3] The combination of clomipramine with tranylcypromine is particularly dangerous. Symptoms suggestive of the serotonin syndrome occurred in an elderly patient due to an interaction between clomipramine and moclobemide, a reversible inhibitor of monoamine oxidase type A (RIMA).[4] Two fatalities due to serotonin syndrome have been reported following overdosage with clomipramine and moclobemide.[5] The syndrome has also developed when a patient was switched from clomipramine to moclobemide with no suitable drug-free interval.[6] A 39-year-old woman developed the serotonin syndrome while taking imipramine with moclobemide, although it was suggested that an excessive dose of the tricyclic may have been ingested accidentally.[7]

The UK Committee on Safety of Medicines (CSM) has warned[8] that enhanced serotonergic effects may result from combination therapy of *SSRIs* with *MAOIs* or other antidepressants. Although such an enhancement may be beneficial in some instances it can produce a life-threatening serotonin syndrome. Such reactions were later reported in patients taking sertraline with MAOIs.[9-11] Three fatalities due to serotonin syndrome have been reported following overdosage with citalopram and moclobemide.[5] One case of serotonin syndrome has been reported after switching from fluoxetine to moclobemide with no suitable drug-free interval.[6] Bakish *et al.*[12] have reported good efficacy and tolerability with combinations of moclobemide and SSRIs. However, Hawley *et al.*[13] reported a high rate of adverse events with these combinations, although as significant improvement in depressive symptoms was observed in some patients, they suggested that the combination of moclobemide with SSRIs deserved consideration as an option for the treatment of refractory depression.

Combination therapy with a *tricyclic antidepressant and an SSRI* has sometimes been used to treat resistant depression. Fluvoxamine[14] and fluoxetine[15] have been reported to increase plasma concentrations of the tricyclic, although to varying degrees. Fluoxetine has been reported to produce three- to fourfold increases in plasma concentrations of desipramine and imipramine. Fluvoxamine has a minimal effect on desipramine plasma levels but produces a three- to fourfold increase in concentrations of imipramine.[16] Plasma-desipramine concentrations are elevated threefold by paroxetine but increases of only 30% are produced by sertraline.[16] However, an inadequate interval of one day between stopping desipramine and starting paroxetine resulted in a case of serotonin syndrome.[6] Serotonin syndrome has also been reported[17] in a patient who received paroxetine and imipramine together and in another given sertraline and amitriptyline.[18] A threefold increase in concentrations of trimipramine resulting in sedation and orthostatic hypotension has been reported[19] in 2 patients treated concomitantly with paroxetine. Additionally, norfluoxetine, the active metabolite of fluoxetine, has a long half-life and is responsible for the continuing interaction with tricyclics for several days or weeks after fluoxetine has been withdrawn. Citalopram was reported to have no effect on plasma-tricyclic concentrations in one patient although antidepressant effects were augmented.[20]

Lithium and *tryptophan* have been used to augment the effect of other antidepressants in refractory depression. Phenelzine has been used successfully in combination with lithium and tryptophan[21] in patients with treatment-resistant chronic depression although such a regimen has probably been used since the reports of the eosinophilia-myalgia syndrome associ-

ated with tryptophan (see p.311). There have, however, been several case reports of reactions similar to the serotonin syndrome in patients receiving MAOIs together with tryptophan.[22,23] Although lithium is often added to tricyclic antidepressant therapy in patients with refractory depression, epileptic seizures have been reported in a patient receiving amitriptyline when lithium was added.[24] Serotonin syndrome has been reported[25] in a patient given clomipramine and lithium. Severe neurotoxicity has been reported[26,27] in some patients receiving lithium and tricyclic or tetracyclic antidepressants together; adverse effects included tremor, memory impairment, disorganised thinking, and auditory hallucinations. One manufacturer of lithium preparations also reports symptoms of nephrogenic diabetes in patients receiving these combinations. By 1989 the CSM had received 19 reports of adverse reactions in patients treated with fluvoxamine and lithium; 5 reports concerned convulsions and 1 hyperthermia.[8] Tremor has been reported when lithium was given with paroxetine,[28] and in general the risk of CNS toxicity is increased when lithium is administered together with fluoxetine, fluvoxamine, paroxetine, or sertraline. There has been a report[29] of a fatality when fluoxetine was replaced by tranylcypromine and tryptophan with no drug-free period; the patient was also receiving other drugs concurrently.

Use of the serotonin and noradrenaline reuptake inhibitor (SNRI) *venlafaxine with tricyclic antidepressants* has been associated with increased antimuscarinic adverse effects.[30,31] Similar adverse effects have occurred in patients given *venlafaxine and the SSRI* fluoxetine;[31] serotonin syndrome has been reported in a patient who received venlafaxine and paroxetine.[6] The combination of *venlafaxine with MAOIs* is contra-indicated by the manufacturers of venlafaxine because of the risk of life-threatening adverse reactions. Serious adverse reactions have been reported when venlafaxine was combined with isocarboxazid,[32] moclobemide,[6] phenelzine,[33] or tranylcypromine.[34]

Trazodone is chemically unrelated to other antidepressants but does have serotonergic actions. Serotonin syndrome has been reported when trazodone was combined with the SSRI paroxetine.[35]

Serotonin syndrome has been reported[36] in a patient who took *nefazodone* and *fluoxetine* together. There has been a similar report[37] in a patient who received *paroxetine* 2 days after finishing gradual withdrawal from over 6 months of treatment with nefazodone.

In a report[38] of an interaction between *hypericum* and *paroxetine*, a 50-year-old woman was found incoherent, groggy, and slow-moving after self-administering a single dose of paroxetine while taking hypericum; recovery was uneventful. Concomitant administration of hypericum and the SSRIs may potentiate their serotonergic effects and increase the incidence of adverse reactions. The CSM has advised that patients should stop taking hypericum if treatment with an SSRI is necessary.[39] Symptoms of serotonin syndrome have also been reported when *hypericum* and *nefazodone* were taken concomitantly.[40]

1. Katona CLE, Barnes TRE. Pharmacological strategies in depression. *Br J Hosp Med* 1985; **34:** 168–71.
2. Beaumont G. Drug interactions with clomipramine (Anafranil). *J Int Med Res* 1973; **1:** 480–4.
3. Graham PM, *et al.* Combination monoamine oxidase inhibitor/tricyclic antidepressant interaction. *Lancet* 1982; **ii:** 440.
4. Spigset O, *et al.* Serotonin syndrome caused by a moclobemide-clomipramine interaction. *BMJ* 1993; **306:** 248.
5. Neuvonen PJ, *et al.* Five fatal cases of serotonin syndrome after moclobemide-citalopram or moclobemide-clomipramine overdoses. *Lancet* 1993; **342:** 1419.
6. Chan BSH, *et al.* Serotonin syndrome resulting from drug interactions. *Med J Aust* 1998; **169:** 523–5.
7. Brodribb TR, *et al.* Efficacy and adverse effects of moclobemide. *Lancet* 1994; **343:** 475.
8. Committee on Safety of Medicines. Fluvoxamine and fluoxetine-interaction with monoamine oxidase inhibitors, lithium and tryptophan. *Current Problems* 26 1989. Correction. *ibid.* 27 1989 [hypothermia should have read hyperthermia].
9. Brannan SK, *et al.* Sertraline and isocarboxazid cause a serotonin syndrome. *J Clin Psychopharmacol* 1994; **14:** 144–5.
10. Graber MA, *et al.* Sertraline-phenelzine drug interaction: a serotonin syndrome reaction. *Ann Pharmacother* 1994; **28:** 732–5.
11. Corkeron MA. Serotonin syndrome — a potentially fatal complication of antidepressant therapy. *Med J Aust* 1995; **163:** 481–2.
12. Bakish D, *et al.* Moclobemide and specific serotonin re-uptake inhibitor combination treatment of resistant anxiety and depressive disorders. *Hum Psychopharmacol Clin Exp* 1995; **10:** 105–9.
13. Hawley CJ, *et al.* Combining SSRIs and moclobemide. *Pharm J* 1996; **257:** 506.
14. Bertschy G, *et al.* Fluvoxamine-tricyclic antidepressant interaction: an accidental finding. *Eur J Clin Pharmacol* 1991; **40:** 119–20.
15. Westermeyer J. Fluoxetine-induced tricyclic toxicity: extent and duration. *J Clin Pharmacol* 1991; **31:** 388–92.
16. Ereshefsky L, *et al.* Antidepressant drug interactions and the cytochrome P450 system: the role of cytochrome P450 2D6. *Clin Pharmacokinet* 1995; **29** (suppl 1): 10–19.
17. Weiner AL, *et al.* Serotonin syndrome: case report and review of the literature. *Conn Med* 1997; **61:** 717–21.
18. Alderman CP, Lee PC. Serotonin syndrome associated with combined sertraline-amitriptyline treatment. *Ann Pharmacother* 1996; **30:** 1499–1500.
19. Leinonen E, *et al.* Paroxetine increases serum trimipramine concentration: a report of two cases. *Hum Psychopharmacol Clin Exp* 1995; **10:** 345–7.
20. Baettig D, *et al.* Tricyclic antidepressant plasma levels after augmentation with citalopram: a case study. *Eur J Clin Pharmacol* 1993; **44:** 403–5.

21. Barker WA, *et al.* The Newcastle chronic depression study: results of a treatment regime. *Int Clin Psychopharmacol* 1987; **2:** 261–72.
22. Pare CMB. Potentiation of monoamine oxidase inhibitors by tryptophan. *Lancet* 1963; **ii:** 527–8.
23. Price WA, *et al.* Serotonin syndrome: a case report. *J Clin Pharmacol* 1986; **26:** 77–8.
24. Solomon JG. Seizures during lithium-amitriptyline therapy. *Postgrad Med* 1979; **66:** 145–8.
25. Kojima H, *et al.* Serotonin syndrome during clomipramine and lithium treatment. *Am J Psychiatry* 1993; **150:** 1897.
26. Austin LS, *et al.* Toxicity resulting from lithium augmentation of antidepressant treatment in elderly patients. *J Clin Psychiatry* 1990; **51:** 344–5.
27. Lafferman J, *et al.* Lithium augmentation for treatment-resistant depression in the elderly. *J Geriatr Psychiatry Neurol* 1988; **1:** 49–52.
28. Zaninelli R, *et al.* Changes in quantitatively assessed tremor during treatment of major depression with lithium augmented by paroxetine or amitriptyline. *J Clin Psychopharmacol* 2001; **21:** 190–8.
29. Kline SS, *et al.* Serotonin syndrome versus neuroleptic malignant syndrome as a cause of death. *Clin Pharm* 1989; **8:** 510–14.
30. Benazzi F. Anticholinergic toxic syndrome with venlafaxine-desipramine combination. *Pharmacopsychiatry* 1998; **31:** 36–7.
31. Benazzi F. Venlafaxine drug-drug interactions in clinical practice. *J Psychiatry Neurosci* 1998; **23:** 181–2.
32. Klysner R, *et al.* Toxic interaction of venlafaxine and isocarboxazid. *Lancet* 1995; **346:** 1298–9.
33. Heister MA, *et al.* Serotonin syndrome induced by administration of venlafaxine and phenelzine. *Ann Pharmacother* 1996; **30:** 84.
34. Hodgman MJ. Serotonin syndrome due to venlafaxine and maintenance tranylcypromine therapy. *Hum Exp Toxicol* 1997; **16:** 14–17.
35. Reeves RR, *et al.* Serotonin syndrome produced by paroxetine and low-dose trazodone. *Psychosomatics* 1995; **36:** 159.
36. Smith DL, Wenegrat BG. A case report of serotonin syndrome associated with combined nefazodone and fluoxetine. *J Clin Psychiatry* 2000; **61:** 146.
37. John L, *et al.* Serotonin syndrome associated with nefazodone and paroxetine. *Ann Emerg Med* 1997; **29:** 287–9.
38. Gordon JB. SSRIs and St. John's Wort: possible toxicity? *Am Fam Physician* 1998; **57:** 950, 953.
39. Committee on Safety of Medicines/Medicines Control Agency. Reminder: St John's wort (Hypericum perforatum) interactions. *Current Problems* 2000; **26:** 6–7.
40. Lantz MS, *et al.* St. John's Wort and antidepressant drug interactions in the elderly. *J Geriatr Psychiatry Neurol* 1999; **12:** 7–10.

Antiepileptics. Antidepressants may antagonise the activity of antiepileptics by lowering the convulsive threshold. Treatment with *carbamazepine* should be avoided with or within 2 weeks of MAOIs.

Antimigraine drugs. For the effect of MAOIs on serotonin (5-HT$_1$) agonists, see under Sumatriptan, p.457.

Antineoplastics. For the effect of MAOIs on *altretamine*, see p.506.

Dopaminergics. For the effect of MAOIs on *amantadine*, see p.1162, on *levodopa*, see p.1171, and on *selegiline*, see p.1177.

General anaesthetics. The problems that may be encountered with MAOIs and general anaesthetics are discussed under Anaesthesia in Precautions, above.

Insulin. For the effect of MAOIs on Insulin, see p.328.

Neuromuscular blockers. For the effects of MAOIs on *suxamethonium*, see p.1342. Problems that may be encountered with MAOIs and neuromuscular blockers used during anaesthesia are discussed under Precautions, above.

Opioid analgesics. The problems that may be encountered with MAOIs and opioid analgesics used during anaesthesia are discussed under Precautions, above.

Respiratory stimulants. For the effect of MAOIs on *doxapram*, see p.1509.

Pharmacokinetics

Phenelzine is readily absorbed from the gastrointestinal tract reaching peak plasma concentrations 2 to 4 hours after ingestion. It is metabolised in the liver and is excreted in the urine almost entirely in the form of metabolites.

Uses and Administration

Monoamine oxidase inhibitors (MAOIs) inhibit the action of monoamine oxidase, the enzyme responsible for the metabolism of several biogenic amines. Monoamine oxidase exists in two forms: type A and type B. Monoamine oxidase type A preferentially de-aminates, by oxidation, adrenaline, noradrenaline, and serotonin whereas monoamine oxidase type B preferentially metabolises benzylamine and phenylethylamine; dopamine and tyramine are de-aminated by both forms of the enzyme. The traditional MAOIs such as phenelzine, iproniazid, isocarboxazid, nialamide, and tranylcypromine are inhibitors of both types; apart from tranylcypromine, all are hydrazine derivatives and bind irreversibly. Selective inhibitors include selegiline (p.1177), an irreversible inhibitor of monoamine oxidase type B used in the

treatment of Parkinson's disease. Clorgiline is an irreversible selective type A inhibitor. Reversible inhibitors of monoamine oxidase type A (RIMAs) include brofaromine, moclobemide, and toloxatone. Antidepressant activity appears to reside predominantly with inhibition of monoamine oxidase type A although the mode of action of these drugs in depression is not fully understood. Advantages claimed for selective inhibitors are fewer or less severe side-effects than those experienced with non-selective inhibitors. As tyramine is de-aminated by both monoamine oxidase types A and B, inhibiting only one of the enzymes allows for continued, albeit reduced, de-amination. Thus the dietary precautions that need to be observed with non-selective inhibitors of both monoamine oxidase types A and B are less stringent with the selective inhibitors.

Phenelzine and other antidepressant MAOIs are used in the treatment of atypical depression, particularly where phobic features or associated anxiety are present, or in patients who have not responded to other antidepressants. However, the risks associated with irreversible non-selective MAOIs usually mean that other antidepressants are preferred. Up to a month may elapse before an antidepressant response is obtained with MAOIs. After a response has been obtained maintenance therapy may need to be continued for at least 4 to 6 months to avoid relapse on discontinuation of therapy. MAOI therapy is not generally indicated for children. Care should be taken in elderly patients because of an increased susceptibility to adverse effects. Moreover, therapy with the non-selective inhibitors is particularly unsuitable for patients considered unable to adhere to the strict dietary requirements necessary for its safe usage.

Phenelzine is given by mouth as the sulfate in doses equivalent to phenelzine 15 mg three times daily; if no response has been obtained after 2 weeks the dosage may be increased to 15 mg four times daily; severely depressed patients in hospital may be given up to 30 mg three times daily. Once a response has been obtained the dosage may be gradually reduced for maintenance therapy; some patients may continue to respond to 15 mg on alternate days.

Phenelzine should be withdrawn gradually to reduce the risk of withdrawal symptoms.

Anxiety disorders. MAOIs have been used in the treatment of *anxiety disorders*. MAOIs appear to be effective in blocking *panic attacks* (see p.649). They also appear to be effective in *social phobias* (see under Phobic Disorders, p.649) and can improve anticipatory anxiety and functional disability. The major treatment for *post-traumatic stress disorder* (p.650) is psychotherapy but MAOIs can help to reduce traumatic recollections and nightmares and to repress flashbacks.

References.
1. Buigues J, Vallejo J. Therapeutic response to phenelzine in patients with panic disorder and agoraphobia with panic attacks. *J Clin Psychiatry* 1987; **48:** 55–9.
2. Frank JB, *et al.* A randomized clinical trial of phenelzine and imipramine for posttraumatic stress disorder. *Am J Psychiatry* 1988; **145:** 1289–91.
3. Heimberg RG, *et al.* Cognitive behavioural group therapy vs phenelzine therapy for social phobia: 12 week outcome. *Arch Gen Psychiatry* 1998; **55:** 1133–41.

Depression. As discussed on p.271 there is very little difference in efficacy between the different groups of antidepressant drugs, and choice is often made on the basis of adverse effects. MAOIs are rarely used as first-choice antidepressants because of the dangers of dietary and drug interactions. Even in depressed patients with atypical, hypochondriacal, hysterical, or phobic features, for which MAOIs are particularly effective, it is often recommended that another antidepressant type should be tried first. Reversible inhibitors of monoamine oxidase type A (RIMAs) offer an alternative to the MAOIs and less strict dietary restrictions are necessary. They may be an effective first choice in a wide range of depressive disorders, although their relative efficacy in atypical depression remains to be established.

Combination therapy with differing classes of antidepressants, including the MAOIs, has been used in the treatment of drug-resistant depression. However, such therapy may result in enhanced adverse reactions or interactions and is considered unsuitable or controversial by some workers. For further details, see Antidepressants under Interactions, above.

Hyperactivity. When drug therapy is required for attention deficit hyperactivity disorder (p.1505), initial treatment is usually with a central stimulant. MAOIs have been used success-

fully but problems with dietary restriction and potential drug interactions have limited their use.

Migraine. A number of drugs have been used for the prophylaxis of migraine (p.449), although propranolol or pizotifen are generally preferred. Antidepressants such as the tricyclics can be useful alternatives when these drugs are ineffective or unsuitable. MAOIs are best reserved for severe cases refractory to other forms of prophylactic treatment.

Preparations

BP 2001: Phenelzine Tablets;
USP 25: Phenelzine Sulfate Tablets.

Proprietary Preparations (details are given in Part 3)
Austral.: Nardil; ***Belg.:*** Nardelzine; ***Canad.:*** Nardil; ***Irl.:*** Nardil; ***Israel:*** Nardil; ***NZ:*** Nardil; ***UK:*** Nardil; ***USA:*** Nardil.

Pirlindole   (14854-c)

Pirlindole *(rINN)*.
2,3,3a,4,5,6-Hexahydro-8-methyl-1*H*-pyrazino[3,2,1-*jk*]carbazole.
$C_{15}H_{18}N_2 = 226.3$.
CAS — 60762-57-4.

Profile

Pirlindole has been given in doses of up to a maximum of 400 mg daily by mouth in the treatment of depression.

Preparations

Proprietary Preparations (details are given in Part 3)
Spain: Lifril†.

Pivagabine   (15915-r)

Pivagabine *(rINN)*.
4-Pivalamidobutyric acid.
$C_9H_{17}NO_3 = 187.2$.
CAS — 69542-93-4.
ATC — N06AX15.

Profile

Pivagabine has been used as an antidepressant.

Preparations

Proprietary Preparations (details are given in Part 3)
Ital.: Tonerg†; Zenit†.

Protriptyline Hydrochloride   (2534-j)

Protriptyline Hydrochloride *(BANM, USAN, rINNM)*.
MK-240.   3-(5*H*-Dibenzo[*a,d*]cyclohept-5-enyl)propyl(methyl)amine hydrochloride.
$C_{19}H_{21}N,HCl = 299.8$.
CAS — 438-60-8 (protriptyline); 1225-55-4 (protriptyline hydrochloride).
Pharmacopoeias. In *Br.* and *US.*

Pharmacopoeial description

BP 2001: A white to yellowish-white, odourless or almost odourless, powder. Freely soluble in water; in alcohol, and in chloroform; practically insoluble in ether. A 1% solution in water has a pH of 5.0 to 6.5.

USP 25: A white to yellowish powder. Is odourless or has not more than a slight odour. Soluble 1 in 2 of water, 1 in 3.5 of alcohol, and 1 in 2.5 of chloroform; practically insoluble in ether. pH of a 1% solution in water is between 5.0 and 6.5.

Adverse Effects, Treatment, and Precautions

As for tricyclic antidepressants in general (see Amitriptyline, p.273).

Since protriptyline may have some stimulant properties anxiety and agitation may occur more frequently; cardiovascular effects such as tachycardia and hypotension may also be more frequent than with other tricyclics. Photosensitivity rashes have been noted more commonly with protriptyline than with other tricyclic antidepressants and patients taking it should avoid direct sunlight.

Interactions

For interactions associated with tricyclic antidepressants, see Amitriptyline, p.276.

Pharmacokinetics

Protriptyline is well but slowly absorbed after oral administration, peak plasma concentrations being achieved after several hours.

Paths of metabolism of protriptyline include *N*-oxidation and hydroxylation. Protriptyline is excreted in the urine, mainly in the form of its metabolites, either free or in conjugated form. Protriptyline is widely distributed throughout the body and extensively bound to plasma and tissue protein. Protriptyline has been estimated to have a very prolonged elimination half-life ranging from 55 to 198 hours, which may be further prolonged in overdosage.

Uses and Administration

Protriptyline is a dibenzocycloheptatriene tricyclic antidepressant with actions and uses similar to those of amitriptyline (p.278). It has considerably less sedative properties than other tricyclics and may have a stimulant effect, thus making it particularly suitable for apathetic and withdrawn patients; its antimuscarinic properties are moderate.

In the treatment of depression, protriptyline hydrochloride is given by mouth in doses of 5 to 10 mg three or four times daily. It has been suggested that, because of its potential stimulant activity, any dosage increases should be added to the morning dose first and if insomnia occurs the last dose should be given no later than mid-afternoon. Higher doses of up to 60 mg daily may be required in severely depressed patients. A suitable initial dose for adolescents and the elderly is 5 mg three times daily; close monitoring of the cardiovascular system has been recommended if the dose exceeds a total of 20 mg daily in elderly subjects.

Protriptyline should be withdrawn gradually to reduce the risk of withdrawal symptoms.

Preparations

BP 2001: Protriptyline Tablets;
USP 25: Protriptyline Hydrochloride Tablets.

Proprietary Preparations (details are given in Part 3)
Canad.: Triptil; *Denm.:* Concordin; *Irl.:* Concordin; *Swed.:* Concordin; *UK:* Concordin†; *USA:* Vivactil.

Quinupramine (13204-x)

Quinupramine (rINN).
LM-208.   10,11-Dihydro-5-(quinuclidin-3-yl)-5H-dibenz[b,f]azepine.
$C_{21}H_{24}N_2 = 304.4$.
CAS — 31721-17-2.
ATC — N06AA23.

Profile
Quinupramine is a tricyclic antidepressant (see Amitriptyline, p.273). It has been given by mouth or by intravenous infusion in doses of 5 to 15 mg daily in the treatment of depression.

Quinupramine should be withdrawn gradually to reduce the risk of withdrawal symptoms.

Preparations

Proprietary Preparations (details are given in Part 3)
Aust.: Kevopril; *Fr.:* Kinupril†.

Reboxetine Mesilate (20430-f)

Reboxetine Mesilate (BANM, rINNM).
FCE-20124 (reboxetine or reboxetine mesilate); PNU-155950E; Reboxetine Mesylate (USAN). (±)-(2RS)-2-[(αRS)-α-(2-Ethoxyphenoxy)benzyl]morpholine methanesulphonate.
$C_{19}H_{23}NO_3,CH_4O_3S = 409.5$.
CAS — 71620-89-8; 98769-81-4 (both reboxetine); 98769-82-5; 98769-84-7 (both reboxetine mesilate).

Reboxetine mesilate 5.23 mg is approximately equivalent to 4 mg of reboxetine.

Adverse Effects

Side-effects reported with reboxetine include insomnia, increased sweating, dizziness, postural hypotension, paraesthesia, impotence, and dysuria. Vertigo, dry mouth, constipation, tachycardia, and urinary retention (mainly in men) have also been reported. Reduced plasma-potassium concentrations have been observed in elderly patients following prolonged administration.

Hyponatraemia, possibly as a result of inappropriate secretion of antidiuretic hormone, has been associated with the use of antidepressants, particularly in the elderly.

Effects on the endocrine system. A report[1] of *hyponatraemia*, thought to be associated with reboxetine therapy and to be due to the syndrome of inappropriate antidiuretic hormone secretion, in an elderly patient.
1. Ranieri P, *et al.* Reboxetine and hyponatremia. *N Engl J Med* 2000; 342: 215–16.

Precautions

Reboxetine should be used with caution in patients with renal or hepatic impairment. It should also be used under close supervision in patients with bipolar disorder, urinary retention, benign prostatic hyperplasia, glaucoma, or a history of epilepsy or cardiac disorders.

Patients should be closely monitored during early therapy until improvement in depression is observed because suicide is an inherent risk in depressed patients. For further details, see under Depression, p.271.

Ability to perform tasks requiring motor or cognitive skills or judgement may be impaired by reboxetine and patients, if affected, should not drive or operate machinery.

Interactions

Reboxetine should not be taken together with, or within two weeks of discontinuing an MAOI; at least one week should elapse after discontinuing reboxetine therapy before starting any drug liable to provoke a serious reaction (e.g. phenelzine). Increases in blood pressure may occur when reboxetine and ergotamine are administered together. Caution should be exercised when reboxetine is given with other drugs that lower blood pressure because postural hypotension has occurred with reboxetine. Clinical data on interactions with reboxetine are limited but the manufacturer advises that concomitant administration with drugs that may have the potential to inhibit its elimination such as the azole antifungals (e.g. ketoconazole), macrolide antibiotics (e.g. erythromycin), or fluvoxamine should be avoided. Reboxetine in high concentrations has been shown *in vitro* to inhibit the cytochrome P450 isoenzymes CYP3A4 and CYP2D6. It should therefore be used with caution together with drugs metabolised by these isoenzymes and with a narrow therapeutic margin such as antiarrhythmics, antipsychotics, ciclosporin, and tricyclic antidepressants. The possibility of hypokalaemia if reboxetine is given with potassium-depleting diuretics should also be considered.

Pharmacokinetics

Reboxetine is well absorbed from the gastrointestinal tract with peak plasma levels occurring after about 2 hours. Plasma protein binding is about 97% (92% in elderly subjects). Reboxetine is metabolised by dealkylation, hydroxylation, and oxidation followed by glucuronide or sulfate conjugation. Elimination is mainly via urine (78%) with 10% excreted as unchanged drug. The plasma elimination half-life is 13 hours. Data from *animal* studies indicate that reboxetine crosses the placenta and is distributed into breast milk.

◊ References.
1. Dostert P, *et al.* Review of the pharmacokinetics and metabolism of reboxetine, a selective noradrenaline reuptake inhibitor. *Eur Neuropsychopharmacol* 1997; 7 (suppl 1): S23–S35.
2. Fleishaker JC. Clinical pharmacokinetics of reboxetine, a selective norepinephrine reuptake inhibitor for the treatment of patients with depression. *Clin Pharmacokinet* 2000; 39: 413–27.

Uses and Administration

Reboxetine is a selective and potent inhibitor of the reuptake of noradrenaline; it also has a weak effect on serotonin reuptake. Reboxetine has no significant affinity for muscarinic receptors. It is given by mouth as the mesilate for the treatment of depression with doses expressed as reboxetine. The daily dose of reboxetine is 8 mg in two divided doses, which may be increased after 3 to 4 weeks, if necessary, to 10 mg daily; the maximum daily dose should not exceed 12 mg. Lower initial doses of 4 mg daily in two divided doses are recommended in hepatic or renal impairment; doses may be increased thereafter according to tolerance.

◊ References.
1. Berzewski H, *et al.* Efficacy and tolerability of reboxetine compared with imipramine in a double-blind study in patients suffering from major depressive episodes. *Eur Neuropsychopharmacol* 1997; 7 (suppl 1): S37–S47.
2. Anonymous. Reboxetine—another new antidepressant. *Drug Ther Bull* 1998; 36: 86–8.
3. Montgomery SA. The place of reboxetine in antidepressant therapy. *J Clin Psychiatry* 1998; 59 (suppl 14): 26–9.
4. Massana J, *et al.* Reboxetine: a double-blind comparison with fluoxetine in major depressive disorder. *Int Clin Psychopharmacol* 1999; 14: 73–80.
5. Versiani M, *et al.* Reboxetine, a unique selective NRI, prevents relapse and recurrence in long-term treatment of major depressive disorder. *J Clin Psychiatry* 1999; 60: 400–406.
6. Holm KJ, Spencer CM. Reboxetine: a review of its use in depression. *CNS Drugs* 1999; 12: 65–83.
7. Scates AC, Doraiswamy PM. Reboxetine: a selective norepinephrine reuptake inhibitor for the treatment of depression. *Ann Pharmacother* 2000; 34: 1302–12.

Preparations

Proprietary Preparations (details are given in Part 3)
Aust.: Edronax; *Belg.:* Edronax; *Denm.:* Edronax; *Fin.:* Edronax; *Ger.:* Edronax; *Irl.:* Edronax; *Ital.:* Davedax; Edronax; *Mex.:* Edronax; *Norw.:* Edronax; *Port.:* Edronax; *S.Afr.:* Edronax; *Spain:* Norebox; *Swed.:* Edronax; *UK:* Edronax.

Sertraline Hydrochloride (18681-x)

Sertraline Hydrochloride (BANM, USAN, rINNM).
CP-51974-01; CP-51974-1. (1S,4S)-4-(3,4-Dichlorophenyl)-1,2,3,4-tetrahydro-1-naphthyl(methyl)amine hydrochloride.
$C_{17}H_{17}Cl_2N,HCl = 342.7$.
CAS — 79617-96-2 (sertraline); 79559-97-0 (sertraline hydrochloride).

Sertraline hydrochloride 56 mg is approximately equivalent to 50 mg of sertraline.

Adverse Effects, Treatment, and Precautions
As for SSRIs in general (see Fluoxetine, p.284).

Interactions
For interactions associated with SSRIs, see Fluoxetine, p.287.

Pharmacokinetics
Sertraline is slowly absorbed from the gastrointestinal tract with peak plasma concentrations occurring about 4.5 to 8.5 hours after ingestion. It undergoes extensive first-pass metabolism in the liver. The main pathway is demethylation to *N*-desmethylsertraline which is inactive; further metabolism and glucuronide conjugation occurs. Sertraline is widely distributed throughout body tissues and is highly bound (about 98%) to plasma proteins. The plasma elimination half-life of sertraline is reported to be 24 to 26 hours. Sertraline is excreted in approximately equal amounts in the urine and faeces, mainly as metabolites. Sertraline is distributed into breast milk (see Breast Feeding under Precautions in Fluoxetine, p.286).

◊ References.
1. Démolis J-L, *et al.* Influence of liver cirrhosis on sertraline pharmacokinetics. *Br J Clin Pharmacol* 1996; 42: 394–7.
2. Preskorn SH, ed. Sertraline: a pharmacokinetic profile. *Clin Pharmacokinet* 1997; 32 (suppl 1): 1–55.

Uses and Administration
Sertraline, a naphthaleneamine derivative, is an SSRI with actions and uses similar to those of fluoxetine (p.288). It is given by mouth as sertraline hydrochloride as a single dose in the morning or evening. Doses are expressed in terms of sertraline.

In the treatment of **depression**, the usual initial dose of sertraline is 50 mg daily increased, if necessary, in increments of 50 mg at intervals of at least a week to a maximum of 200 mg daily.

In the treatment of **obsessive-compulsive disorder** the usual initial dose of sertraline is 50 mg daily. In the treatment of **panic disorder** with or without agoraphobia and **post-traumatic stress disorder**, the usual initial dose is 25 mg daily increased after one week to 50 mg daily. Thereafter, doses in all these disorders may be increased, if necessary, in increments of 50 mg at intervals of at least a week to a maximum of 200 mg daily.

Sertraline is also given for the treatment of obsessive-compulsive disorder in children and adolescents aged 6 years and over. In children aged 6 to 12 years the usual initial dose is 25 mg once daily; adolescents may be started on 50 mg once daily. Increases in doses, if necessary, are similar to those in adults; however, the lower body-weights of children should be considered in order to avoid excessive doses.

Once the optimal therapeutic response is obtained dosage should be reduced to the lowest effective level for maintenance.

Lower or less frequent doses are recommended in patients with significant hepatic impairment, although some manufacturers recommend that sertraline should not be used at all. Caution is advised in patients with renal impairment.

Sertraline should be withdrawn gradually to reduce the risk of withdrawal symptoms.

◊ Reviews.
1. Murdoch D, McTavish D. Sertraline: a review of its pharmacodynamic and pharmacokinetic properties, and therapeutic potential in depression and obsessive-compulsive disorder. *Drugs* 1992; **44:** 604–24.
2. Grimsley SR, Jann MW. Paroxetine, sertraline, and fluvoxamine: new selective serotonin reuptake inhibitors. *Clin Pharm* 1992; **11:** 930–57.

Anxiety disorders. Sertraline has been given in a variety of anxiety disorders including obsessive-compulsive disorder (p.649), panic attacks (p.649), social phobia (see under Phobic Disorders, p.649), and post-traumatic stress disorder (p.650). References.
1. Jenike MA, *et al.* Sertraline in obsessive-compulsive disorder: a double-blind comparison with placebo. *Am J Psychiatry* 1990; **147:** 923–8.
2. Chouinard G, *et al.* Results of a double-blind placebo controlled trial of a new serotonin uptake inhibitor, sertraline, in the treatment of obsessive-compulsive disorder. *Psychopharmacol Bull* 1990; **26:** 279–84.
3. Greist J, *et al.* Double-blind parallel comparison of three dosages of sertraline and placebo in outpatients with obsessive-compulsive disorder. *Arch Gen Psychiatry* 1995; **52:** 289–95.
4. Katzelnick DJ, *et al.* Sertraline for social phobia: a double-blind, placebo-controlled crossover study, *Am J Psychiatry* 1995; **152:** 1368–71.
5. Brady KT, *et al.* Sertraline treatment of comorbid posttraumatic stress disorder and alcohol dependence. *J Clin Psychiatry* 1995; **56:** 502–5.
6. March JS, *et al.* Sertraline in children and adolescents with obsessive-compulsive disorder: a multicenter randomized controlled trial. *JAMA* 1998; **280:** 1752–6.
7. Londborg PD, *et al.* Sertraline in the treatment of panic disorder. A multi-site, double-blind, placebo-controlled, fixed-dose investigation. *Br J Psychiatry* 1998; **173:** 54–60.
8. Brady K, *et al.* Efficacy and safety of sertraline treatment of post-traumatic stress disorder: a randomized controlled trial. *JAMA* 2000; **283:** 1837–44.

Depression. As discussed on p.271, there is very little difference in efficacy between the different groups of antidepressant drugs, and choice is often made on the basis of adverse effect profile. SSRIs such as sertraline are widely used as an alternative to the older tricyclics as they have fewer unpleasant side-effects and are safer in overdosage. References.
1. Haider A, *et al.* Clinical effect of converting antidepressant therapy from fluoxetine to sertraline. *Am J Health-Syst Pharm* 1995; **52:** 1317–19.
2. Bennie EH, *et al.* A double-blind multicenter trial comparing sertraline and fluoxetine in outpatients with major depression. *J Clin Psychiatry* 1995; **56:** 229–37.
3. Stowe ZN, *et al.* Sertraline in the treatment of women with postpartum major depression. *Depression* 1995; **3:** 49–55.
4. Keller MB, *et al.* Maintenance phase efficacy of sertraline for chronic depression: a randomized controlled trial. *JAMA* 1998; **280:** 1665–72.

Headache. For reference to the use of SSRIs, including sertraline, in the management of various types of headache, see under Fluoxetine, p.289.

Premenstrual syndrome. Sertraline in doses ranging from 50 to 150 mg daily throughout the menstrual cycle has produced beneficial effects in controlling both the psychological and somatic symptoms of women with premenstrual syndrome.[1-3] Administration of sertraline in doses of 50 or 100 mg daily solely during the luteal phase was also of benefit.[4,5] For a discussion of the overall management of premenstrual syndrome, see p.1475.
1. Freeman EW, *et al.* Sertraline versus desipramine in the treatment of premenstrual syndrome: an open-label trial. *J Clin Psychiatry* 1999; **57:** 7–11.
2. Yonkers KA, *et al.* Sertraline in the treatment of premenstrual dysphoric disorder. *Psychopharmacol Bull* 1996; **32:** 41–6.
3. Yonkers KA, *et al.* Symptomatic improvement of premenstrual dysphoric disorder with sertraline treatment: a randomized controlled trial. *JAMA* 1997; **278:** 983–8.
4. Young SA, *et al.* Treatment of premenstrual dysphoric disorder with sertraline during the luteal phase: a randomized, double-blind, placebo-controlled crossover trial. *J Clin Psychiatry* 1998; **59:** 76–80.
5. Jermain DM, *et al.* Luteal phase sertraline treatment for premenstrual dysphoric disorder: results of a double-blind, placebo-controlled, crossover study. *Arch Fam Med* 1999; **8:** 328–32.

Sexual dysfunction. Impotence or ejaculatory problems have been reported as adverse effects of SSRIs (see Effects on Sexual Function in Adverse Effects of Fluoxetine, p.285). Such properties of the SSRIs have been studied as a potential form of treatment for men with premature ejaculation. Significant improvements were noted in a placebo-controlled trial[1] of sertraline involving 52 men with self-reported premature ejaculation.
1. Mendels J, *et al.* Sertraline treatment for premature ejaculation. *J Clin Psychopharmacol* 1995; **15:** 341–6.

Preparations

Proprietary Preparations (details are given in Part 3)
Aust.: Gladem; Tresleen; Zoloft†; *Austral.:* Zoloft; *Belg.:* Serlain; *Braz.:* Zoloft; *Canad.:* Zoloft; *Denm.:* Zoloft; *Fin.:* Zoloft; *Fr.:* Zoloft; *Ger.:* Gladem; Zoloft; *Hong Kong:* Zoloft; *Irl.:* Lustral; *Israel:* Lustral; *Ital.:* Serad; Tatig; Zoloft; *Mex.:* Altruline; *Neth.:* Zoloft; *Norw.:* Zoloft; *NZ:* Zoloft; *Port.:* Zoloft; *S.Afr.:* Zoloft;

Singapore: Zoloft; *Spain:* Aremis; Besitran; Sealdin; *Swed.:* Zoloft; *Switz.:* Gladem; Zoloft; *Thai.:* Zoloft; *UK:* Lustral; *USA:* Zoloft.

Teniloxazine   (2991-c)
Teniloxazine (rINN).
Sufoxazine; Y-8894. (±)-2-{[(α-2-Thienyl-o-tolyl)oxy]methyl}morpholine.
$C_{16}H_{19}NO_2S = 289.4.$
CAS — 62473-79-4.

Profile
Teniloxazine has antidepressant properties and has also been studied for use in the management of dementia.

◊ References.
1. Ogura C, *et al.* Clinical pharmacology of a new antidepressant, Y-8894 in healthy young and elderly volunteers. *Br J Clin Pharmacol* 1987; **23:** 537–43.
2. Orlando R, *et al.* The pharmacokinetics of teniloxazine in healthy subjects and patients with hepatic cirrhosis. *Br J Clin Pharmacol* 1995; **39:** 445–8.
3. Aguglia E, *et al.* Comparison of teniloxazine and piracetam in Alzheimer-type or vascular dementia. *Curr Ther Res* 1995; **56:** 250–7.

Tianeptine Sodium   (17007-n)
Tianeptine Sodium (rINNM).
The sodium salt of 7-[(3-chloro-6,11-dihydro-6-methyldibenzo[c,f][1,2]thiazepin-11-yl)amino]heptanoic acid S,S-dioxide.
$C_{21}H_{25}ClN_2NaO_4S = 459.9.$
CAS — 66981-73-5 (tianeptine).

Profile
Tianeptine sodium is an antidepressant reported to act by increasing (rather than inhibiting) the presynaptic reuptake of serotonin. It is given by mouth in doses of 12.5 mg three times daily in the treatment of depression (p.271). Doses should be reduced to a total of 25 mg daily in elderly patients and those with renal impairment, but it has been stated that no dose modification is necessary in patients with chronic alcoholism or cirrhosis.

Isolated cases of hepatitis have been reported during treatment with tianeptine.

◊ References.
1. Royer RJ, *et al.* Tianeptine and its main metabolite: pharmacokinetics in chronic alcoholism and cirrhosis. *Clin Pharmacokinet* 1989; **16:** 186–91.
2. Carlhant D, *et al.* Pharmacokinetics and bioavailability of tianeptine in the elderly. *Drug Invest* 1990; **2:** 167–72.
3. Demotes-Mainard F, *et al.* Pharmacokinetics of the antidepressant tianeptine at steady state in the elderly. *J Clin Pharmacol* 1991; **31:** 174–8.
4. Wilde MI, Benfield P. Tianeptine: a review of its pharmacodynamic and pharmacokinetic properties, and therapeutic efficacy in depression and coexisting anxiety and depression. *Drugs* 1995; **49:** 411–39.

Asthma. Tianeptine has been reported to improve symptoms in patients with asthma.[1] It was thought that reduction of raised levels of free serotonin found in such patients contributed to the beneficial effect of tianeptine.
1. Lechin F, *et al.* The serotonin uptake-enhancing drug tianeptine suppresses asthmatic symptoms in children: a double-blind, crossover, placebo-controlled study. *J Clin Pharmacol* 1998; **38:** 918–25.

Preparations
Proprietary Preparations (details are given in Part 3)
Fr.: Stablon; *Mex.:* Stablon; *Port.:* Stablon; *Thai.:* Stablon.

Toloxatone   (3229-y)
Toloxatone (rINN).
5-(Hydroxymethyl)-3-m-tolyl-2-oxazolidinone.
$C_{11}H_{13}NO_3 = 207.2.$
CAS — 29218-27-7.
ATC — N06AG03.

Profile
Toloxatone is a reversible inhibitor of monoamine oxidase type A (RIMA) (see Moclobemide, p.299). It is used as an antidepressant in doses of 200 mg three times daily by mouth.

◊ References.
1. Benedetti MS, *et al.* Pharmacokinetics of toloxatone in man following intravenous and oral administrations. *Arzneimittelforschung* 1982; **32:** 276–80.
2. Lemoine P, Mirabaud C. A double-blind comparison of moclobemide and toloxatone in out-patients presenting a major depressive disorder. *Psychopharmacology (Berl)* 1992; **106** (suppl): S118–S119.

Preparations
Proprietary Preparations (details are given in Part 3)
Fr.: Humoryl; *Ital.:* Umoril†.

Tranylcypromine Sulfate   (2537-k)
Tranylcypromine Sulfate (rINNM).
SKF-385; Transamine Sulphate; Tranylcypromine Sulphate (BANM). (±)-trans-2-Phenylcyclopropylamine sulphate.
$(C_9H_{11}N)_2,H_2SO_4 = 364.5.$
CAS — 155-09-9 (tranylcypromine); 13492-01-8 (tranylcypromine sulfate).
Pharmacopoeias. In Br.

Tranylcypromine sulfate 13.7 mg is approximately equivalent to 10 mg of tranylcypromine.

Pharmacopoeial description
BP 2001: A white or almost white crystalline powder; odourless or with a faint odour of cinnamaldehyde. Soluble in water; very slightly soluble in alcohol and in ether; insoluble in chloroform.

Adverse Effects, Treatment, and Precautions
As for MAOIs in general (see Phenelzine, p.303).

Tranylcypromine has a stimulant action and insomnia is a common side-effect if it is taken in the evening.

Hypertensive reactions are more likely to occur with tranylcypromine than with other MAOIs, but severe liver damage occurs less frequently. Tranylcypromine should not be used in patients with hyperthyroidism.

Dependence. Dependence on tranylcypromine with tolerance has been reported in patients receiving high doses with or without a history of previous substance abuse. For further details, see Withdrawal under Precautions in Phenelzine, p.305.

Effects on the cardiovascular system. Although orthostatic hypotension is the more common effect of MAOIs on blood pressure, hypertension can occur. A hypertensive crisis has been described in two patients after only one dose of tranylcypromine.[1,2] In the first case it was thought possible that an autointeraction may have occurred between tranylcypromine and amfetamine to which it is partly metabolised. In the second case the provocation of hypertension led to the finding of a previously undiagnosed phaeochromocytoma and it was suggested this may have been a possibility in previous reports of hypertension induced by MAOIs.
1. Gunn J, *et al.* Hypertensive crisis and broad complex bradycardia after a single dose of monoamine oxidase inhibitor. *BMJ* 1989; **298:** 964.
2. Cook RF, Katritsis D. Hypertensive crisis precipitated by a monoamine oxidase inhibitor in a patient with phaeochromocytoma. *BMJ* 1990; **300:** 614.

Porphyria. Tranylcypromine is considered to be unsafe in patients with porphyria because it has been shown to be porphyrinogenic in *animals*.

Interactions
For interactions associated with MAOIs, see Phenelzine, p.305.
The concomitant administration of clomipramine with tranylcypromine is particularly hazardous.

Pharmacokinetics
Tranylcypromine is readily absorbed from the gastrointestinal tract, peak plasma concentrations occurring about 1 to 3 hours after ingestion. It is excreted in the urine mainly in the form of metabolites. Tranylcypromine has a reported plasma elimination half-life of about 2.5 hours.

◊ In 9 depressed patients, tranylcypromine absorption was rapid after oral dosing.[1] Absorption was biphasic in 7. Elimination was also rapid, with an elimination half-life of 1.54 to 3.15 hours. From 2 to 7 hours after dosing, standing systolic and diastolic blood pressures were lowered, and standing pulse was raised. The onset of the effect on standing systolic blood pressure correlated with the time of peak plasma tranylcypromine concentration. Maximum orthostatic drop of blood pressure and rise in pulse rate occurred 2 hours after dosing. Mean plasma-tranylcypromine concentrations correlated with mean orthostatic drop of systolic blood pressure and rise of pulse rate. Patients experiencing clinically significant hypotensive reactions to tranylcypromine may benefit from changes in their dose regimen aimed at minimising peak concentrations.
1. Mallinger AG, *et al.* Pharmacokinetics of tranylcypromine in patients who are depressed: relationship to cardiovascular effects. *Clin Pharmacol Ther* 1986; **40:** 444–50.

Uses and Administration
Tranylcypromine, a cyclopropylamine derivative, is an MAOI with actions and uses similar to those of phenelzine (p.307). It produces a less prolonged inhibition of the enzymes than phenelzine.

Tranylcypromine is used in the treatment of depression, but as discussed on p.271, the risks associated with traditional non-selective MAOIs such as tranylcypromine usually mean that other antidepressants are preferred. It is given by mouth as the sulfate in doses equivalent to tranylcypromine 10 mg in the morning and 10 mg in the afternoon; if the response is inadequate after a week, 10 mg may be given additionally at midday; a dosage of 30 mg daily should only be exceeded with caution, although some authorities have allowed a maximum dose of 60 mg daily. Once a satisfactory response has been obtained the dosage may be gradually reduced for maintenance; some patients may continue to respond to 10 mg daily.

Tranylcypromine should be withdrawn gradually to reduce the risk of withdrawal symptoms.

Preparations

BP 2001: Tranylcypromine Tablets.

Proprietary Preparations (details are given in Part 3)
Austral.: Parnate; *Braz.:* Parnate; *Canad.:* Parnate; *Ger.:* Jatrosom N; Parnate†; *Irl.:* Parnate; *NZ:* Parnate; *S.Afr.:* Parnate; *Spain:* Parnate; *UK:* Parnate; *USA:* Parnate.

Multi-ingredient: *Braz.:* Stelapar; *Irl.:* Parstelin; *Ital.:* Parmodalin; *UK:* Parstelin†.

Trazodone Hydrochloride (2541-y)

Trazodone Hydrochloride *(BANM, USAN, rINNM).*
AF-1161. 2-[3-(4-*m*-Chlorophenylpiperazin-1-yl)propyl]-1,2,4-triazolo[4,3-*a*]pyridin-3(2*H*)-one hydrochloride.
$C_{19}H_{22}ClN_5O,HCl = 408.3$.
CAS — 19794-93-5 (trazodone); 25332-39-2 (trazodone hydrochloride).
Pharmacopoeias. In Br. and US.

Pharmacopoeial description

BP 2001: A white or almost white crystalline powder. Soluble in water; sparingly soluble in alcohol; practically insoluble in ether. A 1% solution in water has a pH of 3.9 to 4.5. Store in airtight containers. Protect from light.

USP 25: A white to off-white crystalline powder. Sparingly soluble in water and in chloroform. Store in airtight containers. Protect from light.

Adverse Effects and Treatment

Trazodone has sedative properties and drowsiness may initially occur but usually disappears on continuing treatment. Other side-effects occasionally reported include dizziness, headache, nausea and vomiting, weakness, weight loss, tremor, dry mouth, bradycardia or tachycardia, orthostatic hypotension, oedema, constipation, diarrhoea, blurred vision, restlessness, confusional states, insomnia, and skin rash. Although some of these effects are typical of antimuscarinic activity it is reported that trazodone has little antimuscarinic activity compared with tricyclic antidepressants. *Animal* studies have also indicated that trazodone is less cardiotoxic than the tricyclics. Priapism has been reported on a number of occasions.

Agranulocytosis, thrombocytopenia, and anaemia have been reported rarely. Adverse effects on hepatic function, including jaundice and hepatocellular damage, which may sometimes be severe, have also been reported rarely.

Hyponatraemia possibly due to inappropriate secretion of antidiuretic hormone has been associated with the use of antidepressants, particularly in the elderly.

Symptoms of overdosage include drowsiness, dizziness, vomiting, priapism, respiratory arrest, seizures, and ECG changes. Treatment of overdosage involves gastric lavage followed by the administration of activated charcoal and symptomatic and supportive therapy.

Effects on the cardiovascular system. Although trazodone is considered to cause fewer adverse cardiovascular reactions than the tricyclic antidepressants, side-effects have, nevertheless, been reported in individual patients. In therapeutic doses it has been associated with heart block in a patient with pre-existing cardiovascular disease,[1] as well as in a patient with no ECG abnormalities.[2] Similarly, ventricular arrhythmias have been associated with therapeutic doses of trazodone both in patients with a history of cardiac problems,[3,4] and with no history of cardiac abnormalities.[5] Atrial fibrillation has been reported in a patient with ischaemic heart disease.[6]

1. Rausch JL, *et al.* Complete heart block following a single dose of trazodone. *Am J Psychiatry* 1984; **141:** 1472–3.
2. Lippmann S, *et al.* Trazodone cardiotoxicity. *Am J Psychiatry* 1983; **140:** 1383.
3. Janowsky D, *et al.* Ventricular arrhythmias possibly aggravated by trazodone. *Am J Psychiatry* 1983; **140:** 796–7.
4. Vlay SC, Friedling S. Trazodone exacerbation of VT. *Am Heart J* 1983; **106:** 604.
5. Johnson BA. Trazodone toxicity. *Br J Hosp Med* 1985; **33:** 298.
6. White WB, Wong SHY. Rapid atrial fibrillation associated with trazodone hydrochloride. *Arch Gen Psychiatry* 1985; **42:** 424.

Effects on the eyes. A patient receiving clomipramine and trazodone by mouth noted excessive blinking whenever the dose of trazodone exceeded or equalled that of clomipramine.[1] When trazodone, but not clomipramine, was withdrawn, blinking became normal within 3 weeks.

1. Cooper MA, Dening TR. Excessive blinking associated with combined antidepressants. *BMJ* 1986; **293:** 1243.

Effects on the liver. A mixed hepatocellular-cholestatic liver enzyme pattern has been reported in a patient after about 3 weeks of treatment with trazodone in doses of up to 500 mg

daily.[1] The enzyme abnormalities returned to normal 4 weeks after trazodone was discontinued but it was suggested that liver enzyme values should be monitored during the first 4 weeks of therapy. A similar case apparently presenting as obstructive jaundice and hepatocellular inflammation, in which the patient had only been receiving 50 mg daily for 2 weeks, has also been described.[2] It was believed that the patient suffered an idiosyncratic drug reaction to trazodone. Further reports of trazodone-induced liver injury include an elderly patient who developed chronic active hepatitis after receiving trazodone 150 mg daily for approximately 8 months.[3] A case of fatal hepatic necrosis reported in another elderly patient was considered to be due to treatment with trazodone and antipsychotics.[4] The authors of the report[4] noted that up to August 1991 the UK Committee on Safety of Medicines had received 14 reports of adverse effects on the liver associated with trazodone including one episode of fatal hepatic necrosis.

1. Chu AG, *et al.* Trazodone and liver toxicity. *Ann Intern Med* 1983; **99:** 128–9.
2. Sheikh KH, Nies AS. Trazodone and intrahepatic cholestasis. *Ann Intern Med* 1983; **99:** 572.
3. Beck PL, *et al.* Chronic active hepatitis associated with trazodone therapy. *Ann Intern Med* 1993; **118:** 791–2.
4. Hull M, *et al.* Fatal hepatic necrosis associated with trazodone and neuroleptic drugs. *BMJ* 1994; **309:** 378.

Effects on mental state. There have been reports of mania,[1,2] and paranoid psychosis with hallucinations[3] associated with the use of trazodone in depressed patients; delirium[4] in patients with bulimia nervosa; and possible psychosis or hypomania[5] in a patient receiving trazodone-tryptophan treatment of aggression.

1. Warren M, Bick PA. Two case reports of trazodone-induced mania. *Am J Psychiatry* 1984; **141:** 1103–4.
2. Arana GW, Kaplan GB. Trazodone-induced mania following desipramine-induced mania in major depressive disorders. *Am J Psychiatry* 1985; **142:** 386.
3. Kraft TB. Psychosis following trazodone administration. *Am J Psychiatry* 1983; **140:** 1383–4.
4. Damlouji NF, Ferguson JM. Trazodone-induced delirium in bulimic patients. *Am J Psychiatry* 1984; **141:** 434–5.
5. Patterson BD, Srisopark MM. Severe anorexia and possible psychosis or hypomania after trazodone-tryptophan treatment of aggression. *Lancet* 1989; **i:** 1017.

Effects on sexual function. Trazodone is notable for the number of reports of priapism associated with its use.[1,2] In most cases, priapism occurred during treatment with standard doses after 1 to 3 weeks of therapy. Several patients required surgery and recovery was not always complete.[1] A review[3] of priapism induced by psychotropic drugs proposed that the effect was related to blockade of alpha-adrenoceptors in the absence of sufficient antimuscarinic activity, criteria which the pharmacological profile of trazodone fulfills.

Trazodone has been tried in the treatment of impotence (see Sexual Dysfunction in Uses, below).

Inhibition of ejaculation has also been reported in one man[4] and an increase in libido in women[5] and men.[6] There has also been a report of trazodone-associated priapism of the clitoris.[7]

1. Committee on Safety of Medicines. Priapism and trazodone (Molipaxin). *Current Problems 13* 1984.
2. Anonymous. Priapism with trazodone (Desyrel). *Med Lett Drugs Ther* 1984; **26:** 35.
3. Patel AG, *et al.* Priapism associated with psychotropic drugs. *Br J Hosp Med* 1996; **55:** 315–19.
4. Jones SD. Ejaculatory inhibition with trazodone. *J Clin Psychopharmacol* 1984; **4:** 279–81.
5. Gartrell N. Increased libido in women receiving trazodone. *Am J Psychiatry* 1986; **143:** 781–2.
6. Sullivan G. Increased libido in three men treated with trazodone. *J Clin Psychiatry* 1988; **49:** 202–3.
7. Pescatori ES, *et al.* Priapism of the clitoris: a case report following trazodone use. *J Urol (Baltimore)* 1993; **149:** 1557–9.

Effects on the skin. Individual reports of adverse dermatological reactions to trazodone have included leucocytoclastic vasculitis,[1] erythema multiforme,[2] and exacerbation of psoriasis.[3]

1. Mann SC, *et al.* Leukocytoclastic vasculitis secondary to trazodone treatment. *J Am Acad Dermatol* 1984; **10:** 699–70.
2. Ford HE, Jenike MA. Erythema multiforme associated with trazodone therapy: case report. *J Clin Psychiatry* 1985; **46:** 294–5.
3. Barth JH, Baker H. Generalized pustular psoriasis precipitated by trazodone in the treatment of depression. *Br J Dermatol* 1986; **115:** 629–30.

Epileptogenic effect. Tonic-clonic seizures related to trazodone therapy have been reported in 2 patients[1,2] with no previous history of seizure disorders.

1. Bowdan ND. Seizure possibly caused by trazodone hydrochloride. *Am J Psychiatry* 1983; **140:** 642.
2. Lefkowitz D, *et al.* Seizures and trazodone therapy. *Arch Gen Psychiatry* 1985; **42:** 523.

Overdosage. Reviews have indicated that the incidence of serious toxicity from trazodone overdose alone was low compared with tricyclic antidepressant overdose.[1-4]

In one review covering 149 overdose cases,[1] only 10 deaths had been reported and in only one case was trazodone the sole agent reported to be ingested; in this case autopsy revealed an acute myocardial infarction after the patient was stable. The remaining 9 patients also had histories of ingestion of unknown quantities of alcohol, benzodiazepines, or other sedative-hypnotics that may have contributed to their demise. In the surviving 139 patients, 2 cases of respiratory arrest, one case of priapism, one occurrence of seizure, 2 cases of right bundle branch block, one

case of atrioventricular block, and one T-wave inversion were reported. The remaining patients had minor CNS-depressant effects.

In the second review[2] no fatalities occurred in 39 of 88 cases of overdosage where trazodone alone was ingested. However 9 deaths occurred in the remaining 49 cases where trazodone was ingested with other drugs or alcohol.

For a discussion of choice of antidepressant with respect to safety in overdosage, see under Depression, p.271.

1. Hassan E, Miller DD. Toxicity and elimination of trazodone after overdose. *Clin Pharm* 1985; **4:** 97–100.
2. Gamble DE, Peterson LG. Trazodone overdose: four years of experience from voluntary reports. *J Clin Psychiatry* 1986; **47:** 544–6.
3. Crome P, Ali C. Clinical features and management of self-poisoning with newer antidepressants. *Med Toxicol* 1986; **1:** 411–20.
4. Gallant DM. Antidepressant overdose: symptoms and treatment. *Psychopathology* 1987; **20** (suppl 1): 75–81.

Precautions

Trazodone should be used with caution in patients with cardiovascular disorders, such as ischaemic heart disease and its use is not recommended in the immediate recovery phase after myocardial infarction. Similarly, it should be used with caution in patients with epilepsy and severe hepatic or renal insufficiency. Trazodone should be discontinued immediately if patients develop signs of hepatic dysfunction or blood dyscrasias. Patients developing inappropriate or prolonged penile erections should discontinue trazodone immediately.

Patients should be closely monitored during early antidepressant therapy until improvement in depression is observed because suicide is an inherent risk in depressed patients. For further details, see under Depression, p.271.

Drowsiness is often experienced at the start of trazodone antidepressant therapy and patients, if affected, should not drive or operate machinery.

As with other antidepressants, trazodone therapy should be withdrawn gradually.

Breast feeding. In a study of 6 lactating women each given a single 50-mg dose of trazodone, it was concluded that exposure of babies to trazodone via breast milk is very small.[1] However, trazodone has been reported to form an active metabolite and it was not known to what extent this metabolite distributed into breast milk.

1. Verbeeck RK, *et al.* Excretion of trazodone in breast milk. *Br J Clin Pharmacol* 1986; **22:** 367–70.

Porphyria. Trazodone hydrochloride is considered to be unsafe in patients with porphyria because it has been shown to be porphyrinogenic in *animals*.

Interactions

Trazodone should not be given to patients receiving MAOIs or for at least 14 days after their discontinuation. It has also been recommended that any drug liable to provoke a serious reaction (e.g. phenelzine) should not be given within one week after the discontinuation of trazodone therapy. For further details, see Antidepressants under Interactions of Phenelzine, p.306.

It is considered unlikely that trazodone will alter the effects of antihypertensives such as guanethidine; some interaction may, however, occur with clonidine. The dose of other antihypertensives may need to be reduced if administered concomitantly with trazodone.

The sedative effects of trazodone may be enhanced by concurrent administration with alcohol or other CNS depressants. The potential for interaction between trazodone and general anaesthetics exists and some manufacturers recommend that trazodone should be stopped before elective surgery for as long as clinically feasible.

Trazodone may increase plasma concentrations of digoxin and some manufacturers recommend monitoring concentrations if used concurrently with trazodone.

Anticoagulants. For the effect of trazodone on *warfarin*, see p.995.

Antiepileptics. Antidepressants may antagonise the activity of antiepileptics by lowering the convulsive threshold.

Trazodone may increase plasma concentrations of *carbamazepine* (see p.344) and *phenytoin* (see p.360). Some manufacturers recommend monitoring concentrations of phenytoin if used with trazodone.

Pharmacokinetics

Trazodone is readily absorbed from the gastrointestinal tract although absorption is affected by food. When trazodone is taken shortly after a meal there may be an increase in the amount absorbed, a decrease in the maximum concentration, and a lengthening in the time to maximum concentration compared with the fasting state; peak plasma concentrations occur about one hour after administration when taken on an empty stomach and after about 2 hours when taken with food. Protein binding is reported to be about 89 to 95%.

Trazodone is extensively metabolised in the liver and paths of metabolism include *N*-oxidation and hydroxylation. The metabolite *m*-chlorophenylpiperazine is active in *animals*. Trazodone is excreted predominantly in the urine almost entirely in the form of its metabolites, either in free or in conjugated form: some is excreted in the faeces via biliary elimination. The elimination of trazodone from the plasma is biphasic, with a terminal elimination half-life of 5 to 9 hours.

Small amounts of trazodone are distributed into breast milk (see under Breast Feeding in Precautions, above).

◊ References.
1. Bayer AJ, *et al.* Pharmacokinetic and pharmacodynamic characteristics of trazodone in the elderly. *Br J Clin Pharmacol* 1983; **16**: 371–6.

Uses and Administration

Trazodone is a triazolopyridine antidepressant chemically unrelated to other classes of antidepressants. It blocks the reuptake of serotonin at presynaptic neurones and also has an action at 5-HT$_1$ receptors. Unlike the tricyclic antidepressants, trazodone does not inhibit the peripheral reuptake of noradrenaline, although it may indirectly facilitate neuronal release. Trazodone blocks central α_1-adrenoceptors and appears to have no effect on the central reuptake of dopamine. It does not appear to have very significant antimuscarinic properties, but has a marked sedative action. Trazodone is used as the hydrochloride.

Trazodone hydrochloride is given by mouth for the treatment of **depression** in doses of 150 mg daily initially; total daily dosage may be increased by 50 mg every 3 or 4 days up to 300 to 400 mg daily if necessary. The daily dosage may be divided throughout the day after food or be given as a single dose at night. Divided daily dosages of up to 600 mg may be given in severe depression in hospitalised patients. A suggested initial dose in elderly and other susceptible patients is 100 mg daily, and total daily doses above 300 mg are unlikely to be needed in these patients.

In the treatment of **anxiety** (p.649), trazodone hydrochloride is given in an initial dose of 75 mg daily by mouth increasing to 300 mg daily if necessary.

As with other antidepressants, trazodone should be withdrawn gradually.

Depression. As discussed on p.271, there is very little difference in efficacy between the different groups of antidepressant drugs, and choice is often made on the basis of adverse effect profile. Trazodone has a different biochemical profile from both the tricyclics and the SSRIs.
References.
1. Weisler RH, *et al.* Comparison of bupropion and trazodone for the treatment of major depression. *J Clin Psychopharmacol* 1994; **14**: 170–9.

Disturbed behaviour. Trazodone has produced beneficial results[1-3] when tried in various disorders for the control of symptoms such as agitation, aggression, and disruptive behaviour (see p.650). Although adverse effects such as sedation and orthostatic hypotension can occur with trazodone and may be particularly problematical in the elderly, some[4] consider that, in the management of dementia, trazodone might be worth trying in nonpsychotic patients with disturbed behaviour, especially those with mild symptoms or those intolerant of or unresponsive to antipsychotics.
1. Pasion RC, Kirby SG. Trazodone for screaming. *Lancet* 1993; **341**: 970.

The symbol † denotes a preparation no longer actively marketed

2. Lebert F, *et al.* Behavioral effects of trazodone in Alzheimer's disease. *J Clin Psychiatry* 1994; **55**: 536–8.
3. Sultzer DL, *et al.* A double-blind comparison of trazodone and haloperidol for treatment of agitation in patients with dementia. *Am J Geriatr Psychiatry* 1997; **5**: 60–9.
4. American Psychiatric Association. Practice guideline for the treatment of patients with Alzheimer's disease and other dementias of late life. *Am J Psychiatry* 1997; **154** (suppl): 1–39.

Sexual dysfunction. Priapism can occur as an adverse effect of trazodone (see Effects on Sexual Function in Adverse Effects, above) and this has led to trials of oral trazodone for the treatment of erectile dysfunction (p.1663). Positive responses have been reported, either in conjunction with yohimbine[1] or alone.[2] However, this has not been borne out by controlled studies.[3]
1. Montorsi F, *et al.* Effect of yohimbine-trazodone on psychogenic impotence: a randomized, double-blind, placebo-controlled study. *Urology* 1994; **44**: 732–6.
2. Lance R, *et al.* Oral trazodone as empirical therapy for erectile dysfunction: a retrospective review. *Urology* 1995; **46**: 117–20.
3. Costabile RA, Spevak M, Oral trazodone is not effective therapy for erectile dysfunction: a double-blind, placebo controlled trial. *J Urol (Baltimore)* 1999; **161**: 1819–22.

Substance dependence. The antidepressant and anxiolytic properties of trazodone have been reported to have been useful when tried in patients experiencing withdrawal syndromes from cocaine (p.1310)[1] or benzodiazepines (p.675).[2]
1. Small GW, Purcell JJ. Trazodone and cocaine abuse. *Arch Gen Psychiatry* 1985; **42**: 524.
2. Ansseau M, De Roeck J. Trazodone in benzodiazepine dependence. *J Clin Psychiatry* 1993; **54**: 189–91.

Preparations

USP 25: Trazodone Hydrochloride Tablets.

Proprietary Preparations (details are given in Part 3)
Aust.: Trittico; *Belg.:* Trazolan; *Canad.:* Desyrel; *Trazorel; Fin.:* Azona; *Ger.:* Thombran; *Hong Kong:* Trittico; *Irl.:* Molipaxin; *Israel:* Depyrel; Trazodil; *Ital.:* Trittico; *Mex.:* Sideril; *Neth.:* Trazolan; *Port.:* Trazone; Triticum; *S.Afr.:* Molipaxin; *Spain:* Deprax; *Switz.:* Trittico; *Thai.:* Desirel; *UK:* Molipaxin; *USA:* Desyrel.

Trimipramine   (2538-a)

Trimipramine *(BAN, USAN, rINN)*.

IL-6001; 7162-RP; Trimeprimine. Dimethyl{3-(10,11-dihydro-5*H*-dibenz[*b,f*]azepin-5-yl-2-methyl)propyl}amine.
$C_{20}H_{26}N_2 = 294.4$.
CAS — 739-71-9.
ATC — N06AA06.

Trimipramine Maleate   (2539-t)

Trimipramine Maleate *(BANM, USAN, rINNM)*.

Trimipramine Hydrogen Maleate; Trimipramini Maleas.
$C_{20}H_{26}N_2,C_4H_4O_4 = 410.5$.
CAS — 521-78-8.
Pharmacopoeias. In *Eur.* (see p.vi).

Trimipramine maleate 34.9 mg is approximately equivalent to 25 mg of trimipramine.

Pharmacopoeial description
Ph. Eur.: A white or almost white crystalline powder. Slightly soluble in water and in alcohol; practically insoluble in ether. Protect from light.

Adverse Effects, Treatment, and Precautions

As for tricyclic antidepressants in general (see Amitriptyline, p.273).

Porphyria. Trimipramine is considered to be unsafe in patients with porphyria although there is conflicting experimental evidence of porphyrinogenicity.

Interactions

For interactions associated with tricyclic antidepressants, see Amitriptyline, p.276.

Pharmacokinetics

Trimipramine is readily absorbed after oral administration, peak plasma concentrations being obtained in 2 hours. It is metabolised in the liver to its major metabolite desmethyltrimipramine, which is active. Trimipramine is excreted in the urine mainly in the form of its metabolites. It is extensively bound to plasma proteins. The plasma elimination half-life is reported to be about 23 hours.

◊ References.
1. Abernethy DR, *et al.* Trimipramine kinetics and absolute bioavailability: use of gas-liquid chromatography with nitrogen-phosphorus detection. *Clin Pharmacol Ther* 1984; **35**: 348–53.
2. Maurer H. Metabolism of trimipramine in man. *Arzneimittelforschung* 1989; **39**: 101–3.
3. Musa MN. Nonlinear kinetics of trimipramine in depressed patients. *J Clin Pharmacol* 1989; **29**: 746–7.

Uses and Administration

Trimipramine is a dibenzazepine tricyclic antidepressant with actions and uses similar to those of amitriptyline (p.278). It has marked antimuscarinic and sedative properties.

In the treatment of depression, trimipramine is given by mouth as the maleate in usual initial doses equivalent to 50 to 75 mg of trimipramine daily, gradually increased as necessary to 150 to 300 mg daily. The recommended initial dose for the elderly in the UK is 30 to 75 mg daily, gradually increased as necessary. In the USA, the elderly and adolescents may be given 50 mg daily initially followed by gradual increments as necessary up to a maximum of 100 mg daily. Trimipramine may be given in divided doses during the day, but since it has a prolonged half-life, once-daily dosage regimens are also suitable, usually given at night.

Trimipramine has also been given orally as the hydrochloride and intramuscularly as the mesilate.

Trimipramine should be withdrawn gradually to reduce the risk of withdrawal symptoms.

Preparations

BP 2001: Trimipramine Tablets.

Proprietary Preparations (details are given in Part 3)
Aust.: Stangyl; *Austral.:* Surmontil; *Belg.:* Surmontil; *Canad.:* Apo-Trimip; Novo-Tripramine; Rhotrimine; Surmontil; *Denm.:* Surmontil; *Fin.:* Surmontil; *Fr.:* Surmontil; *Ger.:* Herphonal; Stangyl; *Hong Kong:* Apo-Trimip; Surmontil; *Irl.:* Surmontil; *Israel:* Surmontil; *Ital.:* Surmontil; *Neth.:* Surmontil; *Norw.:* Surmontil; *NZ:* Surmontil; Tripress; *Port.:* Surmontil; *S.Afr.:* Surmontil; Tydamine; *Spain:* Surmontil; *Swed.:* Surmontil; *Switz.:* Surmontil; *UK:* Surmontil; *USA:* Surmontil.

Tryptophan   (664-p)

Tryptophan *(USAN, rINN)*.

L-Tryptophan; Tryptophanum; W. L-2-Amino-3-(indol-3-yl)propionic acid.
$C_{11}H_{12}N_2O_2 = 204.2$.
CAS — 73-22-3.
ATC — N06AX02.
Pharmacopoeias. In *Eur.* (see p.vi), *Jpn*, and *US.*
Fr. also includes DL-Tryptophan.

Pharmacopoeial description
Ph. Eur.: A white or almost white crystalline or amorphous powder. Sparingly soluble in water; slightly soluble in alcohol; practically insoluble in ether; dissolves in dilute mineral acids and in dilute solutions of alkali hydroxides. Protect from light.
USP 25: White to slightly yellowish-white crystals or crystalline powder. Soluble in hot alcohol and in dilute hydrochloric acid. pH of a 1% solution in water is between 5.5 and 7.0.

Adverse Effects
Tryptophan-containing products have been associated with the eosinophilia-myalgia syndrome; for further details, see below. Other side-effects that have been reported include nausea, headache, lightheadedness, and drowsiness.

An increased incidence of bladder tumours has been reported in *mice* given L-tryptophan orally as well as in cholesterol pellets embedded in the bladder lumen.

Eosinophilia-myalgia syndrome. In late 1989 the first notification linking the eosinophilia-myalgia syndrome with the use of tryptophan-containing products was made in the USA.[1] There followed a number of similar published case reports from the USA, Europe, and Japan. Reviews of tryptophan-associated eosinophilia-myalgia syndrome have noted that by early 1990 over 1500 cases were known in the USA.[2,3] In early 1990 the Centers for Disease Control in the USA summarised the features and known reports concerning the syndrome.[4] As the name implies the characteristic features are an intense eosinophilia together with disabling fatigue and muscle pain, although multisystem organ involvement and inflammatory disorders affecting the joints, skin, connective tissue, lungs, heart, and liver have also been recorded. Symptoms have generally developed over several weeks and the syndrome has occurred in patients who had been receiving tryptophan for many years previously with no untoward effect. In most patients slow and gradual improvement in the degree of eosinophilia and other clinical manifestations has followed the withdrawal of tryptophan, but in some patients the disease has progressed despite withdrawal and there have been fatalities.[5-7] The inflammatory condition has necessitated the use of corticosteroids in some patients.

The eosinophilia-myalgia syndrome has been reported in patients taking both tryptophan-containing prescription products for depression and non-prescription dietary supplements for a number of disorders including insomnia, the premenstrual syndrome, and stress; it does not appear to have occurred in patients receiving amino-acid preparations containing tryptophan as part of total parenteral nutrition regimens. The recognition of this syndrome led to the withdrawal of tryptophan-containing products or severe restrictions being imposed upon their use in many countries during 1990.

Various theories were proposed as to the reason for the association of tryptophan with this syndrome. Confusion existed because the reports implicated a very wide range of products from different manufacturers. More recent evidence, however, appears to have confirmed that contaminated tryptophan has originated from a single manufacturer in Japan.[8-10] Bulk tryptophan is imported from Japan for manufacture into finished pharmaceutical dosage forms and it was noted in one of these reports[9] that a single product was often found to contain two or more lots of powdered tryptophan that were blended together during the production of tablets or capsules. Many trace contaminants have been found in batches of tryptophan associated with the syndrome.[11] One contaminant has been identified as 1,1'-ethylidenebis(tryptophan).[12] Its inclusion in bulk tryptophan powder appeared to coincide with alterations in the manufacturing conditions that involved a change in the strain of *Bacillus amyloliquefaciens* used in the fermentation process and a reduction in the amount of charcoal used for purification.[9] Other investigations indicated the presence of bacitracin-like peptides in batches of the contaminated tryptophan.[13] However, further work[14] has provided only weak support for an association between the syndrome and any one particular contaminant and the causative agent remains to be confirmed. Nonetheless, since the syndrome only appeared to be associated with tryptophan from one manufacturer, tryptophan preparations were reintroduced in the UK in 1994 for restricted use under carefully monitored conditions.[15]

1. Anonymous. Eosinophilia-myalgia syndrome—New Mexico. *MMWR* 1989; **38:** 765–7.
2. Troy JL. Eosinophilia-myalgia syndrome. *Mayo Clin Proc* 1991; **66:** 535–8.
3. Milburn DS, Myers CW. Tryptophan toxicity: a pharmacoepidemiologic review of eosinophilia-myalgia syndrome. *DICP Ann Pharmacother* 1991; **25:** 1259–62.
4. Kilbourne EM, *et al.* Interim guidance on the eosinophilia-myalgia syndrome. *Ann Intern Med* 1990; **112:** 85–6.
5. Anonymous. Eosinophilia-myalgia syndrome associated with ingestion of L-tryptophan—United States, through August 24, 1990. *JAMA* 1990; **264:** 1655.
6. Kaufman LD, *et al.* Clinical follow-up and immunogenetic studies of 32 patients with eosinophilia-myalgia syndrome. *Lancet* 1991; **337:** 1071–4.
7. Hertzman PA, *et al.* The eosinophilia-myalgia syndrome: status of 205 patients and results of treatment 2 years after onset. *Ann Intern Med* 1995; **122:** 851–5.
8. Slutsker L, *et al.* Eosinophilia-myalgia syndrome associated with exposure to tryptophan from a single manufacturer. *JAMA* 1990; **264:** 213–17.
9. Belongia EA, *et al.* An investigation of the cause of the eosinophilia-myalgia syndrome associated with tryptophan use. *N Engl J Med* 1990; **323:** 357–65.
10. Varga J, *et al.* The cause and pathogenesis of the eosinophilia-myalgia syndrome. *Ann Intern Med* 1992; **116:** 140–7.
11. Hill RH, *et al.* Contaminants in L-tryptophan associated with eosinophilia myalgia syndrome. *Arch Environ Contam Toxicol* 1993; **25:** 134–42.
12. Mayeno AN, *et al.* Characterization of "peak E", a novel amino acid associated with eosinophilia-myalgia syndrome. *Science* 1990; **250:** 1707–8.
13. Barnhart ER, *et al.* Bacitracin-associated peptides and contaminated L-tryptophan. *Lancet* 1990; **336:** 742.
14. Philen RM, *et al.* Tryptophan contaminants associated with eosinophilia-myalgia syndrome. *Am J Epidemiol* 1993; **138:** 154–9.
15. Committee on Safety of Medicines/Medicines Control Agency. L-Tryptophan (Optimax): limited availability for resistant depression. *Current Problems* 1994; **20:** 2.

Precautions

Tryptophan has been associated with eosinophilia-myalgia syndrome and it is therefore recommended that patients receiving tryptophan should be closely monitored with particular care being paid to eosinophil counts, haematological changes, and muscle symptomatology.

Patients taking tryptophan may experience drowsiness and, if affected, they should not drive or operate machinery. For further details of the effects of antidepressant therapy on driving see under Amitriptyline, p.276.

Abnormal metabolism of tryptophan may occur in patients with pyridoxine deficiency and tryptophan is thus sometimes given with pyridoxine supplements.

Interactions

Although tryptophan has been given as additional therapy to patients receiving MAOIs in the belief that clinical efficacy may be improved, it should be noted that the adverse effects of either drug may also be potentiated. For further details, see Antidepressants under Interactions of Phenelzine, p.306.

Use of tryptophan with drugs that inhibit the reuptake of serotonin may exacerbate the adverse effects of the latter and precipitate the serotonin syndrome (p.304).

There have been occasional reports of sexual disinhibition in patients taking tryptophan in conjunction with phenothiazines or benzodiazepines.

For a report of tryptophan reducing blood concentrations of levodopa, see Nutritional Agents under Interactions for Levodopa, p.1172.

Pharmacokinetics

Tryptophan is readily absorbed from the gastrointestinal tract. Tryptophan is extensively bound to plasma albumin. It is metabolised in the liver by tryptophan pyrrolase. Metabolites include hydroxytryptophan, which is then converted to serotonin,

and kynurenine derivatives. Some tryptophan is converted to nicotinic acid and nicotinamide. Pyridoxine and ascorbic acid are cofactors in the decarboxylation and hydroxylation respectively of tryptophan; pyridoxine apparently prevents the accumulation of the kynurenine metabolites.

◊ References.
1. Green AR, *et al.* The pharmacokinetics of L-tryptophan following its intravenous and oral administration. *Br J Clin Pharmacol* 1985; **20:** 317–21.

Uses and Administration

Tryptophan is an amino acid which is an essential constituent of the diet. Tryptophan and DL-tryptophan have been used as dietary supplements.

Tryptophan is a precursor of serotonin. Because CNS depletion of serotonin is considered to be involved in depression, tryptophan has been used in its treatment. Although it has been given alone, evidence of effectiveness is scant and tryptophan has generally been used as adjunctive therapy in depression. Pyridoxine and ascorbic acid are involved in the metabolism of tryptophan to serotonin (see Pharmacokinetics, above) and have sometimes been given concomitantly.

In many countries preparations containing tryptophan have either been withdrawn from the market or their availability severely restricted or limited because of its association with the eosinophilia-myalgia syndrome. In the UK tryptophan is restricted to use by hospital specialists only as an adjunct to other antidepressant medication for patients with severe and disabling depressive illness of more than 2 years' continuous duration who have failed to respond to an adequate trial of standard antidepressant drug treatment.

In the treatment of depression the usual dose of tryptophan is 1 g given three times daily, but some patients may require up to 6 g daily in divided doses. Lower doses may be required in the elderly especially those with renal or hepatic impairment.

Depression. Tryptophan has only weak antidepressant properties itself but it has been used in combination with other antidepressants in the belief that it would potentiate their effects. Although beneficial effects have been reported in some patients given tryptophan with tricyclic antidepressants or MAOIs, alone or with lithium, evidence of efficacy is mainly limited to case reports and small controlled studies.[1,2]

Since the publication of reports linking the use of tryptophan with the eosinophilia-myalgia syndrome (see under Adverse Effects, above) preparations containing tryptophan for depression have either been withdrawn from the market or their use severely restricted as in the UK[3] and many other countries. For details of UK restrictions see Uses and Administration, above. For a discussion of the treatment of depression, see p.271.

1. Barker WA, *et al.* The Newcastle chronic depression study: results of a treatment regime. *Int Clin Psychopharmacol* 1987; **2:** 261–72.
2. Smith S. Tryptophan in the treatment of resistant depression—a review. *Pharm J* 1998; **261:** 819–21.
3. Committee on Safety of Medicines/Medicines Control Agency. L-Tryptophan (Optimax): limited availability for resistant depression. *Current Problems* 1994; **20:** 2.

Dietary supplementation. The use of tryptophan as a dietary supplement has been reviewed.[1] However, because of its association with the eosinophilia-myalgia syndrome (see under Adverse Effects, above), the addition of tryptophan to food intended for human consumption is prohibited in some countries.
1. Li Wan Po A, Maguire T. Tryptophan: useful dietary supplement or a health hazard? *Pharm J* 1990; **244:** 484–5.

Insomnia. Tryptophan, sometimes in the form of dietary supplements, has enjoyed some popularity for the treatment of insomnia (p.652). However, the point has been made that in comparison with other hypnotics such as the benzodiazepines, the effects of tryptophan have been more difficult to substantiate and enthusiasm for tryptophan has waned considerably amongst sleep researchers.[1] It should also be noted that since the publication of reports linking the use of tryptophan with the eosinophilia-myalgia syndrome (see under Adverse Effects, above) preparations indicated for insomnia have been withdrawn from the market in many countries.
1. Lahmeyer HW. Tryptophan for insomnia. *JAMA* 1989; **262:** 2748.

Preparations

Proprietary Preparations (details are given in Part 3)
Aust.: Kalma; *Canad.:* Tryptan; *Ger.:* Ardeytropin; Kalma; *UK:* Optimax.
Multi-ingredient: *Fr.:* Vita-Dermacide; *Irl.:* Optimax; *Spain:* Calcioretard; *USA:* PDP Liquid Protein.

Venlafaxine Hydrochloride (10487-d)

Venlafaxine Hydrochloride (BANM, USAN, rINNM).
Wy-45030. (RS)-1-(2-Dimethylamino-1-p-methoxyphenylethyl)cyclohexanol hydrochloride.
$C_{17}H_{27}NO_2,HCl = 313.9$.
CAS — 93413-69-5 (venlafaxine); 99300-78-4 (venlafaxine hydrochloride).

Venlafaxine hydrochloride 28.3 mg is approximately equivalent to 25 mg of venlafaxine.

Adverse Effects and Treatment

Adverse effects that have been reported most frequently with venlafaxine include nausea, headache, insomnia, somnolence, dry mouth, dizziness, constipation, sexual dysfunction, asthenia, sweating, and nervousness. Other adverse effects have included anorexia, dyspepsia, abdominal pain, anxiety, urinary frequency, visual disturbances, vasodilatation, vomiting, tremor, paraesthesia, chills, palpitations, weight gain, increased serum cholesterol, agitation, and skin rashes. Convulsions have also been reported. Reversible increases in liver enzymes have also been noted. Orthostatic hypotension has been noted occasionally. Dose-related increases in blood pressure have been observed in some patients. There are occasional reports of ecchymosis or bleeding disorders. Activation of mania or hypomania has occasionally been reported.

Hyponatraemia possibly due to inappropriate secretion of antidiuretic hormone has been associated with the use of antidepressants, particularly in the elderly.

In overdosage, the symptoms that have been reported include lethargy, somnolence, ECG changes, cardiac arrhythmias, and seizures. Treatment of overdosage includes consideration of the use of activated charcoal or gastric lavage followed by symptomatic and supportive therapy. Dialysis, haemoperfusion, exchange perfusion, and measures to increase urine production are considered unlikely to be of benefit.

Effects on the liver. Acute hepatitis developed in a 44-year-old woman approximately 6 months after starting venlafaxine;[1] she recovered once venlafaxine was withdrawn. In another report,[2] acute hepatitis developed in a 78-year-old man about a month after venlafaxine was added to therapy. Again, symptoms resolved when the drug was discontinued.

For a report of hepatotoxicity in patients taking venlafaxine subsequent to an attempted overdose with sertraline, see p.285.
1. Horsmans Y, *et al.* Venlaxafine-associated [sic] hepatitis. *Ann Intern Med* 1999; **130:** 944.
2. Cardona X, *et al.* Venlafaxine-associated hepatitis. *Ann Intern Med* 2000; **132:** 417.

Neuroleptic malignant syndrome. For mention of neuroleptic malignant syndrome developing when venlafaxine was added to treatment with antipsychotics see under Interactions in Chlorpromazine, p.664.

Overdosage. Although the newer antidepressants such as venlafaxine are said to be safer in overdose than the tricyclic antidepressants, rare serious events including seizures and ECG changes[1-3] have occurred. In some cases, death has ensued.[4]
1. White CM, *et al.* Seizure resulting from a venlafaxine overdose. *Ann Pharmacother* 1997; **31:** 178–80.
2. Coorey AN, Wenck DJ. Venlafaxine overdose. *Med J Aust* 1998; **168:** 523.
3. Blythe D, Hackett LP. Cardiovascular and neurological toxicity of venlafaxine. *Hum Exp Toxicol* 1999; **18:** 309–13.
4. Banham NDG. Fatal venlafaxine overdose. *Med J Aust* 1998; **169:** 445, 448.

Precautions

Venlafaxine should be used with caution in patients with moderate to severe hepatic or renal impairment and dosage adjustment may be necessary. Caution is also advised in those with a history of myocardial infarction or unstable heart disease, or whose condition might be exacerbated by an increase in heart rate. Blood pressure monitoring may be advisable. Venlafaxine should also be used with caution in patients with a history of epilepsy and should be discontinued in any patient developing a seizure. It should also be used cautiously in patients with a history of hypomania or mania. Patients with raised intra-ocular pressure or at risk of angle-closure glaucoma should be monitored closely. Patients who develop a rash, urticaria, or related allergic reaction with venlafaxine should be advised to contact their doctor.

Patients should be closely monitored during early antidepressant therapy until improvement in depression is observed because suicide is an inherent risk in depressed patients. For further details, see under Depression, p.271.

As with other antidepressants, venlafaxine may impair performance of skilled tasks and, if affected, patients should not drive or operate machinery. Patients, especially the elderly, should be warned of the risk of dizziness or unsteadiness due to orthostatic hypotension.

Symptoms reported on abrupt discontinuation or dose reduction of venlafaxine therapy include fatigue, headache, nausea, vomiting, dizziness, dry mouth, diarrhoea, insomnia, nervousness, confusion, paraesthesia, sweating, and vertigo. It is therefore recommended that venlafaxine should be withdrawn gradually over at least one week after more than one week's therapy and the patient monitored to minimise the risk of withdrawal reactions.

Withdrawal. Case reports[1,2] of withdrawal reactions to venlafaxine.

1. Anonymous. Venlafaxine withdrawal reactions. *Med J Aust* 1998; **169:** 91–2.
2. Johnson H, et al. Withdrawal reaction associated with venlafaxine. *BMJ* 1998; **317:** 787.

Interactions
Venlafaxine should not be used concomitantly with MAOIs and at least 14 days should elapse between discontinuation of an MAOI and starting treatment with venlafaxine. At least 7 days should elapse between stopping venlafaxine and starting any drug liable to provoke a serious reaction (e.g. phenelzine). For further details, see Antidepressants under Interactions of Phenelzine, p.306.

Cimetidine inhibits the hepatic metabolism of venlafaxine but not its active metabolite *O*-desmethylvenlafaxine, which is present in the plasma in much greater concentrations. The manufacturer, therefore, recommends that when cimetidine and venlafaxine are used together clinical monitoring may only be necessary in elderly patients and in those with hepatic impairment or pre-existing hypertension.

◊ Conversion of venlafaxine to its equally active metabolite *O*-desmethylvenlafaxine is mediated by the cytochrome P450 isoenzyme CYP2D6. Although the potential exists for drugs which inhibit or act as a substrate for this enzyme to affect plasma concentrations of venlafaxine and its active metabolite the manufacturers consider that as the total amount of active compounds is not affected no dosage adjustment is usually necessary for venlafaxine. Venlafaxine itself is considered to be a relatively weak inhibitor of CYP2D6.

Antipsychotics. For mention of neuroleptic malignant syndrome developing in patients who received venlafaxine concomitantly with antipsychotics see under Interactions in Chlorpromazine, p.664.

Selegiline. Although it is generally recommended that venlafaxine should not be started for at least 14 days after discontinuation of an MAOI, there is a report[1] of serotonin syndrome developing when a patient began venlafaxine treatment 15 days after stopping selegiline, which is an MAO type B inhibitor.

1. Gitlin MJ. Venlafaxine, monoamine oxidase inhibitors, and the serotonin syndrome. *J Clin Psychopharmacol* 1997; **17:** 66–7.

Pharmacokinetics
Venlafaxine is readily absorbed from the gastrointestinal tract. Following oral administration it undergoes extensive first-pass metabolism in the liver mainly to the active metabolite *O*-desmethylvenlafaxine; formation of *O*-desmethylvenlafaxine is mediated by the cytochrome P450 isoenzyme CYP2D6. Other metabolites include *N*-desmethylvenlafaxine and *N,O*-didesmethylvenlafaxine. Peak plasma concentrations of venlafaxine and *O*-desmethylvenlafaxine appear about 2 and 4 hours after administration, respectively. Protein binding of venlafaxine and *O*-desmethylvenlafaxine is low. The mean elimination half-life of venlafaxine and *O*-desmethylvenlafaxine is about 5 and 11 hours, respectively. Venlafaxine is excreted predominately in the urine, mainly in the form of its metabolites, either free or in conjugated form; about 2% is excreted in the faeces.

◊ References.
1. Troy SM, et al. The pharmacokinetics of venlafaxine when given in a twice-daily regimen. *J Clin Pharmacol* 1995; **35:** 404–9.
2. Troy SM, et al. Pharmacokinetics and effect of food on the bioavailability of orally administered venlafaxine. *J Clin Pharmacol* 1997; **37:** 954–61.
3. Ball SE, et al. Venlafaxine: in vitro inhibition of CYP2D6 dependent imipramine and desipramine metabolism; comparative studies with selected SSRIs, and effects on human hepatic CYP3A4, CYP2C9 and CYP1A2. *Br J Clin Pharmacol* 1997; **43:** 619–26.

Distribution into breast milk. In one study[1] both venlafaxine and its metabolite *O*-desmethylvenlafaxine were detected

in breast milk in significant quantities and there were measurable concentrations of desmethylvenlafaxine in the infants' plasma.

1. Ilett KF, et al. Distribution and excretion of venlafaxine and O-desmethylvenlafaxine in human milk. *Br J Clin Pharmacol* 1998; **45:** 459–62.

Renal impairment. The mean terminal disposition half-life of venlafaxine was prolonged from a mean of 3.8 hours in 18 healthy subjects to 5.8 hours in 12 patients with mild to moderate renal impairment (creatinine clearance 10 to 70 mL per minute) and 10.6 hours in patients requiring haemodialysis;[1] corresponding values for *O*-desmethylvenlafaxine, the active major metabolite of venlafaxine, were 11.8, 16.8, and 28.5 hours, respectively. Because of the large intersubject variability the change in disposition for venlafaxine and its active metabolite was evident only in patients with a creatinine clearance of less than 30 mL per minute; drug clearance in these patients was reduced by about 55% and half-life more than doubled. It was calculated that for these patients half the usually daily dose could be given once daily.

1. Troy SM, et al. The effect of renal disease on the disposition of venlafaxine. *Clin Pharmacol Ther* 1994; **56:** 14–21.

Uses and Administration
Venlafaxine, a phenylethylamine derivative, is a serotonin and noradrenaline reuptake inhibitor (SNRI); it also weakly inhibits dopamine reuptake. It is reported to have little affinity for muscarinic, histaminergic, or α_1-adrenergic receptors *in vitro*.

Venlafaxine is used in the treatment of **depression**. It is given by mouth as the hydrochloride; doses are expressed in terms of venlafaxine. The initial daily dose is 75 mg in two or three divided doses with food, which may be increased, if necessary, after several weeks to 150 mg daily. Some countries permit further increases to a maximum daily dose of 225 mg; increases should be made at intervals of not less than 4 days. Severely depressed or hospitalised patients may require an initial daily dose of 150 mg increased, if necessary, by up to 75 mg every 2 to 3 days to a maximum daily dose of 375 mg; the dosage should then be gradually reduced. Modified-release preparations are available for once daily dosing.

Venlafaxine is also used, as a modified-release preparation, in the treatment of **generalised anxiety disorder**. The recommended initial dose is 75 mg once daily by mouth. In the USA it is suggested that some patients may be best begun with 37.5 mg daily for 4 to 7 days initially; dosage may subsequently be adjusted, at intervals of at least 4 days, up to a maximum of 225 mg daily. Venlafaxine should be withdrawn gradually if there is no response after 8 weeks.

Patients with renal or hepatic impairment may require a reduced dose. It has been suggested that for patients with moderate renal or hepatic impairment, the dose should be reduced by half and given once daily.

Venlafaxine should be withdrawn gradually to reduce the risk of withdrawal symptoms.

◊ Reviews.
1. Montgomery SA. Venlafaxine: a new dimension in antidepressant pharmacotherapy. *J Clin Psychiatry* 1993; **54:** 119–26.
2. Anonymous. Venlafaxine—a new antidepressant. *Med Lett Drugs Ther* 1994; **36:** 49–50.
3. Ellingrod VL, Perry PJ. Venlafaxine: a heterocyclic antidepressant. *Am J Hosp Pharm* 1994; **51:** 3033–46.
4. Holliday SM, Benfield P. Venlafaxine: a review of its pharmacology and therapeutic potential in depression. *Drugs* 1995; **49:** 280–94.
5. Morton WA, et al. Venlafaxine: a structurally unique and novel antidepressant. *Ann Pharmacother* 1995; **29:** 387–95.
6. Baldwin DS. Venlafaxine. *Prescribers' J* 1999; **39:** 242–7.

Anxiety disorders. Venlafaxine is used in the treatment of generalised anxiety disorder; it may be of use in a variety of other types of anxiety disorders including the treatment of obsessive-compulsive disorder (p.649), panic attacks (p.649), and social phobia (see under Phobic Disorders, p.649).

References.
1. Ananth J, et al. Venlafaxine for treatment of obsessive-compulsive disorder. *Am J Psychiatry* 1995; **152:** 1832.
2. Geracioti TD. Venlafaxine treatment of panic disorder: a case series. *J Clin Psychiatry* 1995; **56:** 408–10.
3. Rauch SL, et al. Open treatment of obsessive-compulsive disorder with venlafaxine: a series of ten cases. *J Clin Psychopharmacol* 1996; **16:** 81–4.
4. Pollack MH, et al. Venlafaxine for panic disorder: results from a double-blind, placebo-controlled study. *Psychopharmacol Bull* 1996; **32:** 667–70.
5. Altamura AC, et al. Venlafaxine in social phobia: a study in selective serotonin reuptake inhibitor non-responders. *Int Clin Psychopharmacol* 1999; **14:** 239–45.
6. Davidson JR, et al. Efficacy, safety, and tolerability of venlafaxine extended release and buspirone in outpatients with generalized anxiety disorder. *J Clin Psychiatry* 1999; **60:** 528–35.

Depression. As discussed on p.271, there is very little difference in efficacy between the different groups of antidepressant drugs, and choice is often made on the basis of adverse effect profile. SSRIs are widely used as an alternative to the older tricyclics as they have fewer unpleasant side-effects and are safer in overdosage. Similar properties also favour the use of serotonin and noradrenaline reuptake inhibitors such as venlafaxine.

References.
1. Schweizer E, et al. Placebo-controlled trial of venlafaxine for the treatment of major depression. *J Clin Psychopharmacol* 1991; **11:** 233–6.
2. Mendels J, et al. Efficacy and safety of b i d doses of venlafaxine in a dose-response study. *Psychopharmacol Bull* 1993; **29:** 169–74.
3. Schweizer E, et al. Comparison of venlafaxine and imipramine in the acute treatment of major depression in outpatients. *J Clin Psychiatry* 1994; **55:** 104–8.
4. Cunningham LA, et al. A comparison of venlafaxine, trazodone, and placebo in major depression. *J Clin Psychopharmacol* 1994; **14:** 99–106.
5. Shrivastava RK, et al. Long-term safety and clinical acceptability of venlafaxine and imipramine in outpatients with major depression. *J Clin Psychopharmacol* 1994; **14:** 322–9.
6. Derivan A, et al. Venlafaxine: measuring the onset of antidepressant action. *Psychopharmacol Bull* 1995; **31:** 439–47.
7. Anonymous. Three new antidepressants. *Drug Ther Bull* 1996; **34:** 65–8.

Hyperactivity. When drug therapy is indicated for attention deficit hyperactivity disorder (p.1505) initial treatment is usually with a central stimulant. Antidepressants may be used for patients who fail to respond to, or who are intolerant of, central stimulants and venlafaxine has been reported[1,2] to be effective in a small number of adult patients.

1. Hedges D, et al. An open trial of venlafaxine in adult patients with attention deficit hyperactivity disorder. *Psychopharmacol Bull* 1995; **31:** 779–83.
2. Adler LA, et al. Open-label trial of venlafaxine in adults with attention deficit disorder. *Psychopharmacol Bull* 1995; **31:** 785–8.

Pain. There are reports of benefit from the use of venlafaxine in patients with painful diabetic neuropathy,[1,2] or neuropathic pain of unknown cause.[3]

1. Davis JL, Smith RL. Painful peripheral diabetic neuropathy treated with venlafaxine HCl extended release capsules. *Diabetes Care* 1999; **22:** 1909–10.
2. Kiayias JA, et al. Venlafaxine HCl in the treatment of painful peripheral diabetic neuropathy. *Diabetes Care* 2000; **23:** 699.
3. Sumpton JE, Moulin DE. Treatment of neuropathic pain with venlafaxine. *Ann Pharmacother* 2001; **35:** 557–9.

Preparations
Proprietary Preparations (details are given in Part 3)
Aust.: Efectin; Efexor; Trewilor; *Austral.:* Efexor; *Belg.:* Efexor; *Canad.:* Effexor; *Denm.:* Efexor; *Fin.:* Efexor; *Fr.:* Effexor; *Ger.:* Trevilor; *Hong Kong:* Efexor; *Irl.:* Efexor; *Israel:* Efexor; *Ital.:* Efexor; *Mex.:* Efexor; *Neth.:* Efexor; *Norw.:* Efexor; *NZ:* Efexor; *Port.:* Efexor; *S.Afr.:* Efexor; *Singapore:* Efexor; *Spain:* Dobupal; Vandral; *Swed.:* Efexor; *Switz.:* Efexor; *UK:* Efexor; *USA:* Effexor.

Viloxazine Hydrochloride (2540-I)
Viloxazine Hydrochloride (BANM, USAN, rINNM).
ICI-58834. 2-(2-Ethoxyphenoxymethyl)morpholine hydrochloride.
$C_{13}H_{19}NO_3,HCl = 273.8$.
CAS — 46817-91-8 (viloxazine); 35604-67-2 (viloxazine hydrochloride).

Viloxazine hydrochloride 57.7 mg is approximately equivalent to 50 mg of viloxazine.

Adverse Effects
Nausea is commonly associated with viloxazine therapy, and vomiting and headache may also occur. Viloxazine has been associated with fewer antimuscarinic side-effects such as dry mouth, disturbance of accommodation, tachycardia, constipation, and difficulty with micturition than the tricyclic antidepressants. Exacerbation of anxiety, agitation, drowsiness, confusion, ataxia, dizziness, insomnia, tremor, paraesthesia, sweating, musculoskeletal pain, mild hypertension, skin rashes, convulsions, and jaundice with elevated aminotransferases have also been reported less frequently.

It has also been stated that cardiac arrhythmias and severe hypotension are less likely to occur with viloxazine than with tricyclic antidepressants in high doses or in overdosage.

Epileptogenic effect. In a review[1] of 6 cases of convulsive seizures during treatment with viloxazine notified to the UK Committee on Safety of Medicines, and 2 other cases from Japan, critical study of the patients' histories suggested a possible causal connection in only 2. It was concluded that even if viloxazine did possess convulsive properties like other antidepressants, it was probably less epileptogenic than conventional tricyclics and was not contra-indicated in epileptics.

1. Edwards JG, Glen-Bott M. Does viloxazine have epileptogenic properties? *J Neurol Neurosurg Psychiatry* 1984; **47:** 960–4.

Precautions
Although antimuscarinic and cardiotoxic effects may be less common than with tricyclic antidepressants, similar precautions may apply (see p.275). Viloxazine should be given with care to patients with hepatic or renal insufficiency, or cardiovascular disease. Caution is necessary in patients with epilepsy.

Patients should be carefully monitored during treatment until improvement in depression is observed, as suicide is an inherent risk in depressed patients. For further details, see under Depression, p.271.

Viloxazine is not recommended in patients who are breast feeding.

Viloxazine should be withdrawn gradually to reduce the risk of withdrawal symptoms such as malaise, headache, and vomiting.

Impaired alertness may be experienced with viloxazine antidepressant therapy and patients, if affected, should not drive or operate machinery. For further details of the effects of antidepressant therapy on driving see under Amitriptyline, p.276.

If surgery is required the anaesthetist should be informed that the patient has received viloxazine (see also Anaesthesia under Amitriptyline, p.275).

Migraine. Mention has been made that viloxazine may occasionally precipitate attacks in migrainous patients and in these circumstances should be discontinued.[1]

1. Nightingale S. Management of migraine. *Prescribers' J* 1985; **25:** 129–34.

Porphyria. Viloxazine hydrochloride is considered to be unsafe in patients with porphyria because it has been shown to be porphyrinogenic in *animals*.

Interactions

Viloxazine should not be given to patients receiving MAOIs or for at least 14 days after their discontinuation. It has also been recommended that any drug liable to provoke a serious reaction (e.g. phenelzine) should not be given within one week after discontinuation of viloxazine therapy. Viloxazine may diminish the effects of antihypertensives, such as guanethidine, debrisoquine, and betanidine; some interaction may also occur with clonidine and, in general, blood pressure should be monitored when viloxazine is prescribed with antihypertensive therapy. Interactions may occur with drugs that undergo hepatic metabolism increasing their plasma concentrations. The dosage of drugs such as phenytoin, carbamazepine, and theophylline may therefore need to be reduced, but it should also be noted that viloxazine has caused convulsions. Since viloxazine appears to have some influence on brain dopamine metabolism it should be given with caution to patients receiving levodopa. The CNS depressant action of alcohol may be enhanced by concurrent administration of viloxazine.

Pharmacokinetics

Viloxazine is readily absorbed from the gastrointestinal tract and extensively metabolised. The principal paths of metabolism of viloxazine include hydroxylation and conjugation. Viloxazine is excreted in the urine, mainly in the form of its metabolites, either free or in conjugated form.

Unlike the tricyclic antidepressants, viloxazine has a short plasma half-life of about 2 to 5 hours.

Viloxazine is distributed into breast milk.

Uses and Administration

Viloxazine is a bicyclic antidepressant. It does not have marked antimuscarinic or sedative properties. Like the tricyclic antidepressants (see Amitriptyline, p.273), viloxazine is an inhibitor of the reuptake of noradrenaline; it may also enhance the release of serotonin from neuronal stores.

Viloxazine is given for the treatment of depression (p.271) by mouth as the hydrochloride in usual doses equivalent to viloxazine 300 mg daily. If necessary, the dose may be increased to 600 mg daily if tolerated. The initial dose for the elderly or patients with hepatic or renal impairment is 100 mg daily cautiously increased if necessary. Viloxazine hydrochloride may also be given by intravenous infusion.

Viloxazine should be withdrawn gradually to reduce the risk of withdrawal symptoms.

Preparations

Proprietary Preparations (details are given in Part 3)
Aust.: Vivarint†; *Belg.:* Vivalan; *Fr.:* Vivalan; *Ger.:* Vivalan; *Ital.:* Vicilan; *Port.:* Vivalan; *Spain:* Vivarint; *UK:* Vivalan†.

Antidiabetics

This chapter describes diabetes mellitus and its management with antidiabetics. The oral drugs included in this chapter are classified in Table 1, below; insulin, which is given parenterally, is discussed on p.324 and classified in Table 2, p.326.

Diabetes mellitus

Diabetes mellitus is a group of disorders of carbohydrate metabolism in which the action of insulin is diminished or absent through altered secretion, decreased insulin activity, or a combination of both factors. It is characterised by hyperglycaemia. As the disease progresses tissue or vascular damage ensues leading to severe complications such as retinopathy, nephropathy, neuropathy, cardiovascular disease, and foot ulceration.

Diabetes mellitus may be categorised into several types but the two major types are type 1 (insulin-dependent diabetes mellitus; IDDM) and type 2 (non-insulin-dependent diabetes mellitus; NIDDM). The term juvenile-onset diabetes has sometimes been used for type 1 and maturity-onset diabetes for type 2. Malnutrition-related diabetes is no longer considered a separate entity (see Effects of Cassava, under Starch, p.1380).

Type 1 diabetes mellitus is present in patients who have little or no endogenous insulin secretory capacity and who therefore require exogenous insulin therapy for survival. This form of the disease has an auto-immune basis in most cases, and usually develops before adulthood. The associated hypoinsulinaemia and hyperglucagonaemia put such patients at risk of ketosis and ketoacidosis.

In **type 2 diabetes mellitus** the disease typically develops in later life. Insulin secretion may appear normal or even excessive (and type 2 patients are thus less prone to ketosis) but it is insufficient to compensate for insulin resistance. Obesity is present in the majority of type 2 patients; non-obese patients tend to have low insulin secretory capacity (although not as low as in type 1 diabetes) rather than appreciable insulin resistance.

Diagnosis of diabetes mellitus. Diagnosis is based upon blood-glucose concentrations exceeding set values under specified conditions.[1-4] Diabetes mellitus is likely if the glucose concentration in a random sample of venous plasma is 11.1 mmol or more per litre. If there are accompanying symptoms of increased thirst and urine volume, recurrent infections and weight loss, the presence of marked hyperglycaemia is considered diagnostic of diabetes. In the absence of symptoms or if the elevation of blood-glucose concentration is less marked (more often the case with type 2 than with type 1 diabetes), the diagnosis needs to be confirmed either by repeated sampling or by an **oral glucose tolerance test** (OGTT). This test consists of an overnight fast followed by measurement of the fasting blood-glucose concentration, then the administration of a 75-g oral glucose load (in children 1.75 g per kg body-weight up to a maximum of 75 g), and further measurement of the blood-glucose concen-

tration two hours later. Diagnostic values for measurements in venous whole blood are greater than or equal to 6.1 mmol per litre for the fasting state and 10.0 mmol per litre after the glucose load. The corresponding values for capillary whole blood are 6.1 and 11.1 mmol per litre, and for venous plasma 7.0 and 11.1 mmol per litre.[5] There has been some confusion at an international level as to whether the glucose load should be 75 g of the anhydrous form or the monohydrate. Sources at WHO have therefore suggested that the form should be standardised as 75 g of anhydrous glucose (anhydrous dextrose), which would be equivalent to 82.5 g of the monohydrate (glucose BP; dextrose monohydrate). The threshold for the diagnosis of diabetes has recently been lowered from a fasting plasma glucose concentration of 7.8 mmol per litre,[5] to reflect an increased risk of microvascular disease in patients with concentrations of 7.0 mmol per litre or more. However, there has been some concern about the lack of agreement between these newer criteria and the previous ones, which may result in alterations in prevalence of diabetes.[6,7]

Other diagnostic methods, such as measurement of glycosylated haemoglobin have been investigated.[8] There is also some interest in using antibodies to insulin, to islet cells, or to the enzyme glutamic acid decarboxylase, as predictive tests for those patients likely to develop diabetes mellitus.[9]

Once the presence of diabetes has been confirmed the distinction between type 1 and type 2 is made on clinical grounds.

Management of diabetes mellitus.

- DIETARY MODIFICATION. Dietary control is important in both type 1 and type 2 diabetes, and in the latter, possibly in association with increased exercise (see below), may sometimes correct the condition, at least temporarily. Reducing dietary sugar is not the only aim. Correction of obesity is desirable in all patients and in those with type 2 diabetes it will remove one of the factors associated with insulin resistance. Anorectic drugs are not effective in promoting weight loss in these patients.[10] A high fibre intake may also lower blood-glucose concentrations and additional fibre is sometimes taken in the form of guar gum (see p.324). The influence of diet on diabetes is such that all diabetic patients need to be aware of the composition of foods and to be able to make adjustments to their diet, especially to counteract treatment-induced hypoglycaemia. Controversy continues, however, as to the optimum composition of the diet in diabetics, and in particular as to what the relative contribution of calories from fat and from carbohydrate should be.

- EXERCISE. All diabetic patients should be encouraged to exercise, according to their age and physical capability.[5] Exercise improves metabolism and enhances the action of insulin on the tissues. It is also a useful component of any weight reduction programme although diet is more effective in promoting weight loss and metabolic control.[10]

- ORAL ANTIDIABETICS. If patients with type 2 diabetes have not achieved suitable control after about 3 months of dietary modification and increased physical activity, then oral antidiabetics (oral hypoglycaemics) may be tried. The two major classes are the *sulfonylureas* and the *biguanides*. Sulfonylureas act mainly by increasing endogenous insulin secretion, while biguanides act chiefly by decreasing hepatic gluconeogenesis and increasing peripheral utilisation of glucose. Both types function only in the presence of some endogenous insulin production. More recently developed classes of oral antidiabetics include the *alpha-glucosidase inhibitors*, the *meglitinides*, and the *thiazolidinediones* (see Table 1). Alpha-glucosidase inhibitors act by delaying the absorption of glucose from the gastrointestinal tract; meglitinides increase endogenous insulin secretion; and thiazolidinediones appear to increase insulin sensitivity.

Oral treatment of type 2 diabetes in non-obese patients is usually begun with a sulfonylurea. Chlorpropamide and glibenclamide have long half-lives and hence an increased tendency to cause hypoglycaemia, although a large study[11] reported that hypoglycaemic episodes were less frequent with chlorpropamide than glibenclamide. These 2 drugs are best avoided in the elderly;

a sulfonylurea with a short half-life, such as gliclazide, gliquidone, or tolbutamide, should be used instead.

There is evidence that the use of low-dose sulfonylurea therapy in patients with diagnosed type 2 diabetes but near-normoglycaemia due to early remission (the so-called honeymoon period) can delay the onset of hyperglycaemia.[12]

Sulfonylureas can cause weight gain and obese patients are preferably treated with the biguanide metformin rather than with a sulfonylurea. Results from the UK Prospective Diabetes Study (UKPDS) have suggested that the use of metformin to provide intensive blood-glucose control in overweight diabetic patients substantially reduced the risk of diabetes-related endpoints such as myocardial infarction, stroke, amputation, renal failure, blindness, and death.[13] Metformin is as effective as the sulfonylureas in terms of blood-glucose control and is less likely to cause hypoglycaemia,[13] but has a rare tendency to cause lactic acidosis in patients with renal impairment, in whom it should not be used.

Drug treatment may also involve an alpha-glucosidase inhibitor such as acarbose or miglitol. These have a small but significant effect in lowering blood glucose and do not cause hypoglycaemia when used alone, but they can cause intolerable gastrointestinal effects. Meglitinides such as repaglinide and nateglinide are a new chemical class of antidiabetics which act similarly to sulfonylureas; repaglinide has a rapid onset and short duration of action and is administered with meals. The thiazolidinediones, such as pioglitazone or rosiglitazone, appear to increase insulin sensitivity and have been the subject of much interest for type 2 diabetes and insulin resistance, but hepatotoxicity has limited the use of troglitazone.

Should treatment with one of the oral antidiabetics fail then a different type or in some instances combinations of different types may produce improvement. Alarming evidence[13] of an increased risk of death in UKPDS patients given intensive therapy with metformin in combination with a sulfonylurea was not borne out by further analysis, and this combination is widely used. In patients in whom such combinations fail or are contra-indicated, pioglitazone or rosiglitazone may be combined with metformin or a sulfonylurea as an alternative to progressing to insulin. Biguanides may also be added to meglitinide therapy. Alpha-glucosidase inhibitors may improve diabetes control when used as an adjunct to sulfonylureas or biguanides. Guar gum may also be used as an adjunct to any of the oral hypoglycaemics to enhance the improvement in blood-glucose control.

Patients with type 2 diabetes who cannot be controlled adequately by oral therapy and diet need insulin either in addition to or in place of oral therapy. Type 2 diabetes is a progressive disease, and about 30% of those on sulfonylureas will be transferred to insulin treatment within 4 years, a change which now tends to be made earlier owing to increasingly strict criteria for glycaemic control (tight control of blood glucose has now been shown to decrease the risk of complications, see Diabetic Complications, below). There is evidence that therapy with insulin and a sulfonylurea is more effective than therapy with insulin alone in type 2 patients.[14] Biguanides and alpha-glucosidase inhibitors may also be combined with insulin. As insulin therapy is associated with more hypoglycaemic episodes and a greater tendency to weight gain it remains reasonable to begin with oral therapy in type 2 diabetes before proceeding to insulin.[15]

Insulin is also substituted for oral treatment to provide cover during periods of severe stress, as in severe infection, trauma, or major surgery. Type 2 patients who become pregnant should also be switched from oral therapy to insulin (see Pregnancy, below).

- INSULIN THERAPY. While insulin may not be a necessary part of the treatment of type 2 diabetes, it is essential in the treatment of patients with type 1, since they have little or no endogenous insulin secretory capacity.

The aim of insulin therapy is to achieve the best possible control of blood-glucose concentrations without the risk of the hypoglycaemia that can occur if too fine a degree of control is attempted. Tight control of blood-glucose concentrations can reduce the long-

Table 1. Classification of oral antidiabetics.

Aldose Reductase Inhibitors	*Sulfonylureas*
Epalrestat	Acetohexamide
Sorbinil	Carbutamide
Tolrestat	Chlorpropamide
Alpha Glucosidase Inhibitors	Glibenclamide
Acarbose	Glibornuride
Emiglitate	Gliclazide
Miglitol	Glimepiride
Voglibose	Glipizide
	Gliquidone
Biguanides	Glisentide
Buformin	Glisolamide
Metformin	Glisoxepide
Phenformin	Glyclopyramide
	Glycyclamide
Meglitinides	Tolazamide
Nateglinide	Tolbutamide
Repaglinide	
	Thiazolidinediones
Miscellaneous	Pioglitazone
Glybuzole	Rosiglitazone
Glymidine	Troglitazone
Guar Gum	
Midaglizole	

term complications of diabetes such as retinopathy, nephropathy, and neuropathy (see Diabetic Complications, below) but in some patients (such as the elderly, or those who lack motivation) it may be better merely to alleviate symptoms rather than attempt tight control. Exercise and dietary discipline are necessary to maintain normal sensitivity to insulin.

Insulin may be of beef or pork origin, or it may be human insulin produced by gene technology or by modification of porcine insulin. Human and porcine insulin are less immunogenic than bovine insulin and where possible most newly diagnosed type 1 patients are now given human insulin. Modified insulin analogues such as insulin lispro are now available.

Insulin is available in a range of preparations offering a short, intermediate, or long action on subcutaneous injection. Insulin dosage schedules make use of the varying durations of action, for example by incorporating a short-acting and intermediate-acting insulin into a daily schedule. Most patients with type 1 diabetes require two or three injections of insulin daily, or with intensive regimens even more. A once-daily regimen can be used if the patient is simply to be kept asymptomatic; this may also be successful in patients with type 2 diabetes not satisfactorily controlled by oral antidiabetics.

The various types of insulin may also be given intramuscularly but the subcutaneous route is usually preferred. Soluble insulin can also be given intravenously. Details of insulin administration are given on p.330.

- IMMUNOSUPPRESSION. Many patients with type 1 diabetes experience a temporary improvement in pancreatic beta-cell function soon after initial treatment with insulin. This produces a period of remission known as the honeymoon period during which a small dose of insulin is sufficient to maintain good control. Attempts to prolong the honeymoon period have included tight control immediately following diagnosis and also, given the probable auto-immune nature of the condition, administration of an immunosuppressant.[16-20]

- PANCREATIC TRANSPLANTATION. Transplantation of the whole pancreas in patients with type 1 diabetes poorly controlled by insulin therapy has led to insulin-independence, and has usually been carried out in association with kidney transplantation (see also Other Organs, under Organ and Tissue Transplantation, p.504).[21-23] Transplantation of pancreatic islet cells has been investigated as an alternative.[22-27] However, few patients to date have remained independent of insulin within a year of islet-cell transplantation.[27] Results in *animals* have suggested that a reasonable degree of glycaemic control may be achievable long term without immunosuppression, using a vascularised 'artificial pancreas' containing allogeneic or even xenogeneic islet cells.[28]

- OTHER DRUG TREATMENTS. Various other drugs have been tried for diabetes mellitus, particularly when conventional therapy has proved unsuccessful. Addition of the amylin analogue *pramlintide* to insulin therapy has improved glycaemic control in patients with type 1 and type 2 diabetes.[29,30] Other approaches under investigation include inhibition of fatty acid oxidation or the use of β_3-adrenoceptor agonists (selective agonists of β-receptors thought to be associated with lipolysis and thermogenesis) to stimulate energy expenditure.[31] *Mecasermin* (insulin-like growth factor I; IGF-1) has been shown to improve metabolic control in patients with type 1 insulin resistance and insulin resistance (and in some type 2 patients).[32,33] *Glucagon-like peptide 1* (GLP-1; insulinotropin) improves glycaemic control in type 2 patients.[34] Improvements in insulin sensitivity have also been seen in insulin-resistant type 2 patients treated with a haemodialysate of calf blood,[35] while in other studies improved insulin sensitivity was seen following treatment with the *vanadium* salt, vanadyl sulfate,[36] or *chromium* supplementation.[37]

- PROPHYLAXIS. Because overt diabetes is the culmination of a prolonged process methods to delay or prevent its development are being investigated, either by modifying risk factors in populations or groups, or by targeting individuals thought to be at high risk. Strategies under consideration for the prevention of type 1 diabetes include avoidance of cows' milk proteins (thought to be a possible environmental trigger) during infancy;[38] administration of free radical scavengers such as nicotinamide;[39] administration of prophylactic insulin[40,41] (or possibly of oral antidiabetics) to allow 'beta cell rest'; encouraging the development of anti-

gen tolerance, for example by the oral administration of antigens such as insulin, glutamic acid decarboxylase, or heat shock protein[41-43] (a similar approach using subcutaneous antigen has apparently extended the honeymoon period in *animal* studies[44]); or by immunosuppression (see above) or immunomodulation with agents such as BCG vaccine,[45] although some have found the latter ineffective.[46] Preventive strategies for insulin resistance and type 2 diabetes have tended to focus on weight loss and dietary modification. However, prophylactic drug therapy may be possible: a study with troglitazone in nondiabetic obese subjects demonstrated reduced insulin resistance, and improved glucose tolerance in those in whom it was impaired.[47,48]

Monitoring of therapy. Monitoring of therapy is an integral part of the management of the diabetic patient. Detection of urinary glucose has generally been superseded by the monitoring of blood glucose (see Glucose Tests, p.1616). For adequate diabetic control, the aim is to reduce fasting blood-glucose concentrations to within the range 3.3 to 5.6 mmol per litre of venous whole blood, and postprandial concentrations to below 10 mmol per litre.[5] Many patients monitor their blood-glucose concentrations regularly at home and this is essential for intensified insulin regimens when tight control is required. The value of self-monitoring of blood-glucose concentrations in type 2 patients is more debatable.[49] Detection of urinary ketones is useful in diabetics prone to ketosis; this is usually performed in clinics. Diabetic clinics also measure the degree of haemoglobin glycosylation (HbA_1 or HbA_{1c}) as an indicator of longer term blood-glucose control and hence the risk of complications (see Diabetic Complications, below). More recently the advanced glycation end-product (AGE) of haemoglobin has also been found to be a useful indicator of long-term blood glucose control.[50] Techniques for continuous monitoring of blood glucose are under investigation,[51,52] as are noninvasive or minimally invasive methods.[53]

Pregnancy. Adverse pregnancy outcomes, including spontaneous abortion and congenital malformation, are more common in diabetic than in nondiabetic women. Improved management of the pregnant diabetic patient, particularly early in pregnancy, lessens the incidence of such events,[54,55] but an increased risk still exists.[56] Diabetic women are advised to plan their pregnancies so that glycaemic control can be improved before conception. Some may need to avoid pregnancy (most commonly because of renal disease),[57] but management has improved sufficiently for this to be rare.[55]

Insulin is the preferred treatment in pregnancy,[58] even in women with type 2 diabetes; patients taking oral antidiabetics should therefore be switched to insulin. Insulin regimens are similar to those in nonpregnant patients, the dose being adjusted according to regular blood-glucose measurements. Insulin requirements may decrease during the first trimester but they increase during the latter two, reaching about twice prepregnancy requirements at term; they then fall once labour has begun and fall again after delivery.[58]

Pregnant diabetic patients are at risk of nocturnal hypoglycaemia owing to continued fetal glucose consumption while the mother is in a relatively fasting state. They are also prone to diabetic ketoacidosis which must be treated with great urgency because of the high risk of fetal loss.

Gestational diabetes, that is diabetes which develops during pregnancy, may usually be impaired glucose tolerance associated with pregnancy.[59] It is not clear whether treatment of gestational glucose intolerance significantly decreases perinatal mortality or birth-weight.[60] There is, therefore, disagreement about the benefits of universal screening for gestational glucose intolerance.[59-62] Many women with gestational diabetes may be managed by diet alone or, if necessary, also with insulin. Some workers, however, have advocated prophylactic administration of insulin to women who could be managed by diet alone, in view of the metabolic effects of insulin.[63]

Surgery. Insulin-dependent diabetics who require surgery may be managed with a continuous intravenous insulin infusion.[64] Insulin is given as normal the night before operation, and switched to either a variable-rate infusion via a syringe pump, together with a 5 or 10% glucose drip (with potassium chloride, provided the patient is not hyperkalaemic), or to a combined insulin-glucose infusion, on the day of operation. (Many anaesthetists prefer insulin and a sodium chloride infusion if blood glucose is already high.[65]) Subsequent conversion back

to subcutaneous insulin should be undertaken before breakfast, giving the first subcutaneous dose 30 minutes before stopping continuous infusion. Non-insulin-dependent patients should have any oral treatment omitted on the day of operation, and may be given insulin by a similar regimen if control is poor or deteriorates as can happen with major surgery.

1. Meltzer S, et al. 1998 clinical practice guidelines for the management of diabetes in Canada. Can Med Assoc J 1998; 159 (suppl 8): S1–S29.
2. WHO. Definition, diagnosis and classification of diabetes mellitus and its complications. Geneva: WHO, 1999.
3. Colman PG, et al. New classification and criteria for diagnosis of diabetes mellitus. Med J Aust 1999; 170: 375–8.
4. American Diabetes Association. Report of the Expert Committee on the Diagnosis and Classification of Diabetes Mellitus. Diabetes Care 2001; 24 (suppl 1): S5–S20.
5. WHO. Diabetes mellitus: report of a WHO study group. WHO Tech Rep Ser 727 1985.
6. DECODE Study Group. Will new diagnostic criteria for diabetes mellitus change phenotype of patients with diabetes? Reanalysis of European epidemiological data. BMJ 1998; 317: 371–5.
7. Wahl PW, et al. Diabetes in older adults: comparison of 1997 American Diabetes Association classification of diabetes mellitus with 1985 WHO classification. Lancet 1998; 352: 1012–15.
8. McCance DR, et al. Comparison of tests for glycated haemoglobin and fasting and two hour plasma glucose concentrations as diagnostic methods for diabetes. BMJ 1994; 308: 1323–8.
9. Palmer JP. What is the best way to predict IDDM? Lancet 1994; 343: 1377–8.
10. Brown SA, et al. Promoting weight loss in type II diabetes. Diabetes Care 1996; 19: 613–24.
11. United Kingdom Prospective Diabetes Study Group. United Kingdom prospective diabetes study (UKPDS) 13: relative efficacy of randomly allocated diet, sulphonylurea, insulin, and metformin in patients with newly diagnosed non-insulin dependent diabetes followed for three years. BMJ 1995; 310: 83–8.
12. Banerji MA, et al. Prolongation of near-normoglycemic remission in black NIDDM subjects with chronic low-dose sulfonylurea treatment. Diabetes 1995; 44: 466–70.
13. UK Prospective Diabetes Study Group. Effect of intensive blood-glucose control with metformin on complications in overweight patients with type 2 diabetes (UKPDS 34). Lancet 1998; 352: 854–65. Correction. ibid.; 1558.
14. Johnson JL, et al. Efficacy of insulin and sulfonylurea combination therapy in type II diabetes: a meta-analysis of the randomized placebo-controlled trials. Arch Intern Med 1996; 156: 259–64.
15. United Kingdom Prospective Diabetes Study Group. United Kingdom Prospective Diabetes Study 24: a 6-year, randomized, controlled trial comparing sulfonylurea, insulin, and metformin therapy in patients with newly diagnosed type 2 diabetes that could not be controlled with diet therapy. Ann Intern Med 1998; 128: 165–75.
16. Pozzilli P, Maclaren NK. Immunotherapy at clinical diagnosis of insulin-dependent diabetes: an approach still worth considering. Trends Endocrinol Metab 1993; 4: 101–5.
17. Bougneres PF, et al. Factors associated with early remission of type I diabetes in children treated with cyclosporine. N Engl J Med 1988; 318: 663–70.
18. The Canadian-European Randomized Control Trial Group. Cyclosporin-induced remission of IDDM after early intervention: association of 1 yr of cyclosporin treatment with enhanced insulin secretion. Diabetes 1988; 37: 1574–82.
19. Harrison LC, et al. Increase in remission rate in newly diagnosed type I diabetic subjects treated with azathioprine. Diabetes 1985; 34: 1306–8.
20. Yilmaz MT, et al. Immunoprotection in spontaneous remission of type 1 diabetes: long-term follow-up results. Diabetes Res Clin Pract 1993; 19: 151–62.
21. Remuzzi G, et al. Pancreas and kidney/pancreas transplants: experimental medicine or real improvement? Lancet 1994; 343: 27–31.
22. Robertson RP. Pancreatic and islet transplantation for diabetes—cures or curiosities? N Engl J Med 1992; 327: 1861–8.
23. Ryan EA. Pancreas transplants: for whom? Lancet 1998; 351: 1072–3. Correspondence. ibid.; 352: 65–6.
24. Pyzdrowski KL, et al. Preserved insulin secretion and insulin dependence in recipients of islet autografts. N Engl J Med 1992; 327: 220–6.
25. Gores PF, et al. Insulin independence in type I diabetes after transplantation of unpurified islets from single donor with 15-deoxyspergualin. Lancet 1993; 341: 19–21.
26. Soon-Shiong P, et al. Insulin independence in a type 1 diabetic patient after encapsulated islet transplantation. Lancet 1994; 343: 950–1.
27. Weir GC, Bonner-Weir S. Scientific and political impediments to successful islet transplantation. Diabetes 1997; 46: 1247–56.
28. Maki T, et al. Novel delivery of pancreatic islet cells to treat insulin-dependent diabetes mellitus. Clin Pharmacokinet 1995; 28: 471–82.
29. Thompson RG, et al. Effects of pramlintide, an analog of human amylin, on plasma glucose profiles in patients with IDDM: results of a multicenter trial. Diabetes 1997; 46: 632–6.
30. Thompson RG, et al. Pramlintide, a synthetic analog of human amylin, improves the metabolic profile of patients with type 2 diabetes using insulin. Diabetes Care 1998; 21: 987–93.
31. Petrie JR, Donnelly R. New pharmacological approaches to insulin and lipid metabolism. Drugs 1994; 47: 701–10.
32. Moses AC, et al. Insulin-like growth factor I (rhIGF-I) as a therapeutic agent for hyperinsulinemic insulin-resistant diabetes mellitus. Diabetes Res Clin Pract 1995; 28(suppl): S185–S194.
33. Acerini CL, et al. Randomised placebo-controlled trial of human recombinant insulin-like growth factor I plus intensive insulin therapy in adolescents with insulin-dependent diabetes mellitus. Lancet 1997; 350: 1199–1204.
34. Todd JF, et al. Glucagon-like peptide-1 (GLP-1): a trial of treatment in non-insulin-dependent diabetes mellitus. Eur J Clin Invest 1997; 27: 533–6.
35. Jacob S, et al. Improvement of glucose metabolism in patients with type II diabetes after treatment with a hemodialysate. Arzneimittelforschung 1996; 46: 269–72.
36. Cohen N, et al. Oral vanadyl sulfate improves hepatic and peripheral insulin sensitivity in patients with non-insulin-dependent diabetes mellitus. J Clin Invest 1995; 95: 2501–9.

37. Anderson RA, *et al.* Elevated intakes of supplemental chromium improve glucose and insulin variables in individuals with type 2 diabetes. *Diabetes* 1997; **46:** 1786–91.
38. Åkerblom HK. Diabetes and cows' milk. *Lancet* 1996; **348:** 1656–7.
39. Pozzilli P, *et al.* Meta-analysis of nicotinamide treatment in patients with recent-onset IDDM. *Diabetes Care* 1996; **19:** 1357–63.
40. Keller RJ, *et al.* Insulin prophylaxis in individuals at high risk of type 1 diabetes. *Lancet* 1993; **341:** 927–8.
41. Alberti KGMM. Preventing insulin dependent diabetes mellitus. *BMJ* 1993; **307:** 1435–6.
42. Williams G. IDDM: long honeymoon, sweet ending. *Lancet* 1994; **343:** 684–5.
43. Jones DB, Armstrong NW. Peptide therapy for diabetes. *Lancet* 1994; **343:** 1168–9.
44. Elias D, Cohen IR. Peptide therapy in NOD mice. *Lancet* 1994; **343:** 704–6.
45. Shehadeh N, *et al.* Effect of adjuvant therapy on development of diabetes in mouse and man. *Lancet* 1994; **343:** 706–7.
46. Pozzilli P, *et al.* BCG vaccine in insulin-dependent diabetes mellitus. *Lancet* 1997; **349:** 1520–1.
47. Nolan JJ, *et al.* Improvement in glucose tolerance and insulin resistance in obese subjects treated with troglitazone. *N Engl J Med* 1994; **331:** 1188–93.
48. Keen H. Insulin resistance and the prevention of diabetes mellitus. *N Engl J Med* 1994; **331:** 1226–7.
49. Tattersall R. Self monitoring of blood glucose concentrations by non-insulin dependent diabetic patients. *BMJ* 1992; **305:** 1171–2.
50. Wolffenbuttel BHR, *et al.* Long-term assessment of glucose control by haemoglobin-AGE measurement. *Lancet* 1996; **347:** 513–15.
51. Pickup JC. Sampling and sensing blood glucose. *Lancet* 1993; **342:** 1068.
52. Bolinder J, *et al.* Long-term continuous glucose monitoring with microdialysis in ambulatory insulin-dependent diabetic patients. *Lancet* 1993; **342:** 1080–5.
53. Marwick C. Development of noninvasive methods to monitor blood glucose levels in people with diabetes. *JAMA* 1998; **280:** 312–3.
54. Steel JM, *et al.* Can prepregnancy care of diabetic women reduce the risk of abnormal babies? *BMJ* 1990; **301:** 1070–4.
55. Steel JM, Johnstone FD. Guidelines for the management of insulin-dependent diabetes mellitus in pregnancy. *Drugs* 1996; **52:** 60–70.
56. Casson IF, *et al.* Outcomes of pregnancy in insulin dependent diabetic women: results of a five year population cohort study. *BMJ* 1997; **315:** 275–8.
57. Pearson JF. Pregnancy and complicated diabetes. *Br J Hosp Med* 1993; **49:** 739–42.
58. Crombach G, *et al.* Insulin use in pregnancy: clinical pharmacokinetic considerations. *Clin Pharmacokinet* 1993; **24:** 89–100.
59. Jarrett RJ. Gestational diabetes: a non-entity? *BMJ* 1993; **306:** 37–8.
60. Ales KL, Santini DL. Should all pregnant women be screened for gestational glucose intolerance? *Lancet* 1989; **i:** 1187–91.
61. Mazze RS, Krogh CL. Gestational diabetes mellitus: now is the time for detection and treatment. *Mayo Clin Proc* 1992; **67:** 995–1002.
62. Hoffman L, *et al.* Gestational diabetes mellitus—management guidelines [of] the Australasian Diabetes in Pregnancy Society. *Med J Aust* 1998; **169:** 93–7.
63. Thompson DJ, *et al.* Prophylactic insulin in the management of gestational diabetes. *Obstet Gynecol* 1990; **75:** 960–4.
64. Jacober SJ, Sowers JR. An update on perioperative management of diabetes. *Arch Intern Med* 1999; **159:** 2405–11.
65. Eldridge AJ, Sear JW. Peri-operative management of diabetic patients: any changes for the better since 1985? *Anaesthesia* 1996; **51:** 45–51.

Diabetic complications

Much of the increased mortality and morbidity seen in diabetic patients is the result of various complications which develop with increasing duration of disease, particularly when glycaemic control is poor. Such complications may originate from increased glycation of proteins and other biological macromolecules in the hyperglycaemic environment, or from increased accumulation of sorbitol and other polyols via the aldose reductase pathway, but other factors play an important role in determining susceptibility. At the *macrovascular* level, diabetics are prone to hypertension and ischaemic heart disease, and heart disease is a major cause of death; control of blood pressure is now seen as being as important as glycaemic control in patients with type 2 diabetes. *Microvascular* tissue damage is an important factor in the development of diabetic nephropathy and retinopathy; it may also contribute to the other major complication, diabetic neuropathy. Collagen abnormalities are also seen. Diabetics with poor glycaemic control also have an increased liability to severe bacterial or fungal infection. Sometimes several factors may interact; thus neuropathy, infection, and impaired blood flow due to macro- or microvascular disease may all play a role in the development of diabetic foot disease, a complication which can ultimately lead to amputation.

Prevention of diabetic complications. Much attention has been focussed on whether strict or tight glycaemic control can modify the development or progression of diabetic complications. In general, the longer-term studies have provided more encouraging results than initial results indicated, and meta-analysis of such studies[1] has suggested that intensive regimens may prevent microvascular complications.

The Diabetes Control and Complications Trial (DCCT)[2] confirmed this view in type 1 diabetes. It compared in selected patients the effects of conventional insulin therapy with those of continuous subcutaneous insulin infusion or multiple-injection regimens, on the development and progression of complications. The intensive treatment was aimed at keeping preprandial blood-glucose concentrations between 3.9 and 6.7 mmol per litre, postprandial concentrations at less than 10 mmol per litre, a weekly 3 a.m. measurement at greater than 3.6 mmol per litre, and the monthly glycosylated haemoglobin measurement at less than 6.05%. Intensive insulin therapy reduced the development and progression of retinopathy; it also reduced the occurrence of microalbuminuria, albuminuria, and clinical neuropathy. The major disadvantage of intensive insulin therapy was a threefold greater risk of hypoglycaemia; weight gain was also significantly greater.

While it is accepted that some patients will benefit from intensive insulin therapy, this approach requires caution in patients at risk of hypoglycaemia. Also such intensive treatment may not always be necessary, for example in patients known to maintain good control by conventional dosage schedules, or where improvement can be obtained by setting achievable targets and improving patient education.[3] However, intensive therapy can help sustain endogenous insulin secretion in type 1 diabetes, which is associated with improved metabolic control;[4] this would support initiation of intensive insulin therapy at an early stage.

The reports of the UK Prospective Diabetes Study (UKPDS) have provided similar evidence in patients with type 2 diabetes. This study has examined the benefits of intensive therapy, using a variety of drugs together with diet and exercise. Intensive therapy, which aimed at producing fasting plasma-glucose concentrations of below 6 mmol per litre, substantially decreased the risk of microvascular complications (particularly retinopathy). There was no difference in benefit between intensive therapy with sulfonylureas and with insulin.[5] Metformin also produced benefit in the overweight patients who received it.[6] The UKPDS did not provide unequivocal evidence of a reduction in macrovascular disease with improved glycaemic control, although there was some suggestion of a reduction in risk of myocardial infarction (in line with a small earlier Japanese study[7]). However, it did show that vigorous control of blood pressure, using captopril or atenolol as the first-line drugs, reduced the risk of both macrovascular and microvascular complications,[8,9] suggesting that this should have a high priority in the treatment of type 2 diabetes.

Diabetic eye disease. Diabetic patients are prone to potentially blinding eye disease, usually in the form of cataract or diabetic retinopathy. Cataract generally requires surgical extraction, particular care being taken to avoid infection. Diabetic retinopathy may take a 'background', non-proliferative form, or become a more serious proliferative retinopathy associated with neovascularisation, vitreous haemorrhage and retinal detachment.

Although strict glycaemic control has been shown to reduce the risk of developing retinopathy,[2,5] once proliferative retinopathy has developed, glycaemic control is not adequate to prevent worsening.[10] Moreover, transient early worsening may occur in patients transferred to more intensive regimens.[11]

Aldose reductase inhibitors such as epalrestat and sorbinil have been investigated for the prevention of retinopathy, but despite some benefits results have generally been unimpressive.[12] The benefits of antiplatelet drugs are also unclear; aspirin, dipyridamole, and ticlopidine appear to reduce the development of microaneurysms in diabetic patients,[13,14] but aspirin has not been shown to prevent the development of retinopathy.[15]

Once proliferative retinopathy has developed photocoagulation using an argon laser or a xenon arc is effective in limiting progression, while vitrectomy may be helpful for vitreous haemorrhage and retinal detachment. Interferon alfa-2a has been reported to slow the progression of proliferative diabetic retinopathy in 3 patients,[16] although all 3 experienced haemorrhage within 6 weeks of stopping the drug. Epoetin has also proved of benefit in a few patients,[17] and it has been suggested that oxpentifylline [pentoxifylline] should be investigated.[18] Results from a large European study (EUCLID) demonstrated a reduction in the progression of retinopathy in patients with type 1 diabetes treated with an ACE inhibitor, lisinopril.[19] Improvement in retinal hard exudates has been

seen in patients given the low-molecular-weight heparinoid danaparoid sodium.[20]

Diabetic nephropathy. Nephropathic changes associated with microvascular disease develop in up to 30% of patients with type 1 diabetes and up to 40% of those with type 2 disease; diabetic nephropathy, of which the first clinical sign is albuminuria, is one of the major causes of end-stage renal disease (p.1185).

Results from the DCCT indicate that strict glycaemic control reduces the incidence of microalbuminuria in type 1 diabetes,[2] and a smaller reduction was seen in the UKPDS in patients with type 2 diabetes.[5] However, while good control may prevent development of the initial lesion, it is not clear whether it can prevent progression in patients who are already microalbuminuric. Some studies, including the DCCT, have suggested that this is the case;[2,7] others have failed to confirm it.[21]

Another approach is dietary protein restriction (see Renal Failure, p.1351), which appears from a number of small studies to have a beneficial effect on disease progression.[22,23]

The most important approach to slowing the progression of diabetic nephropathy is aggressive antihypertensive control.[8,24,25] Although meta-analysis[26] has suggested that ACE inhibitors have an antiproteinuric effect over and above their antihypertensive properties, results from the UKPDS showed no difference between the effects of an ACE inhibitor and a beta blocker in reducing microalbuminuria in type 2 diabetics with hypertension.[9] Beneficial effects have also been reported when ACE inhibitors are given to patients with microalbuminuria but without hypertension,[26-31] and it has been recommended that such patients receive ACE inhibitors, initially in small doses, to slow the progression of renal disease.[24] Some consider that small decreases in blood pressure associated with such therapy may be responsible for the benefit.[9] ACE inhibition also had a modest renal protective effect in normotensive diabetics with normal urinary albumin excretion,[32] and such use requires further study.

The aldose reductase inhibitors have been investigated for their effects on nephropathy, but results have been, at best, ambiguous; a study in microalbuminuric patients given tolrestat did show a decrease in urinary albumin excretion but this was concomitant with a decrease in the (initially raised) glomerular filtration rate.[33] Pimagedine, which inhibits the formation of glycosylated end products, is also under investigation.

Diabetic neuropathy. A variety of peripheral neuropathies are common complications of diabetes mellitus. The intensity and extent of neurological abnormalities are proportional to the degree and duration of hyperglycaemia. Neuropathic symptoms include symmetrical sensory loss, particularly in the feet and lower limbs; the various features of autonomic neuropathy including gastroparesis, postural hypotension, impotence, and gustatory sweating; pain and cranial nerve palsy associated with mononeuropathies; and acute, painful, sensory neuropathy.

Results from the DCCT indicated that strict glycaemic control could substantially reduce the occurrence of clinical neuropathy in patients with type 1 diabetes,[2,34] a result which was not duplicated in the UKPDS in patients with type 2 diabetes.[5]

Although some studies have suggested that aldose reductase inhibitors such as epalrestat[35] and tolrestat[36] can reduce the severity of diabetic neuropathy, larger scale analysis has apparently failed to demonstrate any benefit. Interesting preliminary results have suggested that ACE inhibitors may also have benefits in diabetic neuropathy.[37,38] Recombinant human nerve growth factor is being investigated.[39]

Other management of diabetic neuropathy is essentially symptomatic. The pain, which can be severe, may be managed with tricyclic antidepressants; mexiletine, carbamazepine, and topical capsaicin may also be tried, as discussed on p.5.

Diabetic gastroparesis may respond to prokinetic drugs such as metoclopramide, cisapride, or domperidone;[40] an alternative is to try erythromycin.[41] Diarrhoea may respond to tetracycline (see below), while postural hypotension should be managed conventionally (see p.1070) although care may be required in the use of elastic stockings in patients with impaired blood flow to the feet. Results from a study using the antoxidant thioctic acid have suggested some improvement in cardiac autonomic neuropathy.[42]

Diarrhoea. Diabetic patients may develop intermittent bouts of watery diarrhoea, increasing in frequency as the condition worsens; autonomic neuropathy and abnormalities of digestion and bowel flora may play a role.[43] Beneficial results have been reported from the use of clonidine,[44,45] and of octreotide,[46,47] but a conventional antidiarrhoeal drug (usually codeine or diphenoxylate) or a broad spectrum antibacterial (especially tetracycline) may also be effective. The mechanism of action of tetracycline in diabetic diarrhoea is uncertain, but it has been suggested that one or two doses of tetracycline should be the first line of treatment.[48]

Foot disease. Various types of diabetic tissue damage, including circulatory impairment, neuropathy, collagen changes, and increased susceptibility to infection, may contribute to the foot lesions to which diabetics are prone. Ulceration and tissue necrosis at pressure-points may be followed by infection, gangrene, and sepsis. Management involves drainage and debridement of dead and infected tissue, and the use of antibiotics if necessary: broad spectrum cover should be given intravenously if there is systemic infection, and adapted once the results of bacteriological culture are available.[49] Local antiseptic therapy may be helpful, especially for infections with *Pseudomonas* or *Proteus* spp. Neuropathic skin ulcers of the lower extremities have responded to a platelet-derived growth factor, becaplermin.[50] Strict control of blood glucose is important and insulin should be given as required. Effective pain relief, together with bed rest, may be required, and surgical reconstruction to improve blood supply may be helpful in some cases. Ultimately, some patients require amputation of all or part of the foot. Preventive care, with regular visits to a chiropodist, is therefore particularly important.

Heart disease. Most damage to the cardiac tissue in diabetic patients is due to accelerated ischaemic heart disease. Hypertension and hyperlipidaemias, both of which are prevalent in diabetes mellitus, contribute to this process. Symptoms of angina pectoris may be less marked or absent in diabetic patients. Management of ischaemic heart disease is, however, similar in diabetic and non-diabetic patients (see Angina Pectoris, p.791), except that if a beta blocker is given it should be a selective one. Diabetic patients are more likely than non-diabetics to die after myocardial infarction, but it has been shown that treatment with an insulin-glucose infusion after myocardial infarction, followed by subcutaneous insulin for at least 3 months, improves long-term survival in patients with both type 1 and type 2 diabetes.[51] Despite concerns about the use of aspirin in diabetics there is evidence for its value for the secondary prevention of cardiovascular disease and for primary prevention in patients at high risk.[52-54] There is some suggestion that higher than usual doses (300 mg rather than 75 to 100 mg daily) may be required in diabetics.[52]

Diabetics may also develop a form of restrictive cardiomyopathy in the absence of ischaemic heart disease. Again, the condition is managed similarly to cardiomyopathy in non-diabetic patients (see p.796).

Cardiac autonomic neuropathy has been reported to be improved by thioctic acid (see Diabetic Neuropathy, above).

Hyperlipidaemias. Insulin plays an important role in lipid metabolism and deficient insulin action means that diabetics are prone to hypertriglyceridaemia and have a blood-lipid profile associated with an increased risk of atherosclerosis, and hence of macrovascular complications. To reduce the risk of such complications good glycaemic control, dietary advice and where necessary the use of lipid regulating drugs (see p.800) are necessary. The American Diabetes Association recommends that LDL cholesterol concentrations should be below 2.6 mmol per litre, HDL cholesterol concentrations more than 1.15 mmol per litre, and triglyceride concentrations less than 2.3 mmol per litre.[55] When necessary statins, such as simvastatin,[56] should be used to lower LDL cholesterol. Nicotinic acid has been used to raise HDL cholesterol concentrations,[57] but it can exacerbate hyperglycaemia.[55] Fibrates may therefore be used as an alternative, and can also be used to lower triglyceride concentrations.[55]

Hypertension. Hypertension is twice as common in the diabetic as in the non-diabetic population, and is associated with both macrovascular complications and microvascular disease (especially diabetic nephropathy). Management of hypertension in diabetics follows the same principles as in the general population, but it should be treated aggressively with a view to retarding development of complications,[8,58-61] and the threshold for drug treatment and the treatment goal are lower than in non-diabetic patients (see Hypertension, p.802). All of the main groups of antihypertensive drugs may be used although an ACE inhibitor, such as ramipril,[62] or a beta blocker may be effective in reducing complications.[8,9] Low-dose diuretic therapy has also been shown to be beneficial.[63] The calcium-channel blocker felodipine was effective in the subset of diabetics in one study[64] but other studies have suggested that calcium-channel blockers are less effective than ACE inhibitors, or may even increase cardiovascular adverse events (see under Nifedipine, p.942).

1. Wang PH, *et al.* Meta-analysis of effects of intensive blood-glucose control on late complications of type I diabetes. *Lancet* 1993; **341:** 1306–9.
2. The Diabetes Control and Complications Trial Research Group. The effect of intensive treatment of diabetes on the development and progression of long-term complications in insulin-dependent diabetes mellitus. *N Engl J Med* 1993; **329:** 977–86.
3. Short R. Implementing the lessons of DCCT. *Diabetic Med* 1994; **11:** 220–8.
4. The Diabetes Control and Complications Trial Research Group. Effect of intensive therapy on residual β-cell function in patients with type 1 diabetes in the Diabetes Control and Complications Trial: a randomized, controlled trial. *Ann Intern Med* 1998; **128:** 517–23.
5. UK Prospective Diabetes Study Group. Intensive blood-glucose control with sulphonylureas or insulin compared with conventional treatment and risk of complications in patients with type 2 diabetes (UKPDS 33). *Lancet* 1998; **352:** 837–53.
6. UK Prospective Diabetes Study (UKPDS) Group. Effect of intensive blood-glucose control with metformin on complications in overweight patients with type 2 diabetes (UKPDS 34). *Lancet* 1998; **352:** 854–65. Correction. *ibid.*; 1558.
7. Ohkubo Y, *et al.* Intensive insulin therapy prevents the progression of diabetic microvascular complications in Japanese patients with non-insulin-dependent diabetes mellitus: a randomized prospective 6-year study. *Diabetes Res Clin Pract* 1995; **28:** 103–17.
8. UK Prospective Diabetes Study Group. Tight blood pressure control and risk of macrovascular and microvascular complications in type 2 diabetes: UKPDS 38. *BMJ* 1998; **317:** 703–13.
9. UK Prospective Diabetes Study Group. Efficacy of atenolol and captopril in reducing risk of macrovascular and microvascular complications in type 2 diabetes: UKPDS 39. *BMJ* 1998; **317:** 713–20.
10. Esmatjes E, *et al.* Long-term evolution of diabetic retinopathy and renal function after pancreas transplantation. *Transplant Proc* 1992; **24:** 12–13.
11. Henricsson M, *et al.* The effect of glycaemic control and the introduction of insulin therapy on retinopathy in non-insulin-dependent diabetes mellitus. *Diabetic Med* 1997; **14:** 123–31.
12. Sorbinil Retinopathy Trial Research Group. A randomized trial of sorbinil, an aldose reductase inhibitor, in diabetic retinopathy. *Arch Ophthalmol* 1990; **108:** 1234–44.
13. The DAMAD Study Group. Effect of aspirin alone and aspirin plus dipyridamole in early diabetic retinopathy: a multicenter randomized controlled clinical trial. *Diabetes* 1989; **38:** 491–8.
14. The TIMAD Study Group. Ticlopidine treatment reduces the progression of nonproliferative diabetic retinopathy. *Arch Ophthalmol* 1990; **108:** 1577–83.
15. Early Treatment Diabetic Retinopathy Study Research Group. Effects of aspirin treatment on diabetic retinopathy: ETDRS report number 8. *Ophthalmology* 1991; **98** (suppl): 757–65.
16. Skowsky WR, *et al.* A pilot study of chronic recombinant interferon-alfa 2a for diabetic proliferative retinopathy: metabolic effects and ophthalmologic effects. *J Diabetes Complications* 1996; **10:** 94–9.
17. Friedman EA. Erythropoietin in diabetic macular edema and renal insufficiency. *Am J Kidney Dis* 1995; **26:** 202–8.
18. Sebag J, *et al.* Effects of pentoxifylline on choroidal blood flow in nonproliferative diabetic retinopathy. *Angiology* 1994; **45:** 429–33.
19. Chaturvedi N, *et al.* Effect of lisinopril on progression of retinopathy in normotensive people with type 1 diabetes. *Lancet* 1998; **351:** 28–31.
20. van der Pijl JW, *et al.* Effect of danaparoid sodium on hard exudates in diabetic retinopathy. *Lancet* 1997; **350:** 1743–5.
21. Microalbuminuria Collaborative Study Group, United Kingdom. Intensive therapy and progression to clinical albuminuria in patients with insulin dependent diabetes mellitus and microalbuminuria. *BMJ* 1995; **311:** 973–7.
22. Pedrini MT. The effect of dietary protein restriction on the progression of diabetic and nondiabetic renal diseases: a meta-analysis. *Ann Intern Med* 1996; **124:** 627–32.
23. Waugh NR, Robertson AM. Protein restriction for diabetic renal disease (updated 16 May 2000). Available in The Cochrane Library; Issue 3. Oxford: Update Software; 2001.
24. Mogensen CE, *et al.* Prevention of diabetic renal disease with special reference to microalbuminuria. *Lancet* 1995; **346:** 1080–4.
25. Savage MW, *et al.* Therapeutic options in diabetic renal disease and hypertension. *Br J Hosp Med* 1995; **54:** 429–34.
26. Kasiske BL, *et al.* Effect of antihypertensive therapy on the kidney in patients with diabetes: a meta-regression analysis. *Ann Intern Med* 1993; **118:** 129–38.
27. Laffel LMB, *et al.* The beneficial effect of angiotensin-converting enzyme inhibition with captopril on diabetic nephropathy in normotensive IDDM patients with microalbuminuria. *Am J Med* 1995; **99:** 497–504.
28. Ravid M, *et al.* Long-term stabilizing effect of angiotensin-converting enzyme inhibition on plasma creatinine and on proteinuria in normotensive type II diabetic patients. *Ann Intern Med* 1993; **118:** 577–81.
29. Mathiesen ER, *et al.* Randomised controlled trial of long term efficacy of captopril on preservation of kidney function in normotensive patients with insulin dependent diabetes and microalbuminuria. *BMJ* 1999; **319:** 24–5.
30. The EUCLID Study Group. Randomised placebo-controlled trial of lisinopril in normotensive patients with insulin-dependent diabetes and normoalbuminuria or microalbuminuria. *Lancet* 1997; **349:** 1787–92.
31. Lovell HG. Angiotensin converting enzyme inhibitors in normotensive diabetic patients with microalbuminuria (updated 9 May 2001). Available in The Cochrane Library; Issue 3. Oxford: Update Software; 2001.
32. Ravid M, *et al.* Use of enalapril to attenuate decline in renal function in normotensive, normoalbuminuric patients with type 2 diabetes mellitus: a randomized controlled trial. *Ann Intern Med* 1998; **128:** 982–8.
33. Passariello N, *et al.* Effect of aldose reductase inhibitor (tolrestat) on urinary albumin excretion rate and glomerular filtration rate in IDDM subjects with nephropathy. *Diabetes Care* 1993; **16:** 789–95.
34. The Diabetes Control and Complications Trial Research Group. The effect of intensive diabetes therapy on measures of autonomic nervous system function in the Diabetes Control and Complications Trial (DCCT). *Diabetologia* 1998; **41:** 416–23.
35. Uchida N, *et al.* Effect of 24 weeks of treatment with epalrestat, an aldose reductase inhibitor, on peripheral neuropathy in patients with non-insulin-dependent diabetes mellitus. *Clin Ther* 1995; **17:** 460–6.
36. Boulton AJM, *et al.* A multicentre trial of the aldose-reductase inhibitor, tolrestat, in patients with symptomatic diabetic neuropathy. *Diabetologia* 1990; **33:** 431–7.
37. Reja A, *et al.* Is ACE inhibition with lisinopril helpful in diabetic neuropathy? *Diabetic Med* 1995; **12:** 307–9.
38. Malik RA, *et al.* Effect of angiotensin-converting-enzyme (ACE) inhibitor trandolapril on human diabetic neuropathy: randomised double-blind controlled trial. *Lancet* 1998; **352:** 1978–81.
39. Apfel SC, *et al.* Recombinant human nerve growth factor in the treatment of diabetic polyneuropathy. *Neurology* 1998; **51:** 695–702.
40. Drenth JPH, Engels LGJB. Diabetic gastroparesis: a critical reappraisal of new treatment strategies. *Drugs* 1992; **44:** 537–53.
41. Richards RD, *et al.* The treatment of idiopathic and diabetic gastroparesis with acute intravenous and chronic oral erythromycin. *Am J Gastroenterol* 1993; **88:** 203–7.
42. Ziegler D, *et al.* Effects of treatment with the antioxidant α-lipoic acid on cardiac autonomic neuropathy in NIDDM patients: a 4-month randomized controlled multicenter trial (DEKAN study). *Diabetes Care* 1997; **20:** 369–73.
43. Ogbonnaya KI, Arem R. Diabetic diarrhea: pathophysiology, diagnosis, and management. *Arch Intern Med* 1990; **150:** 262–7.
44. Fedorak RN, *et al.* Treatment of diabetic diarrhea with clonidine. *Ann Intern Med* 1985; **102:** 197–9.
45. Sacerdote A. Topical clonidine for diabetic diarrhea. *Ann Intern Med* 1986; **105:** 139.
46. Michaels PE, Cameron RB. Octreotide is cost-effective therapy in diabetic diarrhea. *Arch Intern Med* 1991; **151:** 349–50.
47. Mourad FH, *et al.* Effective treatment of diabetic diarrhoea with somatostatin analogue, octreotide. *Gut* 1992; **33:** 1578–80.
48. Clark CM, Lee DA. Prevention and treatment of the complications of diabetes mellitus. *N Engl J Med* 1995; **332:** 1210–17.
49. West NJ. Systemic antimicrobial treatment of foot infections in diabetic patients. *Am J Health-Syst Pharm* 1995; **52:** 1199–1207.
50. Wieman TJ, *et al.* Efficacy and safety of a topical gel formulation of recombinant human platelet-derived growth factor-BB (becaplermin) in patients with chronic neuropathic diabetic ulcers: a phase III randomized placebo-controlled double-blind study. *Diabetes Care* 1998; **21:** 822–7.
51. Malmberg K, *et al.* Prospective randomised study of intensive insulin treatment on long term survival after acute myocardial infarction in patients with diabetes mellitus. *BMJ* 1997; **314:** 1512–15.
52. Yudkin JS. Which diabetic patients should be taking aspirin? *BMJ* 1995; **311:** 641–2.
53. American Diabetes Association. Aspirin therapy in diabetes. *Diabetes Care* 1997; **20:** 1772–3.
54. Grundy SM, *et al.* Diabetes and cardiovascular disease: a statement for healthcare professionals from the American Heart Association. *Circulation* 1999; **100:** 1134–46.
55. American Diabetes Association. Management of dyslipidemia in adults with diabetes. *Diabetes Care* 1999; **22:** (suppl 1): S56–9.
56. Haffner SM, *et al.* Reduced coronary events in simvastatin-treated patients with coronary heart disease and diabetes or impaired fasting glucose levels: subgroup analyses in the Scandinavian Simvastatin Survival Study. *Arch Intern Med* 1999; **159:** 2661–7.
57. Elam MB, *et al.* Effect of niacin on lipid and lipoprotein levels and glycemic control in patients with diabetes and peripheral arterial disease. The ADMIT study: a randomized trial. *JAMA* 2000; **284:** 1263–70.
58. Fatourechi V, *et al.* A practical guideline for management of hypertension in patients with diabetes. *Mayo Clin Proc* 1996; **71:** 53–8.
59. Haffner SM, *et al.* Mortality from coronary heart disease in subjects with type 2 diabetes and in nondiabetic subjects with and without prior myocardial infarction. *N Engl J Med* 1998; **339:** 229–34.
60. Barnett AH. Diabetes and hypertension. *Br Med Bull* 1994; **50:** 397–407.
61. Gilbert RE, *et al.* Diabetes and hypertension: Australian Diabetes Society position statement. *Med J Aust* 1995; **163:** 372–5.
62. Heart Outcomes Prevention Evaluation (HOPE) study investigators. Effects of ramipril on cardiovascular and microvascular outcomes in people with diabetes mellitus: results of the HOPE study and MICRO-HOPE substudy. *Lancet* 2000; **355:** 253–9. Correction. *ibid.*; **356:** 860.
63. Curb JD, *et al.* Effect of diuretic-based antihypertensive treatment on cardiovascular disease risk in older diabetic patients with isolated systolic hypertension. *JAMA* 1996; **276:** 1886–92. Correction. *ibid.* 1997; **277:** 1356.
64. Hansson L, *et al.* Effects of intensive blood-pressure lowering and low-dose aspirin in patients with hypertension: principal results of the Hypertension Optimal Treatment (HOT) randomised trial. *Lancet* 1998; **351:** 1755–62.

Diabetic emergencies

Hypoglycaemia. The most frequent complication of insulin therapy is hypoglycaemia and patients taking insulin need to be educated about its cause, symptoms, and treatment. Most patients can recognise the early warning signs of hypoglycaemia and by taking sugar immediately can prevent more serious symptoms developing. Comatose patients need to be given intravenous glucose or, if this is not practicable, subcutaneous, intramuscular, or intravenous glucagon (although glucose is still required if there is no response within 10 minutes). Hypoglycaemia can also develop in patients taking oral antidiabetics, notably the sulfonylureas.

Some patients report loss of the warning signs of hypoglycaemia after transferring from animal to human insulin and these patients, if appropriate, may need to be transferred back to animal insulin. However, the most significant factor in loss of hypoglycaemic warning signs may be exposure to hypoglycaemia itself; a study found that total avoidance of hypoglycaemic episodes for 3 weeks while maintaining glycaemic control restored awareness.[1] Loss of hypoglycaemic awareness, which appears to be due to an adaptive conservation of glucose uptake in the brain,[2] is liable to be a particular problem in patients receiving intensive therapy. In a single-dose study, caffeine 250 mg improved awareness of hypoglycaemia compared with placebo.[3]

For further details on the treatment of insulin-induced hypoglycaemia, see p.325.

Diabetic ketoacidosis is caused by an absolute or relative lack of insulin and commonly occurs after noncompliance or failure to adjust insulin dosage in the presence of factors such as infection that increase insulin requirements (see Precautions for Insulin, p.328). Failure of an insulin pump can be a cause.[4] Also pregnant diabetic women are more prone to development of diabetic ketoacidosis.

Diabetic ketoacidosis is characterised by hyperglycaemia, hyperketonaemia, and acidaemia, with subsequent dehydration and electrolyte abnormalities. Onset may be rapid, or insidious over many days. Initial presenting symptoms such as thirst, polyuria, fatigue, and weight loss are those of any newly presenting type 1 diabetic; they then progress to nausea, vomiting, abdominal pain, and impaired consciousness or coma, and, if untreated, death.[4,5]

Diabetic ketoacidosis is a medical emergency and should be treated immediately with fluid replacement and insulin.[4-7] Fluid requirements depend on the needs of the individual; over vigorous fluid replacement without severe dehydration carries the risk of precipitating cerebral oedema.[5-7]

Soluble insulin should also be administered immediately. Large doses were formerly thought necessary, but lower dose regimens accompanied by adequate hydration have since been shown to be preferable.[4] Insulin resistance in diabetic ketoacidosis is generally exacerbated by hyperosmolarity and other confounding factors, and insulin therapy is therefore most effective when preceded or accompanied by adequate fluid and electrolyte replacement.[4] In the UK, the *British National Formulary* considers that administration of insulin should preferably be by intravenous infusion, with the intramuscular route used if facilities for intravenous infusion are not available. However, in the USA some consider that an intravenous bolus followed by subcutaneous injection may be appropriate in certain patients.[4] Intramuscular or subcutaneous injection are not appropriate in patients with hypovolaemic shock due to poor tissue perfusion.[4] Where the response to insulin is inadequate the intravenous route is generally required[4] and the rate of infusion may be doubled on an hourly basis until an appropriate response is seen. A case report has suggested that mecasermin may be useful if there is insulin resistance.[8]

When the blood-glucose concentration has fallen to about 12.5 mmol per litre the dose of insulin may be reduced by about half and glucose is administered intravenously,[4] usually in a strength of 5% with saline although in rare cases a glucose strength of 10% may be necessary.[4] The administration of glucose enables insulin to be continued in order to clear ketone bodies without inducing hypoglycaemia. Once glucose concentrations have been controlled and acidosis has completely cleared, subcutaneous injections of insulin can be begun;[5] but intravenous insulin should not be stopped before subcutaneous administration has begun.

Total body stores of potassium are depleted in patients with diabetic ketoacidosis. Insulin deficiency appears to be the main initiating factor for hyperkalaemia in diabetic ketoacidosis.[9] Although patients may present with raised, normal, or decreased serum-potassium concentrations, the concentrations will start to fall with the correction of acidosis. Potassium is added to the infusion fluid after initial fluid expansion and once insulin therapy is commenced.[4] In hyperkalaemic patients, potassium is administered once serum concentrations have fallen to within normal limits.[4,5] In the rare patient presenting with hypokalaemia potassium replacement should be

The symbol † denotes a preparation no longer actively marketed

begun before insulin therapy and the latter withheld until potassium concentrations have risen to normal values.[4]

Intravenous bicarbonate is now generally reserved for patients with severe acidaemia; a common practice[4,5] is to give isotonic bicarbonate to those with a pH of less than 7.0 with the aim of raising the pH to 7.1.

Phosphate concentrations are affected in a similar manner to potassium concentrations in the ketoacidotic state, but there is less agreement on the need for routine phosphate administration. Phosphate concentrations should be monitored and phosphate administered if clinically significant hypophosphataemia occurs.[4,5]

The precipitating cause of diabetic ketoacidosis should also be identified and managed appropriately.

Hyperosmolar hyperglycaemic state or hyperosmolar hyperglycaemic nonketotic coma (HONK) occurs mainly in elderly patients with type 2 diabetes and though much less common than diabetic ketoacidosis it carries a higher mortality. Patients may present in coma with severe hyperglycaemia but with minimal ketosis; dehydration and renal impairment are common.[4] Treatment is similar to that of diabetic ketoacidosis (see above), although potassium requirements are lower and large amounts of fluid and less insulin may be required; some suggest the use of hypotonic fluid if necessary.[10] There is an increased likelihood of thrombotic events, so prophylactic anticoagulation should be considered.

1. Cranston I, *et al.* Restoration of hypoglycaemia awareness in patients with long-duration insulin-dependent diabetes. *Lancet* 1994; **344:** 283–7.
2. Boyle PJ, *et al.* Brain glucose uptake and unawareness of hypoglycaemia in patients with insulin-dependent diabetes mellitus. *N Engl J Med* 1995; **333:** 1726–31.
3. Debrah K, *et al.* Effect of caffeine on recognition of and physiological responses to hypoglycaemia in insulin-dependent diabetes. *Lancet* 1996; **347:** 19–24.
4. Kitabchi AE, *et al.* Management of hyperglycemic crises in patients with diabetes. *Diabetes Care* 2001; **24:** 131–53.
5. Lebovitz HE. Diabetic ketoacidosis. *Lancet* 1995; **345:** 767–72.
6. Adrogué HJ, *et al.* Salutary effects of modest fluid replacement in the treatment of adults with diabetic ketoacidosis: use in patients without extreme volume deficit. *JAMA* 1989; **262:** 2108–13.
7. Johnston D. Fluid replacement in diabetic ketoacidosis. *BMJ* 1992; **305:** 522.
8. Usala A-L, *et al.* Brief report: treatment of insulin-resistant diabetic ketoacidosis with insulin-like growth factor I in an adolescent with insulin-dependent diabetes. *N Engl J Med* 1992; **327:** 853–7.
9. Anonymous. Hyperkalaemia in diabetic ketoacidosis. *Lancet* 1986; **ii:** 845–6.
10. Wright AD. Diabetic emergencies in adults. *Prescribers' J* 1989; **29:** 147–54.

Acarbose (12304-c)

Acarbose (BAN, USAN, rINN).

Bay-g-5421. O-{4-Amino-4,6-dideoxy-N-[(1S,4R,5S,6S)-4,5,6-trihydroxy-3-hydroxymethylcyclohex-2-enyl]-α-D-glucopyranosyl}-(1→4)-O-α-D-glucopyranosyl-(1→4)-D-glucopyranose.
$C_{25}H_{43}NO_{18}$ = 645.6.
CAS — 56180-94-0.
ATC — A10BF01.

Adverse Effects

Acarbose may cause gastrointestinal disturbances, including flatulence due to bacterial action on non-absorbed carbohydrate in the colon. Abdominal distension, diarrhoea, and pain may occur. A decreased dosage of acarbose together with improved dietary habits may reduce these adverse effects. Hepatotoxicity may occur and may necessitate a reduction in dosage or withdrawal of the drug. Skin reactions have occurred rarely.

◊ The manufacturers reported that the incidence of adverse effects with acarbose was lower in a postmarketing surveillance study than in previous clinical trials;[1] this was held to represent better tailoring of individual doses to patient tolerability.

1. Spengler M, Cagatay M. The use of acarbose in the primary-care setting: evaluation of efficacy and tolerability of acarbose by postmarketing surveillance study. *Clin Invest Med* 1995; **18:** 325–31.

Effects on the liver. Reports of hepatocellular liver damage, with jaundice and elevated serum aminotransferases, in patients receiving acarbose.[1-3] Symptoms resolved on discontinuation of the drug.

1. Andrade RJ, *et al.* Hepatic injury caused by acarbose. *Ann Intern Med* 1996; **124:** 931.
2. Carrascosa M, *et al.* Acarbose-induced acute severe hepatotoxicity. *Lancet* 1997; **349:** 698–9.
3. Fujimoto Y, *et al.* Acarbose-induced hepatic injury. *Lancet* 1998; **351:** 340.

Precautions

Acarbose is contra-indicated in inflammatory bowel disease, particularly where there is associated ulceration, and in gastrointestinal obstruction or patients predisposed to it. It should be avoided in conditions which may deteriorate as a result of increased gas formation, such as hernia.

Acarbose is also contra-indicated in patients with hepatic impairment and liver enzyme values should be monitored at high doses.

Acarbose is not appropriate for pregnant patients or for those who are breast feeding.

If hypoglycaemia should develop in a patient receiving acarbose it needs to be treated with glucose, since the action of acarbose inhibits the hydrolysis of disaccharides.

Interactions

Acarbose may enhance the effects of other antidiabetics, including insulin, and may necessitate a reduction in their dosage. Concomitant administration of gastrointestinal adsorbents and digestive enzyme preparations may diminish the effects of acarbose and should be avoided. Neomycin and colestyramine may enhance the effects of acarbose and a reduction in its dosage may be required.

Pharmacokinetics

Following oral administration of acarbose, the majority of active unchanged drug remains in the lumen of the gastrointestinal tract to exert its pharmacological activity and is metabolised by intestinal enzymes and by the microbial flora. Ultimately about 35% of a dose is absorbed in the form of metabolites. Acarbose is excreted in the urine and faeces.

Uses and Administration

Acarbose is an inhibitor of alpha glucosidases, especially sucrase. Through this action it retards the digestion and absorption of carbohydrates in the small intestine and hence reduces the increase in blood-glucose concentrations after a carbohydrate load. It is given by mouth in the treatment of type 2 diabetes mellitus (p.315) either alone or combined with a sulfonylurea, biguanide, or insulin. Acarbose is given in a usual dose of 25 or 50 mg three times daily, immediately before food; treatment may be begun with 25 or 50 mg daily to minimise gastrointestinal disturbance. Doses up to 100 to 200 mg three times daily may be given if necessary. Some benefit has also been demonstrated when acarbose is used to supplement insulin therapy in type 1 diabetes mellitus.

Acarbose has also been studied for the treatment of reactive hypoglycaemia, the dumping syndrome, and certain types of hyperlipoproteinaemia.

◊ References.

1. Anonymous. Acarbose for non-insulin-dependent diabetes mellitus. *Drug Ther Bull* 1994; **32:** 51–3.
2. Chiasson J-L, *et al.* The efficacy of acarbose in the treatment of patients with non-insulin-dependent diabetes mellitus: a multi-center controlled clinical trial. *Ann Intern Med* 1994; **121:** 928–35.
3. Coniff RF, *et al.* Multicenter, placebo-controlled trial comparing acarbose (BAY g 5421) with placebo, tolbutamide, and tolbutamide-plus-acarbose in non-insulin-dependent diabetes mellitus. *Am J Med* 1995; **98:** 443–51.
4. Spengler M, Cagatay M. The use of acarbose in the primary-care setting: evaluation of efficacy and tolerability of acarbose by postmarketing surveillance study. *Clin Invest Med* 1995; **18:** 325–31.
5. Salvatore T, Giugliano D. Pharmacokinetic-pharmacodynamic relationships of acarbose. *Clin Pharmacokinet* 1996; **30:** 94–106.
6. Anonymous. Acarbose for diabetes mellitus. *Med Lett Drugs Ther* 1996; **38:** 9–10.
7. Hoffman J, Spengler M. Efficacy of 24-week monotherapy with acarbose, metformin, or placebo in dietary-treated NIDDM patients: the Essen-II study. *Am J Med* 1997; **103:** 483–90.
8. Hollander P, *et al.* Acarbose in the treatment of type 1 diabetes. *Diabetes Care* 1997; **20:** 248–53.
9. Buse J, *et al.* The PROTECT study: final results of a large multicenter postmarketing study in patients with type 2 diabetes. *Clin Ther* 1998; **20:** 257–69.
10. Holman RR, *et al.* A randomized double-blind trial of acarbose in type 2 diabetes shows improved glycemic control over 3 years (UK Prospective Diabetes Study 44). *Diabetes Care* 1999; **22:** 960–4.

Preparations

Proprietary Preparations (details are given in Part 3)
Aust.: Glucobay; *Austral.:* Glucobay; *Belg.:* Glucobay; *Braz.:* Glucobay; *Canad.:* Prandase; *Denm.:* Glucobay; *Fin.:* Glucobay;

320 Antidiabetics

Fr.: Glucor; *Ger.:* Glucobay; *Hong Kong:* Glucobay; *Irl.:* Glucobay; *Israel:* Prandase; *Ital.:* Glicobase; Glucobay; *Mex.:* Glucobay; *Neth.:* Glucobay; *Norw.:* Glucobay; *NZ:* Glucobay; *Port.:* Glucobay; *S.Afr.:* Glucobay; *Singapore:* Glucobay; *Spain:* Glucobay; Glumida; *Swed.:* Glucobay; *Switz.:* Glucobay; *Thai.:* Glucobay; *UK:* Glucobay; *USA:* Precose.

Acetohexamide (7213-j)

Acetohexamide *(BAN, USAN, rINN).*

Compound 33006. 1-(4-Acetylbenzenesulphonyl)-3-cyclohexylurea.

$C_{15}H_{20}N_2O_4S = 324.4.$

CAS — 968-81-0.

ATC — A10BB31.

Pharmacopoeias. In *Jpn,* and *US.*

Pharmacopoeial description

USP 25: A white, practically odourless, crystalline powder. Practically insoluble in water and in ether; soluble 1 in 230 of alcohol and 1 in 210 of chloroform; soluble in pyridine and in dilute solutions of alkali hydroxides.

Profile

Acetohexamide is a sulfonylurea antidiabetic (p.334). Its duration of action is 12 hours or more. It is given by mouth in the treatment of type 2 diabetes mellitus (p.315) in a usual initial dose of 250 mg daily before breakfast. The daily dose may then be increased by 250 to 500 mg at intervals of 5 to 7 days, to a maintenance dose of up to 1.5 g daily; increasing the dose above 1.5 g daily does not usually lead to further benefit. Doses in excess of 1 g daily may be taken in 2 divided doses, before the morning and evening meals.

Preparations

USP 25: Acetohexamide Tablets.

Proprietary Preparations (details are given in Part 3)
Canad.: Dimelor†; *Hong Kong:* Dimelor; *S.Afr.:* Dimelor; *USA:* Dymelor.

Biguanide Antidiabetics (17495-w)

Adverse Effects

Gastrointestinal adverse effects including anorexia, nausea, and diarrhoea may occur with biguanides; patients may experience a metallic taste and there may be weight loss. Absorption of various substances including vitamin B_{12} may be impaired.

Hypoglycaemia is rare with a biguanide given alone, although it may occur if other contributing factors or drugs are present.

Lactic acidosis, sometimes fatal, has occurred with biguanides, primarily with phenformin. When it has occurred with metformin most cases have been in patients whose condition contra-indicated the use of the drug, particularly those with renal impairment.

Phenformin has been implicated in the controversial reports of excessive cardiovascular mortality associated with oral hypoglycaemic therapy (see under Sulfonylureas, Effects on the Cardiovascular System, p.334).

◊ A review of the adverse effects of biguanide therapy.[1]

1. Paterson KR, *et al.* Undesired effects of biguanide therapy. *Adverse Drug React Acute Poisoning Rev* 1984; 3: 173–82.

Effects on the blood. Megaloblastic anaemia has occurred with biguanide therapy (see Malabsorption, under Effects on the Gastrointestinal Tract, below). A case of metformin-induced haemolysis resulting in hyperbilirubinaemia and jaundice has also been described.[1]

1. Lin K-D, *et al.* Metformin-induced hemolysis with jaundice. *N Engl J Med* 1998; 339: 1860–1.

Effects on the gastrointestinal tract. DIARRHOEA. In a retrospective survey,[1] 30 of 265 diabetic patients reported diarrhoea or alternating diarrhoea and constipation, comprising: 11 of 54 taking metformin; 9 of 45 taking metformin with a sulfonylurea; 3 of 53 taking a sulfonylurea only; 5 of 78 on insulin therapy; 2 of 35 on diet alone. Among 150 nondiabetic controls 12 reported diarrhoea.

1. Dandona P, *et al.* Diarrhea and metformin in a diabetic clinic. *Diabetes Care* 1983; 6: 472–4.

MALABSORPTION. Megaloblastic anaemia due to vitamin B_{12} malabsorption in a 58-year-old woman was associated with long-term treatment with metformin.[1]

In a survey of diabetic patients receiving biguanide therapy,[2] malabsorption of vitamin B_{12} was observed in 14 of 46 diabetics taking metformin or phenformin; metformin was more

commonly to blame. Withdrawal of the drug resulted in normal absorption in only 7 of the 14.

1. Callaghan TS, *et al.* Megaloblastic anaemia due to vitamin B_{12} malabsorption associated with long-term metformin treatment. *BMJ* 1980; 280: 1214–15.
2. Adams JF, *et al.* Malabsorption of vitamin B_{12} and intrinsic factor secretion during biguanide therapy. *Diabetologia* 1983; 24: 16–18.

Effects on the liver. A report of severe cholestatic hepatitis attributed to metformin.[1]

1. Babich MM, *et al.* Metformin-induced acute hepatitis. *Am J Med* 1998; 104: 490–2.

Hypersensitivity. Vasculitis and pneumonitis in a 59-year-old woman was associated with administration of metformin.[1] Symptoms improved on withdrawal of metformin, but reappeared on its reintroduction.

1. Klapholz L, *et al.* Leucocytoclastic vasculitis and pneumonitis induced by metformin. *BMJ* 1986; 293: 483.

Hypoglycaemia. The UK manufacturers of metformin state that hypoglycaemia does not occur with metformin alone, even in overdosage, although it may occur if given with alcohol or other hypoglycaemics. Interim results from the UK Prospective Diabetes Study,[1] however, indicate that metformin therapy was associated with fewer hypoglycaemic episodes than sulfonylurea or insulin treatment, but more than with diet alone. One or more hypoglycaemic episodes were reported in 6% of the patients receiving the biguanide in this study, although only 1 patient had a severe episode.

1. United Kingdom Prospective Diabetes Study Group. United Kingdom prospective diabetes study (UKPDS) 13: relative efficacy of randomly allocated diet, sulphonylurea, insulin, or metformin in patients with newly diagnosed non-insulin dependent diabetes followed for 3 years. *BMJ* 1995; 310: 83–8.

Lactic acidosis. References to lactic acidosis associated with use of biguanide antidiabetics.[1-12] Most recent reports implicate metformin, the most widely used biguanide, although cases of phenformin-associated lactic acidosis still occur.[10,11] From 1995, when metformin was introduced in the USA, until June 1996, the FDA had received reports of metformin-associated lactic acidosis in 66 patients,[12] the diagnosis being confirmed in 47. This represented a rate of about 5 cases per 100 000. Almost all patients with confirmed lactic acidosis had 1 or more risk factors such as cardiac or chronic hypoxic pulmonary disease, or renal insufficiency.

1. Anonymous. Biguanides and lactic acidosis in diabetics. *BMJ* 1977; 2: 1436.
2. Misbin RI. Phenformin-associated lactic acidosis: pathogenesis and treatment. *Ann Intern Med* 1977; 87: 591–5.
3. Bergman U, *et al.* Epidemiology of adverse drug reactions to phenformin and metformin. *BMJ* 1978; 2: 464–6.
4. Korhonen T, *et al.* Biguanide-induced lactic acidosis in Finland. *Eur J Clin Pharmacol* 1979; 15: 407–10.
5. McGuiness ME, Talbert RL. Phenformin-induced lactic acidosis: a forgotten adverse drug reaction. *Ann Pharmacother* 1993; 27: 1183–7.
6. Monson JP. Metformin and lactic acidosis. *Prescribers' J* 1993; 33: 170–3.
7. Wilholm B-E, Myrhed M. Metformin-associated lactic acidosis in Sweden 1977–1991. *Eur J Clin Pharmacol* 1993; 44: 589–91.
8. Khan IH, *et al.* Severe lactic acidosis in patient receiving continuous ambulatory peritoneal dialysis. *BMJ* 1993; 307: 1056–7.
9. Pearlman BL, *et al.* Metformin-associated lactic acidosis. *Am J Med* 1996; 101: 109–10.
10. Rosand J, *et al.* Fatal phenformin-associated lactic acidosis. *Ann Intern Med* 1997; 127: 170.
11. Enia G, *et al.* Lactic acidosis induced by phenformin is still a public health problem in Italy. *BMJ* 1997; 315: 1466–7.
12. Misbin RI, *et al.* Lactic acidosis in patients with diabetes treated with metformin. *N Engl J Med* 1998; 338: 265–6.

Pancreatitis. References to acute pancreatitis associated with phenformin.

1. Wilde H. Pancreatitis and phenformin. *Ann Intern Med* 1972; 77: 324.
2. Chase HS, Mogan GR. Phenformin-associated pancreatitis. *Ann Intern Med* 1977; 87: 314–15.

Treatment of Adverse Effects

Acute poisoning with biguanides may lead to the development of lactic acidosis (p.1180) and calls for intensive supportive therapy. Glucose or glucagon may be required for hypoglycaemia, the general management of which is outlined in Insulin, p.325.

Precautions

Biguanides are inappropriate for patients with diabetic coma and ketoacidosis, or for those with severe infection, trauma, or other severe conditions where the biguanide is unlikely to control the hyperglycaemia; insulin should be administered in such situations. Biguanides should not be given to patients with even mild impairment of renal function, as it may predispose patients to lactic acidosis, and renal function should be monitored throughout therapy. Biguanides should also not be given to patients with heart failure, recent myocardial infarction, dehydration, alcoholism, hepatic impairment, or any other condition likely to predispose to lactic acidosis. Biguanides should be temporarily stopped 48 hours before exam-

inations using contrast media because of the risk of contrast media-induced renal impairment.

Insulin is preferred for the treatment of diabetes in pregnancy.

Owing to the possibility of decreased vitamin B_{12} absorption, annual monitoring of vitamin B_{12} concentrations is advisable during long-term treatment.

Driving. In the UK, patients with diabetes mellitus treated with insulin or oral hypoglycaemics are required to notify their condition to the Driver and Vehicle Licensing Agency, who then assess their fitness to drive. Patients treated with oral hypoglycaemics are generally allowed to retain standard driving licences; those treated with insulin receive restricted licences which must be renewed (with appropriate checks) every 1 to 3 years. Patients should be warned of the dangers of hypoglycaemic attacks while driving, and should be counselled in appropriate management of the situation (stopping driving as soon as it is safe to do so, taking carbohydrate immediately, and quitting the driving seat and removing the ignition key from the car) should such an event occur. Patients who have lost hypoglycaemic awareness, or have frequent hypoglycaemic episodes, should not drive. In addition, eyesight must be adequate (field of vision of at least 120°) for a licence to be valid. Patients treated with diet or oral hypoglycaemics are normally allowed to hold vocational driving licences for heavy goods vehicles or passenger carrying vehicles; those treated with insulin may not drive such vehicles, and are restricted in driving some other vehicles such as small lorries and minibuses.

1. British Diabetic Association (Diabetes UK). *Information sheet: driving and diabetes: Aug 2001.* Available at: http://www.diabetes.org.uk/info/inform/drive.doc (accessed 13/09/01).

Interactions

Use of a biguanide concomitantly with other drugs that lower blood-glucose concentrations increases the risk of hypoglycaemia, while drugs that increase blood glucose may reduce the effect of biguanide therapy.

In general fewer drug interactions have been reported with biguanides than with sulfonylureas. Alcohol may increase the risk of lactic acidosis as well as of hypoglycaemia. Care should be taken if biguanides are given concomitantly with drugs that may impair renal function.

Anticoagulants. For the effect of metformin on *phenprocoumon,* see Antidiabetics, p.995.

Cimetidine. Cimetidine administration resulted in increased plasma-metformin concentrations in 7 healthy subjects.[1] The renal clearance of metformin was reduced; competition for proximal tubular secretion was considered responsible. A reduction in metformin dosage may be required in patients taking metformin and cimetidine concomitantly in order to reduce the risk of lactic acidosis.

1. Somogyi A, *et al.* Reduction of metformin renal tubular secretion by cimetidine in man. *Br J Clin Pharmacol* 1987; 23: 545–51.

Ketotifen. Platelet counts in 10 diabetic patients receiving biguanides fell (markedly in 3 patients) when they were also given ketotifen.[1] Counts returned to normal a few days after the end of ketotifen therapy. However, the investigators did not consider the effect clinically significant.

1. Doleček R. Ketotifen in the treatment of diabetics with various allergic conditions. *Pharmatherapeutica* 1981; 2: 568–74.

Sulfonylureas. For reference to an apparent increase in mortality with an intensive regimen of metformin plus a sulfonylurea, see p.336.

Uses and Administration

The biguanide antidiabetics are a class of antidiabetic drugs given by mouth in the treatment of type 2 diabetes mellitus (p.315). They are used to supplement treatment by diet modification when such modification has not proved effective on its own. In addition, because biguanides are not associated with weight gain they are preferred in obese patients. Although sulfonylureas (p.334) may be preferred in non-obese patients, a biguanide is often added or given instead to patients who are not responding to a sulfonylurea.

The mode of action of biguanides is not clear. They do not stimulate insulin release but require that some insulin be present in order to exert their hypoglycaemic effect. Possible mechanisms of action include delay in the absorption of glucose from the gastrointestinal tract, an increase in insulin sensitivity and glucose uptake into cells, and inhibition of hepatic gluconeogenesis. Biguanides do not usually lower blood-glucose concentrations in non-diabetic subjects.

Hyperlipidaemias. The effect of biguanides on lipid metabolism is unclear although some studies have demonstrated a lowering of blood concentrations of very low-density-lipoprotein cholesterol and total cholesterol.[1] Such effects may be beneficial in the long-term treatment of type 2 diabetes mellitus with concomitant lipid disorders.[2,3] For a discussion of the treatment of hyperlipidaemias, see p.800.

1. Schäfer G. Biguanides: a review of history, pharmacodynamics and therapy. *Diabete Metab* 1983; **9:** 148–63.
2. Rains SGH, *et al.* The reduction of low density lipoprotein cholesterol by metformin is maintained with long-term therapy. *J R Soc Med* 1989; **82:** 93–4.
3. Lalor BC, *et al.* Placebo-controlled trial of the effects of guar gum and metformin on fasting blood glucose and serum lipids in obese, type 2 diabetic patients. *Diabetic Med* 1990; **7:** 242–5.

Polycystic ovary syndrome. For discussion of the potential of metformin in polycystic ovary syndrome, see p.333.

Buformin (14764-j)

Buformin (USAN, pINN).
DBV; W-37. 1-Butylbiguanide.
$C_6H_{15}N_5 = 157.2$.
CAS — 692-13-7 (buformin); 1190-53-0 (buformin hydrochloride).
ATC — A10BA03.

Profile
Buformin is a biguanide antidiabetic (p.320). It is given by mouth in the treatment of type 2 diabetes mellitus (p.315) in doses of up to 300 mg daily. The hydrochloride has also been used.

Preparations
Proprietary Preparations (details are given in Part 3)
Spain: Silubin; *Switz.:* Silubin.

Carbutamide (7215-c)

Carbutamide (BAN, rINN).
BZ-55; Ca-1022; Glybutamide; U-6987. 1-Butyl-3-sulphanilylurea.
$C_{11}H_{17}N_3O_3S = 271.3$.
CAS — 339-43-5.
ATC — A10BB06.
Pharmacopoeias. In It.

Profile
Carbutamide is a sulfonylurea antidiabetic (p.334). It is given by mouth in the treatment of type 2 diabetes mellitus (p.315) in single daily doses of 0.5 to 1 g, but is more toxic than chlorpropamide.

Preparations
Proprietary Preparations (details are given in Part 3)
Aust.: Invenol†; *Fr.:* Glucidoral.

Chlorpropamide (7216-k)

Chlorpropamide (BAN, rINN).
Chlorpropamidum. 1-(4-Chlorobenzenesulphonyl)-3-propylurea.
$C_{10}H_{13}ClN_2O_3S = 276.7$.
CAS — 94-20-2.
ATC — A10BB02.
Pharmacopoeias. In Chin., Eur. (see p.vi), Jpn, Pol., and US.

Pharmacopoeial description
Ph. Eur.: A white, crystalline powder. It exhibits polymorphism. Practically insoluble in water; soluble in alcohol; freely soluble in acetone and in dichloromethane; dissolves in dilute solutions of alkali hydroxides. Protect from light.
USP 25: A white crystalline powder having a slight odour. Practically insoluble in water; soluble in alcohol; sparingly soluble in chloroform.

Adverse Effects and Treatment
As for sulfonylureas in general, p.334.
Chlorpropamide may be more likely than other sulfonylureas to induce a syndrome of inappropriate secretion of antidiuretic hormone characterised by water retention, hyponatraemia, and CNS effects. Patients receiving chlorpropamide may develop facial flushing after drinking alcohol.

Precautions
As for sulfonylureas in general, p.335.
Chlorpropamide should be avoided in the elderly and in renal or hepatic impairment because its long half-life increases the risk of hypoglycaemia. Some manufacturers recommend that chlorpropamide should not be used in patients with severe impairment of thyroid function. The antidiuretic effect of chlorpropa-

mide may cause problems in patients with conditions associated with fluid retention.

Porphyria. Chlorpropamide has been associated with acute attacks of porphyria and is considered unsafe in porphyric patients.

Interactions
As for sulfonylureas in general, p.335.
Chlorpropamide may produce profound facial flushing in association with alcohol ingestion.

Pharmacokinetics
Chlorpropamide is readily absorbed from the gastrointestinal tract and is extensively bound to plasma proteins. The half-life is about 35 hours. About 80% of a dose is metabolised in the liver; metabolites and unchanged drug are excreted in the urine. Chlorpropamide crosses the placenta and has been detected in breast milk.

Uses and Administration
Chlorpropamide is a sulfonylurea antidiabetic (p.334). It has a duration of action of at least 24 hours, and is given by mouth in the treatment of type 2 **diabetes mellitus** (p.315) in an initial daily dose of 250 mg as a single dose with breakfast. It is usual to adjust this dose after 5 to 7 days to achieve an optimum maintenance dose which is usually in the range 100 to 500 mg daily; increasing the dose above 500 mg is unlikely to produce further benefit. Although a reduced dose range has been proposed for the elderly, use of chlorpropamide is inadvisable in this group.
Chlorpropamide, though not the other sulfonylureas, is also sometimes used in cranial **diabetes insipidus** (p.1273). It has been reported to act by sensitising the renal tubules to antidiuretic hormone. The dose has to be carefully adjusted to minimise the risk of hypoglycaemia. An initial dose of 100 mg daily, adjusted if necessary to a maximum of 350 mg daily has been recommended, although doses of up to 500 mg daily have been used.

Diabetes mellitus. Patients with type 2 diabetes whose blood glucose is adequately controlled at first by sulfonylureas often eventually experience treatment failure and loss of diabetic control. Results from the UK Prospective Diabetes Study[1] have suggested that the 6-year failure rate was higher in patients treated with glibenclamide (48%) than in those given chlorpropamide (40%). This difference was equivalent to delaying the requirement for additional therapy for a year in chlorpropamide-treated patients.

1. Matthews DR, *et al.* UKPDS 26: sulphonylurea failure in non-insulin-dependent diabetic patients over six years. *Diabetic Med* 1998; **15:** 297–303.

Preparations
BP 2001: Chlorpropamide Tablets;
USP 25: Chlorpropamide Tablets.
Proprietary Preparations (details are given in Part 3)
Austral.: Diabinese; *Belg.:* Diabinese; *Braz.:* Diabinese; *Canad.:* Diabinese; Novo-Propamide†; *Fr.:* Diabinese†; *Hong Kong:* Diabinese†; *Irl.:* Diabinese; *Israel:* Diabinese; *Ital.:* Diabemide; Diabexan†; *Mex.:* Deavynfar; Diabiclor; Diabinese; Insogen; *Norw.:* Diabinese†; *S.Afr.:* Diabinese; Diabitex; Hypomide; *Singapore:* Chlomide; Diabinese; Propamide; *Spain:* Diabinese; *Swed.:* Diabinese; *Switz.:* Diabinese†; *Thai.:* Diabeedol; Diabinese; Dibecon; Glycemin; Propamide; *UK:* Diabinese†; Glymese; *USA:* Diabinese.
Multi-ingredient: *Ital.:* Bidiabe; Pleiamide; *Mex.:* Insogen Plus; Mellitron; Obinese; *Switz.:* Diabiformine.

Emiglitate (18830-k)

Emiglitate (BAN, rINN).
Bay-o-1248. Ethyl 4-(2-[(2R,3R,4R,5S)-3,4,5-trihydroxy-2-(hydroxymethyl)piperidino]ethoxy)benzoate.
$C_{17}H_{25}NO_7 = 355.4$.
CAS — 80879-63-6.

Profile
Emiglitate is an alpha-glucosidase inhibitor similar in action to acarbose (p.319). It is given by mouth and has been investigated for the management of diabetes mellitus.

◊ References.
1. Lembcke B, *et al.* Inhibition of sucrose- and starch-induced glycaemic and hormonal responses by the α-glucosidase inhibitor emiglitate (BAY o 1248) in healthy volunteers. *Eur J Clin Pharmacol* 1991; **41:** 561–7.

Epalrestat (2905-h)

Epalrestat (rINN).
ONO-2235. 5-[(Z,E)-β-Methylcinnamilidene]-4-oxo-2-thioxo-3-thiazolidineacetic acid.
$C_{15}H_{13}NO_3S_2 = 319.4$.
CAS — 82159-09-9.

Profile
Epalrestat is an aldose reductase inhibitor similar in action to tolrestat (p.337). It is given by mouth for the treatment of diabetic complications including neuropathy (p.317).

◊ References.
1. Goto Y, *et al.* A placebo-controlled double-blind study of epalrestat (ONO-2235) in patients with diabetic neuropathy. *Diabetic Med* 1993; **10** (suppl 2): 39S–43S.
2. Ucluda K, *et al.* Effect of 24 weeks of treatment with epalrestat, an aldose reductase inhibitor, on peripheral neuropathy in patients with non-insulin-dependent diabetes mellitus. *Clin Ther* 1995; **17:** 460–6.

Preparations
Proprietary Preparations (details are given in Part 3)
Jpn: Kinedak.

Glibenclamide (7217-a)

Glibenclamide (BAN, rINN).
Glibenclamidum; Glybenclamide; Glybenzcyclamide; Glyburide (USAN); HB-419; U-26452. 1-{4-[2-(5-Chloro-2-methoxybenzamido)ethyl]benzenesulphonyl}-3-cyclohexylurea.
$C_{23}H_{28}ClN_3O_5S = 494.0$.
CAS — 10238-21-8.
ATC — A10BB01.
NOTE. The name glibornuride has frequently but erroneously been applied to glibenclamide.
Pharmacopoeias. In Chin., Eur. (see p.vi), Int., Jpn, Pol., and US.

Pharmacopoeial description
Ph. Eur.: A white or almost white, crystalline powder. Practically insoluble in water and in ether; slightly soluble in alcohol and in methyl alcohol; sparingly soluble in dichloromethane; dissolves in dilute solutions of alkali hydroxides.
USP 25: Store in airtight containers.

Adverse Effects, Treatment, and Precautions
As for sulfonylureas in general, p.334.

◊ For a suggestion that the failure rate in type 2 diabetics treated with glibenclamide may be higher than that for those treated with chlorpropamide, see Diabetes Mellitus under Uses and Administration of Chlorpropamide, p.321.

Effects on the blood. References.
1. Nataas OB, Nesthus I. Immune haemolytic anaemia induced by glibenclamide in selective IgA deficiency. *BMJ* 1987; **295:** 366–7.

Hypoglycaemia. Severe hypoglycaemia may occur in any patient treated with any sulfonylurea (see p.335); this potentially life-threatening complication requires prolonged and energetic treatment.[1] Glibenclamide has a relatively prolonged duration of action and appears to cause severe hypoglycaemia more often than shorter-acting sulfonylureas such as tolbutamide.
In a review[2] of 57 instances of hypoglycaemia associated with glibenclamide the median age of patients affected was 70 years; only one was less than 60 years old. Median daily dosage was 10 mg. Coma or disturbed consciousness was observed in 46 patients. Ten of these remained comatose despite alleviation of their hypoglycaemia and died up to 20 days after presentation. In discussing their review, the authors reported that, including the present series of 57 cases, there had been published reports on 101 severe hypoglycaemias with glibenclamide, 14 with a fatal outcome.
There has been a report[3] of hypoglycaemic coma associated with the inhalation of glibenclamide by a worker at a pharmaceutical plant.

1. Ferner RE, Neil HAW. Sulphonylureas and hypoglycaemia. *BMJ* 1988; **296:** 949–50.
2. Asplund K, *et al.* Glibenclamide-associated hypoglycaemia: a report on 57 cases. *Diabetologia* 1983; **24:** 412–17.
3. Albert F, *et al.* Hypoglycaemia by inhalation. *Lancet* 1993; **342:** 47–8.

Porphyria. Glibenclamide has been associated with acute attacks of porphyria and is considered unsafe in porphyric patients.

Interactions
As for sulfonylureas in general, p.335.

Pharmacokinetics
Glibenclamide is readily absorbed from the gastrointestinal tract, peak plasma concentrations usually occurring within 2 to 4 hours, and is extensively bound to plasma proteins. Absorption may be slower in

hyperglycaemic patients and may differ according to the particle size of the preparation used. It is metabolised, almost completely, in the liver, the principal metabolite being only very weakly active. Approximately 50% of a dose is excreted in the urine and 50% via the bile into the faeces.

◊ References.
1. Coppack SW, *et al.* Pharmacokinetic and pharmacodynamic studies of glibenclamide in non-insulin dependent diabetes mellitus. *Br J Clin Pharmacol* 1990; **29:** 673–84.
2. Jaber LA, *et al.* The pharmacokinetics and pharmacodynamics of 12 weeks of glyburide therapy in obese diabetics. *Eur J Clin Pharmacol* 1993; **45:** 459–63.
3. Hoffman A, *et al.* The effect of hyperglycaemia on the absorption of glibenclamide in patients with non-insulin-dependent diabetes mellitus. *Eur J Clin Pharmacol* 1994; **47:** 53–5.
4. Rydberg T, *et al.* Concentration-effect relations of glibenclamide and its active metabolites in man: modelling of pharmacokinetics and pharmacodynamics. *Br J Clin Pharmacol* 1997; **43:** 373–81.

Uses and Administration
Glibenclamide is a sulfonylurea antidiabetic (p.334). It is given by mouth in the treatment of type 2 diabetes mellitus (p.315) and has a duration of action of up to 24 hours.

The usual initial dose of conventional formulations in type 2 diabetes mellitus is 2.5 to 5 mg daily with breakfast, adjusted every 7 days by increments of 2.5 mg daily up to 15 mg daily. Although increasing the dose above 15 mg is unlikely to produce further benefit, doses of up to 20 mg daily have been given. Doses greater than 10 mg daily may be given in 2 divided doses. Because of the relatively long duration of action of glibenclamide, it is best avoided in the elderly.

In some countries micronised preparations of glibenclamide are available, in which the drug is formulated with a smaller particle size, and which have enhanced bioavailability. The usual initial dose of one such preparation (Glynase, USA) is 1.5 to 3 mg daily, adjusted every 7 days by increments of 1.5 mg, up to a usual maximum of 12 mg daily. Doses greater than 6 mg daily may be given in 2 divided doses.

Action. Proceedings of a symposium on the mechanism of action of glibenclamide.[1]
1. Gavin JR, ed. Glyburide: new insights into its effects on the beta cell and beyond. *Am J Med* 1990; **89** (suppl 2A): 1–53S.

EFFECTS ON THE HEART. A reduced incidence of ventricular fibrillation has been reported in diabetics treated with glibenclamide who develop myocardial infarction, compared with those receiving other treatments or with nondiabetic patients with myocardial infarction.[1] However, some evidence has also suggested that sulfonylureas may impair the adaptive responses of the heart to ischaemia—see p.334.
1. Lomuscio A, *et al.* Effects of glibenclamide on ventricular fibrillation in non-insulin-dependent diabetes with acute myocardial infarction. *Coron Artery Dis* 1994; **5:** 767–71.

Preparations
BP 2001: Glibenclamide Tablets;
USP 25: Glyburide Tablets.

Proprietary Preparations (details are given in Part 3)
Aust.: Dia-Eptal; Euglucon; Gewaglucon; Gilemal; Glucobene; Neogluconin; Normoglucon; Semi-Euglucon; *Austral.:* Daonil; Euglucon†; Glimel; Semi-Daonil; *Belg.:* Bevoren; Daonil; Euglucon; *Braz.:* Aglucil; Daonil; Euglucon; Lisaglucon; *Canad.:* Dia-Beta; Euglucon; Gen-Glybe; *Denm.:* Daonil; Euglucon; Hexaglucon; *Fin.:* Daonil; Euglamin; Euglucon; Origlucon; Semi-Euglucon; *Fr.:* Daonil; Euglucan; Hemi-Daonil; Miglucan; *Ger.:* Azuglucon; Bastiverit; Dia-BASF; duraglucon N; Euglucon N; Glib; Glib-ratiopharm; Gliben; Gliben-Azu; Gliben-Puren N; Glibenbeta; Glibendoc; Glibenhexal; Glimidstada; Gluco-Tablinen†; Gluconorm; Glucoremed; Glukoreduct; Glukovital; glycolande N; Humedia; Maninil; Praeciglucon; Semi-Euglucon N; Semi-Gliben-Puren N; *Hong Kong:* Calabren; Daonil; Euglucon; GBN; Gliboral; Glimel; Melix; Semi-Euglucon; *Irl.:* Daonil; Melbetese†; Semi-Daonil; *Israel:* Daonil; Glibetic; Gluben; *Ital.:* Daonil; Euglucon; Gliben; Gliboral; *Jpn:* Euglucon†; *Mex.:* Daonil; Dibetid; Euglucon; Glibenil; Glicoxem; Glifarcal; Glucal; Glucoven; Nadib; Norboral; Reglusan; Salugliben; *Neth.:* Daonil; Euglucon†; Hemi-Daonil; Semi-Euglucon†; *Norw.:* Daonil; Euglucon; NZ: Daonil; Gliben; Semi-Daonil; *Port.:* Daonil; Euglucon; Semi-Daonil; Semi-Euglucon; *S.Afr.:* Cliniben†; Daonil; Euglucon; Glyben; Glycomin; Melix†; Semi-Daonil†; *Singapore:* Clamide; Daonil; Dibelet; Euglucon; GBN; Glibemid; Glibesyn; Glimide; *Spain:* Daonil; Euglucon; Glucolon; Norglicem; *Swed.:* Daonil; Euglucon; GBN; gli-basan; Glibesifar; Melix; Semi-Euglucon; *Switz.:* Daonil; Diabetamide; Euglucon; Semi-Euglucon; *Thai.:* Benclamin; BNIL; Cytagon; Daonil; Debtan; Diabenol; Dibelet; Diclanil; Euglucon; Gliben; Glibesyn; Glibetic; Glibic; Gluconil; Gluzo; Med-Glionil; Semi-Euglucon; Sugril; *UAE:* Glynase; *UK:* Calabren; Daonil; Diabetamide; Euglucon; Malix; Semi-Daonil; *USA:* DiaBeta; Glynase; Micronase.

Multi-ingredient: *Ital.:* Bi-Euglucon; Bi-Euglucon M; Gliben F; Glibomet; Gliconorm; Gliformin; Glucomide; Suguan; Suguan

M; *Mex.:* Bi-Euglucon M; Dabex G; Glinorboral; Sil-Norboral; *USA:* Glucovance.

Glibornuride (7218-t)
Glibornuride (BAN, USAN, rINN).
Ro-6-4563. 1-[(2S,3R)-2-Hydroxyborn-3-yl]-3-tosylurea; 1-[(2S,3R)-2-Hydroxyborn-3-yl]-3-*p*-tolylsulphonylurea.
$C_{18}H_{26}N_2O_4S = 366.5.$
CAS — 26944-48-9.
ATC — A10BB04.

NOTE. The name glibornuride has frequently but erroneously been applied to glibenclamide.

Profile
Glibornuride is a sulfonylurea antidiabetic (p.334). It is given by mouth in the treatment of type 2 diabetes mellitus (p.315) in doses of 12.5 to 75 mg daily; up to 100 mg daily has occasionally been given. Daily doses of 50 mg or more are given in 2 divided doses.

Preparations
Proprietary Preparations (details are given in Part 3)
Aust.: Gluborid; Glutril; *Fr.:* Glutril; *Ger.:* Gluborid; Glutril; *Switz.:* Gluborid; Glutril.

Gliclazide (7220-y)
Gliclazide (BAN, rINN).
Gliclazidum; Glyclazide; SE-1702. 1-(3-Azabicyclo[3.3.0]oct-3-yl)-3-tosylurea; 1-(3-Azabicyclo[3.3.0]oct-3-yl)-3-*p*-tolylsulphonylurea.
$C_{15}H_{21}N_3O_3S = 323.4.$
CAS — 21187-98-4.
ATC — A10BB09.
Pharmacopoeias. In *Eur.* (see p.vi).

Pharmacopoeial description
Ph. Eur.: A white or almost white powder. Practically insoluble in water; slightly soluble in alcohol; sparingly soluble in acetone; freely soluble in dichloromethane.

Adverse Effects, Treatment, and Precautions
As for sulfonylureas in general, p.334.

It has been suggested that gliclazide may be suitable for use in patients with renal impairment, but careful monitoring of blood-glucose concentration is essential. The UK manufacturers recommend that it should not be used in patients with severe renal impairment.

Interactions
As for sulfonylureas in general, p.335.

Pharmacokinetics
Gliclazide is readily absorbed from the gastrointestinal tract. It is extensively bound to plasma proteins. The half-life is about 10 to 12 hours. Gliclazide is extensively metabolised in the liver to metabolites that have no significant hypoglycaemic activity. Metabolites and a small amount of unchanged drug are excreted in the urine.

◊ References.
1. Kobayashi K, *et al.* Pharmacokinetics of gliclazide in healthy and diabetic subjects. *J Pharm Sci* 1984; **73:** 1684–7.

Uses and Administration
Gliclazide is a sulfonylurea antidiabetic (p.334). It is given by mouth in the treatment of type 2 diabetes mellitus (p.315) and has a duration of action of 12 hours or more. Because its effects are less prolonged than those of chlorpropamide or glibenclamide it may be more suitable for elderly patients, who are prone to hypoglycaemia with longer-acting sulfonylureas. The usual initial dose is 40 to 80 mg daily, gradually increased, if necessary, up to 320 mg daily. Doses of more than 160 mg daily are given in 2 divided doses. A modified release tablet is also available: the usual initial dose is 30 mg once daily, increased if necessary up to a maximum of 120 mg daily.

◊ References.
1. Holmes B, *et al.* Gliclazide: a preliminary review of its pharmacodynamic properties and therapeutic efficacy in diabetes mellitus. *Drugs* 1984; **27:** 301–27.

2. Palmer KJ, Brogden RN. Gliclazide: an update of its pharmacological properties and therapeutic efficacy in non-insulin-dependent diabetes mellitus. *Drugs* 1993; **46:** 92–125.
3. Mailhot J. Efficacy and safety of gliclazide in the treatment of non-insulin-dependent diabetes mellitus: a Canadian multicenter study. *Clin Ther* 1993; **15:** 1060–8.

Preparations
BP 2001: Gliclazide Tablets.

Proprietary Preparations (details are given in Part 3)
Aust.: Diamicron; *Austral.:* Diamicron; Glyade; *Belg.:* Diamicron; *Braz.:* Diamicron; *Canad.:* Diamicron; *Denm.:* Diamicron; *Fr.:* Diamicron; Glycemirex; *Ger.:* Diamicron; *Hong Kong:* Diamicron; *Irl.:* Diabrezide; Diamicron; *Ital.:* Diabrezide; Diamicron; *Mex.:* Diamicron; *Neth.:* Diamicron; *NZ:* Diamicron; *Port.:* Diamicron; *S.Afr.:* Diamicron; Glycron; Ziclin; *Singapore:* Diamicron; Glimicron; Glucozide; Medoclazide; Sun-Glizide; *Spain:* Diamicron; *Switz.:* Diamicron; *Thai.:* Cadicon; Diabeside; Diaclaron; Dialoc; Diamexon; Diamicron; Glicron; Glucozide; Glycon; Serviclazide; *UAE:* Glyzide; *UK:* Diaglyk; Diamicron.

Glimepiride (2804-x)
Glimepiride (BAN, USAN, rINN).
Hoe-490. 1-({*p*-[2-(3-Ethyl-4-methyl-2-oxo-3-pyrroline-1-carboxamido)ethyl]phenyl}sulfonyl)-3-(*trans*-4-methylcyclohexyl)urea.
$C_{24}H_{34}N_4O_5S = 490.6.$
CAS — 93479-97-1.
ATC — A10BB12.

Adverse Effects, Treatment, and Precautions
As for sulfonylureas in general, p.334. In some countries hepatic and haematological monitoring is recommended in patients receiving glimepiride.

Interactions
As for sulfonylureas in general, p.335.

Pharmacokinetics
Glimepiride is completely absorbed from the gastrointestinal tract. Peak plasma concentrations occur in 2 to 3 hours, and it is highly protein bound. The drug is extensively metabolised to two main metabolites, a hydroxy derivative and a carboxy derivative. The half-life after multiple doses is about 9 hours. Approximately 60% of a dose is eliminated in the urine and 40% in the faeces.

Uses and Administration
Glimepiride is a sulfonylurea antidiabetic (p.334). It is given by mouth for the treatment of type 2 diabetes mellitus (p.315). Doses of 1 to 2 mg daily by mouth initially may be increased if necessary to 4 mg daily for maintenance. The maximum recommended dose is 6 mg in the UK and 8 mg in the USA.

◊ References.
1. Langtry HD, Balfour JA. Glimepiride: a review of its use in the management of type 2 diabetes mellitus. *Drugs* 1998; **55:** 563–84.
2. Campbell RK. Glimepiride: role of a new sulfonylurea in the treatment of type 2 diabetes mellitus. *Ann Pharmacother* 1998; **32:** 1044–52.

Preparations
Proprietary Preparations (details are given in Part 3)
Aust.: Amaryl; *Austral.:* Amaryl; *Belg.:* Amarylle; *Denm.:* Amaryl; *Fr.:* Amarel; *Ger.:* Amaryl; *Hong Kong:* Amaryl; *Irl.:* Amaryl; *Ital.:* Amaryl; *Mex.:* Amaryl; *Neth.:* Amaryl; *Norw.:* Amaryl; *Port.:* Amaryl; *S.Afr.:* Amaryl; *Singapore:* Amaryl; *Spain:* Amaryl; Roname; *Swed.:* Amaryl; *Switz.:* Amaryl; *Thai.:* Amaryl; *UK:* Amaryl; *USA:* Amaryl.

Multi-ingredient: *Ital.:* Solosa.

Glipizide (7222-z)
Glipizide (BAN, USAN, pINN).
CP-28720; Glipizidum; Glydiazinamide; K-4024. 1-Cyclohexyl-3-{4-[2-(5-methylpyrazine-2-carboxamido)ethyl]benzenesulphonyl}urea.
$C_{21}H_{27}N_5O_4S = 445.5.$
CAS — 29094-61-9.
ATC — A10BB07.
Pharmacopoeias. In *Eur.* (see p.vi) and *US.*

Pharmacopoeial description
Ph. Eur.: A white or almost white crystalline powder. Practically insoluble in water and in alcohol; sparingly soluble in acetone; soluble in dichloromethane. It dissolves in dilute solutions of alkali hydroxides.
USP 25: Store in airtight containers. Protect from light.

Adverse Effects, Treatment, and Precautions
As for sulfonylureas in general, p.334.

Porphyria. Glipizide has been associated with acute attacks of porphyria and is considered unsafe in porphyric patients.

Interactions
As for sulfonylureas in general, p.335.

Antacids. *Magnesium hydroxide* and *sodium bicarbonate* have been reported to increase the rate of absorption, although not the total amount absorbed, of a dose of glipizide in healthy subjects.[1,2] No such effect was seen with *aluminium hydroxide*.[2]

1. Kivisto KT, Neuvonen PJ. Enhancement of absorption and effect of glipizide by magnesium hydroxide. *Clin Pharmacol Ther* 1991; **49:** 39–43.
2. Kivisto KT, Neuvonen PJ. Differential effects of sodium bicarbonate and aluminium hydroxide on the absorption and activity of glipizide. *Eur J Clin Pharmacol* 1991; **40:** 383–6.

Pharmacokinetics
Glipizide is readily absorbed from the gastrointestinal tract with peak plasma concentrations occurring 1 to 3 hours after a single dose. It is extensively bound to plasma proteins and has a half-life of approximately 2 to 4 hours. It is metabolised mainly in the liver and excreted chiefly in the urine, largely as inactive metabolites.

Uses and Administration
Glipizide is a sulfonylurea antidiabetic (p.334). It is given by mouth in the treatment of type 2 diabetes mellitus (p.315) and has a duration of action of up to 24 hours. The usual initial dose is 2.5 to 5 mg daily given as a single dose 15 to 30 minutes before breakfast. Dosage may be adjusted at intervals of several days by amounts of 2.5 to 5 mg daily, to a maximum of 20 mg daily. Doses up to 40 mg daily have been used, but see below. Doses larger than 15 mg daily are given in two divided doses before meals. Modified-release formulations of glipizide are available in some countries; one such preparation (Glucotrol XL, USA) is given in doses of 5 to 10 mg daily as a single dose with breakfast.

Administration. Although glipizide may be given in doses up to a maximum of 40 mg daily, evidence for the benefits of high doses is scanty. A small study in patients with type 2 diabetes mellitus found that not only did increases in glipizide doses to more than 10 mg daily produce little or no benefit, but that the higher doses were associated with reduced rises in plasma-insulin concentrations and a lesser reduction in plasma-glucose concentrations.[1] There is, however, some evidence that glycaemic control and insulin sensitivity can be improved by the use of a modified-release rather than a conventional formulation of glipizide.[2,3]

1. Stenman S, *et al.* What is the benefit of increasing the sulfonylurea dose? *Ann Intern Med* 1993; **118:** 169–72.
2. Berelowitz M, *et al.* Comparative efficacy of once-daily controlled-release formulation of glipizide and immediate-release glipizide in patients with NIDDM. *Diabetes Care* 1994; **17:** 1460–4.
3. Leaf E, King JO. Patient outcomes after formulary conversion from immediate-release to extended-release glipizide tablets. *Am J Health-Syst Pharm* 1999; **56:** 454–6.

Preparations
BP 2001: Glipizide Tablets;
USP 25: Glipizide Tablets.

Proprietary Preparations (details are given in Part 3)
Aust.: Glibenese; Minidiab; *Austral.:* Melizide; Minidiab; *Belg.:* Glibenese; Minidiab; *Braz.:* Minidiab; *Denm.:* Glibenese; Minidiab; *Fin.:* Apamid; Glibenese; Melizid; Minidiab; *Fr.:* Minidiab; Ozidia; *Ger.:* Glibenese†; *Hong Kong:* Glidiab; Glucotrol; Minidiab; *Irl.:* Glibenese; *Israel:* Gluco-Rite; *Ital.:* Minidiab; *Mex.:* Glupital; Minodiab; *Neth.:* Glibenese; Norw.:* Apamid; Minidiab; *NZ:* Glipid; Minidiab; *Port.:* Minidiab; *S.Afr.:* Minidiab; *Singapore:* Diasef; Melizide; Minidiab; *Spain:* Glibenese; Minodiab; *Swed.:* Apamid; Glibenese†; Glipiscand; Mindiab; *Switz.:* Glibenese; *Thai.:* Diasef; Dipazide; Glygen; Melizide; Minidiab; *UK:* Glibenese; Minodiab; *USA:* Glucotrol.

Gliquidone (7223-c)
Gliquidone *(BAN, rINN).*
ARDF-26. 1-Cyclohexyl-3-{4-[2-(3,4-dihydro-7-methoxy-4,4-dimethyl-1,3-dioxo-2(1*H*)-isoquinolyl)ethyl]benzenesulphonyl}urea.
$C_{27}H_{33}N_3O_6S = 527.6$.
CAS — 33342-05-1.
ATC — A10BB08.
Pharmacopoeias. In Br.

Pharmacopoeial description
BP 2001: A white or almost white powder. Practically insoluble in water; slightly soluble in alcohol and in methyl alcohol; soluble in acetone; freely soluble in dimethylformamide.

Adverse Effects, Treatment, and Precautions
As for sulfonylureas in general, p.334.

Since renal excretion plays little part in the elimination of gliquidone, it has been suggested that it may be suitable in patients with renal impairment, but careful monitoring of blood-glucose concentration is essential. The UK manufacturers recommend that it should not be used in patients with severe renal impairment.

Interactions
As for sulfonylureas in general, p.335.

Pharmacokinetics
Gliquidone is readily absorbed from the gastrointestinal tract. It is extensively bound to plasma proteins and has a half-life of approximately 1.5 hours. It is extensively metabolised in the liver, the metabolites having no significant hypoglycaemic effect, and is eliminated chiefly in the faeces via the bile; only about 5% of a dose is excreted in the urine.

The symbol † denotes a preparation no longer actively marketed

Uses and Administration
Gliquidone is a sulfonylurea antidiabetic (p.334). It is given by mouth in the treatment of type 2 diabetes mellitus (p.315) in a usual initial dosage of 15 mg daily given as a single dose up to 30 minutes before breakfast. Dosage may be adjusted by increments of 15 mg to a usual dose of 45 to 60 mg daily in 2 or 3 unequally divided doses, the largest dose being taken in the morning with breakfast. Single doses above 60 mg and daily doses above 180 mg are not recommended.

Preparations
BP 2001: Gliquidone Tablets.
Proprietary Preparations (details are given in Part 3)
Aust.: Glurenorm; *Belg.:* Glurenorm; *Ger.:* Glurenorm; *Ital.:* Glurenor; *Port.:* Glurenor; *Spain:* Glurenor; *Thai.:* Glurenor; *UK:* Glurenorm.

Glisentide (12786-b)
Glisentide *(rINN).*
Glipentide. 1-Cyclopentyl-3-[*p*-(2-o-anisamidoethyl)benzenesulphonyl]urea.
$C_{22}H_{27}N_3O_5S = 445.5$.
CAS — 32797-92-5.

Profile
Glisentide is a sulfonylurea antidiabetic (p.334). It is given by mouth in the treatment of type 2 diabetes mellitus (p.315) in doses of 2.5 to 20 mg daily.

Preparations
Proprietary Preparations (details are given in Part 3)
Spain: Staticum.

Glisolamide (12787-v)
Glisolamide *(rINN).*
1-Cyclohexyl-3-{*p*-[2-(5-methylisoxazole-3-carboxamido)ethyl]benzenesulphonyl}urea.
$C_{20}H_{26}N_4O_5S = 434.5$.
CAS — 24477-37-0.

Profile
Glisolamide is a sulfonylurea antidiabetic (p.334). It is given by mouth in the treatment of type 2 diabetes mellitus (p.315) in doses of 5 to 20 mg daily.

Preparations
Proprietary Preparations (details are given in Part 3)
Ital.: Diabenor.

Glisoxepide (7224-k)
Glisoxepide *(BAN, rINN).*
Bay-b-4231; FBB-4231; Glisoxepid; RP-22410. 1-(Perhydroazepin-1-yl)-3-{4-[2-(5-methylisoxazole-3-carboxamido)ethyl]benzenesulphonyl}urea.
$C_{20}H_{27}N_5O_5S = 449.5$.
CAS — 25046-79-1.
ATC — A10BB11.

Profile
Glisoxepide is a sulfonylurea antidiabetic (p.334). It is given by mouth in the treatment of type 2 diabetes mellitus (p.315) in a usual initial dose of 2 to 4 mg daily at breakfast, increased if necessary to up to 16 mg daily in divided doses.

Preparations
Proprietary Preparations (details are given in Part 3)
Aust.: Pro-Diaban; *Ger.:* Pro-Diaban.

Glybuzole (7225-a)
Glybuzole *(rINN).*
AN-1324; Désaglybuzole; RP-7891. *N*-(5-*tert*-Butyl-1,3,4-thiadiazol-2-yl)benzenesulphonamide.
$C_{12}H_{15}N_3O_2S_2 = 297.4$.
CAS — 1492-02-0.

Profile
Glybuzole is an oral antidiabetic with a structure distinct from that of the sulfonylureas, biguanides, or sulfonamidopyrimidines.

Glyclopyramide (7226-t)
Glyclopyramide *(rINN).*
1-(4-Chlorobenzenesulphonyl)-3-(pyrrolidin-1-yl)urea.
$C_{11}H_{14}ClN_3O_3S = 303.8$.
CAS — 631-27-6.

Profile
Glyclopyramide is a sulfonylurea antidiabetic (p.334). It has been given by mouth in the treatment of type 2 diabetes mellitus.

Glycyclamide (7227-x)
Glycyclamide *(rINN).*
Gliciclamide; K-38; K-386; Tolcyclamide. 1-Cyclohexyl-3-tosylurea; 1-Cyclohexyl-3-*p*-tolylsulphonylurea.
$C_{14}H_{20}N_2O_3S = 296.4$.
CAS — 664-95-9.

Profile
Glycyclamide is a sulfonylurea antidiabetic (p.334). It is given by mouth in the treatment of type 2 diabetes mellitus.

Preparations
Proprietary Preparations (details are given in Part 3)
Ital.: Diaborale.

Glymidine Sodium (7228-r)
Glymidine Sodium *(BAN, USAN, rINN).*
Glycodiazine; Glymidine; SH-717. *N*-[5-(2-Methoxyethoxy)pyrimidin-2-yl]benzenesulphonamide sodium.
$C_{13}H_{14}N_3NaO_4S = 331.3$.
CAS — 3459-20-9 (glymidine sodium); 339-44-6 (glymidine).
ATC — A10BC01.

Profile
Glymidine sodium is a sulfonamidopyrimidine antidiabetic; its actions and uses are similar to those of the sulfonylureas (p.334) and it has been given by mouth in the treatment of type 2 diabetes mellitus.

Guar Gum (5427-l)
E412; Guar Flour; Guar Galactomannan; Jaguar Gum.
CAS — 9000-30-0.
ATC — A10BX01.
Pharmacopoeias. In Eur. (see p.vi). Also in USNF.

Pharmacopoeial description
Ph. Eur.: Guar is obtained by grinding the endosperms of the seeds of *Cyamopsis tetragonolobus*. It consists mainly of guar galactomannan. Guar is a white or almost white powder, yielding a mucilage of variable viscosity when dissolved in water. Practically insoluble in alcohol.
Guar Galactomannan is a yellowish-white powder. It is soluble in cold and hot water; practically insoluble in organic solvents. Its main components are polysaccharides composed of D-galactose and D-mannose at molecular ratios of 1:1.4 to 1:2. The molecules consist of a linear main chain of β-(1→4)-glycosidically linked mannopyranoses and single α-(1→6)-glycosidically linked galactopyranoses.
USNF 20: A gum obtained from the ground endosperms of *Cyamopsis tetragonolobus* (Leguminosae). It consists chiefly of a high-molecular-weight hydrocolloidal polysaccharide, a galactomannan, composed of galactan and mannan units combined through glycosidic linkages. It is a white to yellowish-white, practically odourless, powder. Dispersible in hot or cold water forming a colloidal solution.

Adverse Effects and Precautions
Guar gum can cause gastrointestinal disturbance with flatulence, diarrhoea, or nausea, particularly at the start of treatment.

Because guar gum swells on contact with liquid it should always be washed down carefully with water and should not be taken immediately before going to bed. It should not be used in patients with oesophageal disease or intestinal obstruction.

Interactions
Guar gum may retard the absorption of other drugs given concomitantly; where this is likely to pose a problem the other drug should be taken at least an hour before administration of guar gum.

Uses and Administration
Guar gum is used in diabetes mellitus (p.315) as an adjunct to treatment with diet, insulin, or oral antidiabetics since it results in some reduction in both postprandial and fasting blood-glucose concentrations. It is given with or immediately before meals in doses of 5 g usually three times daily. Adverse gastrointestinal effects may be decreased by initial administration of 5 g once daily. Each dose of guar gum granules should be taken stirred in about 200 mL of a cold drink. Alternatively it can be sprinkled over or mixed with food which must be taken accompanied by about 200 mL of fluid. Guar gum has also been incorporated into various foods.

Guar gum is also used to slow gastric emptying in some patients with the dumping syndrome (p.1203). It is being investigated in the treatment of hyperlipidaemias.

Guar gum is also used as a thickening and suspending agent, and as a tablet binder.

◊ Guar gum is an example of a soluble fibre.[1] On contact with water it forms a highly viscous gel, the viscosity of which varies with such factors as its plant source or the form in which it is administered.[2]

Fibres such as guar gum reduce postprandial and fasting blood-glucose concentrations as well as plasma-insulin concentrations in healthy subjects and diabetic patients.[1,3,4] Such reductions in blood-glucose concentrations and in glycosylated haemoglobin have been demonstrated in both type 1 and type 2 **diabetes,** but they have generally been small.[3] Possible mechanisms for these effects of guar gum include a delay in gastric emptying,[1,3-5] decreased small-bowel motility,[1,4] decreased glucose absorption resulting from increased viscosity of the contents of the gastrointestinal tract,[1,3] or inhibition of gastrointestinal hormones.[3]

Guar gum also lowers serum total cholesterol and low-density-lipoprotein (LDL) cholesterol concentrations; high-density-lipoprotein (HDL) cholesterol and triglyceride concentrations appear to be unaffected.[4] The most likely mechanism is binding of bile acids, reducing their enterohepatic circulation in a similar way to bile-acid sequestrants.[3,4] When used alone in patients with **hypercholesterolaemia** guar gum has generally produced a modest reduction in plasma-cholesterol and LDL-cholesterol concentrations although some studies have been unable to demonstrate an effect. A few studies have suggested that the cholesterol-lowering effect is attenuated after 8 to 12 weeks of treatment but a long-term study observed a 17% decrease in total serum cholesterol that was maintained for 24 months.[6] Preliminary studies have shown further reductions in cholesterol and LDL-cholesterol concentrations on addition of guar gum to therapy with other lipid regulating drugs. The usual treatment of hyperlipidaemias is discussed on p.800.

There have been suggestions that guar gum reduces appetite by promoting a feeling of fullness, but a meta-analysis has indicated that it is not effective for reducing body weight.[7] Products containing guar gum have, however, been promoted as **slimming aids.** Their use cannot be advocated because of the risk of tablets swelling before reaching the stomach and causing oesophageal obstruction.

1. Hockaday TDR. Fibre in the management of diabetes 1: natural fibre useful as part of total dietary prescription. *BMJ* 1990; **300:** 1334–6.
2. Ellis PR, *et al.* Guar gum: the importance of reporting data on its physico-chemical properties. *Diabetic Med* 1986; **3:** 490–1.
3. Anonymous. Guar gum: of help to diabetics? *Drug Ther Bull* 1987; **25:** 65–7.
4. Todd PA, *et al.* Guar gum: a review of its pharmacological properties, and use as a dietary adjunct in hypercholesterolaemia. *Drugs* 1990; **39:** 917–28.
5. Tattersall R, Mansell P. Fibre in the management of diabetes 2: benefits of fibre itself are uncertain. *BMJ* 1990; **300:** 1336–7.
6. Salenius J-P, *et al.* Long term effects of guar gum on lipid metabolism after carotid endarterectomy. *BMJ* 1995; **310:** 95–6.
7. Pittler MH, Ernst E. Guar gum for body weight reduction: meta-analysis of randomized trials. *Am J Med* 2001; **110:** 724–30.

Preparations

Proprietary Preparations (details are given in Part 3)
Austral.: Benefiber; *Fin.:* Guarem; *Ger.:* Glucotard†; Guar Verlan; Lejguar; *Hong Kong:* Guarem; *Irl.:* Guarem; *Israel:* Guarem; *Spain:* Biotropic†; Fibraguar; Plantaguar; *Switz.:* Leiguar; Lubo; *UK:* Guarem; Resource Benefiber.

Multi-ingredient: *Belg.:* Mucipulgite; *Fr.:* Moxydar; Mucipulgite; Mulkine; *Ital.:* Cruscasohn; Resource Gelificata; *Port.:* Fibra Light; *Switz.:* Demosvelte N†; Mucipulgite; *UK:* Lipolest.

Insulin (7202-e)

Insulinum.

CAS — 9004-10-8 (insulin; neutral insulin); 11070-73-8 (bovine insulin); 12584-58-6 (porcine insulin); 11061-68-0 (human insulin); 8063-29-4 (biphasic insulin); 9004-21-1 (globin zinc insulin); 68859-20-1 (insulin argine); 8049-62-5 (insulin zinc suspensions); 53027-39-7 (isophane insulin); 9004-17-5 (protamine zinc insulin); 116094-23-6 (insulin aspart); 9004-12-0 (dalanated insulin); 51798-72-2 (bovine insulin defalan); 11091-62-6 (porcine insulin defalan); 160337-95-1 (insulin glargine); 133107-64-9 (insulin lispro).

ATC — A10AB01 (human); A10AB02 (beef); A10AB03 (pork); A10AB04 (lispro); A10AC01 (human); A10AC02 (beef); A10AC03 (pork); A10AC04 (lispro); A10AD01 (human); A10AD02 (beef); A10AD03 (pork); A10AD04 (lispro); A10AE01 (human); A10AE02 (beef); A10AE03 (pork).

Pharmacopoeias. Most pharmacopoeias define a variety of insulin preparations. See also below.

Definitions and Terminology

Insulin is a hormone produced by the beta cells of the islets of Langerhans of the pancreas and consists of 2 chains of amino acids, the A and B chains, connected by 2 disulfide bridges. Insulin produced by different species conforms to the same basic structure but has different sequences of amino acids in the chains. **Porcine insulin** ($C_{256}H_{381}N_{65}O_{76}S_6 = 5777.5$) differs from **human insulin** ($C_{257}H_{383}N_{65}O_{77}S_6 = 5807.6$) in only one amino acid in the B chain whereas **bovine insulin** ($C_{254}H_{377}N_{65}O_{75}S_6 = 5733.5$) differs from human insulin not only in this same amino acid in the B chain but also in 2 amino acids in the A chain.

The precursor of insulin in the pancreas is proinsulin which is a single polypeptide chain incorporating both the A and B chains of insulin connected by a peptide termed the C-peptide (or connecting-peptide). Although the insulins of various species may be similar in composition the proinsulins are not, in that the sequence and number of amino acids in the C-peptide may vary considerably.

Insulin (USP 25) is of either bovine or porcine origin; the USP 25 also allows mixed bovine and porcine origin. **Bovine Insulin** and **Porcine Insulin** are separate monographs in the Ph. Eur. **Human Insulin** (Ph. Eur.) is produced either by the enzymatic modification and suitable purification of porcine insulin or by recombinant DNA technology in micro-organisms. **Insulin Human** (USP 25) is produced similarly.

Early commercial insulins were obtained by extraction from bovine or porcine or mixed bovine and porcine pancreases and were purified by recrystallisation only. Insulins obtained by such methods were often termed '**conventional insulins**' to distinguish them from insulins which have undergone further purification processes. An extract which has been recrystallised only once can be separated into 3 components or fractions termed the 'a', 'b', and 'c' components. The 'a' component consists of high molecular weight substances and is only usually found in very impure preparations since repeated recrystallisation will remove most of it. The 'b' component consists largely of proinsulin and insulin dimers, and the 'c' component consists of insulin, insulin esters, arginine insulin, and desamidoinsulin. Other pancreatic peptides such as glucagon, pancreatic polypeptide, somatostatin, and vasoactive intestinal peptide are also usually found in products which have not undergone further purification. Gel filtration will substantially reduce the content of proinsulin but will not significantly reduce the content of insulin derivatives or pancreatic peptides; products purified by gel filtration are often termed '**single-peak insulins**'. Addition of ion-exchange chromatography to the purification methods will further reduce the proinsulin content and also reduce the contamination by insulin derivatives and pancreatic peptides. In the UK '**highly purified insulins**' and '**monocomponent insulins**' are terms sometimes applied to insulins which have undergone both gel filtration and ion-exchange chromatography. In the USA the FDA has designated the term '**purified insulins**' for preparations similarly prepared and containing less than 10 ppm of proinsulin.

Much of the insulin now produced has an amino-acid sequence identical to that of human insulin. **Human insulin (emp)** is produced by the enzymatic modification of insulin obtained from the porcine pancreas; it is also sometimes called **semisynthetic human insulin.** The term **human insulin (crb)** is used for insulin produced by the chemical combination of A and B chains which have been obtained from bacteria genetically modified by recombinant DNA technology. **Human insulin (prb)** is produced from proinsulin obtained from bacteria genetically modified by recombinant DNA technology. **Human insulin (pyr)** is insulin produced from a precursor obtained from a yeast genetically modified by recombinant DNA technology. Human insulin obtained by recombinant

DNA technology is sometimes termed **biosynthetic human insulin.**

Insulin or human insulin is supplied in a variety of forms in solution or suspension for injection (see Table 2, p.326). Crystalline insulin may be prepared for therapeutic use merely by making a solution, either of acidic or neutral pH. **Soluble insulin** or '**neutral insulin**' is a short-acting preparation that can be given intravenously if necessary to cover emergencies. Soluble formulations are sometimes referred to as '**regular insulin**' or '**unmodified insulin**'; these names reflect the fact that the preparation has not been formulated in order to prolong the duration of action of the insulin.

In order to prolong the duration of action of insulin, preparations may be formulated as suspensions in 2 general ways. The first involves complexing insulin with a protein from which it is slowly released; examples are **protamine zinc insulin**, which contains an excess of protamine, and **isophane insulin** (NPH insulin), which contains equimolecular amounts of insulin and protamine. The second method of prolonging the action of insulin is to modify the particle size and the various **insulin zinc suspensions** are in this category.

Biphasic insulins are mixtures providing for both immediate and prolonged action.

Chemical modification of the insulin molecule has resulted in insulins such as **dalanated insulin** (prepared by the removal of the C-terminal alanine from the B chain of insulin), **insulin defalan** (prepared by the removal of the terminal phenylalanine), and **sulfated insulin**, but these insulins have not been widely used.

More recently, recombinant DNA technology has enabled production of insulin analogues with altered pharmacokinetic profiles. **Insulin lispro** is one such analogue, in which the B28 and B29 amino acid residues of human insulin are replaced with lysine and proline. It is available as a rapidly acting alternative to soluble insulin and as an intermediate-acting complex with protamine. Other insulin analogues include **insulin glargine** (HOE-901), a long-acting form used for once-daily administration, and a variety of others such as **insulin aspart**; further information on these can be found under Insulin Analogues and Proinsulin under Uses, below.

Stability and Storage

Insulin in powder form should be stored in airtight containers and protected from light. Storage at a low temperature is also recommended. The Ph. Eur. advises storage at a temperature of −20° while the USP 25 requires storage at −10° to −25°. It is stressed that this temperature is for the powder and not for the preparations; preparations should not be subjected to storage conditions that lead to freezing.

Both the Ph. Eur. and the USP 25 recommend that insulin preparations be stored in a refrigerator at 2° to 8°, protected from light, and not be allowed to freeze. It is recognised that patients may not follow such stringent storage guidelines and most manufacturers of commercial insulin preparations consider that storage by the patient at a temperature of up to 25° would be acceptable for up to one month. Patients should still be advised not to expose their vials or cartridges to excessive heat or sunlight.

It is advisable to shake suspensions gently before a dose is withdrawn.

Adsorption. The adsorption of insulin onto glass and plastics used in giving sets has been decreased by the addition of albumin or polygeline to insulin solutions. Some workers consider this to be unnecessary since in practice insulin adsorption is not a major problem.[1,2] Running approximately 10 mL of the insulin solution through the intravenous tubing before beginning the infusion has been suggested by some.[2]

1. Alberti KGMM. Diabetic emergencies. *Br Med Bull* 1989; **45:** 242–63.
2. Sanson TH, Levine SN. Management of diabetic ketoacidosis. *Drugs* 1989; **38:** 289–300.

Aggregation. For discussion of the problems of insulin aggregation, see Intensive Administration Regimens under Uses, below.

Units

One unit of *bovine insulin* is contained in 0.03891 mg of the first International Standard (1986). One unit of *porcine insulin* is contained in 0.03846 mg of the first

International Standard (1986). One unit of *human insulin* is contained in 0.03846 mg of the first International Standard (1986).

Adverse Effects

The most frequent complication of insulin therapy is hypoglycaemia, the speed of onset and duration of which may vary according to the type of preparation used and the route of administration. It is usually associated with an excessive dosage of insulin, the omission of a meal by the patient, or increased physical activity. Patients, especially the elderly or those with tightly controlled diabetes or diabetes of long standing, may not experience the typical early warning symptoms of a hypoglycaemic attack. There have been reports of hypoglycaemia, sometimes with decreased warning symptoms, in patients changing from animal (especially bovine) to human insulin (see under Hypoglycaemia, below). Symptoms of hypoglycaemia resulting from increased sympathetic activity include hunger, pallor, sweating, palpitations, anxiety, and tremulousness. Other symptoms include headache, visual disturbances such as blurred or double vision, slurred speech, paraesthesia of the mouth and fingers, alterations in behaviour, and impaired mental or intellectual ability. If untreated, hypoglycaemia may lead to convulsions and coma which should not be confused with hyperglycaemic coma.

Insulin, administered subcutaneously, may cause either lipoatrophy or lipohypertrophy. Lipoatrophy appears to occur less frequently with purified insulins than with conventional insulins; if it has occurred, it may be reversed by the injection of a purer animal insulin or human insulin into and around the atrophied site. Lipohypertrophy is usually associated with repeated injections at the same site and may usually be overcome by rotating the site of injection, although it should be remembered that absorption of insulin may vary from different anatomical areas. Prolonged insulin therapy may result in weight gain.

Insulin may occasionally cause local or systemic hypersensitivity reactions. Local reactions, characterised by erythema and pruritus at the injection site, usually disappear with continued treatment. Generalised hypersensitivity may produce urticaria, angioedema, and very rarely anaphylactic reactions; if continued therapy with insulin is essential hyposensitisation procedures may need to be performed. Again, hypersensitivity reactions are observed less frequently with purified than with conventional insulins and porcine insulin is less immunogenic than bovine insulin. Although hypersensitivity reactions have been reported in patients transferred from animal to human insulins, there are only isolated reports of such reactions in patients treated exclusively with human insulin.

Many patients treated with insulin, either animal or human insulin, develop antibodies but the clinical significance of this is not entirely clear.

◊ Of patients who received intensive insulin therapy for type 1 diabetes as part of the Diabetes Control and Complications Trial, those who experienced the greatest weight gain also had increased blood concentrations of triglycerides and low-density-lipoprotein cholesterol, and lowered high-density-lipoprotein cholesterol.[1] These lipid changes, together with higher blood pressure, increased waist-to-hip ratio, and greater insulin requirements, were held to be similar to the symptoms of insulin resistance and to indicate a possible increased risk of macrovascular disease. Results from the UK Prospective Diabetes Study indicated that type 2 diabetic patients treated with insulin had greater weight gain than those managed with other therapies,[2] but demonstrated no evidence of harmful cardiovascular effects.

For discussion of some of the specific problems associated with continuous infusion of insulin, see Intensive Administration Regimens under Uses, below.

1. Purnell JQ, *et al.* Effect of excessive weight gain with intensive therapy of type 1 diabetes on lipid levels and blood pressure: results from the DCCT. *JAMA* 1998; **280**: 140–6. Correction. *ibid.*; 1484.
2. UK Prospective Diabetics Study (UKPDS) Group. Intensive blood-glucose control with sulphonylureas or insulin compared with conventional treatment and risk of complications in patients with type 2 diabetes (UKPDS 33). *Lancet* 1998; **352**: 837–53.

The symbol † denotes a preparation no longer actively marketed

Antibody formation. A review of human insulin including a discussion on the clinical importance of insulin antibodies.[1] Both pork and human insulin are definitely less immunogenic than beef insulin producing fewer circulating insulin antibodies, but several studies have indicated no detectable change in antibody concentrations on switching from pork to human insulin or *vice versa*. Antibodies cause lipoatrophy and are responsible for the substantial insulin resistance seen in some patients, but with purified pork insulin in common use, both events became rare. Interest has been revived in the possible contribution of antibodies in modifying metabolic control. In the short term and under hospital conditions, they are known to prolong the intravenous half-life of injected insulin and to delay the appearance in the circulation of a subcutaneously administered bolus dose. Patients with moderate concentrations of antibodies are also reported to show delay in recovery from induced hypoglycaemia, but on the other hand to lose control less quickly after insulin withdrawal and thus may be relatively protected from ketoacidosis.

1. Pickup J. Human insulin. *BMJ* 1986; **292**: 155–7.

Effects on the liver. For a report of hepatomegaly occurring after insulin overdosage, see under Abuse, in Precautions, below.

Effects on the skin. Delayed pressure urticaria, in the form of large wheals occurring 4 to 6 hours after prolonged pressure, and lasting for up to 24 hours, was seen in a patient with type 1 diabetes within 6 months of changing from animal to human insulin.[1] The condition improved following a switch back to insulin of animal origin, and became aggravated again following a second attempt to switch to human insulin.

1. Payne CMER, *et al.* True delayed pressure urticaria induced by human Monotard insulin. *Br J Dermatol* 1996; **134**: 184.

Hypersensitivity. Hypersensitivity reactions to insulin preparations may be caused not only by the insulin itself, but also by other components of the formulation such as zinc[1] or protamine.[2]

See also under Antibody Formation, above and under Precautions, below.

1. Feinglos MN, Jegasothy BV. "Insulin" allergy due to zinc. *Lancet* 1979; **i**: 122–4.
2. Sánchez MB, *et al.* Protamine as a cause of generalised allergic reactions to NPH insulin. *Lancet* 1982; **i**: 1243.

HYPOSENSITISATION. Following failure of standard hyposensitisation measures in a patient with cutaneous hypersensitivity to insulin, hyposensitisation was attempted by giving insulin by mouth.[1] Aspirin 1.3 g three times daily by mouth was also given to antagonise vascular mediators of the reaction. After one week subsequent hyposensitisation using insulin by injection was successful. When the patient stopped taking aspirin after 8 months the original hypersensitivity reactions recurred; aspirin was then given permanently in a dose of 1.3 g twice daily.

1. Holdaway IM, Wilson JD. Cutaneous insulin allergy responsive to oral desensitisation and aspirin. *BMJ* 1984; **289**: 1565–6.

Hypoglycaemia. Hypoglycaemia is the major adverse effect of insulin treatment with severe hypoglycaemic episodes in up to a third of all insulin-treated patients at some point in their lives. Moves towards more intensive insulin therapy, in order to reduce the development of diabetic complications, increase the risk of hypoglycaemic episodes.[1,2] This may be connected with the fact that patients maintaining strict glycemic control are prone to 'hypoglycaemia unawareness' in which the normal adrenergic counter-response to hypoglycaemia (characterised by symptoms such as pallor, sweating, and tremor) is reduced or lost,[3] so that hypoglycaemia can develop without warning. Such a loss of awareness of impending hypoglycaemia also seems to develop in diabetics as disease duration increases.[4] One of the primary factors in reducing awareness of hypoglycaemia is that repeated hypoglycaemic episodes seem to trigger an adaptive conservation of glucose concentrations in the brain, resulting in higher central than peripheral blood glucose values;[5] avoidance of hypoglycaemia helps restore awareness.

When recombinant human insulin became generally available in the late 1980s a number of patients complained of a loss of awareness of impending hypoglycaemia following transfer to human insulin,[6,7] and there were reports of severe or even fatal hypoglycaemia occurring in patients who had been well stabilised on animal insulins.[6-8]

This was, and remains, a somewhat controversial area. Despite some small studies suggesting a problem,[9-12] others failed to find evidence of a difference between animal and human insulins.[13-15] However, most commentators appear to consider that patients should continue to have access to animal insulins if desired, and that those well maintained on animal insulin should not be transferred to human insulin without appropriate clinical grounds,[4,8,16-18] and then only with careful monitoring. There has also been concern about possible long-term sequelae of hypoglycaemic episodes on the CNS. However, a recent report on patients participating in the Diabetes Control and Complications Trial (DCCT) suggested that the increased risk of hypoglycaemia seen with intensive therapy was not associated with neuropsychological impairment.[19]

For the treatment of insulin-induced hypoglycaemia, see below.

1. The Diabetes Control and Complications Trial Research Group. The effect of intensive treatment of diabetes on the development and progression of long-term complications in insulin-dependent diabetes mellitus. *N Engl J Med* 1993; **329**: 977–86.

2. Egger M, *et al.* Risk of adverse effects of intensified treatment in insulin-dependent diabetes mellitus: a meta-analysis. *Diabetic Med* 1997; **14**: 919–28.
3. Widom B, Simonson DC. Glycemic control and neuropsychologic function during hypoglycemia in patients with insulin-dependent diabetes mellitus. *Ann Intern Med* 1990; **112**: 904–12.
4. Everett J, Kerr D. Changing from porcine to human insulin. *Drugs* 1994; **47**: 286–96.
5. Cranston I, *et al.* Restoration of hypoglycaemia awareness in patients with long-duration insulin-dependent diabetes. *Lancet* 1994; **344**: 283–7.
6. Teuscher A, Berger WG. Hypoglycaemia unawareness in diabetics transferred from beef/porcine insulin to human insulin. *Lancet* 1987; **ii**: 382–5.
7. Pickup J. Human insulin: problems with hypoglycaemia in a few patients. *BMJ* 1989; **299**: 991–3.
8. Gale EAM. Hypoglycaemia and human insulin. *Lancet* 1989; **ii**: 1264–6.
9. Berger W, *et al.* Warning symptoms of hypoglycaemia during treatment with human and porcine insulin in diabetes mellitus. *Lancet* 1989; **i**: 1041–4.
10. Heine RJ, *et al.* Responses to human and porcine insulin in healthy subjects. *Lancet* 1989; **ii**: 946–9.
11. Egger M, *et al.* Risk of severe hypoglycaemia in insulin treated diabetic patients transferred to human insulin: a case control study. *BMJ* 1991; **303**: 617–21.
12. Egger M, *et al.* Influence of human insulin on symptoms and awareness of hypoglycaemia: a randomised double blind crossover trial. *BMJ* 1991; **303**: 622–6.
13. Colagiuri S, *et al.* Double-blind crossover comparison of human and porcine insulins in patients reporting lack of hypoglycaemia awareness. *Lancet* 1992; **339**: 1432–5.
14. Patrick AW, *et al.* Human insulin and awareness of acute hypoglycaemic symptoms in insulin-dependent diabetes. *Lancet* 1991; **338**: 528–32.
15. Maran A, *et al.* Double blind clinical and laboratory study of hypoglycaemia with human and porcine insulin in diabetic patients reporting hypoglycaemia unawareness after transferring to human insulin. *BMJ* 1993; **305**: 167–71.
16. Gerich JE. Unawareness of hypoglycaemia and human insulin. *BMJ* 1992; **305**: 324–5.
17. Williams G, Patrick AW. Human insulin and hypoglycaemia: burning issue or hot air? *BMJ* 1992; **305**: 355–7.
18. Teuscher A, Kiln MR. Patient-empowerment and free insulin market. *Lancet* 1994; **344**: 1299–1300.
19. The Diabetes Control and Complications Trial Research Group. Effects of intensive diabetes treatment on neuropsychological function in adults in the Diabetes Control and Complications Trial. *Ann Intern Med* 1996; **124**: 379–88.

Oedema. Severe, acute oedema is a rare adverse effect of insulin treatment, occurring most often at the initiation of therapy.[1-3] It should be distinguished from chronic and subacute forms of oedema which may be complications of the diabetic disease process.[2,3] Possible mechanisms of acute oedema are sodium retention resulting from a direct action of insulin on the renal tubule or an effect of insulin on vascular permeability.[1,3] The oedema usually responds to a decrease in insulin dosage.

1. Bleach NR, *et al.* Insulin oedema. *BMJ* 1979; **2**: 177–8.
2. Lawrence JR, Dunnigan MG. Diabetic (insulin) oedema. *BMJ* 1979; **2**: 445.
3. Evans DJ. Insulin oedema. *Postgrad Med J* 1986; **62**: 665–8.

Treatment of Insulin-induced Hypoglycaemia

In the conscious and cooperative patient hypoglycaemia is treated by the oral administration of a readily absorbable form of carbohydrate, such as sugar lumps or a glucose-based drink and all diabetics should always carry a suitable sugar source by way of precaution.

If hypoglycaemic coma occurs, the *British National Formulary* recommends that 50 mL of a 20% solution of glucose or 25 mL of glucose 50% should be given intravenously (some sources in the USA have recommended up to 50 mL of glucose 50%). Glucose 10% may be used but larger volumes are required. Occasionally this may need to be repeated and an intravenous infusion of glucose initiated. If after about one hour, blood-glucose concentrations are normal and the patient has failed to regain consciousness, the possibility of cerebral oedema should be considered. In situations where the intravenous administration of glucose is impractical or not feasible, glucagon 0.5 to 1 mg by subcutaneous, intramuscular, or intravenous injection may arouse the patient sufficiently to allow oral glucose to be given. If the patient fails to respond to glucagon within about 10 to 15 minutes, then glucose has to be given intravenously despite any impracticalities.

Following a return to consciousness, carbohydrates by mouth may need to be given until the action of insulin has ceased which, for preparations with a relatively long duration of action such as isophane insulin, some insulin zinc suspensions, and protamine zinc insulin, may be several hours.

326 Antidiabetics

Table 2. Ph. Eur., BP, and USP insulin preparations.

Type	Ph. Eur./BP/USP Title	Synonyms	Description	pH	Common classification	Approximate action profile after subcutaneous administration		
						Onset	Time to peak	Duration
Soluble insulins (also known as regular or unmodified insulin)	Soluble Insulin Injection (Ph. Eur.)	Neutral Insulin Neutral Insulin Injection Soluble Insulin Insulin Injection	Solution of bovine, porcine, or human insulin	6.9 to 7.8	Short-acting	30 minutes to 1 hour	2 to 5 hours	6 to 8 hours
	Insulin Injection (USP 25)		Solution of bovine or porcine insulin	7.0 to 7.8				
	Insulin Human Injection (USP 25)		Solution of human insulin	7.0 to 7.8				
Biphasic insulins	Biphasic Insulin Injection (Ph. Eur.)	Biphasic Insulin	Suspension of crystals containing bovine insulin in a solution of porcine insulin	6.6 to 7.2				
	Biphasic Isophane Insulin Injection (Ph. Eur.)	Biphasic Isophane Insulin	Buffered suspension of porcine insulin or human insulin complexed with protamine sulfate or other suitable protamine, in a solution of porcine insulin or human insulin respectively.	6.9 to 7.8				
Insulin suspensions	Isophane Insulin Injection (Ph. Eur.)	Isophane Insulin Isophane Insulin (NPH) Isophane Protamine Insulin Injection	Suspension of bovine, porcine, or human insulin complexed with protamine sulfate or another suitable protamine. Contains 300 to 600μg of protamine sulfate per 100 units of insulin	6.9 to 7.8	Intermediate-acting	Within 2 hours	4 to 12 hours	Up to 24 hours
	Isophane Insulin Suspension (USP 25)		Buffered aqueous suspension of zinc-insulin (bovine or porcine) crystals and protamine sulfate, combined in a manner such that the solid phase of the suspension consists of crystals composed of insulin, protamine, and zinc	7.0 to 7.8				
	Isophane Insulin Human Suspension (USP 25)		Buffered aqueous suspension of zinc-insulin human crystals and protamine sulfate, combined in such a manner that the solid phase of the suspension consists of crystals composed of insulin human, protamine, and zinc	7.0 to 7.5				
	Insulin Zinc Injectable Suspension (Amorphous) (Ph. Eur.)	Amorph. I.Z.S. Insulin Semilente Insulin Zinc Suspension (Amorphous)	Suspension of bovine, porcine, or human insulin complexed with a suitable zinc salt; the insulin is in a form practically insoluble in water	6.9 to 7.8				
	Prompt Insulin Zinc Suspension (USP 25)		Buffered aqueous suspension of bovine or porcine insulin modified by the addition of a suitable zinc salt in a manner such that the solid phase is amorphous	7.0 to 7.8				

Table 2. Ph. Eur., BP, and USP insulin preparations.

Type	Ph. Eur./BP/USP Title	Synonyms	Description	pH	Common classification	Approximate action profile after subcutaneous administration		
						Onset	Time to peak	Duration
Insulin suspensions *cont*	Insulin Zinc Injectable Suspension (Ph. Eur.)	Insulin Lente I.Z.S. I.Z.S. (Mixed) Insulin Zinc Suspension (Mixed) Insulin Zinc Suspension	Suspension of bovine or porcine, or a mixture of bovine and porcine, or human insulin with a suitable zinc salt; the insulin is in a form practically insoluble in water. It may be produced by mixing Insulin Zinc Injectable Suspension (Amorphous) (Ph. Eur.) and Insulin Zinc Injectable Suspension (Crystalline) (Ph. Eur.) in a ratio of 3 to 7	6.9 to 7.8				
	Insulin Zinc Suspension (USP 25)	Insulin Zinc	Buffered aqueous suspension of bovine or porcine insulin modified by the addition of a suitable zinc salt in a manner such that the solid phase of the suspension consists of a mixture of approximately 3 parts of amorphous insulin to 7 parts of crystalline insulin	7.0 to 7.8	Intermediate or long-acting	2 to 3 hours	6 to 15 hours	Up to 30 hours
	Insulin Human Zinc Suspension (USP 25)		Buffered aqueous suspension of human insulin modified by the addition of a suitable zinc salt in a manner such that the solid phase of the suspension consists of a mixture of approximately 3 parts of amorphous insulin to 7 parts of crystalline insulin	7.0 to 7.8				
	Insulin Zinc Injectable Suspension (Crystalline) (Ph. Eur.)	Cryst. I.Z.S. Insulin Ultralente Insulin Zinc Suspension (Crystalline)	Suspension of bovine, porcine, or human insulin complexed with a suitable zinc salt; the insulin is in a form practically insoluble in water	6.9 to 7.8				
	Protamine Zinc Insulin Injection (BP 2001)	Protamine Zinc Insulin	Buffered suspension of bovine, porcine, or human insulin complexed with protamine sulfate or another suitable protamine and zinc chloride or another suitable zinc salt	6.9 to 7.8	Long-acting	4 hours	10 to 20 hours	Up to 36 hours
	Extended Insulin Zinc Suspension (USP 25)		Buffered aqueous suspension of bovine or porcine insulin modified by the addition of a suitable zinc salt in a manner such that the solid phase is predominantly crystalline	7.0 to 7.8				
	Extended Insulin Human Zinc Suspension (USP 25)		Buffered aqueous suspension of human insulin modified by the addition of a suitable zinc salt in a manner such that the solid phase of the suspension is predominantly crystalline	7.0 to 7.8				

Carbohydrate. A comparative study[1] of 7 different preparations of oral carbohydrate for the treatment of hypoglycaemia in the conscious patient found no significant difference in effectiveness between glucose or sucrose in solution or tablet form; a hydrolysed polysaccharide solution containing glucose, maltose, and various more complex saccharides (Glucidex 19) was also roughly comparable. However, a glucose gel and orange juice were each less effective in treating hypoglycaemia.

1. Slama G, et al. The search for an optimized treatment of hypoglycemia: carbohydrates in tablets, solution, or gel for the correction of insulin reactions. Arch Intern Med 1990; 150: 589–93.

Glucagon. A discussion of the relative merits of parenteral glucose and glucagon in unconscious hypoglycaemic patients[1] suggested that glucagon should be encouraged as first-line treatment, although in practice (see above) parenteral glucose is usually preferred. The effect of glucagon relies upon the patient having adequate liver glycogen stores, which may not always be the case.

1. Gibbins RL. Treating hypoglycaemia in general practice. BMJ 1993; 306: 600–1.

Overdose. The requirements for glucose are greater and more prolonged when hypoglycaemia is caused by insulin overdosage rather than therapeutic doses.[1] Correction of insulin-induced hypokalaemia may also be required. Surgical excision of tissue at the site of injection has been used for massive overdose of a long-acting insulin.[2,3]

1. Roberge RJ, et al. Intentional massive insulin overdosage: recognition and management. Ann Emerg Med 1993; 22: 228–34.
2. Campbell IW, Ratcliffe JG. Suicidal insulin overdose managed by excision of insulin injection site. BMJ 1982; 285: 408–9.
3. Levine DF, Bulstrode C. Managing suicidal insulin overdose. BMJ 1982; 285: 974–5.

Precautions

Dosage requirements of insulin may be altered by many factors. Increased doses are usually necessary during infection, emotional stress, accidental or surgical trauma, puberty, and the latter two trimesters of pregnancy, and decreased doses are usually necessary in patients with impaired renal or liver function or during the first trimester of pregnancy. Following initiation and stabilisation of therapy in newly diagnosed diabetic patients, a temporary decrease in requirements may also occur (the so-called honeymoon period).

Because of the possibility of differing responses to insulins from different species, care is recommended to avoid the inadvertent change from insulin of one species to another. Reduction in insulin dosage may be required on transfer from animal (especially bovine insulin) to human insulin. Hypoglycaemic problems associated with a change to human insulin are discussed under Adverse Effects, above. Care is also necessary during excessive exercise; hypoglycaemia caused by metabolic effects and increased insulin absorption is the usual response, but hyperglycaemia may sometimes occur.

The use of insulin necessitates monitoring of therapy, such as the testing of blood or urine for glucose concentrations and the urine for ketones, by the patient.

Drugs which have an effect on blood-glucose concentrations may alter glycaemic control with consequent need for a change in insulin dose (see under Interactions, below).

CAUTION. *Biphasic insulin, insulin zinc suspensions, isophane insulin, protamine zinc insulin, and insulin glargine should never be given intravenously and they are not suitable for the emergency treatment of diabetic ketoacidosis.*

Abuse. Transient recurrent hepatomegaly associated with hypoglycaemia was associated with the surreptitious administration of additional insulin injections in an insulin-dependent diabetic. Increased storage of glycogen in the liver resulting from insulin excess was considered responsible for the hepatomegaly.[1]

Decreased plasma C-peptide concentrations or the presence of anti-insulin antibodies may be used to confirm insulin abuse as a cause of hypoglycaemia in patients who have never been treated with insulin medically.[2] Insulin has been abused by bodybuilders and other sportspersons;[3,4] severe brain damage after prolonged neuroglycopenia has resulted.[3]

1. Asherov J, et al. Hepatomegaly due to self-induced hyperinsulinism. Arch Dis Child 1979; 54: 148–9.
2. Grunberger G, et al. Factitious hypoglycemia due to surreptitious administration of insulin: diagnosis, treatment, and long-term follow-up. Ann Intern Med 1988; 108: 252–7.
3. Elkin SL, et al. Bodybuilders find it easy to obtain insulin to help them in training. BMJ 1997; 314: 1280.
4. Honour JW. Misuse of natural hormones in sport. Lancet 1997; 349: 1786.

Accelerated absorption. Factors such as a hot bath, sauna, or use of a sunbed have been reported to accelerate the absorption of subcutaneous injection, presumably by an increase in skin blood flow.[1-4] There may, therefore, be a risk of hypoglycaemia.[4]

1. Koivisto VA. Sauna-induced acceleration in insulin absorption from subcutaneous injection site. BMJ 1980; 280: 1411–13.
2. Cüppers HJ, et al. Sauna-induced acceleration in insulin absorption? BMJ 1980; 281: 307.
3. Koivisto VA. Sauna-induced acceleration in insulin absorption. BMJ 1980; 281: 621–2.
4. Husband DJ, Gill GV. "Sunbed seizures": a hypoglycaemic hazard for insulin-dependent diabetics. Lancet 1984; ii: 1477.

Adrenocortical insufficiency. A report of 2 cases of recurrent severe hypoglycaemia in type 1 diabetics which persisted despite a reduction in insulin doses and proved to be due to Addison's disease.[1] Insulin requirements rose again in both patients following replacement therapy with fludrocortisone and hydrocortisone.

1. Armstrong L, Bell PM. Addison's disease presenting as reduced insulin requirement in insulin dependent diabetes. BMJ 1996; 312: 1601–2.

Driving. In the UK, patients with diabetes mellitus treated with insulin or oral hypoglycaemics are required to notify their condition to the Driver and Vehicle Licensing Agency, who then assess their fitness to drive. Patients treated with oral hypoglycaemics are generally allowed to retain standard driving licences; those treated with insulin receive restricted licences which must be renewed (with appropriate checks) every 1 to 3 years. Patients should be warned of the dangers of hypoglycaemic attacks while driving, and should be counselled in appropriate management of the situation (stopping driving as soon as it is safe to do so, taking carbohydrate immediately, and quitting the driving seat and removing the ignition key from the car) should such an event occur. Patients who have lost hypoglycaemic awareness, or have frequent hypoglycaemic episodes, should not drive. In addition, eyesight must be adequate (field of vision of at least 120°) for a licence to be valid. Patients treated with diet or oral hypoglycaemics are normally allowed to hold vocational driving licences for heavy goods vehicles or passenger carrying vehicles; those treated with insulin may not drive such vehicles, and are restricted in driving some other vehicles such as small lorries and minibuses.[1] Regulations in other countries differ widely.[2]

1. British Diabetic Association (Diabetes UK). Information sheet: driving and diabetes: Aug 2001. Available at: http://www.diabetes.org.uk/info/inform/drive.doc (accessed 13/09/01).
2. DiaMond Project Group on Social Issues. Global regulations on diabetics treated with insulin and their operation of commercial motor vehicles. BMJ 1993; 307: 250–3.

Exercise. A discussion of the metabolic effects of exercise and the precautions to be taken by the exercising type 1 diabetic.[1]

1. Greenhalgh PM. Competitive sport and the insulin-dependent diabetic patient. Postgrad Med J 1990; 66: 803–6.

Hypersensitivity to protamine. A retrospective survey has indicated that patients receiving isophane insulin, which contains protamine, have an increased risk of severe reactions simulating anaphylaxis when protamine is used to reverse systemic heparinisation after cardiac catheterisation.[1] A mechanism involving IgE and IgG antibodies to protamine has been proposed.[2]

See also Hypersensitivity under Adverse Effects, above.

1. Stewart WJ, et al. Increased risk of severe protamine reactions in NPH insulin-dependent diabetics undergoing cardiac catheterization. Circulation 1984; 70: 788–92.
2. Weiss ME, et al. Association of protamine IgE and IgG antibodies with life-threatening reactions to intravenous protamine. N Engl J Med 1989; 320: 886–92.

Infections. Decreased requirements of insulin, added to the dialysate, occurred in 6 diabetic patients undergoing continuous ambulatory peritoneal dialysis for chronic renal failure during episodes of severe bacterial peritonitis.[1] This was contrary to the increased insulin requirements exhibited by most diabetic patients during severe infections and probably resulted from increased absorption of insulin due to mesothelial damage.

1. Henderson IS, et al. Decreased intraperitoneal insulin requirements during peritonitis on continuous ambulatory peritoneal dialysis. BMJ 1985; 290: 1474.

Menstruation. Discussion on the control of diabetes during the menstrual cycle and the possible need to adjust insulin dosage regularly around the time of menstruation.[1]

1. Magos A, Studd J. Effects of the menstrual cycle on medical disorders. Br J Hosp Med 1985; 33: 68–77.

Morning hyperglycaemia. Morning hyperglycaemia may be the result of mere waning of subcutaneously injected insulin. It may also be rebound hyperglycaemia (posthypoglycaemic hyperglycaemia or the Somogyi phenomenon) occurring after an episode of nocturnal hypoglycaemia. Morning hyperglycaemia has also been observed without antecedent hypoglycaemia even during constant intravenous infusion of insulin, when the waning of previously injected insulin would not be a factor and this is commonly referred to as the dawn phenomenon. Clinically, it is important to distinguish between the dawn phenomenon, simple waning of previously injected insulin, and rebound hyperglycaemia as a cause of early-morning hyperglycaemia because their treatment differs. Management of the dawn phenomenon and insulin waning generally consists of adjusting the evening dose of insulin to provide additional coverage between 4 a.m. and 7 a.m. Management of rebound hyper-

glycaemia consists of reducing insulin doses or providing additional late-evening carbohydrate, or both, to avoid nocturnal hypoglycaemia. Mistaking rebound hyperglycaemia for the dawn phenomenon or mere waning of injected insulin could result in more serious nocturnal hypoglycaemia, if evening doses of insulin were increased.[1]

1. Cryer PE, Gerich JE. Glucose counterregulation, hypoglycemia, and intensive insulin therapy in diabetes mellitus. N Engl J Med 1985; 313: 232–41.

Pregnancy. For discussion of the precautions necessary in the management of diabetes mellitus during pregnancy, see p.315. There has been a report of 2 cases of fetal malformation in the offspring of well-controlled diabetic women who received *insulin lispro*.[1] However, the incidence of fetal malformation is increased in infants of women with diabetes. Although the use of insulin lispro is not recommended during pregnancy the manufacturers were aware of 19 live births among women treated with insulin lispro, 1 of which exhibited a congenital abnormality.[2]

1. Diamond T, Kormas N. Possible adverse fetal effect of insulin lispro. N Engl J Med 1997; 337: 1009.
2. Anderson JH, et al. Possible adverse fetal effect of insulin lispro. N Engl J Med 1997; 337: 1010.

Renal impairment. See under Infections, above.

Smoking. Smoking has been reported to decrease the absorption of insulin and may contribute to metabolic instability in diabetic patients.[1] Dosage adjustment may be necessary.

1. Miller LG. Recent developments in the study of the effects of cigarette smoking on clinical pharmacokinetics and clinical pharmacodynamics. Clin Pharmacokinet 1989; 17: 90–108.

Surgery. For a discussion of the management of diabetes mellitus during surgery, see p.315.

Transmission of prion disease. Studies of cattle with proven bovine spongiform encephalopathy (BSE) have not detected infectivity in the pancreas, from which bovine insulin is derived.[1]

1. Wickham EA. Potential transmission of BSE via medicinal products. BMJ 1996; 312: 988–9.

Travelling. Advice for the diabetic patient when travelling, including adjustment of insulin dosage when crossing time zones.[1,2] Since insulin solution or suspension must not be frozen, it should not be carried in the luggage hold of an aircraft.

1. Barry M, Bia F. Advice for the traveling diabetic. JAMA 1989; 261: 1799.
2. Sane T, et al. Adjustment of insulin doses of diabetic patients during long distance flights. BMJ 1990; 301: 421–2.

Interactions

Many drugs have an effect on blood-glucose concentrations and may alter insulin requirements. Drugs with hypoglycaemic activity or which may decrease insulin requirements include ACE inhibitors, alcohol, anabolic steroids, aspirin, beta blockers (which may also mask the warning signs of hypoglycaemia), disopyramide, fenfluramine, guanethidine, some MAOIs, mebendazole, octreotide, some tetracyclines, and the tricyclic antidepressant amitriptyline.

On the other hand, increased requirements of insulin may possibly be seen with chlordiazepoxide, chlorpromazine, some calcium-channel blockers such as diltiazem or nifedipine, corticosteroids, diazoxide, lithium, thiazide diuretics, and thyroid hormones.

Both increased and decreased requirements may occur with cyclophosphamide, isoniazid, and oral contraceptives.

ACE inhibitors. Although ACE inhibitors are favoured for use in diabetic patients with hypertension or evidence of incipient nephropathy or both, they may increase insulin sensitivity and thus decrease insulin requirements when given concomitantly.[1,2] The need for oral antidiabetics may also be decreased.

1. Ferriere M, et al. Captopril and insulin sensitivity. Ann Intern Med 1985; 102: 134–5.
2. McMurray J, Fraser DM. Captopril, enalapril, and blood glucose. Lancet 1986; i: 1035.

Alcohol. Severe hypoglycaemic episodes have been reported in type 1 diabetics following heavy drinking episodes.[1,2] Alcohol inhibits gluconeogenesis, and its effects are therefore likely to be greatest if taken without food; however, it seems to be generally agreed that diabetics need not abstain from a moderate alcohol intake with meals.

1. Arky RA, et al. Irreversible hypoglycemia. JAMA 1968; 206: 575–8.
2. Potter J, et al. Insulin induced hypoglycaemia in an accident and emergency department: the tip of an iceberg? BMJ 1982; 285: 1180–2.

Aspirin. Aspirin produces a modest decrease in blood-glucose concentrations but a significant interaction at conventional analgesic doses appears to be unlikely. One study in children with type 1 diabetes found an average 15% decrease in blood glucose values following treatment with aspirin 1.2 to 2.4 g daily for 3 days, but there were no significant changes in insulin requirements.[1] However, high doses of aspirin can reduce or even replace the insulin dose required.[2] Other salicylates might be expected to have similar properties.

1. Kaye R, *et al.* Antipyretics in patients with juvenile diabetes mellitus. *Am J Dis Child* 1966; **112:** 52–5.
2. Reid J, Lightbody TD. The insulin equivalence of salicylate. *BMJ* 1959; **1:** 897.

Beta blockers. There are a few reports of severe hypoglycaemia in patients, including insulin-treated diabetics, who were given *propranolol* or *pindolol*;[1-3] there is also a report of an interaction with *timolol* given as eye drops.[4] Some evidence exists of an interaction with *metoprolol*,[5] but little evidence for some of the more selective beta blockers. Because of the effects of beta blockers on the sympathetic nervous system the usual premonitory signs of hypoglycaemia may not occur, allowing a severe episode to develop before the patient is aware and able to counter it.

1. Kotler MN, *et al.* Hypoglycaemia precipitated by propranolol. *Lancet* 1966; **ii:** 1389–90.
2. McMurtry RJ. Propranolol, hypoglycemia, and hypertensive crisis. *Ann Intern Med* 1974; **80:** 669–70.
3. Samii K, *et al.* Severe hypoglycaemia due to beta-blocking drugs in haemodialysis patients. *Lancet* 1976; **i:** 545–6.
4. Angelo-Nielsen K. Timolol topically and diabetes mellitus. *JAMA* 1980; **244:** 2263.
5. Newman RJ. Comparison of propranolol, metoprolol, and acebutolol on insulin-induced hypoglycaemia. *BMJ* 1976; **2:** 447–9.

Calcium-channel blockers. Diabetes worsened in an insulin-treated diabetic when given *diltiazem*.[1] The resultant intractable hyperglycaemia improved when the drug was withdrawn, and recurred, although at a more manageable level, when diltiazem was restarted at a lower dose. There are also reports of a diabetogenic effect of *nifedipine*.[2,3] However, reports of significant disturbances of metabolic control appear to be uncommon.

1. Pershadsingh HA, *et al.* Association of diltiazem therapy with increased insulin resistance in a patient with type I diabetes mellitus. *JAMA* 1987; **257:** 930–1.
2. Bhatnagar SK, *et al.* Diabetogenic effects of nifedipine. *BMJ* 1984; **289:** 19.
3. Heyman SN, *et al.* Diabetogenic effect of nifedipine. *DICP Ann Pharmacother* 1989; **23:** 236–7.

Interferons. A report of markedly increased insulin requirements developing in a previously well controlled diabetic following treatment with *interferon alfa 2a*.[1] Insulin requirements rapidly fell once interferon therapy was discontinued.

1. Campbell S, *et al.* Rapidly reversible increase in insulin requirement with interferon. *BMJ* 1996; **313:** 92.

Oral contraceptives. Both increases and decreases (mainly the former) in insulin requirements have been reported in insulin-dependent diabetics given various oral contraceptives.[1] However, it appears that in most cases the effects of a hormonal contraceptive on diabetic control are modest or insignificant: one study suggests that progestogen-only and combined oral contraceptives in general have little effect.[2]

1. Zeller WJ, *et al.* Verträglichkeit von hormonalen Ovulationskemmern bei Diabetikerinnen. *Arzneimittelforschung* 1974; **24:** 351–7.
2. Rådberg T, *et al.* Oral contraception in diabetic women: diabetes control, serum and high density lipoprotein lipids during low-dose progestogen, combined oestrogen/progestogen and non-hormonal contraception. *Acta Endocrinol (Copenh)* 1981; **98:** 246–51.

Pharmacokinetics

Insulin has no hypoglycaemic effect when administered by mouth since it is inactivated in the gastrointestinal tract.

It is fairly rapidly absorbed from subcutaneous tissue following injection and although the half-life of unmodified insulin in blood is very short (being only a matter of minutes), the duration of action of most preparations is considerably longer due to their formulation (for further details see Uses and Administration, below). The rate of absorption from different anatomical sites may be different depending on local blood flow, with absorption from the abdomen being faster than that from the arm, and that from the arm faster than from buttock or thigh. Absorption may also be increased by exercise. The absorption of insulin after intramuscular administration is more rapid than that following subcutaneous administration. Human insulin may be absorbed slightly faster from subcutaneous tissue than porcine or bovine insulin.

Insulin is rapidly metabolised, mainly in the liver but also in the kidneys and muscle tissue. In the kidneys it is reabsorbed in the proximal tubule and either returned to venous blood or metabolised, with only a small amount excreted unchanged in the urine.

◊ For discussion of factors which may affect the absorption of insulin, see under Precautions, Accelerated Absorption, above, and Uses, Administration Routes, below.

Resistance to Insulin

The term insulin resistance has traditionally been used to describe a state in which diabetic patients exhibit considerably increased insulin requirements. It is now used in a much wider sense, and is for instance also applied to patients in whom a subnormal biological response to insulin can be demonstrated, although many of these patients do not apparently present difficulties in their clinical management. Insulin resistance is found particularly in obese patients; resistance to endogenous insulin is thought to be linked to the development of type 2 diabetes in such patients. Insulin resistance is frequently associated with lipid disorders, hypertension, and ischaemic heart disease. In women, it may also be linked to polycystic ovary syndrome.

Insulin resistance of the type manifested by greatly increased insulin requirements may be due to a variety of factors, including antibody formation (see under Adverse Effects, above) and inadequate absorption of insulin from subcutaneous sites. A few patients with severe insulin resistance have responded to insulin lispro (see Insulin Analogues and Proinsulin under Uses, below).

Mecasermin (insulin-like growth factor) has been observed to reverse hyperglycaemia and ketoacidosis in patients with insulin resistance (see p.1297).

◊ References.

1. Moller DE, Flier JS. Insulin resistance—mechanisms, syndromes, and implications. *N Engl J Med* 1991; **325:** 938–48.
2. Eckel RH. Insulin resistance: an adaptation for weight maintenance. *Lancet* 1992; **340:** 1452–3.
3. Clausen JO, *et al.* Insulin resistance: interactions between obesity and a common variant of insulin receptor substrate-1. *Lancet* 1995; **346:** 397–402.
4. Davidson MB. Clinical implications of insulin resistance syndromes. *Am J Med* 1995; **99:** 420–6.
5. Krentz AJ. Insulin resistance. *BMJ* 1996; **313:** 1385–9. Correction. *ibid.* 1997; **314:** 134.

Uses and Administration

Insulin is a hormone that plays a key role in regulating carbohydrate, protein, and fat metabolism. The main stimulus for its secretion is glucose, although many other factors including amino acids, catecholamines, cortisol, glucagon, and growth hormone and its hypothalamic release-inhibiting hormone (somatostatin), are involved in its regulation. The secretion of insulin is not constant and peaks occur in response to the intake of food.

The major effects of insulin on carbohydrate homoeostasis follow its binding to specific cell-surface receptors on insulin-sensitive tissues, notably the liver, muscles, and adipose tissue. It inhibits hepatic glucose production and enhances peripheral glucose disposal thereby reducing blood-glucose concentration. It also inhibits lipolysis thereby preventing the formation of ketone bodies.

Therapy with insulin is essential for the long-term survival of all patients with type 1 diabetes mellitus. It may also be necessary in some patients with type 2 disease. The management of diabetes mellitus and the role of insulin in type 1 and type 2 disease is discussed on p.315. Insulin is generally the treatment chosen for all types of diabetes mellitus during pregnancy.

Choice of insulin. The different types of insulin and their formulations are described under Definitions, above. In some countries including the UK the commercially available preparations have been standardised to a single strength containing 100 units per mL; a strength of 40 units per mL is still available in some other countries, and in others concentrated injections (500 units per mL) are available to enable high doses to be given subcutaneously in a small volume. All formulations can be given by subcutaneous injection, most by intramuscular injection, but only soluble insulins can be given by the intravenous route. The long-term management of diabetic patients usually involves the subcutaneous route. Syringes and needles for subcutaneous injection are preferably disposable. Pen-injector devices which hold the insulin in cartridge form and meter the required dose are be-

coming increasingly popular. Soluble insulin is often given by the intraperitoneal route to patients on continuous ambulatory peritoneal dialysis.

The various formulations of insulin are classified, according to their duration of action after subcutaneous injection, as short-, intermediate-, or long-acting. The exact duration of action for any particular preparation, however, is variable and may depend upon factors such as interindividual variation, the patient's antibody status, whether the insulin is of human or animal origin, the dose, and the site of injection. *Short-acting* insulins are the soluble insulins, which have an onset after about 30 minutes to 1 hour, a peak activity at about 2 to 5 hours, and a duration of about 6 to 8 hours. Some analogues, such as insulins lispro and aspart, are also short-acting. *Intermediate-acting* insulins include biphasic insulins, isophane insulins, and amorphous insulin zinc suspensions. In general these have an onset within about 2 hours, peak activity after about 4 to 12 hours, and a duration of up to 24 hours. Commercially available mixtures of soluble insulins and isophane insulins have activities which would normally place them within the intermediate-acting category. Mixed insulin zinc suspensions may be classified as either *intermediate- or long-acting* as the duration of action may be up to 30 hours; the onset of action is generally 2 to 3 hours and the time to peak activity 6 to 15 hours. *Long-acting* insulins include crystalline insulin zinc suspensions and protamine zinc insulins. These generally have an onset after about 4 hours, a peak activity at about 10 to 20 hours, and a duration of up to 36 hours. The insulin analogue insulin glargine is also long-acting. Following intramuscular injection, the onset of action of all insulins is generally more rapid and the duration of action shorter.

The type of formulation, its dose, and the frequency of administration are chosen to suit the needs of the individual patient. Whatever the formulation, human insulin is generally used for all newly diagnosed diabetics.

Control. The dosage of insulin must be determined for each patient and although a precise dose range cannot be given a total dose in excess of about 80 units daily would be unusual and may indicate the presence of a form of insulin resistance. The dose should be adjusted as necessary according to the results of regular monitoring of blood concentrations (or occasionally urine concentrations) of glucose by the patient.

The WHO has recommended that the glucose concentration of venous whole blood under fasting conditions should be kept within the range of 3.3 to 5.6 mmol per litre (60 to 100 mg per 100 mL) and after meals should not be allowed to exceed 10 mmol per litre (180 mg per 100 mL); blood-glucose concentrations should not be allowed to fall below 3 mmol per litre (55 mg per 100 mL). In practice it seems to be generally acceptable for patients to aim for blood-glucose concentrations between 4 and 10 mmol per litre, with the understanding that occasional variations outside this range may occur. It should be remembered that the glucose concentrations in venous plasma, venous whole blood, and capillary whole blood may be slightly different. Control may also be determined by monitoring of glycosylated haemoglobin concentrations; ideally the aim is an HbA_{1c} level of less than 7% or an HbA_1 of less than 8.8%, compared with normal ranges of 4 to 6% and 5 to 7.5% respectively. Insulin requirements may be altered by various factors (see Precautions, above). The aim of any regimen should be to achieve the best possible control of blood glucose by attempting to mimic as closely as possible the pattern of optimum endogenous insulin secretion. Many **regimens** involve the use of a short-acting soluble insulin together with an intermediate-acting insulin, such as isophane insulin or mixed insulin zinc suspension. Such a combination is often given twice daily with about two-thirds of the total daily requirement given before breakfast and the remaining third before the evening meal. It may sometimes be necessary, though, to give 3 or 4 injections daily to achieve good control and this typically involves the administration of a soluble insulin before meals together with an intermediate- or long-acting insulin given usually in the evening. A once-daily injection of an intermediate- or long-acting insulin is now generally considered to be acceptable only for those patients with type 2 diabetes mellitus who still retain some endogenous insulin secretion but nevertheless require insulin therapy, or for those patients with type 1 disease unable to cope satisfactorily with more intensive regimens. If a more intensive regimen is desired, **continuous subcutaneous infusion** may be employed using soluble insulin in an infusion pump. This delivers a constant basal infusion of insulin supplying about half of the total daily requirements, the remainder being provided by patient-activated bolus doses before each meal. The technique has a limited place in the management of diabetes; patients using it need to be well-motivated, reliable, and able to monitor their own blood glucose, and must have access to expert advice at all times. Formulations in which the insulin is in suspension are not suitable for administration by continuous subcutaneous infusion and some brands of soluble insulin are unsuitable for this purpose because of the risk of precipitation in the pump catheter.

Ketoacidosis. Insulin is also an essential part of the emergency management of diabetic ketoacidosis, see Diabetic Emergencies, below. Only short-acting soluble insulins should be used. Treatment includes adequate fluid replacement, usually by infusing sodium chloride 0.9% initially, and the administration of potassium salts to prevent or correct hypokalaemia. Insulin should be given by continuous intravenous infusion if possible, although other routes have also been used—for details of regimens see Diabetic Emergencies, under Diabetes Mellitus, below. Since insulin normally corrects hyperglycaemia before ketosis it is usually necessary to continue administration of insulin once normoglycaemia has been achieved but to change the rehydration fluid to glucose-saline so that the additional glucose prevents the development of hypoglycaemia.

◊ General reviews of insulin and its use.[1-7] It has been suggested that the plethora of insulin preparations available might sensibly be reduced,[7] although others dispute this.[8]

1. Brogden RN, Heel RC. Human insulin: a review of its biological activity, pharmacokinetics and therapeutic use. *Drugs* 1987; **34:** 350–71.
2. Fisher BM. Choosing an insulin. *Prescribers' J* 1988; **28:** 138–43 and 169 (correction).
3. Anonymous. Human insulins: an update. *Drug Ther Bull* 1989; **27:** 21–4.
4. Home PD, et al. Insulin treatment: a decade of change. *Br Med Bull* 1989; **45:** 92–110.
5. Zinman B. The physiologic replacement of insulin: an elusive goal. *N Engl J Med* 1989; **321:** 363–70.
6. MacPherson JN, Feely J. Insulin. *BMJ* 1990; **300:** 731–6.
7. Anonymous. Insulin preparations—time to rationalise. *Drug Ther Bull* 1996; **34:** 11–14.
8. von Kriegstein E, et al. Need for many types of insulin. *Lancet* 1996; **347:** 1045.

Administration. ADMINISTRATION ROUTES. The long-term management of diabetic patients usually involves injection by the **subcutaneous** route. The advice to diabetics has been to inject their insulin using a full-depth perpendicular injection.[1] In many non-obese patients, however, such a technique may result in inadvertent intramuscular injection.[1,2] Since insulin is absorbed more rapidly after intramuscular than subcutaneous administration, such a change between routes may lead to greater day to day variability in blood-glucose control. In particular, overnight control may be inadequate if intermediate-acting preparations such as isophane insulin are used.[1] Some workers therefore consider that extended-action insulins should be injected at an angle into a raised skin fold. Although injection of soluble insulin into muscle may produce a more physiological action profile, until more data are available a technique that ensures subcutaneous administration may be prudent with soluble insulins as well.[1]

The anatomic *site* of subcutaneous insulin injection is usually rotated in an attempt to decrease local adverse effects (see Adverse Effects, above). However, the rate of absorption varies between sites and such a practice may also contribute to day-to-day variability in blood-glucose concentrations.[3] For example, large variations in blood-glucose concentrations have been reported following subcutaneous injection into the thigh.[4] Some workers have suggested rotation of injection sites within

an anatomic region, or possibly use of the same anatomic region for injections given at a specific time of day.[3]

Jet injectors deliver insulin at high pressure across the skin into the subcutaneous tissue without use of a needle.[5-7] The greater dispersion obtained gives more rapid absorption of short- and intermediate-acting insulins and consequently reduces the total duration of action.[5,7] Delayed pain and bleeding may be a problem.[5,7] Despite having been available for some years, there is little information about their benefits and risks[7] and they are not widely used.[7] However, results in a small study in women with gestational diabetes have suggested that jet injection may be associated with less variation in postprandial blood-glucose concentration and a lower incidence of insulin antibodies.[9]

Insulin preparations may also be administered by **intramuscular** injection. Absorption is more rapid than from a subcutaneous injection. However, exercise may produce considerable variations in insulin absorption after intramuscular administration.[1] Soluble insulins may be given **intravenously**; this route is used in diabetic ketoacidosis, and also in surgery and labour.[10] Intermittent pulsed intravenous insulin therapy added to a conventional subcutaneous regimen has been reported to improve symptoms of postural hypotension[11] and hypertension.[12]

The subcutaneous and intravenous routes, and, rarely, the intramuscular route have all been used for the continuous administration of insulin (see Intensive Administration Regimens, below).

Formulations of insulin for **intranasal** administration are under investigation,[6,13,14] and have been tried in type 1[15,16] and type 2[17,18] diabetes. Absorption enhancers have been used to facilitate uptake of insulin from the nasal mucosa and local adverse effects are dependent, in part, on their irritancy.

Devices for delivering insulin to the lungs via oral **inhalation** are being developed. Aerosolised insulin generated by a nebuliser was effective in a small study in patients with type 2 diabetes.[19]

Endogenous insulin is delivered into the portal venous system, and then passes immediately to the liver where a large fraction of the insulin is extracted. The above routes of administration all deliver insulin into the peripheral circulation, with the risk of peripheral hyperinsulinaemia which has been considered a risk factor for atherosclerotic complications.[20] Administration of insulin via the **intraperitoneal** or **oral** routes may overcome this problem to some extent. Peritoneal insulin is used routinely in diabetics undergoing chronic ambulatory peritoneal dialysis, but has also been used for continuous administration (see Intensive Administration Regimens, below). Various formulations of insulin for oral delivery are also under investigation.[6] Some success in controlling blood-glucose concentrations has been achieved in a limited number of diabetics using a microemulsion of insulin in a lipid phase of similar composition to chylomicra.[21] **Rectal** administration of insulin has also been tried.[6,22]

1. Thow J, Home P. Insulin injection technique: depth of injection is important. *BMJ* 1990; **301:** 3–4.
2. Frid A, Linden B. Where do lean diabetics inject their insulin? A study using computed tomography. *BMJ* 1986; **292:** 1638.
3. Bantle JP, et al. Rotation of the anatomic regions used for insulin injections and day-to-day variability of plasma glucose in type 1 diabetic subject. *JAMA* 1990; **263:** 1802–6.
4. Henriksen JE, et al. Impact of injection sites for soluble insulin on glycaemic control in type 1 (insulin-dependent) diabetic patients treated with a multiple insulin injection regimen. *Diabetologia* 1993; **36:** 752–8.
5. Anonymous. Jet injection of insulin. *Lancet* 1985; **i:** 1140.
6. Chien YW, Banga AK. Potential developments in systemic delivery of insulin. *Drug Dev Ind Pharm* 1989; **15:** 1601–34.
7. MacPherson JN, Feely J. Insulin. *BMJ* 1990; **300:** 731–6.
8. Pickup J. The pursuit of perfect control in diabetes: better insulin better delivered. *BMJ* 1988; **297:** 929–31.
9. Jovanovic-Peterson L, et al. Jet-injected insulin is associated with decreased antibody production and postprandial glucose variability when compared with needle-injected insulin in gestational diabetic women. *Diabetes Care* 1993; **16:** 1479–84.
10. Home PD, et al. Insulin treatment: a decade of change. *Br Med Bull* 1989; **45:** 92–110.
11. Aoki TT, et al. Chronic intermittent intravenous insulin therapy corrects orthostatic hypotension of diabetes. *Am J Med* 1995; **99:** 683–4.
12. Aoki TT, et al. Effect of chronic intermittent intravenous insulin therapy on antihypertensive medication requirements in IDDM subjects with hypertension and nephropathy. *Diabetes Care* 1995; **18:** 1260–5.
13. Pontiroli AE, et al. Intranasal drug delivery: potential advantages and limitations from a clinical pharmacokinetic perspective. *Clin Pharmacokinet* 1989; **17:** 299–307.
14. Illum L, Davis SS. Intranasal insulin: clinical pharmacokinetics. *Clin Pharmacokinet* 1992; **23:** 30–41.
15. Salzman R, et al. Intranasal aerosolized insulin: mixed-meal studies and long-term use in type I diabetes. *N Engl J Med* 1985; **312:** 1078–84.
16. Lassmann-Vague V, et al. Preprandial intranasal insulin. *Lancet* 1988; **i:** 367–8.
17. Coates PA, et al. Intranasal insulin: the effects of three dose regimens on postprandial glycaemic profiles in type II diabetic subjects. *Diabetic Med* 1995; **12:** 235–9.
18. El-Etr M, et al. Preprandial intranasal insulin as adjuvant therapy in type II diabetics. *Lancet* 1987; **ii:** 1085–6.
19. Laube BL, et al. Preliminary study of the efficacy of insulin aerosol delivered by oral inhalation in diabetic patients. *JAMA* 1993; **269:** 2106–9.
20. Zinman B. The physiologic replacement of insulin: an elusive goal. *N Engl J Med* 1989; **321:** 363–70.
21. Cho YW, Flynn M. Oral delivery of insulin. *Lancet* 1989; **ii:** 1518–19.
22. Nishihata T, et al. Effectiveness of insulin suppositories in diabetic patients. *J Pharm Pharmacol* 1989; **41:** 799–801.

INSULIN ANALOGUES AND PROINSULIN. Recombinant-DNA technology has enabled the production of insulin analogues with altered pharmacokinetic profiles.[1] Most of the insulin in pharmaceutical preparations is in the form of hexamers, which requires time to dissociate before absorption from a subcutaneous site. Substitution of amino-acid residues at the monomer-monomer interface has produced monomeric insulin analogues that retain the biological activity of insulin.[1] Good results have been reported with an analogue, **insulin lispro**, in which the B28 and B29 residues are replaced with lysine and proline. This analogue is commercially available and has been widely reviewed.[2-6] In comparative studies of insulin lispro versus soluble insulin given before meals to patients also receiving a long-acting insulin, insulin lispro was reported to result in good glycaemic control, and could be given immediately before meals (5 to 15 minutes) rather than 20 to 40 minutes before as with soluble insulin. There is a suggestion that it may result in fewer severe hypoglycaemic episodes in such patients.[7] However, an analysis of 10 clinical trials did not find any difference between insulin lispro and neutral insulin (Humulin R) with respect to overall adverse effects or development of long-term diabetic complications.[8] A few cases of response to insulin lispro in patients with severe insulin resistance have been reported.[9,10] Insulin lispro has been complexed with protamine to produce an intermediate-acting form, which is available as a biphasic preparation.[11] **Insulin aspart** is another short-acting insulin analogue, with aspartic acid substituted for proline at position B28.[12,13] It is also used immediately before meals and controls postprandial blood glucose concentrations at least as well as regular human insulin.[13,14]

Protein engineering has also been used to produce a range of soluble insulins with absorption half-lives greater than 24 hours and hence a prolonged action.[1,15] Development has been slower than with the rapid-acting analogues,[1] but the long-acting basal insulin **insulin glargine** is now licensed for once-daily use.[16] It is available as a solution at pH 4; following subcutaneous administration and neutralisation by tissue buffering processes, microprecipitates are formed that slowly release insulin glargine over 24 hours with no pronounced peak in concentration or in metabolic activity. Controlled studies have reported insulin glargine to be at least as effective as once- or twice-daily human isophane insulin in producing glycaemic control as part of a basal-bolus regimen,[17] and to be associated with fewer hypoglycaemic episodes.[18-20]

Proinsulin (the natural precursor of insulin) appears to be more active than insulin in suppressing the hepatic production rather than the peripheral uptake of glucose.[15,21] It has therefore been studied particularly in patients with type 2 diabetes mellitus. However, development by some manufacturers has been suspended because of a higher rate of adverse cardiac effects in patients treated with proinsulin than in controls.[15]

1. Barnett AH, Owens DR. Insulin analogues. *Lancet* 1997; **349:** 47–51. Correction. *ibid.;* 656.
2. Anonymous. Lispro, a rapid-onset insulin. *Med Lett Drugs Ther* 1996; **38:** 97–8.
3. Campbell RK, et al. Insulin lispro: its role in the treatment of diabetes mellitus. *Ann Pharmacother* 1996; **30:** 1263–71.
4. Holleman F, Hoekstra JBL. Insulin lispro. *N Engl J Med* 1997; **337:** 176–83.
5. Anonymous. Humalog—a new insulin analogue. *Drug Ther Bull* 1997; **35:** 57–8.
6. Wilde MI, McTavish D. Insulin Lispro: a review of its pharmacological properties and therapeutic use in the management of diabetes mellitus. *Drugs* 1997; **54:** 597–614.
7. Brunelle RL, et al. Meta-analysis of the effect of insulin lispro on severe hypoglycemia in patients with type 1 diabetes. *Diabetes Care* 1998; **21:** 1726–31.
8. Glazer NB, et al. Safety of insulin lispro: pooled data from clinical trials. *Am J Health-Syst Pharm* 1999; **56:** 542–7.
9. Henrichs HR, et al. Severe insulin resistance treated with insulin lispro. *Lancet* 1996; **348:** 1248.
10. Lahtela JT, et al. Severe antibody-mediated human insulin resistance: successful treatment with the insulin analog lispro. *Diabetes Care* 1997; **20:** 71–3.
11. Heise T, et al. Time-action profiles of novel premixed preparations of insulin lispro and NPL insulin. *Diabetes Care* 1998; **21:** 800–3.
12. Simpson KL, Spencer CM. Insulin aspart. *Drugs* 1999; **57:** 759–65.
13. Setter SM, et al. Insulin aspart: a new rapid-acting insulin analog. *Ann Pharmacother* 2000; **34:** 1423–31.
14. Raskin P, et al. Use of insulin aspart, a fast-acting insulin analog, as the mealtime insulin in the management of patients with type 1 diabetes. *Diabetes Care* 2000; **23:** 583–8.
15. Zinman B. The physiologic replacement of insulin: an elusive goal. *N Engl J Med* 1989; **321:** 363–70.
16. Gillies PS, et al. Insulin glargine. *Drugs* 2000; **59:** 253–60.
17. Raskin P, et al. A 16-week comparison of the novel insulin analog insulin glargine (HOE 901) and NPH human insulin used with insulin lispro in patients with type 1 diabetes. *Diabetes Care* 2000; **23:** 1666–71.
18. Ratner RE, et al. Less hypoglycemia with insulin glargine in intensive insulin therapy for type 1 diabetes. *Diabetes Care* 2000; **23:** 639–43.
19. Pieber TR, et al. Efficacy and safety of HOE 901 versus NPH insulin in patients with type 1 diabetes. *Diabetes Care* 2000; **23:** 157–62.
20. Yki-Järvinen H, et al. Less nocturnal hypoglycemia and better post-dinner glucose control with bedtime insulin glargine compared with bedtime NPH insulin during insulin combination therapy in type 2 diabetes. *Diabetes Care* 2000; **23:** 1130–6.
21. Goran EA. Human proinsulin—a new therapeutic agent? *Pharm J* 1986; **236:** 667.

INTENSIVE ADMINISTRATION REGIMENS. Intensive regimens for insulin administration aim to mimic more closely the physiological insulin pattern in which a basal insulin concentration is supplemented by a preprandial boost of insulin.[1-5] Such intensive regimens are used to provide tight control in an attempt to avoid long-term complications (see p.317).

In multiple-injection regimens, the basal insulin is provided by an injection of intermediate- or long-acting insulin given usually at night. Soluble insulin is administered before each main meal, perhaps with a pen-injector device.[6] Systems for continuous administration may be designed on an open-loop or closed-loop delivery system. Open-loop systems comprise an infusion pump with the infusion rate programmed or controlled manually according to manual blood-glucose monitoring. Closed-loop systems (the 'artificial pancreas') consist of an insulin pump, a glucose sensor, and a computer for analysis of blood-glucose data. Systems for continuous administration have most commonly used the subcutaneous route, but intraperitoneal, intravenous, or intramuscular infusion have also been used.

The most extensively investigated open-loop system is continuous subcutaneous insulin infusion using an external pump. A battery-powered pump infuses soluble insulin via a subcutaneous catheter which is resited every 1 to 3 days. A background infusion is given at a predetermined rate, and preprandial bolus doses given using an override switch or manual entry.[7] Complications include erythema, abscess, or cellulitis at the injection site and, rarely, systemic infection, hypersensitivity reactions to components of the administration set, pump malfunction, adsorption of insulin or preservative on to the administration set, or catheter obstruction.[7] Pump therapy increases the risk of ketoacidosis and intensive regimens are associated with decreased hypoglycaemic awareness and more severe hypoglycaemic episodes.[8] If the pump fails, the onset of ketoacidosis may be more rapid and more likely to be associated with dangerous hyperkalaemia than with conventional administration regimens because there is no depot of insulin.[5]

Further development of open-loop delivery systems has been in the design of implantable insulin pumps. The first pumps delivered insulin at a constant basal rate, but variable-rate models, such as the programmable implantable medication system (PIMS) are now available.[2,9] One of the major problems with implantable pumps has been the tendency for insulin to aggregate on prolonged exposure to body heat, movement, and contact with hydrophobic surfaces.[2] Insulin aggregates may occlude pumps and tubing,[2,9] and studies have suggested that their prolonged infusion may induce amyloidosis.[9] Insulin aggregation has been decreased by the development of insulin preparations containing calcium, glycerol, bicarbonate, or, most successfully, poloxamer.[2,9] Insulin pumps are implanted subcutaneously, usually in the abdomen, but the catheter is usually placed peritoneally or intravenously.[2,9] Glycaemic control has been good;[10,11] a French multicentre study involving 224 patients found that glycosylated haemoglobin fell on average from 7.4 to 6.8% six months after implantation.[12] Specific problems with hypoglycaemia or ketoacidosis do not appear to have been identified,[9–11] and indeed there is some evidence that the postprandial insulin profile is better and hypoglycaemia less frequent, in patients using implantable pumps for intraperitoneal or intravenous delivery compared with those receiving continuous subcutaneous infusion from an external pump.[13] Complications include mechanical failure of the system, infection (particularly of the implantation site) and skin necrosis over the implant. Peritoneal catheters may become obstructed by omental tissue.[9–11]

Closed-loop continuous insulin infusion systems are generally confined to research and experimental work. External pumps are used since no glucose sensor suitable for implantation has yet been developed.[9] (However, results in *animals* have suggested that an alternative to such systems may be a vascularised artificial pancreas containing islet cells.[14])

Intensified insulin regimens have the advantage of improving the patient's lifestyle and allowing flexibility in timing of meals. However, careful dietary control must still be maintained and regular monitoring of blood-glucose concentrations is an important component of such regimens. Therefore patients must be well-motivated, reliable, and able to monitor their own blood glucose, and must have access to expert 24-hour help.[4–7] Although there are reports of success with intensive administration regimens in brittle (labile) diabetics,[15] these patients are generally unlikely to benefit from such regimens.[5]

1. Fisher BM. Choosing an insulin. *Prescribers' J* 1988; **28:** 138–43 and 169 (correction).
2. Pickup J. The pursuit of perfect control in diabetes: better insulin better delivered. *BMJ* 1988; **297:** 929–31.
3. Home PD, *et al.* Insulin treatment: a decade of change. *Br Med Bull* 1989; **45:** 92–110.
4. Zinman B. The physiologic replacement of insulin: an elusive goal. *N Engl J Med* 1989; **321:** 363–70.
5. MacPherson JN, Feely J. Insulin. *BMJ* 1990; **300:** 731–6.
6. Anonymous. Insulin pen: mightier than syringe? *Lancet* 1989; **i:** 307–8.
7. Anonymous. Continuous subcutaneous insulin infusion. *JAMA* 1989; **262:** 1239–43.
8. Egger M, *et al.* Risk of adverse effects of intensified treatment in insulin-dependent diabetes mellitus: a meta-analysis. *Diabetic Med* 1997; **14:** 919–28.
9. Anonymous. Continuous peritoneal insulin infusion and implantable insulin infusion pumps for diabetic control. *JAMA* 1989; **262:** 3195–8.
10. Point Study Group. One-year trial of a remote-controlled implantable insulin infusion system in type I diabetic patients. *Lancet* 1988; **ii:** 866–9.

11. Saudek CD, *et al.* A preliminary trial of the programmable implantable medication system for insulin delivery. *N Engl J Med* 1989; **321:** 574–9.
12. Broussolle C, *et al.* French multicentre experience of implantable insulin pumps. *Lancet* 1994; **343:** 514–15.
13. Nathan DM, *et al.* Postprandial insulin profiles with implantable pump therapy may explain decreased frequency of severe hypoglycemia, compared with intensive subcutaneous regimens, in insulin-dependent diabetes mellitus patients. *Am J Med* 1996; **100:** 412–17.
14. Maki T, *et al.* Novel delivery of pancreatic islet cells to treat insulin-dependent diabetes mellitus. *Clin Pharmacokinet* 1995; **28:** 471–82.
15. Wood DF, *et al.* Management of "brittle" diabetes with a preprogrammable implanted pump delivering intraperitoneal insulin. *BMJ* 1990; **301:** 1143–4.

MIXING OF INSULINS. There are studies indicating that the rapid effect of soluble insulin may be lost if mixed in the syringe immediately prior to injection with insulins containing high concentrations of free zinc.[1,2] Insulin manufacturers recommend immediate injection of mixtures prepared in the syringe; if delay is unavoidable a consistent routine is advised. The shorter-acting insulin should be drawn into the syringe first to prevent contamination of the vial by the longer-acting preparation. Insulins from different manufacturers should not be mixed since formulation differences, such as the buffer or preservative used, may render them incompatible.[3]

1. Mühlhauser I, *et al.* Miscibility of human and bovine ultralente insulin with soluble insulin. *BMJ* 1984; **289:** 1656–7.
2. Heine RJ, *et al.* Mixing short and intermediate acting insulins in the syringe: effect on postprandial blood glucose concentrations in type I diabetics. *BMJ* 1985; **290:** 204–5.
3. Fisher BM. Choosing an insulin. *Prescribers' J* 1988; **28:** 138–43. Correction. *ibid.;* 169.

Diabetes mellitus. Insulin is the mainstay of the treatment of **type 1 diabetes mellitus.** For a discussion of the treatment of diabetes mellitus, including the contexts in which insulin is used, see p.315. The possible role of tight glycaemic control with insulin to prevent the development of microvascular and macrovascular complications in patients with type 1 diabetes is discussed on p.317, while further discussion of specific regimens and approaches to insulin therapy is given under Administration, above.

DIABETIC EMERGENCIES. As discussed on p.318, **diabetic ketoacidosis** and hyperosmolar hyperglycaemic state are medical emergencies and should be treated immediately with fluid replacement and insulin. Potassium, and possibly phosphate, replacement may also be required, but bicarbonate should not be given unless acidaemia is very severe. In the *UK* the *British National Formulary* recommends that insulin be given by intravenous infusion for diabetic ketoacidosis, as a solution of soluble insulin 1 unit per mL via an infusion pump. An infusion rate of 6 units per hour in adults and 0.1 units per kg bodyweight per hour in children is recommended initially, with the rate doubled or quadrupled if the blood glucose concentration fails to decrease by about 5 mmol per litre per hour. When blood glucose concentrations have fallen to 10 mmol per litre the infusion rate can be reduced to 3 units per hour in adults or about 0.02 units per kg per hour in children, and continued, together with glucose 5% to prevent hypoglycaemia, until ketone bodies have been cleared and the patient is ready to take food by mouth. The insulin infusion should not be stopped before subcutaneous insulin has been started. Potassium chloride is included in the infusion as appropriate to prevent insulin-induced hypokalaemia. If facilities for intravenous infusion are not available the insulin is given by intramuscular injection: in adults an initial loading dose of 20 units intramuscularly is followed by 6 units intramuscularly every hour until the blood glucose concentration falls to 10 mmol per litre, when the dose is given every 2 hours. Late hypoglycaemia due to insulin accumulation should be watched for and managed appropriately.

In the *USA* the intramuscular or subcutaneous route have been used as alternatives to intravenous insulin administration, together with other appropriate management. One successful set of protocols for insulin dosage in diabetic ketoacidosis is as follows:[1] an initial intravenous bolus of 0.15 units per kg is followed by infusion of 0.1 units per kg per hour; if blood glucose does not fall by about 2.5 to 3.5 mmol per litre in the first hour the infusion rate is doubled every hour until this rate of decline is achieved. (A similar insulin regimen has proved effective in patients with hyperosmolar hyperglycaemic state.[1]) When given by the intramuscular or subcutaneous routes an initial bolus of 0.4 units per kg is divided and given half by the intravenous route and half either intramuscularly or subcutaneously as appropriate. This is followed by 0.1 units per kg every hour intramuscularly or subcutaneously; if response is inadequate it is accompanied by an intravenous bolus of 10 units until blood glucose falls by 2.5 to 3.5 mmol per litre. In children intravenous infusion of 0.1 units per kg per hour is recommended, or if intravenous infusion is impractical an initial intravenous bolus of 0.1 units per kg followed by 0.1 units per kg per hour either intramuscularly or subcutaneously. Treatment is continued at this rate until acidosis is cleared, when the rate is decreased to 0.05 units per kg per hour until subcutaneous insulin treatment can be begun.[1]

1. Kitabchi AE, *et al.* Management of hyperglycemic crises in patients with diabetes. *Diabetes Care* 2001; **24:** 131–53.

TYPE 2 DIABETES MELLITUS. Traditionally the use of insulin in patients with type 2 diabetes has tended to be reserved for those who cannot be controlled by diet and oral antidiabetics alone.[1,2]

Given the possible association between circulating insulin and atherosclerotic cardiovascular symptoms[3] there has been some concern about the administration of exogenous insulin to insulin-resistant patients who are already hyperinsulinaemic. Furthermore, patients switched to insulin tend to gain weight[2] which is undesirable in a frequently obese patient group.

Insulin is nonetheless being used more frequently in type 2 patients. This is largely because of a trend toward more intensive regimens designed to produce tighter glycaemic control, on the hypothesis that, as in patients with type 1 disease, this will reduce the development and progression of diabetic complications. Results from the UK Prospective Diabetes Study,[4–6] show that insulin is an effective option in type 2 diabetes, and confirm both the value of intensive therapy in retarding microvascular complications,[6] and that oral therapy should be used before insulin in patients with primary diet failure.[7]

In order to minimise the dose of insulin required, and any risks it may entail, it has been suggested that insulin therapy in type 2 diabetes should be combined with other measures including oral hypoglycaemic drugs.[8] There has long been debate about the value of combined therapy, but a recent meta-analysis indicated that glycaemic control was better, and insulin requirements lower, in type 2 diabetics who received insulin with a sulfonylurea.[9]

For further discussion of the management of type 2 diabetes mellitus see p.315.

1. Tattersall RB, Scott AR. When to use insulin in the maturity onset diabetic. *Postgrad Med J* 1987; **63:** 859–64.
2. Taylor R. Insulin for the non-insulin dependent? *BMJ* 1988; **296:** 1015–16.
3. Stern MP. Do non-insulin-dependent diabetes mellitus and cardiovascular disease share common antecedents? *Ann Intern Med* 1996; **124** (suppl): 110–16.
4. United Kingdom Prospective Diabetes Study Group. United Kingdom prospective diabetes study (UKPDS) 13: relative efficacy of randomly allocated diet, sulphonylurea, insulin, or metformin in patients with newly diagnosed non-insulin-dependent diabetes followed for three years. *BMJ* 1995; **310:** 83–8.
5. Turner R, *et al.* United Kingdom Prospective Diabetes Study 17: a 9-year update of a randomized, controlled trial on the effect of improved metabolic control on complications in non-insulin-dependent diabetes mellitus. *Ann Intern Med* 1996; **124** (suppl): 136–45.
6. UK Prospective Diabetes Study Group. Intensive blood-glucose control with sulphonylureas or insulin compared with conventional treatment and risk of complications in patients with type 2 diabetes (UKPDS 33). *Lancet* 1998; **352:** 837–53.
7. United Kingdom Prospective Diabetes Study Group. United Kingdom Prospective Diabetes Study 24: a 6-year, randomized, controlled trial comparing sulfonylurea, insulin, and metformin therapy in patients with newly diagnosed type 2 diabetes that could not be controlled with diet therapy. *Ann Intern Med* 1998; **128:** 165–75.
8. Henry RR. Glucose control and insulin resistance in non-insulin-dependent diabetes mellitus. *Ann Intern Med* 1996; **124** (suppl): 97–103.
9. Johnson JL, *et al.* Efficacy of insulin and sulfonylurea combination therapy in type II diabetes: a meta-analysis of the randomized placebo-controlled trials. *Arch Intern Med* 1996; **156:** 259–64.

Diagnosis and testing. PITUITARY FUNCTION. Insulin-induced hypoglycaemia has been used to provide a stressful stimulus in order to assess hypothalamic-pituitary function. The insulin stress or insulin tolerance test has been used as a standard test for assessment of growth hormone or corticotropin deficiency. However, it is unpleasant, expensive, and not without risk, and is contra-indicated in patients with angina, heart failure, cerebrovascular disease, or epilepsy; some workers recommend its use only when results of alternative tests are equivocal,[1,2] and it should only be performed in specialist units under strict surveillance.[3]

1. Clayton RN. Diagnosis of adrenal insufficiency. *BMJ* 1989; **298:** 271–2.
2. Stewart PM, *et al.* A rational approach for assessing the hypothalamic-pituitary-adrenal axis. *Lancet* 1988; **1:** 1208–10.
3. Hindmarsh PC, Swift PGF. An assessment of growth hormone provocation tests. *Arch Dis Child* 1995; **72:** 362–8.

Hyperkalaemia. Insulin promotes the intracellular uptake of potassium. It is therefore used in the management of moderate to severe hyperkalaemia, when it is given with glucose (see p.1182).

Liver disorders. References[1,2] to the use of insulin and glucagon in the treatment of liver disorders based on their reported hepatotrophic effect. However, a small randomised study[3] found no benefit from insulin and glucagon infusions in fulminant hepatic failure.

1. Baker AL, *et al.* A randomized clinical trial of insulin and glucagon infusion for treatment of alcoholic hepatitis: progress report in 50 patients. *Gastroenterology* 1981; **81:** 1410–14.
2. Jaspan JB, *et al.* Insulin and glucagon infusion in the treatment of liver failure. *Arch Intern Med* 1984; **144:** 2075–8.
3. Harrison PM, *et al.* Failure of insulin and glucagon infusion to stimulate liver regeneration in fulminant hepatic failure. *J Hepatol* 1990; **10:** 332–6.

Myocardial infarction. Discussions on the effects of insulin with glucose and potassium in the ischaemic heart including its effect in reducing blood free fatty acids have been emphasised and its potential benefits in left ventricular failure and cardiogenic shock.[1,2] Glucose-insulin-potassium solutions have been investigated in only small numbers of patients with acute myocardial infarction although a meta-analysis[3] of randomised controlled studies performed before the widespread use of thrombolytics found a reduction in mortality in recipients of these solutions;

following a small pilot study with similar findings,[4] a larger study is now underway. Insulin-glucose infusion followed by multiple daily subcutaneous insulin injections has been reported to reduce mortality in diabetics who suffered a myocardial infarction.[5,6]

For the conventional management of myocardial infarction see p.805.

1. Opie LH. Glucose and the metabolism of ischaemic myocardium. *Lancet* 1995; **345:** 1520–1.
2. Taegtmeyer H, *et al.* Metabolic support for the postischaemic heart. *Lancet* 1995; **345:** 1552–5.
3. Fath-Ordoubadi F, Beatt KJ. Glucose-insulin-potassium therapy for treatment of acute myocardial infarction: an overview of randomized placebo-controlled trials. *Circulation* 1997; **96:** 1152–6.
4. Díaz R, *et al.* Metabolic modulation of acute myocardial infarction: the ECLA Glucose-Insulin-Potassium Pilot Trial. *Circulation* 1998; **98:** 2227–34.
5. Malmberg K, *et al.* Randomized trial of insulin-glucose infusion followed by subcutaneous insulin treatment in diabetic patients with acute myocardial infarction (DIGAMI Study): effects on mortality at 1 year. *J Am Coll Cardiol* 1995; **26:** 57–65.
6. Malmberg K, *et al.* Prospective randomised study of intensive insulin treatment on long term survival after acute myocardial infarction in patients with diabetes mellitus. *BMJ* 1997; **314:** 1512–15.

Neonatal hyperglycaemia. Hyperglycaemia is common in very immature neonates, although hypoglycaemia is more common in neonates born to diabetic mothers. Neonatal hyperglycaemia has been treated by glucose restriction until glucose tolerance improves. However, the use of an insulin infusion can allow normal glucose administration to continue.[1] It was suggested that insulin was best administered intravenously in a separate, easily titratable solution because of the frequent fluctuations of requirement in these infants. An alternative approach, namely subcutaneous injection of a long-acting insulin, has been reported to result in less fluctuation of blood-glucose concentrations,[2] and hence easier management.

1. Binder ND, *et al.* Insulin infusion with parenteral nutrition in extremely low birth weight infants with hyperglycemia. *J Pediatr* 1989; **114:** 273–80.
2. Mitamura R, *et al.* Ultralente insulin treatment of transient neonatal diabetes mellitus. *J Pediatr* 1996; **128:** 268–70.

Overdosage with calcium-channel blockers. Continuous infusion of insulin 0.5 units per kg body-weight per hour, together with glucose as required to maintain euglycaemia, has been reported to be of value in the management of overdosage with calcium-channel blockers when conventional therapy has failed.[1]

1. Boyer EW, Shannon M. Treatment of calcium-channel-blocker intoxication with insulin infusion. *N Engl J Med* 2001; **344:** 1721–2.

Preparations

BP 2001: Protamine Zinc Insulin Injection;
Ph. Eur.: Biphasic Insulin Injection; Biphasic Isophane Insulin Injection; Insulin Zinc Injectable Suspension; Insulin Zinc Injectable Suspension (Amorphous); Insulin Zinc Injectable Suspension (Crystalline); Isophane Insulin Injection; Soluble Insulin Injection;
USP 25: Extended Insulin Human Zinc Suspension; Extended Insulin Zinc Suspension; Insulin Human Injection; Insulin Human Zinc Suspension; Insulin Injection; Insulin Zinc Suspension; Isophane Insulin Human Suspension; Isophane Insulin Suspension; Prompt Insulin Zinc Suspension.

Proprietary Preparations (details are given in Part 3)
Aust.: Actrapid HM; Depot-Insulin; Humalog; Humalog Mix 25 and 50; Huminsulin Basal; Huminsulin Long; Huminsulin Normal; Huminsulin Profil I, II, III, and IV; Huminsulin Ultralong; Insulatard HM; Insuman Basal; Insuman Comb 15, 25, and 50; Insuman Infusat; Insuman komb Typ 15, Typ 25, and Typ 50; Insuman Rapid; Komb-Insulin; Lente MC; Mixtard HM 10/90, 15/85, 20/80, 30/70, 40/60, and 50/50; Monotard HM; Ultratard HM; Velosulin HM; *Austral.:* Actrapid; Humalog; Humalog Mix 25; Humulin 20/80, 30/70 and 50/50; Humulin L; Humulin NPH; Humulin R; Humulin UL; Hypurin Isophane; Hypurin Neutral; Insulin 2†; Isotard MC; Lente MC†; Mixtard 20/80, 30/70, 50/50; Monotard; NovoRapid; Protamine Zinc Insulin MC†; Protaphane; Ultralente MC†; Ultratard; *Belg.:* Actrapid HM; Humaject 20/80, 30/70, 40/60, 50/50; Humaject NPH; Humaject Regular; Humalog; Humuline 20/80, 30/70, 40/60, 50/50; Humuline Long; Humuline NPH; Humuline Regular; Humuline Ultralong; Insulatard HM; Lente MC; Mixtard HM 10/90, 20/80, 40/60, 50/50; Monotard HM; Ultralente MC†; Ultratard HM; Velosuline Humanum†; *Braz.:* Actrapid MC; Biohulin 70/30 and 80/20; Biohulin L; Biohulin NPH; Biohulin R; Biohulin Ultralenta; Humulin 70/30, 80/20, and 90/10; Humulin Lenta; Humulin NPH; Humulin Regular; Iolin NPH; Iolin Regular; Monolin NPH; Monolin Regular; Monotard MC; Neosulin Lenta; Neosulin NPH; Neosulin Regular; Novolin 70/30; Novolin L; Novolin N; Novolin R; Protaphane HM; *Canad.:* Humalog; Humulin 10/90, 20/80, 30/70, 40/60, and 50/50; Humulin L; Humulin N; Humulin R; Humulin U; Iletin II Pork Lente; Iletin II Pork NPH; Iletin II Pork Regular; Iletin Lente; Iletin NPH; Iletin Regular; Novolin 10/90, 20/80, 30/70, 40/60, 50/50; Novolin Lente; Novolin NPH; Novolin Toronto; Novolin Ultralente; *Denm.:* Actrapid; Humalog; Humalog Mix 25 and 50; Humulin Mix 30/70; Humulin NPH; Humulin Regular; Humutard Ultra; Insulatard; Mixtard 10/90, 20/80, 30/70, 40/60, and 50/50; Monotard; NovoRapid; Velosulin; *Fin.:* Actrapid; Humalog; Humalog Mix 25 and 50; Humulin Mix 30/70; Humulin NPH; Humulin Regular; Humutard; Humutard Ultra; Insulin Lente MC; Insulin Lyht; Insulin Pitka; Insuman Basal; Insuman Comb 25; Insuman Infusat; Insuman Rapid; Mixtard 10/90, 20/80, 30/70, 40/60, and 50/50; Monotard; NovoRapid; Protaphan; Ultratard; Velosulin; *Fr.:* Actrapid HM; Endopancrine

100†; Endopancrine 40†; Endopancrine Protamine†; Endopancrine Zinc Protamine†; Humalog; Humalog Mix 25 and 50; Insulatard HM; Insuline Semi Tardum†; Insuline Tardum MX†; Insuline Ultra Tardum†; Insuman Basal; Insuman Comb 15, 25, and 50; Insuman Infusat; Insuman Intermediaire 100%†; Insuman Intermediaire 25/75†; Insuman Rapid; Lente MC†; Lillypen Profil 10, 20, 30, and 40; Lillypen Protamine Isophane; Lillypen Rapide; Mixtard 10, 20, 30, 40, and 50 HM; Monotard HM; Orgasuline 30/70; Orgasuline NPH; Orgasuline Rapide; Rapitard MC†; Semilente MC†; Ultralente MC†; Ultratard HM; Umuline Profil 10, 20, 30, 40, and 50; Umuline Protamine Isophane (NPH); Umuline Rapide; Umuline Zinc; Umuline Zinc Compose; *Ger.:* Actraphane HM 10/90, 20/80, 30/70, 40/60, 50/50; Actrapid HM; B-Insulin; Basal-H-Insulin†; Berlinsulin H 10/90, 20/80, 30/70, 40/60, 50/50; Berlinsulin H Basal; Berlinsulin H Normal; Depot-H-Insulin†; Depot-H15-Insulin†; Depot-Insulin; Depot-Insulin S; H-Insulin†; H-Tronin; Humalog; Huminsulin; Huminsulin Basal; Huminsulin Long†; Huminsulin Normal; Huminsulin Profil II and III; Huminsulin Ultralong†; Insulatard Human; Insulatard MC; Insulin S; Insulin SNC; Insuman Basal; Insuman Comb 15, 25, and 50; Insuman Rapid; Komb-H-Insulin†; Komb-Insulin; Komb-Insulin S; L-Insulin; L-Insulin SNC; Lente; Mixtard; Mixtard Human†; Monotard HM; NovoRapid; Protaphan HM; Rapitard†; Semilente; Ultralente†; Ultratard HM; Velasulin; Velasulin Human; Velasulin MC; *Hong Kong:* Actrapid HM; Actrapid MC; Humalog; Humulin 70/30; Humulin L; Humulin N; Humulin R; Mixtard 10, 20, 30, 40, and 50 HM; Monotard HM; Monotard MC; Protaphane HM; Protaphane MC; Ultratard HM; *Irl.:* Actrapid; Humalog; Humalog Mix 25 and 50; Humulin I; Humulin Lente; Humulin M2, M3, M4; Humulin S; Humulin Zn; Insulatard; Insuman Comb 15, 25, and 50; Insuman Rapid; Mixtard 10, 20, 30, 40, and 50; Monotard; NovoRapid; Ultratard; *Israel:* Actrapid; Humulin 70/30, 80/20; Humulin N; Humulin R; Humulin U; *Ital.:* Actraphane 10/90, 20/80, 30/70, 40/60, 50/50; Actrapid; Bio-Insulin 10/90, 20/80, 30/70, and 50/50; Bio-Insulin L; Bio-Insulin R; Bio-Insulin U; Humalog; Humulin 10/90, 20/80, 30/70, 40/60, and 50/50; Humulin I; Humulin L; Humulin R; Humulin U; Monotard; Protaphane HM; Ultratard; *Jpn:* Humacart 3/7; *Mex.:* Anilusin; Humalog; Humanilusin; Humulin 70/30, 80/20; Humulin L; Humulin N; Humulin R; Insulex; Novolin 30/70; Novolin L; Novolin N; Novolin R; *Neth.:* Actrapid; Humaject 10/90, 20/80, 30/70, 40/60, 50/50; Humaject NPH; Humaject Regular; Humalog; Humalog Mix 25; Humuline 10/90, 20/80, 30/70, 40/60, 50/50; Humuline NPH; Humuline Regular; Humuline Zink†; Insulatard; Insuman Basal; Insuman Comb 15, 25, and 50; Insuman Rapid; Isuhuman Basal†; Isuhuman Comb 15, Comb 25, Comb 50†; Isuhuman Infusat; Isuhuman Rapid†; Mixtard 10/90, 20/80, 30/70, 40/60, 50/50; Monotard; NovoRapid; Ultratard; Velosulin; *Norw.:* Actrapid; Humalog; Humalog Mix 25; Humulin Mix 30/70; Humulin NPH; Humulin Regular; Insulatard; Insulin Basal; Insulin Infusat; Insulin Komb 25/75; Insulin Rapid; Mixtard 10/90, 20/80, 30/70, 40/60, 50/50; Monotard; Ultratard; Velosulin; *NZ:* Actrapid; Humalog; Humulin 80/20 and 70/30; Humulin L; Humulin N; Humulin R; Humulin U; Mixtard 30 or 50; Monotard; PenMix 10, 20, 30, 40, or 50; Protaphane; Ultratard; *Port.:* Actrapid; Humalog; Humulin Lenta; Humulin M1, M2, M3, M4; Humulin NPH; Humulin Regular; Humulin Ultralenta; Insulatard; Isuhuman Basal; Isuhuman Comb 25; Isuhuman Rapid; Mixtard 10, 20, 30, 40, and 50 HM; Monotard; Ultratard; *S.Afr.:* Actraphane HM; Actrapid HM; Humulin Mix 30/70; Humulin NPH; Humulin R; Humulin U†; Mixtard 20/80, 40/60; Monotard HM; Protaphane HM; Ultratard HM; *Singapore:* Actrapid; Humalog; Humulin 30/70; Humulin L; Humulin N; Humulin R; Insulatard HM; Mixtard 20, 30, 50 HM; Monotard HM; Ultratard HM; *Spain:* Actrapid; Humalog; Humaplus 10/90, 20/80, 30/70, 40/60, 50/50; Humaplus NPH; Humaplus Regular; Humulina 10:90, 20:80, 30:70, 40:60, 50:50; Humulina Lenta; Humulina NPH; Humulina Regular; Humulina Ultralenta; Insulatard NPH; Lente MC; Mixtard 10, 20, 30, 40, and 50; Mixtard 30/70; Monotard; Ultratard; *Swed.:* Actrapid; Humalog; Humulin Mix 30/70; Humulin NPH; Humulin Regular; Humutard†; Insulatard; Insuman Basal; Insuman Comb 25; Insuman Infusat; Insuman Rapid; Isuhuman Basal†; Isuhuman Comb 25/75, 50/50†; Isuhuman Infusat†; Isuhuman Rapid†; Mixtard 10/90, 20/80, 30/70, 40/60, 50/50; Monotard; Novo Rapid; Ultratard; Velosulin; *Switz.:* Actrapid HM; Actrapid MC; Humalog; Huminsulin Basal (NPH); Huminsulin Long; Huminsulin Normal; Huminsulin Profil I, II, III, and IV; Huminsulin Ultralong; Insulatard HM; Insulatard MC; Insuman Basal; Insuman Comb 15, 25, and 50; Insuman Infusat; Insuman Rapid; Lente MC; Mixtard 30 MC; Mixtard HM 10, 20, 30, 40, 50; Monotard HM; NovoRapid; Rapitard MC†; Semilente MC; Ultralente MC†; Ultratard HM; Velosulin HM; Velosulin MC†; *Thai.:* Actrapid HM; Humalog; Humulin 70/30, 80/20; Humulin N; Humulin R; Insulatard; Mixtard 20, 30, 50 HM; Monotard HM; Ultratard HM; *UAE:* Jusline 70/30; Jusline N; Jusline R; *UK:* Humaject I; Humaject M1, M2, M3, M4, M5; Humaject S; Humalog; Humalog Mix 25 and 50; Human Actraphane†; Human Actrapid; Human Initard 50/50†; Human Insulatard; Human Mixtard 10, 20, 30, 40, and 50; Human Monotard; Human Ultratard; Human Velosulin; Humulin I; Humulin Lente; Humulin S; Humulin Zn; Humulin M2, M3, M5; Hypurin 30/70; Hypurin Isophane; Hypurin Lente; Hypurin Neutral; Hypurin Protamine Zinc; Initard 50/50†; Insuman Basal; Insuman Comb 15, 25, and 50; Insuman Rapid; Lentard MC†; NovoRapid; PenMix 10/90, 20/80, 30/70, 40/60, 50/50†; Pork Actrapid; Pork Insulatard; Pork Mixtard 30; Rapitard MC†; Semitard MC†; Velosulin†; *USA:* Humalog; Humalog Mix 75/25 and 50/50; Humulin 50/50, 70/30; Humulin L; Humulin N; Humulin R; Humulin U Ultralente; Lantus; Lente; Lente Iletin I†; Lente Iletin II; Lente L†; Novolin 70/30; Novolin L; Novolin N; Novolin R; NovoLog; NPH Iletin I†; NPH Iletin II; Regular Iletin I†; Regular Iletin II; Ultralente; Velosulin Human BR.

Metformin Hydrochloride (7231-c)

Metformin Hydrochloride (*BANM, USAN, rINNM*).
LA-6023; La-6023 (metformin); Metformini Hydrochloridum.
1,1-Dimethylbiguanide hydrochloride.
$C_4H_{11}N_5,HCl = 165.6$.
CAS — 657-24-9 (metformin); 1115-70-4 (metformin hydrochloride).
Pharmacopoeias. In *Eur.* (see p.vi) and *Pol.*

Pharmacopoeial description

Ph. Eur.: White crystals. Freely soluble in water; slightly soluble in alcohol; practically insoluble in acetone and in dichloromethane.

Adverse Effects, Treatment, and Precautions

As for biguanides in general, p.320.

Interactions

As for biguanides in general, p.320.

Pharmacokinetics

Metformin hydrochloride is slowly and incompletely absorbed from the gastrointestinal tract; the absolute bioavailability of a single 500-mg dose is reported to be about 50 to 60%, although this is reduced somewhat if taken with food. Following absorption plasma protein binding is negligible, and it is excreted unchanged in the urine. The plasma elimination half-life is reported to range from about 2 to 6 hours after oral administration.

◊ References.
1. Scheen AJ. Clinical pharmacokinetics of metformin. *Clin Pharmacokinet* 1996; **30:** 359–71.
2. Sambol NC, *et al.* Pharmacokinetics and pharmacodynamics of metformin in healthy subjects and patients with noninsulin-dependent diabetes mellitus. *J Clin Pharmacol* 1996; **36:** 1012–21.

Uses and Administration

Metformin hydrochloride is a biguanide antidiabetic (p.320). It is given by mouth in the treatment of type 2 diabetes mellitus (p.315), and is the drug of first choice in obese patients. Initial dosage is 500 mg two or three times daily or 850 mg once or twice daily with or after meals, gradually increased if necessary to 2 to 3 g daily; doses above 2 g daily are associated with an increased incidence of gastrointestinal adverse effects.

Metformin is also used as the chlorophenoxyacetate and as the embonate.

◊ General references.
1. Dunn CJ, Peters DH. Metformin: a review of its pharmacological properties and therapeutic use in non-insulin-dependent diabetes mellitus. *Drugs* 1995; **49:** 721–49.
2. Anonymous. Metformin for non-insulin-dependent diabetes mellitus. *Med Lett Drugs Ther* 1995; **37:** 41–2.
3. Bailey CJ, Turner RC. Metformin. *N Engl J Med* 1996; **334:** 574–9.
4. Melchior WR, Jaber LA. Metformin: an antihyperglycemic agent for treatment of type II diabetes. *Ann Pharmacother* 1996; **30:** 158–64.
5. Davidson MB, Peters AL. An overview of metformin in the treatment of type 2 diabetes mellitus. *Am J Med* 1997; **102:** 99–110.
6. Klepser TB, Kelly MW. Metformin hydrochloride: an antihyperglycemic agent. *Am J Health-Syst Pharm* 1997; **54:** 893–903. Correction. *ibid.*; 1335.

Action. A review of the action of metformin[1] considered that although a number of possible mechanisms have been suggested (see p.320), the major action of metformin lay in increasing glucose transport across the cell membrane in skeletal muscle. There is also some evidence *in vitro* that it can inhibit the formation of advanced glycosylation end-products.[2]

1. Klip A, Leiter LA. Cellular mechanism of action of metformin. *Diabetes Care* 1990; **13:** 696–704.
2. Tanaka Y, *et al.* Inhibitory effect of metformin on formation of advanced glycation end products. *Curr Ther Res* 1997; **58:** 693–7.

Diabetes mellitus. Results of the United Kingdom Prospective Diabetes Study (UKPDS) demonstrated that intensive blood glucose control with metformin reduces the risk of diabetic complications and death in overweight patients with type 2 diabetes.[1] The study also generated some concern regarding intensive therapy with metformin plus a sulfonylurea (see p.336) but this was not borne out on further analysis and such combinations are widely used. Metformin is also used in combination with the glitazones, or with insulin in patients requiring combined or more intensive therapy.

1. UK Prospective Diabetes Study Group. Effect of intensive blood-glucose control with metformin on complications in overweight patients with type 2 diabetes (UKPDS 34). *Lancet* 1998; **352:** 854–65.

Polycystic ovary syndrome. It has been suggested that hyperinsulinism may play a pathogenetic role in stimulating the abnormal androgen production from the ovary seen in women with polycystic ovary syndrome (PCOS, p.1276). Two small studies have reported an improvement in androgen concentrations concomitant with a decrease in serum insulin following metformin treatment in women with the syndrome.[1,2] Similar effects and improvements in menstrual patterns, ovulation rate, and hirsutism have been reported[3] to have been obtained in other small studies. However, another study was unable to demonstrate a reduction in either insulin or circulating androgen concentrations when metformin was given.[4] Combination of metformin with clomifene appears to improve ovulatory response, compared with clomifene alone, in women with PCOS; metformin also increased the rate of spontaneous ovulation.[5] Some consider that current evidence supported a trial of metformin in patients with anovulation, androgen excess, and vascular risk factors but because of the lack of data on long-term safety such use should be supervised by an endocrinologist or a physician with suitable expertise.[3]

1. Velazquez EM, et al. Metformin therapy in polycystic ovary syndrome reduces hyperinsulinemia, insulin resistance, hyperandrogenemia, and systolic blood pressure, while facilitating normal menses and pregnancy. *Metabolism* 1994; **43:** 647–54.
2. Nestler JE, Jakubowicz DJ. Decreases in ovarian cytochrome P450c17α activity and serum free testosterone after reduction of insulin secretion in polycystic ovary syndrome. *N Engl J Med* 1996; **335:** 617–23.
3. Norman RJ, et al. Metformin and intervention in polycystic ovary syndrome. *Med J Aust* 2001; **174:** 580–3.
4. Ehrmann DA, et al. Effects of metformin on insulin secretion, insulin action, and ovarian steroidogenesis in women with polycystic ovary syndrome. *J Clin Endocrinol Metab* 1997; **82:** 524–30.
5. Nestler JE, et al. Effects of metformin on spontaneous and clomiphene-induced ovulation in the polycystic ovary syndrome. *N Engl J Med* 1998; **338:** 1876–80.

Preparations

BP 2001: Metformin Tablets.

Proprietary Preparations (details are given in Part 3)
Aust.: Diabetex; Glucophage; Meglucon; Orabet; *Austral.:* Diabex; Diaformin; Glucohexal; Glucomet; Glucophage; Novomet; *Belg.:* Glucophage; *Braz.:* Glifage; Glucoformin; *Canad.:* Glucophage; Glycon; *Denm.:* Glucophage; Orabet; *Fin.:* Diformin; Glucophage; Metformin; Oramet; *Fr.:* Eddia†; Glucinan; Glucophage; Glymax; Metfirex; Stagid; *Ger.:* Biocos; Diabesin; Diabetase; espa-formin; Glucobon; Glucophage S; Mediabet; Meglucon; Mescorit; Met; Metfogamma; Siofor; Thiabet; *Hong Kong:* Diaformin; Glucophage; Melbin; *Irl.:* Glucophage; *Israel:* Apophage; Glucomin; Glucophage; Glufor; *Ital.:* Glucophage; Metbay; Metforal; Metiguanide; *Mex.:* Dabex; Dimefor; Glucophage; *Neth.:* Glucophage; *Norw.:* Glucophage; Orabet; *NZ:* Glucomet; Glucophage; Metomin; *Port.:* Glucophage; Risidon; Stagid; *S.Afr.:* Dextin; Glucophage; *Singapore:* Diabetmin; Diamin; Glucophage; Glycoran; *Spain:* Dianben; Glucophage†; *Swed.:* Glucophage; Gluformin; Glustress; Gluzolyte; Maformin; ME-F; Meformed; Metfor-500; Metfron; Miformin; Pocophage; Poli-Formin; Prophage; Serformin; Siamformet; *UK:* Glucamet; Glucophage; Orabet; *USA:* Glucophage.

Multi-ingredient: *Ital.:* Bi-Euglucon M; Glibomet; Gliconorm; Glucomide; Glucosulfa; Pleiamide; Suguan M; *Mex.:* Bi-Euglucon M; Dabex G; Insogen Plus; Obinese; *Switz.:* Diabiformine; *USA:* Glucovance.

Midaglizole (3694-z)

Midaglizole (rINN).

DG-5128. (±)-2-[α-(2-Imidazolin-2-ylmethyl)benzyl]pyridine.

$C_{16}H_{17}N_3 = 251.3.$
$CAS — 66529-17-7.$

Profile

Midaglizole has been investigated as an antidiabetic. A proposed mode of action is stimulation of insulin secretion by antagonism of alpha$_2$-adrenoceptors. Midaglizole has also been investigated as a bronchodilator in asthma.

◊ References.
1. Kawazu S, et al. Initial phase II clinical studies on midaglizole (DG-5128). *Diabetes* 1987; **36:** 221–6.
2. Yoshie Y, et al. The inhibitory effect of a selective α$_2$-adrenergic receptor antagonist on moderate- to severe-type asthma. *J Allergy Clin Immunol* 1989; **84:** 747–52.
3. Nomura M, et al. Pharmacokinetics of midaglizole, a new hypoglycaemic agent in healthy subjects. *Biopharm Drug Dispos* 1990; **11:** 701–13.

Miglitol (18829-n)

Miglitol (BAN, USAN, pINN).

Bay-m-1099. (2R,3R,4R,5S)-1-(2-Hydroxyethyl)-2-(hydroxymethyl)piperidine-3,4,5-triol.

$C_8H_{17}NO_5 = 207.2.$
$CAS — 72432-03-2.$
$ATC — A10BF02.$

Adverse Effects and Precautions

As for alpha-glucosidase inhibitors in general (see Acarbose, p.319). Skin rash may occur. Miglitol should be used with caution in patients with renal impairment.

Interactions

As for alpha-glucosidase inhibitors in general (see Acarbose, p.319). Miglitol may reduce the bioavailability of propranolol and ranitidine.

Pharmacokinetics

Miglitol is completely absorbed at a dose of 25 mg, but only 50 to 70% is absorbed at a dose of 100 mg. It is not metabolised, and is excreted unchanged in the urine.

Uses and Administration

Miglitol is an alpha-glucosidase inhibitor similar in action to acarbose (p.319). It is given by mouth in the management of type 2 diabetes mellitus (p.315), alone or in combination with a sulfonylurea. Usual initial doses are 25 mg three times daily with meals, increased if necessary to a maximum of 100 mg three times daily.

◊ References.
1. Campbell LK, et al. Miglitol: assessment of its role in the treatment of patients with diabetes mellitus. *Ann Pharmacother* 2000; **34:** 1291–1301.
2. Scott LJ, Spencer CM. Miglitol: a review of its therapeutic potential in type 2 diabetes mellitus. *Drugs* 2000; **59:** 521–49.

Preparations

Proprietary Preparations (details are given in Part 3)
Aust.: Diastabol; *Fin.:* Diastabol; *Fr.:* Diastabol; *Ger.:* Diastabol; *Port.:* Diastabol; *Spain:* Diastabol; Plumarol; *Swed.:* Diastabol; *Switz.:* Diastabol; *USA:* Glyset.

Nateglinide (9668-z)

Nateglinide (USAN, rINN).

A-4166; AY-4166; DJN-608; SDZ-DJN-608; Senaglinide; YM-026. (−)-N-[(trans-4-Isopropylcyclohexyl)carbonyl]-D-phenylalanine.

$C_{19}H_{27}NO_3 = 317.4.$
$CAS — 105816-04-4.$

Adverse Effects and Precautions

Nateglinide can cause hypoglycaemia, back and joint pain, and dizziness. Hypersensitivity reactions and transient elevations in liver enzymes may occur rarely.

Interactions

As with other oral antidiabetics, the efficacy of nateglinide may be affected by drugs independently increasing or decreasing blood glucose concentrations (see Sulfonylureas, p.335).

Pharmacokinetics

Nateglinide is rapidly absorbed after oral administration, with peak plasma concentrations occurring within one hour and an absolute bioavailability of 73%. Nateglinide is 98% bound to plasma proteins. It is predominantly metabolised by cytochrome P450 isoenzyme CYP2C9, and to a lesser extent by CYP3A4. The parent drug and metabolites are mainly excreted in the urine but about 10% is eliminated in the faeces. The elimination half-life is about 1.5 hours.

Uses and Administration

Nateglinide, like repaglinide (p.334), is a meglitinide antidiabetic used in the treatment of type 2 diabetes mellitus (p.315). It lowers blood-glucose concentrations by stimulating insulin release from the pancreas. It is given by mouth up to 30 minutes before meals in doses of 60 or 120 mg three times daily. This may be increased to 180 mg three times daily if necessary. Nateglinide is also given in similar doses in combination with metformin in type 2 diabetes not adequately controlled by metformin alone.

◊ References.
1. Dunn CJ, Faulds D. Nateglinide. *Drugs* 2000; **60:** 607–15.
2. Hanefeld M, et al. Rapid and short-acting mealtime insulin secretion with nateglinide controls both prandial and mean glycemia. *Diabetes Care* 2000; **23:** 202–7.
3. Horton ES, et al. Nateglinide alone and in combination with metformin improves glycemic control by reducing mealtime glucose levels in type 2 diabetes. *Diabetes Care* 2000; **23:** 1660–5.

Preparations

Proprietary Preparations (details are given in Part 3)
UK: Starlix; *USA:* Starlix.

Phenformin Hydrochloride (7232-k)

Phenformin Hydrochloride (BANM, pINNM).

Fenformina Cloridrato. 1-Phenethylbiguanide hydrochloride.

$C_{10}H_{15}N_5,HCl = 241.7.$
$CAS — 114-86-3 (phenformin); 834-28-6 (phenformin hydrochloride).$
Pharmacopoeias. In Chin. and Pol.

Profile

Phenformin hydrochloride is a biguanide antidiabetic (p.320). Although it is generally considered to be associated with an unacceptably high incidence of lactic acidosis, often fatal, it is still available in some countries for the treatment by mouth of type 2 diabetes mellitus.

Phenformin was implicated in the controversial reports of excess cardiovascular mortality associated with oral hypoglycaemic therapy (see under Sulfonylureas, Effects on the Cardiovascular System, p.334).

Preparations

Proprietary Preparations (details are given in Part 3)
Braz.: Debei; *Mex.:* Azucaps; Debeone; *Port.:* Debeina.
Multi-ingredient: *Ital.:* Bi-Euglucon; Bidiabe; Gliben F; Gliformin; Suguan.

Pimagedine (17309-z)

Pimagedine (rINN).

GER-11 (pimagedine hydrochloride). Aminoguanidine.

$CH_6N_4 = 74.09.$
$CAS — 79-17-4.$

NOTE. Pimagedine Hydrochloride is *USAN*.

Profile

Pimagedine reportedly inhibits the formation of glycosylated proteins (advanced glycosylation end-products) and has other actions including inhibition of aldose reductase. It is under investigation for the prevention of diabetic complications (p.317).

◊ References.
1. Corbett JA, et al. Aminoguanidine, a novel inhibitor of nitric oxide formation, prevents diabetic vascular dysfunction. *Diabetes* 1992; **41:** 552–6.
2. Wolffenbuttel BHR, Huijberts MSP. Aminoguanidine, a potential drug for the treatment of diabetic complications. *Neth J Med* 1993; **42:** 205–8.

Pioglitazone Hydrochloride (10380-l)

Pioglitazone Hydrochloride (BANM, USAN, rINNM).

AD-4833 (pioglitazone); U-72107A; U-72107E (pioglitazone). (±)-5-{p-[2-(5-Ethyl-2-pyridyl)ethoxy]benzyl}-2,4-thiazolidinedione hydrochloride.

$C_{19}H_{20}N_2O_3S,HCl = 392.9.$
$CAS — 111025-46-8 (pioglitazone); 112529-15-4 (pioglitazone hydrochloride).$

Adverse Effects and Precautions

As for Rosiglitazone, p.334. Other adverse effects reported include upper respiratory-tract infections, haematuria, myalgia, and visual disturbances.

In the UK, concomitant use of pioglitazone with insulin is considered to be contra-indicated, because of a possibly increased risk of heart failure. However, in the USA, pioglitazone is licensed for combination therapy with insulin.

Pharmacokinetics

Pioglitazone is rapidly absorbed after oral administration. Peak plasma concentrations are obtained within 2 hours and bioavailability exceeds 80%. Pioglitazone is more than 99% bound to plasma proteins. It is extensively metabolised by cytochrome P450 isoenzymes CYP3A4 and CYP2C9 to both active and inactive metabolites. It is excreted in urine and faeces and has a plasma half-life of up to 7 hours. The active metabolites have a half-life of up to 24 hours.

Uses and Administration

Pioglitazone is a thiazolidinedione oral antidiabetic similar to troglitazone (p.337). In the UK it is licensed for use in combination with metformin, or where this is inappropriate, a sulfonylurea. In the USA and some other countries it may also be given as monotherapy, or in combination with insulin (see also Adverse Effects and Precautions, above). It is used in the management of type 2 diabetes mellitus (p.315). It is given in a usual dose of 15 to 30 mg daily, which may be increased in patients on pioglitazone monotherapy to a maximum of 45 mg daily if necessary.

◊ References.
1. Gillies PS, Dunn CJ. Pioglitazone. *Drugs* 2000; **60:** 333–43.

Preparations

Proprietary Preparations (details are given in Part 3)
Austral.: Actos; *UK:* Actos; *USA:* Actos.

Pramlintide (15583-k)

Pramlintide (BAN, USAN, rINN).

AC-137; AC-0137 (pramlintide or pramlintide acetate); Tripro-amylin.

$CAS — 151126-32-8 (pramlintide); 196078-30-5 (pramlintide acetate).$

Profile

Pramlintide is an analogue of amylin, a pancreatic peptide

The symbol † denotes a preparation no longer actively marketed

thought to play a role in the regulation of glucose homoeostasis. Pramlintide is under investigation in the management of diabetes mellitus (p.315).

◊ References.
1. Kolterman OG, et al. Reduction of postprandial hyperglycemia in subjects with IDDM by intravenous infusion of AC137, a human amylin analogue. Diabetes Care 1995; 18: 1179–82.
2. Thompson RG, et al. Pramlintide: a human amylin analogue reduced postprandial plasma glucose, insulin, and C-peptide concentrations in patients with type 2 diabetes. Diabetic Med 1997; 14: 547–55.
3. Thompson RG, et al. Effects of pramlintide, an analog of human amylin, on plasma glucose profiles in patients with IDDM: results of a multicenter trial. Diabetes 1997; 46: 632–6.
4. Thompson RG, et al. Pramlintide, a synthetic analog of human amylin, improves the metabolic profile of patients with type 2 diabetes using insulin. Diabetes Care 1998; 21: 987–93.

Repaglinide (15410-t)

Repaglinide (BAN, USAN, rINN).

AG-EE-6232W; AG-EE-623-ZW. (+)-2-Ethoxy-α-{[(S)-α-isobutyl-o-piperidinobenzyl]carbamoyl}-p-toluic acid; (S)-2-Ethoxy-4-{[1-(o-piperidinophenyl)-3-methylbutyl]carbamoylmethyl}benzoic acid.
$C_{27}H_{36}N_2O_4 = 452.6$.
CAS — 135062-02-1.
ATC — A10BX02.

Adverse Effects and Precautions
Repaglinide may cause gastrointestinal adverse effects including abdominal pain, diarrhoea, constipation, nausea, and vomiting. Hypoglycaemia (usually mild), hypersensitivity rashes and urticaria, and elevated liver enzyme values may occur.

Precautions are similar to those which apply with the shorter-acting sulfonylurea hypoglycaemics (p.335).

Interactions
As with other oral antidiabetics, the efficacy of repaglinide may be affected by drugs independently increasing or decreasing blood glucose concentrations (see Sulfonylureas, p.335).

Cytochrome P450 isoenzyme CYP3A4 inducers such as rifampicin and phenytoin may decrease the effect of repaglinide. In vitro studies suggest that drugs that inhibit CYP3A4 may increase the effect of repaglinide.

◊ References.
1. Hatorp V, Thomsen MS. Drug interaction studies with repaglinide: repaglinide on digoxin or theophylline pharmacokinetics and cimetidine on repaglinide pharmacokinetics. J Clin Pharmacol 2000; 40: 184–92.
2. Niemi M, et al. Rifampin decreases the plasma concentrations and effects of repaglinide. Clin Pharmacol Ther 2000; 68: 495–500.

Pharmacokinetics
Repaglinide is rapidly absorbed from the gastrointestinal tract, with peak plasma concentrations occurring within 1 hour. The mean bioavailability is about 60%. Repaglinide is highly bound to plasma proteins, and has a plasma elimination half-life of about 1 hour. It undergoes almost complete hepatic metabolism involving the cytochrome P450 isoenzyme CYP3A4. The metabolites, which are inactive, are excreted in the bile.

Uses and Administration
Repaglinide is a meglitinide antidiabetic used for the treatment of type 2 diabetes mellitus (p.315). It has a chemical structure different from that of the sulfonylureas, but appears to have a similar mode of action.

Repaglinide is given by mouth up to 30 minutes before meals, in usual initial doses of 0.5 mg; initial doses of 1 or 2 mg are usually given to patients who have had previous hypoglycaemic treatment. The dose may be adjusted, at intervals of 1 to 2 weeks, up to a maximum of 4 mg before meals; a total of 16 mg daily should not be exceeded. Repaglinide is also given in combination with metformin in type 2 diabetes not adequately controlled by metformin alone.

◊ References.
1. Wolfenbuttel BHR, et al. Effects of a new oral hypoglycaemic agent, repaglinide, on metabolic control in sulfonylurea-treated patients with NIDDM. Eur J Clin Pharmacol 1993; 45: 113–16.
2. Anonymous. Repaglinide for type 2 diabetes mellitus. Med Lett Drugs Ther 1998; 40: 55–6.
3. Wolffenbuttel BH, Landgraf R. A 1-year multicenter randomized double-blind comparison of repaglinide and glyburide for the treatment of type 2 diabetes. Diabetes Care 1999; 22: 463–7.
4. Moses RG, et al. Flexible meal-related dosing with repaglinide facilitates glycemic control in therapy-naive type 2 diabetes. Diabetes Care 2001; 24: 11–15.

Preparations

Proprietary Preparations (details are given in Part 3)
Aust.: NovoNorm; Austral.: Novonorm; Canad.: Gluconorm; Denm.: NovoNorm; Fin.: NovoNorm; Fr.: NovoNorm; Ger.: NovoNorm; Irl.: NovoNorm; Ital.: NovoNorm; Neth.: NovoNorm; Norw.: NovoNorm; NZ: NovoNorm; S.Afr.: NovoNorm; Singapore: NovoNorm; Spain: NovoNorm; Swed.: NovoNorm; Thai.: NovoNorm; UK: NovoNorm; USA: Prandin.

Rosiglitazone Maleate (20162-a)

Rosiglitazone Maleate (BANM, USAN, rINNM).

BRL-49653-C. (±)-5-{p-[2-(Methyl-2-pyridylamino)ethoxy]benzyl}-2,4-thiazolidinedione maleate (1:1).
$C_{18}H_{19}N_3O_3S,C_4H_4O_4 = 473.5$.
CAS — 155141-29-0 (rosiglitazone maleate); 122320-73-4 (rosiglitazone).
ATC — A10BG02.

Adverse Effects and Precautions
Rosiglitazone may cause hypoglycaemia, headache, weight gain, and anaemia. It may also cause dizziness, gastrointestinal disturbances, muscle cramps, dyspnoea, pruritus, and hypercholesterolaemia.

Rosiglitazone can cause oedema, which may worsen or precipitate heart failure. It should therefore be used with caution in patients with a history of oedema or heart failure. Concomitant use with insulin is considered to be contra-indicated, because of a possibly increased risk of heart failure. Liver function should be monitored periodically as there have been isolated reports of liver dysfunction, and the drug should be used with caution in patients with hepatic impairment.

Pharmacokinetics
Rosiglitazone is well absorbed from the gastrointestinal tract following oral dosing. Peak plasma concentrations are achieved within 1 hour and the bioavailability is 99%. It is 99.8% bound to plasma proteins. Rosiglitazone is extensively metabolised, almost exclusively by the cytochrome P450 isoenzyme CYP2C8. It is excreted in the urine and faeces, and has a half-life of 3 to 4 hours.

Uses and Administration
Rosiglitazone is a thiazolidinedione oral antidiabetic (see Troglitazone, p.337) used for the treatment of type 2 diabetes mellitus (p.315). In the UK it is licensed for use with metformin, or where this is inappropriate, a sulfonylurea. In the USA and some other countries it is also licensed as monotherapy. The usual initial dose is 4 mg per day, given in a single or two divided doses. The dose may be increased to a maximum of 8 mg per day if necessary after 8 to 12 weeks.

◊ References.
1. Barman Balfour JA, Plosker GL. Rosiglitazone. Drugs 1999; 57: 921–30.
2. Nolan JJ, et al. Rosiglitazone taken once daily provides effective glycaemic control in patients with type 2 diabetes mellitus. Diabetic Med 2000; 17: 287–94.
3. Fonseca V, et al. Effect of metformin and rosiglitazone combination therapy in patients with type 2 diabetes mellitus: a randomized controlled trial. JAMA 2000; 283: 1695–1702.
4. Lebovitz HE, et al. Rosiglitazone monotherapy is effective in patients with type 2 diabetes. J Clin Endocrinol Metab 2001; 86: 280–8.

Preparations

Proprietary Preparations (details are given in Part 3)
Austral.: Avandia; Irl.: Avandia; Thai.: Avandia; UK: Avandia; USA: Avandia.

Sorbinil (16992-t)

Sorbinil (BAN, USAN, rINN).

CP-45634. (S)-6-Fluorospiro(chroman-4,4'-imidazolidine)-2',5'-dione.
$C_{11}H_9FN_2O_3 = 236.2$.
CAS — 68367-52-2.

Profile
Sorbinil is an aldose reductase inhibitor similar in action to tolrestat (p.337). It was tried mainly in the treatment of diabetic retinopathy and neuropathy, with conflicting results.

Severe skin reactions have been reported.

◊ References.
1. Sorbinil Retinopathy Trial Research Group. A randomized trial of sorbinil, an aldose reductase inhibitor, in diabetic retinopathy. Arch Ophthalmol 1990; 108: 1234–44.
2. Sorbinil Retinopathy Trial Research Group. The sorbinil retinopathy trial; neuropathy results. Neurology 1993; 43: 1141–9.

Sulfonylurea Antidiabetics (17475-g)

Adverse Effects
Gastrointestinal disturbances such as nausea, vomiting, heartburn, anorexia, diarrhoea, and a metallic taste may occur with sulfonylureas and are usually mild and dose-dependent; increased appetite and weight gain may occur. Skin rashes and pruritus may occur and photosensitivity has been reported. Rashes are usually hypersensitivity reactions and may progress to more serious disorders (see below). Facial flushing may develop in patients receiving sulfonylureas, particularly chlorpropamide, when alcohol is consumed (see under Interactions, below).

Hypoglycaemia may occur 4 or more hours after food; this is usually an indication of overdosage and is relatively uncommon. Hypoglycaemia is more likely with long-acting sulfonylureas such as chlorpropamide and glibenclamide, which have been associated with severe, prolonged, and sometimes fatal hypoglycaemia.

Other severe effects may be manifestations of a hypersensitivity reaction. They include altered liver enzyme values and cholestatic jaundice, leucopenia, thrombocytopenia, aplastic anaemia, agranulocytosis, haemolytic anaemia, erythema multiforme or the Stevens-Johnson syndrome, exfoliative dermatitis, and erythema nodosum.

The sulfonylureas, particularly chlorpropamide, occasionally induce a syndrome of inappropriate secretion of antidiuretic hormone (SIADH) characterised by water retention, hyponatraemia, and CNS effects. However, some sulfonylureas, such as glibenclamide, glipizide, and tolazamide are also stated to have mild diuretic actions.

Work on tolbutamide has suggested that the sulfonylureas might be associated with an increase in cardiovascular mortality; this has been the subject of considerable debate (see Effects on the Cardiovascular System, below).

◊ Reviews.
1. Paice BJ, et al. Undesired effects of the sulphonylurea drugs. Adverse Drug React Acute Poisoning Rev 1985; 4: 23–36.
2. Harrower ADB. Comparative tolerability of sulphonylureas in diabetes mellitus. Drug Safety 2000; 22: 313–20.

Effects on the cardiovascular system. A multicentre study carried out under the University Group Diabetes Program (UGDP) reported an increased incidence in mortality from cardiovascular complications in diabetic patients given tolbutamide as compared with those treated with diet alone or insulin;[1] a similar increase was also noted in patients given phenformin.[2] The reports from the UGDP aroused prolonged controversy which was not entirely settled by detailed reassessment of relevant studies.[3] Eventually in 1984 the FDA made it a requirement that sulfonylurea oral antidiabetics be labelled with a specific warning about the possibility of increased cardiovascular mortality associated with the use of these drugs.[4] Subsequently the cardiovascular effects of the sulfonylureas were reviewed by Huupponen.[5] More recently it has been hypothesised that the action of the sulfonylureas in preventing the opening of ATP-sensitive potassium channels in the myocardium may abolish adaptive changes (ischaemic preconditioning) that protect the heart against ischaemic insult.[6] However, results from the UK Prospective Diabetes Study did not demonstrate any adverse cardiovascular effects associated with sulfonylurea therapy.[7]

1. University Group Diabetes Program. Effects of hypoglycemic agents on vascular complications in patients with adult-onset diabetes III: clinical implications of UGDP results. JAMA 1971; 218: 1400–10.
2. University Group Diabetes Program. Effects of hypoglycemic agents on vascular complications in patients with adult-onset diabetes IV: a preliminary report on phenformin results. JAMA 1971; 217: 777–84.
3. Report of the Committee for the Assessment of Biometric Aspects of Controlled Trials of Hypoglycemic Agents. JAMA 1975; 231: 583–600.
4. FDA. Class labeling for oral hypoglycemics. FDA Drug Bull 1984; 14: 16–17.
5. Huupponen R. Adverse cardiovascular effects of sulphonylurea drugs: clinical significance. Med Toxicol 1987; 2: 190–209.
6. Yellon DM, et al. Angina reassessed: pain or protector? Lancet 1996; 347: 1159–62.
7. UK Prospective Diabetes Study (UKPDS) Group. Intensive blood-glucose control with sulphonylureas or insulin compared with conventional treatment and risk of complications in patients with type 2 diabetes (UKPDS 33). Lancet 1998; 352: 837–53.

Effects on the eyes. When a diabetic patient who had experienced bilateral visual loss for several months and who had been taking chlorpropamide for one year stopped treatment, visual acuity improved and colour vision rapidly returned.[1] A

5-day challenge with chlorpropamide resulted in a mild decrease in acuity followed by return to baseline values when treatment was again stopped. Drug-induced optic neuropathy was considered to have occurred. There is also a report of a patient with type 2 diabetes mellitus who developed myopia two days after starting treatment with glibenclamide 10 mg daily.[2] Visual difficulties resolved a few days after stopping glibenclamide.

1. Wymore J, Carter JE. Chlorpropamide-induced optic neuropathy. *Arch Intern Med* 1982; **142:** 381.
2. Teller J, *et al.* Accommodation insufficiency induced by glybenclamide. *Ann Ophthalmol* 1989; **21:** 275–6.

Effects on the kidneys. A report in one patient of the nephrotic syndrome in association with chlorpropamide therapy.[1] Serological testing and renal biopsy demonstrated that the glomerular lesions were of an immune-complex nature. Both the nephrotic syndrome and the glomerulonephritis resolved after treatment was stopped. The patient also developed a skin eruption, hepatitis, and eosinophilia.

1. Appel GB, *et al.* Nephrotic syndrome and immune complex glomerulonephritis associated with chlorpropamide therapy. *Am J Med* 1983; **74:** 337–42.

Effects on the liver. Chlorpropamide was implicated[1] in 8 of 53 cases of drug-induced acute liver disease admitted to a hospital in Jamaica over the years 1973 to 1988. Hepatocanalicular cholestasis occurred in 5 cases and diffuse necrosis in 3. One patient with massive hepatic necrosis died. Intrahepatic cholestasis,[2] and an acute hepatitis-like syndrome[3] have been described in patients receiving glibenclamide.

1. Lee MG, *et al.* Drug-induced acute liver disease. *Postgrad Med J* 1989; **65:** 367–70.
2. Wongpaitoon V, *et al.* Intrahepatic cholestasis and cutaneous bullae associated with glibenclamide therapy. *Postgrad Med J* 1981; **57:** 244–6.
3. Goodman RC, *et al.* Glyburide-induced hepatitis. *Ann Intern Med* 1987; **106:** 837–9.

Effects on the thyroid. See under Precautions, below.

Hypoglycaemia. Severe hypoglycaemia may occur in any patient treated with any sulfonylurea; this potentially life-threatening complication requires prolonged and energetic treatment.[1] Sulfonylureas with a prolonged duration of action such as chlorpropamide and glibenclamide appear to cause severe hypoglycaemia more often than shorter-acting drugs such as tolbutamide. Experience with newer drugs is limited.

A review of 1418 cases of drug-induced hypoglycaemia reported since 1940 has shown that sulfonylureas (especially chlorpropamide and glibenclamide), either alone or with a second antidiabetic or potentiating drug, account for 63% of all cases.[2] A study of sulfonylurea use in nearly 14,000 patients aged 65 years or older confirmed that chlorpropamide and glibenclamide were associated with hypoglycaemia. However, glipizide caused significantly fewer cases than glibenclamide.[3]

An analysis,[4] of 185 children reported to 10 regional poison centres in the USA after ingesting sulfonylureas found that hypoglycaemia developed only in 56. A lack of hypoglycaemia during the first 8 hours after ingestion was predictive of a benign outcome, and it was recommended that suspected cases be observed for 8 hours with frequent blood glucose monitoring. Children who developed signs of hypoglycaemia, or in whom blood glucose fell below 3.3 mmol per litre could be given intravenous glucose if necessary.

See also under Abuse, below.

1. Ferner RE, Neil HAW. Sulphonylureas and hypoglycaemia. *BMJ* 1988; **296:** 949–50.
2. Seltzer HS. Drug-induced hypoglycaemia. *Endocrinol Metab Clin North Am* 1989; **18:** 163–83.
3. Shorr RI, *et al.* Individual sulfonylureas and serious hypoglycemia in older people. *J Am Geriatr Soc* 1996; **44:** 751–5.
4. Spiller HA, *et al.* Prospective multicenter study of sulfonylurea ingestion in children. *J Pediatr* 1997; **131:** 141–6.

Treatment of Adverse Effects

In acute poisoning the stomach should be emptied and/or activated charcoal administered. Hypoglycaemia should be treated with urgency; the general management of hypoglycaemia is described under insulin (see p.325). The patient should be observed over several days in case hypoglycaemia recurs.

◊ References.

1. Spiller HA. Management of antidiabetic medication in overdose. *Drug Safety* 1998; **19:** 411–24.

Precautions

Sulfonylureas should not be used in type 1 diabetes mellitus. Use in type 2 diabetes mellitus is contra-indicated in patients with ketoacidosis and in those with severe infection, trauma, or other severe conditions where the sulfonylurea is unlikely to control the hyperglycaemia; insulin should be administered in such situations.

Insulin is also preferred for treatment during pregnancy. Some sulfonylureas are distributed into breast milk and the class of drugs should be avoided during breast feeding.

The symbol † denotes a preparation no longer actively marketed

Sulfonylureas with a long half-life such as chlorpropamide or glibenclamide are associated with an increased risk of hypoglycaemia. They should therefore be avoided in patients with impairment of renal or hepatic function, and a similar precaution would tend to apply in other groups with an increased susceptibility to this effect, such as the elderly, debilitated or malnourished patients, and those with adrenal or pituitary insufficiency. Irregular mealtimes, missed meals, changes in diet, or prolonged exercise may also provoke hypoglycaemia. Where a sulfonylurea needs to be used in patients at increased risk of hypoglycaemia, a short-acting drug such as tolbutamide, gliquidone, or gliclazide may be preferred; these three sulfonylureas, being principally inactivated in the liver, are perhaps particularly suitable in renal impairment, although careful monitoring of blood-glucose concentration is essential.

Abuse. A report of severe hypoglycaemia, at first thought to be due to insulinoma but later found to be due to nesidioblastosis [proliferation of the islet cells], in a woman covertly taking chlorpropamide.[1]

1. Rayman G, *et al.* Hyperinsulinaemic hypoglycaemia due to chlorpropamide-induced nesidioblastosis. *J Clin Pathol* 1984; **37:** 651–4.

Administration. It has been suggested that continuously high plasma concentrations of sulfonylureas may lead to the development of tolerance, and that therefore the maximum recommended doses should be reduced.[1]

1. Melander A, *et al.* Is there a concentration-effect relationship for sulphonylureas? *Clin Pharmacokinet* 1998; **34:** 181–8.

Driving. In the UK, patients with diabetes mellitus treated with insulin or oral hypoglycaemics are required to notify their condition to the Driver and Vehicle Licensing Agency, who then assess their fitness to drive. Patients treated with oral hypoglycaemics are generally allowed to retain standard driving licences; those treated with insulin receive restricted licences which must be renewed (with appropriate checks) every 1 to 3 years. Patients should be warned of the dangers of hypoglycaemic attacks while driving, and should be counselled in appropriate management of the situation (stopping driving as soon as it is safe to do so, taking carbohydrate immediately, and quitting the driving seat and removing the ignition key from the car) should such an event occur. Patients who have lost hypoglycaemic awareness, or have frequent hypoglycaemic episodes, should not drive. In addition, eyesight must be adequate (field of vision of at least 120°) for a licence to be valid. Patients treated with diet or oral hypoglycaemics are normally allowed to hold vocational driving licences for heavy goods vehicles or passenger carrying vehicles; those treated with insulin may not drive such vehicles, and are restricted in driving some other vehicles such as small lorries and minibuses.

1. British Diabetic Association (Diabetes UK). *Information sheet: driving and diabetes:* Aug 2001. Available at: http://www.diabetes.org.uk/info/inform/drive.doc (accessed 13/09/01).

Porphyria. Sulfonylureas have been associated with acute attacks of porphyria and are considered unsafe in porphyric patients.

Thyroid disorders. There are conflicting reports concerning the effects of sulfonylureas on thyroid function, with some studies suggesting an increased incidence of thyroid dysfunction in patients treated with tolbutamide or chlorpropamide,[1] while other suggest no antithyroid action.[2,3] Some manufacturers consequently recommend that chlorpropamide be avoided in patients with severe impairment of thyroid function. Changes in thyroid function may conversely affect glycaemic control—for mention of the possible effects of thyroid hormones on sulfonylurea requirements see under Interactions, below.

1. Hunton RB, *et al.* Hypothyroidism in diabetics treated with sulphonylurea. *Lancet* 1965; **ii:** 449–51.
2. Burke G, *et al.* Effect of long-term sulfonylurea therapy on thyroid function in man. *Metabolism* 1967; **16:** 651–7.
3. Feely J, *et al.* Antithyroid effect of chlorpropamide? *Hum Toxicol* 1983; **2:** 149–53.

Interactions

Numerous interactions have been reported with the sulfonylureas, largely representing either pharmacokinetic interactions (due to the displacement of the antidiabetic from plasma proteins or alteration in its metabolism or excretion) or pharmacological interactions with drugs having an independent effect on blood glucose. In the former class most reports concern older sulfonylureas such as chlorpropamide and tolbutamide, although the possibility of such reactions with newer drugs should be borne in mind.

A diminished hypoglycaemic effect, possibly requiring an increased dose of sulfonylurea, has been seen or might be expected on theoretical grounds with adrenaline [epinephrine], aminoglutethimide, chlor-

promazine, corticosteroids, diazoxide, oral contraceptives, rifamycins, and thiazide diuretics.

An increased hypoglycaemic effect has occurred or might be expected with ACE inhibitors, alcohol, allopurinol, some analgesics (notably azapropazone, phenylbutazone, and the salicylates), azole antifungals (fluconazole, ketoconazole, and miconazole), chloramphenicol, cimetidine, clofibrate and related compounds, coumarin anticoagulants, halofenate, heparin, MAOIs, octreotide (although this may also produce hyperglycaemia), ranitidine, sulfinpyrazone, sulfonamides (including co-trimoxazole), tetracyclines, tricyclic antidepressants, and thyroid hormones.

Beta blockers have been reported both to increase hypoglycaemia and to mask the typical sympathetic warning signs. There are sporadic and conflicting reports of a possible interaction with calcium-channel blockers, but overall any effect seems to be of little clinical significance.

In addition to producing hypoglycaemia alcohol can interact with chlorpropamide to produce an unpleasant flushing reaction. Such an effect is rare with other sulfonylureas and alcohol.

◊ General references.

1. O'Byrne S, Feely J. Effects of drugs on glucose tolerance in non-insulin-dependent diabetics (part I). *Drugs* 1990; **40:** 6–18.
2. O'Byrne S, Feely J. Effects of drugs on glucose tolerance in non-insulin-dependent diabetics (part II). *Drugs* 1990; **40:** 203–19.
3. Girardin E, *et al.* Hypoglycémies induites par les sulfamides hypoglycémiants. *Ann Med Interne (Paris)* 1992; **143:** 11–17.

ACE inhibitors. There are sporadic reports of marked hypoglycaemia developing in patients taking a sulfonylurea who are given an ACE inhibitor (mainly *captopril* or *enalapril*),[1-3] and 2 case-control studies have indicated that the combination is associated with an increased risk of developing severe hypoglycaemia.[4,5] However, other studies have failed to find much evidence of a problem.[6-9]

1. McMurray J, Fraser DM. Captopril, enalapril, and blood glucose. *Lancet* 1986; **i:** 1035.
2. Rett K, *et al.* Hypoglycemia in hypertensive diabetic patients treated with sulfonylureas, biguanides, and captopril. *N Engl J Med* 1988; **319:** 1609.
3. Arauz-Pacheco C, *et al.* Hypoglycemia induced by angiotensin-converting enzyme inhibitors in patients with non-insulin-dependent diabetes receiving sulfonylurea therapy. *Am J Med* 1990; **89:** 811–13.
4. Herings RMC, *et al.* Hypoglycaemia associated with use of inhibitors of angiotensin converting enzyme. *Lancet* 1995; **345:** 1195–8.
5. Morris AD, *et al.* ACE inhibitor use is associated with hospitalization for severe hypoglycemia in patients with diabetes. *Diabetes Care* 1997; **20:** 1363–7.
6. Ferriere M, *et al.* Captopril and insulin sensitivity. *Ann Intern Med* 1985; **102:** 134–5.
7. Passa P, *et al.* Enalapril, captopril, and blood glucose. *Lancet* 1986; **i:** 1447.
8. Winocour P, *et al.* Captopril and blood glucose. *Lancet* 1986; **ii:** 461.
9. Shorr RI, *et al.* Antihypertensives and the risk of serious hypoglycemia in older persons using insulin or sulfonylureas. *JAMA* 1997; **278:** 40–3.

Alcohol. Sulfonylurea-induced alcohol intolerance is seen mainly but not exclusively with chlorpropamide; this is similar to the disulfiram-alcohol interaction, although it is not clear whether the mechanism is the same. Since the main symptom of the reaction (facial flushing) appears to occur more commonly in diabetic than non-diabetic subjects, it has been proposed that this symptom could be used as a diagnostic test for a certain subset of patients with type 2 diabetes mellitus.[1,2] However, some have not considered the test to be sufficiently specific[3-6] and despite a great deal having been published on the chlorpropamide-alcohol flushing test (CPAF), its value remains poorly defined. Alcohol, as well as provoking a flushing reaction with chlorpropamide, has been reported both to increase and to decrease the half-life of tolbutamide depending on whether the alcohol administration was acute or chronic.[7] Alcohol may also have a variable effect of its own on blood-glucose concentrations; there is a general tendency to increased hypoglycaemia when alcohol and sulfonylureas are taken concurrently.[6]

1. Leslie RDG, Pyke DA. Chlorpropamide-alcohol flushing: a dominantly inherited trait associated with diabetes. *BMJ* 1978; **2:** 1519–21.
2. Pyke DA, Leslie RDG. Chlorpropamide-alcohol flushing: a definition of its relation to non-insulin-dependent diabetes. *BMJ* 1978; **2:** 1521–2.
3. de Silva NE, *et al.* Low incidence of chlorpropamide-alcohol flushing in diet-treated, non-insulin-dependent diabetes. *Lancet* 1981; **i:** 128–31.
4. Fui SNT, *et al.* Epidemiological study of prevalence of chlorpropamide alcohol flushing in insulin-dependent diabetics, non-insulin dependent diabetics, and non-diabetics. *BMJ* 1983; **287:** 1509–12.
5. Fui SNT, *et al.* Test for chlorpropamide-alcohol flush becomes positive after prolonged chlorpropamide treatment in insulin-dependent and non-insulin-dependent diabetics. *N Engl J Med* 1983; **309:** 93–6.

6. Lao B, *et al.* Alcohol tolerance in patients with non-insulin-dependent (type 2) diabetes treated with sulphonylurea derivatives. *Arzneimittelforschung* 1994; **44:** 727–34.
7. Sellers EM, Holloway MR. Drug kinetics and alcohol ingestion. *Clin Pharmacokinet* 1978; **3:** 440–52.

Analgesics. *Phenylbutazone*[1,2] and related drugs such as *azapropazone*[3] have been associated with acute hypoglycaemic episodes when given to patients receiving sulfonylureas (in most reports, tolbutamide). Other analgesics may enhance the hypoglycaemic effect of sulfonylureas, including *indobufen*,[4] *fenclofenac*,[5] and the *salicylates*.[6,7]

1. Tannenbaum H, *et al.* Phenylbutazone-tolbutamide drug interaction. *N Engl J Med* 1974; **290:** 344.
2. Dent LA, Jue SG. Tolbutamide-phenylbutazone interaction. *Drug Intell Clin Pharm* 1976; **10:** 711.
3. Andreasen PB, *et al.* Hypoglycaemia induced by azapropazone-tolbutamide interaction. *Br J Clin Pharmacol* 1981; **12:** 581–3.
4. Elvander-Ståhl E, *et al.* Indobufen interacts with the sulphonylurea, glipizide, but not with the β-adrenergic receptor antagonists, propranolol and atenolol. *Br J Clin Pharmacol* 1984; **18:** 773–8.
5. Allen PA, Taylor RT. Fenclofenac and thyroid function tests. *BMJ* 1980; **281:** 1642.
6. Richardson T, *et al.* Enhancement by sodium salicylate of the blood glucose lowering effect of chlorpropamide—drug interaction or summation of similar effects? *Br J Clin Pharmacol* 1986; **22:** 43–8.
7. Kubacka RT, *et al.* Effects of aspirin and ibuprofen on the pharmacokinetics and pharmacodynamics of glyburide in healthy subjects. *Ann Pharmacother* 1996; **30:** 20–6.

Antibacterials. *Chloramphenicol* markedly inhibits the metabolism of tolbutamide and increases its half-life,[1] which can result in hypoglycaemia. Sulfonamides,[2] including *co-trimoxazole*,[3,4] may also enhance the hypoglycaemic effects of the sulfonylureas, while *rifampicin* (and probably other rifamycins) can enhance the metabolism and decrease the effect of tolbutamide, chlorpropamide,[5,6] and glibenclamide[7] and dosage of the hypoglycaemic drug may need to be increased. The effects on glipizide appear to be less pronounced.[7]

1. Christensen LK, Skovsted L. Inhibition of drug metabolism by chloramphenicol. *Lancet* 1969; **ii:** 1397–9.
2. Soeldner JS, Steinke J. Hypoglycemia in tolbutamide-treated diabetes: report of two cases with measurement of serum insulin. *JAMA* 1965; **193:** 148–9.
3. Wing LMH, Miners JO. Cotrimoxazole as an inhibitor of oxidative drug metabolism: effects of trimethoprim and sulphamethoxazole separately and combined on tolbutamide disposition. *Br J Clin Pharmacol* 1985; **20:** 482–5.
4. Johnson JF, Dobmeier ME. Symptomatic hypoglycemia secondary to a glipizide-trimethoprim/sulfamethoxazole drug interaction. *DICP Ann Pharmacother* 1990; **24:** 250–1.
5. Syvälahti EKG, *et al.* Rifampicin and drug metabolism. *Lancet* 1974; **ii:** 232–3.
6. Self TH, Morris T. Interaction of rifampin and chlorpropamide. *Chest* 1980; **77:** 800–1.
7. Niemi M, *et al.* Effects of rifampin on the pharmacokinetics and pharmacodynamics of glyburide and glipizide. *Clin Pharmacol Ther* 2001; **69:** 400–406.

Anticoagulants. *Dicoumarol* increases serum concentrations and therefore the hypoglycaemic effects of tolbutamide, and possibly chlorpropamide. In addition, sulfonylureas may affect anticoagulant function (p.995).

Antiepileptics. For references to *phenytoin* toxicity when tolbutamide or tolazamide was given concurrently, see under Phenytoin p.360.

Antifungals. Increased plasma concentrations of tolbutamide have been reported when *fluconazole* was given concomitantly,[1] but there was no evidence of hypoglycaemia, and no hypoglycaemic symptoms were seen in 29 women receiving gliclazide or glibenclamide who were given fluconazole or *clotrimazole* for vulvovaginitis.[2] However, there are reports of hypoglycaemia in a patient who took fluconazole with glipizide,[3] and similar interactions have been reported for *ketoconazole* (with tolbutamide, in healthy subjects),[4] and *miconazole* (with tolbutamide, in a diabetic),[5] suggesting that such combinations should be regarded with caution.

1. Lazar JD, Wilner DK. Drug interactions with fluconazole. *Rev Infect Dis* 1990; **12** (suppl 3): S327–S333.
2. Rowe BR, *et al.* Safety of fluconazole in women taking oral hypoglycaemic agents. *Lancet* 1992; **339:** 255–6.
3. Fournier JP, *et al.* Coma hypoglycémique chez une patiente traitée par glipizide et fluconazole: une possible interaction? *Therapie* 1992; **47:** 446–7.
4. Krishnaiah YSR, *et al.* Interaction between tolbutamide and ketoconazole in healthy subjects. *Br J Clin Pharmacol* 1994; **37:** 205–7.
5. Meurice JC, *et al.* Interaction miconazole et sulfamides hypoglycémiants. *Presse Med* 1983; **12:** 1670.

Metformin. Results apparently suggesting increased mortality in patients who received intensive drug therapy with metformin in combination with a sulfonylurea were reported by the UK Prospective Diabetes Study.[1] This was considered to be artefactual, since it was not confirmed by epidemiological analysis, and such combinations are widely used in practice, but some concern remains and further study is needed.

1. UK Prospective Diabetes Study Group. Effect of intensive blood-glucose control with metformin on complications in overweight patients with type 2 diabetes (UKPDS 34). *Lancet* 1998; **352:** 854–65. Correction. *ibid.;* 1558.

Thyroid hormones. It has been suggested that initiation of thyroid replacement therapy may increase the requirement for insulin or oral antidiabetic drugs in diabetic patients,[1] which would not seem unreasonable given the stimulant effects of thyroid hormones on metabolic function. Patients stabilised on long-term thyroid replacement therapy are, however, unlikely

to be at risk. For a discussion of the mooted effects of sulfonylureas on thyroid function, see Precautions, above.

1. Refetoff S. Thyroid hormone therapy. *Med Clin North Am* 1975; **59:** 1147–62.

Pharmacokinetics

◊ Reviews.

1. Marchetti P, Navalesi R. Pharmacokinetic-pharmacodynamic relationships of oral hypoglycaemic agents: an update. *Clin Pharmacokinet* 1989; **16:** 100–28.

Uses and Administration

The sulfonylurea antidiabetics are a class of antidiabetic drugs given by mouth in the treatment of type 2 diabetes mellitus (p.315). They are used to supplement treatment by diet modification when such modification has not proved effective on its own, although metformin is preferred in patients who are obese.

Sulfonylureas appear to have several modes of action, apparently mediated by inhibition of ATP-sensitive potassium channels. Initially, secretion of insulin by functioning islet beta cells is increased. However, insulin secretion subsequently falls again but the hypoglycaemic effect persists and may be due to inhibition of hepatic glucose production and increased sensitivity to any available insulin; this may explain the observed clinical improvement in glycaemic control. The duration of action of sulfonylureas is variable; drugs such as gliclazide and tolbutamide are relatively short-acting (approximately 12 and 10 hours respectively) while chlorpropamide has a prolonged action (over 24 hours).

Sulfonylurea therapy may be combined with metformin or other oral hypoglycaemics in patients who fail to respond to a single type of drug; such combination therapy is usually tried (in the absence of contra-indications) before considering transfer to insulin therapy.

Tolazamide (7233-a)

Tolazamide (BAN, USAN, rINN).

NSC-70762; U-17835. 1-(Perhydroazepin-1-yl)-3-tosylurea; 1-(Perhydroazepin-1-yl)-3-*p*-tolylsulphonylurea.

$C_{14}H_{21}N_3O_3S = 311.4$.
CAS — 1156-19-0.
ATC — A10BB05.
Pharmacopoeias. In *Br., Jpn,* and *US.*

Pharmacopoeial description

BP 2001: A white or almost white, odourless or almost odourless, crystalline powder. Very slightly soluble in water; slightly soluble in alcohol; soluble in acetone; freely soluble in chloroform.

USP 25: A white or off-white crystalline powder, odourless or having a slight odour. Very slightly soluble in water; slightly soluble in alcohol; soluble in acetone; freely soluble in chloroform.

Adverse Effects, Treatment, and Precautions

As for sulfonylureas in general, p.334.

◊ Tolazamide has been associated with acute attacks of porphyria and is considered unsafe in porphyric patients.

Interactions

As for sulfonylureas in general, p.335.

Pharmacokinetics

Tolazamide is slowly absorbed from the gastrointestinal tract, peak plasma concentrations occurring 4 to 8 hours after a dose by mouth, and is extensively bound to plasma proteins. It has a half-life of about 7 hours. It is metabolised in the liver to metabolites with some hypoglycaemic activity. About 85% of an oral dose is excreted in the urine, chiefly as metabolites.

Uses and Administration

Tolazamide is a sulfonylurea antidiabetic (p.334). It is given by mouth in the treatment of type 2 diabetes mellitus (p.315) and has a duration of action of at least 10 hours and sometimes up to 20 hours. The usual initial dose in type 2 diabetes mellitus is 100 to 250 mg daily by mouth given as a single dose with breakfast and increased if necessary at weekly intervals by 100 to 250 mg usually to a maximum of 1 g daily; no further benefit is likely to be gained with higher doses. Doses of 500 mg or more daily may be given in divided doses.

Preparations

BP 2001: Tolazamide Tablets;
USP 25: Tolazamide Tablets.

Proprietary Preparations (details are given in Part 3)
Irl.: Tolanase†; **Neth.:** Tolinase†; **Swed.:** Tolinase†; **UK:** Tolanase†; **USA:** Tolinase.

Tolbutamide (7234-t)

Tolbutamide (BAN, rINN).

Butamidum; Tolbutamidum; Tolglybutamide. 1-Butyl-3-tosylurea; 1-Butyl-3-*p*-tolylsulphonylurea.

$C_{12}H_{18}N_2O_3S = 270.3$.
CAS — 64-77-7 (tolbutamide); 473-41-6 (tolbutamide sodium).
ATC — A10BB03; V04CA01.
Pharmacopoeias. In *Chin., Eur.* (see p.vi), *Int., Jpn, Pol.,* and *US.*

Tolbutamide sodium 1.08 g is approximately equivalent to 1 g of tolbutamide.

Pharmacopoeial description

Ph. Eur.: A white crystalline powder. Practically insoluble in water; soluble in alcohol and in acetone; slightly soluble in ether. It dissolves in dilute solutions of alkali hydroxides.

USP 25: A white or practically white, practically odourless, crystalline powder. Practically insoluble in water; soluble in alcohol and in chloroform.

Adverse Effects, Treatment, and Precautions

As for sulfonylureas in general, p.334. Tolbutamide was implicated in the controversial reports of excess cardiovascular mortality associated with oral hypoglycaemic therapy (see under Sulfonylureas, Effects on the Cardiovascular System, p.334).

Thrombophlebitis has occurred following the intravenous injection of tolbutamide sodium; too rapid injection may cause a transient sensation of heat in the vein.

It has been suggested that tolbutamide may be suitable for use in patients with renal impairment, but careful monitoring of blood-glucose concentration is essential. The UK manufacturers recommend that it should not be used in patients with severe renal impairment.

Porphyria. Tolbutamide has been associated with acute attacks of porphyria and is considered unsafe in porphyric patients.

Interactions

As for sulfonylureas in general, p.335.

Pharmacokinetics

Tolbutamide is readily absorbed from the gastrointestinal tract and is extensively bound to plasma proteins; the half-life is generally within the range of 4 to 7 hours but may be considerably longer. Tolbutamide is metabolised in the liver by hydroxylation mediated by the cytochrome P450 isoenzyme CYP2C9. It is excreted in the urine chiefly as metabolites with little hypoglycaemic activity. Tolbutamide has been detected in breast milk.

Uses and Administration

Tolbutamide is a sulfonylurea antidiabetic (p.334). It is given by mouth in the treatment of type 2 diabetes mellitus (p.315) and has a duration of action of about 10 hours.

The usual initial dose by mouth in type 2 diabetes mellitus may range from 1 to 2 g daily, given either as a single dose with breakfast or, more usually, in divided doses. Maintenance doses usually range from 0.25 to 2 g daily. Although it is unlikely that the response will be improved by increasing the dose further, daily doses of 3 g have been given.

Tolbutamide sodium ($C_{12}H_{17}N_2NaO_3S = 292.3$) has sometimes been used in the diagnosis of insulinoma as well as other pancreatic disorders including diabetes mellitus. The equivalent of 1 g of tolbutamide is given by intravenous injection as a 5% solution usually over 2 to 3 minutes.

Diagnosis and testing. References.

1. McMahon MM, *et al.* Diagnostic interpretation of the intravenous tolbutamide test for insulinoma. *Mayo Clin Proc* 1989; **64:** 1481–8.
2. Marks V. Diagnosis and differential diagnosis of hypoglycemia. *Mayo Clin Proc* 1989; **64:** 1558–61.

Preparations

BP 2001: Tolbutamide Tablets;
USP 25: Tolbutamide for Injection; Tolbutamide Tablets.

Proprietary Preparations (details are given in Part 3)
Aust.: Rastinon; **Austral.:** Rastinon; **Belg.:** Rastinon†; **Canad.:** Novo-Butamide†; Orinase†; **Denm.:** Arcosal; **Fr.:** Dolipol†; **Ger.:**

Artosin†; Orabet; Rastinon†; **Hong Kong:** Diatol; Rastinon; **Irl.:** Rastinon†; **Israel:** Orsinon; **Ital.:** Rastinon†; **Mex.:** Dabetil; Diatelan; Diaval; Flusan; Ifumelus; Ipoglusan; Rastinon; **Neth.:** Artosin†; Rastinon; **NZ:** Diatol; **S.Afr.:** Rastinon†; **Spain:** Rastinon; **Switz.:** Rastinon†; **UK:** Glyconon; Rastinon†; **USA:** Orinase; Orinase Diagnostic; Tol-Tab†.

Multi-ingredient: *Ital.:* Glucosulfa.

Tolrestat   (17014-d)

Tolrestat *(BAN, USAN, rINN).*

AY-27773.   N-[6-Methoxy-5-trifluoromethyl-1-naphthyl(thiocarbonyl)]-N-methylglycine.

$C_{16}H_{14}F_3NO_3S = 357.3.$
CAS — 82964-04-3.
ATC — A10XA01.

Profile
Tolrestat inhibits the enzyme aldose reductase which catalyses the conversion of glucose to sorbitol. It has been suggested that accumulation of sorbitol in certain cells, occurring only in conditions of hyperglycaemia and resulting in a hyperosmotic effect, may be involved in the pathogenesis of some diabetic complications. Aldose reductase inhibitors have no influence on blood-glucose concentrations.

Tolrestat was investigated in the management of diabetic complications, but was subsequently withdrawn by the manufacturers following reports of poor efficacy and adverse effects on the liver.

Troglitazone   (17121-m)

Troglitazone *(BAN, USAN, rINN).*

CI-991; CS-045; GR-92132X. (±)-all-rac-5-{p-[(6-Hydroxy-2,5,7,8-tetramethyl-2-chromanyl)methoxy]benzyl}-2,4-thiazolidinedione.

$C_{24}H_{27}NO_5S = 441.5.$
CAS — 97322-87-7.
ATC — A10BG01.

Adverse Effects and Precautions
Troglitazone has been associated with severe hepatic reactions, sometimes fatal, which has led to its withdrawal in a number of countries. Regular monitoring of liver function during therapy, and withdrawal of the drug in any patient who develops jaundice or signs of liver dysfunction, is required. It should not be given to patients with pre-existing moderate or severe elevations of liver enzyme values, or active liver disease. Increased plasma volume has been reported in healthy subjects given troglitazone: it should be used with caution in patients with heart failure. Other adverse effects reported in patients receiving troglitazone include dizziness, headache, fatigue, musculoskeletal pain, and nausea and vomiting. There is no evidence of hypoglycaemia associated with the use of troglitazone alone.

Effects on the liver. The UK Committee on Safety of Medicines[1] was aware of over 130 cases of hepatic reactions to troglitazone worldwide as of December 1997, although only 1 had been in the UK. There had been 6 deaths. The average time to the onset of the reaction was 3 months, but the frequency of these reactions, and the existence of risk factors predisposing to them, were unclear. The manufacturers had voluntarily withdrawn the drug in the UK.

The US manufacturer and the FDA recommended[2] a schedule for routine monitoring of liver function in November 1997 and revised this again in December 1997. It was estimated that 2% of patients treated with troglitazone would have elevated liver enzyme values necessitating discontinuation of the drug. The FDA[3] had received 560 reports of troglitazone-associated hepatotoxicity by June 1998. There were 24 cases of hepatic failure which were likely to have been caused by the drug; 21 patients died and 3 patients received transplants. More intensive liver function monitoring recommendations were made by the US manufacturer again in July 1998 and in June 1999. Subsequently the manufacturer withdrew the drug in Australia, Japan, and the USA in March 2000.

1. Committee on Safety of Medicines/Medicines Control Agency. Troglitazone (Romozin) withdrawn. *Current Problems* 1997; **23:** 13.
2. Anonymous. Troglitazone and liver injury. *WHO Drug Inf* 1998; **12:** 13.
3. Misbin RI. Troglitazone-associated hepatic failure. *Ann Intern Med* 1999; **130:** 330.

Interactions
Troglitazone may enhance the hypoglycaemic effects of sulfonylureas; dosage adjustment may be necessary. There is a possibility that troglitazone may enhance the metabolism of drugs metabolised by cytochrome P450 isoenzyme CYP3A4, including some oral contraceptives and terfenadine.

Ciclosporin. For the effect of troglitazone on blood concentrations of ciclosporin see Hypoglycaemic Drugs, p.522.

Colestyramine. Colestyramine markedly impaired the absorption of troglitazone when the 2 drugs were given concomitantly.[1]

1. Young MA, *et al.* Concomitant administration of cholestyramine influences the absorption of troglitazone. *Br J Clin Pharmacol* 1998; **45:** 37–40.

Pharmacokinetics
Troglitazone is rapidly absorbed following oral administration, with peak plasma concentrations 1 to 3 hours after a dose. Bioavailability is about 53%; absorption is markedly increased in the presence of food. In the body, troglitazone is more than 99% bound to plasma albumin. It is extensively metabolised in the liver and excreted largely in faeces as metabolites; small amounts of metabolites are excreted in urine. Plasma elimination half-life ranges from 10 to 39 hours.

Uses and Administration
Troglitazone is a thiazolidinedione oral antidiabetic which is thought to act by increasing receptor sensitivity to insulin. It has been given by mouth for the treatment of type 2 diabetes mellitus (p.315) in usual doses of 200 to 400 mg daily (maximum 600 mg daily) with food, although as mentioned above it has been withdrawn in a number of countries owing to hepatotoxicity.

◊ Reviews.
1. Anonymous. Troglitazone for non-insulin-dependent diabetes mellitus. *Med Lett Drugs Ther* 1997; **39:** 49–51.
2. Spencer CM, Markham A. Troglitazone. *Drugs* 1997; **54:** 89–101.
3. Chen C. Troglitazone: an antidiabetic agent. *Am J Health-Syst Pharm* 1998; **55:** 905–25.
4. Plosker GL, Faulds D. Troglitazone: a review of its use in the management of type 2 diabetes mellitus. *Drugs* 1999; **57:** 409–38.
5. Parulkar AA, *et al.* Nonhypoglycemic effects of thiazolidinediones. *Ann Intern Med* 2001; **134:** 61–71.

Preparations
Proprietary Preparations (details are given in Part 3)
Austral.: Rezulin†; **Jpn:** Noscal†; **Mex.:** Rezulin; **UK:** Romozin†; **USA:** Rezulin†.

Voglibose   (15399-k)

Voglibose *(USAN, rINN).*

A-71100; AO-128. 3,4-Dideoxy-4-{[2-hydroxy-1-(hydroxymethyl)ethyl]amino}-2-C-(hydroxymethyl)-D-epi-inositol.

$C_{10}H_{21}NO_7 = 267.3.$
CAS — 83480-29-9.
ATC — A10BF03.

Profile
Voglibose is an inhibitor of alpha-glucosidase with general properties similar to those of acarbose (p.319). It is used in the treatment of diabetes mellitus (p.315) in doses of 200 to 300 μg by mouth three times daily before meals.

Preparations
Proprietary Preparations (details are given in Part 3)
Jpn: Basen; **Thai.:** Basen.

Antiepileptics

This chapter describes antiepileptic drugs and their use in the management of epilepsy, status epilepticus, and other convulsive disorders. The main antiepileptics are

- Acetylureas: Phenacemide
- Barbiturates: Phenobarbital, primidone
- Benzodiazepines: Clonazepam
- GABA analogues: Gabapentin, vigabatrin
- Hydantoins: Phenytoin
- Iminostilbenes: Carbamazepine
- Succinimides: Ethosuximide
- Miscellaneous: Felbamate, lamotrigine, topiramate, valproate.

Epilepsy

Definitions and classification. An epileptic seizure has been defined as a paroxysmal discharge of cerebral neurones accompanied by clinical phenomena apparent to the patient or to an observer. The phenomena may be of a motor, sensory, or autonomic nature and there may also be impairment or complete loss of consciousness. Motor disturbances may include convulsions, which are involuntary, violent, and spasmodic or prolonged contraction of skeletal muscles. The word 'fit' is often used colloquially to describe an epileptic seizure. Epilepsy is defined as a condition characterised by a recurrence of such seizures. A patient should not be described as having epilepsy until a second non-febrile seizure occurs.

Effective management of a patient with epilepsy requires a detailed and accurate classification of seizure types. The following is a broad account of the classification of seizures, epilepsies, and epileptic syndromes based on the views of the Commission on Classification and Terminology of the International League Against Epilepsy in 1981[1] and 1989.[2]

- **Partial seizures** (focal seizures or localisation-related seizures) are epileptic seizures in which the neuronal discharges remain localised in one area of the brain. The phenomena associated with such a seizure depend on the site of origin of the discharge. If there is no loss of consciousness, the seizure is known as a *simple partial seizure* and includes Jacksonian epilepsy, which may be associated with motor or sensory disturbances. If there is impaired consciousness the seizure is referred to as a *complex partial seizure*. Partial seizures were formerly referred to as psychomotor epilepsy or temporal lobe epilepsy, but the terms are not synonymous and should be avoided. Partial seizures may become *secondarily generalised seizures* if the neuronal discharge spreads to involve the entire brain.
- **Generalised seizures** are characterised by neuronal discharges involving both cerebral hemispheres simultaneously from the outset. Subclassifications are based on the presence or absence of different types of convulsions. *Absences* (petit mal) are generalised seizures occurring in children characterised by a sudden loss of consciousness lasting for a few seconds. There is usually accompanying motor activity which may vary in degree from eyelid blinking to more extensive clonic body movements. *Atypical absence seizures* are those with a slower onset and longer duration. *Myoclonic seizures* are epileptic seizures in which the motor manifestation is myoclonus (see below). *Clonic seizures* are characterised by loss of consciousness, autonomic symptoms, and rhythmic clonic contractions of all muscles. *Tonic seizures* are also associated with loss of consciousness and autonomic symptoms accompanied by tonic contraction of the limbs. *Tonic-clonic seizures* (grand mal) are characterised by disordered contraction of muscles. During the tonic phase, all the

muscles go into spasm followed up to a minute later by rhythmic clonic contractions. Finally, the patient enters a deep stupor followed by a period of confusion as consciousness is regained. *Atonic seizures* are characterised by loss of postural tone; the head sags or the patient falls down.

Within the categories of partial and generalised epilepsies, seizures have also been classified as idiopathic in which no cause can be identified; symptomatic in which the seizures are associated with diagnosable underlying disorders; or cryptogenic in which the epilepsies are known or suspected to be symptomatic but the cause is not clear. Localisation-related syndromes include Rolandic and occipital epilepsies (both idiopathic), while generalised idiopathic syndromes include childhood absence epilepsies, juvenile myoclonic epilepsy, and the cryptogenic or symptomatic generalised syndromes include infantile spasms (as for example in West's syndrome), Lennox-Gastaut syndrome, and epilepsy with myoclonic absences.

- A third **unclassified** category covers undetermined epilepsies and epileptic syndromes.
- **Special syndromes** include conditions such as febrile convulsions (see below) in which seizures are related to specific situations.

It has been suggested that classification based on seizure type is the most useful in choice of antiepileptic drug whereas the syndrome classification has more benefits in deciding an overall therapeutic strategy and assessing long-term prognosis.

Status epilepticus is generally recognised as a seizure lasting more than 30 minutes or several distinct episodes without restoration of consciousness in between (see below).

Other convulsive disorders include alcohol withdrawal syndrome, eclampsia and pre-eclampsia, myoclonus, neonatal seizures, and porphyria, and are discussed below.

Starting antiepileptic therapy. A single seizure does not constitute epilepsy and therefore does not necessarily warrant immediate treatment with antiepileptics. The decision to start antiepileptic therapy should be based on whether the risks of further seizures outweigh the risks of treatment. Starting antiepileptic therapy too early means that the patient may be unnecessarily exposed to the adverse effects of the drugs used, and may have social implications if erroneously diagnosed, such as the loss of a patient's driving licence. However, the implications of delaying treatment must also be considered. Although there has long been concern that seizures may damage the brain and intellectual capabilities, or even cause death, there are insufficient data to support these claims. Status epilepticus rather than individual seizures or seizure frequency may be responsible for brain injury or death, although the risks of a newly diagnosed epileptic patient developing status epilepticus are unknown. The most compelling reasons for treatment are risk of personal injury or causing injury to others during a seizure, and the psychosocial consequences of untreated epilepsy such as low self-esteem, anxiety, and domestic and employment difficulties.

Whether antiepileptic therapy should be started early to improve prognosis or delayed or avoided altogether remains contentious.[3,4] There has been a long-held belief that seizures beget seizures, and that untreated epilepsy would have a poor prognosis. Nevertheless, there is still uncertainty, especially in childhood, over whether or not antiepileptics can alter the natural progression of epilepsy.

Differences in reported risks in seizure recurrence may be attributable to differences in methodology as well as different important risk factors in the populations studied; also, few studies have followed up patients for more than 2 to 4 years. In a prospective study[5] of children identified at the time of a first unprovoked seizure, the risk of recurrence after 8 years of follow-up was found to be less than 50%. Furthermore, a decelerating disease process with successively longer intervals between seizures has been shown[6] in untreated children with newly diagnosed tonic-clonic seizures followed up for 2 years. Sadzot[7] pointed out that epidemiological studies conducted in untreated patients in developing countries do not support the assumption that repeated seizures exacerbate epilepsy. Results from another study[8] suggested that seizure

control or the prospects for and success of eventual withdrawal of therapy is little influenced by the number of pretreatment seizures up to 10 seizures; above this number there was a reduced chance of completely controlling seizures. However, experimental evidence would suggest that certain seizure types can have a detrimental effect on prognosis,[9] and one study[10] found that patients treated immediately after a first tonic-clonic seizure had a lower 2-year risk of recurrence than patients who were only started on treatment after a recurrence. Epilepsy is a heterogeneous disorder and further prospective studies on larger homogeneous groups are needed, as well as identification of the factors that contribute to the development of chronic and intractable seizures, in order to make firm conclusions.[7]

Some neurologists do not treat a first seizure but prefer to wait for evidence of recurrence unless clinical features such as more than one seizure type or a neurological deficit predispose to poor seizure control. However, it should be borne in mind that the first attack of many non-convulsive seizures may go undetected. Furthermore, as single partial seizures appear to occur less frequently than single generalised tonic-clonic seizures, many neurologists assume that the first detected attack of a non-convulsive seizure is in fact one of multiple seizures and institute treatment.

Choice of antiepileptic. Once a decision to treat has been made, the choice of antiepileptic is determined primarily by its effectiveness against the type of seizures experienced and its potential adverse effects.[11-20] Monotherapy is preferable to a multiple-drug regimen and treatment is therefore initiated with a single drug, increasing the dose gradually until seizures are brought under control or adverse effects become unacceptable. If treatment with the first drug fails, it is preferable to try alternative single first-line antiepileptics before giving combinations of drugs. The change-over from one antiepileptic to another should be made cautiously, withdrawing the first drug only when the new regimen has been largely established. If combinations are necessary in intractable cases, regimens should avoid the inclusion, where possible, of sedating drugs such as the barbiturates or benzodiazepines. Furthermore, drugs with different modes of action should be selected, to reduce the risk that adverse effects will be additive. Many antiepileptics interact with each other through complex mechanisms and dosage adjustments may be necessary to maintain plasma concentrations within the therapeutic range; plasma monitoring is often advisable with combination therapy.

Simple and complex **partial seizures** with or without **secondary generalisation** may be treated with *carbamazepine*, *phenytoin* or *valproate*; the response rate is somewhat lower than for tonic-clonic seizures associated with primary generalised epilepsy (see below). There is some evidence in favour of carbamazepine as the first choice in partial seizures.[21] *Lamotrigine* has been shown to be of equal efficacy to carbamazepine as monotherapy for partial seizures with or without secondary generalisation. In some countries *oxcarbazepine* is becoming more widely accepted as an effective and safe alternative to carbamazepine.[22] *Phenobarbital* or *primidone* are used less often; sedation can be a problem. *Acetazolamide*, *clobazam*, or *clonazepam*, or one of the newer antiepileptics such as *gabapentin*, *levetiracetam*, *tiagabine*, *topiramate*, or *vigabatrin*, may be tried as adjunctive therapy in refractory cases. Calcium-channel blockers such as flunarizine, nifedipine, and nimodipine have been studied with equivocal results in patients with refractory epilepsy, particularly those with partial seizures.

The drugs used most often to treat **generalised** tonic-clonic seizures are *carbamazepine, lamotrigine, phenytoin,* or *valproate*. For tonic-clonic seizures as part of the syndrome of primary generalised epilepsy, valproate is the drug of choice, although a meta-analysis was unable to establish evidence for this.[21] *Phenobarbital* and *primidone* may also be used, but sedation might be a problem. In refractory cases, *vigabatrin* may be tried, or a combination of valproate and lamotrigine (or failing this, *topiramate*) has been proposed.[20]

The drugs of choice for **absence seizures** are *ethosuximide* or *valproate*, both of which appear to be equally effective.[23] Since absence seizures occur primarily in children the precautions concerning valproate hepatotoxicity apply, and some prefer ethosuximide despite its potentially serious adverse effects (see p.348). However, where absence seizures are associated with tonic-clonic seizures valproate is the drug of choice since it is effective in both conditions; valproate is also preferred for atypical absence seizures.

Valproate is normally the drug of choice for **myoclonic seizures**, including those associated with juvenile myoclonic epilepsy.[24,25] *Clonazepam* is also used alone or in combination with valproate[26] but its sedative side-effects and the development of tolerance limit its use.[27] *Ethosuximide* and *mesuximide* have also been used. Some forms of myoclonus may respond to *lamotrigine* but others may be exacerbated.[25]

In **catamenial epilepsy** (epilepsy associated with menstruation) seizures can be predicted and intermittent therapy with *clobazam* may be useful.

The **Lennox-Gastaut syndrome** begins in early childhood and is particularly difficult to treat because multiple seizure types co-exist; seizures rarely remit entirely. *Valproate* is most frequently used[28] because of its broad spectrum of activity and *lamotrigine* is also effective. *Phenytoin, phenobarbital,* and *carbamazepine* may be useful for tonic or tonic-clonic seizures, but they may exacerbate absence or myoclonic seizures. *Benzodiazepines* have also been used although development of tolerance is a problem. *Felbamate, topiramate,* and *vigabatrin* have also been shown to be effective.

Infantile spasms (as for example in **West's syndrome**) are generally unresponsive to conventional antiepileptics.[29,30] *Corticotropin* and *corticosteroids* have been commonly used but they are associated with frequent and severe adverse effects, and there is controversy over whether they have a better effect on long-term outcome than antiepileptics. *Vigabatrin* is effective either as adjunctive treatment or monotherapy. Many consider that it should replace corticotropin or corticosteroids as the treatment of choice,[31-35] despite the risk of visual field defects,[36] although others disagree.[37,38] However, vigabatrin may offer the best first option in the treatment of infantile spasms due to tuberous sclerosis.[39] Other drugs that have been used include *nitrazepam* and *valproate*. *Felbamate* and *lamotrigine* have also been shown to be effective for infantile spasms,[40] as has *topiramate*.[41]

Choice of antiepileptics in children. The use of antiepileptics in general in children has been reviewed.[40,42,43] Again, appropriate treatment depends on seizure type, but there is a lack of evidence to support many therapeutic choices,[43,44] in part because of the difficulties in undertaking trials in this population. In addition, children may be particularly susceptible to some adverse effects, including effects on behaviour, cognition, and development; behavioural problems have been associated particularly with phenobarbital.[45] Where control is not achieved with one antiepileptic others should be tried,[43,46] although the chances of remission are reduced somewhat.[46] Dietary modification (the ketogenic diet) may also be tried.

Withdrawal of antiepileptic therapy. The possibility of withdrawal of antiepileptic therapy arises in patients who achieve prolonged seizure-free periods. Concern over the potential adverse effects of antiepileptic therapy clearly makes withdrawal attractive; however, the practical and social consequences of seizure recurrence may be considerable (for example, loss of driving licence and restricted employment prospects).

Several studies have addressed the prognosis for relapse following antiepileptic withdrawal in children in remission. Long-term follow-up in children whose therapy was withdrawn after seizures had been controlled for several years found that about 25 to 30% had seizure recurrence, in most cases within 2 years of withdrawal.[47,48] Another group reported a higher relapse rate when therapy was withdrawn after 1 year (46%) compared with 3 years (29%);[49] analysis by seizure type suggested that this was due particularly to a difference in outcome in children with complex partial seizures.[50] Another prospective study found that the remission rate may be as high as 80% among the general population of epileptic children (containing fewer refractory cases than those seen in epilepsy centres).[51]

There has been some uncertainty as to whether these results can be extrapolated to adults.[52] A meta-analysis[53] that included 25 studies and 5354 patients (children and adults) found the overall rate of relapse in seizure-free patients following discontinuation of antiepileptic therapy was 25% at 1 year and 29% at 2 years. There was a higher risk for relapse in adolescent- and adult-onset epilepsy compared with childhood-onset epilepsy.

Although these findings indicate that it is often possible to withdraw therapy successfully, it is more difficult to offer an individual prognosis. Some consider that most adult patients whose livelihood or lifestyle depends on their being seizure-free would be ill advised to contemplate drug withdrawal.[54] Epilepsy of long duration before remission is achieved,[47,55] refractory epilepsy[55] or combined seizure types,[47] cerebral pathology[56] or mental or neurological deficit[57] may all increase the risk of relapse, and, as previously mentioned, there is a greater likelihood of relapse in adolescent- and adult-onset epilepsy. Seizure type also seems to be important in most studies, with partial seizures associated with a higher risk of relapse,[55] particularly if secondarily generalised;[55] the risk may also be increased in patients with a history of tonic-clonic seizures but the findings of studies are conflicting.[54] Withdrawal of treatment in juvenile myoclonic epilepsy is generally considered inappropriate as up to 90% of patients who are in remission will relapse if treatment is withdrawn.[58,59] Abnormal EEG before withdrawal is also reported in many studies, including the previously quoted meta-analysis,[53] to be prognostic of a poor outcome but this is not universally accepted.[56] One group[49] found that in children who demonstrated abnormal EEG activity the overall risk of relapse on discontinuation of therapy was only slightly higher than in patients with no such activity, although certain abnormal activities were associated with higher relapse rates than others.

Treatment with more than one antiepileptic is a risk factor for poor prognosis on withdrawal.[54,60] One study has suggested that the type of drug withdrawn is significant, with a poorer prognosis for patients on valproate.[55] Interestingly, however, another study in patients receiving *combination* antiepileptic therapy, as opposed to monotherapy, indicated that a significant increase in seizures was more likely when the carbamazepine component was withdrawn.[61] It should be remembered that withdrawal of hepatic enzyme-inducing antiepileptics can result in changes in serum concentrations of other concomitantly administered antiepileptics.[62]

Limited data suggest that the longer the duration of remission before withdrawal, the lower the risk of relapse.[60] In practice seizure control for at least 2 to 3 years before withdrawal is attempted appears to be considered mandatory,[56,63] although some suggest that this may not be necessary with all seizure types.[50]

Several strategies for predicting the likely outcome after withdrawal of antiepileptic therapy in individuals have been published.[59,64,65] Recognising that epilepsy is a heterogeneous disorder, scoring systems to allow for various risk factors have been devised.[59,64]

When a decision to withdraw is made, it is agreed that drug withdrawal should be gradual to reduce the risk of provoking withdrawal seizures. Drugs should be withdrawn one at a time[66] but there is no agreement on the optimum rate of withdrawal for individual drugs. Shorvon[66] suggested that withdrawal of carbamazepine, barbiturates, or benzodiazepines should be carried out slowly whereas it may be possible to discontinue phenytoin or valproate quickly (over a few days in hospital) if necessary. Exacerbation of seizures may be brought under control by re-establishing the drug being withdrawn. Although it has been suggested that withdrawal over a long period may reduce the relapse rate, one study in children indicated no significant difference in seizure recurrence rate when various antiepileptics including barbiturates were withdrawn over 6 weeks or 9 months.[67]

1. Commission on Classification and Terminology of the International League against Epilepsy. Proposal for revised clinical and electroencephalographic classification of epileptic seizures. *Epilepsia* 1981; **22**: 489–501.
2. Commission on Classification and Terminology of the International League against Epilepsy. Proposal for revised classification of epilepsies and epileptic syndromes. *Epilepsia* 1989; **30**: 389–99.
3. Reynolds EH. Do anticonvulsants alter the natural course of epilepsy?: treatment should be started as early as possible. *BMJ* 1995; **310**: 176–7.
4. Chadwick D. Do anticonvulsants alter the natural course of epilepsy?: case for early treatment is not established. *BMJ* 1995; **310**: 177–8.
5. Shinnar S, *et al*. The risk of seizure recurrence after a first unprovoked afebrile seizure in childhood: an extended follow-up. *Pediatrics* 1996; **98**: 216–25.
6. van Donselaar CA, *et al*. Clinical course of untreated tonic-clonic seizures in childhood: prospective, hospital based study. *BMJ* 1997; **314**: 401–4.
7. Sadzot B. Epilepsy: a progressive disease? *BMJ* 1997; **314**: 391–2.
8. Camfield C, *et al*. Does the number of seizures before treatment influence ease of control or remission of childhood epilepsy?: not if the number is 10 or less. *Neurology* 1996; **46**: 41–4.
9. O'Donoghue M, Sander JWAS. Does early anti-epileptic drug treatment alter the prognosis for remission of the epilepsies? *J R Soc Med* 1996; **89**: 245–8.
10. First Seizure Trial Group. Randomized clinical trial on the efficacy of antiepileptic drugs in reducing the risk of relapse after a first unprovoked tonic-clonic seizure. *Neurology* 1993; **43**: 478–83.
11. Anonymous. Drugs for epilepsy. *Med Lett Drugs Ther* 1995; **37**: 37–40.
12. Sabers A, Gram L. Drug treatment of epilepsy in the 1990s: achievements and new developments. *Drugs* 1996; **52**: 483–93.
13. Brodie MJ, Dichter MA. Antiepileptic drugs. *N Engl J Med* 1996; **334**: 168–75.
14. Britton JW, So EL. Selection of antiepileptic drugs: a practical approach. *Mayo Clin Proc* 1996; **71**: 778–86.
15. Wallace SJ, *et al*. Epilepsy—a guide to medical treatment 1: antiepileptic drugs. *Hosp Med* 1998; **59**: 379–87.
16. Dichter MA, Brodie MJ. New antiepileptic drugs. *N Engl J Med* 1996; **334**: 1583–90.
17. Stephen LJ, Brodie MJ. New drug treatments for epilepsy. *Prescribers' J* 1998; **38**: 98–106.
18. Devinsky O. Patients with refractory seizures. *N Engl J Med* 1999; **340**: 1565–70.
19. Feely M. Drug treatment of epilepsy. *BMJ* 1999; **318**: 106–9.
20. Smith D, Chadwick D. The management of epilepsy. *J Neurol Neurosurg Psychiatry* 2001; **70** (suppl 2): ii15–ii21.
21. Marson AG, *et al*. Carbamazepine versus valproate monotherapy for epilepsy (updated 30 May 2001). Available in The Cochrane Library; Issue 3. Oxford: Update Software; 2001.
22. Perucca E. The new generation of antiepileptic drugs: advantages and disadvantages. *Br J Clin Pharmacol* 1996; **42**: 531–43.
23. Mikati MA, Browne TR. Comparative efficacy of antiepileptic drugs. *Clin Neuropharmacol* 1988; **11**: 130–40.
24. Timmings PL, Richens A. Juvenile myoclonic epilepsy. *BMJ* 1992; **305**: 4–5.
25. Wallace SJ. Myoclonus and epilepsy in childhood: a review of treatment with valproate, ethosuximide, lamotrigine and zonisamide. *Epilepsy Res* 1998; **29**: 147–54.
26. Anonymous. Diagnosing juvenile myoclonic epilepsy. *Lancet* 1992; **340**: 759–60.
27. Ashton H. Guidelines for the rational use of benzodiazepines: when and what to use. *Drugs* 1994; **48**: 25–40.
28. Schmidt D, Bourgeois B. A risk-benefit assessment of therapies for Lennox-Gastaut syndrome. *Drug Safety* 2000; **22**: 467–77.
29. Appleton RE. Infantile spasms. *Arch Dis Child* 1993; **69**: 614–18.
30. Haines ST, Casto DT. Treatment of infantile spasms. *Ann Pharmacother* 1994; **28**: 779–91.
31. Vigevano F, Cilio MR. Vigabatrin versus ACTH as first-line treatment for infantile spasms: a randomized, prospective study. *Epilepsia* 1997; **38**: 1270–4.
32. Granstrom ML, *et al*. Treatment of infantile spasms: results of a population-based study with vigabatrin as the first drug for spasms. *Epilepsia* 1999; **40**: 950–7.
33. Cossette P, *et al*. ACTH versus vigabatrin therapy in infantile spasms: a retrospective study. *Neurology* 1999; **52**: 1691–4.
34. Appleton RE. Guideline may help in prescribing vigabatrin. *BMJ* 1998; **317**: 1322. Full version: http://www.bmj.com/cgi/content/full/317/7168/1322
35. Appleton RE, *et al*. Randomised, placebo-controlled study of vigabatrin as first-line treatment of infantile spasms. *Epilepsia* 1999; **40**: 1627–33.
36. Vigabatrin Paediatric Advisory Group. Guideline for prescribing in children has been revised. *BMJ* 2000; **320**: 1404–5.
37. Lux AL, *et al*. Revised guideline for prescribing vigabatrin in children: guideline's claim about infantile spasms is not based on appropriate evidence. *BMJ* 2001; **322**: 236–7.
38. Riikonen RS. Steroids or vigabatrin in the treatment of infantile spasms? *Pediatr Neurol* 2000; **23**: 403–8.
39. Hancock E, Osborne JP. Vigabatrin in the treatment of infantile spasms in tuberous sclerosis: literature review. *J Child Neurol* 1999; **14**: 71–4.
40. Morton LD, Pellock JM. Diagnosis and treatment of epilepsy in children and adolescents. *Drugs* 1996; **51**: 399–414.
41. Glauser TA, *et al*. Long-term response to topiramate in patients with West syndrome. *Epilepsia* 2000; **41** (suppl 1): S91–4.
42. Zupanc ML. Update on epilepsy in pediatric patients. *Mayo Clin Proc* 1996; **71**: 899–916.
43. Neville BGR. Epilepsy in childhood. *BMJ* 1997; **315**: 924–30.
44. Appleton RE. The new antiepileptic drugs. *Arch Dis Child* 1996; **75**: 256–62. Correction. *ibid.* 1997; **76**: 81.
45. de Silva M, *et al*. Randomised comparative monotherapy trial of phenobarbitone, phenytoin, carbamazepine, or sodium valproate for newly diagnosed childhood epilepsy. *Lancet* 1996; **347**: 709–13.
46. Camfield PR, *et al*. If a first antiepileptic drug fails to control a child's epilepsy, what are the chances of success with the next drug? *J Pediatr* 1997; **131**: 821–4.
47. Thurston JH, *et al*. Prognosis in childhood epilepsy. *N Engl J Med* 1982; **306**: 831–6.
48. Shinnar S, *et al*. Discontinuing antiepileptic medication in children with epilepsy after two years without seizures. *N Engl J Med* 1985; **313**: 976–80.
49. Andersson T, *et al*. A comparison between one and three years of treatment in uncomplicated childhood epilepsy: a prospective study: II: the EEG as predictor of outcome after withdrawal of treatment. *Epilepsia* 1997; **38**: 225–32.
50. Braathen G, *et al*. Comparison between one and three years of treatment in uncomplicated childhood epilepsy: a prospective study: I: outcome in different seizure types. *Epilepsia* 1996; **37**: 822–32.
51. Bouma PAD, *et al*. Discontinuation of antiepileptic therapy: a prospective study in children. *J Neurol Neurosurg Psychiatry* 1987; **50**: 1579–83.
52. Pedley TA. Discontinuing antiepileptic drugs. *N Engl J Med* 1988; **318**: 982–4.
53. Berg AT, Shinnar S. Relapse following discontinuation of antiepileptic drugs: a meta-analysis. *Neurology* 1994; **44**: 601–8.
54. Anonymous. Antiepileptic drug withdrawal—hawks or doves? *Lancet* 1991; **337**: 1193–4.
55. Callaghan N, *et al*. Withdrawal of anticonvulsant drugs in patients free of seizures for two years: a prospective study. *N Engl J Med* 1988; **318**: 942–6.
56. Chadwick D. Drug withdrawal and epilepsy: when and how? *Drugs* 1988; **35**: 579–83.
57. Emerson R, *et al*. Stopping medication in children with epilepsy: predicators of outcome. *N Engl J Med* 1981; **304**: 1125–9.
58. Anonymous. Diagnosing juvenile myoclonic epilepsy. *Lancet* 1992; **340**: 759–60.
59. Medical Research Council Antiepileptic Drug Withdrawal Study Group. Prognostic index for recurrence of seizures after remission of epilepsy. *BMJ* 1993; **306**: 1374–8.

60. Medical Research Council Antiepileptic Drug Withdrawal Study Group. Randomised study of antiepileptic drug withdrawal in patients in remission. *Lancet* 1991; **337:** 1175–80.
61. Duncan JS, *et al.* Discontinuation of phenytoin, carbamazepine, and valproate in patients with active epilepsy. *Epilepsia* 1990; **31:** 324–33.
62. Duncan JS, *et al.* Effects of discontinuation of phenytoin, carbamazepine, and valproate on concomitant antiepileptic medication. *Epilepsia* 1991; **32:** 101–15.
63. Anonymous. Withdrawing antiepileptic drugs. *Drug Ther Bull* 1989; **27:** 29–30.
64. Camfield C, *et al.* Outcome of childhood epilepsy: a population-based study with a simple predictive scoring system for those treated with medication. *J Pediatr* 1993; **122:** 861–8.
65. Shinnar S, *et al.* Discontinuing antiepileptic drugs in children with epilepsy: a prospective study. *Ann Neurol* 1994; **35:** 534–45.
66. Shorvon SD. Medical assessment and treatment of chronic epilepsy. *BMJ* 1991; **302:** 363–6.
67. Tennison MB, *et al.* Discontinuing antiepileptic drugs in children with epilepsy: a comparison of a six-week and a nine-month taper period. *N Engl J Med* 1994; **330:** 1407–10.

Cognition. The relationship between cognitive impairment, antiepileptic drugs, and epilepsy is complex and poorly understood; psychosocial and environmental factors may also contribute.[1] Children are particularly vulnerable to cognitive impairment, which can develop insidiously and therefore be overlooked. Many studies, including comparative studies, have assessed the effects of antiepileptics on cognitive function, but the results have often been variable. A major difficulty has been to distinguish subtle effects of drug therapy on mental function, if they exist, from those of sedation or the effect of the disease itself or its underlying pathology.[1,2]

Although subtle effects on cognition have been most commonly reported with barbiturate antiepileptics such as phenobarbital, they may also occur with other antiepileptics, and in adults as well as children. Benzodiazepines, phenobarbital, and primidone are most frequently linked to sedative effects and behavioural problems whereas phenytoin, carbamazepine, and valproate are less problematic. Studies of effects on cognition have been conducted in healthy adults in an effort to separate any confounding factors of epilepsy and seizures, and standard antiepileptics have been shown to impair cognition in people with and without epilepsy. Results from recent studies in both groups have demonstrated that at therapeutic serum concentrations phenobarbital, phenytoin, carbamazepine, oxcarbazepine, and valproate have similar adverse effects on cognitive function,[1,3] although there is also evidence that phenobarbital has the greatest potential for adverse cognitive and behavioural effects.[1] Most of the newer antiepileptics appear to be better tolerated, although zonisamide and topiramate produce some cognitive impairment. There is also limited evidence that gabapentin, lamotrigine, and vigabatrin may enhance cognitive function. However, further data are required for the newer antiepileptics before a definitive assessment can be made.[1,4]

There is wide interindividual variation in the effects that antiepileptics have on cognitive function; in some patients the effects may become apparent at low serum levels, whereas other tolerate high serum levels without apparent untoward effect.[4] Variable results from studies mean that it is difficult to make comparisons. It is, however, generally agreed that phenobarbital is less desirable for use in children than other antiepileptics.

Most studies on the adverse effects of antiepileptics on cognitive function have had methodological flaws and have involved small numbers of patients; recommendations for future research have been made.[5] Future studies should assess antiepileptic use in different epileptic patient populations.[4]

In view of the potential effect of antiepileptics on cognition, the Committee on Drugs of the American Academy of Pediatrics[6] has made a number of recommendations, that include the following

- the relative influence of each antiepileptic on cognitive and behavioural function should be considered along with all other potential adverse effects;
- the child's behaviour and academic progress should be monitored through routine questioning of parents and teachers as well as by the physician's own observations of cognitive function, mood, and behaviour;
- should behavioural or cognitive changes occur in relation to starting antiepileptic therapy, the need for medication and/or possible alteration of medication must be reassessed.

1. Kwan P, Brodie MJ. Neuropsychological effects of epilepsy and antiepileptic drugs. *Lancet* 2001; **357:** 216–22.
2. Prevey ML, *et al.* Complex partial and secondarily generalized seizure patients: cognitive functioning prior to treatment with antiepileptic medication. *Epilepsy Res* 1998; **30:** 1–9.

3. Kälviäinen R, *et al.* Cognitive adverse effects of antiepileptic drugs: incidence, mechanisms and therapeutic implications. *CNS Drugs* 1996; **5:** 358–68.
4. Devinsky O. Cognitive and behavioral effects of antiepileptic drugs. *Epilepsia* 1995; **36** (suppl 2): S46–S65.
5. Aldenkamp AP, Vermeulen J. Phenytoin and carbamazepine: differential effects on cognitive function. *Seizure* 1995; **4:** 95–104.
6. Committee on Drugs of the American Academy of Pediatrics. Behavioral and cognitive effects of anticonvulsant therapy. *Pediatrics* 1995; **96:** 538–40.

Driving. Driving by patients with epilepsy is generally regulated[1,2] and restricted to those whose seizures are adequately controlled. Also, antiepileptic drugs may produce CNS-related adverse effects, including dizziness and drowsiness, that could impair a patient's ability to drive a vehicle or operate machinery, particularly during the initial stages of therapy.

In the UK,[3] patients suffering from epilepsy may drive a motor vehicle (but not a heavy goods or public service vehicle) provided that they have had a seizure-free period of 1 year, or, if subject to attacks only while asleep, have established a 3-year period without awake attacks. It is recommended that patients should not drive during withdrawal of antiepileptic drugs, or for 6 months afterwards.

1. Berg AT, Engel J. Restricted driving for people with epilepsy. *Neurology* 1999; **52:** 1306–7.
2. Ooi WW, Gutrecht JA. International regulations for automobile driving and epilepsy. *J Travel Med* 2000; **7:** 1–4.
3. Driver and Vehicle Licensing Agency. At a glance: a guide for medical practitioners. Available at: http://www.dvla.gov.uk/at_a_glance/ch1_neurological.htm (accessed 25/10/01).

Pregnancy and breast feeding. The management of epilepsy during pregnancy may present problems for both the mother and the fetus.[1-6]

The incidence of spontaneous abortion and still-births increases in women with epilepsy although the reason is unknown. A single generalised seizure does not usually pose clinical problems for the fetus, but both mother and fetus are at risk of serious trauma from maternal falls and intra-uterine deaths have been reported. Status epilepticus is associated with significant mortality in mother and fetus. The frequency of seizures increases during pregnancy in some women; this may be related to hormonal or other factors such as lack of sleep, but one of the main reasons is likely to be decreased plasma-antiepileptic concentrations due to changes in drug clearance and binding as pregnancy progresses.

Although more than 90% of pregnant women receiving antiepileptic therapy will deliver normal infants, unequivocal teratogenic risks have been identified for all the major antiepileptics.[7] The risk appears to increase when 2 or more drugs are given together. Untreated epilepsy itself has been associated with an increase in fetal abnormalities,[8] although to a lesser degree than with antiepileptics. This does not appear to be associated with maternal seizures during pregnancy and, since some of these effects were also described before the use of antiepileptics became widespread, there may be a relationship with a genetic component of epilepsy.[7,8] A variety of syndromes, including craniofacial and digital abnormalities and, less commonly, cleft lip and palate, have been described with *carbamazepine, phenobarbital, phenytoin, primidone, trimethadione,* and *valproate*; congenital heart disease, microcephaly, and developmental delay may also occur with some antiepileptics. Specific syndromes have previously been ascribed to individual antiepileptics such as the 'fetal hydantoin syndrome' with phenytoin, but now it is recognised that there is some degree of overlap between the effects seen with different drugs, and the broader term 'fetal antiepileptic drug syndrome' is therefore considered to be more appropriate by some.[7,8] In some cases, the milder dysmorphic features become less apparent as the child grows older. There is still insufficient data to determine which of the older antiepileptics is more teratogenic.[7] Neural tube defects are associated with valproate and carbamazepine and the risk of spina bifida has been calculated[9-11] to be about 1%, which is about 20 times the rate in the general population. Analysis of data[12] from 5 prospective studies showed that there was a dose-response relationship between maternal use of valproate and the development of major congenital abnormalities; in particular, daily doses above 1 g were associated with a significantly increased risk. Additional problems that may occur with some antiepileptic therapies include neonatal sedation and drug dependence with phenobarbital (see p.355) and benzodiazepines if given close to term. Neonatal bleeding is associated with the enzyme-inducing antiepileptics carbamazepine, phenobarbital, and phenytoin, and has also been reported with valproate and other antiepileptics. Little is known of the effects of the newer antiepileptics

on the fetus, although the manufacturers have reported congenital anomalies in the offspring of some mothers using *vigabatrin* during pregnancy and teratogenicity with *topiramate* and *vigabatrin* in *animals*. There appears to be little evidence of teratogenic potential for *felbamate, gabapentin,* or *lamotrigine* in *animal* studies to date, although there is a theoretical risk with lamotrigine because, like valproate, it is a folate antagonist. However, zonisamide has been found to be teratogenic in *animal* studies.

Patients with epilepsy who wish to become pregnant require specialist advice. Withdrawal of antiepileptic therapy may be an option if the patient has been seizure-free for at least 2 years (for further details of drug withdrawal, see above); resumption of therapy may be considered after the end of the first trimester. If antiepileptics are to be continued throughout pregnancy, monotherapy is preferred using the lowest possible effective dose, although doses may have to be increased in response to changes in drug disposition during pregnancy, with the necessary readjustments being made after delivery. Since there is a risk of fetal malformations with all the established antiepileptics, and a lack of data for the newer ones, it is generally considered that as long as there is good seizure control there is little to be gained from changing a pregnant patient's antiepileptic treatment. However high daily doses of valproate (more than 1 g daily) should be avoided if possible, and peak plasma concentrations may be reduced by dividing the daily dose over 3 or 4 administrations. If a patient becomes pregnant while taking carbamazepine, phenytoin, or valproate she should be counselled regarding the risk of neural tube and other defects and should be offered antenatal screening. Adequate supplementation of folic acid is advised before pregnancy and during the first trimester to counteract the risk of neural tube defects; it has been suggested that women receiving antiepileptics should be given folic acid in similar doses to those used in women who have previously given birth to an infant with neural tube defects (for further details, see Neural Tube Defects under Folic Acid, p.1362). Although folic acid can reduce serum-phenytoin concentrations this does not appear to be a problem in practice (see p.362).

To counteract the risk of neonatal bleeding associated with carbamazepine, phenobarbital, and phenytoin, prophylactic vitamin K_1 is recommended for the mother from 36 weeks' gestation, and then for the neonate after delivery (for further details, see under Haemorrhagic Disease of the Newborn, p.1397), although the justification of prophylactic maternal administration has been challenged[13] in the face of available evidence.

Status epilepticus occurring during pregnancy should be treated in the same way as for the general population (see below). First seizures occurring during the second half of pregnancy may be part of eclampsia (see below) and should be differentiated from epilepsy.

Antiepileptics are generally distributed into breast milk (although this information is not always known for the newer ones), but for most of the older established drugs, the concentrations are lower than in maternal plasma, and **breast feeding** is considered to be safe for these antiepileptics when given in usual doses, with the possible exception of the barbiturates and ethosuximide.[1-3,14] Problems of neonatal sedation may occur with the benzodiazepines and barbiturates (including primidone)[1] and breast feeding should be avoided when possible. Ethosuximide is distributed in significant amounts into breast milk and breast feeding should be avoided; hyperexcitability and poor suckling have been reported in the infant. There is little data for the new antiepileptics regarding breast feeding, and therefore the manufacturers recommend that breast feeding should be avoided.

1. Brodie MJ. Management of epilepsy during pregnancy and lactation. *Lancet* 1990; **336:** 426–7.
2. Delgado-Escueta AV, Janz D. Consensus guidelines: preconception counseling, management, and care of the pregnant woman with epilepsy. *Neurology* 1992; **42** (suppl 5): 149–160.
3. Anonymous. Epilepsy and pregnancy. *Drug Ther Bull* 1994; **32:** 49–51.
4. Cleland PG. Management of pre-existing disorders in pregnancy: epilepsy. *Prescribers' J* 1996; **36:** 102–109.
5. Quality Standards Subcommittee of the American Academy of Neurology. Practice parameter: management issues for women with epilepsy (summary statement). *Neurology* 1998; **51:** 944–8.
6. Nulman I, *et al.* Treatment of epilepsy in pregnancy. *Drugs* 1999; **57:** 535–44.
7. Finnell RH, *et al.* Teratogenicity of antiepileptic drugs. In: Levy RH, *et al.* eds. *Antiepileptic drugs.* 4th ed. New York: Raven Press, 1995; 209–30.
8. Gaily E, *et al.* Minor anomalies in offspring of epileptic mothers. *J Pediatr* 1988; **112:** 520–9.
9. Lindhout D, Schmidt D. In-utero exposure to valproate and neural tube defects. *Lancet* 1986; **i:** 1392–3.

10. Oakeshott P, Hunt GM. Valproate and spina bifida. *BMJ* 1989; **298:** 1300–1.
11. Rosa FW. Spina bifida in infants of women treated with carbamazepine during pregnancy. *N Engl J Med* 1991; **324:** 674–7.
12. Samrén EB, *et al.* Maternal use of antiepileptic drugs and the risk of major congenital malformations: a joint European prospective study of human teratogenesis associated with maternal epilepsy. *Epilepsia* 1997; **38:** 981–90.
13. Hey E. Effect of maternal anticonvulsant treatment on neonatal blood coagulation. *Arch Dis Child Fetal Neonatal Ed* 1999; **81:** F208–F210.
14. Hägg S, Spigset O. Anticonvulsant use during lactation. *Drug Safety* 2000; **22:** 425–40.

Status epilepticus

Status epilepticus has been arbitrarily defined as a prolonged seizure, or a period of repeated seizures without restoration of normal consciousness in between, lasting for more than 30 minutes,[1] although it has been suggested that in practice prolonged or repeated seizure activity lasting more than 5 to 10 minutes can be regarded as status epilepticus and requires treatment.[2-4] Any type of seizure can lead to status epilepticus but generalised tonic-clonic status epilepticus is the most common and most dangerous type.[2,3] The longer seizures continue, the more difficult they are to control and the higher the morbidity and mortality; permanent neuronal damage can occur after 30 minutes of seizure activity.

Initial treatment consists of supporting respiration, including the provision of oxygen, and maintaining blood pressure. The aim is then to terminate the seizures as quickly as possible. Antiepileptic treatment differs slightly between centres and countries,[1-10] but in most cases treatment is started with *diazepam* to abort the attack followed by phenytoin (or alternatively phenobarbital, clomethiazole, or paraldehyde) to prevent recurrence. Diazepam is given by intravenous injection or as a rectal solution. (Rectal diazepam has also been used in the home setting to treat acute repetitive seizures,[11] which may evolve into status epilepticus.) Some prefer *lorazepam* to diazepam as the initial benzodiazepine[4] because it combines rapid onset with prolonged duration of antiepileptic action. Other benzodiazepines used have included *clonazepam* and *midazolam*.

Once control of seizures is obtained *phenytoin sodium* may be given intravenously with monitoring of blood pressure and ECG. *Fosphenytoin sodium* is a prodrug of phenytoin sodium and has the advantage that it may be administered at a faster rate of intravenous infusion. Phenytoin has been considered to be more appropriate than a benzodiazepine for the management of status epilepticus or recurrent seizures in patients with head injuries or other acute neurological lesions. Phenytoin carries a lower risk of respiratory failure or loss of consciousness, and results in a longer-lasting control of seizures.[12] Alternatively, intravenous *phenobarbital sodium* may be given if the patient has not recently received oral phenobarbital or primidone; careful observation of respiration is mandatory as a large dose of diazepam may have been given previously.[1] Some workers have suggested that using phenobarbital for the initial treatment of convulsive status epilepticus might be at least as effective, safe, and practical as using diazepam with phenytoin,[13] but others consider that phenytoin is again to be preferred as causing less CNS and respiratory depression.[4] Other alternatives include *clomethiazole edisilate* by intravenous infusion or *paraldehyde* rectally or by deep intramuscular injection. Another option is to give *lignocaine [lidocaine]* intravenously.

If the above measures do not control seizures, anaesthesia should be instituted with a short-acting barbiturate such as *thiopental*, and the patient ventilated;[1,5] *pentobarbital* is used similarly.[2,3,7] Other anaesthetics have been tried in the treatment of intractable convulsive status epilepticus including *etomidate, isoflurane, midazolam*, and *propofol*.[3,5,7]

If cerebral neoplasm or arteritis is suspected high-dose *dexamethasone* therapy is started, provided meningitis or cerebral abscess is absent.[1] Alcoholics are given intravenous *thiamine*.[1,5] Pyridoxine may be tried in children under 3 years of age with established convulsive status epilepticus, in case the seizures are pyridoxine dependent or responsive.[4]

Valproate administered intravenously in a small study was found to be effective in controlling status epilepticus of various types including that associated with generalised tonic-clonic and myoclonic seizures.[14]

The treatment of partial status epilepticus is similar to that of generalised tonic-clonic status epilepticus.[3] However, epilepsia partialis continua (continuous clonic movements of a limited part of the body) may be refrac-tory to standard antiepileptics; it may respond to treatment with high doses of *corticosteroids*.[1]

Intravenous benzodiazepines are usually used for the initial treatment of absence status epilepticus[3] followed by oral administration of valproate or *ethosuximide*. Valproate is considered to be the drug of choice for the prevention of recurrence of absence status epilepticus.[15]

1. Brodie MJ. Status epilepticus in adults. *Lancet* 1990; **336:** 551–2.
2. Working Group on Status Epilepticus. Treatment of convulsive status epilepticus: recommendations of the Epilepsy Foundation of America's Working Group on Status Epilepticus. *JAMA* 1993; **270:** 854–9.
3. Bauer J, Elger CE. Management of status epilepticus in adults. *CNS Drugs* 1994; **1:** 26–44.
4. The Status Epilepticus Working Party. The treatment of convulsive status epilepticus in children. *Arch Dis Child* 2000; **83:** 415–19.
5. Anonymous. Stopping status epilepticus. *Drug Ther Bull* 1996; **34:** 73–5.
6. Rylance GW. Treatment of epilepsy and febrile convulsions in children. *Lancet* 1990; **336:** 488–91.
7. Cascino GD. Generalized convulsive status epilepticus. *Mayo Clin Proc* 1996; **71:** 787–92.
8. Shorvon S. Tonic clonic status epilepticus. *J Neurol Neurosurg Psychiatry* 1993; **56:** 125–34.
9. Tasker RC. Emergency treatment of acute seizures and status epilepticus. *Arch Dis Child* 1998; **79:** 78–83.
10. Lowenstein DH, Alldredge BK. Status epilepticus. *N Engl J Med* 1998; **338:** 970–6.
11. Akinbi MS, Welty TE. Benzodiazepines in the home treatment of acute seizures. *Ann Pharmacother* 1999; **33:** 99–102.
12. Eldridge PR, Punt JAG. Risks associated with giving benzodiazepines to patients with acute neurological injuries. *BMJ* 1990; **300:** 1189–90.
13. Shaner DM, *et al.* Treatment of status epilepticus: a prospective comparison of diazepam and phenytoin versus phenobarbital and optional phenytoin. *Neurology* 1988; **38:** 202–7.
14. Giroud M, *et al.* Use of injectable valproic acid in status epilepticus: a pilot study. *Drug Invest* 1993; **5:** 154–9.
15. Berkovic SF, *et al.* Valproate prevents the recurrence of absence status. *Neurology* 1989; **39:** 1294–7.

Other convulsive disorders

Disorders that feature convulsions or epileptic seizures but are not considered to be forms of epilepsy are described below.

Alcohol withdrawal syndrome. For a discussion of the management of seizures associated with alcohol withdrawal syndrome, see p.1131.

Eclampsia and pre-eclampsia. Pre-eclampsia is a hypertensive disorder occurring in pregnancy that entails increased blood pressure together with proteinuria, and sometimes abnormal coagulation and liver function, and oedema; it may progress to eclampsia, which is a convulsive phase. The treatment of pre-eclampsia and eclampsia is primarily aimed at reducing hypertension (see Hypertension in Pregnancy, under Hypertension, p.802) and treating or preventing resultant seizures. Whether the treatment of the hypertension alone is sufficient to prevent the progression of pre-eclampsia to eclampsia is a matter of debate.[1] The management of seizures associated with eclampsia has been discussed.[2,3] It is difficult to identify those patients who will experience eclamptic seizures. Some give *antiepileptics* prophylactically to all women with advanced pre-eclampsia, but this is considered greatly to increase the risk of major adverse effects; others reserve antiepileptics for those who have had a first seizure. 'Lytic cocktails' consisting of chlorpromazine, pethidine, and/or promethazine have been used in some countries in the management of pre-eclampsia and imminent eclampsia but they result in heavy sedation and the use of phenothiazines is generally not recommended late in pregnancy.

Eclampsia in the UK has been treated with *diazepam, clomethiazole,* or *phenytoin*. However, for many years *magnesium sulfate* has been the preferred treatment of eclampsia in the USA and studies[4-6] have shown it to be more effective and to cause fewer adverse effects. A meta-analysis[7] of 9 randomised trials involving 2390 patients with pre-eclampsia and 1743 patients with eclampsia concluded that magnesium sulfate was more effective than phenytoin or no therapy in prevention of seizures in pre-eclamptic patients. In eclamptic patients, magnesium sulfate was superior to phenytoin, diazepam, or a lytic cocktail in terms of seizure recurrence. Thus, many in the UK now consider magnesium sulfate to be the preferred drug for the treatment of eclampsia.[8-12] However, its role for the prevention of eclampsia in pre-eclamptic patients is less clear,[8,11,12] although it is still considered the drug of choice if a prophylactic anticonvulsant is to be used.[12] A systematic review[13] considered that there was insufficient evidence to establish the benefits and hazards of anticonvulsants for women with pre-eclampsia, but concluded that magnesium sulfate appeared to be the best choice if an anticonvulsant were needed. Some commentators have suggested,[14] in the light of evidence of possible neonatal toxicity, that magnesium sulfate should be restricted to use in eclampsia or more severe pre-eclampsia.

1. Ramsay MM, *et al.* Are anticonvulsants necessary to prevent eclampsia. *Lancet* 1994; **343:** 540–1.
2. Redman CWG, Roberts JM. Management of pre-eclampsia. *Lancet* 1993; **341:** 1451–4.
3. Mushambi MC, *et al.* Recent developments in the pathophysiology and management of pre-eclampsia. *Br J Anaesth* 1996; **76:** 133–48.
4. Dommisse J. Phenytoin sodium and magnesium sulphate in the management of eclampsia. *Br J Obstet Gynaecol* 1990; **97:** 104–9.
5. The Eclampsia Trial Collaborative Group. Which anticonvulsant for women with eclampsia?: evidence from the Collaborative Eclampsia Trial. *Lancet* 1995; **345:** 1455–63. Correction. *ibid.;* **346:** 258.
6. Lucas MJ, *et al.* A comparison of magnesium sulfate with phenytoin for the prevention of eclampsia. *N Engl J Med* 1995; **333:** 201–5.
7. Chien PFW, *et al.* Magnesium sulphate in the treatment of eclampsia and pre-eclampsia: an overview of the evidence from randomised trials. *Br J Obstet Gynaecol* 1996; **103:** 1085–91.
8. Anthony J, *et al.* Role of magnesium sulfate in seizure prevention in patients with eclampsia and pre-eclampsia. *Drug Safety* 1996; **15:** 188–99.
9. Robson SC. Magnesium sulphate: the time of reckoning. *Br J Obstet Gynaecol* 1996; **103:** 99–102.
10. Duley L. Magnesium sulphate regimens for women with eclampsia: messages from the Collaborative Eclampsia Trial. *Br J Obstet Gynaecol* 1996; **103:** 103–5.
11. Gülmezoglu AM, Duley L. Use of anticonvulsants in eclampsia and pre-eclampsia: survey of obstetricians in the United Kingdom and Republic of Ireland. *BMJ* 1998; **316:** 975–6.
12. Walker JJ. Pre-eclampsia. *Lancet* 2000; **356:** 1260–5.
13. Duley L, *et al.* Anticonvulsants for women with pre-eclampsia (updated 28 October 1999). Available in The Cochrane Library; Issue 3. Oxford: Update Software; 2001.
14. Bennett P, Edwards D. Use of magnesium sulphate in obstetrics. *Lancet* 1997; **350:** 1491.

Febrile convulsions. Febrile convulsions have been defined[1] as epileptic seizures occurring between the ages of 6 months to 5 years and associated with a fever arising from an infectious illness outside the CNS. They usually occur during the rising phase of fever early in the course of the infection and are not considered to be a form of epilepsy.[2]

Febrile convulsions are considered to be benign if limited to a single tonic or tonic-clonic seizure lasting less than 15 minutes without any focal characteristics.[2] About one-third of children who have a benign febrile convulsion will experience a recurrence.[1,2] The risk of developing epilepsy is low, but nevertheless it is 2 to 3 times greater than the risk in the population as a whole.[2] Unless they are recurrent, benign febrile convulsions need only simple treatment to lower body temperature[1,2] such as that described under Fever and Hyperthermia, p.8.

Prolonged febrile convulsions lasting longer than 15 minutes and associated with some focal characteristics are not considered to be benign and further increase the risk of developing epilepsy.[2] When they are prolonged or recurrent they are treated with *diazepam* intravenously, or as a rectal solution, to prevent possible brain damage resulting from continued seizure activity, although any such effect appears to be rare.[3]

The prophylactic administration of *antiepileptics* to children thought to be at risk of recurrence of febrile convulsions remains controversial. Many consider that even if recurrences can be prevented there is no evidence that the risk of developing epilepsy is reduced.[1,2,4] A working group of the Royal College of Physicians and the British Paediatric Association considered that pooled analyses of studies of the prophylactic use of *phenobarbital* or *sodium valproate* showed that long-term prophylaxis was rarely indicated.[1] Although some workers have demonstrated that intermittent prophylaxis with phenobarbital or diazepam[5] given at the onset of and during fever could prevent recurrence of febrile convulsions, the working group did not recommend their routine use in this way.[1] Other workers have found that administration of paracetamol as an antipyretic and the use of diazepam for intermittent prophylaxis failed to prevent recurrences of febrile convulsions.[6] A later meta-analysis[7] concluded that neither continuous nor intermittent prophylaxis could be recommended as the benefits did not outweigh the potential adverse effects, a view endorsed by the American Academy of Pediatrics.[8]

1. Joint Working Group of the Research Unit of the Royal College of Physicians and the British Paediatric Association. Guidelines for the management of convulsions with fever. *BMJ* 1991; **303:** 634–6.
2. Smith MC. Febrile seizures: recognition and management. *Drugs* 1994; **47:** 933–44.
3. Verity CM. Do seizures damage the brain? The epidemiological evidence. *Arch Dis Child* 1998; **78:** 78–84.
4. Knudsen FU, *et al.* Long term outcome of prophylaxis for febrile convulsions. *Arch Dis Child* 1996; **74:** 13–18.

5. Rosman NP, *et al.* A controlled trial of diazepam administered during febrile illnesses to prevent recurrence of febrile seizures. *N Engl J Med* 1993; **329:** 79–84.
6. Uhari M, *et al.* Effect of acetaminophen and of low intermittent doses of diazepam on prevention of recurrences of febrile seizures. *J Pediatr* 1995; **126:** 991–5.
7. Rantala H, *et al.* A meta-analytic review of the preventative treatment of recurrences of febrile seizures. *J Pediatr* 1997; **131:** 922–5.
8. American Academy of Pediatrics. Practice parameter: long-term treatment of the child with simple febrile seizures. *Pediatrics* 1999; **103:** 1307–9.

Myoclonus. Myoclonus consists of brief, involuntary, jerky movements of sudden onset which may be focal, segmental, or generalised, and are caused by muscular contractions (positive myoclonus) or inhibitions (negative myoclonus). The term 'myoclonus' is non-specific and classification is important in order to decide on treatment:[1] physiological (in normal subjects); essential (no known cause); epileptic (seizures dominate); or symptomatic (encephalopathy dominates and there are many causes including storage diseases, neurodegenerative syndromes, toxic and drug-induced syndromes, and hypoxia).

Myoclonus may also be subdivided into cortical, reticular, or spinal forms. Cortical myoclonus is considered to be a subset of epilepsy and responds best to antiepileptics, usually *valproate* and/or *clonazepam*; *piracetam* is also used, usually as adjunctive therapy. In epileptic myoclonus, epileptic seizures (myoclonic seizures in which the motor manifestation is myoclonus) dominate. Their treatment is discussed under Epilepsy, above. Reticular myoclonus is usually caused by anoxia or acute encephalopathy and may be treated with *clonazepam* or *serotonin*. Posthypoxic myoclonus occurring after hypoxic coma may respond to *oxitriptan* or *serotonin* combined with *carbidopa*; antiepileptics may help. Essential myoclonus may benefit from clonazepam.

1. Caviness JN. Myoclonus. *Mayo Clin Proc.* 1996; **71:** 679–88.

Neonatal seizures. Neonatal seizures differ from epilepsy and the definitions in the international classification of epilepsy and epileptic syndromes (see above) do not apply. They are frequently subtle and difficult to recognise. Causes include asphyxia, glucose or electrolyte imbalance, infection, CNS or cerebrovascular lesions, inborn errors of metabolism, and drug withdrawal or intoxication.

Neonatal seizures represent a neurological emergency in the newborn and rapid diagnosis and treatment is essential. Infusion of glucose or electrolytes may be of benefit. Current practice involves administration of antiepileptic drugs to control seizures, although there is no consensus on their use. *Phenobarbital* and *phenytoin* are the most widely used. Some consider phenobarbital to be the mainstay of treatment for all types of seizures in neonates, although response rates are variable. If seizures persist, phenytoin may be added to therapy. Other drugs that have been tried include *carbamazepine, benzodiazepines,* and *primidone.* Pyridoxine dependent seizures can be abolished by regular administration of large doses of the vitamin (see p.1387).
References.

1. Zupanc ML. Update on epilepsy in pediatric patients. *Mayo Clin Proc* 1996; **71:** 899–916.
2. Morton LD, Pellock JM. Diagnosis and treatment of epilepsy in children and adolescents. *Drugs* 1996; **51:** 399–414.
3. Singh B, *et al.* Treatment of neonatal seizures with carbamazepine. *J Child Neurol* 1996; **11:** 378–82.
4. Evans D, Levene M. Neonatal seizures. *Arch Dis Child Fetal Neonatal Ed* 1998; **78:** F70–F75.
5. Painter MJ, *et al.* Phenobarbital compared with phenytoin for the treatment of neonatal seizures. *N Engl J Med* 1999; **341:** 485–9.

Porphyria. Convulsions may occur at the peak of an attack of acute porphyria (p.1011) but usually disappear as the attack resolves and therapy should be aimed at the underlying disease. However, some patients continue to experience convulsions while in remission and their management poses a major therapeutic problem as all the first-line antiepileptics have been associated with acute attacks.[1] Barbiturates (*phenobarbital, primidone*), hydantoins (*phenytoin, ethotoin*), and *carbamazepine* are considered unsafe, as are *sultiame* and *progabide.* There is limited evidence that the *benzodiazepines, sodium valproate,* and probably *valpromide* are porphyrinogenic but status epilepticus has been treated successfully with intravenous *diazepam.* Seizure prophylaxis may be undertaken as a calculated risk using sodium valproate or *clonazepam* if considered essential. *Magnesium sulfate* is safe. *Clomethiazole* is also probably safe. *Gabapentin* and *vigabatrin* have each been tried in a few patients without ill-effect, although there has been a report of a bullous skin eruption in a patient with porphyria cutanea

tarda given vigabatrin.[2] Other antiepileptics such as the succinimides (*ethosuximide, mesuximide, phensuximide*) and oxazolidinediones (*paramethadione, trimethadione*) are considered to be unsafe.

1. Gorchein A. Drug treatment in acute porphyria. *Br J Clin Pharmacol* 1997; **44:** 427–34.
2. Hommel L, *et al.* Acute bullous skin eruption after treatment with vigabatrine. *Dermatology* 1995; **191:** 181.

4-Amino-3-hydroxybutyric Acid (12360-n)

Buxamin; Gabob.
$C_4H_9NO_3 = 119.1.$
CAS — 352-21-6.

Profile
Aminohydroxybutyric acid has been claimed to be of value in a variety of neurological disorders including as an adjunct in the treatment of epilepsy. It should be distinguished from its isomer 3-amino-4-hydroxybutyric acid (Gobab) which is reported to possess anti-inflammatory and antifungal activity.

Preparations
Proprietary Preparations (details are given in Part 3)
Braz.: Gamibetal; **Ital.:** Gamibetal; **Mex.:** Gamibetal; **Port.:** Gabomade; Gamibetal; **Spain:** Bogil.

Multi-ingredient: Braz.: Gamibetal Complex; **Ital.:** Gamibetal Complex; Gamibetal Plus; Parvisedil; **Port.:** Gabisedil; Gamibetal Compositum; **Spain:** Cefabol; Disfil; Gamalate B6; Pertranquil; Redutona.

Barbexaclone (12418-m)

Barbexaclone (*rINN*).
Compound of (–)-N,α-Dimethylcyclohexaneethylamine with 5-ethyl-5-phenylbarbituric acid .
$C_{12}H_{12}N_2O_3,C_{10}H_{21}N = 387.5.$
CAS — 4388-82-3.
ATC — N03AA04.

Profile
Barbexaclone is a compound of levopropylhexedrine (p.1514) with phenobarbital (p.355). It is used in the treatment of various types of epilepsy (p.338). Usual adult doses are 200 to 400 mg daily given by mouth in divided doses.

Preparations
Proprietary Preparations (details are given in Part 3)
Aust.: Maliasin; **Braz.:** Maliasin; **Ger.:** Maliasin; **Ital.:** Maliasin; **Switz.:** Maliasin.

Beclamide (6604-r)

Beclamide (*BAN, rINN*).
Benzchlorpropamide; Chlorethylphenamide. N-Benzyl-3-chloropropionamide.
$C_{10}H_{12}CINO = 197.7.$
CAS — 501-68-8.
ATC — N03AX30.

Profile
Beclamide has been used as an antiepileptic for the control of tonic-clonic and simple partial seizures (p.338). It has also been used for the management of behaviour disorders (p.650).

Preparations
Proprietary Preparations (details are given in Part 3)
Spain: Posedrine†.

Carbamazepine (6605-f)

Carbamazepine (*BAN, USAN, rINN*).
Carbamazepinum; G-32883. 5H-Dibenz[b,f]azepine-5-carboxamide.
$C_{15}H_{12}N_2O = 236.3.$
CAS — 298-46-4.
ATC — N03AF01.

Pharmacopoeias. In Chin., Eur. (see p.vi), Int., Jpn, Pol., and US.

Pharmacopoeial description
Ph. Eur.: A white or almost white crystalline powder. It exhibits polymorphism. Very slightly soluble in water; sparingly soluble in alcohol and in acetone; freely soluble in dichloromethane. Store in airtight containers.

USP 25: A white or off-white powder. Practically insoluble in water; soluble in alcohol and in acetone. Store in airtight containers.

Incompatibility. Carbamazepine suspension should be mixed with an equal volume of diluent before nasogastric administration as undiluted suspension is adsorbed onto polyvinyl chloride nasogastric tubes.[1]
The FDA have received a report of a patient who passed an orange rubbery mass in his faeces the day after taking a carbamazepine suspension (Tegretol) followed immediately by chlorpromazine solution (Thorazine). Subsequent testing showed that mixing the same carbamazepine suspension with a

thioridazine hydrochloride solution (Mellaril) also resulted in the precipitation of a rubbery orange mass.
1. Clark-Schmidt AL, *et al.* Loss of carbamazepine suspension through nasogastric feeding tubes. *Am J Hosp Pharm* 1990; **47:** 2034–7.

Stability. FDA studies indicate that carbamazepine tablets could lose up to one-third of their effectiveness if stored in humid conditions.[1] This appears to be due to formation of a dihydrate form which leads to hardening of the tablet resulting in poor dissolution and absorption.[2] As the dihydrate has also been detected after storage under ambient conditions some suggest that storage with silica gel sachets may be necessary to avoid physical deterioration of carbamazepine tablets.[2]

1. Anonymous. Moisture hardens carbamazepine tablets, FDA finds. *Am J Hosp Pharm* 1990; **47:** 958.
2. Lowes MMJ. More information on hardening of carbamazepine tablets. *Am J Hosp Pharm* 1991; **48:** 2130–1.
3. Wang JT, *et al.* Effects of humidity and temperature on in vitro dissolution of carbamazepine tablets. *J Pharm Sci* 1993; **82:** 1002–5.

Adverse Effects

Fairly common side-effects of carbamazepine, particularly in the initial stages of therapy, include dizziness, drowsiness, and ataxia. These effects may be minimised by starting therapy with a low dose. Drowsiness and disturbances of cerebellar and oculo-motor function (with ataxia, nystagmus, and diplopia) are also symptoms of excessive plasma concentrations of carbamazepine, and may disappear with continued treatment at reduced dosage.

Gastrointestinal symptoms are reported to be less common, and include dry mouth, abdominal pain, nausea and vomiting, anorexia, and diarrhoea or constipation.

Generalised erythematous rashes may be severe and may necessitate withdrawal of treatment. Photosensitivity reactions, urticaria, exfoliative dermatitis, toxic epidermal necrolysis, erythema multiforme and the Stevens-Johnson syndrome, and systemic lupus erythematosus have also been reported.

Occasional reports of blood disorders include agranulocytosis, aplastic anaemia, eosinophilia, persistent leucopenia, leucocytosis, thrombocytopenia, and purpura. Lymphadenopathy, splenomegaly, pneumonitis, abnormalities of liver and kidney function, and cholestatic jaundice have occurred. Some or all of these symptoms as well as fever and rashes may represent a generalised hypersensitivity reaction to carbamazepine.

Hyponatraemia, and sometimes oedema, have occurred. Other adverse effects reported include paraesthesia, headache, arrhythmias and heart block, heart failure, impotence, male infertility, gynaecomastia, galactorrhoea, and dystonias and dyskinesias with asterixis. Rectal administration has resulted in local irritation.

Overdosage may be manifested by many of the adverse effects listed above, especially those on the CNS, and may result in stupor, coma, convulsions, respiratory depression, and death.

In rare cases, carbamazepine has been reported to exacerbate seizures in patients suffering from mixed-type epilepsy—see Precautions, below.

Congenital malformations have been reported in infants born to women who received carbamazepine during pregnancy.

Effects on the blood. Occasional reports of fatal haematological reactions associated with carbamazepine led the manufacturers to recommend extensive blood monitoring during therapy. However, because of the rarity of blood disorders due to carbamazepine these recommendations were questioned and the manufacturers subsequently modified their guidelines (see Precautions, below).
Case reports and studies of carbamazepine's haematological effects have been reviewed.[1] The incidence of haematological reactions to carbamazepine has been estimated to range between 1:10 800 and 1:38 000 per year while one group reported the rate of bone marrow suppression to be between 1:10 000 and 1:50 000 cases. The incidence of aplastic anaemia has been calculated to be 1:200 000 per year. Another investigator indicated that 2.2 deaths per million exposures were associated with aplastic anaemia and agranulocytosis. However, of 27 reports of aplastic anaemia (16 fatal) associated with carbamazepine many were found to have had co-incidental disease or were receiving multiple-drug therapy. Benign or clinically insignificant leucopenia has occurred, usually during the first 3

months of treatment, in about 12% of children and 7% of adults but in most patients this resolved despite continuation of therapy. Mild transient thrombocytopenia has occurred in about 2% of patients; transient eosinophilia has also occurred.

The reviewers[1] suggested that all patients should have blood and platelet counts before treatment. Patients with low white cell and neutrophil counts were at risk of developing leucopenia and should be monitored every 2 weeks for the first 1 to 3 months. If counts fell further the dose should be reduced or treatment discontinued if necessary. It should be noted that some authorities doubt the practical value of routine monitoring: in particular, aplastic anaemia, agranulocytosis, and thrombocytopenia have a rapid onset and are best monitored by instructing the patient to report warning symptoms (see Precautions, below).

For a discussion of the effects of antiepileptics, including carbamazepine, on serum folate, see under Phenytoin, p.358.

1. Sobotka JL, et al. A review of carbamazepine's hematologic reactions and monitoring recommendations. DICP Ann Pharmacother 1990; 24: 1214–19.

Effects on bone. For the effects of antiepileptics including carbamazepine on bone and on calcium and vitamin D metabolism, see under Phenytoin, p.358.

Effects on the endocrine system. There have been a number of reports of *hyponatraemia* or *water intoxication* in patients receiving carbamazepine.[1-6] One review[7] states that although hyponatraemia occurs in 10 to 15% of patients taking carbamazepine, it is seldom symptomatic or severe enough to cause fluid retention. However, care should be taken to distinguish the confusion, dizziness, nausea and headache of water intoxication from side-effects due to the central and gastrointestinal effects of the drug.[2] The mechanism is uncertain; although some studies suggest an increase in secretion of antidiuretic hormone,[3,4,6] others indicate the reverse,[5,8] and the fact that the hyponatraemic effects of carbamazepine can be partly reversed by demeclocycline[5] is cited as evidence for an effect on the kidney, either directly upon the distal tubule or by increasing sensitivity to the effects of antidiuretic hormone.

Carbamazepine may reduce serum concentrations of *thyroid* hormones through enzyme induction—see under Interactions of Thyroxine [levothyroxine], p.1527.

For mention of the effects of antiepileptics on *sexual function* in male epileptic patients, see under Phenytoin, p.358.

1. Henry DA, et al. Hyponatraemia during carbamazepine treatment. BMJ 1977; 1: 83–4.
2. Stephens WP, et al. Water intoxication due to carbamazepine. BMJ 1977; 1: 754–5.
3. Ashton MG, et al. Water intoxication associated with carbamazepine treatment. BMJ 1977; 1: 1134–5.
4. Smith NJ, et al. Raised plasma arginine vasopressin concentration in carbamazepine-induced water intoxication. BMJ 1977; 2: 804.
5. Ballardie FW, Mucklow JC. Partial reversal of carbamazepine-induced water intolerance by demeclocycline. Br J Clin Pharmacol 1984; 17: 763–5.
6. Sørensen PS, Hammer M. Effects of long-term carbamazepine treatment on water metabolism and plasma vasopressin concentration. Eur J Clin Pharmacol 1984; 26: 719–22.
7. Mucklow J. Selected side-effects 2: carbamazepine and hyponatraemia. Prescribers' J 1991; 31: 61–4.
8. Stephens WP, et al. Plasma arginine vasopressin concentrations and antidiuretic action of carbamazepine. BMJ 1978; 1: 1445–7.

Effects on the eyes. On rare occasions lenticular opacities have been associated with carbamazepine.[1] Retinotoxicity associated with long-term carbamazepine use has been reported[2] in 2 patients. Following discontinuation of the drug visual function and retinal morphological changes improved.

1. Anonymous. Adverse ocular effects of systemic drugs. Med Lett Drugs Ther 1976; 18: 63–4.
2. Nielsen NV, Syversen K. Possible retinotoxic effect of carbamazepine. Acta Ophthalmol (Copenh) 1986; 64: 287–90.

Effects on the heart. A review[1] of reports of cardiac effects associated with carbamazepine revealed that patients could be divided into 2 distinct groups based on their symptoms. One group consisted mainly of young patients with non life-threatening sinus tachycardia following carbamazepine overdosage while the other group was composed of older female patients with potentially life-threatening bradycardia or atrioventricular block associated with therapeutic or modestly raised blood concentrations of carbamazepine. However, there has been a report of fatal syncope, probably due to ventricular asystole, in a 20-year-old patient.[2] Carbamazepine should be avoided in patients who develop conduction abnormalities, or who have conditions such as myotonic dystrophy in which conduction abnormalities are likely.[1]

Elevation of ventricular and atrial stimulation thresholds was reported in a 59-year-old man with a permanent dual-chamber pacemaker, 5 days after starting carbamazepine for mania.[3]

For a report of carbamazepine producing fatal eosinophilic myocarditis, see under Hypersensitivity, below.

1. Kasarkis EJ, et al. Carbamazepine-induced cardiac dysfunction: characterization of two distinct clinical syndromes. Arch Intern Med 1992; 152: 186–91.
2. Stone S, Lange LS. Syncope and sudden unexpected death attributed to carbamazepine in a 20-year-old epileptic. J Neurol Neurosurg Psychiatry 1986; 49: 1460–1.
3. Ambrosi P, et al. Carbamazepine and pacing threshold. Lancet 1993; 342: 365.

The symbol † denotes a preparation no longer actively marketed

Effects on the liver. A report in 1990 commented that of 499 reports of unwanted effects of carbamazepine on the liver about half comprised only abnormal results from liver function tests;[1] however, deaths have occurred from liver failure[1,2] or hepatic necrosis.[3]

Hepatotoxicity may form part of the antiepileptic hypersensitivity syndrome reported with carbamazepine (see below).

1. Hadžić N, et al. Acute liver failure induced by carbamazepine. Arch Dis Child 1990; 65: 315–17.
2. Zucker P, et al. Fatal carbamazepine hepatitis. J Pediatr 1977; 91: 667–8.
3. Smith DW, et al. Fatal hepatic necrosis associated with multiple anticonvulsant therapy. Aust N Z J Med 1988; 18: 575–81.

Effects on mental function. Carbamazepine therapy has been associated in a few patients with the development of acute psychotic and paranoid symptoms[1-3] and with phobias[2] and mood disturbances, including mania[4] and melancholia.[5] One case of acute paranoid psychosis was associated with the addition of carbamazepine to long-term sodium valproate therapy in a patient subsequently diagnosed as having a schizotypal personality.[3] The problems of antiepileptic therapy adversely affecting cognition are discussed on p.340.

1. Berger H. An unusual manifestation of Tegretol® (carbamazepine) toxicity. Ann Intern Med 1971; 74: 449–50.
2. Mathew G. Psychiatric symptoms associated with carbamazepine. BMJ 1988; 296: 1071.
3. McKee RJW, et al. Acute psychosis with carbamazepine and sodium valproate. Lancet 1989; i: 167.
4. Reiss AL, O'Donnell DJ. Carbamazepine-induced mania in two children: case report. J Clin Psychiatry 1984; 45: 272–4.
5. Gardner DL, Cowdry RW. Development of melancholia during carbamazepine treatment in borderline personality disorder. J Clin Psychopharmacol 1986; 6: 236–9.

Effects on the nervous system. ASEPTIC MENINGITIS. Aseptic meningitis has developed in a patient with Sjögren's syndrome given carbamazepine. It abated when the drug was withdrawn and symptoms recurred on rechallenge.[1] Aseptic meningitis has also been associated with carbamazepine in a patient without Sjögren's syndrome.[2]

1. Hilton E, Stroh EM. Aseptic meningitis associated with administration of carbamazepine. J Infect Dis 1989; 159: 363–4.
2. Simon LT, et al. Carbamazepine-induced aseptic meningitis. Ann Intern Med 1990; 112: 627–8.

EXTRAPYRAMIDAL EFFECTS. References to extrapyramidal effects associated with carbamazepine.

1. Crosley CJ, Swender PT. Dystonia associated with carbamazepine administration: experience in brain-damaged children. Pediatrics 1979; 63: 612–15.
2. Jacome D. Carbamazepine-induced dystonia. JAMA 1979; 241: 2263.
3. Joyce RP, Gunderson CH. Carbamazepine-induced orofacial dyskinesia. Neurology 1980; 30: 1333–4.
4. Neglia JP, et al. Tics and vocalizations in children treated with carbamazepine. Pediatrics 1984; 73: 841–4.

Effects on the skin. Rashes occurring with carbamazepine may form part of an antiepileptic hypersensitivity syndrome (see below). In one report,[1] erythema multiforme followed substitution of a generic for a proprietary brand of carbamazepine. Skin lesions resolved when the patient stopped taking the generic formulation and did not recur when the proprietary brand was restarted. A 6-year-old boy developed Stevens-Johnson syndrome 5 weeks after carbamazepine was added to valproic acid, which he had been taking as sole antiepileptic therapy for several weeks.[2] Carbamazepine was discontinued and the patient eventually made a full recovery; administration of valproic acid was continued because it was not thought to be the causative agent (but see under Valproate, p.367).

1. Busch RL. Generic carbamazepine and erythema multiforme: generic-drug nonequivalency. N Engl J Med 1989; 321: 692–3.
2. Keating A, Blahunka P. Carbamazepine-induced Stevens-Johnson syndrome in a child. Ann Pharmacother 1995; 29: 538–9.

Hypersensitivity. An antiepileptic hypersensitivity syndrome, comprising fever, rash, and lymphadenopathy and less commonly hepatosplenomegaly and eosinophilia, has been associated with some antiepileptic drugs including carbamazepine.[1-3] Although a literature search[1] was only able to find 20 published cases to 1986, 22 cases had been reported to the Australian Adverse Drug Reactions Advisory Committee between 1975 and 1990. Some have estimated the incidence at 1 in 1000 to 1 in 10 000 new exposures to aromatic anticonvulsants.[2,3] However the true incidence is uncertain due to variations in presentation and reporting. Most reactions occurred within 30 days of the start of carbamazepine administration,[1] although symptoms may occur anywhere between 1 and 8 weeks after exposure.[2] In previously sensitised individuals the reactions may occur within 1 day of rechallenge.

Carbamazepine antibodies were detected in an 8-year-old child who developed symptoms of serum sickness including fever, skin rash, oedema, and lymphadenopathy during treatment with carbamazepine.[4] Hypersensitivity to carbamazepine with multisystem effects clinically resembling a mononucleosis syndrome was reported in a 15-year-old boy 2 weeks after starting monotherapy with carbamazepine.[5] All symptoms resolved after discontinuation of carbamazepine and treatment with prednisone.

A hypersensitivity reaction producing fatal eosinophilic myocarditis has been reported in a 13-year-old patient; initial symptoms mimicked scarlet fever.[6]

Generalised erythroderma with renal, hepatic, and bone-marrow failure (characterised by hypercellularity and dyserythropoiesis) has been reported[7] in an 81-year-old man 50 days after starting carbamazepine therapy. Symptoms recurred following an inadvertent rechallenge. The presence of underlying lymphoproliferative disease may have potentiated the severe drug-induced reaction.

For references to successful desensitisation in patients sensitive to carbamazepine, see Hypersensitivity Reactions under Treatment of Adverse Effects, below.

1. Anonymous. Anticonvulsants and lymphadenopathy. WHO Drug Inf 1991; 5: 11.
2. Knowles SR, et al. Anticonvulsant hypersensitivity syndrome: incidence, prevention and management. Drug Safety 1999; 21: 489–501.
3. Bessmertny O, et al. Antiepileptic hypersensitivity syndrome in children. Ann Pharmacother 2001; 35: 533–8.
4. Hosoda N, et al. Anticarbamazepine antibody induced by carbamazepine in a patient with severe serum sickness. Arch Dis Child 1991; 66: 722–3.
5. Merino N, et al. Multisystem hypersensitivity reaction to carbamazepine. Ann Pharmacother 1994; 28: 402–3.
6. Salzman MB, et al. Carbamazepine and fatal eosinophilic myocarditis. N Engl J Med 1997; 336: 878–9.
7. Lombardi SM, et al. Severe multisystemic hypersensitivity reaction to carbamazepine including dyserythropoietic anemia. Ann Pharmacother 1999; 33: 571–5.

Systemic lupus erythematosus. A review[1] of 80 cases of systemic lupus erythematosus-like syndromes associated with carbamazepine that had been reported to the manufacturer suggested that the frequency of reports (less than 0.001%) was below that for idiopathic lupus. The symptoms due to carbamazepine usually resolved on discontinuation of treatment.

1. Jain KK. Systemic lupus erythematosus (SLE)-like syndromes associated with carbamazepine therapy. Drug Safety 1991; 6: 350–60.

Treatment of Adverse Effects

In the treatment of carbamazepine overdosage repeated doses of activated charcoal may be given by mouth with the aim not only of preventing absorption but also of aiding elimination. Gastric lavage may be considered if undertaken within 1 hour of ingestion. Supportive and symptomatic therapy alone may then suffice, with particular attention to correcting hypoxia and hypotension; haemoperfusion has been suggested for the management of the more severely poisoned patient (but see below).

Hypersensitivity reactions. If the antiepileptic hypersensitivity syndrome develops immediate withdrawal of carbamazepine is recommended. In most cases this is all that is required and does not seem to precipitate an increase in seizures, compared with gradual withdrawal.[1]

Successful desensitisation to carbamazepine was reported[2] in a 12-year-old boy who was sensitive to carbamazepine, sodium valproate, and phenytoin. Starting with a low dose of carbamazepine 0.1 mg daily the dose was doubled, generally every 2 days, up to 100 mg daily. The dose was then gradually increased over 4 weeks to a maintenance dose of 200 mg twice daily. The same technique was used to desensitise 7 patients all of whom developed dramatic skin rashes when first exposed to carbamazepine.[3] Carbamazepine therapy in full doses was achieved without problem in about 6 weeks. Some[4] consider that desensitisation is not to be recommended in patients with full-blown antiepileptic hypersensitivity syndrome.

1. Pirmohamed M, et al. Hypersensitivity to carbamazepine and lamotrigine: clinical considerations. Br J Clin Pharmacol 2000; 49: 519P–520P.
2. Smith H, Newton R. Adverse reactions to carbamazepine managed by desensitisation. Lancet 1985; i: 753.
3. Eames P. Adverse reactions to carbamazepine managed by desensitisation. Lancet 1989; i: 509–10.
4. Knowles SR, et al. Anticonvulsant hypersensitivity syndrome: incidence, prevention and management. Drug Safety 1999; 21: 489–501.

Overdosage. Carbamazepine poisoning and its management has been reviewed.[1,2] Supportive measures such as management of airways, ventilation and monitoring of cardiovascular function and electrolyte balance are most important. Administration of activated charcoal, via a nasogastric tube is effective and should be continued until the patient is free of symptoms.[1] Although charcoal haemoperfusion is also of value, repeated oral doses of activated charcoal seem to be as effective and less invasive. Gastric lavage may be particularly useful in carbamazepine overdosage as the antimuscarinic effects delay gastric emptying. In patients who are comatose or who have lost the gag reflex gastric lavage may be performed via a large-bore orogastric tube following endotracheal intubation.

A report[3] of the use of plasmapheresis in the treatment of an acute overdose of carbamazepine concluded that plasmapheresis removed a very small percentage of the total body load of carbamazepine and could not be recommended.

Death due to carbamazepine overdosage does occasionally occur and the cause reported in two cases was aspiration of gastric contents;[2] the authors considered this to be a major danger of carbamazepine overdosage.

344 Antiepileptics

For a further review of the features and management of poisoning with some antiepileptics, including carbamazepine, see under Phenytoin, p.358.

1. Durelli L, *et al.* Carbamazepine toxicity and poisoning: incidence, clinical features and management. *Med Toxicol Adverse Drug Exp* 1989; **4:** 95–107.
2. Denning DW, *et al.* Death due to carbamazepine self-poisoning: remedies reviewed. *Hum Toxicol* 1985; **4:** 255–60.
3. Kale PB, *et al.* Evaluation of plasmapheresis in the treatment of an acute overdose of carbamazepine. *Ann Pharmacother* 1993; **27:** 866–70.

Precautions

Carbamazepine should be avoided in patients with atrioventricular conduction abnormalities. It should not be given to patients with a history of bone marrow depression. Carbamazepine should be given with caution to patients with a history of blood disorders or haematological reactions to other drugs, or of cardiac, hepatic, or renal disease. Patients or their carers should be told how to recognise signs of blood, liver, and skin toxicity and they should be advised to seek immediate medical attention if symptoms such as fever, sore throat, rash, mouth ulcers, bruising, or bleeding develop. Carbamazepine should be withdrawn, if necessary under cover of a suitable alternative antiepileptic, if leucopenia which is severe, progressive, or associated with clinical symptoms develops. The manufacturers recommend blood counts and hepatic and renal-function tests before starting carbamazepine therapy and periodically during treatment, but UK authorities consider the evidence of practical value unsatisfactory. Clinical monitoring is of primary importance throughout treatment.

Care is required in identifying patients with mixed seizure disorders that include generalised absence or atypical absence seizures, who may be at risk of an increase in generalised seizures if given carbamazepine. It may also exacerbate absence and myoclonic seizures.

Care is required when withdrawing carbamazepine therapy—see also under Uses and Administration, below.

Since carbamazepine has mild antimuscarinic properties caution should be observed in patients with glaucoma or raised intra-ocular pressure; scattered punctate lens opacities occur rarely with carbamazepine and it has been suggested that patients should be examined periodically for eye changes.

Abuse. Overdosage requiring hospital admission has been reported following abuse of carbamazepine.[1]

1. Crawford PJ, Fisher BM. Recreational overdosage of carbamazepine in Paisley drug abusers. *Scott Med J* 1997; **42:** 44–5.

Breast feeding. For comment on antiepileptic therapy and breast feeding, see under Pregnancy on p.340.

Driving. For comment on antiepileptic drugs and driving, see p.340.

Multiple sclerosis. Exacerbation of symptoms of multiple sclerosis has been reported[1] in 5 patients following initiation of carbamazepine therapy for paroxysmal neurological symptoms and pain. There was a close temporal association between starting carbamazepine therapy and worsening of symptoms, followed by resolution when it was discontinued.

1. Ramsaransing G, *et al.* Worsening of symptoms of multiple sclerosis associated with carbamazepine. *BMJ* 2000; **320:** 1113.

Porphyria. Carbamazepine has been associated with acute attacks of porphyria and is considered unsafe in porphyric patients.

Pregnancy. For comments on the management of epilepsy during pregnancy, see p.340.

There is an increased risk of neural tube defects in infants exposed *in utero* to antiepileptics including carbamazepine and a variety of syndromes such as craniofacial and digital abnormalities and, less commonly, cleft lip and palate have been described. Exposure to carbamazepine has been calculated to carry a 1% risk of spina bifida.[1] A 'carbamazepine syndrome' characterised by facial dysmorphic features and mild mental retardation has been described.[2] There is also a risk of neonatal bleeding.

1. Rosa FW. Spina bifida in infants of women treated with carbamazepine during pregnancy. *N Engl J Med* 1991; **324:** 674–7.
2. Ornoy A, Cohen E. Outcome of children born to epileptic mothers treated with carbamazepine during pregnancy. *Arch Dis Child* 1996; **75:** 517–20.

Interactions

There are complex interactions between antiepileptics and toxicity may be enhanced without a corresponding increase in antiepileptic activity. Such interactions are very variable and unpredictable and plasma monitoring is often advisable with combination therapy.

The metabolism of carbamazepine is reported to be less susceptible to inhibition by other drugs than that of phenytoin but a few drugs are reported to inhibit its metabolism, resulting in raised plasma concentrations and associated toxicity.

Carbamazepine is a hepatic enzyme inducer and induces its own metabolism as well as that of a number of other drugs, including some antibacterials (notably, doxycycline), anticoagulants, and sex hormones (notably, oral contraceptives). Carbamazepine and phenytoin may also mutually enhance one another's metabolism. The metabolism of carbamazepine is similarly enhanced by enzyme inducers such as phenobarbital.

◊ General references.

1. Spina E, *et al.* Clinically significant pharmacokinetic drug interactions with carbamazepine: an update. *Clin Pharmacokinet* 1996; **31:** 198–214.

Alcohol. Alcohol may exacerbate the CNS side-effects of carbamazepine.

Analgesics. *Dextropropoxyphene* has been reported to cause substantial elevation of serum-carbamazepine concentrations[1] and carbamazepine toxicity,[1,2] probably due to inhibition of carbamazepine metabolism.[1]

1. Dam M, Christiansen J. Interaction of propoxyphene with carbamazepine. *Lancet* 1977; **ii:** 509.
2. Yu YL, *et al.* Interaction between carbamazepine and dextropropoxyphene. *Postgrad Med J* 1986; **62:** 231–3.

Anthelmintics. For the effect of carbamazepine on *mebendazole* and *praziquantel*, see p.102 and p.107, respectively.

Antibacterials. The antimycobacterial *isoniazid*[1,2] and macrolides such as *troleandomycin*[3,4] and *erythromycin*[4-7] have been reported to cause substantial elevations of serum concentrations of carbamazepine and symptoms of carbamazepine toxicity[1-4,6,7] when given concomitantly with the antiepileptic. *Clarithromycin* has also been reported to increase serum concentrations of carbamazepine.[8]

Carbamazepine may enhance the metabolism of *doxycycline*.[9]

1. Valsalan VC, Cooper GL. Carbamazepine intoxication caused by interaction with isoniazid. *BMJ* 1982; **285:** 261–2.
2. Wright JM, *et al.* Isoniazid-induced carbamazepine toxicity and vice versa. *N Engl J Med* 1982; **307:** 1325–7.
3. Dravet C, *et al.* Interaction between carbamazepine and triacetyloleandomycin. *Lancet* 1977; **i:** 810–11.
4. Mesdjian E, *et al.* Carbamazepine intoxication due to triacetyloleandomycin administration in epileptic patients. *Epilepsia* 1980; **21:** 489–96.
5. Wong YY, *et al.* Effect of erythromycin on carbamazepine kinetics. *Clin Pharmacol Ther* 1983; **33:** 460–4.
6. Hedrick R, *et al.* Carbamazepine-erythromycin interaction leading to carbamazepine toxicity in four epileptic children. *Ther Drug Monit* 1983; **5:** 405–7.
7. Mitsch RA. Carbamazepine toxicity precipitated by intravenous erythromycin. *Drug Intell Clin Pharm* 1989; **23:** 878–9.
8. Albani F, *et al.* Clarithromycin-carbamazepine interaction: a case report. *Epilepsia* 1993; **34:** 161–2.
9. Neuvonen PJ, *et al.* Effect of antiepileptic drugs on the elimination of various tetracycline derivatives. *Eur J Clin Pharmacol* 1975; **9:** 147–54.

Anticoagulants. For the effect of carbamazepine on warfarin, see p.995.

Antidepressants. As with all antiepileptics, antidepressants may antagonise the antiepileptic activity of carbamazepine by lowering the convulsive threshold.

Antidepressants such as *fluoxetine*,[1] *fluvoxamine*,[2] *nefazodone*[3] (and perhaps *trazodone*[4]), and *viloxazine*[5] increase plasma concentrations of carbamazepine and may induce carbamazepine toxicity. A toxic serotonin syndrome (see p.304) has been reported in a patient who received *fluoxetine* and carbamazepine concomitantly.[6] Severe neurotoxicity reported during concomitant therapy with *lithium* and carbamazepine[7,8] may be due to a synergistic effect as reports indicate that either drug was tolerated when not administered with the other and measured plasma concentrations did not indicate overdosage.[8] However, toxic serum concentrations of lithium have also been reported, due to carbamazepine-induced acute renal failure (see p.294).

Because of the structural similarity to tricyclic antidepressants the manufacturers have suggested that carbamazepine should not be given to patients taking an *MAOI* or within 14 days of stopping such treatment.

Hypericum has been shown to induce several drug metabolising enzymes (see p.290) and consequently it might reduce the blood concentrations of carbamazepine leading to an increased risk of seizure.[9]

For the effect of carbamazepine on antidepressants, see Mianserin (p.298) and Amitriptyline (p.277).

1. Pearson HJ. Interaction of fluoxetine with carbamazepine. *J Clin Psychiatry* 1990; **51:** 126.
2. Fritze J, *et al.* Interaction between carbamazepine and fluvoxamine. *Acta Psychiatr Scand* 1991; **84:** 583–4.
3. Ashton AK, Wolin RE. Nefazodone-induced carbamazepine toxicity. *Am J Psychiatry* 1996; **153:** 733.
4. Sánchez Romero A, *et al.* Interaction between trazodone and carbamazepine. *Ann Pharmacother* 1999; **33:** 1370.
5. Scarpello JHB, Cottrell N. Overuse of monitoring of blood concentrations of antiepileptic drugs. *BMJ* 1987; **294:** 1355.
6. Dursun SM, *et al.* Toxic serotonin syndrome after fluoxetine plus carbamazepine. *Lancet* 1993; **342:** 442–3.
7. Andrus PF. Lithium and carbamazepine. *J Clin Psychiatry* 1984; **45:** 525.
8. Chaudhry RP, Waters BGH. Lithium and carbamazepine interaction: possible neurotoxicity. *J Clin Psychiatry* 1983; **44:** 30–1.
9. Committee on Safety of Medicines/Medicines Control Agency. Reminder: St John's wort (Hypericum perforatum) interactions. *Current Problems* 2000; **26:** 6–7.

Antiepileptics. Interactions of varying degrees of clinical significance have been reported between carbamazepine and other antiepileptics.

Serum concentrations of carbamazepine are reported to be reduced by *phenobarbital*, but without loss of seizure control;[1,2] this reduction is probably due to induction of carbamazepine metabolism.

The interaction with *phenytoin* is somewhat more complex and the consequences vary. There is evidence of a lowering of serum-carbamazepine concentrations, presumably due to induction of metabolism by phenytoin;[1-3] in turn carbamazepine has been reported both to lower and increase serum phenytoin—see p.360. Again, these reports do not indicate a loss of seizure control or toxicity resulting from the interaction, although the possibility presumably exists. Gradually withdrawing phenytoin from 2 patients who had been receiving carbamazepine and phenytoin resulted in a dramatic increase in plasma-carbamazepine concentrations;[4] one patient exhibited neurotoxic symptoms. The authors recommended that plasma-carbamazepine monitoring should be carried out whenever phenytoin is discontinued in patients receiving these two drugs together.

Valproic acid produces an increase in serum concentrations of the active epoxide metabolite of carbamazepine. This is usually attributed to inhibition of its hydrolysis by epoxide hydrolase,[5] although an additional proposed mechanism[6] is inhibition of the glucuronidation of carbamazepine-10,11-trans-diol, the compound that the epoxide is converted to under normal circumstances. Adverse effects may be a problem if unusually high epoxide concentrations arise but, in general, this interaction is of limited clinical significance. However, *valpromide*, the amide derivative of valproic acid is a much more powerful inhibitor of epoxide hydrolase than valproic acid,[7-9] and therefore produces greater increases in epoxide plasma concentrations with clinical signs of toxicity.[8] Switching from sodium valproate to valpromide has resulted in toxicity in patients also receiving carbamazepine.[8] Neither valproic acid nor valpromide have any significant effect on plasma concentrations of the parent drug, carbamazepine. *Valnoctamide*, an isomer of valpromide, appears to be at least as potent as valpromide in inhibiting the elimination of the epoxide metabolite of carbamazepine.[10] Valnoctamide is used as an anxiolytic, although it does appear to possess some antiepileptic activity. For a report of acute psychosis associated with the combination of carbamazepine and sodium valproate, see Effects on Mental Function under Adverse Effects, above. For the effects of carbamazepine on valproate, see p.368.

For the effects of carbamazepine on *ethosuximide*, see p.348.

Of the other antiepileptics *stiripentol*[11] has been reported to inhibit carbamazepine metabolism, while *felbamate* causes a significant fall in plasma-carbamazepine concentrations which may require an increase in the dose of carbamazepine.[12] However, another study[13] has shown a significant increase in plasma-concentrations of the active epoxide metabolite, which may counteract the effect of the decrease in plasma concentrations of the parent compound. Neurotoxicity has been observed following use of carbamazepine with *lamotrigine*.[14] The suggestion that this was due to raised concentrations of carbamazepine epoxide was not confirmed in a controlled study in which the 2 drugs were used together safely and effectively.[15] *Progabide* has been reported to increase plasma concentrations of the epoxide metabolite, probably due to inhibition of microsomal epoxide hydrolase.[16] For the effects of carbamazepine on *oxcarbazepine*, see p.354, and on *topiramate*, see p.365.

For interactions with benzodiazepines, see below.

1. Cereghino JJ, *et al.* The efficacy of carbamazepine combinations in epilepsy. *Clin Pharmacol Ther* 1975; **18:** 733–41.
2. Rane A, *et al.* Kinetics of carbamazepine and its 10,11-epoxide metabolite in children. *Clin Pharmacol Ther* 1976; **19:** 276–83.
3. Christiansen J, Dam M. Influence of phenobarbital and diphenylhydantoin on plasma carbamazepine levels in patients with epilepsy. *Acta Neurol Scand* 1973; **49:** 543–6.
4. Chapron DJ, *et al.* Unmasking the enzyme-inducing effects of phenytoin on serum carbamazepine concentrations during phenytoin withdrawal. *Ann Pharmacother* 1993; **27:** 708–11.
5. Kerr BM, Levy RH. Carbamazepine epoxide. In: Levy RH, *et al.* eds. *Antiepileptic drugs.* 4th ed. New York: Raven Press, 1995: 529–41.
6. Bernus I, *et al.* The mechanism of the carbamazepine-valproate interaction in humans. *Br J Clin Pharmacol* 1997; **44:** 21–7.
7. Levy RH. Inhibition of carbamazepine epoxide elimination by valpromide and valproic acid. *Epilepsia* 1986; **27:** 592.
8. Meijer JWA, *et al.* Possible hazard of valpromide-carbamazepine combination therapy in epilepsy. *Lancet* 1984; **i:** 802.

9. Pisani F, *et al.* Effect of valpromide on the pharmacokinetics of carbamazepine-10,11-epoxide. *Br J Clin Pharmacol* 1988; **25:** 611–13.
10. Pisani F, *et al.* Impairment of carbamazepine-10,11-epoxide elimination by valpromide, a valpromide isomer, in healthy subjects. *Br J Clin Pharmacol* 1992; **34:** 85–7.
11. Levy RH, *et al.* Stiripentol level-dose relationship and interaction with carbamazepine in epileptic patients. *Epilepsia* 1985; **26:** 544–5.
12. Albani F, *et al.* Effect of felbamate on plasma levels of carbamazepine and its metabolites. *Epilepsia* 1991; **32:** 130–2.
13. Wagner ML, *et al.* Effect of felbamate on carbamazepine and its major metabolites. *Clin Pharmacol Ther* 1993; **53:** 536–43.
14. Warner T, *et al.* Lamotrigine-induced carbamazepine toxicity: an interaction with carbamazepine-10,11-epoxide. *Epilepsy Res* 1992; **11:** 147–50.
15. Stolarek I, *et al.* Vigabatrin and lamotrigine in refractory epilepsy. *J Neurol Neurosurg Psychiatry* 1994; **57:** 921–4.
16. Kroetz DL, *et al.* In vivo and in vitro correlation of microsomal epoxide hydrolase inhibition by progabide. *Clin Pharmacol Ther* 1993; **54:** 485–97.

Antifungals. Malaise, myoclonus, and trembling are reported[1] to have developed in a patient receiving carbamazepine following the addition of *miconazole* to therapy. Administration of *ketoconazole* was associated with a significant increase in plasma-carbamazepine concentrations in 8 epileptic patients stabilised on carbamazepine;[2] plasma concentrations of the epoxide metabolite were unchanged.

For the effect of carbamazepine on *itraconazole,* see p.388.

1. Loupi E, *et al.* Interactions médicamenteuses et miconazole. *Therapie* 1982; **37:** 437–41.
2. Spina E, *et al.* Elevation of plasma carbamazepine concentrations by ketoconazole in patients with epilepsy. *Ther Drug Monit* 1997; **19:** 535–8.

Antihistamines. *Terfenadine* and carbamazepine are both highly protein bound and therefore may compete for protein binding sites. An 18-year-old woman receiving carbamazepine as an antiepileptic experienced symptoms of neurotoxicity shortly after starting treatment with terfenadine for rhinitis.[1] The concentration of free carbamazepine in the plasma was higher than normal and returned to normal on discontinuation of terfenadine.

1. Hirschfeld S, Jarosinski P. Drug interaction of terfenadine and carbamazepine. *Ann Intern Med* 1993; **118:** 907–8.

Antimalarials. *Chloroquine* and *mefloquine* may antagonise the antiepileptic activity of carbamazepine by lowering the convulsive threshold.

Antiprotozoals. A patient receiving carbamazepine for bipolar disorder developed dizziness, diplopia, and nausea 4 days after the addition of *metronidazole* for diverticulitis.[1]

1. Patterson BD. Possible interaction between metronidazole and carbamazepine. *Ann Pharmacother* 1994; **28:** 1303–4.

Antipsychotics. As with all antiepileptics, antipsychotics may antagonise the antiepileptic activity of carbamazepine by lowering the convulsive threshold. Increased plasma concentrations of carbamazepine epoxide have been reported to occur during concomitant therapy with carbamazepine and *loxapine,* possibly due to induction of carbamazepine metabolism or inhibition of metabolism of the epoxide.[1] Raised serum concentrations of carbamazepine have also been reported in patients receiving *haloperidol.*[2] For the effect of carbamazepine on antipsychotics, see under Chlorpromazine, p.664.

1. Collins DM, *et al.* Potential interaction between carbamazepine and loxapine: case report and retrospective review. *Ann Pharmacother* 1993; **27:** 1180–3.
2. Iwahashi K, *et al.* The drug-drug interaction effects of haloperidol on plasma carbamazepine levels. *Clin Neuropharmacol* 1995; **18:** 233–6.

Antivirals. *Ritonavir* inhibits several microsomal liver enzymes and therefore may potentially increase plasma concentrations of carbamazepine. The manufacturer of ritonavir advises that such combinations may require patient monitoring or should be avoided. Carbamazepine toxicity has been reported[1] in one patient following a severe interaction when ritonavir was given concomitantly.

For the effect of carbamazepine on HIV-protease inhibitors, see p.626.

1. Mateu-de Antonio J, Grau S. Ritonavir-induced carbamazepine toxicity. *Ann Pharmacother* 2001; **35:** 125–6.

Anxiolytics. For a discussion of the potential interaction between carbamazepine and the anxiolytic *valnoctamide,* an isomer of the antiepileptic valpromide, see under Antiepileptics, above.

See also under Benzodiazepines, below.

Benzodiazepines. The metabolism of benzodiazepines may be enhanced in patients who have received long-term therapy with carbamazepine due to induction of hepatic drug-metabolising enzymes; the benzodiazepine plasma concentrations are reduced, its half-life is shorter, and clearance is increased.[1,2] Some benzodiazepines may also affect carbamazepine. One group of workers reported that after addition of *clobazam* to carbamazepine therapy a dose reduction for the latter was required due to increased blood concentrations.[3] In a later study[4] it appeared that clobazam could produce a moderate increase in the metabolism of carbamazepine. The plasma ratio of metabolites of carbamazepine, including carbamazepine-10,11-epoxide, to parent compound was increased in patients taking clobazam and carbamazepine.

1. Dhillon S, Richens A. Pharmacokinetics of diazepam in epileptic patients and normal volunteers following intravenous administration. *Br J Clin Pharmacol* 1981; **12:** 841–4.

2. Lai AA, *et al.* Time-course of interaction between carbamazepine and clonazepam in normal man. *Clin Pharmacol Ther* 1978; **24:** 316–23.
3. Franceschi M, *et al.* Clobazam in drug-resistant and alcoholic withdrawal seizures. *Clin Trials J* 1983; **20:** 119–25.
4. Muñoz JJ, *et al.* The effect of clobazam on steady state plasma concentrations of carbamazepine and its metabolites. *Br J Clin Pharmacol* 1990; **29:** 763–5.

Calcium-channel blockers. Six patients with steady-state carbamazepine concentrations experienced symptoms of neurotoxicity consistent with carbamazepine intoxication within 36 to 96 hours of the administration of the first dose of *verapamil.*[1] In 5 patients, in whom plasma concentrations were measured, there was a mean increase of 46% in total and 33% in free carbamazepine; no effect on the plasma protein binding of carbamazepine was observed. The results suggested that verapamil inhibits the metabolism of carbamazepine to an extent likely to have important clinical repercussions. There has also been a report[2] of a patient in whom *diltiazem,* but not *nifedipine,* precipitated carbamazepine neurotoxicity.

For the effect of carbamazepine on dihydropyridine calcium-channel blockers, see under Nifedipine, p.942.

1. Macphee GJA, *et al.* Verapamil potentiates carbamazepine neurotoxicity: a clinically important inhibitory interaction. *Lancet* 1986; **i:** 700–703.
2. Brodie MJ, Macphee GJA. Carbamazepine neurotoxicity precipitated by diltiazem. *BMJ* 1986; **292:** 1170–1.

Ciclosporin. For the effect of carbamazepine on ciclosporin, see p.521.

Corticosteroids. For the effect of carbamazepine on corticosteroids, see p.1043.

Danazol. Co-administration of *danazol* with carbamazepine has been reported to increase the half-life and decrease clearance of carbamazepine,[1] resulting in increases in plasma-carbamazepine concentrations of up to 100%[1,2] and resultant toxicity in a number of patients.[2]

1. Krämer G, *et al.* Carbamazepine-danazol drug interaction: its mechanism examined by a stable isotope technique. *Ther Drug Monit* 1986; **8:** 387–92.
2. Zielinski JJ, *et al.* Clinically significant danazol-carbamazepine interaction. *Ther Drug Monit* 1987; **9:** 24–7.

Dermatological drugs. In one patient stabilised on carbamazepine therapy addition of *isotretinoin* appeared to reduce plasma concentrations of carbamazepine and its active epoxide metabolite.[1] However, no adverse events were noted during a 6-week period of treatment with isotretinoin.

1. Marsden JR. Effect of isotretinoin on carbamazepine pharmacokinetics. *Br J Dermatol* 1988; **119:** 403–4.

Diuretics. There has been a report of symptomatic hyponatraemia associated with concomitant use of carbamazepine and a diuretic (*hydrochlorothiazide* or *frusemide [furosemide]*—see under Interactions in Frusemide, p.894). Carbamazepine serum concentrations are increased by concomitant administration of *acetazolamide.*[1]

1. McBride MC. Serum carbamazepine levels are increased by acetazolamide. *Ann Neurol* 1984; **16:** 393.

Gastrointestinal drugs. *Cimetidine* is reported to produce a transient increase in plasma-carbamazepine concentrations, followed by a return to pre-cimetidine values within about a week;[1] some increase in side-effects was seen. *Ranitidine* does not appear to affect plasma-carbamazepine concentrations.[2] Neurotoxicity has been observed in a patient receiving carbamazepine and *metoclopramide.*[3]

1. Dalton MJ, *et al.* Cimetidine and carbamazepine: a complex drug interaction. *Epilepsia* 1986; **27:** 553–8.
2. Dalton MJ, *et al.* Ranitidine does not alter single-dose carbamazepine pharmacokinetics in healthy adults. *Drug Intell Clin Pharm* 1985; **19:** 941–4.
3. Sandyk R. Carbamazepine and metoclopramide interaction: possible neurotoxicity. *BMJ* 1984; **288:** 830.

Grapefruit juice. The bioavailability and plasma concentrations of carbamazepine have been reported[1] to be increased by grapefruit juice.

1. Garg SK, *et al.* Effect of grapefruit juice on carbamazepine bioavailability in patients with epilepsy. *Clin Pharmacol Ther* 1998; **64:** 286–8.

Neuromuscular blockers. For the effect of carbamazepine on *suxamethonium,* see p.1342 and on *competitive neuromuscular blockers,* see under Atracurium, p.1334.

Sex hormones. For the effect of carbamazepine on sex hormones in oral contraceptives, see p.1459 and for the possible effect on tibolone, see p.1495.

Theophylline. A decrease in serum-carbamazepine concentrations of about 50% was reported[1] in an epileptic patient given theophylline. The patient experienced seizures and the proposed mechanism was that theophylline had increased the metabolism of carbamazepine.

For the effect of carbamazepine on theophylline, see p.780.

1. Mitchell EA, *et al.* Interaction between carbamazepine and theophylline. *N Z Med J* 1986; **99:** 69–70.

Thyroxine [levothyroxine]. For the effect of carbamazepine on thyroxine [levothyroxine], see p.1527.

Vitamins. The plasma concentration of carbamazepine was increased in 2 patients given *nicotinamide.*[1] For the effect of antiepileptics, including carbamazepine, on *vitamin D* concen-

trations, see Effects on Bone under the Adverse Effects of Phenytoin, p.358.

1. Bourgeois BFD, *et al.* Interactions between primidone, carbamazepine, and nicotinamide. *Neurology* 1982; **32:** 1122–6.

Pharmacokinetics

Carbamazepine is slowly and irregularly absorbed from the gastrointestinal tract. It is extensively metabolised in the liver, notably by the cytochrome P450 isoenzymes CYP3A4 and CYP2C8. One of its primary metabolites, carbamazepine-10,11-epoxide, is also active. Carbamazepine is excreted in the urine almost entirely in the form of its metabolites; some is also excreted in faeces. Elimination of carbamazepine is reported to be more rapid in children and accumulation of the active metabolite may often be higher than in adults.

Carbamazepine is widely distributed throughout the body and is extensively bound (about 75%) to plasma proteins. It induces its own metabolism so that the plasma half-life may be considerably reduced after repeated administration. Estimation of the mean plasma half-life of carbamazepine on repeated administration is about 10 to 20 hours; it appears to be considerably shorter in children than in adults. Moreover, the metabolism of carbamazepine is readily induced by drugs which induce hepatic microsomal enzymes (see under Interactions, above).

Monitoring of plasma concentrations may be performed as an aid in assessing control and the therapeutic range of total plasma-carbamazepine is usually quoted as being about 4 to 12 µg per mL (16 to 50 µmol per litre), although this is subject to considerable variation. It has been suggested by some, but not all investigators, that measurement of free carbamazepine concentrations in plasma may prove more reliable, and measurement of concentrations in saliva or tears, which contain only free carbamazepine, has also been performed.

Carbamazepine crosses the placental barrier and is distributed into breast milk.

The pharmacokinetics of carbamazepine are affected by the concomitant administration of other antiepileptics (see under Interactions, above).

◊ References.
1. Schmidt D, Haenel F. Therapeutic plasma levels of phenytoin, phenobarbital, and carbamazepine: individual variation in relation to seizure frequency and type. *Neurology* 1984; **34:** 1252–5.
2. Bertilsson L, Tomson T. Clinical pharmacokinetics and pharmacological effects of carbamazepine and carbamazepine-10,11-epoxide: an update. *Clin Pharmacokinet* 1986; **11:** 177–98.
3. Gilman JT. Carbamazepine dosing for pediatric seizure disorders: the highs and lows. *DICP Ann Pharmacother* 1991; **25:** 1109–12.
4. Kodama Y, *et al.* In vivo binding characteristics of carbamazepine and carbamazepine-10,11-epoxide to serum proteins in paediatric patients with epilepsy. *Eur J Clin Pharmacol* 1993; **44:** 291–3.
5. Bernus I, *et al.* Early stage autoinduction of carbamazepine metabolism in humans. *Eur J Clin Pharmacol* 1994; **47:** 355–60.
6. Caraco Y, *et al.* Carbamazepine pharmacokinetics in obese and lean subjects. *Ann Pharmacother* 1995; **29:** 843–7.
7. Mahmood I, Chamberlin N. A limited sampling method for the estimation of AUC and C_{max} of carbamazepine and carbamazepine epoxide following a single and multiple dose of a sustained-release product. *Br J Clin Pharmacol* 1998; **45:** 241–6.
8. Cohen H, *et al.* Feasibility and pharmacokinetics of carbamazepine oral loading doses. *Am J Health-Syst Pharm* 1998; **55:** 1134–40.

Uses and Administration

Carbamazepine is a dibenzazepine derivative with antiepileptic and psychotropic properties. It is used to control secondarily generalised tonic-clonic seizures and partial seizures, and in some primary generalised seizures. Carbamazepine is also used in the treatment of trigeminal neuralgia and has been tried with variable success in glossopharyngeal neuralgia and other severe pain syndromes associated with neurological disorders such as tabes dorsalis and multiple sclerosis. Another use of carbamazepine is in the prophylaxis of bipolar disorder unresponsive to lithium.

In the treatment of **epilepsy,** the dose of carbamazepine should be adjusted to the needs of the individual patient to achieve adequate control of seizures; this usually requires total plasma-carbamazepine concentrations of about 4 to 12 µg per mL (16 to 50 µmol per litre). A low initial dose of carbamazepine is recommended to minimise side-effects. The suggested initial oral dose is 100 to 200 mg once or twice daily gradually increased by increments of 100 to 200 mg every 2 weeks to a usual maintenance dose of 0.8 to 1.2 g daily in divided doses; up to 2 g daily may occasionally be necessary. The usual oral dosage in children based on body-weight is 10 to 20 mg per kg daily in divided doses. Alternatively the dose may be expressed in terms of the age of the child and suggested daily doses are: up to 1 year of age, 100 to 200 mg; 1 to 5 years, 200 to 400 mg; 5 to 10 years, 400 to 600 mg; 10 to 15 years, 0.6 to 1 g.

Oral daily doses are divided and carbamazepine is usually given 2 to 4 times daily. A twice-daily regimen may be associated with improved compliance but may produce widely fluctuating plasma-carbamazepine concentrations leading to intermittent side-effects. However, twice-daily administration may be suitable for patients receiving carbamazepine as monotherapy, and without peak-related side-effects. Also modified-release formulations can minimise fluctuations in plasma concentration and may allow effective twice-daily administration. Different preparations vary in bioavailability and it may be prudent to avoid changing the formulation.

The time and manner of taking carbamazepine should be standardised for the patient since variations might affect absorption with consequent fluctuations in the plasma concentrations.

Carbamazepine may be given by the rectal route in doses up to a maximum of 250 mg every 6 hours to patients for whom oral treatment is temporarily not possible. The dosage should be increased by about 25% when changing from an oral formulation to suppositories, and it is recommended that the rectal route should not be used for longer than 7 days.

As with other antiepileptics, withdrawal of carbamazepine therapy or transition to or from another type of antiepileptic therapy should be made gradually to avoid precipitating an increase in the frequency of seizures. For a discussion on whether or not to withdraw antiepileptic therapy in seizure-free patients, see p.338.

In the treatment of **trigeminal neuralgia** the initial dose of carbamazepine is 100 mg once or twice daily by mouth increased gradually as necessary; the usual maintenance dose is 400 to 800 mg daily in 2 to 4 divided doses but up to 1.6 g daily may be required. When pain relief has been obtained attempts should be made to reduce and ultimately discontinue the therapy, until another attack occurs.

For the prophylaxis of **bipolar disorder**, carbamazepine is given in an initial oral dose of 400 mg daily in divided doses, increased gradually as necessary up to a maximum of 1.6 g daily; the usual maintenance dose range is 400 to 600 mg daily.

Administration. A modified-release formulation of carbamazepine can produce a substantial reduction in intra-dose fluctuations in carbamazepine concentrations,[1] and tolerability and seizure control in patients with epilepsy may be improved.[2,3] Such formulations should be considered in patients receiving high doses who suffer intermittent adverse effects, and might also permit a reduction to twice- or even, in some patients, once-daily administration.[2,4] However, bioavailability appears to be slightly less than conventional preparations and dosage adjustments may be required when changing between formulations.[1]

1. McKee PJW, et al. Monotherapy with conventional and controlled-release carbamazepine: a double-blind, double-dummy comparison in epileptic patients. Br J Clin Pharmacol 1991; 32: 99–104.
2. Anonymous. Carbamazepine update. Lancet 1989; ii: 595–7.
3. Ryan SW, et al. Slow release carbamazepine in treatment of poorly controlled seizures. Arch Dis Child 1990; 65: 930–5.
4. McKee PJW, et al. Double dummy comparison between once and twice daily dosing with modified-release carbamazepine in epileptic patients. Br J Clin Pharmacol 1993; 36: 257–61.

Bipolar disorder. Carbamazepine is an alternative to lithium in patients with bipolar disorder (p.271) and seems to be particularly effective in those who have rapid cycling disease with 4 or more affective episodes a year. Although clearly effective in the majority of patients in the short-term,[1,2] at least one study showed a much lower response rate in the long-term[2] and claims that carbamazepine is as effective as lithium in this condition have been criticised.[3] In another study lithium appeared to be more effective than carbamazepine in the acute phase of

mania but there was no significant difference in the follow-up phase;[4] men tended to respond better to carbamazepine than women. Mania appears to respond better than depression.[1] Carbamazepine has been tried in combination with lithium,[1,5] particularly in patients unresponsive to one drug alone. This combination may produce a more rapid response than lithium alone[6] but is associated with a potential risk of serious neurotoxicity—see Antidepressants under Interactions, above.

1. Ballenger JC. The clinical use of carbamazepine in affective disorders. J Clin Psychiatry 1988; 49 (suppl): 13–19.
2. Frankenburg FR, et al. Long-term response to carbamazepine: a retrospective study. J Clin Psychopharmacol 1988; 8: 130–2.
3. Murphy DJ, et al. Carbamazepine in bipolar affective disorder. Lancet 1989; ii: 1151–2.
4. Lusznat RM, et al. Carbamazepine vs lithium in the treatment and prophylaxis of mania. Br J Psychiatry 1988; 153: 198–204.
5. Kramlinger KG, Post RM. Adding lithium carbonate to carbamazepine: antimanic efficacy in treatment-resistant mania. Acta Psychiatr Scand 1989; 79: 378–85.
6. Di Costanzo E, Schifano F. Lithium alone or in combination with carbamazepine for the treatment of rapid-cycling bipolar affective disorder. Acta Psychiatr Scand 1991; 83: 456–9.

Depression. Carbamazepine has been tried[1,2] for the augmentation of antidepressant therapy in the treatment of resistant depression (p.271). However, such combined therapy may lead to interactions—see also Antidepressants under Interactions, above.

1. De la Fuente JM, Mendlewicz J. Carbamazepine addition in tricyclic antidepressant-resistant unipolar depression. Biol Psychiatry 1992; 32: 369–74.
2. Otani K, et al. Carbamazepine augmentation therapy in three patients with trazodone-resistant depression. Int Clin Psychopharmacol 1996; 11: 55–7.

Diabetes insipidus. Cranial diabetes insipidus is usually treated by replacement therapy with antidiuretic hormone (ADH) in the form of desmopressin (see p.1273). Carbamazepine is one of a variety of other drugs that have been tried to promote ADH secretion, although some consider that it is usually ineffective and has unwanted effects.[1,2] Doses of 200 to 400 mg daily by mouth have been given. See also Effects on the Endocrine System under Adverse Effects, above.

1. Seckl J, Dunger D. Postoperative diabetes insipidus. BMJ 1989; 298: 2–3.
2. Singer I, et al. The management of diabetes insipidus in adults. Arch Intern Med 1997; 157: 1293–1301.

Epilepsy. Carbamazepine is one of the drugs of choice for partial seizures with or without secondary generalisation (see p.338). It has been used for some primary generalised seizures, although valproate is the drug of choice, but may exacerbate absence and myoclonic seizures.

Hemifacial spasm. Carbamazepine has been reported to have been of help in the treatment of hemifacial spasm (p.1326).

Hiccup. A protocol for the management of intractable hiccups can be found under Chlorpromazine, p.667. Carbamazepine may be of value for the treatment of neurogenic hiccups such as those that occur in multiple sclerosis.[1] Carbamazepine has also been reported to have been of benefit in 3 patients with diaphragmatic flutter,[2] a rare disorder associated with involuntary contractions of the diaphragm.

1. McFarling DA, Susac JO. Hoquet diabolique: intractable hiccups as a manifestation of multiple sclerosis. Neurology 1979; 29: 797–801.
2. Vantrappen G, et al. High-frequency diaphragmatic flutter: symptoms and treatment by carbamazepine. Lancet 1992; 339: 265–7.

Hyperactivity. When drugs are indicated for attention deficit hyperactivity disorder (p.1505) initial treatment is usually with a central stimulant but meta-analysis of a small number of trials has provided preliminary evidence that carbamazepine may be an effective alternative.[1]

1. Silva RR, et al. Carbamazepine use in children and adolescents with features of attention-deficit hyperactivity disorder: a meta-analysis. J Am Acad Child Adolesc Psychiatry 1996; 35: 352–8.

Lesch-Nyhan syndrome. The severe self-mutilation that occurs in patients with Lesch-Nyhan syndrome (p.667) has been reported to improve in those given antiepileptics such as carbamazepine.[1]

1. Roach ES, et al. Carbamazepine trial for Lesch-Nyhan self-mutilation. J Child Neurol 1996; 11: 476–8.

Movement disorders. Carbamazepine is one of many drugs that have been tried in the symptomatic treatment of chorea (p.650); there have been anecdotal reports of benefit in both non-hereditary[1] and hereditary choreas.[2] Carbamazepine is also among the drugs that have been tried in the treatment of dystonias that have not responded to levodopa or antimuscarinics (p.1173). Although some patients may benefit from carbamazepine, it is not generally recommended because of a relatively low success rate and the possibility of adverse effects.[3] Carbamazepine has also been used in resistant cases of tardive dyskinesia (see under Extrapyramidal Disorders, p.662).

1. Roig M, et al. Carbamazepine: an alternative drug for the treatment of nonhereditary chorea. Pediatrics 1988; 82: 492–5.
2. Roulet E, Deonna T. Successful treatment of hereditary dominant chorea with carbamazepine. Pediatrics 1989; 83: 1077.
3. Anonymous. Dystonia: underdiagnosed and undertreated? Drug Ther Bull 1988; 26: 33–6.

Neonatal seizures. Carbamazepine has been tried in the management of neonatal seizures (p.342).

Neuropathic pain. As well as being used to ease the pain of trigeminal neuralgia (see below) carbamazepine may be of use in other neuropathic pain associated with diabetic neuropathy (p.5). Chronic burning pain in the feet of a former prisoner of war, a result of neuropathic beriberi, was virtually abolished by treatment with carbamazepine 200 mg three times daily.[1]

1. Skelton WP. Neuropathic beriberi and carbamazepine. Ann Intern Med 1988; 109: 598–9.

Psychiatric disorders. Carbamazepine has psychotropic properties and has been tried in the management of several psychiatric disorders, particularly in patients with bipolar disorder (see above). Carbamazepine has also been used with mixed results in various disorders for the control of symptoms such as agitation, aggression, and rage[1-4] (see under Disturbed Behaviour, p.650). It may produce modest benefit when used as an adjunct to antipsychotics in the management of refractory schizophrenia (p.651) but any improvement appears to be related to its mood stabilising effect.[5] However, carbamazepine also has the potential to reduce serum concentrations of antipsychotics, resulting in clinical deterioration (see under Interactions for Chlorpromazine, p.664). Carbamazepine has also been tried[6] in post-traumatic stress disorder (p.650).

1. Mattes JA. Comparative effectiveness of carbamazepine and propranolol for rage outbursts. J Neuropsychiatr Clin Neurosci 1990; 2: 159–64.
2. Gleason RP, Schneider LS. Carbamazepine treatment of agitation in Alzheimer's outpatients refractory to neuroleptics. J Clin Psychiatry 1990; 51: 115–18.
3. Tariot PN, et al. Carbamazepine treatment of agitation in nursing home patients with dementia: a preliminary study. J Am Geriatr Soc 1994; 42: 1160–6.
4. Cueva JE, et al. Carbamazepine in aggressive children with conduct disorder: a double-blind and placebo-controlled study. J Am Acad Child Adolesc Psychiatry 1996; 35: 480–90.
5. Okuma T. Use of antiepileptic drugs in schizophrenia: a review of efficacy and tolerability. CNS Drugs 1994; 1: 269–84.
6. Wolf ME, et al. Posttraumatic stress disorder in Vietnam veterans: clinical and EEG findings; possible therapeutic effects of carbamazepine. Biol Psychiatry 1988; 23: 642–4.

Restless legs syndrome. The aetiology of restless legs syndrome (see Parasomnias, p.653) is obscure and treatment has been largely empirical. In a double-blind study involving 174 patients carbamazepine appeared to be more effective than placebo.[1]

1. Telstad W, et al. Treatment of the restless legs syndrome with carbamazepine: a double blind study. BMJ 1984; 288: 444–6.

Tinnitus. Treatment of tinnitus (p.1316) is difficult, and many drugs have been tried. Although carbamazepine has been reported to be effective in some patients, it is rarely used because of its adverse effects.

Trigeminal neuralgia. Carbamazepine is the drug of choice in the treatment of the acute stages of trigeminal neuralgia (p.8). Satisfactory pain relief may be achieved in 70% or more of patients, although increasingly larger doses may be required and side-effects can be troublesome.

Withdrawal syndromes. Carbamazepine has been tried in the prophylaxis and treatment of various withdrawal syndromes. Reduction in cocaine use associated with carbamazepine treatment was demonstrated in one short-term controlled study,[1] although a review[2] of data from later studies concluded that there is no current evidence to support the use of carbamazepine in the treatment of cocaine dependence (p.1310). It has been reported[3,4] to be of benefit in some patients during benzodiazepine withdrawal but such adjunct therapy is not usually indicated (see p.675). Carbamazepine has been shown[5,6] to be effective in the treatment of symptoms of the alcohol withdrawal syndrome (p.1131) but as there are limited data on its efficacy in preventing associated delirium tremens and seizures it is usually recommended that it should only be used as an adjunct to benzodiazepine therapy. Carbamazepine is also being studied[7] as an aid in the treatment of alcohol dependence.

1. Halikas JA, et al. Cocaine reduction in unmotivated crack users using carbamazepine versus placebo in a short-term, double-blind crossover design. Clin Pharmacol Ther 1991; 50: 81–95.
2. Lima AR, et al. Carbamazepine for cocaine dependence (updated 25 August 2000). Available in The Cochrane Library; Issue 3. Oxford: Update Software; 2001.
3. Schweizer E, et al. Carbamazepine treatment in patients discontinuing long-term benzodiazepine therapy: effects on withdrawal severity and outcome. Arch Gen Psychiatry 1991; 48: 448–52.
4. Klein E, et al. Alprazolam withdrawal in patients with panic disorder and generalized anxiety disorder: vulnerability and effect of carbamazepine. Am J Psychiatry 1994; 151: 1760–6.
5. Malcolm R, et al. Double-blind controlled trial comparing carbamazepine to oxazepam treatment of alcohol withdrawal. Am J Psychiatry 1989; 146: 617–21.
6. Stuppaeck CH, et al. Carbamazepine versus oxazepam in the treatment of alcohol withdrawal: a double-blind study. Alcohol Alcohol 1992; 27: 153–8.
7. Mueller TI, et al. A double-blind, placebo-controlled pilot study of carbamazepine for the treatment of alcohol dependence. Alcohol Clin Exp Res 1997; 21: 86–92.

Preparations

BP 2001: Carbamazepine Tablets;
USP 25: Carbamazepine Extended-Release Tablets; Carbamazepine Oral Suspension; Carbamazepine Tablets.

Proprietary Preparations (details are given in Part 3)
Aust.: Neurotop; Sirtal†; Tegretol; Austral.: Carbium; Tegretol; Teril; Belg.: Tegretol; Braz.: Tegretard; Tegretol; Canad.: Novo-Carbamaz; Tegretol; Denm.: Nordotol; Tardotol†; Tegretol; Tri-

monil; *Fin.:* Neurotol; Tegretol; Trimonil; *Fr.:* Tegretol; *Ger.:* Carba; Carbabeta; Carbaflux; Carbagamma; Carbium; espa-lepsin; Finlepsin; Fokalepsin; Sirtal; Tegretal; Timonil; *Hong Kong:* Tegretol; Teril; Timonil; *Irl.:* Gericarb; Tegretol; Temporol; *Israel:* Carbi; Tegretol; Teril; Timonil; *Ital.:* Tegretol; *Mex.:* Adepril; Carbalan; Carbazep; Carbazina; Carpin; Clostedal; Kezepin; Neugeron; Neurolep; Tegretol; Trantil; Volutol; Zepiken; *Neth.:* Tegretol; *Norw.:* Tegretol; Trimonil; *NZ:* Tegretol; Teril; *Port.:* Tegretol; *S.Afr.:* Carpaz; Degranol; Prozine†; Tegretol; Temporol†; *Singapore:* Neurotop; Tegretol; *Spain:* Tegretol; *Swed.:* Hermolepsin; Tegretol; Trimonil; *Switz.:* Tegretol; Timonil; *Thai.:* Antafit; Carbazene; Carmapine; Carpine; Carzepine; Mapezine; Panitol; Taver; Tegretol; *UAE:* Fitzecalm; *UK:* Carbagen; Epimaz; Tegretol; Teril; Timonil; *USA:* Atretol; Carbatrol; Epitol; Tegretol.

Clonazepam (6606-d)

Clonazepam *(BAN, USAN, rINN)*.

Clonazepamum; Ro-5-4023. 5-(2-Chlorophenyl)-1,3-dihydro-7-nitro-1,4-benzodiazepin-2-one.

$C_{15}H_{10}ClN_3O_3 = 315.7$.

CAS — 1622-61-3.

ATC — N03AE01.

Pharmacopoeias. In Eur. (see p.vi), Jpn, Pol., and US.

Pharmacopoeial description

Ph. Eur.: A slightly yellowish, crystalline powder. Practically insoluble in water; slightly soluble in alcohol and in methyl alcohol; very slightly soluble in ether. Protect from light.

USP 25: A light yellow powder having a faint odour. Insoluble in water; slightly soluble in alcohol and in ether; sparingly soluble in acetone and in chloroform. Store in airtight containers. Protect from light.

Dependence and Withdrawal

As for Diazepam, p.675.

Withdrawal. A study[1] of the withdrawal of clonazepam therapy in 40 epileptic children found that 19 exhibited withdrawal symptoms of increased seizure frequency, either alone or with other symptoms but that this effect was transient. Withdrawal seizures and status may become an obstacle to the removal of useless or even deleterious therapy with clonazepam because the transient nature of these effects is not always recognised. Clonazepam should not be prescribed for more than 3 to 6 months and should be discontinued if clear and lasting therapeutic benefit cannot be demonstrated.

See also under Uses and Administration, below.

1. Specht U, *et al.* Discontinuation of clonazepam after long-term treatment. *Epilepsia* 1989; **30:** 458–63.

Adverse Effects, Treatment, and Precautions

As for Diazepam, p.675.

The principal adverse effect of clonazepam is drowsiness, which occurs in about 50% of all patients on starting therapy. Salivary or bronchial hypersecretion may cause respiratory problems in children.

Care is required when withdrawing clonazepam therapy—see above.

Breast feeding. Benzodiazepines, such as clonazepam, given to the mother may cause neonatal sedation and breast feeding should be avoided. For comments on antiepileptic therapy and breast feeding, see under Pregnancy on p.340.

Driving. For a comment on antiepileptic drugs and driving, see p.340.

Effects on the endocrine system. Precocious development of secondary sexual characteristics occurred in a 15-month-old girl 2 months after starting treatment with clonazepam 500 μg twice daily for convulsions.[1] Symptoms regressed upon withdrawal of clonazepam.

1. Choonara IA, *et al.* Clonazepam and sexual precocity. *N Engl J Med* 1985; **312:** 185.

Effects of sexual function. Sexual dysfunction was reported briefly[1] in male patients receiving clonazepam for the treatment of post-traumatic stress disorder; symptoms resolved when therapy was changed to diazepam.

1. Fossey MD, Hamner MB. Clonazepam induced sexual dysfunction in male veterans with PTSD. *Biol Psychiatry* 1994; **35:** 656.

Extrapyramidal disorders. For reference to extrapyramidal disorders associated with the administration of benzodiazepines including clonazepam, see under Effects on the Nervous System in Diazepam, p.675. However, clonazepam is also used in the treatment of some extrapyramidal disorders as discussed under Uses and Administration, below.

Porphyria. Clonazepam is considered to be unsafe in patients with porphyria although there is conflicting evidence of porphyrinogenicity.

For comments on the use of benzodiazepines in porphyria, see p.342.

Pregnancy. For comments on the management of epilepsy during pregnancy, see p.340.

The symbol † denotes a preparation no longer actively marketed

Interactions

Concomitant administration of hepatic enzyme inducers, such as carbamazepine, phenobarbital, or phenytoin, may accelerate the metabolism of clonazepam. Concomitant intake of alcohol may affect the patient's response to clonazepam. Clonazepam may be expected to have the sedative interactions associated with benzodiazepines in general (see under Interactions of Diazepam, p.677).

Antiarrhythmics. For reference to an interaction between clonazepam and amiodarone, see under Diazepam, p.677.

Antiepileptics. Serum-clonazepam concentrations fell markedly in 4 of 8 children who had *lamotrigine* added to their therapy.[1] For reference to possible interactions between clonazepam and other antiepileptics, see under Diazepam, p.678 and Benzodiazepines under Interactions of Phenytoin, p.361.

1. Eriksson A-S, *et al.* Pharmacokinetic interactions between lamotrigine and other antiepileptic drugs in children with intractable epilepsy. *Epilepsia* 1996; **37:** 769–73.

Pharmacokinetics

Clonazepam is well absorbed following oral administration and peak plasma concentrations have been reported to occur within 4 hours. It is extensively metabolised in the liver, its principal metabolite being 7-aminoclonazepam, which probably has little antiepileptic activity; minor metabolites are the 7-acetamido- and 3-hydroxy- derivatives. It is excreted mainly in the urine almost entirely as its metabolites in free or conjugated form. It is about 86% bound to plasma protein and estimations of its plasma half-life range from about 20 to 40 hours, and occasionally more.

A therapeutic range of plasma concentrations has not been established.

Clonazepam crosses the placental barrier and is distributed into breast milk.

Bioavailability. It has been suggested, on the basis of anecdotal evidence,[1] that there may be differences in bioavailability, and hence in clinical effect, between formulations of clonazepam.

1. Rapaport MH. Clinical differences between the generic and non-generic forms of clonazepam. *J Clin Psychopharmacol* 1997; **17:** 424.

Uses and Administration

Clonazepam is a benzodiazepine derivative similar to diazepam (p.680), with marked antiepileptic properties.

It may be used in the treatment of all types of epilepsy and seizures (p.338) but its usefulness is sometimes limited by the development of tolerance and by sedation, and other antiepileptics are often preferred. It may also be used in myoclonus (p.342) and associated abnormal movements. Clonazepam is also employed for the treatment of panic disorders.

Treatment is initiated with small doses that are progressively increased to an optimum dose according to the response of the patient. In the UK the initial adult dose is 1 mg (500 μg in the elderly) by mouth at night for 4 nights gradually increased over 2 to 4 weeks to a usual maintenance dose of 4 to 8 mg daily in 3 or 4 divided doses; in the USA it is recommended that the total dose should not exceed 20 mg daily. In the UK initial daily doses in children are 250 μg for children up to 5 years of age and 500 μg for children 5 to 12 years of age; usual daily maintenance doses, given in 3 or 4 divided doses, are: infants, 0.5 to 1 mg; children 1 to 5 years, 1 to 3 mg; children 5 to 12 years, 3 to 6 mg. In the USA it is recommended that the total dose should not exceed 200 μg per kg body-weight daily in children. There is little value in routinely monitoring plasma-clonazepam concentrations.

Clonazepam is also used as an alternative to other benzodiazepines in the emergency management of status epilepticus (p.341). The usual dose is 1 mg given by intravenous injection over about 30 seconds or by intravenous infusion, repeated if necessary; the dose in infants and children is 500 μg.

As with other antiepileptics, withdrawal of clonazepam therapy or transition to or from another type of antiepileptic therapy should be made gradually to avoid precipitating an increase in the frequency of seizures. For a discussion on whether or not to with-

draw antiepileptic therapy in seizure-free patients, see p.338 and above.

In the treatment of panic disorders, clonazepam is given in an initial dose of 250 μg twice daily by mouth. This may be increased after 3 days to a total of 1 mg daily; a few patients may benefit from further increases, up to a maximum of 4 mg daily. In order to minimise drowsiness, dosage may be taken as a single dose at bedtime. Withdrawal should again be gradual.

Administration. Serum concentrations of clonazepam following administration via the buccal, intranasal, or intravenous routes were measured in a crossover study[1] in 7 healthy males. The results demonstrated that intranasal clonazepam may offer an alternative to buccal administration in patients with serial seizures but the initial concentrations were too low to recommend its use as an alternative to intravenous clonazepam in the management of status epilepticus. The nasal formulation used in this study contained dimethyl-β-cyclodextrin as a solubiliser and absorption enhancer.

1. Schols-Hendriks MWG, *et al.* Absorption of clonazepam after intranasal and buccal administration. *Br J Clin Pharmacol* 1995; **39:** 449–51.

Anxiety disorders. Clonazepam is used for the treatment of panic attacks with or without agoraphobia (p.649), and a beneficial response has been reported in such patients,[1] suggesting a similar action to alprazolam (p.655).

1. Davidson JRT, Moroz G. Pivotal studies of clonazepam in panic disorder. *Psychopharmacol Bull* 1998; **34:** 169–74.

Depression. Short-term use of clonazepam in low doses has been tried[1] with beneficial results for the augmentation of fluoxetine therapy in the treatment of depression (p.271).

1. Londborg PD, *et al.* Short-term cotherapy with clonazepam and fluoxetine: anxiety, sleep disturbance and core symptoms of depression. *J Affect Disord* 2000; **61:** 73–9.

Extrapyramidal disorders. Clonazepam may be of benefit in some extrapyramidal disorders. It has been tried in the management of patients with *tic disorders* such as *Tourette's syndrome* (p.650) but evidence of efficacy from controlled studies is limited.[1] Some use clonazepam in preference to haloperidol[2] since it does not carry the risk of tardive dyskinesia associated with such antipsychotics. There is also limited evidence of benefit with clonazepam in antipsychotic-induced *akathisia*[3,4] and *tardive dyskinesia*[5] (see under Extrapyramidal Disorders, p.662), and of improvement in *dysarthria* in a study in patients with parkinsonism.[6]

1. Goetz CG. Clonidine and clonazepam in Tourette syndrome. *Adv Neurol* 1992; **58:** 245–51.
2. Truong DD, *et al.* Clonazepam, haloperidol, and clonidine in tic disorders. *South Med J* 1988; **81:** 1103–5.
3. Kutcher S, *et al.* Successful clonazepam treatment of neuroleptic-induced akathisia in older adolescents and young adults: a double-blind, placebo-controlled study. *J Clin Psychopharmacol* 1989; **9:** 403–6.
4. Pujalte D, *et al.* A double-blind comparison of clonazepam and placebo in the treatment of neuroleptic-induced akathisia. *Clin Neuropharmacol* 1994; **17:** 236–42.
5. Thaker GK, *et al.* Clonazepam treatment of tardive dyskinesia: a practical GABAmimetic strategy. *Am J Psychiatry* 1990; **147:** 445–51.
6. Biary N, *et al.* A double-blind trial of clonazepam in the treatment of parkinsonian dysarthria. *Neurology* 1988; **38:** 255–8.

Hiccup. A protocol for the management of intractable hiccups can be found under Chlorpromazine, p.667. Clonazepam might also be of value, especially in neurogenic hiccups.

Parasomnias. Treatment of parasomnias (p.653) including sleep behaviour disorder, restless legs syndrome, and periodic limb movements in sleep is largely empirical, but benzodiazepines such as clonazepam are often employed.[1] Small double-blind studies have provided some evidence for benefit with clonazepam therapy.[2,3]

1. Schenck CH, Mahowald MW. Long-term, nightly benzodiazepine treatment of injurious parasomnias and other disorders of disrupted nocturnal sleep in 170 adults. *Am J Med* 1996; **100:** 333–7.
2. Montagna P, *et al.* Clonazepam and vibration in restless legs syndrome. *Acta Neurol Scand* 1984; **69:** 428–30.
3. Peled R, Lavie P. Double-blind evaluation of clonazepam on periodic leg movements in sleep. *J Neurol Neurosurg Psychiatry* 1987; **50:** 1679–81.

Phantom limb pain. The management of phantom limb pain (p.7) can be difficult, and tricyclic antidepressants and antiepileptics are used for the neuropathic components of the pain. Rapid and marked pain relief was achieved in 2 patients with lancinating phantom limb pain following treatment with clonazepam with or without amitriptyline.[1]

1. Bartusch SL, *et al.* Clonazepam for the treatment of lancinating phantom limb pain. *Clin J Pain* 1996; **12:** 59–62.

Stiff-man syndrome. Clonazepam has been used as an alternative to diazepam in the management of stiff-man syndrome (p.681) and is reported[1] to be effective for familial startle disease, a rare congenital form of stiff-man syndrome.

1. Ryan SG, *et al.* Startle disease, or hyperekplexia: response to clonazepam and assignment of the gene (STHE) to chromosome 5q by linkage analysis. *Ann Neurol* 1992; **31:** 663–8.

Trigeminal neuralgia. Although carbamazepine is the drug of choice in the treatment of trigeminal neuralgia (p.8), clonazepam may be used in carbamazepine-intolerant patients.

Preparations

BP 2001: Clonazepam Injection;
USP 25: Clonazepam Tablets.

Proprietary Preparations (details are given in Part 3)
Aust.: Rivotril; *Austral.:* Paxam; Rivotril; *Belg.:* Rivotril; *Braz.:* Rivotril; *Canad.:* Clonapam; Rivotril; *Denm.:* Rivotril; *Fin.:* Rivatril; *Fr.:* Rivotril; *Ger.:* Antelepsin; *Hong Kong:* Rivotril; *Irl.:* Rivotril; *Israel:* Clonex; Rivotril; *Ital.:* Rivotril; *Mex.:* Kenoket; Rivotril; *Neth.:* Rivotril; *Norw.:* Rivotril; *NZ:* Rivotril; *Port.:* Rivotril; *S.Afr.:* Rivotril; *Singapore:* Rivotril; *Spain:* Rivotril; *Swed.:* Iktorivil; *Switz.:* Rivotril; *Thai.:* Rivotril; *UK:* Rivotril; *USA:* Klonopin.

Ethadione (9445-d)

3-Ethyl-5,5-dimethyl-2,4-oxazolidinedione.
$C_7H_{11}NO_3 = 157.2$.
CAS — 520-77-4.
ATC — N03AC03.

Profile
Ethadione is an oxazolidinedione antiepileptic with actions and uses similar to those of trimethadione (p.366); like trimethadione it appears to owe its action to metabolism to dimethadione. It has been used to treat epilepsy (p.338) in patients with absence seizures resistant to other therapy. Usual initial doses are 500 mg daily by mouth, increased gradually to up to 2 g daily if necessary.

Preparations
Proprietary Preparations (details are given in Part 3)
Aust.: Petidion; *Switz.:* Petidion.

Ethosuximide (6611-x)

Ethosuximide *(BAN, USAN, rINN)*.
CI-366; CN-10395; NSC-64013; PM-671. 2-Ethyl-2-methylsuccinimide.
$C_7H_{11}NO_2 = 141.2$.
CAS — 77-67-8.
ATC — N03AD01.
Pharmacopoeias. In Chin., Eur. (see p.vi), Int., Jpn, and US.

Pharmacopoeial description
Ph. Eur.: A white or almost white powder or waxy solid. Freely soluble in water; very soluble in alcohol, in dichloromethane, and in ether. Protect from light.
USP 25: A white to off-white crystalline powder or waxy solid, having a characteristic odour. Freely soluble in water and in chloroform; very soluble in alcohol and in ether; very slightly soluble in petroleum spirit. Store in airtight containers.

Adverse Effects and Treatment
Gastrointestinal side-effects including nausea, vomiting, anorexia, gastric upset, and abdominal pain occur fairly frequently with ethosuximide. Other side-effects which may occur include headache, fatigue, lethargy, drowsiness, dizziness, ataxia, hiccup, and mild euphoria.

More rarely dyskinesias, personality changes, depression, psychosis, skin rashes, erythema multiforme or Stevens-Johnson syndrome, systemic lupus erythematosus, photophobia, gum hypertrophy, tongue swelling, myopia, and vaginal bleeding have been reported. There are a few reports of blood disorders including eosinophilia, leucopenia, agranulocytosis, thrombocytopenia, pancytopenia, and aplastic anaemia; fatalities have occurred.

Abnormal renal and liver function values have been recorded.

Overdosage. For a review of the features and management of poisoning with some antiepileptics, including ethosuximide, see under Phenytoin, p.358.

Precautions
Ethosuximide should be used with caution in patients with impaired hepatic or renal function. The manufacturers recommend regular hepatic and renal-function tests (and some suggest blood counts) during treatment with ethosuximide, although some authorities question the practical value of such monitoring. Patients or their carers should be told how to recognise signs of blood toxicity and they should be advised to seek immediate medical attention if symptoms such as fever, sore throat, mouth ulcers, bruising, or bleeding develop.

Care is required when withdrawing ethosuximide therapy—see also under Uses and Administration, below.

Breast feeding. Ethosuximide is distributed in significant amounts into breast milk and breast feeding should be avoided; hyperexcitability and poor suckling have been reported in the infant. For comment on antiepileptic therapy and breast feeding, see under Pregnancy and Breast Feeding on p.340.

Driving. For a comment on antiepileptic drugs and driving, see p.340.

Porphyria. Ethosuximide has been associated with acute attacks of porphyria and is considered unsafe in porphyric patients.

Pregnancy. For comments on the management of epilepsy during pregnancy, see p.340.

Interactions
There are complex interactions between antiepileptics and toxicity may be enhanced without a corresponding increase in antiepileptic activity. Such interactions are very variable and unpredictable and plasma monitoring is often advisable with combination therapy.

Antibacterials. *Isoniazid* raises the plasma concentration and increases the risk of toxicity of ethosuximide. Psychotic behaviour has been reported[1] in a patient stabilised on ethosuximide and sodium valproate, after the introduction of *isoniazid*. Serum-ethosuximide concentrations rose substantially until both ethosuximide and isoniazid were discontinued.

1. van Wieringen A, Vrijlandt CM. Ethosuximide intoxication caused by interaction with isoniazid. *Neurology* 1983; 33: 1227–8.

Antidepressants. As with all antiepileptics, antidepressants may antagonise the antiepileptic activity of ethosuximide by lowering the convulsive threshold.

Antiepileptics. Since ethosuximide has a limited spectrum of antiepileptic action, patients with mixed seizure syndromes may require concomitant administration of other antiepileptics. *Carbamazepine, phenobarbital,* and *phenytoin* have all been shown[1] to increase the clearance of ethosuximide and thus reduce plasma concentrations. This interaction is likely to be clinically relevant and higher ethosuximide dosages may be necessary to achieve therapeutic drug levels. Although ethosuximide has been used with *valproic acid* quite frequently, there is little evidence of an interaction. However, in one study 4 of 5 patients receiving a combination regimen including ethosuximide experienced a marked increase in serum ethosuximide concentrations when valproic acid was added,[2] and there is evidence for a decrease in ethosuximide clearance and consequent prolongation in its half-life when the two drugs are given together, although the effect seems to vary between individuals, with some unaffected.[3]

1. Giaccone M, *et al.* Effect of enzyme inducing anticonvulsants on ethosuximide pharmacokinetics in epileptic patients. *Br J Clin Pharmacol* 1996; 41: 575–9.
2. Mattson RH, Cramer JA. Valproic acid and ethosuximide interaction. *Ann Neurol* 1980; 7: 583–4.
3. Pisani F, *et al.* Valproic acid-ethosuximide interaction: a pharmacokinetic study. *Epilepsia* 1984; 25: 229–33.

Antipsychotics. As with all antiepileptics, antipsychotics may antagonise the antiepileptic activity of ethosuximide by lowering the convulsive threshold.

Sex hormones. For the effects of ethosuximide on *oral contraceptives,* see p.1459.

Pharmacokinetics
Ethosuximide is readily absorbed from the gastrointestinal tract and extensively hydroxylated in the liver to its principal metabolite which is reported to be inactive. It is excreted in the urine mainly in the form of its metabolites either free or in conjugated form but about 20% is also excreted as unchanged ethosuximide.

Ethosuximide is widely distributed throughout the body, but is not significantly bound to plasma proteins. A half-life of about 60 hours has been reported for adults with a shorter half-life of about 30 hours in children.

Monitoring of plasma concentrations has been suggested as an aid in assessing control and the therapeutic range of ethosuximide is usually quoted as being 40 to 100 µg per mL (about 300 to 700 µmol per litre); measurement of concentrations in saliva and tears has also been performed.

Ethosuximide crosses the placental barrier, and is distributed into breast milk.

The pharmacokinetics of ethosuximide are affected by the concomitant administration of other antiepileptics (see under Interactions, above).

Uses and Administration
Ethosuximide is a succinimide antiepileptic used in the treatment of absence seizures. It may also be used for myoclonic seizures. Ethosuximide is ineffective against tonic-clonic seizures and may unmask them if given alone in mixed seizure types.

A plasma-ethosuximide concentration of 40 to 100 µg per mL (about 300 to 700 µmol per litre) appears to be generally necessary. The initial dose for adults and children of 6 years and over is 500 mg daily by mouth. The dosage is then adjusted by increments, usually by 250 mg every 4 to 7 days, according to the response of the patient. Control of seizures is usually produced with a daily dose of 1 to 1.5 g, although some patients may require doses of up to 2 g; strict supervision is necessary when the dose exceeds 1.5 g. For children up to 6 years of age the initial dose is 250 mg daily increased gradually in small increments every few days to a usual dose of 20 mg per kg body-weight; one manufacturer recommends that the dose should not exceed 1 g.

As with other antiepileptics, withdrawal of ethosuximide therapy or transition to or from another type of antiepileptic therapy should be made gradually to avoid precipitating an increase in the frequency of seizures. For a discussion on whether or not to withdraw antiepileptic therapy in seizure-free patients, see p.338.

Epilepsy. Ethosuximide is a drug of choice in the treatment of absence seizures; it may also be used for myoclonic, atonic, and tonic seizures but is ineffective in other forms of epilepsy (p.338). Ethosuximide may be administered with other antiepileptics in the treatment of mixed-seizure syndromes that include absences. It has been suggested that ethosuximide may provoke tonic-clonic seizures, but there is not a great deal of evidence for this. One early report indicated that 22 of 85 patients receiving a regimen of ethosuximide, mesuximide, and trimethadione for absence seizures developed tonic-clonic seizures[1] and another of similar vintage reported exacerbation of mixed-seizure types in 7 patients receiving ethosuximide.[2] However, it is known that up to half of all patients with absence seizures experience generalised tonic-clonic seizures at some point[3] and it would presumably be difficult to distinguish such attacks from any putative effect of ethosuximide. Furthermore, ethosuximide is not effective against tonic-clonic seizures, and in patients with mixed-seizure types it might be expected to unmask the non-absence components of the disease.

Ethosuximide has also been tried in the management of absence status epilepticus (p.341).

1. Friedel B, Lempp R. Grand-mal-Provokation bei der Behandlung kindlicher petit-mal mit Oxazolidinen oder Succinimiden und ihre therapeutischen Konsequenzen. *Z Kinderheilk* 1962; 87: 42–51.
2. de Haas AML, Kuilman M. Ethosuximide (α-ethyl-α-methylsuccinimide) and grand mal. *Epilepsia* 1964; 5: 90–6.
3. Sherwin AL. Ethosuximide: clinical use. In: Levy RH, *et al.*, eds. *Antiepileptic drugs* 4th ed. New York: Raven Press, 1995: 667–73.

Preparations
BP 2001: Ethosuximide Capsules; Ethosuximide Oral Solution;
USP 25: Ethosuximide Capsules; Ethosuximide Oral Solution.

Proprietary Preparations (details are given in Part 3)
Aust.: Petinimid; Simatin; Suxinutin; *Austral.:* Zarontin; *Belg.:* Zarontin; *Canad.:* Zarontin; *Denm.:* Zarondan; *Fin.:* Suxinutin; *Fr.:* Zarontin; *Ger.:* Petnidan; Pyknolepsinum†; Suxilep; Suxinutin; *Irl.:* Zarontin; *Israel:* Zarontin; *Ital.:* Zarontin; *Mex.:* Zarontin; *Neth.:* Zarontin; *Norw.:* Zarondan; *NZ:* Zarontin; *S.Afr.:* Zarontin; *Spain:* Zarontin; *Swed.:* Suxinutin; *Switz.:* Petinimid; Suxinutin; *UK:* Emeside; Zarontin; *USA:* Zarontin.

Multi-ingredient: *Aust.:* Acrisuxin; *Switz.:* Acrisuxin†.

Ethotoin (6612-r)

Ethotoin *(BAN, rINN)*.
3-Ethyl-5-phenylhydantoin.
$C_{11}H_{12}N_2O_2 = 204.2$.
CAS — 86-35-1.
ATC — N03AB01.
Pharmacopoeias. In US.

Pharmacopoeial description
USP 25: A white crystalline powder. Insoluble in water; freely soluble in dehydrated alcohol and in chloroform; soluble in ether. Store in airtight containers.

Profile
Ethotoin is a hydantoin antiepileptic with actions similar to those of phenytoin (p.357), but it is reported to be both less toxic and less effective; it is not one of the main drugs used to treat epilepsy (p.338).

Ethotoin has been given by mouth in an initial dosage of up to 1 g daily, increased gradually at intervals of several days to 2 to 3 g daily, given in 4 to 6 divided doses after meals.

◊ A study[1] of the pharmacokinetics of ethotoin given at more convenient intervals of every 8 hours.

1. Browne TR, Szabo GK. A pharmacokinetic rationale for three times daily administration of ethotoin (Peganone). *J Clin Pharmacol* 1989; **29:** 270–1.

Porphyria. Ethotoin has been associated with acute attacks of porphyria and is considered unsafe in porphyric patients.

Preparations

USP 25: Ethotoin Tablets.

Proprietary Preparations (details are given in Part 3)
USA: Peganone.

Felbamate   (2858-e)

Felbamate (USAN, rINN).
AD-03055; W-554. 2-Phenyl-1,3-propanediol dicarbamate.
$C_{11}H_{14}N_2O_4$ = 238.2.
CAS — 25451-15-4.
ATC — N03AX10.

Adverse Effects

The most frequently reported adverse effects with felbamate are anorexia, weight loss, nausea and vomiting, rash, insomnia, headache, dizziness, somnolence, and diplopia. Aplastic anaemia or acute liver failure, sometimes fatal, have occurred rarely, and there have been reports of Stevens-Johnson syndrome.

Effects on the skin. Toxic epidermal necrolysis has been reported[1] in a patient 16 days after she started monotherapy with felbamate for partial complex seizures.

1. Travaglini MT, *et al.* Toxic epidermal necrolysis after initiation of felbamate therapy. *Pharmacotherapy* 1995; **15:** 260–4.

Precautions

Felbamate is contra-indicated in patients with a history of blood disorders or hepatic impairment. It should be used only in the treatment of severe epilepsy refractory to other antiepileptics because of the risk of fatal aplastic anaemia or acute liver failure. Patients or their carers should be advised of the symptoms of aplastic anaemia and be told to report immediately should any such symptoms develop. Complete blood counts should be carried out before the patient starts treatment and regularly during treatment (but see Epilepsy, under Uses and Administration, below). Aplastic anaemia can occur after felbamate has been discontinued so patients should continue to be monitored for some time. Liver function tests are also recommended before commencing and regularly (at 1- to 2-week intervals) during treatment. Felbamate should be discontinued if there is any evidence of bone marrow depression or liver abnormalities. Felbamate should be used with caution in patients with renal impairment. Felbamate may cause photosensitivity reactions and patients should be advised to take protective measures against exposure to UV radiation.

Care is required when withdrawing felbamate therapy—see also under Uses and Administration, below.

Breast feeding. For comment on antiepileptic therapy and breast feeding, see under Pregnancy and Breast Feeding on p.340.

The elderly. Following single doses of felbamate, plasma concentrations and half-lives were greater and mean clearance lower in elderly than in young subjects, whereas pharmacokinetic parameters following multiple dosing schedules were similar.[1] Thus, the elderly may require lower initial doses of felbamate and slower dose titration.

1. Richens A, *et al.* Single and multiple dose pharmacokinetics of felbamate in the elderly. *Br J Clin Pharmacol* 1997; **44:** 129–34.

Pregnancy. For comments on the management of epilepsy during pregnancy, see p.340.

Renal impairment. A single-dose pharmacokinetic study[1] indicated that in patients with renal impairment the initial dose of felbamate may need to be lower and increases made more cautiously than in patients with normal renal function.

1. Glue P, *et al.* Single-dose pharmacokinetics of felbamate in patients with renal dysfunction. *Br J Clin Pharmacol* 1997; **44:** 91–3.

Interactions

The metabolism of felbamate is enhanced by enzyme inducers such as phenytoin or carbamazepine. In con-

trast, the half-life of felbamate may be prolonged by gabapentin. Felbamate inhibits or enhances the metabolism of several other antiepileptics and care is required when it is added to therapy.

◊ For some references to the effect of felbamate on other antiepileptics, see under Carbamazepine, p.344, Phenobarbital, p.356, Phenytoin, p.360, and Valproate p.368.

For the effect of felbamate on warfarin, see p.995.

Pharmacokinetics

Felbamate is well absorbed from the gastrointestinal tract and peak plasma concentrations have been reported 1 to 6 hours after oral administration. Protein binding is reported to be about 22 to 36%. It is partly metabolised in the liver by hydroxylation and conjugation to inactive metabolites. Felbamate is excreted in the urine as metabolites and unchanged drug (40 to 50%); less than 4% appears in the faeces. The elimination half-life is reported to be between 14 and 23 hours. Felbamate has been detected in breast milk.

The pharmacokinetics of felbamate are reported to be linear at the doses used clinically. Therapeutic plasma concentrations have been reported to be between 30 and 80 µg per mL.

◊ See under Precautions (above) for mention of pharmacokinetic studies of felbamate in the elderly and in patients with renal impairment.

Uses and Administration

Felbamate is a carbamate structurally related to meprobamate (p.691). It is used in the treatment of epilepsy.

Felbamate is given to adults as monotherapy or adjunctive therapy for refractory partial seizures with or without secondary generalisation. It is used in children as adjunctive therapy in controlling the seizures associated with the Lennox-Gastaut syndrome. Because of its toxicity felbamate should only be used in severe cases unresponsive to other drugs.

The initial adult dose of felbamate when given as *monotherapy* is 1.2 g daily by mouth in 3 or 4 divided doses. The daily dose should be increased gradually under close supervision; increments of 600 mg every 2 weeks are given according to response, up to 2.4 g daily. Thereafter doses may be further increased to a maximum of 3.6 g daily if necessary.

Similar initial doses are given as *adjunctive* therapy, but the doses of concomitant antiepileptics should be decreased as necessary. Incremental increases of adjunctive felbamate are 1200 mg at weekly intervals. The initial dose in children 2 to 14 years of age is 15 mg per kg body-weight daily in 3 or 4 divided doses increased gradually in increments of 15 mg per kg per day at weekly intervals up to a maximum of 45 mg per kg daily.

As with other antiepileptics, withdrawal of felbamate therapy or transition to or from another type of antiepileptic therapy should be made gradually to avoid precipitating an increase in the frequency of seizures. For a discussion on whether or not to withdraw antiepileptic therapy in seizure-free patients, see p.338.

Epilepsy. Although felbamate was well tolerated in clinical trials, rare but serious adverse effects were noted during early postmarketing use.[1,2] Aplastic anaemia and serious hepatotoxic reactions, sometimes with fatal outcomes, developed in some patients. Patients taking felbamate should have frequent blood counts and monitoring of liver enzymes. However there is no evidence that such monitoring will prevent adverse outcomes; in addition, the risk of aplastic anaemia is thought to decrease after the first year of therapy, and the need for ongoing blood counts is still less clear.[3] Even if detected early, aplastic anaemia and hepatic impairment may not be reversible.[3] Usage in the USA is restricted to patients with refractory partial seizures with or without secondary generalisation or for adjunctive therapy for children with Lennox-Gastaut syndrome. Guidelines on appropriate use have been issued.[3]

The efficacy of felbamate as adjunctive therapy in refractory partial seizures in both adults[4] and children,[5] and in patients with the Lennox-Gastaut syndrome[6,7] has been demonstrated, although there appears to be an increased rate of drug clearance in younger children.[5] Felbamate also appears to be useful as adjunctive therapy in refractory absence seizures.[8]

The overall management of epilepsy is discussed on p.338.

1. Dichter MA, Brodie MJ. New antiepileptic drugs. *N Engl J Med* 1996; **334:** 1583–90.
2. Appleton RE. The new antiepileptic drugs. *Arch Dis Child* 1996; **75:** 256–62.
3. French J, *et al.* The use of felbamate in the treatment of patients with intractable epilepsy. Report of the Quality Standards Subcommittee of the American Academy of Neurology and the American Epilepsy Society. *Epilepsia* 1999; **40:** 803–8.
4. Bourgeois B, *et al.* Felbamate: a double-blind controlled trial in patients undergoing presurgical evaluation of partial seizures. *Neurology* 1993; **43:** 693–6.
5. Carmant L, *et al.* Efficacy of felbamate in therapy for partial epilepsy in children. *J Pediatr* 1994; **125:** 481–6.
6. The Felbamate Study Group in Lennox-Gastaut Syndrome. Efficacy of felbamate in childhood epileptic encephalopathy (Lennox-Gastaut Syndrome). *N Engl J Med* 1993; **328:** 29–33.
7. Dodson WE. Felbamate in the treatment of Lennox-Gastaut syndrome: results of a 12-month open-label study following a randomized clinical trial. *Epilepsia* 1993; **34** (suppl 7): S18–S24.
8. Devinsky O, *et al.* Felbamate for refractory absence seizures. *J Epilepsy* 1994; **7:** 189–94.

Preparations

Proprietary Preparations (details are given in Part 3)
Aust.: Taloxa; **Belg.:** Taloxa; **Fr.:** Taloxa; **Ger.:** Taloxa; **Ital.:** Taloxa; **Neth.:** Taloxa; **Norw.:** Taloxa; **Port.:** Taloxa; **Spain:** Taloxa; **Swed.:** Taloxa; **Switz.:** Taloxa; **USA:** Felbatol.

Fosphenytoin Sodium   (17705-b)

Fosphenytoin Sodium (BANM, USAN, rINNM).
ACC-9653; ACC-9653-010; CI-982 (fosphenytoin or fosphenytoin sodium); PD-135711-15B. 5,5-Diphenyl-3-[(phosphonooxy)methyl]-2,4-imidazolidinedione, disodium salt; 3-(Hydroxymethyl)-5,5-diphenylhydantoin, disodium phosphate (ester); 2,5-Dioxo-4,4-diphenylimidazolidin-1-ylmethyl phosphate disodium.
$C_{16}H_{13}N_2Na_2O_6P$ = 406.2.
CAS — 93390-81-9 (fosphenytoin); 92134-98-0 (fosphenytoin sodium).

Each mmol of fosphenytoin yields one mmol of phenytoin. Fosphenytoin sodium 75 mg is approximately equivalent to phenytoin sodium 50 mg.

Stability. References.

1. Fischer JH, *et al.* Stability of fosphenytoin sodium with intravenous solutions in glass bottles, polyvinyl chloride bags, and polypropylene syringes. *Ann Pharmacother* 1997; **31:** 553–9.

Adverse Effects and Precautions

As for Phenytoin, p.357.

Severe cardiovascular reactions, sometimes fatal, have been reported following intravenous administration of fosphenytoin. Therefore, continuous monitoring of ECG, blood pressure, and respiratory function is recommended during the infusion, and the patient should be kept under observation for at least 30 minutes after the end of the infusion. Hypotension may occur with recommended doses and rates of infusion; a reduction in the infusion rate or discontinuation of therapy may be necessary.

Burning, itching, and paraesthesia, particularly in the groin area, have also been reported following intravenous administration of fosphenytoin; reducing the rate of, or temporarily stopping, the infusion may relieve the discomfort.

Caution should be exercised when administering fosphenytoin to patients in whom phosphate restriction is necessary. The rate of metabolism of fosphenytoin to phenytoin may be increased following intravenous administration to patients with hepatic or renal disease, or in those with hypoalbuminaemia, and consequently there is an increased risk of adverse effects in such patients.

Effects on the cardiovascular system. The UK Committee on the Safety of Medicines[1] stated in May 2000 that worldwide there had been reports of 21 cases of asystole, ventricular fibrillation, or cardiac arrest associated with intravenous administration of fosphenytoin. Of these, 5 cases had received doses or infusion rates greater than recommended. There had also been 34 reports of hypotension, 15 of bradycardia, and 10 of varying degrees of heart block. Most reactions had occurred within 30 minutes of the infusion.

1. Committee on Safety of Medicines/Medicines Control Agency. Fosphenytoin sodium (Pro-Epanutin): serious arrhythmias and hypotension. *Current Problems* 2000; **26:** 1.

Interactions

As for Phenytoin, p.359.

Pharmacokinetics

Plasma concentrations of fosphenytoin are maximal at the end of intravenous infusion and about 30 minutes after intramuscular injection. Protein binding of fosphenytoin is high (95 to 99%) and is saturable; fosphenytoin displaces phenytoin from protein binding sites. Fosphenytoin is completely metabolised to phenytoin; other metabolites include phosphate and formaldehyde. Metabolites of phenytoin are excreted in the urine. For the pharmacokinetics of phenytoin, see p.362.

Uses and Administration

Fosphenytoin is a prodrug of phenytoin (p.357) used similarly as part of the emergency treatment of status epilepticus (p.341). It is also used for the prevention and treatment of post-traumatic seizures (p.363) associated with neurosurgery or head trauma and as a short-term parenteral substitute for oral phenytoin in the management of epilepsy (p.338).

Fosphenytoin is administered in the form of the sodium salt and doses of fosphenytoin sodium are expressed as phenytoin sodium equivalents (PSE); therefore no adjustment in dosage is necessary when substituting fosphenytoin for phenytoin or vice versa. The maximum rate of intravenous infusion of fosphenytoin sodium is 150 mg PSE per minute (or in children over 5 years of age, 3 mg PSE per kg per minute) and should not be exceeded. Continuous monitoring of ECG, blood pressure, and respiratory function is recommended during intravenous infusion. Patients should also be observed for at least 30 minutes after the end of infusion.

In the treatment of tonic-clonic status epilepticus in the UK, the loading dose in PSE administered by intravenous infusion is 15 mg per kg body-weight at a rate of 100 to 150 mg per minute (or in children over 5 years of age, 2 to 3 mg per kg per minute). The intramuscular route is not appropriate for the management of status epilepticus because peak phenytoin concentrations will not be reached quickly enough. The loading dose in PSE for seizures other than in status epilepticus is 10 to 15 mg per kg, given by intramuscular injection or by intravenous infusion at a rate of 50 to 100 mg per minute (or in children over 5 years of age, 1 to 2 mg per kg per minute). Initial maintenance doses for status epilepticus and other seizures are 4 to 5 mg PSE per kg daily given by intramuscular injection or by intravenous infusion at a rate of 50 to 100 mg PSE per minute (or in children over 5 years of age, 1 to 2 mg PSE per kg per minute). Subsequent doses are dependent on patient response and trough plasma-phenytoin concentrations.

Fosphenytoin given intramuscularly or by intravenous infusion may be substituted for oral phenytoin at the same equivalent total daily dose for up to 5 days.

In the USA, loading doses of up to 20 mg PSE per kg are permitted, and maintenance doses are 4 to 6 mg PSE per kg daily.

A lower loading dose and/or infusion rate, and lower or less frequent maintenance dosing may be necessary for elderly patients; the UK manufacturer suggests a reduction in dose or rate of 10 to 25%. Similar reductions are suggested for patients with renal or hepatic impairment or in those with hypoalbuminaemia, except in the treatment of status epilepticus.

Withdrawal of antiepileptic therapy or transition to or from another type of antiepileptic therapy should be made gradually to avoid precipitating an increase in the frequency of seizures. For a discussion on whether or not to withdraw antiepileptic therapy in seizure-free patients, see p.338.

◊ References.
1. Wilder BJ, et al. Safety and tolerance of multiple doses of intramuscular fosphenytoin substituted for oral phenytoin in epilepsy or neurosurgery. Arch Neurol 1996; 53: 764–8.
2. Meek PD, et al. Guidelines for nonemergency use of parenteral phenytoin products: proceedings of an expert panel consensus process. Arch Intern Med 1999; 159: 2639–44.
3. Heafield MTE. Managing status epilepticus: new drug offers real advantages. BMJ 2000; 320: 953–4.
4. DeToledo JC, Ramsay RE. Fosphenytoin and phenytoin in patients with status epilepticus: improved tolerability versus increased costs. Drug Safety 2000; 22: 459–66.

Preparations

Proprietary Preparations (details are given in Part 3)
Canad.: Cerebyx; *Denm.*: Pro-Epanutin; *Fin.*: Pro-Epanutin; *Fr.*: Prodilantin; *Irl.*: Pro-Epanutin; *Neth.*: Pro-Epanutin; *Norw.*: Pro-Epanutin; *Port.*: Pro-Epanutin; *Swed.*: Pro-Epanutin; *UK*: Pro-Epanutin; *USA*: Cerebyx.

Gabapentin (3797-f)

Gabapentin (BAN, USAN, rINN).
CI-945; GOE-3450. 1-(Aminomethyl)cyclohexaneacetic acid.
$C_9H_{17}NO_2 = 171.2$.
CAS — 60142-96-3.
ATC — N03AX12.

Adverse Effects and Precautions

The most commonly reported adverse effects associated with gabapentin are somnolence, dizziness, ataxia, and fatigue. Nystagmus, tremor, diplopia, amblyopia, pharyngitis, dysarthria, weight gain, dyspepsia, amnesia, weakness, paraesthesia, arthralgia, purpura, leucopenia, anxiety, and urinary-tract infection may occur less frequently. Rarely, pancreatitis, altered liver function tests, erythema multiforme, Stevens-Johnson syndrome, rhinitis, nervousness, myalgia, headache, nausea and vomiting, and blood glucose fluctuations in diabetics have been reported.

Gabapentin should be used with caution in patients with a history of psychotic illness. It should also be used with caution in renal impairment; the manufacturer recommends dosage reduction in patients with reduced renal function or those undergoing haemodialysis. False positive readings have been reported with some urinary protein tests in patients taking gabapentin.

Care is required when withdrawing gabapentin therapy—see also under Uses and Administration, below.

Breast feeding. For comment on antiepileptic therapy and breast feeding, see under Pregnancy and Breast Feeding on p.340.

Carcinogenicity. It had been reported[1] that studies on gabapentin had been temporarily stopped in 1990 when pancreatic tumours were seen in *rodent* studies. However, the tumours were benign, occurred only with large doses, and were not thought to relate to humans.
1. Ramsay RE. Clinical efficacy and safety of gabapentin. *Neurology* 1994; **44** (suppl 5): S23–S30.

Driving. For a comment on antiepileptic drugs and driving, see p.340.

Effects on mental state. There have been isolated reports of depression, aggression, confusion, delusions, and hallucinations in patients receiving gabapentin.[1]
1. Anonymous. Gabapentin—a new antiepileptic drug. *Drug Ther Bull* 1994; **32:** 29–30.

Pregnancy. For comments on the management of epilepsy during pregnancy, see p.340.

Interactions

The absorption of gabapentin from the gastrointestinal tract is reduced by antacids and concomitant administration is therefore not recommended. Cimetidine has been reported to reduce the renal clearance of gabapentin but the manufacturers do not consider this to be of clinical importance. For reference to a possible interaction with other antiepileptics, see under Phenytoin, p.360.

Pharmacokinetics

Gabapentin is absorbed from the gastrointestinal tract by means of a saturable mechanism. Following multiple dosing peak plasma concentrations are usually achieved within 2 hours of administration and steady-state achieved within 1 to 2 days. Gabapentin is not appreciably metabolised and most of a dose is excreted unchanged in the urine with the remainder appearing in the faeces. Gabapentin is widely distributed throughout the body but binding to plasma proteins is minimal. The elimination half-life has been reported to be about 5 to 7 hours. Gabapentin is distributed into breast milk.

◊ References.
1. Blum RA, et al. Pharmacokinetics of gabapentin in subjects with various degrees of renal function. *Clin Pharmacol Ther* 1994; **56:** 154–9.
2. Elwes RDC, Binnie CD. Clinical pharmacokinetics of newer antiepileptic drugs: lamotrigine, vigabatrin, gabapentin and oxcarbazepine. *Clin Pharmacokinet* 1996; **30:** 403–15.

In children. A study[1] of the pharmacokinetics of gabapentin following single doses in children aged 1 month to 12 years found that peak plasma concentrations occurred 2 to 3 hours after the dose in all age groups but that the mean value was higher in those older than 5 years than in younger children, and the exposure was calculated to be about 30% less in the younger age group. As a result it was suggested that the initial dose of gabapentin in studies of safety and efficacy should be 40 mg per kg body-weight daily in children aged from 1 month up to 5 years, and 30 mg per kg daily in children aged 5 to 12 years. (For licensed doses, see Uses and Administration, below.)
1. Haig GM, et al. Single-dose gabapentin pharmacokinetics and safety in healthy infants and children. *J Clin Pharmacol* 2001; **41:** 507–14.

Uses and Administration

Gabapentin is an antiepileptic effective in the treatment of partial seizures with or without secondary generalisation and is used as adjunctive therapy in patients unresponsive to or intolerant of standard antiepileptic drugs. It is not generally considered effective for absence seizures. Although gabapentin is an analogue of gamma-aminobutyric acid (GABA), it is neither a GABA agonist nor antagonist and its mechanism of action is unknown. Gabapentin is also used in the treatment of neuropathic pain.

The initial adult dose of gabapentin for the treatment of epilepsy is 300 mg by mouth on the first day of treatment, 300 mg twice daily on the second day, and 300 mg three times daily on the third day; thereafter the dose may be increased in increments of 300 mg daily until effective antiepileptic control is achieved, which is usually within the range of 0.9 to 1.2 g daily. Higher doses up to a maximum of 2.4 g daily may be required in some patients; in the USA, doses of up to 3.6 g daily administered for a short period have been reported to be well tolerated. The total daily dose should be taken in three equally divided doses and the maximum dosage interval should not exceed 12 hours.

The initial dose for children 6 to 12 years of age for the treatment of epilepsy is 10 mg per kg body-weight on the first day of treatment, 20 mg per kg on the second day, and 25 to 35 mg per kg on the third day. Recommended maintenance doses are 900 mg daily for children weighing 26 to 36 kg and 1200 mg daily for those weighing 37 to 50 kg. In the USA, gabapentin is licensed for adjunctive use in children from 3 years of age. An initial dose of 10 to 15 mg per kg daily is recommended, increased over about 3 days to doses of about 40 mg per kg daily in those aged 3 to 4, or 25 to 35 mg per kg daily in those 5 years of age or older. The total daily dose should be taken in three divided doses.

In the treatment of neuropathic pain in adults, doses should be titrated to a maximum of 1.8 g daily in three divided doses, in a similar manner to that recommended for the treatment of epilepsy in adults given above.

Reduced doses are recommended for patients with renal impairment. Suitable maintenance doses are: 600 to 1200 mg daily for patients with a creatinine clearance of 50 to 79 mL per minute; 300 to 600 mg daily for a clearance of 30 to 49 mL per minute; 300 mg on alternate days to 300 mg daily for a clearance of 15 to 29 mL per minute; and 300 mg on alternate days for a clearance of less than 15 mL per minute. The total daily doses should be given in 3 divided doses.

As with other antiepileptics, withdrawal of gabapentin therapy or transition to or from another type of antiepileptic therapy should be made gradually to avoid precipitating an increase in the frequency of seizures. The manufacturers recommend reducing the dose gradually over at least 7 days. For a discussion on whether or not to withdraw antiepileptic therapy in seizure-free patients, see p.338.

Bipolar disorder. Although some preliminary results suggest benefit from gabapentin in patients with bipolar disorder good controlled studies are presently lacking.[1]
1. Letterman L, Markowitz JA. Gabapentin: a review of published experience in the treatment of bipolar disorder and other psychiatric conditions. *Pharmacotherapy* 1999; **19:** 565–72.

Ciguatera poisoning. Gabapentin has relieved some of the neurological symptoms associated with ciguatera poisoning (see Mannitol, p.925).

Epilepsy. Gabapentin is used in epilepsy (p.338) as adjunctive therapy for partial seizures with or without secondary generalisation in patients refractory to standard antiepileptics.[1-5] In double-blind placebo-controlled studies[6-9] in such patients seizure frequency was reduced when gabapentin was added to treatment. Long-term efficacy has been encouraging.[10-12] It appears to have similar efficacy to other adjunctive antiepileptics.[3] However, gabapentin may cause fewer adverse effects and its lack of potential for interactions with other antiepileptics is considered to make it particularly suitable for adjunctive treatment. Dosage is adjusted against clinical response rather than by monitoring blood concentrations. Experience of its use as monotherapy in partial epilepsy[13-15] is limited and its efficacy as adjunctive treatment in generalised seizures also remains to be determined.

Although experience with gabapentin in children is also limited it has been found to be effective as adjunctive therapy in children with refractory partial seizures.[16]

1. Goa KL, Sorkin EM. Gabapentin: a review of its pharmacological properties and clinical potential in epilepsy. *Drugs* 1993; **46:** 409–27.
2. Chadwick D. Gabapentin. *Lancet* 1994; **343:** 89–91.
3. Anonymous. Gabapentin—a new antiepileptic drug. *Drug Ther Bull* 1994; **32:** 29–30.
4. Ramsay RE. Clinical efficacy and safety of gabapentin. *Neurology* 1994; **44** (suppl 5): S23–S30.
5. Andrews CO, Fischer JH. Gabapentin: a new agent for the management of epilepsy. *Ann Pharmacother* 1994; **28:** 1188–96.
6. UK Gabapentin Study Group. Gabapentin in partial epilepsy. *Lancet* 1990; **335:** 1114–17.
7. Sivenius J, *et al.* Double-blind study of gabapentin in the treatment of partial seizures. *Epilepsia* 1991; **32:** 539–42.
8. US Gabapentin Study Group. Gabapentin as add-on therapy in refractory partial epilepsy: a double-blind, placebo-controlled, parallel-group study. *Neurology* 1993; **43:** 2292–8.
9. Anhut H, *et al.* International Gabapentin Study Group. Gabapentin (Neurontin) as add-on therapy in patients with partial seizures: a double-blind, placebo-controlled study. *Epilepsia* 1994; **35:** 795–801.
10. US Gabapentin Study Group. The long-term safety and efficacy of gabapentin (Neurontin®) as add-on therapy in drug-resistant partial epilepsy. *Epilepsy Res* 1994; **18:** 67–73.
11. Sivenius J, *et al.* Long-term safety with gabapentin in patients with drug-resistant epileptic seizures. *Arch Neurol* 1994; **51:** 1047–50.
12. Anhut H, *et al.* Long-term safety and efficacy of gabapentin (Neurontin) as add-on therapy in patients with refractory partial seizures. *J Epilepsy* 1995; **8:** 44–50.
13. Ojemann LM, *et al.* Long-term treatment with gabapentin for partial epilepsy. *Epilepsy Res* 1992; **13:** 159–65.
14. Beydoun A, *et al.* Gabapentin monotherapy II: a 26-week, double-blind, dose-controlled multicenter study of conversion from polytherapy in outpatients with refractory complex partial or secondarily generalized seizures. *Neurology* 1997; **49:** 746–52.
15. Chadwick DW, *et al.* A double-blind trial of gabapentin monotherapy for newly diagnosed partial seizures. *Neurology* 1998; **51:** 1282–8.
16. Appleton R, *et al.* Gabapentin as add-on therapy in children with refractory partial seizures: a 12-week, multicentre, double-blind, placebo-controlled study. *Epilepsia* 1999; **40:** 1147–54.

Headache. Benefit has been reported[1] from the use of gabapentin in the prophylaxis of migraine (p.449).

1. Mathew NT, *et al.* Efficacy of gabapentin in migraine prophylaxis. *Headache* 2001; **41:** 119–128.

Lesch-Nyhan syndrome. The severe self-mutilation that occurs in patients with Lesch-Nyhan syndrome (p.667) has been reported to improve in those given antiepileptics such as gabapentin.[1]

1. McManaman J, Tam DA. Gabapentin for self-injurious behavior in Lesch-Nyhan syndrome. *Pediatr Neurol* 1999; **20:** 381–2.

Motor neurone disease. Interest has been shown in gabapentin as a potential therapy for amyotrophic lateral sclerosis (see Motor Neurone Disease, p.1658) because it may inhibit glutamate formation. Results of one study[1] demonstrated a trend towards a beneficial effect but this requires confirmation from further study.

1. Miller RG, *et al.* Placebo-controlled trial of gabapentin in patients with amyotrophic lateral sclerosis. *Neurology* 1996; **47:** 1383–8.

Multiple sclerosis. Gabapentin has been found to control pain, spasm, and spasticity in patients with multiple sclerosis (p.633).

References.

1. Mueller ME, *et al.* Gabapentin for relief of upper motor neuron symptoms in multiple sclerosis. *Arch Phys Med Rehabil* 1997; **78:** 521–4.
2. Samkoff LM, *et al.* Amelioration of refractory dysesthetic limb pain in multiple sclerosis by gabapentin. *Neurology* 1997; **49:** 304–5.
3. Solaro C, *et al.* An open-label trial of gabapentin treatment of paroxysmal symptoms in multiple sclerosis patients. *Neurology* 1998; **51:** 609–11.
4. Dunevsky A, Perel AB. Gabapentin for relief of spasticity associated with multiple sclerosis. *Am J Phys Med Rehabil* 1998; **77:** 451–4.

Neuropathic pain. Neuropathic pain is often insensitive to opioid analgesics, and various drugs, including antiepileptics, have been tried (see Choice of Analgesic, p.2). Carbamazepine appears to be the antiepileptic most frequently used. There have been anecdotal reports and a few controlled studies of the successful use of gabapentin in the treatment of patients with intractable neuropathic pain,[1] including central pain[2] (see p.5),

postherpetic neuralgia[3] (see p.7), and painful diabetic neuropathy[4,5] (see also p.5).

1. Rosner H, *et al.* Gabapentin adjunctive therapy in neuropathic pain states. *Clin J Pain* 1996; **12:** 56–8.
2. Schachter SC, Sauter MK. Treatment of central pain with gabapentin: case reports. *J Epilepsy* 1996; **9:** 223–5.
3. Rowbotham M, *et al.* Gabapentin for the treatment of postherpetic neuralgia: a randomized controlled trial. *JAMA* 1998; **280:** 1837–42.
4. Backonja M, *et al.* Gabapentin for the symptomatic treatment of painful neuropathy in patients with diabetes mellitus: a randomized controlled trial. *JAMA* 1998; **280:** 1831–6.
5. Morello CM, *et al.* Randomized double-blind study comparing the efficacy of gabapentin with amitriptyline on diabetic peripheral neuropathy pain. *Arch Intern Med* 1999; **159:** 1931–7.

Parkinsonism. While some overall ratings of Parkinson's disease (p.1160) appeared to be improved by gabapentin in a double-blind study involving 19 patients with advanced parkinsonism, improvements in individual signs and symptoms were not significant.[1] It was also reported that 5 of 6 other patients with progressive supranuclear palsy had experienced worsening of their disease when given gabapentin.

1. Olson WL, *et al.* Gabapentin for parkinsonism: a double-blind, placebo-controlled, crossover trial. *Am J Med* 1997; **102:** 60–6.

Preparations

Proprietary Preparations (details are given in Part 3)

Aust.: Neurontin; *Austral.:* Neurontin; *Belg.:* Neurontin; *Canad.:* Neurontin; *Fin.:* Neurontin; *Fr.:* Neurontin; *Ger.:* Neurontin; *Hong Kong:* Neurontin; *Irl.:* Neurontin; *Israel:* Neurontin; *Ital.:* Aclonium; Neurontin; *Mex.:* Neurontin; *Neth.:* Neurontin; *Norw.:* Neurontin; *NZ:* Neurontin; *Port.:* Neurontin; *S.Afr.:* Neurontin; *Singapore:* Neurontin; *Spain:* Equipax; Neurontin; *Swed.:* Neurontin; *Switz.:* Neurontin; *Thai.:* Neurontin; *UK:* Neurontin; *USA:* Neurontin.

Lamotrigine (18658-r)

Lamotrigine (BAN, USAN, rINN).
BW-430C. 6-(2,3-Dichlorophenyl)-1,2,4-triazine-3,5-diyldiamine.
$C_9H_7Cl_2N_5 = 256.1$.
CAS — 84057-84-1.
ATC — N03AX09.

Adverse Effects and Treatment

Skin rashes may occur during therapy with lamotrigine; severe skin reactions including Stevens-Johnson syndrome and toxic epidermal necrolysis have been reported, especially in children, and usually occur within 8 weeks of starting lamotrigine. Symptoms such as fever, malaise, influenza-like symptoms, drowsiness, lymphadenopathy, facial oedema and, rarely, hepatic dysfunction, leucopenia and thrombocytopenia have also been reported in conjunction with rashes as part of a hypersensitivity syndrome. Other adverse effects include angioedema and photosensitivity; diplopia, blurred vision, and conjunctivitis; and dizziness, drowsiness, insomnia, headache, ataxia, tiredness, nausea and vomiting, irritability and aggression, tremor, agitation, and confusion.

◊ The manufacturers report that there have been rare instances of death following a rapidly progressive illness with status epilepticus, multi-organ dysfunction, and disseminated intravascular coagulation in patients receiving therapy with multiple antiepileptics including lamotrigine, although the role of lamotrigine remains to be established. It has been suggested[1] that multi-organ failure and disseminated intravascular coagulation, with associated rhabdomyolysis, are complications of severe convulsive seizures rather than lamotrigine therapy. However, there has been a report[2] of a patient with no history of generalised seizures who developed a syndrome of disseminated intravascular coagulation, rhabdomyolysis, renal failure, maculopapular rash, and ataxia 14 days after lamotrigine was added to her antiepileptic regimen. Two cases of disseminated intravascular coagulation were found in a cohort of 11316 patients involved in prescription-event monitoring of lamotrigine therapy in general practice.[3]

1. Yuen AWC, Bihari DJ. Multiorgan failure and disseminated intravascular coagulation in severe convulsive seizures. *Lancet* 1992; **340:** 618.
2. Schaub JEM, *et al.* Multisystem adverse reaction to lamotrigine. *Lancet* 1994; **344:** 481.
3. Mackay FJ, *et al.* Safety of long-term lamotrigine in epilepsy. *Epilepsia* 1997; **38:** 881–6.

Effects on the blood. Septic shock secondary to leucopenia occurred in a patient when lamotrigine was added to therapy with sodium valproate.[1] There has also been a report of agranulocytosis in a child given high initial doses of monotherapy with lamotrigine.[2] The fall in the blood count was noted several days after lamotrigine had been discontinued due to skin rash. The UK Committee on Safety of Medicines (CSM) subsequently reported[3] that 7 cases of aplastic anaemia, 12 of bone-marrow depression, and 20 of pancytopenia associated with lamotrigine had been received worldwide. Given the extensive

usage of lamotrigine the CSM considered the risk of aplastic anaemia to be small and routine blood monitoring was not recommended. However, prescribers were warned to be alert to symptoms and signs suggestive of bone-marrow depression.

1. Nicholson RJ, *et al.* Leucopenia associated with lamotrigine. *BMJ* 1995; **310:** 504.
2. de Camargo OAK, Bode H. Agranulocytosis associated with lamotrigine. *BMJ* 1999; **318:** 1179.
3. Committee on Safety of Medicines/Medicines Control Agency. Lamotrigine (Lamictal): rare blood dyscrasias. *Current Problems* 2000; **26:** 4.

Effects on the liver. Fatal fulminant hepatic failure has been reported[1] in a patient following addition of lamotrigine to an antiepileptic regimen comprising sodium valproate and carbamazepine.

1. Makin AJ, *et al.* Fulminant hepatic failure induced by lamotrigine. *BMJ* 1995; **311:** 292.

Effects on the skin. Rashes account for withdrawal from therapy in about 2% of those given lamotrigine,[1,2] and serious skin reactions including Stevens-Johnson syndrome and toxic epidermal necrolysis occur in about 1 in 1000 adult patients.[3,4] The main risk factors appear to be concomitant use with valproate, and exceeding the recommended initial dose of lamotrigine or the recommended rate of dose escalation. The risk appears to be greater in children[1,4,5] and has been estimated to be between 1 in 50 and 1 in 300. These skin reactions usually occur within 8 weeks of starting therapy with lamotrigine, but onset as early as the first day and as late as 2 years has been noted.[6] Following continuing reports of serious skin reactions in children UK recommended dosage regimens for children have been revised to further reduce the risk of such reactions.[7]

1. Mackay FJ, *et al.* Safety of long-term lamotrigine in epilepsy. *Epilepsia* 1997; **38:** 881–6.
2. Messenheimer J, *et al.* Safety review of adult clinical trial experience with lamotrigine. *Drug Safety* 1998; **18:** 281–96.
3. Committee on Safety of Medicines/Medicines Control Agency. Lamotrigine (Lamictal) and serious skin reactions. *Current Problems* 1996; **22:** 1.
4. Committee on Safety of Medicines/Medicines Control Agency. Lamotrigine (Lamictal): increased risk of serious skin reactions in children. *Current Problems* 1997; **23:** 8.
5. Mitchell P. Paediatric lamotrigine use hit by rash reports. *Lancet* 1997; **349:** 1080.
6. Adverse Drug Reactions Advisory Committee (ADRAC). Lamotrigine and severe skin reactions. *Aust Adverse Drug React Bull* 1997; **16:** 3.
7. Committee on Safety of Medicines/Medicines Control Agency. Lamotrigine (Lamictal): revised doses for children. *Current Problems* 2000; **26:** 3.

Overdosage. No serious toxicity was observed in a patient who deliberately took an overdose of 1.35 g of lamotrigine and was subsequently treated with gastric lavage and activated charcoal.[1] Symptoms at presentation one hour after ingestion had included nystagmus and muscle hypertonicity. ECG monitoring had revealed widening of the QRS interval. Low-grade fever, erythema, and periorbital oedema suggestive of a hypersensitivity syndrome developed in another patient who inadvertently received lamotrigine 2.7 g daily for 4 days.[2] The patient recovered following corticosteroid treatment and discontinuation of lamotrigine. Generalised tonic-clonic seizures, tremor, muscle weakness, ataxia, and hypertonia were reported[3] in a 2-year-old child following ingestion of 800 mg of lamotrigine. Symptoms resolved within 24 hours following treatment with gastric lavage and activated charcoal, midazolam, and fluids. Plasma-lamotrigine concentrations were at the high adult therapeutic range (3.8 µg per mL) with a slow elimination rate.

For a further review of the features and management of poisoning with some antiepileptics, including lamotrigine, see under Phenytoin, p.358.

1. Buckley NA, *et al.* Self-poisoning with lamotrigine. *Lancet* 1993; **342:** 1552–3.
2. Mylonakis E, *et al.* Lamotrigine overdose presenting as anticonvulsant hypersensitivity syndrome. *Ann Pharmacother* 1999; **33:** 557–9.
3. Briassoulis G, *et al.* Lamotrigine childhood overdose. *Pediatr Neurol* 1998; **19:** 239–42.

Precautions

Lamotrigine should be given with caution to patients with hepatic renal impairment. Patients receiving lamotrigine should be closely monitored and changes in hepatic, renal, and clotting functions looked for. They should be warned to see their doctor immediately if rashes or influenza-like symptoms associated with hypersensitivity develop. Withdrawal of lamotrigine should be considered if rash, fever, influenza-like symptoms, drowsiness, or worsening of seizure control occurs. Care is required when withdrawing lamotrigine therapy—see also under Uses and Administration, below. Abrupt withdrawal should be avoided unless serious skin reactions have occurred. To minimise the risk of developing serious skin reactions, dosage recommendations should not be exceeded. Particular care is needed in patients also receiving valproate—see under Interactions, below. Children's

The symbol † denotes a preparation no longer actively marketed

body-weight should be monitored and the dose reviewed if necessary.

Breast feeding. For comment on antiepileptic therapy and breast feeding, see under Pregnancy and Breast Feeding on p.340.

Driving. For a comment on antiepileptic drugs and driving, see p.340.

Intellectual impairment. Aggressive behaviour has been reported in intellectually impaired patients given lamotrigine.[1] Of 19 such patients given lamotrigine, aggressive behaviour developed in 9; the drug was discontinued in 5, and stopped but reintroduced in a further 2, together with psychiatric management. One patient responded to a reduction in lamotrigine dosage.

1. Beran RG, Gibson RJ. Aggressive behaviour in intellectually challenged patients with epilepsy treated with lamotrigine. *Epilepsia* 1998; **39:** 280–2.

Pregnancy. For comments on the management of epilepsy during pregnancy, see p.340. There appears to be little evidence of teratogenic potential for lamotrigine in *animal* studies to date, although there is a theoretical risk with lamotrigine because it is a folate antagonist.

Renal impairment. Results from a pharmacokinetic study[1] indicated that impaired renal function was likely to have little effect on plasma concentrations of lamotrigine. The drug is mainly cleared by metabolism and although the glucuronide metabolite accumulates it is inactive. Nevertheless, there is limited clinical experience with lamotrigine in such patients and caution was recommended.

1. Wootton R, *et al.* Comparison of the pharmacokinetics of lamotrigine in patients with chronic renal failure and healthy volunteers. *Br J Clin Pharmacol* 1997; **43:** 23–7.

Interactions

There are complex interactions between antiepileptics and toxicity may be enhanced without a corresponding increase in antiepileptic activity. Such interactions are very variable and unpredictable and plasma monitoring is often advisable with combination therapy. The metabolism of lamotrigine is enhanced by the enzyme inducers carbamazepine, phenytoin, phenobarbital, and primidone, and inhibited by valproate (see below).

Analgesics. Concomitant use of *paracetamol* affects the metabolic disposition of lamotrigine but the clinical significance of this interaction remains to be determined.[1] Paracetamol reduced the area under the plasma concentration-time curve for lamotrigine, reduced lamotrigine's half-life, and increased the percentage of lamotrigine recovered in the urine.

1. Depot M, *et al.* Kinetic effects of multiple oral doses of acetaminophen on a single oral dose of lamotrigine. *Clin Pharmacol Ther* 1990; **48:** 346–55.

Antibacterials. Concomitant use of *rifampicin* significantly increased the clearance of lamotrigine.[1] The total urinary excretion of lamotrigine and the amount excreted as glucuronide were significantly higher compared with placebo.

1. Ebert U, *et al.* Effects of rifampicin and cimetidine on pharmacokinetics and pharmacodynamics of lamotrigine in healthy subjects. *Eur J Clin Pharmacol* 2000; **56:** 299–304.

Antiepileptics. *Valproate* can inhibit the metabolism of lamotrigine resulting in increased concentrations of lamotrigine. This effect can be beneficial in the control of certain seizures, although careful monitoring is required as toxicity may occur. Disabling tremor occurred in 3 patients receiving such a combination which resolved when the dose of lamotrigine or valproate was reduced.[1]

Other reported symptoms of toxicity, that resolved on reduction of the lamotrigine dose, were sedation, ataxia, and fatigue.[2] Reversible encephalopathy has been reported[3] when sodium valproate was substituted for phenytoin in a patient also receiving lamotrigine, although her clinical condition had been satisfactory on this new regimen for several months. Symptoms improved when the doses of both valproate and lamotrigine were reduced. Pharmacokinetic studies[4,5] in healthy adults have attempted to elucidate the mechanism of the interaction between lamotrigine and valproate. The clearance of lamotrigine was found to be reduced, and the area under the curve and elimination half-life increased when valproate was administered concomitantly. Renal elimination was not affected and the investigators[4] suggested that there was hepatic competition for glucuronidation between valproate and lamotrigine. However, there was no substantial alteration in the linear kinetics of lamotrigine in the presence of therapeutic plasma concentrations of valproate.[5] Similar observations were made when lamotrigine was added to existing antiepileptic regimens in children,[6] although the clinical relevance of the influence of age on the pharmacokinetics remains to be determined. Both young age and concomitant administration of valproate are risk factors for lamotrigine-induced dermatological toxicity—see Effects on the Skin, above.

For details of dosage reductions required for lamotrigine when given together with valproate, see Uses and Administration, below.

Other antiepileptics also affect plasma concentrations of lamotrigine when given concomitantly. May *et al.*[7] confirmed that, while valproate inhibited its elimination, *carbamazepine, phenytoin,* or *phenobarbital* all markedly induced the elimination of lamotrigine. Others have confirmed a reduction in plasma-lamotrigine concentrations when given with phenytoin and other enzyme-inducing antiepileptics,[8] but analysis of results from another study[9] suggested that the increase in lamotrigine clearance by phenytoin and carbamazepine was of minimal clinical significance. Plasma-lamotrigine concentrations were also significantly reduced when administered concomitantly with mesuximide in 16 young patients (aged 9 to 19 years) with a variety of seizure types and syndromes.[10]

For the effect of lamotrigine on the pharmacokinetics of carbamazepine, see p.344. For a report of severe toxicity occurring with concomitant use of lamotrigine and *oxcarbazepine*, see p.354.

1. Reutens DC, *et al.* Disabling tremor after treatment with lamotrigine. *Lancet* 1993; **342:** 185–6.
2. Pisani F, *et al.* Interaction of lamotrigine with sodium valproate. *Lancet* 1993; **341:** 1224.
3. Hennessy MJ, Wiles CM. Lamotrigine encephalopathy. *Lancet* 1996; **347:** 974–5.
4. Yuen AWC, *et al.* Sodium valproate acutely inhibits lamotrigine metabolism. *Br J Clin Pharmacol* 1992; **33:** 511–13.
5. Anderson GD, *et al.* Bidirectional interaction of valproate and lamotrigine in healthy subjects. *Clin Pharmacol Ther* 1996; **60:** 145–56.
6. Vauzelle-Kervroëdan F, *et al.* Influence of concurrent antiepileptic medication on the pharmacokinetics of lamotrigine as add-on therapy in epileptic children. *Br J Clin Pharmacol* 1996; **41:** 325–30.
7. May TW, *et al.* Serum concentrations of lamotrigine in epileptic patients: the influence of dose and comedication. *Ther Drug Monit* 1996; **18:** 523–31.
8. Battino D, *et al.* Lamotrigine plasma concentrations in children and adults: influence of age and associated therapy. *Ther Drug Monit* 1997; **19:** 620–7.
9. Grasela TH, *et al.* Population pharmacokinetics of lamotrigine adjunctive therapy in adults with epilepsy. *J Clin Pharmacol* 1999; **39:** 373–84.
10. Besag FM, *et al.* Methsuximide lowers lamotrigine blood levels: a pharmacokinetic antiepileptic drug interaction. *Epilepsia* 2000; **41:** 624–7.

Pharmacokinetics

Lamotrigine is well absorbed from the gastrointestinal tract and peak plasma concentrations have been reported 2.5 hours after oral administration. It is widely distributed in the body and is reported to be about 55% bound to plasma protein. It is extensively metabolised in the liver and excreted almost entirely in urine, principally as a glucuronide conjugate. It slightly induces its own metabolism and the half-life at steady state is reported to be about 24 hours. Lamotrigine is distributed into breast milk.

The pharmacokinetics of lamotrigine are affected by the concomitant administration of other antiepileptics (see Interactions, above).

◊ General references.

1. Rambeck B, Wolf P. Lamotrigine clinical pharmacokinetics. *Clin Pharmacokinet* 1993; **25:** 433–43.
2. Elwes RDC, Binnie CD. Clinical pharmacokinetics of newer antiepileptic drugs: lamotrigine, vigabatrin, gabapentin and oxcarbazepine. *Clin Pharmacokinet* 1996; **30:** 403–15.

Therapeutic drug monitoring. In a study of newly diagnosed or poorly controlled epileptic patients[1] there appeared to be little relationship between plasma concentrations of lamotrigine and either its efficacy or the onset of adverse effects. Thus a 'target' range of concentrations for lamotrigine was considered to be inappropriate and routine therapeutic drug monitoring not to be useful.

1. Kilpatrick ES, *et al.* Concentration-effect and concentration-toxicity relations with lamotrigine: a prospective study. *Epilepsia* 1996; **37:** 534–8.

Renal impairment. See under Precautions, above.

Uses and Administration

Lamotrigine, a phenyltriazine compound, is an antiepileptic used as monotherapy and as an adjunct to treatment with other antiepileptics for partial seizures and primary and secondarily generalised tonic-clonic seizures. It is also used for seizures associated with the Lennox-Gastaut syndrome.

In the UK the initial **adult** dose for use as *monotherapy* is 25 mg once daily by mouth for 2 weeks followed by 50 mg once daily for 2 weeks; thereafter the dose is increased by a maximum of 50 to 100 mg every 1 to 2 weeks to usual maintenance doses of 100 to 200 mg daily, given as a single dose or in 2 divided doses. Some patients have required up to 500 mg daily.

The initial adult dose of lamotrigine for use as an *adjunct* to therapy with enzyme-inducing antiepileptics (but *not with valproate*) is 50 mg once daily for 2

weeks followed by 50 mg twice daily for 2 weeks; thereafter the daily dose is increased by a maximum of 100 mg every 1 to 2 weeks to usual maintenance doses of 200 to 400 mg daily given in 2 divided doses. Some patients have required up to 700 mg daily. In adults *taking valproate* the initial dose of lamotrigine is 25 mg every other day for 2 weeks followed by 25 mg once daily for 2 weeks; thereafter the daily dose is increased by a maximum of 25 to 50 mg every 1 to 2 weeks to usual maintenance doses of 100 to 200 mg daily given as a single dose or in 2 divided doses.

The doses above are permitted in the UK in **children** over 12 years of age; the use of lamotrigine as *monotherapy* is not recommended for children under 12 years of age. For children aged 2 to 12 years the initial dose of lamotrigine as an *adjunct* to therapy with enzyme-inducing antiepileptics (but *not with valproate*) is 0.6 mg per kg body-weight daily in 2 divided doses for 2 weeks followed by 1.2 mg per kg daily in 2 divided doses for 2 weeks; thereafter the dose is increased as necessary by a maximum of 1.2 mg per kg every 1 to 2 weeks; usual maintenance doses are 5 to 15 mg per kg daily in 2 divided doses. In children *taking valproate*, the initial dose of lamotrigine is 0.15 mg per kg once daily for 2 weeks followed by 0.3 mg per kg once daily for 2 weeks; thereafter the dose is increased by a maximum of 0.3 mg per kg every 1 to 2 weeks to usual maintenance doses of 1 to 5 mg per kg, which may be given once daily or in 2 divided doses. If the calculated dose for children lies between 2.5 and 5 mg then 5 mg may be given on alternate days for the first 2 weeks of therapy.

If the potential for interaction with adjunctive antiepileptics is unknown, treatment with lamotrigine should be initiated with lower doses such as those used with valproate.

Doses should be reduced by about 50% in patients with moderate hepatic impairment, and by about 75% in severe hepatic impairment.

As with other antiepileptics, withdrawal of lamotrigine therapy or transition to or from another type of antiepileptic therapy should be made gradually to avoid precipitating an increase in the frequency of seizures. For a discussion on whether or not to withdraw antiepileptic therapy in seizure-free patients, see p.338. The manufacturers recommend that the withdrawal of lamotrigine should be tapered over at least 2 weeks.

Bipolar disorder. In a multicentre placebo-controlled study involving 195 patients, lamotrigine 50 or 200 mg daily by mouth produced dose-related improvement in patients with bipolar disorder (p.271) experiencing a major depressive episode.[1] A review[2] of this controlled study as well as earlier case reports and small open trials concluded that lamotrigine is a promising option for the treatment of refractory bipolar disorder. Further data from randomised controlled trials[3-5] continue to suggest benefit.

1. Calabrese JR, *et al.* A double-blind placebo-controlled study of lamotrigine monotherapy in outpatients with bipolar I depression. *J Clin Psychiatry* 1999; **60:** 79–88.
2. Engle PM, Heck AM. Lamotrigine for the treatment of bipolar disorder. *Ann Pharmacother* 2000; **34:** 258–62.
3. Bowden CL, *et al.* Lamotrigine in the treatment of bipolar depression. *Eur Neuropsychopharmacol* 1999; **9** (suppl 4): S113–S117.
4. Calabrese JR, *et al.* A double-blind, placebo-controlled, prophylaxis study of lamotrigine in rapid-cycling bipolar disorder. *J Clin Psychiatry* 2000; **61:** 841–50.
5. Ichim L, *et al.* Lamotrigine compared with lithium in mania: a double-blind randomized controlled trial. *Ann Clin Psychiatry* 2000; **12:** 5–10.

Epilepsy. Lamotrigine is used in the treatment of epilepsy (p.338) refractory to standard antiepileptic therapy. It has been used for both partial and secondarily generalised tonic-clonic seizures.[1-6] About 30% of patients may experience a 50% reduction in seizure frequency and a relatively small percentage will become seizure-free.[4] Some patients may become sufficiently stabilised to allow withdrawal of concomitant antiepileptic therapy.[3] A meta-analysis[7] of randomised, placebo-controlled trials concluded that lamotrigine is effective in reducing the seizure frequency when added to current antiepileptic regimens in patients with refractory partial seizures. Lamotrigine has shown comparable efficacy to carbamazepine as monotherapy for partial seizures with or without secondary generalisation and primary generalised tonic-clonic seizures in newly diagnosed patients.[8] It also appears to be an effective adjunctive treatment in children with the Lennox-Gastaut syndrome.[9,10]

Lamotrigine has also been used for myoclonic seizures. There are anecdotal reports suggesting efficacy in patients with other types of seizures including atypical absence seizures, atonic seizures, primary generalised tonic-clonic seizures, and status epilepticus; preliminary studies of lamotrigine given with valproate for absence seizures[11] and infantile spasms[12] showed promising results. Lamotrigine as adjunctive therapy has been found to be effective and well tolerated in paediatric patients with refractory epilepsy including those with developmental impairment;[13] it was particularly effective in absence and atypical seizures in this open-label study. However, despite all these encouraging views concerning the role of lamotrigine, the authors of a follow-up study[14] were less optimistic. They followed up 124 patients who had participated in an open-label trial of lamotrigine as adjunctive therapy for refractory epilepsy 6 to 8 years earlier and concluded that lamotrigine had only marginal benefit on the long-term prognosis of severe refractory epilepsy.

1. Richens A, Yuen AWC. Overview of the clinical efficacy of lamotrigine. *Epilepsia* 1991; **32** (suppl 2): S13–S16.
2. Brodie MJ. Lamotrigine. *Lancet* 1992; **339:** 1397–1400.
3. Goa KL, *et al.* Lamotrigine: a review of its pharmacological properties and clinical efficacy in epilepsy. *Drugs* 1993; **46:** 152–76.
4. Brodie MJ. Drugs in focus: 10. Lamotrigine. *Prescribers' J* 1993; **33:** 212–16.
5. Gilman JT. Lamotrigine: an antiepileptic agent for the treatment of partial seizures. *Ann Pharmacother* 1995; **29:** 144–51.
6. Anonymous. Lamotrigine for epilepsy. *Med Lett Drugs Ther* 1995; **37:** 21–3.
7. Ramaratnam S, *et al.* Lamotrigine add-on for drug-resistant partial epilepsy (updated 30 May 2001). Available in The Cochrane Library, Issue 3. Oxford: Update Software; 2001.
8. Brodie MJ, *et al.* UK Lamotrigine/Carbamazepine Monotherapy Trial Group. Double-blind comparison of lamotrigine and carbamazepine in newly diagnosed epilepsy. *Lancet* 1995; **345:** 476–9.
9. Donaldson JA, *et al.* Lamotrigine adjunctive therapy in childhood epileptic encephalopathy (the Lennox Gastaut Syndrome). *Epilepsia* 1997; **38:** 68–73.
10. Motte J, *et al.* Lamotrigine for generalized seizures associated with the Lennox-Gastaut syndrome. *N Engl J Med* 1997; **337:** 1807–12. Correction. *ibid.* 1998; **339:** 851–2.
11. Ferrie CD, *et al.* Lamotrigine as an add-on drug in typical absence seizures. *Acta Neurol Scand* 1995; **91:** 200–202.
12. Veggiotti P, *et al.* Lamotrigine in infantile spasms. *Lancet* 1994; **344:** 1375–6.
13. Besag FMC, *et al.* Lamotrigine for the treatment of epilepsy in childhood. *J Pediatr* 1995; **127:** 991–7.
14. Walker MC, *et al.* Long term use of lamotrigine and vigabatrin in severe refractory epilepsy: audit of outcome. *BMJ* 1996; **313:** 1184–5.

Movement disorders. Symptomatic improvement and a trend towards decreased chorea was reported[1] with lamotrigine in a double-blind, placebo-controlled study of 64 patients with Huntington's chorea (p.650) with motor signs of less than 5 years' duration. There was, however, no clear evidence that lamotrigine retarded the progression of early Huntington disease over a period of 30 months.

1. Kremer B, *et al.* Influence of lamotrigine on progress of early Huntington disease: a randomized clinical trial. *Neurology* 1999; **53:** 1000–11.

Neuropathic pain. Lamotrigine was effective when used in conjunction with carbamazepine or phenytoin in the treatment of refractory trigeminal neuralgia[1] (p.8). It has also shown promise in the treatment of pain associated with HIV-related distal sensory neuropathy[2] (p.610). Case reports[3] and a placebo-controlled trial[4] have also indicated that lamotrigine may be effective in central post-stroke pain (p.5).

1. Zakrewska JM, *et al.* Lamotrigine (Lamictal) in refractory trigeminal neuralgia: results from a double-blind placebo controlled crossover study. *Pain* 1997; **73:** 223–30.
2. Simpson DM, *et al.* A placebo-controlled trial of lamotrigine for painful HIV-associated neuropathy. *Neurology* 2000; **54:** 2115–19.
3. Canavero S, Bonicalzi V. Lamotrigine control of central pain. *Pain* 1996; **68:** 179–81.
4. Vestergaard K, *et al.* Lamotrigine for central post-stroke pain: a randomized controlled trial. *Neurology* 2001; **56:** 184–90.

Preparations

Proprietary Preparations (details are given in Part 3)
Aust.: Lamictal; *Austral.:* Lamictal; *Belg.:* Lamictal; *Braz.:* Lamictal; *Canad.:* Lamictal; *Denm.:* Lamictal; *Fin.:* Lamictal; *Fr.:* Lamictal; *Ger.:* Lamictal; *Hong Kong:* Lamictal; *Irl.:* Lamictal; *Israel:* Lamictal; *Ital.:* Lamictal; *Mex.:* Lamictal; *Neth.:* Lamictal; *Norw.:* Lamictal; *NZ:* Lamictal; *Port.:* Lamictal; *S.Afr.:* Lamicitin; *Singapore:* Lamictal; *Spain:* Labileno; Lamictal; *Swed.:* Lamictal; *Switz.:* Lamictal; *Thai.:* Lamictal; *UK:* Lamictal; *USA:* Lamictal.

Levetiracetam (13816-h)

Levetiracetam *(BAN, USAN, rINN).*
S-Etiracetam; ucb-22059; ucb-L059. (S)-2-(2-Oxopyrrolidin-1-yl)butanamide.
$C_8H_{14}N_2O_2 = 170.2.$
CAS — 102767-28-2.

Adverse Effects and Precautions

The most commonly reported adverse effects associated with levetiracetam are somnolence, weakness, and dizziness. Anorexia, diarrhoea, dyspepsia, nausea, ataxia, headache, amnesia, depression, emotional lability, insomnia, aggression, nervousness, tremor, vertigo, diplopia, and rash may occur less frequently.

Levetiracetam should be used with caution in renal impairment; the manufacturer recommends dosage reduction in patients with reduced renal function or those undergoing haemodialysis. Renal function should also be assessed in patients with severe hepatic impairment, and the dose adjusted accordingly. Care is required when withdrawing levetiracetam therapy—see also under Uses and Administration, below.

Breast feeding. For comment on antiepileptic therapy and breast feeding, see under Pregnancy and Breast Feeding on p.340.

Driving. For a comment on antiepileptic drugs and driving, see p.340.

Pregnancy. For comments on the management of epilepsy during pregnancy, see p.340.

Pharmacokinetics

Levetiracetam is readily absorbed from the gastrointestinal tract and peak plasma concentrations are usually achieved within 1.3 hours of oral administration and steady-state achieved after 2 days. Levetiracetam is not extensively metabolised; approximately 25% of the dose is metabolised by hydroxylation and the metabolites are inactive. About 95% of a dose is excreted as unchanged drug and metabolites in the urine. Plasma protein binding is minimal. The plasma elimination half-life has been reported to be about 7 hours.

Uses and Administration

Levetiracetam is an analogue of piracetam (p.1652) used as adjunctive therapy in the treatment of partial seizures with or without secondary generalisation.

The daily dose of levetiracetam is given by mouth in two divided doses. The initial adult dose of levetiracetam is 1 g on the first day of treatment. Thereafter the daily dose may be increased in increments of 1 g every 2 to 4 weeks until effective antiepileptic control is achieved, up to a maximum dose of 3 g daily.

Reduced doses are recommended for patients with renal impairment. Suitable daily doses given in 2 divided doses are: 1 to 2 g for patients with a creatinine clearance of 50 to 79 mL per minute; 0.5 to 1.5 g for a clearance of 30 to 49 mL per minute; 0.5 to 1 g for a clearance of less than 30 mL per minute. In patients with severe liver impairment creatinine clearance may underestimate concomitant renal impairment, and the usual adult dose should be reduced by 50% in those with creatinine clearance of less than 70 mL per minute.

As with other antiepileptics, withdrawal of levetiracetam therapy or transition to or from another type of antiepileptic therapy should be made gradually to avoid precipitating an increase in the frequency of seizures. The manufacturers recommend reducing the daily dose by 1 g every 2 to 4 weeks. For a discussion on whether or not to withdraw antiepileptic therapy in seizure-free patients, see p.338.

◊ References.
1. Dooley M, Plosker GL. Levetiracetam: a review of its adjunctive use in the management of partial onset seizures. *Drugs* 2000; **60:** 871–93.
2. Chaisewikul R, *et al.* Levetiracetam add-on for drug-resistant localization related (partial) epilepsy (updated 28 February 2001). Available in The Cochrane Library; Issue 3. Oxford: Update Software; 2001.

Preparations

Proprietary Preparations (details are given in Part 3)
Irl.: Keppra; *UK:* Keppra; *USA:* Keppra.

Losigamone (11013-x)

Losigamone *(rINN).*
AO-33. (5R*)-5-[(αS*)-o-Chloro-α-hydroxybenzyl]-4-methoxy-2(5H)-furanone.
$C_{12}H_{11}ClO_4 = 254.7.$
CAS — 112856-44-7.

Profile

Losigamone is an antiepileptic under investigation as adjunctive therapy in the treatment of partial seizures.

◊ References
1. Bauer J, *et al.* Losigamone add-on therapy in partial epilepsy: a placebo-controlled study. *Acta Neurol Scand* 2001; **103:** 226–30.

Mephenytoin (6613-f)

Mephenytoin *(BAN, USAN, rINN).*
Mephenetoin; Methantoin; Methoin; NSC-34652; Phenantoin. 5-Ethyl-3-methyl-5-phenylhydantoin.
$C_{12}H_{14}N_2O_2 = 218.3.$
CAS — 50-12-4.
ATC — N03AB04.
Pharmacopoeias. In Aust. and US.

Profile

Mephenytoin is a hydantoin antiepileptic with actions similar to those of phenytoin (p.357), but it is more toxic. Because of its potential toxicity it is not one of the main drugs used in the treatment of epilepsy (p.338) and is given only to patients unresponsive to other treatment. Some of the side-effects of mephenytoin may be due to the metabolite, 5-ethyl-5-phenyl-

hydantoin (also termed nirvanol). Like phenytoin the rate of metabolism of mephenytoin is subject to genetic polymorphism.

Mephenytoin is given in an initial daily dose by mouth of 50 to 100 mg for one week; thereafter the daily dose is increased by 50 to 100 mg at weekly intervals until the optimum dose is reached, which is usually between 200 and 600 mg daily for an adult and 100 and 400 mg daily for a child; daily maintenance doses are usually taken in 3 divided doses.

Porphyria. Mephenytoin has been associated with acute attacks of porphyria and is considered unsafe in porphyric patients.

Preparations

USP 25: Mephenytoin Tablets.

Proprietary Preparations (details are given in Part 3)
Aust.: Epilan; *USA:* Mesantoin.

Mesuximide (6614-d)

Mesuximide *(BAN, rINN).*
Methsuximide; PM-396. N,2-Dimethyl-2-phenylsuccinimide.
$C_{12}H_{13}NO_2 = 203.2.$
CAS — 77-41-8.
ATC — N03AD03.
Pharmacopoeias. In US.

Pharmacopoeial description

USP 25: A white to greyish-white crystalline powder. Is odourless or has a slight odour. Soluble 1 in 350 of water, 1 in 3 of alcohol, 1 in less than 1 of chloroform, and 1 in 2 of ether. Store in airtight containers.

Profile

Mesuximide is a succinimide antiepileptic with actions similar to those of ethosuximide (p.348), but with some activity in complex partial seizures. It is thought to owe its activity to its major metabolite N-desmethylmesuximide. It is usually only given to patients unresponsive to other antiepileptic treatment.

The usual initial dosage is a single dose of 300 mg daily by mouth for the first week, and this is increased by 300 mg at weekly intervals to an optimum dosage, according to the patient's response. The suggested maximum daily dose is 1.2 g in divided doses.

Epilepsy. Mesuximide is used for absence seizures that are refractory to less toxic antiepileptics such as ethosuximide or valproate, which are the usual drugs to try (see p.338). Mesuximide has also been tried in complex partial seizures and myoclonic seizures.

References.
1. Tennison MB, *et al.* Methsuximide for intractable childhood seizures. *Pediatrics* 1991; **87:** 186–9.

Interactions. For the effect of mesuximide on lamotrigine, see p.352.

Porphyria. Mesuximide has been associated with acute attacks of porphyria and is considered unsafe in porphyric patients.

Preparations

USP 25: Methsuximide Capsules.

Proprietary Preparations (details are given in Part 3)
Aust.: Petinutin; *Canad.:* Celontin; *Ger.:* Petinutin; *Israel:* Celontin; *Neth.:* Celontin; *S.Afr.:* Celontin†; *Switz.:* Petinutin; *USA:* Celontin.

Methylphenobarbital (4050-w)

Methylphenobarbital *(BAN, rINN).*
Enphenemalum; Mephobarbital; Methylphenobarbitalum; Methylphenobarbitone; Phemitone. 5-Ethyl-1-methyl-5-phenylbarbituric acid.
$C_{13}H_{14}N_2O_3 = 246.3.$
CAS — 115-38-8.
ATC — N03AA01.
Pharmacopoeias. In Eur. (see p.vi) and US.

Pharmacopoeial description

Ph. Eur.: A white, crystalline powder or colourless crystals. Practically insoluble in water; very slightly soluble in dehydrated alcohol; slightly soluble in ether. It forms water-soluble compounds with alkali hydroxides and carbonates, and with ammonia.

USP 25: A white, odourless, crystalline powder. Slightly soluble in water, in alcohol, and in ether; soluble in chloroform and in solutions of fixed alkali hydroxides and carbonates. Its saturated solution in water is acid to litmus.

Dependence and Withdrawal, Adverse Effects, Treatment, and Precautions

As for Phenobarbital, p.355.

Interactions

As for Phenobarbital, p.355.

Pharmacokinetics

Methylphenobarbital is incompletely absorbed from the gastrointestinal tract. It is demethylated to phenobarbital in the liver.

The symbol † denotes a preparation no longer actively marketed

Uses and Administration

Methylphenobarbital is used similarly to phenobarbital (p.356) in the treatment of epilepsy (p.338). It is given in usual doses of 200 to 400 mg daily by mouth; up to 600 mg daily may be given if required. It has also been used as a sedative.

Preparations

BP 2001: Methylphenobarbital Tablets;
USP 25: Mephobarbital Tablets.

Proprietary Preparations (details are given in Part 3)
Austral.: Prominal; **Spain:** Prominal†; **UK:** Prominal†; **USA:** Mebaral.

Multi-ingredient: Belg.: Mathoine; **Ital.:** Dintoinale; Metinal-Idantoina; Metinal-Idantoina L; **Port.:** Comital L; **Spain:** Comital L†.

Oxcarbazepine (19623-a)

Oxcarbazepine (BAN, rINN).

GP-47680.   10,11-Dihydro-10-oxo-5H-dibenz[b,f]azepine-5-carboxamide.
$C_{15}H_{12}N_2O_2 = 252.3$.
CAS — 28721-07-5.
ATC — N03AF02.

Adverse Effects, Treatment, and Precautions

As for Carbamazepine, p.342.

Skin rashes occur less frequently with oxcarbazepine than with carbamazepine and a large proportion of patients with skin reactions to carbamazepine are able to tolerate oxcarbazepine. However, oxcarbazepine reduces plasma-sodium concentrations to a greater extent than carbamazepine.

Dosage reductions are recommended in renal impairment.

Breast feeding. For comment on antiepileptic therapy and breast feeding, see under Pregnancy and Breast Feeding on p.340.

Hyponatraemia. Hyponatraemia associated with oxcarbazepine appears to be more pronounced at clinical doses of oxcarbazepine than with carbamazepine. Hyponatraemia was reported[1] in 12 of 15 patients in whom oxcarbazepine was substituted for carbamazepine therapy. The fall in plasma-sodium concentrations appeared to be related to the dose of oxcarbazepine. In another report[2] hyponatraemia occurred in 23% of 350 patients whose serum-sodium concentrations were monitored. Most patients remain asymptomatic but some may experience drowsiness, increase in seizure frequency, and impaired consciousness.[3] It has been suggested that serum-sodium concentrations should be measured before the start of therapy but routine repeated determinations may be indicated only in elderly patients or if a high dosage is used.[4] Severe hyponatraemia has been reported[5] in a 12-year-old child during treatment with oxcarbazepine. On reviewing the case notes of 48 other children who had received oxcarbazepine in the same centre, 9 were found to have had hyponatraemia, and the authors suggested that sodium levels should be monitored in paediatric patients.

1. Pendlebury SC, et al. Hyponatraemia during oxcarbazepine therapy. Hum Toxicol 1989; **8:** 337–44.
2. Friis ML, et al. Therapeutic experiences with 947 epileptic outpatients in oxcarbazepine treatment. Acta Neurol Scand 1993; **87:** 224–7.
3. Steinhoff BJ, et al. Hyponatraemic coma under oxcarbazepine therapy. Epilepsy Res 1992; **11:** 67–70.
4. Källviäinen R, et al. Place of newer antiepileptic drugs in the treatment of epilepsy. Drugs 1993; **46:** 1009–24.
5. Borusiak P, et al. Hyponatremia induced by oxcarbazepine in children. Epilepsy Res 1998; **30:** 241–6.

Pregnancy. For comments on the management of epilepsy during pregnancy, see p.340.

Interactions

Plasma concentrations of the active monohydroxy metabolite of oxcarbazepine may be reduced by strong inducers of cytochrome P450 isoenzymes, such as carbamazepine, phenytoin, or phenobarbital. Oxcarbazepine and its active metabolite inhibit the cytochrome P450 isoenzyme CYP2C19, and in high doses may raise plasma concentrations of concomitantly administered phenobarbital or phenytoin. Oxcarbazepine and its metabolite also have the capacity to induce CYP3A4 and CYP3A5 with the possibility of reducing plasma concentrations of drugs such as carbamazepine, dihydropyridine calcium-channel blockers and oral contraceptives.

Antiepileptics. In a study[1] of epileptic patients receiving monotherapy the area under the concentration-time curve for *carbamazepine*, *phenytoin*, or *valproate* was unchanged when oxcarbazepine was added to treatment; only carbamazepine affected the pharmacokinetics of oxcarbazepine, producing a reduction in the area under the curve for the active metabolite hydroxycarbazepine. It was considered that there was unlikely to be any clinically relevant pharmacokinetic interaction if oxcarbazepine was used with any of these antiepileptics, including carbamazepine. However, increases in plasma-phenytoin concentration have been reported following use with oxcarbazepine (see p.360).

There is a case-report of severe toxicity occurring with concomitant use of oxcarbazepine and *lamotrigine*.[2]

1. McKee PJW, et al. A double-blind, placebo-controlled interaction study between oxcarbazepine and carbamazepine, sodium valproate and phenytoin in epileptic patients. Br J Clin Pharmacol 1994; **37:** 27–32.
2. Alving J. Case of severe acute intoxication with oxcarbazepine combined with lamotrigine. Epilepsia 1994; **35** (suppl 7): 72.

Sex hormones. The manufacturers state that oxcarbazepine may reduce the effectiveness of *oral contraceptives* when given concomitantly.

Pharmacokinetics

Oxcarbazepine is well absorbed from the gastrointestinal tract. It is widely distributed in the body and is reported to be about 40% bound to plasma protein. It is rapidly and extensively metabolised in the liver to the principal metabolite 10,11-dihydro-10-hydroxy-carbamazepine, which possesses antiepileptic activity. Oxcarbazepine is excreted in the urine mainly as metabolites; less than 1% is excreted as unchanged drug. The elimination half-life has been reported to be 1.0 to 2.5 hours for oxcarbazepine, and about 8 to 14 hours for the monohydroxy metabolite. Oxcarbazepine and its monohydroxy derivative cross the placental barrier and are distributed into breast milk.

◊ References.

1. Dickinson RG, et al. First dose and steady-state pharmacokinetics of oxcarbazepine and its 10-hydroxy metabolite. Eur J Clin Pharmacol 1989; **37:** 69–74.
2. Patsalos PN, et al. Protein binding of oxcarbazepine and its primary active metabolite, 10-hydroxycarbazepine, in patients with trigeminal neuralgia. Eur J Clin Pharmacol 1990; **39:** 413–15.
3. Kumps A, Wurth C. Oxcarbazepine disposition: preliminary observations in patients. Biopharm Drug Dispos 1990; **11:** 365–70.
4. van Heiningen PNM, et al. The influence of age on the pharmacokinetics of the antiepileptic agent oxcarbazepine. Clin Pharmacol Ther 1991; **50:** 410–19.
5. Elwes RDC, Binnie CD. Clinical pharmacokinetics of newer antiepileptic drugs: lamotrigine, vigabatrin, gabapentin and oxcarbazepine. Clin Pharmacokinet 1996; **30:** 403–15.

Uses and Administration

Oxcarbazepine is a derivative of carbamazepine (p.345) with similar actions. It is used as monotherapy or adjunctive therapy in the treatment of partial seizures with or without secondarily generalised tonic-clonic seizures. The initial dose for monotherapy and adjunctive therapy in adults is 600 mg daily by mouth, given in 2 divided doses. The dose may be increased thereafter, if necessary, in maximum increments of 600 mg daily at approximately weekly intervals until the desired clinical response has been achieved. Maintenance doses are usually in the range of 600 to 1200 mg daily or up to 2400 mg daily if given as adjunctive therapy or in refractory patients switched from other antiepileptics. The recommended initial dose for children over 6 years of age is 8 to 10 mg per kg body-weight by mouth daily, given in 2 divided doses. This may be increased as necessary in maximum increments of 10 mg per kg daily at approximately weekly intervals to a maximum dose of 46 mg per kg daily; usual maintenance doses are around 30 mg per kg daily. In the USA, similar dosage recommendations are given for adjunctive therapy in children over 4 years of age.

Initial doses for patients with renal impairment with a creatinine clearance of less than 30 mL per minute should be half the usual starting dose, increased at weekly intervals or longer.

As with other antiepileptics, withdrawal of oxcarbazepine therapy or transition to or from another type of antiepileptic therapy should be made gradually to avoid precipitating an increase in the frequency of seizures. For a discussion on whether or not to withdraw antiepileptic therapy in seizure-free patients, see p.338.

Epilepsy. Oxcarbazepine is used in the treatment of epilepsy (p.338) and may be a useful alternative in patients unable to tolerate carbamazepine.

The actions and uses of oxcarbazepine have been reviewed.[1-3] The efficacy of oxcarbazepine appears to be similar to that of carbamazepine and it may have a lower propensity to produce adverse effects on the CNS, and allergic reactions, although hyponatraemia is likely to be troublesome. Oxcarbazepine appears to induce hepatic enzymes to a lesser extent than carbamazepine[4,5] and may therefore produce fewer interactions. Oxcarbazepine has a different pharmacokinetic profile to that of carbamazepine and is reduced to a pharmacologically active 10-hydroxy metabolite.[1-3]

In a double-blind trial[6] involving newly diagnosed adult patients, oxcarbazepine was of similar efficacy and tolerability to valproate for partial or generalised tonic-clonic seizures. Oxcarbazepine was of similar efficacy to phenytoin, but was better tolerated in adults and children with newly diagnosed partial or generalised tonic-clonic seizures.[7,8] Further randomised controlled trials (and a small systematic review[9]) have also confirmed the efficacy and tolerability of oxcarbazepine as adjunctive therapy[9,10] or monotherapy[11] in refractory partial seizures in children and adults.

1. Grant SM, Faulds D. Oxcarbazepine: a review of its pharmacology and therapeutic potential in epilepsy, trigeminal neuralgia and affective disorders. Drugs 1992; **43:** 873–88.
2. Källviäinen R, et al. Place of newer antiepileptic drugs in the treatment of epilepsy. Drugs 1993; **46:** 1009–24.
3. Patsalos PN, Sander JWAS. Newer antiepileptic drugs: towards an improved risk-benefit ratio. Drug Safety 1994; **11:** 37–67.
4. Patsalos PN, et al. Dose dependent enzyme induction by oxcarbazepine? Eur J Clin Pharmacol 1990; **39:** 187–8.

5. Larkin JG, et al. Lack of enzyme induction with oxcarbazepine (600 mg daily) in healthy subjects. Br J Clin Pharmacol 1991; **31:** 65–71.
6. Christe W, et al. A double-blind controlled clinical trial: oxcarbazepine versus sodium valproate in adults with newly diagnosed epilepsy. Epilepsy Res 1997; **26:** 451–60.
7. Bill PA, et al. A double-blind controlled clinical trial of oxcarbazepine versus phenytoin in adults with previously untreated epilepsy. Epilepsy Res 1997; **27:** 195–204.
8. Guerreiro MM, et al. A double-blind controlled clinical trial of oxcarbazepine versus phenytoin in children and adolescents with epilepsy. Epilepsy Res 1997; **27:** 205–13.
9. Castillo S, et al. Oxcarbazepine add-on for drug-resistant partial epilepsy (updated 30 May 2001). Available in The Cochrane Library; Issue 3. Oxford: Update Software; 2001.
10. Glauser TA, et al. Adjunctive therapy with oxcarbazepine in children with partial seizures. Neurology 2000; **54:** 2237–44.
11. Beydoun A, et al. Oxcarbazepine monotherapy for partial-onset seizures: a multicenter, double-blind, clinical trial. Neurology 2000; **54:** 2245–51.

Preparations

Proprietary Preparations (details are given in Part 3)
Aust.: Trileptal; **Austral.:** Trileptal; **Braz.:** Trileptal; **Denm.:** Apydan; **Fin.:** Apydan; Trileptal; **Fr.:** Trileptal; **Hong Kong:** Trileptal; **Irl.:** Trileptal; **Israel:** Trileptin; **Ital.:** Trileptal; **Mex.:** Trileptal; **Neth.:** Trileptal; **S.Afr.:** Trileptal; **Switz.:** Trileptal; **UK:** Trileptal; **USA:** Trileptal.

Paramethadione (6615-n)

Paramethadione (BAN, rINN).

5-Ethyl-3,5-dimethyl-1,3-oxazolidine-2,4-dione.
$C_7H_{11}NO_3 = 157.2$.
CAS — 115-67-3.
ATC — N03AC01.

Profile

Paramethadione is an oxazolidinedione antiepileptic with actions similar to those of trimethadione (p.366). Because of its potential toxicity it was given only to patients unresponsive to other antiepileptics.

Porphyria. Paramethadione has been associated with acute attacks of porphyria and is considered unsafe in porphyric patients.

Phenacemide (6616-h)

Phenacemide (BAN, rINN).

Carbamidum Phenylaceticum. (Phenylacetyl)urea.
$C_9H_{10}N_2O_2 = 178.2$.
CAS — 63-98-9.
ATC — N03AX07.

Profile

Phenacemide is an acetylurea antiepileptic which is the straight-chain analogue of a hydantoin. It has been used in the treatment of epilepsy (p.338), especially in complex partial seizures; because of its potential toxicity it was given only to patients unresponsive to other antiepileptics.

Severe adverse effects reported with phenacemide have included psychoses and personality changes, blood disorders including aplastic anaemia, and liver and kidney damage; extreme caution has been advised in giving phenacemide to patients with a history of such disorders.

◊ Serum-creatinine concentrations should not be used as a measure of renal function in patients receiving phenacemide as it can increase creatinine concentrations in the absence of renal impairment.[1]

1. Cahen R, et al. Creatinine metabolism impairment by an anticonvulsant drug, phenacemide. Ann Pharmacother 1994; **28:** 49–51.

Preparations

Proprietary Preparations (details are given in Part 3)
USA: Phenurone†.

Pheneturide (6617-m)

Pheneturide (BAN, rINN).

Ethylphenacemide; S-46. (2-Phenylbutyryl)urea.
$C_{11}H_{14}N_2O_2 = 206.2$.
CAS — 90-49-3.
ATC — N03AX13.

Profile

Pheneturide is an acetylurea antiepileptic used in the treatment of epilepsy (p.338). It is given by mouth in usual daily doses of 300 to 600 mg in 2 to 3 divided doses, up to a maximum of 1.2 g daily.

Preparations

Proprietary Preparations (details are given in Part 3)
Belg.: Laburide; **Switz.:** Benuride†.

Phenobarbital (4060-I)

Phenobarbital (BAN, rINN).

Fenobarbital; Phenemalum; Phenobarbitalum; Phenobarbitone; Phenylethylbarbituric Acid; Phenylethylmalonylurea. 5-Ethyl-5-phenylbarbituric acid.

$C_{12}H_{12}N_2O_3 = 232.2$.

CAS — 50-06-6.

ATC — N03AA02.

Pharmacopoeias. In Chin., Eur. (see p.vi), Int., Jpn, Pol., and US.

Pharmacopoeial description

Ph. Eur.: A white, crystalline powder or colourless crystals. Very slightly soluble in water; freely soluble in alcohol; soluble in ether. It forms water-soluble compounds with alkali hydroxides and carbonates, and with ammonia.

USP 25: White, odourless, glistening, small crystals or a white crystalline powder. It may exhibit polymorphism. Soluble 1 in 1000 of water and 1 in 10 of alcohol; sparingly soluble in chloroform; soluble in ether and in solutions of fixed alkali hydroxides and carbonates. A saturated solution in water has a pH of about 5.

Phenobarbital Sodium (4061-y)

Phenobarbital Sodium (BANM, rINN).

Fenobarbital Sódico; Phenemalnatrium; Phenobarbitalum Natricum; Phenobarbitone Sodium; Sodium Phenylethylbarbiturate; Soluble Phenobarbitone. Sodium 5-ethyl-5-phenylbarbiturate.

$C_{12}H_{11}N_2NaO_3 = 254.2$.

CAS — 57-30-7.

Pharmacopoeias. In Chin., Eur. (see p.vi), Int., Pol., and US.

Phenobarbital sodium is incompatible with many other drugs and phenobarbital may be precipitated from mixtures containing phenobarbital sodium. This precipitation is dependent upon the concentration and the pH, and also on the presence of other solvents.

Pharmacopoeial description

Ph. Eur.: A white, hygroscopic, crystalline powder. Freely soluble in carbon dioxide-free water (a small amount may be insoluble); soluble in alcohol; practically insoluble in dichloromethane and in ether. A 10% solution in water has a pH not greater than 10.2. Store in airtight containers.

USP 25: Flaky crystals, or white crystalline granules, or a white powder. It is odourless and hygroscopic. Very soluble in water; soluble in alcohol; practically insoluble in chloroform and in ether. pH of a 10% solution in water is between 9.2 and 10.2. Solutions decompose on standing. Store in airtight containers.

Dependence and Withdrawal

As for the barbiturates (see Amobarbital, p.655).

Adverse Effects

The most frequent adverse effect following administration of phenobarbital is sedation, but this often becomes less marked with continued administration. Like some of the other antiepileptics, phenobarbital may produce subtle mood changes and impairment of cognition and memory that may not be apparent without testing. Depression may occur.

Prolonged administration may occasionally result in folate deficiency; rarely, megaloblastic anaemia has been reported. There is some evidence that phenobarbital interferes with vitamin D metabolism.

At high doses nystagmus and ataxia may occur and the typical barbiturate-induced respiratory depression may become severe. Overdosage can prove fatal; toxic effects include coma, severe respiratory and cardiovascular depression, with hypotension and shock leading to renal failure. Hypothermia may occur, with associated pyrexia during recovery. Skin blisters (bullae) reportedly occur in about 6% of patients with barbiturate overdose.

Sodium salts of barbiturates have a very high pH in solution, and necrosis has followed subcutaneous injection or extravasation. Intravenous injections can be hazardous and cause hypotension, shock, laryngospasm, and apnoea.

Hypersensitivity reactions occur in a small proportion of patients; skin reactions are reported in 1 to 3% of patients receiving phenobarbital, and are most commonly maculopapular, morbilliform, or scarlatiniform rashes. More severe reactions such as exfoliative dermatitis, Stevens-Johnson syndrome, and toxic epidermal necrolysis are extremely rare. Hepatitis and disturbances of liver function have been reported.

The symbol † denotes a preparation no longer actively marketed

Paradoxical excitement, restlessness, and confusion may sometimes occur in the elderly, and irritability and hyperactivity may occur in children.

Neonatal drug dependence and symptoms resembling vitamin K deficiency have been reported in infants born to mothers who received phenobarbital during pregnancy. Congenital malformations have been reported in children of women who received phenobarbital during pregnancy but the causal role of the drug is a matter of some debate.

Effects on the blood. For the effects of antiepileptics, including phenobarbital, on serum folate, see under Phenytoin, p.358.

Effects on bone. For the effects of antiepileptics including phenobarbital on bone and on calcium and vitamin D metabolism, see under Phenytoin, p.358.

Effects on connective tissue. The use of phenobarbital and primidone has been associated with the development of Dupuytren's contracture, frozen shoulder, Ledderhose's syndrome, Peyronie's disease, fibromas, and general joint pain.[1]

1. Mattson RH, et al. Barbiturate-related connective tissue disorders. Arch Intern Med 1989; **149:** 911–14.

Effects on the endocrine system. For mention of the effects of antiepileptics on *sexual function* in male epileptic patients, see under Phenytoin, p.358.

Barbiturates may reduce serum concentrations of *thyroid* hormones through enzyme induction—see under Interactions of Thyroxine [levothyroxine], p.1527.

Effects on the liver. For mention of the effects of phenobarbital on the liver, see under Phenytoin, p.358.

Effects on mental function. For a review of the effects of antiepileptic therapy including phenobarbital on *cognition*, see p.340.

DEPRESSION. Follow-up of 28 patients aged 6 to 16 who had received phenobarbital or carbamazepine for epilepsy indicated that the rate of major depression was significantly higher in those receiving phenobarbital.[1] Treatment with phenobarbital should be avoided particularly in patients with a personal or family history of an affective disorder and patients who do receive it should be monitored for symptoms of depression.

1. Brent DA, et al. Phenobarbital treatment and major depressive disorder in children with epilepsy: a naturalistic follow-up. Pediatrics 1990; **85:** 1086–91.

Hypersensitivity. An antiepileptic hypersensitivity syndrome, comprising fever, rash, and lymphadenopathy and less commonly lymphocytosis, and liver and other organ involvement, has been associated with some antiepileptic drugs including phenobarbital.[1,2] Some have estimated the incidence at 1 in 1000 to 1 in 10 000 new exposures to aromatic anticonvulsants,[1,2] but the true incidence is unknown due to variations in presentation and reporting. The syndrome occurs most frequently on first exposure to the drug, with initial symptoms starting anywhere between 1 and 8 weeks after exposure. In previously sensitised individuals the reaction may occur within 1 day of rechallenge. The potential for cross-reactivity between carbamazepine, phenobarbital, and phenytoin is approximately 75%, and patients who develop the syndrome, and their close relatives should be warned of the risk associated with use of these antiepileptics.[1]

1. Knowles SR, et al. Anticonvulsant hypersensitivity syndrome: incidence, prevention and management. Drug Safety 1999; **21:** 489–501.
2. Bessmertny O, et al. Antiepileptic hypersensitivity syndrome in children. Ann Pharmacother 2001; **35:** 533–8.

Treatment of Adverse Effects

Following an overdose of a barbiturate, gastric lavage may be considered if undertaken within 1 to 2 hours or if the patient is unconscious. Repeated doses of activated charcoal should be given by mouth with the aim not only of preventing absorption but also of aiding elimination. The prime objectives of management are then intensive symptomatic and supportive therapy with particular attention being paid to the maintenance of cardiovascular, respiratory, and renal functions and to the maintenance of the electrolyte balance.

Charcoal haemoperfusion may be considered for patients with severe refractory poisoning; other methods aimed at the active removal of a barbiturate with a long elimination half-life such as phenobarbital include forced diuresis, haemodialysis, and peritoneal dialysis, but the hazards of such procedures are generally considered to outweigh any purported benefits.

Precautions

Phenobarbital and other barbiturates should be used with care in children and in elderly or debilitated patients, in those in acute pain, and in those with depressive disorders. Also they should be given cautiously to patients with impaired hepatic, renal, or respiratory function and may be contra-indicated when the impairment is severe.

Care is required when withdrawing phenobarbital therapy—see also Uses and Administration, below.

Phenobarbital and other barbiturates cause drowsiness and patients receiving them, if affected, should not take charge of vehicles or machinery where loss of attention could cause accidents.

Breast feeding. For comment on antiepileptic therapy and breast feeding, see under Pregnancy and Breast Feeding on p.340.

Phenobarbital given to the mother may cause neonatal sedation, and breast feeding should be avoided.

Driving. For a comment on antiepileptic drugs and driving, see p.340.

Neonates. Care should be taken when giving phenobarbital orally as the elixir to neonates because regular dosing could result in alcohol toxicity [the BP 2001 formulation contains 38% v/v alcohol].[1] Aqueous preparations are more readily made using the sodium salt than the acid.[2]

1. Colquhoun-Flannery W, Wheeler R. Treating neonatal jaundice with phenobarbitone: the inadvertent administration of significant doses of ethyl alcohol. Arch Dis Child 1992; **67:** 152.
2. Leach F. Treating neonatal jaundice with phenobarbitone: the inadvertent administration of significant doses of ethyl alcohol. Arch Dis Child 1992; **67:** 152.

Porphyria. Phenobarbital has been associated with acute attacks of porphyria and is considered unsafe in porphyric patients.

Pregnancy. For comments on the management of epilepsy during pregnancy, see p.340.

Congenital craniofacial and digital abnormalities and, less commonly, cleft lip and palate have been described with antiepileptics including phenobarbital. In utero exposure to phenobarbital might result in neonatal sedation and drug dependence and also in neonatal bleeding.

Interactions

There are complex interactions between antiepileptics, and toxicity may be enhanced without a corresponding increase in antiepileptic activity. Such interactions are very variable and unpredictable and plasma monitoring is often advisable with combination therapy. Valproate and phenytoin have been reported to cause rises in phenobarbital (and primidone) concentrations in plasma.

The effects of phenobarbital and other barbiturates are enhanced by the concurrent administration of other CNS depressants including alcohol.

Phenobarbital and other barbiturates may reduce the activity of many drugs by increasing the rate of metabolism through induction of drug-metabolising enzymes in liver microsomes.

Analgesics. Administration of *dextropropoxyphene* 65 mg three times daily to 4 epileptic patients stabilised on phenobarbital therapy resulted in increases in serum-phenobarbital concentration ranging from 8 to 29% but the increase was not considered of major importance in the light of the normally accepted therapeutic range for phenobarbital.[1]

For the effect of phenobarbital on *methadone* and *pethidine*, see p.53 and p.76, respectively.

1. Hansen BS, et al. Influence of dextropropoxyphene on steady state serum levels and protein binding of three anti-epileptic drugs in man. Acta Neurol Scand 1980; **61:** 357–67.

Antiarrhythmics. For the effect of phenobarbital on *disopyramide*, *lignocaine [lidocaine]* and *quinidine*, see p.879, p.1314, and p.965, respectively.

Antibacterials. Serum concentrations of phenytoin and phenobarbital in a previously stabilised patient were increased when he took *chloramphenicol* concomitantly.[1] Subsequent monitoring revealed a similar effect when chloramphenicol was taken with phenobarbital alone. In turn, phenobarbital may affect serum concentrations of chloramphenicol (see p.180).

Barbiturates such as phenobarbital and primidone may enhance the metabolism of *doxycycline*.[2]

1. Koup JR, et al. Interaction of chloramphenicol with phenytoin and phenobarbital. Clin Pharmacol Ther 1978; **24:** 571–5.
2. Neuvonen PJ, et al. Effect of antiepileptic drugs on the elimination of various tetracycline derivatives. Eur J Clin Pharmacol 1975; **9:** 147–54.

Anticoagulants. For the effect of barbiturates such as phenobarbital and primidone on warfarin, see p.995.

Antidepressants. As with all antiepileptics, antidepressants may antagonise the antiepileptic activity of phenobarbital by lowering the convulsive threshold.

Hypericum has been shown to induce several drug metabolising enzymes (see p.290) and consequently it might reduce the blood concentrations of phenobarbital leading to an increased risk of seizure.[1]

For the effect of phenobarbital on antidepressants, see Mianserin (p.298) and under Fluoxetine (p.287).

Inhibition of drug-metabolising enzymes by MAOIs may enhance the effects of barbiturates.

1. Committee on Safety of Medicines/Medicines Control Agency. Reminder: St John's wort (Hypericum perforatum) interactions. *Current Problems* 2000; **26:** 6–7.

Antiepileptics. Interactions may occur if phenobarbital is given with other antiepileptics, of which probably the most significant is the interaction with *valproate*. Valproate results in an increase in plasma-phenobarbital concentration that has been reported to range from 17 to 48%,[1] and it may be necessary to reduce the dose of phenobarbital in some patients.[1,2] The mechanism for the increase appears to be inhibition of the metabolism of phenobarbital, resulting in reduced clearance;[2,3] valproate appears to inhibit both the direct *N*-glucosidation of phenobarbital and the *O*-glucuronidation of *p*-hydroxyphenobarbital.[4] However, it is worthy of note that phenobarbital reciprocally increases the clearance of valproate, thus potentially requiring the valproate dose to be adjusted too.[5]

A similarly complex interaction exists between phenobarbital and *phenytoin*. Phenytoin may cause a rise in plasma concentrations of phenobarbital in some patients[6] since the two drugs compete for metabolism by the same enzyme system, but other evidence suggests that where this occurs it is rarely of significant magnitude.[7] Similarly, although phenobarbital induces the metabolism of phenytoin it is also, as stated, a competitive inhibitor and in practice the two effects appear to balance out, with rarely any need for dose adjustment.[7-9] However, dosage adjustment of phenobarbital may be crucial for some patients.[10] Measurement of serum concentrations of phenytoin and phenobarbital in one patient[10] showed that, in her case, large increases in serum-phenobarbital concentrations resulted from concomitant administration of phenytoin; the increases were concentration-dependent.

The GABA-agonist, *progabide* has also been reported to cause a significant increase in phenobarbital concentrations when the two were given together to healthy subjects,[11] and the possibility exists that dosage adjustment might be necessary if progabide were added to phenobarbital therapy.

Neurotoxicity, attributed to an increase in plasma concentrations of phenobarbital, has been observed[12] in one patient receiving phenobarbital and sodium valproate when *felbamate* was added to treatment. The dosage of phenobarbital had already been reduced before treatment with felbamate was started. Data from a pharmacokinetic study[13] indicated that the interaction may result from the inhibition of phenobarbital hydroxylation by felbamate.

Vigabatrin has been reported to lower plasma concentrations of phenobarbital in some patients,[14] although dosage changes were not necessary in these patients.

For the effect of phenobarbital on the metabolism of other antiepileptics, see under Carbamazepine, p.344, Clonazepam, p.347, Ethosuximide, p.348, and Lamotrigine, p.352.

1. Richens A, Ahmad S. Controlled trial of sodium valproate in severe epilepsy. *BMJ* 1975; **4:** 255–6.
2. Patel IH, *et al.* Phenobarbital-valproic acid interaction. *Clin Pharmacol Ther* 1980; **27:** 515–21.
3. Kapetanović IM, *et al.* Mechanism of valproate-phenobarbital interaction in epileptic patients. *Clin Pharmacol Ther* 1981; **29:** 480–6.
4. Bernus I, *et al.* Inhibition of phenobarbitone N-glucosidation by valproate. *Br J Clin Pharmacol* 1994; **38:** 411–16.
5. Perucca E, *et al.* Disposition of sodium valproate in epileptic patients. *Br J Clin Pharmacol* 1978; **5:** 495–9.
6. Morselli PL, *et al.* Interaction between phenobarbital and diphenylhydantoin in animals and in epileptic patients. *Ann N Y Acad Sci* 1971; **179:** 88–107.
7. Eadie MJ, *et al.* Factors influencing plasma phenobarbitone levels in epileptic patients. *Br J Clin Pharmacol* 1977; **4:** 541–7.
8. Cucinell SA, *et al.* Drug interactions in man: lowering effect of phenobarbital on plasma levels of bishydroxycoumarin (Dicumarol) and diphenylhydantoin (Dilantin). *Clin Pharmacol Ther* 1965; **6:** 420–9.
9. Booker HE, *et al.* Concurrent administration of phenobarbital and diphenylhydantoin: lack of an interference effect. *Neurology* 1971; **21:** 383–5.
10. Kuranari M, *et al.* Effect of phenytoin on phenobarbital pharmacokinetics in a patient with epilepsy. *Ann Pharmacother* 1995; **29:** 83–4.
11. Bianchetti G, *et al.* Pharmacokinetic interactions of progabide with other antiepileptic drugs. *Epilepsia* 1987; **28:** 68–73.
12. Gidal BE, Zupanc ML. Potential pharmacokinetic interaction between felbamate and phenobarbital. *Ann Pharmacother* 1994; **28:** 455–8.
13. Reidenberg P, *et al.* Effects of felbamate on the pharmacokinetics of phenobarbital. *Clin Pharmacol Ther* 1995; **58:** 279–87.
14. Browne TR, *et al.* A multicentre study of vigabatrin for drug-resistant epilepsy. *Br J Clin Pharmacol* 1989; **27** (suppl): 95S–100S.

Antifungals. For the effect of phenobarbital on griseofulvin, see p.386, and on itraconazole, see p.388.

Antiprotozoals. For the effect of phenobarbital on metronidazole, see p.595.

Antipsychotics. As with all antiepileptics, antipsychotics may antagonise the antiepileptic activity of phenobarbital by lowering the convulsive threshold.

For the effect of phenobarbital on antipsychotics, see under Chlorpromazine, p.664.

Antivirals. For the possible effect of phenobarbital on HIV-protease inhibitors, see p.626.

Beta blockers. For the effect of barbiturates on beta blockers, see under Anxiolytics and Antipsychotics, p.847.

Calcium-channel blockers. For the effect of phenobarbital on dihydropyridine calcium-channel blockers, see under Nifedipine, p.942, and on verapamil, see p.990.

Cardiac glycosides. Phenobarbital may greatly accelerate the metabolism of digitoxin (p.869).

Ciclosporin. For the effect of phenobarbital on ciclosporin, see p.521.

Corticosteroids. For the effect of phenobarbital on corticosteroids, see p.1043.

Diuretics. Serum-phenobarbital concentrations were raised in 8 of 10 epileptic patients taking phenobarbital and additional antiepileptics when given *frusemide [furosemide]* 40 mg three times daily for 4 weeks.[1] This might have been the cause of drowsiness in 5 of 14 patients, 3 of whom had to discontinue frusemide [furosemide].

1. Ahmad S, *et al.* Controlled trial of frusemide as an antiepileptic drug in focal epilepsy. *Br J Clin Pharmacol* 1976; **3:** 621–5.

Sex hormones. For the effect of phenobarbital on sex hormones in oral contraceptives, see p.1459.

Theophylline. For the effect of phenobarbital on theophylline, see p.780.

Thyroxine [levothyroxine]. For the effects of barbiturates on thyroxine [levothyroxine], see p.1527.

Vaccines. *Influenza* vaccination can cause prolonged rises in serum-phenobarbital concentrations in some patients.[1]

1. Jann MW, Fidone GS. Effect of influenza vaccine on serum anti-convulsant concentrations. *Clin Pharm* 1986; **5:** 817–20.

Vitamins. *Pyridoxine* reduced serum-phenobarbital concentrations in 5 patients.[1] Plasma concentrations of phenobarbital and primidone are possibly reduced by *folic acid* and *folinic acid*. For the effect of antiepileptics, including phenobarbital, on *vitamin D* concentrations, see Effects on Bone under the Adverse Effects of Phenytoin, p.358.

1. Hansson O, Sillanpaa M. Pyridoxine and serum concentration of phenytoin and phenobarbitone. *Lancet* 1976; **i:** 256.

Pharmacokinetics

Like other barbiturates phenobarbital is readily absorbed from the gastrointestinal tract, although it is relatively lipid-insoluble and may require an hour or longer to achieve effective concentrations.

Phenobarbital is about 45% bound to plasma proteins and is only partly metabolised in the liver. About 25% of a dose is excreted in the urine unchanged at normal urinary pH. The plasma half-life is about 90 to 100 hours in adults but is greatly prolonged in neonates, and shorter (about 65 to 70 hours) in children. There is considerable interindividual variation in phenobarbital kinetics.

Monitoring of plasma concentrations has been performed as an aid in assessing control and the therapeutic range of plasma-phenobarbital is usually quoted as being 15 to 40 μg per mL (65 to 170 μmol per litre).

Phenobarbital crosses the placental barrier and is distributed into breast milk.

The pharmacokinetics of phenobarbital are affected by the concomitant administration of other antiepileptics (see under Interactions, above).

Uses and Administration

Phenobarbital is a barbiturate that may be used as an antiepileptic to control partial and generalised tonic-clonic seizures.

The dose should be adjusted to the needs of the individual patient to achieve adequate control of seizures; this usually requires plasma concentrations of 15 to 40 μg per mL (65 to 170 μmol per litre). The usual dose by mouth is 60 to 180 mg daily, taken at night, and a suggested dose for children is up to 8 mg per kg body-weight daily.

Phenobarbital sodium may be given parenterally as part of the emergency management of acute seizures. Doses of 200 mg have been given by intramuscular or subcutaneous injection to adults, repeated after 6 hours if necessary. Children may be given 15 mg per kg body-weight intramuscularly as a loading dose, which may be followed by 5 mg per kg daily by

mouth in divided doses if appropriate. Doubts have been expressed about the efficacy of the intramuscular route owing to the delay in achieving adequate blood concentrations, and the subcutaneous route may cause tissue necrosis.

For the control of status epilepticus in adults, doses of 10 mg per kg may be given intravenously. Injections for intravenous administration should be diluted 1 in 10 and given at a rate not exceeding 100 mg per minute.

As with other antiepileptics, withdrawal of phenobarbital therapy or transition to or from another type of antiepileptic therapy should be made gradually to avoid precipitating an increase in the frequency of seizures. For a discussion on whether or not to withdraw antiepileptic therapy in seizure-free patients, see p.338.

Phenobarbital has also been used as a hypnotic and sedative but drugs such as the benzodiazepines are preferred.

Phenobarbital stimulates the enzymes in hepatic microsomes responsible for the metabolism of some drugs and normal body constituents including bilirubin, and for this reason it has been used to reduce hyperbilirubinaemia in neonatal jaundice.

Phenobarbital magnesium and phenobarbital diethylamine have also been used.

Alcohol withdrawal syndrome. Phenobarbital is used in some centres for the management of alcohol withdrawal syndrome (p.1131), but has a lower safety profile than benzodiazepines (the drugs of choice) and creates the potential for multiple drug interactions. Additionally, a lack of well-defined studies make its role difficult to assess.[1]

1. Rodgers JE, Crouch MA. Phenobarbital for alcohol withdrawal syndrome. *Am J Health-Syst Pharm* 1999; **56:** 175–8.

Cerebral malaria. Phenobarbital is used to prevent convulsions in patients with cerebral malaria (p.428). In an early study[1] a single intramuscular injection of phenobarbital sodium 3.5 mg per kg body-weight, or 200 mg in patients over 60 kg was effective. Since then a dose of 10 to 15 mg per kg has been suggested.[2] Although a single intramuscular dose of phenobarbital 20 mg per kg markedly reduced seizure frequency in young children with cerebral malaria, it was also associated with a doubling of mortality.[3] The frequency of respiratory arrest was higher in the phenobarbital group than in controls given placebo, and mortality was greatly increased in those given phenobarbital who required 3 or more doses of diazepam.[3] The optimal dose, particularly in children, still awaits confirmation.

1. White NJ, *et al.* Single dose phenobarbitone prevents convulsions in cerebral malaria. *Lancet* 1988; **ii:** 64–6.
2. Gilles HM. *Management of severe and complicated malaria.* Geneva: WHO, 1991.
3. Crawley J, *et al.* Effect of phenobarbitone on seizure frequency and mortality in childhood cerebral malaria: a randomized, controlled intervention study. *Lancet* 2000; **355:** 701–6.

Epilepsy. Phenobarbital is used in the treatment of epilepsy (p.338) for partial seizures with or without secondary generalisation and for primary generalised tonic-clonic seizures. It may also be tried for atypical absence, atonic, and tonic seizures but is not effective in absence seizures. However, the usefulness of phenobarbital is limited by problems of sedation in adults and paradoxical excitement in children. There is also concern about its effects on behaviour and cognition in children. Phenobarbital is therefore usually reserved for use in cases unresponsive to other antiepileptics, although some have suggested that its low cost and broad efficacy make it a suitable first-line drug in developing countries.

References.

1. Mattson RH, *et al.* Comparison of carbamazepine, phenobarbital, phenytoin, and primidone in partial and secondarily generalised tonic-clonic seizures. *N Engl J Med* 1985; **313:** 145–51.
2. Heller AJ, *et al.* Phenobarbitone, phenytoin, carbamazepine, or sodium valproate for newly diagnosed adult epilepsy: a randomised comparative monotherapy trial. *J Neurol Neurosurg Psychiatry* 1995; **58:** 44–50.
3. de Silva M, *et al.* Randomised comparative monotherapy trial of phenobarbitone, phenytoin, carbamazepine, or sodium valproate for newly diagnosed childhood epilepsy. *Lancet* 1996; **347:** 709–13.
4. Pal DK, *et al.* Randomised controlled trial to assess acceptability of phenobarbital for childhood epilepsy in rural India. *Lancet* 1998; **351:** 19–23.

Febrile convulsions. Phenobarbital has been used prophylactically in children thought to be at risk of recurrence of febrile convulsions (p.341), but routine use of antiepileptics is no longer recommended.

References.

1. Newton RW. Randomised controlled trials of phenobarbitone and valproate in febrile convulsions. *Arch Dis Child* 1988; **63:** 1189–91.
2. Farwell JR, *et al.* Phenobarbital for febrile seizures: effects on intelligence and on seizure recurrence. *N Engl J Med* 1990; **322:** 364–9. Correction. *ibid.* 1992; **326:** 144.

Neonatal intraventricular haemorrhage. Phenobarbital is one of several drugs that has been tried to prevent the development of neonatal intraventricular haemorrhage (p.723). Initial studies[1-3] of antenatal administration to the mother were promising, but a larger randomised study[4] in 610 women failed to show any effect of antenatal phenobarbital on incidence or severity of intraventricular haemorrhage. Meta-analysis[5] of these and other studies concluded that administration of phenobarbital before preterm birth cannot be recommended for routine clinical practice; strategies for future trials were suggested to improve methodology. Studies of administration to neonates have also shown inconsistent results. A meta-analysis[6] of studies in which phenobarbital was given to preterm neonates as prophylaxis to prevent intraventricular haemorrhage concluded that such postnatal administration cannot be recommended and is associated with an increased need for mechanical ventilation.

1. Kaempf JW, et al. Antenatal phenobarbital for the prevention of periventricular and intraventricular hemorrhage: a double-blind, randomized, placebo-controlled, multihospital trial. *J Pediatr* 1990; **117**: 933–8.
2. Barnes ER, Thompson DF. Antenatal phenobarbital to prevent or minimize intraventricular hemorrhage in the low-birthweight neonate. *Ann Pharmacother* 1993; **27**: 49–52.
3. Thorp JA, et al. Antepartum vitamin K and phenobarbital for preventing intraventricular hemorrhage in the premature newborn: a randomized, double-blind, placebo-controlled trial. *Obstet Gynecol* 1994; **83**: 70–6.
4. Shankaran S, et al. The effect of antenatal phenobarbital therapy on neonatal intracranial hemorrhage in preterm infants. *N Engl J Med* 1997; **337**: 466–71.
5. Crowther CA, Henderson-Smart DJ, et al. Phenobarbital prior to preterm birth for preventing neonatal periventricular haemorrhage (updated 28 February 2001). Available in The Cochrane Library; Issue 3. Oxford: Update Software; 2001.
6. Whitelaw A. Postnatal phenobarbitone for the prevention of intraventricular hemorrhage in preterm infants (updated 13 February 2001). Available in The Cochrane Library; Issue 3. Oxford: Update Software; 2001.

Neonatal opioid dependence. For reference to the use of phenobarbital for the treatment of neonates with opioid abstinence syndrome, see p.67.

Neonatal seizures. Some consider phenobarbital to be the mainstay of treatment for all types of neonatal seizures (p.342). In a study[1] in 120 neonates with clinical seizure activity of varying aetiology, 48 were controlled by an initial intravenous loading dose of phenobarbital 15 to 20 mg per kg body-weight over 10 to 15 minutes, and a further 37 were controlled by sequential bolus doses of phenobarbital 5 to 10 mg per kg every 20 to 30 minutes up to a serum concentration of 40 μg per mL. Of the remaining 35 neonates only 7 responded when the serum-phenobarbital concentration was increased to 100 μg per mL, 13 required addition of a second antiepileptic (phenytoin or lorazepam) and 4 were controlled by addition of a third drug. Phenobarbital alone can effectively control seizures in the majority of neonates with recurrent seizure activity.

Phenobarbital administered prophylactically as a single dose of about 40 mg per kg body-weight intravenously over one hour has also been shown to be effective in reducing the incidence of seizures in 15 infants with severe perinatal asphyxia compared with a control group who only received phenobarbital if there was clinical evidence of seizures.[2] Subsequent follow-up over 3 years suggested that prophylactic phenobarbital might also improve later neurological outcome.[2]

1. Gilman JT, et al. Rapid sequential phenobarbital treatment of neonatal seizures. *Pediatrics* 1989; **83**: 674–8.
2. Hall RT, et al. High-dose phenobarbital therapy in term newborn infants with severe perinatal asphyxia: a randomized, prospective study with three-year follow-up. *J Pediatr* 1998; **132**: 345–8.

Status epilepticus. Phenobarbital given intravenously is an alternative to intravenous phenytoin in the management of status epilepticus (p.341) to prevent the recurrence of seizures once they have been brought under control with a benzodiazepine. Phenobarbital should not be used in patients who have recently received oral phenobarbital or primidone.

One study[1] suggested that phenobarbital might be at least as effective, safe, and practical as diazepam with phenytoin for the initial treatment of convulsive status epilepticus.

1. Shaner DM, et al. Treatment of status epilepticus: a prospective comparison of diazepam and phenytoin versus phenobarbital and optional phenytoin. *Neurology* 1988; **38**: 202–7.

Preparations

BP 2001: Phenobarbital Elixir; Phenobarbital Injection; Phenobarbital Sodium Tablets; Phenobarbital Tablets;
USP 25: Phenobarbital Elixir; Phenobarbital Sodium for Injection; Phenobarbital Sodium Injection; Phenobarbital Tablets; Theophylline, Ephedrine Hydrochloride, and Phenobarbital Tablets.

Proprietary Preparations (details are given in Part 3)
Belg.: Gardenal; **Braz.:** Edhanol; Fenocris; Gardenal; **Denm.:** Fenemal; **Fr.:** Aparoxal; Gardenal; Kaneuron; **Ger.:** Lepinal; Lepinaletten; Luminal; Luminaletten; Phenaemal; Phenaemaletten; **Hong Kong:** Gardenal; **Israel:** Luminal; **Ital.:** Comizial; Gardenale; Luminale; Luminaletten; Neurobiol; **Mex.:** Alepsal; Fenocriz; Sevenal; Sevenaleta; **Norw.:** Fenemal; **NZ:** Gardenal; **Port.:** Bialminal; Luminal; Luminaletas; **S.Afr.:** Gardenal; Lethyl; Sedabarb; **Spain:** Gardenal; Gratusminal; Luminal; Luminaletas; **Swed.:** Fenemal; **Switz.:** Aphenylbarbit; Luminal; **Thai.:** Gardenal; Phenotal; **UK:** Luminal; **USA:** Luminal; Solfoton.

Multi-ingredient: **Belg.:** Epipropane; Spasmosedine†; Vethoine; **Braz.:** Bromosedan; Espasmalgon; Filinasma; Gamibetal Complex; Gratusminal; Piptalake P; Vagostesyl; Gardenale† **Canad.:** Bellergal; Dilantin with Phenobarbitol†; Donnatal; Phenaphen with Codeine; Tedral†; **Fr.:** Alepsal; Anxoral; Atrium†; Dinacode; Enure-

tine†; Natisedine†; Neurocalcium; Nuidor†; Ortenal†; Prenoxan au Phenobarbital†; Sedatonyl†; Sedibaine†; Spasmidenal; Sympaneurol†; Ve ricardine; **Hung.:** Triospan; **Israel:** Pacetal; Philinal; **Ital.:** Bellergil†; Gamibetal Complex; Metinal-Idantoina L; **Port.:** Anti-Asmatico; Comital L; Cosmaxil†; Fluidin Antiasmatico; Fluidin Nocturno†; Hidantina Composta; Prelus†; **S.Afr.:** Adco-Phenobarbitone Vitalet; Analgex-SA; Bellatard; Bellavern†; Bellergal†; Depain Plus†; Donnatal; Garoin†; Menoflush + ¼†; Millerspas; Pedriachol; Propain Forte; Tedral†; Tropax†; **Spain:** Comital L†; Disfil; Distovagal†; Epilantin; Redutona; Solufilina Sedante†; Winasma; **Switz.:** Atrium†; Bellergal; **Thai.:** Bellergal; Benera; Donnatal; Neuramizone; **USA:** Antispasmodic Elixir; Antrocol; Arco-Lase Plus; Barbidonna; Bel-Phen-Ergot S; Bellacane; Bellatal; Bellergal-S; Chardonna-2; Donna-Sed†; Donnamor†; Donnatal; Folergot-DF; Gustase Plus; Hyosophen; Levsin with Phenobarbitone; Lufyllin-EPG; Malatal†; Mudrane; Mudrane GG; Phenerbel-S; Quadrinal; Susano; Tedrigen; Theodrine.

Phensuximide (6618-b)

Phensuximide (BAN, rINN).
N-Methyl-2-phenylsuccinimide.
$C_{11}H_{11}NO_2 = 189.2$.
CAS — 86-34-0.
ATC — N03AD02.
Pharmacopoeias. In US.

Pharmacopoeial description

USP 25: A white to off-white crystalline powder. Is odourless or has not more than a slight odour. Slightly soluble in water; soluble in alcohol; very soluble in chloroform. Store in airtight containers.

Profile

Phensuximide is a succinimide antiepileptic with actions similar to those of ethosuximide (p.348), but it is reported to be less effective.

Porphyria. Phensuximide has been associated with acute attacks of porphyria and is considered unsafe in porphyric patients.

Preparations

USP 25: Phensuximide Capsules.

Phenytoin (6601-a)

Phenytoin (BAN, USAN, rINN).
Diphenylhydantoin; Fenitoina; Phenantoinum; Phenytoinum. 5,5-Diphenylhydantoin; 5,5-Diphenylimidazolidine-2,4-dione.
$C_{15}H_{12}N_2O_2 = 252.3$.
CAS — 57-41-0.
ATC — N03AB02.
Pharmacopoeias. In Eur. (see p.vi), Int., Jpn, Pol., and US.

Phenytoin 92 mg is approximately equivalent to 100 mg of phenytoin sodium (but see also under Uses and Administration, below).

Pharmacopoeial description

Ph. Eur.: A white or almost white, crystalline powder. Practically insoluble in water; sparingly soluble in alcohol; very slightly soluble in dichloromethane. It dissolves in dilute solutions of alkali hydroxides.

USP 25: A white, odourless, powder. Practically insoluble in water; soluble in hot alcohol; slightly soluble in cold alcohol, in chloroform, and in ether. Store in airtight containers.

Phenytoin Sodium (6602-t)

Phenytoin Sodium (BANM, rINNM).
Diphenin; Phenytoinum Natricum; Soluble Phenytoin.
$C_{15}H_{11}N_2NaO_2 = 274.2$.
CAS — 630-93-3.
Pharmacopoeias. In Chin., Eur. (see p.vi), Int., Jpn, Pol., and US.

Pharmacopoeial description

Ph. Eur.: A white, slightly hygroscopic, crystalline powder. Soluble in water and in alcohol; practically insoluble in dichloromethane and in ether. Store in airtight containers.

USP 25: A white, odourless, powder. Is somewhat hygroscopic and on exposure to air gradually absorbs carbon dioxide. Freely soluble in water, the solution usually being somewhat turbid due to partial hydrolysis and absorption of carbon dioxide; soluble in alcohol; practically insoluble in chloroform and in ether. Store in airtight containers.

Incompatibility. Phenytoin sodium only remains in solution when the pH is considerably alkaline (about 10 to 12) and there have been reports of loss of clarity or precipitation of phenytoin crystals when solutions of phenytoin sodium for injection have been mixed with a variety of drugs[1-6] or added to intravenous infusion fluids,[7-10] while binding has been reported following addition to enteral nutrition solutions.[11] A phenytoin precipitate has been reported to occlude implanted central venous access devices following the inadvertent admixture of phenytoin with glucose 5% or glucose in sodium chloride (pH 4);[12,13] it may be successfully cleared by the local instillation of sodium bicarbonate 8.4% to increase the pH of the medium.

1. Misgen R. Compatibilities and incompatibilities of some intravenous solution admixtures. *Am J Hosp Pharm* 1965; **22**: 92–4.
2. Patel JA, Phillips GL. A guide to physical compatibility of intravenous drug admixtures. *Am J Hosp Pharm* 1966; **23**: 409–11.
3. Klamerus KJ, et al. Stability of nitroglycerin in intravenous admixtures. *Am J Hosp Pharm* 1984; **41**: 303–5.
4. Hasegawa GR, Eder JF. Visual compatibility of dobutamine hydrochloride with other injectable drugs. *Am J Hosp Pharm* 1984; **41**: 949–51.
5. Gayed AA, et al. Visual compatibility of diltiazem injection with various diluents and medications during simulated Y-site injection. *Am J Health-Syst Pharm* 1995; **52**: 516–20.
6. Trissel LA, et al. Compatibility of propofol injectable emulsion with selected drugs during simulated Y-site administration. *Am J Health-Syst Pharm* 1997; **54**: 1287–92.
7. Bauman JL, et al. Phenytoin crystallization in intravenous fluids. *Drug Intell Clin Pharm* 1977; **11**: 646–9.
8. Bauman JL, Siepler JK. Intravenous phenytoin (concluded). *N Engl J Med* 1977; **296**: 111.
9. Cloyd JC, et al. Concentration-time profile of phenytoin after admixture with small volumes of intravenous fluids. *Am J Hosp Pharm* 1978; **35**: 45–8.
10. Giacona N, et al. Crystallization of three phenytoin preparations in intravenous solutions. *Am J Hosp Pharm* 1982; **39**: 630–4.
11. Miller SW, Strom JG. Stability of phenytoin in three enteral nutrient formulas. *Am J Hosp Pharm* 1988; **45**: 2529–32.
12. Akinwande KI, Keehn DM. Dissolution of phenytoin precipitate with sodium bicarbonate in an occluded central venous access device. *Ann Pharmacother* 1995; **29**: 707–9.
13. Tse CST, Abdullah R. Dissolving phenytoin precipitate in central venous access device. *Ann Intern Med* 1998; **128**: 1049.

Adverse Effects

Side-effects are fairly frequent in patients receiving phenytoin, but some remit with dose reduction or continued administration. Often reported are lack of appetite, headache, dizziness, transient nervousness, insomnia, and gastrointestinal disturbances such as nausea, vomiting, and constipation. Tenderness and hyperplasia of the gums often occurs, particularly in younger patients. Acne, hirsutism, and coarsening of the facial features may be associated with phenytoin therapy, and may be particularly undesirable in adolescents and women.

Phenytoin toxicity may be manifested as a syndrome of cerebellar, vestibular, and ocular effects, notably nystagmus, diplopia, slurred speech, and ataxia. Mental confusion, sometimes severe, may occur, and dyskinesias and exacerbations of seizure frequency have been noted. Hyperglycaemia has been associated with toxic concentrations.

Overdosage may result in hypotension, coma, and respiratory depression. Hypotension and CNS depression may also follow intravenous administration, if too rapid, as may cardiac arrhythmias and impaired cardiac conduction. Solutions for injection are very alkaline and may result in irritation at the injection site or phlebitis.

Prolonged therapy may produce subtle effects on mental function and cognition, especially in children. In addition there is some evidence that phenytoin interferes with vitamin D and folate metabolism. Rickets and osteomalacia have occurred in a few patients not exposed to adequate sunlight, although the causal role of phenytoin is debatable. A proportion of patients develop peripheral neuropathies, usually mild, and occasional cases of megaloblastic anaemia have been seen.

Mild hypersensitivity reactions are common, with skin rashes, often morbilliform, sometimes accompanied by fever. Bullous, exfoliative, or purpuric rashes may be symptoms of rare but severe reactions such as lupus erythematosus, erythema multiforme, Stevens-Johnson syndrome, or toxic epidermal necrolysis. Eosinophilia, lymphadenopathy, hepatitis, polyarteritis nodosa, and blood disorders such as aplastic anaemia, leucopenia, thrombocytopenia, and agranulocytosis, have occurred rarely; some of these conditions may also represent hypersensitivity reactions.

Hypoprothrombinaemia of the newborn following administration of phenytoin during pregnancy has been reported. Congenital malformations have been seen in the offspring of mothers receiving phenytoin during pregnancy (see under Precautions, below).

Effects on the blood. AGRANULOCYTOSIS. Fatal agranulocytosis has been reported[1] in a patient 17 years after starting therapy with phenytoin and primidone. In the report it was stated that since 1963 the UK Committee on Safety of Medicines had received reports of 3 previous cases of fatal agranulocytosis associated with phenytoin and none associated with primidone. The most likely cause was considered to be a direct toxic effect of phenytoin although other possible mechanisms included the ability of both drugs to produce folate deficiency. For a discussion of the effect of antiepileptics on serum folate, see below.

1. Laurenson IF, et al. Delayed fatal agranulocytosis in an epileptic taking primidone and phenytoin. *Lancet* 1994; **344**: 332–3.

FOLIC ACID DEFICIENCY. Antiepileptic therapy has long been associated with folate deficiency and some studies have suggested that more than half of all patients on long-term therapy with drugs such as phenytoin, phenobarbital, and primidone have subnormal serum-folate concentrations;[1,2] megaloblastic haematopoiesis is often present,[3] but clinical megaloblastic anaemia appears to be rare.

The relative importance of individual antiepileptics in causing folate deficiency and macrocytosis has been difficult to establish, because of the tendency to use combination regimens; with greater emphasis on single drug therapy there is evidence that monotherapy may produce less significant changes.[4,5] Despite suggestions that carbamazepine has relatively little effect on folic acid concentrations, Goggin et al. found its effects to be comparable with those of phenytoin;[5] in this study only valproate had little or no effect on red cell folate concentrations.

The mechanism by which phenytoin and similar antiepileptics reduce serum folate is uncertain; there is good evidence for a reduction in absorption of glutamate both *in vitro*[6] and *in vivo*,[7] but the drugs associated with subnormal serum folate are all enzyme inducers and it has been suggested that enzyme induction and enhanced folate metabolism may also play a role.[2,5] Adverse blood changes also result from hypersensitivity (see below).

1. Horwitz SJ, et al. Relation of abnormal folate metabolism to neuropathy developing during anticonvulsant drug therapy. *Lancet* 1968; **i**: 563–5.
2. Maxwell JD, et al. Folate deficiency after anticonvulsant drugs: an effect of hepatic enzyme induction? *BMJ* 1972; **1**: 297–9.
3. Wickramasinghe SN, et al. Megaloblastic erythropoiesis and macrocytosis in patients on anticonvulsants. *BMJ* 1975; **4**: 136–7.
4. Dellaportas DI, et al. Chronic toxicity in epileptic patients receiving single-drug treatment. *BMJ* 1982; **285**: 409–10.
5. Goggin T, et al. A comparative study of the relative effects of anticonvulsant drugs and dietary folate on the red cell folate status of patients with epilepsy. *Q J Med* 1987; **NS65** (247): 911–9.
6. Hoffbrand AV, Necheles TF. Mechanism of folate deficiency in patients receiving phenytoin. *Lancet* 1968; **ii**: 528–30.
7. Rosenberg IH, et al. Impairment of intestinal deconjugation of dietary folate. *Lancet* 1968; **ii**: 530–2.

Effects on bone. The effects of phenytoin and other antiepileptics on the skeletal system are a matter of some debate. There are numerous reports indicating effects on bone and on calcium and vitamin D metabolism. Therapy with *carbamazepine, phenobarbital,* or *phenytoin* has been found[1] to be associated with reduction in serum-calcium concentration to hypocalcaemic values, significant reduction in 25-hydroxycholecalciferol concentrations, and elevated alkaline phosphatase. In this study, involving 226 outpatients with epilepsy, the association was not seen with *valproate*. The effects were significantly greater in the group of patients receiving polytherapy, and there was limited evidence that these biochemical changes were exacerbated by reduced exposure to sunlight. In contrast, measurements of bone mineral density in one study of 26 children,[2] and in another of 19 children,[3] receiving antiepileptic monotherapy revealed a reduction in density in those taking *valproate* but no reduction with *carbamazepine*.

Nonetheless, despite these findings, reports of clinical osteomalacia are rare.[4] A study in 20 epileptic outpatients who had received antiepileptic therapy for a mean of 14½ years failed to show any clinical evidence of osteomalacia although there was some evidence of altered calcium metabolism.[5] Similarly, osteomalacia was seen in only 1 of 19 elderly inpatients in another study,[6] a rate similar to that previously seen in elderly patients with acute illness not receiving antiepileptic therapy.

1. Gough H, et al. A comparative study of the relative influence of different anticonvulsant drugs, UV exposure and diet on vitamin D and calcium metabolism in out-patients with epilepsy. *Q J Med* 1986; **NS59** (230): 569–77.
2. Sleth RD, et al. Effect of carbamazepine and valproate on bone mineral density. *J Pediatr* 1995; **127**: 256–62.
3. Kafalı G, et al. Effect of antiepileptic drugs on bone mineral density in children between ages 6 and 12 years. *Clin Pediatr (Phila)* 1999; **38**: 93–8.
4. Beghi E, et al. Adverse effects of anticonvulsant drugs: a critical review. *Adverse Drug React Acute Poisoning Rev* 1986; **2**: 63–86.
5. Fogelman I, et al. Do anticonvulsant drugs commonly induce osteomalacia? *Scott Med J* 1982; **27**: 136–42.
6. Harrington MG, Hodkinson HM. Anticonvulsant drugs and bone disease in the elderly. *J R Soc Med* 1987; **80**: 425–7.

Effects on the endocrine system and metabolism. Antiepileptics diminish *sexual potency* and *fertility* in young male epileptics.[1] Phenytoin is excreted in human semen in small quantities and this may possibly affect sperm morphology and motility. Reduced plasma concentrations of free testosterone have been detected in male epileptic patients receiving one or more of the following: carbamazepine, phenytoin, primidone, and sodium valproate.[2] Gynaecomastia has been reported[3] in 5 men receiving long-term antiepileptic treatment; one also complained of impotence but libido was stated to be normal in all 5. Phenytoin was a component of treatment in all patients and was the sole drug used in one.

Phenytoin may cause reversible *hyperglycaemia* at toxic doses but it does not appear to produce long-term effects on glucose tolerance when used in therapeutic doses.[4] Paradoxically, phenytoin has also been reported to improve insulin resistance in some patients.

Phenytoin may reduce serum concentrations of *thyroid* hormones through enzyme induction—see under Interactions of Thyroxine [levothyroxine], p.1527.

1. Anonymous. [A brief summary]. *BMJ* 1979; **2**: 1118.
2. Dana-Haeri J, et al. Reduction of free testosterone by antiepileptic drugs. *BMJ* 1982; **284**: 85–6.
3. Monson JP, Scott DF. Gynaecomastia induced by phenytoin in men with epilepsy. *BMJ* 1987; **294**: 612.
4. Hurel SJ, Taylor R. Drugs and glucose tolerance. *Adverse Drug React Bull* 1995; **174**: 659–62.

Effects on the liver. There have been occasional reports of liver damage, probably due to hypersensitivity (see below), associated with phenobarbital and phenytoin; the authors of an early study suggested that such drugs need not be withdrawn if there were merely transient elevations in transaminase values,[1] but care is needed to distinguish such effects from the early symptoms of the antiepileptic hypersensitivity syndrome.

1. Aiges HW, et al. The effects of phenobarbital and diphenylhydantoin on liver function and morphology. *J Pediatr* 1980; **97**: 22–6.

Effects on the lungs. Pulmonary eosinophilia and acute respiratory failure requiring mechanical ventilation have been reported[1] in a patient receiving phenytoin; other pulmonary symptoms associated with phenytoin were reviewed.

1. Mahatma M, et al. Phenytoin-induced acute respiratory failure with pulmonary eosinophilia. *Am J Med* 1989; **87**: 93–4.

Effects on mental function. For a review of the effects of antiepileptic therapy including phenytoin on cognition, see p.340.

Effects on the skin. Skin reactions produced by phenytoin are discussed under Hypersensitivity, below. Rare, but severe reactions such as Stevens-Johnson syndrome and toxic epidermal necrolysis have also occurred.

For reference to cutaneous manifestations of zinc deficiency, possibly due to chelation with phenytoin, see under Valproate, p.367.

Gingival hyperplasia. Gingival hyperplasia, characterised by inflammation and a marked fibrotic response, may affect up to 50% of patients receiving phenytoin. It usually becomes apparent within the first few months of therapy and is observed more frequently in children; there is no increase in alveolar bone loss. The mechanism underlying its development is unknown, although the main metabolite of phenytoin, 5-(4-hydroxyphenyl)-5-phenylhydantoin, has been implicated.[1-3]

1. Ball DE, et al. Plasma and saliva concentrations of phenytoin and 5-(4-hydroxyphenyl)-5-phenylhydantoin (HPPH) in relation to gingival overgrowth in epileptic patients. *Br J Clin Pharmacol* 1995; **39**: 539P–588P.
2. Ieiri I, et al. Effect of 5-(p-hydroxyphenyl)-5-phenylhydantoin (p-HPPH) enantiomers, major metabolites of phenytoin, on the occurrence of chronic-gingival hyperplasia: in vivo and in vitro study. *Eur J Clin Pharmacol* 1995; **49**: 51–6.
3. Zhou LX, et al. Metabolism of phenytoin by the gingiva of normal humans: the possible role of reactive metabolites of phenytoin in the initiation of gingival hyperplasia. *Clin Pharmacol Ther* 1996; **60**: 191–8.

Hypersensitivity. An antiepileptic hypersensitivity syndrome, comprising fever, rash, and lymphadenopathy and less commonly lymphocytosis, and liver and other organ involvement, has been associated with some antiepileptic drugs including phenytoin.[1-3] Clinical manifestations may include interstitial nephritis, anaemia, interstitial pulmonary infiltrates, thrombocytopenia, eosinophilia, myopathy, and diffuse intravascular coagulation.[1,2] Some have estimated the incidence at 1 in 1000 to 1 in 10 000 new exposures to aromatic anticonvulsants,[2,3] but the true incidence is unknown due to variations in presentation and reporting. The syndrome occurs most frequently on first exposure to the drug, with initial symptoms starting anywhere between 1 and 8 weeks after exposure. The mean interval to onset is 17 to 21 days with phenytoin. In previously sensitised individuals the reaction may occur within 1 day of rechallenge. The potential for cross-reactivity between carbamazepine, phenobarbital, and phenytoin is approximately 75%, and patients who develop the syndrome, and their close relatives should be warned of the risk associated with use of these antiepileptics.[2] An early review[1] of the syndrome in patients taking phenytoin commented that it occurred mainly in black male patients and should not be confused with more common mild general hypersensitivity reactions. More recent evidence does not suggest that ethnic origin predicts differences in risk.[2]

Most cases resolve spontaneously following withdrawal of the drug and symptomatic management. The use of corticosteroids in the management of severe cases remains controversial in the absence of controlled double-blind studies of their effectiveness.[1,2]

Phenytoin-induced pseudolymphoma mimicking cutaneous T-cell lymphoma has also been reported.[2,4] In most cases, symptoms resolve within 7 to 14 days of drug discontinuation, and the condition is not considered premalignant.[2] However, in one report[4] the cutaneous eruption and lymphadenopathy persisted after withdrawal of phenytoin for one year when the patient eventually became asymptomatic.

In a prospective study[5] of 306 patients given phenytoin there was an overall incidence of 8.5% of morbilliform rash, but there was a marked seasonal incidence with most reactions occurring during the summer months. The results did not appear to be due to photosensitivity and might represent seasonal alterations in the immune system.

1. Flowers FP, et al. Phenytoin hypersensitivity syndrome. *J Emerg Med* 1987; **5**: 103–8.
2. Knowles SR, et al. Anticonvulsant hypersensitivity syndrome: incidence, prevention and management. *Drug Safety* 1999; **21**: 489–501.
3. Bessmertny O, et al. Antiepileptic hypersensitivity syndrome in children. *Ann Pharmacother* 2001; **35**: 533–8.
4. Harris DWS, et al. Phenytoin-induced pseudolymphoma: a report of a case and review of the literature. *Br J Dermatol* 1992; **127**: 403–6.
5. Leppik IE, et al. Seasonal incidence of phenytoin allergy unrelated to plasma levels. *Arch Neurol* 1985; **42**: 120–2.

Peripheral neuropathies. Electrophysiological abnormalities following prolonged phenytoin treatment are common, but clinically significant peripheral neuropathy is rare.[1] The neuropathy usually involves sensory nerves and lesions are generally mild and asymptomatic.[2] Much of the reported clinical neuropathy has been associated with multiple drug therapy of epilepsy and with exposure to toxic concentrations of phenytoin.[1] Although an association with folate deficiency has been suggested, a study in 52 patients receiving long-term antiepileptic therapy failed to find any convincing evidence of a relationship between serum-folate concentration and peripheral neuropathy.[3]

1. Bruni J. Phenytoin toxicity. In: Levy RH, et al. eds. *Antiepileptic drugs.* 4th ed. New York: Raven Press, 1995: 345–50.
2. Argov Z, Mastaglia FL. Drug-induced peripheral neuropathies. *BMJ* 1979; **1**: 663–6.
3. Horwitz SJ, et al. Relation of abnormal folate metabolism to neuropathy developing during anticonvulsant drug therapy. *Lancet* 1968; **i**: 563–5.

Treatment of Adverse Effects

Treatment of poisoning with phenytoin tends to be supportive. Repeated doses of activated charcoal should be given by mouth with the aim not only of preventing absorption but also of aiding elimination. If vomiting is severe, charcoal may be given by nasogastric tube. Gastric lavage may be considered if a very large amount has been taken within 1 hour.

◊ Multiple oral doses of activated charcoal may reduce the absorption of phenytoin[1,2] but the degree of clinical benefit is unclear.[3] The value of charcoal haemoperfusion in the management of phenytoin overdosage is debatable. A review of haemoperfusion included data from 2 patients who ingested phenytoin[4] but, although it was suggested that haemoperfusion should contribute significantly to drug removal, results are difficult to evaluate in these patients who had also ingested phenobarbital. An evaluation in a patient who had also taken primidone[5] suggested that, although initial clearance of phenytoin was promising, the system rapidly became saturated and there was little overall benefit. Neither haemodialysis[6] nor peritoneal dialysis[7] is considered worthwhile. A review[3] of the features and management of poisoning with the antiepileptics carbamazepine, ethosuximide, lamotrigine, phenytoin, valproate, and vigabatrin concluded that meticulous supportive care is required; gastric lavage and activated charcoal should be administered within 1 to 2 hours of overdose. Haemodialysis and haemoperfusion are kinetically unfavourable and of doubtful clinical efficacy.

1. Weidle PJ, et al. Multiple-dose activated charcoal as adjunct therapy after chronic phenytoin intoxication. *Clin Pharm* 1991; **10**: 711–14.
2. Dolgin JG, et al. Pharmacokinetic simulation of the effect of multiple-dose activated charcoal in phenytoin poisoning—report of two pediatric cases. *DICP Ann Pharmacother* 1991; **25**: 646–9.
3. Jones AL, Proudfoot AT. Features and management of poisoning with modern drugs used to treat epilepsy. *Q J Med* 1998; **91**: 325–32.
4. Pond S, et al. Pharmacokinetics of haemoperfusion for drug overdose. *Clin Pharmacokinet* 1979; **4**: 329–54.
5. Baehler RW, et al. Charcoal hemoperfusion in the therapy for methsuximide and phenytoin overdose. *Arch Intern Med* 1980; **140**: 1466–8.
6. Rubinger D, et al. Inefficiency of haemodialysis in acute phenytoin intoxication. *Br J Clin Pharmacol* 1979; **7**: 405–7.
7. Czajka PA, et al. A pharmacokinetic evaluation of peritoneal dialysis for phenytoin intoxication. *J Clin Pharmacol* 1980; **20**: 565–9.

Precautions

Phenytoin is metabolised in the liver and should be given with care to patients with impaired liver function. Caution is also advocated in diabetic patients because of the potential effects of phenytoin on blood sugar.

Protein binding may be reduced in certain disease states such as uraemia, and in certain patient populations such as neonates, pregnant women, and the elderly. However, this may be of little clinical significance in itself, provided that hepatic function is not impaired, because the concentration of free (pharmacologically active) drug in the plasma often remains more or less unchanged, due to distribution, metabolism, and excretion. Thus, an alteration in protein binding would not necessarily require a change in dosage of phenytoin to be made although, when plasma concentrations are being monitored, relatively lower total plasma-phenytoin concentrations will be found to be effective since there is less bound (pharmacologically inactive) phenytoin available for measurement.

Intravenous phenytoin must be given slowly and extravasation and intra-arterial administration must be avoided. Phenytoin should not be given intravenously to patients with sinus bradycardia, heart block, or Stokes-Adams syndrome, and should be used with caution in patients with hypotension, heart failure, and myocardial infarction; monitoring of blood pressure and the ECG is recommended during intravenous therapy.

Patients or their carers should be told how to recognise signs of blood or skin toxicity and they should be advised to seek immediate medical attention if symptoms such as fever, sore throat, rash, mouth ulcers, bruising, or bleeding develop. Phenytoin should be withdrawn, if necessary under cover of a suitable alternative antiepileptic, if leucopenia which is severe, progressive, or associated with clinical symptoms develops. It should also be discontinued if a skin rash develops; in the case of mild rashes phenytoin may be reintroduced cautiously, but should be discontinued immediately and permanently if the rash recurs.

Care is required when withdrawing phenytoin therapy—see also under Uses and Administration, below.

Phenytoin may interfere with some tests of thyroid function as it can reduce free and circulating concentrations of tetra-iodothyronine, mainly by enhanced conversion to tri-iodothyronine, and it may also produce lower than normal values for dexamethasone and metyrapone suppression tests.

Breast feeding. For comment on antiepileptic therapy and breast feeding, see under Pregnancy and Breast Feeding on p.340.

Driving. For comment on antiepileptic drugs and driving, see p.340.

Infections. A 52-year-old woman previously well-controlled on phenytoin 400 mg daily suffered phenytoin toxicity after a viral infection;[1] her plasma-phenytoin concentration had increased from 16 µg per mL to 51 µg per mL. Six weeks later she had recovered and was re-stabilised on phenytoin 400 mg daily.

1. Levine M, Jones MW. Toxic reaction to phenytoin following a viral infection. *Can Med Assoc J* 1983; **128:** 1270–1.

AIDS. Renal abnormalities or hypoalbuminaemia associated with AIDS may increase the risk of elevated free phenytoin concentrations and subsequent toxicity. Altered protein binding resulted in marked phenytoin toxicity, with lethargy and seizure-like activity, in an HIV-positive patient with profound hypoalbuminaemia and moderate renal insufficiency.[1] Therapeutic drug monitoring in 21 patients with AIDS indicated that although total serum concentrations of phenytoin were lower than in a reference population, the fraction of unbound drug was higher.[2] These changes might be attributed to hypoalbuminaemia and it was suggested that free rather than total phenytoin concentrations should be measured in HIV-infected patients with hypoalbuminaemia.

Phenytoin itself was associated with reversible hypogammaglobulinaemia in an HIV-positive patient who previously had borderline hypergammaglobulinaemia.[3]

1. Toler SM, *et al.* Severe phenytoin intoxication as a result of altered protein binding in AIDS. *DICP Ann Pharmacother* 1990; **24:** 698–700.
2. Burger DM, *et al.* Therapeutic drug monitoring of phenytoin in patients with the acquired immunodeficiency syndrome. *Ther Drug Monit* 1994; **16:** 616–20.
3. Britigan BE. Diphenylhydantoin-induced hypogammaglobulinemia in a patient infected with human immunodeficiency virus. *Am J Med* 1991; **90:** 524–7.

Porphyria. Phenytoin has been associated with acute attacks of porphyria and is considered unsafe in porphyric patients.

Pregnancy. For comments on the management of epilepsy during pregnancy, see p.340.

There is an increased risk of neural tube defects in infants exposed *in utero* to antiepileptics including phenytoin and a variety of syndromes such as craniofacial and digital abnormalities and, less commonly, cleft lip and palate have been described. Specific syndromes such as the 'fetal hydantoin syndrome' with phenytoin have been linked to individual antiepileptics.

However, there is overlap between the effects seen with different antiepileptics and some consider the broader term 'fetal antiepileptic drug syndrome' to be more appropriate. There is also a risk of neonatal bleeding with phenytoin.

Interactions

There are complex interactions between antiepileptics, and toxicity may be enhanced without a corresponding increase in antiepileptic activity. Such interactions are very variable and unpredictable and plasma monitoring is often advisable with combination therapy.

Since phenytoin is extensively bound to plasma proteins it can be displaced by drugs competing for protein-binding sites, thus liberating more free (pharmacologically active) phenytoin into the plasma. However, elevation of free phenytoin is reported to be of little clinical significance provided hepatic function is not impaired (see Precautions, above). A potentially more serious type of interaction may occur because phenytoin metabolism is saturable: toxic concentrations of phenytoin can develop in patients given drugs which inhibit phenytoin metabolism even to quite a minor degree. Phenytoin is a potent enzyme inducer, and induces the metabolism of a number of drugs, including some antibacterials, anticoagulants, corticosteroids, quinidine, and sex hormones (notably, oral contraceptives). The hypotensive properties of dopamine and the cardiac depressant properties of drugs such as lignocaine [lidocaine] may be dangerously enhanced by intravenous administration of phenytoin.

◊ General references.

1. Nation RL, *et al.* Pharmacokinetic drug interactions with phenytoin. *Clin Pharmacokinet* 1990; **18:** 37–60 and 131–150.

Anaesthetics. A 10-year-old girl with epilepsy who had been treated with phenytoin 100 mg three times daily for 5 years and who had lateral nystagmus developed symptoms of phenytoin intoxication following anaesthesia with *halothane*.[1] The plasma concentration of phenytoin 72 hours after anaesthesia was 41 µg per mL. It was suggested that temporary liver dysfunction was responsible for impaired metabolism of phenytoin.

1. Karlin JM, Kutt H. Acute diphenylhydantoin intoxication following halothane anesthesia. *J Pediatr* 1970; **76:** 941–4.

Analgesics. Various analgesics may interact with phenytoin. *Aspirin* is reported to displace phenytoin from plasma binding[1,2] but there is no evidence of any effect on metabolism and effects are unlikely to be clinically significant.[3,4] *Paracetamol* is reported to have no significant effect on serum-phenytoin concentrations.[4] Alterations of pharmacokinetic parameters have been reported with *bromfenac*, but it was thought unlikely that a change in phenytoin dose would be necessary.[5] Other analgesic and anti-inflammatory drugs may have clinically significant effects. *Phenylbutazone* has been reported to cause an initial decrease in serum phenytoin, followed by an increase;[4] in addition to effects on protein binding it inhibits phenytoin metabolism[6] and severe phenytoin toxicity may result.[7] *Azapropazone* appears to be a competitive inhibitor of phenytoin metabolism and has also been implicated in interactions resulting in toxicity.[8,9] Substantial increases in serum phenytoin have been demonstrated in healthy subjects given *fenyramidol*,[10] indicating a potential for toxicity. There is a single report of toxicity in a patient receiving *ibuprofen* with phenytoin[11] but in a study in 9 healthy subjects, ibuprofen had no effect on the pharmacokinetics of phenytoin.[12]

The opioid analgesic *dextropropoxyphene* has also been reported to affect phenytoin metabolism, with the resultant development of toxic blood-phenytoin concentrations;[13] however, the patient in this case was taking relatively high doses of dextropropoxyphene (650 mg daily). For the effect of phenytoin on *methadone* and *pethidine*, see p.53 and p.76, respectively.

1. Fraser DG, *et al.* Displacement of phenytoin from plasma binding sites by salicylate. *Clin Pharmacol Ther* 1980; **27:** 165–9.
2. Paxton JW. Effects of aspirin on salivary and serum phenytoin kinetics in healthy subjects. *Clin Pharmacol Ther* 1980; **27:** 170–8.
3. Leonard RF, *et al.* Phenytoin-salicylate interaction. *Clin Pharmacol Ther* 1981; **29:** 56–60.
4. Neuvonen PJ, *et al.* Antipyretic analgesics in patients on antiepileptic drug therapy. *Eur J Clin Pharmacol* 1979; **15:** 263–8.
5. Gumbhir-Shah K, *et al.* Evaluation of pharmacokinetic interaction between bromfenac and phenytoin in healthy males. *J Clin Pharmacol* 1997; **37:** 160–8.
6. Andreasen PB, *et al.* Diphenylhydantoin half-life in man and its inhibition by phenylbutazone: the role of genetic factors. *Acta Med Scand* 1973; **193:** 561–4.
7. Kristensen MB. Drug interactions and clinical pharmacokinetics. *Clin Pharmacokinet* 1976; **1:** 351–72.
8. Roberts CJC, *et al.* Anticonvulsant intoxication precipitated by azapropazone. *Postgrad Med J* 1981; **57:** 191–2.
9. Geaney DP, *et al.* Interaction of azapropazone with phenytoin. *BMJ* 1982; **284:** 1373.
10. Solomon HM, Schrogie JJ. The effect of phenyramidol on the metabolism of diphenylhydantoin. *Clin Pharmacol Ther* 1967; **8:** 554–6.

11. Sandyk R. Phenytoin toxicity induced by interaction with ibuprofen. *S Afr Med J* 1982; **62:** 592.
12. Townsend RJ, *et al.* The effects of ibuprofen on phenytoin pharmacokinetics. *Drug Intell Clin Pharm* 1985; **19:** 447–8.
13. Kutt H. Interactions between anticonvulsants and other commonly prescribed drugs. *Epilepsia* 1984; **25** (suppl 2): S118–S131.

Anthelmintics. For report of an interaction between phenytoin and *levamisole* with fluorouracil, see under Antineoplastics, below. For the effect of phenytoin on *mebendazole* and *praziquantel*, see p.102 and p.107, respectively.

Antiarrhythmics. There have been reports of phenytoin toxicity associated with substantial rises in serum-phenytoin concentrations following addition of *amiodarone* to the therapeutic regimen.[1,2] For the effect of phenytoin on amiodarone, see p.837.

For the effect of phenytoin on other antiarrhythmics, see p.879 (disopyramide), p.932 (mexiletine), p.965 (quinidine), and p.1314 (lignocaine [lidocaine]).

1. Gore JM, *et al.* Interaction of amiodarone and diphenylhydantoin. *Am J Cardiol* 1984; **54:** 1145.
2. McGovern B, *et al.* Possible interaction between amiodarone and phenytoin. *Ann Intern Med* 1984; **101:** 650.

Antibacterials. Interactions, some clinically significant, may occur between phenytoin and various antibacterials. Concurrent administration of *chloramphenicol* with phenytoin has resulted in marked[1] to marked[2] elevation of serum-phenytoin concentrations due to inhibition of phenytoin metabolism;[2] toxicity has resulted.[3,4] In turn, phenytoin may affect serum concentrations of chloramphenicol (see p.180).

Phenytoin may enhance the metabolism of *doxycycline*.[5]

There is limited evidence that *erythromycin* decreases phenytoin clearance[6] but this was subject to considerable interindividual variation and is of unknown clinical significance. Results from another study[7] suggested that clarithromycin might also raise phenytoin levels.

The interaction with *isoniazid* is well documented and potentially significant in slow acetylators of isoniazid who may develop raised phenytoin concentrations and signs of toxicity;[8,9] in at least one case, death has resulted.[10] Plasma-isoniazid concentrations may become sufficiently raised in slow acetylators of isoniazid to produce marked inhibition of the hepatic microsomal enzymes responsible for the metabolism of phenytoin.

There are conflicting reports of the effect of *ciprofloxacin* on serum concentrations of phenytoin. While some report no effect[11] others have reported reduced[12-16] or increased[17,18] concentrations of phenytoin in patients given ciprofloxacin. A fall in serum-phenytoin concentrations, and resultant loss of seizure control has been reported in a patient in whom *nitrofurantoin* was added to therapy.[19] The mechanism of this interaction is unknown although a combination of impaired absorption and increased metabolism of the phenytoin was suggested. Something similar was reported in a patient given *oxacillin* in whom plasma-phenytoin concentrations dropped markedly and status epilepticus developed.[20] This effect was thought to be due to impaired phenytoin absorption.

Rifampicin can also reduce plasma-phenytoin concentrations and markedly increase its clearance;[21,22] this is in marked contrast to the effects of isoniazid, and when given together it overrides the effects of isoniazid on phenytoin, even in slow acetylators.[22]

Various sulfonamides are reported to interact with phenytoin, reducing clearance and prolonging half-life: *sulfaphenazole* is reportedly the strongest inhibitor of phenytoin metabolism but *sulfamethizole* also inhibits phenytoin metabolism and the latter has been implicated in producing phenytoin toxicity.[23] *Co-trimoxazole* reportedly inhibits phenytoin metabolism to a modest degree; a case of phenytoin toxicity in a child given co-trimoxazole has been reported[24] but the role of the co-trimoxazole is uncertain since the patient was also receiving sultiame.

See also under Antiprotozoals, below.

1. Koup JR, *et al.* Interaction of chloramphenicol with phenytoin and phenobarbital. *Clin Pharmacol Ther* 1978; **24:** 571–5.
2. Christensen LK, Skovsted L. Inhibition of drug metabolism by chloramphenicol. *Lancet* 1969; **ii:** 1397–9.
3. Ballek RE, *et al.* Inhibition of diphenylhydantoin metabolism by chloramphenicol. *Lancet* 1973; **i:** 150.
4. Rose JQ, *et al.* Intoxication caused by interaction of chloramphenicol and phenytoin. *JAMA* 1977; **237:** 2630–1.
5. Neuvonen PJ, *et al.* Effect of antiepileptic drugs on the elimination of various tetracycline derivatives. *Eur J Clin Pharmacol* 1975; **9:** 147–54.
6. Bachmann K, *et al.* Single dose phenytoin clearance during erythromycin treatment. *Res Commun Chem Pathol Pharmacol* 1984; **46:** 207–17.
7. Burger DM, *et al.* Therapeutic drug monitoring of phenytoin in patients with the acquired immunodeficiency syndrome. *Ther Drug Monit* 1994; **16:** 616–20.
8. Brennan RW, *et al.* Diphenylhydantoin intoxication attendant to slow inactivation of isoniazid. *Neurology* 1970; **20:** 687–93.
9. Kutt H, *et al.* Diphenylhydantoin intoxication: a complication of isoniazid therapy. *Am Rev Respir Dis* 1970; **101:** 377–84.
10. Johnson J, Freeman HL. Death due to isoniazid (INH) and phenytoin. *Br J Psychiatry* 1976; **129:** 511.
11. Slavich IL, *et al.* Grand mal epileptic seizures during ciprofloxacin therapy. *JAMA* 1989; **261:** 558–9.
12. Dillard ML, *et al.* Ciprofloxacin-phenytoin interaction. *Ann Pharmacother* 1992; **26:** 263.
13. Pollak PT, Slayter KL. Hazards of doubling phenytoin dose in the face of an unrecognized interaction with ciprofloxacin. *Ann Pharmacother* 1997; **31:** 61–4.
14. Brouwers PJ, *et al.* Ciprofloxacin-phenytoin interaction. *Ann Pharmacother* 1997; **31:** 498.

15. McLeod R, Trinkle R. Unexpectedly low phenytoin concentration in a patient receiving ciprofloxacin. *Ann Pharmacother* 1998; **32:** 1110–11.
16. Otero M-J, *et al.* Interaction between phenytoin and ciprofloxacin. *Ann Pharmacother* 1999; **33:** 251–2.
17. Schroeder D, *et al.* Effect of ciprofloxacin on serum phenytoin concentrations in epileptic patients. *Pharmacotherapy* 1991; **11:** 276.
18. Hull RL. Possible phenytoin-ciprofloxacin interaction. *Ann Pharmacother* 1993; **27:** 1283.
19. Heipertz R, Pilz H. Interaction of nitrofurantoin with diphenylhydantoin. *J Neurol* 1978; **218:** 297–301.
20. Fincham RW, *et al.* Use of phenytoin serum levels in a case of status epilepticus. *Neurology* 1976; **26:** 879–81.
21. Wagner JC, Slama TG. Rifampin-phenytoin drug interaction. *Drug Intell Clin Pharm* 1984; **18:** 497.
22. Kay L, *et al.* Influence of rifampicin and isoniazid on the kinetics of phenytoin. *Br J Clin Pharmacol* 1985; **20:** 323–6.
23. Siersbaek-Nielsen K, *et al.* Sulfamethizole-induced inhibition of diphenylhydantoin and tolbutamide metabolism in man. *Clin Pharmacol Ther* 1973; **14:** 148.
24. Gillman MA, Sandyk R. Phenytoin toxicity and co-trimoxazole. *Ann Intern Med* 1985; **102:** 559.

Anticoagulants. Serum-phenytoin concentrations have been reported to be markedly elevated by concurrent administration of *dicoumarol*[1,2] and elevated to a lesser extent by *phenprocoumon*;[2] however, although *warfarin* has been implicated in a report of phenytoin toxicity,[3] other evidence suggests that it has no effect on serum-phenytoin concentrations in most patients.[2]

For the effect of phenytoin on anticoagulants such as dicoumarol and warfarin, see p.995.

1. Hansen JM, *et al.* Dicoumarol-induced diphenylhydantoin intoxication. *Lancet* 1966; **ii:** 265–6.
2. Skovsted L, *et al.* The effect of different oral anticoagulants on diphenylhydantoin and tolbutamide metabolism. *Acta Med Scand* 1976; **199:** 513–5.
3. Rothermich NO. Diphenylhydantoin intoxication. *Lancet* 1966; **ii:** 640.

Antidepressants. As with all antiepileptics, antidepressants may antagonise the antiepileptic activity of phenytoin by lowering the convulsive threshold.

Plasma-phenytoin concentrations rose in 2 epileptic patients also receiving *imipramine* 75 mg daily for about 3 months for depression.[1] In one patient the concentration gradually increased over several weeks to more than twice the pretreatment figure and he showed mild signs of phenytoin intoxication which remitted after imipramine was stopped. Increased serum-phenytoin concentration and phenytoin toxicity has been described[2] in one patient, possibly precipitated by addition of *trazodone*; the manufacturers of trazodone recommend monitoring serum-phenytoin concentrations in patients receiving these two drugs concomitantly. Elevated plasma-phenytoin concentrations, in some cases accompanied by signs and symptoms of phenytoin toxicity, have also been reported with *fluoxetine*,[3] *fluvoxamine*,[4] *sertraline*,[5] or *viloxazine*.[6] The manufacturer of *mianserin* recommends that plasma concentrations of phenytoin should be monitored carefully during concomitant therapy.

Hypericum has been shown to induce several drug metabolising enzymes (see p.290) and consequently it might reduce the blood concentrations of phenytoin leading to an increased risk of seizure.[7]

For the effects of phenytoin on antidepressants, see under Amitriptyline (p.277), Fluoxetine (p.287), and Lithium (p.294).

1. Perucca E, Richens A. Interaction between phenytoin and imipramine. *Br J Clin Pharmacol* 1977; **4:** 485–6.
2. Dorn JM. A case of phenytoin toxicity possibly precipitated by trazodone. *J Clin Psychiatry* 1986; **47:** 89–90.
3. Nightingale SL. Fluoxetine labeling revised to identify phenytoin interaction and to recommend against use in nursing mothers. *JAMA* 1994; **271:** 1067.
4. Feldman D, *et al.* Cas clinique d'interaction médicamenteuse entre phénytoïne et fluvoxamine. *J Pharm Clin* 1995; **14:** 296–7.
5. Haselberger MB, *et al.* Elevated serum phenytoin concentrations associated with coadministration of sertraline. *J Clin Psychopharmacol* 1997; **17:** 107–9.
6. Pisani F, *et al.* Elevation of plasma phenytoin by viloxazine in epileptic patients: a clinically significant interaction. *J Neurol Neurosurg Psychiatry* 1992; **55:** 126–7.
7. Committee on Safety of Medicines/Medicines Control Agency. Reminder: St John's wort (Hypericum perforatum) interactions. *Current Problems* 2000; **26:** 6–7.

Antidiabetics. Transient rises in the amount of non-protein-bound phenytoin were observed in 17 patients when *tolbutamide* was given in addition to phenytoin, but none developed signs of intoxication.[1] Toxic symptoms were reported in another patient given phenytoin and tolbutamide concomitantly, although she had tolerated this combination on a previous occasion.[2]

Symptoms of phenytoin toxicity are known to have occurred[1] in one patient receiving *tolazamide* and phenytoin.

For the effect of phenytoin on repaglinide, see p.334.

1. Wesseling H, Mols-Thürkow I. Interaction of diphenylhydantoin (DPH) and tolbutamide in man. *Eur J Clin Pharmacol* 1975; **8:** 75–8.
2. Beech E, *et al.* Phenytoin toxicity produced by tolbutamide. *BMJ* 1988; **297:** 1613–14.

Antiepileptics. Interactions may occur when phenytoin is given concomitantly with other antiepileptics, but these are often variable in their effect and difficult to predict.

For a discussion of the effect of *benzodiazepines* on plasma concentrations of phenytoin, see under Benzodiazepines, below.

Carbamazepine has been generally reported to lower serum-phenytoin concentrations,[1,2] although reports exist of elevated serum-phenytoin concentrations when the two were given concurrently.[3] It should be noted that phenytoin also reduces serum-carbamazepine values—see p.344. These studies have not indicated any loss of seizure control due to this interaction.

For the effects of phenytoin on *ethosuximide*, see p.348.

Felbamate has caused increases in serum-phenytoin concentrations, and in some cases toxicity requiring a reduction in phenytoin dose.[4,5]

Increased plasma concentrations of phenytoin with symptoms of toxicity have been reported in one patient receiving phenytoin, carbamazepine, and clobazam after *gabapentin* was added to treatment.[6]

Phenytoin reduces plasma concentrations of *lamotrigine* as described on p.352.

Phenytoin plasma concentrations may be increased by high doses of *oxcarbazepine* (p.354); the US manufacturer of oxcarbazepine suggests that doses of phenytoin may need to be reduced when high doses of oxcarbazepine are given concomitantly.

Phenobarbital both induces the metabolism of phenytoin and competes with it for metabolism by the same enzyme system; in practice there is rarely sufficient alteration for a change in phenytoin dosage to be necessary.[7-9] For the effect of phenytoin on phenobarbital, see p.356.

Progabide may increase blood-phenytoin concentrations[10] and *stiripentol* appears to produce a dose-dependent reduction in phenytoin clearance.[11]

Sultiame causes substantial increases in plasma-phenytoin concentrations, in some cases resulting in phenytoin toxicity;[12] the dose of phenytoin may therefore require adjustment if these drugs are given together.

Modest increases in plasma-phenytoin concentrations have been observed in some patients when *topiramate* was added to therapy, but it was considered that dosage adjustments were unlikely to be necessary.[13] For the effect of phenytoin on topiramate, see p.365.

The interaction between phenytoin and *valproate* is complex. Valproate displaces phenytoin from serum binding sites and may inhibit its metabolism;[14] the former effect increases the concentration of free drug but reduces total serum phenytoin.[15,16] Most studies seem to suggest that the dose of phenytoin need only rarely be adjusted, but the possibility of loss of seizure control, or phenytoin toxicity, does exist.[14] Interestingly there is some evidence that the interactions may be affected by circadian variations in valproate concentrations.[17] Total plasma-phenytoin concentrations rose significantly in 9 of 11 patients, 2 of whom developed toxic symptoms, when the formulation of sodium valproate that they were receiving concurrently with phenytoin was changed from a standard tablet to a slow-release form.[18] The authors hypothesised that the reduced diurnal fluctuations in plasma-valproate concentrations due to the use of slow-release tablets reduced the displacement interaction between phenytoin and valproate, thereby increasing total plasma-phenytoin concentrations. Phenytoin may also cause a fall in serum concentrations of valproate—see p.368.

Gradual or delayed reductions in plasma-phenytoin concentrations have been observed in several studies in patients given *vigabatrin*;[19] one review[19] states that concentrations have been reduced by 20 to 30%. The manufacturer of vigabatrin considers that this is unlikely to be of clinical significance although in one study the reduction was considered to compromise seizure control.[20]

1. Hansen JM, *et al.* Carbamazepine-induced acceleration of diphenylhydantoin and warfarin metabolism in man. *Clin Pharmacol Ther* 1971; **12:** 539–43.
2. Windorfer A, Sauer W. Drug interactions during anticonvulsant therapy in childhood: diphenylhydantoin, primidone, phenobarbitone, clonazepam, nitrazepam, carbamazepine, and dipropylacetate. *Neuropadiatrie* 1977; **8:** 29–41.
3. Zielinski JJ, *et al.* Carbamazepine-phenytoin interaction: elevation of plasma phenytoin concentration due to carbamazepine comedication. *Ther Drug Monit* 1985; **7:** 51–3.
4. Sheridan PH, *et al.* Open pilot study of felbamate (ADD03055) in partial seizures. *Epilepsia* 1986; **27:** 649.
5. Wilensky AJ, *et al.* Pharmacokinetics of W-554 (ADD 03055) in epileptic patients. *Epilepsia* 1985; **26:** 602–6.
6. Tyndel F. Interaction of gabapentin with other antiepileptics. *Lancet* 1994; **343:** 1363–4.
7. Morselli PL, *et al.* Interaction between phenobarbital and diphenylhydantoin in animals and in epileptic patients. *Ann N Y Acad Sci* 1971; **179:** 88–107.
8. Cucinell SA, *et al.* Drug interactions in man: 1. lowering effect of phenobarbital on plasma levels of bishydroxycoumarin (Dicumarol) and diphenylhydantoin (Dilantin). *Clin Pharmacol Ther* 1965; **6:** 420–9.
9. Booker HE, *et al.* Concurrent administration of phenobarbital and diphenylhydantoin: lack of an interference effect. *Neurology* 1971; **21:** 383–5.
10. Bianchetti G, *et al.* Pharmacokinetic interactions of progabide with other antiepileptic drugs. *Epilepsia* 1987; **28:** 68–73.
11. Levy RH, *et al.* Stiripentol kinetics in epileptic patients: nonlinearity and interactions. *Epilepsia* 1984; **25:** 657.
12. Hansen JM, Koch KM. Drug interactions with valproic acid. *Epilepsia* 1982; **9:** 17–22.
13. Bourgeois BFD. Drug interaction profile of topiramate. *Epilepsia* 1996; **37** (suppl 2): S14–S17.
14. Hansen JM, Koch KM. Drug interactions with valproic acid. *Drugs* 1982; **24:** 543–56.
15. Monks A, Richens A. Effect of single doses of sodium valproate on serum phenytoin levels and protein binding in epileptic patients. *Clin Pharmacol Ther* 1980; **27:** 89–95.

16. Perucca E, *et al.* Interaction between phenytoin and valproic acid: plasma protein binding and metabolic effects. *Clin Pharmacol Ther* 1980; **28:** 779–89.
17. Riva R, *et al.* Time-dependent interaction between phenytoin and valproic acid. *Neurology* 1985; **35:** 510–15.
18. Suzuki Y, *et al.* Interaction between valproate formulation and phenytoin concentrations. *Eur J Clin Pharmacol* 1995; **48:** 61–3.
19. Grant SM, Heel RC. Vigabatrin: a review of its pharmacodynamic and pharmacokinetic properties, and therapeutic potential in epilepsy and disorders of motor control. *Drugs* 1991; **41:** 889–926.
20. Browne TR, *et al.* Vigabatrin for refractory complex partial seizures: multicenter single-blind study with long-term follow-up. *Neurology* 1987; **37:** 184–9.

Antifungals. There have been several reports of interactions, sometimes resulting in phenytoin toxicity, between imidazole antifungals and phenytoin. The drug most frequently implicated is *miconazole*.[1-3] The related triazole antifungal *fluconazole* is also reported to interact with phenytoin,[4-6] possibly due to dose-related inhibition of cytochrome P450 by fluconazole.[4]

Phenytoin can decrease plasma concentrations of azole antifungals such as ketoconazole and itraconazole.

1. Bourgoin B, *et al.* Interaction pharmacocinétique possible phénytoïne-miconazole. *Therapie* 1981; **36:** 347–9.
2. Loupi E, *et al.* Interactions médicamenteuses et miconazole. *Therapie* 1982; **37:** 437–41.
3. Rolan PE, *et al.* Phenytoin intoxication during treatment with parenteral miconazole. *BMJ* 1983; **287:** 1760.
4. Mitchell AS, Holland JT. Fluconazole and phenytoin: a predictable interaction. *BMJ* 1989; **298:** 1315.
5. Howitt KM, Oziemski MA. Phenytoin toxicity induced by fluconazole. *Med J Aust* 1989; **151:** 603–4.
6. Cadle RM, *et al.* Fluconazole-induced symptomatic phenytoin toxicity. *Ann Pharmacother* 1994; **28:** 191–5.

Antigout drugs. The manufacturer of *sulfinpyrazone* states that it displaces phenytoin from its protein-binding sites, and also inhibits microsomal liver enzymes. The net result is an increase in plasma-phenytoin concentrations and a prolonged half-life, which is potentially hazardous.

A case has been described[1] in which reduced doses of phenytoin were necessary to avoid toxicity when *allopurinol* was added to the therapy of a child with the Lesch-Nyhan syndrome. Although the authors thought caution was advisable in using these two drugs together, they did emphasise that overgeneralisation may be dangerous since the child also received other antiepileptics and the contribution his disease may have played was unknown.

1. Yokochi K, *et al.* Phenytoin-allopurinol interaction: Michaelis-Menten kinetic parameters of phenytoin with and without allopurinol in a child with Lesch-Nyhan syndrome. *Ther Drug Monit* 1982; **4:** 353–7.

Antihistamines. A young woman developed drowsiness, ataxia, diplopia, tinnitus, and episodes of occipital headaches associated with vomiting after concomitant administration of phenytoin sodium and *chlorpheniramine [chlorphenamine]*.[1] Chlorpheniramine [chlorphenamine] might have delayed the hepatic metabolism of phenytoin thereby increasing the plasma concentrations.

1. Pugh RNH, *et al.* Interaction of phenytoin with chlorpheniramine. *Br J Clin Pharmacol* 1975; **2:** 173–5.

Antihypertensives. In 2 patients with hypoglycaemia associated with hyperinsulinism, therapeutic serum-phenytoin concentrations could not be achieved while they were also receiving *diazoxide*.[1] It was suggested that an increased rate of metabolism, and possibly a decreased binding, of phenytoin induced by diazoxide might have been responsible.

1. Roe TF, *et al.* Drug interaction: diazoxide and diphenylhydantoin. *J Pediatr* 1975; **87:** 480–4.

Antimalarials. Antimalarials may antagonise the antiepileptic activity of phenytoin by lowering the convulsive threshold.

Antineoplastics. There have been reports of decreased plasma-phenytoin concentrations associated with cancer chemotherapy,[1-4] resulting in some cases in loss of seizure control.[2-4] The effect appears to be due to impaired absorption of phenytoin arising from antineoplastic damage to the gastrointestinal mucosa. In one patient a mean of 32% of an oral dose of phenytoin was absorbed following therapy with *cisplatin*, *vinblastine*, and *bleomycin*; this compared with a reported oral bioavailability of 80% or more.[3] Increased plasma-phenytoin concentrations were reported[5] in one patient when *tacrolimus* was added to existing therapy. Phenytoin was discontinued until levels were within the therapeutic range and then restarted at a lower dose, tacrolimus therapy continuing throughout; phenytoin levels remained stable thereafter.

The US manufacturer of levamisole reports that increased plasma-phenytoin concentrations have been observed in patients taking phenytoin concomitantly with *levamisole* administered as an adjuvant to *fluorouracil* therapy. For the effect of phenytoin on busulfan see under Effects on the Nervous System under Adverse Effects of Busulfan, p.513.

1. Fincham RW, Schottelius DD. Decreased phenytoin levels in antineoplastic therapy. *Ther Drug Monit* 1979; **1:** 277–83.
2. Bollini P, *et al.* Decreased phenytoin level during antineoplastic therapy: a case report. *Epilepsia* 1983; **24:** 75–8.
3. Sylvester RK, *et al.* Impaired phenytoin bioavailability secondary to cisplatinum, vinblastine, and bleomycin. *Ther Drug Monit* 1984; **6:** 302–5.
4. Grossman SA, *et al.* Decreased phenytoin levels in patients receiving chemotherapy. *Am J Med* 1989; **87:** 505–10.
5. Thompson PA, Mosley CA. Tacrolimus-phenytoin interaction. *Ann Pharmacother* 1996; **30:** 544.

Antiprotozoals. Conflicting results have been reported with *metronidazole*: while one study has suggested only minimal effects on phenytoin concentrations and metabolism,[1] another has indicated inhibition of the metabolism of phenytoin.[2] For the effect of phenytoin an metronidazole, see p.595.

1. Jensen JC, Gugler R. Interaction between metronidazole and drugs eliminated by oxidative metabolism. *Clin Pharmacol Ther* 1985; **37:** 407–10.
2. Blyden GT, *et al.* Metronidazole impairs clearance of phenytoin but not of alprazolam or lorazepam. *Clin Pharmacol Ther* 1986; **39:** 181.

Antipsychotics. As with all antiepileptics, antipsychotics may antagonise the antiepileptic activity of phenytoin by lowering the convulsive threshold. Two cases of phenytoin toxicity and elevated plasma-phenytoin concentrations associated with concurrent administration of the phenothiazine *thioridazine* have been reported;[1] but another study indicated that concurrent treatment with *thioridazine*, *chlorpromazine*, or *mesoridazine* reduced serum-phenytoin concentrations.[2]

The non-phenothiazine antipsychotic *loxapine* has also been implicated as producing a fall in serum-phenytoin concentration.[3]

For the effect of phenytoin on antipsychotics in general, see under Chlorpromazine, p.664. For the effect of phenytoin on clozapine, see p.673.

1. Vincent FM. Phenothiazine-induced phenytoin intoxication. *Ann Intern Med* 1980; **93:** 56–7.
2. Haidukewych D, Rodin EA. Effect of phenothiazines on serum antiepileptic drug concentrations in psychiatric patients with seizure disorder. *Ther Drug Monit* 1985; **7:** 401–4.
3. Ryan GM, Matthews PA. Phenytoin metabolism stimulated by loxapine. *Drug Intell Clin Pharm* 1977; **11:** 428–9.

Antivirals. *Zidovudine* may possibly reduce or increase plasma concentrations of phenytoin. There has been a report[1] of markedly decreased serum-phenytoin concentrations resulting in a recurrence of seizure activity in an epileptic patient following initiation of *nelfinavir* as part of antiretroviral therapy.

For the possible effect of phenytoin on HIV-protease inhibitors, see p.626.

1. Honda M, *et al.* A generalized seizure following initiation of nelfinavir in a patient with human immunodeficiency virus type 1 infection, suspected due to interaction between nelfinavir and phenytoin. *Intern Med* 1999; **38:** 302–3.

Anxiolytics. See under Benzodiazepines, below.

Benzodiazepines. The metabolism of benzodiazepines may be enhanced as a result of induction of hepatic drug-metabolising enzymes following long-term therapy with phenytoin. In comparison with healthy subjects, half-lives have been shorter and clearance increased.[1,2]

There are sporadic reports of interactions between phenytoin and benzodiazepines, but the evidence is conflicting. One group of workers[3] found some evidence of elevated plasma concentrations of phenytoin in patients given *diazepam* or *chlordiazepoxide* but, in contrast, another study suggested that these drugs produced a significant fall in serum-phenytoin concentrations.[4] There have been reports suggesting that phenytoin intoxication could result from the impaired metabolism associated with the combination[3,5] but in practice this seems to be very rare. There are similar conflicting reports for *clonazepam*.[6-8]

1. Dhillon S, Richens A. Pharmacokinetics of diazepam in epileptic patients and normal volunteers following intravenous administration. *Br J Clin Pharmacol* 1981; **12:** 841–4.
2. Scott AK, *et al.* Oxazepam pharmacokinetics in patients with epilepsy treated long-term with phenytoin alone or in combination with phenobarbitone. *Br J Clin Pharmacol* 1983; **16:** 441–4.
3. Vajda FJE, *et al.* Interaction between phenytoin and the benzodiazepines. *BMJ* 1971; **1:** 346.
4. Houghton GW, Richens A. The effect of benzodiazepines and pheneturide on phenytoin metabolism in man. *Br J Clin Pharmacol* 1974; **1:** 344P–345P.
5. Kutt H, McDowell F. Management of epilepsy with diphenylhydantoin sodium: dosage regulation for problem patients. *JAMA* 1968; **203:** 969–72.
6. Eeg-Olofsson O. Experiences with Rivotril® in treatment of epilepsy—particularly minor motor epilepsy—in mentally retarded children. *Acta Neurol Scand* 1973; **49** (suppl 53): 29–31.
7. Johannessen SI, *et al.* Lack of effect of clonazepam on serum levels of diphenylhydantoin, phenobarbital and carbamazepine. *Acta Neurol Scand* 1977; **55:** 506–12.
8. Saavedra IN, *et al.* Phenytoin/clonazepam interaction. *Ther Drug Monit* 1985; **7:** 481–4.

Calcium-channel blockers. Raised serum-phenytoin concentration with phenytoin toxicity developed in a patient who had been taking *nifedipine* in addition to phenytoin for 3 weeks;[1] symptoms resolved completely after nifedipine withdrawal. The mechanism of interaction appeared to be complex. Similar effects have been reported with *diltiazem*.[2]

For the effect of phenytoin on dihydropyridine calcium-channel blockers, see under Nifedipine, p.942, and on verapamil, see p.990.

1. Ahmad S. Nifedipine-phenytoin interaction. *J Am Coll Cardiol* 1984; **3:** 1582.
2. Bahls FH, *et al.* Interactions between calcium channel blockers and the anticonvulsants carbamazepine and phenytoin. *Neurology* 1991; **41:** 740–2.

Cardiac glycosides. For the effect of phenytoin on cardiac glycosides, see under Digoxin, p.871.

Ciclosporin. For the effect of phenytoin on ciclosporin, see p.521.

Corticosteroids. Serum concentrations of phenytoin have been elevated[1] or reduced[2,3] following concurrent administration of *dexamethasone* and adjustment of phenytoin dosage may be required.[2,3] For the effect of phenytoin on corticosteroids, see p.1043.

1. Lawson LA, *et al.* Phenytoin-dexamethasone interaction: a previously unreported observation. *Surg Neurol* 1981; **16:** 23–4.
2. Wong DD, *et al.* Phenytoin-dexamethasone: a possible drug-drug interaction. *JAMA* 1985; **254:** 2062–3.
3. Recuenco I, *et al.* Effect of dexamethasone on the decrease of serum phenytoin concentrations. *Ann Pharmacother* 1995; **29:** 935.

Dermatological drugs. For the effect of phenytoin on methoxsalen, see p.1119.

Disulfiram. A well-documented interaction exists between phenytoin and *disulfiram*, which may result in clinical phenytoin toxicity.[1,2] The effect appears to be due to non-competitive inhibition of the metabolism of phenytoin by disulfiram,[2] which results in a substantial increase in phenytoin half-life and a decrease in its clearance.[3]

1. Dry J, Pradalier A. Intoxication par la phénytoïne au cours d'une association thérapeutique avec le disulfirame. *Therapie* 1973; **28:** 799–802.
2. Taylor JW, *et al.* Mathematical analysis of a phenytoin-disulfiram interaction. *Am J Hosp Pharm* 1981; **38:** 93–5.
3. Svendsen TL, *et al.* The influence of disulfiram on the half-life and metabolic clearance rate of diphenylhydantoin and tolbutamide in man. *Eur J Clin Pharmacol* 1976; **9:** 439–41.

Diuretics. Severe osteomalacia in 2 previously active young women taking *acetazolamide* in association with phenytoin or primidone and phenobarbital has been reported.[1]

For the effect of antiepileptics such as phenytoin on frusemide [furosemide], see p.894.

1. Mallette LE. Anticonvulsants, acetazolamide and osteomalacia. *N Engl J Med* 1975; **293:** 668.

Enteral and parenteral nutrition. Therapeutic plasma concentrations of phenytoin may be difficult to achieve in patients receiving enteral or total parenteral nutrition.[1,2] Incompatibility studies which indicate that phenytoin probably binds to components of the feed (see under Incompatibility, above) might explain this interaction when both are given together nasogastrically, but the same effect has also been reported when they were given separately by the intravenous route.[2] A review[3] of case reports and studies concluded that the exact role of enteral feeding in this interaction still remained unclear because of a lack of prospective, randomised, controlled trials performed in patients, rather than in healthy subjects. However, because of the amount of literature describing such a phenomenon, it was considered unlikely to occur just by chance. Monitoring of serum-phenytoin concentrations to guide therapy was recommended, and measures such as staggering phenytoin and enteral feed administration might be considered to minimise the occurrence of this reaction.

1. Summers VM, Grant R. Nasogastric feeding and phenytoin interaction. *Pharm J* 1989; **243:** 181.
2. Messahel FM, *et al.* Does total parenteral nutrition lower serum phenytoin levels? *Curr Ther Res* 1990; **47:** 1017–20.
3. Au Yeung SC, Ensom MH. Phenytoin and enteral feedings: does evidence support an interaction? *Ann Pharmacother* 2000 **34:** 896–905.

Gastrointestinal drugs. Evidence for an interaction between phenytoin and *antacids* is conflicting. Some studies have shown a decrease in the bioavailability of phenytoin given with various antacid mixtures[1,2] but others have failed to find any evidence of reduced absorption.[3] Furthermore even those studies which recorded decreased absorption varied in their results with regard to particular drugs, suggesting for example that calcium carbonate both does[1] and does not[2] reduce phenytoin bioavailability. The clinical significance of this data is uncertain but it has been suggested that if antacids and phenytoin are both required their doses should be spaced several hours apart.[4,5] *Sucralfate*, is also reported to reduce phenytoin absorption.[6]

A well documented interaction exists between phenytoin and *cimetidine*, which produces a dose-dependent reduction in phenytoin clearance[7] and a significant elevation of serum-phenytoin concentration.[8] There are reports of phenytoin toxicity following cimetidine administration to epileptic patients[9,10] including a report of severe granulocytopenia associated with the combination.[11] Although some studies have found that neither *ranitidine*[12] nor *famotidine*[13] appear to affect the pharmacokinetics of phenytoin significantly, there have been isolated reports of raised plasma concentrations of phenytoin associated with concurrent use of ranitidine[14-16] or famotidine.[17]

Omeprazole 40 mg daily can decrease the plasma clearance of phenytoin[18] and increase the area under the serum-phenytoin concentration-time curve,[19] but one study[20] suggests that the dosage of 20 mg daily usually used for peptic ulcer disease is unlikely to produce a clinically significant effect on the steady-state plasma concentrations of phenytoin in patients with epilepsy.

1. Garnett WR, *et al.* Bioavailability of phenytoin administered with antacids. *Ther Drug Monit* 1979; **1:** 435–6.
2. Kulshrestha VK, *et al.* Interaction between phenytoin and antacids. *Br J Clin Pharmacol* 1978; **6:** 177–9.
3. O'Brien LS, *et al.* Failure of antacids to alter the pharmacokinetics of phenytoin. *Br J Clin Pharmacol* 1978; **6:** 176–7.
4. Cacek AT. Review of alterations in oral phenytoin bioavailability associated with formulation, antacids, and food. *Ther Drug Monit* 1986; **8:** 166–71.

5. D'Arcy PF, McElnay JC. Drug-antacid interactions: assessment of clinical importance. *Drug Intell Clin Pharm* 1987; **21:** 607–17.
6. Smart HL, *et al.* The effects of sucralfate upon phenytoin absorption in man. *Br J Clin Pharmacol* 1985; **20:** 238–40.
7. Bartle WR, *et al.* Dose-dependent effect of cimetidine on phenytoin kinetics. *Clin Pharmacol Ther* 1983; **33:** 649–55.
8. Iteogu MO, *et al.* Effect of cimetidine on single-dose phenytoin kinetics. *Clin Pharm* 1983; **2:** 302–4.
9. Phillips P, Hansky J. Phenytoin toxicity secondary to cimetidine administration. *Med J Aust* 1984; **141:** 602.
10. Hetzel DJ, *et al.* Cimetidine interaction with phenytoin. *BMJ* 1981; **282:** 1512.
11. Sazie E, Jaffe JP. Severe granulocytopenia with cimetidine and phenytoin. *Ann Intern Med* 1980; **93:** 151–2.
12. Watts RW, *et al.* Lack of interaction between ranitidine and phenytoin. *Br J Clin Pharmacol* 1983; **15:** 499–500.
13. Sambol NC, *et al.* A comparison of the influence of famotidine and cimetidine on phenytoin elimination and hepatic blood flow. *Br J Clin Pharmacol* 1989; **27:** 83–7.
14. Bramhall D, Levine M. Possible interaction of ranitidine with phenytoin. *Drug Intell Clin Pharm* 1988; **22:** 979–80.
15. Tse CST, *et al.* Phenytoin concentration elevation subsequent to ranitidine administration. *Ann Pharmacother* 1993; **27:** 1448–51.
16. Tse CST, Iagmin P. Phenytoin and ranitidine interaction. *Ann Intern Med* 1994; **120:** 892–3.
17. Shinn AF. Unrecognized drug interactions with famotidine and nizatidine. *Arch Intern Med* 1991; **151:** 814.
18. Gugler R, Jensen JC. Omeprazole inhibits oxidative drug metabolism: studies with diazepam and phenytoin in vivo and 7-ethoxycoumarin in vitro. *Gastroenterology* 1985; **89:** 1235–41.
19. Prichard PJ, *et al.* Oral phenytoin pharmacokinetics during omeprazole therapy. *Br J Clin Pharmacol* 1987; **24:** 543–5.
20. Andersson T, *et al.* A study of the interaction between omeprazole and phenytoin in epileptic patients. *Ther Drug Monit* 1990; **12:** 329–33.

Muscle relaxants. An increase in serum concentrations of phenytoin has been reported[1] in a patient when *tizanidine* was added to therapy.

1. Ueno K, *et al.* Phenytoin-tizanidine interaction. *DICP Ann Pharmacother* 1991; **25:** 1273.

Neuromuscular blockers. For the effect of phenytoin on *suxamethonium*, see p.1342 and on *competitive neuromuscular blockers*, see under Atracurium, p.1334.

Sex hormones. For the effect of phenytoin on sex hormones in oral contraceptives, see p.1459.

Stimulants and anorectics. Although there has been a report of elevated phenytoin and primidone serum concentrations in a 5-year-old following addition of *methylphenidate* to therapy[1] there was no similar elevation in 2 other children receiving phenobarbital and phenytoin in the same report, nor in 11 patients of varying ages given methylphenidate with antiepileptic therapy as part of a controlled study.[2] The likelihood of an interaction seems small in the majority of patients.

1. Garrettson LK, *et al.* Methylphenidate interaction with both anticonvulsants and ethyl biscoumacetate. *JAMA* 1969; **207:** 2053–6.
2. Kupferberg HJ, *et al.* Effect of methylphenidate on plasma anticonvulsant levels. *Clin Pharmacol Ther* 1972; **13:** 201–4.

Theophylline. Although most reports of an interaction between phenytoin and *theophylline* concern effects on theophylline concentrations, one study in 14 healthy subjects suggested that concurrent administration of the two could produce lowered serum-phenytoin concentrations, with a subsequent rise in concentration on discontinuing theophylline.[1] The mechanism was suggested to be enzyme induction by the xanthine resulting in increased phenytoin metabolism.

For the effect of phenytoin on theophylline, see p.780.

1. Taylor JW, *et al.* The interaction of phenytoin and theophylline. *Drug Intell Clin Pharm* 1980; **14:** 638.

Thyroxine [levothyroxine]. For the effects of phenytoin on thyroxine [levothyroxine], see p.1527.

Ticlopidine. Acute phenytoin toxicity has been reported in a well-stabilised 44-year-old patient following introduction of ticlopidine to prevent restenosis after placement of a coronary stent.[1] The patient also received metoprolol, aspirin, and for a short period lovastatin, but inhibition of the cytochrome P450 isoenzyme CYP2C19 by ticlopidine was considered the most likely cause of the patient's elevated serum phenytoin. A similar interaction occurred in a 72-year-old patient,[2] and the authors postulated that, since steady-state plasma concentrations of ticlopidine are almost twofold higher in elderly patients than those in younger patients, the higher ticlopidine concentrations may have played a role in this drug interaction.

1. Donahue SR, *et al.* Ticlopidine inhibition of phenytoin metabolism mediated by potent inhibition of CYP2C19. *Clin Pharmacol Ther* 1997; **62:** 572–7.
2. Klaassen SL. Ticlopidine-induced phenytoin toxicity. *Ann Pharmacother* 1998; **32:** 1295–8.

Vaccines. Contradictory results have been reported for the effects of *influenza vaccine* on serum-phenytoin concentrations. Jann and Fidone[1] reported a significant elevation in total phenytoin concentration following vaccination, which was suggested to be due to interferon induction and concomitant inhibition of cytochrome P450. In contrast, other reports have suggested that any increase in serum-phenytoin concentration was temporary and not significant overall[2] or even that there was a slight fall in serum-phenytoin concentration.[3] One study reported a significant increase in total phenytoin concentration two days after vaccination, followed by a return to previous values but this was accompanied by evidence of a gradual and prolonged fall in free phenytoin concentrations.[4] The possibility of either phenytoin toxicity or loss of seizure control may exist in some epileptic patients given influenza vaccine during phenytoin therapy.[5]

1. Jann MW, Fidone GS. Effect of influenza vaccine on serum anti-convulsant concentrations. *Clin Pharm* 1986; **5:** 817–20.
2. Levine M, *et al.* Increased serum phenytoin concentration following influenza vaccination. *Clin Pharm* 1984; **3:** 505–9.
3. Sawchuk RJ, *et al.* Effect of influenza vaccination on plasma phenytoin concentrations. *Ther Drug Monit* 1979; **1:** 285–8.
4. Smith CD, *et al.* Effect of influenza vaccine on serum concentrations of total and free phenytoin. *Clin Pharm* 1988; **7:** 828–32.
5. Grabenstein JD. Drug interactions involving immunologic agents, part 1. vaccine-vaccine, vaccine-immunoglobulin, and vaccine-drug interactions. *DICP Ann Pharmacother* 1990; **24:** 67–81.

Vitamins. *Pyridoxine* given in large doses produced a reduction in serum-phenytoin concentrations in 7 patients,[1] perhaps reflecting increased activity by pyridoxal phosphate-dependent enzymes involved in phenytoin metabolism.

Correction of antiepileptic-associated folate deficiency with *folic acid* has been reported to result in a decrease in serum-phenytoin concentrations and an increase in seizure frequency.[2,3] The effect has been reported to be most marked in subjects with high initial serum-phenytoin concentrations[4] and is associated with an increased phenytoin metabolism.[5] However, in the majority of patients the effect is unlikely to assume clinical significance,[2,4] and there is some evidence that very low doses of folic acid may be used to maintain normal serum-folate values without an increase in seizure frequency.[3] Information regarding the dual and interdependent interaction between phenytoin and folic acid has been reviewed.[6] Although limited numbers of patients and healthy subjects were involved, evaluation of the data suggested that initiation of phenytoin and folic acid concomitantly prevents decreased folate levels and steady-state concentrations of phenytoin are reached sooner. Plasma concentrations of phenytoin are also possibly reduced by *folinic acid*.

For the effect of antiepileptics, including phenytoin, on *vitamin D* concentrations, see Effects on Bone under Adverse Effects, above.

1. Hansson O, Sillanpaa M. Pyridoxine and serum concentration of phenytoin and phenobarbitone. *Lancet* 1976; **i:** 256.
2. Baylis EM, *et al.* Influence of folic acid on blood-phenytoin levels. *Lancet* 1971; **i:** 62–4.
3. Inoue F. Clinical implications of anticonvulsant-induced folate deficiency. *Clin Pharm* 1982; **1:** 372–3.
4. Furlanut M, *et al.* Effects of folic acid on phenytoin kinetics in healthy subjects. *Clin Pharmacol Ther* 1978; **24:** 294–7.
5. Berg MJ, *et al.* Phenytoin and folic acid interaction: a preliminary report. *Ther Drug Monit* 1983; **5:** 389–94.
6. Lewis DP, *et al.* Phenytoin-folic acid interaction. *Ann Pharmacother* 1995; **29:** 726–35.

Pharmacokinetics

Phenytoin is slowly but almost completely absorbed from the gastrointestinal tract. It is largely insoluble at the acid pH of the stomach, most being absorbed from the upper intestine; the rate of absorption is variable and is reported to be affected by the presence of food. Absorption from the intramuscular site is slower than that from the gastrointestinal tract.

Phenytoin is extensively metabolised in the liver to inactive metabolites, chiefly 5-(4-hydroxyphenyl)-5-phenylhydantoin. The rate of metabolism appears to be subject to genetic polymorphism and may also be influenced by racial characteristics; it is reported to be increased during pregnancy and menstruation and to decrease with age. Phenytoin hydroxylation is saturable and is therefore readily inhibited by drugs that compete for its metabolic pathways; this is also the reason why small increments in dose may produce large rises in plasma concentration. Phenytoin undergoes enterohepatic recycling and is excreted in the urine, mainly as its hydroxylated metabolite, in either free or conjugated form.

Phenytoin is widely distributed throughout the body. It is extensively bound (about 90%) to plasma protein, although this may be reduced in certain disease states and in certain patient populations (see under Precautions, above). It has a very variable, dose-dependent half-life, but the mean plasma half-life appears to be about 22 hours at steady state; because phenytoin inhibits its own metabolism it may sometimes be several weeks before a steady-state plasma-phenytoin concentration is attained.

Monitoring of plasma concentrations may be performed as an aid in assessing control, and the therapeutic range of total plasma-phenytoin concentrations is usually quoted as being 10 to 20 µg per mL (40 to 80 µmol per litre); some patients, however, achieve control at concentrations outside this range. It has been suggested that, because of differences in protein binding, measurement of free phenytoin concentrations in plasma may prove more reliable; measurement of concentrations in saliva, which contains only free phenytoin, has also been performed.

Phenytoin crosses the placental barrier and small amounts are distributed into breast milk.

The pharmacokinetics of phenytoin are affected by the concomitant administration of other antiepileptics (see Interactions, above).

Uses and Administration

Phenytoin is a hydantoin antiepileptic used to control partial and generalised tonic-clonic seizures. It is also used as part of the emergency treatment of status epilepticus and has been used for the prophylactic control of seizures associated with neurosurgery or severe traumatic injury to the head. Phenytoin has also been used in the treatment of trigeminal neuralgia. It is a class Ib antiarrhythmic and has been used to treat cardiac arrhythmias.

Doses may be expressed in terms of phenytoin or phenytoin sodium; although phenytoin 92 mg is approximately equivalent to 100 mg of phenytoin sodium these molecular equivalents are not necessarily biologically equivalent. In the UK an oral suspension of phenytoin 90 mg in 15 mL may be considered approximately equivalent in therapeutic effect to capsules or tablets containing phenytoin sodium 100 mg. In the USA a suspension containing phenytoin 125 mg in 5 mL is available.

For **epilepsy** the dose of phenytoin should be adjusted to the needs of the individual patient to achieve adequate control of seizures, preferably with monitoring of plasma concentrations; in many patients control requires total plasma-phenytoin concentrations of 10 to 20 µg per mL (40 to 80 µmol per litre), but some are controlled at concentrations outside this range. A suggested initial dose by mouth of phenytoin or phenytoin sodium given as a single dose or in divided doses is 3 to 4 mg per kg body-weight daily or 150 to 300 mg daily progressively increased with care to 600 mg daily if necessary; the suggested minimum interval between increments has ranged from about 7 to 10 days. Particular care is needed at higher doses, where saturation of metabolism may mean that a small increment produces a large rise in plasma concentrations. A usual maintenance dose is 200 to 500 mg daily.

A suggested initial dose for children is 5 mg per kg body-weight daily in 2 or 3 divided doses up to a maximum of 300 mg daily; a suggested maintenance dose is 4 to 8 mg per kg daily in divided doses. Young children may require a higher dose per kg body-weight than adults due to more rapid metabolism.

The practice of starting phenytoin therapy with initial small doses means that more than a week may be required before therapeutic plasma concentrations are attained; it has been reported that it may even be several weeks before a steady-state concentration is established. Some have therefore preferred to give an initial loading dose in order to reach the recommended plasma concentrations sooner, with the usual maintenance dosage being instituted 24 hours after the loading dose. Once the patient is stabilised the long half-life of phenytoin may permit the total daily dose to be given in two daily divisions, or perhaps as a single dose, usually at night.

Although clinical evidence is lacking, different brands of phenytoin, as well as different formulations from the same manufacturer, may vary in their bioavailability and patients may need to be restabilised in the event of a change.

In order to lessen gastric irritation, phenytoin should be taken with or after food. The time and manner of taking phenytoin should be standardised for the patient since variations might affect absorption with consequent fluctuations in the plasma concentrations.

As with other antiepileptics, withdrawal of phenytoin therapy or transition to or from another type of antiepileptic therapy should be made gradually to avoid precipitating an increase in the frequency of seizures.

For a discussion on whether or not to withdraw antiepileptic therapy in seizure-free patients, see p.338.

In the treatment of tonic-clonic **status epilepticus** a benzodiazepine such as diazepam is usually given initially intravenously or rectally followed by the administration of phenytoin sodium intravenously. A suggested dose of phenytoin sodium has been 10 to 15 mg per kg body-weight given by slow intravenous injection or by intermittent infusion at a uniform rate of not more than 50 mg per minute. Thereafter maintenance doses of 100 mg by mouth or intravenously are given every 6 to 8 hours; the rate and dose should be reduced according to body-weight. The intravenous dose for neonates is 15 to 20 mg per kg at a rate not exceeding 1 to 3 mg per kg per minute. A suggested dose in children is 15 mg per kg given at a rate of 1 mg per kg per minute, not to exceed 50 mg per minute. Deaths have been caused by the over-rapid intravenous injection of phenytoin sodium and continuous monitoring of the ECG and blood pressure is recommended whenever phenytoin sodium is given intravenously.

Phenytoin sodium is absorbed slowly and erratically from the intramuscular site and therefore intramuscular injections are not appropriate for the emergency arrest of status epilepticus. They may, however, be used in certain situations to maintain or establish therapeutic plasma concentrations of phenytoin in patients who are unconscious or otherwise unable to take phenytoin by mouth. Owing to the slower absorption of phenytoin from intramuscular sites, patients stabilised on the oral route require an increase in the intramuscular dose of about 50%; it is recommended that, if possible, intramuscular injections of phenytoin sodium should not be continued for longer than one week. On transfer back to the oral route the patient should receive 50% of the original oral dose for the same period of time as intramuscular injections were given, to allow for continued absorption of the residual phenytoin in the intramuscular sites. In a patient who has not previously received phenytoin sodium, a suggested intramuscular dose is 100 to 200 mg.

Administration. IN CHILDREN AND NEONATES. A comparison of methods[1] for the prediction of required phenytoin dosage in paediatric patients indicated that all methods produced a sizeable number of predictions with an error of more than 10% and that close monitoring of serum concentrations and clinical status was recommended regardless of the method chosen to adjust dosage. Loughnan *et al.*[2] came to similar conclusions on the need to monitor plasma concentrations of phenytoin in the newborn and young infants.

1. Yuen GJ, *et al.* Phenytoin dosage predictions in paediatric patients. *Clin Pharmacokinet* 1989; **16:** 254–60.
2. Loughnan PM, *et al.* Pharmacokinetic observations of phenytoin in the newborn and young infant. *Arch Dis Child* 1977; **52:** 302–9.

IN THE ELDERLY. Pharmacokinetic studies in elderly patients have shown reduced binding to plasma protein which was not itself an indication for dosage change,[1] but a study showing a decreased metabolism[2] did indicate that elderly patients may need lower doses of phenytoin than younger adults to maintain similar serum concentrations.

1. Patterson M, *et al.* Plasma protein binding of phenytoin in the aged: in vivo studies. *Br J Clin Pharmacol* 1982; **13:** 423–5.
2. Bauer LA, Blouin RA. Age and phenytoin kinetics in adult epileptics. *Clin Pharmacol Ther* 1982; **31:** 301–4.

IN HEPATIC IMPAIRMENT. For comments regarding the administration of phenytoin in hepatic impairment, see Precautions above.

Cardiac arrhythmias. Phenytoin has been given intravenously in the treatment of ventricular arrhythmias (p.794), especially those caused by overdosage with cardiac glycosides, but this use now appears to be obsolete.

A usual dose of phenytoin sodium was 3.5 to 5 mg per kg body-weight administered by slow intravenous injection at a uniform rate of not more than 50 mg per minute, repeated once if necessary.

Eclampsia and pre-eclampsia. Phenytoin has been used for eclampsia but now treatment with magnesium sulfate is preferred, see p.341.

Epidermolysis bullosa. There have been reports[1,2] of a favourable but variable clinical response to phenytoin in patients with recessive dystrophic epidermolysis bullosa (p.1105), a condition for which there is no truly effective treatment. However, a double-blind placebo-controlled study[3] concluded that phenytoin is not an effective treatment and offered no overall benefit when compared with placebo.

1. Bauer EA, et al. Phenytoin therapy of recessive dystrophic epidermolysis bullosa. N Engl J Med 1980; 303: 776–81.
2. Cooper TW, Bauer EA. Therapeutic efficacy of phenytoin in recessive dystrophic epidermolysis. Arch Dermatol 1984; 120: 490–5.
3. Caldwell-Brown D, et al. Lack of efficacy of phenytoin in recessive dystrophic epidermolysis bullosa. N Engl J Med 1992; 327: 163–7.

Epilepsy. Phenytoin is one of the drugs of choice in the treatment of partial seizures with or without secondary generalisation and in primarily generalised tonic-clonic seizures (see p.338). It is also effective in other forms of epilepsy with the exception of absence and myoclonic seizures.

The non-linear pharmacokinetics of phenytoin make it difficult to use, particularly at higher doses, because small increases in doses may produce large rises in plasma concentrations. Phenytoin may be unsuitable for adolescents or for women because of potential coarsening of the facial features, acne, or hirsutism. Gingival hyperplasia and tenderness can also be a problem.

References.

1. Mattson RH, et al. Comparison of carbamazepine, phenobarbital, phenytoin, and primidone in partial and secondarily generalised tonic-clonic seizures. N Engl J Med 1985; 313: 145–51.
2. Heller AJ, et al. Phenobarbitone, phenytoin, carbamazepine, or sodium valproate for newly diagnosed adult epilepsy: a randomised comparative monotherapy trial. J Neurol Neurosurg Psychiatry 1995; 58: 44–50.
3. de Silva M, et al. Randomised comparative monotherapy trial of phenobarbitone, phenytoin, carbamazepine, or sodium valproate for newly diagnosed childhood epilepsy. Lancet 1996; 347: 709–13.

Hiccup. Phenytoin may be of value for the treatment of intractable hiccups,[1] especially those of neurogenic origin. A protocol for the management of intractable hiccups may be found under Chlorpromazine, p.667.

1. Petroski D, Patel AN. Diphenylhydantoin for intractable hiccups. Lancet 1974; i: 739.

Intracerebral haemorrhage. For reference to the use of antiepileptic prophylaxis, usually with phenytoin, in patients following intracerebral haemorrhage, see under Stroke, p.813.

Myotonia. A review[1] of myotonia congenita, a hereditary muscular disorder characterised by symptoms of muscle stiffness especially after rest and when initiating movement. Where treatment is necessary it is usually with phenytoin or procainamide, the former being preferred as being better tolerated.

1. Gutmann L, et al. Myotonia congenita. Semin Neurol 1991; 11: 244–8.

Neonatal seizures. Phenytoin is one of the antiepileptics that may be used in the management of neonatal seizures (p.342).

Post-traumatic seizures. In a double-blind study[1] in patients with serious head trauma, only 7 of 208 assigned to receive phenytoin experienced seizures within 1 week of commencing treatment, compared with 26 of 196 assigned to placebo. On follow-up for 2 years, however, the differences between the groups were not significant. Phenytoin, given in an initial loading dose of 20 mg per kg body-weight intravenously, and subsequently given in doses adequate to maintain a high therapeutic concentration, appeared to reduce the incidence of seizures in the first week after major head trauma but not thereafter. However, in another study involving 86 similar patients only 6% of those who had received phenytoin had developed post-traumatic epilepsy at the 2-year follow-up compared with 42% of the untreated patients.[2] A meta-analysis[3] of these and other controlled studies investigating carbamazepine, phenobarbital, and phenytoin concluded that prophylactic antiepileptics are effective in reducing early seizures. However, there is no evidence that such use of antiepileptics reduces the occurrence of late seizures, or has any effect on death and neurological disability, and there is insufficient evidence to establish the net benefit of prophylactic treatment at any time after injury. Another review[4] reached similar conclusions, and also that phenytoin has the best evidence to support its use in reducing the frequency of early post-traumatic seizures. Guidelines[5] for the use of parenteral phenytoin and fosphenytoin in non-emergency situations, including prevention of post-traumatic seizures, have been suggested. Children with severe, acute neurotrauma were found to have markedly altered protein binding and phenytoin metabolism, and therefore may require increased doses.[6]

1. Temkin NR, et al. A randomized, double-blind study of phenytoin for the prevention of post-traumatic seizures. N Engl J Med 1990; 323: 497–502.
2. Pechadre JC, et al. Prévention de l'épilepsie post-traumatique tardive par phénytoïne dans les traumatismes crâniens graves: suivi durant 2 ans. Presse Med 1991; 20: 841–5.
3. Schierhout G, Roberts I. Anti-epileptic drugs for preventing seizures following acute traumatic brain injury (updated 6 September 2000). Available in the Cochrane Library; Issue 3. Oxford: Update Software; 2001.
4. Chadwick D. Seizures and epilepsy after traumatic brain injury. Lancet 2000; 355: 334–5.
5. Meek PD, et al. Guidelines for nonemergency use of parenteral phenytoin products. Arch Intern Med 1999; 159: 2639–44.
6. Stowe CD, et al. Altered phenytoin pharmacokinetics in children with severe, acute traumatic brain injury. J Clin Pharmacol 2000; 40: 1452–61.

Status epilepticus. Administration of a benzodiazepine is the most usual method used to abort an attack of status epilepticus (p.341). Once seizures have been brought under control, phenytoin may be given by intravenous infusion. Phenytoin has been considered more appropriate than a benzodiazepine for the management of status epilepticus in patients with head injuries or other acute neurological lesions.[1]

1. Eldridge PR, Punt JAG. Risks associated with giving benzodiazepines to patients with acute neurological injuries. BMJ 1990; 300: 1189–90.

Syndrome of inappropriate ADH secretion. Phenytoin has been used occasionally to inhibit pituitary antidiuretic hormone (ADH) secretion in patients with the syndrome of inappropriate ADH secretion (SIADH), the management of which is discussed on p.1277.

Tinnitus. Phenytoin is one of many drugs that have been tried in tinnitus (p.1316), but although it has been reported to be effective in some patients it is rarely used because of problems with adverse effects.

Trigeminal neuralgia. Phenytoin is used alone or added to treatment in trigeminal neuralgia (p.8) in patients unresponsive to or intolerant of carbamazepine.

Withdrawal syndromes. Phenytoin has little place in the management of seizures associated with the *alcohol withdrawal syndrome* (p.1131). Prophylaxis with phenytoin has been shown[1,2] to be ineffective for prevention of recurrent alcohol-related seizures and therefore drugs such as the benzodiazepines or clomethiazole, which are effective both for the treatment and prophylaxis of such seizures, are preferred. Results from a double-blind study[3] indicated that phenytoin was associated with a reduction in *cocaine abuse* compared with placebo. The abuse of cocaine is discussed on p.1309 and treatment of cocaine withdrawal on p.1310.

1. Chance JF. Emergency department treatment of alcohol withdrawal seizures with phenytoin. Ann Emerg Med 1991; 20: 520–2.
2. Rathlev NK, et al. The lack of efficacy of phenytoin in the prevention of recurrent alcohol-related seizures. Ann Emerg Med 1994; 23: 513–8.
3. Crosby RD, et al. Phenytoin in the treatment of cocaine abuse: a double-blind study. Clin Pharmacol Ther 1996; 59: 458–68.

Wounds and ulcers. Phenytoin has been used to promote wound healing (p.1108). Topical application of phenytoin has produced encouraging results in the healing of various types of ulcers[1-5] and large abscess cavities.[6] It has been suggested that phenytoin may reduce bacterial colonisation by changing the pH or by a direct antibacterial effect.[2] The enhanced wound healing may also be due to increased fibroblast proliferation and increased collagen content.[2] Limited absorption from the wound site may occur[7,8] and patients may need to be monitored for signs of toxicity.

1. Muthukumarasamy MG, et al. Topical phenytoin in diabetic foot ulcers. Diabetes Care 1991; 14: 909–11.
2. Pendse AK, et al. Topical phenytoin in wound healing. Int J Dermatol 1993; 32: 214–17.
3. Anstead GM, et al. Phenytoin in wound healing. Ann Pharmacother 1996; 30: 768–75.
4. Adjei O, et al. Phenytoin in the treatment of Buruli ulcer. Trans R Soc Trop Med Hyg 1998; 92: 108–9.
5. Rhodes RS, et al. Topical phenytoin treatment of stage II decubitus ulcers in the elderly. Ann Pharmacother 2001; 35: 675–81.
6. Lodha SC, et al. Role of phenytoin in healing of large abscess cavities. Br J Surg 1991; 78: 105–8.
7. Gore R, et al. Topical phenytoin. Pharm J 1991; 247: 620.
8. Lewis WG, Rhodes RS. Systemic absorption of topical phenytoin sodium. Ann Pharmacother 1994; 28: 961.

Preparations

BP 2001: Phenytoin Capsules; Phenytoin Injection; Phenytoin Oral Suspension; Phenytoin Tablets;
USP 25: Extended Phenytoin Sodium Capsules; Phenytoin Oral Suspension; Phenytoin Sodium Injection; Phenytoin Tablets; Prompt Phenytoin Sodium Capsules.

Proprietary Preparations (details are given in Part 3)
Aust.: Epanutin; Epilan-D; Phenhydan; *Austral.:* Dilantin; *Belg.:* Di-Hydan†; Diphantoine; Epanutin; *Braz.:* Epelin; Hidantal; *Canad.:* Dilantin; *Fin.:* Hydantin; *Fr.:* Di-Hydan; Dilantin; Pyoredol†; *Ger.:* Epanutin; Phenhydan; Zentropil; *Hong Kong:* Dilantin; *Irl.:* Epanutin; *Israel:* Dilantin; Epanutin; *Ital.:* Aurantin; Dintoina; *Jpn:* Aleviatin†; *Mex.:* Epamin; Fenidantion S; Fenitron; Hidantina; Hidantoina; Nuctane; *Neth.:* Epanutin; *Norw.:* Epinat; *NZ:* Dilantin; *Port.:* Hidantina; *S.Afr.:* Epanutin; *Singapore:* Dilantin; *Spain:* Epanutin; Neosidantoina; Sinergina; *Swed.:* Epanutin; Fenantoin; Lehydan; *Switz.:* Epanutin; Epilantine; Phenhydan; *Thai.:* Dilantin; Ditoin; Ditomed; Pepsytoin; *UK:* Epanutin; Pentran†; *USA:* Dilantin.

Multi-ingredient: *Belg.:* Mathoine; Vethoine; *Braz.:* Dialudon; Gamibetal Complex; Taludon; *Canad.:* Dilantin with Phenobarbital†; *Ital.:* Dintoinale; Gamibetal Complex; Metinal-Idantoina; Metinal-Idantoina L; *Port.:* Comital L; Hidantina Composta; *S.Afr.:* Garoin†; *Spain:* Comital L†; Disfil; Epilantin; Redutona.

Pregabalin   (19950-w)

Pregabalin (USAN, rINN).
CI-1008. (S)-3-(Aminomethyl)-5-methylhexanoic acid.
$C_8H_{17}NO_2 = 159.2$.
CAS — 148553-50-8.

Profile
Pregabalin is an antiepileptic under investigation in various

neurological disorders, notably as adjunctive therapy in the treatment of partial seizures.

◊ References.

1. Beydoun AA, et al. Pregabalin add-on trial: a double-blind, multicenter study in patients with partial epilepsy: results from the interim analysis (N = 129). Epilepsia 1999; 40 (suppl 7): 108.
2. French JA, et al. Pregabalin adjunctive therapy in patients with partial seizures. Epilepsia 1999: 40 (suppl 7): 106.

Primidone   (6619-v)

Primidone (BAN, rINN).
Hexamidinum; Primaclone; Primidonum. 5-Ethyl-5-phenylperhydropyrimidine-4,6-dione.
$C_{12}H_{14}N_2O_2 = 218.3$.
CAS — 125-33-7.
ATC — N03AA03.

Pharmacopoeias. In *Chin.*, *Eur.* (see p.vi), *Jpn*, *Pol.*, and *US*.

Pharmacopoeial description

Ph. Eur.: A white or almost white, crystalline powder. Very slightly soluble in water; slightly soluble in alcohol; practically insoluble in ether.

USP 25: A white, odourless, crystalline powder. Soluble 1 in 2000 of water and 1 in 200 of alcohol; very slightly soluble in most organic solvents.

Adverse Effects, Treatment, and Precautions

As for Phenobarbital, p.355. Adverse effects may be more frequent than with phenobarbital. Most patients rapidly develop tolerance to the adverse CNS effects of primidone, including ataxia, drowsiness, headache, nausea and vomiting, nystagmus, and visual disturbances.

Care is required when withdrawing primidone therapy—see also under Uses and Administration, below.

Tremor. It was noted that patients receiving primidone for essential tremor have a high incidence of acute adverse reactions following small initial doses.[1] This could be due to the absence of induced hepatic enzymes in these patients previously not exposed to antiepileptics.

1. Findley LJ, et al. Primidone in essential tremor of the hands and head: a double blind controlled clinical study. J Neurol Neurosurg Psychiatry 1985; 48: 911–15.

Effects on the blood. For a report of delayed agranulocytosis in a patient treated with phenytoin and primidone, see p.357.

Effects on the endocrine system. For mention of the effects of antiepileptics on *sexual function* in male epileptic patients, see under Phenytoin, p.358.

Overdosage. Crystalluria has been reported[1] following acute overdosage of primidone and 7 other reported cases were also reviewed. Based on these few reports, crystalluria appears to be associated with serum-primidone concentrations in excess of 80 μg per mL. There is evidence from 2 reports of renal damage associated with crystal formation *in vivo*. Vigorous hydration, with or without forced alkaline diuresis, is recommended in patients at risk, in order to lessen the potential for renal toxicity and improve elimination.

1. Lehmann DF. Primidone crystalluria following overdose: a report of a case and an analysis of the literature. Med Toxicol 1987; 2: 383–7.

Porphyria. Primidone has been associated with acute attacks of porphyria and is considered unsafe in porphyric patients.

Interactions

Primidone is metabolised in the body in part to phenobarbital and interactions recorded for phenobarbital (p.355) might potentially occur in patients receiving primidone. In addition, enzyme-inducing drugs enhance this metabolism and have the potential to produce elevated phenobarbital concentrations.

Antiepileptics. Both *phenytoin*[1,2] and *carbamazepine*[3] have been reported to enhance the metabolism of primidone to phenobarbital and when primidone was combined with phenytoin there have been instances of phenobarbital toxicity.[2] *Vigabatrin* has been reported[4] to lower plasma concentrations of primidone in some patients, although it is unlikely that dosage changes would be necessary. *Valproate* may increase plasma concentrations of primidone and phenobarbital, but patient response seems to be inconsistent.

1. Reynolds EH, et al. Interaction of phenytoin and primidone. BMJ 1975; 2: 594–5.
2. Fincham RW, Schottelius DD. Primidone: interactions with other drugs. In: Levy RH, et al. (eds). Antiepileptic drugs. (4th ed.) New York: Raven Press, 1995: 467–75.
3. Baciewicz AM. Carbamazepine drug interactions. Ther Drug Monit 1986; 8: 305–17.
4. Browne TR, et al. A multicentre study of vigabatrin for drug-resistant epilepsy. Br J Clin Pharmacol 1989; 27 (suppl 1): 95S–100S.

The symbol † denotes a preparation no longer actively marketed

Pharmacokinetics

Primidone is readily absorbed from the gastrointestinal tract and is reported to have a plasma half-life ranging from 10 to 15 hours, which is shorter than those of its principal metabolites phenylethylmalonamide and phenobarbital, both of which are active. Therapeutic plasma concentrations of primidone have been suggested to be between 5 and 12 μg per mL. It is excreted in urine as unchanged drug (40%) and metabolites.

Primidone is widely distributed but is only partially bound to plasma protein; it has been suggested that it exhibits variable binding of up to about 20%. It crosses the placenta and is distributed into breast milk.

Uses and Administration

Primidone is an antiepileptic that is partially metabolised to phenobarbital (p.356), but is also considered to have some antiepileptic activity in its own right. It may be given to control partial (especially complex partial) and generalised tonic-clonic seizures. Primidone is also used in the management of essential tremor.

In the treatment of **epilepsy** the dose of primidone should be adjusted according to the response of the patient; a limited correlation with plasma concentrations has suggested that concentrations of 5 to 12 μg per mL (23 to 55 μmol per litre) are usually necessary, but some sources suggest that monitoring of phenobarbital concentrations may be adequate.

Suggested initial doses are 125 mg daily by mouth at bedtime increased, if necessary, by 125 mg every 3 days to a total of 500 mg daily given in 2 divided doses. If necessary, the daily dose may be increased further every 3 days by 250 mg in adults up to a maximum of 1.5 g daily given in divided doses; in children under 9 years of age the dose may be increased by increments of 125 mg. Usual maintenance doses in adults and children over 9 years of age are 0.75 to 1.5 g daily. Suggested maintenance doses for children are: up to 2 years, 250 to 500 mg daily; 2 to 5 years, 500 to 750 mg daily; 6 to 9 years, 0.75 to 1 g daily. Maintenance doses are usually given as 2 divided doses.

As with other antiepileptics, withdrawal of primidone therapy or transition to or from another type of antiepileptic therapy should be made gradually to avoid precipitating an increase in the frequency of seizures. For a discussion on whether or not to withdraw antiepileptic therapy in seizure-free patients, see p.338.

For **essential tremor** primidone is given in usual initial doses of 50 mg daily by mouth, increased gradually over 2 to 3 weeks if necessary, to a maximum of 750 mg daily.

Epilepsy. Primidone, like its metabolite phenobarbital, is used in the treatment of epilepsy (p.338) for partial seizures with or without secondary generalisation and for primary generalised tonic-clonic seizures. However, because of problems of sedation, it is usually reserved for use in cases unresponsive to other antiepileptics.

Neonatal apnoea. Methylxanthines such as caffeine and theophylline are the main drugs used in the treatment of neonatal apnoea (p.784) in patients with no underlying seizure disorder; doxapram may be considered as an alternative in patients who do not respond to xanthines. Results from a preliminary study have suggested that adjunctive treatment with primidone[1] may be of value in neonates resistant to xanthine therapy alone.

1. Miller CA, *et al.* The use of primidone in neonates with theophylline-resistant apnea. *Am J Dis Child* 1993; **147:** 183–6.

Neonatal seizures. Primidone has been tried in the management of neonatal seizures (p.342).

Tremor. A beta blocker is often the first drug used in patients with essential tremor who require regular treatment (p.848) but primidone[1] may also be tried. A high incidence of acute adverse reactions has been reported following initial doses (see above). There has been concern that long-term use may produce tolerance to primidone's effects, although a small study has found a reduced response in only a few patients.[2]

1. Koller WC, Royse VL. Efficacy of primidone in essential tremor. *Neurology* 1986; **36:** 121–4.
2. Sasso E, *et al.* Primidone in the long-term treatment of essential tremor: a prospective study with computerized quantitative analysis. *Clin Neuropharmacol* 1990; **13:** 67–76.

Preparations

BP 2001: Primidone Oral Suspension; Primidone Tablets;
USP 25: Primidone Oral Suspension; Primidone Tablets.

Proprietary Preparations (details are given in Part 3)
Aust.: Cyral; Mysoline; **Austral.:** Mysoline; **Belg.:** Mysoline; **Canad.:** Mysoline; **Denm.:** Mysoline; **Fin.:** Mysoline; **Fr.:** Mysoline; **Ger.:** Liskantin; Mylepsinum; Resimatil; **Hong Kong:** Mysoline; **Irl.:** Mysoline; **Israel:** Prysoline; **Ital.:** Mysoline; **Mex.:** Mysoline; **Neth.:** Mysoline; **Norw.:** Mysoline; **NZ:** Mysoline; **Port.:** Mysoline; **S.Afr.:** Mysoline; **Singapore:** Mysoline; **Spain:** Mysoline; **Swed.:** Mysoline; **Switz.:** Mysoline; **UK:** Mysoline; **USA:** Mysoline.

Progabide (16968-t)

Progabide (BAN, USAN, rINN).

Halogabide; SL-76-002. 4-(4′-Chloro-5-fluoro-2-hydroxyben-zhydrylideneamino)butyramide.

$C_{17}H_{16}ClFN_2O_2 = 334.8.$
CAS — 62666-20-0.
ATC — N03AG05.

Profile

Progabide is an analogue of gamma-aminobutyric acid (GABA) and is believed to owe its antiepileptic properties to its action as an agonist at central GABA receptors. It has been used in the treatment of partial and generalised tonic-clonic seizures resistant to other therapy and for myoclonic seizures and in the Lennox-Gastaut and West's syndromes.

Liver disorders, indicated by elevation of liver enzyme values, have been reported to occur in about 9% of patients receiving progabide, usually in the first few months of treatment, and have progressed to jaundice, hepatitis, encephalopathy and death in some patients.

Interactions. For the effects of progabide on other antiepileptics, see Carbamazepine, p.344; Phenobarbital, p.356; and Phenytoin, p.360.

Porphyria. Progabide is considered to be unsafe in patients with porphyria because it has been shown to be porphyrinogenic in *in-vitro* systems.

Preparations

Proprietary Preparations (details are given in Part 3)
Fr.: Gabrene†.

Remacemide Hydrochloride (11035-m)

Remacemide Hydrochloride (USAN, pINNM).

FPL-12924AA (remacemide); FPL-12924AA (remacemide hydrochloride); PR-934-423 (remacemide); PR-934423 (remacemide); PR-934-423A (remacemide or remacemide hydrochloride). (±)-2-Amino-N-(1-methyl-1,2-diphenylethyl)acetamide.

$C_{17}H_{20}N_2O = 268.4.$
CAS — 128298-28-2 (remacemide); 111686-79-4 (remacemide hydrochloride).

Profile

Remacemide is an NMDA antagonist under investigation as adjunctive treatment for refractory epilepsy. It has also been investigated for the treatment of Parkinson's disease and as a neuroprotective drug in ischaemic stroke and for intra-operative cerebral ischaemia.

◊ References.

1. Dyker AG, Lees KR. Remacemide hydrochloride: a double-blind, placebo-controlled, safety and tolerability study in patients with acute ischaemic stroke. *Stroke* 1999; **30:** 1796–1801.
2. Parkinson Study Group. A multicenter randomized controlled trial of remacemide hydrochloride as monotherapy for PD. *Neurology* 2000; **54:** 1583–8.
3. Schachter SC, Tarsy D. Remacemide: current status and clinical applications. *Expert Opin Invest Drugs* 2000; **9:** 871–83.
4. Richens A, *et al.* A placebo-controlled, double-blind cross-over trial of adjunctive one month remacemide hydrochloride treatment in patients with refractory epilepsy. *Seizure* 2000; **9:** 537–43.
5. Chadwick D, *et al.* Remacemide hydrochloride: a placebo-controlled, one month, double-blind assessment of its safety, tolerability and pharmacokinetics as adjunctive therapy in patients with epilepsy. *Seizure* 2000; **9:** 544–50.
6. Shoulson I, *et al.* A randomized, controlled trial of remacemide for motor fluctuations in Parkinson's disease. *Neurology* 2001; **56:** 455–62.

Rufinamide (1220-e)

Rufinamide (BAN, USAN, rINN).

RUF-331. 1-(2,6-Difluorobenzyl)-1H-1,2,3-triazole-4-carboxamide.

$C_{10}H_8F_2N_4O = 238.2.$
CAS — 106308-44-5.

Profile

Rufinamide is an antiepileptic under investigation as adjunctive therapy in the treatment of partial and primary generalised tonic-clonic seizures.

◊ References.

1. Jain KK. An assessment of rufinamide as an anti-epileptic in comparison with other drugs in clinical development. *Expert Opin Invest Drugs* 2000; **9:** 829–40.
2. Palhagen S, *et al.* Rufinamide: a double-blind, placebo-controlled proof of principle trial in patients with epilepsy. *Epilepsy Res* 2001; **43:** 115–24.

Stiripentol (3634-m)

Stiripentol (USAN, rINN).

BCX-2600. 4,4-Dimethyl-1-[(3,4-methylenedioxy)phenyl]-1-penten-3-ol.

$C_{14}H_{18}O_3 = 234.3.$
CAS — 49763-96-4.

Adverse Effects and Precautions

Insomnia, occasional psychotic reactions, and gastrointestinal disturbances have been reported in patients receiving stiripentol.

Interactions

Stiripentol is a potent inhibitor of hepatic microsomal drug metabolism, and interactions are possible when it is given with other drugs.

◊ Stiripentol appears to inhibit several cytochrome P450 isoenzymes, including CYP1A2 and CYP3A4.[1] For interactions of stiripentol with other antiepileptics, see under Carbamazepine, p.344 and Phenytoin, p.360.

1. Tran A, *et al.* Influence of stiripentol on cytochrome P450-mediated metabolic pathways in humans: in vitro and in vivo comparison and calculation of in vivo inhibition constants. *Clin Pharmacol Ther* 1997; **62:** 490–504.

Pharmacokinetics

Stiripentol is incompletely absorbed following oral administration, and undergoes hepatic first-pass metabolism; as a result bioavailability of an oral dose is reported to be only about 20%. Its pharmacokinetics are non-linear, clearance decreasing with increasing dosage. Stiripentol is reported to be more than 99% protein bound. It is extensively metabolised and excreted in urine almost entirely as metabolites. Elimination is biphasic with a rapid initial and a prolonged terminal phase.

Uses and Administration

Stiripentol has been investigated for the treatment of various types of epilepsy. It is thought to be less potent than some conventional antiepileptics, but may reduce their adverse effects when used adjunctively.

Epilepsy. A 24-week study[1] in 10 children demonstrated that stiripentol might be effective as adjunctive therapy for the treatment of atypical absence seizures (p.338). Further studies suggested benefit from adjunctive use in children with partial epilepsy[2] and severe myoclonic epilepsy.[2,3]

1. Farwell JR, *et al.* Stiripentol in atypical absence seizures in children: an open trial. *Epilepsia* 1993; **34:** 305–11.
2. Perez J, *et al.* Stiripentol: efficacy and tolerability in children with epilepsy. *Epilepsia* 1999; **40:** 1618–26.
3. Chiron C, *et al.* Stiripentol in severe myoclonic epilepsy in infancy: a randomised placebo-controlled syndrome-dedicated trial. *Lancet* 2000; **356:** 1638–42.

Sultiame (6621-f)

Sultiame (BAN, rINN).

Riker-594; Sulthiame (USAN). 4-(Tetrahydro-2H-1,2-thiazin-2-yl)benzenesulphonamide, S,S-dioxide.

$C_{10}H_{14}N_2O_4S_2 = 290.4.$
CAS — 61-56-3.
ATC — N03AX03.

Pharmacopoeias. In Jpn.

Profile

Sultiame is a carbonic anhydrase inhibitor that has been used as an antiepileptic in most forms of epilepsy (p.338) except absence seizures. It has usually been given in conjunction with other antiepileptics and it is believed that much of its activity is due to the inhibition of metabolism of the other drugs.

Sultiame has been given by mouth in initial doses of 100 mg twice daily or 50 mg three times daily gradually increased according to response to 200 mg three times daily. A dose of 5 to 10 mg per kg daily, adjusted according to response, has been recommended in Rolandic epilepsy.

Interactions. For the effect of sultiame on phenytoin, see p.360.

Porphyria. Sultiame has been associated with acute attacks of porphyria and is considered unsafe in porphyric patients.

Preparations

Proprietary Preparations (details are given in Part 3)
Austral.: Ospolot; **Ger.:** Ospolot; **Israel:** Ospolot.

Tiagabine Hydrochloride (14669-z)

Tiagabine Hydrochloride *(BANM, USAN, rINNM)*.
Abbott-70569.1; ABT-569; NNC-05-0328; NO-05-0328.
(−)-(R)-1-[4,4-Bis(3-methyl-2-thienyl)-3-butenyl]nipecotic acid hydrochloride.
$C_{20}H_{25}NO_2S_2,HCl = 412.0$.
CAS — 115103-54-3 (tiagabine); 145821-59-6 (tiagabine hydrochloride).

Tiagabine hydrochloride 55 mg is approximately equivalent to 50 mg of tiagabine.

Adverse Effects

The most common adverse effects include dizziness, nervousness, tiredness, somnolence, and tremor. Other reported adverse effects include irritability, confusion, depression, difficulties in concentration, diarrhoea, abdominal pain, nausea, ataxia, emotional lability, and nystagmus. Bruising, rashes, speech difficulties, and an influenza-like syndrome of chills, fever, myalgia, and headache have also been reported. Visual field defects have been reported rarely.

◊ In a meta-analysis[1] of 5 double-blind trials involving approximately 1000 patients receiving tiagabine as adjunctive therapy for refractory partial seizures, discontinuation resulting from adverse effects was infrequent and occurred in 15% of patients receiving tiagabine compared with 5% receiving placebo. Adverse effects were usually associated with dose titration, and were generally mild to moderate in severity, and transient.

1. Leppike IE. Tiagabine: the safety landscape. *Epilepsia* 1995; **36** (suppl 6): S10–S13.

Precautions

Hepatic metabolism of tiagabine is reduced in patients with hepatic impairment, and dosage should therefore be reduced and/or the intervals between doses increased. It should not be used in patients with severely impaired hepatic functions.

Care is required when withdrawing tiagabine therapy—see Uses and Administration, below.

Driving. For comment on antiepileptic drugs and driving, see p.340.

Interactions

There are complex interactions between antiepileptics and toxicity may be enhanced without a corresponding increase in antiepileptic activity. Such interactions are very variable and unpredictable and plasma monitoring is often advisable with combination therapy. The hepatic metabolism of tiagabine is accelerated by concomitant administration of antiepileptics that induce enzymes of the cytochrome P450 system such as carbamazepine, phenobarbital, phenytoin, or primidone. Plasma concentrations of tiagabine may be reduced by up to threefold by concomitant use.

Pharmacokinetics

Tiagabine is readily absorbed after oral administration. Food reduces the rate but not the extent of absorption. The absorption and elimination pharmacokinetics of tiagabine are linear within the therapeutic dosage range.

Tiagabine is widely distributed throughout the body and plasma protein binding is high (96%).

Tiagabine is extensively metabolised in the liver and excreted as metabolites in the faeces or, to a lesser extent, in the urine; less than 2% of a dose is eliminated as unchanged drug. The plasma-elimination half-life is 7 to 9 hours, although this may be reduced to 2 to 3 hours by concomitant administration of liver enzyme-inducing drugs (see also Interactions, above).

◊ References.
1. Gustavson LE, Mengel HB. Pharmacokinetics of tiagabine, a γ-aminobutyric acid-uptake inhibitor, in healthy subjects after single and multiples doses. *Epilepsia* 1995; **36**: 605–11.
2. So EL, *et al.* Pharmacokinetics of tiagabine as add-on therapy in patients taking enzyme-inducing antiepilepsy drugs. *Epilepsy Res* 1995; **22**: 221–6.
3. Snel S, *et al.* The pharmacokinetics of tiagabine in healthy elderly volunteers and elderly patients with epilepsy. *J Clin Pharmacol* 1997; **37**: 1015–20.

The symbol † denotes a preparation no longer actively marketed

Uses and Administration

Tiagabine hydrochloride is a nipecotic acid derivative used in the treatment of epilepsy (p.338) as adjunctive therapy for refractory partial seizures with or without secondary generalisation. It inhibits the uptake of GABA into neuronal and glial cells, and therefore increases the availability of GABA at receptor sites.

In the UK, the initial dose of tiagabine hydrochloride as adjunctive therapy in adults and children over 12 years of age is the equivalent of tiagabine 5 mg twice daily by mouth for 1 week, increased as necessary by weekly increments of 5 to 10 mg daily. The usual maintenance dose is 30 to 45 mg daily, in three divided doses, in patients receiving enzyme-inducing antiepileptics; in patients *not* taking enzyme-inducing drugs an initial maintenance dosage of 15 to 30 mg daily is suggested. Lower initial doses are recommended in the USA. Doses should be taken with food to avoid rapid rises in plasma concentrations, thereby reducing the incidence of adverse effects. The initial daily maintenance dosage in patients with mild to moderate liver impairment should be reduced to 5 to 10 mg given as a single dose or in 2 divided doses.

As with other antiepileptics, withdrawal of tiagabine therapy or transition to or from another type of antiepileptic therapy should be made gradually to avoid precipitating an increase in the frequency of seizures. The manufacturer recommends gradual withdrawal over a period of 2 to 3 weeks. For a discussion on whether or not to withdraw antiepileptic therapy in seizure-free patients, see p.338.

◊ References.
1. Leach JP, Brodie MJ. Tiagabine. *Lancet* 1998; **351**: 203–7.
2. Adkins JC, Noble S. Tiagabine: a review of its pharmacodynamic and pharmacokinetic properties and therapeutic potential in the management of epilepsy. *Drugs* 1998; **55**: 437–60.
3. Luer MS, Rhoney DH. Tiagabine: a novel antiepileptic drug. *Ann Pharmacoter* 1998; **32**: 1173–80.
4. Anonymous. Tiagabine: add-on treatment for partial seizures. *Drug Ther Bull* 2000; **38**: 47–8.

Preparations

Proprietary Preparations (details are given in Part 3)
Aust.: Gabitril; *Austral.:* Gabitril; *Belg.:* Gabitril; *Denm.:* Gabitril; *Fin.:* Gabitril; *Fr.:* Gabitril; *Ger.:* Gabitril; *Irl.:* Gabitril; *Ital.:* Gabitril; *Port.:* Gabitril; *Spain:* Gabitril; *Switz.:* Gabitril; *UK:* Gabitril; *USA:* Gabitril.

Topiramate (3130-h)

Topiramate *(BAN, USAN, rINN)*.
McN-4853; RWJ-17021. 2,3:4,5-Di-*O*-isopropylidene-β-D-fructopyranose sulphamate.
$C_{12}H_{21}NO_8S = 339.4$.
CAS — 97240-79-4.
ATC — N03AX11.

Adverse Effects

Adverse effects associated with topiramate therapy include ataxia, impaired concentration, confusion, dizziness, fatigue, paraesthesia, drowsiness, and difficulties with memory or cognition. Agitation, emotional lability (with mood disorders), and depression may also occur. Other reported adverse effects include abdominal pain, anorexia, asthenia, diplopia, leucopenia, nausea, nystagmus, psychomotor retardation, impaired speech, altered taste, visual disturbances, and weight loss. The risk of developing renal calculi is increased, especially in predisposed patients.

Effects on electrolytes. Metabolic acidosis has been reported[1] in a 52-year-old man with normal renal function receiving topiramate as adjunctive therapy for intractable epilepsy.
1. Wilner A, *et al.* Topiramate and metabolic acidosis. *Epilepsia* 1999; **40**: 792–5.

Effects on the liver. Fulminant liver failure has been reported[1] following an increase in adjunctive topiramate dose in a patient maintained on carbamazepine.
1. Bjøro K, *et al.* Topiramate and fulminant liver failure. *Lancet* 1998; **352**: 1119.

Effects on the nervous system. Hemiparesis that resolved on withdrawal of topiramate has been reported[1] in 2 patients, although both already had compromised neurological function.
1. Stephen LJ, *et al.* Transient hemiparesis with topiramate. *BMJ* 1999; **318**: 845.

Precautions

Topiramate should be used with caution in patients with renal or hepatic impairment. Adequate hydration is recommended to reduce the risk of developing renal calculi, especially in predisposed patients.

Care is required when withdrawing topiramate therapy—see also under Uses and Administration, below.

Driving. For a comment on antiepileptic drugs and driving, see p.340.

Pregnancy. For comments on the management of epilepsy during pregnancy, see p.340.

Interactions

There are complex interactions between antiepileptics and toxicity may be enhanced without a corresponding increase in antiepileptic activity. Such interactions are very variable and unpredictable and plasma monitoring is often advisable with combination therapy.

Antiepileptics. In pharmacokinetic studies[1] *phenytoin* and *carbamazepine* decreased the plasma concentration of topiramate by about 50%.
For the effect of topiramate on phenytoin, see p.360.
1. Bourgeois BFD. Drug interaction profile of topiramate. *Epilepsia* 1996; **37:** (suppl 2): S14–S17.

Cardiac glycosides. For the effect of topiramate on *digoxin*, see p.871.

Sex hormones. For the effects of antiepileptics including topiramate on *oral contraceptives*, see p.1459.

Pharmacokinetics

Topiramate is readily absorbed following oral administration with peak plasma concentrations achieved about 2 hours after a dose. Bioavailability is not affected by the presence of food. The volume of distribution in women is approximately half that in men. Up to 50% of a dose may undergo metabolism in the liver in patients receiving enzyme-inducing drugs concomitantly. It is eliminated chiefly in urine, as unchanged drug and metabolites; mean plasma elimination half-life is about 21 hours. Steady-state concentrations are achieved after about 4 to 8 days in patients with normal renal function. Clearance is decreased in patients with impaired renal or hepatic function, and steady-state plasma concentrations may not be achieved for 10 to 15 days in the former. Children exhibit a higher clearance and shorter elimination half-life than adults.

The pharmacokinetics of topiramate may be affected by the concurrent administration of other antiepileptics (see under Interactions, above).

◊ References.
1. Perucca E, Bialer M. The clinical pharmacokinetics of the newer antiepileptic drugs: focus on topiramate, zonisamide, and tiagabine. *Clin Pharmacokinet* 1996; **31**: 29–46.
2. Glauser TA, *et al.* Topiramate pharmacokinetics in infants. *Epilepsia* 1999; **40**: 788–91.

Uses and Administration

Topiramate, a sulfamate-substituted monosaccharide, is an antiepileptic used as adjunctive therapy for refractory partial seizures with or without secondary generalisation, seizures associated with the Lennox-Gastaut syndrome, and primary generalised tonic-clonic seizures.

An initial dose of topiramate is 25 mg once daily by mouth for one week increased thereafter by increments of 25 to 50 mg at intervals of one to two weeks until the effective dose is reached, which is usually within the range of 200 to 400 mg daily taken in 2 divided doses; some patients may require up to 800 mg daily. Smaller increments or longer intervals between increments may be necessary if patients cannot tolerate the above regimen.

The initial dose for children aged 2 to 16 years is 25 mg nightly for the first week, increased at intervals of one to two weeks by increments of 1 to 3 mg per kg daily, according to response. The recommended dose thereafter is about 5 to 9 mg per kg body-weight daily given in 2 divided doses.

Daily doses of more than 25 mg should be taken in 2 divided doses. Patients with moderate or severe renal impairment take longer to reach steady-state plasma concentrations than patients with normal renal function (see under Pharmacokinetics, above). It has been recommended that doses be halved in such patients.

As with other antiepileptics, withdrawal of topiramate therapy or transition to or from another type of antiepileptic therapy should be made gradually to avoid precipitating an increase in the frequency of seizures. For a discussion on whether or not to withdraw antiepileptic therapy in seizure-free patients, see p.338. The manufacturers have suggested decreasing the dose by 100 mg daily at weekly intervals.

◊ Reviews.
1. Langtry HD, et al. Topiramate: a review of its pharmacodynamic and pharmacokinetic properties and clinical efficacy in the management of epilepsy. Drugs 1997; 54: 752–73.
2. Privitera MD. Topiramate: a new antiepileptic drug. Ann Pharmacother 1997; 31: 1164–73.
3. Markind JE. Topiramate: a new antiepileptic drug. Am J Health-Syst Pharm 1998; 55: 554–62.
4. Sachdeo RC, et al. Topiramate: clinical profile in epilepsy. Clin Pharmacokinet 1998; 34: 335–46.
5. Garnett WR. Clinical pharmacology of topiramate: a review. Epilepsia 2000; 41 (suppl 1): S61–S65.

Epilepsy. Topiramate is used in epilepsy (p.338) as adjunctive therapy for refractory partial seizures;[1,2] monotherapy with topiramate appeared to be safe and effective in one study.[3] Gradual initiation of topiramate therapy improves tolerability without delaying therapeutic response.[4]

Topiramate is also used in patients with the Lennox-Gastaut syndrome[5] and with primary generalised tonic-clonic seizures.[6] It has also been investigated in children with infantile spasms (as for example in West's syndrome)[7] and severe myoclonic epilepsy.[8] A retrospective review[9] of the use of topiramate in such drug-resistant childhood epilepsies concluded that it was efficacious and well tolerated.
1. Ben-Menachem E, et al. Double-blind, placebo-controlled trial of topiramate as add-on therapy in patients with refractory partial seizures. Epilepsia 1996; 37: 539–43.
2. Sharief M, et al. Double-blind, placebo-controlled study of topiramate in patients with refractory partial epilepsy. Epilepsy Res 1996; 25: 217–24.
3. Sachdeo RC, et al. Topiramate monotherapy for partial onset seizures. Epilepsia 1997; 38: 294–300.
4. Biton V, et al. Topiramate titration and tolerability. Ann Pharmacother 2001; 35: 173–9.
5. Sachdeo RC, et al. A double-blind, randomized trial of topiramate in Lennox-Gastaut syndrome. Neurology 1999; 52: 1882–7.
6. Biton V. A randomized, placebo-controlled study of topiramate in primary generalized tonic-clonic seizures. Neurology 1999; 52: 1330–7.
7. Glauser TA, et al. Long-term response to topiramate in patients with West syndrome. Epilepsia 2000; 41 (suppl 1): S91–S94.
8. Nieto-Barrera M, et al. Topiramate in the treatment of severe myoclonic epilepsy in infancy. Seizure 2000; 9: 590–4.
9. Yeung S, et al. Topiramate for drug-resistant epilepsies. Europ J Paediatr Neurol 2000; 4: 31–3.

Other neurological disorders. There have been case reports and pilot studies of the use of topiramate in the treatment of bipolar disorder,[1-3] trigeminal neuralgia,[4] tremor,[5] and binge-eating.[6]
1. Teter CJ, et al. Treatment of affective disorder and obesity with topiramate. Ann Pharmacother 2000; 34: 1262–5.
2. Erfurth A, Kuhn G. Topiramate monotherapy in the maintenance treatment of bipolar I disorder: effects on mood, weight and serum lipids. Neuropsychobiology 2000; 42 (suppl 1): 50–1.
3. McElroy SL, et al. Open-label adjunctive topiramate in the treatment of bipolar disorders. Biol Psychiatry 2000; 47: 1025–33.
4. Zvartau-Hind M, et al. Topiramate relieves refractory trigeminal neuralgia in MS patients. Neurology 2000; 55: 1587–8.
5. Galvez-Jimenez N, Hargreave M. Topiramate and essential tremor. Ann Neurol 2000; 47: 837–8.
6. Shapira NA, et al. Treatment of binge-eating disorder with topiramate: a clinical case series. J Clin Psychiatry 2000; 61: 368–72.

Preparations

Proprietary Preparations (details are given in Part 3)
Aust.: Topamax; *Austral.:* Topamax; *Belg.:* Topamax; *Canad.:* Topamax; *Denm.:* Topimax; *Fin.:* Topimax; *Fr.:* Epitomax; *Ger.:* Topamax; *Hong Kong:* Topamax; *Irl.:* Topamax; *Israel:* Topamax; *Ital.:* Topamax; *Mex.:* Topamax; *Neth.:* Topamax; *Norw.:* Topimax; *NZ:* Topamax; *Port.:* Topamax; *S.Afr.:* Topamax; *Singapore:* Topamax; *Spain:* Topamax; *Swed.:* Topimax; *Switz.:* Topamax; *Thai.:* Topamax; *UK:* Topamax; *USA:* Topamax.

Trimethadione (6622-d)

Trimethadione (BAN, rINN).

Trimetadiona; Trimethadionum; Trimethinum; Troxidone. 3,5,5-Trimethyl-1,3-oxazolidine-2,4-dione.
$C_6H_9NO_3 = 143.1$.
CAS — 127-48-0.
ATC — N03AC02.
Pharmacopoeias. In Eur. (see p.vi), Int. and Jpn.

Pharmacopoeial description
Ph. Eur.: Colourless or almost colourless crystals. Soluble in water; very soluble in alcohol and in ether. Protect from light.

Adverse Effects

Many adverse effects of trimethadione are serious and call for prompt discontinuation of therapy. Common side-effects include drowsiness, which may subside on continuation of therapy, and photophobia and hemeralopia (blurring of vision in bright light), which is more frequent in adults.

Other side-effects include nausea and vomiting, abdominal pain, anorexia, weight loss, hiccups, malaise, insomnia, vertigo, headache, alopecia, paraesthesias, changes in blood pressure, and personality changes. Blood disorders include neutropenia (which does not call for withdrawal of therapy provided that it remains moderate), thrombocytopenia, pancytopenia, agranulocytosis, and aplastic anaemia. Lymphadenopathy, a lupus erythematosus syndrome, the nephrotic syndrome, and hepatitis may also occur. Skin rashes may lead to exfoliative dermatitis and erythema multiforme. A syndrome resembling myasthenia gravis has also been reported.

Symptoms of acute overdosage include drowsiness, nausea, dizziness, ataxia, visual disturbances, and coma.

Characteristic congenital malformations, termed the fetal trimethadione syndrome, have been associated with the use of trimethadione in pregnancy.

Precautions

Trimethadione is contra-indicated in patients with severe hepatic or renal disease or with severe blood disorders. It should be used with caution in patients with disease of the retina or optic nerve and should be withdrawn if scotomata occur. Frequent examinations of blood, urine, and hepatic function should be carried out in patients receiving trimethadione, and therapy should be withdrawn promptly at signs of renal or hepatic dysfunction, severe neutropenia or other blood disorders, or drug hypersensitivity. Trimethadione should also be discontinued, at least temporarily, on the appearance of any skin disorder, however mild.

Care is required when withdrawing trimethadione therapy—see also under Uses and Administration, below. Abrupt withdrawal should be avoided unless serious adverse effects have occurred, in which case substitution by an alternative antiepileptic may be necessary.

Administration of trimethadione in pregnancy has been associated with a high incidence of congenital malformations.

Porphyria. Trimethadione has been associated with acute attacks of porphyria and is considered unsafe in porphyric patients.

Pregnancy. For comments on the management of epilepsy during pregnancy, see p.340.

Pharmacokinetics

Trimethadione is readily absorbed from the gastrointestinal tract and extensively demethylated in the liver to its active metabolite, dimethadione, which is primarily responsible for the activity of trimethadione on chronic administration.

Trimethadione is very slowly excreted in the urine, over a period of several days, almost entirely in the form of dimethadione.

Trimethadione is reported not to be significantly bound to plasma proteins.

Some correlation has been found between plasma concentrations of dimethadione exceeding 700 µg per mL and therapeutic response.

Uses and Administration

Trimethadione is an oxazolidinedione antiepileptic that has been given by mouth in the treatment of absence seizures refractory to other antiepileptics. However, because of its potential toxicity, other antiepileptics are preferred (see under Epilepsy, p.338).

As with other antiepileptics, withdrawal of trimethadione therapy or transition to or from another type of antiepileptic therapy should be made gradually to avoid precipitating an increase in the frequency of seizures. For a discussion on whether or not to withdraw antiepileptic therapy in seizure-free patients, see p.338.

Valproate (10447-z)

Valproate is a generic term applied to valproic acid, its salts and esters.

Valproic Acid (6623-n)

Valproic Acid (BAN, USAN, rINN).
Abbott-44089; Acidum Valproicum. 2-Propylvaleric acid; 2-Propylpentanoic acid.
$C_8H_{16}O_2 = 144.2$.
CAS — 99-66-1.
ATC — N03AG01.
Pharmacopoeias. In Eur. (see p.vi) and US.

Pharmacopoeial description
Ph. Eur.: A colourless or very slightly yellow, slightly viscous, clear liquid. Very slightly soluble in water; miscible with alcohol and with dichloromethane. It dissolves in dilute solutions of alkali hydroxides. Store in airtight containers.

USP 25: A colourless to pale yellow, slightly viscous, clear liquid having a characteristic odour. Slightly soluble in water; freely soluble in alcohol, in acetone, in chloroform, in ether, in methyl alcohol, in benzene, in n-heptane, and in 1N sodium hydroxide; slightly soluble in 0.1N hydrochloric acid. Store in airtight glass, stainless steel, or polyethylene containers.

Sodium Valproate (6608-h)

Sodium Valproate (BANM, rINNM).
Abbott-44090; Natrii Valproas; Valproate Sodium (USAN). Sodium 2-propylvalerate; Sodium 2-propylpentanoate.
$C_8H_{15}NaO_2 = 166.2$.
CAS — 1069-66-5.
Pharmacopoeias. In Chin., Eur. (see p.vi), Int., and Jpn.

Pharmacopoeial description
Ph. Eur.: A white or almost white, hygroscopic, crystalline powder. Very soluble in water; slightly to freely soluble in alcohol. Store in airtight containers.

Valproate Pivoxil (2480-c)

Valproate Pivoxil (rINN).
Hydroxymethyl 2-propylvalerate pivalate.
$C_{14}H_{26}O_4 = 258.4$.
CAS — 77372-61-3.

Valproate Semisodium (16983-a)

Valproate Semisodium (rINN).
Abbott-50711; Divalproex Sodium (USAN); Semisodium Valproate (BAN). 2-Propylvaleric acid—Sodium 2-propylvalerate (1:1); Sodium hydrogen bis(2-propylvalerate) oligomer.
$C_{16}H_{31}NaO_4 = 310.4$.
CAS — 76584-70-8.

Valpromide (6624-h)

Valpromide (rINN).
Dipropylacetamide. 2-Propylvaleramide.
$C_8H_{17}NO = 143.2$.
CAS — 2430-27-5.
ATC — N03AG02.

Adverse Effects

The most frequently reported adverse effects associated with valproate therapy are gastrointestinal disturbances, particularly on initiation of therapy; use of enteric-coated formulations, administration with meals, and commencement of therapy with low doses may minimise symptoms. There may be increased appetite, and weight gain is common.

Less common adverse effects include oedema, headache, reversible prolongation of bleeding time, and thrombocytopenia. Leucopenia and bone marrow depression have been reported. Neurological adverse effects including ataxia, tremor, sedation, lethargy, confusion, and more rarely encephalopathy and coma, have occasionally been reported, although these are often associated with too high a starting dose, increasing doses too rapidly, or concomitant use of other antiepileptics. Very rare cases of extrapyramidal symptoms or reversible dementia associated with cerebral atrophy have been reported. Increased alertness may occur, which is generally considered beneficial, but occasionally aggression, hyperactivity, and behavioural disturbances have been reported. Hearing loss has been reported. There may occasionally be rashes, and, rarely, hirsutism, acne, toxic epidermal necrolysis and Stevens-Johnson syndrome or erythema multiforme. Transient hair loss, sometimes with regrowth of curly hair, has occurred. Irregular periods, amenorrhoea, and gynaecomastia have been reported rarely.

Liver dysfunction including hepatic failure has occasionally been reported, usually in the first few months of treatment, and necessitates valproate withdrawal; there have been fatalities. Elevation of liver enzyme values is common but normally transient and dose-related. Hyperammonaemia has occurred, even in the absence of overt hepatic failure and is sometimes associated with neurological symptoms; hyperglycinaemia has also been reported. Pancreatitis has also been reported; plasma amylase should be measured if there is acute abdominal pain. In a few patients there have been reports of reversible defects in renal tubular function (Fanconi's syndrome).

Congenital malformations have been reported in infants born to women who had received antiepileptics including valproate during pregnancy.

Inflammatory reactions and pain have been reported at the injection site following intravenous administration.

◊ Side-effects were present in 71 of 88 children receiving sodium valproate monotherapy[1] and, although average doses in these patients were significantly higher than in the 17 with no side-effects, no difference in the plasma concentrations was observed between the 2 groups. Behavioural alterations seen in 56 included irritability, longer and deeper sleep, superficial sleep, hyperactivity, being more alert, lassitude, drowsiness, being more sociable, calmness, being happier, absent mindedness, being sadder, aggressiveness, being more skillful, and docility; it was emphasised that stimulatory reactions were as frequent as depressant effects. Digestive disorders occurred in 43 children with anorexia, abdominal pain, and nausea and vomiting being the most frequent; diarrhoea, constipation, an increase in appetite, and a gain in weight also occurred. Neurological changes in the form of tremor, paraesthesia, or ataxia, occurring in only 4 patients, were less frequent than either behavioural or digestive reactions. Miscellaneous reactions including polydipsia, polyuria, diaphoresis, enuresis, hair loss, change in hair colour or texture, and rash were seen in 23 children. Of the 71 children experiencing reactions therapy continued unchanged in 56, was changed in 3 either by altering the pharmaceutical formulation (syrup, tablets, granules), by changing the frequency of dosing, or by reducing the dose in 6, and in the remaining 9 children valproate therapy was discontinued. With the exception of a temporary increase in plasma transaminase concentrations in 2 patients, hepatic or pancreatic dysfunction was not seen.

1. Herranz JL, et al. Side effects of sodium valproate in monotherapy controlled by plasma levels: a study in 88 pediatric patients. Epilepsia 1982; 23: 203–14.

Carnitine deficiency. Carnitine deficiency (p.1356) may occasionally arise during long-term administration of valproate; although it is unclear whether carnitine supplementation is of value in children receiving valproate, some neurologists consider it justified in selected cases.[1]

1. De Vivo DC, et al. L-Carnitine supplementation in childhood epilepsy: current perspectives. Epilepsia 1998; 39: 1216–25.

Effects on the blood. A number of reports have implicated valproate as a cause of occasional neutropenia,[1,2] leucopenia,[3] and thrombocytopenia.[2] A 1-year prospective study involving 45 patients found that absolute neutropenia developed in 12 and thrombocytopenia in 15, but that the disorders were transient and self-limiting.[2] However, neutropenia has occasionally been sufficiently severe to warrant withdrawal of valproate.[4] Red cell aplasia has also been associated with valproate therapy.[5,6] A study[7] involving 30 children indicated that valproate might produce symptoms similar to those of von Willebrand's disease; 19 of the 30 had a history of minor haemorrhage during therapy, and 7 had abnormal bleeding times. They felt that factor VIII therapy may need to be given in patients receiving valproate who undergo surgery or in whom bleeding is severe.

For a discussion of the effects of antiepileptics, including valproate, on serum folate, see under Phenytoin, p.358.

1. Jaeken J, et al. Neutropenia during sodium valproate treatment. Arch Dis Child 1979; 54: 986–7.
2. Barr RD, et al. Valproic acid and immune thrombocytopenia. Arch Dis Child 1982; 57: 681–4.
3. Coulter DL, et al. Valproic acid therapy in childhood epilepsy. JAMA 1980; 244: 785–8.
4. Symon DNK, Russell G. Sodium valproate and neutropenia. Arch Dis Child 1983; 58: 235.
5. MacDougall LG. Pure red cell aplasia associated with sodium valproate therapy. JAMA 1982; 247: 53–4.
6. Watts RG, et al. Valproic acid-induced cytopenias: evidence for a dose-related suppression of hematopoiesis. J Pediatr 1990; 117: 495–9.
7. Kreuz W, et al. Induction of von Willebrand disease type I by valproic acid. Lancet 1990; 335: 1350–1.

Effects on bone. For the effects of antiepileptics including valproate on bone and on calcium and vitamin D metabolism, see under Phenytoin, p.358.

Effects on the endocrine system. *Menstrual disturbances* occurred more frequently with valproate than other antiepileptics in a study of 238 women with epilepsy.[1] The disturbances were attributed to valproate-associated reproductive endocrine disorders, namely polycystic ovaries and elevated serum-testosterone concentrations.

For mention of the effects of antiepileptics on *sexual function* in male epileptic patients, see under Phenytoin, p.358.

1. Isojärvi JIT, et al. Polycystic ovaries and hyperandrogenism in women taking valproate for epilepsy. N Engl J Med 1993; 329: 1383–8.

Effects on the liver. One review[1] of the hepatotoxicity of valproate included an analysis of 42 cases with fatal hepatitis, 3 cases with a Reye's-like syndrome, and 22 instances of hyperammonaemia.

• In 19 clinical trials the incidence of *abnormal serum aminotransferase* activity has ranged from 0 to 44% with an overall incidence of 11% in the 1197 patients monitored; in the non-fatal cases activity was usually between one and three times the upper limit of normal and was not usually, except in the most severe cases, accompanied by rises in serum bilirubin or alkaline phosphatase.

• In the 42 cases of *hepatitis* with a fatal outcome the age at presentation ranged from 2.5 months to 34 years with 69% aged 10 years or less. Below the age of 15 years the proportion of males was 62.5% but above this age it was 30%; the disproportionate vulnerability of young individuals, particularly boys, does not appear to be a reflection of prescribing habits in that age group. In more than two-thirds of these patients with a fatal outcome, prodromal symptoms comprised anorexia and vomiting, loss of epilepsy control, impaired consciousness, and ataxia; in about one-third there were signs of liver damage with fever, jaundice, ascites, peripheral oedema, and easy bruising. In all of the patients hepatic coma developed. In 36 patients on whom data were available the onset of hepatic illness in one-third occurred between 1 and 2 months and in only 2 patients did the onset occur after more than 5 months. Of these 42 patients with fatal hepatotoxicity 36 had received other drugs, mostly antiepileptics, concurrently.

• The 3 children with the *Reye's-like syndrome* all died within 3 weeks of the first occurrence of symptoms as a result of cerebral oedema (2) or aspiration pneumonia (1).

• In the 22 patients with symptomatic *hyperammonaemia*, characterised usually by impaired consciousness and ataxia, but without overt liver disease, withdrawal of valproate resulted in all becoming asymptomatic and biochemical abnormalities returned to normal. Hyperammonaemia has also been reported in asymptomatic patients.

Various hypotheses for the cause of valproate hepatotoxicity have been discussed in detail.

Analysis of deaths in the USA attributed to valproate liver toxicity identified a decline in the incidence of fatalities as use in young children and use concurrently with other antiepileptics declined.[3]

1. Powell-Jackson PR, et al. Hepatotoxicity to sodium valproate: a review. Gut 1984; 25: 673–81.
2. Eadie MJ, et al. Valproate-associated hepatotoxicity and its biochemical mechanisms. Med Toxicol 1988; 3: 85–106.
3. Dreifuss FE, et al. Valproic acid hepatic fatalities: II US experience since 1984. Neurology 1989; 39: 201–7.

Effects on mental function. For a review of the effects of antiepileptic therapy including sodium valproate on cognition, see p.340.

Effects on the nervous system. An *extrapyramidal* syndrome of tremor and rigidity, unresponsive to benzatropine or benzhexol [trihexyphenidyl], developed in a 52-year-old man with schizophrenia given a therapeutic trial of sodium valproate 1 to 2 g daily.[1] Administration of sodium valproate to a man with dystonic movements of the neck and spine produced a severe subjective and objective deterioration in his symptoms which returned to their previous severity on withdrawal of the drug.[2]

A *stuporous state* associated with EEG abnormalities has been described[3,4] during valproate therapy for complex partial or mixed seizure types and it was suggested that in certain forms of epilepsy valproate may exhibit a paradoxical epileptogenic effect. Other findings[5] have argued against an epileptic origin for valproate-induced stupor.

1. Lautin A, et al. Extrapyramidal syndrome with sodium valproate. BMJ 1979; 2: 1035–6.
2. Dick DJ, Saunders M. Extrapyramidal syndrome with sodium valproate. BMJ 1980; 280: 189.
3. Marescaux C, et al. Stuporous episodes during treatment with sodium valproate: report of seven cases. Epilepsia 1982; 23: 297–305.
4. Stecker MM, Kita M. Paradoxical response to valproic acid in a patient with a hypothalamic hamartoma. Ann Pharmacother 1998; 32: 1168–72.
5. Aguglia U, et al. Negative myoclonus during valproate-related stupor: neurophysiological evidence of a cortical non-epileptic origin. Electroencephalogr Clin Neurophysiol 1995; 94: 103–8.

Effects on the pancreas. An early report of 4 cases of pancreatitis associated with valproic acid therapy also reviewed 10 previously published cases.[1] None of the 14 patients, 2 of whom died, suffered other symptoms of a toxic reaction to valproic acid. Pancreatitis was not dose-related and had developed as early as one week and as late as 4.5 years following the introduction of therapy. Symptoms recurred on rechallenge in 6 of 7 patients. However, routine monitoring of serum-amylase concentrations in asymptomatic patients did not seem necessary. In February 1994 the UK Committee on Safety of Medicines commented[2] in a review of drug-induced pancreatitis that they had received 29 reports of pancreatitis, including 2 fatalities, associated with sodium valproate.

1. Wyllie E, et al. Pancreatitis associated with valproic acid therapy. Am J Dis Child 1984; 138: 912–14.
2. Committee on Safety of Medicines/Medicines Control Agency. Drug-induced pancreatitis. Current Problems 1994; 20: 2–3.

Effects on the skin and hair. Five of 250 patients developed curly hair during treatment with sodium valproate 1 g daily;[1] in 3 patients this effect followed temporary alopecia. Another report of hair curling in a patient who received sodium valproate in doses up to 3 g daily for 30 months commented that her hair started to revert to the former straight style 9 months after discontinuing the drug.[2]

Valproate-induced nicotinic-acid deficiency with an associated pellagra-like syndrome has been reported in a young boy;[3] the condition responded dramatically to the administration of nicotinamide.

Reduced serum-zinc concentrations and cutaneous manifestations of zinc deficiency were found in 2 patients receiving antiepileptic drugs.[4] It was postulated that deficiency occurred as a result of chelation by sodium valproate, and possibly phenytoin, in association with malabsorption and that, in one case, malabsorption was initiated by valproate.

Cutaneous vasculitis has been reported[5] in 2 patients taking sodium valproate. The reaction recurred on rechallenge.

Valproate might share the same order of risk as other antiepileptics for the development of Stevens-Johnson syndrome and toxic epidermal necrolysis,[6] although it had previously been regarded as safer in this respect.

1. Jeavons PM, et al. Valproate and curly hair. Lancet 1977; i: 359.
2. Gupta AK. 'Perming' effects associated with chronic valproate therapy. Br J Clin Pract 1988; 42: 75–7.
3. Gillman MA, Sandyk R. Nicotinic acid deficiency induced by sodium valproate. S Afr Med J 1984; 65: 986.
4. Lewis-Jones MS, et al. Cutaneous manifestations of zinc deficiency during treatment with anticonvulsants. BMJ 1985; 290: 603–4.
5. Kamper AM, et al. Cutaneous vasculitis induced by sodium valproate. Lancet 1991; 337: 497–8.
6. Anonymous. Drugs as risk factors in severe cutaneous diseases. WHO Drug Inf 1996; 10: 33–5.

Enuresis. Nocturnal enuresis associated with sodium valproate therapy has been reported[1] in 2 children. Remission of the enuresis was achieved either by reducing or redistributing the doses. Choonara[2] commented that several studies have recorded enuresis as a side-effect of valproate in children, the frequency being between 1 and 7%. The 2 most likely explanations are that it is secondary to a central effect on the thirst centre resulting in polydipsia or is a consequence of the increased depth of sleep associated with valproate.

1. Panayiotopoulos CP. Nocturnal enuresis associated with sodium valproate. Lancet 1985; i: 980–1.
2. Choonara IA. Sodium valproate and enuresis. Lancet 1985; i: 1276.

Treatment of Adverse Effects

Following overdosage the stomach may be emptied by lavage, although it has been suggested that this may be of limited value in view of the rapid absorption of valproic acid and its salts. Supportive therapy alone may then suffice.

◊ Although a variety of active treatments including forced diuresis, naloxone, and haemodialysis or haemoperfusion have been advocated for valproate overdose, supportive measures provided sufficient treatment for a patient who had taken 25 g of sodium valproate.[1] For a further review of the features and management of poisoning with some antiepileptics, including valproate, see under Phenytoin, p.358.

1. Lakhani M, McMurdo MET. Survival after severe self poisoning with sodium valproate. Postgrad Med J 1986; 62: 409–10.

Precautions

Valproate is contra-indicated in patients with pre-existing liver disease or a family history of severe hepatic dysfunction. Children under 3 years of age and those with congenital metabolic disorders, organic brain disease, or severe seizure disorders associated with mental retardation may be at particular risk of hepatotoxicity and the drug should be used with particular caution in these groups. Combination with other antiepileptics, which may also increase the risks of liver damage, should be avoided if possible. Liver function tests should be carried out, particularly in those most at risk, before and during the first 6 months of therapy. Raised liver enzymes are not uncommon during treatment and are usually transient or respond to reduction in dosage, but patients should be reassessed clinically and liver function, including prothrombin time, monitored until they return to normal. An abnormally prolonged prothrombin time, particularly in association with other relevant abnormalities, requires discontinuation of treatment. Treatment should also be discontinued if pancreatitis is diagnosed.

Patients or their carers should be told how to recognise signs of blood and liver toxicity or pancreatitis, and they should be advised to seek immediate medical attention if symptoms develop.

Patients should be monitored for platelet function before major elective surgery; some sources suggest regular monitoring before and during therapy.

Valproate should be used with caution if systemic lupus erythematosus is suspected.

The symbol † denotes a preparation no longer actively marketed

Patients should be warned of the risk of weight gain and appropriate strategies adopted to minimise the effect.

Care is required when withdrawing valproate therapy—see also under Uses and Administration, below.

It should be noted that the protein binding of valproate is saturable and thus shows concentration dependency with significant increases in free drug occurring at high total plasma concentrations.

Because valproate is partly excreted in the form of ketone bodies, it may cause false positives in urine tests for diabetes mellitus.

Dosage adjustments may be necessary in severe renal impairment in accordance with free serum valproate levels.

Breast feeding. Thrombocytopenic purpura and anaemia occurred in a breast-fed infant whose mother was being treated with valproic acid.[1] The baby recovered when breast feeding was stopped. Low serum-valproate levels were detected[2] in 6 breast-fed infants whose mothers had been taking valproate semisodium post partum; no adverse effects were observed in the infants. For comment on antiepileptic therapy and breast feeding, see under Pregnancy and Breast Feeding on p.340.

1. Stahl MMS, et al. Thrombocytopenic purpura and anemia in a breast-fed infant whose mother was treated with valproic acid. J Pediatr 1997; 130: 1001–3.
2. Piontek CM, et al. Serum valproate levels in 6 breastfeeding mother-infant pairs. J Clin Psychiatry 2000; 61: 170–2.

Driving. For a comment on antiepileptic drugs and driving, see p.340.

HIV infection and AIDS. The use of valproic acid in HIV-positive patients has been reviewed.[1] Limited data from several small in-vitro studies have demonstrated that valproic acid may induce viral replication of HIV; some clinicians have therefore suggested increased monitoring of viral load in HIV-positive patients treated with valproic acid.

1. Jennings HR, Romanelli F. The use of valproic acid in HIV-positive patients. Ann Pharmacother 1999; 33: 1113–16.

Porphyria. Valproate is considered to be unsafe in patients with porphyria because it has been shown to be porphyrinogenic in animals or in-vitro systems. There is conflicting evidence of the porphyrinogenicity of valpromide, although it has also been shown to be porphyrinogenic in in-vitro systems.

For comments on the use of valproate in porphyria, see p.342.

Pregnancy. For comments on the management of epilepsy during pregnancy see p.340.

There is an increased risk of neural tube defects in infants exposed in utero to antiepileptics including valproate and a variety of syndromes such as craniofacial and digital abnormalities and, less commonly, cleft lip and palate have been described. In an unselected series[1] of 17 infants whose epileptic mothers had received valproate during pregnancy, 9 had minor abnormalities and of these 5 also had major abnormalities, including congenital heart defect in 4. Neonatal bleeding, attributed to fibrinogen depletion and sometimes fatal, has been reported following exposure in utero to valproate.[2,3] Hypoglycaemia was recorded[4] in 13 of 22 neonates whose mothers had taken valproate during pregnancy. Valproate-withdrawal symptoms, including irritability, jitteriness, hypertonia, seizures, and feeding problems were also noted.

1. Thisted E, Ebbesen F. Malformations, withdrawal manifestations, and hypoglycaemia after exposure to valproate in utero. Arch Dis Child 1993; 69: 288–91.
2. Majer RV, Green PJ. Neonatal afibrinogenaemia due to sodium valproate. Lancet 1987; ii: 740–1.
3. Bavoux F, et al. Neonatal fibrinogen depletion caused by sodium valproate. Ann Pharmacother 1994; 28: 1307.
4. Ebbesen F, et al. Neonatal hypoglycaemia and withdrawal symptoms after exposure in utero to valproate. Arch Dis Child Fetal Neonatal Ed 2000; 83: F124–F129.

Interactions

There are complex interactions between antiepileptics and toxicity may be enhanced without a corresponding increase in antiepileptic activity. Such interactions are very variable and unpredictable and plasma monitoring is often advisable with combination therapy. Caution is recommended when giving valproate with other drugs liable to interfere with blood coagulation, such as aspirin or warfarin. Use with other hepatotoxic drugs should be avoided.

◊ General references.
1. Levy RH, Koch KM. Drug interactions with valproic acid. Drugs 1982; 24: 543–56.

Analgesics. The valproic acid free fraction was reported to be increased, as was the half-life, when aspirin was given concomitantly in a study in 6 epileptic children;[1] this suggests that salicylates may inhibit the metabolism of valproate in addition to displacing it from protein binding sites. Furthermore, salicylates have been associated with an increased risk of Reye's syndrome (p.15) in children, and combination with another

hepatotoxic drug such as valproate is clearly undesirable. In addition, both aspirin and valproate affect blood coagulation and platelet function.

Naproxen has also been reported to produce a slight displacement of protein-bound valproic acid but the effect is probably not sufficiently marked for it to have a clinical effect.[2]

1. Orr JM, et al. Interaction between valproic acid and aspirin in epileptic children: serum protein binding and metabolic effects. Clin Pharmacol Ther 1982; 31: 642–9.
2. Grimaldi R, et al. In vivo plasma protein binding interaction between valproic acid and naproxen. Eur J Drug Metab Pharmacokinet 1984; 9: 359–63.

Antibacterials. A patient receiving valproate therapy was reported[1] to have had raised valproate blood concentrations and symptoms consistent with valproate toxicity during concomitant therapy with erythromycin.

There is a theoretical possibility that carnitine deficiency may be increased in patients receiving pivampicillin and valproate.

Decreases in plasma concentrations of valproic acid to subtherapeutic levels have been noted in 2 patients during concomitant therapy with meropenem and amikacin.[2] Meropenem was regarded as the likely cause of the interaction with valproic acid. Marked reductions in valproate concentrations have also been reported in 3 children given panipenem (with betamipron).[3] Increased serum-valproate concentrations resulting in signs of valproate toxicity occurred in a child after beginning therapy with isoniazid;[4] the child was a slow acetylator of isoniazid and valproate dosage had to be reduced by about 60% to maintain satisfactory concentrations. When isoniazid was subsequently stopped, valproate dosage had to be increased to its previous value in order to maintain a therapeutic effect.

1. Redington K, et al. Erythromycin and valproate interaction. Ann Intern Med 1992; 116: 877–8.
2. De Turck BJG, et al. Lowering of plasma valproic acid concentrations during concomitant therapy with meropenem and amikacin. J Antimicrob Chemother 1998; 42: 563–4.
3. Nagai K, et al. Decrease in serum levels of valproic acid during treatment with a new carbapenem, panipenem/betamipron. J Antimicrob Chemother 1997; 39: 295–6.
4. Jonville AP, et al. Interaction between isoniazid and valproate: a case of valproate overdosage. Eur J Clin Pharmacol 1991; 40: 197–8.

Antidepressants. As with all antiepileptics, antidepressants may antagonise the antiepileptic activity of valproate by lowering the convulsive threshold. For the effect of valproate on amitriptyline, see p.277.

Antiepileptics. The barbiturate antiepileptic phenobarbital is reported to decrease serum-valproate concentrations when given concomitantly,[1] apparently by induction of valproate metabolism.[2] This effect is overshadowed, however, by the marked increase in serum-phenobarbital concentrations caused by valproate inhibition of phenobarbital metabolism—see p.356.

Carbamazepine and phenytoin are also enzyme-inducing drugs and, as might be expected, are reported to increase the metabolism of valproate and decrease the serum concentration of valproate.[3-5] The effect may be clinically significant.[6] The reciprocal effects of valproate on both drugs are complex, with conflicting effects on metabolism and protein binding, and the clinical outcome is difficult to predict. For more details see under Carbamazepine, p.344 and Phenytoin, p.360.

Raised serum concentrations of valproic acid have been reported in patients given felbamate.[7]

Valproate inhibits the metabolism of lamotrigine which may result in serious toxic reactions—see p.352. There is limited evidence that valproic acid may inhibit the metabolism of ethosuximide in some patients—see p.348.

For interactions with benzodiazepines, see under Diazepam, p.678.

1. Perucca E. Pharmacokinetic interactions with antiepileptic drugs. Clin Pharmacokinet 1982; 7: 57–84.
2. Levy RH, Koch KM. Drug interactions with valproic acid. Drugs 1982; 24: 543–56.
3. Panesar SK, et al. The effect of carbamazepine on valproic acid disposition in adult volunteers. Br J Clin Pharmacol 1989; 27: 323–8.
4. Reunanen MI, et al. Low serum valproic acid concentrations in epileptic patients on combination therapy. Curr Ther Res 1980; 28: 456–62.
5. Cramer JA, et al. Variable free and total valproic acid concentrations in sole- and multi-drug therapy. Ther Drug Monit 1986; 8: 411–15.
6. Jann MW, et al. Increased valproate serum concentrations upon carbamazepine cessation. Epilepsia 1988; 29: 578–81.
7. Wagner ML, et al. The effect of felbamate on valproic acid disposition. Clin Pharmacol Ther 1994; 56: 494–502.

Antimalarials. Low serum concentrations of valproate have been reported[1] in patients taking mefloquine. Also, mefloquine and chloroquine may antagonise the antiepileptic activity of valproate by lowering the convulsive threshold.

1. Anonymous. Mefloquine for malaria. Med Lett Drugs Ther 1990; 32: 13–14.

Antineoplastics. A marked reduction in serum-valproate concentration occurred in a 6-year-old child following a high-dose 24-hour infusion of methotrexate.[1]

1. Schröder H, Østergaard JR. Interference of high-dose methotrexate in the metabolism of valproate? Pediatr Hematol Oncol 1994; 11: 445–9.

Antipsychotics. As with all antiepileptics, antipsychotics may antagonise the antiepileptic activity of valproate by lower-

ing the convulsive threshold. For the effect of valproate on clozapine, see p.673.

Antivirals. For the effect of valproate on zidovudine, see p.646.

Benzodiazepines. For interactions between valproate and benzodiazepines, see under Diazepam, p.678.

Colestyramine. Colestyramine may decrease the absorption of valproate.

Gastrointestinal drugs. Administration with an antacid (aluminium and magnesium hydroxides) has been shown to increase significantly the bioavailability of a valproic acid preparation in healthy subjects;[1] other antacids in this study (calcium carbonate and an aluminium magnesium trisilicate mixture) had a lesser, insignificant effect.

Cimetidine significantly increased the half-life and decreased the clearance of sodium valproate in another study;[2] ranitidine had no effect on valproate pharmacokinetics.[2]

These interactions have not been reported to be of clinical significance, although the possibility must exist, particularly in patients on high-dose therapy.

1. May CA, et al. Effects of three antacids on the bioavailability of valproic acid. Clin Pharm 1982; 1: 244–7.
2. Webster LK, et al. Effect of cimetidine and ranitidine on carbamazepine and sodium valproate pharmacokinetics. Eur J Clin Pharmacol 1984; 27: 341–3.

Pharmacokinetics

Valproic acid and its salts are rapidly and completely absorbed from the gastrointestinal tract; the rate, but not the extent, of absorption is delayed by administration with or after food.

Valproic acid is extensively metabolised in the liver, a large part by glucuronidation and the rest by a variety of complex pathways. It does not appear to enhance its own metabolism, but metabolism may be enhanced by other drugs which induce hepatic microsomal enzymes. It is excreted in the urine almost entirely in the form of its metabolites; small amounts are excreted in faeces and expired air.

Valproic acid is extensively bound to plasma protein. The extent of protein binding is concentration dependent and is stated to be about 90 to 95% at total concentrations of 50 µg per mL, falling to about 80 to 85% at 100 µg per mL. Reported half-lives for valproic acid have ranged from about 5 to 20 hours; the shorter half-lives have generally been recorded in epileptic patients receiving multiple drug therapy.

The 'target' range of total plasma-valproic acid is usually quoted as being 40 to 100 µg per mL (280 to 700 µmol per litre) but routine monitoring of plasma concentrations is not generally considered to be of use as an aid to assessing control.

Valproic acid crosses the placental barrier and small amounts are distributed into breast milk.

Valpromide is an amide derivative of valproic acid and its absorption is slower and its bioavailability somewhat less than that of valproic acid. Valpromide is rapidly and almost completely metabolised in the liver to valproic acid.

The pharmacokinetics of valproate are affected by the concomitant administration of other antiepileptics (see under Interactions, above).

◊ References.
1. Zaccara G, et al. Clinical pharmacokinetics of valproic acid—1988. Clin Pharmacokinet 1988; 15: 367–89.
2. Bialer M. Clinical pharmacology of valpromide. Clin Pharmacokinet 1991; 20: 114–22.
3. Cloyd JC, et al. Valproic acid pharmacokinetics in children IV: effects of age and antiepileptic drugs on protein binding and intrinsic clearance. Clin Pharmacol Ther 1993; 53: 22–9.
4. Yukawa E, et al. Population-based investigation of valproic acid relative clearance using nonlinear mixed effects modeling: influence of drug-drug interaction and patient characteristics. J Clin Pharmacol 1997; 37: 1160–7.

Absorption. For a reference to the pharmacokinetics of rectal and oral administration of valproic acid, see under Uses and Administration, below.

Uses and Administration

Valproate, available as valproic acid, its salts and esters, is an antiepileptic used particularly in the treatment of primary generalised seizures, and notably absence and myoclonic seizures, and also for partial seizures. Its actions are complex and its mode of action in epilepsy is not fully understood. Valproate is also used to treat the acute manic phase of bipolar disorder and for the prophylaxis of migraine.

It can be given in a variety of forms including the sodium salts (valproate semisodium and sodium valproate), the amide derivative (valpromide), or as valproic acid. Magnesium valproate has also been tried as has calcium valproate. Valproate should preferably be taken with or after food.

In the treatment of **epilepsy** the dose should be adjusted to the needs of the individual patient to achieve adequate control of seizures. Plasma concentrations of valproate (see Pharmacokinetics, above) are not considered to be a useful index of efficacy and thus their routine monitoring is generally not helpful. A suggested initial oral dose of *sodium valproate* for *adults* is 600 mg daily in 2 divided doses, increased every 3 days by 200 mg daily to a usual range of 1 to 2 g daily (20 to 30 mg per kg body-weight daily); further increases up to a maximum of 2.5 g daily may be necessary if adequate control has not been achieved.

A suggested initial oral dose of sodium valproate for *children* weighing more than 20 kg is 400 mg daily (irrespective of weight) in 2 divided doses, gradually increased until control is achieved, with a usual range of 20 to 30 mg per kg daily; further increases to a maximum of 35 mg per kg daily may be necessary if adequate control has not been achieved. Children weighing less than 20 kg may be given 20 mg per kg daily in 2 divided doses, which may be increased to 40 mg per kg daily in severe cases, but only if it is possible to monitor the patient's plasma-valproate concentrations; it has been recommended that if the dose exceeds 40 mg per kg daily, the patient's clinical chemistry and haematological parameters should also be monitored.

When the oral route is not possible, sodium valproate may be given *intravenously* to initiate therapy or to continue therapy previously given orally. A suggested dose to *initiate* therapy in *adults* is up to 10 mg per kg body-weight by intravenous injection over 3 to 5 minutes followed by intravenous infusion, as necessary, up to a total of 2.5 g daily. The usual intravenous dose for *children* is in the range of 20 to 30 mg per kg daily. If doses in excess of this are required, plasma-valproate concentrations must be monitored, and if the dose exceeds 40 mg per kg daily, clinical chemistry and haematological parameters should also be monitored. To *continue* therapy intravenously doses are the same as the patient's previous oral dose. In the USA, intravenous sodium valproate is given in doses similar to those used for valproic acid by mouth.

A suggested initial oral dose of *valproic acid* is 15 mg per kg daily increased at one-week intervals by 5 to 10 mg per kg daily. The maximum recommended dose of valproic acid in the UK is 30 mg per kg daily whereas in the USA is 60 mg per kg daily. Valproic acid may be given in 2 to 4 divided doses. *Valproate semisodium* is given in similar doses to valproic acid.

The amide derivative of valproic acid, *valpromide*, is also used in some countries. Usual doses have ranged from 600 mg to 1.8 g by mouth daily, in divided doses.

As with other antiepileptics, withdrawal of valproate or transition to or from another type of antiepileptic therapy should be made gradually to avoid precipitating an increase in the frequency of seizures. For a discussion on whether or not to withdraw antiepileptic therapy in seizure-free patients, see p.338.

In the treatment of acute manic episodes of **bipolar disorder**, valproate semisodium is given by mouth in an initial dose equivalent to valproic acid 750 mg daily in divided doses. Thereafter, the dose is increased as rapidly as possible to achieve the optimal response, up to a maximum of 60 mg per kg body-weight daily. Patients receiving doses higher than 45 mg per kg daily should be carefully monitored.

In the prophylaxis of **migraine** valproate semisodium is given by mouth in a dose equivalent to valproic acid 250 mg twice daily; up to 1 g daily may be necessary in some patients.

Administration. The pharmacokinetics of rectal and oral valproic acid have been compared;[1] rectal absorption does not show the slight circadian variation present when the drug is absorbed via the oral route and the rectal route appears to be an effective means of administration.

1. Yoshiyama Y, *et al.* Chronopharmacokinetic study of valproic acid in man: comparison of oral and rectal administration. *J Clin Pharmacol* 1989; **29:** 1048–52.

Bipolar disorder. Valproate, usually as valproate semisodium, is increasingly being used as an alternative to lithium in patients with bipolar disorder (p.271).[1-10] Some consider it to be particularly effective in those who have rapid cycling disease with 4 or more affective episodes a year but a recent meta-analysis[11] considered that any shift in prescribing practice in favour of valproate was not based on reliable evidence of efficacy.

References.

1. Pope HG, *et al.* Valproate in the treatment of acute mania: a placebo-controlled study. *Arch Gen Psychiatry* 1991; **48:** 62–8.
2. Keck PE, *et al.* Valproate oral loading in the treatment of acute mania. *J Clin Psychiatry* 1993; **54:** 305–8.
3. Joffe RT. Valproate in bipolar disorder: the Canadian perspective. *Can J Psychiatry* 1993; **38** (suppl 2): S46–S50.
4. Schaff MR, *et al.* Divalproex sodium in the treatment of refractory affective disorders. *J Clin Psychiatry* 1993; **54:** 380–4.
5. Nurnberg HG, *et al.* Response to anticonvulsant substitution among refractory bipolar manic patients. *J Clin Psychopharmacol* 1994; **14:** 207–9.
6. Anonymous. Valproate for bipolar disorder. *Med Lett Drugs Ther* 1994; **36:** 74–5.
7. Bowden CL, *et al.* Efficacy of divalproex vs lithium and placebo in the treatment of mania. *JAMA* 1994; **271:** 918–24. Correction. *ibid.*; 1830.
8. Stoll AL, *et al.* Neurologic factors predict a favorable valproate response in bipolar and schizoaffective disorders. *J Clin Psychopharmacol* 1994; **14:** 311–13.
9. Swann AC, *et al.* Depression during mania: treatment response to lithium or divalproex. *Arch Gen Psychiatry* 1997; **54:** 37–42.
10. Müller-Oerlinghausen B, *et al.* Valproate as adjunct to neuroleptic medication for the treatment of acute episodes of mania: a prospective, randomized, double-blind, placebo-controlled, multicenter study. *J Clin Psychopharmacol* 2000; **20:** 195–203.
11. Macritchie KAN, *et al.* Valproic acid, valproate and divalproex in the maintenance treatment of bipolar disorder (updated 30 March 2001). Available in The Cochrane Library; Issue 3. Oxford: Update Software; 2001.

Cushing's syndrome. Sodium valproate has been used with metyrapone to reduce cortisol secretion in the management of Cushing's syndrome (p.1272).

Depression. Valproate has been added as a mood stabiliser for augmentation of antidepressant therapy in the treatment of resistant depression (p.271).

Epilepsy. Valproate is one of the drugs of choice in primary generalised tonic-clonic seizures, absence seizures, and myoclonic seizures (see p.338), although evidence for some of these is lacking. It is also the drug of choice in epileptic syndromes such as the Lennox-Gastaut syndrome because of its wide therapeutic spectrum, and it may be useful in infantile spasms. It is often used in partial seizures and controlled trials have suggested similar efficacy to the first-line drugs carbamazepine and phenytoin.

References.

1. Mattson RH, *et al.* A comparison of valproate with carbamazepine for the treatment of complex partial seizures and secondarily generalized tonic-clonic seizures in adults. *N Engl J Med* 1992; **327:** 765–71.
2. Davis R, *et al.* Valproic acid: a reappraisal of its pharmacological properties and clinical efficacy in epilepsy. *Drugs* 1994; **47:** 332–72.
3. Richens A, *et al.* A multicentre trial of valproate and carbamazepine in adult onset epilepsy. *J Neurol Neurosurg Psychiatry* 1994; **57:** 682–7.
4. Verity CM, *et al.* A multicentre comparative trial of sodium valproate and carbamazepine in paediatric epilepsy. *Dev Med Child Neurol* 1995; **37:** 97–108.
5. Beydoun A, *et al.* and the Depakote Monotherapy for Partial Seizures Study Group. Safety and efficacy of divalproex sodium monotherapy in partial epilepsy: a double-blind, concentration-response design clinical trial. *Neurology* 1997; **48:** 182–8.
6. Brodie MJ, Mumford JP. Double-blind substitution of vigabatrin and valproate in carbamazepine-resistant partial epilepsy. *Epilepsy Res* 1999; **34:** 199–205.

Extrapyramidal disorders. Valproate is one of several drugs with GABAergic action that has been tried with encouraging results in the management of tardive dyskinesia (see under Extrapyramidal Disorders on p.662).

Febrile convulsions. Sodium valproate has been used prophylactically in children thought to be at risk of recurrence of febrile convulsions (p.341), but routine use of antiepileptics is no longer recommended.

References.

1. Newton RW. Randomised controlled trials of phenobarbitone and valproate in febrile convulsions. *Arch Dis Child* 1988; **63:** 1189–91.

Headache. Valproate, as valproate semisodium, may be used for the prophylaxis of *migraine* (p.449) in patients refractory to drugs such as propranolol or pizotifen; success has been demonstrated in several studies.[1-5] Valproate has also been shown to be effective and well-tolerated in the prophylaxis of migraine in children aged between 7 and 16 years.[6] Preliminary data from an open-label study suggest that intravenous valproate is

effective and well-tolerated in the treatment of acute migraine attacks.[7]

Valproate has also been tried in the prophylaxis of persistent chronic daily headache including *tension-type headache* (p.450) unresponsive to other drugs.[8]

1. Sørensen KV. Valproate: a new drug in migraine prophylaxis. *Acta Neurol Scand* 1988; **78:** 346–8.
2. Hering R, Kuritzky A. Sodium valproate in the prophylactic treatment of migraine: a double-blind study versus placebo. *Cephalalgia* 1992; **12:** 81–4.
3. Coria F, *et al.* Low-dose sodium valproate in the prophylaxis of migraine. *Clin Neuropharmacol* 1994; **17:** 569–73.
4. Mathew NT, *et al.* Migraine prophylaxis with divalproex. *Arch Neurol* 1995; **52:** 281–6.
5. Kaniecki RG. A comparison of divalproex with propranolol and placebo for the prophylaxis of migraine without aura. *Arch Neurol* 1997; **54:** 1141–5.
6. Caruso JM, *et al.* The efficacy of divalproex sodium in the prophylactic treatment of children with migraine. *Headache* 2000; **40:** 672–6.
7. Mathew NT, *et al.* Intravenous valproate sodium (Depacon) aborts migraine rapidly: a preliminary report. *Headache* 2000; **40:** 720–3.
8. Mathew NT, Ali S. Valproate in the treatment of persistent chronic daily headache: an open label study. *Headache* 1991; **31:** 71–4.

Hiccup. Valproic acid may be of value in the treatment of intractable hiccups,[1] especially those of neurogenic origin. A protocol for the management of intractable hiccups may be found under Chlorpromazine, p.667.

1. Jacobson PL, *et al.* Treatment of intractable hiccups with valproic acid. *Neurology* 1981; **31:** 1458–60.

Migraine. See under Headache, above.

Muscle spasm. The mainstay of management of *spasticity* is physiotherapy and an antispastic drug (see p.1322). Valproate has been tried for its GABAergic activity and case reports[1] of 4 patients with spastic conditions of various aetiologies indicated that the addition of valproate to the existing regimen of antispastic drugs might produce improvements in spasticity and pain; further studies are warranted.

Valproate has also been tried[2] in the management of *stiff-man syndrome* (p.681) unresponsive to diazepam.

1. Zachariah SB, *et al.* Positive response to oral divalproex sodium (Depakote) in patients with spasticity and pain. *Am J Med Sci* 1994; **308:** 38–40.
2. Spehlmann R, *et al.* Improvement of stiff-man syndrome with sodium valproate. *Neurology* 1981; **31:** 1162–3.

Myoclonus. Valproate is used alone or in combination with clonazepam for cortical myoclonus (see p.342).

Psychiatric disorders. Valproate has psychotropic properties and has been used in the management of depression and bipolar disorder (see above). Valproate has also been tried in various disorders for the control of symptoms such as agitation, aggression, and rage[1,2] (see under Disturbed Behaviour, p.650). It has also been reported[3,4] to be efficacious as adjunctive therapy to antipsychotics. It has also been tried in anxiety disorders such as panic attacks[5-7] (p.649), and post-traumatic stress disorder[8] (p.650).

1. Geracioti TD. Valproic acid treatment of episodic explosiveness related to brain injury. *J Clin Psychiatry* 1994; **55:** 416–17.
2. Narayan M, *et al.* Treatment of dementia with behavioral disturbances using divalproex or a combination of divalproex and a neuroleptic. *J Clin Psychiatry* 1997; **58:** 351–4.
3. Wassef AA, *et al.* Randomized, placebo-controlled pilot study of divalproex sodium in the treatment of acute exacerbations of chronic schizophrenia. *J Clin Psychopharmacol* 2000; **20:** 357–61.
4. Grove VE, *et al.* Improvement of Huntington's disease with olanzapine and valproate. *N Engl J Med* 2000; **343:** 973–4.
5. Primeau F, *et al.* Valproic acid and panic disorder. *Can J Psychiatry* 1990; **35:** 248–50.
6. Keck PE, *et al.* Valproate treatment of panic disorder and lactate-induced panic attacks. *Biol Psychiatry* 1993; **33:** 542–6.
7. Woodman CL, Noyes R. Panic disorder: treatment with valproate. *J Clin Psychiatry* 1994; **55:** 134–6.
8. Fesler FA. Valproate in combat-related posttraumatic stress disorder. *J Clin Psychiatry* 1991; **52:** 361–4.

Status epilepticus. Valproate is not usually given in the management of status epilepticus (p.341). However, it has been used in absence status epilepticus once the initial attack has been brought under control with intravenous benzodiazepines[1] and has been considered to be the drug of choice to prevent its recurrence.[2] In a small study it was effective in controlling status epilepticus associated with generalised tonic-clonic and myoclonic seizures.[3] Intravenous valproate decreased clinical seizures in 2 children with refractory generalised convulsive and 1 with nonconvulsive status epilepticus, although one of the former continued to exhibit electrical activity consistent with seizures.[4]

1. Bauer J, Elger CE. Management of status epilepticus in adults. *CNS Drugs* 1994; **1:** 26–44.
2. Berkovic SF, *et al.* Valproate prevents the recurrence of absence status. *Neurology* 1989; **39:** 1294–7.
3. Giroud M, *et al.* Use of injectable valproic acid in status epilepticus: a pilot study. *Drug Invest* 1993; **5:** 154–9.
4. Hovinga CA, *et al.* Use of intravenous valproate in three pediatric patients with nonconvulsive or convulsive status epilepticus. *Ann Pharmacother* 1999; **33:** 579–84.

Trigeminal neuralgia. Although carbamazepine is the drug of choice in the treatment of trigeminal neuralgia (p.8), sodium valproate is an alternative antiepileptic that may be used in carbamazepine-intolerant patients.

Preparations

BP 2001: Sodium Valproate Enteric-coated Tablets; Sodium Valproate Oral Solution; Sodium Valproate Tablets;
USP 25: Divalproex Sodium Delayed-Release Tablets; Valproic Acid Capsules; Valproic Acid Syrup.

Proprietary Preparations (details are given in Part 3)
Aust.: Convulex; Depakine; Depakine Chrono; Leptilanil; **Austral.:** Epilim; Valpro; **Belg.:** Convulex; Depakine; **Braz.:** Depakene; Valpakine; **Canad.:** Depakene; Deproic; Epiject; Epival; **Denm.:** Delepsine; Deprakine; Leptilan; Orfiril; **Fin.:** Absenor; Deprakine; Deprakine Depot; Orfiril; **Fr.:** Depakine; Depakine Chrono; Depakote; Depamide; **Ger.:** Convulex; Convulsofin; Ergenyl; Ergenyl Chrono; Leptilan; Mylproin; Orfiril; **Hong Kong:** Epilim; Orfiril; Valpro; **Irl.:** Epilim; Epilim Chrono; **Israel:** Depalept; Depalept Chrono; Valporal; **Ital.:** Depakin; Depakin Chrono; Depamag; Depamide; **Jpn:** Depakene; Selenica†; **Mex.:** Atemperator; Cryoval; Depakene; Epival; Leptilan; Proteval; Provetal; Valcaps; Valken; Valprosid; **Neth.:** Convulex; Depakine; Depakine Chrono; **Norw.:** Deprakine; Orfiril; **NZ:** Epilim; **Port.:** Depakine; Depakine Chrono; Diplexil; **S.Afr.:** Convulex; Epilim; **Singapore:** Convulex; Encorate; Epilim; **Spain:** Depakine; Depamide; **Swed.:** Absenor; Ergenyl; Orfiril; **Switz.:** Convulex; Depakine; Depakine Chrono; Orfiril; **Thai.:** Depakine; Valparin; **UK:** Convulex; Depakote; Epilim; Epilim Chrono; Orlept; **USA:** Depacon; Depakene; Depakote.

Vigabatrin (17030-d)

Vigabatrin (BAN, USAN, rINN).

4-Amino-5-hexenoic Acid; MDL-71754; RMI-71754; γ-Vinyl Aminobutyric Acid; γ-Vinyl-GABA. 4-Aminohex-5-enoic acid.

$C_6H_{11}NO_2 = 129.2$.

CAS — 60643-86-9.
ATC — N03AG04.

Pharmacopoeias. In Br.

Pharmacopoeial description

BP 2001: A white to almost white powder. Very soluble in water.

Adverse Effects, Treatment, and Precautions

About half of all patients experience adverse effects with vigabatrin. The most common adverse effects associated with vigabatrin therapy are drowsiness and fatigue, although in children excitation and agitation occur more frequently. Other CNS-related adverse effects include dizziness, nervousness, irritability, headache, nystagmus, ataxia, paraesthesia, tremor, and impaired concentration. Less commonly, confusion and memory disturbances have been reported. Other reported adverse effects include weight gain, gastrointestinal disturbances, oedema, alopecia, angioedema, urticaria, and skin rash. Haemoglobin and liver enzyme values may be decreased. Rarely marked sedation, stupor and confusion, together with other symptoms suggestive of encephalopathy, have occurred.

About one-third of all patients receiving vigabatrin have developed irreversible visual field defects, ranging from mild to severe and usually occurring after months or years of therapy. Blurred vision, diplopia, or nystagmus are somewhat less common. Retinal disorders such as peripheral retinal atrophy, or very rarely optic neuritis or atrophy have also been reported (see also below). Visual field function should be assessed before beginning treatment and during routine follow-up (ideally at 6-month intervals), and patients should be warned to report any new visual symptoms that develop during therapy. Vigabatrin should not be used in patients with pre-existing visual field defects.

Psychiatric reactions such as agitation, aggression, depression, and paranoid reactions have occurred in patients with or without a psychiatric history; psychosis or mania have been reported rarely. Patients receiving vigabatrin should be observed carefully for any signs of adverse effects on neurological function. Caution is warranted in patients with a history of psychosis or behavioural problems.

Vigabatrin may exacerbate myoclonic or absence seizures.

Vigabatrin should be given with caution to the elderly and patients with renal impairment.

Care is required when withdrawing vigabatrin therapy—see also under Uses and Administration, below.

Breast feeding. The manufacturers state that breast feeding is not recommended in women receiving vigabatrin. For comment on antiepileptic therapy and breast feeding, see under Pregnancy and Breast Feeding on p.340.

Driving. For a comment on antiepileptic drugs and driving, see p.340.

Particular care should be taken in view of the possible effects of vigabatrin on visual acuity.

Effects on the eyes. A report of 3 patients who developed bilateral severely constricted visual fields 2 to 3 years after vigabatrin was added to their antiepileptic regimens[1] prompted publication of similar anecdotal reports.[2-5] Peripheral retinal atrophy rather than optic nerve damage appeared to be the cause. Symptoms showed no improvement on discontinuation of the drug, although there was no further deterioration. At that time (1997) the manufacturers replied[6] stating that it was a rare occurrence (less than 0.1%) and was being monitored in further clinical trials. The UK Committee on Safety of Medicines (CSM) subsequently stated[7] (in March 1998) that it had received 41 reports of visual field defects since December 1989, which persisted in most cases despite discontinuation of treatment. The evidence suggested that the onset of symptoms varied from 1 month to several years after starting vigabatrin. In most cases, visual field defects have persisted despite discontinuation of vigabatrin.[8,9] Interim results of a Prescription Event Monitoring Study[10] in the UK stated that vigabatrin was considered to be probably or possibly associated with objective evidence of a visual field defect in 0.2% of patients. However, subsequent evidence appears to have confirmed that the incidence of visual field defects is much higher;[11-14] revised product literature issued by the manufacturers in late 1999 indicated that visual field defects occurred in about one-third of all patients receiving vigabatrin.

The CSM now considers[14] that vigabatrin should only be prescribed by a specialist, and only where all other combination therapies have failed. Ophthalmological consultation and visual field assessment should be undertaken before starting vigabatrin and visual field screening repeated at 6-monthly intervals during treatment. Conventional perimetry is unsuitable in patients under 9 years of age, in whom alternative methods should be employed. Opinion amongst some paediatricians[15] is that the risk of developing visual field defects had to be weighed against the potential benefit of seizure control. In very young patients, in whom monitoring of vision was impossible, the benefits of vigabatrin in the treatment of infantile spasms are felt by some to outweigh this risk.[16]

Vigabatrin should not be used in patients with pre-existing visual field defects.[14,15]

1. Eke T, *et al.* Severe persistent visual field constriction associated with vigabatrin. *BMJ* 1997; **314:** 180–1.
2. Wilson EA, Brodie MJ. Severe persistent visual field constriction associated with vigabatrin. *BMJ* 1997; **314:** 1693.
3. Wong ICK, *et al.* Severe persistent visual field constriction associated with vigabatrin. *BMJ* 1997; **314:** 1693–4.
4. Blackwell N, *et al.* Severe persistent visual field constriction associated with vigabatrin. *BMJ* 1997; **314:** 1694.
5. Harding GFA. Severe persistent visual field constriction associated with vigabatrin. *BMJ* 1997; **314:** 1694.
6. Backstrom JT, *et al.* Severe persistent visual field constriction associated with vigabatrin. *BMJ* 1997; **314:** 1694–5.
7. Committee of Safety of Medicines/Medicines Control Agency. Vigabatrin (Sabril) and visual field defects. *Current Problems* 1998; **24:** 1.
8. Hardus P, *et al.* Long term changes in the visual fields of patients with temporal lobe epilepsy using vigabatrin. *Br J Ophthalmol* 2000; **84:** 788–90.
9. Johnson MA, *et al.* Visual function loss from vigabatrin: effect of stopping the drug. *Neurology* 2000; **55:** 40–5.
10. Wilton LV, *et al.* Interim report on the incidence of visual field defects in patients on long term vigabatrin therapy. *Pharmacoepidemiol Drug Safety* 1999; **8** (suppl): S9–S14.
11. Wilton LV, *et al.* Visual field defect associated with vigabatrin: observational cohort study. *BMJ* 1999; **319:** 1165–6.
12. Kälviäinen R, *et al.* Vigabatrin, a gabaergic antiepileptic drug, causes concentric visual field defects. *Neurology* 1999; **53:** 922–6.
13. Lawden MC, *et al.* Visual field defects associated with vigabatrin therapy. *J Neurol Neurosurg Psychiatry* 1999; **67:** 716–22.
14. Committee on Safety of Medicines/Medicines Control Agency. Vigabatrin (Sabril): visual field defects. *Current Problems* 1999; **25:** 13.
15. Appleton RE. Guideline may help in prescribing vigabatrin. *BMJ* 1998; **317:** 1322.
16. Harding GFA. Severe persistent visual field constriction associated with vigabatrin. *BMJ* 1998; **316:** 232–3.

Effects on the liver. Vigabatrin has demonstrated *in-vivo* and *in-vitro* inhibition of plasma-alanine transaminase activity, which may mask signs of early underlying hepatic disease if only transaminase levels are evaluated.[1]

1. Richens A, *et al.* Evidence for both in vivo and in vitro interaction between vigabatrin and alanine transaminase. *Br J Clin Pharmacol* 1997; **43:** 163–8.

Effects on mental function. Behavioural disturbances ranging from irritability and confusion to psychotic reactions have been reported in patients receiving vigabatrin.[1-7] An analysis[8] of adverse effect reports from double-blind controlled studies found that the incidence of psychotic reactions was about 2.5% in vigabatrin treated patients; however, the most common psychiatric reaction was depression, which occurred in 8 to 12% of patients. Symptoms of psychiatric disturbance were often relatively mild. Psychiatric reactions are generally reversible when doses are reduced or gradually discontinued. In 2 patients[9,10] psychosis developed following sudden withdrawal of viga-

batrin; mental state improved when the drug was reinstated. It is not clear whether patients with a history of previous psychiatric disturbances are at greater risk when given vigabatrin.[8,11] Also, using low doses of vigabatrin to start therapy did not reduce the incidence of disturbances.[11]

The problems of antiepileptic therapy adversely affecting cognition are discussed on p.340.

1. Sander JWAS, Hart YM. Vigabatrin and behaviour disturbances. *Lancet* 1990; **335:** 57.
2. Dam M. Vigabatrin and behaviour disturbances. *Lancet* 1990; **335:** 605.
3. Betts T, Thomas L. Vigabatrin and behaviour disturbances. *Lancet* 1990; **335:** 605–6.
4. Johnston SJ. Vigabatrin and behaviour disturbances. *Lancet* 1990; **335:** 606.
5. Robinson MK, *et al.* Vigabatrin and behaviour disturbances. *Lancet* 1990; **336:** 504.
6. Martínez AC, *et al.* Vigabatrin-associated reversible acute psychosis in a child. *Ann Pharmacother* 1995; **29:** 1115–17.
7. Naumann M, *et al.* Bipolar affective psychosis after vigabatrin. *Lancet* 1994; **343:** 606–7.
8. Levinson DF, Devinsky O. Psychiatric adverse events during vigabatrin therapy. *Neurology* 1999; **53:** 1503–11.
9. Ring HA, Reynolds EH. Vigabatrin and behaviour disturbance. *Lancet* 1990; **335:** 970.
10. Brodie MJ, McKee PJW. Vigabatrin and psychosis. *Lancet* 1990; **335:** 1279.
11. Wong ICK. Retrospective study of vigabatrin and psychiatric behavioural disturbances. *Epilepsy Res* 1995; **21:** 227–30.

Effects on the nervous system. Two patients developed disturbances of motor behaviour associated with the addition of vigabatrin to therapy for intractable seizures.[1]

Acute encephalopathy was reported[2] in two patients after starting vigabatrin in addition to carbamazepine; symptoms of stupor, dysphoria, and irritability were present in both and their EEG background activity was slowed. Clinical symptoms could not be related to intoxication with carbamazepine or its epoxide but it was not known whether an interaction between carbamazepine and vigabatrin had caused the acute encephalopathy. In a further report[3] vigabatrin was associated with the development of encephalopathy in 3 patients already receiving a variety of antiepileptic drugs other than carbamazepine; withdrawal of vigabatrin led to full recovery. The authors suggested that acute encephalopathy after vigabatrin may be related to a pre-existing cerebral abnormality.

1. Jongsma MJ, *et al.* Reversible motor disturbances induced by vigabatrin. *Lancet* 1991; **338:** 893.
2. Sälke-Kellermann A, Baier H. Acute encephalopathy with vigabatrin. *Lancet* 1993; **342:** 185.
3. Sharief MK, *et al.* Acute encephalopathy with vigabatrin. *Lancet* 1993; **342:** 619.

Interference with diagnostic tests. Vigabatrin can cause changes in the urinary excretion of amino acids which could be potentially misleading in patients undergoing investigation for metabolic disorders.[1,2]

1. Bonham JR, *et al.* Pyroglutamicaciduria from vigabatrin. *Lancet* 1989; **i:** 1452–3.
2. Shih VE, Tenanbaum A. Aminoaciduria due to vinyl-gaba administration. *N Engl J Med* 1990; **323:** 1353.

Overdosage. For a review of the features and management of poisoning with some antiepileptics, including vigabatrin, see under Phenytoin, p.358.

Porphyria. For comment on the use of vigabatrin in porphyria, see p.342.

Pregnancy. For comments on the management of epilepsy in pregnancy, see p.340.

Little is known of the effects of newer antiepileptics such as vigabatrin on the fetus, although congenital anomalies have been reported in the offspring of some mothers using vigabatrin during pregnancy.

Interactions

There are complex interactions between antiepileptics and toxicity may be enhanced without a corresponding increase in antiepileptic activity. Such interactions are very variable and unpredictable and plasma monitoring is often advisable with combination therapy.

Antiepileptics. For the effect of vigabatrin on plasma concentrations of other antiepileptics, see Phenobarbital, p.356; Phenytoin, p.360; and Primidone, p.363.

Pharmacokinetics

Vigabatrin is well absorbed following oral administration of the racemate; the inactive $R(-)$-enantiomer is reported to be present at much higher plasma concentrations than the active $S(+)$-enantiomer, perhaps indicating a difference in bioavailability. Most of an oral dose is excreted in urine as unchanged drug. The elimination half-life is reported to be 5 to 8 hours. Vigabatrin is not significantly bound to plasma proteins.

There does not appear to be any correlation between plasma concentrations of vigabatrin and its efficacy or toxicity.

Vigabatrin is distributed into breast milk.

◊ References.

1. Rey E, *et al.* Vigabatrin: clinical pharmacokinetics. *Clin Pharmacokinet* 1992; **23:** 267–78.
2. Hoke JF, *et al.* Pharmacokinetics of vigabatrin following single and multiple oral doses in normal volunteers. *J Clin Pharmacol* 1993; **33:** 458–62.
3. Elwes RDC, Binnie CD. Clinical pharmacokinetics of newer antiepileptic drugs: lamotrigine, vigabatrin, gabapentin and oxcarbazepine. *Clin Pharmacokinet* 1996; **30:** 403–15.
4. Vauzelle-Kervroëdan F, *et al.* Pharmacokinetics of the individual enantiomers of vigabatrin in neonates with uncontrolled seizures. *Br J Clin Pharmacol* 1996; **42:** 779–81.
5. Jacqz-Aigrain E, *et al.* Pharmacokinetics of the S(+) and R(−) enantiomers of vigabatrin during chronic dosing in a patient with renal failure. *Br J Clin Pharmacol* 1997; **44:** 183–5.
6. Tran A, *et al.* Vigabatrin: placental transfer in vivo and excretion into breast milk of the enantiomers. *Br J Clin Pharmacol* 1998; **45:** 409–11.

Uses and Administration

Vigabatrin is an analogue of gamma-aminobutyric acid (GABA) that acts as an irreversible inhibitor of GABA-transaminase, the enzyme responsible for the catabolism of GABA. It is used as an adjunctive antiepileptic in patients with resistant partial epilepsy with or without secondary generalisation, unresponsive to other therapy. It is also used as monotherapy for infantile spasms (as for example in West's syndrome).

The recommended initial dose of vigabatrin as *adjunctive therapy* in adults is 1 g daily by mouth, increased if necessary in increments of 0.5 g at weekly intervals to a maximum of 3 g daily. A recommended initial dose in children is 40 mg per kg body-weight daily. Maintenance recommendations according to body-weight range are: 10 to 15 kg body-weight, 0.5 to 1 g daily; 15 to 30 kg, 1 to 1.5 g daily; 30 to 50 kg, 1.5 to 3 g daily; and 50 kg or more, 2 to 3 g daily. For infantile spasms the dose of vigabatrin as *monotherapy* is 50 mg per kg daily, adjusted according to response over 7 days. Up to 150 mg per kg daily has been used in some infants.

Doses may be divided and given twice daily or taken as a single daily dose. Dosage reductions may be required in the elderly and in patients with renal impairment.

As with other antiepileptics, withdrawal of vigabatrin therapy or transition to or from another type of antiepileptic therapy should be made gradually to avoid precipitating an increase in the frequency of seizures. For a discussion on whether or not to withdraw antiepileptic therapy in seizure-free patients, see p.338. It has been recommended that the dose of vigabatrin should be gradually reduced over 2 to 4 weeks.

◊ General references.

1. Gidal BE, *et al.* Vigabatrin: a novel therapy for seizure disorders. *Ann Pharmacother* 1999; **33:** 1277–86.

Epilepsy. Vigabatrin is used in the treatment of epilepsy (p.338) as adjunctive therapy for refractory seizures. Reviews[1-4] of vigabatrin have considered it to be most effective in the treatment of complex partial seizures with or without secondary generalisation; it may, however, exacerbate myoclonic or absence seizures. Efficacy as adjunctive therapy in refractory partial seizures was demonstrated by 2 multicentre studies[5,6] involving 228 patients (including 46 children) and a study[7] involving 52 patients being assessed for epilepsy surgery. However, in a follow-up study[8] of 120 patients who had participated in an open-label trial of vigabatrin as adjunctive therapy for refractory epilepsy 6 to 8 years earlier, it was considered that vigabatrin had had only marginal benefit on the long-term prognosis of severe refractory epilepsy, despite favourable results from the original trial.

Vigabatrin is also of value in infantile spasms (as for example in West's syndrome). In an assessment of vigabatrin as monotherapy in 192 infants with infantile spasms who were followed up for an average of 7.6 months,[9] there was complete cessation of spasms in 131 patients, a decrease in cluster frequency in 37, and no improvement in 24 (including deterioration in one infant). A crossover study comparing vigabatrin with corticotropin in 42 infants found that both drugs produced some benefit.[10] A review of the literature suggested that vigabatrin was particularly effective in infantile spasms associated with tuberous sclerosis;[11] the authors considered that its efficacy might be less in other forms of infantile spasm.[11]

1. Grant SM, Heel RC. Vigabatrin: a review of its pharmacodynamic and pharmacokinetic properties, and therapeutic potential in epilepsy and disorders of motor control. *Drugs* 1991; **41:** 889–926.

2. Brodie M. Drugs in focus I: vigabatrin. *Prescribers' J* 1992; **32:** 21–6.
3. Connelly JF. Vigabatrin. *Ann Pharmacother* 1993; **27:** 197–204.
4. Srinivasan J, Richens A. A risk-benefit assessment of vigabatrin in the treatment of neurological disorders *Drug Safety* 1994; **10:** 395–405.
5. Dalla Bernadina B, *et al.* Efficacy and tolerability of vigabatrin in children with refractory partial seizures: a single-blind dose-increasing study. *Epilepsia* 1995; **36:** 687–91.
6. French JA, *et al.* A double-blind, placebo-controlled study of vigabatrin three g/day in patients with uncontrolled complex partial seizures. *Neurology* 1996; **46:** 54–61.
7. Malmgren K, *et al.* Cost analysis of epilepsy surgery and of vigabatrin treatment in patients with refractory partial epilepsy. *Epilepsy Res* 1996; **25:** 199–207.
8. Walker MC, *et al.* Long term use of lamotrigine and vigabatrin in severe refractory epilepsy: audit of outcome. *BMJ* 1996; **313:** 1184–5.
9. Aicardi J, *et al.* Sabril IS Investigator and Peer Review Groups. Vigabatrin as initial therapy for infantile spasms: a European retrospective survey. *Epilepsia* 1996; **37:** 638–42.
10. Vigevano F, Cilio MR. Vigabatrin versus ACTH as first-line treatment for infantile spasms: a randomized, prospective study. *Epilepsia* 1997; **38:** 1270–4.
11. Hancock E, Osborne JP. Vigabatrin in the treatment of infantile spasms in tuberous sclerosis. *J Child Neurol* 1999; **14:** 71–4.

Metabolic disorders. Vigabatrin, an irreversible inhibitor of GABA-transaminase, has been tried in GABA metabolic disorders not accompanied by epilepsy,[1-4] with ambivalent results. Data from 23 case reports of patients with succinic semialdehyde dehydrogenase deficiency indicated that vigabatrin was clinically beneficial in only about one-third of patients.[4]

1. Jaeken J, *et al.* Vigabatrin in GABA metabolism disorders. *Lancet* 1989; **i:** 1074.
2. Gibson KM, *et al.* Vigabatrin therapy in patient with succinic semialdehyde dehydrogenase deficiency. *Lancet* 1989; **ii:** 1105–6.
3. Stephenson JBP. Vigabatrin for startle-disease with altered cerebrospinal-fluid free gamma-aminobutyric acid. *Lancet* 1992; **340:** 430–1.
4. Gibson KM, *et al.* The clinical phenotype of succinic semialdehyde dehydrogenase deficiency (4-hydroxybutyric aciduria): case reports of 23 new patients. *Pediatrics* 1997; **99:** 567–74.

Stiff-man syndrome. There have been anecdotal reports[1,2] of improvement of stiff-man syndrome (p.681) with vigabatrin in patients unable to tolerate benzodiazepine therapy.

1. Vermeij FH, *et al.* Improvement of stiff-man syndrome with vigabatrin. *Lancet* 1996; **348:** 612.
2. Prevett MC, *et al.* Improvement of stiff-man syndrome with vigabatrin. *Neurology* 1997; **48:** 1133–4.

Preparations

BP 2001: Vigabatrin Oral Powder; Vigabatrin Tablets†.

Proprietary Preparations (details are given in Part 3)
Aust.: Sabril; *Austral.:* Sabril; *Belg.:* Sabril; *Braz.:* Sabril; *Canad.:* Sabril; *Denm.:* Sabrilex; *Fin.:* Sabrilex; *Fr.:* Sabril; *Ger.:* Sabril; *Hong Kong:* Sabril; *Irl.:* Sabril; *Israel:* Sabrilan; *Ital.:* Sabril; *Mex.:* Sabril; *Neth.:* Sabril; *Norw.:* Sabrilex; *NZ:* Sabril; *Port.:* Sabril; *S.Afr.:* Sabril; *Singapore:* Sabril; *Spain:* Sabrilex; *Swed.:* Sabrilex; *Switz.:* Sabril; *UK:* Sabril.

Zonisamide (1668-x)

Zonisamide *(BAN, USAN, rINN)*.

AD-810; CI-912; PD-110843. 1-(1,2-Benzoxazol-3-yl)methanesulphonamide.

$C_8H_8N_2O_3S = 212.2$.

CAS — 68291-97-4.

Adverse Effects

The most common adverse effects with zonisamide have included anorexia, nausea, somnolence, dizziness, headache, and agitation or irritability. Severe skin reactions including Stevens-Johnson syndrome and toxic epidermal necrolysis have occurred rarely, and consideration should be given to withdrawing zonisamide in patients who develop unexplained rash. There have been isolated reports of aplastic anaemia or agranulocytosis. Other adverse effects have included renal calculi (see below), depression, psychosis, psychomotor slowing, reduced concentration, speech or language difficulties, and fatigue. Reduced sweating with hyperthermia has occurred in children.

Renal calculi. Patients treated with zonisamide in the USA and Europe may have had a higher incidence of renal calculi than those treated in Japan. In one US study, 4 of 113 patients (3.5%) receiving long-term treatment with zonisamide developed renal calculi,[1] but a familial relationship was found for 2. In pooled data from earlier studies, renal calculi had been reported in 13 of 700 patients (1.9%) treated in the USA and Europe compared with 2 of 1008 patients (0.2%) in Japan.[2]

1. Patsalos PN, Sander JWAS. Newer antiepileptic drugs: towards an improved risk-benefit ratio. *Drug Safety* 1994; **11:** 37–67.
2. Peters DH, Sorkin EM. Zonisamide: a review of its pharmacodynamic and pharmacokinetic properties, and therapeutic potential in epilepsy. *Drugs* 1993; **45:** 760–87.

Precautions

Zonisamide is a sulfonamide derivative and is therefore contraindicated in patients with a history of hypersensitivity to sulfonamides. It should be used with care in patients with hepatic or renal impairment. Adequate hydration is recommended to increase urine output and try to reduce the risk of developing renal calculi, especially in predisposed patients.

Care is required when withdrawing zonisamide therapy—see also under Uses and Administration below.

Zonisamide has been found to be teratogenic in *animal* studies.

Breast feeding. Although it is not known whether zonisamide is distributed into breast milk, in view of the potential for serious adverse effects in infants from zonisamide, the manufacturers recommend that it should only be used in nursing mothers if the benefits outweigh the risks. For comment on antiepileptic therapy and breast feeding, see under Pregnancy and Breast Feeding on p.340.

Driving. For a comment on antiepileptic drugs and driving, see p.340.

Pregnancy. For comments on the management of epilepsy during pregnancy, see p.340.

Interactions

Use with drugs that induce or inhibit the cytochrome P450 isoenzyme CYP3A4 may alter plasma concentrations of zonisamide. Concomitant administration with carbamazepine, phenytoin, phenobarbital, or valproate reduces the half-life of zonisamide.

Pharmacokinetics

Zonisamide is absorbed from the gastrointestinal tract and peak plasma concentrations are achieved within 2 to 6 hours of oral administration. The presence of food does not affect the bioavailability of zonisamide but the time to reach peak plasma concentrations is delayed. Steady-state concentrations are achieved within 14 days. Plasma protein binding is low but zonisamide is extensively bound to erythrocytes. The plasma elimination half-life is about 63 hours.

Zonisamide undergoes acetylation to *N*-acetylzonisamide and reduction mediated by the cytochrome P450 isoenzyme CYP3A4 to 2-sulfamoylacetylphenol (SAMP). Excretion is mainly in the urine, 35% appearing as unchanged drug, 15% as *N*-acetylzonisamide, and 50% as the glucuronide of SAMP.

◊ References.

1. Kochak GM, *et al.* Steady-state pharmacokinetics of zonisamide, an antiepileptic agent for treatment of refractory complex partial seizures. *J Clin Pharmacol* 1998; **38:** 166–71.
2. Mimaki T. Clinical pharmacology and therapeutic drug monitoring of zonisamide. *Ther Drug Monit* 1998; **20:** 593–7.

Uses and Administration

Zonisamide, a benzisoxazole derivative, is used as an adjunctive antiepileptic in the treatment of partial seizures. The usual initial adult dose is 100 mg given once daily by mouth, increased after at least 2 weeks to 200 mg daily given in one or two divided doses. Thereafter, if necessary, the dose may be further increased by increments of 100 mg at intervals of at least 2 weeks up to 400 mg daily. Doses up to 600 mg daily have been used, but there is no current evidence of an increase in response above 400 mg daily; many of the adverse effects of zonisamide are reported to be more frequent at a dose of 300 mg daily.

As with other antiepileptics, withdrawal of zonisamide therapy or transition to or from another type of antiepileptic therapy should be made gradually to avoid precipitating an increase in the frequency of seizures. For a discussion on whether or not to withdraw antiepileptic therapy in seizure-free patients, see p.338.

Epilepsy. Zonisamide is used in the treatment of refractory epilepsy (p.338). Many studies have been conducted in Japan where clinical experience demonstrated its efficacy mainly in the treatment of partial seizures with or without secondary generalisation.[1,2] Data from studies[3-5] conducted outside Japan have confirmed the efficacy of zonisamide as an adjunct in the treatment of partial epilepsies. Efficacy in primary generalised and mixed-seizure epilepsies appears to be more variable, although it may be of value in refractory myoclonic seizures.[6] Zonisamide might also be of use in the treatment of epileptic syndromes such as Lennox-Gastaut syndrome and West's syndrome, although only a small number of patients with the latter condition have been studied.

1. Peters DH, Sorkin EM. Zonisamide: a review of its pharmacodynamic and pharmacokinetic properties, and therapeutic potential in epilepsy. *Drugs* 1993; **45:** 760–87.
2. Patsalos PN, Sander JWAS. Newer antiepileptic drugs: towards an improved risk-benefit ratio. *Drug Safety* 1994; **11:** 37–67.
3. Leppik IE, *et al.* Efficacy and safety of zonisamide: results of a multicenter study. *Epilepsy Res* 1993; **14:** 165–73.
4. Schmidt D, *et al.* Zonisamide for add-on treatment of refractory partial epilepsy: a European double-blind trial. *Epilepsy Res* 1993; **15:** 67–73.
5. Chadwick DW, Marson AG. Zonisamide add-on for drug-resistant partial epilepsy (updated 30 May 2001). Available in The Cochrane Library; Issue 3. Oxford: Update Software; 2001.
6. Kyllerman M, Ben-Menachen E. Zonisamide for progressive myoclonus epilepsy: long-term observations in seven patients. *Epilepsy Res* 1998; **29:** 109–14.

Preparations

Proprietary Preparations (details are given in Part 3)
Jpn: Excegran; *USA:* Zonegran.

Antifungals

This chapter describes those drugs that are used mainly in the treatment and prophylaxis of fungal infections (mycoses). They include the azole derivatives, including imidazoles (such as ketoconazole) and triazoles (such as fluconazole and itraconazole), the allylamines (naftifine and terbinafine), several polyene antibiotics (including amphotericin B and nystatin), other antifungal antibiotics (for example griseofulvin), and a number of other compounds among them amorolfine, ciclopirox olamine, flucytosine, haloprogin, tolnaftate, and undecenoic acid and its salts.

Choice of Antifungal

Fungi may be classified as either yeasts or moulds according to their appearance and means of growth. Yeast-like fungi involved in infections include *Blastomyces dermatitidis*, *Candida* spp., *Coccidioides immitis*, *Histoplasma capsulatum*, *Sporothrix schenckii*, and the infective agents of chromoblastomycosis. Examples of pathogenic moulds include *Aspergillus* spp., the dermatophytes, and the Mucorales fungi.

Some fungi are true pathogens and can cause disease in any individual. Other fungi such as *Candida* species and *Pneumocystis carinii* (once thought to be a protozoan but now considered to be a fungus) are of low pathogenicity and require an alteration in the normal defence mechanisms for disease to occur; such disease is called opportunistic.

Fungal infections may be classified as **superficial**, affecting only the skin, hair, nails, or mucous membranes, or **systemic**, affecting the body as a whole; systemic infections tend to occur more frequently in immunocompromised individuals such as those with AIDS. Fungal infections may also be described as **local** when they are restricted to one body area, as **invasive** when there is spread into the tissues, or as **disseminated** when the infection has spread from the primary site to other organs throughout the body.

Ideally antifungal treatment should be chosen after the infecting organism has been identified but it is often necessary to start treatment before the pathogen can be cultured and identified especially in immunocompromised patients in whom infections are often rapidly progressive.

The choice of treatment for the important fungal diseases is described below.

Aspergillosis

Aspergillosis is an infection caused by fungi of the genus *Aspergillus*, usually *A. fumigatus* although *A. flavus* and *A. niger* are also important. Aspergillosis is usually acquired by inhalation and most commonly causes non-invasive disease of the respiratory tract. Other sites of infection include the eye following trauma or cataract surgery. Invasive disease of tissues adjacent to the site of infection, for example spread from the paranasal sinus to the orbit, and dissemination to distant organs may occur, predominantly in immunocompromised patients. In severely immunocompromised patients aspergillosis usually presents as severe acute pneumonia. Other organs affected may include the heart (particularly damaged or prosthetic valves), kidneys, bone, brain, liver, and skin.

In general the response of **invasive** aspergillosis to treatment is poor and early initiation of treatment is essential. Surgical excision may be necessary. High intravenous doses of amphotericin B remain the antifungal treatment of choice.[1-4] However, the overall response rate to conventional amphotericin B is reported[3] to be only 30 to 35%, although this may be improved by the use of liposomal amphotericin B.[5-7] Combination therapy with amphotericin B and flucytosine has also been suggested[8] and may be useful in cerebral, meningeal, or endocardial infections.[3] Itraconazole by mouth[4,9] is emerging as the main alternative to amphotericin B. Caspofungin may be used in patients who are refractory to, or intolerant of, other antifungals.

A number of approaches to reducing the incidence of aspergillosis in immunocompromised patients have been discussed, including chemoprophylaxis with either low-dose intravenous, intranasal, or nebulised amphotericin B, or oral itraconazole[10,11] or a combination of these.[12]

Non-invasive forms of aspergillosis include allergic bronchopulmonary aspergillosis, a hypersensitivity reaction to *Aspergillus* usually occurring in asthmatic patients, and aspergilloma, a fungal mass or ball developing within the pulmonary cavity or paranasal sinus.

Allergic bronchopulmonary aspergillosis is usually treated with corticosteroids although oral itraconazole may be a useful adjunct.[4] However, a review concluded that there is insufficient information available to recommend the routine use of azole antifungals.[13] The treatment of **aspergilloma** depends on the severity of symptoms, and includes conservative management, antifungal therapy, or surgical resection. Oral itraconazole or intravenous amphotericin B are the most effective drugs. Direct intracavitary instillation of antifungals may also be useful[4] and has been advocated for patients at particularly high risk of complications.[14] Inhaled amphotericin B aerosol was reported to be poorly tolerated and of little value in preventing invasive pulmonary aspergillosis in granulocytopenic patients.[15]

Chronic locally invasive infections have been reported to respond to prolonged treatment with itraconazole;[16] in this small study, itraconazole produced clinical improvements but not mycological cure.

Aspergillosis of the **eye**, like other fungal eye infections, is difficult to treat; antifungals are generally not well absorbed following topical application and infections extending into the vitreous or anterior chamber require subconjunctival, intra-ocular, and/or systemic treatment. Systemic treatment is necessary for ocular manifestations of disseminated disease. When systemic therapy is required intravenous amphotericin B is usually given; an oral azole compound may be given for less severe infections. For superficial eye infections a number of antifungals, including natamycin, amphotericin B, azole compounds, and sulfadiazine silver have been applied topically alone or as an adjunct to systemic therapy. Surgical excision of infected tissue may be necessary in severe infections.

1. Anonymous. Essential drugs: systemic mycoses. *WHO Drug Inf* 1991; **5:** 129–36.
2. Anonymous. Systemic antifungal drugs. *Med Lett Drugs Ther* 1997; **39:** 86–8.
3. Denning DW. Treatment of invasive aspergillosis. *J Infect* 1994; **28** (suppl 1): 25–33.
4. Stevens DA, *et al.* Practice guidelines for diseases caused by Aspergillus. *Clin Infect Dis* 2000; **30:** 696–709.
5. Ringdén O, *et al.* Efficacy of amphotericin B encapsulated in liposomes (AmBisome) in the treatment of invasive fungal infections in immunocompromised patients. *J Antimicrob Chemother* 1991; **28** (suppl B): 73–82.
6. Chopra R, *et al.* Liposomal amphotericin B (AmBisome) in the treatment of fungal infections in neutropenic patients. *J Antimicrob Chemother* 1991; **28** (suppl B): 93–104.
7. Mills W, *et al.* Liposomal amphotericin B in the treatment of fungal infections in neutropenic patients: a single-centre experience of 133 episodes in 116 patients. *Br J Haematol* 1994; **86:** 754–60.
8. Saral R. Candida and aspergillus infections in immunocompromised patients: an overview. *Rev Infect Dis* 1991; **13:** 487–92.
9. Denning DW, *et al.* NIAID mycoses study group multicenter trial of oral itraconazole therapy for invasive aspergillosis. *Am J Med* 1994; **97:** 135–44. Correction. *ibid.;* 497.
10. Beyer J, *et al.* Strategies in prevention of invasive pulmonary aspergillosis in immunosuppressed or neutropenic patients. *Antimicrob Agents Chemother* 1994; **38:** 911–17.
11. Cafferkey MT. Chemoprophylaxis of invasive pulmonary aspergillosis. *J Antimicrob Chemother* 1994; **33:** 917–24.
12. Todeschini G, *et al.* Oral itraconazole plus nasal amphotericin B for prophylaxis of invasive aspergillosis in patients with hematological malignancies. *Eur J Clin Microbiol Infect Dis* 1993; **12:** 614–18.
13. Wark P, *et al.* Azoles for allergic bronchopulmonary aspergillosis (updated 25 May 2001). Available in The Cochrane Library; Issue 3. Oxford: Update Software; 2001.
14. Kauffman CA. Quandary about treatment of aspergillomas persists. *Lancet* 1996; **347:** 1640.
15. Erjavec Z, *et al.* Tolerance and efficacy of amphotericin B inhalations for prevention of invasive pulmonary aspergillosis in haematological patients. *Eur J Clin Microbiol Infect Dis* 1997; **16:** 364–8.
16. Caras WE, Pluss JL. Chronic necrotizing pulmonary aspergillosis: pathologic outcome after itraconazole therapy. *Mayo Clin Proc* 1996; **71:** 25–30.

Blastomycosis

Blastomycosis (not to be confused with South American blastomycosis, see Paracoccidioidomycosis, below) is an infection caused by the fungus *Blastomyces dermatitidis*. Infection may be through the lungs and is usually followed by dissemination; the skin, skeleton, and genitourinary system often become infected. Blastomycosis has been reported only rarely in patients with AIDS, but when it occurs it may be widely disseminated with CNS involvement and a high mortality.[1]

Intravenous amphotericin B, once the mainstay of treatment, is reserved for severe cases, CNS disease, cases unresponsive to other treatment, and infections in immunocompromised patients.[2] Mild to moderate disease is treated with an oral azole,[2] usually itraconazole, although fluconazole, or ketoconazole may also be effective. Patients with AIDS may require prolonged suppressive treatment, preferably with an oral azole, after a clinical response has been achieved.[1]

1. Pappas PG, *et al.* Blastomycosis in patients with the acquired immunodeficiency syndrome. *Ann Intern Med* 1992; **116:** 847–53.
2. Chapman SW, *et al.* Practice guidelines for the management of patients with blastomycosis. *Clin Infect Dis* 2000; **30:** 679–83.

Candidiasis

Candida spp. are commensal fungi commonly found in the gastrointestinal tract, mouth, and vagina; they become pathogenic only when natural defence mechanisms fail. *C. albicans* is the species most commonly associated with infection, although infections with other species notably *C. glabrata (Torulopsis glabrata)*, *C. krusei*, *C. lusitaniae*, *C. parapsilosis*, and *C. tropicalis* also occur. Predisposing factors for pathogenic *Candida* infection include antibacterial therapy, skin trauma, debility, diabetes mellitus, pregnancy, and immunodeficiency; candidiasis often occurs in patients with HIV infection.

Candidiasis (or candidosis), the general term for pathogenic infection with *Candida* spp., can be superficial, deep local invasive, or disseminated.

Superficial candidiasis includes infection of the oropharynx, vagina, and skin. Oropharyngeal and vulvovaginal infections are commonly known as thrush. Superficial infections can usually be treated topically with an antifungal although the rare chronic mucocutaneous candidiasis syndrome normally requires systemic treatment. Antifungals used topically include amphotericin B, ciclopirox olamine, natamycin, nystatin, terbinafine, and the azole derivatives butoconazole, clotrimazole, econazole, fenticonazole, isoconazole, miconazole, oxiconazole, sulconazole, terconazole, and tioconazole. The choice of drug is determined by the availability of a suitable formulation for the site of infection as well as by toxicity and duration of treatment.

Antiseptics including chlorhexidine and povidone-iodine have anticandidal activity and have been used in **oropharyngeal** infections, although they are toxic if swallowed.[1] Methylrosanilinium chloride has also been used,[2,3] but as well as being cosmetically less acceptable its use has become restricted due to fears over possible carcinogenicity.

Infection involving the **nails** and surrounding tissue is difficult to treat. Chronic paronychia (infection affecting the tissue around the nails) is often resistant to treatment but may respond to prolonged application of topical imidazoles.[1] Onychomycosis (infection affecting the nail itself) generally requires systemic treatment with oral itraconazole.[4]

Oesophageal infections are not normally accessible to topical therapy and should be treated with oral azoles.

Vulvovaginal candidiasis responds well to short courses of treatment (typically 3 to 14 days) with a topical antifungal as a cream or pessary. Single-dose preparations are available for local treatment but may be less effective.[5] In general, uncomplicated vulvovaginal infections in immunocompetent patients will respond to a course of treatment of 7 days or less, while patients with complicated infections usually require treatment for 10 to 14 days.[4,6] In pregnancy a topical imidazole appears to be more effective than nystatin.[7] Treatment for 7 days may be necessary. Single-dose or short-course oral therapy with fluconazole or itraconazole is also effective, but oral treatment of such superficial infections may be reserved for patients who do not respond to, or are intolerant of, topical therapy. Vulvovaginal infections with non-*albicans* species may not respond to azoles and such infections may respond to topical boric acid or topical flucytosine.[4]

Topical therapy of superficial candidiasis in general may not be adequate in immunocompromised patients and oral azole therapy should also be considered in these patients.[8] Patients who either do not respond to or do not tolerate oral therapy, or those at risk of developing disseminated disease, may require intravenous amphotericin B.[2,3,8]

Relapse after treatment of superficial candidiasis is common especially in patients with predisposing factors for infection. Recurrence may result from inadequate initial treatment. (In recurrent vulvovaginal candidiasis re-infection from other body sites or by sexual transmission from an untreated partner is not thought to be implicated.[9,10]) Patients with frequent recurrences usually require systemic treatment. Although long-term or intermittent administration of oral antifungals, usually fluconazole, has been recommended to reduce recurrences in immunocompromised patients,[8,11] and 6-month maintenance therapy has been used in immunocompetent patients with recurrent infections,[5,6,10] there is growing concern over the increasing incidence of drug resistance.[12-16] Secondary prophylaxis in immunocompromised patients is now largely restricted to those with frequent or severe recurrences, including oesophageal infections.[17] Resistance may be a consequence of the selection of resistant strains of *C. albicans* or of intrinsically less sensitive species such as *C. krusei*.[14,18-21] Primary prophylaxis against candidiasis is not recommended for patients with advanced HIV infection.[17]

Preparations, such as yogurt, containing *Lactobacillus* spp. have been used in the treatment and prevention of vaginal candidiasis in an attempt to displace *Candida* from the vagina but evidence to support their use is limited. Other novel treatments have included the adjuvant use of granulocyte-macrophage colony-stimulating factors.[22,23]

Deep and disseminated candidiasis requires systemic antifungal treatment. Intravenous amphotericin B, with or without flucytosine, has been regarded as the initial treatment of choice in most infections, although there has been some concern regarding the use of flucytosine in AIDS patients because of its bone-marrow toxicity. Treatment with an azole such as fluconazole and itraconazole may be an effective alternative. Fluconazole has been shown to be as effective as intravenous amphotericin B.[24,25] Fluconazole is emerging as a first-line option for clinically stable patients with uncomplicated candidaemia, provided that they have not recently been treated with an azole.[26] Fluconazole may also be used in combination with fluconazole in severe infections.[4] However, consensus has not been reached on how to treat patients in an unstable clinical condition or those with non-*albicans* candidal infections,[27] although amphotericin B is often preferred.[4] Fluconazole is preferred for infections with *C. lusitaniae* since many strains are resistant to amphotericin B.[4] As with superficial infections, the emergence of resistant *Candida* is causing concern, especially in intensive care settings and in severely immunocompromised patients.[28] Prophylactic antifungal treatment is not recommended routinely[26,29] although some would consider it in critically ill patients or those receiving bone-marrow transplants at high risk of infection.[4,26] Empirical treatment before confirmation of disseminated

candidiasis has been recommended for patients with heavy colonisation and a deteriorating condition.[26,29]

1. WHO. *WHO model prescribing information: drugs used in skin diseases.* Geneva: WHO, 1997.
2. WHO. *Global programme on AIDS: guidelines for the clinical management of HIV infection in children.* Geneva: WHO, 1993.
3. Garber GE. Treatment of oral candida mucositis infections. *Drugs* 1994; **47:** 734–40.
4. Rex JH, *et al.* Infectious Diseases Society of America. Practice guidelines for the treatment of candidiasis. *Clin Infect Dis* 2000; **30:** 662–78.
5. Anonymous. Drugs for sexually transmitted infections. *Med Lett Drugs Ther* 1999; **41:** 85–90.
6. Centers for Disease Control. 1998 Guidelines for treatment of sexually transmitted diseases. *MMWR* 1998; **47** (RR-1): 1–116.
7. Young GL, Jewell D. Topical treatment for vaginal candidiasis in pregnancy (updated 3 November 2000). Available in The Cochrane Library; Issue 3. Oxford: Update Software; 2001.
8. British Society for Antimicrobial Chemotherapy Working Party. Antifungal chemotherapy in patients with acquired immunodeficiency syndrome. *Lancet* 1992; **340:** 648–51.
9. Working Group of the British Society for Medical Mycology. Management of genital candidiasis. *BMJ* 1995; **310:** 1241–4.
10. Clinical Effectiveness Group, Association of Genitourinary Medicine and the Medical Society for the Study of Venereal Diseases. National guideline for the management of vulvovaginal candidiasis. *Sex Transm Inf* 1999; **75**(suppl 1): S19–S20.
11. Working Party of the British Society for Antimicrobial Chemotherapy. Chemoprophylaxis for candidosis and aspergillosis in neutropenia and transplantation: a review and recommendations. *J Antimicrob Chemother* 1993; **32:** 5–21.
12. Powderly WG. Resistant candidiasis. *AIDS Res Hum Retroviruses* 1994; **10:** 925–9.
13. Sangeorzan JA, *et al.* Epidemiology of oral candidiasis in HIV-infected patients: colonization, infection, treatment, and emergence of fluconazole resistance. *Am J Med* 1994; **97:** 339–46.
14. Johnson EM, Warnock DW. Azole drug resistance in yeasts. *J Antimicrob Chemother* 1995; **36:** 751–5.
15. Baily G. Weekly fluconazole for preventing mucosal candidiasis in HIV infection. *Ann Intern Med* 1997; **127:** 1131.
16. Goldman M, *et al.* Does long-term itraconazole prophylaxis result in in vitro azole resistance in mucosal Candida albicans isolates from persons with advanced human immunodeficiency virus infection? *Antimicrob Agents Chemother* 2000; **44:** 1585–7.
17. Centers for Disease Control. 1999 USPHS/IDSA guidelines for the prevention of opportunistic infections in persons infected with human immunodeficiency virus. *MMWR* 1999; **48** (RR-10): 1–59.
18. Millon L, *et al.* Émergence de Candida glabrata et Candida krusei chez des patients séropositifs pour le VIH atteints de candidose oropharyngée, traités de façon prolongée par le fluconazole. *J Mycol Med* 1994; **4:** 90–2.
19. Law D, *et al.* High prevalence of antifungal resistance in Candida spp from patients with AIDS. *J Antimicrob Chemother* 1994; **34:** 659–68.
20. Denning DW. Can we prevent azole resistance in fungi? *Lancet* 1995; **346:** 454–5.
21. Lewis RE, Klepser ME. The changing face of nosocomial candidemia: epidemiology, resistance, and drug therapy. *Am J Health-Syst Pharm* 1999; **56:** 525–33.
22. Shahar E, *et al.* White cell enhancement in the treatment of severe candidosis. *Lancet* 1995; **346:** 974–5.
23. Capetti A, *et al.* Employment of recombinant human granulocyte-macrophage colony stimulating factor in oesophageal candidiasis in AIDS patients. *AIDS* 1995; **9:** 1378–9.
24. Rex JH, *et al.* A randomized trial comparing fluconazole with amphotericin B for the treatment of candidemia in patients without neutropenia. *N Engl J Med* 1994; **331:** 1325–30.
25. Anaissie EJ, *et al.* Management of invasive candidal infections: results of a prospective, randomized, multicenter study of fluconazole versus amphotericin B and review of the literature. *Clin Infect Dis* 1996; **23:** 964–72.
26. Edwards JE, *et al.* International conference for the development of a consensus on the management and prevention of severe candidal infections. *Clin Infect Dis* 1997; **25:** 43–59.
27. Graybill JR. Editorial response: can we agree on the treatment of candidiasis? *Clin Infect Dis* 1997; **25:** 60–2.
28. Nguyen MH, *et al.* The changing face of candidemia: emergence of non-Candida albicans species and antifungal resistance. *Am J Med* 1996; **100:** 617–23.
29. British Society for Antimicrobial Chemotherapy Working Party. Management of deep Candida infection in surgical and intensive care unit patients. *Intensive Care Med* 1994; **20:** 522–8.

Chromoblastomycosis

Chromoblastomycosis (chromomycosis) is an infection caused by a number of opportunistic fungi, including *Fonsecaea compacta (Phialophora compacta), F. pedrosoi (P. pedrosoi), Phialophora verrucosa, Cladosporium carrionii*, and *Rhinocladiella aquaspersa*, following invasion of skin trauma sites. It occurs worldwide but is more common in tropical and subtropical climates. The disease is characterised by chronic cutaneous and subcutaneous lesions. In its early stages, when lesions are small, surgical excision or cryotherapy are the treatments of choice, although it has been suggested that there is some risk of spreading the lesion during surgery. Drug treatment with itraconazole, alone or in combination with flucytosine, may be used.[1] Saperconazole[2] and terbinafine[3] have also been used with some success. However, recurrence and drug resistance has been a problem with monotherapy. Local heat treatment aids healing and may be useful.

1. WHO. *WHO model prescribing information: drugs used in skin diseases.* Geneva: WHO, 1997.
2. Franco L, *et al.* Saperconazole in the treatment of systemic and subcutaneous mycoses. *Int J Dermatol* 1992; **31:** 725–9.
3. Esterre P, *et al.* Treatment of chromomycosis with terbinafine: preliminary results of an open pilot study. *Br J Dermatol* 1996; **134** (suppl 46): 33–6.

Coccidioidomycosis

Coccidioidomycosis is an infection caused by inhalation of the spores of *Coccidioides immitis*, a fungus found in the soil in arid and semi-desert areas mainly of North, Central, and South America. Patients may experience acute or chronic lung infections, meningitis, and disseminated disease although many infections are subclinical. Common names for the infection include valley fever, desert fever, and desert rheumatism. In endemic areas, coccidioidomycosis is a common opportunistic infection in immunocompromised patients.

Acute pulmonary coccidioidomycosis is usually self-limiting and resolves spontaneously without specific chemotherapy; in 60% of cases the infection is asymptomatic or mild. In some patients the infection progresses to chronic pulmonary coccidioidomycosis with granulomatous lesions, fibrosis, and cavitation. A small proportion of patients develop acute progressive pneumonia which is commonly fatal if untreated, or disseminated disease usually involving the skin, bone, meninges, and joints. Severe pulmonary and disseminated infections are more likely in pregnant women, dark-skinned races, diabetics, and immunocompromised patients.

Antifungal therapy is with either intravenous amphotericin B or an oral azole.[1,2] Treatment is usually reserved for severe or complicated infections or for patients with concurrent risk factors, especially immunosuppression.[2] Ketoconazole, itraconazole, and fluconazole have all been reported to be at least moderately effective in non-meningeal infections.[2] Amphotericin B is generally used for rapidly progressive disease.[2] Fluconazole is effective in meningeal infections and is the most frequently recommended antifungal for this indication,[2] although itraconazole has also produced beneficial responses; intrathecal amphotericin B may also be used, especially in aggressive infections.[2,3] The incidence of relapses following treatment is high, and lifelong therapy is recommended following coccidioidal meningitis.[4] In patients with HIV infection, lifelong suppressive therapy with fluconazole or itraconazole is recommended following treatment of either meningeal or non-meningeal coccidioidomycosis.[5]

1. Stevens DA. Coccidioidomycosis. *N Engl J Med* 1995; **332:** 1077–82.
2. Galgiani JN, *et al.* Infectious Diseases Society of America. Practice guidelines for the treatment of coccidioidomycosis. *Clin Infect Dis* 2000; **30:** 658–61.
3. Anonymous. Systemic antifungal drugs. *Med Lett Drugs Ther* 1997; **39:** 86–8.
4. Dewsnup DH, *et al.* Is it ever safe to stop azole therapy for Coccidioides immitis meningitis? *Ann Intern Med* 1996; **124:** 305–10.
5. Centers for Disease Control. 1999 USPHS/IDSA guidelines for the prevention of opportunistic infections in persons infected with human immunodeficiency virus. *MMWR* 1999; **48** (RR-10): 1–59.

Cryptococcosis

Cryptococcosis is an infection caused by inhalation of the fungus *Cryptococcus neoformans*. It is rare in immunocompetent individuals, but is an important life-threatening disease in immunocompromised patients, especially those with AIDS, in whom it occurs principally as **cryptococcal meningitis**.

Mild infections in immunocompetent patients may resolve without treatment, but oral fluconazole is usually effective if treatment is necessary.[1] Itraconazole is a suitable alternative in patients unable to take fluconazole. In either case, treatment should continue for several months. For more severe disease, amphotericin B may be given alone, or, especially if there is CNS involvement, with flucytosine. Patients may be transferred to oral fluconazole after induction therapy with amphotericin B and flucytosine or may continue on amphotericin B and flucytosine for 6 to 10 weeks.[1] Intrathecal or intraventricular amphotericin B may be used in refractory cases.

Any infection in immunocompromised patients should be treated as for CNS infections in immunocompetent patients, although AIDS-related cryptococcal pneumonia may be treated with oral fluconazole or itraconazole, continued indefinitely. Fluconazole plus flucytosine is another alternative, but the toxicity of this regimen limits its usefulness.[1] Immunocompromised patients require long-term suppressive treatment, typically with oral fluconazole, after a primary course of antifungal therapy, and in patients with HIV infection this should be lifelong.[1,2] Oral itraconazole or intermittent intravenous amphotericin B are alternatives but are generally reserved for patients who cannot take fluconazole.

Antifungals

Primary prophylaxis in patients with HIV infection is not generally recommended since it has not been shown to be more beneficial than treating cryptococcal infections when they occur and may increase the risk of resistance.[2]

1. Saag MS, *et al.* Infectious Diseases Society of America. Practice guidelines for the management of cryptococcal disease. *Clin Infect Dis* 2000; **30**: 710–18.
2. Centers for Disease Control. 1999 USPHS/IDSA guidelines for the prevention of opportunistic infections in persons infected with human immunodeficiency virus. *MMWR* 1999; **48** (RR-10): 1–59.

Dermatophytoses
See under Skin Infections, below.

Endocarditis
Infective endocarditis caused by fungi such as *Aspergillus* or *Candida* is much less common than that caused by bacteria (p.119). Fungal endocarditis is usually treated with intravenous amphotericin B; surgical removal of an infected valve may be required.[1] Long-term survival was reported[2] in a patient with endocarditis due to *C. parapsilosis* who was not suitable for surgery. Treatment was initially with amphotericin B, replaced by fluconazole after 27 days because of renal dysfunction. At the time of publication, the patient remained free of disease having received fluconazole for 26 months.

1. Ellis M. Fungal endocarditis. *J Infect* 1997; **35**: 99–103.
2. Czwerwiec FS, *et al.* Long-term survival after fluconazole therapy of candidal prosthetic valve endocarditis. *Am J Med* 1993; **94**: 545–6.

Eye infections
Fungal infections of the eye are less common than infections with bacteria or viruses, but are usually severe and may lead to loss of vision. Diagnosis may be delayed due to a gradual onset of symptoms and empirical treatment with antibacterials. Infections may involve the cornea (keratitis), the interior of the eye (endophthalmitis), or the orbit and may occur following trauma (including surgery) or systemic disseminated infection. Patients with impaired host resistance such as diabetics or immunocompromised patients are particularly at risk. The most common fungi causing eye infections are *Aspergillus*, *Candida,* and *Fusarium*; others include *Blastomyces*, *Cryptococcus*, and *Sporothrix*. Infections of the orbit usually occur by spread from an infection of the paranasal sinus, commonly mucormycosis or aspergillosis.

Fungal infections of the eye are difficult to treat. Antifungals are generally not well absorbed following topical application and infections extending to the vitreous or anterior chamber require subconjunctival, intra-ocular, and/or systemic treatment. Systemic treatment is necessary for ocular manifestations of disseminated disease. When systemic therapy is required intravenous amphotericin B is usually given; an oral azole compound may be given for less severe infections. Superficial infections may respond to topical treatment. Amphotericin B or natamycin are most commonly used. An azole compound such as miconazole is sometimes used, or flucytosine in combination with another antifungal. Chlorhexidine has also produced promising results. Topical treatment may also be used as an adjunct to systemic therapy. Surgical excision of infected tissue may be necessary in severe infections.

Histoplasmosis
Histoplasmosis is a systemic infection caused by *Histoplasma capsulatum,* a fungus found in the soil in endemic areas, particularly at sites with heavy accumulations of bird or bat excrement. Infection is by inhalation of spores. Two types of histoplasmosis occur: classic histoplasmosis due to infection with *H. capsulatum* var. *capsulatum* and African histoplasmosis due to infection with *H. capsulatum* var. *duboisii.*

The major endemic area for *H. capsulatum* var. *capsulatum* is central USA. In endemic regions most of the population is infected and mild infections are generally asymptomatic. However, acute pulmonary infection can occur. Massive infection can be fatal. Chronic pulmonary histoplasmosis can result in lung fibrosis and cavitation. Histoplasmosis may also present as an acute or chronic disseminated infection involving widespread infiltration of the reticuloendothelial system and is primarily seen in immunodeficient or immunocompromised patients.

Histoplasma capsulatum var. *duboisii* is found in central Africa and causes a chronic disseminated form of histoplasmosis with focal lesions predominantly in skin and bone.

Antifungal therapy for classic or African histoplasmosis is necessary in patients with severe pulmonary infections, chronic fibrotic or cavitary disease, or disseminated infection. Infections which are not life-threatening may be treated with an oral azole in both immunocompetent and immunocompromised patients.[1] Itraconazole is the preferred drug.[1] Ketoconazole is moderately effective but more toxic. Fluconazole is less effective than either itraconazole or ketoconazole but may be the preferred azole in CNS infections where its better penetration may be an advantage.[1] Patients with life-threatening infections or those not responding to oral treatment are given amphotericin B intravenously. Patients with HIV infection should continue maintenance therapy with itraconazole daily or amphotericin B weekly;[1,2] the use of fluconazole for maintenance should be discouraged.[1] Primary prophylaxis with itraconazole is not recommended routinely but may be considered for patients with advanced AIDS at especially high risk of infection due to occupational exposure or residence in a hyperendemic area.[2]

1. Wheat J, *et al.* Infectious Diseases Society of America. Practice guidelines for the management of patients with histoplasmosis. *Clin Infect Dis* 2000; **30**: 688–95.
2. Centers for Disease Control. 1999 USPHS/IDSA guidelines for the prevention of opportunistic infections in persons infected with human immunodeficiency virus. *MMWR* 1999; **48** (RR-10): 1–59.

Infections in immunocompromised patients
Patients with a defective immune system are at special risk of infections, including those caused by fungi. Primary immune deficiency is rare, whereas secondary deficiency is more common; immunosuppressive therapy, cancer and its treatment, HIV infection, and splenectomy may all cause neutropenia and impaired humoral and cellular immunity in varying degrees. Fungi most commonly associated with infection in these patients include *Cryptococcus neoformans* and species of *Aspergillus* and *Candida*. *Pneumocystis carinii*, now considered to have characteristics of fungi, is an important cause of pneumonia in patients with AIDS. In areas in which they are endemic, coccidioidomycosis, histoplasmosis, and *Penicillium marneffei* infections are also more common in immunocompromised patients and a growing number of uncommon organisms including *Fusarium* spp., *Scedosporium* spp., and *Trichosporon* spp. can cause invasive infections. A fungal cause of infection should be considered in immunocompromised patients with fever of unknown origin who have not responded to broad spectrum antibacterials. Fungal infection in patients with immune deficiency usually occurs as a widely disseminated disease and treatment should be commenced as early as possible. If the infection has not been identified, empirical treatment with intravenous amphotericin B has been attempted but the effects of this on overall mortality remain uncertain.

Long-term suppression of fungal infection has been recommended for immunocompromised patients although this might allow development of resistance and the overgrowth of species not susceptible to the antifungals used. This is of particular concern with fluconazole (p.384), one of the drugs that has been most widely used for this purpose. Antifungals are also used in selective digestive tract decontamination (see Intensive Care, p.126).

Treatment and prophylaxis of specific fungal infections in immunocompromised patients is discussed under the appropriate headings—see Aspergillosis, Candidiasis, Coccidioidomycosis, Cryptococcosis, and Histoplasmosis (above), and *Pneumocystis carinii* Pneumonia (below).

References.

1. British Society for Antimicrobial Chemotherapy Working Party. Antifungal chemotherapy in patients with acquired immunodeficiency syndrome. *Lancet* 1992; **340**: 648–51.
2. Working Party of the British Society for Antimicrobial Chemotherapy. Chemoprophylaxis for candidosis and aspergillosis in neutropenia and transplantation: a review and recommendations. *J Antimicrob Chemother* 1993; **32**: 5–21.
3. American Thoracic Society. Fungal infection in HIV-infected persons. *Am J Respir Crit Care Med* 1995; **152**: 816–22.
4. Warnock DW. Fungal complications of transplantation: diagnosis, treatment and prevention. *J Antimicrob Chemother* 1995; **36** (suppl B): 73–90.
5. Meunier F. Targeting fungi: a challenge. *Am J Med* 1995; **99** (suppl 6A): 60S–67S.
6. Hood S, Denning DW. Treatment of fungal infections in AIDS. *J Antimicrob Chemother* 1996; **37** (suppl B): 71–85.
7. Gøtzsche PC, Johansen HK. Meta-analysis of prophylactic or empirical antifungal treatment versus placebo or no treatment in patients with cancer complicated by neutropenia. *BMJ* 1997; **314**: 1238–44.

8. Working Party of the British Society for Antimicrobial Chemotherapy. Therapy of deep fungal infection in haematological malignancy. *J Antimicrob Chemother* 1997; **40**: 779–88.
9. Warnock DW. Fungal infections in neutropenia: current problems and chemotherapeutic control. *J Antimicrob Chemother* 1998; **41** (suppl D): 95–105.
10. Centers for Disease Control. 1999 USPHS/IDSA guidelines for the prevention of opportunistic infections in persons infected with human immunodeficiency virus. *MMWR* 1999; **48** (RR-10): 1–59.
11. Johansen HK, Gøtzsche PC. Amphotericin B versus fluconazole for controlling fungal infections in neutropenic cancer patients (updated 22 May 2001). Available in The Cochrane Library; Issue 3. Oxford: Update Software; 2001.
12. Gotzsche PC, Johansen HK. Routine versus selective antifungal administration for control of fungal infections in patients with cancer (updated 23 February 2001). Available in The Cochrane Library; Issue 2. Oxford: Update Software; 2001.

Meningitis
Fungal diseases associated with meningitis include aspergillosis, candidiasis, coccidioidomycosis, cryptococcosis, and histoplasmosis (see above), although many disseminated fungal infections can involve the CNS, especially in immunocompromised patients. The treatment of each infection is discussed under the appropriate heading, but in general the initial drug of choice in fungal meningitis is intravenous amphotericin B, sometimes with flucytosine.

Mucormycosis
Mucormycosis, a rare but serious infection caused by Mucorales fungi, is a type of zygomycosis, a term which is sometimes used synonymously. Mucormycosis usually occurs in poorly controlled diabetic patients or in immunocompromised patients. Patients receiving desferrioxamine may also be at increased risk of infection (see p.1004). Infections of the mucosa of the respiratory tract or gastrointestinal tract, or of abraded skin, usually with *Rhizopus* or *Rhizomucor* spp., can result in local invasion of deeper tissues including bone and the CNS with extensive tissue destruction. Disseminated disease may also occur.

Amphotericin B intravenously can be effective in mucormycosis and is usually combined with aggressive surgical debridement of infected tissue. Invasive disease is difficult to treat and is usually fatal.

1. Boelaert JR. Mucormycosis (zygomycosis): is there news for the clinician? *J Infect* 1994; **28** (suppl 1): 1–6.

Mycetoma
Mycetoma is seen especially in the tropics and subtropics and involves subcutaneous tissue, bone, and skin. The term Madura foot is used for mycetoma affecting the foot. Organisms enter the tissues via local skin trauma. Mycetomas caused by fungi such as *Madurella mycetomatis*, *M. grisea*, or *Pseudallescheria boydii* are called eumycetomas. Those caused by the filamentous bacteria, actinomycetes, are called actinomycetomas and are discussed on p.130. Eumycetomas are often unresponsive to treatment. Some infections have responded to prolonged treatment with ketoconazole[1,2] and itraconazole has also been tried.[2] Surgical excision may be necessary.

1. Mahgoub ES, Gumaa SA. Ketoconazole in the treatment of eumycetoma due to Madurella mycetomii. *Trans R Soc Trop Med Hyg* 1984; **78**: 376–9.
2. Restrepo A. Treatment of tropical mycoses. *J Am Acad Dermatol* 1994; **31**: S91–S102.

Nail infections
See under Skin Infections, below.

Paracoccidioidomycosis
Paracoccidioidomycosis (South American blastomycosis) is caused by an infection with the fungus *Paracoccidioides brasiliensis*. The disease occurs mainly in inhabitants or former inhabitants of regions of Central and South America and may remain dormant for long periods. Infection is thought to be by inhalation. While most primary infections are subclinical, some may be progressive and severe, particularly in immunocompromised patients. The lungs may be affected, the disease usually presenting as a chronic infection. Disseminated disease affects the skin, mucous membranes, gastrointestinal tract, reticuloendothelial system, and adrenals, and may be either acute or chronic.

Treatment is usually with itraconazole, ketoconazole, or intravenous amphotericin B for patients with severe infection.[1] Sulfonamides are now rarely used. Other azole derivatives may prove effective. There has been a case report describing successful treatment with terbinafine when access to azoles was not possible.[2] Treatment may need to be continued for months or years to prevent relapse.

1. Anonymous. Systemic antifungal drugs. *Med Lett Drugs Ther* 1997; **39:** 86–8.

2. Ollague JM, *et al.* Paracoccidioidomycosis (South American blastomycosis) successfully treated with terbinafine: first case report. *Br J Dermatol* 2000; **143:** 188–91.

Peritonitis

Fungal peritonitis occasionally occurs in patients undergoing continuous ambulatory peritoneal dialysis or abdominal surgery, or in trauma. It is usually caused by yeasts such as *Candida*. Amphotericin B has been the treatment of choice;[1,2] intravenous administration has been preferred to intraperitoneal administration since the latter route is painful.[3] Fluconazole or other azole antifungals or flucytosine may also be effective.[1,4] However, fungal peritonitis is a difficult infection to treat and it has a high morbidity and mortality.[3]

1. Keane WF, *et al.* Peritoneal dialysis-related peritonitis treatment recommendations: 1996 update. *Perit Dial Int* 1996; **16:** 557–73.

2. Johnson CC, *et al.* Peritonitis: update on pathophysiology, clinical manifestations, and management. *Clin Infect Dis* 1997; **24:** 1035–47.

3. Working Party of the British Society for Antimicrobial Chemotherapy. Diagnosis and management of peritonitis in continuous ambulatory peritoneal dialysis. *Lancet* 1987; **i:** 845–9.

4. Aguado JM, *et al.* Successful treatment of candida peritonitis with fluconazole. *J Antimicrob Chemother* 1994; **34:** 847.

Pityriasis versicolor

See under Skin Infections, below.

Pneumocystis carinii pneumonia

Pneumocystis carinii is an opportunistic unicellular pathogen which has been classified both with the protozoa and with the fungi, although more recent evidence suggests that it is probably a fungus. It appears to be acquired by the airborne route, but in persons with normally functioning immune systems clinical infection resolves spontaneously. However, in immunosuppressed patients it can produce interstitial pneumonia with progressive damage to the alveolar walls and accumulation of exudate in the air spaces; if untreated, the disease is almost always fatal. With the advent of AIDS (p.608), *Pneumocystis carinii* pneumonia (PCP) has become an increasing problem.

Co-trimoxazole, dapsone, and pentamidine are currently the most effective drugs for both treatment and prophylaxis. However, there is evidence of the emergence of strains of *P. carinii* potentially resistant to both sulfonamides and dapsone,[1,2] emphasising the need for continuing development of alternative regimens.

Treatment of acute disease is primarily with either co-trimoxazole or pentamidine.[3] Co-trimoxazole is the preferred drug,[4–6] given intravenously in severe infections and orally in mild infections. Intravenous pentamidine is generally reserved for patients who do not respond to or cannot tolerate co-trimoxazole. Combination therapy with co-trimoxazole and pentamidine is not more effective and is potentially more toxic than either drug alone.[7] Some centres prefer trimethoprim with dapsone for second-line therapy[5] although the combination is only effective in patients with mild or moderately severe infections.[6] Dapsone should probably not be used alone for treatment of PCP,[5] but may be useful for prophylaxis (see below). Other alternatives include primaquine plus clindamycin,[8–10] and trimetrexate plus folinic acid.[11,12] Atovaquone may be used to treat mild to moderate infections.[6,13,14] Nebulised pentamidine is occasionally suggested for mild infections but is now generally reserved for prophylaxis (see below). Studies suggest that there is probably little difference in efficacy between these regimens, and ultimately the choice will be based on adverse effects and availability.[10] Although it has been suggested that folinic acid could be administered with co-trimoxazole to reduce the risk of haematotoxicity,[5] increased therapeutic failure has been reported in patients receiving this combination.[15]

Prompt additional treatment with a corticosteroid is now of established value for patients with moderate or severe disease (see p.1056) and is started at the same time as the antipneumocystis treatment is begun.[6] Adjuvant treatment with corticosteroids reduces morbidity and mortality[6] and concerns over corticosteroid-induced immunosuppression have generally not been borne out in practice.

Prophylaxis is used in high-risk patients, especially among those with compromised immunity due to HIV

infection. Primary prophylaxis is attempted in all HIV-infected adults with a CD4+ T lymphocyte count below 200 per μL or those with a history of candidiasis regardless of CD4+ T lymphocyte count.[16] In infants and young children, in whom the CD4+ T lymphocyte count is normally higher than in adults and in whom PCP commonly occurs at CD4+ T lymphocyte counts of greater than 200 per μL, separate guidelines in the USA proposed prophylaxis at age-specific CD4+ T lymphocyte count thresholds.[17] USA guidelines recommend that infants of HIV-positive mothers should receive prophylaxis beginning at 4 to 6 weeks of age and continuing until they are shown to be seronegative, or for at least 1 year initially.[16] However, some children at risk of infection have not received recommended prophylaxis.[18,19] In Europe, clinicians tend to have a less aggressive approach to prophylaxis, with only one-third of clinics offering prophylaxis routinely to all children exposed to HIV while the remaining two-thirds only offer prophylaxis once HIV infection is confirmed or opportunistic infection occurs.[20]

Secondary prophylaxis is given to all patients with a history of PCP. Recommendations for prophylaxis in patients without HIV infection are not widely publicised, but it has been suggested that prophylaxis should be considered for patients who are immunosuppressed due to an underlying disorder or to immunosuppressant drug therapy.[21,22]

Co-trimoxazole by mouth is currently preferred for primary and secondary prophylaxis.[6,16] Pentamidine administered by an appropriate jet nebuliser, dapsone (alone or with pyrimethamine), or atovaquone, are the usual alternatives in patients unable to tolerate co-trimoxazole.[6,16] A meta-analysis found that co-trimoxazole was more effective than dapsone or pentamidine.[23] However, co-trimoxazole is not well tolerated and long-term studies suggest that, on an intention-to-treat basis, the efficacy of dapsone[24] or inhaled pentamidine[24,25] may be comparable, at least in patients with CD4+ T lymphocyte counts of more than 100 per μL. For secondary prophylaxis dapsone was found to be less effective than nebulised pentamidine in a study in patients with AIDS,[26] but the efficacy of regimens for secondary prophylaxis has not yet been fully evaluated. Regimens containing co-trimoxazole or dapsone also protect against toxoplasmosis, an increasingly common opportunistic infection in AIDS patients.[16,27,28]

Co-trimoxazole and dapsone are usually administered daily for prophylaxis of PCP,[16] but intermittent administration has been tried in an attempt to improve tolerance without compromising efficacy. Doses of co-trimoxazole have usually been 960 mg given on three days of each week although 960 mg twice daily on three days each week has also been used; a low dose of 480 mg daily on every day each week is said to be better tolerated than a dose of 960 mg daily on every day each week and equally effective (see under Co-trimoxazole, p.195). Intermittent use of dapsone has involved administration with pyrimethamine on two days each week[29] although such intermittent use may be less effective than other regimens.[30,31] Response to inhaled pentamidine can be influenced by the choice of nebuliser;[32] commonly used nebulisers include the Fisoneb and Respirgard II. Patients receiving inhaled pentamidine may be prone to extrapulmonary *Pneumocystis* infection.[33,34] Other alternative prophylactic regimens include intermittent parenteral administration of pentamidine, pyrimethamine with sulfadoxine, clindamycin with primaquine, trimetrexate, and dapsone with trimethoprim.[6,16]

It may be possible to discontinue primary[35–40] and secondary[35,36,38,40,41] prophylaxis in patients with HIV infection who obtain a sustained response to potent combination antiretroviral therapy with at least partial recovery of immune function.[35–41] However, a study of solid organ transplant recipients[42] suggested that lung transplant recipients were at continued risk of developing PCP and that prophylaxis may need to be continued indefinitely in this group.

1. Mei Q, *et al.* Failure of co-trimoxazole in Pneumocystis carinii infection and mutations in dihydropteroate synthase gene. *Lancet* 1998; **351:** 1631–2.

2. Helweg-Larsen J, *et al.* Effects of mutations in Pneumocystis carinii dihydropteroate synthase gene on outcome of AIDS-associated P carinii pneumonia. *Lancet* 1999; **354:** 1347–51.

3. Masur H. Prevention and treatment of pneumocystis pneumonia. *N Engl J Med* 1992; **327:** 1853–60. Correction. *ibid.* 1993; **328:** 1136.

4. Anonymous. Drugs for parasitic infections. *Med Lett Drugs Ther* 1998; **40:** 1–12.

5. Peters BS, *et al.* Adverse effects of drugs used in the management of opportunistic infections associated with HIV infection. *Drug Safety* 1994; **10:** 439–54.

6. Miller RF, *et al.* Pneumocystis carinii infection: current treatment and prevention. *J Antimicrob Chemother* 1996; **37** (suppl B): 33–53.

7. Glatt AE, Chirgwin K. Pneumocystis carinii pneumonia in human immunodeficiency virus-infected patients. *Arch Intern Med* 1990; **150:** 271–9.

8. Toma E, *et al.* Clindamycin/primaquine versus trimethoprim-sulfamethoxazole as primary therapy for Pneumocystis carinii pneumonia in AIDS: a randomized, double-blind pilot trial. *Clin Infect Dis* 1993; **17:** 178–84.

9. Black JR, *et al.* Clindamycin and primaquine therapy for mild-to-moderate episodes of Pneumocystis carinii pneumonia in patients with AIDS: AIDS Clinical Trials Group 044. *Clin Infect Dis* 1994; **18:** 905–13.

10. Safrin S, *et al.* Comparison of three regimens for treatment of mild to moderate Pneumocystis carinii pneumonia in patients with AIDS: a double-blind, randomized trial of oral trimethoprim-sulfamethoxazole, dapsone-trimethoprim, and clindamycin-primaquine. *Ann Intern Med* 1996; **124:** 792–802.

11. Amsden GW, *et al.* Trimetrexate for Pneumocystis carinii pneumonia in patients with AIDS. *Ann Pharmacother* 1992; **26:** 218–26.

12. Sattler FR, *et al.* Trimetrexate with leucovorin versus trimethoprim-sulfamethoxazole for moderate to severe episodes of Pneumocystis carinii pneumonia in patients with AIDS: a prospective, controlled multicenter investigation of the AIDS Clinical Trials Group Protocol 029/031. *J Infect Dis* 1994; **170:** 165–72.

13. Hughes W, *et al.* Comparison of atovaquone (566C80) with trimethoprim-sulfamethoxazole to treat Pneumocystis carinii pneumonia in patients with AIDS. *N Engl J Med* 1993; **328:** 1521–7.

14. Dohn MN, *et al.* Oral atovaquone compared with intravenous pentamidine for Pneumocystis carinii pneumonia in patients with AIDS. *Ann Intern Med* 1994; **121:** 174–80.

15. Safrin S, *et al.* Adjunctive folinic acid with trimethoprim-sulfamethoxazole for Pneumocystis carinii pneumonia in AIDS patients is associated with an increased risk of therapeutic failure and death. *J Infect Dis* 1994; **170:** 912–7.

16. Centers for Disease Control. 1999 USPHS/IDSA guidelines for the prevention of opportunistic infections in persons infected with human immunodeficiency virus. *MMWR* 1999; **48** (RR-10): 1–59.

17. Centers for Disease Control. 1995 Revised guidelines for prophylaxis against Pneumocystis carinii pneumonia for children infected with or perinatally exposed to human immunodeficiency virus. *MMWR* 1995; **44** (RR-4): 1–11.

18. Kovacs JA, Kovacs AAS. PCP prophylaxis in paediatric HIV infection: time for a change? *Lancet* 1994; **344:** 5–6.

19. Simonds RJ, *et al.* Prophylaxis against Pneumocystis carinii pneumonia among children with perinatally acquired human immunodeficiency virus infection in the United States. *N Engl J Med* 1995; **332:** 786–90.

20. Bernardi S, *et al.* Variable use of therapeutic interventions for children with human immunodeficiency virus type 1 infection in Europe. *Eur J Pediatr* 2000; **159:** 170–5.

21. Sepkowitz KA, *et al.* Pneumocystis carinii pneumonia without acquired immunodeficiency syndrome: more patients, same risk. *Arch Intern Med* 1995; **155:** 1125–8.

22. Yale SH, Limper AH. Pneumocystis carinii pneumonia in patients without acquired immunodeficiency syndrome: associated illnesses and prior corticosteroid therapy. *Mayo Clin Proc* 1996; **71:** 5–13.

23. Ioannidis JP, *et al.* A meta-analysis of the relative efficacy and toxicity of Pneumocystis carinii prophylactic regimens. *Arch Intern Med* 1996; **156:** 177–88.

24. Bozzette SA, *et al.* A randomised trial of three antipneumocystis agents in patients with advanced human immunodeficiency virus infection. *N Engl J Med* 1995; **332:** 693–9.

25. Rizzardi GP, *et al.* Risks and benefits of aerosolized pentamidine and cotrimoxazole in primary prophylaxis of Pneumocystis carinii pneumonia in HIV-1-infected patients: a two-year Italian multicentric randomized controlled trial. *J Infect* 1996; **32:** 123–31.

26. Salmon-Ceron D, *et al.* Lower survival in AIDS patients receiving dapsone compared with aerosolized pentamidine for secondary prophylaxis of Pneumocystis carinii pneumonia. *J Infect Dis* 1995; **172:** 656–64.

27. Girard P-M, *et al.* Dapsone–pyrimethamine compared with aerosolized pentamidine as primary prophylaxis against Pneumocystis carinii pneumonia and toxoplasmosis in HIV infection. *N Engl J Med* 1993; **328:** 1514–20.

28. Torres RA, *et al.* Randomized trial of dapsone and aerosolized pentamidine for the prophylaxis of Pneumocystis carinii pneumonia and toxoplasmosis encephalitis. *Am J Med* 1993; **95:** 573–83.

29. Podzamczer D, *et al.* Intermittent trimethoprim-sulfamethoxazole compared with dapsone-pyrimethamine for the simultaneous primary prophylaxis of pneumocystis pneumonia and toxoplasmosis in patients infected with HIV. *Ann Intern Med* 1995; **122:** 755–61.

30. Souza JP, *et al.* High rates of Pneumocystis carinii pneumonia in allogeneic blood and marrow transplant recipients receiving dapsone prophylaxis. *Clin Infect Dis* 1999; **29:** 1467–71.

31. McIntosh K, *et al.* Toxicity and efficacy of daily vs weekly dapsone for prevention of Pneumocystis carinii pneumonia in children infected with human immunodeficiency virus. *Pediatr Infect Dis J* 1999; **18:** 432–9.

32. Miller R, Steel S. Nebulized pentamidine as prophylaxis for Pneumocystis carinii pneumonia. *J Antimicrob Chemother* 1991; **27:** 153–7.

33. Witt K, *et al.* Dissemination of Pneumocystis carinii in patients with AIDS. *Scand J Infect Dis* 1991; **23:** 691–5.

34. Sha BE, *et al.* Pneumocystis carinii choroiditis in patients with AIDS: clinical features, response to therapy, and outcome. *J Acquir Immune Defic Syndr Hum Retrovirol* 1992; **5:** 1051–8.

35. Schneider MME, *et al.* Discontinuation of prophylaxis for Pneumocystis carinii pneumonia in HIV-1-infected patients treated with highly active antiretroviral therapy. *Lancet* 1999; **353:** 201–3.

36. Weverling GJ, *et al.* Discontinuation of Pneumocystis carinii pneumonia prophylaxis after start of highly active antiretroviral therapy in HIV-1 infection. *Lancet* 1999; **353:** 1293–8.

37. Furrer H, *et al.* Discontinuation of primary prophylaxis against Pneumocystis carinii pneumonia in HIV-1-infected adults treated with combination antiretroviral therapy. *N Engl J Med* 1999; **340:** 1301–6.

38. Yangco BG, *et al.* Discontinuation of chemoprophylaxis against Pneumocystis carinii pneumonia in patients with HIV infection. *Ann Intern Med* 2000; **132:** 201–5.

39. Mussini C, *et al.* Discontinuation of primary prophylaxis for Pneumocystis carinii pneumonia and toxoplasmic encephalitis in human immunodeficiency virus type 1-infected patients: the changes in opportunistic prophylaxis study. *J Infect Dis* 2000; **181**: 1635–42.
40. Lopez Bernaldo de Quiros JC, *et al.* A randomized trial of the discontinuation of primary and secondary prophylaxis against Pneumocystis carinii pneumonia after highly active antiretroviral therapy in patients with HIV infection. *N Engl J Med* 2001; **344**: 159–67.
41. Ledergerber B, *et al.* Discontinuation of secondary prophylaxis against Pneumocystis carinii pneumonia in patients with HIV infection who have a response to antiretroviral therapy. *N Engl J Med* 2001; **344**: 168–74.
42. Gordon SM, *et al.*. Should prophylaxis for Pneumocystis carinii pneumonia in solid organ transplant recipients ever be discontinued? *Clin Infect Dis* 1999; **28**: 240–6.

Protothecosis

Protothecosis is an infection with algae of the *Prototheca* spp., usually *P. wickerhamii*. Infection may follow minor trauma or surgery leading to a chronic skin lesion and occasionally dissemination. There are case reports of amphotericin B with tetracycline[1] or of itraconazole[2] being used successfully in protothecosis.

1. Venezio FR, *et al.* Progressive cutaneous protothecosis. *Am J Clin Pathol* 1982; **77**: 485–93.
2. Tang WYM, *et al.* Cutaneous protothecosis: report of a case in Hong Kong. *Br J Dermatol* 1995; **133**: 479–82.

Respiratory-tract infections

A number of pathogenic fungi enter the body by inhalation and colonise the respiratory tract. Fungal infections of the respiratory tract include aspergillosis, blastomycosis, coccidioidomycosis, cryptococcosis, histoplasmosis, and paracoccidioidomycosis (see above). *Pneumocystis carinii*, now considered to have characteristics of fungi, is an important cause of pneumonia in HIV-infected patients (see above). Other fungi reported to produce respiratory-tract infections mainly in immunocompromised patients include *Candida* spp., *Fusarium* spp., *Penicillium marneffei*, *Pseudoallescheria boydii*, and Zygomycetes such as *Rhizopus arrhizus*. Acute pulmonary fungal infections in immunocompetent individuals are mostly self-limiting conditions that resolve without treatment. Severe, persistent, or progressive infections, or infections in immunocompromised patients, require treatment. Intravenous amphotericin B is usually the drug of choice but mild to moderate infection can be treated with an oral azole such as fluconazole, itraconazole, or ketoconazole. Pulmonary granulomas may require surgical removal. Chronic suppressive treatment is recommended for patients with immunosuppression due to HIV infection.

Skin infections

The most common fungal skin infections are the dermatophytoses, pityriasis versicolor, and candidiasis. The first two are described here; candidiasis is described on p.372. Other fungal skin infections are discussed under the appropriate headings: blastomycosis, chromoblastomycosis, mycetoma, mucormycosis, protothecosis (above), and sporotrichosis (below). Fungal infections that may involve the skin by dissemination include aspergillosis, coccidioidomycosis, cryptococcosis, histoplasmosis, and paracoccidioidomycosis (above). Less common fungi causing skin infections include *Penicillium marneffei*. Sometimes the infection may affect mucous membranes, nails, or subcutaneous tissue, and there can be spread to deeper tissue and dissemination especially in immunosuppressed patients. The term superficial fungal infections includes those involving the skin, nails, and mucous membranes. Antifungal treatment may be topical or systemic.[1,2]

Dermatophytoses (ringworm, tinea) are infections by dermatophytes, a group of fungi which includes soil-dwelling organisms and human and animal pathogens from 3 genera — *Epidermophyton*, *Microsporum*, and *Trichophyton*. Dermatophytoses are encouraged by hot and humid conditions and poor hygiene and occur throughout tropical and temperate regions of the world. Dermatophytoses are classified according to the body site affected. They include

- tinea barbae (beard)
- tinea capitis (scalp)
- tinea corporis (body)
- tinea cruris (groin)
- tinea manuum (hand)
- tinea pedis (athlete's foot)
- tinea unguium (nail)

A chronic infection most commonly seen in the tropics is known as favus (tinea favosa) and a variant of tinea corporis known as tinea imbricata (tokelau) is caused by *T.*

concentricum and is endemic in parts of the Far East and Central and South America. A severe form of dermatophytosis caused by animal pathogens with deep, suppurant, inflammatory lesions is known as kerion.

Deep infections may occur rarely in immunocompromised patients and may spread to involve lymph nodes, liver, and brain, and may be fatal.

Mild localised superficial dermatophytoses of hairless skin sites will often respond to *topical* therapy.[3-5] Non-specific agents that have a long history of topical use include benzoic acid, methylrosanilinium chloride, selenium sulfide, and salicylic acid. Many of these agents are effective, and while some older preparations such as compound benzoic acid ointment may be less cosmetically acceptable than modern products, they still have a role in the treatment of minor infections, particularly in the tropics.[6] However, the use of methylrosanilinium chloride is restricted due to fears over possible carcinogenicity (see p.1150). There are a number of specific topical antifungals that are active against dermatophytes. The azoles used topically include clotrimazole, econazole, ketoconazole, and miconazole. Ciclopirox olamine[7] and the allylamine antifungals naftifine and terbinafine[8] appear to have similar activity. Chlorphenesin, tolnaftate, and undecenoic acid salts are all effective in uncomplicated dermatophytoses, but there are few comparative studies of their relative efficacy. Amorolfine has also been shown to be effective in skin infections, although its major application is in nail infections (see below).

Infections of some body sites respond poorly to topical therapy, as do extensive infections or those in heavily keratinised areas.[4] *Systemic* therapy may be appropriate in these cases as well as in disseminated disease. Griseofulvin, ketoconazole, and itraconazole are the drugs most widely used. Griseofulvin has proved to have few major toxic effects during long-term therapy and is useful for tinea capitis, extensive or disseminated infections, and nail infections in selected patients. However, since it has a narrow spectrum of activity largely confined to the dermatophytes, accurate diagnosis is essential particularly before embarking on a prolonged treatment course when no immediate response is anticipated. Ketoconazole has a broader spectrum of activity, but severe adverse effects can occur on prolonged administration and its place is likely to be taken by itraconazole which appears to produce a rapid response and thus requires shorter treatment periods.[4] Other azoles such as fluconazole may also be effective.[9] Terbinafine has been reported to be more effective than itraconazole in some forms of tinea[10,11] and also requires only short-duration therapy.[12,13] However, efficacy is reported to depend on the infecting organism.[14] Selenium sulfide shampoo may be a useful adjunct to oral therapy for tinea capitis to improve efficacy and limit the spread of infection.[15,16] A suitable topical antifungal is used in individuals suspected of carrying infection.[17]

Infections of the **nails (onychomycoses)** are notoriously difficult to treat.[5,18] Infections of the fingernails take up to 6 months to respond to oral griseofulvin and those of the toenails, a year or longer, but about 60% of nail infections fail to respond or relapse after the initial treatment course. The oral antifungals, terbinafine, itraconazole, and fluconazole, produce persistent antifungal concentrations in the nail more rapidly than griseofulvin.[18,19] Terbinafine and itraconazole have been most widely studied. Both are reported to produce clinical and mycological cures in a high proportion of patients more quickly than griseofulvin — generally after 12 weeks' treatment or less. Long-term follow-up has demonstrated that the response to terbinafine is maintained.[20-22] Terbinafine has been reported to be more effective than itraconazole[23-25] although neither is effective in all patients. Although topical treatments are generally ineffective in nail infections amorolfine applied as a lacquer has produced encouraging results.[26] Another approach has been the dissolution of the nail plate with 40% urea paste, usually in combination with bifonazole.[27]

Pityriasis versicolor (tinea versicolor) is a superficial infection caused by the commensal yeast *Malassezia furfur* (*Pityrosporum orbiculare*). It is more common in tropical than in temperate latitudes and sun exposure may trigger the infection. Pityriasis versicolor will often respond to topical treatment with an azole antifungal or with selenium sulfide. Terbinafine administered topically (but not orally) is an alternative. Immunocompromised patients, including those receiving corticosteroids, may develop extensive infections. In addition, these fungi have caused septicaemia in patients receiving parenteral nutrition.[28]

Severe infections require oral treatment with an azole.[29] Griseofulvin is not effective.

Other infections in which *Malassezia* yeasts are implicated include seborrhoeic dermatitis (p.1107) and pityrosporum folliculitis both of which may present in a more severe form in patients with AIDS. Topical or systemic azole antifungals are effective in these conditions and are the main drugs used. However, relapses are common.[30]

1. Gupta AK, *et al.* Antifungal agents: an overview, part II. *J Am Acad Dermatol* 1994; **30**: 911–33.
2. Piérard GE, *et al.* Treatment and prophylaxis of tinea infections. *Drugs* 1996; **52**: 209–24.
3. Smith EB. Topical antifungal drugs in the treatment of tinea pedis, tinea cruris, and tinea corporis. *J Am Acad Dermatol* 1993; **28**: S24–S28.
4. Degreef HJ, DeDoncker PRG. Current therapy of dermatophytosis. *J Am Acad Dermatol* 1994; **31**: S25–S30.
5. Crawford F, *et al.* Topical treatments for fungal infections of the skin and nails of the foot (updated 3 February 2000). Available in The Cochrane Library; Issue 3. Oxford: Update Software; 2001.
6. Gooskens V, *et al.* Treatment of superficial mycoses in the tropics: Whitfield's ointment versus clotrimazole. *Int J Dermatol* 1994; **33**: 738–42.
7. Bogaert H, *et al.* Multicentre double-blind clinical trials of ciclopirox olamine cream 1% in the treatment of tinea corporis and tinea cruris. *J Int Med Res* 1986; **14**: 210–16.
8. Hart R, *et al.* Systematic review of topical treatments for fungal infections of the skin and nails of the feet. *BMJ* 1999; **319**: 79–82.
9. Faergemann J, *et al.* A multicentre (double-blind) comparative study to assess the safety and efficacy of fluconazole and griseofulvin in the treatment of tinea corporis and tinea cruris. *Br J Dermatol* 1997; **136**: 575–7.
10. Budimulja U, *et al.* A double-blind, randomized, stratified controlled study of the treatment of tinea imbricata with oral terbinafine or itraconazole. *Br J Dermatol* 1994; **130** (suppl 43): 29–31.
11. De Keyser P, *et al.* Two-week oral treatment of tinea pedis, comparing terbinafine (250 mg/day) with itraconazole (100 mg/day): a double-blind, multicentre study. *Br J Dermatol* 1994; **130** (suppl 43): 22–25.
12. Farag A, *et al.* One-week therapy with oral terbinafine in cases of tinea cruris/corporis. *Br J Dermatol* 1994; **131**: 684–6.
13. Hay RJ, *et al.* A comparison of 2 weeks of terbinafine 250 mg/day with 4 weeks of itraconazole 100 mg/day in plantar-type tinea pedis. *Br J Dermatol* 1995; **132**: 604–8.
14. Baudraz-Rosselet F, *et al.* Efficacy of terbinafine treatment of tinea capitis in children varies according to the dermatophyte species. *Br J Dermatol* 1996; **135**: 1011–12.
15. Allen HB, *et al.* Selenium sulfide: adjunctive therapy for tinea capitis. *Pediatrics* 1982; **69**: 81–3.
16. Givens TG, *et al.* Comparison of 1% and 2.5% selenium sulfide in the treatment of tinea capitis. *Arch Pediatr Adolesc Med* 1995; **149**: 808–11.
17. Anonymous. Management of scalp ringworm. *Drug Ther Bull* 1996; **34**: 5–6.
18. Denning DW, *et al.* Fungal nail disease: a guide to good practice (report of a working group of the British Society for Medical Mycology). *BMJ* 1995; **311**: 1277–81.
19. Gupta AK, Scher RK. Oral antifungal agents for onychomycosis. *Lancet* 1998; **351**: 541–2.
20. De Cuyper C. Long-term evaluation of terbinafine 250 and 500 mg daily in a 16-week oral treatment for toenail onychomycosis. *Br J Dermatol* 1996; **135**: 156–7.
21. Bräutigam M, *et al.* Successful treatment of toenail mycosis with terbinafine and itraconazole gives long term benefits. *BMJ* 1998; **317**: 1084.
22. De Cuyper C, Hindryckx PHFB. Long-term outcomes in the treatment of toenail onychomycosis. *Br J Dermatol* 1999; **141** (suppl 56): 15–20.
23. De Backer M, *et al.* A 12-week treatment for dermatophyte toe onychomycosis: terbinafine 250 mg/day vs itraconazole 200 mg/day — a double-blind comparative trial. *Br J Dermatol* 1996; **134** (suppl 46): 16–17.
24. Bräutigam M, *et al.* Randomised double blind comparison of terbinafine and itraconazole for treatment of toenail tinea infection. *BMJ* 1995; **311**: 919–22. Correction. *ibid.*; 1350.
25. Evans EGV, Sigurgeirsson B. Double blind, randomised study of continuous terbinafine compared with intermittent itraconazole in treatment of toenail onychomycosis. *BMJ* 1999; **318**: 1031–5.
26. Reinel D. Topical treatment of onychomycosis with amorolfine 5% nail lacquer: comparative efficacy and tolerability of once and twice weekly use. *Dermatology* 1992; **184** (suppl 1): 21–4.
27. Roberts DT, *et al.* Topical treatment of onychomycosis using bifonazole 1% urea/40% paste. *Ann N Y Acad Sci* 1988; **544**: 586–7.
28. Dankner WM, *et al.* Malassezia fungemia in neonates and adults: complication of hyperalimentation. *Rev Infect Dis* 1987; **9**: 743–53.
29. Goodless DR, *et al.* Ketoconazole in the treatment of pityriasis versicolor: international review of clinical trials. *DICP Ann Pharmacother* 1991; **25**: 395–8.
30. McGrath J, Murphy GM. The control of seborrhoeic dermatitis and dandruff by antipityrosporal drugs. *Drugs* 1991; **41**: 178–84.

Sporotrichosis

Sporotrichosis is a disease caused by *Sporothrix schenckii*, a fungus found in soil and vegetation, and seen in the Americas and Africa. It may be divided into cutaneous or extracutaneous infection. The cutaneous form is the more common. It probably follows entry of the organism through skin abrasions and usually presents as a single skin lesion, although infection may spread along lymphatic channels causing a series of skin lesions. Extracutaneous sporotrichosis usually presents as osteoarticular infection. Pulmonary infections are occasionally seen and, rarely, CNS and ocular infections.

Potassium iodide by mouth has traditionally been used for cutaneous infections although the mode of action is unclear since potassium iodide does not demonstrate antifungal activity *in vitro*. Itraconazole by mouth is also effective[1-3] and is regarded by some[4] as the treatment of choice. Oral treatment with terbinafine[5,6] or fluconazole[7] has been tried and may be effective.

Extracutaneous sporotrichosis is treated with amphotericin B given intravenously or with itraconazole by mouth;[4] fluconazole is an alternative[1] although it is mainly reserved for patients who cannot tolerate amphotericin B or itraconazole.[4]

Lifelong maintenance therapy with itraconazole may be beneficial in patients with AIDS following treatment of a primary infection.[4]

1. Anonymous. Systemic antifungal drugs. *Med Lett Drugs Ther* 1997; **39:** 86–8.
2. Sharkey-Mathis PK, *et al.* Treatment of sporotrichosis with itraconazole. *Am J Med* 1993; **95:** 279–85.
3. Restrepo A, *et al.* Itraconazole therapy in lymphangitic and cutaneous sporotrichosis. *Arch Dermatol* 1986; **122:** 413–17.
4. Kauffman CA, *et al.* Infectious Diseases Society of America. Practice guidelines for the management of patients with sporotrichosis. *Clin Infect Dis* 2000; **30:** 684–7.
5. Hull PR, Vismer HP. Treatment of cutaneous sporotrichosis with terbinafine. *J Dermatol Treat* 1992; **3** (suppl 1): 35–8.
6. Kudoh K, *et al.* Successful treatment of cutaneous sporotrichosis with terbinafine. *J Dermatol Treat* 1996; **7:** 33–5.
7. Castro LGM, *et al.* Successful treatment of sporotrichosis with oral fluconazole: a report of three cases. *Br J Dermatol* 1993; **128:** 352–6.

Tinea

See under Skin Infections, above.

Amorolfine Hydrochloride (15828-f)

Amorolfine Hydrochloride (BANM, rINNM).
Ro-14-4767-000 (amorolfine); Ro-14-4767/002 (amorolfine hydrochloride). (±)-*cis*-2,6-Dimethyl-4-[2-methyl-3-(*p-tert*-pentylphenyl)propyl]morpholine hydrochloride.
$C_{21}H_{35}NO,HCl = 354.0$.
CAS — 78613-35-1 (amorolfine); 78613-38-4 (amorolfine hydrochloride).

NOTE. Amorolfine is USAN.

Adverse Effects

Skin irritation, presenting as erythema, pruritus, or a burning sensation, and, rarely, more severe skin reactions have been reported following topical application of amorolfine.

Antimicrobial Action

Amorolfine is a morpholine derivative with antifungal activity. It appears to act by interfering with the synthesis of sterols essential for the functioning of fungal cell membranes.

Amorolfine is active *in vitro* against a wide variety of pathogenic and opportunistic fungi including dermatophytes, *Blastomyces dermatitidis*, *Candida* spp., *Histoplasma capsulatum*, and *Sporothrix schenckii*. It also has variable activity against *Aspergillus* spp. However, despite its *in vitro* activity, amorolfine is inactive when given systemically and this limits its use to topical application for superficial infections.

Uses and Administration

Amorolfine is a morpholine derivative applied topically as the hydrochloride in the treatment of fungal nail and skin infections (p.376). After topical application, systemic absorption of amorolfine is negligible.

For the treatment of nail infections caused by dermatophytes, yeasts, and moulds a lacquer containing the equivalent of 5% amorolfine is painted onto the affected nail once or sometimes twice weekly until the nail has regenerated. Treatment generally needs to be continued for 6 to 12 months.

For the treatment of skin infections, including dermatophyte infections, a cream containing the equivalent of 0.25% amorolfine is applied once daily until clinical cure is achieved and then for a further 3 to 5 days.

◊ Reviews.
1. Haria M, Bryson HM. Amorolfine: a review of its pharmacological properties and therapeutic potential in the treatment of onychomycosis and other superficial fungal infections. *Drugs* 1995; **49:** 103–20.

The symbol † denotes a preparation no longer actively marketed

Preparations

Proprietary Preparations (details are given in Part 3)
Aust.: Loceryl; *Austral.:* Loceryl; *Belg.:* Loceryl; *Braz.:* Loceryl; *Denm.:* Loceryl; *Fin.:* Loceryl; *Fr.:* Loceryl; *Ger.:* Loceryl; *Hong Kong:* Loceryl; *Irl.:* Loceryl; *Mex.:* Loceryl; *Norw.:* Loceryl; *NZ:* Loceryl; *Port.:* Locetar; *S.Afr.:* Loceryl; *Singapore:* Loceryl; *Spain:* Locetar; Odenil Unas; *Swed.:* Loceryl; *Switz.:* Loceryl; *UK:* Loceryl.

Amphotericin B (2562-a)

Amphotericin B (BANM, rINN).
Amphotericin; Anfotericina B.
$C_{47}H_{73}NO_{17} = 924.1$.
CAS — 1397-89-3.
ATC — A01AB04; A07AA07; G01AA03; J02AA01.
Pharmacopoeias. In Chin., Eur. (see p.vi), Int., Jpn, Pol., and US.

Injections typical of conventional amphotericin B formulations, are a complex of amphotericin B and deoxycholate with suitable buffers which forms a colloidal dispersion when reconstituted. Other formulations of amphotericin B for injection include a liposomal formulation, a colloidal dispersion of amphotericin B and sodium cholesteryl sulfate, and a complex with phospholipids.

Preparation of solutions for injection. Lyophilised formulations for injection are prepared by reconstitution of amphotericin B with sterile water for injection without preservatives, then dilution with glucose injection 5% with a pH above 4.2 to the desired final concentration. Mixture with sodium chloride injection 0.9% would precipitate the amphotericin B.

Incompatibilities. Because of the wide range of incompatibilities reported with conventional amphotericin B preparations it is generally advisable not to mix them with any other drug. Most incompatibilities are caused by precipitation of amphotericin B due to a change in pH or by the disruption of the colloidal suspension. Precipitation can occur if amphotericin B is added to sodium chloride 0.9% or to electrolyte solutions.

Although heparin is generally reported to be compatible with conventional amphotericin B injection care should be taken if heparin flush solutions, which are diluted with sodium chloride solution, are used to maintain the patency of intravenous lines in patients receiving amphotericin B. Flushing the intravenous line with 5% glucose solution has been suggested.

Pharmacopoeial description

Ph. Eur.: A mixture of antifungal polyenes produced by the growth of certain strains of *Streptomyces nodosus* or by any other means. It consists largely of amphotericin B. It occurs as a yellow or orange powder. The potency is not less than 750 units per mg with reference to the dried substance. It contains not more than 10% of tetraenes, or not more than 5% if intended for use in parenteral dosage forms. Practically insoluble in water and in alcohol; soluble in dimethyl sulfoxide and in propylene glycol; slightly soluble in dimethylformamide; very slightly soluble in methyl alcohol. Amphotericin B is inactivated at low pH values. Store at 2° to 8° in airtight containers. Protect from light.

USP 25: A yellow to orange, odourless or practically odourless, powder. It contains not less than 750 µg of $C_{47}H_{73}NO_{17}$ per mg, and, for material intended for oral or topical use, not more than 15% of amphotericin A, both calculated on the dried substance. Insoluble in water, in dehydrated alcohol, in ether, in benzene, and in toluene; soluble in dimethylformamide, in dimethyl sulfoxide, and in propylene glycol; slightly soluble in methyl alcohol. Store at a temperature not exceeding 8° in airtight containers. Protect from light.

◊ References.
1. Kintzel PE, Smith GH. Practical guidelines for preparing and administering amphotericin B. *Am J Hosp Pharm* 1992; **49:** 1156–64.

Compatibility with lipid emulsions. Mixtures of conventional amphotericin B in commercial lipid emulsions have been reported to be unstable,[1-3] although others have reported satisfactory stability.[4-6] In one study[6] vigorous agitation of the mixtures enhanced their stability when compared to gentle mixing.

1. Ericsson O, *et al.* Amphotericin B is incompatible with lipid emulsions. *Ann Pharmacother* 1996; **30:** 298.
2. Ranchère JY, *et al.* Amphotericin B intralipid formulation: stability and particle size. *J Antimicrob Chemother* 1996; **37:** 1165–9.
3. Heide PE. Precipitation of amphotericin B from iv fat emulsion. *Am J Health-Syst Pharm* 1997; **54:** 1449.
4. Lopez RM, *et al.* Stability of amphotericin B in an extemporaneously prepared iv fat emulsion. *Am J Health-Syst Pharm* 1996; **53:** 2724–7.
5. Owens D, *et al.* Stability of amphotericin B 0.05 and 0.5 mg/mL in 20% fat emulsion. *Am J Health-Syst Pharm* 1997; **54:** 683–6.
6. Shadkhan Y, *et al.* The use of commercially available lipid emulsions for the preparation of amphotericin B-lipid admixtures. *J Antimicrob Chemother* 1997; **39:** 655–8. Correction. *ibid.* 1998; **42:** 413.

Adverse Effects

Amphotericin B for intravenous administration was originally only available in a conventional colloidal form; liposomal and other formulations have been developed to reduce toxicity. The following adverse ef-

fects apply to the **conventional** form. Common adverse effects which occur during or following intravenous infusion of amphotericin B include headache, nausea, vomiting, chills, fever, malaise, muscle and joint pains, anorexia, diarrhoea, and gastrointestinal cramp. Hypertension, hypotension, cardiac arrhythmias including ventricular fibrillation and cardiac arrest, skin rashes, anaphylactoid reactions, blurred vision, tinnitus, hearing loss, vertigo, gastrointestinal bleeding, liver disorders, peripheral neuropathy, and convulsions have been reported occasionally.

Nephrotoxicity occurs in almost all patients receiving amphotericin B intravenously. Both tubular and glomerular damage occur; there may be improvement on cessation of therapy, but there is a risk of permanent impairment of renal function, particularly in patients receiving large cumulative doses (over 5 g). Renal tubular acidosis without systemic acidosis may develop. Amphotericin B administration is associated with increased urinary excretion of potassium and magnesium resulting in hypokalaemia and hypomagnesaemia respectively. Uric acid excretion is increased and nephrocalcinosis can occur. Limited data indicate that renal toxicity may be associated with sodium depletion; for strategies to improve sodium load see Nephrotoxicity, below, under Treatment of Adverse Effects, below.

A reversible, normocytic, normochromic anaemia develops in most patients receiving amphotericin B, possibly due to a direct suppressive effect on erythropoietin production. There are rare reports of thrombocytopenia, leucopenia, agranulocytosis, eosinophilia, and coagulation defects.

Leucoencephalopathy has been reported rarely in patients also receiving total body irradiation.

Solutions of amphotericin B irritate the venous endothelium and may cause pain and thrombophlebitis at the injection site. Extravasation may cause tissue damage.

After intrathecal injection amphotericin B may also cause irritation of the meninges, neuropathy with pain, impaired vision, and retention of urine.

Topical application may produce local irritation, pruritus, and skin rash.

In general, adverse effects of **nonconventional** amphotericin B have been similar to those of conventional amphotericin B, but are less frequent and less severe. Brief reversible episodes of renal impairment have been observed but nonconventional formulations have been considered to be safe enough to use in patients with renal impairment who could not be given conventional amphotericin B. Anaphylaxis has been reported rarely.

Alternative formulations. Conventional amphotericin B dispersed in lipid emulsions (such as Intralipid) has been tried as a less expensive alternative to the lipid-based commercial formulations. However, such dispersions have not been shown convincingly to reduce renal toxicity or improve tolerability compared with conventional amphotericin B in glucose solution.[1-5]

1. Sievers TM, *et al.* Safety and efficacy of Intralipid emulsions of amphotericin B. *J Antimicrob Chemother* 1996; **38:** 333–47.
2. Laverdière M, *et al.* Poor immediate tolerability of amphotericin B lipid emulsion in patients with haematological malignancies. *J Antimicrob Chemother* 1997; **40:** 910–12.
3. Schöffski P, *et al.* Safety and toxicity of amphotericin B in glucose 5% or intralipid 20% in neutropenic patients with pneumonia or fever of unknown origin: randomised study. *BMJ* 1998; **317:** 379–84.
4. Nath CE, *et al.* Amphotericin B in children with malignant disease: a comparison of the toxicities and pharmacokinetics of amphotericin B administered in dextrose versus lipid emulsion. *Antimicrob Agents Chemother* 1999; **43:** 1417–23.
5. Nucci M, *et al.* Comparison of the toxicity of amphotericin B in 5% dextrose with that of amphotericin B in fat emulsion in a randomized trial with cancer patients. *Antimicrob Agents Chemother* 1999; **43:** 1445–8.

Effects on the cardiovascular system. Ventricular arrhythmias in 2 patients, resulting in fatal sudden cardiac arrest in 1, were associated with both conventional and liposomal formulations of amphotericin B at conventional doses and infusion rates,[1] but cardiac toxicity is more commonly associated with high doses or rapid infusion rates (see Infusion Rate, under Administration, below). Cardiac arrests in 5 infants and children, fatal in 4 cases, were associated with overdoses of conventional amphotericin B of between 3.8 and 40.8 mg per kg body-weight.[2] An increased risk of arrhythmia and cardiac arrest has been reported in patients with evidence of antimony-induced myocardial damage who were switched to amphotericin B treatment for visceral leishmaniasis.[3] A rest period of at least 10 days was advised before beginning amphotericin B in such patients.

Severe hypertension was associated with infusion of phospholipid-amphotericin B complex in 1 patient.[4]

1. Aguado JM, et al. Ventricular arrhythmias with conventional and liposomal amphotericin. Lancet 1993; 342: 1239.
2. Cleary JD, et al. Amphotericin B overdose in pediatric patients with associated cardiac arrest. Ann Pharmacother 1993; 27: 715–19.
3. Thakur CP. Sodium antimony gluconate, amphotericin, and myocardial damage. Lancet 1998; 351: 1928–9.
4. Rowles DM, Fraser SL. Amphotericin B lipid complex (ABLC)-associated hypertension: case report and review. Clin Infect Dis 1999; 29: 1564–5.

Effects on the eyes. Rapid loss of vision resulting in permanent bilateral blindness occurred in a patient with lupus erythematosus and cryptococcal meningitis after receiving a 1-mg test-dose of amphotericin B.[1] Amphotericin B was considered to be the causative agent as visual disturbances associated with cryptococcal meningitis are usually progressive in nature and acute blindness with normal funduscopic appearance had not previously been reported.

1. Li PKT, Lai KN. Amphotericin B induced ocular toxicity in cryptococcal meningitis. Br J Ophthalmol 1989; 73: 397–8.

Effects on the liver. Amphotericin B has only rarely been associated with adverse effects on the liver. Fatal liver failure was reported in a patient after administration of a total dose of 4.82 g intermittently over one year.[1] The patient had been given a potentially incompatible intravenous admixture of amphotericin B and diphenhydramine.

There have been a few reports of abnormal liver-function tests during amphotericin B therapy;[2,3] in such cases amphotericin B should be discontinued.

1. Carnecchia BM, Kurtzke JF. Fatal toxic reaction to amphotericin B in cryptococcal meningo-encephalitis. Ann Intern Med 1960; 53: 1027–36.
2. Miller MA. Reversible hepatotoxicity related to amphotericin B. Can Med Assoc J 1984; 131: 1245–7.
3. Abajo FJ, Carcas AJ. Amphotericin B hepatotoxicity. BMJ 1986; 293: 1243.

Effects on the lungs. Reports implicating concomitant administration of leucocytes[1] or other blood products[2] in the development of pulmonary reactions in patients receiving amphotericin B have been refuted by the findings of other workers.[3,4] However, a report has indicated that amphotericin B can produce pulmonary toxicity in the absence of blood products.[5] An increased incidence of pulmonary symptoms was noted in patients receiving amphotericin B in lipid emulsion,[6] including acute respiratory distress after initiation of the infusion.

1. Wright DG, et al. Lethal pulmonary reactions associated with the combined use of amphotericin B and leukocyte transfusions. N Engl J Med 1981; 304: 1185–9.
2. Haber RH, et al. Acute pulmonary decompensation due to amphotericin B in the absence of granulocyte transfusions. N Engl J Med 1986; 315: 836.
3. Forman SJ, et al. Pulmonary reactions associated with amphotericin B and leukocyte transfusions. N Engl J Med 1981; 305: 584–5.
4. Bow EJ, et al. Pulmonary complications in patients receiving granulocyte transfusions and amphotericin B. Can Med Assoc J 1984; 130: 593–7.
5. Roncoroni AJ, et al. Bronchiolitis obliterans possibly associated with amphotericin B. J Infect Dis 1990; 161: 589.
6. Schöffski P, et al. Safety and toxicity of amphotericin B in glucose 5% or intralipid 20% in neutropenic patients with pneumonia or fever of unknown origin: randomised study. BMJ 1998; 317: 379–84.

Effects on potassium homoeostasis. In addition to the hypokalaemia known to be associated with amphotericin B and due to increased urinary excretion of potassium, hyperkalaemia has been reported in a patient with severely impaired renal function who received a rapid infusion of amphotericin B (see Infusion Rate, under Administration, below).

Hypersensitivity. Anaphylactoid reactions have occurred with conventional amphotericin B. However, anaphylactic reactions have been associated with liposomal amphotericin B,[1,2] including a report in 2 patients who subsequently tolerated conventional amphotericin B.[1]

1. Laing RBS, et al. Anaphylactic reactions to liposomal amphotericin. Lancet 1994; 344: 682.
2. Torre I, et al. Anaphylactic reaction to liposomal amphotericin B in children. Ann Pharmacother 1996; 30: 1036–7.

Red man syndrome. Red man syndrome (see Vancomycin, p.267) occurred in a patient on 2 occasions following a test-dose of amphotericin B 1 mg.[1]

1. Ellis ME, Tharpe W. Red man syndrome associated with amphotericin B. BMJ 1990; 300: 1468.

Treatment of Adverse Effects

To reduce febrile reactions antipyretics such as aspirin or paracetamol, and antihistamines such as diphenhydramine may be given before the intravenous infusion of conventional amphotericin B. Hydrocortisone given intravenously before or during amphotericin B infusion may reduce febrile reac-

tions. However, corticosteroids should not be given indiscriminately to patients receiving amphotericin B (see Interactions, below) and dosage should be kept to a minimum. In the UK the advice is to give antipyretics or hydrocortisone prophylactically, but only to patients who have previously experienced acute adverse reactions and in whom continued treatment with intravenous amphotericin B is essential. Pethidine has been given intravenously to treat amphotericin B-induced shaking chills. Antiemetics may also be required. Amphotericin B is not removed by haemodialysis. Hypokalaemia and hypomagnesaemia should be corrected, and adequate hydration and sodium supplements may reduce the severity of renal impairment. Liposomal, phospholipid-complexed, or nonconventional colloidal amphotericin B can be substituted for conventional amphotericin B if the latter cannot be tolerated.

Heparin has been added to conventional amphotericin B infusions to reduce the incidence of thrombophlebitis.

◊ The value of prophylaxis against generalised reactions to amphotericin B infusion was questioned after a retrospective study in 397 patients.[1] The most commonly used drugs were diphenhydramine, corticosteroids, paracetamol, and heparin. It was concluded that patients who had experienced an adverse reaction following amphotericin B administration should receive appropriate premedication before subsequent amphotericin B infusions, but that routine premedication was not justified.

1. Goodwin SD, et al. Pretreatment regimens for adverse events related to infusion of amphotericin B. Clin Infect Dis 1995; 20: 755–61.

Anaemia. Amphotericin B appears to produce a normochromic, normocytic anaemia by suppression of erythropoietin production.[1,2] Discontinuation of amphotericin B reverses the suppression but if the anaemia is severe, or treatment with amphotericin B cannot be stopped, blood transfusions may be required. Recombinant erythropoietin may prove an alternative to blood transfusions in patients who need to continue treatment with amphotericin B.

1. MacGregor RR, et al. Erythropoietin concentrations in amphotericin B-induced anemia. Antimicrob Agents Chemother 1978; 14: 270–3.
2. Lin AC, et al. Amphotericin B blunts erythropoietin response to anemia. J Infect Dis 1990; 161: 348–51.

Electrolyte disturbances. It has been suggested[1] that amiloride could ameliorate the hypokalaemia and hypomagnesaemia associated with amphotericin B therapy. However, since amiloride may produce sodium depletion and its own associated renal toxicity this strategy is potentially hazardous. Another report[2] has suggested that spironolactone may be a safe and effective method of preventing hypokalaemia.

1. Wazny LD, Brophy DF. Amiloride for the prevention of amphotericin B-induced hypokalemia and hypomagnesemia. Ann Pharmacother 2000; 34: 94–7.
2. Ural, AU. Comment: spironolactone prevents amphotericin B-induced hypokalemia in neutropenic patients. Ann Pharmacother 2000; 34: 1488.

Nephrotoxicity. There are limited reports indicating that correction of sodium depletion may reverse amphotericin B-induced nephrotoxicity.[1] However, assessment of sodium status and correction of deficiency should precede amphotericin B administration.[2,3] Use of mannitol as a protective agent is controversial and is not recommended.[2-4] Diuretics in general should be avoided[5] although there have been suggestions that potassium-sparing diuretics such as amiloride or spironolactone may be useful in preventing hypokalaemia (see Electrolyte Disturbances, above). Some have recommended supplementation with 150 mmol sodium for suitable patients.[3] However, routine prophylactic administration of sodium is not advised.[6] A randomised study in a small number of patients has suggested that prophylactic sodium supplementation could be beneficial, but that it enhances potassium loss.[7] Administration of amphotericin B on alternate days is widely practised although it has never been proven to reduce nephrotoxicity.[2,3] A review of strategies for limiting the toxicity of amphotericin B concluded that sodium balance should be monitored and sodium replacement implemented if necessary and that, where possible, salt restriction and drugs which potentiate sodium loss or nephrotoxicity should be avoided.[8]

More detailed, liposomal, nonconventional colloidal, and phospholipid-complex formulations have been reported to overcome most problems of chronic nephrotoxicity, even in patients with impaired renal function following previous treatment with conventional amphotericin B (see Alternative Formulations, under Administration, below).

1. Heidemann HT, et al. Amphotericin B nephrotoxicity in humans decreased by salt repletion. Am J Med 1983; 75: 476–81.
2. Warda J, Barriere SL. Amphotericin B nephrotoxicity. Drug Intell Clin Pharm 1985; 19: 25–6.
3. Sabra R, Branch RA. Amphotericin B nephrotoxicity. Drug Safety 1990; 5: 94–108.

4. Bullock WE, et al. Can mannitol reduce amphotericin B nephrotoxicity? Double-blind study and description of a new vascular lesion in kidneys. Antimicrob Agents Chemother 1976; 10: 555–63.
5. Fisher MA, et al. Risk factors for amphotericin B-associated nephrotoxicity. Am J Med 1989; 87: 547–52.
6. Gardner ML, et al. Sodium loading treatment for amphotericin B-induced nephrotoxicity. DICP Ann Pharmacother 1990; 24: 940–6.
7. Llanos A, et al. Effect of salt supplementation on amphotericin B nephrotoxicity. Kidney Int 1991; 40: 302–8.
8. Khoo SH, et al. Administering amphotericin B—a practical approach. J Antimicrob Chemother 1994; 33: 203–13.

Precautions

Although anaphylaxis is rare following intravenous administration of amphotericin B, it is advisable to administer a test dose and then to observe the patient carefully for about 30 minutes before starting treatment. Patients experiencing acute toxic reactions in whom treatment is essential may be given prophylactic treatment, as mentioned under Treatment of Adverse Effects, above, to ameliorate the reactions. To reduce the risk of vein irritation and infusion-related adverse effects, the rate of intravenous infusion of conventional amphotericin B should be slow. For a discussion between infusion rate and adverse effects, see Infusion Rate, under Administration, below. Patients receiving any parenteral form of amphotericin B should be monitored for changes in renal function, liver function, serum electrolytes, and haematological status. If the BUN or creatinine concentrations increase to clinically significant levels amphotericin B therapy should be interrupted or the dose reduced until renal function improves. Alternatively, a nonconventional amphotericin B preparation may be substituted. Treatment should be discontinued if liver function tests are abnormal. Acute pulmonary reactions have been noted in patients receiving amphotericin B during or shortly after leucocyte transfusions. It is advisable to separate these infusions and to monitor pulmonary function in these patients.

Care should be taken not to confuse the dosage regimens for individual preparations, and in particular those of conventional and non-conventional formulations.

Pregnancy. There are case reports of amphotericin B having been used successfully to treat fungal infections in pregnant women without any adverse effects on the infant.[1,2]

1. Ismail MA, Lerner SA. Disseminated blastomycosis in a pregnant woman. Am Rev Respir Dis 1982; 126: 350–3.
2. Peterson CM, et al. Coccidiodal meningitis and pregnancy: a case report. Obstet Gynecol 1989; 73: 835–6.

Interactions

Most interactions have been observed during treatment with conventional amphotericin B. Since non-conventional formulations appear to be less toxic, it may be anticipated that they will produce fewer serious interactions.

Concomitant administration of nephrotoxic antibacterials, ciclosporin or other nephrotoxic immunosuppressants, or parenteral pentamidine may lead to an increased risk of nephrotoxicity. If possible, amphotericin B should not be given to patients receiving antineoplastics. Diuretics should generally be avoided in patients taking amphotericin B. If a diuretic has to be given then volume and electrolyte depletion should be monitored carefully. The potassium-depleting effect of amphotericin B may enhance the effects of neuromuscular blocking drugs and may increase the toxicity of digitalis glycosides; corticosteroids may enhance the depletion of potassium and their immunosuppressive effects may be detrimental in patients with severe fungal infections.

Amphotericin B may increase the toxicity of flucytosine, but the combination is used in severe infections for its synergistic activity. For information on synergistic and antagonistic effects with other antimicrobials, see under Antimicrobial Action, below. Renal excretion of zalcitabine may be reduced by concurrent administration of amphotericin B.

For an increased risk of cardiac arrhythmias and arrest when amphotericin B was given to patients with myocardial damage induced by an antimony compound, see Effects on the Cardiovascular System, under Adverse Effects, above.

Antimicrobial Action

Amphotericin B is a polyene antifungal antibiotic which appears to act mainly by interfering with the permeability of the cell membrane of sensitive fungi by binding to sterols, chiefly ergosterol. It is reported to be fungistatic at concentrations achieved clinically. It is active against *Absidia* spp., *Aspergillus* spp., *Basidiobolus* spp., *Blastomyces dermatitidis*, *Candida* spp., *Coccidioides immitis*, *Conidiobolus* spp., *Cryptococcus neoformans*, *Histoplasma capsulatum*, *Mucor* spp., *Paracoccidioides brasiliensis*, *Rhizopus* spp., *Rhodotorula* spp., and *Sporothrix schenckii*. Minimum inhibitory concentrations range from 0.03 to 1 µg per mL for many of these organisms. Other organisms that have been reported to be sensitive to amphotericin B include the algal *Prototheca* spp. and the protozoa *Leishmania* and *Naegleria*. It is inactive against bacteria (including rickettsia) and viruses.

Some resistant strains of *Candida* have been isolated from immunocompromised patients receiving prolonged treatment with amphotericin B.

Microbiological interactions. Until recently, assessment of antifungal activity has depended largely upon empirical observations based on clinical experience. The development of a standard *in-vitro* method of susceptibility testing should improve the comparability of test results obtained from different laboratories, but the correlation of *in-vitro* results with clinical outcome has still to be determined, especially in relation to drug combinations.[1]

Azoles. Although there have been occasional reports of synergy between amphotericin B and the azole antifungals,[2] greater emphasis has been placed on possible antagonism. Studies *in vitro* have supported theoretical concerns that the action of amphotericin B (which depends on binding to ergosterol in the fungal cell membrane) would be antagonised by azoles (which inhibit ergosterol synthesis).[3,4] *Animal* studies appear to have confirmed antagonism between amphotericin B and the imidazole ketoconazole, but not between amphotericin B and the triazoles fluconazole or itraconazole.[1] Available clinical evidence seems to indicate that azoles given concurrently, or as continuation therapy after induction therapy with amphotericin B, are effective in severe infections although reduced plasma concentrations of itraconazole have been reported in some patients while receiving amphotericin B.[5] However, strains of *Candida albicans* resistant to both amphotericin B and fluconazole have emerged in patients who have received repeated or prolonged courses of fluconazole.[6,7]

Flucytosine. Despite the results of an *in-vitro* study which found antagonism between amphotericin B and flucytosine,[3] this combination is used clinically in severe systemic fungal infections and is generally considered to be synergistic.

Rifamycins. *In-vitro* studies have shown rifampicin[8] or rifabutin[9] to increase the antifungal activity of amphotericin B against various *Aspergillus* spp.[8,9] and *Fusarium*.[9]

Tetracyclines. Minocycline may enhance amphotericin B's activity against *Aspergillus* spp. *in vitro*.[10]

Zidovudine. Amphotericin B may inhibit the metabolism of zidovudine, see p.646.

1. Sugar AM. Use of amphotericin B with azole antifungal drugs: what are we doing? *Antimicrob Agents Chemother* 1995; **39:** 1907–12.
2. Smith D, *et al.* Effect of ketoconazole and amphotericin B on encapsulated and non-encapsulated strains of Cryptococcus neoformans. *Antimicrob Agents Chemother* 1983; **24:** 851–5.
3. Martin E, *et al.* Antagonistic effects of fluconazole and 5-fluorocytosine on candidacidal action of amphotericin B in human serum. *Antimicrob Agents Chemother* 1994; **38:** 1331–8.
4. Sud IJ, Feingold DS. Effect of ketoconazole on the fungicidal action of amphotericin B in Candida albicans. *Antimicrob Agents Chemother* 1983; **23:** 185–7.
5. Pennick GJ, *et al.* Concomitant therapy with amphotericin B and itraconazole: does this combination affect the serum concentration of itraconazole? *Intersci Conf Antimicrob Agents Chemother* 1994; **34:** 39 (A34).
6. Kelly SL, *et al.* Resistance to fluconazole and amphotericin in Candida albicans from AIDS patients. *Lancet* 1996; **348:** 1523–4.
7. Nolte FS, *et al.* Isolation and characterization of fluconazole- and amphotericin B-resistant Candida albicans from blood of two patients with leukemia. *Antimicrob Agents Chemother* 1997; **44:** 196–9.
8. Hughes CE, *et al.* In vitro activities of amphotericin B in combination with four antifungal agents and rifampin against Aspergillus spp. *Antimicrob Agents Chemother* 1984; **25:** 560–2.
9. Clancy CJ, *et al.* Inhibition of RNA synthesis as a therapeutic strategy against Aspergillus and Fusarium: demonstration of in vitro synergy between rifabutin and amphotericin B. *Antimicrob Agents Chemother* 1998; **42:** 509–13.
10. Hughes CE, *et al.* Enhancement of the in vitro activity of amphotericin B against Aspergillus spp. by tetracycline analogs. *Antimicrob Agents Chemother* 1984; **26:** 837–40.

Pharmacokinetics

There is little or no absorption of amphotericin B from the gastrointestinal tract. When administered intravenously in the conventional colloidal form and in the usual increasing dosage regimens, peak plasma concentrations of 0.5 to 4 µg per mL have been reported; the average plasma concentration with maintenance doses of 400 to 600 µg per kg body-weight daily tends to be 0.5 µg per mL. Amphotericin B is reported to be highly bound to plasma proteins and is widely distributed but passes into the CSF only in small quantities. The plasma half-life has been reported to be about 24 hours; with long-term administration the terminal half-life increases to 15 days.

Unchanged amphotericin B is excreted in small amounts slowly in the urine. Traces have been reported to be present in the serum and urine several weeks after completion of treatment. Amphotericin B is not removed by haemodialysis.

The pharmacokinetics of the nonconventional formulations differ considerably from the conventional formulation and from each other.

At the doses used clinically, liposomal amphotericin B produces higher peak plasma concentrations (10 to 35 µg per mL after a dose of 3 mg per kg) than conventional amphotericin B. A colloidal formulation with sodium cholesteryl sulfate produces lower maximum plasma concentrations of between 1 and 2.5 µg per mL after doses of 0.25 to 1.5 mg per kg. At a dose of 5 mg per kg per day, a phospholipid complex formulation is reported to produce mean maximum plasma concentrations of 1.7 µg per mL. *Animal* studies have shown that concentrations in the kidney following the nonconventional formulations are several times lower than those following the conventional formulation.

Children and neonates. Serum-amphotericin B concentrations ranged from 0.78 to 10.02 µg per mL in 12 children (many with leukaemia) aged 4 months to 14 years following the intravenous infusion of conventional amphotericin B 0.25 to 1.5 mg per kg body-weight daily. Serum concentrations did not correlate with dose. The elimination half-life was 18.1 ± 6.65 hours. There was an inverse relationship between age and total clearance, suggesting that children older than 9 years may require lower doses.[1]

The pharmacokinetics of amphotericin B have also been studied in a group of 13 neonates with systemic fungal infections.[2] Conventional amphotericin B was infused over 4 to 6 hours every 24 hours. Ten of the infants started treatment with 100 µg per kg increased over 4 to 6 days to 500 µg per kg. Three infants were started on a dose of 800 µg to 1 mg per kg reduced to 500 µg per kg daily. All infants were maintained on 500 µg per kg daily; total doses ranged from 17.3 to 28.6 mg per kg. Serum-amphotericin B concentrations were measured after the first dose in 3 infants in the first group and 2 in the second; no serum-amphotericin B could be detected in the 3 infants who had received 100 µg per kg. After 5 days' treatment peak serum-amphotericin B concentrations ranged from 0.5 to 4.0 µg per mL and this was considered to be the range that could be achieved with the daily maintenance dose of 500 µg per kg. The elimination half-life was 14.8 hours. Drug elimination between doses was not detected in 4 of the infants; one was in oliguric renal failure and the other 3 had developed increases in serum-creatinine concentrations. CSF-amphotericin B concentrations in 5 of the neonates ranged from 40 to 90% of simultaneous serum concentrations. It was considered that an initial dose of 500 µg per kg was well tolerated and could produce therapeutic serum concentrations more quickly than a regimen which consisted of 100 µg per kg on day one increased over 4 to 6 days to 500 µg per kg daily.

1. Benson JM, Nahata MC. Pharmacokinetics of amphotericin B in children. *Antimicrob Agents Chemother* 1989; **33:** 1989–93.
2. Baley JE, *et al.* Pharmacokinetics, outcome of treatment, and toxic effects of amphotericin B and 5-fluorocytosine in neonates. *J Pediatr* 1990; **116:** 791–7.

Distribution. Amphotericin B concentrations in various organs and tissues were determined in 13 cancer patients who had received conventional amphotericin B before death.[1] Concentrations were determined by high-pressure liquid chromatography (HPLC) and bioassay. Mean recovery by HPLC reported as a percentage of total dose given was liver 27.5%, spleen 5.2%, lungs 3.2%, kidney 1.5%, heart 0.4%, brain 0.3%, and pancreas 0.2%; each organ had a specific accumulation pattern. The mean total recovery was 38.8%. Reported median bile concentration was 7.3 µg per mL. The drug concentrations obtained by bioassay were much lower than those measured by HPLC. As the HPLC-determined concentrations of amphotericin B were higher than the MICs for the pathogens in patients

with candidiasis or aspergillosis, the poor clinical outcome in these patients suggested that amphotericin B in the tissue lacked antifungal activity.

In another study amphotericin B was not detected in the CSF of 4 AIDS patients with cryptococcal meningitis on intravenous maintenance conventional doses of 350 µg to 1.89 mg per kg body-weight given 1 to 7 times weekly.[2] The clinical success of amphotericin B for this indication could not be explained by measurable CSF drug concentrations.

Concentrations of amphotericin B have been measured in fetal-cord serum in an infant and were 37.5% of maternal serum concentration.[3]

1. Collette N, *et al.* Tissue concentrations and bioactivity of amphotericin B in cancer patients treated with amphotericin B-deoxycholate. *Antimicrob Agents Chemother* 1989; **33:** 362–8.
2. Dugoni BM, *et al.* Amphotericin B concentrations in cerebrospinal fluid of patients with AIDS and cryptococcal meningitis. *Clin Pharm* 1989; **8:** 220–1.
3. Ismail MA, Lerner SA. Disseminated blastomycosis in a pregnant woman. *Am Rev Respir Dis* 1982; **126:** 350–3.

Half-life. The terminal half-life for amphotericin B was 15 days in 2 patients on completion of conventional amphotericin B infusion therapy for disseminated histoplasmosis.[1] In another study the half-life was 21.5 hours (based on the exponential phase of disappearance from the blood) in a 65-year-old patient on a maintenance conventional dose of 500 µg per kg body-weight infused over one hour every other day.[2] Serum concentrations appeared to plateau at about 600 nanograms per mL 36 to 48 hours after each dose. This suggested that alternate-day administration might be effective.

1. Atkinson AJ, Bennett JE. Amphotericin B pharmacokinetics in humans. *Antimicrob Agents Chemother* 1978; **13:** 271–6.
2. Hoeprich PD. Elimination half-life of amphotericin B. *J Infect* 1990; **20:** 173–5.

Non-conventional formulations. References.

1. Janknegt R, *et al.* Liposomal and lipid formulations of amphotericin B: clinical pharmacokinetics. *Clin Pharmacokinet* 1992; **23:** 279–91.
2. Adedoyin A, *et al.* Pharmacokinetic profile of ABELCET (amphotericin B lipid complex injection): combined experience from phase I and phase II studies. *Antimicrob Agents Chemother* 1997; **41:** 2201–8.
3. Adedoyin A, *et al.* A pharmacokinetic study of amphotericin B lipid complex injection (Abelcet) in patients with definite or probable systemic fungal infections. *Antimicrob Agents Chemother* 2000; **44:** 2900–2.

Uses and Administration

Amphotericin B is a polyene antifungal antibiotic. It is reported to be fungistatic at concentrations achieved clinically. Amphotericin B is administered by intravenous infusion in the treatment of severe *systemic* fungal infections including aspergillosis, blastomycosis, candidiasis, coccidioidomycosis, cryptococcosis, histoplasmosis, mucormycosis, paracoccidioidomycosis, and sporotrichosis, and is the usual treatment of choice in fungal endocarditis, meningitis, peritonitis, or severe respiratory-tract infections. Many of these infections are most likely to occur in immunocompromised patients. Amphotericin may be given in combination with flucytosine (p.385) in severe infections.

Amphotericin B is also used for the *local* treatment of superficial candidiasis. It is taken by mouth for intestinal candidiasis, sometimes as part of regimens for selective decontamination of the digestive tract in patients at special risk of infection, such as those in intensive care (see p.126).

The role of amphotericin B in the treatment of the above systemic and local infections is discussed under Choice of Antifungal, p.372.

Amphotericin B also has antiprotozoal activity. It is used for primary amoebic meningoencephalitis caused by *Naegleria* spp. and for the treatment of visceral and mucocutaneous leishmaniasis.

Administration and dosage. Amphotericin B is administered by *intravenous* infusion conventionally as a colloidal complex with sodium deoxycholate. There is also a liposomal form and other complexes of amphotericin B available for administration by infusion when conventional amphotericin B is contra-indicated because of toxicity, especially nephrotoxicity. Before starting therapy with any form of intravenous amphotericin B a test dose is usually advised and the patient observed carefully for about 30 minutes.

Details of intravenous administration and dosage vary according to the formulation being used. Therapy has sometimes continued for several months depending on the infection. Doses are expressed in terms of amphotericin B.

- *Conventional amphotericin B* (e.g. Fungizone, UK). After an initial test dose (1 mg infused over 20 to 30 minutes) treatment usually starts with a daily dose of 250 µg per kg body-weight, increased gradually to a maximum of 1 mg per kg daily; in seriously ill patients up to 1.5 mg per kg daily or on alternate days may be necessary. If treatment is stopped for longer than 7 days, it should be resumed at a dose of 250 µg per kg daily and increased gradually. The daily dose is infused over 2 to 4 hours at a concentration of 100 µg per mL in glucose 5%. Slower infusion, over up to 6 hours, may be necessary to reduce the incidence of acute toxic effects.

- *Liposomal amphotericin B* (e.g. AmBisome, UK). After an initial test dose (1 mg infused over 10 minutes), the usual dose is 1 mg per kg daily, increased gradually to 3 mg per kg if necessary. The daily dose is infused over 30 to 60 minutes at a concentration of 200 to 2000 µg per mL in glucose 5%.

- *Sodium cholesteryl sulfate-amphotericin B complex* (e.g. Amphocil, UK). After an initial test dose (2 mg infused over 10 minutes) the usual dose is 1 mg per kg daily, increased gradually to 3 to 4 mg per kg daily if necessary; doses of up to 6 mg per kg daily have been given. The daily dose is infused at a rate of 1 to 2 mg per kg per hour at a concentration of 625 µg per mL in glucose 5%.

- *Phospholipid-amphotericin B complex* (e.g. Abelcet, UK). After an initial test dose (1 mg infused over 15 minutes) the usual dose is 5 mg per kg daily. The daily dose is infused at a rate of 2.5 mg per kg per hour as a diluted suspension containing 1 mg per mL in glucose 5%.

Conventional amphotericin B may be given by *intrathecal* injection to patients with severe meningitis especially when intravenous therapy has been ineffective. Commencing with 25 µg, the dose is gradually increased to the maximum that can be tolerated without excessive discomfort. The usual dosage is 0.25 to 1 mg given two to four times each week.

Amphotericin B is also used *orally* as 10-mg lozenges or as a suspension containing 100 mg per mL for oral or perioral candidiasis. The suspension is given in a dose of 1 mL four times daily; it should be retained in the mouth for as long as possible before swallowing. The lozenges are intended to be dissolved in the mouth and are given four times daily, increased to eight lozenges daily if necessary. Doses of 100 to 200 mg are given four times daily by mouth as tablets or suspension to suppress intestinal *Candida*.

Amphotericin B has been given for candiduria by continuous bladder irrigation daily at a suggested concentration of 50 mg in 1000 mL of sterile water. Intermittent irrigation has also been tried.

Amphotericin B has also been administered into the lung by nebulised solution, into the eye topically or by subconjunctival or intravitreal injection, to the skin by topical application, into body cavities by instillation, and into joint spaces by intra-articular injection.

Administration. ALTERNATIVE FORMULATIONS. A number of lipid formulations of amphotericin B have been developed in an attempt to minimise renal toxicity and acute toxic reactions. Three lipid-based formulations of amphotericin B available commercially in some countries are: liposomes (e.g. AmBisome); a lipid complex with L-α-dimyristoylphosphatidylcholine and L-α-dimyristoylphosphatidylglycerol (e.g. Abelcet); and a colloidal dispersion with sodium cholesteryl sulfate (e.g. Amphocil).[1,2] The aim of reducing renal toxicity has largely been achieved, and in some cases patients unable to tolerate conventional amphotericin B have subsequently been successfully treated with one of the lipid-based formulations. Experience with the liposomal formulation suggests that it also produces fewer acute toxic reactions.[1] Clinical studies with these formulations are generally encouraging,[1-6] but they differ in their pharmacokinetics and dosage and there are few formal comparisons of their efficacy.

Conventional amphotericin B dispersed in lipid emulsions (such as Intralipid) has been tried as a less expensive alternative to these commercial formulations.[7] However, such dispersions require vigorous mixing to incorporate the amphotericin B into the lipid phase and several have been shown to be unstable (see above). While some clinical successes have been achieved, reduced renal toxicity or improved tolerability have not been convincingly demonstrated (see Alternative Formulations, under Adverse Effects, above). There is currently insufficient evidence to recommend their use.[8]

Other novel formulations under investigation include an aggregated form produced by heating conventional amphotericin B injection,[9] a lipid nanosphere-encapsulated form (NS-718),[10,11] and a conjugate with the polysaccharide arabinogalactan.[12]

1. Tollemar J, Ringdén O. Lipid formulations of amphotericin B: less toxicity but at what economic cost? *Drug Safety* 1995; **13:** 207–18.
2. Graybill JR. Lipid formulations for amphotericin B: does the emperor need new clothes? *Ann Intern Med* 1996; **124:** 921–3.
3. de Marie S, *et al.* Clinical use of liposomal and lipid-complexed amphotericin B. *J Antimicrob Chemother* 1994; **33:** 907–16.
4. Coukell AJ, Brogden RN. Liposomal amphotericin B: therapeutic use in the management of fungal infections and visceral leishmaniasis. *Drugs* 1998; **55:** 585–612.
5. Brogden RN, *et al.* Amphotericin-B colloidal dispersion: a review of its use against systemic fungal infections and visceral leishmaniasis. *Drugs* 1998; **56:** 365–83.
6. Johansen HK, Gøtzsche PC. Amphotericin B lipid soluble formulations versus amphotericin B in cancer patients with neutropenia (updated 15 February 2001). Available in The Cochrane Library; Issue 3. Oxford: Update Software; 2001.
7. Cleary JD. Amphotericin B formulated in a lipid emulsion. *Ann Pharmacother* 1996; **30:** 409–12.
8. Sievers TM, *et al.* Safety and efficacy of Intralipid emulsions of amphotericin B. *J Antimicrob Chemother* 1996; **38:** 333–47.
9. Petit C, *et al.* Activity of a heat-induced reformulation of amphotericin B deoxycholate (Fungizone) against Leishmania donovani. *Antimicrob Agents Chemother* 1999; **43:** 390–2.
10. Hossain MA, *et al.* Efficacy of NS-718, a novel lipid nanosphere-encapsulated amphotericin B, against Cryptococcus neoformans. *Antimicrob Agents Chemother* 1998; **42:** 755–64.
11. Hossain MA, *et al.* Attenuation of nephrotoxicity by a novel lipid nanosphere (NS-718) incorporating amphotericin B. *J Antimicrob Chemother* 2000; **46:** 263–8.
12. Falk R, *et al.* A novel injectable water-soluble amphotericin B-arabinogalactan conjugate. *Antimicrob Agents Chemother* 1999; **43:** 1975–81.

INFUSION RATE. Conventional amphotericin B is usually given by intravenous infusion over 2 to 6 hours. A long infusion time is inconvenient for outpatients and often impractical in patients receiving other intravenous medications. This may be overcome by using one of the nonconventional formulations that can be infused over 30 to 120 minutes. Shorter infusion times have been tried with conventional amphotericin B with varying results. In studies in small numbers patients without pre-existing renal impairment rapid infusion over 1 hour was generally no more toxic than infusion over 4 hours in two studies,[1,2] whereas others[3] found infusion over 45 minutes to be more toxic than a 4-hour infusion during the first 5 to 7 days of treatment. Cardiac toxicity reported in patients receiving rapid infusions includes atrial fibrillation in a patient with pre-existing cardiac disease,[2] ventricular fibrillation associated with hyperkalaemia in a patient with severely impaired renal function,[4] and bradycardia[5] and dilated cardiomyopathy[6] in patients without apparent risk factors. Ventricular dysrhythmias were not observed in 27 patients with adequate renal function.[7] In general, there is not sufficient evidence to justify reducing infusion times for conventional amphotericin B to below 2 hours.

Conversely, continuous administration of amphotericin B over 24 hours has resulted in fewer side-effects and a significant reduction in nephrotoxicity compared with infusion over 4 hours.[8]

1. Oldfield EC, *et al.* Randomized, double-blind trial of 1- versus 4-hour amphotericin B infusion durations. *Antimicrob Agents Chemother* 1990; **34:** 1402–6.
2. Cruz JM, *et al.* Rapid intravenous infusion of amphotericin B: a pilot study. *Am J Med* 1992; **93:** 123–30.
3. Ellis ME, *et al.* Double-blind randomized study of the effect of infusion rates on toxicity of amphotericin B. *Antimicrob Agents Chemother* 1992; **36:** 172–9.
4. Craven PC, Gremillion DH. Risk factors of ventricular fibrillation during rapid amphotericin B infusion. *Antimicrob Agents Chemother* 1985; **27:** 868–71.
5. Soler JA, *et al.* Bradycardia after rapid intravenous infusion of amphotericin B. *Lancet* 1993; **341:** 372–3.
6. Arswa EL, *et al.* Amphotericin B-induced dilated cardiomyopathy. *Am J Med* 1994; **97:** 560–2.
7. Bowler WA, *et al.* Risk of ventricular dysrhythmias during 1-hour infusions of amphotericin B in patients with preserved renal function. *Antimicrob Agents Chemother* 1992; **36:** 2542–3.
8. Eriksson U, *et al.* Comparison of effects of amphotericin B deoxycholate infused over 4 or 24 hours: randomised controlled trial. *BMJ* 2001; **322:** 579–82.

Administration in neonates. Although the most appropriate dose of lipid formulations of amphotericin B for low-birth-weight preterm infants has yet to be firmly established reports suggest that it may be safe and effective at doses similar to those used in adults, relative to body weight.[1-3]

1. Scarcella A, *et al.* Liposomal amphotericin B treatment for neonatal fungal infections. *Pediatr Infect Dis J* 1998; **17:** 146–8.
2. Weitkamp J-H, *et al.* Candida infection in very low birth-weight infants: outcome and nephrotoxicity of treatment with liposomal amphotericin B (AmBisome). *Infection* 1998; **26:** 11–15.
3. Walsh TJ, *et al.* Amphotericin B lipid complex in pediatric patients with invasive fungal infections. *Pediatr Infect Dis J* 1999; **18:** 702–8.

Leishmaniasis. The treatment of visceral and mucocutaneous leishmaniasis including the use of amphotericin B is described on p.584.

VISCERAL LEISHMANIASIS. Evidence of declining responsiveness to pentavalent antimonials has led to the evaluation of intravenous amphotericin B as an alternative for first-line therapy. WHO has included liposomal amphotericin B 3 mg per kg body-weight daily on each of 5 consecutive days and a sixth dose 6 days later among the regimens suggested for first-line therapy of Mediterranean visceral leishmaniasis in immunocompetent patients.[1] Amphotericin B is also being evaluated in

other parts of the world. In India, conventional amphotericin B in modest doses (0.5 mg per kg on alternate days) produced good responses both in patients unresponsive to antimonials[2,3] and as first-line therapy.[4] Experience with a higher dose of 1 mg per kg daily for 20 days achieved a 99% cure rate in 938 patients.[5] Liposomal amphotericin B 2 mg per kg daily on 3, 5 or 7 days over a 10-day period all produced clinical cures and minimal toxicity[6] as did amphotericin B lipid complex 1, 2, or 3 mg per kg daily for 5 days,[7] or 5 mg per kg given once or twice,[8] although relapses occurred in some patients taking the lower doses in these latter studies. In Brazil, colloidal amphotericin B with sodium cholesteryl sulfate in a dose of 2 mg per kg daily for 5 days produced cures in 10 patients although 1 subsequently relapsed.[9] A study by WHO[10] suggested that more intensive courses of treatment may be needed in Brazil compared with India and Kenya. Responses to liposomal amphotericin B were reported to be slower in immunocompromised patients, and relapses occurred in 8 of 11 patients despite treatment with liposomal amphotericin B 1.38 to 1.85 mg per kg daily for 21 days.[11] Increasing the dose to 4 mg per kg daily given on 10 days over a 38-day period did not improve the long-term outcome, although initial responses were good.[12]

MUCOCUTANEOUS LEISHMANIASIS. Amphotericin B is used in mucocutaneous leishmaniasis unresponsive to antimonials. Successful treatment with liposomal amphotericin B has been reported.[13]

1. Gradoni L, *et al.* Treatment of Mediterranean visceral leishmaniasis. *Bull WHO* 1995; **73:** 191–7.
2. Giri OP. Amphotericin B therapy in kala-azar. *J Indian Med Assoc* 1993; **91:** 91–3.
3. Mishra M, *et al.* Amphotericin versus pentamidine in antimony-unresponsive kala-azar. *Lancet* 1992; **340:** 1256–7.
4. Mishra M, *et al.* Amphotericin versus sodium stibogluconate in first-line treatment of Indian kala-azar. *Lancet* 1994; **344:** 1599–1600.
5. Thakur CP, *et al.* Amphotericin B deoxycholate treatment of visceral leishmaniasis with newer modes of administration and precautions: a study of 938 cases. *Trans R Soc Trop Med Hyg* 1999; **93:** 319–23.
6. Thakur CP, *et al.* Comparison of three treatment regimens with liposomal amphotericin B (AmBisome) for visceral leishmaniasis in India: a randomized dose-finding study. *Trans R Soc Trop Med Hyg* 1996; **90:** 319–22.
7. Sundar S, *et al.* Short-course, low-dose amphotericin B lipid complex therapy for visceral leishmaniasis unresponsive to antimony. *Ann Intern Med* 1997; **127:** 133–7.
8. Sundar S, *et al.* Treatment of antimony-unresponsive Indian visceral leishmaniasis with ultra-short courses of amphotericin-B-lipid complex. *Ann Trop Med Parasitol* 1998; **92:** 755–64.
9. Dietze R, *et al.* Treatment of kala-azar in Brazil with Amphocil (amphotericin B cholesterol dispersion) for 5 days. *Trans R Soc Trop Med Hyg* 1995; **89:** 309–11.
10. Berman JD, *et al.* Efficacy and safety of liposomal amphotericin B (AmBisome) for visceral leishmaniasis in endemic developing countries. *Bull WHO* 1998; **76:** 25–32.
11. Davidson RN, *et al.* Liposomal amphotericin B (AmBisome) in Mediterranean visceral leishmaniasis: a multi-centre trial. *Q J Med* 1994; **87:** 75–81.
12. Russo R, *et al.* Visceral leishmaniasis in HIV infected patients: treatment with high dose liposomal amphotericin B (AmBisome). *J Infect* 1996; **32:** 133–7.
13. Sampaio RNR, Marsden PD. Mucosal leishmaniasis unresponsive to glucantime therapy successfully treated with AmBisome. *Trans R Soc Trop Med Hyg* 1997; **91:** 77.

Primary amoebic meningoencephalitis. Although amphotericin B is active *in vitro* against *Naegleria fowleri* and has been recommended for the treatment of primary amoebic meningoencephalitis (p.582) caused by this amoeba, there have been few reports of survival after its use. One patient who survived was treated with intravenous and intrathecal amphotericin B.[1] Another survivor received both amphotericin B and miconazole by the intravenous and intrathecal routes, and rifampicin and sulfafurazole by mouth.[2] In a third, aggressive therapy with intravenous and intrathecal amphotericin B together with high-dose oral rifampicin was successful.[3]

1. Anderson K, Jamieson A. Primary amoebic meningoencephalitis. *Lancet* 1972; **i:** 902–3.
2. Seidel JS, *et al.* Successful treatment of primary amebic meningoencephalitis. *N Engl J Med* 1982; **306:** 346–8.
3. Brown RL. Successful treatment of primary amebic meningoencephalitis. *Arch Intern Med* 1991; **151:** 1201–2.

Preparations

BP 2001: Amphotericin Lozenges; Amphotericin Oral Suspension;
USP 25: Amphotericin B Cream; Amphotericin B for Injection; Amphotericin B Lotion; Amphotericin B Ointment.

Proprietary Preparations (details are given in Part 3)
Aust.: Abelcet; AmBisome; Ampho-Moronal; Amphocil; *Austral.:* Abelcet; AmBisome; Fungilin; Fungizone; *Belg.:* AmBisome†; Fungizone; *Braz.:* Fungizon; *Canad.:* Fungizone; *Denm.:* Abelcet; AmBisome; Amphocil; Fungilin; *Fin.:* Abelcet; AmBisome; Fungizone; *Fr.:* Abelcet; AmBisome; Fungizone; *Ger.:* AmBisome; Ampho-Moronal; *Hong Kong:* Abelcet; AmBisome; Fungilin; Fungizone; *Irl.:* Abelcet; AmBisome; Amphocil; Fungizone; *Israel:* AmBisome; Amphocil; Fungilin; Fungizone; *Ital.:* Abelcet; AmBisome; Amphocil; Fungilin; Fungizone; *Mex.:* Amfostat; Amphocil; Candipres; *Neth.:* AmBisome; Amphocil; Fungizone; *Norw.:* Abelcet; Fungizone; *NZ:* AmBisome; Fungilin; Fungizone; *Port.:* Amphocil†; *S.Afr.:* Fungizone; *Singapore:* Abelcet; Amphocil; Fungizone; *Spain:* Abelcet; AmBisome; Amphocil; Funganiline; Fungizona; *Swed.:* Abelcet; AmBisome; Amphocil; Fungizone; *Switz.:* Abelcet; AmBisome; Ampho-Moronal; Fungizone; *Thai.:* AmBisome; Fungizone; *UK:* Abelcet; AmBisome; Amphocil; Fungilin; Fungizone; *USA:* Abelcet; AmBisome; Amphotec; Fungizone.

Multi-ingredient: *Aust.:* Mysteclin; *Braz.:* Talsutin; Tericin AT; *Fr.:* Amphocycline; *Ger.:* Ampho-Moronal V; Ampho-Moronal V

L; Mysteclin; **Hong Kong:** Talsutin; **Ital.:** Anfocort; **S.Afr.:** Mysteclin-V†; Vagmycin; **Spain:** Gine Heyden; Sanicel; Trigon Topico.

Bifonazole (12444-v)

Bifonazole (BAN, USAN, rINN).
Bay-h-4502; Bifonazolum. 1-(α-Biphenyl-4-ylbenzyl)imidazole.
$C_{22}H_{18}N_2 = 310.4$.
CAS — 60628-96-8.
ATC — D01AC10.
Pharmacopoeias. In Eur. (see p.vi) and Jpn.

Pharmacopoeial description
Ph. Eur.: A white or almost white crystalline powder. It exhibits polymorphism. Practically insoluble in water; sparingly soluble in dehydrated alcohol.

Profile
Bifonazole is an imidazole antifungal with a broad spectrum of activity; sensitive fungi include dermatophytes, *Malassezia furfur*, and *Candida* spp. It also has antibacterial activity *in vitro* against some Gram-positive cocci.
Bifonazole is mainly used by topical application in the treatment of fungal skin and nail infections (p.376). It is applied topically once daily as a 1% cream, powder, solution, or gel. Treatment is usually continued for 2 to 4 weeks. More prolonged treatment is necessary for nail infections and bifonazole may be applied initially with a 40% urea paste to soften the nail.
Local reactions including burning and itching have been reported.
The need for caution when using an azole antifungal in pregnant or lactating patients is discussed under Fluconazole, p.383.
◊ References.
1. Lackner TE, Clissold SP. Bifonazole: a review of its antimicrobial activity and therapeutic use in superficial mycoses. *Drugs* 1989; **38:** 204–25.

Preparations
Proprietary Preparations (details are given in Part 3)
Aust.: Fungiderm; Mycosporin†; **Austral.:** Canesten Once Daily; Mycosporin; **Belg.:** Mycospor; **Denm.:** Mycospor†; **Fr.:** Amycor; **Ger.:** Bifomyk; Bifon; Mycospor; **Hong Kong:** Mycospor; **Israel:** Agispor; **Ital.:** Azolmen; Bifazol; **Mex.:** Mycospor; **Neth.:** Mycospor; **Norw.:** Mycospor; **Port.:** Mycospor; Topical; **S.Afr.:** Mycospor; **Spain:** Bifokey; Moldina; Monostop; Mycospor; **Swed.:** Mycosporan; **Thai.:** Mycospor; **UK:** Canesten AF.
Multi-ingredient: Denm.: Mycospor Carbamid†; **Fr.:** Amycor Onychoset; **Ger.:** Mycospor Nagelset; **Israel:** Agispor Onychoset; Comagis; Keratospor; **Mex.:** Mycospor Onicoset; **Norw.:** Mycospor Carbamid†; **Port.:** Mycospor†; **Spain:** Mycospor Onicoset; **Swed.:** Mycosporan Karbamid†.

Bromochlorosalicylanilide (2212-t)

5-Bromo-4′-chlorosalicylanilide; 5-Bromo-N-(4-chlorophenyl)-2-hydroxybenzamide.
$C_{13}H_9BrClNO_2 = 326.6$.
ATC — D01AE01.

Profile
Bromochlorosalicylanilide is a bromsalan antifungal that has been applied topically. Photosensitivity may occur. See also Bromsalans, p.1136.

Preparations
Proprietary Preparations (details are given in Part 3)
Aust.: Multifungin†.
Multi-ingredient: Aust.: Multifungin†.

Buclosamide (2564-x)

Buclosamide (BAN, rINN).
N-Butyl-4-chlorosalicylamide; N-Butyl-4-chloro-2-hydroxybenzamide.
$C_{11}H_{14}ClNO_2 = 227.7$.
CAS — 575-74-6.

Profile
Buclosamide is an antifungal that has been applied topically in association with salicylic acid in the treatment of fungal skin infections. Photosensitivity has occurred.

Preparations
Proprietary Preparations (details are given in Part 3)
Multi-ingredient: Braz.: Jadit.

Butenafine Hydrochloride (17893-n)

Butenafine Hydrochloride (BANM, USAN, rINN).
KP-363. N-(p-tert-Butylbenzyl)-N-methyl-1-naphthalenemethylamine hydrochloride; 4-tert-Butylbenzyl(methyl)(1-naphthalenemethyl)amine hydrochloride.
$C_{23}H_{27}N,HCl = 353.9$.
CAS — 101828-21-1 (butenafine); 101827-46-7 (butenafine hydrochloride).

Profile
Butenafine is a benzylamine antifungal with actions similar to those of the allylamine antifungal terbinafine (p.394). The hydrochloride is used topically as a 1% cream for the treatment of superficial dermatophyte infections (p.376).
◊ Reviews.
1. McNeely W, Spencer CM. Butenafine. *Drugs* 1998; **55:** 405–12.

Preparations
Proprietary Preparations (details are given in Part 3)
Israel: Mentax; **Jpn:** Mentax; **USA:** Mentax.

Butoconazole Nitrate (16554-x)

Butoconazole Nitrate (BANM, USAN, rINN).
RS-35887; RS-35887-00-10-3. 1-[4-(4-Chlorophenyl)-2-(2,6-dichlorophenylthio)butyl]imidazole mononitrate.
$C_{19}H_{17}Cl_3N_2S,HNO_3 = 474.8$.
CAS — 64872-76-0 (butoconazole); 64872-77-1 (butoconazole nitrate).
Pharmacopoeias. In US.

Pharmacopoeial description
USP 25: A white to off-white crystalline powder. Practically insoluble in water; slightly soluble in acetone, in acetonitrile, in dichloromethane, and in tetrahydrofuran; very slightly soluble in ethyl acetate; sparingly soluble in methyl alcohol. Protect from light.

Adverse Effects and Precautions
Local reactions including burning and irritation may occur when butoconazole is applied vaginally.
Intravaginal preparations of butoconazole may damage latex contraceptives and additional contraceptive measures are therefore necessary during local administration.
For information about the use of butoconazole during pregnancy and lactation, see under Pregnancy in Fluconazole, Precautions, p.383.
Effects on the blood. Severe reversible thrombocytopenia was associated with treatment with intravaginal butoconazole in a patient.[1] The patient had previously experienced a drop in white cell count following treatment with intravaginal clotrimazole, suggestive of an idiosyncratic reaction to imidazoles.
1. Maloley PA, *et al.* Severe reversible thrombocytopenia resulting from butoconazole cream. *DICP Ann Pharmacother* 1990; **24:** 143–4.

Antimicrobial Action
Butoconazole is an imidazole antifungal with antimicrobial activity similar to that of ketoconazole (p.389) including activity against *Candida* spp.

Pharmacokinetics
Approximately 5% of a dose of butoconazole is absorbed following vaginal administration. The plasma half-life is 21 to 24 hours.

Uses and Administration
Butoconazole nitrate is an imidazole antifungal used locally in the treatment of vulvovaginal candidiasis (p.372). It is administered intravaginally as a 100-mg pessary or as 5 g of a 2% cream for 3 consecutive nights; a single application of the cream has also been used.

Preparations
USP 25: Butoconazole Nitrate Vaginal Cream.
Proprietary Preparations (details are given in Part 3)
Belg.: Gynomyk; **Fr.:** Gynomyk; **Mex.:** Femstal; **Neth.:** Gynomyk; **USA:** Femstat; Gynazole; Mycelex-3.

Candicidin (2566-f)

Candicidin (BAN, USAN, rINN).
NSC-94219.
CAS — 1403-17-4.
ATC — G01AA04.
A mixture of antifungal heptaenes produced by *Streptomyces griseus*.

Profile
Candicidin is a polyene antibiotic with antifungal actions. It has been used in the treatment of vaginal candidiasis.

Caspofungin Acetate (6630-d)

Caspofungin Acetate (BANM, USAN, rINN).
L-743873; MK-0991. (4R,5S)-5-[(2-Aminoethyl)amino]-N²-(10,12-dimethyltetradecanoyl)-4-hydroxy-L-ornithyl-L-threonyl-trans-4-hydroxy-L-prolyl-(S)-4-hydroxy-4-(p-hydroxyphenyl)-L-threonyl-threo-3-hydroxy-L-ornithyl-trans-3-hydroxy-L-proline cyclic (6→1)-peptide diacetate.
$C_{52}H_{88}N_{10}O_{15},2C_2H_4O_2 = 1213.4$.
CAS — 179463-17-3.

Adverse Effects
Adverse experiences reported with caspofungin have included nausea and vomiting, flushing, fever, and venous complications around the infusion site. Possible histamine-mediated symp-

toms have been rash, facial swelling, pruritus, or sensation of warmth; a case of anaphylaxis is known.

Interactions
Caspofungin concentrations may be reduced if it is administered with other drugs that can induce drug clearance. Such effects have been noted with carbamazepine, dexamethasone, efavirenz, nelfinavir, nevirapine, phenytoin, and rifampicin and an increase in the dose of caspofungin to 70 mg daily should be considered in patients who are taking these drugs and who are not clinically responding.
When caspofungin has been administered with ciclosporin, an increase in the area under the concentration-time curve for caspofungin, as well as increases in hepatic enzymes, were observed and concomitant use of the two drugs is not recommended.
Caspofungin has resulted in decreased blood concentrations of tacrolimus and therapeutic drug monitoring and appropriate dosage adjustments to tacrolimus are recommended.
Caspofungin is not an inhibitor of any enzyme in the cytochrome P450 system.

Pharmacokinetics
Plasma concentrations of caspofungin decline in a polyphasic manner following intravenous infusion. The initial short α-phase occurs immediately post-infusion and is followed by a β-phase with a half-life of 9 to 11 hours; an additional longer γ-phase also occurs with a half-life of 40 to 50 hours. Plasma clearance is dependent on distribution rather than on biotransformation or excretion. There is slow metabolism of caspofungin by hydrolysis and N-acetylation and excretion in faeces and urine.

Uses and Administration
Caspofungin is an antifungal used in the treatment of invasive aspergillosis (p.372) in patients who are refractory to, or intolerant of, other therapy. It acts by inhibiting the synthesis of β-(1,3)-D-glucan, an essential component of the cell wall of susceptible filamentous fungi.
Caspofungin is used as the acetate and is given by slow intravenous infusion over about 1 hour. A loading dose of 70 mg is given on the first day and is followed by 50 mg daily. In patients with moderate hepatic impairment a daily dose of 35 mg should be used after the initial dose of 70 mg; appropriate doses for patients with severe hepatic impairment have not been studied.

Preparations
Proprietary Preparations (details are given in Part 3)
USA: Cancidas.

Chlormidazole Hydrochloride (2569-h)

Chlormidazole Hydrochloride (BANM, rINN).
Clomidazole Hydrochloride. 1-(4-Chlorobenzyl)-2-methylbenzimidazole hydrochloride.
$C_{15}H_{13}ClN_2,HCl = 293.2$.
CAS — 3689-76-7 (chlormidazole); 54118-67-1 (chlormidazole hydrochloride).

Profile
Chlormidazole hydrochloride is an imidazole antifungal used topically in the treatment of fungal infections of the skin.
The need for caution when using an azole antifungal in pregnant or lactating patients is discussed under Fluconazole, p.383.

Preparations
Proprietary Preparations (details are given in Part 3)
Multi-ingredient: Aust.: Myco-Synalar; **Spain:** Myco-Synalar†; **Switz.:** Myco-Synalar.

Chlorphenesin (2570-a)

Chlorphenesin (BAN, pINN).
3-(4-Chlorophenoxy)propane-1,2-diol.
$C_9H_{11}ClO_3 = 202.6$.
CAS — 104-29-0.
ATC — D01AE07.

Profile
Chlorphenesin has antifungal and antibacterial properties. It is applied locally in mild uncomplicated dermatophyte and other cutaneous infections and in vaginal infections.
Chlorphenesin carbamate (p.1327) is used as a skeletal muscle relaxant.

Preparations
Proprietary Preparations (details are given in Part 3)
Aust.: Adermykon; **Austral.:** Nappy Rash Powder; **Canad.:** Mycil; **Ger.:** Soorphenesin.
Multi-ingredient: Aust.: Aleot; **Austral.:** ZSC; **Braz.:** Adermykon-C; Oto Betnovate; **Canad.:** Anivy†.

The symbol † denotes a preparation no longer actively marketed

Ciclopirox Olamine (2572-x)

Ciclopirox Olamine (BANM, USAN, rINNM).
Hoe-296. The 2-aminoethanol salt of 6-Cyclohexyl-1-hydroxy-4-methyl-2-pyridone.
$C_{12}H_{17}NO_2,C_2H_7NO = 268.4$.
CAS — 29342-05-0 (ciclopirox); 41621-49-2 (ciclopirox olamine).
Pharmacopoeias. In Eur. (see p.vi) and US. Eur. also includes Ciclopirox.

Pharmacopoeial description

Ph. Eur.: A white or pale yellow crystalline powder. It exhibits polymorphism. Slightly soluble in water; very soluble in alcohol and in dichloromethane; slightly soluble in ethyl acetate; practically insoluble in cyclohexane. A 1% solution in water has a pH of 8.0 to 9.0. Protect from light.
USP 25: A 1% solution has a pH of 8.0 to 9.0.

Adverse Effects

Irritation and pruritus have been reported after topical application of ciclopirox olamine.

Antimicrobial Action

Ciclopirox olamine has a wide spectrum of antifungal activity. It inhibits most Candida, Epidermophyton, Microsporum, and Trichophyton spp. and is also active against Malassezia furfur. It has some antibacterial activity.

Uses and Administration

Ciclopirox olamine is an antifungal which is applied topically twice daily as a 1% cream, solution, or powder (equivalent to 0.77% ciclopirox) in the treatment of fungal skin infections, including cutaneous candidiasis (p.372), dermatophytosis, and pityriasis versicolor (p.376). It has also been used in the treatment of vaginal candidiasis.

A lacquer containing 8% ciclopirox base is used for nail infections.

◊ References.
1. Jue SG, et al. Ciclopirox olamine 1% cream: a preliminary review of its antimicrobial activity and therapeutic use. Drugs 1985; 29: 330–41.

Preparations

USP 25: Ciclopirox Olamine Cream; Ciclopirox Olamine Topical Suspension.

Proprietary Preparations (details are given in Part 3)
Aust.: Batrafen; **Braz.:** Gino Loprox; Loprox; Micoliv; **Canad.:** Loprox; **Denm.:** Mycofen; **Fr.:** Mycoster; Stiprox; **Ger.:** Batrafen; Nagel Batrafen; **Hong Kong:** Batrafen; **Irl.:** Batrafen; **Israel:** Batrafen; Cicloderm; **Ital.:** Batrafen; Biroxol; Brumixol; Dafnegin; Miclast; Micomicen; Micoxolamina; **Mex.:** Loprox; **Neth.:** Loprox; **NZ:** Batrafen; Nail Batrafen; **Spain:** Aquomin; Batrafen; Ciclochem; Fungowas; Rimafungol†; **Switz.:** Batrafen; Dafnegil Neo; **Thai.:** Loprox; **UK:** Oilatum Shampoo; **USA:** Loprox; Penlac.
Multi-ingredient: Fr.: Stiproxal; **Israel:** Cicloderm-C.

Clodantoin (2568-n)

Clodantoin (BAN, rINN).
Chlordantoin (USAN). 5-(1-Ethylpentyl)-3-(trichloromethylthio)hydantoin; 5-(1-Ethylpentyl)-3-(trichloromethylthio)imidazolidine-2,4-dione.
$C_{11}H_{17}Cl_3N_2O_2S = 347.7$.
CAS — 5588-20-5.
ATC — G01AX01.

Profile

Clodantoin is an antifungal used locally for vulvovaginal infections.

Preparations

Proprietary Preparations (details are given in Part 3)
Multi-ingredient: Spain: Blastoestimulina.

Clotrimazole (2573-r)

Clotrimazole (BAN, USAN, rINN).
Bay-5097; Clotrimazolum; FB-5097. 1-(α-2-Chlorotrityl)imidazole.
$C_{22}H_{17}ClN_2 = 344.8$.
CAS — 23593-75-1.
ATC — A01AB18; D01AC01; G01AF02.

NOTE. Compounded preparations of clotrimazole may be represented by the following names:
- Co-climasone (USP 25)—clotrimazole and betamethasone dipropionate.

Pharmacopoeias. In Chin., Eur. (see p.vi), Jpn, Pol., and US.

Pharmacopoeial description

Ph. Eur.: A white or pale yellow crystalline powder. Practically insoluble in water; soluble in alcohol and in dichloromethane; slightly soluble in ether. Protect from light.
USP 25: A white to pale yellow, crystalline powder. Practically insoluble in water; freely soluble in alcohol, in acetone, in chloroform, and in methyl alcohol. Store in airtight containers.

Adverse Effects and Precautions

Gastrointestinal disturbance, elevation of liver enzymes, dysuria, and mental depression have been reported after administration of clotrimazole by mouth. Local reactions including irritation and a burning sensation may occur in patients treated topically; contact allergic dermatitis has been reported.

Intravaginal preparations of clotrimazole may damage latex contraceptives and additional contraceptive measures are therefore necessary during local administration.

For information about the use of clotrimazole during pregnancy and lactation, see under Pregnancy in Fluconazole, Precautions, p.383.

Antimicrobial Action

Clotrimazole is an imidazole antifungal with antimicrobial activity similar to that of ketoconazole (p.389). A high proportion of fungi sensitive to clotrimazole are inhibited by concentrations of 3 μg per mL. The protozoan Trichomonas vaginalis requires up to 100 μg per mL for inhibition.

Pharmacokinetics

When applied topically clotrimazole penetrates the epidermis but there is little if any systemic absorption. Absorption of 3 to 10% of a dose has been reported following vaginal administration. Clotrimazole is metabolised in the liver to inactive compounds and excreted in the faeces and urine.

Uses and Administration

Clotrimazole is an imidazole antifungal used topically in superficial candidiasis (p.372), and in the skin infections pityriasis versicolor and dermatophytosis (p.376). It may also be used occasionally in the treatment of the protozoal infection trichomoniasis when other drugs are contra-indicated (see p.586).

Clotrimazole is applied topically two or three times daily for 2 to 4 weeks as a 1% cream, lotion, or solution in the treatment of fungal skin infections; a 1% powder may be used in conjunction with the cream or solution and has been applied to prevent re-infection. The 1% solution is also used topically for fungal otitis externa. Clotrimazole is given as pessaries in dosage regimens of 100 mg for 6 days, 200 mg for 3 days, or a single dose of 500 mg in the treatment of vulvovaginal candidiasis; similar doses are given as a 1, 2, or 10% vaginal cream. It may be necessary to treat balanitis in male partners concurrently.

Lozenges of clotrimazole 10 mg are dissolved in the mouth for treatment or prophylaxis of oral candidiasis and may be used five times daily for 14 days. Clotrimazole has also been given by mouth but has now been largely superseded by other azole drugs.

Seborrhoeic dermatitis. Topical preparations containing an imidazole such as clotrimazole, ketoconazole, or miconazole usually together with hydrocortisone are used in the management of seborrhoeic dermatitis (see p.1107).

Sickle-cell disease. Oral clotrimazole has been investigated[1] in the treatment of sickle-cell disease (p.717).

1. Brugnara C, et al. Therapy with oral clotrimazole induces inhibition of the Gardos channel and reduction of erythrocyte dehydration in patients with sickle cell disease. J Clin Invest 1996; 97: 1227–34.

Preparations

BP 2001: Clotrimazole Cream; Clotrimazole Pessaries;
USP 25: Clotrimazole and Betamethasone Dipropionate Cream; Clotrimazole Cream; Clotrimazole Lotion; Clotrimazole Lozenges; Clotrimazole Topical Solution; Clotrimazole Vaginal Tablets.

Proprietary Preparations (details are given in Part 3)
Aust.: Candibene; Canesten; Myko Cordes; Pedikurol; **Austral.:** Canesten; Chemists Own Clozole; Clofeme 3 Day; Clonea; Clozole; Gyne-Lotrimin; Hiderm†; Tinaderm Extra†; **Belg.:** Canesten; Gyno-Canesten; **Braz.:** Canesten; Clomazem; Clotrimix; Dermobene; Gino Clotrimix; Micotrizol; Tricosten; **Canad.:** Canesten; Clotrimaderm; Myclo-Derm; Myclo-Gyne; Neo-Zol; **Denm.:** Canazol; Canesten; **Fin.:** Canesten; Klotricid; **Ger.:** Antifungol; Antimyk; Apocanda†; Aru C; Azutrimazol; Benzoderm Myco; Candazol; Canesten; Canifug; Cloderm; Clotri OPT†; Clotrifug†; Clotrigalen; cutistad†; Dignotrimazol†; durafungol; Fungiderm; Fungizid; Gilt; Gyno-Canesten; Holfungin; Jenamazol†; KadeFungin; Logomed Fungizid-Salbe†; Lokalicid; Mycofug; Mycohaug C†; Myko Cordes; Mykofungin; Mykohaug; Ovis Neu; Pedisafe; Radikal; SD-Hermal; Uromykol; **Hong Kong:** Canesten; Clocreme; Clotri-Denk; Clozole; Cotren; Fungizid; Gyne-Lotremin; Lotremin; **Irl.:** Canesten; **Israel:** Agisten; Baby Agisten; Clotrimaderm; Myco-Hermal; Oralten Troche; **Ital.:** Antimicotico; Canesten; Gyno-Canesten; **Mex.:** Candimon; Canesten; Cinabel; Lotrimin; **Neth.:** Canesten; **Norw.:** Canesten; Fungisten; **NZ:** Canesten; Clocreme; Clotrimaderm; Fungizid; **Port.:** Candid; Canesten; Diomicete; Gino-Canesten; Gino-Lotremine; Lotremine; Pan-Fungex; **S.Afr.:** A-Por; Canalba; Candaspor; Candizole; Canesten; Canex; Clomaderm†; Closcript; Covospor; Dynaspor; Gynezol†; Gyno-Trimaze; Medaspor; Micomisan; Mycoban; Mycohexal; Normospor; Stiemazol†; Trimaze; Xeraspor; **Singapore:** Candazole; Canesten; Clozole; Cotren; Cristan; Gyne-Lotremin; Lotremin; Myco-Hermal; **Spain:** Canesten; Fungidermo; Gine Canesten; Ictan; **Swed.:** Canesten; Clotriferm†; **Switz.:** Acnecolor; Canestene; Clocim; cutistad†; Eurosan; Fungotox; Gromazol; Gyno-Canestene; Imazol; **Thai.:** Canadine; Canazol; Candid; Candinox; Canesten; Clotricin; Comat; Cotren; CST; Defungo; Fungiderm; Gynebo; Klamacin; Nestic; Taraten; Vamazole; Vanesten; **UK:** Abtrim; Athletes Foot Cream; Candiden; Canesten; Canesten Combi; Fungederm; Masnoderm†; Medisport Athlete's Foot; Mycil Gold; Privacom; **USA:** Fungoid†; Gyne-Lotrimin; Lotrimin; Lotrimin AF; Mycelex; Mycelex-7; Mycelex-G†; Prescription Strength Desenex†.

Multi-ingredient: Aust.: Myko Cordes; **Austral.:** Hydrozole; **Belg.:** Lotriderm; **Braz.:** Baycuten; Floregin Composto; **Canad.:** Lotriderm; **Denm.:** Clotrason; **Ger.:** Baycuten; Canesten HC; Fungidexan; Imazol; Imazol comp; Lotricomb; Myko Cordes Plus; **Hong Kong:** Synco-CFN; Triderm; **Irl.:** Canesten HC; Lotriderm; **Israel:** Hydrozole; Polycutan; Triderm; **Ital.:** Desamix Effe; Meclon; **Mex.:** Baycuten N; Quadriderm NF; **NZ:** Lotricomb; **Port.:** Baycuten; Flotiran; Quadriderme; **S.Afr.:** Lotriderm; **Singapore:** Canesten HC; Combiderm; Gentrisone; Neoderm; Triderm; **Spain:** Beta Micoter; Clotrasone; **Switz.:** Imacort; Imazol; Triderm; **Thai.:** Canasone; Canazol-BE; Clotrasone; Fungiderm-B; Gynestin; **UK:** Canesten HC; Lotriderm†; **USA:** Lotrisone.

Copper Naphthenate (5290-e)

CAS — 1338-02-9.

Profile

Copper naphthenate is a topical antifungal used in veterinary medicine.

Croconazole Hydrochloride (1983-p)

Croconazole Hydrochloride (rINNM).
Cloconazole Hydrochloride; 710674-S (croconazole). 1-(1-{o-[(m-Chlorobenzyl)oxy]phenyl}vinyl)imidazole hydrochloride.
$C_{18}H_{15}ClN_2O,HCl = 347.2$.
CAS — 77175-51-0 (croconazole).
Pharmacopoeias. In Jpn.

Profile

Croconazole hydrochloride is an imidazole antifungal used topically in the treatment of superficial cutaneous candidiasis, dermatophytosis, and pityriasis versicolor.

The need for caution when using an azole antifungal in pregnant or lactating patients is discussed under Fluconazole, p.383.

Preparations

Proprietary Preparations (details are given in Part 3)
Aust.: Pilzcin; **Ger.:** Pilzcin; **Jpn:** Pilzcin.

Eberconazole (15271-n)

Eberconazole (rINN).
WAS-2160. (±)-1-(2,4-Dichloro-10,11-dihydro-5H-dibenzo[a,d]cyclohepten-5-yl)imidazole.
$C_{18}H_{14}Cl_2N_2 = 329.2$.
CAS — 128326-82-9.

Profile

Eberconazole is an imidazole antifungal under investigation for the topical treatment of superficial fungal skin infections.

Econazole Nitrate (2579-b)

Econazole Nitrate (BANM, USAN, rINNM).
C-C2470; Econazoli Nitras; R-14827; SQ-13050. (±)-1-[2,4-Dichloro-β-(4-chlorobenzyloxy)phenethyl]imidazole nitrate.
$C_{18}H_{15}Cl_3N_2O,HNO_3 = 444.7$.
CAS — 27220-47-9 (econazole); 24169-02-6 (econazole nitrate); 68797-31-9 ((±)-econazole nitrate).
Pharmacopoeias. In Eur. (see p.vi) and US.

Pharmacopoeial description

Ph. Eur.: A white or almost white crystalline powder. Very slightly soluble in water; slightly soluble in alcohol; sparingly soluble in dichloromethane; practically insoluble in ether; soluble in methyl alcohol. Protect from light.
USP 25: A white or practically white, crystalline powder, with not more than a slight odour. Very slightly soluble in water and in ether; slightly soluble in alcohol; sparingly soluble in chloroform; soluble in methyl alcohol. Protect from light.

Adverse Effects and Precautions

Local reactions including burning and irritation may occur when econazole nitrate is applied topically. Contact dermatitis has been reported rarely.

Intravaginal preparations of econazole may damage latex contraceptives and additional contraceptive measures are therefore necessary during local administration.

For information about the use of econazole during pregnancy and lactation, see under Pregnancy in Fluconazole, Precautions, p.383.

Porphyria. Econazole nitrate has been associated with acute attacks of porphyria and is considered unsafe in porphyric patients.

Antimicrobial Action

Econazole is an imidazole antifungal with antimicrobial activity similar to that of ketoconazole (p.389).

Pharmacokinetics

Absorption is not significant when econazole nitrate is applied to the skin or vagina.

Uses and Administration

Econazole is an imidazole antifungal used topically in the treatment of superficial candidiasis (see p.372) and in dermatophytosis and pityriasis versicolor (see Skin Infections, p.376).

Econazole nitrate is applied topically up to 3 times daily as a 1% cream, lotion, powder, or solution in the treatment of fungal skin infections. Treatment is continued for 2 to 4 weeks. It is also used in the treatment of vaginal candidiasis as pessaries of 150 mg once daily at bedtime for 3 consecutive nights; a single dose of 150 mg in a long-acting formulation has also been used. Intravaginal administration of 5 g of a 1% cream once daily at night has been given for 2 weeks. A 1% cream may be used concurrently for the treatment of vulval infections or balanitis in a male partner.

Econazole nitrate has also been administered as eye or ear drops.

Preparations

BP 2001: Econazole Cream; Econazole Pessaries.

Proprietary Preparations (details are given in Part 3)
Aust.: Gyno-Pevaryl; Pevalip; Pevaryl; *Austral.:* Dermazole; Ecostatin; Pevaryl; *Belg.:* Gyno-Pevaryl; Pevaryl; *Braz.:* Limpele Conjugado; Micostyl; *Canad.:* Ecostatin; *Denm.:* Pevaryl; *Fin.:* Pevaryl; *Fr.:* Dermazol; Fongeryl; Gyno-Pevaryl; Mycoapaisyl; Pevaryl; *Ger.:* Epi-Pevaryl; Epi-Pevaryl Pv; Gyno-Pevaryl; *Hong Kong:* Dermazole; Gyno-Pevaryl; Heads Shampoo; Pevaryl; *Irl.:* Ecostatin; Gyno-Pevaryl; Pevaryl; *Israel:* Gyno-Pevaryl; Pevaryl; *Ital.:* Amicel†; Chemionazolo; Eccelium; Eco Mi; Ecodergin; Ecorex; Ecosteril; Ifenec; Micogin†; Micos; Pargin†; Pevaryl; Polinazolo; *Mex.:* Micostyl; Pevaryl; *Neth.:* Pevaryl; *Norw.:* Pevaryl; *NZ:* Dermazole; Ecostatin; Ecreme; Gyno-Pevaryl; Pevaryl; *Port.:* Gyno-Pevaryl; Pevaryl; *S.Afr.:* Gyno-Pevaryl; Pevaryl; *Singapore:* Dermazole; Ecoderm; Gyno-Pevaryl; Pevaryl; *Spain:* Ecotam; Etramon†; Gyno-Pevaryl; Micospec; Micoseptil†; Pevaryl; *Swed.:* Pevaryl; *Switz.:* Gyno-Pevaryl; Pevaryl; Sebolith; *UK:* Ecostatin; Gyno-Pevaryl; Pevaryl; *USA:* Spectazole.

Multi-ingredient: *Aust.:* Pevaryl; Pevisone; *Belg.:* Pevaryl; *Denm.:* Pevisone; *Fin.:* Pevisone; *Fr.:* Pevisone; *Ger.:* Epi-Pevaryl Heilpaste; Epipevisone; *Hong Kong:* Pevisone; *Israel:* Pevisone; *Ital.:* Pevisone; *Norw.:* Pevisone; *Port.:* Pevisone; *S.Afr.:* Pevisone; *Singapore:* Ecocort; Pevisone; *Swed.:* Pevisone; *Switz.:* Pevaryl; Pevisone; *Thai.:* Ecoderm; Econ; Pevisone; *UK:* Econacort; Pevaryl TC.

Enilconazole   (12690-t)

Enilconazole *(BAN, USAN, rINN).*
R-23979. (±)-1-(β-Allyloxy-2,4-dichlorophenethyl)imidazole.
$C_{14}H_{14}Cl_2N_2O = 297.2.$
CAS — 35554-44-0.

Profile

Enilconazole is an imidazole antifungal that has been used in veterinary medicine as a 0.2% solution for the treatment of fungal skin infections in cattle, horses, and dogs.

Fenticlor   (2580-x)

Fenticlor *(BAN, USAN, rINN).*
D-25; HL-1050; NSC-4112; Ph-549; S-7. 2,2'-Thiobis(4-chlorophenol).
$C_{12}H_8Cl_2O_2S = 287.2.$
CAS — 97-24-5.

The symbol † denotes a preparation no longer actively marketed

Profile

Fenticlor is an antifungal that has been applied topically in the treatment of dermatophyte infections.
Photosensitivity reactions have been reported.

Preparations

Proprietary Preparations (details are given in Part 3)
Multi-ingredient: *Spain:* Dermisdin.

Fenticonazole Nitrate   (16806-n)

Fenticonazole Nitrate *(BANM, USAN, rINNM).*
Fenticonazoli Nitras; Rec-15/1476. (±)-1-[2,4-Dichloro-β-{[p-(phenylthio)benzyl]oxy}phenethyl]imidazole mononitrate.
$C_{24}H_{20}Cl_2N_2OS,HNO_3 = 518.4.$
CAS — 73151-29-8 (fenticonazole nitrate); 72479-26-6 (fenticonazole).
Pharmacopoeias. In Eur. (see p.vi).

Pharmacopoeial description
Ph. Eur.: A white or almost white, crystalline powder. Practically insoluble in water; sparingly soluble in dehydrated alcohol; freely soluble in dimethylformamide and in methyl alcohol. Protect from light.

Adverse Effects and Precautions

Burning and itching have been reported following the application of fenticonazole nitrate.

Intravaginal preparations of fenticonazole may damage latex contraceptives and additional contraceptive measures are therefore necessary during local administration.

The need for caution when using an azole antifungal in pregnant or lactating patients is discussed under Fluconazole, p.383.

Antimicrobial Action

Fenticonazole is an imidazole antifungal active against a range of organisms including dermatophyte pathogens, *Malassezia furfur,* and *Candida albicans.*

Uses and Administration

Fenticonazole nitrate is an imidazole antifungal used locally in the treatment of vulvovaginal candidiasis (p.372). A 200-mg pessary is inserted into the vagina at bedtime for 3 nights or a 600-mg pessary is inserted once only at bedtime. Fenticonazole nitrate is also applied topically for the treatment of fungal skin infections.

Preparations

Proprietary Preparations (details are given in Part 3)
Aust.: Fenizolan; Lomexin; *Fr.:* Lomexin; Terlomexin; *Ger.:* Fenizolan; Lomexin; *Ital.:* Falvin; Fentiderm†; Fentigyn; Lomexin; *S.Afr.:* Lomexin; *Spain:* Laurimic; Lomexin; *Switz.:* Mycodermil; *UK:* Lomexin.

Fluconazole   (18642-y)

Fluconazole *(BAN, USAN, rINN).*
UK-49858. 2-(2,4-Difluorophenyl)-1,3-bis(1H-1,2,4-triazol-1-yl)propan-2-ol.
$C_{13}H_{12}F_2N_6O = 306.3.$
CAS — 86386-73-4.
ATC — D01AC15; J02AC01.

◊ Compatibility and stability studies with fluconazole.
1. Lor E, et al. Visual compatibility of fluconazole with commonly used injectable drugs during simulated Y-site administration. *Am J Hosp Pharm* 1991; **48:** 744–6.
2. Couch P, et al. Stability of fluconazole and amino acids in parenteral nutrient solutions. *Am J Hosp Pharm* 1992; **49:** 1459–62.
3. Hunt-Fugate AK, et al. Stability of fluconazole in injectable solutions. *Am J Hosp Pharm* 1993; **50:** 1186–7.
4. Ishisaka DY. Visual compatibility of fluconazole with drugs given by continuous infusion. *Am J Hosp Pharm* 1994; **51:** 2290 and 2292.

Adverse Effects

Adverse effects reported with fluconazole most commonly affect the gastrointestinal tract and include abdominal pain, diarrhoea, flatulence, nausea, and vomiting. Other adverse effects include headache, dizziness, leucopenia, thrombocytopenia, hyperlipidaemias, and raised liver enzyme values. Serious hepatotoxicity has been reported in patients with severe underlying disease. Anaphylaxis and angioedema have been reported rarely.

Skin reactions are rare but exfoliative cutaneous reactions such as toxic epidermal necrolysis and Stevens-Johnson syndrome have occurred, more commonly in patients with AIDS.

Alopecia. Alopecia has occasionally been reported in patients receiving fluconazole, especially during prolonged treatment.[1,2]
1. Weinroth SE, Tuazon CU. Alopecia associated with fluconazole treatment. *Ann Intern Med* 1993; **119:** 637.
2. Pappas PG, et al. Alopecia associated with fluconazole therapy. *Ann Intern Med* 1995; **123:** 354–7.

Effect on electrolyte balance. Hypokalaemia was associated with fluconazole administration in 3 patients with acute myeloid leukaemia.[1]
1. Kidd C, et al. Hypokalaemia in patients with acute myeloid leukaemia after treatment with fluconazole. *Lancet* 1989; **i:** 1017.

Effects on the heart. Prolonged QT interval and torsade de pointes have been reported in 2 patients receiving fluconazole.[1,2]
1. Wassmann S, et al. Long QT syndrome and torsade de pointes in a patient receiving fluconazole. *Ann Intern Med* 1999; **131:** 797.
2. Tholakanahalli VN, et al. Fluconazole-induced torsade de pointes. *Ann Pharmacother* 2001; **35:** 432–4.

Effects on the liver. Although severe hepatic reactions to fluconazole are rare they have been reported, especially in patients with severe underlying diseases or hepatic dysfunction.[1,2] Elevation of liver enzymes is commonly encountered and there have been reports of jaundice associated with fluconazole treatment.[3,4] Hepatic necrosis has been found rarely post mortem in patients with severe underlying disease who had received fluconazole.
1. Wells C, Lever AML. Dose-dependent fluconazole hepatotoxicity proven on biopsy and rechallenge. *J Infect* 1992; **24:** 111–12.
2. Jacobson MA, et al. Fatal acute hepatic necrosis due to fluconazole. *Am J Med* 1994; **96:** 188–90.
3. Holmes J, Clements D. Jaundice in HIV positive haemophiliac. *Lancet* 1989; **i:** 1027.
4. Franklin IM, et al. Fluconazole-induced jaundice. *Lancet* 1990; **336:** 565.

Precautions

Fluconazole should be used with caution in patients with impaired renal or hepatic function. Abnormalities in haematological, hepatic, and renal function tests have been observed in patients with serious underlying diseases.

Teratogenicity has occurred in *animals* given high doses of fluconazole and its use is not recommended in pregnancy (see under Pregnancy, below). It should not be given to breast-feeding women.

Breast feeding. Fluconazole is distributed into breast milk, achieving concentrations similar to those found in maternal plasma, and its use in breast-feeding mothers is not recommended. Similar recommendations have been made for itraconazole and ketoconazole.

Pregnancy. High (toxic) doses of fluconazole, itraconazole, and ketoconazole have been reported to be teratogenic in *rodents.* Although there is little information about the use of these drugs in human pregnancy there is a report of a woman who had received fluconazole 400 mg daily throughout pregnancy and who gave birth to an infant with severe craniofacial and limb abnormalities.[1] The abnormalities resembled those associated with the Antley-Bixler syndrome, a genetic disorder, but a teratogenic effect could not be excluded. Although prescription-event-monitoring studies of fluconazole did not reveal adverse effects on the fetus,[2-4] congenital abnormalities have occurred in infants whose mothers had received high doses of fluconazole for 3 months or more. Data collected by the manufacturer[5] relating to 198 women exposed to itraconazole during the first trimester of pregnancy indicated that the malformation rate for both exposed women and matched controls was within the expected baseline risk for the general population. Nevertheless, the manufacturers recommend that fluconazole, itraconazole, and ketoconazole should be avoided during pregnancy.

Other azole antifungals including butoconazole, clotrimazole, econazole, miconazole, sulconazole, terconazole, and tioconazole are reported to be embryotoxic but not teratogenic in *rodents* given high doses. Many of these drugs are used topically or intravaginally and the systemic absorption from these routes of administration varies. While these drugs may not necessarily be contra-indicated in pregnancy consideration should be given to these potential risks when choosing antifungal therapy for such patients.
1. Lee BE, et al. Congenital malformations in an infant born to a woman treated with fluconazole. *Pediatr Infect Dis J* 1992; **11:** 1062–4.
2. Rubin PC, et al. Fluconazole and pregnancy: results of a prescription event-monitoring study. *Int J Gynecol Obstet* 1992; **37** (suppl): 25–7.
3. Inman W, et al. Safety of fluconazole in the treatment of vaginal candidiasis: a prescription-event monitoring study, with special reference to the outcome of pregnancy. *Eur J Clin Pharmacol* 1994; **46:** 115–18.

4. Sørensen HT, *et al.* Risk of malformations and other outcomes in children exposed to fluconazole in utero. *Br J Clin Pharmacol* 1999; **48:** 234–8.
5. Bar-Oz B, *et al.* Pregnancy outcome after in utero exposure to itraconazole: a prospective cohort study. *Am J Obstet Gynecol* 2000; **183:** 617–20.

Renal impairment. For dose adjustments in renal impairment, see Uses and Administration, below.

Interactions

In general, fewer interactions are considered to occur with fluconazole than with either itraconazole or ketoconazole.

Concomitant administration of rifampicin with fluconazole results in reduced plasma concentrations of fluconazole. Administration of hydrochlorothiazide and fluconazole has resulted in clinically insignificant increases in plasma-fluconazole concentrations.

Fluconazole may interfere with the metabolism of some drugs if given concomitantly, mainly through inhibition of the cytochrome P450 isoenzymes CYP3A4 and CYP2C9. This may account for the reported increases in plasma concentrations of ciclosporin, midazolam, nortriptyline, phenytoin, rifabutin, sulfonylurea hypoglycaemics, tacrolimus, triazolam, warfarin, and zidovudine; reductions in the production of a toxic metabolite of sulfamethoxazole may occur.

Increases in terfenadine concentrations following high doses of fluconazole have been associated with ECG abnormalities. A similar effect may be anticipated with astemizole. Concurrent administration of fluconazole and cisapride could result in increased cisapride concentrations and associated toxicity. The concomitant use of fluconazole with astemizole, cisapride, or terfenadine should be avoided because of the risk of cardiac arrhythmias. Syncope attributed to increased amitriptyline concentrations has occurred when amitriptyline was given with fluconazole.

Fluconazole may also reduce the clearance of theophylline. The concentration of contraceptive steroids has been reported to be both increased and decreased in patients receiving fluconazole and the efficacy of oral contraceptives may be affected.

◊ Reviews of drug interactions with azole antifungals.
1. Baciewicz AM, Baciewicz FA. Ketoconazole and fluconazole drug interactions. *Arch Intern Med* 1993; **153:** 1970–6.
2. Lomaestro BM, Piatek MA. Update on drug interactions with azole antifungal agents. *Ann Pharmacother* 1998; **32:** 915–28.
3. Venkatakrishnan K, *et al.* Effects of the antifungal agents on oxidative drug metabolism: clinical relevance. *Clin Pharmacokinet* 2000; **38:** 111–80.

Antimicrobial Action

Fluconazole is a triazole antifungal drug which in sensitive fungi inhibits cytochrome P450-dependent enzymes resulting in impairment of ergosterol synthesis in fungal cell membranes. It is active against *Blastomyces dermatitidis*, *Candida* spp., *Coccidioides immitis*, *Cryptococcus neoformans*, *Epidermophyton* spp., *Histoplasma capsulatum*, *Microsporum* spp., and *Trichophyton* spp.

Resistance has developed in some *Candida* spp. following long-term prophylaxis with fluconazole, and cross-resistance with other azoles has been reported.

Microbiological interactions. A synergistic antifungal effect was seen *in vitro* with terbinafine and fluconazole against strains of *Candida albicans.*[1] For effects on the antifungal activity of fluconazole when given with amphotericin B, see p.379.
1. Barchiesi F, *et al.* In vitro activities of terbinafine in combination with fluconazole and itraconazole against isolates of Candida albicans with reduced susceptibility to azoles. *Antimicrob Agents Chemother* 1997; **41:** 1812–14.

Resistance. The emergence of strains of *Candida* spp. resistant to fluconazole is increasingly important, particularly in immunocompromised patients receiving long-term prophylaxis with fluconazole.[1] In addition to resistance in *C. albicans*,[2-4] infections with *C. dubliniensis*,[4] *C. glabrata*, and *C. krusei*, all of which may be less sensitive to fluconazole than *C. albicans*, are becoming more common in these patients,[5,6] and secondary resistance of *C. glabrata* has been reported during fluconazole therapy.[7,8] Resistance to fluconazole is reported to occur more frequently than with ketoconazole or itraconazole and may be related to the widespread use of this drug.[3,6] Cross-resistance with other azoles[9,10] and with amphotericin B[11,12] has been reported.

Fluconazole resistance has also been reported in *Cryptococcus neoformans*[13] and *Histoplasma capsulatum*.[14] Histoplasmosis developed during treatment with fluconazole in a patient with HIV infection.[15] Fluconazole-resistant *C. neoformans* has been isolated from an immunocompetent patient who had not been exposed to azole antifungals previously.[16]
1. Rex JH, *et al.* Resistance of Candida species to fluconazole. *Antimicrob Agents Chemother* 1995; **39:** 1–8.
2. Sandven P, *et al.* Susceptibilities of Norwegian Candida albicans strains to fluconazole: emergence of resistance. *Antimicrob Agents Chemother* 1993; **37:** 2443–8.
3. Johnson EM, *et al.* Emergence of azole drug resistance in Candida species from HIV-infected patients receiving prolonged fluconazole therapy for oral candidosis. *J Antimicrob Chemother* 1995; **35:** 103–14.
4. Ruhnke M, *et al.* Development of simultaneous resistance to fluconazole in Candida albicans and Candida dubliniensis in a patient with AIDS. *J Antimicrob Chemother* 2000; **46:** 291–5.
5. Price MF, *et al.* Fluconazole susceptibilities of Candida species and distribution of species recovered from blood cultures over a 5-year period. *Antimicrob Agents Chemother* 1994; **38:** 1422–4.
6. Odds FC. Resistance of yeasts to azole-derivative antifungals. *J Antimicrob Chemother* 1993; **31:** 463–71.
7. Hitchcock CA, *et al.* Fluconazole resistance in Candida glabrata. *Antimicrob Agents Chemother* 1993; **37:** 1962–5.
8. Miyazaki H, *et al.* Fluconazole resistance associated with drug efflux and increased transcription of a drug transporter gene, PDH1, in Candida glabrata. *Antimicrob Agents Chemother* 1998; **42:** 1695–1701.
9. Martinez-Suarez JV, Rodriguez-Tudela JL. Patterns of in vitro activity of itraconazole and imidazole antifungal agents against Candida albicans with decreased susceptibility to fluconazole from Spain. *Antimicrob Agents Chemother* 1995; **39:** 1512–16.
10. Goldman M, *et al.* Does long-term itraconazole prophylaxis result in in vitro azole resistance in mucosal Candida albicans isolates from persons with advanced immunodeficiency virus infection? *Antimicrob Agents Chemother* 2000; **44:** 1585–7.
11. Kelly SL, *et al.* Resistance to fluconazole and amphotericin in Candida albicans from AIDS patients. *Lancet* 1996; **348:** 1523–4.
12. Nolte FS, *et al.* Isolation and characterization of fluconazole- and amphotericin B-resistant Candida albicans from blood of two patients with leukemia. *Antimicrob Agents Chemother* 1997; **41:** 196–9.
13. Venkateswarlu K, *et al.* Fluconazole tolerance in clinical isolates of Cryptococcus neoformans. *Antimicrob Agents Chemother* 1997; **41:** 748–51.
14. Wheat J, *et al.* Hypothesis on the mechanism of resistance to fluconazole in Histoplasma capsulatum. *Antimicrob Agents Chemother* 1997; **41:** 410–14.
15. Pottage JC, Sha BE. Development of histoplasmosis via human immunodeficiency virus infected patient receiving fluconazole. *J Infect Dis* 1991; **164:** 622–3.
16. Omi-Wasserlauf R, *et al.* Fluconazole-resistant Cryptococcus neoformans isolated from an immunocompetent patient without prior exposure to fluconazole. *Clin Infect Dis* 1999; **29:** 1592–3.

Pharmacokinetics

Fluconazole is well absorbed following oral administration, bioavailability from the oral route being 90% or more of that from the intravenous route. Mean peak plasma concentrations of 6.72 µg per mL have been reported in healthy subjects following a 400-mg oral dose. Peak concentrations are reached within 1 to 2 hours of oral administration. Plasma concentrations are proportional to the dose over a range of 50 to 400 mg. Multiple dosing leads to increases in peak plasma concentrations; steady-state concentrations are reached in 6 to 10 days but may be attained on day 2 if a loading dose is given.

Fluconazole is widely distributed and the apparent volume of distribution is close to that of total body water. Concentrations in breast milk, joint fluid, saliva, sputum, vaginal fluids, and peritoneal fluid are similar to those achieved in plasma. Concentrations in the CSF range from 50 to 90% of plasma concentrations, even in the absence of meningeal inflammation. Protein binding is only about 12%.

About 80% or more of a dose is excreted unchanged in the urine and about 11% as metabolites. The elimination half-life of fluconazole is about 30 hours and is increased in patients with impaired renal function. Fluconazole is removed by dialysis.

◊ Reviews.
1. Debruyne D, Ryckelynck J-P. Clinical pharmacokinetics of fluconazole. *Clin Pharmacokinet* 1993; **24:** 10–27.
2. Debruyne D. Clinical pharmacokinetics of fluconazole in superficial and systemic mycoses. *Clin Pharmacokinet* 1997; **33:** 52–77.

Burns. The mean half-life of fluconazole was decreased to 24.4 hours in 9 patients with burns.[1] Fluconazole clearance was 27.5 mL per minute which was 30% higher than that reported in healthy subjects.
1. Boucher BA, *et al.* Fluconazole pharmacokinetics in burn patients. *Antimicrob Agents Chemother* 1998; **42:** 930–3.

Children and neonates. References.
1. Saxén H, *et al.* Pharmacokinetics of fluconazole in very low birth weight infants during the first two weeks of life. *Clin Pharmacol Ther* 1993; **54:** 269–77.
2. Nahata MC, Brady MT. Pharmacokinetics of fluconazole after oral administration in children with human immunodeficiency virus infection. *Eur J Clin Pharmacol* 1995; **48:** 291–3.

Distribution. Salivary concentrations of fluconazole following oral administration should be adequate for the treatment of oropharyngeal and oesophageal candidiasis[1,2] even in patients with AIDS who may have decreased salivation.[3] Treatment failures are more likely to be due to inadequate dosage or resistant organisms than to decreased salivary secretion.[3]

Pharmacologically active concentrations of fluconazole have been detected in scalp hair[4] and nails[5] following oral treatment with conventional daily administration and with once-weekly administration.
1. Force RW, Nahata MC. Salivary concentrations of ketoconazole and fluconazole: implications for drug efficacy in oropharyngeal and esophageal candidiasis. *Ann Pharmacother* 1995; **29:** 10–15.
2. Koks CHW, *et al.* Pharmacokinetics of fluconazole in saliva and plasma after administration of an oral suspension and capsules. *Antimicrob Agents Chemother* 1996; **40:** 1935–7.
3. Garcia-Hermoso D, *et al.* Fluconazole concentrations in saliva from AIDS patients with oropharyngeal candidosis refractory to treatment with fluconazole. *Antimicrob Agents Chemother* 1995; **39:** 656–60.
4. Yeates R, *et al.* Accumulation of fluconazole in scalp hair. *J Clin Pharmacol* 1998; **38:** 138–43.
5. Faergemann J. Pharmacokinetics of fluconazole in skin and nails. *J Am Acad Dermatol* 1999; **40** (suppl): S14–S20.

HIV-infected patients. Plasma clearance of fluconazole may be lower in patients with HIV infection than in immunocompetent patients, and the half-life may be prolonged.[1,2]
1. Tett S, *et al.* Pharmacokinetics and bioavailability of fluconazole in two groups of males with human immunodeficiency virus (HIV) infection compared with those in a group of males without HIV infection. *Antimicrob Agents Chemother* 1995; **39:** 1835–41.
2. McLachlan AJ, Tett SE. Pharmacokinetics of fluconazole in people with HIV infection: a population analysis. *Br J Clin Pharmacol* 1996; **41:** 291–8.

Uses and Administration

Fluconazole is a triazole antifungal used for superficial mucosal (oropharyngeal, oesophageal, or vaginal) candidiasis and for fungal skin infections. It is also given for systemic infections including systemic candidiasis, coccidioidomycosis, and cryptococcosis, and has been tried in blastomycosis, chromoblastomycosis, histoplasmosis, and sporotrichosis. The place of fluconazole in the treatment of fungal infections is discussed under Choice of Antifungal, p.372.

Fluconazole is given by mouth or intravenous infusion in similar doses. For intravenous infusion it is given as a solution containing 2 mg per mL at a rate of 5 to 10 mL per minute. In the USA, a maximum infusion rate of 200 mg (100 mL) per hour is recommended.

For superficial mucosal candidiasis (other than genital candidiasis) the usual dose of fluconazole in the UK is 50 mg daily by mouth, although 100 mg daily may be given if necessary. Treatment usually continues for 7 to 14 days in oropharyngeal candidiasis (except in severely immunocompromised patients), for 14 days in atrophic oral candidiasis associated with dentures, and for 14 to 30 days in other mucosal candidal infections including oesophagitis. Higher doses are recommended in the USA where an initial dose of fluconazole 200 mg is followed by 100 mg daily and where the minimum treatment period is 14 days for oropharyngeal infection, or a minimum of 21 days and at least 14 days after resolution of symptoms for oesophageal infections; doses of up to 400 mg daily may be used for oesophageal candidiasis if necessary.

Fluconazole 150 mg by mouth as a single dose may be used for vaginal candidiasis or candidal balanitis.

Dermatophytosis, pityriasis versicolor, and *Candida* infections of the skin may be treated with fluconazole 50 mg daily by mouth for up to 6 weeks.

Systemic candidiasis, cryptococcal meningitis, and other cryptococcal infections may be treated with fluconazole by mouth or by intravenous infusion; the initial dose is 400 mg followed by 200 to 400 mg daily. Duration of therapy is based on clinical and mycological response, but is usually at least 6 to 8 weeks in cryptococcal meningitis; in the USA, treatment for 10 to 12 weeks after the CSF cultures become negative is recommended. Fluconazole may also be used in daily doses of 100 to 200 mg orally or intravenously to prevent relapse following a primary course of antifungal treatment for acute cryptococcal meningitis in patients with AIDS.

In immunocompromised patients at risk of fungal infections fluconazole may be given prophylactically in a dose of 50 to 400 mg daily by mouth or by intravenous infusion, although long-term prophylaxis has been associated with the emergence of resistant organisms (see below).

Doses for children over 4 weeks of age are 3 mg per kg daily for superficial infections (a loading dose of 6 mg per kg may be used on the first day if necessary), and 6 to 12 mg per kg daily for systemic infections. For prophylaxis in immunocompromised children, a dose of 3 to 12 mg per kg daily may be given. For infants under 2 weeks of age, all these doses should be given once every 72 hours; for those aged between 2 and 4 weeks, the doses should be given every 48 hours. A maximum dose of 400 mg daily should not be exceeded in children, or 12 mg per kg at appropriate intervals in infants.

Patients with renal impairment may require dosage reduction. Normal loading or initial doses should be given on the first day of treatment and subsequent doses of fluconazole should be adjusted according to creatinine clearance. If the creatinine clearance is more than 50 mL per minute, the standard dose can be given. If the creatinine clearance is less than 50 mL per minute and the patient is not receiving dialysis, half the standard dose can be given. Patients on regular haemodialysis should receive a standard dose of fluconazole after every dialysis session. No dosage adjustment is needed in patients with renal impairment given single-dose therapy.

◊ Reviews of fluconazole.
1. Grant SM, Clissold SP. Fluconazole: a review of its pharmacodynamic and pharmacokinetic properties, and therapeutic potential in superficial and systemic mycoses. *Drugs* 1990; **39:** 877–916. Correction. *ibid.* **40:** 862.
2. Kowalsky SF, Dixon DM. Fluconazole: a new antifungal agent. *Clin Pharm* 1991; **10:** 179–94.
3. Goa KL, Barradell LB. Fluconazole: an update of its pharmacodynamic and pharmacokinetic properties and therapeutic use in major superficial and systemic mycoses in immunocompromised patients. *Drugs* 1995; **50:** 658–90.

Administration. HIGH DOSES. Doses of fluconazole of up to 1000 mg daily have been tried in the treatment of cryptococcal meningitis. In a study of 11 patients who received fluconazole 800 to 1000 mg daily intravenously for 3 weeks then orally until the CSF culture became negative, 6 patients had responded at 10 weeks and another 2 improved clinically.[1] Daily doses of up to 800 mg have been used in blastomycosis[2] and coccidioidomycosis,[3] and doses of 10 mg per kg body-weight daily have been tried in disseminated candidiasis.[4]

Once-weekly treatment with fluconazole has been tried in onychomycosis[5] and tinea capitis.[6]
1. Menichetti F, *et al.* High-dose fluconazole therapy for cryptococcal meningitis in patients with AIDS. *Clin Infect Dis* 1996; **22:** 838–40.
2. Pappas PG, *et al.* Treatment of blastomycosis with higher doses of fluconazole. *Clin Infect Dis* 1997; **25:** 200–5.
3. Galgiani JN, *et al.* Infectious Diseases Society of America. Practice guidelines for the treatment of coccidioidomycosis. *Clin Infect Dis* 2000; **30:** 658–61.
4. Graninger W, *et al.* Treatment of Candida albicans fungaemia with fluconazole. *J Infect* 1993; **26:** 133–46.
5. Scher RK, *et al.* Once-weekly fluconazole (150 mg, 300 mg, or 450 mg) in the treatment of distal subungual onychomycosis of the toenail. *J Am Acad Dermatol* 1998; **38:** S77–S86.
6. Gupta AK, *et al.* Once weekly fluconazole is effective in children in the treatment of tinea capitis: a prospective, multicentre study. *Br J Dermatol* 2000; **142:** 965–8.

INTERMITTENT DOSES. Concern has been expressed about the increasingly widespread use of fluconazole[1] and, in particular, about the impact of continuous fluconazole therapy in immunocompromised patients on the development of resistance (see under Antimicrobial Action, above). Nevertheless, fluconazole remains popular for primary and secondary prophylaxis. Some investigators have suggested the use of intermittent doses[2,3] although this could further increase the risk of infections with resistant organisms.
1. Mangino JE, *et al.* When to use fluconazole. *Lancet* 1995; **345:** 6–7.
2. Singh N, *et al.* Low-dose fluconazole as primary prophylaxis for cryptococcal infection in AIDS patients with CD4 cell counts of ≤ 100/mm³: demonstration of efficacy in a prospective, multicenter trial. *Clin Infect Dis* 1996; **23:** 1282–6.
3. Schuman P, *et al.* Weekly fluconazole for the prevention of mucosal candidiasis in women with HIV infection: a randomized, double-blind, placebo-controlled trial. *Ann Intern Med* 1997; **126:** 689–96.

Preparations

Proprietary Preparations (details are given in Part 3)
Aust.: Diflucan; Fungata; *Austral.:* Diflucan; *Belg.:* Diflucan; *Braz.:* Candizol; Fluconal; Flunazol; Lertus; Triazol; Zoltec; *Canad.:* Diflucan; *Denm.:* Diflucan; *Fin.:* Diflucan; *Fr.:* Triflucan; *Ger.:* Diflucan; Fungata; *Hong Kong:* Diflucan; *Irl.:* Diflucan; *Israel:* Diflucan; Trican; Triflucan; *Ital.:* Biozolene; Diflucan; Elazor; *Mex.:* Afungil; Bioxel; Diflucan; Flukenol; Flukezol; Neofomiral; Oxifungol; Waynazol; Zonal; *Neth.:* Diflucan;

Norw.: Diflucan; *NZ:* Diflucan; *Port.:* Diflucan; *S.Afr.:* Diflucan; *Singapore:* Diflucan; *Spain:* Diflucan; Lavisa; Loitin; Solacap; *Swed.:* Diflucan; *Switz.:* Diflucan; *Thai.:* Biozole; Flucozole; Funa; *UK:* Diflucan; *USA:* Diflucan.

Flucytosine   (2582-f)

Flucytosine (BAN, USAN, rINN).

5-FC; Flucytosinum; Ro-2-9915. 5-Fluorocytosine; 4-Amino-5-fluoropyrimidin-2(1H)-one.

$C_4H_4FN_3O = 129.1$.

CAS — 2022-85-7.
ATC — D01AE21; J02AX01.

Pharmacopoeias. In Eur. (see p.vi), *Int., Jpn,* and US.

A solution of flucytosine for intravenous infusion should be stored between 18° and 25°. Precipitation may occur at lower temperatures and decomposition, with the formation of fluorouracil, at higher temperatures.

Pharmacopoeial description

Ph. Eur.: A white or almost white crystalline powder. Sparingly soluble in water; slightly soluble in dehydrated alcohol; practically insoluble in ether. Protect from light.

USP 25: A white to off-white crystalline powder, odourless or with a slight odour. Sparingly soluble in water; slightly soluble in alcohol; practically insoluble in chloroform and in ether. Store in airtight containers. Protect from light.

◊ References.
1. Biondi L, Nairn JG. Stability studies of 5-fluorocytosine in aqueous solutions. *J Parenter Sci Technol* 1985; **39:** 200–4.
2. Biondi L, Nairn JG. Stability of 5-fluorouracil and flucytosine in parenteral solutions. *Can J Hosp Pharm* 1986; **39:** 60–6.
3. McPhail DC, *et al.* Stability and bioavailability of a flucytosine suspension. *Int J Pharm Pract* 1994; **2:** 235–9.
4. Wintermeyer SM, Nahata MC. Stability of flucytosine in an extemporaneously compounded oral liquid. *Am J Health-Syst Pharm* 1996; **53:** 407–9.

Adverse Effects

Side-effects of flucytosine include nausea, vomiting, diarrhoea, and skin rashes. Less frequently reported side-effects include confusion, hallucinations, convulsions, headache, sedation, and vertigo, and also allergic reactions, toxic epidermal necrolysis, and cardiotoxicity. Alterations in liver function tests are generally dose-related and reversible; hepatotoxicity may also occur. Hypokalaemia may occur. There have been a few reports of peripheral neuropathy.

Bone-marrow depression, especially leucopenia and thrombocytopenia, is associated with blood concentrations of flucytosine greater than 100 µg per mL, with concurrent amphotericin B administration, and with renal impairment. Fatal agranulocytosis and aplastic anaemia have been reported.

Effects on the blood. Bone marrow toxicity associated with flucytosine has been attributed to its conversion to fluorouracil, possibly by intestinal flora.[1]
1. Pirmohamed M, *et al.* The role of active metabolites in drug toxicity. *Drug Safety* 1994; **11:** 114–44.

Precautions

Flucytosine should be administered with great care to patients with renal impairment, or with blood disorders or bone marrow depression. Renal and hepatic function and blood counts should be monitored during therapy (at least weekly in patients with renal impairment or blood disorders). In patients with renal impairment, doses should be reduced and blood concentrations of flucytosine should be checked regularly. Monitoring is best done by measuring trough concentrations; thus blood samples should be taken just before an injection of flucytosine. Care should be taken in patients receiving radiation therapy or other drugs which depress bone marrow.

Flucytosine is teratogenic in *rats* and this should be taken into account if pregnant women or those of child-bearing age are to be treated. It should be avoided during breastfeeding.

AIDS. High incidences of bone marrow toxicity have been reported in patients with AIDS during flucytosine therapy.[1] However, in a study in 381 patients, no additional haematotoxicity was reported in patients receiving amphotericin B plus flucytosine compared with those receiving amphotericin B alone.[2] The toxicity could be minimised by monitoring serum concentrations[3] and the British Society for Antimicrobial Chemotherapy has suggested that these should be maintained within 25 to 50 µg per mL in patients with AIDS.[4]
1. Chuck SL, Sande MA. Infections with Cryptococcus neoformans in the acquired immunodeficiency syndrome. *N Engl J Med* 1989; **321:** 794–9.

2. van der Horst CM, *et al.* Treatment of cryptococcal meningitis associated with the acquired immunodeficiency syndrome. *N Engl J Med* 1997; **337:** 15–21.
3. Viviani MA. Flucytosine—what is its future? *J Antimicrob Chemother* 1995; **35:** 241–4.
4. British Society for Antimicrobial Chemotherapy Working Party. Antifungal chemotherapy in patients with acquired immunodeficiency syndrome. *Lancet* 1992; **340:** 648–51.

Renal impairment. For dosage recommendations, see Uses and Administration, below.

Interactions

Flucytosine is commonly given in combination with amphotericin B. Amphotericin B can cause a deterioration in renal function, which can result in raised flucytosine blood concentrations and increased toxicity. However, the two drugs are generally regarded as having synergistic antifungal activity. Cytarabine has been claimed to reduce blood concentrations of flucytosine and to antagonise its antifungal activity, although the evidence has been limited.

Antimicrobial Action

Flucytosine is a fluorinated pyrimidine antifungal. In susceptible fungi it is converted by cytosine deaminase to fluorouracil which is then incorporated in place of uracil into fungal RNA and disrupts protein synthesis. The activity of thymidilate synthetase is also inhibited and this effect interferes with fungal DNA synthesis.

Flucytosine is active against *Candida* spp., *Cryptococcus neoformans*, *Cladosporium* spp., and *Fonsecaea* spp. Some *Aspergillus* spp. have also been reported to be sensitive. There is synergy between flucytosine and amphotericin B against *Candida* spp. and *Cryptococcus neoformans*.

There is a high incidence of primary resistance to flucytosine among isolates of *Candida* spp. and *Cryptococcus neoformans*. Resistance also develops during treatment with flucytosine and has been reported rarely from combination therapy with flucytosine and amphotericin B.

Microbiological interactions. Although flucytosine is generally regarded as having synergistic activity with amphotericin B, antagonism of the *in vitro* antifungal activity of *amphotericin B* against *Candida* spp. by flucytosine has been reported.[1] Enhanced antifungal activity against *Cryptococcus neoformans* has been reported using a combination of flucytosine and *fluconazole* in *animal* studies.[2,3]
1. Martin E, *et al.* Antagonistic effects of fluconazole and 5-fluorocytosine on candidacidal action of amphotericin B in human serum. *Antimicrob Agents Chemother* 1994; **38:** 1331–8.
2. Larsen RA, *et al.* Effect of fluconazole on fungicidal activity of flucytosine in murine cryptococcal meningitis. *Antimicrob Agents Chemother* 1996; **40:** 2178–82.
3. Nguyen MH, *et al.* Combination therapy with fluconazole and flucytosine in the murine model of cryptococcal meningitis. *Antimicrob Agents Chemother* 1997; **41:** 1120–3.

Pharmacokinetics

Flucytosine is absorbed rapidly and almost completely from the gastrointestinal tract. Bioavailability is reported to be 78 to 89%. After oral doses of 37.5 mg per kg body-weight every 6 hours, peak plasma concentrations of 70 to 80 µg per mL have been achieved within 2 hours; similar concentrations have been achieved but more rapidly, after an intravenous dose. The plasma-flucytosine concentration for optimum response is 25 to 50 µg per mL. Flucytosine is distributed widely through the body tissues and fluids; concentrations in the CSF have been reported to be 65 to 90% of those in serum. About 2 to 4% of flucytosine is protein bound.

About 90% of a dose is excreted unchanged by glomerular filtration; a small amount of flucytosine may be metabolised to fluorouracil. The small amount of an oral dose of flucytosine not absorbed from the gastrointestinal tract is eliminated unchanged in the faeces. The elimination half-life is 2.5 to 6 hours in patients with normal renal function but increases with decreasing renal function. Flucytosine is removed by haemodialysis or peritoneal dialysis.

◊ References.
1. Daneshmend TK, Warnock DW. Clinical pharmacokinetics of systemic antifungal agents. *Clin Pharmacokinet* 1983; **8:** 17–42.
2. Baley JE, *et al.* Pharmacokinetics, outcome of treatment, and toxic effects of amphotericin B and 5-fluorocytosine in neonates. *J Pediatr* 1990; **116:** 791–7.

The symbol † denotes a preparation no longer actively marketed

Uses and Administration

Flucytosine is a fluorinated pyrimidine antifungal used in the treatment of systemic fungal infections. It is mainly used in combination with amphotericin B or fluconazole in the treatment of severe systemic candidiasis and cryptococcal meningitis. It has also been tried in other infections due to susceptible fungi including chromoblastomycosis. The various treatments for the above infections are discussed under Choice of Antifungal, p.372.

Flucytosine is given by *intravenous infusion* as a 1% solution over 20 to 40 minutes. The usual dose is 200 mg per kg body-weight daily in 4 divided doses; a dose of 100 to 150 mg per kg daily may be sufficient in some patients. Dosage should be adjusted to produce plasma concentrations of 25 to 50 µg per mL. This is particularly important in patients with AIDS who are at increased risk of bone marrow toxicity. Parenteral treatment is rarely given for more than 7 days, except for cryptococcal meningitis when it is continued for at least 4 months.

Because flucytosine is mainly excreted by the kidneys, the dose must be adjusted in patients with renal impairment. Doses of 50 mg per kg every 12 hours should be used in patients with a creatinine clearance of 20 to 40 mL per minute and similar doses every 24 hours in patients with a creatinine clearance of 10 to 20 mL per minute. Patients with a creatinine clearance of less than 10 mL per minute may be given a single dose of 50 mg per kg; further doses should then be based on plasma concentrations which should not exceed 80 µg per mL.

Flucytosine is given by *mouth* in usual doses of 50 to 150 mg per kg daily in four divided doses. Again, blood concentrations should be monitored and dosage adjusted in patients with renal impairment to avoid accumulation of the drug.

Flucytosine has been used *topically*, but such use may increase problems of resistance.

◊ Reviews.
1. Viviani MA. Flucytosine—what is its future? *J Antimicrob Chemother* 1995; **35:** 241–4.
2. Summers KK, *et al.* Therapeutic drug monitoring of systemic antifungal therapy. *J Antimicrob Chemother* 1997; **40:** 753–64.
3. Vermes A, *et al.* Flucytosine: a review of its pharmacology, clinical indications, pharmacokinetics, toxicity and drug interactions. *J Antimicrob Chemother* 2000; **46:** 171–9.

Preparations

BP 2001: Flucytosine Tablets;
USP 25: Flucytosine Capsules.

Proprietary Preparations (details are given in Part 3)
Aust.: Ancotil; **Austral.:** Ancotil; **Braz.:** Ancotil; **Denm.:** Ancotil; **Fr.:** Ancotil; **Ger.:** Ancotil; **Hong Kong:** Ancotil; **Irl.:** Alcobon; Ancotil; **Ital.:** Ancotil; **Neth.:** Ancotil†; **Norw.:** Ancotil†; **NZ:** Alcobon; **Singapore:** Ancotil; **Swed.:** Ancotil; **Switz.:** Ancotil; **UK:** Ancotil; **USA:** Ancobon.

Flutrimazole (10991-c)

Flutrimazole *(BAN, rINN)*.

Flutrimazolum; UR-4056. 1-[o-Fluoro-α-(p-fluorophenyl)-α-phenylbenzyl]imidazole; *(RS)*-1-(2,4′-Difluorotrityl)imidazole.
$C_{22}H_{16}F_2N_2 = 346.4$.
CAS — 119006-77-8.
ATC — D01AC16.

Pharmacopoeias. In *Eur.* (see p.vi).

Pharmacopoeial description

Ph. Eur.: A white or almost white powder. Practically insoluble in water; soluble in methyl alcohol; freely soluble in tetrahydrofuran. Protect from light.

Profile

Flutrimazole is an imidazole antifungal used topically in the treatment of superficial fungal infections.

The need for caution when using an azole antifungal in pregnant or lactating patients is discussed under Fluconazole, p.383.

Preparations

Proprietary Preparations (details are given in Part 3)
Spain: Flusporan; Funcenal; Micetal.

Genaconazole (10423-q)

Sch-39304; SM-8668. [R-(R*,R*)]-α-(2,4-Difluorophenyl)-α[1-(methylsulphonyl)ethyl]-1H-1,2,4-triazole-1-ethanol.
$C_{13}H_{15}F_2N_3O_3S = 331.3$.
CAS — 121650-83-7.

Profile

Genaconazole is a triazole antifungal that has been investigated for systemic use.

Griseofulvin (2561-k)

Griseofulvin *(BAN, rINN)*.

Curling Factor; Griseofulvina; Griseofulvinum. (2S,4′R)-7-Chloro-2′,4,6-trimethoxy-4′-methylspiro[benzofuran-2(3H),3′-cyclohexene]-3,6′-dione.
$C_{17}H_{17}ClO_6 = 352.8$.
CAS — 126-07-8.
ATC — D01AA08; D01BA01.

Pharmacopoeias. In *Chin.*, *Eur.* (see p.vi), *Int.*, *Jpn*, *Pol.*, and *US*.

Pharmacopoeial description

Ph. Eur.: An antifungal substance produced by the growth of certain strains of *Penicillium griseofulvum*, or by any other means. It is a white or yellowish-white powder. The particles are generally up to 5 µm in maximum dimension, though larger particles, which may occasionally exceed 30 µm, may be present. It contains 97 to 102% of $C_{17}H_{17}ClO_6$, calculated on the dried substance.

Practically insoluble in water; slightly soluble in dehydrated alcohol and in methyl alcohol; freely soluble in dimethylformamide and in tetrachloroethane.

USP 25: A white to creamy-white, odourless powder, in which particles of the order of 4 µm in diameter predominate. It has a potency of not less than 900 µg of $C_{17}H_{17}ClO_6$ per mg. Very slightly soluble in water; sparingly soluble in alcohol; soluble in acetone, in chloroform, and in dimethylformamide. Store in airtight containers.

Adverse Effects

Side-effects are usually mild and transient and consist of headache, skin rashes and urticaria, dry mouth, an altered sensation of taste, and gastrointestinal disturbances. Angioedema, erythema multiforme, toxic epidermal necrolysis, proteinuria, leucopenia and other blood dyscrasias, oral candidiasis, peripheral neuropathy, photosensitisation, and severe headache have been reported occasionally. Depression, confusion, dizziness, insomnia, and fatigue have also been reported. Griseofulvin may precipitate or aggravate systemic lupus erythematosus.

There have been a few reports of hepatotoxicity attributed to griseofulvin.

Effects on the skin. A report of fatal toxic epidermal necrolysis in a 19-year-old woman.[1] The reaction was attributed to griseofulvin which she had taken for 6 days; she had also received metronidazole for one day. Erythema multiforme occurred in 3 patients taking griseofulvin for 3 to 10 days.[2]

1. Mion G, *et al.* Fatal toxic epidermal necrolysis after griseofulvin. *Lancet* 1989; **ii:** 1331.
2. Rustin MHA, *et al.* Erythema multiforme due to griseofulvin. *Br J Dermatol* 1989; **120:** 455–8.

Precautions

Griseofulvin is contra-indicated in patients with severe liver disease or systemic lupus erythematosus.

Griseofulvin is embryotoxic and teratogenic in *rats*. It is contra-indicated in pregnancy. Women should not become pregnant during, or within 1 month of stopping, griseofulvin treatment. Since griseofulvin may reduce the effectiveness of oral contraceptives, additional contraceptive precautions should be taken during this time. The manufacturers also warn that men receiving griseofulvin should not father children within 6 months of treatment. The warning is based on data from *in-vitro* and *in-vivo* studies using mammalian cells which demonstrated aneuploidy.

Griseofulvin may impair the ability to drive or operate machinery, and has been reported to enhance the effects of alcohol.

Porphyria. Griseofulvin has been associated with acute attacks of porphyria and is considered unsafe in porphyric patients.

Pregnancy. The US manufacturers report isolated cases of conjoined twins following griseofulvin treatment during the first trimester of pregnancy.

Interactions

Phenobarbital has been reported to decrease the gastrointestinal absorption of griseofulvin. Plasma concentrations of griseofulvin have also been reported to be reduced by concomitant administration of drugs that induce metabolising enzymes such as phenylbutazone and hypnotics.

Griseofulvin may increase the rate of metabolism and diminish the effects of some drugs such as coumarin anticoagulants and oral contraceptives.

Griseofulvin may enhance the effects of alcohol.

Alcohol. In addition to reports of griseofulvin enhancing the effects of alcohol, a severe disulfiram-like reaction to alcohol has been reported in a patient taking griseofulvin.[1]

1. Fett DL, Vukov LF. An unusual case of severe griseofulvin-alcohol interaction. *Ann Emerg Med* 1994; **24:** 95–7.

Bromocriptine. For a report that griseofulvin can block the response to bromocriptine, see p.1166.

Salicylates. Griseofulvin has been reported to reduce plasma concentrations of salicylate in a patient taking aspirin, see p.16.

Antimicrobial Action

Griseofulvin is a fungistatic antibiotic which inhibits fungal cell division by disruption of the mitotic spindle structure. It may also interfere with DNA production. It is active against the common dermatophytes, including some species of *Epidermophyton*, *Microsporum*, or *Trichophyton*.

Pharmacokinetics

Absorption of griseofulvin from the gastrointestinal tract is variable and incomplete, but is enhanced by reducing the particle size and by administration with a fatty meal. Peak plasma concentrations are reached within 4 hours and are maintained for 10 to 20 hours.

Griseofulvin is about 84% bound to plasma proteins. It is deposited in keratin precursor cells and is concentrated in the stratum corneum of the skin and in the nails and hair, thus preventing fungal invasion of newly formed cells. Concentrations of 12 to 25 µg per g are maintained in skin during long-term administration, while concurrent plasma concentrations remain at about 1 to 2 µg per mL. Griseofulvin has an elimination half-life of 9 to 24 hours, and is metabolised by the liver mainly to 6-demethylgriseofulvin and its glucuronide conjugate which are excreted in the urine. A large amount of a dose of griseofulvin of reduced particle size appears unchanged in the faeces; less than 1% is excreted unchanged in the urine; some is excreted in the sweat.

Uses and Administration

Griseofulvin is an antifungal administered by mouth in the treatment of dermatophyte infections. It is generally given for such infections that involve the scalp, hair, nails, and skin and which do not respond to topical treatment (see p.376); infections of the soles of the feet, the palms of the hands, and the nails respond slowly.

The usual dose of griseofulvin is 0.5 to 1 g daily in single or divided doses; children may be given 10 mg per kg body-weight daily. These recommended doses are for preparations of griseofulvin of reduced particle size, sometimes known as microcrystalline or microsize griseofulvin, but the doses have been reduced by about one-third when preparations, available in some countries, containing ultramicrocrystalline or ultramicrosize griseofulvin are used. Griseofulvin is probably best given with or after meals.

The duration of treatment depends on the thickness of the keratin layer: 2 to 6 weeks for infections of the hair and skin, up to 6 months for infections of the fingernails, and 12 months or more for infections of the toenails.

Administration. Although griseofulvin is usually given systemically, beneficial responses have been reported with some topical formulations[1,2] in fungal skin infections.

1. Macasaet EN, Pert P. Topical (1%) solution of griseofulvin in the treatment of tinea corporis. *Br J Dermatol* 1991; **124:** 110–11.
2. Aly R, *et al.* Topical griseofulvin in the treatment of dermatophytoses. *Clin Exp Dermatol* 1994; **19:** 43–6.

Non-infective skin disorders. Lichen planus is usually treated with corticosteroids, ciclosporin, or retinoids (see p.1106) but griseofulvin has been suggested as an alternative to topical corticosteroids in erosive disease.[1] However, some researchers have found it to be of no value.[2]

Dramatic responses of pigmented purpuric dermatoses to griseofulvin 500 to 750 mg daily have been reported in 5 patients.[3]

1. Lamey P-J, Lewis MAO. Oral medicine in practice: white patches. *Br Dent J* 1990; **168:** 147–52.
2. Bagan JV, *et al.* Treatment of lichen planus with griseofulvin. *Oral Surg Oral Med Oral Pathol* 1985; **60:** 608–10.
3. Tamaki K, *et al.* Successful treatment of pigmented purpuric dermatosis with griseofulvin. *Br J Dermatol* 1995; **132:** 159–60.

Preparations

BP 2001: Griseofulvin Tablets;
USP 25: Griseofulvin Capsules; Griseofulvin Oral Suspension; Griseofulvin Tablets; Ultramicrosize Griseofulvin Tablets.

Proprietary Preparations (details are given in Part 3)
Aust.: Griseomed; Grisovin; *Austral.:* Fulcin; Griseostatin; Grisovin; *Braz.:* Fulcin; Sporostatin; *Canad.:* Fulvicin; Grisovin FP†; *Denm.:* Fulcin; *Fin.:* Fulcin; *Fr.:* Fulcine†; Grisefuline; *Ger.:* Fulcin S; Gricin; Griseo; Likuden M; *Hong Kong:* Fulcin; Griseostatin; Grisovin; *Irl.:* Fulcin; *Israel:* Grifulin; *Ital.:* Fulcin; Grisovina FP; *Mex.:* Fulcin; Fulvina; Griseoful; Grisovin; *Neth.:* Fulcin†; *Norw.:* Fulcin; Lamoryl†; *NZ:* Grisovin; *Port.:* Fulcin; Grisomicon; Grisovin; *S.Afr.:* Fulcin; Grisovin†; Microcidal; *Singapore:* Erlivin; Fulcin; Grivin; Krisovin; Medofulvin; *Spain:* Fulcin; Greosin; *Swed.:* Fulcin; Lamoryl†; *Switz.:* Fulcin; Grisol; *Thai.:* Fulcin; Grifulvin; Grisflavin; Grisovin; Grivin; Neofulvin; Trivanex; *UK:* Fulcin†; Grisovin; *USA:* Fulvicin; Grifulvin V; Gris-PEG; Grisactin.

Hachimycin (2583-d)

Hachimycin *(BAN, pINN).*
Trichomycin; Trichomycinum.
CAS — 1394-02-1.
ATC — D01AA03; G01AA06; J02AA02.
Pharmacopoeias. In Jpn.

Profile

Hachimycin is a polyene antifungal antibiotic produced by *Streptomyces hachijoensis.* It has been used locally and by mouth in the treatment of candidiasis, in the protozoal infection trichomoniasis, and in some fungal skin infections including those caused by *Trichophyton* spp.

Haloprogin (2585-h)

Haloprogin *(USAN, rINN).*
M-1028; NSC-100071. 3-Iodoprop-2-ynyl 2,4,5-trichlorophenyl ether.
$C_9H_4Cl_3IO = 361.4.$
CAS — 777-11-7.
ATC — D01AE11.

Adverse Effects

Local reactions may occur and include irritation, pruritus, and vesiculation.

Antimicrobial Action

Haloprogin is reported to inhibit *Epidermophyton, Microsporum, Trichophyton,* and *Candida* spp. and *Malassezia furfur.*

Uses and Administration

Haloprogin is an antifungal used in the treatment of dermatophytosis and pityriasis versicolor. It is applied topically as a 1% cream or solution twice daily for 2 to 4 weeks.

Preparations

Proprietary Preparations (details are given in Part 3)
USA: Halotex.

Hydroxystilbamidine Isetionate (2588-v)

Hydroxystilbamidine Isetionate *(BANM, rINNM).*
Hydroxystilbamidine Isethionate. 2-Hydroxystilbene-4,4′-dicarboxamidine bis(2-hydroxyethanesulphonate).
$C_{16}H_{16}N_4O,2C_2H_6O_4S = 532.6.$
CAS — 495-99-8 (hydroxystilbamidine); 533-22-2 (hydroxystilbamidine isetionate).

Profile

Hydroxystilbamidine isetionate is an antifungal formerly used in the treatment of blastomycosis and in the protozoal infection leishmaniasis.

Isoconazole (11423-z)

Isoconazole *(BAN, USAN, rINN).*
Isoconazolum. 1-[2,4-Dichloro-β-(2,6-dichlorobenzyloxy)phenethyl]imidazole.
$C_{18}H_{14}Cl_4N_2O = 416.1.$
CAS — 27523-40-6.
ATC — D01AC05; G01AF07.
Pharmacopoeias. In Eur. (see p.vi).

The symbol † denotes a preparation no longer actively marketed

Pharmacopoeial description

Ph. Eur.: A white or almost white powder. Practically insoluble in water; freely soluble in alcohol; very soluble in methyl alcohol. Protect from light.

Isoconazole Nitrate (12868-g)

Isoconazole Nitrate *(BANM, rINNM).*
Isoconazoli Nitras; R-15454.
$C_{18}H_{14}Cl_4N_2O,HNO_3 = 479.1.$
CAS — 24168-96-5 (isoconazole mononitrate); 40036-10-0 (isoconazole nitrate).
Pharmacopoeias. In Eur. (see p.vi).

Pharmacopoeial description

Ph. Eur.: A white or almost white powder. Very slightly soluble in water; slightly soluble in alcohol; soluble in methyl alcohol. Protect from light.

Adverse Effects and Precautions

Local reactions including burning or itching may occur following the application of isoconazole.

Intravaginal preparations of azole antifungals may damage latex contraceptives and additional contraceptive measures are therefore necessary during local administration of isoconazole.

The need for caution when using an azole antifungal in pregnant or lactating patients is discussed under Fluconazole, p.383.

Antimicrobial Action

Isoconazole is an imidazole antifungal active against a wide spectrum of fungi including *Candida* spp., dermatophytes, and *Malassezia furfur.* It is also active against some Gram-positive bacteria.

Uses and Administration

Isoconazole nitrate is an imidazole antifungal used locally in the treatment of vaginal mycoses, particularly due to *Candida* spp. (p.372) and in fungal skin infections (p.376). For vaginal infections it is usually administered in a single dose of 600 mg or 300 mg daily for 3 days, in the form of pessaries. For skin infections a 2% cream or other topical formulation has been used.

Preparations

BP 2001: Isoconazole Pessaries.

Proprietary Preparations (details are given in Part 3)
Aust.: Gyno-Travogen; Travogen; *Belg.:* Gyno-Travogen†; Travogen; *Braz.:* Gyno Icaden; Gyno-Mycel; Icaden; Mycel; *Fr.:* Fazol; Fazol G; *Ger.:* Travogen; Gyno-Travogen; Travogen; *Hong Kong:* Gyno-Travogen; Travogen; *Israel:* Gyno-Travogen; Isogen; *Ital.:* Isogyn; Travogen; *Mex.:* Icaden; *NZ:* Gyno-Travogen; *Port.:* Gino-Travogen; *Singapore:* Gyno-Travogen; Travogen; *Switz.:* Gyno-Travogen; Travogen; *Thai.:* Nacozil; Travogen; *UK:* Travogyn†.

Multi-ingredient: *Aust.:* Travocort; *Belg.:* Travocort; *Ger.:* Bi-Vaspit; Travocort; *Hong Kong:* Travocort; *Irl.:* Travocort; *Israel:* Isocort; *Ital.:* Travocort; *Mex.:* Scheriderm; *Port.:* Travocort; *S.Afr.:* Travocort; *Singapore:* Travocort; *Switz.:* Travocort; *Thai.:* Travocort.

Itraconazole (18657-x)

Itraconazole *(BAN, USAN, rINN).*
Itraconazolum; Oriconazole; R-51211. (±)-2-sec-Butyl-4-[4-(4-{4-[(2R*,4S*)-2-(2,4-dichlorophenyl)-2-(1H-1,2,4-triazol-1-ylmethyl)-1,3-dioxolan-4-ylmethoxy]phenyl}-piperazin-1-yl)phenyl]-2,4-dihydro-1,2,4-triazol-3-one.
$C_{35}H_{38}Cl_2N_8O_4 = 705.6.$
CAS — 84625-61-6.
ATC — J02AC02.
Pharmacopoeias. In Eur. (see p.vi).

Pharmacopoeial description

Ph. Eur.: A white or almost white powder. Practically insoluble in water; very slightly soluble in alcohol; freely soluble in dichloromethane; sparingly soluble in tetrahydrofuran. Protect from light.

Adverse Effects

The most common adverse effects associated with itraconazole include dyspepsia, abdominal pain, nausea, constipation, diarrhoea (with the oral liquid), headache, and dizziness. Others include allergic reactions such as pruritus, rash, urticaria, and angioedema. Isolated cases of the Stevens-Johnson syndrome have been associated with itraconazole.

An increase in liver enzyme values has occurred in some patients and cases of hepatitis and cholestatic jaundice have been observed, especially in those treated for more than one month. There have been rare cases of liver failure and death.

Heart failure and pulmonary oedema have been reported rarely and serious cardiovascular events including arrhythmias and sudden death have been

attributed to drug interactions in patients receiving itraconazole (see Interactions, below).

Alopecia, oedema, and hypokalaemia have also been associated with prolonged treatment. Menstrual disorders and peripheral neuropathy have been reported in a few patients.

◊ Itraconazole 50 to 400 mg daily for a median of 5 months was considered to be well tolerated in 189 patients with systemic fungal infections.[1] Eighty-six patients had underlying disease including 49 with AIDS, 16 with diabetes, and 23 with malignancy. Nausea and vomiting occurred in 19 patients, hypertriglyceridaemia in 16, hypokalaemia in 11, and elevated liver enzyme values in 13. The role of itraconazole in hypertriglyceridaemia could not be assessed because all the samples were not drawn in the fasting state and hypertriglyceridaemia is a complication of HIV infection. Gynaecomastia occurred in 2 patients, 1 receiving concurrent spironolactone. Rash occurred in 4 patients.

Of 49 patients receiving 100 to 400 mg itraconazole daily for up to 39 months, 23 patients did not experience adverse effects during treatment.[2] Six patients had nausea and vomiting. Five patients developed oedema and 2 developed hypertension; 3 of the patients who developed oedema and 1 who became hypertensive were diabetic. Three patients discontinued itraconazole; 1 due to vomiting, 1 to leucopenia, and 1 to nephrotic syndrome. The patient with nephrotic syndrome had pre-existing oedema and hypertension; the syndrome cleared when itraconazole was discontinued.

1. Tucker RM, *et al.* Adverse events associated with itraconazole in 189 patients on chronic therapy. *J Antimicrob Chemother* 1990; **26:** 561–6.
2. Graybill JR, *et al.* Itraconazole treatment of coccidioidomycosis. *Am J Med* 1990; **89:** 282–90.

Effects on the heart. Between September 1992, when itraconazole was approved in the USA, and April 2001, the FDA had received 58 reports of potential cases of heart failure associated with itraconazole.[1] Twenty-eight patients were admitted to hospital and 13 died. However, a causal relationship was difficult to prove. Overall, 43 patients had risk factors or diseases which might confound an association between the use of itraconazole and development of heart failure. Unpublished studies in *dogs* and humans had suggested a negative inotropic effect with intravenous itraconazole.

In August 2001, the UK Committee on Safety of Medicines (CSM) published a similar alert.[2] By this time, approximately 67 million patients worldwide had received itraconazole and there had been 75 spontaneously reported cases of suspected heart failure and an additional 63 reports of oedema suggestive of heart failure associated with oral formulations; there had been only 1 report of suspected heart failure in the UK. The CSM considered that the risk of heart failure with itraconazole was low, especially in young healthy patients receiving short courses of treatment (e.g. for vulvovaginal candidiasis). However, the risks appeared to be higher for older patients, patients with pre-existing heart disease or risk factors for heart failure, and for those receiving high doses and longer treatment courses (e.g. for onychomycosis).

The CSM[2] therefore advised caution when prescribing itraconazole to patients at risk of heart failure, whereas the FDA[1] contra-indicated it for the treatment of onychomycosis in patients with evidence of ventricular dysfunction.

1. Ahmad SR, *et al.* Congestive heart failure associated with itraconazole. *Lancet* 2001; **357:** 1766–7.
2. Committee on Safety of Medicines. Cardiodepressant effect of itraconazole (Sporanox). *Current Problems* 2001; **27:** 11–12.

Precautions

Itraconazole has caused abnormalities in fetal development in *rodents* and is therefore contra-indicated in pregnancy. Breast feeding while receiving itraconazole is not recommended although only small amounts of itraconazole are distributed into breast milk. For further information, see under Pregnancy in Fluconazole, Precautions, p.383.

Itraconazole should be avoided in patients with liver disease. Liver function should be monitored if treatment lasts more than one month or if there are symptoms suggestive of hepatitis. Treatment should be stopped if abnormal liver function is detected. Plasma-itraconazole concentrations should be monitored in patients with active liver disease and the dosage adjusted if necessary. Dose adjustments may also be required in some patients with renal insufficiency, for example those receiving continuous ambulatory peritoneal dialysis. Intravenous administration is not recommended in patients with a creatinine clearance of less than 30 mL per minute. Itraconazole should be discontinued if neuropathy develops.

Itraconazole should not be used for the treatment of less severe fungal infections such as onychomycosis in patients with evidence of, or a history of, ventricular dysfunction such as heart failure.

Hypochlorhydria, which may be present in patients with AIDS, can reduce absorption of itraconazole. In this case absorption may be improved by administering itraconazole with an acidic drink, such as a cola beverage.

Interactions
Enzyme-inducing drugs such as carbamazepine, isoniazid, nevirapine, phenobarbital, phenytoin, rifabutin, or rifampicin may decrease plasma concentrations of itraconazole. Conversely, enzyme inhibitors such as clarithromycin, erythromycin, indinavir, or ritonavir may increase plasma concentrations of itraconazole. Concomitant administration of drugs that reduce stomach acidity, such as antimuscarinics, antacids, proton pump inhibitors, and histamine H_2-receptor antagonists, may reduce the absorption of itraconazole.

Itraconazole may interfere with drugs metabolised by hepatic microsomal enzymes, especially the cytochrome P450 isoenzyme CYP3A4, hence the warnings that plasma concentrations of astemizole, ciclosporin, cisapride, dihydropyridine calcium-channel blockers, such as felodipine, midazolam, pimozide, quinidine, sildenafil, sirolimus, statins such as atorvastatin, lovastatin or simvastatin, tacrolimus, terfenadine, triazolam, verapamil, and warfarin may be increased. Concentrations of HIV-protease inhibitors such as indinavir or ritonavir may also be increased; itraconazole plasma concentrations may be increased in turn. Other drugs that may be affected include alfentanil, alprazolam, buspirone, busulfan, carbamazepine, diazepam, digoxin, docetaxel, methylprednisolone, oral hypoglycaemics, rifabutin, trimetrexate, and the vinca alkaloids. The efficacy of oral contraceptives might be reduced.

There is a risk of cardiac arrhythmias if itraconazole is used with astemizole, cisapride, dofetilide, pimozide, quinidine, or terfenadine and such combinations should be avoided.

◊ For reviews of drug interactions with azole antifungals, see Fluconazole, p.384.

Metal ions. Didanosine in a formulation containing aluminium and magnesium ion buffering agents could reduce the absorption of itraconazole due to the resultant increase in gastric pH.[1]
1. Moreno F, *et al.* Itraconazole-didanosine excipient interaction. *JAMA* 1993; **269:** 1508.

Antimicrobial Action
Itraconazole is a triazole antifungal drug which in sensitive fungi inhibits cytochrome P450-dependent enzymes resulting in impairment of ergosterol synthesis in fungal cell membranes. It has a slightly wider spectrum of activity than ketoconazole. It is active against *Aspergillus* spp., *Blastomyces dermatitidis*, *Candida* spp., *Coccidioides immitis*, *Cryptococcus neoformans*, *Epidermophyton* spp., *Histoplasma capsulatum*, *Malassezia furfur*, *Microsporum* spp., *Paracoccidioides brasiliensis*, *Sporothrix schenckii*, and *Trichophyton* spp. Itraconazole also has some antiprotozoal activity against *Leishmania* spp.

Acquired resistance to itraconazole is rare but ketoconazole-resistant strains of *Candida albicans* have been found to be cross resistant to itraconazole.

Microbiological interactions. Synergistic antifungal effects were seen *in vitro* with terbinafine and itraconazole against strains of *Candida albicans*[1] and *Scedosporium prolificans*.[2] For effects on the antifungal activity of azoles when given with amphotericin B, see p.379.
1. Barchiesi F, *et al.* In vitro activities of terbinafine in combination with fluconazole and itraconazole against isolates of Candida albicans with reduced susceptibility to azoles. *Antimicrob Agents Chemother* 1997; **41:** 1812–14.
2. Meletiadis J, *et al.* In vitro interaction of terbinafine with itraconazole against clinical isolates of Scedosporium prolificans. *Antimicrob Agents Chemother* 2000; **44:** 470–2.

Resistance. For a discussion of increasing resistance of *Candida* spp. to azoles see Fluconazole, Antimicrobial Action, p.384. Decreased susceptibility to itraconazole and cross-resistance to fluconazole has been reported in *C. albicans* isolat-

ed from patients with AIDS receiving long-term prophylaxis with itraconazole.[1] *Aspergillus fumigatus* resistant to itraconazole has also been identified.[2]
1. Goldman M, *et al.* Does long-term itraconazole prophylaxis result in in vitro azole resistance in mucosal Candida albicans isolates from persons with advanced human immunodeficiency virus infection? *Antimicrob Agents Chemother* 2000; **44:** 1585–7.
2. Denning DW, *et al.* Itraconazole resistance in Aspergillus fumigatus. *Antimicrob Agents Chemother* 1997; **41:** 1364–8.

Pharmacokinetics
Itraconazole is absorbed from the gastrointestinal tract when administered by mouth either as capsules containing itraconazole coated onto sugar spheres or as an oral liquid formulated with hydroxypropyl-β-cyclodextrin. Absorption from the capsule formulation is enhanced by an acidic gastric environment and is greatest when doses are taken with food; absorption from the oral liquid is not dependent on an acid environment, and absorption is greatest in the fasting state. Peak plasma concentrations are achieved between 1.5 and 5 hours after a dose of either formulation, and steady state is reached within 15 days during daily dosing. Peak plasma concentrations at steady state of about 2 μg per mL have been reported following daily doses of 200 mg.

Bioavailability increases with doses of 100 to 400 mg in such a manner as to suggest that itraconazole undergoes saturable metabolism. Itraconazole is highly protein bound; only 0.2% circulates as free drug. Itraconazole is widely distributed but only small amounts diffuse into the CSF. Concentrations attained in the skin, sebum, pus, and many organs and tissues are several times higher than simultaneous plasma concentrations. Therapeutic concentrations of itraconazole remain in the skin and mucous membranes for 1 to 4 weeks after the drug is discontinued. Small amounts are distributed into breast milk.

Itraconazole is metabolised in the liver predominantly by cytochrome P450 isoenzyme CYP3A4. The major metabolite, hydroxyitraconazole, has antifungal activity comparable with that of itraconazole. Itraconazole is also excreted as inactive metabolites in the bile or urine; 3 to 18% is excreted in the faeces as unchanged drug. Small amounts are eliminated in the stratum corneum and hair. Itraconazole is not removed by dialysis.

The elimination half-life following a single 100-mg dose has been reported as 20 hours; the half-life increases to 30 hours with continued administration.

◊ References.
1. Baelaert J, *et al.* Itraconazole pharmacokinetics in patients with renal dysfunction. *Antimicrob Agents Chemother* 1988; **32:** 1595–7.
2. Cauwenbergh G, *et al.* Pharmacokinetic profile of orally administered itraconazole in human skin. *J Am Acad Dermatol* 1988; **18:** 263–8.
3. Zimmermann T, *et al.* Influence of concomitant food intake on the oral absorption of two triazole antifungal agents, itraconazole and fluconazole. *Eur J Clin Pharmacol* 1994; **46:** 147–50.
4. Coronel B, *et al.* Itraconazole concentrations during continuous haemodiafiltration. *J Antimicrob Chemother* 1994; **34:** 448–9.
5. Patterson TF, *et al.* Systemic availability of itraconazole in lung transplantation. *Antimicrob Agents Chemother* 1996; **40:** 2217–20.
6. Zhou H, *et al.* A pharmacokinetic study of intravenous itraconazole followed by oral administration of itraconazole capsules in patients with advanced human immunodeficiency virus infection. *J Clin Pharmacol* 1998; **38:** 593–602.
7. Poirier J-M, Cheymol G. Optimisation of itraconazole therapy using target drug concentrations. *Clin Pharmacokinet* 1998; **35:** 461–73.

Bioavailability. The bioavailability of extemporaneously prepared oral liquid formulations of itraconazole has generally been poor.[1-3] However, a formulation with hydroxypropyl-β-cyclodextrin, which is available commercially, has been shown to have good bioavailability in both healthy subjects[4] and patients.[5-8]
1. Kintzel PE, *et al.* Low itraconazole serum concentrations following administration of itraconazole suspension to critically ill allogeneic bone marrow transplant recipients. *Ann Pharmacother* 1995; **29:** 140–3.
2. Villarreal JD, Erush SC. Bioavailability of itraconazole from oral liquids in question. *Am J Health-Syst Pharm* 1995; **52:** 1707–8.
3. Christensen KJ, *et al.* Relative bioavailability of itraconazole from an extemporaneously prepared suspension and from the marketed capsules. *Am J Health-Syst Pharm* 1998; **55:** 261–5.
4. Barone JA, *et al.* Enhanced bioavailability of itraconazole in hydroxypropyl-β-cyclodextrin solution versus capsules in healthy volunteers. *Antimicrob Agents Chemother* 1998; **42:** 1862–5.

5. Prentice AG, *et al.* Multiple dose pharmacokinetics of an oral solution of itraconazole in autologous bone marrow transplant recipients. *J Antimicrob Chemother* 1994; **34:** 247–52.
6. Prentice AG, *et al.* Multiple dose pharmacokinetics of an oral solution of itraconazole in patients receiving chemotherapy for acute myeloid leukaemia. *J Antimicrob Chemother* 1995; **36:** 657–63.
7. Reynes J, *et al.* Pharmacokinetics of itraconazole (oral solution) in two groups of human immunodeficiency virus-infected adults with oral candidiasis. *Antimicrob Agents Chemother* 1997; **41:** 2554–8.
8. de Repentigny L, *et al.* Repeated-dose pharmacokinetics of an oral solution of itraconazole in infants and children. *Antimicrob Agents Chemother* 1998; **42:** 404–8.

Uses and Administration
Itraconazole is a triazole antifungal given by mouth for the treatment of oropharyngeal and vulvovaginal candidiasis, for pityriasis versicolor, for dermatophytoses unresponsive to topical treatment, and for systemic infections including aspergillosis, blastomycosis, candidiasis, chromoblastomycosis, coccidioidomycosis, cryptococcosis, histoplasmosis, paracoccidioidomycosis, and sporotrichosis. It is also given for the prophylaxis of fungal infections in immunocompromised patients. The place of itraconazole in the treatment of fungal infections is discussed under Choice of Antifungal, p.372.

When given by mouth, itraconazole capsules and oral liquid may not be used interchangeably. Itraconazole oral liquid may be given for oral or oesophageal candidiasis in a dose of 200 mg daily in one or two doses, the liquid being held in the mouth before swallowing. The dose may be doubled in resistant infections. For prophylaxis of systemic fungal infections in immunocompromised patients, a dose of 5 mg per kg body-weight daily in two divided doses is recommended.

The following doses all apply to itraconazole capsules. The dose in oropharyngeal candidiasis is 100 mg (or 200 mg in patients with AIDS or neutropenia) daily by mouth for 15 days. Vulvovaginal candidiasis may be treated with itraconazole 200 mg by mouth twice daily for one day. Pityriasis versicolor may be treated with itraconazole 200 mg daily for 7 days. For dermatophytoses the dose is 100 mg daily for 15 days or 200 mg daily for 7 days in tinea corporis or tinea cruris; doses are 100 mg daily for 30 days or 200 mg twice daily for 7 days in tinea pedis or tinea manuum. For nail infections the dose is 200 mg daily for 3 months or pulse therapy with 200 mg twice daily for 7 days repeated once (for fingernails) or twice (for toenails) after intervals of 21 days.

For systemic infections, itraconazole is given by mouth in usual doses of 100 to 200 mg once daily, increased to 200 mg twice daily for invasive or disseminated infections, including cryptococcal meningitis. In life-threatening infections a loading dose of 200 mg three times daily for 3 days has been given. A dose of 200 mg daily is used for primary or secondary prophylaxis in neutropenic patients or those with AIDS. Absorption may be impaired in these patients and monitoring of plasma concentrations is advised with an increase in dose to 200 mg twice daily if necessary. This higher dose is recommended routinely by some authorities in the USA.

Itraconazole may also be given by intravenous infusion in a dose of 200 mg given twice daily over 1 hour for two days, then 200 mg daily thereafter.

◊ Reviews.
1. Haria M, *et al.* Itraconazole: a reappraisal of its pharmacological properties and therapeutic use in the management of superficial fungal infections. *Drugs* 1996; **51:** 585–620.
2. Stevens DA (ed). Managing fungal infections in the 21st century: focus on itraconazole. *Drugs* 2001; **61** (suppl 1): 1–56.
3. Slain D, *et al.* Intravenous itraconazole. *Ann Pharmacother* 2001; **35:** 720–9.

Administration. Doses of itraconazole 600 mg daily in two divided doses for 3 to 16 months were used in 8 patients with systemic mycoses resistant to conventional therapy.[1] Two patients with AIDS and cryptococcal meningitis failed to respond and two who responded initially later relapsed or developed progressive disease when the dose was reduced. The main adverse effects were hypokalaemia, hypertension, and oedema possibly associated with adrenal suppression.

In a patient with cerebral aspergillosis, itraconazole 800 mg daily for 5 months then 400 mg daily for a further 4½ months produced complete resolution of cerebral lesions.[2]

1. Sharkey PK, *et al.* High-dose itraconazole in the treatment of severe mycoses. *Antimicrob Agents Chemother* 1991; **35:** 707–13.
2. Sánchez C, *et al.* Treatment of cerebral aspergillosis with itraconazole: do high doses improve the prognosis? *Clin Infect Dis* 1995; **21:** 1485–7.

Administration in neonates. Itraconazole was administered to two premature infants with disseminated candidiasis in a dose of 10 mg per kg body-weight daily in two divided doses for 3 or 4 weeks without adverse effects.[1] Treatment was successful in both infants.

1. Bhandari V, Narang A. Oral itraconazole therapy for disseminated candidiasis in low birth weight infants. *J Pediatr* 1992; **120:** 330.

Amoebic infections. Itraconazole has been suggested for *Acanthamoeba* keratitis, when it is given orally in combination with topical miconazole (see p.582).

Leishmaniasis. When systemic therapy is required for the treatment of cutaneous leishmaniasis, pentavalent antimonials are most commonly used (see p.584). The successful use of itraconazole has been reported in a few patients[1-3] but infections with *Leishmania aethiopica* may not respond.[4]

1. Albanese G, *et al.* Cutaneous leishmaniasis: treatment with itraconazole. *Arch Dermatol* 1989; **125:** 1540–2.
2. Pialoux G, *et al.* Cutaneous leishmaniasis in an AIDS patient: cure with itraconazole. *J Infect Dis* 1990; **162:** 1221–2.
3. Dogra J, Saxena VN. Itraconazole and leishmaniasis: a randomised double-blind trial in cutaneous disease. *Int J Parasitol* 1996; **26:** 1413–15.
4. Akuffo H, *et al.* The use of itraconazole in the treatment of leishmaniasis caused by Leishmania aethiopica. *Trans R Soc Trop Med Hyg* 1990; **84:** 532–4.

Trypanosomiasis. Itraconazole may produce beneficial responses in American trypanosomiasis (p.587).

Preparations

Proprietary Preparations (details are given in Part 3)
Aust.: Sporanox; *Austral.:* Sporanox; *Belg.:* Sporanox; *Braz.:* Itranax; Sporanox; Traconal; *Canad.:* Sporanox; *Denm.:* Sporanox; *Fin.:* Sporanox; *Fr.:* Sporanox; *Ger.:* Sempera; Siros; *Hong Kong:* Sporanox; *Irl.:* Sporanox; *Israel:* Sporanox; *Ital.:* Sporanox; Triasporin; *Mex.:* Carexan; Fuzoltec; Isox; Itranax; Sporanox; Zolken; *Neth.:* Trisporal; *Norw.:* Sporanox; *NZ:* Sporanox; *Port.:* Sporanox; *S.Afr.:* Sporanox; *Singapore:* Sporanox; *Spain:* Canadiol; Hongoseril; *Swed.:* Sporanox; *Switz.:* Sporanox; *Thai.:* Sporal; *UK:* Sporanox; *USA:* Sporanox.

Multi-ingredient: *Mex.:* Sporasec.

Ketoconazole   (2589-g)

Ketoconazole (BAN, USAN, rINN).
Ketoconazolum; R-41400. (±)-*cis*-1-Acetyl-4-{4-[2-(2,4-dichlorophenyl)-2-imidazol-1-ylmethyl-1,3-dioxolan-4-ylmethoxy]phenyl}piperazine.
$C_{26}H_{28}Cl_2N_4O_4 = 531.4$.
CAS — 65277-42-1.
ATC — D01AC08; G01AF11; J02AB02.
Pharmacopoeias. In *Eur.* (see p.vi) and *US.*

Pharmacopoeial description

Ph. Eur.: A white or almost white powder. Practically insoluble in water; sparingly soluble in alcohol; freely soluble in dichloromethane; soluble in methyl alcohol. Protect from light.

Adverse Effects

Gastrointestinal disturbances are the most frequently reported adverse effect following the oral administration of ketoconazole. Nausea and vomiting have been reported in about 3% of patients, and abdominal pain in about 1%. These adverse effects are dose-related and may be minimised by giving ketoconazole with food. Asymptomatic, transient elevations in serum concentrations of liver enzymes may occur in about 10% of patients. Hepatitis has been reported and the risk appears to increase if treatment with ketoconazole is continued for longer than 2 weeks; it is usually reversible on discontinuation of ketoconazole but fatalities have occurred. Ketoconazole interferes with steroid biosynthesis and reported adverse endocrine effects include gynaecomastia, oligospermia, menstrual irregularities, and adrenal cortex suppression, especially at high doses.

Other adverse effects include allergic reactions such as urticaria and angioedema, pruritus, rash, alopecia, headache, dizziness, impotence, and somnolence. Thrombocytopenia, paraesthesia, raised intracranial pressure, and photophobia have been reported rarely.

After topical administration of ketoconazole, irritation, dermatitis, or a burning sensation has occurred.

The symbol † denotes a preparation no longer actively marketed

Effects on endocrine function. References.

1. DeFelice R, *et al.* Gynecomastia with ketoconazole. *Antimicrob Agents Chemother* 1981; **19:** 1073–4.
2. Pont A, *et al.* High-dose ketoconazole therapy and adrenal and testicular function in humans. *Arch Intern Med* 1984; **144:** 2150–3.
3. White MC, Kendall-Taylor P. Adrenal hypofunction in patients taking ketoconazole. *Lancet* 1985; **i:** 44–5.
4. Dandona P, *et al.* Non-suppression of cortisol secretion by long term treatment with ketoconazole in patients with acute leukaemia. *J Clin Pathol* 1985; **38:** 677–8.
5. Pillans PI, *et al.* Hyponatraemia and confusion in a patient taking ketoconazole. *Lancet* 1985; **i:** 821–2.
6. McCance DR, *et al.* Acute hypoadrenalism and hepatotoxicity after treatment with ketoconazole. *Lancet* 1987; **i:** 573.
7. Best TR, *et al.* Persistent adrenal insufficiency secondary to low-dose ketoconazole therapy. *Am J Med* 1987; **82:** 676–80.
8. Khosla S, *et al.* Adrenal crisis in the setting of high-dose ketoconazole therapy. *Arch Intern Med* 1989; **149:** 802–4.

Effects on the liver. Transient minor elevations of liver enzymes without clinical signs or symptoms of hepatic disease occur in about 10% of patients given ketoconazole and may occur at any stage of treatment. Although this reaction is not usually clinically important it may signal the onset of more serious hepatic injury and indicates the need for close monitoring of liver function. Symptomatic hepatic reactions are much rarer occurring in less than 0.1% of patients but are potentially fatal. There is usually a hepatocellular pattern of damage and sometimes cholestasis. Patients at increased risk of hepatic injury include those with a history of liver disease, those aged over 50, especially women, and those requiring prolonged treatment. It is important to monitor liver function during treatment as well as to limit the length of treatment. If liver enzyme values continue to rise or jaundice or hepatitis occur, ketoconazole should be withdrawn immediately since fatalities have occurred in patients who continued treatment after signs of hepatic injury developed.

References.

1. Janssen PA, Symoens JE. Hepatic reactions during ketoconazole treatment. *Am J Med* 1983; **74:** 80–5.
2. Lewis JH, *et al.* Hepatic injury associated with ketoconazole therapy. *Gastroenterology* 1984; **86:** 503–13.
3. Lake-Bakaar G, *et al.* Hepatic reactions associated with ketoconazole in the United Kingdom. *BMJ* 1987; **294:** 419–21.
4. García Rodríguez LA, *et al.* A cohort study on the risk of acute liver injury among users of ketoconazole and other antifungal drugs. *Br J Clin Pharmacol* 1999; **48:** 847–52.

Precautions

Since ketoconazole has been reported to cause hepatotoxicity it should not be administered to patients with pre-existing liver disease. Patients receiving ketoconazole should be monitored for symptoms of hepatitis; also, liver function tests should be performed before commencement of treatment with ketoconazole lasting for more than 14 days and then at least monthly throughout treatment.

Ketoconazole has been shown to be teratogenic in *animal* studies and its use is generally not recommended during pregnancy. It should be avoided in breast-feeding women. For further information, see under Pregnancy in Fluconazole, Precautions, p.383.

Hypochlorhydria, which may be present in patients with AIDS, can reduce absorption of ketoconazole. In this case absorption may be improved by administering ketoconazole with an acidic drink, such as a cola beverage.

Porphyria. Ketoconazole is considered to be unsafe in patients with porphyria because it has been shown to be porphyrinogenic in *in-vitro* systems.

Interactions

Concomitant administration of drugs that reduce stomach acidity, such as antimuscarinics, antacids, histamine H_2-antagonists, and proton pump inhibitors, may reduce the absorption of ketoconazole. Absorption of ketoconazole may also be reduced by sucralfate. Concomitant administration of ketoconazole with enzyme-inducing drugs such as rifampicin, isoniazid, or phenytoin may reduce plasma-ketoconazole concentrations. Concentrations of isoniazid and rifampicin may also be reduced by ketoconazole.

Ketoconazole inhibits certain hepatic oxidase enzymes especially the cytochrome P450 isoenzyme CYP3A4 and may account for increases in plasma concentrations of some hepatically metabolised drugs such as alfentanil, the antihistamines astemizole and terfenadine, the benzodiazepines midazolam and triazolam, ciclosporin, cisapride, dihydropyridine calcium-channel blockers, HIV-protease inhibitors such as indinavir or ritonavir (which may increase plasma concentrations of ketoconazole in turn), methylpred-

nisolone, non-nucleoside reverse transcriptase inhibitors including delavirdine and nevirapine, oral anticoagulants, paclitaxel, pimozide, quinidine, sertindole, sildenafil, statins such as lovastatin or simvastatin, tacrolimus, tolbutamide, verapamil, and zidovudine. Other drugs that may be affected include buspirone, busulfan, carbamazepine, digoxin, docetaxel, rifabutin, trimetrexate, and the vinca alkaloids.

There is a risk of cardiac arrhythmias if ketoconazole is used with astemizole, cisapride, pimozide, quinidine or terfenadine and such combinations should be avoided.

A disulfiram-like reaction may occur in patients taking ketoconazole after drinking alcohol. The efficacy of oral contraceptives may be reduced.

◊ For reviews of drug interactions with azole antifungals, see Fluconazole, p.384.

Antimicrobial Action

Ketoconazole is an imidazole antifungal which interferes with ergosterol synthesis and therefore alters the permeability of the cell membrane of sensitive fungi. It is reported to be fungistatic at concentrations achieved clinically. Ketoconazole has a wide spectrum of antimicrobial activity including activity against *Blastomyces dermatitidis*, *Candida* spp., *Coccidioides immitis*, *Epidermophyton floccosum*, *Histoplasma capsulatum*, *Malassezia* spp., *Microsporum canis*, *Paracoccidioides brasiliensis*, *Trichophyton mentagrophytes*, and *T. rubrum*. Some strains of *Aspergillus* spp., *Cryptococcus neoformans*, and *Sporothrix schenckii* are sensitive. MIC values for ketoconazole are dependent on the method used for their determination, and are not always predictive of *in vivo* activity. Ketoconazole has activity against some Gram-positive bacteria and some antiprotozoal activity against *Leishmania* spp. There are rare reports of *Candida albicans* acquiring resistance to ketoconazole.

Microbiological interactions. For the effect of imidazoles and amphotericin B on each other's antimicrobial activity, see Amphotericin B, p.379.

Resistance. For a discussion of increasing resistance of *Candida* spp. to azoles see Fluconazole, Antimicrobial Action, p.384.

Pharmacokinetics

The absorption of ketoconazole from the gastrointestinal tract is variable and increases with decreasing stomach pH. It is recommended that ketoconazole is given with food to increase absorption and reduce gastrointestinal disturbances, although reduced rate and extent of absorption have occurred when given after a meal. Mean peak plasma concentrations of about 3.5 µg per mL have been obtained 2 hours after administration of 200 mg by mouth. Systemic absorption following topical or vaginal application in healthy subjects is minimal. Ketoconazole is more than 90% bound to plasma proteins, mainly albumin. It is widely distributed and appears in breast milk. Penetration into the CSF is poor. The elimination of ketoconazole is reported to be biphasic, with an initial half-life of 2 hours and a terminal half-life of about 8 hours.

Ketoconazole is metabolised in the liver to inactive metabolites. It is excreted as metabolites and unchanged drug chiefly in the faeces; some is excreted in the urine.

◊ References.

1. Daneshmend TK, Warnock DW. Clinical pharmacokinetics of ketoconazole. *Clin Pharmacokinet* 1988; **14:** 13–34.
2. Lelawongs P, *et al.* Effect of food and gastric acidity on absorption of orally administered ketoconazole. *Clin Pharm* 1988; **7:** 228–35.
3. Lake-Bakaar G, *et al.* Gastropathy and ketoconazole malabsorption in the acquired immunodeficiency syndrome (AIDS). *Ann Intern Med* 1988; **109:** 471–3.
4. Daneshmend TK. Diseases and drugs but not food decrease ketoconazole 'bioavailability'. *Br J Clin Pharmacol* 1990; **29:** 783–4.

Uses and Administration

Ketoconazole is an imidazole antifungal administered topically or by mouth. It is given by mouth in chronic mucocutaneous candidiasis, in fungal infections of the gastrointestinal tract, in dermatophyte infections of the skin and fingernails not responding to topical treatment, and in systemic infections including blastomycosis, candidiasis, coccidioidomycosis, histoplasmosis, and paracoccidioidomycosis. It has been given for the prophylaxis of fungal infections in immunocompromised patients although fluconazole or itraconazole are usually preferred. It has been recommended that because of its erratic absorption and slow therapeutic response, ketoconazole should not be used for the treatment of life-threatening fungal infections including fungal meningitis or for severe infections in immunocompromised patients. Also because of the risk of hepatotoxicity with ketoconazole, its use in nonsystemic fungal infections tends to be restricted to serious infections resistant to other treatment.

The place of ketoconazole in the treatment of fungal infections is discussed under Choice of Antifungal, p.372.

The usual oral dose for treatment and prophylaxis of fungal infections is 200 mg once daily taken with food. This may be increased to 400 mg daily if an adequate response is not obtained; in some infections even higher doses have been used. Children may be given approximately 3 mg per kg body-weight daily, or 50 mg for those aged 1 to 4 years and 100 mg for children aged 5 to 12 years. Treatment should usually be continued for 14 days and for at least one week after symptoms have cleared and cultures have become negative. Some infections may require several months' treatment and administering ketoconazole for such prolonged periods may increase the risk of liver toxicity.

A dose of 400 mg once daily for 5 days is used for the treatment of chronic vaginal candidiasis.

Ketoconazole is applied topically as a 2% cream in the treatment of candidal or dermatophyte infections of the skin, or in the treatment of pityriasis versicolor. It is applied once or twice daily and continued for at least a few days after the disappearance of symptoms. A shampoo containing 2% ketoconazole is applied twice weekly for 2 to 4 weeks in the treatment of seborrhoeic dermatitis or once daily for up to 5 days in pityriasis versicolor.

Acanthamoeba infections. Although there is currently no established treatment for granulomatous amoebic encephalitis, ketoconazole may have some activity against the *Acanthamoeba* spp. responsible for this infection and has been applied topically to skin lesions. Ketoconazole has also been suggested for *Acanthamoeba* keratitis (p.582), when it has been given orally in combination with topical miconazole.

Acute respiratory distress syndrome. In two small double-blind, controlled trials,[1,2] the development of acute respiratory distress syndrome (ARDS—p.1046) and mortality rates were lower in high-risk patients who received ketoconazole than in those who received placebo. An accompanying editorial[3] commented that the achievement of adequate blood concentrations appeared to be essential. The mode of action could be associated with inhibition of leukotriene and thromboxane synthesis.[2,3] Nevertheless, in a study in 234 patients,[4] ketoconazole failed to reduce mortality or improve clinical outcomes when given early in the course of ARDS. Some centres have developed guidelines for ketoconazole prophylaxis in patients at risk of ARDS.[5]

1. Slotman GJ, et al. Ketoconazole prevents acute respiratory failure in critically ill surgical patients. *J Trauma* 1988; **28:** 648–54.
2. Yu M, Tomasa G. A double-blind, prospective, randomized trial of ketoconazole, a thromboxane synthetase inhibitor, in the prophylaxis of the adult respiratory distress syndrome. *Crit Care Med* 1993; **21:** 1635–42.
3. Slotman GJ. Ketoconazole: maybe it isn't the magic potion, but ... *Crit Care Med* 1993; **21:** 1642–4.
4. The ARDS Network Authors for the ARDS Network. Ketoconazole for early treatment of acute lung injury and acute respiratory distress syndrome: a randomized controlled trial. *JAMA* 2000; **283:** 1995–2002.
5. Sinuff T, et al. Development, implementation, and evaluation of a ketoconazole practice guideline for ARDS prophylaxis. *J Crit Care* 1999; **14:** 1–6.

Blastomycosis. Although ketoconazole has been replaced by itraconazole as the azole of choice in the treatment of blasto-

mycosis (p.372), it has been used as an alternative in doses of 400 to 800 mg daily.[1]

1. Chapman SW, et al. Practice guidelines for the management of patients with blastomycosis. *Clin Infect Dis* 2000; **30:** 679–83.

Endocrine disorders and malignant neoplasms. Ketoconazole has been reported to impair steroid hormone synthesis[1] and to blunt the response of cortisone to adrenocorticotrophic hormone (ACTH)[2] and has been tried in the management of a number of endocrine disorders.

In **Cushing's syndrome** (p.1272) there have been a few reports of patients responding to ketoconazole in doses of 600 to 1200 mg daily,[3,4] including regression of a metastatic adrenal carcinoma in 1 patient.[5] Definitive treatment is usually aimed at correcting the underlying pathology, and drug therapy often has an adjuvant or palliative role. Good results have been reported from the use of ketoconazole as an adjuvant to pituitary radiotherapy.[6]

Treatment of **hirsutism** is usually with an anti-androgen (see p.1468), but ketoconazole has been tried in small numbers of women at a dose of 300 mg daily[7] or 400 mg daily[8,9] with variable results.

Ketoconazole was reported to produce a beneficial response in 3 boys with a form of **precocious puberty** (p.1277) that does not generally respond to gonadorelin analogues.[10]

The anti-androgenic effects of ketoconazole have also been found useful in the management of **prostatic cancer** (p.497) in selected patients.[11-13] However, the usual dose of ketoconazole of 1200 mg daily given in 3 doses is frequently poorly tolerated, and other drugs are generally preferred.

1. Pont A, et al. Ketoconazole blocks adrenal steroid synthesis. *Ann Intern Med* 1982; **97:** 370–2.
2. White MC, Kendall-Taylor P. Adrenal hypofunction in patients taking ketoconazole. *Lancet* 1985; **i:** 44–5.
3. Angeli A, Frairia R. Ketoconazole therapy in Cushing's disease. *Lancet* 1985; **i:** 821.
4. Shepherd FA, et al. Ketoconazole: use in the treatment of ectopic adrenocorticotropic hormone production and Cushing's syndrome in small-cell lung cancer. *Arch Intern Med* 1985; **145:** 863–4.
5. Contreras P, et al. Regression of metastatic adrenal carcinoma during palliative ketoconazole treatment. *Lancet* 1985; **ii:** 151–2.
6. Estrada J, et al. The long-term outcome of pituitary irradiation after unsuccessful transsphenoidal surgery in Cushing's disease. *N Engl J Med* 1997; **336:** 172–7.
7. Venturoli S, et al. A prospective randomized trial comparing low dose flutamide, finasteride, ketoconazole, and cyproterone acetate-estrogen regimens in the treatment of hirsutism. *J Clin Endocrinol Metab* 1999; **84:** 1304–10.
8. Sonino N, et al. Low-dose ketoconazole treatment in hirsute women. *J Endocrinol Invest* 1990; **13:** 35–40.
9. Venturoli S, et al. Ketoconazole therapy for women with acne and/or hirsutism. *J Clin Endocrinol Metab* 1990; **71:** 335–9.
10. Holland FJ, et al. Ketoconazole in the management of precocious puberty not responsive to LHRH-analogue therapy. *N Engl J Med* 1985; **312:** 1023–8.
11. Williams G, et al. Objective responses to ketoconazole therapy in patients with relapsed progressive prostatic cancer. *Br J Urol* 1986; **58:** 45–51.
12. Lowe FC, Bamberger MH. Indications for use of ketoconazole in management of metastatic prostate cancer. *Urology* 1990; **36:** 541–5.
13. Mahler C, et al. Ketoconazole and liarozole in the treatment of advanced prostatic cancer. *Cancer* 1993; **71:** 1068–73.

Hypercalcaemia. Ketoconazole has been used[1,2] in the treatment of hypercalcaemia (p.1181). It acts by reducing 1,25-dihydroxycholecalciferol concentrations by inhibiting cytochrome P450-dependent 1α-hydroxylation of vitamin D.

1. Yavuz H. Familiar drugs for the treatment of hypercalcemia. *J Pediatr* 1998; **133:** 311.
2. Young C, et al. Hypercalcaemia in sarcoidosis. *Lancet* 1999; **353:** 374.

Leishmaniasis. As discussed on p.584, ketoconazole has been tried as an alternative to conventional first- and second-line therapy for visceral leishmaniasis[1,2] although reports of treatment have not all been favourable.[3,4]

It has also been tried in cutaneous leishmaniasis. A cure rate of 70% was reported in over 100 patients with *Leishmania major* infections treated with ketoconazole 200 to 400 mg daily by mouth for 4 to 6 weeks. Ketoconazole was not considered to be effective in infections due to *L. tropica*, *L. aethiopica*,[5] or *L. guyanensis*.[6] Ketoconazole 600 mg daily for 28 days has produced similar results to sodium stibogluconate intramuscularly for 20 days in patients with cutaneous leishmaniasis due to *L. panamensis*.[7] In a Guatemalan study,[8] ketoconazole was less effective than sodium stibogluconate when cutaneous leishmaniasis was due to *L. braziliensis*, but more effective when *L. mexicana* was the cause.

1. Wali JP, et al. Ketoconazole in treatment of visceral leishmaniasis. *Lancet* 1990; **330:** 810–11.
2. Wali JP, et al. Ketoconazole in the treatment of antimony- and pentamidine-resistant Kala-azar. *J Infect Dis* 1992; **166:** 215–16.
3. Sundar S, et al. Ketoconazole in visceral leishmaniasis. *Lancet* 1990; **336:** 1582–3.
4. Rashid JR, et al. The efficacy and safety of ketoconazole in visceral leishmaniasis. *East Afr Med J* 1994; **71:** 392–5.
5. Weinrauch L, et al. Ketoconazole in cutaneous leishmaniasis. *Br J Dermatol* 1987; **117:** 666–7.
6. Dedet J-P, et al. Failure to cure Leishmania braziliensis guyanensis cutaneous leishmaniasis with oral ketoconazole. *Trans R Soc Trop Med Hyg* 1986; **80:** 176.

7. Saenz RE, et al. Efficacy of ketoconazole against Leishmania braziliensis panamensis cutaneous leishmaniasis. *Am J Med* 1990; **89:** 147–55.
8. Navin TR, et al. Placebo-controlled clinical trial of sodium stibogluconate (Pentostam) versus ketoconazole for treating cutaneous leishmaniasis in Guatemala. *J Infect Dis* 1992; **165:** 528–34.

Seborrhoeic dermatitis. Ketoconazole 2% cream or shampoo is effective[1,2] in seborrhoeic dermatitis (p.1107) where it is usually used together with hydrocortisone.

1. Green CA, et al. Treatment of seborrhoeic dermatitis with ketoconazole II: response of seborrhoeic dermatitis of the face, scalp and trunk to topical ketoconazole. *Br J Dermatol* 1987; **116:** 217–21.
2. Katsambas A, et al. A double-blind trial of treatment of seborrhoeic dermatitis with 2% ketoconazole cream compared with 1% hydrocortisone cream. *Br J Dermatol* 1989; **121:** 353–7.

Preparations

USP 25: Ketoconazole Oral Suspension; Ketoconazole Tablets.

Proprietary Preparations (details are given in Part 3)
Aust.: Beltop†; Fungoral; Nizoral; **Austral.:** Daktagold; Nizoral; Sebizole; **Belg.:** Nizoral; **Braz.:** Arcolan; Candiderm; Candoral; Cetonax; Cetonil; Cetozol; Fungoral; Ketocon; Ketonan; Konazil; Miconan; Norizal; Norizal; **Canad.:** Nizoral; **Denm.:** Nizoral; **Fin.:** Nizoral; **Fr.:** Ketoderm; Nizoral; **Ger.:** Nizoral; Terzolin; **Hong Kong:** Nizoral; **Irl.:** Nizoral; **Israel:** Nizoral; **Ital.:** Nizoral; Triatop; **Mex.:** Akorazol; Conazol; Cremosan; Ehlifung; Eurolat; Fungamizol; Fungazol; Fungoral; Honzil; Kestomicol; Ketofar; Ketomizol; Ketone; Konaderm; Lizovag; Lornazol; Luminovag; Luperzol; Mi-Ke-Sons; Micogal; Micoser; Miketos; Mycodib; Nazolfarm; Nikorazol; Nizoral; Onofin-K; Termizol; Tiniazol; Tocomizol; Toconal; Vagmicor; **Neth.:** Nizoral; **Norw.:** Fungoral; **NZ:** Nizoral; Sebizole; **Port.:** Cesol; Frisolac; Nizoral; Rapamic; Tedol; **S.Afr.:** Nizcreme; Nizoral; Nizovules; Nizshampoo; **Singapore:** Antanazol; Dezoral; Diazon; Ketozole; Mycoral; Nizoral; Spozal; Zorinax; **Spain:** Fungarest; Fungo Hubber; Ketoisdin; Micoticum; Panfungol; **Swed.:** Fungoral; **Switz.:** Nizoral; Terzolin; **Thai.:** AC-FA; Diazon; Fungazol; Fungicide; Funginox; Katsin; Kazinal; Kenalyn; Kenazol; Kenazole; Kenoral; Ketazol; Ketazon; Ketocine; Ketolan; Ketomed; Ketonazole; Ketosil; Konazol; Masarol; Mycella; Ninazol; Nizoral; Nora; Pasalen; Triatop; **UK:** Daktarin Gold; Neutrogena Long Lasting Dandruff Control†; Nizoral; **USA:** Nizoral.

Multi-ingredient: Braz.: Candicort; Capel; Novacort.

Lanoconazole (15901-z)

Lanoconazole (rINN).

Latoconazole; NND-318; TJN-318. (±)-α-[(E)-4-(o-Chlorophenyl)-1,3-dithiolan-2-ylidene]imidazole-1-acetonitrile.
$C_{14}H_{10}ClN_3S_2 = 319.8$.
CAS — 101530-10-3.

Profile

Lanoconazole is an imidazole antifungal that has been used topically in the treatment of fungal skin infections. The need for caution when using an azole antifungal in pregnant or lactating patients is discussed under Fluconazole, p.383.

Preparations

Proprietary Preparations (details are given in Part 3)
Jpn: Astat.

Loflucarban (2576-n)

Loflucarban (rINN).

Clofluonide; Dichlorofluorothiocarbanilide. 3,5-Dichloro-4'-fluorothiocarbanilide.
$C_{13}H_9Cl_2FN_2S = 315.2$.
CAS — 790-69-2.

Profile

Loflucarban is an antibacterial and antifungal that has been used topically in the treatment of dermatophytosis and pyoderma.

Preparations

Proprietary Preparations (details are given in Part 3)
Austral.: Fluonilid†.

Mepartricin (2590-f)

Mepartricin (BAN, USAN, rINN).

Methylpartricin; SN-654; SPA-S-160.
CAS — 11121-32-7.
ATC — A01AB16; D01AA06; G01AA09; G04CX03.

A mixture of the methyl esters of 2 related polyene antibiotics obtained from a strain of *Streptomyces aureofaciens* or by any other means.

Profile

Mepartricin has antifungal and antiprotozoal activity and has been used in vaginal candidiasis and trichomoniasis as pessaries, as a vaginal cream, and as oral tablets. A cream and oral suspension are also available for the treatment of superficial and oral candidiasis. Mepartricin sodium laurilsulfate is also used.

◊ Mepartricin has been given by mouth in the treatment of benign prostatic hyperplasia (see p.1477 for the more usual treatment).

References.

1. Tosto A, *et al.* A double-blind study of the effects of mepartricin in the treatment of obstruction due to benign prostatic hyperplasia. *Curr Ther Res* 1995; **56:** 1270–75.
2. Denis L, *et al.* Double-blind, placebo-controlled trial to assess the efficacy and tolerability of mepartricin in the treatment of BPH. *Prostate* 1998; **37:** 246–52.

Preparations

Proprietary Preparations (details are given in Part 3)
Aust.: Iperplasin; **Belg.:** Montricin†; Tricandil; **Braz.:** Montricin; Orofungin; **Ital.:** Ipertrofan; Montricin; Tricandil; **Port.:** Tricandil.

Multi-ingredient: Braz.: Tricangine-A.

Miconazole (2591-d)

Miconazole *(BAN, rINN)*.

Miconazolum; R-18134. 1-[2,4-Dichloro-β-(2,4-dichlorobenzyloxy)phenethyl]imidazole.
$C_{18}H_{14}Cl_4N_2O = 416.1$.
CAS — 22916-47-8.
ATC — A01AB09; A07AC01; D01AC02; G01AF04; J02AB01; S02AA13.
Pharmacopoeias. In Eur. (see p.vi), Jpn, and US.

Pharmacopoeial description

Ph. Eur.: A white or almost white powder. It exhibits polymorphism. M.p. 83° to 87°. Very slightly soluble in water; soluble in alcohol; freely soluble in methyl alcohol. Protect from light.
USP 25: A white to pale cream powder. M.p. 78° to 82°. Insoluble in water; soluble 1 in 9.5 of alcohol, 1 in 2 of chloroform, 1 in 15 of ether, 1 in 4 of isopropyl alcohol, 1 in 5.3 of methyl alcohol, and 1 in 9 of propylene glycol; freely soluble in acetone and in dimethylformamide. Protect from light.

Incompatibility. Leaching of the potentially toxic plasticising agent diethylhexyl phthalate was reported when solutions containing miconazole were stored in PVC containers.[1]

1. Pearson SD, *et al.* Leaching of diethylhexyl phthalate from polyvinyl chloride containers by selected drugs and formulation components. *Am J Hosp Pharm* 1993; **50:** 1405–9.

Stability. Miconazole in castor oil or arachis oil is stable to dry heat sterilisation at 160° for 90 minutes.[1]

1. Lee RLH. Stability of miconazole on dry heating in vegetable oils. *Aust J Hosp Pharm* 1985; **15:** 233–4.

Miconazole Nitrate (2592-n)

Miconazole Nitrate *(BANM, USAN, rINNM)*.

Miconazoli Nitras; R-14889.
$C_{18}H_{14}Cl_4N_2O,HNO_3 = 479.1$.
CAS — 22832-87-7.
Pharmacopoeias. In Eur. (see p.vi), Int., Jpn, and US.

Pharmacopoeial description

Ph. Eur.: A white or almost white powder. Very slightly soluble in water; slightly soluble in alcohol; practically insoluble in ether; sparingly soluble in methyl alcohol. Protect from light.
USP 25: A white or practically white, crystalline powder, with not more than a slight odour. Soluble 1 in 6250 of water, 1 in 312 of alcohol, 1 in 75 of methyl alcohol, 1 in 525 of chloroform, 1 in 1408 of isopropyl alcohol, 1 in 119 of propylene glycol; freely soluble in dimethyl sulfoxide; soluble in dimethylformamide; insoluble in ether. Protect from light.

Adverse Effects

After administration of miconazole by mouth, nausea and vomiting have been reported, and also diarrhoea (usually on long-term treatment). There have been allergic reactions, rarely, and isolated reports of hepatitis.

Local irritation and sensitivity reactions may occur when miconazole nitrate is used topically; contact dermatitis has been reported.

After the intravenous infusion of miconazole, phlebitis, nausea, vomiting, diarrhoea, anorexia, pruritus, rash, febrile reactions, flushes, drowsiness, and hyponatraemia have been reported. Other effects include hyperlipidaemia, aggregation of erythrocytes, anaemia, and thrombocytosis. Transient tachycardia and other cardiac arrhythmias have followed the rapid intravenous injection of miconazole. Rare adverse effects include acute psychosis, arthralgia, and anaphylaxis. Many of these adverse effects have been associated with the injection vehicle which contains polyethoxylated castor oil (see Polyoxyl Castor Oils, p.1347).

Effects on the heart. Bradycardia, progressing to fatal ventricular fibrillation and cardiac arrest, occurred in a heart transplant patient during intravenous infusion of miconazole for an invasive fungal infection.[1]

1. Coley KC, Crain JL. Miconazole-induced fatal dysrhythmia. *Pharmacotherapy* 1997; **17:** 379–82.

Overdosage. A report[1] of a generalised tonic-clonic convulsion in an infant occurring 10 to 15 minutes after infusion of miconazole. A dose of 500 mg rather than the prescribed dose of 50 mg had inadvertently been administered.

1. Coulthard K, *et al.* Convulsions after miconazole overdose. *Med J Aust* 1987; **146:** 57–8.

Precautions

Miconazole should be avoided in patients with hepatic impairment.

Intravaginal preparations of miconazole may damage latex contraceptives and additional contraceptive measures are therefore necessary during local administration.

Miconazole has been fetotoxic at high doses in *animals* and its use is generally not recommended during pregnancy. For further information, see under Pregnancy in Fluconazole, Precautions, p.383.

When given intravenously the injection should be infused slowly to minimise cardiorespiratory toxicity. Haematocrit, haemoglobin, and serum electrolytes and lipids should be monitored regularly.

Porphyria. Miconazole is considered to be unsafe in patients with porphyria because it has been shown to be porphyrinogenic in *in-vitro* systems.

Interactions

Miconazole can inhibit the metabolism of drugs metabolised by the cytochrome P450 isoenzymes CYP3A4 and CYP2C9, and may thus have effects similar to those of fluconazole (p.384). Miconazole may enhance the activity of oral anticoagulants, sulfonylurea hypoglycaemics, or phenytoin. Adverse effects have been reported when miconazole was given concomitantly with carbamazepine.

There is a risk of cardiac arrhythmias if miconazole is used with astemizole, cisapride, or terfenadine and such combinations should be avoided.

Anticoagulants. The anticoagulant activity of coumarin anticoagulants can be potentiated by miconazole administered orally[1] or intravaginally.[2]

1. Ortín M, *et al.* Miconazole oral gel enhances acenocoumarol anticoagulant activity: a report of three cases. *Ann Pharmacother* 1999; **33:** 175–7.
2. Lansdorp D, *et al.* Potentiation of acenocoumarol during vaginal administration of miconazole. *Br J Clin Pharmacol* 1999; **47:** 223–30.

Antimicrobial Action

Miconazole is an imidazole antifungal with similar antimicrobial activity to that of ketoconazole (p.389). It also has some activity against *Aspergillus* spp., *Cryptococcus neoformans*, *Pseudallescheria boydii*, and some Gram-positive bacteria including staphylococci and streptococci.

Microbiological interactions. A study *in vitro* indicating antimicrobial synergism of miconazole and benzoyl peroxide against *Staphylococcus* spp. and *Propionibacterium acnes*.[1]

For the effect on antifungal activity of giving azoles and amphotericin B together, see p.379.

1. Vanden Bossche H, *et al.* Synergism of the antimicrobial agents miconazole and benzoyl peroxide. *Br J Dermatol* 1982; **107:** 343–8.

Pharmacokinetics

Miconazole is incompletely absorbed from the gastrointestinal tract. Peak plasma concentrations of 1μg per mL are achieved about 4 hours after a dose of 1 g daily. Over 90% is reported to be bound to plasma proteins.

Miconazole is metabolised in the liver to inactive metabolites. From 10 to 20% of an oral dose is excreted in the urine, mainly as metabolites, within 6 days. About 50% of an oral dose may be excreted mainly unchanged in the faeces. The elimination pharmacokinetics of miconazole have been described as triphasic, with a biological half-life of about 24 hours.

Very little miconazole is removed by haemodialysis.

There is little absorption through skin or mucous membranes when miconazole nitrate is applied topically.

◊ Reviews.

1. Daneshmend TK, Warnock DW. Clinical pharmacokinetics of systemic antifungal drugs. *Clin Pharmacokinet* 1983; **8:** 17–42.

Uses and Administration

Miconazole is an imidazole antifungal used as miconazole base or nitrate in the treatment of superficial candidiasis (p.372), and of the skin infections dermatophytosis and pityriasis versicolor (p.376). It has also been given intravenously by infusion in the treatment of disseminated fungal infections, but other azoles are now more commonly used.

Miconazole may be given by mouth in a dose of 15 mg per kg body-weight daily in four divided doses as an oral gel containing 20 mg per g for the treatment of oropharyngeal and intestinal candidiasis. For the treatment of oral lesions the oral gel is applied directly. A sustained release lacquer is available for dentures.

Miconazole nitrate is applied usually twice daily as a 2% cream, lotion, or powder in the treatment of fungal infections of the skin including candidiasis, dermatophytosis, and pityriasis versicolor. In the treatment of vaginal candidiasis, 5 g of a 2% intravaginal cream is inserted into the vagina once daily for 10 to 14 days or twice daily for 7 days. Miconazole nitrate pessaries may be inserted in dosage regimens of 100 mg once daily for 7 or 14 days, 100 mg twice daily for 7 days, 200 or 400 mg daily for 3 days, or in a single dose of 1200 mg.

Acanthamoeba keratitis. Miconazole has been applied topically in *Acanthamoeba* keratitis (p.582) in combination with systemic treatment with either ketoconazole or itraconazole.

Skin disorders. Topical preparations containing an imidazole such as clotrimazole, ketoconazole, or miconazole usually together with hydrocortisone are used in the management of *seborrhoeic dermatitis* (p.1107). A cream containing miconazole nitrate 2% and benzoyl peroxide 5% has been used topically in the treatment of *acne* (p.1103).

Preparations

BP 2001: Miconazole Cream; Miconazole Oromucosal Gel;
USP 25: Miconazole Injection; Miconazole Nitrate Cream; Miconazole Nitrate Topical Powder; Miconazole Nitrate Vaginal Suppositories.

Proprietary Preparations (details are given in Part 3)
Aust.: Daktarin; Gyno-Daktarin; **Austral.:** Chemists Own Zapazole; Daktarin; Fungo; Gyno-Daktarin†; Leuko Fungex Antifungal; Monistat; **Belg.:** Albistat; Daktar; Daktarin; Gyno-Daktarin; **Braz.:** Daktarin; Ginedak; Gyno-Daktarin; Micogyn; Micoless; Vodol; **Canad.:** Micatin; Micozole; Monazole; Monistat; **Denm.:** Brenazol; Brentan; Dumicoat; **Fin.:** Daktarin; Dumicoat; Gyno-Daktarin; Medizol; **Fr.:** Britane; Daktarin; Gyno-Daktar; Gyno-Daktarin; **Ger.:** Amykon; Daktarin; Derma-Mykotral; Dumicoat; Epi-Monistat†; Fungur M; Gyno-Daktar; Gyno-Monistat†; Gyno-Mykotral; InfectoSoor; Micotar; Mykoderm Mund-Gel; Mykotin mono; **Hong Kong:** Daktarin; Fungo; Gyno-Daktarin; **Irl.:** Daktarin; Gyno-Daktarin; **Israel:** Daktarin; Gyno-Daktarin; Pitrion; **Ital.:** Andergin†; Daktarin; Fungiderm†; Micoderm†; Micomax; Miconal; Micotef; Miderm; Nizacol; Pivanozolo; Prilagin; **Mex.:** Aloid; Daktarin; Dermifun; Fungiquim; Gyno-Daktarin; K-Mizol; Lotrimin AF; Micosid; Neomicol; Nimicon; Piat; **Neth.:** Daktarin; Dermacure; Gyno-Daktarin; **Norw.:** Daktar; Dumicoat; **NZ:** Daktarin; Fungo; Gyno-Daktarin; Micozole; Micreme; **Port.:** Daktarin; Gyno-Daktarin; Micane; **S.Afr.:** Daktarin; Gyno-Daktarin; Gynospor; **Singapore:** Candiplas; Daktarin; Decozol; Fungo; Zarin; **Spain:** Daktarin; Fungisdin; **Swed.:** Daktar; Dumicoat; **Switz.:** Daktarin; Dumicoat; Monistat; **Thai.:** Candiplas; Daktarin; Funcort; Fungi-M; Fungisil; Liconar; Micazin; Minaza; Misone; Mysocort; Neomite; Nikarin; Ranozol; Tara; **UAE:** Mikozal; **UK:** Daktarin; Dumicoat†; Femeron†; Gyno-Daktarin; **USA:** Absorbine Antifungal Foot Powder; Ansul Antifungal Foot Powder†; Breezee Mist Antifungal; Femizol-M; Fungoid; Lotrimin AF; M-Zole; Maximum Strength Desenex Antifungal; Micatin; Monistat; Ony-Clear†; Podactin; Prescription Strength Desenex†; Ting; ZeaSorb AF.

Multi-ingredient: Aust.: Acnidazil; Daktacort; **Austral.:** Daktozin; Fungo; **Belg.:** Acnidazil†; Daktacort; Daktozin; **Braz.:** Amplium-G; Fa-Cyl M; Gino Pletil; Ginosutin M; Trinizol M; **Denm.:** Acnidazil†; Brentacort; **Fin.:** Daktacort†; **Ger.:** Acne Plus; Acnidazil†; Decoderm tri; InfectoSoor; Vobaderm; **Hong Kong:** Acnidazil†; **Irl.:** Daktacort; **Israel:** Daktacort; **Ital.:** Acnidazil; **Mex.:** Daktacort; **Neth.:** Acnecure; Acnidazil; Daktacort; **Norw.:** Daktacort; **NZ:** Daktacort; Daktozin; Fungocort; Micreme H; **S.Afr.:** Acneclear; Acnidazil; Daktacort; Trialone; **Singapore:** Betnovate-GM; Betnovate-M; Conazole; Daktacort; Decocort; Hairscience; Tri-Micon; Zaricort; **Spain:** Bexicortil; Brentan; Dermisdin; Nutracel; **Swed.:** Cortimyk; Daktacort; **Switz.:** Acne Creme Plus; Acnidazil†; Daktacort; Decoderm trivalent; Fungisil-T; Kelaplus; Ladocort; Tara-Plus; **UK:** Acnidazil†; Daktacort; Daktacort HC; **USA:** Fungoid HC.

The symbol † denotes a preparation no longer actively marketed

Naftifine Hydrochloride (12995-y)

Naftifine Hydrochloride (BANM, USAN, rINNM).

AW-105-843; Naftifungin Hydrochloride; SN-105-843 (naftifine). (E)-N-Cinnamyl-N-methyl(1-naphthylmethyl)amine hydrochloride.

$C_{21}H_{21}N,HCl = 323.9$.

CAS — 65472-88-0 (naftifine); 65473-14-5 (naftifine hydrochloride).

Pharmacopoeias. In US.

Pharmacopoeial description

USP 25: Store in airtight containers.

Profile

Naftifine hydrochloride is an allylamine derivative (see Terbinafine Hydrochloride, p.394) which is reported to be fungicidal against dermatophytes, but only fungistatic against Candida spp.

Naftifine hydrochloride 1% is applied topically once or twice daily for fungal skin infections particularly dermatophytosis (p.376).

Local reactions such as burning or stinging may occur.

Preparations

USP 25: Naftifine Hydrochloride Cream; Naftifine Hydrochloride Gel.

Proprietary Preparations (details are given in Part 3)
Aust.: Benecut; Exoderil; Canad.: Naftin; Ger.: Exoderil; Hong Kong: Exoderil; Ital.: Suadian; Singapore: Exoderil; Spain: Micosona; USA: Naftin.

Multi-ingredient: Aust.: Exoderil Zinkpaste†; Naftifin Zinkpaste†.

Natamycin (2593-h)

Natamycin (BAN, USAN, pINN).

Antibiotic A-5283; CL-12625; E235; Pimaricin.

$C_{33}H_{47}NO_{13} = 665.7$.

CAS — 7681-93-8.

ATC — A01AB10; A07AA03; D01AA02; G01AA02; S01AA10.

Pharmacopoeias. In Pol. and US.

A polyene antibiotic produced by the growth of Streptomyces natalensis.

Pharmacopoeial description

USP 25: An off-white to cream-coloured powder. It may contain up to 3 moles of water. Practically insoluble in water; soluble in glacial acetic acid and in dimethylformamide; slightly soluble in methyl alcohol. A 1% suspension in water has a pH of 5.0 to 7.5. Store in airtight containers. Protect from light.

Adverse Effects and Precautions

Gastrointestinal disturbances have occurred after the administration of natamycin by mouth. Local application of natamycin has sometimes produced irritation.

Porphyria. Natamycin has been associated with acute attacks of porphyria and is considered unsafe in porphyric patients.

Antimicrobial Action

Natamycin is a polyene antifungal active against Candida and Fusarium spp. In addition it is active against the protozoan Trichomonas vaginalis.

Pharmacokinetics

Natamycin is poorly absorbed from the gastrointestinal tract. It is not absorbed through the skin or mucous membranes when applied topically. Following ocular administration, natamycin is present in therapeutic concentrations in corneal stroma but not in intra-ocular fluid; systemic absorption does not usually occur.

Uses and Administration

Natamycin is a polyene antifungal antibiotic used for the local treatment of candidiasis (p.372) and fungal keratitis (see Eye Infections, p.374). It has also been used in vaginal trichomoniasis (p.586).

A 5% ophthalmic suspension or a 1% ointment of natamycin is used in the treatment of blepharitis, conjunctivitis, or keratitis due to susceptible fungi, including Fusarium solani.

Natamycin is given by mouth for the treatment of intestinal candidiasis in a dose of up to 400 mg daily in divided doses, and as 10-mg lozenges for oral candidiasis.

Natamycin is used topically for fungal skin infections and for candidal and trichomonal infections of the vagina. Natamycin pessaries have been used.

Preparations

USP 25: Natamycin Ophthalmic Suspension.

Proprietary Preparations (details are given in Part 3)
Belg.: Pimafucin†; Fin.: Pimafucin; Ger.: Deronga Heilpaste; Pima Biciron N; Pimafucin; Ital.: Natafucin; S.Afr.: Natacyn; Singapore: Natacyn; Thai.: Natacyn; USA: Natacyn.

Multi-ingredient: Belg.: Pimafucort; Fin.: Pimafucort; Ger.: Pimafucort; Neth.: Pimafucort†; NZ: Pimafucort; Port.: Pimafucort.

Neticonazole Hydrochloride (4989-z)

Neticonazole Hydrochloride (rINNM).

SS-717. (E)-1-{2-(Methylthio)-1-[o-(pentyloxy)phenyl]vinyl}imidazole hydrochloride.

$C_{17}H_{22}N_2OS,HCl = 338.9$.

CAS — 130726-68-0 (neticonazole); 130773-02-3 (neticonazole hydrochloride);.

Profile

Neticonazole hydrochloride is an imidazole antifungal used topically in the treatment of superficial fungal infections. The need for caution when using an azole antifungal in pregnant or lactating patients is discussed under Fluconazole, p.383.

Preparations

Proprietary Preparations (details are given in Part 3)
Jpn: Atolant; Methitoral†; Newral†.

Nifuroxime (2594-m)

Nifuroxime (rINN).

5-Nitro-2-furaldehyde oxime.

$C_5H_4N_2O_4 = 156.1$.

CAS — 6236-05-1.

Profile

Nifuroxime is a nitrofuran antimicrobial that has been used with furazolidone to treat vaginal candidiasis and trichomoniasis.

Preparations

Proprietary Preparations (details are given in Part 3)
Multi-ingredient: Ital.: Ginecofuran†.

Nystatin (2596-v)

Nystatin (BAN, USAN, rINN).

Fungicidin; Nistatina; Nystatinum.

CAS — 1400-61-9.

ATC — A07AA02; D01AA01; G01AA01.

Pharmacopoeias. In Eur. (see p.vi), Int., Pol., and US which specify not less than 4400 units per mg. Also in Jpn which does not specify potency.

Pharmacopoeial description

Ph. Eur.: An antifungal substance produced by the growth of certain strains of Streptomyces noursei. It contains mainly tetraenes, the principal component being nystatin A_1. The potency is not less than 4400 units per mg, calculated with reference to the dried substance. It is a yellow or slightly brownish hygroscopic powder. Very slightly soluble in water; practically insoluble in alcohol and in ether; freely soluble in dimethylformamide; slightly soluble in methyl alcohol. Store in airtight containers at a temperature between 2° and 8°. Protect from light.

USP 25: A substance, or a mixture of two or more substances, produced by the growth of Streptomyces noursei (Streptomycetaceae). It has a potency of not less than 4400 units per mg, or, where intended for use in extemporaneous preparation of oral suspensions, not less than 5000 units per mg. A yellow to light tan, hygroscopic powder, with an odour suggestive of cereals; it is affected by long exposure to light, heat, and air. Practically insoluble in water and in alcohol; insoluble in chloroform, in ether, and in benzene; slightly to sparingly soluble in methyl alcohol, in n-butyl alcohol, and in n-propyl alcohol. A 3% suspension in water has a pH of 6.0 to 8.0. Store in airtight containers. Protect from light.

Adverse Effects

Nausea, vomiting, and diarrhoea have occasionally been reported after the oral administration of nystatin. Oral irritation or sensitisation may occur. Rashes, including urticaria, and rarely the Stevens-Johnson syndrome have been reported. Irritation may occur rarely after the topical use of nystatin.

Effects on the skin. Generalised pustular eruptions were reported in 3 patients following oral administration of nystatin.[1] Subsequent sensitivity testing revealed delayed (type IV) hypersensitivity to nystatin.

1. Küchler A, et al. Acute generalized exanthematous pustulosis following oral nystatin therapy: a report of three cases. Br J Dermatol 1997; 137: 808–11.

Precautions

Intravaginal preparations of nystatin may damage latex contraceptives and additional contraceptive precautions are necessary during treatment.

Antimicrobial Action

Nystatin is a polyene antifungal antibiotic which interferes with the permeability of the cell membrane of sensitive fungi by binding to sterols, chiefly ergosterol. Its main action is against Candida spp.

Pharmacokinetics

Nystatin is poorly absorbed from the gastrointestinal tract. It is not absorbed through the skin or mucous membranes when applied topically.

Administration. In a study in 5 healthy subjects high salivary nystatin concentrations were maintained throughout a 2-hour period during which a controlled-release delivery system was used in the mouth; concentrations exceeded those achieved with a nystatin pastille.[1] However, a further study[2] found that fungicidal nystatin concentrations were maintained in saliva 5 hours after nystatin pastilles had been used, whereas concentrations were undetectable 2 hours after using an oral suspension.

1. Encarnacion M, Chin I. Salivary nystatin concentrations after administration of an osmotic controlled release tablet and a pastille. Eur J Clin Pharmacol 1994; 46: 533–5.
2. Millns B, Martin MV. Nystatin pastilles and suspension in the treatment of oral candidosis. Br Dent J 1996; 181: 209–11.

Uses and Administration

Nystatin is a polyene antifungal antibiotic used for the prophylaxis and treatment of candidiasis of the skin and mucous membranes (see p.372). It has been administered with antibiotics in various regimens to suppress the overgrowth of gastrointestinal flora and as part of selective decontamination regimens (see Intensive Care, p.126).

For the treatment of intestinal or oesophageal candidiasis, nystatin is given in doses of 500 000 or 1 000 000 units by mouth 3 or 4 times daily. In infants and children a dosage of 100 000 units or more may be given 4 times daily.

For the treatment of lesions of the mouth, pastilles or a suspension may be given in a dosage of 100 000 units four times daily. Higher doses of, for example, 500 000 units four times daily, may be needed in immunocompromised patients. The formulation should be kept in contact with the affected area for as long as possible, and patients should avoid taking food or drink earlier than one hour after a dose. In the USA doses of 400 000 to 600 000 units four times daily of the suspension, or 200 000 to 400 000 units four or five times daily as lozenges, are used.

For prophylaxis of intestinal candidiasis in patients receiving broad-spectrum antibiotics, a total dose of 1 000 000 units daily may be given. A suggested prophylactic dose for infants born to mothers with vaginal candidiasis is 100 000 units daily.

For the treatment of vaginal infections nystatin is given in a dosage of 100 000 to 200 000 units daily for 14 days or longer as pessaries or vaginal cream. For cutaneous lesions, ointment, gel, cream, or dusting powder containing 100 000 units per g may be applied 2 to 4 times daily.

A liposomal formulation of nystatin for parenteral administration is under investigation.

◊ Reviews.
1. Gøtzsche PC, Johansen HK. Nystatin prophylaxis and treatment in severely immunodepressed patients (updated 23 May 2001). Available in The Cochrane Library; Issue 3. Oxford: Update Software; 2001.

Preparations

BP 2001: Nystatin Ointment; Nystatin Oral Suspension; Nystatin Pastilles; Nystatin Pessaries; Nystatin Tablets;
USP 25: Nystatin and Triamcinolone Acetonide Cream; Nystatin and Triamcinolone Acetonide Ointment; Nystatin Cream; Nystatin for Oral Suspension; Nystatin Lotion; Nystatin Lozenges; Nystatin Ointment; Nystatin Oral Suspension; Nystatin Tablets; Nystatin Topical Powder; Nystatin Vaginal Suppositories; Nystatin Vaginal Tablets; Nystatin, Neomycin Sulfate, Gramicidin, and Triamcinolone Acetonide Cream; Nystatin, Neomycin Sulfate, Gramicidin, and Triamcinolone Acetonide Ointment; Oxytetracycline and Nystatin Capsules; Oxytetracycline and Nystatin for Oral Suspension; Tetracycline Hydrochloride and Nystatin Capsules.

Proprietary Preparations (details are given in Part 3)
Aust.: Candio; Mycostatin; Austral.: Mycostatin; Nilstat; Belg.: Nilstat; Braz.: Micostatin; Nidazolin; Canad.: Candistatin; Mycostatin; Nadostine; Nilstat; Nyaderm; Denm.: Mycostatin; Fin.: Mycostatin; Fr.: Mycostatine; Ger.: Adiclair; Biofanal; Candio; Cordes Nystatin Soft; Fungireduct; Lederlind; Moronal; Mykoderm Heilsalbe; MykoPosterine N; Mykundex; Mykundex mono; Nystaderm; Hong Kong: Lystin; Mycostatin; Nadostine; Irl.: Mycostatin; Ital.: Mycostatin; Mex.: Bistatin; Micostatin; Nistan; Nistaquim; Nystasan; Norw.: Mycostatin; NZ: Mycostatin; Nilstat; Port.: Mycostatin; S.Afr.: Canstat; Mycostatin; Nystacid; Singapore: Mycostatin; Spain: Mycostatin; Swed.: Mycostatin; Switz.: Candio†; Mycostatin; Rivostatin†; Thai.: Lystin; Mycostatin; UAE: Mikostat; UK: Infestat†; Nyspes; Nystamont; Nystan; Nystatin-Dome; USA: Mycostatin; Nilstat; Nystex; Nystop; Pedi-Dri.

Multi-ingredient: Aust.: Mycostatin V; Mycostatin-Zinkoxid; Topsym polyvalent; Austral.: Aristocomb†; Kenacomb; Mysteclin-V; Otocomb Otic; **Belg.:** Eoline; Flogocid; Mycolog; Polygynax; **Braz.:** Benzevit; Bio-Vagin; Colpagex N; Colpanist; Colpatrin; Colpist MT; Colpistar; Colpistatin; Colpolase; Dermodex; Donnagel; Flagyl Nistatina; Fungimax; Ginometrim; Gynax-N; Naxogin Composto; Omcilon AM; Poliginax; Tricolpex; Trisdazol; Trivagel N; Vagi Biotic; Vagimax; Vagitrin-N; **Canad.:** Flagystatin; Kenacomb; Triacomb; Viaderm-KC; **Denm.:** Kenalog Comp med Mycostatin; **Fin.:** Flagyl Comp; **Fr.:** Auricularum; Myco-Ultralan; Mycolog; Mycomnes†; Polygynax; Polygynax Virgo; Tergynan†; **Ger.:** Aureomycin N; Candio-Hermal Plus; Halog Tri; Jellin polyvalent; Lokalison-antimikrobiell Creme N; Moronal V; Multilind; mykoproct sine†; Mykundex Heilsalbe; Nystaderm comp; Nystalocal; Penanyst; Polygynax; Topsym polyvalent; Volonimat Plus N; **Hong Kong:** Kenacomb; Macmiror Complex; Polygynax; Triacomb; **Irl.:** Flagyl Compak; Kenacomb; Nystaform; Nystaform-HC; Terra-Cortril Nystatin; Timodine; Tinaderm-M; **Israel:** Auricularum; Dermacombin; Kenacomb; **Ital.:** Assocort; Fasigin N; Macmiror Complex; **Mex.:** Decadron Con Nistatina; Dermalog-C; Flagystatin N; Kenacomb; Macmiror Complex V; Promibasol-Plus; Vagitrol-V; **Neth.:** Mycolog; **NZ:** Kenacomb; Kenoid; **Port.:** Dafnegil; Dermovate-NN; Kenacomb; Polygynax; **S.Afr.:** Hiconcil-NS†; Kenacomb; Riostatin; Tetrex-F†; **Singapore:** Flagystatin; Kenacomb; Polygynax; **Spain:** Deltasiton†; Interderm; Intradermo Cort Ant Fung; Milrosina Nistatina; Positon; **Swed.:** Kenacombin Novum; Kenacombin†; **Switz.:** Dafnegil†; Dermovate-NN; Flogocid NN†; Korticoid polyvalent; Multilind; Mycolog; Nystacortone; Nystalocal; Topsym polyvalent; **Thai.:** Dermacombin; Gynoco; Kenacomb; Nystin; Quinradon-N; Vagicin; **UAE:** Panderm; **UK:** Dermovate-NN; Flagyl Compak; Gregoderm; Nystadermal†; Nystaform; Nystaform-HC; Terra-Cortril Nystatin; Timodine; Tinaderm-M; Tri-Adcortyl; Trimovate; **USA:** Myco-Biotic II; Myco-Triacet II; Mycogen II; Mycolog-II; Myconel; Mytrex; NGT; Tri-Statin II.

Omoconazole Nitrate (5542-z)

Omoconazole Nitrate (USAN, rINNM).

10-80-07. (Z)-1-{2,4-Dichloro-β-[2-(p-chlorophenoxy)ethoxy]-α-methylstyryl}imidazole nitrate.

$C_{20}H_{17}Cl_3N_2O_2,HNO_3 = 486.7$.

CAS — 74512-12-2 (omoconazole); 83621-06-1 (omoconazole nitrate).

Profile

Omoconazole nitrate is an imidazole antifungal used locally for fungal skin infections (p.376) and for vaginal candidiasis (p.372). It is applied topically as a 1% cream, powder, or solution in the treatment of cutaneous candidiasis, dermatophytosis, and pityriasis versicolor. For vaginal candidiasis, omoconazole nitrate is given as pessaries in doses of 150 mg daily for 6 days, 300 mg daily for 3 days, or 900 mg as a single dose.

Intravaginal preparations of azoles may damage latex contraceptives.

The need for caution when using an azole antifungal in pregnant or lactating patients is discussed under Fluconazole, p.383.

Preparations

Proprietary Preparations (details are given in Part 3)
Aust.: Azameno†; **Belg.:** Fongarex; **Braz.:** Fongamil; Fongarex; **Ger.:** Fungisan; **Ital.:** Afongan; **Mex.:** Afongan; **Port.:** Afongan†; **Spain:** Afongan†; Fongamil; **Switz.:** Azameno.

Oxiconazole Nitrate (16940-q)

Oxiconazole Nitrate (BANM, USAN, rINNM).

Ro-13-8996; Ro-13-8996/001; Ro-13-8996/000 (oxiconazole); SGD-301-76; ST-813. 2′,4′-Dichloro-2-imidazol-1-ylacetophenone (Z)-O-(2,4-dichlorobenzyl)oxime mononitrate.

$C_{18}H_{13}Cl_4N_3O,HNO_3 = 492.1$.

CAS — 64211-45-6 (oxiconazole); 64211-46-7 (oxiconazole nitrate).

Profile

Oxiconazole nitrate is an imidazole antifungal applied topically as a cream, solution, or powder equivalent to oxiconazole 1% in the treatment of fungal infections of the skin (p.376). It is also given as a pessary in a single dose equivalent to 600 mg of oxiconazole in the treatment of vaginal candidiasis (p.372).

Local reactions including burning and itching have been reported. Intravaginal preparations of azoles may damage latex contraceptives.

The need for caution when using an azole antifungal in pregnant or lactating patients is discussed under Fluconazole, p.383.

◊ Reviews.
1. Jegasothy BV, Pakes GE. Oxiconazole nitrate: pharmacology, efficacy, and safety of a new imidazole antifungal agent. *Clin Ther* 1991; **13:** 126–41.

Preparations

Proprietary Preparations (details are given in Part 3)
Aust.: Gyno Oceral; Gyno-Liderman; Liderman; Oceral; **Braz.:** Oceral; **Canad.:** Oxizole; **Fr.:** Fonx; **Ger.:** Myfungar; Oceral GB; **Mex.:** Gyno-Myfungar; Myfungar; Oxistat; **Spain:** Salongo; **Switz.:** Gyno-Myfungar; Myfungar; Oceral; **USA:** Oxistat.

Parconazole Hydrochloride (6364-r)

Parconazole Hydrochloride (USAN, rINNM).

R-39500. cis-1-{[2-(2,4-Dichlorophenyl)-4-[(2-propynyloxy)methyl]-1,3-dioxolan-2-yl]methyl}-1H-imidazole hydrochloride.

$C_{17}H_{16}Cl_2N_2O_3 \cdot HCl = 403.7$.

CAS — 68685-54-1 (parconazole); 62973-77-7 (parconazole hydrochloride).

Profile

Parconazole is an antifungal used as the hydrochloride in the treatment of gastrointestinal candidiasis in veterinary medicine.

Pentamycin (3000-z)

$C_{35}H_{58}O_{12} = 670.8$.

CAS — 6834-98-6.

ATC — G01AA11.

Profile

Pentamycin is a polyene antifungal obtained from *Streptomyces pentaticus*. It is used in the treatment of vaginal candidiasis and for the protozoal infection trichomoniasis. One or two 3-mg vaginal pessaries are inserted for 5 to 10 consecutive days.

Preparations

Proprietary Preparations (details are given in Part 3)
Switz.: Pentacine.

Propionic Acid (3001-c)

E280; E282 (calcium propionate); E283 (potassium propionate). Propanoic acid.

$C_2H_5 \cdot CO_2H = 74.08$.

CAS — 79-09-4.

Pharmacopoeias. In Fr. Also in USNF.

Pharmacopoeial description

USNF 20: An oily liquid having a slight pungent, rancid odour. Miscible with water, with alcohol, and with various other organic solvents. Store in airtight containers.

Sodium Propionate (3005-x)

E281. Sodium propanoate.

$C_3H_5NaO_2 = 96.06$.

CAS — 137-40-6 (anhydrous sodium propionate); 6700-17-0 (sodium propionate hydrate).

ATC — S01AX10.

Pharmacopoeias. In Br. and Fr. Also in USNF.

Pharmacopoeial description

BP 2001: Colourless deliquescent crystals or a white granular powder; odourless or with a slight characteristic odour. Freely soluble in water; soluble in alcohol.

USNF 20: Colourless transparent crystals or a granular crystalline powder; odourless or with a faint acetic-butyric odour. Deliquescent in moist air. Soluble 1 in 1 of water, 1 in 0.65 of boiling water, and 1 in 24 of alcohol; practically insoluble in chloroform and in ether. Store in airtight containers.

Profile

Propionic acid and its salts are antifungals.

Sodium propionate has been used topically, usually in combination with other antimicrobial agents for the treatment of dermatophyte infections. Eye drops containing sodium propionate have also been used.

Propionic acid and its calcium, sodium, and potassium salts are used in the baking industry as inhibitors of moulds.

Preparations

Proprietary Preparations (details are given in Part 3)
Ital.: Propionat.

Multi-ingredient: Aust.: Dermowund; **Austral.:** Mycoderm; **Braz.:** Andriodermol; Gynax-N; Otosulf; Vagitrin-N; **Canad.:** Amino-Cerv; **Fr.:** Angispray†; Dermacide; Otoralgyl a la phenylephrine; Rhinyl; **Israel:** Otomycin; **S.Afr.:** Neopan; **USA:** Amino-Cerv; Prophyllin.

Protiofate (14254-z)

Protiofate (rINN).

Dipropyl 3,4-dihydroxy-2,5-thiophenedicarboxylate.

$C_{12}H_{16}O_6S = 288.3$.

CAS — 58416-00-5.

ATC — G01AX13.

Profile

Protiofate is a thiophene derivative with antifungal and antiprotozoal activity. It has been used locally in the treatment of vaginal candidiasis and trichomoniasis.

Pyrrolnitrin (3002-k)

Pyrrolnitrin (USAN, rINN).

52230; NSC-107654. 3-Chloro-4-(3-chloro-2-nitrophenyl)pyrrole.

$C_{10}H_6Cl_2N_2O_2 = 257.1$.

CAS — 1018-71-9.

ATC — D01AA07.

Profile

Pyrrolnitrin is an antifungal antibiotic isolated from *Pseudomonas pyrrocinia* and applied topically in the treatment of superficial fungal infections.

Preparations

Proprietary Preparations (details are given in Part 3)
Ital.: Micutrin.

Multi-ingredient: Ital.: Micutrin Beta; **Port.:** Pirrolfungin.

Saperconazole (6498-l)

Saperconazole (BAN, USAN, rINN).

R-66905. 2-sec-Butyl-4-[4-{4-[(2RS,4SR)-2-(2,4-difluorophenyl)-2-(1H-1,2,4-triazol-1-ylmethyl)-1,3-dioxolan-4-ylmethoxy]phenyl}piperazin-1-yl]phenyl]-2,4-dihydro-1,2,4-triazol-3-one.

$C_{35}H_{38}F_2N_8O_4 = 672.7$.

CAS — 110588-57-3.

Profile

Saperconazole is a triazole derivative under investigation for the treatment of systemic fungal infections.

The need for caution when using an azole antifungal in pregnant or lactating patients is discussed under Fluconazole, p.383.

◊ References.
1. Odds FC. Antifungal activity of saperconazole (R66905) in vitro. *J Antimicrob Chemother* 1989; **24:** 533–7.
2. Franco L, *et al.* Saperconazole in the treatment of systemic and subcutaneous mycoses. *Int J Dermatol* 1992; **31:** 725–9.
3. Khoo SH, Denning DW. Cure of chronic invasive sinus aspergillosis with oral saperconazole. *J Med Vet Mycol* 1995; **33:** 63–6.

Sertaconazole Nitrate (17275-r)

Sertaconazole Nitrate (BANM, rINNM).

Sertaconazoli Nitras. (±)-1-{2,4-Dichloro-β-[(7-chlorobenzo[b]thien-3-yl)methoxy]phenethyl}imidazole nitrate.

$C_{20}H_{15}Cl_3N_2OS,HNO_3 = 500.8$.

CAS — 99592-32-2 (sertaconazole); 99592-39-9 (sertaconazole nitrate).

Pharmacopoeias. In Eur. (see p.vi).

Pharmacopoeial description

Ph. Eur.: A white or almost white powder. Practically insoluble in water; sparingly soluble in alcohol and in dichloromethane; soluble in methyl alcohol. Protect from light.

Profile

Sertaconazole nitrate is an imidazole antifungal used topically in the treatment of superficial candidiasis, dermatophytosis, and pityriasis versicolor.

The need for caution when using an azole antifungal in pregnant or lactating patients is discussed under Fluconazole, p.383.

Preparations

Proprietary Preparations (details are given in Part 3)
Braz.: Zalain; **Ger.:** Mykosert; Zalain; **Mon.:** Monazol; **Port.:** Dermofix; **Singapore:** Zalain; **Spain:** Dermofix; Dermoseptic; Gine Zalain; Ginedermofix; Zalain.

Sulconazole Nitrate (16999-m)

Sulconazole Nitrate (BANM, USAN, rINNM).

RS-44872; RS-44872-00-10-3. 1-[2,4-Dichloro-β-(4-chlorobenzyl)thiophenethyl]imidazole nitrate.

$C_{18}H_{15}Cl_3N_2S,HNO_3 = 460.8$.

CAS — 61318-90-9 (sulconazole); 61318-91-0 (sulconazole nitrate).

Pharmacopoeias. In Fr. and US.

Pharmacopoeial description

USP 25: A white to off-white crystalline powder. Soluble 1 in 3333 of water, 1 in 100 of alcohol, 1 in 130 of acetone, 1 in 333 of chloroform, 1 in 286 of dichloromethane, 1 in 2000 of dioxan, 1 in 71 of methyl alcohol, 1 in 10 of pyridine, and 1 in 2000 of toluene. Protect from light.

Adverse Effects and Precautions

Local reactions including burning, itching, and erythema have been reported following sulconazole use.

For information about the use of sulconazole during pregnancy and lactation see under Pregnancy in Fluconazole, Precautions, p.383.

Antimicrobial Action

Sulconazole is an imidazole antifungal with activity against dermatophytes, *Candida* spp., and *Malassezia furfur*.

The symbol † denotes a preparation no longer actively marketed

Uses and Administration

Sulconazole nitrate is an imidazole antifungal applied topically once or twice daily as a 1% cream or solution in the treatment of fungal skin infections including dermatophyte infections and pityriasis versicolor (p.376), and candidiasis (p.372).

◊ Reviews.
1. Benfield P, Clissold SP. Sulconazole: a review of its antimicrobial activity and therapeutic use in superficial dermatomycoses. *Drugs* 1988; **35:** 143–53.

Preparations

Proprietary Preparations (details are given in Part 3)
Belg.: Myk-1; *Fr.:* Myk; *Irl.:* Exelderm; *Ital.:* Exelderm†; *Mex.:* Exelderm; *Neth.:* Myk-1; *UK:* Exelderm; *USA:* Exelderm.

Terbinafine Hydrochloride (14747-y)

Terbinafine Hydrochloride (BANM, rINNM).
SF-86-327 (terbinafine). (E)-6,6-Dimethylhept-2-en-4-ynl(methyl)-(1-naphthylmethyl)amine hydrochloride.
$C_{21}H_{26}ClN = 327.9$.
CAS — 91161-71-6 (terbinafine); 78628-80-5 (terbinafine hydrochloride).
NOTE. Terbinafine is USAN.

Adverse Effects

The most frequent adverse effects following oral administration of terbinafine hydrochloride are gastrointestinal disturbances such as nausea, diarrhoea, and mild abdominal pain. Loss or disturbance of taste may occur and occasionally may be severe enough to lead to anorexia and weight loss. Other frequent adverse effects include headache and skin reactions including rash or urticaria sometimes with arthralgia or myalgia. Severe skin reactions including Stevens-Johnson syndrome and toxic epidermal necrolysis have occurred rarely. Liver dysfunction with isolated reports of cholestasis, hepatitis, and jaundice, has occurred and there have also been rare cases of liver failure, sometimes leading to death or necessitating liver transplantation, in patients both with and without pre-existing liver disease. Other rare adverse effects include malaise, fatigue, and alopecia. Haematological disorders including neutropenia, thrombocytopenia, and agranulocytosis have been reported very rarely.

There may be local reactions after topical use of terbinafine.

◊ Postmarketing surveillance of about 10 000 patients[1] suggested the following incidences of adverse effects to oral terbinafine: gastrointestinal symptoms, 4.7%; dermatological effects, 3.3%; CNS symptoms (commonly headache), 1.8%; taste disturbances, 0.6%; and transient disturbances in liver function, 0.1%. Serious adverse effects possibly or probably related to terbinafine included angioedema, bronchospasm, erythema multiforme, extended stroke, and unilateral leg oedema. Combined data from 25 884 patients from this and 3 further studies[2] generally confirmed these results. Overall, adverse effects were reported in 10.5% of patients and caused treatment to be discontinued in 5.3%. Serious adverse effects probably or possibly related to terbinafine occurred in 12 patients (0.046%).
1. O'Sullivan DP, et al. Postmarketing surveillance of oral terbinafine in the UK: report of a large cohort study. *Br J Clin Pharmacol* 1996; **42:** 559–65.
2. O'Sullivan DP. Terbinafine: tolerability in general medical practice. *Br J Dermatol* 1999; **141** (suppl 56): 21–5.

Effects on the eyes. The US manufacturer has noted that changes in the lens and retina of the eye have sometimes been associated with oral terbinafine, although the significance of these changes was not known.

Effects on the salivary glands. Bilateral parotid swelling was associated with terbinafine therapy in a 38-year-old man.[1] Information from the manufacturer and the UK Committee on Safety of Medicines indicated that this effect had occurred in other patients but was very rare.
1. Torrens JK, McWhinney PH. Parotid swelling and terbinafine. *BMJ* 1998; **316:** 440–1.

Effects on the skin. Serious skin reactions are occasionally reported in patients receiving terbinafine and have included erythema multiforme,[1,2] erythroderma,[1] severe urticaria,[1] pityriasis rosea,[1] worsening of pre-existing psoriasis,[1] acute generalised exanthematous pustulosis,[3] and lupus erythematosus.[4-6] Several of these patients had a history of autoimmune disease[2,6] and it has been suggested that this could be a risk factor for developing severe reactions.[2]
1. Gupta AK, et al. Cutaneous adverse effects associated with terbinafine therapy: 10 case reports and a review of the literature. *Br J Dermatol* 1998; **138:** 529–32.
2. Goeteyn V, et al. Is systemic autoimmune disease a risk factor for terbinafine-induced erythema multiforme? *Br J Dermatol* 2000; **142:** 578–9.

3. Condon CA, et al. Terbinafine-induced acute generalized exanthematous pustulosis. *Br J Dermatol* 1998; **138:** 709–10.
4. Murphy M, Barnes L. Terbinafine-induced lupus erythematosus. *Br J Dermatol* 1998; **138:** 708–9.
5. Brooke R, et al. Terbinafine-induced subacute cutaneous lupus erythematosus. *Br J Dermatol* 1998; **139:** 1132–3.
6. Holmes S, Kemmett D. Exacerbation of systemic lupus erythematosus induced by terbinafine. *Br J Dermatol* 1998; **139:** 1133.

Effects on taste. Disturbance and loss of taste have been reported in about 0.6% of patients receiving terbinafine. While this usually resolves gradually once the drug is withdrawn, persistent impairment of taste has been reported.[1,2]
1. Bong JL, et al. Persistent impairment of taste resulting from terbinafine. *Br J Dermatol* 1998; **139:** 747–8.
2. Duxbury AJ, et al. Persistent impairment of taste associated with terbinafine. *Br Dent J* 2000; **188:** 295–6.

Precautions

Terbinafine should be used with caution in patients with hepatic impairment and liver function tests should be performed in all patients before starting oral therapy. Terbinafine should be discontinued if clinical or biochemical evidence of hepatotoxicity develops; it should also be discontinued if any progressive skin rash occurs. It should not be given during breast feeding.

Psoriasis. It has been suggested that terbinafine may provoke or exacerbate psoriasis,[1] (see also under Effects on the Skin, above), and that it should be avoided in patients with this disorder.
1. Wilson NJE, Evans S. Severe pustular psoriasis provoked by oral terbinafine. *Br J Dermatol* 1998; **139:** 168.

Interactions

Plasma concentrations of terbinafine may be increased by drugs that inhibit its metabolism by cytochrome P450, such as cimetidine, and decreased by drugs that induce cytochrome P450, such as rifampicin. Menstrual disturbances including breakthrough bleeding have been reported in patients taking oral contraceptives and terbinafine.

For the effects of terbinafine on some other drugs, see under ciclosporin (p.521), nortriptyline (p.277), and warfarin (p.995).

Antimicrobial Action

Terbinafine is an allylamine derivative reported to have a broad spectrum of antifungal activity. It is considered to act through inhibition of fungal sterol synthesis. Terbinafine is fungicidal against dermatophytes and some yeasts.

◊ References.
1. Petranyi G, et al. Antifungal activity of the allylamine derivative terbinafine in vitro. *Antimicrob Agents Chemother* 1987; **31:** 1365–8.
2. Schuster I, Ryder NS. Allylamines—mode and selectivity of action compared to azole antifungals and biological fate in mammalian organisms. *J Dermatol Treat* 1990; **1** (suppl 2): 7–9.
3. Clayton YM. Relevance of broad-spectrum and fungicidal activity of antifungals in the treatment of dermatomycoses. *Br J Dermatol* 1994; **130** (suppl 43): 7–8.
4. Leeming JP, et al. Susceptibility of Malassezia furfur subgroups to terbinafine. *Br J Dermatol* 1997; **137:** 764–7.
5. Ryder NS, et al. In vitro activities of terbinafine against cutaneous isolates of Candida albicans and other pathogenic yeasts. *Antimicrob Agents Chemother* 1998; **42:** 1057–61.
6. McGinnis MR, et al. In vitro comparison of terbinafine and itraconazole against Penicillium marneffei. *Antimicrob Agents Chemother* 2000; **44:** 1407–8.

Microbiological interactions. Additive and synergistic activity was reported with terbinafine in combination with fluconazole or itraconazole against strains of *Candida albicans* that had reduced susceptibility to azoles in vitro.[1] Terbinafine was also reported to enhance the activity of azoles against *Scedosporium prolificans*[2] and against the protozoan *Leishmania braziliensis*.[3]
1. Barchiesi F, et al. In vitro activities of terbinafine in combination with fluconazole and itraconazole against isolates of Candida albicans with reduced susceptibility to azoles. *Antimicrob Agents Chemother* 1997; **41:** 1812–14.
2. Meletiadis J, et al. In vitro interaction of terbinafine with itraconazole against clinical isolates of Scedosporium prolificans. *Antimicrob Agents Chemother* 2000; **44:** 470–2.
3. Rangel H, et al. Naturally azole-resistant Leishmania braziliensis promastigotes are rendered susceptible in the presence of terbinafine: comparative study with azole-susceptible Leishmania mexicana promastigotes. *Antimicrob Agents Chemother* 1996; **40:** 2785–91. Correction. *ibid.* 1997; **41:** 496.

Pharmacokinetics

Terbinafine hydrochloride is well absorbed from the gastrointestinal tract. The bioavailability is about 40% because of first-pass hepatic metabolism. Mean peak plasma concentrations of about 1 µg per mL are

reported within 2 hours of a single oral dose of 250 mg. Steady state concentrations are about 25% higher than those seen after a single dose and are reached in 10 to 14 days. Terbinafine is extensively bound to plasma proteins. Terbinafine is distributed into the stratum corneum of the skin, the nail plate, and hair where it reaches concentrations considerably higher than those found in plasma. It appears in breast milk. Less than 5% of a topical dose of terbinafine hydrochloride is absorbed.

Terbinafine is metabolised in the liver to inactive metabolites which are excreted mainly in the urine. A plasma elimination half-life varying from 11 to 36 hours has been reported and a terminal elimination half-life of up to 400 hours in patients receiving prolonged therapy, probably representing elimination from skin and adipose tissue. Fungicidal concentrations in nails are maintained for several weeks after therapy is discontinued. The elimination rate may be altered in patients with liver disease or kidney disease.

◊ References.
1. Kovarik JM, et al. Multiple-dose pharmacokinetics and distribution in tissue of terbinafine and metabolites. *Antimicrob Agents Chemother* 1995; **39:** 2738–41.

Uses and Administration

Terbinafine hydrochloride is an allylamine antifungal given by mouth in the treatment of dermatophyte infections of the skin and nails (p.376). It is also applied to the skin in dermatophytoses, in pityriasis versicolor (p.376), and in cutaneous candidiasis (p.372).

Terbinafine 250 mg as the hydrochloride is given once daily by mouth for 2 to 4 weeks for tinea cruris; treatment may be continued for 6 weeks for tinea pedis infections; a 4-week course is used in tinea corporis infections. A cream or solution containing 1% terbinafine hydrochloride is applied once or twice daily for 1 to 2 weeks to treat tinea corporis and tinea cruris; a 1-week course is recommended for tinea pedis. A 2-week course of treatment is used in cutaneous candidiasis and pityriasis versicolor.

Dermatophyte infections of the nails are treated with terbinafine 250 mg by mouth, as the hydrochloride, once daily for 6 to 12 weeks although longer treatment may be necessary in toe-nail infections.

◊ Reviews.
1. Balfour JA, Faulds D. Terbinafine: a review of its pharmacodynamic and pharmacokinetic properties, and therapeutic potential in superficial mycoses. *Drugs* 1992; **43:** 259–84.
2. Abdel-Rahman SM, Nahata MC. Oral terbinafine: a new antifungal agent. *Ann Pharmacother* 1997; **31:** 445–56.
3. McClellan KJ, et al. Terbinafine: an update of its use in superficial mycoses. *Drugs* 1999; **58:** 179–202.

Administration in children. Although terbinafine has not generally been recommended for use in children it has been tried in children over 2 years of age in doses of 125 mg daily by mouth for those weighing 20 to 40 kg and 62.5 mg daily for those weighing less than 20 kg.[1]
1. Jones TC. Overview of the use of terbinafine (Lamisil) in children. *Br J Dermatol* 1995; **132:** 683–9.

Non-dermatophyte fungal infections. Beneficial responses to oral terbinafine have been reported in candidal nail infections,[1,2] aspergillosis,[3] chromoblastomycosis,[4] and sporotrichosis.[5,6]
1. Nolting S, et al. Terbinafine in onychomycosis with involvement by non-dermatophytic fungi. *Br J Dermatol* 1994; **130** (suppl 43): 16–21.
2. Segal R, et al. Treatment of Candida nail infection with terbinafine. *J Am Acad Dermatol* 1996; **35:** 958–61.
3. Schiraldi GF, et al. Refractory pulmonary aspergillosis: compassionate trial with terbinafine. *Br J Dermatol* 1996; **134** (suppl 46): 25–9.
4. Esterre P, et al. Treatment of chromomycosis with terbinafine: preliminary results of an open pilot study. *Br J Dermatol* 1996; **134** (suppl 46): 33–6.
5. Hull PR, Vismer HP. Treatment of cutaneous sporotrichosis with terbinafine. *J Dermatol Treat* 1992; **3** (suppl 1): 35–8.
6. Kudoh K, et al. Successful treatment of cutaneous sporotrichosis with terbinafine. *J Dermatol Treat* 1996; **7:** 33–5.

Preparations

Proprietary Preparations (details are given in Part 3)
Aust.: Daskil; Lamisil; *Austral.:* Lamisil; *Belg.:* Lamisil; *Braz.:* Lamisil; *Canad.:* Lamisil; *Denm.:* Lamisil; *Fin.:* Lamisil; *Fr.:* Lamisil; *Ger.:* Lamisil; *Hong Kong:* Lamisil; *Irl.:* Lamisil; *Israel:* Lamisil; *Ital.:* Daskil; Lamisil; *Mex.:* Lamisil; *Neth.:* Lamisil; *Norw.:* Lamisil; *NZ:* Lamisil; *Port.:* Daskyl; Lamisil; *S.Afr.:* Lamisil; *Singapore:* Lamisil; *Spain:* Daskil; Lamisil; *Swed.:* Lamisil; *Switz.:* Lamisil; *Thai.:* Lamisil; *UK:* Lamisil; *USA:* Lamisil.

Terconazole (13307-b)

Terconazole (BAN, USAN, rINN).

R-42470; Terconazolum; Triaconazole. 1-{4-[[2-(2,4-Dichlorophenyl)-r-2-(1H-1,2,4-triazol-1-ylmethyl)-1,3-dioxolan-c-4-yl]methoxy]phenyl}-4-isopropylpiperazine.

$C_{26}H_{31}Cl_2N_5O_3 = 532.5$.
CAS — 67915-31-5.
ATC — G01AG02.
Pharmacopoeias. In Eur. (see p.vi).

Pharmacopoeial description

Ph. Eur.: A white or almost white powder. It exhibits polymorphism. Practically insoluble in water; sparingly soluble in alcohol; soluble in acetone; freely soluble in dichloromethane. Protect from light.

Adverse Effects

Local reactions including burning and itching have been reported with vaginal use of terconazole. Other adverse effects have included dysmenorrhoea and abdominal pain. A flu-like syndrome with headache, fever, chills, and hypotension has been reported in some patients and may be more prevalent with vaginal pessaries providing doses larger than 80 mg.

Flu syndrome. References.
1. Moebius UM. Influenza-like syndrome after terconazole. Lancet 1988; ii: 966–7.

Precautions

Intravaginal preparations of terconazole may damage latex contraceptives and additional contraceptive measures are therefore necessary during local administration.

For information about the use of terconazole during pregnancy and lactation, see under Pregnancy in Fluconazole, Precautions, p.383.

Antimicrobial Action

Terconazole is a triazole derivative that binds to fungal cytochrome P450, thus disrupting ergosterol synthesis. Terconazole is active in vitro against Candida spp. and other fungi. It has some antibacterial activity in vitro but not against usual vaginal flora such as lactobacilli.

Pharmacokinetics

Following intravaginal administration, 5 to 16% of terconazole is absorbed. Systemically absorbed drug is metabolised by the liver and excreted in urine and faeces.

Uses and Administration

Terconazole is a triazole antifungal used in the local treatment of vulvovaginal candidiasis (p.372). Intravaginal dosage regimens are terconazole 40 mg (by 0.8% vaginal cream) or 80 mg (by pessary) at bedtime for 3 consecutive nights or 20 mg (by 0.4% cream) at bedtime for 7 consecutive nights.

Preparations

Proprietary Preparations (details are given in Part 3)
Belg.: Gyno-Terazol; **Braz.:** Gyno-Fungistat; Gyno-Fungix; **Canad.:** Terazol; **Denm.:** Terazol†; **Mex.:** Fungistat; **Neth.:** Gyno-Terazol; **S.Afr.:** Terazol†; **Swed.:** Terazol†; **Switz.:** Gyno-Terazol; **USA:** Terazol.

Tioconazole (13348-y)

Tioconazole (BAN, USAN, rINN).

UK-20349. 1-[2,4-Dichloro-β-(2-chloro-3-thenyloxy)phenethyl]imidazole.

$C_{16}H_{13}Cl_3N_2OS = 387.7$.
CAS — 65899-73-2.
ATC — D01AC07; G01AF08.
Pharmacopoeias. In Br. and US.

Pharmacopoeial description

BP 2001: A white or almost white crystalline powder. Very slightly soluble in water; freely soluble in dehydrated alcohol, in acetone, in ethyl acetate, and in methyl alcohol.

USP 25: Store in airtight containers.

Adverse Effects and Precautions

Local reactions to tioconazole including burning, itching, and erythema have been reported.

Intravaginal preparations of tioconazole may damage latex contraceptives and additional contraceptive measures are therefore necessary during local administration.

For information about the use of tioconazole during pregnancy and lactation, see under Pregnancy in Fluconazole, Precautions, p.383.

Hypersensitivity. Tioconazole, an imidazole antifungal widely used in Finland, appeared to be an important cause of contact allergy in that country, since an incidence of more than 1% was reported in patients undergoing routine patch testing.[1] There may be cross-reactivity with other commonly used imidazole derivatives.
1. Heikkilä H, et al. A study of 72 patients with contact allergy to tioconazole. Br J Dermatol 1996; 134: 678–80.

Antimicrobial Action

Tioconazole is an imidazole antifungal with a broad spectrum of activity including action against dermatophytes, Malassezia furfur, and Candida albicans. Tioconazole is active in vitro against some Gram-positive bacteria.

The symbol † denotes a preparation no longer actively marketed

Uses and Administration

Tioconazole is an imidazole antifungal used in the treatment of superficial candidiasis (p.372), and dermatophytoses and pityriasis versicolor (p.376).

For vaginal candidiasis it is used as pessaries or vaginal cream or ointment usually as a single 300-mg dose.

It has been applied topically as a 1% cream, lotion, or powder in the treatment of superficial fungal infections. Tioconazole has also been used for nail infections as a 28% w/w topical solution, although systemic treatment is generally preferred.

◊ Reviews.
1. Clissold SP, Heel RC. Tioconazole: a review of its antimicrobial activity and therapeutic use in superficial mycoses. Drugs 1986; **31:** 29–51.

Preparations

BP 2001: Tioconazole Cream; Tioconazole Nail Solution.

Proprietary Preparations (details are given in Part 3)
Aust.: Gyno-Trosyd†; Trosyd; **Braz.:** Gino Tralen; Tralen; **Canad.:** Gynecure; Trosyd; **Fin.:** Gyno-Trosyd; Trosyd; **Fr.:** Gyno-Trosyd†; Trosyd†; **Ger.:** Fungibacid†; Mykontral; **Hong Kong:** Gyno-Trosyd; Trosyd; **Irl.:** Trosyl; **Ital.:** Trosyd; **NZ:** Gyno-Trosyd; Trosyd; **Port.:** Gino-Trosyd; Trosyd; **S.Afr.:** Gyno-Trosyd; Trosyd; **Singapore:** Gyno-Trosyd; Trosyd; **Spain:** Trosid; **Switz.:** Gyno-Trosyd; Trosyd; **Thai.:** Trosyd; **UK:** Trosyl; **USA:** Vagistat.

Multi-ingredient: Braz.: Cartrax; **Fin.:** Trosycort; **Mex.:** Fasigyn VT.

Tolciclate (3008-d)

Tolciclate (USAN, rINN).

K-9147; KC-9147. O-(1,2,3,4-Tetrahydro-1,4-methano-6-naphthyl) m,N-dimethylthiocarbanilate.

$C_{20}H_{21}NOS = 323.5$.
CAS — 50838-36-3.
ATC — D01AE19.

Profile

Tolciclate is an antifungal with activity against Epidermophyton, Microsporum, and Trichophyton spp. It has been used topically as a 1% cream, lotion, or ointment, or as a 0.5% powder in the treatment of various dermatophyte infections and in pityriasis versicolor.

Preparations

Proprietary Preparations (details are given in Part 3)
Braz.: Tolmicol; **Ger.:** Fungifos; **Hong Kong:** Tolmicen; **Ital.:** Tolmicen; **Mex.:** Kilmicen; **NZ:** Tolmicen; **Port.:** Tolmicen†.

Tolnaftate (3009-n)

Tolnaftate (BAN, USAN, rINN).

Sch-10144; Tolnaftatum. O-2-Naphthyl m,N-dimethylthiocarbanilate.

$C_{19}H_{17}NOS = 307.4$.
CAS — 2398-96-1.
ATC — D01AE18.
Pharmacopoeias. In Eur. (see p.vi), Jpn, and US.

Pharmacopoeial description

Ph. Eur.: A white or yellowish-white powder. Practically insoluble in water; very slightly soluble in alcohol; freely soluble in acetone and in dichloromethane; sparingly soluble in ether. Protect from light.

USP 25: A white to creamy-white, fine powder, with a slight odour. Practically insoluble in water; slightly soluble in alcohol; freely soluble in acetone and in chloroform; sparingly soluble in ether. Store in airtight containers.

Adverse Effects

Skin reactions occur rarely with tolnaftate and include irritation and contact dermatitis.

Antimicrobial Action

Tolnaftate inhibits the growth of the dermatophytes Epidermophyton, Microsporum, Trichophyton spp., and Malassezia furfur, but is not active against Candida spp. or bacteria.

Uses and Administration

Tolnaftate is an antifungal used topically as a 1% gel, solution, powder, or cream in the treatment or prophylaxis of superficial dermatophyte infections and of pityriasis versicolor (see p.376). Tolnaftate is applied twice daily for 2 to 6 weeks. Repeat treatment may be required.

Preparations

USP 25: Tolnaftate Cream; Tolnaftate Gel; Tolnaftate Topical Aerosol; Tolnaftate Topical Powder; Tolnaftate Topical Solution.

Proprietary Preparations (details are given in Part 3)
Aust.: Sorgoran; **Austral.:** Antifungal Foot Deodorant; Curatin; Ringworm Ointment; Tinaderm; Tineafax; **Braz.:** Trinaderm; **Canad.:** Absorbine Antifungal†; Avon Footworks; Pitrex; Scholl Athlete's Foot Preparations; Tinactin; ZeaSorb AF; **Fr.:** Sporiline; **Ger.:** Sorgoa†; Tinatox; Tonoftal; **Hong Kong:** Aftate; **Irl.:** Mycil; **Israel:** Athletes Foot; Pitrex; Tinasol; **Ital.:** Tinaderm; **Mex.:** Excelsior; Tinaderm; Tolnaderm; **NZ:** Tinaderm; **Port.:** Tinaderme; **S.Afr.:** Tinaderm; **Singapore:** Tinaderm; **Spain:** Devorfungi†; Micoisdin; Tinaderm; **Thai.:** Ezon-T; Tono; **UK:** Mycil; Scholl Athlete's Foot; Tinaderm; **USA:** Absorbine

Antifungal†; Aftate; Blis-To-Sol; Breezee Mist Antifungal; Desenex†; Dr Scholl's Athlete's Foot; Dr Scholl's Tritin Antifungal Powder†; Genaspor; NP-27†; Podactin; Quinsana Plus; Tinactin.

Multi-ingredient: Aust.: Focusan†; **Austral.:** Curatin; Mycil; **Braz.:** Quadriderm; Quadrilon; **Canad.:** Absorbine Jr Antifungal; **Hong Kong:** Quadriderm; Triditol-G; **Irl.:** Mycil; Tinaderm-M; **Israel:** Phytoderm Compositum; **S.Afr.:** Quadriderm; **Singapore:** Quadriderm; **Spain:** Cuatroderm; **Switz.:** Quadriderm; **Thai.:** Alber T; Ezon-T; Quadriderm; **UK:** Mycil; Tinaderm-M; **USA:** Absorbine Athletes Foot Care; Dermasept Antifungal; SteriNail†.

Triacetin (3010-k)

Triacetin (rINN).

E1518; Glycerol Triacetate; Glycerolum Triacetas; Glyceryl Triacetate. 1,2,3-Propanetriol triacetate.

$C_9H_{14}O_6 = 218.2$.
CAS — 102-76-1.
Pharmacopoeias. In Eur. (see p.vi) and US.

Pharmacopoeial description

Ph. Eur.: A clear, colourless slightly viscous, oily liquid. Soluble in water; miscible with dehydrated alcohol and with toluene. Store in well-filled containers.

USP 25: A colourless, somewhat oily liquid with a slight, fatty odour. Soluble in water; slightly soluble in carbon disulfide; miscible with alcohol, with chloroform, and with ether. Store in airtight containers.

Profile

Triacetin is reported to possess fungistatic properties based on the liberation of acetic acid. It has been applied topically in the treatment of superficial dermatophyte infections. It has also been used as a plasticiser in oral preparations.

Triacetin may destroy rayon fabric. It should not come into contact with metals.

Preparations

Proprietary Preparations (details are given in Part 3)
Multi-ingredient: Braz.: Acidern; Micosan; **Thai.:** Alber T; Ezon-T.

Undecenoic Acid (3012-t)

Acidum Undecylenicum; 10-Hendecenoic Acid; Undecylenic Acid. Undec-10-enoic acid.

$C_{11}H_{20}O_2 = 184.3$.
CAS — 112-38-9.
ATC — D01AE04.
Pharmacopoeias. In Chin., Eur. (see p.vi), and US.

Pharmacopoeial description

Ph. Eur.: A colourless or pale yellow liquid or a white or very pale yellow crystalline mass. Practically insoluble in water; freely soluble in alcohol, in ether, and in fatty and essential oils. Store in non-metallic containers at a temperature of 8° to 15°. Protect from light.

USP 25: A clear, colourless to pale yellow liquid with a characteristic odour. Practically insoluble in water; miscible with alcohol, with chloroform, with ether, with benzene, and with fixed and volatile oils. Store in airtight containers. Protect from light.

Calcium Undecenoate (16172-g)

Calcium Undecylenate (USAN). Calcium di(undec-10-enoate).

$(C_{11}H_{19}O_2)_2Ca = 406.6$.
Pharmacopoeias. In US.

Pharmacopoeial description

USP 25: A fine white powder with a characteristic odour and no grit. Practically insoluble in water, in cold alcohol, in acetone, in chloroform, and in ether; slightly soluble in hot alcohol.

Zinc Undecenoate (3014-r)

Undecilinato de Zinco; Zinc Undecylenate; Zinci Undecylenas. Zinc di(undec-10-enoate).

$(C_{11}H_{19}O_2)_2Zn = 431.9$.
CAS — 557-08-4.
Pharmacopoeias. In Chin., Eur. (see p.vi), and US.

Pharmacopoeial description

Ph. Eur.: A fine white or almost white powder. Practically insoluble in water, in alcohol, and in ether. Protect from light.

USP 25: A fine, white powder. Practically insoluble in water and in alcohol.

Adverse Effects

Irritation may rarely occur after the topical application of undecenoic acid or its salts.

Antimicrobial Action

Undecenoic acid and its derivatives are active against some pathogenic fungi, including the dermatophytes Epidermophyton, Trichophyton, and Microsporum spp.

Uses and Administration

Undecenoic acid and its zinc salt are applied topically in the prophylaxis and treatment of superficial dermatophytoses, particularly tinea pedis (p.376). Typical concentrations are undecenoic acid 2 to 5% and zinc undecenoate 20%. They are used in creams, ointments, or powders, often in conjunction with each other. Calcium undecenoate is used as a 10 or 15% powder.

Several other salts and derivatives of undecenoic acid including methyl and propyl undecenoate, sodium sulfosuccinated undecenoic acid monoethanolamide, and undecenoic acid monoethanolamide are used similarly.

◊ Reviews.
1. Crawford F, *et al.* Topical treatments for fungal infections of the skin and nails of the foot (updated 3 Feb 2000). Available in The Cochrane Library; Issue 3. Oxford: Update Software; 2001.

Preparations

USP 25: Compound Undecylenic Acid Ointment.

Proprietary Preparations (details are given in Part 3)
Aust.: Mayfung; Pelsana Med; Umadren†; *Canad.:* Caldesene; Cruex†; *Fr.:* Mycodecyl; *Hong Kong:* Mycota; *Irl.:* Caldesene; *Mex.:* Cruex; *Switz.:* Lubex; Turexan Douche; *USA:* Blis-To-Sol; Caldesene; Cruex; Decylenes; Fungoid AF†; Protectol; Undelenic.

Multi-ingredient: *Aust.:* Crino Cordes; Dequafungan; Mycopol; Mykozem†; Pelsana Med; Salvyl; Tineafax†; Umadren†; *Austral.:* Acnederm; Egomycol; Mycoderm; Pedoz; Sebitar; Seborrol; *Belg.:* Pelsano†; *Braz.:* Acidern; Andriodermol; Micosan; Micoz; *Canad.:* Athletes Foot Antifungal†; Cruex†; Desenex; *Fr.:* Micaveen; Mycodecyl; Paps; *Ger.:* Gehwol Fungizid; Gehwol Nagelpilz; Skinman Soft; *Hong Kong:* Acnederm; Sebitar; Seborrol; *Irl.:* Ceanel; Desenex; Genisol; Monphytol†; *Israel:* Fungimon; Pedisol; Pitrisan; Undecyl; *Ital.:* Balta Intimo Soluzione†; Foot Zeta; Genisol; Micofoot; Neo Zeta-Foot†; Propast; *NZ:* Acnederm; Egomycol; Grans Remedy; Sebitar; Seborrol; *Port.:* Edoltar; Micaveen†; *S.Afr.:* AF; Ceanel†; Mycota; Pedil; *Singapore:* Acnederm; Sebitar; *Spain:* Acnosan; *Switz.:* Crimanex; Fungex; Pelsano; Pruri-med; Sebo Shampooing; Turexan Creme; Turexan Emulsion; *UK:* Ceanel; Healthy Feet; Monphytol; Mycota; *USA:* Dermasept Antifungal; Desenex; Gordochom; Pedi-Pro; Phicon-F; SteriNail†.

Voriconazole (18393-I)

Voriconazole *(BAN, rINN).*

UK-109496; Voriconazol. (2R,3S)-2-(2,4-Difluorophenyl)-3-(5-fluoropyrimidin-4-yl)-1-(1,2,4-triazol-1-yl)butan-2-ol.

$C_{16}H_{14}N_5F_3O = 349.3$.

CAS — 137234-62-9.

Profile

Voriconazole is a triazole antifungal under investigation for systemic use.

◊ Reviews.
1. Sabo JA, Abdel-Rahman SM. Voriconazole: a new triazole antifungal. *Ann Pharmacother* 2000; **34:** 1032–43.

Antigout Drugs

This chapter deals with the treatment of gout and hyperuricaemia and the drugs used mainly for these disorders.

Gout and hyperuricaemia
Uric acid is the final product of the metabolism of endogenous and exogenous purine in man. An excess of uric acid, measured in the plasma as sodium urate, constitutes **hyperuricaemia**. This excess may be caused by an overproduction or underexcretion of urate. It may be primary (mainly idiopathic) or secondary to conditions such as some enzyme deficiency states, cancer (and its treatment), renal impairment, and hypertension; other contributing factors include obesity, alcohol, and certain drugs, especially thiazide diuretics.

A patient is usually considered to be hyperuricaemic when plasma-urate concentrations exceed 0.42 mmol per litre (7 mg per 100 mL) in men and 0.36 mmol per litre (6 mg per 100 mL) in women. At these high concentrations there is a risk of crystals of monosodium urate monohydrate being formed and deposited in synovial fluid and various tissues. However, some subjects may have supersaturated plasma-urate concentrations without any crystal deposits, while others may suffer from deposits in the absence of apparent hyperuricaemia.

The presence of urate crystals in the synovial fluid leads to an inflammatory response in the affected joint, often the big toe. The ensuing pain, tenderness, and swelling constitute the symptoms of **acute inflammatory gouty arthritis**. Repeated acute attacks may be associated with a build up of crystal deposits (**tophi**) at various sites including in and around the affected joint. Tophi release urate crystals into the synovial fluid following various stimuli and so cause further acute attacks, leading to **chronic gout**. Intra-articular and peri-articular tophi may cause gradual joint erosion, which, without treatment, results in chronic gouty arthritis. Rarely, the kidney can be affected by urate deposits producing a gouty nephropathy and by uric acid calculi or stones (uric acid nephrolithiasis or urolithiasis).

Treatment

Plasma-urate concentrations may be reduced by control of obesity and modification of diet and alcohol intake. Drug treatment can relieve the pain of acute attacks but more prolonged therapy for hyperuricaemia should be considered only if there are recurrent attacks of gout or there is renal involvement (see under Chronic Gout, below).

Acute gout. An attack of acute inflammatory gouty arthritis is best treated as soon as possible with an NSAID. Aspirin or other salicylates are not suitable since they may increase plasma-urate concentrations. Treatment is started with high doses of an NSAID, the doses being reduced as the patient responds. Usually treatment can be withdrawn within a week. Colchicine has a role in treating patients in whom NSAIDs are contra-indicated. Patients who do not respond to NSAIDs or colchicine, or for whom these drugs are contra-indicated, may be treated with a systemic corticosteroid. Intra-articular corticosteroids are effective in acute monoarticular gout. Drugs used for chronic gout (allopurinol or the uricosurics) should not be started during an acute attack since they can exacerbate and prolong it (see below).

Chronic gout. If the patient suffers frequent acute attacks or develops tophaceous gout, or has renal complications as a result of urate overproduction, then long-term **'interval treatment'** of hyperuricaemia may be needed. Such therapy should not be started during an acute attack, or for 2 to 3 weeks thereafter, as fluctuations in urate concentration, may prolong the existing attack or initiate a new one. Treatment involves inhibiting the production of uric acid with allopurinol or enhancing the urinary excretion of uric acid with a uricosuric such as benzbromarone, probenecid, or sulfinpyrazone. Hyperuricaemia associated with underexcretion of uric acid can be treated with either allopurinol or a uricosuric. Allopurinol is most commonly given as first-line therapy, but may be combined with, or replaced by uricosurics if treatment fails. Hyperuricaemia due to overproduction of urate is treated with allopurinol; such patients excrete more than 700 or 800 mg of uric acid in their urine over 24 hours. Allopurinol should also be used for patients with renal urate deposits or with uric acid renal calculi.

As the plasma-urate concentration falls with either treatment there is mobilisation of urate crystals from established tophi which can trigger further acute attacks of gout. Patients are thus also given **prophylaxis** with an NSAID or colchicine from the start of interval treatment until at least a month after the plasma-urate has been reduced to an acceptable concentration; 3 or 4 months of prophylactic cover appears to be common.

Once the hyperuricaemia is corrected, the patient continues to receive therapy with allopurinol or uricosurics indefinitely. If an acute attack occurs during such maintenance therapy, this therapy should be continued to avoid fluctuations in urate concentration, and the acute attack treated in its own right.

Surgery may have to be considered for patients severely affected by chronic tophaceous gout.

General references to gout and its management are given below.

1. Star VL, Hochberg MC. Prevention and management of gout. *Drugs* 1993; **45:** 212–22.
2. Emmerson BT. The management of gout. *N Engl J Med* 1996; **334:** 445–51.
3. Wood J. Gout and its management. *Pharm J* 1999; **262:** 808–11.
4. Snaith ML. Gout hyperuricaemia, and crystal arthritis. In: Snaith ML, ed. *ABC of rheumatology*. 2nd ed. London: BMJ Publishing Group, 1999.

Allopurinol (1004-m)

Allopurinol (BAN, USAN, rINN).

Allopurinolum; BW-56-158; HPP; NSC-1390. 1H-Pyrazolo[3,4-d]pyrimidin-4-ol; 1,5-Dihydro-4H-pyrazolo[3,4-d]pyrimidin-4-one.

$C_5H_4N_4O = 136.1$.

CAS — 315-30-0 (allopurinol); 17795-21-0 (allopurinol sodium).

ATC — M04AA01.

Pharmacopoeias. In Chin., Eur. (see p.vi), Int., Jpn, Pol., and US.

It is a tautomeric mixture of 1H-pyrazolo[3,4-d]pyrimidin-4-ol and 1,5-dihydro-4H-pyrazolo[3,4-d]pyrimidin-4-one.

Pharmacopoeial description

Ph. Eur.: A white or almost white powder. Very slightly soluble in water and in alcohol; dissolves in dilute solutions of alkali hydroxides.

USP 25: A fluffy white to off-white powder having only a slight odour. Very slightly soluble in water and in alcohol; practically insoluble in chloroform and in ether; soluble in solutions of potassium and sodium hydroxides.

Incompatibility. Allopurinol sodium as a 3 mg per mL solution in 0.9% sodium chloride was visually incompatible with a number of drugs including amikacin sulfate, amphotericin B, carmustine, cefotaxime sodium, chlorpromazine hydrochloride, cimetidine hydrochloride, clindamycin phosphate, cytarabine, dacarbazine, daunorubicin hydrochloride, diphenhydramine hydrochloride, doxorubicin hydrochloride, doxycycline hyclate, droperidol, floxuridine, gentamicin sulfate, haloperidol lactate, hydroxyzine hydrochloride, idarubicin hydrochloride, imipenem with cilastatin sodium, methylprednisolone sodium succinate, metoclopramide hydrochloride, minocycline hydrochloride, mustine [chlormethine] hydrochloride, nalbuphine hydrochloride, netilmicin sulfate, ondansetron hydrochloride, pethidine hydrochloride, prochlorperazine edisilate, promethazine hydrochloride, sodium bicarbonate, streptozocin, tobramycin sulfate, and vinorelbine tartrate.[1]

1. Trissel LA, Martinez JF. Compatibility of allopurinol sodium with selected drugs during simulated Y-site administration. *Am J Hosp Pharm* 1994; **51:** 1792–9.

Adverse Effects
The most common side-effect of allopurinol is skin rash. Rashes are generally maculopapular or pruritic, but more serious hypersensitivity reactions may occur and include exfoliative rashes, the Stevens-Johnson syndrome, and toxic epidermal necrolysis. It is therefore recommended that allopurinol be withdrawn immediately if a rash occurs (see under Precautions, below). Further symptoms of hypersensitivity include fever and chills, lymphadenopathy, leucopenia or leucocytosis, eosinophilia, arthralgia, and vasculitis leading to renal and hepatic damage and, very rarely, epilepsy. These hypersensitivity reactions may be severe, even fatal, and patients with hepatic or renal impairment are at special risk.

Hepatotoxicity and signs of altered liver function may also be found in patients not exhibiting hypersensitivity.

Many other side-effects have been noted rarely and include paraesthesia, peripheral neuropathy, alopecia, hypertension, taste disturbances, nausea, vomiting, abdominal pain, diarrhoea, headache, drowsiness, and vertigo.

Patients with gout may experience an increase in acute attacks on beginning treatment with allopurinol, although attacks usually subside after several months.

◊ A Boston Collaborative Drug Surveillance Program of 29 524 hospitalised patients revealed that, with the exception of skin reactions, of 1835 patients treated with allopurinol 33 (1.8%) experienced adverse effects. These effects were dose-related and the most frequent were haematological (11 patients, 0.6%), diarrhoea (5 patients, 0.3%), and drug fever (5 patients, 0.3%). Hepatotoxicity was reported in 3 patients (0.2%). Two patients developed possible hypersensitivity reactions to allopurinol.[1]
A further analysis involving 1748 outpatients indicated no instances of acute blood disorders, skin diseases, or hypersensitivity that warranted hospital treatment. Liver disease, although found, was considered to be unassociated with allopurinol. There were only 2 patients in whom renal disease could possibly have been caused by allopurinol.[2]
1. McInnes GT, *et al.* Acute adverse reactions attributed to allopurinol in hospitalised patients. *Ann Rheum Dis* 1981; **40:** 245–9.
2. Jick H, Perera DR. Reactions to allopurinol. *JAMA* 1984; **252:** 1411.

Effects on the blood. In addition to the haematological abnormalities of leucopenia, thrombocytopenia, haemolytic anaemia, and clotting abnormalities noted in the Boston Collaborative Drug Surveillance Program,[1] aplastic anaemia has also been reported, sometimes in patients with impaired renal function.[2] One case of pure red cell aplasia has been reported.[3]
1. McInnes GT, *et al.* Acute adverse reactions attributed to allopurinol in hospitalised patients. *Ann Rheum Dis* 1981; **40:** 245–9.
2. Anonymous. Allopurinol and aplastic anaemia. *WHO Drug Inf* 1989; **3:** 26.
3. Lin Y-W *et al.* Acute pure red cell aplasia associated with allopurinol therapy. *Am J Hematol* 1999; **61:** 209–11.

Effects on the eyes. Some case reports have suggested an association between allopurinol use and the development of cataracts,[1] but a detailed ophthalmological survey involving 51 patients who had taken allopurinol failed to confirm this possible adverse effect.[2] However, a large retrospective case-control study in elderly patients concluded that long-term, or high-dose, allopurinol therapy did increase the risk of cataract extraction.[3]
1. Fraunfelder FT, *et al.* Cataracts associated with allopurinol therapy. *Am J Ophthalmol* 1982; **94:** 137–40.
2. Clair WK, *et al.* Allopurinol use and the risk of cataract formation. *Br J Ophthalmol* 1989; **73:** 173–6.
3. Garbe E, *et al.* Exposure to allopurinol and the risk of cataract extraction in elderly patients. *Arch Ophthalmol* 1998; **116:** 1652–6.

Effects on the skin. Skin reactions are the most common side-effects of allopurinol.
An Australian report calculated that of 215 adverse effects noted over a 16-year period 188 (87.4%) were related to the skin or mucous membranes.[1] An analysis by the Boston Collaborative Drug Surveillance Program in the USA, of data on 15 438 patients hospitalised between 1975 and 1982 detected 6 allergic skin reactions attributed to allopurinol among 784 recipients of the drug.[2]
Serious skin reactions to allopurinol may occur as part of a generalised hypersensitivity reaction. A review of the literature between 1970 and the end of 1990 revealed 101 cases of allopurinol hypersensitivity syndrome, 94 of which involved the skin.[3] Skin reactions included erythema multiforme, Stevens-Johnson syndrome, toxic epidermal necrolysis, or a diffuse maculopapular or exfoliative dermatitis; 27 of the 101 patients died. The relative risk of toxic epidermal necrolysis or Stevens-Johnson syndrome occurring with allopurinol was high (calculated to be 5.5) in a case-control study including 13 patients with these cutaneous reactions who had received allopurinol.[4] This risk was not constant over time, being higher during the first 2 months of treatment. During these 2 months the estimated excess risk was 1.5 cases per million users per week.
1. Vinciullo C. Allopurinol hypersensitivity. *Med J Aust* 1984; **141:** 449–50.
2. Bigby M, *et al.* Drug-induced cutaneous reactions. *JAMA* 1986; **256:** 3358–63.
3. Arellano F, Sacristán JA. Allopurinol hypersensitivity syndrome: a review. *Ann Pharmacother* 1993; **27:** 337–43.
4. Roujeau J-C, *et al.* Medication use and the risk of Stevens-Johnson syndrome or toxic epidermal necrolysis. *N Engl J Med* 1995; **333:** 1600–1607.

Hypersensitivity. For mention of the allopurinol hypersensitivity syndrome, see Effects on the Skin, above.

Precautions

Allopurinol should not be used for the treatment of an acute attack of gout; additionally, allopurinol therapy should not be initiated for any purpose during an acute attack. However, allopurinol is continued when acute attacks occur in patients already receiving the drug, and the acute attack is treated separately.

Treatment should be stopped immediately if any skin reactions or other signs of hypersensitivity develop. A cautious reintroduction at a low dose may be attempted when mild skin reactions have cleared; allopurinol should not be reintroduced in those patients who have experienced other forms of hypersensitivity reaction. Dosage should be reduced in renal impairment (see below) and in hepatic impairment; extra monitoring may be necessary. Care is advised in patients being treated for hypertension or cardiac insufficiency, who may have concomitant renal impairment.

To reduce the risk of renal xanthine deposition an adequate fluid intake (2 to 3 litres daily) is required. In addition, a neutral or slightly alkaline urine may be desirable.

Allopurinol should be used with caution in nursing mothers as it has been reported to be distributed into breast milk.

Renal impairment. Excretion of allopurinol and its active metabolite oxipurinol is primarily via the kidneys and therefore the dosage should be reduced if renal function is impaired.

In the USA the manufacturer (Glaxo Wellcome) suggests a daily dose of 200 mg for patients with a creatinine clearance of 10 to 20 mL per minute and a maximum daily dose of 100 mg for a clearance of under 10 mL per minute with consideration being given to a longer dosing interval if the clearance falls below 3 mL per minute.

In the UK the manufacturer (Wellcome) recommends a maximum initial daily dosage of 100 mg for those with impaired renal function, increased only if the response is inadequate. Doses less than 100 mg daily or 100 mg at intervals longer than 1 day are recommended for those with severe renal insufficiency. Because of the imprecision of low creatinine clearance values, they suggest that, if facilities are available for monitoring, the allopurinol dose should be adjusted to maintain plasma-oxipurinol concentrations below 100 μmol per litre (15.2 μg per mL). A suggested alternative dose for patients requiring dialysis two or three times a week is 300 to 400 mg allopurinol immediately after dialysis only.

Interactions

Drugs that can increase uric acid concentrations may decrease the efficacy of allopurinol. Aspirin and the salicylates possess this activity and should generally be avoided in hyperuricaemia and gout. An increase in hypersensitivity reactions, and possibly also other adverse effects, has been reported in patients receiving allopurinol with ACE inhibitors or thiazide diuretics, particularly in patients with impaired renal function.

The metabolism of azathioprine and mercaptopurine is inhibited by allopurinol and their doses should be reduced to one-quarter to one-third of the usual dose when either of them is given with allopurinol to avoid potentially life-threatening toxicity. There have also been reports of allopurinol enhancing the activity of, and possibly increasing the toxicity of, a number of other drugs including some antibacterials, some anticoagulants, some antineoplastics, ciclosporin, some sulfonylurea antidiabetics, theophylline, and vidarabine.

ACE inhibitors. An apparent interaction between allopurinol and *captopril* has been reported in patients with chronic renal failure. In one patient fatal Stevens-Johnson syndrome developed and it was suggested that the reaction was secondary to the introduction of allopurinol potentiated by the presence of captopril.[1] In the second patient hypersensitivity, characterised by fever, arthralgia, and myalgia, occurred and in this case the cause was believed to be captopril, or one of its metabolites, potentiated by the addition of allopurinol.[2] The authors of both reports considered that the combination of allopurinol and captopril should be prescribed with care, especially in patients with chronic renal failure.

1. Pennell DJ, et al. Fatal Stevens-Johnson syndrome in a patient on captopril and allopurinol. Lancet 1984; i: 463.
2. Samanta A, Burden AC. Fever, myalgia, and arthralgia in a patient on captopril and allopurinol. Lancet 1984; i: 679.

Antacids. Allopurinol failed to reduce blood-uric-acid concentrations when administered at the same time as *aluminium*

hydroxide in 3 patients on chronic haemodialysis. However, if allopurinol was given 3 hours before aluminium hydroxide the expected decrease in uric acid concentration did occur.[1]

1. Weissman I, Krivoy N. Interaction of aluminium hydroxide and allopurinol in patients on chronic hemodialysis. Ann Intern Med 1987; 107: 787.

Antibacterials. Although an increased incidence of skin rashes has been noted when allopurinol has been used with *ampicillin* or *amoxicillin*, data currently available are insufficient to confirm whether this is due to allopurinol or not. For further details, see Ampicillin, p.151.

Anticoagulants. For the effect of allopurinol on *dicoumarol, phenprocoumon*, or *warfarin*, see Warfarin, p.995.

Antiepileptics. For a report of allopurinol possibly inhibiting the metabolism of *phenytoin*, see under Antigout Drugs, p.360.

Antigout drugs. Uricosuric drugs are likely to increase the renal elimination of oxipurinol (the major active metabolite of allopurinol). For example, concurrent administration of allopurinol and *benzbromarone* was found to lower plasma concentrations of oxipurinol by some 40%, although plasma concentrations of allopurinol itself were not affected.[1] The interaction was not clinically significant, since the combination was more effective than allopurinol alone in lowering serum concentrations of uric acid. The manufacturer recommends reassessing the dosage of allopurinol on an individual basis when a uricosuric drug is added.

Probenecid has been reported to decrease the clearance of orally administered allopurinol riboside.[2]

1. Müller FO. The effect of benzbromarone on allopurinol/oxypurinol kinetics in patients with gout. Eur J Clin Pharmacol 1993; 44: 69–72.
2. Were JBO, Shapiro TA. Effects of probenecid on the pharmacokinetics of allopurinol riboside. Antimicrob Agents Chemother 1993; 37: 1193–6.

Antineoplastics and immunosuppressants. Allopurinol inhibits the metabolism of *azathioprine* and *mercaptopurine* and marked dosage reduction of these drugs is required if either is given concomitantly with allopurinol (p.510 and p.552, respectively). There are also reports of interactions between allopurinol and other antineoplastics. Mild chronic allopurinol-induced hepatotoxicity has been reported in one male patient to have been exacerbated by *tamoxifen*.[1] Hypersensitivity vasculitis resulting in the death of one patient receiving allopurinol and *pentostatin* has been described. Although it could not be ascertained whether this effect was due to one of the drugs alone or to an interaction it was believed that this combination should not be employed.[2]

For a report of an increased incidence of bone-marrow toxicity in patients given allopurinol with *cyclophosphamide*, see p.528. The effects of allopurinol on *ciclosporin* concentrations (a marked increase) are reported on p.520.

1. Shah KA, et al. Allopurinol hepatotoxicity potentiated by tamoxifen. N Y State J Med 1982; 82; 1745–6.
2. Steinmetz JC, et al. Hypersensitivity vasculitis associated with 2-deoxycoformycin and allopurinol therapy. Am J Med 1989; 86: 499.

Antivirals. For the effect of allopurinol on *didanosine*, see p.618.

Xanthines. For the effect of allopurinol on *theophylline* pharmacokinetics, see p.781.

Pharmacokinetics

Up to 90% of a dose of allopurinol is absorbed from the gastrointestinal tract after oral administration; its plasma half-life is about 1 to 2 hours. Allopurinol's major metabolite is oxipurinol (alloxanthine) which is also an inhibitor of xanthine oxidase with a plasma half-life of about 15 or more hours in patients with normal renal function, although this is greatly prolonged by renal impairment. Both allopurinol and oxipurinol are conjugated to form their respective ribonucleosides. Allopurinol and oxipurinol are not bound to plasma proteins.

Excretion is mainly through the kidney, but it is slow since oxipurinol undergoes tubular reabsorption. About 70% of a daily dose may be excreted in the urine as oxipurinol and up to 10% as allopurinol; prolonged administration may alter these proportions due to allopurinol inhibiting its own metabolism. The remainder of the dose is excreted in the faeces. Allopurinol and oxipurinol have also been detected in breast milk.

◊ References.
1. Murrell GAC, Rapeport WG. Clinical pharmacokinetics of allopurinol. Clin Pharmacokinet 1986; 11: 343–53.
2. McGaurn SP, et al. The pharmacokinetics of injectable allopurinol in newborns with the hypoplastic left heart syndrome. Pediatrics 1994; 94: 820–3.
3. Turnheim K, et al. Pharmacokinetics and pharmacodynamics of allopurinol in elderly and young subjects. Br J Clin Pharmacol 1999; 48: 501–9.

Uses and Administration

Allopurinol is used to treat hyperuricaemia (p.397) associated with chronic gout, acute uric acid nephropathy, recurrent uric acid stone formation, enzyme disorders, and cancer or cancer chemotherapy. It is not used for asymptomatic hyperuricaemia. Allopurinol is also used in the management of renal calculi caused by the deposition of calcium oxalate (in the presence of hyperuricosuria) and of 2,8-dihydroxyadenine (see Renal Calculi, below). It may have the potential to reduce oxidative injury by blocking the production of free radicals and is an ingredient of kidney preservation solutions. In addition allopurinol has antiprotozoal activity and has been used in leishmaniasis and American trypanosomiasis.

Allopurinol is used in **gout and hyperuricaemia** to inhibit the enzyme xanthine oxidase, thus preventing the oxidation of hypoxanthine to xanthine and xanthine to uric acid. The urinary purine load, normally almost entirely uric acid, is thereby divided between hypoxanthine, xanthine, and uric acid, each with its independent solubility. This results in the reduction of urate and uric acid concentrations in plasma and urine, ideally to such an extent that deposits of monosodium urate monohydrate or uric acid are dissolved or prevented from forming. At low concentrations allopurinol acts as a competitive inhibitor of xanthine oxidase and at higher concentrations as a non-competitive inhibitor. However, most of its activity is due to the metabolite oxipurinol which is a non-competitive inhibitor of xanthine oxidase.

Allopurinol is used in patients with chronic gout to correct hyperuricaemia thereby reducing the likelihood of acute attacks and preventing the sequelae of chronic gout. In the initial stages of allopurinol therapy, the release of urate and uric acid from deposits may increase concentrations of these compounds circulating in plasma. This may trigger or exacerbate acute attacks, hence allopurinol should not be started until an acute attack has completely subsided. In addition, it is recommended that treatment should be started with a low dose increased gradually and that an NSAID or colchicine should also be given during the first few months.

A suggested starting dose of allopurinol is 100 mg daily by mouth, gradually increased by 100 mg for example at weekly intervals until the concentration of urate in plasma is reduced to 0.36 mmol per litre (6 mg per 100 mL) or less. A daily dose range of 100 to 300 mg may be adequate for those with mild to moderate gout and up to 600 mg for those with moderately severe tophaceous gout. The maximum recommended daily dose is 800 mg in the USA and 900 mg in the UK. Up to 300 mg may be taken as a single daily dose; larger amounts should be taken in divided doses to reduce the risk of gastric irritation. Taking allopurinol after food will also minimise gastric irritation. Patients should maintain an adequate fluid intake to prevent renal xanthine deposition.

Doses of allopurinol should be reduced in patients with impaired renal function (see under Precautions, above)

When used for the prevention of uric acid nephropathy associated with cancer therapy 600 to 800 mg may be given daily generally for 2 or 3 days and starting before the cancer treatment. A high fluid intake is essential. In hyperuricaemia secondary to cancer or cancer chemotherapy, maintenance doses of allopurinol are similar to those used in gout and are given according to the response.

The main use of allopurinol in children is for hyperuricaemia associated with cancer or cancer chemotherapy or with enzyme disorders. The dosage used may vary: in the UK a dose of 10 to 20 mg per kg bodyweight daily up to a maximum of 400 mg daily is recommended for children under 15 years of age, while in the USA the dose is 150 mg daily for children under 6 years of age and 300 mg daily for those aged 6 to 10 years, adjusted if necessary after 48 hours.

Allopurinol has been given as the sodium salt by intravenous infusion in sodium chloride 0.9% or glucose 5% to patients (usually cancer patients) unable to take allopurinol by mouth. The recommended dose in adults is 200 to 400 mg per m² body-surface daily up to a maximum of 600 mg per day.

Diagnosis and testing. Deficiency of the enzyme ornithine carbamoyltransferase can result in severe CNS dysfunction or even in death, and identification of women at risk of being carriers of this genetic enzyme deficiency has been described.[1] The enzyme deficiency causes carbamoyl phosphate to accumulate, which stimulates the synthesis of orotidine. The test relies on the administration of a single dose of allopurinol, which will, in carriers, greatly increase the urinary excretion of orotidine.

1. Hauser ER, et al. Allopurinol-induced orotidinuria. N Engl J Med 1990; **322:** 1641–5. Correction. ibid. 1997; **336:** 1335.

Duchenne muscular dystrophy. Allopurinol has been used in an attempt to increase the ATP levels in muscle which are depleted in Duchenne muscular dystrophy (p.1054). Although some have reported favourable results,[1-3] double-blind studies[4-6] failed to show any benefit from treatment. Despite these findings, some interest in the use of allopurinol for this disorder has continued.[7]

1. Thomson WHS, Smith I. X-linked recessive (Duchenne) muscular dystrophy (DMD) and purine metabolism: effects of oral allopurinol and adenylate. Metabolism 1978; **27:** 151–63.
2. Thomson WHS, Smith I. Allopurinol in Duchenne's muscular dystrophy. N Engl J Med 1978; **299:** 101.
3. Castro-Gago M, et al. Allopurinol in Duchenne muscular dystrophy. Lancet 1980; **i;** 1358–9.
4. Stern LM, et al. The progression of Duchenne muscular dystrophy: clinical trial of allopurinol therapy. Neurology 1981; **31:** 422–6.
5. Hunter JR, et al. Effects of allopurinol in Duchenne's muscular dystrophy. Arch Neurol 1983; **40:** 294–9.
6. Bertorini TE, et al. Chronic allopurinol and adenine therapy in Duchenne muscular dystrophy: effects on muscle function, nucleotide degradation, and muscle ATP and ADP content. Neurology 1985; **35:** 61–5.
7. Castro-Gago M, et al. Long-term effects of xanthine-oxidase inhibitor (allopurinol) in Duchenne muscular dystrophy. Int Pediatr 1994; **9:** 15–20.

Epilepsy. Reduction in the frequency of seizures has been described in some patients with severe or intractable epilepsy (p.338) when allopurinol was added to their existing antiepileptic therapy.[1-3] Although the mode of action was not known it was noted that the patients were not hyperuricaemic and that allopurinol did not affect plasma concentrations of existing antiepileptics.[1]

1. DeMarco P, Zagnoni P. Allopurinol and severe epilepsy. Neurology 1986; **36:** 1538–9.
2. Tada H, et al. Clinical effects of allopurinol on intractable epilepsy. Epilepsia 1991; **32:** 279–83.
3. Zagnoni PG, et al. Allopurinol as an add-on therapy in refractory epilepsy—a double-blind placebo-controlled randomised study. Epilepsia 1994; **35:** 107–12.

Organ transplantation. Allopurinol 25 mg on alternate days has been added to the immunosuppressive treatment given to the patient after renal transplantation,[1] and is reported to reduce the frequency of acute rejection. One possible explanation for this effect is allopurinol's ability to suppress the production of free radicals (see Oxidative Injury, below). Organ and tissue transplantation, and the more usual drugs used in immunosuppressive regimens are discussed on p.502. It should be noted that allopurinol interacts with azathioprine (see Antineoplastics and Immunosuppressants, under Interactions, above) and ciclosporin (p.520).

1. Chocair P, et al. Low-dose allopurinol plus azathioprine/cyclosporin/prednisolone, a novel immunosuppressive regimen. Lancet 1993; **342:** 83–4.

Oxidative injury. Allopurinol through its inhibition of xanthine oxidase can block the development of superoxide free radicals during reperfusion after an ischaemic episode. Consequently, the ability of allopurinol to reduce oxidative injury has been investigated in a number of clinical situations.

In patients undergoing coronary artery bypass graft surgery, perioperative allopurinol administration reduced the number of ischaemic events and reduced the amount of dopamine required.[1,2] However, allopurinol failed to reduce the incidence of periventricular leucomalacia (thought to represent ischaemic infarction of the developing brain) in preterm infants compared with placebo in a large study.[3] Similarly, allopurinol did not reduce the incidence of infarct extension in patients with acute myocardial infarction.[4]

The possibility that allopurinol limits the production of free radicals has also led to allopurinol sodium being included as an ingredient of the University of Wisconsin (UW) solution, which is used for the preservation of organs for transplantation.[5]

A pilot study using allopurinol showed a beneficial effect on free radical formation, cerebral blood volume, and electrical brain activity in severely asphyxiated newborns.[6]

1. Sisto T, et al. Pretreatment with antioxidants and allopurinol diminishes cardiac onset events in coronary artery bypass grafting. Ann Thorac Surg 1995; **59:** 1519–23.
2. Coghlan JG, et al. Allopurinol pretreatment improves postoperative recovery and reduces lipid peroxidation in patients undergoing coronary artery bypass grafting. J Thorac Cardiovasc Surg 1994; **107:** 248–56.

The symbol † denotes a preparation no longer actively marketed

3. Russell GAB, Cooke RWI. Randomised controlled trial of allopurinol prophylaxis in very preterm infants. Arch Dis Child Fetal Neonatal Ed 1995; **73:** F27–F31.
4. Parmley LF, et al. Allopurinol therapy of ischemic heart disease with infarct extension. Can J Cardiol 1992; **8:** 280–6.
5. Southard JH, Belzer FO. Organ preservation. Annu Rev Med 1995; **46:** 235–47.
6. Van Bel F, et al. Effect of allopurinol on postasphyxial free radical formation, cerebral haemodynamics, and electrical brain activity. Pediatrics 1998; **101:** 185–93.

Protozoal infections. Beneficial results have been reported in patients with visceral leishmaniasis (p.584) when allopurinol was added to their therapy;[1,2] these studies involved patients who either had a poor or no response to antimonial drugs or included untreated patients from areas where unresponsive cases were frequent. Positive results in leishmaniasis have also been described in patients with AIDS.[3,4] Variable responses in American cutaneous leishmaniasis have been reported.[5-7] Some beneficial results have been noted in indeterminate and chronic Chagas' disease (American trypanosomiasis, p.587).[8-10]

The selective antiparasitic action of allopurinol is believed to be due to its incorporation into the protozoal, but not the mammalian, purine salvage pathway. This leads to the formation of 4-aminopyrazolopyrimidine ribonucleotide triphosphate, a highly toxic analogue of adenosine triphosphate, that is incorporated into ribonucleic acid. This action of allopurinol is shared by allopurinol riboside, one of the minor metabolites in man but not by oxipurinol, the major human metabolite. Thus, some studies have been conducted with allopurinol riboside, rather than allopurinol, in an attempt to enhance activity by avoiding host-mediated inactivation.[11]

1. Chunge CN, et al. Visceral leishmaniasis unresponsive to antimonial drugs: successful treatment using a combination of sodium stibogluconate plus allopurinol. Trans R Soc Trop Med Hyg 1985; **79:** 715–18.
2. di Martino L, et al. Low dosage combination of meglumine antimoniate plus allopurinol as first choice treatment of infantile visceral leishmaniasis in Italy. Trans R Soc Trop Med Hyg 1990; **84:** 534–5.
3. Dellamonica P, et al. Allopurinol for treatment of visceral leishmaniasis in patients with AIDS. J Infect Dis 1989; **160:** 904–5.
4. Smith D, et al. Visceral leishmaniasis (kala azar) in a patient with AIDS. J Infect Dis 1989; **3:** 41–3.
5. Martinez S, Marr JJ. Allopurinol in the treatment of American cutaneous leishmaniasis. N Engl J Med 1992; **326:** 741–4.
6. Velez I, et al. Inefficacy of allopurinol as monotherapy for Colombian cutaneous leishmaniasis: a randomized, controlled trial. Ann Intern Med 1997; **126:** 232–6.
7. Martinez S, et al. Treatment of cutaneous leishmaniasis with allopurinol and stibogluconate. Clin Infect Dis 1997; **24:** 165–9.
8. Gallerano RH, et al. Therapeutic efficacy of allopurinol in patients with chronic Chagas' disease. Am J Trop Med Hyg 1990; **43:** 159–66.
9. Sánchez G, et al. Treatment with allopurinol and itraconazole changes lytic activity in patients with chronic, low grade Trypanosoma cruzi infection. Trans R Soc Trop Med Hyg 1995; **89:** 438–9.
10. Apt W, et al. Treatment of chronic Chagas' disease with itraconazole and allopurinol. Am J Trop Med Hyg 1998; **59:** 133–8.
11. Shapiro TA, et al. Pharmacokinetics and metabolism of allopurinol riboside. Clin Pharmacol Ther 1991; **49:** 506–14.

Renal calculi. Patients with recurrent calcium oxalate stones are usually treated with thiazide diuretics (p.910). Allopurinol has been suggested as an alternative, particularly where there is also hyperuricosuria; the recommended dose of allopurinol is 200 to 300 mg per day adjusted on the basis of subsequent 24-hour urinary urate excretion. However, there have been conflicting reports of the value of allopurinol in such patients.[1,2] Allopurinol is also advocated for the management of 2,8-dihydroxyadenine (2,8-DHA) renal stones associated with deficient activity of the enzyme adenine phosphoribosyltransferase.

1. Ettinger B, et al. Randomized trial of allopurinol in the prevention of calcium oxalate calculi. N Engl J Med 1986; **315:** 1386–9.
2. Tiselius H-G, et al. Clinical results of allopurinol treatment in the prevention of calcium oxalate stone formation. J Urol (Baltimore) 1986; **136:** 50–3.

Sarcoidosis. Although corticosteroids remain the mainstay of drug therapy for sarcoidosis (p.1058), and other drugs are very much second line, there is a report[1] of benefit in cutaneous disease from the use of allopurinol.

1. Brechtel B, et al. Allopurinol: a therapeutic alternative for disseminated cutaneous sarcoidosis. Br J Dermatol 1996; **135:** 307–9.

Preparations

BP 2001: Allopurinol Tablets;
USP 25: Allopurinol Tablets.

Proprietary Preparations (details are given in Part 3)
Aust.: Allostad; Allotyrol; Apurin; Gewapurol; Gichtex; Purinol; Urosin; Zyloric; **Austral.:** Allohexal; Allorin; Capurate; Progout; Zygout†; Zyloprim; **Belg.:** Zyloric; **Braz.:** Uricemil; Zyloric; **Canad.:** Novo-Purol†; Zyloprim; **Denm.:** Abopur; Apurin; Hexanurat; **Fin.:** Allonol; Apurin; Arturic; Zyloric; **Fr.:** Zyloric; **Ger.:** Allo; Allo-300-Tablinen†; Allo-Efeka; Allo-Puren; Allobeta; Allohexal†; Allpargin; Bleminol; Cellidrin; dura AL; Foligan; Jenapurinol; Milurit; Pureduct; Remid; Uribenz; Uripurinol; Urosin†; Urtias†; Zyloric; **Hong Kong:** Allorin; Caplenal; Mephanol; Milurit; Progout; Zyloric; **Irl.:** Caplenal; Purinol; Tipuric; Zyloric; **Israel:** Alloril; Żylol; Zyloric; **Ital.:** Allurit; Uricemil; Zyloric; **Mex.:** Atisuril; Labypurol; Oloprim; Unizuric; Zyloprim; **Neth.:** Zyloric; **Norw.:** Allopur; Arturic; Zyloric; **NZ:** Allorin; Progout; Zr 300; Zyloprim; **Pol.:** Alosfar; Uriprim; Zurim; Zyloric†; **S.Afr.:** Abburic†; Be-Uric; Ethipurinol†; Lo-Uric; Lonol; Puricos; Pyrazol†; Ranpuric; Redurate; Urinol†; Urozyl-SR†; Zyloprim; **Singapore:** Allorin; Erloric; Progout; Valeric; Zyloric; **Spain:** Allural; Zyloric; **Swed.:** Zyloric; **Switz.:** allo-basan; Allop-

ur; Cellidrine; Foligan†; Lysuron; Mephanol; Sigapurol; Uredimin†; Uriconorme; Zyloric; **Thai.:** Alinol; Allopin; Allorin; Apnol; Apurol; Loporic; Medoric; Mephanol; Puricin; Puride; Sigapurol; Uricad; Valeric; Xanol; Zyloric; **UK:** Aloral†; Caplenal; Cosuric; Progout; Rimapurinol; Xanthomax; Zyloric; **USA:** Aloprim; Zyloprim.

Multi-ingredient: Aust.: Allobenz; Duovitan; Gichtex plus; Uroplus†; **Belg.:** Comburic; **Fr.:** Desatura†; **Ger.:** Acifugan; Allo.comp.; Allomaron; Harpagin; **Ital.:** Uricodue; **Port.:** Acifugan; **S.Afr.:** Allomaron; **Spain:** Acifugan; Facilit; **Switz.:** Acifugan; **Thai.:** Allomaron;

Benzbromarone (1005-b)

Benzbromarone (BAN, USAN, rINN).

Benzbromaronum; L-2214; MJ-10061. 3,5-Dibromo-4-hydroxyphenyl 2-ethylbenzofuran-3-yl ketone.
$C_{17}H_{12}Br_2O_3 = 424.1$.
CAS — 3562-84-3.
ATC — M04AB03.

Pharmacopoeias. In Eur. (see p.vi) and Jpn.

Pharmacopoeial description

Ph. Eur.: A white or almost white crystalline powder. Practically insoluble in water; sparingly soluble in alcohol; freely soluble in acetone and in dichloromethane. Protect from light.

Adverse Effects

Benzbromarone may cause gastrointestinal side-effects, especially diarrhoea. It may precipitate an acute attack of gout and cause uric acid renal calculi and renal colic. Because rare cases of hepatotoxicity have occurred, some manufacturers recommend monitoring liver function.

Effects on the liver. Benzbromarone-induced liver damage has been reported.[1,2]

1. Van Der Klauw MM, et al. Hepatic injury caused by benzbromarone. J Hepatol 1994; **20:** 376–9.
2. Anonymous. Benzbromarone and hepatitis. WHO Drug Inf 2000; **14:** 29.

Precautions

Benzbromarone should be avoided in patients with moderate or severe renal impairment, in those with uric acid renal calculi, and in those with urinary uric acid excretion rates of greater than 700 mg per 24 hours. Like other uricosurics, treatment with benzbromarone should not be started during an acute attack of gout. Similarly, an adequate fluid intake should be maintained to reduce the risk of uric acid renal calculi; additionally alkalinisation of the urine may be considered.

Interactions

Aspirin and other salicylates antagonise the effect of benzbromarone. Benzbromarone may increase the anticoagulant activity of coumarin oral anticoagulants.

Antigout drugs. For mention of the effects of benzbromarone on the clearance of oxipurinol, the major active metabolite of allopurinol, and the view that this was not clinically significant, see under Interactions of Allopurinol, p.398.

Pharmacokinetics

Benzbromarone is only partially absorbed from the gastrointestinal tract, reaching peak plasma concentrations about 2 to 4 hours after a dose by mouth. Benzbromarone is extensively bound to plasma proteins. It is metabolised in the liver, and is excreted mainly in the faeces; a small amount appears in the urine.

◊ References.
1. Maurer H, Wollenberg P. Urinary metabolites of benzbromarone in man. Arzneimittelforschung 1990; **40:** 460–2.
2. Walter-Sack I, et al. Variation of benzbromarone elimination in man—a population study. Eur J Clin Pharmacol 1990; **39:** 173–6.

Uses and Administration

Benzbromarone is a uricosuric drug which reduces plasma concentrations of uric acid by blocking renal tubular reabsorption. It has been suggested that benzbromarone may also increase the intestinal elimination of uric acid. It is used to treat hyperuricaemia including that associated with chronic gout (p.397).

Benzbromarone is not used to treat acute attacks of gout and may exacerbate and prolong them if given during an attack; treatment should not start therefore until an acute attack has subsided.

The usual dose is 50 to 300 mg daily by mouth. An NSAID or colchicine should be given initially to reduce the risk of precipitating acute gout. An adequate fluid intake should be maintained. Lower doses of benzbromarone (20 or 25 mg) are also used in the form of a combination product with allopurinol.

Preparations

Proprietary Preparations (details are given in Part 3)
Aust.: Uricovac; **Belg.:** Desuric; **Braz.:** Narcaricina; **Fr.:** Desuric; **Ger.:** Narcaricin; **Hong Kong:** Narcaricin; **Mex.:** Desuric; **Neth.:** Desuric; **S.Afr.:** Minuric; **Singapore:** Narcaricin; **Spain:** Urinorm; **Switz.:** Desuric; Obaron; **Thai.:** Narcaricin.

Multi-ingredient: Aust.: Allobenz; Duovitan; Gichtex plus; Uroplus†; **Belg.:** Comburic; **Fr.:** Desatura†; **Ger.:** Acifugan; Allo.comp.; Allomaron; Harpagin; **Port.:** Acifugan; **S.Afr.:** Allomaron; **Spain:** Acifugan; Facilit; **Switz.:** Acifugan; **Thai.:** Allomaron.

Benziodarone (9211-v)

Benziodarone (BAN, rINN).

L-2329. 2-Ethylbenzofuran-3-yl 4-hydroxy-3,5-di-iodophenyl ketone.

$C_{17}H_{12}I_2O_3 = 518.1$.

CAS — 68-90-6.

ATC — C01DX04.

Profile

Benziodarone is a uricosuric drug structurally related to benzbromarone (see above) that is used to reduce hyperuricaemia in chronic gout. It was formerly used as a vasodilator.

Benziodarone has been associated with jaundice and thyroid disorders.

Preparations

Proprietary Preparations (details are given in Part 3)

Spain: Dilafurane.

Multi-ingredient: *Ital.:* Uricodue.

Colchicine (1001-d)

Colchicinum. (S)-N-(5,6,7,9-Tetrahydro-1,2,3,10-tetrameth-oxy-9-oxobenzo[a]heptalen-7-yl)acetamide.

$C_{22}H_{25}NO_6 = 399.4$.

CAS — 64-86-8.

ATC — M04AC01.

Pharmacopoeias. In Chin., Eur. (see p.vi), Int., Jpn, and US.

Chin. also has a monograph for colchicine amide.

An alkaloid obtained from various *Colchicum* spp.

Pharmacopoeial description

Ph. Eur.: A yellowish-white amorphous or crystalline powder. Very soluble in water, rapidly recrystallising from concentrated solutions as the sesquihydrate; freely soluble in alcohol and in chloroform. Protect from light.

USP 25: Pale yellow to pale greenish-yellow amorphous scales, or powder or crystalline powder. Is odourless or nearly so, and darkens on exposure to light. Soluble 1 in 25 of water and 1 in 220 of ether; freely soluble in alcohol and in chloroform. Store in airtight containers. Protect from light.

Adverse Effects and Treatment

The most frequent adverse effects of oral colchicine are those involving the gastrointestinal tract and may be associated with its antimitotic action. Diarrhoea, nausea, vomiting, and abdominal pain are often the first signs of toxicity and are usually an indication that colchicine therapy should be stopped or the dose reduced. Larger doses may cause profuse diarrhoea, gastrointestinal haemorrhage, skin rashes, and renal and hepatic damage.

Rarely, bone marrow depression with agranulocytosis, thrombocytopenia, and aplastic anaemia have occurred on prolonged treatment as have peripheral neuropathy, myopathy, rashes, and alopecia.

Adverse effects after intravenous administration include cardiac arrhythmias and local reactions such as thrombophlebitis and neuritis. Extravasation may cause tissue necrosis.

Symptoms of acute **overdosage** with oral colchicine often do not appear for 2 to 12 hours. The first signs of toxicity may be a feeling of burning and rawness in the mouth and throat and difficulty in swallowing. These are followed by nausea, vomiting, and diarrhoea. The diarrhoea may be severe and haemorrhagic and accompanied by colic and tenesmus. These symptoms, coupled with vascular damage, may lead to dehydration, hypotension, and shock. Multiple organ failure may occur and may be manifest as CNS toxicity, bone marrow depression, hepatocellular damage, muscle damage, respiratory distress, myocardial injury, and renal damage. Death may be due to respiratory depression, cardiovascular collapse, or sepsis. In surviving patients, alopecia, rebound leucocytosis, and stomatitis may occur about 10 days after the acute overdose. The lethal dose varies: 7 mg of colchicine has caused death, yet recovery has occurred after much larger doses.

When treating colchicine overdosage or acute poisoning patients should be carefully monitored for some time to take account of the delayed onset of symptoms. In acute poisoning the stomach may be emptied by lavage; multiple dose activated charcoal should be administered. Treatment is primarily symptomatic and supportive with attention being given to the con-

trol of respiration, maintenance of blood pressure and the circulation, and correction of fluid and electrolyte imbalance.

Effects on the neuromuscular system. Colchicine-induced myoneuropathy may be a common but unrecognised condition in patients with *reduced* renal function who receive usual doses of colchicine.[1] Although both skeletal muscles and peripheral nerves are affected, myopathy is most prominent and associated axonal neuropathy is mild. The condition usually presents with proximal muscle weakness and is always accompanied by elevations in serum creatine kinase concentrations. Withdrawal of colchicine leads to spontaneous remission of these symptoms within a few weeks but resolution of the polyneuropathy is slow. Examination of proximal muscles shows marked abnormal spontaneous activity and, because of the features of the condition, it is often initially misdiagnosed as probable polymyositis or uraemic myopathy.

There has been a report of a patient with *normal* renal function but chronic alcohol-induced liver disease who developed an unusual form of myoneuropathy after receiving only a short course of colchicine. This patient was also taking tolbutamide, the microsomal enzyme-inhibiting activity of which may have exacerbated the toxicity of colchicine.[2]

1. Kuncl RW, *et al.* Colchicine myopathy and neuropathy. *N Engl J Med* 1987; **316:** 1562–8.
2. Besana C, *et al.* Colchicine myoneuropathy. *Lancet* 1987; **ii:** 1271–2.

Overdosage. References.

1. Davies HO, *et al.* Massive overdose of colchicine. *Can Med Assoc J* 1988; **138:** 335–6.
2. Simons RJ, Kingma DW. Fatal colchicine toxicity. *Am J Med* 1989; **86:** 356–7.
3. McIntyre IM, *et al.* Death following colchicine poisoning. *J Forensic Sci* 1994; **39:** 280–6.
4. Hood RL. Colchicine poisoning. *J Emerg Med* 1994; **12:** 171–7.
5. Baud FJ, *et al.* Brief report: treatment of severe colchicine overdose with colchicine-specific Fab fragments. *N Engl J Med* 1995; **332:** 642–5.
6. Critchley JAJH, *et al.* Granulocyte-colony stimulating factor in the treatment of colchicine poisoning. *Hum Exp Toxicol* 1997; **16:** 229–32.
7. Milne ST, Meek PD. Fatal colchicine overdose: report of a case and review of the literature. *Am J Emerg Med* 1998; **16:** 603–8.

Precautions

Colchicine should be given with great care to old and debilitated patients who may be particularly susceptible to cumulative toxicity. It should also be used with caution in patients with cardiac, hepatic, renal, or gastrointestinal disease. Colchicine should generally be avoided in pregnancy since it is known to be teratogenic in *animals* and there have also been some suggestions of a risk of fetal chromosome damage (trisomy 21) in humans.

Colchicine should not be administered by subcutaneous or intramuscular injection as it causes severe local irritation.

Pregnancy. Colchicine is considered to be contra-indicated in pregnancy because of *animal* teratogenicity. However, colchicine has been used during pregnancy in women with familial Mediterranean fever (see under Uses, below).[1] There was no increase in abnormality rate of the newborns and no problems were detected in 130 offspring.

1. Rabinovitch O, *et al.* Colchicine treatment in conception and pregnancy: two hundred thirty-one pregnancies in patients with familial Mediterranean fever. *Am J Reprod Immunol* 1992; **28:** 245–6.

Interactions

Ciclosporin. Several workers have highlighted the need for caution if colchicine is used concomitantly with ciclosporin. Myopathies or rhabdomyolysis, especially in patients with renal impairment, may be a problem with this combination.[1,2] In addition, increased blood-ciclosporin concentrations and nephrotoxicity have developed in a renal transplant patient after the introduction of colchicine therapy.[3]

1. Rumpf KW, Henning HV. Is myopathy in renal transplant patients induced by cyclosporin or colchicine? *Lancet* 1990; **335:** 800–1.
2. Arellano F, Krupp P. Muscular disorders associated with cyclosporin. *Lancet* 1991; **337:** 915.
3. Menta R, *et al.* Reversible acute cyclosporin nephrotoxicity induced by colchicine administration. *Nephrol Dial Transplant* 1987; **2:** 380–1.

Erythromycin. Life-threatening colchicine toxicity has been described after 2 weeks of concomitant use of erythromycin in a patient with hepatic and renal impairment.[1]

1. Caraco Y, *et al.* Acute colchicine intoxication—possible role of erythromycin administration. *J Rheumatol* 1992; **19:** 494–6.

Tolbutamide. For a suggestion that tolbutamide may have exacerbated the toxicity of colchicine in a patient with liver disease, see under Effects on the Neuromuscular System, above.

Pharmacokinetics

Peak plasma concentrations of colchicine are reached within 2 hours of oral administration. Colchicine is partially deacetylated in the liver and the unchanged drug and its metabolites are excreted in the bile and undergo intestinal reabsorption. Colchicine is found in high concentrations in leucocytes, kidneys, the liver, and spleen. Most of the drug is excreted in the faeces but 10 to 20% is excreted in the urine and this proportion rises in patients with liver disorders.

◊ References.

1. Rochdi M, *et al.* Toxicokinetics of colchicine in humans: analysis of tissue, plasma and urine data in ten cases. *Hum Exp Toxicol* 1992; **11:** 510–16.
2. Chappey ON, *et al.* Colchicine disposition in human leukocytes after single and multiple oral administration. *Clin Pharmacol Ther* 1993; **54:** 360–7.
3. Rochdi M, *et al.* Pharmacokinetics and absolute bioavailability of colchicine after iv and oral administration in healthy human volunteers and elderly subjects. *Eur J Clin Pharmacol* 1994; **46:** 351–4.
4. Ferron GM, *et al.* Oral absorption characteristics and pharmacokinetics of colchicine in healthy volunteers after single and multiple doses. *J Clin Pharmacol* 1996; **36:** 874–83.

Uses and Administration

Colchicine is used for the relief of acute gout (p.397) and for the prophylaxis of acute attacks, particularly during the first few months of treatment with allopurinol or uricosurics. Colchicine produces a dramatic response in acute gout, probably by reducing the inflammatory reaction to urate crystals; this effect might be due to several actions including decreased leucocyte mobility. It is not an analgesic and has no effect on blood concentrations of uric acid, or on the excretion of uric acid. Colchicine also has an antimitotic action.

Colchicine has also been used in several other conditions including amyloidosis, Behçet's syndrome, familial Mediterranean fever, idiopathic thrombocytopenic purpura, pericarditis, primary biliary cirrhosis, and pyoderma gangrenosum.

If colchicine is used for acute attacks of **gout**, then treatment should be started as soon as possible and an effect may be expected within 12 hours. The recommended oral dose in the UK is 1 mg initially then 0.5 mg every 2 to 3 hours until pain relief is obtained or gastrointestinal adverse effects occur; the total dose should not exceed 6 mg. At least 3 days should elapse before another course is given. In the USA the dose by mouth is 0.5 to 1.2 mg initially, then 0.5 or 0.6 mg every 1 to 2 hours or 1 or 1.2 mg every 2 hours until pain is relieved or gastrointestinal adverse effects occur; the maximum total dose is 6 mg. Colchicine has sometimes been given intravenously in a dose of 1 or 2 mg over 2 to 5 minutes with additional doses of 0.5 or 1 mg every 6 to 24 hours as required to a total dose of not more than 4 mg in one course; once this amount of colchicine has been given further doses should not then be given by any route for at least 7 days.

When used for the short-term prophylaxis of gout doses by mouth are 0.5 or 0.6 mg one to three times daily.

Consideration should be given to using reduced dosages in patients with mild to moderate renal impairment; it should be avoided or given in reduced doses in severe renal impairment.

Amyloidosis. Colchicine is well known to have a useful role in secondary amyloidosis in familial Mediterranean fever, where results have unexpectedly suggested the possibility of reversing nephropathic changes due to renal amyloid deposition (see below), and it has been used in some other forms of amyloidosis,[1-6] especially when combined with other drugs. The mechanism of the anti-amyloid effect of colchicine is not clear. Amyloidosis and its management are discussed further on p.501.

1. Benson MD. Treatment of AL amyloidosis with melphalan, prednisone, and colchicine. *Arthritis Rheum* 1986; **29:** 683–7.
2. Cohen AS, *et al.* Survival of patients with primary (AL) amyloidosis: colchicine-treated cases from 1976 to 1983 compared with cases seen in previous years (1961 to 1973). *Am J Med* 1987; **82:** 1182–90.
3. Fritz DA, *et al.* Unusual longevity in primary systemic amyloidosis: a 19-year survivor. *Am J Med* 1989; **86:** 245–8.
4. Schattner A, *et al.* Primary amyloidosis with unusual bone involvement: reversibility with melphalan, prednisone, and colchicine. *Am J Med* 1989; **86:** 347–8.

5. Skinner M, *et al.* Treatment of 100 patients with primary amyloidosis: a randomised trial of melphalan, prednisone, and colchicine versus colchicine only. *Am J Med* 1996; **100:** 290–8.
6. Kyle RA, *et al.* A trial of three regimens for primary amyloidosis: colchicine alone, melphalan and prednisone, and melphalan, prednisone, and colchicine. *N Engl J Med* 1997; **336:** 1202–7.

Behçet's syndrome. Behçet's syndrome (p.1047) has been treated with numerous drugs. Where possible, topical treatment of local lesions should be attempted before embarking on systemic therapy. Corticosteroids are favoured for systemic treatment in many countries, but colchicine has also been widely employed. Beneficial responses have been described for most of the symptoms including the ocular and cutaneous manifestations,[1-4] although a systematic review has questioned colchicine's efficacy.[5] The mechanism of action in this condition is believed to be based on the effect on polymorphonuclear leucocytes and other cellular effects.[6] Colchicine has also been used in combination with corticosteroids for acute exacerbations, followed by colchicine maintenance;[7] colchicine with aspirin has also been recommended in acute disease,[8] and colchicine with benzathine benzylpenicillin has been tried.[9]

1. Mizushima Y, *et al.* Colchicine in Behçet's disease. *Lancet* 1977; **ii:** 1037.
2. Miyachi Y, *et al.* Colchicine in the treatment of the cutaneous manifestations of Behçet's disease. *Br J Dermatol* 1981; **104:** 67–9.
3. Benezra D, Cohen E. Treatment and visual prognosis in Behçet's disease. *Br J Ophthalmol* 1986; **70:** 589–92.
4. Masuda K, *et al.* Double-masked trial of cyclosporin versus colchicine and long term open study of cyclosporin in Behçet's disease. *Lancet* 1989; **i:** 1093–6.
5. Saenz A, *et al.* Pharmacotherapy for Behçet's syndrome (updated 30 August 2000). Available in The Cochrane Library; Issue 2. Oxford: Update Software; 2001.
6. Schattner A. Colchicine—expanding horizons. *Postgrad Med J* 1991; **67:** 223–6.
7. Rakover Y, *et al.* Behcet disease: long-term follow-up of three children and review of the literature. *Pediatrics* 1989; **83:** 986–92.
8. Wechsler B, Piette JC. Behçet's disease. *BMJ* 1992; **304:** 1199–1200.
9. Çalgüneri M, *et al.* Effect of prophylactic benzathine penicillin on mucocutaneous symptoms of Behçet's disease. *Dermatology* 1996; **192:** 125–8.

Diffuse parenchymal lung disease. Colchicine is a potential alternative to corticosteroid therapy in patients with cryptogenic fibrosing alveolitis (see Diffuse Parenchymal Lung Disease, p.1050).
References.

1. Douglas WW, *et al.* Colchicine versus prednisolone as treatment of usual interstitial pneumonia. *Mayo Clin Proc* 1997; **72:** 201–9.
2. Douglas WW, *et al.* Colchicine versus prednisone in the treatment of idiopathic pulmonary fibrosis: a randomized prospective study. *Am J Respir Crit Care Med* 1998; **158:** 220–5.

Familial Mediterranean fever. Familial Mediterranean fever (recurrent or paroxysmal polyserositis; periodic disease) is an inherited disorder that primarily affects Sephardic Jews or persons of Arab, Armenian, and Turkish ancestry.[1] It is characterised by attacks of acute abdominal pain, fever, and signs of peritonitis, which resolve spontaneously, usually in 24 to 48 hours. Pleuritic chest pain, arthritis, skin rash, pericarditis, and headache may occur. The most dangerous complication, however, is type AA amyloidosis (see also p.501), which can lead to nephrotic syndrome, renal failure, and death.
Familial Mediterranean fever is treated with colchicine.[1] Although a course of the drug may abort an acute attack if given early enough in its development, most patients receive prophylactic treatment, usually with a daily dose in adults of about 0.5 to 2 mg. Such treatment reduces the frequency of attacks and the development of amyloidosis;[2,3] some reversal of established renal problems may also be possible.[4,5] Some evidence suggests interferon alfa may abort acute attacks.[6]

1. Ben-Chetrit E, Levy M. Familial Mediterranean fever. *Lancet* 1998; **351:** 659–63.
2. Zemer D, *et al.* Colchicine in the prevention and treatment of the amyloidosis of familial Mediterranean fever. *N Engl J Med* 1986; **314:** 1001–5.
3. Majeed HA, *et al.* Long-term colchicine prophylaxis in children with familial Mediterranean fever (recurrent hereditary polyserositis). *J Pediatr* 1990; **116:** 997–9.
4. Zemer D, *et al.* Reversal of the nephrotic syndrome by colchicine in amyloidosis of familial Mediterranean fever. *Ann Intern Med* 1992; **116:** 426.
5. Fak AS, *et al.* Colchicine and secondary amyloidosis. *Ann Intern Med* 1992; **117:** 795–6.
6. Tunca M, *et al.* The efficacy of interferon alpha on colchicine-resistant familial Mediterranean fever attacks: a pilot study. *Br J Rheumatol* 1997; **36:** 1005–8.

Idiopathic thrombocytopenic purpura. Case reports have described a few patients with idiopathic thrombocytopenic purpura (p.1052) who had partial or complete responses to colchicine.[1-3] A trial of colchicine has been suggested in adult patients with disease refractory to standard therapy who also do not respond to danazol or vinca alkaloids.[4]

1. Strother SV, *et al.* Colchicine therapy for refractory idiopathic thrombocytopenic purpura. *Arch Intern Med* 1984; **144:** 2198–2200.
2. Jim RTS. Therapeutic use of colchicine in thrombocytopenia. *Hawaii Med J* 1986; **45:** 221–6.
3. Baker RI, Manoharan A. Colchicine therapy for idiopathic thrombocytopenic purpura—an inexpensive alternative. *Aust N Z J Med* 1992; **19:** 412–13.
4. McMillian R. Therapy for adults with refractory chronic immune thrombocytopenic purpura. *Ann Intern Med* 1997; **126:** 307–14.

Pericarditis. Colchicine produced an improvement in a few patients who required corticosteroid therapy to control recurrent episodes of pericarditis.[1,2] Corticosteroid therapy was withdrawn about 2 months after starting treatment with colchicine and the patients had been free of further attacks for up to 54 months. Subsequent experience has also found colchicine of benefit in treating pericardial inflammation.[3,4] The drug has also been used successfully in children.[5]

1. Rodriguez de la Serna AR, *et al.* Colchicine for recurrent pericarditis. *Lancet* 1987; **ii:** 1517.
2. Guindo J, *et al.* Recurrent pericarditis: relief with colchicine. *Circulation* 1990; **82:** 1117–20.
3. Millaire A, *et al.* Treatment of recurrent pericarditis with colchicine. *Eur Heart J* 1994; **15:** 120–4.
4. Adler Y, *et al.* Colchicine treatment for recurrent pericarditis: a decade of experience. *Circulation* 1998; **97:** 2183–5.
5. Yazigi A, *et al.* Colchicine for pericarditis in children. *Acta Paediatr Scand* 1998; **87:** 603–4.

Primary biliary cirrhosis. Primary biliary cirrhosis (p.501) is a chronic progressive liver disease with no specific treatment, and in general drug therapy has been poor or largely ineffective. Reviewers have noted[1-3] that several trials have been conducted with colchicine, and, although biochemical parameters were improved, a beneficial effect on clinical symptoms or liver histology was not found, and only one study showed improved survival of the patients.[4] A comparative study of colchicine and methotrexate therapy showed that while both drugs improved biochemical test results and symptoms, the response to methotrexate was greater.[5] Some commentators consider that combination therapy with colchicine, methotrexate, and ursodeoxycholic acid may be more promising than single-agent therapy,[6] but others have noted that preliminary experience with such combinations has not been encouraging.[7]

1. Bateson MC. New directions in primary biliary cirrhosis. *BMJ* 1990; **301:** 1290–1.
2. Stavinoha MW, Soloway RD. Current therapy of chronic liver disease. *Drugs* 1990; **39:** 814–40.
3. Neuberger J, *et al.* Primary biliary cirrhosis. *Gut* 1991; **32** (suppl): S73–S78.
4. Kaplan MM, *et al.* A prospective trial of colchicine for primary biliary cirrhosis. *N Engl J Med* 1986; **315:** 1448–54.
5. Kaplan MM, *et al.* A prospective trial of colchicine and methotrexate in the treatment of primary biliary cirrhosis. *Gastroenterology* 1999; **117:** 1173–80.
6. Goddard CJR, Warnes TW. Primary biliary cirrhosis: how should we evaluate new treatments? *Lancet* 1994; **343:** 1305–6.
7. Lim AG. Evaluation of new treatment for primary biliary cirrhosis. *Lancet* 1994; **344:** 61.

Pyoderma gangrenosum. Pyoderma gangrenosum (p.1107) associated with inflammatory bowel disease has been successfully treated with colchicine in 2 patients.[1,2] Colchicine was also of benefit in 3 patients with pyoderma associated with familial Mediterranean fever.[3]

1. Paolini O, *et al.* Treatment of pyoderma gangrenosum with colchicine. *Lancet* 1995; **345:** 1057–8.
2. Rampal P, *et al.* Colchicine in pyoderma gangrenosum. *Lancet* 1998; **351:** 1134–5.
3. Lugassy G, Ronnen M. Severe pyoderma associated with familial Mediterranean fever: favourable response to colchicine in three patients. *Am J Med Sci* 1992; **304:** 29–31.

Preparations

BP 2001: Colchicine Tablets;
USP 25: Colchicine Injection; Colchicine Tablets; Probenecid and Colchicine Tablets.

Proprietary Preparations (details are given in Part 3)
Austral.: Colgout; **Hong Kong:** Colgout; **Mex.:** Colchiquim; Ticolcin; **Thai.:** Colchily; Tolchicine.

Multi-ingredient: Fr.: Colchimax; **Spain:** Colchimax; **USA:** ColBenemid; Proben-C†.

Colchicum   (1003-h)

Colchique.

The dried ripe seeds or dried corm of the meadow saffron, *Colchicum autumnale*.

Profile
Colchicum contains colchicine (p.400) and has been used similarly for the relief of acute gout.
It is also included in several herbal and homoeopathic preparations.

Preparations
Proprietary Preparations (details are given in Part 3)
Ger.: Colchysat.

Multi-ingredient: Fr.: Antigoutteux Rezall†; **Ger.:** Unguentum lymphaticum.

Isobromindione   (12866-b)

Isobromindione (rINN).

5-Bromo-2-phenyl-indan-1,3-dione.
$C_{15}H_9BrO_2 = 301.1$.
CAS — 1470-35-5.
ATC — M04AB04.

Profile
Isobromindione is a uricosuric drug that has been used by mouth in gout and hyperuricaemia. Bromindione used to be given as an anticoagulant.

Preparations

Proprietary Preparations (details are given in Part 3)
Ital.: Uridion†.

Probenecid   (1008-q)

Probenecid (BAN, rINN).
Probenecidum. 4-(Dipropylsulphamoyl)benzoic acid.
$C_{13}H_{19}NO_4S = 285.4$.
CAS — 57-66-9.
ATC — M04AB01.

Pharmacopoeias. In *Chin., Eur.* (see p.vi), *Int., Jpn,* and *US.*

Pharmacopoeial description

Ph. Eur.: A white or almost white crystalline powder or small crystals. Practically insoluble in water; sparingly soluble in dehydrated alcohol; soluble in acetone; slightly soluble in ether.

USP 25: A white or practically white, fine, practically odourless, crystalline powder. Practically insoluble in water and in dilute acids; soluble in alcohol, in acetone, in chloroform, and in dilute alkali.

Adverse Effects

Probenecid may cause nausea, vomiting, anorexia, headache, sore gums, flushing, dizziness, and urinary frequency. Hypersensitivity reactions, with fever, dermatitis, pruritus, urticaria, and, rarely, anaphylaxis, and Stevens Johnson syndrome have occurred. There have been reports of hepatic necrosis, the nephrotic syndrome, and aplastic anaemia. Haemolytic anaemia has also occurred, and may be associated with glucose-6-phosphate dehydrogenase deficiency.

When used in chronic gout, and particularly during the first few months of therapy, probenecid may precipitate acute attacks, and uric acid renal calculi with or without haematuria and renal colic may occur.

In massive overdosage probenecid causes stimulation of the CNS, with convulsions and death from respiratory failure. Severe overdosage should be managed by emesis or lavage and symptomatic treatment.

Precautions

Probenecid therapy should not be started during an acute attack of gout; however treatment is usually continued when acute attacks occur in patients already receiving the drug, and the acute attack is treated separately. Probenecid should not be given to patients with a history of uric acid renal calculi or blood disorders. It is not recommended for children under 2 years of age. Probenecid is also unsuitable for the control of hyperuricaemia secondary to cancer or cancer chemotherapy. It should be used with caution in patients with a history of peptic ulceration. Probenecid should not be used as an antibacterial adjunct in patients with known renal impairment, and it is ineffective in gout in patients with severe renal impairment.

To reduce the risk of uric acid renal calculi in patients with gout an adequate fluid intake (2 to 3 litres daily) is required, and, if necessary, especially during the first few months of treatment, sodium bicarbonate or potassium citrate may be given to render the urine alkaline.

A reducing substance has been found in the urine of some patients taking probenecid, and may give false positive results with some tests for glucose in the urine. Probenecid reduces the excretion of some iodinated contrast media and may interfere with laboratory tests by decreasing the excretion of aminohippuric acid, phenolsulfonphthalein, and sulfobromophthalein.

Abuse. It has been alleged that some athletes using banned anabolic steroids have also been taking probenecid in an attempt to inhibit the urinary excretion of steroid metabolites in order to avoid detection by urine screening tests.[1]

1. Anonymous. Does probenecid mask steroid use? *Pharm J* 1987; **239:** 299.

Porphyria. Probenecid should not be given to patients with porphyria.

Interactions

The dose of probenecid may need to be increased if patients are also given drugs such as *diuretics* or *pyrazinamide* that increase the blood concentration of uric acid. Salicylates, including *aspirin*, and probenecid are mutually antagonistic and should not be given together.

Probenecid may also affect many other drugs given concomitantly. By inhibiting renal tubular secretion, probenecid has the potential to increase the toxicity and/or to enhance the therapeutic efficacy of drugs excreted by that route. In some instances a reduction in dose is essential to counteract an increase in toxicity, as is the case with *methotrexate*. Some combinations, such as that with *ketorolac* should be avoided. Conversely, probenecid may be given with some *antibacterials* such as the penicillins and cephalosporins to increase their effects.

Altered excretion may also increase serum concentrations of other antibacterials (aminosalicylic acid, conjugated sulfonamides, dapsone, meropenem, some quinolones, rifampicin), some *antivirals* (aciclovir, ganciclovir, zalcitabine, zidovudine, and possibly famciclovir), some *benzodiazepines* (adinazolam, lorazepam, and possibly nitrazepam), *captopril,* some *NSAIDs* (diflunisal, indometacin, ketoprofen, meclofenamate, naproxen), *paracetamol,* and *sulfonylurea hypoglycaemic drugs.* The clinical significance of such interactions is not entirely clear although the possibility of the need for a reduction in dosage of these drugs should be borne in mind.

It has been reported that patients receiving probenecid require lower doses of *thiopental* for induction of anaesthesia; induction of anaesthesia may be quicker with *midazolam.*

Reducing the urinary concentration of some drugs could diminish their activity in certain diseases as might happen with *nitrofurantoin* or some *quinolones* in urinary-tract infections and *penicillamine* in cystinuria.

Pharmacokinetics

Probenecid is completely absorbed from the gastrointestinal tract with peak plasma concentrations achieved 2 to 4 hours after a dose. It is extensively bound to plasma proteins (85 to 95%). The plasma half-life is dose-dependent and ranges from less than 5 to more than 8 hours. Probenecid crosses the placenta. It is metabolised by the liver, and excreted in the urine mainly as metabolites. Excretion is increased in alkaline urine.

◊ References.
1. Ho JC, *et al.* Probenecid disposition by parallel Michaelis-Menten and dose-dependent pseudo-first-order processes. *J Pharm Sci* 1986; **75:** 664–8.
2. Emanuelsson B-M, *et al.* Non-linear elimination and protein binding of probenecid. *Eur J Clin Pharmacol* 1987; **32:** 395–401.

Uses and Administration

Probenecid is a uricosuric drug used to treat hyperuricaemia (p.397) associated with chronic gout; it has also been used to treat hyperuricaemia caused by diuretic therapy. It is also used as an adjunct to some antibacterials to reduce their renal tubular excretion and has been given with the antiviral cidofovir (p.617) to reduce nephrotoxicity.

Probenecid is used in **chronic gout and hyperuricaemia** to inhibit the renal tubular reabsorption of uric acid so increasing the urinary excretion of uric acid, lowering plasma-urate concentrations, and eventually reducing urate deposits in the tissues. Probenecid is therefore of value in hyperuricaemia caused by decreased uric acid excretion rather than increased urate production, and is not used for hyperuricaemia associated with cancer or cancer therapy.

Probenecid has no analgesic or anti-inflammatory action and is of no value in acute gout. In the initial stages of probenecid therapy, the release of urate and uric acid from deposits may increase concentrations of these compounds in plasma. This may trigger or exacerbate acute attacks, hence probenecid should not

be started until an acute attack has completely subsided. The risk of an attack occurring during the first few months of treatment with probenecid may be reduced by the concurrent administration of an NSAID or colchicine.

It is usual to start treatment for gout with doses of 250 mg twice daily by mouth increased after a week to 500 mg twice daily and later, if the therapeutic effects are inadequate, by increments of 500 mg every 4 weeks, up to 2 g daily. Probenecid may not be effective in chronic renal impairment particularly when the glomerular filtration rate is less than 30 mL per minute. An adequate fluid intake is required to reduce the risk of uric acid renal calculi.

When the patient has been free from acute attacks for at least 6 months, and provided that the plasma-urate concentration is within acceptable limits, the daily dose may be gradually reduced, by 500 mg every 6 months, to the lowest effective maintenance dose which is then given indefinitely.

Probenecid may also be used as an **adjunct to antibacterial therapy** particularly when treating severe or resistant infections. It reduces the tubular excretion of penicillins and most cephalosporins and may increase their plasma concentrations up to fourfold. The usual dosage for reducing tubular excretion of penicillins and cephalosporins is 500 mg four times daily, or less in elderly patients with suspected renal impairment. When renal impairment is sufficient to retard the excretion of antibacterials, probenecid should not be given concurrently.

The dosage for children over 2 years of age and weighing less than 50 kg is 25 mg per kg bodyweight (700 mg per m^2 body-surface) initially, followed by 10 mg per kg (300 mg per m^2) every 6 hours.

Single doses of probenecid 1 g are given together with an oral antibacterial, or at least 30 minutes before an injected antibacterial, in the single-dose treatment of gonorrhoea.

Preparations

BP 2001: Probenecid Tablets;
USP 25: Ampicillin and Probenecid for Oral Suspension; Probenecid and Colchicine Tablets; Probenecid Tablets.

Proprietary Preparations (details are given in Part 3)
Austral.: Benemid; Pro-Cid; *Canad.:* Benemid; Benuryl; *Fin.:* Probecid; *Fr.:* Benemide; *Irl.:* Benemid; *Mex.:* Benecid; *Neth.:* Benemid†; *Norw.:* Probecid; *NZ:* Benemid; *S.Afr.:* Benemid†; Proben; *Swed.:* Probecid; *Switz.:* Benemid; *Thai.:* Bencid; Benemid; *UK:* Benemid†; *USA:* Benemid; Probalan†.

Multi-ingredient: *USA:* ColBenemid; Proben-C†.

Used as an adjunct in: **Braz.:** Ampicler com Probenecide; Degona; Gonocilin; Gonol; Gonorrels; Probecilin; **Spain:** Blenox; **USA:** Polycillin-PRB†.

Sulfinpyrazone (1009-p)

Sulfinpyrazone (BAN, rINN).

G-28315; Sulfinpyrazonum; Sulphinpyrazone; Sulphoxyphenylpyrazolidine. 1,2-Diphenyl-4-(2-phenylsulphinylethyl)pyrazolidine-3,5-dione.
$C_{23}H_{20}N_2O_3S = 404.5.$
CAS — 57-96-5.
ATC — M04AB02.

Pharmacopoeias. In *Eur.* (see p.vi), *Jpn,* and *US.*

Pharmacopoeial description

Ph. Eur.: A white or almost white powder. Very slightly soluble in water; sparingly soluble in alcohol; slightly soluble in ether; dissolves in dilute solutions of alkali hydroxides. Protect from light.

USP 25: A white to off-white powder. Practically insoluble in water and in petroleum spirit; soluble in alcohol and in acetone; sparingly soluble in dilute alkali.

Adverse Effects

The most frequent adverse effects of sulfinpyrazone involve the gastrointestinal tract, and include nausea, vomiting, and abdominal pain. It may cause gastric bleeding and aggravate existing peptic ulcers. Skin rashes have been reported, and may be associated with a hypersensitivity reaction. Anaemia, agranulocytosis, leucopenia, and thrombocytopenia have been reported rarely as have raised liver enzyme values,

jaundice, and hepatitis, impaired renal function, salt and water retention, and acute renal failure.

When used in chronic gout, particularly during the first few months of treatment, sulfinpyrazone may precipitate acute attacks and there is a risk of uric acid renal calculi developing.

Symptoms of overdosage include hypotension, acute renal failure, arrhythmias, respiratory disorders, convulsions, and coma, as well as gastrointestinal effects. Treatment of overdose may involve gastric lavage where appropriate, followed by symptomatic and supportive therapy.

Effects on the kidneys. Although renal failure has been reported occasionally in patients receiving sulfinpyrazone for gout[1] many of the cases have occurred in patients given the drug after a myocardial infarction.[2,3] Acute renal failure may also occur after overdose or in patients with intravascular volume depletion.[4,5]
1. Durham DS, Ibels LS. Sulfinpyrazone-induced acute renal failure. *BMJ* 1981; **282:** 609.
2. Boelaert J, *et al.* Sulfinpyrazone-induced decrease in renal function: a review of reports with discussion of pathogenesis. *Acta Clin Belg* 1982; **37:** 368–75.
3. Lijnen P, *et al.* Decrease in renal function due to sulfinpyrazone treatment early after myocardial infarction. *Clin Nephrol* 1983; **19:** 143–6.
4. Florkowski CM, *et al.* Acute non-oliguric renal failure secondary to sulphinpyrazone overdose. *J Clin Pharm Ther* 1992; **17:** 71.
5. Walls M, *et al.* Acute renal failure due to sulfinpyrazone. *Am J Med Sci* 1998; **315:** 319–21.

Precautions

Sulfinpyrazone should not be started during an acute attack of gout; however, treatment is usually continued when acute attacks occur in patients already receiving the drug, and the acute attack is treated separately. It should not be given to patients with uric acid renal calculi or peptic ulcer disease or a history of such disorders; use is also contra-indicated in patients with blood dyscrasias or blood coagulation disorders, and in those with severe kidney or liver damage. Sulfinpyrazone should not be given to patients hypersensitive to it or to other pyrazole derivatives such as phenylbutazone; nor should it be given to patients in whom hypersensitivity reactions (including bronchospastic reactions in asthmatics) have been provoked by aspirin or by other drugs with prostaglandin-synthetase inhibiting activity. Sulfinpyrazone is not suitable for the control of hyperuricaemia associated with cancer or cancer chemotherapy. It should be given with care to patients whose renal function is impaired and to those with heart failure.

To reduce the risk of uric acid renal calculi an adequate fluid intake (2 to 3 litres daily) is required; alkalinising the urine with sodium bicarbonate or potassium citrate may also be considered. It is recommended that patients have periodic full blood counts to detect any haematological abnormalities.

Renal-function tests involving aminohippuric acid or phenolsulfonphthalein may be invalidated.

Porphyria. Sulfinpyrazone is contra-indicated in patients with porphyria.

Interactions

Doses of sulfinpyrazone may need to be increased if it is given with other drugs such as *diuretics* or *pyrazinamide* that increase uric acid concentrations. Sulfinpyrazone and salicylates including *aspirin* are mutually antagonistic and should not be used together. There may also be an increased risk of bleeding when sulfinpyrazone is used with other drugs such as aspirin that inhibit platelet function.

Sulfinpyrazone's renal tubular secretion is inhibited by probenecid although with little clinical effect. Since sulfinpyrazone, like probenecid, inhibits the tubular secretion of weak organic acids, interactions can be expected with penicillins although the effect is not considered to be clinically useful.

Sulfinpyrazone can potentiate the action of some drugs. The most significant interaction of this type involves *warfarin, nicoumalone [acenocoumarol],* and possibly other coumarin anticoagulants (p.995). Patients receiving sulfinpyrazone and such an anticoagulant should have their prothrombin times monitored and the anticoagulant dosage reduced as appropriate. Similarly, sulfinpyrazone may potentiate the effects of *phenytoin* (see Antigout Drugs, p.360), and possibly some *sulfonamides* and *sulfonylureas*.

In contrast, sulfinpyrazone may increase the metabolism of *theophylline* (p.781) and diminish its activity.

Pharmacokinetics

Sulfinpyrazone is readily absorbed from the gastrointestinal tract. About 98% of the sulfinpyrazone in the circulation is bound to plasma proteins. It has been reported to have a plasma half-life of about 2 to 4 hours. Sulfinpyrazone is partly metabolised in the liver and some of the metabolites are active. On long-term therapy, sulfinpyrazone appears to induce its own metabolism. Unchanged drug and metabolites are mainly excreted in the urine.

◊ References.
1. Bradbrook ID, *et al.* Pharmacokinetics of single doses of sulphinpyrazone and its major metabolites in plasma and urine. *Br J Clin Pharmacol* 1982; **13:** 177–85.
2. Schlicht F, *et al.* Pharmacokinetics of sulphinpyrazone and its major metabolites after a single dose and during chronic treatment. *Eur J Clin Pharmacol* 1985; **28:** 97–103.

Uses and Administration

Sulfinpyrazone is a uricosuric drug used to treat hyperuricaemia associated with chronic gout (p.397). It also has some antiplatelet activity.

Sulfinpyrazone is used in chronic gout to inhibit the renal tubular reabsorption of uric acid so increasing the urinary excretion of uric acid, lowering plasma-urate concentrations, and eventually reducing urate deposits in the tissues. It is therefore of value in hyperuricaemia caused by decreased uric acid excretion rather than increased urate production and is not used for hyperuricaemia associated with cancer or cancer therapy.

Sulfinpyrazone has little analgesic or anti-inflammatory action and is of no value in acute gout. In the initial stages of treatment with sulfinpyrazone the release of urate and uric acid from deposits may increase concentrations of these compounds in plasma. This may trigger or exacerbate acute attacks, hence sulfinpyrazone should not be given until an acute attack has completely subsided. An NSAID or colchi-cine may be given during the first few months of treatment to reduce the risk of such attacks.

The initial dose of sulfinpyrazone is 100 to 200 mg once or twice daily, taken with meals or milk. This may be gradually increased over 1 to 3 weeks until a daily dosage of 600 mg is reached; up to 800 mg daily may be given if necessary. After the plasma-urate concentration has been controlled, the daily maintenance dose may be reduced to as low as 200 mg. An adequate fluid intake is required to prevent formation of uric acid renal calculi.

Antiplatelet therapy. Sulfinpyrazone inhibits platelet function, thereby inhibiting thrombosis. It has been given after myocardial infarction, at a maintenance dose of 200 mg four times daily. For other antithrombotic indications the drug may be given at a dose of 600 to 800 mg daily in 3 or 4 divided doses. A meta-analysis of trials, conducted by the Antiplatelet Trialists' Collaboration, has shown that sulfinpyrazone reduces the risk of myocardial infarction, stroke, or vascular death in patients at high risk of occlusive vascular disease.[1] Similarly, sulfinpyrazone reduces the risk of occlusion in patients undergoing arterial reperfusion and revascularisation procedures.[2] However, aspirin is the most widely tested antiplatelet therapy, as discussed on p.812.
1. Antiplatelet Trialists' Collaboration. Collaborative overview of randomised trials of antiplatelet therapy—I: prevention of death, myocardial infarction, and stroke by prolonged antiplatelet therapy in various categories of patients. *BMJ* 1994; **308:** 81–106.
2. Antiplatelet Trialists' Collaboration. Collaborative overview of randomised trials of antiplatelet therapy—II: maintenance of vascular graft or arterial patency by antiplatelet therapy. *BMJ* 1994; **308:** 159–68.

Preparations

BP 2001: Sulfinpyrazone Tablets;
USP 25: Sulfinpyrazone Capsules; Sulfinpyrazone Tablets.

Proprietary Preparations (details are given in Part 3)
Aust.: Anturan; ***Austral.:*** Anturan; ***Canad.:*** Anturan†; Novo-Pyrazone†; ***Israel:*** Anturan; ***Ital.:*** Enturen; ***NZ:*** Anturan; SPZ; ***Port.:*** Sulfinona; ***S.Afr.:*** Anturan†; ***Switz.:*** Anturan†; ***UK:*** Anturan; ***USA:*** Anturane.

Tisopurine (1010-n)

Tisopurine *(rINN)*.
MPP. 1*H*-Pyrazolo[3,4-*d*]pyrimidine-4-thiol.
$C_5H_4N_4S = 152.2$.
CAS — 5334-23-6.
ATC — M04AA02.

Profile

Tisopurine, an analogue of allopurinol, is an inhibitor of uric acid synthesis. It is used in the treatment of disorders associated with hyperuricaemia (p.397), including gout, in doses of 100 to 400 mg daily.

Preparations

Proprietary Preparations (details are given in Part 3)
Aust.: Exuracid.

Urate Oxidase (20961-m)

CB-8129; Uricase.
CAS — 9002-12-4.
ATC — M04AX01.

Rasburicase (14002-a)

Rasburicase *(BAN, USAN, rINN)*.
SR-29142.
CAS — 134774-45-1.
ATC — V03AF07.

Profile

Rasburicase is a recombinant form of the enzyme urate oxidase, which oxidises uric acid to allantoin. It is used in the treatment and prophylaxis of severe hyperuricaemia associated with the treatment of malignancy. It is given by intravenous infusion before and during the initiation of chemotherapy, in a dose of 200 μg per kg body-weight daily over 30 minutes. Duration of treatment may vary from 5 to 7 days. Adverse effects reported during treatment with rasburicase include fever, vomiting, and nausea; hypersensitivity reactions have occurred. Rasburicase is contra-indicated in patients with glucose-6-phosphate dehydrogenase deficiency or other cellular metabolic disorders known to cause haemolytic anaemia; hydrogen peroxide, which is produced during oxidation of uric acid to allantoin, can induce haemolytic anaemia in these patients.

The native enzyme has also been used.

Tumour lysis syndrome. Rasburicase was effective in the prophylaxis or treatment of hyperuricaemia in young patients with leukaemia or lymphoma who either presented with abnormally high plasma concentrations of uric acid or had large tumour cell burdens.[1] Treatment was mostly well tolerated; one patient developed nausea and vomiting and one experienced bronchospasm and hypoxaemia 3 hours after infusion. Antibodies to rasburicase were seen in 17 of 121 assessable patients.
1. Pui C-H, *et al.* Recombinant urate oxidase for the prophylaxis or treatment of hyperuricemia in patients with leukaemia or lymphoma. *J Clin Oncol* 2001; **19:** 697–704.

Preparations

Proprietary Preparations (details are given in Part 3)
Fr.: Uricozyme; ***Ital.:*** Uricozyme; ***UK:*** Fasturtec.

The symbol † denotes a preparation no longer actively marketed

Antihistamines

The peripheral effects of histamine are chiefly mediated by 2 sets of receptors termed H_1 and H_2. Those effects which are mediated by the H_1 receptors include the contraction of smooth muscle and the dilatation and increased permeability of the capillaries. The effects of histamine on vascular smooth muscle are mediated by the H_2 as well as the H_1 receptors. Other effects that are mediated by the H_2 receptors include cardiac accelerating effects and, in particular, the stimulating action of histamine on the secretion of gastric acid. An H_3 receptor has also been identified in a number of systems including the CNS and peripheral nerves. It is thought that H_3 receptors are involved in the autoregulation of the release of histamine and other neurotransmitters from neurones.

The term 'antihistamines' is normally reserved for histamine H_1-antagonists and this is the convention used in *Martindale*. H_2-antagonists, typified by cimetidine (p.1216), are described in the chapter on Gastrointestinal Drugs. Presently, H_3-antagonists are being investigated for clinical use.

The older antihistamines are associated with troublesome sedative and antimuscarinic effects, and are often termed 'sedating antihistamines'. The newer antihistamines, which are essentially devoid of these effects, are correspondingly termed 'non-sedating antihistamines' and include acrivastine, astemizole, cetirizine, loratadine, and terfenadine.

On the basis of their chemical structure most antihistamines can be classified into one of 6 groups:

- *Alkylamines:* drugs within this group typically possess significant sedative actions, although paradoxical stimulation can occur, especially in children. They are highly potent H_1-antagonists. Brompheniramine and chlorpheniramine [chlorphenamine] are typical alkylamines; acrivastine is a non-sedating alkylamine antihistamine.
- *Monoethanolamines:* monoethanolamine derivatives have pronounced sedative and antimuscarinic actions but a low incidence of gastrointestinal effects. Examples include clemastine and diphenhydramine.
- *Ethylenediamines:* these antihistamines are selective H_1-antagonists. They cause moderate sedation (despite having weak CNS effects), gastric disturbances, and skin sensitisation. Antazoline and mepyramine are examples.
- *Phenothiazines:* phenothiazine antihistamines have significant sedative, and pronounced antiemetic and antimuscarinic effects. Photosensitivity reactions have occurred. Promethazine is a typical phenothiazine.
- *Piperazines:* this group of antihistamines possesses moderate sedative and significant antiemetic actions. Piperazine derivatives include cetirizine, cyclizine, and hydroxyzine. Cetirizine causes less sedation than other members of this group.

- *Piperidines:* piperidines cause moderate or low sedation and are highly selective for H_1 receptors. Examples include azatadine, cyproheptadine, and the non-sedating antihistamines astemizole, loratadine, and terfenadine.

Although characteristic pharmacological properties have been described for members of each group it should be noted that many of the effects of antihistamines vary as much with each patient as with each drug and that, in particular, some of the newer non-sedating antihistamines may share the chemical structure of a group in which the other members have sedative effects.

◊ References.
1. Hill SJ, *et al.* International Union of Pharmacology. XIII. Classification of histamine receptors. *Pharmacol Rev* 1997; **49:** 253–78.
2. Leurs R, *et al.* Therapeutic potential of histamine H_3 receptor agonists and antagonists. *Trends Pharmacol Sci* 1998; **19:** 177–83.

Hypersensitivity. Hypersensitivity may be defined as an exaggerated or inappropriate immune response causing tissue damage. Hypersensitivity reactions are generally classified into 4 types (types I to IV) although this may be considered an over simplification and more than one type can often be postulated for a patient's hypersensitivity. In each of the 4 types, prior sensitisation of the patient to the specific antigen is required. The term 'allergy' by definition originally covered all types of hypersensitivity reactions as well as the induction of immunity in an individual. Nowadays, the term is more commonly applied to type I hypersensitivity reactions.

Type I, immediate hypersensitivity reactions occur after exposure to an antigen (the allergen) in a sensitised subject; that is, one in whom the initial exposure to the antigen has caused the production of specific antibodies, mainly IgE (immunoglobulin E), which are bound to the surface of mast cells and basophils. At subsequent exposure, antigen binds to antibody resulting in degranulation of mast cells and basophils with release of mediators. These include preformed mediators such as histamine and chemotactic factors, and newly synthesised mediators such as leukotrienes, platelet-activating factor, and prostaglandins. Although type I reactions are usually described as being acute and short-lived, clinically there may often also be a late-phase and more prolonged reaction affecting the skin and bronchi. Examples of type I hypersensitivity reactions discussed below include allergic conjunctivitis, allergic rhinitis, urticaria and angioedema, and anaphylactic shock.

Type II, cell-surface hypersensitivity reactions are caused by the interaction of circulating antibodies, mainly IgG (immunoglobulin G) and IgM (immunoglobulin M), with antigens that are on the surface of specific cells or tissues. This interaction results in activation of complement and of phagocytic and killer cells leading to cell damage or lysis. Type II reactions are responsible for blood transfusion reactions, some drug-induced blood disorders, and many auto-immune disorders.

Type III, immune complex hypersensitivity reactions, are caused by the interaction of fixed or circulating antigens with circulating antibodies, mainly IgG and IgM (either soluble or particulate), resulting in formation of immune complexes. The immune complexes trigger a variety of inflammatory processes including complement activation, mediator release from mast cells and basophils, and platelet aggregation. Examples of type III reactions include serum sickness, some auto-immune and neoplastic disorders, type 2 lepra reactions (p.126), and reactions, particularly in the lung, to some particulate antigens such as micro-organisms.

Type IV, cell-mediated or delayed hypersensitivity reactions, are caused by interaction of an antigen with sensitised T lymphocytes; lymphokines are released by T lymphocytes and inflammation ensues. Type IV reactions usually occur at least 24 hours after contact with the antigen. A type IV reaction is responsible for tuberculin reactions for sensitivity testing, contact dermatitis, and some reactions to chronic infectious disease for example type 1 lepra reactions (p.126).

An **anaphylactoid** (pseudoallergic) reaction produces similar symptoms to those of anaphylaxis (see below), but is caused by direct release of histamine provoked by an unclear, non-immune mechanism. There is thus no re-

quirement for prior exposure to the triggering factor, commonly a drug.

Adverse Effects of Antihistamines

The most common side-effect of the *sedating antihistamines* is CNS depression, with effects varying from slight drowsiness to deep sleep, and including lassitude, dizziness, and incoordination (although paradoxical stimulation may occasionally occur, especially at high doses and in children or the elderly). These sedative effects, when they occur, may diminish after a few days of treatment. A major advantage of the *non-sedating antihistamines* is that they generally cause little or no drowsiness (but see below).

Other side-effects that are more common with the *sedating antihistamines* include headache, psychomotor impairment, and antimuscarinic effects, such as dry mouth, thickened respiratory-tract secretions, blurred vision, urinary difficulty or retention, constipation, and increased gastric reflux. Another major advantage of the *non-sedating antihistamines* is that most have little or no antimuscarinic effect.

Occasional gastrointestinal side-effects of antihistamines include nausea, vomiting, diarrhoea, or epigastric pain. Those with antiserotonin actions, such as cyproheptadine, may cause an increase in appetite with resultant weight gain, whereas anorexia has been reported with some other antihistamines.

Palpitations and arrhythmias have been reported occasionally with most antihistamines, but a major disadvantage of the *non-sedating antihistamines* astemizole and terfenadine is the rare occurrence of hazardous ventricular arrhythmias which has led to important restrictions on their use (see under Precautions, below).

Antihistamines may sometimes cause rashes and hypersensitivity reactions (including bronchospasm, angioedema, and anaphylaxis) and cross-sensitivity to related drugs may occur. Photosensitivity can be a problem, particularly with the phenothiazine antihistamines.

Blood disorders, including agranulocytosis, leucopenia, haemolytic anaemia, and thrombocytopenia, although rare, have been reported. Jaundice has also been observed, particularly with the phenothiazine antihistamines.

Other adverse effects that have been reported with the antihistamines include convulsions, sweating, myalgia, paraesthesias, extrapyramidal effects, tremor, sleep disturbances, depression, confusion, tinnitus, hypotension, and hair loss.

Despite reports suggesting a possibility of human fetal abnormalities resulting from the use of some antihistamines, especially the piperazine derivatives, a causal relationship has largely been rejected; for details see under Precautions, below.

Some antihistamines have been abused for their mental effects.

Antihistamines available as preparations for application to the skin may occasionally cause skin sensitisation; systemic side-effects have been reported after topical application to large areas of the skin.

Overdosage with *sedating antihistamines* is associated with antimuscarinic, extrapyramidal, and CNS effects. When CNS stimulation predominates over CNS depression, which is more likely in children or the elderly, it causes ataxia, excitement, tremors, psychoses, hallucinations, and convulsions; hyperpyrexia may also occur. Deepening coma and cardiorespiratory collapse may follow. In adults, CNS depression is more common with drowsiness, coma, and convulsions, progressing to respiratory failure and cardiovascular collapse. In the case of the *non-sedating antihistamines*, antimuscarinic effects are less marked, but hazardous ventricular arrhythmias (below) may be a special problem with astemizole and terfenadine, even in modest overdoses, and have led to restrictions on their use.

◊ Reviews.
1. Simons FER. H₁-receptor antagonists: comparative tolerability and safety. *Drug Safety* 1994; **10:** 350–80.

Arrhythmias. Ventricular arrhythmias have been reported rarely with astemizole and terfenadine particularly in association with increased blood concentrations. For full details and specific warnings see under Astemizole, p.409, and Terfenadine, p.424.

The suspicion that such life-threatening arrhythmias may be a class effect of the non-sedating antihistamines has so far proven unfounded. Data[1] from the WHO adverse drug reaction database showed that cardiac events had been reported with the 5 most widely prescribed non-sedating antihistamines (acrivastine, astemizole, cetirizine, loratadine, and terfenadine), and an attempt to quantify the risk[2] suggested that use of these drugs was associated overall with a fourfold increase in likelihood of developing ventricular arrhythmias, although the absolute risk remained low. However, other centres[3] have argued that definitive causality has only been proven for astemizole and terfenadine. In addition, a possible mechanism for drug-induced cardiac toxicity has only been demonstrated with astemizole and terfenadine;[4] both drugs have been shown to block cardiac potassium channels *in vitro*, a phenomenon that results in prolongation of the QT interval, which is a risk factor for developing ventricular arrhythmias. Studies[5] with loratadine and cetirizine have demonstrated that neither drug blocked potassium channels *in vitro*.

1. Lindquist M, Edwards IR. Risks of non-sedating antihistamines. *Lancet* 1997; **349:** 1322. Correction. *ibid.;* 1482.
2. de Abajo FJ, García Rodrígues LA. Risk of ventricular arrhythmias associated with nonsedating antihistamine drugs. *Br J Clin Pharmacol* 1999; **47:** 307–13.
3. Himmel MH, *et al.* Dangers of non-sedating antihistamines. *Lancet* 1997; **350:** 69.
4. Salata JJ, *et al.* Cardiac electrophysiological actions of the histamine H₁-receptor antagonists astemizole and terfenadine compared with chlorpheniramine and pyrilamine. *Circ Res* 1995; **76:** 110–19.
5. Woosley RL. Cardiac actions of antihistamines. *Ann Rev Pharmacol Toxicol* 1996; **36:** 233–52.

Reye's syndrome. For criticism of a suggested link in children between antihistamines and Reye's syndrome, see p.15.

Sedation. CNS depression is a common adverse effect of the sedating antihistamines and sedative effects can range from slight drowsiness to deep sleep. Daytime sedation can be a problem especially for those who have to drive or operate machinery. When sedative effects do occur they are most apparent at the start of treatment and often diminish after a few days despite continued administration. Sedation caused by alcohol or other CNS depressants is enhanced. Many studies have attempted to quantify and compare the sedative effects of the older antihistamines, but results vary widely and classifications are difficult to make. Theoretically, the onset, degree, and persistence of sedation depend on factors such as penetration of the blood-brain barrier and on the relative affinity for central and peripheral histamine H₁ receptors. In general, antihistamines of the monoethanolamine and phenothiazine classes cause the most sedation.

In view of these problems, non-sedating antihistamines have been developed. These compounds have poor penetration into the CNS and/or higher affinity for peripheral rather than central histamine H₁ receptors. Studies with acrivastine,[1] astemizole,[2] fexofenadine,[3] loratadine,[4] and terfenadine[5] have generally indicated a lower incidence of sedation and related CNS effects than that observed with older antihistamines and comparable with that of placebo. In a study[6] to compare the effects of acrivastine, terfenadine, and diphenhydramine on driving performance, terfenadine had no significant effect on driving performance. Acrivastine's effects were dose-related, but with little effect at the normal therapeutic dose, whereas diphenhydramine profoundly impaired all the measures of driving performance. In another study,[7] the effects of fexofenadine on driving performance were comparable to placebo. Studies with terfenadine[5] suggest that the incidence of sedation does not increase significantly with increased dose or duration of administration. Cetirizine appears to be more sedating than loratadine or terfenadine but less sedating than older antihistamines; the effect appears to be dose dependent.[8] Limited data with azelastine[9] indicate a similar incidence of drowsiness to that with terfenadine. An incidence of sedation comparable with that caused by terfenadine has also been observed for mequitazine when given in the recommended dosage of 5 mg twice daily.[5] Sedation has, however, occurred after doses of 10 mg twice daily.[10] Other newer antihistamines claimed to produce no troublesome sedation include ebastine, epinastine, mizolastine, and setastine.

A number of studies have indicated that the non-sedating antihistamines do not seem to enhance the effects of alcohol and other CNS depressants.

A few patients treated with non-sedating antihistamines have experienced drowsiness. Therefore it is prudent to exercise caution before driving or operating machinery; the effect of a drug on a particular patient can be ascertained after the first few doses.

1. Bojkowski CJ, *et al.* Acrivastine in allergic rhinitis: a review of clinical experience. *J Int Med Res* 1989; **17** (suppl 2): 54B–68B.

2. Anonymous. Astemizole—another non-sedating antihistamine. *Med Lett Drugs Ther* 1989; **31:** 43–4.
3. Hindmarch I, *et al.* A double-blind, placebo-controlled investigation of the effects of fexofenadine, loratadine and promethazine on cognitive and psychomotor function. *Br J Clin Pharmacol* 1999; **48:** 200–206.
4. Clissold SP, *et al.* Loratadine: a preliminary review of its pharmacodynamic properties and therapeutic efficacy. *Drugs* 1989; **37:** 42–57.
5. McTavish D, *et al.* Terfenadine: an updated review of its pharmacological properties and therapeutic efficacy. *Drugs* 1990; **39:** 552–74.
6. Ramaekers JG, O'Hanlon JF. Acrivastine, terfenadine and diphenhydramine effects on driving performance as a function of dose and time after dosing. *Eur J Clin Pharmacol* 1994; **47:** 261–6.
7. Weiler JM, *et al.* Effects of fexofenadine, diphenhydramine, and alcohol on driving performance: a randomized, placebo-controlled trial in the Iowa driving simulator. *Ann Intern Med* 2000; **132:** 354–63.
8. Spencer CM, *et al.* Cetirizine: a reappraisal of its pharmacological properties and therapeutic use in selected allergic disorders. *Drugs* 1993; **46:** 1055–80.
9. McTavish D, Sorkin EM. Azelastine: a review of its pharmacodynamic and pharmacokinetic properties, and therapeutic potential. *Drugs* 1989; **38:** 778–800.
10. Brandon ML. Newer non-sedating antihistamines: will they replace older agents? *Drugs* 1985; **30:** 377–81.

Precautions for Antihistamines

Drowsiness is a major problem with the *sedating antihistamines* and those affected should not drive or operate machinery; alcohol should be avoided. In the case of *non-sedating antihistamines*, although drowsiness is rare, it can occur and it may affect the performance of skilled tasks.

Because of their antimuscarinic actions the *sedating antihistamines* should be used with care in conditions such as angle-closure glaucoma, urinary retention, prostatic hyperplasia, or pyloroduodenal obstruction; antimuscarinic side-effects are not a significant problem with the *non-sedating antihistamines*.

Occasional reports of convulsions in patients taking antihistamines also calls for caution in patients with epilepsy.

Many antihistamines are excreted in the urine in the form of active metabolites so that dosage reduction may be necessary in renal impairment (see individual monographs for specific advice). Caution is also needed in hepatic impairment, notably with phenothiazine antihistamines (for further details, see under Chlorpromazine on p.661) and, above all, with the *non-sedating antihistamines*, astemizole and terfenadine (hazardous ventricular arrhythmias may occur in the presence of excessive blood concentrations). Other important cautions for astemizole and terfenadine include avoidance of concomitant use of drugs liable to interfere with their hepatic metabolism or otherwise increase the risk of arrhythmias, and contra-indication in patients with cardiac disease, known or suspected prolongation of the QT interval, or hypokalaemia or other electrolyte imbalances. For full details see under Astemizole, p.409, and Terfenadine, p.424.

Antihistamines should not be given to neonates owing to their increased susceptibility to antimuscarinic effects. It has also been recommended that antihistamines, in particular phenothiazines (see Promethazine, p.423 and Trimeprazine, p.426), should be avoided in young children. Elderly patients are also more susceptible to many of the adverse effects of antihistamines and, in particular, their inappropriate use for postural giddiness should be avoided (see Vertigo, below).

Topical preparations containing antihistamines should not be used on broken or eczematous skin.

A number of large studies have failed to demonstrate any strong associations between fetal abnormalities and antihistamines taken during pregnancy (see under Pregnancy, below).

Asthma. Antihistamines have been considered ineffective in the management of asthma despite demonstrated bronchodilator and histamine-blocking effects.[1] There has also been concern that antihistamines may cause airway obstruction (apparently due to bronchoconstriction), and hence their use has often been contra-indicated in patients with asthma. However, antihistamine-induced airway obstruction has rarely been noted clinically and many patients with asthma tolerate concurrent treatment with antihistamines without obvious adverse effects. Therefore the American Academy of Allergy and Immunology has recommended that antihistamines are not contra-indicated

in patients with asthma, unless an adverse reaction has previously been demonstrated and the FDA subsequently removed a warning against the use of over-the-counter antihistamines by people with asthma.[2]

1. Meltzer EO. To use or not to use antihistamines in patients with asthma. *Ann Allergy* 1990; **64:** 183–6.
2. Food and Drug Administration. Cold, cough, allergy, bronchodilator, and antiasthmatic drug products for over-the-counter human use: final monograph for OTC antihistamine drug products: final rule. *Fed Regist* 1992; **57:** 58369–70.

Pregnancy. Considerable anxiety has surrounded the issue of whether there is any risk to the fetus from antiemetic therapy during pregnancy. The most widely studied preparation was Debendox which contained doxylamine, dicyclomine [dicycloverine], and pyridoxine, and was known as Bendectin in some countries. Dicyclomine [dicycloverine] was removed from the preparation in 1976 in the USA and subsequently in other countries, and the product was withdrawn from the market in 1983 because of threatened litigation.[1] By that time Debendox had been used for over 27 years and in over 33 million pregnancies worldwide.[1]

Initial concern came from anecdotal reports of malformations in infants whose mothers had taken Debendox during pregnancy.[2,3] Evidence was found[4] of an association between prenatal exposure to the 3-component formulation of Bendectin and an increased risk of pyloric stenosis and possibly also defective heart valves in a study of 1369 malformed infants and 2968 healthy control cases. Other studies have suggested an increased incidence of oral clefts,[5] gastrointestinal atresia,[6] and genital tract disorders,[7] but generally such increases have been small. No overall pattern of malformations appears to have emerged, and many large studies have failed to confirm an association between doxylamine use and congenital malformations.[8–13]

A prospective study of 11 481 pregnancies found no increased incidence of either severe congenital abnormalities or perinatal mortality rates in women who had been prescribed prochlorperazine, meclozine, cyclizine, or Bendectin during pregnancy, although there was some evidence of an excess number of congenital abnormalities in patients taking trimethobenzamide.[14]

The Collaborative Perinatal Project[15] monitored the mothers of 50 282 children between 1958 and 1965. Of these, 5401 were exposed to antihistamines and 1309 to phenothiazines during the first 4 months of pregnancy. There was no evidence to suggest that exposure to these drugs was related to malformations, although there were slight suggestions of associations between respiratory malformations and pheniramine, inguinal hernia and meclozine, inguinal hernia or genito-urinary malformations and diphenhydramine, and cardiovascular deformities and phenothiazines. A report[16] on the same study found no effects of phenothiazines on perinatal mortality, birth-weight, or IQ scores at the age of 4 years. The Collaborative Perinatal Project also noted a relationship between cardiovascular defects and inguinal hernia and dimenhydrinate exposure.[15]

Both the UK Committee on Safety of Medicines[17] and the FDA in the USA[18] reviewed the literature in 1981 and concluded that while the scientific evidence did not demonstrate an increase in birth defects with the Debendox combination, the risk of teratogenicity could not be completely excluded. There has been a study indicating that vomiting itself is not teratogenic.[19]

A number of other studies have been carried out on meclozine prompted by reports of fetal abnormalities in 10 patients associated with a preparation of meclozine and pyridoxine;[20] these studies have not supported the original reports.[21–23]

1. Merrell Pharmaceuticals. Production of Debendox to stop. *Lancet* 1983; **i:** 1395.
2. Paterson DC. Congenital deformities associated with Bendectin. *Can Med Assoc J* 1977; **116:** 1348.
3. Donnai D, Harris R. Unusual fetal malformations after antiemetics in early pregnancy. *BMJ* 1978; **1:** 691–2.
4. Eskenazi B, Bracken MB. Bendectin (Debendox) as a risk factor for pyloric stenosis. *Am J Obstet Gynecol* 1982; **144:** 919–24.
5. Golding J, *et al.* Maternal anti-nauseants and clefts of lip and palate. *Hum Toxicol* 1983; **2:** 63–73.
6. Jick H, *et al.* First-trimester drug use and congenital disorders. *JAMA* 1981; **246:** 343–6.
7. Gibson GT, *et al.* Congenital anomalies in relation to the use of doxylamine/dicyclomine and other antenatal factors: an ongoing prospective study. *Med J Aust* 1981; **i:** 410–4.
8. Shapiro S, *et al.* Antenatal exposure to doxylamine succinate and dicyclomine hydrochloride (Bendectin) in relation to congenital malformations: perinatal mortality rate, birth weight, and intelligence quotient score. *Am J Obstet Gynecol* 1977; **128:** 480–5.
9. Harron DWG, *et al.* Debendox and congenital malformations in Northern Ireland. *BMJ* 1980; **281:** 1379–81.
10. Fleming DM, *et al.* Debendox in early pregnancy and fetal malformation. *BMJ* 1981; **283:** 99–101.
11. Mitchell AA, *et al.* Birth defects related to Bendectin use in pregnancy 1: Oral clefts and cardiac defects. *JAMA* 1981; **245:** 2311–14.
12. Mitchell AA, *et al.* Birth defects in relation to Bendectin use in pregnancy. *Am J Obstet Gynecol* 1983; **147:** 737–42.
13. Winship KA, *et al.* Maternal drug histories and central nervous system anomalies. *Arch Dis Child* 1984; **59:** 1052–9.
14. Milkovich L, van den Berg BJ. An evaluation of the teratogenicity of certain antinauseant drugs. *Am J Obstet Gynecol* 1976; **125:** 244–8.
15. Heinonen OP, *et al. Birth defects and drugs in pregnancy.* Massachusetts: Publishing Sciences Group, 1977.
16. Slone D, *et al.* Antenatal exposure to the phenothiazines in relation to congenital malformations, perinatal mortality rate, birth weight, and intelligence quotient score. *Am J Obstet Gynecol* 1977; **128:** 486–8.

17. Committee on Safety of Medicines. Data sheet change—Debendox. *Current Problems* 6 1981.
18. Food and Drugs Administration. Indications for Bendectin narrowed. *FDA Drug Bull* 1981; **11** (1).
19. Klebanoff MA, Mills JL. Is vomiting during pregnancy teratogenic? *BMJ* 1986; **292**: 724–6.
20. Watson GI. Meclozine ("Ancoloxin") and foetal abnormalities: preliminary report by the epidemic observation unit of the College of General Practitioners. *BMJ* 1962; **ii**: 1446.
21. Lenz W. How can the teratogenic action of a factor be established in man? *South Med J* 1971; **64** (suppl 1): 41–7.
22. Greenberg G, *et al.* Maternal drug histories and congenital abnormalities. *BMJ* 1977; **2**: 853–6.
23. Shapiro S, *et al.* Meclizine in pregnancy in relation to congenital malformations. *BMJ* 1978; **i**: 483.

Interactions of Antihistamines

Sedating antihistamines may enhance the sedative effects of CNS depressants including alcohol, barbiturates, hypnotics, opioid analgesics, anxiolytic sedatives, and antipsychotics. Sedative interactions apply to a lesser extent with the *non-sedating antihistamines*; they do not appear to potentiate the effects of alcohol, but it should be avoided in excess.

Sedating antihistamines have an additive antimuscarinic action with other antimuscarinic drugs, such as atropine and some antidepressants (both tricyclics and MAOIs).

Potentially hazardous ventricular arrhythmias have occurred when the *non-sedating antihistamines* astemizole and terfenadine have been given concomitantly with drugs liable to interfere with their hepatic metabolism, with other potentially arrhythmogenic drugs including those that prolong the QT interval, or with those likely to cause electrolyte imbalance. For full details see under Astemizole, p.409, and Terfenadine, p.425.

It has been suggested that some *sedating antihistamines* could mask the warning signs of damage caused by ototoxic drugs such as aminoglycoside antibiotics.

Antihistamines may suppress the cutaneous histamine response to allergen extracts and should be stopped several days before skin testing.

Uses of Antihistamines

Histamine H_1-antagonists (termed 'antihistamines' in *Martindale*) diminish or abolish the major actions of histamine in the body by competitive, reversible blockade of histamine H_1-receptor sites on tissues; they do not inactivate histamine or prevent its synthesis, nor, in most cases, its release (although some are claimed to have mast-cell stabilising properties). Histamine H_1 receptors are responsible for vasodilation, increased capillary permeability, flare and itch reactions in the skin, and to some extent for contraction of smooth muscle in the bronchi and gastrointestinal tract.

Many of the *sedating antihistamines* also possess antimuscarinic, adrenaline-antagonising, serotonin-antagonising, and local anaesthetic effects. Some have calcium-channel blocking activity.

Antihistamines are used primarily for the alleviation of conditions such as urticarial rashes and nasal allergy that are characterised by type I hypersensitivity (see above), but by virtue of their associated pharmacological actions they are also used to alleviate the symptoms of a wide range of other conditions (such as pruritus and nausea and vomiting).

The antihistamines can improve or relieve the symptoms of seasonal allergic rhinitis ('hay fever') in a high percentage of patients. They alleviate rhinorrhoea and sneezing (and ocular symptoms such as conjunctivitis) but may be less effective for nasal congestion. The relief obtained is dependent on the severity and nature of the symptoms, being greater in the milder stages. The *non-sedating antihistamines* are preferred for daytime control, but a *sedating antihistamine* may be preferred at night. Antihistamines may also be of value in vasomotor rhinitis, despite the fact that this is not primarily an allergic condition.

Antihistamines are of value in preventing urticaria and are used to treat urticarial rashes and mild angioedema. They are also used as adjuncts to adrenaline [epinephrine] in the emergency treatment of ana-

phylaxis and severe angioedema. The use of an antihistamine is not appropriate for the control of blood transfusion reactions caused by ABO incompatibility.

The *sedating antihistamines* are of value in the alleviation of pruritus both of allergic and of non-allergic origin; they have a major role in pruritus associated with atopic eczema. The *non-sedating antihistamines* do not alleviate pruritus of non-allergic origin owing to their poor penetration of the blood-brain barrier.

Sedating antihistamines have marked antiemetic activity and are used to control nausea and vomiting caused by a variety of vestibular disorders. In the case of motion sickness a sedating antihistamine, such as dimenhydrinate or promethazine, is used if severe drowsiness (or even sleep) is not considered undesirable, but generally a less sedative antihistamine, such as cyclizine, cinnarizine, or meclozine may be preferred. Sedating antihistamines are similarly used to control the vertigo and nausea associated with Ménière's disease and related conditions, with cinnarizine promoted as a specific treatment. Sedating antihistamines also have an important role in the alleviation of the nausea and vomiting of migraine, and buclizine or cyclizine are marketed in some countries in a combination preparation for this purpose; cyproheptadine, which has serotonin antagonist and calcium-channel blocking activity, may be of value in the prophylaxis of migraine. Sedating antihistamines have a very limited role in the short-term management of vomiting of pregnancy and are no longer considered appropriate for nausea alone. *Sedating antihistamines* have also been widely used for premedication in anaesthetic practice and still have a major role in the prevention of postoperative nausea and vomiting.

Some of the antihistamines with very pronounced sedative effects, such as diphenhydramine and promethazine, have been marketed for treatment of occasional insomnia but their long duration of action can cause hangover effects. *Sedating antihistamines* are also widely marketed, often with a decongestant, in compound preparations for the symptomatic treatment of coughs and colds although there is little evidence of value. Some antihistamines are also available as preparations for topical application for the alleviation of insect bites, but there is little evidence of any real value and such use may be associated with sensitisation.

◊ General references.
1. Simons FER, Simons KJ. Clinical pharmacology of new histamine H_1 receptor antagonists. *Clin Pharmacokinet* 1999; **36**: 329–52.
2. Slater JW, *et al.* Second-generation antihistamines: a comparative review. *Drugs* 1999; **57**: 31–47.

Anaesthesia

Phenothiazine antihistamines have been used for anaesthetic premedication (p.1256) and to relieve anxiety during surgical and obstetric procedures, but benzodiazepines are now used more routinely. However, sedating antihistamines such as promethazine and cyclizine do have a role in the control of postoperative vomiting (below). Trimeprazine [alimemazine] is licensed for premedication in children, although when given alone it may cause postoperative restlessness if pain is present.

Anaphylaxis

Anaphylaxis is commonly a type I (immediate) hypersensitivity reaction (see above) to various allergens such as drugs, foods, and insect venoms. A clinically identical reaction can, however, be provoked by some other immune mechanisms, or by non-immune mechanisms (an anaphylactoid reaction). Symptoms of anaphylaxis and anaphylactoid reactions include erythema, pruritus, urticaria, and angioedema; respiratory obstruction may result from oedema of the larynx or epiglottis. Gastrointestinal disturbances, bronchospasm, hypotension, and coma can occur in severe reactions.

Patients with severe anaphylactic or anaphylactoid reactions should be given immediate treatment with adrenaline [epinephrine] (see Anaphylactic Shock, p.832). Addition of a parenteral antihistamine such as

chlorpheniramine [chlorphenamine] maleate or diphenhydramine hydrochloride and a corticosteroid such as hydrocortisone after the acute episode may decrease the duration and severity of symptoms and prevent relapse. The use of antihistamines in treating the symptoms of milder forms of anaphylaxis is discussed under individual symptoms such as Pruritus (below) and Urticaria and Angioedema (below).

Angioedema

See under Urticaria and Angioedema, below.

Asthma

Antihistamines, with the possible exception of ketotifen, appear to have no place in the treatment of asthma (p.757). A meta-analysis[1] of double-blind randomised placebo-controlled trials published since 1980 did not support the use of antihistamines in the treatment of asthma, although the quality of the studies was generally considered to be poor.

1. Van Ganse E, *et al.* Effects of antihistamines in adult asthma: a meta-analysis of clinical trials. *Eur Respir J* 1997; **10**: 2216–24.

Conjunctivitis

Allergic conjunctivitis is a type I hypersensitivity reaction (above). It is usually seasonal but perennial attacks due to allergens such as house dust mites can occur. Itching, tears, and burning are common symptoms and frequently rhinitis (below) will co-exist. Conjunctivitis can also be caused by pathogenic micro-organisms (p.121).

Avoidance of unnecessary exposure to aeroallergens is of prime importance in the management of allergic conjunctivitis. Since a large number of inflammatory mediators are involved in its pathogenesis no single drug will be completely effective. Systemic sedating and non-sedating antihistamines are effective in reducing allergic symptoms and preventing attacks and the choice of drug depends on the degree of sedation required. Ophthalmic antihistamine preparations such as antazoline, azelastine, levocabastine, and olopatadine may also be used for acute attacks. Ophthalmic corticosteroids may reduce inflammation, but use should be restricted to severe cases only and limited to 5 to 7 days' duration because of the risk of local adverse effects such as cataract or raised intra-ocular pressure. Mast-cell stabilisers including lodoxamide, nedocromil, and sodium cromoglicate have been widely used for prophylaxis; some antihistamines also have mast-cell stabilising properties. Ketorolac eye drops are available for the treatment of allergic conjunctivitis. Combined preparations of astringents such as zinc sulfate and sympathomimetics such as naphazoline may also be used for symptomatic relief.

References.
1. Ciprandi G, *et al.* Drug treatment of allergic conjunctivitis: a review of the evidence. *Drugs* 1992; **43**: 154–76.
2. Hingorani M, Lightman S. Therapeutic options in ocular allergic disease. *Drugs* 1995; **50**: 208–21.
3. McGill JI, *et al.* Allergic eye disease mechanisms. *Br J Ophthalmol* 1998; **82**: 1203–14.

Coughs and colds

Sedating antihistamines are frequently used in combination preparations for the treatment of coughs and colds (p.1082 and p.605 respectively). The mechanism of their antitussive action may involve reduction in cholinergic nerve transmission or may simply result from their sedative effects; reduction of nasal secretions may be of value in treating cough caused by postnasal drip. Antihistamines should not be used to treat productive coughs because reduction in bronchial secretions may cause formation of viscid mucus plugs. The sedative effects of antihistamines may prove troublesome for daytime use but may be a short-term advantage for night coughs.

Food allergy

The term food allergy (food hypersensitivity) should be reserved for instances in which an immune mechanism for the reaction is proven, as may occur, for example, with nuts; food intolerance is used to describe a non-immune reaction. Food allergy may be the result of a type I (immediate), or possibly a type III (immune complex), hypersensitivity reaction (see above). Management revolves around the identification of the provoking food allergen and its subsequent avoidance. Individualised diets are designed and patients are educated about possible hidden sources of the allergen. Drug therapy has a very limited role in the prevention of food allergy; oral sodium cromoglicate has been used but efficacy has not been unequivocally established.

Inadvertent exposure to an allergen resulting in anaphylactic shock (p.832) requires immediate treatment with adrenaline [epinephrine]. Milder symptoms may be controlled by antihistamines and corticosteroids. Hyposensitisation plays no role in the routine management of food allergy (see p.1576).

References.
1. Hunter JO. Food allergy and intolerance. *Prescribers' J* 1997; **37:** 193–8.
2. Sampson HA. Food allergy. *JAMA* 1997; **278:** 1888–94.
3. Bindslev-Jensen C. Food allergy. *BMJ* 1998; **316:** 1299–1302.
4. Høst A, *et al.* Dietary products used in infants for treatment and prevention of food allergy: joint statement of the European Society for Paediatric Allergology and Clinical Immunology (ESPACI) Committee on Hypoallergenic Formulas and the European Society for Paediatric Gastroenterology, Hepatology and Nutrition (ESPGHAN) Committee on Nutrition. *Arch Dis Child* 1999; **81:** 80–4.
5. David TJ. Adverse reactions and intolerance to foods. *Br Med Bull* 2000; **56:** 34–50.

Hay fever
Hay fever is a seasonal form of allergic rhinitis in which symptoms of conjunctivitis are also present. Management is symptomatic and therapies used are discussed under Conjunctivitis, above and Rhinitis, below.

Insomnia
Some of the older sedating antihistamines including diphenhydramine and promethazine, have been promoted to the public for occasional insomnia (p.652), although their long duration of action may cause hangover effects. Promethazine was formerly popular for children but the use of hypnotics in this age group is not usually justified. Moreover a possible association between phenothiazines and sudden infant death syndrome (see under the Adverse Effects of Promethazine, p.423) contributed to the recommendation that such antihistamines should not be used in young children.

Ménière's disease
Ménière's disease is a disorder of the labyrinth (the inner ear) characterised by recurrent attacks of vertigo, progressive hearing loss, and worsening tinnitus (p.1316). It usually presents in middle age and may equally affect men and women. The predominant pathological feature is an excess of endolymph fluid producing an increase in pressure in the membranous labyrinth (endolymphatic hydrops). Attacks occur in clusters over a few weeks with periods of remission lasting weeks or months.

The aims of treatment are to alleviate symptoms and preserve hearing if possible. It is therefore important to assess how far the disease has progressed, particularly in terms of hearing loss. In addition to conventional hearing tests, cochlear dysfunction may be assessed pharmacologically. Hypertonic glycerol has been administered orally to reduce the endolymphatic fluid volume by osmotic diuresis, any temporary improvement in hearing indicating reversible impairment. However, this test is associated with side-effects that some consider unacceptable. Urea has been used as an alternative to glycerol. Intravenous acetazolamide has been used diagnostically to increase endolymphatic pressure temporarily in order to produce transient hearing loss in patients in the reversible stages of the disease.

Acute attacks of vertigo in the early stages may be treated with the same drugs used for vertigo of any cause (see below).

Vasodilators have been advocated for maintenance treatment because ischaemia of the labyrinth has been postulated as a factor in the aetiology. Betahistine, a histamine analogue, is used. Restriction of dietary sodium and administration of diuretics, such as chlortalidone, frusemide [furosemide], and hydrochlorothiazide, has also been used traditionally to reduce the amount of fluid in the endolymphatic spaces.

As the disease progresses, vestibular ablation with aminoglycosides may be indicated. Systemic streptomycin has been used but the risk of further hearing loss and other serious adverse effects has limited its use. Intratympanic administration of gentamicin is now preferred, and can improve vertigo in up to 90% of patients, although exacerbation of hearing loss is still a risk, albeit at a lower incidence than that with systemic streptomycin.

Surgical treatment remains an option for patients with Ménière's disease refractory to medical interventions.

References.
1. Saeed SR, *et al.* Ménière's disease. *Br J Hosp Med* 1994; **51:** 603–12.
2. Brookes GB. The pharmacological treatment of Ménière's disease. *Clin Otolaryngol* 1996; **21:** 3–11.
3. Claes J, Van de Heyning PH. Medical treatment of Ménière's disease: a review of literature. *Acta Otolaryngol (Stockh)* 1997; suppl 526: 37–42.
4. Saeed SR. Diagnosis and treatment of Ménière's disease. *BMJ* 1998; **316:** 368–72.
5. Thai-Van H, *et al.* Ménière's disease: pathophysiology and treatment. *Drugs* 2001; **61:** 1089–1102.

Migraine
Antihistamines have a number of uses in the management of migraine (p.449). Those with antiemetic activity such as buclizine and cyclizine are used to alleviate the nausea and vomiting associated with migraine; they are common ingredients of compound analgesic preparations given for the initial treatment of migraine.

Those antihistamines with antiserotonin actions, including cyproheptadine and flunarizine, have been used for the prophylaxis of migraine.

Nausea and vomiting
The management of various types of nausea and vomiting is discussed in detail on p.1206.

The older antihistamines such as cinnarizine, cyclizine, dimenhydrinate, meclozine, and promethazine are among the principal drugs used for **motion sickness**. They are all of similar efficacy but may differ in onset and duration of action and in the extent of side-effects such as drowsiness and antimuscarinic effects. If a sedative effect is desired dimenhydrinate and promethazine are useful, otherwise a slightly less sedating antihistamine such as cinnarizine, cyclizine, or meclozine may be preferred. The aim is prevention of motion sickness since antiemetics are more effective for prophylaxis than for treatment. Antihistamines may be slightly less effective against motion sickness than the antimuscarinic hyoscine (p.468), but are often better tolerated. Non-sedating antihistamines such as astemizole and terfenadine, which penetrate poorly into the CNS, do not appear to be effective against motion sickness.

Diphenhydramine has been included in antiemetic regimens for the control of nausea and vomiting associated with **cancer chemotherapy** to reduce the extrapyramidal reactions associated with metoclopramide; it may also improve overall antiemetic control. Cyclizine is used as an antiemetic in **palliative care**.

Cyclizine is given as a supplement to opioids for premedication and has been effective prophylactically as well as in established **postoperative nausea and vomiting**. Promethazine has also been used for the prevention and treatment of postoperative nausea and vomiting, but has marked sedative effects.

Nausea in the first trimester of **pregnancy** does not require drug therapy, but on rare occasions if vomiting is severe an antihistamine such as promethazine may be required pending specialist advice. See under Precautions for Antihistamines, above, for a discussion of the risks of antiemetic therapy during pregnancy.

Otitis media
Although antihistamines and decongestants, alone or in combination, have been widely used in children for the treatment of symptoms of acute otitis media and associated respiratory symptoms, studies[1,2] have failed to show benefit, and their use is not recommended.[3] Acute otitis media and otitis media with effusion may resolve without treatment although, as discussed on p.132, antibacterials are often given.

1. Cantekin EI, *et al.* Lack of efficacy of a decongestant-antihistamine combination for otitis media with effusion ("secretory" otitis media) in children. *N Engl J Med* 1983; **308:** 297–301.
2. Mandel EM, *et al.* Efficacy of amoxicillin with and without decongestant-antihistamine for otitis media with effusion in children: results of a double-blind, randomized trial. *N Engl J Med* 1987; **316:** 432–7.
3. The Otitis Media Guideline Panel. Managing otitis media with effusion in young children. *Pediatrics* 1994; **94:** 766–73.

Pruritus
The sedating antihistamines are commonly used to relieve pruritus (itching) (p.1106) from a variety of causes. They are effective in relieving pruritus associated with urticaria (below) but are also used for itching associated with dermatoses such as atopic eczema (p.1105), where the degree of benefit is less certain. They are given in the latter to control nocturnal itching and for severe pruritus associated with relapse.

The exact pathophysiology of itching remains unclear.[1-3] Although histamine release is associated with itching in atopic eczema different inflammatory mediators are involved in other dermatoses. The CNS is also thought to play a part in the perception of itch. Hence, the relative roles of CNS sedation and peripheral histamine-receptor blockade in the mode of action of antihistamines in these conditions is a matter of debate. Although sedation has generally been considered the more important, the benefits of sedating antihistamines appear to be less in eczema than in urticaria. In addition, clemastine has been reported to provide no antipruritic benefit, yet it induces significant sedation. Studies with non-sedating antihistamines have been inconclusive; most have indicated no benefit in pruritus associated with atopic eczema, although one has shown a slight benefit from the addition of acrivastine or terfenadine to treatment with a topical corticosteroid and an emollient.[4]

1. Krause L, Shuster S. Mechanism of action of antipruritic drugs. *BMJ* 1983; **287:** 1199–1200.
2. Advenier C, Queille-Roussel C. Rational use of antihistamines in allergic dermatological conditions. *Drugs* 1989; **38:** 634–44.
3. Greaves MW, Wall PD. Pathophysiology of itching. *Lancet* 1996; **348:** 938–40.
4. Doherty V, *et al.* Treatment of itching in atopic eczema with antihistamines with a low sedative profile. *BMJ* 1989; **298:** 96.

Rhinitis
Rhinitis may be allergic or non-allergic in origin. Allergic rhinitis is a type I hypersensitivity reaction (see above); both early (sneezing, rhinorrhoea and nasal congestion) and late (nasal congestion) reactions may be provoked. It may be seasonal (as in hay fever) or perennial and, in some patients, will frequently co-exist with conjunctivitis (above). Non-allergic rhinitis may be divided into eosinophilic non-allergic rhinitis or non-eosinophilic non-allergic rhinitis. The term vasomotor rhinitis has been used to describe the latter although its use is best avoided since no vasomotor dysfunction has been clearly identified.

In the management of **allergic rhinitis**, avoidance of unnecessary exposure to aeroallergens is of prime importance. However in most sufferers this is not possible and some form of drug therapy will be necessary. A large number of inflammatory mediators are involved in the pathogenesis of rhinitis and no single drug is completely effective in the alleviation of symptoms.

- Some antihistamines may nonetheless be useful and any antimuscarinic effect may be of additional value in reducing secretions. They are also useful for controlling nasal itching, sneezing, and ocular symptoms, such as conjunctivitis but are less effective for relief of nasal congestion. Antihistamines are the drugs of choice for the treatment of mild and/or intermittent allergic rhinitis and they are also employed for the management of breakthrough symptoms in those sufferers using prophylactic intranasal corticosteroids or sodium cromoglicate (see below). Since the maximum effect of antihistamines occurs several hours after peak serum concentrations have been obtained, they should be given in anticipation of a reaction to achieve the maximum response. Studies of acrivastine, cetirizine, loratadine, and terfenadine have generally indicated comparable efficacy to that of the older antihistamines. Most antihistamines are unsuitable for topical use in the nose or eye since they are generally ineffective at the concentrations suitable for local therapy; also there is the potential for sensitisation. However, the antazoline salts, azelastine, and levocabastine have been used topically in the nose for control of symptoms. Such preparations are considered less effective than intranasal corticosteroids but probably more effective than cromoglicate.

- The actions of topical corticosteroids in allergic rhinitis include relief of inflammation, a decrease in capillary permeability and in mucus production, and vasoconstriction; they inhibit both the early and late response to allergen exposure. Corticosteroids are first-line treatment for the prophylaxis of moderate and/or persistent allergic rhinitis. In seasonal allergic rhinitis, they should be started at least 2 weeks before the pollen season and taken regularly throughout the season. Those applied intranasally include beclometasone, budesonide, flunisolide, and fluticasone. At recommended dosage, local adverse effects are mild and transient and systemic effects are not a risk; aqueous sprays may cause less local effects than pressurised aerosols. Treatment of allergic rhinitis with oral or parenteral corticosteroids has been reserved for short-term treatment in special circumstances only, although some have contested even this practice.

- Mast-cell stabilisers such as ketotifen, nedocromil, and sodium cromoglicate are thought to act primarily by preventing release of inflammatory mediators from sensitised mast cells through stabilisation of mast-cell membranes. They are an alternative to corticosteroids in the prophylactic treatment of allergic rhinitis and are often preferred to the use of a corticosteroid as first-choice therapy in children. They may also be useful in controlling mild to moderate symptoms.
- Intranasal sympathomimetics such as phenylephrine, naphazoline, oxymetazoline, and xylometazoline may be useful for short-term treatment of allergic rhinitis to relieve severe nasal congestion which can be painful and may impede delivery of sodium cromoglicate or a corticosteroid to the mucosal surfaces. Oral sympathomimetic decongestants such as pseudoephedrine and phenylpropanolamine are less effective than topical sympathomimetics and adverse effects may be troublesome.

Hyposensitisation (see p.1576) is generally only indicated in severe allergic rhinitis when sensitivity testing demonstrates sensitivity to one allergen and when exposure to the allergen is unavoidable or symptomatic treatment has failed.

The management of **non-allergic rhinitis** is similar to that of allergic rhinitis despite different mechanisms being involved in its aetiology. Corticosteroids are often first-line therapy especially if nasal congestion is a dominant feature. The role of antihistamines is more limited; sedating antihistamines are useful in reducing nasal secretions because of their antimuscarinic actions; however, non-sedating antihistamines are relatively ineffective. In patients in whom rhinorrhoea is a particular problem, intranasal administration of the antimuscarinic ipratropium is of value. Although intranasal sympathomimetics have also been used they should generally be avoided because of the risk of rebound congestion. Oral sympathomimetics are largely ineffective.

Other therapies tried include topical capsaicin, to induce local desensitisation, and nasal douching with a saline and sodium bicarbonate solution.

References
1. Horak F. Seasonal allergic rhinitis: newer treatment approaches. *Drugs* 1993; **45:** 518–27.
2. International Rhinitis Management Working Group. International consensus report on the diagnosis and management of rhinitis. *Allergy* 1994; **49** (suppl 19): 1–34.
3. Scadding GK. Chronic non-infectious, non-allergic rhinitis. *Prescribers' J* 1996; **36:** 93–101.
4. Parikh A, Scadding GK. Seasonal allergic rhinitis. *BMJ* 1997; **314:** 1392–5.
5. Naclerio R, Soloman W. Rhinitis and inhalant allergens. *JAMA* 1997; **278:** 1842–8.
6. Durham S. Summer hay fever. *BMJ* 1998; **316:** 843–5.
7. Mackay IS, Durham SR. Perennial rhinitis. *BMJ* 1998; **316:** 917–20.

Urticaria and angioedema

Most patients with urticaria or angioedema (p.1107) derive some benefit from oral antihistamines, especially in relief of pruritus. However, patients who are severely affected, particularly those with laryngeal oedema, are allergic emergencies and require immediate treatment with adrenaline [epinephrine] (see under Anaphylactic Shock, p.832). Also, large doses of antihistamines are sometimes required and urticarias with a type I immunological origin and iatrogenic urticarias respond better than physical urticarias. If attacks of urticaria are frequent, antihistamines may be given prophylactically. Sedating antihistamines such as chlorpheniramine [chlorphenamine] and diphenhydramine have been widely used in the treatment of urticaria but non-sedating antihistamines are now generally preferred. Hydroxyzine has been used particularly in dermographism and cholinergic urticaria. Cyproheptadine has generally been considered the drug of choice for cold urticaria, although appetite stimulation may be a problem.

Some drugs with both H₁-antagonist and mast-cell stabilising actions, such as ketotifen, oxatomide, and azatadine have shown efficacy in the treatment of urticaria; the role of mast-cell stabilisation is unknown.

Topical treatment is rarely effective except for cases of mild urticaria; topical antihistamines carry a risk of sensitisation.

References
1. Advenier C, Queille-Roussel C. Rational use of antihistamines in allergic dermatological conditions. *Drugs* 1989; **38:** 634–44.
2. Greaves MW, Sabroe RA. Allergy and the skin: urticaria. *BMJ* 1998; **316:** 1147–50.

3. Mann KV, *et al.* Nonsedating histamine H₁-receptor antagonists. *Clin Pharm* 1989; **8:** 331–44.
4. Monroe EW. Chronic urticaria: review of nonsedating H₁ antihistamines in treatment. *J Am Acad Dermatol* 1988; **19:** 842–9.
5. Theoharides TC. Histamine₂ (H₂)-receptor antagonists in the treatment of urticaria. *Drugs* 1989; **37:** 345–55.

Vertigo

Vertigo is a symptom of vestibular disorders. It is characterised by a sensation of rotation of the surroundings or of movement of static objects. Dizziness is considered to be a wider term, although some use it as a synonym for vertigo.

A variety of disorders may affect the vestibular system and produce vertigo, including cerebrovascular disorders, epilepsy, head injury, malignant neoplasms, Ménière's disease (above), migraine, multiple sclerosis, and infections. Motion sickness can induce vertigo. Ototoxic drugs may also cause vestibular damage and precipitate vertigo.

Patients suffering from vertigo should undergo thorough investigations to identify any underlying cause. Simple measures to improve the integration of sensory input from visual, proprioceptive, and vestibular receptors may prove effective, especially in the elderly, in whom the inappropriate prescribing of drugs for postural instability needs to be avoided. Such measures include improving visual acuity, balance exercises, and the use of walking aids.

The most widely used drugs for acute vertigo are the antihistamines. They may have a direct action on the inner ear besides acting centrally. Antimuscarinic actions may contribute to their activity; antimuscarinics, especially hyoscine, have a long history of use in vertigo. Antihistamines used in the treatment of vertigo include buclizine, cyclizine, dimenhydrinate, diphenhydramine, meclozine, and promethazine. Cinnarizine and flunarizine are also used for vertigo although they are devoid of any significant antimuscarinic actions; their activity may be due to calcium-channel blockade. Phenothiazines such as prochlorperazine are also used to control any associated vomiting. Benzodiazepines including diazepam have been given in acute severe attacks. However their prolonged use in those with chronic symptoms is of questionable value.

Vasodilators may be of benefit in the treatment of vertigo of vascular aetiology. Parenteral or sublingual histamine was formerly widely used, and betahistine is still advocated especially for vertigo associated with Ménière's disease. Nicotinyl alcohol has also been used.

References
1. Rascol O, *et al.* Antivertigo medications and drug-induced vertigo: a pharmacological review. *Drugs* 1995; **50:** 777–91.
2. Luxon LM. Vertigo: new approaches to diagnosis and management. *Br J Hosp Med* 1996; **56:** 519–20 and 537–41.
3. Luxon LM. Assessment and management of vertigo. *Prescribers' J* 1998; **38:** 87–97.
4. Baloh RW. Vertigo. *Lancet* 1998; **352:** 1841–6.

Acrivastine (16017-a)

Acrivastine (BAN, USAN, rINN).
BW-825C. (E)-3-{6-[(E)-3-Pyrrolidin-1-yl-1-*p*-tolylprop-1-enyl]-2-pyridyl}acrylic acid.
$C_{22}H_{24}N_2O_2 = 348.4$.
CAS — 87848-99-5.
ATC — R06AX18.

Adverse Effects and Precautions

As for the non-sedating antihistamines in general, p.404. It should be given with care in mild renal impairment and avoided in those with a creatinine clearance of less than 50 mL per minute.

Sedation. For a discussion of the sedative effects of antihistamines see p.405.

Interactions

As for the non-sedating antihistamines in general, p.406.

Pharmacokinetics

Acrivastine is well absorbed from the gastrointestinal tract; peak plasma concentrations are achieved in about 1.5 hours. The plasma half-life of acrivastine is about 1.5 hours and the drug does not appear to cross the blood-brain barrier to a significant extent. Acrivastine along with an active metabolite is excreted principally in the urine.

Uses and Administration

Acrivastine is a non-sedating antihistamine structurally related to triprolidine. It does not have any significant sedative or antimuscarinic actions. It is used for the symptomatic relief of allergic conditions such as rhinitis (p.407) and various types of urticaria (p.408) when it is given by mouth in doses of 8 mg three times daily.

Preparations

Proprietary Preparations (details are given in Part 3)
Aust.: Semprex; *Denm.:* Benadryl; Semprex†; *Fin.:* Semprex; *Hong Kong:* Semprex; *Ital.:* Semprex; *Neth.:* Semprex; *S.Afr.:* Semprex; *Singapore:* Semprex; *Swed.:* Semprex; *Switz.:* Semprex; *Thai.:* Semprex; *UK:* Benadryl; Semprex.
Multi-ingredient: *Aust.:* Duact; *Denm.:* Duact; *Fin.:* Duact; *UK:* Benadryl Plus; *USA:* Semprex-D.

Antazoline Hydrochloride (6104-n)

Antazoline Hydrochloride (BANM, rINN).
Antazolini Hydrochloridum; Antazolinium Chloride; Imidamine Hydrochloride; Phenazolinum. N-Benzyl-N-(2-imidazolin-2-ylmethyl)aniline hydrochloride.
$C_{17}H_{19}N_3, HCl = 301.8$.
CAS — 91-75-8 (antazoline); 2508-72-7 (antazoline hydrochloride).
Pharmacopoeias. In *Eur.* (see p.vi) and *Pol.*

Pharmacopoeial description

Ph. Eur.: A white or almost white crystalline powder. Sparingly soluble in water; soluble in alcohol; slightly soluble in dichloromethane.

Antazoline Mesilate (6105-h)

Antazoline Mesilate (BANM, rINN).
Antazoline Mesylate; Antazoline Methanesulphonate; Imidamine Mesylate.
$C_{17}H_{19}N_3, CH_3SO_3H = 361.5$.
CAS — 3131-32-6.

Antazoline Phosphate (6106-m)

Antazoline Phosphate (BANM, rINN).
Imidamine Phosphate.
$C_{17}H_{19}N_3, H_3PO_4 = 363.3$.
CAS — 154-68-7.
Pharmacopoeias. In *US.*

Pharmacopoeial description

USP 25: A white to off-white crystalline powder. Soluble in water; practically insoluble in ether and in benzene; sparingly soluble in methyl alcohol. pH of a 2% solution in water is between 4.0 and 5.0. Store in airtight containers.

Antazoline Sulfate (10003-w)

Antazoline Sulfate (rINNM).
Antazoline Sulphate (BANM); Imidamine Sulphate.
$(C_{17}H_{19}N_3)_2H_2SO_4, 2H_2O = 664.8$.
CAS — 24359-81-7 (anhydrous antazoline sulfate).
NOTE. The above molecular formula is that provided in the *It. P.* Other sources give a molecular formula of $C_{17}H_{19}N_3, H_2SO_4$.
Pharmacopoeias. In *It.*

Adverse Effects and Precautions

As for the antihistamines in general, p.404.

Hypersensitivity. Reports of acute interstitial pneumonitis (with fever, rash, and dyspnoea)[1] and of immune thrombocytopenic purpura[2] were attributed to hypersensitivity reactions following the oral administration of antazoline.
1. Pahissa A, *et al.* Antazoline-induced allergic pneumonitis. *BMJ* 1979; **2:** 1328.
2. Nielsen JL, *et al.* Immune thrombocytopenia due to antazoline (Antistina). *Allergy* 1981; **36:** 517–19.

Uses and Administration

Antazoline, an ethylenediamine derivative, is an antihistamine used topically for the treatment of allergic conjunctivitis (p.426). It is used as the hydrochloride, phosphate, or sulfate in eye drops, most commonly in a concentration of 0.5%; the mesilate has also been used. Antazoline salts are often used with a vasoconstrictor such as naphazoline hydrochloride or nitrate or xylometazoline hydrochloride.

Antazoline hydrochloride is used in a strength of up to 2% in a cream or ointment for the treatment of minor skin irritations, but as with other antihistamines there is a risk of sensitisation. The hydrochloride has also been given by mouth.

Preparations

Proprietary Preparations (details are given in Part 3)
Denm.: Antistina-Privin; *Singapore:* Antistin-Privin; *UK:* Wasp-Eze.
Multi-ingredient: *Aust.:* Histophtal†; *Austral.:* Albalon-A; Allergy Eyes; Antistine-Privine; In A Wink Allergy; Murine Allergy; Optazine A†; *Belg.:* Zincfrin Antihistaminicum; *Braz.:* Albassol; Neo Vastrictol; *Canad.:* Albalon-A Liquifilm; Cooper AR†; Ophtrivin-A; Vasocon-A; Zincfrin-A; *Denm.:* Sesal; *Fin.:* Antis-

tin-Privin; Zincfrin-A; *Ger.:* Allergopos N; Antistin-Privin; Ophtalmin; Spersallerg; *Hong Kong:* Spersallerg; *Irl.:* Otrivine-Antistin; RBC; *Israel:* Antistin-Privin; *Ital.:* Antistin-Privina; Eubetal; *Norw.:* Spersallerg; *NZ:* Albalon-A; Otrivine-Antistin; *Port.:* Alergiftalmina; *S.Afr.:* Albalon-A; Antistin-Privin; Covosan; Gemini; Spersallerg; Zincfrin-A†; *Singapore:* Alergoftal; Spersallerg; *Spain:* Alergoftal; *Swed.:* Antasten-Privin; *Switz.:* Antistin-Privin; Spersallerg; *Thai.:* Antazallerge; Histaoph; Opsa-His; Spersallerg; *UK:* Modantis; Otrivine-Antistin; RBC; *USA:* Antazoline-V; Vasocon-A.

Astemizole   (12403-t)

Astemizole *(BAN, USAN, rINN).*

Astemizolum; R-43512. 1-(4-Fluorobenzyl)-2-{[1-(4-methoxyphenethyl)-4-piperidyl]amino}benzimidazole.

$C_{28}H_{31}FN_4O = 458.6.$
CAS — 68844-77-9.
ATC — R06AX11.
Pharmacopoeias. In Eur. (see p.vi) and US.

Pharmacopoeial description

Ph. Eur.: A white or almost white powder. Practically insoluble in water; soluble in alcohol; freely soluble in dichloromethane and in methyl alcohol. Protect from light.

USP 25: Store in airtight containers.

Adverse Effects and Precautions

As for the non-sedating antihistamines in general, p.404. Increased appetite and weight gain have been reported with astemizole.

Ventricular arrhythmias, including torsade de pointes, have occurred rarely with astemizole, particularly in association with raised blood concentrations (see Arrhythmias below) and as a result the drug has been withdrawn from the market in most countries. To reduce the risk of developing such arrhythmias recommendations were that licensed doses should **not** be exceeded, and that it should be **avoided** in patients with cardiac or significant hepatic disease, with hypokalaemia or other electrolyte imbalance, or with known or suspected prolonged QT interval. The concomitant administration of drugs liable to interfere with the hepatic metabolism of astemizole, of other potentially arrhythmogenic drugs including those that prolong the QT interval, and of drugs likely to cause electrolyte imbalance was **contra-indicated** (see under Interactions below).

Arrhythmias. Although severe life-threatening cardiovascular effects including torsade de pointes and other ventricular arrhythmias were initially reported mainly after substantial overdoses of astemizole, such reactions have also occurred rarely with doses as low as 20 to 30 mg daily and even as low as 10 mg daily in those with possible predisposing factors. There has been a report[1] of astemizole-induced torsade de pointes in a 15-year-old girl who claimed to have taken 10 mg daily for 10 weeks but pharmacokinetic data were more consistent with acute ingestion of higher doses. There have also been several reports of cardiotoxicity following accidental overdosage with astemizole in children.[2-4]

Although the drug is now withdrawn in the UK, recommendations were made by the UK Committee on Safety of Medicines to reduce the risk of developing serious arrhythmias[5-7] (see Adverse Effects above for details). It was considered that astemizole should be discontinued immediately in patients who experience syncope, and appropriate clinical evaluation including ECG monitoring instituted because syncope has preceded or accompanied severe arrhythmias in some cases. Convulsions in patients taking astemizole may also be related to cardiovascular effects.[8]

Studies have suggested that astemizole induces ventricular arrhythmias by inhibiting cardiac potassium channels which results in prolongation of the QT interval, a risk factor for developing arrhythmias.[9] Whether arrhythmias occur with the non-sedating antihistamines in general is uncertain—see p.405.

1. Simons FER, *et al.* Astemizole-induced torsade de pointes. *Lancet* 1988; **ii:** 624.
2. Hoppu K, *et al.* Accidental astemizole overdose in young children. *Lancet* 1991; **338:** 538–40.
3. Tobin JR, *et al.* Astemizole-induced cardiac conduction disturbances in a child. *JAMA* 1991; **266:** 2737–40.
4. Wiley JF, *et al.* Cardiotoxic effects of astemizole overdose in children. *J Pediatr* 1992; **120:** 799–802.
5. Committee on Safety of Medicines. Ventricular arrhythmias due to terfenadine and astemizole. *Current Problems 35* 1992.
6. Committee on Safety of Medicines/Medicines Control Agency. Drug-induced prolongation of the QT interval. *Current Problems* 1996; **22:** 2.
7. Committee on Safety of Medicines/Medicines Control Agency. Astemizole (Hismanal): only available on prescription. *Current Problems* 1999; **25:** 2.
8. Clark A, Love H. Astemizole-induced ventricular arrhythmias: an unexpected cause of convulsions. *Int J Cardiol* 1991; **33:** 165–7.
9. Rankin AC. Non-sedating antihistamines and cardiac arrhythmia. *Lancet* 1997; **350:** 1115–16.

Overdosage. Severe cardiac events have been associated with astemizole overdosage (see under Arrhythmias, above); management is mainly supportive. The absorption of astemizole from the gastrointestinal tract can be prevented by administration of activated charcoal[1] but because astemizole is rapidly absorbed it would need to be given as soon as possible after poi-

soning. Haemodialysis does not appear to increase the clearance of astemizole.

1. Laine K, *et al.* The effect of activated charcoal on the absorption and elimination of astemizole. *Hum Exp Toxicol* 1994; **13:** 502–5.

Porphyria. Astemizole is considered to be unsafe in patients with porphyria because it has been shown to be porphyrinogenic in *in-vitro* systems.

Sedation. For discussion of the sedative effects of antihistamines see p.405.

Interactions

As for the non-sedating antihistamines in general, p.406.

Astemizole should not be given with drugs that inhibit its hepatic metabolism because of the increased risk of serious ventricular arrhythmias. These drugs include the *imidazole and triazole antifungals* such as *ketoconazole* and *itraconazole*, the macrolide antibacterials *clarithromycin, erythromycin, troleandomycin*, and possibly other *macrolides*. Others, similarly to terfenadine (p.425), may include *serotonin reuptake inhibitors, HIV-protease inhibitors, non-nucleoside reverse transcriptase inhibitor antiretrovirals*, and *zileuton*. The metabolism of astemizole may also be inhibited by *grapefruit juice* and concomitant use should be avoided.

Concomitant administration with other potentially arrhythmogenic drugs (including those that prolong the QT interval) such as *antiarrhythmics, tricyclic antidepressants*, the antimalarials *halofantrine* and *quinine, antipsychotics, cisapride*, and the beta blocker *sotalol* should be avoided, as should co-administration of *diuretics* that cause electrolyte imbalances such as hypokalaemia. The use of *terfenadine* and astemizole together is not recommended.

Pharmacokinetics

Absorption of astemizole from the gastrointestinal tract is rapid and is reduced by food. First-pass metabolism is extensive, therefore plasma concentrations of unchanged drug are very low. The plasma concentration of astemizole plus metabolites takes about 4 to 8 weeks to reach steady state. The metabolism of astemizole is mediated through the cytochrome P450 enzyme system by the isoenzymes CYP3A4, CYP2D6, and CYP2A6. The elimination half-life of astemizole and its metabolites at steady state is about 19 days. Unchanged astemizole is highly bound to plasma proteins and does not appear to cross the blood-brain barrier to a significant extent. Desmethyllastemizole, the major metabolite of astemizole, has histamine H_1-receptor-blocking activity. The metabolites of astemizole are excreted slowly in the urine and faeces, and undergo enterohepatic recycling. Virtually none of an oral dose is excreted as unchanged drug.

Uses and Administration

Astemizole, a piperidine derivative, is a non-sedating antihistamine with a very long duration of action. It does not have significant sedative or antimuscarinic actions. Astemizole has been used for the symptomatic relief of allergic conditions including rhinitis (p.407) and conjunctivitis (p.406), and skin disorders such as urticaria (p.408). Preparations of astemizole have now been withdrawn from the market in most countries because of the risk of adverse effects.

Astemizole has been given by mouth in a dose of 10 mg once daily, or 5 mg daily in children aged 6 to 12 years. These doses must not be exceeded because of the risk of cardiac arrhythmias with higher doses.

Preparations

USP 25: Astemizole Tablets.

Proprietary Preparations (details are given in Part 3)
Aust.: Hismanal†; Pollonis†; *Austral.:* Hismanal†; *Belg.:* Hismanal†; *Braz.:* Cilergil; Hismanal†; Hisnot; Histabloc; *Canad.:* Hismanal†; *Denm.:* Hismanal†; *Fr.:* Hismanal†; *Ger.:* Hismanal†; *Irl.:* Hismanal†; *Israel:* Hismanal†; *Ital.:* Hismanal†; Histamen†; *Mex.:* Alerken; Aleztem; Antagon 1; Astemina; Astesen; Aztemin; Biostan; Emdar; Emizol; Farmidal S; Fustermizol; Ginomizol; Henofin; Hismanal†; Histalino; Histaser; Novasten; Urtigen; *Neth.:* Hismanal†; *Port.:* Hismanal†; Perifer H1†; *S.Afr.:* Hismanal†; *Spain:* Alermizol; Esmacen; Hismanal†; Histaminos; Hubermizol; Laridal; Paralergin; Retolen; Rifedot; Rimbol†; Romadin; Simprox; Urdrim; *Switz.:* Hismanal†; *Thai.:* Anhisnon; Astahis; Astem; Astmazol; Dayamin; Hismacon; Hismizol; Hisno; Histema; Irene; Tenon; *UK:* Hismanal†; Polloneze†; *USA:* Hismanal†.

Multi-ingredient: *Aust.:* Hismadrin; *S.Afr.:* Hismanal-D†.

Azatadine Maleate   (6107-b)

Azatadine Maleate *(BANM, USAN, rINNM).*

Sch-10649. 6,11-Dihydro-11-(1-methyl-4-piperidylidene)-5*H*-benzo[5,6]cyclohepta[1,2-*b*]pyridine dimaleate.

$C_{20}H_{22}N_2,2C_4H_4O_4 = 522.5.$
CAS — 3964-81-6 (azatadine); 3978-86-7 (azatadine maleate).
Pharmacopoeias. In US.

Pharmacopoeial description

USP 25: A white to light cream-coloured, odourless powder. Freely soluble in water, in alcohol, in chloroform, and in methyl alcohol; practically insoluble in ether and in benzene.

Adverse Effects and Precautions

As for the sedating antihistamines in general, p.404.

Extrapyramidal effects. An acute dystonic reaction was reported in a patient who had taken azatadine maleate 20 to 30 mg by mouth over a 24-hour period.[1] The condition was reversed by intravenous injection of benzatropine 2 mg.

1. Joske DJL. Dystonic reaction to azatadine. *Med J Aust* 1984; **141:** 449.

Interactions

As for the sedating antihistamines in general, p.406.

Pharmacokinetics

Azatadine maleate is readily absorbed from the gastrointestinal tract and is partly metabolised. Peak plasma concentrations are achieved in about 4 hours. The elimination half-life has been reported to be 9 to 12 hours. Excretion of unchanged drug and metabolites is via the urine.

Uses and Administration

Azatadine maleate is a piperidine derivative closely related to cyproheptadine. It is a sedating antihistamine with a long duration of action; it also has antimuscarinic and antiserotonin properties.

Azatadine maleate is used for the symptomatic relief of allergic conditions including rhinitis (p.407) and urticaria (p.408); it is also used for other pruritic skin disorders as well as reactions to insect bites and stings. It is given by mouth, usually in doses of 1 mg twice daily; if necessary 2 mg twice daily may be given. Children aged 6 to 12 years may be given 0.5 to 1 mg twice daily, and children aged 1 to 6 years, 0.25 mg twice daily.

Preparations

USP 25: Azatadine Maleate Tablets.

Proprietary Preparations (details are given in Part 3)
Austral.: Zadine; *Belg.:* Optimine; *Canad.:* Optimine; *Hong Kong:* Zadine; *Irl.:* Optimine; *Mex.:* Idulamine; *NZ:* Zadine; *S.Afr.:* Optimine†; *Singapore:* Zadine; *Spain:* Lergocil; *UK:* Optimine; *USA:* Optimine.

Multi-ingredient: *Braz.:* Cedrin; *Canad.:* Trinalin; *Mex.:* Trinalin; *Spain:* Atiramin; Idulanex; *USA:* Rynatan; Trinalin.

Azelastine Hydrochloride   (15943-h)

Azelastine Hydrochloride *(BANM, USAN, rINNM).*

A-5610 (azelastine or azelastine hydrochloride); E-0659 (azelastine or azelastine hydrochloride); W-2979M (azelastine or azelastine hydrochloride). 4-(p-Chlorobenzyl)-2-(hexahydro-1-methyl-1*H*-azepin-4-yl)-1(2*H*)-phthalazinone monohydrochloride.

$C_{22}H_{24}ClN_3O,HCl = 418.4.$
CAS — 58581-89-8 (azelastine); 79307-93-0 (azelastine hydrochloride).
Pharmacopoeias. In Br.

Pharmacopoeial description

BP 2001: A white, crystalline powder. Slightly soluble in water; soluble in dehydrated alcohol; practically insoluble in ether, in *n*-hexane, and in toluene. Store in airtight containers. Protect from light.

Adverse Effects and Precautions

As for the antihistamines in general, p.404.

When administered intranasally irritation of the nasal mucosa and taste disturbances have been reported; somnolence, headache, and dry mouth have also been noted in some patients. Taste disturbance can occur after ophthalmic administration.

Sedation. For discussion of the sedative effects of antihistamines see p.405.

Pharmacokinetics

When administered intranasally, approximately 40% of the dose of azelastine reaches the systemic circulation. Elimination is via hepatic metabolism with excretion mainly in the faeces.

◊ Azelastine is rapidly and almost completely absorbed after administration *by mouth*, peak plasma concentrations being achieved in 4 to 5 hours. Azelastine undergoes hepatic metabolism; the major metabolite, demethylazelastine, has antihistamine activity. The elimination half-life of azelastine is about 25 hours, increasing to 35.5 hours after multiple oral doses, possibly as a result of accumulation of the demethyl metabolite. Azelastine and its metabolites are excreted predominantly in the faeces and also in urine.

Uses and Administration

Azelastine hydrochloride is an antihistamine which, in addition to its histamine H_1-receptor-blocking activity, appears to inhibit the release of inflammatory mediators from mast cells. It is used topically in the symptomatic relief of allergic conditions including

The symbol † denotes a preparation no longer actively marketed

rhinitis (p.407) and conjunctivitis (p.406). It is also used in the treatment of non-allergic (vasomotor) rhinitis.

In the treatment of allergic **rhinitis** in adults and children aged 5 years and over, the usual dose in the UK is 140 µg by nasal spray into each nostril twice daily. In the USA, however, 2 sprays of a similar preparation (supplying 137 µg per spray) may be given into each nostril twice daily; children aged 5 years and over may be given 1 spray into each nostril twice daily. In the USA, azelastine is also used in the treatment of non-allergic rhinitis in adults and children aged 12 years and over. The dose is 2 sprays into each nostril twice daily. In **conjunctivitis** in adults and children aged 3 (USA) or 4 (UK) years and over a 0.05% solution is instilled into each eye twice daily; this may be increased to four times daily in severe conditions.

Azelastine hydrochloride has also been given by mouth.

◊ References.
1. McTavish D, Sorkin EM. Azelastine: a review of its pharmacodynamic and pharmacokinetic properties, and therapeutic potential. *Drugs* 1989; **38:** 778–800 (oral and nasal administration).
2. Busse WW, *et al.* Corticosteroid-sparing effect of azelastine in the management of bronchial asthma. *Am J Respir Crit Care Med* 1996; **153:** 122–7 (oral).
3. Wober W, *et al.* Efficacy and tolerability of azelastine nasal spray in the treatment of allergic rhinitis: large scale experience in community practice. *Curr Med Res Opin* 1997; **13:** 617–26 (nasal).
4. McNeely W, Wiseman LR. Intranasal azelastine: a review of its efficacy in the management of allergic rhinitis. *Drugs* 1998; **56:** 91–114.

Preparations

Proprietary Preparations (details are given in Part 3)
Aust.: Allergodil; Lasticom; *Belg.:* Allergodil; *Braz.:* Rino-Lastin; *Denm.:* Allergodil; *Fin.:* Lastin; *Fr.:* Allergodil; *Ger.:* Allergodil; Loxin; Rhinolast†; *Hong Kong:* Azep; *Irl.:* Rhinolast; *Ital.:* Allergodil; *Jpn:* Azeptin†; *Mex.:* Astelin; Az; *Neth.:* Allergodil; *NZ:* Rhinolast; *Port.:* Allergodil; Azep†; *S.Afr.:* Rhinolast; *Singapore:* Azep; *Spain:* Afluon; Alferos†; Corifina; *Swed.:* Lastin; *Switz.:* Allergodil; *Thai.:* Azep; *UK:* Optilast; Rhinolast; *USA:* Astelin; Optivar.

Bamipine (6108-v)

Bamipine *(BAN, rINN)*.
N-Benzyl-N-(1-methyl-4-piperidyl)aniline.
$C_{19}H_{24}N_2 = 280.4$.
CAS — 4945-47-5.
ATC — D04AA15; R06AX01.

Profile
Bamipine is a sedating antihistamine (p.404) with pronounced sedative effects.

Bamipine and its salts are used mainly for the symptomatic relief of allergic conditions such as urticaria (p.408) and in pruritic skin disorders. Bamipine hydrochloride is given by mouth in a dose of 50 to 100 mg three or four times daily. Bamipine, bamipine lactate, and bamipine salicylate have all been applied topically.

Preparations
Proprietary Preparations (details are given in Part 3)
Aust.: Soventol; *Ger.:* Soventol; *Mex.:* Soventol; *Neth.:* Soventol†.
Multi-ingredient: *Aust.:* Multifungin†.

Bepotastine (20138-a)

Bepotastine *(rINN)*.
TAU-284 (bepotastine besilate). (+)-4-{[(S)-p-Chloro-α-2-pyridylbenzyl]oxy}-1-piperidinebutyric acid.
$C_{21}H_{25}ClN_2O_3 = 388.9$.
CAS — 125602-71-3.

Profile
Bepotastine is an antihistamine (p.404) used in the treatment of allergic rhinitis.

Bromazine Hydrochloride (6109-g)

Bromazine Hydrochloride *(BANM, rINNM)*.
Bromodiphenhydramine Hydrochloride. 2-(4-Bromobenzhydryloxy)-NN-dimethylethylamine hydrochloride.
$C_{17}H_{20}BrNO,HCl = 370.7$.
CAS — 118-23-0 (bromazine); 1808-12-4 (bromazine hydrochloride).
Pharmacopoeias. In *US.*

Pharmacopoeial description
USP 25: A white to pale buff-coloured, crystalline powder having no more than a faint odour. Soluble 1 in less than 1 of water, 1 in 2 of alcohol and of chloroform, 1 in 3500 of ether, and 1 in

31 of isopropyl alcohol; insoluble in petroleum spirit. Store in airtight containers.

Profile
Bromazine hydrochloride, a monoethanolamine derivative, is a sedating antihistamine (p.404) with antimuscarinic and marked sedative actions. It is used in combination preparations for the symptomatic treatment of coughs and the common cold (p.406) in a dose by mouth of 12.5 to 25 mg every 4 to 6 hours. The recommended maximum dose in such preparations is 150 mg daily. Children over 6 years of age may be given 6.25 to 12.5 mg every 6 hours.

Preparations
USP 25: Bromodiphenhydramine Hydrochloride Elixir.
Proprietary Preparations (details are given in Part 3)
Multi-ingredient: *Canad.:* Ambenyl†; *USA:* Ambenyl Cough Syrup; Amgenal Cough; Bromotuss with Codeine.

Brompheniramine Maleate (6110-f)

Brompheniramine Maleate *(BANM, rINNM)*.
Brompheniramini Maleas; Parabromdylamine Maleate. (±)-3-(4-Bromophenyl)-NN-dimethyl-3-(2-pyridyl)propylamine hydrogen maleate.
$C_{16}H_{19}BrN_2,C_4H_4O_4 = 435.3$.
CAS — 86-22-6 (brompheniramine); 980-71-2 (brompheniramine maleate).
Pharmacopoeias. In *Eur.* (see p.vi) and *US.*

Incompatibility has been reported with some amidotrizoate, adipiodone, and iotalamate salts.

Pharmacopoeial description
Ph. Eur.: A white or almost white, crystalline powder. Soluble in water; freely soluble in alcohol, in dichloromethane, and in methyl alcohol. A 1% solution in water has a pH of 4.0 to 5.0. Protect from light.
USP 25: A white, odourless, crystalline powder. Soluble 1 in 5 of water, 1 in 15 of alcohol and of chloroform; slightly soluble in ether and in benzene. pH of a 1% solution in water is between 4.0 and 5.0. Store in airtight containers. Protect from light.

Dexbrompheniramine Maleate (6126-q)

Dexbrompheniramine Maleate *(BANM, rINNM)*.
CAS — 2391-03-9.
Pharmacopoeias. In *US.*

Pharmacopoeial description
USP 25: A white, odourless, crystalline powder. It exists in two polymorphic forms, one melting between 106° and 107°, and the other between 112° and 113°; a mixture of the two forms may melt between 105° and 113°. Soluble 1 in 1.2 of water, 1 in 2.5 of alcohol, 1 in 2 of chloroform, and 1 in 3000 of ether. pH of a 1% solution in water is about 5. Store in airtight containers. Protect from light.

Adverse Effects and Precautions
As for the sedating antihistamines in general, p.404.

Effects on the blood. A report[1] that agranulocytosis in a 34-year-old alcoholic man was possibly associated with brompheniramine therapy.
1. Hardin AS, Padilla F. Agranulocytosis during therapy with a brompheniramine-medication. *J Arkansas Med Soc* 1978; **75:** 206–8.

Extrapyramidal disorders. Facial dyskinesias have been reported[1,2] after administration of antihistamines including brompheniramine or dexbrompheniramine maleate.
1. Thach BT, *et al.* Oral facial dyskinesia associated with prolonged use of antihistaminic decongestants. *N Engl J Med* 1975; **293:** 486–7 (brompheniramine maleate, chlorpheniramine maleate, and phenindamine tartrate).
2. Barone DA, Raniolo J. Facial dyskinesia from overdose of an antihistamine. *N Engl J Med* 1980; **303:** 107 (dexbrompheniramine maleate).

Withdrawal. Withdrawal symptoms have been reported[1] following discontinuation of long-term therapy with brompheniramine maleate. A patient had been taking 48 mg almost every day for 20 years and developed tremor, nausea, depression, and apyrexial sweating within 48 hours of stopping treatment; symptoms resolved over the following weeks.
1. Kavanagh GM, *et al.* Withdrawal symptoms after discontinuation of long-acting brompheniramine maleate. *Br J Dermatol* 1994; **131:** 913–14.

Interactions
As for the sedating antihistamines in general, p.406.

Pharmacokinetics
After oral administration brompheniramine maleate appears to be well absorbed from the gastrointestinal tract. Peak plasma concentrations are achieved within about 5 hours. An elimination half-life of about 25

hours has been reported. Unchanged drug and metabolites are excreted primarily in the urine.

◊ References.
1. Simons FER, *et al.* The pharmacokinetics and antihistaminic effects of brompheniramine. *J Allergy Clin Immunol* 1982; **70:** 458–64.
2. Paton DM, Webster DR. Clinical pharmacokinetics of H_1-receptor antagonists (the antihistamines). *Clin Pharmacokinet* 1985; **10:** 477–97.

Uses and Administration
Brompheniramine maleate, an alkylamine derivative, is a sedating antihistamine with antimuscarinic and moderate sedative actions.

Brompheniramine is a racemic mixture; dexbrompheniramine, the dextrorotatory isomer, has approximately twice the activity of brompheniramine by weight. Brompheniramine maleate and dexbrompheniramine maleate are used for the symptomatic relief of allergic conditions, mainly rhinitis (p.407) and conjunctivitis (p.406). They are common ingredients of compound preparations for the symptomatic treatment of coughs and the common cold (p.406).

Brompheniramine maleate is given by mouth usually in doses of 4 to 8 mg three or four times daily. Children up to 3 years of age are given 0.4 to 1 mg per kg body-weight over 24 hours in four divided doses. Children aged 3 to 6 years are given 1 to 2 mg three or four times daily and those aged 6 to 12 years 2 to 4 mg three or four times daily.

Brompheniramine maleate has also been given by subcutaneous, intramuscular, or slow intravenous injection; the dose is usually 10 mg every 8 to 12 hours as necessary and the total parenteral dose should not exceed 40 mg in 24 hours.

Dexbrompheniramine maleate is normally given as an ingredient of decongestant preparations containing pseudoephedrine. The dose of dexbrompheniramine maleate by mouth in these combinations is 2 mg up to four times daily. Children over 6 years can be given 1 mg up to four times a day.

Modified-release oral preparations of brompheniramine maleate or dexbrompheniramine maleate are available in some countries; dosage is specific to a particular formulation.

Preparations
BP 2001: Brompheniramine Tablets;
USP 25: Brompheniramine Maleate Elixir; Brompheniramine Maleate Injection; Brompheniramine Maleate Tablets; Dexbrompheniramine Maleate and Pseudoephedrine Sulfate Oral Solution.

Proprietary Preparations (details are given in Part 3)
Canad.: Dimetane; *Fr.:* Dimegan; *Ger.:* Dimegan†; *Irl.:* Dimotane; *Singapore:* Neo-Meton; *Thai.:* Centapp; Dimetane; *UK:* Dimotane; *USA:* Cophene-B†; Diamine TD†; Dimetane; Lodrane Allergy; Nasahist B†; ND Stat†; Oraminic II; Sinusol-B†; Veltane†.

Multi-ingredient: *Aust.:* Disophrol; *Austral.:* Dimetapp; Dimetapp DM; Dimetapp LA†; *Belg.:* Nasapert; Rinafort; *Braz.:* Bialerge; Dimetapp; Dimetapp Expectorante; Disofrol; *Canad.:* Centracol†; Cold & Allergy; Cold & Allergy Relief; Cough, Cold & Allergy Relief; Decongestant Antihistaminic Syrup; Dimetane Expectorant; Dimetane Expectorant C; Dimetane Expectorant DC; Dimetapp; Dimetapp Chewables; Dimetapp Clear; Dimetapp Cough & Cold Liqui-Gels; Dimetapp DM; Dimetapp Liqui-Gels; Dimetapp Oral Infant Drops; Dimetapp Quick Dissolve; Dimetapp-C; Drixoral; Drixoral Day/Night; Drixtab; Pharmetapp†; Tantapp; *Fin.:* Dimetane Expect; Dimetane Expect DC; Disofrol; Lunerin; *Fr.:* Dimetane; Martigene; Rupton Chronules†; Sebrane Rhume; *Ger.:* Ilvico N†; *Hong Kong:* Brom-PP; Brom-Ramine Compound; Bromphenex; Dime-Time; Dimetapp; Disobrom; Drixoral; ENT; Neosed; *Irl.:* Dimotane Co; Dimotane Expectorant; Dimotapp; Ilvico; *Mex.:* Afrinex; Dimetapp; *Port.:* Constipal; Ilvico N; *S.Afr.:* Dimetapp; Ilvico; *Singapore:* Bromanate; Drixoral; *Spain:* Disofrol; Ilvico; *Swed.:* Disofrol; Lunerin†; *Switz.:* Dimetapp; Disofrol; Rupton Chronules; *Thai.:* AA Cold; Aorinyl; Asiatapp; Bepeno-G; Bluco; Bromavon; Bromesep Elixir; Bromesep Expectorant; Bromped; Bromtussia; Bromtussia DC; Bromtussin; Coldate; Dimetane Expectorant; Dimetane Expectorant DC; Dimetapp; Medimegen; Meditapp; Meditapp Expectorant; Minra; Nartap; Nasosil; Polydine; Postap; Postap Expectorant; Rhinophen-C; Rupton; Stobcon; *UK:* Dimotane Co; Dimotane Expectorant; Dimotane Plus; Dimotapp; Robitussin Night-Time; *USA:* 12 Hour Antihistamine Nasal Decongestant; 12 Hour Cold; Alka-Seltzer Plus Night-Time Cold†; Alka-Seltzer Plus Sinus Allergy†; Allent; Ami-Drixt†; Anaplex DM; Anaplex HD; Andehist; Andehist DM; Brofed; Bromaline Plus†; Bromaline†; Bromanate†; Bromarest DX; Bromatane DX; Bromatapp†; Bromfed; Bromfed-DM; Bromfed-PD; Bromfenex; Bromophen TD†; Bromphen DX Cough; Bromphen†; Brompheniramine Cough; Brompheniramine DC Cough†; Coldec DM; Dallergy-JR; Dexaphen-SA; Dimaphen†; Dimetane DC†; Dimetane Decongestant; Dimetane DX; Dimetapp; Dimetapp Cold & Allergy Chewable†; Dimetapp Cold & Fever; Dimetapp Cold & Flu†; Dimetapp DM; Dimetapp Nighttime Flu; Disobrom; Disophrol; Dristan Allergy; Dristan Cold Maximum Strength Multi-symptom Formula; Drixomed; Drixoral; Drixoral Cold & Allergy; Drixoral Cold & Flu; Drixoral Plus; Endafed; ENT†; Histine DM†; Histinex DM†; Iofed; Iohist DM†; Liqui-Histine DM†; Lodrane; Maximum Strength Dristan Cold; Myphetane DC†; Myphetane DX; Myphetapp†; Partapp TD†; Poly-Histine CS†; Poly-Histine DM†; Respahist; Rondec; Sildec-DM; Siltapp†; Sinadrin Plus; Tamine SR†; Touro A & H; Touro Allergy; Trihist-CS†; Trihist-DM†; ULTRAbrom; Vicks DayQuil Allergy Relief†.

Buclizine Hydrochloride (6111-d)

Buclizine Hydrochloride (BANM, USAN, rINNM).

NSC-25141; UCB-4445. (RS)1-(4-tert-Butylbenzyl)-4-(4-chlorobenzhydryl)piperazine dihydrochloride.

$C_{28}H_{33}ClN_2,2HCl = 505.9$.

CAS — 82-95-1 (buclizine); 129-74-8 (buclizine hydrochloride).

Pharmacopoeias. In Br.

Pharmacopoeial description

BP 2001: A white or slightly yellowish, crystalline powder. Practically insoluble in water; very slightly soluble in alcohol; sparingly soluble in chloroform and in propylene glycol.

Adverse Effects and Precautions

As for the sedating antihistamines in general, p.404.

Interactions

As for the sedating antihistamines in general, p.406.

Uses and Administration

Buclizine hydrochloride, a piperazine derivative, is a sedating antihistamine with antimuscarinic and moderate sedative actions. It is used mainly for its antiemetic action, particularly in the prevention of motion sickness (p.407) and in the treatment of migraine in combination with analgesics (p.449). In some countries it is given in the management of allergic conditions and in pruritic skin disorders (p.407). Buclizine has also been used in the treatment of vertigo (p.408) associated with disorders of the vestibular system, although its value in these conditions remains to be established.

To prevent motion sickness, buclizine hydrochloride is given at least 30 minutes before travelling in a dose of 25 or 50 mg by mouth, which may be repeated, if necessary, after 4 to 6 hours. The usual dose to alleviate nausea is 25 or 50 mg given up to three times daily.

In the treatment of migraine, buclizine hydrochloride is given in usual doses of 12.5 mg at the start of an attack or when one is known to be imminent.

In pruritic skin disorders the usual dose of buclizine hydrochloride is 25 to 50 mg daily.

Preparations

Proprietary Preparations (details are given in Part 3)
Belg.: Longifene; **Braz.:** Buclina; Postafen; **Fr.:** Aphilan; **Hong Kong:** Longifene; **Mex.:** Postavit-B; **Port.:** Buclina; Postafeno; **S.Afr.:** Longifene; **Singapore:** Longifene; **Switz.:** Longifene†; **USA:** Bucladin-S Softab.

Multi-ingredient: Braz.: Apetibe; Apetil; Buclamin; Bucliamin; Buclifen-Vit; Bucliplex; Buclitina; Carnabol; Carnizin; Complevit; Kelavitam; Klizin; Lisinvitan; Nutrimaiz SM; Pepsivit; Pondusvitam; Profol; Propan; Stin; Useton; Vitaler; Vitalisin; Vitamil; **Ger.:** Migralave N; **Hong Kong:** Propan; **Irl.:** Migraleve; **Israel:** Migraleve; **Port.:** Migraleve; **S.Afr.:** Vomifene; **Singapore:** Migraleve; **Spain:** Migraleve; **Switz.:** Hexafene†; Migraleve; **UK:** Migraleve; Migralift†.

Carbinoxamine Maleate (6113-h)

Carbinoxamine Maleate (BANM, rINNM).

2-[4-Chloro-α-(2-pyridyl)benzyloxy]-NN-dimethylethylamine hydrogen maleate.

$C_{16}H_{19}ClN_2O,C_4H_4O_4 = 406.9$.

CAS — 486-16-8 (carbinoxamine); 3505-38-2 (carbinoxamine maleate).

Pharmacopoeias. In US.

Pharmacopoeial description

USP 25: A white, odourless, crystalline powder. Soluble 1 in less than 1 of water, 1 in 1.5 of alcohol and of chloroform, and 1 in 8300 of ether. pH of a 1% solution in water is between 4.6 and 5.1. Store in airtight containers. Protect from light.

Adverse Effects and Precautions

As for the sedating antihistamines in general, p.404.

Interactions

As for the sedating antihistamines in general, p.406.

Uses and Administration

Carbinoxamine maleate, a monoethanolamine derivative, is a sedating antihistamine with antimuscarinic, significant sedative, and serotonin antagonist effects. Carbinoxamine maleate is used for the relief of allergic conditions such as rhinitis (p.407), and is a common ingredient of compound preparations for symptomatic treatment of coughs and the common cold (p.406).

The dose of carbinoxamine maleate by mouth, used alone or in combination preparations, is usually in the range of 2 to 4 mg

three or four times daily. Children may be given half the adult dose. Carbinoxamine polistirex has also been given by mouth.

Preparations

USP 25: Carbinoxamine Maleate Tablets; Pseudoephedrine Hydrochloride, Carbinoxamine Maleate, and Dextromethorphan Hydrobromide Oral Solution.

Proprietary Preparations (details are given in Part 3)
Fr.: Allergefon; **Ger.:** Polistin Pad; Polistin T-Caps; **Thai.:** Histin; Sinumine; **USA:** Histex CT; Histex PD.

Multi-ingredient: Aust.: Capramin; Co-Tylenol; Rhinopront; **Belg.:** Rhinopront; **Braz.:** Afebrin; Gripenil; Iodeto de Potassio Composto; Naldecon; Resprin; Xarope de Iodeto de Potassio Composto; **Fin.:** Tinaroc-Combi; **Fr.:** Humex; **Ger.:** Rhinopront; Rhinotussal; **Hong Kong:** Coritussal; Metoplex; Rhinopront; **Israel:** Rhinovis; **Ital.:** Rondec; Torfan; **Mex.:** Prindex; **S.Afr.:** Coryretard-C†; Rhinotussal†; **Singapore:** Coritussal; Metussa; Rhinopront; **Spain:** Rinomax; Rinoretard; Rondec†; Toscal Compuesto†; Toscal†; **Switz.:** Rhinopront; Rhinotussal; **Thai.:** Nasalgen; Rhinar; Rhinohist; Rhinopront; Rhinotussal; Rondec-DM; **UAE:** Fluzal; **USA:** Andehist; Andehist DM; Carbinoxamine Compound; Carbiset; Carbodec; Carbodec DM; Cardec DM Pediatric; Cardec-S; Cydec; Cydec DM; Histex HC; Palgic DS; Palgic-D; Pseudo-Car DM; Rondamine-DM; Rondec; Rondec-DM; Sildec-DM; Tussafed.

Cetirizine Hydrochloride (18617-l)

Cetirizine Hydrochloride (BANM, USAN, rINNM).

Cetirizini Dihydrochloridum; P-071; UCB-P071. The dihydrochloride of 2-[4-(4-chlorobenzhydryl)piperazin-1-yl]ethoxyacetic acid.

$C_{21}H_{25}ClN_2O_3,2HCl = 461.8$.

CAS — 83881-51-0 (cetirizine); 83881-52-1 (cetirizine hydrochloride).

Pharmacopoeias. In Eur. (see p.vi).

Pharmacopoeial description

Ph. Eur.: A white or almost white powder. Freely soluble in water; practically insoluble in acetone and in dichloromethane. A 5% solution in water has a pH of 1.2 to 1.8. Protect from light.

Adverse Effects and Precautions

As for the non-sedating antihistamines in general, p.404. Reduced dosage is recommended for patients with renal impairment.

Arrhythmias. The ECG effects of cetirizine were studied[1] in normal subjects and administration of doses of up to six times the usual recommended dose did not prolong the QT interval. Additionally, workers from the FDA[2] in the USA and representatives of the manufacturers[3] in Belgium have not found any association so far between cetirizine and the development of ventricular arrhythmias. The fear that arrhythmias might be a class effect of the non-sedating antihistamines is discussed on p.405.

1. Sale ME, et al. The electrocardiographic effects of cetirizine in normal subjects. Clin Pharmacol Ther 1994; 56: 295–301.
2. Himmel MH, et al. Dangers of non-sedating antihistamines. Lancet 1997; 350: 69.
3. Coulie P, et al. Non-sedating antihistamines and cardiac arrhythmias. Lancet 1998; 351: 451.

Effects on the liver. Life-threatening hepatitis developed in a 23-year-old man who had been taking cetirizine long-term for atopic dermatitis.[1] He recovered following treatment with prednisolone.

1. Watanabe M, et al. Severe hepatitis in a patient taking cetirizine. Ann Intern Med 2001; 135: 142–3.

Hypersensitivity. Hypersensitivity reactions manifest as urticaria have been reported with cetirizine.[1,2]

1. Karamfilov T, et al. Cetirizine-induced urticarial reaction. Br J Dermatol 1999; 140: 979–80.
2. Calista D, et al. Urticaria induced by cetirizine. Br J Dermatol 2001; 144: 196.

Sedation. For discussion of the sedative effects of antihistamines see p.405.

Interactions

As for the non-sedating antihistamines in general, p.406. However, some interactions are less likely with cetirizine than with non-sedating antihistamines such as astemizole and terfenadine, since cetirizine appears to have low hepatic metabolism and little arrhythmogenic potential (see Arrhythmias, above).

Anticoagulants. For a report of an interaction between cetirizine and nicoumalone [acenocoumarol], see under Interactions in Warfarin, p.995.

Pharmacokinetics

Cetirizine is rapidly absorbed from the gastrointestinal tract after oral administration, peak plasma concentrations being attained within about one hour. Food delays the time to peak plasma concentrations but does not decrease the amount of drug absorbed. It

is highly bound to plasma proteins and has an elimination half-life of about 10 hours. Cetirizine has been detected in breast milk. Cetirizine is excreted primarily in the urine mainly as unchanged drug. Cetirizine does not appear to cross the blood-brain barrier to a significant extent.

◊ References.
1. Awni WM, et al. Effect of haemodialysis on the pharmacokinetics of cetirizine. Eur J Clin Pharmacol 1990; 38: 67–9.
2. Desager JP, et al. A pharmacokinetic evaluation of the second-generation H₁-receptor antagonist cetirizine in very young children. Clin Pharmacol Ther 1993; 53: 431–5.

Uses and Administration

Cetirizine hydrochloride, a piperazine derivative and metabolite of hydroxyzine (p.419), is described as a non-sedating antihistamine which is long-acting and has some mast-cell stabilising activity. It appears to have a low potential for drowsiness in usual doses and to be virtually free of antimuscarinic activity. It is used for the symptomatic relief of allergic conditions including rhinitis (p.407) and chronic urticaria (p.408).

In adults and children of 6 years and over, cetirizine hydrochloride is given by mouth in a dose of 10 mg once daily or 5 mg twice daily. In children aged 2 to 6 years old a dose of 5 mg once daily or 2.5 mg twice daily may be used for seasonal allergic rhinitis.

In patients with renal impairment it is recommended that the dosage is reduced to half the usual daily dose.

◊ References.
1. Spencer CM, et al. Cetirizine: a reappraisal of its pharmacological properties and therapeutic use in selected allergic disorders. Drugs 1993; 46: 1055–80.
2. Barnes CL, et al. Cetirizine: a new, nonsedating antihistamine. Ann Pharmacother 1993; 27: 464–70.
3. Breneman D, et al. Cetirizine and astemizole therapy for chronic idiopathic urticaria: a double-blind placebo-controlled, comparative trial. J Am Acad Dermatol 1995; 33: 192–8.
4. Breneman DL. Cetirizine versus hydroxyzine and placebo in chronic idiopathic urticaria. Ann Pharmacother 1996; 30: 1075–9.
5. Anonymous. Cetirizine—a new antihistamine. Med Lett Drugs Ther 1996; 38: 21–3.

Preparations

Proprietary Preparations (details are given in Part 3)
Aust.: Zyrtec; **Austral.:** Zyrtec; **Belg.:** Zyrtec; **Braz.:** Cetirizin; Zetir; Zyrtec; **Canad.:** Reactine; Zyrtec; **Denm.:** Zyrtec; **Fin.:** Zyrtec; **Fr.:** Virlix; Zyrtec; **Ger.:** Alerid; Zyrtec; **Hong Kong:** Zyrtec; **Irl.:** Zirtek; **Israel:** Histazine; Zyrtec; **Ital.:** Formistin; Virlix; Zyrtec; **Jpn:** Zyrtec; **Mex.:** Virlix; Zyrtec; **Neth.:** Zyrtec; **Norw.:** Zyrtec; **NZ:** Zyrtec; **Port.:** Virlix; Zyrtec; **S.Afr.:** Zyrtec; **Singapore:** Zyrtec; **Spain:** Alerlisin; Virlix; Voltric; Zyrtec; **Swed.:** Zyrlex; **Switz.:** Zyrtec; **Thai.:** Cetrizet; Cistamine; Triz; Zermed; Zyrex; Zyrtec; Zyrzine; Zytine; **UAE:** Cetralon; **UK:** Zirtek; **USA:** Zyrtec.

Multi-ingredient: Belg.: Cirrus; **Canad.:** Reactine Plus; **Fin.:** Cirrus; **Hong Kong:** Cirrus; **Ital.:** Naristar; **Mex.:** Virlix-D; Zyrtec-D; **Singapore:** Cirrus; **Spain:** Stopcold; **USA:** Zyrtec-D.

Chlorcyclizine Hydrochloride (6114-m)

Chlorcyclizine Hydrochloride (BANM, rINNM).

Chlorcyclizini Hydrochloridum; Chlorcyclizinium Chloride. 1-(4-Chlorobenzhydryl)-4-methylpiperazine hydrochloride.

$C_{18}H_{21}ClN_2,HCl = 337.3$.

CAS — 82-93-9 (chlorcyclizine); 1620-21-9 (chlorcyclizine hydrochloride).

Pharmacopoeias. In Eur. (see p.vi).

Pharmacopoeial description

Ph. Eur.: A white, crystalline powder. Freely soluble in water and in dichloromethane; soluble in alcohol; practically insoluble in ether. A 1% solution in water has a pH of 5.0 to 6.0. Protect from light.

Profile

Chlorcyclizine hydrochloride, a piperazine derivative, is a sedating antihistamine (p.404). It is given by mouth in doses of 50 to 100 mg once or twice daily for the symptomatic relief of hypersensitivity reactions; it is also used as an antiemetic. It has been used at a strength of 2% in topical preparations, although as with other antihistamines, there is a risk of sensitisation.

Chlorcyclizine dibunate (naftoclizine) has been administered as a cough suppressant similarly to sodium dibunate (p.1100).

Preparations

Proprietary Preparations (details are given in Part 3)
Denm.: Trihistan; **Norw.:** Trihistan; **Swed.:** Di-Paralene†.

Multi-ingredient: Fin.: Anervan; **Israel:** Temigran; **Neth.:** Primatour; **Norw.:** Anervan; **Spain:** Diminex Antitusigeno; Diminex Balsamico†; **Swed.:** Anervan; Exolyt; **USA:** Mantadil†.

Chloropyramine Hydrochloride (6135-p)

Chloropyramine Hydrochloride (BANM, rINNM).

Halopyramine Hydrochloride. N-(4-Chlorobenzyl)-N'N'-dimethyl-N-(2-pyridyl)ethylenediamine hydrochloride.

$C_{16}H_{20}ClN_3,HCl = 326.3$.

CAS — 59-32-5 (chloropyramine); 6170-42-9 (chloropyramine hydrochloride).

Profile

Chloropyramine hydrochloride, an ethylenediamine derivative, is an antihistamine (p.404). It has been given by mouth and by injection.

Preparations

Proprietary Preparations (details are given in Part 3)
Hung.: Suprastin; *Mex.:* Avapena.

Chlorpheniramine Maleate (6116-v)

Chlorpheniramine Maleate (BANM).

Chlorphenamine Maleate (BANM, rINNM); Chlorphenamini Maleas; Chlorprophenpyridamine Maleate. (±)-3-(4-Chlorophenyl)-NN-dimethyl-3-(2-pyridyl)propylamine hydrogen maleate.

$C_{16}H_{19}ClN_2,C_4H_4O_4 = 390.9$.

CAS — 132-22-9 (chlorpheniramine [chlorphenamine]); 113-92-8 (chlorpheniramine [chlorphenamine] maleate).

Pharmacopoeias. In Chin., Eur. (see p.vi), Int., Jpn, and US.

Incompatibility has been reported with calcium chloride, kanamycin sulfate, noradrenaline [norepinephrine] acid tartrate, pentobarbital sodium, and meglumine adipiodone.

Pharmacopoeial description

Ph. Eur.: A white, crystalline powder. Freely soluble in water; soluble in alcohol; slightly soluble in ether. Protect from light.

USP 25: A white, odourless, crystalline powder. Soluble 1 in 4 of water and 1 in 10 of alcohol and of chloroform; slightly soluble in ether and in benzene. Its solutions in water have a pH between 4 and 5. Store in airtight containers. Protect from light.

Dexchlorpheniramine Maleate (6127-p)

Dexchlorpheniramine Maleate (BANM, rINNM).

Dexchlorphenamine Maleate; Dexchlorpheniramini Maleas.

CAS — 25523-97-1 (dexchlorpheniramine); 2438-32-6 (dexchlorpheniramine maleate).

Pharmacopoeias. In Eur. (see p.vi), Jpn, and US.

Pharmacopoeial description

Ph. Eur.: A white crystalline powder. Very soluble in water; freely soluble in alcohol, in dichloromethane, and in methyl alcohol. A 1% solution in water has a pH of 4.5 to 5.5. Protect from light.

USP 25: A white, odourless, crystalline powder. Soluble 1 in 1.1 of water, 1 in 2 of alcohol, 1 in 1.7 of chloroform, and 1 in 2500 of ether; slightly soluble in benzene. pH of a 1% solution in water is between 4.0 and 5.0. Store in airtight containers. Protect from light.

Adverse Effects and Precautions

As for the sedating antihistamines in general, p.404. Exfoliative dermatitis may develop. Injections may be irritant and cause transient hypotension or stimulation of the CNS.

Effects on the blood. There are several old and isolated reports of blood dyscrasias after administration of chlorpheniramine [chlorphenamine] maleate; these include agranulocytosis,[1,2] thrombocytopenia,[3] pancytopenia,[4] and aplastic anaemia.[5] Haemolytic anaemia has occurred after administration of dexchlorpheniramine maleate.[6] The association with antihistamine administration has been questioned in some of these cases.[7]

1. Shenfield G, Spry CJF. Unusual cause of agranulocytosis. *BMJ* 1968; ii: 52–3.
2. Hardin AS. Chlorpheniramine and agranulocytosis. *Ann Intern Med* 1988; **108:** 770.
3. Eisner EV, et al. Chlorpheniramine-dependent thrombocytopenia. *JAMA* 1975; **231:** 735–6.
4. Deringer PM, Maniatis A. Chlorpheniramine-induced bone-marrow suppression. *Lancet* 1976; **i:** 432.
5. Kanoh T, et al. Aplastic anaemia after prolonged treatment with chlorpheniramine. *Lancet* 1977; **i:** 546–7.
6. Duran-Suarez JR, et al. The I antigen as an immune complex receptor in a case of haemolytic anaemia induced by an antihistaminic agent. *Br J Haematol* 1981; **49:** 153–4.
7. Spry CJF. Chlorpheniramine-induced bone-marrow suppression. *Lancet* 1976; **i:** 545.

Effects on the senses. Chlorpheniramine [chlorphenamine] has been reported to affect the senses of smell and taste.[1]

1. Schiffman SS. Taste and smell in disease. *N Engl J Med* 1983; **308:** 1275–9.

Extrapyramidal disorders. Facial dyskinesias have been reported[1,2] after administration of chlorpheniramine [chlorphenamine] maleate by mouth.

1. Thach BT, et al. Oral facial dyskinesia associated with prolonged use of antihistaminic decongestants. *N Engl J Med* 1975; **293:** 486–7.
2. Davis WA. Dyskinesia associated with chronic antihistamine use. *N Engl J Med* 1976; **294:** 113.

Interactions

As for the sedating antihistamines in general, p.406.

Antiepileptics. For a report of the effect of chlorpheniramine [chlorphenamine] on phenytoin, see p.360.

Pharmacokinetics

Chlorpheniramine [chlorphenamine] maleate is absorbed relatively slowly from the gastrointestinal tract, peak plasma concentrations occurring about 2.5 to 6 hours after administration by mouth. Bioavailability is low, values of 25 to 50% having been reported. Chlorpheniramine [chlorphenamine] appears to undergo considerable first-pass metabolism. About 70% of chlorpheniramine [chlorphenamine] in the circulation is bound to plasma proteins. There is wide interindividual variation in the pharmacokinetics of chlorpheniramine [chlorphenamine]; values ranging from 2 to 43 hours have been reported for the half-life. Chlorpheniramine [chlorphenamine] is widely distributed in the body, including passage into the CNS.

Chlorpheniramine [chlorphenamine] maleate is extensively metabolised. Metabolites include desmethyl- and didesmethylchlorpheniramine. Unchanged drug and metabolites are excreted primarily in the urine; excretion is dependent on urinary pH and flow rate. Only trace amounts have been found in the faeces.

A duration of action of 4 to 6 hours has been reported; this is shorter than may be predicted from pharmacokinetic parameters.

More rapid and extensive absorption, faster clearance, and a shorter half-life have been reported in children.

◊ References.

1. Rumore MM. Clinical pharmacokinetics of chlorpheniramine. *Drug Intell Clin Pharm* 1984; **18:** 701–7.
2. Paton DM, Webster DR. Clinical pharmacokinetics of H₁-receptor antagonists (the antihistamines). *Clin Pharmacokinet* 1985; **10:** 477–97.

Uses and Administration

Chlorpheniramine [chlorphenamine] maleate, an alkylamine derivative, is a sedating antihistamine that causes a moderate degree of sedation; it also has antimuscarinic activity.

Chlorpheniramine [chlorphenamine] is a racemic mixture; the dextrorotatory isomer, dexchlorpheniramine, has approximately twice the activity of chlorpheniramine [chlorphenamine] by weight.

Chlorpheniramine [chlorphenamine] maleate and dexchlorpheniramine maleate are used for the symptomatic relief of allergic conditions including urticaria and angioedema (p.408), rhinitis (p.407), and conjunctivitis (p.406), and in pruritic skin disorders (p.407). They are common ingredients of compound preparations for symptomatic treatment of coughs and the common cold (p.406). Chlorpheniramine [chlorphenamine] may be administered intravenously as an adjunct in the emergency treatment of anaphylactic shock (p.406).

Chlorpheniramine [chlorphenamine] maleate is given by mouth in doses of 4 mg every 4 to 6 hours up to a maximum of 24 mg daily. Doses for children are: 1 to 2 years, 1 mg twice daily; 2 to 5 years, 1 mg every 4 to 6 hours (maximum 6 mg daily); 6 to 12 years, 2 mg every 4 to 6 hours (maximum 12 mg daily).

Chlorpheniramine [chlorphenamine] maleate may be given by intramuscular, by subcutaneous, or by slow intravenous injection over a period of 1 minute. The usual dose is 10 to 20 mg and the total dose given by these routes in 24 hours should not normally exceed 40 mg. For children, doses of 87.5 µg per kg body-

weight subcutaneously four times daily have been suggested.

Dexchlorpheniramine maleate is given by mouth in doses of 2 mg every 4 to 6 hours up to a maximum of 12 mg daily. Children aged 2 to 5 years may be given 0.5 mg every 4 to 6 hours (maximum 3 mg daily), and those aged 6 to 12 years, 1 mg every 4 to 6 hours (maximum 6 mg daily).

Modified-release oral preparations of chlorpheniramine [chlorphenamine] maleate or dexchlorpheniramine maleate are available in some countries; dosage is specific to a particular formulation.

Chlorpheniramine [chlorphenamine] polistirex (a sulfonated diethenylbenzene-ethenylbenzene copolymer complex) and chlorpheniramine [chlorphenamine] tannate are given by mouth and used similarly to the maleate.

Malaria. Chlorpheniramine [chlorphenamine] may be tried in patients with malaria who experience chloroquine-induced pruritus (see p.433), but additionally it has been shown to have some promise as an adjunct in the treatment of chloroquine-resistant malaria itself. Early studies indicated that chlorpheniramine [chlorphenamine] was only one of a number of drugs that reversed chloroquine resistance *in vitro* in isolates of *Plasmodium falciparum*. Later clinical studies in children in Nigeria demonstrated enhanced efficacy when chlorpheniramine [chlorphenamine] was given with chloroquine.[1-5] The overall management of malaria is discussed on p.428.

1. Sowunmi A, et al. Enhanced efficacy of chloroquine-chlorpheniramine combination in acute uncomplicated falciparum malaria in children. *Trans R Soc Trop Med Hyg* 1997; **91:** 63–7.
2. Sowunmi A, Oduola AMJ. Comparative efficacy of chloroquine/chlorpheniramine combination and mefloquine for the treatment of chloroquine-resistant *Plasmodium falciparum* malaria in Nigerian children. *Trans R Soc Trop Med Hyg* 1997; **91:** 689–93.
3. Sowunmi A, et al. Comparative efficacy of chloroquine plus chlorpheniramine and pyrimethamine/sulfadoxine in acute uncomplicated falciparum malaria in Nigerian children. *Trans R Soc Trop Med Hyg* 1998; **92:** 77–81.
4. Sowunmi A, et al. Comparative efficacy of chloroquine plus chlorpheniramine and halofantrine in acute uncomplicated falciparum malaria in Nigerian children. *Trans R Soc Trop Med Hyg* 1998; **92:** 441–5.
5. Okonkwo CA, et al. Effect of chlorpheniramine on the pharmacokinetics of and response to chloroquine of Nigerian children with falciparum malaria. *Trans R Soc Trop Med Hyg* 1999; **93:** 306–11.

Preparations

BP 2001: Chlorphenamine Injection; Chlorphenamine Oral Solution; Chlorphenamine Tablets;
USP 25: Chlorpheniramine Maleate and Phenylpropanolamine Hydrochloride Extended-release Capsules; Chlorpheniramine Maleate and Phenylpropanolamine Hydrochloride Extended-release Tablets; Chlorpheniramine Maleate and Pseudoephedrine Hydrochloride Extended-release Capsules; Chlorpheniramine Maleate and Pseudoephedrine Hydrochloride Oral Solution; Chlorpheniramine Maleate Extended-release Capsules; Chlorpheniramine Maleate Injection; Chlorpheniramine Maleate Syrup; Chlorpheniramine Maleate Tablets; Dexchlorpheniramine Maleate Syrup; Dexchlorpheniramine Maleate Tablets.

Proprietary Preparations (details are given in Part 3)
Aust.: Polaramin; Polaronil; *Austral.:* Piriton†; Polaramine; *Belg.:* Bronchalene†; Polaramine; *Braz.:* Histamin; Polaramine; *Canad.:* Chlor-Tripolon; Histalon; Novo-Pheniram; Polaramine; *Denm.:* Polaramin; *Fr.:* Polaramine; *Ger.:* Polaronil; *Hong Kong:* Chlorpyrimine; Primat; Piriton; Polaramine; Sprinsol; Uni-Ramine; *Irl.:* Anti-Hist†; Piriton; *Israel:* Ahiston; Anaphyl; *Ital.:* Polamin; Polaramin; Trimeton; *Mex.:* Alerdil; Bioflusin; Blendox; Cloro-Trimeton; Cronal; Polaramine; *Neth.:* Polaramine; *Norw.:* Phenamin; Polaramin; *NZ:* Histafen; Polaramine; *Port.:* Trenelone; *S.Afr.:* Allergex; Allerhist†; Chlor-Trimeton; Chlorhist; Histamed†; Polaramine; *Singapore:* Allerphen; Chlorpyrimine; Piriton; Polaramine; Rhiniramine; *Spain:* Antihistaminico; Polaramine; *Swed.:* Polaramin; *Switz.:* Polaramine; *Thai.:* Allergin; Chlorleate; Chlorpyrimine; Cohistan; Histatapp; Nasamine; Piriton; *UAE:* Chlorohistol; *UK:* Allergy Relief; Calimal; Piriject; Piriton; Pollenase Antihistamine; Rimarin; *USA:* Aller-Chlor; Allergy; Chlo-Amine; Chlor-Pro; Chlor-Trimeton; Chlor†; Chlorate†; Chlorspan†; Dexchlor†; Diabetic Tussin Allergy Relief†; Efidac 24-Chlorpheniramine; Gen-Allerate†; PediaCare Allergy Formula; Pfeiffer's Allergy†; Phenetron†; Poladex†; Polaramine; Ricobid H†; Telachlor†; Teldrin.

Multi-ingredient: numerous preparations are listed in Part 3.

Chlorphenoxamine Hydrochloride (353-c)

Chlorphenoxamine Hydrochloride (BANM, rINNM).

2-(4-Chloro-α-methylbenzhydryloxy)-NN-dimethylethylamine hydrochloride.

$C_{18}H_{22}ClNO,HCl = 340.3$.

CAS — 77-38-3 (chlorphenoxamine); 562-09-4 (chlorphenoxamine hydrochloride).

Profile

Chlorphenoxamine, a congener of diphenhydramine (p.416), has antimuscarinic and antihistaminic properties. It has been used in nausea, vomiting, and vertigo, and was formerly used in the symptomatic treatment of parkinsonism. Chlorphenoxamine has also been used in hypersensitivity reactions.

Preparations

Proprietary Preparations (details are given in Part 3)
Aust.: Systral; **Ger.:** Systral; **Hong Kong:** Systral; **Port.:** Systral†; **Thai.:** Systral.

Multi-ingredient: **Aust.:** Calcilin compositum; Longtussin†; Rodavan†; Spirbon; Systral C; Systrason; **Ger.:** Rodavan; Systral C; **S.Afr.:** Analgen-SA.

Cinnarizine   (6118-q)

Cinnarizine (BAN, USAN, rINN).

Cinnarizinum; 516-MD; R-516; R-1575. 1-Benzhydryl-4-cinnamylpiperazine; (E)-1-(Diphenylmethyl)-4-(3-phenylprop-2-enyl)piperazine.

$C_{26}H_{28}N_2 = 368.5$.
CAS — 298-57-7.
ATC — N07CA02.

Pharmacopoeias. In Eur. (see p.vi), Jpn, and Pol.

Pharmacopoeial description

Ph. Eur.: A white or almost white powder. Practically insoluble in water; slightly soluble in alcohol and in methyl alcohol; soluble in acetone; freely soluble in dichloromethane. Protect from light.

Adverse Effects and Precautions

As for the sedating antihistamines in general, p.404.

There have been rare reports of extrapyramidal symptoms after cinnarizine, sometimes associated with depressive feelings.

High doses of cinnarizine should be used with caution in patients with hypotension because of the possibility of decreasing blood pressure further.

Extrapyramidal disorders. For reference to extrapyramidal disorders associated with the use of cinnarizine, see Flunarizine, p.418.

Hypersensitivity. A report[1] of immunologically-defined lichen planus pemphigoides in a 72-year-old woman taking cinnarizine. Lesions began to clear when treatment was stopped but challenge with cinnarizine provoked severe itching and reactivation of pigmented lesions.

1. Miyagawa S, et al. Lichen planus pemphigoides-like lesions induced by cinnarizine. Br J Dermatol 1985; **112:** 607–13.

Porphyria. Cinnarizine is considered to be unsafe in patients with porphyria because it has been shown to be porphyrinogenic in animals.

Tinnitus. The Spanish System of Pharmacovigilance had received reports[1] of tinnitus associated with calcium-channel blockers; some of the reports, including the one relating to cinnarizine, were in patients also receiving other ototoxic drugs. WHO was said to have additional reports of tinnitus associated with calcium-channel blockers including cinnarizine.

1. Narváez M, et al. Tinnitus with calcium-channel blockers. Lancet 1994; **343:** 1229–30.

Weight gain. There has been a report[1] of weight gain in four patients who had taken cinnarizine for one to two years; in all cases the weight gain was associated with increased appetite.

1. Navarro-Badenes J, et al. Weight-gain associated with cinnarizine. Ann Pharmacother 1992; **26:** 928–30.

Interactions

As for the sedating antihistamines in general, p.406.

Pharmacokinetics

Cinnarizine is absorbed from the gastrointestinal tract, peak plasma concentrations occurring 2 to 4 hours after oral administration. It undergoes metabolism and has a half-life of 3 to 6 hours. Cinnarizine is excreted in the faeces mainly as unchanged drug, and in the urine predominantly as metabolites.

Uses and Administration

Cinnarizine is a piperazine derivative with antihistamine, sedative, and calcium-channel blocking activity. It is used for the symptomatic treatment of nausea and vertigo caused by Ménière's disease and other vestibular disorders (p.408) and for the prevention and treatment of motion sickness (p.407). It is also used in the management of various peripheral and cerebral vascular disorders.

The symbol † denotes a preparation no longer actively marketed

---

In the UK, the usual dose for vertigo and vestibular disorders is 30 mg three times daily by mouth. For motion sickness a dose of 30 mg is taken 2 hours before the start of the journey and 15 mg every 8 hours during the journey if necessary. Children aged 5 to 12 years are given half the adult dose for both indications. In European countries other than the UK, a dose of 75 mg once or twice daily has been given for vertigo and vestibular disorders. Doses of 75 mg may also be given 1 to 3 times daily for cerebrovascular disorders and 2 or 3 times daily for peripheral vascular disorders.

◊ References.

1. Shupak A, et al. Cinnarizine in the prophylaxis of seasickness: laboratory vestibular evaluation and sea study. Clin Pharmacol Ther 1994; **55:** 670–80.

Preparations

Proprietary Preparations (details are given in Part 3)
Aust.: Cinnabene; Pericephal; Stutgeron; **Belg.:** Stugeron; **Braz.:** Antigeron; Cinageron; Cronogeron; Stugeron; Vessel; **Denm.:** Sepan; **Ger.:** Cinnacet; Stutgeron†; **Hong Kong:** Celenid; Corathiem; Stugeron; **Irl.:** Stugeron; **Israel:** Stunarone; **Ital.:** Cinazyn; Stugeron; Toliman; **Mex.:** Cisaken; Stugeron; **Neth.:** Cinnipirine; **Port.:** Cinon; Stugeron; **S.Afr.:** Antimet; Purazine†; Stugeron; **Singapore:** Celenid; Cinnar; Cinnaron; Stugeron; Urizine; **Spain:** Pervasum; Stugeron; **Swed.:** Glanil†; **Switz.:** Cerepar; Cinnageron; Stugeron; **Thai.:** Celenid; Cenai; Cerebroad; Ceremin; Cinerine; Cinnar; Cinnaza; Cinrizine; CN-25; Linazine; Med-Circuron; Medozine; Siarizine; Silicin; Sorebral; Stugeron; Urizine; Vernarin; **UK:** Cinaziere; Stugeron.

Multi-ingredient: **Aust.:** Cinnarplus; **Belg.:** Rinomar; Touristil; **Braz.:** Exit; Sureptil; **Fin.:** Rinomar; **Fr.:** Sureptil; **Ger.:** Arlevert; **Neth.:** Primatour; **Norw.:** Rinomar†; **Spain:** Clinadil; Clinadil Compositum; Diclamina; Ederal; Neorgine†; Ornade†; **Swed.:** Rinomar.

Clemastine Fumarate   (6119-p)

Clemastine Fumarate (BANM, USAN, rINNM).

Clemastini Fumaras; HS-592 (clemastine); Meclastine Fumarate; Mecloprodine Fumarate. (+)-(2R)-2-{2-[(R)-4-Chloro-α-methylbenzhydryloxy]ethyl}-1-methylpyrrolidine hydrogen fumarate.

$C_{21}H_{26}ClNO,C_4H_4O_4 = 460.0$.
CAS — 15686-51-8 (clemastine); 14976-57-9 (clemastine fumarate).
Pharmacopoeias. In Eur. (see p.vi), Jpn, Pol., and US.

Clemastine fumarate 1.34 mg is approximately equivalent to 1 mg of clemastine base.

Pharmacopoeial description

Ph. Eur.: A white or almost white, crystalline powder. Very slightly soluble in water; sparingly soluble in alcohol (70%); slightly soluble in alcohol (50%) and in methyl alcohol. A 10% suspension in water has a pH of 3.2 to 4.2.

USP 25: A colourless to faintly yellow, odourless, crystalline powder. Very slightly soluble in water; very slightly soluble in chloroform; slightly soluble in methyl alcohol. pH of a 10% suspension in water is between 3.2 to 4.2. Store in airtight containers at a temperature not exceeding 25°. Protect from light.

Adverse Effects and Precautions

As for the sedating antihistamines in general, p.404.

Breast feeding. Drowsiness, irritability, and refusal to feed in a 10-week-old breast-fed baby occurred 12 hours after her mother started treatment with clemastine.[1] Clemastine was detected in the mother's breast milk. The baby recovered and was feeding normally on the day after the drug was stopped.

1. Kok THHG, et al. Drowsiness due to clemastine transmitted in breast milk. Lancet 1982; **i:** 914–15.

Porphyria. Clemastine has been associated with acute attacks of porphyria and is considered unsafe in porphyric patients.

Interactions

As for the sedating antihistamines in general, p.406.

Pharmacokinetics

Clemastine fumarate is rapidly and almost completely absorbed from the gastrointestinal tract; peak plasma concentrations are achieved in 2 to 4 hours. Unchanged drug and metabolites are excreted principally in the urine. An elimination half-life of about 21 hours has been reported. Clemastine is distributed into breast milk.

◊ References.

1. Schran HF, et al. The pharmacokinetics and bioavailability of clemastine and phenylpropanolamine in single-component and combination formulations. J Clin Pharmacol 1996; **36:** 911–22.

Uses and Administration

Clemastine fumarate, a monoethanolamine derivative, is a sedating antihistamine with antimuscarinic and moderate sedative properties. It has been reported to have a duration of action of about 10 to 12 hours. It is used for the symptomatic relief of allergic conditions including urticaria and angioedema (p.408), rhinitis (p.407) and conjunctivitis (p.406), and in pruritic skin disorders (p.407).

Doses of clemastine fumarate are expressed in terms of the equivalent amount of clemastine base. The usual dose by mouth is 1 mg twice daily. Up to 6 mg daily has been given, particularly for urticaria and angioedema. Children aged 1 to 3 years may be given 0.25 to 0.5 mg twice daily; those aged 3 to 6 years, 0.5 mg twice daily; and those aged 6 to 12 years 0.5 to 1 mg twice daily.

Clemastine fumarate may be given by intramuscular or slow intravenous injection in a total daily dose equivalent to 2 to 4 mg of clemastine for acute allergic reactions; for prophylaxis 2 mg is given by intravenous injection. The dose for children is 25 μg per kg body-weight daily in two divided doses by intramuscular injection.

Clemastine fumarate has also been used topically, although as with other antihistamines, there is a risk of sensitisation.

Preparations

BP 2001: Clemastine Oral Solution; Clemastine Tablets;
USP 25: Clemastine Fumarate Tablets.

Proprietary Preparations (details are given in Part 3)
Aust.: Tavegyl; **Braz.:** Agasten; **Canad.:** Tavist; **Denm.:** Tavegyl; **Ger.:** Tavegil; **Irl.:** Tavegil; **Ital.:** Tavegil; **Mex.:** Tavist; **Neth.:** Tavegil; **Norw.:** Tavegyl†; **Port.:** Tavegyl; Tavist; **S.Afr.:** Tavegyl; **Spain:** Tavegil; **Swed.:** Tavegyl; **Switz.:** Tavegil; **UK:** Aller-eze†; Tavegil; **USA:** Antihist-1; Contac 12 Hour Allergy; Dayhist-1; Tavist; Tavist Allergy.

Multi-ingredient: **Braz.:** Emistin; **Canad.:** Tavist-D†; **Ger.:** Corto-Tavegil; **Mex.:** Tavist-D; **Spain:** Dexa Tavegil; **UK:** Aller-eze Plus†; **USA:** Antihist-D†; Tavist-D†.

Clemizole Hydrochloride   (6120-n)

Clemizole Hydrochloride (BANM, rINNM).

AL-20. 1-(4-Chlorobenzyl)-2-(pyrrolidin-1-ylmethyl)benzimidazole hydrochloride.

$C_{19}H_{20}ClN_3,HCl = 362.3$.
CAS — 442-52-4 (clemizole); 1163-36-6 (clemizole hydrochloride).

Profile

Clemizole hydrochloride is a sedating antihistamine (p.404). It has been used for the symptomatic relief of allergic conditions, in pruritic skin disorders, and in combination preparations for the treatment of symptoms of the common cold. Clemizole has also been applied topically as the hexachlorophene, the sodium sulfate, and the undecylate derivatives in topical and rectal preparations combined with corticosteroids and local anaesthetics, although as with other antihistamines, there is a risk of sensitisation.

See p.188 for the use of clemizole penicillin.

Preparations

Proprietary Preparations (details are given in Part 3)

Multi-ingredient: **Aust.:** Apracur; Ultraproct; **Austral.:** Scheriproct; Ultraproct; **Belg.:** Scheriproct; **Braz.:** Ultraproct; **Fin.:** Scheriproct; **Hong Kong:** Ultraproct; **Thai.:** Scheriproct.

Clocinizine Hydrochloride   (12583-c)

Clocinizine Hydrochloride (rINNM).

Chlorcinnazine Dihydrochloride. 1-(4-Chlorobenzhydryl)-4-cinnamylpiperazine dihydrochloride.

$C_{26}H_{27}ClN_2,2HCl = 475.9$.
CAS — 298-55-5 (clocinizine).

Profile

Clocinizine hydrochloride, a piperazine derivative, is an antihistamine (p.404) given by mouth in combination preparations for the symptomatic treatment of upper respiratory-tract disorders, often with a decongestant.

Preparations

Proprietary Preparations (details are given in Part 3)

Multi-ingredient: **Belg.:** Denoral; **Fr.:** Denoral; **Hong Kong:** Denoral; **Ital.:** Denoral; **Spain:** Senioral.

Cyclizine (6121-h)

Cyclizine (BAN, rINN).
1-Benzhydryl-4-methylpiperazine.
$C_{18}H_{22}N_2 = 266.4$.
CAS — 82-92-8.
ATC — R06AE03.
Pharmacopoeias. In Br.

Pharmacopoeial description

BP 2001: A white or creamy white, crystalline powder. Practically insoluble in water. It dissolves in most organic solvents and in dilute acids. M.p. about 107°. A saturated solution in water has a pH of 7.6 to 8.6.

Cyclizine Hydrochloride (6122-m)

Cyclizine Hydrochloride (BANM, rINNM).
Cyclizini Hydrochloridum.
$C_{18}H_{22}N_2,HCl = 302.8$.
CAS — 303-25-3.
Pharmacopoeias. In Eur. (see p.vi) and US.

Pharmacopoeial description

Ph. Eur.: A white, crystalline powder. Slightly soluble in water and in alcohol; practically insoluble in ether. A 2% solution in alcohol 2 vol. and water 3 vol. has a pH of 4.5 to 5.5. Protect from light.

USP 25: A white, odourless, crystalline powder or small colourless crystals. Soluble 1 in 115 of water and of alcohol and 1 in 75 of chloroform; insoluble in ether. pH of a 2% solution in alcohol 2 vol. and water 3 vol. is between 4.5 and 5.5. Store in airtight containers. Protect from light.

Cyclizine Lactate (6123-b)

Cyclizine Lactate (BANM, rINNM).
$C_{18}H_{22}N_2,C_3H_6O_3 = 356.5$.
CAS — 5897-19-8.
Pharmacopoeias. Br. includes an injection of cyclizine lactate.

Cyclizine lactate is reported to be incompatible with oxytetracycline hydrochloride, chlortetracycline hydrochloride, benzylpenicillin, and solutions with a pH of 6.8 or more.

Cyclizine Tartrate (10006-y)

Cyclizine Tartrate (BANM, rINNM).
$C_{18}H_{22}N_2,C_4H_6O_6 = 416.5$.

Adverse Effects and Precautions

As for the sedating antihistamines in general, p.404. Cyclizine may aggravate severe heart failure. Hypotension may occur on injection.

Abuse. Cyclizine tablets have been abused either alone or in conjunction with opioids for their euphoric effects.[1-5] They have been taken by mouth or used to make injections. It has been suggested that cyclizine dependence may occur when it is used with opioids in the treatment of chronic pain.[6]

1. Gott PH. Cyclizine toxicity—intentional drug abuse of a proprietary antihistamine. *N Engl J Med* 1968; **279:** 596.
2. Kahn A, Harvey GJ. Increasing misuse of cyclizine. *Pharm J* 1985; **235:** 706.
3. Atkinson MK. Misuse of cyclizine. *Pharm J* 1985; **235:** 773.
4. Halpin D. Misuse of cyclizine. *Pharm J* 1985; **235:** 773.
5. Council of the Pharmaceutical Society of Great Britain. Sales of preparations containing cyclizine. *Pharm J* 1985; **235:** 797.
6. Hughes AM, Coote J. Cyclizine dependence. *Pharm J* 1986; **236:** 130.

Effects on the blood. Agranulocytosis occurred in a patient after six weeks of treatment with cyclizine 50 mg three times daily.[1] The blood count returned to normal once cyclizine was withdrawn.

1. Collier PM. Agranulocytosis associated with oral cyclizine. *BMJ* 1986; **292:** 174.

Effects on the heart. In a study[1] of 11 patients with severe heart failure, cyclizine produced detrimental haemodynamic effects including increased systemic and pulmonary artery pressures and ventricular filling pressures, and negated the vasodilator effects of diamorphine. It was suggested that the use of cyclizine should be avoided in patients with acute myocardial infarction or severe heart failure.

1. Tan LB, et al. Detrimental haemodynamic effects of cyclizine in heart failure. *Lancet* 1988; **i:** 560–1.

Effects on the liver. An 8-year-old girl developed jaundice on 2 occasions after taking cyclizine hydrochloride 25 mg daily by mouth. 'Hypersensitivity hepatitis' was considered responsible.[1]

1. Kew MC, et al. "Hypersensitivity hepatitis" associated with administration of cyclizine. *BMJ* 1973; **2:** 307.

Pregnancy. For discussion of the use of antihistamines in pregnancy, including studies involving cyclizine, see p.405.

Interactions

As for the sedating antihistamines in general, p.406. Cyclizine may counteract the haemodynamic benefits of opioids (see Effects on the Heart, above) and this should be considered before using preparations that contain a combination of cyclizine and an opioid analgesic.

General anaesthetics. For a possible interaction between cyclizine premedication and *barbiturate anaesthetics* see under Thiopental, p.1269.

Pharmacokinetics

Cyclizine is absorbed from the gastrointestinal tract and has an onset of action within two hours. The duration of action is reported to be approximately 4 hours. Cyclizine is metabolised in the liver to the relatively inactive metabolite, norcyclizine. Both cyclizine and norcyclizine have plasma elimination half-lives of 20 hours. Less than 1% of the total oral dose is eliminated in the urine in 24 hours.

Uses and Administration

Cyclizine, a piperazine derivative, is a sedating antihistamine with antimuscarinic activity, although the sedative effects are not marked.

It is used as an antiemetic in the management of nausea and vomiting (p.407) including motion sickness, postoperative nausea and vomiting, after radiotherapy, and in drug-induced nausea and vomiting. It is included as an antiemetic with some opioids, and in combination preparations for the treatment of migraine attacks (p.449). Cyclizine is also used for the symptomatic treatment of vertigo (p.408) caused by Ménière's disease and other vestibular disturbances.

In the management of nausea and vomiting, cyclizine hydrochloride is given by mouth in a usual dose of 50 mg up to three times daily, although up to 200 mg may be given in 24 hours if necessary. For the prevention of motion sickness, the first dose should be given about 30 minutes before travelling. Children aged 6 to 12 years may be given 25 mg up to three times daily.

Cyclizine is given intramuscularly or intravenously as the lactate. Doses of cyclizine lactate are similar to those of cyclizine hydrochloride given by mouth. For the prevention of postoperative nausea and vomiting the first dose of cyclizine lactate should be given about 20 minutes before the anticipated end of surgery.

Cyclizine salts are used as antiemetics in combination with morphine or dipipanone; the use of such fixed-combination opioid preparations is considered to be unsuitable for the prolonged treatment that may be required in palliative care. See also under Interactions, above.

Preparations

BP 2001: Cyclizine Injection; Cyclizine Tablets; Dipipanone and Cyclizine Tablets;
USP 25: Cyclizine Hydrochloride Tablets.

Proprietary Preparations (details are given in Part 3)
Aust.: Echnatol; Fortravel; Marzine†; **Canad.:** Marzine†; **Denm.:** Marzine; **Fin.:** Marzine; **Hong Kong:** Marzine; Valoid; **Irl.:** Valoid; **Norw.:** Marzine; **NZ:** Marzine; Valoid; **S.Afr.:** Aculoid†; Covamet; Emitex; Medazine; Nauzine; Norizine; Ryccard; Triazine; Valoid; **Singapore:** Marzine; **Swed.:** Marzine; **Switz.:** Marzine; **UK:** Valoid; **USA:** Marezine.

Multi-ingredient: Aust.: Echnatol B₆; Migril; **Austral.:** Migral; **Canad.:** Megral; **Fin.:** Vertipam; **Fr.:** Migwell; **Hong Kong:** Migril; Wellconal; **Irl.:** Cyclimorph; Diconal; Migril; Migril†; **Neth.:** Migril; **NZ:** Migril; **S.Afr.:** Cyclimorph; Migril; Wellconal; **Singapore:** Migril; **Spain:** Igril; **Switz.:** Migril; **UK:** Cyclimorph; Diconal; Migril.

Cyproheptadine Hydrochloride

(6124-v)

Cyproheptadine Hydrochloride (BANM, rINNM).
Cyproheptadini Hydrochloridum. 4-(5H-Dibenzo[a,d]cyclohepten-5-ylidene)-1-methylpiperidine hydrochloride sesquihydrate.
$C_{21}H_{21}N,HCl,1½H_2O = 350.9$.
CAS — 129-03-3 (cyproheptadine); 969-33-5 (anhydrous cyproheptadine hydrochloride); 41354-29-4 (cyproheptadine hydrochloride sesquihydrate).
Pharmacopoeias. In Chin., Eur. (see p.vi), Jpn, and US.

Anhydrous cyproheptadine hydrochloride 10 mg is approximately equivalent to 11 mg of cyproheptadine hydrochloride sesquihydrate.

Pharmacopoeial description

Ph. Eur.: A white or slightly yellow, crystalline powder. Slightly soluble in water; sparingly soluble in alcohol; freely soluble in methyl alcohol; practically insoluble in ether. Protect from light.

USP 25: A white to slightly yellow, odourless or practically odourless, crystalline powder. Soluble 1 in 275 of water, 1 in 35 of alcohol, 1 in 26 of chloroform, and 1 in 1.5 of methyl alcohol; practically insoluble in ether.

Adverse Effects and Precautions

As for the sedating antihistamines in general, p.404. Increased appetite and weight gain may occur with cyproheptadine.

Abuse. A report[1] of dependence developing in a patient who had taken approximately 180 mg of cyproheptadine daily by mouth for 5 years.

1. Craven JL, Rodin GM. Cyproheptadine dependence associated with an atypical somatoform disorder. *Can J Psychiatry* 1987; **32:** 143–5.

Effects on the nervous system. Antimuscarinic toxicity manifest by hallucinations and agitation developed in a 9-year-old child taking cyproheptadine 4 mg twice daily for migraine prophylaxis.[1]

1. Watemberg NM, et al. Central anticholinergic syndrome on therapeutic doses of cyproheptadine. *Pediatrics* 1999; **103:** 158–60.

Interference with diagnostic tests. Cyproheptadine reduced hypoglycaemia-induced growth hormone secretion by between 5 and 97% in 8 healthy subjects.[1] It was suggested that if patients receiving cyproheptadine were given a pituitary function test which used growth hormone response to insulin-induced hypoglycaemia, then cyproheptadine therapy should be stopped before the test.

1. Bivens CH, et al. Inhibition of hypoglycaemia-induced growth hormone secretion by the serotonin antagonists cyproheptadine and methysergide. *N Engl J Med* 1973; **289:** 236–9.

Interactions

As for the sedating antihistamines in general, p.406.

Antidepressants. For reports suggesting that cyproheptadine can reduce the effectiveness of *SSRIs*, see under Fluoxetine, p.287.

Pharmacokinetics

After absorption from the gastrointestinal tract, cyproheptadine hydrochloride undergoes almost complete metabolism. Metabolites are excreted principally in the urine as conjugates, and also in the faeces.

Uses and Administration

Cyproheptadine, a piperidine derivative, is a sedating antihistamine with antimuscarinic, serotonin-antagonist, and calcium-channel blocking actions. It is used as the hydrochloride for the symptomatic relief of allergic conditions including urticaria and angioedema (p.408), rhinitis (p.407) and conjunctivitis (p.406), and in pruritic skin disorders (p.407). Other uses include the management of migraine (p.407).

For allergic conditions and pruritus the dose in adults, expressed as anhydrous cyproheptadine hydrochloride, is initially 4 mg three times daily by mouth, adjusted as necessary. The average dose requirement is 12 to 16 mg per day in three or four divided doses, but daily doses of up to 32 mg may occasionally be necessary. The dose for children aged 2 to 6 years is 2 mg two or three times daily increasing to a maximum of 12 mg per day and for children aged 7 to 14 years, 4 mg two or three times daily up to a maximum of 16 mg per day. Cyproheptadine is not recommended in debilitated elderly patients.

A dose of 4 mg is used for both prophylaxis and treatment of migraine and other vascular headaches and may be repeated after 30 minutes; patients who respond usually obtain relief with 8 mg, and this dose should not be exceeded within a 4- to 6-hour period. A maintenance dose of 4 mg may be given every 4 to 6 hours.

Other cyproheptadine salts that have been given by mouth include the acetylaspartate, aspartate, cyclamate, orotate, acephyllinate (7-theophyllineacetate), and the pyridoxal phosphate salt (dihexazine).

Abdominal migraine. Cyproheptadine has been tried in the treatment of children with abdominal migraine (see Pizotifen, p.455).

Angina pectoris. Cyproheptadine was used successfully to treat 2 patients with Prinzmetal's angina (p.791) refractory to standard treatment with calcium-channel blockers and nitrates.[1] Serotonin is an important endocrine mediator of coronary vasospasm and the beneficial effects of cyproheptadine were attributed to its activity as a serotonin antagonist.

1. Schecter AD, et al. Refractory Prinzmetal angina treated with cyproheptadine. Ann Intern Med 1994; 121: 113–14.

Appetite disorders. Cyproheptadine has been widely used as an appetite stimulant, including for anorexia nervosa and cachexia (p.1481), but in the long-term appears to have little value in producing weight gain and such use is no longer generally recommended. There has been concern that cyproheptadine was being promoted and used inappropriately as an appetite stimulant in some developing countries.[1]

1. Anonymous. Cyproheptadine: no longer promoted as an appetite stimulant. WHO Drug Inf 1994; 8: 66.

Carcinoid syndrome. The management of carcinoid tumours (p.483) is largely symptomatic. Cyproheptadine hydrochloride, a serotonin antagonist, has had limited success in relieving symptoms such as diarrhoea but somatostatin analogues may now be preferred.[1] It has been used successfully with fenclonine, aprotinin, methylprednisolone, and antibacterials to prevent complications arising from release of tumour metabolites during hepatic embolisation, a procedure sometimes used to relieve the symptoms of carcinoid syndrome.[2] There have been a few reports of tumour regression, in addition to symptomatic control, after treatment of carcinoid tumours with cyproheptadine.[3,4]

1. Caplin ME, et al. Carcinoid tumour. Lancet 1998; 352: 799–805.
2. Maton PN, et al. Role of hepatic arterial embolisation in the carcinoid syndrome. BMJ 1983; 287: 932–5. Correction to dosage. ibid.; 1664.
3. Harris AL, Smith IE. Regression of carcinoid tumour with cyproheptadine. BMJ 1982; 285: 475.
4. Leitner SP, et al. Partial remission of carcinoid tumor in response to cyproheptadine. Ann Intern Med 1989; 111: 760–1.

Serotonin syndrome. Cyproheptadine has been successfully used to treat the serotonin syndrome (p.304) in patients who have developed the syndrome following overdoses involving serotonergic drugs or who have had their antidepressant therapy changed without an adequate wash-out period.[1,2]

1. Lappin RI, Auchincloss EL. Treatment of the serotonin syndrome with cyproheptadine. N Engl J Med 1994; 331: 1021–2.
2. McDaniel WW. Serotonin syndrome: early management with cyproheptadine. Ann Pharmacother 2001; 35: 870–3.

Sexual dysfunction. Cyproheptadine has been tried in the management of sexual dysfunction induced by SSRIs (see Effects on Sexual Function under Fluoxetine, p.285) but may possibly reduce the effectiveness of the SSRI.

Preparations

BP 2001: Cyproheptadine Tablets;
USP 25: Cyproheptadine Hydrochloride Syrup; Cyproheptadine Hydrochloride Tablets.

Proprietary Preparations (details are given in Part 3)
Aust.: Periactin; **Austral.:** Periactin; **Belg.:** Periactin; **Braz.:** Periatin; **Canad.:** Periactin; **Denm.:** Periactin; **Fr.:** Periactine; **Ger.:** Peritol; **Hong Kong:** Cyprogin; Periactin; **Irl.:** Periactin; **Ital.:** Periactin; **Mex.:** Viternum; **Neth.:** Periactin; **NZ:** Periactin; **Port.:** Periactin; Supersan; Trimetabol; Viternum; **S.Afr.:** Periactin; **Spain:** Klarivitina; Periactin; Viternum; **Swed.:** Periactin; **Switz.:** Periactin; Cyheptine; Cyprogin; Cyprosian; Periactin; Polytab; **UK:** Periactin; **USA:** Periactin.

Multi-ingredient: **Braz.:** Apevitin BC; Ativit; Cobactin; Cobaglobal; Cobavital; Periatin BC; Periavita; Trimetabol; **Hong Kong:** Lybovit; Petina Compound; Tres Orix Forte; **Ital.:** Carpantin; **Mex.:** Ciprolisina; **Spain:** Actilevol Orex†; Anti Anorex Triple; Childrevit; Covitasa B12; Desarrol; Enoton; Glotone; Medenorex; Pantobamin; Pranzo; Stolina; Tonico Juventus; Tres Orix Forte; Trimetabol; Troforex Pepsico; Vita Menal.

Deptropine Citrate   (6125-g)

Deptropine Citrate (BANM, rINNM).

Deptropini Citras; Dibenzheptropine Citrate. (1R,3r,5S)-3-(10,11-Dihydro-5H-dibenzo[a,d]cyclohepten-5-yloxy)tropane dihydrogen citrate.
$C_{23}H_{27}NO,C_6H_8O_7 = 525.6$.
CAS — 604-51-3 (deptropine); 2169-75-7 (deptropine citrate).
Pharmacopoeias. In Eur. (see p.vi).

Pharmacopoeial description

Ph. Eur.: A white or almost white, microcrystalline powder. Very slightly soluble in water and in dehydrated alcohol; practically insoluble in dichloromethane and in ether. A saturated solution in water has a pH of 3.7 to 4.5. Protect from light.

Profile

Deptropine citrate is a sedating antihistamine (p.404) with a marked antimuscarinic action. It was given by mouth mainly in the treatment of respiratory-tract disorders.

Preparations

Proprietary Preparations (details are given in Part 3)
Ital.: Brontin†.

Desloratadine   (20021-v)

Desloratadine (BAN, USAN, rINN).
Sch-34117. 8-Chloro-6,11-dihydro-11-(4-piperidylidene)-5H-benzo[5,6]cyclohepta[1,2-b]pyridine.
$C_{19}H_{19}ClN_2 = 310.8$.
CAS — 100643-71-8.

Profile

Desloratadine, the major, active metabolite of loratadine (p.420), is a non-sedating antihistamine. Desloratadine is used in the symptomatic relief of allergic conditions including rhinitis (p.407) and urticaria (p.408).

In the management of seasonal allergic rhinitis, desloratadine is given by mouth in a dose of 5 mg once daily. Similar doses are recommended for chronic idiopathic urticaria.

◊ References.
1. McClellan K, Jarvis B. Desloratadine. Drugs 2001; 61: 789–96.

Preparations

Proprietary Preparations (details are given in Part 3)
UK: Neoclarityn.

Dimenhydrinate   (6128-s)

Dimenhydrinate (BAN, rINN).
Chloranautine; Dimenhydrinatum; Diphenhydramine Teoclate; Diphenhydramine Theoclate. The diphenhydramine salt of 8-chlorotheophylline .
$C_{17}H_{21}NO,C_7H_7ClN_4O_2 = 470.0$.
CAS — 523-87-5.
Pharmacopoeias. In Chin., Eur. (see p.vi), Jpn, Pol., and US.

Dimenhydrinate has been reported to be incompatible in solution with a wide range of compounds; those most likely to be encountered with dimenhydrinate include: aminophylline, glycopyrronium bromide, hydrocortisone sodium succinate, hydroxyzine hydrochloride, meglumine adipiodone, some phenothiazines, and some soluble barbiturates.

Pharmacopoeial description

Ph. Eur.: A white, crystalline powder or colourless crystals. M.p. 102° to 106°. Slightly soluble in water; freely soluble in alcohol; sparingly soluble in ether. A saturated solution in water has a pH of 7.1 to 7.6.
USP 25: A white, odourless, crystalline powder. Slightly soluble in water; freely soluble in alcohol and in chloroform; sparingly soluble in ether.

Adverse Effects and Precautions

As for the sedating antihistamines in general, p.404.

Effects on the eyes. Dimenhydrinate 100 mg, given at 4-hourly intervals for 3 doses, was found to affect colour discrimination, night vision, reaction time, and stereopsis.[1]

1. Luria SM, et al. Effects of aspirin and dimenhydrinate (Dramamine) on visual processes. Br J Clin Pharmacol 1979; 7: 585–93.

Porphyria. Dimenhydrinate has been associated with acute attacks of porphyria and is considered unsafe in porphyric patients.

Pregnancy. For discussion of the use of antihistamines in pregnancy, including a suggestion of a relationship between cardiovascular defects or inguinal hernia and dimenhydrinate exposure, see p.405.

Interactions

As for the sedating antihistamines in general, p.406.

Uses and Administration

Dimenhydrinate, a monoethanolamine derivative, is a sedating antihistamine with antimuscarinic and significant sedative effects. It is used mainly as an antiemetic in the prevention and treatment of motion sickness (p.407). It is also used for the symptomatic treatment of nausea and vertigo caused by Ménière's disease and other vestibular disturbances (p.408).

The usual dose of dimenhydrinate by mouth is 50 to 100 mg, given 3 or 4 times daily. For the prevention of motion sickness, the first dose should be given at least 30 minutes before travelling. Typical doses for children are: 2 to up to 6 years, 12.5 to 25 mg every 6 to 8 hours to a maximum of 75 mg daily (in some countries lower doses of 6.25 to 12.5 mg are given two or three times daily); 6 to 12 years, 25 to 50 mg every 6 to 8 hours (again lower doses are used in some countries).

Dimenhydrinate may be given parenterally in usual doses of 50 mg, a concentration of 5% being used for intramuscular injection and 0.5% for slow intravenous injection (usually over 2 minutes). Children

have been given dimenhydrinate by intramuscular or slow intravenous injection in a dose of 1.25 mg per kg body-weight four times daily to a maximum of 300 mg daily.

Dimenhydrinate has also been administered by the rectal route.

Preparations

BP 2001: Dimenhydrinate Tablets;
USP 25: Dimenhydrinate Injection; Dimenhydrinate Syrup; Dimenhydrinate Tablets.

Proprietary Preparations (details are given in Part 3)
Aust.: Emedyl; Nausex; Travel-Gum; Vertirosan; **Austral.:** Andrumin†; Dramamine; **Belg.:** Dramamine†; Vagomine; **Braz.:** Dramin; **Canad.:** Anti-Nauseant; Childrens Motion Sickness Liquid; Gravol; Nauseatol; Nausex†; Novo-Dimenate; Travamine; Travel Aid; Travel Tabs; Travelmate†; Traveltabs; **Fr.:** Dramamine; Nausicalm; **Ger.:** Dimen; Logomed Reise-Tabletten†; Mandros Reise†; Monotrean†; Reisegold; Reisetabletten-ratiopharm; RubieMen; Superpep; Vertigo-Vomex; Vomacur; Vomex A; **Hong Kong:** Dimenate; Dramamine; Gravol; Travelgum; **Irl.:** Dramamine; **Israel:** Dramamine; Travamin; **Ital.:** Lomarin; Motozina; Travelgum; Valontan; Xamamina; **Mex.:** Dimetin-F; Dimicaps; Dramamine; Unitril; Vomisin; **Neth.:** Dramamine; **NZ:** Dramamine; **Port.:** Dramamine; Enjomin; Travel-Gum†; Viabom; Vomidrine; **S.Afr.:** Dramamine†; **Singapore:** Dramamine; Novomin; **Spain:** Biodramina; Cinfamar; Contramareo; Travel Well; **Swed.:** Amosyt; **Switz.:** Antemin; Demodenal†; Dramamine; Reise Superpep-K†; Superpep; Trawell; **Thai.:** Denim; Dimeno; Dramamine; Gravol; Motivan; Navamed; Navamine; Vominar; **UAE:** Diznil; **UK:** Dramamine†; **USA:** Calm-X; Dimetabs; Dinate; DMH†; Dramamine; Dramanate; Dramilin†; Dymenate; Hydrate; Marmine†; Tega-Vert†; Triptone; Vertab†.

Multi-ingredient: **Aust.:** Neo-Emedyl; Synkapton; Vertirosan Vitamin B_6; **Austral.:** Travacalm; **Belg.:** R Calm + B6†; **Braz.:** Dramin B-6; Dramin B-6 DL; **Canad.:** Gravergol; **Fr.:** Mercalm; **Ger.:** Arlevert; Migraeflux N; Migraeflux orange N; **Hong Kong:** Gravergol; Rhinocap; **Spain:** Acetuber; Biodramina Cafeina; Cinfamar Cafeina; Saldeva; Salvarina; Sin Mareo x 4; **Switz.:** Agorhino; Antemin compositum; Demodenal compositum; Dragees contre les maux de voyage no 537; Dramamine-compositum; Medramine retard†; Medramine-B6 Rectocaps†; Rhinocap; Viaggio†.

Dimetindene Maleate   (6129-w)

Dimetindene Maleate (BANM, rINNM).
Dimethindene Maleate (USAN); Dimethpyrindene Maleate; Dimethylpyrindene Maleate; Dimetindeni Maleas; NSC-107677; Su-6518. NN-Dimethyl-2-{3-[1-(2-pyridyl)ethyl]-1H-inden-2-yl}ethylamine hydrogen maleate.
$C_{20}H_{24}N_2,C_4H_4O_4 = 408.5$.
CAS — 5636-83-9 (dimetindene); 3614-69-5 (dimetindene maleate).
Pharmacopoeias. In Eur. (see p.vi).

Pharmacopoeial description

Ph. Eur.: A white to almost white, crystalline powder. Slightly soluble in water; soluble in methyl alcohol. Protect from light.

Profile

Dimetindene maleate, an alkylamine derivative, is a sedating antihistamine (p.404); it is mildly sedative and is reported to have mast-cell stabilising properties. It is used for the symptomatic relief of allergic conditions including urticaria and angio-edema (p.408) and rhinitis (p.407), and in pruritic skin disorders (p.407). It is also used in compound preparations for the symptomatic treatment of coughs and the common cold (p.406).

Dimetindene maleate is given by mouth in a dose of 1 to 2 mg three times daily; modified-release preparations are also available. It may also be given by the intravenous route. Dimetindene maleate is applied topically as a 0.1% gel although, as with other antihistamines, there is a risk of sensitisation. It is used in a strength of 0.025% in compound nasal preparations.

Preparations

Proprietary Preparations (details are given in Part 3)
Aust.: Fenistil; **Belg.:** Fenistil; **Ger.:** Fenistil; **Israel:** Fenistil; **Ital.:** Fenistil; **Neth.:** Fenistil; **Norw.:** Fenistil; **Port.:** Fenistil; Neostil; **Spain:** Fenistil; **Switz.:** Fenistil; **Thai.:** Fenistil.

Multi-ingredient: **Aust.:** Trimedil; Vibrocil; **Belg.:** Vibrocil; **Braz.:** Gripen; Trimedal; **Ger.:** Vibrocil; **Hong Kong:** Vibrocil; **Israel:** Vibrocil NF; **Ital.:** Vibrocil; **Port.:** Vibrocil; **S.Afr.:** Vibrocil; Vibrocil-S; **Switz.:** Vibrocil.

Dimetotiazine Mesilate   (6130-m)

Dimetotiazine Mesilate (BANM, rINNM).
Dimethothiazine Mesylate; Fonazine Mesylate (USAN); IL-6302 (dimetotiazine); 8599-RP (dimetotiazine). 10-(2-Dimethylaminopropyl)-NN-dimethylphenothiazine-2-sulphonamide methanesulphonate.
$C_{19}H_{25}N_3O_2S_2,CH_3SO_3H = 487.7$.
CAS — 7456-24-8 (dimetotiazine); 7455-39-2 (dimetotiazine mesilate).

Profile

Dimetotiazine mesilate, a phenothiazine derivative, is a sedating antihistamine (p.404). It has been used for the symptomatic relief of hypersensitivity reactions, in pruritic skin disorders, and in the management of headaches including migraine.

Preparations

Proprietary Preparations (details are given in Part 3)
Mex.: Migristene; *Spain:* Migristene†.

Diphenhydramine (10007-j)

Diphenhydramine (BAN, rINN).
Benzhydramine. 2-Benzhydryloxy-NN-dimethylethylamine.
$C_{17}H_{21}NO = 255.4$.
CAS — 58-73-1.
ATC — D04AA32; R06AA02.
Pharmacopoeias. In Jpn.

Diphenhydramine Citrate (18347-g)

Diphenhydramine Citrate (BANM, rINNM).
Benzhydramine Citrate.
$C_{17}H_{21}NO,C_6H_8O_7 = 447.5$.
CAS — 88637-37-0.
Pharmacopoeias. In US.

Diphenhydramine citrate 15.3 mg is approximately equivalent to diphenhydramine hydrochloride 10 mg.

Pharmacopoeial description
USP 25: Store in airtight containers. Protect from light.

Diphenhydramine Di(acefyllinate) (12669-f)

Benzhydramine Di(acefyllinate); Bietanautine; Diphenhydramine Di(acephyllinate). Diphenhydramine bis(theophyllin-7-ylacetate).
$C_{17}H_{21}NO,2C_9H_{10}N_4O_4 = 731.8$.
CAS — 6888-11-5.

NOTE. The name Etanautine has been applied both to diphenhydramine monoacefyllinate and to ethylbenzhydramine, an antimuscarinic formerly used in the symptomatic treatment of parkinsonism.

Diphenhydramine di(acefyllinate) 25.1 mg is approximately equivalent to diphenhydramine hydrochloride 10 mg.

Diphenhydramine Hydrochloride (6131-b)

Diphenhydramine Hydrochloride (BANM, rINNM).
Benzhydramine Hydrochloride; Dimedrolum; Diphenhydramini Hydrochloridum; Diphenhydraminium Chloride.
$C_{17}H_{21}NO,HCl = 291.8$.
CAS — 147-24-0.
Pharmacopoeias. In Chin., Eur. (see p.vi), Jpn, Pol., and US. Jpn also includes Diphenhydramine Tannate.

Incompatibility has been reported with amphotericin B, cefmetazole sodium, cefalotin sodium, hydrocortisone sodium succinate, some soluble barbiturates, some contrast media, and solutions of alkalis or strong acids.

Pharmacopoeial description
Ph. Eur.: A white or almost white, crystalline powder. Very soluble in water; freely soluble in alcohol; practically insoluble in ether. A 5% solution in water has a pH of 4.0 to 6.0. Protect from light.
USP 25: A white, odourless, crystalline powder. It slowly darkens on exposure to light. Soluble 1 in 1 of water, 1 in 2 of alcohol and of chloroform, and 1 in 50 of acetone; very slightly soluble in ether and in benzene. Its solutions are neutral to litmus. Store in airtight containers. Protect from light.

Adverse Effects and Precautions

As for the sedating antihistamines in general, p.404.

Abuse. Reports of the abuse of diphenhydramine hydrochloride.
1. Anonymous. Is there any evidence that Benylin syrup is addictive? *BMJ* 1979; 1: 459.
2. Smith SG, Davis WM. Nonmedical use of butorphanol and diphenhydramine. *JAMA* 1984; 252: 1010.
3. Feldman MD, Behar M. A case of massive diphenhydramine abuse and withdrawal from use of the drug. *JAMA* 1986; 255: 3119–20.
4. de Nesnera AP. Diphenhydramine dependence: a need for awareness. *J Clin Psychiatry* 1996; 57: 136–7.
5. Dinndorf PA, et al. Risk of abuse of diphenhydramine in children and adolescents with chronic illnesses. *J Pediatr* 1998; 133: 293–5.

Extrapyramidal disorders. Reports of dystonic extrapyramidal reactions to diphenhydramine.
1. Lavenstein BL, Cantor FK. Acute dystonia: an unusual reaction to diphenhydramine. *JAMA* 1976; 236: 291.
2. Santora J, Rozek S. Diphenhydramine-induced dystonia. *Clin Pharm* 1978; 8: 471.
3. Roila F, et al. Diphenhydramine and acute dystonia. *Ann Intern Med* 1989; 111: 92–3.

Overdosage. In an evaluation of 136 cases, one fatal, of intoxication with diphenhydramine, the plasma concentration was correlated with frequency or extent of symptoms.[1] The most common symptom was impaired consciousness; psychosis, seizures, antimuscarinic symptoms such as mydriasis, tachycardia, and tachyarrhythmias, and respiratory failure were also observed. The positive association between dose and frequency and severity of symptoms was confirmed in a more recent study;[2] it was also found that severe symptoms were more likely to occur when 1 g or more of diphenhydramine had been taken.

Another report[3] described a patient with rhabdomyolysis as an effect of oral diphenhydramine overdosage. The liberal application of a lotion containing diphenhydramine produced acute delirium with visual and auditory hallucinations in a 9-year-old boy[4] and similar effects were seen in 3 children with varicella-zoster infection following the topical application of diphenhydramine (2 of these children also received oral diphenhydramine).[5]

1. Köppel C, Tenczer J. Clinical symptomatology of diphenhydramine overdose: an evaluation of 136 cases in 1982 to 1985. *Clin Toxicol* 1987; 25: 53–70.
2. Radovanovic D, et al. Dose-dependent toxicity of diphenhydramine overdose. *Hum Exp Toxicol* 2000; 19: 489–95.
3. Hampel G, et al. Myoglobinuric renal failure due to drug-induced rhabdomyolysis. *Hum Toxicol* 1983; 2: 197–203.
4. Filloux F. Toxic encephalopathy caused by topically applied diphenhydramine. *J Pediatr* 1986; 108: 1018–20.
5. Chan CYJ, Wallander KA. Diphenhydramine toxicity in three children with varicella-zoster infection. *DICP Ann Pharmacother* 1991; 25: 130–2.

Porphyria. Diphenhydramine has been associated with acute attacks of porphyria and is considered unsafe in porphyric patients.

Pregnancy. A pregnant woman who was receiving diphenhydramine hydrochloride 150 mg daily for a pruritic rash gave birth to an infant who developed diarrhoea and generalised tremulousness 5 days later.[1] The delay in appearance of withdrawal symptoms was considered to be due to absence of full activity of glucuronyl conjugating enzymes in the first few days of life.
For discussion of the use of antihistamines in pregnancy, including a suggestion of a relationship between inguinal hernia or genito-urinary malformations and diphenhydramine exposure, see p.405. See also under Interactions, below, for a report of perinatal death possibly associated with temazepam and diphenhydramine.
1. Parkin DE. Probable Benadryl withdrawal manifestations in a new-born infant. *J Pediatr* 1974; 85: 580.

Interactions

As for the sedating antihistamines in general, p.406.

Benzodiazepines. There has been a report[1] suggesting that a reduction in *temazepam* metabolism caused by diphenhydramine may have contributed to perinatal death after ingestion of these drugs by the mother.
1. Kargas GA, et al. Perinatal mortality due to interaction of diphenhydramine and temazepam. *N Engl J Med* 1985; 313: 1417–18.

Pharmacokinetics

Diphenhydramine hydrochloride is well absorbed from the gastrointestinal tract, though high first-pass metabolism appears to affect systemic availability. Peak plasma concentrations are achieved about 1 to 4 hours after administration by mouth. Diphenhydramine is widely distributed throughout the body including the CNS. It crosses the placenta and has been detected in breast milk. Diphenhydramine is highly bound to plasma proteins. Metabolism is extensive. Diphenhydramine is excreted mainly in the urine as metabolites; little is excreted as unchanged drug. The elimination half-life has been reported to range from 2.4 to 9.3 hours.

◊ References.
1. Glazko AJ, et al. Metabolic disposition of diphenhydramine. *Clin Pharmacol Ther* 1974; 16: 1066–76.
2. Paton DM, Webster DR. Clinical pharmacokinetics of H_1-receptor antagonists (the antihistamines). *Clin Pharmacokinet* 1985; 10: 477–97 (includes studies indicating a correlation between plasma concentrations and both antihistaminic and sedative effects).
3. Simons KJ, et al. Diphenhydramine: pharmacokinetics and pharmacodynamics in elderly adults, young adults, and children. *J Clin Pharmacol* 1990; 30: 665–71.
4. Scavone JM, et al. Pharmacokinetics and pharmacodynamics of diphenhydramine 25 mg in young and elderly volunteers. *J Clin Pharmacol* 1998; 38: 603–9.

Uses and Administration

Diphenhydramine, a monoethanolamine derivative, is a sedating antihistamine with antimuscarinic and pronounced sedative properties. It is used for the symptomatic relief of allergic conditions including urticaria and angioedema (p.408), rhinitis (p.407) and conjunctivitis (p.406), and in pruritic skin disorders (p.407). It is also used for its antiemetic properties in the treatment of nausea and vomiting (p.407), particularly in the prevention and treatment of motion sickness (when it should be given at least 30 minutes before travelling), and in the treatment of vertigo of various causes (p.408). Diphenhydramine is used for its antimuscarinic properties in the control of parkinsonism (p.1160) and drug-induced extrapyramidal disorders (p.662) (although the possibility that diphenhydramine itself may cause extrapyramidal symptoms should be remembered). Diphenhydramine has pronounced central sedative properties and may be used as a hypnotic in the short-term management of insomnia (p.407). It is a common ingredient of compound preparations for symptomatic treatment of coughs and the common cold (p.406). Diphenhydramine may be used parenterally as an adjunct in the emergency treatment of anaphylactic shock (p.406) or when oral therapy is not feasible.

For most indications, diphenhydramine hydrochloride is given by mouth in usual doses of 25 to 50 mg three or four times daily. The dose for children is 6.25 to 25 mg three or four times daily, or a total daily dose of 5 mg per kg body-weight may be given in divided doses. The maximum dose in adults and children is 300 mg daily. A dose of 20 to 50 mg may be used as a hypnotic in adults and children over 12 years old.

When oral therapy is not feasible, diphenhydramine hydrochloride may be given by deep intramuscular injection or by intravenous injection using concentrations of 1% or 5%. Usual doses are 10 to 50 mg, although doses of 100 mg have been given. No more than 400 mg should be given in 24 hours. Diphenhydramine hydrochloride is applied topically, usually in preparations containing 1 to 2% although, as with other antihistamines, there is a risk of sensitisation.

Diphenhydramine citrate is given by mouth in a dose of 76 mg at night in combination preparations for its hypnotic action. Diphenhydramine di(acefyllinate) is given by mouth as an antiemetic for the prevention and treatment of motion sickness and of nausea and vomiting; the usual dose is 90 to 135 mg. Other diphenhydramine salts that have been used include the polistirex, the salicylate, and the tannate administered by mouth, the methylbromide given rectally, and the metilsulfate applied topically.

Dimenhydrinate (p.415) is diphenhydramine teoclate and mefenidramium metilsulfate (p.421) is diphenhydramine methylsulfomethylate.

Preparations

BP 2001: Diphenhydramine Oral Solution;
USP 25: Acetaminophen and Diphenhydramine Citrate Tablets; Acetaminophen, Diphenhydramine Hydrochloride, and Pseudoephedrine Hydrochloride Tablets; Diphenhydramine and Pseudoephedrine Capsules; Diphenhydramine Hydrochloride Capsules; Diphenhydramine Hydrochloride Elixir; Diphenhydramine Hydrochloride Injection.

Proprietary Preparations (details are given in Part 3)
Aust.: Dermodrin; Dibondrin; Histaxin; Prurex; *Austral.:* Benadryl†; Nytol; Unisom; *Belg.:* Azaron; Benylin Antihistaminicum; Diphamine; Nuicalm†; R Calm; *Canad.:* Aller-Aide; Allerdryl; Allergy Elixir; Allergy Formula; Allergy Tablets; Allernix; Benadryl; Calmex; Dormex; Dormiphen; Insomnal; Nytol; Sleep Aid; Sleep-Eze D; Sominex; Unisom; Unisom-C†; *Fin.:* Benylan; *Fr.:* Butix; Nautamine; *Ger.:* Benadryl N; Dolestan; Dormigoa N†; Dormutil N; Emesan; Halbmond; Hevert-Dorm; Logomed Beruhigungs-Tabletten†; Logomed Juckreiz†; Lupovalin†; Medapur; nervo OPT N; Nytol; Pellisal-Gel†; Pellit Insektenstich, Pellit Sonnenallergie†; Pheramin N; ratioAllerg; S.8; Sediat; Sedopretten†; Sedovegan Novo; Vivinox Stark†; *Hong Kong:* Benadryl; *Ital.:* Allergan; Benadryl†; Nytol; *Mex.:* Difedram; Difenhistat; Sontedril; Tzoali; Ulcoid; *Neth.:* Benylin-Difenhydraminehydrochloride†; *Port.:* Benaderma; *S.Afr.:* Betasleep; Nytol; *Singapore:* Paxidorm; *Spain:* Benadryl; Dormplus; Neosayomol; Nytol; Sonodor; *Swed.:* Benylan†; Desentol; *Switz.:* Bedorma Nouvelle formulation; Benocten; Benylin Paediatric†; Comprimes somniferes "S"; Comprimes somniferes formule 533; Dobacen; Neo-Synodorm; *Thai.:* Benadryl; *UAE:* Amydramine II; *UK:* Aller-eze; Dreemon; Histergan; Medinex†; Nightcalm; Nytol; Paxidorm; Sleep Aid; Sleepeaze; Sleepia†; *USA:* 40 Winks; Aler-Dryl; AllerMax; Banophen Allergy; Belix†; Ben-Allergin†; Benadryl; Benadryl Itch; Bydramine Cough†; Compoz Night-time Sleep Aid; Dermamycin; Dihydrex†; Diphen AF; Diphen Cough; Diphenhist; Dormarex 2†; Dormin; DPH†; Dytuss; Genahist; Hydramyn†; Hyrexin; Maximum Strength Sleepinal; Maximum Strength Unisom SleepGels; Miles Nervine; MouthKote P/R; Nordryl†; Nytol; Phendry†; Scot-Tussin Allergy; Siladryl; Silphen; Sleep-Ettes D; Sleep-eze 3; Sleepwell 2-nite; Snooze Fast; Sominex; Tusstat; Twilite; Uni-Bent Cough.

Multi-ingredient: numerous preparations are listed in Part 3.

Diphenylpyraline Hydrochloride (6132-v)

Diphenylpyraline Hydrochloride (BANM, rINNM).
4-Benzhydryloxy-1-methylpiperidine hydrochloride.
$C_{19}H_{23}NO$,HCl = 317.9.
CAS — 147-20-6 (diphenylpyraline); 132-18-3 (diphenylpyraline hydrochloride).
Pharmacopoeias. In Br.

Pharmacopoeial description

BP 2001: A white or almost white, odourless or almost odourless powder. Freely soluble in water, in alcohol, and in chloroform; practically insoluble in ether.

Adverse Effects and Precautions

As for the sedating antihistamines in general, p.404.

Interactions

As for the sedating antihistamines in general, p.406.

Pharmacokinetics

◊ References.
1. Graham G, Bolt AG. Half-life of diphenylpyraline in man. J Pharmacokinet Biopharm 1974; **2:** 191–5 (ranged from 24 to 40 hours).

Uses and Administration

Diphenylpyraline hydrochloride, a piperidine derivative, is a sedating antihistamine with antimuscarinic and significant sedative properties.

It is used for the symptomatic relief of allergic conditions including rhinitis (p.407), and in pruritic skin disorders (p.407). It is also used in compound preparations for the symptomatic treatment of coughs and the common cold (p.406).

Diphenylpyraline hydrochloride has been given by mouth in a dose of up to 20 mg daily in 3 or 4 divided doses. Diphenylpyraline and diphenylpyraline hydrochloride have been applied topically although, as with other antihistamines, there is a risk of sensitisation.

Diphenylpyraline teoclate is piprinhydrinate (p.423).

Preparations

Proprietary Preparations (details are given in Part 3)
Ger.: Arbid N.

Multi-ingredient: Aust.: Arbid; Astronautal; Eucillin; Prurimix; Tropoderm; **Belg.:** Bicold; Rhinamide; Tri-Cold†; **Braz.:** Ornatrol; Pelmic; **Cynstop:** Biohisdex DM; Biohisdine DM; Creo-Rectal; Emercreme No 4; Sinugex†; Vito Bronches; **Ger.:** Perdiphen; Proctospre; Templi N; Topoderm N; **S.Afr.:** Actophlem; Eskornade; Solphyllex; Theophen Comp; **Switz.:** Arbid; Proctospre; **UK:** Eskornade.

Doxylamine Succinate (6133-g)

Doxylamine Succinate (BANM, rINNM).
Doxylamine Hydrogen Succinate; Doxylamini Hydrogenosuccinas; Doxylamine Succinate; Histadoxylamine Succinate. NN-Dimethyl-2-[α-methyl-α-(2-pyridyl)benzyloxy]ethylamine hydrogen succinate.
$C_{17}H_{22}N_2O,C_4H_6O_4$ = 388.5.
CAS — 469-21-6 (doxylamine); 562-10-7 (doxylamine succinate).
Pharmacopoeias. In Eur. (see p.vi) and US.

Pharmacopoeial description

Ph. Eur.: A white or almost white powder. Very soluble in water; freely soluble in alcohol.
USP 25: A white or creamy-white powder having a characteristic odour. Soluble 1 in 1 of water, 1 in 2 of alcohol and of chloroform, and 1 in 370 of ether; very slightly soluble in benzene. Protect from light.

Adverse Effects and Precautions

As for the sedating antihistamines in general, p.404. The controversy surrounding the use in pregnancy of combination products of doxylamine is discussed on p.405.

Overdosage. In an evaluation of 109 cases of intoxication with doxylamine,[1] no correlation was found between the amount ingested or plasma concentration and the frequency or extent of symptoms. The most common symptom was impaired consciousness. Psychotic behaviour, seizures, and antimuscarinic symptoms such as tachycardia and mydriasis were also observed. Rhabdomyolysis occurred in one patient and was accompanied by transient impairment of renal function. The same group commented[2] that rhabdomyolysis had been noted in 7 of 442 cases of doxylamine overdosage, with an associated rise in plasma creatine kinase and myoglobinuria, and suggested that doxylamine has a direct toxic effect on striated muscle.
1. Köppel C, et al. Poisoning with over-the-counter doxylamine preparations: an evaluation of 109 cases. Hum Toxicol 1987; **6:** 355–9.
2. Köppel C, et al. Rhabdomyolysis in doxylamine overdose. Lancet 1987; **i:** 442–3.

Interactions

As for the sedating antihistamines in general, p.406.

Pharmacokinetics

Following oral administration of doxylamine succinate peak plasma concentrations occur after 2 to 3 hours. An elimination half-life of about 10 hours has been reported.

The symbol † denotes a preparation no longer actively marketed

◊ References.
1. Friedman H, et al. Clearance of the antihistamine doxylamine: reduced in elderly men but not in elderly women. Clin Pharmacokinet 1989; **16:** 312–16.

Uses and Administration

Doxylamine succinate, a monoethanolamine derivative, is a sedating antihistamine with antimuscarinic and pronounced sedative effects.

Doxylamine succinate is given by mouth for the symptomatic relief of hypersensitivity reactions, in pruritic skin disorders (p.407), as a hypnotic in the short-term treatment of insomnia (p.407), and as an ingredient of compound preparations for symptomatic treatment of coughs and the common cold (p.406).

In general it is no longer used in the management of nausea and vomiting of early pregnancy (see p.405 for the controversy that has surrounded the use in pregnancy of combination products of doxylamine).

Doses of up to 25 mg of doxylamine succinate have been given every 4 to 6 hours to a maximum of 150 mg daily. The usual hypnotic dose is 25 mg at night.

Preparations

USP 25: Acetaminophen, Dextromethorphan Hydrobromide, Doxylamine Succinate, and Pseudoephedrine Hydrochloride Oral Solution; Doxylamine Succinate Syrup; Doxylamine Succinate Tablets.

Proprietary Preparations (details are given in Part 3)
Austral.: Dozile; Restavit; **Belg.:** Mereprine†; **Canad.:** Unisom-2; **Fr.:** Donormyl; Lidene; Mereprine; Noctyl; **Ger.:** Gittalun; Hewedormir forte; Hoggar N; Mereprine; Munleit; SchlafTabs; Sedaplus; **Israel:** Unisom; **NZ:** Dozile; **S.Afr.:** Restwel; Somnil; **Spain:** Donormyl; Dormidina; Duebien; Unisom; **Switz.:** Mereprine†; Sanalepsi N; **USA:** Unisom SleepTabs.

Multi-ingredient: Aust.: Wick Erkaltungs-Saft fur die Nacht; Wick Hustensaft; **Austral.:** Chemists Own Dolased; Dimetapp Cold, Cough & Flu; Fiorinal; Mersyndol; Ordov Migradol; Panadeine Plus; Panalgesic; **Belg.:** Pholco-Mereprine; **Braz.:** Bisolvon Complex; Bronco-Ped; Broncolex; EMS Expectorante; Revenil; Revenil Dospan; Revenil Expectorante; Silencium; Silomat Plus; **Canad.:** Calmydone; Dalmacol; Diclectin; Mercodol with Decapryn; Mersyndol with Codeine; Nighttime Cold & Flu; Nyquil; **Ger.:** Paedisup; Wick Medinait; **Irl.:** Syndol; **Ital.:** Vicks Medinait; **NZ:** Mersyndol; Pryndette; Nausefe; **S.Afr.:** Abflex; Acurate; Adco-Dol; Asic; Betapyn; Cepacol; Dolerax†; Forpyn; Lenapain; Nethaprin Dospan; Nethaprin Expectorant; Nomopain; Paxidal; Pynstop; Sedapain; Sedinol; Syndette; Syndol; Tensopyn†; Xerotens; **Spain:** Cariban; Medinait†; Upsadex; Vicks Medinait; **Switz.:** Vicks Medinait; **UK:** Boots Tension Headache Relief; Syndol; Vicks Medinite; **USA:** Alka-Seltzer Plus Night-Time Cold; All-Nite Cold Formula; Genite; Night Time Cold/Flu Relief; Nite Time Cold Formula; NyQuil Hot Therapy; NyQuil Nighttime Cold/Flu; Nytcold Medicine; Vicks NyQuil LiquiCaps; Vicks NyQuil Multi-Symptom Cold Flu Relief.

Ebastine (2738-m)

Ebastine (BAN, USAN, rINN).
LAS-W-090.   4'-tert-Butyl-4-[4-(diphenylmethoxy)piperidino]butyrophenone.
$C_{32}H_{39}NO_2$ = 469.7.
CAS — 90729-43-4.
ATC — R06AX22.

Profile

Ebastine, a piperidine derivative, is a non-sedating antihistamine (p.404) with a long duration of action. It does not have significant sedative or antimuscarinic actions.

Ebastine is given by mouth for the symptomatic relief of allergic conditions including rhinitis (p.407) and in pruritic skin disorders (p.407). The usual dose is 10 mg daily.

◊ References.
1. Murris-Espin M, et al. Comparison of efficacy and safety of cetirizine and ebastine in patients with perennial allergic rhinitis. Ann Allergy Asthma Immunol 1998; **80:** 399–403.
2. Luria X. Comparative clinical studies with ebastine: efficacy and tolerability. Drug Safety 1999; **21** (suppl 1): 63–7.
3. Hurst M, Spencer CM. Ebastine: an update of its use in allergic disorders. Drugs 2000; **59:** 981–1006.

Preparations

Proprietary Preparations (details are given in Part 3)
Belg.: Estivan; **Denm.:** Kestine; **Fin.:** Kestine; **Hong Kong:** Kestine; **Israel:** Kestine; **Jpn:** Ebastel; **Mex.:** Evastel; **Neth.:** Kestine; **Norw.:** Kestine; **S.Afr.:** Kestine; **Singapore:** Kestine; **Spain:** Bromselon; Ebastel; **Swed.:** Kestine.

Multi-ingredient: Spain: Rino Ebastel; Tundrax.

Embramine Hydrochloride (6134-q)

Embramine Hydrochloride (BANM, rINNM).
Embraminium Chloratum; Mebrophenhydramine Hydrochloride; Mebrophenhydraminium Chloratum. 2-(4-Bromo-α-methylbenzhydryloxy)-NN-dimethylethylamine hydrochloride.
$C_{18}H_{22}BrNO$,HCl = 384.7.
CAS — 3565-72-8 (embramine); 13977-28-1 (embramine hydrochloride).

Profile

Embramine hydrochloride, a monoethanolamine derivative, is a sedating antihistamine (p.404). Embramine hydrochloride

and embramine teoclate have been administered by mouth for their antihistamine and antiemetic properties.

Emedastine Fumarate (6475-v)

Emedastine Fumarate (BANM, rINNM).
AL-3432A; Emedastine Difumarate (USAN). 1-(2-Ethoxyethyl)-2-(hexahydro-4-methyl-1H-1,4-diazepin-1-yl)benzimidazole fumarate (1:2).
$C_{17}H_{26}N_4O,2C_4H_4O_4$ = 534.6.
CAS — 87233-61-2 (emedastine); 87233-62-3 (emedastine fumarate).
Pharmacopoeias. In US.

Pharmacopoeial description

USP 25: A white to faintly yellow crystalline powder. Soluble in water. pH of a 0.2% solution in water is between 3.0 and 4.5. Store in airtight containers. Protect from light.

Adverse Effects and Precautions

As for the antihistamines in general, p.404. Ocular corneal infiltrates, local irritation, photophobia, rhinitis, and headaches have been reported following use of emedastine eye drops. Treatment should be discontinued if corneal infiltrates develop.

Pharmacokinetics

Small amounts of emedastine are absorbed following application to the eye. It is mainly metabolised in the liver to two primary metabolites 5- and 6-hydroxyemedastine which are excreted in the urine along with a small amount of unchanged drug. The elimination half-life of topical emedastine is 10 hours.

Uses and Administration

Emedastine is an antihistamine. It is instilled twice daily as the fumarate as eye drops containing 0.05% for the symptomatic relief of allergic conjunctivitis (p.406).

Preparations

USP 25: Emedastine Ophthalmic Solution.

Proprietary Preparations (details are given in Part 3)
Aust.: Emadine; **Belg.:** Emadine; **Canad.:** Emadine; **Denm.:** Emadine; **Fin.:** Emadine; **Fr.:** Emadine; **Ger.:** Emadine; **Irl.:** Emadine; **Ital.:** Emadine; **Port.:** Emadine; **Swed.:** Emadine; **UK:** Emadine; **USA:** Emadine.

Epinastine Hydrochloride (2906-m)

Epinastine Hydrochloride (rINNM).
WAL-801-Cl.   3-Amino-9,13b-dihydro-1H-dibenz[c,f]imidazo[1,5-a]azepine hydrochloride.
$C_{16}H_{15}N_3$,HCl = 285.8.
CAS — 80012-43-7 (epinastine).

Profile

Epinastine hydrochloride is an antihistamine (p.404) reported to have no significant sedative activity. It has been given by mouth in the management of asthma, allergic rhinitis, and pruritic skin disorders.

Preparations

Proprietary Preparations (details are given in Part 3)
Jpn: Alesion†; **Mex.:** Flurinol.

Fexofenadine Hydrochloride (3887-n)

Fexofenadine Hydrochloride (BANM, USAN, rINNM).
MDL-16455A; Terfenadine Carboxylate Hydrochloride. (±)-p-{1-Hydroxy-4-[4-(hydroxydiphenylmethyl)-piperidino]butyl}-α-methylhydratropic acid hydrochloride.
$C_{32}H_{39}NO_4$,HCl = 538.1.
CAS — 138452-21-8.

Adverse Effects and Precautions

As for the non-sedating antihistamines in general, p.404.

Arrhythmias. A 67-year-old man suffered syncope after taking fexofenadine 180 mg daily for two months.[1] His ECG showed an abnormally prolonged QT interval which shortened once fexofenadine was discontinued, although the interval tended to be long even without drug therapy. Nonetheless rechallenge was positive. The manufacturers of fexofenadine have commented[2] that the patient was at risk of developing arrhythmias before taking the drug.
The ECG effects of fexofenadine have been studied[3] in normal subjects and administration of doses of up to 480 mg daily [4 times the recommended dose for seasonal allergic rhinitis] did

not prolong the QT interval. The fear that arrhythmias might be a class effect of the non-sedating antihistamines is discussed on p.405.

1. Pinto YM, *et al.* QT lengthening and life-threatening arrhythmias associated with fexofenadine. *Lancet* 1999; **353**: 980.
2. Giraud T. QT lengthening and arrhythmias associated with fexofenadine. *Lancet* 1999; **353**: 2072.
3. Pratt CM, *et al.* Cardiovascular safety of fexofenadine HCl. *Am J Cardiol* 1999; **83**: 1451–4.

Interactions

As for the non-sedating antihistamines in general, p.406.

Plasma concentrations of fexofenadine have been increased after the concomitant administration of erythromycin or ketoconazole, but, unlike terfenadine, the manufacturer has stated that this was not associated with adverse effects on the QT interval.

Antacids containing aluminium and magnesium hydroxide have reduced the absorption of fexofenadine.

Pharmacokinetics

Fexofenadine is rapidly absorbed after oral administration with peak plasma concentrations being reached in 2 to 3 hours. It is about 60 to 70% bound to plasma proteins. About 5% of the total dose is metabolised, mostly by the intestinal mucosa, with only 0.5 to 1.5% of the dose undergoing hepatic biotransformation. Elimination half-life of about 14 hours has been reported although this may be prolonged in patients with renal impairment. Excretion is mainly in the faeces with only 10% being present in the urine. Fexofenadine does not appear to cross the blood-brain barrier.

Fexofenadine is a metabolite of terfenadine and as such has been detected in breast milk after the administration of terfenadine.

◊ References.
1. Russell T, *et al.* Pharmacokinetics, pharmacodynamics, and tolerance of single- and multiple-dose fexofenadine hydrochloride in healthy male volunteers. *Clin Pharmacol Ther* 1998; **64**: 612–21.

Uses and Administration

Fexofenadine, an active metabolite of terfenadine (p.424), is a non-sedating antihistamine. It does not possess significant sedative or antimuscarinic actions. Fexofenadine is used as the hydrochloride in the symptomatic relief of allergic conditions including seasonal allergic rhinitis (p.407) and urticaria (p.408).

Fexofenadine hydrochloride is given by mouth in a dose of 120 mg daily either as a single dose or in two divided doses. Higher doses of 180 mg daily are recommended in the UK for urticaria. In the USA, children aged 6 to 11 years old may be given fexofenadine in doses of 30 mg twice daily for the treatment of allergic rhinitis or urticaria.

It has been suggested that patients with renal impairment should receive an initial dose of 60 mg daily.

◊ References.
1. Markham A, Wagstaff AJ. Fexofenadine. *Drugs* 1998; **55**: 269–74.

Preparations

Proprietary Preparations (details are given in Part 3)
Aust.: Telfast; *Austral.:* Telfast; *Belg.:* Telfast; *Canad.:* Allegra; *Denm.:* Telfast; *Fr.:* Telfast; *Ger.:* Telfast; *Hong Kong:* Telfast; *Irl.:* Telfast; *Ital.:* Kalicet; Telfast; *Mex.:* Allegra; *Neth.:* Telfast; *Norw.:* Telfast; *NZ:* Telfast; *Port.:* Telfast; *S.Afr.:* Telfast; *Spain:* Telfast; *Swed.:* Telfast; *Switz.:* Telfast; *Thai.:* Telfast; *UK:* Telfast; *USA:* Allegra.

Multi-ingredient: *Austral.:* Telfast Decongestant; *Canad.:* Allegra-D; *NZ:* Telfast Decongestant; *USA:* Allegra-D.

Flunarizine Hydrochloride (12759-n)

Flunarizine Hydrochloride (BANM, USAN, rINNM).
R-14950. *trans*-1-Cinnamyl-4-(4,4′-difluorobenzhydryl)piperazine dihydrochloride.
$C_{26}H_{26}F_2N_2,2HCl = 477.4$.
CAS — 52468-60-7 (flunarizine); 30484-77-6 (flunarizine hydrochloride).
Pharmacopoeias. In Belg.

Flunarizine hydrochloride 11.8 mg is approximately equivalent to 10 mg of flunarizine.

Adverse Effects and Precautions

As for the sedating antihistamines in general, p.404. Adverse effects observed after administration of flunarizine also include weight gain, extrapyramidal symptoms (sometimes associated with depression), and, rarely, galactorrhoea.

Extrapyramidal disorders. Extrapyramidal motor signs (including parkinsonism, orofacial tardive dyskinesia, and akathisia) have been reported in 12 patients given flunarizine 10 to 40 mg daily for between 3 weeks and 15 months; 11 also had mental depression.[1] Partial or complete improvement of symptoms occurred after withdrawal of flunarizine. There have been other reports of similar effects,[2-4] but the association with flunarizine has not been certain. Some workers have commented that flunarizine is often used in patients at increased risk of depression (migraine and geriatric patients) or extrapyramidal symptoms (geriatric patients)[2,5] or that flunarizine may unmask subclinical idiopathic Parkinson's disease.[5,6]

Extrapyramidal signs, including parkinsonism, have also been associated with the related drug, cinnarizine.[3,4] It has been suggested that such effects may be less likely to occur with cinnarizine than with flunarizine because of its shorter half-life and lower lipophilicity.[3]

1. Chouza C, *et al.* Parkinsonism, tardive dyskinesia, akathisia, and depression induced by flunarizine. *Lancet* 1986; **i:** 1303–4.
2. Meyboom RHB, *et al.* Parkinsonism, tardive dyskinesia, akathisia, and depression induced by flunarizine. *Lancet* 1986; **ii:** 292.
3. Laporte J-R, Capella D. Useless drugs are not placebos: lessons from flunarizine and cinnarizine. *Lancet* 1986; **ii:** 853–4.
4. Laporte J-R, Capella D. Useless drugs are not placebos. *Lancet* 1987; **i:** 1324.
5. Amery W. Side-effects of flunarizine. *Lancet* 1986; **i:** 1497.
6. Benvenuti F, *et al.* Side-effects of flunarizine. *Lancet* 1986; **ii:** 464.

Porphyria. Flunarizine hydrochloride is considered to be unsafe in patients with porphyria because it has been shown to be porphyrinogenic in *in-vitro* systems.

Interactions

As for the sedating antihistamines in general, p.406.

Hepatic enzyme inducers such as carbamazepine, phenytoin, and valproate may interact with flunarizine by increasing its metabolism; an increase in dosage of flunarizine may be required.

Pharmacokinetics

Flunarizine hydrochloride is well absorbed from the gastrointestinal tract, peak plasma concentrations occurring 2 to 4 hours after oral administration. Flunarizine hydrochloride is very lipophilic and is more than 90% bound to plasma proteins. It appears to undergo extensive metabolism; metabolites are excreted principally in the bile. Flunarizine hydrochloride has an elimination half-life of about 18 days.[3]

Uses and Administration

Flunarizine is the difluorinated derivative of cinnarizine. It has antihistamine, sedative, and calcium-channel blocking activity. Flunarizine hydrochloride is used for migraine prophylaxis, for vertigo and vestibular disorders, and for peripheral and cerebral vascular disorders. It has also been tried as adjunctive antiepileptic therapy in patients refractory to standard regimens.

Flunarizine hydrochloride is given by mouth; doses are expressed in terms of the equivalent amount of flunarizine. The usual dose is 5 to 10 mg daily, usually given at night to minimise the effects of drowsiness.

Epilepsy. Flunarizine has demonstrated antiepileptic activity in *animal* models, but the mechanism of action is unclear; calcium entry blockade or an effect on sodium channels has been postulated.[1] Most clinical studies have evaluated its use as adjunctive therapy in epileptic patients with partial seizures resistant to conventional treatment (see p.338). Doses of flunarizine of 15 to 20 mg daily by mouth appeared to provide the best response when given as part of multiple-drug antiepileptic regimens.[1] However, studies using fixed doses of flunarizine have been considered unsatisfactory because of its variable clearance and long elimination half-life. A study using a parallel group design and adjusting doses to achieve a constant plasma concentration of 60 nanograms per mL found flunarizine to have modest antiepileptic efficacy as adjunctive therapy for partial seizures.[2] Even so, others[3] have concluded that the pharmacokinetic profile of flunarizine is too complex for its clinical use as an antiepileptic.

1. Todd PA, Benfield P. Flunarizine: a reappraisal of its pharmacological properties and therapeutic use in neurological disorders. *Drugs* 1989; **38:** 481–99.

2. Pledger GW, *et al.* Flunarizine for treatment of partial seizures: results of a concentration-controlled trial. *Neurology* 1994; **44:** 1830–6.
3. Hoppu K, *et al.* Flunarizine of limited value in children with intractable epilepsy. *Pediatr Neurol* 1995; **13:** 143–7.

Migraine. Flunarizine is used for the prophylaxis of migraine (p.449) in some countries. It reduces the frequency of migraine attacks in both adult and paediatric patients and appears to be at least as effective as several other prophylactic antimigraine drugs including those generally preferred, pizotifen and propranolol.[1-4] However, flunarizine is more likely to be reserved for use when first-line drugs have proved to be ineffective or unsuitable. Doses of flunarizine reported to be used for migraine prophylaxis are 10 mg daily for adults and 5 mg daily for children. Its mode of action in migraine is unclear; possible mechanisms are inhibition of vasospasm induced by mediators such as serotonin and prostaglandins, inhibition of cellular hypoxia, and improved blood viscosity and erythrocyte deformability. Calcium-channel blocking activity might have a role, but evidence for the efficacy of other calcium-channel blockers in migraine prophylaxis (see Nifedipine, p.944) is less convincing than for flunarizine.

Case reports have indicated benefit with flunarizine in the prophylaxis of the rare disorder of alternating hemiplegia in childhood[5,6] but a subsequent study[7] in 12 children did not produce conclusive findings. A later long-term study[8] reported that of 9 children given flunarizine for up to 5 years for hemiplegia 7 showed a reduction in the duration of attacks and 3 had a reduction in the frequency, but only 1 of these obtained a complete cessation of episodes.

The role of antihistamines in general in the management of migraine is discussed briefly on p.407.

1. Todd PA, Benfield P. Flunarizine: a reappraisal of its pharmacological properties and therapeutic use in neurological disorders. *Drugs* 1989; **38:** 481–99.
2. Andersson K-E, Vinge E. β-Adrenoceptor blockers and calcium antagonists in the prophylaxis and treatment of migraine. *Drugs* 1990; **3:** 355–73.
3. Soelberg Sørensen P, *et al.* Flunarizine versus metoprolol in migraine prophylaxis: a double-blind, randomized parallel group study of efficacy and tolerability. *Headache* 1991; **31:** 650–7.
4. Gawel MJ, *et al.* Comparison of the efficacy and safety of flunarizine to propranolol in the prophylaxis of migraine. *Can J Neurol Sci* 1992; **19:** 340–5.
5. Casaer P, Azou M. Flunarizine in alternating hemiplegia in childhood. *Lancet* 1984; **ii:** 579.
6. Curatolo P, Cusmai R. Drugs for alternating hemiplegic migraine. *Lancet* 1984; **i:** 980.
7. Casaer P. Flunarizine in alternating hemiplegia in childhood. An international study in 12 children. *Neuropediatrics* 1987; **18:** 191–5.
8. Silver K, Andermann F. Alternating hemiplegia of childhood: a study of 10 patients and results of flunarizine treatment. *Neurology* 1993; **43:** 36–41.

Tourette's syndrome. A small unblinded study[1] involving 7 patients has suggested that flunarizine is more effective than placebo in the treatment of Tourette's syndrome (see Tics, p.650).

1. Micheli F, *et al.* Treatment of Tourette's syndrome with calcium antagonists. *Clin Neuropharmacol* 1990; **13:** 77–83.

Vertigo. Antihistamines are the mainstay of the treatment of vertigo (p.408). However, their antimuscarinic side-effects may prove troublesome, particularly in the elderly, and they produce central sedation. Flunarizine is a calcium-channel blocker and an antihistamine that is devoid of antimuscarinic properties, although it may produce central sedation.

Preparations

Proprietary Preparations (details are given in Part 3)
Aust.: Amalium, Sibelium; *Belg.:* Sibelium; *Braz.:* Flunarin; Fluvert; Sibelium; Vertix; *Canad.:* Sibelium; *Denm.:* Sibelium; *Fr.:* Sibelium; *Ger.:* Flunavert; Sibelium; *Hong Kong:* Sibelium; *Irl.:* Sibelium; *Ital.:* Flugeral; Flunagen; Fluxarten; Gradient; Issium; Sibelium; Vasculene; *Mex.:* Fasolan; Naſluryl; Sibelium; Sibelium; *Port.:* Sibelium; Vasilium; Zinasen; *S.Afr.:* Sibelium; *Singapore:* Sibelium; *Spain:* Flerudin; Flurpax; Sibelium; *Switz.:* Sibelium; *Thai.:* Cedelate; Floxin; Fludan; Flulium; Flunarium; Flunaza; Flunazine; Fluricin; FNZ; Hexilium; Liberal; Medilium; Poli-Flunarin; Sibelium; Simoyiam; Sobelin; Zelium.

Multi-ingredient: *Braz.:* Vertizine D.

Homochlorcyclizine Hydrochloride (6137-w)

Homochlorcyclizine Hydrochloride (BANM, rINNM).
1-(4-Chlorobenzhydryl)perhydro-4-methyl-1,4-diazepine dihydrochloride.
$C_{19}H_{23}ClN_2,2HCl = 387.8$.
CAS — 848-53-3 (homochlorcyclizine); 1982-36-1 (homochlorcyclizine hydrochloride).
Pharmacopoeias. In Jpn.

Profile

Homochlorcyclizine hydrochloride, a piperazine derivative, is a sedating antihistamine (p.404) with antimuscarinic and moderate sedative properties. It is used for the symptomatic relief of allergic conditions such as urticaria (p.408) and rhinitis (p.407), and in pruritic skin disorders (p.407). It is given by mouth in doses of 10 to 20 mg three times daily.

Preparations

Proprietary Preparations (details are given in Part 3)
Hong Kong: Homoclomin; *Jpn:* Homoclomin; *Thai.:* Homoclomin.

Hydroxyzine Embonate (6138-e)

Hydroxyzine Embonate *(BANM, rINNM).*
Hydroxyzine Pamoate. 2-{2-[4-(4-Chlorobenzhydryl)piperazin-1-yl]ethoxy}ethanol 4,4′-methylenebis(3-hydroxy-2-naphthoate).
$C_{21}H_{27}ClN_2O_2,C_{23}H_{16}O_6 = 763.3$.
CAS — 68-88-2 (hydroxyzine); 10246-75-0 (hydroxyzine embonate).
Pharmacopoeias. In Jpn and US.

Hydroxyzine embonate 170 mg is approximately equivalent to 100 mg of hydroxyzine hydrochloride.

Pharmacopoeial description
USP 25: A light yellow, practically odourless powder. Soluble 1 in more than 1000 of water, of chloroform, and of ether, 1 in 700 of alcohol, 1 in 10 of dimethylformamide, and 1 in 3.5 of 10M sodium hydroxide solution; practically insoluble in methyl alcohol. Store in airtight containers.

Hydroxyzine Hydrochloride (6139-l)

Hydroxyzine Hydrochloride *(BANM, rINNM).*
Hydroxyzini Hydrochloridum.
$C_{21}H_{27}ClN_2O_2,2HCl = 447.8$.
CAS — 2192-20-3.
Pharmacopoeias. In Eur. (see p.vi), Jpn, and US.

Incompatibility has been reported with aminophylline, benzylpenicillin salts, chloramphenicol sodium succinate, dimenhydrinate, doxorubicin hydrochloride (in a liposomal formulation), thioridazine, and some soluble barbiturates.

Pharmacopoeial description
Ph. Eur.: A white or almost white, crystalline, hygroscopic powder. Freely soluble in water and in alcohol; slightly soluble in acetone. Store in airtight containers. Protect from light.
USP 25: A white, odourless, powder. Soluble 1 in 1 of water, 1 in 4.5 of alcohol, and 1 in 13 of chloroform; slightly soluble in acetone; practically insoluble in ether. Store in airtight containers.

Stability. A mixture of hydroxyzine hydrochloride, chlorpromazine hydrochloride, and pethidine hydrochloride stored in glass or plastic syringes was found[1] to be stable for 366 days at 4° and 25°.
1. Conklin CA, *et al.* Stability of an analgesic-sedative combination in glass and plastic single-dose syringes. *Am J Hosp Pharm* 1985; **42:** 339–42.

Adverse Effects and Precautions
As for the sedating antihistamines in general, p.404.
Intramuscular injection of hydroxyzine has been reported to cause marked local discomfort. Intravenous administration has been associated with haemolysis.

◊ Accidental intra-arterial injection of hydroxyzine has led to necrosis of the extremity requiring amputation of the digits of the affected limb.[1]
1. Hardesty WH. Inadvertent intra-arterial injection. *JAMA* 1970; **213:** 872.

Arrhythmias. ECG abnormalities, particularly alterations in T-waves, were associated with anxiolytic doses of hydroxyzine hydrochloride and were similar to those produced by thioridazine and tricyclic antidepressants.[1]
1. Hollister LE. Hydroxyzine hydrochloride: possible adverse cardiac interactions. *Psychopharmacol Comm* 1975; **1:** 61–5.

Effects on sexual function. A 32-year-old man experienced prolonged penile erections (priapism) after taking two separate doses of hydroxyzine for a skin rash.[1] It was suggested that the effect might be due to a hydroxyzine metabolite which was found to be structurally similar to a metabolite of trazodone, a drug known to induce penile erections.
1. Thavundayil JX. *et al.* Prolonged penile erections induced by hydroxyzine: possible mechanism of action. *Neuropsychobiology* 1994; **30:** 4–6.

Effects on the skin. Four children given hydroxyzine hydrochloride for restlessness developed a fixed drug eruption of the penis.[1] All recovered on drug withdrawal and subsequently had positive rechallenges.
1. Cohen HA, *et al.* Fixed drug eruption of the penis due to hydroxyzine hydrochloride. *Ann Pharmacother* 1997; **31:** 327–9.

Liver disorders. A study[1] has suggested that hydroxyzine should only be administered once daily for the relief of pruritus in patients with primary biliary cirrhosis. The mean serum elimination half-lives of hydroxyzine and its metabolite cetirizine in 8 patients with primary biliary cirrhosis were 36.6 and 25.0 hours respectively.
1. Simons FER, *et al.* The pharmacokinetics and pharmacodynamics of hydroxyzine in patients with primary biliary cirrhosis. *J Clin Pharmacol* 1989; **29:** 809–15.

Porphyria. Hydroxyzine has been associated with acute attacks of porphyria and is considered unsafe in porphyric patients.

Interactions
As for the sedating antihistamines in general, p.406.

Pharmacokinetics
Hydroxyzine is rapidly absorbed from the gastrointestinal tract and is metabolised. Metabolites include cetirizine (p.411) which has antihistamine activity. An elimination half-life of about 20 hours has been reported.

◊ References.
1. Paton DM, Webster DR. Clinical pharmacokinetics of H₁-receptor antagonists (the antihistamines). *Clin Pharmacokinet* 1985; **10:** 477–97.

Liver disorders. For reference to a prolonged half-life of hydroxyzine in patients with primary biliary cirrhosis, see under Adverse Effects and Precautions, above.

Uses and Administration
Hydroxyzine, a piperazine derivative, is a sedating antihistamine with antimuscarinic and significant sedative properties; it is also an antiemetic. Its main use is as an anxiolytic (p.649). It is also used as an adjunct to pre- and postoperative medication (p.406) and in the management of pruritus (p.407) and urticaria (p.408) and has been used as an adjunct to opioid analgesia in the management of cancer pain (p.5).

Hydroxyzine may be given by mouth as the hydrochloride or the embonate; doses are expressed in terms of the equivalent amount of hydroxyzine hydrochloride.

The usual doses by mouth in adults are: 50 to 100 mg four times daily for the short-term management of anxiety; for pruritus an initial dose of 25 mg given at night, increased if necessary to 25 mg three or four times daily; and 50 to 100 mg for pre- or postoperative sedation. For pruritus in children over 6 years the initial dose is 15 to 25 mg daily increased if necessary to 50 to 100 mg daily in divided doses; for children 6 months to 6 years old the initial dose is 5 to 15 mg daily increased if necessary to 50 mg daily in divided doses. The pre- or postoperative sedative dose in children is 600 µg per kg body-weight.

Hydroxyzine hydrochloride may also be given by deep intramuscular injection. For prompt control of anxiety or agitation in adults 50 to 100 mg is injected intramuscularly initially, and the dose may be repeated every four to six hours as required. For other indications when oral administration is not practical, the intramuscular dose is 25 to 100 mg for adults and 1.1 mg per kg for children. Hydroxyzine should not be given by intravenous injection since haemolysis may result.

Preparations
USP 25: Hydroxyzine Hydrochloride Injection; Hydroxyzine Hydrochloride Syrup; Hydroxyzine Hydrochloride Tablets; Hydroxyzine Pamoate Capsules; Hydroxyzine Pamoate Oral Suspension.

Proprietary Preparations (details are given in Part 3)
Aust.: Atarax; *Austral.:* Atarax; *Belg.:* Atarax; *Canad.:* Atarax; Multipax†; *Denm.:* Atarax; *Fin.:* Atarax; *Fr.:* Atarax; *Ger.:* AH 3 N; Atarax; Elroquil N; *Hong Kong:* Atarax; *Irl.:* Atarax; *Israel:* Otarex; *Ital.:* Atarax; *Mex.:* Atarax; *Neth.:* Atarax; Navicalm; *Norw.:* Atarax; *NZ:* Serecid; *Port.:* Atarax; *S.Afr.:* Aterax; *Singapore:* Atarax; Phymorax; *Spain:* Atarax; *Swed.:* Atarax; Vistaril†; *Switz.:* Atarax; *Thai.:* Abacus; Antizine; Atano; Atarax; Cerax; Drazine; Hadarax; Histan; Hizin; Honsa; Hydroxin; Masarax; Med-Xyzarax; Taraxin; Trandrozine; *UK:* Atarax; Ucerax; *USA:* Anxanil†; Atarax; E-Vista†; Hyzine†; Quiess†; Rezine†; Vistacon†; Vistaquel†; Vistaril; Vistazine.

Multi-ingredient: *Aust.:* Diligan; *Belg.:* Vesparax†; *Braz.:* Marax; *Ger.:* Diligan; *Neth.:* Vesparax†; *Port.:* Diligan†; Vesparax†; *S.Afr.:* Geratar; Vesparax†; *Spain:* Calmoplex; Difilina Asmorax†; Dolodens; Somatarax; *Swed.:* Histilos; Kombistrat†; *Switz.:* Hexafene†; *USA:* Hydrophed; Marax; Theomax DF.

Isothipendyl Hydrochloride (6140-v)

Isothipendyl Hydrochloride *(BANM, rINNM).*
NN-Dimethyl-1-(pyrido[3,2-b][1,4]benzothiazin-10-ylmethyl)ethylamine hydrochloride.
$C_{16}H_{19}N_3S,HCl = 321.9$.
CAS — 482-15-5 (isothipendyl); 1225-60-1 (isothipendyl hydrochloride).

Profile
Isothipendyl hydrochloride, an azaphenothiazine derivative, is an antihistamine (p.404) that has been applied topically for hypersensitivity and pruritic skin disorders although as with any antihistamine there is a risk of sensitisation. It has also been administered by mouth and by the rectal route.

Preparations
Proprietary Preparations (details are given in Part 3)
Belg.: Andantol; *Braz.:* Andantol; *Fr.:* Apaisyl†; Istamyl†; Sedermyl; *Israel:* Thiodantol; *Ital.:* Calmogel; *Mex.:* Andantol.

Levocabastine Hydrochloride

(15953-b)

Levocabastine Hydrochloride *(BANM, USAN, rINNM).*
Levocabastini Hydrochloridum; R-50547. (−)-trans-1-[cis-4-Cyano-4-(p-fluorophenyl)cyclohexyl]-3-methyl-4-phenylisonipecotic acid hydrochloride.
$C_{26}H_{29}FN_2O_2,HCl = 457.0$.
CAS — 79516-68-0 (levocabastine); 79547-78-7 (levocabastine hydrochloride); 79449-98-2 (cabastine).

NOTE. The racemate of levocabastine, cabastine, is *rINN.*
Pharmacopoeias. In Eur. (see p.vi).

Levocabastine hydrochloride 1.09 mg is approximately equivalent to 1 mg of levocabastine.

Pharmacopoeial description
Ph. Eur.: A white or almost white powder. Practically insoluble in water; slightly soluble in alcohol and in a 0.2% solution of sodium hydroxide; sparingly soluble in methyl alcohol. Protect from light.

Adverse Effects and Precautions
As for the antihistamines in general, p.404. The most common adverse effects reported with levocabastine eye drops are transient stinging and burning of the eyes, urticaria, dyspnoea, drowsiness, and headache. Following nasal administration headache, nasal irritation, somnolence, and fatigue have been noted. The use of levocabastine nasal spray is not recommended in those with significant renal impairment.

Pharmacokinetics
Levocabastine is absorbed following both nasal and ocular administration. Systemic availability has been estimated at 60 to 80% after nasal administration and 30 to 60% after ocular application. However absolute peak plasma concentrations are low. Plasma protein binding is about 55%. An elimination half-life of 35 to 40 hours has been reported for all routes of delivery. Elimination of levocabastine is primarily renal with 70% excreted as unchanged drug and 10% as an inactive acetylglucuronide metabolite; the remaining 20% is excreted unchanged in the faeces.

Trace amounts of levocabastine have been found in breast milk after ocular and nasal administration.

◊ References.
1. Heykants J, *et al.* The pharmacokinetic properties of topical levocabastine: a review. *Clin Pharmacokinet* 1995; **29:** 221–30.

Uses and Administration
Levocabastine, a piperidine derivative, is a long-acting and potent antihistamine with a rapid onset of action. Levocabastine hydrochloride equivalent to 0.05% levocabastine is used topically twice daily as eye drops or as nasal spray in the treatment of allergic conjunctivitis (p.406) and rhinitis (p.407), respectively in adults and children aged 9 years and over. The frequency of the dose in both conditions may be increased to 3 or 4 times daily if necessary. In conjunctivitis it is recommended that treatment should be discontinued if there is no improvement within 3 days.

◊ References.
1. Dechant KL, Goa KL. Levocabastine: a review of its pharmacological properties and therapeutic potential as a topical antihistamine in allergic rhinitis and conjunctivitis. *Drugs* 1991; **41:** 202–24.
2. Noble S, McTavish D. Levocabastine: an update of its pharmacology, clinically efficacy and tolerability in the topical treatment of allergic rhinitis and conjunctivitis. *Drugs* 1995; **50:** 1032–49.

Preparations
Proprietary Preparations (details are given in Part 3)
Aust.: Livostin; *Austral.:* Livostin; *Belg.:* Livostin; *Canad.:* Livostin; *Denm.:* Livostin; *Fin.:* Livostin; *Fr.:* Levophta; *Ger.:* Levophta; Livocab; *Israel:* Livostin; *Ital.:* Levostab; Livostin; *Jpn:* Livostin; *Mex.:* Livostin; *Neth.:* Livocab; *Norw.:* Livostin;

The symbol † denotes a preparation no longer actively marketed

Levocetirizine (20123-e)

Levocetirizine (rINN).

(2-{4-[(R)-p-Chloro-α-phenylbenzyl]-1-piperazinyl}ethoxy)acetic acid.

$C_{21}H_{25}ClN_2O_3 = 388.9.$

CAS — 130018-77-8.

Profile

Levocetirizine is the R-enantiomer of cetirizine (p.411) and is used similarly, as the hydrochloride, for the symptomatic relief of allergic conditions including rhinitis (p.407) and chronic urticaria (p.408).

In adults and children aged 6 years and over, levocetirizine hydrochloride is given by mouth in a dose of 5 mg once daily.

The dose should be reduced in patients with renal impairment: the recommended dose in patients with moderate renal impairment (creatinine clearance 30 to 49 mL per minute) is 5 mg every 2 days; in those with severe impairment, the dose interval should be increased to every 3 days. Patients with end-stage renal disease or receiving dialysis should not be given levocetirizine.

Preparations

Proprietary Preparations (details are given in Part 3)
UK: Xyzal.

Loratadine (18661-c)

Loratadine (BAN, USAN, rINN).

Sch-29851. Ethyl 4-(8-chloro-5,6-dihydro-11H-benzo[5,6]cyclohepta[1,2-b]pyridin-11-ylidene)piperidine-1-carboxylate.

$C_{22}H_{23}ClN_2O_2 = 382.9.$

CAS — 79794-75-5.

ATC — R06AX13.

Adverse Effects and Precautions

As for the non-sedating antihistamines in general, p.404.

Effects on the liver. Two patients[1] developed severe necroinflammatory liver injury after receiving loratadine 10 mg daily for allergic rhinitis. Although both recovered after drug withdrawal, one patient required a liver transplantation and recovery was prolonged.

The manufacturers note that abnormal hepatic function including jaundice, hepatitis, and hepatic necrosis have been reported rarely.

1. Schiano TD, et al. Subfulminant liver failure and severe hepatotoxicity caused by loratadine use. Ann Intern Med 1996; 125: 738–40.

Sedation. For discussion of the sedative effects of antihistamines see p.405.

Interactions

As for the non-sedating antihistamines in general, p.406.

Loratadine is metabolised by cytochrome P450 isoenzymes CYP3A4 and CYP2D6. Therefore concomitant administration of other drugs that inhibit or are metabolised by these hepatic enzymes may result in changes in plasma concentrations of either drug and, possibly, adverse effects. Drugs known to inhibit one or other of these enzymes include cimetidine, erythromycin, ketoconazole, quinidine, fluconazole, and fluoxetine.

◊ Data held on file by the manufacturer show that erythromycin can inhibit the metabolism of loratadine. However, even when given in large doses loratadine does not appear to cause the cardiac conduction disorders associated with the non-sedating antihistamines astemizole (see p.409) and terfenadine (see p.424).[1] Similarly, clarithromycin seemed to inhibit the metabolism of loratadine and its active metabolite descarboethoxyloratadine.[2]

Ketoconazole also appears to be able to inhibit the metabolism of loratadine and at therapeutic doses, is approximately 3 times more inhibitory than erythromycin.[3] However, the concentrations of ketoconazole required are reported to be much higher than those required to inhibit the metabolism of astemizole or terfenadine.

Cimetidine also appears to have an inhibitory effect on the metabolism of loratadine and all 4 drugs also attenuate the clearance of its active metabolite descarboethoxyloratadine although no clinically significant consequences were observed in these studies.[2,3]

1. Affrime MB, et al. Three month evaluation of electrocardiographic effects of loratadine in humans. J Allergy Clin Immunol 1993; 91: 259.

2. Carr RA, et al. Steady-state pharmacokinetics and electrocardiographic pharmacodynamics of clarithromycin and loratadine after individual or concomitant administration. Antimicrob Agents Chemother 1998; 42: 1176–80.

3. Brannan MD, et al. Effects of various cytochrome P450 inhibitors on the metabolism of loratadine. Clin Pharmacol Ther 1995; 57: 193.

Pharmacokinetics

Loratadine is rapidly absorbed from the gastrointestinal tract after oral administration, peak plasma concentrations being attained in about one hour. Bioavailability is increased and time to peak plasma concentrations is delayed when administered with food. Loratadine undergoes extensive metabolism. The major metabolite, descarboethoxyloratadine (desloratadine, see p.415), has potent antihistamine activity. Reported mean elimination half-lives for loratadine and descarboethoxyloratadine are 8.4 and 28 hours respectively. Loratadine is about 98% bound to plasma proteins; descarboethoxyloratadine is less extensively bound. Loratadine and its metabolites have been detected in breast milk, but do not appear to cross the blood-brain barrier to a significant extent. Most of a dose is excreted equally in the urine and faeces, mainly in the form of metabolites.

Renal impairment. The disposition of loratadine does not appear to be significantly altered in patients with severe renal insufficiency and haemodialysis does not appear to be an effective means of removing loratadine or its metabolite descarboethoxyloratadine from the body.[1]

1. Matzke GR, et al. Pharmacokinetics of loratadine in patients with renal insufficiency. J Clin Pharmacol 1990; 30: 364–71.

Uses and Administration

Loratadine, a piperidine derivative related to azatadine, is a long-acting, non-sedating antihistamine with no significant antimuscarinic activity. It is used for the symptomatic relief of allergic conditions including rhinitis (p.407) and chronic urticaria (p.408).

Loratadine is given by mouth in a dose of 10 mg once daily. The US manufacturer recommends that patients with hepatic failure or renal impairment should be given 10 mg on alternate days initially. Children aged 2 to 5 years may be given 5 mg once daily and those aged 6 to 12 years may be given 10 mg once daily.

◊ References.

1. Haria M, et al. Loratadine: a reappraisal of its pharmacological properties and therapeutic use in allergic disorders. Drugs 1994; 48: 617–37.

Preparations

Proprietary Preparations (details are given in Part 3)
Aust.: Clarityn; Loratyn; Austral.: Claratyne; Lorastyne; Belg.: Claritine; Sanelor; Braz.: Alertal; Claritin; Loranil; Canad.: Claritin; Denm.: Clarityn; Versal; Fin.: Clarityn; Fr.: Clarityne; Ger.: Lisino; Hong Kong: Clarityne; Irl.: Clarityn; Israel: Lorastine; Ital.: Alorin; Clarityn; Fristamin; Mex.: Clarityne; Lertamine; Lowadina; Rodakin; Sensibit; Neth.: Allerfre; Claritine; Norw.: Clarityn; Versal†; NZ: Claratyne; Port.: Alertrin†; Claritine; S.Afr.: Clarityne; Loratyne; Polaratyne; Singapore: Clarityne; Spain: Civeran; Clarityne; Optimin; Velodan; Viatine; Swed.: Clarityn; Versal; Switz.: Claritine; Thai.: Aller-Tab; Allerdine; Allersil; Clarityne; Loranox; Loritype; Lorsedin; Lordadine; Ridamin; UAE: Loratin; UK: Clarityn; USA: Claritin.

Multi-ingredient: Aust.: Clarinase; Austral.: Clarinase; Belg.: Clarinase; Braz.: Claritin-D; Canad.: Chlor-Tripolon ND; Claritin Extra; Denm.: Clarinex; Fr.: Clarinase; Hong Kong: Clarinase; Israel: Clarinase; Mex.: Clarinase; Clarityne D; Lertamine-D; NZ: Claratyne Decongestant; Demazin Non-Drowsy; Port.: Claridon; S.Afr.: Clarityne D; Demazin NS; Polaratyne D; Singapore: Clarinase; Spain: Clarinase; Logradin; Narine; Thai.: Clarinase; USA: Claritin-D.

Mebhydrolin (12145-k)

Mebhydrolin (BAN, rINN).

5-Benzyl-1,2,3,4-tetrahydro-2-methyl-γ-carboline.

$C_{19}H_{20}N_2 = 276.4.$

CAS — 524-81-2.

ATC — R06AX15.

Mebhydrolin Napadisilate (6141-g)

Mebhydrolin Napadisilate (BANM, rINN).

Diazolinum; Mebhydrolin Napadisylate; Mebhydrolin Naphthalenedisulphonate; Mebhydrolin naphthalene-1,5-disulphonate.

$(C_{19}H_{20}N_2)_2,C_{10}H_8O_6S_2 = 841.0.$

CAS — 6153-33-9.

Mebhydrolin napadisilate 152 mg is approximately equivalent to 100 mg of mebhydrolin.

Profile

Mebhydrolin, an ethylenediamine derivative, is a sedating antihistamine (p.404) with antimuscarinic and sedative properties. It has been given by mouth as the base or as the napadisilate salt for the symptomatic relief of allergic conditions including urticaria and rhinitis, and in pruritic skin disorders. Granulocytopenia and agranulocytosis have been reported.

Preparations

Proprietary Preparations (details are given in Part 3)
Austral.: Fabahistin†; Ger.: Omeril†; Hong Kong: Incidal; Israel: Cidalin; Ital.: Incidal†; Neth.: Incidal†; S.Afr.: Fabahistin†; Thai.: Dayhist; Incidal; Posidol.

Meclozine Hydrochloride (6142-q)

Meclozine Hydrochloride (BAN, pINNM).

Meclizine Hydrochloride; Meclizinium Chloride; Meclozini Hydrochloridum; Parachloramine Hydrochloride. 1-(4-Chlorobenzhydryl)-4-(3-methylbenzyl)piperazine dihydrochloride.

$C_{25}H_{27}ClN_2,2HCl = 463.9.$

CAS — 569-65-3 (meclozine); 1104-22-9 (anhydrous meclozine hydrochloride); 31884-77-2 (meclozine hydrochloride, monohydrate).

Pharmacopoeias. In Eur. (see p.vi).
US specifies the monohydrate.

Pharmacopoeial description

Ph. Eur.: A yellow or yellowish-white, crystalline powder. Slightly soluble in water; soluble in alcohol and in dichloromethane; practically insoluble in ether. Store in airtight containers.

USP 25: The monohydrate is white or slightly yellowish crystalline powder that has a slight odour. Practically insoluble in water and in ether; freely soluble in chloroform, in pyridine, and in acid-alcohol-water mixtures; slightly soluble in dilute acids and in alcohol. Store in airtight containers.

Adverse Effects and Precautions

As for the sedating antihistamines in general, p.404. For reports of the use of antihistamines, including meclozine, in pregnancy, see p.405.

Interactions

As for the sedating antihistamines in general, p.406.

Uses and Administration

Meclozine hydrochloride, a piperazine derivative, is a sedating antihistamine with antimuscarinic and moderate sedative properties. It is mainly used for its antiemetic action which may last for up to 24 hours. Meclozine hydrochloride is used in the prevention and treatment of nausea and vomiting associated with a variety of conditions including motion sickness (p.407) and for the symptomatic treatment of vertigo (p.408) caused by Ménière's disease and other vestibular disorders. Meclozine hydrochloride has also been used for the symptomatic relief of hypersensitivity reactions and pruritic skin disorders (p.407).

The usual dose of meclozine hydrochloride for motion sickness is 25 to 50 mg by mouth taken about one hour before travelling and repeated every 24 hours if necessary; up to 100 mg daily in divided doses has been given for the treatment of vertigo and vestibular disorders. In the prevention and treatment of motion sickness in children aged 6 to 12 years, 12.5 mg is given once daily; for children aged 2 to 6 years the dose is 6.25 mg once daily.

Both meclozine hydrochloride and meclozine base have been administered by the rectal route; doses are similar to those given by mouth.

Preparations

USP 25: Meclizine Hydrochloride Tablets.

Proprietary Preparations (details are given in Part 3)
Belg.: Agyrax; Postafene; Canad.: Antivert; Bonamine; Denm.: Postafen; Fin.: Postafen; Fr.: Agyrax; Ger.: Bonamine†; Peremesin; Peremesin N; Postadoxin N; Hong Kong: Postafene; Neth.: Suprimal†; Norw.: Peremesin; Postafen; NZ: Sea-Legs; Port.: Navicalm; Spain: Chiclida; Dramine; Marevit; Navicalm; Swed.: Postafen; Switz.: Duremesan; Thai.: Bonamine; UK: Sea-legs; USA: Antivert; Antrizine; Bonine; Dizmiss; Dramamine II; Meni-D; Nico-Vert†; Vergon; Vertin†.

Multi-ingredient: Aust.: Contravert B6; Diligan; Belg.: Postadoxine; Ger.: Diligan; Hong Kong: Navidoxine; Mex.: Bonadoxina; Emediba; Liatriz; Meclifar; Neth.: Emesafene; Neo-Cranimal†; Port.: Diligan†; S.Afr.: Geratar; Singapore: Navidoxine; Swed.: Histilos; Switz.: Duremesan; Itinerol B6.

Mefenidramium Metilsulfate (2750-f)

Mefenidramium Metilsulfate (rINN).

Diphenhydramine Methylsulfomethylate; Diphenhydramine Methylsulphomethylate; Mefenidramium Methylsulfate; Mefenidramium Methylsulphate. [2-(Diphenylmethoxy)ethyl]trimethylammonium methyl sulphate.

$C_{19}H_{27}NO_5S = 381.5$.
CAS — 4858-60-0.

Profile

Mefenidramium metilsulfate, a monoethanolamine derivative, is a sedating antihistamine (p.404). It has antimuscarinic and significant sedative properties. Mefenidramium has been given for the symptomatic relief of hypersensitivity reactions and in pruritic skin disorders.

Mepyramine Hydrochloride (13752-h)

Mepyramine Hydrochloride (BANM, rINNM).

Pyranisamine Hydrochloride; Pyrilamine Hydrochloride. N-p-Anisyl-N'N'-dimethyl-N-(2-pyridyl)ethylenediamine hydrochloride.

$C_{17}H_{23}N_3O,HCl = 321.8$.
CAS — 91-84-9 (mepyramine); 6036-95-9 (mepyramine hydrochloride).

Mepyramine Maleate (6144-s)

Mepyramine Maleate (BANM, rINNM).

Mepyramini Maleas; Pyranisamine Maleate; Pyrilamine Maleate. Mepyramine hydrogen maleate.

$C_{17}H_{23}N_3O,C_4H_4O_4 = 401.5$.
CAS — 59-33-6.
Pharmacopoeias. In Eur. (see p.vi) and US.

Pharmacopoeial description

Ph. Eur.: A white or slightly yellowish, crystalline powder. Very soluble in water; freely soluble in alcohol; very slightly soluble in ether. M.p. 99° to 103°. A 2% solution in water has a pH of 4.9 to 5.2. Protect from light.

USP 25: A white crystalline powder usually having a faint odour. Soluble 1 in 0.5 of water, 1 in 3 of alcohol, 1 in 15 of dehydrated alcohol, and 1 in 2 of chloroform; slightly soluble in ether and in benzene. Its solutions are acid to litmus. Store in airtight containers. Protect from light.

Adverse Effects and Precautions

As for the sedating antihistamines in general, p.404.

Interactions

As for the sedating antihistamines in general, p.406.

Uses and Administration

Mepyramine, an ethylenediamine derivative, is a sedating antihistamine with antimuscarinic and sedative properties. Mepyramine maleate is used for the symptomatic relief of hypersensitivity reactions and in pruritic skin disorders (p.407). Mepyramine maleate is also a common ingredient of compound preparations for the symptomatic treatment of coughs and the common cold (p.406).

Mepyramine maleate has been given by mouth in a dose of 25 to 50 mg three times daily; higher doses have also been used. Mepyramine maleate has also been used in eye drops. In some countries mepyramine maleate is available for parenteral use.

A cream containing 2% mepyramine maleate is used locally for insect bites or stings, and for hypersensitivity and pruritic skin conditions but, as with any antihistamine, there is a risk of sensitisation.

Mepyramine hydrochloride has been administered parenterally or by the rectal route. Mepyramine tannate and mepifylline (mepyramine acephyllinate) have been given by mouth.

Preparations

BP 2001: Mepyramine Tablets;
USP 25: Pyrilamine Maleate Tablets.

Proprietary Preparations (details are given in Part 3)
Austral.: Anthisan†; Relaxa-Tabs; *Hong Kong:* Anthisan; *Irl.:* Anthisan; *Ital.:* Antemesyl; *Mex.:* Fluidasa; *NZ:* Anthisan; *S.Afr.:* Anthisan; Histamed†; Mepyrimal; Pyramine†; Pyriped†; *Spain:* Fluidasa; *UK:* Anthisan.

Multi-ingredient: *Aust.:* Prefrin A; *Austral.:* Hycomine†; Neo-Diophen; *Belg.:* Nortussine; *Braz.:* Adegripan; Alergo Glucalbet; Alersan; Analgex C; Atagripe; Beclase; Cefunk; Conidrin; Engov; Enjoy; Expectussin; Fluviral; Gripefago C; Gripefin; Gripol C; Gripol Composto; Gripsay; Killgrip; Naricin; Naridrin; Nasogrip; Nasopan; Plenogripe; Posdrink; Prenefrin; Subitan; *Canad.:* Antitussive Decongestant Antihistamine Syrup; Bronchodex DM†; Bronchosirum†; Caldomine-DH; Centracol DM; Hycomine; IDM

The symbol † denotes a preparation no longer actively marketed

Solution†; Jack and Jill Cough Syrup; Lemon Time; Midol Extra Strength; Midol Multi-Symptom†; Midol PMS Extra Strength; Pamprin; Pharmacol DM; Pharminicol DM†; Prefrin A; Tantacol DM; Theo-Bronc; Trendar PMS; Triaminic Expectorant DH†; Triaminic†; Triaminicin†; Trisulfaminic; Tussaminic C†; Tussaminic DH†; Tylenol Menstrual; *Fr.:* Nortussine; *Israel:* Aforinol; Alnase; Phenyphrine-Azol; *Ital.:* Antemesyl; Balsamina Kroner; Triaminic; Vasofen; *Mex.:* LM6; *Port.:* Naso Prieulina; Profrin-A†; Solpic; Ugrilon; *S.Afr.:* Antiflu; Ascold†; Bronchiflu; Bronchistop†; Cetamine; Cetrispect†; Codef; Codomill; Colcaps; Coughcod; Docsed; Dykatuss Co; Efcod†; Expectco†; Expectotussin "C"; Flucol†; Histodor; Kiddiekof; Medituss; Metaxol; Monotussin; Prefrin A†; Pyracod†; Triami†; Triaminic; *Spain:* Amplidermis; Pectobal Dextro; Triominic†; *Switz.:* Calpred; Demoderhin†; Demostan N; Escogripp sans codeine; Euceta Pic; Histacyl Compositum; Histacylettes; No Grip†; Stilex; *Thai.:* Antergan; *UK:* Anthisan Plus; Wasp-Eze; *USA:* 4-Way Fast Acting; A-Caine†; Albatussin NN†; Atrohist Pediatric; Calamycin; Codal-DH; Codal DH; Codimal DH; Codimal DM; Codimal PH; Covangesic†; Derma-Pax; Duonate; Gelhist; HC Derma-Pax; Histalet Forte†; Histosal†; Hydrophene DH†; Iohist D†; Kisitan†; Medacote†; Midol Maximum Strength Multi-Symptom Menstrual; Midol PMS; Myci-Spray; ND-Gesic; Pamprin; Phanadex Cough†; Poly-Histine; Poly-Histine D†; Premsyn PMS; Quadra-Hist D†; R-Tanna; R-Tannamine; R-Tannate; R-Tannic-S; Rectagene Medicated Rectal Balm; Rhinatate; Robitussin Night Relief; Rolatuss with Hydrocodone†; Ru-Tuss with Hydrocodone†; Ryna-12 S; Soothaderm; Statuss Green†; Tanoral; Theracaps†; Tri-P†; Tri-Tannate; Triaminic Expectorant DH†; Triaminic Oral Infant†; Tricodene Cough & Cold; Trihist-D†; Triotann; Tritan; Vanex Forte†; Vetuss HC†; Vitanumonyl†.

Mequitazine (6145-w)

Mequitazine (BAN, rINN).

LM-209. 10-(Quinuclidin-3-ylmethyl)phenothiazine.

$C_{20}H_{22}N_2S = 322.5$.
CAS — 29216-28-2.
ATC — R06AD07.

Adverse Effects and Precautions

As for the sedating antihistamines in general, p.404.

Sedation. For discussion of the sedative effects of antihistamines, see p.405. When mequitazine is given in the recommended dosage of 5 mg twice daily the incidence of sedation appears comparable with that of terfenadine. Sedation has, however, occurred after doses of 10 mg twice daily.

Interactions

As for the sedating antihistamines in general, p.406.

Antibacterials. For a report of torsade de pointes in a patient taking *spiramycin* and mequitazine, see p.249.

Pharmacokinetics

After absorption from the gastrointestinal tract, mequitazine is metabolised. Unchanged drug and metabolites are excreted principally in the bile.

Uses and Administration

Mequitazine, a phenothiazine derivative, is a sedating antihistamine with antimuscarinic and mild sedative properties.

Mequitazine is used for the symptomatic relief of allergic conditions including urticaria (p.408), rhinitis (p.407) and conjunctivitis (p.406), and in pruritic skin disorders (p.407). It has been given in usual doses of 5 mg twice daily by mouth.

Preparations

Proprietary Preparations (details are given in Part 3)
Aust.: Metaplexan; *Belg.:* Mircol†; *Braz.:* Primasone; *Fr.:* Butix†; Primalan; Quitadrill; *Ger.:* Metaplexan; *Irl.:* Primalan†; *Ital.:* Primalan; *Neth.:* Mircol†; *Port.:* Primalan; *Spain:* Mircol; *Thai.:* Primalan; *UK:* Primalan†.

Methapyrilene (20146-a)

Methapyrilene (BAN, rINN).

Thenylpyramine.   NN-Dimethyl-N'-(2-pyridyl)-N'-(2-thenyl)ethylenediamine.

$C_{14}H_{19}N_3S = 261.4$.
CAS — 91-80-5 (methapyrilene); 33032-12-1 (methapyrilene fumarate); 135-23-9 (methapyrilene hydrochloride).
ATC — R06AC05.

Profile

Methapyrilene, an ethylenediamine derivative, is an antihistamine that was withdrawn following reports of carcinogenicity in *rats*. It was used as the fumarate or the hydrochloride.

Methdilazine (6148-y)

Methdilazine (BAN, rINN).

10-(1-Methylpyrrolidin-3-ylmethyl)phenothiazine.

$C_{18}H_{20}N_2S = 296.4$.
CAS — 1982-37-2.
ATC — R06AD04.

Methdilazine 7.2 mg is equivalent to approximately 8 mg of methdilazine hydrochloride.

Methdilazine Hydrochloride (6149-j)

Methdilazine Hydrochloride (BANM, rINNM).

$C_{18}H_{20}N_2S,HCl = 332.9$.
CAS — 1229-35-2.
Pharmacopoeias. In US.

Pharmacopoeial description

USP 25: A light tan crystalline powder having a slight characteristic odour. Soluble 1 in 2 of water and of alcohol, 1 in 6 of chloroform, and 1 in 1 of 0.1N hydrochloric acid and of 0.1N sodium hydroxide solution; practically insoluble in ether. pH of a 1% solution in water is between 4.8 and 6.0. Store in airtight containers. Protect from light.

Adverse Effects and Precautions

As for the sedating antihistamines in general, p.404.

Interactions

As for the sedating antihistamines in general, p.406.

Uses and Administration

Methdilazine, a phenothiazine derivative, is a sedating antihistamine with antimuscarinic and sedative activity. Methdilazine is also reported to have serotonin-antagonist properties.

Methdilazine hydrochloride is used for the symptomatic relief of hypersensitivity reactions and particularly for the control of pruritic skin disorders (p.407). A dose of 8 mg has been given by mouth 2 to 4 times daily. Children over 3 years of age have been given half the adult dose. Methdilazine base has been used in similar doses.

Preparations

USP 25: Methdilazine Hydrochloride Syrup; Methdilazine Hydrochloride Tablets.

Proprietary Preparations (details are given in Part 3)
Austral.: Dilosyn; *Denm.:* Tacryl; *USA:* Tacaryl†.

Mizolastine (15293-q)

Mizolastine (BAN, rINN).

SL-85.0324-00. 2-{1-[1-(4-Fluorobenzyl)-1H-benzimidazol-2-yl]-4-piperidyl(methyl)amino}pyrimidin-4(1H)-one.

$C_{24}H_{25}FN_6O = 432.5$.
CAS — 108612-45-9.
ATC — R06AX25.

Adverse Effects and Precautions

As for the non-sedating antihistamines in general, p.404. Mizolastine has only a weak potential to prolong the QT interval and has not been associated with arrhythmias. However, the manufacturers have warned against the use of mizolastine in patients with significant cardiac or hepatic disease, with hypokalaemia or other electrolyte imbalance, or with known or suspected QT prolongation. The concomitant administration of drugs liable to interfere with the hepatic metabolism of mizolastine and of other potentially arrhythmogenic drugs should also be avoided (see under Interactions, below).

Interactions

As for the non-sedating antihistamines in general, p.406. Moderate increases in plasma concentrations of mizolastine have been reported following administration of *erythromycin* and *ketoconazole*; the concurrent use of macrolide antibacterials or systemic imidazole antifungals is contra-indicated by the manufacturer. They also advise against the concurrent use of drugs known to prolong the QT interval, such as *class I and III antiarrhythmics*, with mizolastine.

Other potent inhibitors of or substrates for the hepatic metabolism of mizolastine include *cimetidine, ciclosporin*, and *nifedipine*; caution is advised with concurrent administration.

Pharmacokinetics

Mizolastine is rapidly absorbed from the gastrointestinal tract with peak plasma concentrations being reached after about 1.5 hours. Plasma protein binding is about 98%. The mean elimination half-life is about 13 hours. Mizolastine is mainly metabolised by glucuronidation although other metabolic pathways are involved, including metabolism by the cytochrome P450 isoenzyme CYP3A4, with the formation of inactive hydroxylated metabolites.

◊ References.
1. Rosenzweig P, *et al.* Pharmacodynamics and pharmacokinetics of mizolastine (SL 85.0324), a new nonsedative H_1 antihistamine. *Ann Allergy* 1992; **69:** 135–9.
2. Lebrun-Vignes B, *et al.* Clinical pharmacokinetics of mizolastine. *Clin Pharmacokinet* 2001; **40:** 501–7.

Uses and Administration
Mizolastine is a non-sedating antihistamine with a long duration of action. It does not have significant antimuscarinic actions; it is reported to have mast-cell stabilising properties. Mizolastine is used for the symptomatic relief of allergic conditions including rhinitis (p.407), conjunctivitis (p.406), and skin disorders such as urticaria (p.408). The dose, by mouth, is 10 mg daily.

◊ References.
1. Leynadier F, *et al.* Efficacy and safety of mizolastine in seasonal allergic rhinitis. *Ann Allergy Asthma Immunol* 1996; **76:** 163–8.
2. Brostoff J, *et al.* Efficacy of mizolastine, a new antihistamine, compared with placebo in the treatment of chronic idiopathic urticaria. *Allergy* 1996; **51:** 320–5.
3. Stern MA, *et al.* Can an antihistamine delay appearance of hayfever symptoms when given prior to pollen season? *Allergy* 1997; **52:** 440–4.

Preparations
Proprietary Preparations (details are given in Part 3)
Belg.: Mistamine; Mizollen; **Denm.:** Mistamine; Mizollen; **Fin.:** Mizollen; **Fr.:** Mistaline†; Mizollen; **Ger.:** Mizollen; Zolim; **Irl.:** Mistamine; Mizollen; **Ital.:** Mizollen; Zolistam; **Neth.:** Mistalin; Mizollen; **Port.:** Mistamine; Mizollen; Zolistam; **Spain:** Mistamine; Mizolen; Zolistan; **Swed.:** Mistamine; **Switz.:** Mizollen; **UK:** Mistamine; Mizollen.

Niaprazine (13006-j)
Niaprazine *(rINN).*
1709-CERM. *N*-[3-(4-*p*-Fluorophenylpiperazin-1-yl)-1-methylpropyl]nicotinamide.
$C_{20}H_{25}FN_4O = 356.4.$
CAS — 27367-90-4.
ATC — N05CM16.

Profile
Niaprazine, a piperazine derivative, is an antihistamine (p.404) used in children for its sedative and hypnotic properties. The usual dose by mouth is 1 mg per kg body-weight at night.

Preparations
Proprietary Preparations (details are given in Part 3)
Fr.: Nopron; **Ital.:** Nopron.

Olopatadine Hydrochloride (15042-e)
Olopatadine Hydrochloride *(BANM, USAN, pINNM).*
ALO-4943A; KW-4679. 11-[(Z)-3-(Dimethylamino)propylidene]-6,11-dihydrodibenz[b,e]oxepin-2-acetic acid hydrochloride.
$C_{21}H_{23}NO_3,HCl = 373.9.$
CAS — 113806-05-6 (olopatadine); 140462-76-6 (olopatadine hydrochloride).

Adverse Effects and Precautions
As for the antihistamines in general, p.404. Headache and stinging or burning of the eye have occurred after ocular administration.

Uses and Administration
Olopatadine hydrochloride is an antihistamine with mast-cell stabilising properties. It is used twice daily as eye drops containing the equivalent of 0.1% of olopatadine base in the treatment of allergic conjunctivitis (p.406).

◊ References.
1. Anonymous. Olopatadine for allergic conjunctivitis. *Med Lett Drugs Ther* 1997; **39:** 108–9.

Preparations
Proprietary Preparations (details are given in Part 3)
Canad.: Patanol; **Singapore:** Patanol; **Thai.:** Patanol; **USA:** Patanol.

Oxatomide (13056-n)
Oxatomide *(BAN, USAN, rINN).*
R-35443. 1-[3-(4-Benzhydrylpiperazin-1-yl)propyl]benzimidazolin-2-one.
$C_{27}H_{30}N_4O = 426.6.$
CAS — 60607-34-3.
ATC — R06AE06.

Profile
Oxatomide, a piperazine derivative, is a sedating antihistamine (p.404) that has also been reported to have mast-cell stabilising properties. It is used for the symptomatic relief of allergic conditions including urticaria (p.408), rhinitis (p.407), and conjunctivitis (p.406). Oxatomide is given by mouth as the anhydrous substance or as the monohydrate; doses are expressed as the anhydrous substance. The usual dose is 30 mg twice daily. The hydrate has also been applied topically but, as with other antihistamines, there is a risk of sensitisation.

Effects on the CNS. Acute dystonic reactions and long-lasting impaired consciousness were associated with oxatomide therapy in 6 children.[1] Impaired consciousness varied from lethargy and somnolence to a clinical picture resembling encephalitis and persisted for 2 days or more in three patients. Plasma-oxatomide concentrations were measured in three patients and found to be high, although two of these had been given the recommended dose.
1. Casteels-Van Daele M, *et al.* Acute dystonic reactions and long-lasting impaired consciousness associated with oxatomide in children. *Lancet* 1986; **i:** 1204–5.

Preparations
Proprietary Preparations (details are given in Part 3)
Aust.: Tinset; **Belg.:** Tinset; **Fr.:** Tinset; **Ger.:** Tinset†; **Hong Kong:** Tinset; **Ital.:** Tinset; **Mex.:** Tinset; **Neth.:** Tinset; **Port.:** Tinset; **S.Afr.:** Tinset; **Spain:** Cobiona; Oxatokey; Oxleti†; Tanzal; **Thai.:** Tinset.

Oxomemazine (6151-p)
Oxomemazine *(rINN).*
RP-6847; Trimeprazine SS-Dioxide. 10-(3-Dimethylamino-2-methylpropyl)phenothiazine 5,5-dioxide.
$C_{18}H_{22}N_2O_2S = 330.4.$
CAS — 3689-50-7.
ATC — R06AD08.

Oxomemazine Hydrochloride (6152-s)
Oxomemazine Hydrochloride *(rINNM).*
$C_{18}H_{22}N_2O_2S,HCl = 366.9.$
CAS — 4784-40-1.
Pharmacopoeias. In *Fr.*

Oxomemazine hydrochloride 11.1 mg is approximately equivalent to 10 mg of oxomemazine.

Profile
Oxomemazine, a phenothiazine derivative, is a sedating antihistamine (p.404) used for the symptomatic relief of hypersensitivity reactions and in pruritic skin disorders (p.407). It is also an ingredient of compound preparations for the symptomatic treatment of coughs and the common cold (p.406).
Oxomemazine is given by mouth in doses of 10 to 40 mg daily. It may also be administered by the rectal route in doses similar to those used by mouth. Oxomemazine hydrochloride has been used similarly by mouth.

Preparations
Proprietary Preparations (details are given in Part 3)
Belg.: Doxergan; **Fr.:** Rectoplexil†; **Neth.:** Doxergan†.

Multi-ingredient: Aust.: Aplexil; **Belg.:** Rectoplexil; Toplexil; **Braz.:** Expec; Iodesin; Iodeto de Potassium Composto; Iodobec; KI-Expectorante; Toplexil; **Fr.:** Toplexil; **Israel:** Oxacatin; Toplexil; **Neth.:** Toplexil; **Switz.:** Toplexil.

Phenindamine Tartrate (6153-w)
Phenindamine Tartrate *(BANM, USAN, rINNM).*
Phenindamine Acid Tartrate; Phenindamini Tartras; Phenindaminium Tartrate. 1,2,3,4-Tetrahydro-2-methyl-9-phenyl-2-azafluorene hydrogen tartrate; 2,3,4,9-Tetrahydro-2-methyl-9-phenyl-1H-indeno[2,1-c]pyridine hydrogen tartrate.
$C_{19}H_{19}N,C_4H_6O_6 = 411.4.$
CAS — 82-88-2 (phenindamine); 569-59-5 (phenindamine tartrate).
Pharmacopoeias. In *Br.*

Pharmacopoeial description
BP 2001: A white or almost white, odourless or almost odourless, voluminous powder. Sparingly soluble in water; slightly soluble in alcohol; practically insoluble in chloroform and in ether. A 1% solution in water has a pH of 3.4 to 3.9. Protect from light.

Adverse Effects and Precautions
As for the sedating antihistamines in general, p.404. Phenindamine tartrate may have a stimulant effect in certain individuals; to avoid the possibility of insomnia patients may be advised to take the last dose of the day several hours before retiring.

Interactions
As for the sedating antihistamines in general, p.406.

Uses and Administration
Phenindamine, a piperidine derivative, is a sedating antihistamine; however it may be mildly stimulating in certain individuals. It is used as the tartrate for the symptomatic relief of allergic conditions including urticaria (p.408) and rhinitis (p.407), and as an ingredient of compound preparations for coughs and the common cold (p.406).
Phenindamine tartrate is given by mouth in doses of 25 mg every 4 to 6 hours, up to a maximum of 150 mg daily. Children over 6 years of age have been given half these doses.

Preparations
Proprietary Preparations (details are given in Part 3)
Irl.: Thephorin; **UK:** Thephorin†; **USA:** Nolahist.
Multi-ingredient: Braz.: Superhist; **USA:** Nolamine†; P-V-Tussin.

Pheniramine (14746-l)
Pheniramine *(BAN, rINN).*
Prophenpyridamine. NN-Dimethyl-3-phenyl-3-(2-pyridyl)propylamine.
$C_{16}H_{20}N_2 = 240.3.$
CAS — 86-21-5.
ATC — R06AB05.

Pheniramine Aminosalicylate (10013-l)
Pheniramine *p*-Aminosalicylate; Pheniramine 4-Aminosalicylate; Pheniramine Para-aminosalicylate. Pheniramine 4-amino-2-hydroxybenzoate.
$C_{16}H_{20}N_2,C_7H_7NO_3 = 393.5.$
CAS — 3269-83-8.

Pheniramine Maleate (6154-e)
Pheniramine Maleate *(BANM, USAN, rINNM).*
Pheniramini Maleas; Pheniraminium Maleate; Prophenpyridamine Maleate. Pheniramine hydrogen maleate.
$C_{16}H_{20}N_2,C_4H_4O_4 = 356.4.$
CAS — 132-20-7.
Pharmacopoeias. In *Eur.* (see p.vi) and *US.*

Pharmacopoeial description
Ph. Eur.: A white, crystalline powder. Very soluble in water; freely soluble in alcohol, in dichloromethane, and in methyl alcohol. M.p. 106° to 109°. A 1% solution in water has a pH of 4.5 to 5.5. Protect from light.
USP 25: A white crystalline powder having a faint amine-like odour. Soluble in water and in alcohol. pH of a 1% solution in water is between 4.5 and 5.5.

Adverse Effects and Precautions
As for the sedating antihistamines in general, p.404.

Abuse. References to the abuse of pheniramine by mouth.
1. Jones IH, *et al.* Pheniramine as an hallucinogen. *Med J Aust* 1973; **1:** 382–6.
2. Csillag ER, Landauer AA. Alleged hallucinogenic effect of a toxic overdose of an antihistamine preparation. *Med J Aust* 1973; **1:** 653–4.
3. Buckley NA, *et al.* Pheniramine—a much abused drug. *Med J Aust* 1994; **160:** 188–92.

Pregnancy. For discussion of the use of antihistamines, including pheniramine, in pregnancy, see p.405.

Interactions
As for the sedating antihistamines in general, p.406.

Pharmacokinetics
◊ The pharmacokinetics of pheniramine and its metabolites, *N*-desmethylpheniramine and *N*-didesmethylpheniramine, were investigated in 6 healthy subjects.[1] After oral administration of pheniramine aminosalicylate, peak-plasma pheniramine concentrations were reached in 1 to 2.5 hours. The terminal half-life ranged between 8 and 17 hours after intravenous administration (pheniramine maleate) and 16 and 19 hours after oral administration. The total recovery of pheniramine as unchanged drug and metabolites from the urine was 68 to 94% of the intravenous dose and 70 to 83% of the oral dose.
1. Witte PU, *et al.* Pharmacokinetics of pheniramine (Avil®) and metabolites in healthy subjects after oral and intravenous administration. *Int J Clin Pharmacol Ther Toxicol* 1985; **23:** 59–62.

Uses and Administration
Pheniramine, an alkylamine derivative, is a sedating antihistamine with antimuscarinic and moderate sedative properties.
It is used as the maleate for the symptomatic relief of allergic conditions including urticaria and angioedema (p.408), rhinitis (p.407), and conjunctivitis (p.406), and in pruritic skin disorders (p.407). It has also been used for its antiemetic properties in the prevention and control of motion sickness (p.407). Pheniramine maleate is used as an ingredient of compound preparations for the symptomatic treatment of coughs and the common cold (p.406). It is also used in combination with a decongestant in eye and nasal preparations.
Pheniramine maleate is given by mouth in a dose of 15 to 30 mg two or three times daily. In some countries pheniramine maleate has been administered parenterally.
The aminosalicylate, the hydrochloride, and the tannate have also been used.

Preparations
Proprietary Preparations (details are given in Part 3)
Aust.: Avil; **Austral.:** Avil; Fenamine; **Belg.:** Avil†; **Braz.:** Histalerg Profen; **Ger.:** Avil; **Irl.:** Daneral; **Ital.:** Inhiston; **Mex.:** Histatex; **NZ:** Avil; **S.Afr.:** Avil†; **UAE:** Histol; **UK:** Daneral†.

Multi-ingredient: Aust.: Neo Citran; Peremin; **Austral.:** Avil Decongestant; Naphcon-A; **Braz.:** Claril; Gripefin; **Canad.:** Ak-Vernacon; Antitussive Decongestant Antihistamine Syrup; Bronchodex D; Bronchodex Pediatrique†; Bronchosirum†; Caldomine-DH; Calmylin Ace; Centracol DM; Centracol Pediatrique; Citron Chaud; Citron Chaud DM; Cold Decongestant; Diopticon A; Dristan; Hot Lemon; Hot Lemon Relief; Naphcon-A; Neo Citran; Neo Citran A; Neo Citran Calorie Reduced; Neo Citran DM; Opcon-A; Pharmacol DM; Pharminicol DM†; Pulmorphan; Pulmorphan Pediatrique; Robitussin AC; Robitussin with Codeine; Tantacol DM; Triaminic Expectorant DH†; Triaminic†; Triaminicin†; Tri-sulfaminic; Tussaminic C†; Tussaminic DH†; *Fr.*: Fervex; Tri-aminic†; *Ger.*: Konjunktival Thilo; Rhinosovil; *Hong Kong*: Konjunktival; Naphcon-A; *Irl.*: Triominic; *Israel*: Tussosedan; *Ital.*: Medramil†; Nafcon A; Senodin-AN; Tetramil; Triaminic; Triaminicflu; *Mex.*: Solutina; *NZ*: Naphcon-A; *S.Afr.*: Allertac; Calasthetic; Coff-Up; Degoran; Triami†; Triaminic; *Singapore*: Naphcon-A; *Spain*: Triominic†; *Switz.*: Nasello†; Neo Citran; Neo-Urtisan†; *Thai.*: Naphcon-A; *UK*: Triominic†; *USA*: Ak-Con-A†; Dristan Nasal Spray; Iohist D†; Nafazair A; Naphazole-A†; Naphazoline Plus; Naphcon-A; Naphoptic-A; Ocuhist; Opcon-A; Poly-Histine; Poly-Histine D†; Quadra-Hist D†; Rolatuss with Hydrocodone†; Ru-Tuss with Hydrocodone†; S-T Forte†; Scot-Tussin Original 5-Action; Statuss Green†; Tri-P†; Triaminic Expectorant DH†; Triaminic Oral Infant†; Trihist-D†; Tussirex; Vetuss HC†.

Phenyltoloxamine Citrate (6155-l)

Phenyltoloxamine Citrate *(BANM, rINNM)*.

C-5581H (phenyltoloxamine); Phenyltolyloxamine Citrate; PRN (phenyltoloxamine). 2-(2-Benzylphenoxy)-*NN*-dimethylethylamine dihydrogen citrate.

$C_{17}H_{21}NO, C_6H_8O_7 = 447.5$.

CAS — 92-12-6 (phenyltoloxamine); 1176-08-5 (phenyltoloxamine citrate).

Profile

Phenyltoloxamine citrate, a monoethanolamine derivative, is a sedating antihistamine (p.404). It is usually given by mouth in combination preparations with a decongestant or analgesic. Phenyltoloxamine citrate has been used in nasal preparations. Phenyltoloxamine polistirex has also been administered by mouth.

Preparations

Proprietary Preparations (details are given in Part 3)

Multi-ingredient: *Aust.*: Codipront; Codipront cum Expectorans†; *Belg.*: Afebrin; Naldecon; Sinutab; *Canad.*: Omni-Tuss; Sinutab Sinus & Allergy 12 Hour; Tussionex; *Fr.*: Biocidan; Netux; Rinurel; Rinutan; *Ger.*: Codipront; *Hong Kong*: Codipront; Codipront cum Expectorans; Sinutab; *Israel*: Codivis; *Ital.*: Codipront; *Port.*: Codipront; *S.Afr.*: Adco-Sinal Co; Decon†; Dequa-Flu; Pholtex; Sinustop with Codeine†; Sinustop†; Sinutab; Sinutab with Codeine; Suncodin; *Singapore*: Codipront; *Spain*: Codipront; *Switz.*: Codipront; Codipront cum Expectorans; Ergosanol special a la cafeine; Ergosanol special†; *Thai.*: Codipront; *UK*: Sinutab Nightime; *USA*: Aceta-Gesic; Anabar; Conextan LA; Decongestabs†; Decongestant SR†; Decongestant†; Flextra; Iohist D†; Lobac; Magsal; Major-gesic; Menoplex†; Mobigesic; Momentum; Myogesic†; Naldecon†; Nalex-A; Nalgest†; Nalspan Pediatric†; New Decongestant Pediatric†; Norel Plus†; Percogesic; Phenylgesic; Poly-Histine; Poly-Histine D†; Quadra Hist†; Quadra-Hist D†; Tetra-Mag; Tri-Phen-Chlor TR†; Trihist-D†; Uni-Decon†.

Pimethixene (13118-f)

Pimethixene *(rINN)*.

BP-400; Pimetixene. 9-(1-Methyl-4-piperidylidene)thioxanthene.

$C_{19}H_{19}NS = 293.4$.

CAS — 314-03-4.

ATC — R06AX23.

Profile

Pimethixene is reported to be a sedating antihistamine (p.404) and an inhibitor of serotonin. It is given by mouth to children as a sedative and for the treatment of respiratory disorders.

Preparations

Proprietary Preparations (details are given in Part 3)
Braz.: Muricalm; Sonin; *Fr.*: Calmixene; *Switz.*: Sedosil†.

Multi-ingredient: *Braz.*: Santussal.

Piprinhydrinate (6156-y)

Piprinhydrinate *(BAN, rINN)*.

Diphenylpyraline Teoclate; Diphenylpyraline Theoclate. The diphenylpyraline salt of 8-chlorotheophylline ; 4-Benzhydryloxy-1-methylpiperidine salt of 8-chlorotheophylline .

$C_{19}H_{23}NO, C_7H_7ClN_4O_2 = 496.0$.

CAS — 606-90-6.

Profile

Piprinhydrinate, a piperidine derivative, is an antihistamine (p.404) given by mouth as an ingredient of compound preparations for the symptomatic relief of coughs and the common cold.

Preparations

Proprietary Preparations (details are given in Part 3)
Hong Kong: Plokon; *Thai.*: Plokon.

Multi-ingredient: *Aust.*: Influvidon; *Ger.*: Kolton grippale N.

The symbol † denotes a preparation no longer actively marketed

Promethazine (6101-r)

Promethazine *(BAN, rINN)*.

Dimethyl (1-methyl-2-phenothiazin-10-ylethyl)amine.

$C_{17}H_{20}N_2S = 284.4$.

CAS — 60-87-7.

ATC — D04AA10; R06AD02.

Promethazine Hydrochloride (6102-f)

Promethazine Hydrochloride *(BANM, rINNM)*.

Diprazinum; Proazamine Chloride; Promethazini Hydrochloridum; Promethazinium Chloride.

$C_{17}H_{20}N_2S, HCl = 320.9$.

CAS — 58-33-3.

Pharmacopoeias. In Chin., Eur. (see p.vi), Int., Jpn, Pol., and US.

Solutions of promethazine hydrochloride are incompatible with alkaline substances, which precipitate the insoluble promethazine base. Compounds reported to be incompatible with promethazine hydrochloride include aminophylline, barbiturates, benzylpenicillin salts, carbenicillin sodium, chloramphenicol sodium succinate, chlorothiazide sodium, cefmetazole sodium, cefoperazone sodium, cefotetan disodium, dimenhydrinate, doxorubicin hydrochloride (in a liposomal formulation), frusemide [furosemide], heparin sodium, hydrocortisone sodium succinate, meticillin sodium, morphine sulfate, nalbuphine hydrochloride, and some contrast media and parenteral nutrient solutions.

Pharmacopoeial description

Ph. Eur.: A white or faintly yellowish, crystalline powder. Very soluble in water; freely soluble in alcohol and in dichloromethane. A 10% solution in water has a pH of 4.0 to 5.0. Protect from light.

USP 25: A white to faint yellow, practically odourless, crystalline powder. Slowly oxidises and acquires a blue colour on prolonged exposure to air. Freely soluble in water, in hot dehydrated alcohol, and in chloroform; practically insoluble in acetone, in ether, and in ethyl acetate. pH of a 5% solution in water is between 4.0 to 5.0. Store in airtight containers. Protect from light.

Adsorption. References[1-4] to studies of the adsorption of promethazine hydrochloride onto various glass and plastic containers and infusion systems. Factors affecting the degree of adsorption included the particular material tested and the pH of the solution.

1. Kowaluk EA, *et al.* Interactions between drugs and polyvinyl chloride infusion bags. *Am J Hosp Pharm* 1981; **38:** 1308–14.
2. Kowaluk EA, *et al.* Interactions between drugs and intravenous delivery systems. *Am J Hosp Pharm* 1982; **39:** 460–7.
3. Rhodes RS, *et al.* Stability of meperidine hydrochloride, promethazine hydrochloride, and atropine sulfate in plastic syringes. *Am J Hosp Pharm* 1985; **42:** 112–5.
4. Martens HJ, *et al.* Sorption of various drugs in polyvinyl chloride, glass, and polyethylene-lined infusion containers. *Am J Hosp Pharm* 1990; **47:** 369–73.

Promethazine Teoclate (6103-d)

Promethazine Teoclate *(BAN, rINN)*.

Promethazine Theoclate. The promethazine salt of 8-chlorotheophylline .

$C_{17}H_{20}N_2S, C_7H_7ClN_4O_2 = 499.0$.

CAS — 17693-51-5.

Pharmacopoeias. In Br.

Promethazine teoclate 1.5 mg is approximately equivalent to 1 mg of promethazine hydrochloride.

Pharmacopoeial description

BP 2001: A white or almost white, odourless or almost odourless powder. Very slightly soluble in water; sparingly soluble in alcohol; freely soluble in chloroform; practically insoluble in ether. Protect from light.

Adverse Effects

As for the sedating antihistamines in general, p.404.

Cardiovascular side-effects are more commonly seen after injection, and bradycardia, tachycardia, transient minor increases in blood pressure, and occasional hypotension have all been reported with promethazine hydrochloride. Jaundice and blood dyscrasias have been reported, and extrapyramidal effects may occur at high doses.

Venous thrombosis has been reported at the site of intravenous injections, and arteriospasm and gangrene may follow inadvertent intra-arterial injection.

Overdosage. A toxic neurological syndrome which included CNS depression, acute excitomotor manifestations, ataxia and visual hallucinations, plus peripheral antimuscarinic effects developed in 2 children aged 44 months and 16 months after topical application of a 2% promethazine cream providing between 12.9 and 26 mg per kg body-weight.[1] The older child had also received hydroxyzine 10 mg by mouth 1 hour earlier.

1. Shawn DH, McGuigan MA. Poisoning from dermal absorption of promethazine. *Can Med Assoc J* 1984; **130:** 1460–1.

Sudden infant death syndrome. Although some early reports raised the possibility of an association between the use of phenothiazine antihistamines and the sudden infant death syndrome (SIDS) this has not been confirmed. Following an initial report that 4 of 7 infants with SIDS had been given trimeprazine [alimemazine] before death and that a series of severe apnoeic crises had been observed in the twin of a SIDS victim given promethazine,[1] the same workers studied 52 SIDS victims, 36 near-miss infants (those who had experienced severe unexplained episodes of cyanosis or pallor during sleep), and 175 control subjects to investigate the role of nasopharyngitis and phenothiazines in this syndrome.[2] It was found that there was no difference in the incidence of nasopharyngitis between the 3 groups, but that the proportion of infants given phenothiazines was higher in both the SIDS group (23%) and the near-miss group (22%) than in the control group (2%). In a subsequent study,[3] they found that the incidence of central and obstructive sleep apnoeas was increased in 4 healthy infants given promethazine for 3 days, although the duration of the attacks was unaltered and generally short, with a range of 3 to 10 seconds. A report on behalf of the Commission of the European Communities,[4] stated that no link between sudden deaths in infants and drug administration had been confirmed by national drug monitoring centres. It was likely that the risk of apnoea was associated with all sedative drugs, especially in overdose.[4] Previously, phenothiazine-induced hyperthermia had been proposed as a contributory factor in SIDS.[5]

As recently as 1994 concern has been expressed[6] that promethazine was frequently prescribed for children under 2 years despite recommendations to the contrary. The current view in the UK and USA is that phenothiazine antihistamines such as promethazine and trimeprazine [alimemazine] should not be given to children under 2 years of age, primarily because the safety of such use has not been established.

1. Kahn A, Blum D. Possible role of phenothiazines in sudden infant death. *Lancet* 1979; **ii:** 364–5.
2. Kahn A, Blum D. Phenothiazines and sudden infant death syndrome. *Pediatrics* 1982; **70:** 75–8.
3. Kahn A, *et al.* Phenothiazine-induced sleep apneas in normal infants. *Pediatrics* 1985; **75:** 844–7.
4. Cockfield. Phenergan, Theralene, Algotropyl—drugs responsible for the death of new-born babies. *Off J EC* 1986; **29:** C130/25–6.
5. Stanton AN. Sudden infant death syndrome and phenothiazines. *Pediatrics* 1983; **71:** 986–7.
6. Pollard AJ, Rylance G. Inappropriate prescribing of promethazine in infants. *Arch Dis Child* 1994; **70:** 357.

Precautions

As for the sedating antihistamines in general, p.405.

Intravenous injections of promethazine hydrochloride must be given slowly and extreme care must be taken to avoid extravasation or inadvertent intra-arterial injection, due to the risk of severe irritation. Intramuscular injection may be painful, and it should not be given by subcutaneous injection.

False negative and positive results have been reported with some pregnancy tests.

Anaesthesia. In 8 healthy subjects promethazine 25 mg intravenously decreased lower oesophageal sphincter pressure and increased the incidence of gastro-oesophageal reflux.[1] It might, therefore, increase the risk of regurgitation and aspiration of gastric contents during induction of and recovery from anaesthesia. The effect was attributed to the antimuscarinic properties of promethazine.

1. Brock-Utne JG, *et al.* The action of commonly used antiemetics on the lower oesophageal sphincter. *Br J Anaesth* 1978; **50:** 295–8.

Children. A possible association between phenothiazine sedatives and sudden infant death syndrome has been suggested, but has not been confirmed (see under Adverse Effects, above). The current view in the UK and USA is that promethazine should not be given to children under 2 years of age, primarily because the safety of such use has not been established.

Porphyria. Promethazine is considered to be unsafe in patients with porphyria because it has been shown to be porphyrinogenic in *animals* or *in-vitro* systems.

Pregnancy. For discussion of the use of antihistamines in pregnancy, including studies involving phenothiazines, see p.405.

Renal impairment. Phenothiazine-induced toxic psychosis occurred in a patient with chronic renal failure who had been given promethazine.[1]

1. McAllister CJ, *et al.* Toxic psychosis induced by phenothiazine administration in patients with chronic renal failure. *Clin Nephrol* 1978; **10:** 191–5.

Interactions

As for the sedating antihistamines in general, p.406.

Pharmacokinetics

Promethazine is well absorbed after oral or intramuscular administration. Peak plasma concentrations have been observed 2 to 3 hours after administration by these routes, although there is low systemic bioavailability after oral administration, due to high first-pass metabolism in the liver. Promethazine crosses the blood-brain barrier and the placenta, and is distributed into breast milk. Values ranging from 76 to 93% have been reported for plasma-protein binding. Promethazine undergoes extensive metabolism, predominantly to promethazine sulfoxide, and also to N-desmethylpromethazine. It is excreted slowly via the urine and bile, chiefly as metabolites. Elimination half-lives of 5 to 14 hours have been reported.

◊ References.

1. Taylor G, et al. Pharmacokinetics of promethazine and its sulphoxide metabolite after intravenous and oral administration to man. Br J Clin Pharmacol 1983; 15: 287–93.
2. Paton DM, Webster DR. Clinical pharmacokinetics of H₁-receptor antagonists (the antihistamines). Clin Pharmacokinet 1985; 10: 477–97.
3. Stavchansky S, et al. Bioequivalence and pharmacokinetic profile of promethazine hydrochloride suppositories in humans. J Pharm Sci 1987; 76: 441–5.
4. Strenkoski-Nix LC, et al. Pharmacokinetics of promethazine hydrochloride after administration of rectal suppositories and oral syrup to healthy subjects. Am J Health-Syst Pharm 2000; 57: 1499–1505.

Uses and Administration

Promethazine, a phenothiazine derivative, is a sedating antihistamine with antimuscarinic, significant sedative, and some serotonin-antagonist properties. It is usually given as the hydrochloride or teoclate. Promethazine embonate and promethazine maleate have also been administered by mouth. Promethazine dioxide (dioxopromethazine) has been used as the hydrochloride in eye and nose drops. The antihistamine action has been reported to last for between 4 and 12 hours.

Promethazine hydrochloride is used for the symptomatic relief of allergic conditions including urticaria and angioedema (p.408), rhinitis (p.407) and conjunctivitis (p.406), and in pruritic skin disorders (p.407). It may be administered intravenously as an adjunct in the emergency treatment of anaphylactic shock (p.406).

Promethazine hydrochloride and promethazine teoclate are used for their antiemetic action in the prevention and treatment of nausea and vomiting in conditions such as motion sickness, drug-induced vomiting, and postoperative vomiting (p.407). They are also used for the symptomatic treatment of nausea and vertigo caused by Ménière's disease and other vestibular disorders (p.408). Promethazine hydrochloride is also employed pre- and postoperatively in surgery and obstetrics for its sedative effects and for the relief of apprehension (p.406); it is often given in association with pethidine hydrochloride. Promethazine hydrochloride may be used for night-time sedation (p.407).

Promethazine hydrochloride is a common ingredient of compound preparations for the symptomatic treatment of coughs and the common cold (p.406).

The following doses have been given by mouth. For the treatment of allergic conditions promethazine hydrochloride is usually given in a dose of 25 mg at night increased to 25 mg twice daily if necessary; owing to its pronounced sedative effect it is preferably given at night but an alternative dose is 10 to 20 mg two or three times daily. Promethazine hydrochloride is given in doses of 20 to 50 mg at night for the short-term management of insomnia although its prolonged duration of action can lead to considerable drowsiness the following day. For the prevention of motion sickness promethazine hydrochloride can be given in a dose of 20 or 25 mg the night before travelling followed by a similar dose the following morning if necessary. The teoclate is used similarly. For the prevention of motion sickness the dose of promethazine teoclate is 25 mg at night or 25 mg one to two hours before travelling. For nausea and vomiting arising from causes such as labyrinthitis a dose of 25 mg at night is usually adequate; this may be increased to 50 or 75 mg at night or to 25 mg two or three times daily if necessary to a maximum of 100 mg daily.

In children the following oral doses of promethazine hydrochloride have been recommended. For allergic conditions: 2 to 5 years, 5 to 15 mg daily in one or two divided doses; 5 to 10 years, 10 to 25 mg daily in one or two divided doses. For night sedation: 2 to 5 years, 15 to 20 mg; 5 to 10 years, 20 to 25 mg. For the prevention of motion sickness the following doses of promethazine hydrochloride may be given the night before the journey and repeated on the following morning if necessary: 2 to 5 years, 5 mg; 5 to 10 years, 10 mg. Promethazine teoclate may also be given to children aged 5 to 10 years for the prevention of motion sickness in a dose of 12.5 mg daily, starting either on the night before travelling for long journeys or one to two hours before short journeys. Children aged 5 to 10 years may also receive promethazine teoclate for nausea and vomiting from causes such as labyrinthitis in a dose of 12.5 to 37.5 mg daily.

Promethazine hydrochloride is also administered by the rectal route as suppositories. Doses are similar to those given by mouth.

Promethazine hydrochloride is given parenterally by deep intramuscular injection as a solution of 25 or 50 mg per mL. It may also be given by slow intravenous injection or injected into the tubing of a freely running infusion in a concentration of not more than 25 mg per mL, although it is usually diluted to 2.5 mg per mL. The rate of infusion should not exceed 25 mg per minute. The usual parenteral dose for all indications apart from nausea and vomiting is 25 to 50 mg; a dose of 100 mg should not be exceeded. Doses of 12.5 to 25 mg, repeated at intervals of not less than 4 hours, may be given for the treatment of nausea and vomiting, although not more than 100 mg is usually given in 24 hours.

Children aged 5 to 10 years may be given 6.25 to 12.5 mg of promethazine hydrochloride by deep intramuscular injection.

Promethazine has been used topically to provide relief in hypersensitivity disorders of the skin and for burns but, as with other antihistamines, it may produce skin sensitisation.

Sedation. For reference to the use of lytic cocktails of chlorpromazine, promethazine, and pethidine, and the view that alternatives should be considered in children, see under Pethidine, p.76.

Preparations

BP 2001: Promethazine Hydrochloride Tablets; Promethazine Injection; Promethazine Oral Solution; Promethazine Teoclate Tablets;
USP 25: Promethazine Hydrochloride Injection; Promethazine Hydrochloride Suppositories; Promethazine Hydrochloride Syrup; Promethazine Teoclate Tablets.

Proprietary Preparations (details are given in Part 3)
Aust.: Phenergan; *Austral.:* Avomine; Gold Cross Antihistamine Elixir; Insomn-Eze; Phenergan; *Belg.:* Phenergan; *Braz.:* Fenergan; Fenergan Creme; Pamergan; *Canad.:* Histantil; Phenergan; *Denm.:* Phenergan; *Fr.:* Phenergan; *Ger.:* Atosil; Eusedon mono; Promethawern; Proneurin; Prothanon; *Hong Kong:* Avomine; Phenergan; Synvomin; *Irl.:* Avomine†; Phenergan; *Israel:* Prothiazine; *Ital.:* Allerfen; Duplamin†; Fargan; Farganesse; Fenazil; *Neth.:* Phenergan; *Norw.:* Phenergan; *NZ:* Avomine; Goodnight; Phenergan; *Port.:* Fenergan; *S.Afr.:* Avomine; Brunazine; Daralix; Lenazine; Phenergan; Prohist; Promahist†; Receptozine; *Singapore:* Phenergan; Xepagan; *Spain:* Fenergan Topico; Frinova; Sayomol†; *Swed.:* Lergigan; *Switz.:* Phenergan; *Thai.:* Phenergan; *UAE:* Histaloc; *UK:* Avomine; Phenergan; Phenhalal; Q-Mazine†; Sominex; Ziz; *USA:* Anergan; K-Phen†; Pentazine†; Phenameth†; Phenazine†; Phenergan; Phenoject†; Pro†; Promethegan†; Prorex†; Prothazine†.

Multi-ingredient: *Austral.:* Painstop; Panadol Elixir with Promethazine†; Panquil; Phensedyl; Tixylix Nightime; *Belg.:* Phenergan Expectorant†; *Braz.:* Fenergan Expectorante; Lisador; *Canad.:* Phenergan Expectorant with Codeine†; Phenergan Expectorant†; Phenergan VC Expectorant with Codeine†; Phenergan VC Expectorant†; Promatussin DM; *Fr.:* Algotropyl; Fluisedal; Paxeladine Noctee†; Quintopan Enfant†; Rhinathiol Promethazine; Transmer; Tussisedal; *Ger.:* Prothazin; Thesit P; *Hong Kong:* Dhasedyl; Ephedyl; PEC; Rhinathiol Promethazine; Sedilix DM; Tixylix Nightime; Tripe P; *Irl.:* Night Nurse; Tixylix†; *Israel:* Promethazine Expectorants; Prothiazine Expectorant; *Ital.:* Bronconait; Difmetus Compositum; Nuleron; *NZ:* Coldrex Night Relief; Phensedyl Dry Family Cough; Tixylix; *S.Afr.:* Acustop; Antituss†; Ban Pain; Brunacod; Colcaps; Darosed†; Dequa-Coff; Dimiprol†; Dynapayne; Go-Pain; Goldgesic; Histodor; Infapain Forte; Lenazine Forte; Lentogesic†; Lesspain†; Maxadol; Megapyn; Painagon; Pedigesic†; Pedpain; Phenergan†; Phensedyl; Propain; Pynmed; Salterpyn; Stilpane; Stopayne; Synaleve†; Tenston; Tixylix; Vacudol; Xeramax; *Singapore:* Delix; Dhasedyl; Dhasedyl DM; PCL; Phensedyl; Procodin; Phensedyl; Rhinathiol Promethazine; Sedilix; Sedilix DM; Unisedyl; Walsedyl; *Spain:* Actithiol Antihist; Antihemorroidal; Fenergan

Expectorante; Psicosoma Solucion; Sugarceton†; *Swed.:* Lergigan comp; *Switz.:* Broncatar; Linervidol; Lysedil; Lysedil compositum; Nardyl; Phenergan Expectorant; Rectoquintyl-Promethazine; Rhinathiol Promethazine; *Thai.:* Conadyl; Decos; Nordyl; Nortuss; Phencodin; Phensedyl; Teradyl; *UAE:* Flukit; *UK:* Medised; Night Nurse; Pamergan P100; Phensedyl Plus; Ronpirin Cold Remedy; Tixylix Night-Time; *USA:* Mepergan; Pentazine VC with Codeine; Phenameth DM; Phenergan VC; Phenergan VC with Codeine; Phenergan with Codeine; Phenergan with Dextromethorphan; Pherazine DM; Pherazine VC; Pherazine VC with Codeine; Pherazine with Codeine; Prometh VC Plain; Prometh with Dextromethorphan; Promethazine VC with Codeine; Promethist with Codeine†.

Propiomazine Hydrochloride (6158-z)

Propiomazine Hydrochloride (BANM, rINNM).
Wy-1359 (propiomazine). 1-[10-(2-Dimethylaminopropyl)phenothiazin-2-yl]propan-1-one hydrochloride.
$C_{20}H_{24}N_2OS,HCl = 376.9$.
CAS — 362-29-8 (propiomazine); 1240-15-9 (propiomazine hydrochloride).

NOTE. Propiomazine is USAN.

Propiomazine Maleate (6159-c)

Propiomazine Maleate (BANM, rINNM).
Propiomazine Hydrogen Maleate.
$C_{20}H_{24}N_2OS,C_4H_4O_4 = 456.6$.
CAS — 3568-23-8.

Propiomazine maleate 1.3 mg is approximately equivalent to 1 mg of propiomazine and 1.1 mg of propiomazine hydrochloride.

Adverse Effects and Precautions

As for the sedating antihistamines in general, p.404. Local irritation may occur at the site of intravenous injection of propiomazine hydrochloride and there may be thrombophlebitis.

Interactions

As for the sedating antihistamines in general, p.406.

Uses and Administration

Propiomazine, a phenothiazine derivative, is a sedating antihistamine used for its sedative and antiemetic properties in insomnia (p.407) and nausea and vomiting (p.407).

The maleate is given by mouth as a hypnotic in doses equivalent to 25 to 50 mg of the base at night.

Propiomazine hydrochloride has also been given by intramuscular or slow intravenous injection in doses ranging from 10 to 40 mg for anaesthetic premedication and during surgical and obstetric procedures (p.406). Children weighing up to 27 kg have been given 0.55 to 1.1 mg per kg body-weight intramuscularly or intravenously. Alternatively, those aged 2 to 4 years have been given 10 mg; 4 to 6 years, 15 mg; 6 to 12 years, 25 mg.

Preparations

Proprietary Preparations (details are given in Part 3)
Swed.: Propavan; *USA:* Largon†.

Setastine Hydrochloride (5686-p)

Setastine Hydrochloride (rINNM).
EGYT-2062. 1-{2-[(p-Chloro-α-methyl-α-phenylbenzyl)oxy]-ethyl}hexahydro-1H-azepine hydrochloride.
$C_{22}H_{28}ClNO,HCl = 394.4$.
CAS — 64294-95-7 (setastine).

Profile

Setastine hydrochloride, a derivative of clemastine, is an antihistamine (p.404) claimed to have no sedative activity. It is given by mouth for the symptomatic relief of hypersensitivity disorders in doses of up to 6 mg daily.

Preparations

Proprietary Preparations (details are given in Part 3)
Hung.: Loderix.

Terfenadine (13308-v)

Terfenadine (BAN, USAN, rINN).
MDL-9918; RMI-9918; Terfenadinum. 1-(4-tert-Butylphenyl)-4-[4-(α-hydroxybenzhydryl)piperidino]butan-1-ol.
$C_{32}H_{41}NO_2 = 471.7$.
CAS — 50679-08-8.
ATC — R06AX12.
Pharmacopoeias. In Eur. (see p.vi).

Pharmacopoeial description

Ph. Eur.: A white, crystalline powder. It shows polymorphism. Very slightly soluble in water and in dilute hydrochloric acid; freely soluble in dichloromethane; soluble in methyl alcohol. Protect from light.

Adverse Effects and Precautions

As for the non-sedating antihistamines in general, p.404. Erythema multiforme and galactorrhoea have also been reported.
Ventricular arrhythmias, including torsade de pointes, have occurred rarely with terfenadine, particularly in association with

raised blood concentrations (see Arrhythmias, below). To *reduce the risk* of developing such arrhythmias the recommended dose should **not** be exceeded and terfenadine should be **avoided** in patients with cardiac or significant hepatic disease, with hypokalaemia or other electrolyte imbalance, or with known or suspected prolonged QT interval. The concomitant administration of drugs liable to interfere with the hepatic metabolism of terfenadine, of other potentially antiarrhythmic drugs including those that prolong the QT interval, and of drugs likely to cause electrolyte imbalance is **contra-indicated** (see under Interactions, below). If palpitations, dizziness, syncope, or convulsions occur terfenadine should be withdrawn and the patient investigated for potential arrhythmias.

Alopecia. Hair loss was associated with terfenadine treatment in a 24-year-old patient.[1] Regrowth occurred when treatment was stopped.

1. Jones SK, Morley WN. Terfenadine causing hair loss. *BMJ* 1985; **291:** 940.

Arrhythmias. Ventricular arrhythmias including torsade de pointes have occurred at doses greater than those recommended[1] and also at normal doses in patients whose metabolism of terfenadine is impaired by drugs or by liver disease. Generalised convulsions and a quinine-like effect on the ECG have also been reported after a presumed overdose of terfenadine.[2] Consequently a number of recommendations have been made to *reduce the risk* of developing serious arrhythmias, including those from the UK Committee on Safety of Medicines[3,4] (see Adverse Effects and Precautions, above, for details). Terfenadine should be discontinued immediately, and the patient evaluated for potential arrhythmias, in those who experience syncope, palpitations, dizziness, or convulsions after taking terfenadine.

Studies[5] have suggested that the ventricular arrhythmias are due to terfenadine itself rather than its active metabolite fexofenadine (p.417). Terfenadine has been shown to inhibit cardiac potassium channels which results in prolongation of the QT interval, a risk factor for developing arrhythmias, while the non-sedating antihistamines cetirizine, fexofenadine, and loratadine have had no demonstrable effect[5,6] (see also p.405).

1. MacConnell TJ, Stanners AJ. Torsades de pointes complicating treatment with terfenadine. *BMJ* 1991; **302:** 1469.
2. Davies AJ, *et al.* Cardiotoxic effect with convulsions in terfenadine overdose. *BMJ* 1989; **298:** 325.
3. Committee on Safety of Medicines. Ventricular arrhythmias due to terfenadine and astemizole. *Current Problems 35* 1992.
4. Committee on Safety of Medicines/Medicines Control Agency. Drug-induced prolongation of the QT interval. *Current Problems* 1996; **22:** 2.
5. Woolsey RL, *et al.* Mechanism of the cardiotoxic actions of terfenadine. *JAMA* 1993; **269:** 1532–6.
6. Rankin AC. Non-sedating antihistamines and cardiac arrhythmia. *Lancet* 1997; **350:** 1115–16.

Effects on the liver. Three episodes of acute hepatitis with jaundice occurred in a patient taking terfenadine intermittently over a period of 17 months.[1] Liver function tests returned to normal after interruption of drug administration. Two further cases[2] of cholestatic hepatitis associated with terfenadine administration have been reported. Again, liver function tests returned to normal after drug withdrawal. A study[3] by the Boston Collaborative Drug Surveillance Program of 210 683 patients who had received prescriptions for terfenadine concluded that the use of terfenadine was rarely associated with important idiopathic liver disease. The investigators found only 3 cases of acute liver disease where a causal connection to terfenadine could not be ruled out; all these patients had received a concomitant hepatotoxic drug and had made a full recovery.

1. Larrey D, *et al.* Terfenadine and hepatitis. *Ann Intern Med* 1985; **103:** 634.
2. Sahai A, Villeneuve JP. Terfenadine-induced cholestatic hepatitis. *Lancet* 1996; **348:** 552–3.
3. Myers MW, Jick H. Terfenadine and risk of acute liver disease. *Br J Clin Pharmacol* 1998; **46:** 251–3.

Effects on the nervous system. Non-sedating effects on the CNS have been reported after a single dose of terfenadine;[1] these have included anxiety, palpitations, and insomnia. The UK manufacturers commented that clinical studies suggest that the incidence of such effects is similar to that seen after placebo.[2]

Workers who had described a generalised tonic-clonic seizure in a patient taking terfenadine[3] later reported that the patient had subsequently had a second unprovoked seizure[4] and now considered that terfenadine may not have been the cause of his original seizure. Convulsions have been reported following overdose with terfenadine (see under Arrhythmias, above).

The sedative effects of the older antihistamines and the lack of such effects with the non-sedating antihistamines including terfenadine are discussed under Sedation on p.405.

1. Napke E, Biron P. Nervous reactions after first dose of terfenadine in adults. *Lancet* 1989; **ii:** 615–16.
2. Masheter HC. Nervous reactions to terfenadine. *Lancet* 1989; **ii:** 1034.
3. Tidswell P, d'Assis-Fonseca A. Generalised seizure due to terfenadine. *BMJ* 1993; **307:** 241.
4. Tidswell P, d'Assis-Fonseca A. Generalised seizure due to terfenadine. *BMJ* 1993; **307:** 736.

Hypersensitivity. Terfenadine administration was associated with 108 reports of skin reactions, including rashes, urticaria,

---

angioedema, photosensitivity reactions and peeling of the skin of the hands or feet.[1]

1. Stricker BHCh, *et al.* Skin reactions to terfenadine. *BMJ* 1986; **293:** 536.

Porphyria. Terfenadine has been associated with acute attacks of porphyria and is considered unsafe in porphyric patients.

Interactions

As for the non-sedating antihistamines in general, p.406.

Terfenadine should not be given with drugs that inhibit its hepatic metabolism because of the increased risk of serious ventricular arrhythmias. These drugs include the *triazole* and *imidazole antifungals* such as *itraconazole* and *ketoconazole*, the *macrolide antibacterials* including *clarithromycin*, *erythromycin*, *josamycin*, and *troleandomycin*, the streptogramin antibacterial *quinupristin/dalfopristin*, the serotonin reuptake inhibitors *citalopram*, *fluoxetine*, *fluvoxamine*, *nefazodone*, and *paroxetine*, the HIV-protease inhibitors *indinavir*, *nelfinavir*, *ritonavir*, and *saquinavir*, the non-nucleoside reverse transcriptase inhibitor antiretroviral *efavirenz*, and *zileuton*. The metabolism of terfenadine may also be inhibited by grapefruit juice and concomitant use should be avoided.

Concomitant administration with other potentially arrhythmogenic drugs (including those that prolong the QT interval) such as *antiarrhythmics*, *tricyclic antidepressants*, the antimalarials *halofantrine* and *quinine*, *antipsychotics*, *cisapride*, *probucol*, *pentamidine isetionate*, and the beta blocker *sotalol* should be avoided as should co-administration of *diuretics* that cause electrolyte imbalances especially hypokalaemia. The use of terfenadine and *astemizole* together is not recommended.

◊ General references.

1. Kivistö KT, *et al.* Inhibition of terfenadine metabolism: pharmacokinetic and pharmacodynamic consequences. *Clin Pharmacokinet* 1994; **27:** 1–5.

Antibacterials. Pharmacokinetic studies have demonstrated that the macrolide antibiotics *erythromycin*[1] and *clarithromycin*[2] interfere with the metabolism of terfenadine leading to its accumulation. A high plasma-terfenadine concentration is associated with prolongation of the QT interval, and arrhythmias such as torsade de pointes have been reported in patients treated with therapeutic doses of terfenadine and erythromycin[3] or troleandomycin.[4]

1. Honig PK, *et al.* Changes in the pharmacokinetics and electrocardiographic pharmacodynamics of terfenadine with concomitant administration of erythromycin. *Clin Pharmacol Ther* 1992; **52:** 231–8.
2. Honig P, *et al.* Effect of erythromycin, clarithromycin and azithromycin on the pharmacokinetics of terfenadine. *Clin Pharmacol Ther* 1993; **53:** 161.
3. Biglin KE, *et al.* Drug-induced torsades de pointes: a possible interaction of terfenadine and erythromycin. *Ann Pharmacother* 1994; **28:** 282.
4. Fournier P, *et al.* Une nouvelle cause de torsades de pointes: association terfenadine et troleandomycine. *Ann Cardiol Angeiol (Paris)* 1993; **42:** 249–52.

Antidepressants. Cardiac abnormalities have been reported in 2 patients taking *fluoxetine* and terfenadine concomitantly.[1,2] Similarly, the co-administration of *nefazodone* and terfenadine has resulted in prolongation of the QT interval.[3]

1. Swims MP. Potential terfenadine-fluoxetine interaction. *Ann Pharmacother* 1993; **27:** 1404–5.
2. Marchiando RJ, Cook MD. Probable terfenadine-fluoxetine-associated cardiac toxicity. *Ann Pharmacother* 1995; **29:** 937–8.
3. Abernethy DR, *et al.* Loratadine and terfenadine interaction with nefazodone: both antihistamines associated with QTc prolongation. *Clin Pharmacol Ther* 2001; **69:** 96–103.

Antiepileptics. For reference to an interaction between terfenadine and *carbamazepine*, see p.345.

Antifungals. Pharmacokinetic studies have demonstrated that *itraconazole*[1] and *ketoconazole*[2] interfere with the metabolism of terfenadine leading to its accumulation. A high plasma-terfenadine concentration is associated with prolongation of the QT interval, and arrhythmias such as torsade de pointes have been reported in patients treated with therapeutic doses of terfenadine and ketoconazole[3] or itraconazole.[1,4] While there has been a pharmacokinetic study[5] that suggested that the interaction between terfenadine and *fluconazole* might not be clinically significant, as the mechanism of the interaction appeared to involve the metabolite of terfenadine and did not lead to accumulation of the cardiotoxic parent compound, this may not always be the case. Studies in a small group of patients who exhibited abnormal patterns of terfenadine metabolism demonstrated increases in terfenadine concentrations associated with ECG abnormalities when terfenadine was administered with high doses of fluconazole.[6]

1. Pohjola-Sintonen S, *et al.* Itraconazole prevents terfenadine metabolism and increases risk of torsades de pointes ventricular tachycardia. *Eur J Clin Pharmacol* 1993; **45:** 191–3.
2. Honig PK, *et al.* Terfenadine-ketoconazole interaction: pharmacokinetic and electrocardiographic consequences. *JAMA* 1993; **269:** 1513–18.
3. Monahan BP, *et al.* Torsades de pointes occurring in association with terfenadine use. *JAMA* 1990; **264:** 2788–90.
4. Crane JK, *et al.* Syncope and cardiac arrhythmia due to an interaction between itraconazole and terfenadine. *Am J Med* 1993; **95:** 445–6.
5. Honig PK, *et al.* The effect of fluconazole on the steady-state pharmacokinetics and electrocardiographic pharmacodynamics of terfenadine in humans. *Clin Pharmacol Ther* 1993; **53:** 630–6.
6. Cantilena LR, *et al.* Fluconazole alters terfenadine pharmacokinetics and electrocardiographic pharmacodynamics. *Clin Pharmacol Ther* 1995; **57:** 185.

Calcium-channel blockers. For reference to an interaction between terfenadine and *nifedipine*, see p.942.

Grapefruit juice. A study[1] in healthy subjects given terfenadine and *grapefruit juice* concomitantly for 7 days demonstrated raised plasma-terfenadine concentrations and prolongation of the QT interval. These effects were less pronounced when terfenadine was administered 2 hours before grapefruit juice, but were nevertheless quantifiable in some subjects. In another study QT interval changes were not found in healthy subjects given single doses of terfenadine and grapefruit juice.[2] However the highly variable pharmacokinetics between individuals led the authors to conclude that prolongation of the QT interval was possible following single doses. The probable mechanism of the interaction is inhibition of the metabolism of terfenadine by the cytochrome P450 isoenzyme CYP3A4, although the component of grapefruit juice responsible is as yet unknown.

1. Benton RE, *et al.* Grapefruit juice alters terfenadine pharmacokinetics, resulting in prolongation of repolarization on the electrocardiogram. *Clin Pharmacol Ther* 1996; **59:** 383–8.
2. Rau SE, *et al.* Grapefruit juice-terfenadine single-dose interaction: magnitude, mechanism, and relevance. *Clin Pharmacol Ther* 1997; **61:** 401–9.

Pharmacokinetics

Terfenadine is rapidly absorbed from the gastrointestinal tract; peak plasma concentrations are achieved within about 2 hours. It is a prodrug and undergoes extensive first-pass metabolism in the liver to its active metabolite the carboxylic acid derivative fexofenadine (p.417). The other main metabolite is an inactive piperidine-carbinol derivative. About 97% of terfenadine is bound to plasma proteins; fexofenadine is reported to be less extensively bound. Terfenadine does not appear to cross the blood-brain barrier to a significant extent; limited amounts of fexofenadine, but not the parent drug, have been detected in breast milk. An elimination half-life of 16 to 23 hours has been reported for terfenadine. The metabolites, and traces of unchanged drug, are excreted in the urine and the faeces.

◊ References.

1. Eller MG, *et al.* Pharmacokinetics of terfenadine in healthy elderly subjects. *J Clin Pharmacol* 1992; **32:** 267–71.
2. Lucas BD, *et al.* Terfenadine pharmacokinetics in breast milk in lactating women. *Clin Pharmacol Ther* 1995; **57:** 398–402.

Uses and Administration

Terfenadine, a piperidine derivative, is a non-sedating antihistamine. It does not have significant antimuscarinic actions. It is used for the symptomatic relief of allergic conditions including rhinitis (p.407) and conjunctivitis (p.406) and skin disorders such as urticaria (p.408).

The maximum adult dose of terfenadine is 120 mg daily by mouth given either as 60 mg twice daily or 120 mg in the morning; a starting dose of 60 mg daily in a single dose or in two divided doses is recommended for rhinitis and conjunctivitis. Half the usual daily dose has been suggested for patients with significantly impaired renal function. Children who are over 12 years of age and weigh more than 50 kg may receive the usual adult dosage.

◊ Reviews.

1. McTavish D, *et al.* Terfenadine: an updated review of its pharmacological properties and therapeutic efficacy. *Drugs* 1990; **39:** 552–74.

Preparations

BP 2001: Terfenadine Oral Suspension; Terfenadine Tablets.

Proprietary Preparations (details are given in Part 3)

Aust.: Terlane; Triludan; ***Austral.:*** Teldane; ***Belg.:*** Triludan; ***Braz.:*** Fenasil; Histadane; Pridinol; Teldane; ***Canad.:*** Allergy Relief†; Contac Allergy Formula†; Seldane†; ***Denm.:*** Teldanex; ***Fin.:*** Teldanex; ***Fr.:*** Teldane†; ***Ger.:*** Balkis Spezial†; Fomos†; Hisfedin; Histaterfen†; Logomed Allergie-Tabletten†; Teldane; Terfedura; Terfemundin; Terfium†; Vividrin mit Terfenadin†; ***Hong Kong:*** Histafen; Tamagon; Teldane; ***Irl.:*** Triludan; ***Israel:*** Apoterfin; Ternalin; ***Ital.:*** Allerplus†; Allerzil; Teldane†; Triludan†; ***Mex.:*** Teldane†; ***Neth.:*** Triludan; Norw.: Teldanex; ***Port.:*** Triludan; ***S.Afr.:*** Fendin; Terfenor; Triludan; ***Spain:*** Aldira; Alergist; Cyater; Rapidal; Ternadin; Triludan†; ***Swed.:*** Teldanex; Terfex†; ***Switz.:*** Teldane†; Triludan†; ***Thai.:*** Centerfen; Fenason; Servinadine; Tamagon; Teranic; Terden; Terdine; Terfadine; Terfegen; Terfen; Trexyl; ***UK:*** Aller-eze Clear†; Antihistamine Forte; Boots Hayfever Relief Antihistamine; Histafen; Seldane†; Terfenor Antihistamine; Terfex†; Triludan†; ***USA:*** Seldane†.

Multi-ingredient: ***Aust.:*** Teldafed†; ***Belg.:*** Teldafen†; ***Braz.:*** Teldafen; ***Israel:*** Ternalin-D; ***Port.:*** Trilufen†; ***USA:*** Seldane-D†.

Thenyldiamine Hydrochloride (6165-j)

Thenyldiamine Hydrochloride (*BANM, rINNM*).

Thenyldiaminium Chloride. NN-Dimethyl-N′-(2-pyridyl)-N′-(3-thenyl)ethylenediamine hydrochloride.

$C_{14}H_{19}N_3S,HCl = 297.8$.

CAS — 91-79-2 (thenyldiamine); 958-93-0 (thenyldiamine hydrochloride).

Profile

Thenyldiamine hydrochloride, an ethylenediamine derivative, is an antihistamine (p.404). It is given by mouth as an ingredient of compound preparations for the symptomatic treatment of coughs and the common cold.

The symbol † denotes a preparation no longer actively marketed

Preparations

Proprietary Preparations (details are given in Part 3)
Multi-ingredient: *Braz.:* Asafen; *Ital.:* NTR; *Spain:* Sinefricol.

Thiazinamium Metilsulfate (6166-z)

Thiazinamium Metilsulfate (rINN).

Methylpromethazinium Methylsulfuricum; Thiazinamium Methylsulphate; Wy-460E (thiazinamium chloride). Trimethyl[1-methyl-2-(phenothiazin-10-yl)ethyl]ammonium methyl sulphate.
$C_{19}H_{26}N_2O_4S_2 = 410.6$.
CAS — 2338-21-8 (thiazinamium); 4320-13-2 (thiazinamium chloride); 58-34-4 (thiazinamium metilsulfate).

NOTE. Thiazinamium Chloride is *USAN.*
Pharmacopoeias. In *Fr.*

Profile

Thiazinamium metilsulfate, a phenothiazine derivative, is an antihistamine (p.404) that has been given in combination preparations for respiratory-tract disorders.

Thiethylperazine (17248-a)

Thiethylperazine (BAN, USAN, rINN).

2-Ethylthio-10-[3-(4-methylpiperazin-1-yl)-propyl]phenothiazine.
$C_{22}H_{29}N_3S_2 = 399.6$.
CAS — 1420-55-9.
ATC — R06AD03.

Thiethylperazine Malate (7110-q)

Thiethylperazine Malate (BANM, rINNM).
$C_{22}H_{29}N_3S_2,2C_4H_6O_5 = 667.8$.
CAS — 52239-63-1.

Thiethylperazine malate 10.53 mg is approximately equivalent to 6.3 mg of thiethylperazine.

Thiethylperazine Maleate (7111-p)

Thiethylperazine Maleate (BANM, USAN, rINNM).
GS-95; NSC-130044; Thiethylperazine Dimaleate.
$C_{22}H_{29}N_3S_2,2C_4H_4O_4 = 631.8$.
CAS — 1179-69-7.
Pharmacopoeias. In *Fr., Swiss,* and *US.*

Thiethylperazine maleate 10 mg is approximately equivalent to 6.3 mg of thiethylperazine.

Pharmacopoeial description

USP 25: A yellowish granular powder, odourless or has not more than a slight odour. Soluble 1 in 1700 of water and 1 in 530 of alcohol; practically insoluble in chloroform and in ether; slightly soluble in methyl alcohol. pH of a 0.1% solution in water is between 2.8 and 3.8. Store in airtight containers. Protect from light.

Incompatibility.

Incompatibility has been reported between injections of thiethylperazine maleate and nalbuphine hydrochloride.[1]

1. Jump WG, *et al.* Compatibility of nalbuphine hydrochloride with other preoperative medications. *Am J Hosp Pharm* 1982; **39:** 841–3.

Adverse Effects and Precautions

As for the sedating antihistamines in general, p.404.

Interactions

As for the sedating antihistamines in general, p.406.

Uses and Administration

Thiethylperazine, a phenothiazine derivative with a piperazine side-chain, is a sedating antihistamine used as an antiemetic for the control of nausea and vomiting (p.407) associated with surgical procedures and cancer therapy. It has also been used for the management of vertigo (p.408) and motion sickness although there is some doubt over its efficacy for these indications.

Thiethylperazine is given in usual doses of 10 mg of the *maleate* up to three times daily by mouth; the maleate has also been given rectally. Where oral administration is impractical similar doses of the *malate* may be given by deep intramuscular injection.

Reduced doses of phenothiazines may be required in elderly patients. Thiethylperazine is not recommended for use in children.

Preparations

USP 25: Thiethylperazine Maleate Suppositories; Thiethylperazine Maleate Tablets.

Proprietary Preparations (details are given in Part 3)
Aust.: Torecan; *Ger.:* Torecan; *Ital.:* Torecan; *Mex.:* Torecan; *Neth.:* Torecan†; *Spain:* Torecan; *Swed.:* Torecan; *Switz.:* Torecan; *USA:* Norzine†; Torecan.

Thonzylamine Hydrochloride (6167-c)

Thonzylamine Hydrochloride (BANM, USAN, rINNM).

N-p-Anisyl-N'N'-dimethyl-N-(pyrimidin-2-yl)ethylenediamine hydrochloride.
$C_{16}H_{22}N_4O,HCl = 322.8$.
CAS — 91-85-0 (thonzylamine); 63-56-9 (thonzylamine hydrochloride).

Profile

Thonzylamine hydrochloride, an ethylenediamine derivative, is an antihistamine (p.404) given for the symptomatic relief of hypersensitivity disorders in doses of 50 to 100 mg daily by mouth; a 1% nasal solution and 2.5% ointment are also available. As with other antihistamines, there is a risk of skin sensitisation with the ointment.

Preparations

Proprietary Preparations (details are given in Part 3)
Ital.: Tonamil.

Multi-ingredient: *Ital.:* Ascotodin; Collirio Alfa Antistaminico; Imidazyl Antistaminico; Iristamina; Narlisim; Pupilla Antistaminico; *Port.:* Narizima; *Spain:* Normo Nar.

Tolpropamine Hydrochloride (6168-k)

Tolpropamine Hydrochloride (BANM, rINNM).

NN-Dimethyl-3-phenyl-3-p-tolylpropylamine hydrochloride.
$C_{18}H_{23}N,HCl = 289.8$.
CAS — 5632-44-0 (tolpropamine); 3339-11-5 (tolpropamine hydrochloride).

Profile

Tolpropamine hydrochloride, an alkylamine derivative, is an antihistamine (p.404). It has been used topically for the symptomatic relief of hypersensitivity and pruritic skin disorders although, as with other antihistamines, there is a risk of skin sensitisation.

Preparations

Proprietary Preparations (details are given in Part 3)
Aust.: Pragman.

Trimeprazine Tartrate (6169-a)

Trimeprazine Tartrate (BANM).

Alimemazine Tartrate (BANM, rINNM). NN-Dimethyl-2-methyl-3-(phenothiazin-10-yl)propylamine tartrate.
$(C_{18}H_{22}N_2S)_2,C_4H_6O_6 = 747.0$.
CAS — 84-96-8 (trimeprazine [alimemazine]); 4330-99-8 (trimeprazine [alimemazine] tartrate).
Pharmacopoeias. In *Br., Fr., Jpn,* and *US.*

Trimeprazine [alimemazine] tartrate 25 mg is approximately equivalent to 20 mg of trimeprazine [alimemazine].

Pharmacopoeial description

BP 2001: A white or slightly cream, odourless or almost odourless powder. It darkens on exposure to light. Freely soluble in water and in chloroform; sparingly soluble in alcohol; very slightly soluble in ether. A 2% solution in water has a pH of 5.0 to 6.5. Protect from light.

USP 25: A white to off-white, odourless, crystalline powder. Soluble 1 in 2 of water, 1 in 20 of alcohol, 1 in 5 of chloroform, and 1 in 1800 of ether; very slightly soluble in benzene. Store in airtight containers. Protect from light.

Adverse Effects and Precautions

As for the sedating antihistamines in general, p.404.

Children. There have been reports of adverse effects in children given trimeprazine [alimemazine] tartrate by mouth. Fatal malignant hyperthermia[1] and severe cardiovascular depression[2] have occurred after its use for premedication, and severe respiratory and CNS depression[3] after use as a postoperative sedative. Doses in these 3 reports ranged from 2.4 to 4.4 mg per kg body-weight. A possible association between phenothiazine sedatives and sudden infant death syndrome has also been suggested, but has not been confirmed (see Promethazine Hydrochloride, p.423). Trimeprazine [alimemazine] tartrate is no longer licensed in the UK for short-term sedation in children and it is recommended that it should not be used in infants less than 2 years of age. The maximum recommended dose for premedication for children aged 2 to 7 years is 2 mg per kg body-weight by mouth. There has been a warning[4] that the use of trimeprazine [alimemazine] for deep sedation in diagnostic and therapeutic procedures in children is associated with prolonged drowsiness and that standards of monitoring, starvation, and postprocedural care should be similar to those with general anaesthesia.

1. Moyes DG. Malignant hyperpyrexia caused by trimeprazine. *Br J Anaesth* 1973; **45:** 1163–4.
2. Loan WB, Cuthbert D. Adverse cardiovascular response to oral trimeprazine in children. *BMJ* 1985; **290:** 1548–9.
3. Mann NP. Trimeprazine and respiratory depression. *Arch Dis Child* 1981; **56:** 481–2.
4. Cray SH, Hinton W. Sedation for investigations: prolonged effect of chloral and trimeprazine. *Arch Dis Child* 1994; **71:** 179.

Pregnancy. For a discussion of the use of antihistamines in pregnancy, including studies involving phenothiazines, see p.405.

Interactions

As for the sedating antihistamines in general, p.406.

Uses and Administration

Trimeprazine [alimemazine], a phenothiazine derivative, is a sedating antihistamine with antiemetic activity and pronounced sedative effects. It also has some antimuscarinic actions. It is used mainly for the relief of urticaria (p.408) and pruritus (p.407), and, in the UK, for pre-operative medication in children. Trimeprazine [alimemazine] may also be used in compound preparations for the symptomatic treatment of coughs (p.406).

Trimeprazine [alimemazine] tartrate is administered by mouth; doses in the UK are given as the amount of trimeprazine [alimemazine] tartrate; those in the USA are expressed in terms of the equivalent amount of trimeprazine [alimemazine]. Even allowing for this, lower doses are used in the USA. The adult dose of trimeprazine [alimemazine] tartrate used for the relief of **urticaria** and **pruritus** in the *UK* is 10 mg two or three times daily; up to 100 mg daily has been given in refractory cases. Elderly patients are given 10 mg once or twice daily and children over 2 years of age 2.5 to 5 mg three or four times daily. In the *USA* the adult dose is the equivalent of trimeprazine [alimemazine] 2.5 mg four times daily, or 5 mg twice daily as a modified-release preparation. Children in the USA between 2 and 3 years of age have been given 1.25 mg at night or three times daily; for older children this dose has been increased to 2.5 mg.

The usual recommended dose for **premedication** in children over 2 years is up to 2 mg per kg body-weight given by mouth about one to two hours before the operation.

Anaesthesia. Trimeprazine [alimemazine] tartrate may be used for anaesthetic premedication (see p.406) in children when the oral route of administration is preferred to the more usual parenteral route of other phenothiazine antihistamines. Adverse effects have, however, been reported in children (see under Adverse Effects and Precautions, above), and in the UK trimeprazine [alimemazine] tartrate is not licensed for use in infants less than 2 years of age.

Insomnia. Antihistamines such as trimeprazine [alimemazine] tartrate have been used as alternatives to benzodiazepines for the treatment of insomnia (p.407), particularly for children. However, they are only indicated for short-term use, and antimuscarinic side-effects may prove troublesome.

Regimens involving a short course of trimeprazine [alimemazine] tartrate in high dosage were tried in order to alter the sleep pattern of children with sleeping difficulties.[1,2] Adverse effects have, however, been reported in children (see under Adverse Effects and Precautions, above). The UK product is no longer indicated for short-term sedation in children and should not be used in infants less than 2 years of age.

1. Valman HB. ABC of 1 to 7 (revised): sleep problems. *BMJ* 1987; **294:** 828–30.
2. Anonymous. What can be done for night waking in children? *Lancet* 1987; **ii:** 948–9.

Preparations

BP 2001: Alimemazine Tablets; Paediatric Alimemazine Oral Solution; Strong Paediatric Alimemazine Oral Solution;
USP 25: Trimeprazine Tartrate Syrup; Trimeprazine Tartrate Tablets.

Proprietary Preparations (details are given in Part 3)
Austral.: Chemists Own Peetalix; Vallergan; *Belg.:* Theralene; *Canad.:* Panectyl; *Denm.:* Vallergan†; *Fr.:* Theralene; *Ger.:* Repeltin; *Hong Kong:* Vallergan; *Irl.:* Vallergan; *Neth.:* Nedeltran; *Norw.:* Vallergan; *NZ:* Vallergan; *S.Afr.:* Vallergan; *Spain:* Variargil; *Swed.:* Theralen; *UK:* Vallergan.

Multi-ingredient: *Belg.:* Theralene Pectoral†; *Fr.:* Theralene Pectoral Nourrisson; *Singapore:* Walekof.

Trimethobenzamide Hydrochloride (6170-e)

Trimethobenzamide Hydrochloride (rINNM).

N-[4-(2-Dimethylaminoethoxy)benzyl]-3,4,5-trimethoxybenzamide hydrochloride.
$C_{21}H_{28}N_2O_5,HCl = 424.9$.
CAS — 138-56-7 (trimethobenzamide); 554-92-7 (trimethobenzamide hydrochloride).
Pharmacopoeias. In *US.*

Pharmacopoeial description

USP 25: A white crystalline powder having a slight phenolic odour. Soluble 1 in 2 of water, 1 in 59 of alcohol, 1 in 67 of chloroform, and 1 in 720 of ether; insoluble in benzene.

Adverse Effects and Precautions

As for the sedating antihistamines in general, p.404.
Pain at the site of intramuscular injection and local irritation after rectal administration have been noted.

Pregnancy. For discussion of the use of antihistamines in pregnancy, including some evidence of an excess number of congenital abnormalities in infants born to mothers exposed to trimethobenzamide, see p.405.

Interactions

As for the sedating antihistamines in general, p.406.

Uses and Administration

Trimethobenzamide hydrochloride, a monoethanolamine derivative, is a sedating antihistamine used as an antiemetic in the control of nausea and vomiting (p.407).

The usual dose is 250 mg by mouth or 200 mg by deep intramuscular injection or rectally three or four times daily. Children weighing more than 15 kg have been given 100 to 200 mg three or four times daily by the oral or rectal route. Children weighing less than 15 kg have been given 100 mg three or four times daily by the rectal route.

Preparations

USP 25: Trimethobenzamide Hydrochloride Capsules; Trimethobenzamide Hydrochloride Injection.

Proprietary Preparations (details are given in Part 3)
Mex.: Tigan; *USA:* Arrestin†; T-Gen; Tebamide; Ticon; Tigan; Trimazide.

Multi-ingredient: *USA:* Emergent-Ez; Tigan; Triban.

Tripelennamine Citrate (6171-l)

Tripelennamine Citrate *(BANM, rINNM).*

Tripelennaminium Citrate. *N-Benzyl-N'N'-dimethyl-N-(2-pyridyl)ethylenediamine dihydrogen citrate.*
$C_{16}H_{21}N_3,C_6H_8O_7 = 447.5.$
CAS — 91-81-6 (tripelennamine); 6138-56-3 (tripelennamine citrate).

Tripelennamine citrate 150 mg is approximately equivalent to 100 mg of tripelennamine hydrochloride.

Tripelennamine Hydrochloride (6172-y)

Tripelennamine Hydrochloride *(BANM, rINNM).*

Tripelennaminium Chloride.
$C_{16}H_{21}N_3,HCl = 291.8.$
CAS — 154-69-8.
Pharmacopoeias. In US.

Pharmacopoeial description

USP 25: A white crystalline powder. It slowly darkens on exposure to light. Soluble 1 in 1 of water, 1 in 6 of alcohol and of chloroform, and 1 in 350 of acetone; insoluble in ether, in ethyl acetate, and in benzene. Its solutions are practically neutral to litmus. Protect from light.

Adverse Effects and Precautions

As for the sedating antihistamines in general, p.404.

Abuse. References to the intravenous abuse of tripelennamine alone[1] or with pentazocine in the combination known as T's and blues.[2-4]

1. Addington J, el-Guebaly N. Intravenous tripelennamine abuse in schizophrenia. *Can J Psychiatry* 1996; **41:** 63.
2. Showalter CV. T's and blues: abuse of pentazocine and tripelennamine. *JAMA* 1980; **244:** 1224–5.
3. von Almen WF, Miller JM. "Ts and Blues" in pregnancy. *J Reprod Med* 1986; **31:** 236–9.
4. McGwier BW, *et al.* Acute myocardial infarction associated with intravenous injection of pentazocine and tripelennamine. *Chest* 1992; **101:** 1730–2.

Overdosage. A severe toxic reaction, including agitation, hallucinations, and myoclonic jerks occurred in an 8-year-old child who was sprayed over the trunk and extremities with tripelennamine hydrochloride 2.1375 g in the treatment of severe poison ivy poisoning.[1] It was likely that inhalation of the fine mist of the aerosol spray contributed to the reaction but in this patient the initial reaction began 3 hours after exposure suggesting that percutaneous absorption through the multiple skin lesions probably contributed significantly. The original reaction was inadvertently prolonged by subsequent treatment

with diphenhydramine hydrochloride and promethazine hydrochloride.

1. Schipior PG. An unusual case of antihistamine intoxication. *J Pediatr* 1967; **71:** 589–91.

Interactions

As for the sedating antihistamines in general, p.406.

Uses and Administration

Tripelennamine, an ethylenediamine derivative, is a sedating antihistamine with antimuscarinic and moderate sedative properties. It is used for the symptomatic relief of hypersensitivity reactions.

Tripelennamine hydrochloride is given by mouth in usual doses of 25 to 50 mg every 4 to 6 hours. Higher doses of up to 600 mg daily have been given. A suggested dose of the hydrochloride for children is 5 mg per kg body-weight daily in 4 to 6 divided doses; up to 300 mg daily has been given. Tripelennamine citrate has been used in equivalent doses in an elixir.

Tripelennamine hydrochloride has also been applied topically to the skin, although, as with other antihistamines, there is a risk of sensitisation.

Preparations

USP 25: Tripelennamine Hydrochloride Tablets.

Proprietary Preparations (details are given in Part 3)
Aust.: Azaron; *Canad.:* Pyribenzamine†; Vaginex†; *Fin.:* Etono; *Ger.:* Azaron; Fenistil; *Neth.:* Azaron†; *Spain:* Azaron; *USA:* PBZ; Pelamine†; Vaginex.

Multi-ingredient: *Braz.:* Asmosterona; Gripinex; *Ital.:* Anticorizza; *Spain:* Oxidermiol Antihist; *USA:* Di-Delamine.

Triprolidine Hydrochloride (6173-j)

Triprolidine Hydrochloride *(BANM, rINNM).*

(E)-2-[3-(Pyrrolidin-1-yl)-1-*p*-tolylprop-1-enyl]pyridine hydrochloride monohydrate.
$C_{19}H_{22}N_2,HCl,H_2O = 332.9.$
CAS — 486-12-4 (triprolidine); 550-70-9 (anhydrous triprolidine hydrochloride); 6138-79-0 (triprolidine hydrochloride, monohydrate).
Pharmacopoeias. In Br. and US.

Pharmacopoeial description

BP 2001: A white, odourless or almost odourless, crystalline powder. Freely soluble in water and in alcohol; very soluble in chloroform; practically insoluble in ether.

USP 25: A white crystalline powder, having no more than a slight, but unpleasant, odour. Soluble 1 in 2.1 of water, 1 in 1.8 of alcohol, 1 in 1 of chloroform, and 1 in 2000 of ether. Its solutions are alkaline to litmus. Store in airtight containers. Protect from light.

Adverse Effects and Precautions

As for the sedating antihistamines in general, p.404.

Interactions

As for the sedating antihistamines in general, p.406.

Pharmacokinetics

After absorption from the gastrointestinal tract, triprolidine is metabolised; a carboxylated derivative accounts for about half the dose excreted in the urine. Reported half-lives vary from 3 to 5 hours or more.

◊ General references.

1. Paton DM, Webster DR. Clinical pharmacokinetics of H_1-receptor antagonists (the antihistamines). *Clin Pharmacokinet* 1985; **10:** 477–97.
2. Miles MV, *et al.* Pharmacokinetics of oral and transdermal triprolidine. *J Clin Pharmacol* 1990; **30:** 572–5.

Distribution into breast milk. In a study[1] in 3 women of the excretion of triprolidine and pseudoephedrine, taken by mouth in a combined preparation, triprolidine was found to reach concentrations in breast milk similar to those found in plasma in one subject, and slightly lower than in plasma in the others. It was calculated that 0.06 to 0.2% of the ingested dose was excreted in breast milk over 24 hours. Concentrations of pseudoephedrine in breast milk exceeded those in plasma in all 3 women.

1. Findlay JWA, *et al.* Pseudoephedrine and triprolidine in plasma and breast milk of nursing mothers. *Br J Clin Pharmacol* 1984; **18:** 901–6.

Uses and Administration

Triprolidine hydrochloride, an alkylamine derivative, is a sedating antihistamine with antimuscarinic and mild sedative effects. It is used for the symptomatic relief of allergic conditions including urticaria (p.408) and rhinitis (p.407), and in pruritic skin disorders (p.407). It is often used in combination with pseudoephedrine hydrochloride for rhinitis and in other compound preparations for the symptomatic treatment of coughs and the common cold (p.406).

It is given by mouth, the usual dose for adults being 2.5 mg up to four times daily.

Triprolidine hydrochloride has also been applied topically to the skin although, as with other antihistamines, there is a risk of sensitisation.

Preparations

BP 2001: Triprolidine Tablets;
USP 25: Triprolidine and Pseudoephedrine Hydrochlorides Syrup; Triprolidine and Pseudoephedrine Hydrochlorides Tablets; Triprolidine Hydrochloride Syrup; Triprolidine Hydrochloride Tablets.

Proprietary Preparations (details are given in Part 3)
Aust.: Actidil; Pro-Actidil; *Israel:* Pro-Actidil; *Ital.:* Actidil; *Spain:* Pro-Actidil; *USA:* Myidyl†.

Multi-ingredient: *Austral.:* Actifed; Actifed CC Junior; Codral Daytime/Nightime; Sudafed Sinus Pain & Allergy Relief; *Belg.:* Actifed; *Braz.:* Trifedrin; *Canad.:* Actifed; Actifed DM; Actifed Plus; CoActifed; Cotridin; Cotridin Expectorant; Triprofed†; *Fr.:* Actifed; Actifed Toux Seche; Tussifed†; *Ger.:* Actifed†; Olynth Kombi; *Hong Kong:* Actifed; Actifed Compound; Actifed DM; Cough-EN; Fedac; Fedac Compound; Uni-Fedra Compound; *Irl.:* Actifed; Actifed Chesty; Actifed Compound; *Israel:* Actifed; Actifed Compound; Actifed DM; Actifed Expectorant; Histafed; Histafed Comp; Histafed Expectorant; *Ital.:* Actifed; Actifed Composto; Actigrip; *NZ:* Actifed; Actifed CC Chesty; Actifed CC Dry; Actifed CC Junior; Codral Daytime/Nightime; Sudafed Day/Nightime Relief; *Port.:* Actifed; Dinaxil; *S.Afr.:* Actifed; Actifed Co; Actifed DM; Actigesic; Acuflu-P†; Acugest; Acugest Co; Acugest Expect; Acutussive; Adco-Flupain; Adco-Muco Expect†; Adco-Tussend; Arcana Cough Linctus†; Arcana Expectorant†; Arcanafed†; Betafed; Coff-Rest; Coryx; Emprazil-A†; Endcol Cough Linctus†; Endcol Decongestant†; Fludactil; Fludactil Co; Fludactil Expectorant; Linctifed; Medifed; Merck-Cough Linctus; Merck-Expectorant; Merck-Fed; Neofed; Phendex; Rhinofed†; Sinuclear P; Tixylix Flu; Trifen; *Singapore:* Actifed; Actifed Compound; Actifed DM; Actifed Expectorant; Cough-EN; Fedac; Fedac Compound; Unitifed; Unitifed Compound; *Spain:* Iniston; Iniston Antitusivo; Iniston Expectorante; *Thai.:* Actifed; Actifed Compound; Actifed DM; Actil; Cofed; Consudine; Hiscifed; Med-Actigen; Milafed; Nanafed; Nasolin; Policol; Policold; Profed; Prophedin; Sinusaid; Trifed; Triofed; Tripo; Triprodrine; *UAE:* Sedofan; Sedofan DM; *UK:* Actifed; Actifed Compound; Actifed Expectorant; Benylin Childrens Coughs & Colds; Sudafed Plus; *USA:* Actagen; Actagen-C Cough; Actifed; Actifed Cold & Allergy; Actifed Cold & Sinus; Actifed Plus; Actifed with Codeine†; Allercon; Allerfrim; Allerfrim with Codeine; Allergy Cold†; Allerphed; Aprodine; Aprodine with Codeine; Bayer Select Night Time Cold; Cenafed Plus; Genac; Silafed; Triafed with Codeine†; Triafed; Trifed-C Cough; Trifed†; Triofed; Triposed.

Tritoqualine (13384-k)

Tritoqualine *(rINN).*

L-554. 7-Amino-4,5,6-triethoxy-3-(5,6,7,8-tetrahydro-4-methoxy-6-methyl-1,3-dioxolo[4,5-g]isoquinolin-5-yl)phthalide.
$C_{26}H_{32}N_2O_8 = 500.5.$
CAS — 14504-73-5.
ATC — R06AX21.

Profile

Tritoqualine is stated to inhibit histidine decarboxylase which catalyses the conversion of histidine to histamine. It has the uses of antihistamines (p.404) and has been given by mouth for the symptomatic relief of hypersensitivity reactions and in pruritic skin disorders.

Preparations

Proprietary Preparations (details are given in Part 3)
Aust.: Hypostamin; *Fr.:* Hypostamine; *Ger.:* Inhibostamin.

Antimalarials

This chapter describes the principal drugs used in the treatment and prophylaxis of malaria, one of the most serious protozoal infections in man. An estimated 40% of the world's population may be at risk of malaria; more than 500 million develop clinical infection, which is often very severe, and 1 to 3 million die each year. WHO produces guidelines for its strategic control and the management of malaria is under constant review. In 1998, WHO initiated the 'Roll Back Malaria' project to coordinate action to control the disease, the main objective being to significantly reduce the global malaria burden and to halve the number of deaths due to malaria by 2010. Measures to control malaria include *protection* from mosquito bites, *prophylaxis* with antimalarial drugs, and prompt *treatment* of any infection that develops. They also involve *vector control*; it is now recognised that for many countries vector eradication is an unrealistic aim.

Malaria

Malaria is caused by infection by any of four species of *Plasmodium* protozoa. *P. falciparum* causes falciparum (malignant tertian or subtertian) malaria which is the most serious form of malaria and can be rapidly fatal in non-immune individuals if not treated promptly. The other three species cause what are often termed 'benign' malarias; *P. vivax* causes vivax (benign tertian) malaria which is widespread but rarely fatal, although symptoms during the primary attack can be severe; *P. malariae* causes quartan malaria which is generally mild but can cause fatal nephrosis; and *P. ovale* causes ovale (ovale tertian) malaria which is the least common type of malaria, and produces clinical features similar to *P. vivax*.

The life cycle of *Plasmodium* is complex, comprising a sexual phase (sporogony) in the mosquito (vector) and an asexual phase (schizogony) in man (see Figure 1, below). Infection in man is usually caused by injection of *sporozoites* by the bite of an infected female anopheline mosquito. It may rarely be acquired in other ways such as through blood transfusion, congenitally via the placenta, through needlestick injuries, or after organ transplantation. Following an infected mosquito bite some of the sporozoites rapidly enter liver parenchymal cells where they undergo *exoerythrocytic* or *pre-erythrocytic schizogony*, forming *tissue schizonts* which mature and release thousands of *merozoites* into the blood on rupture of the cell. Some of these merozoites enter erythrocytes where they transform into *trophozoites*. These produce *blood schizonts* which, as they mature, rupture and release merozoites into the circulation which can infect other erythrocytes. This is termed the *erythrocytic cycle* and it is this periodic release of merozoites which is responsible for the characteristic periodicity of the fever in malaria. After several erythrocytic cycles, depending on the type of malaria, some erythrocytic forms develop into sexual *gametocytes*. It is ingestion of infected blood containing gametocytes by a biting female mosquito which allows the life cycle to be completed with the sexual phase in the mosquito. In *P. vivax* and *P. ovale* infections, some of the sporozoites entering the liver cells are thought to enter a latent tissue stage in the form of *hypnozoites* which are responsible for recurrence of malaria caused by these organisms. Recurrences resulting from the persistence of latent tissue forms are often referred to as *relapses* while renewed attacks caused by persistent residual erythrocytic forms are termed *recrudescences*. True relapses do not occur with falciparum or quartan malarias. Patients may sometimes be classified as *non-immune* if they have not previously or recently been exposed to *Plasmodium* infection and as *semi-immune* or *immune* if they have a history of prolonged exposure.

Clinical manifestations of malaria

The clinical symptoms of malaria are varied and non-specific but commonly include fever, fatigue, malaise, headache, myalgia, and sweating. Anaemia is a common complication due to haemolysis and in falciparum malaria serious complications such as acute renal failure, pulmonary oedema, and cerebral dysfunction can occur. Since none of the clinical features of malaria are diagnostic, a definitive diagnosis depends upon the demonstration of parasites in stained blood films. However, antimalarial drug treatment should not be withheld in the absence of positive blood films if there is clinical suspicion of malaria.

Antimalarial drugs

Antimalarial drugs can be classified by the stage of the parasitic life cycle they affect. Thus:

Blood schizontocides act on the erythrocytic stages of the parasite which are directly responsible for the clinical symptoms of the disease. They can produce a clinical cure or suppression of infection by susceptible strains of all four species of malaria parasite, but, since they have no effect on exoerythrocytic forms, do not produce a radical cure of relapsing forms of ovale or vivax malarias.

Tissue schizontocides act on the exoerythrocytic stages of the parasite and are used for causal prophylaxis to prevent invasion of the blood cells, or as anti-relapse drugs to produce radical cures of vivax and ovale malarias.

Gametocytocides destroy the sexual forms of the parasite to interrupt transmission of the infection to the mosquito vector.

Sporontocides have no direct effect on the gametocytes in the human host but prevent sporogony in the mosquito.

Antimalarial drugs can also be classified by the chemical group to which they belong, which in turn determines the stage of the life cycle they affect.- The principal antimalarial drugs, classified according to *drug group* and *activity*, are listed in Table 1 p.429.

The naphthyridine derivative pyronaridine is under investigation for its use as an antimalarial. The quinolone antibacterials, and the 4-piperazinoquinoline derivatives, piperaquine and hydroxypiperaquine, have also been studied for their antimalarial activity. The 9-aminoacridines such as mepacrine are no longer used in the treatment of malaria.

The differing mechanisms of action of antimalarial drugs allow the use of combinations of antimalarials to improve efficacy. Such combinations may have a simple additive effect or, more commonly, the drugs used may potentiate each other, for instance by acting at sequential steps in the parasite's folic acid pathway (e.g. pyrimethamine with sulfadoxine or dapsone). Alternatively, a combination may be complementary, when the drugs involved act against different stages in the life cycle of the parasite (e.g. the use of chloroquine with primaquine to produce radical cure of *P. vivax* or *P. ovale* infections). The rationale behind the use of such combinations may be to enhance efficacy, particularly when drug resistance is a problem (see below), or it may be an attempt to delay the development of resistance to one or more of the drugs concerned.

Resistance of *Plasmodium* to antimalarial drugs, in particular the spread of strains of *P. falciparum* resistant to chloroquine, is of great concern.

Chloroquine resistance in *P. falciparum* now affects most of Asia and the western Pacific islands with evidence of a westward spread. It is well established in South America. Major and alarming changes in susceptibility have occurred in sub-Saharan Africa; chloroquine resistance is now found to varying degrees in almost all endemic countries of Africa and especially in eastern Africa. Central America is the only endemic area yet to report resistance of *P. falciparum* to chloroquine.

Resistance in *P. falciparum* to proguanil and pyrimethamine is apparent in many endemic areas. Cross-resistance between proguanil and pyrimethamine may also occur.

Resistance in *P. falciparum* to the combination pyrimethamine-sulfadoxine (Fansidar) spread rapidly from Thailand to other parts of the world including parts of South America and East Africa. Resistance to quinine, halofantrine, mefloquine, and artemisinin derivatives has also been noted. The emergence of multiple drug resistance in *P. falciparum* makes the selection of effective prophylaxis and treatment difficult.

Resistance in *P. vivax* to chloroquine and primaquine has also been reported in several parts of the world.[1]

A knowledge of the extent of resistance in terms of the geographical distribution and degree of resistance is important for the selection of appropriate control measures and for the development of policies for the rational use of antimalarial drugs. Effective drugs and drug combinations need to be selected according to local patterns of drug resistance. Indiscriminate and uncontrolled use of drugs should be prevented and adequate doses should be given to delay the selection of resistant strains. Malaria control strategies also need to involve other measures such as vector control and health education.

Treatment of malaria

Malaria is a serious and potentially fatal disease, particularly in the case of falciparum malaria (see below) and especially in non-immune individuals; prompt diagnosis and effective treatment are crucial.[2-4] Treatment is with a *blood schizontocide*, selected with due regard to the prevalence of specific patterns of drug resistance in the area of infection. In the case of vivax and ovale malarias (see below) subsequent treatment with a *tissue schizontocide* is needed where it is considered appropriate to prevent relapse.

Antimalarials are generally given by mouth, although in order to obtain a rapid response in patients with severe or complicated malaria (see below) it may be necessary to give parenteral therapy initially, the patient being transferred to oral therapy when feasible.[4]

Treatment of falciparum malaria. In most parts of the world *P. falciparum* is now resistant to chloroquine and therefore, apart from the rare circumstance of exposure

Figure 1. Life cycle of the malaria parasite *Plasmodium*.

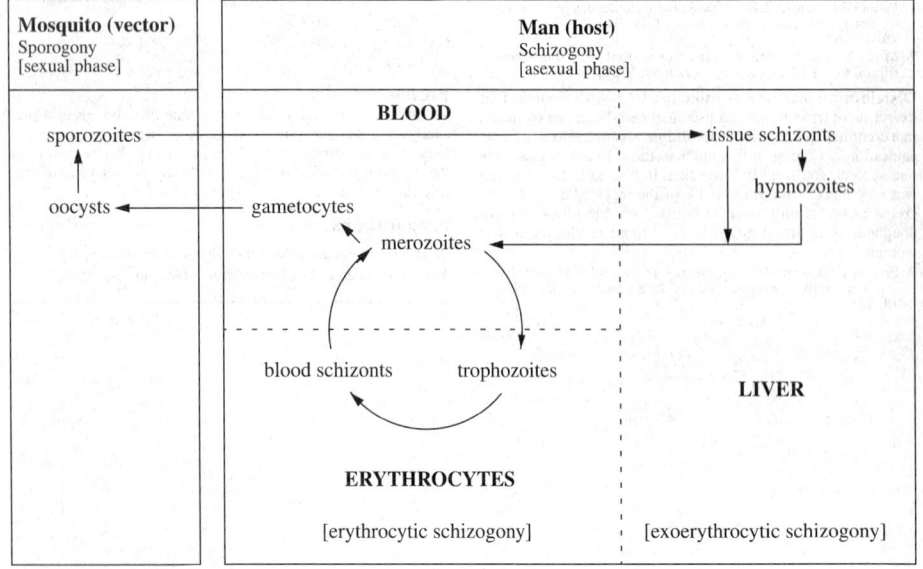

Table 1. Principal antimalarial drugs.

Antimalarial groups	Principal drugs	Activity
4-Methanolquinolines	Cinchona alkaloids Quinine Quinidine	Rapid-acting blood schizontocides. Some gametocytocidal activity.
	Mefloquine	Blood schizontocide.
4-Aminoquinolines	Chloroquine Hydroxychloroquine Amodiaquine	Rapid-acting blood schizontocides. Some gametocytocidal activity.
8-Aminoquinolines	Primaquine Tafenoquine	Tissue schizontocide. Also gametocytocidal activity and some activity at other stages of the parasite's life-cycle.
Biguanides	Proguanil Chlorproguanil	Tissue schizontocides and slow-acting blood schizontocides. Some sporontocidal activity. Dihydrofolate reductase inhibitors.
Diaminopyrimidines	Pyrimethamine	Tissue schizontocide and slow-acting blood schizontocide. Some sporontocidal activity. Dihydrofolate reductase inhibitor. Usually used with antimalarials that inhibit different stages of folate synthesis (sulfonamides or sulfones) to form synergistic combinations.
Dichlorobenzylidines	Lumefantrine	Blood schizontocide.
Hydroxynaphthoquinones	Atovaquone	Blood schizontocide. Usually given in combination with proguanil.
9-Phenanthrenemethanols	Halofantrine	Blood schizontocide.
Sesquiterpene lactones	Artemisinin and its derivatives	Blood schizontocide.
Sulfonamides	Sulfadoxine Sulfametopyrazine	Blood schizontocides. Dihydropteroate and folate synthesis inhibitors. Usually given in combination with pyrimethamine.
Tetracyclines	Doxycycline Tetracycline	Blood schizontocides. Some tissue schizontocidal activity.
Lincosamides	Clindamycin	Blood schizontocide. Some tissue schizontocidal activity.
Sulfones	Dapsone	Blood schizontocide. Folate synthesis inhibitor. Usually given in combination with pyrimethamine.

in one of the few remaining areas of chloroquine sensitivity, chloroquine is **not** suitable for treatment. Instead, in the UK, **uncomplicated falciparum malaria** is treated with:

- quinine *and* (if quinine resistance is known or suspected) followed by *either* pyrimethamine-sulfadoxine (Fansidar) *or* (if Fansidar-resistant) by doxycycline

or alternatively with

- mefloquine

or

- atovaquone-proguanil (Malarone).

It is not necessary to give pyrimethamine-sulfadoxine (Fansidar) or doxycycline after the latter two treatments. Artemisinin derivatives may be used if necessary in difficult cases.

For malaria-endemic areas where there is chloroquine resistance, WHO recommends pyrimethamine-sulfadoxine (Fansidar) or amodiaquine as treatment of choice in uncomplicated malaria (although cross-resistance between chloroquine and amodiaquine has been reported). If either of these options is, or becomes, unsatisfactory then mefloquine, or alternatively quinine, may be used; quinine is usually given in combination with tetracycline or doxycycline to ensure a high cure rate.

To combat the increasing problem of drug-resistant falciparum malaria, WHO has recommended that artemisinin and related compounds should be reserved solely for areas of multidrug-resistant malaria (and should not be used for prophylaxis); in practice, however, they appear to be more widely used. They should be given in combination with another antimalarial and have usually been given with mefloquine, but a number of other combinations have been investigated, of which artemether with lumefantrine, or artesunate with pyrimethamine-sulfadoxine are showing particular promise. If the combination of an artemisinin derivative with pyrimethamine-sulfadoxine (Fansidar) proves safe and effective, it may be used as first-line treatment as a further alternative to chloroquine in areas of chloroquine resistance. Other possible combinations with artemisinin derivatives are with pyronaridine, with chlorproguanil-dapsone, and with atovaquone-proguanil.

In **severe or complicated falciparum malaria** including cerebral malaria, parenteral treatment is required to produce adequate blood concentrations as quickly as possible.[2,4-7] The importance of achieving therapeutic concentrations of antimalarial drugs as early as possible has been emphasised.[8] Chloroquine should be given if the in-

fection is known to be sensitive to it. In chloroquine-resistant malaria, or where sensitivity to chloroquine is not known, quinine is usually given intravenously, starting with a loading dose; intravenous artesunate or intramuscular artemether may alternatively be used; intravenous quinidine may be used if parenteral quinine or artemisinin derivatives are not available. Patients of all ages need to be closely monitored while undergoing parenteral therapy and treatment is changed to an orally administered antimalarial as soon as the patient's condition permits. When there are only minimal health care facilities and parenteral therapy is not possible, artemisinin or artesunate suppositories may be given; the nasogastric route may also be used.[2,4] Supportive therapy in patients with severe or complicated malaria needs to be directed at reducing hyperpyrexia, controlling convulsions, maintaining fluid balance, and correcting hypoglycaemia.[2,4,5] Since iron might be involved in the pathogenesis of cerebral malaria, the iron chelator desferrioxamine has been tried in addition to standard antimalarial therapy, but any benefit is yet to be established and WHO advises against its use.[4] Anecdotal reports of the value of corticosteroids in cerebral malaria have not been substantiated by controlled studies and they have no place in the management of this condition. Other approaches such as the use of hyperimmune serum or monoclonal antibody to tumour necrosis factor have also been unsuccessful.

Treatment of benign malarias. Benign malarias, which are usually caused by *P. vivax* and less commonly by *P. ovale* and *P. malariae*, can be debilitating but are usually less severe than falciparum malaria. Chloroquine is still the drug of choice (but chloroquine-resistant vivax infection has been reported from some areas—notably Papua New Guinea, Indonesia, Myanmar, and Vanuatu). Chloroquine alone is adequate for *P. malariae* infections, but in the case of those caused by *P. vivax* or *P. ovale* a subsequent *radical cure* with a tissue schizontocide, usually primaquine, is needed to avoid the risk of relapse (caused by the presence of latent hypnozoites) months or years after the primary infection. Radical cure is inappropriate for patients living within an endemic area since re-infection is likely and therefore WHO recommends that it should be limited to patients resident in areas where transmission is *very low* or *absent* and to those treated *during an epidemic*; other patients should simply be treated with a further course of chloroquine in the event of relapse or re-infection. *P. vivax* cases that fail to respond to chloroquine may be treated with quinine or mefloquine.

Treatment of malaria during pregnancy. Malaria is especially dangerous during pregnancy and the seriousness of the disease usually outweighs any potential risk from treatment. Although fetal abnormalities have been associated with the use of high doses of chloroquine, extensive clinical experience suggests it is safe; its use may be limited however, due to resistance. Quinine may be used for chloroquine-resistant malaria but care should be taken that patients do not become hypoglycaemic.[5] There may be difficulty if additional drugs are required as opinion varies over their suitability. Intermittent treatment with pyrimethamine-sulfadoxine (Fansidar) (one dose in the second and one dose in the third trimester) may reduce the risk of severe anaemia in late pregnancy in malaria-endemic areas,[9] although there are some concerns over emerging resistance. Moreover, some consider that pyrimethamine combinations should be avoided, especially during the first trimester (see under Pregnancy in Precautions of Pyrimethamine, p.443). the tetracyclines are contra-indicated on dental grounds and the safety of mefloquine, halofantrine, or atovaquone has not been fully assessed although mefloquine is now suggested for prophylactic use from the fourth month of pregnancy. For patients with vivax or ovale malaria during pregnancy radical cure with primaquine should be postponed until after delivery;[5,6] weekly chloroquine can be given during the remaining weeks of pregnancy.

Treatment of splenomegaly syndrome. A small number of individuals infected with *Plasmodium* develop chronic hyperreactive malarial splenomegaly syndrome, an aberrant immunological response formerly known as the tropical splenomegaly syndrome. Traditionally, patients have first received a full course of antimalarial chemotherapy appropriate to the causative species followed by lengthy and probably lifelong chemoprophylaxis.[10] However, a study in 312 patients suggested that pyrimethamine given with folinic acid for 30 days could produce a rapid reduction of splenomegaly which persisted for at least 3 months.[11]

Prophylaxis of malaria

Chemoprophylaxis of malaria may refer to absolute prevention of infection (*causal prophylaxis*) or to suppression of parasitaemia and its symptoms (*clinical prophylaxis*). Causal prophylaxis is provided by tissue schizontocides which destroy the exoerythrocytic forms of the parasite. Clinical prophylaxis is provided by blood schizontocides which, if continued until all exoerythrocytic forms of the parasite are destroyed, will ultimately produce a *suppressive cure*. In *P. falciparum* infections this would be achieved by about a month after the last infected bite, but relapses with *P. vivax* and *P. ovale* may still occur after standard clinical prophylactic regimens due to the presence of latent exoerythrocytic forms (hypnozoites).

The continuing increase in the prevalence of strains of *P. falciparum* resistant to chloroquine and other antimalarials along with growing evidence of toxicity of some regimens make recommendations for malaria prophylaxis increasingly difficult. Absolute protection cannot be guaranteed by any chemoprophylactic regimen currently in use and the importance and effectiveness of methods of avoiding bites from infected mosquitoes such as the use of *protective clothing, bed netting, insect repellents,* and *insecticides* must be stressed.[2,3] WHO recommends[3] the following measures to protect against mosquito bites:

- application of an effective insect repellent to exposed skin between dusk and dawn when mosquitoes commonly bite
- accommodation in buildings with screens over doors and windows
- use of mosquito nets at night, preferably impregnated with pyrethroid insecticides such as permethrin or deltamethrin
- and use of anti-mosquito sprays or insecticide dispensers, or mosquito coils in bedrooms at night.

Studies have demonstrated that pyrethroid-impregnated mosquito nets can reduce mortality substantially.[12] In addition to these measures, travellers should be advised, even if chemoprophylaxis has been taken regularly, to regard **any** fever *after the first week (especially within 3 months)* and for *up to 1 year following possible exposure* as being caused by malaria and to seek medical advice **immediately**. Some authorities advise that travellers should also have antimalarial drugs ready for emergency self-treatment (*standby treatment*) when prompt medical attention is not available.

WHO considers that chemoprophylaxis should be reserved for those at high risk, notably *non-immune visi-*

tors; widespread chemoprophylaxis in *immune or semi-immune* populations is no longer recommended except for women who are *pregnant*. For the elderly, pregnant women, and children, careful consideration should be given as to whether travel to areas where falciparum malaria occurs is absolutely necessary. WHO specifically advises pregnant women not to travel to areas where transmission of *P. falciparum* occurs and also advises against taking babies and young children to malarious areas (particularly where there is transmission of *P. falciparum*).[3] Advice on chemoprophylaxis must be based on a knowledge of the occurrence and susceptibility of malaria strains in specific geographical areas. Local variations due to altitude, seasonal variations in temperature and rainfall, the degree of urbanisation, and many other factors further complicate the issue. WHO collates information provided by national health administrations and regularly publishes this information to assist in advising international travellers on the current situation; similar information is provided at national level by local institutes specialising in tropical diseases. However, the situation is so complex that advice differs. Recommendations issued by various authorities are usually for short-term stays and expert advice should be sought if long-term cover is required.

It is generally recommended that chemoprophylaxis should start about 1 week (or longer for mefloquine) before exposure to malaria, or if this is not possible at the earliest opportunity up to 1 or 2 days before exposure; this is partly to ensure that the patient is able to tolerate the drug. Chemoprophylaxis should continue throughout exposure and generally for at least 4 weeks after leaving the malarious area.

Prophylactic regimens. Depending upon the risk of infection and the availability and standard of local medical care, WHO[3] has made various recommendations concerning chemoprophylaxis and/or standby treatment for non-immune travellers:

- in areas where *P. falciparum* is *absent* or still *sensitive to chloroquine*, travellers can either take chloroquine for prophylaxis or, if the infection risk is *very low*, not take prophylaxis at all
- in areas where *P. falciparum* is *resistant to chloroquine* but with a low risk of infection, chloroquine with proguanil is recommended as it may give some protection against *P. falciparum* and may alleviate the symptoms if an attack does occur; chloroquine given alone will only protect against *P. vivax* in these areas. Mefloquine is recommended as second choice. Again if the infection risk is very low travellers may do without prophylaxis
- in areas of high risk or where there is multidrug resistance, mefloquine is recommended as first choice for prophylaxis, doxycycline is recommended as second choice, and chloroquine with proguanil as third choice. Again if the infection risk is very low travellers may do without prophylaxis. These recommendations are subject to the local patterns of drug resistance.

WHO also recommends that for the small number of travellers who would be unable to obtain prompt medical attention when malaria is suspected (within 24 hours of the onset of symptoms), it may be necessary to provide a course of treatment for self-administration (*standby treatment*). Clear instructions must be given and persons taking standby medication must seek medical advice as soon as possible. Also having completed the standby course they should resume any prophylaxis. The basis upon which the choice of prophylaxis is made (as detailed above) in turn broadly determines the appropriate choice of standby treatment. Thus:

- where *no prophylaxis* is deemed necessary, chloroquine is given for standby treatment in areas where there is chloroquine sensitivity, otherwise standby treatment is with pyrimethamine-sulfadoxine (Fansidar), or with mefloquine, or with quinine
- where prophylaxis is *with chloroquine* (either alone or with proguanil), standby treatment is with pyrimethamine-sulfadoxine (Fansidar), or with mefloquine, or with quinine
- where prophylaxis is *with mefloquine*, standby treatment is with pyrimethamine-sulfadoxine (Fansidar), or with quinine alone, or with quinine plus doxycycline or tetracycline
- where prophylaxis is *with doxycycline*, standby treatment is with mefloquine or with quinine plus tetracycline.

It should be noted that pyrimethamine-sulfadoxine (Fansidar) is appropriate *only for* areas such as India and for

African countries where no resistance to it has been reported.

In the USA recommendations for prophylaxis are provided by the Centers for Disease Control (CDC)[13-15] and other sources.[6] The recommendations for chloroquine-sensitive malaria are similar to those of WHO in that chloroquine alone is advised; hydroxychloroquine is suggested as an alternative. For all areas with chloroquine-resistant malaria, the use of mefloquine alone is recommended with alternatives being either doxycycline or atovaquone-proguanil (Malarone). Pyrimethamine-sulfadoxine (Fansidar) or atovaquone-proguanil (Malarone) are recommended for emergency standby treatment. The use of primaquine is also advocated during the last 2 weeks of prophylaxis to prevent relapses due to *P. vivax* or *P. ovale* in persons returning from prolonged exposure in areas where relapsing malaria is endemic.

UK experts[16] have also published guidelines for the prophylaxis of malaria and, while these are in broad agreement with those of WHO, they also recommend the additional option of atovaquone-proguanil (Malarone) for both prophylaxis and emergency standby treatment. Further options recommended for standby treatment are artemether-lumefantrine (Riamet) or the combined use of quinine with pyrimethamine-sulfadoxine (Fansidar).[16] The UK recommendations also allow the use of pyrimethamine-dapsone (Maloprim) for prophylaxis in restricted circumstances, notably in epileptic patients (see below), but it is not considered a suitable option for most patients.[16]

VACCINES. Malaria vaccines are under development and several are currently undergoing clinical evaluation (see p.1546).

Prophylaxis during pregnancy. The choice of drugs for prophylaxis during pregnancy is limited and whenever possible women who are pregnant or likely to become so should avoid travelling to malarious areas (see also above). In pregnant women who cannot avoid travelling to endemic areas, chloroquine may be given alone for prophylaxis in the few areas where *P. falciparum* is sensitive to chloroquine, or in combination with proguanil where resistance exists.[3] Mefloquine is normally avoided during the first trimester but may be given from the fourth month onwards; pyrimethamine-dapsone (Maloprim) is also contra-indicated in the first trimester. Folate supplements (folic acid 5 mg daily) need to be taken with proguanil and pyrimethamine-dapsone (Maloprim).[16] Doxycycline, atovaquone-proguanil (Malarone), or primaquine are contra-indicated in pregnant women by most experts. In non-pregnant women of child-bearing potential, pregnancy needs to be avoided for 3 months after completing mefloquine prophylaxis and for one week following doxycycline prophylaxis.

Pregnant women living in endemic areas commonly receive malaria chemoprophylaxis as a matter of policy since their susceptibility to the disease, especially among primigravidas, is believed to be increased. Routine prophylaxis has been shown to reduce anaemia and produce a trend towards higher birth-weights and lower perinatal mortality.[17-19] A study of chemoprophylaxis in 1049 pregnancies[20] suggested that multigravidas obtained less benefit than primigravidas and a follow-up study[21] found that the outcome of subsequent pregnancies was similar regardless of whether chemoprophylaxis or placebo had been given in the first pregnancy. This result suggested that it may be possible to restrict chemoprophylaxis to first pregnancies in endemic areas. A review of randomised studies[22] came to a similar conclusion.

Prophylaxis during breast feeding. Breast feeding by mothers taking mefloquine is usually contra-indicated although the amount ingested by the nursing infant may be too small to produce adverse effects. Doxycycline and atovaquone-proguanil (Malarone) are contra-indicated during breast feeding. For other antimalarials it is generally accepted that the amount distributed into breast milk and consumed by nursing infants is too small to be harmful. However, these amounts are also too small to provide adequate protection and breast-fed infants still require chemoprophylaxis.

Prophylaxis in children. Chloroquine and proguanil may be given in scaled down doses to children of all ages but the choice of alternative drugs may be restricted especially in very young children and consideration should be given to whether their travel to malarious areas is absolutely necessary (see also above).

Prophylaxis in epilepsy. In subjects with a history of epilepsy the UK guidelines[16] advise that both chloroquine

and mefloquine are unsuitable for prophylaxis. In areas without chloroquine resistance proguanil alone is recommended. In areas with a high risk of chloroquine resistance atovaquone-proguanil (Malarone) or doxycycline may be considered, but the metabolism of doxycycline may be influenced by antiepileptics. Pyrimethamine-dapsone (Maloprim) is a further alternative; the UK guidelines mention folate supplementation (folic acid 5 mg daily) in those taking pyrimethamine-dapsone with phenytoin or phenobarbital.

Prophylaxis in HIV-infected travellers. HIV-infected travellers may take chloroquine routinely for antimalarial prophylaxis but its potential immunosuppressive effects should be recognised; proguanil, mefloquine, or doxycycline can also be used.[23,24] Although patients with AIDS may be at increased risk of adverse effects to sulfonamides a combination such as pyrimethamine-sulfadoxine (Fansidar) can be used for standby treatment if an alternative is not available.[23,24]

1. Whitby M. Drug resistant Plasmodium vivax malaria. *J Antimicrob Chemother* 1997; **40**: 749–52.
2. WHO. WHO expert committee on malaria: twentieth report. *WHO Tech Rep Ser* 892 2000.
3. WHO. *International travel and health: vaccination requirements and health advice.* Geneva: WHO, 2001.
4. WHO. *Management of severe malaria: a practical handbook.* Geneva: WHO, 2000.
5. Molyneux M, Fox R. Diagnosis and treatment of malaria in Britain. *BMJ* 1993; **306**: 1175–80.
6. Anonymous. Drugs for parasitic infections. *Med Lett Drugs Ther* 1998; **40**: 1–12.
7. WHO. Severe falciparum malaria. *Trans R Soc Trop Med Hyg* 2000; **94** (suppl 1): S1/1–S1/90.
8. White NJ. Not much progress in treatment of cerebral malaria. *Lancet* 1998; **352**: 594–5.
9. Shulman CE, *et al.* Intermittent sulphadoxine-pyrimethamine to prevent severe anaemia secondary to malaria in pregnancy: a randomised placebo-controlled trial. *Lancet* 1999; **353**; 632–6.
10. Cook GC. Prevention and treatment of malaria. *Lancet* 1988; **i**: 32–7.
11. Manenti F, *et al.* Treatment of hyperreactive malarial splenomegaly syndrome. *Lancet* 1994; **343**: 1441–2.
12. Lengeler C. Insecticide-treated bednets and curtains for preventing malaria (updated 29 May 2001). Available in The Cochrane Library; Issue 4. Oxford: Update Software; 2001.
13. Centers for Disease Control. Recommendations for the prevention of malaria among travelers. *MMWR* 1990; **39** (RR-3): 1–10.
14. Centers for Disease Control. Revised dosing regimen for malaria prophylaxis with mefloquine. *MMWR* 1990; **39**: 630.
15. Centers for Disease Control. Change of dosing regimen for malaria prophylaxis with mefloquine. *MMWR* 1991; **40**: 72–3.
16. Bradley DJ, Bannister B. Guidelines for malaria prevention in travellers from the United Kingdom for 2001. *Commun Dis Public Health* 2001; **4**: 84–101.
17. Greenwood AM, *et al.* The distribution of birth weights in Gambian women who received malaria chemoprophylaxis during their first pregnancy and in control women. *Trans R Soc Trop Med Hyg* 1994; **88**: 311–12.
18. Schultz LJ, *et al.* The efficacy of antimalarial regimens containing sulfadoxine-pyrimethamine and/or chloroquine in preventing peripheral and placental Plasmodium falciparum infection among pregnant women in Malawi. *Am J Trop Med Hyg* 1994; **51**: 515–22.
19. Nosten F, *et al.* Mefloquine prophylaxis prevents malaria during pregnancy: a double-blind, placebo-controlled study. *J Infect Dis* 1994; **169**: 595–603.
20. Greenwood BM, *et al.* The effects of malaria chemoprophylaxis given by traditional birth attendants on the course and outcome of pregnancy. *Trans R Soc Trop Med Hyg* 1989; **83**: 589–94.
21. Greenwood AM, *et al.* Can malaria chemoprophylaxis be restricted to first pregnancies? *Trans R Soc Trop Med Hyg* 1994; **88**: 681–2.
22. Garner P, Brabin B. A review of randomized controlled trials of routine antimalarial drug prophylaxis during pregnancy in endemic malarious areas. *Bull WHO* 1994; **72**: 89–99.
23. von Reyn CF, *et al.* International travel and HIV infection. *Bull WHO* 1990; **68**: 251–9.
24. Wilson ME, *et al.* Infections in HIV-infected travelers: risks and prevention. *Ann Intern Med* 1991; **114**: 582–92.

Amodiaquine (16289-t)

Amodiaquine (BAN, rINN).

4-(7-Chloro-4-quinolylamino)-2-(diethylaminomethyl)phenol.
$C_{20}H_{22}ClN_3O = 355.9$.
CAS — 86-42-0.
ATC — P01BA06.
Pharmacopoeias. In *Int.* and *US.*

Pharmacopoeial description

USP 25: Very pale yellow to light tan-yellow, odourless, powder. Practically insoluble in water; slightly soluble in alcohol; sparingly soluble in 1.0N hydrochloric acid. Store in airtight containers.

Amodiaquine Hydrochloride (1374-g)

Amodiaquine Hydrochloride (BANM, rINNM).

Amodiaquini Hydrochloridum. 4-(7-Chloro-4-quinolylamino)-2-(diethylaminomethyl)phenol dihydrochloride dihydrate.
$C_{20}H_{22}ClN_3O,2HCl,2H_2O = 464.8$.
CAS — 69-44-3 (anhydrous amodiaquine hydrochloride); 6398-98-7 (amodiaquine hydrochloride dihydrate).
Pharmacopoeias. In *Fr., Int.,* and *US.*

Amodiaquine base 200 mg is approximately equivalent to 260 mg of amodiaquine hydrochloride.

Pharmacopoeial description

USP 25: A yellow, odourless, crystalline powder. Soluble 1 in 25 of water and 1 in 78 of alcohol; very slightly soluble in chloroform, in ether, and in benzene. Store in airtight containers.

Sorption. For reference to loss of amodiaquine hydrochloride from solutions during membrane filtration, see Chloroquine, p.432.

Adverse Effects and Precautions

As for Chloroquine, p.432, but amodiaquine was associated with hepatitis and a much higher incidence of agranulocytosis when it was used for the prophylaxis of malaria.

◊ Early isolated reports of amodiaquine causing severe neutropenia were usually when it had been used in anti-inflammatory doses for rheumatoid arthritis, but there was a cluster of cases in 1986 associated with its use in malaria prophylaxis.[1] In all, 23 cases of agranulocytosis, 7 of which were fatal, were reported in the UK, USA, and Switzerland during a 12-month period ending March 1986. Nearly all of these patients had used the drug at a dosage of 400 mg weekly and the periods of exposure ranged from 3 to 24 weeks.[1] Some of these patients also had evidence of liver damage[1] and there have been other reports of hepatotoxicity associated with the prophylactic use of amodiaquine.[2] Examination of data submitted to the UK Committee on Safety of Medicines[3] suggested that the frequency of adverse reactions to amodiaquine was about 1 in 1700 for serious reactions, 1 in 2200 for blood disorders, 1 in 15 650 for serious hepatic disorders, and 1 in 15 650 for fatal reactions. In contrast the frequency of agranulocytosis in users in France[4] has been estimated to be 1 in 25 000. Worldwide[4] the risk of severe reactions appears to be between 1 in 1000 and 1 in 5000. The manufacturers reportedly had 42 cases of serious adverse effects during amodiaquine prophylaxis, between 1985 and 1991; there were 28 cases of agranulocytosis (9 deaths) and 14 of hepatitis (3 deaths).[5] Whether there was significantly less risk when amodiaquine was given for treatment of malaria rather than prophylaxis was not certain.[6]

It has been suggested that an immunological reaction to amodiaquine quinone imine, which can be produced by autoxidation among other processes, may partially account for amodiaquine's greater tendency to induce agranulocytosis compared with chloroquine.[7,8]

The acute toxicity of amodiaquine appears to differ from that of chloroquine in that there have been no reports of cardiovascular symptoms following overdosage with amodiaquine[9] but intoxication with amodiaquine is also far less frequent than chloroquine poisoning. However, large doses of amodiaquine have been reported to produce syncope, spasticity, convulsions, and involuntary movements.[9]

1. Anonymous. Amodiaquine and agranulocytosis. *WHO Drug Inf* 1987; **1:** 5–6.
2. Larrey D, *et al.* Amodiaquine-induced hepatitis. *Ann Intern Med* 1986; **104:** 801–3.
3. Phillips-Howard PA, West LJ. Serious adverse drug reactions to pyrimethamine–sulphadoxine, pyrimethamine–dapsone and to amodiaquine in Britain. *J R Soc Med* 1990; **83:** 82–5.
4. Anonymous. Development of recommendations for the protection of short-stay travellers to malaria endemic areas: memorandum from two WHO meetings. *Bull WHO* 1988; **66:** 177–96.
5. Olliaro P, *et al.* Systematic review of amodiaquine treatment in uncomplicated malaria. *Lancet* 1996; **348:** 1196–1201.
6. White NJ. Can amodiaquine be resurrected? *Lancet* 1996; **348:** 1184–5.
7. Winstanley PA, *et al.* The toxicity of amodiaquine and its principal metabolites towards mononuclear leucocytes and granulocyte/monocyte colony forming units. *Br J Clin Pharmacol* 1990; **29:** 479–85.
8. Park BK, Kitteringham NR. Drug–protein conjugation and its immunological consequences. *Drug Metab Rev* 1990; **22:** 87–144.
9. Jaeger A, *et al.* Clinical features and management of poisoning due to antimalarial drugs. *Med Toxicol* 1987; **2:** 242–73.

Pharmacokinetics

Amodiaquine hydrochloride is readily absorbed from the gastrointestinal tract. Amodiaquine is rapidly converted in the liver to the active metabolite desethylamodiaquine, only a negligible amount of amodiaquine being excreted unchanged in the urine. The plasma elimination half-life of desethylamodiaquine has varied from 1 to 10 days or more. Amodiaquine and desethylamodiaquine have been detected in the urine several months after administration.

◊ References.
1. Winstanley P, *et al.* The disposition of amodiaquine in man after oral administration. *Br J Clin Pharmacol* 1987; **23:** 1–7.
2. White NJ, *et al.* Pharmacokinetics of intravenous amodiaquine. *Br J Clin Pharmacol* 1987; **23:** 127–35.
3. Winstanley PA, *et al.* The disposition of amodiaquine in Zambians and Nigerians with malaria. *Br J Clin Pharmacol* 1990; **29:** 695–701.
4. Krishna S, White NJ. Pharmacokinetics of quinine, chloroquine and amodiaquine: clinical implications. *Clin Pharmacokinet* 1996; **30:** 263–99.

Uses and Administration

Amodiaquine is a 4-aminoquinoline antimalarial with an action similar to that of chloroquine (p.435). It is as effective as chloroquine against chloroquine-sensitive strains of *Plasmodium falciparum* and is also effective against some chloroquine-resistant strains, although resistance to amodiaquine has developed and there may be partial cross-resistance between amodiaquine and chloroquine. Because of resistance and the risk of

The symbol † denotes a preparation no longer actively marketed

---

major toxicity amodiaquine is not recommended for the prophylaxis of malaria.

Amodiaquine is given by mouth as the hydrochloride, but doses are expressed in terms of amodiaquine base. For the treatment of falciparum malaria a total dose of 35 mg per kg body-weight has been given over 3 days.

◊ References.
1. Olliaro P, Mussano P. Amodiaquine for treating malaria (updated 29 November 2000). Available in The Cochrane Library; Issue 4. Oxford: Update Software; 2001.
2. McIntosh HM. Chloroquine or amodiaquine combined with sulfadoxine-pyrimethamine for treating uncomplicated malaria (updated 27 August 2001). Available in The Cochrane Library; Issue 4. Oxford: Update Software; 2001.

Preparations

USP 25: Amodiaquine Hydrochloride Tablets.

Proprietary Preparations (details are given in Part 3)
Fr.: Flavoquine.

Amopyroquine Hydrochloride   (1375-q)

Amopyroquine Hydrochloride (*rINNM*).

Amopyroquin Hydrochloride; CI-356; PAM-780; WR-4835. 4-(7-Chloro-4-quinolylamino)-2-(pyrrolidin-1-ylmethyl)phenol dihydrochloride.

$C_{20}H_{20}ClN_3O,2HCl = 426.8$.

CAS — 550-81-2 (amopyroquine); 10350-81-9 (amopyroquine dihydrochloride).

Profile

Amopyroquine is a 4-aminoquinoline antimalarial that is an analogue of amodiaquine (above). It has been administered as the hydrochloride by intramuscular injection or by mouth in the treatment of malaria.

Artemisinin Derivatives   (18783-m)

Artemether   (12024-p)

Artemether (*BAN, rINN*).

Dihydroartemisinin Methyl Ether; Dihydroqinghaosu Methyl Ether; *o*-Methyldihydroartemisinin; SM-224. (3R,5aS,6R,8aS,9R,10S,12R,12aR)-Decahydro-10-methoxy-3,6,9-trimethyl-3,12-epoxy-12H-pyrano[4,3-*j*]-1,2-benzodioxepin.

$C_{16}H_{26}O_5 = 298.4$.

CAS — 71963-77-4.

Artemisinin   (12023-q)

Artemisinin (*rINN*).

Arteannuin; Artemisinine; Huanghuahaosu; Qinghaosu. (3R,5aS,6R,8aS,9R,12S,12aR)-Octahydro-3,6,9-trimethyl-3,12-epoxy-12H-pyrano[4,3-*j*]-1,2-benzodioxepin-10(3H)-one.

$C_{15}H_{22}O_5 = 282.3$.

CAS — 63968-64-9.

Artemotil   (9352-a)

Artemotil (*rINN*).

Arteether; Dihydroartemisinin Ethyl Ether; Dihydroqinghaosu Ethyl Ether; SM-227. (3R,5aS,6R,8aS,9R,10S,12R,12aR)-Decahydro-10-ethoxy-3,6,9-trimethyl-3,12-epoxy-12H-pyrano[4,3-*j*]-1,2-benzodioxepin.

$C_{17}H_{28}O_5 = 312.4$.

CAS — 75887-54-6.

Sodium Artesunate   (5761-m)

Sodium Artesunate (*rINNM*).

Dihydroartemisinin Hemisuccinate Sodium; Dihydroqinghaosu Hemisuccinate Sodium; SM-804. (3R,5aS,6R,8aS,9R,10S,12R,12aR)-Decahydro-3,6,9-trimethyl-3,12-epoxy-12H-pyrano-[4,3-*j*]-1,2-benzodioxepin-10-ol hydrogen succinate sodium.

$C_{19}H_{27}O_8Na = 406.4$.

CAS — 88495-63-0 (artesunate).

Adverse Effects and Precautions

Treatment with artemisinin and its derivatives appears to be generally well tolerated, although there have been reports of mild gastrointestinal disturbance, dizziness, tinnitus, neutropenia, elevated liver enzyme values, and ECG abnormalities including prolongation of the QT interval.

Evidence of severe neurotoxicity has been seen in *animals* given high doses.

◊ General references to adverse effects associated with artemisinin derivatives.
1. Price R, *et al.* Adverse effects in patients with acute falciparum malaria treated with artemisinin derivatives. *Am J Trop Med Hyg* 1999; **60:** 547–55.

Effects on the heart. Bradycardia was reported in 10 of 34 patients who received artemether orally for 4 days.[1]

1. Karbwang J, *et al.* Comparison of oral artemether and mefloquine in acute uncomplicated falciparum malaria. *Lancet* 1992; **340:** 1245–8.

Effects on the nervous system. Neurotoxicity has been reported in *animals* given artemotil or artemether.[1] An in-vitro study[2] has shown that dihydroartemisinin, the metabolite common to all artemisinin derivatives currently used, is neurotoxic. There has been a report[3] of acute cerebellar dysfunction manifesting as ataxia and slurred speech in a patient who took a 5-day course of artesunate by mouth.

1. Brewer TG, *et al.* Neurotoxicity in animals due to arteether and artemether. *Trans R Soc Trop Med Hyg* 1994; **88** (suppl 1): 33–6.
2. Wesche DL, *et al.* Neurotoxicity of artemisinin analogs in vitro. *Antimicrob Agents Chemother* 1994; **38:** 1813–19.
3. Miller LG, Panosian CB. Ataxia and slurred speech after artesunate treatment for falciparum malaria. *N Engl J Med* 1997; **336:** 1328.

Pregnancy. Artesunate or artemether was used to treat multidrug-resistant falciparum malaria in 83 pregnant women in Thailand; of 73 pregnancies resulting in live births none showed evidence of any congenital abnormality.[1] Sixteen of the women had received artesunate during the first trimester; of these, 12 had normal deliveries, 1 was lost to study, and 3 had spontaneous abortions.

No undue adverse effects on the neonates occurred in a study[2] involving 45 women treated for multidrug-resistant malaria during their second or third trimester of pregnancy with either artemether or artemether plus mefloquine.

1. McGready R, *et al.* Artemisinin derivatives in the treatment of falciparum malaria in pregnancy. *Trans R Soc Trop Med Hyg* 1998; **92:** 430–3.
2. Sowunmi A, *et al.* Randomised trial of artemether versus artemether and mefloquine for the treatment of chloroquine/sulfadoxine[sic]-pyrimethamine-resistant falciparum malaria during pregnancy. *J Obstet Gynaecol* 1998; **18:** 322–7.

Interactions

Grapefruit juice. The oral bioavailability of artemether may be increased by concomitant administration of grapefruit juice.

1. van Agtmael MA, *et al.* The effect of grapefruit juice on the time-dependent decline of artemether plasma levels in healthy subjects. *Clin Pharmacol Ther* 1999; **66:** 408–14.

Pharmacokinetics

Peak plasma concentrations have been achieved in about 3 hours after oral administration of artemether, in about 6 hours after intramuscular injection of artemether, and in about 11 hours after rectal administration of artemisinin. Artemisinin and its derivatives are all rapidly hydrolysed to the active metabolite dihydroartemisinin. Reported elimination half-lives have been about 45 minutes after intravenous administration of artesunate, about 4 hours after rectal artemisinin, and about 4 to 11 hours after intramuscular or oral artemether. There is very little published data on the pharmacokinetics of artemotil, but its elimination half-life appears to be longer than that of artemether.

◊ Reviews.
1. White NJ, *et al.* Clinical pharmacokinetics and pharmacodynamics of artemether-lumefantrine. *Clin Pharmacokinet* 1999; **37:** 105–25.
2. Navaratnam V, *et al.* Pharmacokinetics of artemisinin-type compounds. *Clin Pharmacokinet* 2000; **39:** 255–70.

Uses and Administration

Artemisinin is a sesquiterpene lactone isolated from *Artemisia annua*, a herb that has traditionally been used in China for the treatment of malaria. It is a potent and rapidly acting blood schizontocide active against *Plasmodium vivax* and against both chloroquine-sensitive and chloroquine-resistant strains of *P. falciparum*.

Artemisinin and its derivatives are used usually in combination with other antimalarials for the treatment of malaria resistant to conventional drugs.

The following doses are those suggested by WHO for the treatment of malaria in areas of multidrug resistance. For oral administration in uncomplicated falciparum malaria, artemisinin or sodium artesunate may be given as a 3-day course. The dose of artemisinin is 25 mg per kg body-weight on the first day with 12.5 mg per kg on the second and the third days. For artesunate, the initial dose is 5 mg per kg on the first day with 2.5 mg per kg on days two and three. In both cases a single dose of mefloquine 15 mg per kg (or occasionally 25 mg per kg if necessary) is given on the second day to effect clinical cure.

For oral treatment of uncomplicated falciparum malaria, artemether is given in combination with lumefantrine, over a period of 60 hours in a dose of 80 mg administered at diagnosis and repeated after 8, 24, 36, 48 and 60 hours (total dose 480 mg). If the oral artemisinin compounds have to be used alone they should be given for a minimum of 5 days.

For parenteral administration in severe malaria, artemether or artesunate are employed. The loading dose of artemether is 3.2 mg per kg body-weight intramuscularly, followed by 1.6 mg per kg daily for a maximum of 5 days. The loading dose of artesunate is 2.4 mg per kg intravenously, followed at 12 and 24 hours by a dose of 1.2 mg per kg, and then 1.2 mg per kg daily for a maximum of 6 days. For both drugs the patient should be transferred to oral therapy as soon as possible. Additionally a single oral dose of mefloquine should be given to effect clinical cure.

◊ Reviews.
1. de Vries PJ, Dien TK. Clinical pharmacology and therapeutic potential of artemisinin and its derivatives in the treatment of malaria. *Drugs* 1996; **52**: 818–36.
2. McIntosh HM, Olliaro P. Artemisinin derivatives for treating uncomplicated malaria (updated 20 February 2001). Available in The Cochrane Library; Issue 4. Oxford: Update Software; 2001.
3. McIntosh HM, Olliaro P. Artemisinin derivatives for treating severe malaria (updated 29 August 2001). Available in The Cochrane Library; Issue 4. Oxford: Update Software; 2001.

Administration of artemisinin derivatives. To overcome the poor solubility of *artemisinin* in water a number of dosage forms and routes of administration have been tried. Also, several more potent derivatives with more suitable pharmacological properties have been developed,[1-3] notably the methyl ether derivative, *artemether*, and the ethyl ether derivative, *artemotil*, which are more lipid soluble; the sodium salt of the hemisuccinate ester, *sodium artesunate*, which is soluble in water but appears to have poor stability in aqueous solutions; and *sodium artelinate* which is both soluble and stable in water. Other derivatives which have been studied include *arteflene*. Several preparations of artemisinin derivatives are available either commercially or for studies organised by bodies such as WHO.[3] These include oral formulations of artemether, artesunate, artemisinin itself, and *dihydroartemisinin*; intramuscular formulations of artemotil, artemether, and artesunate; intravenous formulations of *artelinic acid* and artesunate; and suppositories of artemisinin and artesunate.
1. Titulaer HAC, *et al.* Formulation and pharmacokinetics of artemisinin and its derivatives. *Int J Pharmaceutics* 1991; **69**: 83–92.
2. WHO. *WHO model prescribing information: drugs used in parasitic diseases.* 2nd ed. Geneva: WHO, 1995.
3. Olliaro PL, Trigg PI. Status of antimalarial drugs under development. *Bull WHO* 1995; **73**: 565–71.

Malaria. Artemisinin and its derivatives have been shown in many studies to be effective in the treatment of both acute uncomplicated and severe malaria, the overall management of which is discussed further on p.428. In an attempt to delay the development of resistance to these compounds, WHO has recommended[1,2] that their use be restricted to the treatment of malaria in areas of documented multidrug resistance and that they should not be used at all for prophylaxis; in practice, however, they appear to be more widely used. Recrudescence rates are high when artemisinin compounds are given alone and they should therefore, when possible, be given with another antimalarial such as mefloquine in order to effect a clinical cure.
In acute uncomplicated malaria the drugs are usually given by mouth. Those used have been artemisinin,[3] artemether[4-9] or artesunate[9-14] usually with mefloquine additionally. Artemether is also used with lumefantrine (see p.438). The combination of artesunate with pyrimethamine-sulfadoxine is under investigation for use as first-line treatment in areas of chloroquine resistance. Artemotil[15] may be given intramuscularly in acute malaria.
Parenteral therapy is generally necessary in severe malaria and good results in multidrug-resistant areas have been obtained with artemether,[16-18] artemotil,[19] or artesunate[18,20] intramuscularly, usually followed by oral mefloquine. Artesunate has also been given intravenously.[18] Rectal administration of artesunate[21] or artemisinin,[18,20] followed by oral mefloquine, has been successful.
Alternatives to standard treatment of cerebral malaria with intravenous quinine have been sought, partly because of the problems associated with giving intravenous infusions in the field. Several studies have shown intramuscular artemether to be effective,[22-24] but the wisdom of such use when there is no multidrug resistance has been severely questioned.[23,24] Also, although artemether has compared favourably with quinine in the treatment of severe (including cerebral) falciparum malaria,[16] in other studies artemether, although an effective alternative to quinine, was either associated with slightly longer coma-recovery times[17,23] or did not reduce mortality significantly compared with quinine.[17,23,25]
1. Anonymous. Artemisinin and its derivatives: use as antimalarials. *WHO Drug Inf* 1993; **7**: 111–13.
2. WHO. *WHO model prescribing information: drugs used in parasitic diseases.* 2nd ed. Geneva: WHO, 1995.

3. Hung LN, *et al.* Single dose artemisinin-mefloquine versus mefloquine alone for uncomplicated falciparum malaria. *Trans R Soc Trop Med Hyg* 1997; **91**: 191–4.
4. Karbwang J, *et al.* Comparison of oral artemether and mefloquine in acute uncomplicated falciparum malaria. *Lancet* 1992; **340**: 1245–8.
5. Bunnag D, *et al.* Artemether-mefloquine combination in multidrug resistant falciparum malaria. *Trans R Soc Trop Med Hyg* 1995; **89**: 213–15.
6. Karbwang J, *et al.* A comparative clinical trial of two different regimens of artemether plus mefloquine in multidrug resistant falciparum malaria. *Trans R Soc Trop Med Hyg* 1995; **89**: 296–8.
7. Karbwang J, *et al.* A comparative clinical trial of artemether and the sequential regimen of artemether-mefloquine in multidrug resistant falciparum malaria. *J Antimicrob Chemother* 1995; **36**: 1079–83.
8. Price RN, *et al.* Artesunate versus artemether in combination with mefloquine for the treatment of multidrug-resistant falciparum malaria. *Trans R Soc Trop Med Hyg* 1995; **89**: 523–7.
9. Bunnag D, *et al.* Artemether or artesunate followed by mefloquine as a possible treatment for multidrug resistant falciparum malaria. *Trans R Soc Trop Med Hyg* 1996; **90**: 415–17.
10. Looareesuwan S, *et al.* Randomized trial of mefloquine-doxycycline, and artesunate-doxycycline for treatment of acute uncomplicated falciparum malaria. *Am J Trop Med Hyg* 1994; **50**: 784–9.
11. Karbwang J, *et al.* Comparison of oral artesunate and quinine plus tetracycline in acute uncomplicated falciparum malaria. *Bull WHO* 1994; **72**: 233–8.
12. Luxemburger C, *et al.* Oral artesunate in the treatment of uncomplicated hyperparasitemic falciparum malaria. *Am J Trop Med Hyg* 1995; **53**: 522–5.
13. Looareesuwan S, *et al.* Comparative clinical trial of artesunate followed by mefloquine in the treatment of acute uncomplicated falciparum malaria: two- and three-day regimens. *Am J Trop Med Hyg* 1996; **54**: 210–13.
14. Price R, *et al.* Artesunate and mefloquine in the treatment of uncomplicated multidrug-resistant hyperparasitaemic falciparum malaria. *Trans R Soc Trop Med Hyg* 1998; **92**: 207–11.
15. Mishra SK, *et al.* Effectiveness of α,β-arteether in acute falciparum malaria. *Trans R Soc Trop Med Hyg* 1995; **89**: 299–301.
16. Karbwang J, *et al.* Comparison of artemether and quinine in the treatment of severe falciparum malaria in south-east Thailand. *Trans R Soc Trop Med Hyg* 1995; **89**: 668–71.
17. Hien TT, *et al.* A controlled trial of artemether or quinine in Vietnamese adults with severe falciparum malaria. *N Engl J Med* 1996; **335**: 76–83.
18. Vinh H, *et al.* Severe and complicated malaria treated with artemisinin, artesunate or artemether in Viet Nam. *Trans R Soc Trop Med Hyg* 1997; **91**: 465–7.
19. Mohanty S, *et al.* α,β-Arteether for the treatment of complicated falciparum malaria. *Trans R Soc Trop Med Hyg* 1997; **91**: 328–30.
20. Phuong CXT, *et al.* Comparison of artemisinin suppositories, intramuscular artesunate and intravenous quinine for the treatment of severe childhood malaria. *Trans R Soc Trop Med Hyg* 1997; **91**: 335–42.
21. Looareesuwan S, *et al.* Efficacy and tolerability of a sequential, artesunate suppository plus mefloquine, treatment of severe falciparum malaria. *Ann Trop Med Parasitol* 1995; **89**: 469–75.
22. Walker O, *et al.* An open randomized comparative study of intramuscular artemether and intravenous quinine in cerebral malaria in children. *Trans R Soc Trop Med Hyg* 1993; **87**: 564–6.
23. Boele van Hensbroek M, *et al.* A trial of artemether or quinine in children with cerebral malaria. *N Engl J Med* 1996; **335**: 69–75.
24. Murphy S, *et al.* An open randomized trial of artemether versus quinine in the treatment of cerebral malaria in African children. *Trans R Soc Trop Med Hyg* 1996; **90**: 298–301.
25. Taylor TE, *et al.* Intramuscular artemether vs intravenous quinine: an open, randomized trial in Malawian children with cerebral malaria. *Trop Med Int Hlth* 1998; **3**: 3–8.

Preparations

Proprietary Preparations (details are given in Part 3)
Fr.: Paluther; Thai.: Plasmotrim.

Multi-ingredient: *Switz.:* Riamet; *UK:* Riamet.

Chloroquine (1371-m)

Chloroquine (BAN, rINN).

Cloroquina. 4-(7-Chloro-4-quinolylamino)pentyldiethylamine; 7-Chloro-4-(4-diethylamino-1-methylbutylamino)quinoline.
$C_{18}H_{26}ClN_3 = 319.9$.
CAS — 54-05-7.
ATC — P01BA01.

Pharmacopoeias. In US.

Pharmacopoeial description

USP 25: A white or slightly yellow, odourless, crystalline powder. M.p. 87° to 92°. Very slightly soluble in water; soluble in chloroform, in ether, and in dilute acids.

Chloroquine Hydrochloride (18496-t)

Chloroquine Hydrochloride (BANM, rINNM).
$C_{18}H_{26}ClN_3, 2HCl = 392.8$.
CAS — 3545-67-3.

Pharmacopoeias. US includes the injection.

Chloroquine hydrochloride 123 mg is approximately equivalent to 100 mg of chloroquine base.

Chloroquine Phosphate (1372-b)

Chloroquine Phosphate (BANM, rINNM).
Chingaminum; Chlorochinium Phosphoricum; Chlorochinum Diphosphoricum; Chloroquini Diphosphas; Chloroquini Phosphas; Fosfato de Cloroquina; Quingamine; SN-7618.
$C_{18}H_{26}ClN_3, 2H_3PO_4 = 515.9$.
CAS — 50-63-5.

Pharmacopoeias. In *Chin., Eur.* (see p.vi), *Int., Pol.,* and *US.*

Chloroquine phosphate 161 mg is approximately equivalent to 100 mg of chloroquine base.

Pharmacopoeial description

Ph. Eur.: A white or almost white, hygroscopic, crystalline powder. It exists in two forms, one melting at about 195° and the other at about 218°. Freely soluble in water; very slightly soluble in alcohol, in ether, and in methyl alcohol. A 10% solution in water has a pH of 3.8 to 4.3. Store in airtight containers. Protect from light.

USP 25: A white, odourless, crystalline powder, which slowly discolours on exposure to light. It exists in two polymorphic forms, one melting between 193° and 195° and the other between 210° and 215°; mixture of the two forms melts between 193° and 215°. Freely soluble in water; practically insoluble in alcohol, in chloroform, and in ether. Its solutions have a pH of about 4.5.

Chloroquine Sulfate (1373-v)

Chloroquine Sulfate (rINNM).
Chloroquine Sulphate (BANM); Chloroquini Sulfas; RP-3377; Sulfato de Cloroquina.
$C_{18}H_{26}ClN_3, H_2SO_4, H_2O = 436.0$.
CAS — 132-73-0 (anhydrous chloroquine sulfate).

Pharmacopoeias. In *Eur.* (see p.vi) and *Int.*

Chloroquine sulfate 136 mg is approximately equivalent to 100 mg of chloroquine base.

Pharmacopoeial description

Ph. Eur.: A white or almost white crystalline powder. Freely soluble in water and in methyl alcohol; very slightly soluble in alcohol; practically insoluble in ether. An 8% solution in water has a pH of 4.0 to 5.0. Store in airtight containers. Protect from light.

Sorption. Various studies using low concentrations of chloroquine phosphate or chloroquine sulfate indicate that chloroquine exhibits pH-dependent binding to several materials used in medical equipment and membrane filters including soda glass and various plastics such as cellulose acetate, cellulose propionate, methacrylate butadiene styrene, polypropylene, PVC, ethylvinyl acetate, and polyethylene.[1-3] Although this effect may not be of relevance at doses used clinically[4] it is considered critical that laboratory workers undertaking assays and sensitivity testing should recognise that significant reductions in concentrations can occur when chloroquine is prepared or stored in equipment made from these materials.[2,3] As the effect of borosilicate glass or polystyrene appears to be minimal it has been suggested that they may be suitable for use in such procedures.[2,3]
Similar sorption has also been reported during membrane filtration of solutions of amodiaquine hydrochloride, mefloquine hydrochloride, or quinine sulfate.[1]
1. Baird JK, Lambros C. Effect of membrane filtration on in vitro activity against Plasmodium falciparum. *Bull WHO* 1984; **62**: 439–44.
2. Yahya AM, *et al.* Binding of chloroquine to glass. *Int J Pharmaceutics* 1985; **25**: 217–23.
3. Yahya AM, *et al.* Investigation of chloroquine binding to plastic materials. *Int J Pharmaceutics* 1986; **34**: 137–43.
4. Martens HJ, *et al.* Sorption of various drugs in polyvinyl chloride, glass, and polyethylene-lined infusion containers. *Am J Hosp Pharm* 1990; **47**: 369–73.

Adverse Effects

Adverse effects experienced with dosage regimens of chloroquine used in the treatment and prophylaxis of malaria are generally less common and less severe than those associated with the larger doses used for prolonged periods in rheumatoid arthritis.

Frequent adverse effects of chloroquine include headache, various skin eruptions, pruritus, and gastrointestinal disturbances such as nausea, vomiting, and diarrhoea. More rarely, mental changes including psychotic episodes, agitation, and personality changes may occur. Convulsions have been reported. Visual disturbances such as blurred vision and difficulties in focusing have occurred but these are more common with larger doses, when they may be associated with keratopathy or retinopathy, as discussed under Effects on the Eyes, below. Keratopathy usually occurs in the form of corneal opacities and is normally reversible when chloroquine is withdrawn. Retinopathy is the most serious adverse effect of chloroquine on the eyes and it can result in severe visual impairment. Changes may be irreversible and can even progress after chloroquine is discontinued. Those taking large doses of chloroquine for prolonged periods appear to be at greatest risk of developing retinopathy. Other uncommon adverse effects from prolonged use include loss of hair, bleaching of hair pigment, bluish-black pigmentation of the mucous membranes and skin, photosensitivity, tinnitus, reduced hearing, nerve deafness, neuromyopathy, and myopathy, including cardiomyopathy.

Blood disorders have been reported rarely. They include aplastic anaemia, reversible agranulocytosis, thrombocytopenia, and neutropenia.

There have also been rare reports of changes in liver function, including hepatitis and abnormal liver function tests.

Parenteral therapy with chloroquine can be hazardous and rapid intravenous administration or the use of large doses can result in cardiovascular toxicity and other symptoms of acute overdosage.

Acute overdosage with chloroquine is extremely dangerous and death can occur within a few hours. Initial effects include headache, gastrointestinal disturbances, drowsiness, and dizziness. Hypokalaemia may occur within a few hours of ingestion of chloroquine. Visual disturbances may be dramatic with a sudden loss of vision. However, the main effect of overdosage with chloroquine is cardiovascular toxicity with hypotension and cardiac arrhythmias progressing to cardiovascular collapse, convulsions, cardiac and respiratory arrest, coma, and death.

Effects on the blood. Aplastic anaemia was associated with the use of chloroquine in 3 patients.[1] Two patients had received treatment over several months and one of these was later found to have acute myeloblastic leukaemia after receiving chloroquine treatment initially for discoid lupus erythematosus, and later for cerebral malaria. In the third patient aplastic anaemia developed 3 weeks after a short course of chloroquine for malaria.

1. Nagaratnam N, et al. Aplasia and leukaemia following chloroquine therapy. Postgrad Med J 1978; 54: 108–12.

Effects on the eyes. The main adverse effects of chloroquine and hydroxychloroquine on the eye are keratopathy and retinopathy.

Keratopathy, characterised by corneal deposits, may occur within a few weeks of starting treatment. However, patients are often asymptomatic and fewer than 50% of affected patients complain of visual symptoms such as photophobia, haloes around lights, or blurred vision. Keratopathy is completely reversible on withdrawal of treatment and is not usually considered to be a contra-indication to continued treatment.[1]

Retinopathy is potentially more serious. The outcome following discontinuation of treatment is unpredictable and changes may be irreversible or may even progress.[2,3] Delayed-onset retinopathy has also been reported in patients many years after cessation of treatment.[4] The reported incidence of retinopathy varies according to the methodology and criteria used.[1,5,6] From studies in patients on long-term antimalarial treatment, it was reported[1] that an accumulation of 100 g of chloroquine [phosphate] (250 mg daily for 1 year) might cause retinopathy; the risk was significantly increased as the total dosage exceeded 300 g. Experience in rheumatology also indicates that the incidence of retinal toxicity is dose-related. While the total cumulative dose, the duration of treatment, and the age of the patient might all affect the incidence of retinal toxicity[7,8] the daily dose might be the most important factor.[9] It has been suggested that the risk of retinal damage is small with daily doses of up to 4.0 mg of chloroquine phosphate per kg body-weight (= chloroquine base approximately 2.5 mg per kg daily) or up to 6.5 mg of hydroxychloroquine sulfate per kg.[9] In obese patients, excessive dosage should be avoided by calculating dosage on the basis of lean body-weight. It appears that retinopathy is rarely, if ever, associated with the weekly dosages of chloroquine recommended for the prophylaxis of malaria.[10,11] In the UK, the Royal College of Ophthalmologists has made recommendations regarding use by rheumatologists and dermatologists. Chloroquine should only be used if hydroxychloroquine or other preferred drugs have failed as there is inadequate data to advise on a safe maximum dose; thus the following recommendations relate only to hydroxychloroquine as no guidelines have been published for chloroquine. Baseline assessment before treatment with hydroxychloroquine is commenced (maximum daily dosage 6.5 mg per kg lean body-weight) should consist of checking renal and hepatic function, questioning the patient about visual impairment not corrected by glasses, and recording near visual acuity. Thereafter, patients should be monitored annually with enquiry about visual symptomatology, rechecking of acuity, and assessment for blurred vision. Patients should be referred to an ophthalmologist if problems are detected either before or during treatment. Those taking long-term hydroxychloroquine should be subject

The symbol † denotes a preparation no longer actively marketed

to occasional ophthalmological review after 5 years' continuous treatment.

1. Bernstein HN. Ophthalmologic considerations and testing in patients receiving long-term antimalarial therapy. Am J Med 1983; 75 (suppl 1A): 25–34.
2. Ogawa S, et al. Progression of retinopathy long after cessation of chloroquine therapy. Lancet 1979; i: 1408.
3. Easterbrook M. Ocular effects and safety of antimalarial agents. Am J Med 1988; 85 (suppl 4A): 23–9.
4. Ehrenfeld M, et al. Delayed-onset chloroquine retinopathy. Br J Ophthalmol 1986; 70: 281–3.
5. Finbloom DS, et al. Comparison of hydroxychloroquine and chloroquine use and the development of retinal toxicity. J Rheumatol 1985; 12: 692–4.
6. Morsman CDG, et al. Screening for hydroxychloroquine retinal toxicity: is it necessary? Eye 1990; 4: 572–6.
7. Elman A, et al. Chloroquine retinopathy in patients with rheumatoid arthritis. Scand J Rheumatol 1976; 5: 161–6.
8. Marks JS, Power BJ. Is chloroquine obsolete in treatment of rheumatic disease? Lancet 1979; i: 371–3.
9. Mackenzie AH. Dose refinements in long-term therapy of rheumatoid arthritis with antimalarials. Am J Med 1983; 75 (suppl 1A): 40–5.
10. Breckenridge A. Risks and benefits of prophylactic antimalarial drugs. BMJ 1989; 299: 1057–8.
11. Lange WR, et al. No evidence for chloroquine-associated retinopathy among missionaries on long-term malaria chemoprophylaxis. Am J Trop Med Hyg 1994; 51: 389–92.

Effects on glucose metabolism. While hypoglycaemia has occurred with quinine (see p.445), it was not generally thought to be associated with chloroquine; however, there has been a report of its occurrence in a patient with reactive hypoglycaemia.[1]

1. Abu-Shakra M, Lee P. Hypoglycemia: an unusual adverse reaction to chloroquine. Clin Exp Rheumatol 1994; 12: 95.

Effects on the heart. Studies in patients with malaria[1] and in healthy subjects[2] indicate that the acute cardiovascular toxicity that may be associated with parenteral administration of chloroquine is related to transiently high plasma concentrations produced during the early part of the distribution phase; these findings appear to confirm that the rate of administration is a major determinant of this toxicity. Cardiac conduction abnormalities, including heart block, have also occurred in patients receiving long-term oral treatment with chloroquine,[3] including use in lupus erythematosus,[4,5] as well as after chloroquine overdosage or abuse.[6] Histological changes in endomyocardial biopsy specimens from 2 patients with cardiomyopathy associated with chloroquine or hydroxychloroquine therapy were found to be virtually identical to those seen in the skeletal muscle of patients with chloroquine-induced myopathy[7] (see also Effects on the Muscles, below).

1. White NJ, et al. Parenteral chloroquine for treating falciparum malaria. J Infect Dis 1987; 155: 192–201.
2. Looareesuwan S, et al. Cardiovascular toxicity and distribution kinetics of intravenous chloroquine. Br J Clin Pharmacol 1986; 22: 31–6.
3. Ogola ESN, et al. Chloroquine related complete heart block with blindness: case report. East Afr Med J 1992; 69: 50–2.
4. Piette J-C, et al. Chloroquine cardiotoxicity. N Engl J Med 1987; 317: 710–11.
5. Baguet J-P, et al. Chloroquine cardiomyopathy with conduction disorders. Heart 1999; 81: 221–3.
6. Ihenacho HNC, Magulike E. Chloroquine abuse and heart block in Africans. Aust N Z J Med 1989; 19: 17–21.
7. Ratliff NB, et al. Diagnosis of chloroquine cardiomyopathy by endomyocardial biopsy. N Engl J Med 1987; 316: 191–3.

Effects on the muscles. In a review[1] of drug-induced myotoxicity, the following points were made with regard to chloroquine. The myopathy induced by chloroquine is characterised by progressive weakness and atrophy of proximal muscles and can develop insidiously after periods of therapy ranging from a few weeks to a few years. There are often mild sensory changes, depression of tendon reflexes, and abnormal nerve conduction studies suggestive of an associated peripheral neuropathy. The myopathy is reversible on withdrawal of treatment but recovery may take several months. Cardiomyopathy may also occur (see under Effects on the Heart, above). Similar effects have been reported with hydroxychloroquine.[2] In a retrospective review of 4405 patients with rheumatic disorders, 214 had received chloroquine or hydroxychloroquine and, of these, 3 developed myopathy.[3]

1. Mastaglia FL. Adverse effects of drugs on muscle. Drugs 1982; 24: 304–21.
2. Estes ML, et al. Chloroquine neuromyotoxicity. Am J Med 1987; 82: 447–55.
3. Avina-Zubieta JA, et al. Incidence of myopathy in patients treated with antimalarials: a report of three cases and a review of the literature. Br J Rheumatol 1995; 34: 166–70.

Effects on the nervous system. Apart from neuropathies (see Effects on the Muscles, above) other adverse effects of chloroquine on the nervous system have included isolated reports of extrapyramidal symptoms and other involuntary movements[1,2] (in patients being treated for malaria), nystagmus[3] (in a patient on prolonged treatment for rheumatoid arthritis), and convulsions[4,5] and nonconvulsive status epilepticus[6] (in patients on malaria prophylaxis).

1. Umez-Eronini EM, Eronini EA. Chloroquine induced involuntary movements. BMJ 1977; 1: 945–6.
2. Singhi S, et al. Chloroquine-induced involuntary movements. BMJ 1977; 2: 520.
3. Marks JS. Motor polyneuropathy and nystagmus associated with chloroquine phosphate. Postgrad Med J 1979; 55: 569.
4. Fish DR, Espir MLE. Convulsions associated with prophylactic antimalarial drugs: implications for people with epilepsy. BMJ 1988; 297: 526–7.

5. Fish DR, Espri MLE. Malaria prophylaxis and epilepsy. BMJ 1988; 297: 1267.
6. Mülhauser P, et al. Chloroquine and nonconvulsive status epilepticus. Ann Intern Med 1995; 123: 76–7.

Effects on the skin. *Pruritus* is frequently reported in patients receiving chloroquine for the treatment of malaria and it may become so severe as to compromise treatment. The onset of itching occurs a few hours after administration but usually remits spontaneously within 72 hours. Although most workers consider that antihistamines are generally ineffective,[1,2] some patients may obtain some relief.[3] The incidence of pruritus is purported to be higher in black patients, but this may only reflect the greater number of black patients surveyed. The aetiology of this reaction is unknown, but the apparent higher incidence in black patients has prompted suggestions that it may have a genetic basis[4] or be related to the affinity of chloroquine for melanin.[2] Chloroquine's main metabolite, monodesethylchloroquine, has also been implicated.[5] A survey[1] in Nigeria found that, of 1100 patients, 74% had pruritus during antimalarial therapy; 61% of these reacted to chloroquine, 30% reacted to amodiaquine, 2.5% to Fansidar (pyrimethamine-sulfadoxine), and 6.5% reacted to all three. In another study in Nigeria,[4] the incidence of pruritus was reported to be 14% (8 of 56 patients) for chloroquine, 27% (14 of 52) for amodiaquine, and 13% (7 of 53) for halofantrine; none of 58 patients receiving quinine or 82 patients receiving mefloquine experienced pruritus.

There have been rare reports of more severe cutaneous reactions associated with chloroquine, including *toxic epidermal necrolysis*,[6,7] *erythema multiforme*,[8] and *Stevens-Johnson syndrome*,[9] although the causal role of chloroquine is not always clear as some of these patients also received other antimalarials, sometimes at an inappropriate dosage. In a more recent case of toxic epidermal necrolysis,[10] chloroquine given alone for malaria prophylaxis was the probable cause. For a discussion including the possible effect of chloroquine on the incidence of erythema multiforme in patients taking pyrimethamine with sulfadoxine, see Adverse Effects with Sulfonamides, under Pyrimethamine, p.443.

1. Ajayi AA, et al. Epidemiology of antimalarial-induced pruritus in Africans. Eur J Clin Pharmacol 1989; 37: 539–40.
2. Osifo NG. Chloroquine-induced pruritus among patients with malaria. Arch Dermatol 1984; 120: 80–2.
3. Okor RS. Responsiveness of chloroquine-induced pruritus to antihistamine therapy—clinical survey. J Clin Pharm Ther 1990; 15: 147–50.
4. Sowunmi A, et al. Pruritus and antimalarial drugs in Africans. Lancet 1989; ii: 213.
5. Essien EE, et al. Chloroquine disposition in hypersensitive and non-hypersensitive subjects and its significance in chloroquine-induced pruritus. Eur J Drug Metab Pharmacokinet 1989; 14: 71–7.
6. Kanwar AJ, Singh OP. Toxic epidermal necrolysis—drug induced. Indian J Dermatol 1976; 21: 73–7.
7. Phillips-Howard PA, Warwick Buckler J. Idiosyncratic reaction resembling toxic epidermal necrolysis caused by chloroquine and Maloprim. BMJ 1988; 296: 1605.
8. Steffen R, Somaini B. Severe cutaneous adverse reactions to sulfadoxine-pyrimethamine in Switzerland. Lancet 1986; i: 610.
9. Bamber MG, et al. Fatal Stevens-Johnson syndrome associated with Fansidar and chloroquine. J Infect 1986; 13: 31–3.
10. Boffa MJ, Chalmers RJG. Toxic epidermal necrolysis due to chloroquine phosphate. Br J Dermatol 1994; 131: 444–5.

Overdosage. For adverse effects associated with chloroquine overdosage, see Treatment of Adverse Effects, below.

Treatment of Adverse Effects

Acute overdosage with chloroquine can be rapidly lethal and intensive symptomatic supportive treatment should be commenced immediately. The first steps should be to maintain adequate respiration and to correct any cardiovascular disturbances. Early administration of adrenaline [epinephrine] with diazepam (see below) may minimise the cardiotoxicity of chloroquine and control the arrhythmias. Activated charcoal may be given by mouth to adults or children who present within one hour of ingesting more than the equivalent of 15 mg per kg body-weight of chloroquine base; activated charcoal may be left in the stomach to limit any further absorption. Other methods to increase the elimination of chloroquine, such as dialysis, are probably of little use.

◊ The clinical features and management of poisoning due to antimalarial drugs, including chloroquine, have been reviewed.[1]

Chloroquine overdosage is the most severe and frequent cause of intoxication with antimalarial drugs and chloroquine is often used for suicide attempts. Severe toxic manifestations may occur within 1 to 3 hours and fatal outcomes usually occur within 2 to 3 hours of drug ingestion. The major clinical symptoms are of neurological, respiratory, and cardiovascular toxicity;[1] death is usually due to cardiac arrest related to the direct effect of chloroquine on the myocardium.[2] Chloroquine has a low safety margin: doses of 20 mg per kg body-weight are considered toxic and 30 mg per kg may be lethal. The mortality rate in some published studies has ranged from 10 to 30%.[1] If gastric lavage is attempted it should be preceded by correction of severe cardiovascular disturbances and institution of artificial ventilation because insertion of the stomach tube may induce sudden cardiac arrest or convulsions; induction of emesis is contra-indicated because of the risk of lung aspiration. Activated charcoal has been recommended to limit absorption of chloroquine that may be left in the gut.[3] There is no evidence to indicate that attempts to increase chloroquine elimination such as acidification of the urine, haemodialysis, peritoneal dialysis, or exchange transfusion, are effective in overdosage. Elimination in the urine is more dependent on haemodynamic status than on infusion of osmotic solutions or acidification. Any clearance achieved by haemoperfusion or haemodialysis is low in comparison with the normal total body clearance.[1]

It is not clear if correction of hypokalaemia is essential, but administration of potassium should be avoided in the initial phases of intoxication when conduction disturbances still exist. The degree of hypokalaemia may be correlated with the severity of chloroquine intoxication and might be useful diagnostically.[4] However, chloroquine-induced hypokalaemia may be due to a transport-dependent mechanism rather than to true potassium depletion and overzealous correction could result in hyperkalaemia.[4]

Since there had been no effective treatment for severe chloroquine poisoning, one group of workers tried treatment with early mechanical ventilation, together with adrenaline [epinephrine] and high doses of diazepam, both given intravenously, to counteract cardiotoxicity, with encouraging results.[2] Diazepam had earlier been shown to decrease the cardiotoxicity of chloroquine in *animal* studies and there had been several clinical reports of beneficial responses. It was considered that routine administration of adrenaline [epinephrine] before the onset of cardiac arrhythmia might be beneficial in the treatment of severe chloroquine poisoning.[2] The manufacturers of chloroquine have suggested giving adrenaline [epinephrine] by intravenous infusion in a dose of 0.25 µg per kg body-weight per minute initially, with increments of 0.25 µg per kg per minute until adequate systolic blood pressure is restored, and diazepam by intravenous infusion in a dose of 2 mg per kg over 30 minutes as a loading dose, followed by 1 to 2 mg per kg per day for up to 2 to 4 days.

1. Jaeger A, *et al*. Clinical features and management of poisoning due to antimalarial drugs. *Med Toxicol* 1987; **2:** 242–73.
2. Riou B, *et al*. Treatment of severe chloroquine poisoning. *N Engl J Med* 1988; **318:** 1–6.
3. Neuvonen PJ, *et al*. Prevention of chloroquine absorption by activated charcoal. *Hum Exp Toxicol* 1992; **11:** 117–20.
4. Clemessy J-L, *et al*. Hypokalaemia related to acute chloroquine ingestion. *Lancet* 1995; **346:** 877–80.

Precautions

Excessive doses of chloroquine and hydroxychloroquine are associated with retinal or visual field changes and the precautions to be observed in order to minimise such toxicity are discussed under Effects on the Eyes in Adverse Effects, above. There may be a temporary effect on visual accommodation.

Care is necessary in administering chloroquine to patients with impaired liver or renal function, or to those with severe gastrointestinal disorders, a history of psoriasis, or neurological disorders, especially a history of epilepsy (see below for advice not to use for malaria prophylaxis). Chloroquine should be used with caution in patients with myasthenia gravis as it may aggravate the condition. Patients with glucose-6-phosphate dehydrogenase deficiency should be observed for haemolytic anaemia during chloroquine treatment. Although there have been reports of fetal abnormalities associated with the use of chloroquine during pregnancy, the risks of malaria are considered to be greater and there appears to be no justification for withholding chloroquine for the treatment or prophylaxis of malaria.

It is important that when chloroquine is given intravenously it should be by slow infusion otherwise severe cardiotoxicity may develop.

Epilepsy. Following reports[1,2] of convulsions associated with the use of chloroquine for malaria prophylaxis in 4 previously healthy patients and in 2 patients with a history of seizures, it has been suggested that prospective travellers who have a history of epilepsy should be warned of the risk. Although it was initially considered[3] that this should not restrict the use of chloroquine in epileptic patients, UK malaria experts have recommended that it should be avoided for malaria prophylaxis.[4]

1. Fish DR, Espir MLE. Convulsions associated with prophylactic antimalarial drugs: implications for people with epilepsy. *BMJ* 1988; **297:** 526–7.
2. Fish DR, Espir MLE. Malaria prophylaxis and epilepsy. *BMJ* 1988; **297:** 1267.
3. Hellgren U, Rombo L. Malaria prophylaxis and epilepsy. *BMJ* 1988; **297:** 1267.
4. Bradley DJ, Bannister B. Guidelines for malaria prevention in travellers from the United Kingdom for 2001. *Commun Dis Public Health* 2001; **4:** 84–101.

Porphyria. Although chloroquine is probably safe in porphyric patients, some authorities consider its use to be contentious. Pyrimethamine is also probably safe in porphyric patients. Other drugs used for prophylaxis, such as dapsone and sulfadoxine and combinations containing them, are definitely contra-indicated in porphyric patients. Quinine is of proven safety in patients with porphyria and cell-culture tests have suggested that proguanil and mefloquine may also be safe.

Chloroquine has been tried in the treatment of porphyria cutanea tarda, but this is considered by some to be hazardous (see under Uses, below).

Pregnancy and breast feeding. There has been concern about the potential teratogenic effects of chloroquine because of a few case reports including defects in hearing and vision.[1] Two of 169 infants born to women who had received chloroquine 300 mg weekly throughout pregnancy had birth defects compared with 4 of 454 control infants whose mothers had not been exposed to antimalarials; the difference was not significant. The data suggested that chloroquine in the recommended prophylactic doses is not a strong teratogen and that its proved antimalarial benefits outweigh any possible risk of low-grade teratogenicity. Also it has been reported that chloroquine prophylaxis during pregnancy did not affect the birth-weight of neonates, compared with a control group.[2]

Chloroquine is distributed into breast milk, but not in an amount adequate to provide chemoprophylaxis against malaria for the infant (see under Pharmacokinetics, below).

1. Wolfe MS, Cordero JF. Safety of chloroquine in chemosuppression of malaria during pregnancy. *BMJ* 1985; **290:** 1466–7.
2. Cot M, *et al*. Effect of chloroquine chemoprophylaxis during pregnancy on birth weight: results of a randomized trial. *Am J Trop Med Hyg* 1992; **46:** 21–7.

Psoriatic arthritis. It is recommended that chloroquine and hydroxychloroquine should not be used in the treatment of psoriatic arthritis as exacerbations of skin lesions can occur. Some patients may go on to develop generalised erythroderma with subsequent exfoliative dermatitis.[1] However, there has been controversy over the reported incidence of this adverse effect.[2,3]

1. Slagel GA, James WD. Plaquenil-induced erythroderma. *J Am Acad Dermatol* 1985; **12:** 857–62.
2. Luzar MJ. Hydroxychloroquine in psoriatic arthropathy: exacerbations of psoriatic skin lesions. *J Rheumatol* 1982; **9:** 462–4.
3. Sayers ME, Mazanec DJ. Use of antimalarial drugs for the treatment of psoriatic arthritis. *Am J Med* 1992; **93:** 474–5.

Renal impairment. Although the elimination of chloroquine is prolonged in renal impairment no dosage adjustment is required in the treatment of malaria. Similarly, dosage reduction is not required for chloroquine prophylaxis except in those with severe renal impairment. Doses tend to be reduced when it is given for longer periods to patients with impaired renal function.

Interactions

There is an increased risk of inducing ventricular arrhythmias if chloroquine is given together with halofantrine (see p.436) or other arrhythmogenic drugs such as amiodarone. There is an increased risk of convulsions when chloroquine is given with mefloquine. The absorption of chloroquine can be reduced by concomitant administration of antacids or kaolin and its metabolism may be inhibited by cimetidine.

Antiepileptics. Chloroquine may antagonise the antiepileptic activity of *carbamazepine* (see p.345) and *valproate* (see p.368).

Antimalarials. Chloroquine should not be used with *halofantrine* since the latter prolongs the QT interval and therefore there is an increased potential to induce arrhythmias (see p.436). Use of chloroquine with *mefloquine* increases the risk of convulsions. Also concurrent use of chloroquine and *proguanil* may increase the incidence of proguanil-associated mouth ulceration.[1] The activity of chloroquine may be affected when it is given with other *antimalarials*. Mixtures of chloroquine with *quinine, mefloquine, amodiaquine, artemisinin,* or *pyrimethamine-sulfadoxine* were antagonistic *in vitro* against *Plasmodium falciparum*.[2] *Quinine* and chloroquine when used together may be antagonistic.[3]

1. Drysdale SF, *et al*. Proguanil, chloroquine, and mouth ulcers. *Lancet* 1990; **335:** 164.
2. Stahel E, *et al*. Antagonism of chloroquine with other antimalarials. *Trans R Soc Trop Med Hyg* 1988; **82:** 221.
3. Hall AP. Quinine and chloroquine antagonism in falciparum malaria. *Trans R Soc Trop Med Hyg* 1973; **67:** 425.

Antimicrobials. Acute dystonic reactions occurred during concomitant therapy with chloroquine and *metronidazole* in a woman who had previously tolerated chloroquine alone.[1] Chloroquine may also reduce the gastrointestinal absorption of *ampicillin* (see p.151).

1. Achumba JI, *et al*. Chloroquine-induced acute dystonic reactions in the presence of metronidazole. *Drug Intell Clin Pharm* 1988; **22:** 308–10.

Ciclosporin. Chloroquine has been reported to increase plasma concentrations of ciclosporin (see p.521).

Digoxin. Hydroxychloroquine has been reported to increase plasma concentrations of digoxin (see p.872).

Gastrointestinal drugs. Patients often wish to take chloroquine with food, antacids, or other gastrointestinal drugs to alleviate gastrointestinal irritation. Administration with *food* may be beneficial as it appears to improve the absorption of chloroquine.[1,2] However, *antacids* or *kaolin* can reduce the absorption of chloroquine and it is therefore recommended that they should be administered at least 4 hours apart.[3,4]

Cimetidine and chloroquine should be used with caution as *cimetidine* can significantly reduce the metabolism and elimination of chloroquine and increase its volume of distribution;[5] *ranitidine* might be more suitable if a histamine H_2-antagonist is required as it appears to have little effect on the pharmacokinetics of chloroquine.[6]

1. Tulpule A, Krishnaswamy K. Effect of food on bioavailability of chloroquine. *Eur J Clin Pharmacol* 1982; **23:** 271–3.
2. Lagrave M, *et al*. The influence of various types of breakfast on chloroquine levels. *Trans R Soc Trop Med Hyg* 1985; **79:** 559.
3. McElnay JC, *et al*. In vitro experiments on chloroquine and pyrimethamine absorption in the presence of antacid constituents or kaolin. *J Trop Med Hyg* 1982; **85:** 153–8.
4. McElnay JC, *et al*. The effect of magnesium trisilicate and kaolin on the in vivo absorption of chloroquine. *J Trop Med Hyg* 1982; **85:** 159–63.
5. Ette EI, *et al*. Chloroquine elimination in humans: effect of low-dose cimetidine. *J Clin Pharmacol* 1987; **27:** 813–16.
6. Ette EI, *et al*. Effect of ranitidine on chloroquine disposition. *Drug Intell Clin Pharm* 1987; **21:** 732–4.

Praziquantel. For mention of possible reduced bioavailability of praziquantel when given with chloroquine, see p.107.

Thyroxine [levothyroxine]. For a report of a possible interaction of chloroquine with thyroxine [levothyroxine], see p.1527.

Vaccines. Although concurrent antimalarial prophylaxis with chloroquine has been reported to reduce the antibody response to *human diploid rabies vaccine* (see p.1560), the immune response to other vaccines used in routine immunisation schedules (tetanus, diphtheria, measles, poliomyelitis, typhoid, and BCG) has not been found to be altered by chloroquine prophylaxis.[1,2]

1. Greenwood BM. Chloroquine prophylaxis and antibody response to immunisation. *Lancet* 1984; **ii:** 402–3.
2. Wolfe MS. Precautions with oral live typhoid (Ty 21a) vaccine. *Lancet* 1990; **336:** 631–2.

Pharmacokinetics

Chloroquine is rapidly and almost completely absorbed from the gastrointestinal tract when given by mouth. Absorption is also rapid following intramuscular or subcutaneous administration. It is widely distributed into body tissues and has a large apparent volume of distribution. It accumulates in high concentrations in some tissues, such as the kidneys, liver, lungs, and spleen and is strongly bound in melanin-containing cells such as those in the eyes and the skin. It also crosses the placenta. Chloroquine is eliminated very slowly from the body and it may persist in tissues for months or even years after discontinuation of therapy.

Chloroquine is extensively metabolised in the liver, mainly to monodesethylchloroquine with smaller amounts of bisdesethylchloroquine (didesethylchloroquinine) and other metabolites being formed. Monodesethylchloroquine has been reported to have some activity against Plasmodium falciparum. Chloroquine and its metabolites are excreted in the urine, with about half of a dose appearing as unchanged drug and about 10% as the monodesethyl metabolite. Chloroquine and its monodesethyl metabolite are both distributed into breast milk.

◊ General references.
1. Krishna S, White NJ. Pharmacokinetics of quinine, chloroquine and amodiaquine; clinical implications. *Clin Pharmacokinet* 1996; **30:** 263–99.
2. Ducharme J, Farinotti R. Clinical pharmacokinetics and metabolism of chloroquine: focus on recent advancements. *Clin Pharmacokinet* 1996; **31:** 257–74.

◊ Chloroquine is rapidly absorbed from the gastrointestinal tract but peak plasma concentrations following oral administration can vary considerably.[1] A mean peak plasma concentration of 76 nanograms per mL has been obtained in healthy adults a mean of 3.6 hours after administration of the equivalent of 300 mg of chloroquine base by mouth as tablets.[2] In children with uncomplicated malaria given the equivalent of 10 mg per kg body-weight peak plasma concentrations of 250 nanograms per mL have been reached after 2 hours;[3] a mean peak of 134 nanograms per mL has been obtained after 5 hours in healthy children given a similar dose.[4] Nasogastric administration has also produced therapeutic concentrations in children with severe falciparum malaria.[5]

Oral bioavailability is increased if chloroquine is taken with food[6,7] and some beverages[8] and may also be affected by the state of health of the patient; mean values have ranged from about 70% in patients with malaria[9] to 78 or 89% in healthy adults.[2] Although oral bioavailability appears to be unaltered in moderately undernourished adults[10] it has been reported that it may be significantly reduced in children with kwashiorkor.[4]

Preliminary studies with chloroquine suppositories indicate that although rectal bioavailability is less than half of that of oral chloroquine, sustained therapeutic concentrations may be achieved.[11]

Absorption is also rapid following subcutaneous or intramuscular injection and mean peak plasma concentrations of chloroquine have been obtained within about 30 minutes.[5,9,12]

Chloroquine has a large apparent volume of distribution. A multicompartmental model appears to be necessary to describe the distribution kinetics of chloroquine.[2,13] Following intravenous administration there is a multi-exponential decline in plasma concentrations as chloroquine distributes out of a central compartment that has been estimated to be several orders of magnitude smaller than the total volume of distribution.[5,14] This slow distribution out of the central compartment produces transiently high cardiotoxic concentrations of chloroquine if the overall rate of parenteral delivery is not carefully controlled.

Reported mean values for protein binding have ranged from about 58 to 64%.[15,16] Chloroquine is also bound to platelets and granulocytes so that the plasma concentration is only 10 to 15% of that in whole blood.[17] If these cells are not removed by gentle centrifugation during analysis, erroneously high plasma concentrations will be reported. Furthermore, as chloroquine concentrations determined in serum are higher than those in plasma, probably due to release of chloroquine from platelets during coagulation, it is crucial to state whether analysis has been done on whole blood, serum, or properly separated plasma.

About 50% of a dose of chloroquine is metabolised in the liver mainly to the N-dealkylated metabolite monodesethylchloroquine; smaller amounts of bisdesethylchloroquine, 7-chloro-4-aminoquinoline, and N-oxidation products are formed. Some of these metabolites may contribute to the cardiotoxicity associated with chloroquine. In one study peak plasma concentrations of 7-chloro-4-aminoquinoline were found to be twice those of unchanged chloroquine despite the fact that only relatively small amounts are formed; this appears to be due to its fast rate of formation and long elimination half-life.[18]

A mean of 42 to 47% of a dose has been reported to be excreted in the urine as unchanged chloroquine and 7 to 12% as monodesethylchloroquine.[2] Various estimates of the terminal elimination half-life of chloroquine range from several days to up to 2 months but its slow release from tissues ensures that small amounts may still be detected after a year.[18,19]

1. Hellgren U, et al. On the question of interindividual variations in chloroquine concentrations. Eur J Clin Pharmacol 1993; 45: 383–5.
2. Gustafsson LL, et al. Disposition of chloroquine in man after single intravenous and oral doses. Br J Clin Pharmacol 1983; 15: 471–9.
3. Adelusi SA, et al. Kinetics of the uptake and elimination of chloroquine in children with malaria. Br J Clin Pharmacol 1982; 14: 483–7.
4. Walker O, et al. Single dose disposition of chloroquine in kwashiorkor and normal children—evidence for decreased absorption in kwashiorkor. Br J Clin Pharmacol 1987; 23: 467–72.
5. White NJ, et al. Chloroquine treatment of severe malaria in children: pharmacokinetics, toxicity, and new dosage recommendations. N Engl J Med 1988; 319: 1493–1500.
6. Tulpule A, Krishnaswamy K. Effect of food on bioavailability of chloroquine. Eur J Clin Pharmacol 1982; 23: 271–3.
7. Lagrave M, et al. The influence of various types of breakfast on chloroquine levels. Trans R Soc Trop Med Hyg 1985; 79: 559.
8. Mahmoud BM, et al. Significant reduction in chloroquine bioavailability following coadministration with the Sudanese beverages aradaib, karkadi and lemon. J Antimicrob Chemother 1994; 33: 1005–9.
9. White NJ, et al. Parenteral chloroquine for treating falciparum malaria. J Infect Dis 1987; 155: 192–201.
10. Tulpule A, Krishnaswamy K. Chloroquine kinetics in the undernourished. Eur J Clin Pharmacol 1983; 24: 273–6.
11. WHO. Severe and complicated malaria. 2nd ed. Trans R Soc Trop Med Hyg 1990; 84 (suppl 2): 1–65.
12. Phillips RE, et al. Divided dose intramuscular regimen and single dose subcutaneous regimen for chloroquine: plasma concentrations and toxicity in patients with malaria. BMJ 1986; 293: 13–16.
13. Frisk-Holmberg M, et al. The single dose kinetics of chloroquine and its major metabolite desethylchloroquine in healthy subjects. Eur J Clin Pharmacol 1984; 26: 521–30.
14. Looareesuwan S, et al. Cardiovascular toxicity and distribution kinetics of intravenous chloroquine. Br J Clin Pharmacol 1986; 22: 31–6.
15. Walker O, et al. Characterization of chloroquine plasma protein binding in man. Br J Clin Pharmacol 1983; 15: 375–7.
16. Ofori-Adjei D, et al. Protein binding of chloroquine enantiomers and desethylchloroquine. Br J Clin Pharmacol 1986; 22: 356–8.
17. Gustafsson LL, et al. Pitfalls in the measurement of chloroquine concentrations. Lancet 1983; i: 126.
18. Ette EI, et al. Pharmacokinetics of chloroquine and some of its metabolites in healthy volunteers: a single dose study. J Clin Pharmacol 1989; 29: 457–62.
19. Gustafsson LL, et al. Chloroquine excretion following malaria prophylaxis. Br J Clin Pharmacol 1987; 24: 221–4.

Distribution into breast milk. Studies[1,2] have suggested that it is safe for mothers to breast feed when they are receiving chloroquine for treatment of malaria. Although chloroquine and its monodesethyl metabolite are distributed into breast milk it has been estimated that the amount that would be con-

sumed by an infant is well below the therapeutic range and separate chemoprophylaxis for the infant is required.

There appears to be no data on the excretion of hydroxychloroquine in milk after doses appropriate for the prevention or treatment of malaria but hydroxychloroquine has been detected in breast milk from 2 mothers receiving doses of 400 mg daily for systemic lupus erythematosus or rheumatoid arthritis.[3,4] One group of workers estimated that, calculated on a body-weight basis, a 9-month-old infant could receive about 2% of a maternal dose via breast feeding.[3]

1. Ogunbona FA, et al. Excretion of chloroquine and desethylchloroquine in human milk. Br J Clin Pharmacol 1987; 23: 473–6.
2. Akintonwa A, et al. Placental and milk transfer of chloroquine in humans. Ther Drug Monit 1988; 10: 147–9.
3. Nation RL, et al. Excretion of hydroxychloroquine in human milk. Br J Clin Pharmacol 1984; 17: 368–9.
4. Østensen M, et al. Hydroxychloroquine in human breast milk. Eur J Clin Pharmacol 1985; 28: 357.

Uses and Administration

Chloroquine is a 4-aminoquinoline antimalarial used in the treatment and prophylaxis of malaria. It has also been used in the treatment of hepatic amoebiasis, lupus erythematosus, light-sensitive skin eruptions, and rheumatoid arthritis.

Chloroquine is used for the prophylaxis and treatment of malaria due to susceptible strains of Plasmodium falciparum, P. ovale, P. vivax, and P. malariae, but widespread resistance in P. falciparum has greatly limited its value. It is a rapid-acting blood schizontocide with some gametocytocidal activity against P. ovale, P. vivax, P. malariae, and immature gametocytes of P. falciparum. Since it has no activity against exoerythrocytic forms, chloroquine does not produce a radical cure of vivax or ovale malarias. The mechanism of action of chloroquine against blood schizonts remains unclear, but it may influence haemoglobin digestion by raising intravesicular pH in malaria parasite cells. It also interferes with synthesis of nucleoproteins by the parasite.

Chloroquine may be given as the phosphate, sulfate, or hydrochloride. Doses are normally expressed in terms of chloroquine base, and as a general guide:

chloroquine base 300 mg is approximately equivalent to chloroquine phosphate 500 mg or chloroquine sulfate 400 mg

chloroquine base 40 mg is approximately equivalent to chloroquine hydrochloride 50 mg

Oral bioavailability is increased when chloroquine is taken with food.

For the treatment of malaria caused by P. vivax, P. ovale, P. malariae, and the few remaining strains of chloroquine-sensitive P. falciparum, the usual total oral dose for adults and children is the equivalent of a total of about 25 mg of chloroquine base per kg body-weight given over 3 days. This total dose is given in a variety of ways. One way is to give 10 mg per kg, followed after 6 to 8 hours by 5 mg per kg, then 5 mg per kg daily for the next 2 days; alternatively, 10 mg per kg may be given daily for the first 2 days and 5 mg per kg on the third day. Sometimes the adult doses are not expressed in terms of body-weight but as 600 mg followed after 6 to 8 hours by 300 mg, then 300 mg daily for the next 2 days. In severe and complicated malaria when the patient is unable to take oral medication and when chloroquine is to be used, then it can be given by injection. The intravenous route is preferred and a slow rate of infusion is essential, the required dose of 25 mg per kg being given in several infusions over 30 to 32 hours as described in further detail under Malaria, below. Should the patient recover sufficiently to be able to take chloroquine by mouth then the intravenous regimen should be halted and oral therapy commenced. It is important to bear in mind that in most parts of the world P. falciparum is now resistant to chloroquine which should not therefore be given for treatment.

For prophylaxis of malaria in areas where P. falciparum is absent or in one of the few remaining areas where it is still sensitive to chloroquine, a dose equivalent to 300 mg of chloroquine base is given once each week, beginning about one week before exposure and continuing throughout, and for at least 4 weeks after, exposure. For children, a weekly dose of

5 mg per kg has been recommended (but see also under Malaria, below). In areas of chloroquine-resistant malaria, but with a low risk of infection, chloroquine is administered with proguanil; where there is a high risk of infection alternative antimalarial regimens are recommended.

In the treatment of hepatic amoebiasis, chloroquine is used with emetine or dehydroemetine. The usual dose is the equivalent of 600 mg of chloroquine base daily for 2 days then 300 mg daily for 2 or 3 weeks. A dose of 6 mg per kg daily up to a maximum of 300 mg daily has been suggested for children.

When chloroquine is used for long-term therapy in conditions such as rheumatoid arthritis or lupus erythematosus, the dosage in obese patients should be calculated on the basis of lean body-weight in order to avoid excessive dosage.

In rheumatoid arthritis, response to treatment may not be apparent for up to 6 months, but if there is no improvement by then treatment should be discontinued. The usual dose is the equivalent of chloroquine base 150 mg daily (maximum 2.5 mg per kg daily) or up to 3 mg per kg daily in children. For further details see under Effects on the Eyes, above.

In discoid and systemic lupus erythematosus (p.1059), chloroquine is used initially at a dose equivalent to 150 mg (maximum 2.5 mg per kg) of base daily, reducing gradually once symptoms have been controlled. Children are given a dose of up to 3 mg per kg daily.

In the management of light-sensitive skin eruptions, adults are given the equivalent of 150 to 300 mg of chloroquine base daily during periods of intense light exposure; children are given up to 3 mg per kg.

Amoebiasis. For a discussion of the treatment of amoebiasis with mention of chloroquine for hepatic amoebiasis, see p.582.

Inflammatory disorders. Chloroquine and hydroxychloroquine possess anti-inflammatory properties and they have been tried or used with some benefit in a range of inflammatory conditions which often have an immunological basis, although they rarely constitute first-line therapy in these disorders. Such conditions include rheumatoid arthritis (see under Hydroxychloroquine, p.437), ulcerative colitis,[1] infantile interstitial pneumonitis,[2,3] asthma,[4] giant cell arteritis,[5] and various skin disorders (see below). The mode of action in these conditions is unclear. Results of studies have been conflicting but it does appear that chloroquine and hydroxychloroquine might have some immunosuppressive effects.[6,7]

1. Mayer L, Sachar DB. Efficacy of chloroquine in the treatment of inflammatory bowel disease. Gastroenterology 1988; 94: A293.
2. Springer C, et al. Chloroquine treatment in desquamative interstitial pneumonia. Arch Dis Child 1987; 62: 76–7.
3. Kerem E, et al. Sequential pulmonary function measurements during treatment of infantile chronic interstitial pneumonitis. J Pediatr 1990; 116: 61–7.
4. Charous BL. Open study of hydroxychloroquine in the treatment of severe symptomatic or corticosteroid-dependent asthma. Ann Allergy 1990; 65: 53–8.
5. Le Guennec P, et al. Management of giant cell arteritis: value of synthetic antimalarial agents: a retrospective study of thirty six patients. Rev Rhum 1994; 61: 423–8.
6. Bygbjerg IC, Flachs H. Effect of chloroquine on human lymphocyte proliferation. Trans R Soc Trop Med Hyg 1986; 80: 231–5.
7. Prasad RN, et al. Immunopharmacology of chloroquine. Trans R Soc Trop Med Hyg 1987; 81: 168–9.

Malaria. The overall treatment and prophylaxis of malaria and the place of chloroquine in current recommendations are discussed on p.428.

TREATMENT. In the treatment of patients with chloroquine-sensitive falciparum malaria studies have found chloroquine to be at least as effective as quinine in both uncomplicated and severe infections.[1,2] However, few areas exist where Plasmodium falciparum remains sensitive to chloroquine. There are also reports of resistance to chloroquine in P. vivax.[3] There is limited evidence that chlorpheniramine [chlorphenamine] might reverse chloroquine resistance in P. falciparum (see p.412).

Treatment with chloroquine is usually by mouth, adults and children being given the equivalent of 25 mg of chloroquine base per kg body-weight over 3 days. Any chloroquine lost through vomiting needs to be replaced by additional doses.[4] Encouraging results have also been obtained in a limited number of patients given the equivalent of 30 mg of chloroquine base per kg by mouth over 2 days in the form of a loading dose of 10 mg per kg followed by two doses of 5 mg per kg at intervals of 6 hours on the first day and two doses of 5 mg per kg at intervals of 12 hours on the second day.[5]

Parenteral therapy may be used if the infection is severe or oral administration is not possible. The parenteral regimen for adults and children recommended by WHO[6] consists of a loading dose equivalent to 10 mg of chloroquine base per kg body-weight given by constant rate intravenous infusion in sodium chloride 0.9% over a period of at least 8 hours and followed by a further three 8-hour infusions each of 5 mg per kg during the next 24 hours. Alternatively the entire course may be given over 30 hours, each infusion of 5 mg per kg being given over 6 hours. There should be close monitoring for hypotension and other signs of cardiovascular toxicity.

The intramuscular or subcutaneous routes have been used if intravenous administration is not possible. Intramuscular or subcutaneous doses for adults and children are 3.5 mg per kg every 6 hours[4,6] or 2.5 mg per kg every 4 hours to a total dose equivalent to 25 mg of the base per kg body-weight.[4]

Whichever parenteral route is used, patients should be transferred to oral therapy as soon as possible and administration continued until a total dose equivalent to 25 mg of the base per kg body-weight has been given.

If injections cannot be given a chloroquine suspension or syrup appears to be well absorbed when given by nasogastric tube even in comatose patients. Rectal administration in young children has also produced promising responses.[7,8]

PROPHYLAXIS. The widespread prevalence of strains of *P. falciparum* resistant to chloroquine has considerably diminished the value of chloroquine for malaria chemoprophylaxis and has made recommendations increasingly complex (see p.428). If chloroquine is used for prophylaxis it is usually administered with proguanil. A dose equivalent to 300 mg of chloroquine base is given by mouth once each week, beginning about one week before exposure and continuing throughout, and for at least 4 weeks after, exposure. Some countries advise the use of 100 mg daily for 6 days a week. For children, a weekly dose of chloroquine base 5 mg per kg body-weight has been recommended, although UK malaria experts[9] have suggested the following prophylactic doses for children based on fractions of the adult dose of 300 mg weekly; under 6.0 kg (0 to 12 weeks of age), one-eighth the adult dose; 6.0 to 9.9 kg (3 to 11 months), one-quarter the adult dose; 10.0 to 15.9 kg (1 year to 3 years 11 months), three-eighths the adult dose; 16.0 to 24.9 kg (4 years to 7 years 11 months), half the adult dose; 25.0 to 44.9 kg (8 years to 12 years 11 months), three-quarters the adult dose; and over 45 kg (13 years and over), the adult dose. They noted that body-weight was a better guide to dosage than age for children over 6 months.

1. Watt G, *et al.* Chloroquine and quinine: a randomized, double-blind comparison of efficacy and side effects in the treatment of Plasmodium falciparum malaria in the Philippines. *Trans R Soc Trop Med Hyg* 1988; **82:** 205–8.
2. White NJ, *et al.* Open comparison of intramuscular chloroquine and quinine in children with severe chloroquine-sensitive falciparum malaria. *Lancet* 1989; **ii:** 1313–16.
3. Whitby M. Drug resistant Plasmodium vivax malaria. *J Antimicrob Chemother* 1997; **40:** 749–52.
4. WHO. *WHO model prescribing information: drugs used in parasitic diseases.* 2nd ed. Geneva: WHO, 1995.
5. Pussard E, *et al.* Efficacy of a loading dose of oral chloroquine in a 36-hour treatment schedule for uncomplicated Plasmodium falciparum malaria. *Antimicrob Agents Chemother* 1991; **35:** 406–9.
6. WHO. *Management of severe malaria: a practical handbook.* Geneva: WHO 2000.
7. Westman L, *et al.* Rectal administration of chloroquine for treatment of children with malaria. *Trans R Soc Trop Med Hyg* 1994; **88:** 446.
8. Antia-Obong OE, *et al.* Chloroquine phosphate suppositories in the treatment of childhood malaria in Calabar, Nigeria. *Curr Ther Res* 1995; **56:** 928–35.
9. Bradley DJ, Bannister B. Guidelines for malaria prevention in travellers from the United Kingdom for 2001. *Commun Dis Public Health* 2001; **4:** 84–101.

Porphyria cutanea tarda. Chloroquine and hydroxychloroquine have been used with some benefit in the treatment of porphyria cutanea tarda (p.1011) and low doses (such as chloroquine phosphate 125 mg or hydroxychloroquine sulfate 200 mg given twice weekly) have been considered by some to be useful in patients unsuitable for phlebotomy[1-3] (but see under Porphyria in Precautions, above). However, the acute increase in urinary porphyrins and fall in hepatic porphyrin content produced by these drugs have been associated with a variable degree of hepatotoxicity[4] and others prefer to use desferrioxamine.[5]

1. Grossman ME, *et al.* Porphyria cutanea tarda. *Am J Med* 1979; **67:** 277–86.
2. Cainelli T, *et al.* Hydroxychloroquine versus phlebotomy in the treatment of porphyria cutanea tarda. *Br J Dermatol* 1983; **108:** 593–600.
3. Ashton RE, *et al.* Low-dose oral chloroquine in the treatment of porphyria cutanea tarda. *Br J Dermatol* 1984; **111:** 609–13.
4. Scholnick PL, *et al.* The molecular basis of the action of chloroquine in porphyria cutanea tarda. *J Invest Dermatol* 1973; **61:** 226–32.
5. Rocchi E. Treatment of porphyria cutanea tarda. *Br J Dermatol* 1987; **116:** 139–40.

Rheumatoid arthritis. For reference to the use of chloroquine in the treatment of rheumatoid arthritis, see under Hydroxychloroquine, p.437.

Sarcoidosis. Chloroquine and hydroxychloroquine have been tried in the management of sarcoidosis (p.1058) as alternatives or adjuncts to corticosteroid therapy.

References.

1. Spiteri MA, *et al.* Lupus pernio: a clinico-radiological study of thirty-five cases. *Br J Dermatol* 1985; **112:** 315–22.

2. O'Leary TJ, *et al.* The effects of chloroquine on serum 1,25-di-hydroxyvitamin D and calcium metabolism in sarcoidosis. *N Engl J Med* 1986; **315:** 727–30.
3. Adams JS, *et al.* Effective reduction in the serum 1,25-dihydroxyvitamin D and calcium concentration in sarcoidosis-associated hypercalcemia with short-course chloroquine therapy. *Ann Intern Med* 1989; **111:** 437–8.
4. DeSimone DP, *et al.* Granulomatous infiltration of the talus and abnormal vitamin D and calcium metabolism in a patient with sarcoidosis: successful treatment with hydroxychloroquine. *Am J Med* 1989; **87:** 694–6.
5. Jones E, Callen JP. Hydroxychloroquine is effective therapy for control of cutaneous sarcoidal granulomas. *J Am Acad Dermatol* 1990; **23:** 487–9.
6. Zic JA, *et al.* Treatment of cutaneous sarcoidosis with chloroquine: review of the literature. *Arch Dermatol* 1991; **127:** 1034–40.

Skin disorders. In addition to their use in lupus erythematosus hydroxychloroquine and chloroquine have been tried in a number of other skin disorders including polymorphic light eruptions,[1] lichen planus[2] (p.1106), cutaneous symptoms of dermatomyositis (p.1057), erythema nodosum,[3,4] and recurrent erythema multiforme (p.1105).

1. Murphy GM, *et al.* Hydroxychloroquine in polymorphic light eruption: a controlled trial with drug and visual sensitivity monitoring. *Br J Dermatol* 1987; **116:** 379–86.
2. Mostafa WZ. Lichen planus of the nail: treatment with antimalarials. *J Am Acad Dermatol* 1989; **20:** 289–90.
3. Alloway JA, Franks LK. Hydroxychloroquine in the treatment of chronic erythema nodosum. *Br J Dermatol* 1995; **132:** 661–2.
4. Jarrett P, Goodfield MJD. Hydroxychloroquine and chronic erythema nodosum. *Br J Dermatol* 1996; **134:** 373.

Preparations

BP 2001: Chloroquine Phosphate Tablets; Chloroquine Sulphate Injection; Chloroquine Sulphate Tablets;
USP 25: Chloroquine Hydrochloride Injection; Chloroquine Phosphate Tablets.

Proprietary Preparations (details are given in Part 3)
Aust.: Resochin; **Austral.:** Chlorquin; Nivaquine†; **Belg.:** Nivaquine; **Braz.:** Palux; **Canad.:** Aralen; **Denm.:** Malarex; **Fin.:** Heliopar; **Fr.:** Nivaquine; **Ger.:** Arthrabas†; Resochin; Weimerquin; **Hong Kong:** Chlorquin; Syncoquin; **Irl.:** Avloclor; Nivaquine†; **Israel:** Aralen; Avloclor; **Mex.:** Aralen; Klorokin; Paluken; **Neth.:** Nivaquine; **NZ:** Nivaquine; **Port.:** Resochina; **S.Afr.:** Anoclor; Daramal; Nivaquine; Plasmoquine; Promal†; **Singapore:** Avloclor; **Spain:** Resochin; **Switz.:** Chlorochin; Nivaquine; Resochine†; **Thai.:** Diroquine; Genocin; P-Roquine; **UK:** Avloclor; Malaviron; Nivaquine; **USA:** Aralen.

Multi-ingredient: *Braz.:* Clopirim; *Fr.:* Savarine; *S.Afr.:* Daraclor†; Daramal-Paludrine.

Chlorproguanil Hydrochloride (1376-p)

Chlorproguanil Hydrochloride (BANM, rINNM).

M-5943. 1-(3,4-Dichlorophenyl)-5-isopropylbiguanide hydrochloride.

$C_{11}H_{15}Cl_2N_5,HCl = 324.6$.

CAS — 537-21-3 (chlorproguanil); 15537-76-5 (chlorproguanil hydrochloride).

Profile
Chlorproguanil is a biguanide antimalarial with actions and uses similar to those of proguanil (p.441). It is sometimes given in combination with a sulfone such as dapsone.

◊ References.

1. Keuter M, *et al.* Comparison of chloroquine, pyrimethamine and sulfadoxine, and chlorproguanil and dapsone as treatment for falciparum malaria in pregnant and non-pregnant women, Kakamega district, Kenya. *BMJ* 1990; **301:** 466–70.
2. Rooth I, *et al.* Proguanil daily or chlorproguanil twice weekly are efficacious against falciparum malaria in a holoendemic area of Tanzania. *J Trop Med Hyg* 1991; **94:** 45–9.
3. Nevill CG, *et al.* Daily chlorproguanil is an effective alternative to daily proguanil in the prevention of Plasmodium falciparum malaria in Kenya. *Trans R Soc Trop Med Hyg* 1994; **88:** 319–20.
4. Winstanley P, *et al.* Chlorproguanil/dapsone for uncomplicated Plasmodium falciparum malaria in young children: pharmacokinetics and therapeutic range. *Trans R Soc Trop Med Hyg* 1997; **91:** 322–7.
5. Amukoye E, *et al.* Chlorproguanil-dapsone: effective treatment for uncomplicated falciparum malaria. *Antimicrob Agents Chemother* 1997; **41:** 2261–4.

Halofantrine Hydrochloride (16829-p)

Halofantrine Hydrochloride (BANM, USAN, rINNM).

Halofantrini Hydrochloridum; WR-171669. (RS)-3-Dibutylamino-1-(1,3-dichloro-6-trifluoromethyl-9-phenanthryl)propan-1-ol hydrochloride; 1,3-Dichloro-α-[2-(dibutylamino)ethyl]-6-trifluoromethyl-9-phenanthrene-methanol hydrochloride.

$C_{26}H_{30}Cl_2F_3NO,HCl = 536.9$.

CAS — 69756-53-2 (halofantrine); 36167-63-2 (halofantrine hydrochloride); 66051-63-6 (±-halofantrine).

Pharmacopoeias. In Eur. (see p.vi).

Pharmacopoeial description
Ph. Eur.: A white or almost white powder. It exhibits polymorphism. Practically insoluble in water; sparingly soluble in alcohol; freely soluble in methyl alcohol. Protect from light.

Adverse Effects and Precautions
Adverse effects associated with halofantrine include diarrhoea, abdominal pain, nausea, vomiting, pruritus, and skin rash. Transient elevation of serum transaminases, intravascular haemolysis, and hypersensitivity reactions have also been reported.

Halofantrine can adversely affect the heart and this is mainly seen as a prolongation of QT interval. Serious ventricular arrhythmias have been reported and fatalities have occurred. As a result it is contra-indicated in patients known to have a prolonged QT interval or those with cardiac disease or a family history of congenital QT prolongation, and also in those with unexplained syncopal attacks, thiamine deficiency, or electrolyte disturbances, or taking other arrhythmogenic drugs (see also under Effects on the Heart, below, and under Interactions, below).

Halofantrine is not recommended during pregnancy or in breast-feeding women. It should not be taken on a full stomach since this increases its bioavailability and thus the risk of toxicity; after taking halofantrine, fatty food should be avoided for 24 hours.

Effects on the blood. Halofantrine has been associated with acute intravascular haemolysis.[1,2]

1. Vachon F, *et al.* Halofantrine and acute intravascular haemolysis. *Lancet* 1992; **340:** 909–10.
2. Mojon M, *et al.* Intravascular haemolysis following halofantrine intake. *Trans R Soc Trop Med Hyg* 1994; **88:** 91.

Effects on the heart. Prolonged PR[1,2] and QT[1-5] intervals have been reported in patients given halofantrine and there are individual reports of fatal cardiac arrest[1,5] and of torsade de pointes.[4] In 1994, the UK Committee on Safety of Medicines[6] noted that QT interval prolongation occurred at recommended doses of halofantrine in the majority of patients and that worldwide there had been 14 reports of cardiac arrhythmias associated with halofantrine; 8 patients were known to have died. To reduce the risk of arrhythmias they stressed that halofantrine should *not* be taken with meals, with other drugs that may induce arrhythmias (e.g. quinine, chloroquine, and mefloquine; tricyclic antidepressants; antipsychotics; certain antiarrhythmics; and the antihistamines terfenadine and astemizole), or with drugs causing electrolyte disturbances. They also stated that it should *not* be administered to patients known to have prolongation of the QT interval or with any form of cardiac disease associated with QT interval prolongation or ventricular arrhythmia (e.g. coronary heart disease, cardiomyopathy, or congenital heart disease). Some workers[2] have suggested ECG screening of all patients before starting treatment with halofantrine. Others[7] found pretreatment ECGs to be poorly predictive of QT lengthening during treatment. Children may experience serious cardiac effects at standard doses.[8]

1. Nosten F, *et al.* Cardiac effects of antimalarial treatment with halofantrine. *Lancet* 1993; **341:** 1054–6.
2. Monlun E, *et al.* Cardiac complications of halofantrine: a prospective study of 20 patients. *Trans R Soc Trop Med Hyg* 1995; **89:** 430–3.
3. Castot A, *et al.* Prolonged QT interval with halofantrine. *Lancet* 1993; **341:** 1541.
4. Monlun E, *et al.* Prolonged QT interval with halofantrine. *Lancet* 1993; **341:** 1541–2.
5. Anonymous. Halofantrine: revised data sheet. *WHO Drug Inf* 1993; **7:** 66–7.
6. Committee on Safety of Medicines/Medicines Control Agency. Cardiac arrhythmias with halofantrine (Halfan). *Current Problems* 1994; **20:** 6.
7. Matson PA, *et al.* Cardiac effects of standard-dose halofantrine therapy. *Am J Trop Med Hyg* 1996; **54:** 229–31.
8. Sowunmi A, *et al.* Cardiac effects of halofantrine in children suffering from acute uncomplicated falciparum malaria. *Trans R Soc Trop Med Hyg* 1998; **92:** 446–8.

Effects on the skin. For a comparison of the incidence of pruritus associated with halofantrine and other antimalarials, see Effects on the Skin under Adverse Effects of Chloroquine, p.433.

Interactions
Halofantrine prolongs the QT interval and should not be administered with other drugs that have the potential to induce cardiac arrhythmias, in particular the antimalarials mefloquine, chloroquine, and quinine, and also tricyclic antidepressants, phenothiazine antipsychotics, some antiarrhythmics (including amiodarone, disopyramide, flecainide, procainamide, quinidine, and the beta blocker sotalol), cisapride, and the antihistamines astemizole and terfenadine. Also, halofantrine should not be given with drugs that cause electrolyte disturbances (such as diuretics).

Pharmacokinetics

Halofantrine is slowly and erratically absorbed following administration by mouth, although it appears in the circulation within about one hour, peak concentrations occurring in 3 to 6 hours. Bioavailability of halofantrine is increased by administration with or after food, particularly food high in fat content, and it must therefore be taken on an empty stomach because of the risk of cardiac toxicity. The elimination half-life of halofantrine varies considerably between individuals, but is generally about 1 to 2 days. Halofantrine is metabolised in the liver, its major metabolite being desbutylhalofantrine which appears to be as active as the parent compound. Excretion of halofantrine is primarily via the faeces.

◊ References.

1. Milton KA, *et al.* Pharmacokinetics of halofantrine in man: effects of food and dose size. *Br J Clin Pharmacol* 1989; **28:** 71–7.
2. Karbwang J, *et al.* Pharmacokinetics of halofantrine in healthy Thai volunteers. *Br J Clin Pharmacol* 1991; **32:** 639–40.
3. Veenendaal JR, *et al.* Pharmacokinetics of halofantrine and N-desbutylhalofantrine in patients with falciparum malaria following a multiple dose regimen of halofantrine. *Eur J Clin Pharmacol* 1991; **41:** 161–4.
4. Karbwang J, Na Bangchang K. Clinical pharmacokinetics of halofantrine. *Clin Pharmacokinet* 1994; **27:** 104–19.
5. Watkins WM, *et al.* Halofantrine pharmacokinetics in Kenyan children with non-severe and severe malaria. *Br J Clin Pharmacol* 1995; **39:** 283–7.
6. Ohrt C, *et al.* Pharmacokinetics of an extended-dose halofantrine regimen in patients with malaria and in healthy volunteers. *Clin Pharmacol Ther* 1995; **57:** 525–32.

Uses and Administration

Halofantrine is a 9-phenanthrenemethanol antimalarial used in the *treatment* of uncomplicated chloroquine-resistant falciparum and of chloroquine-resistant vivax malaria. Halofantrine is a blood schizontocide but has no activity against exoerythrocytic forms. Its value is limited by its unpredictable bioavailability and by cardiotoxicity. It should *not* be used where mefloquine has been used for prophylaxis (see under Malaria, below; and for cardiac hazard, see Effects on the Heart, above). Halofantrine should also *not* be used for malaria prophylaxis and is no longer recommended for standby treatment.

In the treatment of malaria, halofantrine hydrochloride is given by mouth as 3 doses of 500 mg at intervals of 6 hours, on an empty stomach. Dosage for children is based on 24 mg per kg body-weight divided into 3 doses. The following doses are recommended: 23 to 31 kg body-weight, 3 doses of 250 mg at intervals of 6 hours; 32 to 37 kg body-weight, 3 doses of 375 mg at intervals of 6 hours; over 37 kg body-weight, adult dose. A second course should be given after a week.

◊ Reviews.

1. Bryson HM, Goa KL. Halofantrine: a review of its antimalarial activity, pharmacokinetic properties and therapeutic potential. *Drugs* 1992; **43:** 236–58.

Administration. A micronised oral formulation of halofantrine was developed in an attempt to improve bioavailability and allow a smaller administered dose,[1-5] although wide interindividual variation in plasma concentrations was still seen.[1,5] A parenteral dosage form was also evaluated.[5]

1. Fadat G, *et al.* Efficacy of micronized halofantrine in semi-immune patients with acute uncomplicated falciparum malaria in Cameroon. *Antimicrob Agents Chemother* 1993; **37:** 1955–7.
2. Wildling E, *et al.* High dose chloroquine versus micronized halofantrine in chloroquine-resistant Plasmodium falciparum malaria. *J Antimicrob Chemother* 1994; **33:** 871–5.
3. Kremsner PG, *et al.* Comparison of micronized halofantrine with chloroquine-antibiotic combinations for treating Plasmodium falciparum malaria in adults from Gabon. *Am J Trop Med Hyg* 1994; **50:** 790–5.
4. Bouchaud O, *et al.* Clinical efficacy and pharmacokinetics of micronized halofantrine for the treatment of acute uncomplicated falciparum malaria in nonimmune patients. *Am J Trop Med Hyg* 1994; **51:** 204–13.
5. Krishna S, *et al.* Pharmacokinetics, efficacy and toxicity of parenteral halofantrine in uncomplicated malaria. *Br J Clin Pharmacol* 1993; **36:** 585–91.

Malaria. Halofantrine is one of the drugs that may be used for the treatment of falciparum malaria (p.428) where there is chloroquine resistance, but its value is limited by its unpredictable bioavailability and by cardiotoxicity (see Effects on the Heart, above). Halofantrine should not be used in patients in whom mefloquine treatment[1] or prophylaxis[2] has failed since cross-resistance occurs between halofantrine and mefloquine.

The symbol † denotes a preparation no longer actively marketed

Halofantrine should not be used for malaria prophylaxis and is no longer recommended for standby treatment.

1. ter Kuile FO, *et al.* Halofantrine versus mefloquine in treatment of multidrug-resistant falciparum malaria. *Lancet* 1993; **341:** 1044–9.
2. Gay F, *et al.* Cross-resistance between mefloquine and halofantrine. *Lancet* 1990; **336:** 1262.

Preparations

Proprietary Preparations (details are given in Part 3)
Aust.: Halfan†; *Belg.:* Halfan; *Fr.:* Halfan; *Ger.:* Halfan; *Neth.:* Halfan; *Port.:* Halfan; *S.Afr.:* Halfan; *Spain:* Halfan; *Switz.:* Halfan; *UK:* Halfan†; *USA:* Halfan.

Hydroxychloroquine Sulfate   (1380-b)

Hydroxychloroquine Sulfate *(rlNNM)*.
Hydroxychloroquine Sulphate *(BANM)*; Oxichlorochin Sulphate; Sulfato de Hidroxicloroquina; Win-1258-2. 2-{N-[4-(7-Chloro-4-quinolylamino)pentyl]-N-ethylamino}ethanol sulphate.
$C_{18}H_{26}ClN_3O,H_2SO_4 = 434.0$.
CAS — 118-42-3 (hydroxychloroquine); 747-36-4 (hydroxychloroquine sulfate).
Pharmacopoeias. In Br., Port., and US.

Hydroxychloroquine sulfate 100 mg is approximately equivalent to 77 mg of hydroxychloroquine base.

Pharmacopoeial description

BP 2001: A white or almost white, odourless or almost odourless, crystalline powder. Freely soluble in water; practically insoluble in alcohol, in chloroform, and in ether. A 1% solution in water has a pH of 3.5 to 5.5. Protect from light.

USP 25: A white or practically white, odourless, crystalline powder. It exists in two forms, the usual form melting at about 240° and the other form at about 198°. Freely soluble in water; practically insoluble in alcohol, in chloroform, and in ether. Its solutions in water have a pH of about 4.5. Protect from light.

Adverse Effects, Treatment, and Precautions

As for Chloroquine, p.432.

Effects on the eyes. The main adverse effects of chloroquine and hydroxychloroquine on the eye are keratopathy and retinopathy. With respect to retinopathy, precautions should be observed in patients undergoing long-term treatment, as described under Chloroquine on p.433.

Interactions

As for Chloroquine, p.434.

Pharmacokinetics

The pharmacokinetics of hydroxychloroquine are similar to those of chloroquine (see p.434).

◊ References.

1. Tett SE, *et al.* Bioavailability of hydroxychloroquine tablets in healthy volunteers. *Br J Clin Pharmacol* 1989; **27:** 771–9.
2. Miller DR, *et al.* Steady-state pharmacokinetics of hydroxychloroquine in rheumatoid arthritis. *DICP Ann Pharmacother* 1991; **25:** 1302–5.
3. Ducharme J, *et al.* Enantioselective disposition of hydroxychloroquine after a single oral dose of the racemate to healthy subjects. *Br J Clin Pharmacol* 1995; **40:** 127–33.

Uses and Administration

Hydroxychloroquine sulfate is a 4-aminoquinoline antimalarial with actions similar to those of chloroquine (p.435), but is mainly used in the treatment of systemic and discoid lupus erythematosus and rheumatoid arthritis. It has also been used in the treatment of light-sensitive skin eruptions.

Hydroxychloroquine sulfate is given by mouth.

In *lupus erythematosus* and *rheumatoid arthritis*, response to treatment may not be apparent for up to 6 months but if there is no improvement by then, treatment should be discontinued. In the UK, treatment is usually started with 400 mg daily in divided doses with meals. In the USA, recommended initial doses are 400 to 600 mg daily for rheumatoid arthritis and 400 mg once or twice daily for lupus erythematosus. Doses are reduced to the minimum effective dose for maintenance; this is usually 200 to 400 mg daily but should not exceed 6.5 mg per kg body-weight daily (or 400 mg daily whichever is the smaller). To avoid excessive dosage in obese patients, special care is needed to calculate the dosage on the basis of lean body-weight. For further details, see under Effects on the Eyes in Chloroquine, p.433. In children, the minimum effective dose should be used up to a maximum

of 6.5 mg per kg body-weight daily (or 400 mg daily whichever is the smaller).

Hydroxychloroquine sulfate is also used in similar doses for the treatment of *light-sensitive skin eruptions*, but treatment should only be given during periods of maximum exposure to light.

Hydroxychloroquine sulfate may be used in *malaria* both for treatment and prophylaxis, when chloroquine is not available, with the same limitations as for chloroquine. In the USA, the manufacturers recommend for *prophylaxis* of malaria a dose of 400 mg every 7 days; children may be given a weekly prophylactic dose of hydroxychloroquine sulfate 6.5 mg per kg body-weight (up to a maximum of 400 mg). In *treating* an acute malarial attack, a dose of 800 mg has been used, followed after 6 to 8 hours by 400 mg and a further 400 mg on each of the 2 following days; in children, an initial dose of hydroxychloroquine sulfate 13 mg per kg may be given, followed by 6.5 mg per kg 6 hours later and again on the second and third days.

Inflammatory disorders. For the use of hydroxychloroquine and chloroquine in a range of inflammatory conditions, see under Chloroquine, p.435 and under Rheumatoid Arthritis, below.

Lupus erythematosus. One of hydroxychloroquine's main indications is lupus erythematosus (p.1059).

Malaria. The role of chloroquine and potentially therefore of hydroxychloroquine in the treatment and prophylaxis of malaria is discussed on p.428.

Porphyria cutanea tarda. For reference to the use of hydroxychloroquine in the treatment of porphyria cutanea tarda, see under the Uses and Administration of Chloroquine, p.436.

Rheumatoid arthritis. Hydroxychloroquine and chloroquine may be used as antirheumatic drugs in the management of *rheumatoid arthritis* (p.9) in an attempt to suppress the rate of cartilage erosion or alter the course of the disease.[1] These antimalarials are considered to be less effective than the other disease-modifying antirheumatic drugs (DMARDs) but they are usually better tolerated and so may be preferred in patients with milder forms of the disease.[2] Additional benefit has been obtained using antimalarials with other DMARDs especially methotrexate and sulfasalazine,[3,4] although adverse effects may be more common. For reference to precautions to reduce the incidence of retinopathy, see under Effects on the Eyes in Adverse Effects of Chloroquine, p.433.

Generally the lowest effective dose should be used for maintenance to minimise toxicity; for hydroxychloroquine sulfate this should not exceed 6.5 mg per kg lean body-weight daily. Daily doses of 200 or 400 mg are commonly used but one study indicates that there is little advantage in using the higher dose.[5]

Experience with antimalarials to treat *juvenile idiopathic arthritis* (p.9) is limited and the results have been variable.[6,7]

Chloroquine and hydroxychloroquine have also been reported to be of use in *palindromic rheumatism.*[8-10]

1. Suarez-Almazor ME, *et al.* Antimalarials for treating rheumatoid arthritis (updated 29 August 2001). Available in The Cochrane Library; Issue 4. Oxford: Update Software; 2001.
2. HERA Study Group. A randomized trial of hydroxychloroquine in early rheumatoid arthritis: the HERA study. *Am J Med* 1995; **98:** 156–68.
3. Clegg DO, *et al.* Safety and efficacy of hydroxychloroquine as maintenance therapy for rheumatoid arthritis after combination therapy with methotrexate and hydroxychloroquine. *J Rheumatol* 1997; **24:** 1896–1902.
4. O'Dell JR. Triple therapy with methotrexate, sulfasalazine, and hydroxychloroquine in patients with rheumatoid arthritis. *Rheum Dis Clin North Am* 1998; **24:** 465–77.
5. Pavelka K, *et al.* Hydroxychloroquine sulphate in the treatment of rheumatoid arthritis: a double blind comparison of two dose regimens. *Ann Rheum Dis* 1989; **48:** 542–6.
6. Brewer EJ, *et al.* Penicillamine and hydroxychloroquine in the treatment of severe juvenile rheumatoid arthritis. *N Engl J Med* 1986; **314:** 1269–76.
7. Grondin C, *et al.* Slow-acting antirheumatic drugs in chronic arthritis of childhood. *Semin Arthritis Rheum* 1988; **18:** 38–47.
8. Golding DN. D-Penicillamine in palindromic rheumatism. *BMJ* 1976; **2:** 1382–3.
9. Richardson MR, Zalin AM. Treatment of palindromic rheumatism with chloroquine. *BMJ* 1987; **294:** 741.
10. Hanonen P, *et al.* Treatment of palindromic rheumatism with chloroquine. *BMJ* 1987; **294:** 1289.

Sarcoidosis. Chloroquine and hydroxychloroquine have been tried in the management of sarcoidosis (p.1058) as alternatives or adjuncts to corticosteroid therapy. For references to the use of hydroxychloroquine, see under Chloroquine, p.436.

Skin disorders. For reference to the use of hydroxychloroquine in a variety of skin disorders, see under Chloroquine, p.436.

Venous thromboembolism. Standard prophylaxis for surgical patients at high risk of venous thromboembolism (p.817) is usually with an anticoagulant. Hydroxychloroquine has been described by some as an antiplatelet agent[1] and although its mechanism of action is uncertain the incidence of fatal pulmonary embolism has been reduced in patients given hydroxychloroquine prophylactically after total hip replacement;[2] the usual daily divided dose was about 800 mg from the day before surgery until discharge; larger doses had been used.

1. Antiplatelet Trialists' Collaboration. Collaborative overview of randomised trials of antiplatelet therapy—III: reduction in venous thrombosis and pulmonary embolism by antiplatelet prophylaxis among surgical and medical patients. *BMJ* 1994; **308**: 235–46.
2. Loudon JR. Hydroxychloroquine and postoperative thromboembolism after total hip replacement. *Am J Med* 1988; **85**: (suppl 4A): 57–61.

Preparations

BP 2001: Hydroxychloroquine Tablets;
USP 25: Hydroxychloroquine Sulfate Tablets.

Proprietary Preparations (details are given in Part 3)
Aust.: Plaquenil; *Austral.:* Plaquenil; *Belg.:* Plaquenil; *Braz.:* Plaquenil; *Canad.:* Plaquenil; *Denm.:* Ercoquin†; Plaquenil; *Fin.:* Oxiklorin; Plaquenil; *Fr.:* Plaquenil; *Ger.:* Quensyl; *Hong Kong:* Plaquenil; *Irl.:* Plaquenil; *Israel:* Plaquenil; *Ital.:* Plaquenil; *Mex.:* Plaquenil; *Neth.:* Plaquenil; *Norw.:* Ercoquin; Plaquenil; *NZ:* Plaquenil; *Port.:* Plaquinol; *Singapore:* Plaquenil; *Swed.:* Plaquenil; *Switz.:* Plaquenil; *Thai.:* Plaquenil; *UK:* Plaquenil; *USA:* Plaquenil.

Hydroxypiperaquine Phosphate (19318-s)

1,3-Bis[1-(7-chloro-4-quinolyl)-4-piperazinyl]-2-hydroxypropane phosphate.
$C_{29}H_{32}OCl_2N_6.4H_3PO_4 = 943.5$.
CAS — 74351-60-3.

Profile

Hydroxypiperaquine phosphate is a 4-piperazinoquinoline antimalarial which has been reported to be effective in the treatment of vivax malaria and chloroquine-sensitive and chloroquine-resistant falciparum malaria.

Lumefantrine (14735-s)

Lumefantrine (BAN, rINN).

Benflumelol; Benflumetol. 2,7-Dichloro-9-[(4-chlorophenyl)methylene]-α-[(dibutylamino)methyl]-9H-fluorene-4-methanol.
$C_{30}H_{32}Cl_3NO = 528.9$.
CAS — 82186-77-4.

Adverse Effects and Precautions

Adverse effects associated with lumefantrine in combination with artemether commonly include headache, dizziness, sleep disturbance, palpitations, gastrointestinal disturbances, anorexia, pruritus, rash, cough, arthralgia, myalgia, and fatigue.

Pharmacokinetics

Following administration by mouth, the bioavailability of lumefantrine is variable; absorption begins after a lag-time of up to 2 hours and is substantially increased by co-administration with food, particularly meals high in fat. Peak plasma concentrations occur after about 6 to 8 hours. Lumefantrine is almost completely protein bound. It is considered to be metabolised mainly in the liver and is excreted in the faeces. The elimination half-life is reported to be between 4 to 6 days in patients with malaria.

◊ References.
1. White NJ, *et al.* Clinical pharmacokinetics and pharmacodynamics of artemether-lumefantrine. *Clin Pharmacokinet* 1999; **37**: 105–25.
2. Ezzet F, *et al.* Pharmacokinetics and pharmacodynamics of lumefantrine (benflumetol) in acute falciparum malaria. *Antimicrob Agents Chemother* 2000; **44**: 697–704.

Uses and Administration

Lumefantrine is a dichlorobenzylidine derivative given by mouth in combination with artemether (p.431) for the treatment of uncomplicated falciparum malaria. It is a blood schizontocide with a relatively slow onset of action but it has a longer duration of action than artemether.

Lumefantrine is given over a period of 60 hours in a dose of 480 mg, in combination with artemether, administered at diagnosis and repeated after 8, 24, 36, 48, and 60 hours (total dose 2.88 g).

◊ References.
1. von Seidlein L, *et al.* Treatment of African children with uncomplicated falciparum malaria with a new antimalarial drug, CGP 56697. *J Infect Dis* 1997; **176**: 1113–16.
2. van Vugt M, *et al.* Randomized comparison of artemether-benflumetol and artesunate-mefloquine in treatment of multidrug-resistant falciparum malaria. *Antimicrob Agents Chemother* 1998; **42**: 135–9.

3. Hatz C, *et al.* Efficacy and safety of CGP 56697 (artemether and benflumetol) compared with chloroquine to treat acute falciparum malaria in Tanzanian children aged 1-5 years. *Trop Med Int Hlth* 1998; **3**: 498–504.
4. von Seidlein L, *et al.* A randomized controlled trial of artemether/benflumetol, a new antimalarial and pyrimethamine/sulfadoxine in the treatment of uncomplicated falciparum malaria in African children. *Am J Trop Med Hyg* 1998; **58**: 638–44.
5. Looareesuwan S, *et al.* A randomized, double-blind, comparative trial of a new oral combination of artemether and benflumetol (CGP 56697) with mefloquine in the treatment of acute Plasmodium falciparum malaria in Thailand. *Am J Trop Med Hyg* 1999; **60**: 238–43.
6. van Vugt M, *et al.* Efficacy of six doses of artemether-lumefantrine (benflumetol) in multidrug-resistant Plasmodium falciparum malaria. *Am J Trop Med Hyg* 1999; **60**: 936–42.
7. van Vugt M, *et al.* Artemether-lumefantrine for the treatment of multidrug-resistant falciparum malaria. *Trans R Soc Trop Med Hyg* 2000; **94**: 545–8.

Preparations

Proprietary Preparations (details are given in Part 3)
Multi-ingredient: *Switz.:* Riamet; *UK:* Riamet.

Mefloquine Hydrochloride (1381-v)

Mefloquine Hydrochloride (BANM, USAN, rINNM).

Mefloquini Hydrochloridum; Ro-21-5998 (mefloquine); Ro-21-5998/001 (mefloquine hydrochloride); WR-142490 (mefloquine). (RS)-[2,8-Bis(trifluoromethyl)-4-quinolyl]-(SR)-(2-piperidyl)methanol hydrochloride.
$C_{17}H_{16}F_6N_2O,HCl = 414.8$.
CAS — 53230-10-7 (mefloquine); 51773-92-3 (mefloquine hydrochloride).

Pharmacopoeias. In Eur. (see p.vi).

Mefloquine base 250 mg is approximately equivalent to mefloquine hydrochloride 274 mg.

Pharmacopoeial description

Ph. Eur.: A white or slightly yellow, crystalline powder. It shows polymorphism. Very slightly soluble in water; soluble in alcohol; freely soluble in methyl alcohol. Protect from light.

Sorption. For reference to loss of mefloquine hydrochloride from solutions during membrane filtration, see Chloroquine, p.432.

Stability. A report of the photolytic degradation of mefloquine hydrochloride in water.[1]

1. Tønnesen HH, Grislingaas A-L. Photochemical stability of biologically active compounds II: photochemical decomposition of mefloquine in water. *Int J Pharmaceutics* 1990; **60**: 157–62.

Adverse Effects

Since mefloquine has a long elimination half-life, adverse effects may occur or persist up to several weeks after the last dose.

The most frequent adverse effects of mefloquine are nausea, diarrhoea, vomiting, abdominal pain, anorexia, headache, dizziness, loss of balance, somnolence, and sleep disorders, notably insomnia and abnormal dreams.

Neurological or psychiatric disturbances have also been reported with mefloquine and include sensory and motor neuropathies, tremor, ataxia, visual disturbances, tinnitus, convulsions, anxiety, depression, confusion, hallucinations, panic attacks, emotional instability, aggression and agitation, and acute psychosis.

Other adverse effects include skin rashes, pruritus and urticaria, hair loss, muscle weakness, myalgia, liver function disturbances, and very rarely thrombocytopenia and leucopenia. There have been rare occurrences of erythema multiforme and Stevens-Johnson syndrome. Cardiovascular effects have included hypotension, hypertension, tachycardia or palpitations, bradycardia, and other minor ECG changes. There have been isolated cases of atrioventricular block.

◊ The frequencies of adverse effects reported[1] in 134 soldiers who received mefloquine hydrochloride 250 mg weekly for malaria chemoprophylaxis were diarrhoea (48%), nausea (13%), vomiting (2%), headache (13%), and dizziness (7%). All of 7 healthy subjects who received a dose of mefloquine hydrochloride 15 mg per kg body-weight had symptoms which included vertigo, nausea, dizziness, and lightheadedness.[2] The manufacturers report that dizziness has occurred in 24% of patients with malaria treated with 750 mg of mefloquine, in 38% treated with 1000 mg, and in 96% treated with 1500 mg; splitting a dose into two doses given 8 hours apart can reduce the incidence of dizziness.[3] A prospective study involving 3673 patients found that anorexia, nausea, vomiting, dizziness, and sleep disorders were 1.1 to 1.4 times more frequent in patients receiving mefloquine 25 mg per kg for treatment of malaria than in those receiving 15 mg per kg, and that vomiting could

be reduced by 40% if the higher dose was split and given as 15 mg per kg followed by a further 10 mg per kg after 16 to 24 hours.[4] The frequency of adverse effects is reported to be higher in subjects who become dehydrated.[5]

There has been concern that the adverse effects of mefloquine, especially neuropsychiatric reactions, might limit its use for the prophylaxis of malaria, but as discussed under Effects on the Nervous System, below, the incidence of adverse effects does not appear to be greater than with other prophylactic schedules.

1. Arthur JD, *et al.* Mefloquine prophylaxis. *Lancet* 1990; **335**: 972.
2. Patchen LC, *et al.* Neurologic reactions after a therapeutic dose of mefloquine. *N Engl J Med* 1989; **321**: 1415.
3. Stürchler D, *et al.* Neuropsychiatric side effects of mefloquine. *N Engl J Med* 1990; **322**: 1752–3.
4. ter Kuile FO, *et al.* Mefloquine treatment of acute falciparum malaria: a prospective study of non-serious adverse effects in 3673 patients. *Bull WHO* 1995; **73**: 631–42.
5. Perry IC. Malaria prophylaxis. *BMJ* 1995; **310**: 1673.

Effects on the blood. Agranulocytosis was reported[1] in a patient with malaria 48 hours after treatment with a 1250-mg course of mefloquine. The patient had previously taken 250 mg of mefloquine weekly for 7 weeks without side-effects.

1. Hennequin C, *et al.* Agranulocytosis during treatment with mefloquine. *Lancet* 1991; **337**: 984.

Effects on the liver. Acute fatty liver was reported[1] in a patient who had recently received mefloquine 250 mg weekly for 5 weeks for malaria prophylaxis. Symptoms resolved with fluid, electrolyte, and albumin replacement, following discontinuation of mefloquine. In another report,[2] acute elevation of liver transaminases, associated with severe acute hepatitis, occurred in a patient with pre-existing mild hepatic impairment following a 6-week course of mefloquine 250 mg weekly.

1. Grieco A, *et al.* Acute fatty liver after malaria prophylaxis with mefloquine. *Lancet* 1999; **353**: 295–6.
2. Gotsman I, *et al.* Mefloquine-induced acute hepatitis. *Pharmacotherapy* 2000; **20**: 1517–19.

Effects on the nervous system. Neuropsychiatric reactions have been associated with the use of mefloquine although various figures have been reported for their frequency. The UK Committee on Safety of Medicines has quoted[1] figures of 1 in 10 000 to 1 in 20 000 for severe reactions to *prophylactic* doses and similarly the manufacturers report that 1 in 10 000 patients receiving mefloquine prophylaxis will experience serious problems. Others consider that the incidence of serious reactions is extremely low,[2] with a frequency of about 1 in 80 000. The manufacturers have also reported that most reactions in patients taking mefloquine for prophylaxis appear to occur after the first dose and have suggested that monitoring after the first dose could identify 40% of those at risk of neuropsychiatric effects.[3] Some authorities consider that over 75% of such reactions to mefloquine are apparent by the third dose.[4] This may allow for tolerability problems with mefloquine prophylaxis to be identified before travel. There has been much discussion on the comparative tolerability of antimalarials used for chemoprophylaxis. The incidence of adverse events, including neuropsychiatric events, was comparable for mefloquine and chloroquine in 2 uncontrolled questionnaire studies, one in tourists[5] and one in US Peace Corps volunteers.[6] However, in a more recent questionnaire in travellers,[7] although the incidence of reported adverse events was similar for mefloquine and chloroquine plus proguanil, neuropsychiatric adverse events were significantly more common in mefloquine recipients. In two randomised controlled trials,[8,9] both in military personnel, there was no difference between CNS symptoms in those receiving weekly mefloquine and those receiving chloroquine (with or without proguanil). In one of these studies,[9] a subgroup receiving a loading dose of mefloquine daily for 3 days initially had a higher incidence of CNS events. A review[10] of 10 controlled trials found no significant difference in the rates of withdrawal and overall incidence of adverse effects for mefloquine and alternative prophylactic regimens, but mefloquine was more likely than other drugs to cause insomnia and fatigue. Women may be at greater risk of adverse effects than men, and WHO has commented that the occurrence of such adverse effects may mean that only highly motivated occupational subgroups or individuals at high risk of infection with chloroquine-resistant malaria will be willing to continue with mefloquine prophylaxis.[11]

Neuropsychiatric reactions are more frequent following the higher doses of mefloquine used for *treatment* than those used for prophylaxis. Some workers have estimated that overall 1 in 8000 mefloquine users suffers from such reactions, with the incidence 60 times higher after treatment than after prophylaxis.[12] Other workers who have used mefloquine in nearly 14 000 treatments calculated that the overall frequency of serious neuropsychiatric reactions was 1 per 1754 treatments; serious neuropsychiatric reactions therefore appeared to be ten times more probable after treatment than with prophylactic use of mefloquine.[13]

A severe neurological syndrome associated with mefloquine treatment, with agitation, delirium, stupor, hyperpyrexia, mydriasis, and generalised rigors responded rapidly to treatment with physostigmine, suggesting a central anticholinergic aetiology.[14]

A discrete post-malaria neurological syndrome (including an acute confusional state or acute psychosis, convulsions, and tremor) has been observed following recovery from falciparum malaria and there appeared to be a strong association with mefloquine although it was not the only risk factor.[15] Nevertheless the risk was considered unacceptable and the recommendation made[15] that, where there was an effective alternative drug, mefloquine should not be used after initial treatment of severe malaria.

Emergence delirium during recovery from general anaesthesia after mefloquine prophylaxis has been reported in 3 cases.[16]

1. Committee on Safety of Medicines. Mefloquine (Lariam) and neuropsychiatric reactions. *Current Problems* 1996; **22:** 6.
2. Croft AMJ, World MJ. Neuropsychiatric reactions with mefloquine chemoprophylaxis. *Lancet* 1996; **347:** 326.
3. Stürchler D, *et al.* Neuropsychiatric side effects of mefloquine. *N Engl J Med* 1990; **322:** 1752–3.
4. Bradley DJ, Bannister B. Guidelines for malaria prevention in travellers from the United Kingdom for 2001. *Commun Dis Public Health* 2001; **4:** 84–101.
5. Steffen R, *et al.* Mefloquine compared with other malaria chemoprophylactic regimens in tourists visiting East Africa. *Lancet* 1993; **341:** 1299–1303.
6. Lobel HO, *et al.* Long-term malaria prophylaxis with weekly mefloquine. *Lancet* 1993; **341:** 848–51.
7. Barrett PJ, *et al.* Comparison of adverse events associated with use of mefloquine and combination of chloroquine and proguanil as antimalarial prophylaxis: postal and telephone survey of travellers. *BMJ* 1996; **313:** 525–8. Correspondence. *ibid.*; 1552–4.
8. Croft AMJ, *et al.* Side effects of mefloquine prophylaxis for malaria: an independent randomized controlled trial. *Trans R Soc Trop Med Hyg* 1997; **91:** 199–203.
9. Boudreau E, *et al.* Tolerability of prophylactic Lariam regimens. *Trop Med Parasitol* 1993; **44:** 257–65.
10. Croft A, Garner P. Mefloquine to prevent malaria: a systematic review of trials. *BMJ* 1997; **315:** 1412–16. Correspondence. *ibid.* 1998; **316:** 1980–1.
11. Anonymous. Mefloquine effectiveness impaired by high withdrawal rates. *WHO Drug Inf* 1998; **12:** 7–8.
12. Weinke T, *et al.* Neuropsychiatric side effects after the use of mefloquine. *Am J Trop Med Hyg* 1991; **45:** 86–91.
13. Luxemburger C, *et al.* Mefloquine for multidrug-resistant malaria. *Lancet* 1991; **338:** 1268.
14. Speich R, Haller A. Central anticholinergic syndrome with the antimalarial drug mefloquine. *N Engl J Med* 1994; **331:** 57–8.
15. Mai NTH, *et al.* Post-malaria neurological syndrome. *Lancet* 1996; **348:** 917–21.
16. Gullahorn GM, *et al.* Anaesthesia emergence delirium after mefloquine prophylaxis. *Lancet* 1993; **341:** 632.

Effects on the oesophagus. Oesophageal ulceration in one patient and discomfort in another 4 was attributed to swallowing mefloquine tablets with insufficient fluid.[1]

1. Phillips M. Antimalarial mefloquine. *Med J Aust* 1994; **161:** 227–8.

Effects on the skin. Single cases of Stevens-Johnson syndrome,[1] severe facial lesions,[2] exfoliative dermatitis,[3] toxic epidermal necrolysis,[4] and cutaneous vasculitis[5] have been associated with use of mefloquine for malaria prophylaxis.

For a comparison of the incidence of pruritus induced by various antimalarials, see under Chloroquine, p.433.

1. Van den Enden E, *et al.* Mefloquine-induced Stevens-Johnson syndrome. *Lancet* 1991; **337:** 683.
2. Shlim DR. Severe facial rash associated with mefloquine. *JAMA* 1991; **266:** 2560.
3. Martin GJ, *et al.* Exfoliative dermatitis during malarial prophylaxis with mefloquine. *Clin Infect Dis* 1993; **16:** 341–2.
4. McBride SR, *et al.* Fatal toxic epidermal necrolysis associated with mefloquine antimalarial prophylaxis. *Lancet* 1997; **349:** 101.
5. White AC, *et al.* Cutaneous vasculitis associated with mefloquine. *Ann Intern Med* 1995; **123:** 894.

Overdosage. Cardiac, hepatic, and neurological symptoms have been reported in a patient who inadvertently received 5.25 g of mefloquine over 6 days.[1] All symptoms disappeared rapidly when mefloquine was discontinued.

1. Bourgeade A, *et al.* Intoxication accidentelle à la méfloquine. *Presse Med* 1990; **19:** 1903.

Precautions

Tasks requiring fine coordination such as driving should not be undertaken during treatment with mefloquine or for at least 3 weeks afterwards; in the case of prophylactic use, care should be exercised while taking mefloquine and for at least 3 weeks after stopping it. The use of mefloquine for malaria prophylaxis is contra-indicated in patients with a history of psychiatric (including depression) or convulsive disorders and in those with severe hepatic impairment. Mefloquine is teratogenic in *animals* and its use during pregnancy is best avoided; however, in areas of chloroquine-resistant *Plasmodium falciparum*, WHO and UK authorities suggest that mefloquine may be taken for malaria prophylaxis from the fourth month of pregnancy. It is recommended that women should also avoid becoming pregnant during, and for 3 months after, mefloquine use and that mothers should not breast feed while taking mefloquine. Mefloquine should be used with caution in patients with renal impairment and in those with cardiac conduction disorders.

Porphyria. For a discussion of the problems of the use of antimalarials in patients with porphyria and a comment that mefloquine may be safe for use in such patients, see under Precautions for Chloroquine, p.434.

Pregnancy. The manufacturers of mefloquine report that it is teratogenic in *rodents*. There is limited information on its effects in humans. One study in Thailand cited by WHO[1] found no difference between mefloquine and quinine in pregnancy outcome, but the numbers of treated patients who were in their first trimester were very small and its use should be kept to a minimum in that stage of pregnancy. Further spontaneous reports of exposure to mefloquine during the first trimester of pregnancy collected by the manufacturer revealed 24 fetal abnormalities and 17 spontaneous or missed abortions in 358 pregnancies, although a causal relationship was not established,[2] and a later study by the manufacturer involving 1627 reports of exposure during pregnancy appeared to show a similar incidence of congenital malformation to that in offspring of unexposed women.[3] In 53 army service women who inadvertently used mefloquine in pregnancy, and for whom pregnancy outcome was known, there were 17 elective abortions, 12 spontaneous abortions, one molar pregnancy, and 23 healthy live births, with no major congenital malformations.[4] The rate of spontaneous abortions was considered high.[4] A prospective cohort study involving 236 pregnant women who received an antimalarial in the first trimester did not demonstrate an increased risk of spontaneous abortion or anomaly in women who took mefloquine compared with other antimalarials, and the rate of spontaneous abortion was comparable with background rates.[5]

Confidence in the safety of mefloquine has increased, and mefloquine is now considered suitable for malaria prophylaxis in the second and third trimesters by both WHO[6] and authorities in the UK.[7] It should be avoided in the first trimester unless the risk of withholding mefloquine is considered greater, and pregnancy should be avoided during and for 3 months after prophylactic use.

1. WHO. Practical chemotherapy of malaria: report of a WHO scientific group. *WHO Tech Rep Ser 805* 1990.
2. Palmer KJ, *et al.* Mefloquine: a review of its antimalarial activity, pharmacological properties and therapeutic efficacy. *Drugs* 1993; **45:** 430–75.
3. Vanhauwere B, *et al.* Post-marketing surveillance of prophylactic mefloquine (Lariam®) use in pregnancy. *Am J Trop Med Hyg* 1998; **58:** 17–21.
4. Smoak BL, *et al.* The effects of inadvertent exposure of mefloquine chemoprophylaxis on pregnancy outcomes and infants of US Army service women. *J Infect Dis* 1997; **176:** 831–3.
5. Phillips-Howard PA, *et al.* Safety of mefloquine and other antimalarial agents in the first trimester of pregnancy. *J Travel Med* 1998; **5:** 121–6.
6. WHO. *International travel and health: vaccination requirements and health advice.* Geneva: WHO, 2001.
7. Bradley DJ, Bannister B. Guidelines for malaria prevention in travellers from the United Kingdom for 2001. *Commun Dis Public Health* 2001; **4:** 84–101.

Interactions

Halofantrine should not be given with or after mefloquine because of the increased potential to induce hazardous cardiac arrhythmias, as discussed on p.436. There is an increased risk of convulsions when mefloquine is administered with chloroquine or quinine.

Alcohol. There has been a case report[1] of a patient who experienced neuropsychiatric disturbances after consuming a large quantity of alcohol in conjunction with mefloquine; subsequent abstention from alcohol led to complete reversal of the reactions.

1. Wittes RC, Saginur R. Adverse reaction to mefloquine associated with ethanol ingestion. *Can Med Assoc J* 1995; **152:** 515–17.

Antibacterials. Studies in healthy subjects have indicated that *ampicillin*[1] or *tetracycline*,[2] could increase blood concentrations of mefloquine.

1. Karbwang J, *et al.* Effect of ampicillin on mefloquine pharmacokinetics in Thai males. *Eur J Clin Pharmacol* 1991; **40:** 631–3.
2. Karbwang J, *et al.* Effect of tetracycline on mefloquine pharmacokinetics in Thai males. *Eur J Clin Pharmacol* 1992; **43:** 567–9.

Antidepressants. The manufacturers of mefloquine state that theoretically in patients taking tricyclic antidepressants co-administration of mefloquine may contribute to prolongation of the QT interval.

Antiepileptics. For the effect of mefloquine on *valproate*, see p.368. For its effect on *carbamazepine*, see p.345.

Antihistamines. The co-administration of mefloquine with antihistamines may contribute to the prolongation of QT intervals; however, this is not considered to be an absolute contra-indication.

Antimalarials. It is well established that the use of *halofantrine* with or after mefloquine is contra-indicated because of the risk of hazardous cardiac arrhythmias. Mefloquine and other related compounds such as *quinine*, *quinidine*, and *chloroquine* may be given concomitantly only under close medical supervision because of possible additive cardiac toxicity; there is also an increased risk of convulsions.

A study in healthy subjects indicated that concurrent administration of *primaquine* could increase blood concentrations of

mefloquine and might increase the incidence of adverse effects due to mefloquine,[1] but others reported no such interaction.[2]

1. MacLeod CM, *et al.* Interaction of primaquine with mefloquine in healthy males. *J Clin Pharmacol* 1990; **30:** 841.
2. Karbwang J, *et al.* Pharmacokinetics of mefloquine in the presence of primaquine. *Eur J Clin Pharmacol* 1992; **42:** 559–60.

Antipsychotics. The co-administration of mefloquine with *phenothiazines* or *pimozide* may contribute to prolonged QT intervals, although this is not considered to be an absolute contra-indication.

Cardiovascular drugs. It has been recommended that extreme caution should be exercised in the use of mefloquine in patients also taking *antiarrhythmics*, *beta blockers*, *calcium-channel blockers*, or *digitalis*, until more was known about the risks of cardiotoxicity. More recently, WHO malaria prophylaxis guidelines[1] considered, in the light of information currently available, that although co-administration of mefloquine with *antiarrhythmics*, *beta blockers*, and *calcium-channel blockers*, might contribute to prolongation of QT intervals, it was not absolutely contra-indicated. Nevertheless an increased risk of ventricular arrhythmias has been reported when mefloquine is used concomitantly with *amiodarone*.
Cardiopulmonary arrest has occurred after a single dose of mefloquine in a patient who was taking *propranolol*.[2]

1. WHO. *International travel and health: vaccination requirements and health advice.* Geneva: WHO, 2001.
2. Anonymous. Mefloquine for malaria. *Med Lett Drugs Ther* 1990; **32:** 13–14.

Metoclopramide. Concomitant administration of metoclopramide may increase plasma concentrations of mefloquine.[1]

1. Na Bangchang K, *et al.* The effect of metoclopramide on mefloquine pharmacokinetics. *Br J Clin Pharmacol* 1991; **32:** 640–1.

Vaccines. The manufacturers state that mefloquine-induced attenuation of immunisation produced by oral live *typhoid vaccines* cannot be excluded and therefore vaccination with such live vaccines should be completed at least 3 days before taking mefloquine.

Pharmacokinetics

The pharmacokinetics of mefloquine may be altered by malaria infection in a manner similar to those of quinine, the main effects being reductions in both its volume of distribution and its overall clearance.

Mefloquine is well absorbed from the gastrointestinal tract but there is marked interindividual variation in the time required to achieve peak plasma concentrations. Mefloquine is about 98% bound to plasma proteins and high concentrations have been reported in red blood cells. It is widely distributed throughout the body. Mefloquine has a long elimination half-life; mean values of about 21 days have been reported for some patients, although like other pharmacokinetic data on mefloquine there is considerable variation in reported figures. Subtherapeutic concentrations of mefloquine may persist in the blood for several months. Mefloquine is metabolised in the liver. Little of a dose is excreted in the urine and animal studies suggest excretion of mefloquine and its metabolites is mainly in the bile and faeces.

Mefloquine is distributed into breast milk in small amounts.

◊ Reviews of pharmacokinetic studies of mefloquine reveal considerable interindividual variation for several pharmacokinetic parameters and some evidence that there might be pharmacokinetic differences between ethnic groups.[1,2] Mefloquine is well absorbed by healthy subjects and by patients with uncomplicated malaria following oral administration.[3,4] In patients with complicated malaria adequate blood concentrations have been obtained using nasogastric administration but this route cannot be relied upon for seriously ill patients[5] as absorption may be incomplete.[1] Mefloquine has a large apparent volume of distribution but this is reduced in the presence of malaria.[6,7] In children who received mefloquine with sulfadoxine and pyrimethamine as tablets crushed and mixed with a glucose syrup, maximum blood-mefloquine concentrations were higher and reached in a shorter time compared with equivalent doses in adults.[8] In pregnant women with uncomplicated malaria blood concentrations were lower than in non-pregnant women and the apparent volume of distribution was larger.[9] Once-weekly prophylactic doses of mefloquine resulted in steady-state conditions at about 10 doses with no evidence of subsequent accumulation.[10] The manufacturer has stated that mefloquine is about 98% bound to plasma proteins.
Mefloquine is metabolised in the liver[11] largely into 2,8-bis(trifluoromethyl)-4-quinoline carboxylic acid [Ro-21-5104][12] but this metabolite appears to be inactive against *Plasmodium falciparum*.[13] Only a small percentage of a dose is excreted in the urine[14] and studies in *animals* suggest excretion of mefloquine and its metabolites is primarily in the bile and faeces.[1] Mefloquine has an extremely long plasma elimination half-life; again there is considerable interindividual variation and mean values

The symbol † denotes a preparation no longer actively marketed

ranging from 13.9 to 27.5 days have been quoted, the smaller figure of the range referring to a formulation that did not provide as good absorption as the preparation now in use.[1]

Mefloquine is distributed into breast milk, but a single dose study in 2 women[15] indicated that the concentration of mefloquine in milk was only a small proportion of that seen in plasma.

1. Karbwang J, White NJ. Clinical pharmacokinetics of mefloquine. *Clin Pharmacokinet* 1990; **19:** 264–79.
2. Palmer KJ, *et al.* Mefloquine: a review of its antimalarial activity, pharmacokinetic properties and therapeutic efficacy. *Drugs* 1993; **45:** 430–75.
3. Karbwang J, *et al.* The pharmacokinetics of mefloquine when given alone or in combination with sulphadoxine and pyrimethamine in Thai male and female subjects. *Eur J Clin Pharmacol* 1987; **32:** 173–7.
4. Looareesuwan S, *et al.* Studies of mefloquine bioavailability and kinetics using a stable isotope technique: a comparison of Thai patients with falciparum malaria and healthy caucasian volunteers. *Br J Clin Pharmacol* 1987; **24:** 37–42.
5. Chanthavanich P, *et al.* Intragastric mefloquine is absorbed rapidly in patients with cerebral malaria. *Am J Trop Med Hyg* 1985; **34:** 1028–36.
6. Juma FD, Ogeto JO. Mefloquine disposition in normals and in patients with severe Plasmodium falciparum malaria. *Eur J Drug Metab Pharmacokinet* 1989; **14:** 15–17.
7. Karbwang J, *et al.* A comparison of the pharmacokinetics of mefloquine in healthy Thai volunteers and in Thai patients with falciparum malaria. *Eur J Clin Pharmacol* 1988; **35:** 677–80.
8. Singhasivanon V, *et al.* Pharmacokinetic study of mefloquine in Thai children aged 5-12 years suffering from uncomplicated falciparum malaria treated with MSP or MSP plus primaquine. *Eur J Drug Metab Pharmacokinet* 1994; **19:** 27–32.
9. Na Bangchang K, *et al.* Mefloquine pharmacokinetics in pregnant women with acute falciparum malaria. *Trans R Soc Trop Med Hyg* 1994; **88:** 321–3.
10. Pennie RA, *et al.* Steady state pharmacokinetics of mefloquine in long-term travellers. *Trans R Soc Trop Med Hyg* 1993; **87:** 459–62.
11. WHO. Severe and complicated malaria. 2nd ed. *Trans R Soc Trop Med Hyg* 1990; **84** (suppl 2): 1–65.
12. Panisko DM, Keystone JS. Treatment of malaria—1990. *Drugs* 1990; **39:** 160–89.
13. Håkanson A, *et al.* Comparison of the activity in vitro of mefloquine and two metabolites against Plasmodium falciparum. *Trans R Soc Trop Med Hyg* 1990; **84:** 503–4.
14. Schwartz DE, *et al.* Urinary excretion of mefloquine and some of its metabolites in African volunteers at steady state. *Chemotherapy* 1987; **33:** 305–8.
15. Edstein MD, *et al.* Excretion of mefloquine in human breast milk. *Chemotherapy* 1988; **34:** 165–9.

Uses and Administration

Mefloquine is a 4-methanolquinoline antimalarial related to quinine. It is a blood schizontocide effective against all forms of malaria including chloroquine- or multidrug-resistant strains of *Plasmodium falciparum*, although some strains are naturally resistant to mefloquine. It is used for the treatment of uncomplicated falciparum malaria and chloroquine-resistant vivax malaria, and also for malaria prophylaxis. Mefloquine is also used following treatment with an artemisinin derivative for acute uncomplicated malaria, to reduce the risk of recrudescence.

Mefloquine is administered by mouth as the hydrochloride but variation in the way doses for mefloquine are expressed could lead to confusion. In the UK and elsewhere doses are expressed in terms of the base and a dose of 250 mg base is approximately equivalent to 274 mg of mefloquine hydrochloride. In the USA doses are expressed in terms of the hydrochloride and a dose of 250 mg is therefore approximately equivalent to only 228 mg of mefloquine base. Doses in the USA could therefore be about 10% less than elsewhere.

Doses recommended in the UK are as follows. For the *treatment of malaria*, mefloquine base 20 to 25 mg per kg body-weight (up to a maximum of 1.5 g) as a single dose or preferably in 2 or 3 divided doses 6 to 8 hours apart. For the *prophylaxis of malaria*, a dose of mefloquine base 250 mg once weekly in adults and children over 45 kg. Children weighing 5 to 19 kg (age 3 months to 5 years) may be given one-quarter the adult dose; those weighing 20 to 30 kg (6 to 8 years), half the adult dose; and those weighing 31 to 45 kg (9 to 14 years), three-quarters the adult dose. Prophylaxis should be started 1 to 3 weeks before exposure and continued for 4 weeks after leaving the malarious area.

For other dosage recommendations, see under Malaria, below.

Malaria. The overall treatment and prophylaxis of malaria and the place of mefloquine in current recommendations are discussed on p.440.

TREATMENT. Clinical studies have shown mefloquine to be effective in the treatment of chloroquine- or multidrug-resistant fal-

ciparum malaria. It is also effective in benign malarias, but is not normally required since they usually respond to chloroquine.

Mefloquine is widely considered to be a suitable alternative to regimens using quinine for the treatment of chloroquine-resistant or multidrug-resistant strains of *Plasmodium falciparum*.[1-4] It may also be used in combination with an artemisinin derivative in regions of greatest multidrug resistance (see p.432). Other combinations are also being evaluated.[5,6]

As there is no parenteral formulation of mefloquine currently available it can only be used in patients who can take oral medication and is therefore unsuitable for sole treatment in severe infections. Mefloquine has produced adequate blood concentrations following nasogastric administration, but this route cannot be relied upon in seriously ill patients.[7] If mefloquine is given to patients after parenteral administration of quinine, it is recommended that a period of 12 hours should be allowed after the last dose of quinine to avoid toxicity.

In the UK, the recommended dose for the treatment of malaria is the equivalent of 20 to 25 mg of mefloquine base per kg body-weight, as a single dose or preferably in two or three divided doses 6 to 8 hours apart, to a maximum of 1.5 g. The manufacturers recommend a lower dose of 15 mg per kg for the partially immune. In the USA, the manufacturers recommend 1250 mg of mefloquine hydrochloride given as a single dose. WHO has recommended a dose of mefloquine base of 15 mg per kg (up to a maximum of 1000 mg). In areas of multidrug-resistant malaria a dose of 25 mg per kg[8,9] has been shown to improve the response, and this dose is now recommended by WHO[10] for standby treatment in such areas (see below).

Mefloquine is one of the antimalarial drugs recommended by some experts to be carried as a *standby* for the emergency treatment of malaria. The adult dose recommended by WHO[10] for self-treatment is 15 mg per kg as a single dose, or 25 mg per kg (given as 15 mg per kg followed by 10 mg per kg 6 to 24 hours later) in areas of mefloquine resistance. In the USA mefloquine is not recommended for self-treatment.[11]

PROPHYLAXIS. It had been hoped that mefloquine could be reserved for the treatment of malaria, but increasing drug resistance to chemoprophylactic regimens has led to it being widely used for malaria prophylaxis. WHO recommends[10] that mefloquine should only be used in high-risk areas where chloroquine-resistant malaria is prevalent and authorities in the UK[12] and USA[13] endorse this. The equivalent of 250 mg of mefloquine base is given every week, starting 1 to 3 weeks before departure, and continuing throughout the period of exposure and for 4 weeks after leaving the malarious area. Starting mefloquine prophylaxis 2 to 3 weeks before exposure allows for detection of possible adverse effects before travelling (see Effects on the Nervous System, above, for concerns about neurotoxicity). It is now considered that mefloquine prophylaxis can be given for periods of up to one year instead of the previous limit of 3 months.

Mefloquine is considered to be suitable[10] for prophylaxis in women from the fourth month of pregnancy, although it should be avoided during the first trimester and pregnancy should be avoided during and for three months after stopping the drug.

Recommended dosages of mefloquine for prophylaxis in children have generally been based on 5 mg per kg body-weight as a single weekly dose in children over 15 kg body-weight[2] and above the age of 2 years. However, the doses now usually used in the UK[12] for infants and children over 5 kg body-weight and above 3 months of age are as follows: 6 to 15.9 kg (3 months to 3 years 11 months), one-quarter the adult dose; 16 to 24.9 kg (4 years to 7 years 11 months), half the adult dose; 25 to 44.9 kg (8 years to 12 years 11 months), three-quarters the adult dose. Similarly, WHO[10] recommends: 5 to 12 kg (3 to 23 months), one-quarter the adult dose; 13 to 16 kg (2 to 3 years), one-third the adult dose; 17 to 24 kg (4 to 7 years), half the adult dose; 25 to 35 kg (8 to 10 years), three-quarters the adult dose; 36 to 50 kg (11 to 13 years), the adult dose.

In the event of breakthrough malaria during malaria prophylaxis there may be a delay of up to several months before the onset of symptoms in contrast to that seen with other forms of prophylaxis.[14] Mefloquine should not be used for treatment if it has been used for prophylaxis.

1. WHO. WHO expert committee on malaria: twentieth report. *WHO Tech Rep Ser 892* 2000.
2. WHO. *WHO model prescribing information: drugs used in parasitic diseases.* 2nd ed. Geneva: WHO, 1995.
3. Molyneux M, Fox R. Diagnosis and treatment of malaria in Britain. *BMJ* 1993; **306:** 1175–80.
4. Anonymous. Drugs for parasitic infections. *Med Lett Drugs Ther* 1998; **40:** 1–12.
5. Looareesuwan S, *et al.* Randomized trial of mefloquine-doxycycline, and artesunate-doxycycline for treatment of acute uncomplicated falciparum malaria. *Am J Trop Med Hyg* 1994; **50:** 784–9.
6. Looareesuwan S, *et al.* Randomized trial of mefloquine-tetracycline and quinine-tetracycline for acute uncomplicated falciparum malaria. *Acta Trop (Basel)* 1994; **57:** 47–53.
7. Chanthavanich P, *et al.* Intragastric mefloquine is absorbed rapidly in patients with cerebral malaria. *Am J Trop Med Hyg* 1985; **34:** 1028–36.
8. ter Kuile FO, *et al.* High-dose mefloquine in the treatment of multidrug-resistant falciparum malaria. *J Infect Dis* 1992; **166:** 1393–1400.
9. Smithuis FM, *et al.* Comparison of two mefloquine regimens for treatment of Plasmodium falciparum malaria on the northeastern Thai-Cambodian border. *Antimicrob Agents Chemother* 1993; **37:** 1977–81.
10. WHO. *International travel and health: vaccination requirements and health advice.* Geneva: WHO, 2001.
11. Centers for Disease Control. Recommendations for the prevention of malaria among travelers. *MMWR* 1990; **39** (RR-3): 1–10.
12. Bradley DJ, Bannister B. Guidelines for malaria prevention in travellers from the United Kingdom for 2001. *Commun Dis Public Health* 2001; **4:** 84–101.
13. Centers for Disease Control. Change of dosing regimen for malaria prophylaxis with mefloquine. *MMWR* 1991; **40:** 72–3.
14. Day JH, Behrens RH. Delay in onset of malaria with mefloquine prophylaxis. *Lancet* 1995; **345:** 398.

Preparations

Proprietary Preparations (details are given in Part 3)

Aust.: Lariam; *Austral.:* Lariam; *Belg.:* Lariam; *Braz.:* Mephaquin Lactab; *Canad.:* Lariam; *Denm.:* Lariam; *Fin.:* Lariam; *Fr.:* Lariam; *Ger.:* Lariam; *Hong Kong:* Lariam; Mephaquin; *Irl.:* Lariam; *Israel:* Lariam; Mephaquin; *Ital.:* Lariam; *Neth.:* Lariam; *Norw.:* Lariam; *NZ:* Lariam; *Port.:* Mephaquin; *S.Afr.:* Lariam; Mefliam; *Singapore:* Lariam; Mephaquine; *Swed.:* Lariam; *Switz.:* Lariam; Mephaquine; *Thai.:* Mephaquin; *UK:* Lariam; *USA:* Lariam.

Multi-ingredient: *Switz.:* Fansimef.

Piperaquine Phosphate (19666-g)

Piperaquini Phosphas; 13228-RP. 1,3-Bis[1-(7-chloro-4-quinolyl)-4'-piperazinyl]propane.

$C_{29}H_{32}Cl_2N_6,4H_3PO_4,4H_2O = 999.6.$

Pharmacopoeias. In Chin.

Profile

Piperaquine phosphate is a 4-piperazinoquinoline derivative which has been studied in the treatment and prophylaxis of falciparum malaria.

Primaquine Phosphate (1387-e)

Primaquine Phosphate (BANM, rINNM).

Difosfato de Primaquina; Primachina Fosfato; Primachini Phosphas; Primaquine Diphosphate; Primaquini Diphosphas; Primaquinum Phosphoricum; SN-13,272. (RS)-8-(4-Amino-1-methylbutylamino)-6-methoxyquinoline diphosphate.

$C_{15}H_{21}N_3O,2H_3PO_4 = 455.3.$

CAS — 90-34-6 (primaquine); 63-45-6 (primaquine phosphate).

Pharmacopoeias. In Chin., Eur. (see p.vi), Int., and US.

Primaquine base 7.5 mg is approximately equivalent to 13.2 mg of primaquine phosphate.

Pharmacopoeial description

Ph. Eur.: An orange crystalline powder. Soluble in water; practically insoluble in alcohol and in ether. Protect from light.

USP 25: An orange-red, odourless, crystalline powder. Soluble 1 in 15 of water; insoluble in chloroform and in ether. Its solutions are acid to litmus. Protect from light.

Adverse Effects

Adverse effects with therapeutic doses of primaquine are usually minimal but abdominal pain and gastric distress are more common if administered on an empty stomach. Larger doses may cause nausea and vomiting. Methaemoglobinaemia may occur occasionally. Haemolytic anaemia can occur in persons with a deficiency of glucose-6-phosphate dehydrogenase (G6PD) (see below). Other uncommon effects include mild anaemia and leucocytosis. Hypertension and cardiac arrhythmias have been reported on rare occasions. Primaquine may rarely produce leucopenia or agranulocytosis, usually following overdosage. Other effects associated with overdosage include gastrointestinal symptoms, haemolytic anaemia, and methaemoglobinaemia with cyanosis.

◊ A wide range of side-effects has been reported following the use of primaquine[1] but some, including pruritus and disturbances of visual accomodation, are considered to be inadequately documented or doubtfully attributed to the drug.

Acute intravascular haemolysis is the most serious toxic hazard of primaquine, especially in people with G6PD deficiency, other defects of the erythrocytic pentose phosphate pathway of glucose metabolism, or some types of haemoglobinopathy. In individuals with G6PD deficiency the severity of haemolysis is directly related to the degree of deficiency and to the quantity of primaquine administered. In patients with the African variant the standard course of primaquine generally produces a moderate and self-limiting anaemia, while in those with the Mediterranean and related Asian variants, haemolysis can result in progressive haemoglobinaemia and haemoglobinuria which can be fatal. Whenever possible, therapy with primaquine should be delayed until the acute stage of malaria has been brought under control by a blood schizontocide because of the risk of inducing haemolysis and compromising the gastrointestinal tolerance of therapy.

1. Clyde DF. Clinical problems associated with the use of primaquine as a tissue schizontocidal and gametocytocidal drug. *Bull WHO* 1981; **59:** 391–5.

Precautions
Primaquine should be administered cautiously to acutely ill patients with any serious systemic disease characterised by a tendency to granulocytopenia such as rheumatoid arthritis or lupus erythematosus. It should also be used with care in patients with glucose-6-phosphate dehydrogenase deficiency. Primaquine should be withdrawn if signs of haemolysis or methaemoglobinaemia occur and the blood count should be monitored periodically.

Pregnancy. Radical cure of vivax or ovale malarias with primaquine should be delayed in pregnant women until after delivery.[1]

1. Panisko DM, Keystone JS. Treatment of malaria—1990. *Drugs* 1990; **39:** 160–89.

Interactions
Primaquine should not be used with drugs liable to induce haemolysis or bone marrow depression. Theoretically, mepacrine may increase the plasma concentrations of primaquine resulting in a higher risk of toxicity, and it has been recommended that these drugs should not be used together.

Antimalarials. The pharmacokinetics of primaquine were not altered by *mefloquine* in healthy subjects,[1] although the effect of primaquine on mefloquine pharmacokinetics is uncertain (see under Mefloquine, p.439). In a study in patients with malaria, *quinine* reduced the plasma concentrations of primaquine, although the clinical importance of the interaction was unclear.[1]

1. Edwards G, *et al.* Interactions among primaquine, malaria infection and other antimalarials in Thai subjects. *Br J Clin Pharmacol* 1993; **35:** 193–8.

Pharmacokinetics
Primaquine is readily absorbed from the gastrointestinal tract. Peak plasma concentrations occur about 1 to 2 hours after a dose is taken and then rapidly diminish with a reported elimination half-life of 3 to 6 hours. It is widely distributed into body tissues.

Primaquine is rapidly metabolised in the liver, its major metabolite being carboxyprimaquine, and little unchanged drug is excreted in the urine. Carboxyprimaquine accumulates in the plasma on repeated administration.

◊ References.

1. Fletcher KA, *et al.* Studies on the pharmacokinetics of primaquine. *Bull WHO* 1981; **59:** 407–12.
2. White NJ. Clinical pharmacokinetics of antimalarial drugs. *Clin Pharmacokinet* 1985; **10:** 187–215.
3. Mihaly GW, *et al.* Pharmacokinetics of primaquine in man, I: studies of the absolute bioavailability and effects of dose size. *Br J Clin Pharmacol* 1985; **19:** 745–50.
4. Ward SA, *et al.* Pharmacokinetics of primaquine in man, II: comparison of acute vs chronic dosage in Thai subjects. *Br J Clin Pharmacol* 1985; **19:** 751–5.
5. Bhatia SC, *et al.* Pharmacokinetics of primaquine in patients with P. vivax malaria. *Eur J Clin Pharmacol* 1986; **31:** 205–10.
6. Rønn A, Bygbjerg I. Unexpected high primaquine concentrations in acutely ill malaria patients. *Lancet* 1993; **341:** 305.

Uses and Administration
Primaquine is an 8-aminoquinoline antimalarial which is effective as a tissue schizontocide against intrahepatic forms of all types of malaria parasite and is used to produce radical cure of vivax and ovale malarias.

When used for radical cure of vivax and ovale malarias, a course of treatment with a blood schizontocide must be given first to kill any erythrocytic parasites. Primaquine phosphate is then given by mouth, usually in a dose equivalent to 15 mg of the base daily for 14 days but higher doses or longer courses may be required to overcome resistance in some strains of *P. vivax* (see below); WHO has advised that a treatment period of 21 days should be used to achieve radical cure in most of South-East Asia and Oceania. A dose for children is 250 µg per kg body-weight daily for 14 days.

Regimens of 30 mg (children 500 to 750 µg per kg) once every 7 days for 8 weeks have been suggested to minimise haemolysis in patients with glucose-6-

phosphate dehydrogenase deficiency (but see Adverse Effects and Precautions, above).

Primaquine is also gametocytocidal and a single dose of 30 to 45 mg has been suggested to prevent transmission of falciparum malaria particularly in areas where there is potential for re-introduction of malaria.

Primaquine is also used in the treatment of *Pneumocystis carinii* pneumonia in AIDS patients in combination with clindamycin.

Malaria. The overall treatment and prophylaxis of malaria and the place of primaquine in current recommendations are described on p.428.

Despite the generally successful use of primaquine for radical cure of benign malarias,[1,2] there has been a report[3] of a patient weighing 84 kg who had relapse of vivax malaria after treatment including primaquine 15 mg given daily for 21 days; no further symptoms occurred after a second course of 15 mg given daily for 3 months. It was suggested that a daily dose of 15 mg might be inadequate for patients weighing more than 50 kg and that patients with vivax malaria who have relapsed after the standard course of primaquine and possibly those with vivax malaria acquired in South-East Asia or Melanesia should receive a total dose of 6 mg per kg body-weight in daily doses of 15 to 22.5 mg. A report from Thailand,[4] where primaquine-resistant strains of *Plasmodium vivax* are increasing, showed that a dose of primaquine 22.5 mg daily for 14 days was safe and more effective in preventing relapses than 15 mg daily in patients with an average body-weight of about 51 kg. There have been several other reports of primaquine-resistant *P. vivax*,[5-8] and the suggestion has been made that higher doses of primaquine (15 mg twice daily for 14 days, to give a total dose of 6 mg per kg assuming a body-weight of 70 kg) should be considered wherever the vivax malaria was acquired.[8]

Variable responses to primaquine in the Amazonian region were attributed to considerable variation in the content of primaquine both between and within batches of tablets; primaquine content ranged from 19 to 168% of the labelled content.[9]

In the USA, the CDC have suggested the use of primaquine during the last 2 weeks of prophylaxis to prevent relapses due to *P. vivax* or *P. ovale* in persons returning from prolonged exposure in areas where relapsing malaria is endemic.[10]

Primaquine has also been tried for prophylaxis of falciparum and vivax malaria; use for a year produced effective cover and was well tolerated by Javanese men without G6PD deficiency.[11] It was also effective for prophylaxis in Colombian military personnel; it was noted that primaquine prophylaxis could be stopped 1 week after departing the endemic area.[12]

1. WHO. *WHO model prescribing information: drugs used in parasitic diseases.* 2nd ed. Geneva: WHO, 1995.
2. Molyneux M, Fox R. Diagnosis and treatment of malaria in Britain. *BMJ* 1993; **306:** 1175–80.
3. Luzzi GA, *et al.* Treatment of primaquine-resistant Plasmodium vivax malaria. *Lancet* 1992; **340:** 310.
4. Bunnag D, *et al.* High dose of primaquine in primaquine resistant vivax malaria. *Trans R Soc Trop Med Hyg* 1994; **88:** 218–19.
5. Collins WE, Jeffrey GM. Primaquine resistance in Plasmodium vivax. *Am J Trop Med Hyg* 1996; **55:** 243–9.
6. Signorini L, *et al.* Short report: primaquine-tolerant Plasmodium vivax in an Italian traveler from Guatemala. *Am J Trop Med Hyg* 1996; **55:** 472–3.
7. Smoak BL, *et al.* Plasmodium vivax infections in US Army troops: failure of primaquine to prevent relapse in studies from Somalia. *Am J Trop Med Hyg* 1997; **56:** 231–4.
8. Doherty JF, *et al.* Treatment of Plasmodium vivax malaria—time for a change? *Trans R Soc Trop Med Hyg* 1997; **91:** 76.
9. Petralanda I. Quality of antimalarial drugs and resistance to Plasmodium vivax in Amazonian region. *Lancet* 1995; **345:** 1433.
10. Centers for Disease Control. Recommendations for the prevention of malaria among travelers. *MMWR* 1990; **39** (RR-3): 1–10.
11. Fryauff DJ, *et al.* Randomised placebo-controlled trial of primaquine for prophylaxis of falciparum and vivax malaria. *Lancet* 1995; **346:** 1190–3.
12. Soto J, *et al.* Primaquine prophylaxis against malaria in nonimmune Colombian soldiers: efficacy and toxicity. *Ann Intern Med* 1998; **129:** 241–4.

Pneumocystis carinii pneumonia. Primaquine with clindamycin is used in the treatment of *Pneumocystis carinii* pneumonia as an alternative to co-trimoxazole or pentamidine (see p.375). Treatment has usually lasted 3 weeks, with primaquine being given by mouth in daily doses equivalent to 30 mg of the base, and clindamycin usually being given intravenously in doses of 600 mg four times daily or 300 to 450 mg four times daily by mouth.[1]

A randomised multicentre study[2] compared the use of a combination of primaquine (30 mg daily) and clindamycin (600 mg three times daily) with co-trimoxazole and with a combination of dapsone and trimethoprim in 181 AIDS patients who had confirmed mild to moderate *Pneumocystis carinii* pneumonia. Primaquine-clindamycin was as effective as the other two regimens, although the authors suggested that the combination might be best avoided in patients with severe myelosuppression.

Primaquine with clindamycin is not normally recommended for prophylaxis although there are reports of it being tried.[3]

1. Anonymous. Drugs for parasitic infections. *Med Lett Drugs Ther* 1998; **40:** 1–12.

2. Safrin S, *et al.* Comparison of three regimens for treatment of mild to moderate Pneumocystis carinii pneumonia in patients with AIDS: a double-blind, randomized trial of oral trimethoprim-sulfamethoxazole, dapsone-trimethoprim, and clindamycin-primaquine. *Ann Intern Med* 1996; **124:** 792–802.
3. Kay R, DuBois RE. Clindamycin/primaquine therapy and secondary prophylaxis against Pneumocystis carinii pneumonia in patients with AIDS. *South Med J* 1990; **83:** 403–4.

Preparations
USP 25: Primaquine Phosphate Tablets.

Proprietary Preparations (details are given in Part 3)
Austral.: Primacin.

Proguanil Hydrochloride (1388-I)

Proguanil Hydrochloride (*BANM, rINNM*).

Bigumalum; Chloriguane Hydrochloride; Chloroguanide Hydrochloride; Proguanide Hydrochloride; Proguanili Hydrochloridum; RP-3359; SN-12,837. 1-(4-Chlorophenyl)-5-isopropylbiguanide hydrochloride.

$C_{11}H_{16}ClN_5,HCl = 290.2$.

CAS — 500-92-5 (proguanil); 637-32-1 (proguanil hydrochloride).

Pharmacopoeias. In *Br.* and *It.*

Pharmacopoeial description
BP 2001: A white, odourless or almost odourless, crystalline powder. Slightly soluble in water, more soluble in hot water; sparingly soluble in alcohol; practically insoluble in chloroform and in ether. Protect from light.

Stability. Although the BP 2001 directs that proguanil hydrochloride should be protected from light, stability studies[1,2] suggest that it is a very stable compound with only small amounts of its major decomposition product 4-chloroaniline being formed during thermal and photochemical stress.

1. Owoyale JA, Elmarakby ZS. Effect of sunlight, ultraviolet irradiation and heat on proguanil. *Int J Pharmaceutics* 1989; **50:** 219–21.
2. Taylor RB, *et al.* A chemical stability study of proguanil hydrochloride. *Int J Pharmaceutics* 1990; **60:** 185–90.

Adverse Effects and Precautions
Apart from mild gastric intolerance, diarrhoea, and some reports of aphthous ulceration there appear to be few adverse effects associated with usual doses of proguanil hydrochloride. Haematological changes have been reported in patients with severe renal impairment. Overdosage may produce epigastric discomfort, vomiting, and renal irritation leading to haematuria.

Proguanil should be used with caution in patients with renal impairment; dosage should be reduced accordingly (see under Uses and Administration, below).

Proguanil may be taken during pregnancy, but UK authorities recommend that folate supplements (folic acid 5 mg daily) should also be given.

◊ Until 1985 proguanil was generally taken in a dose of 100 mg daily for malaria prophylaxis with few adverse effects. Although no serious adverse effects have been reported since the dose was increased to 200 mg daily, and it began to be used with chloroquine, there have been an increasing number of reports of reversible aphthous ulceration.[1] Chloroquine may exacerbate this effect.[2] There has also been a report of reversible alopecia in women and scaling of the skin in both men and women using proguanil.[3]

Megaloblastic anaemia and pancytopenia were associated with proguanil accumulation in 2 patients with renal failure receiving usual doses.[4]

1. Peto TEA. Toxicity of antimalarial drugs. *J R Soc Med* 1989; **82** (suppl 17): 30–4.
2. Drysdale SF, *et al.* Proguanil, chloroquine, and mouth ulcers. *Lancet* 1990; **335:** 164.
3. Hanson SN, *et al.* Hairloss and scaling with proguanil. *Lancet* 1989; **1:** 225.
4. Boots M, *et al.* Megaloblastic anemia and pancytopenia due to proguanil in patients with chronic renal failure. *Clin Nephrol* 1982; **18:** 106–8.

Porphyria. For a discussion of the problems of the use of antimalarials in patients with porphyria and a comment that proguanil may be safe for use in such patients, see under Precautions for Chloroquine, p.434.

Interactions
Fluvoxamine. Fluvoxamine can virtually abolish[1] the metabolism of proguanil to its active metabolite cycloguanil via an inhibitory effect on the cytochrome P450 isoenzyme CYP2C19.

1. Jeppesen U, *et al.* The CYP2C19 catalyzed bioactivation of proguanil is abolished during fluvoxamine intake. *Eur J Clin Pharmacol* 1997; **52** (suppl): A134.

The symbol † denotes a preparation no longer actively marketed

Warfarin. For a report of haematuria and high prothrombin ratio in a patient stabilised on warfarin who took proguanil for malaria prophylaxis, see p.995.

Pharmacokinetics

Proguanil is readily absorbed from the gastrointestinal tract following administration by mouth, peak plasma concentrations occurring within about 4 hours. Proguanil is metabolised in the liver to the active metabolite cycloguanil. Peak plasma concentrations of cycloguanil occur approximately one hour after those of the parent drug. The elimination half-lives of both proguanil and cycloguanil are about 20 hours. Approximately 40 to 60% of proguanil is eliminated in the urine, of which 60% is unchanged and 30% cycloguanil. There is also some elimination via the faeces. Proguanil is distributed into breast milk in small amounts (which are not adequate to provide chemoprophylaxis for the infant).

◊ Early studies found proguanil to be well absorbed from the gastrointestinal tract with peak plasma concentrations occurring about 4 hours after administration.[1] In more recent studies, peak plasma concentrations of proguanil have been achieved within 2 to 4 hours.[2-4] Plasma protein binding for proguanil is stated to be 75%.[5] Proguanil is metabolised in the liver[3] to the active metabolite cycloguanil and to *p*-chlorophenylbiguanide which is inactive. Peak plasma concentrations of cycloguanil have been reported to occur about 5.3 hours after administration of proguanil.[4] Unlike proguanil and *p*-chlorophenylbiguanide, cycloguanil is not concentrated in erythrocytes and thus concentrations of cycloguanil in plasma and whole blood are similar.[4] The elimination half-lives for proguanil and cycloguanil are reported to be around 20 hours.[3,4] A review of early studies states that between 40 and 60% of a dose of proguanil was found to be excreted in the urine, 60% of this as the unchanged drug, 30% as cycloguanil, and 8% as *p*-chlorophenylbiguanide.[1] About 10% of a dose was excreted in the faeces.[1] However, these values can vary greatly and wide interindividual variations in the ability to metabolise proguanil to cycloguanil have been reported.[3,6,7] Malaria prophylaxis with proguanil might be less effective in poor metabolisers although this has not been proved conclusively[8] and, anyway, other factors such as lack of protection against mosquitoes and sensitivity of the malaria parasite might be more important.[9] Plasma concentrations of cycloguanil may be reduced in the third trimester of pregnancy.[10]

1. White NJ. Clinical pharmacokinetics of antimalarial drugs. *Clin Pharmacokinet* 1985; **10:** 187–215.
2. Kelly JA, *et al.* The kinetics of proguanil during prophylaxis. *Trans R Soc Trop Med Hyg* 1986; **80:** 338.
3. Watkins WM, *et al.* Variability in the metabolism of proguanil to the active metabolite cycloguanil in healthy Kenyan adults. *Trans R Soc Trop Med Hyg* 1990; **84:** 492–5.
4. Wattanagoon Y, *et al.* Single dose pharmacokinetics of proguanil and its metabolites in healthy subjects. *Br J Clin Pharmacol* 1987; **24:** 775–80.
5. Jaeger A, *et al.* Clinical features and management of poisoning due to antimalarial drugs. *Med Toxicol* 1987; **2:** 242–73.
6. Ward SA, *et al.* Inter-subject variability in the metabolism of proguanil to the active metabolite cycloguanil in man. *Br J Clin Pharmacol* 1989; **27:** 781–7.
7. Helsby NA, *et al.* The multiple dose pharmacokinetics of proguanil. *Br J Clin Pharmacol* 1993; **35:** 653–6.
8. Mberu EK, *et al.* Japanese poor metabolizers of proguanil do not have an increased risk of malaria chemoprophylaxis breakthrough. *Trans R Soc Trop Med Hyg* 1995; **89:** 658–9.
9. Skjelbo E, *et al.* Chloroguanide metabolism in relation to the efficacy in malaria prophylaxis and the S-mephenytoin oxidation in Tanzanians. *Clin Pharmacol Ther* 1996; **59:** 304–11.
10. Wangboonskul J, *et al.* Single dose pharmacokinetics of proguanil and its metabolites in pregnancy. *Eur J Clin Pharmacol* 1993; **44:** 247–51.

Uses and Administration

Proguanil is a biguanide compound which has little antimalarial activity until metabolised in the body to the active antimalarial drug cycloguanil. Cycloguanil, like pyrimethamine, inhibits plasmodial dihydrofolate reductase and thus disrupts synthesis of nucleic acids in the parasite. Cycloguanil is active against pre-erythrocytic forms and is a slow-acting blood schizontocide. It also has some sporontocidal activity, rendering the gametocytes non-infective to the mosquito vector.

The value of proguanil is limited by the rapid development of resistance.

Proguanil is used as the hydrochloride for the chemoprophylaxis of malaria, in association with chloroquine or with atovaquone. The schizontocidal activity of cycloguanil on erythrocytic forms is too slow for cycloguanil or proguanil to be used alone for the treatment of malaria, but proguanil hydrochloride is given in combination with atovaquone for the treatment of uncomplicated falciparum malaria.

For prophylaxis of malaria in combination with chloroquine the usual adult daily dose of proguanil hydrochloride is 200 mg taken after food. For prophylaxis in combination with atovaquone 250 mg, the daily dose of proguanil hydrochloride is 100 mg. It is generally recommended that chemoprophylaxis for travellers should start one week before exposure to malaria, but if this is not possible it can be started 1 to 2 days prior to travel. Administration should continue throughout exposure and for at least 4 weeks (1 week when proguanil is given with atovaquone) after leaving a malarious area. For children's prophylactic doses, see under Administration in Children, below.

For the treatment of uncomplicated falciparum malaria, adult doses are proguanil hydrochloride 400 mg together with atovaquone 1000 mg, each by mouth as a single dose for 3 consecutive days. Children weighing 11 to 20 kg are given one-quarter the adult dose; those weighing 21 to 30 kg, half the adult dose; those weighing 31 to 40 kg, three-quarters the adult dose; and children over 40 kg, the adult dose.

Cycloguanil was formerly administered as an oily suspension of the embonate by intramuscular injection.

Administration in children. Dosage recommendations for proguanil (in association with chloroquine) for *malaria prophylaxis* in children have varied. A daily dose of proguanil hydrochloride 3 mg per kg body-weight has been recommended,[1,2] although UK malaria experts[1] have suggested the following prophylactic doses for children based on fractions of the adult dose of 200 mg daily:

• under 6.0 kg body-weight (0 to 12 weeks of age): one-eighth the adult dose
• 6 to 9.9 kg (3 to 11 months): one-quarter the adult dose
• 10 to 15.9 kg (1 year to 3 years 11 months): three-eighths the adult dose
• 16 to 24.9 kg (4 years to 7 years 11 months): half the adult dose
• 25 to 44.9 kg (8 years to 12 years 11 months): three-quarters the adult dose
• 45 kg and over (13 years or more): the adult dose

They noted that body-weight was a better guide to dosage than age for children over 6 months.

For doses of proguanil in combination with atovaquone for the *treatment* of malaria in children, see above. Atovaquone-proguanil (Malarone) is not licensed in the UK for *prophylaxis* in persons under 40 kg body-weight.

1. Bradley DJ, Bannister B. Guidelines for malaria prevention in travellers from the United Kingdom for 2001. *Commun Dis Public Health* 2001; **4:** 84–101.
2. WHO. *International travel and health: vaccination requirements and health advice.* Geneva: WHO, 2001.

Administration in renal impairment. Proguanil is excreted by the kidneys and should be given in reduced dosage or avoided in patients with renal impairment. The following doses have been recommended based on creatinine clearance (CC):

• creatinine clearance 20 to 59 mL per minute, 100 mg daily
• 10 to 19 mL per minute, 50 mg every other day
• less than 10 mL per minute, up to 50 mg once weekly

Malaria. The overall treatment and prophylaxis of malaria and the place of proguanil in current recommendations are discussed on p.428.

TREATMENT. Proguanil alone is not suitable for the treatment of malaria. However, a combination of proguanil with atovaquone (Malarone) can be effective for the treatment of acute uncomplicated falciparum malaria,[1] including that produced by multidrug-resistant strains.[2] The combination has also been reported to be effective in benign malarias,[3] including *P. vivax* malaria in association with primaquine.[4]

PROPHYLAXIS. Proguanil has been used alone for the prophylaxis of malaria in very low risk areas of North Africa and the Middle East, but is more often given with chloroquine. However, the widespread prevalence of resistant strains of *Plasmodium falciparum* has considerably diminished the value of this regimen and has made recommendations for malaria prophylaxis increasingly complex. Studies using proguanil with a sulfonamide for chemoprophylaxis of malaria in Thailand produced encouraging results.[5,6] More recent studies have found proguanil in combination with atovaquone (Malarone) to be effective for prophylaxis in both adults[7] and children[8] living in endemic areas and in non-immune persons temporarily residing in endemic areas.[9]

1. Radloff PD, *et al.* Atovaquone and proguanil for Plasmodium falciparum malaria. *Lancet* 1996; **347:** 1511–14.
2. Sabchareon A, *et al.* Efficacy and pharmacokinetics of atovaquone and proguanil in children with multidrug-resistant Plasmodium falciparum malaria. *Trans R Soc Trop Med Hyg* 1998; **92:** 201–6.
3. Radloff PD, *et al.* Atovaquone plus proguanil is an effective treatment for Plasmodium ovale and P. malariae malaria. *Trans R Soc Trop Med Hyg* 1996; **90:** 682.

4. Looareesuwan S, *et al.* Atovaquone and proguanil hydrochloride followed by primaquine for treatment of Plasmodium vivax malaria in Thailand. *Trans R Soc Trop Med Hyg* 1999; **93:** 637–40.
5. Pang LW, *et al.* Malaria prophylaxis with proguanil and sulfisoxazole in children living in a malaria endemic area. *Bull WHO* 1989; **67:** 51–8.
6. Karwacki JJ, *et al.* Proguanil-sulphonamide for malaria prophylaxis. *Trans R Soc Trop Med Hyg* 1990; **84:** 55–7.
7. Shanks GD, *et al.* Efficacy and safety of atovaquone/proguanil as suppressive prophylaxis for Plasmodium falciparum malaria. *Clin Infect Dis* 1998; **27:** 494–9.
8. Lell B, *et al.* Randomised placebo-controlled study of atovaquone plus proguanil for malaria prophylaxis in children. *Lancet* 1998; **351:** 709–13.
9. Høgh B, *et al.* Atovaquone-proguanil versus chloroquine-proguanil for malaria prophylaxis in non-immune travellers: a randomised, double-blind study. *Lancet* 2000; **356:** 1888–94.

Preparations

BP 2001: Proguanil Tablets.

Proprietary Preparations (details are given in Part 3)
Aust.: Paludrine; Austral.: Paludrine; *Belg.:* Paludrine; *Canad.:* Paludrine; *Denm.:* Paludrine; *Fin.:* Paludrine; *Fr.:* Paludrine; *Ger.:* Paludrine; *Irl.:* Paludrine; *Israel:* Paludrin; *Ital.:* Paludrine; *Neth.:* Paludrine; *Norw.:* Paludrine; *NZ:* Paludrine; *Port.:* Paludrine; *S.Afr.:* Paludrine; *Singapore:* Paludrine; *Swed.:* Paludrine; *Switz.:* Paludrine; *UK:* Paludrine.

Multi-ingredient: *Aust.:* Malarone; *Austral.:* Malarone; *Belg.:* Malarone; *Canad.:* Malarone; *Denm.:* Malarone; *Fr.:* Malarone; Savarine; *Ger.:* Malarone; *S.Afr.:* Daramal-Paludrine; *Singapore:* Malarone; *Swed.:* Malarone; *Switz.:* Malarone; *UK:* Malarone; *USA:* Malarone.

Pyrimethamine (1389-y)

Pyrimethamine *(BAN, rINN)*.

BW-50-63; Pirimetamina; Pyrimethaminum; RP-4753. 5-(4-Chlorophenyl)-6-ethylpyrimidine-2,4-diyldiamine.
$C_{12}H_{13}ClN_4 = 248.7$.
CAS — 58-14-0.
ATC — P01BD01.

Pharmacopoeias. In Chin., Eur. (see p.vi), *Int.,* and *US.*

Pharmacopoeial description

Ph. Eur.: An almost white crystalline powder or colourless crystals. Practically insoluble in water; slightly soluble in alcohol; very slightly soluble in ether. Protect from light.

USP 25: A white, odourless, crystalline powder. Practically insoluble in water; soluble 1 in 200 of alcohol and 1 in 125 of chloroform; slightly soluble in acetone. Store in airtight containers. Protect from light.

Adverse Effects and Treatment

Administration of pyrimethamine for prolonged periods, as used to be the case when it was *given alone* for the prophylaxis of malaria, can cause depression of haematopoiesis due to interference with folic acid metabolism. Skin rashes and hypersensitivity reactions also occurred.

Larger doses, such as those used in the treatment of toxoplasmosis, may cause gastrointestinal symptoms such as atrophic glossitis, abdominal pain, and vomiting; haematological effects such as megaloblastic anaemia, leucopenia, thrombocytopenia, and pancytopenia are also more likely to occur. CNS effects including headache, dizziness, and insomnia have also been reported.

Pulmonary eosinophilia has been reported in patients receiving pyrimethamine *in combination with other antimalarials.* Severe and sometimes fatal reactions have occurred when pyrimethamine has been used with *sulfadoxine* (Fansidar), including erythema multiforme and the Stevens-Johnson syndrome, and toxic epidermal necrolysis; there have also been isolated reports of hepatic toxicity. Agranulocytosis occurs more frequently when pyrimethamine is used with *dapsone* (Maloprim) and fatalities have been reported.

Acute overdosage with pyrimethamine can cause gastrointestinal effects and CNS stimulation with vomiting, excitability, and convulsions. Tachycardia, respiratory depression, circulatory collapse, and death may follow. Treatment of overdosage is symptomatic.

Adverse effects with dapsone. Between 1972 and 1988 the UK Committee on Safety of Medicines received 76 reports of reactions that were attributed to the use of pyrimethamine with dapsone (Maloprim) of which 40 (53%) were considered to be serious including 6 deaths.[1] The incidence was estimated to be 1 in 9100 for serious reactions and 1 in 60 200 for fatalities. Serious blood disorders including agranulocytosis, granulocytopenia, or leucopenia occurred in 15 patients (estimated incidence of 1 in 20 000), five of whom died. The other death was in a patient with myocarditis. Three patients had cyanosis due to methaemoglobinaemia. Respiratory disorders such as pulmonary eosinophilia, influenza-like syndrome, and dyspnoea occurred in 6 patients. In 4 patients skin disorders were the principal effect and included epidermal necrolysis, angioedema, and bullous eruptions. Hepatic disorders were also reported in 4 patients. Three women using pyrimethamine-dapsone during pregnancy delivered malformed babies, one of them being stillborn. Other effects in 4 patients included convulsions, exacerbated epilepsy, pancreatitis, or a generalised allergic reaction.

A review[2] of 21 cases of agranulocytosis associated with pyrimethamine-dapsone concluded that, although agranulocytosis can occur very rarely in patients taking pyrimethamine or dapsone alone, agranulocytosis due to the combination appears to be caused by an idiosyncratic reaction to dapsone exacerbated by the concurrent administration of pyrimethamine. Of the 18 individuals for whom dosage was certain, 12 had been taking one tablet of pyrimethamine-dapsone twice weekly. The recommended dose is one tablet taken once weekly. Of the 9 patients who died, 6 had been taking one tablet twice weekly and one patient had taken one tablet once weekly; the dosage was uncertain in the remaining patients. The time of onset of symptoms had been 7 to 9 weeks after starting therapy in 16 of 19 of the patients.

Some consider that pyrimethamine with dapsone may produce some degree of immunosuppression and render users more susceptible to common infections. A higher incidence of non-specific upper respiratory-tract infections occurred in military recruits receiving the combination than in those not receiving antimalarial prophylaxis.[3]

Pulmonary eosinophilia has also occurred in patients taking pyrimethamine with dapsone, but, as there have also been similar reports of pulmonary toxicity in patients taking pyrimethamine with sulfadoxine (see below) or pyrimethamine with chloroquine, it has been suggested that pyrimethamine is probably the causative agent.[4]

1. Phillips-Howard PA, West LJ. Serious adverse drug reactions to pyrimethamine–sulphadoxine, pyrimethamine–dapsone and to amodiaquine in Britain. *J R Soc Med* 1990; **83:** 82–5.
2. Hutchinson DBA, *et al.* Agranulocytosis with Maloprim: review of cases. *Hum Toxicol* 1986; **5:** 221–7.
3. Lee PS, Lau EYL. Risk of acute non-specific upper respiratory tract infections in healthy men taking dapsone–pyrimethamine for prophylaxis against malaria. *BMJ* 1988; **296:** 893–5.
4. Davidson AC, *et al.* Pulmonary toxicity of malaria prophylaxis. *BMJ* 1988; **297:** 1240–1.

Adverse effects with sulfonamides. Severe and potentially fatal cutaneous reactions such as erythema multiforme and the Stevens-Johnson syndrome, and toxic epidermal necrolysis have been associated with the combined use of pyrimethamine with sulfadoxine (Fansidar) for malaria prophylaxis. The reported incidence of these reactions has varied with surveys in the UK,[1] USA,[2] and Sweden[3] yielding similar results and a survey from Switzerland[4] finding a much lower incidence. The overall rate of serious reactions to pyrimethamine–sulfadoxine in the UK has been estimated to be 1 in 2100. The estimates for severe cutaneous reactions were 1 in 4900 in the UK, 1 in 5000 to 1 in 8000 in the USA, 1 in 10 000 in Sweden, and 1 in 150 000 in Switzerland and the death rates were 1 in 11 100 in the UK, 1 in 11 000 to 1 in 25 000 in the USA, and 1 in 35 000 in Sweden; no fatalities were reported in Switzerland. Workers on the Swiss survey[4] had suggested that the high incidence of cutaneous reactions reported in the USA might have been due to concurrent therapy with chloroquine but this has been disputed.[5] The authors of the UK survey[1] suggested that the lower incidence reported in Switzerland may have been due to the different methods used to estimate the amount of drug usage. Whether this toxicity is due to the combined use of pyrimethamine and sulfadoxine is unclear as the estimated frequency of fatal reactions associated with the use of sulfadoxine alone in Mozambique[6] was 1 in 50 000.

There have been isolated reports of other severe or life-threatening reactions associated with the use of pyrimethamine-sulfadoxine when used alone or with chloroquine, including hepatotoxicity[7-9] (estimated incidence of 1 in 11 100 in the UK[1]), fatal multisystem toxicity,[10] drug fever and photodermatitis,[11] agranulocytosis,[11] and erythroderma resembling Sézary syndrome.[12] Severe pulmonary reactions have also occurred[3,13] but as similar reactions have also been reported when pyrimethamine has been used with other antimalarials including dapsone it has been suggested that pyrimethamine is the causative agent (see Adverse Effects with Dapsone, above). Hyperammonaemia and carnitine deficiency with deterioration in mental status has been reported in a patient receiving pyrimethamine and sulfadiazine for the treatment of toxoplasmosis.[14]

Severe megaloblastic anaemia in a patient receiving pyrimethamine and sulfadiazine for toxoplasmosis of the CNS[15] was treated by withdrawal of pyrimethamine and oral administration of folinic acid, together with a single platelet infusion.

For a comparison of the incidence of pruritus induced by various antimalarials including pyrimethamine with sulfadoxine, see Effects on the Skin under Chloroquine, p.433.

1. Phillips-Howard PA, West LJ. Serious adverse drug reactions to pyrimethamine–sulphadoxine, pyrimethamine–dapsone and to amodiaquine in Britain. *J R Soc Med* 1990; **83:** 82–5.
2. Miller KD, *et al.* Severe cutaneous reactions among American travelers using pyrimethamine–sulfadoxine (Fansidar®) for malaria prophylaxis. *Am J Trop Med Hyg* 1986; **35:** 451–8.

3. Hellgren U, *et al.* Adverse reactions to sulphadoxine–pyrimethamine in Swedish travellers: implications for prophylaxis. *BMJ* 1987; **295:** 365–6.
4. Steffen R, Somaini B. Severe cutaneous adverse reactions to sulfadoxine–pyrimethamine in Switzerland. *Lancet* 1986; **i:** 610.
5. Rombo L, *et al.* Does chloroquine contribute to the risk of serious adverse reactions to Fansidar? *Lancet* 1985; **ii:** 1298–9.
6. Hernborg A. Stevens-Johnson syndrome after mass prophylaxis with sulfadoxine for cholera in Mozambique. *Lancet* 1985; **ii:** 1072–3.
7. Lazar HP, *et al.* Fansidar and hepatic granulomas. *Ann Intern Med* 1985; **102:** 722.
8. Wejstal R, *et al.* Liver damage associated with Fansidar. *Lancet* 1986; **i:** 854–5.
9. Zitelli BJ, *et al.* Fatal hepatic necrosis due to pyrimethamine–sulfadoxine (Fansidar). *Ann Intern Med* 1987; **106:** 393–5.
10. Selby CD, *et al.* Fatal multisystemic toxicity associated with prophylaxis with pyrimethamine and sulfadoxine (Fansidar). *BMJ* 1989; **290:** 113–14.
11. Olsen VV, *et al.* Serious reactions during malaria prophylaxis with pyrimethamine–sulfadoxine. *Lancet* 1982; **ii:** 994.
12. Langtry JAA, *et al.* Erythroderma resembling Sézary syndrome after treatment with Fansidar and chloroquine. *BMJ* 1986; **292:** 1107–8.
13. Svanbom M, *et al.* Unusual pulmonary reaction during short term prophylaxis with pyrimethamine–sulfadoxine (Fansidar). *BMJ* 1984; **288:** 1876.
14. Sekas G, Harbhajan PS. Hyperammonemia and carnitine deficiency in a patient receiving sulfadiazine and pyrimethamine. *Am J Med* 1993; **95:** 112–13.
15. Chute JP, *et al.* Severe megaloblastic anemia complicating pyrimethamine therapy. *Ann Intern Med* 1995; **122:** 884–5.

Overdosage. Reports of overdosage with pyrimethamine in infants.

1. Akinyanju O, *et al.* Pyrimethamine poisoning. *BMJ* 1973; **4:** 147–8.
2. Elmalem J, *et al.* Les accidents graves lors de la prescription de pyriméthamine chez les nourrissons traités pour une toxoplasmose. *Therapie* 1985; **40:** 357–9.

Precautions

Pyrimethamine may aggravate subclinical folic acid deficiency and it should not be given to patients with conditions associated with folate deficiency such as megaloblastic anaemia. Blood counts are required with prolonged treatment, and when large doses of pyrimethamine are used, as in the treatment of toxoplasmosis, blood counts should be checked twice weekly. Folinic acid, which does not interfere with the action of pyrimethamine against malaria or toxoplasmosis, has been given to prevent haematological toxicity due to pyrimethamine and its use is especially recommended if pyrimethamine is given during pregnancy (folic acid may be used as an alternative to folinic acid in malaria, but it interferes with the action of pyrimethamine against toxoplasmosis). Even if given with a folate supplement, some authorities consider pyrimethamine to be contra-indicated at least during the first trimester of pregnancy (see also under Pregnancy, below).

Pyrimethamine should be given with caution to patients with renal or hepatic impairment. When patients with convulsive disorders need to receive large doses, as in the treatment of toxoplasmosis, it is recommended that small starting doses should be used.

When pyrimethamine is administered with sulfonamides or dapsone the general precautions applicable to those drugs should also be observed (see under Sulfamethoxazole, p.254 and under Dapsone, p.197) and treatment should be discontinued immediately if any skin reactions, sore throat, or shortness of breath occurs.

Breast feeding. Pyrimethamine is distributed into breast milk[1] but as no adverse effects have been reported in breast-fed infants, some experts consider breast feeding to be compatible with the use of pyrimethamine for malaria prophylaxis.[2,3] However, administration of other folate antagonists to the infant should be avoided. The large doses of pyrimethamine used for treating toxoplasmosis may distribute into breast milk in sufficient quantities to interfere with folic acid metabolism in nursing infants.

1. Edstein MD, *et al.* Excretion of chloroquine, dapsone and pyrimethamine in human milk. *Br J Clin Pharmacol* 1986; **22:** 733–5.
2. Bennett PN, ed. *Drugs and human lactation.* Amsterdam: Elsevier, 1988.
3. American Academy of Pediatrics, Committee on Drugs. The transfer of drugs and other chemicals into human milk. *Pediatrics* 2001; **108:** 776–89.

Porphyria. For a discussion of the problems of the use of antimalarials in patients with porphyria and a comment that pyrimethamine is probably safe for use in such patients, see under Precautions for Chloroquine, p.434.

Pregnancy. There have been concerns over the use of pyrimethamine during pregnancy as it has been shown to be teratogenic in *animal* studies.[1] In one report severe congenital de-

fects in a stillborn infant were attributed to the use of pyrimethamine in early pregnancy[2] but the association was considered to be questionable.[3] Other instances of congenital malformations with pyrimethamine and dapsone are given under Adverse Effects with Dapsone, above.

WHO considers that pyrimethamine combinations may be used after the first trimester of pregnancy in the treatment of toxoplasmosis,[4] and that pyrimethamine-sulfadoxine may be used for intermittent treatment in high-risk malaria-endemic regions.[5] UK experts[6] consider that pyrimethamine with dapsone (Maloprim) can be used cautiously for malaria prophylaxis after the first trimester if a visit to an area of transmission is unavoidable; a folate supplement (folic acid 5 mg daily) should be given.

1. Anonymous. Pyrimethamine combinations in pregnancy. *Lancet* 1983; **ii:** 1005–7. Correction. *ibid.*; 1378.
2. Harpey J-P, *et al.* Teratogenicity of pyrimethamine. *Lancet* 1983; **ii:** 399.
3. Smithells RW, Sheppard S. Teratogenicity of Debendox and pyrimethamine. *Lancet* 1983; **ii:** 623–4.
4. WHO. *WHO model prescribing information: drugs used in parasitic diseases.* 2nd ed. Geneva: WHO, 1995.
5. WHO. WHO expert committee on malaria: twentieth report. *WHO Tech Rep Ser* 892 2000.
6. Bradley DJ, Bannister B. Guidelines for malaria prevention in travellers from the United Kingdom for 2001. *Commun Dis Public Health* 2001; **4:** 84–101.

Interactions

Administration of pyrimethamine with other folate antagonists such as co-trimoxazole, trimethoprim, methotrexate, or phenytoin may exacerbate bone marrow depression.

Lorazepam. Signs of mild liver toxicity in 2 of 5 subjects who received lorazepam and pyrimethamine appeared to confirm earlier suspicions that concomitant administration of these drugs could cause hepatotoxicity. Both patients tolerated each drug when given separately.[1]

1. Briggs M, Briggs M. Pyrimethamine toxicity. *BMJ* 1974; **1:** 40.

Zidovudine. Studies *in vitro* and in *animals* suggest that zidovudine could reduce the effectiveness of pyrimethamine in the treatment of toxoplasmic encephalitis.[1] Furthermore, the dose of zidovudine may need to be altered if these drugs are used together as there has been a report that pyrimethamine with sulfadoxine (Fansidar) prolonged the serum half-life of zidovudine.[2]

1. Israelski DM, *et al.* Zidovudine antagonizes the action of pyrimethamine in experimental infection with Toxoplasma gondii. *Antimicrob Agents Chemother* 1989; **33:** 30–4.
2. Klein RS. Prophylaxis of opportunistic infections in individuals infected with HIV. *AIDS* 1989; **3** (suppl 1): S161–S173.

Pharmacokinetics

Pyrimethamine is almost completely absorbed from the gastrointestinal tract and peak plasma concentrations of about 200 nanograms per mL are obtained 2 to 6 hours after oral administration of 25 mg by mouth. It is mainly concentrated in the kidneys, lungs, liver, and spleen and about 80 to 90% is bound to plasma proteins.

It is metabolised in the liver and slowly excreted via the kidney, the average half-life in plasma being about 4 days. Several metabolites have been detected in the urine. Pyrimethamine crosses the placenta. It is distributed into breast milk (see under Breast Feeding in Precautions, above).

◊ References.

1. White NJ. Clinical pharmacokinetics of antimalarial drugs. *Clin Pharmacokinet* 1985; **10:** 187–215.
2. Cook IF, *et al.* Race-linked differences in serum concentrations of dapsone, monoacetyldapsone and pyrimethamine during malaria prophylaxis. *Trans R Soc Trop Med Hyg* 1986; **80:** 897–901.
3. Weiss LM, *et al.* Pyrimethamine concentrations in serum and cerebrospinal fluid during treatment of acute toxoplasma encephalitis in patients with AIDS. *J Infect Dis* 1988; **157:** 580–3.
4. Edstein MD, *et al.* Multiple-dose pharmacokinetics and in vitro antimalarial activity of dapsone plus pyrimethamine (Maloprim®) in man. *Br J Clin Pharmacol* 1990; **30:** 259–65.
5. Hellgren U, *et al.* Plasma concentrations of sulfadoxine-pyrimethamine, mefloquine and its main metabolite after regular malaria prophylaxis for two years. *Trans R Soc Trop Med Hyg* 1991; **85:** 356–7.
6. Winstanley PA, *et al.* The disposition of oral and intramuscular pyrimethamine/sulphadoxine in Kenyan children with high parasitaemia but clinically non-severe falciparum malaria. *Br J Clin Pharmacol* 1992; **33:** 143–8.
7. Newton CRJC, *et al.* A single dose of intramuscular sulfadoxine-pyrimethamine as an adjunct to quinine in the treatment of severe malaria: pharmacokinetics and efficacy. *Trans R Soc Trop Med Hyg* 1993; **87:** 207–10.
8. Jacobson JM, *et al.* Pyrimethamine pharmacokinetics in human immunodeficiency virus-positive patients seropositive for Toxoplasma gondii. *Antimicrob Agents Chemother* 1996; **40:** 1360–5.
9. Klinker H, *et al.* Plasma pyrimethamine concentrations during long-term treatment for cerebral toxoplasmosis in patients with AIDS. *Antimicrob Agents Chemother* 1996; **40:** 1623–7.
10. Trenque T, *et al.* Human maternofoetal distribution of pyrimethamine-sulphadoxine. *Br J Clin Pharmacol* 1998; **45:** 179–80.

The symbol † denotes a preparation no longer actively marketed

Uses and Administration

Pyrimethamine is a diaminopyrimidine antimalarial used in the treatment and prophylaxis of malaria, in combination with a sulfonamide or dapsone. It is also used with a sulfonamide in the treatment of toxoplasmosis. Pyrimethamine with sulfadoxine has been tried in the treatment of actinomycetoma and for prophylaxis of *Pneumocystis carinii* pneumonia. Pyrimethamine alone or with sulfadoxine has also been tried in the treatment of isosporiasis.

Pyrimethamine exerts its antimalarial activity by inhibiting plasmodial dihydrofolate reductase thus indirectly blocking the synthesis of nucleic acids in the malaria parasite. It is active against pre-erythrocytic forms and is also a slow-acting blood schizontocide. It also has some sporontocidal activity; it does not prevent the formation of gametocytes but renders them non-infective to the mosquito vector. It is mainly effective against *Plasmodium falciparum* but has some activity against *P. vivax*.

The development of plasmodial resistance has rendered obsolete the use of pyrimethamine on its own in malaria. Combinations of pyrimethamine with long-acting sulfonamides, such as sulfadoxine or sulfametopyrazine, or with dapsone are now used, although resistance has also developed to them.

For *treatment of chloroquine-resistant or multidrug-resistant falciparum malaria*, pyrimethamine is usually given in combination with a long-acting sulfonamide, often following a course of quinine. Pyrimethamine in combination with sulfadoxine in a fixed dose ratio of 1 to 20 (Fansidar) is usually given by mouth. A single dose of pyrimethamine 75 mg with sulfadoxine 1.5 g is usually recommended. The dose should not be repeated for at least 7 days. The combination of pyrimethamine with sulfadoxine may also be administered intramuscularly. Suggested oral doses for children are: 5 to 10 kg body-weight, 12.5 mg pyrimethamine and 250 mg sulfadoxine; 11 to 20 kg, 25 mg pyrimethamine and 500 mg sulfadoxine; 21 to 30 kg, 37.5 mg pyrimethamine and 750 mg sulfadoxine; 31 to 45 kg, 50 mg pyrimethamine and 1 g sulfadoxine. A combination of pyrimethamine with sulfametopyrazine is used similarly.

The combination of pyrimethamine with a sulfonamide, again usually sulfadoxine, may also be used in specified areas as *standby treatment* for malaria. For this purpose doses are similar to those given for standard treatment as described above.

For *prophylaxis of malaria*, a combined preparation of pyrimethamine and dapsone in a fixed ratio of 1 to 8 (Maloprim) is still occasionally used in areas of chloroquine or multidrug resistance, although mefloquine is now generally preferred. The usual dose for adults is pyrimethamine 12.5 mg and dapsone 100 mg as a single weekly dose. Suggested doses for children are: 6 to 15.9 kg (3 months to 3 years 11 months), one-quarter the adult dose; 16 to 24.9 kg (4 years to 7 years 11 months), half the adult dose; 25 to 44.9 kg (8 years to 12 years 11 months), three-quarters the adult dose; 45 kg and over (13 years or more), adult dose. It is generally recommended that prophylaxis for travellers should start about one week before exposure to malaria and should continue throughout exposure and for at least 4 weeks after leaving a malarious area.

Pyrimethamine administered with a sulfonamide such as sulfadiazine is used in the *treatment of toxoplasmosis*. Alternatively, pyrimethamine may be given with clindamycin in AIDS patients with toxoplasmosis unable to tolerate a sulfonamide. For details of dosage regimens used, see below.

Isosporiasis. Isosporiasis (p.584) usually responds well to treatment with co-trimoxazole, but there is a high incidence of recurrence in immunocompromised patients, such as those with AIDS, and some form of maintenance therapy is generally required. Co-trimoxazole 960 mg given three times weekly or pyrimethamine 25 mg with sulfadoxine 500 mg given weekly were found to be equally effective maintenance regimens.[1] Pyrimethamine given alone in daily doses of 50 to 75 mg with

folate therapy may be of use in the treatment of patients sensitive to sulfonamides.[2]

1. Pape JW, *et al.* Treatment and prophylaxis of Isospora belli infection in patients with the acquired immunodeficiency syndrome. *N Engl J Med* 1989; **320:** 1044–7.
2. Weiss LM, *et al.* Isospora belli infection: treatment with pyrimethamine. *Ann Intern Med* 1988; **109:** 474–5.

Malaria. The overall treatment and prophylaxis of malaria and the place of pyrimethamine-sulfadoxine (Fansidar) and pyrimethamine-dapsone (Maloprim) in current recommendations are discussed on p.428.

TREATMENT. Resistance to combinations of pyrimethamine with sulfadoxine or sulfametopyrazine is now widespread, particularly in South-East Asia and South America and more recently in East and Central Africa; however, pyrimethamine-sulfadoxine still has a role in practice in the treatment of falciparum malaria in endemic areas.[1,2] It may be given in the treatment of falciparum malaria following a course of quinine, if quinine resistance is known or suspected. A formulation of pyrimethamine with sulfadoxine for intramuscular administration has been studied[3-6] but its role in the treatment of falciparum malaria is not clear. WHO considers that a combination of mefloquine with pyrimethamine and sulfadoxine offers no therapeutic advantage over mefloquine alone and does not recommend this combination for treatment or for prophylaxis. The efficacy and safety of a combination of artesunate and pyrimethamine-sulfadoxine is under investigation[1]

PROPHYLAXIS. Owing to the development of resistance pyrimethamine is not effective on its own for prophylaxis.[7] Although resistance has developed to pyrimethamine with dapsone,[8] and the combination has been largely superseded by mefloquine, it remains useful for prophylaxis in some areas where other drugs are ineffective.[9] Chloroquine may be given in addition. The risk of toxicity with pyrimethamine in combination with a sulfonamide is considered too high for prophylactic use[9] but it may still be used in specified areas for standby treatment.[10]

1. WHO. WHO expert committee on malaria: twentieth report. *WHO Tech Rep Ser* 892 2000.
2. WHO. *Management of severe malaria: a practical handbook.* Geneva: WHO, 2000.
3. Harinasuta T, *et al.* Parenteral Fansidar® in falciparum malaria. *Trans R Soc Trop Med Hyg* 1988; **82:** 694.
4. Salako LA, *et al.* Parenteral sulphadoxine–pyrimethamine (Fansidar®): an effective and safe but under used method of antimalarial treatment. *Trans R Soc Trop Med Hyg* 1990; **84:** 641–3.
5. Simão F, *et al.* Comparison of intramuscular sulfadoxine-pyrimethamine and intramuscular quinine for the treatment of falciparum malaria in children. *Trans R Soc Trop Med Hyg* 1991; **85:** 341–4.
6. Newton CRJC, *et al.* A single dose of intramuscular sulfadoxine-pyrimethamine as an adjunct to quinine in the treatment of severe malaria: pharmacokinetics and efficacy. *Trans R Soc Trop Med Hyg* 1993; **87:** 207–10.
7. Nahlen BL, *et al.* Lack of efficacy of pyrimethamine prophylaxis in pregnant Nigerian women. *Lancet* 1989; **ii:** 830–4.
8. Cook IF. Inadequate prophylaxis of malaria with dapsone-pyrimethamine. *Med J Aust* 1985 **142:** 340–2.
9. Bradley DJ, Bannister B. Guidelines for malaria prevention in travellers from the United Kingdom for 2001. *Commun Dis Public Health* 2001; **4:** 84–101.
10. WHO. *International travel and health: vaccination requirements and health advice.* Geneva: WHO, 2001.

Mycetoma. For reference to the use of pyrimethamine as part of the treatment of actinomycetoma, see under Mycetoma, p.130.

Pneumocystis carinii pneumonia. For a mention of pyrimethamine in combination with dapsone or sulfadoxine for the prophylaxis of *Pneumocystis carinii* pneumonia, and a discussion of conventional prophylaxis and treatment, see p.375.

Toxoplasmosis. Pyrimethamine is given, usually in conjunction with sulfadiazine, in the treatment of toxoplasmosis (p.585). Folinic acid is also given to counteract the megaloblastic anaemia associated with these drugs. A suggested dosage regimen is pyrimethamine 50 to 200 mg daily with sulfadiazine 250 to 1000 mg every 6 hours for one or two days, then pyrimethamine 25 to 50 mg daily with sulfadiazine 125 to 500 mg every 6 hours for 2 to 4 weeks, or 4 to 6 weeks if the patient is immunocompromised. A suggested dose of pyrimethamine for children is 1 mg per kg body-weight daily for 1 to 3 days, then 0.5 mg per kg daily for 4 to 6 weeks, given with usual paediatric doses of sulfadiazine. Treatment may continue for 6 months to 1 year in infants with congenital toxoplasmosis.

Patients with AIDS may be given a loading dose of 100 to 200 mg pyrimethamine daily with sulfadiazine 500 to 1500 mg every 6 hours for one or two days, and then 50 to 100 mg pyrimethamine daily with the same dose of sulfadiazine for 3 to 6 weeks. Maintenance treatment for AIDS patients with pyrimethamine 25 to 50 mg daily and sulfadiazine 250 to 1000 mg every 6 hours may continue indefinitely. Pyrimethamine with clindamycin is an alternative in patients unable to tolerate a sulfonamide.

Other drugs tried in combination with pyrimethamine with promising results include azithromycin,[1] clarithromycin,[2] and doxycycline.[3,4]

Alternative regimens tried for long-term maintenance therapy in patients with AIDS include pyrimethamine plus sulfadiazine given twice weekly[5,6] or pyrimethamine alone in doses of 25 mg[7] or 50 mg[8] daily or 50 mg three times weekly.[9] However, results from a study involving 396 patients suggested that

the mortality rate was higher in those receiving pyrimethamine 25 mg three times weekly for primary prophylaxis than in those receiving placebo.[10] Pyrimethamine with dapsone given once a week can provide effective prophylaxis but was not well tolerated.[11] Pyrimethamine with sulfadoxine, also given once weekly, has produced promising results in bone-marrow transplant recipients.[12]

1. Saba J, *et al.* Pyrimethamine plus azithromycin for treatment of acute toxoplasmic encephalitis in patients with AIDS. *Eur J Clin Microbiol Infect Dis* 1993; **12:** 853–6.
2. Fernandez-Martin J, *et al.* Pyrimethamine-clarithromycin combination therapy of acute Toxoplasma encephalitis in patients with AIDS. *Antimicrob Agents Chemother* 1991; **35:** 2049–52.
3. Morris JT, Kelly JW. Effective treatment of cerebral toxoplasmosis with doxycycline. *Am J Med* 1992; **93:** 107–8.
4. Hagberg L, *et al.* Doxycycline and pyrimethamine for toxoplasmic encephalitis. *Scand J Infect Dis* 1993; **25:** 157–60.
5. Pedrol E, *et al.* Central nervous system toxoplasmosis in AIDS patients: efficacy of an intermittent maintenance therapy. *AIDS* 1990; **4:** 511–17.
6. Podzanczer D, *et al.* Twice-weekly maintenance therapy with sulfadiazine-pyrimethamine to prevent recurrent toxoplasmic encephalitis in patients with AIDS. *Ann Intern Med* 1995; **123:** 175–80.
7. Murphy K, *et al.* Pyrimethamine alone as long-term suppressive therapy in cerebral toxoplasmosis. *Am J Med* 1994; **96:** 95–6.
8. de Gans J, *et al.* Pyrimethamine alone as maintenance therapy for central nervous system toxoplasmosis in 38 patients with AIDS. *J Acquir Immune Defic Syndr Hum Retrovirol* 1992; **5:** 137–42.
9. Leport C, *et al.* Pyrimethamine for primary prophylaxis of toxoplasmic encephalitis in patients with human immunodeficiency virus infection: a double-blind, randomized trial. *J Infect Dis* 1996; **173:** 91–7.
10. Jacobson MA. *et al.* Primary prophylaxis with pyrimethamine for toxoplasmic encephalitis in patients with advanced human immunodeficiency virus disease: results of a randomized trial. *J Infect Dis* 1994; **169:** 384–94.
11. Opravil M, *et al.* Once-weekly administration of dapsone/pyrimethamine vs. aerosolized pentamidine as combined prophylaxis for Pneumocystis carinii pneumonia and toxoplasmic encephalitis in human immunodeficiency virus-infected patients. *Clin Infect Dis* 1995; **20:** 531–41.
12. Foot ABM, *et al.* Prophylaxis of toxoplasmosis infection with pyrimethamine/sulfadoxine (Fansidar) in bone marrow transplant recipients. *Bone Marrow Transplant* 1994; **14:** 241–5.

Preparations

BP 2001: Pyrimethamine Tablets;
USP 25: Pyrimethamine Tablets; Sulfadoxine and Pyrimethamine Tablets.

Proprietary Preparations (details are given in Part 3)
Aust.: Daraprim; **Austral.:** Daraprim; **Belg.:** Daraprim; **Braz.:** Daraprim; **Canad.:** Daraprim; **Fr.:** Malocide; **Ger.:** Daraprim; **Irl.:** Daraprim; **Israel:** Daraprim; **Mex.:** Daraprim; **Neth.:** Daraprim; **S.Afr.:** Daraprim; **Spain:** Daraprim; **Swed.:** Daraprim†; **Switz.:** Daraprim; **Thai.:** Daraprim; **UK:** Daraprim; **USA:** Daraprim.

Multi-ingredient: Aust.: Fansidar†; **Austral.:** Fansidar; Maloprim†; **Belg.:** Fansidar†; **Braz.:** Clopirim; Fansidar; Periodine Anti-Malarico; **Canad.:** Fansidar; **Denm.:** Fansidar; **Fr.:** Fansidar; **Irl.:** Fansidar; Maloprim; **Israel:** Fansidar; **Ital.:** Metakelfin; **Neth.:** Fansidar†; **S.Afr.:** Daraclor†; Fansidar; Maloprim; **Singapore:** Madomine; **Swed.:** Fansidar†; **Switz.:** Fansidar; Fansimef; **Thai.:** Vivaxine; **UK:** Fansidar; Maloprim; **USA:** Fansidar.

Pyronaridine Phosphate (329-c)

Malaridine Phosphate. 7-Chloro-2-methoxy-10-[3,5-bis(pyrrolidinomethyl)-4-hydroxyanilino]benzo-[*b*]-1,5-naphthyridine phosphate.

$C_{29}H_{32}ClN_5O_2,4H_3PO_4 = 910.0$.
CAS — 74847-35-1 (pyronaridine); 76748-86-2 (pyronaridine phosphate).
Pharmacopoeias. In Chin.

Profile

Pyronaridine is a naphthyridine derivative used in China in the treatment of vivax malaria and chloroquine-resistant falciparum malaria. Its use in Africa and Thailand is also under investigation. Pyronaridine has been given as the phosphate by mouth or by intramuscular or intravenous injection.

◊ References.

1. Shao B-R. A review of antimalarial drug pyronaridine. *Chin Med J* 1990; **103:** 428–34.
2. Shao B-R, *et al.* A 5-year surveillance of sensitivity in vivo of Plasmodium falciparum to pyronaridine/sulfadoxine/pyrimethamine in Diaolou area, Hainan province. *Southeast Asian J Trop Med Public Health* 1991; **22:** 65–7.
3. Chen C, *et al.* Studies on a new antimalarial compound: pyronaridine. *Trans R Soc Trop Med Hyg* 1992; **86:** 7–10.
4. Winstanley P. Pyronaridine: a promising drug for Africa? *Lancet* 1996; **347:** 2–3.
5. Ringwald P, *et al.* Randomised trial of pyronaridine versus chloroquine for acute uncomplicated falciparum malaria in Africa. *Lancet* 1996; **347:** 24–8.
6. Looareesuwan S, *et al.* Pyronaridine. *Lancet* 1996; **347:** 1189–90.
7. Anonymous. Pyronaridine: yet another promising antimalarial substance from China. *WHO Drug Inf* 1996; **10:** 9–10.
8. Looareesuwan S, *et al.* Clinical study of pyronaridine for the treatment of acute uncomplicated falciparum malaria in Thailand. *Am J Trop Med Hyg* 1996; **54:** 205–9.
9. Ringwald P, *et al.* Efficacy of oral pyronaridine for the treatment of acute uncomplicated falciparum malaria in African children. *Clin Infect Dis* 1998; **26:** 946–53.

Quinine   (1398-j)

Quinine *(BAN)*.

Chinina; Chininum; Quinina. (8S,9R)-6′-Methoxycinchonan-9-ol; (αR)-α-(6-Methoxy-4-quinolyl)-α-[(2S,4S,5R)-(5-vinylquinuclidin-2-yl)]methanol.

$C_{20}H_{24}N_2O_2 = 324.4$.

CAS — 130-95-0 *(anhydrous quinine)*.

ATC — P01BC01.

Pharmacopoeias. It. specifies the trihydrate.

The chief alkaloid of various species of *Cinchona* (Rubiaceae). It is an optical isomer of quinidine. **Protect** from light.

Quinine Bisulfate   (1391-q)

Chininum Bisulfuricum; Neutral Quinine Sulphate; Quinine Acid Sulphate; Quinine Bisulphate *(BANM)*; Quinini Bisulfas.

$C_{20}H_{24}N_2O_2,H_2SO_4,7H_2O = 548.6$.

CAS — 549-56-4 *(anhydrous quinine bisulfate)*.

Pharmacopoeias. In Aust., Br., and Int.

Quinine bisulfate 169 mg is approximately equivalent to 100 mg of anhydrous quinine.

Pharmacopoeial description

BP 2001: Colourless crystals or a white crystalline powder. It effloresces in dry air. Freely soluble in water; sparingly soluble in alcohol. A 1% solution in water has a pH of 2.8 to 3.4. Protect from light.

Quinine Dihydrochloride   (1393-s)

Quinine Dihydrochloride *(BANM)*.

Chinini Dihydrochloridum; Neutral Quinine Hydrochloride; Quinine Acid Hydrochloride; Quinini Dihydrochloridum.

$C_{20}H_{24}N_2O_2,2HCl = 397.3$.

CAS — 60-93-5.

Pharmacopoeias. In Aust., Br., and Int.

Quinine dihydrochloride 122 mg is approximately equivalent to 100 mg of anhydrous quinine.

Pharmacopoeial description

BP 2001: A white or almost white powder. Very soluble in water; freely soluble in alcohol. A 3% solution in water has a pH of 2.0 to 3.0. Protect from light.

Quinine Ethyl Carbonate   (1394-w)

Euquinina; Euquinine; Quinine Etabonate.

$C_{23}H_{28}N_2O_4 = 396.5$.

CAS — 83-75-0.

Pharmacopoeias. In Jpn.

Quinine ethyl carbonate 122 mg is approximately equivalent to 100 mg of anhydrous quinine.

Quinine Hydrobromide   (1395-e)

Quinine Hydrobromide *(BANM)*.

Basic Quinine Hydrobromide; Chinini Bromidum; Quinine Monohydrobromide.

$C_{20}H_{24}N_2O_2,HBr,H_2O = 423.3$.

CAS — 549-49-5 *(anhydrous quinine hydrobromide)*.

Pharmacopoeias. In Fr.

Quinine hydrobromide 130 mg is approximately equivalent to 100 mg of anhydrous quinine.

Quinine Hydrochloride   (1396-l)

Quinine Hydrochloride *(BANM)*.

Basic Quinine Hydrochloride; Chinini Hydrochloridum; Chininii Chloridum; Chininum Chloratum; Chininum Hydrochloricum; Quinine Monohydrochloride; Quinini Hydrochloridum.

$C_{20}H_{24}N_2O_2,HCl,2H_2O = 396.9$.

CAS — 130-89-2 *(anhydrous quinine hydrochloride)*; 6119-47-7 *(quinine hydrochloride dihydrate)*.

Pharmacopoeias. In Eur. (see p.vi), Int., Jpn, and Pol.

Quinine hydrochloride 122 mg is approximately equivalent to 100 mg of anhydrous quinine.

Pharmacopoeial description

Ph. Eur.: Colourless, fine, silky needles, often grouped in clusters. Soluble in water; freely soluble in alcohol. A 1% solution in water has a pH of 6.0 to 6.8. Protect from light.

Quinine Sulfate   (1390-g)

Basic Quinine Sulphate; Chinini Sulfas; Chininum Sulfuricum; Quinine Sulphate *(BANM)*; Quinini Sulfas.

$(C_{20}H_{24}N_2O_2)_2,H_2SO_4,2H_2O = 782.9$.

CAS — 804-63-7 *(anhydrous quinine sulfate)*; 6119-70-6 *(quinine sulfate dihydrate)*.

Pharmacopoeias. In Eur. (see p.vi), Int., Jpn, and US.

Quinine sulfate 121 mg is approximately equivalent to 100 mg of anhydrous quinine.

Pharmacopoeial description

Ph. Eur.: A white or almost white, crystalline powder or fine, colourless needles. Slightly soluble in water; sparingly soluble in boiling water and in alcohol. A 1% suspension in water has a pH of 5.7 to 6.6. Protect from light.

The symbol † denotes a preparation no longer actively marketed

---

USP 25: It is the sulfate of an alkaloid obtained from the bark of species of *Cinchona*. White, odourless, fine needle-like crystals, usually lusterless, making a light and readily compressible mass. It darkens on exposure to light. Soluble 1 in 500 of water and 1 in 120 of alcohol; sparingly soluble in water at 100°; slightly soluble in chloroform; freely soluble in alcohol at 80° and in a mixture of 2 parts of chloroform and one part of dehydrated alcohol; very slightly soluble in ether; Its saturated solution in water is neutral or alkaline to litmus. Protect from light.

Sorption. For reference to loss of quinine sulfate from solutions during membrane filtration, see Chloroquine, p.432.

Adverse Effects

Administration of quinine or its salts in usual therapeutic doses may give rise to a train of symptoms known as cinchonism, characterised in its mild form by tinnitus, impaired hearing, headache, nausea, and disturbed vision, with, in its more severe manifestations, vomiting, abdominal pain, diarrhoea, and vertigo.

Cinchonism may also occur after small doses in patients hypersensitive to quinine, but urticaria and flushing of the skin with intense pruritus are the most frequent reactions seen in these patients. Other effects include fever, skin rashes, and dyspnoea. Angioedema may also occur and asthma can be precipitated. Thrombocytopenia and other blood disorders have been reported. Thrombocytopenic purpura has been associated with quinine hypersensitivity. Haemoglobinuria occurs rarely.

Other adverse effects of quinine include hypoglycaemia, hypoprothrombinaemia, and renal failure.

The main symptoms of overdosage, which can be fatal, include gastrointestinal effects, oculotoxicity, CNS disturbances, and cardiotoxicity. Visual disturbances including sudden blindness are usually slowly reversible but there may be residual damage. Overdosage is discussed in detail below. Quinine can produce cardiovascular toxicity similar to that seen with quinidine including conduction disturbances, arrhythmias, anginal symptoms, and hypotension leading to cardiac arrest and circulatory failure. Severe or even fatal cardiovascular toxicity can result from rapid intravenous administration of quinine.

Large amounts of quinine can induce abortion; congenital malformations, particularly of the optic and auditory nerves, have been reported after failure to induce abortion with quinine. However, quinine should not be withheld from pregnant women with life-threatening malaria (see also under Pregnancy in Precautions, below).

Intramuscular injections of quinine can be irritant and have caused pain, focal necrosis, and abscess formation; tetanus has developed in some patients (see under Malaria in Uses and Administration, below).

Effects on the blood. Between 1966 and 1975 the Swedish Adverse Drug Reaction Committee received 43 reports of *thrombocytopenia* attributable to quinine or quinidine[1] and the Boston Collaborative Drug Surveillance Program had 11 similar reports in patients studied between 1972 and 1981.[2] The FDA in the USA subsequently received details of 2 fatalities due to quinine-induced thrombocytopenia.[3] Quinine-induced thrombocytopenia appears to be a hypersensitivity reaction and beverages containing quinine as a bitter in concentrations as low as 20 μg per mL have precipitated thrombocytopenic purpura in previously sensitised individuals.[4]

Although quinine can cause *haemolysis*, there is some doubt over the traditional view that irregular dosage with quinine predisposes patients with malaria to *blackwater fever*, a syndrome of severe haemolytic anaemia, haemoglobinuria, oliguria, and renal failure.[5] Some of the patients affected may have had glucose-6-phosphate dehydrogenase deficiency.[5] Haemolyticuraemic syndrome[6-8] and pancytopenia with coagulopathy and renal impairment[9,10] have also been associated with the use of quinine.

There have also been reports of *disseminated intravascular coagulation*, including one fatality, following the use of quinine by patients with quinine hypersensitivity.[11-13] In one case[13] the hypersensitivity reaction closely mimicked septic shock. There have been isolated reports of *agranulocytosis* due to quinine.[14]

1. Böttiger LE, *et al.* Drug-induced blood dyscrasias. *Acta Med Scand* 1979; **205:** 457–61.
2. Danielson DA, *et al.* Drug-induced blood disorders. *JAMA* 1984; **252:** 3257–60.
3. Freiman JP. Fatal quinine-induced thrombocytopenia. *Ann Intern Med* 1990; **112:** 308–9.
4. Murray JA, *et al.* Bitter lemon purpura. *BMJ* 1979; **2:** 1551–2.

---

5. WHO. Severe and complicated malaria. 2nd ed. *Trans R Soc Trop Med Hyg* 1990; **84** (suppl 2): 1–65.
6. Hagley MT, *et al.* Hemolytic-uremic syndrome associated with ingestion of quinine. *Am J Nephrol* 1992; **12:** 192–5.
7. Gottschall JL, *et al.* Quinine-induced immune thrombocytopenia with hemolytic uremic syndrome: clinical and serological findings in nine patients and review of literature. *Am J Hematol* 1994; **47:** 283–9.
8. McDonald SP, *et al.* Quinine-induced hemolytic uremic syndrome. *Clin Nephrol* 1997; **47:** 397–400.
9. Maguire RB, *et al.* Recurrent pancytopenia, coagulopathy, and renal failure associated with multiple quinine-dependent antibodies. *Ann Intern Med* 1993; **119:** 215–17.
10. Schmitt SK, Tomford JW. Quinine-induced pancytopenia and coagulopathy. *Ann Intern Med* 1994; **120:** 90–1.
11. Spearing RL, *et al.* Quinine-induced disseminated intravascular coagulation. *Lancet* 1990; **336:** 1535–7.
12. Barr E, *et al.* Recurrent acute hypersensitivity to quinine. *BMJ* 1990; **301:** 323.
13. Schattner A. Quinine hypersensitivity simulating sepsis. *Am J Med* 1998; **104:** 488–90.
14. Sutherland R, *et al.* Quinine-induced agranulocytosis: toxic effect of quinine bisulphate on bone marrow cultures in vitro. *BMJ* 1977; **1:** 605–7.

Effects on the ears. Although ototoxicity such as tinnitus or deafness is known to be a possible adverse effect of quinine, reversible hearing loss may also occur. While one group of workers[1] found the reduction in auditory acuity to be greatest at higher frequencies, another group[2] have found that hearing loss was generally equal across the range of frequencies tested and appeared to be related to the plasma concentration of quinine.

1. Roche RJ, *et al.* Quinine induces reversible high-tone hearing loss. *Br J Clin Pharmacol* 1990; **29:** 780–2.
2. Karlsson KK, *et al.* Audiometry as a possible indicator of quinine plasma concentration during treatment of malaria. *Trans R Soc Trop Med Hyg* 1990; **84:** 765–7.

Effects on the eyes. Oculotoxicity following overdosage with quinine is well recognised (see below), but there has also been a report of blindness in two patients occurring during supposedly routine therapy.[1]

1. Waddell K. Blindness from quinine as an antimalarial. *Trans R Soc Trop Med Hyg* 1996; **90:** 331–2.

Effects on glucose metabolism. Hypoglycaemia is now recognised to be a frequent complication encountered in falciparum malaria and it is often associated with a poor prognosis. Children, pregnant women, and patients with severe disease appear to be particularly at risk. It is important to recognise that hypoglycaemia may be the cause of coma rather than cerebral malaria. Hypoglycaemia may also be induced by antimalarial therapy; first episodes of hypoglycaemia have been detected after patients received quinine[1-3] or quinidine[4] intravenously although others have not found that quinine led to the development of hypoglycaemia.[5,6]

Quinine has also been reported to induce hypoglycaemia during treatment for leg cramps.[7]

1. White NJ, *et al.* Severe hypoglycemia and hyperinsulinemia in falciparum malaria. *N Engl J Med* 1983; **309:** 61–6.
2. Okitolonda W, *et al.* High incidence of hypoglycaemia in African patients treated with intravenous quinine for severe malaria. *BMJ* 1987; **295:** 716–18.
3. Looareesuwan S, *et al.* Quinine and severe falciparum malaria in late pregnancy. *Lancet* 1985; **ii:** 4–8.
4. Phillips RE, *et al.* Hypoglycaemia and antimalarial drugs: quinidine and release of insulin. *BMJ* 1986; **292:** 1319–21.
5. Taylor TE, *et al.* Blood glucose levels in Malawian children before and during the administration of intravenous quinine for severe falciparum malaria. *N Engl J Med* 1988; **319:** 1040–7.
6. Kawo NG, *et al.* The metabolic effects of quinine in children with severe and complicated Plasmodium falciparum malaria in Dar es Salaam. *Trans R Soc Trop Med Hyg* 1991; **85:** 711–13.
7. Limburg PJ, *et al.* Quinine-induced hypoglycemia. *Ann Intern Med* 1993; **119:** 218–19.

Effects on the heart. Cardiotoxicity following overdosage with quinine is well recognised, and prolongation of the QT interval has been noted with therapeutic doses. There has also been a report[1] of fatal ventricular fibrillation with QT prolongation in an elderly patient who received standard doses of quinine by slow intravenous infusion for falciparum malaria. It was noted that the patient had some prolongation of the QT interval before starting quinine and also that her free quinine concentrations were unusually high despite total quinine concentrations considered to be within the therapeutic range.

1. Bonington A, *et al.* Fatal quinine cardiotoxicity in the treatment of falciparum malaria. *Trans R Soc Trop Med Hyg* 1996; **90:** 305–7.

Effects on the kidneys. See Effects on the Blood, above.

Effects on the liver. Although hepatitis has been associated with quinidine therapy (see p.965) there appear to be few reports of hepatotoxicity due to quinine usage. Granulomatous hepatitis has been reported in 2 patients taking quinine[1,2] but the diagnosis in the first of these cases was challenged as the histological findings were considered to be more indicative of non-specific reactive hepatitis.[3] Hepatotoxicity due to quinine hypersensitivity has been reported in another patient.[4] Symptoms of hepatotoxicity occurred within 24 hours in a further patient taking quinine for nocturnal leg cramps.[5]

1. Katz B, *et al.* Quinine-induced granulomatous hepatitis. *BMJ* 1983; **286:** 264–5.
2. Mathur S, *et al.* Quinine induced granulomatous hepatitis and vasculitis. *BMJ* 1990; **300:** 613.
3. Nirodi NS. Quinine induced granulomatous hepatitis. *BMJ* 1983; **286:** 647.

4. Punukollu RC, *et al.* Quinine hepatotoxicity: an underrecognized or rare phenomenon? *Arch Intern Med* 1990; **150**: 1112–13.
5. Farver DK, Lavin MN. Quinine-induced hepatotoxicity. *Ann Pharmacother* 1999; **33**: 32–4.

Effects on the skin. Urticaria, cutaneous flushing, various skin rashes, and pruritus are the commonest symptoms of hypersensitivity reactions to quinine.

Topical contact with quinine may cause contact as well as photocontact allergy, but quinine can also induce photosensitivity reactions following systemic administration.[1,2] Photosensitivity associated with quinine intake from excessive consumption of tonic water has been reported.[3] There have also been reports of eczematous dermatitis,[1] oedema and erythema,[4] and lichen planus.[4] Both phototoxic[4] and photoallergic[1] mechanisms have been suggested. Fatal cutaneous vasculitis related to quinine treatment for nocturnal cramps has been reported.[5]

For a comparison of the incidence of pruritus induced by various antimalarials, see under Chloroquine, p.433.

1. Ljunggren B, Sjövall P. Systemic quinine photosensitivity. *Arch Dermatol* 1986; **122**: 909–11.
2. Ljunggren B, *et al.* Systemic quinine photosensitivity with photoepicutaneous cross-reactivity to quinidine. *Contact Dermatitis* 1992; **26**: 1–4.
3. Wagner GH, *et al.* 'I'll have mine with a twist of lemon': quinine photosensitivity from excessive intake of tonic water. *Br J Dermatol* 1994; **131**: 734–5.
4. Ferguson J, *et al.* Quinine induced photosensitivity: clinical and experimental studies. *Br J Dermatol* 1987; **117**: 631–40.
5. Price EJ, *et al.* Quinine-induced cutaneous vasculitis. *Br J Clin Pract* 1992; **46**: 138–9.

Hypersensitivity. For reference to hypersensitivity reactions associated with quinine, see Effects on the Blood, Effects on the Liver, and Effects on the Skin, above.

Overdosage. Cinchonism may occur with therapeutic doses of quinine and symptoms include nausea, vomiting, tinnitus, deafness, headache, vasodilatation, and slightly disturbed vision. These symptoms may also occur in acute overdosage, but the visual disorders may be severe and there may be CNS disturbances and cardiotoxicity. A lethal dose or lethal plasma-quinine concentration has not been established but fatalities have been reported[1] in adults after doses of 2 to 8 g and in children after 1 g.

An analysis[2] of 165 cases of acute quinine poisoning revealed that: 21% had no symptoms, nausea with or without vomiting occurred in 47%, visual disturbances in 42%, tinnitus in 38%, other auditory disturbances in 23%, sinus tachycardia in 23%, and other ECG abnormalities in 8%. Mild impairment of consciousness was reported in 14% of the patients while 7 (4%) patients had deeper grades of coma. Of the 5 patients who died, 4 developed intractable ventricular arrhythmias and the fifth had a Jacksonian fit followed by cardiac arrest.

The effects of oculotoxicity may include blurred vision, defective colour perception, visual field constriction, and total blindness.[2,3] The onset of symptoms may vary from a few hours to a day or more after ingestion.[2,3] Suggested mechanisms for quinine's oculotoxicity include an action on the retinal vasculature to produce ischaemia or a direct toxic effect on the retina.[1] Visual loss in one group of patients[3] was associated with plasma-quinine concentrations in excess of 10 μg per mL. However, in another group plasma-quinine concentrations were considered to be an imprecise guide to predicting visual disturbances.[2] The speed and degree of visual recovery varies. Of 70 patients with visual disturbances following quinine poisoning, 39 subsequently complained of a period of total blindness.[2] Permanent visual deficits remained in 19 of these but no patient had permanent bilateral blindness. All of the 31 patients who had had blurred vision recovered full visual acuity.

It is considered that the actions of quinine on the myocardium are similar to those of quinidine but that it is less potent.[1] Sinus tachycardia and minor ECG changes are the most common cardiovascular effects. Conduction abnormalities and ventricular dysrhythmias may occur with severe poisoning. Ventricular tachycardia is mostly associated with cardiogenic shock or circulatory collapse. Hypokalaemia may also occur.[1]

1. Jaeger A, *et al.* Clinical features and management of poisoning due to antimalarial drugs. *Med Toxicol* 1987; **2**: 242–73.
2. Boland ME, *et al.* Complications of quinine poisoning. *Lancet* 1985; **i**: 384–5.
3. Dyson EH, *et al.* Death and blindness due to overdose of quinine. *BMJ* 1985; **291**: 31–3.

Treatment of Adverse Effects

In acute overdosage with quinine or its salts multiple doses of activated charcoal may be given to adults or children who present within one hour of ingesting more than the equivalent of 15 mg per kg body-weight of quinine base; gastric lavage may also be considered for use in adults. Other measures aimed at enhancing the elimination of quinine are largely ineffective. Treatment is mostly symptomatic with attention being given to maintaining blood pressure, respiration, and renal function, and to treating arrhythmias.

Vasodilators and stellate ganglion block have been used to prevent or reverse visual impairment but there is little evidence to support their use.

◊ It has been suggested that, as quinine has antimuscarinic effects, gastric emptying may be delayed and considerable amounts of drug might be removed from the stomach beyond the usual 4 hours.[1] Others consider that gastric lavage is of doubtful value as quinine is rapidly absorbed and vomiting has often occurred before admission.[2] However, studies in healthy subjects and poisoned patients suggest that oral administration of charcoal may increase the elimination of quinine.[3,4] Other methods of increasing elimination are probably ineffective. In a study involving 16 patients with quinine poisoning forced acid diuresis, haemodialysis, haemoperfusion, or plasma exchange were all found to be ineffective in increasing quinine elimination.[5]

Stellate ganglion block has been recommended to prevent or reverse retinal damage, the rationale being that quinine-induced oculotoxicity might arise from retinal arteriolar constriction. However, clinical studies have failed to find sufficient improvement to justify its use.[6,7] There has been a report of the intravenous administration of nitrates producing beneficial responses in 2 patients.[8]

1. Boland M, Volans G. ABC of poisoning: miscellaneous drugs. *BMJ* 1984; **289**: 1361–5.
2. Jaeger A, *et al.* Clinical features and management of poisoning due to antimalarial drugs. *Med Toxicol* 1987; **2**: 242–73.
3. Lockey D, Bateman DN. Effect of oral activated charcoal on quinine elimination. *Br J Clin Pharmacol* 1989; **27**: 92–4.
4. Prescott LF, *et al.* Treatment of quinine overdosage with repeated oral charcoal. *Br J Clin Pharmacol* 1989; **27**: 95–7.
5. Bateman DN, *et al.* Pharmacokinetics and clinical toxicity of quinine overdosage: lack of efficacy of techniques intended to enhance elimination. *Q J Med* 1985; **54**: 125–31.
6. Boland ME, *et al.* Complications of quinine poisoning. *Lancet* 1985; **i**: 384–5.
7. Dyson EH, *et al.* Quinine amblyopia: is current management appropriate? *J Toxicol Clin Toxicol* 1985–6; **23**: 571–8.
8. Moore D, *et al.* Research into quinine ocular toxicity. *Br J Ophthalmol* 1992; **76**: 703.

Precautions

Quinine and its salts are contra-indicated in patients with a history of hypersensitivity to quinine or quinidine and in patients with tinnitus or optic neuritis. They should not be used in the presence of haemolysis. They should be used with caution in patients with atrial fibrillation, cardiac conduction defects, or heart block. Quinine should be avoided in patients with myasthenia gravis as it may aggravate their condition.

Pregnancy in a patient with malaria is not generally regarded as a contra-indication to the use of quinine.

As quinine has been implicated in precipitating blackwater fever it is generally contra-indicated in patients who have already suffered an attack. Quinine may also cause haemolysis in some types of glucose-6-phosphate dehydrogenase deficiency and should be used with care.

It is important that when quinine is given intravenously it should be given by slow infusion and the patient observed closely for signs of cardiotoxicity. Blood-glucose concentrations should also be monitored. Problems that have been associated with intramuscular administration are discussed under Malaria in Uses and Administration, below.

Breast feeding. Although quinine is distributed into breast milk in small amounts[1] the American Academy of Pediatrics considers that the use of quinine is probably compatible with breast feeding.[2]

1. Phillips RE, *et al.* Quinine pharmacokinetics and toxicity in pregnant and lactating women with falciparum malaria. *Br J Clin Pharmacol* 1986; **21**: 677–83.
2. American Academy of Pediatrics, Committee on Drugs. The transfer of drugs and other chemicals into human milk. *Pediatrics* 2001; **108**: 776–89.

Liver disease. See under Pharmacokinetics, below.

Porphyria. For a discussion of the problems of the use of antimalarials in patients with porphyria and a comment that quinine is considered to be safe for use in such patients, see under Precautions for Chloroquine, p.434.

Pregnancy. The use of quinine in large doses as an abortifacient in the past has led to concern over its use during pregnancy but no evidence of an oxytocic effect was found when it was used to treat severe falciparum malaria in women in the third trimester of pregnancy.[1]
Congenital abnormalities including damage to the auditory and optic nerves have been seen, usually following attempted abortions, but WHO[2] considers quinine to be safe when used in normal therapeutic doses during pregnancy. Jitteriness attributed to quinine withdrawal has been reported in an infant whose mother had drunk large quantities of tonic water containing quinine during the last 17 weeks of pregnancy.[3]
As malaria infection is potentially serious during pregnancy and poses a threat to the mother and fetus, there appears to be little justification for withholding treatment in the absence of a suitable alternative. However, pregnant patients treated for malaria are at special risk from hypoglycaemia exacerbated or caused by quinine-induced hyperinsulinaemia (see under Effects on Glucose Metabolism in Adverse Effects, above) and should be managed appropriately.

1. Looareesuwan S, *et al.* Quinine and severe falciparum malaria in late pregnancy. *Lancet* 1985; **ii**: 4–8.
2. WHO. *WHO model prescribing information: drugs used in parasitic diseases.* 2nd ed. Geneva: WHO, 1995.
3. Evans ANW, *et al.* The ingestion by pregnant women of substances toxic to the foetus. *Practitioner* 1980; **224**: 315–19.

Renal impairment. See under Pharmacokinetics, below.

Interactions

As quinine shares many of the actions of quinidine, interactions seen between quinidine and other drugs (see p.965) might also occur with quinine. Both have actions on skeletal muscle and may potentiate the effects of drugs with neuromuscular-blocking activity (see under Antiarrhythmics on p.1334). There is an increased risk of inducing ventricular arrhythmias if quinine is given together with halofantrine (see p.436) or other arrhythmogenic drugs such as amiodarone, the antihistamines astemizole and terfenadine, cisapride, and the antipsychotic pimozide. There may be an increased risk of convulsions when quinine is administered with mefloquine.

Amantadine. For a report of quinine reducing renal clearance of amantadine, see p.1162.

Anticoagulants. Quinine can cause hypoprothrombinaemia and thereby enhance the effect of anticoagulants. In one report, reductions in *warfarin* dosage were necessary after ingestion of large amounts of tonic water containing quinine (see p.995).

Antimalarials. Quinine and *chloroquine* may be antagonistic when used for falciparum malaria (see p.434). For a report of quinine reducing plasma concentrations of *primaquine*, see p.441.

Ciclosporin. For a report of quinine decreasing plasma concentrations of ciclosporin, see p.521.

Digoxin. Quinidine has been reported to increase serum-digoxin concentrations (see p.871) and quinine has reduced total body clearance of digoxin (see p.872).

Flecainide. For a report of quinine inhibiting the metabolism of flecainide, see p.891.

Histamine H₂-antagonists. *Cimetidine* has been reported to reduce the clearance of quinine and prolong its elimination half-life in a study in healthy subjects; no significant effect was seen with *ranitidine*.[1]

1. Wanwimolruk S, *et al.* Effects of cimetidine and ranitidine on the pharmacokinetics of quinine. *Br J Clin Pharmacol* 1986; **22**: 346–50.

Rifampicin. Elimination of quinine has been reported to increase in patients also receiving rifampicin.[1]

1. Wanwimolruk S, *et al.* Marked enhancement by rifampicin and lack of effect of isoniazid on the elimination of quinine in man. *Br J Clin Pharmacol* 1995; **40**: 87–91.

Tobacco smoking. A single-dose study in healthy subjects has suggested that blood concentrations of quinine are lower in heavy smokers than in non-smokers, potentially impairing efficacy.[1]

1. Wanwimolruk S, *et al.* Cigarette smoking enhances the elimination of quinine. *Br J Clin Pharmacol* 1993; **36**: 610–14.

Pharmacokinetics

The pharmacokinetics of quinine are altered significantly by malaria infection, the major effects being reductions in both its apparent volume of distribution and its clearance.

Quinine is rapidly and almost completely absorbed from the gastrointestinal tract and peak concentrations in the circulation are attained about 1 to 3 hours after oral administration of the sulfate or bisulfate. Plasma protein binding is about 70% in healthy subjects and rises to 90% or more in patients with malaria. Quinine is widely distributed throughout the body. Concentrations attained in the CSF of patients with cerebral malaria have been reported to be about 2 to 7% of those in the plasma.

Quinine is extensively metabolised in the liver and rapidly excreted mainly in the urine. Estimates of the proportion of unchanged quinine excreted in the urine vary from less than 5 to 20%. Excretion is increased in acid urine. The elimination half-life is about 11 hours in healthy subjects but may be prolonged in patients with malaria. Small amounts of quinine also appear in the bile and saliva.

Quinine crosses the placenta and is distributed into breast milk (see Breast Feeding, above).

◊ References.

1. White NJ. Clinical pharmacokinetics of antimalarial drugs. *Clin Pharmacokinet* 1985; **10**: 187–215.
2. Supanaranond W, *et al.* Disposition of oral quinine in acute falciparum malaria. *Eur J Clin Pharmacol* 1991; **40**: 49–52.
3. Wanwimolruk S, *et al.* Pharmacokinetics of quinine in young and elderly subjects. *Trans R Soc Trop Med Hyg* 1991; **85**: 714–17.
4. Dyer JR, *et al.* The pharmacokinetics and pharmacodynamics of quinine in the diabetic and non-diabetic elderly. *Br J Clin Pharmacol* 1994; **38**: 205–12.
5. Sowunmi A, Salako LA. Effect of dose size on the pharmacokinetics of orally administered quinine. *Eur J Clin Pharmacol* 1996; **49**: 383–6.
6. Krishna S, White NJ. Pharmacokinetics of quinine, chloroquine and amodiaquine: clinical implications. *Clin Pharmacokinet* 1996; **30**: 263–99.
7. Boele van Hensbroek M, *et al.* Quinine pharmacokinetics in young children with severe malaria. *Am J Trop Med Hyg* 1996; **54**: 237–42.
8. Zhang H, *et al.* Evidence for involvement of human CYP3A in the 3-hydroxylation of quinine. *Br J Clin Pharmacol* 1997; **43**: 245–52.
9. Viriyayudhakorn S, *et al.* Pharmacokinetics of quinine in obesity. *Trans R Soc Trop Med Hyg* 2000; **94**: 425–8.

Administration in liver disease. Reduced clearance of quinine and prolonged elimination half-life have been reported in patients with acute hepatitis B given a single intravenous dose.[1] The results suggested that quinine accumulation following multiple doses could be greater in patients with hepatitis, even once hepatic function had returned to normal. In another study[2] patients with moderate chronic liver disease were given quinine by mouth; the half-life was prolonged but total clearance was not affected.

1. Karbwang J, *et al.* The pharmacokinetics of quinine in patients with hepatitis. *Br J Clin Pharmacol* 1993; **35**: 444–6.
2. Auprayoon P, *et al.* Pharmacokinetics of quinine in chronic liver disease. *Br J Clin Pharmacol* 1995; **40**: 494–7.

Administration in renal impairment. As urinary clearance comprises only 20% of total clearance of quinine, it appears that high plasma concentrations reported in patients with severe falciparum malaria and acute renal failure may be related more to the severity of the malaria, and associated pharmacokinetic changes, than to any reduction in the glomerular filtration rate.[1] There were significant changes in the pharmacokinetics of quinine in 6 patients with chronic renal failure following a single oral dose.[2] The changes included a prolonged half-life, but there was no clear relationship between severity of renal failure and the degree of impairment of quinine clearance.

1. White NJ. Clinical pharmacokinetics of antimalarial drugs. *Clin Pharmacokinet* 1985; **10**: 187–215.
2. Rimchala P, *et al.* Pharmacokinetics of quinine in patients with chronic renal failure. *Eur J Clin Pharmacol* 1996; **49**: 497–501.

Uses and Administration

Quinine is a cinchona alkaloid and a 4-methanolquinoline antimalarial which is a rapid-acting blood schizontocide with activity against *Plasmodium falciparum*, *P. vivax*, *P. ovale*, and *P. malariae*. It is active against the gametocytes of *P. malariae* and *P. vivax*, but not against mature gametocytes of *P. falciparum*. The precise mechanism of action of quinine is unclear but it may interfere with lysosome function or nucleic acid synthesis in the malaria parasite. Since it has no activity against exoerythrocytic forms, quinine does not produce a radical cure in vivax or ovale malarias. The increasing spread of resistance to chloroquine has been responsible for the re-emergence of quinine as an important drug in the treatment of falciparum malaria. Quinine is not generally used for malaria prophylaxis.

Quinine is also used to treat the protozoal infection babesiosis and for the relief of nocturnal leg cramps.

Quinine has mild analgesic and antipyretic properties and is sometimes included in preparations used for the symptomatic relief of the common cold and influenza; additional salts that have been used for this purpose include the camsilate and the gluconate.

Quinine is also used as a bitter and a flavour.

For the *treatment of malaria* quinine is given by mouth, usually as the sulfate, hydrochloride, or dihydrochloride, or parenterally as the dihydrochloride; quinine ethyl carbonate is sometimes used for oral administration because, unlike other quinine salts which are intensely bitter, it is tasteless. They all contain approximately the same amount of quinine and any of them can be used when the dose is cited in terms of "quinine salt"; this is not the case for the bisulfate which contains a correspondingly smaller amount of quinine. Quinine formate is sometimes used for parenteral administration.

A course of treatment with quinine for falciparum malaria usually lasts 7 days and in uncomplicated infections treatment should preferably be given by the oral route. The usual oral dose is 600 mg of quinine salt given every 8 hours for 7 days. For children a dose of 10 mg of quinine salt per kg body-weight given every 8 hours for 7 days has been recommended.

In severe or complicated falciparum malaria or when the patient is unable to take oral medication, quinine should be given parenterally by slow intravenous infusion, but this can be hazardous and patients generally need monitoring, particularly for signs of cardiotoxicity. Therapy should be changed to oral administration as soon as possible to complete the course. To obtain therapeutic concentrations rapidly with parenteral therapy, quinine is often given in an initial loading dose followed by maintenance doses. Recommended dosage regimens for intravenous administration include an initial loading dose of 20 mg of quinine dihydrochloride per kg (up to a maximum of 1.4 g) given over 4 hours with maintenance infusions being started 8 hours later, calculated from the start of the previous infusion. Alternatively, in intensive care units, an initial loading dose of 7 mg per kg may be given over 30 minutes followed immediately by the first of the maintenance infusions. Maintenance infusions consist of 10 mg per kg (up to a maximum of 700 mg) given over 4 hours every 8 to 12 hours. A loading dose should not be given if the patient has received quinine, quinidine, mefloquine, or halofantrine, during the previous 24 hours. If parenteral therapy is required for more than 48 hours the maintenance dose of quinine dihydrochloride should be reduced to 5 to 7 mg per kg. If intravenous infusion is not possible quinine dihydrochloride has been given intramuscularly where doses, including the loading dose, are the same as those used for intravenous administration; it should be diluted in sodium chloride 0.9% to a concentration of 60 to 100 mg of the dihydrochloride per mL, and the total dose divided between two administration sites, preferably each anterior thigh (not the buttock). However, intramuscular administration can be irritant and there have been concerns regarding its safety and efficacy (see under Malaria, below).

When used for the *relief of nocturnal leg cramps*, quinine is given at night in a dose of 200 to 300 mg by mouth of the sulfate or bisulfate. Quinine benzoate has also been used.

Babesiosis. Although there is no established specific treatment for babesiosis (p.583), a combination of quinine and clindamycin has been used for *Babesia microti* infections.[1-3] Suggested doses[3] are quinine 650 mg three times daily by mouth with clindamycin 1.2 g twice daily intravenously or 600 mg three times daily by mouth; treatment is continued for 7 days. Children may be given quinine 25 mg per kg body-weight daily plus clindamycin 20 to 40 mg per kg daily, both by mouth in 3 divided doses. Quinine with azithromycin was reported to be effective in a patient who had not responded to quinine with clindamycin.[4]

1. Wittner M, *et al.* Successful chemotherapy of transfusion babesiosis. *Ann Intern Med* 1982; **96**: 601–4.
2. Anonymous. Clindamycin and quinine treatment for Babesia microti infections. *MMWR* 1983; **32**: 65–6, 72.
3. Anonymous. Drugs for parasitic infections. *Med Lett Drugs Ther* 1998; **40**: 1–12.
4. Shaio MF, Yang KD. Response of babesiosis to a combined regimen of quinine and azithromycin. *Trans R Soc Trop Med Hyg* 1997; **91**: 214–15.

Flavouring. The Joint FAO/WHO Expert Committee on Food Additives concluded that quinine levels in soft drinks of up to 100 mg per litre (as quinine base) were not of toxicological concern.[1] However, because of the possibility of hypersensitivity reactions in some individuals, the committee recommended that consumers be informed of the presence of quinine in food or beverages.

1. FAO/WHO. Evaluation of certain food additives and contaminants: forty-first report of the joint FAO/WHO expert committee on food additives. *WHO Tech Rep Ser 837* 1993.

Malaria. Quinine has an important role in the treatment of falciparum malaria (see p.428) being used where there is chloroquine or multidrug *Plasmodium falciparum* resistance,[1-4] and also (in view of the widespread problem of *P. falciparum* resistance) where the infective species is not known, or if the infection is mixed. Ideally treatment should be with one of the quinine salts given by mouth when a dose of 600 mg of quinine

salt for adults or 10 mg per kg body-weight for children is given every 8 hours for 7 days. However, to reduce quinine-related adverse effects and thereby improve compliance, a 3-day course of quinine salt combined with either 7 days of a tetracycline or a single dose of pyrimethamine-sulfadoxine (Fansidar) or clindamycin for 3 days may be considered in regions without quinine resistance. The dose of quinine salt applies to the hydrochloride, dihydrochloride, sulfate, and ethyl carbonate, but not to the bisulfate. Any quinine lost through vomiting within one hour after oral administration should be replaced by additional doses.[1]

The oral route may not provide effective treatment in severe infection and in such cases quinine should be given as the dihydrochloride by slow intravenous infusion, with the patient being observed closely, particularly for any signs of cardiotoxicity.[4] Loading doses of quinine are often used to obtain therapeutic blood concentrations as soon as possible in severely ill patients but they should not be given to patients who have received quinine, quinidine, mefloquine, or halofantrine, within the previous 24 hours.

WHO[4] recommends that an initial loading dose of 20 mg of quinine dihydrochloride per kg [up to a maximum of 1.4 g] be given intravenously over 4 hours followed 8 hours after the start of the loading dose by maintenance infusions of 10 mg per kg given over 4 hours and repeated every 8 hours (sometimes the interval may be every 12 hours). Alternatively, in intensive care units, a loading dose of 7 mg per kg body-weight may be given by intravenous infusion over 30 minutes followed immediately by the first of the maintenance infusions. The loading and maintenance doses given above were found to be necessary in Thailand where the MIC of quinine for local strains of *Plasmodium falciparum* was around 10 µg per mL. In some areas where *P. falciparum* is more sensitive to quinine a regimen consisting of a loading dose of 10 mg per kg and maintenance doses of 5 mg per kg, given at 12-hour intervals, might also produce adequate plasma concentrations. A regimen suggested for young children in Africa with severe malaria consisted of a 15 mg per kg loading dose of quinine dihydrochloride given by intravenous infusion over 2 hours, followed by maintenance doses of 10 mg per kg every 12 hours.[5] This regimen was challenged however, on the basis that it might result in under-treatment of the disease.[6] In another study in African children with cerebral malaria,[7] a loading dose of quinine dihydrochloride 20 mg per kg given intravenously over the first 4 hours (followed by maintenance doses of 10 mg per kg intravenously, over 4 hours, every 8 hours for 3 days, and then orally for 4 days) was judged to be more effective than a similar regimen without a loading dose. Whichever regimen is chosen, patients are transferred to oral therapy as soon as possible, at a dose of 10 mg of quinine salt per kg every 8 hours, and treatment continued until a total of at least 7 days of therapy has been given.[4] However, if patients still require parenteral therapy after 48 hours it has been suggested that maintenance doses should be reduced to 5 to 7 mg per kg.[4] If intravenous formulations of quinine are unavailable quinidine may be used as an alternative; for further details see under the Uses and Administration of Quinidine, p.966.

If facilities for administration by intravenous infusion, including monitoring, are not available WHO[4] recommends that quinine should be given by deep intramuscular injection. A loading dose of 20 mg of quinine dihydrochloride per kg may be given by injection in divided sites followed by injections of 10 mg per kg every 8 hours; a dose interval of 12 hours has also been employed. Patients should be transferred to oral therapy as soon as possible. The use of the intramuscular route has been controversial because of concerns over safety and efficacy. However, some studies have demonstrated that it can safely be used in adults and children with severe infections.[8-11] Intramuscular injections of quinine can be irritant and have caused pain, focal necrosis, and abscess formation; fatal tetanus has developed in some patients.[12] It has been suggested that some such reactions may be related to the use of preparations formulated in urethane or other irritant substances. Diluted solutions of quinine dihydrochloride 60 mg per mL adjusted to neutral pH appear to be less painful than the usual undiluted preparation of 300 mg per mL.

If facilities do not exist to administer quinine parenterally then patients with severe malaria should receive quinine by mouth or nasogastric tube. Rectal administration has also been suggested.[13]

Quinine as formerly standardised used to contain a higher concentration of cinchona alkaloids and there might be synergy between mixtures of these alkaloids.[14] In practice no advantage has been demonstrated by such mixtures over quinine alone in the treatment of chloroquine-resistant falciparum malaria.[15]

1. WHO. *WHO model prescribing information: drugs used in parasitic diseases.* 2nd ed. Geneva: WHO, 1995.
2. Molyneux M, Fox R. Diagnosis and treatment of malaria in Britain. *BMJ* 1993; **306**: 1175–80.
3. Anonymous. Drugs for parasitic infections. *Med Lett Drugs Ther* 1998; **40**: 1–12.
4. WHO. *Management of severe malaria: a practical handbook.* Geneva: WHO, 2000.
5. Winstanley PA, *et al.* Towards optimal regimens of parenteral quinine for young African children with cerebral malaria: unbound quinine concentrations following a simple loading dose regimen. *Trans R Soc Trop Med Hyg* 1994; **88**: 577–80.
6. White NJ. Optimal regimens of parenteral quinine. *Trans R Soc Trop Med Hyg* 1995; **89**: 462–3.

7. van der Torn M, *et al.* Loading dose of quinine in African children with cerebral malaria. *Trans R Soc Trop Med Hyg* 1998; **92:** 325–31.
8. Wattanagoon Y, *et al.* Intramuscular loading dose of quinine for falciparum malaria: pharmacokinetics and toxicity. *BMJ* 1986; **293:** 11–13. Correction. *ibid.*; 362.
9. Mansor SM, *et al.* The safety and kinetics of intramuscular quinine in Malawian children with moderately severe falciparum malaria. *Trans R Soc Trop Med Hyg* 1990; **84:** 482–7.
10. Waller D, *et al.* The pharmacokinetic properties of intramuscular quinine in Gambian children with severe falciparum malaria. *Trans R Soc Trop Med Hyg* 1990; **84:** 488–91.
11. Schapira A, *et al.* Comparison of intramuscular and intravenous quinine for the treatment of severe and complicated malaria in children. *Trans R Soc Trop Med Hyg* 1993; **87:** 299–302.
12. Yen LM, *et al.* Role of quinine in the high mortality of intramuscular injection tetanus. *Lancet* 1994; **344:** 786–7.
13. Barennes H. Is intrarectal injectable quinine a safe alternative to intramuscular injectable quinine? *Trop Doct* 1994; **24:** 32–3.
14. Druilhe P, *et al.* Activity of a combination of three cinchona bark alkaloids against Plasmodium falciparum in vitro. *Antimicrob Agents Chemother* 1988; **32:** 250–4.
15. Bunnag D, *et al.* A combination of quinine, quinidine and cinchonine (LA 40221) in the treatment of chloroquine resistant falciparum malaria in Thailand: two double-blind trials. *Trans R Soc Trop Med Hyg* 1989; **83:** 66.

Muscle spasm. Quinine (usually as quinine sulfate or bisulfate) has traditionally been used for nocturnal cramps (p.1322) but there has been concern over its efficacy and potential for adverse effects, especially in the elderly. In the USA, for example, the FDA ruled that quinine products should no longer be used for the management of nocturnal cramps.[1,2] Meta-analyses[3,4] concluded that although quinine was effective in the treatment of nocturnal cramps in ambulatory patients the risk of serious adverse effects should be borne in mind. It was recommended that patients should be closely monitored while the efficacy of quinine is assessed over a period of at least 4 weeks.

Some[5] have recommended that treatment be stopped every 3 months to see whether it was still needed.

Haemodialysis-induced cramp has been reported to respond to treatment with quinine.[6,7]

1. FDA. Drug products for the treatment and/or prevention of nocturnal leg muscle cramps for over-the-counter human use. *Fed Regist* 1994; **59:** 43234–52.
2. Nightingale SL. Quinine for nocturnal leg cramps. *ACP J Club* 1995; **123:** 86.
3. Man-Son-Hing M, Wells G. Meta-analysis of efficacy of quinine for treatment of nocturnal leg cramps in elderly people. *BMJ* 1995; **310:** 13–17.
4. Man-Son-Hing M, *et al.* Quinine for nocturnal leg cramps: a meta-analysis including unpublished data. *J Gen Intern Med* 1998; **13:** 600–606.
5. Anonymous. Quinine for nocturnal leg cramps? *Drug Ther Bull* 1996; **34:** 7–8.
6. Kaji DM, *et al.* Prevention of muscle cramps in haemodialysis patients by quinine sulphate. *Lancet* 1976; **ii:** 66–7.
7. Roca AO, *et al.* Dialysis leg cramps; efficacy of quinine versus vitamin E. *ASAIO J* 1992; **38:** M481–M485.

Preparations

BP 2001: Quinine Bisulphate Tablets; Quinine Sulphate Tablets; *USP 25:* Quinine Sulfate Capsules; Quinine Sulfate Tablets.

Proprietary Preparations (details are given in Part 3)
Austral.: Biquinate; Myoquin; Quinate; Quinbisul; Quinoctal; Quinsul; *Braz.:* Impalud; Paluquina; *Denm.:* Kinin; *Fr.:* Quinoforme; Surquina; *Ger.:* Limptar N; Sagittaproct; *NZ:* Q200; Q300; Quinoc; *Swed.:* Kinin; *Switz.:* Circonyl N†; *Thai.:* Genin; *USA:* Night Leg Cramp Relief†.

Multi-ingredient: *Aust.:* Dilatol-Chinin; Iromin Chinin C; Limptar; Seltoc; Togal; *Belg.:* Eugrippine†; Spasmosedine†; *Braz.:* Monotrean; Paludil; *Fin.:* Crampiton; Relapamil; *Fr.:* Arsiquinoforme†; Dinacode; Hexaquine; Pholcones†; Quinimax; Quinisedine; Tussipax a l'Euquinine†; *Ger.:* Antiphlebin†;

Limptar; Togal; *Irl.:* Anadin; *Ital.:* Monotrean; *Neth.:* Aflukin C†; *NZ:* Nicobrevin; *Port.:* Broncosil; Bronquico; Recto Bronco Tosse†; Transbronquina Rectal; *S.Afr.:* Cetamine; Ilvico; *Spain:* Brota Rectal Bals; *Switz.:* Limptar†; *UK:* Nicobrevin; Ronpirin APCQ.

Tafenoquine (20244-x)

Tafenoquine *(BAN, rINN)*.

WR-238605. (±)-8-[(4-Amino-1-methylbutyl)amino]-2,6-dimethoxy-4-methyl-5-[(α,α,α-trifluoro-*m*-tolyl)oxy]quinoline; (*RS*)-*N*⁴-[2,6-Dimethoxy-4-methyl-5-(3-trifluoromethylphenoxy)quinolin-8-yl]pentane-1,4-diamine.

$C_{24}H_{28}F_3N_3O_3 = 463.5.$
CAS — *106635-80-7*.

Profile

Tafenoquine is an 8-aminoquinoline antimalarial. It acts as a tissue schizontocide and is under investigation as the succinate for the radical cure and prevention of relapse in vivax malaria. It may also have a role in the prophylaxis of falciparum malaria.

◊ References.

1. Brueckner RP, *et al.* First-time-in-humans safety and pharmacokinetics of WR 238605, a new antimalarial. *Am J Trop Med Hyg* 1998; **58:** 645–9.
2. Walsh DS, *et al.* Randomized dose-ranging study of the safety and efficacy of WR 238605 (Tafenoquine) in the prevention of relapse of Plasmodium vivax malaria in Thailand. *J Infect Dis* 1999; **180:** 1282–7.
3. Lell B, *et al.* Malaria chemoprophylaxis with tafenoquine: a randomised study. *Lancet* 2000; **355:** 2041–5.

Antimigraine Drugs

This chapter reviews the management of headache, in particular, migraine and cluster headache, and the drugs used mainly for their treatment. The mechanisms of head pain or headache are not fully understood but may involve neurovascular changes (as in migraine and cluster headache), muscle contraction (tension headache), nerve lesions (neuralgias), direct head injury, infection (meningitis), or referred pain (sinusitis, toothache, eye disorders). Headache is also an adverse effect of many drugs including, paradoxically, those used to treat it. The International Headache Society has published guidelines to aid the diagnosis of the various headache types. Patients may have more than one headache disorder and require separate treatment for each.

◊ References.
1. Headache Classification Committee of the International Headache Society. Classification and diagnostic criteria for headache disorders, cranial neuralgias and facial pain. *Cephalalgia* 1988; **8** (suppl 7): 1–96.

Analgesic-induced headache
Overuse of analgesics and other drugs such as ergotamine or caffeine to treat headache can lead to dependence and paradoxical chronic daily headache in headache-prone patients; such headaches do not appear to occur when these drugs are used to treat other disorders.[1] Such analgesic-induced headaches, also referred to as rebound headaches or analgesic abuse headaches, are relieved by withdrawal of the offending drug, but the primary headache may still persist. Furthermore, abrupt discontinuation can exacerbate headache and produce other symptoms of withdrawal. This may then lead the patient to resume treatment to relieve the headache thereby setting up a vicious circle.

Analgesic-induced headache can be difficult to treat. Options for outpatient treatment include either gradual or abrupt withdrawal of the overused analgesic, sometimes together with substitution by a long-acting NSAID or intramuscular dihydroergotamine.[2,3] However, withdrawal symptoms may persist for up to 2 weeks and detoxification may require hospitalisation; intravenous metoclopramide and repetitive intravenous dihydroergotamine may be required to control nausea and vomiting and intractable headache, respectively. General advice on the prevention of analgesic-induced headache has included limiting the frequency of administration of analgesics and the avoidance of compound and opioid analgesics.[1,2]

1. Olesen J. Analgesic headache. *BMJ* 1995; **310:** 479–80.
2. Silberstein SD, Young WB. Analgesic rebound headache. *Drug Safety* 1995; **13:** 133–44.
3. Zed PJ, et al. Medication-induced headache: overview and systematic review of therapeutic approaches. *Ann Pharmacother* 1999; **33:** 61–72.

Cluster headache
Cluster headache (migrainous neuralgia, histaminic cephalalgia, Horton's syndrome) is of unknown aetiology but may be neurovascular in origin. Patients experience one or more short-lived attacks of intense unilateral head pain, usually at the same time of day (often at night). The period during which attacks may occur is called a cluster period; it may last several weeks. Restlessness during the attacks appears to be a characteristic feature of cluster headache. In the typical episodic form of cluster headache, cluster periods are followed by periods of remission lasting for months or years but in the more rare chronic form, patients may have cluster periods lasting for more than a year or with very short periods of remission in between. Substances such as alcohol or glyceryl trinitrate can precipitate headache attacks during cluster periods, but not during periods of remission.

The **treatment** of individual acute attacks during a cluster period is difficult because the headache is short-lived and analgesics administered by the oral route are unlikely to be absorbed fast enough to produce much benefit. Inhalation of 100% oxygen is rapid and effective in aborting attacks, but because of practical difficulties other treatments such as inhaled ergotamine or subcutaneous sumatriptan are more likely to be used. Dihydroergotamine is also effective but generally requires administration by injection and is usually reserved for use in emergency settings. Intranasal instillation of lignocaine [lidocaine] has been reported to be effective in aborting attacks but does not appear to be widely used.

Since individual attacks are difficult to treat it is probably more effective to manage cluster headache by **prophylaxis** once a cluster period has started. Several drugs have been used to prevent attacks. Ergotamine is used for prevention in episodic cluster headache when it is given by mouth or rectally for limited periods of up to 2 weeks. It is often given for only 5 to 6 days in each week, which allows the patient to assess whether the cluster period has ended. Other drugs that have been used, either alone or with ergotamine, include verapamil, lithium carbonate, and prednisolone. Lithium may be particularly useful for the chronic form of the disorder. Methysergide and pizotifen have also been tried.

Chronic paroxysmal hemicrania is a rare variant of cluster headache in which patients experience numerous attacks every day for years. One of its features, which may be diagnostic, is its invariable response to indometacin.

References.
1. Kudrow L. Treatment of cluster headache. *Headache Q* 1993; **4** (suppl 2): 42–7.
2. Kumar KL, Cooney TG. Headaches. *Med Clin North Am* 1995; **79:** 261–86.

Migraine
Migraine is characterised by recurrent attacks of headache which typically last 4 to 72 hours. Attacks persisting for longer than 72 hours are referred to as status migrainosus. The headache is usually a unilateral pulsating pain that is aggravated by movement and is usually of sufficient severity to disturb or prevent daily activities. It is frequently accompanied by nausea, vomiting, or other gastrointestinal disturbances and there may be photophobia and phonophobia. Migraine with aura (classic migraine) is characterised by an aura consisting of visual or sensory symptoms that lasts less than an hour. The headache usually follows the aura directly, or within 1 hour, but may begin simultaneously with the aura. In addition, aura can occur without headache. Migraine without aura (common migraine) is the more common form occurring in about 75% of patients with migraine. Premonitory symptoms may occur before a migraine attack (with or without aura). Familial hemiplegic migraine is a rare syndrome in which migraine with aura may be preceded or accompanied by aphasia, confusion, and hemiparesis. Basilar migraine is another rare form of migraine with aura in which there may be disturbances of the brain stem or occipital lobes accompanied by symptoms such as impairment of consciousness, vertigo, ataxia, dysarthria, and diplopia.

Migraine is described as a neurovascular headache. Traditionally, intracranial vasoconstriction was considered responsible for the aura and extracranial vasodilatation for the headache. However, it appears that vascular events may be secondary to neuropathic changes and the liberation of vasoactive substances including serotonin (5-HT), catecholamines, histamine, kinins, neuropeptides, and prostaglandins.

There are several factors which may precipitate migraine attacks. These include anxiety, physical and emotional stress, a change in sleep pattern, bright lights, fasting, some foods, and menstruation. Migraine may also be precipitated by drugs including combined oral contraceptives and oestrogens, and glyceryl trinitrate. The frequency of migraine attacks can be reduced if such precipitating factors can be identified and avoided. Quiet, darkness, and sleep can ease an attack, with sleep heralding recovery.

Treatment. There is evidence that therapy tailored to the severity of individual disease from the outset (stratified care) is preferable to beginning with simple analgesics and adjusting treatment subsequently according to response (step strategy).

Simple analgesics (paracetamol or aspirin and other NSAIDs) are effective if taken at the earliest signs of an attack. Weak opioid analgesics such as codeine are sometimes included in oral compound analgesic preparations, but many consider that opioids are best avoided, especially in patients who experience frequent headaches. Other drugs used with analgesics in antimigraine preparations have included the sympathomimetic vasoconstrictor isometheptene and sedatives such as dichloralphenazone.

If the initial treatment of migraine is delayed, absorption of oral drugs may be compromised by gastric stasis and nausea and vomiting, which commonly develop as the at-

tack progresses. Antiemetics are often included in compound antimigraine preparations; those commonly used include buclizine, cyclizine, and the prokinetic drugs metoclopramide and domperidone. Prokinetic drugs also have the advantage of promoting gastric emptying and normal peristalsis. Dispersible and effervescent analgesic preparations are preferable because of their more rapid absorption. If nausea and vomiting is prominent rectal administration may be necessary.

Attacks not responding to simple analgesics or NSAIDs may be treated with specific antimigraine drugs such as the selective serotonin (5-HT$_1$) agonists (e.g. sumatriptan) and the ergot derivatives ergotamine and dihydroergotamine; poor absorption and adverse effects limit the use of ergot derivatives and selective serotonin (5-HT$_1$) agonists are generally preferred.

Sumatriptan was the first serotonin (5-HT$_1$) agonist developed and is available for oral, intranasal, or subcutaneous use. A single dose is usually administered at the first sign of a migraine attack, but it is also effective if used during the established headache phase of an attack. There is some evidence that it is not effective if administered in the aura phase of migraine with aura. Some patients experience recurrence of the headache within 24 to 48 hours, and often respond to a second dose. Other available selective serotonin (5-HT$_1$) agonists include almotriptan, naratriptan, rizatriptan, and zolmitriptan, which may all be given orally.

If ergotamine is used it should be given at the first warning of an attack; the earlier it is given, the more effective the treatment. Since its oral bioavailability is poor and may be reduced further during a migraine attack, ergotamine has sometimes been administered in sublingual or rectal preparations or by oral inhaler. Ergotamine can also exacerbate nausea and vomiting necessitating antiemetics such as metoclopramide or domperidone; if nausea and vomiting becomes severe the phenothiazine antiemetics chlorpromazine or prochlorperazine may be given. Dihydroergotamine may be of use if parenteral treatment is required; it can also be given intranasally but there is less experience with this route.

Patients who rapidly develop severe migraine may be given dihydroergotamine or sumatriptan parenterally. If there is no response to these drugs dopamine antagonists such as metoclopramide, chlorpromazine, or prochlorperazine given parenterally may be effective in relieving the pain of acute migraine attacks. Prolonged attacks (status migrainosus) may require intravenous administration of dihydroergotamine with metoclopramide. Other drugs that may be given alone or in combination include prochlorperazine, chlorpromazine, corticosteroids, or pethidine. Lignocaine [lidocaine] has been given intravenously for the emergency treatment of migraine; intranasal lignocaine [lidocaine] has also been tried. The opioid agonist-antagonist butorphanol, administered by nasal spray, has been advocated, but its place in therapy, if any, remains to be established.

Prophylactic treatment should be considered for patients in whom abortive measures are ineffective or migraine attacks occur frequently, or for those with less frequent but severe or prolonged attacks. Some recommend prophylaxis if attacks occur more often than once or twice a month. Prophylaxis can reduce the severity and/or frequency of attacks but does not eliminate them completely and patients still need additional abortive or symptomatic treatment. Drugs suggested for prophylaxis have a range of actions which reflects uncertainty over the pathogenesis of migraine. It is important to give prophylactic drugs for an adequate period before assessing their efficacy. Once an optimum effect has been achieved the need for continuing prophylaxis should be reviewed at intervals of about 3 to 6 months.

The main prophylactic drugs are beta blockers, pizotifen, and tricyclic antidepressants. Propranolol is considered by many to be the prophylactic drug of choice. Lethargy appears to be the most common adverse effect. Other beta blockers reported to be effective are those that, like propranolol, possess no intrinsic sympathomimetic activity, which include atenolol, metoprolol, nadolol, and timolol. The potential for beta blockers to interact with some serotonin (5-HT$_1$) agonists and ergotamine should be borne in mind. Pizotifen, an antihistamine and serotonin antagonist, is one of the main alternatives to propranolol. Drowsiness and increased appetite with weight gain may be a problem, although these may be overcome to some extent by gradual increases in dose and administration at night. Tricyclic antidepressants, particularly amitriptyline, given in gradually increasing doses at night are useful for preventing migraine, especially in patients who also have depression or tension-type headache, although antimuscarinic side-effects may occur.

Other drugs have been used for the prophylaxis of migraine: of the drugs with calcium-channel blocking activity, flunarizine appears to be effective and verapamil may be useful, but evidence for the efficacy of other calcium-channel blockers such as diltiazem, nifedipine, or nimodipine is less convincing; valproate, a gamma-aminobutyric acid (GABA) agonist, may be effective; NSAIDs may be worth trying. The use of methysergide, a potent serotonin antagonist, has declined because of serious side-effects, in particular retroperitoneal fibrosis. MAOIs such as phenelzine have been used occasionally but are best reserved for severe cases refractory to other forms of prophylactic treatment. Cyproheptadine, an antihistamine and serotonin antagonist, has been used for migraine prophylaxis, particularly in children. Other drugs used for the prophylaxis of migraine have included clonidine, cyclandelate, indoramin, and feverfew, and the ergot derivatives lisuride and metergoline. Promising results have been seen with riboflavin; magnesium (as the citrate) may also be of use.

References.
1. Lance JW. Treatment of migraine. *Lancet* 1992; **339:** 1207–9.
2. MacGregor EA. Prescribing for migraine. *Prescribers' J* 1993; **33:** 50–8.
3. Solomon GD. Therapeutic advances in migraine. *J Clin Pharmacol* 1993; **33:** 200–209.
4. Welch KMA. Drug therapy of migraine. *N Engl J Med* 1993; **329:** 1476–83.
5. Kumar KL, Cooney TG. Headaches. *Med Clin North Am* 1995; **79:** 261–86.
6. Goadsby PJ, Olesen J. Diagnosis and management of migraine. *BMJ* 1996; **312:** 1279–83.
7. Capobianco DJ, *et al.* An overview of the diagnosis and pharmacologic treatment of migraine. *Mayo Clin Proc* 1996; **71:** 1055–66.
8. Pryse-Phillips WEM, *et al.* Guidelines for the diagnosis and management of migraine in clinical practice. *Can Med Assoc J* 1997; **156:** 1273–87.
9. Ferrari MD. Migraine. *Lancet* 1998; **351:** 1043–51.
10. Anonymous. Managing migraine. *Drug Ther Bull* 1998; **36:** 41–4.
11. Anonymous. New "triptans" and other drugs for migraine. *Med Lett Drugs Ther* 1998; **40:** 97–100.
12. Diener H-C, *et al.* A practical guide to the management and prevention of migraine. *Drugs* 1998; **56:** 811–24.
13. Bartleson JD. Treatment of migraine headaches. *Mayo Clin Proc* 1999; **74:** 702–8.
14. Tfelt-Hansen P, *et al.* Triptans in migraine: a comparative review of pharmacology, pharmacokinetics and efficacy. *Drugs* 2000; **60:** 1259–87.
15. Lipton RB, *et al.* Stratified care vs step care strategies for migraine: the Disability in Strategies of Care (DISC) study, a randomised trial. *JAMA* 2000; **284:** 2599–2605.

Post-dural puncture headache

For the management of headache associated with lumbar puncture or spinal anaesthesia, see Post-dural Puncture Headache under Local Anaesthetics, p.1303.

Tension-type headache

Tension-type headaches, also referred to as muscle-contraction headaches, are probably the commonest form of headache. They are characterised by bilateral pain, which unlike migraine is continuous and non-pulsatile. The pain is often described by the patient as feeling like a tight band pressed around the head. Headaches of this type may be precipitated by many factors including psychosocial stress or muscular stress. Many patients also have associated symptoms of anxiety or depression. Also tension-type headaches and migraine frequently co-exist when they are often referred to as combination or mixed headaches. Some patients may only experience isolated acute attacks of tension-type headache (episodic tension-type headache), but others may develop chronic tension-type headache which is difficult to treat.

Treatment is aimed at removing the underlying causes where these can be identified. Simple massage may help if muscle contraction is a prominent component of the pain. Non-opioid analgesics, such as aspirin or other NSAIDs and paracetamol, may be tried for individual acute attacks of headache, but analgesic overuse must be avoided as this can lead to chronic headache resistant to other measures (see Analgesic-induced Headache, above). Opioids alone or in combination preparations with other analgesics should be avoided. Hypnotics or sedatives have sometimes been used in combination preparations with analgesics in the management of tension-type headache which disrupts sleep but, because of the potential for abuse, they should be avoided in chronic

headaches. Muscle relaxants appear to have little place in the management of tension-type headache; although some patients may respond results are generally disappointing. Prophylaxis is preferable to regular short-term use of analgesics in controlling chronic tension-type headache. Tricyclic antidepressants, particularly amitriptyline, are generally considered as first choice, although benefit is rarely complete. The mode of action is unclear and appears to be independent of any antidepressant action. In most cases, improvement is seen with low doses, but full antidepressant doses are necessary in the presence of underlying depression. Addition of a beta blocker such as propranolol may sometimes be of benefit for patients with some migraine features. Other drugs that have been tried include valproate.

References.
1. Clough C. Non-migrainous headaches: classification and management. *BMJ* 1989; **299:** 70–2.
2. Olesen J, Schoenen J, eds. *Tension-type headache: classification, mechanisms, and treatment.* New York: Raven Press, 1993.
3. Silberstein SD. Tension-type and chronic daily headache. *Neurology* 1993; **43:** 1644–9.
4. Kumar KL, Cooney TG. Headaches. *Med Clin North Am* 1995; **79:** 261–86.
5. Anonymous. Management of tension-type headache. *Drug Ther Bull* 1999; **37:** 41–4.

Almotriptan Malate (20397-j)

Almotriptan Malate (BANM, USAN, rINNM).
LAS-31416 (almotriptan); PNU-180638E (almotriptan malate). 1-[({3-[2-(Dimethylamino)ethyl]indol-5-yl}methyl)sulfonyl]pyrrolidine malate (1:1).
$C_{17}H_{25}N_3O_2S,C_4H_6O_5 = 469.6.$
CAS — 154323-57-6 (almotriptan); 181183-52-8 (almotriptan malate).

Almotriptan malate 17.5 mg is approximately equivalent to 12.5 mg of almotriptan.

Adverse Effects and Precautions

As for Sumatriptan, p.456.

Almotriptan should not be used in patients with severe hepatic impairment since clearance is likely to be markedly impaired, and should be given with caution to patients with mild to moderate degrees of hepatic impairment. The dose of almotriptan should be reduced in patients with severe renal impairment.

The manufacturer recommends caution during breast feeding; distribution of almotriptan and its metabolites into milk has been reported in *rats*.

Interactions

As for Sumatriptan, p.457.

Pharmacokinetics

After oral administration, peak plasma-almotriptan concentrations are obtained in about 1 to 3 hours, with a bioavailability of about 70%. Protein binding is about 35%. Almotriptan is metabolised, primarily by monoamine oxidase type A to the inactive indole acetic acid derivative and to a lesser extent by cytochrome P450 isoenzymes CYP3A4 and CYP2D6 to the inactive gamma-aminobutyric acid derivative. More than 75% of an oral dose is excreted in the urine and the remainder in faeces. Approximately 40 to 50% of the dose in the urine and 5% in the faeces is excreted as unchanged drug. The plasma elimination half-life is about 3.5 hours in healthy subjects, increasing to about 7 hours in severe renal impairment.

Distribution into milk has been demonstrated in studies in *rats*.

Uses and Administration

Almotriptan malate is a selective serotonin (5-HT₁) agonist with actions and uses similar to those of sumatriptan (p.457). It is used for the acute treatment of the headache phase of migraine attacks. It should not be used prophylactically. Almotriptan is given by mouth as the malate, and doses are expressed in terms of the base.

The usual initial dose of almotriptan is 12.5 mg in the UK and 6.25 or 12.5 mg in the USA. If this is ineffective, a second dose should not be taken for the same attack. If the headache recurs within 24 hours, a second dose may be taken after an interval of at least 2 hours. No more than 2 doses should be taken in a 24-hour period. In patients with hepatic impairment or severe renal impairment, no more than 12.5 mg should be taken in 24 hours; a starting dose of 6.25 mg may be used. Almotriptan is contra-indicated in patients with severe hepatic disease.

◊ References.
1. Holm KJ, Spencer CM. Almotriptan. *CNS Drugs* 1999; **11:** 159–64.
2. Pascual J, *et al.* Consistent efficacy and tolerability of almotriptan in the acute treatment of multiple migraine attacks: results of a large, randomized, double-blind, placebo-controlled study. *Cephalalgia* 2000; **20:** 588–96.
3. Cabarrocas X, *et al.* Long-term efficacy and safety of oral almotriptan: interim analysis of a 1-year open study. *Headache* 2001; **41:** 57–62.

Preparations

Proprietary Preparations (details are given in Part 3)
UK: Almogran; *USA:* Axert.

Alpiropride (11925-j)

Alpiropride (rINN).
(±)-N-[(1-Allyl-2-pyrrolidinyl)methyl]-4-amino-5-(methylsulfamoyl)-o-anisamide.
$C_{17}H_{26}N_4O_4S = 382.5.$
CAS — 81982-32-3.

Profile

Alpiropride is a dopamine antagonist that was formerly given by mouth for the treatment and prophylaxis of migraine.

Dihydroergotamine (11340-l)

Dihydroergotamine (BAN, rINN).
(5'S,8R)-5'-Benzyl-9,10-dihydro-12'-hydroxy-2'-methyl-3',6',18-trioxoergotaman.
$C_{33}H_{37}N_5O_5 = 583.7.$
CAS — 511-12-6.
ATC — N02CA01.

Dihydroergotamine Mesilate (1504-d)

Dihydroergotamine Mesilate (BANM, rINNM).
Dihydroergotamine Mesylate (USAN); Dihydroergotamine Methanesulphonate; Dihydroergotamini Mesilas. (5'S,8R)-5'-Benzyl-9,10-dihydro-12'-hydroxy-2'-methyl-3',6',18-trioxoergotaman methanesulphonate.
$C_{33}H_{37}N_5O_5,CH_4O_3S = 679.8.$
CAS — 6190-39-2.
Pharmacopoeias. In *Eur.* (see p.vi), *Jpn, Pol.,* and *US.*

Pharmacopoeial description

Ph. Eur.: Colourless crystals or a white or almost white crystalline powder. Slightly soluble in water and in alcohol; sparingly soluble in methyl alcohol. A 0.1% solution in water has a pH of 4.4 to 5.4. Protect from light.

USP 25: A white to slightly yellowish powder, or off-white to faintly red powder, having a faint odour. Soluble 1 in 125 of water, 1 in 90 of alcohol, 1 in 175 of chloroform, and 1 in 2600 of ether. pH of a 0.1% solution in water is between 4.4 and 5.4. Protect from light.

Dihydroergotamine Tartrate (1505-n)

Dihydroergotamine Tartrate (BANM, rINNM).
Dihydroergotamini Tartras.
$(C_{33}H_{37}N_5O_5)_2,C_4H_6O_6 = 1317.4.$
CAS — 5989-77-5.
Pharmacopoeias. In *Eur.* (see p.vi).

Pharmacopoeial description

Ph. Eur.: Colourless crystals or a white or almost white crystalline powder. Very slightly soluble in water; sparingly soluble in alcohol. A 0.1% suspension in water has a pH of 4.0 to 5.5. Protect from light.

Adverse Effects and Treatment

As for Ergotamine Tartrate, p.452, although vasoconstriction may be less pronounced and the frequency of nausea and vomiting lower with dihydroergotamine mesilate than with ergotamine tartrate. Dihydroergotamine does not appear to produce physical dependence.

Effects on the cardiovascular system. There are conflicting reports on the risk of vasospasm in patients given dihydroergotamine with heparin for thromboembolism prophylaxis. Vasospastic or necrotic reactions have been reported on several occasions during such therapy.[1-4] In an Austrian study of 147 290 patients given drug prophylaxis for thromboembolism, complications attributable to ergotism were seen in 142 of 61 092 (0.23%) who received dihydroergotamine and heparin.[5] Others,[6] however, observed only one case of vasospasm in 5100 trauma patients (0.02%) given the combination. In 1989 the Swedish Adverse Drug Reactions Advisory Committee reported[7] that up to the end of September 1987 the manufacturer had received 201 reports of vasospastic reactions associated with the use of Orstanorm (dihydroergotamine + lignocaine [lidocaine]) with heparin. Permanent damage occurred in 59% of these patients. Vasospastic reactions had occurred more frequently in patients who had undergone surgery for trauma and the prognosis for such patients was generally poorer than for others. Since the risk of permanent damage appeared to be related to treatment length the Committee recommended that this preparation should not be given for more than 7 days. The possibility of such reactions and the contra-indications of dihydroergotamine should be borne in mind when employing this form of prophylaxis (see Venous Thromboembolism, under Uses, below).

1. van den Berg E, *et al.* Ergotism leading to threatened limb amputation or to death in two patients given heparin-dihydroergotamine prophylaxis. *Lancet* 1982; **i:** 955–6.
2. van den Berg E, *et al.* Vascular spasm during thromboembolism prophylaxis with heparin-dihydroergotamine. *Lancet* 1982; **ii:** 268–9.
3. Monreal M, *et al.* Skin and muscle necrosis during heparin-dihydroergotamine prophylaxis. *Lancet* 1984; **ii:** 820.

4. Kilroy RA, *et al.* Vascular spasm during heparin-dihydroergotamine prophylaxis. *Clin Pharm* 1987; **6**: 575–7.
5. Gatterer R. Ergotism as complication of thromboembolic prophylaxis with heparin and dihydroergotamine. *Lancet* 1986; **ii**: 638–9.
6. Schlag G, *et al.* Risk/benefit of heparin-dihydroergotamine thromboembolic prophylaxis. *Lancet* 1986; **ii**: 1465.
7. Swedish Adverse Drug Reaction Advisory Committee. Dihydroergotamine + lidocaine – vasospasm. *Bull Swed Adverse Drug React Advisory Committee* 1989; (54): 1.

Fibrosis. For reference to fibrosis associated with the administration of dihydroergotamine, see Methysergide Maleate, p.454.

Precautions

As for Ergotamine Tartrate, p.452. Contra-indications and precautions in cardiovascular disorders resemble those which apply for serotonin (5-HT$_1$) agonists (see Sumatriptan Succinate, p.456).

Porphyria. Dihydroergotamine has been associated with acute attacks of porphyria and is considered unsafe in porphyric patients.

Interactions

Interactions involving those ergot alkaloids used primarily in the management of migraine are discussed under ergotamine (p.452). References specific to dihydroergotamine may be found there under the headings Antibacterials and Glyceryl Trinitrate. Concurrent administration of other vasoconstrictive drugs, including supplementary antimigraine treatment with ergotamine or sumatriptan, should be avoided.

Pharmacokinetics

Peak plasma-dihydroergotamine concentrations have been attained within about 2 to 3 hours after oral administration, about 30 minutes after intramuscular injection, about 15 to 45 minutes after subcutaneous injection, and about 45 to 55 minutes after administration by intranasal spray. However, the bioavailability of dihydroergotamine after oral administration is very low; values ranging from less than 0.1 to 1.5% have been reported. Although dihydroergotamine is incompletely absorbed from the gastrointestinal tract, the low bioavailability is considered to be determined primarily by extensive first-pass hepatic metabolism. It is 93% bound to plasma proteins.

Dihydroergotamine undergoes extensive metabolism, the major metabolite, 8′-β-hydroxydihydroergotamine, being pharmacologically active. Plasma concentrations of this metabolite are greater than those of dihydroergotamine. A further oxidation step produces 8′,10′-dihydroxydihydroergotamine which is also pharmacologically active. Other metabolites are also formed. Most of a dose is excreted as metabolites, mainly in the bile; 5 to 10% is excreted in the urine of which only trace amounts are of unchanged drug. The elimination of dihydroergotamine is biphasic; half-lives of about 1 to 2 hours and 22 to 32 hours have been reported for the 2 phases, respectively.

◊ References.

1. Bobik A, *et al.* Low oral bioavailability of dihydroergotamine and first-pass extraction in patients with orthostatic hypotension. *Clin Pharmacol Ther* 1981; **30**: 673–9.
2. Little PJ, *et al.* Bioavailability of dihydroergotamine in man. *Br J Clin Pharmacol* 1982; **13**: 785–90.
3. Lindblad B, *et al.* The pharmacokinetics of subcutaneous dihydroergotamine with and without a dextran 70 infusion. *Eur J Clin Pharmacol* 1983; **24**: 813–18.
4. Maurer G, Frick W. Elucidation of the structure and receptor binding studies of the major primary, metabolite of dihydroergotamine in man. *Eur J Clin Pharmacol* 1984; **26**: 463–70.
5. Müller-Schweinitzer E. Pharmacological actions of the main metabolites of dihydroergotamine. *Eur J Clin Pharmacol* 1984; **26**: 699–705.
6. Aellig WH, Rosenthaler J. Venoconstrictor effects of dihydroergotamine after intranasal and intramuscular administration. *Eur J Clin Pharmacol* 1986; **30**: 581–4.
7. de Marées H, *et al.* Relationship between the venoconstrictor activity of dihydroergotamine and its pharmacokinetics during acute and chronic oral dosing. *Eur J Clin Pharmacol* 1986; **30**: 685–9.
8. Humbert H, *et al.* Human pharmacokinetics of dihydroergotamine administered by nasal spray. *Clin Pharmacol Ther* 1996; **60**: 265–75.

Uses and Administration

Dihydroergotamine is a semisynthetic ergot alkaloid that has weaker oxytocic and vasoconstrictor effects than ergotamine (p.453). Its activity as a 5-HT$_1$ ago-

The symbol † denotes a preparation no longer actively marketed

nist is believed to contribute to its antimigraine action. It is used in the treatment of migraine and cluster headache, and in the treatment of orthostatic hypotension. It has also been used for the prophylaxis of venous thromboembolism (see below).

Dihydroergotamine is commonly used as the mesilate and is usually given by subcutaneous, intramuscular, or intravenous injection, although it may also be given as a nasal spray or by mouth.

For the treatment of migraine and to terminate an acute attack of cluster headache, dihydroergotamine mesilate is usually given by subcutaneous or intramuscular injection in doses of 1 mg repeated, if necessary, after 30 to 60 minutes up to a maximum daily dose of 3 mg. If a more rapid effect is desired it may be administered intravenously in doses of 0.5 mg up to a maximum daily dose of 2 mg. The total weekly dose given by any route of injection should not exceed 6 mg. The usual nasal dose of dihydroergotamine mesilate for an acute attack of migraine is 0.5 mg sprayed into each nostril as a 0.4% solution followed after 15 minutes by an additional 0.5 mg in each nostril. A total intranasal dose of 2 mg per attack should not be exceeded. The maximum dose in 24 hours is 2 mg, and in a 7-day period is 8 mg. In some countries it is given by mouth; up to 10 mg daily has been given by mouth for the treatment of acute attacks of migraine. Lower oral doses have been given in some countries for migraine prophylaxis.

Dihydroergotamine mesilate has also been used alone or with etilefrine hydrochloride (p.888) in the treatment of orthostatic hypotension in usual doses of up to 10 mg daily by mouth in divided doses.

Dihydroergotamine tartrate has been used for indications similar to those of the mesilate.

Analgesic-induced headache. Dihydroergotamine may be used in the treatment of analgesic-induced headache (p.449), including symptoms of ergotamine withdrawal.

Migraine and cluster headache. Sumatriptan is often the treatment of choice to abort acute attacks of migraine (p.449) that do not respond to simple analgesic preparations; parenteral dihydroergotamine is an alternative for patients who develop severe or refractory migraine.[1,2] Dihydroergotamine is used similarly in the treatment of cluster headache (p.449), usually in emergency settings, where it is given to patient individual headache attacks. Although dihydroergotamine is usually given by injection, preparations for intranasal[3,4] administration are also available; in some countries, it is given orally. In a comparative study, relief of migraine was slower after subcutaneous dihydroergotamine than after subcutaneous sumatriptan, but headache recurred less often.[5] In another study, intranasal dihydroergotamine was not as effective as subcutaneous sumatriptan.[4]

1. Scott AK. Dihydroergotamine: a review of its use in the treatment of migraine and other headaches. *Clin Neuropharmacol* 1992; **15**: 289–96.
2. Silberstein SD, Young WB. Safety and efficacy of ergotamine tartrate and dihydroergotamine in the treatment of migraine and status migrainosus. *Neurology* 1995; **45**: 577–84.
3. Ziegler D, *et al.* Dihydroergotamine nasal spray for the acute treatment of migraine. *Neurology* 1994; **44**: 447–53.
4. Touchon J, *et al.* A comparison of subcutaneous sumatriptan and dihydroergotamine nasal spray in the acute treatment of migraine. *Neurology* 1996; **47**: 361–5.
5. Winner P, *et al.* A double-blind study of subcutaneous dihydroergotamine vs subcutaneous sumatriptan in the treatment of acute migraine. *Arch Neurol* 1996; **53**: 180–4.

Orthostatic hypotension. Dihydroergotamine may be of use in patients with refractory orthostatic hypotension (p.1070). It is sometimes used in preparations with sympathomimetics such as etilefrine. After parenteral administration of dihydroergotamine, standing blood pressure is increased, but total peripheral resistance and supine blood pressure are also increased.[1] It does not prevent postprandial hypotension, presumably because it does not constrict the splanchnic veins, although the administration of caffeine with dihydroergotamine may overcome this problem. The main disadvantage of dihydroergotamine, however, is that it is ineffective, or at best weakly effective, when given by mouth although there has been some evidence that oral ergotamine tartrate may be of value.

Dihydroergotamine has also been suggested for use in the prevention of hypotension associated with epidural anaesthesia,[2] the usual management of which is discussed under Treatment of Adverse Effects, p.1303. It has also been tried in the management of hypotension associated with haemodialysis.[3]

1. Anonymous. Management of orthostatic hypotension. *Lancet* 1987; **i**: 197–8.

2. Mattila M, *et al.* Dihydroergotamine in the prevention of hypotension associated with extradural anaesthesia. *Br J Anaesth* 1985; **57**: 976–82.
3. Milutinovic S. Dihydroergotamin in der Behandlung von Patienten mit symptomatischer Hypotonie während Dauerhämodialyse. *Arzneimittelforschung* 1987; **37**: 554–6.

Venous thromboembolism. Standard prophylaxis for surgical patients at high risk of venous thromboembolism is usually with heparin (p.817). Dihydroergotamine can reduce venous stasis by vasoconstriction of capacitance vessels and has enhanced postoperative prophylaxis when used in association with heparin.[1] A suggested dose is dihydroergotamine mesilate 500 μg with heparin 5000 units, both given subcutaneously 2 hours before surgery. This regimen has then been given every 8 to 12 hours for 5 to 14 days depending on the risk of thrombosis. Some workers have investigated the use of dihydroergotamine with low-molecular-weight heparin fractions. Such a combination has been demonstrated to be of similar efficacy to dihydroergotamine with heparin[2,3] but might offer a more convenient dosing schedule. However, although dihydroergotamine might enhance the effect of heparin, a US National Institutes of Health consensus conference warned of the potential risk associated with its vasoconstrictive effects, and the contra-indications to its use.[4] In 1989 the Swedish Adverse Drug Reactions Advisory Committee recommended that dihydroergotamine with heparin should not be given for more than 7 days (see Effects on the Cardiovascular System, under Adverse Effects, above).

1. Lindblad B. Prophylaxis of postoperative thromboembolism with low dose heparin alone or in combination with dihydroergotamine: a review. *Acta Chir Scand* 1988; (suppl 543): 31–42.
2. Sasahara AA, *et al.* Low molecular weight heparin plus dihydroergotamine for prophylaxis of postoperative deep vein thrombosis. *Br J Surg* 1986; **73**: 697–700.
3. Haas S, *et al.* Prophylaxis of deep vein thrombosis in high risk patients undergoing total hip replacement with low molecular weight heparin plus dihydroergotamine. *Arzneimittelforschung* 1987; **37**: 839–43.
4. Consensus conference. Prevention of venous thrombosis and pulmonary embolism. *JAMA* 1986; **256**: 744–9.

Preparations

USP 25: Dihydroergotamine Mesylate Injection.

Proprietary Preparations (details are given in Part 3)
Aust.: Adhaegon; Detemes; Dihydergot; Divegal; Ergont; Ergovasan; Migranal; *Austral.:* Dihydergot; *Belg.:* Diergo; Dihydergot; Dystonal; Ikaran†; *Braz.:* Dihydergot; *Canad.:* Migranal; *Fin.:* Orstanorm; *Fr.:* Ikaran; Seglor; Tamik; *Ger.:* Agit; Angionorm; Clavigrenin; DET MS; DET MS spezial; DHE; Dihydergot; Dihytamin; Endophlebant; Ergomimet; Ergont; ergotam; Tonopres†; Verladyn; *Hong Kong:* Tamik; *Ital.:* Diidergot; Ikaran; Migranal; Seglor; *Neth.:* Dihydergot; Port.: Dihydergot; Seglor; *S.Afr.:* Dihydergot; *Spain:* Dihydergot; Tenuatina†; *Swed.:* Migranal; Orstanorm; *Switz.:* Dihydergot; Ergotonine; Ikaran; *Thai.:* Poligot; *UK:* Migranal†; *USA:* DHE; Migranal.

Multi-ingredient: *Aust.:* Agilan; Cedanon†; Defluina; Dihydergot; Effortil comp; Embolex; Hypodyn; Tonopan; Troparin compositum†; Veno; Venotop; *Braz.:* Cefalium; Cefaliv; Parcel; Tonopan; Vasofluina; *Fr.:* Diergo; *Ger.:* Agit plus; Dihydergot plus; Effortil plus; Embolex NM; Ergo-Lonarid PD; Ergolefrin; Ergomimet plus; Optalidon special NOC; Venelbin†; *Mex.:* Parsel; Tonopan; *Norw.:* Dihydergot†; *Spain:* Tonopan; *Switz.:* Dihydergot; Dihydergot plus; Effortil plus; Tonopan.

Eletriptan (18395-j)

Eletriptan *(BAN, rINN)*.

UK-116044. (R)-2-[3-(1-Methylpyrrolidin-2-ylmethyl)indol-5-yl]ethyl phenyl sulfone.

$C_{22}H_{26}N_2O_2S = 382.5$.

CAS — 143322-58-1 (eletriptan); 177834-92-3 (eletriptan hydrobromide).

NOTE. Eletriptan Hydrobromide is *USAN*.

Profile

Eletriptan is a selective serotonin (5-HT$_1$) agonist with actions similar to those of sumatriptan (p.456). It is used for the acute treatment of the headache phase of migraine attacks. It should not be used prophylactically. Eletriptan is given by mouth as the hydrobromide, but doses are expressed in terms of the base. The usual initial dose is 40 mg; if this is ineffective a second dose should not be taken for the same attack. If the headache recurs within 24 hours a second dose may be taken after an interval of at least 2 hours. Doses may be increased to 80 mg in patients who fail to respond to a trial of the lower dose. In patients with mild to moderate renal impairment an initial dose of 20 mg is recommended, increased if necessary to a maximum of 40 mg. Eletriptan is contra-indicated in patients with severe renal or severe hepatic impairment.

◊ References.

1. Pitei D, Hettiarachchi J. Efficacy of eletriptan in treating women with menstrually associated migraine and women on oral contraceptives or hormone replacement therapy. *Obstet Gynecol* 2000; **95** (suppl 1): S32.

Preparations

Proprietary Preparations (details are given in Part 3)
UK: Relpax.

Ergotamine Tartrate (1508-b)

Ergotamine Tartrate (BANM, rINNM).

Ergotamini Tartras. (5'S)-12'-Hydroxy-2'-methyl-5'-benzylergotaman-3',6',18-trione tartrate; (5'S)-12'-Hydroxy-2'-methyl-3',6',18-trioxo-5-benzylergotaman (+)-tartrate.

$(C_{33}H_{35}N_5O_5)_2,C_4H_6O_6 = 1313.4$.

CAS — 113-15-5 (ergotamine); 379-79-3 (ergotamine tartrate).

Pharmacopoeias. In Chin., Eur. (see p.vi), Int., Jpn, Pol., and US.

Pharmacopoeial description

Ph. Eur.: Slightly hygroscopic, colourless crystals or a white or almost white crystalline powder. It may contain 2 molecules of methanol of crystallisation. Slightly soluble in alcohol; practically insoluble in ether. Aqueous solutions slowly become cloudy owing to hydrolysis; this may be prevented by the addition of tartaric acid. A 0.25% suspension in water has a pH of 4.0 to 5.5. Store in airtight glass containers at a temperature of 2° to 8°. Protect from light.

USP 25: Colourless odourless crystals or a white or yellowish-white crystalline powder. Soluble 1 in about 3200 of water, but soluble 1 in about 500 of water in the presence of a slight excess of tartaric acid; soluble 1 in 500 of alcohol. Store at a temperature not exceeding 8°. Protect from light.

Stability in solution. References.
1. Kreilgård B, Kisbye J. Stability of ergotamine tartrate in aqueous solution. *Arch Pharm Chemi (Sci)* 1974; **2:** 1–13 and 38–49.

Adverse Effects

The adverse effects of ergotamine may be attributed either to its effects on the CNS, or to vasoconstriction of blood vessels and possible thrombus formation.

After therapeutic doses nausea and vomiting commonly occur as a result of the direct emetogenic effect of ergotamine; some patients may also experience abdominal pain. Weakness and muscle pains in the extremities and numbness and tingling of the fingers and toes may occur. There may occasionally be localised oedema and itching in hypersensitive patients. Treatment should be stopped if symptoms of vasoconstriction develop. Susceptible patients, especially those with severe infections, liver disease, kidney disease, or occlusive peripheral vascular disease, may show signs of acute or chronic poisoning with normal doses of ergotamine.

Symptoms of acute overdosage include nausea, vomiting, diarrhoea, extreme thirst, coldness, tingling, and itching of the skin, a rapid and weak pulse, hypotension, shock, confusion, convulsions, and unconsciousness; fatalities have been reported. Further symptoms of peripheral vasoconstriction or of cardiovascular disturbances, as seen in chronic ergotamine poisoning, may also occur but be delayed.

In chronic poisoning or ergotism, resulting from therapeutic overdosage or the use of ergotamine in susceptible patients, severe circulatory disturbances may develop. The extremities, especially the feet and legs, become numb, cold, tingling, and pale or cyanotic, with muscle pain; there may be no pulse in the affected limb. Eventually gangrene develops in the toes and sometimes the fingers. Anginal pain, tachycardia or bradycardia, and hypertension or hypotension have been reported. Myocardial infarction has occurred rarely. Pleural and peritoneal fibrosis may occur with excessive use. Chronic, intractable headache (rebound headache) may occur and is also a major withdrawal symptom following the development of ergotamine dependence (see under Precautions, below). Other adverse effects include confusion and convulsions. On rare occasions symptoms of vasoconstriction of blood vessels in the brain, eye, intestines, and kidneys occur. Anorectal ulceration sometimes leading to rectal necrosis and stenosis has been reported after excessive use of suppositories containing ergotamine.

Effects on the cardiovascular system. Reports of adverse cardiovascular effects associated with ergotamine, including mention of fatalities.
1. Joyce DA, Gubbay SS. Arterial complications of migraine treatment with methysergide and parenteral ergotamine. *BMJ* 1982; **285:** 260–1.
2. Corrocher R, et al. Multiple arterial stenoses in chronic ergot toxicity. *N Engl J Med* 1984; **310:** 261.
3. Fisher PE, et al. Ergotamine abuse and extra-hepatic portal hypertension. *Postgrad Med J* 1985; **61:** 461–3.

4. Deviere J, et al. Ischemic pancreatitis and hepatitis secondary to ergotamine poisoning. *J Clin Gastroenterol* 1987; **9:** 350–2.
5. Galer BS, et al. Myocardial ischemia related to ergot alkaloids: a case report and literature review. *Headache* 1991; **31:** 446–50.
6. Redfield MM, et al. Valve disease associated with ergot alkaloid use: echocardiographic and pathologic correlations. *Ann Intern Med* 1992; **117:** 50–2.
7. Lazarides MK, et al. Severe facial ischaemia caused by ergotism. *J Cardiovasc Surg* 1992; **33:** 383–5.
8. Hillis W, MacIntyre PD. Drug reactions: sumatriptan and chest pain. *Lancet* 1993; **341:** 1564–5. Correction. *ibid.;* **342:** 1310.

Fibrosis. For reference to fibrosis associated with the administration of ergotamine tartrate, see Methysergide Maleate, p.454.

Treatment of Adverse Effects

Treatment of acute poisoning with ergotamine is symptomatic. Following recent ingestion the stomach may be emptied by lavage; activated charcoal may be used to reduce absorption. In chronic poisoning, withdrawal of ergotamine may be all that is required in some patients.

In both acute and chronic poisoning, attempts must be made to maintain an adequate circulation to the affected parts in order to prevent the onset of gangrene. In severe arterial vasospasm vasodilators such as sodium nitroprusside by intravenous infusion have been given; heparin and dextran 40 have also been advocated to minimise the risk of thrombosis. Analgesics may be required for severe ischaemic pain.

◊ Sodium nitroprusside has been administered in severe ergotamine poisoning for its vasodilating and hypotensive actions; it should therefore be used with care if hypotension is a symptom of poisoning. It is usually given by intravenous infusion[1-4] although there have also been reports of intra-arterial infusion for ergotamine-induced ischaemia;[5,6] for details of precautions to be observed, see p.971.
Many other drugs have been used in the treatment of circulatory disturbances induced by ergotamine. These include captopril by mouth[7] and alprostadil by intra-arterial infusion.[8,9]
For reference to the ergotamine withdrawal syndrome see Dependence under Precautions, below.
1. Carliner NH, et al. Sodium nitroprusside treatment of ergotamine-induced peripheral ischemia. *JAMA* 1974; **277:** 308–9.
2. Andersen PK, et al. Sodium nitroprusside and epidural blockade in the treatment of ergotism. *N Engl J Med* 1977; **296:** 1271–3.
3. Eurin B, et al. Ergot and sodium nitroprusside. *N Engl J Med* 1978; **298:** 632–3.
4. Carr P. Self-induced myocardial infarction. *Postgrad Med J* 1981; **57:** 654–5.
5. O'Dell CW, et al. Sodium nitroprusside in the treatment of ergotism. *Radiology* 1977; **124:** 73–4.
6. Whitsett TL, et al. Nitroprusside reversal of ergotamine-induced ischemia. *Am Heart J* 1978; **96:** 700.
7. Zimran A, et al. Treatment with captopril for peripheral ischaemia induced by ergotamine. *BMJ* 1984; **288:** 364.
8. Levy JM, et al. Prostaglandin E₁ for alleviating symptoms of ergot intoxication: a case report. *Cardiovasc Intervent Radiol* 1984; **7:** 28–30.
9. Horstmann R, et al. Kritische Extremitätenischämie durch Ergotismus: Behandlung mit intraarterieller Prostaglandin-E₁-Infusion. *Dtsch Med Wochenschr* 1993; **118:** 1067–71.

Precautions

Ergotamine tartrate is contra-indicated in patients with severe or uncontrolled hypertension, severe or persistent sepsis, peripheral vascular disease, ischaemic heart disease, hyperthyroidism, or impaired hepatic or renal function. Ergotamine tartrate should be administered with care to patients with anaemia. It is contra-indicated in pregnancy because of its oxytocic effect (see also below). Ergotamine tartrate should be avoided in nursing mothers; the distribution of unchanged drug and metabolites into breast milk presents a risk of ergotism in the infant and repeated doses of ergotamine may impair lactation.

Patients should be warned to keep within the recommended dosage. Some symptoms of overdosage may mimic those of migraine. Numbness or tingling of the extremities generally indicates that ergotamine should be discontinued. Although ergotamine is used for limited periods in the prevention of episodic cluster headache, it should not be administered prophylactically in other circumstances, as prolonged use may give rise to gangrene. Ergotamine dependence has occurred following regular use of ergotamine tartrate even if dosage recommendations are adhered to (see below).

Dependence. Ergotamine dependence can develop insidiously when ergotamine tartrate is used for more than 2 days a week, even if total daily or weekly dosage recommendations are observed.[1] Individual reports indicate a state of addiction

characterised by a predictable and irresistible pattern of drug usage, the development of tolerance to adverse effects, and a syndrome of withdrawal on discontinuing the drug. Ergotamine-dependent patients suffer from daily, or almost daily, migraine headaches, often referred to as 'analgesic-induced headaches' or 'rebound headaches', which are only alleviated by ergotamine. An intensifying headache in association with autonomic disturbances occurs within 24 to 48 hours of withdrawal of ergotamine and may continue for 72 hours or longer. As with other analgesic-induced headaches (p.449), supportive and symptomatic measures should be taken to treat the withdrawal syndrome.
1. Saper JR. Ergotamine dependency—a review. *Headache* 1987; **27:** 435–8.

Porphyria. Ergotamine tartrate has been associated with acute attacks of porphyria and is considered unsafe in porphyric patients.

Pregnancy. Ergotamine is contra-indicated in pregnancy because of its oxytocic effect. Jejunal atresia has been reported[1] in an infant born prematurely to a woman who had taken ergotamine tartrate 6 to 8 mg daily, as Cafergot tablets, throughout her pregnancy.
Accidental administration of ergotamine 2 mg in the form of a Cafergot suppository to a patient at 39 weeks of pregnancy caused uterine contractions and fetal tachycardia.[2] An emergency caesarean section was undertaken because of suspected placental abruption but no clear signs of retroplacental haemorrhage were found. The neonate recovered quickly after delivery and had developed normally during the next 10 years.
1. Graham JM, et al. Jejunal atresia associated with Cafergot ingestion during pregnancy. *Clin Pediatr (Phila)* 1983; **22:** 226–8.
2. de Groot ANJA, et al. Ergotamine-induced fetal stress: review of side effects of ergot alkaloids during pregnancy. *Eur J Obstet Gynecol Reprod Biol* 1993; **51:** 73–7.

Interactions

The vasoconstrictor effects of ergotamine are enhanced by sympathomimetics such as adrenaline [epinephrine]. There is also an increased risk of peripheral vasoconstriction during concomitant administration of ergotamine and beta blockers. Administration of ergotamine with a macrolide antibiotic such as erythromycin has produced ergotism. There is also a risk of ergotism if ergotamine is given with the HIV-protease inhibitors amprenavir, indinavir, nelfinavir, ritonavir, and possibly saquinavir. Ergotamine should not be given until at least 6 hours after stopping a serotonin (5-HT₁) agonist such as sumatriptan, since there is an additional risk of prolonged vasospastic reactions (see also p.457). Conversely, a delay is advised before starting a serotonin agonist in patients who have been receiving ergotamine: sumatriptan or rizatriptan should not be given until at least 24 hours, and zolmitriptan until at least 6 hours, after stopping the use of preparations containing ergotamine.

Antibacterials. Acute reactions ranging from minor ergotism[1] to severe vasospasm[2] have been reported in patients given erythromycin in addition to ergotamine. There is also a report of acute ergotism in 2 patients receiving ergotamine tartrate and troleandomycin.[3] The theoretical possibility exists that there may be a similar interaction with azithromycin. Ergotism has also been reported in patients receiving erythromycin[4] or troleandomycin[5] in conjunction with dihydroergotamine.
1. Lagier G, et al. Un cas d'ergotisme mineur semblant en rapport avec une potentialisation de l'ergotamine par l'éthylsuccinate d'érythromycine. *Therapie* 1979; **34:** 515–21.
2. Ghali R, et al. Erythromycin-associated ergotamine intoxication: arteriophysiologic and electrophysiologic analysis of a rare cause of severe ischemia of the lower extremities and associated ischemic neuropathy. *Ann Vasc Surg* 1993; **7:** 291–6.
3. Matthews NT, Havill JH. Ergotism with therapeutic doses of ergotamine tartrate. *N Z Med J* 1979; **89:** 476–7.
4. Leroy F, et al. Dihydroergotamine-erythromycin-induced ergotism. *Ann Intern Med* 1988; **109:** 249.
5. Franco A, et al. Ergotisme aigu par association dihydroergotamine-triacétyloléandomycine. *Nouv Presse Med* 1978; **7:** 205.

Antimigraine drugs. Arterial occlusion has been reported[1] in 2 patients taking methysergide and a high parenteral dosage of ergotamine concomitantly for cluster headache; the combination should be avoided. Administration of ergotamine as supplementary antimigraine medication in patients receiving dihydroergotamine is not recommended.
For reports of arterial vasoconstriction in patients taking beta blockers and antimigraine drugs, see below. See also above for a comment on the risk of vasospastic reactions with serotonin (5-HT₁) agonists such as sumatriptan.
1. Joyce DA, Gubbay SS. Arterial complications of migraine treatment with methysergide and parenteral ergotamine. *BMJ* 1982; **285:** 260–1.

Antivirals. Reports of ergotism in 5 patients who received concomitant treatment with combination antiviral treatment for HIV infection and ergotamine. It was suggested that the ergotism might have been caused by inhibition of ergotamine metabolism by ritonavir in 3 cases,[1-3] indinavir in one,[4] and nelfinavir[5] in the other.

The metabolism of ergot alkaloids may be inhibited by efavirenz (p.620).

1. Caballero-Granado FJ, et al. Ergotism related to concurrent administration of ergotamine tartrate and ritonavir in an AIDS patient. Antimicrob Agents Chemother 1997; 41: 1207.
2. Montero A, et al. Leg ischemia in a patient receiving ritonavir and ergotamine. Ann Intern Med 1999; 130: 329–30.
3. Liandet L, et al. Severe ergotism associated with interaction between ritonavir and ergotamine. BMJ 1999; 318: 771.
4. Rosenthal E, et al. Ergotism related to concurrent administration of ergotamine tartrate and indinavir. JAMA 1999; 281: 987.
5. Mortier E, et al. Ergotism related to interaction between nelfinavir and ergotamine. Am J Med 2001; 110: 594.

Beta blockers. Peripheral vasoconstriction was reported in a patient with migraine after addition of propranolol to regular use of Cafergot suppositories twice daily.[1] This combination has been used without complication by other workers who suggested that ergotism caused by excessive dosage of ergotamine tartrate, rather than an interaction between ergotamine and propranolol, was responsible.[2] However, arterial vasoconstriction has been reported after concomitant use of methysergide and propranolol and of oxprenolol and ergotamine.[3] Such combinations should therefore be used with caution.

1. Baumrucker JF. Drug interaction—propranolol and Cafergot. N Engl J Med 1973; 288: 916–17.
2. Diamond S. Propranolol and ergotamine tartrate. N Engl J Med 1973; 289: 159.
3. Venter CP, et al. Severe peripheral ischaemia during concomitant use of beta blockers and ergot alkaloids. BMJ 1984; 289: 288–9.

Glyceryl trinitrate. Glyceryl trinitrate has been reported to increase the oral bioavailability and plasma concentrations of dihydroergotamine in patients with orthostatic hypotension.[1]

1. Bobik A, et al. Low oral bioavailability of dihydroergotamine and first-pass extraction in patients with orthostatic hypotension. Clin Pharmacol Ther 1981; 30: 673–9.

Tacrolimus. Ergotamine may inhibit the metabolism of tacrolimus (see p.570).

Pharmacokinetics

Absorption from the gastrointestinal tract after administration by mouth is poor and may be further decreased by the occurrence of gastric stasis during migraine attacks. Bioavailability of ergotamine is also diminished by a high first-pass hepatic metabolism. Ergotamine has been given rectally or by inhalation in an attempt to overcome these effects with some improvement in rate and/or extent of absorption but bioavailability is still of the order of 5% or less. Absorption of sublingual ergotamine is very poor. There is considerable interindividual variation in the bioavailability of ergotamine, regardless of the route of administration. Caffeine is sometimes included in oral and rectal preparations of ergotamine to improve the latter's absorption, although whether it does so is not clear. Drugs such as metoclopramide are sometimes given with the aim of alleviating gastric stasis to improve absorption of ergotamine.

Ergotamine is metabolised extensively in the liver, the majority of metabolites being excreted in the bile. About 4% of a dose is excreted in the urine. Ergotamine or its metabolites have been detected in breast milk. Some of the metabolites are pharmacologically active. The elimination of ergotamine is biphasic; half-lives of about 2 hours and 21 hours have been reported for the 2 phases respectively.

◊ References.
1. Schmidt R, Fanchamps A. Effect of caffeine on intestinal absorption of ergotamine in man. Eur J Clin Pharmacol 1974; 7: 213–16.
2. Eadie MJ. Ergotamine pharmacokinetics in man: an editorial. Cephalalgia 1983; 3: 135–8.
3. Perrin VL. Clinical pharmacokinetics of ergotamine in migraine and cluster headache. Clin Pharmacokinet 1985; 10: 334–52.

Uses and Administration

Ergotamine is an alkaloid derived from ergot (p.1608). It has marked vasoconstrictor effects, and may have a partial agonist action at serotonin (5-HT) receptors; it also has a powerful oxytocic action on the uterus, although less so than ergometrine (p.1607). It is used in migraine and cluster headache, and has been tried in orthostatic hypotension.

Ergotamine is commonly used as the tartrate. It is usually given by mouth, but has also been given sublingually, rectally, and by oral inhalation. It was formerly given by subcutaneous or intramuscular injection. Caffeine is sometimes given with ergotamine tartrate with the intention of improving the lat-

ter's absorption, although whether it does so is not clear. Antiemetics such as cyclizine hydrochloride are sometimes included in combination preparations with ergotamine tartrate.

Ergotamine is used in migraine unresponsive to non-opioid analgesics. However, its adverse effects limit how much it can be used and prevent its use for prophylaxis. It is most effective when administered as early as possible in a migraine attack, preferably during the prodromal phase.

The usual dose is 1 to 2 mg of ergotamine tartrate by mouth, repeated, if necessary, half an hour later. Usually not more than 6 mg should be given in 24 hours, although some manufacturers recommend not more than 4 mg in 24 hours and others not more than 8 mg per attack. The recommended minimum interval between successive 24-hour courses is 4 days, with the additional restriction of the total weekly dose being limited to a maximum of 12 mg, although some manufacturers recommend a lower weekly limit of 8 mg. It is also recommended that patients should receive no more than 2 courses per month. Similar doses may be given sublingually.

Ergotamine tartrate may also be given rectally as suppositories, especially if the oral route is not effective or not practicable. The rectal dose of ergotamine tartrate is 2 mg repeated, if necessary, one hour later. Usually, not more than 4 mg should be given in 24 hours and not more than 8 mg in one week with an interval of at least 4 days between successive 24-hour courses.

A more rapid onset of action may be achieved by oral inhalation. One dose containing 360 µg of ergotamine tartrate may be inhaled at the onset of the attack and repeated, if necessary, at 5-minute intervals. Not more than 6 inhalation doses should be taken in 24 hours and not more than 12 in one week with an interval of at least 5 days between successive 24-hour courses.

Ergotamine is used in patients with cluster headache to treat individual attacks of headache but since such attacks are short-lived oral inhalation may be preferable to oral, sublingual, or rectal routes. Doses used are similar to those given to treat migraine. It has also been used to prevent headache attacks during cluster periods, when it is usually given daily in low doses for up to 2 weeks, either by mouth or rectally (see below).

Migraine and cluster headache. Ergotamine was formerly one of the main drugs used to treat acute attacks of migraine (p.449) unresponsive to antimigraine preparations containing non-opioid analgesics, but triptan serotonin (5-HT1) agonists such as sumatriptan are now preferred. Since ergotamine may exacerbate the nausea and vomiting that commonly develops as a migraine attack progresses it is often necessary to give an antiemetic as well. Poor oral bioavailability may be reduced further during a migraine attack and ergotamine has sometimes been given sublingually, rectally, or by inhalation. Adverse effects limit how much ergotamine can be used for an individual attack and prevent the long-term use that would be required for migraine prophylaxis.

Ergotamine may be used similarly in cluster headache (p.449) to treat individual headaches during a cluster period. Since such attacks are short-lived administration by oral inhalation may be more effective than other routes. Ergotamine is also used in low doses given by mouth or rectally for limited periods of up to 2 weeks in the prophylaxis of cluster headache during a cluster period. Regimens that have been tried for such prophylaxis include 1 to 2 mg of ergotamine tartrate given 1 to 2 hours before an expected attack or 1 to 2 hours before bedtime for nocturnal attacks. The total maximum dose of ergotamine tartrate that may be given weekly for the prevention of cluster headache is less well established than for the treatment of migraine. Ergotamine is often given for only 5 to 6 days in each week, which allows the patient to assess whether the cluster period has ended.

References.
1. Silberstein SD, Young WB. Safety and efficacy of ergotamine tartrate and dihydroergotamine in the treatment of migraine and status migrainosus. Neurology 1995; 45: 577–84.

Orthostatic hypotension. Ergotamine and dihydroergotamine might be of use in patients with refractory orthostatic hypotension (p.1070). Ergotamine is believed[1] to be less selective than dihydroergotamine (p.451) in its actions and affects both venous capacitance and peripheral resistance.[2,3] However, the oral bioavailability of ergotamine is greater[2] than that of dihy-

droergotamine and there have also been some reports of successful treatment with inhaled ergotamine.[3,4]

1. Anonymous. Management of orthostatic hypotension. Lancet 1987; i: 197–8.
2. Ahmad RAS, Watson RDS. Treatment of postural hypotension: a review. Drugs 1990; 39: 74–85.
3. Tonkin AL, Wing LMH. Hypotension: assessment and management. Med J Aust 1990; 153: 474–85.
4. Stumpf JL, Mitrzyk B. Management of orthostatic hypotension. Am J Hosp Pharm 1994; 51: 648–60.

Preparations

BP 2001: Ergotamine Sublingual Tablets;
USP 25: Ergotamine Tartrate and Caffeine Suppositories; Ergotamine Tartrate and Caffeine Tablets; Ergotamine Tartrate Inhalation Aerosol; Ergotamine Tartrate Injection; Ergotamine Tartrate Tablets.

Proprietary Preparations (details are given in Part 3)
Aust.: Ergokapton; **Austral.:** Ergodryl Mono; **Braz.:** Enxak; Gynergene; **Canad.:** Ergomar; **Ger.:** ergo sanol spezial N; Ergo-Kranit mono; Migrexa; RubieNex mono; **Irl.:** Lingraine; **Ital.:** Ergotan; **S.Afr.:** Ergate†; **Thai.:** Ergosia; Gynaemine; **UK:** Lingraine†; Medihaler-Ergotamine†; **USA:** Ergomar.

Multi-ingredient: Aust.: Avamigran; Cafergot; Migril; Pansecoff†; Synkapton; **Austral.:** Cafergot; Ergodryl; Migral; **Belg.:** Cafergot; **Braz.:** Cafergot; Migrane; Ormigrein; **Canad.:** Bellergal; Cafergot; Cafergot-PB; Ergodryl; Gravergol; Megral; Wigraine†; **Denm.:** Ergokoffin; Gynergen Comp; **Fr.:** Gynergene Cafeine; Migwell; **Ger.:** Avamigran N; Cafergot N; Ergo-Kranit; Ergoffin; Migratan S; RubieNex spezial; **Hong Kong:** Cafergot; Gravergol; Migril; **Irl.:** Cafergot; Migranat; Migril; **Israel:** Cafergot; Temigran; **Ital.:** Bellergil†; Cafergot; Virdex; **Mex.:** Cafergot; Ergocaf; Sydolil; Trinergot; **Neth.:** Cafergot; Migril†; Neo-Cranimal†; **Norw.:** Anervan; Cafergot Comp†; Cafergot†; **NZ:** Cafergot; Ergodryl; Migril; **Port.:** Avamigran; Migretil; **S.Afr.:** Bellergal†; Cafergot; Cafergot-PB; Migril; **Singapore:** Cafergot; Migril; **Spain:** Cafergot; Cafergot-PB; Distovagal†; Hemicraneal; Igril; **Swed.:** Anervan; **Switz.:** Bellagolin; Bellergal; Cafergot; Cafergot-PB; Ergosanol a la cafeine; Ergosanol special a la cafeine; Ergosanol special†; Migrexa; Migril; **Thai.:** Avamigran; Bellergal; Benera; Cafergot; Degran; Neuramizone; Poligot-CF; Polygot; **UK:** Cafergot; Migril; **USA:** Bel-Phen-Ergot S; Bellergal-S; Cafatine; Cafatine-PB; Cafergot; Cafetrate†; Ercaf; Folergot-DF; Migergot†; Phenerbel-S; Wigraine.

Feverfew   (16808-m)

Camomille (Grande); Tanaceti Parthenii Herba.

Pharmacopoeias. In *Eur.* (see p.vi). Also in *USNF* which also describes Powdered Feverfew.

Pharmacopoeial description

Ph. Eur.: The dried, whole or fragmented aerial parts of *Tanacetum parthenium*. It contains not less than 0.2% of parthenolide ($C_{15}H_{20}O_3 = 248.3$), calculated with reference to the dried drug. It has a camphoraceous odour. Protect from light.

USNF 20: Feverfew consists of the dried leaves of *Tanacetum parthenium* (Asteraceae), collected when the plant is in flower. Store in a dry place. Protect from light.

Adverse Effects and Precautions

Mouth ulceration and soreness have been reported following ingestion of feverfew, and may be due to sensitisation; if they occur feverfew should be discontinued. Contact dermatitis has been reported. Feverfew is reputed to have abortifacient properties and it is suggested that preparations should not be used in pregnancy.

Uses and Administration

Feverfew is a traditional herbal remedy used in the prophylactic treatment of migraine. Its effects have been attributed to the plant's content of sesquiterpene lactones, notably parthenolide. A preparation of the dried leaf powder, which has been standardised to provide a minimum of 0.2% parthenolide, is available in some countries. A suggested dose is 125 or 250 mg daily by mouth.

Migraine. Feverfew is a traditional herbal remedy used in the management of migraine (p.449).[1] Studies of standardised preparations of the freeze-dried powdered leaf have produced variable results in preventing or ameliorating migraine attacks,[2-4] and systematic reviews[5,6] suggest that its effectiveness in preventing migraine remains to be established.

1. Berry M. Feverfew. Pharm J 1994; 253: 806–8.
2. Johnson ES, et al. Efficacy of feverfew as prophylactic treatment of migraine. BMJ 1985; 291: 569–73.
3. Murphy JJ, et al. Randomised double-blind placebo controlled trial of feverfew in migraine prevention. Lancet 1988; ii: 189–92.
4. de Weerdt CJ, et al. Herbal medicines in migraine prevention: randomized double-blind placebo-controlled crossover trial of a feverfew preparation. Phytomedicine 1996; 3: 225–30.
5. Vogler BK, et al. Feverfew as a preventive treatment for migraine: a systematic review. Cephalalgia 1998; 18: 704–8.
6. Pittler MH, et al. Feverfew for preventing migraine (updated 27 February 2001). Available in The Cochrane Library; Issue 2. Oxford: Update Software; 2001.

Rheumatoid arthritis. Feverfew has been used as a herbal medicine for the treatment of arthritis. Although it has anti-inflammatory activity *in vitro*, feverfew was found to be ineffective in rheumatoid arthritis.[1]

1. Pattrick M, et al. Feverfew in rheumatoid arthritis: a double blind, placebo controlled study. Ann Rheum Dis 1989; 48: 547–9.

The symbol † denotes a preparation no longer actively marketed

Preparations

Proprietary Preparations (details are given in Part 3)
Austral.: Herbal Headache Relief; *Canad.:* Tanacet; *UK:* Tanacet.
Multi-ingredient: *Austral.:* Extralife Arthri-Care; Extralife Migrai-Care.

Frovatriptan (1885-g)

Frovatriptan (BAN, rINN).

SB-209509AX (frovatriptan or frovatriptan succinate); VML-251 (frovatriptan or frovatriptan succinate). (6R)-5,6,7,8-Tetrahydro-6-methylaminocarbazole-3-carboxamide.
$C_{14}H_{17}N_3O = 243.3$.
CAS — 158747-02-5 (frovatriptan); 158930-17-7 (frovatriptan succinate monohydrate).
NOTE. Frovatriptan Succinate is USAN.

Profile

Frovatriptan is a serotonin (5-HT$_1$) agonist with actions similar to those of sumatriptan (p.456). It is used for the acute treatment of migraine attacks.

Preparations

Proprietary Preparations (details are given in Part 3)
USA: Frova.

Methysergide Maleate (1513-n)

Methysergide Maleate (BANM, rINNM).

1-Methyl-D-lysergic Acid Butanolamide Maleate. N-[1-(Hydroxymethyl)propyl]-1-methyl-D-lysergamide hydrogen maleate; 9,10-Didehydro-N-[1-(hydroxymethyl)propyl]-1,6-dimethylergoline-8β-carboxamide hydrogen maleate.
$C_{21}H_{27}N_3O_2,C_4H_4O_4 = 469.5$.
CAS — 361-37-5 (methysergide); 129-49-7 (methysergide maleate).
NOTE. Methysergide is USAN.
Pharmacopoeias. In Br., Swiss, and US.

Methysergide maleate 1.33 mg is approximately equivalent to 1 mg of methysergide.

Pharmacopoeial description

BP 2001: A white or almost white crystalline powder which may have a yellow or pink tinge; odourless or almost odourless. Slightly soluble in water and in methyl alcohol; practically insoluble in chloroform and in ether. A 0.2% solution in water has a pH of 3.7 to 4.7. Store at a temperature of 2° to 8°. Protect from light.

USP 25: A white to yellowish-white or reddish-white, crystalline powder. Is odourless or has not more than a slight odour. Soluble 1 in 200 of water and 1 in 165 of alcohol; soluble 1 in 3400 of chloroform; practically insoluble in ether. pH of a 1 in 500 solution is between 3.7 and 4.7. Store in airtight containers at a temperature of 2° to 8°. Protect from light.

Adverse Effects

Gastrointestinal effects such as nausea, vomiting, heartburn, and abdominal pain are common on initial treatment with methysergide maleate, as are dizziness and drowsiness. Other CNS effects reported include ataxia, insomnia, weakness, restlessness, lightheadedness, euphoria, and hallucinations. Peripheral or localised oedema, leg cramps, and weight gain have occurred and there have been occasional reports of skin rashes, loss of hair, joint and muscle pain, neutropenia, and eosinophilia. Orthostatic hypotension and tachycardia have been observed.

Arterial spasm has occurred in some patients with manifestations such as paraesthesia of the extremities and anginal pain, similar to those reported with ergotamine (p.452); if such symptoms occur methysergide should be withdrawn, although rebound headaches may be experienced if it is withdrawn suddenly. Vascular insufficiency of the lower limbs may represent arterial spasm or fibrotic changes. Retroperitoneal fibrosis, with obstruction of abdominal blood vessels and ureters, pleuropulmonary fibrosis, and fibrotic changes in heart valves have occurred in patients on long-term treatment. Methysergide must be withdrawn immediately if fibrosis occurs. Retroperitoneal fibrosis is usually reversible, but other fibrotic changes are less readily reversed.

Fibrosis. Fibrosis has been associated with the long-term use of methysergide maleate. In one early report[1] in 27 patients retroperitoneal fibrosis was attributed to daily administration of methysergide for periods of 9 to 54 months in doses ranging from 2 to 28 mg daily. There was partial or complete regression of fibrosis in 13 of the patients whose treatment was withdrawn. Improvement usually began within a few days, in some cases with the aid of prednisone. The other 14 patients were treated by surgery; those few who continued taking methysergide had difficult postoperative courses. Cardiac murmurs occurred in 7 patients, and regressed wholly or partially in 3 after therapy was stopped. Fibrotic changes affecting the aorta, heart valves, and pulmonary tissues occurred in a few of the patients. Others have reported the development of endocardial fibrosis indicated by cardiac murmurs in 48 patients receiving methysergide.[2] The murmurs gradually regressed in 27 when methysergide was discontinued. Retroperitoneal fibrosis was present in 9 patients and pleuropulmonary fibrosis in 2. Fibro-

sis of the iliac vein has been described in one patient.[3] A few cases of retroperitoneal fibrosis associated with ergotamine tartrate or dihydroergotamine have been noted.[1] These 2 drugs have also been implicated in a few other cases of retroperitoneal fibrosis or other fibrotic disorders in patients taking high doses for long periods.[4-7]

1. Graham JR, *et al.* Fibrotic disorders associated with methysergide therapy for headache. *N Engl J Med* 1966; **274:** 359–68.
2. Bana DS, *et al.* Cardiac murmurs and endocardial fibrosis associated with methysergide therapy. *Am Heart J* 1974; **88:** 640–55.
3. Bucci JA, Manoharan A. Methysergide-induced retroperitoneal fibrosis: successful outcome and two new laboratory features. *Mayo Clin Proc* 1997; **72:** 1148–50.
4. Lepage-Savary D, Vallières A. Ergotamine as a possible cause of retroperitoneal fibrosis. *Clin Pharm* 1982; **1:** 179–80.
5. Damstrup L, Jensen TT. Retroperitoneal fibrosis after long-term daily use of ergotamine. *Int Urol Nephrol* 1986; **18:** 299–301.
6. Robert M, *et al.* Fibrotic processes associated with long-term ergotamine therapy. *N Engl J Med* 1984; **311:** 601 and 602.
7. Malaquin F, *et al.* Pleural and retroperitoneal fibrosis from dihydroergotamine. *N Engl J Med* 1989; **321:** 1760.

Treatment of Adverse Effects

As for Ergotamine Tartrate, p.452. Methysergide maleate should be withdrawn immediately if fibrosis develops. Corticosteroids can be used to treat fibrosis, although surgery may be required.

Precautions

As for Ergotamine Tartrate, p.452. In addition, methysergide maleate is contra-indicated in valvular heart disease, pulmonary and collagen diseases, diseases of the urinary tract, phlebitis and cellulitis of the lower extremities, and debilitated states. It should be used with caution in patients with peptic ulcer because it may increase gastric acidity. Patients should be closely supervised. Methysergide maleate should not be given continuously for more than 6 months and should normally be withdrawn gradually (see Uses, below). However, it should be withdrawn immediately if symptoms of fibrosis or arterial spasm develop.

Porphyria. Methysergide is considered to be unsafe in patients with porphyria because it has been shown to be porphyrinogenic in *animals* or *in-vitro* systems.

Interactions

Interactions involving those ergot alkaloids used primarily in the management of migraine are discussed under ergotamine (p.452). References specific to methysergide may be found there under the headings Antimigraine Drugs and Beta Blockers.

Pharmacokinetics

Methysergide maleate is rapidly absorbed from the gastrointestinal tract with maximum plasma concentrations being obtained within about one hour of ingestion. Methysergide undergoes extensive first-pass hepatic metabolism to methylergometrine (p.1635). Methysergide is excreted in the urine as unchanged drug and metabolites.

◊ References.

1. Bredberg U, *et al.* Pharmacokinetics of methysergide and its metabolite methylergometrine in man. *Eur J Clin Pharmacol* 1986; **30:** 75–7.

Uses and Administration

Methysergide maleate is a semisynthetic ergot alkaloid. It is a potent serotonin antagonist and, compared with ergotamine, has only feeble vasoconstrictor and oxytocic effects. It may be used prophylactically in the management of severe recurrent migraine (p.449) and in the prevention of headache attacks during cluster periods (p.449), although its use has declined because of adverse effects. It is ineffective in the treatment of acute attacks.

Methysergide maleate is given by mouth in a dosage equivalent to 2 to 6 mg of methysergide base daily in divided doses with meals. It is suggested that treatment should be started with 1 mg at bedtime and doses increased gradually over about 2 weeks; the minimum effective dose should be used. In the USA and some other countries doses are expressed in terms of the maleate, a usual dose of which is 4 to 8 mg daily. Careful and regular observation of the patient is essential because of the high incidence of side-effects and it is recommended that treatment should only be carried out under hospital supervision. If treatment still proves to be ineffective after 3 weeks, further administration is unlikely to be of benefit. Treatment should not be continued for more than 6 months, after which it should be gradually withdrawn over 2 or 3 weeks and then discontinued for at least a month for reassessment. Some consider that treatment courses should not exceed 3 months without a break.

Methysergide maleate has also been used to control diarrhoea associated with carcinoid syndrome (p.483) in high doses equivalent to 12 to 20 mg of methysergide daily.

As a serotonin antagonist, methysergide might be expected to help reverse the serotonin syndrome (p.304).

Preparations

BP 2001: Methysergide Tablets;
USP 25: Methysergide Maleate Tablets.

Proprietary Preparations (details are given in Part 3)
Austral.: Deseril; *Belg.:* Deseril; *Braz.:* Deserila; *Canad.:* Sansert; *Fr.:* Desernil; *Ger.:* Deseril; *Irl.:* Deseril; *Ital.:* Deserril†; *Neth.:* Deseril; *S.Afr.:* Deseril; *Switz.:* Deseril; *UK:* Deseril; *USA:* Sansert.

Naratriptan Hydrochloride (17247-k)

Naratriptan Hydrochloride (BANM, USAN, rINNM).

GR-85548A (naratriptan hydrochloride); GR-85548X (naratriptan). N-Methyl-3-(1-methyl-4-piperidyl)indole-5-ethanesulfonamide hydrochloride.
$C_{17}H_{25}N_3O_2S,HCl = 371.9$.
CAS — 121679-13-8 (naratriptan); 121679-19-4 (naratriptan hydrochloride); 143388-64-1 (naratriptan hydrochloride).

Naratriptan hydrochloride 1.11 mg is approximately equivalent to 1 mg of naratriptan.

Adverse Effects and Precautions

As for Sumatriptan, p.456.

Naratriptan should not be used in patients with severe hepatic or renal impairment (creatinine clearance less than 15 mL per minute) and should be used with caution in more moderate degrees of renal or hepatic impairment. Patients with hypersensitivity to sulfonamides may theoretically exhibit a similar reaction to naratriptan.

Analgesic-induced headache. For a report of an association between naratriptan and analgesic-induced headache, see under Adverse Effects of Sumatriptan, p.456.

Interactions

As for Sumatriptan, p.457.

Pharmacokinetics

Following oral administration, peak plasma-naratriptan concentrations are observed at 2 to 3 hours, and bioavailability is reported to be 63% in men and 74% in women. Plasma protein binding is 29%. Naratriptan undergoes some hepatic metabolism by a wide range of cytochrome P450 isoenzymes. It is predominantly excreted in the urine with 50% of a dose being recovered as unchanged drug and 30% as inactive metabolites. The elimination half-life is 6 hours, and is significantly prolonged in patients with renal or hepatic impairment.

Uses and Administration

Naratriptan is a selective serotonin (5-HT$_1$) agonist with actions and uses similar to those of sumatriptan (p.457). It is used for the acute treatment of migraine attacks, and should be administered as soon as possible after onset of migraine headache. It should not be used prophylactically. It is given by mouth as the hydrochloride, and doses are expressed in terms of the base.

The recommended initial dose of naratriptan in the UK is 2.5 mg, and in the USA is 1 or 2.5 mg. If no response is obtained with the initial dose, a second dose should not be taken for the same attack. If symptoms recur following an initial response, the dose may be repeated after an interval of 4 hours, to a maximum of 5 mg in any 24-hour period. In patients with mild to moderate hepatic or renal impairment, the recommended maximum dose in 24 hours is 2.5 mg and a low starting dose should be considered.

Migraine. References.

1. Klassen A, *et al.* Naratriptan is effective and well tolerated in the acute treatment of migraine: results of a double-blind, placebo-controlled, parallel-group study. *Headache* 1997; **37:** 640–5.
2. Mathew NT, *et al.* Naratriptan is effective and well tolerated in the acute treatment of migraine: results of a double-blind, placebo-controlled, crossover study. *Neurology* 1997; **49:** 1485–90.
3. Bomhof MAM, *et al.* Tolerability and efficacy of naratriptan tablets with long-term treatment (6 months). *Cephalalgia* 1998; **18:** 33–7.
4. Sheftell F, *et al.* Low migraine headache recurrence with naratriptan: clinical parameters related to recurrence. *Headache* 2000; **40:** 103–10.
5. Stark S, *et al.* Naratriptan efficacy in migraineurs who respond poorly to oral sumatriptan. *Headache* 2000; **40:** 513–20.
6. Luciani R, *et al.* Prevention of migraine during prodrome with naratriptan. *Cephalalgia* 2000; **20:** 122–6.
7. Gobel H, *et al.* Comparison of naratriptan and sumatriptan in recurrence-prone migraine patients. *Clin Ther* 2000; **8:** 981–9.
8. Heywood J, *et al.* Tolerability and efficacy of naratriptan tablets in the acute treatment of migraine attacks for 1 year. *Cephalalgia* 2000; **20:** 470–4.

Preparations

Proprietary Preparations (details are given in Part 3)
Aust.: Antimigrain; Naramig; *Austral.:* Naramig; *Belg.:* Naramig; *Canad.:* Amerge; *Denm.:* Naragran; *Fin.:* Naramig; *Fr.:* Naramig; *Ger.:* Naramig; *Israel:* Naramig; *Mex.:* Naramig; *Neth.:*

Naramig; *Norw.:* Naramig; *Port.:* Naramig; *S.Afr.:* Naramig; *Singapore:* Naramig; *Spain:* Naramig; *Swed.:* Naramig; *Switz.:* Naramig; *Thai.:* Naramig; *UK:* Naramig; *USA:* Amerge.

Oxetorone Fumarate (13059-b)

Oxetorone Fumarate *(USAN, rINNM)*.

L-6257. 3-(6,12-Dihydrobenzofuro[3,2-c][1]benzoxepin-6-ylidene)-*NN*-dimethylpropylamine hydrogen fumarate.

$C_{21}H_{21}NO_2,C_4H_4O_4 = 435.5$.

CAS — 26020-55-3 (oxetorone); 34522-46-8 (oxetorone fumarate).

Profile

Oxetorone fumarate is an antihistamine and serotonin antagonist used in the treatment of migraine (p.449) and cluster headache (p.449) in doses of up to 180 mg daily by mouth. Oxetorone was reported to have induced hyperplastic changes in breast tissue and the uterine endometrium of *rodents*.

Preparations

Proprietary Preparations (details are given in Part 3)
Belg.: Nocertone; *Fr.:* Nocertone.

Pizotifen (14855-k)

Pizotifen *(BAN, rINN)*.

BC-105; Pizotyline *(USAN)*. 9,10-Dihydro-4-(1-methylpiperidin-4-ylidene)-4*H*-benzo[4,5]cyclohepta[1,2-*b*]thiophene.

$C_{19}H_{21}NS = 295.4$.

CAS — 15574-96-6.

ATC — N02CX01.

Pharmacopoeias. In Chin.

Pizotifen Malate (6157-j)

Pizotifen Malate *(BANM, rINNM)*.

Pizotifen Hydrogen Malate; Pizotyline Malate. 9,10-Dihydro-4-(1-methylpiperidin-4-ylidene)-4*H*-benzo[4,5]cyclohepta[1,2-*b*]thiophene hydrogen malate.

$C_{19}H_{21}NS,C_4H_6O_5 = 429.5$.

CAS — 5189-11-7.

Pharmacopoeias. In Br.

Pizotifen malate 1.45 mg is approximately equivalent to 1 mg of pizotifen.

Pharmacopoeial description

BP 2001: A white or slightly yellowish-white, odourless or almost odourless, crystalline powder. Very slightly soluble in water; slightly soluble in alcohol and in chloroform; sparingly soluble in methyl alcohol. Protect from light.

Adverse Effects and Precautions

As for the sedating antihistamines in general, see p.404. Increased appetite and weight gain may occur with pizotifen. Drowsiness may be troublesome.

◊ Of 47 patients with severe migraine given pizotifen 1 to 2 mg daily adverse effects were recorded in 22 patients.[1] These reactions included weight increase (15), muscle pain or cramps (3), heavy legs or restless legs (3), fluid retention (3), drowsiness (2), more frequent milder headaches (2), facial flushing (1), reduced libido (1), exacerbation of epilepsy (1), and dreaming (2). Adverse effects necessitating withdrawal from the study occurred in 11 patients.

1. Peet KMS. Use of pizotifen in severe migraine: a long-term study. *Curr Med Res Opin* 1977; **5:** 192–9.

Interactions

As for the sedating antihistamines in general, see p.406.

Antihypertensives. Following a report[1] of loss of blood pressure control when treatment with pizotifen was started in a patient receiving debrisoquine the manufacturer suggested that since pizotifen had a similar chemical structure to the tricyclic antidepressants it might antagonise the actions of adrenergic neurone blockers in a similar manner.

1. Bailey RR. Antagonism of debrisoquine sulphate by pizotifen (Sandomigran). *N Z Med J* 1976; **1:** 449.

Pharmacokinetics

Pizotifen is well absorbed from the gastrointestinal tract, peak plasma concentrations occurring approximately 5 hours after a single oral dose. Over 90% is bound to plasma proteins. Pizotifen undergoes extensive metabolism. Over half of a dose is excreted in the urine, chiefly as metabolites; a significant proportion is excreted in the faeces. The primary metabolite of pizotifen (*N*-glucuronide conjugate) has a long elimination half-life of about 23 hours.

The symbol † denotes a preparation no longer actively marketed

Uses and Administration

Pizotifen is a sedating antihistamine (p.406) that has strong serotonin antagonist and weak antimuscarinic properties. It also antagonises the action of tryptamine. Pizotifen is used, usually as the malate, for the prophylaxis of migraine and for the prevention of headache attacks during cluster periods. It is not effective in treating an acute attack. Doses of pizotifen malate are expressed in terms of the equivalent amount of the base. The usual adult dose is 1.5 mg daily by mouth either in three divided doses or as a single dose at night. Gradual increase from an initial dose of 0.5 mg may help to avoid undue drowsiness. Doses in individual patients may vary from 0.5 mg up to a maximum of 4.5 mg daily. Not more than 3 mg should be given as a single dose. Up to 1.5 mg daily in divided doses (maximum single dose of 1 mg at night) has been recommended for children.

Pizotifen hydrochloride has also been used in the management of migraine.

Abdominal migraine. The term abdominal migraine has been proposed by some workers for a syndrome in children consisting of recurrent episodes of midline abdominal pain lasting for many hours.[1,2] There is usually a family history of migraine. Patients commonly wish to lie down and try to sleep, and the pain is severe enough to disrupt normal activities. Other symptoms include pallor, anorexia, nausea, and vomiting. Sleep, and sometimes vomiting, terminate the attack.

However the existence of this syndrome is not universally recognised and is a matter of debate.[2,3] In 1988 the Headache Classification Committee of the International Headache Society[4] were unable to include abdominal migraine as a separate syndrome in their classification of headache and related conditions since they were unable to propose diagnostic criteria to differentiate it from a number of similar childhood periodic syndromes. Nonetheless, in a recent study[5] pizotifen was found to be effective for the prophylaxis of abdominal pain in children considered to have this disorder. Children with abdominal migraine may also benefit from prophylactic treatment with propranolol or cyproheptadine.[6]

1. Symon DNK, Russell G. Abdominal migraine: a syndrome defined. *Cephalalgia* 1986; **6:** 223–8.
2. Symon DNK. Is there a place for "abdominal migraine" as a separate entity in the IHS classification? Yes! *Cephalalgia* 1992; **12:** 345–6.
3. Hockaday JM. Is there a place for "abdominal migraine" as a separate entity in the IHS classification? NO! *Cephalalgia* 1992; **12:** 346–8.
4. Headache Classification Committee of the International Headache Society. Classification and diagnostic criteria for headache disorders, cranial neuralgias and facial pain. *Cephalalgia* 1988; **8** (suppl 7): 1–96.
5. Symon DNK, Russell G. Double blind placebo controlled trial of pizotifen syrup in the treatment of abdominal migraine. *Arch Dis Child* 1995; **72:** 48–50.
6. Worawattanakul M, *et al.* Abdominal migraine: prophylactic treatment and follow-up. *J Pediatr Gastroenterol Nutr* 1999; **28:** 37–40.

Migraine and cluster headache. Pizotifen is one of the main alternatives to propranolol for the prophylaxis of migraine (p.449). It has also been tried in the management of cluster headache (p.449) to prevent headache attacks during a cluster period.

References.

1. Bellavance AJ, Meloche JP. A comparative study of naproxen sodium, pizotyline and placebo in migraine prophylaxis. *Headache* 1990; **30:** 710–15.

Preparations

BP 2001: Pizotifen Tablets.

Proprietary Preparations (details are given in Part 3)
Aust.: Sandomigran; *Austral.:* Sandomigran; *Belg.:* Sandomigran; *Braz.:* Sandomigran; *Canad.:* Sandomigran; *Denm.:* Sandomigrin; *Fr.:* Sanmigran; *Ger.:* Mosegor; *Sandomigran; *Hong Kong:* Sandomigran; *Irl.:* Sanmigran; *Israel:* Sandomigran; *Ital.:* Sandomigran; *Neth.:* Sandomigran; *Norw.:* Sandomigrin†; *NZ:* Sandomigran; *S.Afr.:* Sandomigran; *Spain:* Mosegor; *Swed.:* Sandomigrin; *Switz.:* Mosegor; *Thai.:* Anorsia; Mosegor; Pizomed; Zofen; *UK:* Sanmigran.

Rizatriptan Benzoate (3685-j)

Rizatriptan Benzoate *(BANM, USAN, pINNM)*.

MK-462; MK-0462. 3-[2-(Dimethylamino)ethyl]-5-(1*H*-1,2,4-triazol-1-ylmethyl)indole monobenzoate; Dimethyl{2-[5-(1*H*-1,2,4-triazol-1-ylmethyl)indol-3-yl]ethyl}amine monobenzoate.

$C_{15}H_{19}N_5,C_7H_6O_2 = 391.5$.

CAS — 144034-80-0 (rizatriptan); 145202-66-0 (rizatriptan benzoate).

Rizatriptan benzoate 14.54 mg is approximately equivalent to 10 mg of rizatriptan.

Adverse Effects and Precautions

As for Sumatriptan, p.456. Toxic epidermal necrolysis has also been reported with rizatriptan.

Rizatriptan should not be used in patients with severe hepatic or renal impairment and should be given with caution to patients with more moderate degrees of renal or hepatic impairment.

Breast feeding. Studies *in rats* indicated a high distribution of rizatriptan into milk. The manufacturer recommends that infant exposure be minimised by avoiding breast feeding for 24 hours after treatment.

Interactions

As for Sumatriptan, p.457. Propranolol increases plasma-rizatriptan concentrations and it is recommended that lower doses of rizatriptan should be used in patients receiving this combination (see Uses and Administration, below).

Pharmacokinetics

After oral administration, peak plasma-rizatriptan concentrations are obtained in about 1 to 1.5 hours or 1.6 to 2.5 hours depending on the formulation. Bioavailability is about 40 to 45%. Food may delay the time to peak-plasma concentrations of the tablet formulation by about 1 hour. Plasma protein binding is low (14%).

Rizatriptan is metabolised, primarily by monoamine oxidase type A to the inactive indole acetic acid derivative. The active metabolite *N*-monodesmethyl-rizatriptan is formed to a minor degree; other minor metabolites are also produced. About 14% of an oral dose is excreted in the urine as unchanged rizatriptan, 51% as the indole acetic acid metabolite, and 1% as *N*-monodesmethyl-rizatriptan. The plasma half-life is about 2 to 3 hours.

◊ References.

1. Sciberras DG, *et al.* Initial human experience with MK-462 (rizatriptan): a novel 5-HT$_{1D}$ agonist. *Br J Clin Pharmacol* 1997; **43:** 49–54.
2. Lee Y, *et al.* Pharmacokinetics and tolerability of oral rizatriptan in healthy male and female volunteers. *Br J Clin Pharmacol* 1999; **47:** 373–8.
3. Goldberg MR, *et al.* Rizatriptan, a novel 5-HT$_{1B/1D}$ agonist for migraine: single- and multiple-dose tolerability and pharmacokinetics in healthy subjects. *J Clin Pharmacol* 2000; **40:** 74–83.

Uses and Administration

Rizatriptan is a selective serotonin (5-HT$_1$) agonist with actions and uses similar to those of sumatriptan (p.457) but appears to have a faster onset of action. It is used for the acute treatment of the headache phase of migraine attacks. It should not be used prophylactically. Rizatriptan is administered as the benzoate, and doses are expressed in terms of the base.

A usual initial dose of rizatriptan is 10 mg by mouth. If this is ineffective, a second dose should not be taken for the same attack. If the headache recurs, a further dose of 10 mg may be taken after an interval of at least 2 hours. The recommended maximum dose in 24 hours is 20 mg in the UK and 30 mg in the USA.

In patients with mild to moderate hepatic or renal impairment, the dose of rizatriptan should be reduced to 5 mg. If the headache recurs, a further dose of 5 mg may be taken after an interval of at least 2 hours. The recommended maximum dose in 24 hours in these patients is 10 mg in the UK and 15 mg in the USA. Similar dosage reductions for rizatriptan are also recommended in patients receiving propranolol concomitantly, but it is also recommended that the administration of the 2 drugs should be separated by at least 2 hours.

Migraine. References.

1. Visser WH, *et al.* Rizatriptan vs sumatriptan in the acute treatment of migraine: a placebo-controlled, dose-ranging study. *Arch Neurol* 1996; **53:** 1132–7.
2. Gijsman H, *et al.* Double-blind, placebo-controlled, dose-finding study of rizatriptan (MK-462) in the acute treatment of migraine. *Cephalalgia* 1997; **17:** 647–51.
3. Ahrens SP, *et al.* Efficacy and safety of rizatriptan wafer for the acute treatment of migraine. *Cephalalgia* 1999; **19:** 525–30.
4. Dahlof C, *et al.* Rizatriptan in the treatment of migraine. *Clin Ther* 1999; **11:** 1823–36.
5. Dooley M, Faulds D. Rizatriptan: a review of its efficacy in the management of migraine. *Drugs* 1999; **58:** 699–723. Correction. *ibid.* 2000; **59:** 179.

6. Adelman JU, *et al.* Rizatriptan tablet versus wafer: patient preference. *Headache* 2000; **40:** 371–2.
7. Mathew NT, *et al.* Treatment of nonresponders to oral sumatriptan with zolmitriptan and rizatriptan: a comparative open trial. *Headache* 2000; **40:** 464–5.
8. Silberstein SD, *et al.* Rizatriptan in the treatment of menstrual migraine. *Obstet Gynecol* 2000; **96:** 237–42.

Preparations

Proprietary Preparations (details are given in Part 3)
Aust.: Maxalt; *Belg.:* Maxalt; *Canad.:* Maxalt; *Denm.:* Maxalt; *Fin.:* Maxalt; *Ger.:* Maxalt; *Israel:* Rizalt; *Ital.:* Maxalt; Rizaliv; *Mex.:* Maxalt; *Neth.:* Maxalt; *Norw.:* Maxalt; *NZ:* Maxalt; *Port.:* Maxalt; *S.Afr.:* Maxalt; *Spain:* Maxalt; *Swed.:* Maxalt; *UK:* Maxalt; *USA:* Maxalt.

Sumatriptan Succinate (3945-a)

Sumatriptan Succinate (BANM, USAN, rINNM).
GR-43175C; GR-43175X (sumatriptan); Sumatriptani Succinas.
3-(2-Dimethylaminoethyl)indol-5-yl-*N*-methylmethanesulphonamide succinate.
$C_{14}H_{21}N_3O_2S,C_4H_6O_4 = 413.5$.
CAS — 103628-46-2 (sumatriptan); 103628-47-3 (sumatriptan hemisuccinate); 103628-48-4 (sumatriptan succinate).

Pharmacopoeias. In Eur. (see p.vi).

Sumatriptan succinate 69.99 mg is approximately equivalent to 50 mg of sumatriptan.

Pharmacopoeial description

Ph. Eur.: A white or almost white powder. Freely soluble in water; practically insoluble in dichloromethane; sparingly soluble in methyl alcohol. A 1% solution in water has a pH of 4.5 to 5.3. Protect from light.

Stability. Oral liquid preparations of sumatriptan 5 mg/mL (as the succinate salt) prepared from crushed sumatriptan succinate tablets in 3 different syrups were stable for at least 21 days when stored at 4° and protected from light.[1]

1. Fish DN, *et al.* Stability of sumatriptan succinate in extemporaneously prepared oral liquids. *Am J Health-Syst Pharm* 1997; **54:** 1619–22.

Adverse Effects

The most commonly reported adverse effects of serotonin (5-HT$_1$) agonists such as sumatriptan include dizziness, flushing, weakness, drowsiness, and fatigue. Nausea and vomiting may occur. Pain or sensations of tingling, heaviness, heat, pressure, or tightness have also been commonly reported, and can affect any part of the body including the throat and chest, and may be intense. These symptoms may be due to vasospasm, which on rare occasions has resulted in severe cardiovascular events including cardiac arrhythmias, myocardial ischaemia, or myocardial infarction. There have been isolated reports of associated cerebrovascular events in patients receiving sumatriptan. Transient increases in blood pressure may occur soon after treatment. Hypotension, bradycardia or tachycardia, and palpitations have been reported. Visual disturbances have also occurred.

Sumatriptan has occasionally been associated with minor disturbances in liver function. There have also been rare reports of seizures with sumatriptan. Hypersensitivity reactions ranging from skin rashes to, more rarely, anaphylaxis have occurred.

Transient pain at the injection site is common after subcutaneous sumatriptan administration; stinging, burning, erythema, bruising, and bleeding have also been reported. Irritation of the nasal mucosa and throat and epistaxis have been reported after intranasal sumatriptan administration.

◊ In a Dutch postmarketing survey[1] completed by 1187 patients who had taken sumatriptan the most common adverse reactions attributed to sumatriptan were paraesthesia (reported by 11.7% of patients), dizziness (8.1%), feeling of heaviness (8.0%), chest pain (7.9%), nausea and/or vomiting (7.3%), drowsiness/sedation (7.0%), flushing (5.1%), fatigue (4.6%), pressure in throat (3.3%), headache (3.1%), injection site reaction (3.0%), palpitations (2.8%), abdominal pain (2.6%), muscle pain (2.4%), and dyspnoea (2.2%).

1. Ottervanger JP, *et al.* Adverse reactions attributed to sumatriptan: a postmarketing study in general practice. *Eur J Clin Pharmacol* 1994; **47:** 305–9.

Analgesic-induced headache. Sumatriptan may have a similar risk of misuse to that associated with analgesics and ergotamine compounds in patients with analgesic-induced headache (p.449). There have been reports[1-3] of patients using one or more daily doses of sumatriptan to control migraine. Many of the patients had a history of abuse of other antimi-

graine drugs and were using sumatriptan to prevent recurrence of headache. Whether misuse of sumatriptan was due to addiction or rebound headache as seen with ergotamine, is unknown. A postmarketing study in 952 patients receiving sumatriptan found that 36 of the patients (4%) used sumatriptan daily or more than 10 times a week. This overuse was related to poor efficacy and not to rebound headache.[4] One study[5] and an anecdotal report[6] suggest that, rather than producing euphoria or other effects associated with drugs of abuse such as morphine, sumatriptan is more likely to be associated with dysphoria and apathetic sedation.

The development of analgesic-induced headache has also been reported with naratriptan and zolmitriptan.[7]

1. Osborne MJ, *et al.* Is there a problem with long term use of sumatriptan in acute migraine? *BMJ* 1994; **308:** 113.
2. Kaube H, *et al.* Sumatriptan. *BMJ* 1994; **308:** 1573–4.
3. Gaist D, *et al.* Misuse of sumatriptan. *Lancet* 1994; **344:** 1090.
4. Ottervanger JP, *et al.* Pattern of sumatriptan use and overuse in general practice. *Eur J Clin Pharmacol* 1996; **50:** 353–5.
5. Sullivan JT, *et al.* Psychoactivity and abuse potential of sumatriptan. *Clin Pharmacol Ther* 1992; **52:** 635–42.
6. Bakshi R, Yan-Go FL. Prolonged marijuana-like dysphoria after subcutaneous sumatriptan. *Ann Pharmacother* 1996; **30:** 683.
7. Limmroth V, *et al.* Headache after frequent use of serotonin agonists zolmitriptan and naratriptan. *Lancet* 1999; **353:** 378.

Effects on the cardiovascular system. About 10 months after sumatriptan injection had been made available commercially, the UK Committee on Safety of Medicines reported that it had received 34 reports of pain or tightness in the chest and 2 reports of myocardial ischaemia associated with this injection.[1] The Netherlands Centre for Monitoring of Adverse Reactions to Drugs reported about that time that it had received 12 reports of chest or anginal pain mostly associated with oral sumatriptan.[2] A later postmarketing survey based on data from Dutch general practitioners identified chest pain in 1.3% of 1727 patients,[3] a figure considered to be lower than that seen in earlier studies, but in a subsequent questionnaire completed by 1187 of these patients 7.9% reported chest pain.[4] The Australian Adverse Drug Reactions Advisory Committee (ADRAC)[5] stated in December 1994 that they had received 114 reports of chest pain since sumatriptan had been marketed in mid 1992. Most patients had recovered quickly but 2 had died. The first developed a fatal myocardial infarction after coronary artery dissection but the causal relation between this and taking sumatriptan was unclear. The second patient who had hypertrophic obstructive cardiomyopathy developed ventricular fibrillation a few hours after the onset of chest pain and this led to fatal cardiac arrest.

One group of workers[6] who studied the effect of sumatriptan 16 mg given subcutaneously suggested that the symptoms of chest pain might be due to an effect of sumatriptan on oesophageal function, but others have argued against this suggestion.[7] ADRAC[5] considered that the reaction in the 28 reports of throat tightness they had received by December 1994 was a different reaction to that of chest pain, and probably resulted from changes in oesophageal motility.

Several reports have provided details of individual cases of the adverse cardiovascular effects of sumatriptan including arrhythmias,[8] acute myocardial infarction,[9-13] and unstable angina.[14] Most of these reports concerned subcutaneous sumatriptan administration, but in one myocardial infarction occurred after oral administration.[11] Ventricular tachycardia following subcutaneous sumatriptan has been reported in 2 patients.[8] In the first patient the ventricular fibrillation following immediately after the sumatriptan injection would have been fatal but for rapid treatment with DC shock. In another report[9] a 47-year-old woman experienced chest pain after each of 3 subcutaneous injections of sumatriptan 6 mg for acute attacks of cluster headache. On the third occasion the patient was admitted to hospital and was diagnosed as having an acute myocardial infarction. In this instance, the patient did not have a history of ischaemic heart disease or Prinzmetal's angina, or any predisposing conditions. Atrial fibrillation associated with sumatriptan use has also been reported.[15]

A review[16] of published reports on chest pain as well as relevant data held by the UK manufacturer considered that the risk of myocardial ischaemia following vasoconstriction induced by sumatriptan was small. However, the contra-indications and cautions given under Precautions, below, should be observed.

1. Committee on Safety of Medicines. Sumatriptan (Imigran) and chest pain. *Current Problems 34* 1992.
2. Stricker BHC. Coronary vasospasm and sumatriptan. *BMJ* 1992; **305:** 118.
3. Ottervanger JP, *et al.* Postmarketing study of cardiovascular adverse reactions associated with sumatriptan. *BMJ* 1993; **307:** 1185.
4. Ottervanger JP, *et al.* Adverse reactions attributed to sumatriptan: a postmarketing study in general practice. *Eur J Clin Pharmacol* 1994; **47:** 305–9.
5. Boyd IW, Rohan AP. Sumatriptan-induced chest pain. *Lancet* 1994; **344:** 1704–5.
6. Houghton LA, *et al.* Is chest pain after sumatriptan oesophageal in origin? *Lancet* 1994; **344:** 985–6.
7. Hood S, *et al.* Sumatriptan-induced chest pain. *Lancet* 1994; **344:** 1500–1.
8. Curtin T, *et al.* Cardiorespiratory distress after sumatriptan given by injection. *BMJ* 1992; **305:** 713–14.
9. Ottervanger JP, *et al.* Transmural myocardial infarction with sumatriptan. *Lancet* 1993; **341:** 861–2.
10. Kelly KM. Cardiac arrest following use of sumatriptan. *Neurology* 1995; **45:** 1211–13.

11. O'Connor P, Gladstone P. Oral sumatriptan-associated transmural myocardial infarction. *Neurology* 1995; **45:** 2274–6.
12. Mueller L, *et al.* Vasospasm-induced myocardial infarction with sumatriptan. *Headache* 1996; **36:** 329–31.
13. Main ML *et al.* Cardiac arrest and myocardial infarction immediately after sumatriptan injection. *Ann Intern Med* 1998; **128:** 874.
14. Walton-Shirley M, *et al.* Unstable angina pectoris associated with Imitrex therapy. *Cathet Cardiovasc Diagn* 1995; **34:** 188.
15. Morgan DR, *et al.* Atrial fibrillation associated with sumatriptan. *BMJ* 2000; **321:** 275.
16. Hillis WS, MacIntyre PD. Drug reactions: sumatriptan and chest pain. *Lancet* 1993; **341:** 1564–5. Correction. *ibid.*; **342:** 1310.

Effects on the cerebrovascular system. Various adverse cerebrovascular effects have been reported after the use of subcutaneous sumatriptan including hemiparesis,[1] stroke,[2,3] and intracerebral haemorrhage.[4]

1. Luman W, Gray RS. Adverse reactions associated with sumatriptan. *Lancet* 1993; **341:** 1091–2.
2. Cavazos J, *et al.* Sumatriptan-induced stroke in sagittal sinus thrombosis. *Lancet* 1994; **343:** 1105–6.
3. Meschia JF, *et al.* Reversible segmental cerebral arterial vasospasm and cerebral infarction: possible association with excessive use of sumatriptan and Midrin. *Arch Neurol* 1998; **55:** 712–14.
4. Edwards KR, *et al.* Intracerebral hemorrhage associated with sumatriptan. *Headache* 1995; **35:** 309.

Effects on the gastrointestinal tract. Severe ischaemic colitis associated with sumatriptan use has been reported in 8 patients.[1] A further five episodes of mesenteric ischaemia occurred in 2 patients, each within hours of sumatriptan administration.[2] Three of these episodes in one patient were associated with doses of sumatriptan above the recommended daily maximum.

Oesophageal constriction or throat tightness has been reported in some patients taking sumatriptan and may be due to a direct effect on the oesophagus. See Effects on the Cardiovascular System, above.

1. Knudsen JF, *et al.* Ischemic colitis and sumatriptan use. *Arch Intern Med* 1998; **158:** 1946–8.
2. Liu JJ, Ardolf JC. Sumatriptan-associated mesenteric ischemia. *Ann Intern Med* 2000; **132:** 597.

Effects on the respiratory system. See under Asthma in Precautions, below.

Hypersensitivity. Reactions to sumatriptan such as skin rashes and, more rarely, anaphylaxis have been noted by the manufacturer. Published reports include a case of angioedema occurring in a patient 5 minutes after subcutaneous administration of sumatriptan,[1] and urticaria occurring 20 to 24 hours after oral or subcutaneous sumatriptan.[2]

1. Dachs R, Vitillo J. Angioedema associated with sumatriptan administration. *Am J Med* 1995; **99:** 684–5.
2. Pradalier A, *et al.* Delayed urticaria with sumatriptan. *Cephalalgia* 1996; **16:** 280–1.

Precautions

Sumatriptan and other serotonin (5-HT$_1$) agonists should only be used where there is a clear diagnosis of migraine or cluster headache and care should be taken to exclude other potentially serious neurological conditions. They should not be used prophylactically and should not be administered to patients with basilar or hemiplegic migraine.

Serotonin (5-HT$_1$) agonists are contra-indicated in patients with uncontrolled hypertension, ischaemic heart disease (coronary artery disease), a history of myocardial infarction, coronary vasospasm (Prinzmetal's angina), peripheral vascular disease, or a previous cerebrovascular accident or transient ischaemic attack. Unrecognised cardiovascular disease should be excluded before the use of serotonin (5-HT$_1$) agonists in postmenopausal women, men over 40 years of age, and those with risk factors for ischaemic heart disease (see below). If chest pain and tightness occur during use, appropriate investigations should be performed.

Drowsiness may follow treatment with serotonin (5-HT$_1$) agonists and patients thus affected should not drive or operate machinery.

Sumatriptan should be used with caution in patients with hepatic or renal impairment, and should generally be avoided if these are severe.

Sumatriptan injection should not be given intravenously because of the increased risk of producing coronary vasospasm. There have been rare reports of seizures following use of sumatriptan and it should therefore be used with caution in patients with a history of epilepsy or other conditions predisposing to seizures. Patients with hypersensitivity to sulfonamides may exhibit a similar reaction to sumatriptan.

◊ Patients with risk factors for ischaemic heart disease such as diabetes, hypertension, hypercholesterolaemia, obesity, and a strong family history of atheroma, as well as postmenopausal women, men over 40 years of age, and smokers should be given their first dose of sumatriptan under medical supervision.[1]

1. Hillis WS, MacIntyre PD. Drug reactions: sumatriptan and chest pain. *Lancet* 1993; **341:** 1564–5. Correction. *ibid.*; **342:** 1310.

Asthma. The manufacturers reviewed data from more than 75 clinical studies of sumatriptan involving 12 701 patients and reported[1] that the incidence of adverse events related to asthma did not differ between patients with or without asthma. Earlier there had been concern over the safety of sumatriptan in patients with asthma following 2 reports of bronchospasm and a report of a patient with asthma who died during a study of sumatriptan although the patient had not received sumatriptan in the month before her death.

1. Lloyd DK, Pilgrim AJ. The safety of sumatriptan in asthmatic migraineurs. *Cephalalgia* 1993; **13:** 201–4.

Breast feeding. The distribution of sumatriptan into breast milk following a 6-mg subcutaneous dose has been studied in 5 lactating mothers.[1] The mean total recovery of sumatriptan in breast milk was estimated to be 14.4 μg or 0.24% of the dose. It was calculated that on a weight adjusted basis an infant could receive a maximum of 3.5% of the maternal dose. The manufacturers have suggested that infant exposure can be minimised by avoiding breast feeding for 24 hours after treatment.

1. Wojnar-Horton RE, *et al.* Distribution and excretion of sumatriptan in human milk. *Br J Clin Pharmacol* 1996; **41:** 217–21.

Cerebrovascular disorders. A patient with a superior sagittal sinus thrombosis who presented with headache and was misdiagnosed as having migraine variant developed a cortical stroke within minutes of a second 6-mg subcutaneous injection of sumatriptan.[1] The authors of the report emphasised the importance of establishing a diagnosis of typical migraine or cluster headache before using sumatriptan and cautioned against its use in any patient who may have unstable cerebrovascular disease or raised intracranial pressure. They also pointed out that there was no clinical evidence that a second injection would relieve a headache when the initial injection had been ineffective.

1. Cavazos J, *et al.* Sumatriptan-induced stroke in sagittal sinus thrombosis. *Lancet* 1994; **343:** 1105–6.

Interactions

Sumatriptan and other serotonin (5-HT₁) agonists should not be given with ergotamine or related compounds (including methysergide) since there is an increased risk of vasospastic reactions. In addition, a delay is advised before starting a serotonin (5-HT₁) agonist in patients who have been receiving ergotamine or related compounds: sumatriptan, almotriptan, or rizatriptan should not be given until at least 24 hours, and zolmitriptan until at least 6 hours, after stopping the use of preparations containing ergotamine. Conversely, ergotamine should not be given until 6 hours after stopping these drugs. Serotonin (5-HT₁) agonists should not be given together.

It is recommended that sumatriptan or rizatriptan should not be used with, and for 2 weeks after stopping, an MAOI. Opinion varies on the concomitant use of zolmitriptan and inhibitors of monoamine oxidase type A such as moclobemide. In the UK the manufacturers recommend that the maximum dose of zolmitriptan should be reduced when used with inhibitors of monoamine oxidase type A whereas in the USA the manufacturers contraindicate such combinations. There is a theoretical possibility that the use of serotonin (5-HT₁) agonists with selective serotonin reuptake inhibitors may increase the risk of serotonin syndrome, but see under Antidepressants, below.

◊ Oral sumatriptan appeared to delay gastric emptying and might affect the absorption of co-administered drugs, as judged by its delaying effect on paracetamol absorption in migraine patients.[1]

1. Rani PU, *et al.* Sumatriptan delays paracetamol absorption in migraine patients. *Clin Drug Invest* 1996; **11:** 300–304.

Antidepressants. Sumatriptan and rizatriptan are metabolised predominantly by monoamine oxidase type A and the manufacturers advise that patients taking *MAOIs*, including reversible selective type A inhibitors such as moclobemide, should not be given these serotonin (5-HT₁) agonists. Clearance of zolmitriptan was decreased after administration of moclobemide; therefore, a reduced dose of zolmitriptan is advised if the drug is used concomitantly with an inhibitor of monoamine oxidase type A. SSRIs such as fluoxetine may also interact with serotonin (5-HT₁) agonists with an increased risk of serotonin syndrome (p.304), and it has been suggested that *lithium* and sumatriptan may interact similarly. However, a review of the concomitant use of sumatriptan with MAOIs, SSRIs, or lithium found little evidence of an increased risk of serotonin syndrome.[1] It was concluded that most patients tolerate the combination of sumatriptan and an SSRI or lithium without incidence. However, it was suggested that the combination of su-

matriptan and an MAOI should continue to be avoided until further data supporting its safety becomes available. The manufacturers of zolmitriptan advise a reduction in dosage if it is given with fluvoxamine as the latter may inhibit zolmitriptan metabolism through its effects on the cytochrome P450 CYP1A2 isoenzyme. Increased serotonergic effects with increased incidence of adverse effects have been reported following the concomitant administration of *hypericum* (St. John's Wort) with triptans.[2] Patients should be advised to stop taking hypericum if treatment with a serotonin (5-HT₁) agonist is necessary.

1. Gardner DM, Lynd LD. Sumatriptan contraindications and the serotonin syndrome. *Ann Pharmacother* 1998; **32:** 33–8.
2. Committee on Safety of Medicines/Medicines Control Agency. Reminder: St John's wort (Hypericum perforatum) interactions. *Current Problems* 2000; **26:** 6–7.

Antimigraine drugs. The efficacy and tolerability of subcutaneous sumatriptan in the acute treatment of migraine did not appear to be affected in patients already taking dihydroergotamine orally for migraine prophylaxis.[1] However, the bioavailability of dihydroergotamine after oral administration is low and it could not be assumed that it was safe to use parenteral dihydroergotamine and sumatriptan concomitantly.[2] The use of sumatriptan as supplementary antimigraine medication following dihydroergotamine is not recommended; the concomitant use of sumatriptan and ergotamine or other related compounds is also considered contra-indicated (see above).

It is recommended that sumatriptan should not be given until at least 24 hours after stopping ergotamine or related compounds. Acute myocardial infarction has been reported[3] in a premenopausal woman with controlled hypertension and no known coronary artery disease after subcutaneous use of sumatriptan within a few hours of taking methysergide by mouth.

1. Henry P, *et al.* Subcutaneous sumatriptan in the acute treatment of migraine in patients using dihydroergotamine as prophylaxis. *Headache* 1993; **33:** 432–5.
2. Campbell JK. *Headache* 1993; **33:** 435 [editor's comment].
3. Liston H, *et al.* The association of the combination of sumatriptan and methysergide in myocardial infarction in a premenopausal woman. *Arch Intern Med* 1999; **159:** 511–13.

Antipsychotics. For reference to a potential interaction between sumatriptan and loxapine, see Chlorpromazine, p.664.

Pharmacokinetics

Sumatriptan is rapidly but incompletely absorbed following oral administration and undergoes first-pass metabolism, resulting in a low absolute bioavailability of about 14%. Peak plasma concentrations following oral administration are achieved in about 2 hours. Bioavailability is much higher (96%) following subcutaneous administration with peak concentrations occurring within 25 minutes. Bioavailability after intranasal administration is 16% relative to subcutaneous administration, with peak concentrations occurring in 1 to 1.5 hours. Plasma protein binding is low at about 14 to 21%.

The elimination half-life of sumatriptan is about 2 hours. Sumatriptan is extensively metabolised in the liver predominantly by monoamine oxidase type A and is excreted mainly in the urine as the inactive indole acetic acid derivative and its glucuronide. Sumatriptan and its metabolites also appear in the faeces. Small amounts of sumatriptan are distributed into breast milk (see above).

◊ Reviews.

1. Scott AK. Sumatriptan clinical pharmacokinetics. *Clin Pharmacokinet* 1994; **27:** 337–44.
2. Lacey LF, *et al.* Single dose pharmacokinetics of sumatriptan in healthy volunteers. *Eur J Clin Pharmacol* 1995; **47:** 543–8.

Uses and Administration

Sumatriptan is a selective serotonin agonist which acts at 5-HT₁ receptors and produces vasoconstriction of cranial arteries. It is used for the acute treatment of migraine attacks and of cluster headache. It should not be used prophylactically. It may be administered by mouth or subcutaneously as the succinate and intranasally as the base. Doses are expressed in terms of sumatriptan base.

For the acute treatment of **migraine** sumatriptan should be administered as soon as possible after the onset of the headache phase, but efficacy is independent of the duration of the attack before starting treatment. If no response is obtained with the initial dose by any route, a second dose should not be given for the same attack.

The recommended initial dose by mouth in the UK is 50 mg, although some patients may require 100 mg. A 50-mg dose is considered suitable for patients with

hepatic impairment. A clinical response can be expected after about 30 minutes. If there is a response but the migraine returns, further doses may be given provided that there is a minimum interval of 2 hours between doses and that not more than 300 mg is taken in any 24-hour period. In the USA a lower initial dose of 25 mg may be used, although some patients require 50 or 100 mg. This may be followed by a second dose of up to 100 mg if a satisfactory response has not been obtained after 2 hours provided that the total daily dose does not exceed the recommended maximum of 200 mg.

When administered intranasally a clinical response can be expected in 15 minutes. The recommended initial dose of sumatriptan in the UK is 20 mg administered into one nostril; 10 mg may be effective in some patients and in the USA, the recommended initial dose is 5, 10, or 20 mg. If symptoms recur, a second dose may be given in the next 24 hours, at least 2 hours after the first dose. Not more than 40 mg should be used in a 24-hour period.

Sumatriptan may be self-administered by subcutaneous injection in a single dose of 6 mg when a clinical response may be expected after 10 to 15 minutes. If symptoms recur, a second dose of 6 mg may be injected at least one hour after the first dose; not more than 12 mg should be given in a 24-hour period.

For the acute treatment of **cluster headache,** sumatriptan succinate is given by subcutaneous injection in similar doses to those used for migraine.

Migraine and cluster headache. The use of sumatriptan in the treatment of cluster headache (p.449) and migraine (p.449) has been reviewed.[1-5]

In **migraine** serotonin (5-HT₁) agonists are preferred to ergotamine for the treatment of acute attacks unresponsive to non-opioid analgesics. Sumatriptan has been shown to be effective when given orally,[6] subcutaneously,[7,8] or intranasally,[9] but there are few comparative studies with other antimigraine drugs. A comparative review[10] of the triptans suggested tentatively that in recommended doses eletriptan might give better headache relief than sumatriptan by mouth, whereas naratriptan and frovatriptan seemed less effective; other oral triptans were roughly comparable to sumatriptan, although rizatriptan seems to have a faster onset of action. No oral triptan has been shown to be more effective than subcutaneous sumatriptan. In one study[11] sumatriptan given orally was found to be more effective than ergotamine with caffeine, but in others[12,13] it was only of similar efficacy to aspirin compounds given with metoclopramide and was associated with more adverse effects. In another study, oral sumatriptan was of similar efficacy to the NSAID tolfenamic acid.[14] Subcutaneous sumatriptan had a faster onset of action but a higher headache recurrence rate than subcutaneous dihydroergotamine in one study.[15] Subcutaneous sumatriptan was more effective than intranasal dihydroergotamine.[16]

One review[5] noted that 50 to 69% of patients given sumatriptan orally, and 62 to 78% given sumatriptan intranasally, obtained relief of their headache within 2 hours, and 56 to 80% had relief within one hour when sumatriptan was given subcutaneously. About 21 to 57% of patients who initially respond to sumatriptan have a recurrence of their headache within 24 to 48 hours; this may be related in part to its short half-life. Such recurrences usually respond to a second dose[17,18] but studies indicate that if a first dose is ineffective subsequent doses for the same attack are of no benefit.[7,8,17] Sumatriptan is considered[19] to be effective when given at any time once the headache phase of migraine has started but prior administration during migraine aura appears to be of little benefit since it does not affect the aura or prevent or delay the development of headache.[20] Repeated or long-term use does not appear to be associated with reduced efficacy.[21,22] For reports of an association between sumatriptan and analgesic-induced headache, see under Adverse Effects, above.

Sumatriptan's effectiveness appears to be maintained in menses-related migraine, a condition which is considered to be less responsive to treatment than nonmenstrual migraine.[23]

Experience of use in children has been reported.[24] Results of a randomised, placebo-controlled study[25] in adolescents aged 12 to 17 years showed evidence of efficacy, tolerability, and safety in this age group; it was felt that the nasal spray might be particularly well suited for adolescent use.

Subcutaneous sumatriptan has also been shown to be effective in relieving acute attacks of headache in patients with **cluster headache.** In studies about 75% of patients have obtained relief within 15 minutes of a 6-mg subcutaneous injection;[26,27] the use of higher doses was found to be of no advantage. Long term efficacy appears to be maintained[28] but the significance of the transient increase in the frequency of attacks seen in some patients remains to be determined.[29] It does not appear to be effective for the prevention of headache during cluster peri-ods.[30]

1. Fullerton T, Gengo FM. Sumatriptan: a selective 5-hydroxytryp-tamine receptor agonist for the acute treatment of migraine. *Ann Pharmacother* 1992; **26**: 800–8.
2. Anonymous. Sumatriptan for migraine. *Med Lett Drugs Ther* 1992; **34**: 91–3.
3. Hsu VD. Sumatriptan: a new drug for vascular headache. *Clin Pharm* 1992; **11**: 919–29.
4. Bateman DN. Sumatriptan. *Lancet* 1993; **341**: 221–4.
5. Perry CM, Markham A. Sumatriptan: an updated review of its use in migraine. *Drugs* 1998; **55**: 889–922.
6. Goadsby PJ, *et al.* Oral sumatriptan in acute migraine. *Lancet* 1991; **338**: 782–3.
7. Cady RK, *et al.* Treatment of acute migraine with subcutaneous sumatriptan. *JAMA* 1991; **265**: 2831–21.
8. The Subcutaneous Sumatriptan International Study Group. Treatment of migraine attacks with sumatriptan. *N Engl J Med* 1991; **325**: 316–21.
9. Ryan R. Sumatriptan nasal spray for the acute treatment of mi-graine: results of two clinical studies. *Neurology* 1997; **49**: 1225–30.
10. Tfelt-Hansen P, *et al.* Triptans in migraine: a comparative re-view of pharmacology, pharmacokinetics and efficacy. *Drugs* 2000; **60**: 1259–87.
11. The Multinational Oral Sumatriptan and Cafergot Comparative Study Group. A randomized, double-blind comparison of su-matriptan and cafergot in the acute treatment of migraine. *Eur Neurol* 1991; **31**: 314–22.
12. The Oral Sumatriptan and Aspirin plus Metoclopramide Com-parative Study Group. A study to compare oral sumatriptan with oral aspirin plus oral metoclopramide in the acute treatment of migraine. *Eur Neurol* 1992; **32**: 177–84.
13. Tfelt-Hansen P, *et al.* The effectiveness of combined oral lysine acetylsalicylate and metoclopramide compared with oral su-matriptan for migraine. *Lancet* 1995; **346**: 923–6.
14. Myllylä VV, *et al.* Tolfenamic acid rapid release versus su-matriptan in the acute treatment of migraine: comparable effect in a double-blind, randomized, controlled, parallel-group study. *Headache* 1998; **38**: 201–7.
15. Winner P, *et al.* A double-blind study of subcutaneous dihydro-ergotamine vs subcutaneous sumatriptan in the treatment of acute migraine. *Arch Neurol* 1996; **53**: 180–4.
16. Touchon J, *et al.* A comparison of subcutaneous sumatriptan and dihydroergotamine nasal spray in the acute treatment of mi-graine. *Neurology* 1996; **47**: 361–5.
17. Ferrari MD, *et al.* Oral sumatriptan: effect of a second dose, and incidence and treatment of headache recurrences. *Cephalalgia* 1994; **14**: 330–8.
18. Dahlöf C. Headache recurrence after subcutaneous sumatriptan and early treatment. *Lancet* 1992; **340**: 909.
19. Ferrari MD. Sumatriptan in the treatment of migraine. *Neurolo-gy* 1993; **43** (suppl 3): S43–S47.
20. Bates D, *et al.* Sumatriptan during the migraine aura. *Neurology* 1994; **44**: 1587–92.
21. Cady RK, *et al.* Efficacy of subcutaneous sumatriptan in repeat-ed episodes of migraine. *Neurology* 1993; **43**: 1363–8.
22. Tansey MJB, *et al.* Long-term experience with sumatriptan in treatment of migraine. *Eur Neurol* 1993; **33**: 310–15.
23. Solbach MP, Waymer RS. Treatment of menstruation-associated migraine headache with subcutaneous sumatriptan. *Obstet Gynecol* 1993; **82**: 769–72.
24. Linder SL. Subcutaneous sumatriptan in the clinical setting: the first 50 consecutive patients with acute migraine in a pediatric neurology office practice. *Headache* 1996; **36**: 419–22.
25. Winner P, *et al.* A randomized, double-blind, placebo-controlled study of sumatriptan nasal spray in the treatment of acute mi-graine in adolescents. *Pediatrics* 2000; **106**: 989–997.
26. The Sumatriptan Cluster Headache Study Group. Treatment of acute cluster headache with sumatriptan. *N Engl J Med* 1991; **325**: 322–6.
27. Ekbom K, *et al.* Subcutaneous sumatriptan in the acute treat-ment of cluster headache: a dose comparison study. *Acta Neurol Scand* 1993; **88**: 63–9.
28. Ekbom K, *et al.* Cluster headache attacks treated for up to three months with subcutaneous sumatriptan (6 mg). *Cephalalgia* 1995; **15**: 230–6.
29. Hardebo JE. Subcutaneous sumatriptan in cluster headache: a time study of the effect on pain and autonomic symptoms. *Head-ache* 1993; **33**: 18–21.
30. Monstad I, *et al.* Preemptive oral treatment with sumatriptan during a cluster period. *Headache* 1995; **35**: 607–13.

Preparations

Proprietary Preparations (details are given in Part 3)

Aust.: Imigran; *Austral.:* Imigran; *Belg.:* Imitrex; *Braz.:* Imigran; Migril; Sumax; *Canad.:* Imitrex; *Denm.:* Imigran; *Fin.:* Imigran; *Fr.:* Imigrane; Imiject; *Ger.:* Imigran; *Hong Kong:* Imigran; *Irl.:* Imigran; *Israel:* Imitrex; *Ital.:* Imigran; Sumigrene; *Mex.:* Imi-gran; *Neth.:* Imigran; *Norw.:* Imigran; *NZ:* Imigran; *Port.:* Dil-etan; *S.Afr.:* Imigran; *Singapore:* Imigran; *Spain:* Arcoiran; Imigran; Novelian; *Swed.:* Imigran; *Switz.:* Imigran; *Thai.:* Imigran; *UK:* Imigran; *USA:* Imitrex.

Zolmitriptan   (17598-k)

Zolmitriptan *(BAN, USAN, rINN)*.

311C90. (S)-4-{3-[2-(Dimethylamino)ethyl]indol-5-ylmethyl}-1,3-oxazolidin-2-one.

$C_{16}H_{21}N_3O_2 = 287.4$.

CAS — 139264-17-8.
ATC — N02CC03.

Adverse Effects and Precautions

As for Sumatriptan, p.456. Zolmitriptan should also be avoided in patients with Wolff-Parkinson-White syndrome or arrhythmias associated with accessory cardiac conduction pathways. The dose of zol-mitriptan should be reduced in patients with moderate to severe hepatic impairment.

Analgesic-induced headache. For a report of an association between zolmitriptan and analgesic-induced headache, see un-der Adverse Effects of Sumatriptan, p.456.

Hepatic impairment. A study[1] has indicated that while there is no need to reduce the size of the initial dose of zol-mitriptan in patients with moderate or severe hepatic impair-ment, accumulation may occur with repeated administration in patients with severe hepatic impairment and their total daily dosage should be reduced (see Uses and Administration, be-low).

1. Dixon R, *et al.* Effect of hepatic impairment on the pharmacoki-netics of zolmitriptan. *J Clin Pharmacol* 1998; **38**: 694–701.

Ischaemia. A spinal cord lesion related to the use of zol-mitriptan has been reported in a 50-year-old woman;[1] clinical features suggested that the lesion was an ischaemic infarct.

1. Vijayan N, Peacock JH. Spinal cord infarction during use of zol-mitriptan: a case report. *Headache* 2000; **40**: 57–60.

Renal impairment. Although renal clearance of zolmitriptan and its metabolites was reduced in one study[1] in patients with moderate to severe renal impairment, the resulting effect was thought unlikely to be of clinical importance and adjustment of zolmitriptan dosage in patients with renal impairment was con-sidered unnecessary.

1. Gillotin C, *et al.* No need to adjust the dose of 311C90 (zol-mitriptan), a novel anti-migraine treatment in patients with renal failure not requiring dialysis. *Int J Clin Pharmacol Ther* 1997; **35**: 522–6.

Interactions

As for Sumatriptan, p.457. It is recommended that the maximum dose of zolmitriptan in 24 hours should be reduced in patients receiving cimetidine (see under Uses and Administration, below). Opinion varies on the concomitant use of zolmitriptan and inhibitors of monoamine oxidase type A such as moclobemide. In the UK the manufacturers recommend that the maxi-mum dose of zolmitriptan should be reduced when used with inhibitors of monoamine oxidase type A whereas in the USA the manufacturers contraindicate such combinations. A similar reduction in zol-mitriptan dosage is anticipated if it is given with drugs, such as fluvoxamine and ciprofloxacin, that in-hibit the cytochrome P450 isoenzyme CYP1A2. Zol-mitriptan should not be used within 12 hours of other serotonin (5-HT$_1$) agonists.

◊ References.

1. Dixon R, *et al.* The metabolism of zolmitriptan: effects of an in-ducer and an inhibitor of cytochrome P450 on its pharmacokinet-ics in healthy volunteers. *Clin Drug Invest* 1998; **15**: 515–22.

Beta blockers. *Propranolol* increased plasma-zolmitriptan concentrations in a study in 12 healthy volunteers, but the changes were not thought to be clinically important, therefore dosage adjustment of zolmitriptan in patients taking pro-pranolol for migraine prophylaxis was not considered neces-sary.[1]

1. Peck RW, *et al.* The interaction between propranolol and the nov-el antimigraine agent zolmitriptan (311C90). *Br J Clin Pharma-col* 1997; **44**: 595–9.

Pharmacokinetics

The absolute bioavailability of zolmitriptan following oral administration is about 40 to 50%, and peak-plas-ma concentrations are achieved in about 1.5 to 3.5 hours depending on the formulation. Plasma protein binding is low (about 25%). Zolmitriptan undergoes hepatic metabolism, principally to the indole acetic acid, and also the *N*-oxide and *N*-desmethyl ana-logues. The *N*-desmethyl metabolite (183C91) was more active than the parent compound in *animal* stud-ies, and would be expected to contribute to the thera-peutic effect of zolmitriptan. The primary metabolism of zolmitriptan is mediated mainly by the cytochrome P450 isoenzyme CYP1A2 while monoamine oxidase type A is responsible for further metabolism of the *N*-desmethyl metabolite. Over 60% of a dose is excreted in the urine, mainly as the indole acetic acid, and about 30% appears in the faeces, mainly as unchanged drug. The elimination half-life is 2.5 to 3 hours, and is prolonged in patients with liver disease.

◊ References.

1. Seaber E, *et al.* The tolerability and pharmacokinetics of the nov-el antimigraine compound 311C90 in healthy male volunteers. *Br J Clin Pharmacol* 1996; **41**: 141–7.
2. Dixon R, *et al.* The pharmacokinetics and effects on blood pres-sure of multiple doses of the novel anti-migraine drug zol-mitriptan (311C90) in healthy volunteers. *Br J Clin Pharmacol* 1997; **43**: 273–81.
3. Seaber E, *et al.* The absolute bioavailability and metabolic dis-position of the novel antimigraine compound zolmitriptan (311C90). *Br J Clin Pharmacol* 1997; **43**: 579–87.
4. Peck RW, *et al.* The pharmacodynamics and pharmacokinetics of the 5HT$_{1B/1D}$-agonist zolmitriptan in healthy young and elderly men and women. *Clin Pharmacol Ther* 1998; **63**: 342–53.
5. Seaber EJ. *et al.* The absolute bioavailability and effect of food on the pharmacokinetics of zolmitriptan in healthy volunteers. *Br J Clin Pharmacol* 1998; **46**: 433–9.
6. Dixon R, *et al.* A comparison of the pharmacokinetics and toler-ability of the novel antimigraine compound zolmitriptan in ado-lescents and adults. *J Child Adolesc Psychopharmacol* 1999; **9**: 35–42.

Uses and Administration

Zolmitriptan is a selective serotonin (5-HT$_1$) agonist with actions and uses similar to those of sumatriptan (p.457). It is used for the acute treatment of migraine attacks. Zolmitriptan should not be used prophylacti-cally. It should be administered as early as possible after the onset of migraine headache, but efficacy is independent of the duration of the attack before start-ing treatment.

The recommended initial dose in the UK is 2.5 mg. If symptoms persist or return within 24 hours, a second dose may be taken not less than 2 hours after the first dose. The maximum dose of zolmitriptan in 24 hours is 15 mg; in those with moderate or severe hepatic im-pairment a reduced maximum dose of 5 mg in 24 hours is recommended. A similar reduction is recom-mended in those taking cimetidine concurrently; in patients taking zolmitriptan while receiving an inhib-itor of monoamine oxidase type A, the maximum dose of zolmitriptan in 24 hours should be 7.5 mg. If a patient does not achieve satisfactory relief with an initial dose of 2.5 mg, subsequent attacks may be treated with initial doses of 5 mg.

Recommended doses in the USA are somewhat low-er; the initial dose is 1.25 to 2.5 mg with a maximum dose of 10 mg in 24 hours. A single dose of less than 2.5 mg is recommended for patients with hepatic im-pairment.

Doses may need to be reduced in patients receiving other drugs that inhibit the metabolism of zol-mitriptan (see under Interactions, above).

Migraine. References.

1. Rapoport AM, *et al.* Optimizing the dose of zolmitriptan (Zomig, 311C90) for the acute treatment of migraine: a multi-center, double-blind, placebo-controlled dose range-finding study. *Neurology* 1997; **49**: 1210–18.
2. Solomon GD, *et al.* Clinical efficacy and tolerability of 2.5 mg zolmitriptan for the acute treatment of migraine. *Neurology* 1997; **49**: 1219–26.
3. Anonymous. Zolmitriptan for migraine. *Med Lett Drugs Ther* 1998; **40**: 27–8.
4. The International 311C90 Long-term Study Group. The long-term tolerability and efficacy of oral zolmitriptan (Zomig, 311C90) in the acute treatment of migraine: an international study. *Headache* 1998; **38**: 173–83.
5. Spencer CM, *et al.* Zolmitriptan: a review of its use in migraine. *Drugs* 1999; **58**: 347–74.
6. Tepper SJ, *et al.* A long-term study to maximise migraine relief with zolmitriptan. *Curr Med Res Opin* 1999; **15**: 254–71.
7. Tuchman M, *et al.* Zolmitriptan provides consistent migraine re-lief when used in the long-term. *Curr Med Res Opin* 1999; **15**: 272–81.
8. Mauskop A, *et al.* Zolmitriptan is effective for the treatment of persistent and recurrent migraine headache. *Curr Med Res Opin* 1999; **15**: 282–9.
9. Bahra A, *et al.* Oral zolmitriptan is effective in the acute treat-ment of cluster headache. *Neurology* 2000; **54**: 1832–9.
10. Mathew NT, *et al.* Treatment of nonresponders to oral su-matriptan with zolmitriptan and rizatriptan: a comparative open trial. *Headache* 2000; **40**: 464–5.

Preparations

Proprietary Preparations (details are given in Part 3)

Aust.: Zomig; *Austral.:* Zomig; *Belg.:* Zomig; *Canad.:* Zomig; *Denm.:* Zomig; *Fin.:* Zomig; *Fr.:* Zomig; *Ger.:* AscoTop; *Hong Kong:* Zomig; *Irl.:* Zomig; *Israel:* Zomig; *Ital.:* Zomig; *Mex.:* Zomig; *Neth.:* Zomig; *Norw.:* Zomig; *Port.:* Zomig; *S.Afr.:* Zomig; *Singapore:* Zomig; *Spain:* Zomig; *Swed.:* Zomig; *Switz.:* Zomig; *Thai.:* Zomig; *UK:* Zomig; *USA:* Zomig.

Antimuscarinics

Antimuscarinic drugs are competitive inhibitors of the actions of acetylcholine at the muscarinic receptors of autonomic effector sites innervated by parasympathetic (cholinergic postganglionic) nerves, as well as being inhibitors of the action of acetylcholine on smooth muscle lacking cholinergic innervation. They have also been described as parasympatholytic, atropinic, atropine-like, and as anticholinergic, although the latter term should encompass compounds that also have antinicotinic actions.

Antimuscarinics can be classified as tertiary amine or quaternary ammonium compounds. The naturally occurring alkaloids such as atropine, hyoscine, and hyoscyamine are tertiary amines, that is they have a tertiary nitrogen atom; semisynthetic derivatives or synthetic antimuscarinics may be either tertiary (e.g. homatropine or benzhexol [trihexyphenidyl]) or quaternary ammonium (e.g. homatropine methylbromide or ipratropium) compounds. At least 5 different pharmacologically identifiable types of **muscarinic receptor** (M_1, M_2, M_3, M_4, and M_5) have been described as have 5 different molecular forms (m_1, m_2, m_3, m_4, and m_5) of these receptors. While the traditional antimuscarinics appear to be relatively non-specific, newer compounds like pirenzepine and telenzepine have a selective action on the M_1 receptors within ganglia supplying cholinergic postganglionic nerves to the gastrointestinal tract. At therapeutic doses tertiary amine antimuscarinics have little effect on the actions of acetylcholine at nicotinic receptors. However, the quaternary ammonium antimuscarinics exhibit a greater degree of antinicotinic potency, and some of their side-effects at high doses are due to ganglionic blockade; excessively high doses may even produce neuromuscular block. There are also pharmacokinetic differences between tertiary amine and quaternary ammonium antimuscarinics. Quaternary ammonium compounds are less lipid soluble than tertiary amines; their gastrointestinal absorption is poor and they do not readily pass the blood-brain barrier or conjunctiva.

Antimuscarinics can produce a wide range of effects at therapeutic doses. The **peripheral** antimuscarinic effects that are produced as the dose increases are: decreased production of secretions from the salivary, bronchial, and sweat glands; dilatation of the pupils (mydriasis) and paralysis of accommodation (cycloplegia); increased heart rate; inhibition of micturition and reduction in gastrointestinal tone; and inhibition of gastric acid secretion. As for **central** effects, with the exception of hyoscine, which causes CNS depression at therapeutic doses, tertiary amines stimulate the medulla and higher cerebral centres producing mild central vagal excitation and respiratory stimulation. At toxic doses all tertiary amines, including hyoscine, cause stimulation of the CNS with restlessness, disorientation, hallucinations, and delirium. As the dose increases stimulation is followed by central depression and death from respiratory paralysis. Synthetic tertiary amines are less potent in their central

effects than natural tertiary amines; quaternary ammonium compounds have negligible central effects.

These actions of antimuscarinics have led to their use in a variety of clinical conditions.

◊ References.
1. Goyal RK. Muscarinic receptor subtypes: physiology and clinical implications. *N Engl J Med* 1989; **321:** 1022–9.
2. Caulfield MP. Muscarinic receptors—characterization, coupling and function. *Pharmacol Ther* 1993; **58:** 319–79.
3. Caulfield MP, Birdsall NJM. International Union of Pharmacology. XVII. Classification of muscarinic acetylcholine receptors. *Pharmacol Rev* 1998; **50:** 279–90.

Anaesthesia
Antimuscarinics, including *atropine, hyoscine,* and *glycopyrronium,* have been used pre-operatively to inhibit salivation and excessive secretions of the respiratory tract during anaesthesia (p.1256). This use is less important now that less irritating anaesthetics are used. Atropine and glycopyrronium are given to reduce intra-operative bradycardia and hypotension induced by drugs such as suxamethonium, halothane, or propofol, or following vagal stimulation. Glycopyrronium causes less tachycardia than atropine when given intravenously. When hyoscine is used as a premedicant it also provides some amnesia, sedation, and antiemesis but, unlike atropine, may cause bradycardia rather than tachycardia. Atropine or glycopyrronium is also used before, or with, anticholinesterases such as neostigmine to prevent their muscarinic adverse effects (see p.1420).

Cardiac disorders
The cardiac uses of *atropine* are discussed on p.462.

Colic pain
Antimuscarinics may relieve painful spasms of the biliary and genito-urinary systems and have been used in biliary or renal (ureteral) colic, although, as discussed on p.5, analgesics are normally used. However, an antispasmodic should be given with morphine and its derivatives in patients with biliary disorders to counteract painful spasms of the sphincter of Oddi which may be produced by the opioid. See Gastrointestinal Disorders (below) for reference to gastrointestinal spasm.

Dystonias
Antimuscarinics such as benzhexol [trihexyphenidyl] have been used in the management of dystonias (p.1173). The high doses which may be required are tolerated much better by children and adolescents than by adults.

Extrapyramidal disorders
See Dystonias (above) and Parkinsonism, including drug-induced extrapyramidal disorders (below).

Eye disorders
See under Mydriasis and Cycloplegia (below).

Gastrointestinal disorders
Antimuscarinics have been used to relieve **spasms** of the gastrointestinal tract in diverticular disease (p.1203), dyspepsia (p.1204), and irritable bowel syndrome (p.1206); they are no longer considered appropriate for use in infant colic (see Gastrointestinal Spasm, p.1204; see above for use in other forms of colic). Antimuscarinics have also been tried in an attempt to relax the smooth muscle in oesophageal spasm (p.1208), although results are often disappointing. They should be avoided in patients with oesophageal reflux because of a tendency to relax the oesophageal sphincter.

Antimuscarinics have been used for their antisecretory effects in the treatment of **peptic ulcer disease** (p.1208), generally as adjuncts to other antiulcer drugs. *Pirenzepine,* a selective antimuscarinic, was considered to have the advantage over nonselective antimuscarinics of fewer adverse effects.

Hyoscine is one of the principal drugs used to prevent **motion sickness** (see under Nausea and Vomiting, p.1206). It may be given by mouth for short-term protection or transdermally from controlled release systems for a prolonged duration of action.

Hyperhidrosis
Antimuscarinics such as *diphemanil metilsulfate, glycopyrronium bromide,* and *hyoscine hydrobromide* have been applied topically as alternatives to aluminium salts in the treatment of hyperhidrosis (p.1105). Side-effects of antimuscarinics administered by mouth generally preclude their use by this route, although oral *propantheline* has been used successfully.

Micturition disorders
Normal micturition — awareness of the need to void urine as a result of bladder filling, postponement of urination until convenient, and the ability to empty the bladder voluntarily — is controlled by the smooth detrusor muscle of the bladder (innervated predominantly by parasympathetic nerves) and the external sphincter (sympathetic innervation). During urination parasympathetic stimulation causes the detrusor muscle to contract while reduced sympathetic tone allows the external sphincter to relax. Micturition disorders can occur through local effects on the bladder or urethra or may result through disturbances of their nervous control. They include nocturnal enuresis, urinary incontinence, and urinary retention. The terms 'neurogenic bladder' and 'neuropathic bladder' are used loosely to describe any bladder dysfunction resulting from any neurological disturbance.

Nocturnal enuresis. Involuntary discharge of urine during sleep, termed nocturnal enuresis (bed-wetting), is a normal occurrence in young children, but may persist in up to 5% by the age of 10 years. Nonpharmacological approaches to treatment include bladder retention training, motivational therapy, and behaviour modification or conditioning therapy using moisture-sensitive alarms. Drug therapy may initially produce a more rapid response, but training and the use of alarms has generally appeared to be more effective and to have a lower relapse rate. Although preparations are available to treat children as young as 5 years of age many consider drug therapy to be inappropriate for children under 7 years. Drug therapy is probably most useful for intermittent use on special occasions such as sleeping away from home or when added to treatment in children who fail to respond to nonpharmacological methods alone. The long-term use of drugs for enuresis is controversial.

Administration of *desmopressin* at night can be effective in the short-term control of nocturnal enuresis and many now consider it to be the drug of choice in terms of safety. However, it should not be given when enuresis is due to polydipsia as desmopressin may provoke water intoxication and convulsions due to hyponatraemia.

Of the tricyclic antidepressants most experience has been with *imipramine*. Their mechanism of action in nocturnal enuresis is unclear. It may be partly the result of their antimuscarinic and antispasmodic actions.

Antimuscarinics such as *oxybutynin* reduce uninhibited bladder contractions, but although they may be of benefit in diurnal enuresis they are rarely of benefit in nocturnal enuresis alone.

References.
1. Marcovitch H. Treating bed wetting. *BMJ* 1993; **306:** 536.
2. Rappaport L. The treatment of nocturnal enuresis—where are we now? *Pediatrics* 1993; **92:** 465–6.
3. Mark SD, Frank JD. Nocturnal enuresis. *Br J Urol* 1995; **75:** 427–34.
4. Monda JM, Husmann DA. Primary nocturnal enuresis: a comparison among observation, imipramine, desmopressin acetate and bed-wetting alarm systems. *J Urol (Baltimore)* 1995, **154:** 745–8.
5. Burke JR, *et al.* A comparison of amitriptyline, vasopressin and amitriptyline with vasopressin in nocturnal enuresis. *Pediatr Nephrol* 1995; **9:** 438–40.
6. Tietjen DN, Husmann DA. Nocturnal enuresis: a guide to evaluation and treatment. *Mayo Clin Proc* 1996; **71:** 857–62.
7. Owens RG, Karram MM. Comparative tolerability of drug therapies used to treat incontinence and enuresis. *Drug Safety* 1998; **19:** 123–39.

Urinary incontinence and retention. Urinary incontinence is defined as an involuntary loss of urine which is objectively demonstrable and a social or hygienic problem. Nocturnal enuresis is discussed above. Depending on the cause patients may have symptoms of urinary frequency, nocturia, urgency, dribbling, or dysuria. Classifications of incontinence vary but the main types include: stress incontinence, urge incontinence, and overflow incontinence (a consequence of urinary retention). The term functional incontinence is used when the patient's condition is due to impaired mobility or mental function. It is important to determine the type and, where possible, cause of urinary incontinence before attempting treatment. Urinary-tract infections, constipation, and benign prostatic hyperplasia may mimic or cause the symptoms of urinary incontinence and should be excluded.

Stress incontinence is the commonest form of incontinence in women. The patient usually has urethral sphincter incompetence and loss of urine is associated with increases in intra-abdominal pressure such as may occur on standing or coughing. Treatment may be with nonpharmacological measures such as pelvic floor exercises, electrical stimulation, or biofeedback, and the use of devices such as vaginal cones; with surgery; or with drugs. Some consider that drug therapy has little part in the treatment of stress incontinence. Alpha-adrenoceptor agonists such as *ephedrine, phenylpropanolamine,* and *pseudoephedrine* have been used to increase tone in the muscles of the urethra and at the base of the bladder; they may be helpful when used prophylactically in certain stress situations, but long-term experience has been mostly disappointing. *Oestrogens* used with an alpha-adrenoceptor agonist such as phenylpropanolamine appear to be effective and this combination may be of use for postmenopausal women with mild stress incontinence; unfortunately addition of a progestogen to treatment to reduce the risk of endometrial carcinoma in women with an intact uterus might exacerbate the incontinence. The value of oestrogens used without an alpha-adrenoceptor agonist is less clear. Intra-urethral injections of *collagen* or *polytef* appear to be effective, but there are concerns over migration and granuloma formation with polytef.

In **urge incontinence**, also known as unstable bladder or detrusor instability, uninhibited contractions of the detrusor muscle occur without warning and overcome urethral sphincter resistance. Micturition occurs despite any attempt the patient might make to prevent it. Urge incontinence is the most common form of incontinence in the elderly and is often refractory to treatment. The cause is usually unknown and these cases are referred to as being due to **idiopathic detrusor instability**. When there is overt neurological disease, such as upper motor neurone lesions in spinal cord injury or multiple sclerosis, the term **detrusor hyperreflexia** is used. Reduction of excessive fluid intake and avoidance of drinks containing alcohol or caffeine may control mild symptoms of urge incontinence. Physiotherapy and behaviour therapy including bladder drill, biofeedback, hypnotherapy, acupuncture, and electrical stimulation may help. No drug treatment has been found to be universally effective. Drugs with antimuscarinic activity have been used to relax the detrusor muscle by inhibiting unstable detrusor muscle contractions but the incidence of adverse effects can be high. As these drugs can increase bladder volume they should not be used in patients with urinary retention. The antimuscarinic *oxybutynin* also has direct smooth muscle relaxant properties and is considered by some to be the most useful drug, but adverse effects are common. *Tolterodine* and *propiverine* have been introduced as alternatives to oxybutynin. *Flavoxate* has also been used but appears to be less effective than oxybutynin. *Propantheline,* although once widely used, is not recommended for routine use due to its low response rate and a high incidence of side-effects. *Emepronium* was once popular but is now considered to be of limited use. *Tricyclic antidepressants* have also been used in urge incontinence because of their antimuscarinic activity but their main use has been in nocturnal enuresis and nocturia (see above). *Desmopressin* is also mainly used in nocturnal enuresis and nocturia. Evidence regarding the use of *oestrogens* is inconclusive, but they may be useful in the adjunctive treatment of postmenopausal women with symptoms of urgency, frequency, and nocturia. Injection of *botulinum A toxin* into the detrusor muscle may be effective in the treatment of detrusor hyperreflexia which is resistant to antimuscarinics. Surgery is reserved for intractable cases.

Urge incontinence can also be due to abnormalities in bladder sensation; the causes of **sensory urgency** are often unknown but may be due to conditions such as urinary-tract infections or interstitial cystitis. Bladder retraining techniques and antimuscarinic therapy have been suggested when no underlying disorder can be identified.

Patients with **overflow incontinence** suffer from a continuous or frequent dribbling of urine as a consequence of an overdistended bladder produced by **urinary retention**. It may result from some form of urethral blockage or may be associated with drug treatment or conditions that reduce detrusor contractions or interfere with relaxation of the urethra. Overflow incontinence is uncommon in women and most patients are elderly men with urethral blockage due to benign prostatic hyperplasia (p.1477). However, urinary retention may also occur postpartum or postoperatively. Treatment depends on the underlying condition. Catheterisation is used to relieve acute painful urinary retention or when no cause can be found. Surgical procedures or dilatation are often used to correct any mechanical outflow obstruction. Alpha-adrenoceptor blocking drugs such as *alfuzosin, doxazosin, indoramin, prazosin, tamsulosin,* and *terazosin* may be given to patients waiting for surgery or to those unfit for surgery. They decrease outflow resistance and improve bladder emptying. Patients with detrusor hypotonicity have been given parasympathomimetics such as *bethanechol, carbachol,* and *distigmine* to increase detrusor muscle contractions but there have been doubts about their efficacy. Parasympathomimetics have also been used for the management of postoperative urinary retention, but have been superseded by catheterisation.

References.

1. International Continence Society Standardization Committee. The standardization of terminology of lower urinary tract function. *Br J Obstet Gynaecol* 1990; **97** (suppl 6): 1–16.
2. Battock TM, Castleden CM. Pharmacological treatment of urinary incontinence. *Br Med Bull* 1990; **46**: 147–55.
3. Cardozo L. Urinary incontinence in women: have we anything new to offer? *BMJ* 1991; **303**: 1453–7.
4. Anonymous. Non-surgical treatment of stress incontinence. *Lancet* 1992; **340**: 643–4.
5. Eckford SD, Keane DP. Management of detrusor instability. *Br J Hosp Med* 1993; **49**: 282–5.
6. Wise BG, Cardozo LD. Urinary urgency in women. *Br J Hosp Med* 1993; **50**: 243–50.
7. Richmond D. The incontinent woman: 2. *Br J Hosp Med* 1993; **50**: 490–2.
8. Resnick NM. Urinary incontinence. *Lancet* 1995; **346**: 94–9.
9. Owens RG, Karram MM. Comparative tolerability of drug therapies used to treat incontinence and enuresis. *Drug Safety* 1998; **19**: 123–39.
10. Chutka DS, Takahashi PY. Urinary incontinence in the elderly: drug treatment options. *Drugs* 1998; **56**: 587–95.
11. Scientific Committee of the First International Consultation on Incontinence. Assessment and treatment of urinary incontinence. *Lancet* 2000; **355**: 2153–8.

Mydriasis and cycloplegia

Drugs that dilate the pupil (mydriatics) and paralyse accommodation (cycloplegics) are used topically in the examination of the eye and other ophthalmic procedures, in the management of inflammatory conditions of the eye to treat or prevent the formation of adhesions between the lens and the iris (see Uveitis, p.1060), and in strabismus (p.1414).

Mydriasis can be achieved by paralysis of the pupillary constrictor muscles (which is how antimuscarinics act) or by stimulation of the dilator muscles (which is how sympathomimetics act). Cycloplegia results from paralysis of the ciliary muscles (antimuscarinics, but not sympathomimetics, have this effect).

Antimuscarinics used in ophthalmology vary in onset and duration of action. *Atropine* can take up to 40 minutes or more to produce mydriasis, which persists for at least 7 days; it takes 1 to 3 hours to produce cycloplegia and 6 to 12 days for recovery of accommodation. *Hyoscine* has a shorter duration of action than atropine, although the effects may still persist for 3 to 7 days. For ophthalmic procedures, antimuscarinics such as *homatropine, cyclopentolate,* or *tropicamide,* which have a more rapid onset and shorter duration of action than atropine, may be preferable. Tropicamide has the shortest duration of action with recovery occurring in up to 6 hours. The effects of cyclopentolate may last for 24 hours. Recovery following administration of homatropine may take up to 3 days. However, cycloplegia with homatropine may be incomplete and for young children (who are often resistant to the action of homatropine), cyclopentolate or atropine may be preferred.

The sympathomimetic most commonly used topically is *phenylephrine* but *hydroxyamfetamine* is also used in some countries. They are often used with an antimuscarinic to enhance mydriasis especially in patients who might respond poorly to antimuscarinics alone, such as those with dark irides or diabetes or those who are receiving prolonged miotic therapy. *Adrenaline [epinephrine]* has been used for maintenance of mydriasis during ophthalmic surgery.

The local anaesthetic *cocaine* also has an independent mydriatic effect but because of concern over corneal toxicity it is now little used in ophthalmology.

Miosis (pupil constriction) resistant to conventional mydriatics often develops during ocular surgery, possibly due to the release of prostaglandins and other substances associated with trauma. *NSAIDs* are prostaglandin synthetase inhibitors and have been tried before ocular surgery to prevent or reduce intra-operative miosis. They do not possess intrinsic mydriatic properties.

Parkinsonism

Antimuscarinics are used in Parkinson's disease (idiopathic or primary parkinsonism) and drug-induced parkinsonism. Those most commonly used are the tertiary amines, *benzhexol [trihexyphenidyl], benzatropine, orphenadrine,* and *procyclidine*. In Parkinson's disease (p.1160), antimuscarinics are generally used in the early stages when the condition is mild and tremor is the predominant symptom, as they provide little benefit in bradykinesia. They can also reduce the sialorrhoea experienced by patients with this disease but can aggravate other associated conditions such as constipation or dementia. Antimuscarinics may also be used later as adjuvant therapy to levodopa such as in patients with refractory tremor or dystonias.

Although antimuscarinics may provide relief from the extrapyramidal symptoms that occur as side-effects of antipsychotic therapy (see p.662), they do not relieve the symptoms of tardive dyskinesia and should be discontinued if it develops.

Respiratory-tract disorders

The parasympathetic nervous system is involved in regulating bronchomotor tone; antimuscarinics have potent bronchodilatory activity and may be used in the management of bronchospasm. *Ipratropium* and *oxitropium* by inhalation are used in chronic bronchitis (p.759) and are at least as effective as beta₂ agonists. They may also be added to an existing regimen of inhaled short-acting beta₂ agonist plus regular high-dose inhaled corticosteroid in severe chronic asthma, and are used in severe acute asthma exacerbations (p.757).

Atropine and *glycopyrronium* have been used.

References.

1. Gross NJ, Skorodin MS. Role of the parasympathetic system in airway obstruction due to emphysema. *N Engl J Med* 1984; **311**: 421–5.

Rhinitis

The antimuscarinic drug ipratropium is used intranasally for the treatment of rhinitis (see p.767).

Vertigo

Antihistamines are the mainstay of the treatment of vertigo (p.408), although the antimuscarinic drug *hyoscine* is effective in the prophylaxis and treatment of vertigo and nausea associated with vestibular disorders, such as Ménière's disease (p.407). See also motion sickness under Nausea and Vomiting (p.469).

Atropine   (331-w)

Atropine (BAN).
(±)-Hyoscyamine. (1R,3r,5S,8r)-Tropan-3-yl (RS)-tropate.
C₁₇H₂₃NO₃ = 289.4.
CAS — 51-55-8.
ATC — A03BA01; S01FA01.
Pharmacopoeias. In Swiss and US.

An alkaloid which may be obtained from solanaceous plants, or prepared by synthesis.

Pharmacopoeial description

USP 25: White crystals, usually needle-like, or white crystalline powder. Soluble 1 in 460 of water, 1 in 90 of water at 80°, 1 in 2 of alcohol, 1 in 1 of chloroform, and 1 in 25 of ether; soluble in glycerol. Its saturated solution in water is alkaline to phenolphthalein. Store in airtight containers. Protect from light.

Atropine Methobromide   (332-e)

Atropine Methobromide (BANM).
Atropine Methylbromide; Methylatropine Bromide; Methylatropini Bromidum; Methylatropinium Bromatum; Mydriasine.
(1R,3r,5S)-8-Methyl-3-[(±)-tropoyloxy]tropanium bromide.
C₁₈H₂₆BrNO₃ = 384.3.
CAS — 2870-71-5.
Pharmacopoeias. In Eur. (see p.vi).

Pharmacopoeial description

Ph. Eur.: Colourless crystals or a white crystalline powder. Freely soluble in water; sparingly soluble in alcohol; practically insoluble in ether. Protect from light.

Atropine Methonitrate (333-I)

Atropine Methonitrate (BANM, rINN).

Atrop. Methonit.; Atropini Methonitras; Methylatropine Nitrate (USAN); Methylatropini Nitras. (1R,3r,5S)-8-Methyl-3-[(±)-tropoyloxy]tropanium nitrate.
$C_{18}H_{26}N_2O_6 = 366.4$.
CAS — 52-88-0.
Pharmacopoeias. In Eur. (see p.vi).

Aqueous solutions are unstable; stability is enhanced in acid solutions of pH below 6.

Pharmacopoeial description

Ph. Eur.: A white, crystalline powder or colourless crystals. Freely soluble in water; soluble in alcohol; practically insoluble in ether. Protect from light.

Atropine Sulfate (335-j)

Atrop. Sulph.; Atropine Sulphate (BANM); Atropini Sulfas.
$(C_{17}H_{23}NO_3)_2,H_2SO_4,H_2O = 694.8$.
CAS — 55-48-1 (anhydrous atropine sulfate); 5908-99-6 (atropine sulfate monohydrate).

NOTE. Compounded preparations of atropine sulfate may be represented by the following names:
• Co-phenotrope (BAN)—atropine sulfate 1 part and diphenoxylate hydrochloride 100 parts (w/w).

ATR is a code approved by the BP 2001 for use on single unit dose eye drops containing atropine sulfate where the individual container may be too small to bear all the appropriate labelling information.
Pharmacopoeias. In Chin., Eur. (see p.vi), Int., Jpn, Pol., and US.

Pharmacopoeial description

Ph. Eur.: A white, crystalline powder or colourless crystals. Very soluble in water; freely soluble in alcohol; practically insoluble in ether. A 2% solution in water has a pH of 4.5 to 6.2. Protect from light.

USP 25: Odourless, colourless crystals or white crystalline powder. It effloresces in dry air. Soluble 1 in 0.5 of water, 1 in 2.5 of boiling water, 1 in 5 of alcohol, and 1 in 2.5 of glycerol. Store in airtight containers.

Incompatibility. Incompatibility between atropine sulfate and hydroxybenzoate preservatives has been observed,[1] resulting in a total loss of the atropine in 2 to 3 weeks.
1. Deeks T. Oral atropine sulphate mixtures. Pharm J 1983; 230: 481.

Adverse Effects

The pattern of adverse effects seen with atropine and other antimuscarinics can mostly be related to their pharmacological actions at muscarinic and, at high doses, nicotinic receptors (see p.459). These effects are dose-related and are usually reversible when therapy is discontinued. The **peripheral** side-effects of atropine and other antimuscarinics are a consequence of their inhibitory effect on muscarinic receptors within the autonomic nervous system. At therapeutic doses, adverse effects include dryness of the mouth with difficulty in swallowing and talking, thirst, reduced bronchial secretions, dilatation of the pupils (mydriasis) with loss of accommodation (cycloplegia) and photophobia, flushing and dryness of the skin, transient bradycardia followed by tachycardia, with palpitations and arrhythmias, and difficulty in micturition, as well as reduction in the tone and motility of the gastrointestinal tract leading to constipation. Some of the **central** side-effects of atropine and other tertiary antimuscarinics seen at toxic doses (see below) may also occur at therapeutic doses.

In **overdosage**, the peripheral effects become more pronounced and other symptoms such as hyperthermia, hypertension, increased respiratory rate, and nausea and vomiting may occur. A rash may appear on the face or upper trunk. Toxic doses also cause CNS stimulation marked by restlessness, confusion, excitement, ataxia, incoordination, paranoid and psychotic reactions, hallucinations and delirium, and occasionally seizures. However, in severe intoxication, central stimulation may give way to CNS depression, coma, circulatory and respiratory failure, and death.

There is considerable variation in susceptibility to atropine; recovery has occurred even after 1 g, whereas deaths have been reported from doses of 100 mg or less for adults and 10 mg for children.

Quaternary ammonium antimuscarinics, such as atropine methobromide or methonitrate and propantheline bromide, have some ganglion-blocking activity and high doses may cause postural hypotension and

impotence; in toxic doses non-depolarising neuromuscular block may be produced.

Systemic toxicity may be produced by the **local** instillation of antimuscarinic eye drops, particularly in children and in the elderly. Prolonged administration of atropine to the eye may lead to local irritation, hyperaemia, oedema, and conjunctivitis. An increase in intra-ocular pressure may occur, especially in patients with angle-closure glaucoma.

Hypersensitivity to atropine is not uncommon and may occur as conjunctivitis or a skin rash.

Effects on body temperature. Atropine can cause hyperthermia as a result of inhibition of sweating. This may be attenuated by atropine's ability to dilate cutaneous blood vessels. However, there has been a report of hypothermia in a 14-year-old feverish patient following intravenous administration of atropine.[1]
For reports of fatal heat stroke in patients receiving an antimuscarinic and an antipsychotic concomitantly, see under Interactions in Benzatropine, p.463.
1. Lacouture PG, et al. Acute hypothermia associated with atropine. Am J Dis Child 1983; 137: 291–2.

Effects on the eyes. In addition to the expected ocular effects of atropine there have been instances of acute angle-closure glaucoma in patients receiving nebulised atropine.[1]
1. Berdy GJ, et al. Angle closure glaucoma precipitated by aerosolized atropine. Arch Intern Med 1991; 151: 1658–60.

Effects on the gastrointestinal tract. A report of paralytic ileus in a 77-year-old man with Parkinson's disease who had been receiving atropine sulfate by mouth to control excess salivation.[1]
1. Beatson N. Atropine and paralytic ileus. Postgrad Med J 1982; 58: 451–3.

Effects on the heart. Atropine sulfate to a total of 1 mg per 70 kg body-weight given intravenously to 79 patients before surgery produced arrhythmias in over 20% of patients but particularly frequently in the young.[1] Atrioventricular dissociation was the most common disturbance in adults and in children atrial rhythm disturbances were common. In another study[2] premedication including atropine or glycopyrronium given intramuscularly resulted in a significantly greater incidence of tachycardia during anaesthetic induction and intubation compared with controls who received no antimuscarinic drug. Patients who received glycopyrronium also had a higher incidence of tachycardia during surgery than the controls. No significant difference in bradycardia or extrasystoles was found in the atropine- or the glycopyrronium-treated patients. Atrial fibrillation has been reported in 2 elderly glaucoma patients following post-surgical application of atropine ointment or eye drops to the eye.[3]
1. Dauchot P, Gravenstein JS. Effects of atropine on the electrocardiogram in different age groups. Clin Pharmacol Ther 1971; 12: 274–80.
2. Shipton EA, Roelofse JA. Effects on cardiac rhythm of premedication with atropine or glycopyrrolate. S Afr Med J 1984; 66: 287–8.
3. Merli GJ, et al. Cardiac dysrhythmias associated with ophthalmic atropine. Arch Intern Med 1986; 146: 45–7.

Effects on mental function. A study[1] in patients with Parkinson's disease and healthy control subjects suggested that although short-term memory was impaired in patients receiving long-term antimuscarinic therapy the effect was reversible on discontinuation.
See also under Benzhexol [trihexyphenidyl] (p.464) and under Oxybutynin (p.471).
1. Van Herwaarden G, et al. Short-term memory in Parkinson's disease after withdrawal of long-term anticholinergic therapy. Clin Neuropharmacol 1993; 16: 438–43.

Hypersensitivity. A report[1] of anaphylactic shock developing in a 38-year-old woman following an intravenous injection of atropine.
1. Aguilera L, et al. Anaphylactic reaction after atropine. Anaesthesia 1988; 43: 955–7.

Overdosage. Reports of atropine poisoning or overdosage have included a respiratory therapist[1] who had given 10 atropine sulfate aerosol treatments in the preceding 24 hours and children who had taken overdoses of a preparation containing diphenoxylate and atropine.[2]
1. Larkin GL. Occupational atropine poisoning via aerosol. Lancet 1991; 337: 917.
2. McCarron MM, et al. Diphenoxylate-atropine (Lomotil) overdose in children: an update (report of eight cases and review of the literature). Pediatrics 1991; 87: 694–700.

Treatment of Adverse Effects

If a patient presents within an hour of an overdose of atropine by mouth the stomach may be emptied or activated charcoal given to reduce absorption. Supportive therapy should be given as required.

Physostigmine has been tried for antimuscarinic poisoning (see p.1422) but such use can be hazardous and is not generally recommended. Diazepam may be given to control marked excitement and convulsions;

phenothiazines should not be given as they may exacerbate antimuscarinic effects. Antiarrhythmics are not recommended if arrhythmias develop; hypoxia and acidosis should be corrected and sodium bicarbonate may be given even if acidosis is not present.

Precautions

Atropine needs to be used with caution in children and the elderly (who may be more susceptible to its adverse effects). It is contra-indicated in patients with prostatic enlargement, in whom it may lead to urinary retention, and in those with paralytic ileus or pyloric stenosis. In patients with ulcerative colitis its use may lead to ileus or megacolon, and its effects on the lower oesophageal sphincter may exacerbate reflux. Caution is generally advisable in any patient with diarrhoea. It should not be given to patients with myasthenia gravis except to reduce adverse muscarinic effects of an anticholinesterase.

Atropine should not be given to patients with angle-closure glaucoma or with a narrow angle between the iris and the cornea, since it may raise intra-ocular pressure and precipitate an acute attack. Acute angle-closure glaucoma has been reported in patients receiving nebulised atropine. Some recommend that atropine eye drops should not be used in infants aged less than 3 months due to the possible association between the induced cycloplegia and the development of amblyopia. Systemic reactions have followed the absorption of atropine from eye drops; overdosage is less likely if the eye ointment is used. In the event of blurred vision following topical administration of atropine to the eye patients should not drive or operate machinery. Systemic administration of antimuscarinics may also cause blurred vision, dizziness, and other effects that may impair a patient's ability to perform skilled tasks such as driving.

Because of the risk of provoking hyperthermia, atropine should not be given to patients, especially children, when the ambient temperature is high. It should also be used cautiously in patients with fever.

Atropine and other antimuscarinics need to be used with caution in conditions characterised by tachycardia such as thyrotoxicosis, heart failure, and in cardiac surgery, where they may further accelerate the heart rate. Care is required in patients with acute myocardial infarction, as ischaemia and infarction may be made worse, and in patients with hypertension.

Atropine may cause confusion, especially in the elderly. Reduced bronchial secretion caused by systemic administration of atropine may be associated with the formation of mucous plugs.

In the treatment of parkinsonism, increases in dosage and transfer to other forms of treatment should be gradual and antimuscarinic should not be withdrawn abruptly. Minor reactions may be controlled by reducing the dose until tolerance has developed.

Persons with Down's syndrome appear to have an increased susceptibility to some of the actions of atropine, whereas those with albinism may have a reduced susceptibility.

Interactions

The effects of atropine and other antimuscarinics may be enhanced by the concomitant administration of other drugs with antimuscarinic properties, such as amantadine, some antihistamines, phenothiazine antipsychotics, and tricyclic antidepressants. Inhibition of drug-metabolising enzymes by MAOIs may possibly enhance the effects of antimuscarinics. The reduction in gastric motility caused by antimuscarinics may affect the absorption of other drugs. Antimuscarinics and parasympathomimetics may counteract each others effects.

Pharmacokinetics

Atropine is readily absorbed from the gastrointestinal tract; it is also absorbed from mucous membranes, the eye, and to some extent through intact skin. It is rapidly cleared from the blood and is distributed throughout the body. It crosses the blood-brain barrier. It is incompletely metabolised in the liver and is excreted in the urine as unchanged drug and metabolites. A half-life of about 4 hours has been reported. Atropine crosses the placenta and traces appear in breast milk.

Quaternary ammonium salts of atropine, such as the methonitrate, are less readily absorbed after oral administration. They are highly ionised in body fluids and being poorly soluble in lipids they do not readily cross the blood-brain barrier.

Pregnancy. Studies of the pharmacokinetics of atropine in mother and fetus in late pregnancy[1-3] indicated that atropine rapidly crosses the placenta. However, whereas peak concentrations of atropine in fetal cord blood were reached about 5 minutes after intravenous administration, the maximum effect on fetal heart rate occurred after about 25 minutes.

1. Barrier G, et al. La pharmacocinétique de l'atropine chez la femme enceinte et le foetus en fin de grossesse. Anesth Analg Reanim 1976; 33: 795–800.
2. Onnen I, et al. Placental transfer of atropine at the end of pregnancy. Eur J Clin Pharmacol 1979; 15: 443–6.
3. Kanto J, et al. Placental transfer and pharmacokinetics of atropine after a single maternal intravenous and intramuscular administration. Acta Anaesthesiol Scand 1981; 25: 85–8.

Uses and Administration

Atropine is a tertiary amine antimuscarinic alkaloid with both central and peripheral actions (see p.459). It is usually given as the sulfate. It first stimulates and then depresses the CNS and has antispasmodic actions on smooth muscle and reduces secretions, especially salivary and bronchial secretions; it also reduces perspiration, but has little effect on biliary or pancreatic secretion. Atropine depresses the vagus and thereby increases the heart rate. When given by mouth atropine reduces smooth-muscle tone and diminishes gastric and intestinal motility but has little effect on gastric secretion in usual therapeutic doses. Quaternary ammonium derivatives, such as the methonitrate, have less effect on the CNS but strong ganglion-blocking activity.

Atropine is used for a variety of purposes, including: in anaesthetic practice as a premedicant and to counteract the muscarinic effects of anticholinesterases such as neostigmine and other parasympathomimetics; as an antispasmodic in gastrointestinal disorders; as an adjunct to opioid analgesics for the symptomatic relief of biliary or renal colic; to treat bradycardia; to treat or prevent bronchospasm; and in the treatment of poisoning with mushrooms that contain muscarine and in organophosphorus pesticide poisoning. Atropine is used topically as a mydriatic and cycloplegic in ophthalmology.

See under headings below for details of dosage and administration of atropine and its derivatives in specific indications.

Anaesthesia. The role of antimuscarinics in anaesthesia is discussed on p.459.

Atropine has been given as a premedicant before general anaesthesia to diminish the risk of vagal inhibition of the heart and to reduce salivary and bronchial secretions. For premedication 300 to 600 µg of atropine sulfate may be given by subcutaneous or intramuscular injection, usually 30 to 60 minutes before anaesthesia. Alternatively 300 to 600 µg of atropine sulfate may be given intravenously immediately before induction of anaesthesia. Atropine sulfate may also be given in combination with up to 10 mg morphine sulfate by subcutaneous or intramuscular injection about an hour before anaesthesia. Suitable paediatric premedication doses of atropine sulfate are: 100 µg subcutaneously or intramuscularly for children weighing up to 3 kg; 200 µg for children weighing 7 to 9 kg; 300 µg for children weighing 12 to 16 kg; and children weighing over 20 kg may be given the adult dose.

To counteract the muscarinic effects of anticholinesterases when they are used to reverse the effects of competitive muscle relaxants (see Neostigmine, p.1420) adults are given atropine sulfate 0.6 to 1.2 mg by intravenous injection before or with the anticholinesterase. Neonates and infants may be given a dose of 20 µg per kg body-weight.

Anoxic seizures. A reflex anoxic seizure is a paroxysmal event triggered by a noxious stimulus which, by vagal stimulation, causes pronounced bradycardia or cardiac arrest and consequent relative cerebral ischaemia.[1] Certain features of the attack may lead to a misdiagnosis of epilepsy. To avoid confusion with epileptic seizures (p.338), reflex anoxic seizures have also been called white or type 2 breath holding attacks. Depending

on the degree of vagal hypersensitivity or noxious stimulus, attacks may occur infrequently or several times a day.

Infants and young children are mainly affected, however, the condition usually resolves by early childhood. It is generally benign and children do not suffer cardiac or cerebral damage. Treatment is seldom necessary, but atropine has been advocated to prevent vagal hypersensitivity in those children with frequent, persistent attacks. As atropine may require frequent administration with an attendant risk of overdosage, transdermal hyoscine has been tried as an alternative.[2]

1. Appleton RE. Reflex anoxic seizures. BMJ 1993; 307: 214–5.
2. Palm L, Blennow G. Transdermal anticholinergic treatment of reflex anoxic seizures. Acta Paediatr Scand 1985; 74: 803–4.

Cardiac disorders. Atropine depresses the vagus and thereby increases the heart rate. It is therefore used in a variety of disorders or circumstances in which bradyarrhythmias occur. It is frequently used in sudden onset bradyarrhythmias and although it may also be employed for the initial treatment of chronic arrhythmias (p.794), cardiac pacing is generally preferred for long-term control. Examples of acute use include the prevention and treatment of arrhythmias associated with anaesthesia (see above), the treatment of other drug-induced arrhythmias, and in cardiac arrest due to asystole or electromechanical dissociation (pulseless electrical activity—p.790). Atropine sulfate has been used in the management of bradycardia after acute myocardial infarction; however, caution is required, as atropine may exacerbate ischaemia or infarction in these patients.

International guidelines[1] for advanced life support in adults recommend doses of atropine sulfate in asystole and electromechanical dissociation, of 1 mg intravenously, repeated every 3 to 5 minutes to a total of 0.04 mg per kg body-weight. UK guidelines[2] for adults recommend a single dose of 3 mg intravenously or 6 mg via an endotracheal tube.

In **bradycardia**, atropine is given in doses of 0.5 to 1 mg intravenously repeated every 3 to 5 minutes to a total dose of 0.04 mg per kg body-weight.[2]

If an intravenous line cannot be established, atropine can be given via an endotracheal tube; 2 to 3 times the intravenous dose should be given, diluted in 10 mL of sterile water or sodium chloride 0.9%.

1. The American Heart Association in collaboration with the International Committee on Resuscitation (ILCOR). International guidelines 2000 for cardiopulmonary resuscitation and emergency cardiovascular care: a consensus on science. Circulation 2000; 102 (suppl I): I1–I384. [Also published in Resuscitation 2000; 46: 3–447.]
2. Resuscitation Council (UK). Resuscitation Guidelines 2000. Available at: http://www.resus.org.uk/pages/guide.htm (accessed 15/08/01).

Colic pain. Atropine has been used as an adjunct to opioid analgesics for symptomatic relief of biliary or renal colic (see p.690).

Eye disorders. Atropine is used to produce mydriasis and cycloplegia (p.460) for ophthalmic examination. One local application can take up to 40 minutes or more to produce mydriasis, which lasts for a week or more; marked paralysis of accommodation is obtained in 1 to 3 hours with recovery in 6 to 12 days. However, other antimuscarinics such as cyclopentolate, homatropine, or tropicamide may be preferred because they have a more rapid onset and shorter duration of action than atropine. Atropine is also used in the management of uveitis and iritis, and in strabismus. It is used in the treatment of iritis and uveitis to immobilise the ciliary muscle and iris and to prevent or break down adhesions. Because of its powerful cycloplegic action atropine is also used in the determination of refraction in children below the age of 6 and in children with convergent strabismus (p.1414).

In the treatment of **inflammatory eye disorders** such as uveitis or iritis (p.1060), the dose of atropine sulfate for adults is 1 or 2 drops of a 0.5 or 1% solution instilled into the eye(s) up to four times daily. The dose in children is 1 or 2 drops of a 0.5% solution (or one drop of a 1% solution) instilled up to three times daily. For **refraction** in adults the dose is one drop of a 1% solution of atropine sulfate; this may be instilled either twice daily for 1 or 2 days before the procedure or on a single occasion one hour before the procedure. In children the dose for refraction is 1 or 2 drops of a 0.5% solution (or one drop of a 1% solution) instilled twice daily for 1 to 3 days before the procedure, with a further dose given one hour before the procedure. An ophthalmic ointment of atropine sulfate 1% may be preferred for children under 5 years of age and particularly in infants under 3 months of age who are at increased risk of systemic effects with eye drops. Some recommend that atropine sulfate should not be used in the eyes of children younger than 3 months of age due to a possible association between the cycloplegia produced and the development of amblyopia.

Atropine borate has also been used in ophthalmic preparations.

References.

1. Stolovitch C, et al. Atropine cycloplegia: how many instillations does one need? J Pediatr Ophthalmol Strabismus 1992; 29: 175–6.
2. Foley-Nolan A, et al. Atropine penalisation versus occlusion as the primary treatment for amblyopia. Br J Ophthalmol 1997; 81: 54–7.

Gastrointestinal disorders. Antimuscarinics may be used in gastrointestinal disorders (see p.459) because of their marked inhibitory effect on gastrointestinal motility and their

antisecretory effects. Atropine (as the sulfate or quaternary derivatives such as the methobromide or methonitrate) has been used to reduce smooth-muscle tone and diminish motility, but has little effect on gastric secretion at usual therapeutic doses (about 200 µg of atropine sulfate). It has been tried as an adjunct to the treatment of benign gastric and duodenal ulcers and the antispasmodic action of atropine has been used to facilitate radiological examination of the gut. Atropine sulfate has also been used in the treatment of irritable bowel syndrome. Atropine oxide hydrochloride is also used for gastrointestinal disorders.

Poisoning. Atropine is used in the management of overdosage or poisoning due to various substances with muscarinic actions. It is used to overcome the effects of accumulation of acetylcholine produced by anticholinesterase compounds including organophosphorus pesticides,[1,2] chemical warfare nerve gases,[3] and parasympathomimetics such as neostigmine. It is also used to antagonise the effects of cholinomimetic substances in the treatment of overdosage with parasympathomimetics such as bethanechol and in the treatment of poisoning with mushrooms that contain muscarine. Atropine blocks the action of these compounds at muscarinic receptors reversing bradycardia and decreasing tracheobronchial secretions, bronchoconstriction, intestinal secretions, and intestinal motility.

In the treatment of poisoning with organophosphorus pesticides or chemical warfare nerve gases atropine sulfate may be given to adults in an initial dose of 2 mg or more intramuscularly or intravenously every 10 to 30 minutes until muscarinic effects disappear or signs of atropine toxicity are seen. In severe cases injections have been given as often as every 5 minutes in some centres. In moderate to severe poisoning a state of atropinisation is usually maintained for at least 2 days and continued for as long as symptoms are evident. In severely poisoned patients this may entail prolonged treatment.[4,5] As large amounts of atropine may be required it is important to use a preservative-free preparation to avoid the potential toxicity associated with administration of excess quantities of preservatives such as benzyl alcohol or chlorobutanol. Since atropine is ineffective against any nicotinic effects of these compounds a cholinesterase reactivator such as pralidoxime (p.1020) may be used as an adjunct.

The use of atropine in poisoning or overdosage with other compounds having muscarinic actions is similar to that for organophosphorus pesticides but the duration of treatment necessary is usually shorter. An initial dose of 0.5 to 1 mg given subcutaneously or intravenously and repeated every 2 hours may be adequate for overdosage with cholinomimetics such as bethanechol.

1. Karalleidde L, Senanayake N. Organophosphorus insecticide poisoning. Br J Anaesth 1989; 63: 736–50.
2. Lotti M. Treatment of acute organophosphate poisoning. Med J Aust 1991; 154: 51–5.
3. Anonymous. Prevention and treatment of nerve gas poisoning. Med Lett Drugs Ther 1990; 32: 103–5.
4. Golsousidis H, Kokkas V. Use of 19 590 mg of atropine during 24 days of treatment, after a case of unusually severe parathion poisoning. Hum Toxicol 1985; 4: 339–40.
5. Afzaal S, et al. High dose atropine in organophosphorus poisoning. Postgrad Med J 1990; 66: 70–1.

Respiratory-tract disorders. Although atropine is a potent bronchodilator its use in the management of reversible airways obstruction has largely been replaced by other antimuscarinics (see p.460). It is sometimes used in combination preparations with antihistamines and decongestants for the symptomatic relief of symptoms of the common cold.

References.

1. Sur S, et al. A random double-blind trial of the combination of nebulized atropine methylnitrate and albuterol in nocturnal asthma. Ann Allergy 1990; 65: 384–8.
2. Vichyanond P, et al. Efficacy of atropine methylnitrate alone and in combination with albuterol in children with asthma. Chest 1990; 98: 637–42.

Preparations

BP 2001: Atropine Eye Drops; Atropine Eye Ointment; Atropine Injection; Atropine Tablets; Morphine and Atropine Injection;
USP 25: Atropine Sulfate Injection; Atropine Sulfate Ophthalmic Ointment; Atropine Sulfate Ophthalmic Solution; Atropine Sulfate Tablets; Diphenoxylate Hydrochloride and Atropine Sulfate Oral Solution; Diphenoxylate Hydrochloride and Atropine Sulfate Tablets.

Proprietary Preparations (details are given in Part 3)
Austral.: Atropt; *Belg.:* Stellatropine; *Canad.:* Atropisol; *Fin.:* Oftan Atropin; *Fr.:* Chibro-Atropine; Genatropine; *Ger.:* Atropinol; Dysurgal N; Noxenur S; *Israel:* Atropspan; *Ital.:* Liotropina†; *Mex.:* Atro Grin; Tropyn Z; *NZ:* Atropt; *Port.:* Atropocil; *S.Afr.:* Spersatropine†; *Switz.:* Bellafit N; Skiatropine; *USA:* AtroPen; Atropisol; Ocu-Tropine; Sal-Tropine.

Multi-ingredient: *Aust.:* Causat†; Dysurgal; Ichtho-Bellol; Lactolavol; Myocardon; Noxenur; Perphyllon; *Austral.:* Contac; Donnagel; Donnalix; Donnatab; Neo-Diophen; *Braz.:* Enterotonus; Espasmocron; Tonaton; Vagostesyl; *Canad.:* Diban; Donnatal; *Ger.:* Angiocardyl N†; Causat B12 N; Causat N; Dilaudid-Atropin; Eupond†; Ichtho-Bellol; Ichtho-Bellol compositum S; Mydrial-Atropin; *Hong Kong:* Virulex Forte; *Israel:* Patropin; Spasmalgin; *Ital.:* Cardiostenol; Deltamidrina; Genatrop; *Mex.:* Redotex NF; *Port.:* Cosmaxil†; *S.Afr.:* Allertac; Bellatard; Bellaven†; Colstat; Donnatal; Dyrosol; Famucaps; Millerspas; Telament†; Tropax†; Virobis; *Spain:* Abdominol; Derbitan Antibiotico†; Laxo Vian†; Midriati; Rubia Paver; Sulmetin Papaver; Sulmetin Papaverina; Tabletas Quimpe; *Swed.:* Dilaudid-Atropin; *Switz.:* Brosol; Dilaudid-Atropin; Dolopyrine†; Nardyl; Spasmosol; Viaggio†; **Thai.:** Alkamine; Diolin; Donnatal; Droximag; Stomac; **UK:** Actonorm; **USA:** Antispasmodic Elixir; Antrocol; Arco-Lase Plus; Atrohist Plus†; Atropine and Demerol; Atrosept; Barbidonna; Bellatal; Deconhist LA†; Dolsed; Donna-Sed†; Donnamor†; Donnatal; Emergent-Ez; Hyosophen; Malatal†; Phenahist-TR†; Phenchlor SHA†; Prosed/DS; Ru-Tuss†; Stahist; Susano; Trac Tabs 2X; UAA; Uridon Modified; Urised.

Used as an adjunct in: **Austral.:** Lofenoxal; Lomotil; **Belg.:** Reasec†; **Braz.:** Lomotil; **Canad.:** Lomotil; **Denm.:** Retardin; **Fr.:** Diarsed; **Ger.:** Reasec†; **Hong Kong:** Dhamotil; Lomotil; **Irl.:** Lomotil; **Ital.:** Reasec†; **Mex.:** Lomotil; **NZ:** Diastop; Lomotil; **Port.:** Lomotil†; **S.Afr.:** Eldox; Lomotil; **Singapore:** Dhamotil; Erlotyl; Lomotil; Remodil; **Switz.:** Lyspafen†; Reasec; **Thai.:** Dilomil; Ditropine; Lomotil; **UAE:** Intard; **UK:** Diarphen†; Lomotil; Lotharin; Tropergen; **USA:** Enlon-Plus; Logen; Lomotil; Lonox; Motofen; Neostigmine Min-I-Mix.

Belladonna (339-a)

Belladona; Belladone; Deadly Nightshade; Tollkirschen.

Pharmacopoeias. Eur. (see p.vi) and US include a monograph for Belladonna Leaf. Chin. includes Belladonna Herb.
Eur. also includes Prepared Belladonna Leaf and Standardised Belladonna Leaf Dry Extract.
Aust. also includes Belladonna Root. Jpn includes only Belladonna Root.

Pharmacopoeial description

Ph. Eur.: Belladonna Leaf (Belladonnae Folium; Belladonna Herb (BP 2001)) consists of the dried leaf, or dried leaf and flowering, and occasionally fruit-bearing, tops of *Atropa belladonna*. It contains not less than 0.30% of total alkaloids, calculated as hyoscyamine. The alkaloids consist mainly of hyoscyamine together with smaller amounts of hyoscine. It has a slightly nauseous odour. Protect from light.

Prepared Belladonna (Belladonnae Pulvis Normatus; Prepared Belladonna Herb (BP 2001)) is belladonna leaf powder adjusted to an alkaloidal content of 0.28 to 0.32% of total alkaloids, calculated as hyoscyamine. Store in airtight containers. Protect from light.

Standardised Belladonna Leaf Dry Extract (Belladonnae Folii Extractum Siccum Normatum) is produced from belladonna leaf. It contains not less than 0.95% and not more than 1.05% of total alkaloids, calculated as hyoscyamine. A hygroscopic brown or greenish powder. Store in airtight containers. Protect from light.

NOTE. The BP 2001 directs that when Belladonna Herb, Belladonna Leaf, or Powdered Belladonna Herb is prescribed, Prepared Belladonna Herb be dispensed.

USP 25: Belladonna Leaf consists of the dried leaf and flowering or fruiting top of *Atropa belladonna* (Solanaceae). It yields not less than 0.35% of the alkaloids of belladonna leaf. When moistened, its odour is slight, somewhat tobacco-like. Avoid long exposure to direct sunlight. Protect powdered Belladonna Leaf from light.

Stability in mixtures. Atropine in belladonna preparations was unstable at alkaline pH and would quickly be degraded in mixtures with a pH above 7.[1] Such mixtures in the BPC 1973 included Aluminium Hydroxide and Belladonna Mixture, Cascara and Belladonna Mixture, and Magnesium Trisilicate and Belladonna Mixture.
1. *PSGB Lab Report P/71/9* 1971.

Adverse Effects, Treatment, and Precautions
As for Atropine Sulfate, p.461.

Interactions
As for antimuscarinics in general (see Atropine Sulfate, p.461).

Uses and Administration
Belladonna has the actions of atropine (p.461). Belladonna herb and its preparations have been used for their antimuscarinic actions in a wide range of conditions, including the relief of gastrointestinal and urinary-tract disorders associated with smooth muscle spasm, but they are generally regarded as an outmoded form of treatment.

Belladonna liniments and plasters have been used as counterirritants for the relief of pain but there is little evidence that they have a beneficial effect and side-effects have occurred.

Belladonna is used in homoeopathic medicine.

Preparations
BP 2001: Belladonna Tincture; Standardised Belladonna Leaf Dry Extract;
USP 25: Belladonna Extract; Belladonna Extract Tablets; Belladonna Tincture.

Proprietary Preparations (details are given in Part 3)
Aust.: Bellanorm; **Austral.:** Atrobel; **Ger.:** Belladonnysat Burger; Tremoforat; **USA:** Bellafoline†.

Multi-ingredient: Aust.: Bellasthman†; Tampositorien mit Belladonna; **Belg.:** Baume Dalet†; Calmant Martou†; Colimax; Escouflaire†; Eucalyptine Pholcodine Le Brun; Folcodex; Gastrofilm; Gloceda; Grains de Vals; Hemosedan; Sanicolax†; Sirop Toux du Larynx†; Solucamphre†; **Braz.:** Acridin; Antispasmin; Atroveran; Atrovex; Bismubell; Bisuisan; Bromosedan; Bronquidex; Calminex S; Cessatosse; Cynaridol; Cystex; Dorveran; Efedronal; Espasmolex; Espasmosan; Espasmosan Composto; Etaverol; Gotas Hepaticas; Gotas Nican; Hemovirtu's Pomada; Hepato-Flux; Hepatobyl; Hepavirmo; Neutracido; Ormigrein; Pilulas Ross; Pulmoiodo; Pyelodion; Regran; Revulsan; Salicilato de Bismuto Composto; Solvobil; Teutoss; Tussifen; Xarope de Caraguata + Bromoformio; **Canad.:** Bellergal; Cafergot-PB; Rheumalan;

The symbol † denotes a preparation no longer actively marketed

---

Wigraine†; **Fin.:** Tannopon; **Fr.:** Bronpax†; Gastrosedyl†; Gelumaline; Humex; Mucinum†; Peter's Sirop†; Sirop Pectoral adulte†; Suppomaline; **Ger.:** Dalet Med Balsam; **Hong Kong:** Contac; Rheogen; **Israel:** Laxative; Laxative Comp; **Ital.:** Antiemorroidali; Antispasmina Colica; Bellergil†; Farmospasmina; Lassatina; Neo-Heparbil†; **Mex.:** Chofabol; **Neth.:** Abdijsiroop (Akker-Siroop)†; **Norw.:** Cafergot Comp†; **Port.:** Anti-Gripe; Antispasmina Colica; Anucet; Calmo; Codoforme; Diacol; Fluidin Antiasmatico; Fluidin Infantil; Lactucol; Migretil; Servetinal; Vaporil; **S.Afr.:** Bellergal†; Cafergot-PB; Diastat†; Peter Pote's†; Rectosan 'A'†; **Spain:** Alofedina; Boldolaxin; Broncovital; Cafergot-PB; Carminativo Juventus; Crislaxo; Digestovital; Distovagal†; Dolokey; Laxante Bescansa Aloico; Medecitral; Menabil Complex; Servetinal†; Sin Mareo x 4; Takata; Tanagel; **Switz.:** Ajaka†; Aloinophen†; Bellagotin; Bellergal; Bromocod N; Bronchalin†; Bronchofluid†; Cafergot-PB; Demo elixir pectoral N; Demo sirop contre la toux†; Dragees laxatives no 510†; Escotussin; Lysedil; Lysedil compositum; Nican; Phol-Tux; Physiolax†; Phytolax; Saintbois nouvelle formule; Sirop pectoral DP2, DP3†; Solucamphre†; Spedro†; Tavolax†; Thymodrosin†; **Thai.:** Belacid; Bellergal; Benera; Contac; Diolin; Neuramizone; **UK:** Bellocarb†; Enterosan†; Opazimes; **USA:** B & O Supprettes No. 15A; B & O Supprettes No. 16A; Bel-Phen-Ergot S; Bellergal-S; Butibel; Cafatine-PB; Chardonna-2; Folergot-DF; Phenerbel-S; Respa-ARM†; Wyanoids†.

Benzatropine Mesilate (344-z)

Benzatropine Mesilate (BANM, rINNM).
Benzatropine Methanesulfonate; Benztropine Mesylate. (1R,3r,5S)-3-Benzhydryloxytropane methanesulphonate.
$C_{21}H_{25}NO,CH_4O_3S = 403.5$.
CAS — 86-13-5 (benzatropine); 132-17-2 (benzatropine mesilate).
Pharmacopoeias. In Br. and US.

Pharmacopoeial description
BP 2001: A white, odourless or almost odourless, crystalline powder. Very soluble in water; freely soluble in alcohol; practically insoluble in ether.

USP 25: A white, slightly hygroscopic, crystalline powder. Very soluble in water; freely soluble in alcohol; very slightly soluble in ether. Store in airtight containers.

Adverse Effects, Treatment, and Precautions
As for Atropine Sulfate, p.461. Drowsiness may be severe in some patients and patients so affected should not drive or operate machinery. Benzatropine may also produce severe mental disturbances and excitement.

Effects on the heart. Paradoxical sinus bradycardia in a patient with depression and psychotic symptoms was attributed to benzatropine since it persisted despite modification to other treatment and resolved only when benzatropine was withdrawn.[1]
1. Voinov H, *et al.* Sinus bradycardia related to the use of benztropine mesylate. *Am J Psychiatry* 1992; **149:** 711.

Interactions
As for antimuscarinics in general (see Atropine Sulfate, p.461).

Antidepressants. A report[1] of 5 patients who developed delirium while taking an antipsychotic, a SSRI, and benzatropine suggested that there might be an interaction between SSRIs and benzatropine.
1. Roth A, *et al.* Delirium associated with the combination of a neuroleptic, an SSRI, and benztropine. *J Clin Psychiatry* 1994; **55:** 492–5.

Antipsychotics. Fatal heat stroke has been reported[1,2] in patients receiving benzatropine and antipsychotic drugs following exposure to an ambient temperature of over 29°. Paralytic ileus, sometimes fatal, has also been documented in patients taking benzatropine mesilate and antipsychotics together.[3]
1. Stadnyk AN, Glezos JD. Drug-induced heat stroke. *Can Med Assoc J* 1983; **128:** 957–9.
2. Tyndel F, Labonté R. Drug-facilitated heat stroke. *Can Med Assoc J* 1983; **129:** 680.
3. Wade LC, Ellenor GL. Combination mesoridazine- and benztropine mesylate-induced paralytic ileus: two case reports. *Drug Intell Clin Pharm* 1980; **14:** 17–22.

Uses and Administration
Benzatropine mesilate is a tertiary amine antimuscarinic with actions and uses similar to those of benzhexol [trihexyphenidyl] (p.464); it also has antihistaminic properties.

Benzatropine is used for the symptomatic treatment of parkinsonism (p.460), including the alleviation of the extrapyramidal syndrome induced by drugs such as phenothiazines, but, like other antimuscarinics, is of no value against tardive dyskinesias.

Benzatropine mesilate is given by mouth or, if necessary, by intramuscular or intravenous injection.

In idiopathic parkinsonism benzatropine mesilate is usually given by mouth in an initial daily dose of 0.5 to 1 mg. Its actions are cumulative, and may not be manifest for several days after beginning therapy. Patients with post-encephalitic parkinsonism often tolerate an initial dose of 2 mg. The dose may be gradually increased by 500 µg every 5 to 6 days to a maximum of 6 mg daily until the optimum dose for each individual patient is reached. Maintenance therapy may be given as a single daily dose at bedtime or in divided doses 2 to 4 times daily.

In the management of drug-induced extrapyramidal disorders doses of 1 to 4 mg once or twice daily have been given orally or parenterally. Therapy may be withdrawn after one to two weeks to assess whether it is still necessary.

In an emergency, benzatropine mesilate may be injected intramuscularly or intravenously in a dose of 1 to 2 mg; intramuscular administration is reported to produce an effect as quickly as intravenous administration, so the latter is rarely necessary.

Benzatropine has also been given as the hydrochloride.

Preparations
BP 2001: Benzatropine Injection; Benzatropine Tablets;
USP 25: Benztropine Mesylate Injection; Benztropine Mesylate Tablets.

Proprietary Preparations (details are given in Part 3)
Aust.: BETE; Cogentin; **Austral.:** Cogentin; **Canad.:** Cogentin; **Denm.:** Cogentin; **Ger.:** Cogentinol; **Hong Kong:** Cogentin; **Irl.:** Cogentin; **Norw.:** Cogentin; **NZ:** Cogentin; **Port.:** Cogentin; **Swed.:** Cogentin; **Thai.:** Cogentin; Phatropine; **UK:** Cogentin; **USA:** Cogentin.

Benzhexol Hydrochloride (342-y)

Benzhexol Hydrochloride (BANM).
Trihexyphenidyl Hydrochloride (BANM, rINNM); Cloridrato de Triexilfenidila; Cyclodolum; Trihexyphenidyli Hydrochloridum; Trihexyphenidylium Chloratum. 1-Cyclohexyl-1-phenyl-3-piperidinopropan-1-ol hydrochloride.
$C_{20}H_{31}NO,HCl = 337.9$.
CAS — 144-11-6 (benzhexol [trihexyphenidyl]); 52-49-3 (benzhexol [trihexyphenidyl] hydrochloride).
Pharmacopoeias. In Chin., Eur. (see p.vi), Int., Jpn, Pol., and US.

Pharmacopoeial description
Ph. Eur.: A white crystalline powder. Slightly soluble in water; sparingly soluble in alcohol and in dichloromethane. A 1% solution in water has a pH of 5.2 to 6.2.

USP 25: A white or slightly off-white, crystalline powder, having not more than a very faint odour. Slightly soluble in water; soluble in alcohol and in chloroform. Store in airtight containers.

Adverse Effects, Treatment and Precautions
As for Atropine Sulfate, p.461. In some patients, such as those with arteriosclerosis or a history of drug idiosyncrasy, benzhexol [trihexyphenidyl] may produce severe mental disturbances, excitement, nausea, and vomiting; such patients should be allowed to develop a tolerance by starting with a small initial dose and gradually increasing it until an effective level is reached.

Abuse. Benzhexol [trihexyphenidyl] hydrochloride has been abused for its euphoric effect[1] especially by psychiatric patients.[2] However, its abuse potential in schizophrenic patients has been questioned[3] and its unpleasant antimuscarinic effects tend to limit its repeated use.[4]
1. Crawshaw JA, Mullen PE. A study of benzhexol abuse. *Br J Psychiatry* 1984; **145:** 300–3.
2. Pullen GP, *et al.* Anticholinergic drug abuse: a common problem? *BMJ* 1984; **289:** 612–13.
3. Goff DC, *et al.* A placebo-controlled trial of trihexyphenidyl in unmedicated patients with schizophrenia. *Am J Psychiatry* 1994; **151:** 429–31.
4. WHO. WHO committee on drug dependence: twenty-ninth report. *WHO Tech Rep Ser 856* 1995.

Effects on the heart. Paradoxical sinus bradycardia developed in a schizophrenic patient after receiving benzhexol [trihexyphenidyl] for extrapyramidal side-effects due to antipsychotic medication.[1] Normal sinus rhythm was restored after benzhexol [trihexyphenidyl] was discontinued. The patient had previously received benzhexol [trihexyphenidyl] and suffered bradycardia which at the time was attributed to haloperidol.
1. Blumensohn R, *et al.* Bradycardia due to trihexyphenidyl hydrochloride. *Drug Intell Clin Pharm* 1986; **20:** 786–7.

Effects on mental function. Benzhexol [trihexyphenidyl] 2 mg by mouth significantly impaired memory function compared with placebo in a study in 13 elderly patients.[1] Impairment of memory has also been observed in patients with Parkinson's disease given antimuscarinics such as benzhexol [trihexyphenidyl].[2] However, impairment may be reversible on discontinuation of the antimuscarinic (see Atropine, p.461).

1. Potamianos G, Kellett JM. Anti-cholinergic drugs and memory: the effects of benzhexol on memory in a group of geriatric patients. *Br J Psychiatry* 1982; **140**: 470–2.
2. Sadeh M, *et al.* Effects of anticholinergic drugs on memory in Parkinson's disease. *Arch Neurol* 1982; **39**: 666–7.

Overdosage. A 34-year-old woman developed a toxic reaction with widely dilated pupils, dry skin, and visual hallucinations within 24 hours of taking about 300 mg of benzhexol [trihexyphenidyl] hydrochloride with suicidal intent.[1] After 3 to 4 days the hallucinations were replaced by illusions; complete recovery occurred after a week, with no special treatment.

1. Ananth JV, *et al.* Toxic psychosis induced by benzhexol hydrochloride. *Can Med Assoc J* 1970; **103**: 771.

Withdrawal. A 61-year-old woman who had taken benzhexol [trihexyphenidyl] 6 mg daily for a year for Parkinson's disease developed encephalopathy and miosis on two occasions when treatment was abruptly withdrawn.[1] Slowly tapered withdrawal avoided these effects.

1. Johkura K, *et al.* Trihexyphenidyl withdrawal encephalopathy. *Ann Neurol* 1997; **41**: 133–4.

Interactions

As for antimuscarinics in general (see Atropine Sulfate, p.461).

Chlorpromazine. For the effect of benzhexol [trihexyphenidyl] on plasma concentrations of chlorpromazine, see under Antiparkinsonian Drugs, p.665.

Pharmacokinetics

Benzhexol [trihexyphenidyl] hydrochloride is well absorbed from the gastrointestinal tract and has been stated to exert an effect within 1 hour of a dose by mouth.

Half-life. The reported half-life of benzhexol [trihexyphenidyl] has varied according to the assay method used. Values reported when using radioreceptor and chromatographic techniques have ranged from about 1 to more than 24 hours[1] and from 10 to 29 hours,[2] respectively, but the sensitivity and specificity of these methods has been criticised.[3] With a more recently developed radio immunoassay it was found that following oral administration there was an initial elimination phase with an estimated half-life of 5.33 hours followed by a terminal elimination phase with an estimated half-life of 32.7 hours.

1. Burke RE, Fahn S. Pharmacokinetics of trihexyphenidyl after short-term and long-term administration to dystonic patients. *Ann Neurol* 1985; **18**: 35–40.
2. Garbarg S, *et al.* Comparaison pharmacoclinique de deux formes galéniques de trihexyphénidyle. *Encephale* 1983; **IX**: 167–74.
3. He H, *et al.* Development and application of a specific and sensitive radioimmunoassay for trihexyphenidyl to a pharmacokinetic study in humans. *J Pharm Sci* 1995; **84**: 561–7.

Uses and Administration

Benzhexol [trihexyphenidyl] hydrochloride is a tertiary amine antimuscarinic with actions similar to those of atropine (p.462). It also has a direct antispasmodic action on smooth muscle.

Benzhexol [trihexyphenidyl] hydrochloride is employed in the symptomatic treatment of parkinsonism, including the alleviation of the extrapyramidal syndrome induced by drugs such as phenothiazines, but, like other antimuscarinics, is of no value against tardive dyskinesias. It has been used in the treatment of dystonias.

In idiopathic parkinsonism, benzhexol [trihexyphenidyl] hydrochloride is given in 3 or 4 divided doses daily before or with food. The usual initial dose of 1 mg daily is gradually increased over a period of several days by increments of 2 mg to 6 to 10 mg daily according to the response of the patient; for advanced cases, 12 to 15 mg daily or even more may be needed. As a rule, postencephalitic patients tolerate and require the larger doses; elderly patients may require smaller doses.

Usual doses for drug-induced extrapyramidal symptoms lie within the range of 5 to 15 mg daily, although as little as 1 mg daily may be sufficient in some cases.

Antimuscarinic treatment of parkinsonism should never be terminated suddenly and it is usual when changing from one drug to another to withdraw one in small amounts while gradually increasing the dose of the other.

Benzhexol [trihexyphenidyl] hydrochloride may be given with other drugs used for the relief of parkinsonism, such as levodopa, but the dose of each drug may need to be reduced.

Extrapyramidal disorders. Antimuscarinics such as benzhexol [trihexyphenidyl] can be effective when used in the management of dystonias (p.1173).[1] However, adults tolerate antimuscarinics less well than children and adolescents and for these patients it is often not possible to achieve the high doses that may be required for control.[2] Side-effects may be limited by starting with a low dose such as benzhexol [trihexyphenidyl] 2.5 mg twice daily and increasing by 2.5 mg daily every one or two weeks to the maximum tolerable, which in some young patients might be as much as 180 mg daily.

1. Burke RE, *et al.* Torsion dystonia: a double-blind, prospective trial of high-dosage trihexyphenidyl. *Neurology* 1986; **36**: 160–4.
2. Marsden CD, Quinn NP. The dystonias. *BMJ* 1990; **300**: 139–44.

Parkinsonism. For the use of antimuscarinics, such as benzhexol [trihexyphenidyl], in the symptomatic treatment of parkinsonism, see p.460.

Preparations

BP 2001: Trihexyphenidyl Tablets;
USP 25: Trihexyphenidyl Hydrochloride Elixir; Trihexyphenidyl Hydrochloride Extended-release Capsules; Trihexyphenidyl Hydrochloride Tablets.

Proprietary Preparations (details are given in Part 3)
Aust.: Artane; *Austral.:* Artane; *Belg.:* Artane; *Braz.:* Artane; *Canad.:* Apo-Trihex; Artane†; Novo-Hexidyl†; *Denm.:* Peragit; *Fin.:* Artane; *Fr.:* Artane; Parkinane; *Ger.:* Artane; Parkopan; *Hong Kong:* Apo-Trihex; Artandyl; Artane; *Irl.:* Artane; *Israel:* Artane; Partane; *Ital.:* Artane; *Mex.:* Hipokinon; Kexidil; *Neth.:* Artane; *Port.:* Artane; *S.Afr.:* Artane; *Singapore:* Apo-Trihex; B-Hex; *Spain:* Artane; *Swed.:* Pargitan; *Switz.:* Artane; *Thai.:* Aca; Acamed; Artane; Pozhexol; Tridyl; *UK:* Artane†; Broflex; *USA:* Artane†; Trihexy.

Multi-ingredient: *Ger.:* Spasman; *Spain:* Largatrex.

Biperiden (346-k)

Biperiden (BAN, rINN).

1-(Bicyclo[2.2.1]hept-5-en-2-yl)-1-phenyl-3-piperidinopropan-1-ol.

$C_{21}H_{29}NO = 311.5$.

CAS — 514-65-8.

ATC — N04AA02.

Pharmacopoeias. In Int. and US.

Pharmacopoeial description

USP 25: A white, practically odourless, crystalline powder. Practically insoluble in water; sparingly soluble in alcohol; freely soluble in chloroform. Protect from light.

Biperiden Hydrochloride (347-a)

Biperiden Hydrochloride (BANM, rINNM).

Biperideni Hydrochloridum.

$C_{21}H_{29}NO,HCl = 347.9$.

CAS — 1235-82-1.

Pharmacopoeias. In Eur. (see p.vi), Int., Jpn, and US.

Pharmacopoeial description

Ph. Eur.: A white, crystalline powder. Slightly soluble in water and in alcohol; very slightly soluble in dichloromethane; practically insoluble in ether. A 0.2% solution in water has a pH of 5.0 to 6.5. Store in airtight containers. Protect from light.

USP 25: A white, practically odourless, crystalline powder. Slightly soluble in water, in alcohol, in chloroform, and in ether; sparingly soluble in methyl alcohol. Protect from light.

Biperiden Lactate (348-t)

Biperiden Lactate (BANM, rINNM).

$C_{21}H_{29}NO,C_3H_6O_3 = 401.5$.

CAS — 7085-45-2.

Pharmacopoeias. US includes Biperiden Lactate Injection.

Adverse Effects, Treatment, and Precautions

As for Atropine Sulfate, p.461.

Parenteral administration may be followed by slight transient hypotension. Biperiden may cause drowsiness and patients so affected should not drive or operate machinery.

Abuse. A report[1] of abuse of biperiden in psychiatric patients.

1. Pullen GP, *et al.* Anticholinergic drug abuse: a common problem? *BMJ* 1984; **289**: 612–13.

Interactions

As for antimuscarinics in general (see Atropine Sulfate, p.461).

Pharmacokinetics

Biperiden is readily absorbed from the gastrointestinal tract, but bioavailability is only about 30% suggesting that it undergoes extensive first-pass metabolism. Biperiden has an elimination half-life of about 20 hours.

◊ References.

1. Hollmann M, *et al.* Biperiden effects and plasma levels in volunteers. *Eur J Clin Pharmacol* 1984; **27**: 619–21.
2. Grimaldi R, *et al.* Pharmacokinetic and pharmacodynamic studies following the intravenous and oral administration of the antiparkinsonian drug biperiden to normal subjects. *Eur J Clin Pharmacol* 1986; **29**: 735–7.

Uses and Administration

Biperiden is a tertiary amine antimuscarinic with actions and uses similar to those of benzhexol [trihexyphenidyl] (p.464) but with more potent antinicotinic properties.

Biperiden is used in the symptomatic treatment of parkinsonism (p.460), including the alleviation of the extrapyramidal syndrome induced by drugs such as phenothiazines, but, like other antimuscarinics, is of no value against tardive dyskinesias.

Biperiden is administered by mouth as the hydrochloride and by injection as the lactate.

In the UK, the initial dose by mouth is 1 mg of the hydrochloride twice daily, gradually increased over several days according to the needs of the patient. The usual optimum maintenance dosage varies from 3 to 12 mg daily in divided doses. The dose of the lactate given by intramuscular or slow intravenous injection is 2.5 to 5 mg as a single dose to a maximum of 20 mg in 24 hours.

In the USA, the initial dose by mouth for idiopathic parkinsonism is 2 mg of the hydrochloride three or four times daily increased according to the needs of the patient to a maximum of 16 mg in 24 hours. The dose for drug-induced extrapyramidal symptoms is 2 mg of the hydrochloride by mouth one to three times daily or 2 mg of biperiden lactate given by intramuscular or slow intravenous injection and repeated every 30 minutes if needed up to a maximum of 4 doses in 24 hours.

Preparations

USP 25: Biperiden Hydrochloride Tablets; Biperiden Lactate Injection.

Proprietary Preparations (details are given in Part 3)
Aust.: Akineton; *Austral.:* Akineton; *Belg.:* Akineton; *Braz.:* Akineton; *Canad.:* Akineton; *Denm.:* Akineton; *Fin.:* Akineton; Ipsatol; *Fr.:* Akineton; *Ger.:* Akineton; Desiperiden†; Norakin N; *Irl.:* Akineton; *Israel:* Dekinet; *Ital.:* Akineton; *Mex.:* Akineton; Roloken; *Neth.:* Akineton; *Norw.:* Akineton; *Port.:* Akineton; *S.Afr.:* Akineton; *Singapore:* Akineton; *Spain:* Akineton; *Swed.:* Akineton; *Switz.:* Akineton; *Thai.:* Akineton; *UK:* Akineton; *USA:* Akineton.

Bornaprine Hydrochloride (349-x)

Bornaprine Hydrochloride (BANM, rINNM).

3-Diethylaminopropyl 2-phenylbicyclo[2.2.1]heptane-2-carboxylate hydrochloride.

$C_{21}H_{31}NO_2,HCl = 365.9$.

CAS — 20448-86-6 (bornaprine); 26908-91-8 (bornaprine hydrochloride).

Profile

Bornaprine hydrochloride is a quaternary ammonium antimuscarinic with actions and uses similar to those of benzhexol [trihexyphenidyl] (p.463). It is used in the symptomatic treatment of parkinsonism (p.460), but it is claimed to be mainly effective against tremor. It is given by mouth in initial doses of 2 mg daily gradually increased to 6 to 12 mg daily according to the response of the patient.

Preparations

Proprietary Preparations (details are given in Part 3)
Aust.: Sormodren; *Ger.:* Sormodren; *Ital.:* Sormodren; *Mex.:* Sormodren.

Butropium Bromide (350-y)

Butropium Bromide (rINN).

(−)-(1R,3r,5S)-8-(4-Butoxybenzyl)-3-[(S)-tropoyloxy]tropanium bromide.

$C_{28}H_{38}BrNO_4 = 532.5$.

CAS — 29025-14-7.

Pharmacopoeias. In Jpn.

Profile
Butropium bromide is a quaternary ammonium antimuscarinic with peripheral effects similar to those of atropine (p.461). It has been used in the symptomatic treatment of visceral spasms.

Preparations
Proprietary Preparations (details are given in Part 3)
Hong Kong: Coliopan; *Jpn:* Coliopan†; *Singapore:* Coliopan.

Buzepide Metiodide (351-j)
Buzepide Metiodide (rINN).
Diphexamide Iodomethylate; FI-6146; Metazepium Iodide; R-661. 1-(3-Carbamoyl-3,3-diphenylpropyl)-1-methylperhydroazepinium iodide.
$C_{23}H_{31}IN_2O = 478.4$.
CAS — 15351-05-0.

Profile
Buzepide metiodide is a quaternary ammonium antimuscarinic with peripheral effects similar to those of atropine (p.461). It has been given with other compounds for upper respiratory-tract disorders and in gastrointestinal disorders with smooth muscle spasm.

Preparations
Proprietary Preparations (details are given in Part 3)
Multi-ingredient: *Belg.:* Denoral; *Fr.:* Denoral†; Vesadol; *Hong Kong:* Denoral; *Ital.:* Denoral.

Ciclonium Bromide (4095-d)
Ciclonium Bromide (rINN).
Asta-3746.   Diethylmethyl{2-[(α-methyl-α-5-norbornen-2-yl-benzyl)oxy]ethyl}ammonium bromide.
$C_{22}H_{34}BrNO = 408.4$.
CAS — 29546-59-6.

Profile
Ciclonium bromide is an antimuscarinic used in the treatment of gastrointestinal and urinary-tract disorders.

Preparations
Proprietary Preparations (details are given in Part 3)
Thai.: Adamon.

Cimetropium Bromide (1702-g)
Cimetropium Bromide (rINN).
DA-3177; Hyoscine-N-(cyclopropylmethyl) Bromide. 8-(Cyclopropylmethyl)-6β,7β-epoxy-3α-hydroxy-1αH,5αH-tropanium bromide, (−)-(S)-tropate.
$C_{21}H_{28}BrNO_4 = 438.4$.
CAS — 51598-60-8.
ATC — A03BB05.

Profile
Cimetropium bromide is a quaternary ammonium antimuscarinic with peripheral effects similar to those of atropine (p.461). It has been used as an antispasmodic in the treatment of gastrointestinal disorders (p.459) in usual doses of 50 mg two or three times daily by mouth or by rectal suppository. It has also been given intramuscularly or intravenously in usual doses of 5 mg.

◊ References.
1. Gullo L, *et al.* Inhibition of caerulein-induced gall bladder emptying by cimetropium bromide in humans. *Eur J Clin Pharmacol* 1989; **37:** 483–6.
2. Dobrilla G, *et al.* Longterm treatment of irritable bowel syndrome with cimetropium bromide: a double blind placebo controlled clinical trial. *Gut* 1990; **31:** 355–8.
3. Marzio L, *et al.* Effect of cimetropium bromide on esophageal motility and transit in patients affected by primary achalasia. *Dig Dis Sci* 1994; **39:** 1389–94.

Preparations
Proprietary Preparations (details are given in Part 3)
Ital.: Alginor.

Clidinium Bromide (354-k)
Clidinium Bromide (BAN, USAN, rINN).
Ro-2-3773. 3-Benziloyloxy-1-methylquinuclidinium bromide.
$C_{22}H_{26}BrNO_3 = 432.4$.
CAS — 7020-55-5 (clidinium); 3485-62-9 (clidinium bromide).
Pharmacopoeias. In US.

Pharmacopoeial description
USP 25: A white or nearly white, practically odourless, crystalline powder. Soluble in water and in alcohol; slightly soluble in ether and in benzene. Store in airtight containers. Protect from light.

Profile
Clidinium bromide is a quaternary ammonium antimuscarinic with peripheral effects similar to those of atropine (p.461). It is used alone or with chlordiazepoxide in the symptomatic treatment of peptic ulcer disease and other gastrointestinal disorders

The symbol † denotes a preparation no longer actively marketed

---

(p.459). The usual dose of clidinium bromide is 2.5 to 5 mg three or four times daily before meals and at bedtime.

Preparations
USP 25: Chlordiazepoxide Hydrochloride and Clidinium Bromide Capsules.
Proprietary Preparations (details are given in Part 3)
USA: Quarzan†.
Multi-ingredient: *Aust.:* Librax†; *Belg.:* Librax†; *Canad.:* Apo-Chlorax; Corium†; Librax; *Fin.:* Librax; *Fr.:* Librax; *Hong Kong:* Bralix; Librax; *Israel:* Librax; Nirvaxal; *Ital.:* Librax; *Port.:* Librax; *S.Afr.:* Librax; *Singapore:* Apo-Chlorax; Chlobax; Librax; Medocalm; *Swed.:* Librax†; *Switz.:* Librax; *Thai.:* Kenspa; Liblan; Librax; Pobrax; Tumax; *USA:* Clindex; Librax; Lidox†.

Cyclodrine Hydrochloride (9269-d)
GT-92. 2-Diethylaminoethyl 2-(1-hydroxycyclopentyl)-2-phenylacetate hydrochloride.
$C_{19}H_{29} \cdot NO_2,HCl = 355.9$.
CAS — 52109-93-0 (cyclodrine); 78853-39-1 (cyclodrine hydrochloride).

Profile
Cyclodrine is an analogue of cyclopentolate (below). It has been used as the hydrochloride in eye drops to produce mydriasis and cycloplegia.

Cyclopentolate Hydrochloride
(355-a)

Cyclopentolate Hydrochloride (BANM, rINNM).
Cloridrato de Ciclopentolato; Cyclopentolati Hydrochloridum. 2-Dimethylaminoethyl 2-(1-hydroxycyclopentyl)-2-phenylacetate hydrochloride.
$C_{17}H_{25}NO_3,HCl = 327.8$.
CAS — 512-15-2 (cyclopentolate); 5870-29-1 (cyclopentolate hydrochloride).

NOTE. CYC is a code approved by the BP 2001 for use on single unit doses of eye drops containing cyclopentolate hydrochloride where the individual container may be too small to bear all the appropriate labelling information. PHNCYC is a similar code approved for eye drops containing phenylephrine hydrochloride and cyclopentolate hydrochloride.
Pharmacopoeias. In Eur. (see p.vi), Jpn, and US.

Pharmacopoeial description
Ph. Eur.: A white, crystalline powder. Very soluble in water; freely soluble in alcohol. A 1% solution in water has a pH of 4.5 to 5.5.
USP 25: A white crystalline powder, which develops a characteristic odour on standing. Very soluble in water; freely soluble in alcohol; insoluble in ether. pH of a 1% solution in water is between 4.5 and 5.5. Store at a temperature not exceeding 8° in airtight containers.

Adverse Effects, Treatment, and Precautions
As for Atropine Sulfate, p.461.

Eye drops of cyclopentolate hydrochloride may cause temporary irritation.

◊ Ten of 66 patients who received one drop of 2% cyclopentolate eye drops in each eye developed systemic toxicity of mild to moderate severity; 9 of the 10 were female.[1] Toxic signs included physical weakness, nausea, lightheadedness, changes in emotional attitude, unprovoked weeping, and loss of equilibrium; tachycardia was always present but changes in blood pressure were insignificant. Spontaneous recovery occurred within 1 hour to several days.

As with atropine, it has been recommended that cyclopentolate eye drops should not be used during the first 3 months of life because of the possible association with development of amblyopia. Systemic toxicity has also been reported in neonates following ocular administration of cyclopentolate.[2]

A 4-year-old boy with cerebral palsy and paraplegia suffered tonic-clonic seizures, facial flushing, and tachycardia 70 minutes after one drop of a 1% cyclopentolate solution was instilled into each eye to dilate his pupils.[3] The child had no history of convulsions and had received 1% cyclopentolate eye drops on 2 previous occasions without incident.

1. Awan KJ. Adverse systemic reactions of topical cyclopentolate hydrochloride. *Ann Ophthalmol* 1976; **8:** 695–8.
2. Bauer CR, *et al.* Systemic cyclopentolate (Cyclogyl) toxicity in the newborn infant. *J Pediatr* 1973; **92:** 501–5.
3. Fitzgerald DA, *et al.* Seizures associated with 1% cyclopentolate eyedrops. *J Paediatr Child Health* 1990; **26:** 106–7.

Abuse. A report[1] of abuse of cyclopentolate eye drops by 2 patients. One of the patients who had been instilling 200 to 400 drops of cyclopentolate into both eyes daily for about 4 months, presumably for its CNS effects, experienced intense nausea, vomiting, weakness, and tremors on withdrawal.

1. Sato EH, *et al.* Abuse of cyclopentolate hydrochloride (Cyclogyl) drops. *N Engl J Med* 1992; **326:** 1363–4.

Hypersensitivity. Two children developed hypersensitivity reactions shortly after the instillation of 1% cyclopentolate hydrochloride eye drops into each eye.[1] Both children initially had a facial rash but in one of them the rash later spread to include the arms and legs and was accompanied by mild breathlessness.

1. Jones LWJ, Hodes DT. Possible allergic reactions to cyclopentolate hydrochloride: case reports with literature review of uses and adverse reactions. *Ophthalmic Physiol Opt* 1991; **11:** 16–21.

Interactions
As for antimuscarinics in general (see Atropine Sulfate, p.461).

Uses and Administration
Cyclopentolate hydrochloride is a tertiary amine antimuscarinic with actions similar to those of atropine (p.461). It is used as eye drops to produce mydriasis and cycloplegia (p.460) for ophthalmic diagnostic procedures and also in the treatment of uveitis and iritis (p.1060). It acts more quickly than atropine and has a shorter duration of action; the maximum mydriatic effect is produced 30 to 60 minutes after instillation, and may persist for up to 24 hours; the maximum cycloplegic effect is produced within 25 to 75 minutes and accommodation recovers within 6 to 24 hours.

For diagnostic procedures, 1 drop of a 0.5% solution of cyclopentolate hydrochloride repeated after about 5 to 15 minutes is usually sufficient for adults. Higher strengths have been used. For children 1 or 2 drops of a 1% solution are instilled similarly, although some recommend that strengths greater than 0.5% should not be used in infants and that cyclopentolate should not be used at all during the first 3 months of life.

In the treatment of uveitis and iritis 1 or 2 drops of a 0.5% solution of cyclopentolate hydrochloride are instilled into the eye(s) up to four times daily.

Deeply pigmented eyes are more resistant to pupillary dilatation and may require the use of a 1% solution.

Preparations
BP 2001: Cyclopentolate Eye Drops;
USP 25: Cyclopentolate Hydrochloride Ophthalmic Solution.
Proprietary Preparations (details are given in Part 3)
Austral.: Cyclogyl; *Belg.:* Cyclopentol; *Braz.:* Cicloplegico; *Canad.:* Cyclogyl; Diopentolate; *Denm.:* Cyclogyl; *Fin.:* Oftan Syklo; *Fr.:* Skiacol; *Ger.:* Zykolat-EDO; *Irl.:* Mydrilate; *Ital.:* Ciclolux; *Neth.:* Cyclogyl†; Cyclomydri†; *NZ:* Cyclogyl; *Port.:* Ciclopegicedol; Midriodavi; *S.Afr.:* Cyclogyl; *Singapore:* Cyclogyl; *Spain:* Ciclople†; Cicloplejic; Cicloplejico; *Swed.:* Cyclogyl; *Switz.:* Cyclogyl; *Thai.:* Cyclogyl; *UK:* Mydrilate; *USA:* Ak-Pentolate; Cyclogyl; Cylate†; Ocu-Pentolate; Pentolair.
Multi-ingredient: *S.Afr.:* Cyclomydril; *Singapore:* Cyclomydril; *USA:* Cyclomydril.

Darifenacin (17411-y)
Darifenacin (BAN, rINN).
UK-88525.   (S)-1-[2-(2,3-Dihydro-5-benzofuranyl)ethyl]-α,α-diphenyl-3-pyrrolidineacetamide.
$C_{28}H_{30}N_2O_2 = 426.6$.
CAS — 133099-04-4 (darifenacin); 133099-07-7 (darifenacin hydrobromide).

Profile
Darifenacin is a selective M_3 antimuscarinic under investigation in the treatment of urinary incontinence. It is also being studied in irritable bowel syndrome.

◊ References.
1. Rosario DJ, *et al.* A pilot study of the effects of multiple doses of the M3 muscarinic receptor antagonist darifenacin on ambulatory parameters of detrusor activity in patients with detrusor instability. *Neurourol Urodyn* 1995; **14:** 464–5.

Dexetimide Hydrochloride (358-r)
Dexetimide Hydrochloride (BANM, rINNM).
Dexbenzetimide Hydrochloride; R-16470. (+)-(S)-2-(1-Benzyl-4-piperidyl)-2-phenylglutarimide hydrochloride; (+)-(S)-3-(1-Benzyl-4-piperidyl)-3-phenylpiperidine-2,6-dione hydrochloride.
$C_{23}H_{26}N_2O_2,HCl = 398.9$.
CAS — 21888-98-2 (dexetimide); 21888-96-0 (dexetimide hydrochloride).
NOTE. Dexetimide is *USAN*.

Profile
Dexetimide is a tertiary antimuscarinic with actions similar to those of benzhexol [trihexyphenidyl] (p.463). It has been used as the hydrochloride to alleviate drug-induced extrapyramidal

symptoms, but, like other antimuscarinics, it is of no value against tardive dyskinesias. It has been given in once daily doses of 0.5 to 1 mg by mouth; it has also been given by intramuscular injection.

Preparations

Proprietary Preparations (details are given in Part 3)
Belg.: Tremblex; *Neth.*: Tremblex.

Dicyclomine Hydrochloride (360-z)

Dicyclomine Hydrochloride *(BANM)*.
Dicycloverine Hydrochloride *(BANM, rINNM)*; Cloridrato de Dicicloverina; Dicycloverini Hydrochloridum. 2-Diethylaminoethyl bicyclohexyl-1-carboxylate hydrochloride.
$C_{19}H_{35}NO_2,HCl = 345.9$.
CAS — 77-19-0 *(dicyclomine [dicycloverine])*; 67-92-5 *(dicyclomine [dicycloverine] hydrochloride)*.
Pharmacopoeias. In Eur. (see p.vi) and US.

Pharmacopoeial description

Ph. Eur.: A white or almost white, crystalline powder. It shows polymorphism. Soluble in water; freely soluble in alcohol and in dichloromethane. A 1% solution in water has a pH of 5.0 to 5.5.
USP 25: A fine white, practically odourless, crystalline powder. Soluble 1 in 13 of water, 1 in 5 of alcohol, 1 in 2 of chloroform and of glacial acetic acid, and 1 in 770 of ether. pH of a 1% solution in water is between 5.0 and 5.5.

Adverse Effects, Treatment, and Precautions

As for Atropine Sulfate, p.461. Dicyclomine [dicycloverine] hydrochloride should not be given to infants younger than 6 months of age.

Apnoea. Reports of severe apnoea in infants aged 5 to 10 weeks associated with the administration of dicyclomine [dicycloverine].
1. Williams J, Watkin-Jones R. Dicyclomine: worrying symptoms associated with its use in some small babies. *BMJ* 1984; **288:** 901.
2. Edwards PDL. Dicyclomine in babies. *BMJ* 1984; **288:** 1230.
3. Spoudeas H, Shribman S. Dicyclomine in babies. *BMJ* 1984; **288:** 1230.

Pregnancy. For a review of the risks to the fetus of antiemetic therapy during pregnancy, with particular reference to Debendox (Bendectin: dicyclomine [dicycloverine] with doxylamine and pyridoxine), see under Antihistamines on p.405.

Interactions

As for antimuscarinics in general (see Atropine Sulfate, p.461).

Uses and Administration

Dicyclomine [dicycloverine] hydrochloride is a tertiary amine antimuscarinic with effects similar to but weaker than those of atropine (p.461); it also has a direct antispasmodic action.

Dicyclomine [dicycloverine] is used in gastrointestinal spasm, particularly that associated with the irritable bowel syndrome. For adults, 10 to 20 mg of dicyclomine [dicycloverine] hydrochloride is given 3 times daily; in the USA, up to 40 mg four times daily has been recommended where adverse effects permit. Children aged 6 months to 2 years may be given 5 to 10 mg up to 3 or 4 times daily; doses are usually given 15 minutes before meals. Children aged 2 to 12 years may be given 10 mg three times daily.

Dicyclomine [dicycloverine] hydrochloride may be given intramuscularly in doses of 20 mg given 4 times daily to patients in whom oral therapy is temporarily impractical, but should not be used for longer than 1 to 2 days.

Preparations

BP 2001: Dicycloverine Oral Solution; Dicycloverine Tablets;
USP 25: Dicyclomine Hydrochloride Capsules; Dicyclomine Hydrochloride Injection; Dicyclomine Hydrochloride Syrup; Dicyclomine Hydrochloride Tablets.

Proprietary Preparations (details are given in Part 3)
Austral.: Merbentyl; *Braz.*: Bentyl; *Canad.*: Bentylol; Formulex; Lomine; *Irl.*: Merbentyl; *Israel*: Notensyl; *Mex.*: Bentyl; Diclomin; *NZ*: Merbentyl; *Port.*: Optimal; *S.Afr.*: Clomin; Medicyclomine; Merbentyl; *Spain*: Bentylol†; *Thai.*: Clomin; Dicomin; *UK*: Merbentyl; *USA*: Antispas; Bentyl†; Byclomine; Di-Spaz†; Dibent; Dilomine†; Or-Tyl.
Multi-ingredient: *Braz.*: Anacidron; Gastricin; Gastromag; Kolantyl; *Canad.*: Spasmo Nil†; *Hong Kong*: Colimix; Crema-U; Veragel; *Irl.*: Kolanticon; *Ital.*: Merankol Pastiglie; *Port.*: Nausefe; *S.Afr.*: Alkalite D; Alumite; Asic; Betaclomin; Co-Gel†; Dynagastrin; Gelumen; Kaoneo†; Kolantyl; Medigel; Microgel;

Neutragel; Nu-Gel; pH 550; Propan Gel-S; Remotrox; Spasmogel; *Singapore*: Colimix; Tocid; Veragel DMS; *Spain*: Colchimax; Neocolan; *Thai.*: Berclomine; Biodan; Cymine; Difemic; Kremil-S; Mainnox; Med-Anspasmic; Veragel; *UK*: Diarrest; Kolanticon.

Diethazine Hydrochloride (361-c)

Diethazine Hydrochloride *(BANM, rINNM)*.
Diaethazinium Chloratum; Eazamine Hydrochloride; RP-2987. 10-(2-Diethylaminoethyl)phenothiazine hydrochloride.
$C_{18}H_{22}N_2S,HCl = 334.9$.
CAS — 60-91-3 *(diethazine)*; 341-70-8 *(diethazine hydrochloride)*.
Pharmacopoeias. In Fr.

Profile

Diethazine hydrochloride is an antimuscarinic with actions similar to those of profenamine hydrochloride (p.473), but it is more toxic and bone marrow depression may occur. It has been used in the treatment of parkinsonism.

Difemerine Hydrochloride (362-k)

Difemerine Hydrochloride *(rINNM)*.
UP-57. 2-Dimethylamino-1,1-dimethylethyl benzilate hydrochloride.
$C_{20}H_{25}NO_3,HCl = 363.9$.
CAS — 80387-96-8 *(difemerine)*; 70280-88-5 *(difemerine hydrochloride)*.

Profile

Difemerine hydrochloride is an antimuscarinic with effects similar to those of atropine (p.461) and was used in the symptomatic treatment of visceral spasms.

Dihexyverine Hydrochloride (363-a)

Dihexyverine Hydrochloride *(USAN, rINNM)*.
Dihexiverine Hydrochloride; JL-1078. 2-Piperidinoethyl bicyclohexyl-1-carboxylate hydrochloride.
$C_{20}H_{35}NO_2,HCl = 358.0$.
CAS — 561-77-3 *(dihexyverine)*; 5588-25-0 *(dihexyverine hydrochloride)*.

Profile

Dihexyverine hydrochloride is an antimuscarinic with effects similar to those of atropine (p.461). It is given in the symptomatic treatment of gastrointestinal spasm in daily doses of 20 to 60 mg by mouth or 50 to 150 mg rectally. It has also been given in doses of 10 mg by intramuscular injection.

Preparations

Proprietary Preparations (details are given in Part 3)
Fr.: Spasmodex.

Dimevamide (15840-a)

Dimevamide *(rINN)*.
Aminopentamide. α-[2-(Dimethylamino)propyl]-α-phenylbenzeneacetamide.
$C_{19}H_{24}N_2O = 296.4$.
CAS — 60-46-8.
Pharmacopoeias. US includes Aminopentamide Sulfate.

Profile

Dimevamide is a tertiary amine and has been used as an antimuscarinic.

Preparations

Proprietary Preparations (details are given in Part 3)
Multi-ingredient: *S.Afr.*: Kantrexil.

Diphemanil Metilsulfate (364-t)

Diphemanil Metilsulfate *(BAN, rINN)*.
Diphemanil Methylsulfate; Diphemanil Methylsulphate; Diphenmethanil Methylsulphate; Vagophemanil Methylsulphate. 4-Benzhydrylidene-1,1-dimethylpiperidinium methylsulphate.
$C_{20}H_{24}N,CH_3SO_4 = 389.5$.
CAS — 62-97-5.

Profile

Diphemanil metilsulfate is a quaternary ammonium antimuscarinic with peripheral effects similar to those of atropine (p.461). It is used topically as a 2% cream or powder to treat hyperhidrosis (excessive sweating).

Diphemanil metilsulfate, given by mouth, has been investigated for the treatment of symptomatic bradycardia in infants.

◊ References.
1. Vidal AM, *et al.* Pharmacokinetics of diphemanil methylsulphate in healthy subjects. *Eur J Clin Pharmacol* 1992; **42:** 689–91.
2. Vidal AM, *et al.* Pharmacokinetics of diphemanil methylsulphate in infants. *Eur J Clin Pharmacol* 1993; **45:** 89–91.
3. Pariente-Khayat A, *et al.* Pharmacokinetics of diphemanil methylsulphate in neonates and in premature infants. *Eur J Clin Pharmacol* 1996; **50:** 429–30.

Preparations

Proprietary Preparations (details are given in Part 3)
Austral.: Prantal; *Ital.*: Prantal; *NZ*: Prantal.

Drofenine Hydrochloride (11601-k)

Drofenine Hydrochloride *(pINNM)*.
Hexahydroadiphenine Hydrochloride. 2-(Diethylamino)ethyl α-phenylcyclohexaneacetate hydrochloride.
$C_{20}H_{31}NO_2,HCl = 353.9$.
CAS — 1679-76-1 *(drofenine)*; 548-66-3 *(drofenine hydrochloride)*.
Pharmacopoeias. In Belg. and Swiss.

Profile

Drofenine hydrochloride is an antimuscarinic available in preparations for the treatment of visceral spasms.

Preparations

Proprietary Preparations (details are given in Part 3)
Multi-ingredient: *Aust.*: Spasmoplus; *Belg.*: Spasmo-Cibalgine†; Spasmoplus; *Ger.*: Spasmo-Cibalgin compositum S; Spasmo-Cibalgin S; *Ital.*: Spasmo-Cibalgina; *Mex.*: Espasmo Cibalgina; *Switz.*: Lunadon; Sonotryl†; Spasmo-Cibalgin; Spasmo-Cibalgin comp.

Emepronium Bromide (365-x)

Emepronium Bromide *(BAN, rINN)*.
Ethyldimethyl(1-methyl-3,3-diphenylpropyl)ammonium bromide.
$C_{20}H_{28}BrN = 362.3$.
CAS — 27892-33-7 *(emepronium)*; 3614-30-0 *(emepronium bromide)*.

Emepronium Carrageenate (18635-j)

Emepronium Carrageenate *(BAN)*.

Adverse Effects, Treatment, and Precautions

As for Atropine Sulfate, p.461.
To avoid oesophageal ulceration, tablets of emepronium bromide should always be swallowed with an adequate volume of water, and patients should always be in the sitting or standing position while, and for 10 to 15 minutes after, taking the tablets. Emepronium is contra-indicated in patients with symptoms or signs of oesophageal obstruction or with pre-existing oesophagitis.

Buccal and oesophageal ulceration. Tablet-induced oesophageal damage is widely recognised and is related to direct mucosal injury by the medication. Emepronium bromide has been frequently implicated in this type of mucosal injury, although it rarely results in stricture formation.[1]
1. McCord GS, Clouse RE. Pill-induced esophageal strictures: clinical features and risk factors for development. *Am J Med* 1990; **88:** 512–18.

Interactions

As for antimuscarinics in general (see Atropine Sulfate, p.461).

Pharmacokinetics

Emepronium is incompletely absorbed from the gastrointestinal tract and is mainly excreted unchanged in the urine and faeces. It does not readily cross the blood-brain barrier at therapeutic doses.

Uses and Administration

Emepronium is a quaternary ammonium antimuscarinic with peripheral effects similar to those of atropine (p.461). It is used mainly in the treatment of urinary frequency and incontinence (p.459). A usual dose by mouth is 200 mg of the bromide, or its equivalent as the carrageenate, three times daily.

Preparations

Proprietary Preparations (details are given in Part 3)
Aust.: Cetiprin; *Braz.*: Cetiprin; *Denm.*: Cetiprin; *Fin.*: Cetiprin Novum; *Ger.*: Uro-Ripirin; *Hong Kong*: Cetiprin Novum; *Irl.*: Cetiprin; *Neth.*: Cetiprin; *Norw.*: Cetiprin; *NZ*: Cetiprin; *Spain*: Hexanium†; *Swed.*: Cetiprin; *Switz.*: Cetiprin.

Eucatropine Hydrochloride (369-n)

Eucatropine Hydrochloride *(BANM, rINNM)*.
Clorhidrato de Euftalmina; Eucatropinium Chloride. 1,2,2,6-Tetramethyl-4-piperidyl mandelate hydrochloride.
$C_{17}H_{25}NO_3,HCl = 327.8$.
CAS — 100-91-4 *(eucatropine)*; 536-93-6 *(eucatropine hydrochloride)*.
Pharmacopoeias. In US.

Pharmacopoeial description

USP 25: A white, odourless, granular powder. Very soluble in water; freely soluble in alcohol and in chloroform; insoluble in ether. Its solutions are neutral to litmus. Store in airtight containers. Protect from light.

Profile

Eucatropine hydrochloride is a tertiary amine antimuscarinic that has been used as a mydriatic. It has little or no effect on accommodation.

Preparations

USP 25: Eucatropine Hydrochloride Ophthalmic Solution.

Fentonium Bromide (370-k)

Fentonium Bromide *(rINN)*.

Fa-402; Fentonii Bromidum; Ketocilium; *N*-(4-Phenylphenacyl)-1-hyoscyaminium Bromide; Z-326. (–)-(1*R*,3*r*,5*S*)-8-(4-Phenylphenacyl)-3-[(*S*)-tropyloxy]tropanium bromide.
$C_{31}H_{34}BrNO_4 = 564.5$.
CAS — 5868-06-4.

Profile

Fentonium bromide is a quaternary ammonium antimuscarinic with peripheral effects similar to those of atropine (p.461). It has been used to relieve visceral spasms.

Preparations

Proprietary Preparations (details are given in Part 3)
Mex.: Ulcesium.

Flavoxate Hydrochloride (5233-h)

Flavoxate Hydrochloride *(BANM, USAN, rINNM)*.

DW-61; NSC-114649; Rec-7-0040. 2-Piperidinoethyl 3-methyl-4-oxo-2-phenyl-4*H*-chromene-8-carboxylate hydrochloride.
$C_{24}H_{25}NO_4,HCl = 427.9$.
CAS — 15301-69-6 (flavoxate); 3717-88-2 (flavoxate hydrochloride).

Pharmacopoeias. In Br. and Jpn.

Pharmacopoeial description

BP 2001: A white or almost white crystalline powder. Slightly soluble in water and in alcohol; slightly soluble in dichloromethane. Protect from light.

Adverse Effects, Treatment, and Precautions

As for Atropine Sulfate, p.461.

Adverse effects of flavoxate hydrochloride include increased intra-ocular pressure, difficulty in ocular accommodation, and blurred vision. There may be dry mouth, gastrointestinal disturbances and hypersensitivity reactions. Other adverse effects include headache, sedation, vertigo, dysuria, and confusion, particularly in the elderly. Tachycardia and palpitations have also been reported. Leucopenia has been reported rarely.

Interactions

As for antimuscarinics in general (see Atropine Sulfate, p.461).

Pharmacokinetics

Flavoxate is readily absorbed from the gastrointestinal tract and rapidly metabolised, about 50 to 60% of a dose being excreted in the urine within 24 hours as methyl flavone carboxylic acid.

Uses and Administration

Flavoxate hydrochloride is described as a smooth muscle relaxant but it also has antimuscarinic effects; it is a tertiary amine. It is used for the symptomatic relief of pain, urinary frequency, and incontinence associated with inflammatory disorders of the urinary tract. It is also used for the relief of vesico-urethral spasms resulting from instrumentation or surgery. A usual dose is 200 mg by mouth three times daily.

Urinary incontinence. Flavoxate is indicated mainly in the treatment of urge incontinence (p.459). Results of studies have sometimes been disappointing,[1-4] although side-effects are said to be less marked than those seen with other antimuscarinics such as oxybutynin.

1. Stanton SL. A comparison of emepronium bromide and flavoxate hydrochloride in the treatment of urinary incontinence. *J Urol (Baltimore)* 1973; **110:** 529–32.
2. Meyhoff HH, *et al.* Placebo—the drug of choice in female motor urge incontinence? *Br J Urol* 1983; **55:** 34–7.
3. Robinson JM, Brocklehurst JC. Emepronium bromide and flavoxate hydrochloride in the treatment of urinary incontinence associated with detrusor instability in elderly women. *Br J Urol* 1983; **55:** 371–6.
4. Chapple CR, *et al.* Double-blind, placebo-controlled, cross-over study of flavoxate in the treatment of idiopathic detrusor instability. *Br J Urol* 1990; **66:** 491–4.

Preparations

BP 2001: Flavoxate Tablets.

Proprietary Preparations (details are given in Part 3)
Aust.: Urispas; *Belg.:* Urispas; *Braz.:* Genurin-S; *Canad.:* Urispas; *Denm.:* Urispadol; *Fr.:* Urispas; *Ger.:* Spasuret; *Hong Kong:* Genurin; Urispas; *Irl.:* Urispas; *Ital.:* Genurin; *Jpn:* Bladderon; *Mex.:* Bladuril; *Neth.:* Urispas; *Port.:* Urispas; *S.Afr.:* Urispas; *Singapore:* Cleanxate; Genurin; *Spain:* Uronid; *Switz.:* Urispas; *Thai.:* Flavorin; Spasuri; U-Spa; Uroxate; *UK:* Urispas; *USA:* Urispas.

Multi-ingredient: *Ital.:* Cistalgan.

Flutropium Bromide (2157-v)

Flutropium Bromide *(rINN)*.

Ba-598BR. (8*r*)-8-(2-Fluoroethyl)-3α-hydroxy-1α*H*,5α*H*-tropanium bromide benzilate.
$C_{24}H_{29}BrFNO_3 = 478.4$.
CAS — 63516-07-4.

Profile

Flutropium bromide is a quaternary ammonium antimuscarinic with peripheral effects similar to those of atropine (p.461). It has bronchodilator properties and has been investigated for the treatment of respiratory-tract disorders.

Glycopyrronium Bromide (371-a)

Glycopyrronium Bromide *(BAN, rINN)*.

AHR-504; Glycopyrrolate *(USAN)*. 3-(α-Cyclopentylmandeloyloxy)-1,1-dimethylpyrrolidinium bromide.
$C_{19}H_{28}BrNO_3 = 398.3$.
CAS — 596-51-0.

Pharmacopoeias. In US.

Incompatible with alkalis.

Pharmacopoeial description

USP 25: A white, odourless, crystalline powder. Soluble 1 in 4.2 of water, 1 in 30 of alcohol, 1 in 260 of chloroform, and 1 in 35 000 of ether. Store in airtight containers.

Stability. Investigation of the compatibility of glycopyrronium bromide with infusion solutions and additives showed that the stability of glycopyrronium bromide is questionable above a pH of 6, owing to ester hydrolysis.[1]

1. Ingallinera TS, *et al.* Compatibility of glycopyrrolate injection with commonly used infusion solutions and additives. *Am J Hosp Pharm* 1979; **36:** 508–10. Correction. *ibid.*; 745.

Adverse Effects, Treatment, and Precautions

As for Atropine Sulfate, p.461.

Renal impairment. A comparison[1] of the pharmacokinetics of intravenous glycopyrronium in 11 uraemic and 7 control patients indicated that the renal elimination of glycopyrronium is considerably prolonged in patients with uraemia. The mean amount of a dose excreted in the urine within 3 hours of administration was 0.7% in the uraemic patients and 50% in the control patients; 24-hour excretion was 7% and 65% respectively. The authors of the study concluded that repeated or large doses of glycopyrronium should be avoided or perhaps the drug should not be used in patients with uraemia.

1. Kirvelä M, *et al.* Pharmacokinetics of glycopyrronium in uraemic patients. *Br J Anaesth* 1993; **71:** 437–9.

Interactions

As for antimuscarinics in general (see Atropine Sulfate, p.461).

Pharmacokinetics

Glycopyrronium bromide is poorly absorbed from the gastrointestinal tract; about 10 to 25% has been stated to be absorbed after an oral dose. Glycopyrronium bromide penetrates the blood-brain barrier only poorly. Glycopyrronium is excreted in bile and urine.

◊ References.

1. Kaltiala E, *et al.* The fate of intravenous [³H]glycopyrrolate in man. *J Pharm Pharmacol* 1974; **26:** 352–4.
2. Ali-melkkilä TM, *et al.* Pharmacokinetics of IM glycopyrronium. *Br J Anaesth* 1990; **64:** 667–9.
3. Rautakorpi P, *et al.* Pharmacokinetics of glycopyrrolate in children. *J Clin Anesth* 1994; **6:** 217–20.

Uses and Administration

Glycopyrronium bromide is a quaternary ammonium antimuscarinic with peripheral effects similar to those of atropine (p.461). Following intramuscular administration, onset of effects is within 15 to 30 minutes; vagal blocking effects last for 2 to 3 hours and antisialagogue effects persist for up to 7 hours. Following intravenous administration, onset of actions occurs within one minute.

Glycopyrronium bromide is used similarly to atropine in anaesthetic practice. It has also been used in the iontophoretic treatment of hyperhidrosis and as an adjunct in the treatment of peptic ulcer disease.

See under headings below for details of dosage and administration of glycopyrronium in specific indications.

Anaesthesia. Glycopyrronium bromide is given as a premedicant before general anaesthesia (see p.459) to diminish the risk of vagal inhibition of the heart and to reduce salivary and bronchial secretions. It is given in doses of 200 to 400 μg intravenously or intramuscularly before the induction of anaesthesia; alternatively, it may be given in a dose of 4 to 5 μg per kg body-weight to a maximum of 400 μg. If necessary, similar or lower doses may be given intravenously during the operation and repeated if required. A suggested dosage for premedication in children is 4 to 8 μg per kg intravenously or intramuscularly to a maximum of 200 μg.

Glycopyrronium bromide is given before or with anticholinesterases to counteract their muscarinic effects when they are used to reverse the effects of competitive muscle relaxants (see Neostigmine Metilsulfate, p.1420). The dose is glycopyrronium bromide 200 μg intravenously per 1 mg of neostigmine (or per 5 mg of pyridostigmine); alternatively, it may be given in a dose of 10 to 15 μg per kg intravenously with neostigmine 50 μg per kg. A suggested dosage for children is 10 μg per kg intravenously with neostigmine 50 μg per kg. Glycopyrronium bromide can be administered mixed in the same syringe with the anticholinesterase, and it has been suggested that greater cardiovascular stability results from this method of administration.

Gastrointestinal disorders. Antimuscarinics, including glycopyrronium bromide, have a limited role in the treatment of gastrointestinal spasms and as an adjunct in the treatment of peptic ulcer disease (see p.459).

As an adjunct in the treatment of peptic ulcer disease the usual initial dose of glycopyrronium bromide is 3 to 6 mg daily by mouth in divided doses adjusted according to response to a maximum of 8 mg daily; a maintenance dose of 1 mg twice daily is often adequate. Doses of 100 to 200 μg have been given by intramuscular or intravenous injection.

Hyperhidrosis. Adverse effects generally preclude oral use of antimuscarinics for the management of hyperhidrosis (p.459), but some, such as glycopyrronium, have been applied topically as alternatives to aluminium salts.

In studies involving 22 patients with the Frey syndrome (localised flushing and sweating on eating) glycopyrronium bromide as 1 and 2% cream or roll-on solution gave good control of symptoms;[1] patients tended to prefer the roll-on lotion as it was easier to apply. Topical hyoscine as 0.25, 1, or 3% solution or cream also gave control of sweating, but was associated with a much higher incidence of side-effects. Patients with diabetic gustatory sweating have also noted a reduction in the frequency and severity of episodes after applying glycopyrronium 0.5% cream.[2]

Glycopyrronium bromide has also been used as a 0.05% solution in the iontophoretic treatment of hyperhidrosis.

1. Hays LL, *et al.* The Frey syndrome: a simple, effective treatment. *Otolaryngol Head Neck Surg* 1982; **90:** 419–25.
2. Shaw JE, *et al.* A randomised controlled trial of topical glycopyrrolate, the first specific treatment for diabetic gustatory sweating. *Diabetologia* 1997; **40:** 299–301.

Palliative care. Glycopyrronium bromide is used in palliative care as an alternative to hyoscine in patients requiring continuous subcutaneous infusion to reduce excessive respiratory secretions. A dose of 0.6 to 1.2 mg may be given over 24 hours.

Respiratory-tract disorders. Antimuscarinics have potent bronchodilatory activity and may be used in the management of reversible airways obstruction as discussed on p.460, although glycopyrronium is not one of the main ones used.
References.

1. Schroeckenstein DC, *et al.* Twelve-hour bronchodilation in asthma with a single aerosol dose of the anticholinergic compound glycopyrrolate. *J Allergy Clin Immunol* 1988; **82:** 115–19.
2. Gilman MJ, *et al.* Comparison of aerosolized glycopyrrolate and metaproterenol in acute asthma. *Chest* 1990; **98:** 1095–8.
3. Cydulka RK, Emerman CL. Effects of combined treatment with glycopyrrolate and albuterol in acute exacerbation of chronic obstructive pulmonary disease. *Ann Emerg Med* 1995; **25:** 470–3.

Preparations

USP 25: Glycopyrrolate Injection; Glycopyrrolate Tablets.

Proprietary Preparations (details are given in Part 3)
Aust.: Robinul; *Austral.:* Robinul; *Belg.:* Robinul; *Canad.:* Robinul; *Denm.:* Robinul; *Fin.:* Gastrodyn; Robinul; *Ger.:* Robinul; *Hong Kong:* Robinul; *Irl.:* Robinul; *Neth.:* Robinul; *Norw.:* Robinul; *NZ:* Robinul; *S.Afr.:* Robinul; *Swed.:* Robinul; *Switz.:* Robinul; *UK:* Robinul; *USA:* Robinul.

Multi-ingredient: *Fin.:* Gastrodyn comp.

Used as an adjunct in: *Belg.:* Robinul-Neostigmine; *Denm.:* Robinul-Neostigmin; *Fin.:* Glycostigmin; Robinul-Neostigmine; *Irl.:* Robinul-Neostigmine; *Norw.:* Robinul-Neostigmine; *Swed.:* Robinul-Neostigmine; *Switz.:* Robinul-Neostigmine; *UK:* Robinul-Neostigmine.

Homatropine (373-x)

Homatropine (BAN).
(1R,3r,5S)-Tropan-3-yl (RS)-mandelate.
$C_{16}H_{21}NO_3 = 275.3$.
CAS — 87-00-3.
ATC — S01FA05.

Homatropine Hydrobromide (374-r)

Homatropine Hydrobromide (BANM).
Homatr. Hydrobrom.; Homatropini Hydrobromidum; Homatropinium Bromide; Homatropinum Bromatum; Omatropina Bromidrato; Oxtolyltropine Bromide; Tropyl Mandelate Hydrobromide.
$C_{16}H_{21}NO_3, HBr = 356.3$.
CAS — 51-56-9.

NOTE. HOM is a code approved by the BP 2001 for use on single unit doses of eye drops containing homatropine hydrobromide where the individual container may be too small to bear all the appropriate labelling information.
Pharmacopoeias. In Eur. (see p.vi), Int., Jpn, Pol., and US.

Pharmacopoeial description

Ph. Eur.: A white, crystalline powder or colourless crystals. Freely soluble in water; sparingly soluble in alcohol; very slightly soluble in ether. A 5% solution in water has a pH of 5.0 to 6.5. Protect from light.
USP 25: White crystals or a white crystalline powder. Soluble 1 in 6 of water, 1 in 40 of alcohol, and 1 in 420 of chloroform; insoluble in ether. pH of a 2% solution in water is between 5.7 and 7.0. Store in airtight containers. Protect from light.

Homatropine Methylbromide (375-f)

Homatropine Methylbromide (BANM, rINN).
Homatropine Methobromide; Homatropini Methylbromidum; Methylhomatropinium Bromatum; Methylhomatropinium Bromide. (1R,3r,5S)-3-[(±)-Mandeloyloxy]-8-methyltropanium bromide.
$C_{16}H_{21}NO_3, CH_3Br = 370.3$.
CAS — 80-49-9.
Pharmacopoeias. In Eur. (see p.vi), Int., and US.

Pharmacopoeial description

Ph. Eur.: A white, crystalline powder or colourless crystals. Freely soluble in water; soluble in alcohol; practically insoluble in ether. A 5% solution in water has a pH of 4.5 to 6.5. Protect from light.
USP 25: A white, odourless, powder that slowly darkens on exposure to light. Very soluble in water; freely soluble in alcohol and in acetone containing about 20% of water; practically insoluble in acetone and in ether. pH of a 1% solution in water is between 4.5 and 6.5. Store in airtight containers. Protect from light.

Adverse Effects, Treatment, and Precautions

As for Atropine Sulfate, p.461.

Ophthalmic use. Antimuscarinic toxicity (including ataxia, restlessness, excitement, hallucinations) has been reported in children[1] and the elderly[2,3] following administration of homatropine eye drops.

1. Hoefnagel D. Toxic effects of atropine and homatropine eyedrops in children. N Engl J Med 1961; 264: 168–71.
2. Reid D, Fulton JD. Tachycardia precipitated by topical homatropine. BMJ 1989; 299: 795–6.
3. Tune LE, et al. Anticholinergic delirium caused by topical homatropine ophthalmologic solution: confirmation by anticholinergic radioreceptor assay in two cases. J Neuropsychiatr Clin Neurosci 1992; 4: 195–7.

Interactions

As for antimuscarinics in general (see Atropine Sulfate, p.461).

Uses and Administration

Homatropine is a tertiary amine antimuscarinic with effects similar to those of atropine (p.461). It is used as the hydrobromide, also a tertiary amine, to produce mydriasis and cycloplegia (p.460); its actions are more rapid and of shorter duration than those of atropine, but it is less potent and has a relatively weak cycloplegic effect. In general, onset of action is between 30 and 60 minutes, and recovery within 1 to 3 days. Homatropine hydrobromide is generally used as a 1, 2, or 5% ophthalmic solution. For the determination of refraction, one or two drops may be instilled, repeated if necessary 5 or 10 minutes later. In the treatment of uveitis (p.1060), one or two drops may be instilled two or three times a day, or up to every 3 to 4 hours if required.

Homatropine has also been used as the quaternary ammonium methobromide derivative in the treatment of gastrointestinal spasm and as an adjunct in peptic ulcer disease.

Preparations

BP 2001: Homatropine Eye Drops;
USP 25: Homatropine Hydrobromide Ophthalmic Solution; Homatropine Methylbromide Tablets.

Proprietary Preparations (details are given in Part 3)
Braz.: Novatropina; **Mex.:** Hemogrin Al; Homasedin; Homatropil; Homo; Infafren Simple; Pasmolit; **Port.:** Homatrocil; **Spain:** Coliriocilina Homatrop; Homatrop.

Multi-ingredient: Austral.: Hycomine†; **Braz.:** Analgosedan; Atapec; Belacodid; Diapool; Enterobion; Enteropen; Espasmal-gon; Espasmo Colic; Espasmo Luftal; Espasmobel; Etaverol; Filinasma; Glotil; H-Sal; Linadin; Marsonil; Migrane; Naquinto; Plasmocolit; Plenocedan; Pulmoformil; Sedalene; Somasedin; Spasmotropin; Tebasedan; Tropinal; Vagoplex; **Hung.:** Neotroparin; **Mex.:** Coralzul; Fuzotyl; Sultroquin; **Port.:** Fluidin Nocturno†; **Spain:** Bleukawine†; Cortenema; **Thai.:** Polyenzyme-I; **USA:** Gustase Plus; Hycodan; Hydromet; Hydropane; Tussigon.

Hyoscine (11415-z)

Hyoscine (BAN).
Scopolamine. (–)-(1S,3s,5R,6R,7S,8s)-6,7-Epoxy-3[(S)-tropoyloxy] tropane.
$C_{17}H_{21}NO_4 = 303.4$.
CAS — 51-34-3.
ATC — A04AD01; N05CM05; S01FA02.

Hyoscine Butylbromide (376-d)

Hyoscine Butylbromide (BANM).
Butylscopolamine Bromide; N-Butylscopolammonium Bromide; Butylscopolamonii Bromidum; Hyoscine-N-butyl Bromide; Hyoscini Butylbromidum; Scopolamine N-Butyl Bromide; Scopolamine Butylbromide. (–)-(1S,3s,5R,6R,7S,8r)-6,7-Epoxy-8-butyl-3-[(S)-tropoyloxy]tropanium bromide.
$C_{21}H_{30}BrNO_4 = 440.4$.
CAS — 149-64-4.
Pharmacopoeias. In Eur. (see p.vi) and Jpn.

Pharmacopoeial description

Ph. Eur.: A white or almost white, crystalline powder. Freely soluble in water and in dichloromethane; sparingly soluble in dehydrated alcohol. A 5% solution in water has a pH of 5.5 to 6.5.

Hyoscine Hydrobromide (377-n)

Hyoscine Hydrobromide (BANM).
Bromhidrato de Escopolamina; Hyoscini Hydrobromidum; Ioscina Bromidrato; Scopolamine Bromhydrate; Scopolamine Hydrobromide; Scopolamini Hydrobromidum. (–)-(1S,3s,5R,6R,7S)-6,7-Epoxytropan-3-yl (S)-tropate hydrobromide trihydrate.
$C_{17}H_{21}NO_4, HBr, 3H_2O = 438.3$.
CAS — 114-49-8 (anhydrous hyoscine hydrobromide); 6533-68-2 (hyoscine hydrobromide trihydrate).

NOTE. HYO is a code approved by the BP 2001 for use on single unit doses of eye drops containing hyoscine hydrobromide where the individual container may be too small to bear all the appropriate labelling information.
Pharmacopoeias. In Chin., Eur. (see p.vi), Jpn, Pol., and US.

Pharmacopoeial description

Ph. Eur.: A white, efflorescent, crystalline powder or colourless crystals. Freely soluble in water; soluble in alcohol; practically insoluble in ether. A 5% solution in water has a pH of 4.0 to 5.5. Store below 15° in well-filled airtight containers of small capacity. Protect from light.
USP 25: Colourless or white crystals, or white granular powder. Is odourless and slightly efflorescent in dry air. Soluble 1 in 1.5 of water and 1 in 20 of alcohol; slightly soluble in chloroform; insoluble in ether. pH of a 5% solution in water is between 4.0 and 5.5. Store in airtight containers. Protect from light.

Hyoscine Methobromide (378-h)

Hyoscine Methobromide (BAN).
Epoxymethamine Bromide; Hyoscine Methylbromide; Methscopolamine Bromide; Scopolamine Methobromide; Scopolamine Methylbromide. (–)-(1S,3s,5R,6R,7S)-6,7-Epoxy-8-methyl-3-[(S)-tropoyloxy]tropanium bromide.
$C_{18}H_{24}BrNO_4 = 398.3$.
CAS — 155-41-9.

Hyoscine Methonitrate (379-m)

Hyoscine Methonitrate (BANM).
Hyoscine Methylnitrate; Methscopolamine Nitrate; Methylhyoscini Nitras; Methylscopolamini Nitras; Scopolamine Methonitrate; Scopolamine Methylnitrate. (–)-(1S,3s,5R,6R,7S)-6,7-Epoxy-8-methyl-3-[(S)-tropoyloxy]tropanium nitrate.
$C_{18}H_{24}N_2O_7 = 380.4$.
CAS — 6106-46-3.
Pharmacopoeias. In Aust. and It.

Adverse Effects, Treatment, and Precautions

As for Atropine Sulfate, p.461. In contrast to atropine, hyoscine produces central depression at therapeutic doses and symptoms include drowsiness and fatigue. Toxic doses of hyoscine produce stimulation of the CNS in a similar manner to atropine. However, hyoscine does not stimulate the medullary centres and therefore does not produce the increases in respiration rate or blood pressure seen with atropine. Hyoscine may produce CNS stimulation rather than depression at therapeutic doses if used in the presence of pain without opioid analgesics; symptoms include excitement, restlessness, hallucinations, or delirium.

Patients who experience drowsiness should not drive or operate machinery. Caution has been advised in elderly patients and in patients with impaired metabolic, liver, or kidney function, as adverse CNS effects have been stated to be more likely in these patients. There have been rare reports of an increase in frequency of seizures in epileptic patients.

The quaternary derivatives, such as the butylbromide, methobromide, or methonitrate, do not readily cross the blood-brain barrier, so central effects are rare.

Effects on the eyes. ANISOCORIA. Although bilateral mydriasis has been observed concomitantly with the use of transdermal hyoscine, development of a unilateral fixed dilated pupil (anisocoria) may be due to contamination of a finger with hyoscine in applying the device, and then rubbing the eye.[1-4]

1. Chiaramonte JS. Cycloplegia from transdermal scopolamine. N Engl J Med 1982; 306: 174.
2. Lepore FE. More on cycloplegia from transdermal scopolamine. N Engl J Med 1982; 307: 824.
3. McCrary JA, Webb NR. Anisocoria from scopolamine patches. JAMA 1982; 248: 353–4.
4. Bienia RA, et al. Scopolamine skin-disks and anisocoria. Ann Intern Med 1983; 99: 572–3.

GLAUCOMA. A report[1] of 2 cases of angle-closure glaucoma precipitated by transdermal hyoscine.

1. Fraunfelder FT. Transdermal scopolamine precipitating narrow-angle glaucoma. N Engl J Med 1982; 307: 1079.

STRABISMUS. Strabismus developed in a 4-year-old boy during treatment with transdermal hyoscine patches for drooling.[1] The strabismus resolved shortly after discontinuation of hyoscine.

1. Good WV, Crain LS. Esotropia in a child treated with a scopolamine patch for drooling. Pediatrics 1996; 97: 126–7.

Effects on mental function. There have been reports of psychotic reactions associated with the transdermal administration of hyoscine.[1-3] Psychotic reactions have also occurred following instillation of hyoscine eye drops.[4]

1. Osterholm RK, Camoriano JK. Transdermal scopolamine psychosis. JAMA 1982; 247: 3081.
2. Rodysill KJ, Warren JB. Transdermal scopolamine and toxic psychosis. Ann Intern Med 1983; 98: 561.
3. MacEwan GW, et al. Psychosis due to transdermally administered scopolamine. Can Med Assoc J 1985; 133: 431–2.
4. Barker DB, Solomon DA. The potential for mental status changes associated with systemic absorption of anticholinergic ophthalmic medications: concerns for the elderly. DICP Ann Pharmacother 1990; 24: 847–50.

Effects on the skin. Contact dermatitis occurred in 16 men being treated for seasickness with transdermal hyoscine for 6 weeks to 15 months.[1]

1. Gordon CR, et al. Allergic contact dermatitis caused by transdermal hyoscine. BMJ 1989; 298: 1220–1.

Porphyria. Hyoscine butylbromide has been associated with acute attacks of porphyria and is considered unsafe in porphyric patients.

Pregnancy. A report[1] of hyoscine toxicity in a neonate born to a mother who had received a total of 1.8 mg of hyoscine in divided doses with pethidine and levorphanol prior to delivery. The neonate was lethargic, barrel chested, and had a heart rate of 200 beats per minute. Symptoms subsided following physostigmine 100 μg given intramuscularly.

1. Evens RP, Leopold JC. Scopolamine toxicity in a newborn. Pediatrics 1980; 66: 329–30.

Withdrawal. Dizziness and nausea occurred three days after removal of a hyoscine transdermal delivery system. The patient had been using the transdermal patches to prevent seasickness during a 10-day cruise.[1]

1. Meyboom RHB. More on Transderm Scop patches. N Engl J Med 1984; 311: 1377.

Interactions

As for antimuscarinics in general (see Atropine Sulfate, p.461).

The sedative effect of hyoscine may be enhanced by alcohol or other CNS depressants.

Pharmacokinetics

Hyoscine is readily absorbed from the gastrointestinal tract following oral doses of the hydrobromide. It is almost entirely metabolised, probably in the liver; only a small proportion of an oral dose has been reported to be excreted unchanged in the urine. It crosses the blood-brain barrier and has been stated to cross the placenta. Hyoscine is also well absorbed following application to the skin.

The quaternary derivatives, such as the butylbromide or methobromide, are poorly absorbed from the gastrointestinal tract and do not readily pass the blood-brain barrier.

◊ References.
1. Ebert U, *et al.* Pharmacokinetics and pharmacodynamics of scopolamine after subcutaneous administration. *J Clin Pharmacol* 1998; **38:** 720–6.

Uses and Administration

Hyoscine is a tertiary amine antimuscarinic with central and peripheral actions (see p.459). It is a more powerful suppressant of salivation than atropine, and usually slows rather than increases heart rate, especially in low doses. Its central action differs from that of atropine in that it depresses the cerebral cortex and produces drowsiness and amnesia. Hyoscine hydrobromide is also a tertiary amine, whereas hyoscine butylbromide, hyoscine methobromide, and hyoscine methonitrate are quaternary ammonium derivatives.

Hyoscine and hyoscine hydrobromide are used in the management of motion sickness and other forms of nausea and vomiting; hyoscine hydrobromide is also given as a premedicant in anaesthesia, and to produce mydriasis and cycloplegia. Hyoscine butylbromide and other quaternary ammonium derivatives are used in conditions associated with visceral spasms. In addition, hyoscine methobromide has been employed as an adjunct in the treatment of peptic ulcer disease.

Other hyoscine salts or derivatives that have been used include hyoscine borate, hyoscine hydrochloride, and hyoscine oxide hydrobromide.

See under headings below for details of dosage and administration of hyoscine and its salts in specific indications.

Anaesthesia. The role of antimuscarinics, including hyoscine, in anaesthesia is discussed on p.459. For the use of hyoscine in the prevention of postoperative nausea and vomiting, see below.

For premedication hyoscine hydrobromide is injected subcutaneously or intramuscularly in doses of 200 to 600 µg, usually in association with papaveretum about half to one hour before induction of general anaesthesia.

Anoxic seizures. For mention of the use of transdermal hyoscine as an alternative to atropine in the management of reflex anoxic seizures in children, see p.462.

Cardiac disorders. Although hyoscine is not one of the conventional therapies for heart failure (p.798) or myocardial infarction (p.805), low-dose transdermal hyoscine can increase cardiac vagal activity and thereby reduce the autonomic imbalance seen in patients with these conditions.[1-3]

1. Casadei B, *et al.* Low doses of scopolamine increase cardiac vagal tone in the acute phase of myocardial infarction. *Circulation* 1993; **88:** 353–7.
2. La Rovere MT, *et al.* Scopolamine improves autonomic balance in advanced congestive heart failure. *Circulation* 1994; **90:** 838–43.
3. Venkatesh G, *et al.* Double blind placebo controlled trial of short term transdermal scopolamine on heart rate variability in patients with chronic heart failure. *Heart* 1996; **76:** 137–43.

Colic pain. Hyoscine has been used as an adjunct to opioid analgesics for symptomatic relief of biliary or renal colic (see p.459).

Dysmenorrhoea. Hyoscine has been used for its antispasmodic action in the treatment of dysmenorrhoea. Usual doses of 20 mg of hyoscine butylbromide are given by mouth four times daily.

Eye disorders. Hyoscine hydrobromide is used in the eye for its mydriatic and cycloplegic actions (p.460) usually in a concentration of 0.25%. It has a faster onset and shorter duration of action than atropine although the effects may still persist for up to 3 to 7 days. It may be useful for patients who are hypersensitive to atropine.

Gastrointestinal disorders. Hyoscine has been used to relieve the pain of smooth muscle spasm associated with the gastrointestinal tract (p.459). In such conditions usual doses of 20 mg of hyoscine butylbromide are administered intramuscularly or intravenously, repeated after 30 minutes if necessary, up to a maximum of 100 mg daily; alternatively, 10 mg may be given by mouth three times daily, increased to 20 mg four times daily if necessary. Children aged 6 to 12 years may be given 10 mg three times daily by mouth. Hyoscine may also be useful as an antispasmodic in endoscopy and radiological procedures of the gastrointestinal tract.[1] Hyoscine has been used as an adjunct in the treatment of peptic ulcer disease. Its antiemetic effect is discussed under Nausea and Vomiting, below.

1. Goei R, *et al.* Use of antispasmodic drugs in double contrast barium enema examination: glucagon or Buscopan? *Clin Radiol* 1995; **50:** 553–7.

Hyperhidrosis. Adverse effects of antimuscarinics given orally generally preclude their use by this route for the management of hyperhidrosis (p.459), but some, such as hyoscine, have been applied topically as alternatives to aluminium salts. Hyoscine hydrobromide applied as a 3% cream was successful in reducing gustatory sweating, consisting of flushing and sweating over the right mandible during eating, in a patient who had previously undergone surgical excision of the right submandibular salivary gland.[1]

1. Bailey BMW, Pearce DE. Gustatory sweating following submandibular salivary gland removal. *Br Dent J* 1985; **158:** 17–18.

Nausea and vomiting. Hyoscine is an effective agent in the prevention of **motion sickness** and is one of the principal drugs used. It may be given by mouth for short-term protection or transdermally from controlled-release systems for a prolonged duration of action.

A usual dose of hyoscine hydrobromide by mouth is 300 µg taken 30 minutes before a journey, followed by 300 µg every 6 hours if required up to a maximum of 3 doses in 24 hours. Children aged 4 to 10 years may be given 75 to 150 µg and those over 10 years, 150 to 300 µg. Hyoscine is also given via a transdermal delivery system (Scopoderm, UK) which is placed behind the ear and supplies 1 mg over 3 days. The patch may be used in adults and children aged 10 years and over and should be applied 5 to 6 hours before travelling or on the preceding evening and removed at the end of the journey.

An intranasal formulation of hyoscine hydrobromide is under investigation for the treatment and prevention of motion sickness.

Transdermal hyoscine has been used in adults and children for the prevention of **postoperative nausea and vomiting**.

Hyoscine hydrobromide has also been given by intravenous, subcutaneous, or intramuscular injection for its antiemetic effect in a usual dose of 300 to 600 µg.

The other drugs used in the management of motion sickness and postoperative nausea and vomiting are discussed on p.1206.

References.
1. Dahl E, *et al.* Transdermal scopolamine, oral meclizine, and placebo in motion sickness. *Clin Pharmacol Ther* 1984; **36:** 116–20.
2. Doyle E, *et al.* Prevention of postoperative nausea and vomiting with transdermal hyoscine in children using patient-controlled analgesia. *Br J Anaesth* 1994; **72:** 72–6.
3. Honkavaara P. Effect of transdermal hyoscine on nausea and vomiting during and after middle ear surgery under local anaesthesia. *Br J Anaesth* 1996; **76:** 49–53.

Palliative care. Hyoscine hydrobromide is used in palliative care to reduce excessive respiratory secretions. A dose of 0.4 to 0.6 mg may be given by subcutaneous injection every 4 to 8 hours. Alternatively 0.6 to 2.4 mg may be given over 24 hours by continuous subcutaneous infusion. Care should be taken to avoid the discomfort of a dry mouth.

Urinary incontinence. Various antimuscarinics have been used in the management of urge incontinence (p.459) but the incidence of adverse effects can be high. Results of a small study[1] suggested that transdermal hyoscine might be of benefit in females with detrusor instability.

1. Muskat Y, *et al.* The use of scopolamine in the treatment of detrusor instability. *J Urol (Baltimore)* 1996; **156:** 1989–90.

Vertigo. Hyoscine has a long history of use in the management of vertigo, although other drugs are now preferred (p.408).

Preparations

BP 2001: Hyoscine Butylbromide Injection; Hyoscine Butylbromide Tablets; Hyoscine Eye Drops; Hyoscine Injection; Hyoscine Tablets;
USP 25: Scopolamine Hydrobromide Injection; Scopolamine Hydrobromide Ophthalmic Ointment; Scopolamine Hydrobromide Ophthalmic Solution; Scopolamine Hydrobromide Tablets.

Proprietary Preparations (details are given in Part 3)
Aust.: Buscopan; Scopoderm; *Austral.:* Buscopan; Kwells; Travacalm HO; *Belg.:* Buscopan; *Braz.:* Algexin; Buscopan; *Canad.:* Buscopan; Transderm-V; *Denm.:* Buscopan; Scopoderm; *Fin.:* Buscopan; Scopoderm; *Fr.:* Genoscopolamine†; Scopoderm TTS; *Ger.:* Boro-Scopol; BS-ratiopharm; Buscolysin; Buscopan; espabutyl†; Scopoderm TTS; Spasman scop; Spasmowern; *Hong Kong:* Buscopan; Busopin; Copan; Dhacopan; Holopon; Hysopan; *Irl.:* Buscopan; Kwells; *Ital.:* Buscopan; Transcop; *Mex.:* Alpin; Buscapina; Busina; Buticina; Butiral; Cryopina; Espacil; Espasantral; Hiosinotil; Lemophar; Selpiran-S; Tilosin; *Neth.:* Buscopan; Scopoderm TTS; *Norw.:* Buscopan; Scopoderm; *NZ:* Buscopan; Scopoderm TTS; *Port.:* Buscopan; Vagotrope-S; *S.Afr.:* Buscopan; Hyospasmol; Scopex; Scopoderm TTS†; *Singapore:* Buscopan; Colospan; Dhacopan; Hyomide; Scopoderm TTS; Spasmoliv; Vacopan; *Spain:* Buscapina; Vorigeno; *Swed.:* Buscopan; Scopoderm; *Switz.:* Buscopan; Scopoderm TTS; *Thai.:* Antispa; Bacotan; Buscono; Buscopan; Butyl; Cencopan; Eralga; Hybutyl; Hyostan; Hyozin; Hytic; Kanin; Scopas; Spasgone-H; Vacopan; *UAE:* Scopinal; *UK:* Buscopan; Joy-Rides; Kwells; Scopoderm TTS; Travel Calm; *USA:* Pamine; Scopace; Transderm Scop.

Multi-ingredient: *Aust.:* Asthma; Buscopamol; Buscopan Compositum; Modiscop; *Austral.:* Contac; Donnagel; Donnalix; Donnatab; Travacalm; *Belg.:* Buscopan Compositum; Spasma; *Braz.:* Bioscina; Buscopan Composto; Buscopan Plus; Dorspan; Ductopan; Espasmodid Composto; Sedobion; Tropinal; Vagoplex; *Canad.:* Diban; Donnatal; *Ger.:* Buscopan Plus; Oragallin S†; *Hong Kong:* Crema-U; Virulex Forte; *Ital.:* Buscopan Compositum; Spasmeridan; *Mex.:* Buscapina Compositum; Buscapina Compositum N; Busconet; Busprina; Colepren; Donodol

Compuesto; Escapin-N; Espacil Compuesto; Retodol Compositum; Selpiran; *Port.:* Buscopan Compositum N; *S.Afr.:* Allertac; Bellatard; Bellavern†; Buscopan Compositum; Donnatal; Dyka-D; Millerspas; Respinol; Respinol Compound; Scopex Co†; Tropax†; Virobis; *Spain:* Buscapina Compositum; Midriati; Nolotil Compositum; Oragalin Espasmolitico; Psico Blocan; Urogobens Antiespasmo†; *Swed.:* Spasmofen; *Switz.:* Nardyl; Viaggio†; *Thai.:* Buscopan Plus; Donnatal; Pacopan; Spasgone; Unigan; *UK:* Feminax; *USA:* AH-chew; AlleRx; Antispasmodic Elixir; Atrohist Plus†; Barbidonna; Bellatal; DA Chewable; DA II; Dallergy; Deconhist LA†; Dehistine; Donna-Sed†; Donnamor†; Donnatal; Dura-Vent/DA; Ex-Histine; Extendryl; Hista-Vent DA; Histor-D Timecelles; Hyosophen; Malatal†; Mescolor; Murocoll-2; Omnihist LA; Pannaz; Phenacon†; Phenahist-TR†; Phenchlor SHA†; Prehist D; Rescon-MX; Ru-Tuss†; Stahist; Susano; Xiral.

Hyoscyamine (381-x)
Hyoscyamine (BAN).
(–)-Hyoscyamine; *l*-Hyoscyamine. (–)-(1R,3r,5S)-Tropan-3-yl (S)-tropate.
$C_{17}H_{23}NO_3 = 289.4$.
CAS — 101-31-5.
ATC — A03BA03.
Pharmacopoeias. In US.

An alkaloid obtained from various solanaceous plants. It is the laevo-isomer of atropine into which it can be converted by heating or by the action of alkali.

Pharmacopoeial description
USP 25: A white crystalline powder. M.p. 106° to 109°. Slightly soluble in water and in benzene; freely soluble in alcohol, in chloroform, and in dilute acids; sparingly soluble in ether. Its solutions are alkaline to litmus. Store in airtight containers. Protect from light.

Hyoscyamine Hydrobromide (382-r)
Hyoscyamine Hydrobromide (BANM).
Bromidrato de Hiosciamina; Hyoscyamine Bromhydrate.
$C_{17}H_{23}NO_3,HBr = 370.3$.
CAS — 306-03-6.
Pharmacopoeias. In US.

Pharmacopoeial description
USP 25: White, odourless, crystals or crystalline powder. M.p. not less than 149°. Freely soluble in water; soluble 1 in 2.5 of alcohol, 1 in 1.7 of chloroform, and 1 in 2300 of ether. pH of a 5% solution in water is about 5.4. Store in airtight containers. Protect from light.

Hyoscyamine Sulfate (383-f)
Hyoscyamine Sulphate (BANM); Hyoscyamini Sulfas; Hyoscyaminum Sulfuricum; Iosciamina Solfato.
$(C_{17}H_{23}NO_3)_2,H_2SO_4,2H_2O = 712.8$.
CAS — 620-61-1 (anhydrous hyoscyamine sulfate); 6835-16-1 (hyoscyamine sulfate dihydrate).
Pharmacopoeias. In Eur. (see p.vi) and US.

Pharmacopoeial description
Ph. Eur.: A white, crystalline powder or colourless needles. M.p. about 203° with decomposition. Very soluble in water; sparingly soluble or soluble in alcohol; practically insoluble in ether. A 2% solution in water has a pH of 4.5 to 6.2. Store in airtight containers. Protect from light.
USP 25: White, odourless, crystals or crystalline powder. M.p. not less than 200°. Soluble 1 in 0.5 of water and 1 in 5 of alcohol; practically insoluble in ether. pH of a 1% solution in water is about 5.3. Store in airtight containers. Protect from light.

Adverse Effects, Treatment, and Precautions
As for Atropine Sulfate, p.461.

Interactions
As for antimuscarinics in general (see Atropine Sulfate, p.461).

Uses and Administration
Hyoscyamine is a tertiary amine antimuscarinic with the actions of atropine (p.461), which is racemic hyoscyamine; hyoscyamine, the laevo-isomer, has approximately twice the potency of atropine since the dextro-isomer has only very weak antimuscarinic activity. Hyoscyamine is used mainly in the relief of conditions associated with visceral spasm. It has also been given for rhinitis and was formerly used in the treatment of parkinsonism.

Hyoscyamine is given in usual doses of 150 to 300 µg up to four times daily by mouth, but it is more usually employed as the sulfate; the hydrobromide is also used. Suggested doses of hyoscyamine sulfate are 125 to 250 µg by mouth or sublingually every four hours as needed, up to a maximum of 1.5 mg in 24 hours. Modified-release oral preparations of hyoscyamine sulfate are available in some countries; dosage is specific to a particular formulation. Hyoscyamine sulfate has also been given by injection.

Preparations

USP 25: Hyoscyamine Sulfate Elixir; Hyoscyamine Sulfate Injection; Hyoscyamine Sulfate Oral Solution; Hyoscyamine Sulfate Tablets; Hyoscyamine Tablets.

Proprietary Preparations (details are given in Part 3)
Canad.: Levsin; *Denm.:* Egazil; *Fin.:* Egazil; *Neth.:* Egacene; *Norw.:* Egazil; *Swed.:* Egazil; *USA:* A-Spas; Anaspaz; Cystospaz; Cystospaz-M; Donnamar; ED-SPAZ; Gastrosed; Levbid; Levsin; Levsinex; NuLev; Symax.

Multi-ingredient: *Aust.:* Normensan; *Austral.:* Contac; Donnagel; Donnalix; Donnatab; *Braz.:* Analverin; Tropinal; *Canad.:* Diban; Donnatal; *Ital.:* Antispasmina Colica; *S.Afr.:* Allertac; Bellatard; Bellavern†; Donnatal; Millerspas; Tropax†; *Switz.:* Bronchalin†; Nardyl; Viaggio†; *Thai.:* Belloid; Spasmo; *USA:* Antispasmodic Elixir; Arco-Lase Plus; Atrohist Plus†; Atrosept; Barbidonna; Bellacane; Bellatal; Deconhist LA†; Dolsed; Donna-Sed†; Donnamor†; Donnatal; Hyosophen; Levsin with Phenobarbitone; Malatal†; Phenahist-TR†; Phenchlor SHA†; Prosed/DS; Pyridium Plus; Ru-Tuss†; Stahist; Susano; Trac Tabs 2X; UAA; Uridon Modified; Urimar-T; Urimax; Urised; Urisedamine; Urogesic Blue.

Hyoscyamus   (384-d)

Banotu; Beleño; Bilsenkraut; Giusquiamo; Henbane; Hyoscy.; Hyoscyami; Jusquiame; Jusquiame Noire; Meimendro.

Pharmacopoeias. Chin. specifies only the seeds.

Hyoscyamus Leaf consists of the dried leaf, or the dried leaf and flowering, and occasionally fruit-bearing, tops of *Hyoscyamus niger.* The alkaloids consist mainly of hyoscyamine with varying amounts of hyoscine.

Profile

Hyoscyamus has peripheral and central effects similar to those of atropine (p.461); its preparations have been used mainly for the relief of visceral spasm. The fresh whole flowering plant (*Hyoscyamus niger*) has been used in herbal and homoeopathic medicine.

Preparations

Proprietary Preparations (details are given in Part 3)
Aust.: Kelosoft; *Switz.:* Kelosoft.

Multi-ingredient: *Belg.:* Escouflaire†; Sanicolax†; *Braz.:* Anevrase; Atroveran; Atrovex; Dorveran; Espasmalgon; Espasmolex; Expectolu; Glicodin; MM Expectorante; Sedatux; Subitan; *Denm.:* Zink-Calmitol; *Fr.:* Asthmalgine†; Baume Dalet†; Broncorinol toux seches; Creme Rap; Gastrosedyl†; Laccoderme a l'huile de cade; Thiosedal†; *Ger.:* Unguentum lymphaticum; *Spain:* Laxo Vian†; *Switz.:* Baby Liberol†; Gouttes contre la toux "S"; Keli-med; Kernosan Huile de Massage†; Liberol†; Sirop S contre la toux et la bronchite; *UK:* Onopordon Comp B.

Isopropamide Iodide   (387-m)

Isopropamide Iodide (BAN, rINN).

(3-Carbamoyl-3,3-diphenylpropyl)di-isopropylmethylammonium iodide.

$C_{23}H_{33}IN_2O = 480.4$.
CAS — 7492-32-2 (isopropamide); 71-81-8 (isopropamide iodide).

Pharmacopoeias. In US.

Isopropamide iodide 1.36 mg is approximately equivalent to 1 mg of isopropamide.

Pharmacopoeial description

USP 25: A white to pale yellow crystalline powder. Soluble 1 in 50 of water, 1 in 10 of alcohol, and 1 in 5 of chloroform; very slightly soluble in ether and in benzene. Protect from light.

Profile

Isopropamide iodide is a quaternary ammonium antimuscarinic with peripheral effects similar to those of atropine (p.461). It has been used as an adjunct in the treatment of peptic ulcer disease, in the relief of gastrointestinal and urinary-tract disorders associated with smooth muscle spasm, in rhinitis, and for the relief of symptoms of colds.

Isopropamide bromide has been used similarly.

Preparations

USP 25: Isopropamide Iodide Tablets.

Proprietary Preparations (details are given in Part 3)
Belg.: Priamide†.

Multi-ingredient: *Aust.:* Stelabid†; Vesalium; *Belg.:* Rinomar; Vesalium†; *Braz.:* Descon AP; *Canad.:* Stelabid; *Fr.:* Enuretine†; *Hung.:* Bispan; Triospan; *Irl.:* Stelabid; *Ital.:* Fluvalass; Raffreddoremed; Valtrax; *Mex.:* Stelabid; *S.Afr.:* Stelabid†; *Spain:* Ornade.

Mecloxamine Citrate   (11607-d)

Mecloxamine Citrate (rINNM).

2-[1-(4-Chlorophenyl)-1-phenylethoxy]-N,N-dimethyl-1-propanamine citrate.

$C_{19}H_{24}ClNO,C_6H_8O_7 = 510.0$.
CAS — 5668-06-4 (mecloxamine); 56050-03-4 (mecloxamine citrate).

Profile

Mecloxamine citrate is reported to have antimuscarinic properties and has been used for its antiemetic action in antimigraine preparations.

Preparations

Proprietary Preparations (details are given in Part 3)
Multi-ingredient: *Aust.:* Avamigran.

Mepenzolate Bromide   (390-r)

Mepenzolate Bromide (BAN, rINN).

Mepenzolate Methylbromide; Mepenzolone Bromide. 3-Benziloyloxy-1,1-dimethylpiperidinium bromide.

$C_{21}H_{26}BrNO_3 = 420.3$.
CAS — 25990-43-6 (mepenzolate); 76-90-4 (mepenzolate bromide).

Pharmacopoeias. In Jpn.

Profile

Mepenzolate bromide is a quaternary ammonium antimuscarinic with peripheral actions similar to those of atropine (p.461). It has been used in the relief of gastrointestinal disorders associated with smooth muscle spasm and as an adjunct in the treatment of peptic ulcer disease. It is given in doses of 25 to 50 mg three or four times daily.

Preparations

Proprietary Preparations (details are given in Part 3)
Swed.: Cantil; *USA:* Cantil.

Methanthelinium Bromide   (391-f)

Methanthelinium Bromide (BAN, pINN).

Dixamonum Bromidum; Methantheline Bromide; MTB-51; SC-2910. Diethylmethyl[2-(xanthen-9-ylcarbonyloxy)ethyl]ammonium bromide.

$C_{21}H_{26}BrNO_3 = 420.3$.
CAS — 5818-17-7 (methanthelinium); 53-46-3 (methanthelinium bromide).

Profile

Methanthelinium bromide is a quaternary ammonium antimuscarinic with peripheral effects similar to those of atropine (p.461). It has been used as an adjunct in the treatment of peptic ulcer disease, in gastrointestinal disorders associated with smooth muscle spasm, and in the management of urinary incontinence. A usual dose is 50 to 100 mg by mouth four times daily.

Preparations

Proprietary Preparations (details are given in Part 3)
Ger.: Vagantin; *USA:* Banthine†.

Methylbenactyzium Bromide   (8150-d)

Methylbenactyzium Bromide (rINN).

Benactyzine Methobromide. Diethyl(2-hydroxyethyl)methylammonium bromide benzilate.

$C_{21}H_{28}BrNO_3 = 422.4$.
CAS — 3166-62-9.

Pharmacopoeias. In Jpn.

Profile

Methylbenactyzium bromide, a derivative of benactyzine (p.280), is an antimuscarinic with effects similar to those of atropine (p.461). It has been given by mouth for the treatment of gastrointestinal spasm and nocturnal enuresis.

Preparations

Proprietary Preparations (details are given in Part 3)
Multi-ingredient: *Aust.:* Anxiolit plus.

Metixene Hydrochloride   (392-d)

Metixene Hydrochloride (BANM, rINNM).

Methixene Hydrochloride (USAN); Methixene Hydrochloride Monohydrate; Metixeni Hydrochloridum; NSC-78194; SJ-1977. 9-(1-Methyl-3-piperidylmethyl)thioxanthene hydrochloride monohydrate.

$C_{20}H_{23}NS,HCl,H_2O = 363.9$.
CAS — 4969-02-2 (metixene); 1553-34-0 (anhydrous metixene hydrochloride); 7081-40-5 (metixene hydrochloride monohydrate).

Pharmacopoeias. In Eur. (see p.vi).

Pharmacopoeial description

Ph. Eur.: A white or almost white, crystalline or fine crystalline powder. Soluble in water, in alcohol, and in dichlorometh-

---

ane; practically insoluble in ether. A 1.8% solution in water has a pH of 4.4 to 5.8. Protect from light.

Profile

Metixene hydrochloride is a tertiary antimuscarinic with actions similar to those of atropine (p.461); it also has antihistaminic and direct antispasmodic properties.

It is used for the symptomatic treatment of parkinsonism (p.460), including the alleviation of the extrapyramidal syndrome induced by other drugs such as phenothiazines, but, like other antimuscarinics, it is of no value against tardive dyskinesias. The usual dose by mouth of metixene hydrochloride is 2.5 mg three times daily initially, gradually increased according to the response of the patient to a total of 15 to 60 mg daily in divided doses.

Metixene hydrochloride has also been used in preparations to relieve gastrointestinal spasms.

Preparations

Proprietary Preparations (details are given in Part 3)
Ger.: Metixen; Tremarit; *Ital.:* Tremaril; *Swed.:* Tremoquil.

Multi-ingredient: *Braz.:* Dilubrin; Espasmo Novozyme; Flenalgin; *Port.:* Espasmo Canulase; *S.Afr.:* Spasmo-Canulase; *Spain:* Espasmo Canulasa†; *Switz.:* Gillazyme plus†; Spasmo-Canulase.

Octatropine Methylbromide   (393-n)

Octatropine Methylbromide (BAN, rINN).

Anisotropine Methobromide; Anisotropine Methylbromide (USAN). (1R,3r,5S)-8-Methyl-3-(2-propylvaleryloxy)tropanium bromide.

$C_{17}H_{32}BrNO_2 = 362.3$.
CAS — 80-50-2.

Pharmacopoeias. In It.

Profile

Octatropine methylbromide is a quaternary ammonium antimuscarinic with peripheral actions similar to those of atropine (p.461). It is used in doses of 50 mg three times daily as an adjunct in the treatment of peptic ulcer disease. It is also used in doses of 10 mg three or four times daily by mouth to relieve visceral spasms.

Preparations

Proprietary Preparations (details are given in Part 3)
Spain: Vapin.

Multi-ingredient: *Ital.:* Valpinax; *Spain:* Vapin Complex.

Orphenadrine Citrate   (394-h)

Orphenadrine Citrate (BANM, rINNM).

Mephenamine Citrate; Orphenadin Citrate; Orphenadrini Citras. (RS)-Dimethyl[2-(2-methylbenzhydryloxy)ethyl]amine dihydrogen citrate.

$C_{18}H_{23}NO,C_6H_8O_7 = 461.5$.
CAS — 83-98-7 (orphenadrine); 4682-36-4 (orphenadrine citrate).
ATC — M03BC01.

Pharmacopoeias. In Eur. (see p.vi) and US.

Orphenadrine citrate 100 mg is approximately equivalent to 66 mg of orphenadrine hydrochloride.

Pharmacopoeial description

Ph. Eur.: A white or almost white powder. Sparingly soluble in water; slightly soluble in alcohol. Protect from light.

USP 25: A white, practically odourless, crystalline powder. Sparingly soluble in water; slightly soluble in alcohol; insoluble in chloroform, in ether, and in benzene. Store in airtight containers. Protect from light.

Orphenadrine Hydrochloride   (395-m)

Orphenadrine Hydrochloride (BANM, rINNM).

BS-5930; Mephenamine Hydrochloride; Orphenadin Hydrochloride; Orphenadrini Hydrochloridum. (RS)-Dimethyl[2-(2-methylbenzhydryloxy)ethyl]amine hydrochloride.

$C_{18}H_{23}NO,HCl = 305.8$.
CAS — 341-69-5.
ATC — N04AB02.

Pharmacopoeias. In Eur. (see p.vi).

Pharmacopoeial description

Ph. Eur.: A white or almost white crystalline powder. Freely soluble in water and in alcohol. Protect from light.

Adverse Effects, Treatment, and Precautions

As for Atropine Sulfate, p.461. Orphenadrine may cause insomnia.

Abuse. A 23-year-old schizophrenic man, whose treatment included orphenadrine 100 mg three times daily, obtained illicit supplies and increased the dose for euphoric effect.[1] On one occasion he had an epileptic convulsion after a 600-mg dose.

1. Shariatmadari ME. Orphenadrine dependence. *BMJ* 1975; **3:** 486.

Overdosage. A report[1] of acute poisoning with orphenadrine following massive overdosage in a schizophrenic patient, who responded to intensive supportive treatment, including large doses of adrenaline [epinephrine], dopamine, and dobutamine to restore blood pressure following asystole. Between 1977 and 1980 twelve deaths due to orphenadrine were recorded by the UK National Poisons Unit.

1. Clarke B, *et al.* Acute poisoning with orphenadrine. *Lancet* 1985; **i:** 1386.

Porphyria. Orphenadrine has been associated with acute attacks of porphyria and is considered unsafe in porphyric patients.

Interactions

As for antimuscarinics in general (see Atropine Sulfate, p.461).

Chlorpromazine. For the effect of orphenadrine on plasma concentrations of chlorpromazine, see under Antiparkinsonian Drugs, p.665.

Dextropropoxyphene. A suggested interaction between orphenadrine and dextropropoxyphene was open to question.[1,2]

1. Pearson RE, Salter FJ. Drug interaction? — orphenadrine with propoxyphene. *N Engl J Med* 1970; **282:** 1215.
2. Puckett WH, Visconti JA. Orphenadrine and propoxyphene (cont.). *N Engl J Med* 1970; **283:** 544.

Pharmacokinetics

Orphenadrine is readily absorbed from the gastrointestinal tract and is almost completely metabolised to at least 8 metabolites. It is mainly excreted in the urine as metabolites and small amounts of unchanged drug.

Half-life. While the mean elimination half-life of orphenadrine in 5 healthy subjects given a single dose of the hydrochloride was found to be 15.5 hours, elimination half-lives of 30.5 and 40 hours were calculated in 2 patients who had received repeated oral administration.[1]

1. Labout JJM, *et al.* Difference between single and multiple dose pharmacokinetics of orphenadrine hydrochloride in man. *Eur J Clin Pharmacol* 1982; **21:** 343–50.

Uses and Administration

Orphenadrine, which is a congener of diphenhydramine (p.416) without sharing its soporific effect, is a tertiary amine antimuscarinic with actions and uses similar to those of benzhexol [trihexyphenidyl] (p.464). It also has weak antihistaminic and local anaesthetic properties.

Orphenadrine is used as the hydrochloride in the symptomatic treatment of **parkinsonism**, including the alleviation of the extrapyramidal syndrome induced by drugs such as phenothiazines, but, like other antimuscarinics, is of no value against tardive dyskinesias. The initial dose of orphenadrine hydrochloride is 150 mg daily in divided doses gradually increased by 50 mg every 2 or 3 days according to the response of the patient; the usual maintenance dose is in the range of 150 to 300 mg daily, but some patients may require a total of up to 400 mg daily. Orphenadrine hydrochloride has also been given intramuscularly.

Orphenadrine is also used as the citrate to relieve pain due to **skeletal muscle spasm**. It is given by mouth in a dose of 100 mg twice daily or by intramuscular or slow intravenous (over 5 minutes) injection in a dose of 60 mg which has been repeated every 12 hours.

Since the elderly are more susceptible to the adverse effects of antimuscarinics a reduced dose is usually recommended.

Hiccup. Orphenadrine citrate has been used in some countries for the treatment of intractable hiccup. A protocol for the management of intractable hiccups may be found under Chlorpromazine, p.667.

Muscle spasm. References to the use of orphenadrine in the management of leg cramps and other painful conditions associated with skeletal muscle spasm.

1. Latta D, Turner E. An alternative to quinine in nocturnal leg cramps. *Curr Ther Res* 1989; **45:** 833–7.
2. Hunskaar S, Donnell D. Clinical and pharmacological review of the efficacy of orphenadrine and its combination with paracetamol in painful conditions. *J Int Med Res* 1991; **19:** 71–87.

The symbol † denotes a preparation no longer actively marketed

Preparations

BP 2001: Orphenadrine Hydrochloride Tablets;
USP 25: Orphenadrine Citrate Injection.

Proprietary Preparations (details are given in Part 3)
Aust.: Norflex†; *Austral.:* Disipal†; Norflex; *Belg.:* Disipal; Norflex; *Canad.:* Disipal; Norflex; Orfenace; *Denm.:* Disipal; Lysantin; Norflex; *Fin.:* Norflex; *Ger.:* Norflex; *Irl.:* Disipal; *Israel:* Flexin; *Ital.:* Disipal; *Mex.:* Norflex; *Norw.:* Disipal; *NZ:* Disipal; Norflex; *Port.:* Norflex†; *S.Afr.:* Disipal; Norflex; *Singapore:* Norflex; *Swed.:* Disipal; Norflex; *Switz.:* Norflex†; *Thai.:* Orfenal; *UK:* Biorphen; Disipal; Norflex†; *USA:* Banflex; Flexoject; Flexon; Myolin†; Myophen†; Norflex.

Multi-ingredient: *Aust.:* Neodolpasse; Norgesic; *Austral.:* Norgesic; *Braz.:* Algiflex; Anapirol; Dorflex; Doricin; Flexdor; Recilugo; Rielex; *Canad.:* Norgesic; *Fin.:* Dolan; Norgesic; *Ger.:* Norgesic N; *Hong Kong:* Norgesic; *Irl.:* Norgesic; *Israel:* Muscol; Norgesic; *Mex.:* Norflex Plus; *NZ:* Norgesic; *Port.:* Norgesic†; *S.Afr.:* Besemax; Norgesic; *Singapore:* Anarex; Norgesic; Norphen; *Swed.:* Norgesic; *Switz.:* Norgesic†; *Thai.:* Med-Myolax; Muscol; Myodrine; Myoflex; Myopar; Myosic; Neosec; Norgesic; Norgic; Norphen; Nurasic; Orflex; Orpar; Poli-Relaxane; Polydol; Relar; Rena; *UAE:* Muscadol; *USA:* Norgesic; Orphengesic.

Oxybutynin Hydrochloride (396-b)

Oxybutynin Hydrochloride (BANM, rINNM).

5058; MJ-4309-1; Oxybutynin Chloride (USAN); Oxybutynini Hydrochloridum. 4-Diethylaminobut-2-ynyl α-cyclohexylmandelate hydrochloride.

$C_{22}H_{31}NO_3,HCl = 393.9.$

CAS — 5633-20-5 (oxybutynin); 1508-65-2 (oxybutynin hydrochloride).

Pharmacopoeias. In Eur. (see p.vi) and US.

Pharmacopoeial description

Ph. Eur.: A white or almost white, crystalline powder. Freely soluble in water and in alcohol; soluble in acetone; slightly soluble in cyclohexane. Protect from light.

USP 25: A white, practically odourless, crystalline powder. Freely soluble in water and in alcohol; soluble in acetone; very soluble in chloroform and in methyl alcohol; slightly soluble in ether; very slightly soluble in hexane.

Adverse Effects, Treatment, and Precautions

As for Atropine Sulfate, p.461.

Animal studies have shown reproductive toxicity with high doses of oxybutynin, hence the recommendation that it should be avoided during pregnancy; caution should also be observed during breast feeding.

Effects on body temperature. A 76-year-old man taking oxybutynin hydrochloride 5 mg three times daily suffered heatstroke on a day when the ambient temperature was about 37°. He had had a similar febrile episode the previous summer while taking oxybutynin.[1]

1. Adubofour KO, *et al.* Oxybutynin-induced heatstroke in an elderly patient. *Ann Pharmacother* 1996; **30:** 144–7.

Effects on the gastrointestinal tract. Reflux oesophagitis has been reported[1] in a 36-year-old woman with cerebral palsy and hiatus hernia who had taken oxybutynin for 5 years to prevent urinary incontinence. Symptoms of gastro-oesophageal reflux resolved when oxybutynin was discontinued.

1. Lee M, Sharifi R. Oxybutynin-induced reflux esophagitis. *DICP Ann Pharmacother* 1990; **24:** 583–5.

Effects on mental function. Oxybutynin was associated with the development of acute confusional states in 4 patients with Parkinson's disease and some cognitive impairment.[1]

1. Donnellan CA, *et al.* Oxybutynin and cognitive dysfunction. *BMJ* 1997; **315:** 1363–4.

Night terrors. Night terrors have been reported in 5 patients taking oxybutynin.[1] Four of the patients were young children and the fifth was an elderly woman. Rechallenge was positive in 2 cases.

1. Valsecia ME, *et al.* New adverse effect of oxybutynin: "night terror". *Ann Pharmacother* 1998; **32:** 506.

Overdosage. A report[1] of a 34-year-old woman who ingested 100 mg of oxybutynin. The main symptoms were antimuscarinic effects and included drowsiness, hallucinations, dilatation of pupils, and urinary retention. Tachycardia resolved shortly after admission to hospital but ventricular ectopic beats and bigeminy persisted for over 24 hours. The patient recovered with symptomatic treatment.

1. Banerjee S, *et al.* Poisoning with oxybutynin. *Hum Exp Toxicol* 1991; **10:** 225–6.

Porphyria. Oxybutynin hydrochloride is considered to be unsafe in patients with porphyria because it has been shown to be porphyrinogenic in *animals* or *in-vitro* systems.

Interactions

As for antimuscarinics in general (see Atropine Sulfate, p.461).

Itraconazole. Concomitant use of itraconazole and oxybutynin resulted in moderate increases of serum concentrations of the latter.[1] However, concentrations of the active metabolite, *N*-desethyloxybutynin, were virtually unchanged and the interaction was considered to be of minor clinical significance.

1. Lukkari E, *et al.* Itraconazole moderately increases serum concentrations of oxybutynin but does not affect those of the active metabolite. *Eur J Clin Pharmacol* 1997; **52:** 403–6.

Pharmacokinetics

Following oral administration of oxybutynin, peak plasma concentrations are reached within one hour. It undergoes extensive first-pass metabolism and systemic bioavailability has been reported to be only 6%. A half-life of 2 to 3 hours has been reported. *N*-desethyloxybutynin is an active metabolite. Oxybutynin has been detected in breast milk. Evidence suggests that it may cross the blood-brain barrier.

◊ References.
1. Douchamps J, *et al.* The pharmacokinetics of oxybutynin in man. *Eur J Clin Pharmacol* 1988; **35:** 515–20.
2. Pietzko A, *et al.* Influences of trospium chloride and oxybutynin on quantitative EEG in healthy volunteers. *Eur J Clin Pharmacol* 1994; **47:** 337–43.

Uses and Administration

Oxybutynin hydrochloride is a tertiary amine antimuscarinic with actions similar to those of atropine (p.461); it also has direct effects on smooth muscle. It is used for the management of urinary frequency, urgency, and incontinence in neurogenic bladder disorders and in idiopathic detrusor instability and for nocturnal enuresis, as an adjunct to nonpharmacological therapy.

Usual doses of oxybutynin hydrochloride are 5 mg two or three times daily by mouth, increased to 5 mg four times daily if required. In elderly patients lower doses of 2.5 or 3 mg twice daily initially, increased to 5 mg twice daily if necessary, may be adequate. A modified-release preparation of oxybutynin hydrochloride is also available. It is given once daily in an initial dose of 5 mg, increased by 5 mg per week if necessary, up to a maximum of 30 mg daily.

In children over 5 years of age, oxybutynin is used for neurogenic bladder disorders and nocturnal enuresis in an initial dose of 2.5 or 3 mg twice daily by mouth increased to 5 mg two or three times daily according to response. For nocturnal enuresis the last dose is usually given before bedtime. However, some authorities consider that drug therapy for nocturnal enuresis is not appropriate in children under 7 years of age.

◊ Reviews.
1. Robinson TG, Castelden CM. Oxybutynin hydrochloride. *Prescribers' J* 1994; **34:** 27–30.

Nocturnal enuresis. Antimuscarinics such as oxybutynin reduce uninhibited bladder contractions but, although they may be of use in diurnal enuresis, they are rarely of benefit in nocturnal enuresis (p.459) alone. Oxybutynin did not appear to be effective in treating primary nocturnal enuresis in children with normal bladders.[1]

1. Lovering JS, *et al.* Oxybutynin efficacy in the treatment of primary enuresis. *Pediatrics* 1988; **82:** 104–6.

Urinary incontinence. In addition to its antimuscarinic effect, oxybutynin has a direct antispasmodic effect which also contributes to reducing the number of uninhibited bladder contractions in urge incontinence (see p.459). It is effective when given by mouth[1-3] and some consider it to be the drug of choice.[4] However, frequent adverse effects may limit its use. Direct instillation of oxybutynin into the bladder has also been tried.[5,6]

Oxybutynin has also been studied in detrusor hyperreflexia[7] but, as most of these studies do not distinguish in their analyses between patients with neurogenic and non-neurogenic incontinence, its value remains to be determined.

1. Riva D, Casolati E. Oxybutynin chloride in the treatment of female idiopathic bladder instability: results from double blind treatment. *Clin Exp Obstet Gynecol* 1984; **11:** 37–42.
2. Moore KH, *et al.* Oxybutynin hydrochloride (3 mg) in the treatment of women with idiopathic detrusor instability. *Br J Urol* 1990; **66:** 479–85.
3. Tapp AJS, *et al.* The treatment of detrusor instability in postmenopausal women with oxybutynin chloride: a double blind placebo controlled study. *Br J Obstet Gynaecol* 1990; **97:** 521–6.
4. Yarker YE, *et al.* Oxybutynin: a review of its pharmacodynamic and pharmacokinetic properties, and its therapeutic use in detrusor instability. *Drugs Aging* 1995; **6:** 243–62.

5. Weese DL, *et al.* Intravesical oxybutynin chloride: experience with 42 patients. *Urology* 1993; **41:** 527–30.
6. Szollar SM, Lee SM. Intravesical oxybutynin for spinal cord injury patients. *Spinal Cord* 1996; **34:** 284–7.
7. Thüroff J, *et al.* Randomized, double-blind, multicenter trial on treatment of frequency, urgency and incontinence related to detrusor hyperactivity: oxybutynin versus propantheline versus placebo. *J Urol (Baltimore)* 1991; **145:** 813–17.

Preparations

BP 2001: Oxybutynin Tablets;
USP 25: Oxybutynin Chloride Syrup; Oxybutynin Chloride Tablets.

Proprietary Preparations (details are given in Part 3)
Aust.: Ditropan; *Austral.:* Ditropan; *Belg.:* Ditropan; Driptane; *Canad.:* Ditropan; Nu-Oxybutyn; Oxybutyn; *Fin.:* Cystrin; Ditropan; *Fr.:* Ditropan; Driptane; *Ger.:* Dridase; Oxybugamma; Oxybuton; Oxymedin; Spasyt; *Hong Kong:* Ditropan; *Irl.:* Cystrin; Ditropan; Renamel; *Israel:* Novitropan; *Ital.:* Ditropan; *Mex.:* Tavor; *Neth.:* Dridase; *NZ:* Ditropan; *Port.:* Ditropan; *S.Afr.:* Ditropan; *Spain:* Ditropan; Dresplan; *Swed.:* Ditropan; *Switz.:* Ditropan; *Thai.:* Diutropan; *UK:* Cystrin; Ditropan; Promictuline†; *USA:* Ditropan.

Oxyphencyclimine Hydrochloride (397-v)

Oxyphencyclimine Hydrochloride (BANM, rINNM).
1,4,5,6-Tetrahydro-1-methylpyrimidin-2-ylmethyl α-cyclohexylmandelate hydrochloride.
$C_{20}H_{28}N_2O_3,HCl = 380.9$.
CAS — 125-53-1 (oxyphencyclimine); 125-52-0 (oxyphencyclimine hydrochloride).

Profile

Oxyphencyclimine hydrochloride is a tertiary amine antimuscarinic with effects similar to those of atropine (p.461). It was used as an adjunct in the treatment of peptic ulcer disease and for the relief of smooth muscle spasms in gastrointestinal disorders.

Preparations

Proprietary Preparations (details are given in Part 3)
Hong Kong: Daricon; *Neth.:* Daricon†; *Thai.:* Daricon; MedSpastic; Oxyno; Proclimine.

Multi-ingredient: *Hong Kong:* RUDD-U; *Swed.:* Kombistrat†.

Oxyphenonium Bromide (398-g)

Oxyphenonium Bromide (BAN, rINN).
Oxphenonii Bromidum; Oxyphenonium Bromatum. 2-(α-Cyclohexylmandeloyloxy)ethyldiethylmethylammonium bromide.
$C_{21}H_{34}BrNO_3 = 428.4$.
CAS — 14214-84-7 (oxyphenonium); 50-10-2 (oxyphenonium bromide).
Pharmacopoeias. In Pol.

Profile

Oxyphenonium bromide is a quaternary ammonium antimuscarinic with peripheral effects similar to those of atropine (p.461). It has been given by mouth to relieve visceral spasms.

Preparations

Proprietary Preparations (details are given in Part 3)
S.Afr.: Spastrex.

Penthienate Bromide (402-s)

Penthienate Bromide (BANM).
Penthienate Methobromide. 2-[2-Cyclopentyl-2-(2-thienyl)glycoloyloxy]ethyldiethylmethylammonium bromide.
$C_{18}H_{30}BrNO_3S = 420.4$.
CAS — 22064-27-3 (penthienate); 60-44-6 (penthienate bromide).

Profile

Penthienate bromide is a quaternary ammonium antimuscarinic with peripheral effects similar to those of atropine (p.461). It was used as an adjunct in the treatment of peptic ulcer disease and to relieve smooth muscle spasms in gastrointestinal disorders. It has also been tried in urinary incontinence.

◊ References.
1. Coombes GM, Millard RJ. Urinary urge incontinence: randomised crossover trials of penthienate versus placebo and propantheline. *Med J Aust* 1996; **165:** 473–6.

Phenamazide Hydrochloride (19980-c)

Phenamacide Hydrochloride. (±)-α-Aminobenzeneacetic acid 3-methylbutyl ester hydrochloride.
$C_{13}H_{19}NO_2,HCl = 257.8$.
CAS — 84580-27-8 (phenamazide); 31031-74-0 (phenamazide hydrochloride).

Profile

Phenamazide is an antimuscarinic with actions similar to those of atropine (p.461). It has been used as the hydrochloride in the treatment of visceral spasms in doses of up to 75 mg daily in divided doses.

Preparations

Proprietary Preparations (details are given in Part 3)
Ger.: Aklonin.

Pipenzolate Bromide (404-e)

Pipenzolate Bromide (BAN, rINN).
Pipenzolate Methylbromide. 3-Benziloyloxy-1-ethyl-1-methylpiperidinium bromide.
$C_{22}H_{28}BrNO_3 = 434.4$.
CAS — 13473-38-6 (pipenzolate); 125-51-9 (pipenzolate bromide).
Pharmacopoeias. In It.

Profile

Pipenzolate bromide is a quaternary ammonium antimuscarinic with peripheral actions similar to those of atropine (p.461). It has been used as an adjunct in the treatment of gastrointestinal disorders characterised by smooth muscle spasm.

Preparations

Proprietary Preparations (details are given in Part 3)
Ger.: Ila-med m; *Mex.:* Expal; Poliptal; Propedil.
Multi-ingredient: *Mex.:* Finprob; *S.Afr.:* Pedirachol.

Piperidolate Hydrochloride (405-l)

Piperidolate Hydrochloride (BANM, rINNM).
1-Ethyl-3-piperidyl diphenylacetate hydrochloride.
$C_{21}H_{25}NO_2,HCl = 359.9$.
CAS — 82-98-4 (piperidolate); 129-77-1 (piperidolate hydrochloride).

Profile

Piperidolate hydrochloride is a tertiary amine antimuscarinic with effects similar to those of atropine (p.461). It has been given in the symptomatic treatment of smooth muscle spasm associated with gastrointestinal disorders.

Preparations

Proprietary Preparations (details are given in Part 3)
Mex.: Dactil-OB.
Multi-ingredient: *Braz.:* Dactil-OB.

Pipethanate Ethobromide (13123-t)

Pipethanate Ethobromide (rINNM).
Ethylpipethanate Bromide; Piperilate Ethobromide. 1-(2-Benziloyloxyethyl)-1-ethylpiperidinium bromide.
$C_{23}H_{30}BrNO_3 = 448.4$.
CAS — 4546-39-8 (pipethanate); 23182-46-9 (pipethanate ethobromide).

Profile

Pipethanate ethobromide is an antimuscarinic with actions similar to those of atropine (p.461). It has been used in the symptomatic treatment of visceral spasms in doses by mouth of up to 160 mg daily in divided doses. Pipethanate ethobromide has also been given intramuscularly or intravenously in doses of 10 to 20 mg daily and rectally in doses of 60 or 120 mg daily.

Preparations

Proprietary Preparations (details are given in Part 3)
Ital.: Spalgin†; Spasmodene; Spasmodil; *Jpn:* Panpurol; *Thai.:* Panpurol.

Pirenzepine Hydrochloride (13129-h)

Pirenzepine Hydrochloride (BANM, USAN, rINNM).
LS-519 (pirenzepine); LS-519-Cl2; Pirenzepini Dihydrochloridum Monohydricum. 5,11-Dihydro-11-(4-methylpiperazin-1-ylacetyl)pyrido[2,3-b][1,4]benzodiazepin-6-one dihydrochloride monohydrate.
$C_{19}H_{21}N_5O_2,2HCl,H_2O = 442.3$.
CAS — 28797-61-7 (pirenzepine); 29868-97-1 (pirenzepine hydrochloride).
Pharmacopoeias. In Eur. (see p.vi).

Pharmacopoeial description

Ph. Eur.: A white or yellowish crystalline powder. Freely soluble in water; very slightly soluble in dehydrated alcohol; practically insoluble in dichloromethane; slightly soluble in methyl alcohol. A 10% solution in water has a pH of 1.0 to 2.0. Protect from light.

Adverse Effects and Precautions

Dry mouth and blurred vision have been reported but other side-effects associated with antimuscarinics (see Atropine Sulfate, p.461) are stated to be less likely to occur with pirenzepine because of its selective action on the gastric mucosa and poor penetration across the blood-brain barrier. Pirenzepine should be used with caution in patients with renal impairment, particularly those with end-stage renal failure.

Effects on the blood. Thrombocytopenia in one patient and agranulocytosis in another was probably associated with the administration of pirenzepine.[1]
1. Stricker BHC, *et al.* Blood disorders associated with pirenzepine. *BMJ* 1986; **293:** 1074.

Interactions

As for antimuscarinics in general (see Atropine Sulfate, p.461).

Pharmacokinetics

Pirenzepine is absorbed from the gastrointestinal tract but the bioavailability is reported to be only about 20 to 30% being decreased to about 10 to 20% when taken with food. Very little pirenzepine is metabolised. About 10% of an oral dose is excreted unchanged in the urine, the remainder being excreted in the faeces.

Pirenzepine has an elimination half-life of about 12 hours and is about 12% bound to plasma proteins. Diffusion across the blood-brain barrier is poor and only minimal amounts are stated to be present in breast milk.

◊ References.
1. Tanswell P, *et al.* Absolute bioavailability of pirenzepine in intensive care patients. *Eur J Clin Pharmacol* 1990; **38:** 265–8.

Renal impairment. The renal clearance and total plasma clearance of pirenzepine may be significantly reduced in patients with renal insufficiency,[1,2] with clearance decreasing proportionately with renal impairment. The half-life of pirenzepine is increased with reported values ranging from 14 to 20 hours.[1-3] Plasma concentrations of pirenzepine may be reduced by up to about 50% during haemodialysis.[2,3]
1. Krakamp B, *et al.* Steady-state intravenous pharmacokinetics of pirenzepine in patients with hepatic insufficiency and combined renal- and hepatic insufficiency. *Eur J Clin Pharmacol* 1989; **36:** 71–3.
2. Krakamp B, *et al.* Steady-state intravenous pharmacokinetics of pirenzepine in patients with differing degrees of renal dysfunction. *Eur J Clin Pharmacol* 1989; **36:** 75–8.
3. MacGregor T, *et al.* Oral pharmacokinetics of pirenzepine in patients with chronic renal insufficiency, failure, and maintenance haemodialysis. *Eur J Clin Pharmacol* 1990; **38:** 405–6.

Uses and Administration

Pirenzepine is a selective M_1 tertiary amine antimuscarinic which displays a preferential action on the gastric mucosa thus causing a reduction in the secretion of gastric acid; it also reduces the secretion of pepsin. At therapeutic doses it has few other antimuscarinic actions.

Pirenzepine hydrochloride has been used in the management of peptic ulcer disease (p.459) in a usual dose of 50 mg two or three times daily by mouth for 4 to 6 weeks.

◊ Reviews.
1. Carmine AA, Brogden RN. Pirenzepine: a review of its pharmacodynamic and pharmacokinetic properties and therapeutic efficacy in peptic ulcer disease and other allied diseases. *Drugs* 1985; **30:** 85–126.

Preparations

Proprietary Preparations (details are given in Part 3)
Aust.: Gastrozepin; *Ger.:* durapirenz†; Gastri-P†; Gastricur; Gastrozepin; Pirehexal†; Ulcoprotect; Ulcosafe; Ulgescum†; *Israel:* Ulcepin; *Ital.:* Duogastral; Frazim; Gastrol; Gastropiren; Gastrosed; Gastrozepin; Ulcin; Ulcopir†; *Mex.:* Gastropin; *Neth.:* Abrinac†; *Port.:* Gastrozepina; *S.Afr.:* Gastrozepin†; *Switz.:* Gastrozepine†; piren-basan; *Thai.:* Cevanil.

Poldine Metilsulfate (407-j)

Poldine Metilsulfate (BAN, pINN).
IS-499; McN-R-726-47; Poldine Methosulphate; Poldine Methylsulfate (USAN); Poldine Methylsulphate. 2-Benziloyloxymethyl-1,1-dimethylpyrrolidinium methylsulphate.
$C_{21}H_{26}NO_3,CH_3O_4S = 451.5$.
CAS — 596-50-9 (poldine); 545-80-2 (poldine metilsulfate).
Pharmacopoeias. In Br.

Pharmacopoeial description

BP 2001: A white odourless or almost odourless crystalline powder. Freely soluble in water; soluble in alcohol; slightly soluble in chloroform. A 1% solution in water has a pH of 5.0 to 7.0.

Profile

Poldine metilsulfate is a quaternary ammonium antimuscarinic with peripheral actions similar to those of atropine (p.461) and has been used in the management of gastrointestinal disorders, including peptic ulcer disease.

Preparations

BP 2001: Poldine Tablets.

Proprietary Preparations (details are given in Part 3)
UK: Nacton†.

Prifinium Bromide (409-c)

Prifinium Bromide (rINN).

PDB; Pyrodifenium Bromide. 3-Diphenylmethylene-1,1-diethyl-2-methylpyrrolidinium bromide.

$C_{22}H_{28}BrN = 386.4.$
$CAS — 10236-81-4$ (prifinium); 4630-95-9 (prifinium bromide).
ATC — A03AB18.

Profile

Prifinium bromide is a quaternary ammonium antimuscarinic with peripheral effects similar to those of atropine (p.461). It is structurally related to diphemanil metilsulfate (p.466).

Prifinium bromide is used to relieve visceral spasms. Oral doses usually range from 45 to 120 mg daily in divided doses; higher doses have sometimes been employed. It has also been administered rectally in a dose of 60 mg three or four times daily, or by subcutaneous, intramuscular, or intravenous injection in a dose of 7.5 to 15 mg.

Preparations

Proprietary Preparations (details are given in Part 3)
Fr.: Riabal; Ital.: Riabal; Jpn: Padrin; Mex.: Anespas; Thai.: Riabal.

Procyclidine Hydrochloride (410-s)

Procyclidine Hydrochloride (BANM, rINNM).

Procyclidini Hydrochloridum. 1-Cyclohexyl-1-phenyl-3-(pyrrolidin-1-yl)propan-1-ol hydrochloride.

$C_{19}H_{29}NO,HCl = 323.9.$
$CAS — 77-37-2$ (procyclidine); 1508-76-5 (procyclidine hydrochloride).
Pharmacopoeias. In Br. and US.

Pharmacopoeial description

BP 2001: A white, odourless or almost odourless, crystalline powder. Sparingly soluble in water; soluble in alcohol; practically insoluble in acetone and in ether. A 1% solution in water has a pH of 4.5 to 6.5.

USP 25: A white crystalline powder, having a moderate characteristic odour. Soluble 1 in 35 of water, 1 in 9 of alcohol, 1 in 6 of chloroform, and 1 in 11 000 of ether; insoluble in acetone. pH of a 1% solution in water is between 5.0 and 6.5. Store in a dry place in airtight containers. Protect from light.

Adverse Effects, Treatment, and Precautions

As for Atropine Sulfate, p.461.

Abuse. A report[1] of 2 cases of abuse of procyclidine by adolescents.

1. McGucken RB, et al. Teenage procyclidine abuse. Lancet 1985; i: 1514.

Interactions

As for antimuscarinics in general (see Atropine Sulfate, p.461).

Pharmacokinetics

Procyclidine hydrochloride is absorbed from the gastrointestinal tract and disappears rapidly from the tissues. Procyclidine given intravenously acts within 5 to 20 minutes and has a duration of effect of up to 4 hours.

◊ References.
1. Whiteman PD, et al. Pharmacokinetics and pharmacodynamics of procyclidine in man. Eur J Clin Pharmacol 1985; 28: 73–8.

Uses and Administration

Procyclidine hydrochloride is a tertiary amine antimuscarinic with actions and uses similar to those of benzhexol [trihexyphenidyl] (p.464). It is used for the symptomatic treatment of parkinsonism (p.460), including the alleviation of the extrapyramidal syndrome induced by drugs such as phenothiazines, but, like other antimuscarinics, is of no value against tardive dyskinesias.

The initial dose of 2.5 mg three times daily by mouth may be increased gradually by 2.5 to 5 mg every 2 or 3 days until the optimum maintenance dose, usually 20 to 30 mg daily in 3 (or occasionally 4) divided doses, is reached; daily doses of up to 60 mg have occasionally been required. In emergency, 5 to 10 mg may be given by intravenous injection; higher doses have sometimes been used. The intramuscular route has also been employed when 5 to 10 mg has been given as one injection, repeated if necessary after 20 minutes to a maximum of 20 mg daily.

The symbol † denotes a preparation no longer actively marketed

Preparations

BP 2001: Procyclidine Injection; Procyclidine Tablets;
USP 25: Procyclidine Hydrochloride Tablets.
Proprietary Preparations (details are given in Part 3)
Aust.: Kemadrin; Austral.: Kemadrin; Belg.: Kemadrin; Canad.: Kemadrin; Procyclid; Denm.: Kemadrin; Ger.: Osnervan; Irl.: Kemadrin; Israel: Kemadrin; Ital.: Kemadrin; Neth.: Kemadrin; NZ: Kemadrin; Spain: Kemadren; Swed.: Kemadrin†; Switz.: Kemadrin; UK: Arpicolin; Kemadrin; Muscinil; USA: Kemadrin.

Profenamine Hydrochloride (367-f)

Profenamine Hydrochloride (BANM, rINNM).

Cloridrato de Profenamina; Ethopropazine Hydrochloride; Isothazine Hydrochloride; Profenamini Hydrochloridum; Prophenamini Chloridum. 10-(2-Diethylaminopropyl)phenothiazine hydrochloride.

$C_{19}H_{24}N_2S,HCl = 348.9.$
$CAS — 522-00-9$ (profenamine); 1094-08-2 (profenamine hydrochloride).

Adverse Effects, Treatment, and Precautions

As for Atropine Sulfate, p.461.

Drowsiness and confusion are common in patients taking profenamine; patients so affected should not drive or operate machinery. Profenamine may also cause muscle cramps, paraesthesia, and a sense of heaviness in the limbs, epigastric discomfort, and nausea.

Profenamine is a phenothiazine derivative—for adverse effects associated with phenothiazines, see Chlorpromazine, p.660.

Breast feeding. A report[1] of profenamine distributed into the milk of lactating mothers.
1. Rowan JJ. Excretion of drugs in milk. Pharm J 1976; 217: 184–7.

Interactions

As for antimuscarinics in general (see Atropine Sulfate, p.461).

Uses and Administration

Profenamine hydrochloride is a phenothiazine derivative with antimuscarinic, adrenergic-blocking, antihistaminic, local anaesthetic and ganglion-blocking properties. It has been used in the symptomatic treatment of parkinsonism (p.460), including the alleviation of the extrapyramidal syndrome induced by drugs such as other phenothiazine compounds, but, like other compounds with antimuscarinic properties, is of no value against tardive dyskinesias. It has been used in a usual dose of 50 mg up to 3 times daily by mouth initially, gradually increased to up to 500 mg or more daily in divided doses, according to the response of the patient.

Preparations

Proprietary Preparations (details are given in Part 3)
Canad.: Parsitan.

Propantheline Bromide (411-w)

Propantheline Bromide (BAN, rINN).

Bromuro de Propantelina; Propanthelini Bromidum. Di-isopropylmethyl[2-(xanthen-9-ylcarbonyloxy)ethyl]ammonium bromide.

$C_{23}H_{30}BrNO_3 = 448.4.$
$CAS — 298-50-0$ (propantheline); 50-34-0 (propantheline bromide).
Pharmacopoeias. In Chin., Eur. (see p.vi), Jpn, and US.

Pharmacopoeial description

Ph. Eur.: A white or yellowish-white, slightly hygroscopic powder. Very soluble in water, in alcohol, and in dichloromethane. Store in airtight containers.

USP 25: White or practically white, odourless, crystals. Very soluble in water, in alcohol, and in chloroform; practically insoluble in ether and in benzene.

Adverse Effects, Treatment, and Precautions

As for Atropine Sulfate, p.461. Contact dermatitis has been reported following topical application of propantheline bromide.

Buccal and oesophageal ulceration. Severe buccal mucosal ulceration has been reported[1] in a 95-year-old woman as a result of retaining emepronium bromide tablets in her mouth, and recurred on administration of propantheline bromide tablets.
1. Huston GJ, et al. Anticholinergic drugs, buccal ulceration and mucosal potential difference. Postgrad Med J 1978; 54: 331–2.

Interactions

As for antimuscarinics in general (see Atropine Sulfate, p.461).

Pharmacokinetics

Propantheline bromide is incompletely absorbed from the gastrointestinal tract and bioavailability is

reported to be reduced by food; it is extensively metabolised in the small intestine before absorption. Propantheline is eliminated mainly in the urine as metabolites and less than 10% as unchanged drug. The duration of action is about 6 hours.

Uses and Administration

Propantheline bromide is a quaternary ammonium antimuscarinic with peripheral effects similar to those of atropine (p.461). It has been used in the management of spasm of the gastrointestinal tract and as an adjunct in the treatment of peptic ulcer disease (p.459). The usual initial dose is 15 mg by mouth three times daily before meals and 30 mg at bedtime; doses of up to 120 mg per day may be needed in some patients. In mild cases or elderly patients, doses of 7.5 mg three times daily may be sufficient.

Propantheline bromide has been used in the treatment of adult enuresis or urinary incontinence (p.459) in doses of 15 to 30 mg two or three times daily.

Hyperhidrosis. Some antimuscarinics, including propantheline, have been applied topically in the treatment of hyperhidrosis (p.459). Side-effects of antimuscarinics administered by mouth generally preclude their use by this route, although there is a report of oral propantheline being used successfully to control excessive sweating in 2 patients with spinal cord injuries.[1]
1. Canaday BR, Stanford RH. Propantheline bromide in the management of hyperhidrosis associated with spinal cord injury. Ann Pharmacother 1995; 29: 489–92.

Preparations

BP 2001: Propantheline Tablets;
USP 25: Propantheline Bromide Tablets.
Proprietary Preparations (details are given in Part 3)
Austral.: Pro-Banthine; Belg.: Pro-Banthine†; Canad.: Pro-Banthine; Propanthel; Denm.: Ercoril†; Fr.: Pro-Banthine†; Irl.: Pro-Banthine†; Israel: Pro-Banthine; Mex.: Bropantil; Propantel; Neth.: Pro-Banthine†; NZ: Pro-Banthine; S.Afr.: Pro-Banthine; Swed.: Ercotina†; Switz.: Ercorax Roll-on†; Pro-Banthine†; UK: Pro-Banthine; USA: Pro-Banthine.
Multi-ingredient: Hong Kong: Crema-U; Ital.: Lexil.

Propiverine Hydrochloride (17897-v)

Propiverine Hydrochloride (BANM, rINNM).

BUP-4 (propiverine). 1-Methyl-4-piperidyl diphenylpropoxyacetate hydrochloride.

$C_{23}H_{29}NO_3,HCl = 403.9.$
$CAS — 60569-19-9$ (propiverine); 54556-98-8 (propiverine hydrochloride).

Adverse Effects, Treatment, and Precautions

As for Atropine Sulfate, p.461. Hypotension and drowsiness may also occur with propiverine. Propiverine is contra-indicated in patients with hepatic disorders (but see below) or severe renal impairment. Liver enzyme values should be monitored in patients receiving long-term therapy. Skeletal retardation has occurred in the offspring of animals given high doses of propiverine during pregnancy and therefore its use is not recommended during pregnancy.

Hepatic impairment. Although the manufacturers of propiverine do not recommend its use in patients with hepatic disorders, some workers[1] suggest that on pharmacokinetic grounds it may be given to those with mild to moderate hepatic impairment at recommended doses without increasing the risk of adverse effects.
1. Siepmann M, et al. Pharmacokinetics and safety of propiverine in patients with fatty liver disease. Eur J Clin Pharmacol 1998; 54: 767–71.

Interactions

As for antimuscarinics in general (see Atropine Sulfate, p.461). Hypotension may occur in patients treated with propiverine and isoniazid. Drowsiness may be enhanced by drugs with CNS-depressant properties.

Pharmacokinetics

Propiverine is absorbed from the gastrointestinal tract and peak plasma concentrations are achieved about 2.3 hours after oral administration. It undergoes extensive first-pass metabolism and the average absolute bioavailability is reported to be about 41%. Plasma concentrations of the principal metabolite, the N-oxide, greatly exceed those of the parent compound. Protein binding is about 90% for propiverine and 60% for the N-oxide metabolite. Propiverine and its metabolites are excreted in the urine, bile, and faeces. The elimination half-life is about 20 hours.

Uses and Administration

Propiverine hydrochloride is a tertiary antimuscarinic with actions similar to those of atropine (p.461). It is used for the management of urinary frequency, urgency, and incontinence (p.459) in neurogenic bladder disorders and in idiopathic detrusor instability. Usual doses of propiverine hydrochloride are 15 mg two or three times daily by mouth, increased to 4 times daily if required. In elderly frail patients doses of 15 mg twice daily, increased to 3 times daily if necessary, may be advisable. A daily dose of 1 mg per kg body-weight should not be exceeded.

◊ References.
1. Haustein KO, Huller G. On the pharmacokinetics and metabolism of propiverine in man. *Eur J Drug Metab Pharmacokinet* 1988; **13:** 81–90.

Preparations
Proprietary Preparations (details are given in Part 3)
Ger.: Mictonetten; Mictonorm; *UK:* Detrunorm.

Stramonium (413-l)

Datura; Estramonio; Inferno; Jamestown Weed; Jimson Weed; Stechapfel; Stramoine; Thornapple.

NOTE. The terms Datura, Datura Herb, and Datura Leaf have been applied to preparations of various species of the genus Datura including *Datura metel*.

Pharmacopoeias. *Eur.* (see p.vi) includes a monograph for Stramonium Leaf and Prepared Stramonium.

Pharmacopoeial description
Ph. Eur.: Stramonium Leaf (Stramonii Folium) consists of the dried leaf or the dried leaf, flowering tops and occasionally fruit-bearing tops of *Datura stramonium* and its varieties. It contains not less than 0.25% of total alkaloids, calculated as hyoscyamine. The alkaloids consist mainly of hyoscyamine with a small quantity of hyoscine. It has an unpleasant odour. Protect from light and moisture.

Prepared Stramonium (Stramonii Pulvis Normatus) is stramonium leaf powder adjusted to contain 0.23 to 0.27% of total alkaloids, calculated as hyoscyamine. Store in airtight containers. Protect from light.

The BP 2001 directs that when stramonium leaf or powdered stramonium leaf is prescribed, prepared stramonium shall be dispensed.

Adverse Effects, Treatment, and Precautions
As for Atropine Sulfate, p.461.

Abuse. Some reports[1-3] of poisoning following abuse of *Datura stramonium* or its preparations.
1. Gowdy JM. Stramonium intoxication: review of symptomatology in 212 cases. *JAMA* 1972; **221:** 585–7.
2. Shervette RE, *et al.* Jimson 'Loco' weed abuse in adolescents. *Pediatrics* 1979; **63:** 520–3.
3. Anonymous. Jimson weed poisoning—Texas, New York, and California, 1994. *MMWR* 1995; **44:** 41–4.

Effects on the eyes. A report[1] of anisocoria (unequal dilatation of the pupils) in a patient following accidental entry of a piece of jimson weed *(Datura stramonium)* into the eye while gardening.
1. Savitt DL, *et al.* Anisocoria from Jimsonweed. *JAMA* 1986; **255:** 1439–40.

Uses and Administration
Stramonium has the actions of atropine (p.461). It has been given with other drugs in oral and rectal dosage forms for respiratory-tract disorders. It has also been smoked in cigarettes or burnt in powders and the fumes inhaled but the irritation produced by the fumes may aggravate bronchitis.

Stramonium has been used in homoeopathic medicine.

Preparations
Proprietary Preparations (details are given in Part 3)
Multi-ingredient: *Austral.:* Potassium Iodide and Stramonium Compound; *Belg.:* Escouflaire†; *Braz.:* Teutoss; *Spain:* Balsamo Analgesic Karmel†.

Telenzepine (3637-g)

Telenzepine (rINN).

4,9-Dihydro-3-methyl-[(4-methyl-1-piperazinyl)acetyl]-10*H*-thieno[3,4-*b*][1,5]-benzodiazepin-10-one.
$C_{19}H_{22}N_4O_2S = 370.5$.
CAS — 80880-90-6.

Profile
Telenzepine is reported to be a selective M_1 antimuscarinic and has been investigated for its ability to reduce gastric acid secretion in the management of peptic ulcer disease.

◊ References.
1. Londong W, *et al.* Telenzepine is at least 25 times more potent than pirenzepine—a dose response and comparative secretory study in man. *Gut* 1987; **28:** 888–95.
2. Simon B, *et al.* 3 mg Telenzepin nocte in der Therapie der benignen Ulcus-ventriculi-erkrankung: eine doppelblinde Vergleichsstudie mit 300 mg Ranitidin nocte. *Z Gastroenterol* 1990; **28** 90–3.

Terodiline Hydrochloride (13310-f)

Terodiline Hydrochloride (BANM, USAN, rINNM).
N-tert-Butyl-1-methyl-3,3-diphenylpropylamine hydrochloride.
$C_{20}H_{27}N,HCl = 317.9$.
CAS — 15793-40-5 (terodiline); 7082-21-5 (terodiline hydrochloride).

Profile
Terodiline hydrochloride is an antimuscarinic with actions similar to those of atropine (p.461); it is also reported to possess calcium-channel blocking activity. It was formerly used for the relief of urinary incontinence. However, in 1991 the manufacturer withdrew terodiline from all countries because of its association with cardiac arrhythmias.

◊ References.
1. Committee on Safety of Medicines. Withdrawal of terodiline (Micturin, Kabi Pharmacia Ltd). *Current Problems* 32 1991.
2. Stewart DA, *et al.* Terodiline causes polymorphic ventricular tachycardia due to reduced heart rate and prolongation of QT interval. *Eur J Clin Pharmacol* 1992; **42:** 577–80.

Tiemonium Iodide (418-k)

Tiemonium Iodide (BAN, rINN).

TE-114. 4-[3-Hydroxy-3-phenyl-3-(2-thienyl)propyl]-4-methylmorpholinium iodide.
$C_{18}H_{24}INO_2S = 445.4$.
CAS — 6252-92-2 (tiemonium); 144-12-7 (tiemonium iodide).
ATC — A03AB17.

Tiemonium Metilsulfate (16217-m)

Tiemonium Methylsulphate. 4-[3-Hydroxy-3-phenyl-3-(2-thienyl)propyl]-4-methyl-morpholinium methylsulphate.
$C_{19}H_{27}NO_6S_2 = 429.6$.
CAS — 6504-57-0.

Profile
Tiemonium iodide and tiemonium metilsulfate are quaternary ammonium antimuscarinics with peripheral effects similar to those of atropine (p.461) and are used in the relief of visceral spasms.

Tiemonium iodide is used in a usual dose of 100 mg twice daily by mouth. A dose of 5 mg has been given by intramuscular or slow intravenous injection.

Tiemonium metilsulfate is given in a dose of 100 to 300 mg daily in divided doses by mouth. A dose of 5 mg has been given three times daily by intramuscular or slow intravenous injection. Tiemonium metilsulfate has also been given as a rectal suppository in daily doses of 20 to 40 mg.

Preparations
Proprietary Preparations (details are given in Part 3)
Belg.: Visceralgine; *Fr.:* Visceralgine.

Multi-ingredient: *Belg.:* Asodal; Visceralgine Compositum; *Fr.:* Colchimax; Visceralgine Forte; *Ger.:* Coffalon.

Timepidium Bromide (13346-e)

Timepidium Bromide (rINN).

SA-504. 3-[Di-(2-thienyl)methylene]-5-methoxy-1,1-dimethyl-piperidinium bromide monohydrate.
$C_{17}H_{22}BrNOS_2H_2O = 418.4$.
CAS — 35035-05-3.
ATC — A03AB19.
Pharmacopoeias. In Jpn.

Profile
Timepidium bromide is a quaternary ammonium antimuscarinic with peripheral actions similar to those of atropine (p.461). It has been given by mouth or by injection for the symptomatic treatment of visceral spasms.

Urinary metabolites of timepidium may cause a reddish coloration of the urine.

Preparations
Proprietary Preparations (details are given in Part 3)
Jpn: Sesden; *Singapore:* Sesden.

Tolterodine Tartrate (15401-a)

Tolterodine Tartrate (BANM, USAN, rINNM).

Kabi-2234 (tolterodine); PNU-200583E; Tolterodine L-Tartrate. (+)-(*R*)-2-{α-[2-(Diisopropylamino)ethyl]benzyl}-*p*-cresol tartrate.
$C_{22}H_{31}NO,C_4H_6O_6 = 475.6$.
CAS — 124937-51-5 (tolterodine); 124937-52-6 (tolterodine tartrate).

Adverse Effects, Treatment, and Precautions
As for Atropine Sulfate, p.461. Tolterodine should be used with caution in patients with hepatic or renal impairment. *Animal* studies have shown that high doses may cause fetal toxicity, hence the recommendation that tolterodine should be avoided during pregnancy.

Interactions
As for antimuscarinics in general (see Atropine Sulfate, p.461). There is a theoretical risk of interactions between tolterodine and other drugs metabolised by or inhibiting cytochrome P450 isoenzymes CYP2D6 or CYP3A4. The US manufacturers advise that the dose of tolterodine should not exceed 1 mg twice daily in patients receiving potent CYP3A4 inhibitors such as

the macrolide antibiotics erythromycin or clarithromycin, and the antifungals ketoconazole, itraconazole, or miconazole; UK product information recommends against such combinations.

Pharmacokinetics
Peak plasma concentrations of tolterodine occur 1 to 3 hours after a dose by mouth. Tolterodine is mainly metabolised by the cytochrome P450 isoenzyme CYP2D6 to the active 5-hydromethyl derivative (DD-01); in a minority of poor metabolisers tolterodine is metabolised by CYP3A4 isoenzymes to its inactive N-dealkylated derivative. Tolterodine is excreted primarily in the urine with about 17% appearing in the faeces; less than 1% of a dose is excreted as unchanged drug.

◊ References.
1. Brynne N, *et al.* Pharmacokinetics and pharmacodynamics of tolterodine in man: a new drug for the treatment of urinary bladder overactivity. *Int J Clin Pharmacol Ther* 1997; **35:** 287–95.
2. Brynne N, *et al.* Influence of CYP2D6 polymorphism on the pharmacokinetics and pharmacodynamics of tolterodine. *Clin Pharmacol Ther* 1998; **63:** 529–39.

Uses and Administration
Tolterodine tartrate is a tertiary antimuscarinic with actions similar to those of atropine (p.461); it is claimed to have a greater selectivity for the muscarinic receptors of the bladder. Tolterodine is used in the management of urinary frequency, urgency, and incontinence in detrusor instability (p.459). Usual doses of tolterodine tartrate are 2 mg twice daily by mouth; modified-release preparations are given in a usual dose of 4 mg once daily. Doses of 1 mg twice daily (or 2 mg daily as a modified-release preparation) are recommended in patients with hepatic impairment or in those experiencing troublesome adverse effects or receiving drugs that inhibit the cytochrome P450 isoenzyme CYP3A4 (see Interactions, above).

◊ References.
1. Hills CJ, *et al.* Tolterodine. *Drugs* 1998; **55:** 813–20.
2. Abrams P, *et al.* Tolterodine, a new antimuscarinic agent: as effective but better tolerated than oxybutynin in patients with an overactive bladder. *Br J Urol* 1998; **81:** 801–10.

Preparations
Proprietary Preparations (details are given in Part 3)
Aust.: Detrusitol; *Belg.:* Detrusitol; *Canad.:* Detrol; *Denm.:* Detrusitol; *Fin.:* Detrusitol; *Fr.:* Detrusitol; *Ger.:* Detrusitol; *Hong Kong:* Detrusitol; *Irl.:* Detrusitol; *Israel:* Detrusitol; *Ital.:* Detrusitol; *Mex.:* Detrusitol; *Neth.:* Detrusitol; *Norw.:* Detrusitol; *NZ:* Detrusitol; *Port.:* Detrusitol; *S.Afr.:* Detrusitol; *Singapore:* Detrusitol; *Spain:* Detrusitol; Urotrol; *Swed.:* Detrusitol; *Switz.:* Detrusitol; *Thai.:* Detrusitol; *UK:* Detrusitol; *USA:* Detrol.

Tridihexethyl Chloride (421-l)

Tridihexethyl Chloride (BAN).

(3-Cyclohexyl-3-hydroxy-3-phenylpropyl)triethylammonium chloride.
$C_{21}H_{36}ClNO = 354.0$.
CAS — 60-49-1 (tridihexethyl); 4310-35-4 (tridihexethyl chloride); 125-99-5 (tridihexethyl iodide).

NOTE. Tridihexethyl Iodide is *rINN*.

Profile
Tridihexethyl chloride is a quaternary ammonium antimuscarinic with peripheral effects similar to those of atropine (p.461). It has been used as an adjunct in the treatment of peptic ulcer disease.

Preparations
Proprietary Preparations (details are given in Part 3)
USA: Pathilon†.

Tropatepine Hydrochloride (13385-a)

Tropatepine Hydrochloride (rINNM).

SD-1248-17. 3-(Dibenzo[*b,e*]thiepin-11(6*H*)-ylidene)tropane hydrochloride.
$C_{22}H_{23}NS,HCl = 370.0$.
CAS — 27574-24-9 (tropatepine); 27574-25-0 (tropatepine hydrochloride).

Profile
Tropatepine hydrochloride is an antimuscarinic with actions and uses similar to those of benzhexol [trihexyphenidyl] (p.463). It is used in the management of parkinsonism, including the alleviation of extrapyramidal symptoms induced by drugs such as phenothiazines, but, like other antimuscarinics, it is of no value in tardive dyskinesias. Tropatepine hydrochloride is given in usual doses of 10 to 30 mg daily by mouth; it is also given intramuscularly or by slow intravenous injection in doses of 10 to 20 mg daily.

Preparations
Proprietary Preparations (details are given in Part 3)
Fr.: Lepticur.

Tropicamide (424-z)

Tropicamide (BAN, USAN, rINN).

Bistropamide; Ro-1-7683; Tropicamidum. N-Ethyl-N-(4-pyri-dylmethyl)tropamide.

$C_{17}H_{20}N_2O_2 = 284.4$.
CAS — 1508-75-4.
ATC — S01FA06.

NOTE. TRO is a code approved by the BP 2001 for use on single unit doses of eye drops containing tropicamide where the individual container may be too small to bear all the appropriate labelling information.

Pharmacopoeias. In Eur. (see p.vi), Jpn, and US.

Pharmacopoeial description

Ph. Eur.: A white or almost white, crystalline powder. Slightly soluble in water; freely soluble in alcohol and in dichloromethane. Protect from light.

USP 25: A white or practically white crystalline powder, odourless or having not more than a slight odour. Slightly soluble in water; freely soluble in chloroform and in solutions of strong acids. Store in airtight containers. Protect from light.

Adverse Effects, Treatment, and Precautions

As for Atropine Sulfate, p.461.

◊ References.
1. Vuori M-L, et al. Systemic absorption and anticholinergic activity of topically applied tropicamide. J Ocul Pharmacol 1994; **10:** 431–7.

Interactions

As for antimuscarinics in general (see Atropine Sulfate, p.461).

Uses and Administration

Tropicamide is a tertiary amine antimuscarinic with actions similar to those of atropine (p.461). It is used as eye drops to produce mydriasis and cycloplegia (p.460). It has a more rapid onset and a shorter duration of effect than atropine: mydriasis is produced within 20 to 40 minutes of instillation and usually lasts for about 6 hours; cycloplegia is maximal within about 30 minutes and is short-lasting, with complete recovery of accommodation normally within 6 hours. Tropicamide has been reported to be inadequate for cycloplegia in children.

To produce **mydriasis,** 1 or 2 drops of a 0.5% solution are instilled 15 to 20 minutes before examination of the eye. To produce **cycloplegia** 1 or 2 drops of a 1% solution are required, repeated after 5 minutes; a further drop may be necessary to prolong the effect after 20 to 30 minutes.

Alzheimer's disease. Tropicamide has been studied for use in the differential diagnosis of Alzheimer's disease (see Dementia, p.1412). Excessive pupil dilatation in response to tropicamide eye drops occurred in patients with signs and symptoms of Alzheimer's disease.[1] However, a double-blind placebo-controlled study[2] in similar patients and healthy subjects indicated that this was not a reliable diagnostic test for Alzheimer's disease.

1. Gómez-Tortosa E, et al. Pupil response to tropicamide in Alzheimer's disease and other neurodegenerative disorders. Acta Neurol Scand 1996; **94:** 104–9.
2. Graff-Radford NR, et al. Tropicamide eyedrops cannot be used for reliable diagnosis of Alzheimer's disease. Mayo Clin Proc 1997; **72:** 495–504.

Preparations

BP 2001: Tropicamide Eye Drops;
USP 25: Tropicamide Ophthalmic Solution.

Proprietary Preparations (details are given in Part 3)
Aust.: Mydriaticum; **Austral.:** Mydriacyl; **Belg.:** Mydriaticum†; Tropicol†; **Braz.:** Mydriacyl; **Canad.:** Diotrope; Mydriacyl; **Denm.:** Mydriacyl; **Fr.:** Mydriaticum; **Ger.:** Mydriaticum; Mydrum; **Hong Kong:** Mydriacyl; Mydriaticum; **Irl.:** Mydriacil; **Israel:** Mydramide; **Ital.:** Tropimil; Visumidriatic; **Mex.:** Myriacyl; **Norw.:** Mydrian; **NZ:** Mydriacyl; **Port.:** Tropicil Top; **S.Afr.:** Mydriacyl; Mydriaticum; **Singapore:** Mydriacyl; **Swed.:** Mydriacyl; **Switz.:** Mydriaticum; **Thai.:** Mydriacyl; **UK:** Mydriacyl; **USA:** Mydral; Mydriacyl; Ocu-Tropic; Opticyl; Tropi-Storz†; Tropicacyl.

Multi-ingredient: Canad.: Diophenyl-T; **Hong Kong:** Mydrin-P; **Ital.:** Visumidriatic Antiflogistico†; Visumidriatic Fenilefrina; **USA:** Paremyd.

Tropine Benzilate Hydrochloride (17601-t)

Benztropeine Hydrochloride. 1αH,5αH-Tropan-3α-ol benzilate hydrochloride.

$C_{22}H_{25}NO_3,HCl = 387.9$.
CAS — 3736-36-5 (tropine benzilate); 1674-94-8 (tropine benzilate hydrochloride).

Profile

Tropine benzilate hydrochloride is an antimuscarinic that has been used as an antispasmodic in the treatment of gastrointestinal spasms.

Trospium Chloride (5246-q)

Trospium Chloride (BAN, rINN).

3α-Benziloyloxynortropane-8-spiro-1′-pyrrolidinium chloride.
$C_{25}H_{30}ClNO_3 = 428.0$.
CAS — 10405-02-4.

Adverse Effects, Treatment, and Precautions

As for Atropine Sulfate, p.461. Trospium should be used with caution in patients with hepatic or mild to moderate renal impairment, and avoided in those with severe renal impairment. Animal studies have shown that trospium crosses the placenta and is distributed into breast milk; the manufacturer therefore recommends that caution should be observed during pregnancy and breast feeding.

Interactions

As for antimuscarinics in general (see Atropine Sulfate, p.461).

Pharmacokinetics

Following oral administration of trospium chloride, peak plasma concentrations are reached at 4 to 6 hours. The bioavailability of trospium chloride is reduced by the simultaneous intake of food, especially with a high fat content. Trospium is excreted in the urine mainly as unchanged drug; about 10% appears as the spiroalcohol. The terminal elimination half-life has been reported to be between 10 and 20 hours. The mean half-life has been reported to be prolonged twofold in patients with severe renal impairment (creatinine clearance between 8 and 32 mL per minute). Trospium has been reported to cross the placenta and has been detected in the milk of rats.

◊ For reference to the bioavailability of trospium chloride after intravesical instillation, see below.

Uses and Administration

Trospium chloride is a quaternary ammonium antimuscarinic with actions similar to those of atropine (p.461). It is used for the management of urinary frequency, urgency, and incontinence in detrusor instability or detrusor hyperreflexia.

Usual doses are 20 mg twice daily by mouth before meals on an empty stomach. The need for continued treatment should be assessed at regular intervals of 3 to 6 months. Doses should be reduced to 20 mg daily or on alternate days in patients with a creatine clearance of 10 to 30 mL per minute.

Trospium chloride has also been used as an antispasmodic in genito-urinary tract disorders.

It has also been given by intramuscular or slow intravenous injection, and rectally.

◊ References.
1. Madersbacher H, et al. Trospium chloride versus oxybutynin: a randomized, double-blind, multicentre trial in the treatment of detrusor hyper-reflexia. Br J Urol 1995; **75:** 452–6.
2. Walter P, et al. Bioavailability of trospium chloride after intravesical instillation in patients with neurogenic lower urinary tract dysfunction: a pilot study. Neurourol Urodyn 1999; **18:** 447–53.
3. Cardozo L, et al. Efficacy of trospium chloride in patients with detrusor instability: a placebo-controlled, randomized, double-blind, multicentre clinical trial. BJU Int 2000; **85:** 659–64.
4. Fusgen I, Hauri D. Trospium chloride: an effective option for medical treatment of bladder overactivity. Int J Clin Pharmacol Ther 2000; **38:** 223–34.

Preparations

Proprietary Preparations (details are given in Part 3)
Aust.: Rekont†; Spasmolyt; **Ger.:** Spasmex; Spasmo-Lyt; Spasmo-Rhoival TC; Spasmo-Urgenin TC; Trospi; **Spain:** Spasmosarto†; Uraplex; **Switz.:** Spasmo-Urgenine Neo; **Thai.:** Spasmo-Lyt; **UK:** Regurin.

Multi-ingredient: Aust.: Spasmo-Urgenin; **Port.:** Spasmo-Urgenin; **S.Afr.:** Spasmo-Urgenin; **Spain:** Spasmo-Urgenin; **Thai.:** Spasmo-Urgenin.

Valethamate Bromide (425-c)

Diethylmethyl[2-(3-methyl-2-phenylvaleryloxy)ethyl]ammonium bromide.
$C_{19}H_{32}BrNO_2 = 386.4$.
CAS — 16376-74-2 (valethamate); 90-22-2 (valethamate bromide).

Profile

Valethamate bromide is a quaternary ammonium antimuscarinic with peripheral effects similar to those of atropine (p.461). It has been given by mouth, by injection or rectally in the symptomatic treatment of visceral spasms.

Preparations

Proprietary Preparations (details are given in Part 3)
Ger.: Epidosin†.

Xenytropium Bromide (11617-h)

Xenytropium Bromide (rINN).

N-399. 8-(p-Phenylbenzyl)atropinium bromide.
$C_{30}H_{34}BrNO_3 = 536.5$.
CAS — 511-55-7.

Profile

Xenytropium bromide is reported to have antimuscarinic properties; it has been given by mouth in preparations for the management of gastrointestinal disorders.

Preparations

Proprietary Preparations (details are given in Part 3)
Multi-ingredient: Aust.: Spasmo Gallosanol†; **Ger.:** Spasmo Gallo Sanol N†.

Zamifenacin (15972-q)

Zamifenacin (BAN, rINN).

UK-76654-2 (zamifenacin fumarate). (R)-3-(Diphenylmethoxy)-1-[3,4-(methylenedioxy)phenetyl]piperidine.
$C_{27}H_{29}NO_3 = 415.5$.
CAS — 127308-82-1 (zamifenacin); 127308-98-9 (zamifenacin fumarate).

Profile

Zamifenacin is an antimuscarinic with a selective action at M_3 receptors. It is under investigation for the treatment of irritable bowel syndrome and motion sickness.

◊ References.
1. Golding JF, Stott JRR. Comparison of the effects of a selective muscarinic receptor antagonist and hyoscine (scopolamine) on motion sickness, skin conductance and heart rate. Br J Clin Pharmacol 1997; **43:** 633–7.

Antineoplastics and Immunosuppressants

Antineoplastic drugs are used in the treatment of malignant neoplasms when surgery or radiotherapy is not possible or has proved ineffective, as an adjunct to surgery or radiotherapy, or, as in leukaemia, as the initial treatment. Therapy with antineoplastics is notably successful in a few malignant conditions and may be used to palliate symptoms and prolong life in others.

The two main groups of cytotoxic drugs used in the treatment of malignant disease are the alkylating agents and the antimetabolites. Nitrogen mustards, ethyleneimine compounds, and alkyl sulfonates are the main **alkylating agents**. Other compounds with an alkylating action are the various nitrosoureas. Cisplatin and dacarbazine appear to act similarly.

The **antimetabolites** may be subdivided into folic acid, purine, or pyrimidine antagonists.

Several natural products, or their derivatives, are used for their actions as **mitotic inhibitors**; they include the vinca alkaloids, the derivatives of podophyllotoxin, taxanes, and camptothecin derivatives such as irinotecan and topotecan.

Some **antibiotics** interfere with nucleic acids and are effective as antineoplastics.

Also described in this section are **other drugs** which act by various routes to affect the growth and proliferation of malignant cells.

In recent years considerable interest has focused on immunological approaches to the treatment of malignant disease and a number of monoclonal antibodies have been, or are being, developed. The use of biological response modifiers such as interleukins continues to be the subject of investigation and attempts to develop vaccines against individual neoplasms also continue.

Glucocorticoids (see Corticosteroids, p.1044) are used in association with antineoplastics in the treatment of malignant disease, especially in acute leukaemias and lymphomas. Other agents used in antineoplastic therapy include sex hormones (p.1452) and radiopharmaceuticals (p.1448).

Adverse Effects

The acute effects of antineoplastic administration frequently include nausea and vomiting, often via a central mechanism, and sometimes extremely severe. In addition, many of these compounds are irritant or vesicant, and produce local pain, irritation, and inflammation at the administration site; extravasation may lead to ulceration and necrosis. Hypersensitivity reactions may also occur.

However, many of the adverse effects of antineoplastics are an extension of their therapeutic action, which is not selective for malignant cells but affects all rapidly-dividing cells: antineoplastic therapy is made possible only by increased sensitivity or less effective recovery of malignant cells compared with normal cells, and administration is carefully controlled and timed, and, where possible, localised, to maximise the differences.

In consequence, adverse effects may be expected from most antineoplastics in tissues where normal cell division is fairly rapid, e.g. the bone-marrow, lymphoreticular tissue, gastrointestinal mucosa, skin, and gonads, as well as in the fetus. The effects may not manifest for days or weeks, depending both on the agents used and the rate of division in the tissue concerned, and may sometimes be cumulative. Perhaps the most common serious effect, and one which has frequently limited the doses that can be given, is bone-marrow depression. Because of their effects on the various types of white blood cell many antineoplastics also cause profound suppression of normal immunity, and patients may be at greatly increased risk of severe and disseminated infection.

The rapid destruction of large numbers of cells during antineoplastic therapy of certain highly sensitive tumours, and the consequent release of breakdown products, may also lead to problems with hyperuricaemia and acute renal failure due to uric acid nephropathy (the 'tumour lysis syndrome').

Additionally, some drugs may have specific toxicities which are not necessarily related to their therapeutic action, such as cardiotoxicity due to anthracycline antibiotics, nephrotoxicity with cisplatin, or the effects of bleomycin on the lung.

In the very long term, patients who have undergone successful antineoplastic chemotherapy may develop secondary malignancies, suggesting that antineoplastics may themselves be carcinogenic. In addition, most are potentially mutagenic and teratogenic, and administration in pregnancy, particularly in the first trimester, may lead to fetal abortion, stunting, or malformation.

Carcinogenicity. Although it is difficult to control for a possible effect of the primary disease, there is clear evidence that some antineoplastic drugs may themselves be carcinogenic.[1] Most convincingly associated with secondary malignancies are the various *alkylating agents*,[2-5] including the nitrosoureas.[6] The secondary disease appears to manifest most frequently as leukaemia,[3-8] particularly acute myeloid leukaemia, although solid tumours have been reported such as bladder cancer following cyclophosphamide treatment,[9] and a variety of solid cancers after treatment for Hodgkin's disease,[10] (although radiotherapy rather than chemotherapy may be chiefly responsible for these[11]). It has been suggested by some workers that cyclophosphamide is less leukaemogenic than melphalan or busulfan,[4,12] and there is a suggestion that the risk may be particularly high with lomustine,[6] but others consider that there is little difference in carcinogenic effect between the different alkylating agents.[3]

There is little evidence of carcinogenicity associated with antimetabolites such as methotrexate, although it has been suggested that they may act as co-carcinogens,[2] and immunosuppression associated with their use may allow the development of Epstein-Barr virus-related lymphoma.[13,14] Fludarabine therapy has been reported to be associated with the development of myelodysplasia and acute myeloid leukaemias.[15] Other drugs that have been associated with the development of secondary malignancies are procarbazine,[5,16] podophyllotoxin derivatives such as etoposide,[17-19] and, in particular, teniposide;[12] platinum derivatives such as carboplatin[20,21] and cisplatin;[21] and combinations of cisplatin with doxorubicin,[4] and possibly other anthracycline-based regimens.[22] Agents such as the platinum and podophyllotoxin derivatives which act as DNA topoisomerase II inhibitors have been suggested to be associated particularly with acute myeloid leukaemias.[20,23]

Immunosuppression with azathioprine, ciclosporin, and corticosteroids has also been associated with the development of malignancies,[24-26] although in immunosuppressed patients the characteristic neoplasms are lymphomas and skin cancers, including Kaposi's sarcoma.[26] Infection with Epstein-Barr virus after transplantation appears to play a role in the development of lymphoproliferative disorders in immunosuppressed patients.[27,28] Skin cancer may be a particular risk in immunosuppressed patients with a history of high sun exposure.[29]

Estimates of risk have varied very widely between studies, and have been calculated in various ways, making direct comparison impossible. The risk may depend not only on the chemotherapy regimen, but also the type of secondary malignancy considered.[30] Some workers consider that secondary acute myeloid neoplasia will occur in at least 1% of patients receiving conventional chemotherapy for childhood acute lymphoblastic leukaemia,[17,31] and others have suggested that over 10 years between 5% and 15% of patients treated with alkylating agents will develop cancer, a substantial excess over expected figures.[32] A study of patients receiving high-dose chemotherapy followed by stem cell transplantation found the 5-year cumulative risk of myelodysplasia or acute myeloblastic leukaemia to be 14%, which agreed with previous estimates ranging from 4 to 18%.[15] Several factors appear to influence the risk: treatment-associated myeloid neoplasia is more likely in patients given a higher cumulative dose,[3,5,6,19,33] in splenectomised patients,[5] and in older rather than younger patients.[3,8,15,34] (After transplantation, however, the risk of lymphoproliferative disorders is greater in younger than in older patients,[28] and a study of the survival of young patients with Hodgkin's disease found that the risk of solid tumours, particularly breast cancer, increased with decreasing age at first treatment.[30]) One study in patients treated for Hodgkin's disease in childhood found the risk of secondary neoplasia to be considerably greater in girls than boys.[35]

Although some studies suggest that risk is increased when chemotherapy is combined with radiotherapy,[1,8,36] others do not,[3-6] and the effect of the combination continues to be a matter of debate.[37,38]

In many cases the risk of secondary malignancy is far less than that of undertreating, or of failing to treat, the primary disease.[7,39] However, secondary malignancies may be more resistant to treatment and more aggressive than primary disease,[40] and the risk of inducing malignant neoplasia is certainly a consideration in the use of alkylating agents and immunosuppressants to treat non-malignant disease,[32] and is an increasing challenge in the design of suitable treatment regimens for primary neoplastic disease.[7]

1. Curtis RE, et al. Risk of leukemia associated with the first course of cancer treatment: an analysis of the surveillance, epidemiology, and end results program experience. J Natl Cancer Inst 1984; 72: 531–44.
2. Lien EJ, Ou X-C. Carcinogenicity of some anticancer drugs—a survey. J Clin Hosp Pharm 1985; 10: 223–42.
3. Pedersen-Bjergaard J, et al. Risk of therapy-related leukaemia and preleukaemia after Hodgkin's disease: relation to age, cumulative dose of alkylating agents, and time from chemotherapy. Lancet 1987; ii: 83–8.
4. Kaldor JM, et al. Leukemia following chemotherapy for ovarian cancer. N Engl J Med 1990; 322: 1–6.
5. Kaldor JM, et al. Leukemia following Hodgkin's disease. N Engl J Med 1990; 322: 7–13.
6. Devereux S, et al. Leukaemia complicating treatment for Hodgkin's disease: the experience of the British National Lymphoma Investigation. BMJ 1990; 301: 1077–80.
7. Williams CJ. Leukaemia and cancer chemotherapy. BMJ 1990; 301: 73–4.
8. Pui C-H. Myeloid neoplasia in children treated for solid tumours. Lancet 1990; 336: 417–21.
9. Pedersen-Bjergaard J, et al. Carcinoma of the urinary bladder after treatment with cyclophosphamide for non-Hodgkin's lymphoma. N Engl J Med 1988; 318: 1028–32.
10. Swerdlow AJ, et al. Risk of second primary cancers after Hodgkin's disease by type of treatment: analysis of 2864 patients in the British National Lymphoma Investigation. BMJ 1992; 304: 1137–43.
11. Bhatia S, et al. Breast cancer and other second neoplasms after childhood Hodgkin's disease. N Engl J Med 1996; 334: 745–51.
12. Hawkins MM, et al. Epipodophyllotoxins, alkylating agents, and radiation and risk of secondary leukaemia after childhood cancer. BMJ 1992; 304: 951–8.
13. Kamel OW, et al. Brief report: reversible lymphomas associated with Epstein-Barr virus occurring during methotrexate therapy for rheumatoid arthritis and dermatomyositis. N Engl J Med 1993; 328: 1317–21.
14. Niesvizky R, et al. Epstein-Barr virus-associated lymphoma after treatment of macroglobulinemia with cladribine. N Engl J Med 1999; 341: 55.
15. Micallef INM, et al. Therapy-related myelodysplasia and secondary acute myelogenous leukaemia after high-dose therapy with autologous hematopoietic progenitor-cell support for lymphoid malignancies. J Clin Oncol 2000; 18: 947–55.
16. Lee IP, Dixon RL. Mutagenicity, carcinogenicity and teratogenicity of procarbazine. Mutat Res 1978; 55: 1–14.
17. Pui C-H, et al. Secondary acute myeloid leukemia in children treated for acute lymphoid leukemia. N Engl J Med 1989; 321: 136–42.
18. Meadows AT, et al. Potential long-term toxic effects in children treated for acute lymphoblastic leukemia. N Engl J Med 1989; 321: 1830.
19. Pedersen-Bjergaard J, et al. Increased risk of myelodysplasia and leukaemia after etoposide, cisplatin, and bleomycin for germ-cell tumours. Lancet 1991; 338: 359–63.
20. Snowden JA, et al. Acute promyelocytic leukaemia after treatment for seminoma with carboplatin. Lancet 1994; 344: 1361.
21. Travis LB, et al. Risk of leukemia after platinum-based chemotherapy for ovarian cancer. N Engl J Med 1999; 340: 351–7.
22. Levine MN, et al. Randomized trial of intensive cyclophosphamide, epirubicin, and fluorouracil chemotherapy compared with cyclophosphamide, methotrexate, and fluorouracil in premenopausal women with node-positive breast cancer. J Clin Oncol 1998; 16: 2651–8.
23. Smith MA, et al. Secondary leukemia or myelodysplastic syndrome after treatment with epipodophyllotoxins. J Clin Oncol 1999; 17: 569–77.
24. Maize JC. Skin cancer in immunosuppressed patients. JAMA 1977; 237: 1857–8.
25. Kinlen LJ, et al. Collaborative United Kingdom-Australasian study of cancer in patients treated with immunosuppressive drugs. BMJ 1979; 2: 1461–6.
26. Li PKT, et al. The complications of newer transplant antirejection drugs: treatment with cyclosporin A, OKT3, and FK 506. Adverse Drug React Acute Poisoning Rev 1990; 9: 123–55.
27. Starzl TE, et al. Reversibility of lymphomas and lymphoproliferative lesions developing under cyclosporin-steroid therapy. Lancet 1984; i: 583–7.
28. Boyle GJ, et al. Posttransplantation lymphoproliferative disorders in pediatric thoracic organ recipients. J Pediatr 1997; 131: 309–13.
29. Boyle P, et al. Cancer, warts, and sunshine in renal transplant patients: a case-control study. Lancet 1984; i: 702–5.
30. van Leeuwen FE, et al. Long-term risk of second malignancy in survivors of Hodgkin's disease treated during adolescence or young adulthood. J Clin Oncol 2000; 18: 487–97.
31. Pui C-H, et al. Potential long-term toxic effects in children treated for acute lymphoblastic leukemia. N Engl J Med 1989; 321: 1830–1.
32. Althouse R, et al. Cyclophosphamide in chronic active hepatitis. BMJ 1979; 1: 1630–1.
33. Boice JD, et al. Leukemia after adjuvant chemotherapy with semustine (methyl-CCNU)—evidence of a dose-response effect. N Engl J Med 1986; 314: 119–20.
34. Pedersen-Bjergaard J, et al. Incidence of acute nonlymphocytic leukemia, preleukemia, and acute myeloproliferative syndrome up to 10 years after treatment of Hodgkin's disease. N Engl J Med 1982; 307: 965–71.
35. Tarbell NJ, et al. Sex differences in risk of second malignant tumours after Hodgkin's disease in childhood. Lancet 1993; 341: 1428–32.
36. Krikorian JG, et al. Occurrence of non-Hodgkin's lymphoma after therapy for Hodgkin's disease. N Engl J Med 1979; 300: 452–8.
37. Prosnitz LR. Leukemia after treatment of ovarian cancer or Hodgkin's disease. N Engl J Med 1990; 322: 1819–20.
38. Coltman CA, Dahlberg S. Leukemia after treatment of ovarian cancer or Hodgkin's disease. N Engl J Med 1990; 322: 1820.
39. Macleod AM, Catto GRD. Cancer after transplantation. BMJ 1988; 297: 4–5.
40. Neugut AI, et al. Poor survival of treatment-related acute nonlymphocytic leukemia. JAMA 1990; 264: 1006–8.

EFFECTS ON CHROMOSOMES. Visible chromosome gaps, breaks, and structural rearrangements are found in blood lymphocytes from patients who have received substantial doses of combination chemotherapy, and the changes persist for years after the end of treatment. A more sensitive, if transient, measure of genetic damage is the increased rate of sister chromatid exchange (SCE) that occurs with even quite small doses of cytotoxic drugs.[1] Evidence from a study[2] in patients given chlorambucil suggests that as the dose increases so the capacity of the cells to cope with induced genetic damage is progressively exceeded, and thus SCE frequency reflects cumulative toxicity throughout the course of treatment.

In patients who develop acute myeloid leukaemia following antineoplastic therapy, the most common chromosomal losses involve chromosomes 5, 7, or both; a balanced translocation involving chromosomes 11 and 16 is closely associated with treatment using topoisomerase II inhibitors.[3]

See also under Effects on Reproductive Potential, below.

1. Anonymous. Drugs that can cause cancer. Lancet 1984; i: 261–2.
2. Palmer RG, et al. Chlorambucil-induced chromosome damage to human lymphocytes is dose-dependent and cumulative. Lancet 1984; i: 246–9.
3. Rowley JD, et al. Chromosomal translocations in secondary acute myeloid leukemia. N Engl J Med 1996; 334: 601–3.

Effects on the bladder. Cyclophosphamide (p.528) and ifosfamide (p.546) are the antineoplastics most frequently associated with adverse effects on the bladder, but see also Busulfan, p.513, Chlorambucil, p.517, and Mitomycin, p.558.

Effects on the blood. BONE-MARROW DEPRESSION. Bone-marrow depression, or myelosuppression, is common to the majority of cytotoxic antineoplastics, and is probably the single most important dose-limiting adverse effect, although its significance has been somewhat reduced in recent years by the availability of colony-stimulating factors, and the development of techniques such as peripheral blood stem cell transfusion.

The formation and development of blood cells takes place in the bone marrow. A common progenitor, the pluripotent stem cell, gives rise to 3 major cell lines from which red cells, white cells, and platelets are derived. All the cellular elements of blood may be affected by antineoplastic therapy, resulting in pancytopenia, but in many cases the toxicity appears to be greater for particular cell types. In addition, the different cell types have very different half-lives in the circulation. White blood cells and platelets tend to have the shortest half-lives in circulation. Hence the most usual manifestation of bone-marrow depression is leucopenia with a consequent increased risk of infection, and thrombocytopenia is also fairly common. Erythrocytes have the longest life (about 120 days) and anaemia is somewhat less frequent, and may be associated with megaloblastic changes in the bone marrow.

The onset, duration, and severity of bone marrow depression vary considerably with different antineoplastics. Little or only relatively mild myelosuppression seems to occur with conventional regimens of bleomycin (p.512), mitotane (p.559), streptozocin (p.569), and vincristine (p.579). Megaloblastic anaemia occurring with hydroxyurea [hydroxycarbamide] (p.544) may be treatable by blood transfusions, if necessary, without interrupting therapy.

Many of the alkylating agents are associated with severe and sometimes irreversible bone-marrow depression, particularly at high doses. Busulfan (p.513) and the nitrosoureas such as lomustine (p.550) pose a particular problem because the nadir of white-blood cell and platelet counts may not be reached for up to 6 weeks after a dose. Although high doses of antineoplastic generally produce greater and more rapid bone-marrow toxicity, with some agents, such as thiotepa (p.574), the relationship of toxicity to dose is very variable. These drugs affect both resting and actively cycling stem cells.

Many antimetabolites are also associated with myelosuppression and some such as cytarabine (p.530) may produce megaloblastic anaemia in addition to leucopenia and thrombocytopenia. Cytarabine has a biphasic effect on granulocytes, producing an initial nadir about 7 to 9 days after a dose, and a second and more severe one after 15 to 24 days. Unlike alkylating agents, antimetabolites affect actively proliferating, but not resting, stem cells. Cladribine (p.527) and fludarabine (p.539) produce a prolonged and profound lymphopenia.

Of the other drugs mitomycin (p.558) and procarbazine (p.566) in particular have both been associated with prolonged, delayed myelosuppression. Recovery from the bone-marrow toxicity of mitomycin may take months and about 25% of cases do not recover. Cisplatin (p.525) and anthracyclins such as doxorubicin (p.535) are myelosuppressant, although other toxic effects may be more important in determining dose, but myelosuppression is dose-limiting with carboplatin (p.515). Cisplatin-induced renal toxicity may lead to anaemia by decreasing erythropoietin production. Bone marrow depression is also a significant adverse effect of vinblastine (p.578) vindesine, and vinorelbine, although the effects of vincristine on the bone marrow are much less marked, as mentioned above. Neutropenia is common with the camptothecin derivatives irinotecan (p.549) and topotecan (p.575) and can be dose-limiting.

For further details, see under the individual monographs.

See also Effects on Immune Response, below.

Effects on body-weight. Although the effects of antineoplastics on the gastrointestinal tract (below) may lead to anorexia, malabsorption, and malnutrition, and hence to weight loss, antineoplastic therapy for breast cancer has also been associated with weight gain, sometimes dramatic.[1] Weight gain appeared to be more likely in premenopausal women, in those receiving multidrug regimens, and in those treated for longer periods of time. Weight gain was also noted after long-term follow-up of paediatric leukaemia patients.[2,3]

Concurrent use of corticosteroids may also lead to weight gain.

1. Denmark-Wahnefried W, et al. Why women gain weight with adjuvant chemotherapy for breast cancer. J Clin Oncol 1993; 11: 1418–29.
2. Birkebæk NH, Clausen N. Height and weight pattern up to 20 years after treatment for acute lymphoblastic leukaemia. Arch Dis Child 1998; 79: 161–4.
3. Nysom K, et al. Degree of fatness after treatment for acute lymphoblastic leukaemia in childhood. J Clin Endocrinol Metab 1999; 84: 4591–6.

Effects on bones and joints. Osteoporosis occurs as both an acute[1] and late complication of chemotherapy, but as multicomponent regimens are used and because the pathogenesis of osteoporosis is likely to be multifactorial, it is difficult to assess the impact of individual drugs.[2] It is clear, however, that chemotherapy which causes hypogonadism decreases bone mineral density in the majority of patients.[2] This includes regimens for a variety of neoplasms, including breast, prostate and testicular cancers, lymphomas, and haematological malignancies. In particular, regimens containing cyclophosphamide, mustine [chlormethine], busulfan, or procarbazine may cause ovarian insufficiency and therefore have the potential to lead to osteoporosis in females. Males may be protected from the effects of pronounced hypogonadism, as the cells that produce testosterone only replicate slowly.[2]

In addition, several drugs may exert direct effects on the bone. Methotrexate has been found to increase bone resorption and inhibit bone formation to produce a massive uncoupling of bone turnover.[2] Other drugs, including ciclosporin and doxorubicin have been shown to be toxic to bone in animals.

Corticosteroids are believed to cause bone loss by decreasing osteoblast activity, an effect which may be alleviated by chlorambucil. Surprisingly, corticosteroids have not been implicated in bone loss for most chemotherapy regimens, perhaps because the duration of treatment is short.[2]

A study in children receiving chemotherapy for leukaemia has suggested that the effects of chemotherapy on gastrointestinal and renal handling of nutrients may lead to alterations in calcium and magnesium homoeostasis and hence to abnormal turnover of bone mineral.[3] Renal phosphate loss following damage to the renal tubule caused by ifosfamide can lead to osteomalacia.[2]

1. Arikoski P, et al. Reduced bone density at completion of chemotherapy for a malignancy. Arch Dis Child 1999; 80: 143–8.
2. Pfeilschifter J, Diel IJ. Osteoporosis due to cancer treatment: pathogenesis and management. J Clin Oncol 2000; 18: 1570–93.
3. Atkinson SA, et al. Mineral homeostasis and bone mass in children treated for acute lymphoblastic leukemia. J Pediatr 1989; 114: 793–800.

Effects on the cardiovascular system. THROMBOEMBOLISM. There have been numerous reports which suggest that combination antineoplastic chemotherapy may be associated with thromboembolic events, including angina pectoris,[1] deep-vein thrombosis,[2,3] pulmonary embolism,[2-4] and stroke,[5] sometimes with fatal results.[3-5] Arterial thromboses have also occurred.[5,6] Patients with malignant disease are already at increased risk of thromboembolism, but results of a study in women with breast cancer suggest that the risk is further increased in patients receiving chemotherapy.[7] Several reports have implicated the combinations of bleomycin with a vinca alkaloid and another agent such as cisplatin or etoposide.[1,3,4,6] Such combinations are widely used for testicular cancer and have also been implicated in producing Raynaud's syndrome,[8,9] although there is no evidence of a relationship between the two forms of toxicity,[3] but reports of thrombosis are not confined to such regimens.[2,3,5] Toxic effects on vascular endothelium have been proposed as a possible mechanism for these effects;[2,6] there is also evidence that chemotherapy further elevates an already increased coagulant activity in the blood of cancer patients, an increase which can be diminished by heparin.[10] In men with germ cell cancer there is some evidence that those with liver metastases, or receiving high-dose dexamethasone as antiemetic therapy, are at increased risk of thromboembolic complications.[11]

Thromboembolic complications may also be associated with the indwelling catheters used to provide vascular access for antineoplastic therapy;[12] low-dose warfarin prophylaxis may reduce the risk.[13]

For a discussion of the cardiotoxicity of antineoplastics see Effects on the Heart, below.

1. Rodriguez J, et al. Angina pectoris following cisplatin, etoposide, and bleomycin in a patient with advanced testicular cancer. Ann Pharmacother 1995; 29: 138–9.
2. Cantwell BMJ, et al. Thromboses and thromboemboli in patients with lymphoma during cytotoxic chemotherapy. BMJ 1988; 297: 179–80.
3. Cantwell BMJ, et al. Thromboembolic events during combination chemotherapy for germ cell malignancy. Lancet 1988; ii: 1086–7.
4. Hall MR, et al. Thromboembolic events during combination chemotherapy for germ cell malignancy. Lancet 1988; ii: 1259.
5. Wall JG, et al. Arterial thrombosis associated with adjuvant chemotherapy for breast carcinoma: a Cancer and Leukemia Group B study. Am J Med 1989; 87: 501–4.
6. Garstin IWH, et al. Arterial thrombosis after treatment with bleomycin and cisplatin. BMJ 1990; 300: 1018.
7. Levine MN, et al. The thrombogenic effect of anticancer drug therapy in women with stage II breast cancer. N Engl J Med 1988; 318: 404–7.
8. Vogelzang NJ, et al. Raynaud's phenomenon: a common toxicity after combination chemotherapy for testicular cancer. Ann Intern Med 1981; 95: 288–92.
9. Pechère M, et al. Fingertip necrosis during chemotherapy with bleomycin, vincristine and methotrexate for HIV-related Kaposi's sarcoma. Br J Dermatol 1996; 134: 378–9.
10. Edwards RL, et al. Heparin abolishes the chemotherapy-induced increase in plasma fibrinopeptide A levels. Am J Med 1990; 89: 25–8.
11. Weijl NI, et al. Thromboembolic events during chemotherapy for germ cell cancer: a cohort study and review of the literature. J Clin Oncol 2000; 18: 2169–78.
12. Anderson AJ, et al. Thrombosis: the major Hickman catheter complication in patients with solid tumor. Chest 1989; 95: 71–5.
13. Bern MM, et al. Very low doses of warfarin can prevent thrombosis in central venous catheters: a randomized prospective trial. Ann Intern Med 1990; 112: 423–8.

Effects on electrolytes. It has been suggested that cancer chemotherapy and its complicating opportunistic infection exposes some patients to a combination of treatments likely to produce hypomagnesaemia, including: drug-induced loss of appetite; increased gastrointestinal magnesium loss due to vomiting and diarrhoea; impaired intestinal absorption due to drug-induced mucosal damage; and a direct magnesium-losing effect on the kidney of certain drugs such as cisplatin and some antibacterials.[1] Hypoparathyroidism and associated hypocalcaemia and hypomagnesaemia have been reported in patients receiving chemotherapy for acute leukaemias,[2] and it has been suggested that such changes in electrolyte homoeostasis may result in abnormal bone turnover (see Effects on Bones and Joints, above). Release of the contents of cells destroyed by chemotherapy is well-known to be associated with hyperuricaemia (below) but has also produced hyperphosphataemia, hyperkalaemia, and hypocalcaemia.[3,4]

Disturbances of electrolyte homoeostasis have been reported particularly with cisplatin (p.525), cyclophosphamide (p.528), and ciclosporin (p.518).

1. Brenton DP, Gordon TE. Fluid and electrolyte disorders: magnesium. Br J Hosp Med 1984; 32: 60–9.
2. Freedman DB, et al. Hypoparathyroidism and hypocalcaemia during treatment for acute leukaemia. BMJ 1982; 284: 700–2.
3. Kanfer A, et al. Extreme hyperphosphataemia causing acute anuric nephrocalcinosis in lymphosarcoma. BMJ 1979; 1: 1320–1.
4. Chasty RC, Liu-Yin JA. Acute tumour lysis syndrome. Br J Hosp Med 1993; 49: 488–92.

Effects on the gastrointestinal tract. Apart from anorexia, and nausea and vomiting (see below), many antineoplastics produce gastrointestinal disturbances. Mucosal inflammation (mucositis), notably as stomatitis and sometimes proctitis, is quite common, as are mucosal cellular changes, xerostomia, impaired absorption, and diarrhoea. In some cases gastrointestinal damage may progress to ulceration, haemorrhage, and perforation. Antimetabolites affecting pyrimidine metabolism, such as cytarabine (p.530) and fluorouracil (p.540), and the antifolates such as methotrexate (p.553), seem to be particularly associated with severe gastrointestinal effects, especially at high doses, but there appear to be few antineoplastics that do not cause some degree of gastrointestinal disturbance. Irinotecan (p.549) can produce both an initial transient diarrhoea related to cholinergic stimulation, and more severe prolonged diarrhoea with a delayed onset which may be dose limiting and potentially fatal. Use with radiotherapy may increase the toxicity of some drugs on the gastrointestinal tract. The neutropenia induced by many antineoplastic regimens may lead to secondary gastrointestinal effects, such as stomatitis and gastrointestinal inflammation, associated with infection.

CLOSTRIDIUM DIFFICILE INFECTION. Antineoplastic therapy has occasionally been associated with the development of Clostridium difficile-induced gastrointestinal disease, even in the absence of concomitant antibacterial therapy.[1] Most patients had received multiple drug regimens. Methotrexate, fluorouracil, cyclophosphamide, and doxorubicin have all been associated with a number of cases but this may simply reflect the frequency of their use. For discussion of the treatment of such disease, see Antibiotic-associated Colitis, p.122

1. Anand A, Glatt AE. Clostridium difficile infection associated with antineoplastic chemotherapy: a review. Clin Infect Dis 1993; 17: 109–13.

MUCOSITIS. The suffering associated with oral mucositis is by far the worst part of treatment for many patients undergoing curative chemotherapy or bone-marrow transplantation, and for those undergoing oral radiotherapy.[1] Apart from pain and dysphagia the ulcerated mucosa provides a portal of entry for infection; loss of weight and malnutrition may further impair immune function, and if symptoms are severe enough the treatment cycle may have to be interrupted. Before the patient starts any intensive chemotherapy or local or systemic radiotherapy the oral cavity must be assessed with a view to eliminating sources of infection and chronic irritation.

1. Calman FMB, Langdon J. Oral complications of cancer. BMJ 1991; 302: 485–6.

NAUSEA AND VOMITING. Nausea and vomiting are common side-effects of antineoplastic therapy, and for many patients, represent a major drawback to treatment. Once experienced, anticipatory vomiting may occur at the sight of medical staff, or a needle. The problem may be severe enough in some cases to hinder or completely prevent further treatment.

Antineoplastic or cytotoxic drugs may induce vomiting by both a central action on the chemoreceptor trigger zone and a peripheral action on the gastrointestinal tract. Several neurotransmitters have been implicated over the years including acetylcholine, histamine, enkephalins, dopamine, and serotonin or 5-hydroxytryptamine (5-HT). The cerebral cortex is probably responsible for anticipatory vomiting. Antineoplastics may not all induce emesis by a common pathway, but 5-HT$_3$-receptor mechanisms are clearly important in the pathogenesis of acute cisplatin-associated vomiting. This was suspected when the antiemetic metoclopramide, a dopamine antagonist, was found to have serotonin (5-HT) antagonist activity at the high doses used against cisplatin emesis and confirmed when specific 5-HT$_3$ antagonists such as ondansetron proved to be effective. Different mechanisms are probably involved in delayed emesis since 5-HT$_3$ antagonists are less effective.

Some patients are more susceptible to emesis than others. The emetic potential of antineoplastics also varies in terms of severity and incidence. Emetogenicity may depend to some extent on the dose, route, and schedule of administration. Some combination therapy has resulted in a higher incidence of vomiting than would be expected from the constituents. Vomiting may be very severe with cisplatin, dacarbazine, dactinomycin, mustine [chlormethine], high-dose cyclophosphamide, and streptozocin, and occurs in most patients. Moderate vomiting is likely with the taxanes, doxorubicin, and more modest doses of cyclophosphamide, and high-dose methotrexate, while vinca alkaloids, fluorouracil, lower doses of methotrexate, chlorambucil, bleomycin, and etoposide have low emetogenic potential.

The onset and duration of vomiting also varies from drug to drug. With cisplatin the onset may be between 4 and 8 hours following a dose, while the duration may be up to 48 hours or occasionally even longer; a persistent feeling of nausea, and sometimes vomiting, lasting for several days may also occur. After mustine [chlormethine], vomiting may begin within a half to 2 hours, whereas after cyclophosphamide there may be a latent interval of 9 to 18 hours, but in both cases vomiting is generally less prolonged than with cisplatin. Acute emesis (that occurring within 24 hours) has generally been easier to control than delayed emesis (that occurring more than 24 hours after chemotherapy) or anticipatory emesis.

The management of chemotherapy-induced nausea and vomiting is discussed on p.1206.

Effects on the heart. The cardiotoxicity of antineoplastics has been reviewed.[1] Cardiotoxicity is the major dose-limiting toxicity with anthracyclines such as doxorubicin and daunorubicin, manifesting most seriously as drug-induced cardiomyopathy, which is frequently fatal, and for which no specific treatment exists. Some of the newer anthracycline analogues such as epirubicin or idarubicin were developed to be less toxic to the heart, although this has not always been easy to prove in controlled studies. Cardiotoxicity has also been associated with other antineoplastics, although less frequently. High-dose cyclophosphamide or ifosfamide may produce myocarditis, arrhythmias, and congestive heart failure, sometimes delayed by up to 2 weeks, while fluorouracil has been associated with angina pectoris and myocardial infarction, perhaps due to a combination of vasospastic effects and activation of coagulation. Amsacrine has been associated with arrhythmias, sometimes fatal. Occasional reports of cardiotoxicity associated with busulfan, carmustine, cisplatin, cytarabine, etoposide, mitomycin, paclitaxel, pentostatin, and vincristine also exist.

For a discussion of the thromboembolic events seen with antineoplastics see Effects on the Cardiovascular System, above.

1. Pai VB, Nahata MC. Cardiotoxicity of chemotherapeutic agents: incidence, treatment and prevention. Drug Safety 2000; 22: 263–302.

Effects on immune response. Lymphocytes are produced by stem cells in the bone marrow and at other sites, including the thymus, and are involved in humoral and cell-mediated immunity. Most antineoplastics have a depressant effect on bone marrow (see Effects on the Blood, above) and many have immunosuppressant properties although the degree of suppression varies and may depend on the dose and schedule of administration used. Immunosuppression decreases the patient's resistance to infection and has also been implicated in the development of malignancies (see Carcinogenicity, above). In an early study of immunisation of patients with Hodgkin's disease using dodecavalent pneumococcal vaccine, antibody response was profoundly impaired in patients who had received intensive radiotherapy and/or chemotherapy.[1] Some impairment persisted for at least 4 years after the completion of intensive combined therapy.

The length of time after onset of immunosuppression in transplant patients correlates with the type of infection acquired.[2] In the first few months local bacterial infections predominate. After about 1 month of immunosuppression Aspergillus infections become more common, while between 3 weeks and 4 months after transplantation cytomegalovirus infection (both primary and reactivated) occurs in 20 to 40% of those at risk. Pneumocystis carinii pneumonia is uncommon immediately after transplantation, more usually occurring after months or years. Infection in transplant patients tends to occur in or near the transplanted organ.

For a discussion on the effects of immunosuppressant therapy on the immune response and the infections associated with it, see Corticosteroids, p.1041.

1. Siber GR, et al. Impaired antibody response to pneumococcal vaccine after treatment for Hodgkin's disease. N Engl J Med 1978; 299: 442–8.
2. Anonymous. Immunosuppressive drugs and their complications. Drug Ther Bull 1994; 32: 66–70.

Effects on the kidneys. Nephrotoxicity is well-recognised as an adverse effect of ciclosporin (p.519), cisplatin (p.525), ifosfamide (p.546), and methotrexate (p.554), but renal toxicity may occur with other antineoplastics including the nitrosoureas, mitomycin (due to haemolytic-uraemic syndrome), azacitidine, gemcitabine, and pentostatin.[1]

1. Kintzel PE. Anticancer drug-induced kidney disorders: incidence, prevention and management. Drug Safety 2001; 24: 19–38.

Effects on the liver. Occasional reports of hepatotoxicity exist for many antineoplastics and immunosuppressants including aminoglutethimide (p.507), azathioprine (p.510), busulfan (p.513), dacarbazine (p.531), dactinomycin (p.532), doxorubicin (p.535), floxuridine (p.539), hydroxyurea [hydroxycarbamide] (p.544), methotrexate (p.554), mitomycin (p.558), mitozantrone [mitoxantrone] (p.559), sparfosic acid with fluorouracil (p.569), tamoxifen (p.571), and tioguanine (p.575). However, the relationship of the drug to the adverse effect is not always easy to establish.

An early but detailed review suggested that methotrexate, mercaptopurine, azathioprine, cytarabine, carmustine, streptozocin, asparaginase, and plicamycin could probably be classified as hepatotoxic. There was considered to be insufficient evidence to classify fluorouracil, cyclophosphamide, busulfan, dacarbazine, the anthracyclines, the vinca alkaloids, and the podophyllum derivatives as hepatotoxic, although this classification was not definitive.[1] Liver toxicity may not be confined to patients: one report described 3 cases of liver damage in nurses working on an oncology ward.[2]

1. Ménard DB, et al. Antineoplastic agents and the liver. Gastroenterology 1980; 78: 142–64.
2. Sotaniemi EA, et al. Liver damage in nurses handling cytostatic agents. Acta Med Scand 1983; 214: 181–9.

Effects on the lungs. Lung injury occurs in about 10% of all patients who receive bleomycin, with death in 1 to 2%. The changes in the lung are diffuse and include fibrosis of the alveolar septa, chronic pneumonitis, and enlargement of the type II alveolar lining cells with bizarre alteration of the nucleus; clinically, the reaction presents as non-productive cough and dyspnoea, often with fever, and develops over days to weeks. The reaction is dose-related, being more likely at total doses over 450 000 IU (450 USP units), although it has occurred at much lower doses, and is more common in elderly patients.[1] Hypersensitivity pneumonitis, which is more amenable to treatment, has also been reported.[2]

Pulmonary damage has also been reported in association with an increasing number of antineoplastics apart from bleomycin.[3] Among the alkylating agents cyclophosphamide has been reported to produce lung injury in less than 1% of cases, although this may be increased where it is a component of combination regimens or where it is combined with radiotherapy. Busulfan may produce lung toxicity including insidious pulmonary fibrosis in as many as 4% of patients, usually developing several years after initiation of therapy, and with increased risk the longer that therapy lasts. A few reports exist of interstitial pneumonitis and fibrosis associated with chlorambucil and melphalan, but these appear to be extremely rare. The prognosis in patients with alkylating-agent-induced fibrosis is often poor, with mortality rates of around 50%.

The antimetabolite methotrexate can produce symptoms similar to hypersensitivity pneumonitis in up to 7% of patients, sometimes with pleuritis and acute respiratory failure due to pulmonary oedema, but it is not clear whether a true hypersensitivity mechanism is involved, and symptoms are usually reversible even without discontinuing therapy. High-dose cytarabine has also been associated with pulmonary oedema, while azathioprine has been associated with a few cases of interstitial pneumonitis and fibrosis.

Other antineoplastics known to be associated with pulmonary toxicity include mitomycin (usually in less than 10% of patients though the incidence may be much higher in combination regimens); the vinca alkaloids (generally in combination, and usually producing acute respiratory failure); chlorozotocin; procarbazine; and possibly teniposide. The nitrosoureas, and particularly carmustine, have also emerged as pulmonary toxins. Carmustine has been associated with an insidious chronic pulmonary fibrosis, which in some early studies occurred in as many as 30% of patients and had a high mortality. Symptoms are associated particularly with cumulative doses in excess of about 1.4 g per m^2 body-surface, although toxicity has occurred at cumulative doses as low as 240 mg per m^2 The onset of symptoms may be very delayed: some workers reported fibrosis occurring up to 17 years after treatment in patients who received carmustine as children.[4] Potentially life-threatening pneumonitis has occurred in patients receiving thoracic radiotherapy in association with gemcitabine (p.543).

1. Rosenow EC, et al. Pulmonary disease in the immunocompromised host. Mayo Clin Proc 1985; 60: 473–87.
2. Holoye PY, et al. Bleomycin hypersensitivity pneumonitis. Ann Intern Med 1978; 88: 47–9.
3. Twohig KJ, Matthay RA. Pulmonary effects of cytotoxic agents other than bleomycin. Clin Chest Med 1990; 11: 31–54.
4. O'Driscoll BR, et al. Active lung fibrosis up to 17 years after chemotherapy with carmustine (BCNU) in childhood. N Engl J Med 1990; 323: 378–82.

Effects on mental function. Combination chemotherapy has been associated with psychiatric morbidity (anxiety, depression, behavioural changes) in both adults[1] and children.[2] It has been pointed out that patients receiving cancer chemotherapy inevitably suffer emotional distress, associated in part with the adverse effects of treatment. Patients should be fully informed of aims and likely outcomes of treatment, and adverse effects minimised, in order to keep emotional distress to a minimum.[3]

A number of individual antineoplastics and immunosuppressants have been associated with mental symptoms including chlorambucil (p.517), methotrexate (p.554), mitotane (p.559), and the vinca alkaloids (p.578). In many cases such symptoms can be attributed to direct central neurotoxicity (see also under Effects on the Nervous System, below).

1. Maguire GP, et al. Psychiatric morbidity and physical toxicity associated with adjuvant chemotherapy after mastectomy. BMJ 1980; 281: 1179–80.
2. Dolgin MJ, et al. Behavioral distress in pediatric patients with cancer receiving chemotherapy. Pediatrics 1989; 84: 103–10.
3. Brinkley D. Emotional distress during cancer chemotherapy. BMJ 1983; 286: 663–4.

Effects on the nervous system. Neurotoxic effects have been reported for many antineoplastics, including altretamine (p.506), asparaginase (p.509), busulfan (p.513), carboplatin (p.515), carmustine (p.516), chlorambucil (p.517), ciclosporin (p.518), cisplatin (p.525), cladribine (p.527), cytarabine (p.530), etanidazole (p.538), etoposide (p.538), fludarabine (p.539), fluorouracil (p.541), hydroxyurea [hydroxycarbamide] (p.544), ifosfamide (p.546), lomustine (p.550), methotrexate (p.554), misonidazole (p.557), mitotane (p.559), mitozantrone [mitoxantrone] (p.559), mustine [chlormethine] (p.561), oxaliplatin (p.563), paclitaxel (p.563), pentostatin (p.564), procarbazine (p.566), sparfosic acid (p.569), tacrolimus (p.569), tegafur (p.573), vinblastine (p.578), vincristine (p.579), and vindesine (p.580). In some cases these effects may be associated with particular routes such as the intrathecal. See under the individual monographs for further details. Radiotherapy can also cause damage to the nervous system so combination of the two modalities may lead to additive effects.

EFFECTS ON THE EARS. Several antineoplastics have been associated with ototoxicity,[1] including vincristine and vinblastine, but cisplatin in particular is associated with high-frequency hearing loss and tinnitus. In addition, agents such as the nitrogen mustards and bleomycin are potentially ototoxic.

1. Huang MY, Schacht J. Drug-induced ototoxicity: pathogenesis and prevention. Med Toxicol Adverse Drug Exp 1989; 4: 452–67.

Effects on reproductive potential. CHROMOSOMES. If patients are fertile after treatment with antineoplastics, no significant increase has been seen in fetal chromosome damage, fetal abnormality, or the abortion rate. Several small or medium-sized studies have failed to show any increase in congenital abnormalities or miscarriage rate in the offspring of patients who have received chemotherapy,[1-4] although one study did show an increased risk of abnormal offspring in patients with Hodgkin's disease who received both chemotherapy and irradiation. Another study, while finding no overall link between chemotherapy and the incidence of congenital abnormality did suggest an increased incidence of heart defects in children born to mothers who received dactinomycin,[4] but this was not subsequently confirmed in a larger group.[5] A large case-control study carried out in Canada, and involving over 85 000 parents of children with congenital anomalies, also has failed to confirm a higher incidence of congenital abnormality in the offspring of patients treated with radiotherapy or alkylating agents.[6] However, despite these generally reassuring results, it has been suggested that women should delay conception for a year after cessation of chemotherapy to allow mature ova which might have been damaged to be eliminated.[7]

See also Effects on Chromosomes under Carcinogenicity, above.

1. Rustin GJS, et al. Pregnancy after cytotoxic chemotherapy for gestational trophoblastic tumours. BMJ 1984; 288: 103–6.
2. Li FP, et al. Offspring of patients treated for cancer in childhood. J Natl Cancer Inst 1979; 62: 1193–7.
3. Holmes GE, Holmes FF. Pregnancy outcome of patients treated for Hodgkin's disease: a controlled study. Cancer 1978; 41: 1317–22.

4. Green DM, et al. Congenital anomalies in children of patients who received chemotherapy for cancer in childhood and adolescence. N Engl J Med 1991; 325: 141–6.
5. Byrne J, et al. Absence of birth defects in offspring of women treated with dactinomycin. N Engl J Med 1992; 326: 137.
6. Dodds L, et al. Case-control study of congenital anomalies in children of cancer patients. BMJ 1993; 307: 164–8.
7. Walden PAM, Bagshawe KD. Pregnancies after chemotherapy for gestational trophoblastic tumours. Lancet 1979; ii: 1241.

GONADS. The effects of drugs, including cytotoxic drugs, on the gonads have been reviewed.[1-4] In male patients, antineoplastic drugs may damage the seminiferous tubules, resulting in testicular atrophy with decreased sperm count and motility. Testosterone secretion may also be reduced after damage to Leydig cells. Chlorambucil, cyclophosphamide, mustine [chlormethine], busulfan, procarbazine, and the nitrosoureas have all been associated with testicular germ cell depletion. The total cumulative dose and the duration of treatment are important factors determining the degree of damage. Methotrexate, fluorouracil, and mercaptopurine appear less toxic than alkylating agents.

In women, cytotoxic drugs act on the ovary to produce loss of primordial follicles with failure of ovulation, oligomenorrhoea or amenorrhoea, and failure of endocrine function resulting in loss of libido and menopausal symptoms. As in men, reports of gonadal dysfunction are associated particularly with alkylating agents. The degree of damage and its reversibility depend partly on the drug and its dose but more on the age of the woman at the time of treatment, with older women (35 to 40 or over) being more sensitive, probably a reflection of the decrease in oocyte numbers with age. Ovarian suppression with oral contraceptives to protect the ovary from damage has been tried, but its effectiveness is not confirmed. Gonadotrophin-releasing hormone analogues are also under investigation for their potential protective effects.

Severe gonadal dysfunction in both men and women has been associated with combination chemotherapy regimens for Hodgkin's disease. Mustine [chlormethine] and procarbazine are thought to be mainly responsible for the infertility produced. There is some evidence that the ABVD regimen (doxorubicin, bleomycin, vinblastine, and dacarbazine) results in less damage to gonadal cells than the MOPP regimen (mustine [chlormethine], vincristine, procarbazine, and prednisone). Prolonged gonadal dysfunction has also been seen in patients given combination chemotherapy for acute lymphoblastic leukaemia; girls appear to be at less risk than boys, especially if treated in the prepubertal period.

1. Beeley L. Drug-induced sexual dysfunction and infertility. Adverse Drug React Acute Poisoning Rev 1984; 3: 23–42.
2. Parkinson M, Bateman N. Disorders of sexual function caused by drugs. Prescribers' J 1994; 34: 183–90.
3. Goldman S, Johnson FL. Effects of chemotherapy and irradiation on the gonads. Endocrinol Metab Clin North Am 1993; 22: 617–29.
4. Kovacs GT, Stern K. Reproductive aspects of cancer treatment: an update. Med J Aust 1999; 170: 495–7.

SEXUAL FUNCTION. Loss of libido and decline in sexual performance seem to be relatively common in men receiving combination chemotherapy,[1,2] and may persist after chemotherapy has ended.[1] However, it may sometimes be difficult to distinguish the effects of chemotherapy from those of the disease and the patient's reaction to it: at least one study has shown that gonadal function is disturbed in patients with Hodgkin's disease before treatment.[2] Evidence for decreased libido in women is harder to find, but failure of endocrine function after chemotherapy may lead to loss of libido and menopausal symptoms.[3]

1. Chapman RM, et al. Cyclical combination chemotherapy and gonadal function: retrospective study in males. Lancet 1979; i: 285–9.
2. Chapman RM, et al. Male gonadal dysfunction in Hodgkin's disease: a prospective study. JAMA 1981; 245: 1323–8.
3. Shalet SM. Effects of cancer chemotherapy on gonadal function of patients. Cancer Treat Rev 1980; 7: 141–52.

Effects on the skin. Alopecia occurs with many antineoplastics, and may be severe with doxorubicin, the nitrosoureas, taxanes, and cyclophosphamide. The alkylating agents and some antibiotic antineoplastics are often associated with hyperpigmentation, most commonly of skin, although pigmentation of nails, hair, and teeth has occurred. Some drugs, such as the taxanes, cause dystrophic changes in the nails. Certain drugs may interact with ultraviolet light or x-ray radiation to enhance its effects on the skin and may cause radiation recall, photosensitivity, or, in the case of methotrexate, reactivation of ultraviolet burns. Hypersensitivity to antineoplastics may produce cutaneous reactions including allergic rashes, angioedema, and pruritus. In addition to the above there may be local reactions to irritant and vesicant drugs following extravasation. Finally, certain drugs are associated with specific dermatological reactions: bleomycin may produce hyperkeratotic and sclerotic lesions, dactinomycin is associated with an erythematous papular or pustular rash mimicking septic emboli, fluorouracil may produce inflammation of solar keratoses, and plicamycin is associated with a distinctive flushing phenomenon. A palmar-plantar erythrodysesthesia syndrome has been seen with fluorouracil (p.541) and a number of other antineoplastics.

See also Effects on the Gastrointestinal Tract, above, and Local Toxicity, below. References may also be found under individual monographs.

Hyperuricaemia. Overproduction of purines is a known complication of antineoplastic therapy and may result in hyperuricaemia (p.397). Hyperuricaemia is also an important part of the tumour lysis syndrome—see below.

Local toxicity. Local toxicity due to intravenous cancer chemotherapy may include local irritation, extravasation necrosis, and hypersensitivity.[1] Venous irritation, presenting as vasospasm and pain or endothelial chemical burn of the vessel, resulting in a painful, streaky, long-lasting sterile phlebitis, may be due to the drug, or, as with carmustine, due to the diluent (alcohol). Irritation and phlebitis have been reported particularly with fluorouracil, carmustine, bisantrene, vinorelbine, and mustine [chlormethine].

Up to 6% of patients treated with peripheral intravenous chemotherapy may experience extravasation, usually with pain, erythema, and swelling at the site of injection. Severe necrosis requiring surgical intervention may develop, particularly with antibiotic antineoplastics such as doxorubicin. For a discussion of extravasation and its management, including those drugs most commonly associated with problems, see Extravasation, p.480.

Local hypersensitivity reactions, usually self-limiting, may occur: it is important to distinguish such reactions from extravasation. In contrast to the latter, there is no swelling at the injection site, and pain is felt as a dull ache along the course of the vein, as opposed to the stinging commonly noted following extravasation.

1. Brigden ML, Barnett JB. Local toxicity of cancer chemotherapy—practical considerations. Can J Hosp Pharm 1986; 39: 96–9.

Tumour lysis syndrome. The tumour lysis syndrome represents a biochemical disturbance following massive release of cellular breakdown products from tumour cells sensitive to therapy. The amount of breakdown products is sufficient to overwhelm normal excretory and metabolic mechanisms for their clearance, and the cardinal features of the syndrome are hyperkalaemia, hyperuricaemia, and hyperphosphataemia accompanied by hypocalcaemia. Clinical symptoms may include urate nephropathy or nephrocalcinosis leading to renal impairment, and cardiac arrhythmias associated with the potassium abnormalities. The syndrome is seen particularly when bulky chemosensitive disease is present, and may be more likely in patients with pre-existing renal impairment or hyperuricaemia. The most frequent cases are in patients with Burkitt's or lymphoblastic lymphoma, or an acute leukaemia. Of patients with solid tumours, reports have implicated those with germ-cell tumours, small-cell lung cancer, or neuroblastoma although, surprisingly, the syndrome has also been reported in patients with breast cancer, which is normally less rapidly responsive to chemotherapy.

References.

1. Chasty RC, Liu-Yin JA. Acute tumour lysis syndrome. Br J Hosp Med 1993; 49: 488–92.
2. Kalemkerian GP, et al. Tumor lysis syndrome in small cell carcinoma and other solid tumors. Am J Med 1997; 103: 363–7.

Treatment of Adverse Effects

Intensive supportive care may be necessary to prevent or control the adverse effects of antineoplastic therapy. Antiemetic therapy should be given to reduce, and if possible prevent, nausea and vomiting, since once experienced it may become a conditioned response, and may not respond to antiemetics. Intensive oral care is desirable to minimise the effects of stomatitis while corticosteroids, and if necessary nutritional supplements, may be of some help in patients with anorexia.

Techniques attempting to prevent the occurrence of alopecia have met with varying success (see below). Scalp tourniquets and ice-packs have been used to minimise concentrations of antineoplastics in the scalp after intravenous injection. However, such methods may allow the development of a cancer-cell sanctuary and should not be used in patients with leukaemia or other conditions with circulating malignant cells.

Of particular importance is the management of bone-marrow depression. Recent interest has focused on the use of colony-stimulating factors (see below) to promote the formation of replacement blood elements. Active measures may be necessary to combat infection and bleeding. Transfusions of blood products may be required; granulocyte transfusions have been given for infections unresponsive to antibiotics, although their value is a matter of debate, while transfusion of blood platelets or use of growth factors such as oprelvekin (interleukin-11) may be of value in preventing thrombocytopenia-induced bleeding.

Extravasation of antineoplastics can pose serious problems and its treatment is controversial (see below). Infusion should be stopped immediately once extravasation is noticed and any drug remaining at the site aspirated if possible. Ice-packs are often applied, although warm moist soaks have been advocated for some drugs such as the vinca alkaloids, and some, but not all, centres suggest local injection of a corticosteroid. If ulceration occurs plastic surgery may be required. The value of specific antidotes is not proven.

Hyperuricaemia secondary to tumour lysis in patients with leukaemias or lymphomas can be prevented by the addition of allopurinol to treatment schedules, and by adequate hydration and, if necessary, alkalinisation of the urine. Good hydration is also important to minimise the nephrotoxic effects of drugs such as cisplatin and methotrexate.

Specific treatments exist for the toxicity of certain antineoplastics (for example the use of calcium folinate to reduce methotrexate toxicity, or mesna to control the bladder toxicity of cyclophosphamide or ifosfamide). For further details of the treatment of specific adverse effects see under the individual monographs.

Alopecia. Attempts to prevent or reduce chemotherapy-induced alopecia have relied on either restriction of scalp blood flow with a tourniquet or the use of local hypothermia. Following early reports of benefit[1,2] a scalp tourniquet was applied 5 minutes before administration in patients receiving doxorubicin, cyclophosphamide, and vincristine or teniposide, and was left in position for 20 minutes.[3] Alopecia occurred in 12 of 37 patients so treated, but in 22 of 31 controls. However, the tourniquet was uncomfortable: 5 patients originally assigned to the tourniquet group could not tolerate it.

Several studies have investigated the use of local scalp cooling.[4-6] Of 33 patients in whom ice-packs were applied to the scalp 5 minutes before injections of doxorubicin, and left in place for 30 minutes after injection, 20 maintained good protection against hair loss over 6 to 8 months of treatment, although the benefit decreased with time and was less at higher doses.[4] The results may also depend on the degree of cooling achieved, and the drug regimen used:[5] most studies have concentrated on doxorubicin, which is a potent producer of alopecia, but which is quite rapidly cleared. Vincristine also produces alopecia which, it has been suggested, is less likely to be prevented because of the drug's more prolonged clearance from the circulation,[5] although vincristine-induced alopecia has reportedly been reduced using a tourniquet.[1] There is also concern that restricting access of the antineoplastic to the scalp may create a sanctuary for circulating malignant cells, thus precluding the use of these techniques in patients with conditions such as leukaemias.[4]

In the USA commercial distribution of cooling caps designed to produce localised scalp hypothermia was halted by the FDA in 1990 because of concerns about their effectiveness and their potential to create sanctuary sites and interfere with drug distribution elsewhere in the body. However, they continue to be available in many countries.

For reference to the use of minoxidil to decrease the duration of alopecia following doxorubicin-containing chemotherapy, see p.935.

1. O'Brien R, *et al.* Scalp tourniquet to lessen alopecia after vincristine. *N Engl J Med* 1970; **283:** 1469.
2. Lyons AR. Prevention of hair loss by head-band during cytotoxic therapy. *Lancet* 1974; **i:** 354.
3. Pesce A, *et al.* Scalp tourniquet in the prevention of chemotherapy-induced alopecia. *N Engl J Med* 1978; **298:** 1204–5.
4. Dean JC, *et al.* Prevention of doxorubicin-induced hair loss with scalp hypothermia. *N Engl J Med* 1979; **301:** 1427–9.
5. Gregory RP, *et al.* Prevention of doxorubicin-induced alopecia by scalp hypothermia: relation to degree of cooling. *BMJ* 1982; **284:** 1674.
6. Guy R, *et al.* Scalp cooling by thermocirculator. *Lancet* 1982; **i:** 937–8.

Bone-marrow depression. Use of granulocyte or granulocyte-macrophage colony-stimulating factors (G-CSF or GM-CSF), alone or in combination with autologous bone-marrow transplants, or peripheral blood stem-cells,[1] can markedly reduce the period of neutropenia after high-dose chemotherapy regimens.[2,3] Recombinant thrombopoietin,[4] interleukin-3, interleukin-6, and interleukin-11 have been evaluated for their ability to increase platelet numbers *in vivo* and the latter is now available as oprelvekin, which can reduce chemotherapy-induced thrombocytopenia.[5,6] Erythropoietin may be used to reduce requirements for transfusion of red cells, and preliminary results suggest that it may also potentiate the effects of colony-stimulating factors.[7] Interleukin-1α and macrophage colony-stimulating factor (M-CSF) have also been investigated in the prevention or treatment of thrombocytopenia,[8,9] and stem cell factor has been tried for use in mobilising and transplanting peripheral stem cells.[10]

The American Society of Clinical Oncology has issued detailed guidelines for the use of colony-stimulating factors (CSFs) in patients receiving chemotherapy.[11] These point out that in current practice infectious mortality resulting from febrile neutropenia is rare, and that the incidence with common chemotherapy regimens seldom exceeds 25 to 40% in previously untreated patients; however, episodes of febrile neutropenia prolong hospital stay, expose the patient to further interventions, and may result in delay or dose-reduction of further chemotherapy cycles. Unfortunately, although colony-stimulating factors can markedly reduce the incidence of febrile neutropenia, there was little evidence of improved clinical outcomes from the use of CSFs in most situations.

- Use of colony-stimulating factors for **primary prophylaxis** in previously untreated patients should not normally be considered except where bone-marrow compromise or comorbidity indicated a patient at high risk (and even here the evidence for improved clinical outcome was modest).
- There was no evidence of clinical benefit from the use of colony-stimulating factors in **secondary prophylaxis**. In patients with a previous episode of febrile neutropenia the usual option (except where it would compromise the chances of cure) was dose reduction of the chemotherapy regimen.
- For adjunctive **treatment** of episodes of neutropenia, it was recommended that CSFs should not be routinely used for patients who were *afebrile*; there was also strong and consistent evidence against routine use for uncomplicated fever and neutropenia in *febrile* patients. Use might be considered in high-risk patients with febrile neutropenia.
- Although CSFs could permit **increased dose-intensity** of chemotherapy, this was considered only justified within the context of a clinical trial, since increased dose-intensity had not been shown to improve survival or quality of life in most studies outside the haematological malignancies. Use in patients receiving combined **chemoradiotherapy** was not recommended.
- In patients with **haematological malignancies**, CSFs should be considered after induction chemotherapy in patients with acute myeloid leukaemias who were aged 55 or over, and after initial induction or postremission chemotherapy in patients with acute lymphoblastic leukaemia; a subset of patients with myelodysplastic syndrome might also benefit, but use in patients with refractory or relapsed myeloid leukaemia was not thought to be of benefit.
- CSFs were recommended as adjuncts to **progenitor cell transplantation** to help mobilise peripheral blood stem cells and to speed engraftment.
- Although the guidelines in adults were held to be generally applicable to **children**, it was recognised that there were differences of emphasis in practice and that CSFs tended to be used more often for prophylaxis in children than was recommended in adults, and less often for uncomplicated fever and neutropenia.

The field is still developing, with new growth factors being discovered, and their ultimate place in oncology remains to be determined.

For details on the management of infections in neutropenic patients, see p.125.

1. Anonymous. Peripheral stem cells made to work. *Lancet* 1992; **339:** 648–9.
2. Khwaja A, Goldstone AH. Haemopoietic growth factors. *BMJ* 1991; **302:** 1164–5.
3. Steward WP. Granulocyte and granulocyte-macrophage colony-stimulating factors. *Lancet* 1993; **342:** 153–7. Correction. *ibid.*: 679.
4. Vadhan-Raj S, *et al.* Recombinant human thrombopoietin attenuates carboplatin-induced severe thrombocytopenia and the need for platelet transfusions in patients with gynecologic cancer. *Ann Intern Med* 2000; **132:** 364–8.
5. Gordon MS, *et al.* A phase I trial of recombinant human interleukin-11 (neumega rhIL-11 growth factor) in women with breast cancer receiving chemotherapy. *Blood* 1996; **87:** 3615–24.
6. Isaacs C, *et al.* Randomized placebo-controlled study of recombinant human interleukin-11 to prevent chemotherapy-induced thrombocytopenia in patients with breast cancer receiving dose-intensive cyclophosphamide and doxorubicin. *J Clin Oncol* 1997; **15:** 3368–77.
7. Pierelli L, *et al.* Erythropoietin addition to granulocyte colony-stimulating factor abrogates life-threatening neutropenia and increases peripheral-blood progenitor-cell mobilization after epirubicin, paclitaxel, and cisplatin combination chemotherapy: results of a randomized comparison. *J Clin Oncol* 1999; **17:** 1288–95.
8. Smith JW, *et al.* The effects of treatment with interleukin-1α on platelet recovery after high-dose carboplatin. *N Engl J Med* 1993; **328:** 756–61.
9. Hatake K, *et al.* Macrophage colony-stimulating factor and platelet recovery after chemotherapy. *Lancet* 1993; **341:** 963.
10. Moskowitz CH, *et al.* Recombinant methionyl human stem cell factor and filgrastim for peripheral blood progenitor cell mobilization and transplantation in non-Hodgkin's lymphoma patients: results of a phase I/II trial. *Blood* 1997; **89:** 3136–47.
11. Ozer H, *et al.* 2000 Update of recommendations for the use of hematopoietic colony-stimulating factors: evidence-based, clinical practice guidelines. *J Clin Oncol* 2000; **18:** 3558–85.

Extravasation. Extravasation is the leakage of a vesicant or irritant drug into subcutaneous tissue during parenteral administration. This can result in ulceration and severe necrosis in some cases if not dealt with promptly. It is a particular problem with vesicant antineoplastics such as amsacrine, the anthracyclines (doxorubicin and its derivatives), carmustine, dacarbazine, dactinomycin, mitomycin, mustine [chlormethine], plicamycin, streptozocin, the taxanes (docetaxel and paclitaxel), and the vinca alkaloids. Carboplatin, methotrexate, mitozantrone [mitoxantrone], and the podophyllotoxin derivatives (etoposide and teniposide) are examples of irritant drugs which may also cause problems.

Measures to prevent the occurrence of extravasation include giving vesicant or irritant drugs via a central line, or peripherally via a recently sited cannula; vesicants are generally given by intravenous injection into a fast-running infusion. Glyceryl trinitrate patches may be used to dilate veins where venous access is a problem. The site of administration should be regularly checked, and the patient asked to report any untoward sensations.

If extravasation should occur the infusion should be stopped immediately and as much as possible of the infiltrating drug removed by aspiration. Beyond this, however, the management of extravasation is not well standardised and there has been disagreement as to the most appropriate course; there is little data from controlled studies and much practice is based on anecdotal reports and individual experience. Intravenous and subcutaneous injection of a corticosteroid (usually hydrocortisone) has been advocated, although some consider it ineffective or possibly even disadvantageous. Topical application of a 1% hydrocortisone cream to inflamed skin has also been suggested, and antihistamines and, if necessary, analgesics, may be given by mouth. In most cases application of a cold dressing or ice pack is appropriate. However, following extravasation of the taxanes, vinca alkaloids, or cisplatin the use of warm packs with hyaluronidase to enhance uptake from the skin has been recommended; a similar procedure has been suggested for large volume extravasations of the podophyllotoxin derivatives.

The use of specific antidotes is a particularly contentious area, since few are clinically validated and some (such as the use of sodium bicarbonate 8.4% for anthracycline extravasations) may do more harm than good. Brief infiltration of a less concentrated (2.1%) sodium bicarbonate solution, followed after a few minutes by aspiration, is still, however, advocated by some in the management of extravasations of the anthracyclines, carmustine, and plicamycin. Better accepted in the management of anthracycline and mitomycin extravasation is the topical application of dimethyl sulfoxide every 6 hours or so, sometimes alternated with hydrocortisone 1% cream. Sodium thiosulfate 3 or 4% has been used to infiltrate the site of extravasations of cisplatin, dactinomycin, or mustine [chlormethine].

The role of surgery is also important. It is unequivocally necessary in cases where other methods had failed to prevent evolving tissue damage, but there is some dispute as to the role of early surgery to remove drug-laden tissue and prevent the development of more serious ulceration and necrosis. Techniques of saline flushout and liposuction have been developed for removing drug and non-viable tissue while preserving overlying skin.

Some references to the management of extravasation are given below.

1. Brigden ML, Barnett JB. Local toxicity of cancer chemotherapy—practical considerations. *Can J Hosp Pharm* 1986; **39:** 96–9.
2. Dorr RT. Antidotes to vesicant chemotherapy extravasations. *Blood Rev* 1990; **4:** 41–60.
3. Stanley A. Managing complications of chemotherapy. In: Allwood M, *et al.*, eds. *The Cytotoxics Handbook*. 3rd ed. Oxford: Radcliffe Medical Press, 1997: 105–24.
4. Gault DT. Extravasation injuries. *Br J Plast Surg* 1993; **46:** 91–6.
5. Bertelli G. Prevention and management of extravasation of cytotoxic drugs. *Drug Safety* 1995; **12:** 245–55.

Mucositis. A number of drugs have been tried for the prophylaxis of mucositis caused by antineoplastic therapy, both directly and indirectly (due to neutropenia and infection).[1] Some reviewers consider that sucralfate, chlorhexidine and benzydamine are effective drugs,[1] but a large meta-analysis found that only local cooling with ice chips had any significant benefit in mucositis.[2] Some drugs that have been tried with less success include allopurinol, betacarotene, dinoprostone, glutamine, molgramostim, oxpentifylline [pentoxifylline], silver nitrate, and anti-fungal lozenges.[1,2] Given the number of variables involved in the development of mucositis it was thought unlikely that any one prophylactic regimen would prove suitable for all patients.[1]

1. Verdi CJ. Cancer therapy and oral mucositis: an appraisal of drug prophylaxis. *Drug Safety* 1993; **9:** 185–95.
2. Clarkson JE, *et al.* Interventions for preventing oral mucositis or oral candidiasis for patients with cancer receiving chemotherapy (excluding head and neck cancer) (updated 30 August 2000). Available in The Cochrane Library; Issue 4. Oxford: Update Software; 2000.

Nausea and vomiting. For a detailed discussion of the management of chemotherapy-induced nausea and vomiting, see p.1206.

Precautions

In view of their severe toxicity and possible carcinogenicity these drugs should generally be reserved for severe or life-threatening disease, and it is widely suggested that their use and administration should be confined to experienced staff in specialised centres.

Immunosuppression and bone-marrow depression are features of most of these drugs and their use is associated with an increased risk of infections caused by pathogenic or opportunistic micro-organisms, and a reduced capacity to cope with them. Those drugs which are immunosuppressant should not be given, where possible, to patients with acute infections, and dosage reduction or withdrawal should be considered if infection develops, until the infection has been controlled. For cautions regarding the use of vaccines in patients receiving these drugs see Interactions, below. For discussion of the treatment of infections in immunosuppressed patients, see p.125. Special care is necessary in debilitated patients.

Blood counts and measurement of haemoglobin concentrations should be carried out routinely to help predict the onset of bone-marrow depression. Great caution is needed when the marrow is already depressed following radiotherapy or therapy with other antineoplastics, and modification of dosage regimens may be required.

Although positive evidence of teratogenicity in humans is not available for all antineoplastic agents, pregnancy should be avoided in women receiving antineoplastics: in particular they should not be given, if possible, during the first trimester. Mothers receiving antineoplastic therapy should not breast feed. Because some regimens may result in permanent infertility in male patients the storage of semen samples before such therapy may be desirable.

Many antineoplastic drugs are vesicant or irritant. Care must be taken to avoid extravasation since severe pain and tissue damage may ensue. They must be handled with great care and contact with skin and eyes avoided; they should not be inhaled. In many countries official or professional guidelines on precautions for the safe handling of cytotoxic drugs have been issued.

For precautions specific to particular drugs, see under the individual monographs.

Administration in the elderly. Concern has been expressed by workers in a number of countries that neoplastic disorders in the elderly are undertreated because of an impression that these diseases are less aggressive, and the effects of chemotherapy more likely to be severe, in this age group.[1-3] Although there is a suggestion that haematopoietic reserve is reduced with increasing age, which might lead to greater sensitivity to myelosuppression in the elderly,[2] old people vary as much as any other group in their response to drugs, and the consensus is that they should not be excluded from any form of treatment on the grounds of age alone.[1] However, there have been few studies of chemotherapy specifically in elderly patients,[3] and selection of a suitable dosage regimen is more difficult in consequence.

1. Ganz PA. Does (or should) chronologic age influence the choice of cancer treatment? *Oncology (Huntingt)* 1992; **6** (suppl 2): 45-9.
2. Kimmick GG, et al. Cancer chemotherapy in older adults: a tolerability perspective. *Drugs Aging* 1997; **10:** 34-49.
3. Balducci L, Beghe' C. Cancer and age in the USA. *Crit Rev Oncol Hematol* 2001; **37:** 137-45.

Contraception. Immunosuppressive treatment contra-indicates the use of an intra-uterine device for contraception.[1]

1. Anonymous. Medical factors in contraceptive choice. *Drug Ther Bull* 1986; **24:** 73-6.

Handling and disposal. Many antineoplastics are potent and potentially highly toxic drugs, which must be handled with due care. In many countries official or professional guidelines are available for the handling, reconstitution, and disposal of antineoplastic agents, and most centres or institutions in which these drugs are used will have individual handling policies based on these.[1]

Recommendations generally include:

• that these drugs be reconstituted by trained personnel;
• that reconstitution take place in designated areas, designed to protect personnel and the environment—for example, the use of safety cabinets;
• that protective clothing be worn, including gloves, eye protection, and masks if necessary (it should be noted that gloves may vary in their resistance to penetration, depending upon their thickness, the material of which they are made, and the drug in question. Double gloving has been recommended for dealing with major spillages, and for handling amsacrine, carmustine, mustine [chlormethine], and thiotepa in particular[1,2]);
• that waste should be disposed of carefully in suitable separate containers, clearly labelled as to their contents (it should be noted that the patient's body fluids and excreta may contain appreciable amounts of antineoplastic agents, and it has been suggested that they and materials such as bed linen contaminated with them should also be treated as hazardous waste[3,4]);

• that adequate procedures should be in place for accidental contamination due to spillages;
• that staff exposure to antineoplastic agents be recorded and monitored;
• that pregnant staff should avoid handling these agents if possible.

1. Allwood M, Wright P, eds. *The Cytotoxics Handbook.* 3rd ed. Oxford: Radcliffe Medical Press, 1997.
2. Connor TH. Permeability of nitrile rubber, latex, polyurethane, and neoprene gloves to 18 antineoplastic drugs. *Am J Health-Syst Pharm* 1999; **56:** 2450-3.
3. Harris J, Dodds LJ. Handling waste from patients receiving cytotoxic drugs. *Pharm J* 1985; **235:** 289-91.
4. Cass Y, Musgrave CF. Guidelines for the safe handling of excreta contaminated by cytotoxic agents. *Am J Hosp Pharm* 1992; **49:** 1957-8.

Pregnancy. Antineoplastics may be used during pregnancy for their immunosuppressant properties in auto-immune disease, and for the treatment of cancer, which can complicate 1 in 1000 pregnancies.[1,2] Although the use of potentially teratogenic drugs would normally be avoided during pregnancy, the risk to the mother of inadequate treatment may outweigh whatever risks exist of abnormality in the fetus.[1] The highest incidence of adverse effects appears to occur following exposure during the first trimester:[1,2] approximately 10-20% fetuses exposed to cytotoxics during this period have major malformations, compared with 3% in the general population.[1] Anomalies may be found in the heart, neural tube, eye, ear, palate, haematopoietic system, and genital tract.[2] The risk of fetal malformations following exposure during the second and third trimesters is probably no higher than the background rate, but there may still be an increased risk of still-birth, fetal growth restriction, premature birth and maternal or fetal myelosuppression.[1,2] The delayed effects of antineoplastics on development have not been well-documented, but retardation of growth, development, and intellect have been reported, and maternal antineoplastic therapy has been implicated in a case of childhood neuroblastoma and papillary thyroid cancer.[1] The highest risk seems to be associated with alkylating agents and antimetabolites, in particular aminopterin, fluorouracil, and methotrexate.[1-3] The vinca alkaloids and doxorubicin may entail less risk,[2] although the former have produced malformations in *animals*.[1] Other drugs reported to be teratogenic or potentially teratogenic include azathioprine,[3] busulfan,[1] chlorambucil,[1,3] cyclophosphamide,[1,3] cytarabine,[1] mercaptopurine,[3] mustine [chlormethine],[1] and the podophyllotoxin derivatives.[1]

There are no specific dosage recommendations for the administration of antineoplastics during pregnancy, but physiological changes occurring in the mother can alter the pharmacokinetics of drugs.[1,2] This could potentially increase the toxicity of the antineoplastic, or decrease its efficacy.[2] Myelosuppressive chemotherapy should be avoided 3 weeks before the anticipated delivery so that the mother is neither neutropenic nor thrombocytopenic.[1,2] The timing of delivery is also critical for the neonate, as chemotherapy administered shortly before delivery may not be eliminated through the placenta, prolonging exposure in the newborn.[1]

There has also been concern that long-term occupational exposure to antineoplastics might have an adverse effect on the fetus of pregnant health-care workers: a study in 650 Finnish nurses found that women who experienced fetal loss were more than twice as likely to have had first trimester exposure to antineoplastic drugs as women who successfully gave birth.[4] These results have been criticised on the grounds that such results are not generally seen in cancer patients,[5,6] who presumably are exposed to much higher doses of antineoplastic agents. However, similar results were seen in a cross-sectional analysis of 7094 pregnancies involving 2815 nursing and pharmacy staff.[7] Another study[8] has suggested that the rate of ectopic pregnancy may be increased in nurses occupationally exposed to antineoplastics, but the small number of ectopic pregnancies involved (15 in 734 pregnancies) means that the association with antineoplastics may be due to chance, and again, such an effect does not appear to have been reported in women treated with antineoplastic agents.

See also Effects on Reproductive Potential, above.

1. Buekers TE, Lallas TA. Chemotherapy in pregnancy. *Obstet Gynecol Clin North Am* 1998; **25:** 323-9.
2. Falkenberry SS. Cancer in pregnancy. *Surg Oncol Clin N Am* 1998; **7:** 375-97.
3. Østensen M, Ramsey-Goldman R. Treatment of inflammatory rheumatic disorders in pregnancy: what are the safest treatment options? *Drug Safety* 1998; **19:** 389-410.
4. Selevan SG, et al. A study of occupational exposure to antineoplastic drugs and fetal loss in nurses. *N Engl J Med* 1985; **313:** 1173-8.
5. Kalter H. Antineoplastic drugs and spontaneous abortion in nurses. *N Engl J Med* 1986; **314:** 1048-9.
6. Mulvihill JJ, Stewart KR. Antineoplastic drugs and spontaneous abortion in nurses. *N Engl J Med* 1986; **314:** 1049.
7. Valanis B, et al. Occupational exposure to antineoplastic agents: self-reported miscarriages and stillbirths among nurses and pharmacists. *J Occup Environ Med* 1999; **41:** 632-8.
8. Saurel-Cubizolles MJ, et al. Ectopic pregnancy and occupational exposure to antineoplastic drugs. *Lancet* 1993; **341:** 1169-71.

Interactions

Because of their effects on the gastrointestinal mucosa antineoplastics have the potential to interfere with the absorption of other drugs given by mouth. Anti-

neoplastics and immunosuppressants may reduce the response to vaccines, and there is a possibility of generalised infection with live vaccines. The concomitant use of live vaccines should generally be avoided.

Many antineoplastics are inhibitors of certain isoenzymes of cytochrome P450 and some antineoplastics are also metabolised by these enzymes, and in consequence the possibility of interactions between antineoplastics, or between antineoplastics and concomitant medication, cannot be discounted.

Interactions affecting specific drugs are covered under the individual monographs.

◊ References.
1. Le Blanc GA, Waxman DJ. Interaction of anticancer drugs with hepatic monooxygenase enzymes. *Drug Metab Rev* 1989; **20:** 395-439.
2. Loadman PM, Bibby MC. Pharmacokinetic drug interactions with anticancer drugs. *Clin Pharmacokinet* 1994; **26:** 486-500.
3. Kivistö KT, et al. The role of human cytochrome P450 enzymes in the metabolism of anticancer agents: implications for drug interactions. *Br J Clin Pharmacol* 1995; **40:** 523-30.
4. Mignat C. Clinically significant drug interactions with new immunosuppressive agents. *Drug Safety* 1997; **16:** 267-78.

Antiepileptics. Retrospective review of outcomes in children treated for acute lymphoblastic leukaemia indicated that long-term antiepileptic therapy increased the clearance of several antileukaemic drugs and reduced the efficacy of therapy.[1]

1. Relling MV, et al. Adverse effect of anticonvulsants on efficacy of chemotherapy for acute lymphoblastic leukaemia. *Lancet* 2000; **356:** 285-90.

Effects on other drugs. Antineoplastics and/or immunosuppressants have been reported to affect a number of drugs including:

• digoxin (reduced absorption or increased effect, see p.872)
• oral anticoagulants (increased or decreased effect, see Warfarin, p.995)
• phenytoin (increased or decreased effect, see p.360)
• suxamethonium (prolonged effect, see p.1342)
• vaccines (decreased response, see p.1530).

Action

Much of the development of cancer chemotherapy has been based on an understanding of the way in which tumour cells grow, and the way in which the drugs affect this growth.

After cell division the daughter cells enter a period of growth, G_1, which lasts for different lengths of time in different tissues. This is followed by a period of DNA synthesis, S, in which the amount of chromosomal material is doubled, then a postsynthetic, or premitotic, phase, G_2, then finally by mitotic cell division, M. As an alternative to re-entering the cycle, the products of cell division may enter a kinetically-dormant, nonproliferative stage, G_0, although it is not clear if this differs fundamentally from the G_1 phase, nor what recruits such 'resting' cells back into the cell cycle.

The rate of cell division varies for different tumours; the doubling time for Burkitt's lymphoma and acute lymphoblastic leukaemia is less than 5 days, whereas the mean doubling time for seminoma is about 20 days, that for small-cell lung cancer about 50 days, and those for colon cancer and advanced breast cancer about 100 and 150 days respectively. The range of reported doubling times may also vary widely for a particular tumour type. The majority of common cancers increase very slowly in size in comparison with sensitive normal tissues, including those from which they derive, and the rate may decrease further in large tumours. This difference allows normal cells to recover more quickly than malignant ones from chemotherapy, and is the rationale behind current cyclic dosage schedules. The lethal body tumour burden is reached when the tumour cell mass approaches or exceeds 1×10^{12} cells, equivalent to about 1 kg of tissue, and representing about 40 doublings.

Cell killing by cytotoxic agents is generally a first order process, so a given dose or course of antineoplastic kills a fixed percentage of tumour cells rather than a fixed number. Thus an agent which killed 99% of tumour cells would leave behind 10^{10} cells from a tumour containing 10^{12} cells, but only 10^2 cells from one containing 10^4, reinforcing the importance of treating malignant neoplasms as early as possible.

Cytotoxic drugs act to damage the reproductive integrity of cells. Some are active at a particular stage of the cell cycle. The antimetabolites all act at various points to interfere with DNA synthesis, as does hydroxyurea [hydroxycarbamide], and are thus active against cells in S phase, while the vinca alkaloids inhibit microtubular function and act on cells in phase M. Other drugs such as the alkylating agents, the anthracyclines, and cisplatin are not phase-specific, but since their actions are dependent at least in part on damaging DNA they are more effective against proliferating cells, particularly in S phase. It is now thought that many antineoplastics exert their ultimate effect by inducing cellular apoptosis (programmed cell death). Some drugs, such as bleomycin or vinblastine also have the property of arresting the cycle in a particular phase, and attempts have been made to synchronise tumour cell division in this way, to maximise the number of cells in a sensitive phase when a particular drug is used. However, in practice this approach has been less successful than early experimental results suggested.

Some drugs used in the treatment of neoplasms do not attack the tumour cells directly but are given in order to increase cell vulnerability to other modalities: these include radiosensitisers (which have proved of only limited benefit to date), and photosensitisers such as porfimer sodium, which are employed in photodynamic therapy (PDT) using lasers.

Apart from attacking cell division, increased understanding of the molecular biology of tumour cells has begun to open the possibility of other approaches to the treatment of malignant neoplasms. These include inducing tumour cells to differentiate into non-malignant forms, manipulation of cellular apoptosis and signal transduction, inhibiting the expression of abnormal growth factors, telomerases and other oncogene products (including the use of ribozymes or of 'antisense' compounds which inhibit oncogenic messenger RNA), control of tumour growth through inhibition of angiogenesis, prevention or inhibition of metastasis, and stimulating the immune system to recognise and attack tumour cells. Gene therapy (p.1614) is another form of treatment under consideration. However, such approaches remain largely experimental at present.

◊ References.
1. Masson E, Zamboni WC. Pharmacokinetic optimisation of cancer chemotherapy: effect on outcomes. *Clin Pharmacokinet* 1997; **32:** 324–43.
2. Mahler C, *et al.* Clinical pharmacokinetics of the antiandrogens and their efficacy in prostate cancer. *Clin Pharmacokinet* 1998; **34:** 405–417.
3. Njar VCO, Brodie AMH. Comprehensive pharmacology and clinical efficacy of aromatase inhibitors. *Drugs* 1999; **58:** 233–55.
4. Drummond DC, *et al.* Optimizing liposomes for delivery of chemotherapeutic agents to solid tumours. *Pharmacol Rev* 1999; **51:** 691–743.
5. van den Bongard HJGD, *et al.* Pharmacokinetically guided administration of chemotherapeutic agents. *Clin Pharmacokinet* 2000; **39:** 345–67.
6. Kamen BA, *et al.* High-time chemotherapy or high time for low dose. *J Clin Oncol* 2000; **18:** 2935–7.

◊ References to investigational modes of cancer therapy.
1. Culver KW, *et al.* Gene therapy for solid tumors. *Br Med Bull* 1995; **51:** 192–204.
2. Kiehntopf M, *et al.* Clinical applications of ribozymes. *Lancet* 1995; **345:** 1027–31.
3. Haber DA. Telomeres, cancer, and immortality. *N Engl J Med* 1995; **332:** 955–6.
4. Skuse GR, Ludlow JW. Tumor suppressor genes in disease and therapy. *Lancet* 1995; **345:** 902–6.
5. Houghton AN. On course for a cancer vaccine. *Lancet* 1995; **345:** 1384–5.
6. Baltz JK. Vaccines in the treatment of cancer. *Am J Health-Syst Pharm* 1995; **52:** 2574–85.
7. Askari FK, McDonnell WM. Antisense-oligonucleotide therapy. *N Engl J Med* 1996; **334:** 316–18.
8. Harris AL. Antiangiogenesis for cancer therapy. *Lancet* 1997; **349** (suppl II): 13–15.
9. Shu S, *et al.* Tumor immunology. *JAMA* 1997; **278:** 1972–81.
10. Weichselbaum RR, Kufe D. Gene therapy of cancer. *Lancet* 1997; **349** (suppl II): suppl.
11. Martin LA, *et al.* Genetic prodrug activation therapy. *Lancet* 1997; **349:** 1793–4.
12. Gescher A, *et al.* Suppression of tumour development by substances derived from the diet—mechanisms and clinical implications. *Br J Clin Pharmacol* 1998; **45:** 1–12.
13. Sikic BI. New approaches in cancer treatment. *Ann Oncol* 1999; **10** (suppl 6): 149–53.
14. Knuth A, *et al.* Cancer immunotherapy in clinical oncology. *Cancer Chemother Pharmacol* 2000; **46** (suppl): S46–51.
15. Nelson AR, *et al.* Matrix metalloproteinases: biologic activity and clinical implications. *J Clin Oncol* 2000; **18:** 1135–49.
16. Diel IJ. Antitumour effects of bisphosphonates: first evidence and possible mechanisms. *Drugs* 2000; **59:** 391–9.

17. Noonberg SB, Benz CC. Tyrosine kinase inhibitors targeted to the epidermal growth factor receptor subfamily: role as anticancer agents. *Drugs* 2000; **59:** 753–67.
18. Vile RG, *et al.* Cancer gene therapy: hard lessons and new courses. *Gene Ther* 2000; **7:** 2–8.
19. Bodey B, *et al.* Failure of cancer vaccines: the significant limitations of this approach to immunotherapy. *Anticancer Res* 2000; **20:** 2665–76.
20. Green MC, *et al.* Monoclonal antibody therapy for solid tumors. *Cancer Treat Rev* 2000; **26:** 269–86.

Resistance

Resistance to antineoplastics is one of the greatest limitations to the use of chemotherapy in malignant disease. Resistance may be intrinsic to the tumour or may be acquired during chemotherapy, which effectively acts to select resistant cells from a heterogeneous population; the latter is one reason that relapses, or malignancies in heavily-pretreated patients, may be particularly difficult to treat.

The mechanisms of resistance in cancer cells are complex and imperfectly understood, but appear to include:
• hypoxia and imperfect drug penetration in the centre of large, solid tumours
• the small proportion of cells actively dividing and thus vulnerable to antineoplastics (particularly in slow-growing tumours)
• decreased cellular uptake or increased efflux of antineoplastic
• increased metabolic breakdown or decreased activation of antineoplastic
• increased expression of target enzymes
• metabolism via alternative biochemical pathways to those blocked by the antineoplastic
• more efficient repair of damaged DNA
• possibly the expression of genes which inhibit drug-induced apoptosis.

Several of these mechanisms may be in operation at one time. Much interest has been expressed in the potential use of drugs which can modulate or inhibit mechanisms of resistance, and in particular in compounds such as valspodar, verapamil, quinidine, and ciclosporin, which have the ability to block the action of p-glycoprotein, a membrane glycoprotein which acts as an efflux pump for a range of cytotoxic substances and which is responsible for the multi-drug resistant (MDR) phenotype. However, for sustained benefit it seems likely that several agents would be required, each to overcome a different mechanism of resistance, and it would be necessary to ensure that toxicity of antineoplastics to normal cells was not also enhanced.

If the emergence of heritable resistant phenotypes is a natural part of tumour-cell biology (the Goldie-Coldman hypothesis) it implies that the larger and older the tumour, the more likely is resistance to occur. This would confirm the benefits of surgery and radiotherapy to shrink the primary tumour, and of starting chemotherapy as soon as possible after (a preferably early) diagnosis.

◊ Reviews of antineoplastic resistance.
1. Booser DJ, Hortobagyi GN. Anthracycline antibiotics in cancer therapy: focus on drug resistance. *Drugs* 1994; **47:** 223–58.
2. Ling V. P-Glycoprotein: its role in drug resistance. *Am J Med* 1995; **99** (suppl 6A): 31S–34S.
3. Kaye SB. Clinical drug resistance: the role of factors other than P-glycoprotein. *Am J Med* 1995; **99** (suppl 6A): 44S–44S.
4. Holmes J. Multidrug resistance as a cause of cytotoxic drug failure. *Pharm J* 1996; **257:** 294–6.
5. Dumontet C, Sikic BI. Mechanisms of action of and resistance to antitubulin agents: microtubule dynamics, drug transport, and cell death. *J Clin Oncol* 1999; **17:** 1061–70.
6. Sikic BI. Modulation of multidrug resistance: a paradigm for translational clinical research. *Oncology (Huntingt)* 1999; **13:** 183–7.

◊ Some drugs have been reported to partially abolish multidrug resistance to antineoplastics *in vitro*.[1] These include verapamil, its enantiomers and analogues such as Ro-11-2933; other calcium-channel blockers including prenylamine, diltiazem, nifedipine analogues such as nicardipine and niludipine, and bepridil; various phenothiazines and thioxanthenes including trifluoperazine and the *trans*-isomer of flupentixol, which lacks dopamine-antagonist properties and the consequent extrapyramidal effects; structural analogues of the anthracyclines and vinca alkaloids; progesterone and other steroid hormones, as well as, to some extent, anti-oestrogens such as tamoxifen; ciclosporin and various of its nonimmunosuppressive ana-

logues (such as valspodar); and various miscellaneous agents including amiodarone, quinidine, propranolol, reserpine, yohimbine, dipyridamole, erythromycin, cefoperazone, and ceftriaxone.

However, despite reported effects on resistance *in vitro* clinical results may be less impressive: studies in which verapamil was added to therapy for small cell lung cancer[2] or multiple myeloma[3] failed to demonstrate any benefit.

1. Ford JM, Hait WN. Pharmacology of drugs that alter multidrug resistance in cancer. *Pharmacol Rev* 1990; **42:** 155–99.
2. Milroy R, *et al.* A randomised clinical study of verapamil in addition to combination chemotherapy in small cell lung cancer. *Br J Cancer* 1993; **68:** 813–18.
3. Dalton WS, *et al.* A phase III randomized study of oral verapamil as a chemosensitizer to reverse drug resistance in patients with refractory myeloma: a Southwest Oncology Group Study. *Cancer* 1995; **75:** 815–20.

Choice of Antineoplastic

Role of chemotherapy

In 1994, in a consultation document on cancer chemotherapy,[1] WHO considered that 24 drugs could be considered essential for the rational management of malignant neoplasms.

In 1999, WHO updated the list of essential drugs.[2] The new list divides drugs into 3 categories:
• 17 essential drugs that are used to treat curable cancers or cancers for which the cost-benefit ratio clearly favours drug treatment (bleomycin, *chlorambucil*, cisplatin, cyclophosphamide, *cytarabine*, dactinomycin, daunorubicin, doxorubicin, etoposide, fluorouracil, mercaptopurine, methotrexate, prednisolone, procarbazine, tamoxifen, vinblastine, and vincristine) [note: drugs in italics in this list were not in the previous 1994 list]
• 12 drugs that may have advantages in certain clinical situations (*busulfan, carboplatin, flutamide,* folinic acid, *gonadorelin analogues, interferon alfa, melphalan, megestrol,* mitomycin, *mitozantrone [mitoxantrone], paclitaxel, and vinorelbine)* [note: drugs in italics in this list were not in the previous 1994 list]
• 13 drugs judged as currently not essential for the effective delivery of cancer care (aminoglutethimide, anastrozole, altretamine, carmustine, dacarbazine, docetaxel, epirubicin, gemcitabine, ifosfamide, irinotecan, lomustine, raltitrexed, and topotecan). [note: none of these drugs, except dacarbazine, were in the previous 1994 list.]

Drugs that were in the 1994 list that are no longer in the 1999 list are asparaginase, cladribine, hydroxyurea [hydroxycarbamide], mustine [chlormethine], and levamisole. WHO considers that for some tumours such as hepatocellular carcinoma and lung cancer the development of effective prevention programmes through hepatitis B immunisation and tobacco control is of greater priority than therapy in the immediate future.[2]

Despite the real benefits achieved in selected conditions, reassessment of the role and value of chemotherapy for malignant neoplasms has led a number of oncologists to express the view that it has not lived up to its promise. Braverman[3] suggested in 1991 that for many or most patients medical management should be confined to symptom management and enrolment in a hospice programme, with a considerable reduction in the prescription of antineoplastics and a confinement of studies to agents with novel mechanisms of action, or refinement of regimens known to be effective, a view he has since reiterated.[4] Similar views have been expressed by others during the 1980s and 90s, pointing out the failure of treatment for most common adult tumours,[5] and suggesting that widespread use of chemotherapy is not justified outside clinical trials or specialised centres.[6,7] Bailar and Smith, in a statistical review in 1986, suggested that the 'war against cancer' was being lost, and that concentration on prevention rather than treatment might produce more promising results.[8] Despite acknowledging some areas of progress, an update of this review including data up to the end of 1994 came to the same conclusion.[9] Others have also pointed out the failure to adequately address methods for cancer prevention.[10]

Such views have naturally provoked controversy, and others consider that developments in the use of adjuvant and intensive regimens, as well as the continuing development of new agents, are significant and should not be denigrated.[11-15] However, the frequent reference to the hoped-for benefits of a greatly-improved knowledge of the molecular biology of cancer, and in particular the use of biological response modifiers,[12,16] or gene therapy,[17] does seem to concede that present chemotherapeutic regimens could be improved. Whether dose intensification is one appropriate route for improvement is a matter of some debate,[18,19] and, so far, clear evidence of effectiveness has been reported only for certain leukaemias and lymphomas.[2]

It has been suggested that perhaps attempts to destroy cancer cells are based on a false analogy between oncology and microbiology, and that a more appropriate goal would be the restoration of mechanisms of cellular control, enabling the patient to live with their cancer. Understanding of malignancy as a process, involving complex interactions between the malignant cell and its environment, in which intervention may be feasible to restore regulation of cellular growth, offers a potentially useful approach to cancer treatment. Although such an approach remains largely theoretical at present,[10,20,21] some drugs currently available, such as imatinib and trastuzumab, offer glimpses of its potential.

1. WHO. Essential drugs for cancer chemotherapy. *Bull WHO* 1994; **72:** 693–8.
2. Sikora K, *et al.* Essential drugs for cancer therapy: a World Health Organization consultation. *Ann Oncol* 1999; **10:** 385–90.
3. Braverman AS. Medical oncology in the 1990s. *Lancet* 1991; **337:** 901–2.
4. Braverman AS. Chemotherapeutic failure: resistance or insensitivity? *Ann Intern Med* 1993; **118:** 630–2.
5. Kearsley JH. Cytotoxic chemotherapy for common adult malignancies: the emperor's new clothes revisited? *BMJ* 1986; **293:** 871–6.
6. Milsted RAV, *et al.* Cancer chemotherapy—what have we achieved? *Lancet* 1980; **i:** 1343–6.
7. Mead GM. Chemotherapy for solid tumours: routine treatment not yet justified. *BMJ* 1995; **310:** 246–7.
8. Bailar JC, Smith EM. Progress against cancer? *N Engl J Med* 1986; **314:** 1226–32.
9. Bailar JC, Gornik HL. Cancer undefeated. *N Engl J Med* 1997; **336:** 1569–74.
10. Sporn MB. The war on cancer. *Lancet* 1996; **347:** 1377–81.
11. Tobias JS. Medical oncology in the 1990s. *Lancet* 1991; **337:** 1220.
12. Chabner BA, Rothenberg ML. Medical oncology in the 1990s. *Lancet* 1991; **338:** 576–7.
13. Chabner BA. Biological basis for cancer treatment. *Ann Intern Med* 1993; **118:** 633–7.
14. Cunningham D. Chemotherapy for solid tumours; important progress in treatment. *BMJ* 1995; **310:** 247–8.
15. Kramer BS, Klausner RD. Grappling with cancer—defeatism versus the reality of progress. *N Engl J Med* 1997; **337:** 931–4.
16. Malpas JS. Oncology. *Postgrad Med J* 1990; **66:** 80–93.
17. Lemoine NR, Sikora K. Interventional genetics and cancer treatment. *BMJ* 1993; **306:** 665–6.
18. Hryniuk W. Will increases in dose intensity improve outcome: pro. *Am J Med* 1995; **99** (suppl 6A): 69S–70S.
19. Souhami RL. Will increases in dose intensity improve outcome: con. *Am J Med* 1995; **99** (suppl 6A): 71S–76S.
20. Astrow AB. Rethinking cancer. *Lancet* 1994; **343:** 494–5.
21. Schipper H, *et al.* A new biological framework for cancer research. *Lancet* 1996; **348:** 1149–51.

Management of malignant disease
Carcinoid tumours and other secretory neoplasms. All neoplastic cells have some abnormalities of metabolism, and many secrete characteristic metabolic products. Where the substance secreted has hormonal or pharmacological properties profound clinical effects may result, particularly since secretion is generally unregulated by normal homoeostatic mechanisms. Examples of syndromes associated with such secretory neoplasms include acromegaly (p.1271), Cushing's syndrome (p.1272), hyperprolactinaemia (p.1274), and other endocrine disorders associated with pituitary adenomas; phaeochromocytoma (p.810); and carcinoid syndrome and the various syndromes associated with pancreatic endocrine tumours. Multiple endocrine neoplasia type 1 (MEN1) is an inherited condition in which many tumours occur in often more than one endocrine organ; tumours in this disorder are often secretory.

Carcinoid syndrome. Carcinoid tumours occur mainly in the gastrointestinal tract or lungs (bronchi), although they occasionally arise in other organs with a common embryological origin. Although they are relatively common, accounting for about 30% of all small bowel tumours, symptomatic carcinoid syndrome is rare, both because the tumours vary in their behaviour depending on their embryological origin and because the liver is capable of metabolising those tumour products which are secreted into the portal circulation; only if the carcinoid tumour secretes into the systemic circulation, notably after metastasis to the liver, do symptoms occur. Tumours of embryological foregut origin, usually found in the lung or stomach, predominantly secrete histamine or serotonin (5-HT); mid-gut tumours, with a usual primary site in the terminal ileum, are the most likely to metastasise and produce carcinoid syndrome, and predominantly secrete serotonin; hind-gut tumours, commonly benign, do not secrete active substances.

The characteristic symptoms of carcinoid syndrome include episodic flushing of the face and upper trunk (which may be provoked by alcohol, food, or stress), secretory diarrhoea, wheezing and dyspnoea, weight loss, pellagra, painful hepatomegaly, and right-sided valvular heart disease, which sometimes progresses to right heart failure and death.

The management of carcinoid tumours usually involves surgical resection, and this can be curative, particularly if the primary tumour has not metastasised.[1-3] Antineoplastic chemotherapy has only limited benefit,[1] except perhaps in patients with atypical variants of carcinoid tumours.[2] There is some evidence that treatment with interferon alfa can stabilise the disease or occasionally produce tumour regression,[3] but adverse effects have limited its use.[2] Hepatic arterial embolisation to destroy the blood supply of hepatic metastases has produced symptomatic palliation, but its effects are temporary.[1,2] Results may be better in combination with systemic chemotherapy in selected patients.[4] Antineoplastics such as doxorubicin have also been administered into the hepatic artery for treating hepatic metastases.[2]

For symptomatic relief of carcinoid syndrome somatostatin analogues such as octreotide or lanreotide are highly effective and are the treatment of choice.[1-3] The availability of depot intramuscular preparations has simplified treatment, removing the need for multiple daily subcutaneous injections. However, with prolonged use a few patients develop resistance even to the highest doses.[1] Octreotide is also used in the perioperative management of these patients to treat or prevent carcinoid crisis, when it may be administered intravenously.[1,5] Other drugs that reduce the effects of serotonin that have been tried include cyproheptadine, ondansetron, ketanserin, and methysergide.[1]

Apart from such specific pharmacological therapies, antidiarrhoeals such as codeine phosphate and loperamide are sometimes helpful in controlling diarrhoea. Wheezing (bronchoconstriction) and heart failure are managed conventionally. Supplementation with nicotinamide is advisable to prevent pellagra. It is also important to avoid provocative factors such as stress, alcohol, and particular foods.[1]

Pancreatic endocrine tumours. Neoplasms of the pancreatic islet cells (pancreatic endocrine tumours) are uncommon compared with those of the exocrine pancreas (see Malignant Neoplasms of the Pancreas, p.497). Pancreatic endocrine tumours, whether benign or malignant, often secrete clinically significant amounts of hormone; the hormone secreted, and hence the resultant clinical syndrome, depends on which of the several types of hormone-secreting islet cells is the origin of the tumour (for example, insulinomas arise in islet beta cells).[6] Primary therapy for solitary pancreatic endocrine tumours is surgical resection; metastatic tumours may require a combination of symptomatic drug therapy, chemotherapy, radiotherapy, and surgical debulking. The most frequently used antineoplastic is streptozocin, either alone or combined with other drugs such as fluorouracil or doxorubicin.[6,7] Chlorozotocin is also active.[7] As with carcinoid tumours, hepatic metastases may be treated with hepatic artery embolisation.[3,4,6] Somatostatin analogues and interferon alfa may be used to control symptoms of pancreatic endocrine tumours.[3] Other therapies depend on the specific tumour type. In patients with **insulinoma** (tumours originating in the islet beta cells) excessive insulin secretion results in hypoglycaemia. Where surgical resection is not feasible or not successful diazoxide may be used to control hypoglycaemia. Beneficial results have also been achieved with octreotide. Intake of frequent small meals containing complex carbohydrates is also important.[6] Up to 90% of insulinomas are benign and do not metastasise. In **glucagonoma** the primary neoplasm derives from the alpha cell[6] and the clinical syndrome (a characteristic skin rash known as necrolytic migratory erythema, diabetes mellitus or glucose intolerance, weight loss, and anaemia) results from excessive glucagon secretion. Surgical resection is indicated for localised disease but 50 to 80% of cases have metastasised at presentation. Octreotide usually decreases glucagon secretion and improves symptoms. Another well characterised syndrome results from tumours which release vasoactive intestinal polypeptide (VIP). Such **vipomas** result in profound but intermittent secretory diarrhoea, with consequent hypokalaemia and acidosis;[6] the syndrome is sometimes known as pancreatic cholera. Metabolic imbalances should be corrected by fluid and electrolyte supplementation. Octreotide controls the secretory diarrhoea, and it may be useful for symptom control before surgery as well as for palliation in metastatic disease. About 80% of vipomas are malignant.[6]

Of the other pancreatic endocrine tumours **gastrinoma** is the commonest: it results in Zollinger-Ellison syndrome, the treatment of which is discussed on p.1209. Rarer tumours include **somatostatinoma** and **PPoma** (secreting pancreatic polypeptide).[6]

1. Caplin ME, *et al.* Carcinoid tumour. *Lancet* 1998; **352:** 799–805.
2. Kulke MH, Mayer RJ. Carcinoid tumors. *N Engl J Med* 1999; **340:** 858–68.
3. Öberg K. Advances in chemotherapy and biotherapy of endocrine tumours. *Curr Opin Oncol* 1998; **10:** 58–65.
4. Moertel CG, *et al.* The management of patients with advanced carcinoid tumors and islet cell carcinomas. *Ann Intern Med* 1994; **120:** 302–9.
5. Veall GRQ, *et al.* Review of the anaesthetic management of 21 patients undergoing laparotomy for carcinoid syndrome. *Br J Anaesth* 1994; **72:** 335–41.
6. Sharma V, Lynn JA. Rare tumours 1: the management of rare endocrine tumours of the pancreas. *CME Oncol* 1999; **1:** 85–92.
7. Moertel CG, *et al.* Streptozocin-doxorubicin, streptozocin-fluorouracil, or chlorozotocin in the treatment of advanced islet-cell carcinoma. *N Engl J Med* 1992; **326:** 519–23.

Gestational trophoblastic tumours. The gestational trophoblastic diseases arise from the trophoblast, the first tissue to differentiate in the early embryo, and thus are associated with conception and pregnancy and affect women of reproductive age. They may be divided into molar pregnancy (complete or partial hydatidiform mole), invasive mole (chorioadenoma destruens), choriocarcinoma, and placental site trophoblastic tumour. A persistent gestational trophoblastic tumour (invasive mole or choriocarcinoma) may develop in about 25% of women after evacuation of a complete molar pregnancy, and about 2 to 4% after a partial molar pregnancy.[1] Choriocarcinoma may also occur after normal delivery, abortion, or ectopic pregnancy. All these tumours secrete human chorionic gonadotrophin (hCG), and measurement of the urinary or serum concentrations, which are generally proportional to the total tumour mass, is important in diagnosis of disease and monitoring of treatment.

The trophoblastic tumours vary in aggressiveness but some, such as choriocarcinoma, are highly invasive and rapidly fatal if untreated; however, appropriate treatment, based on the perceived risk category, can result in an excellent prognosis. Prognostic factors for increased risk include high titres of hCG, liver or brain metastases, and failure of previous single-agent chemotherapy as well as, perhaps, greater age. With current treatment, including local irradiation for metastases, virtually 100% of patients with localised disease should be cured, as are over 70% of patients with more advanced stages.

Prophylactic chemotherapy has been used in women considered at particular risk of persistent gestational trophoblastic tumour after evacuation of a complete molar pregnancy, but the practice is controversial.[1]

In patients who develop low- or moderate-risk choriocarcinoma or invasive mole, the treatment of choice is single-agent chemotherapy with methotrexate or dactinomycin.[1-3] The combination EMA-CO (etoposide, methotrexate, dactinomycin, cyclophosphamide, and vincristine) is the current preferred treatment in high-risk patients.[1,3,4] A combination of methotrexate, dactinomycin, and either cyclophosphamide or chlorambucil was the preferred combination in the past. Drugs that may be used in salvage regimens include cisplatin and bleomycin.[3,4]

Brain or liver metastases are generally treated by local irradiation.

Patients with placental site trophoblastic tumour, which is relatively insensitive to chemotherapy, may be best treated by hysterectomy in the early stages.[1] In high-risk patients, a platinum-based regimen is preferred to EMA-CO.[3]

1. Berkowitz RS, Goldstein DP. Chorionic tumors. *N Engl J Med* 1996; **335:** 1740–8.
2. Homesley HD. Single-agent therapy for nonmetastatic and low-risk gestational trophoblastic disease. *J Reprod Med* 1998; **43:** 69–74.
3. Newlands ES, *et al.*. Recent advances in gestational trophoblastic disease. *Hematol Oncol Clin North Am* 1999; **13:** 225–44.
4. Lurain JR. Management of high-risk gestational trophoblastic disease. *J Reprod Med* 1998; **43:** 44–52.

Histiocytic syndromes. Histiocytic syndromes cover a broad range of proliferative disorders of histiocytes (macrophages and dendritic cells), for which the classification and diagnostic criteria are evolving.[1] Langerhans-cell histiocytosis (histiocytosis X) is one such disorder characterised by proliferation of CD1 positive Langerhans cells (a form of dendritic cell).[1] Terms that were formerly used for different clinical manifestations of Langerhans-cell histiocytosis include eosinophilic granuloma, Hand-Schüller-Christian disease, and Letterer-

Siwe syndrome,[1-3] but these are now considered obsolete.[1] Langerhans-cell histiocytosis mainly presents in childhood, and is of uncertain aetiology: it is not clear whether it should be considered a malignancy.

The clinical presentation of Langerhans-cell histiocytosis is highly variable.[2-5] The classic feature is single or multiple bone lesions, and skin lesions may also occur (restricted disease).[3,5] The disorder may also involve visceral organs, ultimately causing dysfunction of the liver, lungs, or bone marrow (extensive or multisystem disease). Sequelae to the disease include diabetes insipidus, growth failure, and orthopaedic handicap.[3,4] The morbidity and prognosis depends upon the number of organ systems involved, and whether normal function of these organs is affected. Patients with restricted disease have a generally benign course, and single lesions often regress spontaneously. However, if a bone lesion does not resolve, or risks causing fracture or deformity before it resolves, or is causing disabling symptoms, it may be treated with curettage, intralesional corticosteroids, or radiotherapy.[3,5] Similarly, single skin lesions may be allowed to resolve without treatment or treated with methoxsalen plus UV light (PUVA) or topical mustine [chlormethine]. Multiple bone lesions may be treated with single-agent chemotherapy.[5]

In more extensive disease the prognosis is not as good, mainly due to organ dysfunction.[3-5] Systemic chemotherapy has been widely used, because the disease tends to be progressive in these patients, but its degree of benefit is uncertain[2-5] and some consider it primarily of value for palliation.[2] A comparative study of the effects of vinblastine or etoposide, both of which have been widely used in moderate- to high-risk patients, was initiated in 1991,[6] and showed a response rate of about 65%.[5] To see if these results can be improved on, a randomised trial of combination chemotherapy has been started.[5] In patients who have not responded to combination chemotherapy, a number of treatments may be considered including ciclosporin,[5] the nucleoside analogues cladribine or pentostatin,[7] and bone marrow transplantation.[4,5] Anti-CD1 monoclonal antibodies[8] may offer improved therapeutic or diagnostic options in the future.

1. Favara BE, et al.. Contemporary classification of histiocytic disorders. The WHO Committee on Histiocytic/Reticulum Cell Proliferations and Reclassification Working Group of the Histiocyte Society. Med Pediatr Oncol 1997; 29: 157–66.
2. Komp DM. Concepts in staging and clinical studies for treatment of Langerhans' cell histiocytosis. Semin Oncol 1991; 18: 18–23.
3. Egeler RM, D'Angio GJ. Langerhans cell histiocytosis. J Pediatr 1995; 127: 1–11.
4. The French Langerhans' Cell Histiocytosis Study Group. A multicentre retrospective survey of Langerhans' cell histiocytosis: 348 cases observed between 1983 and 1993. Arch Dis Child 1996; 75: 17–24.
5. Ladisch S. Langerhans cell histiocytosis. Curr Opin Hematol 1998; 5: 54–8.
6. Ladisch S, et al. LCH-I: a randomized trial of etoposide vs vinblastine in disseminated Langerhans cell histiocytosis. Med Pediatr Oncol 1994; 23: 107–10.
7. Weitzman S, et al. Nucleoside analogues in the therapy of Langerhans cell histiocytosis: a survey of members of the Histiocyte Society and review of the literature. Med Pediatr Oncol 1999; 33: 476–81.
8. Kelly K, et al. CD1 antibody immunolocalisation in Langerhans' cell histiocytosis. Lancet 1993; 342: 367–8.

Leukaemias, acute. The acute leukaemias are malignancies affecting haematopoietic precursor cells. They are relatively rare (about 1 to 3 cases per 100 000 of population), and of uncertain cause in the majority of cases, although radiation, carcinogenic substances, or oncogenic retroviruses have been implicated in some types, and certain individuals appear to have a genetic predisposition to these diseases.

Following the initiating event or events the progeny of the affected cell do not differentiate normally but proliferate in an uncontrolled fashion. The result is the accumulation in the blood and bone marrow of immature cell types (blasts) at the expense of normal functional blood cells.

The acute leukaemias may be broadly divided into **acute lymphoblastic leukaemia** (ALL), in which the neoplastic proliferation affects lymphoid cell lines, and the **acute myeloid leukaemias** (AML), variously known as acute myelogenous leukaemias or acute non-lymphoblastic leukaemias, which affect myeloid cell lines. These broad groups can be divided in various ways. ALL is subdivided by an immunophenotypic classification that distinguishes disease of B- and T-cell lineage; it was formerly divided morphologically into L1, L2, and L3 subtypes. For AML the French-American-British (FAB) classification has been widely used. This distinguishes, by lineage and estimated degree of differentiation:

M0, undifferentiated AML

M1, AML with minimal maturation

M2, AML with maturation

M3, acute promyelocytic leukaemia

M4, acute myelomonocytic leukaemia

M5, acute monocytic leukaemia

M6, erythroid leukaemia

M7, megakaryocytic leukaemia.

However, knowledge of the genotype, via cytogenetic or molecular analysis, is becoming increasingly important in the treatment of leukaemia. Consequently, a revised classification system has been proposed under the auspices of WHO, which uses a combination of morphology, immunophenotype, genetic, and clinical features. In this classification, AML is divided into 4 main groups: AML with recurrent cytogenic translocations; AML with myelodysplasia-related features; therapy-related AML; and AML not otherwise specified.[1] In this classification, acute lymphoblastic leukaemias and lymphoblastic lymphomas are considered to be a single disease with different presentations.

Acute leukaemia usually presents with anaemia, infection (due to granulocytopenia), and bleeding (mainly due to thrombocytopenia). Onset is usually rapid with ALL, although AML may be preceded by myelodysplasia lasting months or years. Bone pain, and enlargement of liver, spleen and lymph nodes due to infiltration of leukaemic cells may occur. Other organs may also be affected, and various metabolic disturbances, including hyperuricaemia, hyponatraemia, and hypokalaemia may be present.

If untreated the acute leukaemias are normally fatal, usually within months. However, these malignancies are among those in which medical treatment can make a substantial difference to life expectancy, and in some cases a permanent remission may be effected.

1. Harris NL, et al. World Health Organization classification of neoplastic diseases of the hematopoietic and lymphoid tissues: report of the clinical advisory committee meeting–Airlie House, Virginia, November 1997. J Clin Oncol 1999; 17: 3835–49.

ACUTE LYMPHOBLASTIC LEUKAEMIA. With current chemotherapy regimens, long-term disease free survival can be achieved in 70 to 80% of children and 20 to 40% of adults with acute lymphoblastic leukaemia (ALL). While there is a lack of consensus on some prognostic factors, it is generally accepted that age less than 1 year or greater than 10 years, and high white cell count at the time of diagnosis indicate patients at higher risk of relapse. These factors probably reflect the presence of specific genotypes. The genotype with the worst prognosis is BCR-ABL t(9;22), which generates the Philadelphia chromosome; this occurs in 3 to 5 % of children and 25% of adults with ALL.

Standard treatment regimens for T-cell and precursor B-cell ALL consist of 2 to 3 years of therapy divided into several phases: a short induction phase; an intensification (consolidation) phase; therapy for prophylaxis of CNS disease, starting during the induction phase, and sometimes continuing for an extended period; and a prolonged continuation (maintenance) phase, sometimes including re-induction therapy.[1-3] Treatment for mature B-cell ALL (Burkitt cell leukaemia) is different in terms of the drugs used, and the maintenance phase is not required.[2,3]

The aim of **induction therapy** is to induce complete remission, and a slow early response to this therapy has been reported to be an indicator of poor prognosis.[3] Standard induction regimens include vincristine and a corticosteroid (prednisolone or prednisone, or dexamethasone), plus asparaginase in children and an anthracycline such as doxorubicin in adults. However, it is now accepted that better remission rates and more prolonged remissions can be achieved with more intensive induction therapy using 4 to 5 drugs—often vincristine, a corticosteroid, asparaginase, and an anthracycline, with or without cyclophosphamide. The use of dexamethasone, rather than prednisolone, in the induction regimen appears to yield improved event-free survival and a lower incidence of CNS relapse.[4,5] However, some have reported a higher incidence of fatal sepsis with the use of dexamethasone.[6] For mature B-cell ALL, a 2- to 8-month intensive regimen of high-dose cyclophosphamide, high-dose methotrexate, and cytarabine is commonly used, sometimes with the addition of ifosfamide and/or etoposide.[3]

About 60% of children and 35% of adults who achieve an initial remission will subsequently relapse with meningeal involvement unless **CNS therapy** directed at the sanctuary sites in the meninges is undertaken. Effective prophylaxis can reduce the incidence of CNS relapse to around 2 to 5%.[3,5] Standard therapy consists of cranial irradiation and intrathecal methotrexate. However, concerns regarding the neurotoxicity of cranial irradiation and its ability to cause secondary brain tumours have led to the investigation of chemotherapy alone, particularly in children.[3-5] Regimens include intrathecal methotrexate combined with high-dose systemic methotrexate, and triple intrathecal chemotherapy with methotrexate, cytarabine and a corticosteroid. These regimens are started during induction therapy and continued intermittently for an extended period. Cranial irradiation may still be required in high-risk patients.[5]

Intensification (consolidation) therapy involves continuation of intensive chemotherapy regimens after the achievement of complete remission. Drugs used in intensification regimens include high-dose cytarabine, etoposide, teniposide, high-dose methotrexate, mercaptopurine, tioguanine, and the antineoplastics used in induction regimens; often 4- to 5-drug combinations are used. The UKALL Trial X showed that addition of intensification therapy at 5 and 20 weeks from the beginning of induction, (using cytarabine, etoposide, tioguanine, and daunorubicin), produced 5-year disease-free survival of 71% compared with 57% in those who received only maintenance therapy.[7] Benefit was seen even in children considered at low risk of treatment failure. Further intensification may benefit those children with a slow response to initial therapy and high-risk of relapse.[8] The value of intensification therapy in adults is less certain, but it appears to result in a longer duration of remission.[2,3]

Continuation (maintenance) therapy is generally given for some 2 to 3 years after remission;[1-3] in the UK treatment is continued for 100 weeks from diagnosis.[9] The standard combination of drugs consists of daily mercaptopurine, weekly methotrexate, and prednisolone and vincristine monthly. Three years rather than two years of maintenance therapy is associated with a lower risk of relapse but not a markedly different survival rate.[10] Many protocols provide for periods of **re-induction** therapy (repeating induction therapy) alternating with standard maintenance,[3] and such intensive therapy is associated with an absolute improvement of about 4% in long-term survival.[10] It has been suggested that individualisation of methotrexate dosage to take account of the patient's ability to clear the drug can improve the outcome.[11]

It is generally agreed that patients who maintain remission for 4 years after the end of maintenance therapy are at little risk of relapse and may be regarded as effectively cured.

Patients who relapse after stopping treatment can usually be brought to **second remission**, often by a repeat of their original induction therapy. However, if relapse occurs during treatment the prognosis is poor, and chemotherapy is unlikely to bring lasting benefit.

The role of **stem-cell transplantation** in the treatment of ALL is a matter of some controversy. Bone-marrow transplantation is associated with significant mortality and morbidity, and the relapse rate of ALL after transplantation is significant, with overall survival generally being similar to that for intensive chemotherapy in unselected patients. Consequently, allogeneic transplantation is usually reserved for patients who do not have a complete remission with induction therapy, and those who are in second remission after relapse.[2,3,12] Transplantation during first remission is considered for patients with Philadelphia-positive ALL, since these patients have a very poor prognosis.[12,13] The lack of suitable HLA-matched family donors has led to the investigation of autologous purged marrow, or the use of marrow from mismatched family donors; however, generally neither of these options has proved more effective than chemotherapy.[13,14] The use of matched unrelated donors has shown some promise,[3,12] and the use of cord blood or peripheral blood stem cells is under investigation.

1. Rivera GK, et al. Treatment of acute lymphoblastic leukemia: 30 years' experience at St Jude Children's Research Hospital. N Engl J Med 1993; 329: 1289–95.
2. Kantarjian HM. Adult acute lymphocytic leukemia: critical review of current knowledge. Am J Med 1994; 97: 176–84.
3. Pui C-H, Evans WE. Acute lymphoblastic leukemia. N Engl J Med 1998; 339: 605–15.
4. Veerman AJP, et al. High cure rate with a moderately intensive treatment regimen in non-high-risk childhood acute lymphoblastic leukemia: results of protocol ALL VI from the Dutch Childhood Leukemia Study Group. J Clin Oncol 1996; 14: 911–18.
5. Pui C-H. Acute lymphoblastic leukemia in children. Curr Opin Oncol 2000; 12: 3–12.

6. Hurwitz CA, *et al.* Substituting dexamethasone for prednisolone complicates remission induction in children with acute lymphoblastic leukemia. *Cancer* 2000; **88:** 1964–9.
7. Chessells JM, *et al.* Intensification of treatment and survival in all children with lymphoblastic leukaemia: results of UK Medical Research Council trial UKALL X. *Lancet* 1995; **345:** 143–8.
8. Nachman JB, *et al.* Augmented post-induction therapy for children with high-risk acute lymphoblastic leukemia and a slow response to initial therapy. *N Engl J Med* 1998; **338:** 1663–7.
9. Chessells JM. Maintenance treatment and shared care in lymphoblastic leukaemia. *Arch Dis Child* 1995; **73:** 368–73.
10. Childhood ALL Collaborative Group. Duration and intensity of maintenance chemotherapy in acute lymphoblastic leukaemia: overview of 42 trials involving 12000 randomised children. *Lancet* 1996; **347:** 1783–8.
11. Evans WE, *et al.* Conventional compared with individualized chemotherapy for childhood acute lymphoblastic leukemia. *N Engl J Med* 1998; **338:** 499–505.
12. Finiewicz KJ, Larson RA. Dose-intensive therapy for adult acute lymphoblastic leukemia. *Semin Oncol* 1999; **26:** 6–20.
13. Aricò M, *et al.* Outcome of treatment in children with Philadelphia chromosome-positive acute lymphoblastic leukemia. *N Engl J Med* 2000; **342:** 998–1006.
14. Borgmann A, *et al.* Autologous bone-marrow transplants compared with chemotherapy for children with acute lymphoblastic leukaemia in a second remission: a matched-pair analysis. *Lancet* 1995; **346:** 873–6.

ACUTE MYELOID LEUKAEMIAS. Treatment of acute myeloid leukaemias (AML) is problematic because normal stem-cell precursors are sensitive to the agents used, and therapy aimed at myeloid leukaemic clones results in destruction of part of the normal stem-cell pool.

Induction of remission is usually possible with intensive chemotherapy. Complete remission has been stated to be achievable in up to 80% of younger patients and about 50% of older patients (who form the majority of those with AML), but patients suffer severe neutropenia during induction and remission rate is to some extent dependent upon the standard of supportive care. Remission rates are lower in those with adverse prognostic factors such as poor performance status, AML secondary to myelodysplasia or antineoplastics, high white cell count, features of multidrug resistance, and unfavourable cytogenetics.[1] Established regimens are based on cytarabine with the anthracycline daunorubicin.[1-3] The first successful regimens also included tioguanine, and some centres continue to use it; although most consider that it gives no additional advantage and have dropped it from induction protocols, it may offer some benefit in older patients (see below). Idarubicin may be preferred to daunorubicin, especially in younger patients.[1,4] Mitozantrone [mitoxantrone] is another alternative to daunorubicin.[1] Addition of etoposide to induction protocols of cytarabine and daunorubicin appears to improve results in younger patients,[5] but in older patients an induction regimen which added tioguanine was found to be more effective than one with etoposide.[6] As in acute lymphoblastic leukaemia (see above) there is a trend towards the use of more intensive induction regimens. Use of high-dose cytarabine (with daunorubicin and etoposide) has been reported to improve the duration of first remission and disease-free survival compared with standard doses of cytarabine.[7] Equally the timing of induction cycles may be important: intensive timing (where the second cycle was given 10 days after the first) has improved disease-free survival, despite more toxicity-related deaths, compared with the standard interval of 14 days or more.[8] Haematopoietic growth factors such as filgrastim and molgramostim may be used to accelerate recovery after induction regimens, although their role has not yet been clearly defined.[1] Once remission is induced, further treatment (**postremission therapy**) is essential in preventing relapse.[1,3] Options include further chemotherapy, or allogeneic or autologous bone marrow transplantation. Long-term survival of about 50% may be possible with these options when used in patients in first remission. However, which option to use is controversial. The most successful chemotherapy regimens use high-dose cytarabine for up to 4 courses, and appear to be comparable to bone marrow transplantation in terms of survival.[9,10] Consequently, some advocate a policy of intensive postremission chemotherapy, reserving transplantation for subsequent relapse, particularly for patients with favourable cytogenetics.[11] The MRC AML10 Trial,[12] however, demonstrated additional benefit from autologous bone-marrow transplantation when used after intensive postremission chemotherapy, and it was suggested that while reserving transplantation for salvage therapy in children and patients with good-risk disease was appropriate, in older patients and those with standard risk it might be better to employ the procedure in first remission.

Where possible, induction and postremission therapy is the treatment of choice in AML.[1,3] However, where debility or concomitant medical conditions make intensive therapy impossible in the elderly, palliative treatment with oral hydroxyurea [hydroxycarbamide] or etoposide is often given, while idarubicin or low-dose subcutaneous cytarabine may also be of benefit.[2] Good results have been reported with a combination of idarubicin and etoposide in elderly patients.[13] Another option for elderly patients who are not able to receive chemotherapy is the toxin-linked monoclonal antibody gemtuzumab ozogamicin.

Acute promyelocytic leukaemia (APL) is a subtype of AML accounting for 10% of AML cases in adults. It is important to distinguish APL from other forms, since unlike other subtypes standard therapy is tretinoin differentiation therapy. Over 90% of patients with APL can achieve complete remission following treatment with tretinoin.[14,15] However the duration of remission is short unless consolidation, usually with an anthracycline- and cytarabine-based regimen, is given subsequently. The combination of tretinoin followed by chemotherapy has been shown to result in improved survival compared with chemotherapy alone.[15,16] Newer regimens include chemotherapy with tretinoin for induction, followed by chemotherapy for consolidation.[15,17] Prolonged maintenance therapy (intermittent tretinoin plus continuous mercaptopurine and methotrexate for 2 years) also appears to reduce the rate of relapse in APL.[17] Although maintenance with tretinoin alone has been reported to be of benefit,[16] resistance generally develops with continuous treatment.[17] The synthetic retinoid, tamibarotene (AM-80), has been used to induce remission in patients who relapsed following successful remission induction with tretinoin.[18] Low doses of arsenic trioxide have also been effective in inducing complete remission in patients with APL who have relapsed.[19,20]

The efficacy of tretinoin appears to be achievable only because the characteristic chromosomal abnormalities in APL result in an abnormal retinoic acid receptor. The development of agents which can effect differentiation in other forms of AML, and indeed in other neoplasms, seems likely to be a long and difficult task.

Among other experimental therapies under investigation for AML, the use of antisense oligonucleotides aimed at abnormal genes are considered promising. Whether inhibitors of multidrug resistance, such as the ciclosporin analogue valspodar, are able to reverse resistance to antineoplastics is also being investigated.

1. Löwenberg B, *et al.* Acute myeloid leukemia. *N Engl J Med* 1999; **341:** 1051–62. Correction. *ibid.*; 1484.
2. Burnett AK, Eden OB. The treatment of acute leukaemia. *Lancet* 1997; **349:** 270–5.
3. Hiddemann W, *et al.* Management of acute myeloid leukemia in elderly patients. *J Clin Oncol* 1999; **17:** 3569–76.
4. The AML Collaborative Group. A systematic collaborative overview of randomized trials comparing idarubicin with daunorubicin (or other anthracyclines) as induction therapy for acute myeloid leukaemia. *Br J Haematol* 1998; **103:** 100–109.
5. Bishop JF, *et al.* Etoposide in acute nonlymphocytic leukaemia. *Blood* 1990; **75:** 27–32.
6. Goldstone AH, *et al.* Attempts to improve treatment outcomes in acute myeloid leukemia (AML) in older patients: the results of the United Kingdom Medical Research Council AML11 trial. *Blood* 2001; **98:** 1302–11.
7. Bishop JF, *et al.* A randomized study of high-dose cytarabine in induction in acute myeloid leukemia. *Blood* 1996; **87:** 1710–17.
8. Woods WG, *et al.* Timed sequential therapy improves postremission outcome in acute myeloid leukemia: a report from the Children's Cancer Group. *Blood* 1996; **87:** 4979–89.
9. Mayer RJ, *et al.* Intensive postremission chemotherapy in adults with acute myeloid leukemia. *N Engl J Med* 1994; **331:** 896–903.
10. Cassileth PA, *et al.* Chemotherapy compared with autologous or allogeneic bone marrow transplantation in the management of acute myeloid leukemia in first remission. *N Engl J Med* 1998; **339:** 1649–56.
11. Edenfield WJ, Gore SD. Stage-specific application of allogeneic and autologous marrow transplantation in the management of acute myeloid leukemia. *Semin Oncol* 1999; **26:** 21–34.
12. Burnett AK, *et al.* Randomised comparison of addition of autologous bone-marrow transplantation to intensive chemotherapy for acute myeloid leukaemia in first remission: results of MRC AML 10 trial. *Lancet* 1998; **351:** 700–8.
13. Jackson GH, *et al.* The use of an all oral chemotherapy (idarubicin and etoposide) in the treatment of acute myeloid leukaemia in the elderly: a report of toxicity and efficacy. *Leukemia* 1997; **11:** 1193–6.
14. Warrell RP, *et al.* Acute promyelocytic leukaemia. *N Engl J Med* 1993; **329:** 177–89.
15. Fenaux P, Degos L. Treatment of acute promyelocytic leukaemia. *Clin Haematol* 1996; **9:** 107–28.
16. Tallman MS, *et al.* All trans-retinoic acid in acute promyelocytic leukemia. *N Engl J Med* 1997; **337:** 1021–8. Correction. *ibid.*; 1639.
17. Fenaux P, *et al.* A randomized comparison of all transretinoic acid (ATRA) followed by chemotherapy and ATRA plus chemotherapy and the role of maintenance therapy in newly diagnosed acute promyelocytic leukemia. *Blood* 1999; **94:** 1192–1200.
18. Tobita T, *et al.* Treatment with a new synthetic retinoid, Am80, of acute promyelocytic leukemia relapsed from complete remission induced by all-trans retinoic acid. *Blood* 1997; **90:** 967–73.
19. Soignet SL, *et al.* Complete remission after treatment of acute promyelocytic leukemia with arsenic trioxide. *N Engl J Med* 1998; **339:** 1341–8.
20. Niu C, *et al.* Studies on treatment of acute promyelocytic leukemia with arsenic trioxide: remission induction, follow-up, and molecular monitoring in 11 newly diagnosed and 47 relapsed acute promyelocytic leukemia patients. *Blood* 1999; **94:** 3315–24.

Leukaemias, chronic. The chronic leukaemias may be broadly divided into those in which the neoplastic proliferation affects lymphoid cell lines, and those affecting the myeloid cell lines.

Chronic leukaemias affecting the *lymphoid cell lines* include chronic lymphocytic leukaemia (CLL), which is B-cell in about 95% of cases and T-cell in about 5%, and hairy cell leukaemia, which affects B-cells. The revised European-American lymphoma classification,[1] and a proposed WHO classification of haematological malignancies,[2] consider lymphoid leukaemias and lymphomas of the same cell type to be one disease with different clinical presentations. Thus B-cell CLL is the same disease as B-cell small lymphocytic lymphoma.

Chronic neoplasms affecting the *myeloid cell lines* include the myeloproliferative disorders chronic myeloid leukaemia (which is Philadelphia chromosome (Ph^1) positive), polycythaemia vera, and primary (essential) thrombocythaemia, and the myelodysplastic syndromes. All of these may undergo transformation to acute myeloid leukaemia.

1. Harris NL, *et al.* A revised European-American classification of lymphoid neoplasms: a proposal from the International Lymphoma Study Group. *Blood* 1994; **84:** 1361–92.
2. Harris NL, *et al.* World Health Organization classification of neoplastic diseases of the hematopoietic and lymphoid tissues: report of the clinical advisory committee meeting–Airlie House, Virginia, November 1997. *J Clin Oncol* 1999; **17:** 3835–49.

CHRONIC LYMPHOCYTIC LEUKAEMIA. Chronic lymphocytic leukaemia (CLL) typically occurs in people over 50 years of age, and accounts for 30% of leukaemias in the West although it is rarer in the Far East. The clinical course is variable: low-risk patients (Rai stage O; Binet stage A) have a median survival of about 14 years, while high-risk patients (Rai stage III/IV; Binet stage C) have a median survival of about 2.5 years; median survival in the intermediate stages is about 6 years.[1]

In patients at low risk and those at intermediate risk with indolent disease cytotoxic chemotherapy is usually deferred until signs and symptoms of disease progression occur.[1-3] In these patient groups, trials of immediate versus deferred chemotherapy for early-stage CLL have shown no significant advantage, or disadvantage, for immediate chemotherapy in terms of 10-year survival.[4] Patients with high-risk or progressive disease are usually treated with immediate chemotherapy.

When therapy is required, it is essentially symptomatic and palliative. Continuous or intermittent chlorambucil has been most widely used, and is given for as long as the patient responds; response rates range from about 40 to 70%.[1] Although chlorambucil is usually combined with a corticosteroid (prednisone or prednisolone), there is now some doubt as to whether this has a real advantage over chlorambucil alone.[1,3,4] Corticosteroid therapy is, however, the treatment of choice where patients present with cytopenias due to an immune mechanism.[1] Combination chemotherapy does not appear to offer any advantage over chlorambucil alone.[4] The most commonly used combinations are cyclophosphamide and prednisone or prednisolone plus either vincristine (COP or CVP) or the anthracycline doxorubicin (CAP), or both (CHOP).

Once initial therapy has failed, the preferred second-line therapy is the nucleoside analogue fludarabine.[1,3,5] Fludarabine is also being investigated as initial therapy,[3] and response rates have been found to be higher than with chlorambucil.[6] Similarly, a comparison of fludarabine with CAP (cyclophosphamide, doxorubicin, and prednisone) found fludarabine to give improved response rates in patients with advanced disease.[7] Cladribine may also be used for CLL refractory to alkylating agents. In patients who fail treatment with conventional therapy, the anti-CD52 antibody alemtuzumab has produced responses.[8]

Patients may require supportive care for systemic complications of CLL. Hypogammaglobulinaemia is common, and the chief cause of infections.[9] Normal immunoglobulin may reduce the infection rate in these patients but it is not clear that it improves survival.[1] If infection occurs broad spectrum antibacterials will be required. Colony-stimulating factors and erythropoietin may be useful for associated cytopenias.

Recent results from patients given bone-marrow transplants after chemoradiotherapy have suggested for the first time the possibility of cure in CLL, but this approach must still be considered experimental.[1,10]

1. Rozman C, Montserrat E. Chronic lymphocytic leukemia. *N Engl J Med* 1995; **333:** 1052–7. Correction. *ibid.*; 1515.
2. Cheson BD, *et al.* National Cancer Institute-sponsored working group guidelines for chronic lymphocytic leukemia: revised guidelines for diagnosis and treatment. *Blood* 1996; **87:** 4990–7.
3. Kalil N, Cheson BD. Chronic lymphocytic leukemia. *Oncologist* 1999; **4:** 352–69.
4. CLL Trialists' Collaborative Group. Chemotherapeutic options in chronic lymphocytic leukemia: a meta-analysis of the randomized trials. *J Natl Cancer Inst* 1999; **91:** 861–8.
5. National Institute for Clinical Excellence. Guidance on the use of fludarabine for B-cell chronic lymphocytic leukaemia (issued September 2001). Available at: http://www.nice.org.uk/pdf/NICEfludarab_E_29guidance.pdf
6. Rai KR, *et al.* Fludarabine compared with chlorambucil as primary therapy for chronic lymphocytic leukemia. *N Engl J Med* 2000; **343:** 1750–7.
7. The French Cooperative Group on CLL, *et al.* Multicentre prospective randomised trial of fludarabine *versus* cyclophosphamide, doxorubicin, and prednisone (CAP) for treatment of advanced-stage chronic lymphocytic leukaemia. *Lancet* 1996; **347:** 1432–8.
8. Osterborg A, *et al.* Phase II multicenter study of human CD52 antibody in previously treated chronic lymphocytic leukemia. *J Clin Oncol* 1997; **15:** 1567–74.
9. Morrison VA. The infectious complications of chronic lymphocytic leukemia. *Semin Oncol* 1998; **25:** 98–106.
10. Khouri IF, *et al.* Hematopoietic stem cell transplantation for chronic lymphocytic leukemia. *Curr Opin Hematol* 1998; **5:** 454–9.

CHRONIC MYELOID LEUKAEMIA. Chronic myeloid (myelogenous) or chronic granulocytic leukaemia (CML) is a rare disease, occurring usually in older patients, and representing about 15% of all adult leukaemias. It is associated in over 90% of cases with the presence in blood cells of an abnormal chromosome, the Philadelphia chromosome (Ph[1]). The median survival for patients with Ph[1]-positive disease is about 5 to 6 years, while in Ph[1]-negative disease (atypical CML) median survival is only about 25 months.[1] Some classification systems consider atypical CML to be a separate disease.

During the **chronic phase**, which may last for several years, standard palliative therapy has been with busulfan or hydroxyurea [hydroxycarbamide].[1-3] Both drugs produce haematological remissions in up to 80% of patients, but do not affect disease progression or induce cytogenetic remissions.[1-3] Hydroxyurea [hydroxycarbamide] is somewhat more effective, and better tolerated, than busulfan.[4] However, evidence from a number of randomised trials has demonstrated that interferon alfa is associated with improved survival compared with busulfan or hydroxyurea [hydroxycarbamide],[5] and interferon alfa has now become the treatment of choice in the chronic phase of CML in patients unsuitable for allogeneic bone-marrow transplantation.[1-3] Some 70 or 80% of patients treated with interferon experience a haematological response, and about 30% seem to undergo suppression of the Ph[1]-positive clone, a response associated with more prolonged survival. The optimum dosage for such therapy has yet to be determined.[5] In efforts to improve the cytogenetic response rate further, interferon alfa has been combined with other therapies. Promising results have been seen with the combination of interferon alfa with cytarabine: this combination produced increased suppression of the Ph[1]-positive clone, and increased survival at 3 years.[6] The tyrosine kinase inhibitor imatinib is also being used. Investigational agents in the chronic phase of CML include homoharringtonine, and a long-acting interferon, polyethylene glycol interferon.[3]

The use of allogeneic bone marrow transplantation (BMT) early in the chronic phase has the potential for cure of CML due to a graft-versus-leukaemia effect. Thus, in suitable patients (younger patients with HLA-matched sibling donors), allogeneic BMT should be considered as first-line therapy.[1-3] The exact timing of the procedure after diagnosis is controversial; however, there is evidence that it should be performed within 2 years.[3] Investigational procedures include matched unrelated BMT, and purged autologous BMT.[3] Purging strategies include the use of antisense oligonucleotides. Options in patients who relapse following BMT include a second transplant or the use of donor lymphocyte infusions, or interferon alfa.[3]

The onset of the subsequent **transformed phase** is unpredictable and may present as rapid onset of a blast cell crisis with the behaviour of an acute leukaemia, or a more gradual appearance of blast cells accompanied by gradual resistance to previous treatment (accelerated phase).[1-3] Transformation may produce lymphoblastic (25 to 30% of patients) or myeloblastic or undifferentiated cells (66 to 75% of patients), and the disease may then be treated as acute lymphoblastic or myeloid leukaemia, but cure, or even remission of long duration, is not generally possible with current chemotherapy regimens.[1,3]

Patients with lymphoid blastic-phase disease have a better chance of response (60%) than those with myeloid blastic-phase disease (20 to 30%).[3] Investigational agents in the myeloid blastic-phase include decitabine.[3,7] High response rates and some prolonged responses have been seen in Ph[1]-positive patients with myeloid blast crisis who were treated with imatinib.[8]

1. Cortes JE, *et al.* Chronic myelogenous leukemia: a review. *Am J Med* 1996; **100:** 555–70.
2. Sawyers CL. Chronic myeloid leukemia. *N Engl J Med* 1999; **340:** 1330–40.
3. Faderl S, *et al.* Chronic myelogenous leukemia: biology and therapy. *Ann Intern Med* 1999; **131:** 207–19.
4. Hehlmann R, *et al.* Randomized comparison of busulfan and hydroxyurea in chronic myelogenous leukemia: prolongation of survival by hydroxyurea. *Blood* 1993; **82:** 398–407.
5. Chronic Myeloid Leukemia Trialists' Collaborative Group. Interferon alfa *versus* chemotherapy for chronic myeloid leukemia: a meta-analysis of seven randomized trials. *J Natl Cancer Inst* 1997; **89:** 1616–20.
6. Guilhot F, *et al.* Interferon alfa-2b combined with cytarabine *versus* interferon alone in chronic myelogenous leukemia. *N Engl J Med* 1997; **337:** 223–9.
7. Sacchi S, *et al.* Chronic myelogenous leukemia in nonlymphoid blastic phase: analysis of the results of first salvage therapy with three different treatment approaches for 162 patients. *Cancer* 1999; **86:** 2632–41.
8. Druker BJ, *et al.* Activity of a specific inhibitor of the BCR-ABL tyrosine kinase in the blast crisis of chronic myeloid leukemia and acute lymphoblastic leukemia with the Philadelphia chromosome. *N Engl J Med* 2001; **344:** 1038–42.

HAIRY-CELL LEUKAEMIA. Hairy-cell leukaemia is a rare, chronic, B-cell lymphoproliferative disorder marked by the presence of white blood cells with prominent cytoplasmic villi, pancytopenia, and splenomegaly. Many patients are asymptomatic and there is no clear advantage to early treatment before symptoms appear.[1,2] When treatment is required, splenectomy was formerly used as initial therapy, but response duration tended to be short. Interferon alfa-2a or -2b given for one year produces at least a partial response in most cases[1] but patients have a tendency to relapse once therapy is discontinued. Better results have been reported with the purine analogues cladribine and pentostatin, and these have now emerged as first-line treatments for this disease.[1,2] Durable complete remission rates of 50% or more are seen after relatively short courses of therapy,[3-6] and toxicity is generally acceptable (pentostatin has produced severe toxicity at higher doses but is less toxic in the doses required for hairy-cell leukaemia). They do not appear to show cross-resistance, and cladribine has been used successfully in patients resistant to, or intolerant of, pentostatin.[7] There is a report of remission from the use of rituximab in a patient with refractory disease.[8]

1. Gollard R, *et al.* The optimal management of hairy cell leukemia. *Drugs* 1995; **49:** 921–31.
2. Tallman MS, *et al.* Treatment of hairy-cell leukemia: current views. *Semin Hematol* 1999; **36:** 155–63.
3. Kane BJ, *et al.* Pentostatin: an adenosine deaminase inhibitor for the treatment of hairy cell leukemia. *Ann Pharmacother* 1992; **26:** 939–47.
4. Saven A, Piro L. Newer purine analogues for the treatment of hairy-cell leukemia. *N Engl J Med* 1994; **330:** 691–7.
5. Cheson BD, *et al.* Treatment of hairy cell leukemia with 2-chlorodeoxyadenosine via the group C protocol mechanism of the National Cancer Institute: a report of 979 patients. *J Clin Oncol* 1998; **16:** 3007–3015.
6. Grever M, *et al.* Randomized comparison of pentostatin *versus* interferon alfa-2a in previously untreated patients with hairy cell leukemia: an intergroup study. *J Clin Oncol* 1995; **13:** 974–82.
7. Saven A, Piro LD. Complete remissions in hairy cell leukemia with 2-chlorodeoxyadenosine after failure with 2'deoxycoformycin. *Ann Intern Med* 1993; **119:** 278–83.
8. Zinzani PL, *et al.* Efficacy of rituximab in hairy cell leukemia treatment. *J Clin Oncol* 2000; **18:** 3875–7.

MYELODYSPLASTIC SYNDROMES. Myelodysplastic syndromes are low-grade neoplasms of haematopoietic stem cells characterised by ineffective haematopoiesis that results in anaemia, neutropenia, or thrombocytopenia in various combinations. They have been described as smouldering leukaemia or preleukaemia and transformation to acute myeloid leukaemia occurs in some patients. The clinical course of myelodysplastic syndromes is variable, and a precise individual determination of prognostic score is important in planning treatment.[1-3] In the few younger patients with suitable HLA-matched siblings, allogeneic bone marrow transplantation has curative potential.[1-4] Patients who are likely to have an indolent course are best treated conservatively with observation and supportive care (transfusions, antibacterials, and epoetins plus filgrastim or molgramostim).[1-4] The treatment of progressive or advanced myelodysplastic syndromes or those that have transformed to acute myeloid leukaemia (AML) may involve intensive chemotherapy similar to that for AML (see p.485), but remission rates are lower.[1,2] However, many patients are elderly with poor performance status, and are unable to tolerate intensive chemotherapy. Low-intensity chemotherapy (low-dose

cytarabine, azacitidine, or decitabine) may be tried in such patients,[3] but has had limited success.[5] A variety of antineoplastics and immunomodulating agents are being investigated for use in myelodysplastic syndromes with a poor prognosis, including topotecan, decitabine, and amifostine.[2,3] Attempts to induce cellular differentiation have generally been disappointing.[1,5]

1. Oscier DG. The myelodysplastic syndromes. *BMJ* 1997; **314:** 883–6.
2. Heaney ML, Golde DW. Myelodysplasia. *N Engl J Med* 1999; **340:** 1649–60.
3. Greenberg P, *et al.* NCCN practice guidelines for the myelodysplastic syndromes. *Oncology* 1998; **12:** 53–80.
4. Provan D. Myelodysplastic syndromes. *Prescribers' J* 1997; **37:** 17–23.
5. Aul C, Gatterman N. The role of low-dose chemotherapy in myelodysplastic syndromes. *Leuk Res* 1992; **16:** 207–15.

POLYCYTHAEMIA VERA. Polycythaemia vera (polycythaemia rubra vera) is a myeloproliferative disorder, apparently due to an abnormal stem cell clone, which results in increased red cell mass and packed cell volume, and is often associated with increases in white cell and platelet counts and splenomegaly. It is a disease of later life, with a median age at presentation of about 60 years. Patients may present with microvascular occlusion, marked by conditions such as erythromelalgia (burning pain and erythema of the hands and feet), paraesthesia, or migraine; and arterial or venous thrombosis (e.g. cerebrovascular accident, myocardial infarction, pulmonary embolism). The risk for thrombosis is highest in patients with a prior history of thrombosis and in those aged over 60 years. Other symptoms include pruritus, characteristically exacerbated by warmth, and hyperuricaemia. In up to 20% of patients the disease eventually enters a spent phase marked by fibrosis and marrow hypoplasia, and about 5% of patients have transformation to acute leukaemia (this is increased by some therapies). Median survival is in the region of 8 to 16 years.

The mainstay of treatment is periodic phlebotomy to maintain the packed cell volume within normal values.[1-3] This may be all that is required in younger patients at low risk of thrombosis. In patients at high risk of thrombosis, including those who have a high phlebotomy requirement, some form of myelosuppressive therapy may be considered as a supplement to phlebotomy. Chlorambucil, which was formerly used for this purpose, has largely been discontinued because of a high incidence of leukaemia in patients so treated.[1] In patients with a life expectancy of less than 10 years, radioactive phosphorus-32 is probably appropriate, and produces good results with few immediate adverse effects.[1,3] However, like the alkylating agents it is associated with an increased risk of secondary malignancies. In younger patients requiring myelosuppressive therapy hydroxyurea [hydroxycarbamide],[1,3] or in some countries pipobroman also,[4] have been preferred because they were considered to have lower risk of inducing leukaemia. However, there is some evidence[4] that they too may have leukaemogenic potential (see also Carcinogenicity, under Hydroxyurea, p.544). Non-cytotoxic therapies that have been shown to be effective include interferon alfa.[5] This may be preferred in younger patients requiring treatment.[3]

Symptoms resulting from microvascular occlusion can be controlled by the use of low-dose aspirin (less than about 80 mg per day).[3] Anagrelide, another antiplatelet agent, has also been tried in polycythaemia vera. Whether these antiplatelet agents can prevent thrombosis in early polycythaemia is being investigated.[6]

1. Berk PD, *et al.* Therapeutic recommendations in polycythaemia vera based on Polycythaemia Vera Study Group protocols. *Semin Hematol* 1986; **23:** 132–43.
2. Smith AG. Polycythaemia and its management. *Prescribers' J* 1994; **34:** 142–51.
3. Tefferi A. The Philadelphia chromosome negative chronic myeloproliferative disorders: a practical overview. *Mayo Clin Proc* 1998; **73:** 1177–84.
4. Najean Y, Rain JD. Treatment of polycythemia vera: the use of hydroxyurea and pipobroman in 292 patients under the age of 65 years. *Blood* 1997; **90:** 3370–7.
5. Lengfelder E, *et al.* Interferon α in the treatment of polycythemia vera. *Ann Hematol* 2000; **79:** 103–9.
6. Michiels JJ, *et al.* Diagnosis and treatment of polycythemia vera and possible future study designs of the PVSG. *Leuk Lymphoma* 2000; **36:** 239–53.

PRIMARY THROMBOCYTHAEMIA. Primary thrombocythaemia (essential thrombocythaemia) is a rare myeloproliferative disorder with abnormal platelet production resulting in elevated platelet counts. It occurs mainly during later life and unlike other myeloproliferative disorders, is associated with generally near-normal life expectancy.[1] However, microvascular occlusion marked by conditions such as erythromelalgia (burning pain and erythema of the hands and feet), paraesthesia, or migraine, and arterial or venous thrombosis (e.g. cerebrovascular accident, myocardial infarction, pulmonary embolism) may occur. The risk for thrombosis is highest in patients with a prior history of thrombosis and in those aged over 60 years. In less than 10% of patients the disease eventually enters a spent phase marked by fibrosis and marrow hypoplasia, or transforms to acute leukaemia.

Asymptomatic patients and those at low risk of thrombosis are generally not treated, but the specific risks considered to warrant treatment are controversial.[1-4] Symptoms resulting from microvascular occlusion can be controlled by the use of low-dose aspirin (less than about 80 mg per day). In patients at risk of thrombosis, drugs that lower platelet counts are used, including cytotoxics.[1,4] Phosphorus-32 and alkylating agents such as busulfan are not much used now because of their known potential to induce leukaemia. Hydroxyurea [hydroxycarbamide] has been shown to reduce thrombotic events, and has tended to be preferred because it was considered to have lower risk of inducing leukaemia. However, there is now some evidence that it too may have leukaemogenic potential (see Carcinogenicity, under Hydroxyurea, p.544). The increased risk of leukaemia from therapy is particularly relevant in younger patients for whom non-cytotoxic drugs may be preferred. Non-cytotoxic therapies that have been shown to reduce platelet counts (but for which there are currently no comparative data on incidence of thrombotic events) include anagrelide[5] and interferon alfa.[6]

1. Tefferi A. The Philadelphia chromosome negative chronic myeloproliferative disorders: a practical overview. Mayo Clin Proc 1998; 73: 1177–84.
2. van Genderen PJJ, Michiels JJ. Primary thrombocythemia: diagnosis, clinical manifestations and management. Ann Hematol 1993; 67: 57–62.
3. Tefferi A, Hoagland HC. Issues in the diagnosis and management of essential thrombocythemia. Mayo Clin Proc 1994; 69: 651–5.
4. Bentley MA, et al. Essential thrombocythaemia. Med J Aust 1999; 171: 210–13.
5. Anonymous. Anagrelide for essential thrombocythemia. Med Lett Drugs Ther 1997; 39: 120.
6. Elliott MA, Tefferi A. Interferon-alpha therapy in polycythemia vera and essential thrombocythemia. Semin Thromb Hemost 1997; 23: 463–72.

Lymphomas. The malignant lymphomas are neoplastic disorders of the lymphoreticular cells. These cells are primarily located in the lymph nodes, but because of their wide distribution in the body lymphomas may arise in extranodal and extralymphatic tissues such as lung, gastrointestinal tract, and skin.

The term covers a heterogeneous group of diseases, comprising two main subgroups: Hodgkin's disease, and the non-Hodgkin's lymphomas (NHL). The cellular origin of Hodgkin's disease is uncertain; the non-Hodgkin's lymphomas are monoclonal malignancies arising from B cells in about 80% of cases, with the remainder from cells of T lineage and from undifferentiated cells.

Management of patients with malignant lymphoma is largely determined by interpretation of histological features, and, especially for NHL by an allocation of subtype and grade. Various classification systems have been proposed for NHL of which the National Cancer Institute Working Formulation has been widely used.[1] Under the Working Formulation, NHL are divided into *low grade*, including small lymphocytic, follicular small cleaved cell, and follicular mixed small cleaved and large cell lymphoma; *intermediate grade*, including follicular large cell, diffuse large cell, diffuse small cleaved cell, and diffuse mixed types; and *high grade*, including large cell immunoblastic, lymphoblastic, and small non-cleaved cell (including Burkitt's) lymphomas. More recently the International Lymphoma Study Group has proposed a revised European-American Lymphoma (REAL) classification,[2] and this has subsequently also been published under the auspices of WHO.[3] It is based on a division into B-cell, T-cell and natural killer cell, and Hodgkin's neoplasms. In this classification, B-cell lymphomas include B-cell small lymphocytic lymphoma, MALT lymphoma, follicular lymphoma (35% of adult NHL, rare in children), diffuse large B-cell lymphoma (30% of adult NHL, 5% of NHL in children), and Burkitt's lymphoma (rare in adults; 30% of NHL in children) and Waldenström's macroglobulinaemia (lymphoplasmacytic lymphoma). Plasma-cell myeloma (multiple myeloma) is also a B-cell neoplasm. T-cell lymphomas include precursor T-cell lymphoblastic lymphoma (rare in adults; 45% of NHL in children) and mycosis fungoides; and Hodgkin's lymphoma is subdivided into nodular lymphocyte-predominant and classical (nodular sclerosis and mixed cellularity) forms.

1. Anonymous. Lymphoma classification—where now? Lancet 1992; 339: 1084–5.
2. Harris NL, et al. A revised European-American classification of lymphoid neoplasms: a proposal from the International Lymphoma Study Group. Blood 1994; 84: 1361–92.
3. Harris NL, et al. World Health Organization classification of neoplastic diseases of the hematopoietic and lymphoid tissues: report of the clinical advisory committee meeting–Airlie House, Virginia, November 1997. J Clin Oncol 1999; 17: 3835–49.

HODGKIN'S DISEASE. Hodgkin's disease (Hodgkin's lymphoma) is characterised histologically by the presence of a particular type of giant cell, the Reed-Sternberg cell. It is more common in males than in females, and in the West is seen particularly in young adults and in the elderly, although the age distribution differs elsewhere.

It usually presents as painless enlargement of one or more lymph nodes, particularly in the neck or axillae. About a third of all patients also have constitutional symptoms of fever, weight loss, and night sweats, which carry adverse prognostic significance. In advanced disease, signs of organ infiltration may occur, as may infectious complications. The mass of the tumour may result in compression of vital organs.

Hodgkin's disease can be treated by radiotherapy or chemotherapy or both, and the choice of treatment depends on the volume and histological subtype of the tumour, the age of the patient, and, particularly, the stage of the disease.[1-5] The Ann Arbor classification recognises 4 stages:

• Stage I, with involvement of a single lymph node region or extralymphatic site
• Stage II, in which spread is restricted to lymph nodes and sites on one side of the diaphragm only
• Stage III, involving spread on both sides of the diaphragm with possible splenic and extralymphatic involvement
• Stage IV, where the patient has diffuse or disseminated disease in one or more extralymphatic organs or tissues.

Stages are subclassified A or B according to the absence or presence respectively of the aforementioned constitutional symptoms. Survival rates following treatment for Hodgkin's disease are generally excellent, and there is increasing emphasis on better tailoring therapy to decrease early and late treatment-related morbidity while not compromising survival.[3,5]

There is some debate about the treatment of early stage disease (stages I, II, and IIIA). Radiotherapy alone has been the treatment of choice in adult patients with limited early disease, especially in those with good prognosis. However, there has been much interest in adjuvant chemotherapy (combined modality treatment) to try to improve disease free survival, reduce doses and volumes of radiotherapy, and avoid the need for surgical staging. Combined modality treatment has gained acceptance in adults with poor-risk early stage disease,[6] and is preferred in children,[5] although the evidence to support this is scanty.[7] A comprehensive meta-analysis of adjuvant chemotherapy in patients with early-stage disease found a reduced risk of resistant or recurrent disease, but this did not translate to an improvement in 10-year survival.[8]

Chemotherapy alone is generally considered to be the treatment of choice in advanced disease (stages IIIB and IV), although the value of adding radiotherapy has still been debated. A meta-analysis of combined modality therapy in advanced disease found no survival benefit from additional radiotherapy, although it may have a role in initial bulky or residual disease.[9] There are currently a number of 4-drug standard regimens available and the choice lies between one of these, alternating cycles of 2 different regimens, or a hybrid cycle that involves giving 7 or 8 drugs in the same course of treatment.[2] However, the single most important factor governing the outcome of chemotherapy is thought to be dose intensity of the drugs given. Complete remission can be achieved in 80 to 95% of patients with such regimens; although some subsequently relapse, salvage chemotherapy is reported to bring the overall cure rate to about 75%.[1] The earliest of the successful 4-drug regimens was combination chemotherapy with mustine [chlormethine], vincristine, procarbazine, and prednisone or prednisolone (MOPP) introduced by DeVita and colleagues.[10] No combination regimen has yet been conclusively shown to be more effective than MOPP, in terms of survival but a number of MOPP-variant regimens exist which may be as effective and less toxic; these include substitution of chlorambucil for mustine [chlormethine] (LOPP), vinblastine for vincristine (MVPP), and both of these changes in one regimen (ChlVPP). An alternative to the MOPP-based regimens exists in a non-cross resistant combination of doxorubicin, bleomycin, vinblastine, and dacarbazine (ABVD), introduced by Bonadonna and colleagues,[11] which has been found to be as effective as MOPP with a reduced risk of inducing sterility. It is not clear whether ABVD is in fact superior to MOPP for the treatment of Hodgkin's disease.[1,2] Better results have been reported with ABVD alone, and with MOPP/ABV(D), than with MOPP alone, but such comparisons have been criticised on the grounds that the dose-intensity of the MOPP regimen has often been suboptimal.[2] More recent attempts to improve the results of ABVD or MOPP have centred on dose intensified hybrid regimens. The German Hodgkin's Lymphoma study group have found early improved results with a hybrid regimen of bleomycin, etoposide, doxorubicin, cyclophosphamide, vincristine, procarbazine, and prednisone (BEA/COPP).[3,12] In the USA, the Stanford V regimen (doxorubicin, vinblastine, mustine [chlormethine], vincristine, bleomycin, etoposide and prednisone, with consolidative radiotherapy) is being studied.[4,12]

Salvage treatment options for patients who relapse depend on the initial treatment and the interval between treatment and relapse. Patients who are candidates for salvage therapy can be divided into 4 groups:

• those initially treated with radiotherapy who have a recurrence, in whom standard chemotherapy regimens are effective
• those who never achieve complete remission with standard chemotherapy, in whom prognosis is very poor, and who are candidates for an intensive salvage regimen with autologous stem-cell or bone-marrow transplantation
• those whose original remission lasted for over a year, of whom about a quarter will respond to re-treatment with standard therapy, but in whom intensive salvage regimens may be considered
• and those whose remission is short, less than one year, in whom standard chemotherapy may be used to reduce tumour volume before intensive therapy and bone- marrow rescue.[2]

A common intensive salvage regimen consists of carmustine, etoposide, cytarabine, and melphalan (BEAM). Immunotherapies under investigation for Hodgkin's disease include monoclonal antibodies to CD25, CD30, or CD16/CD30.[12]

1. Longo DL. The use of chemotherapy in the treatment of Hodgkin's disease. Semin Oncol 1990; 17: 716–35.
2. DeVita VT, Hubbard SM. Hodgkin's disease. N Engl J Med 1993; 328: 560–5.
3. Wolf J, et al. Issues in the treatment of Hodgkin's disease. Curr Opin Oncol 1998; 10: 396–402.
4. National Comprehensive Cancer Network. NCCN practice guidelines for Hodgkin's disease. Oncology 1999; 13: 78–110.
5. Hudson MM, Donaldson SS. Treatment of pediatric Hodgkin's lymphoma. Semin Hematol 1999; 36: 313–23.
6. Cosset JM, et al. Combined modality treatment for poor prognosis stages I and II Hodgkin's disease. Semin Radiat Oncol 1996; 6: 185–95.
7. Louw G, Pinkerton CR. Interventions for early stage Hodgkin's disease in children (updated 13 November 2000). Available in The Cochrane Library; Issue 4. Oxford: Update Software; 2001.
8. Specht L, et al. Influence of more extensive radiotherapy and adjuvant chemotherapy on long-term outcome of early-stage Hodgkin's disease: a meta-analysis of 23 randomized trials involving 3888 patients. J Clin Oncol 1998; 16: 830–43.
9. Loeffler M, et al. Meta-analysis of chemotherapy versus combined modality treatment trials in Hodgkin's disease. J Clin Oncol 1998; 16: 818–29.
10. DeVita VT, et al. Combination chemotherapy in the treatment of advanced Hodgkin's disease. Ann Intern Med 1970; 73: 881–95.
11. Bonadonna G, et al. Combination chemotherapy of Hodgkin's disease with adriamycin, bleomycin, vinblastine, and imidazole carboxamide versus MOPP. Cancer 1975; 36: 252–9.
12. Engert A, et al. Treatment of advanced Hodgkin's lymphoma: standard and experimental approaches. Semin Hematol 1999; 36: 282–9.

NON-HODGKIN'S LYMPHOMAS. The non-Hodgkin's lymphomas are a heterogeneous group of malignancies which vary considerably in their behaviour, prognosis, and management.[1-9] A variety of classifications have been used. The National Cancer Institute Working Formulation, which identifies 10 basic types, classified as low-, intermediate-, or high-grade, has been widely used, although more recently the revised American-European lymphoma (REAL) classification has come into use (see Lymphomas, above). The non-Hodgkin's lymphomas include Burkitt's lymphoma (a high-grade lymphoma), MALT lymphoma (a low-grade lymphoma), and mycosis fungoides (a cutaneous T-cell lymphoma which does not fit well into the Working Formulation classification), all of which are discussed separately.

The usual presentation of lymphomas is lymphadenopathy, which in low-grade lymphoma may develop insidiously over a long period. There may be constitutional symptoms of fever, night sweats, and weight loss. Extranodal involvement may occur, as may various symptoms due to organ compression by the tumour mass.

Lymphomas of T-cell origin have a worse prognosis than B-cell lymphomas of the same type, and excess tumour bulk, involvement of bone marrow or gastrointestinal tract, and elevated serum-lactic dehydrogenase concentrations are also adverse prognostic factors. Staging is of somewhat less importance as a determinant of treatment and prognosis than in Hodgkin's disease.

About 40% of all lymphomas seen in North America and western Europe are *indolent* and of low grade; **follicular lymphoma** is the commonest form.[8] They typically present at an advanced stage in a patient aged 50 to 60 years, and follow a fairly chronic course, with a median survival of 7 or more years, although some undergo transformation to aggressive forms. They are difficult to manage and, if advanced, rarely curable. In the few patients with limited disease at presentation, radiotherapy may achieve long-term freedom from disease.[1] In more advanced disease treatment has not been shown to affect survival, and a conservative approach of withholding treatment until symptoms require it is considered viable.[8] For similar reasons, when treatment is required, single agent therapy with chlorambucil or cyclophosphamide, sometimes with a corticosteroid such as prednisone or prednisolone in the initial stages, is preferred. Patients treated with more aggressive chemotherapy tend to have remission earlier but the remissions do not last longer than those achieved more slowly with single agent therapy. Nonetheless, because of the poor ultimate prognosis, particularly in younger patients, a number of protocols of intensive chemotherapy similar to those tried for aggressive lymphomas (below) have been used. Autologous bone-marrow or stem-cell transplantation is also being investigated.[10] The use of interferons with chemotherapy for remission induction or as 'maintenance', has produced conflicting results, and their role remains to be established.

Relapse of low-grade lymphomas is generally inevitable. Although further remissions can be achieved with standard treatment, the response rate and duration of remission tends to decrease.[3] Alternative therapies such as the use of cladribine, fludarabine, the anti-CD20 antibody rituximab, or toxin-linked or radiolabelled monoclonal antibodies such as iodine (^{131}I) tositumomab offer some promise. The low-grade lymphomas are also at the centre of attempts to develop antitumour vaccines against the lymphomatous clone. Such an approach is currently limited in lymphoma by the need to create a new vaccine for each patient.[11] Another novel and promising approach is the use of an antisense oligonucleotide specific for *BCL-2*, a gene which is often overexpressed on tumour cells including lymphomas, and is responsible for cell resistance to apoptosis; a preliminary study[12] (mostly in patients with low-grade lymphomas) has demonstrated tumour regression and symptomatic improvement after *BCL-2* antisense therapy.

Intermediate- to high-grade lymphomas, of which **diffuse large B-cell lymphoma** (DLCL) is the most common form,[5,6] are *aggressive*, and survival is measured in months in untreated patients. However, unlike indolent lymphomas, they are potentially curable with intensive therapy. DLCL occurs most commonly in patients aged 50 to 60 years, but also occurs in children. Up to 20% of patients with aggressive lymphomas have localised disease at presentation, and combined modality treatment with a brief course of CHOP (cyclophosphamide, doxorubicin, vincristine, and prednisolone) followed by involved field radiotherapy is the treatment of choice.[5,13] Combination chemotherapy is the treatment of choice in advanced aggressive lymphomas: cure can be achieved in about 35% of patients. Many of the regimens used have included the vinca alkaloids and doxorubicin with alkylating agents: CHOP and CVP (cyclophosphamide, vincristine, and prednisone) have been widely used.[5,6] More intensive third generation regimens such as MACOP-B (an intensive 12-week programme of cyclic methotrexate, doxorubicin, cyclophosphamide, vincristine, prednisone, and bleomycin), m-BACOD (with dexamethasone rather than prednisone), and ProMACE-CytaBOM (prednisone, doxorubicin, cyclophosphamide, etoposide, cytarabine, bleomycin, vincristine, and methotrexate), were then developed, and showed initial promising results. However, randomised studies have failed to show any advantage for these third generation regimens over the less toxic and simpler CHOP regimen, and CHOP is once again considered the standard of care.[5,6] High-dose chemotherapy with autologous bone-marrow transplantation has been tried for initial therapy in patients with diffuse aggressive non-Hodgkin's lymphoma,

but remains investigational.[10] However, in patients who relapse after successful initial therapy, high-dose chemotherapy with radiotherapy followed by autologous bone-marrow transplantation or peripheral blood stem cell transplantation has a role in patients less than 60 years of age.[5,10] In one randomised study, it was superior to the conventional salvage regimen, DHAP (dexamethasone, high-dose cytarabine, and cisplatin).[14]

High-grade lymphomas such as **precursor T-lymphoblastic lymphoma** (T-LBL) and Burkitt's lymphoma (see below) are *highly aggressive* and untreated patients survive only weeks. They occur principally in children and young adults, and are often widely disseminated with bone marrow, peripheral blood, and CNS involvement. In children with lymphoblastic lymphoma, good results have been seen with protocols based on those used for high-risk acute lymphoblastic leukaemia (see above), including the use of CNS prophylaxis.[3,7] It is unclear whether a similar approach would be beneficial in adults with lymphoblastic leukaemia: CHOP continues to be widely used, with generally poor results.[7] Transplantation is an option in lymphoblastic lymphoma.[10]

1. O'Reilly SE, Connors JM. Non-Hodgkin's lymphoma I: characterisation and treatment. *BMJ* 1992; **304:** 1682–6.
2. O'Reilly SE, Connors JM. Non-Hodgkin's lymphoma II: management problems. *BMJ* 1992; **305:** 39–42.
3. Armitage JO. Treatment of non-Hodgkin's lymphoma. *N Engl J Med* 1993; **328:** 1023–30.
4. Johnson PWM. The high grade non-Hodgkin's lymphomas. *Br J Hosp Med* 1995; **53:** 14–19.
5. Martelli M, *et al.* Current guidelines for the management of aggressive non-Hodgkin's lymphoma. *Drugs* 1997; **53:** 957–72.
6. Miller TP. Management of intermediate-grade lymphomas. *Oncology* 1998; **12** (suppl 8): 35–9.
7. Magrath IT. Management of high-grade lymphomas. *Oncology* 1998; **12** (suppl 8): 40–8.
8. Peterson BA. Current treatment of follicular low-grade lymphomas. *Semin Oncol* 1999; **26** (suppl 14): 2–11.
9. Hauke RJ, Armitage JO. A new approach to non-Hodgkin's lymphoma. *Intern Med* 2000; **39:** 197–208.
10. Morrison VA, Peterson BA. High-dose therapy and transplantation in non-Hodgkin's lymphoma. *Semin Oncol* 1999; **26:** 84–98.
11. Hamblin TJ. From dendritic cells to tumour vaccines. *Lancet* 1996; **347:** 705–6.
12. Webb A, *et al.* BCL-2 antisense therapy in patients with non-Hodgkin lymphoma. *Lancet* 1997; **349:** 1137–41.
13. Miller TP, *et al.* Chemotherapy alone compared with chemotherapy plus radiotherapy for localized intermediate- and high-grade non-Hodgkin's lymphoma. *N Engl J Med* 1998; **339:** 21–6.
14. Philip T, *et al.* Autologous bone marrow transplantation as compared with salvage chemotherapy in relapses of chemotherapy-sensitive non-Hodgkin's lymphoma. *N Engl J Med* 1995; **333:** 1540–5.

AIDS-related lymphomas. Between 3 and 10% of AIDS patients will develop aggressive non-Hodgkin's lymphoma at some stage of their illness, usually diffuse large cell lymphoma (see above) or small non-cleaved lymphoma (Burkitt's lymphoma—see below).[1-4] About 50% of these are associated with the presence of Epstein-Barr virus. The other common lymphoma in AIDS patients is primary CNS lymphoma, which is invariably associated with Epstein-Barr virus.[1,4] More recently a new type of AIDS-related lymphoma has been identified, termed primary effusion lymphoma or body cavity based lymphoma,[3,4] which is associated with human herpes virus 8. The introduction of highly active antiretroviral therapy for HIV infection (p.610) may reduce the risk of lymphomas by improving immune function,[3,4] but, conversely, may increase the incidence by allowing patients to survive long enough for lymphoma to develop.[3] There is some evidence of tumour response when antiretroviral therapy is started in a patient who already has a lymphoma.[4,5]

A few patients with AIDS-related non-Hodgkin's lymphomas present with localised disease, and may benefit from radiotherapy, but most have disseminated disease, often extranodal, at presentation.[1-4] The common chemotherapy regimens used are similar to those used in non-HIV infected patients, combining cyclophosphamide, vincristine, doxorubicin, and corticosteroids (CHOP), and sometimes additional drugs such as bleomycin, methotrexate, and cytarabine (e.g. m-BACOD).[4] However, although standard dose or even intensive chemotherapy regimens have been used successfully in selected patients, in general patients with AIDS tolerate chemotherapy poorly, and intensive regimens may even shorten their survival. A low-dose modification of m-BACOD has produced responses and survival comparable to standard dose m-BACOD,[6] and low-dose chemotherapy is likely to be preferred in patients with relatively poor immune function (CD4 cell count less than 200 per mm³). The use of colony-stimulating factors with low or standard dose chemotherapy has been suggested to be helpful. However, the prognosis for patients with poor

immune status remains poor, and median survival remains about 5 to 8 months.[1]

Primary CNS lymphoma has a very poor prognosis in patients with HIV infection, with a median survival of 3 months. Palliative radiotherapy is commonly used.[3,4]

1. Schulz TF, *et al.* HIV infection and neoplasia. *Lancet* 1996; **348:** 587–91.
2. Denton AS, *et al.* AIDS-related lymphoma: an emerging epidemic. *Br J Hosp Med* 1996; **55:** 282–8.
3. Tulpule A, Levine A. AIDS-related lymphoma. *Blood Rev* 1999; **13:** 147–50.
4. Hermans P. Opportunistic AIDS-associated malignancies in HIV-infected patients. *Biomed Pharmacother* 2000; **54:** 32–40.
5. Harrington WJ, *et al.* Azothymidine and interferon-α are active in AIDS-associated small non-cleaved cell lymphoma but not large-cell lymphoma. *Lancet* 1996; **348:** 833.
6. Kaplan LD, *et al.* Low-dose compared with standard-dose m-BACOD chemotherapy for non-Hodgkin's lymphoma associated with human immunodeficiency virus infection. *N Engl J Med* 1997; **336:** 1641–8.

Burkitt's lymphoma. Burkitt's lymphoma is a small non-cleaved cell lymphoma (SNCL) of B-cell origin, which is highly aggressive and is seen particularly in children; the rare cases in adults are most often associated with immunodeficiency such as AIDS. There is an endemic form occurring in equatorial Africa, which is associated with Epstein-Barr virus and commonly involves the jaws and other facial bones.

The primary mode of treatment for Burkitt's lymphoma is chemotherapy. Regimens are generally based on cyclophosphamide, in various combinations with methotrexate, cytarabine, vincristine, doxorubicin, etoposide, and prednisone or prednisolone. Ifosfamide may be substituted for cyclophosphamide. The duration and intensity of chemotherapy depends on the stage at diagnosis.[1] Some groups use an initial phase of low-intensity chemotherapy to reduce the risk of tumour lysis syndrome.[2,3] Cytarabine and methotrexate may also be given intrathecally for CNS prophylaxis in advanced disease.[2,3]

In children complete remission is common and prognosis good: probability of long-term disease-free survival is usually greater than 80%. Prognosis has been less good in adults, but with the increasing use of more intensive regimens similar to those used in children, is improving. About half of all adult cases are reported to be curable with intensive chemotherapy regimens, and it is possible that even more intensive regimens coupled with bone-marrow transplantation or the use of colony-stimulating factors may improve results further.[2,4]

1. Magrath IT. Management of high-grade lymphomas. *Oncology* 1998; **12** (suppl 8): 40–8.
2. Patte C, *et al.* Therapy of Burkitt and other B-cell acute lymphoblastic leukaemia and lymphoma: experience with the LMB protocols of the SFOP (French Paediatric Oncology Society) in children and adults. *Clin Haematol* 1994; **7:** 339–48.
3. Reiter A, *et al.* Non-Hodgkin's lymphomas of childhood and adolescence: results of a treatment stratified for biologic subtypes and stage: a report of the Berlin-Frankfurt-Münster Group. *J Clin Oncol* 1995; **13:** 359–72.
4. Straus DJ, *et al.* Small non-cleaved-cell lymphoma (undifferentiated lymphoma, Burkitt's type) in American adults: treatment designed for acute lymphoblastic leukemia. *Am J Med* 1991; **90:** 328–37.

MALT lymphoma. Marginal zone B-cell lymphomas of mucosa-associated lymphoid tissue (MALT) occur most commonly in the stomach, but may also occur in the salivary gland, breast, thyroid, eye, or lung. They tend to be indolent and remain localised for long periods of time, but can transform to a more aggressive type.

Gastric MALT lymphoma accounts for 40% of gastric lymphomas. It has aroused considerable recent interest because of an association with *Helicobacter pylori* infection.[1,2] The bacterium stimulates the formation of MALT in the stomach, which normally lacks organised lymphoid tissue, and there is evidence that it indirectly stimulates tumour growth. Eradication of *H. pylori* infection using antibacterial and antisecretory therapy, as described in Peptic Ulcer Disease, p.1208, has been shown to result in regression of gastric MALT lymphoma in a number of patients.[3-5] Increasing experience of the use of *H. pylori* eradication indicates that the lymphoma regression after eradication can take up to 14 months; eradication suppresses but does not necessarily eradicate the neoplastic clone; only lymphomas limited to the mucosa or submucosa regress after eradication; and that lymphoma recurrence can occur.[6] Thus, patients who are *H. pylori*-positive with early stage primary gastric MALT lymphomas may be treated solely with *H. pylori* eradication regimens and long-term endoscopic follow-up. The best treatment for patients without *H. pylori* infection, those whose tumours do not respond to eradication, and those with more advanced tumour stage at presentation remains to be established, but options include radiation, surgery, or chemotherapy.[7]

It has been suggested that screening for and eradication of *H. pylori* is worth investigating as a means of preventing gastric cancer.[8]

Non-gastrointestinal low-grade MALT lymphomas have been treated with surgery or radiation therapy if localised, and with single-agent or combination chemotherapy (similar to that used for other low-grade non-Hodgkin's lymphomas—see above) if advanced.[9]

1. Wotherspoon AC, *et al.* Helicobacter pylori-associated gastritis and primary B-cell gastric lymphoma. *Lancet* 1991; **338:** 1175–6.
2. Parsonnet J, *et al.* Helicobacter pylori infection and gastric lymphoma. *N Engl J Med* 1994; **330:** 1267–71.
3. Wotherspoon AC, *et al.* Regression of primary low-grade B-cell gastric lymphoma of mucosa-associated lymphoid tissue type after eradication of Helicobacter pylori. *Lancet* 1993; **342:** 575–7.
4. Wotherspoon AC, *et al.* Antibiotic treatment for low-grade gastric MALT lymphoma. *Lancet* 1994; **343:** 1503.
5. Cammarota G, *et al.* Prevention and treatment of low-grade B-cell primary gastric lymphoma by anti-H pylori therapy. *J Clin Gastroenterol* 1995; **21:** 118–22.
6. Isaacson PG. Gastric MALT lymphoma: from concept to cure. *Ann Oncol* 1999; **10:** 637–45.
7. Schechter NR, Yahalom J. Low-grade MALT lymphoma of the stomach: a review of treatment options. *Int J Radiat Oncol Biol Phys* 2000; **46:** 1093–1103.
8. Peterson WL, *et al.* Helicobacter pylori-related disease. *Arch Intern Med* 2000; **160:** 1285–91.
9. Zinzani PL, *et al.* Nongastrointestinal low-grade mucosa-associated lymphoid tissue lymphoma: analysis of 75 patients. *J Clin Oncol* 1999; **17:** 1254–8.

Mycosis fungoides. Mycosis fungoides is the most common of the cutaneous T-cell lymphomas. It is considered to have 3 stages: a premycotic erythematous or patch phase, characterised by a pruritic rash resembling psoriasis, which may persist for years or even decades; an infiltrative or plaque phase, in which some patches become thickened, darker plaques with marked T-cell infiltration; and a tumour phase where lesions enlarge and ulcerate. Ultimately there may be visceral involvement or potentially fatal sepsis secondary to skin breakdown. A variant of mycosis fungoides presents as widespread pruritic erythroderma, accompanied by abnormal T-cells in the blood, and is known as the Sézary syndrome.

There are many therapeutic options for mycosis fungoides, but few have been evaluated in controlled trials. Treatment depends on disease stage and spread.[1-6] Patients with limited and slowly progressive patch phase disease may be managed just with emollients and topical antipruritics, together with UVB irradiation,[2] given their good prognosis (median survival similar to age-matched controls). Some recommend the use of corticosteroids.[4,5] Alternatively, patients may be treated with topical mustine [chlormethine] or carmustine, or with methoxsalen plus ultraviolet light (PUVA).[3,5] In patients with clearly localised patches, or isolated patches that have failed to respond to other treatments, local external beam irradiation may be used.[3]

As in limited disease, the initial therapy for patients with widespread patch/plaque phase disease is topical, with mustine [chlormethine] or PUVA being used.[2,3] Patients who fail to respond to a single agent may be treated with combinations such as PUVA and interferon alfa or synthetic retinoids (isotretinoin, acitretin). Some advocate the use of total skin electron beam therapy as a first-line therapy for infiltrated plaques,[3] but some reserve it for patients with tumour phase disease.[2]

In the tumour phase, options include total skin electron beam therapy, followed by adjuvant therapy such as topical mustine [chlormethine], or PUVA with interferon alfa or retinoids.[3] Systemic chemotherapy may be used for palliation in recalcitrant disease, particularly if there is extracutaneous involvement.[2,3] Options include single-agent methotrexate, etoposide, or vinblastine; nucleoside analogues such as fludarabine or pentostatin have also been tried. Combination regimens include CHOP (cyclophosphamide, doxorubicin, vincristine, and prednisone), CVP (CHOP without doxorubicin) or CAVE (cyclophosphamide, doxorubicin, vincristine, and etoposide).

Mycosis fungoides with erythrodermic features is treated similarly except that skin irradiation tends to be avoided or used in very low doses as it causes severe desquamation.[3] Extracorporeal photopheresis may be useful for disease with erythrodermic features.[2,3]

Newer therapies for persistent or recurrent mycosis fungoides include the interleukin-2 fusion toxin denileukin diftitox,[5,6] and bexarotene, a new retinoid analogue.[5]

1. Bunn PA, *et al.* Systemic therapy of cutaneous T-cell lymphomas (mycosis fungoides and the Sézary syndrome). *Ann Intern Med* 1994; **121:** 592–602.
2. Lorincz AL. Cutaneous T-cell lymphoma (mycosis fungoides). *Lancet* 1996; **347:** 871–6.
3. Kim YH, Hoppe RT. Mycosis fungoides and the Sézary syndrome. *Semin Oncol* 1999; **26:** 276–89.
4. Zackheim HS. Cutaneous T cell lymphoma: update of treatment. *Dermatology* 1999; **199:** 102–5.
5. Duvic M, Cather JC. Emerging new therapies for cutaneous T-cell lymphoma. *Dermatol Clin* 2000; **18:** 147–56.
6. Siegel RS, *et al.* Primary cutaneous T-cell lymphoma: review and current concepts. *J Clin Oncol* 2000; **18:** 2908–25.

Waldenström's macroglobulinaemia. Waldenström's macroglobulinaemia (primary macroglobulinaemia) is a clinical syndrome associated with lymphoplasmacytic lymphoma in which the abnormal lymphocytes secrete a monoclonal serum paraprotein of immunoglobulin M type resulting in increased plasma viscosity. Patients are mainly elderly, and more often male. Although often asymptomatic, patients can present with weakness and fatigue, anaemia, hepatosplenomegaly, lymphadenopathy, or the hyperviscosity syndrome (characterised by oronasal bleeding, visual disturbances and retinal haemorrhage, neurological disturbances such as headache, vertigo, peripheral neuropathy, and hearing loss, and, rarely, heart failure).

Asymptomatic patients require no treatment and may remain stable for some years. Where treatment is required it has usually been with the alkylating agent chlorambucil or, more recently, with the nucleoside analogues cladribine or fludarabine.[1,2] Concomitant plasmapheresis may be performed to reduce plasma viscosity. When disease stabilises treatment may be discontinued and reinstituted on relapse. Although no randomised studies have been conducted, combination chemotherapy does not appear to produce better responses than single-agent chlorambucil.[1,2] Investigational drugs include interferon alfa and rituximab.

1. Dimopoulos MA, *et al.* Waldenström's macroglobulinemia: clinical features, complications, and management. *J Clin Oncol* 2000; **18:** 214–26.
2. Gertz MA, *et al.* Waldenström's macroglobulinemia. *Oncologist* 2000; **5:** 63–7.

PLASMA CELL NEOPLASMS. *Multiple myeloma.* Multiple myeloma (myelomatosis) is a lymphoproliferative disorder of B-cell origin, involving the development of an abnormal plasma-cell precursor. It occurs predominantly in the elderly, and accounts for only 1% or less of all malignancies. It is more common in black than in white patients and in men than in women.

The proliferation of the abnormal clone tends to suppress normal haematopoiesis, resulting in anaemia and immunosuppression, with an increased risk of serious infection. Perhaps the most characteristic complication, however, is skeletal destruction, apparently due to release of an osteoclast stimulating factor, resulting in osteoporosis, lytic lesions and fractures, and bone pain, as well as consequent hypercalcaemia. In addition, the plasma cells release large quantities of monoclonal immunoglobulins, known as paraproteins, which can produce a hyperviscosity syndrome and in some cases may interfere with platelet function. Renal failure of various causes and neurological problems due to compression are also common.

Multiple myeloma is not curable with presently-available treatment, and therapy is concerned with prolongation of survival and alleviation of symptoms.[1-6] Those patients with stable, indolent or smouldering myeloma, or benign monoclonal gammopathy, are followed carefully but not treated until overt progressive disease occurs.

In patients with overt disease, chemotherapy with the aim of inducing remission and prolonging survival, is the treatment of choice. The standard first-line regimen has long been a combination of oral melphalan and corticosteroids, usually prednisolone or prednisone, particularly in elderly and frail patients. This regimen produces an objective response in about half of all patients, and prolongs median survival to between 19 and 39 months.[2] The contribution of corticosteroids to the regimen is controversial although their palliative effects are invaluable;[2] however, high-dose dexamethasone given alone has been reported to be effective in producing remissions.[3,7] More intensive first-line combination regimens are also used, particularly in younger, fitter patients. Examples include the ABCM regimen (doxorubicin, carmustine, cyclophosphamide, and melphalan), alternating combinations of VMCP (vincristine, melphalan, cyclophosphamide, and prednisone) with VBAP (vincristine, carmustine, doxorubicin, and prednisone), the VAD regimen (vincristine, doxorubicin, and dexamethasone), and the M2 protocol (vincristine, carmustine, melphalan, cyclophosphamide, and prednisolone).[1-3,5,6] However, meta-analysis has not shown these combination regimens to be more effective than melphalan and prednisolone or prednisone in terms of survival,[8] although response rates may be higher and occur more rapidly, and some disa-

greement remains about the optimum induction regimen.[1-3,6] The failure of conventional chemotherapy to produce long-term remissions has led to the investigation of high-dose melphalan with autologous bone-marrow or peripheral stem-cell rescue, either as initial therapy or in patients in remission or with stable disease after initial therapy. One study[9] has found some survival benefit from this approach, and other studies are ongoing. Patients who are potential candidates for high-dose therapy with peripheral stem-cell rescue after initial therapy should have their exposure to myelosuppressive drugs such as alkylating agents and nitrosoureas in first-line regimens limited to avoid compromising stem-cell harvest.[5] Maintenance chemotherapy has not been shown convincingly to improve total duration of remissions or survival.[1,2,6] Maintenance treatment with interferon alfa after conventional chemotherapy has been reported to improve remission duration, but most studies have not shown an improvement in survival,[4,6] and toxicity may be a problem. One small study[10] showed benefit for maintenance interferon alfa after bone marrow transplantation.

In patients who fail to respond to initial treatment, or who subsequently relapse, various regimens have been tried. Salvage regimens for progressive disease include VAD with the addition of cyclophosphamide, EDAP (etoposide, dexamethasone, cytarabine, and cisplatin), and high-dose cyclophosphamide.[5,6] About 60 to 70% of patients who relapse later than 6 months after stopping first-line therapy will respond to re-use of the initial regimen.[6] More recently, preliminary results have shown thalidomide to be active against refractory myeloma.[11]

Although chemotherapy aimed at the myelomatous clone will produce symptomatic relief as disease is brought under control, supportive and symptomatic care is also important. Some bisphosphonates have been found to be effective in reducing skeletal complications,[12,13] and are recommended in those patients with bone disease.[5] Radiotherapy is used for impending fracture or impending spinal cord compression, and is often effective in relieving uncontrolled bone pain.[5] A high fluid intake is essential in patients with renal dysfunction or hypercalcaemia (for the appropriate management of the latter, see p.1181). Vigorous antibacterial treatment may be required if infection occurs (see Infections in Immunocompromised Patients, p.125) and plasma exchange may alleviate the hyperviscosity syndrome.[5]

1. MacLennan ICM, *et al.* Multiple myeloma. *BMJ* 1994; **308:** 1033–6.
2. Newland AC. Management of multiple myeloma. *Prescribers' J* 1994; **34:** 102–10.
3. Alexanian R, Dimopoulos M. The treatment of multiple myeloma. *N Engl J Med* 1994; **330:** 484–9.
4. Bataille R, Harousseau J-L. Multiple myeloma. *N Engl J Med* 1997; **336:** 1657–64.
5. National Comprehensive Cancer Network. NCCN practice guidelines for multiple myeloma. *Oncology (Huntingt)* 1998; **12:** 317–51.
6. Huang Y-W, *et al.* Current drug therapy for multiple myeloma. *Drugs* 1999; **57:** 485–506.
7. Alexanian R, *et al.* Primary dexamethasone treatment of multiple myeloma. *Blood* 1992; **80:** 887–90.
8. Myeloma Trialists' Collaborative Group. Combination chemotherapy versus melphalan plus prednisone as treatment for multiple myeloma: an overview of 6,633 patients from 27 randomized trials. *J Clin Oncol* 1998; **16:** 3832–42.
9. Attal M, *et al.* A prospective, randomized trial of autologous bone marrow transplantation and chemotherapy in multiple myeloma. *N Engl J Med* 1996; **335:** 91–7.
10. Cunningham D, *et al.* A randomized trial of maintenance interferon following high-dose chemotherapy in multiple myeloma: long-term follow-up results. *Br J Haematol* 1998; **102:** 495–502.
11. Singhal S, *et al.* Antitumor activity of thalidomide in refractory multiple myeloma. *N Engl J Med* 1999; **341:** 1565–71.
12. Lahtinen R, *et al.* Randomised, placebo-controlled multicentre trial of clodronate in multiple myeloma. *Lancet* 1992; **340:** 1049–52. Correction. *ibid.*; 1420.
13. Berenzon JR, *et al.* Long-term pamidronate treatment of advanced multiple myeloma patients reduces skeletal events. *J Clin Oncol* 1998; **16:** 593–602.

Malignant effusions. The amount of interstitial fluid is normally regulated by a complex equilibrium between capillary filtration, osmotic pressure, and physical hydrostatic or hydraulic forces. Malignant neoplasms can disturb this equilibrium by obstruction of capillary or lymphatic drainage as well as causing active exudation of additional fluid following metastatic implantation. Malignant effusions are associated most often with lung, breast, and ovarian malignancies and lymphomas. Symptoms vary, and the fluid build-up may be asymptomatic; both pleural and pericardial effusions can produce cough, pleuritic chest pain, and dyspnoea and pericardial effusions may progress to cardiac tamponade. Peritoneal effusions may lead to malignant ascites. The primary aim of treatment for malignant effusions is effective palliation of symptoms, and depends in part on the tumour type, patient performance status, and prognosis.[1-6] If the tumour is chemosensitive, systemic chemotherapy may resolve the effusion. Simple fluid drainage (thoracentesis or pericardiocentesis) will relieve symptoms until fluid build-up recurs, and in patients with very poor prognosis (life expectancy less than 1 month), may suffice for palliation.

In malignant ascites, paracentesis is usually necessary but spironolactone may be of benefit in some patients. In other patients with refractory tumours, fluid drainage followed by sclerotherapy is likely to be preferred. The principle involved is the instillation of an irritant agent into the pleural or pericardial cavity to promote inflammatory and fibrotic changes which result in the membranes adhering together and abolition of the space between the membranes in which fluid accumulates. In the case of pleural effusions, success of sclerotherapy is dependent on adequate fluid drainage beforehand and full re-expansion of the lung to bring the pleural surfaces together. Intrapleural thrombolytics such as streptokinase have been used to improve fluid drainage in cases of loculation of the effusion.[6]

Many drugs have been used for sclerotherapy, and the most common are a tetracycline (doxycycline or tetracycline 500 mg), bleomycin (60 000 IU or 60 USP units), or talc (2 to 10 g). There are no clear data from large randomised studies to guide the choice between these three, and opinions on the preferred option differ.[1,4-6] Following drainage of the effusions the sclerosant is instilled in a small volume (20 to 50 mL) of liquid through the drainage tube. Talc may be also administered as a powder insufflation (rather than slurry), but this involves a surgical procedure under general anaesthesia. Sclerotherapy results in painful inflammation, and local anaesthetics or analgesics should be given. For patients who fail sclerotherapy, or for whom this is not considered suitable, there are various surgical options to manage effusions.[1-6]

1. Andrews CO, Gora ML. Pleural effusions: pathophysiology and management. Ann Pharmacother 1994; 28: 894–903.
2. Vaitkus PT, et al. Treatment of malignant pericardial effusion. JAMA 1994; 272: 59–64.
3. Shepherd FA. Malignant pericardial effusion. Curr Opin Oncol 1997; 9: 170–4.
4. Light RW, Vargas FS. Pleural sclerosis for the treatment of pneumothorax and pleural effusion. Lung 1997; 175: 213–23.
5. Grossi F, et al. Management of malignant pleural effusions. Drugs 1998; 55: 47–58.
6. Erasmus JJ, Patz EF. Treatment of malignant pleural effusions. Curr Opin Pulm Med 1999; 5: 250–5.

Malignant neoplasms of the bladder. Cancer of the bladder is the fourth or fifth most common cancer in Europe and the USA, where over 90% of bladder cancers are transitional cell in type. About two-thirds of all cases occur in men, and the median age at diagnosis is 65 years. Known risk factors include smoking and exposure to aniline dyes. In countries where it is endemic, schistosomiasis is an important cause of squamous cell bladder cancer. Most patients present with haematuria; there may also be urinary frequency or dysuria.

Urothelial tumours fall into two major groups, superficial and invasive, which differ in prognosis and management.[1-7] About 70 to 80% of cases at presentation are superficial (non-muscle invasive), and 20 to 30% are invasive.

Of the superficial tumours, about 70% are low-grade transitional cell carcinomas confined to the mucosa (Ta), and have a low risk of progression to muscle invasive disease and a 50% chance of recurrence. Most of the remainder are higher-grade transitional cell carcinomas that have invaded the submucosa (T1), and a small percentage are high-grade carcinoma in situ (CIS). These high-grade tumours have a high risk of progression to muscle invasive disease, and a 50 to 90% chance of recurrence. The standard initial treatment for primary or recurrent superficial disease is surgery, in the form of transurethral resection. In an attempt to prolong remission and reduce the recurrence rate various antineoplastics have been instilled into the bladder after complete resection (prophylactic or adjuvant intravesical therapy). Effective agents include doxorubicin, epirubicin, mitomycin and thiotepa. These have been shown to increase the disease-free interval, but not to reduce the risk of progression to invasive disease, nor to prolong survival.[8] Good results have also been reported with intravesical BCG, which is at least as effective as chemotherapy by the intravesical route, and in some studies has produced lower recurrence rates.[9,10] Currently, it is considered reasonable to use no adjuvant intravesical therapy in patients with primary resected low-grade tumours.[4,6] Adjuvant intravesical therapy with an antineoplastic or perhaps BCG[11] is recommended for patients with recurrent Ta tu-

mours or primary higher grade T1, and BCG is generally preferred to antineoplastics in primary CIS.[4,6,7] Maintenance intravesical BCG therapy for CIS has been suggested.[4] Other agents under investigation for intravesical therapy include bropirimine, interferon alfa, and valrubicin, and photodynamic therapy using intravesical 5-aminolaevulinic acid has been tried. In recurrent or persistent superficial disease with high risk of progression, cystectomy is usually preferred.[4,6]

Management of invasive bladder cancer that has not yet metastasised is a matter of some controversy,[1,3] but conventional therapy has revolved around radical surgery, radiotherapy, or a combination of the two. However, such conventional therapy offers a 5-year survival rate of 50% or less.[3] In consequence, alternatives, including the use of systemic chemotherapy before, or in combination with, cystectomy or radiotherapy, have been tried. The optimal regimen remains to be defined but regimens incorporating cisplatin and methotrexate, such as M-VAC (methotrexate, vinblastine, doxorubicin, and cisplatin), appear to be widely used. Such therapy has produced delays in recurrence of disease, but evidence for improved survival appears to be lacking. For example, a recent large study comparing neo-adjuvant therapy using CMV (cisplatin, methotrexate, and vinblastine) before cystectomy or radiotherapy, found this regimen to result in a higher response rate, but not to significantly prolong survival.[12]

Patients with unresectable or metastatic disease, or who subsequently develop metastatic disease, are usually treated with systemic chemotherapy.[4] For patients with good prognosis, a combination regimen such as M-VAC or CMV may be used. Various combinations of gemcitabine or ifosfamide, paclitaxel, and cisplatin are under investigation,[4] and gemcitabine plus cisplatin has been shown to provide similar survival advantage to MVAC with better tolerability: some now consider that it should be the preferred regimen in advanced disease.[13]

1. Dawson C, Whitfield H. Urological malignancy—II: urothelial tumours. BMJ 1996; 312: 1090–4.
2. Hall RR. Superficial bladder cancer. BMJ 1994; 308: 910–13.
3. Parker CC, Huddart RA. Management of invasive bladder cancer. Br J Hosp Med 1996; 56: 213–18.
4. National Comprehensive Cancer Network. NCCN urothelial cancer practice guidelines. Oncology 1998; 12: 225–271.
5. van der Meijden APM. Bladder cancer. BMJ 1998; 317: 1366–9.
6. Otto T, et al. Therapy of superficial bladder carcinomas. Urol Int 1999; 63: 32–9.
7. Smith JA, et al. The American Urological Association. Bladder Cancer Clinical Guidelines Panel summary report on the management of nonmuscle invasive bladder cancer (stages Ta, T1 and TIS). J Urol (Baltimore) 1999; 162: 1697–1701.
8. Pawinski A, et al. A combined analysis of European Organization for Research and Treatment of Cancer, and Medical Research Council randomised clinical trials for the prophylactic treatment of stage TaT1 bladder cancer. J Urol (Baltimore) 1996; 156: 1934–40.
9. Moss JT, Kadmon D. BCG and the treatment of superficial bladder cancer. DICP Ann Pharmacother 1991; 25: 1355–67.
10. Alexandroff AB, et al. BCG immunotherapy of bladder cancer: 20 years on. Lancet 1999; 353: 1689–94.
11. Shelley MD, et al. Intravesical bacillus Calmette-Guerin in Ta and T1 bladder cancer (updated 15 August 2000). Available in The Cochrane Library; Issue 4. Oxford: Update Software; 2001.
12. International Collaboration of Trialists. Neoadjuvant cisplatin, methotrexate, and vinblastine chemotherapy for muscle-invasive bladder cancer: a randomised controlled trial. Lancet 1999; 354: 533–40. Correction. ibid.; 1650.
13. von der Maase H, et al. Gemcitabine and cisplatin versus methotrexate, vinblastine, doxorubicin, and cisplatin in advanced or metastatic bladder cancer: results of a large, randomized, multinational, multicenter, phase III study. J Clin Oncol 2000; 17: 3068–77.

Malignant neoplasms of the bone. Solid cancers frequently metastasise to the skeleton and metastatic bone disease is a common problem with cancers of the breast, prostate, and lung. Bone metastases are often responsible for cancer pain (the general management of which is discussed on p.5) and also result in immobility, bone fractures, bone-marrow failure, spinal cord compression, and hypercalcaemia.[1] The most common sites of metastasis are the spine, hip, and femur. Primary bone malignancies are rare, and are usually sarcomas (p.500). Multiple myeloma (p.489) also produces bone involvement.

Management of **bone metastases** is essentially palliative since cure is rarely possible.[1,2] External beam radiotherapy is the best treatment for localised metastatic bone pain, with responses occurring in over 70% of patients. Radiation delivered by bone seeking isotopes such as samarium-153 or strontium-89 is an alternative.[3,4] Intravenous bisphosphonates are of benefit in patients with severe bone pain that is too widespread for local use of radiotherapy and does not respond to other analgesics.[2]

Structural weakness secondary to extensive bone loss may require structural support.[1,2] Surgical fixation or stabilisation may be undertaken to treat or prevent fractures.

Surgical excision and reconstruction with methylmethacrylate bone cement may also be required.

Bone metastases cause local osteolysis and various inhibitors of bone resorption have been tried, not only to correct hypercalcaemia of malignancy (p.1181), but also to relieve bone pain and reduce the risk of fractures. Several randomised trials in patients with metastatic bone disease from breast cancer or multiple myeloma have shown 25 to 50% reductions in skeletal events with the use of the bisphosphonates, clodronate or pamidronate.[2,5] Various organisations have produced guidelines to suggest which patients are best treated with bisphosphonates.[2,6] The clearest evidence is in patients who already have lytic destruction of bone. There is much interest in the use of bisphosphonates to prevent the development of bone metastases. However, preliminary evidence of their efficacy is conflicting,[7] and further large controlled trials are considered warranted.[2,6]

Systemic antineoplastic therapy should also be given if the primary tumour is chemosensitive. Endocrine treatment is usually preferred for patients with breast and prostatic cancers, and can produce useful control of symptoms from bone metastases.[1,2] Patients who also have visceral metastases or who have hormone resistant tumours should probably be treated with cytotoxic antineoplastics.[2]

1. Aaron AD. The management of cancer metastatic to bone. JAMA 1994; 272: 1206–9.
2. The Breast Specialty Group of the British Association of Surgical Oncology. The management of metastatic bone disease in the United Kingdom. Eur J Surg Oncol 1999; 25: 3–23.
3. Nightengale B, et al. Strontium chloride Sr89 for treating pain from metastatic bone disease. Am J Health-Syst Pharm 1995; 52: 2189–95.
4. McEwan AJB. Use of radionuclides for the palliation of bone metastases. Semin Radiat Oncol 2000; 10: 103–114.
5. Bloomfield DJ. Should bisphosphonates be part of the standard therapy of patients with multiple myeloma or bone metastases from other cancers? An evidence-based review. J Clin Oncol 1998; 16: 1218–25.
6. Hillner BE, et al. American Society of Clinical Oncology guideline on the role of bisphosphonates in breast cancer. J Clin Oncol 2000; 18: 1378–91.
7. Diel IJ, Mundy GR. Bisphosphonates in the adjuvant treatment of cancer: experimental evidence and first clinical results. Br J Cancer 2000; 82: 1381–6.

Malignant neoplasms of the brain. Most primary brain malignancies are gliomas, such as astrocytoma and glioblastoma multiforme. The frequency and natural history of brain tumours differ between children and adults. Low-grade astrocytomas, and medulloblastomas are the commonest primary brain tumours in children and anaplastic astrocytomas and glioblastoma multiforme are the most common in adults. However, metastatic brain cancer is the most common cause of intracranial tumours in adults, being up to ten times more common than primary brain tumours. The cancers that most frequently metastasise to the brain are lung cancer, breast cancer, and melanoma. CNS involvement in patients with acute leukaemia (p.484) or lymphoma (p.487) is also quite common.

The symptoms of primary and metastatic cranial neoplasms are those of local pressure and damage to the brain (such as focal seizures and visual field defects), of displacement of brain structures (like oculomotor paresis with tentorial herniation) and of raised intracranial pressure (such as impaired consciousness and papilloedema). The single most frequent symptom is headache, which is seen in about 60% of cases.

The mainstay of treatment for most primary brain tumours is surgery to relieve compression and cerebral oedema, establish diagnosis, and where feasible resect as much of the tumour as possible.[1-6] The combination of high-dose corticosteroids and computed tomography has reduced the morbidity of surgery, both for biopsy and excision. For benign tumours (such as pilocytic astrocytomas) resection may be curative, and even for malignant tumours (such as anaplastic astrocytomas, glioblastoma multiforme, and medulloblastomas) there is evidence that extensive resection prolongs survival. Adjuvant radiotherapy is widely used after surgical resection for malignant tumours in adults and children. Surgery alone or combined with radiotherapy is also used for single brain metastases.[7] For multiple brain metastases, most patients are treated with radiotherapy and corticosteroids. Radiosurgery is an investigational technique developed to reduce the radiation dose received by normal brain tissue. Radioactive implants (brachytherapy) are also being investigated.

The role of adjuvant chemotherapy for primary brain malignancies has been less certain, in part because of the difficulty in finding drugs that can cross the blood-brain barrier; the nitrosoureas such as carmustine and lomustine have been the drugs most frequently used, because of their lipid solubility. The PCV regimen, in which procarbazine, lomustine, and vincristine are given, is now generally preferred to single-agent nitrosoureas in the treatment of gliomas after surgical resection and radiation therapy.[4] In young children chemotherapy may be used as a stopgap measure to delay, or reduce the frequency of, radiotherapy, which can cause neurodevelopmental damage.[1,2,5] Studies in children under 3 years of age given combination chemotherapy regimens (often including cyclophosphamide, vincristine, cisplatin or carboplatin, and etoposide or methotrexate), after surgical resection of tumour found that radiotherapy could be safely delayed in most and that a few children might never require it.[5] Adjuvant chemotherapy (for example, vincristine and lomustine with or without cisplatin) has also been used to allow a reduction in radiation therapy in children aged between 3 and 10 years.[5] This chemotherapy regimen has also been used in children with poor-risk medulloblastoma.

Since present regimens for primary brain tumours are far from optimal, alternatives continue to be tried.[8] Newer antineoplastics include temozolomide and topoisomerase inhibitors such as irinotecan. Newer delivery techniques include implantation of biodegradable polymers impregnated with carmustine (which has been shown to improve survival in patients with malignant glioma), and the transient disruption of the blood-brain barrier to allow cytotoxics to cross. Other investigational treatments include thalidomide, lymphokine-activated killer cells, antisense oligonucleotides, and the use of gene therapy.[8,9] The most commonly investigated experimental technique for gene therapy involves the incorporation of the herpes simplex thymidine kinase gene into tumour cells via a retrovirus; such transduced tumour cells can then activate, and be killed by, the antiviral agent ganciclovir.[8]

The value of chemotherapy in cerebral metastatic disease remains to be defined:[7] the primary tumour may be intrinsically resistant to chemotherapy, or metastasis may develop despite treatment of the primary tumour, which will encourage the selection of resistant species. Furthermore, although the blood-brain barrier may not be completely intact in these patients, allowing some passage of antineoplastics into the brain, drug delivery of the less lipid-soluble drugs to cerebral metastases may not be sufficient, or sufficiently consistent, to produce a response. Nonetheless cerebral metastases of some chemosensitive primary tumours may respond to therapy.

1. Black PM. Brain tumors. *N Engl J Med* 1991; **324:** 1471–6 and 1555–64.
2. Pollack IF. Brain tumors in children. *N Engl J Med* 1994; **331:** 1500–7.
3. Bliss P, Brada M. The management of gliomas. *Br J Hosp Med* 1996; **55:** 82–3.
4. Kaba SE, Kyritsis AP. Recognition and management of gliomas. *Drugs* 1997; **53:** 235–44.
5. Packer RJ. Childhood medulloblastoma: progress and future challenges. *Brain Dev* 1999; **21:** 75–81.
6. DeAngelis LM. Brain tumours. *N Engl J Med* 2001; **344:** 114–23.
7. Davey P. Brain metastases. *Curr Probl Cancer* 1999; **23:** 59–98.
8. Avgeropoulos NG, Batchelor TT. New treatment strategies for malignant gliomas. *Oncologist* 1999; **4:** 209–24.
9. Jinnah HA, Friedmann T. Gene therapy and the brain. *Br Med Bull* 1995; **51:** 138–48.

Malignant neoplasms of the breast. Cancer of the breast is the most common malignant neoplasm in women. The disease is rare under the age of 25, and increases in incidence with age, although the rate of increase slows after the menopause. Risk factors include a family history (women with inherited *BRCA1* or *BRCA2* mutations are at higher risk), and reproductive hormonal factors such as early menarche, late menopause, nulliparity, and older age at birth of first child. Oral contraceptives and postmenopausal HRT are also associated with a small excess risk (see Carcinogenicity, Breast, on p.1453 and p.1461 respectively).

Ductal carcinoma in situ (DCIS) is a tumour localised to the breast ducts with no evidence of invasion. Invasive breast cancer can be divided into three main groups: early breast cancer (operable, primary, stage I/II); locally advanced disease (inoperable local, stage III); or advanced disease (metastatic; stage IV). Breast cancer is an extremely heterogeneous disorder, and the clinical course is consequently very variable; such factors as patient age and menopausal status, tumour size and grade, involvement of axillary lymph nodes or skin, and presence of hormone receptors within the tumour may be a guide to the extent and aggressiveness of disease, and hence have prognostic significance for treatment.[1-5]

Up to one-third of breast cancers detected by mammography screening are **ductal carcinomas in situ** (DCIS). The natural history of this cancer, which was rarely diagnosed before the use of mammography, is not fully understood, and there is controversy about its treatment.[6] Mastectomy was the standard treatment, but it is now felt that the majority of women with DCIS are candidates for breast conserving surgery. However, in contrast to invasive breast cancer, outcomes after mastectomy have not been directly compared with breast conserving surgery. There is good evidence that the use of radiotherapy after breast conserving surgery for DCIS reduces the risk of local recurrence and development of invasive disease. There is also evidence that the addition of tamoxifen further reduces the risk.[7] Currently there are no universally accepted prognostic factors for DCIS to allow tailoring of therapy to individual risk. Therefore decisions on therapy are based on the extent of the lesion, surgical margins, clinical judgement, and patient preference.[6]

In patients with **early disease** (stage I or II; a relatively small tumour with no or limited nodal involvement) the prognosis is fairly good. Primary treatment is surgical.[2,3,5] Breast conserving surgery followed by postoperative radiotherapy has been shown to have equivalent local recurrence rates and 10-year survival (about 60%) to mastectomy.[8] The use of postoperative radiotherapy after breast conserving surgery reduces local recurrence rates, but does not appear to affect overall survival.[8,9] Radiotherapy is not usually used after mastectomy, but there are some studies indicating that it may have additional benefits in patients at high risk of recurrence.[10,11]

Further adjuvant therapy with cytotoxic chemotherapy or hormonal manipulations such as tamoxifen and ovarian ablation by surgery, radiotherapy, or gonadorelin analogues has been given to try to eradicate the micrometastases which cause relapses. Overviews of a large number of trials by the Early Breast Cancer Trialists' Collaborative Group (EBCTCG) have confirmed the benefits of adjuvant therapy and attempted to determine which women derive most benefit and which regimens are most effective.[12-15] In these analyses, chemotherapy or hormonal therapy has been shown to have benefits in all women with early breast cancer, regardless of age and nodal status. However, the absolute benefits were greater in women with node-positive disease, and chemotherapy tended to have greater benefits in younger women. The analyses also indicate that the benefits of chemotherapy and tamoxifen are likely to be independent and probably additive. Adjuvant systemic therapy is now considered for all women with early breast cancer, except perhaps those with the lowest risk of recurrence.[3,5] The choice between adjuvant chemotherapy and hormonal therapy or a combination of both is less clear. Chemotherapy is preferred for both pre- and postmenopausal women with negative oestrogen receptor status.[3,5] For women at moderate or high risk of recurrence (e.g. node positive) who are oestrogen receptor positive, chemotherapy with or without tamoxifen may be used. For women at low risk of recurrence with oestrogen receptor positive disease, either tamoxifen or chemotherapy may be considered. Ovarian ablation by surgery or radiotherapy may be considered instead of chemotherapy in premenopausal women with oestrogen receptor positive disease.[5] The most commonly used adjuvant *chemotherapy* regimen has been cyclophosphamide, methotrexate, and fluorouracil (CMF). Other suitable regimens include anthracycline-based combinations such as fluorouracil, doxorubicin, and cyclophosphamide (FAC or CAF) and doxorubicin plus cyclophosphamide (AC). Epirubicin may be used as an alternative to doxorubicin. Anthracycline regimens have been used particularly in women with node-positive disease.[5] The EBCTG analysis[13] found that 3 to 6 months of combination chemotherapy in women aged under 50 could produce reductions in risk of recurrence and mortality of around 35% and 27% respectively. Moreover, the benefits were not confined to this age group: in older women chemotherapy reduced the risks of recurrence and death by about 20% and 8 to 14% (depending on age) respectively.[13] More prolonged chemotherapy had no greater benefit than treatment for 3 to 6 months, and there was some evidence that anthracycline-containing regimens produced more benefit than those without.[13]

Investigational regimens for adjuvant chemotherapy include the sequential use of paclitaxel and AC. The optimum sequencing of surgery, radiotherapy, and chemotherapy is also being investigated. One study found that giving chemotherapy first followed by radio-

therapy produced better overall results than the reverse order.[16] The use of neoadjuvant chemotherapy before surgery in locally advanced disease (see below) has led to its investigation in early disease. While studies have shown its use allows an increase in breast-conserving surgery, there is no clear evidence of an improvement in disease-free or overall survival.[17] Reducing dose intensity results in poorer survival, and this has led to the hypothesis that higher doses may offer more benefit, particularly in patients at high risk of recurrence. However, despite positive reports from phase II trials of high-dose chemotherapy with stem-cell support, and the widespread use of such therapy, particularly in the USA, recent randomised trials have failed to show any benefit of high-dose over standard dose therapy.[18]

In women with oestrogen-receptor positive tumours, the EBCTG analysis showed that 5 years of *hormonal therapy* with tamoxifen was associated with reductions in risk of disease recurrence and death of 50% and 28% respectively.[14] However, the effects of tamoxifen were small in women with oestrogen-receptor negative tumours,[14] and tamoxifen is no longer recommended in women with known oestrogen receptor-negative disease.[3,10,11] The optimum duration of tamoxifen remains to be determined, but more than 5 years' treatment did not appear to confer any additional benefits. An EBCTG analysis has also shown that premenopausal women (but not postmenopausal women) also benefit from ovarian ablation by surgery or radiotherapy.[12,15] Investigational therapies include the newer oestrogen antagonists such as the aromatase inhibitors, and the use of ovarian ablation with gonadorelin analogues combined with tamoxifen and/or chemotherapy.

In locally advanced breast cancer (stage III) the few patients for whom initial surgery is feasible may be treated as those with high-risk early breast cancer (see above). However, for most patients initial therapy is combination chemotherapy, with or without hormonal therapy.[5] Chemotherapy usually results in sufficient tumour shrinkage to allow surgical management.[5] Radiotherapy and additional chemotherapy and tamoxifen are used after surgery.

The aims of therapy in **advanced disease** (stage IV) are palliation and prolongation of life; cure is generally not possible with current regimens,[1,3,5] and it is often appropriate to select therapy on the basis of its adverse effects, to achieve optimal risk/benefit ratios.[19] The choice of initial therapy is between hormonal treatment and combination chemotherapy. *Hormonal therapy* is likely to be favoured in patients with oestrogen receptor-positive tumours, postmenopausal status, long disease-free interval since primary treatment for early breast cancer, and disease limited to bone or soft tissues. *Chemotherapy* is preferred for oestrogen receptor-negative tumours and for aggressive disease, particularly where metastasis is to critical visceral sites such as the liver, or where there has been a short disease-free interval since treatment for early breast cancer. Chemotherapy is also used after failure of second or third-line hormonal treatment. Tamoxifen is probably still the first option for hormonal therapy although results of comparative trials with aromatase inhibitors suggest that this may change. For patients who relapse during or after treatment with tamoxifen, selective aromatase inhibitors such as anastrozole or letrozole are the preferred second-line option in postmenopausal women and ovarian ablation or progestogens in premenopausal women. Progestogens such as medroxyprogesterone acetate are as effective as tamoxifen but not as well tolerated. Ovarian ablation with gonadorelin analogues may be tried. Other anti-oestrogens, such as toremifene have been investigated for first- or second-line treatment. Options for combination chemotherapy include CMF, FAC, or related regimens. The prior use of adjuvant chemotherapy for early breast cancer is likely to influence the response to further treatment. In patients with anthracycline-resistant disease the taxanes, paclitaxel and docetaxel, are favoured for second-line treatment, with vinorelbine often reserved for third-line treatment.[3] Other active agents include capecitabine, gemcitabine, mitozantrone [mitoxantrone], mitomycin, and raltitrexed.[3,5] In cancers which overexpress HER2 (human epidermal growth factor receptor-2), the anti-HER2 monoclonal antibody trastuzumab is an option for chemotherapy-resistant disease. Trastuzumab is also being investigated in combination with various antineoplastics; improved responses have been shown when trastuzumab was combined with an anthracycline and cyclophosphamide, or with paclitaxel.[20] Higher response rates have been achieved by intensive regimens, combined with autologous bone-marrow transplants or stem cells in some studies. However, the results of randomised trials have been disappointing, with no improvement in survival with the use of stem-cell supported high-dose therapy in metastatic breast cancer.[18,21]

The use of bisphosphonates in women with bone metastases reduces bone pain and skeletal complications such as fracture, spinal cord compression, and hypercalcaemia (see Malignant Neoplasms of the Bone, above). Radiotherapy is also used for bone pain, and for the treatment of brain metastases (see Malignant Neoplasms of the Brain, above).

1. Leonard RCF, *et al.* Metastatic breast cancer. *BMJ* 1994; **309:** 1501–4.
2. Allum WH, Smith IE. Carcinoma of the breast. *Br J Hosp Med* 1995; **54:** 255–8.
3. Hortobagyi GN. Treatment of breast cancer. *N Engl J Med* 1998; **339:** 974–84.
4. Buzdar AU, Hortobagyi GN. Breast cancer. *Cancer Chemother Biol Response Modif* 1999; **18:** 435–69.
5. National Comprehensive Cancer Network. Update: NCCN practice guidelines for the treatment of breast cancer. *Oncology* 1999; **13:** 41–66.
6. Schwartz GF, *et al.* Consensus conference on the treatment of in situ ductal carcinoma of the breast, April 22-25, 1999. *Cancer* 2000; **88:** 946–54.
7. Fisher B, *et al.* Tamoxifen in treatment of intraductal breast cancer: National Surgical Adjuvant Breast and Bowel Project B-24 randomised controlled trial. *Lancet* 1999; **353:** 1993–2000.
8. Early Breast Cancer Trialists' Collaborative Group. Effects of radiotherapy and surgery in early breast cancer: an overview of the randomized trials. *N Engl J Med* 1995; **333:** 1444–55. Correction. *ibid.* 1996; **334:** 1003.
9. Early Breast Cancer Trialists' Collaborative Group. Favourable and unfavourable effects on long-term survival of radiotherapy for early breast cancer: an overview of the randomised trials. *Lancet* 2000; **355:** 1757–70.
10. Overgaard M, *et al.* Postoperative radiotherapy in high-risk premenopausal women with breast cancer who receive adjuvant chemotherapy. *N Engl J Med* 1997; **337:** 949–55.
11. Ragaz J, *et al.* Adjuvant radiotherapy and chemotherapy in node-positive premenopausal women with breast cancer. *N Engl J Med* 1997; **337:** 956–62.
12. Early Breast Cancer Trialists' Collaborative Group. Systematic treatment of early breast cancer by hormonal, cytotoxic, or immune therapy: 133 randomised trials involving 31 000 recurrences and 24 000 deaths among 75 000 women. *Lancet* 1992; **339:** 1–15 and 71–85.
13. Early Breast Cancer Trialists' Collaborative Group. Polychemotherapy for early breast cancer: an overview of the randomised trials. *Lancet* 1998; **352:** 930–42.
14. Early Breast Cancer Trialists' Collaborative Group. Tamoxifen for early breast cancer (updated 28 August 2001). Available in The Cochrane Library; Issue 4. Oxford: Update Software; 2001.
15. Early Breast Cancer Trialists' Collaborative Group. Ovarian ablation for early breast cancer (updated 28 August 2001). Available in The Cochrane Library; Issue 4. Oxford: Update Software; 2001.
16. Recht A, *et al.* The sequencing of chemotherapy and radiation therapy after conservative surgery for early-stage breast cancer. *N Engl J Med* 1996; **334:** 1356–61.
17. Wolff AC, Davidson NE. Primary systemic therapy in operable breast cancer. *J Clin Oncol* 2000; **18:** 1558–69.
18. Bergh J. Where next with stem-cell-supported high-dose therapy for breast cancer. *Lancet* 2000; **355:** 944–5.
19. Fossati R, *et al.* Cytotoxic and hormonal treatment for metastatic breast cancer: a systematic review of published randomized trials involving 31510 women. *J Clin Oncol* 1998; **16:** 3439–60.
20. Slamon DJ, *et al.* Use of chemotherapy plus a monoclonal antibody against HER2 for metastatic breast cancer that overexpresses HER2. *N Engl J Med* 2001; **344:** 783–92.
21. Lippman ME. High-dose chemotherapy plus autologous bone marrow transplantation for metastatic breast cancer. *N Engl J Med* 2000; **342:** 1119–20.

PROPHYLAXIS. The recognition of factors increasing the risk of breast cancer, and particularly the identification of specific genes that confer a high risk, has led to increasing urgency to find effective ways of preventing the disease. Current options, other than regular screening to detect the cancer at early stages, include surgery (prophylactic mastectomy and/or oophorectomy), drug therapy (below), and possibly some life-style modifications.[1] No option affords complete protection, and there are no clear data on the overall risks and benefits of each approach. Various groups have produced recommendations for the management of hereditary breast cancer to aid in decision making.[2-5]

Treatment with tamoxifen as part of the adjuvant management of early breast cancer is associated with a reduced risk of developing cancer in the other breast (see above). In view of the difficulty of treating breast cancer once it develops this led to the suggestion that prophylactic tamoxifen might prevent the development of breast cancer in women at risk, and to various trials to test this hypothesis. These studies were not without controversy, given the different risk/benefit for tamoxifen use in healthy women as opposed to women with breast cancer. The first study to be reported was the US National Surgical Adjuvant Breast and Bowel Project (NSABP) P-1 trial,[6] which randomised 13 388 women to 5 years' treatment with tamoxifen or placebo. Participants were either aged 60 years or older, had a history of lobular carcinoma in situ, or had a 5-year predicted risk of develop-

ing breast cancer of greater than 1.66% (as assessed by number of first-degree relatives with breast cancer, number of previous breast biopsies, presence of atypical hyperplasia, and reproductive factors). In this study there was a highly significant 49% reduction in the occurrence of invasive breast cancer in women receiving tamoxifen (21.4 cancers prevented per 1000 women treated). The incidence of non-invasive breast cancer was reduced to a similar extent. Tamoxifen reduced the incidence of oestrogen-receptor positive, but not oestrogen-receptor negative, tumours. Adverse effects of tamoxifen included a modest increase in the risk of endometrial cancer and vascular events (stroke and pulmonary embolism). Preliminary results from 2 smaller randomised European trials did not confirm the benefit of tamoxifen in breast cancer prevention. The British trial[7] was in women with a first-degree family history of breast cancer, and their median age was younger than in the US trial. The Italian trial[8] was in hysterectomised women with no particular risk for breast cancer, and because of its size may not have been sufficiently powered to detect an effect of tamoxifen. Both the European trials, but not the US trial, allowed hormone replacement therapy to be used. None of the trials assessed the incidence of the BRCA1 and 2 genes in the participants, and it is therefore not known if tamoxifen can reduce the risk of breast cancer in patients with these mutations. It is also unclear whether tamoxifen could improve overall survival or is merely delaying the development of breast cancer. Because the US trial was unblinded and all women were allowed to receive tamoxifen, it will not be possible to gain survival data from this trial. Another large placebo-controlled trial is ongoing, and it is hoped this may provide answers to some of these questions. Until then, it is likely there will be continued disagreement on whether tamoxifen should be used for primary prevention, and if so, in whom, and for how long. Various groups have produced assessments of the prophylactic use of tamoxifen.[9-11]

Another anti-oestrogen, raloxifene, has reportedly shown a reduction in breast cancer risk while its effects on osteoporosis were being studied; further data are required.[9]

Other candidates for the prevention of breast cancer include plant oestrogens (phytoestrogens) such as those in soya. Epidemiological evidence suggests that diets high in these compounds may be protective. It was thought that retinoids may also be protective, but a secondary prevention trial of fenretinide failed to show any benefit.[12]

Various life-style modifications have the potential to reduce breast cancer risk based on epidemiological data. These include weight loss, increase in exercise, and dietary factors.[1] These may be proposed as part of an approach to a healthy life-style, but their real value in reducing breast cancer risk is unproven.

1. Chlebowski RT. Reducing the risk of breast cancer. *N Engl J Med* 2000; **343:** 191–8.
2. Burke W, *et al.* Recommendations for follow-up care of individuals with an inherited predisposition to cancer: BRCA1 and BRCA2. *JAMA* 1997; **277:** 997–1003.
3. Eisinger F, *et al.* Recommendations for medical management of hereditary breast and ovarian cancer: the French National Ad Hoc Committee. *Ann Oncol* 1998; **9:** 939–50.
4. Møller P, *et al.* Guidelines for follow-up of women at high risk for inherited breast cancer: consensus statement from the Biomed 2 Demonstration Programme on Inherited Breast Cancer. *Dis Markers* 1999; **15:** 207–11.
5. Eisen A, *et al.* Prophylactic surgery in women with a hereditary predisposition to breast and ovarian cancer. *J Clin Oncol* 2000; **18:** 1980–95.
6. Fisher B, *et al.* Tamoxifen for prevention of breast cancer: report of the National Surgical Adjuvant Breast and Bowel Project P-1 study. *J Natl Cancer Inst* 1998; **90:** 1371–88.
7. Powles T, *et al.* Interim analysis of the incidence of breast cancer in the Royal Marsden Hospital tamoxifen randomised chemoprevention trial. *Lancet* 1998; **352:** 98–101.
8. Veronesi U, *et al.* Prevention of breast cancer with tamoxifen: preliminary findings from the Italian randomised trial among hysterectomised women. *Lancet* 1998; **352:** 93–7.
9. Chlebowski RT, *et al.* American Society of Clinical Oncology technology assessment on breast cancer risk reduction strategies: tamoxifen and raloxifene. *J Clin Oncol* 1999; **17:** 1939–55.
10. American College of Obstetricians and Gynecologists. ACOG committee opinion; tamoxifen and the prevention of breast cancer in high-risk women. *Int J Gynecol Obstet* 2000; **68:** 73–5.
11. Anonymous. Pas de tamoxifène en prévention primaire du cancer du sein. *Rev Prescr* 1999; **19:** 775–8.
12. Veronesi U, *et al.* Randomized trial of fenretinide to prevent second breast malignancy in women with early breast cancer. *J Natl Cancer Inst* 1999; **91:** 1847–56.

MALIGNANT NEOPLASMS OF THE MALE BREAST. Breast cancer can occur in men, although it has a much lower incidence than in women. Risk factors are not well understood, but it may sometimes be associated with abnormalities of sex hormone metabolism, including those acquired through liver disease or testicular trauma. In addition, the inherited mutation BRCA2, which is associated with an increased risk of breast cancer in women, also increases the risk of breast cancer in men. Breast cancer

in men occurs at a slightly older median age than in women (60 to 70 years), and is more likely to be oestrogen-receptor positive. Survival by stage appears to be similar to that in women.

Treatment is similar to that for women.[1-5] Primary management is mastectomy and axillary lymph node dissection. Because of the rarity of the disease large controlled trials are lacking but studies in limited numbers of men and extrapolation from results in women suggest that adjuvant therapy should be considered on the same basis as for women. Radiotherapy may be used to reduce the rate of local recurrence in those considered at high risk. Adjuvant tamoxifen or chemotherapy may also be used, with tamoxifen being the most common. Chemotherapy is probably more appropriate in those with oestrogen-receptor negative tumours, locally advanced disease, or positive nodes. In advanced metastatic disease tamoxifen is generally the first choice treatment. Combination chemotherapy with cyclophosphamide, methotrexate and fluorouracil (CMF) or cyclophosphamide, doxorubicin, and fluorouracil (CAF) is reserved for unresponsive or relapsing disease. Hormonal ablation by adrenalectomy or orchidectomy is also effective, but has become less popular since the advent of tamoxifen.

1. Jaiyesimi IA, *et al.* Carcinoma of the male breast. *Ann Intern Med* 1992; **117:** 771–7.
2. Nagadowska MM, Fentiman IS. Male breast cancer. *Br J Hosp Med* 1993; **49:** 104–10.
3. Donegan WL, Redlich PN. Breast cancer in men. *Surg Clin North Am* 1996; **76:** 343–63.
4. Ravandi-Kashani F, Hayes TG. Male breast cancer: a review of the literature. *Eur J Cancer* 1998; **34:** 1341–7.
5. Jepson AS, Fentiman IS. Male breast cancer. *Int J Clin Pract* 1998; **52:** 571–6.

Malignant neoplasms of the cervix. Cancer of the uterine cervix is one of the most common cancers in women, accounting for about 12% of all female malignancies. It is associated with vaginal intercourse and the presence of human papilloma virus; high-risk types of the virus (HPV-16 and 18) that produce proteins E6 and E7 inactivate host tumour suppressor proteins and thus encourage malignant transformation. Smoking and long-term use of oral contraceptives (p.1453) may also be risk factors. Widespread screening has meant that in many women the disease has been detected in the preinvasive or early stages, when the prognosis is excellent to good.

Preinvasive cervical lesions (cervical intraepithelial neoplasia; CIN) may resolve spontaneously if low-grade, and may be monitored by repeat screening.[1,2] High-grade CIN (cervical dysplasia) and cervical carcinoma in situ may progress to invasive carcinoma and are usually treated with loop electrosurgical excision, laser vaporisation, or cryotherapy. Conization of the cervix (cone biopsy) may be used to rule out the presence of invasive disease. Investigational therapies include photodynamic therapy, and topical fluorouracil.

Invasive cervical cancers are mostly squamous cell in origin (80 to 90%), with 10 to 20% being adenocarcinoma. Invasive cervical cancers may be divided into early-stage (I and IIA), locally advanced (stages IIB to IVA), and metastatic (IVB). The earliest stage of invasive cervical cancer may be treated by conization of the cervix (which maintains fertility) or simple hysterectomy.[1,2] Other early-stage cancers may be treated by surgery (radical hysterectomy) or by radiotherapy. Some patients treated with surgery may require adjuvant radiotherapy. Recent evidence also indicates that patients with poor prognostic factors have better survival if cisplatin-based chemotherapy is added to radiotherapy.[3] Regimens used include cisplatin alone, or cisplatin combined with fluorouracil. Hydroxyurea [hydroxycarbamide] has also been used by some centres, but is less effective than cisplatin.[3] Patients with locally advanced cervical cancer are usually treated with primary radiation therapy,[1] and should also probably receive concurrent cisplatin-based chemotherapy.[3] The evidence for chemotherapy is stronger for stage IIB than for stages III/IVA. Neoadjuvant chemotherapy (chemotherapy before radiotherapy) has been tried, but does not appear to be beneficial.[3] Treatment for metastatic disease consists of palliative radiotherapy and/or chemotherapy with cisplatin;[1] cisplatin with paclitaxel is under investigation. Ifosfamide and bleomycin have also been used. Antineoplastics under investigation for the treatment of invasive cervical cancer include carboplatin, gemcitabine, and irinotecan. The use of human papilloma virus proteins E6 and E7 as targets for a therapeutic or prophylactic vaccine is also under investigation.[4]

1. Cannistra SA, Niloff JM. Cancer of the uterine cervix. *N Engl J Med* 1996; **334:** 1030–8.

2. Miller AB, *et al.* Report on consensus conference on cervical cancer screening and management. *Int J Cancer* 2000; **86:** 440–7.
3. Thomas GM. Concurrent chemotherapy and radiation for locally advanced cervical cancer: the new standard of care. *Semin Radiat Oncol* 2000; **10:** 44–50.
4. Murakami M, *et al.* Human papillomavirus vaccines for cervical cancer. *J Immunother* 1999; **22:** 212–18.

Malignant neoplasms of the endometrium. Cancer of the endometrium is a disease primarily of postmenopausal women, and is more common in developed than developing countries. Most of the risk factors for endometrial cancer are associated with increased oestrogen exposure. Factors resulting in increased endogenous exposure include obesity, anovulatory infertility, and late menopause. Exogenous factors include use of oestrogens without progestogens for hormone replacement therapy (p.1461), and tamoxifen therapy (see Carcinogenicity, p.571). Postmenopausal vaginal bleeding is the most common sign of endometrial cancer, and allows the disease to be diagnosed at an early stage when the prognosis is good (80% of women have early stage disease at presentation). In menopausal or premenopausal women, diagnosis may be delayed because abnormal bleeding patterns may not be so obvious. Most endometrial cancers are adenocarcinomas. A small percentage are clear-cell or serous carcinomas, which are highly aggressive and have a poorer prognosis. Endometrial hyperplasia is generally regarded as a precancerous lesion; endometrial hyperplasia with cytological atypia, in particular, is associated with progression to adenocarcinoma.

Surgery (hysterectomy and oophorectomy) is the primary therapy for endometrial cancers that are stage I to III.[1-3] No further treatment is required in women with stage I disease who are at low risk of recurrence. In those with stage I disease and a higher risk of recurrence, adjuvant brachytherapy or pelvic radiation are used. In all other women, adjuvant radiotherapy is given, the field being tailored depending on the disease stage. Adjuvant progestogen therapy has not been shown to be effective.[4] There are a few studies of adjuvant chemotherapy in women at high risk of recurrence, but further data from randomised trials are required to assess its role.[5] For women with advanced disease (stage IV), systemic therapy with progestogens or cytotoxic chemotherapy can be considered, although response rates are only up to 30%. Progestogens are likely to be preferred because of their better tolerability. Well-differentiated tumours, long disease-free interval, and positive hormone receptor status are factors that suggest increased response to progestogens. When progestogens are ineffective, chemotherapy may be tried. The agents of choice are probably doxorubicin, cisplatin or carboplatin, and cyclophosphamide. Investigational therapies include paclitaxel, dactinomycin, gonadorelin analogues such as goserelin, and anastrozole.[3]

1. Rose PG. Endometrial carcinoma. *N Engl J Med* 1996; **335:** 640–9. Correction. *ibid.* 1997; **336:** 1335.
2. Semple D. Endometrial cancer. *Br J Hosp Med* 1997; **57:** 260–2.
3. Chen L-M, *et al..* Endometrial cancer: recent developments in evaluation and treatment. *Oncology* 1999; **13:** 1665–70.
4. Martin-Hirsch PL, *et al.* Progestagens for endometrial cancer (updated 29 November 2000). Available in The Cochrane Library; Issue 1. Oxford: Update Software; 2001.
5. Pustilnik T, Burke TW. Adjuvant chemotherapy for high-risk endometrial cancer. *Semin Radiat Oncol* 2000; **10:** 23–8.

Malignant neoplasms of the eye. Tumours of the orbit of the eye in adults are most commonly metastases from primary lesions elsewhere in the body, usually in the breast or lung,[1] and local radiotherapy (external beam radiation or plaque radiotherapy) may be required for control of visual symptoms unresponsive to chemotherapeutic treatment of primary disease.[1]

Primary eye tumours are rare. In children, the most common intra-ocular tumour is retinoblastoma (see below), and the most common orbital tumour is rhabdomyosarcoma (see Soft-tissue Sarcomas, below). In adults, primary CNS lymphoma can originate in the eye (ocular lymphoma), and is treated with radiotherapy to the globe. However, the most common primary ocular cancer in adults is **intra-ocular melanoma** (posterior uveal melanoma), which accounts for 80% of all primary ocular cancers. Treatment options for small ocular melanomas include observation or local treatment (radiation, cryotherapy, local resection, photocoagulation, or hyperthermia).[2,3] Large melanomas are treated by removal of the eye (enucleation). Treatment of medium-sized tumours is controversial, with some preferring treatments that preserve vision, and some enucleation. At present there are no good data to support the use of adjuvant chemotherapy. In the few patients with metastatic uveal melanoma, resection and intra-arterial chemotherapy or

chemoembolisation may be used for isolated hepatic metastases.[3] Most of the combination chemotherapy regimens for palliative therapy have included dacarbazine.[3] Ocular surface neoplasms (lesions of the conjunctival or corneal epithelium) are usually treated with local excision. Where surgery is not feasible, topical application of mitomycin (0.04%) or fluorouracil (1%) has been tried.[4]

1. Shields CL. Plaque radiotherapy for the management of uveal metastasis. *Curr Opin Ophthalmol* 1998; **9:** 31–7.
2. Shields JA, Shields CL. Current management of posterior uveal melanoma. *Mayo Clin Proc* 1993; **68:** 1196–1200.
3. Wöll E, *et al.*. Uveal melanoma: natural history and treatment options for metastatic disease. *Melanoma Res* 1999; **9:** 575–81.
4. Majmudar PA, Epstein RJ. Antimetabolites in ocular surface neoplasia. *Curr Opin Ophthalmol* 1998; **9:** 35–9.

Malignant neoplasms of the gastrointestinal tract. Considered as a whole (and excluding skin cancers, which are often poorly registered) the gastrointestinal tract is the most frequent site of malignancies in the world's population, although the frequencies of the various types of gastrointestinal cancer vary greatly from country to country. Direct exposure to various environmental carcinogens is thought to play an important role in many of these cancers. Treatment may include surgery, radiotherapy, and chemotherapy, but the prognosis in most forms of gastrointestinal cancer is not encouraging.

Oesophageal cancer has perhaps the greatest variation in incidence between different geographical regions of any cancer, and is endemic in many parts of the world. The two major histological types are squamous cell carcinoma and adenocarcinoma. Squamous cell carcinoma is strongly associated with tobacco and alcohol use, and may occur as a second primary tumour in patients with tumours of the upper aerodigestive tract (see Malignant Neoplasms of the Head and Neck, below). Adenocarcinoma is more common in non-endemic regions, and is associated with Barrett's oesophagus (see Gastro-oesophageal Reflux Disease, p.1204). Oesophageal cancer usually develops as a growth or ulcerative lesion of the oesophagus with extensive infiltration of the mucosa and invasion of neighbouring structures. Lymphatic and blood-borne metastasis occurs at a relatively early stage. Symptoms of pain and dysphagia due to obstruction occur late and disease is usually well advanced at diagnosis.

Surgical resection is the preferred primary treatment in stage I oesophageal cancer. In general, in patients with localised disease, the choice is between surgery and primary chemoradiotherapy (with fluorouracil plus cisplatin or mitomycin), which appear to give equivalent results.[1,2] Because the overall 5-year survival rate in patients with operable tumours is only 5 to 20%, there has been great interest in adjuvant treatment (pre-operative or postoperative).[3] There is no clear evidence that pre-operative radiotherapy alone improves survival.[4] However, there is conflicting evidence on the value of chemoradiotherapy or chemotherapy used before surgery, with some trials showing improved survival, and others no additional benefit.[3] Meta-analysis has not shown benefit to date,[5] but this approach requires continued evaluation in clinical trials.[1] In half to two-thirds of patients the disease is too advanced at presentation for anything but palliation. Those with poor performance status should be offered supportive care.[1] This may include brachytherapy, laser therapy, or photodynamic therapy with photosensitisers such as porfimer sodium to relieve obstruction. In those patients with good performance status, chemotherapy may offer some palliation of the disease. Standard options include cisplatin-based or fluorouracil-based combinations.[1] Investigational drugs include paclitaxel and irinotecan.[1]

Cancer of the stomach is the most common non-skin cancer worldwide, with particularly high incidence in the Far East, Russia, and parts of Latin America, although the incidence is declining almost everywhere. Over 90% of malignant gastric neoplasms are adenocarcinomas. Less frequent gastric neoplasms include lymphomas (see MALT lymphoma, above) and carcinoid tumours (see above). Dietary factors, such as high consumption of salted or smoked foods, are thought to play a role in the development of gastric cancer. *Helicobacter pylori* infection, and resultant gastritis, plays a role in gastric lymphomas, and may also be a factor in gastric cancer. However, it is not yet known if elimination of *Helicobacter pylori* infection will prove useful in preventing the development of gastric cancer.[6]

Early disease is relatively asymptomatic or produces non-specific gastrointestinal symptoms such as dyspepsia. There is concern that the use of antisecretory drugs for these symptoms may delay the diagnosis of gastric

cancer (see Gastric Carcinoma, under Omeprazole Precautions, p.1240). Gastric epithelial dysplasia is a premalignant condition, and warrants follow-up and possible surgical intervention. Similarly, persistent gastric ulcers may be malignant. More advanced disease may produce discomfort or pain, anaemia, weight loss, and anorexia; obstruction, haemorrhage, and perforation may develop. Extension to the liver and pancreas, and lymphatic and blood-borne (portal) metastases may occur. The overall prognosis is not good, and 5-year survival rates are only 5 to 10%.

Surgery is the mainstay of treatment for early disease,[1,7-9] and is all that is required for stage I. Survival rates are poorer in other stages of locoregional disease, and various adjuvant approaches have been tried. Gastric cancer is relatively chemoresistant, and both an early and more recent meta-analysis of postoperative chemotherapy have failed to show a significant survival benefit.[10,11] Similarly adjuvant radiotherapy alone has not improved survival. More promising results have been obtained with combined chemoradiotherapy (most often with fluorouracil) after surgery. Thus, some recommend the use of adjuvant chemoradiotherapy after resection in the case of positive margins.[1] In addition, this is also an option for the primary treatment of inoperable locoregional disease.[1]

Treatment for advanced disease is purely palliative, and options include supportive care with or without chemotherapy.[1,8,9] Supportive care includes the relief of luminal obstruction with, for example, photodynamic therapy. Chemotherapy may have substantial palliative effect and modest survival gains, and may be considered in those with good performance status. Fluorouracil alone produces responses in up to 20% of patients. Despite doubts about the superiority of combination chemotherapy over single agents fluorouracil, doxorubicin, and mitomycin (FAM) has been widely used. Other combinations include the substitution of cisplatin or methotrexate for mitomycin (FAC and FAMTX, respectively) and the use of epirubicin instead of doxorubicin, (e.g. ECF—epirubicin, cisplatin, and fluorouracil). Investigational drugs include paclitaxel and various oral agents such as etoposide, and fluorouracil derivatives. A study comparing FAMTX with fluorouracil plus cisplatin or a regimen of etoposide, fluorouracil and folinic acid found that all 3 had only modest clinical benefits,[12] and no agreement on standard care exists at present.[13,14]

Cancers of the colon and rectum are very common in developed areas such as the USA and western Europe, but rare among African and Asian populations. Various genetic and dietary factors are thought to be related to development of the disease.[15] Inherited predisposition syndromes include familial adenomatous polyposis and hereditary non-polyposis colorectal cancer.[16] Most large bowel cancers arise within pre-existing intestinal polyps. Over 50% occur in the rectum and about 20% in the sigmoid colon. There may be direct invasion of neighbouring structures and metastatic spread to the lymph nodes, and to lungs, bone, and in particular, liver. Signs and symptoms include blood in the stools, altered bowel habit, anaemia, and weight loss; there may be local obstruction (depending on location) or perforation.

The first-line treatment for early-stage and locally-advanced disease (stages I to III; Dukes A to C) is surgery. Although complete surgical resection is possible in up to 80% of cases at the time of diagnosis, about 50% ultimately die of recurrent disease. Because of this, there has been much research in the use of adjuvant therapies. Local recurrence is more likely to occur with rectal cancers than colon cancers, since anatomical constraints make surgical removal of rectal tumours more difficult. Therefore, the use of local adjuvant (pre- or postoperative) radiotherapy has been extensively studied.[17] Many consider the use of postoperative radiotherapy (combined with adjuvant chemotherapy) to be the standard of care in patients with Dukes B and C (stage II and III) rectal cancer considered at high risk of local relapse. There is some evidence that pre-operative radiotherapy is more effective than postoperative, but further studies are required.[17] Adjuvant chemotherapy, usually based on fluorouracil, is also widely used, both in rectal and colon cancer. In locally advanced colon and rectal cancer (Dukes C; stage III), the use of adjuvant systemic fluorouracil-based therapy has been shown to improve survival,[18-20] and is considered the standard of care.[21-23] The case for adjuvant therapy in stage II colon and rectal cancer is less clear,[24] and its use should preferably be within clinical trials.[23]

Various approaches have been studied to improve the efficacy of fluorouracil adjuvant therapy. Fluorouracil is only effective against actively dividing cells, and there is some evidence that maximising the chances of exposure, by giving prolonged fluorouracil infusions, may improve the results of adjuvant therapy compared with bolus administration. Another approach is the use of biochemical modulators such as folinic acid (see also Administration under Fluorouracil, p.542).[23] Continuing research suggests that fluorouracil combined with low-dose folinic acid may become the preferred regimen.[25]

Newer antineoplastics such as oxaliplatin, irinotecan, and capecitabine, which have been used for palliative therapy, are also under investigation for adjuvant treatment.[23] Reports of improved survival with the adjuvant use of edrecolomab, a murine monoclonal antibody directed against an epithelial cell surface glycoprotein,[26,27] do not seem to have been borne out. Another potential approach is the adjuvant use of intraportal chemotherapy directed at the liver, one of the commonest sites of metastasis for colon cancer. In a meta-analysis of 10 studies,[28] the reduction in hepatic metastases with intraportal vein chemotherapy given for about 1 week after surgery was not significant, although there was a trend towards increased 5-year survival. It was concluded that additional trial evidence was required.[28]

Palliative treatments for advanced colorectal cancer (stage IV; metastatic disease) include surgery, radiotherapy, or chemotherapy.[15,29] In patients with isolated hepatic metastases, these may be surgically resected, or intrahepatic arterial chemotherapy may be considered (see Malignant Neoplasms of the Liver, below). In other patients with advanced colorectal cancer, palliative chemotherapy has resulted in modest survival benefits:[30] the combination of systemic fluorouracil with folinic acid has been recommended as standard chemotherapy. There is evidence that the addition of folinic acid improves the efficacy of fluorouracil in this setting,[31] and that continuous infusion of fluorouracil is more effective than bolus administration.[32] Irinotecan monotherapy is used as second-line therapy after failure of fluorouracil and has improved survival. It is also being investigated for first-line use in combination with fluorouracil.[33] Raltitrexed is also an option for the second-line treatment of advanced colorectal cancer. Oral alternatives to parenteral fluorouracil have been investigated, and include capecitabine, UFT (tegafur combined with uracil), and fluorouracil combined with eniluracil. Also under investigation is the platinum derivative oxaliplatin, which has been used alone and in combination with fluorouracil and folinic acid.[34] Various biological agents have been investigated. Interferon alfa has not proved effective as a modulator of fluorouracil. Anti-idiotype vaccines, gene therapy, and antisense therapy are under investigation.[29]

PROPHYLAXIS. Various drugs and dietary factors have been shown in epidemiological studies to be associated with a reduced risk of colorectal cancer, and some of these have been investigated in prospective randomised trials.[35] Aspirin and NSAIDs are the most widely studied. In short-term randomised trials, both sulindac and celecoxib have reduced the size and number of colonic polyps in patients with familial adenomatous polyposis. However, prophylactic surgical removal of the colon is still considered the standard of care for these patients.[35,36] Calcium supplementation has shown a moderate reduction in the formation of new adenomas in patients with a history of colorectal adenomas. Despite the epidemiological evidence for dietary fibre, a number of large randomised trials of fibre supplements or high-fibre diets have not found any reduction in the formation of new adenomas in patients with a history of colorectal adenomas. Antioxidant vitamins have also been investigated, but evidence for their benefit is conflicting (see Prophylaxis of Malignant Neoplasms, p.1353). Other potential chemopreventive agents on the basis of epidemiological evidence include folic acid, and menopausal HRT.[35]

An important component of the care of patients with inherited predisposition to colon cancer is regular screening.[36] Various screening methods are also under investigation for use in normal risk individuals.[37]

Cancers of the anal canal mucosa are most commonly squamous cell carcinomas. Risk factors include immunosuppression, genital human papillomavirus infection, and sexual activity. Combined chemotherapy and radiotherapy is the usual primary treatment.[38] Fluorouracil is commonly used, sometimes in combination with mitomycin, and the combination of fluorouracil and cisplatin is being investigated. For patients who do not respond, or

who subsequently relapse, surgical resection with the formation of a colostomy is preferred. There is no standard therapy for metastatic disease.[38]

1. National Comprehensive Cancer Network. NCCN practice guidelines for upper gastrointestinal carcinomas. *Oncology* 1998; **12:** 179–223. Correction. *ibid.* 1999; **13:** 259.
2. Minsky BD. Carcinoma of the esophagus. Part 1: primary therapy. *Oncology* 1999; **13:** 1225–32 and 1235–6.
3. Minsky BD. Carcinoma of the esophagus. Part 2: adjuvant therapy. *Oncology* 1999; **13:** 1415–27.
4. Arnott SJ, *et al.* Preoperative radiotherapy for esophageal carcinoma (updated 15 June 2001). Available in The Cochrane Library; Issue 4. Oxford: Update Software; 2001.
5. Malthaner R, Fenlon D. Preoperative chemotherapy for resectable thoracic esophageal cancer (updated 20 November 2001). Available in The Cochrane Library; Issue 4. Oxford: Update Software; 2001.
6. Scheiman JM, Cutler AF. Helicobacter pylori and gastric cancer. *Am J Med* 1999; **106:** 222–6.
7. Thompson GB, *et al.* Adenocarcinoma of the stomach: are we making progress? *Lancet* 1993; **342:** 713–18.
8. Fuchs CS, Mayer RJ. Gastric carcinoma. *N Engl J Med* 1995; **333:** 32–41.
9. Hendlisz A, Bleiberg H. Diagnosis and treatment of gastric cancer. *Drugs* 1995; **49:** 711–20.
10. Hermans J, *et al.* Adjuvant therapy after curative resection for gastric cancer: meta-analysis of randomised trials. *J Clin Oncol* 1993; **11:** 1441–7.
11. Earle CC, Maroun JA. Adjuvant chemotherapy after curative resection for gastric cancer in non-Asian patients: revisiting a meta-analysis of randomised trials. *Eur J Cancer* 1999; **35:** 1059–64.
12. Vanhoefer U, *et al.* Final results of a randomized phase III trial of sequential high-dose methotrexate, fluorouracil, and doxorubicin versus etoposide, leucovorin, and fluorouracil versus infusional fluorouracil and cisplatin in advanced gastric cancer: a trial of the European Organization for Research and Treatment of Cancer Gastrointestinal Tract Cancer Cooperative Group. *J Clin Oncol* 2000; **18:** 2648–57.
13. Ross PJ, *et al.* ECF in gastric cancer. *J Clin Oncol* 2000; **18:** 3874–5.
14. Ajani JA. Standard chemotherapy for gastric carcinoma: is it a myth? *J Clin Oncol* 2000; **18:** 4001–2.
15. Bodger K. Colorectal cancer. *J R Coll Physicians Lond* 2000; **34:** 197–201.
16. Midgley R, Kerr D. Colorectal cancer. *Lancet* 1999; **353:** 391–9.
17. Minsky BD. Adjuvant therapy of rectal cancer. *Semin Oncol* 1999; **26:** 540–4.
18. International Multicentre Pooled Analysis of Colon Cancer Trials (IMPACT) Investigators. Efficacy of adjuvant fluorouracil and folinic acid in colon cancer. *Lancet* 1995; **345:** 939–44.
19. Dube S, *et al.* Adjuvant chemotherapy in colorectal carcinoma: results of a meta-analysis. *Dis Colon Rectum* 1997; **40:** 35–41.
20. Midgley RSJ, Kerr DJ. Adjuvant therapy. *BMJ* 2000; **321:** 1208–11.
21. NIH Consensus Panel. Adjuvant therapy for patients with colon and rectal cancer. *JAMA* 1990; **264:** 1444–50.
22. Seventh King's Fund Forum. Cancer of the colon and rectum consensus statement. *Br J Surg* 1990; **77:** 1063–5.
23. Moore HCF, Haller DG. Adjuvant therapy of colon cancer. *Semin Oncol* 1999; **26:** 545–55.
24. IMPACT B2 Investigators. Efficacy of adjuvant fluorouracil and folinic acid in B2 colon cancer. *J Clin Oncol* 1999; **17:** 1356–63.
25. QUASAR Collaborative Group. Comparison of fluorouracil with additional levamisole, higher-dose folinic acid, or both, as adjuvant chemotherapy for colorectal cancer: a randomised trial. *Lancet* 2000; **355:** 1588–96.
26. Riethmüller G, *et al.* Randomised trial of monoclonal antibody for adjuvant therapy of resected Dukes' C colorectal carcinoma. *Lancet* 1994; **343:** 1177–83.
27. Riethmüller G, *et al.* Monoclonal antibody therapy for resected Dukes' C colorectal cancer: seven-year outcome of a multicentre randomised trial. *J Clin Oncol* 1998; **16:** 1788–94.
28. Liver Infusion Meta-analysis Group. Portal vein chemotherapy for colorectal cancer: a meta-analysis of 4000 patients in 10 studies. *J Natl Cancer Inst* 1997; **89:** 497–505.
29. Ross PJ, Cunningham D. Chemotherapy of metastatic bowel cancer. *Br J Hosp Med* 1996; **55:** 263–6.
30. Best L, *et al.* Palliative chemotherapy for advanced or metastatic colorectal cancer (updated 30 August 2000). Available in The Cochrane Library; Issue 4. Oxford: Update Software; 2001.
31. Advanced Colorectal Cancer Meta-analysis Project. Modulation of fluorouracil by leucovorin in patients with advanced colorectal cancer: evidence in terms of response rate. *J Clin Oncol* 1992; **10:** 896–903.
32. Meta-analysis Group in Cancer. Efficacy of intravenous continuous infusion of fluorouracil compared with bolus administration in advanced colorectal cancer. *J Clin Oncol* 1998; **16:** 301–308.
33. Saltz LB, *et al.* Irinotecan plus fluorouracil and leucovorin for metastatic colorectal cancer. *N Engl J Med* 2000; **343:** 905–14.
34. de Gramont A, *et al.* Leucovorin and fluorouracil with or without oxaliplatin as first-line treatment in advanced colorectal cancer. *J Clin Oncol* 2000; **18:** 2938–47.
35. Jänne PA, Mayer RJ. Chemoprevention of colorectal cancer. *N Engl J Med* 2000; **342:** 1960–8.
36. King JE, *et al.* Care of patients and their families with familial adenomatous polyposis. *Mayo Clin Proc* 2000; **75:** 57–67.
37. Rhodes JM. Colorectal cancer screening in the UK: joint position statement by the British Society of Gastroenterology, the Royal College of Physicians, and the Association of Coloproctology of Great Britain and Ireland. *Gut* 2000; **46:** 746–8.
38. Ryan DP, *et al.* Carcinoma of the anal canal. *N Engl J Med* 2000; **342:** 792–800.

Malignant neoplasms of the head and neck. Cancers of the head and neck are classically defined as those of the mucosal surfaces of the upper aerodigestive tract and include neoplasms of the oral cavity (accounting for 40%), pharynx (15%), and larynx (25%). The majority are squamous cell carcinomas, and the highest incidence is in men aged over 50 years. Overall, cancers of the head and neck account for about 5% of all malignant neoplasms in the West, but are the most common causes in other parts of the world. The major risk factor for these

cancers is the use of tobacco (whether chewed, inhaled, or smoked). Alcohol acts synergistically with tobacco to increase the risk. Endemic nasopharyngeal cancer in parts of India, China, and North Africa is associated with Epstein-Barr virus and the consumption of salt-cured fish.

Premalignant lesions include leucoplakia and erythroplakia, and these can progress to invasive cancer. About one-third of cancers are diagnosed at early stages (I and II), and the rest are usually locally advanced (stage III and IVA). Although early-stage disease can be successfully treated, there is a high incidence of second primary cancers in the head and neck, lung, or oesophagus. Therefore, there is interest in the development of chemopreventive agents to reduce this risk. Fewer than 30% of patients with locally advanced disease are cured.

Surgery or radiotherapy are the mainstays of treatment for early-stage cancers of the oral cavity and the oropharynx.[1-4] The choice is often debated, since both are equally effective, but have different complications. Radiotherapy is preferred for early-stage nasopharyngeal carcinoma, which is anatomically unresectable,[1-3,5] and for carcinoma of the larynx (vocal cords), to preserve the voice.[1-3]

For locally advanced disease, if surgery is used as primary therapy, adjuvant radiotherapy may be used.[1,3] There has also been great interest in the use of chemotherapy in addition to radiotherapy in patients with locally advanced tumours with the aim of improving cure rates, or avoiding the need for surgery and thereby allowing organ preservation. Some recommend this as standard for nasopharyngeal cancer,[3,5] and for cancers involving the larynx to preserve this organ.[3,6] A recent meta-analysis[7] showed only a small overall survival benefit for chemotherapy (4%) in locally advanced head and neck cancers. Further analysis by timing of chemotherapy suggested that there was no significant benefit for adjuvant or neoadjuvant therapy (except perhaps for neoadjuvant therapy with fluorouracil and a platinum compound), but that concomitant or alternating chemo-radiotherapy did offer significant benefits. The authors noted that trials in progress should help to confirm the benefit of combined therapy, and an optimum regimen.[7] Data from 3 trials of larynx preservation using chemotherapy/radiotherapy in patients with locally advanced disease showed a non-significant negative effect in the chemotherapy arm.[7] The authors concluded that laryngeal preservation should remain investigational.[7]

Palliative chemotherapy in metastatic or recurrent disease is likely to be with cisplatin or methotrexate.[1,3,6] Combination regimens such as cisplatin and fluorouracil or cisplatin, bleomycin, and methotrexate, with or without a vinca alkaloid, produce more responses but survival is not definitively improved.[3,6] The choice of best supportive care or single-agent or combination chemotherapy should be dictated by the patient's performance status, as the benefits of chemotherapy are limited.[3] Other active antineoplastics include paclitaxel, docetaxel, and gemcitabine. Also under investigation is local injection of cisplatin in a gel formulation containing adrenaline [epinephrine], and photodynamic therapy with temporfin. Biological approaches being investigated include a monoclonal epidermal growth factor receptor antibody (cetuximab, C-225) and various gene therapies.

Chemoprevention is also under investigation. Isotretinoin reduced the occurrence of second primary tumours in one study,[8] and reversed oral premalignant lesions (leukoplakia) in another.[9] However, it is not well tolerated, and alternative retinoids and other drugs are being considered.[10]

1. Vokes EE, *et al.* Head and neck cancer. *N Engl J Med* 1993; **328:** 184–94.
2. Tobias JS. Cancer of the head and neck. *BMJ* 1994; **308:** 961–6.
3. National Comprehensive Cancer Network. NCCN practice guidelines for head and neck cancer. *Oncology* 1998; **12:** 39–147.
4. Zakrzewska JM. Oral cancer. *BMJ* 1999; **318:** 1051–4.
5. Vokes EE, *et al.* Nasopharyngeal carcinoma. *Lancet* 1997; **350:** 1087–91.
6. Catimel G. Head and neck cancer: guidelines for chemotherapy. *Drugs* 1996; **51:** 73–88.
7. Pignon JP, *et al.* Chemotherapy added to locoregional treatment for head and neck squamous-cell carcinoma: three meta-analyses of updated individual data. *Lancet* 2000; **355:** 949–55. Correction. *ibid.*; 1650.
8. Hong WK, *et al.* Prevention of second primary tumors with isotretinoin in squamous-cell carcinoma of the head and neck. *N Engl J Med* 1990; **323:** 795–801.
9. Lippman SM, *et al.* Comparison of low-dose isotretinoin with beta carotene to prevent oral carcinogenesis. *N Engl J Med* 1993; **328:** 15–20.
10. Armstrong WB, Meyskens FL. Chemoprevention of head and neck cancer. *Otolaryngol Head Neck Surg* 2000; **122:** 728–35.

Malignant neoplasms of the kidney. Cancer of the kidney is relatively uncommon. About 80% of such cancers in adults are renal cell carcinoma, with the remainder mostly cancer of the renal pelvis. The disease is about twice as common in men as in women. Risk factors include smoking, obesity, and phenacetin use. Disease is often clinically silent; there may however be haematuria, flank and back pain, and a palpable mass in the flank or abdomen. About 45% of patients have early-stage disease at presentation (I and II), 25% have locally advanced disease (stage III), and 30% metastatic disease (stage IV). The most common sites for metastases are the lung, liver, and bone, although unusual sites for metastases are a common feature of renal cancer.

The main treatment for early-stage disease is surgery, usually radical nephrectomy although partial nephrectomy may be considered in some patients.[1-3] Radical nephrectomy is also used in selected patients with stage III disease. After radical nephrectomy 20 to 30% of patients with localised tumours will relapse, usually at distant sites.[1,3] This suggests that adjuvant therapy could be useful in reducing the risk of relapse.[2] However, radiotherapy is not beneficial, and no systemic therapy has been shown to reduce relapse (interferon alfa is not effective).[2,3] Standard care therefore remains close observation.[3]

In metastatic disease, nephrectomy may be considered in a few patients for palliation of symptoms. In addition, nephrectomy and surgical removal of solitary metastases may be appropriate in some patients.[1,3] In patients with minimal disease volume and good performance status, cytokine therapy with interleukin-2 or interferon alfa may be considered.[2,3] These cytokines have resulted in overall response rates of 10 to 20%, with a few long-term responses.[3] Meta-analysis has suggested a modest survival benefit for interferon alfa but the use of interleukin-2 has not been validated in appropriate comparative studies.[4] In other patients, supportive care remains the mainstay of therapy for metastatic disease.[3] Renal cell carcinoma is largely resistant to chemotherapy with currently available antineoplastics, and hormonal therapy with progestogens has also had poor success.[1,2] The most extensively studied antineoplastics are vinblastine and floxuridine. However, a review of 83 studies involving 4542 patients and over 70 different drugs found that only floxuridine and fluorouracil appeared to have even modest activity.[5] No antineoplastic can be considered standard in the treatment of metastatic disease.[1,6]

Investigational approaches include attempts to improve the response rates to interleukin-2 and interferon alfa by combining them together, or with antineoplastics or retinoids.[2] There are also attempts to improve the tolerability of interleukin-2 by the use of continuous infusion and the use of lower doses given by the subcutaneous route.[2]

Because of the treatment resistance of renal cell carcinoma, there is an urgent need to develop innovative approaches. Various options in early phase development include radiolabelled monoclonal antibodies, allogeneic dendritic cell vaccines, and angiogenesis inhibitors.[2,7]

1. Motzer RJ, et al. Renal-cell carcinoma. N Engl J Med 1996; 335: 865–75.
2. Vogelzang NJ, Stadler WM. Kidney cancer. Lancet 1998; 352: 1691–6.
3. National Comprehensive Cancer Network. NCCN practice guidelines for kidney cancer. Oncology 1998; 12: 396–412.
4. Coppin C, et al. Immunotherapy for advanced renal cell cancer (updated 13 June 2000). Available in The Cochrane Library; Issue 1. Oxford: Update Software; 2001.
5. Yagoda A, et al. Chemotherapy for advanced renal-cell carcinoma: 1983-1993. Semin Oncol 1995; 22: 42–60.
6. Amato RJ. Chemotherapy for renal cell carcinoma. Semin Oncol 2000; 27: 177–86.
7. Berg WJ, et al. Novel investigative approaches for advanced renal cell carcinoma. Semin Oncol 2000; 27: 234–9.

WILMS' TUMOUR. In children most cases of renal tumours are due to Wilms' tumour (nephroblastoma). This is one of the most frequent solid tumours in childhood with a peak incidence between 1 and 5 years of age and accounting for about 6% of all childhood malignancies. The usual presentation is an asymptomatic abdominal mass; abdominal pain is less frequent and haematuria occurs only in about a quarter of patients. Metastasis in advanced disease is usually to the lungs and liver. Most primary tumours occur in one kidney, but some 5% involve both kidneys.

Unlike other forms of renal cancer Wilms' tumour responds well to chemotherapy. The basis of treatment is surgery, combined with chemotherapy, and if necessary radiotherapy. Precise management varies with disease stage and also varies between different study groups.[1-5]

The US National Wilms' Tumour Study (NWTS) group and some other groups recommend initial surgery (nephrectomy) to confirm diagnosis and perform precise staging.[1,2,4] Conversely, others, including the European Société Internationale d'Oncologie Pédiatrique (SIOP), use neoadjuvant chemotherapy to reduce the tumour size thereby facilitating surgery.[3] Overall survival for patients treated by either approach is very similar, being more than 90% for patients with favourable histology. The aim of the various study protocols has been to identify low-risk children who require less intensive therapy, and those with poor prognosis who require more intensive therapy or alternative investigative regimens.

Current SIOP neoadjuvant chemotherapy consists of 4 weeks of dactinomycin and vincristine for clinically localised disease, and 6 weeks of dactinomycin, vincristine, and epirubicin for metastatic disease.[3,5] Adjuvant chemotherapy regimens for disease with favourable histology are broadly similar between NWTS and SIOP.[3-5] In early disease, chemotherapy consists of vincristine combined with dactinomycin; in more advanced disease radiotherapy, and an anthracycline (doxorubicin or epirubicin) are added. Patients with unfavourable histology and stage I disease are treated the same as those with favourable histology early-stage disease.[5] Combination adjuvant chemotherapy regimens for other patients with unfavourable histology, who have a poorer prognosis, include other drugs such as etoposide, carboplatin, and an alkylating agent (cyclophosphamide or ifosfamide), which may be combined with an anthracycline or vincristine.[3-5] The duration of adjuvant chemotherapy is dependent on the disease stage. In children with recurrent disease survival is usually poor: salvage rates of about 20 to 30% have been reported for those with favourable histology. A regimen of cyclophosphamide, carboplatin, and etoposide is being investigated.[5] Bilateral Wilms' tumour is not usually treated with primary bilateral nephrectomy because of the need to retain renal function. It may be biopsied to assess histology and stage and then treated with neoadjuvant chemotherapy.[4,5] Surgery is then performed, preserving as much of the kidneys as is possible. Survival has been reported to be comparable with that in other patients.[4] Because of these results, some have suggested the use of partial nephrectomy in patients with small unilateral tumours.[4]

1. Mehta MP, et al. Treatment of Wilms' tumour: current recommendations. Drugs 1991; 42: 766–80.
2. Green DM, et al. The treatment of Wilms tumor: results of the National Wilms Tumor Studies. Hematol Oncol Clin North Am 1995; 9: 1267–74.
3. de Kraker J, et al. Preoperative strategies in the management of Wilms tumor. Hematol Oncol Clin North Am 1995; 9: 1275–85.
4. Haase GM, Ritchey ML. Nephroblastoma. Semin Pediatr Surg 1997; 6: 11–16.
5. Suryanarayan K, Marina N. Wilms' tumour: optimal treatment strategies. Drugs 1998; 56: 597–605.

Malignant neoplasms of the liver. Hepatocellular carcinoma (hepatoma) accounts for more than 90% of primary liver cancers. It is uncommon in northern Europe and America but is the most common cancer among men in large parts of Africa and Asia. The incidence in men ranges from 2 to 8 times that in women. Chronic infection with hepatitis B or hepatitis C virus is by far the most important factor associated with development of liver cancer, although other risk factors include ingestion of foodstuffs contaminated with aflatoxins (see p.1574), alcoholic liver disease, haemochromatosis, and the long-term use of anabolic steroids (see under Testosterone, p.1492) and, rarely, combined oral contraceptives, (see p.1454). Over 70% of patients with hepatocellular carcinoma have cirrhosis of the liver.

Clinical manifestations of liver cancer include increasing obstructive jaundice, pain, malaise, and the presence of an epigastric mass; there may be metastasis to the lungs, kidney, bones, brain or other sites, or invasion of local structures.

Although early diagnosis may be improved by screening at-risk groups, few patients have their tumours identified at a stage allowing prolongation of survival with surgical resection or liver transplantation.[1-4] Liver transplantation may be considered in those patients with very small tumours (stage I) and who have advanced cirrhosis and are therefore not suitable for surgical resection. Patients with larger tumours or more advanced stages of disease are not candidates for transplantation because of the high rates of recurrence in the transplanted liver. Surgical resection is considered in patients with no cirrhosis or mild liver impairment whose tumours are considered resectable (stages I to III). However, recurrence rates are high, and 5-year survival is about 30%. Because of this there

has been interest in adjuvant therapy. Preliminary results from one comparative study found a reduction in recurrence and increased survival with a single dose of iodine-131-labelled iodised oil injected into the hepatic artery within 6 to 8 weeks of surgery.[5] However, a meta-analysis of 8 further studies found no evidence that any of the regimens of adjuvant or neoadjuvant therapy they included were of benefit in improving survival or disease-free survival.[6] Hepatocellular carcinoma is relatively resistant to chemotherapy, and adjuvant chemotherapy remains investigational. In patients who have small tumours and are not candidates for surgery or transplantation, percutaneous intratumoral alcohol injection is an option.

Most patients present with advanced stage cancer and significant liver impairment. There are currently no effective treatments to prolong survival in these patients, and options include palliative medical treatments or supportive care.[2,4,7] Systemic chemotherapy has been tried in unresectable disease, but has no standard role. Treatment with doxorubicin alone has been associated with a response rate of 3 to 30% and no increase in survival,[2,4,7] and this has not been bettered by combination chemotherapy. Doxorubicin has also been given by intra-arterial infusion into the hepatic artery, as have fluorouracil, floxuridine, and other agents such as cisplatin and mitomycin. Prolonging the duration of contact and promoting ischaemia of the tumour by temporary occlusion of the artery with substances such as gelatine foam (chemo-embolisation) has also been tried. Although use of these local administration techniques may give higher response rates than systemic therapy, there is no evidence of an improvement in survival,[2,4,7] and their role in the treatment of hepatocellular carcinoma remains to be established. Other options that have been tried include interferon alfa and tamoxifen. Despite some positive data for tamoxifen, a recent large randomised clinical trial failed to show any benefit for therapy at conventional doses (40 mg daily).[8] Adoptive immunotherapy, using activated T-cells cultured with interleukin-2 and a monoclonal anti-CD3 antibody, has been reported to lower recurrence after resection.[9]

In contrast to the poor response of hepatocellular carcinoma to therapy, better progress has been made in strategies for its prevention.[3] Neonatal vaccination against hepatitis B has dramatically decreased the incidence of chronic infection in children in Taiwan, and reduced the incidence of hepatocellular carcinoma. This may be a more promising approach in areas where the disease is common. There is evidence that interferon alfa may delay or prevent the development of hepatocellular carcinoma in cirrhotic patients with hepatitis C infection.[10] Chemoprevention may also be a useful approach after surgical resection: use of a synthetic retinoid, polyprenoic acid, was found to reduce the development of second primary tumours after resection.[11,12]

The liver is the most common site of metastatic disease.[13] For most malignancies the presence of liver metastases is indicative of generalised dissemination, but isolated metastatic liver disease commonly occurs in colorectal cancer (see Malignant Neoplasms of the Gastrointestinal Tract, above) and rarer cancers such as some neuroendocrine tumours (see Carcinoid Tumours, above). In contrast to disseminated disease, treatment of such isolated liver metastases can prolong survival.[13] Surgical resection is the preferred treatment if feasible. Palliative or cytoreductive surgery is beneficial in hepatic metastases from neuroendocrine tumours because of their slow growth. Combining resection with adjuvant hepatic arterial or systemic chemotherapy is under investigation for colorectal liver metastases. Unresectable colorectal liver metastases have been treated with systemic and or hepatic arterial chemotherapy, with modest survival benefits.[14]

1. Haydon GH, Hayes PC. Hepatocellular carcinoma. Br J Hosp Med 1995; 53: 74–80.
2. Colleoni M, et al. Practical considerations in the treatment of hepatocellular carcinoma. Drugs 1998; 55: 367–82.
3. Schafer DF, Sorrell MF. Hepatocellular carcinoma. Lancet 1999; 353: 1253–7.
4. Badvie S. Hepatocellular carcinoma. Postgrad Med J 2000; 76: 4–11.
5. Lau WY, et al. Adjuvant intra-arterial iodine-131-labelled lipiodol for resectable hepatocellular carcinoma: a prospective randomised trial. Lancet 1999; 353: 797–801.
6. Chan ES-Y, et al. Neoadjuvant and adjuvant therapy for operable hepatocellular carcinoma (updated 29 August 2000). Available in The Cochrane Library; Issue 1. Oxford: Update Software; 2001.
7. Mathurin P, et al. Review article: overview of medical treatments in unresectable hepatocellular carcinoma-an impossible meta-analysis? Aliment Pharmacol Ther 1998; 12: 111–126.
8. Cancer of the Liver Italian Programme Group. Tamoxifen in treatment of hepatocellular carcinoma: a randomised controlled trial. Lancet 1998; 352: 17–20.

9. Takayama T, *et al.* Adoptive immunotherapy to lower postsurgical recurrence rates of hepatocellular carcinoma: a randomised trial. *Lancet* 2000; **356:** 802–7. Correction. *ibid.*; 1690.
10. Baffis V, *et al.* Use of interferon for prevention of hepatocellular carcinoma in cirrhotic patients with hepatitis B or hepatitis C virus infection. *Ann Intern Med* 1999; **131:** 696–701.
11. Muto Y, *et al.* Prevention of second primary tumors by an acyclic retinoid, polyprenoic acid, in patients with hepatocellular carcinoma. *N Engl J Med* 1996; **334:** 1561–7.
12. Muto Y, *et al.* Prevention of second primary tumors by an acyclic retinoid in patients with hepatocellular carcinoma. *N Engl J Med* 1999; **340:** 1046–7.
13. Choti MA, Bulkley GB. Management of hepatic metastases. *Liver Transpl Surg* 1999; **5:** 65–80.
14. Thirion P, *et al.* Survival impact of chemotherapy in patients with colorectal metastases confined to the liver: a re-analysis of 1458 non-operable patients randomised in 22 trials and 4 meta-analyses. *Ann Oncol* 1999; **10:** 1317–20.

Malignant neoplasms of the lung. Lung cancer is the most common non-skin cancer in the developed countries and the second most common overall worldwide. About 20 to 25% of all lung cancers are small cell lung cancers (SCLC) derived from endocrine cells in the bronchial mucosa; the remainder, comprising chiefly squamous cell carcinomas (40 to 45% of cases), adenocarcinoma (25 to 30%), and large-cell carcinoma (about 10%), are known collectively as non-small cell lung cancer (NSCLC). More than 80% of all lung cancers are associated with tobacco smoking, and there is also evidence that exposure to the cigarette smoke of others can increase the risk in non-smokers. Other risk factors may include occupational exposure to substances such as asbestos, and the effects of environmental toxins such as air pollutants.

Symptoms due to a lesion in a main bronchus (the most common site) include persistent cough, dyspnoea, haemoptysis, weight loss and sometimes chest pain. Metastatic spread is common, and may affect sites such as brain, liver, and bone. It occurs early with adenocarcinoma and SCLC, but late with squamous cell carcinoma.

Disease staging plays an important role in determining treatment. The management of small cell lung cancer differs significantly from that of non-small cell types.

The mainstay of treatment for **small cell lung cancer** is multi-agent chemotherapy.[1-3] Adjuvant thoracic radiotherapy is commonly used in patients with limited stage disease, and has been shown to improve survival.[4] The optimum scheduling of chemotherapy and radiotherapy is unknown, with some advocating radiotherapy after chemotherapy,[1] and others radiotherapy concurrently with chemotherapy.[3] Surgical resection has been used in patients with limited stage disease, either alone or combined with other therapies, but it is not currently considered standard therapy.[1,3] Around 80% of patients with small cell lung cancer respond to primary therapy, with slightly better response in those with limited disease (confined to one hemithorax) than those with extensive disease. Despite these impressive responses, resistance and relapse almost always occur; the median survival is improved by treatment, but long-term survival is very poor, with about 10 to 20% of patients with limited disease and 5% of those with extensive disease surviving 2 years from the start of the treatment. The most commonly used chemotherapy regimens for limited disease are etoposide and cisplatin (EP or PE), cyclophosphamide, doxorubicin, and vincristine (CAV), cyclophosphamide, doxorubicin, and etoposide (CAE or ACE), and ifosfamide, carboplatin, and etoposide (ICE).[1-3] Various options for dose-intensification have been studied but there is no consistent evidence of improved survival, and such treatments remain investigational.[1,3] Similar combination regimens are used for extensive disease, but because of poor performance status, less aggressive treatments are sometimes used.[1,3] Oral etoposide was widely considered a useful palliative option, but the results of randomised controlled trials have shown slightly worse palliation of symptoms and reduced survival when compared with intravenous combination chemotherapy.[1,3]

One of the most common sites for recurrence is the brain, and prophylactic cranial irradiation may be considered in an attempt to prevent this.[1-3] A recent meta-analysis[5] has confirmed that prophylactic cranial irradiation reduces the risk of brain recurrence and improves survival in patients in complete remission.

The value of chemotherapy in relapsed disease depends in part on the duration of remission before relapse, with greater responses the longer the remission.[3] If cisplatin-based therapy was not used for initial treatment, this may be considered for second-line treatment.[3] Another option for second-line treatment is topotecan. Palliative radiotherapy may also be given.[1,3]

Other drugs under investigation for the treatment of small cell lung cancer include altretamine, the taxanes, irinotecan, vinorelbine, and gemcitabine.[2,3]

In contrast to small cell disease, about 20 to 25% of patients with **non-small cell lung cancer** present with tumour localised to the lung (generally stage I and II), and the treatment of choice in such cases is surgery.[1,2,6] In patients with resectable disease who have medical contra-indications to surgery, radical radiotherapy is used with curative intent. More advanced disease is also treated with radiotherapy, although in disseminated disease this is purely palliative. About 25 to 40% of patients resected for localised disease are still alive after 5 years, while 5-year survival is 4 to 8% in locally advanced disease and less than 1% in disseminated disease. Because of these poor results there has been great interest in the role of adjuvant therapies. In early-stage disease, use of radiotherapy after complete resection has been shown to result in worse survival than surgery alone,[7] and is not recommended.[1,2] Conversely, some recommend[1,6] that post-operative radiotherapy be considered if there is residual disease after surgery, although there is a lack of good evidence for a reduction in local recurrence in this setting. Chemotherapy is also being investigated as an adjuvant to surgery and/or radiotherapy. In early-stage disease, there is currently insufficient evidence to recommend chemotherapy either before or after surgery.[1,2] In patients with locally-advanced disease that is potentially operable, neoadjuvant chemotherapy may increase survival, and requires further investigation.[1,2] Similarly, in this group there is some evidence that cisplatin-based post-operative therapy improves survival, but that alkylating agent-based therapy decreases survival.[8] In patients with unresectable locally advanced disease (stage IIIB), the use of cisplatin-based chemotherapy either before or concurrently with radiotherapy has resulted in a modest increase in survival according to the findings of a number of meta-analyses[8-10] and subsequent clinical trials.[11] The issue of sequencing requires further study, nonetheless induction chemotherapy is considered an option for treatment in this group.[1,2,12] Various combinations have been used including cisplatin plus vinblastine or vindesine, carboplatin plus paclitaxel, and mitomycin, ifosfamide, plus cisplatin.

Chemotherapy may also be used for advanced metastatic disease (stage IV), which is detected in 40 to 50% of patients at presentation. Various meta-analyses have shown a modest improvement in survival and symptom control in patients receiving chemotherapy compared with those receiving best supportive care.[8,13,14] The use of cisplatin-based chemotherapy resulted in an increase in median survival of 6 weeks, and an increase in 1-year survival of 10%.[8] To date no particular regimen has been identified as superior, and it remains appropriate to enrol patients in clinical trials.[1] Regimens include cisplatin combined with either etoposide, gemcitabine, vinblastine, vinorelbine, or paclitaxel,[2,12] or triple regimens such as mitomycin, vindesine, and cisplatin (MVP) or mitomycin, ifosfamide, and cisplatin (MIC). In the UK, gemcitabine, paclitaxel, or vinorelbine are recommended for first-line treatment, combined with platinum-based chemotherapy where tolerated with the choice of drug depending on patient characteristics, adverse effects, and institutional and individual preferences.[15] Drugs that have shown benefit in patients failing cisplatin-based therapy include docetaxel and gemcitabine.[2]

Photodynamic therapy, with porfimer sodium, may be considered for the palliative treatment of bronchial obstruction. (Photodynamic therapy may also be used as an alternative to surgery in patients with very early-stage (in situ) endobronchial non-small cell lung cancer.[16])

Despite the recent advances in chemotherapy for non-small cell lung cancer, the median survival for this disease remains poor, and there is a need to identify alternative approaches to treatment. Those in preclinical development include gene therapy with the tumour suppressor gene p53 (which is abnormal in up to 75% of patients), monoclonal antibodies against epidermal growth factors, and angiogenesis inhibitors.

Given the poor prognosis of lung cancers, and the high incidence of secondary primaries in patients curatively treated for early-stage disease, there has been great interest in **prophylaxis**. The most important factor in primary and secondary prevention is cessation of tobacco smoking, for which a number of interventions may be tried (see Smoking Cessation, p.1642). Diets rich in fruit and vegetables have been associated with a lower incidence of malignant disease, and have prompted the investiga-

tion of antioxidant vitamins. However, primary prevention studies in those at risk of lung cancer have failed to show any benefit for vitamin supplements, and in the case of betacarotene, an increase in lung cancer was seen in those most at risk (see Prophylaxis of Malignant Neoplasms, p.1353).

Metastatic lung disease. The lung is the second most frequent site for metastatic disease, occurring in about 30% of cancer patients. Surgical resection may be used to treat pulmonary metastases when there are no effective systemic therapies, no extrapulmonary metastases, the pulmonary metastasis is completely resectable, and the patient is able to undergo surgery.[17] Specific cancers for which surgical resection of pulmonary metastases is considered include soft-tissue sarcoma, osteosarcoma, and sometimes breast cancer.

1. The Royal College of Radiologists Clinical Oncology Information Network. Guidelines on the non-surgical management of lung cancer. *Clin Oncol* 1999; **11:** S1–S53.
2. Hoffman PC, *et al.* Lung cancer. *Lancet* 2000; **355:** 479–85.
3. Adjei AA, *et al.* Current guidelines for the management of small cell lung cancer. *Mayo Clin Proc* 1999; **74:** 809–16.
4. Pignon JP, *et al.* A meta-analysis of thoracic radiotherapy for small cell lung cancer. *N Engl J Med* 1992; **327:** 1618–24.
5. Aupérin A, *et al.* Prophylactic cranial irradiation for patients with small-cell lung cancer in complete remission. *N Engl J Med* 1999; **341:** 476–84.
6. Bastin KT, Curley R. Non-small-cell lung carcinoma: current and future therapeutic management. *Drugs* 1995; **49:** 362–75.
7. PORT Meta-analysis Trialists Group. Postoperative radiotherapy in non-small-cell lung cancer: systematic review and meta-analysis of individual patient data from nine randomised controlled trials. *Lancet* 1998; **352:** 257–63.
8. Non-small Cell Lung Cancer Collaborative Group. Chemotherapy for non-small cell lung cancer (updated 29 November 2000). Available in The Cochrane Library; Issue 1. Oxford: Update Software; 2001.
9. Pritchard RS, Anthony SP. Chemotherapy plus radiotherapy compared with radiotherapy alone in the treatment of locally advanced, unresectable, non-small-cell lung cancer: a meta-analysis. *Ann Intern Med* 1996; **125:** 723–9. Correction. *ibid.* 1997; **126:** 670.
10. Marino P, *et al.* Randomized trials of radiotherapy alone versus combined chemotherapy and radiotherapy in stages IIIa and IIIb nonsmall cell lung cancer. *Cancer* 1995; **76:** 593–601.
11. Movsas B. Innovative treatment strategies in locally advanced and/or unresectable non-small cell lung cancer. *Cancer Control* 2000; **7:** 25–34.
12. American Society of Clinical Oncology. Clinical practice guidelines for the treatment of unresectable non-small-cell lung cancer. *J Clin Oncol* 1997; **15:** 2996–3018.
13. Souquet PJ, *et al.* Polychemotherapy in advanced non small cell lung cancer: a meta-analysis. *Lancet* 1993; **342:** 19–21.
14. Lilenbaum RC, *et al.* Single agent versus combination chemotherapy in patients with advanced nonsmall cell lung carcinoma: a meta-analysis of response, toxicity, and survival. *Cancer* 1998; **82:** 116–26.
15. National Institute for Clinical Excellence. Guidance on the use of docetaxel, paclitaxel, gemcitabine and vinorelbine for the treatment of non-small cell lung cancer (issued June 2001). Available at: http//www.nice.org.uk/article.asp?a=17378
16. Sheski FD, Mathur PN. Endoscopic treatment of early-stage lung cancer. *Cancer Control* 2000; **7:** 35–44.
17. Downey RJ. Surgical treatment of pulmonary metastases. *Surg Oncol Clin N Am* 1999; **8:** 341–54.

Malignant neoplasms of the ovary. Ovarian cancers account for about 5% of all malignancies in women. The most common form (90% of cases) is **epithelial ovarian cancer**, which ranks as fourth in the leading causes of cancer deaths in women. The lethality of this disease is related to the absence of symptoms in the majority of women during its early stages: in about three-quarters of all patients disease is advanced at diagnosis and has spread to the peritoneum or beyond. It is predominantly a disease of older women, the median age at diagnosis being 63 years. The risk of epithelial ovarian cancer appears to be related to the number of ovulatory cycles a women has in her lifetime, thus nulliparity increases the risk, whereas multiparity, breast feeding, and combined oral contraceptives (p.1454) decrease the risk. Other risk factors are a family history (particularly when associated with the BRCA1 gene), and possibly fertility drugs (see Clomifene, p.1466), perineal talc use (p.1124), and menopausal hormone replacement therapy (p.1462).

The primary treatment for epithelial ovarian cancer is surgical removal of womb, ovaries and fallopian tubes, and omentum, together with debulking of any remaining gross disease.[1-6] The use of adjuvant chemotherapy depends on disease stage.

The minority of patients who have localised disease at diagnosis have a good prognosis. Patients with well differentiated early disease (stage IA and IB) have a 5-year disease-free survival of some 90 to 98%; adjuvant therapy has not been shown to improve survival in this group, and less extensive surgery may be possible without greatly affecting survival. In those subgroups with poorly differentiated or more extensive localised disease (stage IC and II) postoperative platinum-based chemotherapy is usually considered appropriate. Adjuvant intraperitoneal phosphorus-32 and oral melphalan have also been used.

Prognosis is less good in patients with advanced disease (stage III and IV), who presently form the majority at diagnosis. Patients with extra-pelvic disease or positive nodes who have only minimal residual disease after surgery have a 5-year survival rate of less than 30% but in patients with distant metastases or suboptimal debulking there is a less than 10% chance of long-term survival. A wide range of adjuvant regimens have been tried in advanced ovarian cancer, often based on platinum derivatives, alkylating agents, and sometimes also anthracyclines. Combinations of cisplatin or carboplatin with cyclophosphamide (CP) and sometimes doxorubicin (CAP) have been widely used. In 1991, a meta-analysis[7] failed to reach any definite conclusions about the relative benefits of differing chemotherapeutic regimens, but did suggest that immediate treatment was better than delaying until relapse, that platinum-based regimens were probably better than those without a platinum derivative, that combination regimens were better than single-agent platinum where the doses were equivalent, and that carboplatin was as effective as cisplatin. A subsequent updated analysis[8] by the same group reached similar conclusions. Two similar analyses in 1991 and 1992 suggested that regimens of cisplatin, doxorubicin, and cyclophosphamide offered a survival advantage over cisplatin with cyclophosphamide alone.[9,10] Subsequent to these analyses, a large randomised study (ICON2) was instigated to compare carboplatin alone with cyclophosphamide, doxorubicin and cisplatin. This study[11] found no difference in progression-free or overall survival (median 33 months) between the 2 treatment arms, and single-agent carboplatin was less toxic. In the early 1990's, the finding of significant activity for paclitaxel in ovarian cancer led to various studies incorporating this drug. Two studies[12,13] comparing cisplatin plus cyclophosphamide with cisplatin plus paclitaxel found improved overall survival for the paclitaxel-containing arm (median 38 and 35 months versus 24 and 25 months). Substitution of carboplatin for cisplatin results in similar overall survival,[14] and subsequently a number of reviews and guidelines have recommended paclitaxel plus cisplatin or carboplatin as the first-line adjuvant treatment of ovarian cancer.[4,5] The UK's National Institute for Clinical Excellence has made a similar recommendation.[15] Conversely, another study[16] found cisplatin alone (100 mg per m^2) to be no different to cisplatin (75 mg per m^2) plus paclitaxel (135 mg per m^2) in terms of overall survival (median 30 versus 26 months) and progression-free survival, although cisplatin alone was poorly tolerated. This study also contained a single-agent paclitaxel arm (200 mg per m^2), which had poorer progression-free survival, but similar overall survival (26 months) to the other arms. Preliminary results of a further study (ICON3) have also reportedly failed to demonstrate an improvement in progression-free or overall survival for carboplatin plus paclitaxel compared with carboplatin alone or CAP.

Investigational therapies in the adjuvant setting include interval surgical debulking in those with suboptimal debulking at primary surgery,[1,3] and intraperitoneal chemotherapy in those with minimal residual disease after primary surgery.[14]

In patients with recurrent disease, the choice of therapy depends on the time since initial therapy and the drugs used.[17] Relapse occurring more than 6 months after initial therapy is potentially platinum-sensitive and may be re-treated with the initial therapy. In patients who are potentially not sensitive to platinum derivatives, paclitaxel may be used if it was not used previously. Other drugs with second-line activity include topotecan,[18] liposomal doxorubicin, and altretamine. Investigational agents include gemcitabine, oral etoposide, ifosfamide, and tamoxifen.[17]

PROPHYLAXIS. The identification of genes conferring an inherited predisposition to ovarian cancer, and the difficulty in identifying the disease and its poor prognosis has led to increased interest in prevention. Oral contraceptives are known to be protective in the general population, and there is some evidence they are protective in carriers of the BRCA1 gene.[19] Prophylactic oophorectomy may be considered in women with BRCA1 mutations after childbearing or at age 35 years.[20,21] The risk/benefit ratio of this procedure is not known, and a few women who undergo this procedure subsequently develop a primary peritoneal cancer.

Ovarian germ-cell cancers account for less than 3% of ovarian cancers and typically occur in women aged 20 to 30 years. Unlike epithelial ovarian cancer, most patients present with early disease, and even in advanced disease, combination chemotherapy can be curative.[22] Conservative fertility-sparing surgery is the primary therapy. Adjuvant chemotherapy is used except in those with stage I disease able to undergo frequent follow-up. Commonly used regimens are similar to those used in male germ-cell tumours such as bleomycin, etoposide, and cisplatin (BEP) or vinblastine, bleomycin, and cisplatin (VBP).[6]

1. Cannistra SA. Cancer of the ovary. *N Engl J Med* 1993; **329:** 1550–9.
2. Lorigan PC, *et al.* Current drug treatment guidelines for epithelial ovarian cancer. *Drugs* 1996; **51:** 571–84.
3. NIH Consensus Development Panel on Ovarian Cancer. Ovarian cancer: screening, treatment, and follow-up. *JAMA* 1995; **273:** 491–7.
4. Society of Gynecologic Oncologists. Practice guidelines: ovarian cancer. *Oncology (Huntingt)* 1998; **12:** 129–33.
5. American College of Obstetricians and Gynecologists. ACOG educational bulletin: ovarian cancer. *Int J Gynaecol Obstet* 1998; **63:** 301–10.
6. Anthoney DA, Kaye SB. Epithelial ovarian cancer. *Prescribers' J* 1999; **39:** 65–71.
7. Advanced Ovarian Cancer Trialists Group. Chemotherapy in advanced ovarian cancer: an overview of randomised clinical trials. *BMJ* 1991; **303:** 884–9.
8. Advanced Ovarian Cancer Trialists Group. Chemotherapy for advanced ovarian cancer (updated 25 May 2001). Available in The Cochrane Library; Issue 4. Oxford: Update Software; 2001.
9. Fanning J, *et al.* Meta-analysis of cisplatin, doxorubicin, and cyclophosphamide versus cisplatin and cyclophosphamide chemotherapy of ovarian carcinoma. *Obstet Gynecol* 1992; **80:** 954–60.
10. Ovarian Cancer Meta-analysis Project. Cyclophosphamide plus cisplatin versus cyclophosphamide, doxorubicin, and cisplatin chemotherapy of ovarian carcinoma: a meta-analysis. *J Clin Oncol* 1991; **9:** 1668–74.
11. The ICON Collaborators. ICON2: randomised trial of single-agent carboplatin against three-drug combination of CAP (cyclophosphamide, doxorubicin, and cisplatin) in women with ovarian cancer. *Lancet* 1998; **352:** 1571–76.
12. McGuire WP, *et al.* Cyclophosphamide and cisplatin compared with paclitaxel and cisplatin in patients with stage III and stage IV ovarian cancer. *N Engl J Med* 1996; **334:** 1–6.
13. Stuart G *et al.* Updated analysis shows a highly significant improved overall survival (OS) for cisplatin-paclitaxel as first line treatment of advanced ovarian cancer: mature results of the EORTC-GCCG, NO-COVA, NCIC CTG and Scottish Intergroup trial. *Proc ASCO* 1998; **17:** 361a.
14. Herrin VE, Thigpen JT. Chemotherapy for ovarian cancer: current concepts. *Semin Surg Oncol* 1999; **17:** 181–8.
15. National Institute for Clinical Excellence. Guidance on the use of taxanes for ovarian cancer (reviewed March 2001). Available at: http://www.nice.org.uk/Docref.asp?d=15948
16. Muggia FM, *et al.* Phase III randomized study of cisplatin versus paclitaxel versus cisplatin and paclitaxel in patients with suboptimal stage III or IV ovarian cancer: a Gynecologic Oncology Group study. *J Clin Oncol* 2000; **18:** 106–115.
17. Markman M, Bookman MA. Second-line treatment of ovarian cancer. *Oncologist* 2000; **5:** 26–35.
18. National Institute for Clinical Excellence. Guidance on the use of topotecan for the treatment of advanced ovarian cancer (issued August 2001). Available at: http://www.nice.org.uk/article.asp?a=18692
19. Narod SA, *et al.* Oral contraceptives and the risk of hereditary ovarian cancer. *N Engl J Med* 1998; **339:** 424–8.
20. Burke W, *et al.* Recommendations for follow-up care of individuals with an inherited predisposition to cancer: BRCA1 and BRCA2. *JAMA* 1997; **277:** 997–1003.
21. Eisinger F, *et al.* Recommendations for medical management of hereditary breast and ovarian cancer: the French National Ad Hoc Committee. *Ann Oncol* 1998; **9:** 939–50.
22. Bridgewater JA, Rustin GJS. Management of non-epithelial ovarian tumours. *Oncology* 1999; **57:** 89–98.

Malignant neoplasms of the pancreas. Pancreatic adenocarcinoma (cancer of the exocrine pancreas) accounts for about 95% of pancreatic tumours. A very small percentage of pancreatic tumours arise in the endocrine pancreas, and have different clinical features and treatment. They are considered under Carcinoid Tumours and Other Secretory Neoplasms, above. Although rare below the age of 30 the incidence of pancreatic adenocarcinoma rises steadily with age; overall, it accounts for about 3% of all cancers, but is the fifth leading cause of cancer deaths. Pancreatic adenocarcinoma is ductal in origin and metastasises early to the lymph nodes, and by the time of diagnosis more than half of all patients have liver metastases, more than a quarter have peritoneal seeding, and a third have invasion of the duodenum causing ulceration. The most frequent symptom at presentation in patients with cancer of the pancreatic head is jaundice, often with other symptoms indicative of obstruction of the bile duct. In lesions of the body and tail of the pancreas severe and relentless pain may develop. Diabetes mellitus is a manifestation of the disease, but there is also some evidence that it may be a predisposing factor. About 30% of pancreatic cancers are probably due to tobacco smoking.

Pancreatic adenocarcinoma has a very poor prognosis because of its usually advanced stage at diagnosis and lack of effective therapies.[1-4] Apart from a small number of patients with resectable carcinoma of the head of the pancreas, in whom radical surgery results in a 5-year survival of about 10 to 20% most patients with pancreatic adenocarcinoma will be dead within 1 year. Adjuvant therapy with irradiation and fluorouracil may be considered in those with resectable disease,[2-4] as there is some evidence[5] that it optimises the chance for long-term survival. In patients with symptomatic localised unresectable disease, palliative radiotherapy alone or combined with chemotherapy may be used. There is interest in neoadjuvant chemoradiotherapy to improve resectability rates in locally advanced disease, but this remains investigational.[3,5] In patients with advanced (metastatic) disease, supportive care alone remains appropriate. Palliative chemotherapy may be considered, but currently there is no standard therapy and benefits are modest (pancreatic adenocarcinoma is a chemoresistant tumour).[2-4] Single-agent fluorouracil has been used most extensively. Combination regimens, such as FAM (fluorouracil, doxorubicin, mitomycin) SMF (streptozocin, mitomycin, fluorouracil), and FAP (fluorouracil, doxorubicin, cisplatin), have not proved more effective than fluorouracil alone.[2,3] More recently, gemcitabine has become available; in 1 study this improved survival over fluorouracil by 5 weeks but with more adverse events.[6] Various therapies are being investigated for advanced pancreatic cancer including somatostatin analogues, other hormonal strategies, and biological therapies.[7] A preliminary study suggested that flutamide (an anti-androgen) may be beneficial.[8]

1. Carter DC. Clinical features and management of carcinoma of the pancreas. *Br J Hosp Med* 1995; **54:** 459–64.
2. Rosewicz S, Wiedenmann B. Pancreatic carcinoma. *Lancet* 1997; **349:** 485–9.
3. Sporn JR. Practical recommendations for the management of adenocarcinoma of the pancreas. *Drugs* 1999; **57:** 69–79.
4. DiMagno EP, *et al.* American Gastroenterological Association medical position statement: epidemiology, diagnosis, and treatment of pancreatic ductal adenocarcinoma. *Gastroenterology* 1999; **117:** 1463–84.
5. Ghaneh P, *et al.* Adjuvant therapy for pancreatic cancer. *World J Surg* 1999; **23:** 937–45.
6. Burris HA, *et al.* Improvements in survival and clinical benefit with gemcitabine as first-line therapy for patients with advanced pancreas cancer: a randomized trial. *J Clin Oncol* 1997; **15:** 2403–13.
7. Rosenberg L. Pancreatic cancer: a review of emerging therapies. *Drugs* 2000; **59:** 1071–89.
8. Greenway BA. Effect of flutamide on survival in patients with pancreatic cancer: results of a prospective, randomised, double blind, placebo controlled trial. *BMJ* 1998; **316:** 1935–8.

Malignant neoplasms of the prostate. Prostatic cancer is the most commonly diagnosed malignancy in men in the western world, and the second most common cause of cancer deaths in men: about one in 6 men can be expected to develop clinically evident carcinoma of the prostate during his lifetime. The incidence rises steadily with age. More than 95% of all prostate cancer is adenocarcinoma, which begins as a hard mass in the peripheral portion of the gland and infiltrates surrounding tissues slowly. Metastasis may occur in advanced disease, notably to bone. Presenting symptoms of advanced disease are usually those of urinary outflow obstruction, or pelvic or back pain due to bone metastases. However, as a result of the slow rate of tumour growth and usually advanced age at diagnosis, many patients die of other illnesses without having suffered significant disability from the cancer.

Controversy exists regarding all aspects of the management of prostate cancer, from screening to the best treatment for each stage of the disease. Much of this is because of the lack of clear data to guide treatment decisions. Factors that guide treatment decisions include the extent (stage) of the tumour, tumour grade (Gleason score), the patient's life expectancy (based on age and comorbid conditions), and patient preference.[1-6]

There is great controversy over the value of screening for early disease by detection of prostate specific antigen (PSA), and other tests, because of the uncertainties regarding interpretation of the test results, and controversy over the management of asymptomatic early localised disease.[7,8] Screening studies are currently underway.

In patients with localised disease, detected incidentally or by screening, the choices are radical prostatectomy, radical radiotherapy, or deferred treatment (watchful waiting). There is currently no evidence to suggest one form of therapy is more effective than another, except perhaps for poorly differentiated tumours, which have a faster rate of progression and may benefit from earlier therapy.[6] Because of the lack of differences in efficacy, treatment morbidity and patient preferences are particularly important. Adverse effects of surgery include impotence and incontinence, and for radiotherapy, radiation proctitis, impotence and incontinence, and these complications may be severe in up to 5% of patients.[6] In medically fit patients with a life expectancy of 10 years or more many clinicians would consider radical prostatectomy or radiotherapy with curative intent,[1-3,6] although it should be noted that these patients are the ones for whom treatment complications are likely to have the most impact on quality of life.[6] In men with a life expectancy of less than 10 years and with low-grade tumours, there is a definite role for deferring treatment.[2,3,6] Interstitial implantation of radioisotopes (brachytherapy) or cryosurgery are also options for localised disease, but are less well investigated.[9] In patients who undergo radical surgery and who are found to have positive margins, adjuvant radiotherapy or hormonal therapy is being investigated.[9]

For patients with locally advanced disease, options include radiotherapy with or without neoadjuvant or adjuvant hormonal therapy, hormonal treatment alone, or, in those who are asymptomatic, deferred treatment.[3,6] Although radiotherapy alone produces good local control, most patients eventually develop metastatic disease. There is increasing evidence that the use of hormonal therapy before or after radiotherapy improves disease-free, and possibly overall, survival.[10] Deferred treatment was less effective than immediate treatment in one study,[11] but the form of follow-up for deferred treatment was not regulated. In patients for whom deferred treatment is considered, close surveillance is required.

PSA may be used to monitor the efficacy of therapy and detect biochemical relapse,[9] but the interpretation of the test and when to instigate further treatment in patients with no clinical evidence of disease is controversial.

For patients with metastatic disease cure is not possible and therapy is aimed at prolonging survival and palliating symptoms. The basis of therapy is hormonal manipulation: about 80% of patients will respond to such therapy, but resistance eventually develops. The first choice is either orchidectomy or a gonadorelin analogue, which have been shown to be equally effective.[6,12]

An alternative to orchidectomy or gonadorelin analogues is the use of an anti-androgen (such as flutamide, nilutamide, or bicalutamide) alone. However, there is some evidence that these may be less effective and cause more treatment withdrawals (due to gastrointestinal intolerance),[12] although they may have less adverse effect on libido. Although historically oestrogens such as diethylstilbestrol have been used in patients with prostate cancer they are now less favoured because of their cardiovascular adverse effects.

The combined use of anti-androgens such as flutamide with ablation of testicular androgen production (by surgery or gonadorelin analogues) has the advantage of blocking the effects of adrenal androgen production as well (maximal or complete androgen blockade). An early meta-analysis[13] seemed to indicate that this approach did not produce a better survival rate compared with conventional castration, and an update of this meta-analysis[14] confirmed that any survival advantage from maximum androgen blockade using nonsteroidal anti-androgens was likely to be in the region of 3%.

In patients who relapse after or during hormonal therapy second-line hormonal therapy (with, for example, aminoglutethimide, prednisolone, or megestrol) produces responses in about 15% of patients. One potentially beneficial manoeuvre in patients treated with anti-androgens is withdrawal of the drug, as some patients experience a paradoxical response to this. Chemotherapy for recurrent hormone-refractory prostate cancer is still undergoing clinical trials and has no routine place in therapy. Some patients with soft-tissue disease may benefit from an anthracycline.[6] Mitozantrone [mitoxantrone] has resulted in improved palliation and quality of life, but did not improve survival.[15] Various other drugs are being investigated, including estramustine in combination with vinblastine, etoposide, or docetaxel.[16] Interesting preliminary results have indicated that a herbal combination preparation, PC-SPES, in wide use as a complementary medicine, may have beneficial effects in both androgen-dependent and androgen-independent disease.[17] Although suramin originally showed promise, more recent results were less favourable, and it appears its development has been discontinued. Bone metastases are usually treated with palliative radiotherapy (see p.490). Bone-targeted therapy with strontium-89 has been tried,[18] and gene therapy is under investigation.[19]

Because of the difficulties involved in managing prostate cancer there has been interest in the concept of disease *prophylaxis*. Studies with finasteride, which has produced variable results in the management of prostate disease, have been initiated to examine whether 5 mg daily can help reduce the incidence of prostatic cancer in men aged over 55 years. However, 1 small study in men at

high risk of prostate cancer showed little evidence to support such use.[20] There is preliminary evidence that selenium (see p.1375) or vitamin E (see p.1353) supplementation may reduce the risk of prostate cancer.

1. Dearnaley DP. Cancer of the prostate. *BMJ* 1994; **308:** 780–4. Correction. *ibid.*; 975.
2. Catalona WJ. Management of cancer of the prostate. *N Engl J Med* 1994; **331:** 996–1004. Correction. *ibid.*; **332:** 335–6.
3. Frydenberg M, *et al.* Prostate cancer diagnosis and management. *Lancet* 1997; **349:** 1681–7.
4. Rosenthal MA. Management of metastatic prostate cancer. *Med J Aust* 1998; **169:** 46–50.
5. Moffat LEF. Therapeutic choices in prostate cancer. *Prescribers' J* 1999; **39:** 16–23.
6. The Royal College of Radiologists' Clinical Oncology Information Network and British Association of Urological Surgeons. Guidelines on the management of prostate cancer. *Clin Oncol* 1999; **11:** S53–S88.
7. Adami H-O, *et al.* Ethics of a prostate cancer screening trial. *Lancet* 1994; **343:** 958–60.
8. American College of Physicians. Screening for prostate cancer. *Ann Intern Med* 1997; **126:** 480–4.
9. Garnick MB, Fair WR. Prostate cancer: emerging concepts. *Ann Intern Med* 1996; **125:** 118–25 and 205–12.
10. Vicini FA, *et al.* The role of androgen deprivation in the definitive management of clinically localized prostate cancer treated with radiation therapy. *Int J Radiat Oncol Biol Phys* 1999; **43:** 707–13.
11. Medical Research Council Prostate Cancer Working Party Investigators Group. Immediate versus deferred treatment for advanced prostatic cancer: initial results of the Medical Research Council Trial. *Br J Urol* 1997; **79:** 235–46.
12. Seidenfeld J, *et al.* Single-therapy androgen suppression in men with advanced prostate cancer: a systematic review and meta-analysis. *Ann Intern Med* 2000; **132:** 566–77.
13. Prostate Cancer Trialists' Collaborative Group. Maximum androgen blockade in advanced prostate cancer: an overview of 22 randomised trials with 3283 deaths in 5710 patients. *Lancet* 1995; **346:** 265–9.
14. Prostate Cancer Trialists' Collaborative Group. Maximum androgen blockade in advanced prostate cancer: an overview of the randomised trials. *Lancet* 2000; **355:** 1491–8.
15. Tannock IF, *et al.* Chemotherapy with mitoxantrone plus prednisone or prednisone alone for symptomatic hormone-resistant prostate cancer: a Canadian randomized trial with palliative end points. *J Clin Oncol* 1996; **14:** 1756–64.
16. Oh WK. Chemotherapy for patients with advanced prostate carcinoma: a new option for therapy. *Cancer* 2000; **88** (12 suppl): 3015–21.
17. Small EJ, *et al.* Prospective trial of the herbal supplement PC-SPES in patients with progressive prostate cancer. *J Clin Oncol* 2000; **18:** 3595–3603.
18. Tu S-M, *et al.* Bone-targeted therapy for advanced androgen-independent carcinoma of the prostate: a randomised phase II trial. *Lancet* 2001; **357:** 336–41.
19. Harrington KJ, *et al.* Gene therapy for prostate cancer: current status and future prospects. *J Urol (Baltimore)* 2001; **166:** 1220–33.
20. Cote RJ, *et al.* The effect of finasteride on the prostate gland in men with elevated serum prostate-specific antigen levels. *Br J Cancer* 1998; **78:** 413–18.

Malignant neoplasms of the skin. Basal cell carcinoma is the most common form of skin cancer, accounting for about 80% of cases. The second most common skin cancer is squamous cell carcinoma. These 2 types of carcinoma (collectively referred to as nonmelanoma skin cancers) are the most common malignancies among white populations, but because many are not recorded the exact incidence is uncertain and they are often omitted from calculations of the relative frequency of malignancy. A small but increasing proportion of all skin cancers are melanomas, arising from melanocytes (pigment cells). Other cancers that manifest in the skin include cutaneous T-cell lymphomas (see Mycosis Fungoides, above) and Kaposi's sarcoma (see below).

Nonmelanoma and melanoma skin cancers are related to solar radiation, and the incidence is greatest in those regions where light-skinned populations live closest to the equator. Individuals at particular risk include those with fair skin, blue eyes, red hair, a tendency to freckle, and to burn rather than tan. Use of methoxsalen with ultraviolet light (PUVA) has also been associated with an increased incidence of skin cancers (see p.1119). Other risk factors for nonmelanoma skin cancers include various inherited disorders such as xeroderma pigmentosum and albinism. Immunosuppressive therapy, as used after solid organ transplantation, is associated with a very large increase in risk of squamous cell carcinoma.

PROPHYLAXIS. Although nonmelanoma and melanoma skin cancers are related to solar radiation, and measures to reduce sun exposure are therefore advocated for prophylaxis, the relationship appears to differ between the types.
- Squamous cell carcinoma and its precursor lesions are clearly linked to cumulative chronic sun exposure.[1,2] These lesions are more common on frequently exposed skin (head, neck, and back of hands), and are more common in individuals with outdoor occupations. In addition, there is evidence that regular sunscreen use (see p.1516) can reduce the incidence of new actinic keratoses and increase remission of existing lesions,[3] and reduce incident squamous cell carcinomas.[4]

- Although basal cell carcinomas are also common on sun-exposed skin (head and neck), it appears that they may be more related to a history of severe sunburns, particularly in childhood and adolescence, rather than to cumulative sun exposure.[1] In 1 study,[4] there was no difference in incidence of basal cell carcinomas between sunscreen users and non-users.
- Cutaneous melanoma is more common on skin exposed to the sun occasionally (particularly the legs in women, and the back in men), and appears to be more common in indoor than outdoor workers. This suggests that intermittent sun exposure may be more risky than regular exposure for this cancer.[1,2,5] In addition, preliminary evidence suggests that spending more time in the sun could offset any protective effect of sunscreens.[5]

In addition to sun protection measures, chemoprevention has been investigated as a means of reducing the incidence of squamous and basal cell cancers, particularly in those most at risk. Retinoids such as acitretin, etretinate, and isotretinoin have been shown to reduce the incidence of new squamous cell carcinomas in individuals with xeroderma pigmentosum, and in renal transplant recipients.[6] Conversely, neither betacarotene (p.1353) nor selenium (p.1375) has reduced the incidence of squamous or basal cell carcinomas in patients previously treated for these disorders. There is some evidence that a low-fat diet may reduce the incidence of actinic keratosis in patients with a history of nonmelanoma skin cancer.[7]

1. Anonymous. Do sunscreens prevent skin cancer? *Drug Ther Bull* 1998; **36:** 49–51.
2. Bruce AJ, Brodland DG. Overview of skin cancer detection and prevention for the primary care physician. *Mayo Clin Proc* 2000; **75:** 491–500.
3. Thompson SC, *et al.* Reduction of solar keratoses by regular sunscreen use. *N Engl J Med* 1993; **329:** 1147–51.
4. Green A, *et al.* Daily sunscreen application and betacarotene supplementation in prevention of basal-cell and squamous-cell carcinomas of the skin: a randomised controlled trial. *Lancet* 1999; **354:** 723–9.
5. Finkel E. Sorting the hype from the facts in melanoma. *Lancet* 1998; **351:** 1866.
6. Craven NM, Griffiths CEM. Retinoids in the management of non-melanoma skin cancer and melanoma. *Cancer Surv* 1996; **26:** 267–88.
7. Black HS, *et al.* Effect of a low-fat diet on the incidence of actinic keratosis. *N Engl J Med* 1994; **330:** 1272–5.

BASAL CELL AND SQUAMOUS CELL CARCINOMA. The great majority of skin cancers are basal cell carcinomas, which are completely curable if diagnosed early and treated appropriately. Although they rarely metastasise, they have a tendency to be locally destructive. The remainder are mainly squamous cell carcinomas, which, although curable when treated early, have a greater risk of metastatic spread. Common precursor lesions for squamous cell carcinoma are **actinic keratosis** (solar keratosis) and **Bowen's disease** (squamous cell carcinoma in situ).

Treatments for actinic keratosis and Bowen's disease include topical agents such as fluorouracil 5%, cryosurgery, photodynamic therapy (with aminolaevulinic acid), and surgical methods such as excision or curettage. The choice of treatment depends on the site of the lesion and its size, evidence for efficacy, ease of application, and availability.[1]

Treatment options for superficial low-risk basal cell carcinomas include curettage and electrodessication or cryosurgery.[2-5] Topical fluorouracil may be used for superficial lesions in some instances and photodynamic therapy is being investigated. For other histological types or superficial tumours at high-risk sites, and for most squamous cell carcinomas, excision with post-operatively determined margins or Mohs' micrographic surgery (tumour margins examined during the procedure) is more appropriate.[2-6] Radiotherapy is an alternative in patients at risk of surgical complications or where surgery would be difficult or extensive.

The prognosis with appropriate treatment is good, with more or less 100% cure rates in early disease, and 70 to 75% 5-year disease free survival even with local node involvement. However, about 50% of patients will subsequently develop another skin cancer,[2] and regular monitoring to detect this as early as possible is desirable. In addition, patients should be educated about sun protection measures, and chemoprevention with retinoids may be appropriate for some high-risk patients (see Prophylaxis, in Malignant Neoplasms of the Skin, above).

1. Cox NH, *et al.* Guidelines for management of Bowen's disease. *Br J Dermatol* 1999; **141:** 633–41.
2. Preston DS, Stern RS. Nonmelanoma cancers of the skin. *N Engl J Med* 1992; **327:** 1649–62.
3. Marks R, Motley RJ. Skin cancer: recognition and treatment. *Drugs* 1995; **50:** 48–61.

4. Goldberg LH. Basal cell carcinoma. *Lancet* 1996; **347:** 663–7.
5. Telfer NR, *et al.* Guidelines for the management of basal cell carcinoma. *Br J Dermatol* 1999; **141:** 415–23.
6. Marks R. Squamous cell carcinoma. *Lancet* 1996; **347:** 735–8.

MELANOMA. Although cutaneous melanoma is rare it is the most aggressive skin cancer, accounting for the majority of all skin cancer deaths. Melanoma may arise in apparently normal skin or from an existing naevus. Early signs of a naevus that may indicate development of a melanoma are change in size, shape, or colour. Other signs include itching, ulceration, and bleeding. The most common site in women is the legs, and in men the back. For a discussion of sun protection measures in the prevention of melanoma, see Prophylaxis, in Malignant Neoplasms of the Skin, above.

Surgical resection is the mainstay of curative treatment for melanomas.[1-5] About 50% of patients present with a localised primary lesion less than 1.5 mm in depth (stage I), and this has a 5-year survival of 90% with surgical resection alone. Most other patients have a primary lesion greater than 1.5 mm (stage II) or with regional lymph node metastases (stage III), and their outlook is poorer with 5-year survival rates of about 50% and 30%, respectively.[3] Because of the high risk of recurrence after surgery in these patients, there is great interest in adjuvant therapies.[2-4] The most commonly used adjuvant treatment is interferon alfa, which is the subject of ongoing clinical trials.[4] Of the studies reported so far, interferon has shown a clinical benefit in terms of relapse-free survival, but the effect on overall survival is less clear.[6-8] Isolated limb perfusion with melphalan has been used as adjuvant therapy, but a randomised trial failed to show any survival benefit for this compared with surgery alone.[9] Similarly, systemic chemotherapy has not proved useful in the adjuvant setting.[3] Various melanoma vaccines (e.g. GM2 ganglioside, autologous melanoma-associated antigens) are being investigated for adjuvant use,[10] but high-dose interferon alfa has been shown to produce greater clinical benefit than vaccination with GM2.[8] Isolated recurrences are treated with surgical resection.

About 2 to 5% of patients present with metastatic melanoma (stage IV), and they have a 5-year survival of less than 5%.[3] There is no evidence to show that any systemic treatments are better than best supportive care in these patients.[11] Because of this, surgery is still considered an option, and a few patients may survive long term after resection of isolated metastases. Of the antineoplastics tried, dacarbazine, with a response rate of 15 to 25%, is the most commonly used single agent. The orally active analogue temozolomide produces similar responses,[12] and is an alternative. Nitrosoureas (such as carmustine, lomustine, and semustine), vindesine, and cisplatin have also been tried. Various combination regimens have been used, one of the most common being the Dartmouth regimen (dacarbazine, cisplatin, carmustine, and tamoxifen). However, a recent randomised study found that this regimen was no more effective than dacarbazine alone.[13] Similarly, although tamoxifen was thought to potentiate the action of cytotoxics in melanoma, this has not been supported by recent well-designed studies.[3]

Cytokines such as interferon alfa and interleukin-2 have similar activity to chemotherapy in metastatic melanoma.[2,3] There is interest in combining cytotoxic chemotherapy with these cytokines, but so far, this approach has not improved overall survival.[2,3] Various melanoma vaccines are also being investigated in metastatic or recurrent disease,[10] as is gene therapy.

1. National Comprehensive Cancer Network. NCCN melanoma practice guidelines. *Oncology (Huntingt)* 1998; **12:** 153–77.
2. Cohen GL, Falkson CI. Current treatment options for malignant melanoma. *Drugs* 1998; **55:** 791–9.
3. Jackson DP, Patel PM. The current place of systemic therapy in the treatment of malignant melanoma. *CME Oncology* 1998; **1:** 4–8.
4. Hall PN, *et al.* Therapeutic trends in cutaneous melanoma. *Hosp Med* 1999; **60:** 39–43.
5. Australian Cancer Network/National Health and Medical Research Council. The management of cutaneous melanoma. Available at: http://www.health.gov.au/nhmrc/publicat/pdf/cp68.pdf (accessed 02/04/01).
6. Hancock BW, *et al.* Adjuvant interferon-alpha in malignant melanoma: current status. *Cancer Treat Rev* 2000; **26:** 81–9.
7. Kirkwood JM, *et al.* High- and low-dose interferon alfa-2b in high-risk melanoma: first analysis of intergroup trial E1690/S9111/C9190. *J Clin Oncol* 2000; **18:** 2444–58.
8. Kirkwood JM, *et al.* High-dose interferon alfa-2b significantly prolongs relapse-free and overall survival compared with the GM2-KLH/QS-21 vaccine in patients with resected stage IIB-III melanoma: results of intergroup trial E1694/S9512/C509801. *J Clin Oncol* 2001; **19:** 2370–80.
9. Koops HS, *et al.* Prophylactic isolated limb perfusion for localized, high-risk limb melanoma: results of a multicenter randomized phase III trial. *J Clin Oncol* 1998; **16:** 2906–12.

10. Brinckerhoff LH, *et al.* Melanoma vaccines. *Curr Opin Oncol* 2000; **12:** 163–73.
11. Crosby T, *et al.* Systemic treatments for metastatic cutaneous melanoma (updated 23 February 2000). Available in The Cochrane Library; Issue 4. Oxford: Update Software; 2001.
12. Middleton MR, *et al.* Randomized phase III study of temozolomide versus dacarbazine in the treatment of patients with advanced metastatic malignant melanoma. *J Clin Oncol* 2000; **18:** 158–66.
13. Chapman PB, *et al.* Phase III multicenter randomized trial of the Dartmouth regimen versus dacarbazine in patients with metastatic melanoma. *J Clin Oncol* 1999; **17:** 2745–51.

Malignant neoplasms of the testis.

Testicular cancer only accounts for about 1% of all male malignancies but it is the most common cancer in young men. Patients with a history of cryptorchidism are at increased risk. About 95% of testicular tumours arise in germ cells, and 40% or so of these are pure seminomas. The remainder are collectively known as nonseminomatous germ cell tumours (NSGCT) in the WHO classification, and are commonly of mixed cell types with or without a seminoma component. Nonseminomatous tumours have been referred to as teratomas in the British classification system, but this term has a more specific meaning in the WHO classification.[1]

Metastasis first occurs to the lymph nodes, then, in advanced disease, to distant sites such as lung, liver, brain, and bones. The leading symptom is a hard, painless swelling of the testis, but once metastasis occurs the patient may present with back pain (due to enlargement of retroperitoneal lymph nodes), cough, dyspnoea, gynaecomastia due to chorionic gonadotrophin production, or weight loss.

Surgical removal of the testis (orchidectomy) when diagnosis is confirmed is fundamental to the treatment of all types of testicular cancer, but further therapy depends upon the disease type and stage.[2-5]

In patients with **nonseminomatous** disease with the tumour confined to the testis (stage I), options for postorchidectomy management include surveillance and a short course of adjuvant chemotherapy. With surveillance, about 20 to 30% of patients will relapse and are subsequently treated with curative chemotherapy. Surveillance is thus not appropriate for patients who are unable to undergo regular follow-up, or who have prognostic factors suggesting a high risk of relapse such as vascular or lymphatic invasion. In the UK, these patients would be treated with adjuvant chemotherapy with 2 cycles of standard BEP (bleomycin, etoposide, and cisplatin), which will prevent relapse in the vast majority of cases.[4] In the USA, retroperitoneal lymph-node dissection may be carried out to further stage the disease before making a decision regarding surveillance or adjuvant chemotherapy.[3] If resected nodes are clear, patients undergo surveillance, but if they involve tumour (stage II) the decision to give adjuvant chemotherapy is based on the degree of nodal involvement and the ability of the patient to undergo regular follow-up.[3]

Where metastasis to the lymph nodes (stage II) or beyond (stage III) has occurred, standard postorchidectomy therapy is now combination chemotherapy with BEP, which has largely replaced the effective but more toxic PVB regimen (cisplatin, vinblastine, and bleomycin).[5,6] Based on serum markers and the presence or absence of non-pulmonary visceral metastases, patients with metastatic disease can be categorised into good, intermediate, and poor-risk groups, with 5-year survival rates of 92%, 80%, and 50%, respectively after 4 cycles of standard BEP.[4] Consequently, there has been interest in minimising the treatment in patients with good prognosis in order to reduce long-term morbidity. In such patients, 3 cycles of BEP, or 4 cycles of cisplatin and etoposide alone, may be adequate.[3,5] The substitution of carboplatin for cisplatin has resulted in a 10% lower relapse-free survival, and slightly reduced overall survival, and is not usually recommended,[5] although some have reported good results with such a regimen in children.[7] There is evidence that overall survival is improved by increased dose-intensity of etoposide and perhaps bleomycin.[8] Standard management in the UK for patients with intermediate-risk disease is 4 cycles of BEP, while those with poor-risk disease receive 4 to 6 cycles.[4] Patients with poor-risk disease may be offered more intensive chemotherapy such as accelerated therapy, dose escalation with use of haematopoietic growth factors, or high-dose chemotherapy with stem-cell support, with the aim of improving responses. So far, those intensive treatments evaluated in randomised clinical trials have not proved more effective than BEP, and have often been more toxic.[5] Various trials are ongoing.[5] Secondary resection of residual tumour after chemotherapy is commonly undertaken.

Patients who fail, or who relapse after, standard chemotherapy have a poor prognosis, with an overall survival of only 20 to 30%.[4,5] Commonly used salvage regimens include cisplatin, ifosfamide, and etoposide or vinblastine. High-dose chemotherapy with stem-cell support may also be considered.[4,5] Newer drugs with activity in relapsed disease include paclitaxel and gemcitabine.[5]

Seminoma is extremely sensitive to radiation, and adjuvant radiotherapy is the treatment of choice after orchidectomy in limited disease (stage I).[3-5] About three-quarters of patients have stage I disease at diagnosis and cure rates are between 95 and 100%. However, seminoma also responds very well to chemotherapy and adjuvant single-agent carboplatin is currently being compared with adjuvant radiotherapy for stage I disease.[4,5] Patients with greater than stage IIB seminoma have a 20 to 30% relapse rate after adjuvant radiotherapy, and adjuvant chemotherapy is preferred.[3-5] Standard regimens are BEP (3 cycles for good prognosis patients and 4 cycles for others[4]), or cisplatin with etoposide, which produce survival rates of approximately 90%.

1. Read G. Modern management for testicular teratoma. *Br J Hosp Med* 1996; **56:** 218–21.
2. Bosl GJ, Motzer RJ. Testicular germ-cell cancer. *N Engl J Med* 1997; **337:** 242–53. Correction. *ibid.*, 1403.
3. National Comprehensive Cancer Network. NCCN practice guidelines for testicular cancer. *Oncology (Huntingt)* 1998; **12:** 417–62.
4. Dearnaley DP, *et al.* Managing testicular cancer. *BMJ* 2001; **322:** 1583–8.
5. Hartmann JT, *et al.* Diagnosis and treatment of patients with testicular germ cell cancer. *Drugs* 1999; **58:** 257–81.
6. Culine S, Droz J-P. Comparative tolerability of chemotherapy regimens for germ cell cancer. *Drug Safety* 2000; **22:** 373–88.
7. Mann JR, *et al.* The United Kingdom Children's Cancer Study Group's second germ cell tumor study: carboplatin, etoposide, and bleomycin are effective treatment for children with malignant extracranial germ cell tumours, with acceptable toxicity. *J Clin Oncol* 2000; **18:** 3809–18.
8. Toner GC, *et al.* Comparison of two standard chemotherapy regimens for good-prognosis germ-cell tumours: a randomised trial. *Lancet* 2001; **357:** 739–45.

Malignant neoplasms of the thymus.

Thymomas are tumours of the mediastinum, arising from thymic tissue. They are rare, and most commonly present in patients between 40 and 60 years of age. Thymoma originates from the epithelium of the thymus but may also contain a lymphocyte component, which is probably not neoplastic. Up to 50% of patients are asymptomatic, and others have local symptoms such as cough, chest pain, dyspnoea, and obstruction of the vena cava; paraneoplastic syndromes such as myasthenia gravis, red cell aplasia, and hypogammaglobulinaemia may also develop.

Thymomas are classified as non-invasive (encapsulated, stage I), invasive (localised, stage II; extensive, stage III and IVa), and metastatic (IVb). The majority of patients present with non-invasive disease, and can be treated solely by surgical resection with low recurrence rates and long-term survival approaching 100%.[1,2] Patients with invasive disease have a higher risk of recurrence, even if the tumour is completely resected, and they are usually treated with adjuvant radiotherapy.[1,2]

In patients with unresectable invasive disease, radiotherapy alone has been used, but high recurrence rates are seen.[1,2] There is currently interest in combined modality approaches to improve survival in this group.[2] For example, neoadjuvant chemotherapy followed by surgical resection then adjuvant radiotherapy with or without further chemotherapy is being investigated. Chemotherapy regimens used in this approach are similar to those used in metastatic disease.

The role of therapies in recurrent or metastatic disease is not well established because of its rarity.[1,2] Various case series and phase II trials have shown that the tumour is chemosensitive. The demonstration that cisplatin had activity against thymoma has led to much interest in cisplatin-containing regimens such as cisplatin, doxorubicin, and cyclophosphamide (PAC), and the same drugs with addition of vincristine.[1,2] Ifosfamide is also active as a single agent against thymoma, and has been given with cisplatin and etoposide.[1,2] Corticosteroids have been added to some regimens, and may be useful where the lymphocytic component of disease is marked, although whether this represents an antineoplastic effect has been questioned.[1] Interleukin-2 has not proved beneficial.[2] There is some evidence that thymomas possess somatostatin receptors, and there have been a few reports of the benefit of octreotide.[1]

1. Loehrer PJ, *et al.* Thymomas: current experience and future directions in therapy. *Drugs* 1993; **45:** 477–87.
2. Thomas CR, *et al.* Thymoma: state of the art. *J Clin Oncol* 1999; **17:** 2280–9.

Malignant neoplasms of the thyroid. Thyroid cancer accounts for only about 1% of all malignancies. The incidence is reportedly higher in women than men, in patients who received irradiation of the thyroid during childhood, and in populations where goitre is endemic. The natural history varies with the cell type and degree of differentiation. Well-differentiated papillary or follicular tumours (which constitute about 70% and 15% of cases, respectively) are very slow to grow and metastasise, sometimes persisting for years with little change in size and extent, although they may prove more aggressive in children. In contrast medullary carcinomas (5 to 10% of cases), which develop from the cells responsible for calcitonin secretion, and undifferentiated (anaplastic) tumours (5%) metastasise early and follow a much more rapid and aggressive course. About 25% of medullary cancers are hereditary, including those due to multiple endocrine neoplasia type 2.

The well-differentiated types usually present as a thyroid nodule, although most nodules are not malignant, while with anaplastic tumours there is usually bulky disease and often difficulty in breathing due to encroachment on the tracheal lumen.

In patients with **well-differentiated tumours** total or partial thyroidectomy is the treatment of choice.[1] This may be followed by a course of iodine-131 to destroy any residual tumour, although in low-risk patients the prognosis after surgery alone is so favourable that iodine-131 is not usually recommended.[1] Thyroxine [levothyroxine] treatment should be given to all patients to suppress thyroid stimulating hormone (TSH) production, and must be continued for life.[1,2] Ten-year survival of up to 75% in patients with follicular tumours and up to 90% with papillary tumours has been seen.[2] Disease recurrence is commonly treated with further surgery and ablative iodine-131 therapy.[1]

In patients with **medullary cancers** total thyroidectomy and neck dissection are indicated, followed by thyroxine [levothyroxine] treatment. Ten-year survival of 60 to 70% has been reported.[2,3] Prophylactic thyroidectomy may be considered in patients with a hereditary predisposition to medullary cancer.[3] Resection may relieve symptoms in patients with **anaplastic tumours**, but cure is impossible and treatment is purely palliative, with survival measured in months.[2,4] Neither medullary[3] nor anaplastic tumours[2] are sensitive to iodine-131. External radiation therapy has been used for palliation. Chemotherapy has been tried in anaplastic thyroid cancer, as well as in unresponsive disease of other cell types, with limited benefit. Drugs tried, often in combination regimens, include cisplatin, cyclophosphamide, bleomycin, dacarbazine, doxorubicin, fluorouracil, paclitaxel, and vincristine.[2-4]

1. Schlumberger MJ. Papillary and follicular thyroid carcinoma. *N Engl J Med* 1998; **338:** 297–306.
2. O'Doherty MJ, Coakley AJ. Drug therapy alternatives in the treatment of thyroid cancer. *Drugs* 1998; **55:** 801–12.
3. Heshmati HM, *et al.* Advances and controversies in the diagnosis and management of medullary thyroid carcinoma. *Am J Med* 1997; **103:** 60–69.
4. Ain KB. Anaplastic thyroid carcinoma: a therapeutic challenge. *Semin Surg Oncol* 1999; **16:** 64–9.

Neuroblastoma. Neuroblastoma accounts for about 7% of all childhood malignancies overall but is probably the most frequent neoplasm in the first year of life. Three-quarters of all cases present before the age of 5 years. The tumour is derived from cells of the neural crest, and may occur anywhere within the sympathetic nervous system, notably the sympathetic ganglia and the adrenal medulla. It is characterised by a diversity of clinical behaviour ranging from spontaneous remission to rapid metastatic progression and death. Sites of metastasis include lymph nodes, bone marrow, liver, and skin. Adverse prognostic factors include age over 1 year at diagnosis, stage IV (distant metastases), and amplification of the oncogene MYCN.

Progress in the treatment of neuroblastoma over the last 20 years has increased 10-year survival to about 60% overall, although in patients with disseminated disease the gains have been modest.[1] In those with localised disease (stage I or II) surgical resection alone is appropriate, with good long-term survival prospects. In addition, asymptomatic infants less than one year of age with localised tumours and limited dissemination (stage IV special) usually experience a high rate of tumour regression, and can be considered for surgical resection then close observation.[1] Low-dose chemotherapy generally arrests tumour progression should this occur. In those with lo-

calised but unresectable disease (stage II and III), subtotal surgical resection may be followed by standard-dose chemotherapy.[1] Chemotherapy regimens include cyclophosphamide and doxorubicin, sometimes with vincristine for good prognosis patients, and with the addition of cisplatin and etoposide (or teniposide) for poorer prognosis patients. Further surgery may be undertaken, with further chemotherapy and/or radiotherapy used in those with residual disease.[1] Disseminated disease (stage IV) and tumours with adverse prognostic features such as MYCN amplification are often more resistant to chemotherapy, and more intensive therapy is used.[1,2] Surgery and radiation therapy may also be combined with chemotherapy. Regimens used for remission induction include cyclophosphamide, doxorubicin, cisplatin, etoposide or teniposide, and vincristine. Another option is cisplatin, etoposide, and vindesine alternating with vincristine, dacarbazine, ifosfamide, and doxorubicin.[1] After remission induction, consolidation with myeloablative chemotherapy and autologous stem cell or bone marrow rescue may be used. Maintenance therapy with oral cyclophosphamide is being investigated. Isotretinoin and monoclonal antibodies are also being investigated for their ability to maintain remissions after chemotherapy.[1] Targeted radiation, using iodine-131-labelled *m*-iodobenzylguanidine, which is actively taken up by cells synthesising catecholamines, may be used for scanning, and is also being investigated for treatment.[3]

1. Berthold F, Hero B. Neuroblastoma: current drug therapy recommendations as part of the total treatment approach. *Drugs* 2000; **59:** 1261–77.
2. Katzenstein HM, Cohn SL. Advances in the diagnosis and treatment of neuroblastoma. *Curr Opin Oncol* 1998; **10:** 43–51.
3. Meller S. Targeted radiotherapy for neuroblastoma. *Arch Dis Child* 1997; **77:** 389–91.

Retinoblastoma. Retinoblastoma is the most common eye tumour in children and accounts for about 3% of all childhood malignancies (for other malignant neoplasms of the eye, see above). In 60 to 70% of cases the tumour is sporadic and non-hereditary, producing a unilateral, unifocal lesion. In the remaining 30 to 40% of cases there is an abnormal tumour suppressor gene (RB1) inherited: these tumours are typically bilateral and are sometimes associated with an intracranial neuroblastic tumour (trilateral retinoblastoma or pinealoblastoma). In addition, patients with the hereditary form are at very high risk of secondary primary malignancies, particularly osteosarcoma and soft tissue sarcomas. The most common manifestations of retinoblastoma are leukocoria (white pupil), strabismus (squint) and nystagmus. Retinoblastoma is confined to the eye(s) (intra-ocular) at presentation in about 80% of patients, although the majority have extensive disease within the eye. Nevertheless, 5-year disease-free survival after treatment in these patients is greater than 90%. The remainder of patients with extra-ocular disease in the tissues around the eye or with metastatic spread to the CNS and beyond, have a poor 5-year survival of less than 10% despite treatment.

The aim of treatment for intra-ocular retinoblastoma is to cure the disease, and to preserve as much vision as possible.[1-3] In patients with unilateral tumours, enucleation (removal of the eye) is the standard primary treatment when there is no expectation of useful vision (e.g. extensive disease within the eye). In bilateral retinoblastoma, standard treatment was enucleation of the advanced eye and external beam radiation therapy in the less advanced eye. However, there is increasing use of therapies to preserve the eye and to reduce the use of external radiotherapy which further increases the risk of secondary malignancies.[2,3] These include chemotherapy to reduce the tumour size (chemoreduction) and local treatments such as cryotherapy, thermotherapy, and plaque radiotherapy. Chemotherapy regimens used include carboplatin and etoposide (or teniposide) with or without vincristine.[3] Ciclosporin has also been included to overcome the multidrug resistance gene, p-glycoprotein.[3]

Patients who undergo enucleation and who are found to have optic nerve involvement (micrometastatic retinoblastoma) are at high risk of recurrence. Although there is no consensus on further treatment, these patients are often treated with adjuvant chemotherapy (cyclophosphamide, doxorubicin, and vincristine) or radiotherapy.[3]

Patients with orbital extension or distant metastases are treated with chemotherapy.[3] Regimens typically include doxorubicin, cyclophosphamide, and vincristine, and may include carboplatin and etoposide. Although such combination chemotherapy may produce a response it is rarely curative in such advanced disease. Intrathecal

chemotherapy with methotrexate and sometimes also cytarabine and dexamethasone may be combined with surgery and radiotherapy for CNS involvement or trilateral retinoblastoma.

1. Zucker JM, *et al.* Retinoblastoma. *Eur J Cancer* 1998; **34:** 1045–9.
2. Shields CL, Shields JA. Recent developments in the management of retinoblastoma. *J Pediatr Ophthalmol Strabismus* 1999; **36:** 8–18.
3. Finger PT, *et al.* Chemotherapy for retinoblastoma: a current topic. *Drugs* 1999; **58:** 983–96.

Sarcomas. The sarcomas are tumours arising from mesodermal cells which form the bone and connective tissue (as opposed to carcinomas, which arise from ectodermal and endodermal cells, and leukaemias and lymphomas which arise from the bone marrow and immune system).

Sarcomas are uncommon, and vary considerably in their sites, presentation, and prognosis. The primary malignancies of bone include osteosarcoma and Ewing's sarcoma, which most often occur in older children and adolescents, and chondrosarcoma which is most common in later life. Soft tissue sarcomas include those of fibrous tissue (fibrosarcoma), skeletal muscle (rhabdomyosarcoma), smooth muscle (leiomyosarcoma), adipose tissue (liposarcoma), and blood vessels (a group which includes Kaposi's sarcoma).

BONE SARCOMA. The commonest primary malignant tumour of bone is **osteosarcoma** (osteogenic sarcoma) which accounts for about 3 to 4% of all childhood malignancies. It is composed of malignant osteoblasts which form an osteoid matrix within which new bone formation may occur. Most osteosarcomas are aggressive high-grade malignancies which destroy overlying cortical bone and invade adjacent soft tissue, as well as spreading along the medulla. Metastasis, almost exclusively via the vascular system to the lungs and other distant sites, is usual and occurs early.

The primary therapy is surgery, with an increasing trend to more conservative, limb-sparing operations rather than amputation. Adjuvant chemotherapy is an important component of therapy, however, as metastasis of the tumour is common.[1,2] The most widely used combination is doxorubicin and cisplatin, sometimes with high-dose methotrexate and folinic acid rescue. Ifosfamide and cyclophosphamide are also used.[1-3] Chemotherapy is often commenced prior to surgery to attack micrometastases, shrink the primary tumour and enable evaluation of the tumour response.[3] Current aggressive treatment regimens can result in long-term relapse-free survival rates of 70%, although patients with overt metastatic disease at presentation have a poorer prognosis.[3]

Like osteosarcoma, **Ewing's sarcoma** is seen mainly in adolescents and older children. It is a round cell tumour that most commonly arises in the pelvis or the long bones of the limbs. There may be diffuse erosion of the bone and marked periosteal reaction. It spreads through the medullary cavity, and metastases to lung and other bones are common.

Unlike most bone sarcomas this is highly radiosensitive, so radiotherapy is frequently used to control local disease. The role of surgery has been controversial, but as adjuvant chemotherapy has increased survival to over 50%, limb-sparing surgery is gaining popularity.[2] The majority of patients will have micrometastatic disease, and therefore adjuvant chemotherapy remains essential.[3] In the USA, good results have been achieved with a combination of etoposide and ifosfamide added to intermittent high-dose vincristine, doxorubicin or dactinomycin or both, and cyclophosphamide.[1-3] These aggressive treatment regimens are not without risk; a significant proportion of successfully treated patients develop secondary cancers, such as radiation-induced sarcomas or treatment-related leukaemias, as well as anthracycline-induced cardiomyopathy.[1] Although multimodal therapy has improved survival, the prognosis for patients with overt metastatic disease remains poor; survival has been estimated to be only 20 to 30%.[3] Myeloablative therapy followed by stem cell transplantation has met with limited success in patients with metastatic disease at diagnosis.[1]

Chemotherapy appears to have little place in the treatment of other bone sarcomas such as **chondrosarcoma** or **osteoclastoma**; it has been employed in high-grade **fibrosarcomas** and in **histiocytoma** but its value is uncertain.

1. Arndt CAS, Crist WM. Common musculoskeletal tumors of childhood and adolescence. *N Engl J Med* 1999; **341:** 342–52.

2. Yaw KM. Pediatric bone tumors. *Semin Surg Oncol* 1999; **16:** 173–83.
3. Russell EC, *et al.* Lymphomas and bone marrow tumors: clinical presentation, management, and potential late effects of current treatment strategies. *Adolesc Med* 1999; **10:** 419–35.

KAPOSI'S SARCOMA. Kaposi's sarcoma is a tumour of endothelial or spindle cell origin. In its classical form it manifests as red or violet cutaneous lesions of the limbs in elderly men, usually of Jewish or Mediterranean ancestry. An endemic form is also seen in certain areas of Africa.[1] Lesions may eventually affect the whole of the skin, upper airways, gastrointestinal tract, lungs, and lymph nodes, but in general disease is only very slowly progressive, and may require no treatment. Patients receiving immunosuppressive therapy may be at greater risk of developing Kaposi's sarcoma, particularly if they are from ethnic groups that are susceptible to the classic or endemic forms of the disease.[1] In recent years an epidemic form of the disease has appeared in patients with disease due to HIV infection. HIV-associated Kaposi's sarcoma is more aggressive, with a greater tendency to disseminated and metastatic disease.

A novel herpesvirus (human herpesvirus 8, HHV8) has been implicated in the pathogenesis of Kaposi's sarcoma. HHV8 induces changes in endothelial cells that make them more susceptible to inflammatory cytokines and angiogenesis.[2] Some antivirals, such as cidofovir and to a lesser extent foscarnet and ganciclovir, have shown activity against HHV8 *in vitro*, but they have not been equally successful in treating Kaposi's sarcoma *in vivo*. Treatment with highly active antiretroviral therapy has greatly reduced the occurrence of Kaposi's sarcoma in AIDS patients, and may cause regression of milder forms of the disease, but this is thought to be due to improvements in immune function rather than a direct effect on Kaposi's sarcoma.[3] The development of Kaposi's sarcoma is likely to be multifactorial, and as infection with HHV8 alone does not produce disease, and the replication of HHV8 in sarcoma cells is low, antiviral therapy alone is unlikely to be sufficient to control symptoms.[3]

Patients with classic or endemic Kaposi's sarcoma are often treated with surgery or radiotherapy of individual lesions.[1] Extensive or recurrent disease may be treated with vinca alkaloids, bleomycin, doxorubicin, and dacarbazine, alone or in combination.[1] Etoposide and interferon alfa have also been tried.[1] There is a report of the control of non-epidemic Kaposi's sarcoma by the use of dapsone in two patients.[4] Patients with immunosuppression-associated Kaposi's sarcoma may receive similar treatment to those with the classic form, or preferably by alteration of the immunosuppressive regimen if this can be done without graft loss.[1]

The epidemic form of Kaposi's sarcoma is associated with HIV infection, and seen particularly in homosexual patients. In the early stages, highly active antiretroviral therapy may resolve the immunosuppression and therefore control Kaposi's sarcoma, but the response is unpredictable, so specific therapy is often needed.[1] Localised disease may be managed with cryotherapy or radiotherapy, but intralesional vinblastine, interferon alfa, and topical alitretinoin are also used.[2] Photodynamic therapy, using tin ethyletiopurpurin as the photosensitiser, has also been tried.[5] There is a report of a good response to perilesional injection of granulocyte-macrophage colony-stimulating factor,[6] and platelet factor 4, an inhibitor of the growth of vascular epithelium, has been investigated for local and systemic use.

Systemic chemotherapy is generally reserved for patients with more extensive disease or mucosal or visceral involvement. In patients with a CD4 cell count of 200 cells per μL or above, treatment with interferon alfa, in combination with zidovudine, has been advocated by some, but systemic chemotherapy is the treatment of choice.[1-3] The main combination regimens use a vinca alkaloid and bleomycin, with or without doxorubicin.[2,3] Liposomal formulations of doxorubicin and daunorubicin have produced response rates of 40-85% and may be less toxic than conventional chemotherapy;[2,3] many now consider a liposomal anthracycline the drug of choice in extensive disease.[1,2] Paclitaxel is also used as a single agent in advanced disease.[2,3]

Control of Kaposi's sarcoma has been reported in a few patients given high-dose intramuscular chorionic gonadotrophin,[7] but tumour regression ceased and regrowth occurred when dosage was reduced or withdrawn. Although a subsequent study (using lower doses) was discontinued due to toxicity and lack of benefit,[8] others have noted that different preparations may vary in their activity against the tumour (suggesting that it is not chorionic

gonadotrophin itself but some impurity that is active) and have confirmed a benefit following intralesional injection.[9,10] Some results suggest the impurity in question may be a ribonuclease.[11] Other lines of investigation include the use of sulfated polysaccharide peptidoglycans, various other inhibitors of angiogenesis (including captopril[12]), thalidomide, and the retinoids.[13]

1. Antman K, Chang Y. Kaposi's sarcoma. *N Engl J Med* 2000; **342:** 1027–38.
2. Mitsuyasu RT. Update on the pathogenesis and treatment of Kaposi sarcoma. *Curr Opin Oncol* 2000; **12:** 174–80.
3. Hermans P. Opportunistic AIDS-associated malignancies in HIV-infected patients. *Biomed Pharmacother* 2000; **54:** 32–40.
4. De Haas ERM, *et al.* Non-HIV-related Kaposi's sarcoma suppressed by dapsone. *Br J Dermatol* 1996; **135:** 813–14.
5. Allison RR, *et al.* Tin ethyl etiopurpurin-induced photodynamic therapy for the treatment of human immunodeficiency virus-associated Kaposi's sarcoma. *Curr Ther Res* 1998; **59:** 23–7.
6. Boente P, *et al.* Local peri-lesional therapy with rhGM-CSF for Kaposi's sarcoma. *Lancet* 1993; **341:** 1154.
7. Harris PJ. Treatment of Kaposi's sarcoma and other manifestations of AIDS with human chorionic gonadotropin. *Lancet* 1995; **346:** 118–19.
8. Bower M, *et al.* Human chorionic gonadotrophin for AIDS-related Kaposi's sarcoma. *Lancet* 1995; **346:** 642.
9. Gill PS, *et al.* The effects of preparations of human chorionic gonadotropin on AIDS-related Kaposi's sarcoma. *N Engl J Med* 1996; **335:** 1261–9. Correction. *ibid.* 1997; **336:** 670 and 1115.
10. Gill PS, *et al.* Intralesional human chorionic gonadotropin for Kaposi's sarcoma. *N Engl J Med* 1997; **336:** 1188.
11. Griffiths SJ, *et al.* Ribonuclease inhibits Kaposi's sarcoma. *Nature* 1997; **390:** 568.
12. Vogt B, Frey FJ. Inhibition of angiogenesis in Kaposi's sarcoma by captopril. *Lancet* 1997; **349:** 1148.
13. Denton AS, *et al.* Management of pulmonary Kaposi's sarcoma: new perspectives. *Br J Hosp Med* 1995; **53:** 345–50.

SOFT-TISSUE SARCOMA. Soft tissue sarcomas are a group of malignant tumours that originate from mesenchymal stem cells. **Rhabdomyosarcoma** is the commonest soft-tissue sarcoma in childhood, and is thought to arise from progenitor cells for skeletal muscle found throughout the body. The most frequent sites are the head and neck, genito-urinary tract, and extremities. The tumour spreads at an early stage into adjacent tissues and regional lymph nodes, and about 20% of patients have metastatic disease at diagnosis, most frequently in the lungs.

Effective treatment of rhabdomyosarcoma requires a combination of surgery, radiotherapy, and chemotherapy. Complete surgical excision is to be preferred, but where this is impossible wide-field irradiation should be given. Adjuvant chemotherapy is frequently used to control micrometastatic disease and has increased recurrence-free survival.[1,2] Most regimens employ doxorubicin, with various combinations of ifosfamide, etoposide, cisplatin, dactinomycin, dacarbazine, cyclophosphamide, and vincristine.[1,3] Although doxorubicin and ifosfamide are considered to be the most active drugs, there is no consensus on the optimal drug regimen or dose.[1,2]

1. Bishop JM, Lorigan P. Systemic therapy of soft tissue sarcomas. *CME Oncol* 1999; **1:** 81–4.
2. Sarcoma Meta-analysis Collaboration. Adjuvant chemotherapy for localised resectable soft tissue sarcoma in adults (updated 2 August 2001). Available in The Cochrane Library; Issue 4. Oxford: Update Software; 2001.
3. Seynaeve C, Verweij J. High-dose chemotherapy in adult sarcomas: no standard yet. *Semin Oncol* 1999; **26:** 119–33.

Choice of Immunosuppressant

Amyloidosis. Amyloidosis refers to a group of conditions characterised by accumulation of a waxy proteinaceous infiltrate within body tissues. Various forms are known, including AL amyloidosis, in which the amyloid is derived from immunoglobulin light chains, ATTR amyloidosis, in which it is derived from transthyretin, and AA amyloidosis, which is most often secondary to chronic inflammation, such as that associated with rheumatoid arthritis and tuberculosis.[1] Amyloidosis may also be secondary to malignant disease. Familial Mediterranean fever (see p.401) is associated with AA amyloidosis.

Symptoms vary, depending on where the amyloid is deposited, and may include nephrotic syndrome and renal failure, peripheral neuropathy, carpal tunnel syndrome, restrictive cardiomyopathy leading to heart failure, gastrointestinal bleeding, malabsorption, protein-losing enteropathy, polyarthritis, skin nodules, and macroglossia (due to deposition in the tongue).

Management depends to some extent upon the type of amyloidosis involved, and the site, but no agent or combination of agents is unequivocally effective. Colchicine is extremely effective at preventing renal deterioration in patients with familial Mediterranean fever,[2,3] but is not considered to be of benefit in other forms of amyloidosis.[1,4] Amyloidosis may respond to chemotherapy.[4,5] Melphalan plus prednisone is the standard therapy, and has been shown to increase median survival in amyloidosis patients. Such combined regimens are more effective

than colchicine alone in AL amyloidosis,[6] and survival has been reported to be slightly better in patients treated with melphalan and prednisone than in similar patients given these drugs with colchicine.[7] Alternatively, cycles of vincristine, doxorubicin, and dexamethasone may be effective, but patients with cardiac amyloidosis may be at increased risk of anthracycline toxicity. High-dose dexamethasone has also been tried, although its value is controversial, and 4'-iodo-4'-deoxydoxorubicin has been investigated.[1,5] High-dose chemotherapy with autologous peripheral blood stem cell transplantation is gaining popularity.[4,5] Although the therapy is very toxic, good results have been reported in selected patients. Local application or oral administration of dimethyl sulfoxide has also been tried.

Symptomatic management is also important. Care must be taken to avoid digitalis toxicity when cardiac amyloid is present, as well as to avoid salt and water depletion through injudicious use of diuretics. Calcium-channel blockers and beta blockers should be avoided.[1] The intractable diarrhoea that can occur due to autonomic neuropathy or infiltration of the gastrointestinal tract may respond to octreotide.[8] Renal transplantation may be considered in end-stage renal failure due to amyloidosis, but unless amyloid production has been stopped disease is likely to recur in the new kidney. Cardiac transplantation, and subsequent chemotherapy with epirubicin, carmustine, and cyclophosphamide to suppress the underlying disease and control amyloid deposition in the graft has also been described.[9] Liver transplantation is the definitive therapy for patients with ATTR amyloidosis.[1]

1. Falk, RH, *et al.* The systemic amyloidoses. *N Engl J Med* 1997; **337:** 898–909.
2. Zemer D, *et al.* Colchicine in the prevention and treatment of the amyloidosis of familial Mediterranean fever. *N Engl J Med* 1986; **314:** 1001–5.
3. Majeed HA. *et al.* Long-term colchicine prophylaxis in children with familial Mediterranean fever (recurrent hereditary polyserositis). *J Pediatr* 1990; **116:** 997–9.
4. Gertz MA, *et al.* Amyloidosis: recognition, confirmation, prognosis and therapy. *Mayo Clin Proc* 1999; **74:** 490–4.
5. Sezer O, *et al.* New therapeutic approaches in primary systemic AL amyloidosis. *Ann Hematol* 2000; **79:** 1–6.
6. Skinner M, *et al.* Treatment of 100 patients with primary amyloidosis: a randomized trial of melphalan, prednisone, and colchicine versus colchicine only. *Am J Med* 1996; **100:** 290–8.
7. Kyle RA. A trial of three regimens for primary amyloidosis: colchicine alone, melphalan and prednisone, and melphalan, prednisone, and colchicine. *N Engl J Med* 1997; **336:** 1202–7.
8. Yam LT, Oropilla SB. Octreotide for diarrhea in amyloidosis. *Ann Intern Med* 1991; **115:** 577.
9. Hall R, *et al.* Cardiac transplantation for AL amyloidosis. *BMJ* 1994; **309:** 1135–7.

Asthma. Immunosuppressant drugs do not play a role in the regular management of asthma (p.757). In individual patients requiring oral corticosteroids for chronic severe asthma immunosuppressants have however been investigated for their anti-inflammatory and corticosteroid-sparing properties. Both ciclosporin (see p.524) and methotrexate (see p.556) have shown some benefit, but their toxicity is of concern.

Blood disorders, non-malignant. For the use of immunosuppressants in aplastic anaemia, see p.715.

Diabetes mellitus. For a discussion of diabetes mellitus and its treatment, including the experimental use of immunosuppressants, see p.315. See also under Organ and Tissue Transplantation, below.

Gastrointestinal disorders. INFLAMMATORY BOWEL DISEASES. A number of immunosuppressants have been tried in inflammatory bowel disease (p.1205), with some success, but the mainstays of drug therapy remain the aminosalicylates and the corticosteroids. Immunosuppressants may be valuable in some circumstances for their corticosteroid-sparing effect and for chronic active disease refractory to other treatments.

Liver disorders, non-malignant. For a discussion of the role of immunosuppressants, and particularly azathioprine, in the management of chronic active hepatitis, see p.1048.

PRIMARY BILIARY CIRRHOSIS. Primary biliary cirrhosis is a chronic liver disease of unknown aetiology which develops due to progressive destruction of small and intermediate bile ducts within the liver, subsequently evolving to fibrosis and cirrhosis. Over 90% of patients are female, usually aged between 40 and 60 years. The disease is thought to be auto-immune in nature, perhaps triggered by a micro-organism in the environment, and most patients exhibit autoantibodies to mitochondria. Development of such antibodies may be evident in patients with primary biliary cirrhosis before disease is clinically apparent.[1] Symptoms include pruritus, fatigue, jaundice, hepatomegaly, hypercholesterolaemia leading to xanthoma formation, and in late disease portal hypertension, bleeding oesophageal varices and liver failure may develop. Impaired calcium and vitamin D absorption may result in osteomalacia or osteoporosis, and there may be accumulation of copper in the liver. Various other disorders including rheumatoid arthritis, scleroderma, renal tubular acidosis, thyroiditis, and Sjögren's syndrome may be associated with primary biliary cirrhosis.[2]

The disease is slowly progressive, with a mean survival of 8 years for symptomatic patients, and 16 years for asymptomatic individuals.[3] The disease is thought to have an auto-immune component and various attempts have been made to modify the disease process, but to date none has proven unequivocally successful. The best-studied treatment for primary biliary cirrhosis is ursodeoxycholic acid, which is thought to replace toxic endogenous bile acids, stimulate bile acid secretion, and exert local immunosuppressive and cytoprotective effects.[4,5] Ursodeoxycholic acid was thought to delay disease progression and the need for liver transplantation, but a recent meta-analysis has disputed this assumption and some reviewers do not recommend its use.[6,7] It is still prescribed by many workers, however, who consider that long-term therapy (≥ 4 years) will have a beneficial effect on liver histology.[5] Both penicillamine and azathioprine have been used in primary biliary cirrhosis, but trials have failed to show any benefit from treatment[3] and their use has declined. Corticosteroids, colchicine, ciclosporin, chlorambucil, and methotrexate have also been tried with more success, but toxicity has restricted their use. They may be of benefit when administered in conjunction with ursodeoxycholic acid to patients with advanced disease, but the optimum combination and regimen has yet to be defined.[3-5]

Symptomatic treatment includes the use of bile acid sequestrants, such as colestyramine, to treat both pruritus and hypercholesterolaemia. Ursodeoxycholic acid may also improve pruritus in up to 40% of patients, and rifampicin, phenobarbital, and opioid antagonists are used as second-line therapies.[4,5] Vitamin D and calcium supplementation will prevent osteomalacia; supplementation with vitamins K and A may also be necessary.[4,5]

In patients in whom disease progresses to liver failure the ultimate therapy is liver transplantation.[2] Disease can recur after transplantation, but with little short-term adverse clinical effect.[4,5,8]

1. Metcalf JV, et al. Natural history of early primary biliary cirrhosis. Lancet 1996; 348: 1399–1402.
2. Kaplan MM. Primary biliary cirrhosis. N Engl J Med 1996; 335: 1570–80.
3. Heathcote EJ. Evidence-based therapy of primary biliary cirrhosis. Eur J Gastroenterol Hepatol 1999; 11: 607–15.
4. Prince MI, Jones DE. Primary biliary cirrhosis: new perspectives in diagnosis and treatment. Postgrad Med J 2000; 76: 199–206.
5. Poupon R, Poupon RE. Treatment of primary biliary cirrhosis. Baillieres Best Pract Res Clin Gastroenterol 2000; 14: 615–28.
6. Goulis J, et al. Randomised controlled trials of ursodeoxycholic-acid therapy for primary biliary cirrhosis: a meta-analysis. Lancet 1999 354: 1053–60.
7. Anonymous. Ursodeoxycholic acid for primary biliary cirrhosis. Drug Ther Bull 1999; 37: 30–2.
8. Neuberger J. Primary biliary cirrhosis. Lancet 1997; 350: 875–9.

Lung disorders, non-malignant. DIFFUSE PARENCHYMAL LUNG DISEASE. Corticosteroids are the mainstay of treatment for diffuse parenchymal lung disease (p.1050) such as cryptogenic fibrosing alveolitis, usually in combination with azathioprine (or occasionally cyclophosphamide).

Neurological disorders. MULTIPLE SCLEROSIS. Immunosuppressants have been tried in the treatment of multiple sclerosis (p.633), although in some studies the benefit obtained may have been outweighed by toxicity.

MYASTHENIA GRAVIS. Patients with myasthenia gravis (p.1414) who require immunosuppression are usually treated with corticosteroids. Azathioprine is used mainly in myasthenia gravis for its corticosteroid-sparing effect but may also be of use when corticosteroids are contra-indicated or when response to corticosteroids alone is insufficient. Other immunosuppressants which have been tried similarly include ciclosporin, cyclophosphamide, and methotrexate.

Ocular disorders, non-malignant. Immunosuppressants have been used with some success in a variety of ocular disorders with inflammatory or immunological components. In *scleritis* and *uveitis* (see p.1058 and p.1060) necessitating treatment corticosteroids, given topically, intra-ocularly, or systemically are widely used, but in unresponsive disease, or in patients with unaccept-

able side-effects at the required dose of corticosteroids, immunosuppressants such as azathioprine, chlorambucil, cyclophosphamide, or methotrexate, may be given.[1,2] In necrotising scleritis it has been suggested that immunosuppressant therapy should be the initial choice, as therapeutic failure is very common with less aggressive regimens.[3] Immunosuppressants are particularly valuable in the management of the ocular lesions of *Behçet's disease, rheumatoid arthritis,* or *Wegener's granulomatosis*,[2] (see p.1047, p.9, and p.1060, respectively). Ciclosporin is also of value in both scleritis[1] and uveitis,[2,4] and has proved useful as an alternative to cyclophosphamide or azathioprine when combined with corticosteroids in the management of both ocular and vascular symptoms of *Cogan's syndrome*[5] (p.1049). However, nephrotoxicity remains a potential problem with systemic ciclosporin,[4] and in this respect a report of response in refractory corneal ulcers secondary to rheumatic disease, oculomucocutaneous syndrome, or *Sjögren's syndrome* following treatment with 2% ciclosporin eye drops is of interest.[6]

In *Graves' ophthalmopathy*, (see under Hyperthyroidism, p.1519), immunosuppressants have been tried with equivocal results; benefit has however been reported from the use of ciclosporin with prednisone.[7,8]

1. Wakefield D, McCluskey P. Cyclosporin therapy for severe scleritis. Br J Ophthalmol 1989; 73: 743–6.
2. Herman DC. Endogenous uveitis: current concepts of treatment. Mayo Clin Proc 1990; 65: 671–83.
3. Sainz de la Maza M, et al. An analysis of therapeutic decision for scleritis. Ophthalmology 1993; 100: 1372–6.
4. de Vries J, et al. Cyclosporin in the treatment of severe chronic idiopathic uveitis. Br J Ophthalmol 1990; 74: 344–9.
5. Allen NB, et al. Use of immunosuppressive agents in the treatment of severe ocular and vascular manifestations of Cogan's syndrome. Am J Med 1990; 88: 296–301.
6. Zierhut M, et al. Topical treatment of severe corneal ulcers with cyclosporin A. Graefes Arch Clin Exp Ophthalmol 1989; 227: 30–5.
7. Kahaly G, et al. Ciclosporin and prednisone v prednisone in treatment of Graves' ophthalmopathy: a controlled, randomized and prospective study. Eur J Clin Invest 1986; 16: 415–22.
8. Prummel MF, et al. Prednisone and cyclosporine in the treatment of severe Graves' ophthalmopathy. N Engl J Med 1989; 321: 1353–9.

Organ and tissue transplantation. Although surgical techniques suitable for the removal of organs and tissues from a donor, and their engraftment into a host, have existed for many years, such grafts would not normally survive for long. The host's CD4 T-cells recognise foreign antigens from donor cells. These are encoded mainly on highly polymorphic loci within the major histocompatibility complex located on the short arm of chromosome 6. A CD4 cell is subsequently activated by antigen-presenting cells to secrete interleukin-2 and induce T-cell proliferation. Activated T-cells then mediate a rejection response, by increasing the activity and function of B-cells, cytotoxic CD8 T-cells, and macrophages, either directly, or by cytokine release. Only from the 1960s with the development of drugs capable of attenuating or suppressing this response, did transplantation start to become a feasible mode of treatment.

The drugs available vary in their mechanisms of action, and are often combined for optimum effect. The glucocorticoids act at several points in the immune cascade, including antigen recognition and production of lymphokines. Ciclosporin and newer polypeptide immunosuppressants such as tacrolimus prevent formation of cytotoxic T-cells by inhibiting calcineurin activation, an important step in the release of interleukin-2 from helper T-cells, while polyclonal or monoclonal antilymphocyte antibodies such as antilymphocyte immunoglobulin and muromonab CD3 bind to and deplete T-cell populations. Anti-proliferative drugs such as azathioprine, mycophenolate mofetil, methotrexate, and cyclophosphamide act by preventing cell division of lymphocytes. Sirolimus is an anti-proliferative drug that inhibits the T-cell response to cytokines.

Immunosuppressant regimens may be divided into those aimed at

• prevention of rejection in the early period after transplantation
• long-term maintenance prophylaxis
• treatment of acute episodes of rejection.

In bone marrow transplantation, where an immunologically competent tissue is transplanted, it is the donor cells which attack host tissues (graft versus host disease), and immunosuppression is required for prophylaxis of this condition.

Because of the critical nature of the early stage, when the organ or tissue must recover normal function, and perhaps to permit better long-term tolerance, initial immu-

nosuppressant regimens tend to use higher doses than maintenance therapy. Standard protocols are usually based around ciclosporin or tacrolimus, combined with corticosteroids and an anti-proliferative agent. Where appropriate, a 7- to 14-day course of antilymphocyte antibodies is added to the standard regimen for induction. This is usually only required in individuals at increased risk of acute rejection, such as children or patients with a previous transplant or pregnancy, multiple blood transfusions, or a poor HLA-matching. However it also enables delayed introduction of ciclosporin or tacrolimus in patients with post-transplant tubular necrosis.

Since immunosuppressant therapy must in most cases be given for the lifetime of the graft, in long-term maintenance the toxicity of the drugs used, and the risks of infection and neoplasia, must be considered. Doses and numbers of agents used tend to be reduced, and in particular there is a tendency to taper or sometimes even eliminate the doses of corticosteroids used in maintenance regimens because of the potential sequelae of prolonged corticosteroid use.

The use of less intensive maintenance regimens must be balanced against the risk of an acute rejection episode, and the likelihood of its responding to therapy. High-dose corticosteroids and polyclonal or monoclonal antilymphocyte antibodies often play a role in the rescue therapy of patients with acute rejection episodes, although much depends upon the severity of the reaction, and whether such episodes have occurred previously.

The management of immunosuppression for the transplantation of particular organs is discussed in more detail below. With the use of suitable immunosuppressant regimens long-term graft survival can be obtained following transplantation of heart, kidney or liver; the transplantation of other organs such as bowel, lung, or pancreas remains more experimental. Ultimately, however, the complications of chronic rejection are likely to lead to loss of the graft: the induction of specific tolerance to the donor organ remains the goal of much research. In allogeneic bone marrow transplantation, where the aim of immunosuppression is prevention of graft versus host disease rather than rejection, immunosuppressant therapy can often be tapered off and eventually withdrawn.

Much recent interest has been aroused by the possibility of organ transplants from *animals*, genetically modified to reduce complement-mediated hyperacute rejection. It is not clear whether such xenotransplantation will require modified immunosuppressive regimens.

◊ References.

1. Denton MD, et al. Immunosuppressive strategies in transplantation. Lancet 1999; 353: 1083–91.
2. Harlan DM, Kirk AD. The future of organ and tissue transplantation: can T-cell costimulatory pathway modifiers revolutionize the prevention of graft rejection? JAMA 1999; 282: 1076–82.
3. Hong JC, Kahan BD. Immunosuppressive agents in organ transplantation: past, present, and future. Semin Nephrol 2000; 20: 108–25.

HAEMATOPOIETIC STEM CELLS. Haematopoietic stem cell transplantation is used in the treatment of a variety of malignancies, notably in the acute leukaemias and lymphomas; to permit the use of very high-dose chemotherapy in the management of some solid tumours (bone marrow rescue); and to treat some other serious disorders affecting the bone marrow, such as aplastic anaemia and the haemoglobinopathies.[1] Two types of haematopoietic stem cell transplant are in use: in autologous transplantation, the patient's own stem cells are harvested from bone marrow or peripheral blood, while in allogeneic transplantation stem cells are harvested from the bone marrow, peripheral blood or umbilical cord blood of a healthy donor matched for HLA type.[2] Traditionally, bone marrow cells were used, but the use of peripheral blood cells and umbilical cord blood is increasing.[3] Peripheral blood stem cell use is convenient as collection does not require hospitalisation and general anaesthesia for the donor. Clinical trials have demonstrated more rapid engraftment of neutrophils and platelets compared with bone marrow transplants.[3] Umbilical cord blood is mainly used for transplants in children, since the total number of stem cells in a donation often falls short of the levels deemed necessary for engraftment in an adult. Use of umbilical cord blood is associated with slightly delayed engraftment, but a lower risk of graft versus host disease.

With autologous transplants problems of compatibility do not arise, but if abnormal cell clones are present in the marrow (as in leukaemia) they may be transferred back into the patient and cause disease relapse. Contamination is less of a problem with peripheral blood stem cells.[4]

Allogeneic bone-marrow transplants require immuno-suppression but it can usually be withdrawn after about 6 months.[5-7] The need is for suppression of graft-versus-host disease (see below), in which the donor immune system attacks host cells, until a new immunological balance is achieved.

The patient is normally prepared by conditioning with total body irradiation, or myeloablative chemotherapy with agents such as cyclophosphamide or busulfan, or more often both, in order to destroy host bone marrow cells. In autologous procedures, harvesting of bone marrow or peripheral blood must be carried out before conditioning. Bone marrow is aspirated from the donor, and infused into the recipient via an indwelling catheter or directly into a peripheral vein. Peripheral blood stem cells are collected by cell separation after mobilisation, which is best achieved by a combination of chemotherapy and granulocyte or granulocyte-macrophage colony-stimulating factor.[3] Prophylactic cover with antimicrobials and normal immunoglobulins is recommended to prevent infection.[5]

In addition to such supportive care, patients who have received allogeneic transplants require immunosuppressive therapy aimed at the prevention of **graft-versus-host disease** (GVHD). GVHD is usually characterised as acute or chronic depending on the manifestations, and the time of presentation (by convention acute disease occurs within a hundred days of transplantation, and chronic disease after this time, although in practice there is considerable overlap). The organ systems primarily affected are skin, liver, and gastrointestinal tract. Both forms are marked by maculopapular rashes, which in severe disease may progress to bullous lesions and epidermal necrolysis. Liver disease may include cholestatic jaundice (usually in the acute form) and hepatitis; symptoms may need to be distinguished from the veno-occlusive disease which sometimes complicates bone-marrow transplantation and may relate to the pre-transplant conditioning regimen (the latter may respond to treatment with antithrombin III[8] or defibrotide[9]). Ursodeoxycholic acid has been investigated for the prophylaxis of hepatic complications.[10] The primary symptom of gastrointestinal GVHD is diarrhoea, often severe and painful. In patients with chronic GVHD other manifestations may include arthritis, mucositis, lung disease, and scleroderma.

Various drugs have been used for the prophylaxis of graft-versus-host disease following allogeneic bone-marrow transplantation, but most modern regimens are based on ciclosporin. Although GVHD still occurs in many ciclosporin-treated patients, morbidity is much reduced and survival improved. Various combination regimens have been tried for prophylaxis, particularly ciclosporin or tacrolimus with methotrexate, but also combinations with other drugs including antilymphocyte immunoglobulins, corticosteroids, trimetrexate, fludarabine and sirolimus.[7,11] Monoclonal antibodies have also been used to produce T-cell depletion or reduce the effects of circulating cytokines.[7,11,12] Acute GVHD is usually treated by the addition of corticosteroids to the prophylactic regimen until symptoms are controlled, followed by gradual tapering of the dose. Mycophenolate mofetil, antilymphocyte immunoglobulins, monoclonal antibodies such as zolimomab aritox, and thalidomide have also been tried.[7,11] Chronic GVHD requires long-term immunosuppression, and combination therapy results in increased disease-free survival.[7] Ciclosporin, with or without a corticosteroid is commonly used,[7,11] but thalidomide and azathioprine have also been tried.[7] PUVA therapy has been used in refractory cutaneous GVHD and extracorporeal photopheresis has been investigated.[7] Octreotide is recommended for the symptomatic treatment of diarrhoea.[13,14]

However, a degree of acute graft-versus-host disease may be desirable in some stem cell transplants, since it can result in a 'graft-versus malignancy' effect which reduces relapse. Indeed, many leukaemia patients who relapse following allogeneic transplant can be reinduced into remission by an additional infusion of donor lymphocytes.[15] Consequently, too effective an immunosuppressant regimen may not always be desirable, and leukaemic patients given bone marrow transplants purged of T cells, which virtually abolishes GVHD, do not have a better survival rate than those given conventional prophylaxis (engraftment too is reduced in the absence of all T cells). The observation of graft versus malignancy effects has led to the development of low-dose non-myeloablative preparative regimens (with or without donor lymphocyte infusions) for elderly or

more sensitive patients who might have been unable to receive the standard aggressive therapy.[2,15]

1. Goldman JM, et al. Allogeneic and autologous transplantation for haematological diseases, solid tumours and immune disorders: current practice in Europe in 1998. *Bone Marrow Transplant* 1998; **21:** 1–7.
2. Lennard AL, Jackson GH. Stem cell transplantation. *BMJ* 2000; **321:** 433–7.
3. Demirer T, et al. Peripheral blood stem cell mobilization for high-dose chemotherapy. *J Hematother* 1999; **8:** 103–13.
4. Nemunaitis J. A comparative review of colony-stimulating factors. *Drugs* 1997; **54:** 709–29.
5. Rowe JM, et al. Recommended guidelines for the management of autologous and allogeneic bone marrow transplantation: a report from the Eastern Cooperative Oncology Group (ECOG). *Ann Intern Med* 1994; **120:** 143–58.
6. Duncombe A. Bone marrow and stem cell transplantation. *BMJ* 1997; **314:** 1179–82.
7. Flowers MED, et al. Pathophysiology and treatment of graft-versus-host disease. *Hematol Oncol Clin North Am* 1999; **13:** 1091–1112.
8. Morris JD, et al. Antithrombin-III for the treatment of chemotherapy-induced organ dysfunction following bone marrow transplantation. *Bone Marrow Transplant* 1997; **20:** 871–8.
9. Chopra R, et al. Defibrotide for the treatment of hepatic veno-occlusive disease: results of the European compassionate-use study. *Br J Haematol* 2000; **111:** 1122–9.
10. Essell JH, et al. Ursodiol prophylaxis against hepatic complications of allogeneic bone marrow transplantation: a randomized, double-blind, placebo-controlled trial. *Ann Intern Med* 1998; **128:** 975–81.
11. Hiscott A, McLellan DS. Graft-versus-host disease in allogeneic bone marrow transplantation: the role of monoclonal antibodies in prevention and treatment. *Br J Biomed Sci* 2000; **57:** 163–9.
12. Ferrara JLM, et al. Monoclonal antibody and receptor antagonist therapy for GVHD. *Cancer Treat Res* 1999; **101:** 331–68.
13. Ippoliti C, et al. Use of octreotide in the symptomatic management of diarrhea induced by graft-versus-host disease in patients with hematologic malignancies. *J Clin Oncol* 1997; **15:** 3350–4.
14. Kornblau S, et al. Management of cancer treatment-related diarrhea: issues and therapeutic strategies. *J Pain Symptom Manage* 2000; **19:** 118–29.
15. Champlin R, et al. Reinventing bone marrow transplantation: reducing toxicity using nonmyeloablative, preparative regimens and induction of graft-versus-malignancy. *Curr Opin Oncol* 1999; **11:** 87–95.

HEART. Marked improvements have been seen in outcome following heart transplantation since the introduction of ciclosporin, which has resulted in a reduced incidence and severity of rejection episodes. The current 1-year survival rate is now approximately 80%.[1]

A common **immunosuppressive regimen** consists of triple therapy with ciclosporin, azathioprine and corticosteroids.[1] Some centres use induction therapy with antilymphocyte immunoglobulins or muromonab-CD3,[1,2] which increases the risk of infection and lymphoproliferative disorders, but does delay the first rejection episode and allows transplantation in higher risk groups. In addition, it enables ciclosporin administration to be delayed in patients with initial poor renal function and corticosteroids to be discontinued as maintenance therapy in some groups of patients:[1,2] it has been suggested that the high doses of corticosteroids employed increase the risk of cardiac adverse events in the longer term.[3]

There does not seem to be any significant difference in efficacy between tacrolimus and ciclosporin in heart transplant patients.[1,4] Mycophenolate mofetil has shown some benefit over azathioprine in triple therapy, but it is not yet known whether suggestions of a decrease in the incidence of subsequent coronary artery disease are correct.[1,4] Substituting cyclophosphamide for azathioprine for 6 weeks after transplantation is reported to reduce the development of anti-muromonab-CD3 antibodies from induction therapy.[5]

In the early post-transplant period, the most significant **causes of morbidity** are infection and rejection episodes.[1] Co-trimoxazole is used to protect against *Pneumocystis carinii* infection, and ganciclovir as prophylaxis against cytomegalovirus.[1] Rejection is usually treated with corticosteroids, but a variety of drugs have been used for corticosteroid-resistant cases.[1] Antilymphocyte immunoglobulins, mycophenolate mofetil, adjunctive methotrexate, total lymphoid irradiation and photopheresis have all been tried,[1,4] but the treatment of choice is muromonab-CD3.[4] Newer drugs under investigation include sirolimus and basiliximab.[4]

In the late post-transplant period, malignancy and coronary artery disease are the most significant problems.[1,6] Coronary artery disease affects up to 10% of patients at 1 year, and approximately 50% at 5 years post-transplant. It is thought to be mainly an immunological response, but can be accelerated by the classical risk factors of dyslipidaemia, obesity, glucose intolerance, and smoking, as well as by postoperative cytomegalovirus infection.[1] Calcium-channel blockers and statins (HMG-CoA reductase inhibitors) have been used to decrease the incidence of

coronary artery disease,[6] but it has remained a difficult complication to treat.

Improved surgical techniques and the use of ciclosporin have also made possible successful combined heart-lung transplants,[7,8] although these may require enhanced immunosuppression to prevent obliterative bronchiolitis,[9] a possible manifestation of chronic rejection.

1. Hunt SA. Current status of cardiac transplantation. *JAMA* 1998; **280:** 1692–8.
2. Wahlers T. Cytolytic induction therapy in heart and lung transplantation: the protagonist opinion. *Transplant Proc* 1998; **30:** 1100–3.
3. Mehra MR, et al. The prognostic impact of immunosuppression and cellular rejection on cardiac allograft vasculopathy: time for a reappraisal. *J Heart Lung Transplant* 1997; **16:** 743–51.
4. Kobashigawa JA. Advances in immunosuppression for heart transplantation. *Adv Card Surg* 1998; **10:** 155–74.
5. Taylor DO, et al. A prospective, randomized comparison of cyclophosphamide and azathioprine for early rejection prophylaxis after cardiac transplantation: decreased sensitization to OKT3. *Transplantation* 1994; **58:** 645–9.
6. Valantine-von Kaeppler HA. Prevention of chronic heart allograft rejection. *Transplant Proc* 1999; **31:** 1288–4.
7. Scott J, et al. Heart-lung transplantation for cystic fibrosis. *Lancet* 1988; **ii:** 192–4.
8. Smyth RL, et al. Early experience with heart-lung transplantation. *Arch Dis Child* 1989; **64:** 1225–30.
9. Glanville AR, et al. Obliterative bronchiolitis after heart-lung transplantation: apparent arrest by augmented immunosuppression. *Ann Intern Med* 1987; **107:** 300–4.

KIDNEY. The transplantation of kidneys is now established as the ultimate therapy for end-stage renal disease. There is no single generally accepted immunosuppressant regimen, and different centres have achieved good results with a variety of strategies.[1] Therapy should be tailored to the individual patient. A number of factors affect the intensity of immunotherapy required, including the donor source (living or cadaveric) and degree of HLA histocompatibility, and the age, race and panel reactive antibody titre of the recipient.[1] A widely used approach consists of **triple therapy** with ciclosporin, azathioprine, and prednisolone.[1-4] Triple therapy is popular because it allows lower doses of nephrotoxic ciclosporin, and the eventual tapering or even elimination of corticosteroids in some patients.[1] Azathioprine has been replaced by mycophenolate mofetil in a number of institutions, as it may result in fewer acute rejection episodes. However, there is no evidence that this will improve long-term graft survival.[1-4] Tacrolimus has also been substituted for ciclosporin for the same reason, but it has been associated with an increase in the incidence of diabetes mellitus.[1-3] There are limited data comparing the microemulsion form of ciclosporin with tacrolimus, and it is not clear which is more effective.[3] There is some evidence of synergism between sirolimus and ciclosporin, but this requires further study.[2,3]

Sequential quadruple therapy is also used. Induction therapy with antilymphocyte immunoglobulin or muromonab-CD3 is administered postoperatively, in addition to triple therapy. The antibodies are discontinued once good graft function is achieved.[1] The regimen may improve long-term graft survival in patients with delayed graft function.[4] However, such strongly immunosuppressive regimens may increase the risk of cytomegalovirus and other infections and some centres have reverted to the use of triple therapy.[5] There is some evidence that the incidence of complications is lower with antilymphocyte immunoglobulin than with muromonab-CD3.[6] The more specific anti-interleukin-2-receptor antibodies basiliximab,[7] daclizumab,[8] and inolimomab[9] have also been added to initial therapy and appear to reduce the incidence of rejection episodes without increased toxicity.[4]

As immunosuppressant regimens have developed the role of **corticosteroids** has come to be questioned, mainly because of the adverse effects associated with their prolonged use.[10] Studies indicate that corticosteroid withdrawal is feasible in many patients initially receiving triple therapy,[1,3] although there is debate about the long-term consequences of this for graft survival.[10] Some centres go further and avoid the use of corticosteroids at all stages, preferring ciclosporin-based regimens supplemented with drugs such as antithymocyte immunoglobulins or muromonab-CD3, and mycophenolate mofetil.[11] It is unclear which approach gives the best results, and whether all patients would benefit or only selected groups.

Where an **acute rejection** episode occurs treatment is likely to be with high-dose corticosteroids, or with drugs such as antilymphocyte or antithymocyte immunoglobulins, or muromonab-CD3, which are potent and effective reversers of rejection.[1] European guidelines recommend that the antibody preparations be reserved for corticosteroid-resistant rejection or more severe episodes,[4] but approaches remain varied.[1] Ciclosporin and azathioprine are ineffective in treating established rejection. Anti-interleukin-2-receptor antibodies may be of potential benefit in reversing rejection episodes. Other drugs such as tacrolimus,[12] mycophenolate mofetil,[13,14] and gusperimus,[15] have been found to be effective in reversing acute rejection episodes. There has also been evidence that asymptomatic cytomegalovirus infection may be associated with episodes of late acute rejection;[16] ganciclovir is reported to improve graft function in such circumstances. Unfortunately there is little that can be done about **chronic rejection**, which eventually progresses to graft failure,[17] although there is a suggestion that mycophenolate mofetil can delay this process.[18]

The results that can be achieved with existing regimens are good in the short to medium term, with a one-year cadaveric **graft survival** of 80 to 90% and a 10-year survival of 50% reported by most centres.[2] Morbidity and mortality have improved following reductions in cardiac, vascular and infectious complications, but there has been no decrease in death from malignancy, and the risk of developing cancer has been estimated to be approximately 100% by 30 years post-transplant.[19] Although newer drugs have decreased the incidence of acute rejection, there is only limited evidence that this has improved longer-term graft survival.[20-22] Present therapy is clearly not ideal, and studies are continuing with newer drugs to determine the optimum regimens for intermediate and long-term survival. A variety of substances not conventionally regarded as immunosuppressants have also been added to conventional regimens in an attempt to increase their efficacy or reduce their toxicity. These include allopurinol and prostaglandins, or the use of calcium-channel blockers or fish oil[23] to reduce ciclosporin toxicity.

1. First MR. Clinical application of immunosuppressive agents in renal transplantation. *Surg Clin North Am* 1998; **78**: 61–76.
2. Ponticelli C, *et al.* Renal transplantation, past, present and future. *J Nephrol* 1999; **12** (suppl 2): S105–S110.
3. Gonin JM. Maintenance immunosuppression: new agents and persistent dilemmas. *Adv Ren Replace Ther* 2000; **7**: 95–116.
4. EBPG Expert Group on Renal Transplantation. European best practice guidelines for renal transplantation (part 1). *Nephrol Dial Transplant* 2000; **15** (suppl 7): 1–85.
5. Verran D, *et al.* Quadruple immunosuppression in renal allografts—the Auckland experience. *N Z Med J* 1991; **104**: 517–18.
6. Bock HA, *et al.* A randomized prospective trial of prophylactic immunosuppression with ATG-Fresenius versus OKT3 after renal transplantation. *Transplantation* 1995; **59**: 830–40.
7. Nashan B, *et al.* Randomised trial of basiliximab versus placebo for control of acute cellular rejection in renal allograft recipients. *Lancet* 1997; **350**: 1193–8. Correction. *ibid.*; 1484.
8. Vincenti F, *et al.* Interleukin-2-receptor blockade with daclizumab to prevent acute rejection in renal transplantation. *N Engl J Med* 1998; **338**: 161–5.
9. Van Gelder T, *et al.* A double-blind, placebo-controlled study of monoclonal anti-interleukin-2 receptor antibody (BT563) administration to prevent acute rejection after kidney transplantation. *Transplantation* 1995; **60**: 248–52.
10. Tarantino A, *et al.* Corticosteroids in kidney transplant recipients: safety issues and timing of discontinuation. *Drug Safety* 1995; **13**: 145–56.
11. Birkeland SA. Steroid-free immunosuppression in renal transplantation. *Lancet* 1998; **348**: 1105–6.
12. Jordan ML, *et al.* Tacrolimus rescue therapy for renal allograft rejection—five year experience. *Transplantation* 1997; **63**: 223–8.
13. European Mycophenolate Mofetil Cooperative Study Group. Placebo-controlled study of mycophenolate mofetil combined with cyclosporin and corticosteroids for prevention of acute rejection. *Lancet* 1995; **345**: 1321–5.
14. Mycophenolate Mofetil Renal Refractory Rejection Study Group. Mycophenolate mofetil for the treatment of refractory, acute, cellular renal transplant rejection. *Transplantation* 1996; **61**: 722–9.
15. Matas AJ, *et al.* Pilot evaluation of 15-deoxyspergualin for refractory acute renal transplant rejection. *Clin Transplant* 1994; **8**: 116–19.
16. Reinke P, *et al.* Late-acute renal allograft rejection and symptomless cytomegalovirus infection. *Lancet* 1994; **344**: 1737–8.
17. Collier St J, Calne R. Practical problems in immunosuppression: kidney and liver transplants. *Prescribers' J* 1991; **31**: 122–7.
18. Laskon DA, *et al.* The incidence of subsequent acute rejection following the treatment of refractory renal allograft rejection with mycophenolate mofetil (RS61443). *Transplantation* 1994; **57**: 640–3.
19. Mathew TH. Optimal long-term immunotherapy protocols. *Transplant Proc* 1999; **31**: 1102–3.
20. Szczech LA, *et al.* The effect of antilymphocyte induction therapy on renal allograft survival: a meta-analysis of individual patient-level data. *Ann Intern Med* 1998; **128**: 817–26.
21. Ojo AO, *et al.* Mycophenolate mofetil reduces late renal allograft loss independent of acute rejection. *Transplantation* 2000; **69**: 2405–9.
22. Hariharan S, *et al.* Improved graft survival after renal transplantation in the United States, 1988 to 1996. *N Engl J Med* 2000; **342**: 605–12.
23. van der Heide JJH, *et al.* Effect of dietary fish oil on renal function and rejection in cyclosporine-treated recipients of renal transplants. *N Engl J Med* 1993; **329**: 769–73.

LIVER. Marked improvements have occurred in the outcome and reliability of liver transplantation in recent years, and it is now seen as a useful option in end-stage liver disease and some metabolic disorders.

Current immunosuppressive regimens generally combine ciclosporin or tacrolimus with a corticosteroid and azathioprine or mycophenolate mofetil (triple therapy), and with such regimens it is possible to avoid acute rejection episodes in the majority of cases.[1] Double therapy with ciclosporin or tacrolimus and corticosteroids is also used.[2] Addition of an antibody to triple therapy reduces rejection rates by about half,[3] although prophylactic antiviral therapy against cytomegalovirus is advisable. Inolimomab is also reported to be effective, in combination with ciclosporin and low-dose corticosteroids,[4] or with triple therapy, where it is reported to be more effective than antilymphocyte immunoglobulin.[5]

Most acute rejection episodes occur during the first 3 to 6 months of therapy.[2] Corticosteroids are used in the first-line treatment of acute rejection. Muromonab-CD3 has been used for corticosteroid-resistant episodes, but tacrolimus is increasingly preferred, as it is equally effective at reversing rejection and may also prevent recurrent rejection episodes.[1,6] Mycophenolate mofetil is used in patients not responding to conventional therapies, but there have been no controlled trials to determine its efficacy.[6] Chronic rejection is harder to treat. Corticosteroids are generally ineffective, and tacrolimus is the most effective drug available.[6]

The main problems encountered with liver transplants are infection in the early post-transplant period, recurrent disease (particularly viral recurrence), and adverse effects due to immunosuppressants.[7]

Sepsis is an important cause of death in the early post-transplant period.[7] Patients at increased risk, including those with malnutrition, fulminant liver failure, or renal insufficiency, require particularly cautious immunosuppression and more aggressive antibacterial and antifungal prophylaxis regimens.

Recurrence of hepatitis B infection is common. Although the introduction of hepatitis B immunoglobulins and lamivudine have improved the prospects for these patients, combination antiviral therapy and a modified immunosuppression protocol are usually needed.[1,7,8] Hepatitis C recurrence is almost universal in infected patients, with a probable reduction in long-term graft survival.[1,8]

Nephrotoxicity from ciclosporin or tacrolimus can be a significant problem after long-term therapy. Long-term renal function is affected by the function in the early post-transplant period, so serum creatinine concentrations at 1 and 3 months are often used to predict toxicity.[1] Antilymphocyte antibodies may be used post-transplant to delay the introduction of ciclosporin or tacrolimus and avoid early post-transplant renal dysfunction.[7] Cardiovascular complications may follow metabolic abnormalities such as diabetes mellitus, hypertension, hyperlipidaemia, and obesity. Malignancy may occur following prolonged immunosuppression.[8]

The one-year survival after liver transplantation is currently more than 80% using ciclosporin-based regimens.[1,8] The incidence of chronic rejection is only about 5%. Acute rejection appears to have little effect on long-term graft survival;[7,8] only if late or corticosteroid-resistant are episodes correlated with poorer outcome.[7] The liver induces more tolerance and liver transplant recipients usually require less immunosuppression than other solid organ transplant patients.[7] Up to 85% of patients can be withdrawn from corticosteroids within a few months of transplantation, and some centres have performed liver transplants without the use of corticosteroids.[2,7] Patients with underlying auto-immune hepatitis or inflammatory bowel disease may be relatively refractory to corticosteroid withdrawal.[2] It may be feasible to reduce or stop all immunosuppression in up to 40 to 50% of long-term stable liver transplant patients.[7]

1. McMaster P, *et al.* Liver transplantation: changing goals in immunosuppression. *Transplant Proc* 1998; **30**: 1819–21.
2. Everson GT, *et al.* Early steroid withdrawal in liver transplantation is safe and beneficial. *Liver Transpl Surg* 1999; 5 (suppl 1): S48–57.
3. McVicar JP, *et al.* Induction immunosuppressive therapy is associated with a low rejection rate after liver transplantation. *Clin Transplant* 1997; **11**: 328–33.
4. Nashan B, *et al.* Immunoprophylaxis with a monoclonal anti-IL-2 receptor antibody in liver transplant patients. *Transplantation* 1996; **61**: 546–54.
5. Langrehr JM, *et al.* A prospective randomized trial comparing interleukin-2 receptor antibody versus antithymocyte globulin as part of a quadruple immunosuppressive induction therapy following orthotopic liver transplantation. *Transplantation* 1997; **63**: 1772–81.
6. Millis JM. Treatment of liver allograft rejection. *Liver Transpl Surg* 1999; 5 (suppl 1): S98–106.
7. Pirenne J, Koshiba T. Present status and future prospects in liver transplantation. *Int Surg* 1999; **84**: 297–304.
8. Neuberger J. Liver transplantation. *J Hepatol* 2000; **32** (suppl 1): 198–207.

LUNG. Lung transplantation may be tried for end stage pulmonary disease such as pulmonary hypertension, cystic fibrosis, emphysema, and pulmonary fibrosis.[1] Immunosuppressant therapy is usually with a triple therapy regimen of ciclosporin or tacrolimus, azathioprine or mycophenolate mofetil, and a corticosteroid.[2-4] Antilymphocyte immunoglobulin or muromonab-CD3 may be added in the early post-transplant period but evidence that this decreases the incidence of graft rejection is lacking.[4] Acute rejection occurs more frequently with lung transplants than with other solid organ transplants; the prevalence has been estimated to range from 60 to 100%.[5] High doses of intravenous corticosteroids are generally used to control acute episodes of rejection (although some doubt their efficacy[6]). Several other drugs have been tried for corticosteroid-resistant episodes, including tacrolimus, inhaled ciclosporin,[7] antilymphocyte immunoglobulins and muromonab-CD3.[5] The main complication encountered in the long term is chronic rejection manifesting as bronchiolitis obliterans syndrome (obliterative bronchiolitis). This is characterised by progressive airway obstruction and occurs in 30 to 50% of transplant recipients. The frequency and severity of acute rejection episodes are the main risk factors for the development of bronchiolitis obliterans, but cytomegalovirus infection, airway ischaemia and HLA mismatching also play a part.[4] The syndrome is often refractory to immunosuppressants[4,5] and the prognosis is poor, with 40% mortality within 2 years of diagnosis.[4]

With better regimens and greater experience survival rates of 75% or more 1 to 2 years after lung transplantation have been reported from some centres.[2,8] However, 5-year survival is still less than 50% and it is hoped that newer drugs such as mycophenolate mofetil and sirolimus may improve long-term survival.[9]

1. Peters SG, *et al.* Lung transplantation: selection of patients and analysis of outcome. *Mayo Clin Proc* 1997; **72**: 85–8.
2. Midthun DE, *et al.* Medical management and complications in the lung transplant recipient. *Mayo Clin Proc* 1997; **72**: 175–84.
3. Noyes BE, *et al.* Experience with pediatric lung transplantation. *J Pediatr* 1994; **124**: 261–8.
4. Arcasoy SM, Kotloff RM. Lung transplantation. *N Engl J Med* 1999; **340**: 1081–91.
5. van den Berg JWK, *et al.* New immunosuppressive drugs and lung transplantation: last or least? *Thorax* 1999; **54**: 550–3.
6. Kesten S, *et al.* Treatment of presumed and proven acute rejection following six months of lung transplant survival. *Am J Respir Crit Care Med* 1995; **152**: 1321–4.
7. Keenan RJ, *et al.* Efficacy of inhaled cyclosporine in lung transplant recipients with refractory rejection: correlation of intragraft cytokine gene expression with pulmonary function and histologic characteristics. *Surgery* 1995; **118**: 385–91.
8. Weinberger SE. Recent advances in pulmonary medicine. *N Engl J Med* 1993; **328**: 1462–70.
9. Briffa N, Morris RE. Immunosuppressive drugs after lung transplantation. *BMJ* 1998; **316**: 719–20.

OTHER ORGANS. Transplantation of the *pancreas* may be considered in some diabetic patients. In the vast majority of cases, pancreatic grafts have been transplanted together with a kidney in patients with end-stage diabetic nephropathy, which provides better graft survival than transplanting the pancreas alone,[1] although solitary pancreatic transplants may be becoming more acceptable.[2] Overall patient survival in the USA has been estimated to be 92% at 1 year and 81% at 5 years, with graft survival of 76% and 61% at 1 and 5 years, respectively.[2] Advances in surgical and preservation techniques, together with new immunosuppressants, have helped to improve survival in recent years.[1,2] The pancreas is a highly immunogenic organ, so extensive immunosuppression is required. Standard treatment often consists of quadruple induction therapy, using antilymphocyte immunoglobulins or muromonab CD3, followed by maintenance therapy with ciclosporin, corticosteroids and azathioprine.[2] Tacrolimus has been substituted for ciclosporin in certain cases, and mycophenolate mofetil has replaced azathioprine in some regimens.[2,3]

Pancreatic transplantation facilitates normal carbohydrate metabolism and has the potential to improve patient survival and reduce the incidence of diabetic nephropathy. However, there has been concern over the long-term effects of immunosuppression,[2,4] and whether islet-cell autoantibodies might produce diabetes in the transplanted graft (although this is certainly not inevitable with adequate immunosuppression).[2,5] One possible alternative to complete pancreatic transplantation is an *islet-cell* graft. These have rarely been successful,[1] but the use of carefully prepared islet cells and a modified immunosuppressant protocol consisting of low-dose tacrolimus with sirolimus and daclizumab has shown promise in a preliminary study.[6] See also under Diabetes Mellitus, p.315.

Transplantation of the *small bowel* is becoming more common, especially in children.[7] Combined liver and small intestine transplants are used for patients with TPN dependence and irreversible intestinal or liver failure, while intestine-only transplants tend to be used for intestinal failure in patients with severe progressive complications of parenteral nutrition.[7] Overall patient and graft survival is about 50% at 5 years post-transplant, but substantial morbidity occurs and acute rejection and infections are common. Tacrolimus is the basis of the standard immunosuppressive regimen;[7] tapered corticosteroid doses and prostaglandins are also given. Muromonab-CD3 is used for severe rejection episodes and ciclosporin, cyclophosphamide, mycophenolate mofetil and azathioprine have been used if tacrolimus toxicity occurs.[7]

For reference to the use of immunosuppressants to treat graft rejection after *corneal* transplant see Corneal Graft Rejection, under Uses of Corticosteroids, p.1049.

1. Robertson RP, *et al.* Pancreas and islet transplantation for patients with diabetes. *Diabetes Care* 2000; **23:** 112–16.
2. Stratta RJ. Review of immunosuppressive usage in pancreas transplantation. *Clin Transplant* 1999; **13:** 1–12.
3. Gruessner RWG, *et al.* A multicenter analysis of the first experience with FK506 for induction and rescue therapy after pancreas transplantation. *Transplantation* 1996; **61:** 261–73.
4. Kumar A, *et al.* Combined kidney and pancreatic transplantation. *BMJ* 1999; **318:** 886–7.
5. Tydén G, *et al.* Recurrence of autoimmune diabetes mellitus in recipients of cadaveric pancreatic grafts. *N Engl J Med* 1996; **335:** 860–3.
6. Shapiro AMJ, *et al.* Islet transplantation in seven patients with type 1 diabetes mellitus using a glucocorticoid-free immunosuppressive regimen. *N Engl J Med* 2000; **343:** 230–8.
7. Thompson JS. Intestinal transplantation: experience in the United States. *Eur J Pediatr Surg* 1999; **9:** 271–3.

Renal disorders, non-malignant. Corticosteroids and immunosuppressants, usually in the form of cyclophosphamide, are commonly used in the treatment of glomerular kidney disease (p.1051).

Rheumatic disorders. RHEUMATOID ARTHRITIS. A variety of antirheumatic drugs including gold salts, penicillamine, hydroxychloroquine, sulfasalazine, and immunosuppressants may be given to patients with rheumatoid arthritis (p.9) in an attempt to modify the course of the disease. There is little agreement concerning the choice of such disease-modifying antirheumatic drugs (DMARDs).

The most widely used immunosuppressant is probably low-dose methotrexate, which produced clear short-term clinical benefits in patients unresponsive to gold or penicillamine;[1,2] although doubts exist about its ability to prevent radiological disease progression,[1,3-6] this is also true for other DMARDs.[7] There is also considerable concern about the potential toxicity, particularly to the liver, of long-term treatment.[8,9]

The role of other immunosuppressants in rheumatoid arthritis is more debatable. Azathioprine has been used, but is reported to be no more effective than DMARDs and significantly more toxic;[10] it may however be useful with prednisone in rheumatoid vasculitis.[11] Cyclophosphamide[12] is generally reserved for patients with concomitant severe vasculitis, because of its long-term toxicity. Leflunomide is being investigated, but was slightly less effective than methotrexate in one study.[13] Ciclosporin appears to be effective,[14,15] but nephrotoxicity has been a problem;[14] starting at low doses, and not exceeding a dose of 5 mg per kg body-weight daily may help to minimise nephrotoxic effects.[14] Use of ciclosporin with methotrexate has produced clinical improvement in patients who had only partial responses to methotrexate alone,[16] but some investigators found that a combination of methotrexate, ciclosporin and intra-articular corticosteroids was no more effective than standard DMARD therapy.[17]

1. Nordstrom DM, *et al.* Pulse methotrexate therapy in rheumatoid arthritis: a controlled prospective roentgenographic study. *Ann Intern Med* 1987; **107:** 797–801.
2. Tugwell P, *et al.* Methotrexate in rheumatoid arthritis: impact on quality of life assessed by traditional standard-item and individualized patient preference health status questionnaires. *Arch Intern Med* 1990; **150:** 59–62.
3. Weinstein J. Methotrexate in rheumatoid arthritis. *Ann Intern Med* 1988; **108:** 640.
4. Nordstrom DM, *et al.* Methotrexate in rheumatoid arthritis. *Ann Intern Med* 1988; **108:** 640–1.
5. Boerbooms AMT, *et al.* Pulse methotrexate therapy in rheumatoid arthritis. *Ann Intern Med* 1988; **108:** 905.
6. Nordstrom D, *et al.* Pulse methotrexate therapy in rheumatoid arthritis. *Ann Intern Med* 1988; **108:** 905.
7. Kushner I. Does aggressive therapy of rheumatoid arthritis affect outcome. *J Rheumatol* 1989; **16:** 1–4.
8. Whiting-O'Keefe QE, *et al.* Methotrexate and histologic hepatic abnormalities: a meta-analysis. *Am J Med* 1991; **90:** 711–16.

9. Tugwell P, *et al.* Methotrexate in rheumatoid arthritis: feedback on American College of Physicians guidelines. *Ann Intern Med* 1989; **110:** 581–3.
10. Suarez-Almazor ME, *et al.* Azathioprine for rheumatoid arthritis (updated 29 August 2001). Available in The Cochrane Library; Issue 4. Oxford: Update Software; 2001.
11. Heurkens AHM, *et al.* Prednisone plus azathioprine treatment in patients with rheumatoid arthritis complicated by vasculitis. *Arch Intern Med* 1991; **151:** 2249–54.
12. Suarez-Almazor ME, *et al.* Cyclophosphamide for treating rheumatoid arthritis (updated 29 August 2001). Available in The Cochrane Library; Issue 4. Oxford: Update Software; 2001.
13. Emery P, *et al.* A comparison of the efficacy and safety of leflunomide and methotrexate for the treatment of rheumatoid arthritis. *Rheumatology* 2000; **39:** 655–65.
14. Yocum DE, *et al.* Cyclosporin A in severe, treatment-refractory rheumatoid arthritis: a randomized study. *Ann Intern Med* 1988; **109:** 863–9.
15. Tugwell P, *et al.* Low-dose cyclosporin versus placebo in patients with rheumatoid arthritis. *Lancet* 1990; **335:** 1051–5.
16. Tugwell P, *et al.* Combination therapy with cyclosporine and methotrexate in severe rheumatoid arthritis. *N Engl J Med* 1995; **333:** 137–41.
17. Proudman SM, *et al.* Treatment of poor-prognosis early rheumatoid arthritis. *Arthritis Rheum* 2000; **43:** 1809–19.

Sarcoidosis. Where drug therapy is required for sarcoidosis (p.1058), corticosteroids are the usual treatment. In patients in whom these are ineffective or poorly tolerated, cytotoxic immunosuppressants have been given, with variable results. Methotrexate has perhaps been most useful,[1,2] but other agents including azathioprine, chlorambucil, and ciclosporin, have been tried.[3]

1. Webster GF, *et al.* Methotrexate therapy in cutaneous sarcoidosis. *Ann Intern Med* 1989; **111:** 538–9.
2. Soriano FG, *et al.* Neurosarcoidosis: therapeutic success with methotrexate. *Postgrad Med J* 1990; **66:** 142–3.
3. Muthiah MM, Macfarlane JT. Current concepts in the management of sarcoidosis. *Drugs* 1990; **40:** 231–7.

Scleroderma. The term scleroderma has been used for both systemic sclerosis, a multisystem disease characterised by collagen proliferation and fibrosis throughout the body, and for localised fibrotic changes of the skin (morphea) without involvement of other organs. Systemic sclerosis is an uncommon disease which has been linked to various environmental toxins as well as to genetic factors. Vascular involvement produces Raynaud's syndrome, which usually precedes any skin changes and there may be ulceration or ischaemic changes of the digits. A long history of Raynaud's syndrome before skin changes occur suggests a more indolent course (limited cutaneous disease) as opposed to the more aggressive diffuse cutaneous form. Skin oedema is followed by thickening and tightening of the skin of hands and face, and sometimes limbs and trunk, before progressing to atrophy and contractures. There may be decreased gastrointestinal motility, dysphagia and gastro-oesophageal reflux, arthritis, muscle weakness, and cardiac involvement. Among the most serious potential symptoms, which may result in death, are pulmonary disease and renal failure with malignant hypertension.

There is a paucity of adequately controlled trials for scleroderma; no treatment has been clearly demonstrated to affect the progression of the disease, and much management is essentially symptomatic. Immunosuppressants are probably appropriate in the early oedematous stages of diffuse scleroderma, followed by an antifibrotic drug such as penicillamine or an interferon.[1,2] Many immunosuppressive drugs have been tried, but their toxicities may limit their use. Cyclophosphamide is used for lung complications, and ciclosporin, tacrolimus and methotrexate may also be used by some workers.[2] Antilymphocyte immunoglobulins have been tried as an induction therapy in early stages of the disease.[2] Other novel immunosuppressive strategies include bone marrow ablation followed by peripheral blood stem cell transplantation, photopheresis with a psoralen, and the induction of oral tolerance with native bovine type I collagen.[2]

Penicillamine has been widely used as an antifibrotic drug, but its efficacy has never been proven. Interferons alfa and gamma showed promising results in early trials, but larger scale studies have failed to confirm any benefit.[2] Some drugs are being investigated for their anti-fibrotic properties, including halofuginone, minocycline and relaxin.[2] There is some evidence that oxidative stress is involved in the pathogenesis of scleroderma, so antioxidants like probucol may also be useful.[2] Other drugs that have been investigated include potassium aminobenzoate, sulfasalazine, and thymopentin.

Many patients will require therapy for organ-specific symptoms. Systemic antihistamines relieve itching in the early stages of the disease. Treatment of secondary Raynaud's syndrome (p.809) may involve vasodilators such as calcium-channel blockers, topical nitrates and ACE inhibitors but is liable to be more difficult than in primary

disease; intravenous prostaglandins may be used for severe attacks.[2,3] ACE inhibitors have substantially improved the prognosis for patients with renal scleroderma,[2,3] but over 30% of patients will still require renal replacement therapy.[2] Intravenous epoprostenol may help the microvascular lesion, and is often administered from diagnosis.[2] Lung fibrosis is treated with cyclophosphamide, sometimes combined with prednisolone, while calcium-channel blockers and intravenous iloprost may be used for pulmonary hypertension.[2] Proton pump inhibitors such as omeprazole sometimes in combination with prokinetic drugs, are extremely effective for oesophageal involvement, and broad spectrum antibiotics are helpful for small bowel bacterial overgrowth.[2,3] Cardiac involvement may be underdiagnosed;[2] NSAIDS or corticosteroids have been advocated for pericarditis,[3] although both must be used with care in scleroderma because of the risk of exacerbating renal and other problems.[2]

1. Fine LG, *et al.* Systemic sclerosis: current pathogenetic concepts and future prospects for targeted therapy. *Lancet* 1996; **347:** 1453–8.
2. Denton CP, Black CM. Scleroderma and related disorders: therapeutic aspects. *Baillieres Best Pract Res Clin Rheumatol* 2000; **14:** 17–35.
3. Rasaratnam I, Ryan PFJ. Systemic sclerosis and the inflammatory myopathies. *Med J Aust* 1997; **166:** 322–7.

Skin and connective-tissue disorders, non-malignant. Immunosuppressants are used in various skin and connective tissue disorders, including Behçet's syndrome (p.1047), eczema (p.1105), pemphigus and pemphigoid (p.1106), polymyositis (p.1057), psoriasis (p.1106), systemic lupus erythematosus (p.1059), and the various vasculitic syndromes (p.1060). See also Scleroderma, above.

Aceglatone (12305-k)

Aceglatone (rINN).

D-Glucaric acid 1,4:6,3-dilactone diacetate.

$C_{10}H_{10}O_8 = 258.2.$

$CAS — 642-83-1.$

Profile

Aceglatone inhibits the activity of β-glucuronidase and has an anti-inflammatory action. It has been given by mouth to prevent relapse after surgery for carcinoma of the bladder. Adverse effects have included anorexia, gastric discomfort, dry skin, and pigmentation.

Aclarubicin Hydrochloride (12318-f)

Aclarubicin Hydrochloride (BANM, rINNM).

Aclacinomycin A Hydrochloride; NSC-208734 (aclarubicin). Methyl (1R,2R,4S)-4-(O-{2,6-dideoxy-4-O-[(2R,6S)-tetrahydro-6-methyl-5-oxopyran-2-yl]-α-L-*lyxo*-hexopyranosyl}-(1→4)-2,3,6-trideoxy-3-dimethylamino-L-*lyxo*-hexopyranosyloxy)-2-ethyl-1,2,3,4,6,11-hexahydro-2,5,7-trihydroxy-6,11-dioxonaphthacene-1-carboxylate hydrochloride.

$C_{42}H_{53}NO_{15}, HCl = 848.3.$

$CAS — 57576-44-0 (aclarubicin).$

NOTE. Aclarubicin is *USAN*.

Pharmacopoeias. In Jpn.

The hydrochloride of an anthracycline antineoplastic antibiotic isolated from *Streptomyces galilaeus*. Aclarubicin hydrochloride 1.04 mg is approximately equivalent to 1 mg of aclarubicin.

Stability. In a study of the stability of anthracycline antineoplastic agents in 4 infusion fluids—glucose 5%, sodium chloride 0.9%, lactated Ringer's injection, and a commercial infusion fluid—stability appeared to be partly related to pH; aclarubicin was most stable in sodium chloride injection, with a pH of 6.2, and any increase or decrease in pH appeared to affect stability adversely.[1]

1. Poochikian GK, *et al.* Stability of anthracycline antitumor agents in four infusion fluids. *Am J Hosp Pharm* 1981; **38:** 483–6.

Adverse Effects, Treatment, and Precautions

As for Doxorubicin Hydrochloride, p.535. Alopecia and cardiotoxicity may be less pronounced than with doxorubicin. Bone-marrow depression is dose-limiting, with platelet counts reaching a nadir 1 to 2 weeks after administration, while leucopenia is greatest after 2 to 3 weeks; recovery generally occurs within 4 weeks. Myelosuppression may be particularly severe in patients who have received mitomycin or a nitrosourea.

◊ It has become apparent in the course of clinical studies that aclarubicin is not devoid of cardiotoxicity.[1] A strikingly high incidence of ECG changes has been observed, but, although acute cardiotoxicity occurs, the chronic cardiomyopathy classically associated with the anthracyclines (see p.535) appears to be a rare event. Alopecia is also rare, although gastrointestinal disturbances and mucositis are as common or more common than with doxorubicin.

1. Warrell RP. Aclacinomycin A: clinical development of a novel anthracycline antibiotic in the haematological cancers. *Drugs Exp Clin Res* 1986; **12:** 275–82.

Uses and Administration

Aclarubicin is an anthracycline antibiotic with antineoplastic actions similar to those of the other anthracyclines (see Doxorubicin Hydrochloride, p.536), although it inhibits RNA synthesis more strongly than DNA synthesis. It is used as the hydrochloride in the treatment of malignant blood disorders, such as acute myeloid leukaemia (p.485). The usual initial dose as a single agent is the equivalent of 175 to 300 mg of base per m^2 body-surface, given divided over 3 to 7 consecutive days, by intravenous infusion over 30 to 60 minutes. Where appropriate and tolerated, maintenance doses of the equivalent of 25 to 100 mg of aclarubicin per m^2 may be given as a single infusion every 3 to 4 weeks. The total dose that can be given over the patient's life-time depends upon cardiological status but most patients have not received more than 400 mg per m^2. Dosages may need to be reduced when given as part of a combination regimen.

◊ A review of studies in patients with relapsed acute non-lymphoblastic leukaemia confirmed the activity of aclarubicin, with reported complete remission rates of the order of 12 to 24%.[1] Doses varied from 10 to 30 mg per m^2 body-surface daily to higher doses of 75 to 120 mg per m^2 for 2 to 4 days; in general a total dose of about 300 mg per m^2 appeared to be necessary to induce remission. Less information is available concerning activity in acute lymphoblastic leukaemia, but response rates were lower than those in acute myeloid leukaemia. Results in the malignant lymphomas were generally disappointing.

1. Warrell RP. Aclacinomycin A: clinical development of a novel anthracycline antibiotic in the haematological cancers. *Drugs Exp Clin Res* 1986; **12:** 275–82.

Preparations

Proprietary Preparations (details are given in Part 3)
Aust.: Aclaplastin; *Ger.:* Aclaplastin; *UK:* Aclacin.

AE-941 (20856-h)

Profile

AE-941 is an angiogenesis inhibitor derived from shark cartilage extract. It is being studied for the treatment of various malignant neoplasms, including those of the lung and kidney. It is also being investigated for the treatment of psoriasis.

Alemtuzumab (18904-t)

Alemtuzumab *(BAN, rINN)*.
Campath-1; Campath-1H.
CAS — 216503-57-0.

Adverse Effects and Precautions

Alemtuzumab has been associated with severe and prolonged myelosuppression; fatalities have occurred. Pancytopenia, neutropenia, thrombocytopenia, and haemolytic anaemia (including auto-immune thrombocytopenia and anaemia) have been reported. Single doses greater than 30 mg, or cumulative weekly doses greater than 90 mg should not be used, because of the increased incidence of pancytopenia. Complete blood and platelet counts should be measured weekly during alemtuzumab therapy, and more frequently if anaemia, neutropenia, or thrombocytopenia occur; treatment should be discontinued if severe myelosuppression or evidence of haematological toxicity are seen.

Alemtuzumab can cause serious infusion-related reactions, including hypotension, rigors, fever, chills, shortness of breath, bronchospasm, and rash. Gradual increase of the dose is required at the initiation of therapy, and after any interruption of therapy for 7 days or more. Pre-medication with an oral antihistamine and paracetamol should also be used, particularly before the first dose, and with dose increases.

Other adverse effects include nausea and vomiting, diarrhoea, headache, and arthralgia.

Alemtuzumab is contra-indicated for patients with active systemic infection, or underlying immunodeficiency.

Uses and Administration

Alemtuzumab is a humanised form of campath-1, a rat monoclonal antibody to the CD52 antigen found on lymphocytes. Alemtuzumab is used in the treatment of B-cell chronic lymphocytic leukaemia (p.485) resistant to conventional chemotherapy. The dose of alemtuzumab must be increased gradually to avoid infusion-related reactions (see above). The initial dose is 3 mg daily, given as an intravenous infusion over 2 hours. When this dose is tolerated, the dose is gradually increased until 10 mg daily can be tolerated. A maximum maintenance dose of 30 mg given three times per week on alternate days can then be used for up to 12 weeks. The dose should be modified according to haematological toxicity.

Alemtuzumab has been tried in patients with lymphomas and lymphoproliferative disorders, and has also been investigated for the prevention of graft-versus-host disease. It has been tried

with variable results in auto-immune disorders including vasculitis and rheumatoid arthritis, and multiple sclerosis.

◊ References.
1. Hale G, *et al.* Remission induction in non-Hodgkin lymphoma with reshaped human monoclonal antibody campath-1H. *Lancet* 1988; **ii:** 1394–9.
2. Mathieson PW, *et al.* Monoclonal-antibody therapy in systemic vasculitis. *N Engl J Med* 1990; **323:** 250–4.
3. Lim SH, *et al.* Differential response in a patient treated with campath-1H monoclonal antibody for refractory non-Hodgkin lymphoma. *Lancet* 1993; **341:** 432–3.
4. Poynton CH, *et al.* Adverse reactions to campath-1H monoclonal antibody. *Lancet* 1993; **341:** 1037.
5. Lockwood CM, *et al.* Long-term remission of intractable systemic vasculitis with monoclonal antibody therapy. *Lancet* 1993; **341:** 1620–2.
6. Isaacs JD, *et al.* Monoclonal antibody therapy of chronic intraocular inflammation using campath-1H. *Br J Ophthalmol* 1995; **79:** 1054–5.
7. Weinblatt ME, *et al.* Campath-1H, a humanized monoclonal antibody, in refractory rheumatoid arthritis: an intravenous dose-escalation study. *Arthritis Rheum* 1995; **38:** 1589–94.
8. Osterborg A, *et al.* Phase II multicenter study of human CD52 antibody in previously treated chronic lymphocytic leukemia. *J Clin Oncol* 1997; **15:** 1567–74.
9. Coles AJ, *et al.* Pulsed monoclonal antibody treatment and autoimmune thyroid disease in multiple sclerosis. *Lancet* 1999; **354:** 1691–5.
10. Dyer MJ. The role of CAMPATH-1 antibodies in the treatment of lymphoid malignancies. *Semin Oncol* 1999; **26** (suppl 14): 52–7.
11. Dick AD, *et al.* Campath-1H therapy in refractory ocular inflammatory disease. *Br J Ophthalmol* 2000; **84:** 107–9.

Preparations

Proprietary Preparations (details are given in Part 3)
UK: MabCampath; *USA:* Campath.

Alitretinoin (15789-p)

Alitretinoin *(BAN, USAN, rINN)*.
AGN-192013; ALRT-1057; LG-100057; LGD-1057; NSC-659772; 9-cis-Retinoic Acid. (2E,4E,6Z,8E)-3,7-Dimethyl-9-(2,6,6-trimethyl-1-cyclohexen-1-yl)-2,4,6,8-nonatetraenoic acid.
$C_{20}H_{28}O_2 = 300.4$.
CAS — 5300-03-8.
ATC — L01XX22.

Profile

Alitretinoin is a retinoid related to tretinoin (p.1126). It is used topically, as a 0.1% gel, in the management of Kaposi's sarcoma. It is applied directly to the lesions twice daily, increasing to up to 4 times daily if tolerated. Local skin toxicity may occur, in particular erythema and oedema, and in some patients this may be dose-limiting.

Alitretinoin is also under investigation by mouth in acute promyelocytic leukaemia and some other malignancies.

◊ References.
1. Miller WH, *et al.* 9-cis Retinoic acid induces complete remission but does not reverse clinically acquired retinoid resistance in acute promyelocytic leukemia. *Blood* 1995; **85:** 3021–7.
2. Weber C, Dumont E. Pharmacokinetics and pharmacodynamics of 9-cis-retinoic acid in healthy men. *J Clin Pharmacol* 1997; **37:** 566–74.
3. Walmsley S, *et al.* Treatment of AIDS-related cutaneous Kaposi's sarcoma with topical alitretinoin (9-cis-retinoic acid) gel. *J Acquir Immune Defic Syndr* 1999; **22:** 235–46.

Preparations

Proprietary Preparations (details are given in Part 3)
Canad.: Panretin; *USA:* Panretin.

Altretamine (1838-f)

Altretamine *(BAN, USAN, rINN)*.
Hexamethylmelamine; HMM; NSC-13875; WR-95704. 2,4,6-Tris(dimethylamino)-1,3,5-triazine; N^2,N^2,N^4,N^4,N^6,N^6-Hexamethyl-1,3,5-triazine-2,4,6-triamine.
$C_9H_{18}N_6 = 210.3$.
CAS — 645-05-6.
ATC — L01XX03.
Pharmacopoeias. In US.

Pharmacopoeial description

USP 25: A white crystalline powder. Insoluble in water; soluble in chloroform.

◊ CAUTION. *Altretamine is irritant; avoid contact with skin and mucous membranes.*

Adverse Effects, Treatment, and Precautions

For a general outline see Antineoplastics, p.476, p.479, and p.480.

Bone-marrow depression is usually moderate, manifesting as leucopenia and thrombocytopenia, and may require dosage reduction; blood counts should be monitored regularly. Nausea and vomiting are common and usually moderate although they may be

dose-limiting. Prolonged or high-dose therapy may be associated with neurotoxicity, both peripheral (neuropathies) and central (ataxia, depression, confusion, drowsiness, and hallucinations); neurological examination should be performed regularly and administration interrupted or the dose reduced as appropriate. Renal toxicity may also be dose-limiting. Other rare adverse effects include rashes, anaemia, alopecia, and hepatic toxicity.

Interactions

For a general outline of antineoplastic drug interactions, see p.481. Concomitant administration with pyridoxine appears to reduce the activity of altretamine.

Antidepressants. Severe and potentially life-threatening orthostatic hypotension developed in 3 patients who received amitriptyline or imipramine concurrently with altretamine and in a fourth patient who took phenelzine and altretamine concurrently.[1] One patient was able to tolerate a combination of the antineoplastic with nortriptyline.

1. Bruckner HW, Schleifer SJ. Orthostatic hypotension as a complication of hexamethylmelamine antidepressant interaction. *Cancer Treat Rep* 1983; **67:** 516.

Pharmacokinetics

Altretamine is well absorbed from the gastrointestinal tract following oral administration, but is rapidly demethylated in the liver producing variation in plasma-altretamine concentrations. The principal metabolites are pentamethylmelamine and tetramethylmelamine, which are excreted in urine. The elimination half-life has been reported to be 4 to 10 hours.

◊ References.
1. Darmia G, D'Incalci M. Clinical pharmacokinetics of altretamine. *Clin Pharmacokinet* 1995; **28:** 439–48.

Uses and Administration

Altretamine is an antineoplastic agent structurally similar to the alkylating agent tretamine (triethylenemelamine) although its mode of action may be different. It is given by mouth in the treatment of ovarian carcinoma (p.496). Altretamine has also been tried in lung cancer. The usual dose as a single agent in ovarian cancer is 260 mg per m^2 body-surface daily in four divided doses, for 14 days out of a 28-day cycle. Up to 12 cycles may be administered. Therapy should be interrupted, and subsequently restarted at a lower dose of 200 mg per m^2 daily, if the white cell count falls below 2000 per mm^3 or the platelet count below 75 000 per mm^3, or if neurotoxic or intolerable gastrointestinal symptoms occur. Lower doses are also used in combination regimens.

◊ Reviews.
1. Hansen LA, Hughes TE. Altretamine. *DICP Ann Pharmacother* 1991; **25:** 146–52.
2. Anonymous. Altretamine for ovarian cancer. *Med Lett Drugs Ther* 1991; **33:** 76–7.
3. Lee CR, Faulds D. Altretamine: a review of its pharmacodynamic and pharmacokinetic properties, and therapeutic potential in cancer chemotherapy. *Drugs* 1995; **49:** 932–53.

Preparations

USP 25: Altretamine Capsules.

Proprietary Preparations (details are given in Part 3)
Austral.: Hexalen; *Canad.:* Hexalen; *Fr.:* Hexastat†; *Hong Kong:* Hexastat; *Israel:* Hexalen; *Ital.:* Hexastat†; *Neth.:* Hexastat†; *Norw.:* Hexalen; Hexastat†; *Spain:* Hexinawas†; *Swed.:* Hexalen; *UK:* Hexalen; *USA:* Hexalen.

Aminoglutethimide (1803-e)

Aminoglutethimide *(BAN, rINN)*.
Ba-16038. 2-(4-Aminophenyl)-2-ethylglutarimide; 3-(4-Aminophenyl)-3-ethylpiperidine-2,6-dione.
$C_{13}H_{16}N_2O_2 = 232.3$.
CAS — 125-84-8.
Pharmacopoeias. In Eur. (see p.vi) and US.

Pharmacopoeial description

Ph. Eur.: A white or slightly yellow, crystalline powder. Practically insoluble in water; freely soluble in acetone; soluble in methyl alcohol.

USP 25: A white or creamy-white, fine, crystalline powder. Very slightly soluble in water; readily soluble in most organic solvents. It forms water-soluble salts with strong acids. The pH of a 0.1% solution in dilute methyl alcohol (1 in 20) is between 6.2 and 7.3.

Adverse Effects

The most frequent adverse effects reported with aminoglutethimide include drowsiness, lethargy, and skin rashes (sometimes with fever); these generally diminish after the first 6 weeks of therapy. Dizziness and nausea occasionally occur. Leucopenia, thrombocytopenia, agranulocytosis, or severe pancytopenia have occurred rarely. Adrenal insufficiency may rarely occur, and there have been reports of other endocrine disturbances including hypothyroidism, and virilisation. Other rare effects include ataxia, headache, depression, gastrointestinal disturbances, and orthostatic hypotension.

Overdosage may lead to CNS depression and impairment of consciousness, electrolyte disturbances, and respiratory depression.

Effects on lipids. Aminoglutethimide has been reported to produce raised serum-cholesterol concentrations in patients with breast cancer,[1,2] although not, apparently, in those with Cushing's disease.[3] However, the significance of this rise is uncertain in the context of the other biochemical changes which aminoglutethimide may provoke.[2]

1. Bonneterre J, et al. Aminoglutethimide-induced hypercholesterolaemia. *Lancet* 1984; **i:** 912–13.
2. Ceci G, et al. Aminoglutethimide and serum cholesterol. *Lancet* 1984; **ii:** 358.
3. Kasperlik-Zaluska A, Migdalska B. Aminoglutethimide and serum cholesterol. *Lancet* 1984; **ii:** 358.

Effects on the liver. Aminoglutethimide has been associated with reports of cholestatic jaundice, accompanied by rash[1,2] and fever,[2] and probably due to an idiosyncratic hypersensitivity reaction.[1] It has been suggested that liver function tests should be carried out in patients receiving aminoglutethimide who develop fever and eruptions.[2]

1. Gerber SB, Miller KB. Cholestatic jaundice and aminoglutethimide. *Ann Intern Med* 1982; **97:** 138.
2. Perrault DJ, Domovitch E. Aminoglutethimide and cholestasis. *Ann Intern Med* 1984; **100:** 160.

Effects on the lungs. Pulmonary infiltrates in a patient who developed progressive dyspnoea on commencing therapy with aminoglutethimide were found to be due to diffuse alveolar damage and haemorrhage; thrombocytopenia was present but prothrombin and bleeding times were normal. The patient's gas exchange and chest radiographs improved on discontinuation of aminoglutethimide and institution of corticosteroid therapy.[1]

1. Rodman DM, et al. Aminoglutethimide, alveolar damage, and hemorrhage. *Ann Intern Med* 1986; **105:** 633.

Lupus. A report of systemic lupus erythematosus induced by aminoglutethimide in one patient.[1]

1. McCraken M, et al. Systemic lupus erythematosus induced by aminoglutethimide. *BMJ* 1980; **281:** 1254.

Precautions

Aminoglutethimide inhibits adrenal steroid production and supplementary glucocorticoid therapy with hydrocortisone must normally be given, although supplementation may not be necessary in patients with Cushing's syndrome. Some patients also require a mineralocorticoid. It has been suggested that aminoglutethimide should be temporarily withdrawn in patients who undergo shock or trauma, or develop intercurrent infection.

Blood counts and serum electrolytes should be regularly monitored during aminoglutethimide therapy and periodic monitoring of liver and thyroid function is recommended.

Aminoglutethimide should not be given during pregnancy as pseudohermaphroditism may occur in the fetus.

Aminoglutethimide may cause drowsiness: patients so affected should not drive or operate machinery.

Porphyria. Aminoglutethimide has been associated with acute attacks of porphyria and is considered unsafe in porphyric patients.

Interactions

The rate of metabolism of some drugs is increased by aminoglutethimide; patients receiving concomitant therapy with warfarin or other coumarin anticoagulants, with theophylline, with tamoxifen, or with oral hypoglycaemic agents, may require increased dosages of these drugs. The metabolism of dexamethasone is also accelerated, which limits its value for corticosteroid supplementation in patients receiving aminoglutethimide. Concomitant administration of diuretics may lead to hyponatraemia, while alcohol may potentiate the central effects of aminoglutethimide.

◊ For reference to an increase in the clearance of *digitoxin* by aminoglutethimide, see p.869, and for reference to increased clearance of *theophylline* in patients given aminoglutethimide, see p.781. Aminoglutethimide has also been reported to reduce serum concentrations of some *progestogens* (see p.1489). For the effects of aminoglutethimide on *anticoagulants*, see under Warfarin, p.995.

Pharmacokinetics

Aminoglutethimide is well absorbed following oral administration with peak plasma concentrations occurring after 1 to 4 hours. It is metabolised in the liver, primarily to N-hydroxylaminoglutethimide and N-acetylaminoglutethimide, and appears to induce its own metabolism. The half-life, which is reported to be about 13 hours after the administration of a single dose, is decreased to around 9 hours after about 2 weeks of continuous therapy. Aminoglutethimide is excreted in urine,

about half a dose being excreted unchanged and the remainder as metabolites. Only about 20 to 25% of a dose is bound to plasma protein.

◊ A study of the single- and multiple-dose pharmacokinetics of aminoglutethimide in 17 patients demonstrated that the plasma half-life had a mean value of 15.5 hours after single-dose administration but fell to 8.9 hours during multiple-dose therapy.[1] This marked reduction in half-life could largely be attributed to a decrease in the volume of distribution; auto-induction of metabolism may be of less importance in decreasing half-life than has been previously suggested.

1. Lønning PE, et al. Single-dose and steady-state pharmacokinetics of aminoglutethimide. *Clin Pharmacokinet* 1985; **10:** 353–64.

Uses and Administration

Aminoglutethimide is an analogue of glutethimide (p.686) and was formerly used for its weak anticonvulsant properties. Aminoglutethimide blocks the production of adrenal steroids and acts as an aromatase inhibitor to block the conversion of androgens to oestrogens (the major source of oestrogens in women without ovarian function). It has been used in the treatment of metastatic breast cancer (p.491) in postmenopausal or oophorectomised women, in doses of 250 mg up to four times daily by mouth. Aminoglutethimide has also been used in similar doses as palliative treatment in men with advanced prostatic cancer (p.497). Replacement therapy with a corticosteroid must also be given, usually hydrocortisone 20 to 30 mg daily in divided doses (see Adrenocortical Insufficiency, p.1046 for a description of corticosteroid replacement therapy).

Aminoglutethimide is used in similar or higher doses in the treatment of Cushing's syndrome (p.1272); up to 2 g daily may be needed. Corticosteroid supplementation may not be required in these patients.

The *dextro*-isomer of aminoglutethimide, dexaminoglutethimide has also been investigated.

Preparations

BP 2001: Aminoglutethimide Tablets;
USP 25: Aminoglutethimide Tablets.

Proprietary Preparations (details are given in Part 3)
Aust.: Orimeten; **Austral.:** Cytadren; **Belg.:** Orimeten; **Braz.:** Orimeten; **Canad.:** Cytadren†; **Fr.:** Orimetene; **Ger.:** Orimeten; Rodazol; **Hong Kong:** Orimeten; **Irl.:** Orimetene; **Israel:** Orimetene; **Ital.:** Orimeten; **Neth.:** Orimeten; **Norw.:** Orimeten†; **NZ:** Cytadren; **S.Afr.:** Aminoblastin†; Orimeten; **Spain:** Orimeten; **Swed.:** Orimeten; **Switz.:** Orimeten; **UK:** Orimeten; **USA:** Cytadren.

5-Aminolaevulinic Acid (14918-c)

ALA; 5-ALA; δ-Aminolaevulinic Acid.

NOTE. Aminolevulinic Acid Hydrochloride is USAN.

Profile

5-Aminolaevulinic acid is a naturally occurring haem precursor, which is metabolised in the body to protoporphyrin IX and then to haem. It has been used as a photosensitiser by oral or topical application, in combination with phototherapy, in the treatment of superficial malignant or premalignant lesions of the skin (p.498) and bladder (p.490), and non-malignant skin disorders such as psoriasis. Methyl 5-aminolaevulinate is also used.

In the treatment of actinic keratoses, for example, 5-aminolaevulinic acid may be applied to the lesions as a 20% solution of the hydrochloride, and followed, 14 to 18 hours later, by illumination with blue wavelength light sufficient to supply a dose of 10 J per cm². Treatment may be repeated once after 8 weeks if necessary. Patients should avoid sunlight or bright light sources for at least 40 hours after application.

◊ 5-Aminolaevulinic acid has been used topically for superficial malignant or premalignant lesions of the skin usually as a preparation containing 10 to 30%.[1,2] It has also been used topically in non-malignant skin conditions such as psoriasis.[3] An intravesical solution has been instilled into the bladder in the management of superficial bladder cancer.[4] Photodynamic therapy using oral 5-aminolaevulinic acid 60 mg per kg bodyweight as the photosensitiser has also been used to treat Barrett's oesophagus,[5] and other gastrointestinal tumours.[6,7] 5-Aminolaevulinic acid has been reviewed.[8]

1. Svanberg K, et al. Photodynamic therapy of non-melanoma malignant tumours of the skin using topical δ-amino levulinic acid sensitization and laser irradiation. *Br J Dermatol* 1994; **130:** 743–51.
2. Jeffes EW, et al. Photodynamic therapy of actinic keratosis with topical 5-aminolevulinic acid: a pilot dose-ranging study. *Arch Dermatol* 1997; **133:** 727–32.
3. Collins P, et al. The variable response of plaque psoriasis after a single treatment with topical 5-aminolaevulinic acid photodynamic therapy. *Br J Dermatol* 1997; **137:** 743–9.
4. Kriegmair M, et al. Early clinical experience with 5-aminolaevulinic acid for the photodynamic therapy of superficial bladder cancer. *Br J Urol* 1996; **77:** 667–71.
5. Barr J, et al. Eradication of high-grade dysplasia in columnar-lined (Barrett's) oesophagus by photodynamic therapy with endogenously generated protoporphyrin IX. *Lancet* 1996; **348:** 584–5.
6. Grant WE, et al. Photodynamic therapy of oral cancer: photosensitisation with systemic aminolaevulinic acid. *Lancet* 1993; **342:** 147–8.

7. Regula J, et al. Photosensitisation and photodynamic therapy of oesophageal, duodenal, and colorectal tumours using 5 aminolaevulinic acid induced protoporphyrin IX—a pilot study. *Gut* 1995; **36:** 67–75.
8. Peng Q, et al. 5-Aminolaevulinic acid-based photodynamic therapy: clinical research and future challenges. *Cancer* 1997; **79:** 2282–308.

Preparations

Proprietary Preparations (details are given in Part 3)
USA: Levulan Kerastick.

Amonafide (19508-z)

Amonafide (rINN).

M-FA-142. 3-Amino-N-[2-(dimethylamino)ethyl]naphthalimide.

$C_{16}H_{17}N_3O_2 = 283.3$.
CAS — 69408-81-7.

Profile

Amonafide has been investigated as an antineoplastic in a variety of malignant neoplasms including those of the endometrium, cervix, head and neck, and lung, but appears to have limited activity.

◊ References.
1. Evans WK, et al. Phase II study of amonafide: results of treatment and lessons learned from the study of an investigational agent in previously untreated patients with extensive small-cell lung cancer. *J Clin Oncol* 1990; **8:** 390–5.
2. Malviya VK, et al. Phase II trial of amonafide in patients with advanced metastatic or recurrent endometrial adenocarcinoma. A Southwest Oncology Group study. *Am J Clin Oncol* 1994; **17:** 37–40.
3. Asburg R, et al. A phase II trial of amonafide in patients with nonsquamous cell carcinoma of the cervix. A Gynecologic Oncology Group study. *Am J Clin Oncol* 1997; **20:** 626–7.
4. Leaf AN, et al. An ECOG phase II study of amonafide in unresectable or recurrent carcinoma of the head and neck (PB390). Eastern Cooperative Oncology Group. *Invest New Drugs* 1997; **15:** 165–72.

Amsacrine (12374-q)

Amsacrine (BAN, USAN, pINN).

Acridinyl Anisidide; m-AMSA; CI-880; NSC-249992. 4'-(Acridin-9-ylamino)methanesulphon-m-anisidide.

$C_{21}H_{19}N_3O_3S = 393.5$.
CAS — 51264-14-3.
ATC — L01XX01.

Incompatibility. Amsacrine is incompatible with 0.9% sodium chloride injection and with other chloride-containing solutions,[1,2] apparently because of the poor solubility of the hydrochloride salt in aqueous solution.[2] Amsacrine reacts with certain plastics.[1]

1. D'Arcy PF. Reactions and interactions in handling anticancer drugs. *Drug Intell Clin Pharm* 1983; **17:** 532–8.
2. Trissel LA, et al. Visual compatibility of amsacrine with selected drugs during simulated Y-site injection. *Am J Hosp Pharm* 1990; **47:** 2525–8.

Adverse Effects, Treatment, and Precautions

For a general outline see Antineoplastics, p.476, p.479, and p.480.

Bone-marrow depression is usually dose-limiting and may be severe. The nadir of the white cell count has been reported at about 12 days after treatment, with recovery usually by the 25th day. Pancytopenia may occur. Nausea and vomiting (mild to moderate), stomatitis (mild to life-threatening), and alopecia may occur. Grand mal seizures, renal dysfunction, hepatotoxicity, and cardiotoxicity, have been reported. Amsacrine is irritant: there may be phlebitis and local tissue necrosis particularly with administration of high concentrations.

Amsacrine should be given with caution to patients with liver or kidney disease, who may require dosage adjustments.

Interactions

For a general outline of antineoplastic drug interactions, see p.481. Concomitant use of diuretics or nephrotoxic drugs such as the aminoglycosides may theoretically increase the risk of cardiotoxicity with amsacrine by precipitating hypokalaemia.

Pharmacokinetics

Amsacrine is poorly absorbed following oral administration. When given intravenously it has a reported terminal half-life of about 5 to 8 hours. It is metabolised in the liver and excreted primarily in the bile, mostly as metabolites. It is reported to be about 98% protein bound.

Uses and Administration

Amsacrine is an antineoplastic agent that appears to act by intercalation with DNA and inhibition of nucleic acid synthesis. It may also exert an action on cell membranes. Cells in G2 or S phases may be most sensitive to its actions.

It is used for the induction and maintenance of remission in adult acute leukaemias, particularly acute myeloid leukaemia (p.485).

Amsacrine is prepared as a solution in lactic acid and dimethylacetamide, and is given, diluted in glucose 5%, by intravenous infusion over 60 to 90 minutes.

For the induction of remission, amsacrine may be given in a dose of 90 mg per m² body-surface daily for 5 to 8 days, de-

---

The symbol † denotes a preparation no longer actively marketed

pending on clinical response. Courses may be repeated at 2- to 4-week intervals according to response, and the dose may be increased to 120 mg per m² daily in subsequent courses if tolerated. Maintenance doses of 150 mg per m² as a single dose or divided over 3 consecutive days have been given every 3 to 4 weeks, adjusted if necessary according to response.

Complete blood counts should be performed regularly, and cardiac, liver, kidney, and CNS function should be monitored.

Doses should be reduced by 20 to 30% in patients with impaired hepatic or renal function.

Preparations

Proprietary Preparations (details are given in Part 3)
Austral.: Amsidyl; *Belg.:* Amsidine; *Canad.:* Amsa P-D; *Denm.:* Amekrin; *Fin.:* Amekrin; *Fr.:* Amsidine†; *Ger.:* Amsidyl; *Irl.:* Amsidine; *Neth.:* Amsidine; *Norw.:* Amekrin; *NZ:* Amsidyl; *Swed.:* Amekrin; *Switz.:* Amsidyl; *UK:* Amsidine.

Anastrozole (14549-q)

Anastrozole (BAN, USAN, rINN).

ICI-D1033; ZD-1033. 2,2′-Dimethyl-2,2′-[5-(1H-1,2,4-triazol-1-ylmethyl)-1,3-phenylene]bis(propiononitrile); α,α,α′,α′-Tetramethyl-5-(1H-1,2,4-triazol-1-ylmethyl)-*m*-benzenediacetonitrile.

$C_{17}H_{19}N_5 = 293.4$.
CAS — 120511-73-1.
ATC — L02BG03.

Adverse Effects and Precautions

The most frequent adverse effects are gastrointestinal disturbances including anorexia, nausea and vomiting, and diarrhoea; asthenia; hot flushes; dizziness; drowsiness; headache; and rash. Other reported effects include hair thinning, vaginal dryness or bleeding, oedema, myalgia and arthralgia, fever, weight gain, leucopenia, and a flu-like syndrome. Abnormalities in liver enzyme values, thrombophlebitis, and increases in total cholesterol, have occurred in some patients receiving anastrozole.

The use of anastrozole is contra-indicated in premenopausal women (particularly in pregnancy). It is not known whether it can be safely given to patients with moderate or severe hepatic impairment, or severe renal impairment.

Pharmacokinetics

Anastrozole is rapidly and almost completely absorbed from the gastrointestinal tract following oral administration, with peak plasma concentrations occurring within about 2 hours. Food decreases the rate of absorption, though this is not considered clinically significant. Anastrozole is 40% bound to plasma proteins. It is metabolised in the liver, and excreted in urine, chiefly as metabolites. The terminal elimination half-life is about 50 hours, and steady-state concentrations are achieved after about 7 days in patients receiving once-daily doses.

Uses and Administration

Anastrozole is a potent and selective nonsteroidal inhibitor of the aromatase (oestrogen synthetase) system, which converts adrenal androgens to oestrogens in peripheral tissue. It is used in the treatment of advanced or locally advanced breast cancer (p.491) in postmenopausal women in a dose of 1 mg daily. Responses are unlikely in patients with oestrogen receptor-negative disease.

◊ References.
1. Anonymous. Anastrozole for metastatic breast cancer. *Med Lett Drugs Ther* 1996; **38:** 61–2.
2. Buzdar A, *et al.* Anastrozole, a potent and selective aromatase inhibitor, versus megestrol acetate in postmenopausal women with advanced breast cancer: results of overview analysis of two phase III trials. *J Clin Oncol* 1996; **14:** 2000–11.
3. Bonneterre J, *et al.* Anastrozole versus tamoxifen as first-line therapy for advanced breast cancer in 668 postmenopausal women: results of the Tamoxifen or Arimidex Randomized Group Efficacy and Tolerability study. *J Clin Oncol* 2000; **18:** 3748–57.

Preparations

Proprietary Preparations (details are given in Part 3)
Aust.: Arimidex; *Austral.:* Arimidex; *Belg.:* Arimidex; *Canad.:* Arimidex; *Denm.:* Arimidex; *Fin.:* Arimidex; *Fr.:* Arimidex; *Ger.:* Arimidex; *Hong Kong:* Arimidex; *Irl.:* Arimidex; *Israel:* Arimidex; *Ital.:* Arimidex; *Mex.:* Arimidex; *Neth.:* Arimidex; *Norw.:* Arimidex; *NZ:* Arimidex; *Port.:* Arimidex; *S.Afr.:* Arimidex; *Singapore:* Arimidex; *Spain:* Arimidex; *Swed.:* Arimidex;

Switz.: Arimidex; *Thai.:* Arimidex; *UK:* Arimidex; *USA:* Arimidex.

Ancitabine Hydrochloride (1824-c)

Ancitabine Hydrochloride (rINNM).

Ancytabine Hydrochloride; Cyclocytidine Hydrochloride; NSC-145668. 2,2′-Anhydro-(1-β-D-arabinofuranosyl)cytosine hydrochloride.

$C_9H_{11}N_3O_4,HCl = 261.7$.
CAS — 31698-14-3 (ancitabine); 10212-25-6 (ancitabine hydrochloride).

Profile

Ancitabine hydrochloride is an antineoplastic that is hydrolysed slowly to cytarabine (p.530) *in vivo*. It has been used in acute myeloid and other leukaemias.

Antilymphocyte Immunoglobulins

(1808-c)

Antilymphocyte immunoglobulins are polyclonal antibodies to human lymphocytes produced by the purification of sera from appropriately immunised animals. The term antilymphocyte immunoglobulin (ALG; lymphocyte immune globulin) implies a product raised against all lymphocyte subsets. The term antithymocyte immunoglobulin (Antithymocyte gammaglobulin; Antithymocyte, Globulin; ATG) implies specificity for T-cells (thymus lymphocytes or thymocytes). However, in practice the nomenclature does not seem to be used consistently, and both terms tend to be used for antibodies raised against T-cells. Nomenclature normally includes an indication of the animal source of the immunoglobulin e.g. antithymocyte immunoglobulin (horse), or antithymocyte immunoglobulin (rabbit).

In addition to the purified immunoglobulins the native sera (antilymphocyte serum and antithymocyte serum, sometimes referred to as lymphocytic antiserum and thymitic antiserum) have also been used as immunosuppressants.

Adverse Effects and Precautions

Antilymphocyte immunoglobulins contain foreign proteins and hypersensitivity reactions are common, although the fact that these preparations are usually given with other immunosuppressants may help to reduce the incidence of reactions. Hypersensitivity may be manifested as fever and chills or shivering, nausea, tachycardia, and hypotension, and dermatological reactions including rash, pruritus, and urticaria; anaphylaxis may occur in up to 1% of patients. Skin rashes and arthralgia may represent serum sickness.

Other adverse effects may include headache, dizziness, muscle pain, gastrointestinal disturbances, and dyspnoea. As well as lymphocytopenia patients may experience leucopenia and thrombocytopenia, usually transient. Nephrotoxicity has been reported. Thrombophlebitis is common following intravenous administration and administration into a vein with a rapid blood flow is recommended.

Antilymphocyte preparations are contra-indicated in hypersensitive patients, and patients should be tested for sensitivity before administration. Facilities for management of anaphylaxis (see p.832) should be available during treatment, and the patient should be observed continuously.

Infection. A study[1] in renal transplant patients given an immunosuppressive regimen comprising azathioprine and prednisone, with or without antithymocyte immunoglobulin, found that those who received antithymocyte immunoglobulin were more likely to have herpesvirus infections and inverted T-cell subset ratios. Regimens containing antithymocyte immunoglobulin may also increase infection with cytomegalovirus and Epstein-Barr virus.

1. Schooley RT, *et al.* Association of herpesvirus infections with T-lymphocyte-subset alterations, glomerulopathy, and opportunistic infections after renal transplantation. *N Engl J Med* 1983; **308:** 307–13.

Uses and Administration

Antilymphocyte immunoglobulins are antibodies, raised in *animals*, which act against lymphocytes, and in particular against T-cells, to produce suppression of cell-mediated immunity.

They may be added to existing immunosuppressant regimens to treat acute rejection episodes in patients who have undergone organ or tissue transplantation. Alternatively, they may be given prophylactically as part of a combination immunosuppressant regimen

with other agents such as azathioprine, corticosteroids, and ciclosporin (so-called 'quadruple' therapy). For discussion of the role of antilymphocyte immunoglobulins in transplantation, see p.502 *et seq.*

Antilymphocyte immunoglobulins have also been used in the treatment of aplastic anaemia (p.715) in patients unsuitable for bone-marrow transplantation, and have been tried in other immunological disorders.

Different antilymphocyte preparations may vary in their activity, as may different lots of the same preparation. However, doses in transplantation have usually ranged from 10 to 30 mg of equine immunoglobulin per kg body-weight daily, given as a slow intravenous infusion diluted in 250 to 500 mL or more of sodium chloride 0.9%, or other suitable diluent. It has been recommended that the final dilution should contain no more than 1 mg of immunoglobulin per mL and be given over 4 hours or more, via an in-line filter.

◊ Antithymocyte immunoglobulin derived from *rabbits* has been found to be more effective than the equine product in preventing renal graft rejection.[1]

1. Gaber AO, *et al.* Results of the double-blind, randomized, multicenter, phase III clinical trial of Thymoglobulin versus Atgam in the treatment of acute graft rejection episodes after renal transplantation. *Transplantation* 1998; **66:** 29–37.

Preparations

Proprietary Preparations (details are given in Part 3)
Aust.: ATG†; *Austral.:* Atgam; *Belg.:* ATG; Atgam; Lymphoglobuline; Thymoglobuline; *Braz.:* Gat Globulina Antitimocitaria; Thymoglobuline; *Canad.:* Atgam; *Denm.:* Thymoglobuline; *Fr.:* Lymphoglobuline; Thymoglobuline; *Ger.:* Lymphoglobulin; Thymoglobuline; *Hong Kong:* ATG; Atgam; Lymphoglobuline; Thymoglobuline; *Israel:* ATG-S; Atgam; Lymphoglobuline; Thymoglobuline; *Ital.:* Lymphoglobuline; Uman-Gal E†; *Neth.:* Lymphoglobuline; *NZ:* Atgam; *S.Afr.:* Lymphoglobuline; Thymoglobuline; *Singapore:* Atgam; *Spain:* Atgam†; Linfoglobulina; *Switz.:* ATG; Atgam; Lymphoglobuline; Thymoglobuline; *Thai.:* ATG; Lymphoglobuline; Thymoglobuline; *USA:* Atgam.

Antineoplaston A10 (18767-m)

3-Phenylacetylamino-2,6-piperidinedione.
$C_{13}H_{14}N_2O_3 = 246.3$.

Profile

Antineoplaston A10 is one of a group of peptide derivatives isolated from blood and urine that has been investigated for the treatment of breast cancer and other malignant neoplasms although its value has been questioned (see below).

◊ A critical review of the antineoplastons.[1] Most work has been done with antineoplaston A10, which is insoluble in aqueous solutions, and its derivatives antineoplaston AS2.5 (phenylacetylglutamine), and antineoplaston AS2.1 (a 4:1 mixture of phenylacetic acid and phenylacetylglutamine), which have not been independently shown to be active against cancer.

Later references[2-4] suggest that interest in the antineoplastons nonetheless continues.

1. Green S. Antineoplastons: an unproved cancer therapy. *JAMA* 1992; **267:** 2924–8.
2. Tsuda H, *et al.* Quick response of advanced cancer to chemoradiation therapy with antineoplastons. *Oncol Rep* 1998; **5:** 597–600.
3. Buckner JC, *et al.* Phase II study of antineoplastons A10 (NSC 648539) and AS2-1 (NSC 620261) in patients with recurrent glioma. *Mayo Clin Proc* 1999; **74:** 137–45.
4. Badria F, *et al.* Immune modulatory potentials of antineoplaston A-10 in breast cancer patients. *Cancer Lett* 2000; **157:** 57–63.

Asparaginase (1823-z)

Asparaginase (USAN).

L-Asparaginase; L-Asparagine Amidohydrolase; MK-965; NSC-109229; Re-82-TAD-15.
CAS — 9015-68-3.
ATC — L01XX02.

NOTE. Colaspase and crisantaspase are BAN for asparaginase obtained from cultures of *Escherichia coli* and *Erwinia chrysanthemi* (*E. carotovora*) respectively.

Asparaginase should be stored at 2° to 8° (see also Stability, below). **Incompatible** with rubber. The manufacturers recommend that it should not be mixed with other drugs.

Pegaspargase (15343-n)

Pegaspargase (USAN, rINN).

PEG-L-asparaginase. A conjugate of colaspase with a polyethylene glycol of molecular weight 5000; Monomethoxypolyethylene glycol succinimidyl L-asparaginase.
CAS — 130167-69-0.

Pegaspargase should be stored at 2° to 8°.

Stability. Although asparaginase was routinely kept under refrigeration,[1] information from a manufacturer (Merck Sharp & Dohme) indicated that it would remain stable for 48 hours at 15° to 30°. The manufacturer of pegaspargase states it should not be used if stored at room temperature for more than 48 hours.

1. Vogenberg FR, Souney PF. Stability guidelines for routinely refrigerated drug products. *Am J Hosp Pharm* 1983; **40:** 101–2.

Units

One unit of asparaginase splits 1 μmol of ammonia from L-asparagine in 1 minute under standard conditions.

Adverse Effects

Asparaginase may produce anaphylaxis and other hypersensitivity reactions including fever, rashes, and bronchospasm, due to its protein nature; there does not appear to be cross-sensitivity between asparaginase derived from *Escherichia coli* and that from *Erwinia chrysanthemi*. Hypersensitivity to pegaspargase is less common, but about 30% of patients hypersensitive to the native enzyme experience hypersensitivity to pegaspargase treatment.

Liver function abnormalities occur in many patients, and there may be decreased blood concentrations of fibrinogen and clotting factors, alterations in blood lipids and cholesterol, and hypoalbuminaemia. Hyperammonaemia, due to the production of ammonia from asparagine, may occur. Uraemia, and occasionally renal failure, have been reported frequently. Pancreatitis may occur and may be fatal: there may also be hyperglycaemia due to decreased insulin production, and death from ketoacidosis has occurred.

Gastrointestinal disturbances, including nausea and vomiting, and CNS disturbances, including drowsiness, depression, coma, hallucinations, and a Parkinson-like syndrome, have also been reported. Transient bone-marrow depression has occurred rarely, as has marked leucopenia.

Effects on the blood. Both haemorrhage[1] (including intracranial haemorrhage[2]) and thrombosis[1,3] have been reported following asparaginase therapy, but overt symptoms seem to be relatively rare, perhaps because falls in antithrombin III are counteracted by the decrease in plasma coagulation factors.[3]

1. Priest JR, *et al.* A syndrome of thrombosis and hemorrhage complicating L-asparaginase therapy for childhood acute lymphoblastic leukemia. *J Pediatr* 1982; **100:** 984–9.
2. Lederman GS. Stroke due to treatment with L-asparaginase in an adult. *N Engl J Med* 1982; **307:** 1643.
3. Pitney WR, *et al.* Antithrombin III deficiency during asparaginase therapy. *Lancet* 1980; **i:** 493–4.

Precautions

Asparaginase is contra-indicated in patients with pancreatitis, and should be avoided in pregnancy. It should be given cautiously to patients with impaired liver function. Facilities for the management of anaphylaxis (see p.832) should be available during treatment. Some manufacturers recommend an intradermal test dose at the start of asparaginase treatment to check for hypersensitivity, as described under Uses, below, although such tests may not always be predictive. Re-treatment with asparaginase may be associated with an increased risk of allergic reactions. Serum amylase concentrations should be monitored regularly as should blood glucose concentrations. Asparaginase has been reported to interfere with tests of thyroid function by transient reduction of concentrations of thyroxine-binding globulin.

Interactions

If asparaginase is given before, rather than after, methotrexate the activity of the latter may be reduced (see below). Vincristine neurotoxicity may possibly be increased by concurrent administration with intravenous asparaginase.

Methotrexate. Asparaginase inhibits protein synthesis and cell replication, and therefore may interfere with the action of drugs such as methotrexate that require cell replication for their antineoplastic effect.[1] It has been suggested that a 24-hour interval between methotrexate and a subsequent dose of asparaginase permits at least an additive therapeutic effect.[2]

1. Jolivet J, *et al.* Prevention of methotrexate cytotoxicity by asparaginase inhibition of methotrexate polyglutamate formation. *Cancer Res* 1985; **45:** 217–20.

2. Capizzi RL. Asparaginase-methotrexate in combination chemotherapy: schedule-dependent differential effects on normal versus neoplastic cells. *Cancer Treat Rep* 1981; **65** (suppl 4): 115–21.

Pharmacokinetics

Following intravenous injection the plasma half-life of the native enzyme has varied from about 8 to 30 hours; half-lives of up to 49 hours may be seen after intramuscular dosage. The mean half-life of pegaspargase is reported to be 5.7 days. Asparaginase is found in the lymph at about 20% of the concentration in plasma. There is virtually no diffusion into the CSF. Little is excreted in the urine.

Uses and Administration

Asparaginase is an enzyme which acts by breaking down the amino acid L-asparagine to aspartic acid and ammonia. It interferes with the growth of those malignant cells which, unlike most healthy cells, are unable to synthesise L-asparagine for their metabolism, but resistance to its action develops fairly rapidly. Its action is reportedly specific for the G_1 phase of the cell cycle.

Asparaginase is used mainly for the induction of remissions in acute lymphoblastic leukaemia (p.484). Regimens vary but it may be given intravenously in a dose of 1000 units per kg body-weight daily for 10 days following treatment with vincristine and prednisone or prednisolone, or intramuscularly in a dose of 6000 units per m^2 body-surface given every third day for 9 doses during treatment with vincristine and prednisone or prednisolone. Alternatively, in patients hypersensitive to the native enzyme it may be given as pegaspargase, in doses of 2500 units per m^2 every 14 days, preferably by intramuscular injection although the intravenous route may also be used. In patients with a body-surface less than 0.6 m^2 a dose of 82.5 units of pegaspargase per kg body-weight, given every 14 days, is recommended.

Asparaginase is not generally used alone as an induction agent but doses of 200 units per kg daily have been given intravenously for 28 days to adults and children. If pegaspargase is used alone doses are the same as for combination regimens. Children appear to tolerate asparaginase better than adults.

Although not entirely reliable, an intradermal test dose of about 2 units has been recommended in the USA before treatment with asparaginase, or where more than a week has elapsed between doses. Desensitisation has been advocated if no alternative antineoplastic treatment is available. The incidence of hypersensitivity is lower in patients given pegaspargase, and a test dose is not advocated.

When administered intravenously a solution of asparaginase in Water for Injections or sodium chloride 0.9% should be given over not less than 30 minutes through a running infusion of sodium chloride 0.9% or glucose 5%. When given intramuscularly no more than 2 mL of a solution in sodium chloride 0.9% should be injected at a single site.

◊ References.
1. Anonymous. Pegaspargase for acute lymphoblastic leukemia. *Med Lett Drugs Ther* 1995; **37:** 23–4.
2. Holle LM. Pegaspargase: an alternative? *Ann Pharmacother* 1997; **31:** 616–24.

Preparations

Proprietary Preparations (details are given in Part 3)

Austral.: Leunase; *Belg.:* Paronal; *Braz.:* Elspar; *Canad.:* Kidrolase; Oncaspar; *Denm.:* Erwinase; *Fin.:* Erwinase; *Fr.:* Kidrolase; *Ger.:* Erwinase; Oncaspar; *Hong Kong:* Elspar; Leunase; *Israel:* Kidrolase; *Ital.:* Crasnitin†; *Jpn:* Leunase; *Mex.:* Leunase; Serasa; *NZ:* Erwinase; Leunase; *S.Afr.:* Laspar; *Singapore:* Leunase; *Swed.:* Erwinase; Leunase; *Thai.:* Erwinase; Leunase; *UK:* Erwinase; *USA:* Elspar; Oncaspar.

Azacitidine (1809-k)

Azacitidine (USAN, rINN).

5-Azacytidine; Ladakamycin; NSC-102816; U-18496. 4-Amino-1-β-D-ribofuranosyl-1,3,5-triazin-2(1H)-one.

$C_8H_{12}N_4O_5 = 244.2$.

CAS — 320-67-2.

Profile

Azacitidine is an antimetabolite antineoplastic with general properties similar to those of cytarabine (p.530). It also inhibits cellular pyrimidine synthesis. It has been used mainly in the treatment of acute myeloid leukaemia (p.485).

Azathioprine (1812-I)

Azathioprine (BAN, USAN, rINN).

Azathioprinum; BW-57322; NSC-39084. 6-(1-Methyl-4-nitroimidazol-5-ylthio)purine.

$C_9H_7N_7O_2S = 277.3$.

CAS — 446-86-6.

ATC — L04AX01.

NOTE. The abbreviation AZT, which has sometimes been used for azathioprine, has also been used to denote the antiviral zidovudine.

Pharmacopoeias. In Eur. (see p.vi), Int., Jpn, Pol., and US.

Pharmacopoeial description

Ph. Eur.: A pale yellow powder. Practically insoluble in water and in alcohol; soluble in dilute solutions of alkali hydroxides; sparingly soluble in dilute mineral acids. Protect from light.

USP 25: A pale yellow, odourless powder. Insoluble in water; very slightly soluble in alcohol and in chloroform; sparingly soluble in dilute mineral acids; soluble in dilute solutions of alkali hydroxides. Store in airtight containers. Protect from light.

Adverse Effects and Treatment

For a general outline see Antineoplastics and Immunosuppressants, p.476 and p.479.

Dose-related bone-marrow depression may be manifested as leucopenia or less often thrombocytopenia or anaemia, and may occasionally be delayed. Macrocytic, including megaloblastic, anaemia has occurred. Azathioprine has also been associated with the development of liver damage; it has been suggested that cholestatic symptoms may be due to the mercaptopurine moiety. Rarely, delayed and potentially fatal veno-occlusive liver disease has occurred.

Other side-effects associated with azathioprine include gastrointestinal disturbances, reversible alopecia, and symptoms including rashes, muscle and joint pains, fever, rigors, pneumonitis, pancreatitis, tachycardia, renal dysfunction, and hypotension, some or all of which may represent hypersensitivity reactions.

Solutions for injection are irritant.

◊ References.
1. Lawson DH, *et al.* Adverse effects of azathioprine. *Adverse Drug React Acute Poisoning Rev* 1984; **3:** 161–71.

Carcinogenicity. Immunosuppression, including that with azathioprine, may be associated with an increased risk of certain neoplasms in transplant recipients (see p.476) and less so in patients with rheumatoid arthritis.[1] Conversely, a study in 755 patients given azathioprine for inflammatory bowel disease and followed for up to 29 years failed to show any increased risk of neoplasia.[2]

A synergistic clastogenic effect has been noted with azathioprine and long-wave ultraviolet light.

1. Silman AJ, *et al.* Lymphoproliferative cancer and other malignancy in patients with rheumatoid arthritis treated with azathioprine: a 20 year follow up study. *Ann Rheum Dis* 1988; **47:** 988–92.
2. Connell WR, *et al.* Long-term neoplasia risk after azathioprine treatment in inflammatory bowel disease. *Lancet* 1994; **343:** 1249–52.

Effects on the blood. The degree of neutropenia in patients receiving mercaptopurine has been reported to correlate negatively with the concentration of the metabolite tioguanine nucleotide in erythrocytes,[1] and it has been suggested that measurement of metabolite concentrations in erythrocytes,[2] or activity of the enzyme thiopurine methyltransferase,[3-6] permits prediction of those individuals likely to experience severe bone-marrow toxicity with mercaptopurine and the related drugs tioguanine and azathioprine. However, not all studies have found such correlations,[7] therefore effects on the bone marrow with this class of drugs are probably multifactorial,[8] and low activity of other enzymes such as lymphocyte 5-nucleotidase,[9] and other factors, may contribute to toxicity.

1. Lennard L, *et al.* Childhood leukaemia: a relationship between intracellular 6-mercaptopurine metabolites and neutropenia. *Br J Clin Pharmacol* 1983; **16:** 359–63.
2. Maddocks JL, *et al.* Azathioprine and severe bone marrow depression. *Lancet* 1986; **i:** 156.
3. Schütz E, *et al.* Azathioprine-induced myelosuppression in thiopurine methyltransferase deficient renal transplant recipient. *Lancet* 1993; **341:** 436.
4. Lennard L, *et al.* Congenital thiopurine methyltransferase deficiency and 6-mercaptopurine toxicity during treatment for acute lymphoblastic leukaemia. *Arch Dis Child* 1993; **69:** 577–9.

The symbol † denotes a preparation no longer actively marketed

5. Jackson AP, et al. Thiopurine methyltransferase levels should be measured before commencing patients on azathioprine. Br J Dermatol 1997; **136:** 133–4.
6. Black AJ, et al. Thiopurine methyltransferase genotype predicts therapy-limiting severe toxicity from azathioprine. Ann Intern Med 1998; **129:** 716–18.
7. Boulieu R, et al. Intracellular thiopurine nucleotides and azathioprine myelotoxicity in organ transplant patients. Br J Clin Pharmacol 1997; **43:** 116–18.
8. Soria-Royer C, et al. Thiopurine-methyl-transferase activity to assess azathioprine myelotoxicity in renal transplant recipients. Lancet 1993; **341:** 1593–4.
9. Kerstens PJSM, et al. 5-Nucleotidase and azathioprine-related bone-marrow toxicity. Lancet 1993; **342:** 1245–6.

Effects on the liver. A review[1] of drug-related hepatotoxicity noted that azathioprine has been associated with hepatocanalicular cholestasis, in which the interference with bile flow is combined with hepatocyte damage, and with several hepatic vascular disorders, including focal sinusoidal dilatation, peliosis, and veno-occlusive disease.

1. Sherlock S. The spectrum of hepatotoxicity due to drugs. Lancet 1986; **ii:** 440–4.

Hypersensitivity. A report of 5 patients with acute allergic reactions associated with azathioprine.[1] In 2 of these patients, who had undergone renal transplantation, the symptoms (interstitial nephritis) were initially mistaken for acute rejection episodes.

1. Parnham AP, et al. Acute allergic reactions associated with azathioprine. Lancet 1996; **348:** 542–3.

Precautions

For reference to the precautions necessary with antineoplastics and immunosuppressants in general, see p.480. Regular monitoring of blood counts is required. Patients with renal or hepatic impairment require more frequent monitoring of blood counts and reduced doses; liver function tests should be performed in hepatic impairment. Azathioprine should generally be avoided in pregnancy (see below).

Pregnancy and breast feeding. Despite reports of chromosomal aberrations[1] or fetal growth retardation[2] in the offspring of mothers who received azathioprine during pregnancy, there seems to be little evidence that azathioprine is teratogenic in humans.[1,3-5] Given the nature of the severe chronic conditions for which azathioprine is generally used, discontinuing therapy in patients who become pregnant may not be necessary or desirable, but it seems prudent to avoid its use where possible during pregnancy. Leucopenia has been reported in neonates whose mothers received azathioprine during pregnancy.[6] Azathioprine is distributed into breast milk; it has been recommended that mothers receiving azathioprine should not breastfeed.

1. The Registration Committee of the European Dialysis and Transplant Association. Successful pregnancies in women treated by dialysis and kidney transplantation. Br J Obstet Gynaecol 1980; **87:** 839–45.
2. Pirson Y, et al. Retardation of fetal growth in patients receiving immunosuppressive therapy. N Engl J Med 1985; **313:** 328.
3. Hou S. Retardation of fetal growth in patients receiving immunosuppressive therapy. N Engl J Med 1985; **313:** 328.
4. Whittle MJ, Hanretty KP. Prescribing in pregnancy: identifying abnormalities. BMJ 1986; **293:** 1485–8.
5. Alstead EM, et al. Safety of azathioprine in pregnancy in inflammatory bowel disease. Gastroenterology 1990; **99:** 443–6.
6. Davison JM, et al. Maternal azathioprine therapy and depressed haemopoiesis in the babies of renal allograft patients. Br J Obstet Gynaecol 1985; **92:** 233–9.

Interactions

For a general outline of antineoplastic and immunosuppressant drug interactions, see p.481. The effects of azathioprine are enhanced by allopurinol and the dose of azathioprine should be reduced to one-third to one-quarter of the usual dose when allopurinol is given concomitantly.

◊ In addition to being affected by allopurinol, azathioprine may itself affect other drugs including the following:

• competitive neuromuscular blockers (potentiation, see under Immunosuppressants on p.1335)
• vaccines (reduced response or generalised infection, see p.1530)
• warfarin (inhibition, see Antineoplastics, p.995).

Gastrointestinal drugs. For mention of 5-aminosalicylates inhibiting the metabolism of thiopurine antineoplastics such as azathioprine, and increasing their toxicity, see Mercaptopurine, p.552.

Pharmacokinetics

Azathioprine is well absorbed from the gastrointestinal tract when given by mouth. After oral or intravenous administration it disappears rapidly from the circulation and is extensively metabolised to mercaptopurine (which is then further metabolised—see p.552). Both azathioprine and mercaptopurine are about 30% bound to plasma proteins. About 10% of a dose of azathioprine is reported to be split between the sulfur and the purine ring to give 1-methyl-4-nitro-5-thioimidazole. The proportion of different metabolites is reported to vary between patients. Metabolites and small amounts of unchanged azathioprine and mercaptopurine are eliminated in the urine.

◊ Although plasma concentrations of 6-thiouric acid (the inactive product of mercaptopurine, and hence of azathioprine) can be readily measured in patients who have been receiving azathioprine, they are of little value in therapeutic drug monitoring.[1] The active moieties are the tioguanine nucleotides formed intracellularly, which appear to have extremely long half-lives,[2] and mean erythrocyte concentrations of which appear to vary considerably between individuals.[2]

1. Chan GLC, et al. Pharmacokinetics of 6-thiouric acid and 6-mercaptopurine in renal allograft recipients after oral administration of azathioprine. Eur J Clin Pharmacol 1989; **36:** 265–71.
2. Chan GLC, et al. Azathioprine metabolism: pharmacokinetics of 6-mercaptopurine, 6-thiouric acid and 6-thioguanine nucleotides in renal transplant patients. J Clin Pharmacol 1990; **30:** 358–63.

Uses and Administration

Azathioprine is a cytotoxic immunosuppressant with similar actions to those of mercaptopurine (p.552), to which it is converted in the body. Its effects may not be seen for several weeks after administration. It is given by mouth, but in patients in whom oral use is not feasible it may be given by slow intravenous injection or by infusion as azathioprine sodium.

Azathioprine is mainly used as an immunosuppressant for the prevention of rejection in **organ and tissue transplantation** (p.502). The dose for this purpose varies from 1 to 5 mg per kg body-weight daily and depends partly on the regimen employed. Higher doses are used initially, adjusted according to clinical response and haematological tolerance.

Azathioprine is also used in a wide variety of conditions that are considered to have an auto-immune component as indicated by the references given below. The usual dose of azathioprine in these conditions is in the range of 1 to 3 mg per kg body-weight daily by mouth.

Use of azathioprine in conjunction with a corticosteroid (p.1044) may have a corticosteroid-sparing effect.

Blood counts should be carried out regularly during treatment and azathioprine withdrawn or the dosage reduced at the first indication of bone-marrow depression.

Blood disorders, non-malignant. Immunosuppressants such as azathioprine are occasionally tried in auto-immune haemolytic anaemia (p.716) refractory to other treatment and may permit reduction of corticosteroid dosage. Similarly in patients with idiopathic thrombocytopenic purpura (p.1052), immunosuppressants may be tried as a last resort.

Connective-tissue and muscular disorders. Azathioprine is one of many agents tried for disease control in Behçet's syndrome (p.1047). It is used similarly in polymyositis and systemic lupus erythematosus (see p.1057 and p.1059 respectively) and in the former condition combined therapy with azathioprine and a corticosteroid has been found to be better than a corticosteroid alone for maintenance long-term.[1] However, there is also some evidence that methotrexate may be more effective in refractory polymyositis than azathioprine.[2]

1. Bunch TW. Prednisone and azathioprine for polymyositis: long-term followup. Arthritis Rheum 1981; **24:** 45–8.
2. Joffe MM, et al. Drug therapy of the idiopathic inflammatory myopathies: predictors of response to prednisone, azathioprine, and methotrexate and a comparison of their efficacy. Am J Med 1993; **94:** 379–87.

Inflammatory bowel disease. Azathioprine or its metabolite mercaptopurine are used to induce remission in chronically active inflammatory bowel disease (p.1205), and to maintain remission, particularly in Crohn's disease.[1-3] They have a useful corticosteroid-sparing effect. In patients who have been in remission for 4 years, it may be possible to stop treatment.[4] The onset of benefit from oral azathioprine may be delayed for several months. One study[5] reported that a more rapid response could be achieved with an intravenous loading dose but a later study failed to confirm this.[6]

1. Lamers CB, et al. Azathioprine: an update on clinical efficacy and safety in inflammatory bowel disease. Scand J Gastroenterol 1999; **230** (suppl): 111–15.
2. Sandborn W, et al. Azathioprine or 6-mercaptopurine for inducing remission of Crohn's disease (updated 23 November 1998). Available in The Cochrane Library; Issue 2. Oxford: Update Software; 2000.
3. Pearson DC, et al. Azathioprine for maintaining remission of Crohn's disease (updated 24 September 1999). Available in The Cochrane Library; Issue 2. Oxford: Update Software; 2000.

4. Bouhnik Y, et al. Long-term follow-up of patients with Crohn's disease treated with azathioprine or 6-mercaptopurine. Lancet 1996; **347:** 215–19.
5. Sandborn WJ. An intravenous loading dose of azathioprine decreases the time to response in patients with Crohn's disease. Gastroenterology 1995; **109:** 1808–17.
6. Sandborn WJ. Lack of effect of intravenous administration on time to respond to azathioprine for steroid-treated Crohn's disease: North American Azathioprine Study Group. Gastroenterology 1999; **117:** 527–35.

Liver disorders, non-malignant. Azathioprine has been widely used with corticosteroids to produce and maintain remission of chronic active hepatitis,[1-6] as discussed on p.1048, and such combination therapy, which also permits a reduction in corticosteroid dosage, is generally thought to be more effective than azathioprine alone.[2,4] Patients successfully maintained in remission for at least a year on azathioprine with a corticosteroid can subsequently be maintained on azathioprine (at a higher dose of 2 mg per kg body-weight daily) alone.[7] Results in patients with primary biliary cirrhosis (p.501) have been more equivocal, and initial studies did not indicate much benefit from azathioprine,[8,9] although a later study did seem to indicate improved survival and disease retardation.[10]

1. Stavinoha MW, Soloway RD. Current therapy of chronic liver disease. Drugs 1990; **39:** 814–40.
2. Giusti G, et al. Immunosuppressive therapy in chronic active hepatitis (CAH): a multicentric retrospective study on 867 patients. Hepatogastroenterology 1984; **31:** 24–9.
3. Vegnente A, et al. Duration of chronic active hepatitis and the development of cirrhosis. Arch Dis Child 1984; **59:** 330–5.
4. Stellon AJ, et al. Randomised controlled trial of azathioprine withdrawal in autoimmune chronic active hepatitis. Lancet 1985; **i:** 668–70.
5. Brunner G, Hopf U. Relapse after azathioprine withdrawal in autoimmune chronic active hepatitis. Lancet 1985; **i:** 1216.
6. Czaja AJ. Drug therapy in the management of type 1 autoimmune hepatitis. Drugs 1999; **57:** 49–68.
7. Johnson PJ. Azathioprine for long-term maintenance of remission in autoimmune hepatitis. N Engl J Med 1995; **333:** 958–63.
8. Heathcote J, et al. A prospective controlled trial of azathioprine in primary biliary cirrhosis. Gastroenterology 1976; **70:** 656–60.
9. Crowe J, et al. Azathioprine in primary biliary cirrhosis: a preliminary report of an international trial. Gastroenterology 1980; **78:** 1005–10.
10. Christensen E, et al. Beneficial effect of azathioprine and prediction of prognosis in primary biliary cirrhosis: final results of an international trial. Gastroenterology 1985; **89:** 1084–91.

Lung disorders, non-malignant. Although corticosteroids remain the mainstay of treatment for the various forms of diffuse parenchymal lung disease (p.1050) including cryptogenic fibrosing alveolitis (CFA), there is some evidence that combined therapy with azathioprine improves survival in the latter condition,[1] and the British Thoracic Society now recommends that initial treatment of CFA should be with oral prednisolone plus azathioprine 2 to 3 mg per kg body-weight.[2]

1. Raghu G, et al. Azathioprine combined with prednisone in the treatment of idiopathic pulmonary fibrosis: a prospective double-blind, randomized, placebo-controlled clinical trial. Am Rev Respir Dis 1991; **144:** 291–6.
2. British Thoracic Society. The diagnosis, assessment and treatment of diffuse parenchymal lung disease in adults. Thorax 1999; **54** (suppl 1): S1–S30.

Neuromuscular disorders. Azathioprine may be used for its corticosteroid-sparing properties[1,2] in patients who require corticosteroid treatment for myasthenia gravis (p.1414). It may also be of use when corticosteroids are contra-indicated or when response to corticosteroids alone is insufficient.[3] Azathioprine is not usually used alone because it may be several months before any beneficial effect is seen. Studies have also indicated modest benefit from azathioprine[4,5] in patients with multiple sclerosis (p.633). It has been suggested that the benefits are too slight to justify the toxicity of the required doses,[6] but it has also been pointed out that in terms of relapse reduction azathioprine appears as effective as newer treatments such as interferon beta.[7]

1. Mantegazza R, et al. Azathioprine as a single drug or in combination with steroids in the treatment of myasthenia gravis. J Neurol 1988; **235:** 449–53.
2. Palace J, et al. A randomized double-blind trial of prednisolone alone or with azathioprine in myasthenia gravis. Neurology 1998; **50:** 1778–83.
3. Gajdos P, et al. Myasthenia Gravis Clinical Study Group. A randomised clinical trial comparing prednisone and azathioprine in myasthenia gravis: results of the second interim analysis. J Neurol Neurosurg Psychiatry 1993; **56:** 1157–63.
4. British and Dutch Multiple Sclerosis Azathioprine Trial Group. Double-masked trial of azathioprine in multiple sclerosis. Lancet 1988; **ii:** 179–83.
5. Ellison GW, et al. A placebo-controlled, randomized, double-masked, variable dosage, clinical trial of azathioprine with and without methylprednisolone in multiple sclerosis. Neurology 1989; **39:** 1018–26.
6. Yudkin PL, et al. Overview of azathioprine treatment in multiple sclerosis. Lancet 1991; **338:** 1051–5.
7. Palace J, Rothwell P. New treatments and azathioprine in multiple sclerosis. Lancet 1997; **350:** 261.

Ocular disorders, non-malignant. For mention of the use of azathioprine in various disorders characterised by ocular lesions such as scleritis or uveitis, see p.502.

Psoriatic arthritis. Azathioprine may be useful for severe or progressive cases of psoriatic arthritis (see under Spondyloarthropathies, p.10) when the arthritis is not controlled by physical therapy and NSAIDs.

Rheumatoid arthritis. Although azathioprine may be beneficial in rheumatoid arthritis (p.9) in the short-term, it is no more effective than other disease-modifying antirheumatic drugs (DMARDs) and its toxicity is significantly more severe.[1] It may however be useful in patients with severe disease unresponsive to other DMARDs especially in those with extra-articular manifestations such as vasculitis.[2]

1. Suarez-Almazor ME, et al. Azathioprine for rheumatoid arthritis (updated 28 October 1999). Available in The Cochrane Library; Issue 1. Oxford: Update Software; 2000.
2. Heurkens AHM, et al. Prednisone plus azathioprine treatment in patients with rheumatoid arthritis complicated by vasculitis. Arch Intern Med 1991; 151: 2249–54.

Sarcoidosis. Cytotoxic immunosuppressants such as azathioprine have been tried in patients with sarcoidosis (p.1058) who do not respond to or cannot tolerate corticosteroids.

Skin disorders, non-malignant. Like other immunosuppressants, azathioprine has been tried in various refractory skin disorders, notably in pemphigus (see below). Other conditions in which it has been tried include atopic eczema,[1-3] nodular prurigo,[4] chronic actinic dermatitis,[1] pyoderma gangrenosum,[2] and erythema multiforme[2,5] as well as in the skin manifestations of systemic disorders such as dermatomyositis and lupus erythematosus.

1. Younger IR, et al. Azathioprine in dermatology. J Am Acad Dermatol 1991; 25: 281–6.
2. Tan BB, et al. Azathioprine in dermatology: a survey of current practice in the UK. Br J Dermatol 1997; 136: 351–5.
3. Lear JT, et al. A retrospective review of the use of azathioprine in severe atopic dermatitis. Br J Dermatol 1996; 135 (suppl 47): 38.
4. Lear JT, et al. Nodular prurigo responsive to azathioprine. Br J Dermatol 1996; 134: 1151.
5. Schofield JK, et al. Recurrent erythema multiforme: clinical features and treatment in a large series of patients. Br J Dermatol 1993; 128: 542–5.

PEMPHIGUS AND PEMPHIGOID. Corticosteroids are the main treatment for blistering in pemphigus and pemphigoid (p.1106). Immunosuppressive therapy, including azathioprine,[1] has been used in combination with corticosteroids to permit a reduction in corticosteroid dosage. However, it has been suggested that evidence for the corticosteroid-sparing effect is lacking and that immunosuppressants should be reserved for patients who cannot tolerate corticosteroids or in whom they are contra-indicated.[2]

1. Aberer W, et al. Azathioprine in the treatment of pemphigus vulgaris: a long-term follow-up. J Am Acad Dermatol 1987; 16: 527–33.
2. Bystryn J-C, Steinman NM. The adjuvant therapy of pemphigus: an update. Arch Dermatol 1996; 132: 203–12.

Vasculitic syndromes. Azathioprine has been tried in a number of the vasculitic syndromes, including giant cell arteritis (p.1050), microscopic polyangiitis (p.1056), Churg-Strauss syndrome (p.1049), and Wegener's granulomatosis (p.1060). In general it is most useful in maintenance for its corticosteroid-sparing effect. Cyclophosphamide tends to be preferred where a more aggressive regimen is required, as in some combinations for induction of remission.

Preparations

BP 2001: Azathioprine Tablets;
USP 25: Azathioprine Sodium for Injection; Azathioprine Tablets.

Proprietary Preparations (details are given in Part 3)
Aust.: Imurek; *Austral.:* Azahexal; Azamun; Imuran; Thioprine; *Belg.:* Imuran; *Braz.:* Imuran; *Canad.:* Imuran; *Denm.:* Imurel; *Fin.:* Azamun; Imuprin; Imurel; *Fr.:* Imurel; *Ger.:* Azafalk; Imurek; Zytrim; *Hong Kong:* Imuran; *Irl.:* Azopine; Imuran; *Israel:* Azopi; Imuran; *Mex.:* Aseroprim; Azatrilem; Imuran; Satedon; Tiosalprin; *Neth.:* Imuran; Imuran; *Norw.:* Azamun; Imuran; Thioprine; *Port.:* Imuran; *S.Afr.:* Azapress; Imuran; *Singapore:* Imuran; *Spain:* Imurel; *Swed.:* Imurel; *Switz.:* Imurek; *Thai.:* Imuran; *UK:* Azamune†; Berkaprine†; Immunoprin; Imuran; Oprisine†; *USA:* Imuran.

Multi-ingredient: *Ger.:* Azamedac.

Basiliximab (9707-g)

Basiliximab (BAN, USAN, rINN).
SDZ-CHI-621.
CAS — 179045-86-4.
ATC — L04AA09.

Profile

Basiliximab is a chimeric murine/human monoclonal antibody similar to daclizumab (p.532) that functions as an interleukin-2 receptor antagonist by binding to the alpha chain (CD25 antigen) of the interleukin-2 receptor on the surface of activated T-lymphocytes. It is used in the prevention of acute graft rejection episodes in patients undergoing renal transplantation as part of an immunosuppressive regimen that includes ciclosporin and corticosteroids. The recommended adult dose is 20 mg by intravenous infusion given over 20 to 30 minutes, given within 2 hours before surgery and repeated once after 4 days. In the UK, children under 35 kg body-weight may receive 10 mg, repeated after 4 days. In the USA, children 2 years of age or older may receive 12 mg per m² body-surface, up to a maximum single dose of 20 mg, at the same intervals.

Renal transplantation. A course of basiliximab reduced the incidence of acute rejection episodes in the first year after renal

The symbol † denotes a preparation no longer actively marketed

transplantation (p.503) compared with placebo, but there was no difference in graft survival.[1,2]

1. Nashan B, et al. Randomised trial of basiliximab versus placebo for control of acute cellular rejection in renal allograft recipients. Lancet 1997; 350: 1193–8. Correction. ibid.; 1484.
2. Kahan BD, et al. Reduction of the occurrence of acute cellular rejection among renal allograft recipients treated with basiliximab, a chimeric anti-interleukin-2-receptor monoclonal antibody. Transplantation 1999; 67: 276–84.

Preparations

Proprietary Preparations (details are given in Part 3)
Austral.: Simulect; *Belg.:* Simulect; *Denm.:* Simulect; *Fin.:* Simulect; *Fr.:* Simulect; *Ger.:* Simulect; *Hong Kong:* Simulect; *Irl.:* Simulect; *Ital.:* Simulect; *Mex.:* Simulect; *Neth.:* Simulect; *Norw.:* Simulect; *NZ:* Simulect; *Port.:* Simulect; *S.Afr.:* Simulect; *Singapore:* Simulect; *Spain:* Simulect; *Swed.:* Simulect; *Switz.:* Simulect; *Thai.:* Simulect; *UK:* Simulect; *USA:* Simulect.

Batimastat (14528-h)

Batimastat (BAN, USAN, rINN).
BB-94. (2S,3R)-5-Methyl-3-{[(αS)-α-(methylcarbamoyl)phenethyl]carbamoyl}-2-[(2-thienylthio)methyl]hexanohydroxamic acid; (2S,3R)-N¹-Hydroxy-3-isobutyl-N⁴-[(S)-α-(methylcarbamoyl)phenethyl]-2-(2-thienylthiomethyl)succinamide.
$C_{23}H_{31}N_3O_4S_2 = 477.6$.
CAS — 130370-60-4.

Profile

Batimastat is an inhibitor of matrix metalloproteinases, enzymes which are thought to play a role in the metastasis of cancer cells. It has been investigated in a variety of malignant disorders.

Bexarotene (20193-h)

Bexarotene (BAN, USAN, rINN).
LG-100069; LGD-1069. p-[1-(5,6,7,8-Tetrahydro-3,5,5,8,8-pentamethyl-2-naphthyl)vinyl]benzoic acid.
$C_{24}H_{28}O_2 = 348.5$.
CAS — 153559-49-0.

Profile

Bexarotene is an agonist at the retinoid X receptor, which is involved in the regulation of cell differentiation and proliferation. It is used in the treatment of cutaneous T-cell lymphoma, in a usual dose of 300 mg per m² daily by mouth, adjusted according to toxicity. For the topical treatment of refractory disease a 1% gel may be applied on alternate days for the first week, gradually increased to up to 4 times daily, depending on tolerance.

The main adverse effects noted after oral therapy include hyperlipidaemia, hypothyroidism, leucopenia, headache, oedema, altered liver function, rash, and pruritus. Bexarotene capsules and gel should not be used during pregnancy because of the risk of fetal malformation.

◊ References.
1. Anonymous. Bexarotene (Targretin) for cutaneous T-cell lymphoma. Med Lett Drugs Ther 2000; 42: 31–2.

Preparations

Proprietary Preparations (details are given in Part 3)
USA: Targretin.

Bicalutamide (7259-v)

Bicalutamide (BAN, USAN, rINN).
ICI-176334. (RS)-4'-Cyano-α',α',α'-trifluoro-3-(4-fluorophenyl-sulphonyl)-2-hydroxy-2-methylpropiono-m-toluidide.
$C_{18}H_{14}F_4N_2O_4S = 430.4$.
CAS — 90357-06-5.
ATC — L02BB03.

Adverse Effects and Precautions

As for Flutamide, p.542.

Cardiovascular effects including angina, arrhythmias, and ECG changes have been reported rarely.

◊ There is some evidence that bicalutamide is associated with a lower incidence of diarrhoea than flutamide.[1]

1. Schellhammer P, et al. A controlled trial of bicalutamide versus flutamide, each in combination with luteinizing hormone-releasing hormone analogue therapy, in patients with advanced prostate cancer. Urology 1995; 45: 745–52.

Interactions

As for Flutamide, p.542. Bicalutamide inhibits various cytochrome P450 isoenzymes, particularly CYP3A4, in vitro, and the manufacturer recommends that terfenadine, astemizole and cisapride, or other drugs with a narrow therapeutic index, should not be given with bicalutamide.

Pharmacokinetics

Bicalutamide is well absorbed following oral administration. It undergoes extensive metabolism in the liver, the active R-enantiomer predominantly by oxidation, the inactive S-enantiomer primarily by glucuronidation. It is excreted as metabolites in urine and faeces. The half-life of the R-enantiomer is about 5.8 days, and may be prolonged still further in severe hepatic impairment. The S-enantiomer is cleared more rapidly. Bicalutamide is about 96% bound to plasma proteins.

Uses and Administration

Bicalutamide is a nonsteroidal anti-androgen with actions and uses similar to those of flutamide (p.542). It is used by mouth in the palliative treatment of advanced prostatic cancer (p.497). When used with a gonadorelin analogue the usual dose is 50 mg daily; treatment should be started at least 3 days before commencing the gonadorelin analogue to suppress any flare reaction. A similar dose is used with surgical castration starting on the same day as surgery. Bicalutamide may also be given as monotherapy in men with localised or locally advanced non-metastatic disease at a dose of 150 mg daily.

◊ References.
1. Anonymous. Bicalutamide for prostate cancer. Med Lett Drugs Ther 1996; 38: 56–7.
2. Schellhammer P, et al. A controlled trial of bicalutamide versus flutamide, each in combination with luteinizing hormone-releasing hormone analogue therapy, in patients with advanced prostate cancer. Urology 1995; 45: 745–52.
3. Schellhammer PF, et al. Clinical benefits of bicalutamide compared with flutamide in combined androgen blockade for patients with advanced prostatic carcinoma: final report of a double-blind, randomized, multicenter trial. Urology 1997; 50: 330–6.
4. Iversen P, et al. Casodex (bicalutamide) 150-mg monotherapy compared with castration in patients with previously untreated nonmetastatic prostate cancer: results from two multicenter randomized trials at a median follow-up of 4 years. Urology 1998; 51: 389–96.
5. Goa KL, Spencer CM. Bicalutamide in advanced prostate cancer: a review. Drugs Aging 1998; 12: 401–22.
6. Tyrrell CJ, et al. A randomised comparison of 'Casodex' (bicalutamide) 150 mg monotherapy versus castration in the treatment of metastatic and locally advanced prostate cancer. Eur Urol 1998; 33: 447–56.

Preparations

Proprietary Preparations (details are given in Part 3)
Aust.: Casodex; *Austral.:* Cosudex; *Belg.:* Casodex; *Canad.:* Casodex; *Denm.:* Casodex; *Fin.:* Casodex; *Fr.:* Casodex; *Ger.:* Casodex; *Hong Kong:* Casodex; *Irl.:* Casodex; *Israel:* Casodex; *Ital.:* Casodex; *Mex.:* Casodex; *Neth.:* Casodex; *Norw.:* Casodex; *Port.:* Casodex; *S.Afr.:* Casodex; *Singapore:* Casodex; *Spain:* Casodex; *Swed.:* Casodex; *Switz.:* Casodex; *Thai.:* Casodex; *UK:* Casodex; *USA:* Casodex.

Bisantrene Hydrochloride (18846-h)

Bisantrene Hydrochloride (USAN, rINNM).
ADAH; ADCA; CL-216942; NSC-337766, Orange Crush. 9,10-Anthracenedicarboxaldehyde bis(2-imidazolin-2-ylhydrazone) dihydrochloride.
$C_{22}H_{22}N_8, 2HCl = 471.4$.
CAS — 78186-34-2 (bisantrene); 71439-68-4 (bisantrene hydrochloride).

Profile

Bisantrene is a cell-cycle non-specific antineoplastic agent which is believed to act by intercalation with DNA. It has been used as the hydrochloride in the treatment of acute myeloid leukaemias relapsed or refractory to other therapy.

Bleomycin Sulfate (1815-z)

Bleomycin Sulfate (USAN, pINNM).
Bleomycin Sulphate (BANM); Bleomycini Sulfas.
CAS — 11056-06-7 (bleomycin); 9041-93-4 (bleomycin sulfate).

Pharmacopoeias. In Eur. (see p.vi), Int., Jpn, and US.
Int. and Jpn also include Bleomycin Hydrochloride. Chin. includes Bleomycin Hydrochloride for Injection.

The manufacturers of bleomycin state that it should be protected from light.

Pharmacopoeial description
Ph. Eur.: The sulfate of a mixture of glycopeptides obtained by the growth of *Streptomyces verticillus* or by any other means; the two principal components of the mixture are N^1-[3-(dimethylsulphonio)propyl]bleomycinamide (bleomycin A_2) and N^1-4-(guanidinobutyl)bleomycinamide (bleomycin B_2). A white or yellowish-white, very hygroscopic powder. It loses not more than 3% of its weight when dried. Very soluble in water; slight-

ly soluble in dehydrated alcohol; practically insoluble in acetone and in ether. A 0.5% solution in water has a pH of 4.5 to 6.0. Store in airtight containers at a temperature of 2° to 8°.

USP 25: The sulfate salt of a mixture of basic cytotoxic glycopeptides, produced by the growth of *Streptomyces verticillus* or produced by other means. It has a potency of not less than 1.5 units and not more than 2.0 units per mg. It contains between 55% and 70% of bleomycin A_2 and between 25% and 32% of bleomycin B_2; the content of bleomycin B_4 is not more than 1%. The combined percentage of bleomycin A_2 and B_2 is not less than 90%. A cream-coloured, amorphous powder. It loses no more than 6% of its weight when dried. Very soluble in water. A solution in water containing 10 units per mL has a pH of 4.5 to 6.0. Store in airtight containers.

Incompatibility. Dorr and colleagues have reported a loss of bleomycin activity when bleomycin sulfate solutions were mixed with solutions of carbenicillin, cefazolin or cefalotin sodium, nafcillin sodium, benzylpenicillin sodium, methotrexate, mitomycin, hydrocortisone sodium succinate, aminophylline, ascorbic acid, or terbutaline.[1] D'Arcy has summarised the interactions of bleomycin as the chelation of divalent and trivalent cations (especially copper), inactivation by compounds containing sulfhydryl groups, and precipitation by hydrophobic anions; solutions of bleomycin should not be mixed with solutions of essential amino acids, riboflavin, dexamethasone, or frusemide [furosemide].[2]

1. Dorr RT, et al. Bleomycin compatibility with selected intravenous medications. J Med 1982; **13:** 121–30.
2. D'Arcy PF. Reactions and interactions in handling anticancer drugs. Drug Intell Clin Pharm 1983; **17:** 532–8.

Stability. Bleomycin sulfate appears to be equally stable in plastic or glass,[1,2] despite some earlier studies suggesting loss of potency in plastic.[3,4] There is some evidence[5] that bleomycin is more stable in sodium chloride 0.9% than dextrose 5%, and sodium chloride 0.9% is the diluent recommended by the manufacturer.

1. De Vroe C, et al. A study on the stability of three antineoplastic drugs and on their sorption by iv delivery systems and end-line filters. Int J Pharmaceutics 1990; **65:** 49–56.
2. Stajich GV, et al. In vitro evaluation of bleomycin-induced cell lethality from plastic and glass containers. DICP Ann Pharmacother 1991; **25:** 14–16.
3. Benvenuto JA, et al. Stability and compatibility of antitumor agents in glass and plastic containers. Am J Hosp Pharm 1981; **38:** 1914–18.
4. Adams J, et al. Instability of bleomycin in plastic containers. Am J Hosp Pharm 1982; **39:** 1636.
5. Koberda M, et al. Stability of bleomycin sulfate reconstituted in 5% dextrose injection or 0.9% sodium chloride injection stored in glass vials or polyvinyl chloride containers. Am J Hosp Pharm 1990; **47:** 2528–9.

Units

8910 units of bleomycin complex A_2/B_2 are contained in 5 mg of bleomycin complex in one ampoule of the first International Reference Preparation (1980). The Ph. Eur. specifies a potency of not less than 1500 international units (IU) per mg, calculated with reference to the dried substance. These units differ from those used by the USP: Bleomycin Sulfate (USP 25) contains 1.5 to 2.0 units of bleomycin in each mg. A change in the labelling of preparations in the UK, from units equivalent to those of the USP to international units in line with the Ph. Eur., resulted in an apparent but artefactual increase in UK doses by a factor of 1000.

In some countries doses were *formerly* described in terms of mg-potency, where 1 mg-potency corresponded to 1 unit. In the original preparation 1 mg-potency was equivalent to 1 mg-weight but improvements in purification of the product led to a situation in which ampoules labelled as containing 15 mg (i.e. 15 units) contained far fewer mg-weight of bleomycin.

Adverse Effects and Treatment

For a general outline see Antineoplastics, p.476 and p.479.

The most frequent side-effects with bleomycin involve the skin and mucous membranes and include rash, erythema, pruritus, vesiculation, hyperkeratosis, nail changes, alopecia, hyperpigmentation, striae, and stomatitis. Fever is also common, and acute anaphylactoid reactions with hyperpyrexia and cardiorespiratory collapse have been reported in about 1% of patients with lymphoma. There is little depression of the bone marrow. Local reactions and thrombophlebitis may occur at the site of parenteral administration.

The most serious delayed effect is pulmonary toxicity; interstitial pneumonitis and fibrosis occurs in about 10% of patients and produces an overall mortal-

ity rate of 1% of patients treated with bleomycin (see also Effects on the Lungs, p.478). Pulmonary toxicity is more likely in elderly patients and those given total doses greater than 400 000 IU (400 USP units). It is also more likely in patients who have had previous radiotherapy to the chest. For the suggestion that pulmonary toxicity may be potentiated by concomitant use of cisplatin or colony-stimulating factors, see under Interactions, below.

Effects on the nails. A patient developed blistering and ulceration after injection of bleomycin into periungual warts, and many nails fell off.[1] A previous set of injections, 1 month before, had caused only mild pain. Two years later the patient still had complete loss of the nail in one finger, which had also developed Raynaud's phenomenon, and partial loss of nails on 3 other digits.
1. Czarnecki D. Bleomycin and periungual warts. Med J Aust 1984; **141:** 40.

Effects on the vascular system. Although reports of thromboembolic disorders and Raynaud's syndrome have been associated with use of bleomycin in combination regimens, particularly with cisplatin and the vinca alkaloids (see Effects on the Cardiovascular System, p.477) there is some evidence for an association of Raynaud's syndrome with the use of bleomycin alone.[1,2]
See also Effects on the Nails, above.
1. Sundstrup B. Raynaud's phenomenon after bleomycin treatment. Med J Aust 1978; **2:** 266.
2. Adone R, Arlet P. Bleomycin and Raynaud's phenomenon. Ann Intern Med 1984; **100:** 770.

Precautions

For reference to the precautions necessary with antineoplastics and immunosuppressants, see p.480.

Bleomycin should be used with caution in the elderly, in patients with renal impairment or pulmonary infection or pre-existing impairment of pulmonary function, and in those who have received radiotherapy, particularly to the thorax. Patients should undergo regular chest X-rays. If these show infiltrates, or if basal lung crepitations occur, bleomycin should be stopped.

In view of the risk of an anaphylactoid reaction it has been suggested that patients with lymphomas should receive a test dose of 1000 or 2000 IU (1 or 2 USP units) initially.

AIDS. Cutaneous adverse effects occurred in 12 of 50 patients being treated with bleomycin for AIDS-associated Kaposi's sarcoma and increased in severity until bleomycin was withdrawn.[1] Bleomycin should be stopped in people with AIDS if cutaneous side-effects are seen, and rechallenge should be avoided. However, the incidence of side-effects did not appear to be higher in these patients than in cancer patients, and patients with AIDS seem to be less sensitive to bleomycin than to antibacterials such as co-trimoxazole and penicillins.
1. Caumes E, et al. Cutaneous side-effects of bleomycin in AIDS patients with Kaposi's sarcoma. Lancet 1990; **336:** 1593.

Diving. Since the partial pressure of oxygen in the inspired air of a scuba diver increases with increasing depth, a theoretical possibility exists of a toxic [pulmonary] reaction to oxygen in bleomycin-treated patients who subsequently go diving, and such a risk would increase with the depth and duration of each dive.[1]
1. Zanetti CL. Scuba diving and bleomycin therapy. JAMA 1990; **264:** 2869.

Handling and disposal. *Urine* produced for up to 72 hours after a dose of bleomycin should be handled wearing protective clothing.[1]
1. Harris J, Dodds LJ. Handling waste from patients receiving cytotoxic drugs. Pharm J 1985; **235:** 289–91.

Interactions

For a general outline of antineoplastic drug interactions, see p.481. There may be an increased risk of pulmonary toxicity in patients given bleomycin who receive oxygen, for example as part of a general anaesthetic procedure; a reduction in inspired oxygen concentration is recommended.

Cisplatin. Enhanced pulmonary toxicity, in some cases fatal, has been reported in patients given bleomycin and cisplatin,[1-3] presumably because cisplatin-induced renal failure led to a decrease in bleomycin elimination. It seems reasonable to assume that similar interactions might occur if bleomycin were given with other nephrotoxic agents. It has been suggested that apart from a decrease in bleomycin dosage if nephrotoxicity occurs with such a combination, administration of bleomycin by constant infusion rather than intermittent bolus might increase the therapeutic to toxic ratio.[1]
1. Bennett WM, et al. Fatal pulmonary bleomycin toxicity in cisplatin-induced acute renal failure. Cancer Treat Rep 1980; **64:** 921–4.

2. van Barneveld PWC, et al. Influence of platinum-induced renal toxicity on bleomycin-induced pulmonary toxicity in patients with disseminated testicular carcinoma. Oncology 1984; **41:** 4–7.
3. Brodsky A, et al. Stevens-Johnson syndrome, respiratory distress and acute renal failure due to synergic bleomycin-cisplatin toxicity. J Clin Pharmacol 1989; **29:** 821–3.

Colony-stimulating factors. An increased incidence of pulmonary toxicity has been reported in patients receiving bleomycin as part of the ABVD regimen (with doxorubicin, vinblastine, and dacarbazine) who were given granulocyte colony-stimulating factor to alleviate neutropenia.[1] Another case of rapidly developing and fatal pneumonitis in a patient given BEP (bleomycin, etoposide, and cisplatin) with granulocyte colony-stimulating factor has been reported.[2] However, analysis of two randomised controlled trials failed to show increased pulmonary toxicity when granulocyte colony-stimulating factor was added to bleomycin therapy.[3,4]
1. Matthews JH. Pulmonary toxicity of ABVD chemotherapy and G-CSF in Hodgkin's disease: possible synergy. Lancet 1993; **342:** 988.
2. Dirix LY, et al. Pulmonary toxicity and bleomycin. Lancet 1994; **344:** 56.
3. Bastion Y, et al. Possible toxicity with the association of G-CSF and bleomycin. Lancet 1994; **343:** 1221–2.
4. Bastion Y, Coiffier B. Pulmonary toxicity of bleomycin: is G-CSF a risk factor? Lancet 1994; **344:** 474.

Pharmacokinetics

Bleomycin is thought to be poorly absorbed from the gastrointestinal tract. Following parenteral administration some 60 to 70% of a dose has been reported to be excreted in urine as active drug. Enzymic degradation of bleomycin occurs, primarily in plasma, the liver and other organs, and to a much lesser extent in skin and lungs. Elimination is biphasic: mean initial and terminal half-lives of 0.5 and 4 hours respectively have been reported after an intravenous bolus. Elimination may be more prolonged after intravenous infusion and mean half-lives of 1.3 and 9 hours respectively have been reported. Bleomycin does not cross the blood-brain barrier but appears to cross the placenta.

◊ References.
1. Alberts DS, et al. Bleomycin pharmacokinetics in man I: intravenous administration. Cancer Chemother Pharmacol 1978; **1:** 177–81.
2. Broughton A, et al. Clinical pharmacology of bleomycin following intravenous infusion as determined by radioimmunoassay. Cancer 1977; **40:** 2772–8.
3. Yee GC, et al. Bleomycin disposition in children with cancer. Clin Pharmacol Ther 1983; **33:** 668–73.

Uses and Administration

Bleomycin is an antineoplastic antibiotic which binds to DNA and causes strand scissions. It is widely used to treat malignant disease; particularly squamous cell carcinomas, including those of the cervix and external genitalia, oesophagus, skin, and head and neck; Hodgkin's disease and other lymphomas; malignant neoplasms of the testis, and malignant effusions. It has also been tried in other malignancies, including carcinoma of the bladder, lung, and thyroid, and some sarcomas, including Kaposi's sarcoma.

Bleomycin is often used with other antineoplastics, notably with doxorubicin, vinblastine, and dacarbazine (ABVD) for Hodgkin's disease, and with etoposide and cisplatin (BEP) in testicular tumours. Bleomycin is given by either the intramuscular, intravenous, or subcutaneous route. It may also be given intra-arterially or instilled intrapleurally or intraperitoneally. If intramuscular injections are painful they may be given in a 1% solution of lignocaine [lidocaine].

• *Doses are calculated in terms of units of the base but the* **units** *used for preparations in the UK, which were formerly equivalent to those of the USP, are now international units (IU) equivalent to those of the Ph. Eur. (see Units, above). Since 1000 IU is equivalent to 1 USP unit, UK doses now appear to be 1000 times greater than those previously in use, or than those in use in the USA, and care is recommended in evaluating the literature.*

In the UK the licensed dose as a single agent for **squamous cell** or **testicular tumours** is 15 000 IU (15 USP units) three times a week, or 30 000 IU twice a week, by intramuscular or intravenous injection, although in practice treatment of malignancy will generally be with combination regimens. This may be repeated, at usual intervals of 3 to 4 weeks, up to a total cumulative dose of 500 000 IU. The dose and total cumulative dose should be reduced in those over

60 years of age (see below). Doses should be adjusted according to tolerance, and may need to be adjusted as part of combination chemotherapy. Continuous intravenous infusion at a rate of 15 000 IU per 24 hours for up to 10 days or 30 000 IU per 24 hours for up to 5 days may also be used. In patients with **lymphoma** a dose of 15 000 IU once or twice weekly by intramuscular injection has been suggested, to a total dose of 225 000 IU. Again, dosage should be reduced in older patients and in combination regimens if necessary. In the treatment of **malignant effusions** a solution of 60 000 IU in 100 mL of sodium chloride 0.9% may be instilled into the affected serous cavity. Treatment may be repeated as necessary up to a total cumulative dose of 500 000 IU depending on the patient's age. Local anaesthetics or analgesics are given concomitantly.

In the USA recommended doses for **lymphomas** as well as **squamous cell** and **testicular** neoplasms are 250 to 500 IU per kg body-weight (0.25 to 0.5 USP units per kg), or 10 000 to 20 000 IU per m² body-surface (10 to 20 USP units per m²), given once or twice weekly. A test dose of 1000 or 2000 IU (1 or 2 USP units) initially, or for the first two doses, has been suggested in patients with lymphoma. In patients with Hodgkin's disease, once a 50% response has been achieved it may be maintained with 1000 IU (1 USP unit) of bleomycin daily, or 5000 IU (5 USP units) weekly.

In the UK, manufacturers suggest that a total dose of 500 000 IU (500 USP units) should not be exceeded. Total cumulative dose should not exceed 300 000 IU in those aged 60 to 69 years, 200 000 IU in those 70 to 79, and 100 000 IU in those 80 and over; the weekly dose should be no more than 30 000 and 15 000 IU respectively in the latter 2 groups. In the USA the recommended maximum total dose is 400 000 IU (400 USP units); it is generally agreed that patients receiving 400 000 IU or more are at increased risk of pulmonary toxicity (see Adverse Effects, above).

Dosage should be reduced in patients with renal impairment.

Leucoplakia. Leucoplakia is used to describe a white patch or plaque in the mouth which cannot be otherwise characterised: such lesions are of concern because they may be pre-malignant (see also Malignant Neoplasms of the Head and Neck, p.494). It should be distinguished from oral hairy leucoplakia which is associated with HIV infection. Where active treatment is desirable small, easily accessible lesions can be removed surgically; for the treatment of extensive patches or those in which surgery would be difficult topical bleomycin may be dissolved in dimethyl sulfoxide and applied at a dose of 15 000 IU daily for 10 consecutive days.[1] Clinical response to this form of treatment is good and can give sustained effects on long-term follow-up. Chemoprevention with retinoids or betacarotene is under investigation for patients with leucoplakia.[2]

1. Lamey P-J, Lewis MAO. Oral medicine in practice: white patches. *Br Dent J* 1990; **168:** 147–52.
2. Boyle P, *et al.* Oral cancer: necessity for prevention strategies. *Lancet* 1993; **342:** 1129.

Malignant effusions. Bleomycin is used for the sclerotherapy of malignant pleural and pericardial effusions (p.489).

Malignant neoplasms. Bleomycin is employed in regimens for the management of Hodgkin's disease and non-Hodgkin's lymphomas (see p.487, p.487, and p.488), and for germ-cell tumours of the ovary and testis (see p.496, and p.499), as well as for some other malignancies including those of the head and neck (p.494), and Kaposi's sarcoma (p.501).

Pneumothorax. In a patient with AIDS and *Pneumocystis carinii* pneumonia who developed pneumothorax, instillation of bleomycin into each pleural cavity was successful in resolving the pneumothorax after tetracycline sclerotherapy failed to do so.[1]

1. Hnatiuk OW, *et al.* Bleomycin sclerotherapy for bilateral pneumothoraces in a patient with AIDS. *Ann Intern Med* 1990; **113:** 988–90.

Warts. A number of studies have examined the local use of bleomycin sulfate to treat severe or resistant warts (p.1108) of the common, plane, plantar, eponychial, and mosaic types, usually by intralesional injection.[1-3] At the doses used adverse effects, other than pain at the injection site,[1-3] do not seem to be common; however, nail dystrophy and Raynaud's phenomenon have been reported (see under Effects on the Nails, under Adverse Effects, above). Bleomycin has also been applied as a pressure-sensitive adhesive tape,[4] and various techniques for the improvement of intralesional administration have been investigated.[5,6]

1. Shumack PH, Haddock MJ. Bleomycin: an effective treatment for warts. *Australas J Dermatol* 1979; **20:** 41–2.
2. Bunney MH, *et al.* The treatment of resistant warts with intralesional bleomycin: a controlled clinical trial. *Br J Dermatol* 1984; **111:** 197–207.
3. Munkvad M, *et al.* Locally injected bleomycin in the treatment of warts. *Dermatologica* 1983; **167:** 86–9.
4. Takigawa M, *et al.* Treatment of viral warts with pressure-sensitive adhesive tape containing bleomycin sulfate. *Arch Dermatol* 1985; **121:** 1108.
5. Munn SE, *et al.* A new method of intralesional bleomycin therapy in the treatment of recalcitrant warts. *Br J Dermatol* 1996; **135:** 969–71.
6. van der Velden EM, *et al.* Dermatography with bleomycin as a new treatment for verrucae vulgaris. *Int J Dermatol* 1997; **36:** 145–50.

Preparations

BP 2001: Bleomycin Injection;
USP 25: Bleomycin for Injection.

Proprietary Preparations (details are given in Part 3)
Austral.: Blenoxane; *Braz.:* Blenoxane; *Canad.:* Blenoxane; *Ger.:* Bleo-cell; *Jpn:* Bleo; Bleo-S; *Mex.:* Blanoxan; Bleolem; *NZ:* Blenoxane; *Port.:* Blio; *S.Afr.:* Blenoxane; *Thai.:* Bleolem; *UK:* Bleo; *USA:* Blenoxane.

Brequinar Sodium (1739-t)

Brequinar Sodium (*USAN, rINNM*).
DuP-785; NSC-368390. Sodium 6-fluoro-2-(2'-fluoro-4-biphenylyl)-3-methyl-4-quinolinecarboxylate.
$C_{23}H_{14}F_2NO_2Na = 397.3$.
CAS — 96187-53-0 (brequinar); 96201-88-6 (brequinar sodium).

Profile

Brequinar sodium is an inhibitor of pyrimidine metabolism with potent immunosuppressant properties that has been investigated for the prevention and treatment of rejection episodes following organ and tissue transplantation and for treating various cancers.

◊ References.
1. Arteaga CL, *et al.* Phase I clinical and pharmacokinetic trial of brequinar sodium (DuP-785; NSC-368390). *Cancer Res* 1989; **49:** 4648–53.
2. Murphy MP, Morris RE. Brequinar sodium (Dup 785) is a highly potent antimetabolite immunosuppressant that suppresses heart allograft rejection. *Med Sci Res* 1991; **19:** 835–6.
3. Jaffee BD, *et al.* The unique immunosuppressive activity of brequinar sodium. *Transplant Proc* 1993; **25** (suppl 2): 19–22.
4. Cramer DV. Brequinar sodium. *Transplant Proc* 1996; **28:** 960–3.
5. Joshi AS, *et al.* Phase I safety and pharmacokinetic studies of brequinar sodium after single ascending oral doses in stable renal, hepatic, and cardiac allograft recipients. *J Clin Pharmacol* 1997; **37:** 1121–8.

Bropirimine (18707-j)

Bropirimine (*BAN, USAN, rINN*).
ABPP; U-54461; U-54461S. 2-Amino-5-bromo-6-phenyl-4(3H)-pyrimidinone.
$C_{10}H_8BrN_3O = 266.1$.
CAS — 56741-95-8.

Profile

Bropirimine is reported to have immunomodulatory actions, possibly due to the induction of interferons. It has been investigated in the management of carcinoma in situ of the bladder (p.490).

◊ References.
1. Sarosdy MF, *et al.* Oral bropirimine immunotherapy of bladder carcinoma in situ after prior intravesical bacille Calmette-Guerin. *Urology* 1998; **51:** 226–31.

Broxuridine (1816-c)

Broxuridine (*rINN*).
Bromodeoxyuridine; BUDR; NSC-38297. 5-Bromo-2'-deoxyuridine; 5-Bromo-1-(2-deoxy-β-D-ribofuranosyl)pyrimidine-2,4(1H,3H)-dione.
$C_9H_{11}BrN_2O_5 = 307.1$.
CAS — 59-14-3.

Profile

Broxuridine is a thymidine analogue which acts as a radiosensitiser to enhance the effects of radiotherapy. It is also reported to possess antiviral activity. A related compound brivudine (p.616) is used as an antiviral.

Broxuridine has been given by intra-arterial infusion, in association with radiotherapy and other antineoplastic agents, in the treatment of tumours of the brain, head, and neck. It has also been used diagnostically.

◊ References.
1. Freese A, *et al.* The application of 5-bromodeoxyuridine in the management of CNS tumors. *J Neurooncol* 1994; **20:** 81–95.
2. Phillips TL, *et al.* Results of a randomized comparison of radiotherapy and bromodeoxyuridine with radiotherapy alone for brain metastases: report of RTOG trial 89-05. *Int J Radiat Oncol Biol Phys* 1995; **33:** 339–48.

Busulfan (1817-k)

Busulfan (*BAN, rINN*).
Bussulfam; Busulfanum; Busulphan; CB-2041; GT-41; Myelosan; NSC-750; WR-19508. Tetramethylene di(methanesulphonate); Butane-1,4-diol di(methanesulphonate).
$C_6H_{14}O_6S_2 = 246.3$.
CAS — 55-98-1.
ATC — L01AB01.

Pharmacopoeias. In *Chin., Eur.* (see p.vi), *Int., Jpn, Pol.,* and *US.*

Pharmacopoeial description

Ph. Eur.: A white or almost white, crystalline powder. Very slightly soluble in water, in alcohol, and in ether; freely soluble in acetone and in acetonitrile. Store in airtight containers. Protect from light.

USP 25: A white, crystalline powder. Very slightly soluble in water; slightly soluble in alcohol; soluble 1 in 45 of acetone. Store in airtight containers.

◊ CAUTION. *Busulfan is irritant; avoid contact with skin and mucous membranes.*

Adverse Effects and Treatment

For a general outline see Antineoplastics, p.476 and p.479.

The major side-effect of busulfan with standard doses is bone-marrow depression, manifest as leucopenia, thrombocytopenia, and sometimes, anaemia. The nadir of the granulocyte count usually occurs after about 10 to 30 days with recovery occurring over up to 5 months, but busulfan has sometimes caused irreversible or extremely-prolonged bone-marrow depression.

Hyperpigmentation is common, and in a few cases after long-term therapy may be part of a syndrome simulating Addison's disease.

Rarely, progressive interstitial pulmonary fibrosis, known as 'busulfan lung', can occur on prolonged treatment. Gastrointestinal disturbances are rare at usual therapeutic doses but may be dose-limiting where high doses are given before bone-marrow transplantation. Other rare adverse effects include dry skin and other skin reactions, liver damage, gynaecomastia, cataract formation, and, at high doses, CNS effects including convulsions.

Busulfan may result in impaired fertility and gonadal function. As with other alkylating agents, it is potentially carcinogenic and teratogenic.

Effects on the bladder. Haemorrhagic cystitis occurred in a patient who had received prolonged therapy with busulfan.[1]

1. Pode D, *et al.* Busulfan-induced hemorrhagic cystitis. *J Urol (Baltimore)* 1983; **130:** 347–8.

Effects on the liver. Jaundice in the terminal phase of chronic granulocytic leukaemia in a 31-year-old man was attributed to busulfan which had been taken for 6 years, in a report by Underwood and others.[1] Foadi and colleagues have also reported busulfan toxicity involving the liver in a patient who had taken busulfan for 54 months,[2] while hepatitis possibly associated with busulfan therapy has also been reported by Morris and Guthrie.[3] Dose-dependent veno-occlusive disease has been reported in up to about 20% of patients receiving high-dose busulfan before bone-marrow transplantation.[4]

1. Underwood JCE, *et al.* Jaundice after treatment of leukaemia with busulphan. *BMJ* 1971; **1:** 556–7.
2. Foadi MD, *et al.* Portal hypertension in a patient with chronic myeloid leukaemia. *Postgrad Med J* 1977; **53:** 267–9.
3. Morris L, Guthrie T. Busulfan-induced hepatitis. *Am J Gastroenterol* 1988; **83:** 682–3.
4. Vassal G, *et al.* Busulfan and veno-occlusive disease of the liver. *Ann Intern Med* 1990; **112:** 881.

Effects on the nervous system. High-dose busulfan, used in conditioning regimens for bone-marrow transplantation, has been associated with the development of convulsions,[1-4] both generalised[1,3,4] and myoclonic.[2,4] As a result, the use of prophylactic antiepileptic therapy has been suggested as a component of such regimens.[1,3,4] However, some do not consider the routine use of prophylactic antiepileptics justified,[5] and the potential for phenytoin to increase the metabolism of busulfan, thereby possibly decreasing its myeloablative efficacy, has been pointed out.[6] In addition, phenytoin plasma concentrations have been found to be subtherapeutic in patients who developed convulsions despite a standard prophylactic dose,[4] and the regimen was subsequently adjusted to take account of plasma concentrations. Clobazam has been suggested as an alternative to phenytoin for prophylaxis of busulfan-induced seizures.[7] The UK manufacturer Glaxo Wellcome recommends the use of prophylactic anticonvulsants, and prefers a benzodiazepine to phenytoin. However, Orphan Medical in the USA state that the recommended dose of their parenteral product is based on the use of phenytoin, and that if other anticonvulsants are used a 15% increase in plasma-busulfan may be expected, with increased risk of toxicity.

1. Marcus RE, Goldman JM. Convulsions due to high-dose busulphan. *Lancet* 1984; **ii:** 1463.
2. Martell RW, *et al.* High-dose busulfan and myoclonic epilepsy. *Ann Intern Med* 1987; **106:** 173.
3. Sureda A, *et al.* High-dose busulfan and seizures. *Ann Intern Med* 1989; **111:** 543–4.
4. Grigg AP, *et al.* Busulphan and phenytoin. *Ann Intern Med* 1989; **111:** 1049–50. Correction. *ibid.*; **112:** 313.
5. Hugh-Jones K, Shaw PJ. No convulsions in children on high-dose busulphan. *Lancet* 1985; **i:** 220.
6. Fitzsimmons WE, *et al.* Anticonvulsants and busulfan. *Ann Intern Med* 1990; **112:** 552–3.
7. Schwarer AP, *et al.* Clobazam for seizure prophylaxis during busulfan chemotherapy. *Lancet* 1995; **346:** 1238.

Effects on the skin. For the effect of radiotherapy in activating skin lesions in busulfan-treated patients, see under Precautions, below.

Precautions

For reference to the precautions necessary with antineoplastics and immunosuppressants, see p.480. Careful attention should be given to monitoring blood counts during therapy. These should initially be monitored at least weekly during standard dose therapy. With high dose therapy blood counts should be monitored daily, as should liver function. Prophylactic anticonvulsants should be used during high dose therapy (see Effects on the Nervous System, above).

Busulfan should be discontinued if lung toxicity develops. In patients with possible lung toxicity, the use of oxygen may accentuate this; if anaesthesia is required the concentration of oxygen should be minimised.

Porphyria. Busulfan is considered to be unsafe in patients with porphyria because it has been shown to be porphyrinogenic in *animals.*

Radiotherapy. Severe cutaneous reactions occurred in patients given radiotherapy at least 30 days after combined chemotherapy with high-dose busulfan.[1]

It is possible that subsequent radiotherapy could augment subclinical lung injury caused by busulfan.

1. Vassal G, *et al.* Radiosensitisation after busulfan. *Lancet* 1987; **i:** 571.

Interactions

For a general outline of antineoplastic drug interactions, see p.481. Phenytoin increases the clearance of busulfan (see Effects on the Nervous System, above).

Antifungals. Concomitant administration of *itraconazole* with busulfan resulted in a decrease in the clearance of busulfan; fluconazole had no such effect.[1] Busulfan doses may need to be decreased if itraconazole is given concomitantly.

1. Buggia I, *et al.* Itraconazole can increase systemic exposure to busulfan in patients given bone marrow transplantation. *Anticancer Res* 1996; **16:** 2083–8.

Antineoplastics. *Tioguanine* combined with busulfan has resulted in oesophageal varices and abnormal liver function tests.[1]

1. Key NS, *et al.* Oesophageal varices associated with busulfan-thioguanine combination therapy for chronic myeloid leukaemia. *Lancet* 1987; **ii:** 1050–2.

Interferons. For reports of severe cytopenia in patients receiving busulfan and *interferon alfa,* see p.629.

Pharmacokinetics

Busulfan is readily absorbed from the gastrointestinal tract and rapidly disappears from the blood with a half-life of 2 to 3 hours. It is extensively metabolised, and excreted in the urine almost entirely as sulfur-containing metabolites. It crosses the blood-brain barrier.

◊ Results of a study of the pharmacokinetics of high-dose busulfan in 5 patients receiving 1 mg per kg body-weight by mouth every six hours for 4 days showed that the mean elimination half-life decreased from about 3.4 hours after the first dose to about 2.3 hours after the final dose, suggesting that busulfan may induce its own metabolism.[1]

1. Hassan M, *et al.* Pharmacokinetic and metabolic studies of high-dose busulphan in adults. *Eur J Clin Pharmacol* 1989; **36:** 525–30.

Uses and Administration

Busulfan is an antineoplastic with a cell-cycle nonspecific alkylating action unlike that of the nitrogen mustards, and having a selective depressant action on bone marrow. In small doses, it depresses granulocytopoiesis and to a lesser extent thrombocytopoiesis but has little effect on lymphocytes. With larger dos-

es, severe bone-marrow depression eventually ensues.

Because of its selective action, busulfan has been used in the palliative treatment of chronic myeloid leukaemia (p.486). It provides symptomatic relief with a reduction in spleen size and a general feeling of well-being. The fall in leucocyte count is usually accompanied by a rise in the haemoglobin concentration. Permanent remission is not induced and resistance to its beneficial effects gradually develops.

Busulfan may be used in patients with polycythaemia vera (p.486) and in some patients with myelofibrosis and primary thrombocythaemia (p.486). It is also used at high doses as part of a conditioning regimen to prepare patients for bone-marrow transplantation, a procedure discussed on p.502.

The usual initial dosage of busulfan in **chronic myeloid leukaemia** is 60 µg per kg body-weight daily by mouth, up to a maximum single daily dose of 4 mg. This is continued until the white cell count has fallen to between 15 000 and 25 000 per mm^3 (typically 12 to 20 weeks). It should be discontinued earlier if the platelet count falls below 100 000 per mm^3. Higher doses may be given if the response after 3 weeks is inadequate but this increases the risk of irreversible damage to the bone marrow and calls for special vigilance. Complete blood counts should be made at least every week and the trends followed closely; if haemorrhagic tendencies occur or there is a steep rise in the white cell count indicating severe bone-marrow depression, busulfan should be withdrawn until marrow function has returned.

Once an initial remission has been attained treatment is discontinued and not resumed until the white cell count returns to 50 000 per mm^3. If this occurs within 3 months continuous maintenance treatment with a usual dose of 0.5 to 2 mg daily may be given.

In patients with **polycythaemia vera** the usual dose is 4 to 6 mg daily by mouth, continued for 4 to 6 weeks with careful monitoring of blood counts. Further courses are given when relapse occurs, or alternatively maintenance therapy may be given at half the dose required for induction. Doses of 2 to 4 mg daily have been given for **essential thrombocythaemia** or myelofibrosis.

In conditioning regimens for **bone-marrow transplantation** busulfan has been given in usual doses of 3.5 to 4 mg per kg daily in divided doses for 4 days by mouth (total dose 14 to 16 mg per kg), in association with cyclophosphamide, for ablation of the recipient's bone marrow. When given by intravenous infusion in a regimen with phenytoin (see Effects on the Nervous System, above), a recommended dose is 3.2 mg per kg ideal body-weight daily for 4 days (total dose 12.8 mg per kg); actual body-weight is used for the calculation if it is less than the ideal weight. The daily dose is given as 4 infusions of 0.8 mg per kg at intervals of 6 hours; each dose should be diluted in sodium chloride 0.9% or glucose 5% to a final concentration of about 0.5 mg per mL, and administered over 2 hours using an infusion pump.

◊ References.
1. Buggia I, *et al.* Busulfan. *Ann Pharmacother* 1994; **28:** 1055–62.

Preparations

BP 2001: Busulfan Tablets;
USP 25: Busulfan Tablets.

Proprietary Preparations (details are given in Part 3)
Aust.: Myleran; **Austral.:** Myleran; **Belg.:** Myleran; **Braz.:** Mielucin; Myleran; **Canad.:** Busulfex; Myleran; **Fr.:** Myleran; **Ger.:** Myleran; **Hong Kong:** Myleran; **Irl.:** Myleran; **Israel:** Myleran; **Ital.:** Misulban; Myleran; **Mex.:** Myleran; **Neth.:** Myleran; **Norw.:** Myleran†; **NZ:** Myleran; **Port.:** Myleran; **S.Afr.:** Myleran; **Singapore:** Myleran; **Swed.:** Myleran; **Switz.:** Myleran; **Thai.:** Myleran; **UK:** Myleran; **USA:** Busulfex; Myleran.

Capecitabine (17817-l)

Capecitabine (*BAN, USAN, rINN*).

Ro-09-1978/000. Pentyl 1-(5-deoxy-β-D-ribofuranosyl)-5-fluoro-1,2-dihydro-2-oxo-4-pyrimidinecarbamate.

$C_{15}H_{22}FN_3O_6 = 359.4.$
CAS — 154361-50-9; 158798-73-3.
ATC — L01BC06.

Adverse Effects and Precautions

As for Fluorouracil, p.540. Diarrhoea, nausea and vomiting, stomatitis, palmar-plantar syndrome (erythema and desquamation of hands and feet), dermatitis, and bone-marrow depression have all been reported. Hyperbilirubinaemia has occurred. Capecitabine should be used with care in patients with renal impairment; doses should be reduced in moderate renal impairment and use is contra-indicated in those with severe impairment (creatinine clearance below 30 mL per minute).

Effects on the eyes. A report of severe ocular irritation with corneal deposits and impaired visual acuity in 2 patients who received capecitabine.[1] Symptoms resolved within several weeks of discontinuing the drug.

1. Walkhom B, *et al.* Severe ocular irritation and corneal deposits associated with capecitabine use. *N Engl J Med* 2000; **343:** 740–1.

Interactions

As for Fluorouracil, p.541. The manufacturer has received reports of altered prothrombin times in patients on warfarin given capecitabine.

Pharmacokinetics

Capecitabine is readily absorbed from the gastrointestinal tract, with peak plasma concentrations occurring at about 1.5 hours. Food reduces the rate and extent of absorption. Capecitabine is hydrolysed in the liver to 5'-deoxy-5-fluorocytidine, which is then converted to 5'-deoxy-5-fluorouridine and subsequently to 5-fluorouracil in body tissues. 5-Fluorouracil is further metabolised, as discussed on p.541.

◊ References.
1. Reigner B, *et al.* Effect of food on the pharmacokinetics of capecitabine and its metabolites following oral administration in cancer patients. *Clin Cancer Res* 1998; **4:** 941–8.

Uses and Administration

Capecitabine is a prodrug that is converted to fluorouracil (p.541) in body tissues following oral administration. It is given by mouth for the treatment of metastatic breast and colorectal cancer (p.491 and p.493 respectively). The recommended daily dose is 2.5 g per m^2 body-surface, in 2 divided doses about 12 hours apart with food; doses are given for 2 weeks, followed by a 1-week rest period. Doses should be modified in subsequent cycles according to toxicity. In patients with moderate renal impairment (creatinine clearance 30 to 50 mL per minute) initial doses should be reduced to 1.875 g per m^2 daily. Capecitabine is contra-indicated in patients with more severe renal impairment.

Capecitabine is also under investigation in the treatment of other malignancies.

◊ References.
1. Budman DR, *et al.* Preliminary studies of a novel oral fluoropyrimidine carbamate: capecitabine. *J Clin Oncol* 1998; **16:** 1795–1802.
2. Blum JL, *et al.* Multicenter phase II study of capecitabine in paclitaxel-refractory metastatic breast cancer. *J Clin Oncol* 1999; **17:** 485–93.
3. Hoff PM, *et al.* Comparison of oral capecitabine versus intravenous fluorouracil plus leucovorin as first-line treatment in 605 patients with metastatic colorectal cancer: results of a randomized phase III study. *J Clin Oncol* 2001; **19:** 2282–92.

Preparations

Proprietary Preparations (details are given in Part 3)
Austral.: Xeloda; **Canad.:** Xeloda; **NZ:** Xeloda; **S.Afr.:** Xeloda; **Singapore:** Xeloda; **Switz.:** Xeloda; **Thai.:** Xeloda; **UK:** Xeloda; **USA:** Xeloda.

Caracemide (3408-c)

Caracemide (*USAN, pINN*).

NSC-253272. N-Acetyl-N,O-bis(methylcarbamoyl)hydroxylamine.

$C_6H_{11}N_3O_4 = 189.2.$
CAS — 81424-67-1.

Profile

Caracemide is an inhibitor of nucleic acid and protein synthesis that has been investigated as an antineoplastic.

Carbetimer (3410-w)

Carbetimer (*USAN, pINN*).

Carboxyimamidate; N-137. Maleic anhydride polymer with ethylene, reaction product with ammonia.
CAS — 82230-03-3.

Profile

Carbetimer has been investigated as an antineoplastic.

◊ References.
1. Hanauske AR, *et al.* Phase I clinical trial of carbetimer. *Cancer Res* 1988; **48:** 5353–7.
2. Ardalan B, *et al.* Carbetimer: a re-evaluation of a drug with a novel mechanism of action. *Cancer Treat Rev* 1991; **18:** 73–83.

Carboplatin (16564-f)

Carboplatin (BAN, USAN, rINN).

Carboplatinum; CBDCA; JM-8; NSC-241240. cis-Diammine(cyclobutane-1,1-dicarboxylato)platinum.

$C_6H_{12}N_2O_4Pt = 371.2$.

CAS — 41575-94-4.

ATC — L01XA02.

Pharmacopoeias. In Eur. (see p.vi) and US.

Incompatible with aluminium.

Pharmacopoeial description

Ph. Eur.: A colourless, crystalline powder. Sparingly soluble in water; very slightly soluble in alcohol and in acetone. Protect from light.

USP 25: A 1% solution in water has a pH of 5.0 to 7.0. Store in airtight containers. Protect from light.

Stability. About 5% of the initial carboplatin concentration was lost over 24 hours when solutions were diluted in sodium chloride 0.9% and stored at 25°; lesser degrees of degradation were seen at lower sodium chloride concentrations, but carboplatin was apparently stable over this period if diluted with glucose 5%.[1] The authors suggested that chloride-containing infusion solutions are not suitable for carboplatin, not only because of the loss of active drug but because of the possibility that conversion to cisplatin may be occurring, with a risk of increased toxicity.[1] This has been contested by the manufacturers (Bristol-Myers, USA), who found that only 0.5% or 0.7%, depending on formulation, of a carboplatin solution in sodium chloride 0.9%, had been converted to cisplatin after 24 hours.[2] However, the total degradation of carboplatin was not measured. In another study, Allsopp and colleagues calculated the time to 5% degradation of carboplatin at 25° as 29.2 hours in sodium chloride 0.9% compared with 52.7 hours in water.[3] They concluded that carboplatin should not be diluted in sodium chloride 0.9% when intended for continuous infusion over a prolonged period.[3] Carboplatin in glucose 5% was reported to be stable for 7 days at 25° in polyvinyl chloride bags when protected from light.[4]

1. Cheung Y-W, et al. Stability of cisplatin, iproplatin, carboplatin, and tetraplatin in commonly used intravenous solutions. Am J Hosp Pharm 1987; 44: 124–30.
2. Perrone RK, et al. Extent of cisplatin formation in carboplatin admixtures. Am J Hosp Pharm 1989; 46: 258–9.
3. Allsopp MA, et al. The degradation of carboplatin in aqueous solutions containing chloride or other selected nucleophiles. Int J Pharmaceutics 1991; 69: 197–210.
4. Diaz Amador F, et al. Stability of carboplatin in polyvinyl chloride bags. Am J Health-Syst Pharm 1998; 55: 602, 604.

Adverse Effects, Treatment, and Precautions

As for Cisplatin, p.525; nephrotoxicity and gastrointestinal toxicity are less severe than with cisplatin but it is more myelosuppressive. A reversible myelosuppression is the dose-limiting toxicity; platelet counts reach a nadir between 14 and 21 days after a dose, with recovery within 35 days, but recovery from leucopenia may be slower. Myelosuppression may be more severe and prolonged in patients with impaired renal function. Carboplatin should therefore be given at reduced doses to these patients and should be avoided if creatinine clearance is 20 mL per minute or less. Weekly blood counts and regular renal-function tests are recommended in all patients during therapy. Neurological function including assessment of hearing should also be monitored.

◊ Analysis by the manufacturers of the adverse effects of carboplatin, in studies involving 710 patients.[1] Myelosuppression was the dose-limiting toxicity: leucopenia occurred in 55% of the evaluable patients. Leucopenia and thrombocytopenia result in symptomatic events such as infection or bleeding in a minority of patients. Anaemia was frequent (59%) and required transfusional support in about one-fifth of the patients. Nephrotoxicity and serum electrolyte loss were much less of a problem; no high-volume fluid hydration or electrolyte supplementation was given during treatment. Vomiting occurred in about half the patients, and a further 25% had nausea without vomiting. Peripheral neurotoxicity was reported in 6% of evaluable patients and clinical ototoxicity occurred in only 8 cases (about 1%), but see also Effects on the Ears, below. Increases in liver enzyme values have also been reported, as well as, more rarely, alopecia, skin rash, a flu-like syndrome, and local effects at the injection site.

1. Canetta R, et al. Carboplatin: the clinical spectrum to date. Cancer Treat Rev 1985; 12 (suppl A): 125–36.

Effects on the ears. Carboplatin is less ototoxic than cisplatin, but ototoxicity is still common with carboplatin when used in high doses, for example, as part of conditioning regimens for bone marrow transplantation.[1,2] There was some evidence that sodium thiosulfate reduced carboplatin-induced hearing loss,

when carboplatin was used for CNS malignancy[3] (see also Prophylaxis, under cisplatin, p.525).

1. Freilich RJ, et al. Hearing loss in children with brain tumors treated with cisplatin and carboplatin-based high-dose chemotherapy with autologous bone marrow rescue. Med Pediatr Oncol 1996; 26: 95–100.
2. Parsons SK, et al. Severe ototoxicity following carboplatin-containing conditioning regimen for autologous marrow transplantation for neuroblastoma. Bone Marrow Transplant 1998; 22: 669–74.
3. Neuwelt EA, et al. First evidence of otoprotection against carboplatin-induced hearing loss with a two-compartment system in patients with central nervous system malignancy using sodium thiosulfate. J Pharmacol Exp Ther 1998; 286: 77–84.

Effects on the eyes. Cortical blindness developed in 2 patients with impaired renal function receiving high-dose carboplatin;[1] although 10 cases of visual disturbances in patients receiving carboplatin had been reported to the manufacturers, none of these had sudden blindness and it was thought that the effect represented CNS toxicity in the presence of poor renal excretion. It was concluded that it was unwise to give high-dose carboplatin to patients whose glomerular filtration rate is less than 50 mL per minute.

1. O'Brien MER, et al. Blindness associated with high-dose carboplatin. Lancet 1992; 339: 558.

Effects on the kidneys. Although carboplatin is reported to be much less nephrotoxic than cisplatin it is not devoid of adverse effects on the kidney. Salt wasting nephropathy (similar to that seen with cisplatin),[1] and decreased creatinine clearance[2] and glomerular filtration rate[3] have occurred, as has acute renal failure in 2 patients given intraperitoneal carboplatin[4] (although these patients had been heavily pretreated with cisplatin). It has been suggested that renal toxicity may be more likely at cumulative carboplatin doses of about 750 mg per square metre body-surface or more,[3] and there is some evidence to suggest that intensive hydration may ameliorate nephrotoxic effects.[2]

1. Welborn J, et al. Renal salt wasting and carboplatinum. Ann Intern Med 1988; 108: 640.
2. Reed E, Jacob J. Carboplatin and renal dysfunction. Ann Intern Med 1989; 110: 409.
3. Smit EF, et al. Carboplatin and renal function. Ann Intern Med 1989; 110: 1034.
4. McDonald BR, et al. Acute renal failure associated with the use of intraperitoneal carboplatin: a report of two cases and review of the literature. Am J Med 1991; 90: 386–91.

Hypersensitivity. In one series, 12% of 205 patients treated with carboplatin developed a hypersensitivity reaction after a median of 8 courses of platinum therapy.[1] Symptoms were at least moderately severe in half of the patients. Reactions to cisplatin would be anticipated in patients who have been previously sensitised to carboplatin—for 1 such case see p.526.

1. Markman M, et al. Clinical features of hypersensitivity reactions to carboplatin. J Clin Oncol 1999; 17: 1141–5.

Interactions

As for Cisplatin, p.526.

Pharmacokinetics

Following intravenous administration carboplatin exhibits a biphasic elimination and is excreted primarily in the urine, about 70% of a dose being excreted within 24 hours, almost all unchanged. The terminal half-life of intact carboplatin is reported to be about 3 to 6 hours. Platinum from carboplatin slowly becomes protein bound, and is subsequently excreted with a half-life of 5 days or more.

◊ References.

1. van der Vijgh WJF. Clinical pharmacokinetics of carboplatin. Clin Pharmacokinet 1991; 21: 242–61.

Uses and Administration

Carboplatin is an analogue of cisplatin with similar actions and uses (see p.526). It is used in the treatment of advanced ovarian cancers and of small-cell lung cancer, both alone and combined with other antineoplastics. It has also been tried as an alternative to cisplatin in other solid tumours (see below).

Carboplatin is given by intravenous infusion over 15 minutes to 1 hour. In the UK an initial dose of 400 mg per m² body-surface has been recommended as a single agent in previously untreated patients with normal renal function, reduced by 20 to 25% (300 to 320 mg per m²) in patients who have previously been treated with myelosuppressive therapy or who have poor performance status. In the USA an initial dose of 360 mg per m² has been suggested as a single agent in previously untreated patients with recurrent disease. An initial dose of 300 mg per m² has been suggested when used in combination with cyclophosphamide in previously untreated patients. Dosage adjustments are necessary in patients with renal impairment and when

carboplatin is given as part of a combination regimen. The dose in mg may be calculated using the Calvert formula as described under Administration, below. Subsequent doses should be adjusted according to the nadir of the white-blood cell and platelet counts, and should not be given more frequently than every 4 weeks.

◊ A preliminary review[1] of carboplatin, concluded that it was active in ovarian cancer (p.496), with similar responses to those seen with cisplatin; its activity in small-cell lung cancer (p.496), seminoma, and squamous cell carcinomas of the head and neck seemed likely to be comparable, whereas results in gastrointestinal and breast cancers, lymphoma and leukaemias, melanoma, mesothelioma, renal carcinoma, and sarcoma were, generally unimpressive. A subsequent review[2] suggested that in testicular cancer, where there was a prospect of cure, cisplatin, which appeared to give better results in some studies should be preferred. However, in ovarian cancer, where treatment was largely palliative, carboplatin had the advantage of being better tolerated. A further review[3] of randomised studies concurred that carboplatin was equivalent to cisplatin in suboptimally debulked ovarian cancer and extensive-stage small-cell lung cancer, and was inferior to cisplatin in testicular cancer. It was also concluded that carboplatin was inferior to cisplatin in head and neck and oesophageal cancers. There was insufficient comparative evidence for other cancers for which cisplatin has a role.

1. Wagstaff AJ, et al. Carboplatin: a preliminary review of its pharmacodynamic and pharmacokinetic properties and therapeutic efficacy in the treatment of cancer. Drugs 1989; 37: 162–90.
2. Anonymous. Cisplatin or carboplatin for ovarian and testicular cancer? Drug Ther Bull 1994; 32: 62–3.
3. Go RS, Adjei AA. Review of the comparative pharmacology and clinical activity of cisplatin and carboplatin. J Clin Oncol 1999; 17: 409–22.

Administration. Pharmacokinetic studies by Calvert and colleagues[1] have indicated that the dose of carboplatin to produce a desired area under the concentration-time curve (AUC) could be calculated, based on the patient's glomerular filtration rate (GFR), as:

$$\text{Dose in mg} = \text{target AUC} \times (\text{GFR} + 25)$$

It should be noted that the resultant dose is given in mg and not in mg per m² body-surface. This formula was found to be useful in patients with higher than normal as well as reduced GFR. Suggested target AUCs were 5 mg per mL per minute in previously treated patients and 7 mg per mL per minute in those who had not previously received chemotherapy. In combination therapy the appropriate AUC value depended on the other drugs used: an AUC of 4.5 mg per mL per minute gave acceptable results when carboplatin was combined with bleomycin and etoposide for testicular teratoma.

However, determination of GFR may be a problem: clearance of technetium-99m-labelled diethylenetriamine penta-acetic acid (DTPA) or chromium-51-labelled edetic acid is more accurate than 24-hour creatinine clearance, with the first of these more convenient than the second.[2] (It has been suggested that creatinine clearance should not be used to estimate GFR for the Calvert equation.[3]) Nonetheless, radioisotopic determination of GFR is still an elaborate procedure, and may be less accurate in children than adults.[4] Chatelut and colleagues have proposed formulae for determining clearance of carboplatin in both adults[5] and children.[4]

It has been suggested that the Calvert and Chatelut formulae are not sufficiently accurate for use in children, or in adults with very severe renal impairment. Bayesian methods are the technique of choice where serum carboplatin concentrations can be monitored.[3] However, a study in children showed that dosage based on determination of the GFR results in more consistent carboplatin exposure than administration based on body-surface area.[6]

1. Calvert AH, et al. Carboplatin dosage: prospective evaluation of a simple formula based on renal function. J Clin Oncol 1989; 7: 1748–56.
2. Millward MJ, et al. Carboplatin dosing based on measurement of renal function—experience at the Peter MacCallum Cancer Institute. Aust N Z J Med 1996; 26: 372–9.
3. Duffull SB, Robinson BA. Clinical pharmacokinetics and dose optimisation of carboplatin. Clin Pharmacokinet 1997; 33: 161–83.
4. Chatelut E, et al. Population pharmacokinetics of carboplatin in children. Clin Pharmacol Ther 1996; 59: 436–43.
5. Chatelut E, et al. Prediction of carboplatin clearance from standard morphological and biological patient characteristics. J Natl Cancer Inst 1995; 87: 573–80.
6. Thomas H, et al. Prospective validation of renal-function-based carboplatin dosing in children with cancer: a United Kingdom Children's Cancer Study Group Trial. J Clin Oncol 2000; 18: 3614–21.

Preparations

BP 2001: Carboplatin Injection;
USP 25: Carboplatin for Injection.

Proprietary Preparations (details are given in Part 3)
Aust.: Carbosol; Paraplatin; **Belg.:** Paraplatin; **Braz.:** Paraplatin; **Canad.:** Paraplatin; **Denm.:** Carbosin; Paraplatin; **Fin.:** Carbosin; Paraplatin; **Fr.:** Paraplatine; **Ger.:** Carboplat; Ribocarbo; **Hong Kong:** Paraplatin; **Irl.:** Paraplatin; **Israel:** Paraplatin; **Ital.:** Paraplatin; **Mex.:** Blastocarb; Carboplat; Carbotec; Displata; Novoplat; Paraplatin; **Neth.:** Paraplatin; **Norw.:** Carbosin; Paraplatin; **NZ:** Carbosin; Paraplatin; **Port.:** Nealorin; Novoplatinum; **S.Afr.:** Car-

The symbol † denotes a preparation no longer actively marketed

bosin; Paraplatin; *Spain:* Ercar; Nealorin; Paraplatin; Platinwas; *Swed.:* Paraplatin; *Switz.:* Paraplatine; *Thai.:* Carbosin; Kemocarb; Paraplatin; *UK:* Paraplatin; *USA:* Paraplatin.

Carboquone (1818-a)

Carboquone (rINN).

Carbazilquinone. 2,5-Bis(aziridin-1-yl)-3-(2-hydroxy-1-methoxyethyl)-6-methyl-*p*-benzoquinone carbamate.

$C_{15}H_{19}N_3O_5 = 321.3$.

CAS — 24279-91-2.
ATC — L01AC03.

Profile

Carboquone is an alkylating agent that has been used in the treatment of a variety of malignant neoplasms including those of the lung, stomach, and ovary; it has also been used in lymphomas and in chronic myeloid leukaemia. It has been given by the intravenous or intra-arterial route, or by mouth.

Preparations

Proprietary Preparations (details are given in Part 3)
Jpn: Esquinon†.

Carmofur (18912-t)

Carmofur (rINN).

HCFU. 5-Fluoro-*N*-hexyl-3,4-dihydro-2,4-dioxo-1-(2*H*)-pyrimidinecarboxamide.

$C_{11}H_{16}FN_3O_3 = 257.3$.

CAS — 61422-45-5.
ATC — L01BC04.

Pharmacopoeias. In Jpn.

Profile

Carmofur is an orally active derivative of fluorouracil (p.540) and has similar actions. It is used in the adjuvant treatment of colorectal cancer. Carmofur has been associated with the development of neurological disorders including leucoencephalopathy.

◊ References.

1. Yamada T, *et al.* Leukoencephalopathy following treatment with carmofur: a case report and review of the Japanese literature. *Asia Oceania J Obstet Gynaecol* 1989; **15:** 161–8.
2. Sugimachi K, *et al.* Postoperative chemotherapy for colorectal cancer by combining 5-fluorouracil infusion and 1-hexylcarbamoyl-5-fluorouracil administration after curative resection. *Cancer* 1996; **77:** 36–43.

Preparations

Proprietary Preparations (details are given in Part 3)
Fin.: Mirafur.

Carmustine (1819-t)

Carmustine (BAN, USAN, rINN).

BCNU; BiCNU; Carmustinum; NSC-409962; WR-139021. 1,3-Bis(2-chloroethyl)-1-nitrosourea.

$C_5H_9Cl_2N_3O_2 = 214.0$.

CAS — 154-93-8.
ATC — L01AD01.

Pharmacopoeias. In Eur. (see p.vi).

Pharmacopoeial description

Ph. Eur.: A yellowish, granular powder. Very slightly soluble in water; freely soluble in dehydrated alcohol; very soluble in dichloromethane and in ether. It melts at about 31° with decomposition. Store at a temperature of 2° to 8° in airtight containers. Protect from light.

Stability. The manufacturers state that, when reconstituted, resulting carmustine solutions (undiluted or further diluted in sodium chloride 0.9% or glucose 5%) are stable for 8 hours at room temperature, or 24 hours at 2° to 8°, when protected from light. There is some evidence that carmustine interacts with plastic giving sets and containers, and the manufacturer recommends the use of polythene or glass.

A study by Colvin and colleagues has indicated that diluted solutions of carmustine undergo increased degradation in the presence of sodium bicarbonate, with only 73% of the original concentration of carmustine remaining after 90 minutes, much of the loss being in the first 15 minutes.[1]

1. Colvin M, *et al.* Stability of carmustine in the presence of sodium bicarbonate. *Am J Hosp Pharm* 1980; **37:** 677–8.

Adverse Effects and Treatment

For a general outline see Antineoplastics, p.476 and p.479. Delayed and cumulative bone-marrow depression is the most frequent and serious side-effect of intravenous carmustine. Platelets and leucocytes are mainly affected with platelet nadirs occurring at 4 to 5 weeks after administration and leucocyte nadirs at 5 to 6 weeks after administration; although thrombocytopenia is usually more severe, leucopenia may also be dose-limiting. Other side-effects include pulmo-

nary fibrosis (mainly but not exclusively at high cumulative doses—see also Effects on the Lungs, p.478), renal and hepatic damage, and optic neuritis. Nausea and vomiting, beginning up to 2 hours after a dose, is common but can be reduced by prophylactic antiemetic therapy. Venous irritation may follow intravenous injection and transient hyperpigmentation has been noted after contact of a solution with the skin. Flushing of the skin and suffusion of the conjunctiva may occur following rapid intravenous infusion.

Convulsions, cerebral oedema, and various neurological symptoms have been reported in patients given carmustine-containing polymer implants; abnormalities of wound healing at the site of implantation, and an increased incidence of intracranial infection have also been reported.

As with other alkylating agents, carmustine is potentially carcinogenic, mutagenic, and teratogenic.

Effects on the eyes. Ocular toxicity has been reported in patients receiving carmustine,[1,2] and seems to be more likely following administration into the carotid artery,[1,2] although it was also seen following high-dose intravenous therapy. There is some evidence that the alcohol diluent used to prepare carmustine solutions may contribute to the retinopathy.[2]

1. Shingleton BJ, *et al.* Ocular toxicity associated with high-dose carmustine. *Arch Ophthalmol* 1982; **100:** 1766–72.
2. Greenberg HS, *et al.* Intra-arterial BCNU chemotherapy for treatment of malignant gliomas of the central nervous system. *J Neurosurg* 1984; **61:** 423–9.

Extravasation. For mention of the use of sodium bicarbonate as a specific antidote following carmustine extravasation, see under Treatment of Adverse Effects of Antineoplastics, p.480.

Precautions

For reference to the precautions necessary with antineoplastics and immunosuppressants, see p.480. Carmustine should be used with extreme caution in children, who are at particular risk of severe delayed pulmonary toxicity. It should also be used with caution in patients with reduced lung function. Lung function should be monitored before and frequently during therapy. Blood counts should be monitored weekly during therapy, and for at least 6 weeks after the last dose. Renal and hepatic function should also be monitored periodically.

Handling and disposal. Carmustine has been shown to permeate latex, PVC, and rubber gloves, the degree of permeation tending to increase with time,[1,2] up to an equilibrium value.[2] The permeation rate appears not to depend solely on glove thickness and material, and may be different for different gloves made from the same material.[2] The time for initial penetration was reported to vary between 4.7 and 66.0 minutes in one study,[2] and gloves could be chosen accordingly depending on the anticipated length of exposure. Double-gloving, particularly with thicker PVC gloves, may offer some additional protection.[1]

1. Connor TH, *et al.* Permeability of latex and polyvinyl chloride gloves to carmustine. *Am J Hosp Pharm* 1984; **41:** 676–9.
2. Thomas PH, Fenton-May V. Protection offered by various gloves to carmustine exposure. *Pharm J* 1987; **238:** 775–7.

Interactions

For a general outline of antineoplastic drug interactions, see p.481.

Cimetidine. Reductions in white cell counts and platelet counts well below those normally attributed to treatment with carmustine alone were seen in 6 of 8 patients receiving their first course of carmustine and steroids in association with cimetidine given prophylactically,[1] and in 9 patients in a further study.[2]

1. Selker RG, *et al.* Bone-marrow depression with cimetidine plus carmustine. *N Engl J Med* 1978; **299:** 834.
2. Volkin RL, *et al.* Potentiation of carmustine-cranial irradiation-induced myelosuppression by cimetidine. *Arch Intern Med* 1982; **142:** 243–5.

Pharmacokinetics

Following intravenous administration, carmustine is rapidly metabolised, and no intact drug is detectable after 15 minutes; metabolites have a much longer half-life and are presumed to be responsible for its activity. It is primarily excreted in the urine; some is also excreted as carbon dioxide, via the lungs. Carmustine readily crosses the blood-brain barrier, appearing in cerebrospinal fluid in substantial concentrations almost immediately after intravenous injection.

Uses and Administration

Carmustine is a cell-cycle phase non-specific antineoplastic belonging to the nitrosourea group of compounds, which are considered to function as alkylating agents. It is used in the treatment of brain tumours, and in combination chemotherapy for multiple myeloma, and may be given as second-line therapy in Hodgkin's disease, and some other malignancies (see below).

Carmustine is given by intravenous infusion over 1 to 2 hours in sodium chloride 0.9% or glucose 5%, either as a single dose of 150 to 200 mg per m² body-surface or divided into doses of 75 to 100 mg per m² given on 2 successive days. Lower doses are usually given in combination therapy, except for conditioning before stem-cell transplantation. Doses may be repeated every 6 weeks provided that blood counts have returned to acceptable levels. Subsequent doses must be adjusted according to the haematological response.

Polymer implants containing carmustine have been developed for implantation into the brain in the localised treatment of malignant glioma. Each implant contains 7.7 mg of carmustine: up to 8 such implants are inserted into the cavity left by surgical removal of the tumour.

Administration. In a multicentre study[1] in patients with recurrent malignant glioma, biodegradable poly(carboxyphenoxypropane/sebacic acid)anhydride polymer (BIODEL) wafers containing carmustine 7.7 mg or placebo were implanted into the brain after tumour resection to a maximum dose of 8 wafers. The effects of treatment favoured the carmustine implant; 59 of 112 patients given placebo implants were dead at 6 months, compared with 44 of 110 given carmustine implants, with a median survival of 23 and 31 weeks, respectively.

1. Brem H, *et al.* Placebo-controlled trial of safety and efficacy of intraoperative controlled delivery by biodegradable polymers of chemotherapy for recurrent gliomas. *Lancet* 1995; **345:** 1008–12.

Amyloidosis. For mention of chemotherapy with epirubicin, cyclophosphamide, and carmustine to suppress amyloidosis after cardiac transplantation, see p.501.

Malignant neoplasms. Carmustine has been used in chemotherapeutic regimens for a number of malignancies. Because of its ability to pass the blood-brain barrier it has been extensively used in malignant neoplasms of the brain, the management of which is discussed further on p.490. Other conditions in which it has been employed, include malignant melanoma (p.499), Hodgkin's disease (p.487), and multiple myeloma (p.489).

Mycosis fungoides. Topical application of carmustine has been used successfully[1-3] in early mycosis fungoides (p.489). Erythema and telangiectasia were the most frequent side-effects.

1. Zackheim HS, *et al.* Topical carmustine (BCNU) for mycosis fungoides and related disorders: a 10-year experience. *J Am Acad Dermatol* 1983; **9:** 363–74.
2. Zackheim HS, *et al.* Topical carmustine (BCNU) for cutaneous T cell lymphoma: a 15-year experience in 143 patients. *J Am Acad Dermatol* 1990; **22:** 802–10.
3. Zackheim HS. Topical carmustine (BCNU) for patch/plaque mycosis fungoides. *Semin Dermatol* 1994; **13:** 202–6.

Preparations

Proprietary Preparations (details are given in Part 3)
Aust.: Carmubris; *Austral.:* BiCNU; *Belg.:* Becenun; *Canad.:* BiCNU; Gliadel; *Denm.:* Becenun†; *Fr.:* BiCNU; Gliadel; *Ger.:* Carmubris; *Hong Kong:* BiCNU; *Irl.:* BiCNU; *Israel:* BiCNU; Gliadel; *Mex.:* BiCNU; *Norw.:* Becenun†; *NZ:* BiCNU; Gliadel; *Port.:* Gliadel; *S.Afr.:* BiCNU; *Singapore:* BiCNU; Gliadel; *Spain:* Nitrourean; *Swed.:* Becenun†; *Thai.:* BiCNU; *UK:* BiCNU; *USA:* BiCNU; Gliadel.

Chlorambucil (1820-l)

Chlorambucil (BAN, rINN).

CB-1348; Chlorambucilum; Chloraminophene; Chlorbutinum; NSC-3088; WR-139013. 4-[4-Bis(2-chloroethyl)aminophenyl]butyric acid.

$C_{14}H_{19}Cl_2NO_2 = 304.2$.

CAS — 305-03-3.
ATC — L01AA02.

Pharmacopoeias. In Eur. (see p.vi), Int., Pol., and US.

In the UK, the manufacturers recommend that tablets of chlorambucil be stored at 2° to 8° and kept dry. In the USA, the manufacturer recommends they be stored at 15° to 25° in a dry place.

Pharmacopoeial description

Ph. Eur.: A white, crystalline powder. Practically insoluble in water; freely soluble in alcohol and in acetone. Protect from light.

USP 25: An off-white, slightly granular powder. M.p. 65° to 69°. Very slightly soluble in water; soluble 1 in 2 of acetone; soluble in dilute alkali. Store in airtight containers. Protect from light.

◊ CAUTION. *Chlorambucil is irritant; avoid contact with skin and mucous membranes.*

Adverse Effects and Treatment

For a general outline see Antineoplastics, p.476 and p.479.

A reversible progressive lymphocytopenia tends to develop during treatment with chlorambucil. Neutropenia may continue to develop up to 10 days after the last dose. Irreversible bone-marrow depression can occur particularly when the total dosage for the course approaches 6.5 mg per kg body-weight.

Other reported adverse effects include gastrointestinal disturbances, hepatotoxicity, skin rashes (rarely Stevens-Johnson syndrome or toxic epidermal necrolysis), peripheral neuropathy, and central neurotoxicity, including seizures. Interstitial pneumonia and pulmonary fibrosis have occurred; the latter is usually reversible but fatalities have been recorded. Chlorambucil in high doses may produce azoospermia and amenorrhoea; sterility has developed particularly when chlorambucil has been given to boys at or before puberty.

Overdosage may result in pancytopenia and in neurotoxicity, including agitation, ataxia, and grand mal seizures.

Like other alkylating agents, chlorambucil is potentially mutagenic, teratogenic, and carcinogenic, and an increased incidence of acute leukaemias and other secondary malignancies has been reported in patients who have received the drug.

Effects on the bladder. Chlorambucil-induced cystitis was reported in a 73-year-old woman given 2 mg daily for over 2 years for the treatment of lymphocytic lymphoma.[1]
1. Daoud D, *et al.* Sterile cystitis associated with chlorambucil. *Drug Intell Clin Pharm* 1977; **11:** 491.

Effects on the eyes. Visual impairment and optic atrophy in a patient who had been receiving chlorambucil for five years to control non-Hodgkin's lymphoma were thought to be due to the drug,[1] although ocular effects are extremely rare with chlorambucil.
1. Yiannakis PH, Larner AJ. Visual failure and optic atrophy associated with chlorambucil therapy. *BMJ* 1993; **306:** 109.

Effects on mental function. CNS toxicity, manifesting as lethargy, confusion, coma, convulsions, restlessness, and hallucinations, was dose-limiting in 4 of 30 patients in a phase-I study of high-dose chlorambucil.[1]
1. Blumenreich MS, *et al.* A phase I trial of chlorambucil administered in short pulses in patients with advanced malignancies. *Cancer Invest* 1988; **6:** 371–5.

Precautions

For reference to the precautions necessary with antineoplastics and immunosuppressants, see p.480. Chlorambucil should not be administered, or should be given with great care and at reduced doses, for at least 4 weeks after treatment with radiotherapy or other antineoplastic agents unless only low doses of radiation have been given to parts remote from the bone marrow and the neutrophil and platelet counts are not depressed. The dose should be reduced if there is lymphocytic involvement of the bone marrow or if it is hypoplastic. Chlorambucil should be given with care to patients with impaired renal function; the manufacturers state that consideration should also be given to dose reduction in patients with gross hepatic dysfunction. Regular blood counts are required during therapy.

Handling and disposal. Urine produced for up to 48 hours after a dose of chlorambucil should be handled wearing protective clothing.[1]
1. Harris J, Dodds LJ. Handling waste from patients receiving cytotoxic drugs. *Pharm J* 1985; **235:** 289–91.

Porphyria. Chlorambucil is considered to be unsafe in patients with porphyria because it has been shown to be porphyrinogenic in *animals.*

The symbol † denotes a preparation no longer actively marketed

Interactions

For a general outline of antineoplastic and immunosuppressant drug interactions, see p.481.

Pharmacokinetics

Chlorambucil is rapidly and almost completely absorbed from the gastrointestinal tract following oral doses and is reported to have a terminal half-life in plasma of about 1.5 hours. It is extensively metabolised in the liver, primarily to active phenylacetic acid mustard, which has a slightly longer plasma half-life of about 2.5 hours, and which like chlorambucil also undergoes some spontaneous degradation to further derivatives. Chlorambucil and its metabolites are extensively protein bound. It is excreted in the urine almost entirely as metabolites with less than 1% unchanged.

Uses and Administration

Chlorambucil is an antineoplastic derived from mustine [chlormethine] (p.561) and has a similar mode of action. It acts on lymphocytes and to a lesser extent on neutrophils and platelets. Chlorambucil is most valuable in those conditions associated with the proliferation of white blood cells, especially lymphocytes, and is used in the treatment of chronic lymphocytic leukaemia and lymphomas, including Hodgkin's disease. It is also used in Waldenström's macroglobulinaemia and has been given in hairy-cell leukaemia, carcinoma of the breast and ovary and gestational trophoblastic tumours. Although formerly widely used in the management of polycythaemia vera it has largely been superseded.

Chlorambucil also has immunosuppressant properties and has been given in various auto-immune disorders including amyloidosis, Behçet's syndrome, glomerular kidney disease, primary biliary cirrhosis, polymyositis, rheumatoid arthritis, and sarcoidosis.

The use of chlorambucil in these disorders is discussed further elsewhere, as indicated by the cross-references given below.

Chlorambucil is better tolerated than mustine [chlormethine] hydrochloride and serious bone-marrow toxicity is not usually a problem with normal doses. When used as an antineoplastic, chlorambucil is administered by mouth in usual initial doses of 100 to 200 µg per kg body-weight daily (usually 4 to 10 mg once daily), for 4 to 8 weeks. A dose of 100 µg per kg daily may be adequate for the treatment of non-Hodgkin's lymphoma; 150 µg per kg daily until the total leukocyte count falls below 10 000 per mm³ may be used in chronic lymphocytic leukaemia; and in Hodgkin's disease, 200 µg per kg daily is usually required. Lower doses may be given as part of a combination regimen. If lymphocytic infiltration of the bone marrow is present or if the bone marrow is hypoplastic, the daily dose should not exceed 100 µg per kg. Alternatively, high-dose chlorambucil may be given intermittently. For example, in chronic lymphocytic leukaemia it may be given in an initial single dose of 400 µg per kg increased by 100 µg per kg at each 2- or 4-week dose interval until control of lymphocytosis is achieved or toxicity occurs.

Once a remission has been established the patient may receive continuous maintenance with 30 to 100 µg per kg body-weight daily. However, short intermittent courses appear to be safer and are generally preferred for maintenance.

In patients with Waldenström's macroglobulinaemia chlorambucil may be given in an initial dose of 6 to 12 mg daily by mouth until leucopenia develops. Maintenance therapy with doses of 2 to 8 mg daily may then be given indefinitely.

Total and differential white cell counts and haemoglobin examinations are recommended each week during treatment with chlorambucil.

Amyloidosis. Chlorambucil may be of use in preserving kidney function in patients with amyloidosis,[1,2] the management of which is discussed in more detail on p.501.
1. Bergland K, *et al.* Alkylating cytostatic treatment in renal amyloidosis secondary to rheumatic disease. *Ann Rheum Dis* 1987; **46:** 757–62.
2. David J, Woo P. Reactive amyloidosis. *Arch Dis Child* 1992; **67:** 258–61.

Connective-tissue and muscular disorders. Chlorambucil has been used as a corticosteroid-sparing agent in patients with Behçet's syndrome (p.1047). It has occasionally been tried in polymyositis (p.1057). In both these conditions, the potential benefits must be weighed against the possibility of toxicity.

Kidney disorders, non-malignant. Chlorambucil has been used in some forms of glomerular kidney disease (p.1051). In minimal change nephropathy, in which cytotoxics are reserved for the most severe cases because of fears about toxicity, cyclophosphamide is generally preferred to chlorambucil because it is perceived as entailing somewhat less risk, but chlorambucil has been used with corticosteroids in patients with membranous nephropathy.[1-3]
1. Ponticelli C, *et al.* Methylprednisolone plus chlorambucil as compared with methylprednisolone alone for the treatment of idiopathic membranous nephropathy. *N Engl J Med* 1992; **327:** 599–603.
2. Reichert LJM, *et al.* Preserving renal function in patients with membranous nephropathy: daily oral chlorambucil compared with intermittent monthly pulses of cyclophosphamide. *Ann Intern Med* 1994; **121:** 328–33.
3. Ponticelli C, *et al.* A 10-year follow-up of a randomized study with methylprednisolone and chlorambucil in membranous nephropathy. *Kidney Int* 1995; **48:** 1600–4.

Liver disorders, non-malignant. No treatment has proven unequivocally successful in the management of primary biliary cirrhosis (p.501). Chlorambucil is one of a number of agents for which reports of benefit exist.[1]
1. Hoofnagle JH, *et al.* Randomized trial of chlorambucil for primary biliary cirrhosis. *Gastroenterology* 1986; **91:** 1327–34.

Malignant neoplasms. Chlorambucil is used in the management of a number of haematological malignancies including chronic lymphocytic leukaemia (p.485), Hodgkin's disease (p.487), indolent low-grade non-Hodgkin's lymphoma (p.487), and Waldenström's macroglobulinaemia (p.489). It was formerly used in polycythaemia vera (p.486) but is now largely superseded. Chlorambucil may also be used in malignant neoplasms of the ovary (p.496).

Ocular disorders, non-malignant. As mentioned on p.502 chlorambucil is one of the immunosuppressants that may be considered for patients with uveitis or scleritis unresponsive to corticosteroids in tolerable doses.

Rheumatoid arthritis. Chlorambucil has been used for its immunosuppressant properties in a few patients with severe rheumatoid arthritis (especially with vasculitis) who have failed to respond to other drugs. However the use of cytotoxic immunosuppressants other than methotrexate is considered debatable, as mentioned in the discussion of rheumatoid arthritis on p.9.

Sarcoidosis. Where drug therapy is required for sarcoidosis (p.1058), corticosteroids are the usual treatment. Chlorambucil is one of a number of cytotoxic immunosuppressants that have been tried, with variable results, as a second-line therapy.

Preparations

BP 2001: Chlorambucil Tablets;
USP 25: Chlorambucil Tablets.

Proprietary Preparations (details are given in Part 3)
Aust.: Leukeran; *Austral.:* Leukeran; *Belg.:* Leukeran; *Braz.:* Leukeran; *Canad.:* Leukeran; *Denm.:* Leukeran; *Fin.:* Leukeran; *Ger.:* Leukeran; *Hong Kong:* Leukeran; *Irl.:* Leukeran; *Israel:* Leukeran; *Ital.:* Leukeran; Linfolysin; *Mex.:* Leukeran; *Mon.:* Chloraminophene; *Neth.:* Leukeran; *Norw.:* Leukeran; *NZ:* Leukeran; *Port.:* Leukeran; *S.Afr.:* Leukeran; *Singapore:* Leukeran; *Spain:* Leukeran; *Swed.:* Leukeran; *Switz.:* Leukeran; *Thai.:* Leukeran; *UK:* Leukeran; *USA:* Leukeran.

Chlorozotocin (1821-y)

DCNU; NSC-178248. 2-[3-(2-Chloroethyl)-3-nitrosoureido]-2-deoxy-D-glucopyranose.
$C_9H_{16}ClN_3O_7 = 313.7$.
CAS — 54749-90-5.

Profile

Chlorozotocin is an analogue of the antineoplastic streptozocin (p.569) and has been reported to have little diabetogenic effect. It has been tried as an antineoplastic, notably in pancreatic endocrine tumours (p.483). Renal toxicity has occurred.

◊ References.
1. Baker JJ, *et al.* Renal-failure anemia and nitrosourea therapy. *N Engl J Med* 1979; **301:** 662.
2. Bukowski RM, *et al.* Phase II trial of chlorozotocin and fluorouracil in islet cell carcinoma: a Southwest Oncology Group study. *J Clin Oncol* 1992; **10:** 1914–8.

Chromomycin (18961-v)

CAS — 7059-24-7 (chromomycin A₃).

Profile

Chromomycin is an antibiotic complex produced by *Streptomyces griseus* and comprising chiefly chromomycin A_3 (aburamycin B; toyomycin). It has been given parenterally for its antineoplastic properties in the management of malignant neoplasms. Nephrotoxicity, hypocalcaemia, liver disorders, and thrombophlebitis are among the adverse effects reported.

Ciclosporin (1882-m)

Ciclosporin (*rINN*).

27-400; Ciclosporinum; Cyclosporin (*BAN*); Cyclosporin A; Cyclosporine (*USAN*); OL-27-400. Cyclo[-[4-(*E*)-but-2-enyl-*N*,4-dimethyl-L-threonyl]-L-homoalanyl-(*N*-methylglycyl)-(*N*-methyl-L-leucyl)-L-valyl-(*N*-methyl-L-leucyl)-L-alanyl-D-alanyl-(*N*-methyl-L-leucyl)-(*N*-methyl-L-leucyl)-(*N*-methyl-L-valyl)-].

$C_{62}H_{111}N_{11}O_{12} = 1202.6$.

CAS — 59865-13-3.

ATC — L04AA01.

Pharmacopoeias. In Eur. (see p.vi), Jpn, and US.

Pharmacopoeial description

Ph. Eur.: A substance produced by *Beauveria nivea* (=*Tolypocladium inflatum* Gams) or obtained by any other means. A white or almost white powder; practically insoluble in water; freely soluble in dehydrated alcohol and in dichloromethane. Store in airtight containers. Protect from light.

USP 25: A white to almost white powder. Practically insoluble in water; soluble in alcohol, in acetone, in chloroform, in dichloromethane, in ether, and in methyl alcohol; slightly soluble in saturated hydrocarbons. Store in airtight containers. Protect from light.

Incompatibility. The plasticiser diethylhexyl phthalate, which is a possible carcinogen, was leached from PVC containers by ciclosporin preparations containing polyethoxylated castor oil.[1] Such preparations should not be given through PVC tubing nor stored in PVC containers. Polysorbate 80 which is an excipient in other ciclosporin preparations, also leached plasticiser from PVC,[1] and similar precautions would apply to preparations so formulated.

1. Pearson SD, Trissel LA. Leaching of diethylhexyl phthalate from polyvinyl chloride containers by selected drugs and formulation components. *Am J Hosp Pharm* 1993; **50:** 1405–9.

Stability. Ciclosporin was stable over 72 hours following dilution in glucose 5% or glucose/amino-acid solutions and storage at room temperature in the dark; similar stability was seen following dilution in lipid emulsion, but dilutions in sodium chloride 0.9% were considered to be stable only for 8 hours.[1] In all cases miscibility in the diluent was poor and vigorous shaking was required after addition to produce even distribution of ciclosporin. An extemporaneously compounded paste produced from ciclosporin oral solution (Sandimmun) in an oral gel base was found to be stable[2] for at least 31 days in aluminium-lined ointment tubes stored at 2° to 37°.

1. McLeod HL, *et al.* Stability of cyclosporin in dextrose 5%, NaCl 0.9%, dextrose/amino acid solution, and lipid emulsion. *Ann Pharmacother* 1992; **26:** 172–5.
2. Ghnassia LT, *et al.* Stability of cyclosporin in an extemporaneously compounded paste. *Am J Health-Syst Pharm* 1995; **52:** 2204–7.

Adverse Effects and Treatment

Nephrotoxicity, manifesting as raised serum creatinine and urea, is the major adverse effect of ciclosporin and occurs in approximately one-third of all patients. It is related to drug-plasma concentrations and is usually reversible on reduction of the dose. In renal graft recipients episodes of nephrotoxicity may be difficult to distinguish from graft rejection. Interstitial fibrosis may develop during long-term therapy.

Other frequent adverse effects include hypertension, gastrointestinal disturbances, hepatotoxicity, hypertrichosis, hyperplasia of the gums, tremor and burning sensations in the extremities. Occasionally, headaches, hyperlipidaemias, rashes, anaemia, electrolyte disturbances (hyperkalaemia, hypomagnesaemia), weight increase, oedema, pancreatitis, neuropathy, paraesthesia, hyperuricaemia, and convulsions have been reported.

Anaphylactoid reactions have occurred following intravenous administration; it has been suggested that these represent a reaction to the polyethoxylated castor oil vehicle of the intravenous preparation.

There is an increased incidence of development of certain malignancies in patients receiving ciclosporin therapy.

Alopecia. Although ciclosporin is more often associated with reports of hypertrichosis, there have been cases of alopecia areata developing in patients receiving ciclosporin,[1] sometimes with complete hair loss (alopecia universalis).[2,3]

1. Davies MG, Bowers PW. Alopecia areata arising in patients receiving cyclosporin immunosuppression. *Br J Dermatol* 1995; **132:** 835–6.
2. Monti M, *et al.* Alopecia universalis in liver transplant patients treated with cyclosporin. *Br J Dermatol* 1995; **133:** 663–4.
3. Parodi A, *et al.* Alopecia universalis and cyclosporin A. *Br J Dermatol* 1996; **135:** 657.

Carcinogenicity. Like other forms of immunosuppression (see p.476) the use of ciclosporin is associated with an increased incidence of malignancy, notably lymphoma,[1] and also skin cancer and Kaposi's sarcoma. The manufacturers have stated that of an estimated 5550 transplant patients who had been treated with ciclosporin by February 1984, lymphoproliferative disorders had been reported in 40; this represented an overall incidence of 0.7%, varying from 0.2 to 8% in different series.[2] In 1991, a report of 12 cases of lymphoproliferative disorders among 132 paediatric liver graft recipients, estimated the incidence at about 2.8% per year for the first 6 years after transplantation, giving a cumulative risk of nearly 20% after 7 years.[3] There is evidence that the incidence of malignancy is related to dose,[2,4,5] and is greater when ciclosporin is used with other potent immunosuppressants.[2] In addition, the incidence of malignancy varies geographically, possibly reflecting environmental triggers and genetic susceptibility.[6]

It has been suggested that these lymphomas represent proliferation of B-cells under the influence of Epstein-Barr virus, a process normally prevented by the T-cells which are specifically inhibited by ciclosporin.[3,7] The resultant, usually polyclonal, lymphoproliferative tumours appear to regress on prompt excision of the affected tissue and reduction or discontinuation of the immunosuppressant regimen, in most cases without graft loss.[8] However, the need for vigilance and rapid response to these conditions has been stressed, since the responsive polyclonal disorder may evolve into a monoclonal, frankly malignant form; where the presentation is indistinguishable from a classic non-Hodgkins lymphoma the prognosis is much less good.[3] Interestingly, use of lower dose ciclosporin regimens appears to maintain normal elimination of Epstein-Barr virus-infected B-cells by specific T-cells,[9] and may lead to a reduced incidence of malignancy compared with earlier results.[4,5,9]

The risk of skin cancers in ciclosporin recipients is increased by the exposure to sunlight.[10] Prophylactic retinoid therapy may prevent skin cancer in patients with renal transplants.[11]

There is no clear evidence that ciclosporin is associated with an increased incidence of malignancy compared with other immunosuppressants, although in one study dysplastic skin lesions were found in 14 of 64 transplant patients receiving ciclosporin compared with 3 of 33 previous similar patients who had received azathioprine.[12] However, such comparisons are difficult, not least because many transplant patients tend to have received multiple immunosuppressant agents.

1. Penn I. Cancers following cyclosporine therapy. *Transplantation* 1987; **43:** 32–5.
2. Beveridge T, *et al.* Lymphomas and lymphoproliferative lesions developing under cyclosporin therapy. *Lancet* 1984; **i:** 788.
3. Malatack JJ, *et al.* Orthotopic liver transplantation, Epstein-Barr virus, cyclosporine, and lymphoproliferative disease: a growing concern. *J Pediatr* 1991; **118:** 667–75.
4. Kahan BD. Cyclosporine. *N Engl J Med* 1990; **322:** 1531.
5. Dantal J, *et al.* Effect of long-term immunosuppression in kidney-graft recipients on cancer incidence: randomised comparison of two cyclosporine regimens. *Lancet* 1998; **351:** 623–8.
6. Newstead CG. Assessment of risk of cancer after renal transplantation. *Lancet* 1998; **351:** 610–11.
7. Anonymous. Lymphoma in organ transplant recipients. *Lancet* 1984; **i:** 601–3.
8. Starzl TE, *et al.* Reversibility of lymphomas and lymphoproliferative lesions developing under cyclosporin-steroid therapy. *Lancet* 1984; **i:** 583–7.
9. Crawford DH, Edwards JMB. Immunity to Epstein-Barr virus in cyclosporin A-treated renal allograft recipients. *Lancet* 1982; **i:** 1469–70.
10. Boyle J, *et al.* Cancer, warts, and sunshine in renal transplant patients: a case-control study. *Lancet* 1984; **i:** 702–5.
11. Bavinck JN, *et al.* Prevention of skin cancer and reduction of keratotic skin lesions during acitretin therapy in renal transplant recipients: a double-blind, placebo-controlled study. *J Clin Oncol* 1995; **13:** 1933–8.
12. Shuttleworth D, *et al.* Epidermal dysplasia and cyclosporine therapy in renal transplant patients: a comparison with azathioprine. *Br J Dermatol* 1989; **120:** 551–4.

Dysmorphic changes. There was pronounced coarsening of facial features in 11 children who were treated with prednisone and ciclosporin for renal transplantation and followed up for more than 6 months.[1] The changes resembled those seen with phenytoin therapy.

1. Reznik VM, *et al.* Changes in facial appearance during cyclosporin treatment. *Lancet* 1987; **i:** 1405–7.

Effects on the blood. Erythraemia[1,2] and thrombocytosis[3] have both been reported in ciclosporin treatment, both of which may contribute to **thromboembolic complications.** One retrospective study reported 17 thromboembolic events (pulmonary embolism, renal-vein or deep-vein thrombosis, or haemorrhoidal thrombosis) in 13 of 90 renal allograft recipients treated with ciclosporin and corticosteroids, compared with only 1 episode of superficial thrombophlebitis in 90 similar patients treated with an azathioprine-based regimen,[4] although other workers dispute that the incidence of

thromboembolic events is any greater after ciclosporin than azathioprine,[5-7] and one group found the reverse.[8]

Other effects that have been associated with ciclosporin therapy include cases of the haemolytic-uraemic syndrome,[9] and thrombocytopenia,[10] or leucopenia.[11]

1. Tatman AJ, *et al.* Erythraemia in renal transplant recipients treated with cyclosporin. *Lancet* 1988; **i:** 1279.
2. Innes A, *et al.* Cyclosporin and erythraemia. *Lancet* 1988; **ii:** 285.
3. Itami N, *et al.* Thrombocytosis after cyclosporin therapy in child with nephrotic syndrome. *Lancet* 1988; **ii:** 1018.
4. Vanrenterghem Y, *et al.* Thromboembolic complications and haemostatic changes in cyclosporin-treated cadaveric kidney allograft recipients. *Lancet* 1985; **i:** 999–1002.
5. Bergentz S-E, *et al.* Venous thrombosis and cyclosporin. *Lancet* 1985; **ii:** 101–2.
6. Zazgornik J, *et al.* Venous thrombosis and cyclosporin. *Lancet* 1985; **ii:** 102.
7. Choudhury N, *et al.* Thromboembolic complications in cyclosporin-treated kidney allograft recipients. *Lancet* 1985; **ii:** 606.
8. Allen RD, *et al.* Venous thrombosis and cyclosporin. *Lancet* 1985; **ii:** 1004.
9. Bonser RS, *et al.* Cyclosporin-induced haemolytic uraemic syndrome in liver allograft recipient. *Lancet* 1984; **ii:** 1337.
10. Dejong DJ, Sayler DJ. Possible cyclosporine-associated thrombocytopenia. *DICP Ann Pharmacother* 1990; **24:** 1007.
11. Michel F, *et al.* Bone marrow toxicity of cyclosporin in a kidney transplant patient. *Lancet* 1986; **ii:** 394.

Effects on the cardiovascular system. The principal cardiovascular adverse effect of ciclosporin is **hypertension.** This may be severe,[1] appears to be dose-related,[1,2] and is particularly common in recipients of cardiac or heart-lung grafts.[3,4] There may be an association with low serum-magnesium concentrations.[5] A variety of mechanisms have been suggested to contribute to ciclosporin-induced hypertension, including impaired sodium excretion,[6] enhanced sympathetic nervous activity,[3,7] effects on renal prostaglandin metabolism,[2] and direct damage to endothelial cells[8] with release of the potent vasoconstrictor endothelin.[9] Thus hypertension may occur independently of nephrotoxicity,[2,7] and may be difficult to treat with conventional antihypertensive regimens.[6] Currently, calcium-channel blockers are the preferred class of antihypertensives for hypertension that develops after transplantation.[1] It is important to choose one that does not interact with ciclosporin (see below).[1] Beta blockers and labetalol may also be used. Diuretics are usually avoided. For mention of the ability of calcium-channel blockers to ameliorate the nephrotoxic effects of ciclosporin, see Effects on the Kidneys, below. Occasionally, hypertension may be irreversible.[2,10] Raynaud's syndrome has been reported with ciclosporin.[11] For a discussion of possible thromboembolic complications, see Effects on the Blood, above.

1. Textor SC, *et al.* Cyclosporine-induced hypertension after transplantation. *Mayo Clin Proc* 1994; **69:** 1182–93.
2. Porter GA, *et al.* Cyclosporine-associated hypertension. *Arch Intern Med* 1990; **150:** 280–3.
3. Scherrer U, *et al.* Cyclosporine-induced sympathetic activation and hypertension after heart transplantation. *N Engl J Med* 1990; **323:** 693–9.
4. Weidle PJ, Vlasses PH. Systemic hypertension associated with cyclosporine: a review. *Drug Intell Clin Pharm* 1988; **22:** 443–51.
5. June CH, *et al.* Correlation of hypomagnesemia with the onset of cyclosporine-associated hypertension in marrow transplant patients. *Transplantation* 1986; **41:** 47–51.
6. Weinman EJ. Cyclosporine-associated hypertension. *Am J Med* 1989; **86:** 256–7.
7. Mark AL. Cyclosporine, sympathetic activity, and hypertension. *N Engl J Med* 1990; **323:** 748–50.
8. Zaal MJW, *et al.* Is cyclosporin toxic to endothelial cells? *Lancet* 1988; **ii:** 956–7.
9. Deray G, *et al.* Increased endothelin level after cyclosporine therapy. *Ann Intern Med* 1991; **114:** 809.
10. Sennesael JJ, *et al.* Hypertension and cyclosporine. *Ann Intern Med* 1986; **104:** 729.
11. Deray G, *et al.* Cyclosporin and Raynaud phenomenon. *Lancet* 1986; **ii:** 1092–3.

Effects on the gastrointestinal tract. There have been reports[1,2] of severe non-specific colitis associated with both elevated[1] and therapeutic[2] blood or serum concentrations of ciclosporin.

1. Innes A, *et al.* Cyclosporin toxicity and colitis. *Lancet* 1988; **ii:** 957. Correction. *ibid.*; 1094.
2. Bowen JRC, Sahi S. Cyclosporin induced colitis. *BMJ* 1993; **307:** 484.

Effects on glucose tolerance. There is some evidence that ciclosporin, particularly in high doses, may be associated with reduced insulin production,[1] impaired glucose tolerance,[2] and occasional overt diabetes mellitus,[3,4] although ciclosporin has also been tried, with some apparent benefit, in the treatment of recent-onset diabetes mellitus (for mention of the use of immunosuppressants in diabetes mellitus, see p.315). The incidence of fasting hyperglycaemia has been estimated at about 8% in ciclosporin-treated renal transplant recipients, compared with about 5% in those given an azathioprine-based regimen.[4]

1. Scott JP, Higenbottam TW. Adverse reactions and interactions of cyclosporin. *Med Toxicol* 1988; **3:** 107–27.
2. Gunnarsson R, *et al.* Deterioration in glucose metabolism in pancreatic transplant recipients given cyclosporin. *Lancet* 1983; **ii:** 571–2.
3. Bending JJ. Diabetogenic effect of cyclosporin. *BMJ* 1987; **294:** 401–2.
4. Yagisawa T, *et al.* Deterioration in glucose metabolism in cyclosporine-treated kidney transplant recipients and rats. *Transplant Proc* 1986; **18:** 1548–51.

Effects on the kidneys. The use of ciclosporin is associated with nephrotoxicity, characterised by fluid retention, increased serum creatinine and urea concentrations, and a fall in glomerular filtration rate, and decreased sodium and potassium excretion.[1,2] Extremely high intravenous doses (21 mg per kg body-weight per 24 hours for 60 hours) have been reported to be associated with fatal acute tubular necrosis.[3] In renal graft recipients it may be difficult to distinguish nephrotoxicity from graft rejection.[1] Symptoms are usually chronic, dose-related, and reversible,[1] and increase with the duration of exposure.[2] Prolonged administration has been associated with progressive irreversible renal dysfunction in heart transplant patients,[4] despite maintenance of plasma ciclosporin concentrations below 400 ng per mL, the value above which nephrotoxicity is more frequent;[1] however, impairment of renal function has been reported to be reversible in psoriatic patients who had received low-dose ciclosporin for 5 years.[5] It has been pointed out that with current regimens, which tend to use low doses of ciclosporin, the majority of transplant and other patients receiving ciclosporin long-term tolerate the drug without evidence of progressive nephrotoxicity.[5-7]

There is some evidence suggesting that the renal effects are due to a toxic metabolite,[8,9] thus, total ciclosporin and metabolite concentrations, as given by radio-immunoassay, may be more helpful in predicting toxicity than concentration of the parent drug alone.[8]

In addition to these chronic changes ciclosporin has also been associated with a syndrome of acute renal failure, occurring shortly after beginning treatment.[2,10] It has been proposed that this is due to arteriolar vasoconstriction secondary to inhibition of renal prostaglandin synthesis, with serious consequences in patients with clinical conditions in which prostaglandin-induced renal vasodilatation is necessary to maintain glomerular perfusion.[10] Such a mechanism would be in line with suggestions that inhibition of prostaglandin E_2 or prostacyclin synthesis may play a role in the development of chronic ciclosporin-induced nephrotoxicity.[11-13] However, endothelin has also been proposed as a causative agent,[14] and the relationship between the renal and vascular effects of ciclosporin has been a matter of some debate.[2]

A variety of agents have been given in an attempt to ameliorate the nephrotoxic effects of ciclosporin in patients who have undergone transplantation, including calcium-channel blockers (see under diltiazem, p.877, nifedipine, p.945, and verapamil, p.992), clonidine, co-dergocrine,[15-17] omega-3 triglycerides,[18] and misoprostol and other prostaglandin analogues.[19,20] Although benefits have been reported with some of these drugs, hydration, careful monitoring of ciclosporin concentrations, and the use where possible of low-dose or intermittent regimens of ciclosporin appear to remain the major means of keeping nephrotoxicity to a minimum. Calcium-channel blockers are used if hypertension occurs (see Effects on the Cardiovascular System, above).

1. Bennett WM, Pulliam JP. Cyclosporine nephrotoxicity. *Ann Intern Med* 1983; **99:** 851–4.
2. Scott JP, Higenbottam TW. Adverse reactions and interactions of cyclosporin. *Med Toxicol* 1988; **3:** 107–27.
3. Schechter P. Acute tubular necrosis following high-dose cyclosporine A therapy. *Eur J Clin Pharmacol* 1996; **49:** 521–3.
4. Myers BD, *et al.* Cyclosporine-associated chronic nephropathy. *N Engl J Med* 1984; **311:** 699–705.
5. Powles AV, *et al.* Renal function after 10 years' treatment with cyclosporin for psoriasis. *Br J Dermatol* 1998; **138:** 443–9.
6. Burke JF, *et al.* Long-term efficacy and safety of cyclosporine in renal-transplant recipients. *N Engl J Med* 1994; **331:** 358–63.
7. Leaker B, Cairns HS. Clinical aspects of cyclosporin nephrotoxicity. *Br J Hosp Med* 1994; **52:** 529–34.
8. Leunissen KML, *et al.* Cyclosporine metabolites and nephrotoxicity. *Lancet* 1986; **ii:** 1398.
9. Lucey MR, *et al.* Cyclosporin toxicity at therapeutic blood levels and cytochrome P-450 IIIA. *Lancet* 1990; **335:** 11–15.
10. Praga M, *et al.* Cyclosporine-induced acute renal failure in the nephrotic syndrome. *Ann Intern Med* 1987; **107:** 786–7.
11. Duarte R. Cyclosporine: renal effects and prostacyclin. *Ann Intern Med* 1985; **102:** 420.
12. Adu D, *et al.* Cyclosporine and prostaglandins. *Ann Intern Med* 1985; **103:** 303.
13. Stahl RAK, *et al.* Cyclosporine and renal prostaglandin E_2 production. *Ann Intern Med* 1985; **103:** 474.
14. Cairns HS, *et al.* Endothelin and cyclosporin nephrotoxicity. *Lancet* 1988; **ii:** 1496–7.
15. Heinrichs DA, *et al.* The effects of co-dergocrine on cyclosporin A pharmacokinetics and pharmacodynamics. *Br J Clin Pharmacol* 1987; **24:** 117–18.
16. Nussenblatt RB, *et al.* Hydergine and cyclosporin nephrotoxicity. *Lancet* 1986; **i:** 1220–1.
17. Kho TL, *et al.* Hydergine and reversibility of cyclosporin nephrotoxicity. *Lancet* 1986; **ii:** 394–5.
18. Stoof TJ, *et al.* Does fish oil protect renal function in cyclosporin-treated psoriasis patients? *Br J Dermatol* 1990; **123:** 535.
19. Moran M, *et al.* Prevention of acute graft rejection by the prostaglandin E_1 analogue misoprostol in renal-transplant recipients treated with cyclosporine and prednisone. *N Engl J Med* 1990; **322:** 1183–8.
20. Di Palo FQ, *et al.* Role of a prostaglandin E_1 analogue in the prevention of acute graft rejection by cyclosporine. *N Engl J Med* 1990; **323:** 832.

Effects on lipids. Marked **hyperlipidaemia** has been associated with ciclosporin therapy, with notable increases reported in low-density lipoprotein cholesterol,[1,2] and triglycerides.[2] Webb and colleagues reported an increase in lipoprotein (a),[3] but this was disputed.[4-6] Ciclosporin has been reported to have greater effects on lipids than azathioprine[7] or tacrolimus[8] post-transplantation. Lipid-lowering drugs are used to decrease hypercholesterolaemia in transplant patients.

1. Luke DR, *et al.* Longitudinal study of cyclosporine and lipids in patients undergoing bone marrow transplantation. *J Clin Pharmacol* 1990; **30:** 163–9.
2. Ballantyne CM, *et al.* Effects of cyclosporine therapy on plasma lipoprotein levels. *JAMA* 1989; **262:** 53–6.
3. Webb AT, *et al.* Does cyclosporin increase lipoprotein(a) concentrations in renal transplant recipients? *Lancet* 1993; **341:** 268–70.
4. Kronenberg F, *et al.* Cyclosporin and serum lipids in renal transplant recipients. *Lancet* 1993; **341:** 765.
5. Segarra A, *et al.* Cyclosporin and serum lipids in renal transplant recipients. *Lancet* 1993; **341:** 766.
6. Hunt BJ, *et al.* Does cyclosporin affect lipoprotein(a) concentrations? *Lancet* 1994; **343:** 119–20.
7. Van den Dorpel MA, *et al.* Conversion from cyclosporine A to azathioprine treatment improves LDL oxidation in kidney transplant recipients. *Kidney Int* 1997; **51:** 1608–12.
8. Taylor DO, *et al.* A randomized, multicenter comparison of tacrolimus and cyclosporine immunosuppressive regimens in cardiac transplantation: decreased hyperlipidemia and hypertension with tacrolimus. *J Heart Lung Transplant* 1999; **18:** 336–45.

Effects on the nervous system. Adverse effects of ciclosporin on the CNS include tremor,[1-3] ataxia,[1-3] confusion[1,2] or agitation,[2] mental depression,[3] flushing, headache and sleep disturbances,[2] lethargy,[1,2,4] or coma[2,4] (in one case coma persisted for 44 days),[5] convulsions,[2,3,6-9] leucoencephalopathy,[2,5,6] cortical blindness,[2,6] and spasticity or paralysis of the limbs.[1,2] Convulsions have sometimes been associated with hypertension and fluid retention,[8] but this is by no means always the case.[6,7] Severe CNS toxicity has been stated to vary in incidence from 0.1% in renal transplant patients to about 1.6% in bone-marrow transplant recipients.[9] There is some evidence for an association of serious neurological effects with low total serum-cholesterol concentrations,[2] and the use of the intravenous formulation.[2] Neurotoxicity may also be associated with the concomitant administration of lipid solutions.[10] An association with hypomagnesaemia has also been proposed[3] but may just represent concomitant nephrotoxicity.[11] Convulsions may be more likely or more severe in patients with a familial history of epilepsy,[12] subclinical aluminium overload,[13] or who are given concomitant high-dose corticosteroids.[14,15] The mechanism of toxicity is unknown but may be associated with disturbance of the blood-brain barrier;[7,9,16] it has been suggested that the metabolite M-17, or possibly other metabolites, are responsible for neurotoxicity.[4] Although neurotoxicity usually manifests within a month of beginning treatment, it may be delayed, and in one case occurred only after 3 years of ciclosporin therapy.[17]

1. Atkinson K, *et al.* Cyclosporine-associated central-nervous-system toxicity after allogeneic bone-marrow transplantation. *N Engl J Med* 1984; **310:** 527.
2. de Groen PC, *et al.* Central nervous system toxicity after liver transplantation: the role of cyclosporine and cholesterol. *N Engl J Med* 1987; **317:** 861–6.
3. Thompson CB, *et al.* Association between cyclosporin neurotoxicity and hypomagnesaemia. *Lancet* 1984; **ii:** 1116–20.
4. Kunzendorf U, *et al.* Cyclosporin metabolites and central-nervous-system toxicity. *Lancet* 1988; **i:** 1223.
5. Berden JHM, *et al.* Severe central-nervous-system toxicity associated with cyclosporin. *Lancet* 1985; **i:** 219–20.
6. Hughes RL. Cyclosporine-related central nervous system toxicity in cardiac transplantation. *N Engl J Med* 1990; **323:** 420–1.
7. Gottrand F, *et al.* Cyclosporine neurotoxicity. *N Engl J Med* 1991; **324:** 1744–5.
8. Joss DV, *et al.* Hypertension and convulsions in children receiving cyclosporin A. *Lancet* 1982; **i:** 906.
9. Krupp P, *et al.* Encephalopathy associated with fat embolism induced by solvent for cyclosporin. *Lancet* 1989; **i:** 168–9.
10. De Klippel N. Cyclosporin leukoencephalopathy induced by intravenous lipid solution. *Lancet* 1992; **339:** 1114.
11. Allen RD, *et al.* Cyclosporin and magnesium. *Lancet* 1985; **i:** 1283–4.
12. Velu T, *et al.* Cyclosporin-associated fatal convulsions. *Lancet* 1985; **i:** 219.
13. Nordal KP, *et al.* Aluminium overload, a predisposing condition for epileptic seizures in renal-transplant patients treated with cyclosporin. *Lancet* 1985; **ii:** 153–4.
14. Durrant S, *et al.* Cyclosporin A, methylprednisolone, and convulsions. *Lancet* 1982; **ii:** 829–30.
15. Bogaerts MA, *et al.* Cyclosporin, methylprednisolone, and convulsions. *Lancet* 1982; **ii:** 1216–17.
16. Sloane JP, *et al.* Disturbance of blood-brain barrier after bone-marrow transplantation. *Lancet* 1985; **ii:** 280–1.
17. Welge-Lüssen UC, Gerhartz HH. Late onset of neurotoxicity with cyclosporin. *Lancet* 1994; **343:** 293.

Effects on skeletal muscle. Ciclosporin has been associated with a number of reports of myopathy.[1-4] The manufacturer noted that 29 cases had been reported by December 1990, which appeared to be divided into cases of toxic or non-specific myopathy, or mild sensory motor neuropathy, which were generally dose-related; and rhabdomyolysis, often, but not always, associated with concomitant medication with lovastatin or colchicine.[5] Rhabdomyolysis has also been reported with concomitant use of other statins and ciclosporin, see Lipid Regulating Drugs, under Interactions, below.

1. Noppen M, *et al.* Cyclosporine and myopathy. *Ann Intern Med* 1987; **107:** 945–6.
2. Goy J-J. Myopathy as possible side-effect of cyclosporin. *Lancet* 1989; **i:** 1446–7.
3. Grezard O, *et al.* Cyclosporin-induced muscular toxicity. *Lancet* 1990; **335:** 177.
4. Fernandez-Sola J, *et al.* Reversible cyclosporin myopathy. *Lancet* 1990; **335:** 362–3.
5. Arellano F, Krupp P. Muscular disorders associated with cyclosporin. *Lancet* 1991; **337:** 915.

Hyperplasia. Ciclosporin is well known to be associated with the development of gingival hyperplasia or gingival overgrowth: one review[1] has estimated the incidence at about 30% in transplant patients, while noting that reported values in the literature range from about 7 to 70%. The presence of dental plaque may exacerbate the response,[1] and the concomitant administration of nifedipine (which can itself produce hyperplasia) may produce very much greater overgrowth.[2] Good oral hygiene is important in preventing or reducing the development of gingival overgrowth.[1] Overgrowth is generally reversible following dosage reduction or withdrawal of ciclosporin; where this is not feasible, surgical excision is the recommended treatment.[1] However, improvement or resolution of the overgrowth has also been reported following a course of azithromycin in a case series[3] and in a controlled study.[4] Similar benefit has been reported for metronidazole in some patients,[5,6] but not others.[7]

Enlargement of the papillae of the tongue has also occurred in association with ciclosporin.[8]

1. Brunet L, *et al.* Gingival enlargement induced by drugs. *Drug Safety* 1996; **15:** 219–31.
2. Slavin J, Taylor J. Cyclosporin, nifedipine, and gingival hyperplasia. *Lancet* 1987; **ii:** 739.
3. Jugglà A, *et al.* The use of azithromycin for cyclosporin-induced gingival overgrowth. *Br J Dermatol* 1998; **138:** 198–9.
4. Nash MM, Zaltman JS. Efficacy of azithromycin in the treatment of cyclosporine-induced gingival hyperplasia in renal transplant recipients. *Transplantation* 1998; **65:** 1611–5.
5. Wong W, *et al.* Resolution of cyclosporin-induced gingival hypertrophy with metronidazole. *Lancet* 1994; **343:** 986.
6. Cecchin E, *et al.* Treatment of cyclosporine-induced gingival hypertrophy. *Ann Intern Med* 1997; **126:** 409–10.
7. Aufricht C, *et al.* Oral metronidazole does not improve cyclosporine A-induced gingival hyperplasia. *Pediatr Nephrol* 1997; **11:** 552–5.
8. Silverberg NB, *et al.* Lingual fungiform papillae hypertrophy with cyclosporin A. *Lancet* 1996; **348:** 967.

Hypersensitivity. Anaphylactoid reactions in 5 of 21 patients given intravenous ciclosporin infusions were found to be associated with improper mixing of the ciclosporin concentrate, which has a polyethoxylated castor oil vehicle, with the infusion solution.[1] It was concluded that this had led to an initial bolus of polyethoxylated castor oil which had triggered the anaphylactic reactions. Subsequent study indicated that peak concentrations of up to 9 times the intended concentration of ciclosporin and polyethoxylated castor oil were present in the first 10 minutes of a poorly mixed infusion.[2]

1. Liau M, *et al.* High incidence of anaphylactoid reactions to iv cyclosporin A caused by improper dissolution of Cremophor EL. *Clin Pharmacol Ther* 1995; **57:** 209.
2. Liau-Chu M, *et al.* Mechanism of anaphylactoid reactions: improper preparation of high-dose intravenous cyclosporine leads to bolus infusion of Cremophor EL and cyclosporine. *Ann Pharmacother* 1997; **31:** 1287–91.

Hyperuricaemia. Ciclosporin therapy may be associated with marked hyperuricaemia,[1-3] which may lead (predominantly in male patients[1]) to episodes of severe gouty arthritis.[1-3] It has been suggested that ciclosporin specifically reduces urate clearance by the kidney independently of its effects on glomerular filtration.[4,5] Treatment of ciclosporin-induced gout may be difficult since interactions with NSAIDs may lead to enhanced kidney toxicity[5] and patients who are also receiving azathioprine may experience increased bone-marrow toxicity if given allopurinol.[6]

1. Lin H-Y, *et al.* Cyclosporine-induced hyperuricemia and gout. *N Engl J Med* 1989; **321:** 287–92.
2. Kahl LE, *et al.* Gout in the heart transplant recipient: physiologic puzzle and therapeutic challenge. *Am J Med* 1989; **87:** 289–94.
3. Burack DA, *et al.* Hyperuricemia and gout among heart transplant recipients receiving cyclosporine. *Am J Med* 1992; **92:** 141–6.
4. Noordzij TC, *et al.* Cyclosporine-induced hyperuricemia and gout. *N Engl J Med* 1990; **322:** 335.
5. Farge D, *et al.* Hyperuricemia and gouty arthritis in heart transplant recipients. *Am J Med* 1990; **88:** 553.
6. Figg WD. Cyclosporine-induced hyperuricemia and gout. *N Engl J Med* 1990; **332:** 334–5.

Overdosage. Anxiety, diarrhoea, vomiting, and perspiration, with weak and irregular pulse, occurred in a patient accidentally injected with 250 mg (estimated 6.25 mg per kg body-weight) of ciclosporin.[1] The patient subsequently developed atrial fibrillation, which was treated with digoxin, and in the following 36 hours showed signs of slight renal insufficiency. Two days later no adverse effects were apparent. Atrial fibrillation also developed in another patient accidentally administered 1 g of oral ciclosporin microemulsion.[2] No adverse renal, hepatic, or neurological effects were seen in a third patient who took 25 g of ciclosporin over 8 days.[3] There was a mild increase in blood pressure and other symptoms included burning sensations in the mouth and the extremities, dysgeusia, facial flushing, and gastrointestinal disturbances. Symptoms resolved within 2 weeks of stopping ciclosporin.

For reference to fatal tubular necrosis in a patient who received 21 mg per kg body-weight of ciclosporin per 24 hours for 60 hours, see under Effects on the Kidneys, above.

1. Wallemacq PE, Lesne ML. Accidental massive IV administration of cyclosporine in man. *Drug Intell Clin Pharm* 1985; **19:** 29–30.
2. LoVecchio FA, Goltz HR. Atrial fibrillation following acute overdose with oral cyclosporine. *Ann Pharmacother* 2000; **34:** 405.
3. Baumhefner RW, *et al.* High cyclosporin overdose with favourable outcome. *Lancet* 1987; **ii:** 332.

Precautions

Regular monitoring of renal and hepatic function, blood pressure, and serum electrolytes (chiefly potassium) is required in patients receiving ciclosporin. Serum lipids should also be monitored. Monitoring of plasma ciclosporin concentrations is mandatory in transplant patients. Dosage adjustment may frequently be necessary in patients with renal impairment or other factors affecting plasma ciclosporin concentrations. Care is required in patients with hyperuricaemia, and intravenous formulations should be given cautiously to those who have previously received parenteral drugs formulated in polyethoxylated castor oil, or to those with a history of allergic reactions.

Ciclosporin should not be used to treat atopic dermatitis, psoriasis, or rheumatoid arthritis in patients with abnormal renal function, uncontrolled hypertension, uncontrolled infections, or malignancy. An exception is patients with treated malignant or pre-malignant lesions of the skin who may receive ciclosporin as a last resort for psoriasis. Psoriatic patients should not be given concomitant ultraviolet irradiation and should avoid excessive sun exposure.

The commercially available oral formulations of ciclosporin differ in their bioavailability, and patients should not be transferred from one to another without appropriate monitoring.

◊ An oral microemulsion formulation of ciclosporin, with improved bioavailability (see Absorption under Pharmacokinetics, below), has been made available commercially, and patients being undergone conversion from the old formulation (initially on a 1:1 basis by weight, with monitoring of resultant ciclosporin concentrations and subsequent dosage adjustment). However, Bennett and colleagues[1,2] have questioned the wisdom of such routine conversion: they reported 3 patients with biopsy-proven rejection of stable renal grafts following conversion from the old to the new formulation, despite high trough ciclosporin concentrations. They also noted nephrotoxicity following conversion in 3 other patients. Although other physicians consider the new formulation superior,[3,4] there are some with experiences that seem to support the doubts of Bennett,[5,6] and he has pointed out[7] that the evidence suggests that the two formulations are equivalent in efficacy.

1. Bennett WM, et al. Which ciclosporin formulation? Lancet 1996; 348: 205.
2. Olyaei AJ, et al. Switching between cyclosporin formulations: what are the risks? Drug Safety 1997; 16: 366–73.
3. Johnston A, Holt DW. Which cyclosporin formulation? Lancet 1996; 348: 1175.
4. Pollard S. Which cyclosporin formulation? Lancet 1996; 348: 1175–6.
5. Filler G, Ehrich J. Which cyclosporin formulation? Lancet 1996; 348: 1176–7.
6. Gennery A, et al. Which cyclosporin formulation? Lancet 1996; 348: 1177.
7. Bennet WM. Which cyclosporin formulation? Lancet 1996; 348: 1176.

Porphyria. Ciclosporin is considered to be unsafe in patients with porphyria because it has been shown to be porphyrinogenic in *animals*.

Pregnancy and breast feeding. Ciclosporin has been used successfully in pregnant women. However, in common with other immunosuppressants, fetal growth retardation may be a significant problem.[1-4] Patients with hypertension or graft dysfunction are more likely to have adverse outcomes, so patients should have stable graft function and be on maintenance therapy before considering pregnancy.[1,2] Serum ciclosporin concentrations may fall during pregnancy,[2,3,5] but although frequent monitoring is necessary, the suppressed auto-immune state of pregnancy may protect against rejection episodes.[5] Ciclosporin should be used at the lowest possible dose to maintain efficacy, and one review has recommended that the daily dose should be kept below 5 mg per kg body-weight.[3]

One case of osseous malformation, resulting in hypoplasia of the right leg has been reported in an infant born to a ciclosporin-treated mother.[6]

The American Academy of Pediatrics considers that ciclosporin may possibly suppress the immune system in a nursing infant.[7] However, a study[8] in the breast-fed infants of 7 women receiving ciclosporin found that the amounts ingested produced undetectable blood concentrations in the infants. In another case it was estimated that a breast-fed infant received less than 0.1 mg per kg body-weight of ciclosporin daily.[9]

1. Armenti VT, et al. Variables affecting birthweight and graft survival in 197 pregnancies in cyclosporine-treated female kidney transplant recipients. Transplantation 1995; 59: 476–9.
2. Armenti VT, et al. National Transplantation Pregnancy Registry (NTPR): cyclosporine dosing and pregnancy outcome in female renal transplant recipients. Transplant Proc 1996; 28: 2111–12.
3. Huynh LA, Min DI. Outcomes of pregnancy and the management of immunosuppressive agents to minimize fetal risks in organ transplant patients. Ann Pharmacother 1994; 28: 1355–6.

4. Lamarque V, et al. Analysis of 629 pregnancy outcomes in transplant recipients treated with Sandimmun. Transplant Proc 1997; 29: 2480.
5. Thomas AG, et al. The effect of pregnancy on cyclosporine levels in renal allograft patients. Obstet Gynecol 1997; 90: 916–19.
6. Pujals JM, et al. Osseous malformation in baby born to woman on cyclosporin. Lancet 1989; i: 667.
7. American Academy of Pediatrics Committee on Drugs. The transfer of drugs and other chemicals into human milk. Pediatrics 2001; 108: 776–89.
8. Nyberg G, et al. Breast feeding during treatment with cyclosporin. Transplantation 1998; 65: 253–5.
9. Thiru Y, et al. Successful breast feeding while mother was taking cyclosporin. BMJ 1997; 315: 463.

Interactions

Ciclosporin is extensively metabolised in the liver and plasma-ciclosporin concentrations may be affected by inducers or competitive inhibitors of hepatic enzymes, particularly cytochrome P450 isoenzyme CYP3A4. For example, carbamazepine, phenytoin, phenobarbital, rifampicin, and other inducers of hepatic enzymes may cause lowered plasma concentrations of ciclosporin, and increased plasma concentrations have been reported following concurrent administration of ketoconazole, erythromycin, some calcium-channel blockers, sex hormones, corticosteroids and grapefruit juice. In transplant patients frequent measurement of plasma ciclosporin and, if necessary, ciclosporin dosage adjustment is required, particularly during the introduction or withdrawal of other drugs.

Concurrent administration of statins may increase the risk of myopathy and rhabdomyolysis. Potassium-sparing diuretics should be avoided because of the risk of hyperkalaemia, and patients receiving ciclosporin should avoid a high dietary intake of potassium. The risk of gingival hyperplasia may be increased by nifedipine.

During treatment with ciclosporin, vaccination may be less effective, and the use of live vaccines should generally be avoided.

Care should be taken when ciclosporin is given concomitantly with other nephrotoxic drugs.

◊ Reviews of the interactions of ciclosporin.

1. Yee GC, McGuire TR. Pharmacokinetic drug interactions with cyclosporin. Clin Pharmacokinet 1990; 19: 319–32 and 400–15.
2. Lake KD, Canafax DM. Important interactions of drugs with immunosuppressive agents used in transplant recipients. J Antimicrob Chemother 1995; 36 (suppl B): 11–22.
3. Campana C, et al. Clinically significant drug interactions with cyclosporin: an update. Clin Pharmacokinet 1996; 30: 141–79.

Allopurinol. A patient who had been receiving maintenance doses of ciclosporin for some years, with consistent whole-blood trough concentrations of around 130 nanograms per mL at doses of 175 mg twice daily experienced a rise in ciclosporin concentrations to 410 nanograms per mL following 2 months of treatment with allopurinol 200 mg daily.[1] Ciclosporin concentrations returned to their previous levels over several weeks following discontinuation of allopurinol, and rose again on rechallenge. Dosage of ciclosporin was then reduced. A low dose of allopurinol has been added to a ciclosporin-containing immunosuppressive regimen, see p.399.

1. Gorrie M, et al. Allopurinol interaction with cyclosporin. BMJ 1994; 308: 113.

Antibacterials. AMINOGLYCOSIDES. Increased nephrotoxicity has been reported with the concomitant use of aminoglycosides with ciclosporin.[1,2] However, a retrospective analysis in 21 patients given ciclosporin for allogeneic bone-marrow transplant, in whom aminoglycosides were used if fever and neutropenia developed, showed no greater incidence of nephrotoxicity than in 20 autologous bone-marrow recipients who did not receive ciclosporin, suggesting that these drugs can be given together provided careful monitoring is maintained.[3]

1. Termeer A, et al. Severe nephrotoxicity cause by the combined use of gentamicin and cyclosporine in renal allograft recipients. Transplantation 1986; 42: 220–1.
2. Morales JM, et al. Reversible acute renal toxicity by toxic synergic effect between gentamicin and cyclosporine. Clin Nephrol 1988; 29: 272.
3. Chandrasekar PH, Cronin SM. Nephrotoxicity in bone marrow transplant recipients receiving aminoglycoside plus cyclosporine or aminoglycoside alone. J Antimicrob Chemother 1991; 27: 845–9.

CHLORAMPHENICOL. A couple of cases of marked rises in plasma-ciclosporin concentrations have been reported when chloramphenicol was given concurrently.[1,2]

1. Steinfort CL, McConachy KA. Cyclosporin-chloramphenicol drug interaction in a heart-lung transplant recipient. Med J Aust 1994; 161: 455.
2. Bui LL, Huang DD. Possible interaction between cyclosporine and chloramphenicol. Ann Pharmacother 1999; 33: 252–3.

MACROLIDES. There are a number of reports of markedly raised blood concentrations of ciclosporin when given with *erythromycin*.[1-4] The mechanism involved appears to represent a combination of decreased hepatic metabolism of ciclosporin and increased gastrointestinal absorption.[5] Similar elevations of ciclosporin concentrations have been noted following concomitant use of other macrolide antibiotics, including *clarithromycin*,[6-8] *josamycin*,[9,10] *midecamycin*,[11] *midecamycin acetate*,[12] and the structurally-related streptogramin, *pristinamycin*.[13] Small increases in ciclosporin concentrations have been seen with *roxithromycin*.[14] An increase in ciclosporin concentrations was attributed to *azithromycin* in 1 patient,[15] but a study in 6 patients found no effect.[16] *Spiramycin* does not appear to affect the pharmacokinetics of ciclosporin.[17,18]

1. Ptachcinski RJ, et al. Effect of erythromycin on cyclosporine levels. N Engl J Med 1985; 313: 1416–17.
2. Martell R, et al. The effects of erythromycin in patients treated with cyclosporine. Ann Intern Med 1986; 104: 660–1.
3. Wadhwa NK, et al. Interaction between erythromycin and cyclosporine in a kidney and pancreas allograft recipient. Ther Drug Monit 1987; 9: 123–5.
4. Gupta SK, et al. Cyclosporin-erythromycin interaction in renal transplant patients. Br J Clin Pharmacol 1989; 27: 475–81.
5. Ignoffo RJ, Kim LE. Erythromycin and cyclosporine drug interaction. DICP Ann Pharmacother 1991; 25: 30–1.
6. Ferrari SL, et al. The interaction between clarithromycin and cyclosporine in kidney transplant recipients. Transplantation 1994; 58: 725–7.
7. Treille S, et al. Kidney graft dysfunction after drug interaction between clarithromycin and cyclosporin. Nephrol Dial Transplant 1996; 11: 1192–3.
8. Sábada B, et al. Concurrent clarithromycin and cyclosporin A treatment. J Antimicrob Chemother 1998; 42: 393–5.
9. Kreft-Jais C, et al. Effect of josamycin on plasma cyclosporine levels. Eur J Clin Pharmacol 1987; 32: 327–8.
10. Azanza JR, et al. Possible interaction between cyclosporine and josamycin: a description of three cases. Clin Pharmacol Ther 1992; 51: 572–5.
11. Alfonso I, et al. Interaction between cyclosporine A and midecamycin. Eur J Clin Pharmacol 1997; 52: 79–80.
12. Couet W, et al. Effect of ponsinomycin on cyclosporin pharmacokinetics. Eur J Clin Pharmacol 1990; 39: 165–7.
13. Garraffo R, et al. Pristinamycin increases cyclosporin blood levels. Med Sci Res 1987; 15: 461.
14. Billaud EM, et al. Interaction between roxithromycin and cyclosporin in heart transplant patients. Clin Pharmacokinet 1990; 19: 499–502.
15. Ljutic D, Rumboldt Z. Possible interaction between azithromycin and cyclosporin: a case report. Nephron 1995; 70: 130.
16. Gomez E, et al. Interaction between azithromycin and cyclosporin? Nephron 1996; 73: 724.
17. Vernillet L, et al. Lack of effect of spiramycin on cyclosporin pharmacokinetics. Br J Clin Pharmacol 1989; 27: 789–94.
18. Kessler M, et al. Lack of effect of spiramycin on cyclosporin pharmacokinetics. Br J Clin Pharmacol 1990; 29: 370–1.

PENICILLINS. Decreased plasma-ciclosporin concentrations and effect were seen in one patient given *nafcillin*.[1] Conversely, another study reported increased nephrotoxicity with the concomitant use of ciclosporin and nafcillin without an apparent increase in ciclosporin concentrations.[2]

1. Veremis SA, et al. Subtherapeutic cyclosporine concentrations during nafcillin therapy. Transplantation 1987; 43: 913–15.
2. Jahansouz F, et al. Potentiation of cyclosporine nephrotoxicity by nafcillin in lung transplant recipients. Transplantation 1993; 55: 1045–8.

QUINOLONES. A number of reports have indicated that the quinolone *ciprofloxacin* has no effect on the pharmacokinetics of ciclosporin.[1-3] However, there is a report of enhanced nephrotoxicity without a change in ciclosporin concentrations in one patient given ciprofloxacin,[4] and another report showing both enhanced nephrotoxicity and increased ciclosporin concentrations.[5] Furthermore, a small case-control study suggested an increase in transplant rejection with ciprofloxacin.[6] *Norfloxacin* has been reported to decrease clearance and increase blood concentrations of ciclosporin in paediatric patients,[7] probably by inhibition of ciclosporin metabolism. *Levofloxacin* did not alter ciclosporin pharmacokinetics in healthy volunteers.[8]

1. Hooper TL, et al. Ciprofloxacin: a preferred treatment for legionella infections in patients receiving cyclosporin A. J Antimicrob Chemother 1988; 22: 952–3.
2. Tan KKC, et al. Co-administration of ciprofloxacin and cyclosporin: lack of evidence for a pharmacokinetic interaction. Br J Clin Pharmacol 1989; 28: 185–7.
3. Krüger HU, et al. Investigation of potential interaction of ciprofloxacin with cyclosporine in bone marrow transplant recipients. Antimicrob Agents Chemother 1990; 34: 1048–52.
4. Elston RA, Taylor J. Possible interaction of ciprofloxacin with cyclosporin A. J Antimicrob Chemother 1988; 21: 679–80.
5. Nasir M, et al. Interaction between ciclosporin and ciprofloxacin. Nephron 1991; 57: 245–6.
6. Wrishko RE, et al. Investigation of a possible interaction between ciprofloxacin and cyclosporine in renal transplant patients. Transplantation 1997; 64: 996–9.
7. McLellan RA, et al. Norfloxacin interferes with cyclosporine disposition in pediatric patients undergoing renal transplantation. Clin Pharmacol Ther 1995; 58: 322–7.
8. Doose DR, et al. Levofloxacin does not alter cyclosporine disposition. J Clin Pharmacol 1998; 38: 90–93.

RIFAMYCINS. The antimycobacterial antibiotic *rifampicin* has been associated with marked decreases in blood-ciclosporin concentrations when given concomitantly,[1-3] and has resulted in graft rejection.[1,3] Although it has been assumed that this effect represents induction of the hepatic metabolism of ciclosporin by rifampicin, there is some suggestion that rifampicin may decrease the absorption of ciclosporin or induce intestinal metabolism, resulting in reduced bioavailability.[4] Topical application of *rifamycin* has also been associated with a decrease in blood-ciclosporin concentrations in another patient;[5] ciclosporin concentrations rose immediately after withdrawal of rifamycin, suggesting that the effect was not due to enzyme induction.

1. Langhoff E, Madsen S. Rapid metabolism of cyclosporin and prednisone in kidney transplant patient receiving tuberculostatic treatment. *Lancet* 1983; **ii:** 1031.
2. Daniels NJ, *et al.* Interaction between cyclosporin and rifampicin. *Lancet* 1984; **ii:** 639.
3. Allen RDM, *et al.* Cyclosporin and rifampicin in renal transplantation. *Lancet* 1985; **i:** 980.
4. Hebert MF, *et al.* Bioavailability of cyclosporine with concomitant rifampin administration is markedly less than predicted by hepatic enzyme induction. *Clin Pharmacol Ther* 1992; **52:** 453–7.
5. Renoult E, *et al.* Effect of topical rifamycin SV treatment on cyclosporin A blood levels in a renal transplant recipient. *Eur J Clin Pharmacol* 1991; **40:** 433–4.

STREPTOGRAMINS. Increased plasma concentrations of ciclosporin have occurred following therapy with quinupristin/dalfopristin.

SULFONAMIDES. Intravenous, but not oral, therapy with *sulfadimidine* and *trimethoprim* has been associated with falls in ciclosporin concentrations to subtherapeutic values.[1,2] Oral *sulfadiazine* has had a similar effect.[3] Conversely, *trimethoprim* and *cotrimoxazole* can cause rises in serum creatinine, and therefore may contribute to ciclosporin-induced nephrotoxicity.[4,5]

1. Wallwork J, *et al.* Cyclosporin and intravenous sulphadimidine and trimethoprim therapy. *Lancet* 1983; **i:** 366–7.
2. Jones DK, *et al.* Serious interaction between cyclosporin A and sulphadimidine. *BMJ* 1986; **292:** 728–9.
3. Spes CH, *et al.* Sulfadiazine therapy for toxoplasmosis in heart transplant recipients decreases cyclosporine concentration. *Clin Invest* 1992; **70:** 752–4.
4. Thompson JF, *et al.* Nephrotoxicity of trimethoprim and cotrimoxazole in renal allograft recipients treated with cyclosporine. *Transplantation* 1983; **36:** 204–6.
5. Ringden O, *et al.* Nephrotoxicity by co-trimoxazole and cyclosporin in transplanted patients. *Lancet* 1984; **i:** 1016.

TETRACYCLINES. The manufacturers state that the tetracycline *doxycycline* is suspected of increasing ciclosporin concentrations, but the evidence for this seems to be scant.

Antidepressants. Administration of *fluoxetine* to a patient receiving ciclosporin as part of an immunosuppressant regimen after cardiac transplantation was associated with a subsequent marked increase in ciclosporin trough blood concentrations to approximately twice their original value, necessitating a reduction in ciclosporin dosage.[1] Following subsequent withdrawal of fluoxetine, ciclosporin concentrations fell, and dosage had to be increased again. However, a study in 13 other patients receiving ciclosporin with fluoxetine failed to find any evidence that the antidepressant altered ciclosporin concentrations.[2]

1. Horton RC, Bonser RS. Interaction between cyclosporin and fluoxetine. *BMJ* 1995; **311:** 422.
2. Strouse TB, *et al.* Fluoxetine and cyclosporine in organ transplantation: failure to detect significant drug interactions or adverse clinical events in depressed organ recipients. *Psychosomatics* 1996; **37:** 23–30.

HYPERICUM. Ciclosporin plasma levels are reduced by concomitant administration of hypericum. This has lead to acute rejection episodes in transplant patients,[1-3] and the two drugs should not be administered together.[4]

1. Ruschitzka F, *et al.* Acute heart transplant rejection due to Saint John's wort. *Lancet* 2000; **355:** 548–9.
2. Breidenbach T, *et al.* Drug interaction of St John's wort with cyclosporin. *Lancet* 2000; **355:** 1912.
3. Barone GW, *et al.* Drug interaction between St John's wort and cyclosporine. *Ann Pharmacother* 2000; **34:** 1013–16.
4. Committee on Safety of Medicines/Medicines Control Agency. Reminder: St John's wort (Hypericum perforatum) interactions. *Current Problems* 2000; **26:** 6–7.

Antiepileptics. The antiepileptics *carbamazepine*,[1,2] *phenobarbital*,[3] and *phenytoin*,[4] which are all inducers of hepatic cytochrome P450, have been associated with a reduction in blood-ciclosporin concentrations when given concomitantly. *Valproate* has been successfully used in ciclosporin-treated patients without apparent interaction.[1,2]

1. Hillebrand G, *et al.* Valproate for epilepsy in renal transplant recipients receiving cyclosporine. *Transplantation* 1987; **43:** 915–16.
2. Schofield OMV, *et al.* Cyclosporin A in psoriasis: interaction with carbamazepine. *Br J Dermatol* 1990; **122:** 425–6.
3. Carstensen H, *et al.* Interaction between cyclosporin A and phenobarbitone. *Br J Clin Pharmacol* 1986; **21:** 550–1.
4. Freeman DJ, *et al.* Evaluation of cyclosporin-phenytoin interaction with observations on cyclosporin metabolites. *Br J Clin Pharmacol* 1984; **18:** 887–93.

Antifungals. The imidazole *ketoconazole* is a potent inhibitor of hepatic cytochrome P450 and is recognised to result in markedly increased blood-ciclosporin concentrations when the two drugs are given concomitantly.[1-4] The interaction has been employed, similarly to the calcium-channel blockers (see below), to permit therapeutic blood concentrations of ciclosporin to be achieved at lower doses;[5,6] however, the procedure may result in considerable variations in ciclosporin pharmacokinetics, and has been criticised on several grounds.[7] A similar interaction appears to occur with the related drug *itraconazole*,[8] and there is a single report of such an interaction with *miconazole*.[9] However, although such an interaction has also been reported with *fluconazole*,[10] a small study has failed to note any signifi-

cant interaction;[11,12] it has been suggested that an interaction may take place only at high doses of fluconazole.[13]

Increased nephrotoxicity may occur if ciclosporin is given concomitantly with *amphotericin B*,[14] while liposomal amphotericin B has been reported possibly to exacerbate ciclosporin neurotoxicity.[15] There is a report of decreased ciclosporin concentrations following addition of *griseofulvin* to an immunosuppressant regimen in one patient.[16] Modest decreases have also been seen in ciclosporin concentrations when *terbinafine* was given.[17]

1. Ferguson RM, *et al.* Ketoconazole, cyclosporin metabolism, and renal transplantation. *Lancet* 1982; **ii:** 882–3.
2. Dieperink H, Møller J. Ketoconazole and cyclosporin. *Lancet* 1982; **ii:** 1217.
3. Shepard JH, *et al.* Cyclosporine-ketoconazole: a potentially dangerous drug-drug interaction. *Clin Pharm* 1986; **5:** 468.
4. Gomez DY, *et al.* The effects of ketoconazole on the intestinal metabolism and bioavailability of cyclosporine. *Clin Pharmacol Ther* 1995; **58:** 15–19.
5. First MR, *et al.* Concomitant administration of cyclosporin and ketoconazole in renal transplant recipients. *Lancet* 1989; **ii:** 1198–1201.
6. Keogh A, *et al.* Ketoconazole to reduce the need for cyclosporine after cardiac transplantation. *N Engl J Med* 1995; **333:** 628–33.
7. Frey FJ. Concomitant cyclosporin and ketoconazole. *Lancet* 1990; **335:** 109–10.
8. Kramer MR, *et al.* Cyclosporine and itraconazole interaction in heart and lung transplant recipients. *Ann Intern Med* 1990; **113:** 327–9.
9. Horton CM, *et al.* Cyclosporine interactions with miconazole and other azole-antimycotics: a case report and review of the literature. *J Heart Lung Transplant* 1992; **11:** 1127–32.
10. Collignon P, *et al.* Interaction of fluconazole with cyclosporin. *Lancet* 1989; **i:** 1262.
11. Krüger HU, *et al.* Absence of significant interaction of fluconazole with cyclosporin. *J Antimicrob Chemother* 1989; **24:** 781–6.
12. Ehninger G, *et al.* Interaction of fluconazole with cyclosporin. *Lancet* 1989; **ii:** 104–5.
13. López-Gil JA. Fluconazole-cyclosporine interaction: a dose-dependent effect? *Ann Pharmacother* 1993; **27:** 427–30.
14. Kennedy MS, *et al.* Acute renal toxicity with combined use of amphotericin B and cyclosporine after marrow transplantation. *Transplantation* 1983; **35:** 211–15.
15. Ellis ME, *et al.* Is cyclosporin neurotoxicity enhanced in the presence of liposomal amphotericin B? *J Infect* 1994; **29:** 106–7.
16. Abu-Romeh SH, *et al.* Cyclosporin A and griseofulvin: another drug interaction. *Nephron* 1991; **58:** 237.
17. Lo ACY, *et al.* The interaction of terbinafine and cyclosporine A in renal transplant patients. *Br J Clin Pharmacol* 1997; **43:** 340–1.

Antimalarials. A large rise in serum-ciclosporin concentration was seen on 2 occasions in a renal graft recipient when *chloroquine* was added to his medication for malaria prophylaxis.[1] *Quinine* has also been reported to affect ciclosporin concentrations, in this case reducing them.[2]

1. Finielz P, *et al.* Interaction between cyclosporin and chloroquine. *Nephron* 1993; **65:** 333.
2. Tan HW, Ch'ng SL. Drug interaction between cyclosporin A and quinine in a renal transplant patient with malaria. *Singapore Med J* 1991; **32:** 189–90.

Antineoplastics. Elevated plasma-ciclosporin concentrations and an increased incidence of nephrotoxic effects and hypertension have been reported in patients receiving ciclosporin for psoriasis who had been previously,[1] or concurrently,[2] treated with *methotrexate*. Conversely, methotrexate has been used effectively with reduced-dose ciclosporin in graft-versus-host disease.[3] Severe renal failure has been reported when standard oral doses of ciclosporin were given after high-dose intravenous *melphalan* (used as a bone-marrow conditioning agent before allogeneic bone-marrow transplantation).[4]

Ciclosporin increases plasma-*doxorubicin* concentrations and toxicity (see p.535), and has been used to increase oral absorption of paclitaxel (see p.564). For the effects of ciclosporin on the pharmacokinetics of *teniposide*, see p.574.

Ciclosporin and its analogues have been given with antineoplastics for their ability to inhibit the P-glycoprotein cellular pump responsible for multidrug resistance, thus resulting in raised intracellular concentrations of the other drug.

1. Powles AV, *et al.* Cyclosporin toxicity. *Lancet* 1990; **i:** 610.
2. Korstanje MJ, *et al.* Cyclosporine and methotrexate: a dangerous combination. *J Am Acad Dermatol* 1990; **23:** 320–1.
3. Stockschlaeder M, *et al.* A pilot study of low-dose cyclosporin for graft-versus-host prophylaxis in marrow transplantation. *Br J Haematol* 1992; **80:** 49–54.
4. Morgenstern GR, *et al.* Cyclosporin interaction with ketoconazole and melphalan. *Lancet* 1982; **ii:** 1342.

Antivirals. For a report of mutual elevations in the area under the plasma concentration-time curves for ciclosporin and the HIV-protease inhibitor *saquinavir*, see Indinavir, p.626.

Basiliximab. There has been a report of altered ciclosporin requirements in paediatric renal graft patients treated with basiliximab,[1] but others have failed to note such an effect in similar patients,[2] and whether an interaction exists is unclear.

1. Strehlan J, *et al.* Interleukin-2-receptor antibody-induced alterations of ciclosporin dose requirements in paediatric transplant recipients. *Lancet* 2000; **356:** 1327–8.
2. Vester U, *et al.* Basiliximab in paediatric liver-transplant recipients. *Lancet* 2001; **357:** 388–9.

Cardiovascular drugs. ACE INHIBITORS. There may be an increased risk of hyperkalaemia when ACE inhibitors are used with ciclosporin. Acute renal failure has been reported in 2 patients receiving ciclosporin after renal transplantation follow-

ing administration of *enalapril*.[1] Renal function recovered when the ACE inhibitor was withdrawn.

1. Murray BM, *et al.* Enalapril-associated acute renal failure in renal transplants: possible role of cyclosporine. *Am J Kidney Dis* 1990; **16:** 66–9.

ANTIARRHYTHMICS. Marked rises in serum-ciclosporin concentrations despite reductions in dose have been noted in recipients of heart or heart-lung transplants following treatment with *amiodarone*.[1,2] A similar rise in serum ciclosporin has also been seen in a patient given both ciclosporin and *propafenone*.[3]

1. Mamprin F, *et al.* Amiodarone-cyclosporin interaction in cardiac transplantation. *Am Heart J* 1992; **123:** 1725–6.
2. Egami J, *et al.* Increase in cyclosporine levels due to amiodarone therapy after heart and heart-lung transplantation. *J Am Coll Cardiol* 1993; **21:** 141A.
3. Spes CH, *et al.* Ciclosporin-propafenone interaction. *Klin Wochenschr* 1990; **68:** 872.

ANTICOAGULANTS. Treatment with *warfarin* for deep-vein thrombosis in a patient maintained on ciclosporin 3 mg per kg body-weight daily for pure red cell aplasia resulted in a relapse of the latter and a significant fall in ciclosporin blood concentrations.[1] Increase in the ciclosporin dose to 7 mg per kg body-weight daily restored control of the aplasia but resulted in a marked increase in prothrombin activity requiring an increase in warfarin dosage. The results suggest that each drug interferes with the activity of the other. The influence of the patient's other medications (including phenobarbital and folic acid), if any, is unknown.

1. Snyder DS. Interaction between cyclosporine and warfarin. *Ann Intern Med* 1988; **108:** 311.

ANTIPLATELET DRUGS. *Ticlopidine* decreased serum ciclosporin concentrations in isolated cases,[1,2] but a study in 20 heart transplant patients failed to show any interaction between ciclosporin and low-dose ticlopidine.[3]

1. Birmelé B, *et al.* Interaction of cyclosporin and ticlopidine. *Nephrol Dial Transplant* 1991; **6:** 150–1.
2. Verdejo A, *et al.* Probable interaction between cyclosporin A and low dose ticlopidine. *BMJ* 2000; **320:** 1037.
3. Boissonnat P, *et al.* A drug interaction study between ticlopidine and cyclosporin in heart transplant recipients. *Eur J Clin Pharmacol* 1997; **53:** 39–45.

BETA BLOCKERS. Ciclosporin plasma-concentrations increased when *carvedilol* was added to treatment regimens of 21 renal transplant patients.[1] Considerable interindividual variation was seen, so it is recommended that ciclosporin concentrations be monitored carefully if the drugs are used together.

1. Kaijser M, *et al.* Elevation of cyclosporin A blood levels during carvedilol treatment in renal transplant patients. *Clin Transplant* 1997; **11:** 577–81.

CALCIUM-CHANNEL BLOCKERS. The calcium-channel blockers *diltiazem*,[1,2] *nicardipine*,[3,4] and *verapamil*[5] have all been associated with increases in ciclosporin concentrations in blood when given concomitantly. It has been suggested that such an interaction can be made use of, permitting effective ciclosporin concentrations to be maintained at lower doses.[6] In addition, there is some evidence of mitigation of ciclosporin-induced nephrotoxicity when calcium-channel blockers are given concomitantly (see Effects on the Kidneys, above), and they are useful for ciclosporin-induced hypertension (see Effects on the Cardiovascular System, above). However, some caution is required: one report has pointed out that diltiazem does not increase ciclosporin concentrations in all cases,[7] while others have found that concomitant administration alters the pattern of ciclosporin metabolites, and that pharmacokinetic changes are greater in female than in male patients.[8] Therefore, some prefer a calcium-channel blocker that does not alter ciclosporin pharmacokinetics for hypertension and renal protection. *Nifedipine* has not been shown to increase blood-ciclosporin concentrations.[5] For a report of increased nifedipine toxicity with ciclosporin see Immunosuppressants, p.943. In addition, administration of nifedipine with ciclosporin may exacerbate the problem of gingival hyperplasia—see Hyperplasia, under Adverse Effects, above. Other calcium-channel blockers that do not appear to affect ciclosporin pharmacokinetics include *felodipine*[9] and *isradipine*.[10] Ciclosporin concentrations have been reported to increase[11] and to remain unchanged[12] with *amlodipine*.

1. Brockmöller J, *et al.* Pharmacokinetic interaction between cyclosporin and diltiazem. *Eur J Clin Pharmacol* 1990; **38:** 237–42.
2. Bourge RC, *et al.* Diltiazem-cyclosporine interaction in cardiac transplant recipients: impact on cyclosporine dose and medication costs. *Am J Med* 1991; **90:** 402–4.
3. Todd P, *et al.* Nicardipine interacts with cyclosporin. *Br J Dermatol* 1989; **121:** 820.
4. Kessler M, *et al.* Influence of nicardipine on renal function and plasma cyclosporin in renal transplant patients. *Eur J Clin Pharmacol* 1989; **36:** 637–8.
5. Tortorice KL, *et al.* The effects of calcium channel blockers on cyclosporine and its metabolites in renal transplant patients. *Ther Drug Monit* 1990; **12:** 321–8.
6. Sketris IS, *et al.* Effect of calcium-channel blockers on cyclosporine clearance and use in renal transplant patients. *Ann Pharmacother* 1994; **28:** 1227–31.
7. Jones TE, Morris RG. Diltiazem does not always increase blood cyclosporin concentration. *Br J Clin Pharmacol* 1996; **42:** 642–4.
8. Bleck JS, *et al.* Diltiazem increases blood concentrations of cyclized cyclosporine metabolites resulting in different cyclosporine metabolite patterns in stable male and female renal allograft recipients. *Br J Clin Pharmacol* 1996; **41:** 551–6.
9. Cohen DJ, *et al.* Influence of oral felodipine on serum cyclosporine concentrations. *Clin Transplant* 1994; **8:** 541–5.

10. Endresen L, *et al.* Lack of effect of the calcium antagonist israd-ipine on cyclosporine pharmacokinetics in renal transplant pa-tients. *Ther Drug Monit* 1991; **13**: 490–5.
11. Pesavento TE, *et al.* Amlodipine increases cyclosporin levels in hypertensive renal transplant patients: results of a prospective study. *J Am Soc Nephrol* 1996; **7**: 831–5.
12. Toupance O, *et al.* Antihypertensive effect of amlodipine and lack of interference with cyclosporine metabolism in renal transplant recipients. *Hypertension* 1994; **24**: 297–300.

CLONIDINE. Addition of clonidine to the regimen of a 3-year-old child who had developed hypertension after a renal transplant resulted in a marked increase in whole blood ciclosporin con-centrations, despite a reduction in ciclosporin dose.[1] Withdraw-al of clonidine resulted in a rapid fall in ciclosporin concentrations.

1. Gilbert RD, *et al.* Interaction between clonidine and cy-closporine A. *Nephron* 1995; **71**: 105.

DIURETICS. Enhanced nephrotoxicity, without apparent change in ciclosporin blood concentrations, has been seen in individual patients following addition of *metolazone*[1] or *amiloride* with *chlorothiazide*[2] to their regimen. Severe nephrotoxicity, result-ing in loss of graft function, has been seen in a renal transplant patient given *mannitol* with ciclosporin;[3] graft function recov-ered on withdrawal of the diuretic.

1. Christensen P, Leski M. Nephrotoxic drug interaction between metolazone and cyclosporin. *BMJ* 1987; **294**: 578.
2. Deray G, *et al.* Enhancement of cyclosporin nephrotoxicity by diuretic therapy. *Clin Nephrol* 1989; **32**: 47.
3. Brunner FP, *et al.* Mannitol potentiates cyclosporine nephrotox-icity. *Clin Nephrol* 1986; **25** (suppl 1): 3130–6.

Colchicine. Concurrent administration of ciclosporin and col-chicine may result in myopathy—see Effects on Skeletal Mus-cle, under Adverse Effects, above. For reports of adverse ef-fects and increased serum-ciclosporin concentrations follow-ing concurrent therapy with colchicine, see also p.400.

Corticosteroids. It has been suggested that concurrent use of ciclosporin and corticosteroids increases plasma concentra-tions of both drugs, but not all studies support this—see Antine-oplastics and Immunosuppressants, p.1043.

Gastrointestinal drugs. Administration of *cisapride* to renal transplant recipients being treated with ciclosporin has been re-ported to increase peak ciclosporin concentrations and increase the speed of absorption.[1] *Cimetidine*,[2,3] *ranitidine*,[2] or *famoti-dine*,[3] do not appear to affect ciclosporin pharmacokinetics.

1. Finet L, *et al.* Effects of cisapride on the intestinal absorption of cyclosporine in renal transplant recipients. *Gastroenterology* 1991; **100**: A209.
2. Barri YM, *et al.* Cimetidine or ranitidine in renal transplant pa-tients receiving cyclosporine. *Clin Transplant* 1996; **10**: 34–8.
3. Shaefer MS, *et al.* Evaluation of the pharmacokinetic interaction between cimetidine or famotidine and cyclosporine in healthy men. *Ann Pharmacother* 1995; **29**: 1088–91.

Grapefruit juice. Grapefruit juice increases the bioavailabil-ity of oral,[1–4] but not intravenous[4] ciclosporin, resulting in marked increases in blood-ciclosporin concentrations. The oral microemulsion formulation of ciclosporin is also affected.[5] The effect appears to be due to inhibition of cytochrome P450 en-zymes in the gut wall by substances present in grapefruit juice,[3] resulting in transiently reduced ciclosporin metabolism. Al-though it has been suggested that the effect might be used sim-ilarly to that of calcium-channel blockers or ketoconazole in reducing the required dose of ciclosporin,[2] others have pointed out that grapefruit juice is not standardised and its effects are variable.[6]

1. Proppe DG, *et al.* Influence of chronic ingestion of grapefruit juice on steady-state blood concentrations of cyclosporine A in renal transplant patients with stable graft function. *Br J Clin Pharmacol* 1995; **39**: 337–8.
2. Yee GC, *et al.* Effect of grapefruit juice on blood cyclosporin concentration. *Lancet* 1995; **345**: 955–6.
3. Hollander AAMJ, *et al.* The effect of grapefruit juice on cy-closporine and prednisone metabolism in transplant patients. *Clin Pharmacol Ther* 1995; **57**: 318–24.
4. Ducharme MP, *et al.* Disposition of intravenous and oral cy-closporine after administration with grapefruit juice. *Clin Phar-macol Ther* 1995; **57**: 485–91.
5. Ku Y-M, *et al.* Effect of grapefruit juice on the pharmacokinetics of microemulsion cyclosporine and its metabolite in healthy vol-unteers: does the formulation difference matter? *J Clin Pharma-col* 1998; **38**: 959–65.
6. Johnston A, Holt DW. Effect of grapefruit juice on blood cy-closporin concentration. *Lancet* 1995; **346**: 122–3.

Hypoglycaemic drugs. Concurrent administration of *gliben-clamide* with ciclosporin in 6 patients was associated with a mean 57% increase in the steady-state plasma concentration of ciclosporin, suggesting that dosage adjustment may become necessary when these drugs are given concomitantly.[1]

Troglitazone decreased ciclosporin-blood concentrations by 32%, necessitating an increase in ciclosporin dosage.[2]

1. Islam SI, *et al.* Possible interaction between cyclosporine and glibenclamide in posttransplant diabetic patients. *Ther Drug Monit* 1996; **18**: 624–6.
2. Burgess SJ, *et al.* Effect of troglitazone on cyclosporine whole blood levels. *Transplantation* 1998; **66**: 272–3.

Lipid regulating drugs. A study in 10 renal transplant recip-ients indicated that concomitant use of ciclosporin and *probu-col* markedly reduced the whole blood and plasma concentrations of the former in 9 of them, compared with use of ciclosporin alone.[1] Concurrent administration of *bezafibrate* has been reported to result in increased blood concentrations of ciclosporin and resultant nephrotoxicity.[2]

In 1 study, *simvastatin* increased the unbound fraction of ciclosporin in the blood, resulting in a modest increase in ap-parent ciclosporin clearance.[3] In turn, ciclosporin can markedly increase simvastatin concentrations in plasma.[4] In other stud-ies, ciclosporin concentrations were unaffected by *cerivasta-tin*,[5] *lovastatin*,[6] and *pravastatin*,[6,7] but each of the statins showed increases in plasma concentrations. In the case of lov-astatin, this lead to accumulation of the drug,[6] and there are reports of rhabdomyolysis with concurrent administration of ciclosporin and lovastatin—see Effects on Skeletal Muscle, un-der Adverse Effects, above, and also under Lovastatin, p.923. Similar reports have occurred with *simvastatin*,[8,9] and *atorvastatin*[10] and this may be a class effect for statins, see p.970.

1. Gallego C, *et al.* Interaction between probucol and cyclosporine in renal transplant patients. *Ann Pharmacother* 1994; **28**: 940–3.
2. Hirai M, *et al.* Elevated blood concentrations of cyclosporine and kidney failure after bezafibrate in renal graft recipient. *Ann Pharmacother* 1996; **30**: 883–4.
3. Akhlaghi F, *et al.* Effect of simvastatin on cyclosporine unbound fraction and apparent blood clearance in heart transplant recipi-ents. *Br J Clin Pharmacol* 1997; **44**: 537–42.
4. Arnadottir M, *et al.* Plasma concentration profiles of simvastatin 3-hydroxy-3-methyl-glutaryl-coenzyme A reductase inhibitory activity in kidney transplant recipients with and without ciclosporin. *Nephron* 1993; **65**: 410–13.
5. Mück W, *et al.* Increase in cerivastatin systemic exposure after single and multiple dosing in cyclosporine-treated kidney trans-plant recipients. *Clin Pharmacol Ther* 1999; **65**: 251–61.
6. Olbricht C, *et al.* Accumulation of lovastatin, but not pravasta-tin, in the blood of cyclosporine-treated kidney graft patients after multiple doses. *Clin Pharmacol Ther* 1997; **62**: 311–21.
7. Regazzi MB, *et al.* Altered disposition of pravastatin following concomitant drug therapy with cyclosporin A transplant recipi-ents. *Transplant Proc* 1993; **25**: 2732–4.
8. Blaison G, *et al.* Rhabdomyolyse causée par la simvastatine chez un transplanté cardiaque sous ciclosporine. *Rev Med In-terne* 1992; **13**: 61–3.
9. Meier C, *et al.* Rhabdomyolyse bei mit Simvastatin und Ciclosporin behandelten Patienten: Rolle der aktivität des Cyto-chrom-P450-Enzymsystems der Leber. *Schweiz Med Wochen-schr* 1995; **125**: 1342–6.
10. Maltz HC, *et al.* Rhabdomyolysis associated with concomitant use of atorvastatin and cyclosporine. *Ann Pharmacother* 1999; **33**: 1176–9.

Muromonab-CD3. Treatment of acute rejection of kidney grafts in 10 patients using muromonab-CD3 resulted in in-creases in mean trough ciclosporin concentrations, despite a re-duction in ciclosporin dosage.[1] Once muromonab-CD3 was withdrawn the ciclosporin dosage had to be increased again to provide adequate concentrations.

1. Vrahnos D, *et al.* Cyclosporin levels during OKT3 treatment of acute renal allograft rejection. *Pharmacotherapy* 1991; **11**: 278.

NSAIDs. Raised serum-ciclosporin trough concentrations, to-gether with small increases in serum creatinine and BUN con-centrations, followed the administration of *sulindac* to a previously-stabilised renal graft recipient taking an immuno-suppressive regimen including ciclosporin.[1] Increased renal impairment was seen when sulindac or *naproxen* were added to ciclosporin therapy in patients with rheumatoid arthritis.[2] Ne-phrotoxicity, in the absence of significantly raised blood-ciclosporin concentrations, has been reported in other patients given *diclofenac* concomitantly with ciclosporin.[3] Ciclosporin may also increase plasma-diclofenac concentrations, see p.31. In general, because of the known potential of NSAIDs to ad-versely affect renal function, careful monitoring of renal func-tion is advised if these drugs are added to ciclosporin therapy or their dosages altered.

1. Sesin GP, *et al.* Sulindac-induced elevation of serum cy-closporine concentration. *Clin Pharm* 1989; **8**: 445–6.
2. Altman RD, *et al.* Interaction of cyclosporine A and nonsteroidal anti-inflammatory drugs on renal function in patients with rheu-matoid arthritis. *Am J Med* 1992; **93**: 396–402.
3. Branthwaite JP, Nicholls A. Cyclosporin and diclofenac interac-tion in rheumatoid arthritis. *Lancet* 1991; **337**: 252.

Octreotide. A marked reduction in ciclosporin serum con-centrations was seen in 10 diabetic patients with pancreatic transplants when octreotide was given concomitantly;[1] it was suggested that if these 2 drugs are given together the oral dos-age of ciclosporin needs to be increased on average by 50%.

1. Landgraf R, *et al.* Effect of somatostatin analogue (SMS 201-995) on cyclosporine levels. *Transplantation* 1987; **44**: 724–5.

Orlistat. A reduction in ciclosporin concentrations to subther-apeutic levels has been reported[1,2] in transplant recipients fol-lowing concomitant administration of orlistat. It was postulated[2] that the interaction was as a result of reduced ab-sorption of ciclosporin in the presence of orlistat.

1. Nägele H, *et al.* Effect of orlistat on blood cyclosporin concen-tration in an obese heart transplant patient. *Eur J Clin Pharmacol* 1999; **55**: 667–9.
2. Colman E, Fossler M. Reduction in blood cyclosporine concen-trations by orlistat. *N Engl J Med* 2000; **342**: 1141–2.

Retinoids. Following a report of increased whole-blood ciclosporin concentrations and nephrotoxicity in a patient giv-en *etretinate* with ciclosporin, *in-vitro* results indicated that etretinate inhibited hepatic microsomal metabolism of ciclosporin, as did *acitretin* and *isotretinoin*.[1] However, a study failed to find evidence of such an interaction *in vitro*.[2]

1. Shah IA, *et al.* The effects of retinoids and terbinafine on the human hepatic microsomal metabolism of cyclosporin. *Br J Der-matol* 1993; **129**: 395–8.
2. Webber IR, Back DJ. Effect of etretinate on cyclosporin metab-olism in vitro. *Br J Dermatol* 1993; **128**: 42–4.

Sex hormones. Raised ciclosporin concentrations in blood have been seen when therapy with *danazol*,[1] *methyltestoster-one*,[2] or *norethisterone*[1] was given concurrently with ciclo-sporin, and clinical evidence of both nephrotoxicity[1,2] and hepatotoxicity[2] has been seen. Severe hepatotoxicity and raised plasma-ciclosporin trough values also resulted when an oral contraceptive containing *levonorgestrel* and *ethinylestradiol* was taken by a woman receiving ciclosporin;[3] she had taken the same contraceptive before beginning ciclosporin without ill-ef-fects.

1. Ross WB, *et al.* Cyclosporin interaction with danazol and nore-thisterone. *Lancet* 1986; **i**: 330.
2. Møller BB, Ekelund B. Toxicity of cyclosporine during treat-ment with androgens. *N Engl J Med* 1985; **313**: 1416.
3. Deray G, *et al.* Oral contraceptive interaction with cyclosporin. *Lancet* 1987; **i**: 158.

Sirolimus. For the effect of ciclosporin on the pharmacokinet-ics of sirolimus, see p.568.

Tacrolimus. Tacrolimus inhibits ciclosporin metabolism *in vitro*[1] but did not alter the pharmacokinetics of intravenous ciclosporin in 7 liver transplant patients.[2] However, there is a possibility of increased nephrotoxicity when the drugs are ad-ministered together, so the manufacturers recommend avoiding concurrent use.

1. Venkataramanan R, *et al.* Pharmacokinetics of FK 506 in trans-plant patients. *Transplant Proc* 1991; **23**: 2736–40.
2. Jain AB, *et al.* Pharmacokinetics of cyclosporine and nephrotox-icity in orthotopic liver transplant patients rescued with FK 506. *Transplant Proc* 1991; **23**: 2777–9.

Vaccines. Efficacy of immunoprophylaxis may be expected to be diminished during ciclosporin therapy, and administration of live virus vaccines, in particular, is contra-indicated in im-munocompromised patients.[1] Further, there is some evidence that antigens administered during ciclosporin therapy may in-duce tolerance, which might result in increased susceptibility to the diseases one wishes to protect against.

1. Grabenstein JD, Baker JR. Comment: cyclosporine and vaccina-tion. *Drug Intell Clin Pharm* 1985; **19**: 679–80.

Vitamins. For reference to increased absorption of ciclosporin when given with a water-soluble macrogol derivative of *vita-min E*, see Absorption, under Pharmacokinetics, below.

Pharmacokinetics

The pharmacokinetics of ciclosporin are variable and difficult to determine. Results vary depending on the use of a HPLC assay or a radio-immunoassay, and values obtained by the two methods are not strictly comparable.

Absorption of conventional formulations of ciclosporin from the gastrointestinal tract is variable and incomplete. An oral microemulsion formulation with improved absorption characteristics is available and is more rapidly and completely absorbed, with peak concentrations achieved about 1.5 to 2 hours af-ter a dose.

Ciclosporin is widely distributed throughout the body. Distribution in the blood is concentration-de-pendent, with between 41 and 58% in erythrocytes and 10 to 20% in leucocytes; the remainder is found in plasma, about 90% protein-bound, mostly to lipo-protein. Because of distribution into blood cells whole blood concentrations are higher than, and not comparable with, plasma concentrations; where peak plasma concentrations are reported to be approxi-mately 1 nanogram per mL (by specific HPLC assay) for each mg of oral ciclosporin, whole blood concen-trations for each mg range from about 1.4 to 2.7 nanograms per mL. Ciclosporin is reported to cross the placenta, and to be distributed into breast milk.

Clearance from the blood is biphasic. The terminal elimination half-life of an oral dose is reported to range from about 5 to 20 hours; clearance in children is more rapid.

Ciclosporin is extensively metabolised in the liver and primarily excreted in faeces via the bile. About 6% of a dose is reported to be excreted in urine, less than 0.1% unchanged.

Absorption. Ingestion of conventional formulations of ciclosporin with food may increase its bioavailability, although the effect only appears to be significant when the meal is high in fat;[1] ingestion with food and added bile acids may also in-crease absorption moderately.[2] Administration with a micelle-forming macrogol derivative of vitamin E (tocofersolan) has also been reported to markedly increase ciclosporin absorp-tion.[3,4]

Because of the problems of variable oral absorption, an oral microemulsion has been developed which offers greatly im-proved and more predictable bioavailability,[5–9] particularly in liver transplant patients with impaired bile flow.[5-7] It should be noted that the formulation of this microemulsion in fact includes a vitamin E compound.

However, a recent study[10] has suggested that contrary to previous assumptions, conventional formulations of ciclosporin are quite well absorbed, and that the low bioavailability is due to extensive cytochrome-mediated metabolism in the gut wall (see also Metabolism, below). If this were the case, the improved bioavailability seen with the microemulsion formulation is presumably less to do with improved absorption than with protection from such metabolism.

1. Gupta SK, et al. Effect of food on the pharmacokinetics of cyclosporine in healthy subjects following oral and intravenous administration. J Clin Pharmacol 1990; 30: 643–53.
2. Lindholm A, et al. The effect of food and bile acid administration on the relative bioavailability of cyclosporin. Br J Clin Pharmacol 1990; 29: 541–8.
3. Sokol RJ, et al. Improvement of cyclosporin absorption in children after liver transplantation by means of water-soluble vitamin E. Lancet 1991; 338: 212–15.
4. Chang T, et al. The effect of water-soluble vitamin E on cyclosporine pharmacokinetics in healthy volunteers. Clin Pharmacol Ther 1996; 59: 297–303.
5. Trull AK, et al. Cyclosporin absorption from microemulsion formulation in liver transplant recipient. Lancet 1993; 341: 433.
6. Sketris IS, et al. Increased cyclosporin bioavailability from a microemulsion formulation in a liver transplant recipient. Ann Pharmacother 1994; 28: 962–3.
7. Trull AK, et al. Absorption of cyclosporin from conventional and new microemulsion oral formulations in liver transplant recipients with external biliary diversion. Br J Clin Pharmacol 1995; 39: 627–31.
8. van den Borne BEEM, et al. Relative bioavailability of a new oral form of cyclosporin A in patients with rheumatoid arthritis. Br J Clin Pharmacol 1995; 39: 172–5.
9. Friman S, Bäckman L. A new microemulsion formulation of cyclosporin: pharmacokinetic and clinical features. Clin Pharmacokinet 1996; 30: 181–93.
10. Wu C-Y, et al. Differentiation of absorption and first-pass gut and hepatic metabolism in humans: studies with cyclosporine. Clin Pharmacol Ther 1995; 58: 492–7.

Metabolism. Evidence has been seen in vitro[1] and in vivo[2-4] that the low oral bioavailability of ciclosporin is due to first-pass metabolism in the gastrointestinal tract rather than the liver.

1. Tjia JF, et al. Cyclosporin metabolism by the gastrointestinal mucosa. Br J Clin Pharmacol 1991; 31: 344–6.
2. Kolars JC, et al. First-pass metabolism of cyclosporin by the gut. Lancet 1991; 338: 1488–90.
3. Hoppu K, et al. Evidence for pre-hepatic metabolism of oral cyclosporine in children. Br J Clin Pharmacol 1991; 32: 477–81.
4. Wu C-Y, et al. Differentiation of absorption and first-pass gut and hepatic metabolism in humans: studies with cyclosporine. Clin Pharmacol Ther 1995; 58: 492–7.

Monitoring drug concentrations. Considerable debate has attended the necessity for therapeutic monitoring of ciclosporin concentrations and also on the questions of which assay methods to use and whether to measure drug concentrations in whole blood or plasma.

Before the introduction of specific monoclonal radio-immunoassay the HPLC assay for ciclosporin had the advantage of being specific for the parent compound, and some workers suggested it to be the method of choice.[1,2] However, it is a more complex procedure, is not universally available, and is slower to perform than radio-immunoassay.[1,3-5] Specific monoclonal radio-immunoassays are now widely available; a comparative study of specific and non-specific radio-immunoassays, HPLC, and polyclonal fluorescence polarisation immunoassay (FPIA) found that the specific assays, used on whole blood samples, gave the best correlation with clinical events.[6]

Because the distribution of ciclosporin between blood cells and plasma is temperature-dependent, plasma concentrations may be twice as high at 37° as at 21°.[7] The temperature at which samples are stored and processed may therefore considerably influence results. In consequence, measurement of drug concentrations in whole blood is to be preferred.[1,3,4,8] However, many, particularly early, clinical studies have given plasma or serum concentrations, which makes comparison of literature data difficult. This problem is compounded by a considerable degree of variation between laboratories,[9,10] even when the same technique is used,[10] and by circadian variations in ciclosporin metabolism which mean that samples should be taken at the same time of day.[11]

Because of the variability in results caused by difficulties in monitoring it has proved difficult to determine precisely the ciclosporin concentrations associated with therapeutic benefit and toxicity,[1,3-5] and it has been suggested that measurement of the therapeutic concentrations is unnecessary (provided the patient's clinical condition and renal function are monitored) when low-dose ciclosporin is being given (for example, in psoriasis).[12] However, others consider that it is always critical that ciclosporin blood trough concentrations are regularly measured,[13,14] in addition to other monitoring. It has been suggested[15] that trough ciclosporin concentrations, measured by a specific method in whole blood, should not be less than 150 nanograms per mL during the first month after renal transplantation, although lower concentrations are subsequently acceptable; trough concentrations of 250 to 300 nanograms per

mL are recommended in the 3 months following liver transplantation.

1. Ptachcinski RJ, et al. Cyclosporine concentration determinations for monitoring and pharmacokinetic studies. J Clin Pharmacol 1986; 26: 358–66.
2. Varghese Z, et al. How to measure cyclosporin. Lancet 1984; i: 1407–8.
3. Faynor SM, et al. Therapeutic drug monitoring of cyclosporine. Mayo Clin Proc 1984; 59: 571–2.
4. Burkle WS. Cyclosporine pharmacokinetics and blood level monitoring. Drug Intell Clin Pharm 1985; 19: 101–5.
5. Rodighiero V. Therapeutic drug monitoring of cyclosporin: practical applications and limitations. Clin Pharmacokinet 1989; 16: 27–37.
6. Lindholm A, et al. A prospective study of cyclosporine concentration in relation to its therapeutic effect and toxicity after renal transplantation. Br J Clin Pharmacol 1990; 30: 443–52.
7. Dieperink H. Temperature dependency of cyclosporin plasma levels. Lancet 1983; i: 416.
8. Bandini G, et al. Measuring cyclosporin in plasma. Lancet 1983; i: 762.
9. Moyer TP. Measurement of cyclosporine: a challenge to the professional laboratory organizations. Ther Drug Monit 1985; 7: 123–4.
10. Johnston A, et al. The United Kingdom Cyclosporin Quality Assessment Scheme. Ther Drug Monit 1986; 8: 200–4.
11. Venkataramanan R, et al. Diurnal variation in cyclosporine kinetics. Ther Drug Monit 1986; 8: 380–1.
12. Feutren G, et al. Cyclosporin monitoring in psoriasis. Lancet 1990; 335: 866–7.
13. Gupta AK, et al. Short-term changes in renal function, blood pressure, and electrolyte levels in patients receiving cyclosporine for dermatologic disorders. Arch Intern Med 1991; 151: 356–62.
14. Dumont RJ, Ensom MHH. Methods for clinical monitoring of ciclosporin in transplant patients. Clin Pharmacokinet 2000; 38: 427–41.
15. Lindholm A. Therapeutic monitoring of cyclosporin—an update. Eur J Clin Pharmacol 1991; 41: 273–83.

Uses and Administration

Ciclosporin is a powerful immunosuppressant which appears to act specifically on lymphocytes, mainly helper T-cells. It inhibits the activation of calcineurin, an important step in the production of lymphokines including interleukin-2, resulting in a depression of cell-mediated immune response. Unlike cytotoxic immunosuppressants such as cyclophosphamide it has little effect on bone marrow.

Ciclosporin is used, usually combined with corticosteroids (and often with other immunosuppressants), in organ and tissue transplantation for the prophylaxis of graft rejection, or in the management of graft rejection in patients previously treated with other immunosuppressants. It is also used in severe forms of atopic dermatitis, psoriasis, or rheumatoid arthritis, usually when conventional therapy is ineffective or inappropriate, and is used in nephrotic syndrome.

Ciclosporin has been tried in various other diseases considered to have an auto-immune component as indicated by the cross-references given below; they include aplastic anaemia, asthma, Behçet's syndrome, chronic active hepatitis, multiple sclerosis, myasthenia gravis, sarcoidosis, scleritis or uveitis, scleroderma, and various skin disorders.

Ciclosporin is given by mouth as liquid-filled capsules or as an oily solution, which may be diluted with milk or fruit juice (not grapefruit) immediately before administration to improve palatability. Microemulsion formulations with improved bioavailability are available in a number of countries. When changing between preparations, the initial dose of the new formulation should be the same (mg for mg), and should subsequently be adjusted as necessary based on blood-ciclosporin concentrations, serum creatinine, and blood pressure monitoring. The daily dose of ciclosporin is taken in 2 divided doses, although the conventional formulation is sometimes given as a single daily dose.

In **organ transplantation** the usual initial dose of ciclosporin is 10 to 15 mg per kg body-weight daily, beginning 4 to 12 hours before transplantation, and continued for 1 to 2 weeks; lower initial doses may be given in combination with other immunosuppressants (e.g. with corticosteroids or as part of 'triple' or 'quadruple' therapy). Dosage may subsequently be reduced gradually to a daily maintenance dose of 2 to 6 mg per kg.

Kidney function and blood pressure should be monitored regularly, as well as blood concentrations of ciclosporin (see Monitoring Drug Concentrations, above), and dosage should be adjusted as necessary. Hepatic function should also be monitored.

Ciclosporin may also be given intravenously, at one-third of the oral dose, in patients in whom oral administration is not feasible. It is given by slow intravenous infusion over 2 to 6 hours, the 5% concentrate being diluted 1:20 or 1:100 in sodium chloride 0.9% or glucose 5%, to give a 0.05 to 0.25% solution of ciclosporin. Because of the risk of anaphylactoid reactions, which have been attributed to the polyethoxylated castor oil vehicle, patients should be transferred to oral therapy as soon as possible.

For the prevention of graft rejection in **bone-marrow transplantation** and prevention and treatment of graft-versus-host disease an initial dose of 3 to 5 mg per kg daily by the intravenous route is recommended, continued for up to 2 weeks until maintenance by mouth, in doses of 12.5 mg per kg daily can be instituted. This dose is continued for at least 3 to 6 months, then gradually reduced until ciclosporin is withdrawn altogether; this may take up to a year after transplantation.

In the treatment of **psoriasis**, ciclosporin may be given in usual initial doses of 2.5 mg per kg daily (a maximum of 5 mg per kg daily is recommended in the UK and 4 mg per kg daily in the USA), in 2 divided doses by mouth, reduced once remission is achieved to the lowest effective maintenance dose. Treatment should be discontinued if there is insufficient response within 6 weeks to the maximum dose. A similar dosage range may be given for a maximum of 8 weeks in the treatment of severe **atopic dermatitis**.

In **rheumatoid arthritis** ciclosporin may be given by mouth in initial daily doses of 2.5 mg per kg, divided into two doses, for a period of 6 or 8 weeks. If the clinical effect is insufficient dosage may then be increased to a maximum of 4 mg per kg daily; if there is no response after 3 months, treatment should then be discontinued.

For **nephrotic syndrome** secondary to glomerular kidney disease (minimal change nephropathy, focal glomerulosclerosis, or membranous nephropathy) dosage of ciclosporin depends on age and renal function. To induce remission in patients with normal renal function 5 mg per kg daily may be given to adults and 6 mg per kg daily to children, in 2 divided doses by mouth. In patients with renal impairment the initial dose should not exceed 2.5 mg per kg daily. Treatment may be discontinued if there is no response after 3 months (or 6 months in patients with membranous nephropathy). In patients who do respond, maintenance doses should be gradually reduced to the minimum effective value. Ciclosporin can inhibit the P-glycoprotein cellular pump responsible for multidrug resistance, and has been given with antineoplastics to raise their intracellular concentrations.

Nonimmunosuppressive ciclosporin analogues such as valspodar are being investigated for their ability to reverse multidrug resistance.

Administration. It has been suggested that calculating doses in mg per kg body-weight may not be the best way to achieve the desired blood concentrations of ciclosporin.[1] Retrospective study of 1071 renal transplant recipients indicated that blood ciclosporin concentrations were not significantly correlated with patient weight, the best prediction of trough blood concentration being given by the formula:

Blood concentration (nanograms/mL) = dose in mg/day × (1.34 + 0.00011 × days after transplant − 0.0049 × height in cm)

This formula appeared useful in predicting blood concentrations in prospective studies; from the seventh day after transplantation target trough concentrations could be expected to be about 0.3 times the daily ciclosporin dose in mg.

1. Bock HA, et al. Weight-independent dosing of cyclosporine—an alternative to the mg/kg doctrine. Transplantation 1994; 57: 1484–9.

INHALATION. Aerosolised ciclosporin given by inhalation has proved effective in the management of acute graft rejection in lung transplantation.[1] Ciclosporin was administered at a dose of 100 to 300 mg daily via a nebuliser, in addition to continued systemic therapy with ciclosporin or tacrolimus, azathioprine and prednisone. Liposomal formulations are under investigation for the aerosolised administration of ciclosporin.

1. Keenan RJ, et al. Efficacy of inhaled cyclosporine in lung transplant recipients with refractory rejection: correlation of intragraft cytokine gene expression with pulmonary function and histologic characteristics. Surgery 1995; 118: 385–91.

ORAL. A review of the newer microemulsion formulation of ciclosporin.[1] For discussion of the potential problems involved in converting from conventional to microemulsion oral formulations see under Precautions, above.

1. Noble S, Markham A. Cyclosporin: a review of the pharmacokinetic properties, clinical efficacy and tolerability of a microemulsion-based formulation (Neoral). *Drugs* 1995; **50**: 924–41.

Aplastic anaemia. Ciclosporin alone or combined immunosuppression with ciclosporin and antilymphocyte immunoglobulins is used in patients with aplastic anaemia when bone marrow transplantation is unsuitable (see p.715).

Asthma. Ciclosporin is being considered as a potential treatment for some cases of asthma (p.757). A controlled study in patients with chronic severe asthma requiring long-standing oral corticosteroid treatment found that addition of ciclosporin in an initial dose of 5 mg per kg body-weight daily to their regimen resulted in significant improvement in lung function and a reduced frequency of disease exacerbation, compared with placebo.[1] The results were interesting because of the improvement in what had been considered 'irreversible' airflow obstruction. A subsequent study from the same centre involving 39 patients with severe corticosteroid-dependent asthma found that low-dose ciclosporin by mouth (an initial dose of 5 mg per kg body-weight daily) permitted a reduction in the daily dosage of prednisolone, from a median of 10 to 3.5 mg daily.[2]

1. Alexander AG, *et al.* Trial of cyclosporin in corticosteroid-dependent chronic severe asthma. *Lancet* 1992; **339**: 324–8.
2. Lock SH, *et al.* Double-blind, placebo-controlled study of cyclosporin A as a corticosteroid-sparing agent in corticosteroid-dependent asthma. *Am J Respir Crit Care Med* 1996; **153**: 509–14.

Behçet's syndrome. Ciclosporin has been tried[1] in Behçet's syndrome, see p.1047.

1. Masuda K, *et al.* Double-masked trial of cyclosporin versus colchicine and long-term open study of cyclosporin in Behçet's disease. *Lancet* 1989; **i**: 1093–6.

Cogan's syndrome. Ciclosporin has been used in conjunction with corticosteroids for severe Cogan's syndrome with large-vessel vasculitis (see p.1049).

Diabetes mellitus. Immunosuppressants have been used in attempts to prolong the so called 'honeymoon period' in recently diagnosed diabetics (p.315). Ciclosporin has apparently produced modest benefits in such a context,[1-3] but its overall value remains to be determined.

1. Bougneres PF, *et al.* Factors associated with early remission of type 1 diabetes in children treated with cyclosporine. *N Engl J Med* 1988; **318**: 663–70.
2. The Canadian-European Randomized Control Trial Group. Cyclosporin-induced remission of IDDM after early intervention: association of 1 yr of cyclosporin treatment with enhanced insulin secretion. *Diabetes* 1988; **37**: 1574–82.
3. Carel JC, *et al.* Cyclosporine delays but does not prevent clinical onset in glucose intolerant pre-type 1 diabetic children. *J Autoimmun* 1996; **9**: 739–45.

Dry eye. Topical ciclosporin has been tried[1,2] for keratoconjunctivitis sicca (dry eye—see p.1498).

1. Laibovitz RA, *et al.* Pilot trial of cyclosporine 1% ophthalmic ointment in the treatment of keratoconjunctivitis sicca. *Cornea* 1993; **12**: 315–23.
2. Tauber J. The Cyclosporine Study Group. A dose-ranging clinical trial to assess the safety and efficacy of cyclosporine ophthalmic emulsion in patients with keratoconjunctivitis sicca. *Adv Exp Med Biol* 1998; **438**: 969–72.

Eczema. Ciclosporin is effective in atopic eczema (atopic dermatitis),[1-3] where it is employed as adjunctive therapy (see p.1105). It is generally reserved for short-term treatment (up to 8 weeks) in patients with severe disease unresponsive to all conventional therapies, although reports have described long-term use in adult patients.[4-6] Ciclosporin has been used for both short courses[7,8] and continuous therapy in children.[9] Responses have also been reported in severe eczematisation associated with Darier's disease[10] (p.1104).

1. van Joost T, *et al.* Cyclosporin in atopic dermatitis: a multicentre placebo-controlled study. *Br J Dermatol* 1994; **130**: 634–40.
2. Munro CS, *et al.* Maintenance treatment with cyclosporin in atopic eczema. *Br J Dermatol* 1994; **130**: 376–80.
3. Granlund H, *et al.* Cyclosporin in atopic dermatitis: time to relapse and effect of intermittent therapy. *Br J Dermatol* 1995; **132**: 106–12.
4. Sepp N, Fritsch PO. Can cyclosporin A induce permanent remission of atopic eczema? *Br J Dermatol* 1993; **128**: 213–16.
5. Pryce DW, *et al.* Safety and efficacy of longer-term lower-dose cyclosporin A therapy. *Br J Dermatol* 1994; **130**: 681–9.
6. Berth-Jones J, *et al.* Long-term efficacy and safety of cyclosporin in severe adult atopic eczema. *Br J Dermatol* 1996; **135** (suppl 47): 26.
7. Zaki I, *et al.* Treatment of severe atopic dermatitis in childhood with cyclosporin. *Br J Dermatol* 1996; **135** (suppl 48): 21–4.
8. Berth-Jones J, *et al.* Cyclosporin in severe childhood atopic dermatitis: a multicenter study. *J Am Acad Dermatol* 1996; **34**: 1016–21.
9. Harper JI, *et al.* Cyclosporin for severe childhood atopic dermatitis: short course versus continuous therapy. *Br J Dermatol* 2000; **142**: 52–8.
10. Shahidullah H, *et al.* Darier's disease: severe eczematization successfully treated with cyclosporin. *Br J Dermatol* 1994; **131**: 713–16.

Glaucoma. Topical ciclosporin has produced some encouraging results[1] when used as an adjunct to reduce formation of scar tissue and improve outcome of glaucoma filtering surgery (p.1413).

1. Turaçli E, *et al.* A comparative clinical trial of mitomycin C and cyclosporin A in trabeculectomy. *Eur J Ophthalmol* 1996; **6**: 398–401.

Glomerular kidney disease. Ciclosporin has been tried in a number of forms of glomerular kidney disease (p.1051) but use has been cautious because of fears about nephrotoxicity. Nonetheless, responses have been seen in patients with corticosteroid-resistant minimal change nephropathy,[1,2] focal glomerulosclerosis,[1,2] and membranous nephropathy.[3,4]

1. Nyrop M, Olgaard K. Cyclosporin A treatment of severe steroid resistant nephrotic syndrome in adults. *J Intern Med* 1990; **227**: 65–8.
2. Niaudet P, *et al.* Steroid-resistant idiopathic nephrotic syndrome and ciclosporin. *Nephron* 1991; **57**: 481.
3. Rostoker G, *et al.* Cyclosporin in idiopathic steroid-resistant membranous glomerulonephritis. *Lancet* 1989; **ii**: 975–6.
4. Cattran DC, *et al.* A controlled trial of cyclosporine in patients with progressive membranous nephropathy. *Kidney Int* 1995; **47**: 1130–5.

Hepatitis. In chronic active hepatitis (p.1048), some evidence suggests that ciclosporin may offer an alternative therapy in patients with severe auto-immune (non-viral) disease where corticosteroids alone or with azathioprine do not suffice.
References.
1. Mistilis SP, *et al.* Cyclosporin, a new treatment for autoimmune chronic active hepatitis. *Med J Aust* 1985; **143**: 463–5.
2. Sherman KE, *et al.* Cyclosporine in the management of corticosteroid-resistant type 1 autoimmune chronic active hepatitis. *J Hepatol* 1994; **21**: 1040–7.
3. Debray D, *et al.* Efficacy of cyclosporin A in children with type 2 autoimmune hepatitis. *J Pediatr* 1999; **135**: 111–14.

Histiocytic syndromes. As mentioned in the discussion on p.483 ciclosporin has been reported to produce benefit in patients with advanced Langerhans-cell histiocytosis.

Inflammatory bowel disease. Ciclosporin has been tried with variable success as a second-line drug in inflammatory bowel disease (p.1205). Intravenous high-dose ciclosporin has shown some efficacy in refractory ulcerative colitis,[1,2] and may also be useful if given by enema.[3] However, benefit in Crohn's disease is less clear. Although intravenous therapy is reportedly useful in healing refractory fistulae,[4] lower oral doses have produced disappointing results in adults and children with chronic active Crohn's disease,[5,6] and for maintenance of remission.[7]

1. Lichtiger S, *et al.* Cyclosporine in severe ulcerative colitis refractory to steroid therapy. *N Engl J Med* 1994; **330**: 1841–5.
2. Hyde GM, *et al.* Intravenous cyclosporin as rescue therapy in severe ulcerative colitis: time for a reappraisal? *Eur J Gastroenterol Hepatol* 1998; **10**: 411–13.
3. Sandborn WJ, *et al.* Cyclosporine enemas for treatment-resistant, mildly to moderately active, left-sided ulcerative colitis. *Am J Gastroenterol* 1993; **88**: 640–5.
4. Hanauer SB, Smith MB. Rapid closure of Crohn's disease fistulas with continuous intravenous cyclosporin A. *Am J Gastroenterol* 1993; **88**: 646–9.
5. Nicholls S, *et al.* Cyclosporin as initial treatment for Crohn's disease. *Arch Dis Child* 1994; **71**: 243–7.
6. Stange EF, *et al.* European trial of cyclosporine in chronic active Crohn's disease: a 12-month study. *Gastroenterology* 1995; **109**: 774–82.
7. Feagan BG, *et al.* Low-dose cyclosporine for the treatment of Crohn's disease. *N Engl J Med* 1994; **330**: 1846–51.

Lichen planus. Lichen planus is a skin disorder generally controlled with corticosteroids (see p.1106), although ciclosporin has also been used. Ciclosporin has been given successfully in relatively low doses (3 to 5 mg per kg body-weight by mouth) to produce remission of severe lichen planus,[1] but such therapy may be associated with the development of hypertension and impairment of renal function. Topical application of ciclosporin oral solution as a mouthwash for oral lichen planus has been tried, but results have been variable.[2-7] One such study failed to note any benefit long-term from either ciclosporin mouthwash or corticosteroid oral paste.[7]

1. Pigatto PD, *et al.* Cyclosporin A for treatment of severe lichen planus. *Br J Dermatol* 1990; **121**: 121–3.
2. Eisen D, *et al.* Cyclosporin wash for oral lichen planus. *Lancet* 1990; **335**: 535–6.
3. Eisen D, *et al.* Effect of topical cyclosporine rinse on oral lichen planus: a double-blind analysis. *N Engl J Med* 1990; **323**: 290–4.
4. Levell NJ, *et al.* Lack of effect of cyclosporin mouthwash in oral lichen planus. *Lancet* 1991; **337**: 796–7.
5. Ho VC, Conklin RJ. Effect of topical cyclosporine rinse on oral lichen planus. *N Engl J Med* 1991; **325**: 435.
6. Porter SR, *et al.* The efficacy of topical cyclosporin in the management of desquamative gingivitis due to lichen planus. *Br J Dermatol* 1993; **129**: 753–5.
7. Sieg P, *et al.* Topical cyclosporin in oral lichen planus: a controlled, randomized prospective trial. *Br J Dermatol* 1995; **132**: 790–4.

Lupus nephritis. As mentioned on p.1059, ciclosporin has been investigated for systemic lupus erythematosus, particularly lupus nephritis,[1,2] but controlled trials are needed.

1. Fu LW, *et al.* Clinical efficacy of cyclosporin A Neoral in the treatment of paediatric lupus nephritis with heavy proteinuria. *Br J Rheumatol* 1998; **37**: 217–21.
2. Tam LS, *et al.* Long-term treatment of lupus nephritis with cyclosporin A. *Q J Med* 1998; **91**: 573–80.

Multiple sclerosis. As noted on p.633, immunosuppressants, including ciclosporin,[1,2] have produced modest benefit in patients with multiple sclerosis. However, it has been concluded

that the scanty benefits of therapy are outweighed by the toxicity of the doses required.

1. Rudge P, *et al.* Randomised double blind controlled trial of cyclosporin in multiple sclerosis. *J Neurol Neurosurg Psychiatry* 1989; **52**: 559–65.
2. The Multiple Sclerosis Study Group. Efficacy and toxicity of cyclosporine in chronic progressive multiple sclerosis: a randomized, double-blinded, placebo-controlled clinical trial. *Ann Neurol* 1990; **27**: 591–605.

Muscular dystrophies. A study in 15 boys with Duchenne muscular dystrophy (p.1054) given ciclosporin 5 mg per kg body-weight daily by mouth in divided doses, adjusted according to trough serum concentrations of ciclosporin, found that muscular force generation was improved during treatment, but declined again once treatment ceased.[1] The clinical significance, if any, of this effect remains to be established.

1. Sharma KR, *et al.* Cyclosporine increases muscular force generation in Duchenne muscular dystrophy. *Neurology* 1993; **43**: 527–32.

Myasthenia gravis. Ciclosporin may be of use as an alternative to azathioprine in the management of myasthenia gravis (p.1414) for its corticosteroid-sparing effect[1] or when patients are intolerant of or unresponsive to corticosteroids and azathioprine. It appears to be of similar efficacy to azathioprine[2] with a more rapid effect but serious adverse effects such as nephrotoxicity may limit its use.

1. Tindall RSA, *et al.* A clinical therapeutic trial of cyclosporine in myasthenia gravis. *Ann N Y Acad Sci* 1993; **681**: 539–51.
2. Schalke BCG, *et al.* Cyclosporin A vs azathioprine in the treatment of myasthenia gravis: final results of a randomized, controlled double-blind clinical trial. *Neurology* 1988; **38** (suppl 1): 135.

Organ and tissue transplantation. Ciclosporin has greatly improved the prospects for successful organ and tissue transplantation, and is a mainstay of regimens used to prevent rejection of solid organ grafts as well as being used for the prevention of graft-versus-host disease in bone marrow transplantation. For more detailed discussion of organ and tissue transplantation and the role of ciclosporin, see p.502. Ciclosporin has also occasionally been used for corneal graft rejection (p.1049) in high-risk patients, where corticosteroids alone are insufficient.

Pemphigus. Although pemphigus is usually treated with corticosteroids (see p.1106), ciclosporin has also been tried in a few patients with pemphigus vulgaris.[1]

1. Luisi AF, Stoukides CA. Cyclosporine for the treatment of pemphigus vulgaris. *Ann Pharmacother* 1994; **28**: 1183–5.

Polymyositis and dermatomyositis. Ciclosporin has been tried[1,2] in refractory polymyositis and dermatomyositis (see p.1057).

1. Heckmatt J, *et al.* Cyclosporin in juvenile dermatomyositis. *Lancet* 1989; **i**: 1063–6.
2. Lueck CJ, *et al.* Cyclosporin in the management of polymyositis and dermatomyositis. *J Neurol Neurosurg Psychiatry* 1991; **54**: 1007–8.

Primary biliary cirrhosis. In primary biliary cirrhosis (p.501) some benefit has been reported with ciclosporin,[1] but there are problems with toxicity.

1. Lombard M, *et al.* Cyclosporin A treatment in primary biliary cirrhosis: results of a long-term placebo controlled trial. *Gastroenterology* 1993; **104**: 519–26.

Psoriasis. Ciclosporin is used to induce remission or prevent relapse in severe refractory psoriasis (p.1106).
References.
1. Ellis CN, *et al.* Cyclosporine improves psoriasis in a double-blind study. *JAMA* 1986; **256**: 3110–16.
2. Laburte C, *et al.* Efficacy and safety of oral cyclosporin A (CyA; Sandimmun) for long-term treatment of chronic severe plaque psoriasis. *Br J Dermatol* 1994; **130**: 366–75.
3. Berth-Jones J, *et al.* Treatment of psoriasis with intermittent short course cyclosporin (Neoral): a multicentre study. *Br J Dermatol* 1997; **136**: 527–30.
4. Ho VC, *et al.* Intermittent short courses of cyclosporin (Neoral) for psoriasis unresponsive to topical therapy: a 1-year multicentre, randomized study. *Br J Dermatol* 1999; **141**: 283–91.

Psoriatic arthritis. Ciclosporin is used in the management of severe refractory psoriasis (see above). One study[1] has shown that low-dose ciclosporin effectively improves not only skin lesions, but also joint complaints in psoriatic arthritis (see under Spondyloarthropathies, p.10).

1. Mahrle G, *et al.* Anti-inflammatory efficacy of low-dose cyclosporin A in psoriatic arthritis. A prospective multicentre study. *Br J Dermatol* 1996; **135**: 752–7.

Pyoderma gangrenosum. There have been reports[1-3] of responses to ciclosporin in patients with pyoderma gangrenosum (p.1107).

1. Schmitt EC, *et al.* Pyoderma gangrenosum treated with low-dose cyclosporin. *Br J Dermatol* 1993; **128**: 230–1.
2. Fearfield LA, *et al.* Pyoderma gangrenosum associated with Takayasu's arteritis responding to cyclosporin. *Br J Dermatol* 1999; **141**: 339–43.
3. Sassolas B, *et al.* Pyoderma gangrenosum with pathergic phenomenon in pregnancy. *Br J Dermatol* 2000; **142**: 827–8.

Rheumatoid arthritis. Various disease-modifying antirheumatic drugs (DMARDs) are used in rheumatoid arthritis (p.9) in an attempt to modify the disease process. Ciclosporin has produced responses in active disease,[1-4] and there is some evidence that it can slow radiological progression of disease[4] as well as providing symptomatic relief. There has been some concern about associated nephrotoxicity,[1] but the use of low-dose regimens may help to minimise this. Ciclosporin has also been combined with other disease-modifying antirheumatic drugs, and a combination of ciclosporin with methotrexate has reportedly produced responses in patients unresponsive to methotrexate alone.[5] International consensus recommendations exist for the use of ciclosporin in rheumatoid arthritis.[6] These suggest that the use of ciclosporin may be considered in patients who are candidates for DMARDs and who do not have risk factors such as malignancy, uncontrolled hypertension, renal dysfunction, cytopenias, or marked disorder of liver function. They recommend a starting dose of between 2.5 and 3.0 mg per kg body-weight daily, increased if necessary after 4 to 8 weeks, in increments of 0.5 or 1 mg per kg at 1 to 2 month intervals, up to a maximum of 5 mg per kg daily, particular care being taken at doses over 4 mg per kg daily. Once the patient's disease has been stable for at least 3 months the daily dose should be decreased monthly or bimonthly in increments of 0.5 mg per kg to the lowest effective dose. If it is only partially effective after 3 months at the maximum tolerable dose another medication should be considered instead or in addition; if there is no response to the maximum tolerable dose after 3 months, ciclosporin should be discontinued. Patients should be carefully monitored before and during therapy.

1. Yocum DE, et al. Cyclosporin A in severe, treatment-refractory rheumatoid arthritis: a randomized study. *Ann Intern Med* 1988; **109:** 863–9.
2. Tugwell P, et al. Low-dose cyclosporin versus placebo in patients with rheumatoid arthritis. *Lancet* 1990; **335:** 1051–5.
3. Landewé RBM, et al. A randomized, double-blind, 24-week controlled study of low-dose cyclosporine versus chloroquine for early rheumatoid arthritis. *Arthritis Rheum* 1994; **37:** 637–43.
4. Førre Ø, et al. Radiologic evidence of disease modification in rheumatoid arthritis patients treated with cyclosporine: results of a 48-week multicenter study comparing low-dose cyclosporine with placebo. *Arthritis Rheum* 1994; **37:** 1506–12.
5. Tugwell P, et al. Combination therapy with cyclosporine and methotrexate in severe rheumatoid arthritis. *N Engl J Med* 1995; **333:** 137–41.
6. Panayi GS, Tugwell P. The use of cyclosporin A microemulsion in rheumatoid arthritis: conclusions of an international review. *Br J Rheumatol* 1997; **36:** 808–11.

Sarcoidosis. Corticosteroids are the usual therapy for symptomatic sarcoidosis (p.1058), and other agents are very much second-line; ciclosporin is one of a number of immunosuppressants that have been tried with variable results.

Scleritis. Ciclosporin is used alone or with corticosteroids in the treatment of scleritis (see p.1058).

Scleroderma. There are a few reports of responses to ciclosporin in patients with scleroderma, although as discussed on p.505 the use of immunosuppressants remains experimental in this condition.

Uveitis. Ciclosporin is used in refractory posterior uveitis, see p.1060.

Preparations

USP 25: Cyclosporine Capsules; Cyclosporine Injection; Cyclosporine Oral Solution.

Proprietary Preparations (details are given in Part 3)
Aust.: Sandimmun; *Austral.:* Neoral; Sandimmun; *Belg.:* Neoral-Sandimmun; Sandimmun; *Braz.:* Sandimmun; *Canad.:* Neoral; Sandimmune; *Denm.:* Sandimmun; *Fin.:* Sandimmun; *Fr.:* Neoral; Sandimmun; *Ger.:* Sandimmun; *Hong Kong:* Sandimmun; *Irl.:* Neoral; Sandimmun; *Israel:* Sandimmun; *Ital.:* Sandimmun; *Mex.:* Colosina; Immulem; Sandimmun; *Neth.:* Sandimmune; *Norw.:* Sandimmun; *NZ:* Neoral; Sandimmun; *Port.:* Sandimmun; *S.Afr.:* Sandimmun; *Singapore:* Sandimmun Neoral; *Spain:* Sandimmun; *Swed.:* Sandimmun; *Switz.:* Neoral; Sandimmun; *Thai.:* Consupren; Sandimmun; *UK:* Neoral; Sandimmun; Sangcya†; *USA:* Gengraf; Neoral; Sandimmune.

Cisplatin (1822-j)

Cisplatin (BAN, USAN, rINN).
CDDP; Cisplatina; Cisplatinum; Cis-platinum; DDP; *cis*-DDP; NSC-119875; Peyrone's Salt; Platinum Diamminodichloride. *cis*-Diamminedichloroplatinum.
$(NH_3)_2.PtCl_2 = 300.0.$
CAS — 15663-27-1.
ATC — L01XA01.

Pharmacopoeias. In *Chin.*, *Eur.* (see p.vi), *Int.*, and *US.*

Incompatible with aluminium.

Pharmacopoeial description
Ph. Eur.: A yellow powder or yellow or orange-yellow crystals. Slightly soluble in water; practically insoluble in alcohol; sparingly soluble in dimethylformamide. A 0.1% solution in sodium chloride 0.9% has a pH of 4.5 to 6.0 immediately after preparation. Store in airtight containers. Protect from light.
USP 25: Store in airtight containers. Protect from light.

Incompatibility. Cisplatin is rapidly degraded in the presence of bisulfite or metabisulfite,[1,2] and admixture with preparations containing these as preservatives may result in loss of activity.[2] Sodium bicarbonate may also increase the loss of cisplatin from solution, and in some cases may cause precipitation.[3] The stability of cisplatin when mixed with fluorouracil is reported to be limited, with 10% loss of cisplatin in 1.2 to 1.5 hours.[4] Mixtures with etoposide in 0.9% sodium chloride injection formed a precipitate if mannitol and potassium chloride were

present as additives, but not when the diluent was 5% glucose with 0.45% sodium chloride.[5] Turbidity has been reported within 4 hours of mixing 0.1% solutions of cisplatin and thiotepa in 5% glucose.[6] Cisplatin exhibits variable incompatibility with paclitaxel, depending on the paclitaxel concentration and the temperature.[7]

1. Hussain AA, et al. Reaction of cis-platinum with sodium bisulfite. *J Pharm Sci* 1980; **69:** 364–5.
2. Garren KW, Repta AJ. Incompatibility of cisplatin and Reglan Injectable. *Int J Pharmaceutics* 1985; **24:** 91–9.
3. Hincal AA, et al. Cis-platin stability in aqueous parenteral vehicles. *J Parenter Drug Assoc* 1979; **33:** 107–16.
4. Stewart CF, Fleming RA. Compatibility of cisplatin and fluorouracil in 0.9% sodium chloride injection. *Am J Hosp Pharm* 1990; **47:** 1373–7.
5. Stewart CF, Hampton EM. Stability of cisplatin and etoposide in intravenous admixtures. *Am J Hosp Pharm* 1989; **46:** 1400–4.
6. Trissel LA, Martinez JF. Compatibility of thiotepa (lyophilized) with selected drugs during simulated Y-site administration. *Am J Health-Syst Pharm* 1996; **53:** 1041–5.
7. Zhang Y, et al. Compatibility and stability of paclitaxel combined with cisplatin and with carboplatin in infusion solutions. *Ann Pharmacother* 1997; **31:** 1465–70.

Stability. Decomposition of cisplatin in aqueous solutions is primarily due to reversible substitution of water for chloride, and its stability is enhanced in sodium chloride solutions because of the excess of chloride ions available.[1,2] A solution in 0.9% sodium chloride injection has been reported to lose 3% of the drug in less than one hour and to remain stable at this equilibrium value for 24 hours at room temperature.[1] Stability is decreased if exposed to intense light, but the effect of normal lighting conditions is apparently smaller.[1,2] It has been recommended that admixtures of cisplatin with mannitol and magnesium sulfate (in glucose 5% with sodium chloride 0.45%) stored at room temperature in polyvinyl chloride bags should be used within 48 hours, but may be stored for 4 days at 4° or frozen and stored at −15° for up to 30 days.[3] However, solutions containing 600 μg per mL or more of cisplatin precipitate out when refrigerated and are slow to redissolve.[1]

1. Greene RF, et al. Stability of cisplatin in aqueous solution. *Am J Hosp Pharm* 1979; **36:** 38–43.
2. Hincal AA, et al. Cis-platin stability in aqueous parenteral vehicles. *J Parenter Drug Assoc* 1979; **33:** 107–16.
3. LaFollette JM, et al. Stability of cisplatin admixtures in polyvinyl chloride bags. *Am J Hosp Pharm* 1985; **42:** 2652.

Adverse Effects and Treatment

For a general outline see Antineoplastics, p.476 and p.479.

Severe nausea and vomiting occur in most patients during treatment with cisplatin; nausea may persist for up to a week.

Serious toxic effects on the kidneys, bone marrow, and ears have been reported in up to about one third of patients given a single dose of cisplatin; the effects are generally dose-related and cumulative.

Damage to the renal tubules may be evident during the second week after a dose of cisplatin and renal function must return to normal before further cisplatin is given. Adequate hydration, and use of osmotic diuretics such as mannitol to increase urine volume and thus decrease the urinary concentration of platinum, can reduce the incidence of nephrotoxicity. Electrolyte disturbances, particularly hypomagnesaemia and hypocalcaemia, may occur, possibly as a result of renal tubular damage. Hyperuricaemia is also seen.

Bone-marrow depression may be severe with higher doses of cisplatin. Nadirs in platelet and leucocyte counts occur between days 18 and 23 and most patients recover by day 39; anaemia is commonly seen and may be partly related to decreased production of erythropoietin following renal damage.

Ototoxicity may be more severe in children. It can be manifest as tinnitus, loss of hearing in the high frequency range, and occasionally deafness or vestibular toxicity. Other neurological effects reported include peripheral neuropathies, loss of taste, and seizures. Ocular toxicities include optic neuritis, papilloedema, and cerebral blindness.

Anaphylactoid reactions and cardiac abnormalities have occurred.

Platinum derivatives are potentially mutagenic and teratogenic, and there is some evidence they may be associated with the development of secondary leukaemias—see p.476.

Effects on the blood. Cisplatin-induced anaemia appears to be disproportionate to the effects on other blood cells, and to correlate with renal tubular dysfunction.[1] It may therefore be due to an erythropoietin deficiency state resulting from cispla-

tin-induced renal tubular damage. Haemolysis has also been reported.[2]

1. Wood PA, Hrushesky WJ. Cisplatin-associated anemia: an erythropoietin deficiency syndrome *J Clin Invest* 1995; **95:** 1650–9.
2. Rothmann SA, Weick JK. Cisplatin toxicity for erythroid precursors. *N Engl J Med* 1981; **304:** 360.

THROMBOEMBOLISM. For discussion of thromboembolic events possibly associated with cisplatin-containing chemotherapy regimens see Effects on the Cardiovascular System, p.477.

Effects on electrolytes. Renal-magnesium wasting and, less commonly, symptomatic hypomagnesaemia occurs with cisplatin therapy.[1-3] Adding magnesium to the pre- and posthydration fluids has been suggested.[3] When hypocalcaemia is also present, tetany may result,[2,4] although this has responded to electrolyte infusion without the need to interrupt chemotherapy.[2] Cisplatin therapy may also be associated with significant hypokalaemia[2] and hyponatraemia.[5,6]
See also Effects on the Kidneys, below.

1. Schilsky RL, Anderson T. Hypomagnesemia and renal magnesium wasting in patients receiving cisplatin. *Ann Intern Med* 1979; **90:** 929–31.
2. Winkler CF, et al. Cisplatin and renal magnesium wasting. *Ann Intern Med* 1979; **91:** 502.
3. Lajer H, Daugaard G. Cisplatin and hypomagnesemia. *Cancer Treat Rev* 1999; **25:** 47–58.
4. Stuart-Harris R, et al. Tetany associated with cis-platin. *Lancet* 1980; **ii:** 1303.
5. Hutchison FN, et al. Renal salt wasting in patients treated with cisplatin. *Ann Intern Med* 1988; **108:** 21–5.
6. Mariette X, et al. Cisplatin and hyponatremia. *Ann Intern Med* 1988; **108:** 770–1.

Effects on the kidneys. Nephrotoxicity is a well established adverse effect of cisplatin, may be dose-limiting, and can manifest as acute or chronic renal failure, polyuria, or chronic hypomagnesaemia.[1] The mechanism appears to involve primarily damage to the proximal renal tubule; selective magnesium loss may be due to a specific membrane or transport system abnormality. Sulfhydryl metabolism and oxidative stress play a role in toxicity, and measures that reduce glutathione depletion and scavenge intracellular free oxygen radicals have been tried in an attempt to modulate nephrotoxicity.[1-3] However, the primary measures for reducing renal damage have been aggressive hydration with chloride-containing solutions, and the use of mannitol (see also Prophylaxis, below). It has been suggested that cisplatin may mobilise lead accumulated in bone and cause temporary accumulation in the kidney, with concomitant toxicity,[4] but this has been vigorously disputed.[5-7]
See also under Effects on Electrolytes, above.

1. Anand AJ, Bashey B. Newer insights into cisplatin nephrotoxicity. *Ann Pharmacother* 1993; **27:** 1519–25.
2. Meyer KB, Madias NE. Cisplatin nephrotoxicity. *Miner Electrolyte Metab* 1994; **20:** 201–13.
3. Kuhlmann MK, et al. Insights into potential cellular mechanisms of cisplatin nephrotoxicity and their clinical application. *Nephrol Dial Transplant* 1997; **12:** 2478–80.
4. El-Sharkawi AM, et al. Unexpected mobilisation of lead during cisplatin chemotherapy. *Lancet* 1986; **ii:** 249–50.
5. Tothill P, et al. Is lead mobilised by cisplatin? *Lancet* 1989; **ii:** 333.
6. Tothill P, et al. Mobilisation of lead by cisplatin. *Lancet* 1989; **ii:** 1342.
7. Hainsworth IR, Morgan WD. Plasma lead and cisplatin. *Lancet* 1989; **ii:** 624.

PROPHYLAXIS. Hydration with 1 to 2 litres of fluid before treatment, and infusion of cisplatin in a further 2 litres of infusion fluid containing an osmotic diuretic such as mannitol reduces the nephrotoxicity of cisplatin, but does not abolish it. Maintaining adequate hydration and urinary output post-treatment is also important. Administering cisplatin over 6 to 8 hours rather than 1 to 2 hours may also decrease renal toxicity.
Sulfur-containing nucleophiles can inactivate cisplatin, and have therefore been investigated for their chemoprotective potential. Amifostine is a prodrug which is selectively activated by normal tissue, and has been shown to protect normal tissue (principally the kidney) against the cytotoxicity of cisplatin without affecting antitumour activity (for references, see p.1002). Glutathione (p.1010) is a similar agent, which may be selectively taken up by kidney and neural tissue. Sodium thiosulfate does not show selective activation or uptake, and its use is therefore limited to situations where cisplatin is given locally (e.g. intraperitoneal[1]) or directly (e.g. intra-arterial).

1. Howell SB, et al. Intraperitoneal cisplatin with systemic thiosulfate protection. *Ann Intern Med* 1982; **97:** 845–51.

Effects on the nervous system. The features of cisplatin-induced peripheral neuropathy are consistent with damage predominantly to sensory fibres, with numbness, tingling, and decreased vibratory sensation and deep tendon reflexes, progressing in severe cases to disabling sensory ataxia.[1] The toxicity is dose-dependent, with symptoms usually appearing in patients who have received cumulative doses of 300 to 600 mg per square metre body-surface, although individuals vary in susceptibility. Neuropathy is reversible but recovery may take a year or more. The pathophysiology is unknown. Peripheral neuropathy can be a dose-limiting toxicity for cisplatin and agents such as Org-2766 (a corticotropin analogue) and amifostine (p.1001) have been investigated for their potential in protecting peripheral nerves.[1,2] Glutathione is also under investigation for the prevention of neurotoxicity (see p.1010). Autonomic neuropathy, with, in some cases, consequent postural hypotension, has also been described following treatment with

The symbol † denotes a preparation no longer actively marketed

cisplatin-containing regimens.[3] Apart from ototoxicity, cisplatin has also been associated with central neurotoxicity, including focal encephalopathy, seizures, aphasia, confusion, agitation, and cortical blindness.[4-7] It has been suggested that the mechanism of focal encephalopathy may be vascular,[5] although this is uncertain.

1. Mollman JE. Cisplatin neurotoxicity. *N Engl J Med* 1990; **322**: 126–7.
2. Alberts DS, Noel JK. Cisplatin-associated neurotoxicity: can it be prevented? *Anticancer Drugs* 1995; **6**: 369–83.
3. Richardson P, Cantwell BMJ. Autonomic neuropathy after cisplatin based chemotherapy. *BMJ* 1990; **300**: 1466–7.
4. Gorman DJ, *et al.* Focal encephalopathy after cisplatin therapy. *Med J Aust* 1989; **150**: 399–401.
5. Lindeman G, *et al.* Cisplatin neurotoxicity. *N Engl J Med* 1990; **323**: 64–5.
6. Philip PA, *et al.* Convulsions and transient cortical blindness after cisplatin. *BMJ* 1991; **302**: 416.
7. Higa GM, *et al.* Severe, disabling neurologic toxicity following cisplatin retreatment. *Ann Pharmacother* 1995; **29**: 134–7.

Extravasation. For discussion of the management of extravasation, including mention of the potential use of sodium thiosulfate in cisplatin extravasation, see under Treatment of the Adverse Effects of Antineoplastics, p.480.

Hypersensitivity. Anaphylactoid reactions to intravenous cisplatin generally appear within a few minutes of administration and have manifested as facial oedema, wheezing, tachycardia, and hypotension.[1] A high incidence of anaphylactoid reaction has also been seen following intravesical instillation in patients with bladder cancer,[2] but intraperitoneal or intrapleural administration does not seem to be associated with an enhanced risk of hypersensitivity,[3] although anaphylactoid reactions have occurred when cisplatin is given intraperitoneally.[4] Anaphylactoid symptoms and ischaemia of the hands accompanied severe exfoliative dermatitis in a patient on the second cycle of cisplatin-based chemotherapy;[5] she had earlier experienced exfoliative dermatitis associated with carboplatin. Palmar-plantar erythema has also occurred.[6]

1. Von Hoff DD, *et al.* Allergic reactions to cis platinum. *Lancet* 1976; **i**: 90.
2. Denis L. Anaphylactic reactions to repeated intravesical instillation with cisplatin. *Lancet* 1983; **i**: 1378–9.
3. Markman M. No increase in allergic reactions with intracavitary administration of cisplatin. *Lancet* 1984; **ii**: 1164.
4. Hebert ME, *et al.* Anaphylactoid reactions with intraperitoneal cisplatin. *Ann Pharmacother* 1995; **29**: 260–3.
5. Lee TC, *et al.* Severe exfoliative dermatitis associated with hand ischemia during cisplatin therapy. *Mayo Clin Proc* 1994; **69**: 80–2.
6. Vakalis D, *et al.* Acral erythema induced by chemotherapy with cisplatin. *Br J Dermatol* 1998; **139**: 750–1.

Nausea and vomiting. For discussion of the treatment of antineoplastic-induced nausea and vomiting, see under Nausea and Vomiting, p.1206.

Precautions

For reference to the precautions necessary with antineoplastics and immunosuppressants, see p.480. Cisplatin is generally contra-indicated in patients with renal or hearing impairment, or bone-marrow depression. Renal and neurological function and hearing should be monitored during treatment, and regular blood counts performed. Adequate hydration and urinary output must be maintained before, and for 24 hours after, administration.

Handling and disposal. Methods for the destruction of *cisplatin wastes* by reduction with zinc powder under acidic conditions or by reaction with ditiocarb sodium have been described.[1] Residue produced by the degradation of cisplatin by either method showed no mutagenicity *in vitro*.

Urine produced for up to 7 days after a dose of cisplatin should be handled wearing protective clothing.[2]

1. Castegnaro M, *et al.*, eds. Laboratory decontamination and destruction of carcinogens in laboratory wastes: some antineoplastic agents. *IARC Scientific Publications 73.* Lyon: WHO/International Agency for Research on Cancer, 1985.
2. Harris J, Dodds LJ. Handling waste from patients receiving cytotoxic drugs. *Pharm J* 1985; **235**: 289–91.

Radiotherapy. Enhanced ototoxicity has been reported in patients given cisplatin for brain tumours who had also received cranial irradiation.[1,2]

1. Granowetter L, *et al.* Enhanced cis-platinum neurotoxicity in pediatric patients with brain tumors. *J Neurooncol* 1983; **1**: 293–7.
2. Mahoney DH, *et al.* Ototoxicity with cisplatin therapy. *J Pediatr* 1983; **103**: 1006.

Interactions

For a general outline of antineoplastic drug interactions, see p.481. The concomitant use of other nephrotoxic or ototoxic drugs may exacerbate the adverse effects of cisplatin. The effects of cisplatin on renal function may also affect the pharmacokinetics of other drugs excreted by the renal route.

Antibacterials. Although the use of cisplatin with other nephrotoxic or ototoxic drugs requires great caution, there is some evidence that aminoglycosides can be used in patients who have recently received cisplatin if appropriate supportive care is available.[1]

1. Cooper BW, *et al.* Renal dysfunction during high-dose cisplatin therapy and autologous hematopoietic stem cell transplantation: effect of aminoglycoside therapy. *Am J Med* 1993; **94**: 497–504.

Antineoplastics. The ototoxicity of cisplatin was reportedly enhanced by concomitant use of ifosfamide,[1] an agent which is not ototoxic when given alone, although it does have nephrotoxic potential, making reports of increased nephrotoxicity in patients who have received both unsurprising.[2,3]

For a report of increased toxicity with etoposide, see p.538.

1. Meyer WH, *et al.* Ifosfamide and exacerbation of cisplatin-induced hearing loss. *Lancet* 1993; **341**: 754–5.
2. Rossi R, Ehrich JHH. Partial and complete de Toni-Debré-Fanconi syndrome after ifosfamide chemotherapy of childhood malignancy. *Eur J Clin Pharmacol* 1993; **44** (suppl 1): S43–S45.
3. Martinez F, *et al.* Ifosfamide nephrotoxicity: deleterious effect of previous cisplatin administration. *Lancet* 1996; **348**: 1100–1.

Cardiovascular drugs. A patient whose renal function was unaffected by cisplatin alone developed nephrotoxicity when given cisplatin and antihypertensive therapy with frusemide [furosemide], hydralazine, diazoxide, and propranolol.[1] Previous results in *animals* suggest that frusemide [furosemide] may aggravate cisplatin nephrotoxicity, while the other antihypertensives might have contributed to a transient fall in renal-blood flow with resultant increased renal-tubular cisplatin concentration.

1. Markman M, Trump DL. Nephrotoxicity with cisplatin and antihypertensive medications. *Ann Intern Med* 1982; **96**: 257.

Gastrointestinal drugs. For mention of 2 retrospective studies, 1 showing a decreased area under the plasma-concentration time curve of high-dose cisplatin with *ondansetron* and the other an increase, see p.528.

Pharmacokinetics

After intravenous administration cisplatin disappears from the plasma in a biphasic manner and half-lives of 25 to 49 minutes and 58 to 73 hours have been reported for total platinum. The majority of the platinum from a dose is rapidly bound to plasma protein. Cisplatin is concentrated in the liver, kidneys, and large and small intestines. Penetration into the CNS appears to be poor. Excretion is mainly in the urine but is incomplete and prolonged: up to about 50% of a dose has been reported to be excreted in urine over 5 days, and platinum may be detected in tissue for several months afterwards. Cisplatin is well-absorbed following intraperitoneal administration.

◊ A review of the pharmacokinetics of some antineoplastics, including cisplatin.[1] Most pharmacokinetic studies have measured total platinum but cisplatin is believed to be non-enzymatically transformed into 1 or more metabolites, which are protein bound; only the non-bound fraction has more than minimal cytotoxic activity. Protein-bound platinum species represent more than 90% of the dose by 2 to 4 hours after administration. Although total platinum has a bi-exponential decline with a prolonged terminal half-life of 58 to 96 hours the non-bound active form has a much more rapid decline with an initial phase half-life of 8 to 30 minutes and a terminal half-life of 40 to 48 minutes. By 4 to 5 hours, unbound cisplatin accounts for less than 2 to 3% of the total circulating platinum. Excretion is primarily renal, with an initial period of rapid output followed within 4 hours by a decline in renal clearance due to protein binding. There is evidence to suggest that the unbound drug may be actively secreted by the renal tubules. The fraction of a dose excreted in urine increases with increased length of infusion. Faecal excretion is probably insignificant, although the drug is found in bile.

1. Balis FM, *et al.* Clinical pharmacokinetics of commonly used anticancer drugs. *Clin Pharmacokinet* 1983; **8**: 202–32.

Distribution into breast milk. The platinum concentration in breast milk of a patient receiving chemotherapy was 0.9 µg per mL and the concentration in plasma was 0.8 µg per mL.[1] Although most of the platinum in breast milk is probably protein-bound the authors consider that a mother should not breast feed while receiving cisplatin chemotherapy.

1. de Vries EGE, *et al.* Excretion of platinum into breast milk. *Lancet* 1989; **i**: 497. Correction. *ibid.*; 798.

Uses and Administration

The antineoplastic cisplatin is a platinum-containing complex which may act similarly to the alkylating agents. Its antineoplastic actions are cell-cycle non-specific and are dependent upon its *cis* configuration. Although it causes immunosuppression, stimulation of the host immune response against the tumour has been suggested as contributing to its antineoplastic action.

Cisplatin is of value in the treatment of metastatic tumours of the testis, usually as a major component of combination chemotherapy regimens, and particularly in combination with bleomycin and etoposide (BEP). It is also used in metastatic ovarian tumours, lung cancer, and advanced bladder cancer, and has been reported to be active against a wide range of other solid tumours, as indicated by the cross references given below.

Cisplatin is administered by intravenous infusion in sodium chloride 0.9% or sodium chloride and glucose. It is usually given as a single dose of 50 to 120 mg per m² body-surface every 3 to 4 weeks in the treatment of ovarian and bladder cancers. Lower doses are generally used for combination chemotherapy regimens than for single agent therapy. A dose of 20 mg per m² daily for 5 days every 3 weeks has been employed in combination chemotherapy of testicular tumours.

The manufacturers recommend that cisplatin is administered in 2 litres of chloride-containing infusion fluid over at least 1 to 2 hours, and that an infusion time of 6 to 8 hours may further reduce the toxicity. In practice, other regimens may be used at expert centres: for example, doses of up to 100 mg (about 60 mg per m² in an adult) of cisplatin are reportedly dissolved in as little as 250 mL of sodium chloride 0.9% and infused over 30 minutes, provided the patient has acceptable renal function and is well hydrated.

To aid diuresis and protect the kidneys, 37.5 g of mannitol (e.g. 375 mL of mannitol 10%) is usually added to the infusion or is infused separately immediately before cisplatin. In order to initiate diuresis the patient is usually hydrated by the infusion of 1 to 2 litres of a suitable fluid over several hours before the administration of cisplatin. Adequate hydration must also be maintained for up to 24 hours after a dose. Renal, haematological, auditory, and neurological function should be monitored during therapy, and administration adjusted accordingly.

Cisplatin has also been administered by the intra-arterial and intraperitoneal routes, and by instillation into the bladder. It is also being investigated as a liposomal formulation, and as a collagen-based injectable gel containing cisplatin and adrenaline [epinephrine] to localise the effect, MPI-5010.

Various analogues of cisplatin have been developed or investigated including those with fewer adverse effects (e.g. carboplatin, p.515; nedaplatin, p.562), an altered spectrum of activity (oxaliplatin, p.563), or activity following oral administration (satraplatin, p.568).

Action. The pharmacology of inorganic compounds, including cisplatin has been reviewed.[1] The cytotoxicity of cisplatin appears to be related to its hydrolysis in the body. The aquated form, *cis*-Pt(NH₃)₂(H₂0)(OH)⁺, is very reactive, and can also form hydroxyl-bridged dimers and trimers. Selective killing of tumour cells is probably due to attack on the guanine- and cytosine-rich regions of DNA, producing damage which is repairable by normal cells. Platinum crosslinks between DNA strands are not now thought to be important cytotoxic events. It has also been suggested that platinum binding to guanine activates the base so that it can form abnormal base pairs, resulting in unwinding of DNA.

1. Sadler PJ. Inorganic pharmacology. *Chem Br* 1982; **18**: 182–8.

Administration. Various adjustments to the administration of cisplatin have been suggested in an attempt to improve effectiveness while reducing toxicity.

Hydration before and after a dose of cisplatin, together with the use of mannitol to promote diuresis, is now standard (see Uses and Administration, above). Higher doses of cisplatin (up to 200 mg per m² body-surface per treatment cycle) have been successfully given by infusion in hypertonic sodium chloride, accompanied by intensive hydration.[1,3] However, while such a regimen may limit nephrotoxicity, other toxic effects, such as peripheral neuropathy, are not prevented;[1-4] myelosuppression may be less if the total dose is given in 2 divided doses rather than divided over 5 days.[2]

Toxicity has been reported to be reduced when cisplatin was given by continuous intra-arterial[5] or intravenous[6] infusion. It has also been suggested that giving cisplatin in the evening rather than the morning results in less damage to renal function, apparently because of circadian variations in urine production.[7]

A suggested alternative way to increase the platinum dose without crippling toxicity has been the combination of cisplatin and carboplatin.[8]

Various drugs have been investigated to reduce toxicity, including amifostine, glutathione, and thiosulfate, as discussed under

Effects on the Kidneys, and Effects on the Nervous System, above.

1. Ozols RF, *et al.* High-dose cisplatin in hypertonic saline. *Ann Intern Med* 1984; **100:** 19–24.
2. Gandara DR, *et al.* Cisplatin dose intensity in non-small cell lung cancer: phase II results of a day 1 and day 8 high-dose regimen. *J Natl Cancer Inst* 1989; **81:** 790–4.
3. Bagley CM, *et al.* High-dose cisplatin therapy for cancer of the ovary: neurotoxicity. *Ann Intern Med* 1985; **102:** 719.
4. Ozols RF, Young RC. High-dose cisplatin therapy for cancer of the ovary: neurotoxicity. *Ann Intern Med* 1985; **102:** 719.
5. Jacobs SC, *et al.* Intraarterial cisplatin infusion in the management of transitional cell carcinoma of the bladder. *Cancer* 1989; **64:** 388–91.
6. Salem P, *et al.* Cis-diamminedichloroplatinum (II) by 5-day continuous infusion: a new dose schedule with minimal toxicity. *Cancer* 1984; **53:** 837–40.
7. Hrushesky WJM, *et al.* Circadian time dependence of cisplatin urinary kinetics. *Clin Pharmacol Ther* 1982; **32:** 330–9.
8. Piccart MJ, *et al.* Cisplatin combined with carboplatin: a new way of intensification of platinum dose in the treatment of advanced ovarian cancer. *J Natl Cancer Inst* 1990; **82:** 703–7.

Malignant neoplasms. Cisplatin is used in the management of many solid malignancies, notably those of the bladder, cervix, lung, ovary, and testis, as discussed on p.490, p.492, p.496, p.496, and p.499 respectively. Other malignancies where cisplatin may be employed, as discussed in the introduction to this chapter, include non-Hodgkin's lymphomas (p.487), tumours of brain (p.490), endometrium (p.493), upper gastrointestinal tract (p.493), head and neck (p.494), and thymus (p.499), neuroblastoma (p.500), and sarcoma of bone and soft tissue (p.500 and p.501).

Preparations

BP 2001: Cisplatin Injection;
USP 25: Cisplatin for Injection.

Proprietary Preparations (details are given in Part 3)
Aust.: Abiplatin; Platiblastin; Platinol; *Belg.:* Platinol; Platistine; *Braz.:* Cisplatyl; Platiran; Platistine; *Canad.:* Platinol; *Denm.:* Citosin; Lederplatin; Platinol; *Fin.:* Platinol; *Fr.:* Cisplatyl; *Ger.:* Platiblastin; Platinex; *Israel:* Abiplatin; Cisplatyl; Platinex; Platinol; Platosin; *Ital.:* Citoplatino; Platamine; Platinex; Pronto Platamine; *Jpn:* Randa†; *Mex.:* Blastolem; Niyaplat; Plastistil; Platinol; Seroplatin; Tecnoplatin; Tisplal; *Neth.:* Platinol; *Norw.:* Platinol; Platistine; *NZ:* Platamine; *Port.:* Faulplatin; *S.Afr.:* Abiplatin; Platamine; Platosin; *Spain:* Neoplatin; Placis; Platistil; *Swed.:* Lederplatin†; Platinol; Platistin†; *Switz.:* Platiblastin-S; Platinol; *Thai.:* Kemoplat; Platinol; Platosin; *UK:* Platinex; *USA:* Platinol.

Cladribine   (4849-m)

Cladribine *(BAN, USAN, rINN).*
2-Chlorodeoxyadenosine; RWJ-26251; RWJ-26251-000. 2-Chloro-2′-deoxyadenosine.
$C_{10}H_{12}ClN_5O_3 = 285.7$.
CAS — 4291-63-8.
ATC — L01BB04.

Stability. Cladribine shows increased degradation in glucose 5%, therefore this diluent should not be used. Cladribine in sodium chloride 0.9% is stable for at least 24 hours at room temperature and ambient lighting in PVC infusion containers.

The manufacturers recommend that cladribine should be stored at 2° to 8° and protected from light.

Adverse Effects and Treatment

For a general outline see Antineoplastics, p.476 and p.479.

Cladribine produces severe myelosuppression, with neutropenia, anaemia, and thrombocytopenia. Transfusion of blood products may be required. Prolonged CD4 lymphopenia with a nadir at 4 to 6 months also occurs. Prolonged bone-marrow hypocellularity may occur, although it is not clear if this is due to the drug or underlying disease. Haemolytic anaemia has also been reported.

Other adverse effects include fever, fatigue, malaise, mild nausea and gastrointestinal disturbances, rashes, pruritus, purpura, headache, dizziness, cough, dyspnoea, oedema, and tachycardia.

Very high doses of cladribine have been associated with severe renal and nervous system toxicity as well as myelosuppression. Severe neurotoxicity is rare at currently recommended doses, but confusion, neuropathy, ataxia, insomnia, and somnolence have occurred.

Carcinogenicity. As with some other antimetabolites (see p.476), Epstein-Barr virus-related lymphoma has been reported after cladribine therapy.[1]

1. Niesvizky R, *et al.* Epstein-Barr virus-associated lymphoma after treatment of macroglobulinemia with cladribine. *N Engl J Med* 1999; **341:** 55.

Precautions

For the precautions necessary with antineoplastics, see p.480. Careful haematological monitoring is recommended, especially during the first 4 to 8 weeks of therapy. Renal and hepatic function should also be monitored.

Pharmacokinetics

Plasma-cladribine concentrations are reported to decline multi-exponentially after intravenous infusion, with terminal half-lives ranging from 3 to 22 hours. Cladribine is extensively distributed and penetrates into the CNS. It is about 20% bound to plasma proteins. Cladribine is phosphorylated within cells by deoxycytidine kinase to form cytotoxic nucleotides.

◊ References.
1. Liliemark J. The clinical pharmacokinetics of cladribine. *Clin Pharmacokinet* 1997; **32:** 120–31.

Uses and Administration

Cladribine is a purine antimetabolite antineoplastic which inhibits DNA synthesis and repair particularly in lymphocytes and monocytes. It is used for the treatment of lymphoid malignancies including hairy-cell leukaemia (p.486) and chronic lymphocytic leukaemia (p.485). It has been tried in indolent low-grade non-Hodgkin's lymphomas (p.487) including mycosis fungoides (p.489), histiocytic syndromes (p.483), and in Waldenström's macroglobulinaemia (p.489).

The recommended dose of cladribine in hairy-cell leukaemia is a single course of 90 µg per kg bodyweight (3.6 mg per m² body-surface) daily for 7 days by continuous intravenous infusion. Higher doses have been given but may be associated with more severe toxicity (see Adverse Effects, above). If the patient does not respond to the initial course, they are unlikely to respond to further doses.

For the treatment of chronic lymphocytic leukaemia the recommended dose is 120 µg per kg (4.8 mg per m²) daily for 5 consecutive days of a 28-day cycle; the infusion is given over 2 hours. Response should be determined every 2 cycles, and once maximum response has occurred a further 2 cycles of treatment are recommended, up to a maximum of 6 cycles. Patients who do not respond with a lymphocyte reduction of 50% or more after 2 cycles should not receive further therapy.

The use of cladribine by mouth in chronic lymphocytic leukaemia is under investigation.

Cladribine has also been tried in the management of multiple sclerosis (see below).

◊ Reviews.
1. Beutler E. Cladribine (2-chlorodeoxyadenosine). *Lancet* 1992; **340:** 952–6.
2. Bryson HM, Sorkin EM. Cladribine: a review of its pharmacodynamic and pharmacokinetic properties and therapeutic potential in haematological malignancies. *Drugs* 1993; **46:** 872–94.
3. Baltz JK, Montello MJ. Cladribine for the treatment of hematologic malignancies. *Clin Pharm* 1993; **12:** 805–13.
4. Saven A, Piro LD. 2-Chlorodeoxyadenosine: a newer purine analog active in the treatment of indolent lymphoid malignancies. *Ann Intern Med* 1994; **120:** 784–91.

Multiple sclerosis. Cladribine has shown some promising early results in multiple sclerosis (p.633).
References.
1. Sipe JC, *et al.* Cladribine in treatment of chronic progressive multiple sclerosis. *Lancet* 1994; **344:** 9–13.
2. Romine JS, *et al.* A double-blind, placebo-controlled, randomized trial of cladribine in relapsing-remitting multiple sclerosis. *Proc Assoc Am Physicians* 1999; **111:** 35–44.
3. Rice GPA, *et al.* Cladribine and progressive MS: clinical and MRI outcomes of a multicenter controlled trial. *Neurology* 2000; **54:** 1145–55.

Preparations

Proprietary Preparations (details are given in Part 3)
Aust.: Leustatin; *Austral.:* Leustatin; *Braz.:* Leustatin; *Canad.:* Leustatin; *Denm.:* Leustatin; *Fin.:* Leustatin; *Fr.:* Leustatine; *Ger.:* Leustatin; *Hong Kong:* Leustatin; *Ital.:* Leustatin; *Neth.:* Leustatin; *Norw.:* Leustatin; *NZ:* Leustatin; *S.Afr.:* Leustatin; *Spain:* Leustatin; *Swed.:* Leustatin; *Switz.:* Leustatin; *Thai.:* Leustatin; *UK:* Leustat; *USA:* Leustatin.

Corynebacterium parvum   (12609-w)

C. parvum; NSC-220537; *Propionibacterium acnes.*

Profile

Inactivated *Corynebacterium parvum* has been used in the treatment of malignant effusions, and has been tried as an adju-

---

vant to cancer chemotherapy for its immunostimulant properties. It has also been used in the treatment of musculoskeletal and joint disorders.

Fever and pain have occurred after intracavitary injection. There have been reports of nephrotoxicity following intravenous use.

Preparations

Proprietary Preparations (details are given in Part 3)
Braz.: Corymunun; *Ger.:* Arthrokehlan A.

Crisnatol Mesilate   (4868-g)

Crisnatol Mesilate *(rINNM).*
BW-A770U (crisnatol); BW-A770U (crisnatol mesilate); Crisnatol Mesylate *(USAN).*
CAS — 96389-68-3 (crisnatol); 96389-69-4 (crisnatol mesilate).

Profile

Crisnatol is reported to act as a topoisomerase inhibitor and an intercalator of DNA. It has been investigated for its antineoplastic properties, notably for malignant neoplasms of the brain.

Cyclophosphamide   (1825-k)

Cyclophosphamide *(BAN, rINN).*
B-518; Ciclofosfamida; Cyclophosphamidum; Cyclophosphanum; NSC-26271; WR-138719. 2-[Bis(2-chloroethyl)amino]perhydro-1,3,2-oxazaphosphorinan 2-oxide monohydrate.
$C_7H_{15}Cl_2N_2O_2P,H_2O = 279.1$.
CAS — 6055-19-2 (cyclophosphamide monohydrate); 50-18-0 (anhydrous cyclophosphamide).
ATC — L01AA01.

Pharmacopoeias. In Chin., Eur. (see p.vi), Int., Jpn, Pol., and US.

53.45 mg of cyclophosphamide expressed as the monohydrate is equivalent to 50 mg of anhydrous cyclophosphamide.

Pharmacopoeial description

Ph. Eur.: A white or almost white, crystalline powder. Soluble in water and freely soluble in alcohol; slightly soluble in ether. A freshly prepared 2% solution in water has a pH of 4.0 to 6.0.

USP 25: A white, crystalline powder. It liquefies upon loss of its water of crystallisation. Soluble in water and in alcohol. A 1% solution in water has a pH of 3.9 to 7.1 when determined 30 minutes after preparation. Store in airtight containers at 2° to 30°.

Adverse Effects and Treatment

For a general outline see Antineoplastics, p.476 and p.479. The major dose-limiting effect is myelosuppression. After single doses the nadir of the white cell count may occur in around 1 to 2 weeks with full recovery usually in 3 to 4 weeks. Thrombocytopenia and anaemia may occur but tend to be less common and less severe.

Haemorrhagic cystitis may develop after high or prolonged dosage, and can be life-threatening. Adequate hydration to maintain urine output at 100 mL per hour and administration of mesna (see p.1012) are generally recommended in an attempt to reduce urotoxicity. If mesna is used, frequent emptying of the bladder should be avoided. Doses of cyclophosphamide should be administered early in the day.

Alopecia occurs in about 20% of patients given low doses and in practically all patients given high doses. Hair loss starts after 3 weeks of treatment but regrowth is usually evident after 3 months, even with continued treatment. Hyperpigmentation of skin, especially that of the palms and soles, and of the nails, has been reported.

Nausea and vomiting commonly occur, and may be reduced by prophylactic antiemetics. Mucositis may also occur.

Other adverse effects include a syndrome resembling inappropriate secretion of antidiuretic hormone (which may require diuretic therapy), disturbances of carbohydrate metabolism, gonadal suppression (common and occasionally resulting in sterility), interstitial pulmonary fibrosis, and, especially at high doses, cardiotoxicity.

Cyclophosphamide, in common with other alkylating agents, has carcinogenic, mutagenic, and teratogenic potential and secondary malignancies have occurred in patients given previous antineoplastic therapy including cyclophosphamide—see p.476.

Effects on the bladder. *Sterile haemorrhagic cystitis,* believed to be secondary to renal excretion of alkylating metabolites, has occurred following high-dose infusions of cyclophosphamide, or after prolonged low-dose-administration.[1-3] The cystitis appears to result from chronic inflammation leading to fibrosis and telangiectasia of the bladder epithelium; haemorrhage may become life-threatening if drug administration is continued.[1] Symptoms may be delayed, and have been reported to occur up to 6 months after discontinuation of the drug.[4] An increased incidence of cystitis when patients on a high-dose cyclophosphamide regimen were transferred from one brand to another has been reported,[5] apparently because one was labelled in terms of the anhydrous substance and one as the monohydrate, resulting in a 6.4% difference in the content of active substance.[6]

Vigorous hydration (increasing urine output and thus diluting the excreted metabolites), or the use of mesna, may prevent the occurrence of cystitis. Where bleeding occurs, an initial trial of diathermy, and then alum instillation, should probably be made before progressing to the instillation of more toxic agents such as formaldehyde solution, or silver nitrate, or the use of more problematic non-drug techniques.[7] Prostaglandins instilled into the bladder may also be effective in controlling haemorrhagic cystitis.[8-10]

In addition to the shorter term effects, cyclophosphamide has been reported to be associated with the development of *bladder carcinoma.*[3,11-14] A history of cyclophosphamide-induced cystitis may be associated with an increased risk of bladder carcinoma[3,11] but some studies have not found a link,[13] and bladder malignancies can develop in patients who have not experienced cystitis while receiving cyclophosphamide.[12] For a discussion of the carcinogenic effects of antineoplastics, including cyclophosphamide, see p.476.

1. Bender RA, *et al.* Antineoplastic drugs: clinical pharmacology and therapeutic use. *Drugs* 1978; **16:** 46–87.
2. Spiers ASD, *et al.* Haemorrhagic cystitis after low-dose cyclophosphamide. *Lancet* 1983; **i:** 1213–14.
3. Talar-Williams C, *et al.* Cyclophosphamide-induced cystitis and bladder cancer in patients with Wegener granulomatosis. *Ann Intern Med* 1996; **124:** 477–84.
4. Armstrong B, *et al.* Delayed cystitis due to cyclophosphamide. *N Engl J Med* 1979; **300:** 45.
5. Shaw IC, *et al.* Difference in bioactivity between two preparations of cyclophosphamide. *Lancet* 1983; **i:** 709.
6. Hilgard P, *et al.* Bioactivity of cyclophosphamide preparations. *Lancet* 1983; **i:** 1436.
7. Bullock N, Whitaker RH. Massive bladder haemorrhage. *BMJ* 1985; **291:** 1522–3.
8. Mohiuddin J, *et al.* Treatment of cyclophosphamide-induced cystitis with prostaglandin E₂. *Ann Intern Med* 1984; **101:** 142.
9. Miller LJ, *et al.* Treatment of cyclophosphamide-induced hemorrhagic cystitis with prostaglandins. *Ann Pharmacother* 1994; **28:** 590–4.
10. Ippoliti C, *et al.* Intravesicular carboprost for the treatment of hemorrhagic cystitis after marrow transplantation. *Urology* 1995; **46:** 811–15.
11. Wall RL, Clausen KP. Carcinoma of the urinary bladder in patients receiving cyclophosphamide. *N Engl J Med* 1975; **293:** 271–3.
12. Plotz PH, *et al.* Bladder complications in patients receiving cyclophosphamide for systemic lupus erythematosus or rheumatoid arthritis. *Ann Intern Med* 1979; **91:** 221–3.
13. Pedersen-Bjergaard J, *et al.* Carcinoma of the urinary bladder after treatment with cyclophosphamide for non-Hodgkin's lymphoma. *N Engl J Med* 1988; **318:** 1028–32.
14. Travis LB, *et al.* Bladder cancer after chemotherapy for non-Hodgkin's lymphoma. *N Engl J Med* 1989; **321:** 544–5.

Effects on the blood. Amifostine has been reported to protect against the myelosuppressive effects of cyclophosphamide, and may be used to reduce neutropenia-related infection associated with the combination of cyclophosphamide and cisplatin (see p.1001).

Effects on carbohydrate metabolism. Acute onset type 1 diabetes occurred in a patient treated with cyclophosphamide, doxorubicin, vincristine and prednisone (CHOP), and was thought to be due to the cyclophosphamide.[1]

1. Atlan-Gepner C, *et al.* A cyclophosphamide-induced autoimmune diabetes. *Lancet* 1998; **352:** 373–4.

Effects on electrolytes. Water intoxication has been reported following administration of cyclophosphamide,[1-4] usually in high doses (30 to 50 mg per kg body-weight or more) although symptoms have been reported after a dose of 20 mg per kg in a patient with renal disease,[3] and in another patient with systemic lupus erythematosus but apparently normal renal function who received 10 mg per kg.[4] One case of severe hyponatraemia leading to convulsions and death has been reported.[5] Symptoms resemble the syndrome of inappropriate antidiuretic hormone secretion (SIADH)[5] but plasma concentrations of antidiuretic hormone do not appear to be raised in these patients.[3]

1. DeFronzo RA, *et al.* Water intoxication in man after cyclophosphamide therapy: time course and relation to drug activation. *Ann Intern Med* 1973; **78:** 861–9.

2. Green TP, Mirkin BL. Prevention of cyclophosphamide-induced antidiuresis by furosemide infusion. *Clin Pharmacol Ther* 1981; **29:** 634–42.
3. Bressler RB, Huston DP. Water intoxication following moderate-dose intravenous cyclophosphamide. *Arch Intern Med* 1985; **145:** 548–9.
4. McCarron MO, *et al.* Water intoxication after low dose cyclophosphamide. *BMJ* 1995; **311:** 292.
5. Harlow PJ, *et al.* A fatal case of inappropriate ADH secretion induced by cyclophosphamide therapy. *Cancer* 1979; **44:** 896–8.

Effects on the eyes. Recurrent transient myopia was induced by intravenous bolus administration of cyclophosphamide in an adolescent with systemic lupus erythematosus, apparently due to increased hydration of the lens of the eye.[1]

1. Arranz JA, *et al.* Cyclophosphamide-induced myopia. *Ann Intern Med* 1992; **116:** 92–3.

Effects on reproductive potential. Severe gonadal failure with transient or permanent azoospermia is common in men treated with cyclophosphamide. Suppression of germ-cell function with intramuscular testosterone in 5 men during cyclophosphamide therapy for nephrotic syndrome was associated with a more rapid return of spermatogenesis compared with 10 patients who did not receive the androgen.[1]

1. Masala A, *et al.* Use of testosterone to prevent cyclophosphamide-induced azoospermia. *Ann Intern Med* 1997; **126:** 292–5.

Effects on the skin. An erythematous pruritic rash, similar to the palmar-plantar syndrome but occurring on the dorsal surfaces of the hands and feet, occurred 6 days after the first high dose of cyclophosphamide in a patient being prepared for bone-marrow transplantation.[1] Previous cyclophosphamide-containing chemotherapy did not produce this reaction. The symptoms improved somewhat on treatment with triamcinolone ointment, and subsequently desquamation of the hands occurred with decreased purplish discoloration and oedema of the feet. There has also been a report of 2 patients who developed Stevens-Johnson syndrome, with some features suggestive of overlapping toxic epidermal necrolysis.[2]

1. Matsuyama JR, Kwok KK. A variant of the chemotherapy-associated erythrodysesthesia syndrome related to high-dose cyclophosphamide. *DICP Ann Pharmacother* 1989; **23:** 776–9.
2. Assier-Bonnet H, *et al.* Stevens-Johnson syndrome induced by cyclophosphamide: report of two cases. *Br J Dermatol* 1996; **135:** 864–6.

Hypersensitivity. Occasional anaphylaxis has been reported with cyclophosphamide;[1] analysis of data by the Boston Collaborative Drug Surveillance Program detected only one allergic skin reaction among 210 patients given cyclophosphamide, resulting in a calculated incidence of 4.8 reactions per 1000 recipients.[2]

1. Jones JB, *et al.* Cyclophosphamide anaphylaxis. *DICP Ann Pharmacother* 1989; **23:** 88–9.
2. Bigby M, *et al.* Drug-induced cutaneous reactions: a report from the Boston Collaborative Drug Surveillance Program on 15 438 consecutive inpatients, 1975 to 1982. *JAMA* 1986; **256:** 3358–63.

Precautions

For reference to the precautions necessary with antineoplastics and immunosuppressants, see p.480.

Cyclophosphamide should not be given to patients with bone-marrow aplasia, acute infection, or drug- or radiation-induced urothelial toxicity. It should be given with care to those with diabetes mellitus. Care is also needed in elderly or debilitated patients, or those with renal or hepatic impairment or who have undergone adrenalectomy. Liberal fluid intake and frequent micturition are advised to reduce the risk of cystitis but care must be taken to avoid water retention and intoxication. Urine should be examined regularly for red cells, which may precede haemorrhagic cystitis. The haematological profile should be monitored regularly.

The use of cyclophosphamide in pregnancy should be avoided where possible. Mothers taking cyclophosphamide should avoid breast feeding.

Handling and disposal. *Residues* of cyclophosphamide or ifosfamide destroyed using alkaline hydrolysis in the presence of dimethylformamide showed no mutagenicity *in vitro.*[1] An alternative method, involving refluxing of cyclophosphamide with hydrochloric acid, neutralising, and then reacting with sodium thiosulfate, was effective for the degradation of cyclophosphamide, but residues from ifosfamide were still highly mutagenic *in vitro* and this second method should therefore not be used to degrade ifosfamide.

Urine and faeces produced for up to 72 hours and 5 days respectively after an oral dose of cyclophosphamide should be handled wearing protective clothing.[2] As cyclophosphamide was present in sweat and saliva, protective clothing was advised for 72 hours after a dose when bathing the patient or carrying out oral procedures.

1. Castegnaro M, *et al.*, eds. Laboratory decontamination and destruction of carcinogens in laboratory wastes: some antineoplastic agents. *IARC Scientific Publications 73.* Lyon: WHO/International Agency for Research on Cancer, 1985.
2. Harris J, Dodds LJ. Handling waste from patients receiving cytotoxic drugs. *Pharm J* 1985; **235:** 289–91.

Porphyria. Cyclophosphamide is considered to be unsafe in patients with porphyria because it has been shown to be porphyrinogenic in *animals.*

Interactions

For a general outline of antineoplastic drug interactions, see p.481. Since cyclophosphamide must undergo hepatic metabolism before it is active, interactions are possible with drugs that inhibit or stimulate the mixed function oxidase enzymes responsible. There may be an increased risk of cardiotoxicity in patients who have also received doxorubicin or other cardiotoxic drugs.

Allopurinol. Although the Boston Collaborative Drug Surveillance Program reported an increased incidence of bone-marrow depression in patients who received allopurinol with cyclophosphamide than in those receiving cyclophosphamide without allopurinol (15 of 26 compared with only 6 of 32),[1] a subsequent study in patients receiving combination chemotherapy, including cyclophosphamide, for lymphomas failed to find any difference in the nadirs of the platelet and white blood cell counts in cycles in which allopurinol was given concomitantly.[2] Although allopurinol pretreatment resulted in a longer cyclophosphamide half-life in 4 of 26 patients given cyclophosphamide urinary excretion of cyclophosphamide was unchanged.[3] A longer cyclophosphamide half-life was also seen in a study in children who had received allopurinol.[4]

1. Boston Collaborative Drug Surveillance Program. Allopurinol and cytotoxic drugs: interaction in relation to bone marrow depression. *JAMA* 1974; **227:** 1036–40.
2. Stolbach L, *et al.* Evaluation of bone marrow toxic reaction in patients treated with allopurinol. *JAMA* 1982; **247:** 334–6.
3. Bagley CM, *et al.* Clinical pharmacology of cyclophosphamide. *Cancer Res* 1973; **33:** 226–33.
4. Yule SM, *et al.* Cyclophosphamide pharmacokinetics in children. *Br J Clin Pharmacol* 1996; **41:** 13–19.

Antibacterials. Administration of chloramphenicol prior to cyclophosphamide prolonged the mean cyclophosphamide serum half-life from 7.5 to 11.5 hours and reduced the peak activity in all of 5 subjects.[1] Administration of sulfaphenazole prior to cyclophosphamide significantly inhibited the rate of biotransformation of cyclophosphamide in 2 of 7 subjects and enhanced it in 2; it remained unchanged in 3.

1. Faber OK, *et al.* The effect of chloramphenicol and sulphaphenazole on the biotransformation of cyclophosphamide in man. *Br J Clin Pharmacol* 1975; **2:** 281–5.

Anticoagulants. For reference to the interaction of cyclophosphamide with warfarin, see p.995.

Barbiturates. Although patients receiving cyclophosphamide developed higher peak plasma concentrations of active cyclophosphamide metabolites when given enzyme-inducing agents such as barbiturates, the active metabolites also disappeared rapidly.[1]

1. Bagley CM, *et al.* Clinical pharmacology of cyclophosphamide. *Cancer Res* 1973; **33:** 226–33.

Chlorpromazine. The half-life of cyclophosphamide was approximately 200% greater in 2 children who were receiving chlorpromazine concurrently than in children who were not receiving the phenothiazine.[1]

1. Yule SM, *et al.* Cyclophosphamide pharmacokinetics in children. *Br J Clin Pharmacol* 1996; **41:** 13–19.

Colony-stimulating factors. Fatal respiratory insufficiency associated with alveolar fibrosis developed in an infant given cyclophosphamide and doxorubicin followed by filgrastim.[1] Since pulmonary toxicity with cyclophosphamide is normally associated with high cumulative doses it was suggested that in this case the effects might have been exacerbated by the granulocyte colony-stimulating factor. (The pulmonary toxicity of bleomycin has also been suggested to be exacerbated by colony-stimulating factors, as discussed on p.512).

1. van Woensel JBM, *et al.* Acute respiratory insufficiency during doxorubicin, cyclophosphamide, and G-CSF therapy. *Lancet* 1994; **344:** 759–60.

Corticosteroids. Single doses of prednisone have been found to inhibit the activation of cyclophosphamide but after longer-term treatment the rate of activation has increased.[1] A study in children found that pretreatment with dexamethasone was associated with increased clearance of cyclophosphamide and a decrease in its half-life relative to children who had not received the corticosteroid.[2]

1. Faber OK, Mouridsen HT. Cyclophosphamide activation and corticosteroids. *N Engl J Med* 1974; **291:** 211.
2. Yule SM, *et al.* Cyclophosphamide pharmacokinetics in children. *Br J Clin Pharmacol* 1996; **41:** 13–19.

Gastrointestinal drugs. In a retrospective study in patients receiving high-dose cyclophosphamide, cisplatin, and carmustine,[1] the area under the plasma-concentration time curve (AUC) for cyclophosphamide (measured as the parent compound) was 17% lower when *ondansetron* rather than prochlorperazine was added to the antiemetic regimen. In addition, the AUC for cisplatin was 10% higher with the ondansetron regimen. In a similar study,[2] the AUCs for both cyclophosphamide and cisplatin were lower in patients receiving an antiemetic regimen including ondansetron rather than prochlorperazine. The authors of both studies noted that the relevance of these findings to toxicity and antitumour effect of the antineoplastics remained to be determined.

1. Gilbert CJ, *et al.* Pharmacokinetic interaction between ondansetron and cyclophosphamide during high-dose chemotherapy for breast cancer. *Cancer Chemother Pharmacol* 1998; **42**: 497–503.
2. Cagnoni PJ, *et al.* Modification of the pharmacokinetics of high-dose cyclophosphamide and cisplatin by antiemetics. *Bone Marrow Transplant* 1999; **24**: 1–4.

NSAIDs. A report of acute life-threatening water intoxication in a patient given low-dose cyclophosphamide concomitantly with *indometacin*.[1] The patient had previously received treatment with cyclophosphamide (for multiple myeloma) without significant adverse effect.

1. Webberley MJ, Murray JA. Life-threatening acute hyponatraemia induced by low-dose cyclophosphamide and indomethacin. *Postgrad Med J* 1989; **65**: 950–2.

Suxamethonium. For reference to a possible interaction between cyclophosphamide and suxamethonium, see under Suxamethonium Chloride, p.1342.

Pharmacokinetics

Following oral administration, cyclophosphamide is well absorbed from the gastrointestinal tract with a bioavailability greater than 75%. It is widely distributed in the tissues and crosses the blood-brain barrier. It undergoes activation by the mixed function oxidase systems in the liver. The initial metabolites are 4-hydroxycyclophosphamide and its acyclic tautomer, aldophosphamide, which both undergo further metabolism; aldophosphamide may undergo non-enzymatic conversion to active phosphoramide mustard. Acrolein is also produced and may be responsible for bladder toxicity. Cyclophosphamide is excreted principally in urine, as metabolites and some unchanged drug. It crosses the placenta, and is found in breast milk.

◊ Reviews.
1. Grochow LB, Colvin M. Clinical pharmacokinetics of cyclophosphamide. *Clin Pharmacokinet* 1979; **4**: 380–94.
2. Moore MJ. Clinical pharmacokinetics of cyclophosphamide. *Clin Pharmacokinet* 1991; **20**: 194–208.
3. Boddy AV, Yule SM. Metabolism and pharmacokinetics of oxazaphosphorines. *Clin Pharmacokinet* 2000; **38**: 291–304.

Absorption. Cyclophosphamide was detected in the urine of 5 patients following application to intact skin, demonstrating that cyclophosphamide can be absorbed via this route.[1] Absorption continued after the site of application had been cleaned, suggesting that cyclophosphamide had penetrated subcutaneous lipid and was slowly released to the circulation from this depot. Cyclophosphamide was also identified in the urine of 2 oncology nurses but appeared more quickly than in patients, suggesting a faster route of absorption, perhaps by inhalation of aerosols generated during dissolution of the drug.

1. Hirst M, *et al.* Occupational exposure to cyclophosphamide. *Lancet* 1984; **i**: 186–8.

Uses and Administration

Cyclophosphamide is an antineoplastic that is converted in the body to active alkylating metabolites with properties similar to those of mustine [chlormethine] (p.561). It also possesses marked immunosuppressant properties.

Cyclophosphamide is widely used, often in combination with other agents, in the treatment of a variety of malignant diseases as indicated by the cross-references below. It is employed for Burkitt's and other non-Hodgkin's lymphomas, multiple myeloma, and mycosis fungoides. It is also used in the treatment of gestational trophoblastic tumours and malignancies of the breast, endometrium, lung, and ovary; in childhood malignancies such as neuroblastoma, retinoblastoma, Wilms' tumour; and sarcomas.

The immunosuppressant properties of cyclophosphamide have been used in tissue and organ transplantation. It has also been used in the management of various disorders thought to have an auto-immune component including amyloidosis, Behçet's syndrome, glomerular kidney disease, idiopathic thrombocytopenic purpura, interstitial lung disease, polymyositis, scleroderma, systemic lupus erythematosus, and various vasculitic syndromes including the Churg-Strauss syndrome, polyarteritis nodosa, and Wegener's granulomatosis, as indicated by the cross references below.

Cyclophosphamide is usually given by mouth or intravenous injection.

In the BP 2001 the potency of Cyclophosphamide Injection is expressed in terms of the equivalent amount of anhydrous cyclophosphamide whereas the potency of Cyclophosphamide Tablets is given in terms of the monohydrate; the USP 25 expresses potency in terms of anhydrous cyclophosphamide for both injection and tablets. Confusion has arisen when patients were changed from a preparation in which the content was expressed as the monohydrate to one in which it was expressed as the anhydrous substance (see Effects on the Bladder, above). *Doses below are given in terms of anhydrous cyclophosphamide.*

The dosage given depends on the disease being treated, the condition of the patient including the state of the bone marrow, and the concomitant use of radiotherapy or other chemotherapy, and may vary considerably. The white cell count is usually used to guide appropriate dosing. In the UK an example of a low-dose regimen is cyclophosphamide 2 to 6 mg per kg body-weight weekly as a single intravenous dose or in divided doses by mouth; a moderate-dose regimen might be 10 to 15 mg per kg weekly as a single intravenous dose. An example of a high-dose regimen is 20 to 40 mg per kg as a single intravenous dose every 10 to 20 days, although higher doses have been used. The use of mesna is generally recommended with single doses of cyclophosphamide over 2 g, but one manufacturer suggests its use with doses as low as 10 mg per kg.

In the USA, an initial dose of 40 to 50 mg per kg has been licensed for single agent therapy of malignancy, given intravenously in divided doses over 2 to 5 days although in practice treatment of malignancy will generally be with combination regimens. Other intravenous regimens include 3 to 5 mg per kg twice weekly or 10 to 15 mg per kg every 7 to 10 days. Alternatively, 1 to 5 mg per kg daily has been given orally.

A daily oral dose of 2 to 3 mg per kg body-weight has been used in children with minimal change nephropathy leading to the nephrotic syndrome, in whom corticosteroids have been unsuccessful.

In patients who are to undergo bone-marrow transplantation very high doses of cyclophosphamide such as 60 mg per kg daily for 2 to 4 days may be given as part of the conditioning regimen.

Cyclophosphamide has also been given intramuscularly, intraperitoneally, and intrapleurally, as well as intra-arterially, and by local perfusion (but passage through the liver is required for its activation—see Pharmacokinetics, above). A liquid preparation of cyclophosphamide for oral use may be prepared using the powder for injection.

Regular blood counts are essential during therapy with cyclophosphamide and treatment should be withdrawn or delayed if leucopenia or thrombocytopenia becomes severe. Patients should be adequately hydrated and urine output maintained.

Amyloidosis. Although there is no unequivocally effective treatment for amyloidosis (p.501), cyclophosphamide may reduce the decline in renal function;[1] it has also been used in combination with epirubicin and carmustine to suppress the disease in a patient who had undergone heart transplantation for cardiac amyloid.[2]

1. Berglund K, *et al.* Alternating cytostatic treatment in renal amyloidosis secondary to rheumatic disease. *Ann Rheum Dis* 1987; **46**: 757–62.
2. Hall R, *et al.* Cardiac transplantation for AL amyloidosis. *BMJ* 1994; **309**: 1135–7.

Blood disorders, non-malignant. Cyclophosphamide has been used in patients with idiopathic thrombocytopenic purpura (p.1052), but cytotoxic immunosuppressants tend to be a treatment of last resort. Responses generally occur within 8 weeks.[1] In patients with refractory, life-threatening disease high-dose cyclophosphamide,[1] or if that is unsuccessful, combination chemotherapy including cyclophosphamide, which has produced responses in a few patients,[2] may be tried.

1. McMillan R. Therapy for adults with refractory chronic immune thrombocytopenic purpura. *Ann Intern Med* 1997; **126**: 307–14.
2. Figueroa M, *et al.* Combination chemotherapy in refractory immune thrombocytopenic purpura. *N Engl J Med* 1993; **328**: 1226–9.

Cogan's syndrome. For reference to the use of cyclophosphamide in combination with corticosteroids for Cogan's syndrome, see p.1049.

Connective tissue and muscular disorders. Cyclophosphamide is one of a number of immunosuppressants that have

been tried for disease control in Behçet's syndrome (p.1047); such agents may permit a reduction in the use of corticosteroids, although they carry their own risks of toxicity. In polymyositis (p.1057), however, there is some debate about the value of cyclophosphamide as a second-line drug in corticosteroid-unresponsive disease, and the role of immunosuppressants other than azathioprine or methotrexate is poorly defined. In patients with systemic lupus erythematosus (p.1059), cyclophosphamide has been used with some success for severe disease or disease refractory to corticosteroids alone, and appears to be more effective than corticosteroids for lupus nephritis.

Kidney disorders, non-malignant. Cyclophosphamide is used with corticosteroids in the treatment of a number of forms of glomerular kidney disease (p.1051). In minimal change nephropathy, cyclophosphamide 2 to 3 mg per kg body-weight daily for 8 weeks may be added to a course of corticosteroid therapy in relapsing disease;[1-3] addition of cyclophosphamide to corticosteroid therapy also improves the prospect of remission in focal glomerulosclerosis. Oral cyclophosphamide helps to stabilise progressive disease in patients with membranous nephropathy[4] although intermittent intravenous pulses are reported to be ineffective.[5] Such treatment is usually reserved for those whose disease is severe and progressive enough to justify it. Cyclophosphamide has been given with methylprednisolone for rapidly progressive glomerulonephritis,[6] and has been used as part of the aggressive management of renal lesions in Goodpasture's syndrome.

1. Trompeter RS, *et al.* Long-term outcome for children with minimal-change nephrotic syndrome. *Lancet* 1985; **i**: 368–70.
2. Melvin T, Bennett W. Management of nephrotic syndrome in childhood. *Drugs* 1991; **42**: 30–51.
3. Boulton-Jones M. Management of nephrotic syndrome. *Prescribers' J* 1993; **33**: 96–102. Correction *ibid.*; 176.
4. Falk RJ, *et al.* Treatment of progressive membranous glomerulopathy: a randomized trial comparing cyclophosphamide and corticosteroids with corticosteroids alone. *Ann Intern Med* 1992; **116**: 438–45.
5. Reichert LJM, *et al.* Preserving renal function in patients with membranous nephropathy: daily oral chlorambucil compared with intermittent monthly pulses of cyclophosphamide. *Ann Intern Med* 1994; **121**: 328–33.
6. Bruns FJ, *et al.* Long-term follow-up of aggressively treated idiopathic rapidly progressive glomerulonephritis. *Am J Med* 1989; **86**: 400–6.

Liver disorders, non-malignant. For mention of the use of cyclophosphamide in auto-immune hepatitis inadequately controlled by corticosteroids and azathioprine see Chronic Active Hepatitis, p.1048.

Lung disorders, non-malignant. Cyclophosphamide may be useful in combination with corticosteroid therapy in patients with cryptogenic fibrosing alveolitis, as mentioned under Diffuse Parenchymal Lung Disease, p.1050.

Malignant neoplasms. Cyclophosphamide is one of the most widely used drugs for the chemotherapy of malignancy, and mention of its role may be found in the discussions of the management of gestational trophoblastic tumours (p.483); the non-Hodgkin's lymphomas, including AIDS-related lymphoma, Burkitt's lymphoma, and mycosis fungoides (p.487, p.488, p.488, p.489); malignancies of the brain (p.490), breast (p.491), endometrium (p.493), lung (p.496), ovary (p.496) and thymus (p.499); multiple myeloma (p.489); Wilms' tumour, neuroblastoma, and retinoblastoma (p.495, p.500, and p.500 respectively); and sarcomas of bone (p.500) and rhabdomyosarcoma (p.501).

Neuromuscular disorders. Cyclophosphamide has been tried in myasthenia gravis (p.1414) in patients who require immunosuppressants but are intolerant of or unresponsive to corticosteroids and azathioprine. In multiple sclerosis (p.633), the benefits of immunosuppressants such as cyclophosphamide are slight, and outweighed by the toxicity of the required doses. However, moderate dose cyclophosphamide has been employed in conjunction with the 'Gorski manoeuvre' (multiple plasma exchange to reduce antibody titres, a thymic extract to recruit memory cells into division, and then 2 doses of cyclophosphamide after 24 and 48 hours).

References.
1. The Canadian Cooperative Multiple Sclerosis Study Group. The Canadian cooperative trial of cyclophosphamide and plasma exchange in progressive multiple sclerosis. *Lancet* 1991; **337**: 441–6.
2. Currier RD, *et al.* Cyclophosphamide and plasma exchange in multiple sclerosis. *Lancet* 1991; **337**: 1034.
3. Hobbs JR. Controversy in treatment of multiple sclerosis. *Lancet* 1991; **338**: 193–4.

Ocular disorders, non-malignant. Immunosuppressive agents, including cyclophosphamide, have, as mentioned on p.502, been used in scleritis and uveitis unresponsive to corticosteroids in tolerable doses. Cyclophosphamide with a corticosteroid is also reported to be of value in ocular cicatricial pemphigoid,[1] although treatment may not completely prevent cicatrisation.

1. Elder MJ, *et al.* Role of cyclophosphamide and high dose steroid in ocular cicatricial pemphigoid. *Br J Ophthalmol* 1995; **79**: 264–6.

Organ and tissue transplantation. Cyclophosphamide is used in high doses, usually with busulfan or irradiation, in conditioning regimens for bone-marrow transplantation (p.502), and has been tried as part of immunosuppressant regimens following transplantation of heart grafts (p.503).

Paraquat poisoning. For reference to the use of cyclophosphamide in paraquat poisoning, see p.1435.

Pemphigus and pemphigoid. Corticosteroids are the main treatment for blistering in pemphigus and pemphigoid (p.1106). Immunosuppressive therapy, including cyclophosphamide,[1,2] has been used in combination with corticosteroids to permit a reduction in corticosteroid dosage. However, it has been suggested that evidence for the corticosteroid-sparing effect is lacking and that immunosuppressants should be reserved for patients who cannot tolerate corticosteroids or in whom they are contra-indicated.[3]

1. Pandya AG, Sontheimer RD. Treatment of pemphigus vulgaris with pulse intravenous cyclophosphamide. *Arch Dermatol* 1992; **128:** 1626–30.
2. Itoh T, *et al.* Successful treatment of bullous pemphigoid with pulsed intravenous cyclophosphamide. *Br J Dermatol* 1996; **134:** 931–3.
3. Bystryn J-C, Steinman NM. The adjuvant therapy of pemphigus: an update. *Arch Dermatol* 1996; **132:** 203–12.

Rheumatoid arthritis. Cyclophosphamide has been used as a disease-modifying antirheumatic drug in rheumatoid arthritis (p.9), usually in patients with severe disease unresponsive to other drugs; its severe toxicity limits its usefulness.[1] It is of most value in controlling antibody-mediated systemic complications of the disease such as vasculitis[2] through inhibition of B-cell function.

1. Suarez-Almazor ME, *et al.* Cyclophosphamide for rheumatoid arthritis (updated 28 October 1999). Available in The Cochrane Library; Issue 1. Oxford: Update Software; 2000.
2. Choy E, Kingsley G. How do second-line agents work? *Br Med Bull* 1995; **51:** 472–92.

Scleroderma. As discussed on p.505 the role of drug treatment for scleroderma is not well determined, but cyclophosphamide may perhaps be useful combined with a corticosteroid for patients with lung involvement.

Vasculitic syndromes. Treatment of the systemic vasculitides has revolved around the use of corticosteroids and cyclophosphamide. The benefits are uncertain in polyarteritis nodosa (p.1056) and Takayasu's arteritis (p.1060), but the benefits of combined therapy are generally accepted in Churg-Strauss syndrome (p.1049) and microscopic polyangiitis (p.1056), and cyclophosphamide is the mainstay of effective treatment of Wegener's granulomatosis (p.1060). A number of administration regimens are in use; in particular intermittent high-dose intravenous ('pulsed') administration is being evaluated in comparison with continuous therapy.[1]

1. Richmond R, *et al.* Optimisation of cyclophosphamide therapy in systemic vasculitis. *Clin Pharmacokinet* 1998; **34:** 79–90.

Preparations

BP 2001: Cyclophosphamide Injection; Cyclophosphamide Tablets;
USP 25: Cyclophosphamide for Injection; Cyclophosphamide Tablets.

Proprietary Preparations (details are given in Part 3)
Aust.: Endoxan; *Austral.:* Cycloblastin; Endoxan; *Belg.:* Cycloblastine; Endoxan; *Braz.:* Enduxan; Genuxal; *Canad.:* Cytoxan; Procytox; *Denm.:* Carloxan; Sendoxan; *Fin.:* Sendoxan; *Fr.:* Endoxan; *Ger.:* Cyclo-cell; Cyclostin; Endoxan; *Hong Kong:* Endoxan; *Israel:* Cytophosphan; Cytoxan; *Ital.:* Endoxan; *Mex.:* Fosfaseron; Genoxal; Ledoxina; *Neth.:* Cycloblastine†; Endoxan; *Norw.:* Sendoxan; *NZ:* Cycloblastin; Cytoxan; Endoxan; *Port.:* Endoxan; *S.Afr.:* Cycloblastin; Endoxan; *Singapore:* Alkyloxan; Endoxan; *Spain:* Cicloxal†; Genoxal; *Swed.:* Sendoxan; *Switz.:* Endoxan; *Thai.:* Endoxana; *UK:* Endoxana; *USA:* Cytoxan; Neosar.

Cytarabine (1826-a)

Cytarabine *(BAN, USAN, rINN).*
Arabinosylcytosine; Ara-C; Cytarabinum; Cytosine Arabinoside; NSC-63878 (cytarabine hydrochloride); U-19920; U-19920A (cytarabine hydrochloride); WR-28453. 1-β-D-Arabinofuranosylcytosine; 4-Amino-1-β-D-arabinofuranosylpyrimidin-2(1H)-one.
$C_9H_{13}N_3O_5 = 243.2$.
CAS — 147-94-4 (cytarabine); 69-74-9 (cytarabine hydrochloride).
ATC — L01BC01.

Pharmacopoeias. In Eur. (see p.vi), *Int., Jpn,* and *US.*
Chin. includes the hydrochloride.

Pharmacopoeial description
Ph. Eur.: A white or almost white, crystalline powder. Freely soluble in water; very slightly soluble in alcohol and in dichloromethane. Store in airtight containers. Protect from light.

USP 25: An odourless, white to off-white, crystalline powder. Freely soluble in water; slightly soluble in alcohol and in chloroform. Protect from light.

Incompatibility. Although cytarabine has been stated in the literature to be incompatible with solutions of fluorouracil[1,2] and methotrexate[1] some studies have reported it to be stable for some hours when mixed with the latter.[3]

1. D'Arcy PF. Reactions and interactions in handling anticancer drugs. *Drug Intell Clin Pharm* 1983; **17:** 532–8.

2. McRae MP, King JC. Compatibility of antineoplastic, antibiotic and corticosteroid drugs in intravenous admixtures. *Am J Hosp Pharm* 1976; **33:** 1010–13.
3. Cheung Y-W. Stability of cytarabine, methotrexate sodium, and hydrocortisone sodium succinate admixtures. *Am J Hosp Pharm* 1984; **41:** 1802–6.

Adverse Effects, Treatment, and Precautions

For general discussions see Antineoplastics, p.476, p.479, and p.480.

The major dose-limiting adverse effect of cytarabine is bone-marrow depression, manifest as leucopenia (particularly granulocytopenia), thrombocytopenia, and anaemia, sometimes with striking megaloblastic changes. Myelosuppression appears to be more evident after continuous infusions. Leucopenia is biphasic, with a nadir at 7 to 9 days after a dose and another, more severe, at 15 to 24 days. The nadir of the platelet count occurs at about 12 to 15 days. Recovery generally occurs in a further ten days.

Gastrointestinal disturbances may occur: nausea and vomiting may be more severe when doses are given rapidly (but other adverse effects are reported to be worse when the drug is given by infusion). Other adverse effects reported include hepatic dysfunction, renal dysfunction, neurotoxicity, bleeding complications, rashes, oral and anal ulceration, gastrointestinal haemorrhage, oesophagitis, and conjunctivitis. A syndrome of bone and muscle pain, fever, malaise, conjunctivitis, and rash, sometimes described as 'flu-like', has been reported 6 to 12 hours after cytarabine administration, which may be treated or prevented with corticosteroid therapy. Anaphylactoid reactions have occurred rarely. There may be local pain, cellulitis, and thrombophlebitis at the site of injection.

Intrathecal administration of the liposomal cytarabine formulation commonly causes chemical arachnoiditis manifesting as neck stiffness or pain, nausea, vomiting, headache, and fever. Dexamethasone should be used prophylactically to reduce the incidence and severity of this complication. Other rare adverse effects include encephalopathy, and focal seizures. Intrathecal administration of conventional cytarabine formulations has rarely been associated with severe spinal cord toxicity, necrotising encephalopathy, blindness, and other neurotoxicities. If used intrathecally, preservative-free diluents must be used.

High-dose therapy has been associated with particularly severe gastrointestinal and CNS effects, including severe ulceration of the gastrointestinal tract, pneumatosis cystoides leading to peritonitis, necrotising colitis and bowel necrosis, peripheral neuropathy, and cerebral and cerebellar dysfunction, with personality changes, somnolence, and coma. There may also be corneal toxicity leading to punctate keratitis and haemorrhagic conjunctivitis, sepsis, liver abscess, severe skin rash leading to desquamation, alopecia, and cardiac disorders including pericarditis and fatal cardiomyopathy. Pulmonary oedema, sometimes fatal, has occurred.

Cytarabine is teratogenic in *animals* (but see Pregnancy, below).

In addition to frequent white blood cell and platelet counts, blood-uric acid should be monitored because of the risk of hyperuricaemia secondary to lysis of neoplastic cells, and renal and hepatic function should be periodically assessed. Cytarabine should be given with care to patients with impaired liver function; dosage reduction may be necessary.

◊ The toxicity of cytarabine has been reviewed.[1] The principal toxicity of standard dosage regimens is myelosuppression but bleeding complications and gastrointestinal toxicity are also major problems at standard doses. With the high-dose regimens neurological toxicity may be dose-limiting: severe and sometimes irreversible symptoms have been seen in 10 to 10% of patients receiving a cumulative dose of 36 g per square metre body-surface. Ocular toxicity may occur in up to 80% of patients at the highest doses. Since cytarabine toxicity is largely dose-related low-dose therapy is generally well tolerated, even in elderly patients, who are more susceptible: its only significant toxicity is myelosuppression.

1. Stentoft J. The toxicity of cytarabine. *Drug Safety* 1990; **5:** 7–27.

Effects on the nervous system. Although paraplegia has been reported with intrathecal cytarabine[1] (see also under Benzyl Alcohol, p.1135) and peripheral neuropathy has occurred in a patient who had received only conventional intravenous doses,[2] the majority of cases of neurotoxicity associated with cytarabine appear to be in patients given high-dose regimens.[3-7] Although some cases have manifested as demyelinating peripheral neuropathy,[3,4] including a syndrome of painful legs and involuntary movements in the toes which showed some response to carbamazepine,[3] most studies have reported in particular a syndrome of cerebellar toxicity,[5-8] with symptoms such as dysarthria, nystagmus, and ataxia. Toxicity appears to be dose-related: in one series[5] CNS toxicity occurred in none of 12 patients given total doses of up to 24 g per m[2] body-surface of cytarabine, 3 of 19 receiving 36 g per m[2], and 1 of 12 given 48 g per m[2], none of which were life-threatening or irreversible, whereas 4 of 6 given 54 g per m[2] (as 4.5 g per m[2] every 12 hours for 12 doses) developed neurotoxicity, which was fatal in one and irreversible in another. However, persistent, severe cerebellar toxicity has also been reported in a patient who had received a total dose of only 36 g per m[2] (as 3 g per m[2] every 12 hours).[8] There is some evidence[6] that patients aged over 50, and those who have recently received conventional-dose cytarabine[7] may be at increased risk. Intracranial hypertension (pseudotumour cerebri) has occurred rarely.[9]

1. Saleh MN, *et al.* Intrathecal cytosine arabinoside-induced acute, rapidly reversible paralysis. *Am J Med* 1988; **86:** 729–30.
2. Russell JA, Powles RL. Neuropathy due to cytosine arabinoside. *BMJ* 1974; **4:** 652–3.
3. Malapert D, Degos JD. Jambes douloureuses et orteils instables: neuropathie induite par la cytarabine. *Rev Neurol (Paris)* 1989; **145:** 869–71.
4. Nevill TJ, *et al.* Horner's syndrome and demyelinating peripheral neuropathy caused by high-dose cytosine arabinoside. *Am J Hematol* 1989; **32:** 314–15.
5. Lazarus HM, *et al.* Central nervous system toxicity of high-dose systemic cytosine arabinoside. *Cancer* 1981; **48:** 2577–82.
6. Graves T, Hooks MA. Drug-induced toxicities associated with high-dose cytosine arabinoside infusions. *Pharmacotherapy* 1989; **9:** 23–8.
7. Barnett MJ, *et al.* Neurotoxicity of high-dose cytosine arabinoside. *Prog Exp Tumor Res* 1985; **29:** 117–41.
8. Dworkin LA, *et al.* Cerebellar toxicity following high-dose cytosine arabinoside. *J Clin Oncol* 1985; **3:** 613–16.
9. Fort JA, Smith LD. Pseudotumor cerebri secondary to intermediate-dose cytarabine HCl. *Ann Pharmacother* 1999; **33:** 576–8.

Effects on the skin. A syndrome of pain and erythema of the palms and soles, progressing to bullae and desquamation, has been seen in patients receiving intermediate- or high-dose cytarabine.[1,2] The syndrome is similar to the palmar-plantar syndrome reported in patients receiving chemotherapy not including cytarabine,[3] although some considered the two forms of toxicity distinct.[4] Cutaneous small vessel necrotising vasculitis has been reported after high-dose therapy with cytarabine.[5]

1. Baer MR, *et al.* Palmar-plantar erythrodysesthesia and cytarabine. *Ann Intern Med* 1985; **102:** 556.
2. Peters WG, Willemze R. Palmar-plantar skin changes and cytarabine. *Ann Intern Med* 1985; **103:** 805.
3. Lokich JJ, Moore C. Chemotherapy-associated palmar-plantar erythrodysesthesia syndrome. *Ann Intern Med* 1984; **101:** 798–800.
4. Vogelzang NJ, Ratain MJ. Cancer chemotherapy and skin changes. *Ann Intern Med* 1985; **103:** 303–4.
5. Ahmed I, *et al.* Cytosine arabinoside-induced vasculitis. *Mayo Clin Proc* 1998; **73:** 239–42.

Pregnancy. Although there has been a report of limb and ear deformities in the infant of a woman given cytarabine at the estimated time of conception and 4 to 8 weeks later,[1] no congenital abnormalities were noted in 17 infants, 5 therapeutic abortions, and one still-birth (following pre-eclamptic toxaemia) resulting from over 20 known cases in which cytarabine was given during pregnancy.[2]

1. Wagner VM, *et al.* Congenital abnormalities in baby born to cytarabine treated mother. *Lancet* 1980; **ii:** 98–9.
2. Morgenstern G. Cytarabine in pregnancy. *Lancet* 1980; **ii:** 259.

Interactions

For a general outline of antineoplastic drug interactions, see p.481.

Antifungals. Cytarabine has been reported to inhibit the action of *flucytosine*—see p.385.

Antineoplastics. Acute pancreatitis has been reported in patients given cytarabine who had previously received *asparaginase* therapy.[1] Subclinical damage to the pancreas by asparaginase may have rendered it susceptible to cytarabine.

For a report of hepatic dysfunction associated with the combined use of cytarabine and *daunorubicin* see under Daunorubicin Hydrochloride, p.533.

Administration of cytarabine after *fludarabine* is reported to result in a fivefold increase in intracellular cytarabine concentrations in leukaemic cells,[2] producing improved clinical response rates.

1. Altman AJ, *et al.* Acute pancreatitis in association with cytosine arabinoside therapy. *Cancer* 1982; **49:** 1384–6.
2. Avramis VI, *et al.* Pharmacokinetic and pharmacodynamic studies of fludarabine and cytosine arabinoside administered as loading boluses followed by continuous infusions after a phase I/II study in pediatric patients with relapsed leukemias. *Clin Cancer Res* 1998; **4:** 45–52.

Pharmacokinetics

Cytarabine is not effective by mouth due to rapid deamination in the gastrointestinal tract; less than 20% of an oral dose is absorbed. After intravenous injection it disappears rapidly from the plasma with an initial half-life of about 10 minutes; the terminal elimination half-life ranges from 1 to 3 hours. It is converted by phosphorylation to an active form which is rapidly deaminated, mainly in the liver and the kidneys, to inactive 1-β-D-arabinofuranosyluracil (uracil arabinoside, ara-U). The majority of an intravenous dose is excreted in the urine within 24 hours, mostly as the inactive metabolite with about 10% as unchanged cytarabine.

There is only moderate diffusion of cytarabine across the blood-brain barrier following intravenous injection, but, because of low deaminase activity in the CSF, concentrations achieved after continuous intravenous infusion or intrathecal injection are maintained for longer in the CSF than are those in plasma, with a terminal elimination half-life of 3.5 hours. After intrathecal administration of the liposomal formulation, a terminal elimination half-life of 100 to 263 hours was seen. Cytarabine also crosses the placenta.

◊ References.
1. Ho DHW, Frei E. Clinical pharmacology of 1-β-D-arabinofuranosyl cytosine. *Clin Pharmacol Ther* 1971; **12:** 944–54.
2. van Prooijen R, *et al.* Pharmacokinetics of cytosine arabinoside in acute myeloid leukemia. *Clin Pharmacol Ther* 1977; **21:** 744–50.
3. Harris AL, *et al.* Pharmacokinetics of cytosine arabinoside in patients with acute myeloid leukaemia. *Br J Clin Pharmacol* 1979; **8:** 219–27.
4. Slevin ML, *et al.* The pharmacokinetics of subcutaneous cytosine arabinoside in patients with acute myelogenous leukaemia. *Br J Clin Pharmacol* 1981; **12:** 507–10.

Uses and Administration

Cytarabine, a pyrimidine nucleoside analogue, is an antimetabolite antineoplastic which inhibits the synthesis of deoxyribonucleic acid. Its actions are specific for the S phase of the cell cycle. It also has antiviral and immunosuppressant properties. Cytarabine is one of the mainstays of the treatment of acute myeloid leukaemias, together with an anthracycline and tioguanine, (see p.485), and is used for the prophylaxis of meningeal leukaemia, as well as in regimens for consolidation, in patients with acute lymphoblastic leukaemia (p.484). It has also been investigated in the blast crisis of chronic myeloid leukaemia (p.486) and the myelodysplasias (p.486) (see also Administration, below). It may also be used in salvage regimens for Hodgkin's disease (p.487), as part of the complex regimens sometimes employed in aggressive intermediate- and high-grade non-Hodgkin's lymphomas (p.487), and for meningeal lymphoma.

Cytarabine is given by the intravenous route. Higher doses can be tolerated when given by rapid injection rather than slow infusion, because of the rapid clearance of cytarabine, but there is little evidence of clinical advantage for either route. Cytarabine may be given by the intrathecal route for leukaemic or lymphomatous meningitis.

For the induction of remission in adults and children with acute leukaemias a wide variety of dosage regimens have been used: 100 mg per m² body-surface twice daily by rapid intravenous injection, or 100 mg per m² daily by continuous intravenous infusion, have often been employed. These doses are generally given for 5 to 10 days, depending on therapeutic response and toxicity. Children reportedly tolerate high doses better than adults.

For maintenance 75 to 100 mg per m² once weekly, or 1 to 1.5 mg per kg once or twice weekly have been given intravenously or subcutaneously; other regimens have been used.

In the treatment of refractory disease high-dose regimens have been employed, with cytarabine given in doses of up to 3 g per m² every 12 hours for up to 6 days. These doses should be given by intravenous infusion over at least 1 hour.

In leukaemic meningitis cytarabine has been given intrathecally, often in a dose of 10 to 30 mg per m²

The symbol † denotes a preparation no longer actively marketed

body-surface every 2 to 4 days; it has also been used prophylactically. A liposomal formulation is available in some countries for intrathecal administration and permits less frequent dosing because of its longer duration of action. The recommended dose for lymphomatous meningitis is 50 mg intrathecally every 2 weeks for 5 doses then every 4 weeks for 5 doses.

White cell and platelet counts should be determined regularly during treatment with cytarabine and therapy should be stopped immediately if the count falls rapidly or to low values.

Administration. INTRATHECAL. Intrathecal administration of the liposomal formulation of cytarabine results in prolonged drug exposure when compared with intrathecal administration of the conventional formulation (see Pharmacokinetics, above). In a randomised study,[1] the liposomal formulation administered once every 2 weeks gave a higher response rate and improved Karnofsky score compared with the conventional formulation administered twice a week in patients with lymphomatous meningitis secondary to lymphoma.
1. Glantz MJ, *et al.* Randomized trial of a slow-release versus a standard formulation of cytarabine for the intrathecal treatment of lymphomatous meningitis. *J Clin Oncol* 1999; **17:** 3110–16.

LOW-DOSE THERAPY. Because of suggestions that low doses of cytarabine might induce differentiation and maturation of leukaemic cells, low-dose therapy (usually 5 to 10 mg per m² body-surface twice daily) has been tried in patients with myelodysplastic syndrome and acute myeloid leukaemia.[1] Although complete remission may occur in about 20% of patients with myelodysplastic syndromes a similar proportion succumb to treatment-related mortality, and remissions do not appear to be particularly long-lasting. Bone marrow suppression may be marked even at these doses. It is not clear whether the effects of low-dose cytarabine are due to differentiation or cytotoxicity.
1. Aul C, Gattermann N. The role of low-dose chemotherapy in myelodysplastic syndrome. *Leuk Res* 1992; **16:** 207–15.

Leucoencephalopathy. There are anecdotal reports[1-3] of marked improvement in patients with progressive multifocal leucoencephalopathy secondary to AIDS or chemotherapy-induced immunosuppression following intravenous or intrathecal cytarabine. However, a randomised multicentre study[4] has indicated that cytarabine was ineffective and has no role in this condition (see also Infections in Immunocompromised Patients, p.611).
1. O'Riordan T, *et al.* Progressive multifocal leukoencephalopathy-remission with cytarabine. *J Infect* 1990; **20:** 51–4.
2. Portegies P, *et al.* Response to cytarabine in progressive multifocal leucoencephalopathy in AIDS. *Lancet* 1991; **337:** 680–1.
3. Nicoli F, *et al.* Efficacy of cytarabine in progressive multifocal leucoencephalopathy in AIDS. *Lancet* 1992; **339:** 306.
4. Hall CD, *et al.* Failure of cytarabine in progressive multifocal leukoencephalopathy associated with human immunodeficiency virus infection. *N Engl J Med* 1998; **338:** 1345–51.

Preparations

BP 2001: Cytarabine Injection;
USP 25: Cytarabine for Injection.

Proprietary Preparations (details are given in Part 3)
Aust.: Alexan; Cytosar; *Austral.:* Cytosar-U; *Belg.:* Cytosar; *Braz.:* Alexan; Aracytin; *Canad.:* Cytosar; *Denm.:* Arabine; Cytosar; *Fin.:* Arabine; *Fr.:* Aracytine; Cytarbel†; *Ger.:* Alexan; ARA-cell; Udicil; *Hong Kong:* Alexan; Cytosar; *Irl.:* Cytosar; *Israel:* Cytosar; Cytovis; *Ital.:* Aracytin; Erpalfa; *Jpn:* Cylocide; Starasid†; *Mex.:* Alexan; Laracit; Medsara; Serotabir; *Neth.:* Cytosar; *Norw.:* Cytosar; *NZ:* Cytosar-U; *Port.:* Alexan†; Citaloxan; Cytosar; *S.Afr.:* Alexan; Cytosar; *Singapore:* Alexan; Cytosar; *Swed.:* Alexan†; Arabine; Cytosar; *Switz.:* Alexan†; Cytosar; *Thai.:* Alexan; Cytosar-U; *UK:* Cytosar; *USA:* Cytosar-U; DepoCyt.

Dacarbazine   (1827-t)

Dacarbazine (BAN, USAN, rINN).

DIC; DTIC; Imidazole Carboxamide; NSC-45388; WR-139007. 5-(3,3-Dimethyltriazeno)imidazole-4-carboxamide.
$C_6H_{10}N_6O = 182.2.$
CAS — 4342-03-4.
ATC — L01AX04.
Pharmacopoeias. In Br. and US.

Pharmacopoeial description
BP 2001: A colourless or pale yellow, crystalline powder. Slightly soluble in water and in alcohol. Store at 2° to 8°. Protect from light.

USP 25: Store in airtight containers at 2° to 8°. Protect from light.

◊ CAUTION. *Dacarbazine is irritant; avoid contact with skin and mucous membranes.*

Incompatibility. Dacarbazine has been reported to be incompatible with hydrocortisone sodium succinate but not with the sodium phosphate.[1] It has been reported to be incompatible

with heparin,[2] although only with concentrated dacarbazine solutions (25 mg per mL).
1. Dorr RT. Incompatibilities with parenteral anticancer drugs. *Am J Intravenous Ther* 1979; **6:** 42–52.
2. Nelson RW, *et al.* Visual incompatibility of dacarbazine and heparin. *Am J Hosp Pharm* 1987; **44:** 2028.

Stability. References to the photodegradation of dacarbazine solution.[1-3] Dacarbazine is more sensitive to direct sunlight than to artificial lighting or diffuse daylight.
1. Stevens MFG, Peatey L. Photodegradation of solutions of the antitumour drug DTIC. *J Pharm Pharmacol* 1978; **30** (suppl): 47P.
2. Horton JK, Stevens MFG. Search for drug interactions between the antitumour agent DTIC and other cytotoxic agents. *J Pharm Pharmacol* 1979; **31** (suppl): 64P.
3. Kirk B. The evaluation of a light-protecting giving set. *Intensive Therapy Clin Monit* 1987; **8:** 78–86.

Adverse Effects, Treatment, and Precautions

For general discussions see Antineoplastics, p.476, p.479, and p.480.

Leucopenia and thrombocytopenia with dacarbazine, although usually moderate, may be severe. The nadir of the white cell count usually occurs 21 to 25 days after a dose. Anorexia, nausea, and vomiting occur in more than 90% of patients initially but tolerance may develop after repeated doses. Less frequent adverse effects include diarrhoea, skin reactions, alopecia, an influenza-like syndrome, facial flushing and paraesthesia, and rare but potentially fatal hepatotoxicity. There may be local pain at the injection site; extravasation produces pain and tissue damage. Anaphylaxis has occurred occasionally.

Dacarbazine should be used with caution in hepatic and renal impairment, and consideration given to reducing the dose. Haematological monitoring is required during therapy.

Effects on the liver. Based on experience in more than 100 patients it was reported in 1982 that the spectrum of adverse hepatic effects with dacarbazine was broader than previously documented cases of vasculitis leading to acute hepatic failure and death had suggested.[1] Necrosis may be associated with venous thrombosis or occur without signs of inflammation; granulomatous hepatitis has occurred, as has a case of acute toxic hepatitis during the first course of dacarbazine. Morphological studies suggested that dacarbazine may exert a toxic effect on the microfilamentous cytoskeleton of the hepatocytes.
1. Dancygier H, *et al.* Dacarbazine (DTIC)-induced human liver injury. *Gut* 1982; **23:** A447.

Interactions

For a general outline of antineoplastic drug interactions, see p.481.

Levodopa. For a report of dacarbazine reducing the effects of levodopa, see Antineoplastics, p.1171.

Pharmacokinetics

Dacarbazine is poorly absorbed from the gastrointestinal tract. Following intravenous injection it is rapidly distributed with an initial plasma half-life of about 20 minutes; the terminal half-life is reported to be about 5 hours. The volume of distribution is larger than body water content, suggesting localisation in some body tissues, probably mainly the liver. Only about 5% is bound to plasma protein. It crosses the blood-brain barrier to a limited extent with concentrations in cerebrospinal fluid about 14% of those in plasma. Dacarbazine is extensively metabolised in the liver; the major metabolite appears to be 5-aminoimidazole-4-carboxamide (AIC). About half of a dose is excreted unchanged in the urine by tubular secretion.

Uses and Administration

Dacarbazine is a cell-cycle non-specific antineoplastic that is thought to function as an alkylating agent after it has been activated in the liver. Dacarbazine is used mainly in the treatment of metastatic malignant melanoma (p.499). It is also given to patients with Hodgkin's disease (p.487), notably in combination with doxorubicin, bleomycin, and vinblastine (ABVD), and may be given in neuroblastoma (p.500), and in the treatment of soft-tissue and Kaposi's sarcomas (p.501, and p.501) and other tumours.

It is given intravenously in doses of 2 to 4.5 mg per kg body-weight daily for 10 days, repeated at intervals of

4 weeks, or 200 to 250 mg per m^2 body-surface daily for 5 days, repeated at intervals of 3 weeks. For melanoma it can also be given in a dose of 850 mg per m^2 by intravenous infusion at 3-week intervals. In the treatment of Hodgkin's disease doses of 150 mg per m^2 daily for 5 days repeated every 4 weeks, or 375 mg per m^2 every 15 days have been given in association with other agents. Injections may be given over one to two minutes. The reconstituted solution has been further diluted with up to 300 mL of glucose 5% or sodium chloride 0.9% and given by infusion over 15 to 30 minutes.

Preparations

BP 2001: Dacarbazine Injection;
USP 25: Dacarbazine for Injection.

Proprietary Preparations (details are given in Part 3)
Aust.: DTIC-Dome; ***Austral.:*** DTIC; ***Belg.:*** DTIC-Dome; ***Canad.:*** DTIC; ***Fin.:*** Dacatic; ***Fr.:*** Deticene; ***Ger.:*** Detimedac; DTIC†; ***Hong Kong:*** Deticene; ***Irl.:*** DTIC-Dome; ***Israel:*** Deticene; ***Ital.:*** Deticene; ***Mex.:*** Asercit; Deticene; ***Neth.:*** Deticene; ***NZ:*** DTIC-Dome; ***Port.:*** Deticene; Fauldetic; ***S.Afr.:*** DTIC-Dome; ***Spain:*** DTIC-Dome†; ***Swed.:*** DTIC; ***Switz.:*** DTIC; ***UK:*** DTIC-Dome; ***USA:*** DTIC-Dome.

Daclizumab (17621-d)

Daclizumab *(BAN, USAN, rINN).*

Dacliximab; Humanised Anti-Tac Antibody; Ro-24-7375.

CAS — 152923-56-3.

ATC — L04AA08.

The manufacturers recommend that daclizumab be stored between 2° and 8°.

Adverse Effects and Precautions

Severe hypersensitivity reactions have occurred rarely; facilities for the treatment of such reactions should be available during use.

Pharmacokinetics

The recommended regimen of daclizumab (see below) should result in serum concentrations sufficient to saturate interleukin-2 receptors for more than 90 days. The terminal elimination half-life of daclizumab has ranged from 11 to 38 days.

Uses and Administration

Daclizumab is a humanised monoclonal murine antibody that functions as an interleukin-2 receptor antagonist by binding to the alpha chain (CD25 antigen, Tac subunit) of the interleukin-2 receptor on the surface of activated T-lymphocytes. It is used in the prevention of acute graft rejection following kidney transplantation as part of an immunosuppressive regimen that includes ciclosporin and corticosteroids. It is given in a dose of 1 mg per kg body-weight intravenously over 15 minutes within 24 hours before surgery and repeated at intervals of 2 weeks for a total of 5 doses. Daclizumab is also under investigation for its immunosuppressant properties in other forms of transplantation and in various diseases with an auto-immune component.

◊ Reviews.

1. Wiseman LR, Faulds D. Daclizumab: a review of its use in the prevention of acute rejection in renal transplant recipients. *Drugs* 1999; **58:** 1029–42.

Organ and tissue transplantation. Daclizumab reduced the incidence of acute rejection episodes in the first 6 months after renal transplantation (p.503) when compared with placebo, but did not affect the graft survival rate.[1,2] Compared with placebo, daclizumab improved patient survival when added to double therapy (ciclosporin plus corticosteroids),[2] but this effect was not seen when daclizumab was added to triple therapy (ciclosporin, corticosteroids, plus azathioprine).[1]

Daclizumab has been investigated in the prevention of acute rejection following cardiac transplantation.[3]

1. Vincenti F, *et al.* Interleukin-2-receptor blockade with daclizumab to prevent acute rejection in renal transplantation. *N Engl J Med* 1998; **338:** 161–5.
2. Nashan B, *et al.* Reduction of acute renal allograft rejection by daclizumab. *Transplantation* 1999; **67:** 110–15.
3. Beniaminovitz A, *et al.* Prevention of rejection in cardiac transplantation by blockade of the interleukin-2 receptor with a monoclonal antibody. *N Engl J Med* 2000; **342:** 613–19.

Psoriasis. A report[1] of a response to daclizumab in a patient with severe intractable psoriasis.

1. Wohlrab J, *et al.* Treatment of recalcitrant psoriasis with daclizumab. *Br J Dermatol* 2001; **144:** 209–10.

Preparations

Proprietary Preparations (details are given in Part 3)
Aust.: Zenapax; ***Austral.:*** Zenapax; ***Belg.:*** Zenapax; ***Denm.:*** Zenapax; ***Fin.:*** Zenapax; ***Fr.:*** Zenapax; ***Ger.:*** Zenapax; ***Neth.:*** Zenapax; ***NZ:*** Zenapax; ***Port.:*** Zenapax; ***Singapore:*** Zenapax; ***Swed.:*** Zenapax; ***Switz.:*** Zenapax; ***Thai.:*** Zenapax; ***UK:*** Zenapax; ***USA:*** Zenapax.

Dactinomycin (1802-w)

Dactinomycin *(BAN, USAN, rINN).*

Actinomycin C_1; Actinomycin D; Meractinomycin; NSC-3053.
$N^{2.1},N^{2'.1'}$-(2-Amino-4,6-dimethyl-3-oxo-3*H*-phenoxazine-1,9-diyldicarbonyl)bis[threonyl-D-valylprolyl(*N*-methylglycyl)(*N*-methylvaline) 1.5–3.1-lactone].

$C_{62}H_{86}N_{12}O_{16}$ = 1255.4.

CAS — 50-76-0.

ATC — L01DA01.

Pharmacopoeias. In *Chin., Int., Jpn, Pol.,* and *US.*

An antineoplastic antibiotic produced by the growth of *Streptomyces chrysomallus* and other species of *Streptomyces.*

Cactinomycin (actinomycin C; HBF-386; NSC-18268) is a mixture of dactinomycin (actinomycin D) (10%), actinomycin C_2 (45%), and actinomycin C_3 (45%).

Pharmacopoeial description

USP 25: A bright red, somewhat hygroscopic, crystalline powder, affected by light and heat. It has a potency of not less than 950 and not more than 1030 μg per mg, calculated on the dried basis. Soluble in water at 10° and slightly soluble in water at 37°; freely soluble in alcohol; very slightly soluble in ether. Store at a temperature not exceeding 40° in airtight containers. Protect from light.

◊ CAUTION. *Dactinomycin is irritant; avoid contact with skin and mucous membranes.*

Adsorption. Dactinomycin binds to cellulose ester filters,[1] and such filtration should be avoided.[2] Although it has been suggested that significant amounts of drug may be adsorbed to glass or plastic,[3] dactinomycin is reportedly compatible with glass and PVC infusion containers,[4] and administration into the tubing of a fast-running intravenous infusion is the recommended manner of administration—see Uses and Administration, below.

1. Kanke M, *et al.* Binding of selected drugs to a "treated" inline filter. *Am J Hosp Pharm* 1983; **40:** 1323–8.
2. D'Arcy PF. Reactions and interactions in handling anticancer drugs. *Drug Intell Clin Pharm* 1983; **17:** 532–8.
3. Rapp RP, *et al.* Guidelines for the administration of commonly-used intravenous drugs—1984 update. *Drug Intell Clin Pharm* 1984; **18:** 218–32.
4. Benvenuto JA, *et al.* Stability and compatibility of antitumor agents in glass and plastic containers. *Am J Hosp Pharm* 1981; **38:** 1914–18.

Adverse Effects, Treatment, and Precautions

For general discussions see Antineoplastics, p.476, p.479, and p.480.

Apart from nausea and vomiting adverse effects are often delayed, beginning 2 to 4 days after the completion of a course of treatment and reaching a maximum after 1 to 2 weeks. Fatalities have occurred. Bone-marrow depression and gastrointestinal effects (including nausea and vomiting) may prove dose-limiting. Bone-marrow depression is apparent 1 to 7 days after therapy and may be manifest first as thrombocytopenia; the nadir of the platelet and white cell counts usually occurs within 14 to 21 days, with recovery in 21 to 25 days. Other adverse effects include oral and gastrointestinal effects such as stomatitis, diarrhoea, and proctitis; fever, malaise, hypocalcaemia, erythema, myalgia, alopecia, and kidney and liver abnormalities. Anaphylactoid reactions have occurred. Dactinomycin is very irritant and extravasation results in severe tissue damage.

The effects of radiotherapy are enhanced by dactinomycin and severe reactions may follow the concomitant use of high doses. Erythema and pigmentation of the skin may occur in areas previously irradiated. An increase in incidence of second primary tumours has been seen in patients treated with radiation and dactinomycin.

Dactinomycin should not be given to patients with varicella, as severe and even fatal systemic disease may occur. Its use is best avoided in infants under 1 year as they are reported to be highly susceptible to the toxicity of dactinomycin. Blood counts and renal and hepatic function should be monitored frequently.

Effects on the liver. Although doses below about 50 μg per kg body-weight or 1.5 mg per m^2 body-surface do not seem to be associated with an unacceptable degree of hepatotoxicity,[1] administration of dactinomycin as a single dose of 60 μg per kg (about 1.8 mg per m^2) every 3 weeks to children with Wilms' tumour has been associated with a high incidence of severe hepatotoxicity;[2] reduction of this dose to 45 μg per kg every 3 weeks reduced the incidence of hepatotoxicity to one similar to that seen with a standard regimen of 15 μg per kg daily for 5 successive days.[3] Other workers have not seen such a high incidence of hepatotoxicity with doses of 60 μg per kg (despite some raised liver enzyme values), but in this case the high dose was given only every 6 weeks.[4] In general, it is recommended that dactinomycin be given with caution to children with a history of antecedent liver damage, including abdominal irradiation or recent halothane anaesthesia.[1]

1. Pritchard J, *et al.* Hepatotoxicity of actinomycin-D. *Lancet* 1989; **i:** 168.
2. D'Angio GJ. Hepatotoxicity with actinomycin D. *Lancet* 1987; **ii:** 104.
3. D'Angio GJ. Hepatotoxicity and actinomycin D. *Lancet* 1990; **335:** 1290.
4. de Camargo B. Hepatotoxicity and actinomycin D. *Lancet* 1990; **335:** 1290.

Interactions

For a general outline of antineoplastic drug interactions, see p.481.

Pharmacokinetics

Following intravenous administration dactinomycin is rapidly distributed with high concentrations in bone marrow and nucleated cells. It undergoes only minimal metabolism and is slowly excreted in urine and bile. The terminal plasma half-life is reported to be about 36 hours. It does not cross the blood-brain barrier but is thought to cross the placenta.

Uses and Administration

Dactinomycin is a highly toxic antibiotic with antineoplastic properties. It inhibits the proliferation of cells in a cell-cycle non-specific way by forming a stable complex with DNA and interfering with DNA-dependent RNA synthesis. It may enhance the cytotoxic effects of radiotherapy (see also Adverse Effects, above). Dactinomycin also has immunosuppressant properties.

It has been used, usually with other drugs or radiotherapy, in the treatment of Wilms' tumour (p.495), gestational trophoblastic tumours (p.483), and sarcomas such as rhabdomyosarcoma (p.501) and Ewing's sarcoma (p.500).

The usual adult dose is 500 μg intravenously, daily, for a maximum of 5 days. The usual dose for children is 15 μg per kg daily for 5 days; alternatively, a total of 2.5 mg per m^2 of body-surface may be given over a period of 7 days. In both adults and children, a second course may be given after 3 or more weeks if there are no signs of residual toxic effects. The daily dose for adults and children should not exceed 15 μg per kg body-weight, or 400 to 600 μg per m^2 body-surface. Lower doses may be given where dactinomycin is combined with other antineoplastics or with radiotherapy. Localised administration using an isolation-perfusion technique has permitted the use of higher doses, 50 μg per kg being suggested for an isolated lower extremity and 35 μg per kg for an upper extremity.

Great care must be taken to avoid extravasation and administration should, for preference, be into the tubing of a fast-running intravenous infusion. Platelet and white cell counts should be performed daily to detect bone-marrow depression; if either count shows a marked decrease the drug should be withheld until recovery occurs.

Preparations

USP 25: Dactinomycin for Injection.

Proprietary Preparations (details are given in Part 3)
Aust.: Cosmegen; ***Austral.:*** Cosmegen; ***Belg.:*** Lyovac Cosmegen; ***Braz.:*** Cosmegen; ***Canad.:*** Cosmegen; ***Fin.:*** Cosmegen; ***Ger.:*** Lyovac Cosmegen; ***Hong Kong:*** Cosmegen; ***Irl.:*** Cosmegen; ***Ital.:*** Cosmegen; ***Mex.:*** Ac-De; ***Neth.:*** Lyovac Cosmegen; ***Norw.:*** Cosmegen; ***NZ:*** Cosmegen; ***S.Afr.:*** Cosmegen; ***Swed.:*** Cosmegen; ***Switz.:*** Cosmegen; ***Thai.:*** Cosmegen; ***UK:*** Cosmegen; ***USA:*** Cosmegen.

Daunorubicin Hydrochloride (1828-x)

Daunorubicin Hydrochloride (BANM, USAN, rINNM).

Cloridrato de Daunorrubicina; Daunomycin Hydrochloride; Daunorubicini Hydrochloridum; FI-6339 (daunorubicin); NDC-0082-4155; NSC-82151; RP-13057 (daunorubicin); Rubidomycin Hydrochloride. (1S,3S)-3-Acetyl-1,2,3,4,6,11-hexahydro-3,5,12-trihydroxy-10-methoxy-6,11-dioxonaphthacen-1-yl 3-amino-2,3,6-trideoxy-α-L-lyxo-pyranoside hydrochloride; (8S-cis)-8-Acetyl-10-[(3-amino-2,3,6-trideoxy-α-L-lyxo-hexopyranosyl)]oxy-7,8,9,10-tetrahydro-6,8,11-trihydroxy-1-methoxy-5,12-naphthacenedione hydrochloride.

$C_{27}H_{29}NO_{10}$,HCl = 564.0.

CAS — 20830-81-3 (daunorubicin); 23541-50-6 (daunorubicin hydrochloride).

Pharmacopoeias. In Eur. (see p.vi) and US.

Daunorubicin hydrochloride 21.4 mg is approximately equivalent to 20 mg daunorubicin.

Pharmacopoeial description

Ph. Eur.: The hydrochloride of a substance produced by certain strains of Streptomyces coeruleorubidus or S. peucetius or obtained by any other means. It is manufactured by methods designed to minimise or eliminate the presence of histamine. An orange-red, hygroscopic, crystalline powder. It contains between 95 and 102% of the hydrochloride (anhydrous and solvent-free basis). Freely soluble in water and in methyl alcohol; slightly soluble in alcohol; practically insoluble in acetone. A 0.5% solution in water has a pH of 4.5 to 6.5. Store in airtight containers. Protect from light.

USP 25: An orange-red, hygroscopic, crystalline powder. It has a potency equivalent to not less than 842 and not more than 1030 μg of the base per mg. Freely soluble in water and in methyl alcohol; slightly soluble in alcohol; practically insoluble in acetone; very slightly soluble in chloroform. A 0.5% solution in water has a pH of 4.5 to 6.5. Store at a temperature not exceeding 40° in airtight containers. Protect from light.

◊ CAUTION. Daunorubicin hydrochloride is irritant; avoid contact with skin and mucous membranes.

Incompatibility. Daunorubicin is incompatible with heparin sodium,[1] and has also been reported to be incompatible with a solution of dexamethasone sodium phosphate.

1. D'Arcy PF. Reactions and interactions in handling anticancer drugs. Drug Intell Clin Pharm 1983; 17: 532–8.

Stability. In a study of the stability of anthracycline antineoplastic agents in 4 infusion fluids (glucose 5%, sodium chloride 0.9%, lactated Ringer's injection, and a commercial infusion fluid) daunorubicin hydrochloride was stable in all 4, the percentage remaining after 24 hours being 98.5%, 97.4%, 94.7%, and 95.4% respectively. Stability appeared to be partly related to pH; daunorubicin was more stable as the pH of the mixture became more acidic, with the best stability in glucose 5% with a pH of 4.5.[1] Although daunorubicin solutions are degraded by light, the effect is reported not to be significant at concentrations of 500 μg per mL or above; however, below this concentration precautions should be taken to protect solutions from light, and storage should be in polyethylene or polypropylene containers to minimise adsorptive losses.[2] It has been suggested that formulation with the food colouring Scarlet GN, which absorbs light over the same spectral region as daunorubicin, would stabilise daunorubicin solutions to light.[3]

Liposomal daunorubicin should be diluted with glucose 5% solution as aggregation of the liposomes may result with sodium chloride. In addition, the manufacturers advise that liposomal daunorubicin not be mixed with substances containing benzyl alcohol or other detergent-like molecules, which can lead to premature rupture of the liposomes.

1. Poochikian GK, et al. Stability of anthracycline antitumor agents in four infusion fluids. Am J Hosp Pharm 1981; 38: 483–6.
2. Wood MJ, et al. Photodegradation of doxorubicin, daunorubicin and epirubicin measured by high-performance liquid chromatography. J Clin Pharm Ther 1990; 15: 291–300.
3. Thoma K, Klimek R. Photostabilization of drugs in dosage forms without protection from packaging materials. Int J Pharmaceutics 1991; 67: 169–75.

Adverse Effects, Treatment, and Precautions

As for Doxorubicin, p.535 and p.535.

Cardiotoxicity is more likely when the total cumulative dose of daunorubicin exceeds 550 mg per m² body-surface in adults, or 300 mg per m² in children. The manufacturers of liposomal daunorubicin recommend determining ventricular ejection fraction after cumulative doses of 320 mg per m², and every 160 mg per m² thereafter. Daunorubicin should be used in reduced doses in hepatic and renal impairment.

Liposomal formulations of daunorubicin may be associated with a reduced potential for local tissue

necrosis although current clinical experience is limited and such toxicity remains a possibility. An acute syndrome of back pain, flushing, and chest tightness may occur during infusion.

Effects on the heart. For a discussion of the cardiotoxicity of anthracyclines, and its management, see Doxorubicin, p.535.

Effects on the skin. A report of the development of red-brown erythematous hyperpigmentation in a patient given a 3-day course of daunorubicin;[1] the pigmentation subsequently lightened and disappeared within 6 weeks, but recurred on subsequent readministration of the drug.

1. Kelly TM, et al. Hyperpigmentation with daunorubicin therapy. Arch Dermatol 1984; 120: 262–3.

Handling and disposal. For a method for the destruction of daunorubicin in wastes see under Doxorubicin, p.535.

Interactions

As for Doxorubicin, p.535.

Antineoplastics. Hepatic dysfunction was reported in 13 patients who had received daunorubicin 180 to 450 mg per m² body-surface.[1] Eleven of the patients had also received tioguanine, cytarabine, or vincristine, or combinations of these antineoplastics. Other studies had suggested that doxorubicin might enhance the hepatotoxicity of mercaptopurine, and a similar interaction could be involved in the possible hepatotoxicity of daunorubicin, tioguanine, cytarabine, and other antineoplastics.

1. Penta JS, et al. Hepatotoxicity of combination chemotherapy for acute myelocytic leukemia. Ann Intern Med 1977; 87: 247–8.

Pharmacokinetics

After intravenous injection, daunorubicin is rapidly distributed into body tissues, particularly the liver, lungs, kidneys, spleen, and heart with an initial distribution half-life of about 45 minutes. It is rapidly metabolised in the liver, and is excreted in bile and urine as unchanged drug and metabolites. The major metabolite, daunorubicinol, has antineoplastic activity. Up to 25% of a dose is excreted in urine in an active form over several days (the plasma elimination half-lives of daunorubicin and its major metabolite are reported to be 18.5 and 26.7 hours respectively); an estimated 40% is excreted in bile. Daunorubicin does not appear to cross the blood-brain barrier, but crosses the placenta.

The pharmacokinetics of liposomal doxorubicin are significantly different from those of the conventional drug formulation, with a decreased uptake by normal tissues (although tumour neovasculature is reported to have increased permeability to the liposomes), and a terminal half-life of 4 to 5 hours.

Uses and Administration

Daunorubicin is an antineoplastic anthracycline antibiotic closely related to doxorubicin (p.534). It forms a stable complex with DNA and interferes with the synthesis of nucleic acids. Daunorubicin is a cell-cycle non-specific agent, but its cytotoxic effects are most marked on cells in the S phase. Daunorubicin also has antibacterial and immunosuppressant properties. It is used with other antineoplastics to induce remissions in acute leukaemias. Daunorubicin is given in association with vincristine, prednisolone (or prednisone), and cyclophosphamide and/or asparaginase in acute lymphoblastic leukaemia (see p.484) and with cytarabine and tioguanine in acute myeloid leukaemias (see p.485). It has also been tried in some other malignancies. A liposomal formulation of daunorubicin has been developed for use in the management of Kaposi's sarcoma in patients with AIDS (see also p.501).

Daunorubicin is usually given as the hydrochloride, but doses are expressed in terms of the base.

In combination treatment regimens for adult acute leukaemia, the usual dose is 30 to 45 mg per m² body-surface daily for 2 to 3 days, administered as a solution in sodium chloride 0.9% into a fast-running infusion of sodium chloride or glucose. Courses may be repeated after 3 to 6 weeks. A dose of 25 mg per m²

has been given intravenously once a week, in combination regimens, to children with acute lymphoblastic leukaemia.

The total cumulative dose in adults should not exceed 550 mg per m²; in patients who have received radiotherapy to the chest it may be advisable to limit the total dose to about 400 mg per m². Lower limits apply in children: a total cumulative dose of no more than 300 mg per m², or in children aged under 2 years 10 mg per kg body-weight, is recommended. Dosage should be reduced in patients with impaired hepatic or renal function on the basis of serum bilirubin and creatinine concentrations.

In the treatment of Kaposi's sarcoma, liposomal daunorubicin is given intravenously every 2 weeks starting with a dose of 40 mg per m², and continued for as long as disease control can be maintained. It is diluted with glucose 5% (sodium chloride 0.9% should not be used) and given over 30 to 60 minutes.

Blood counts should be determined frequently during treatment as daunorubicin has a potent effect on bone-marrow function. Cardiac function should be monitored at regular intervals to detect signs of cardiotoxicity.

Preparations

USP 25: Daunorubicin Hydrochloride for Injection.

Proprietary Preparations (details are given in Part 3)
Aust.: Daunoblastin; DaunoXome; **Austral.:** DaunoXome; **Belg.:** Cerubidine; DaunoXome†; **Braz.:** Daunoblastina; **Canad.:** Cerubidine; **Denm.:** Cerubidin; DaunoXome; **Fin.:** DaunoXome; **Fr.:** Cerubidine; DaunoXome; **Ger.:** Daunoblastin; DaunoXome; **Hong Kong:** Daunoblastina; **Irl.:** Cerubidin; **Israel:** Cerubidine; **Ital.:** Daunoblastina; DaunoXome; **Mex.:** Rubilem; **Neth.:** Cerubidine; DaunoXome; **Norw.:** Cerubidin; **NZ:** Cerubidine; **Port.:** Daunoblastina; **S.Afr.:** Cerubidin; Daunoblastin; **Singapore:** Daunoblastina; **Spain:** Daunoblastina; DaunoXome; **Swed.:** Cerubidin; DaunoXome; **Switz.:** Cerubidine; DaunoXome; **UK:** Cerubidin; DaunoXome; **USA:** Cerubidin; DaunoXome.

Decitabine (10963-l)

Decitabine (BAN, USAN, rINN).

5-Aza-2′-deoxycytidine; DAC; NSC-127716. 4-Amino-1-(2-deoxy-β-D-erythro-pentofuranosyl)-1,3,5-triazin-2(1H)-one.

$C_8H_{12}N_4O_4$ = 228.2.

CAS — 2353-33-5.

Profile

Decitabine is an antineoplastic antimetabolite structurally related to cytarabine (see p.530). It has been tried in the treatment of acute leukaemias and some solid tumours.

◊ References.

1. Momparler RL, et al. Pilot phase I-II study on 5-aza-2′-deoxycytidine (decitabine) in patients with metastatic lung cancer. Anti-cancer Drugs 1997; 8: 358–68.
2. Kantarjian HM, et al. Results of decitabine therapy in the accelerated and blastic phases of chronic myelogenous leukemia. Leukemia 1997; 11: 1617–20.

Denileukin Diftitox (20135-z)

Denileukin Diftitox (USAN, rINN).

DAB389IL2; LY-335348.

CAS — 173146-27-5.

Profile

Denileukin diftitox is a recombinant interleukin fusion toxin comprised of interleukin-2 linked to the A and B fragments of diphtheria toxin. It is given by intravenous infusion for the management of persistent or recurrent cutaneous T-cell lymphoma (see Mycosis Fungoides, p.489), in patients whose malignant cells express the CD25 interleukin-2 receptor. The recommended dose is 9 or 18 μg per kg body-weight daily, given over 15 minutes or more, for 5 consecutive days every 3 weeks. Infusion reactions, gastrointestinal disturbances, chills, and fever are common; vascular leak syndrome and severe hypersensitivity reactions including anaphylaxis have occurred. Other adverse effects include hypoalbuminaemia, infections, and thrombotic events.

◊ References.

1. Olsen E, et al. Pivotal phase III trial of two dose levels of denileukin diftitox for the treatment of cutaneous T-cell lymphoma. J Clin Oncol 2001; 19: 376–88.

Preparations

Proprietary Preparations (details are given in Part 3)
USA: Ontak.

The symbol † denotes a preparation no longer actively marketed

Diaziquone (19066-v)

Diaziquone (USAN, rINN).

Aziridinylbenzoquinone; AZQ; CI-904; NSC-182986. Diethyl 2,5-bis-(1-aziridinyl)-3,6-dioxo-1,4-cyclohexadiene-1,4-dicarbamate.

$C_{16}H_{20}N_4O_6 = 364.4$.

CAS — 57998-68-2.

Profile

Diaziquone has been investigated as an antineoplastic in the treatment of malignant brain tumours and acute myeloid leukaemia. Adverse effects include bone marrow suppression, manifesting chiefly as leucopenia and thrombocytopenia, gastrointestinal disturbances, and alopecia. Anaphylactoid reactions have occurred.

◊ References.
1. Castleberry RP, et al. Aziridinylbenzoquinone (AZQ) in the treatment of recurrent pediatric brain and other malignant solid tumours: a Pediatric Oncology Group phase II study. Invest New Drugs 1990; 8: 401–6.
2. Schold SC, et al. Randomized comparison of diaziquone and carmustine in the treatment of adults with anaplastic glioma. J Clin Oncol 1993; 11: 77–83.
3. Lee EJ, et al. An evaluation of combinations of diaziquone, etoposide and mitoxantrone in the treatment of adults with relapsed or refractory acute myeloid leukemia: results of 8722, a randomized phase II study conducted by Cancer and Leukemia Group B. Leukemia 1998; 12: 139–43.

Didemnin B (19075-g)

NSC-325319.

$C_{57}H_{89}N_7O_{15} = 1112.4$.

Profile

The didemnins are biologically active peptides extracted from a marine sea squirt of the genus Trididemnum. They possess antineoplastic and antiviral properties; didemnin B is reported to be more active than didemnin A or didemnin C and has been investigated as an antineoplastic, although results have not generally been favourable. Nausea and vomiting are dose-limiting; myelosuppression, cardiac and renal toxicity, liver dysfunction, other gastrointestinal disturbances, myalgia, fatigue, and phlebitis may occur. Hypersensitivity reactions, possibly due to the polyethoxylated castor oil vehicle, are common.

Docetaxel (14634-b)

Docetaxel (BAN, USAN, rINN).

RP-56976. (2R,3S)-N-Carboxy-3-phenylisoserine, N-tert-butyl ester, 13-ester with 5β-20-epoxy-1,2α,4,7β,10β,13α-hexahydroxytax-11-en-9-one 4-acetate 2-benzoate; tert-Butyl {(1S,2S)-2-[(2S,5R,7S,10R,13S)-4-acetoxy-2-benzoyloxy-1,7,10-trihydroxy-9-oxo-5,20-epoxytax-11-en-13-yloxycarbonyl]-2-hydroxy-1-phenylethyl}carbamate.

$C_{43}H_{53}NO_{14} = 807.9$.

CAS — 114977-28-5 (anhydrous docetaxel); 148408-66-6 (docetaxel trihydrate).

ATC — L01CD02.

Adverse Effects, Treatment, and Precautions

As for Paclitaxel, p.563. Anaemia and skin reactions are common and may be severe. Fluid retention, resulting in oedema, ascites, pleural and pericardial effusion, and weight gain, is also common, and may be cumulative; premedication with a corticosteroid can reduce fluid retention as well as the severity of hypersensitivity reactions.

Docetaxel should not be used in patients hypersensitive to polysorbate 80, which is contained in the formulation. Patients with hepatic impairment show increased sensitivity to toxic effects of docetaxel, and should be given the drug with great care and in reduced doses, if at all.

Effects on the eyes. For reference to a report of glaucoma possibly related to docetaxel, see Paclitaxel, p.563.

Effects on the gastrointestinal tract. Ischaemic colitis has occurred in women treated with docetaxel, some of whom also received vinorelbine, which may have exacerbated this complication.[1,2]
1. Ibrahim NK, et al. Colitis associated with docetaxel-based chemotherapy in patients with metastatic breast cancer. Lancet 2000; 355: 281–3.
2. de Matteis A, et al. Intestinal side-effects of docetaxel/vinorelbine combination. Lancet 2000; 355: 1098–9.

Effects on the musculoskeletal system. For reference to a case of docetaxel-induced myalgia successfully treated with gabapentin, see Paclitaxel, p.563.

Interactions

For a general outline of antineoplastic drug interactions, see p.481.

◊ Docetaxel is metabolised by cytochrome P450 isoenzyme CYP3A, and theoretically has the potential to interact with other drugs that are inhibitors or inducers of this enzyme.[1]
1. Royer I, et al. Metabolism of docetaxel by human cytochromes P450: interactions with paclitaxel and other antineoplastic drugs. Cancer Res 1996; 56: 58–65.

Pharmacokinetics

Following intravenous administration docetaxel is rapidly distributed to body tissues. Docetaxel is more than 95% bound to plasma proteins. It is extensively metabolised via hepatic cytochrome P450 isoenzyme CYP3A and excreted chiefly in the faeces as metabolites. Only about 6% of a dose is excreted in urine. The terminal elimination half-life is about 11 hours. Clearance is reduced in patients with mild to moderate hepatic impairment.

◊ References.
1. Bruno R, et al. Pharmacokinetic and pharmacodynamic properties of docetaxel: results of phase I and phase II trials. Am J Health-Syst Pharm 1997; 54 (suppl 2): S16–S19.
2. Clarke SJ, Rivory LP. Clinical pharmacokinetics of docetaxel. Clin Pharmacokinet 1999; 36: 99–114.

Uses and Administration

Docetaxel is a semisynthetic taxane similar to paclitaxel (see p.564). It is manufactured from a taxane precursor derived from the needles of the European yew tree Taxus baccata. Docetaxel is used for locally advanced or metastatic breast cancer (p.491) and non-small cell lung cancer (p.496), after failure of prior chemotherapy. It is also being investigated in various other malignant neoplasms including prostate cancer and the palliative treatment of cancers of the head and neck.

Docetaxel is administered by intravenous infusion in glucose 5% or sodium chloride 0.9% at a concentration not exceeding 0.74 mg per mL. Infusion is normally over 1 hour. The recommended dose for breast cancer is 60 to 100 mg per m^2 body-surface once every 3 weeks, and that for non-small cell lung cancer is 75 mg per m^2 once every 3 weeks. Premedication with an oral corticosteroid for 3 days starting 1 day before docetaxel is recommended.

Regular blood counts are required, and dosage in subsequent courses should be reduced in patients who experience severe or febrile neutropenia, or severe cutaneous reactions or peripheral neuropathy. A 25% initial dosage reduction has been recommended for monotherapy in moderate hepatic impairment, and hepatic function should be monitored; use should be avoided if possible in severe hepatic impairment.

◊ References. For references to taxanes as a class, see Paclitaxel, p.564.
1. Anonymous. Docetaxel (Taxotere) for advanced breast cancer. Med Lett Drugs Ther 1996; 38: 78–8.
2. Leahy M, Howell A. Docetaxel. Br J Hosp Med 1997; 57: 141–4.
3. Tankanow RM. Docetaxel: a taxoid for the treatment of metastatic breast cancer. Am J Health-Syst Pharm 1998; 55: 1777–91.
4. Figgit DP, Wiseman LR. Docetaxel: an update of its use in advanced breast cancer. Drugs 2000; 59: 621–51.
5. Shepherd FA, et al. Prospective randomized trial of docetaxel versus best supportive care in patients with non-small-cell lung cancer previously treated with platinum-based chemotherapy. J Clin Oncol 2000; 18: 2095–2103.

Preparations

Proprietary Preparations (details are given in Part 3)

Aust.: Taxotere; Austral.: Taxotere; Belg.: Taxotere; Braz.: Taxotere; Canad.: Taxotere; Denm.: Taxotere; Fin.: Taxotere; Fr.: Taxotere; Ger.: Taxotere; Hong Kong: Taxotere; Irl.: Taxotere; Israel: Taxotere; Ital.: Taxotere; Jpn: Taxotere; Mex.: Taxotere; Neth.: Taxotere; Norw.: Taxotere; NZ: Taxotere; Port.: Taxotere; S.Afr.: Taxotere; Singapore: Taxotere; Spain: Taxotere; Swed.: Taxotere; Switz.: Taxotere; Thai.: Taxotere; UK: Taxotere; USA: Taxotere.

Doxifluridine (19107-r)

Doxifluridine (rINN).

5′-Deoxy-5-fluorouridine; 5-DFUR; FUDR; Ro-21-9738.

$C_9H_{11}FN_2O_5 = 246.2$.

CAS — 3094-09-5.

Profile

Doxifluridine is an antineoplastic which probably acts through its conversion in the body to fluorouracil (p.540). It is given in

the management of malignant neoplasms of the breast (p.491) and gastrointestinal tract (p.493), and of other solid tumours. It has also been given by the intravenous route.

Pharmacokinetics. Doxifluridine is metabolised to fluorouracil and 5,6-dihydrofluorouracil. It is orally active with a bioavailability of 34 to 47%.

References.
1. Sommadossi J-P, et al. Kinetics and metabolism of a new fluoropyrimidine, 5′-deoxy-5-fluorouridine, in humans. Cancer Res 1983; 43: 930–3.
2. Van Der Heyden SAM, et al. Pharmacokinetics and bioavailability of oral 5′-deoxy-5-fluorouridine in cancer patients. Br J Clin Pharmacol 1999; 47: 351–6.

Preparations

Proprietary Preparations (details are given in Part 3)
Jpn: Furtulon.

Doxorubicin Hydrochloride (1831-z)

Doxorubicin Hydrochloride (BANM, rINNM).

Adriamycin Hydrochloride; Cloridrato de Doxorrubicina; Doxorubicini Hydrochloridum; FI-106 (doxorubicin); 3-Hydroxyacetyldaunorubicin Hydrochloride; 14-Hydroxydaunorubicin Hydrochloride; NSC-123127. 8-Hydroxyacetyl (8S,10S)-10-[(3-amino-2,3,6-trideoxy-α-L-lyxo-hexopyranosyl)oxy]-6,8,11-trihydroxy-1-methoxy-7,8,9,10-tetrahydronaphthacene-5,12-dione hydrochloride.

$C_{27}H_{29}NO_{11},HCl = 580.0$.

CAS — 23214-92-8 (doxorubicin); 25316-40-9 (doxorubicin hydrochloride).

NOTE. Doxorubicin is USAN. In many countries the name 'Adriamycin' is a trade-mark.

Pharmacopoeias. In Eur. (see p.vi), Int., Jpn, Pol., and US.

Pharmacopoeial description

Ph. Eur.: The hydrochloride of a substance isolated from certain strains of Streptomyces coeruleorubidus or S. peucetius or obtained by any other means. It contains between 98% and 102% of the hydrochloride, calculated on the anhydrous substance. An orange-red, hygroscopic, crystalline powder. Soluble in water; slightly soluble in methyl alcohol. A 0.5% solution in water has a pH of 4.0 to 5.5. Store in airtight containers.

USP 25: A red-orange, hygroscopic, crystalline powder. It contains not less than 98% and not more than 102% of $C_{27}H_{29}NO_{11}$,HCl, calculated on the anhydrous, solvent-free basis. Soluble in water, in sodium chloride 0.9%, and in methyl alcohol; practically insoluble in chloroform, in ether, and in other organic solvents. A 0.5% solution in water has a pH of 4.0 to 5.5. Store in airtight containers.

◊ CAUTION. Doxorubicin hydrochloride is irritant; avoid contact with skin and mucous membranes.

Incompatibility. Admixture of doxorubicin hydrochloride with cefalotin sodium, dexamethasone, diazepam, or hydrocortisone sodium succinate is reported to result in immediate precipitation;[1] similarly precipitation has occurred when doxorubicin hydrochloride was mixed with frusemide [furosemide] or heparin sodium.[2] A mixture of fluorouracil or aminophylline with doxorubicin hydrochloride is reported to darken in colour from red to purple, indicating degradation of doxorubicin.[1] For mention of the compatibility of doxorubicin with paclitaxel, see p.563.

Liposomal doxorubicin differs in its incompatibilities from conventional formulations: whereas the latter are reportedly incompatible with allopurinol, cefepime, and ganciclovir, there was no visual evidence of this with the liposomal formulation. However, it was incompatible with a number of drug solutions including amphotericin B, docetaxel, gallium nitrate, hydroxyzine hydrochloride, metoclopramide hydrochloride, miconazole, mitozantrone [mitoxantrone] hydrochloride, morphine sulfate and some other opioids, paclitaxel, sodium bicarbonate, and some antibacterials.[3]
1. Dorr RT. Incompatibilities with parenteral anticancer drugs. Am J Intravenous Ther 1979; 6: 42–52.
2. Cohen MH, et al. Drug precipitation within IV tubing: a potential hazard of chemotherapy administration. Cancer Treat Rep 1985; 69: 1325–6.
3. Trissel LA, et al. Compatibility of doxorubicin hydrochloride liposome injection with selected other drugs during simulated Y-site administration. Am J Health-Syst Pharm 1997; 54: 2708–13.

Stability. Although sensitive to light at low concentrations, doxorubicin is not subject to significant photodegradation at clinical concentrations and special precautions to protect solutions from light during administration do not appear to be necessary.[1,2] Solutions in sodium chloride solution 0.9% were reported[3] to be stable for 24 days when stored in PVC minibags at 25° and for even longer if stored in minibags or polypropylene syringes at 4°. Stability in solution seems to be partly related to pH, with doxorubicin becoming more stable at acid pH.[3-5] A fall in pH of the solution also significantly decreases the loss of doxorubicin by adsorption and precipitation onto the surface of a positively-charged in-line filter.[6]

The liposomal doxorubicin formulation should be diluted only with glucose 5%. If not used immediately, it may be stored for 24 hours at 2° to 8°.

1. Tavoloni N, et al. Photolytic degradation of adriamycin. J Pharm Pharmacol 1980; 32: 860–2.
2. Wood MJ, et al. Photodegradation of doxorubicin, daunorubicin and epirubicin measured by high-performance liquid chromatography. J Clin Pharm Ther 1990; 15: 291–300.
3. Wood MJ, et al. Stability of doxorubicin, daunorubicin and epirubicin in plastic syringes and minibags. J Clin Pharm Ther 1990; 15: 279–89.
4. Poochikian GK, et al. Stability of anthracycline antitumor agents in four infusion fluids. Am J Hosp Pharm 1981; 38: 483–6.
5. Beijnen JH, et al. Stability of anthracycline antitumour agents in infusion fluids. J Parenter Sci Technol 1985; 39: 220–2.
6. Francomb MM, et al. Effect of pH on the adsorption of cytotoxic drugs to a 96 hour intravenous filter. Pharm J 1991; 247: R26.

Adverse Effects and Treatment

For general discussions see Antineoplastics, p.476 and p.479.

Doxorubicin and other anthracyclines cause pronounced bone-marrow depression, which may be dose-limiting. White blood cell count reaches a nadir 10 to 15 days after administration and usually recovers by about 21 days after a dose.

The anthracyclines may produce cardiac toxicity, both as an acute, usually transient disturbance of cardiac function marked by ECG abnormalities and, sometimes, arrhythmias; and as a delayed, sometimes fatal, irreversible congestive heart failure, which may occur suddenly. Severe cardiotoxicity is more likely in adults receiving total cumulative doses of doxorubicin greater than 450 to 550 mg per m^2 body-surface, and may occur months or even years after administration.

Gastrointestinal disturbances including moderate or sometimes severe nausea and vomiting, stomatitis, and, more rarely, facial flushing, conjunctivitis, and lachrymation may occur. Doxorubicin and other anthracyclines are very irritant and thrombophlebitis and streaking of the skin over the vein used for injection has been reported; extravasation is serious and may produce extensive local necrosis and ulceration. Alopecia occurs in the majority of patients. The urine may be coloured red. Occasional hypersensitivity reactions may occur. Hyperuricaemia may occur due to tumour lysis syndrome.

Combination therapy including doxorubicin has rarely been associated with secondary acute non-lymphoblastic leukaemia (see also Carcinogenicity, p.476).

Formulations of liposomal doxorubicin may be associated with a reduced potential for local tissue necrosis, and possibly a reduced incidence of cardiotoxicity, although current clinical experience is limited, and such toxicity remains a possibility. Conversely, palmar-plantar erythrodysesthesia appears to be more common, and may be dose-limiting. In addition, an acute pseudo-allergic reaction may be seen on initial infusion, but generally resolves on slowing or temporarily discontinuing the infusion.

Effects on the heart. Cardiotoxicity has been a major factor in limiting the use of the anthracyclines, doxorubicin and daunorubicin.[1-5] Toxicity is essentially of 2 kinds: acute, usually reversible ECG changes, including a wide range of arrhythmias, and a delayed, usually irreversible dose-related cardiomyopathy, resulting in congestive heart failure.[3-5] The latter may be further subdivided into chronic effects, occurring up to about a year after administration, and late-onset toxicity occurring years after treatment.[4] Delayed toxicity may be fatal in as many as 60% of patients who develop it.[2]

The single most important determinant of cardiac toxicity appears to be *cumulative dose*, with the risk of toxicity becoming ever greater at cumulative doxorubicin doses above 550 mg per m^2 body-surface[2] or daunorubicin doses of 600 mg per m^2 or more.[1] However, patients vary widely in sensitivity,[4] and these values represent relatively arbitrary choices on a continuum of risk: there is no single safe dose.[2] Even at doses which produce no symptoms, subclinical myocardial damage may occur, and in children this may result in diminished cardiac reserve and heart disease in later life.[3,6,7] The *dosage schedule* also appears to be important; relatively-high single doses on an infrequent schedule (presumably resulting in higher peak concentrations) appear to be more cardiotoxic than lower, weekly doses, or continuous infusion.[2,3,5,8-10] Cardiotoxicity is also reported to be more likely in *children and elderly* patients, and in those

who have received prior *radiotherapy* to the chest.[1-5] There is reason to believe that previous *cardiovascular disease* may also increase the risk,[2-4] although such patients are commonly excluded from studies of anthracycline therapy.[2] *Females* may be at greater risk than males.[11] Use with cyclophosphamide, trastuzumab, or *other antineoplastics* with cardiotoxic potential may increase the likelihood of cardiomyopathy.

The late development of cardiac toxicity is a source of some concern: although in one study the mean time to development of symptoms was 33 days after administration, with a range of 0 to 231 days,[2] several reports have indicated that late cardiac failure may occur up to 18 years after anthracycline therapy.[4,12,13]

PREVENTION. Given that doxorubicin-induced cardiac failure has been reported to occur in between 0.4 and 9% of all recipients, and that the fatality rate is high, much effort has gone into ways of predicting and preventing anthracycline-induced cardiotoxicity. Although ECG changes are commonly monitored, most of the changes are not predictive of cardiomyopathy and severe cardiac toxicity can occur without ECG changes. However, a persistent reduction in the voltage of the QRS wave is generally indicative of the need to perform further tests. Non-invasive cardiac monitoring, by means of echocardiography or radionuclide angiography, is useful in predicting the development of cardiomyopathy, but may give normal results until damage is quite advanced; sensitivity may be improved with exercise stress tests.[3-5] Endomyocardial biopsy is the most sensitive indicator of cardiotoxicity, but it is invasive and not widely available. The Childrens Cancer Study Group[14] has issued guidelines for monitoring using ECG, echocardiography, and radionuclide angiocardiography in patients receiving anthracyclines. The role of such techniques in predicting late-onset cardiotoxicity remains to be clarified.[4]

Dexrazoxane (p.1006) has shown some protective effect against the cardiotoxicity of doxorubicin and other anthracyclines, and is used to reduce cardiomyopathy in women receiving doxorubicin for metastatic breast cancer.

Alteration of the dosage schedule to weekly rather than three-weekly dosage, or the use of continuous infusion, has also been advocated as a way of reducing doxorubicin cardiotoxicity,[8-10] as has administration of anthracyclines formulated in liposomes.[4]

Several anthracycline derivatives have been developed with the aim of reducing the inherent cardiotoxicity of this class of compounds, including aclarubicin (p.505), epirubicin (p.537), and mitozantrone [mitoxantrone] (p.559). However, although this strategy has met with some success, almost all these compounds exhibit some degree of cardiotoxicity.

TREATMENT. The result of treatment for such cardiotoxicity has generally been poor. Options have included digoxin, diuretics, low-salt diet, and bed rest. However, beta blockers may be useful, and results in patients with epirubicin-induced cardiotoxicity[15] have indicated that treatment with an ACE inhibitor can improve cardiac function and survival. Study is underway to determine whether ACE inhibitors can also prevent the initial toxicity if given immediately after an anthracycline.[16] Heart transplantation has been used.[5]

1. Von Hoff DD, et al. Daunomycin-induced cardiotoxicity in children and adults: a review of 110 cases. Am J Med 1977; 62: 200–8.
2. Von Hoff DD, et al. Risk factors for doxorubicin-induced congestive heart failure. Ann Intern Med 1979; 91: 710–17.
3. Hale JP, Lewis IJ. Anthracyclines: cardiotoxicity and its prevention. Arch Dis Child 1994; 71: 457–62.
4. Shan K, et al. Anthracycline-induced cardiotoxicity. Ann Intern Med 1996; 125: 47–58.
5. Singal PK, Lliskovic N. Doxorubicin-induced cardiomyopathy. N Engl J Med 1998; 339: 900–905.
6. Yeung ST, et al. Functional myocardial impairment in children treated with anthracyclines for cancer. Lancet 1991; 337: 816–18.
7. Lipschultz SE, et al. Late cardiac effects of doxorubicin therapy for acute lymphoblastic leukemia in childhood. N Engl J Med 1991; 324: 808–15.
8. Legha SS, et al. Reduction of doxorubicin cardiotoxicity by prolonged continuous intravenous infusion. Ann Intern Med 1982; 96: 133–9.
9. Torti FM, et al. Reduced cardiotoxicity of doxorubicin delivered on a weekly schedule: assessment by endomyocardial biopsy. Ann Intern Med 1983; 99: 745–9.
10. Lum BL, et al. Doxorubicin: alteration of dose scheduling as a means of reducing cardiotoxicity. Drug Intell Clin Pharm 1985; 19: 259–64.
11. Lipshultz SE, et al. Female sex and higher drug dose as risk factors for late cardiotoxic effects of doxorubicin therapy for childhood cancer. N Engl J Med 1995; 332: 1738–43.
12. Goorin AM, et al. Initial congestive heart failure, six to ten years after doxorubicin chemotherapy for childhood cancer. J Pediatr 1990; 116: 144–7.
13. Steinherz LJ, et al. Cardiac toxicity 4 to 20 years after completing anthracycline therapy. JAMA 1991; 266: 1672–7.
14. Steinherz LJ, et al. Guidelines for cardiac monitoring of children during and after anthracycline therapy: report of the Cardiology Committee of the Childrens Cancer Study Group. Pediatrics 1992; 89: 942–9.
15. Jensen BV, et al. Treatment with angiotensin-converting-enzyme inhibitor for epirubicin-induced dilated cardiomyopathy. Lancet 1996; 347: 297–9.
16. Jensen BV, et al. Angiotensin-converting enzyme inhibitor for epirubicin-induced dilated cardiomyopathy. Lancet 1996; 347: 1485.

Effects on the liver. Hepatitis and non-specific hepatocellular damage has been reported in patients receiving doxorubicin as part of combination therapy.[1] A characteristic hepatotoxicity

can also be produced by the combination of radiotherapy with doxorubicin.[2]

1. Avilés A, et al. Hepatic injury during doxorubicin therapy. Arch Pathol Lab Med 1984; 108: 912–13.
2. Price LA. Surviving malignant disease: medical and oncological aspects. Br J Hosp Med 1983; 30: 8–12.

Effects on the skin. For specific reference to treatment of alopecia caused by doxorubicin, and for extravasation, see p.480.

Precautions

For a general discussion see Antineoplastics, p.480.

Doxorubicin and other anthracyclines are generally contra-indicated in patients with heart disease. The total cumulative dose should be limited, and cardiac function should be monitored during treatment (see Effects on the Heart, above). Blood counts should be monitored and doses should not be repeated while there is bone-marrow depression or ulceration of the mouth. Doxorubicin should be given with great care in reduced doses to patients with hepatic impairment; dosage reduction may also be necessary in children and the elderly. Extravasation results in severe tissue damage and doxorubicin and other anthracyclines should not be given by intramuscular or subcutaneous injection. The adverse effects of irradiation may be enhanced by doxorubicin and skin reactions previously induced by radiotherapy may recur; the maximum cumulative dose should be reduced to no more than 400 mg per m^2 in patients who have received radiotherapy to the chest or heart. Different liposomal formulations may not be interchangeable with conventional formulations, or with each other.

Handling and disposal. A method for the destruction of doxorubicin or daunorubicin *wastes* using sulfuric acid and potassium permanganate.[1] Residues produced by degradation of daunorubicin by this method showed no mutagenicity *in vitro*; some mutagenicity was seen with high concentrations of residues from doxorubicin.

Urine and faeces produced for up to 7 days after a dose of doxorubicin should be handled wearing protective clothing.[2]

1. Castegnaro M, et al., eds. Laboratory decontamination and destruction of carcinogens in laboratory wastes; some antineoplastic agents. IARC Scientific Publications 73. Lyon: WHO/International Agency for Research on Cancer, 1985.
2. Harris J, Dodds LJ. Handling waste from patients receiving cytotoxic drugs. Pharm J 1985; 235: 289–91.

Pregnancy and lactation. Although doxorubicin has been reported not to be present in detectable amounts in amniotic fluid[1,2] it has been found in fetal tissue (liver, kidney, and lungs) at concentrations several times those in maternal plasma,[2] indicating that it does pass the placenta.

The American Academy of Pediatrics considers that doxorubicin may possibly suppress the immune system in a nursing infant.[3]

1. Roboz J, et al. Does doxorubicin cross the placenta? Lancet 1979; ii: 1382–3.
2. D'Incalci M, et al. Transplacental passage of doxorubicin. Lancet 1983; i: 75.
3. American Academy of Pediatrics Committee on Drugs. The transfer of drugs and other chemicals into human milk. Pediatrics 2001; 108: 776–89.

Interactions

For a general outline of antineoplastic drug interactions, see p.481. The cumulative dose of doxorubicin should be reduced in patients who have received other cardiotoxic drugs such as daunorubicin or cyclophosphamide.

Antibacterials. Hypersensitivity reactions to doxorubicin or daunorubicin have been reported in 2 patients with recent exposure to *clindamycin*, one of whom had exhibited hypersensitivity to that antibiotic.[1] The possibility of cross-sensitivity between anthracyclines and clindamycin should be considered.

1. Arena FP, Sherlock S. Doxorubicin hypersensitivity and clindamycin. Ann Intern Med 1990; 112: 150.

Antineoplastics and immunosuppressants. Administration of doxorubicin with or after agents such as *streptozocin*[1] or *methotrexate*,[2] which can impair hepatic function, has resulted in increased doxorubicin toxicity, possibly due to reduced hepatic clearance. A high incidence of cardiotoxicity (manifest as congestive heart failure) has been reported in patients who received doxorubicin in association with *paclitaxel* (which also has cardiotoxic effects).[3] Any interaction may be schedule dependent.[4] Similarly an increased incidence of cardiotoxicity has been seen when *trastuzumab* was given with or after doxorubicin.[5]

Increased plasma-doxorubicin concentrations and myelotoxicity have occurred when *ciclosporin* was used to modulate tumour resistance.[6] Severe neurological toxicity occurred in another patient given doxorubicin after long-term ciclosporin therapy.[7] It has been suggested that the use of ciclosporin or its analogues such as valspodar to modulate doxorubicin resistance should be undertaken with caution.[8]

For a suggestion that doxorubicin might enhance the hepatotoxicity of *mercaptopurine*, see under Daunorubicin Hydrochloride, p.533.

1. Anonymous. Two drugs may not be better than one. *JAMA* 1976; **236:** 913.
2. Robertson JH, *et al.* Toxicity of doxorubicin and methotrexate in osteogenic sarcoma. *BMJ* 1976; **1:** 23.
3. Gianni L, *et al.* Paclitaxel by 3-hour infusion in combination with bolus doxorubicin in women with untreated metastatic breast cancer: high antitumor efficacy and sequence-finding study. *J Clin Oncol* 1995; **13:** 2688–99.
4. Danesi R, *et al.* Pharmacokinetic optimisation of treatment schedules for anthracyclines and paclitaxel in patients with cancer. *Clin Pharmacokinet* 1999; **37:** 195–211.
5. Sparano JA. Cardiac toxicity of trastuzumab (Herceptin): implications for the design of adjuvant trials. *Semin Oncol* 2001; **28** (suppl 3): 20–7.
6. Rushing DA, *et al.* The effects of cyclosporine on the pharmacokinetics of doxorubicin in patients with small cell lung cancer. *Cancer* 1994; **74:** 834–41.
7. Barbui T, *et al.* Neurological symptoms and coma associated with doxorubicin administration during chronic cyclosporin therapy. *Lancet* 1992; **339:** 1421.
8. Beck WT, Kuttesch JF. Neurological symptoms associated with cyclosporin plus doxorubicin. *Lancet* 1992; **340:** 496.

Pharmacokinetics

Following intravenous injection, doxorubicin is rapidly cleared from the blood, and distributed into tissues including lungs, liver, heart, spleen, and kidneys. It undergoes rapid metabolism in the liver to metabolites including the active metabolite doxorubicinol (adriamycinol). About 40 to 50% of a dose is stated to be excreted in bile within 7 days, of which about half is as unchanged drug. Only about 5% of a dose is excreted in urine within 5 days. It does not cross the blood-brain barrier but may cross the placenta and is distributed into breast milk. The disappearance of doxorubicin from the blood is triphasic: mean half-lives are 12 minutes, 3.3 hours and about 30 hours.

The pharmacokinetics of liposomal formulations are somewhat different from the conventional drug. The use of macrogols in the surface layer of the liposomes (pegylation) reduces removal of liposomes by macrophages. This results in prolonged circulation in the plasma, with relatively little tissue distribution, but tumour neovasculature is reported to permit penetration of liposomes into tumour tissue. Pharmacokinetics are reported to be biphasic with mean half-lives of 5 hours and 55 hours respectively. A non-pegylated liposomal formulation also exists and is reported to produce higher peak plasma concentrations of total doxorubicin than conventional formulations, but lower free (not liposome-encapsulated) concentrations. Clearance is reduced, and peak plasma concentrations of doxorubicinol delayed.

◊ References.
1. Speth PAJ, *et al.* Clinical pharmacokinetics of doxorubicin. *Clin Pharmacokinet* 1988; **15:** 15–31.
2. Rushing DA, *et al.* The disposition of doxorubicin on repeated dosing. *J Clin Pharmacol* 1993; **33:** 698–702.
3. Piscitelli SC, *et al.* Pharmacokinetics and pharmacodynamics of doxorubicin in patients with small cell lung cancer. *Clin Pharmacol Ther* 1993; **53:** 555–61.

Uses and Administration

Doxorubicin is an anthracycline antineoplastic antibiotic which may act by forming a stable complex with DNA and interfering with the synthesis of nucleic acids. It is a cell-cycle non-specific agent but is most active against cells in S phase. It also has actions on cell membranes, and immunosuppressant properties. It is an effective antineoplastic against a wide range of tumours as indicated by the cross-references given below. Doxorubicin is used, often in association with other antineoplastics, in the treatment of Hodgkin's disease, non-Hodgkin's lymphomas, bone and soft-tissue sarcomas, neuroblastoma, Wilms' tumour, and malignant neoplasms of the bladder, breast, lung, ovary, and thyroid. It has also been used in a wide variety of other tumours. Liposomal doxorubicin is used in the management of Kaposi's sarcoma in patients with AIDS and metastatic ovarian cancer.

Doxorubicin hydrochloride is administered intravenously by injecting a solution in sodium chloride 0.9% into a fast-running infusion of sodium chloride

0.9% or glucose 5% over 3 minutes or more. When used as a single agent, the dose is 60 to 75 mg per m^2 body-surface, or 1.2 to 2.4 mg per kg body-weight, once every 3 weeks. Alternatively, doses of 20 to 25 mg per m^2 have been given daily for 3 days every 3 weeks, although dividing the dose in this way may increase the incidence of mucositis. A regimen of 20 mg per m^2 as a single weekly dose may be used, and is reported to be associated with a lower incidence of cardiotoxicity.

Doses may need to be reduced if doxorubicin is given with other antineoplastics: a dose of 30 to 40 mg per m^2 every 3 weeks has been suggested. Doses should also be halved in patients with moderate liver dysfunction (serum-bilirubin concentrations of 12 to 30 µg per mL); those with severe impairment (serum bilirubin greater than 30 µg per mL) should be given a quarter of the usual dose.

The maximum total dose should not exceed 450 to 550 mg per m^2; in patients who have received radiotherapy to the chest, or other cardiotoxic drugs, it may be advisable to further limit the total dose.

In the management of AIDS-related Kaposi's sarcoma pegylated liposomal doxorubicin is given in a dose of 20 mg per m^2 infused over 30 minutes once every 2 to 3 weeks. For the treatment of ovarian cancer, the suggested dose of this liposomal formulation is 50 mg per m^2 infused over 1 hour once every 4 weeks. In both conditions, treatment should be continued for as long as the patient responds satisfactorily and tolerates treatment. The pegylated liposomal formulation should be diluted only with glucose 5%.

A non-pegylated liposomal formulation is also available. It is given in the treatment of metastatic breast cancer in doses of 60 to 75 mg per m^2 every 3 weeks, in combination with cyclophosphamide. Doses are given by intravenous infusion over 1 hour, diluted in sodium chloride 0.9% or glucose 5%.

Blood counts should be made routinely during treatment with doxorubicin and cardiac function should be monitored at regular intervals for early signs of cardiotoxicity.

Doxorubicin has also been instilled into the bladder in the local treatment of malignant neoplasms. For this purpose 50 mL of a 1 mg per mL solution is instilled into the bladder for one hour once a month. Doxorubicin has been given intra-arterially.

◊ Reviews and studies of liposomal formulations.
1. Working PK, Dayan AD. CPMP Preclinical Expert Report: Caelyx (Stealth liposomal doxorubicin HCL). *Hum Exp Toxicol* 1996; **15:** 752–85.
2. Coukell AJ, Spencer CM. Polyethylene glycol-liposomal doxorubicin: a review of its pharmacodynamic and pharmacokinetic properties, and therapeutic efficacy in the management of AIDS-related Kaposi's sarcoma. *Drugs* 1997; **53:** 520–38.
3. Batist G, *et al.* Reduced cardiotoxicity and preserved antitumor efficacy of liposome-encapsulated doxorubicin and cyclophosphamide compared with conventional doxorubicin and cyclophosphamide in a randomized, multicenter trial of metastatic breast cancer. *J Clin Oncol* 2001; **19:** 1444–54.
4. Gordon AN, *et al.* Recurrent epithelial ovarian carcinoma: a randomized phase III study of pegylated liposomal doxorubicin versus topotecan. *J Clin Oncol* 2001; **19:** 3312–22.

Amyloidosis. For mention of the use of doxorubicin in patients with amyloidosis (and of the increased risk this may carry in cardiac amyloidosis) see p.501.

Malignant neoplasms. Doxorubicin plays a major role in combination regimens for chemotherapy of solid malignancies; it is often employed for tumours of the breast and lung (see p.491 and p.496) and for Wilms' tumour and neuroblastoma or retinoblastoma in children (see p.495, p.500, and p.500) but has been used for malignancies of the bladder (p.490); for various gynaecological cancers including those of the endometrium, and ovary (see p.493, and p.496); for cancer of the liver, stomach, and pancreas (p.495, p.493, p.497); and for neoplasms of prostate, and thymus (p.497 and p.499). It is also used in the treatment of sarcomas of bone and soft-tissue (see p.500 and p.501) and liposomal doxorubicin is used in patients with Kaposi's sarcoma (see p.501).

In addition, doxorubicin is a component of the ABVD regimen used to treat Hodgkin's disease (p.487) and is part of the CHOP regimen used for non-Hodgkin's lymphoma (p.487). Doxorubicin is also used in Burkitt's lymphoma (p.488), mycosis fungoides (p.489), and the lymphomas associated with AIDS (see p.488). It has been employed in chronic lymphocytic leukaemia as part of the CHOP regimen (though with uncertain benefit—see p.485) and in multiple myeloma (p.489).

Preparations

BP 2001: Doxorubicin Injection;
USP 25: Doxorubicin Hydrochloride for Injection; Doxorubicin Hydrochloride Injection.

Proprietary Preparations (details are given in Part 3)
Aust.: Adriblastin; Caelyx, *Austral.:* Caelyx; Doxorubin; *Belg.:* Adriblastina; Caelyx; *Braz.:* Adriblastina; Rubex; *Canad.:* Caelyx; *Denm.:* Caelyx; Doxorubin; *Fin.:* Caelyx; *Fr.:* Adriblastine; Caelyx; *Ger.:* Adriblastin; Adrimedac; Caelyx; DOXO-cell; Ribodoxo-L; *Hong Kong:* Caelyx; Israel: Adriblastina; Caelyx; *Ital.:* Adriblastina; Caelyx; *Mex.:* Adriblastina; Caelyx; Doxolem; Doxotec; *Neth.:* Adriblastina; Caelyx; *Norw.:* Caelyx; *NZ:* Doxorubin; *Port.:* Adriblastina; Caelyx; Fauldoxo; *S.Afr.:* Adriblastina; Caelyx; *Singapore:* Caelyx; *Spain:* Caelyx; Farmiblastina; *Swed.:* Caelyx; *Switz.:* Adriblastin; Caelyx; *Thai.:* Adriblastina; Adrim; Doxolem; *UK:* Caelyx; *USA:* Doxil; Rubex.

Droloxifene (2796-y)

Droloxifene *(USAN, rINN).*

3-Hydroxytamoxifen; K-21060E. *(E)*-α-{p-[2-(Dimethylamino)ethoxy]phenyl}-α'-ethyl-3-stilbenol.
$C_{26}H_{29}NO_2 = 387.5.$
CAS — 82413-20-5.

Profile

Droloxifene is a selective oestrogen receptor modulator related to tamoxifen (p.571) and with similar general properties. It has been investigated in the hormonal treatment and prophylaxis of breast cancer and is under study for osteoporosis.

Echinomycin (19121-t)

NSC-526417; Quinomycin A.
$C_{51}H_{64}N_{12}O_{12}S_2 = 1101.3.$
CAS — 512-64-1.

Profile

Echinomycin is an antibiotic derived from *Streptomyces echinatus* which is reported to intercalate with DNA, and which has been investigated as an antineoplastic. Nausea and vomiting may be dose-limiting; other adverse reactions include mild thrombocytopenia, liver dysfunction, fever, and hypersensitivity reactions.

Edatrexate (10981-j)

Edatrexate *(USAN, rINN).*

CGP-30694. N-(p-{1-[(2,4-Diamino-6-pteridinyl)methyl]propyl}benzoyl)-L-glutamic acid.
$C_{22}H_{25}N_7O_5 = 467.5.$
CAS — 80576-83-6.

Profile

Edatrexate is an analogue of methotrexate (p.553) and has similar general properties. It is under investigation as an antineoplastic in the treatment of various malignant neoplasms. Mucositis may be dose limiting.

◊ References.
1. Souhami RL, *et al.* Phase II study of edatrexate in stage III and IV non-small cell lung cancer. *Cancer Chemother Pharmacol* 1992; **30:** 465–8.
2. Lee JS, *et al.* Improved therapeutic index by leucovorin of edatrexate, cyclophosphamide, and cisplatin regimen for non-small cell lung cancer. *J Natl Cancer Inst* 1992; **84:** 1039–40.
3. Schornagel JH, *et al.* Randomized phase III trial of edatrexate versus methotrexate in patients with metastatic and/or recurrent squamous cell carcinoma of the head and neck: a European Organization for Research and Treatment of Cancer Head and Neck Cancer Cooperative Group study. *J Clin Oncol* 1995; **13:** 1649–55.
4. Dreicer R, *et al.* A phase II trial of edatrexate in patients with advanced renal cell carcinoma: an Eastern Cooperative Oncology Group study. *Am J Clin Oncol* 1997; **20:** 251–3.
5. D'Andrea G, *et al.* Phase I study of escalating doses of edatrexate in combination with paclitaxel in patients with metastatic breast cancer. *Clin Cancer Res* 1999; **5:** 275–9.
6. Kindler HL, *et al.* Edatrexate (10-ethyl-deaza-aminopterin) (NSC 626715) with or without leucovorin rescue for malignant mesothelioma: sequential phase II trials by the cancer and leukemia group B. *Cancer* 1999; **86:** 1985–91.

Edrecolomab (15646-c)

Edrecolomab *(USAN, rINN).*

17-1A Antibody; C1; Monoclonal Antibody 17-1A.
CAS — 156586-89-9.
ATC — L01XC01.

Profile

Edrecolomab is a monoclonal antibody of murine origin directed at epithelial cell surface glycoproteins that has been used as adjuvant therapy following surgery in patients with colorectal cancer (p.493), although reports of improved survival do not seem to have been borne out. It has been given by intravenous infusion over 2 hours, in an initial dose of 500 mg, followed by 4 further doses of 100 mg at monthly intervals. The drug is of murine origin and most patients develop antibodies following administration. Hypersensitivity reactions, including anaphylactic reactions, have occurred.

It has also been tried for other malignant neoplasms including pancreatic cancer and advanced breast cancer.

◊ References.
1. Riethmüller G, et al. Randomised trial of monoclonal antibody for adjuvant therapy of resected Dukes' C colorectal carcinoma. Lancet 1994; 343: 1177–83.
2. Riethmüller G, et al. Monoclonal antibody therapy for resected Dukes' C colorectal cancer: seven-year outcome of a multicenter randomized trial. J Clin Oncol 1998; 16: 1788–94.
3. Adkins JC, Spencer CM. Edrecolomab (monoclonal antibody 17-1A). Drugs 1998; 56: 619–26.

Preparations
Proprietary Preparations (details are given in Part 3)
Ger.: Panorex.

Elliptinium Acetate (18634-y)
Elliptinium Acetate (BAN, rINN).
HME; NSC-264137. 9-Hydroxy-2,5,11-trimethyl-6H,2H-pyrido[4,3-b]carbazolium acetate.
$C_{20}H_{20}N_2O_3 = 336.4$.
CAS — 58337-35-2.

Profile
Elliptinium acetate is an antineoplastic which was formerly used in the treatment of metastatic breast cancer.

Eniluracil (20091-t)
Eniluracil (BAN, USAN, rINN).
776C85. 5-Ethynyluracil.
$C_6H_4N_2O_2 = 136.1$.
CAS — 59989-18-3.

Profile
Eniluracil inactivates the enzyme dihydropyrimidine dehydrogenase, which plays an important role in fluorouracil metabolism. Eniluracil increases the bioavailability of fluorouracil, particularly when the latter is given by mouth. It has been investigated as an adjunct to fluorouracil therapy in the treatment of colorectal, breast, and pancreatic cancer.

Enloplatin (15005-g)
Enloplatin (USAN, rINN).
CL-287110. cis-(1,1-Cyclobutane dicarboxylato)[tetrahydro-4H-pyran-4,4-bis(methylamine)]platinum.
$C_{13}H_{22}N_2O_5Pt = 481.4$.
CAS — 111523-41-2.

Profile
Enloplatin is a platinum derivative with general properties similar to those of cisplatin (p.525). It has been studied as an antineoplastic in the treatment of a variety of malignant neoplasms.

◊ References.
1. Weiss RB, Christian MC. New cisplatin analogues in development: a review. Drugs 1993; 46: 360–77.
2. Kudelka AP, et al. A phase II and pharmacokinetic study of enloplatin in patients with platinum refractory advanced ovarian carcinoma. Anticancer Drugs 1997; 8: 649–56.

Enocitabine (19135-h)
Enocitabine (rINN).
Behenoyl Cytarabine; Behenoylcytosine Arabinoside; BH-AC; NSC-239336. N-(1-β-D-Arabinofuranosyl-1,2-dihydro-2-oxo-4-pyrimidinyl)docosanamide.
$C_{31}H_{55}N_3O_6 = 565.8$.
CAS — 55726-47-1.

Profile
Enocitabine is an antineoplastic that is converted in the body to cytarabine (p.530). It has been used similarly in the treatment of acute leukaemias.

Epirubicin Hydrochloride (16631-k)
Epirubicin Hydrochloride (BANM, USAN, rINNM).
4'-Epiadriamycin Hydrochloride; 4'-Epidoxorubicin Hydrochloride; Epirubicini Hydrochloridum; IMI-28; Pidorubicin Hydrochloride. (8S,10S)-10-(3-Amino-2,3,6-trideoxy-α-L-arabinohexopyranosyloxy)-8-glycolloyl-7,8,9,10-tetrahydro-6,8,11-trihydroxy-1-methoxynaphthacene-5,12-dione hydrochloride.
$C_{27}H_{29}NO_{11},HCl = 580.0$.
CAS — 56420-45-2 (epirubicin); 56390-09-1 (epirubicin hydrochloride).
Pharmacopoeias. In Eur. (see p.vi).

The manufacturers state that epirubicin is **incompatible** with heparin or fluorouracil and with alkali.

Pharmacopoeial description
Ph. Eur.: A substance obtained by chemical transformation of a substance produced by certain strains of Streptomyces peucetius. An orange-red powder. Soluble in water and in methyl alcohol; slightly soluble in dehydrated alcohol; practically insoluble in acetone. A 0.5% solution in water has a pH of 4.0 to 5.5. Store at 2° to 8° in airtight containers. Protect from light.

Stability. Epirubicin was not subject to significant photodegradation at clinical concentrations,[1,2] and special precautions to protect solutions from light during administration do not appear to be necessary. However, photodegradation may be significant at lower concentrations (below 500 µg per mL).[1]
1. Wood MJ, et al. Photodegradation of doxorubicin, daunorubicin and epirubicin measured by high-performance liquid chromatography. J Clin Pharm Ther 1990; 15: 291–300.
2. Pujol M, et al. Stability study of epirubicin in NaCl 0.9% injection. Ann Pharmacother 1997; 31: 992–5.

Adverse Effects, Treatment, and Precautions
As for Doxorubicin Hydrochloride, p.535. Cardiotoxicity and myelotoxicity may be less than with doxorubicin. Cardiotoxicity is more likely when the cumulative dose exceeds 0.9 to 1 g per m² body-surface.

Effects on the heart. For further discussion of the cardiotoxicity of anthracyclines, see under Adverse Effects of Doxorubicin, p.535.

Interactions
Antineoplastics. Increased exposure to epirubicin, and a consequent increase in myelotoxicity, has been reported in patients given epirubicin after paclitaxel, compared with patients who received epirubicin before paclitaxel.[1] Similar interactions have been seen when paclitaxel was given before other anthracyclines.[2]
1. Venturini M, et al. Sequence effect of epirubicin and paclitaxel treatment on pharmacokinetics and toxicity. J Clin Oncol 2000; 18: 2116–25.
2. Danesi R, et al. Pharmacokinetic optimisation of treatment schedules for anthracyclines and paclitaxel in patients with cancer. Clin Pharmacokinet 1999; 37: 195–211.

Cimetidine. Cimetidine increased the formation of the active metabolite of epirubicin in a study in 8 patients; there was also a substantial increase in systemic exposure to unchanged epirubicin.[1] The mechanisms and potential clinical significance of the interaction were unclear.
1. Murray LS, et al. The effect of cimetidine on the pharmacokinetics of epirubicin in patients with advanced breast cancer: preliminary evidence of a potentially common drug interaction. Clin Oncol 1998; 10: 35–8.

Pharmacokinetics
Following intravenous administration epirubicin is rapidly and extensively distributed into body tissues, and undergoes metabolism in the liver, with the formation of epirubicinol (13-hydroxyepirubicin) and appreciable amounts of glucuronide derivatives. Epirubicin is eliminated mainly in bile, with a terminal plasma elimination half-life of about 30 to 40 hours. About 10% of a dose is recovered in urine within 48 hours. Epirubicin does not cross the blood-brain barrier.

◊ References.
1. Morris RG, et al. Disposition of epirubicin and metabolites with repeated courses to cancer patients. Eur J Clin Pharmacol 1991; 40: 481–7.
2. Robert J. Clinical pharmacokinetics of epirubicin. Clin Pharmacokinet 1994; 26: 428–38.

Uses and Administration
Epirubicin is an anthracycline antibiotic with antineoplastic actions similar to those of doxorubicin (p.536). It has been tried, alone or in combination with other antineoplastics, in acute leukaemias, lymphomas, multiple myeloma, and in solid tumours including cancer of the bladder (p.490), breast (p.491), cervix (p.492), and gastrointestinal tract (p.493).

Epirubicin hydrochloride is administered intravenously by injecting a solution in sodium chloride 0.9% or Water for Injections into a fast-running infusion of sodium chloride 0.9% or glucose 5% over 3 to 5 minutes, or by infusion up over to 30 minutes. It is given as a single agent in usual doses of 60 to 90 mg per m² body-surface as a single dose every 3 weeks; this dose may be divided over 2 or 3 days if desired. High-dose regimens, of 120 mg or more per m² every 3 weeks, and 45 mg per m² for 3 consecutive days every 3 weeks have been used. A regimen of 20 mg as a single weekly dose has also been tried and is reported to be associated with lower toxicity. Doses should be reduced if epirubicin is given with other antineoplastics, and should be halved in patients with moderate liver dysfunction (serum bilirubin concentrations of 14 to 30 µg per mL), while those with severe liver impairment (serum bilirubin greater than 30 µg per mL) should be given a quarter of the usual dose. Reduced doses are also recommended in those whose bone-marrow function is impaired by age or previous chemotherapy or radiotherapy.

A total cumulative dose of 0.9 to 1 g per m² should not generally be exceeded, because of the risk of cardiotoxicity.

Epirubicin has also been given by intravesical instillation in the local treatment of bladder cancer. Instillation of 50 mg weekly as a 0.1% solution for 8 weeks has been suggested, reduced to 30 mg weekly if chemical cystitis develops; for carcinoma in-situ, the dose may be increased, if tolerated, to 80 mg weekly. For the prophylaxis of recurrence in patients who have undergone transurethral resection, 50 mg weekly for 4 weeks, followed by 50 mg instilled once a month for 11 months is the suggested regimen.

Blood counts should be made routinely during treatment with epirubicin and cardiac function should be carefully monitored. Liver function should be assessed before and if possible during therapy.

◊ References.
1. Plosker GL, Faulds D. Epirubicin: a review of its pharmacodynamic and pharmacokinetic properties, and therapeutic use in cancer chemotherapy. Drugs 1993; 45: 788–856.
2. Coukell AJ, Faulds D. Epirubicin: an updated review of its pharmacodynamic and pharmacokinetic properties and therapeutic efficacy in the management of breast cancer. Drugs 1997; 53: 453–82.

Amyloidosis. For reference to a regimen including epirubicin used to control disease in a patient with amyloidosis, see p.501.

Preparations
Proprietary Preparations (details are given in Part 3)
Aust.: Farmorubicin; *Austral.:* Pharmorubicin; *Belg.:* Farmorubicine; *Braz.:* Farmorubicina; *Canad.:* Pharmorubicin; *Denm.:* Farmorubicin; *Fin.:* Farmorubicine; *Fr.:* Farmorubicine; *Ger.:* Farmorubicin; *Hong Kong:* Pharmorubicin; *Irl.:* Pharmorubicin; *Israel:* Farmorubicin; *Ital.:* Farmorubicina; *Mex.:* Epilem; Farmorubicin; *Neth.:* Farmorubicine; *Norw.:* Farmorubicin; *NZ:* Pharmorubicin; *Port.:* Farmorubicina; *S.Afr.:* Farmorubicin; *Spain:* Farmorubicina; *Swed.:* Farmorubicin; *Switz.:* Farmorubicin; *Thai.:* Farmorubicin; *UK:* Pharmorubicin; *USA:* Ellence.

Estramustine Sodium Phosphate (1832-c)
Estramustine Sodium Phosphate (BANM, rINNM).
Estramustine Phosphate Sodium (USAN); NSC-89199 (estramustine phosphate); Ro-21-8837/001; Ro-22-2296/000 (estramustine). Estra-1,3,5(10)-triene-3,17β-diol 3-[bis(2-chloroethyl)carbamate] 17-(disodium phosphate); Disodium 3-[bis(2-chloroethyl)-carbamoyloxy]estra-1,3,5(10)-trien-17β-yl orthophosphate.
$C_{23}H_{30}Cl_2NNa_2O_6P = 564.3$.
CAS — 2998-57-4 (estramustine); 4891-15-0 (estramustine phosphate); 52205-73-9 (estramustine sodium phosphate).
Pharmacopoeias. In Br.

Pharmacopoeial description
BP 2001: A white or almost white powder. Freely soluble in water and in methyl alcohol; very slightly soluble in dehydrated alcohol and in chloroform. A 0.5% solution in water has a pH of 8.5 to 10.0. Protect from light.

Adverse Effects, Treatment, and Precautions
Oestrogenic side-effects are fairly common, and may include gynaecomastia, fluid retention, and cardiovascular effects. Gastrointestinal disturbances, hepatic dysfunction, loss of libido, hypersensitivity reactions, and occasionally leucopenia and thrombocytopenia may occur. Estramustine is contra-indicated in patients with peptic ulceration and severe hepatic or cardiovascular disease. Diabetes mellitus may be exacerbated, and it should be given with care to patients with disorders such as congestive heart failure, epilepsy, hypertension, and migraine which may be adversely affected by additional fluid retention. Care is also required in patients with conditions predisposing to hypercalcaemia, and serum calcium should be monitored in hypercalcaemic patients.
Estramustine should not be given with milk products or products high in calcium, which may interfere with its absorption.

Pharmacokinetics
About 75% of a dose of estramustine sodium phosphate is absorbed from the gastrointestinal tract. It is concentrated in prostatic tissue. The phosphate moiety appears to be lost in the gastrointestinal tract, liver, and phosphatase-rich tissue such as the prostate and estramustine is found in the body mainly as its 17-keto analogue, estromustine. Following breakage of the carbamate linkage the oestrogenic and alkylating moieties are excreted independently.

Uses and Administration

Estramustine is a combination of estradiol and normustine and has weaker oestrogenic activity than estradiol and weaker antineoplastic activity than most other alkylating agents. Estramustine phosphate is given by mouth as the disodium salt in the treatment of advanced prostatic carcinoma (see also p.497); it has been used with meglumine by intravenous injection.

The usual initial dosage by mouth is the equivalent of 560 mg of estramustine phosphate daily in divided doses; the dose may later be adjusted to between 140 mg and 1.4 g daily according to the response and gastrointestinal tolerance. It should be given not less than 1 hour before or 2 hours after meals. In the USA a dose of 14 mg per kg body-weight or 600 mg per m^2 body-surface, daily in divided doses, is usually employed.

◊ References.
1. Bergenheim AT, Henriksson R. Pharmacokinetics and pharmacodynamics of estramustine phosphate. *Clin Pharmacokinet* 1998; **34:** 163–72.

Preparations

BP 2001: Estramustine Phosphate Capsules.

Proprietary Preparations (details are given in Part 3)
Aust.: Estracyt; *Austral.:* Estracyt†; *Belg.:* Estracyt; *Canad.:* Emcyt; *Denm.:* Estracyt; *Fr.:* Estracyt; *Ger.:* cellmustin; Estracyt; Multosin; Prostamustin; *Irl.:* Estracyt; *Ital.:* Estracyt; *Jpn:* Estracyt; *Mex.:* Emcyt; *Neth.:* Estracyt; *Norw.:* Estracyt; *S.Afr.:* Estracyt; *Spain:* Estracyt; *Swed.:* Estracyt; *Switz.:* Estracyt; *UK:* Estracyt; *USA:* Emcyt.

Etanidazole (1798-q)

Etanidazole (USAN, rINN).

NSC-301467; SR-2508. *N*-(2-Hydroxyethyl)-2-nitroimidazole-1-acetamide.

$C_7H_{10}N_4O_4 = 214.2$.

CAS — 22668-01-5.

Profile

Etanidazole is a radiosensitiser structurally related to metronidazole, and which is under investigation as an adjunct to radiotherapy in the treatment of cancer. Peripheral neuropathy may be dose-limiting.

◊ References.
1. Lee DJ, *et al.* Results of an RTOG phase III trial (RTOG 85-27) comparing radiotherapy plus etanidazole with radiotherapy alone for locally advanced head and neck carcinomas. *Int J Radiat Oncol Biol Phys* 1995; **32:** 567–76.
2. Eschwege F, *et al.* Results of a European randomized trial of etanidazole combined with radiotherapy in head and neck carcinomas. *Int J Radiat Oncol Biol Phys* 1997; **39:** 275–81.

Etoposide (1834-a)

Etoposide (BAN, USAN, rINN).

EPEG; Etoposidum; NSC-141540; VP-16; VP-16-213. 4′-Demethylepipodophyllotoxin 9-[4,6-*O*-(*R*)-ethylidene-β-D-glucopyranoside]; (5S,5aR,8aS,9R)-9-(4,6-*O*-Ethylidene-β-D-glucopyranosyloxy)-5,8,8a,9-tetrahydro-5-(4-hydroxy-3,5-dimethoxyphenyl)-isobenzofuro[5,6-*f*][1,3]benzodioxol-6(5a*H*)-one.

$C_{29}H_{32}O_{13} = 588.6$.

CAS — 33419-42-0.

ATC — L01CB01.

NOTE. The trivial name epipodophyllotoxin has occasionally been used incorrectly for this derivative.

Pharmacopoeias. In *Eur.* (see p.vi) and *US*.

Pharmacopoeial description

Ph. Eur.: A white or almost white, crystalline powder. Practically insoluble in water; slightly soluble in alcohol and in dichloromethane; sparingly soluble in methyl alcohol. Store in airtight containers.

USP 25: A fine, white to off-white, crystalline powder. Very slightly soluble in water; slightly soluble in alcohol, in chloroform, in dichloromethane, and in ethyl acetate; sparingly soluble in methyl alcohol. Store in airtight containers. Protect from light.

Incompatibility. For reference to precipitation when mannitol or potassium chloride was added to mixtures of etoposide and cisplatin in sodium chloride injection, see Cisplatin, p.525.

Adverse Effects, Treatment, and Precautions

For general discussions see Antineoplastics, p.476, p.479, and p.480.

The dose-limiting toxicity with etoposide is myelosuppression, predominantly manifesting as leucopenia, but also thrombocytopenia, and sometimes anaemia. The nadir of the granulocyte count usually occurs 7 to 14 days after a dose, with recovery by about 21 days. Nausea and vomiting are common; there may also be anorexia, diarrhoea, and stomatitis. Gastrointestinal toxicity may be more common after

oral administration. Reversible alopecia may occur in about two-thirds of all patients. Peripheral or central neuropathies, including transient cortical blindness, have been reported rarely, as have hypersensitivity or anaphylactoid reactions, apnoea, fever, rashes and skin pigmentation, pruritus, and dysphagia. Disturbances of liver function have been reported, mainly at high doses. There have been occasional reports of cardiotoxicity. Local irritation and thrombophlebitis may occur at the site of injection. Care should be taken to avoid extravasation although tissue damage (possibly associated with the vehicle) is rare.

Following rapid intravenous administration hypotension may occur; etoposide should be given by infusion over at least 30 minutes. Etoposide should not be given to patients with severe hepatic dysfunction nor by intracavitary administration.

Some of the adverse effects associated with intravenous administration of etoposide may be due to the formulation of the vehicle.

There is evidence that etoposide may be associated with the development of secondary leukaemias—see Carcinogenicity, p.476.

Effects on the nervous system. A report of an acute dystonic reaction in a child given etoposide as part of a combined maintenance regimen for acute lymphoblastic leukaemia;[1] the patient had been receiving the same regimen uneventfully for over a year but symptoms (which responded to diphenhydramine) recurred on rechallenge with etoposide.

1. Ascher DP, Delaney RA. Acute dystonia from etoposide. *Drug Intell Clin Pharm* 1988; **22:** 41–2.

Handling and disposal. Urine and faeces produced for up to 4 and 7 days respectively after a dose of etoposide should be handled wearing protective clothing.[1]

1. Harris J, Dodds LJ. Handling waste from patients receiving cytotoxic drugs. *Pharm J* 1985; **235:** 289–91.

Hypersensitivity. A report of a hypersensitivity reaction to etoposide and a review of 92 further reactions.[1] Hypersensitivity reactions to intravenous etoposide are characterised by one or more of: hypotension, bronchospasm, flushing, exanthema, dyspnoea, fever, chills, tachycardia, tightness in the chest, cyanosis, and hypertension. Although originally stated to be rare, some investigators have reported an incidence of up to about 50%, particularly in younger patients. (Hypersensitivity reactions to teniposide appear to be more frequent than with etoposide, perhaps because the former is formulated with polyethoxylated castor oil whereas the latter is not.) The mechanism of reactions to etoposide is uncertain but may be non-immunogenic as reducing the rate of infusion may prevent reactions, as may reducing etoposide concentration in the infusion solution. Hypersensitivity appears to have been reported less frequently with the oral formulation.

1. Hoetelmans RMW, *et al.* Hypersensitivity reactions to etoposide. *Ann Pharmacother* 1996; **30:** 367–71.

Interactions

For a general outline of antineoplastic drug interactions, see p.481.

Antineoplastics and immunosuppressants. Administration of etoposide 2 days after a dose of *cisplatin* was associated with a marked decrease in etoposide clearance and an increase in toxicity, compared with the same dose given 21 days after a dose of cisplatin, in a study involving 17 children.[1] There was no evidence of a persistent decrease in etoposide clearance associated with the cumulative dose of cisplatin, however.

High-dose *ciclosporin* therapy was found to increase the exposure to etoposide by 80%, and to reduce etoposide clearance by 38%. Leucopenia was increased. Etoposide doses should be halved when the drug is given with high-dose ciclosporin.[2]

1. Relling MV, *et al.* Etoposide pharmacokinetics and pharmacodynamics after acute and chronic exposure to cisplatin. *Clin Pharmacol Ther* 1994; **56:** 503–11.
2. Lum BL, *et al.* Alteration of etoposide pharmacokinetics and pharmacodynamics by cyclosporine in a phase I trial to modulate drug resistance. *J Clin Oncol* 1992; **10:** 1635–42.

Pharmacokinetics

Following administration by mouth absorption is variable, but on average about 50% of the dose of etoposide is absorbed. The pharmacokinetics of etoposide are subject to considerable interindividual variation. It is rapidly distributed, and concentrations in plasma fall in a biphasic manner, with a terminal half-life of 4 to 11 hours. It is about 94% bound to plasma protein. Etoposide is excreted in urine and faeces as unchanged drug and metabolites: about 45% of a dose is reported to be excreted in urine over 72 hours. It

crosses the blood-brain barrier poorly; concentrations in CSF are 1 to 10% of those in plasma.

Metabolism. Studies *in vitro* suggested that metabolic activation of etoposide by oxidation into the *O*-quinone derivative might play an essential role in its activity against DNA.[1]

1. van Maanen JMS, *et al.* Metabolic activation of anti-tumour agent VP 16-213. *Hum Toxicol* 1986; **5:** 136.

Uses and Administration

Etoposide is a semisynthetic derivative of podophyllotoxin with antimitotic and antineoplastic properties; it inhibits DNA synthesis and is most active against cells in the late S and G_2 phases of the cell cycle.

It is used, usually in combination with other antineoplastics, in the treatment of tumours of the testis, and cancers of the lung. It has also been tried in other solid tumours including those of the brain, gastrointestinal tract, ovary, and thymus, and some childhood neoplasms; in lymphomas and acute leukaemias, and in the treatment of Kaposi's sarcoma associated with AIDS. These uses are discussed further under Choice of Antineoplastic, as indicated by the cross-references given below.

It is given by slow intravenous infusion over at least 30 minutes, as a solution in sodium chloride 0.9% or glucose 5% injection. In the UK the manufacturers recommend that the concentration of the infusion should not exceed 250 µg per mL, to avoid the risk of the drug crystallising out of solution, but in the USA an upper limit of 400 µg per mL is regarded as acceptable. Etoposide phosphate, a prodrug with improved solubility in water, has been developed. Intravenous doses are calculated in terms of etoposide, and are identical to those of the base, but it may be given in concentrations up to the equivalent of 20 mg etoposide per mL.

The usual dose is 50 to 120 mg of etoposide per m^2 body-surface daily for 5 days. Somewhat lower doses have been suggested in lung cancer. Alternatively, 100 mg per m^2 has been given on alternate days to a total of 300 mg per m^2. Double the dose given intravenously may be given when etoposide is taken by mouth. Courses may be repeated after 3 to 4 weeks.

Blood disorders, non-malignant. For reference to the use of combination chemotherapy, including etoposide, in a few patients with refractory idiopathic thrombocytopenic purpura, see p.1052.

Histiocytic syndromes. Systemic chemotherapy is often tried in patients with extensive Langerhans-cell histiocytosis (p.483), although its value is uncertain. Etoposide is one of the drugs widely used for this purpose.

Hypereosinophilic syndrome. Etoposide has been reported to produce clinical responses in patients with the hypereosinophilic syndrome.[1]

1. Bourrat E, *et al.* Etoposide for treating the hypereosinophilic syndrome. *Ann Intern Med* 1994; **121:** 899–900.

Malignant neoplasms. Etoposide has been used for a variety of solid tumours: in particular it is part of curative regimens used in the treatment of testicular cancer and germ-cell tumours of the ovary (see p.499 and p.496), and is used with cisplatin and other drugs in the treatment of lung cancer (p.496). Other solid neoplasms in which it is sometimes employed include those of the brain (p.490), stomach (p.493), and thymus (p.499), as well as in neuroblastoma (p.500), retinoblastoma (p.500), and rhabdomyosarcoma (p.501); it has also formed part of systemic regimens for bone sarcomas (p.500), disseminated Kaposi's sarcoma (see p.501), and gestational trophoblastic tumours (p.483). Etoposide is used in regimens for Hodgkin's disease (see p.487); it is also sometimes used in aggressive intermediate- and high-grade non-Hodgkin's lymphomas (p.487), and may produce short-term responses in mycosis fungoides (p.489). Etoposide may have benefits when added to induction protocols for acute myeloid leukaemia (p.485), and when used as part of consolidation therapy in acute lymphoblastic leukaemia (p.484).

Vasculitic syndromes. For mention of the use of etoposide to induce remission in patients with Wegener's granulomatosis resistant to standard therapy with cyclophosphamide and corticosteroids, see p.1060.

Preparations

BP 2001: Etoposide Capsules; Etoposide Intravenous Infusion; **USP 25:** Etoposide Capsules; Etoposide Injection.

Proprietary Preparations (details are given in Part 3)
Aust.: Abiposid; Cehaposid†; Exitop; Vepesid; *Austral.:* Etopophos; Vepesid; *Belg.:* Etopophos; Vepesid; *Braz.:* Vepesid; *Canad.:* Vepesid; *Denm.:* Eposid; Etopofos; Vepesid; *Fin.:* Etopofos; Exitop; Vepesid; *Fr.:* Celltop; Etopophos; Vepeside; *Ger.:* ETO CS; Eto-Gry; Etomedac; Etopophos; Exitop; Ri-

boposid; Vepesid; *Hong Kong:* Vepesid; *Irl.:* Etopophos; Vepesid; *Israel:* Etopophos; Vepesid; *Ital.:* Lastet; Vepesid; *Jpn:* Lastet†; *Mex.:* Etopos; Kenazol; Lastet; Seroposide; Vepesid; VP-Tec; *Neth.:* Etopophos; Vepesid; *Norw.:* Eposin; Etopofos; Vepesid; *NZ:* Etopophos; Vepesid; *Port.:* Lastet; *S.Afr.:* Eposin; Etopophos; Vepesid; *Singapore:* Vepesid; *Spain:* Eposin; Lastet; Vepesid; *Swed.:* Eposin; Etopophos; Exitop; Vepesid; *Switz.:* Etopophos; Vepesid; *Thai.:* Fytosid; Vepesid; *UK:* Etopophos; Vepesid; *USA:* Etopophos; Toposar; Vepesid.

Everolimus (20621-g)

Everolimus (*rINN*).

(3S,6R,7E,9R,10R,12R,14S,15E,17E,19E,21S,23S,26R,27R,34aS)-9,10,12,13,14,21,22,23,24,25,26,27,32,33,34,34a-Hexadecahydro-9,27-dihydroxy-3-{(1R)-2-[(1S,3R,4R)-4-(2-hydroxyethoxy)-3-methoxycyclohexyl]-1-methylethyl}-10,21-dimethoxy-6,8,12,14,20,26-hexamethyl-23,27-epoxy-3H-pyrido[2,1-c][1,4]oxaazacyclohentriacontine-1,5,11,28,29(4H,6H,31H)-pentone.
$C_{53}H_{83}NO_{14} = 958.2.$
CAS — 159351-69-6.

Profile
Everolimus is a derivative of sirolimus (p.568). It is under investigation for its immunosuppressant properties in organ transplantation.

◊ References.
1. Kovarik JM, *et al.* Longitudinal assessment of everolimus in de novo renal transplant recipients over the first post-transplant year: pharmacokinetics, exposure-response relationships, and influence on cyclosporine. *Clin Pharmacol Ther* 2001; **69:** 48–56.

Exemestane (15427-v)

Exemestane (*BAN, rINN*).
FCE-24304. 6-Methyleneandrosta-1,4-diene-3,17-dione.
$C_{20}H_{24}O_2 = 296.4.$
CAS — 107868-30-4.
ATC — L02BG06.

Profile
Exemestane is a selective inhibitor of the aromatase (oestrogen synthase) system, similar to formestane (p.543). It is used in the treatment of advanced breast cancer (p.491), in women who are no longer responsive to anti-oestrogen therapy. The recommended dose is 25 mg daily by mouth.

◊ References.
1. Clemett D, Lamb HM. Exemestane: a review of its use in postmenopausal women with advanced breast cancer. *Drugs* 2000; **59:** 1279–96.
2. Kaufmann M, *et al.* Exemestane is superior to megestrol acetate after tamoxifen failure in postmenopausal women with advanced breast cancer: results of a phase III randomized double-blind trial. *J Clin Oncol* 2000; **18:** 1399–1411.
3. Lønning PE, *et al.* Activity of exemestane in metastatic breast cancer after failure of nonsteroidal aromatase inhibitors: a phase II trial. *J Clin Oncol* 2000; **18:** 2234–44.

Preparations
Proprietary Preparations (details are given in Part 3)
Austral.: Aromasin; *Denm.:* Aromasin; *Fin.:* Aromasin; *Ger.:* Aromasin; *Irl.:* Aromasin; *Ital.:* Aromasin; *Neth.:* Aromasin; *Port.:* Aromasin; *Swed.:* Aromasin; *UK:* Aromasin; *USA:* Aromasin.

Exisulind (17469-p)

Exisulind (*rINN*).
FGN-1; Sulindac Sulfone. 5-Fluoro-2-methyl-1-[(Z)-p-(methylsulfonyl)benzylidene]indene-3-acetic acid.
$C_{20}H_{17}FO_4S = 372.4.$
CAS — 59973-80-7.

Profile
Exisulind is a sulfone metabolite of sulindac (p.85) that is reported to induce apoptosis in cancerous and precancerous cells. It has been studied for the treatment of familial adenomatous polyposis, with variable results. It is also being investigated for the prevention and treatment of a variety of malignant neoplasms, including those of the prostate and lung.

◊ References.
1. Stoner GD, *et al.* Sulindac sulfone induced regression of rectal polyps in patients with familial adenomatous polyposis. *Adv Exp Med Biol* 1999; **470:** 45–53.
2. van Stolk R, *et al.* Phase I trial of exisulind (sulindac sulfone, FGN-1) as a chemopreventive agent in patients with familial adenomatous polyposis. *Clin Cancer Res* 2000; **6:** 78–89.

Fadrozole Hydrochloride (11128-p)

Fadrozole Hydrochloride (*USAN, rINNM*).
CGS-16949 (fadrozole); CGS-16949A. (±)-p-(5,6,7,8-Tetrahydroimidazo[1,5-a]pyridin-5-yl)benzonitrile monohydrochloride.
$C_{14}H_{13}N_3,HCl = 259.7.$
CAS — 102676-47-1 (fadrozole); 102676-96-0 (fadrozole hydrochloride).

The symbol † denotes a preparation no longer actively marketed

Profile
Fadrozole hydrochloride is an inhibitor of the aromatase (oestrogen synthetase) system and is used for the endocrine therapy of breast cancer. It has been given in doses of 1 mg twice daily by mouth.

◊ References.
1. Stein RC, *et al.* Preliminary study of the treatment of advanced breast cancer in postmenopausal women with aromatase inhibitor CGS 16949A. *Cancer Res* 1990; **50:** 1381–4.
2. Miller WR. Oestrogens and breast cancer: biological considerations. *Br Med Bull* 1990; **47:** 470–83.
3. Buzdar AU, *et al.* Fadrozole HCl (CGS-16949A) versus megestrol acetate treatment of postmenopausal patients with metastatic breast carcinoma: results of two randomized double blind controlled multiinstitutional trials. *Cancer* 1996; **77:** 2503–13.
4. Thurlimann B, *et al.* First-line fadrozole HCl (CGS 16949A) versus tamoxifen in postmenopausal women with advanced breast cancer: prospective randomised trial of the Swiss Group for Clinical Cancer Research SAKK 20/88. *Ann Oncol* 1996; **7:** 471–9.

Fenretinide (19171-g)

Fenretinide (*USAN, rINN*).
4-Hydroxyphenylretinamide; McN-R-1967. *all-trans*-4'-Hydroxyretinanilide.
CAS — 65646-68-6.

Profile
Fenretinide is a retinoid derivative given by mouth and being studied in the treatment of breast and prostate cancer and some other malignancies. It has also been tried in oral lichen planus and leucoplakia.

◊ A study of fenretinide for the treatment of psoriasis was discontinued before any therapeutic effect was observed as 2 of 8 patients developed night blindness and 2 developed severe toxic erythema.[1] Fenretinide is being studied for the treatment of breast cancer[2] and cutaneous malignancies but early results have been disappointing and night blindness and mucocutaneous effects have also been associated with this use.[3] However, a combination of tamoxifen and fenretinide, given intermittently, has been reported to be well tolerated.[4] Fenretinide has been investigated[5,6] for the prevention of breast cancer (p.492), but a large randomised study of secondary prevention failed to show any benefit.[5]
1. Kingston TP, *et al.* Visual and cutaneous toxicity during N-(4-hydroxyphenyl) retinamide therapy for psoriasis. *Clin Exp Dermatol* 1986; **11:** 624–7.
2. Baum M, *et al.* Prospects for the chemoprevention of breast cancer. *Br Med Bull* 1991; **47:** 493–503.
3. Modiano MR, *et al.* Phase II study of fenretinide (N-[4-hydroxyphenyl]retinamide) in advanced breast cancer and melanoma. *Invest New Drugs* 1990; **8:** 317–19.
4. Cobleigh MA, *et al.* Phase I/II trial of tamoxifen with or without fenretinide, an analog of vitamin A, in women with metastatic breast cancer. *J Clin Oncol* 1993; **11:** 474–7.
5. Veronesi U, *et al.* Randomized trial of fenretinide to prevent second breast malignancy in women with early breast cancer. *J Natl Cancer Inst* 1999; **91:** 1847–56.
6. Conley B, *et al.* Pilot trial of the safety, tolerability, and retinoid levels of N-(4-hydroxyphenyl) retinamide in combination with tamoxifen in patients at high risk for developing invasive breast cancer. *J Clin Oncol* 2000; **18:** 275–83.

Floxuridine (1835-t)

Floxuridine (*USAN, rINN*).
5-Fluorouracil Deoxyriboside; FUDR; NSC-27640; WR-138720. 2'-Deoxy-5-fluorouridine; 5-Fluoro-2'-deoxyuridine; 1-(2-Deoxy-β-D-ribofuranosyl)-5-fluoropyrimidine-2,4(1H,3H)-dione.
$C_9H_{11}FN_2O_5 = 246.2.$
CAS — 50-91-9.
Pharmacopoeias. In *US*.

Pharmacopoeial description
USP 25: Store in airtight containers. Protect from light.

Adverse Effects, Treatment, and Precautions
As for Fluorouracil, p.540. Adverse reactions following intra-arterial infusion commonly include local reactions, thromboembolic complications, and infection, bleeding, or blockage of the catheter. Erythema, stomatitis, and gastrointestinal disturbances are relatively common. There have also been signs of liver dysfunction.

Effects on the liver. Serious biliary toxicity has been reported in over half of all patients receiving hepatic arterial infusions of floxuridine, usually manifesting as sclerosing cholangitis or acalculous cholecystitis;[1] as a result some surgeons routinely remove the gallbladder at the time of infusion pump implantation.[2] Floxuridine infusions have also been associated with a case of fatal progressive cirrhosis of the liver in the absence of overt cholestasis.[3]
1. Sherlock S. The spectrum of hepatotoxicity due to drugs. *Lancet* 1986; **ii:** 440–4.
2. Anonymous. An implanted infusion pump for chemotherapy of liver metastases. *Med Lett Drugs Ther* 1984; **26:** 89–90.
3. Pettavel J, *et al.* Fatal liver cirrhosis associated with long-term arterial infusion of floxuridine. *Lancet* 1986; **ii:** 1162–3.

Interactions
As for Fluorouracil, p.541.

Pharmacokinetics
Floxuridine is poorly absorbed from the gastrointestinal tract and it is usually given by injection. Floxuridine is metabolised mainly in the liver to fluorouracil following rapid injection. When given by slow intra-arterial infusion, more of the drug is metabolised to floxuridine monophosphate, resulting in greater inhibition of DNA synthesis. It is excreted as carbon dioxide via the lungs; some is excreted, as unchanged drug and metabolites, in urine. Floxuridine crosses the blood-brain barrier to some extent and is found in CSF.

Uses and Administration
Floxuridine is an antineoplastic which acts as an antimetabolite similarly to fluorouracil. When it is administered by rapid injection it acts as fluorouracil, but when given by slow intra-arterial infusion, more of the drug is metabolised to floxuridine monophosphate (F-dump), resulting in greater inhibition of DNA synthesis.

Floxuridine is used in the palliative treatment of hepatic metastases of colorectal cancer—see Malignant Neoplasms of the Liver, p.495. It has been tried in some other solid neoplasms. Doses of 100 to 600 μg per kg body-weight daily are given by continuous arterial infusion, usually with the aid of an infusion pump, until toxicity occurs.

White cell and platelet counts should be carried out regularly during therapy and treatment should be stopped if the white cell count falls rapidly or falls to below 3500 per mm^3, if the platelet count falls below 100 000 per mm^3, or if major adverse effects occur.

◊ References.
1. Fordy C, *et al.* Hepatic arterial floxuridine as second-line treatment for systemic fluorouracil-resistant colorectal liver metastases. *Br J Cancer* 1998; **78:** 1058–60.
2. Kemeny N, *et al.* Hepatic arterial infusion of chemotherapy after resection of hepatic metastases from colorectal cancer. *N Engl J Med* 1999; **341:** 2039–48.
3. Lorenz M, Muller HH. Randomized, multicenter trial of fluorouracil plus leucovorin administered either via hepatic arterial or intravenous infusion versus fluorodeoxyuridine administered via hepatic arterial infusion in patients with nonresectable liver metastases from colorectal carcinoma. *J Clin Oncol* 2000; **18:** 243–54.
4. Fiorentini G, *et al.* Locoregional therapy for liver metastases from colorectal cancer: the possibilities of intraarterial chemotherapy, and new hepatic-directed modalities. *Hepatogastroenterology* 2001; **48:** 305–12.

Preparations
USP 25: Floxuridine for Injection.

Proprietary Preparations (details are given in Part 3)
Singapore: FUDR; *USA:* FUDR.

Fludarabine Phosphate (19183-w)

Fludarabine Phosphate (*BAN, USAN, rINNM*).
2-F-ara-AMP; Fludarabine Monophosphate; 2-Fluoro-ara-AMP; NSC-312887. 9-β-D-Arabinofuranosyl-2-fluoroadenine 5'-dihydrogenphosphate.
$C_{10}H_{13}FN_5O_7P = 365.2.$
CAS — 21679-14-1 (fludarabine); 75607-67-9 (fludarabine phosphate).

Adverse Effects, Treatment, and Precautions
For general discussions see Antineoplastics, p.476, p.479, and p.480.

Bone-marrow suppression from fludarabine is dose-limiting, manifesting as leucopenia, thrombocytopenia, and anaemia; the nadir of the white cell and platelet counts usually occurs after about 2 to 3 weeks. Myelosuppression can be severe and cumulative and prolonged lymphopenia with concomitant risk of opportunistic infections may occur.

Other adverse effects include fever, chills, cough, dyspnoea, pneumonia, gastrointestinal disturbances, stomatitis, oedema, the tumour lysis syndrome, skin rashes, haemolytic anaemia, haemorrhagic cystitis, and neurological disturbances including peripheral neuropathy, agitation, confusion, visual disturbances, and coma. High doses have been associated with progressive encephalopathy and blindness.

Dosage should be reduced in renal impairment and fludarabine should not be given if creatinine clearance is less than 30 mL per minute. It should also be avoided in patients with decompensated haemolytic anaemia.

◊ A review[1] of patients treated with fludarabine-containing regimens showed that therapy was associated with a variety of serious infections including listeriosis, *Pneumocystis carinii* pneumonia mycobacterial infections and opportunistic fungal and viral infections. The risk was exacerbated by previous or concomitant corticosteroid therapy. Prophylactic therapy with co-trimoxazole, triazole antifungals, aciclovir and colony-stimulating factors was recommended in at-risk patients.

A study in patients with chronic lymphocytic leukaemia who were treated with fludarabine found that there was no significantly increased risk of secondary malignancy following therapy, despite the immunosuppressive properties of this drug.[2]

1. Anaissie EJ, et al. Infections in patients with chronic lymphocytic leukaemia treated with fludarabine. *Ann Intern Med* 1998; **129:** 559–66.
2. Cheson BD, et al. Second malignancies as a consequence of nucleoside analog therapy for chronic lymphoid leukaemias. *J Clin Oncol* 1999; **17:** 2454–60.

Effects on the nervous system. Progressive cerebral dysfunction due to leucoencephalopathy developed 6 months after a course of fludarabine in usual doses for chronic lymphocytic leukaemia.[1] The patient became comatose and died 8 weeks after onset of the neurological symptoms.

1. Zabernigg A, et al. Late-onset fatal neurological toxicity of fludarabine. *Lancet* 1994; **344:** 1780.

Graft-versus-host disease. Transfusion-associated graft-versus-host disease has been reported following administration of blood products in patients treated with fludarabine.[1] Fludarabine-treated patients should receive irradiated red cells and platelets (to inactivate any viable T-cells) if they require a transfusion.

1. Williamson LM, et al. Fludarabine treatment and transfusion-associated graft-versus-host disease. *Lancet* 1996; **348:** 472–3.

Interactions

Increased pulmonary toxicity has been reported in patients given concomitant therapy with fludarabine and pentostatin. Administration with cytarabine may reduce the metabolic activation of fludarabine but results in increased intracellular concentrations of cytarabine—see p.530. The therapeutic efficacy of fludarabine may also be reduced by concomitant administration of dipyridamole and other inhibitors of adenosine uptake.

Aminoglycosides. A report of severe ototoxicity when a short course of gentamicin was given to a patient who had recently completed a course of fludarabine.[1]

1. O'Brien RK, Sparling TG. Gentamicin and fludarabine ototoxicity. *Ann Pharmacother* 1995; **29:** 200–1.

Corticosteroids. For a suggestion that use of fludarabine with corticosteroids may increase the risk of infection, see above.

Pharmacokinetics

After intravenous administration, fludarabine phosphate is rapidly dephosphorylated to fludarabine which is taken up by lymphocytes and rephosphorylated to the active triphosphate nucleotide. Peak intracellular concentrations of fludarabine triphosphate are seen about 4 hours after a dose.

Clearance of fludarabine from the plasma is triphasic with a terminal half-life of about 10 to 30 hours. Elimination is mostly via renal excretion: 60% of a dose is excreted in the urine within 24 hours. The pharmacokinetics of fludarabine exhibit considerable interindividual variation.

◊ References.

1. Johnson SA. Clinical pharmacokinetics of nucleoside analogues: focus on haematological malignancies. *Clin Pharmacokinet* 2000; **39:** 5–26.

Uses and Administration

Fludarabine is a fluorinated nucleotide analogue of the antiviral vidarabine (p.643) which acts as a purine antagonist antimetabolite. It is used for its antineoplastic properties in the treatment of chronic lymphocytic leukaemia. Fludarabine phosphate is given by bolus injection or by intravenous infusion over 30 minutes in a usual dose of 25 mg per m² body-surface daily for five consecutive days. Alternatively it may be given by mouth in a dose of 40 mg per m² daily for 5 consecutive days. Courses may be repeated every 28 days, usually for up to 6 cycles.

Haematological function should be monitored regularly; the dosage may need to be reduced, or further courses delayed, if blood counts indicate severe or persistent myelosuppression. Doses should be reduced by up to 50% in patients with mild to moderate renal impairment (creatinine clearance between 30

and 70 mL per minute); the drug should not be given in more severe renal impairment.

◊ General references.

1. Adkins JC, et al. Fludarabine: an update of its pharmacology and use in the treatment of haematological malignancies. *Drugs* 1997; **53:** 1005–37.

Malignant neoplasms. Fludarabine is the preferred second-line therapy for chronic lymphocytic leukaemia once initial alkylating agent therapy fails,[1] and is being investigated for initial therapy (see p.485). It has also been tried in other malignancies. Listed below are some references to the use of fludarabine phosphate for the treatment of chronic lymphocytic leukaemia,[2,3] and its potential activity against a variety of other malignancies, including indolent low-grade non-Hodgkin's lymphoma[4] (p.487), mycosis fungoides,[5] heavy chain disease,[6] prolymphocytic leukaemia,[7,8] hairy cell leukaemia,[9] and Waldenström's macroglobulinaemia.[10]

1. National Institute for Clinical Excellence. Guidance on the use of fludarabine for B-cell chronic lymphocytic leukaemia (issued September 2001). Available at: http://www.nice.org.uk/pdf/NICEfludarab_E_29guidance.pdf
2. Keating MJ, et al. Clinical experience with fludarabine in leukaemia. *Drugs* 1994; **47** (suppl 6): 39–49.
3. French Cooperative Group on CLL, et al. Multicentre prospective randomised trial of fludarabine versus cyclophosphamide, doxorubicin, and prednisone (CAP) for treatment of advanced-stage chronic lymphocytic leukaemia. *Lancet* 1996; **347:** 1432–8.
4. Hiddemann W, Pott-Hoeck C. Fludarabine in the management of malignant lymphomas. *Drugs* 1994; **66** (suppl 6): 50–60.
5. Kuzel TM, et al. Mycosis fungoides: time to define the best therapy. *J Natl Cancer Inst* 1990; **82:** 183–5.
6. Agrawal S, et al. First report of fludarabine in gamma-heavy chain disease. *Br J Haematol* 1994; **88:** 653–5.
7. Smith OP, Mehta AB. Fludarabine monophosphate for prolymphocytic leukaemia. *Lancet* 1990; **336:** 820.
8. Kantarjian HM, et al. Efficacy of fludarabine, a new adenine nucleoside analogue, in patients with prolymphocytic leukemia and the prolymphocytoid variant of chronic lymphocytic leukemia. *Am J Med* 1991; **90:** 223–8.
9. Kantarjian HM, et al. Fludarabine therapy in hairy cell leukemia. *Cancer* 1991; **67:** 1291–3.
10. Dimopoulos MA, et al. Fludarabine therapy in Waldenström's macroglobulinemia. *Am J Med* 1993; **95:** 49–52.

Preparations

Proprietary Preparations (details are given in Part 3)

Aust.: Fludara; **Austral.:** Fludara; **Belg.:** Fludara; **Canad.:** Fludara; **Denm.:** Fludara; **Fin.:** Fludara; **Fr.:** Fludara; **Ger.:** Fludara; **Israel:** Fludara; **Ital.:** Fludara; **Mex.:** Fludara; **Neth.:** Fludara; **Norw.:** Fludara; **NZ:** Fludara; **Port.:** Fludara; **S.Afr.:** Fludara; **Singapore:** Fludara; **Spain:** Beneflur; **Swed.:** Fludara; **Switz.:** Fludara; **Thai.:** Fludara; **UK:** Fludara; **USA:** Fludara.

Fluorouracil (1836-x)

Fluorouracil (BAN, USAN, rINN).

5-Fluorouracil; Fluorouracilo; Fluorouracilum; 5-FU; NSC-19893; Ro-2-9757; WR-69596. 5-Fluoropyrimidine-2,4(1H,3H)-dione.

$C_4H_3FN_2O_2 = 130.1$.

CAS — 51-21-8.
ATC — L01BC02.

Pharmacopoeias. In Eur. (see p.vi), Int., Jpn, and US.

Pharmacopoeial description

Ph. Eur.: A white or almost white, crystalline powder. Sparingly soluble in water; slightly soluble in alcohol; practically insoluble in ether. A 1% solution in water has a pH of 4.5 to 5.0. Protect from light.

USP 25: A white to practically white, practically odourless, crystalline powder. Sparingly soluble in water; slightly soluble in alcohol; practically insoluble in chloroform and in ether. Store in airtight containers. Protect from light.

◊ CAUTION. *Fluorouracil is irritant; avoid contact with skin and mucous membranes.*

Incompatibility. Preparations of fluorouracil are alkaline, and compatibility problems may be expected with acidic drugs and preparations, or those which are unstable in the presence of alkali. Fluorouracil is reported to be incompatible with cytarabine,[1] diazepam,[2] doxorubicin[2] (and presumably other anthracyclines which are unstable at alkaline pH) and calcium folinate;[3] although it has been stated to be incompatible with methotrexate[1] a study of the long-term stability of an admixture of the 2 drugs in sodium chloride (0.9%) injection suggests otherwise.[4]

1. McRae MP, King JC. Compatibility of antineoplastic, antibiotic and corticosteroid drugs in intravenous admixtures. *Am J Hosp Pharm* 1976; **33:** 1010–13.
2. Dorr RT. Incompatibilities with parenteral anticancer drugs. *Am J Intravenous Ther* 1979; **6:** 42–52.
3. Trissel LA, et al. Incompatibility of fluorouracil with leucovorin calcium or levoleucovorin calcium. *Am J Health-Syst Pharm* 1995; **52:** 710–15.
4. Vincké BJ, et al. Extended stability of 5-fluorouracil and methotrexate solutions in PVC containers. *Int J Pharmaceutics* 1989; **54:** 181–9.

Stability. Despite one report that fluorouracil had limited stability when dissolved in 5% glucose injection at room temperature (10% loss from solution in 43 hours when stored in PVC and in only 7 hours when stored in glass),[1] others found such a

solution to be stable for at least 16 weeks when stored in PVC at 5°.[2] When stored at room temperature in PVC, solutions of fluorouracil may be subject to evaporative loss of water, which slowly increases their concentration.[2,3] Results of a study of fluorouracil and methotrexate admixtures in 0.9% sodium chloride solution suggest that extended stability (up to 13 weeks) is possible in this diluent at 5° in PVC bags.[3] Commercial solutions of fluorouracil for injection have been reported to be stable for 7 days at 37° in a portable infusion pump, although at 25° one brand showed evidence of precipitation.[4] Fluorouracil solutions may be incompatible with synthetic elastomers: microscopic precipitation has been reported as soon as 4 hours after placement into polyisoprene reservoirs of elastomeric infusers and in polypropylene syringes with an elastomeric joint.[5] (Some authorities have questioned the validity of this finding.[6,7])

1. Benvenuto JA, et al. Stability and compatibility of antitumor agents in glass and plastic containers. *Am J Hosp Pharm* 1981; **38:** 1914–18.
2. Quebbeman EJ, et al. Stability of fluorouracil in plastic containers used for continuous infusion at home. *Am J Hosp Pharm* 1984; **41:** 1153–6.
3. Vincké B, et al. Extended stability of 5-fluorouracil and methotrexate solutions in PVC containers. *Int J Pharmaceutics* 1989; **54:** 181–9.
4. Stiles ML, et al. Stability of fluorouracil administered through four portable infusion pumps. *Am J Hosp Pharm* 1989; **46:** 2036–40.
5. Corbrion V, et al. Precipitation of fluorouracil in elastomeric infusers with a polyisoprene reservoir and in polypropylene syringes with an elastomeric joint. *Am J Health-Syst Pharm* 1997; **54:** 1845–8.
6. Trissel LA. Fluorouracil precipitate. *Am J Health-Syst Pharm* 1998; **55:** 1314–15.
7. Allwood MC. Fluorouracil precipitate. *Am J Health-Syst Pharm* 1998; **55:** 1315–16.

Adverse Effects and Treatment

For general discussions see Antineoplastics, p.476 and p.479.

The main adverse effects of fluorouracil are on the bone marrow and the gastrointestinal tract, and may be dose-limiting. Toxicity is schedule dependent: reducing the rate of injection to a slow infusion is associated with less haematological toxicity but does not decrease gastrointestinal toxicity. With protracted continuous infusion in particular, the palmar-plantar erythrodysesthesia syndrome (erythema and painful desquamation of the hands and feet) may occur. Gastrointestinal toxicity may be exacerbated if fluorouracil is given with folinic acid.

Leucopenia, thrombocytopenia, stomatitis, gastrointestinal ulceration and bleeding, diarrhoea, or haemorrhage from any site, are signs that treatment should be stopped. The nadir of the white cell count may occur from 7 to 20 days after a dose, and counts usually return to normal after about 30 days. Thrombocytopenia is usually at a maximum 7 to 17 days after a dose. Anaemia may also occur. Nausea and vomiting, rashes, and alopecia are common. Ocular irritation, central neurotoxicity (notably cerebellar ataxia), and myocardial ischaemia have occurred.

Local inflammatory and photosensitivity reactions have occurred following topical use. Dermatitis and, rarely, erythema multiforme have been reported.

Effects on the eyes. Systemic fluorouracil therapy has been associated with various types of ocular toxicity including several cases of excessive lachrymation and watering of the eyes,[1] in one patient associated with symptoms suggesting fibrosis of the tear duct,[1] and possibly representing local irritation due to the presence of fluorouracil in tear fluid[2] although symptoms have not always resolved on discontinuing the drug.[1] More seriously a case of bilateral total corneal epithelial erosion has been described.[3] Optic neuropathy, culminating in near blindness, has also occurred in a patient receiving fluorouracil as part of a combination regimen.[4] Severe ulceration and corneal abscess with hyopyon has followed local injection of fluorouracil into the eye in a diabetic patient with idiopathic band keratopathy.[5]

1. Haidak DJ, et al. Tear-duct fibrosis (dacryostenosis) due to 5-fluorouracil. *Ann Intern Med* 1978; **88:** 657.
2. Christophidis N, et al. Lacrimation and 5-fluorouracil. *Ann Intern Med* 1978; **89:** 574.
3. Hirsh A, et al. Bilateral total corneal epithelial erosion as a side effect of cytotoxic therapy. *Br J Ophthalmol* 1990; **74:** 638.
4. Adams JW, et al. Recurrent acute toxic optic neuropathy secondary to 5-FU. *Cancer Treat Rep* 1984; **68:** 565–6.
5. Hickey-Dwyer M, Wishart PK. Serious corneal complication of 5-fluorouracil. *Br J Ophthalmol* 1993; **77:** 250–1.

Effects on the heart. Life-threatening cardiotoxicity (arrhythmias, ventricular tachycardia, and cardiac arrest, secondary to transmural ischaemia) has been reported to occur in 0.55% of patients given fluorouracil,[1] although the incidence of angina and less severe cardiotoxicity associated with coronary artery spasm may be higher.[1-3] Possible risk factors include pre-existing heart disease or mediastinal radiotherapy and administration by prolonged infusion, but symptoms can also occur in patients without these risk factors.[2-4] Therefore, at present, it is not possible to reliably predict patients at risk.[5]

1. Keefe DL, *et al.* Clinical cardiotoxicity of 5-fluorouracil. *J Clin Pharmacol* 1993; **33**: 1060–70.
2. McLachlan SA, *et al.* The spectrum of 5-fluorouracil cardiotoxicity. *Med J Aust* 1994; **161**: 207–9.
3. Anand AJ. Fluorouracil cardiotoxicity. *Ann Pharmacother* 1994; **28**: 374–8.
4. Hannaford R. Sudden death associated with 5-fluorouracil. *Med J Aust* 1994; **161**: 225.
5. Becker K, *et al.* Cardiotoxicity of the antiproliferative compound fluorouracil. *Drugs* 1999; **57**: 475–84.

Effects on the liver. For reference to hepatotoxicity following administration of fluorouracil with sparfosic acid, see p.569.

Effects on the nervous system. Central neurotoxicity, including cerebellar ataxia, confusion, disorientation, and emotional lability is reported to occur rarely in patients receiving fluorouracil, although the incidence may be increased with high-dose or intensive regimens. Patients with disorders of pyrimidine metabolism may be at increased risk of neurotoxicity.[1-3] It has also been suggested that fluorouracil may produce neurotoxicity by causing thiamine deficiency, and that thiamine may be used to treat it.[4]

1. Tuchman M, *et al.* Familial pyrimidinemia and pyrimidinuria associated with severe fluorouracil toxicity. *N Engl J Med* 1985; **313**: 245–9.
2. Stéphan F, *et al.* Depressed hepatic dihydropyrimidine dehydrogenase activity and fluorouracil-related toxicities. *Am J Med* 1995; **99**: 685–8.
3. Takimoto C, *et al.* Reversible 5-fluorouracil-associated encephalopathy in a dihydropyrimidine dehydrogenase (DPD) deficient patient. *Clin Pharmacol Ther* 1996; **59**: 161.
4. Pirzada NA, *et al.* Fluorouracil-induced neurotoxicity. *Ann Pharmacother* 2000; **34**: 35–8.

Effects on the skin. In addition to reports of fluorouracil-associated dermatitis and photosensitivity a syndrome of erythema, pain, and desquamation of the skin of palms and soles has been reported[1,2] (the 'palmar-plantar erythrodysesthesia syndrome'). Although particularly associated with administration by continuous infusion[1,2] the syndrome may also occur following bolus doses.[3,4] Symptoms generally respond to discontinuation of the drug, but addition of oral pyridoxine to chemotherapy regimens has been reported to prevent or resolve symptoms,[5] as has application of a nicotine patch in one patient.[6]

Rash and confusion developing in an elderly man with malabsorption and poor nutritional intake who received fluorouracil for a biliary-tract tumour was diagnosed as pellagra.[7] Symptoms responded to nicotinic acid therapy.

1. Lokich JJ, Moore C. Chemotherapy-associated palmar-plantar erythrodysesthesia syndrome. *Ann Intern Med* 1984; **101**: 798–800.
2. Feldman LD, Ajani JA. Fluorouracil-associated dermatitis of the hands and feet. *JAMA* 1985; **254**: 3479.
3. Atkins JN. Fluorouracil and the palmar-plantar erythrodysesthesia syndrome. *Ann Intern Med* 1985; **102**: 419.
4. Curran CF, Luce JK. Fluorouracil and palmar-plantar erythrodysesthesia. *Ann Intern Med* 1989; **111**: 858.
5. Vukelja SJ, *et al.* Pyridoxine for the palmar-plantar erythrodysesthesia syndrome. *Ann Intern Med* 1989; **111**: 688–9.
6. Kingsley EC. 5-Fluorouracil dermatitis prophylaxis with a nicotine patch. *Ann Intern Med* 1994; **120**: 813.
7. Stevens HP, *et al.* Pellagra secondary to 5-fluorouracil. *Br J Dermatol* 1993; **128**: 578–80.

Precautions

For general discussions see Antineoplastics, p.480. Fluorouracil should be given with care to weak or malnourished patients, to those with a history of heart disease, or to those with hepatic or renal insufficiency. Blood cell counts should be determined frequently during therapy.

Topical fluorouracil should not be used on mucous membranes. There is a possibility of increased absorption if used excessively or on ulcerated or inflamed skin. Occlusive dressings may increase inflammatory actions. Exposure to sunlight during treatment should be avoided.

Handling and disposal. Urine and faeces produced for up to 48 hours and 5 days respectively after an oral dose of fluorouracil should be handled wearing protective clothing.[1]

1. Harris J, Dodds LJ. Handling waste from patients receiving cytotoxic drugs. *Pharm J* 1985; **235**: 289–91.

Metabolic disorders. For reference to increased neurotoxicity in patients with a defect of pyrimidine metabolism given fluorouracil, see under Effects on the Nervous System, above.

Interactions

For a general discussion of antineoplastic drug interactions, see p.481. The actions of fluorouracil may be modified by the concomitant administration of some other drugs including allopurinol, folinic acid, methotrexate, and metronidazole (see also under Administration, below).

Antineoplastics. For reference to the effect of fluorouracil on the action of *paclitaxel*, see Antineoplastics, p.564. For the increased risk of haemolytic-uraemic syndrome that may be seen if fluorouracil is used with *mitomycin*, see Effects on the Kidneys, p.558.

Antiprotozoals. *Metronidazole* increased the toxicity of fluorouracil in patients with colorectal cancer, apparently by reducing the clearance of the antineoplastic. No enhanced antineoplastic effect was seen with the combination *in vitro*.[1]

1. Bardakji Z, *et al.* 5-Fluorouracil–metronidazole combination therapy in metastatic colorectal cancer. *Cancer Chemother Pharmacol* 1986; **18**: 140–4.

Antivirals. Co-administration of *interferon alfa-2b* with fluorouracil has been reported to produce a marked increase in the initial plasma concentration of fluorouracil and a decrease in fluorouracil clearance.[1]

Severe leucopenia, leading to death in some cases, has been reported in patients who received fluorouracil or fluorouracil prodrugs (such as tegafur) with *sorivudine*, an antiviral developed for herpes zoster.[2,3] A metabolite of sorivudine appears to inhibit dihydropyrimidine dehydrogenase, the primary enzyme responsible for the inactivation of fluorouracil.[3]

1. Czejka MJ, *et al.* Clinical pharmacokinetics of 5-fluorouracil: influence of the biomodulating agents interferon, dipyridamole and folic acid alone and in combination. *Arzneimittelforschung* 1993; **43**: 387–90.
2. Yawata M. Deaths due to drug interaction. *Lancet* 1993; **342**: 1166.
3. Diasio RB. Sorivudine and 5-fluorouracil; a clinically significant drug-drug interaction due to inhibition of dihydropyrimidine dehydrogenase. *Br J Clin Pharmacol* 1998; **46**: 1–4.

Gastrointestinal drugs. Pretreatment with *cimetidine* for 4 weeks led to increased plasma concentrations of fluorouracil following intravenous and oral administration in 6 patients.[1] The effect was probably due to a combination of hepatic enzyme inhibition and reduced hepatic blood flow. No such effect was seen following single doses of cimetidine in 5 patients or pretreatment for just 1 week in 6. Care is required in patients taking both drugs simultaneously.

1. Harvey VJ, *et al.* The influence of cimetidine on the pharmacokinetics of 5-fluorouracil. *Br J Clin Pharmacol* 1984; **18**: 421–30.

Pharmacokinetics

Absorption of fluorouracil from the gastrointestinal tract is unpredictable and fluorouracil is usually given intravenously. Little is absorbed when fluorouracil is applied to healthy skin.

After intravenous injection fluorouracil is cleared rapidly from plasma with a mean half-life of about 16 minutes. It is distributed throughout body tissues and fluids including crossing the blood-brain barrier to appear in the cerebrospinal fluid, and disappears from the plasma within about 3 hours. Within the target cell fluorouracil is converted to 5-fluorouridine monophosphate and floxuridine monophosphate (5-fluorodeoxyuridine monophosphate), the former undergoing conversion to the triphosphate which can be incorporated into RNA while the latter inhibits thymidylate synthetase. About 15% of an intravenous dose is excreted unchanged in the urine within 6 hours. The remainder is inactivated primarily in the liver and is catabolised via dihydropyrimidine dehydrogenase similarly to endogenous uracil. A large amount is excreted as respiratory carbon dioxide; urea and other metabolites are also produced.

◊ The plasma concentrations of fluorouracil during continuous intravenous infusion are reported to undergo circadian variations of as much as 50% of the mean, peak concentrations occurring in the middle of the night.[1] The variation may be due to a circadian variation in the activity of the enzyme dihydropyrimidine dehydrogenase in blood,[2] but striking interpatient variations in peak concentrations of fluorouracil and peak enzyme activity suggest that any adjustment of infusion times would need to be individualised.[2] It has been suggested that pharmacokinetic monitoring should be investigated as a means of individualizing fluorouracil doses with the aim of improving efficacy and reducing toxicity.[3]

1. Petit E, *et al.* Circadian rhythm-varying plasma concentration of 5-fluorouracil during a five-day continuous venous infusion at a constant rate in cancer patients. *Cancer Res* 1988; **48**: 1676–9.
2. Harris BE, *et al.* Relationship between dihydropyrimidine dehydrogenase activity and plasma 5-fluorouracil levels with evidence for circadian variation of enzyme activity and plasma drug levels in cancer patients receiving 5-fluorouracil by protracted continuous infusion. *Cancer Res* 1990; **50**: 197–201.
3. Young AM, *et al.* Can pharmacokinetic monitoring improve clinical use of fluorouracil? *Clin Pharmacokinet* 1999; **36**: 391–8.

Uses and Administration

Fluorouracil, a pyrimidine analogue, is an antineoplastic that acts as an antimetabolite to uracil. After intracellular conversion to the active deoxynucleotide it interferes with the synthesis of DNA by blocking the conversion of deoxyuridylic acid to thymidylic acid by the cellular enzyme thymidylate synthetase. It can also interfere with RNA synthesis.

Fluorouracil is used alone or in combination in the adjuvant and palliative treatment of gastrointestinal cancer. In this setting it may be combined with folinic acid (see Administration, below). Fluorouracil is often used with cyclophosphamide and methotrexate or doxorubicin in the adjuvant treatment of breast cancer. It may also be used in the palliation of other malignant neoplasms such as those of the head and neck, liver, and pancreas. In addition, it may be used topically for treating malignant or premalignant lesions of the skin. Its use in these malignancies is further discussed under Choice of Antineoplastic as indicated by the cross-references given below.

A wide range of dosage regimens has been used. Although it is most often given in combination regimens for the treatment of malignancy many of the licensed dosage regimens relate to single-agent use. Such licensed regimens include:

• by *intravenous injection*, usual doses of 12 mg per kg body-weight daily (to a maximum of 0.8 to 1 g daily) for 3 or 4 days. If there is no evidence of toxicity, this may be followed after 1 day by 6 mg per kg on alternate days for 3 or 4 further doses. An alternative schedule is to give 15 mg per kg intravenously once a week throughout the course. The course may be repeated after 4 to 6 weeks or maintenance doses of 5 to 15 mg per kg may be given weekly.

• by *intravenous infusion*, usual doses of 15 mg per kg daily (to a maximum of 1 g daily) being infused in 500 mL of sodium chloride 0.9% or glucose 5% over 4 hours and repeated on successive days until toxicity occurs or a total of 12 to 15 g has been given. *Continuous infusion* may also be used. The course may be repeated after 4 to 6 weeks.

• by continuous *intra-arterial infusion*, in doses of 5 to 7.5 mg per kg daily (regional perfusion).

• by *mouth*, although the parenteral route is generally preferred a dose of 15 mg per kg, to a maximum of 1 g, has been given once weekly for maintenance.

A variety of regimens have also been used in combination with folinic acid. One suggested regimen is 200 mg per m² body-surface of folinic acid (as calcium folinate) by slow intravenous injection followed immediately by an intravenous bolus of fluorouracil 370 mg per m²; the treatment is given daily for 5 consecutive days, and may be repeated after 21 to 28 days. Lower doses of folinic acid (20 mg per m²) followed by fluorouracil 425 mg per m² for 5 consecutive days, repeated every 4 to 5 weeks (the Mayo regimen) has also been used. A third, widely-used protocol (the de Gramont regimen) employs an initial dose of 200 mg per m² of folinic acid, followed by fluorouracil 400 mg per m² as an initial intravenous bolus injection and then 600 mg per m² by continuous intravenous infusion. This dosage is given for 2 consecutive days every 2 weeks.

The white cell count should be determined frequently during treatment with fluorouracil and therapy stopped immediately if the count falls rapidly or falls to below 3500 per mm³, if the platelet count falls below 100 000 per mm³, or if severe adverse effects occur. Doses should be reduced by up to half in patients with poor nutritional status, impaired bone-marrow, hepatic, or renal function, and within 30 days of major surgery.

Fluorouracil is used topically in the treatment of solar (actinic) keratoses and other superficial tumours and premalignant conditions of the skin including Bowen's disease and superficial basal cell carcinomas. For actinic keratosis it is usually applied as a 1 or 5% cream or as a 1 to 5% solution in propylene glycol once or twice daily for 2 to 4 weeks; the higher strength may be applied for at least 3 to 6 weeks for superficial basal cell carcinomas.

Therapeutic implants containing fluorouracil in a controlled-release protein matrix have been investigated. Such a preparation, comprising fluorouracil 3% in a collagen gel basis, together with adrenaline [epinephrine] to enhance local retention, has been used for the treatment of condylomata acuminata (genital warts) by intralesional intradermal injection.

Administration. Modulation of fluorouracil by various drugs has been tried in an effort to enhance its effects, particularly in the treatment of colorectal cancer (p.493). Examples of modulators used include folinic acid, interferon alfa, levamisole, and methotrexate.

Folinic acid has been extensively used to modulate the effects of fluorouracil, and has become the agent of choice. Various regimens have been used, modifying the fluorouracil schedule (continuous infusion versus bolus), folinic acid dose (low-dose versus high-dose) and the regimen frequency (monthly, bi-monthly, or weekly). Despite numerous studies, the optimum regimen in terms of efficacy and tolerability has yet to be determined. In the adjuvant setting, a recent large-scale randomised trial[1] found no difference in efficacy between low-dose and high-dose folinic acid when added to fluorouracil administered either once weekly for 30 doses, or for 5 consecutive days per month over 6 months. Fluorouracil and low-dose folinic acid may therefore become the preferred regimen in the adjuvant setting. In the palliation of advanced disease, meta-analyses have revealed the value of the addition of folinic acid to fluorouracil,[2] and the use of infusions rather than bolus fluorouracil,[3] in terms of response rates. However, the data for low-dose folinic acid versus high-dose are less clear.[4] In 1 randomised trial,[5] a bimonthly infusion regimen of fluorouracil plus high-dose folinic acid (the de Gramont regimen[6]) was more effective than a monthly bolus regimen of fluorouracil plus low-dose folinic acid. Further studies comparing the effect of high- and low-dose folinic acid added to the same schedule of continuous infusion fluorouracil are required.

Interferon alfa also appears to modify the actions of fluorouracil (see also under Interactions, above), and has been investigated in combination with fluorouracil and folinic acid. Although some early results were promising, recent randomised controlled trials have failed to show any benefit for the addition of interferon alfa to fluorouracil or fluorouracil plus folinic acid.[7] It is not clear whether interferon beta will prove of any greater benefit.

Based on the results of early adjuvant trials, *levamisole* was used as standard therapy to modulate fluorouracil, particularly in the USA. However, more recent trials indicate that levamisole is no more effective than placebo when added to fluorouracil,[1] or to fluorouracil plus folinic acid.[8]

Methotrexate has also been used to modulate fluorouracil. Meta-analysis of several studies of fluorouracil preceded by methotrexate found that the combination doubled the response rate to fluorouracil in metastatic colorectal cancer and produced some survival benefits.[9] (Combination in the reverse order, i.e. methotrexate preceded by fluorouracil, may reduce methotrexate toxicity—see under Treatment of Adverse Effects, p.554.)

1. QUASAR Collaborative Group. Comparison of fluorouracil with additional levamisole, higher-dose folinic acid, or both, as adjuvant chemotherapy for colorectal cancer: a randomised trial. *Lancet* 2000; **355:** 1588–96.
2. Advanced Colorectal Cancer Meta-analysis Project. Modulation of fluorouracil by leucovorin in patients with advanced colorectal cancer: evidence in terms of response rate. *J Clin Oncol* 1992; **10:** 896–903.
3. Meta-analysis Group in Cancer. Efficacy of intravenous continuous infusion of fluorouracil compared with bolus administration in advanced colorectal cancer. *J Clin Oncol* 1998; **16:** 301–8.
4. Rustum YM, et al. Rationale for treatment design: biochemical modulation of 5-fluorouracil by leucovorin. *Cancer J Sci Am* 1998; **4:** 12–18.
5. de Gramont A, et al. Randomized trial comparing monthly low-dose leucovorin and fluorouracil bolus with bimonthly high-dose leucovorin and fluorouracil bolus plus continuous infusion for advanced colorectal cancer: a French Intergroup study. *J Clin Oncol* 1997; **15:** 808–15.
6. de Gramont A, et al. A review of GERCOD trials of bimonthly leucovorin plus 5-fluorouracil 48-h continuous infusion in advanced colorectal cancer: evolution of a regimen. *Eur J Cancer* 1998; **34:** 619–26.
7. Makower D, Wadler S. Interferons as biomodulators of fluoropyrimidines in the treatment of colorectal cancer. *Semin Oncol* 1999; **26:** 663–71.
8. Wolmark N, et al. Clinical trial to assess the relative efficacy of fluorouracil and leucovorin, fluorouracil and levamisole, and fluorouracil, leucovorin, and levamisole in patients with Dukes' B and C carcinoma of the colon: results from National Surgical Adjuvant Breast and Bowel Project C-04. *J Clin Oncol* 1999; **17:** 3553–9.
9. Advanced Colorectal Cancer Meta-analysis Project. Meta-analysis of randomized trials testing the biochemical modulation of fluorouracil by methotrexate in metastatic colorectal cancer. *J Clin Oncol* 1994; **12:** 960–9.

Darier's disease. Two patients with resistant Darier's disease (p.1104) receiving long-term oral retinoid therapy responded to treatment with topical fluorouracil applied as a 1% cream once daily.[1] There was complete clearance of skin lesions after 3 weeks of treatment.

1. Knulst AC, et al. Topical 5-fluorouracil in the treatment of Darier's disease. *Br J Dermatol* 1995; **133:** 463–6.

Glaucoma. A regimen of subconjunctival injections of fluorouracil is effective in improving the outcome of glaucoma filtering surgery[1-3] in selected patients when used as an adjunct to prevent the formation of scar tissue (see p.1413). However, in view of the increased risk of late-onset conjunctival wound leaks caution has been suggested in its use in eyes with a good

prognosis.[3] Although one study[4] found that fluorouracil improved the success rate of combined glaucoma filtering surgery and cataract surgery earlier studies had failed to demonstrate any advantage.[5,6] A meta-analysis[7] of these and 2 other studies concluded that fluorouracil reduced the risk of surgical failure of trabeculectomy in eyes at high risk of failure, and in those undergoing surgery for the first time, but noted that the methodological quality of the studies was not high, and that this practice has largely been superseded by the use of intra-operative mitomycin.

Intraoperative topical application of fluorouracil has been tried as an alternative to subconjunctival injection with conflicting results.[8,9]

1. Ophir A, Ticho U. A randomized study of trabeculectomy and subconjunctival administration of fluorouracil in primary glaucomas. *Arch Ophthalmol* 1992; **110:** 1072–5.
2. Goldenfeld M, et al. 5-Fluorouracil in initial trabeculectomy: a prospective, randomized, multicenter study. *Ophthalmology* 1994; **101:** 1024–9.
3. The Fluorouracil Filtering Surgery Study Group. Five-year follow-up of the Fluorouracil Filtering Surgery Study. *Am J Ophthalmol* 1996; **121:** 349–66.
4. Gandolfi SA, Vecchi M. 5-Fluorouracil in combined trabeculectomy and clear-cornea phacoemulsification with posterior chamber intraocular lens implantation: a one-year randomized, controlled clinical trial. *Ophthalmology* 1997; **104:** 181–6.
5. Wong PC, et al. 5-Fluorouracil after primary combined filtration surgery. *Am J Ophthalmol* 1994; **117:** 149–54.
6. O'Grady JM, et al. Trabeculectomy, phacoemulsification, and posterior chamber lens implantation with and without 5-fluorouracil. *Am J Ophthalmol* 1993; **116:** 594–9.
7. Wormald R, et al. Post-operative 5-fluorouracil for glaucoma surgery (updated 30 May 2001). Available in The Cochrane Library; Issue 4. Oxford: Update Software, 2001.
8. Egbert PR, et al. A prospective trial of intraoperative fluorouracil during trabeculectomy in a black population. *Am J Ophthalmol* 1993; **116:** 612–16.
9. Lachkar Y, et al. Trabeculectomy with intraoperative sponge 5-fluorouracil in Afro-Caribbeans. *Br J Ophthalmol* 1997; **81:** 555–8.

Malignant neoplasms. Fluorouracil plays an important role in the adjuvant treatment of gastrointestinal cancer, as discussed on p.493, and is widely used in adjuvant regimens for early breast cancer (p.491). It may also be employed in the management of a wide variety of other malignancies including pancreatic endocrine tumours (p.483), cancers of the cervix (p.492) and head and neck (p.494), liver metastases (p.495), and tumours of the exocrine pancreas (p.497). In addition, it is sometimes applied topically as part of the management of malignant or pre-malignant lesions of the skin (p.498), or surface neoplasia of the eye (p.493).

Toxoplasmosis. For mention of the use of fluorouracil with clindamycin to treat cerebral toxoplasmosis, see p.585.

Warts. Fluorouracil has been used, as a 1% or, more usually, a 5% cream or solution in the treatment of genital warts (condylomata acuminata),[1-4] and has been tried as an adjuvant to laser therapy in severe papillomavirus-associated vulvar disease,[5] with variable results. A preparation of fluorouracil 3% in a collagen gel base, together with adrenaline [epinephrine] as a local vasoconstrictor, has been tried by injection into genital warts.[6] For a discussion of the various agents, including cytotoxics such as fluorouracil employed to produce destruction of warts, see p.1108.

1. Adler MW, Mindel A. Genital infections. *Br Med Bull* 1985; **41:** 361–6.
2. Anonymous. Interferon for treatment of genital warts. *Med Lett Drugs Ther* 1988; **30:** 70–2.
3. Davis AJ, Emans SJ. Human papilloma virus infection in the pediatric and adolescent patient. *J Pediatr* 1989; **115:** 1–9.
4. Pride GL. Treatment of large lower genital tract condylomata acuminata with topical 5-fluorouracil. *J Reprod Med* 1990; **35:** 384–7.
5. Reid R, et al. Superficial laser vulvectomy IV: extended laser vaporization and adjunctive 5-fluorouracil therapy of human papillomavirus-associated vulvar disease. *Obstet Gynecol* 1990; **76:** 439–48.
6. Anonymous. Injectable gel for genital warts. *Pharm J* 1996; **257:** 13.

Preparations

BP 2001: Fluorouracil Cream; Fluorouracil Injection;
USP 25: Fluorouracil Cream; Fluorouracil Injection; Fluorouracil Topical Solution.

Proprietary Preparations (details are given in Part 3)

Austral.: Efudix; Fluoroplex; *Belg.:* Efudix; Fluroblastine; *Canad.:* Adrucil; Efudex; Fluoroplex†; *Denm.:* Flurablastin; *Fin.:* Flurablastin; *Fr.:* Efudix; *Ger.:* Actino-Hermal; Efudix; Fluroblastin; O-fluor; Ribofluor; *Irl.:* Efudix; *Israel:* Efudix; Fluracedyl; *Ital.:* Efudix; *Mex.:* Efudix; Fiverocil; Flurox; Rhonuracil; *Neth.:* Efudix†; *Norw.:* Flurablastin; Fluracedyl; *NZ:* Efudix; *Port.:* Cinkef-U; *S.Afr.:* Efudix; Fluroblastin; *Singapore:* Efudix; *Spain:* Efudix; *Swed.:* Flurablastin; Fluracedyl; *Switz.:* Efudix; *Thai.:* Efudix; Fivoflu; *UK:* AccuSite†; Efudix; Fluoroplex; *USA:* Adrucil; Efudex; Fluoroplex.

Multi-ingredient: *Braz.:* Efurix; *Ger.:* Verrumal; *Hong Kong:* Verrumal; *Israel:* Verrumal; Verucid; *Port.:* Verrucare; Verrumal; *Singapore:* Verrumal; *Switz.:* Verrumal; *Thai.:* Verrumal.

Flutamide (9050-b)

Flutamide (*BAN, USAN, rINN*).
Flutamidum; Sch-13521. α′,α′,α′-Trifluoro-4′-nitroisobutyro-*m*-toluidide; α,α,α-Trifluoro-2-methyl-4′-nitro-*m*-propionotoluidide.
$C_{11}H_{11}F_3N_2O_3 = 276.2$.
CAS — 13311-84-7.
ATC — L02BB01.
Pharmacopoeias. In Eur. (see p.vi) and US.

Pharmacopoeial description

Ph. Eur.: A pale yellow, crystalline powder. Practically insoluble in water; freely soluble in alcohol and in acetone. Protect from light.

USP 25: A pale yellow, crystalline powder. Practically insoluble in water, in liquid paraffin, and in petroleum spirit; freely soluble in acetone, in ethyl acetate, and in methyl alcohol; soluble in chloroform and in ether. Store in airtight containers. Protect from light.

Adverse Effects and Precautions

The most frequently reported adverse effects with flutamide are reversible gynaecomastia or breast tenderness, sometimes accompanied by galactorrhoea. Nausea, vomiting, diarrhoea, increased appetite, and sleep disturbances may occur. There have been reports of skin reactions, including epidermal necrolysis, and of liver damage, sometimes fatal. Other adverse effects reported in patients receiving flutamide include anaemias, haemolysis, headache, dizziness, malaise, blurred vision, anxiety, depression, decreased libido, discoloration of urine, and hypertension.

Flutamide should be used with care in patients with cardiovascular disease because of the possibility of fluid retention. Regular liver function testing is recommended in all patients: therapy should be discontinued or dosage reduced if there is evidence of hepatotoxicity.

Effects on the blood. A report of methaemoglobinaemia attributed to flutamide.[1]

1. Schott AM, et al. Flutamide-induced methemoglobinemia. *DICP Ann Pharmacother* 1991; **25:** 600–1.

Effects on the liver. Hepatitis occurred in a 79-year-old man receiving flutamide 750 mg daily as sole therapy following a prostatectomy,[1] but a subsequent study[2] in 1091 patients receiving flutamide 250 mg three times daily as part of a regimen for prostate cancer found marked signs of liver damage only in 4, of whom only 2 had clinical evidence of liver toxicity. In the USA, the FDA had received reports of 46 patients with hepatotoxicity associated with flutamide up to December 1994. Of these patients, 20 died from progressive liver disease.[3]

1. Hart W, Stricker BHC. Flutamide and hepatitis. *Ann Intern Med* 1989; **110:** 943–4.
2. Gomez J-L, et al. Incidence of liver toxicity associated with the use of flutamide in prostate cancer patients. *Am J Med* 1992; **92:** 465–70.
3. Wysowski DK, Fourcroy JL. Flutamide hepatotoxicity. *J Urol (Baltimore)* 1996; **155:** 209–12. Correction ibid: 396.

Effects on the skin. A report of photosensitivity reactions in 2 patients receiving flutamide.[1]

1. Fujimoto M, et al. Photosensitive dermatitis induced by flutamide. *Br J Dermatol* 1996; **135:** 496–7.

Interactions

Flutamide may increase the effect of warfarin, see Antineoplastics, p.995. For a general outline of antineoplastic drug interactions see p.481.

Pharmacokinetics

Flutamide is reported to be rapidly and completely absorbed from the gastrointestinal tract with peak plasma concentrations occurring 1 hour after a dose. It is rapidly and extensively metabolised; the major metabolite (2-hydroxyflutamide) possesses anti-androgenic properties. The half-life of the metabolite is about 6 hours. Both flutamide and 2-hydroxyflutamide are more than 90% bound to plasma proteins. Excretion is predominantly in the urine with only minor amounts appearing in the faeces.

◊ References.

1. Radwanski E, et al. Single and multiple dose pharmacokinetic evaluation of flutamide in normal geriatric volunteers. *J Clin Pharmacol* 1989; **29:** 554–8.

Uses and Administration

Flutamide is a nonsteroidal compound with anti-androgenic properties which appears to act by inhibiting the uptake and/or binding of androgens in target tissues. It is used, usually in combination with gonadorelin analogues, in the palliative treatment of prostatic carcinoma (p.497). The usual dose by mouth is 250 mg three times daily. When used in combination therapy the UK manufacturers recommend that flutamide treatment be started at least 3 days before the gonadorelin analogue to suppress any 'flare' reaction; however, in the USA the manufacturers recommend beginning treatment with both agents simultaneously for optimum effect.

Congenital adrenal hyperplasia. For mention of the use of flutamide with testolactone to block androgenic effects in congenital adrenal hyperplasia, see p.1049.

Hirsutism. Anti-androgens (usually cyproterone or spironolactone) are widely used for the drug treatment of hirsutism (p.1468). Flutamide has no particular advantage in this context;[1,2] one study has found flutamide to be more effective than spironolactone in inhibiting hirsutism,[3] but another found them to be of similar efficacy,[4] and the risk of hepatotoxicity with flutamide is a problem.[2]

1. Rittmaster RS. Hyperandrogenism—what is normal? *N Engl J Med* 1992; **327**: 194–6.
2. Rittmaster RS. Hirsutism. *Lancet* 1997; **349**: 191–5.
3. Cusan L, *et al.* Comparison of flutamide and spironolactone in the treatment of hirsutism: a randomized controlled trial. *Fertil Steril* 1994; **61**: 281–7.
4. Erenus M, *et al.* Comparison of the efficacy of spironolactone versus flutamide in the treatment of hirsutism. *Fertil Steril* 1994; **61**: 613–6.

Malignant neoplasms. Androgen blockade, which may include the use of flutamide, is used in the management of metastatic hormone-responsive prostate cancer (p.497); once the cancer begins to progress despite such therapy, discontinuation of flutamide occasionally produces paradoxical disease regression. Promising preliminary results have also followed the use of flutamide in patients with adenocarcinoma of the pancreas (p.497).

Preparations
USP 25: Flutamide Capsules.

Proprietary Preparations (details are given in Part 3)
Aust.: Flutabene; Fugerel; *Austral.:* Eulexin; Flutamin; Fugerel; *Belg.:* Eulexin; Flutaplex; *Braz.:* Eulexin; Tecnoflut; *Canad.:* Euflex; *Denm.:* Eulexin; Flutacan; Flutaplex; Profamid; *Fin.:* Eulexin; Profamid; *Fr.:* Eulexine; Prostadirex; *Ger.:* Apimid; Flumid; Fluta; Fluta-cell; Fluta-Gry; Flutamex; Fugerel; Prostica; Prostogenat; Testac†; Testotard; *Hong Kong:* Flutan; Fugerel; *Irl.:* Drogenil; *Israel:* Eulexin; *Ital.:* Drogenil; Eulexin; *Mex.:* Eulexin; Fluken; Flulem; Tafenil; *Neth.:* Drogenil; Eulexin; *Norw.:* Eulexin; *NZ:* Eulexin; Flutamin; Flutol; *Port.:* Draxon; Eulexin; *S.Afr.:* Eulexin; *Singapore:* Fugerel; *Spain:* Eulexin; Grisetin; Oncosal; Prostacur; *Swed.:* Eulexin; Flutacan; *Switz.:* Flucinome; *Thai.:* Flutan; Fugerel; *UK:* Chimax; Drogenil; *USA:* Eulexin.

Formestane   (19307-g)

Formestane *(BAN, rINN)*.
CGP-32349; 4-Hydroxyandrostenedione; 4-OHA; 4-OHAD. 4-Hydroxyandrost-4-ene-3,17-dione.
$C_{19}H_{26}O_3 = 302.4$.
CAS — 566-48-3.
ATC — L02BG02.

Adverse Effects, Treatment, and Precautions
The most frequent adverse effects of formestane are local irritation and pain at the site of injection. Patients may experience hot flushes due to oestrogen deprivation. Other occasional or rare adverse effects include rashes and pruritus, alopecia or hypertrichosis, drowsiness, dizziness, emotional lability, oedema of the leg, thrombophlebitis, vaginal spotting or bleeding, gastrointestinal disturbances, pelvic or muscle cramps, arthralgia, exacerbation of bone pain, and a vasovagal reaction. Hypersensitivity reactions to the drug or the formulation have occurred.

Care should be taken to avoid intravascular injection. Injection into or near the sciatic nerve may result in pain and nerve trauma. Caution is required if patients drive or operate machinery.

Effects on carbohydrate metabolism. Recurrent hypoglycaemic episodes developed in a diabetic patient previously well maintained on gliclazide following addition of formestane to treatment for metastatic breast cancer.[1] Episodic hypoglycaemia continued following dosage reduction, and eventually withdrawal, of gliclazide, suggesting that the effect was not simply an interaction with the sulfonylurea.

1. Brankin E, *et al.* Hypoglycaemia associated with formestane treatment. *BMJ* 1997; **314**: 869.

Pharmacokinetics
Following intramuscular administration formestane is reported to form a depot which slowly releases active drug into the systemic circulation; maximum plasma concentrations occur about 30 to 48 hours after a single dose and then decline fairly rapidly over 2 to 4 days before declining more slowly, with an apparent elimination half-life of 5 to 6 days. The systemic uptake has been estimated at 20 to 25% of the dose in 14 days. Formestane is about 85% bound to plasma protein in the circulation. It is metabolised by conjugation to the inactive glucuronide: less than 1% of the dose is excreted in urine unchanged.

Uses and Administration
Formestane is an inhibitor of the aromatase (oestrogen synthetase) system which is responsible for the production of oestrogens from androgens. It is used for its anti-oestrogenic properties in the endocrine treatment of advanced breast cancer in postmenopausal women (p.491).

It is given by intramuscular injection, as an aqueous suspension, in doses of 250 mg every 2 weeks. Injections should be given into each buttock alternately.

◊ Reviews.
1. Wiseman LR, McTavish D. Formestane: a review of its pharmacodynamic and pharmacokinetic properties and therapeutic potential in the management of breast cancer and prostatic cancer. *Drugs* 1993; **45**: 66–84.
2. Anonymous. Formestane for advanced breast cancer in postmenopausal women. *Drug Ther Bull* 1993; **31**: 85–7.

Preparations
Proprietary Preparations (details are given in Part 3)
Aust.: Lentaron; *Belg.:* Lentaron†; *Canad.:* Lentaron†; *Denm.:* Lentaron; *Fr.:* Lentaron; *Ger.:* Lentaron; *Hong Kong:* Lentaron; *Irl.:* Lentaron; *Israel:* Lentaron; *Ital.:* Lentaron; *Neth.:* Lentaron; *Port.:* Lentaron; *S.Afr.:* Lentare; *Spain:* Lentaron; *Switz.:* Lentaron; *UK:* Lentaron†.

Fotemustine   (3682-e)

Fotemustine *(BAN, rINN)*.
S-10036.   (±)-Diethyl {1-[3-(2-chloroethyl)-3-nitrosoureido]ethyl}phosphonate.
$C_9H_{19}ClN_3O_5P = 315.7$.
CAS — 92118-27-9.
ATC — L01AD05.

Profile
Fotemustine is a nitrosourea derivative (see Carmustine, p.516). It is used in the treatment of disseminated malignant melanoma, particularly where cerebral metastases are present (p.499) and has been tried in primary malignancies of the brain (p.490). It is given by intravenous infusion in usual doses of 100 mg per m² body-surface weekly for 3 weeks to induce remission, followed after 4 to 6 weeks, if blood counts permit, by maintenance dosage with 100 mg per m² every 3 weeks. Liver function should be monitored regularly during induction treatment. Regular blood counts should be taken and treatment withheld if granulocyte counts are below 2000 per mm³ or platelet counts less than 100 000 per mm³. Bone-marrow suppression may be delayed, with the nadir of the white cell counts 5 or 6 weeks after administration. Solutions for infusion must be freshly prepared and protected from light.

◊ References.
1. Pujol JL, *et al.* Phase II study of nitrosourea fotemustine as single-drug chemotherapy in poor-prognosis non-small-cell lung cancer. *Br J Cancer* 1994; **69**: 1136–40.
2. Kleeberg UR, *et al.* Palliative therapy of melanoma patients with fotemustine: inverse relationship between tumour load and treatment effectiveness. A multicentre phase II trial of the EORTC-Melanoma Cooperative Group (MCG). *Melanoma Res* 1995; **5**: 195–200.
3. Rougier P, *et al.* Fotemustine in patients with advanced gastric cancer, a phase II trial from the EORTC-GITCCG. *Eur J Cancer* 1996; **32A**: 1432–3.
4. Pontes L, *et al.* Isolated limb perfusion with fotemustine after chemosensitization with dacarbazine in melanoma. *Melanoma Res* 1997; **7**: 417–9.
5. Mohr P, *et al.* Combined treatment of stage IV melanoma patients with amifostine and fotemustine—a pilot study. *Melanoma Res* 1998; **8**: 166–9.
6. Marzolini C, *et al.* Pharmacokinetics of temozolomide in association with fotemustine in malignant melanoma and malignant glioma patients: comparison of oral, intravenous, and hepatic intra-arterial administration. *Cancer Chemother Pharmacol* 1998; **42**: 433–40.

Preparations
Proprietary Preparations (details are given in Part 3)
Aust.: Muphoran; *Austral.:* Muphoran; *Fr.:* Muphoran; *Hong Kong:* Muphoran; *Israel:* Muphoran.

Fulvestrant   (11817-w)

Fulvestrant *(BAN, USAN, rINN)*.
ICI-182780; ZD-9238. 7α-[9-(4,4,5,5,5-Pentafluoropentylsulfinyl)nonyl]estra-1,3,5(10)-triene-3,17β-diol.
$C_{32}H_{47}F_5O_3S = 606.8$.
CAS — 129453-61-8.

Profile
Fulvestrant is an oestrogen antagonist that is under investigation for the treatment of advanced breast cancer.

◊ References.
1. Howell A, *et al.* ICI 182,780 (Faslodex): development of a novel, pure antioestrogen. *Cancer* 2000; **89**: 817–25.
2. Curran M, Wiseman L. Fulvestrant. *Drugs* 2001; **61**: 807–13.

Gemcitabine Hydrochloride   (12197-g)

Gemcitabine Hydrochloride *(BANM, USAN, rINNM)*.
LY-188011 (gemcitabine). 4-Amino-1-(2-deoxy-2,2-difluoro-β-D-ribofuranosyl)pyrimidin-2(1H)-one hydrochloride; 2′-Deoxy-2′,2′-difluorocytidine hydrochloride.
$C_9H_{11}F_2N_3O_4$,HCl = 299.7.
CAS — 95058-81-4 (gemcitabine); 122111-03-9 (gemcitabine hydrochloride).

Gemcitabine hydrochloride 1.14 mg is approximately equivalent to 1 mg of gemcitabine.

Adverse Effects, Treatment, and Precautions
As for Cytarabine, p.530; myelotoxicity is, however, reported to be modest even at high doses, although rashes and influenza-like symptoms are relatively common. Oedema (including pulmonary oedema), hypotension, dyspnoea, and alopecia have also been reported. Gemcitabine may produce somnolence: patients so affected should not drive or operate machinery. Severe toxicity, in the form of potentially life-threatening oesophagitis and pneumonitis has been seen in patients given radical radiotherapy to the thorax in association with gemcitabine. It should be used with caution in patients with impaired renal or hepatic function. Haemolytic-uraemic syndrome has been reported and has led to irreversible renal failure; gemcitabine should be discontinued at the first signs of microangiopathic haemolytic anaemia.

Effects on the nervous system. A report of autonomic neuropathy associated with gemcitabine therapy.[1] Symptoms resolved 4 weeks after stopping therapy.
1. Dormann AJ, *et al.* Gemcitabine-associated autonomic neuropathy. *Lancet* 1998; **351**: 644.

Pharmacokinetics
Following intravenous administration gemcitabine is rapidly cleared from the blood and metabolised by cytidine deaminase in the liver, kidney, blood, and other tissues. Clearance is approximately 30% lower in women than in men. Almost all of the dose is excreted in urine as 2′-deoxy-2′,2′-difluorouridine (dFdU), only about 1% being found in the faeces. Intracellular metabolism produces mono-, di-, and triphosphate metabolites, the latter two active. The half-life of gemcitabine ranges from 42 to 94 minutes depending on age or gender. The intracellular half-life of the triphosphate is stated to range from 0.7 to 12 hours.

◊ References.
1. Johnson SA. Clinical pharmacokinetics of nucleoside analogues: focus on haematological malignancies. *Clin Pharmacokinet* 2000; **39**: 5–26.

Uses and Administration
Gemcitabine is an analogue of cytarabine (p.530) which is metabolised intracellularly to active diphosphate and triphosphate nucleosides, which inhibit DNA synthesis and induce apoptosis. It is primarily active against cells in S-phase. It is given in the management of solid tumours including those of the bladder, lung, and pancreas (see p.490, p.496, and p.497, respectively). It is also being tried in cancers of the breast, cervix, and ovary.

Gemcitabine is given intravenously as the hydrochloride; doses are calculated in terms of the base. Doses are reconstituted in sodium chloride 0.9% injection. The concentration of the infusion solution should not exceed the equivalent of 40 mg of gemcitabine per mL. The recommended initial dose is the equivalent of 1 g of gemcitabine per m^2 body-surface, by infusion over 30 minutes. The dose may be repeated at weekly intervals adjusted according to response and toxicity.

In the treatment of pancreatic cancer, an initial course of up to 7 doses at weekly intervals may be given, followed after a one-week recovery period by a regimen of infusions once weekly for 3 consecutive weeks out of 4.

In the treatment of non-small cell lung cancer and bladder cancer, gemcitabine is usually given in combination with cisplatin. The recommended dose of gemcitabine above is given once weekly for 3 weeks, followed by a one-week rest period. Alternatively the equivalent of 1.25 g of gemcitabine per m^2 may be administered on days 1 and 8 of a 21-day cycle to patients with lung cancer. Doses are adjusted according to toxicity.

◊ References.
1. Michael M, Moore M. Clinical experience with gemcitabine in pancreatic carcinoma. *Oncology (Huntingt)* 1997; **11:** 1615–22.
2. Hui YF, Reitz J. Gemcitabine: a cytidine analogue active against solid tumors. *Am J Health-Syst Pharm* 1997; **54:** 162–70.
3. Noble S, Goa KL. Gemcitabine: a review of its pharmacology and clinical potential in non-small cell lung cancer and pancreatic cancer. *Drugs* 1997; **54:** 447–72.
4. Rosell R, *et al.* The activity of gemcitabine plus cisplatin in randomized trials in untreated patients with advanced non-small cell lung cancer. *Semin Oncol* 1998; **25:** (suppl 9): 27–34.
5. Thomas A, Steward WP. Gemcitabine: a major advance? *Ann Oncol* 1998; **9:** 1265–7.

Preparations

Proprietary Preparations (details are given in Part 3)
Aust.: Gemzar; *Austral.:* Gemzar; *Belg.:* Gemzar; *Canad.:* Gemzar; *Denm.:* Gemzar; *Fin.:* Gemzar; *Fr.:* Gemzar; *Ger.:* Gemzar; *Hong Kong:* Gemzar; *Israel:* Gemzar; *Ital.:* Gemzar; *Mex.:* Gemzar; *Neth.:* Gemzar; *Norw.:* Gemzar; *NZ:* Gemzar; *Port.:* Gemzar; *S.Afr.:* Gemzar; *Singapore:* Gemzar; *Spain:* Gemzar; *Swed.:* Gemzar; *Switz.:* Gemzar; *Thai.:* Gemzar; *UK:* Gemzar; *USA:* Gemzar.

Gemtuzumab Ozogamicin (18580-z)

Gemtuzumab Ozogamicin *(USAN, rINNM)*.
CDP-771; CMA-676; Gemtuzumab Zogamicin; WAY-CMA-676.
CAS — 220578-59-6.

Profile

Gemtuzumab ozogamicin is a recombinant humanized monoclonal antibody conjugated with calicheamicin, a cytotoxic antibiotic. The antibody binds specifically to the CD33 antigen, which is expressed on leukaemic myeloblasts but not normal haematopoietic stem cells. Gemtuzumab ozogamicin is used for the second-line treatment of CD33-positive acute myeloid leukaemia in elderly patients who are unable to tolerate conventional chemotherapy. The recommended dose is 9 mg per m^2 given by intravenous infusion over 2 hours, repeated after 14 days.

Myelosuppression is common, and thrombocytopenia may be prolonged. Infusion-related reactions (including fever, chills, dyspnoea, and hypotension) and hypersensitivity may occur; prophylactic administration of an antihistamine and paracetamol is recommended. Hepatotoxicity has also been reported.

◊ References.
1. Anonymous. Gemtuzumab for relapsed acute myeloid leukemia. *Med Lett Drugs Ther* 2000; **42:** 67–8.

Preparations

Proprietary Preparations (details are given in Part 3)
USA: Mylotarg.

Gusperimus Hydrochloride (3060-b)

Gusperimus Hydrochloride *(rINNM)*.
BMS-181173; BMY-42215-1; Deoxyspergualin Hydrochloride; 15-Deoxyspergualin Hydrochloride; Gusperimus Trihydrochloride *(USAN)*; NKT-01; NSC-356894. (±)-*N*-[({4-[(3-Aminopropyl)amino]butyl}carbamoyl)hydroxymethyl]-7-guanidinoheptanamide trihydrochloride.
$C_{17}H_{37}N_7O_3,3HCl$ = 496.9.
CAS — 104317-84-2 (*gusperimus*); 89149-10-0 (*gusperimus*); 85468-01-5 (*gusperimus hydrochloride*).

Profile

Gusperimus is a guanidine derivative with immunosuppressant activity. It inhibits both cell-mediated and antibody-mediated immunity. It is used in the treatment of graft rejection and has been investigated in the management of graft-versus-host disease. For mention of its role in reversing acute graft rejection in kidney transplantation, see p.503.

Gusperimus is used as the hydrochloride. A dose of 3 to 5 mg of gusperimus hydrochloride per kg body-weight daily for 7 days, given by intravenous infusion over 3 hours, has been suggested in the treatment of acute renal graft rejection. Treatment may be continued for a further 3 days if required.

Adverse effects reported with gusperimus include bone-marrow depression, numbness of face and extremities, headache, gastrointestinal disturbances, alterations in liver enzyme values, and facial flushing. Rapid injection should be avoided as studies in *animals* suggest that excessive plasma concentrations associated with bolus administration may produce hypotension and respiratory depression.

◊ References.
1. Amemiya H, *et al.* A novel rescue drug, 15-deoxyspergualin: first clinical trials for recurrent graft rejection in renal recipients. *Transplantation* 1990; **49:** 337–43.
2. Suzuki S, *et al.* Clinical application of 15-deoxyspergualin for treatment of acute graft rejection following renal transplantation. *Transplant Proc* 1990; **22:** 1615–17.
3. Groth CG, *et al.* Deoxyspergualin for liver graft rejection. *Lancet* 1990; **336:** 626.
4. Gores PF, *et al.* Insulin independence in type 1 diabetes after transplantation of unpurified islets from single donor with 15-deoxyspergualin. *Lancet* 1993; **341:** 19–21.
5. Matas AJ, *et al.* Pilot evaluation of 15-deoxyspergualin for refractory acute renal transplant rejection. *Clin Transplant* 1994; **8:** 116–19.
6. Chan G, *et al.* Pharmacokinetics of deoxyspergualin in repeat renal transplant patients. *Clin Pharmacol Ther* 1995; **57:** 219.

Preparations

Proprietary Preparations (details are given in Part 3)
Jpn: Spanidin.

Homoharringtonine (19300-f)

NSC-141633. Cephalotaxine 2-(methoxycarbonylmethyl)-2,6-dihydroxy-5-methylheptanoate.
$C_{29}H_{39}NO_9$ = 545.6.
Pharmacopoeias. In Chin.

Profile

Homoharringtonine is an alkaloid derived from the tree *Cephalotaxus harringtonia*, and related species. It is thought to act at the ribosome to inhibit protein synthesis and is most active against cells in stage G_1. It has been tried as an antineoplastic in the treatment of acute myeloid leukaemias (p.485) and other neoplastic disorders. Some benefit has also been seen in chronic myeloid leukaemia (p.486).

The related compounds harringtonine, isoharringtonine, and deoxyharringtonine have also been investigated.

Reported adverse effects of homoharringtonine include severe hypotension, cardiac arrhythmias, myelosuppression, gastrointestinal disturbances, alopecia, rashes, and hyperglycaemia.

◊ References.
1. Feldman E, *et al.* Homoharringtonine is safe and effective for patients with acute myelogenous leukemia. *Leukemia* 1992; **6:** 1185–8.
2. Feldman EJ, *et al.* Homoharringtonine in patients with myelodysplastic syndrome (MDS) and MDS evolving to acute myeloid leukemia. *Leukemia* 1996; **10:** 40–2.
3. Kantarjian HM, *et al.* Homoharringtonine and low-dose cytarabine in the management of late chronic-phase chronic myelogenous leukemia. *J Clin Oncol* 2000; **18:** 3513–21.

Hydroxyurea (1839-d)

Hydroxyurea *(BAN, USAN)*.
Hydroxycarbamide *(BAN, rINN)*; Hydroxycarbamidum; NSC-32065; SQ-1089; WR-83799.
$NH_2.CO.NHOH$ = 76.05.
CAS — 127-07-1.
ATC — L01XX05.
Pharmacopoeias. In Eur. (see p.vi) *and US.*

Pharmacopoeial description

Ph. Eur.: A white or almost white, hygroscopic, crystalline powder. It exhibits polymorphism. Soluble in water; practically insoluble in alcohol. Store in airtight containers. Protect from light.

USP 25: A white to off-white powder. It is somewhat hygroscopic and decomposes in the presence of moisture. Freely soluble in water and in hot alcohol. Store in airtight containers in a dry atmosphere.

Adverse Effects, Treatment, and Precautions

For general discussions see Antineoplastics, p.476, p.479, and p.480.

Bone-marrow suppression, including megaloblastic changes, is the main adverse effect of hydroxyurea [hydroxycarbamide]. The erythema caused by irradiation may be exacerbated by hydroxyurea [hydroxycarbamide]. Other side-effects reported have included gastrointestinal disturbances, impairment of renal function, pulmonary oedema, dermatological reactions, alopecia, and neurological reactions such as headache, dizziness, drowsiness, disorientation, hallucinations, and convulsions.

The haemoglobin concentration, white cell and platelet counts, and hepatic and renal function should be determined repeatedly during treatment. Treatment should be interrupted if the white cell count drops to less than 2000 to 2500 per mm^3 or the platelet count to less than 80 000 to 100 000 per mm^3. If anaemia occurs when hydroxyurea [hydroxycarbamide] is used as an antineoplastic, it may be corrected by transfusions of whole blood without stopping therapy. If anaemia (haemoglobin less than 4.5 g per 100 mL or reticulocyte count less than 80 000 per mm^3) occurs when hydroxyurea [hydroxycarbamide] is used for sickle-cell disease, therapy should be interrupted. Megaloblastic changes are usually self-limiting.

Hydroxyurea [hydroxycarbamide] should be used with caution in patients with impaired renal function. The elderly may be more sensitive to the adverse effects of hydroxyurea [hydroxycarbamide]. Pre-existing anaemia should be corrected before beginning therapy with hydroxyurea [hydroxycarbamide].

Carcinogenicity. Secondary leukaemias have occurred in patients receiving hydroxyurea [hydroxycarbamide] for myeloproliferative disorders, although the extent to which this is due to the treatment or the underlying disorder is unknown.

Skin cancers have also been associated with hydroxyurea [hydroxycarbamide] therapy. These are often multiple and include both squamous cell and basal cell carcinomas.

References.
1. Liozon E, *et al.* Is treatment with hydroxyurea leukemogenic in patients with essential thrombocythemia? An analysis of three new cases of leukaemic transformation and review of the literature. *Hematol Cell Ther* 1997; **39:** 11–18.
2. Pearson TC, *et al.* Leukemic transformation in polycythemia vera. *Blood* 1998; **92:** 1837–8.
3. De Simone C, *et al.* Multiple squamous cell carcinomas of the skin during long-term treatment with hydroxyurea. *Eur J Dermatol* 1998; **8:** 114–15.
4. Best PJM, Petitt RM. Multiple skin cancers associated with hydroxyurea therapy. *Mayo Clin Proc* 1998; **73:** 961–3.

Effects on the liver. A report of self-limited hepatitis and a flu-like syndrome in a patient receiving hydroxyurea [hydroxycarbamide].[1] Symptoms recurred when the patient was rechallenged with the drug.
1. Heddle R, Calvert AF. Hydroxyurea induced hepatitis. *Med J Aust* 1980; **1:** 121.

Effects on the skin. Reports of skin reactions with hydroxyurea [hydroxycarbamide] include hyperpigmentation of the skin,[1] and of nails (melanonychia).[2]

Hydroxyurea [hydroxycarbamide] therapy has been associated with scaly erythematous skin lesions resembling those of dermatomyositis.[3-5] Such lesions usually occur after several years of hydroxyurea [hydroxycarbamide] treatment and the course is usually benign. However, withdrawal of hydroxyurea [hydroxycarbamide] is usually necessary for healing or improvement, in which case resolution may take several months.[4,5] Hydroxyurea [hydroxycarbamide] may also cause painful leg ulcers, which may require treatment discontinuation.[6] Leg ulcers often coexist with dermatomyositis-like eruptions and may be caused by the same mechanism.[7]

Skin cancers have also occurred, see Carcinogenicity above.
1. Majumdar G, *et al.* Reversible hyperpigmentation associated with high dose hydroxyurea. *BMJ* 1990; **300:** 1468.
2. Adams-Graves P, *et al.* Hydroxyurea in sickle cell disease. *N Engl J Med* 1996; **334:** 333–4.
3. Senet P, *et al.* Hydroxyurea-induced dermatomyositis-like eruption. *Br J Dermatol* 1995; **133:** 455–9.
4. Bahadoran P, *et al.* Pseudo-dermatomyositis induced by long-term hydroxyurea therapy: report of two cases. *Br J Dermatol* 1996; **134:** 1161–2.
5. Daoud MS, *et al.* Hydroxyurea dermopathy: a unique lichenoid eruption complicating long-term therapy with hydroxyurea. *J Am Acad Dermatol* 1997; **36:** 178–82.
6. Best PJ, *et al.* Hydroxyurea-induced leg ulceration in 14 patients. *Ann Intern Med* 1998; **128:** 29–32.
7. Suehiro M, *et al.* Hydroxyurea dermopathy with a dermatomyositis-like eruption and a large leg ulcer. *Br J Dermatol* 1998; **139:** 748–9.

Handling and disposal. Urine produced for up to 48 hours after a dose of hydroxyurea [hydroxycarbamide] should be handled wearing protective clothing.[1]
1. Harris J, Dodds LJ. Handling waste from patients receiving cytotoxic drugs. *Pharm J* 1985; **235:** 289–91.

Interactions

For a general discussion of antineoplastic drug interactions, see p.481.

Pharmacokinetics

Hydroxyurea [hydroxycarbamide] is readily absorbed from the gastrointestinal tract and distributed throughout the body. Peak plasma concentrations are reached within 2 hours. Up to 50% of a dose is metabolised by the liver; hydroxyurea [hydroxycarbamide] is excreted in urine as metabolites and unchanged drug. Some is excreted as carbon dioxide via the lungs. About 80% of a dose is reported to be excreted in the urine within 12 hours. Hydroxyurea [hydroxycarbamide] crosses the blood-brain barrier and the placenta, and is distributed into breast milk.

◊ References.

1. Gwilt PR, Tracewell WG. Pharmacokinetics and pharmacodynamics of hydroxyurea. *Clin Pharmacokinet* 1998; **34**: 347–58.

Uses and Administration

Hydroxyurea [hydroxycarbamide] is an antineoplastic that may cause inhibition of DNA synthesis by acting as a ribonucleotide reductase inhibitor. It is S-phase specific. Hydroxyurea [hydroxycarbamide] is used in the treatment of chronic myeloid leukaemia (p.486), and may be used in the myeloproliferative disorders polycythaemia vera (p.486) and primary (essential) thrombocythaemia (p.486). Hydroxyurea [hydroxycarbamide] has been tried, often combined with radiotherapy, in some solid malignancies such as tumours of the cervix, head and neck, and ovary. Hydroxyurea [hydroxycarbamide] has also been found to be of benefit in the haemoglobinopathies, particularly in sickle-cell disease (see below).

In the treatment of malignancies, hydroxyurea [hydroxycarbamide] is given by mouth in a single dose of 20 to 30 mg per kg body-weight daily or in a single dose of 60 to 80 mg per kg every third day. If a beneficial effect is evident after 6 weeks, therapy may be continued indefinitely. In sickle-cell disease initial doses of 15 mg per kg daily are suggested, increased if necessary by 5 mg per kg daily every 12 weeks according to response and blood counts, up to a maximum of 35 mg per kg daily.

Blood counts and hepatic and renal function should be monitored during therapy; treatment may need to be interrupted if leucopenia or thrombocytopenia occur (see Adverse Effects, Treatment, and Precautions, above).

Haemoglobinopathies. Hydroxyurea [hydroxycarbamide] is considered a promising treatment for the haemoglobinopathies. Hydroxyurea [hydroxycarbamide] can stimulate fetal haemoglobin production, which in turn can reduce haemoglobin polymerisation and the numbers of deformed, dense, and damaged erythrocytes. In adult patients with **sickle-cell disease** (p.717), a randomised controlled study produced evidence that hydroxyurea [hydroxycarbamide] in initial doses of 15 mg per kg daily, adjusted according to response and tolerance to up to 35 mg per kg daily, reduced the rate of sickle-cell crisis compared with placebo.[1] A report in 2 adults has suggested that hydroxyurea [hydroxycarbamide] might reverse splenic dysfunction.[2] Despite some concerns about giving a potential carcinogen to children, preliminary studies in paediatric populations have also reported evidence of benefit in terms of decreased hospitalisation[3] and sickle-cell crisis.[4] Hydroxyurea [hydroxycarbamide] may be an alternative to blood transfusions in children who have had a stroke.[5]

It has been suggested that combination of hydroxyurea [hydroxycarbamide] with erythropoietin might enhance the production of fetal haemoglobin, but results from studies of the combination have been conflicting.[6,7]

There appear to have been few studies of hydroxyurea [hydroxycarbamide] specifically in **thalassaemia** (p.718). Hydroxyurea [hydroxycarbamide] in initial doses of 8.2 to 10.3 mg per kg daily by mouth, increased until toxicity occurred did produce increases in fetal haemoglobin in 3 patients, but these were not sustained.[8] Conversely, sustained responses in 8 patients were seen in another study.[9] In addition, there is a report of sustained responses to therapy with sodium phenylbutyrate and hydroxyurea [hydroxycarbamide] in 2 siblings with thalassaemia major.[10]

1. Charache S, *et al.* Effect of hydroxyurea on the frequency of painful crises in sickle cell anemia. *N Engl J Med* 1995; **332**: 1317–22.
2. Claster S, Vichinsky E. First report of reversal of organ dysfunction in sickle cell anemia by the use of hydroxyurea: splenic regeneration. *Blood* 1996; **88**: 1951–3.
3. Scott JP, *et al.* Hydroxyurea therapy in children severely affected with sickle cell disease. *J Pediatr* 1996; **128**: 820–8.
4. Jayabose S, *et al.* Clinical and hematologic effects of hydroxyurea in children with sickle cell anemia. *J Pediatr* 1996; **129**: 559–65.
5. Ware RE, *et al.* Hydroxyurea as an alternative to blood transfusions for the prevention of recurrent stroke in children with sickle cell disease. *Blood* 1999; **94**: 3022–6.

The symbol † denotes a preparation no longer actively marketed

6. Goldberg MA, *et al.* Treatment of sickle cell anemia with hydroxyurea and erythropoietin. *N Engl J Med* 1990; **323**: 366–72.
7. Rodgers GP, *et al.* Augmentation by erythropoietin of the fetal-hemoglobin response to hydroxyurea in sickle-cell disease. *N Engl J Med* 1993; **328**: 73–80.
8. Hajjar FM, Pearson HA. Pharmacologic treatment of thalassemia intermedia with hydroxyurea. *J Pediatr* 1994; **125**: 490–2.
9. Loukopoulos D, *et al.* Hydroxyurea therapy in thalassemia. *Ann N Y Acad Sci* 1998; **30**: 120–8.
10. Olivieri NF, *et al.* Treatment of thalassaemia major with phenylbutyrate and hydroxyurea. *Lancet* 1997; **350**: 491–2.

HIV infection and AIDS. Studies *in vitro* indicate that hydroxyurea [hydroxycarbamide] (and other hydroxamates) act synergistically with didanosine (p.618) to suppress the replication of HIV and prevent its cytopathic effects.[1,2] A number of studies of such a combination are in progress. In 25 HIV-positive patients given didanosine 200 mg twice daily, together with hydroxyurea [hydroxycarbamide] 15 mg per kg body-weight daily in 2 divided doses, all patients showed a drop in viral load and an increase in CD4+ lymphocyte count.[3] Viraemia was not detectable in 13 of 24 patients evaluated at 6 months and 10 of 20 patients evaluated at 1 year. In 2 of these patients who subsequently received no antiviral treatments for 1 year there was no viral rebound, although some proviral DNA was detected.[4] In another study in 6 patients, didanosine 200 mg twice daily together with hydroxyurea [hydroxycarbamide] 250 mg four times daily (suggested to be a better regimen because of the short half-life of hydroxyurea [hydroxycarbamide]) produced a sharp decrease in viraemia, which was maintained for up to 72 weeks.[5] A rebound occurred in 1 patient on interrupting treatment but viral replication was again suppressed when treatment was restarted. Combination of hydroxyurea [hydroxycarbamide] with didanosine and indinavir[6] or stavudine[7] has also been tried. A controlled trial of the latter combination indicated significantly enhanced activity when the antivirals were combined with hydroxyurea [hydroxycarbamide] rather than placebo.[7] However, toxicity may prove to be a problem—although this controlled trial reported good tolerance of the combination another study (ACTG 5025) was terminated due to the high risk of toxicity.[8] For further discussion of the management of HIV infection and AIDS, see p.608.

1. Lori F, *et al.* Hydroxyurea as an inhibitor of human immunodeficiency virus-type 1 replication. *Science* 1994; **266**: 801–5.
2. Malley SD, *et al.* Suppression of HIV production in resting lymphocytes by combining didanosine and hydroxamate compounds. *Lancet* 1994; **343**: 1292.
3. Vila J, *et al.* 1-year follow-up of the use of hydroxycarbamide and didanosine in HIV infection. *Lancet* 1996; **848**: 203–4.
4. Vila J, *et al.* Absence of viral rebound after treatment of HIV-infected patients with didanosine and hydroxycarbamide. *Lancet* 1997; **350**: 635–6.
5. Lori F, *et al.* Long-term suppression of HIV-1 by hydroxyurea and didanosine. *JAMA* 1997; **277**: 1437–8.
6. Lisziewicz J, *et al.* HIV-1 suppression by early treatment with hydroxyurea, didanosine, and a protease inhibitor. *Lancet* 1998; **352**: 199–200.
7. Rutschmann OT, *et al.* A placebo-controlled trial of didanosine plus stavudine, with and without hydroxyurea, for HIV infection. *AIDS* 1998; **12**: F71–7.
8. Gibbs MA, Sorensen SJ. Hydroxyurea in the treatment of HIV-1. *Ann Pharmacother* 2000; **34**: 89–93.

Psoriasis. An immunosuppressant (usually methotrexate or ciclosporin) may be useful in patients with severe refractory psoriasis (p.1106). Hydroxyurea [hydroxycarbamide] has also been tried, although experience is limited.[1,2]

1. Layton AM, *et al.* Hydroxyurea in the management of therapy resistant psoriasis. *Br J Dermatol* 1989; **121**: 647–53.
2. Smith CH, *et al.* Use of hydroxyurea in psoriasis. *Clin Exp Dermatol* 1999; **24**: 2–6.

Preparations

BP 2001: Hydroxycarbamide Capsules;
USP 25: Hydroxyurea Capsules.

Proprietary Preparations (details are given in Part 3)

Austral.: Hydrea; *Belg.:* Hydrea; *Braz.:* Hydrea; *Canad.:* Hydrea; *Fin.:* Hydrea; *Fr.:* Hydrea; *Ger.:* Litalir, Syrea; *Hong Kong:* Hydrea; *Irl.:* Hydrea; *Israel:* Hydrea; *Ital.:* Onco-Carbide; *Mex.:* Hydrea; Oxeron; *Neth.:* Hydrea; *NZ:* Hydrea; *S.Afr.:* Hydrea; *Singapore:* Hydrea; *Spain:* Hydrea; *Swed.:* Hydrea; *Switz.:* Litalir; *Thai.:* Hydrea; *UK:* Hydrea; *USA:* Droxia; Hydrea; Mylocel.

Idarubicin Hydrochloride (12058-a)

Idarubicin Hydrochloride (BANM, USAN, rINNM).

4-Demethoxydaunorubicin Hydrochloride; IMI-30; NSC-256439 (idarubicin). (7S,9S)-9-Acetyl-7-(3-amino-2,3,6-trideoxy-α-L-lyxo-hexopyranosyloxy)-7,8,9,10-tetrahydro-6,9,11-trihydroxynaphthacene-5,12-dione hydrochloride.
$C_{26}H_{27}NO_9$,HCl = 534.0.

CAS — 58957-92-9 (idarubicin); 57852-57-0 (idarubicin hydrochloride).

Pharmacopoeias. In US.

Pharmacopoeial description

USP 25: A 0.5% solution in water has a pH between 5.0 and 6.5. Store in airtight containers.

Adverse Effects, Treatment, and Precautions

As for Doxorubicin Hydrochloride, p.535. Raised liver enzymes and bilirubin occur in about 20 to 30% of patients. Severe enterocolitis with perforation has been reported rarely. A cumulative total dose limit of 400 mg per m^2 body-surface has been recommended for oral therapy, although it has been suggested that idarubicin may be associated with less cardiotoxicity than doxorubicin. Doses should be reduced in patients with renal or hepatic impairment; idarubicin should probably be avoided if hepatic impairment is severe enough to produce serum bilirubin concentrations of 50 µg per mL or above, and some consider it should not be used if serum bilirubin is above 20 µg per mL.

Pharmacokinetics

Following intravenous administration idarubicin is rapidly distributed into body tissues and extensively tissue bound, with a volume of distribution which may be in excess of 2000 litres. It is extensively metabolised, both in the liver and extrahepatically; the principal metabolite, idarubicinol (13-dihydroidarubicin) has equal antineoplastic activity. Peak concentrations of idarubicin and idarubicinol in bone marrow and nucleated blood cells are 400 (idarubicin) and 200 (idarubicinol) times greater than those in plasma; cellular concentrations of drug and metabolite decline with apparent terminal half-lives of 15 and 72 hours respectively, whereas plasma half-lives are reported to be 20 to 22 hours and about 45 hours respectively. Idarubicin is excreted in bile, and to a lesser extent in urine, as unchanged drug and metabolites.

Idarubicin is also absorbed following oral administration, but estimates of its oral bioavailability vary from about 20 to 50%.

◊ References.

1. Robert J. Clinical pharmacokinetics of idarubicin. *Clin Pharmacokinet* 1993; **24**: 275–88.

Uses and Administration

Idarubicin is an anthracycline antibiotic with antineoplastic actions similar to those of doxorubicin (p.536). It is used as the hydrochloride, alone or in combination with other drugs, for the induction of remission in patients with acute myeloid leukaemias (p.485). It is also used as a second-line treatment in acute lymphoblastic leukaemia (p.484), and advanced breast cancer (p.491). It has been tried in multiple myeloma (p.489) and non-Hodgkin's lymphoma (p.487).

Idarubicin hydrochloride is given by intravenous injection (reconstituted with Water for Injections) into a fast-running infusion of 0.9% sodium chloride or 5% glucose over 5 to 15 minutes. The suggested dose in adult acute myeloid leukaemia is 12 mg per m^2 body-surface daily for 3 days, in combination with cytarabine. A similar dose, as a single agent, has been given in acute lymphoblastic leukaemia. An alternative dosage schedule in acute myeloid leukaemia is 8 mg per m^2 given daily for 5 days. In children with acute lymphoblastic leukaemia a dose of 10 mg per m^2 daily for 3 days as a single agent has been suggested. When the intravenous route cannot be employed, idarubicin hydrochloride may be given by mouth. A suggested dose in adult acute myeloid leukaemia is 30 mg per m^2 daily for 3 days as a single agent, or 15 to 30 mg per m^2 daily in combination with other drugs.

In patients with refractory late breast cancer idarubicin hydrochloride has been given by mouth in doses of 45 mg per m^2, as a single dose or divided over 3 consecutive days; the treatment may be repeated every 3 or 4 weeks depending on the haematological recovery.

Blood counts should be performed frequently in patients receiving idarubicin, and monitoring of cardiac, hepatic, and renal function is recommended. Doses should be reduced in patients with hepatic or renal impairment (see Adverse Effects, Treatment, and Precautions, above). In patients who receive a second course of idarubicin dosage should be reduced by 25% if severe mucositis developed with the first course.[3]

◊ The actions and uses of idarubicin have been reviewed.[1] A study in leukaemia cells *in vitro* suggested that idarubicin was more active than a conventional anthracycline, daunorubicin, against cells with the multidrug resistance (MDR) phenotype.[2] A collaborative overview of randomised trials for acute myeloid leukaemia found that idarubicin-based therapy achieved better remission rates and overall survival than daunorubicin-based regimens.[3]

1. Cersosimo RJ. Idarubicin: an anthracycline antineoplastic agent. *Clin Pharm* 1992; **11:** 152–67.
2. Berman E, McBride M. Comparative cellular pharmacology of daunorubicin and idarubicin in human multidrug-resistant leukaemia cells. *Blood* 1992; **79:** 3267–73.
3. AML Collaborative Group. A systematic collaborative overview of randomised trials comparing idarubicin with daunorubicin (or other anthracyclines) as induction therapy for acute myeloid leukaemia. *Br J Haematol* 1998; **103:** 100–9.

Preparations

USP 25: Idarubicin Hydrochloride for Injection.

Proprietary Preparations (details are given in Part 3)

Aust.: Zavedos; *Austral.:* Zavedos; *Belg.:* Zavedos; *Braz.:* Zavedos; *Canad.:* Idamycin; *Denm.:* Zavedos; *Fin.:* Zavedos; *Fr.:* Zavedos; *Ger.:* Zavedos; *Hong Kong:* Zavedos; *Irl.:* Zavedos; *Israel:* Zavedos; *Ital.:* Zavedos; *Mex.:* Idamycin; *Neth.:* Zavedos; *Norw.:* Zavedos; *NZ:* Zavedos; *Port.:* Zavedos; *S.Afr.:* Zavedos; *Singapore:* Zavedos; *Spain:* Zavedos; *Swed.:* Zavedos; *Switz.:* Zavedos; *Thai.:* Zavedos; *UK:* Zavedos; *USA:* Idamycin.

Idoxifene (17090-I)

Idoxifene (BAN, USAN, rINN).

CB-7432; SB-223030. (E)-I-{2-[4-(1-p-Iodophenyl-2-phenyl-but-1-enyl)phenoxy]ethyl}pyrrolidine.

$C_{28}H_{30}INO = 523.4$.

CAS — 116057-75-1.

Profile

Idoxifene is an analogue of tamoxifen (p.571) with similar general properties. It has been investigated in the endocrine treatment of breast cancer and osteoporosis.

Ifosfamide (1840-c)

Ifosfamide (BAN, USAN, rINN).

Ifosfamidum; Iphosphamide; Isophosphamide; MJF-9325; NSC-109724; Z-4942. 3-(2-Chloroethyl)-2-(2-chloroethylamino)perhydro-1,3,2-oxazaphosphorinane 2-oxide.

$C_7H_{15}Cl_2N_2O_2P = 261.1$.

CAS — 3778-73-2.

ATC — L01AA06.

Pharmacopoeias. In *Eur.* (see p.vi) and *US*.

Pharmacopoeial description

Ph. Eur.: A white or almost white, hygroscopic, fine crystalline powder. Soluble in water; freely soluble in dichloromethane. Store in airtight containers.

USP 25: A white, crystalline powder. M.p. about 40°. Freely soluble in water; very soluble in alcohol, in methyl alcohol, in isopropyl alcohol, in dichloromethane, and in ethyl acetate; very slightly soluble in hexanes. A 10% solution in water has a pH of between 4.0 and 7.0. Store in airtight containers at a temperature not exceeding 25°.

Stability. Ifosfamide undergoes a reversible chemical re-arrangement in aqueous solution, which is sensitive to changes in pH.[1] The ratio of these compounds to one another in biological fluids may have a bearing on the toxicity and efficacy of ifosfamide.

1. Küpfer A, *et al.* Intramolecular rearrangement of ifosfamide in aqueous solutions. *Lancet* 1990; **335:** 1461.

Incompatibility. Ifosfamide appears to be compatible when mixed in solution with mesna.[1,2] However, ifosfamide appears to be incompatible with benzyl alcohol used as a preservative in Water for Injections: solutions made up with water preserved in this way became turbid, with the formation of aqueous and oily phases, at concentrations of ifosfamide greater than 60 mg per mL.[3]

1. Shaw IC, Rose JWP. Infusion of ifosphamide plus mesna. *Lancet* 1984; **i:** 1353–4.
2. Rowland CG, *et al.* Infusion of ifosfamide plus mesna. *Lancet* 1984; **ii:** 468.
3. Behme RJ, *et al.* Incompatibility of ifosfamide with benzyl-alcohol-preserved bacteriostatic water for injection. *Am J Hosp Pharm* 1988; **45:** 627–8.

Adverse Effects, Treatment, and Precautions

As for Cyclophosphamide, p.527. Toxic effects on the urinary tract may be more severe with ifosfamide and may involve the kidneys as well as the bladder. Central nervous system side-effects have been reported, especially confusion and lethargy.

Effects on the heart. Severe myocardial depression, with heart failure and ventricular arrhythmias, has been reported in patients receiving high-dose ifosfamide.[1] Symptoms were reversible with appropriate treatment in most cases although one patient died of cardiogenic shock.

1. Quezado ZMN, *et al.* High-dose ifosfamide is associated with severe, reversible cardiac dysfunction. *Ann Intern Med* 1993; **118:** 31–6.

Effects on the kidneys. In addition to its effects on the bladder ifosfamide may be associated with serious nephrotoxicity. Both proximal and distal tubular damage,[1,2] and to a lesser extent glomerular effects,[2] are seen, and the Fanconi syndrome (with development of hypophosphataemic rickets in a number of children),[2-6] and nephrogenic diabetes insipidus[1,6] may result. Progressive chronic renal failure after high-dose ifosfamide has been described.[7] Life-threatening hypokalaemia possibly due to a renal lesion has also occurred.[8] Results in *rats* suggest that generation of toxic metabolites within the kidney itself may be responsible, and that repairable renal damage occurs after the first dose, which is aggravated by repeated toxic insults.[9] This is in agreement with clinical results, since although renal damage has been seen after a single dose, perhaps representing an idiosyncratic reaction,[10,11] most cases have been in children receiving relatively high doses long-term. Renal damage appears to persist after withdrawal of ifosfamide in these patients and may be largely irreversible.[12]

A combination of younger age and high cumulative doses of ifosfamide was found to convey the highest risk of toxicity, but concomitant use of cisplatin may also increase the risk.[13] The maximum safe dose of ifosfamide remains controversial.[13-15] It has been suggested that cumulative doses of 100 g of ifosfamide per m² body-surface or more should be avoided in children in an attempt to reduce the incidence of nephrotoxicity,[14] although subsequent reviews have suggested that lower cumulative doses may be toxic, especially in younger children.[13,15]

1. Skinner R, *et al.* Nephrotoxicity after ifosfamide. *Arch Dis Child* 1990; **65:** 732–8.
2. Burk CD, *et al.* Ifosfamide-induced renal tubular dysfunction and rickets in children with Wilms tumor. *J Pediatr* 1990; **117:** 331–5.
3. Skinner R, *et al.* Hypophosphataemic rickets after ifosfamide treatment in children. *BMJ* 1989; **298:** 1560–1.
4. Newbury-Ecob RA, Barbor PRH. Hypophosphataemic rickets after ifosfamide treatment. *BMJ* 1989; **299:** 258.
5. Newbury-Ecob RA, *et al.* Ifosfamide-induced Fanconi syndrome. *Lancet* 1989; **i:** 1328.
6. Skinner R, *et al.* Nephrotoxicity of ifosfamide in children. *Lancet* 1989; **ii:** 159.
7. Krämer A, *et al.* Progressive renal failure in two breast cancer patients after high-dose ifosfamide. *Lancet* 1994; **334:** 1569.
8. Husband DJ, Watkin SW. Fatal hypokalaemia associated with ifosfamide/mesna chemotherapy. *Lancet* 1988; **i:** 1116.
9. Graham MI. A proposed mechanism for isophosphamide-induced kidney toxicity. *Hum Toxicol* 1985; **4:** 545–6.
10. Heney D, *et al.* Acute ifosfamide-induced tubular toxicity. *Lancet* 1989; **ii:** 103–4.
11. Devalck C, *et al.* Acute ifosfamide-induced proximal tubular toxic reaction. *J Pediatr* 1991; **118:** 325–6.
12. Heney D, *et al.* Progressive renal toxicity due to ifosfamide. *Arch Dis Child* 1991; **66:** 966–70.
13. Loebstein R, *et al.* Risk factors for long-term outcome of ifosfamide-induced nephrotoxicity in children. *J Clin Pharmacol* 1999; **39:** 454–61.
14. Skinner R, *et al.* Risk factors for ifosfamide nephrotoxicity in children. *Lancet* 1996; **348:** 578–80.
15. Loebstein R, Koren G. Ifosfamide-induced nephrotoxicity in children: critical review of predictive risk factors. *Pediatrics* 1998; **101:** 1067.

Effects on the nervous system. The administration of ifosfamide (with mesna for urothelial protection) may be associated with the development of severe encephalopathy, with EEG abnormalities, disorientation, hallucinations, catatonia, and coma; occasionally central nervous system depression has led to circulatory collapse and death.[1,2] The effect has been suggested to be due to a metabolite, perhaps chloroacetaldehyde,[3] a hypothesis with which the increased incidence of encephalopathy after oral rather than intravenous administration may agree.[4,5] Others suggest that the dechloroethylated metabolites may contribute, and in particular the R-enantiomer of 3-dechloroethyl-ifosfamide which is a metabolite of *S*-ifosfamide.[6] There is some uncertainty about the contributory role of mesna, if any: encephalopathy has not been seen when mesna is given with cyclophosphamide,[7] and has been seen when ifosfamide is given alone,[5] but an exacerbatory role for mesna cannot be ruled out,[8] perhaps via its chelating properties.[1,7] A nomogram has been proposed to identify patients at greatest risk of toxicity,[9,10] such as those with renal or hepatic impairment,[9] although doubts have been raised as to its general applicability,[11] and it has also been suggested that administration should be by continuous infusion over several days where possible, since this route has by far the lowest incidence of encephalopathy (7%, versus 26% with intravenous bolus and 43% with oral administration).[4] Care may also be required when giving other antineoplastics to patients who have experienced encephalopathy after ifosfamide, since a case of encephalopathy following bleomycin (not normally associated with neurotoxicity) has been reported in such a patient.[12]

Preliminary reports suggest that intravenous or oral administration of methylene blue [methylthioninium chloride] may prevent or reverse signs of encephalopathy.[13,14] It was proposed that ifosfamide neurotoxicity was due to derangement of mitochondrial metabolism, and that the process was reversed by methylene blue [methylthioninium chloride].[13]

1. Meanwell CA, *et al.* Encephalopathy associated with ifosphamide/mesna therapy. *Lancet* 1985; **i:** 406–7.
2. Cantwell BMJ, Harris AL. Ifosfamide/mesna and encephalopathy. *Lancet* 1985; **i:** 752.
3. Goren MP, *et al.* Dechloroethylation of ifosfamide and neurotoxicity. *Lancet* 1986; **ii:** 1219–20.
4. Cerny T, *et al.* Ifosfamide by continuous infusion to prevent encephalopathy. *Lancet* 1990; **335:** 175.
5. Lewis LD, Meanwell CA. Ifosfamide pharmacokinetics and neurotoxicity. *Lancet* 1990; **335:** 175–6.
6. Wainer IW, *et al.* Ifosfamide stereoselective dichloroethylation [sic] and neurotoxicity. *Lancet* 1994; **343:** 982–3.
7. Osborne RJ, Slevin ML. Ifosfamide, mesna, and encephalopathy. *Lancet* 1985; **i:** 1398–9.
8. Pinkerton R, *et al.* Ifosfamide, mesna, and encephalopathy. *Lancet* 1985; **i:** 1399.
9. Meanwell CA, *et al.* Avoiding ifosfamide/mesna encephalopathy. *Lancet* 1986; **ii:** 406.
10. Perren TJ, *et al.* Encephalopathy with rapid infusion ifosfamide/mesna. *Lancet* 1987; **i:** 390–1.
11. McCallum AK. Ifosfamide/mesna encephalopathy. *Lancet* 1987; **i:** 987. Correction. *ibid.;* 1048.
12. Atherton P, *et al.* Drug-induced encephalopathy after previous ifosfamide treatment. *Lancet* 1988; **ii:** 1084.
13. Küpfer A, *et al.* Prophylaxis and reversal of ifosfamide encephalopathy with methylene-blue. *Lancet* 1994; **343:** 763–4.
14. Zuhan GB, *et al.* Methylene blue for ifosfamide-associated encephalopathy. *N Engl J Med* 1995; **332:** 1239–40.

Handling and disposal. A study[1] found that ifosfamide 8% solution penetrated all of 4 brands of latex glove and one PVC glove, although the diffusion rate was 4 or more times slower than through cadaver skin. Permeation was greater through the PVC glove than the latex gloves, partly due to its lesser thickness, although permeation was not dependent on thickness alone and varied between gloves of the same brand as well as between brands. They recommended that latex gloves of a suitable brand should be worn when handling ifosfamide, and changed at least every 2 hours. For reference to a method for the destruction of ifosfamide waste, see under Cyclophosphamide, p.528.

1. Corlett SA, *et al.* Permeation of ifosfamide through gloves and cadaver skin. *Pharm J* 1991; **247:** R39.

Interactions

◊ For reference to the effects of ifosfamide on oral anticoagulants, see under Warfarin Sodium, p.995. For a report of the enhancement of cisplatin-induced ototoxicity and nephrotoxicity, see under Cisplatin, p.526.

Pharmacokinetics

Ifosfamide is normally given intravenously, although it is well absorbed from the gastrointestinal tract. The pharmacokinetics of ifosfamide are reported to exhibit considerable interindividual variation. Although the manufacturers state that a mean terminal elimination half-life of about 15 hours has been reported following a single high-dose intravenous bolus, most studies at lower doses appear to have recorded elimination half-lives of about 4 to 8 hours. Following repeated doses (fractionated therapy) there is a decrease in the elimination half-life, apparently due to autoinduction of metabolism. It is extensively metabolised, chiefly by mixed function oxidases in the liver, to a variety of active and inactive metabolites; there is some evidence that metabolism is saturated at very high doses. It is excreted largely in urine, as unchanged drug and metabolites.

◊ General references.

1. Wagner T. Ifosfamide clinical pharmacokinetics. *Clin Pharmacokinet* 1994; **26:** 439–56.
2. Boddy AV, Yule SM. Metabolism and pharmacokinetics of oxazaphosphorines. *Clin Pharmacokinet* 2000; **38:** 291–304.

◊ In a study in 20 patients receiving intravenous ifosfamide over 3 or 5 days, the median elimination half-life of ifosfamide was 3.85 hours in patients under 60 years of age compared with 6.03 hours in those over age 60;[1] this difference appeared to be due to an increased volume of distribution in the older age group. The autoinduction of metabolism typically seen with multiple doses of ifosfamide was not affected by age.

In another study the half-life of the *S*-enantiomer of ifosfamide was found to be 5.98 hours after an intravenous bolus of the racemate, compared with 7.12 hours for the *R*-enantiomer.[2]

1. Lind MJ, *et al.* The effect of age on the pharmacokinetics of ifosfamide. *Br J Clin Pharmacol* 1990; **30:** 140–3.
2. Corlett SA, *et al.* Pharmacokinetics of ifosfamide and its enantiomers following a single 1h intravenous infusion of the racemate in patients with small cell lung carcinoma. *Br J Clin Pharmacol* 1995; **39:** 452–5.

◊ The increased clearance seen over time during a 5-day cycle of ifosfamide treatment, due to increased metabolism, was not sustained over the 21 days between cycles, but was reproducible and of similar magnitude in the subsequent cycle.[1]

1. Lewis LD. A study of 5 day fractionated ifosfamide pharmacokinetics in consecutive treatment cycles. *Br J Clin Pharmacol* 1996; **42:** 179–86.

Uses and Administration

Ifosfamide is an alkylating agent with properties similar to those of cyclophosphamide (p.529), of which it is a congener. It is used in the treatment of a variety of solid tumours including those of the cervix, lung, ovary, testis, and thymus, as well as in sarcoma and in the treatment of lymphomas. For further mention of these uses see the cross-references given below.

Ifosfamide is given intravenously, either by injection as a solution diluted to less than 4%, or by infusion. It is usually given in a total dose of 8 to 12 g per m^2 body-surface divided over 3 to 5 days, although a dose of 6 g per m^2 divided over 5 days has been recommended in the USA; alternatively, courses comprising 5 to 6 g per m^2, to a maximum of 10 g, have been given as a single 24-hour infusion. Courses may be repeated at intervals of 2 to 4 weeks, depending on the blood count. Oral administration of ifosfamide has also been studied.

Ifosfamide should be administered in association with mesna (below), and adequate hydration should be maintained, to avoid urological toxicity; fluid intake should not be less than 2 litres daily.

The isomeric form dexifosfamide (D-4809) is also being studied, as is a combination of ifosfamide with methylene blue [methylthioninium chloride].

Administration. Mesna (p.1011) can combine with urotoxic ifosfamide metabolites in the kidney to form stable and non-toxic compounds. It is therefore given prophylactically with ifosfamide. It has a shorter half-life than ifosfamide so repeated administration is needed to provide adequate protection of the bladder. A common schedule uses intravenous mesna at 60% of the ifosfamide dose, divided into 3 doses given with, or 15 minutes before, ifosfamide, then 4 and 8 hours after ifosfamide administration. Mesna may also be given orally, but higher doses are required.

1. Siu LL, Moore MJ. Use of mesna to prevent ifosfamide-induced urotoxicity. *Support Care Cancer* 1998; **6:** 144–54.

Malignant neoplasms. Ifosfamide may be used as an alternative to cyclophosphamide in lymphomas such as Burkitt's lymphoma (p.488). It is also used in a variety of solid neoplasms, including in palliative regimens for advanced cervical cancer (p.492); in the treatment of lung cancer (p.496); in ovarian cancer (p.496) and second-line and salvage regimens for testicular cancer (p.499); in thymoma (p.499); in adjuvant therapy for bone sarcomas (p.500) and rhabdomyosarcoma (p.501).

Preparations

USP 25: Ifosfamide for Injection.

Proprietary Preparations (details are given in Part 3)
Aust.: Holoxan; *Austral.:* Holoxan; *Belg.:* Holoxan; *Braz.:* Holoxane; *Canad.:* Ifex; *Denm.:* Holoxan; *Fin.:* Holoxan; *Fr.:* Holoxan; *Ger.:* Holoxan; IFO-cell; *Hong Kong:* Holoxan; *Israel:* Ifoxan; *Ital.:* Holoxan; *Mex.:* Holoxan; Ifolem; Ifomida; Ifoxan; Seromida; *Neth.:* Holoxan; *Norw.:* Holoxan; *NZ:* Holoxan; *Port.:* Holoxan; *S.Afr.:* Holoxan; *Singapore:* Holoxan; *Spain:* Tronoxal; *Swed.:* Holoxan; *Switz.:* Holoxan; *Thai.:* Holoxan; *UK:* Mitoxana; *USA:* Ifex.

Ilmofosine   (2954-e)

Ilmofosine *(USAN, rINN).*

BM-41440.   (±)-3-(Hexadecylthio)-2-(methoxymethyl)propyl hydrogen phosphate choline hydroxide inner salt.
$C_{26}H_{56}NO_5PS$ = 525.8.
CAS — 83519-04-4; 89315-55-9.

Profile
Ilmofosine is a phospholipid derivative similar to miltefosine (p.557) that has been investigated for its antineoplastic properties. Gastrointestinal disturbances may be dose-limiting.

Imatinib Mesilate   (20599-n)

Imatinib Mesilate *(pINNM).*

Imatinib Mesylate; STI-571. α-(4-Methyl-1-piperazinyl)-3′-{[4-(3-pyridyl)-2-pyrimidinyl]amino}-p-tolu-   p-toluidide   methanesulfonate.
$C_{29}H_{31}N_7O,CH_4O_3S$ = 589.7.
CAS — 152459-95-5 (imatinib).

Profile
Imatinib mesilate is a tyrosine kinase inhibitor that is used in the treatment of chronic myeloid leukaemia (p.486). It is given orally at a dose equivalent to 600 mg of the base daily to patients with blast crisis or accelerated phase leukaemia. The dose may be increased to 400 mg twice daily if necessary. Patients in chronic phase who have not responded to interferon alfa therapy may be given 400 mg daily, increased to 600 mg

daily if required. Doses should be taken with food, and accompanied by plenty of water, to minimise gastric irritation.

Adverse effects include nausea, vomiting, oedema, and muscle cramps. Neutropenia, thrombocytopenia and hepatotoxicity may occur; blood counts and liver function should be monitored regularly. Severe fluid retention can occur, which may result in pleural and pericardial effusion, pulmonary oedema, and ascites. The long-term effects of therapy remain to be determined.

Promising initial results have been seen from the investigational use of imatinib to treat gastrointestinal stromal tumours.

◊ References.
1. O'Dwyer ME, Druker BJ. Status of bcr-abl tyrosine kinase inhibitors in chronic myelogenous leukemia. *Curr Opin Oncol* 2000; **12:** 594–7.
2. Druker BJ, *et al.* Efficacy and safety of a specific inhibitor of the BCR-ABL tyrosine kinase in chronic myeloid leukemia. *N Engl J Med* 2001; **344:** 1031–7.
3. Druker BJ, *et al.* Activity of a specific inhibitor of the BCR-ABL tyrosine kinase in the blast crisis of chronic myeloid leukemia and acute lymphoblastic leukemia with the Philadelphia chromosome. *N Engl J Med* 2001; **344:** 1038–42.
4. Joensuu H, *et al.* Effect of the tyrosine kinase inhibitor STI571 in a patient with a metastatic gastrointestinal stromal tumor. *N Engl J Med* 2001; **344:** 1052–6.

Adverse Effects. A report of acute generalised exanthematous pustulosis in a patient receiving imatinib[1] The authors noted that severe skin reactions had been reported in some other patients receiving the drug, and speculated that the effect might be dose-dependent and related to its pharmacological action.
1. Brouard M, Saurat J-H. Cutaneous reactions to STI571. *N Engl J Med* 2001; **345:** 618–19.

Preparations

Proprietary Preparations (details are given in Part 3)
UK: Glivec; *USA:* Gleevec.

Improsulfan Tosilate   (12846-d)

Improsulfan Tosilate *(rINNM).*

Improsulfan Tosylate; NSC-140117; 864T; Yoshi-864. Iminodipropyl dimethanesulphonate 4-toluenesulphonate.
$C_8H_{19}NO_6S_2,C_7H_8O_3S$ = 461.6.
CAS — 13425-98-4 (improsulfan); 32784-82-0 (improsulfan tosilate).

Profile
Improsulfan is an alkylating agent related to busulfan (p.513). It has been used as the tosilate in the management of chronic myeloid leukaemia.

Inolimomab   (17632-m)

Inolimomab *(rINN).*

BT-563.
CAS — 152981-31-2.

Profile
Inolimomab is a murine/human monoclonal antibody similar to daclizumab (p.532) that is an interleukin-2 receptor antagonist at the alpha chain (CD25). It is under investigation for its immunosuppressant properties in the treatment and prevention of rejection episodes following organ transplantation (p.502).

◊ References.
1. Otto G, *et al.* Monoclonal antibody to interleukin-2 receptor in liver graft rejection. *Lancet* 1990; **335:** 1596–7.
2. Otto G, *et al.* Monoclonal anti-CD25 for acute rejection after liver transplantation. *Lancet* 1991; **338:** 519.
3. van Gelder T, *et al.* Reversal of graft rejection with monoclonal anti-interleukin-2 receptor. *Lancet* 1992; **339:** 873.
4. Neuhaus P, *et al.* Comparison of quadruple immunosuppression after liver transplantation with ATG or IL-2 receptor antibody. *Transplantation* 1993; **55:** 1320–7.
5. Iberer F, *et al.* Clinical experience with a monoclonal interleukin-2 receptor antibody (BT 563) for rejection therapy after orthotopic heart transplantation. *Transplant Proc* 1994; **26:** 3237–9.
6. Carl S, *et al.* Effect of anti-IL-2-receptor monoclonal antibody BT563 in treatment of acute interstitial renal rejection. *Transplant Proc* 1995; **27:** 854–5.
7. Lemmens HP, *et al.* Interleukin-2 receptor antibody vs ATG for induction immunosuppression after liver transplantation: initial results of a prospective randomized trial. *Transplant Proc* 1995; **27:** 1140–1.

Interleukin-2   (16854-s)

BG-8301 (teceleukin); Epidermal Thymocyte Activating Factor; ETAF; IL-2; T-cell Growth Factor.

A naturally-occurring 133-amino-acid glycoprotein with a molecular weight of about 15 000. It is available from natural sources or as a product of recombinant DNA technology (rIL-2).

In addition to aldesleukin (below) modified forms of interleukin-2 produced by recombinant DNA technology have included celmoleukin and teceleukin.

Aldesleukin   (12027-e)

Aldesleukin *(BAN, USAN, rINN).*

Des-alanyl-1, Serine-125 Human Interleukin-2; Recombinant Interleukin-2; 125-L-Serine-2–133-interleukin 2 (human reduced).
CAS — 110942-02-4.
ATC — L03AC01.

Aldesleukin (modified human recombinant interleukin-2) is produced by recombinant DNA technology using an *Escherichia coli* strain containing an analogue of the human interleukin-2 gene. It differs from native interleukin-2 in that it is not glycosylated, it has no N-terminal alanine, and it has serine substituted for cysteine at position 125.

Incompatibility. Aldesleukin 33 800 units per mL in glucose 5% lost significant biological activity when mixed with a variety of other drugs including ganciclovir sodium, lorazepam, pentamidine isetionate, prochlorperazine edisilate, and promethazine hydrochloride.[1] However, the incompatibility was not detectable by spectrophotometric methods and only lorazepam was visually incompatible, suggesting that these methods may be invalid for assessing the compatibility of proteins.
1. Alex S, *et al.* Compatibility and activity of aldesleukin (recombinant interleukin-2) in presence of selected drugs during simulated Y-site administration: evaluation of three methods. *Am J Health-Syst Pharm* 1995; **52:** 2423–6.

Stability. Aldesleukin lost 75 to 100% of activity when reconstituted with glucose 5% or sodium chloride 0.9% in a plastic syringe and administered over 24 hours with a syringe driver.[1,2] Loss of activity was not seen if aldesleukin was reconstituted with water alone[2] or with the addition of albumin.[1,2] It was suggested that loss of activity could be suspected because of lack of toxicity,[1,2] and that the lack of toxicity in some published studies could be due to this.[1,3] However, the authors of these studies indicated that they had reconstituted aldesleukin with albumin.[4,5] Reconstitution with low concentrations of albumin has been recommended to avoid bioavailability problems,[1,4,6] and was recommended by the manufacturer in the UK when the licensed dosage regimen was by continuous infusion. However, it is not recommended by the manufacturer for subcutaneous use (UK) or for short intravenous infusion (US). The US manufacturer indicates that dilution outside of a specified range results in increased variability in drug delivery. Dilution with sodium chloride 0.9% is not recommended because increased aggregation occurs.
1. Miles DW, *et al.* Reconstitution of interleukin 2 with albumin for infusion. *Lancet* 1990; **335:** 1602–3.
2. Vlasveld LT, *et al.* Reconstitution of interleukin-2. *Lancet* 1990; **336:** 446.
3. Miles DW, *et al.* Toxicity and reconstitution of recombinant interleukin-2 with albumin. *Lancet* 1991; **338:** 1464.
4. Franks CR. Reconstitution of interleukin-2. *Lancet* 1990; **336:** 445–6.
5. Hamblin T. Reconstitution of interleukin-2 with albumin for infusion. *Lancet* 1990; **336:** 251.
6. Lamers CHJ, *et al.* Bioavailability of interleukin-2 after reconstitution with albumin. *Lancet* 1992; **340:** 241.

Units

100 units of human interleukin-2 are contained in one ampoule of the first International Standard Preparation (1987). The activity of interleukin-2 has also been expressed in Nutley and Cetus units: 100 international units is reportedly equivalent to about 83.3 Nutley units and to about 16.7 Cetus units. According to the manufacturers, 18 million international units of aldesleukin are equivalent to 1.1 mg of protein.

Adverse Effects and Treatment

Toxicity is related to dose and route of administration and is often severe; fatalities have been recorded. Decreased vascular resistance and increased capillary permeability (the 'capillary leak syndrome') is common in patients given aldesleukin, and results in hypotension, reduced organ perfusion, and oedema. The incidence and severity of this syndrome is lower after subcutaneous than intravenous administration. Fluid replacement may be necessary to treat the resultant hypovolaemia and dopamine or other pressor agents may be needed to help maintain organ perfusion. Capillary leak syndrome may also be associated with cardiac effects including tachycardia, angina, myocardial infarction; respiratory effects such as dyspnoea, pulmonary oedema, and respiratory failure; renal abnormalities including uraemia and oliguria or anuria; and confusion, disorientation, and drowsiness. Raised liver enzymes, nausea and vomiting, diarrhoea, fever and flu-like symptoms (malaise, rigors, and myalgia), rashes, pruritus, anaemia, and thrombocytopenia, are also relatively common. Paracetamol (but not NSAIDs, see Effects on the Kidneys, below) may be used prophylactically for fever. Antiemetics and antidiarrhoeals may also be required. Antihistamines may benefit some patients with pruritic rash. Injection site reactions are common after subcutaneous administration; necrosis has occurred.

◊ References.
1. Sundin DJ, Wolin MJ. Toxicity management in patients receiving low-dose aldesleukin therapy. *Ann Pharmacother* 1998; **32:** 1344–52.

Bacterial infections. The incidence of sepsis and bacteraemia is increased in patients receiving interleukin-2 via intravenous catheters,[1,2] and possibly subcutaneously,[3] although others have not found this to be the case.[4,5] The increased incidence of nonopportunistic bacterial infection may be a particular problem in patients with AIDS who are treated with interleukin-2.[6] The mechanism is uncertain, but may be related to impairment of neutrophil function by the cytokine.[7]
1. Snydman DR, *et al.* Nosocomial sepsis associated with interleukin-2. *Ann Intern Med* 1990; **112:** 102–7.
2. Shiloni E, *et al.* Interleukin-2 therapy, central venous catheters, and nosocomial sepsis. *Ann Intern Med* 1990; **112:** 882–3.
3. Jones AL, *et al.* Infectious complications of subcutaneous interleukin-2 and interferon-alpha. *Lancet* 1992; **339:** 181–2.
4. Buter J, *et al.* Infection after subcutaneous interleukin-2. *Lancet* 1992; **339:** 552.
5. Schomburg AG, *et al.* Cytokines and infection in cancer patients. *Lancet* 1992; **339:** 1061.
6. Murphy PM, *et al.* Marked disparity in incidence of bacterial infections in patients with the acquired immunodeficiency syndrome receiving interleukin-2 or interferon-γ. *Ann Intern Med* 1988; **108:** 36–41.
7. Klempner MS, *et al.* An acquired chemotactic defect in neutrophils from patients receiving interleukin-2 immunotherapy. *N Engl J Med* 1990; **322:** 959–65.

Effects on endocrine function. It has been suggested that patients with adrenal metastases may be particularly susceptible to adrenal haemorrhage and consequent failure during interleukin therapy.[1] Results also suggested that lack of endogenous steroid production may increase the risk of early severe interleukin-2 toxicity.[1]

Effects on thyroid function have also been reported, with the development of hypothyroidism[2-4] and goitre.[3]
1. VanderMolen LA, *et al.* Adrenal insufficiency and interleukin-2 therapy. *Ann Intern Med* 1989; **111:** 185.
2. Atkins MB, *et al.* Hypothyroidism after treatment with interleukin-2 and lymphokine-activated killer cells. *N Engl J Med* 1988; **318:** 1557–63.
3. van Liessum PA, *et al.* Hypothyroidism and goitre during interleukin-2 therapy without LAK cells. *Lancet* 1989; **i:** 224.
4. Sauter NP, *et al.* Transient thyrotoxicosis and persistent hypothyroidism due to acute autoimmune thyroiditis after interleukin-2 and interferon-α therapy for metastatic carcinoma: a case report. *Am J Med* 1992; **92:** 441–4.

Effects on the kidneys. Intravenous aldesleukin therapy was associated with varying degrees of acute renal dysfunction in almost all patients of 99 consecutive patients.[1] The clinical syndrome of hypotension, oliguria, fluid retention, and associated azotaemia with intense tubular avidity for filtered sodium all support prerenal acute renal failure as the cause of renal dysfunction. However, renal function values returned to baseline levels within 7 days in 62% of patients and in 95% by 30 days. Patients with elevated pretreatment serum-creatinine values, particularly those aged over 60 years, and those who had previously undergone a nephrectomy, were at risk of more severe and prolonged changes in renal function, and might be particularly vulnerable to the use of indometacin for associated fever and chills, which could potentiate renal impairment through its effects on intrarenal prostaglandin production.
1. Belldegrun A, *et al.* Effects of interleukin-2 on renal function in patients receiving immunotherapy for advanced cancer. *Ann Intern Med* 1987; **106:** 817–22.

Precautions

Aldesleukin should be given with great care, if at all, to patients with pre-existing cardiac or pulmonary disease, and those with severe renal or hepatic impairment. It should be avoided in patients with CNS metastases or seizure disorders.

Risk factors for toxicity and poor response include performance status of 1 or greater, 2 or more metastatic sites, and a period of less than 24 months between diagnosis of primary tumour and consideration for aldesleukin therapy. The manufacturer in the UK considers that aldesleukin should not be used to treat metastatic renal cell carcinoma in patients with all three of these risk factors.

Aldesleukin may exacerbate auto-immune diseases, and should be used with caution in patients with these conditions. Bacterial infections should be adequately treated before beginning therapy. Aldesleukin may exacerbate effusions from serosal surfaces, and these should generally be treated before aldesleukin therapy.

Vital signs, blood counts, renal and hepatic function, serum electrolytes, and pulmonary and cardiac function should be monitored during therapy.

Activity. For mention of the loss of activity when aldesleukin was given by continuous infusion without albumin, see Stability above.

Inflammatory bowel disease. Two patients with a history of Crohn's disease had a recurrence of the condition when given aldesleukin. It was suggested that interleukin-2 should be contra-indicated in such patients.[1]
1. Sparano JA, *et al.* Symptomatic exacerbation of Crohn disease after treatment with high-dose interleukin-2. *Ann Intern Med* 1993; **118:** 617–18.

Psoriasis. Exacerbations of psoriasis developed in 3 patients during therapy with aldesleukin alone or with lymphokine-activated killer cells. The psoriatic symptoms remitted with topical therapy.[1]
1. Lee RE, *et al.* Interleukin 2 and psoriasis. *Arch Dermatol* 1988; **124:** 1811–15.

Interactions

Corticosteroids (which reduce some of the adverse effects of interleukin-2 administration) may also reduce its antineoplastic properties: concomitant administration should generally be avoided.

Antivirals. For the effect of interleukin-2 on plasma concentrations of indinavir, see p.627.

NSAIDs. NSAIDs are effective in preventing or reducing fever and myalgia caused by interleukin-2. However, there is concern that they could exacerbate renal toxicity (see also Effects on the Kidneys, above). Administration of concomitant *indometacin* to patients receiving interleukin-2 led to more severe weight gain, oliguria, and azotaemia in 1 study.[1] However, *ibuprofen* was used successfully to reduce interleukin-2 toxicity in another study.[2]
1. Sosman JA, *et al.* Repetitive weekly cycles of interleukin-2 II: clinical and immunologic effects of dose, schedule, and addition of indometacin. *J Natl Cancer Inst* 1988; **80:** 1451–61.
2. Eberlein TJ, *et al.* Ibuprofen causes reduced toxic effects of interleukin 2 administration in patients with metastatic cancer. *Arch Surg* 1989; **124:** 542–7.

Pharmacokinetics

After intravenous bolus administration, the serum distribution and elimination half-lives of aldesleukin are 13 and 85 minutes, respectively. After subcutaneous administration, the absorption half-life is 45 minutes and the elimination half-life is 5.3 hours, while bioavailability ranges between 35 and 47%.

Aldesleukin is metabolised to amino acids by the kidneys.

◊ References.
1. Anderson PM, Sorenson MA. Effects of route and formulation on clinical pharmacokinetics of interleukin-2. *Clin Pharmacokinet* 1994; **27:** 19–31.
2. Piscitelli SC, *et al.* Pharmacokinetics and pharmacodynamics of subcutaneous interleukin-2 in HIV-infected patients. *Pharmacotherapy* 1996; **16:** 754–9.
3. Kirchner GI, *et al.* Pharmacokinetics of recombinant human interleukin-2 in advanced renal cell carcinoma patients following subcutaneous application. *Br J Clin Pharmacol* 1998; **46:** 5–10.

Uses and Administration

Interleukin-2 is a lymphokine which stimulates the proliferation of T-lymphocytes and thus amplifies immune response to an antigen; it also has actions on B-lymphocytes, and induces the production of interferon-γ and the activation of natural killer cells. Interleukin-2 is used in the immunotherapy of metastatic renal cell carcinoma in selected patients (see p.495). It is also used in melanoma (p.499), and has been tried in non-Hodgkin's lymphoma and acute non-lymphoblastic leukaemia.

Interleukin-2 is usually given by intravenous infusion or subcutaneous injection of one of its recombinant forms, such as aldesleukin.

A variety of dosage regimens have been tried. In the UK, the recommended dose of aldesleukin for metastatic renal cell carcinoma is 18 million units administered subcutaneously once daily for 5 days, followed by 2 days rest for the first week. For the next 3 weeks, 18 million units is then administered on days 1 and 2 of each week, and 9 million units on days 3 to 5 of each week, followed by 2 days rest. This 4-week cycle may be repeated after an interval of 1 week. Administration may be delayed or the dose reduced if the regimen is not tolerated.

Aldesleukin was formerly given by intravenous infusion, in similar doses, but such administration is no longer advocated in the UK.

However, in the USA, aldesleukin is given by intravenous infusion for metastatic renal cell carcinoma or melanoma. The recommended dose is an infusion of 600 000 units per kg body-weight over 15 minutes, every 8 hours for up to 14 doses. This 5-day cycle is repeated after 9 days. Further courses may be given at intervals of at least 7 weeks in patients who respond. Doses should be withheld for toxicity.

Interleukin-2 has also been given in adoptive immunotherapy with lymphokine-activated killer (LAK) cells or tumour-infiltrating lymphocytes (TIL), which are harvested from the patient, activated *ex vivo*, and then re-infused.

Interleukin-2 is also being tried in patients with HIV infection and AIDS in an attempt to restore immune response (see below) and has been given in some other infections or immune diseases.

Other interleukins are under investigation (see also Interleukin-1, p.1623). Conjugates of interleukin-2 with macrogol (PEG-IL2; pegaldesleukin) have also been investigated and liposome-encapsulated interleukin-2 has also been investigated for the treatment of brain and CNS tumours.

◊ Reviews.
1. Winkelhake JL, Gauny SS. Human recombinant interleukin-2 as an experimental therapeutic. *Pharmacol Rev* 1990; **42:** 1–28.
2. Kintzel PE, Calis KA. Recombinant interleukin-2: a biological response modifier. *Clin Pharm* 1991; **10:** 110–28.
3. Whittington R, Faulds D. Interleukin-2: a review of its pharmacological properties and therapeutic use in patients with cancer. *Drugs* 1993; **46:** 446–514.
4. Aulitzky WE, *et al.* Interleukins: clinical pharmacology and therapeutic use. *Drugs* 1994; **48:** 667–77.
5. Noble S, Goa K. Aldesleukin (recombinant interleukin-2): a review of its pharmacological properties, clinical efficacy and tolerability in patients with metastatic melanoma. *BioDrugs* 1997; **7:** 394–422.

HIV infection and AIDS. Interleukin-2 was reported to partially restore the deficient proliferation response and natural killer cell activity of lymphocytes from persons with AIDS (p.608) when added *in vitro*. A number of studies have therefore examined the potential benefits of adding interleukin-2 to the treatment of patients with HIV infection. Following earlier pilot studies, studies of antiretroviral therapy plus interleukin-2 have shown it to produce a much greater increase in CD4 cell counts than antiretroviral therapy alone,[1-5] even where therapy included highly active antiretroviral therapy (HAART). The clinical benefits of such combined therapy have not yet, however, been demonstrated.

Although teceleukin has been tried[1] most studies of interleukin-2 therapy in HIV have used aldesleukin. Doses and routes of administration have varied: in general doses seem to have ranged from 6 to 18 million units daily by intravenous infusion, or 3 to 30 million units daily subcutaneously, given in most cases for a 5-day cycle every 8 weeks. Subcutaneous administration appears to be as effective as intravenous, and is more convenient.[2] There is evidence that 5-day dose cycles of 4.5 or 7.5 million units twice daily by subcutaneous injection are effective, whereas cycles with a lower dose of 1.5 million units twice daily are not.[3,6] However, others have reported benefit from a dose as low as 3 million units daily in combination with HAART in patients with advanced disease.[7]

Adverse effects are common, particularly at higher doses and with intravenous infusion rather than subcutaneous administration.[5] However, concerns about a potential stimulant effect on viral replication with a consequent increase in viral load do not seem to have been borne out,[2-5] and some studies have reported reduced viral loads in interleukin-treated patients.[4]

The macrogol conjugate of interleukin-2, PEG-IL2, has also been investigated in this context, but results have been disappointing, since it appears markedly less effective than aldesleukin in stimulating CD4 counts.[2,8]
1. Bartlett JA, *et al.* Coadministration of zidovudine and interleukin-2 increases absolute CD4 cells in subjects with Walter Reed stage 2 human immunodeficiency virus infection: results of ACTG protocol 042. *J Infect Dis* 1998; **178:** 1170–3.
2. Levy Y, *et al.* Comparison of subcutaneous and intravenous interleukin-2 in asymptomatic HIV-1 infection: a randomised controlled trial. *Lancet* 1999; **353:** 1923–9.
3. Losso MH, *et al.* A randomized, controlled, phase II trial comparing escalating doses of subcutaneous interleukin-2 plus antiretrovirals versus antiretrovirals alone in human immunodeficiency virus-infected patients with CD4+ cell counts ≥350/mm³. *J Infect Dis* 2000; **181:** 1614–21.
4. Davey RT, *et al.* Immunologic and virologic effects of subcutaneous interleukin 2 in combination with antiretroviral therapy: a randomized controlled trial. *JAMA* 2000; **284:** 183–9.
5. Piscitelli SC, *et al.* A risk-benefit assessment of interleukin-2 as an adjunct to antiviral therapy in HIV infection. *Drug Safety* 2000; **22:** 19–31.

6. Davey RT, *et al.* A randomized trial of high- versus low-dose subcutaneous interleukin-2 outpatient therapy for early human immunodeficiency virus type 1 infection. *J Infect Dis* 1999; **179:** 849–58.

7. Arnó A, *et al.* Efficacy of low-dose subcutaneous interleukin-2 to treat advanced human immunodeficiency virus type 1 in persons with ≤250/μL CD4 T cells and undetectable plasma virus load. *J Infect Dis* 1999; **180:** 56–60.

8. Carr A, *et al.* Outpatient continuous intravenous interleukin-2 or subcutaneous, polyethylene glycol-modified interleukin-2 in human immunodeficiency virus-infected patients: a randomized, controlled, multicenter study. *J Infect Dis* 1998; **178:** 992–9.

Leishmaniasis. Encouraging preliminary results were seen in 3 patients with disseminated cutaneous leishmaniasis (p.584) who received injections of interleukin-2 180 000 units into their lesions on 3 occasions at 48-hour intervals. There was an influx of T-cells and monocytes into the injected lesions, and a marked reduction in parasite numbers.[1] These results were analogous to those seen in patients with lepromatous leprosy, in whom local injection of interleukin-2 can reconstitute a cell-mediated immune response leading to an extensive reduction in bacterial load at the site of injection.[2]

1. Akuffo H, *et al.* Administration of recombinant interleukin-2 reduces the local parasite load of patients with disseminated cutaneous leishmaniasis. *J Infect Dis* 1990; **161:** 775–80.

2. Kaplan G, *et al.* The reconstitution of cell-mediated immunity in the cutaneous lesions of lepromatous leprosy by recombinant interleukin-2. *J Exp Med* 1989; **169:** 893–907.

Leprosy. See under Leishmaniasis, above.

Vaccine immunoadjuvant. Interleukin-2 250 000 units intramuscularly 4 hours after vaccination for hepatitis B improved immune response in 10 haemodialysis patients who had previously failed to respond to several attempts at hepatitis B vaccination.[1] Protective antibody titres developed in 6, and one showed seroconversion but at low titres, whereas in 8 similar patients given the vaccine alone only one showed any seroconversion. However, another study in which subcutaneous injection of 1 million units of interleukin-2 was given to 27 uraemic patients 5 minutes after hepatitis B injection failed to demonstrate any difference in seroconversion rate compared with 25 further patients given placebo.[2]

1. Meuer SC, *et al.* Low-dose interleukin-2 induces systemic immune responses against HBsAg in immunodeficient non-responders to hepatitis B vaccination. *Lancet* 1989; **i:** 15–18.

2. Jungers P, *et al.* Randomised placebo-controlled trial of recombinant interleukin-2 in chronic uraemic patients who are non-responders to hepatitis B vaccine. *Lancet* 1994; **344:** 856–7.

Preparations

Proprietary Preparations (details are given in Part 3)

Aust.: Proleukin; *Austral.:* Proleukin; *Canad.:* Proleukin; *Denm.:* Proleukin; *Fr.:* Macrolin; *Ger.:* Proleukin; *Hong Kong:* Proleukin; *Israel:* Proleukin; *Ital.:* Proleukin; *Mex.:* Proleukin; *Neth.:* Proleukin; *Port.:* Proleukin; *Singapore:* Proleukin; *Spain:* Proleukin; *Switz.:* Proleukin; *UK:* Proleukin; *USA:* Proleukin.

Irinotecan Hydrochloride (19006-c)

Irinotecan Hydrochloride (BANM, USAN, rINNM).

CPT-11 (irinotecan); U-101440E. (+)-7-Ethyl-10-hydroxycamptothecine 10-[1,4′-bipiperidine]-1′-carboxylate hydrochloride trihydrate; (S)-4,11-Diethyl-3,4,12,14-tetrahydro-4-hydroxy-3,14-dioxo-1*H*-pyrano[3′,4′:6′,7′]indolizino[1,2-b]quinolin-9-yl [1,4′-dipiperidine]-1′-carboxylate hydrochloride trihydrate.

$C_{33}H_{38}N_4O_6,HCl,3H_2O = 677.2$.

CAS — 97682-44-5 (irinotecan); 136572-09-3 (irinotecan hydrochloride trihydrate).

Adverse Effects, Treatment, and Precautions

For general discussions, see Antineoplastics, p.476, p.479, and p.480. Neutropenia and diarrhoea may be dose-limiting in patients receiving irinotecan. The nadir of the white cell count usually occurs about 8 days after a dose, with recovery by about day 22. Anaemia also occurs and, less commonly, thrombocytopenia. Gastrointestinal disturbances are common: acute diarrhoea, occurring within 24 hours of administration, may be part of a cholinergic syndrome which can also include sweating, hypersalivation, abdominal cramps, lachrymation, and miosis. These symptoms can be controlled with atropine. However a more severe, prolonged diarrhoea may occur, beginning more than 24 hours after a dose, and can be life-threatening; prompt management with high-dose loperamide and fluid replacement is required (see below), and irinotecan treatment should be interrupted and any further doses reduced. Other adverse effects include nausea and vomiting, weakness, alopecia, and skin reactions.

Irinotecan should not be given to patients with inflammatory bowel disease. The risk of diarrhoea may be increased in the elderly and in patients who have received radiotherapy to the abdomen or pelvis.

Severe toxicity resulting in an increased number of deaths has been reported from the combination of irinotecan with fluorouracil and folinic acid (see under Interactions, below).

Effects on the gastrointestinal system. Acute diarrhoea occurring as part of a cholinergic syndrome is rarely severe. The syndrome is usually treated or prevented with atropine, but pretreatment with hyoscine butylbromide has also been tried.[1] In contrast, delayed diarrhoea can be dose-limiting or even fatal in some patients. Standard treatment involves fluid and electrolyte replacement and a high-dose loperamide regimen consisting of 4 mg loperamide immediately after the first loose stool, then 2 mg every 2 hours until 12 hours after the last liquid stool. The high-dose therapy should not be given for more than 48 hours and should never be given prophylactically. Other treatments have been tried,[2-5] including glutamine,[4] budesonide,[3] and acetorphan.[2]

1. Zampa G, Magnolfi E. Premedication for irinotecan. *J Clin Oncol* 2000; **18:** 237.

2. Saliba F, *et al.* Pathophysiology and therapy of irinotecan-induced delayed-onset diarrhea in patients with advanced colorectal cancer: a prospective assessment. *J Clin Oncol* 1998; **16:** 2745–51.

3. Lenfers BHM, *et al.* Substantial activity of budesonide in patients with irinotecan (CPT-11) and 5-fluorouracil induced diarrhea and failure of loperamide treatment. *Ann Oncol* 1999; **10:** 1251–3.

4. Savarese D, *et al.* Glutamine for irinotecan diarrhea. *J Clin Oncol* 2000; **18:** 450–1.

5. Ychou M, *et al.* Randomized comparison of prophylactic antidiarrheal treatment versus no prophylactic antidiarrheal treatment in patients receiving CPT-11 (irinotecan) for advanced 5-FU-resistant colorectal cancer: an open-label multicenter phase II study. *Am J Clin Oncol* 2000; **23:** 143–8.

Interactions

Antineoplastics. Although previously reported to be effective, and not associated with excessive toxicity,[1] a regimen combining irinotecan with bolus *fluorouracil* and folinic acid was found to be associated with an excess of early deaths in 2 further studies, which were consequently terminated.[2] Deaths were associated with a variety of events including dehydration (due to diarrhoea, nausea, and vomiting), neutropenia, and sepsis. It has been suggested that combination of irinotecan with fluorouracil by continuous infusion might be better tolerated.[3]

1. Saltz LB, *et al.* Irinotecan plus fluorouracil and leucovorin for metastatic colorectal cancer. *N Engl J Med* 2000; **343:** 905–14.

2. Sargent DJ, *et al.* Recommendation for caution with irinotecan, fluorouracil, and leucovorin for colorectal cancer. *N Engl J Med* 2001; **345:** 144–5.

3. Ledermann JA, *et al.* Recommendation for caution with irinotecan, fluorouracil, and leucovorin for colorectal cancer. *N Engl J Med* 2001; **345:** 145–6.

Pharmacokinetics

Following intravenous administration irinotecan is metabolised by carboxyesterase in body tissues to active SN-38. It exhibits biphasic or triphasic pharmacokinetics, with a terminal half-life of about 14 hours. Only about 20% of a dose is excreted in urine within 24 hours.

◊ References.

1. Chabot GG. Clinical pharmacokinetics of irinotecan. *Clin Pharmacokinet* 1997; **33:** 245–59.

Uses and Administration

Irinotecan is a derivative of the alkaloid camptothecin, obtained from the shrub *Camptotheca acuminata*. The camptothecin derivatives are inhibitors of the enzyme topoisomerase I which inhibit nucleic acid synthesis by interfering with the coiling and uncoiling of DNA during replication. This action is specific for S-phase.

Irinotecan is used, alone or in combination with fluorouracil, in the treatment of metastatic colorectal cancer (p.493). It has been tried in the management of other solid tumours including those of the lung (p.496).

It is given as the hydrochloride, by intravenous infusion. In the treatment of refractory colorectal malignancies one suggested dose regimen is 125 mg of irinotecan hydrochloride per m² body-surface infused over 90 minutes once a week for 4 weeks, followed by a 2-week rest period. Additional courses may be given if required, with doses modified according to toxicity. Another regimen requires administration of an initial dose of 350 mg per m² over 30 to 90 minutes

repeated every 3 weeks and adjusted according to toxicity.

Irinotecan hydrochloride may also be given as part of a combination regimen with fluorouracil and folinic acid in the first-line treatment of metastatic colorectal cancer. The irinotecan component of the course is administered at a dose of 180 mg per m² over 30 to 90 minutes every 2 weeks for 3 doses; alternatively, 125 mg per m² may be given weekly for 4 doses. (For reference to toxicity from such combinations see under Interactions, above.)

◊ References.

1. Wiseman LR, Markham A. Irinotecan: a review of its pharmacological properties and clinical efficacy in the management of advanced colorectal cancer. *Drugs* 1996; **52:** 606–23.

2. Cersosimo RJ. Irinotecan: a new antineoplastic agent for the management of colorectal cancer. *Ann Pharmacother* 1998; **32:** 1324–33.

3. Siu LL, Rowinsky EK. A risk-benefit assessment of irinotecan in solid tumours. *Drug Safety* 1998; **18:** 395–417.

4. Rougier P, *et al.* Randomised trial of irinotecan versus fluorouracil by continuous infusion after fluorouracil failure in patients with metastatic colorectal cancer. *Lancet* 1998; **352:** 1407–12. Correction *ibid*; 1634.

5. Cunningham D, *et al.* Randomised trial of irinotecan plus supportive case versus supportive care alone after fluorouracil failure for patients with metastatic colorectal cancer. *Lancet* 1998; **352:** 1413–18.

6. Van Cutsem E, Blijham GH. Irinotecan versus infusional 5-fluorouracil: a phase III study in metastatic colorectal cancer following failure on first-line 5-fluorouracil. *Semin Oncol* 1999; **26:** (suppl 5): 13–20.

7. Douillard JY, *et al.* Irinotecan combined with fluorouracil compared with fluorouracil alone as first-line treatment for metastatic colorectal cancer: a multicentre randomised trial. *Lancet* 2000; **355:** 1041–7.

Preparations

Proprietary Preparations (details are given in Part 3)

Austral.: Camptosar; *Belg.:* Campto; *Canad.:* Camptosar; *Denm.:* Campto; *Fin.:* Campto; *Fr.:* Campto; *Ger.:* Campto; *Hong Kong:* Campto; *Irl.:* Campto; *Israel:* Campto; *Ital.:* Campto; *Mex.:* Camptosar; *Neth.:* Campto; *Norw.:* Campto; *NZ:* Camptosar; *Port.:* Campto; *S.Afr.:* Campto; *Singapore:* Campto; *Spain:* Campto; *Swed.:* Campto; *Switz.:* Campto; *Thai.:* Campto; *UK:* Campto; *USA:* Camptosar.

Leflunomide (10839-p)

Leflunomide (BAN, USAN, rINN).

HWA-486; SU-101. α,α,α-Trifluoro-5-methyl-4-isoxazolecarboxy-p-toluidide.

$C_{12}H_9F_3N_2O_2 = 270.2$.

CAS — 75706-12-6.

Adverse Effects, Treatment and Precautions

The main adverse effects seen with leflunomide are hypertension, gastrointestinal disturbances, weight loss, headache, dizziness, asthenia, paraesthesia, joint disorders and synovitis, alopecia, eczema, and dry skin. Leucopenia may occur. Hypersensitivity reactions may occur and a few cases of Stevens-Johnson syndrome or toxic epidermal necrolysis have been reported. Hepatotoxicity has occurred. It is usually mild and reversible but rare cases of severe liver disease, including acute hepatic necrosis, have been observed particularly in the first 6 months of therapy.

The active metabolite of leflunomide, A771726, has a half-life of about 2 weeks. Consequently the adverse effects of leflunomide may continue even after therapy has been terminated. When severe reactions occur, a drug washout procedure (see below) may be required.

Leflunomide should not be given to immunocompromised patients or to patients with severe infections or impaired renal or hepatic function. It should be avoided in pregnancy and if patients become pregnant while taking the drug, a washout procedure should be performed. Blood pressure and blood counts should be monitored regularly during therapy.

Liver enzyme values should be checked before beginning therapy and at monthly or more frequent intervals during the first 6 months of treatment; subsequent monitoring should be carried out at 8-week intervals. Dosage should be reduced if moderate elevations of liver enzyme values occur; for more severe elevations leflunomide should be discontinued and washout procedures initiated.

◊ If serious adverse effects occur during leflunomide therapy, the manufacturers recommend that a drug washout procedure is performed. This may also be considered if a patient becomes pregnant while taking the drug, or if it is necessary to swap to another DMARD treatment.

For the washout procedure, either 8 g colestyramine is given 3 times daily or 50 g of activated charcoal is given 4 times daily. Therapy is normally continued for 11 days, but should be repeated until verified plasma concentrations of the primary metabolite A771726 are below 20 nanograms per mL.

Interactions

Concomitant use of other hepatotoxic drugs should be avoided; if a patient is to be transferred to treatment with another hepa-

The symbol † denotes a preparation no longer actively marketed

550 Antineoplastics and Immunosuppressants

totoxic antirheumatic drug such as methotrexate a drug wash-out procedure (above) should be performed first.

Pharmacokinetics

Following oral administration leflunomide undergoes first-pass metabolism to A771726, which is responsible for the majority of the *in vivo* activity. The bioavailability of leflunomide after oral administration ranges from 82 to 95%. Peak plasma concentrations of the active metabolite may occur from 1 to 24 hours after administration.

A771726 has an elimination half-life of approximately 2 weeks, which is thought to be mainly due to enterohepatic recycling. Colestyramine or activated charcoal are able to interrupt recycling and can therefore accelerate drug elimination.

A771726 is more than 99% bound to plasma proteins. It is metabolised in the gut wall and the liver. Approximately 43% of a dose is eliminated in the urine, mainly as glucuronides, and 48% is eliminated in the faeces via the bile.

Uses and Administration

Leflunomide has immunosuppressant and antiproliferative properties. It is used as a disease-modifying antirheumatic drug in the treatment of active rheumatoid arthritis (p.9), and is being investigated in the management of various solid neoplasms.

Because of the long half-life of the principal metabolite a loading dose is required to reach steady-state concentrations relatively rapidly. Therapy for rheumatoid arthritis should be initiated with a loading dose of 100 mg leflunomide by mouth daily for 3 days. The maintenance dose is 10 to 20 mg daily. The therapeutic effect usually starts after 4 to 6 weeks of therapy and further improvements may occur for up to 6 months.

◊ References.
1. Smolen JS, et al. Efficacy and safety of leflunomide compared with placebo and sulphasalazine in active rheumatoid arthritis: a double-blind, randomised, multicentre trial. Lancet 1999; 353: 259–66.
2. Hudes G. Signaling inhibitors in the clinic: new agents and new challenges. J Clin Oncol 1999; 17: 1093–4.
3. Strand V, et al. Treatment of active rheumatoid arthritis with leflunomide compared with placebo and methotrexate. Arch Intern Med 1999; 159: 2542–50.
4. Prakash A, Jarvis B. Leflunomide: a review of its use in active rheumatoid arthritis. Drugs 1999; 58: 1137–64.
5. Emery P, et al. A comparison of the efficacy and safety of leflunomide and methotrexate for the treatment of rheumatoid arthritis. Rheumatology 2000; 39: 655–65.

Preparations

Proprietary Preparations (details are given in Part 3)
Austral.: Arava; *Denm.:* Arava; *Fin.:* Arava; *Fr.:* Arava; *Ger.:* Arava; *Irl.:* Arava; *Neth.:* Arava; *Swed.:* Arava; *Switz.:* Arava; *UK:* Arava; *USA:* Arava.

Letrozole (17432-a)

Letrozole (BAN, USAN, rINN).
CGS-20267. 4,4′-(1H-1,2,4-Triazol-1-ylmethylene)dibenzonitrile.
$C_{17}H_{11}N_5 = 285.3$.
CAS — 112809-51-5.
ATC — L02BG04.
Pharmacopoeias. In US.

Pharmacopoeial description

USP 25: A white to yellowish, crystalline powder. Practically insoluble in water; slightly soluble in alcohol; freely soluble in dichloromethane. Store in airtight containers.

Profile

Letrozole is a nonsteroidal inhibitor of the aromatase (oestrogen synthetase) system, similar to anastrozole (p.508). It is used in the first- or second-line treatment of advanced breast cancer (p.491) in postmenopausal women. It may also be given as neoadjuvant (pre-operative) therapy to those with localised hormone-receptor positive disease, to allow subsequent breast-conserving surgery. The recommended dose is 2.5 mg daily by mouth.

◊ References.
1. Lamb HM, Adkins JC. Letrozole: a review of its use in postmenopausal women with advanced breast cancer. Drugs 1998; 56: 1125–40.
2. Dombernowsky P, et al. Letrozole, a new oral aromatase inhibitor for advanced breast cancer: double-blind randomized trial showing a dose effect and improved efficacy and tolerability compared with megestrol acetate. J Clin Oncol 1998; 16: 453–61.
3. Gershanovich M, et al. Letrozole, a new oral aromatase inhibitor: randomised trial comparing 2.5 mg daily, 0.5 mg daily and aminoglutethimide in postmenopausal women with advanced breast cancer. Ann Oncol 1998; 9: 639–45.
4. Chaudri HA, Trunet PF. Letrozole: updated duration of response. J Clin Oncol 1999; 17: 3859–60.
5. Mouridsen H, et al. Superior efficacy of letrozole versus tamoxifen as first-line therapy for postmenopausal women with advanced breast cancer: results of a phase III study of the International Letrozole Breast Cancer Group. J Clin Oncol 2001; 19: 2596–2606.
6. Ellis MJ, et al. Letrozole is more effective neoadjuvant endocrine therapy than tamoxifen for ErbB-1 and/or ErbB-2-positive, estrogen receptor-positive primary breast cancer: evidence from a phase III randomized trial. J Clin Oncol 2001; 19: 3808–16.

Preparations

USP 25: Letrozole Tablets.
Proprietary Preparations (details are given in Part 3)
Aust.: Femara; *Austral.:* Femara; *Belg.:* Femara; *Canad.:* Femara; *Denm.:* Femar; *Fin.:* Femar; *Fr.:* Femara; *Ger.:* Femara; *Hong Kong:* Femara; *Irl.:* Femara; *Israel:* Femara; *Ital.:* Femara; *Neth.:* Femara; *Norw.:* Femar; *NZ:* Femara; *Port.:* Femara; *S.Afr.:* Femara; *Singapore:* Femara; *Spain:* Femara; *Swed.:* Femar; *Switz.:* Femara; *Thai.:* Femara; *UK:* Femara; *USA:* Femara.

Lithium Gamolenate (17722-v)

EF-13; LiGLA; Lithium Gammalinolenate.

Profile

Lithium gamolenate is a derivative of gamolenic acid (p.1613) which has been investigated for its antineoplastic properties, notably in the treatment of pancreatic cancer (p.497). It has also been investigated in patients with HIV infection.

◊ References.
1. Fearon KC, et al. An open-label phase I/II dose escalation study of the treatment of pancreatic cancer using lithium gammalinolenate. Anticancer Res 1996; 16: 867–74.

Lobaplatin (15418-b)

Lobaplatin (rINN).
D-19466. cis-[trans-1,2-Cyclobutanebis(methylamine)][(S)-lactato-O¹,O¹]platinum.
$C_9H_{18}N_2O_3Pt = 397.3$.
CAS — 135558-11-1.

Profile

Lobaplatin is an analogue of cisplatin (p.525) which has been investigated for its antineoplastic properties. Thrombocytopenia is reported to be dose-limiting. It may be active against some cancer cells resistant to cisplatin or carboplatin.

◊ References.
1. Weiss RB, Christian MC. New cisplatin analogues in development: a review. Drugs 1993; 6: 360–77.
2. Gietema JA, et al. A phase I study of 1,2-diamminomethyl-cyclobutane-platinum (II) lactate (D-19466; lobaplatin) administered daily for 5 days. Br J Cancer 1993; 67: 396–401.
3. Manegold C, et al. Lobaplatin (D-19466) in patients with advanced non-small-cell lung cancer: a trial of the association for medical oncology (AIO) phase II study group. Onkologie 1996; 19: 248–51.
4. Fiebig HH, et al. Phase II clinical trial of lobaplatin (D-19466) in pretreated patients with small-cell lung cancer. Onkologie 1996; 19: 328–32.
5. Sternberg CN, et al. Lobaplatin in advanced urothelial tract tumors. Ann Oncol 1997; 8: 695–6.
6. Welink J, et al. Pharmacokinetics and pharmacodynamics of lobaplatin (D-19466) in patients with advanced solid tumors, including patients with impaired renal or liver function. Clin Cancer Res 1999; 5: 2349–58.

Lomustine (1841-k)

Lomustine (BAN, USAN, rINN).
CCNU; Lomustinum; NSC-79037; RB-1509; WR-139017. 1-(2-Chloroethyl)-3-cyclohexyl-1-nitrosourea.
$C_9H_{16}ClN_3O_2 = 233.7$.
CAS — 13010-47-4.
ATC — L01AD02.
Pharmacopoeias. In Chin. and Eur. (see p.vi).

Pharmacopoeial description

Ph. Eur.: A yellow, crystalline powder. Practically insoluble in water; soluble in alcohol; freely soluble in acetone and in dichloromethane. Protect from light.

Adverse Effects, Treatment, and Precautions

As for Carmustine, p.516, although bone-marrow depression may be even more delayed with lomustine. Neurological reactions such as confusion and lethargy have been reported.

Handling and disposal. A method for the destruction of lomustine *waste* by reaction with hydrobromic acid in glacial acetic acid[1] The residue produced by the degradation of lomustine by this method showed no mutagenicity. This method is not suitable for the degradation of carmustine, semustine, or PCNU.

1. Castegnaro M, et al., eds. Laboratory decontamination and destruction of carcinogens in laboratory wastes: some antineoplastic agents. IARC Scientific Publications 73. Lyon: WHO/International Agency for Research on Cancer, 1985.

Overdosage. A patient who inadvertently received 200 mg of lomustine for 7 days instead of a single 200 mg dose developed pancytopenia and subsequent multiorgan dysfunction including liver dysfunction, abdominal pain, pulmonary toxicity with tachypnoea and hypoxaemia, and CNS toxicity leading to confusion and disorientation.[1] Although the white cell count recovered other signs of toxicity did not and the patient

developed fever and hypotension and died 59 days after the initial dose of lomustine. In another case of accidental overdose, a 30-year old female received a cumulative dose of 28 mg per kg body-weight over 7 days.[2] Severe myelosuppression developed soon after the overdose and lasted for 50 days. The patient was treated with granulocyte colony-stimulating factor and antibiotic cover, norethisterone (to prevent menstruation), and acetylcysteine (to protect against organ toxicity). Gastrointestinal necrosis occurred, and liver enzymes remained elevated even after recovery from the overdose, but the patient survived and her tumour regressed without further chemotherapy.

1. Trent KC, et al. Multiorgan failure associated with lomustine overdose. Ann Pharmacother 1995; 29: 384–6.
2. Abele M, et al. CCNU overdose during PCV chemotherapy for anaplastic astrocytoma. J Neurol 1998; 245: 236–8.

Interactions

For a general outline of antineoplastic drug interactions, see p.481.

Theophylline. Leucopenia and thrombocytopenia in a 45-year-old woman were believed to have been secondary to an interaction between theophylline and lomustine.[1]

1. Zeltzer PM, Feig SA. Theophylline-induced lomustine toxicity. Lancet 1979; ii: 960–1.

Pharmacokinetics

Lomustine is absorbed from the gastrointestinal tract and is rapidly metabolised, with peak plasma concentrations of metabolites occurring within 4 hours of a dose by mouth. Metabolites have a prolonged plasma half-life reported to range from 16 to 48 hours. Active metabolites readily cross the blood-brain barrier and appear in the cerebrospinal fluid in concentrations higher than those in plasma. About half a dose is excreted as metabolites in the urine within 24 hours and about 75% is excreted within 4 days.

Uses and Administration

Lomustine is a nitrosourea with actions and uses similar to those of carmustine (p.516). It has been used in the treatment of brain tumours (p.490) and resistant or relapsed Hodgkin's disease and other lymphomas (p.487), and also lung cancer (p.496), malignant melanoma (p.499), and various solid tumours.

Lomustine is given by mouth to adults and children as a single dose usually of 120 to 130 mg per m² body-surface; division of the dose over 3 consecutive days may reduce gastrointestinal effects. A dose of 100 mg per m² should be given to patients with compromised bone-marrow function. Doses are also generally reduced when lomustine is given as part of a combination regimen. Providing blood counts have returned to acceptable levels, that is, platelets above 100 000 per mm³ and leucocytes above 4000 per mm³, doses may be repeated every 6 to 8 weeks, and should be adjusted according to the haematological response.

Preparations

BP 2001: Lomustine Capsules.

Proprietary Preparations (details are given in Part 3)
Austral.: CeeNU; *Belg.:* Cecenu†; *Braz.:* Citostal; *Canad.:* CeeNU; *Fr.:* Belustine†; *Ger.:* Cecenu; *Hong Kong:* Belustine; CeeNU; *Israel:* CeeNU; *Ital.:* Belustine†; *Mex.:* CeeNU; *NZ:* CeeNU; *S.Afr.:* CeeNU†; *Singapore:* CeeNU; *Spain:* Belustine†; *Swed.:* Lucostine†; *Switz.:* Prava; *Thai.:* CeeNU; *UK:* CCNU; *USA:* CeeNU.

Lonidamine (19416-e)

Lonidamine (BAN, rINN).
AF-1890; Diclondazolic Acid. 1-(2,4-Dichlorobenzyl)indazole-3-carboxylic acid.
$C_{15}H_{10}Cl_2N_2O_2 = 321.2$.
CAS — 50264-69-2.
ATC — L01XX07.

Profile

Lonidamine is an antineoplastic that is thought to act by inhibiting mitochondrial function in tumour cells. It may be given by mouth in the treatment of various solid neoplasms, including those of the lung, breast, prostate, and brain, in usual doses of 450 to 900 mg daily, in 3 divided doses. Myalgia is common, and may be dose-limiting. Other adverse effects include testicular pain, auditory dysfunction, gastrointestinal disturbances, drowsiness, weakness, and conjunctivitis with photophobia, but it is reported to lack myelosuppressive effects and not to cause stomatitis or alopecia.

◊ References.
1. Putzolu S, Taddei I. New perspectives in anticancer therapy: a review on lonidamine. Drugs Today 1989; 25: 195–209.

2. De Lena M, *et al.* Revertant and potentiating activity of lonidamine in patients with ovarian cancer previously treated with platinum. *J Clin Oncol* 1997; **15:** 3208–13.

3. De Marinis F, *et al.* The role of vindesine and lonidamine in the treatment of elderly patients with advanced non-small cell lung cancer: a phase III randomized FONICAP trial. *Tumori* 1999; **85:** 177–82.

4. Pacini P, *et al.* FEC (5-fluorouracil, epidoxorubicin and cyclophosphamide) versus EM (epidoxorubicin and mitomycin-C) with or without lonidamine as first-line treatment for advanced breast cancer: a multicentric randomised study. Final results. *Eur J Cancer* 2000; **36:** 966–75.

Preparations

Proprietary Preparations (details are given in Part 3)

Ital.: Doridamina.

Mafosfamide (18785-v)

Mafosfamide (rINN).

(±)-2-({2-[Bis(2-chloroethyl)amino]tetrahydro-2*H*-1,3,2-oxazaphosphorin-4-yl}thio)ethanesulphonic acid *P*-cis oxide.

$C_9H_{19}Cl_2N_2O_5PS_2 = 401.3$.

CAS — 88859-04-5.

Profile

Mafosfamide is a derivative of cyclophosphamide (p.527) that has been used to treat bone marrow for transplantation.

Marimastat (17715-g)

Marimastat (BAN, USAN, rINN).

BB-2516. (2S,3R)-3-{(S)-[2,2-Dimethyl-1-(methylcarbamoyl)propyl]carbamoyl}-2-hydroxy-5-methylhexanohydroxamic acid.

$C_{15}H_{29}N_3O_5 = 331.4$.

CAS — 154039-60-8.

Profile

Like batimastat (p.511) marimastat is an inhibitor of matrix metalloproteinases, enzymes which are thought to play a role in the metastasis of cancer cells. It has been investigated by mouth in various malignant disorders, but with little success.

◊ Reviews.

1. Heath EI, Grochow LB. Clinical potential of matrix metalloprotease inhibitors in cancer therapy. *Drugs* 2000; **59:** 1043–55.

◊ It was suggested that the alterations in tumour markers reported in patients with ovarian cancer given marimastat might be artefactual;[1] however, at the time the manufacturers considered that these and further results in patients with pancreatic, prostatic, and colorectal cancers were evidence of genuine activity.[2] Subsequent studies have failed to show benefit with marimastat in patients with malignant neoplasms, and further development has reportedly been suspended.

In healthy subjects given doses between 25 and 800 mg by mouth marimastat was reportedly well tolerated and rapidly absorbed, with peak drug concentrations achieved within 3 hours of a dose, and mean half-life of the order of 8 to 10 hours.[3]

1. Gore M, *et al.* Tumour marker levels during marimastat therapy. *Lancet* 1996; **348:** 263.
2. Millar A, *et al.* Tumour marker levels during marimastat therapy. *Lancet* 1996; **348:** 263–4.
3. Millar AW, *et al.* Results of single and repeat dose studies of the oral matrix metalloproteinase inhibitor marimastat in healthy male volunteers. *Br J Clin Pharmacol* 1998; **45:** 21–6.

Masoprocol (13920-h)

Masoprocol (USAN, rINN).

CHX-10; CHX-100; Mesonordihydroguaiaretic Acid; meso-NDGA. meso-4,4'-(2,3-Dimethyltetramethylene)dipyrocatechol.

CAS — 27686-84-6.

ATC — L01XX10.

Profile

Masoprocol is a 5-lipoxygenase inhibitor isolated from the plant *Larrea divaricata*. It is reported to have antineoplastic activity. It has been used in the topical treatment of actinic (solar) keratoses. Local irritation and contact dermatitis have occurred.

Actinic keratoses. Application of a cream containing masoprocol 10% twice daily for 14 to 28 days appeared to be effective in the treatment of actinic keratoses (p.498) but of 113 patients evaluated 25 had to discontinue treatment because of local adverse effects such as erythema, flaking, itching, burning, oedema, dryness, soreness, or bleeding.[1]

1. Olsen EA, *et al.* A double-blind, vehicle-controlled study evaluating masoprocol cream in the treatment of actinic keratoses on the head and neck. *J Am Acad Dermatol* 1991; **24:** 738–43.

Preparations

Proprietary Preparations (details are given in Part 3)

USA: Actinex†.

The symbol † denotes a preparation no longer actively marketed

---

Melphalan (1843-t)

Melphalan (BAN, USAN, rINN).

CB-3025; NSC-8806 (melphalan hydrochloride); PAM; Phenylalanine Mustard; Phenylalanine Nitrogen Mustard; L-Sarcolysine; WR-19813. 4-Bis(2-chloroethyl)amino-L-phenylalanine.

$C_{13}H_{18}Cl_2N_2O_2 = 305.2$.

CAS — 148-82-3.

ATC — L01AA03.

NOTE. Merphalan (CB-3007; NSC-14210; sarcolysine) is the racemic form of melphalan; Medphalan (CB-3026; NSC-35051) is the D-isomer of melphalan.

Pharmacopoeias. In *Br., Jpn,* and *US.*

Pharmacopoeial description

BP 2001: A white or almost white, odourless or almost odourless, powder. It loses not more than 7% of its weight on drying. Practically insoluble in water, in chloroform, and in ether; slightly soluble in methyl alcohol; dissolves in dilute mineral acids. Store at a temperature not exceeding 25°. Protect from light.

USP 25: An off-white to buff powder with a faint odour. Practically insoluble in water, in chloroform, and in ether; slightly soluble in alcohol and in methyl alcohol; soluble in dilute mineral acids. Store in airtight, glass containers. Protect from light.

Stability. A study of the stability of melphalan 40 and 400 μg per mL in infusion fluids reported that the time for a 10% loss of drug at 20° in sodium chloride injection (0.9%) was 4.5 hours, compared with 2.9 hours in lactated Ringer's injection, which has a considerably lower chloride ion content, and only 1.5 hours in glucose injection (5%).[1] At 25° the corresponding figures were 2.4, 1.5, and 0.6 hours, and at 37° they were 0.6, 0.4, and 0.3 hours. It was concluded that melphalan is sufficiently stable at 20° in sodium chloride injection to permit infusion, but that increased temperature and decreased chloride ion concentration were associated with faster degradation rates.[1] Another study recommended that solutions of melphalan be handled at temperatures above 5° for the minimum time but found that a solution containing 20 μg per mL in 0.9% sodium chloride could be stored for at least 6 months at −20° without significant deterioration.[2] A more recent study, while recommending storage at 4° from preparation of the admixture until the infusion began, considered that administration at a room temperature of 20° or below, and use of hypertonic (3%) saline as a diluent, would be sufficient to allow prolonged infusion.[3] The practicalities of such a procedure were not addressed.

1. Tabibi SE, Cradock JC. Stability of melphalan in infusion fluids. *Am J Hosp Pharm* 1984; **41:** 1380–2.
2. Bosanquet AG. Stability of melphalan solutions during preparation and storage. *J Pharm Sci* 1985; **74:** 348–51.
3. Pinguet F, *et al.* Effect of sodium chloride concentration and temperature on melphalan stability during storage and use. *Am J Hosp Pharm* 1994; **51:** 2701–4.

Adverse Effects and Treatment

For general discussions see Antineoplastics, p.476 and p.479.

The onset of neutropenia and thrombocytopenia is variable; the nadir of bone-marrow depression usually occurs at 2 to 3 weeks after starting treatment with melphalan, with recovery after 4 to 5 weeks.

Skin rashes and hypersensitivity reactions, including anaphylaxis, may occur. Cardiac arrest has been reported in association with such effects. Gastrointestinal disturbances may sometimes occur, particularly at high doses where diarrhoea, vomiting, and stomatitis may become dose-limiting. Haemolytic anaemia, vasculitis, and pulmonary fibrosis have been reported. Suppression of ovarian function is common in premenopausal women; temporary or permanent sterility may occur in male patients. As with other alkylating agents, melphalan also has carcinogenic, mutagenic, and teratogenic potential.

Overdosage. A 12-month old child given melphalan 140 mg (a tenfold overdose) intravenously developed pronounced lymphopenia within 24 hours but had no other significant adverse effects until the 7th day, when neutropenia, thrombocytopenia, oral ulceration, and diarrhoea developed.[1] Bone marrow recovered within 40 days. Treatment was by vigorous hyperalimentation and close surveillance during the period of suppression and the patient subsequently remained well 9 months afterwards, without complications.

1. Coates TD. Survival from melphalan overdose. *Lancet* 1984; **ii:** 1048.

Precautions

For general discussions see Antineoplastics, p.480.

Care is required in patients with impaired renal function (see Uses and Administration, below).

Handling and disposal. *Urine and faeces* produced for up to 48 hours and 7 days respectively after a dose of melphalan by mouth should be handled wearing protective clothing.[1]

1. Harris J, Dodds LJ. Handling waste from patients receiving cytotoxic drugs. *Pharm J* 1985; **235:** 289–91.

Interactions

Concomitant administration of nalidixic acid with high-dose intravenous melphalan in children has resulted in fatal haemorrhagic enterocolitis.

Ciclosporin. For reference to enhanced toxicity when melphalan was given with ciclosporin, see under Ciclosporin, p.521.

Food. The bioavailability of oral melphalan is significantly reduced, by up to 45%, by concomitant administration with food. Some recommend that melphalan should not be taken with food, and that if administration is switched from after to before food patients should be monitored for increased toxicity.[1]

1. Nathan C, Betmouni R. Melphalan: avoid with food. *Pharm J* 1996; **257:** 264.

Interferons. For the effect of interferon alfa on the pharmacokinetics of melphalan, see under Pharmacokinetics, below.

Pharmacokinetics

Absorption of melphalan from the gastrointestinal tract is variable; the mean bioavailability is reported to be 56% but it may range from 25 to 89%. Absorption is reduced by the presence of food (see above). Following absorption it is rapidly distributed throughout body water with a volume of distribution of about 0.5 litres per kg body-weight, and has been reported to be inactivated mainly by spontaneous hydrolysis. About 50 to 60% of an absorbed dose has been stated to be protein bound initially, increasing to 80 to 90% after 12 hours. The terminal plasma half-life of melphalan has been reported to be of the order of 30 to 150 minutes. Melphalan is excreted in the urine, about 10% as unchanged drug.

Effect of temperature. The fever caused by concomitant administration of interferon alfa with melphalan resulted in a reduction in the area under the plasma concentration-time curve (AUC) in 10 patients although the peak plasma concentration and time to peak concentration were not affected.[1] The effect was thought to represent increased chemical reactivity of melphalan at the elevated temperature.

1. Ehrsson H, *et al.* Oral melphalan pharmacokinetics: influence of interferon-induced fever. *Clin Pharmacol Ther* 1990; **47:** 86–90.

Uses and Administration

Melphalan is an antineoplastic that acts as a bifunctional alkylating agent. It is used mainly in the treatment of multiple myeloma. Melphalan has also been given to patients with carcinoma of the breast and ovary, neuroblastoma, Hodgkin's disease, and in polycythaemia vera, and has been administered by intra-arterial regional perfusion for malignant melanoma and soft-tissue sarcomas. See also the cross-references given below.

Melphalan is usually given by mouth; it is also administered intravenously. By mouth, it may be given as a single daily dose or in divided doses. Therapy should be interrupted if the platelet count falls below 100 000 per mm³ or the white cell count below 3000 per mm³. During administration of melphalan, frequent blood counts are essential. Dosage should be adjusted according to haematological response. It should be given with great caution if the neutrophil count has recently been depressed by chemotherapy or radiotherapy.

Numerous conventional-dose regimens have been tried for the treatment of multiple myeloma and there is still uncertainty as to the best schedule. **Oral** dosage regimens include: 150 μg per kg body-weight daily in divided doses for 4 to 7 days; or melphalan 250 μg per kg daily for 4 days; or 6 mg daily for 2 to 3 weeks. Melphalan is usually combined with corticosteroids. Courses are followed by a rest period of up to 6 weeks to allow recovery of haematological function and are then repeated, or maintenance therapy may be instituted, usually with a daily dose of 1 to 3 mg, or up to 50 μg per kg. For optimum effect, therapy is usually adjusted to produce a moderate leucopenia, with white cell counts in the range 3000 to 3500 per mm^3.

In the treatment of breast cancer, doses of 150 μg per kg daily or 6 mg per m^2 body-surface daily for 5 days have been given, repeated every 6 weeks. Doses of 200 μg per kg daily for 5 days every 4 to 8 weeks have been given to patients with ovarian carcinoma.

In patients with polycythaemia vera, doses of 6 to 10 mg daily for 5 to 7 days, and then 2 to 4 mg daily, have been used for remission induction; a dose of 2 to 6 mg once a week has been used for maintenance.

Melphalan is also given **intravenously**; a single dose of 1 mg per kg, repeated in 4 weeks if the platelet and neutrophil counts permit, has been given in ovarian adenocarcinoma. It may be infused in sodium chloride injection (0.9%) or injected into the tubing of a fast-running drip; when given by infusion the time from reconstitution of the solution to completion of infusion should not exceed 1.5 hours and prolonged infusions should be carried out with several batches of solution, each freshly prepared. In multiple myeloma, the usual intravenous dose is 400 μg per kg or 16 mg per m^2, infused over 15 to 20 minutes, at 4-week intervals if toxicity permits.

High-dose melphalan has been given intravenously in some malignancies: doses of 100 to 240 mg per m^2 have been cited in neuroblastoma, and 100 to 200 mg per m^2 in multiple myeloma, generally followed by autologous stem cell rescue, which becomes essential where doses exceed 140 mg per m^2.

Melphalan may be given by **local perfusion** in the management of melanoma and soft-tissue sarcomas. A typical dosage range for upper extremity perfusions is 0.6 to 1 mg per kg, whereas for lower extremity perfusions doses of 0.8 to 1.5 mg per kg (in melanoma) or 1.0 to 1.4 mg per kg (in sarcoma) are typically used.

The hydrochloride has also been used.

The dose of intravenous melphalan should be reduced by 50% in patients with moderate to severe **renal impairment** and dosage reduction should be considered when administering it by mouth. High dose regimens are not recommended in patients with moderate to severe renal impairment.

Amyloidosis. For reference to the use of melphalan in amyloidosis, see p.501.

Bone disorders, non-malignant. A patient with fibrogenesis imperfecta ossium, a progressive abnormality of bone structure leading to bone pain and fractures, responded to treatment with melphalan 10 mg and prednisolone 20 mg daily, in 7-day courses.[1]

1. Stamp TCB, et al. Fibrogenesis imperfecta ossium: remission with melphalan. Lancet 1985; i: 582–3.

Malignant neoplasms. The important role played by melphalan in the management of multiple myeloma is discussed on p.489. Melphalan is also used as part of salvage regimens for relapsed Hodgkin's disease (see p.487), in the adjuvant chemotherapy of breast cancer (p.491), in ovarian cancer (p.496), childhood neuroblastoma (p.500) and for local perfusion of melanoma (p.499).

Preparations

BP 2001: Melphalan Injection; Melphalan Tablets;
USP 25: Melphalan Tablets.

Proprietary Preparations (details are given in Part 3)
Aust.: Alkeran; *Austral.*: Alkeran; *Belg.*: Alkeran; *Braz.*: Alkeran; *Canad.*: Alkeran; *Denm.*: Alkeran; *Fin.*: Alkeran; *Fr.*: Alkeran; *Ger.*: Alkeran; *Hong Kong*: Alkeran; *Irl.*: Alkeran; *Israel*: Alkeran; *Ital.*: Alkeran; *Mex.*: Alkeran; *Neth.*: Alkeran; *Norw.*: Alkeran; *NZ*: Alkeran; *Port.*: Alkeran; *S.Afr.*: Alkeran; *Singapore*: Alkeran; *Swed.*: Alkeran; *Switz.*: Alkeran; *Thai.*: Alkeran; *UK*: Alkeran; *USA*: Alkeran.

Menogaril (19470-k)

Menogaril (USAN, rINN)

NSC-269148; 7-Omen; U-52047. (2R,3S,4R,5R,6R,11R,13R)-4-(Dimethylamino)-3,4,5,6,11,12,13,14-octahydro-3,5,8,10,13-pentahydroxy-11-methoxy-6,13-dimethyl-2,6-epoxy-2H-naphthaceno[1,2-b]oxocin-9,16-dione; 7-(R)-O-methylnogarol.
C$_{28}$H$_{31}$NO$_{10}$ = 541.5.
CAS — 71628-96-1.

Profile
Menogaril is an anthracycline derivative related to doxorubicin (p.534) but which may not act by intercalation of DNA.

◊ **References.**
1. Mazurek C, et al. Phase I clinical and pharmacokinetic study of menogaril (7-con-O-methylnogarol) in previously treated patients with acute leukaemia. Invest New Drugs 1993; **11:** 313–22.
2. Dutcher JP, et al. A phase II study of menogaril (7R-O-methylnogarol) in patients with relapsed/refractory acute myeloid leukemia: a study of the Eastern Cooperative Oncology Group. Leukemia 1995; **9:** 1638–42.
3. Moore DF, et al. Phase II trial of menogaril in non-Hodgkin's lymphomas: a Southwest Oncology Group trial. Invest New Drugs 1999; **17:** 169–72.

Mercaptopurine (1844-x)

Mercaptopurine (BAN, rINN)

Mercaptopurinum; NSC-755; 6MP; Purinethiol; WR-2785. 6-Mercaptopurine monohydrate; Purine-6-thiol monohydrate; 1,7-Dihydro-6H-purine-6-thione monohydrate.
C$_5$H$_4$N$_4$S,H$_2$O = 170.2.
CAS — 6112-76-1 (mercaptopurine monohydrate); 50-44-2 (anhydrous mercaptopurine).
ATC — L01BB02.
Pharmacopoeias. In Chin., Eur. (see p.vi), Jpn, Pol., and US.

Pharmacopoeial description
Ph. Eur.: A yellow, crystalline powder. Practically insoluble in water and in ether; slightly soluble in alcohol; dissolves in solutions of alkali hydroxides; Protect from light.

USP 25: A yellow, odourless or practically odourless, crystalline powder. Insoluble in water, in acetone, and in ether; soluble in hot alcohol and in dilute alkali solutions; slightly soluble in 2N sulfuric acid.

Adverse Effects, Treatment, and Precautions
For general discussions see Antineoplastics, p.476, p.479, and p.480.

Bone-marrow depression with mercaptopurine may be delayed; hypoplasia may occur. Mercaptopurine is less toxic to the gastrointestinal tract than the folic acid antagonists or fluorouracil but gastrointestinal disturbances may occur. Hepatotoxicity has been reported, with cholestatic jaundice and necrosis, sometimes fatal. Gastrointestinal and hepatic toxicity are reported to be more frequent in adults than in children, and are more likely at higher doses. Crystalluria with haematuria has been observed rarely as have skin disorders including hyperpigmentation. Fever may occur.

Mercaptopurine is potentially carcinogenic and mutagenic; an increased incidence of abortion has occurred in women given mercaptopurine during the first trimester of pregnancy.

Mercaptopurine should be used with care in patients with impaired hepatic or renal function. Hepatic function should be monitored periodically.

Effects on the blood. Measurement of the activity of thiopurine methyltransferase or the concentration of its substrate, tioguanine nucleotide, has been suggested as a way of predicting those individuals likely to experience severe myelotoxicity with mercaptopurine and related drugs (see Azathioprine, p.509).

Effects on the pancreas. Pancreatitis occurred in 13 of 396 patients given mercaptopurine for inflammatory bowel disease.[1] Symptoms resolved on withdrawal but recurred in 7 who were re-challenged with mercaptopurine or azathioprine.

1. Present DH, et al. 6-Mercaptopurine in the management of inflammatory bowel disease: short- and long-term toxicity. Ann Intern Med 1989; **111:** 641–9.

Handling and disposal. A method for the destruction of mercaptopurine or tioguanine in wastes by oxidation with potassium permanganate in sulfuric acid.[1] Residues produced by this method had no mutagenic activity. Urine and faeces produced for up to 48 hours and 5 days, respectively after a dose of mercaptopurine should be handled wearing protective clothing.[2]

1. Castegnaro M, et al, eds. Laboratory decontamination and destruction of carcinogens in laboratory wastes: some antineoplastic agents. IARC Scientific Publications 73. Lyon: WHO/International Agency for Research on Cancer, 1985.
2. Harris J, Dodds LJ. Handling waste from patients receiving cytotoxic drugs. Pharm J 1985; **235:** 289–91.

Porphyria. Mercaptopurine has been associated with acute attacks of porphyria and is considered unsafe in porphyric patients.

Interactions
Mercaptopurine should be given with particular caution in combination with other drugs known to be hepatotoxic. The effects of mercaptopurine are enhanced by allopurinol and the dose of mercaptopurine should be reduced to one-third to one-quarter of the usual dose when allopurinol is given concomitantly.

Allopurinol. Mercaptopurine plasma concentrations were markedly increased by allopurinol when mercaptopurine was given by mouth but not when it was given intravenously.[1] The results appear to indicate that allopurinol inhibits the first-pass metabolism of mercaptopurine.

1. Zimm S, et al. Inhibition of first-pass metabolism in cancer chemotherapy: interaction of 6-mercaptopurine and allopurinol. Clin Pharmacol Ther 1983; **34:** 810–17.

Anticoagulants. For reference to mercaptopurine diminishing the activity of warfarin, see Warfarin Sodium, p.995.

Doxorubicin. For a suggestion that doxorubicin might enhance the hepatotoxicity of mercaptopurine, see under Daunorubicin Hydrochloride, p.533.

Gastrointestinal drugs. The enzyme thiopurine methyltransferase was inhibited by sulfasalazine and mesalazine in vitro, raising the possibility of an interaction in patients treated simultaneously with an aminosalicylate and a thiopurine such as mercaptopurine or azathioprine.[1] Myelotoxicity has been reported in a patient receiving mercaptopurine concomitantly with olsalazine.[2] Similarly, severe pancytopenia has occurred in a 13-year-old boy when azathioprine was added to mesalazine therapy.[3]

1. Szumlanski C, Weinshilboum RM. Sulfasalazine inhibition of thiopurine methyltransferase: possible mechanism for interaction with 6-mercaptopurine and azathioprine. Br J Clin Pharmacol 1995; **39:** 456–9.
2. Lewis LD, et al. Olsalazine and 6-mercaptopurine-related bone marrow suppression: a possible drug-drug interaction. Clin Pharmacol Ther 1997; **62:** 464–75.
3. Chouragui JP, et al. Azathioprine toxicity in a child with ulcerative colitis: interaction with mesalazine. Gastroenterology 1996; **110** (suppl): A883.

Methotrexate. Concurrent administration of mercaptopurine and low-dose methotrexate by mouth resulted in an increase in mean peak plasma concentrations of mercaptopurine of 26% compared with administration of the same dose of mercaptopurine alone in a study in 14 patients with acute lymphoblastic leukaemia.[1] The effect was probably due to inhibition of the first-pass metabolism of mercaptopurine by methotrexate, which is a potent inhibitor of xanthine oxidase. Although the resultant increase in mercaptopurine concentrations was unlikely to be significant in this case, higher doses of methotrexate given concurrently with mercaptopurine might be cause for concern.

1. Balis FM, et al. The effect of methotrexate on the bioavailability of oral 6-mercaptopurine. Clin Pharmacol Ther 1987; **41:** 384–7.

Pharmacokinetics
Mercaptopurine is variably and incompletely absorbed from the gastrointestinal tract; about 50% of an oral dose has been reported to be absorbed, but the absolute bioavailability is somewhat lower, probably due to gastrointestinal or first-pass metabolism, and is also subject to wide interindividual variation. Once absorbed it is widely distributed throughout body water and tissues. Plasma half-lives ranging from about 20 to 90 minutes have been reported after intravenous injection and the drug is not found in plasma after about 8 hours but this is of limited significance since mercaptopurine is activated intracellularly by conversion to nucleotide derivatives which persist for much longer. It is rapidly and extensively metabolised in the liver, by methylation and oxidation as well as by the formation of inorganic sulfates. Considerable amounts are oxidised to thiouric acid by the enzyme xanthine oxidase. It is excreted in urine as metabolites and some unchanged drug; about half an oral dose has been recovered in 24 hours. A small proportion is excreted over several weeks.

Mercaptopurine crosses the blood-brain barrier to some extent and is found in the CSF, but only in subtherapeutic concentrations.

Uses and Administration
Mercaptopurine is an antineoplastic that acts as an antimetabolite. It is an analogue of the natural purines hypoxanthine and adenine. After the intracellular conversion of mercaptopurine to active nucleotides, including thioinosinic acid, it appears to exhibit a variety of actions including interfering with nucleic acid synthesis. It also has immunosuppressant properties. Its actions are specific for cells in S phase.

Mercaptopurine is used, usually with other agents, in the treatment of leukaemia. It induces remissions in acute lymphoblastic and myeloid leukaemias (p.484 and p.485, respectively) but other agents are generally preferred and mercaptopurine is chiefly employed in maintenance programmes, commonly in association with methotrexate. It may also be effective in chronic myeloid leukaemia (p.486). There is cross-resistance between mercaptopurine and tioguanine (p.575).

Mercaptopurine has been used for its immunosuppressant properties in the treatment of various autoimmune disorders such as inflammatory bowel disease but has been largely replaced by azathioprine.

Mercaptopurine is administered by mouth. The usual initial antineoplastic dose for children and adults is 2.5 mg per kg body-weight or 50 to 75 mg per m^2 body-surface daily but the dosage varies according to individual response and tolerance. If there is no clinical improvement and no evidence of white-cell depression after 4 weeks, the dose may be cautiously increased up to 5 mg per kg daily. In maintenance schedules the dose may vary from 1.5 to 2.5 mg per kg daily. Blood counts should be taken at least once a week and if there is a steep fall in the white cell count or severe bone-marrow depression the drug should be withdrawn immediately. Therapy may be resumed carefully if the white cell count remains constant for 2 or 3 days or rises.

It has been administered intravenously as mercaptopurine sodium. Thioinosine (mercaptopurine riboside) has also been used.

Administration. There is evidence[1] that the maintenance dosage of mercaptopurine should be tailored individually to achieve an appropriate systemic exposure in children with acute lymphoblastic leukaemia (although this would involve determining mercaptopurine pharmacokinetics in each child). Improvements in survival since 1980 may be associated with changes in the prescribing of mercaptopurine which have resulted in greater cumulative doses being given;[2] some children may have been undertreated in the past because of variations in the pharmacokinetics of mercaptopurine (particularly boys, who tolerate mercaptopurine better than girls,[3] but who have a poorer prognosis).[2] The concentration of tioguanine nucleotide metabolites in the erythrocytes has been shown to be directly related to the risk of relapse in children with acute lymphoblastic leukaemia.[4] Thiopurine methyltransferase activity (which results in methylation and inactivation of mercaptopurine rather than the formation of active nucleotides) may play a substantial role in this variation,[5] but titration of the dose of mercaptopurine until myelotoxicity occurs may prevent the problem:[2] despite gaps in therapy caused by more frequent drug withdrawal, it appears to result in greater accumulation of tioguanine nucleotides in the cells.[6]

1. Koren G, *et al.* Systemic exposure to mercaptopurine as a prognostic factor in acute lymphocytic leukemia in children. *N Engl J Med* 1990; **323:** 17–21.
2. Hale JP, Lilleyman JS. Importance of 6-mercaptopurine dose in lymphoblastic leukaemia. *Arch Dis Child* 1991; **66:** 462–6.
3. Lilleyman JS, *et al.* Childhood lymphoblastic leukaemia: sex difference in 6-mercaptopurine utilization. *Br J Cancer* 1984; **49:** 703–7.
4. Lilleyman JS, Lennard L. Mercaptopurine metabolism and risk of relapse in childhood lymphoblastic leukaemia. *Lancet* 1994; **343:** 1188–90.
5. Lennard L, *et al.* Genetic variation in response to 6-mercaptopurine for childhood acute lymphoblastic leukaemia. *Lancet* 1990; **336:** 225–9.
6. Lennard L, *et al.* Mercaptopurine in childhood leukaemia: the effects of dose escalation on thioguanine nucleotide metabolites. *Br J Clin Pharmacol* 1996; **42:** 525–7.

Inflammatory bowel disease. Mercaptopurine has been reported to be of benefit in ulcerative colitis[1,2] and Crohn's disease,[3,4] although azathioprine has generally been preferred (see p.510).

1. Adler DJ, Korelitz BI. The therapeutic efficacy of 6-mercaptopurine in refractory ulcerative colitis. *Am J Gastroenterol* 1990; **85:** 717–21.
2. George J, *et al.* The long-term outcome of ulcerative colitis treated with 6-mercaptopurine. *Am J Gastroenterol* 1996; **91:** 1711–14.
3. Present DH, *et al.* Treatment of Crohn's disease with 6-mercaptopurine: a long-term randomized, double-blind study. *N Engl J Med* 1980; **302:** 981–7.
4. Sandborn W, *et al.* Azathioprine or 6-mercaptopurine for inducing remission of Crohn's disease (updated 15 June 2001). Available in The Cochrane Library; Issue 4. Oxford: Update Software; 2001.

Polymyositis. Mercaptopurine has been tried in a few patients with polymyositis but has not been formally assessed (see p.1057).

Preparations

BP 2001: Mercaptopurine Tablets;
USP 25: Mercaptopurine Tablets.

Proprietary Preparations (details are given in Part 3)
Aust.: Puri-Nethol; *Austral.:* Puri-Nethol; *Belg.:* Puri-Nethol; *Braz.:* Mercaptina; Puri-Nethol; *Canad.:* Puri-Nethol; *Fr.:* Puri-Nethol; *Ger.:* Mercap†; Puri-Nethol; *Hong Kong:* Puri-Nethol; *Irl.:* Puri-Nethol; *Israel:* Puri-Nethol; *Ital.:* Ismipur; Puri-Nethol; *Mex.:* Flocofil; Puri-Nethol; *Neth.:* Puri-Nethol; *Norw.:* Puri-Nethol; *NZ:* Puri-Nethol; *S.Afr.:* Puri-Nethol; *Singapore:* Puri-Nethol; *Swed.:* Puri-Nethol; *Switz.:* Puri-Nethol; *Thai.:* Puri-Nethol; *UK:* Puri-Nethol; *USA:* Puri-Nethol.

Methotrexate (9550-n)

Methotrexate (BAN, USAN, rINN).
Amethopterin; 4-Amino-4-deoxy-10-methylpteroyl-L-glutamic Acid; 4-Amino-10-methylfolic Acid; CL-14377; α-Methopterin; Methotrexatum; Metotrexato; MTX; NSC-740; WR-19039. N-{4-[(2,4-Diamino-6-pteridinylmethyl)methylamino]benzoyl}-L-glutamic acid.
$C_{20}H_{22}N_8O_5 = 454.4$.
CAS — 59-05-2.
ATC — L01BA01.
Pharmacopoeias. In *Chin., Eur.* (see p.vi), *Int., Jpn,* and *US.*

Pharmacopoeial description
Ph. Eur.: Methotrexate contains between 98% and 102% of $C_{20}H_{22}N_8O_5$, calculated with reference to the anhydrous substance. A yellow or orange, hygroscopic, crystalline powder. It contains not more than 13% of water. Practically insoluble in water, in alcohol, and in dichloromethane; dissolves in dilute solutions of mineral acids and of alkali hydroxides and carbonates. Store in airtight containers. Protect from light.
USP 25: Methotrexate is a mixture of 4-amino-10-methylfolic acid and closely related substances; it contains not less than 98% and not more than 102% of $C_{20}H_{22}N_8O_5$, calculated on the anhydrous basis. A yellow or orange-brown crystalline powder. It contains not more than 12% of water. Practically insoluble in water, in alcohol, in chloroform, and in ether; freely soluble in dilute solutions of alkali hydroxides and carbonates; slightly soluble in 6N hydrochloric acid. Store in airtight containers. Protect from light.

Methotrexate Sodium (1845-r)

Methotrexate Sodium (BANM, rINNM).
Methotrexate Disodium.
$C_{20}H_{20}N_8Na_2O_5 = 498.4$.
CAS — 7413-34-5 (methotrexate disodium); 15475-56-6 (methotrexate sodium, xNa).
Pharmacopoeias. *US* includes under the title Methotrexate for Injection.

Methotrexate sodium 16.5 mg is approximately equivalent to 15 mg of methotrexate.

Pharmacopoeial description
USP 25: Protect from light.

◊ CAUTION. *Methotrexate is irritant; avoid contact with skin and mucous membranes.*

Incompatibility. Methotrexate sodium has been reported to be incompatible with cytarabine, fluorouracil, and prednisolone sodium phosphate;[1] however, another study suggests it is compatible with fluorouracil.[2] Furthermore a mixture of methotrexate sodium with cytarabine and hydrocortisone sodium succinate in various infusion fluids has been reported to be visually compatible for at least 8 hours at 25°, although precipitation did occur on storage for several days.[3]

1. McRae MP, King JC. Compatibility of antineoplastic, antibiotic and corticosteroid drugs in intravenous admixtures. *Am J Hosp Pharm* 1976; **33:** 1010–13.
2. Vincké BJ, *et al.* Extended stability of 5-fluorouracil and methotrexate solutions in PVC containers. *Int J Pharmaceutics* 1989; **54:** 181–9.
3. Cheung Y-W, *et al.* Stability of cytarabine, methotrexate sodium, and hydrocortisone sodium succinate admixtures. *Am J Hosp Pharm* 1984; **41:** 1802–6.

Stability to light. Methotrexate undergoes photodegradation when stored in the light in diluted solutions,[1] although undiluted commercial preparations are reported to show negligible photodegradation.[1] The bicarbonate ion catalyses this reaction and such admixtures should be avoided if possible, although they may be stable in light for 12 hours. Storage of solutions diluted in 0.9% sodium chloride injection in PVC bags was reported to protect against photodegradation although the length of the study was only 4 hours.[2] Photodegradation can take place under normal lighting, but is more rapid in direct sunlight, with about 11% drug loss from a 1 mg per mL solution after 7 hours; storage under normal lighting resulted in little change in drug concentration over 24 hours with a decrease of up to 12% by 48 hours.[3] Loss was greatest from unprotected polybutadiene tubing, with almost 80% drug loss in 48 hours.

1. Chatterji DC, Gallelli JF. Thermal and photolytic decomposition of methotrexate in aqueous solutions. *J Pharm Sci* 1978; **67:** 526–31.
2. Dyvik O, *et al.* Methotrexate in infusion solutions—a stability test for the hospital pharmacy. *J Clin Hosp Pharm* 1986; **11:** 343–8.
3. McElnay JC, *et al.* Stability of methotrexate and vinblastine in burette administration sets. *Int J Pharmaceutics* 1988; **47:** 239–47.

Adverse Effects

For general discussions see Antineoplastics, p.476.

The most common dose-related toxic effects of methotrexate are on the bone marrow and gastrointestinal tract. Bone-marrow depression can occur abruptly, and leucopenia, thrombocytopenia, and anaemia may all occur. The nadir of the platelet and white-blood cell counts is usually around 5 to 10 days after a bolus dose, with recovery between about 14 to 28 days, but some sources suggest that leucocytes may exhibit an early fall and rise, followed by a second nadir and recovery, within this period. Ulceration of the mouth and gastrointestinal disturbances are also early signs of toxicity: stomatitis and diarrhoea during treatment indicate that it may need to be interrupted, otherwise haemorrhagic enteritis, intestinal perforation, and death may follow.

Methotrexate therapy is associated with liver damage, both acute (notably after high doses) and, more seriously, chronic (generally after long-term administration). Hepatic fibrosis and cirrhosis may develop without obvious signs of hepatotoxicity, and have led to eventual death.

Other adverse effects include renal failure and tubular necrosis following high doses, pulmonary reactions including life-threatening interstitial lung disease, skin reactions (sometimes severe), alopecia, and ocular irritation. Neurotoxicity may be seen: leucoencephalopathy, paresis, demyelination are associated particularly with intrathecal administration and are more likely when cranial irradiation is also given. Intrathecal administration may also produce arachnoiditis, an acute syndrome of headache, nuchal rigidity, back pain, and fever. Other rarer reactions may include megaloblastic anaemia, osteoporosis, precipitation of diabetes, arthralgias, necrosis of soft tissue and bone, and anaphylaxis.

Methotrexate may cause defective oogenesis and spermatogenesis, and fertility may be impaired (this may be reversible). Like other folate inhibitors it is teratogenic, and it has been associated with fetal deaths. Lymphomas (generally reversible on withdrawal of treatment) have occasionally been reported with methotrexate therapy, although the association has been questioned (see Carcinogenicity, below).

Carcinogenicity. There are reports of lymphomas associated with low-dose methotrexate therapy for rheumatic disorders,[1-3] which in some cases have been associated with concomitant Epstein-Barr virus infection.[2] Transitional cell bladder cancer has also been associated with such therapy.[4] However, a retrospective analysis involving 16 263 patients with rheumatoid arthritis found no evidence of a relationship between the use of methotrexate as an antirheumatic and the development of haematological malignancy.[5] Nonetheless, the spontaneous remission of lymphoma after withdrawal of methotrexate in some patients seems to support an association, and further study is required.[6] The carcinogenic risk with antimetabolites such as methotrexate has generally been considered less than with alkylating agents (p.476).

1. Zimmer-Galler I, Lie JT. Choroidal infiltrates as the initial manifestation of lymphoma in rheumatoid arthritis after treatment with low-dose methotrexate. *Mayo Clin Proc* 1994; **69:** 258–61.
2. Kamel OW, *et al.* Brief report: reversible lymphomas associated with Epstein-Barr virus occurring during methotrexate therapy for rheumatoid arthritis and dermatomyositis. *N Engl J Med* 1993; **328:** 1317–21.
3. Viraben R, *et al.* Reversible cutaneous lymphoma occurring during methotrexate therapy. *Br J Dermatol* 1996; **135:** 116–18.
4. Millard RJ, McCredie S. Bladder cancer in patients on low-dose methotrexate and corticosteroids. *Lancet* 1994; **343:** 1222–3.
5. Moder KG, *et al.* Hematologic malignancies and the use of methotrexate in rheumatoid arthritis: a retrospective study. *Am J Med* 1995; **99:** 276–81.
6. Georgescu L, Paget SA. Lymphoma in patients with rheumatoid arthritis: what is the evidence of a link with methotrexate? *Drug Safety* 1999; **20:** 475–87.

Effects on the blood. Although serious and sometimes fatal blood dyscrasias are a well-known consequence of high-dose methotrexate therapy the UK Committee on Safety of Medicines[1] stated in September 1997 that it was also aware of 83 reports of blood dyscrasias associated with low-dose methotrexate used to treat psoriasis or rheumatoid arthritis; there were 36 fatalities. Many of the cases had contributing factors such as advanced age, renal impairment, or concomitant use of interacting drugs.

1. Committee on Safety Medicines/Medicines Control Agency. Blood dyscrasias and other ADRs with low-dose methotrexate. *Current Problems* 1997; **23:** 12.

MEGALOBLASTIC ANAEMIA. Megaloblastic anaemia, usually with marked macrocytosis, has been reported in mainly elderly patients receiving long-term weekly methotrexate therapy.[1,2] It has been suggested that therapy should be withdrawn if the mean corpuscular volume exceeds 106 femtolitres.[1] Symptoms appear to be associated with folate depletion by methotrexate,[2-4] probably due to increased excretion,[5] and in one case megaloblastic anaemia developed following embarkation on a weight-reducing diet poor in folate.[3] Folate supplementation, conversely, may permit continuation of methotrexate therapy with resolution of the anaemia.[4]

1. Dodd HJ, et al. Megaloblastic anaemia in psoriatic patients treated with methotrexate. Br J Dermatol 1985; 112: 630.
2. Dahl MGC. Folate depletion in psoriatics on methotrexate. Br J Dermatol 1984; 111 (suppl 26): 18.
3. Fulton RA. Megaloblastic anaemia and methotrexate treatment. Br J Dermatol 1986; 114: 267–8.
4. Oxholm A, Thomsen K. Megaloblastic anaemia and methotrexate treatment. Br J Dermatol 1986; 114: 268–9.
5. Duhra P, et al. Intestinal folate absorption in methotrexate treated psoriatic patients. Br J Dermatol 1988; 119: 327–32.

Effects on the kidneys. High dose methotrexate therapy can result in supersaturation of the urine with methotrexate and its metabolites leading to crystal formation.[1] These crystals can cause intravenal obstruction and are a factor in the development of acute renal failure. Risk factors for crystal formation are acid urine, volume depletion, and renal impairment.

1. Perazella MA. Crystal-induced acute renal failure. Am J Med 1999; 106: 459–65.

Effects on the liver. Methotrexate is well established as a cause of hepatotoxicity including periportal fibrosis when given in relatively high doses as an antineoplastic, and it has become clear that its long-term use in lower doses for disorders such as psoriasis and rheumatoid arthritis can also be associated with liver toxicity.[1] There has been some difficulty in these patients in distinguishing the effects of the drug from the effects of the disease, but there is good evidence that the risk is increased in patients given doses on a daily rather than a weekly regimen, and in those with a high alcohol intake.[1] Pre-existing liver disease, obesity (especially if associated with diabetes mellitus), renal impairment, and increasing total cumulative dose may also increase the risk of hepatotoxicity.[1] A lower incidence of hepatotoxicity in patients with rheumatoid arthritis (compared with older studies in patients with psoriasis) may be due to improved dosage regimens and greater awareness of the risks.[1]

In order to minimise the risks of serious liver damage various guidelines and recommendations have been issued for the use of methotrexate in psoriasis and rheumatoid arthritis, and the appropriate monitoring. For patients with *psoriasis*, US guidelines[2] recommend a liver biopsy at the beginning of treatment and after each cumulative dose of 1 to 1.5 g, together with monitoring of alanine aminotransferase (ALT), aspartate aminotransferase (AST), alkaline phosphatase, bilirubin, and albumin. Practice in the UK has been similar, although recommendations on biopsy are less firm.[3] The need to repeat routine liver biopsies has been questioned.[4] In patients with *rheumatoid arthritis* US guidelines[5] suggest an initial biopsy only in patients with a history of excessive alcohol consumption, persistently abnormal AST values or chronic hepatitis B or C infection. All patients should undergo monitoring of liver enzyme values (AST and ALT) and albumin every 4 to 8 weeks, and a biopsy should be performed if 5 of 9 or 6 of 12 measurements of AST are elevated in a 12-month interval; if liver changes are moderate to severe, methotrexate should be discontinued.

The UK Committee on Safety of Medicines advised in 1997 that liver-function tests (together with blood count and renal-function testing) should be performed before beginning long-term low-dose methotrexate therapy and repeated weekly until therapy was stabilised, and thereafter every 2 to 3 months.[6]

1. West SG, et al. Methotrexate hepatotoxicity. Rheum Dis Clin North Am 1997; 23: 883–915.
2. Roenigk HH, et al. Methotrexate in psoriasis: revised guidelines. J Am Acad Dermatol 1988; 19: 145–6.
3. Research Unit of the Royal College of Physicians of London, et al. Guidelines for management of patients with psoriasis. BMJ 1991; 303: 829–35.
4. Boffa MJ, et al. Sequential liver biopsies during long-term methotrexate treatment for psoriasis: a reappraisal. Br J Dermatol 1995; 133: 774–8.
5. Kremer JM, et al. Methotrexate for rheumatoid arthritis: suggested guidelines for monitoring liver toxicity. Arthritis Rheum 1994; 37: 316–28.
6. Committee on Safety of Medicines/Medicines Control Agency. Blood dyscrasias and other ADRs with low-dose methotrexate. Current Problems 1997; 23: 12.

Effects on the lungs. A retrospective review[1] involving 130 patients with rheumatoid arthritis treated with methotrexate found adverse bronchopulmonary effects had occurred in 12: in 4 cases this was considered to be hypersensitivity pneumonitis, whereas in the remainder lung disease was attributed to infection. Intensive care measures were required in all 4 patients with hypersensitivity pneumonitis, despite which 2 died. One patient with infectious lung disease also required hospitalisation. The authors pointed out that pulmonary complications warranted vigilance, and methotrexate should be withdrawn in these patients at the first signs of respiratory intolerance. A multicentre case-control study which examined 29 cases of methotrexate-induced lung injury among rheumatoid arthritis patients reported a number of risk factors.[2] These included age over 60 years, pleuropulmonary disease (or to a lesser extent other extra-articular disease), previous use of other disease-modifying antirheumatic drugs, and low serum-albumin; an as-

sociation with smoking, nonsedentary occupations, and diabetes mellitus was also noted.

1. Hilliquin P, et al. Occurrence of pulmonary complications during methotrexate therapy in rheumatoid arthritis. Br J Rheumatol 1996; 35: 441–5.
2. Alarcón GS, et al. Risk factors for methotrexate-induced lung injury in patients with rheumatoid arthritis: a multicenter, case-control study. Ann Intern Med 1997; 127: 356–64.

Effects on mental function. Children who had received intrathecal methotrexate with cranial irradiation for the prophylaxis of CNS leukaemia, had a significant intellectual deficit compared with their siblings.[1] There was no corresponding significant reduction in IQ in a group of children who had received systemic chemotherapy and radiotherapy when compared with their sibling controls. The results suggest that intrathecal methotrexate and cranial irradiation cause intellectual problems, particularly on the higher, more complex and integrated intellectual functions, and that the repercussions are greater in younger children. Subsequent results in these patients indicated that although the lowering of IQ had persisted, it had not progressed since the original study.[2]

A further study confirmed the adverse neurological effects of leukaemia treatment, and its effects on IQ, and did not find a reduced radiation dose to be any less toxic.[3] Neurotoxicity appeared to be greater when systemic therapy with intramuscular rather than oral methotrexate was given with CNS prophylaxis. A study in 20 patients receiving intermittent oral methotrexate for psoriasis found no evidence of psychological impairment.[4]

1. Twaddle V, et al. Intellectual function after treatment for leukaemia or solid tumours. Arch Dis Child 1983; 58: 949–52.
2. Twaddle V, et al. Intellect after malignancy. Arch Dis Child 1986; 61: 700–2.
3. Chessells JM, et al. Neurotoxicity in lymphoblastic leukaemia: comparison of oral and intramuscular methotrexate and two doses of radiation. Arch Dis Child 1990; 65: 416–22.
4. Duller P, van de Kerkhof PCM. The impact of methotrexate on psycho-organic functioning. Br J Dermatol 1985; 113: 503–4.

Effects on the nervous system. Intrathecal methotrexate is associated with a spectrum of neurotoxic reactions.[1] Acute arachnoiditis and meningismus can develop within hours of administration. The incidence is dose-related and usually subsides within a few days. A subacute form of toxic reaction, characterised by varying degrees of paresis, is generally associated with multiple intrathecal injections and apparently results from prolonged elevation of methotrexate concentrations in the CSF. Paraplegia has been reported, but appears to be rare, and decreasing in incidence with improved drug preparation and monitoring of drug concentrations in CSF. There is also a more delayed syndrome, occurring months to years after treatment, and characterised by necrotising leucoencephalopathy. The syndrome may begin insidiously, and progress to dementia, confusion, ataxia, seizures, and eventual stupor. The effects are dose-related and occur particularly when intrathecal methotrexate in doses greater than 50 mg is combined with cranial irradiation and systemic methotrexate therapy. A late feature may be calcification of the necrotic brain tissue. Not all patients develop this severe encephalopathy but minor neurological injuries, presenting as mild ataxia, seizures, or perceptual disorders, have been reported in at least half the patients in some studies.

See also under Effects on Mental Function, above.

1. Goldberg ID, et al. Nervous system toxic effects of cancer therapy. JAMA 1982; 247: 1437–41.

CEREBRAL OEDEMA. A case of acute cerebral oedema associated with haematoma in a patient given intrathecal methotrexate as part of a combination regimen has been reported by Hughes and Lane.[1] However, the attribution of the symptoms to methotrexate has been questioned.[2,3]

1. Hughes PJ, Lane RJM. Acute cerebral oedema induced by methotrexate. BMJ 1989; 298: 1315.
2. Ellis SJ. Acute cerebral oedema induced by methotrexate. BMJ 1989; 299: 122–3.
3. Enevoldson TP. Acute cerebral oedema induced by methotrexate. BMJ 1989; 299: 516.

Effects on the skin. Methotrexate therapy may be associated with erythematous rashes,[1,2] bullae,[2,3] skin ulceration and necrosis consistent with toxic epidermal necrolysis,[2,3] desquamation,[1] exacerbation of photosensitivity reactions,[4] and purpuric skin lesions due to vasculitis.[5,6] Reactivation of sunburn has also been reported.[7]

1. Doyle LA, et al. Erythema and desquamation after high-dose methotrexate. Ann Intern Med 1983; 98: 611–12.
2. Reed KM, Sober AJ. Methotrexate-induced necrolysis. J Am Acad Dermatol 1983; 8: 677–9.
3. Lawrence CM, Dahl MGC. Cutaneous necrosis associated with methotrexate treatment for psoriasis. Br J Dermatol 1982; 107 (suppl 22): 24.
4. Nedorost ST, et al. Drug-induced photosensitivity reaction. Arch Dermatol 1989; 125: 433–4.
5. Marks CR, et al. Small-vessel vasculitis and methotrexate. Ann Intern Med 1984; 100: 916.
6. Navarro M, et al. Leukocytoclastic vasculitis after high-dose methotrexate. Ann Intern Med 1986; 105: 471–2.
7. Mallory SB, Berry DH. Severe reactivation of sunburn following methotrexate use. Pediatrics 1986; 78: 514–15.

Hypersensitivity. A report of anaphylactic reactions in 2 patients given high-dose methotrexate.[1] See also under Effects on the Lungs, above.

1. Klimo P, Ibrahim E. Anaphylactic reaction induced by high doses in high doses as an adjuvant treatment of osteogenic sarcoma. Cancer Treat Rep 1981; 65: 725.

Treatment of Adverse Effects

For general guidelines, see p.479.

Folinic acid neutralises the immediate toxic effects of methotrexate on the bone marrow. It is given as calcium folinate by mouth, intramuscularly, by intravenous bolus injection, or by infusion. When overdosage is suspected the dose of calcium folinate should be at least as high as that of methotrexate and should be administered as soon as possible; further doses are given as required preferably based on serum methotrexate concentrations. Calcium folinate should be continued until serum- methotrexate concentrations fall below 0.05 to 0.1 μmol per litre, which may necessitate prolonged treatment in patients with delayed elimination. Other dosage regimens, given intramuscularly or by mouth, may be appropriate for more modest toxicity associated with conventional doses of methotrexate. For details, see under Calcium Folinate, p.1363.

Folinic acid is usually given in association with high-dose methotrexate regimens to prevent damage to normal tissue ('folinic acid rescue') and this is discussed in Uses and Administration, below.

An adequate flow of alkaline urine should be maintained following high doses of methotrexate to prevent precipitation of methotrexate or its metabolites in the renal tubules; in addition to adequate hydration, the use of acetazolamide or sodium bicarbonate is recommended.

◊ A discussion of the selection of the appropriate route of administration for folinic acid rescue.[1] The general objective is to give folinic acid (as calcium folinate) at doses which maintain plasma concentrations of reduced folates at a level equivalent to or greater than the plasma-methotrexate concentration. In any clinical situation suggesting impaired gastrointestinal function calcium folinate should be given by injection. Although absorption of intramuscular doses is relatively complete and rapid the intravenous route is usually preferable for other reasons, such as a reduced risk of bleeding at injection sites. In the absence of impaired gastrointestinal function, and where there are no concomitant risk factors for methotrexate toxicity, the oral route may be used provided that methotrexate concentrations are expected to be less than 1 μmol per L. For very high dose methotrexate regimens it is generally appropriate to begin folinic acid rescue intravenously to ensure adequate initial therapy, but the majority of the dosage regimen can generally be given orally.

1. Rodman JH, Crom WR. Selecting an administration route for leucovorin rescue. Clin Pharm 1989; 8: 617,21.

◊ Pretreatment with fluorouracil is reported to reduce the toxicity of subsequent methotrexate administration to a degree sufficient to permit high-dose methotrexate administration without the need for folinic acid rescue.[1] Methotrexate has also been given before fluorouracil to modulate its activity (see Administration, in Fluorouracil, p.542).

The acute neurotoxic effects of methotrexate have been reported to be relieved by intravenous aminophylline or oral theophylline in some children.[2]

For reference to the ineffectiveness of diltiazem in preventing the nephrotoxicity due to high-dose methotrexate, see Kidney Disorders, under Diltiazem p.876.

For evidence that colestyramine might decrease serum-methotrexate concentrations, see Interactions, below.

1. White RM. 5-Fluorouracil modulates the toxicity of high dose methotrexate. J Clin Pharmacol 1995; 35: 1156–65.
2. Bernini JC, et al. Aminophylline for methotrexate-induced neurotoxicity. Lancet 1995; 345: 544–7.

Precautions

For general discussions see p.480.

Methotrexate should be used with great care in patients with bone-marrow, hepatic, or renal impairment. It should also be used cautiously in ulcerative disorders of the gastrointestinal tract, and in the elderly and the very young. Pleural or ascitic effusions may act as a depot for methotrexate and produce enhanced toxicity, and should be drained before treatment. Methotrexate should not be used to treat rheumatoid arthritis or psoriasis in patients with alcoholism, liver disease or abnormal liver function tests, or in those with significant renal impairment, immunodeficiency, or blood disorders. A test dose has been recommended.

Regular monitoring of haematological, renal, and hepatic function, and gastrointestinal toxicity is advisable. Treatment should be interrupted if myelosuppression, diarrhoea, or stomatitis occur. In patients receiving low-dose methotrexate for psoriasis or rheumatoid arthritis full blood counts and renal and liver function tests should be performed before starting treatment and repeated regularly thereafter (for discussion of guidelines for monitoring in these patients see Effects on the Liver, above). Treatment should be interrupted if myelosuppression, stomatitis, or any abnormality of liver function is detected. Dyspnoea or cough may be a sign of pulmonary toxicity and may require treatment discontinuation. Patients or their carers should report any symptoms or signs suggestive of infection, especially sore throat.

With high-dose regimens, plasma concentrations of methotrexate should be monitored. Maintenance of an adequate flow of alkaline urine is essential (see Treatment of Adverse Effects, above).

Methotrexate is a potent teratogen and should be avoided in pregnancy. The *British National Formulary* advises that conception should be avoided for at least 6 months after therapy. Women receiving methotrexate should not breast feed.

Blood products. Enhanced toxicity was seen in 2 of 14 patients receiving methotrexate by 24-hour infusion when packed red cells were transfused immediately after the methotrexate infusion.[1] Erythrocytes act as reservoirs for methotrexate and probably resulted in the prolonged high serum-methotrexate concentrations seen in these patients. Great care should be exercised whenever packed red blood cells and methotrexate are given concurrently.

1. Yap AKL, *et al.* Methotrexate toxicity coincident with packed red cell transfusions. *Lancet* 1986; **ii:** 641.

Handling and disposal. Methods for the destruction of methotrexate *wastes* by oxidation with potassium permanganate and sulfuric acid, by oxidation with aqueous alkaline potassium permanganate, or by oxidation with sodium hypochlorite.[1] The first method may also be used for dichloromethotrexate. Residues produced by the degradation of methotrexate by these methods showed no mutagenicity *in vitro*.
Urine and faeces produced for up to 72 hours and 7 days respectively after a dose of methotrexate should be handled wearing protective clothing.[2]

1. Castegnaro M, *et al.* eds. Laboratory decontamination and destruction of carcinogens in laboratory wastes: some antineoplastic agents. *IARC Scientific Publications 73.* Lyon: WHO/International Agency for Research on Cancer, 1985.
2. Harris J, Dodds LJ. Handling waste from patients receiving cytotoxic drugs. *Pharm J* 1985; **235:** 289–91.

Hepatitis. Reactivation of hepatitis B infection, with the development of hepatocellular necrosis and fulminant hepatic failure requiring liver transplantation, developed on discontinuation of low-dose methotrexate therapy in a patient with rheumatoid arthritis who was also an asymptomatic chronic hepatitis B carrier.[1] It was suggested that all patients being considered for low-dose methotrexate therapy should be screened for the presence of serum HBsAg before beginning therapy.

1. Flowers MA, *et al.* Fulminant hepatitis as a consequence of reactivation of hepatitis B virus infection after discontinuation of low-dose methotrexate therapy. *Ann Intern Med* 1990; **112:** 381–2.

Porphyria. Methotrexate is considered to be unsafe in patients with porphyria because it has been shown to be porphyrinogenic in *animals*.

PUVA. Of a total of 94 patients with psoriasis and 38 with mycosis fungoides treated with PUVA therapy (methoxsalen and ultraviolet light) 2 psoriatics who received concomitant methotrexate and PUVA therapy developed skin cancers.[1] It was suggested that the combination of methotrexate and PUVA may be synergistic in inducing cutaneous malignancy.

1. Fitzsimons CP, *et al.* Synergistic carcinogenic potential of methotrexate and PUVA in psoriasis. *Lancet* 1983; **i:** 235–6.

Radiation. Analysis of neutrophil counts for 18 months in children with acute lymphoblastic leukaemia showed that methotrexate-induced neutropenia was significantly greater in patients given CNS irradiation and was considered to have contributed to 3 of 5 deaths during remission.[1]
For the role of cranial irradiation and intrathecal methotrexate in producing neurotoxicity, see Effects on the Nervous System, above.

1. Report to the Medical Research Council of the Working Party on Leukaemia in Childhood. Analysis of treatment in childhood leukaemia: 1—predisposition to methotrexate-induced neutropenia after craniospinal irradiation. *BMJ* 1975; **3:** 563–6.

Interactions

For a general outline of antineoplastic drug interactions, see p.481. The effects of methotrexate may be enhanced by concurrent use of drugs that decrease its renal excretion, such as NSAIDs and salicylates, probenecid, and some penicillins. Fatal toxicity has occurred in patients given NSAIDs concurrently with methotrexate (see below). Severe toxicity has occurred rarely when co-trimoxazole was given with methotrexate. Use with other hepatotoxic or nephrotoxic agents may increase the risk of toxicity. Folic acid and its derivatives may decrease the effectiveness of methotrexate, although they are often used in combination to reduce methotrexate toxicity (see Treatment of Adverse Effects, above).

Animal studies suggested methotrexate toxicity may be increased by chloramphenicol, para-aminobenzoic acid, and hypoglycaemics, but there does not appear to be any evidence of this clinically.

Antibacterials. The oral *aminoglycosides* neomycin[1] and paromomycin[2] have been reported to reduce the gastrointestinal absorption of methotrexate. Various *penicillins* have been reported to decrease the clearance of methotrexate quite markedly,[3,4] although *ceftazidime* may not.[4] Methotrexate toxicity has been reported in a patient receiving low-dose methotrexate following a course of *tetracycline*.[5] The *sulfonamides* such as sulfafurazole and sulfamethoxazole may displace methotrexate from binding sites[6] and reduce renal clearance.[7] Megaloblastic pancytopenia has been reported on a number of occasions when methotrexate was given concomitantly with *co-trimoxazole*;[8,9] possible mechanisms involved include an additive antifolate effect, in addition to the effect of the sulfamethoxazole component.

1. Shen DD, Azarnoff DL. Clinical pharmacokinetics of methotrexate. *Clin Pharmacokinet* 1978; **3:** 1–13.
2. Cohen MH, *et al.* Effect of oral prophylactic broad spectrum nonabsorbable antibiotics on the gastrointestinal absorption of nutrients and methotrexate in small cell bronchogenic carcinoma patients. *Cancer* 1976; **38:** 1556.
3. Bloom EJ, *et al.* Delayed clearance (CL) of methotrexate (MTX) associated with antibiotics and antiinflammatory agents. *Clin Res* 1986; **34:** 560A.
4. Yamamoto K, *et al.* Delayed elimination of methotrexate associated with piperacillin administration. *Ann Pharmacother* 1997; **31:** 1261–2.
5. Turck M. Successful psoriasis treatment then sudden 'cytotoxicity'. *Hosp Pract* 1984; **19:** 175–6.
6. Liegler DG, *et al.* The effect of organic acids on renal clearance of methotrexate in man. *Clin Pharmacol Ther* 1969; **10:** 849–57.
7. Ferrazzini G, *et al.* Interaction between trimethoprim-sulfamethoxazole and methotrexate in children with leukemia. *J Pediatr* 1990; **117:** 823–6.
8. Liddle BJ, Marsden JR. Drug interactions with methotrexate. *Br J Dermatol* 1989; **120:** 582–3.
9. Jeurissen ME, *et al.* Pancytopenia and methotrexate with trimethoprim-sulfamethoxazole. *Ann Intern Med* 1989; **111:** 261.

Antiepileptics. For mention of the reduction in serum-valproate concentration produced by methotrexate see p.368.

Antineoplastics and immunosuppressants. Enhanced methotrexate toxicity might be expected with nephrotoxic agents such as *cisplatin* which could reduce methotrexate excretion by impairing renal function. Sequential use of methotrexate and *fluorouracil* may result in synergistic enhancement of effect (see Administration, in Fluorouracil, p.542), and equally, fluorouracil before methotrexate may reduce its toxicity (see under Treatment of Adverse Effects, above), but if *asparaginase* (p.509) is given before methotrexate the cytotoxic effect of methotrexate may be reduced. For a report of enhanced toxicity with *ciclosporin* in patients who have received methotrexate see p.521.
Methotrexate may increase the bioavailability of *mercaptopurine* by interference with first-pass metabolism (see p.552).

Colestyramine. Serum-methotrexate concentrations were markedly reduced in 2 patients given colestyramine to treat methotrexate toxicity.[1] Colestyramine appears to bind methotrexate and reduce its enterohepatic recirculation.

1. Erttmann R, Landbeck G. Effect of oral cholestyramine on the elimination of high-dose methotrexate. *J Cancer Res Clin Oncol* 1985; **110:** 48–50.

Nitrous oxide. Severe unpredictable myelosuppression and stomatitis have been attributed to the use of nitrous oxide anaesthesia in patients receiving methotrexate, potentiating the effects of methotrexate on folate metabolism.[1] The effect could be reduced by the use of folinic acid rescue.

1. Goldhirsch A, *et al.* Methotrexate/nitrous-oxide toxic interaction in perioperative chemotherapy for early breast cancer. *Lancet* 1987; **ii:** 151.

NSAIDs. Severe, and in some cases fatal, aggravation of methotrexate toxicity has been reported when it was given with various NSAIDs including aspirin and other salicylates,[1,2] azapropazone,[3] diclofenac,[4] indometacin,[4,5] and ketoprofen.[6] The mechanism is uncertain but may include both displacement of methotrexate from protein-binding sites or an effect of NSAIDs on the kidney resulting in reduced methotrexate excretion.[6,7] Naproxen has been reported not to affect the pharmacokinetics of methotrexate,[8] but a fatal interaction has nonetheless been reported.[9] Despite the risks, some commentators have pointed out that methotrexate and NSAIDs are frequently prescribed together in the treatment of rheumatoid arthritis,[10,11] and that provided this is done with caution, in low doses, and patients are appropriately monitored and cautioned to avoid additional 'over-the-counter' analgesics, such combi-

nations need not be contra-indicated. A study in patients receiving low-dose methotrexate for rheumatoid arthritis suggested that flurbiprofen, ketoprofen, or piroxicam did not influence methotrexate clearance.[12]
Manufacturers of methotrexate generally contra-indicate the use of NSAIDs concomitantly with high-dose methotrexate.

1. Baker H. Intermittent high dose oral methotrexate therapy in psoriasis. *Br J Dermatol* 1970; **82:** 65–9.
2. Zuik M, Mandel MA. Methotrexate-salicylate interaction: a clinical and experimental study. *Surg Forum* 1975; **26:** 567–9.
3. Daly HM, *et al.* Methotrexate toxicity precipitated by azapropazone. *Br J Dermatol* 1986; **114:** 733–5.
4. Gabrielli A, *et al.* Methotrexate and nonsteroidal anti-inflammatory drugs. *BMJ* 1987; **294:** 776.
5. Maiche AG. Acute renal failure due to concomitant action of methotrexate and indomethacin. *Lancet* 1986; **i:** 1390.
6. Thyss A, *et al.* Clinical and pharmacokinetic evidence of a life-threatening interaction between methotrexate and ketoprofen. *Lancet* 1986; **i:** 256–8.
7. Furst DE, *et al.* Effect of aspirin and sulindac on methotrexate clearance. *J Pharm Sci* 1990; **79:** 782–6.
8. Stewart CF, *et al.* Coadministration of naproxen and low-dose methotrexate in patients with rheumatoid arthritis. *Clin Pharmacol Ther* 1990; **47:** 540–6.
9. Singh RR, *et al.* Fatal interaction between methotrexate and naproxen. *Lancet* 1986; **i:** 1390.
10. Tully M. NSAIDs. *Pharm J* 1991; **247:** 746.
11. Zachariae H. Methotrexate and nonsteroidal anti-inflammatory drugs. *Br J Dermatol* 1992; **126:** 95.
12. Tracy TS, *et al.* Methotrexate disposition following concomitant administration of ketoprofen, piroxicam and flurbiprofen in patients with rheumatoid arthritis. *Br J Clin Pharmacol* 1994; **37:** 453–6.

Omeprazole. Elevated serum concentrations of methotrexate have been reported when it was given to a patient also receiving omeprazole.[1] The effect was not seen with subsequent cycles of methotrexate therapy once omeprazole had been discontinued.

1. Reid T, *et al.* Impact of omeprazole on the plasma clearance of methotrexate. *Cancer Chemother Pharmacol* 1993; **33:** 82–4.

Probenecid. Probenecid can result in three- or fourfold increases in serum-methotrexate concentrations when given concurrently,[1,2] presumably by inhibiting renal excretion of methotrexate.

1. Aherne GW, *et al.* Prolongation and enhancement of serum methotrexate concentrations by probenecid. *BMJ* 1978; **1:** 1097–9.
2. Howell SB, *et al.* Effect of probenecid on cerebrospinal fluid methotrexate kinetics. *Clin Pharmacol Ther* 1979; **26:** 641–6.

Retinoids. An increased risk of hepatotoxicity has been reported when methotrexate and *etretinate* are given concurrently,[1] possibly due to increased plasma concentrations of methotrexate.[2,3]

1. Zachariae H. Dangers of methotrexate/etretinate combination therapy. *Lancet* 1988; **i:** 422.
2. Harrison PV, *et al.* Methotrexate and retinoids in combination for psoriasis. *Lancet* 1987; **ii:** 512.
3. Larsen FG, *et al.* Interaction of etretinate with methotrexate pharmacokinetics in psoriatic patients. *J Clin Pharmacol* 1990; **30:** 802–7.

Pharmacokinetics

When given in low doses, methotrexate is rapidly absorbed from the gastrointestinal tract, but higher doses are less well absorbed. It is also rapidly and completely absorbed following intramuscular administration. Peak serum concentrations are achieved in 1 to 2 hours after an oral dose, and 30 to 60 minutes after an intramuscular one.

Methotrexate is distributed to tissues and extracellular fluid with a steady-state volume of distribution of 0.4 to 0.8 litres per kg body-weight; it penetrates ascitic fluid and effusions which may act as a depot and thus enhance toxicity. Clearance from plasma is reported to be triphasic, with a terminal elimination half-life of between 3 and 10 hours after doses less than 30 mg per m^2 body-surface or 8 to 15 hours after high-dose parenteral therapy. It is about 50% bound to plasma protein. Methotrexate enters the cells in part by an active transport mechanism and is bound as polyglutamate conjugates: bound drug may remain in the body for several months, particularly in the liver.

Only small or insignificant amounts cross the blood-brain barrier and enter the CSF following oral or parenteral administration although this may be increased by giving higher doses; however, following intrathecal doses there is significant passage into the systemic circulation.

Methotrexate has been detected in very small amounts in saliva and breast milk. It crosses the placenta.

Methotrexate does not appear to undergo significant metabolism at low doses; following high-dose therapy the 7-hydroxy metabolite has been detected. Methotrexate may be partly metabolised by the intestinal flora after oral administration. It is excreted primarily in the urine, by glomerular filtration and active tubular secretion. Small amounts are excreted in bile and found in faeces; there is some evidence for enterohepatic recirculation.

Considerable interindividual variation exists in the pharmacokinetics of methotrexate: those patients in whom clearance is delayed are at increased risk of toxicity.

◊ References.
1. Shen DD, Azarnoff DL. Clinical pharmacokinetics of methotrexate. *Clin Pharmacokinet* 1978; **3:** 1–13.
2. Balis FM, *et al.* Clinical pharmacokinetics of commonly used anticancer drugs. *Clin Pharmacokinet* 1983; **8:** 202–32.
3. Wang Y-M, Fujimoto T. Clinical pharmacokinetics of methotrexate in children. *Clin Pharmacokinet* 1984; **9:** 335–48.
4. Witter FR. Clinical pharmacokinetics in the treatment of rheumatoid arthritis in pregnancy. *Clin Pharmacokinet* 1993; **25:** 444–9.
5. Bannwarth B, *et al.* Clinical pharmacokinetics of low-dose pulse methotrexate in rheumatoid arthritis. *Clin Pharmacokinet* 1996; **30:** 194–210.

Uses and Administration

Methotrexate is an antineoplastic which acts as an antimetabolite of folic acid. It also has immunosuppressant properties. Within the cell, folic acid is reduced to dihydrofolic and then tetrahydrofolic acid. Methotrexate competitively inhibits the enzyme dihydrofolate reductase and prevents the formation of tetrahydrofolate which is necessary for purine and pyrimidine synthesis and consequently the formation of DNA and RNA. It is most active against cells in the S phase of the cell cycle but its actions on protein and nucleic acid synthesis slow the entry of cells into S phase and so are to some extent self-limiting. Folinic acid (the 5-formyl derivative of tetrahydrofolic acid), or the nucleoside thymidine, have been given after high doses to bypass the block in tetrahydrofolate production in normal cells and prevent the adverse effects of methotrexate. A suggested schedule for *folinic acid rescue* is described under Calcium Folinate, p.1363. (See also under Treatment of Adverse Effects, above). Methotrexate, in very high doses, followed by folinic acid rescue, is used in treating some malignant diseases.

Methotrexate is used in the management of acute lymphoblastic leukaemia. It is seldom used for the induction of remission but is employed in maintenance programmes and in the prophylaxis and treatment of meningeal leukaemia. It may be used for Burkitt's and other non-Hodgkin's lymphomas. In the solid neoplasms it is an important part of curative regimens for choriocarcinoma and other gestational trophoblastic tumours, and for the adjuvant therapy of osteosarcoma and breast cancer. It may also be used in malignant neoplasms of the bladder and head and neck, and a variety of other neoplasms, as indicated by the cross references given below.

Methotrexate is of value in the treatment of psoriasis but because of the risks associated with this use, it should only be given when the disease is severe and has not responded to other forms of treatment. It is used widely as a disease-modifying antirheumatic drug in rheumatoid arthritis. Methotrexate may be used to prevent graft-versus-host disease after bone marrow transplantation and may be used as a cytotoxic immunosuppressant and corticosteroid-sparing agent in a variety of non-malignant diseases.

Methotrexate has a role in the management of ectopic pregnancy (see below).

Methotrexate may be given by mouth as the base or the sodium salt, or by injection as the sodium salt Doses are calculated in terms of methotrexate. The doses and regimens employed vary enormously, and may need to be adjusted according to bone-marrow or other toxicity. Doses larger than 100 mg are usually given partly or wholly by intravenous infusion over not more than 24 hours.

A common dose for maintenance therapy of acute lymphoblastic leukaemia is 15 mg per m² body-surface once or twice weekly, by mouth or intramuscularly, with other agents such as mercaptopurine. Alternatively, 2.5 mg per kg body-weight may be giv-

en intravenously every 14 days. Meningeal leukaemia may be treated by the intrathecal injection of 12 mg per m² body-surface (maximum 15 mg) once or twice weekly; alternatively a regimen based on the age of the patient has been recommended, with children under the age of 1 year receiving 6 mg, 8 mg for those 1 year of age, 10 mg in 2-year-olds, and 12 mg in those 3 years of age or older. Intrathecal doses have also sometimes been given prophylactically to patients with lymphoblastic leukaemia in association with intrathecal cytarabine and hydrocortisone. Methotrexate in intravenous doses of about 500 mg per m², followed by folinic acid rescue, may also produce effective concentrations in the CSF and has been used for meningeal leukaemia.

Choriocarcinoma has been treated with doses of 15 to 30 mg daily by mouth or intramuscularly for 5 days repeated after an interval of 1 week or more, for 3 to 5 courses. Alternatively 0.25 to 1 mg per kg body-weight up to a maximum of 60 mg has been given intramuscularly every 48 hours for 4 doses, followed by folinic acid rescue, and repeated at intervals of 7 days for 4 or more courses. Combination chemotherapy may be necessary in patients with metastases.

Doses of 10 to 60 mg per m² are employed in the treatment of breast cancer, often in combination with cyclophosphamide and fluorouracil.

In advanced lymphosarcoma doses of 0.625 to 2.5 mg per kg daily have been suggested in combination with other antineoplastics. Alternatively, higher doses of up to 30 mg per kg have been given, followed by folinic acid rescue. For Burkitt's lymphoma 10 to 25 mg of methotrexate has been given daily by mouth for 4 to 8 days, repeated after an interval of 7 to 10 days, while patients with mycosis fungoides may be given 2.5 to 10 mg daily by mouth to induce remission; alternatively 50 mg may be given weekly as a single dose or two divided doses, by intramuscular injection.

Very high doses, in the range 12 to 15 g per m² have been given by intravenous infusion, followed by folinic acid, as part of combined adjuvant therapy in patients with osteosarcoma. High-dose regimens have been tried in a variety of other malignancies, including carcinoma of the lung and of the head and neck.

Single weekly doses of 10 to 25 mg may be given by mouth or by intramuscular or intravenous injection in the treatment of psoriasis and adjusted by response. Other, more frequent, regimens have been used but a weekly dosage regimen appears to be less hepatotoxic than a daily one. In the treatment of rheumatoid arthritis doses of 7.5 mg by mouth once weekly are used, adjusted by response and not exceeding 20 mg per week.

It is essential that blood counts and tests of renal and liver function should be made before, during, and after each course of treatment with methotrexate (see Precautions, above).

Asthma. Various immunosuppressants, including methotrexate, have been tried for their anti-inflammatory and corticosteroid-sparing properties in chronic asthma (p.757), but because of fears about toxicity are largely reserved for certain patients dependent upon systemic corticosteroids. Results of individual studies with methotrexate have been conflicting, but it appears that some patients may benefit from the corticosteroid-sparing effects of methotrexate.[1,2] However, other reviewers considered that the reduction in corticosteroid dose was insufficient to offset the adverse effects of methotrexate.[3] Methotrexate therapy must be given for at least 3 months for an adequate assessment of efficacy.

1. Shulimzon TR, Shiner RJ. A risk-benefit assessment of methotrexate in corticosteroid-dependent asthma. *Drug Safety* 1996; **15:** 283–90.
2. Marin MG. Low-dose methotrexate spares steroid usage in steroid-dependent asthmatic patients: a meta-analysis. *Chest* 1997; **112:** 29–33.
3. Davies H, *et al.* Methotrexate as a steroid sparing agent for asthma in adults (updated 6 July 1999). Available in The Cochrane Library; Issue 4. Oxford: Update Software; 1999.

Connective tissue and muscular disorders. Reports in a limited number of patients indicate that methotrexate given once weekly in low to moderate doses may be of benefit in patients with systemic lupus erythematosus, (p.1059), with benefit reported particularly for joint[1] and mucocutaneous[2]

symptoms. Benefit was also reported in 2 of 4 patients with discoid lupus erythematosus refractory to hydroxychloroquine.[3]

Methotrexate therapy has been investigated[4] for its potential corticosteroid-sparing properties in polymyalgia rheumatica (p.1056). It is widely employed in rheumatoid arthritis (see below) and in polymyositis (p.1057), and has been tried in Cogan's syndrome (p.1049).

1. Wilson K, Abeles M. A 2 year, open ended trial of methotrexate in systemic lupus erythematosus. *J Rheumatol* 1994; **21:** 1674–7.
2. Bottomley WW, Goodfield M. Methotrexate for the treatment of severe mucocutaneous lupus erythematosus. *Br J Dermatol* 1995; **133:** 311–14.
3. Bottomley WW, Goodfield MJD. Methotrexate for the treatment of discoid lupus erythematosus. *Br J Dermatol* 1995; **133:** 655–6.
4. Ferraccioli G, *et al.* Methotrexate in polymyalgia rheumatica: preliminary results of an open, randomized study. *J Rheumatol* 1996; **23:** 624–8.

Ectopic pregnancy. Ectopic pregnancy occurs when the fertilised ovum implants outside the uterus, usually in the fallopian tube itself (tubal pregnancy). The problem is increasingly encountered in some developed countries such as the USA, thanks in part to improved diagnostic techniques.[1] Although ectopic pregnancies may spontaneously abort early, without clinical sequelae, the potential adverse effects are serious, ranging from pelvic pain and bleeding at 5 to 6 weeks of gestation (indistinguishable from spontaneous abortion), to potentially fatal intra-abdominal haemorrhage later in the course of an otherwise asymptomatic pregnancy. Laparoscopic surgery remains the standard treatment.[1-3] In some countries non-surgical methods are increasing in popularity. Perhaps the most experience of the latter has been with methotrexate. Management with intramuscular methotrexate may be appropriate for selected women with small unruptured tubal pregnancies who are haemodynamically stable, have low serum-chorionic gonadotrophin concentrations, and lack contra-indications to methotrexate use.[2-5] Surgery is preferred where there is cardiac activity in the conceptus, since a living embryo increases resistance to methotrexate.[4,5] Many studies have used a variable dose regimen of 1 mg per kg body-weight on 4 alternate days, with folinic acid rescue.[1] Early reports suggested that excellent results could also be obtained with a single dose of 50 mg per m² body-surface,[6] but in contrast to the variable dose regimen, which had similar efficacy to surgery, a systematic review has indicated that single-dose therapy has a high failure rate:[7] the authors of this review considered that it should be reserved for clinical trials. Methotrexate has also been given in combination with oral mifepristone.[8] Methotrexate has been given successfully by local injection direct into the ectopic, although the success rate is lower than with systemic methotrexate or surgery.[8]

Systemic methotrexate (with folinic acid rescue) has also been reported to be effective in resolving persistent ectopic pregnancy unsuccessfully treated with surgery.

The role of other agents in the management of ectopic pregnancy is less well established. Local instillation of glucose 50% into unruptured tubes is reported to be more effective than the other major alternative, prostaglandin therapy[9] (in this case with dinoprost injected into the gestational sac, sulprostone intramuscularly, and oestrogens for luteolysis). Whether glucose therapy will prove to be as effective as, and produce less tubal damage than, methotrexate remains a matter of debate.

1. Pisarska MD, *et al.* Ectopic pregnancy. *Lancet* 1998; **351:** 1115–20.
2. Tay JI, *et al.* Ectopic pregnancy. *BMJ* 2000; **320:** 916–9.
3. Hajenius PJ, *et al.* Interventions for tubal ectopic pregnancy (updated 28 May 2001). Available in The Cochrane Library; Issue 4. Oxford: Update Software; 2001.
4. Lipscomb GH, *et al.* Predictors of success of methotrexate treatment in women with tubal ectopic pregnancies. *N Engl J Med* 1999; **341:** 1974–8.
5. American College of Obstetricians and Gynecologists. ACOG practice bulletin: medical management of tubal pregnancy. Number 3, December 1998. *Int J Gynecol Obstet* 1999; **65:** 97–103.
6. Stovall TG, Ling FW. Single-dose methotrexate: an expanded clinical trial. *Am J Obstet Gynecol* 1993; **168:** 1759–65.
7. Parker J, *et al.* A systematic review of single-dose intramuscular methotrexate for the treatment of ectopic pregnancy. *Aust N Z J Obstet Gynaecol* 1998; **38:** 145–50.
8. Gazvani MR. Modern management of ectopic pregnancy. *Br J Hosp Med* 1996; **56:** 597–9.
9. Lang PF, *et al.* Conservative treatment of ectopic pregnancy with local injection of hyperosmolar glucose solution or prostaglandin-F₂α: a prospective randomised study. *Lancet* 1990; **336:** 78–81.

Inflammatory bowel disease. Methotrexate (given intramuscularly once weekly in a dose of 25 mg) was reported to improve symptoms and reduce corticosteroid requirements in a large controlled study in patients with chronic active Crohn's disease.[1] Smaller studies have also reported modest benefit for oral methotrexate 12.5 to 22.5 mg per week compared with placebo in this group of patients.[2,3] Subcutaneous methotrexate has also been used.[4] A review[5] concluded that low-dose methotrexate could be recommended for induction of remission and for its corticosteroid-sparing effect in refractory and corticosteroid-dependent Crohn's disease, although the precise indications, dose, and route for its use were still unclear. The value of methotrexate in ulcerative colitis is also uncertain, although benefits have been seen in some patients.[4,6] However, one study in active ulcerative colitis found no significant differences between oral methotrexate 12.5 mg per week and placebo.[7] For a discussion of inflammatory bowel disease, see p.1205.

1. Feagan BG, *et al.* Methotrexate for the treatment of Crohn's disease. *N Engl J Med* 1995; **332**: 292–7.
2. Oren R, *et al.* Methotrexate in chronic active Crohn's disease: a double-blind, randomized, Israeli multicenter trial. *Am J Gastroenterol* 1997; **92**: 2203–9.
3. Arora S, *et al.* Methotrexate in Crohn's disease: results of a randomized, double-blind, placebo-controlled trial. *Hepatogastroenterology* 1999; **46**: 1724–9.
4. Egan LJ, *et al.* A randomized dose-response and pharmacokinetic study of methotrexate for refractory inflammatory Crohn's disease and ulcerative colitis. *Aliment Pharmacol Ther* 1999; **13**: 1597–1604.
5. Egan LJ, Sandborn WJ. Methotrexate for inflammatory bowel disease: pharmacology and preliminary results. *Mayo Clin Proc* 1996; **71**: 69–80.
6. Kozarek RA. Methotrexate for refractory Crohn's disease: preliminary answers to definitive questions. *Mayo Clin Proc* 1996; **71**: 104–5.
7. Oren R, *et al.* Methotrexate in chronic active ulcerative colitis: a double-blind, randomized, Israeli multicenter trial. *Gastroenterology* 1996; **110**: 1416–21.

Malignant neoplasms. Methotrexate is extensively used in the management of malignant disease. In acute lymphoblastic leukaemia it is used for maintenance therapy, and intrathecally for prophylaxis of CNS relapse, as discussed on p.484, while it also forms part of a number of regimens used for Burkitt's and other aggressive, intermediate- to high-grade non-Hodgkin's lymphomas (see p.488 and p.487), including mycosis fungoides (p.489) and those associated with AIDS (p.488). In the solid neoplasms it is an important part of curative regimens for gestational trophoblastic tumours (p.483), the adjuvant therapy of osteosarcoma (p.500) and is used in regimens for tumours of the bladder (p.490), brain (p.490), breast (p.491), gastrointestinal tract (p.493), and head and neck (p.494).

Multiple sclerosis. Results suggest that methotrexate 7.5 mg by mouth weekly may be of benefit in slowing the progression of multiple sclerosis.[1] Although, as discussed on p.633, the results of studies of immunosuppressant therapy in this condition have tended to be disappointing, it has been pointed out that benefit was assessed differently in the methotrexate study,[2] which may have a bearing on its more favourable conclusions.

1. Goodkin DE, *et al.* Low-dose (7.5 mg) oral methotrexate reduces the rate of progression in chronic progressive multiple sclerosis. *Ann Neurol* 1995; **37**: 30–40.
2. Whitaker JN, *et al.* Clinical outcomes and documentation of partial beneficial effects of immunotherapy for multiple sclerosis. *Ann Neurol* 1995; **37**: 5–6.

Myasthenia gravis. Methotrexate has been tried in the management of myasthenia gravis (p.1414) in patients who require immunosuppression but are intolerant of or unresponsive to corticosteroids and azathioprine.

Organ and tissue transplantation. For reference to the use of methotrexate (usually with ciclosporin) in bone marrow transplantation, see p.502.

Primary biliary cirrhosis. Like other agents used for primary biliary cirrhosis (p.501) methotrexate has been associated with biochemical improvement but evidence of clinical and in particular histological improvement is harder to demonstrate, and the toxicity of immunosuppressants such as methotrexate is problematic.

Psoriatic arthritis. Methotrexate may be useful for severe or progressive cases of psoriatic arthritis (see under Spondyloarthropathies, p.10) when the arthritis is not controlled by physical therapy and NSAIDs, although toxicity may limit long-term use in some patients.

Rheumatoid arthritis. Therapy of rheumatoid arthritis (p.9) is conventionally begun with an analgesic and an NSAID for symptomatic relief, to which a disease-modifying antirheumatic drug (DMARD) is subsequently added in an attempt to retard the disease process. Methotrexate or sulfasalazine tend to be the most widely used of such DMARDs.[1] A meta-analysis has confirmed that methotrexate has significant benefit in the short-term treatment of the disease.[2] Methotrexate has also been tried in combination with ciclosporin,[3] and with hydroxychloroquine and sulfasalazine.[4]

Methotrexate may be of benefit in juvenile idiopathic arthritis (p.9).[5]

Methotrexate may also be of value in the management of associated uveitis (p.1060).

1. Anonymous. Modifying disease in rheumatoid arthritis. *Drug Ther Bull* 1998; **36**: 3–6.
2. Suarez-Almazor ME, *et al.* Methotrexate for rheumatoid arthritis (updated 28 October 1999). Available in The Cochrane Library; Issue 1. Oxford: Update Software; 2000.
3. Tugwell P, *et al.* Combination therapy with cyclosporine and methotrexate in severe rheumatoid arthritis. *N Engl J Med* 1995; **333**: 137–41.
4. O'Dell JR, *et al.* Treatment of rheumatoid arthritis with methotrexate alone, sulfasalazine and hydroxychloroquine, or a combination of all three medications. *N Engl J Med* 1996; **334**: 1287–91.
5. Ravelli A, *et al.* Radiologic progression in patients with juvenile chronic arthritis treated with methotrexate. *J Pediatr* 1998; **133**: 262–5.

Sarcoidosis. Where therapy is required for sarcoidosis (p.1058) corticosteroids are the first choice of drug; methotrexate is one of the preferred second-line immunosuppressants.

References.

1. Webster GF, *et al.* Methotrexate therapy in cutaneous sarcoidosis. *Ann Intern Med* 1989; **111**: 538–9.
2. Soriano FG, *et al.* Neurosarcoidosis: therapeutic success with methotrexate. *Postgrad Med J* 1990; **66**: 142–3.
3. Lower EE, Baughman RP. Prolonged use of methotrexate for sarcoidosis. *Arch Intern Med* 1995; **155**: 846–51.
4. Baughman RP, Lower EE. A clinical approach to the use of methotrexate for sarcoidosis. *Thorax* 1999; **54**: 742–6.

Scleroderma. Although there is evidence of benefit with methotrexate in patients with scleroderma, immunosuppressant therapy is generally considered experimental as indicated in the discussion on p.505.

References.

1. van der Hoogen FH, *et al.* Comparison of methotrexate with placebo in the treatment of systemic sclerosis: a 24 week randomized double-blind trial, followed by a 24 week observational trial. *Br J Rheumatol* 1996; **35**: 364–72.

Skin disorders, non-malignant. Methotrexate is widely used in the treatment of severe refractory psoriasis. As discussed on p.1106 the aim of such therapy is to bring the disease under control, enabling a return to other therapy. For use in psoriatic arthritis see above. Methotrexate is also used in conjunction with corticosteroids in the management of pemphigus and pemphigoid (p.1106) but its value has been questioned.[1]

1. Carson PJ, *et al.* Influence of treatment on the clinical course of pemphigus vulgaris. *J Am Acad Dermatol* 1996; **34**: 645–52.

Termination of pregnancy. Methotrexate has been investigated as an alternative to mifepristone in combination with misoprostol for the termination of pregnancy (p.1439). Intramuscular methotrexate followed 3 days later by intravaginal misoprostol was more effective than misoprostol alone for termination at 56 days or less;[1] the combination was reported to be less successful after 57 to 63 days' gestation.[2] Later studies[3,4] however found the combination to be safe and effective in terminating pregnancies up to 63 days' gestation; in these the misoprostol was administered up to 7 days after the methotrexate. Oral methotrexate is also effective.[5-7]

1. Creinin MD, Vittinghoff E. Methotrexate and misoprostol vs misoprostol alone for early abortion: a randomized controlled trial. *JAMA* 1994; **272**: 1190–5.
2. Creinin MD. Methotrexate and misoprostol for abortion at 57-63 days gestation. *Contraception* 1994; **50**: 511–15.
3. Hausknecht RU. Methotrexate and misoprostol to terminate early pregnancy. *N Engl J Med* 1995; **333**: 537–40.
4. Creinin MD, *et al.* A randomized trial comparing misoprostol three and seven days after methotrexate for early abortion. *Am J Obstet Gynecol* 1995; **173**: 1578–84.
5. Creinin MD. Oral methotrexate and vaginal misoprostol for early abortion. *Contraception* 1996; **54**: 15–18.
6. Creinin MD, *et al.* Medical abortion with oral methotrexate and vaginal misoprostol. *Obstet Gynecol* 1997; **90**: 611–16.
7. Carbonell JLL, *et al.* Oral methotrexate and vaginal misoprostol for early abortion. *Contraception* 1998; **57**: 83–8.

Wegener's granulomatosis. For the use of methotrexate in Wegener's granulomatosis see p.1060.

Preparations

BP 2001: Methotrexate Injection; Methotrexate Tablets;
USP 25: Methotrexate for Injection; Methotrexate Injection; Methotrexate Tablets.

Proprietary Preparations (details are given in Part 3)
Aust.: Abitrexate; *Austral.:* Ledertrexate; Methoblastin; *Belg.:* Ledertrexate; Methoblastine; *Braz.:* Metrotex; *Canad.:* Rheumatrex; *Denm.:* Emthexate; *Fin.:* Emthexat; Trexan; *Fr.:* Ledertrexate; Novatrex; *Ger.:* Farmitrexat; Lantarel; Metex; MTX; Otrexat; *Israel:* Abitrexate; Emthexate; *Mex.:* Ledertrexate; Medsatrexate; Methoblastin; Rhodamer; Texate; Trexeron; Trixilem; Xaken; *Neth.:* Ledertrexate; *Norw.:* Emthexat; *NZ:* Emthexate; Ledertrexate; Methoblastin; *Port.:* Fauldexato; *S.Afr.:* Abitrexate; Emthexate; Methoblastin; *Singapore:* Emthexate; MTX; *Spain:* Emthexate; Swed.: Emthexat; *Thai.:* Abitrexate; Emthexate; Trixilem; *UK:* Maxtrex; *USA:* Abitrexate†; Folex†; Rheumatrex; Trexall.

Miboplatin (15907-r)

Miboplatin (*rINN*).

(–)-*cis*-[(*R*)-2-(Aminomethyl)pyrrolidine](1,1-cyclobutanedicarboxylato)platinum.

$C_{11}H_{18}N_2O_4Pt = 437.3$.
CAS — 103775-75-3.

Profile
Miboplatin is a platinum derivative which is reported to have properties similar to carboplatin (p.515) and has been used for its antineoplastic properties.

◊ References.

1. Weiss RB, Christian MC. New cisplatin analogues in development: a review. *Drugs* 1993; **46**: 360–77.

Miltefosine (11021-x)

Miltefosine (*BAN, rINN*).

D-18506; HDPC; Hexadecylphosphocholine. [2-(Trimethylammonio)ethyl][hexadecyloxyphosphonate].

$C_{21}H_{46}NO_4P = 407.6$.
CAS — 58066-85-6.
ATC — L01XX09.

Profile
Miltefosine is a phospholipid derivative which is structurally related to the phospholipid components of the cell membrane and is thought to exert its antineoplastic actions by disruption of cell-membrane function. A 6% solution is applied once or twice daily as a topical antineoplastic agent for skin metastases of breast cancer. Miltefosine has also been tried by mouth for various malignant neoplasms and for the treatment of visceral leishmaniasis.

Leishmaniasis. Miltefosine, given by mouth in doses of 100 to 150 mg daily, appears to be of benefit[1,2] in the treatment of visceral leishmaniasis (p.584).

1. Sundar S, *et al.* Trial of oral miltefosine for visceral leishmaniasis. *Lancet* 1998; **352**: 1821–3.
2. Jha TK, *et al.* Miltefosine, an oral agent, for the treatment of Indian visceral leishmaniasis. *N Engl J Med* 1999; **341**: 1795–1800.

Malignant neoplasms. References to the use of topical miltefosine in breast cancer (p.491).

1. Clive S, Leonard RCF. Miltefosine in recurrent cutaneous breast cancer. *Lancet* 1997; **349**: 621–2.
2. Clive S, *et al.* Miltefosine as a topical treatment for cutaneous metastases in breast carcinoma. *Cancer Chemother Pharmacol* 1999; **44** (suppl): S29–30.
3. Terwogt JM, *et al.* Phase II trial of topically applied miltefosine solution in patients with skin-metastasized breast cancer. *Br J Cancer* 1999; **79**: 1158–61.

Preparations
Proprietary Preparations (details are given in Part 3)
Fin.: Miltex; *Fr.:* Miltex; *Ger.:* Miltex; *Spain:* Miltex; *Swed.:* Miltex.

Misonidazole (12966-p)

Misonidazole (*BAN, USAN, rINN*).

NSC-261037; Ro-7-0582. 3-Methoxy-1-(2-nitroimidazol-1-yl)propan-2-ol.

$C_7H_{11}N_3O_4 = 201.2$.
CAS — 13551-87-6.

Profile
Misonidazole is a radiosensitiser structurally related to metronidazole (p.594) and shares some of the same properties. It has been investigated as an adjunct to radiotherapy in the treatment of cancer. Misonidazole may produce dose-related peripheral neuropathy, and at high doses, encephalopathy.

◊ References.

1. Huncharek M. Meta-analytic re-evaluation of misonidazole in the treatment of high grade astrocytoma. *Anticancer Res* 1998; **18**: 1935–9.
2. Grigsby PW, *et al.* Irradiation with or without misonidazole for patients with stages IIIB and IVA carcinoma of the cervix: final results of RTOG 80-05. Radiation Therapy Oncology Group. *Int J Radiat Oncol Biol Phys* 1999; **44**: 513–17.

Mitobronitol (1847-d)

Mitobronitol (*BAN, rINN*).

DBM; Dibromomannitol; NSC-94100; R-54; WR-220057. 1,6-Dibromo-1,6-dideoxy-D-mannitol.

$C_6H_{12}Br_2O_4 = 308.0$.
CAS — 488-41-5.
ATC — L01AX01.
Pharmacopoeias. In Br.

Pharmacopoeial description
BP 2001: A white or almost white crystalline solid. Slightly soluble in water, in alcohol, and in acetone; practically insoluble in chloroform. Protect from light.

Profile
Mitobronitol is an antineoplastic which appears to act as an alkylating agent, perhaps by epoxide formation. It has been used in the management of thrombocythaemia, both primary, and secondary to chronic myeloid leukaemia or polycythaemia vera.

The usual dose is 250 mg daily by mouth until the platelet count falls to acceptable levels. Intermittent dosage has been given for maintenance therapy, adjusted according to the blood count. Frequent examination of the blood should be performed during treatment.

Mitobronitol is well absorbed from the gastrointestinal tract and is excreted through the liver into the bile, with reabsorption from the small intestine. It is eliminated as unchanged drug and some bromine-containing metabolites in the urine over several days.

◊ Long-term follow-up of a cooperative study[1] involving 350 patients with polycythaemia vera and treated with mitobronitol found that of 113 patients followed for over 10 years, 68 had survived, and there were no deaths due to acute myeloid leukaemia. Among the 168 living and 69 dead patients who had been followed for between 2 and 10 years there were 7 cases of acute myeloid leukaemia. The frequency of this leukaemia was less than that observed with other chemotherapy regimens and it was thought possible that mitobronitol had an advantage not only over the already discarded chlorambucil but also over phosphorus-32 or busulfan in rarely inducing acute myeloid leukaemia.

For a discussion of the usual management of polycythaemia vera, see p.486.

1. Kelemen E, *et al.* Decreasing risk of leukaemia during prolonged follow-up after mitobronitol therapy for polycythaemia vera. *Lancet* 1987; **ii:** 625.

Preparations

BP 2001: Mitobronitol Tablets.

Proprietary Preparations (details are given in Part 3)
Aust.: Myelobromol; *UK:* Myelobromol.

Mitoguazone Dihydrochloride (13502-q)

Mitoguazone Dihydrochloride *(rINNM).*
Methyl-GAG; Methylglyoxal Bisguanylhydrazone (mitoguazone); MGBG; NSC-32946. 1,1'-[(Methylethanediylidene)dinitrilo]diguanidine dihydrochloride.
$C_5H_{12}N_8,2HCl = 257.1$.
CAS — 459-86-9 (mitoguazone); 7059-23-6 (mitoguazone dihydrochloride).

Profile

Mitoguazone is an antineoplastic which may exert its cytotoxic effects by its ability to inhibit polyamine biosynthesis. It was formerly given as the dihydrochloride monohydrate, by intravenous infusion in doses of 80 to 300 mg daily, for 3 to 5 days, in the treatment of acute myeloid leukaemias (p.485). It may also be given by intramuscular injection. Mitoguazone has also been tried, as the dihydrochloride or the acetate, in the treatment of solid tumours and lymphomas.

Mitoguazone may produce hypoglycaemia and should be administered dissolved in glucose-containing infusion fluids; sugar may be taken by mouth if hypoglycaemia develops during infusion. Granulocytopenia and thrombocytopenia are generally mild and reversible on stopping treatment. Gastrointestinal effects frequently occur.

◊ References.
1. Von Hoff DD. MGBG: teaching an old drug new tricks. *Ann Oncol* 1994; **5:** 487–93.

Mitolactol (1849-h)

Mitolactol *(rINN).*
DBD; Dibromodulcitol; NSC-104800; WR-138743. 1,6-Dibromo-1,6-dideoxy-D-galactitol.
$C_6H_{12}Br_2O_4 = 308.0$.
CAS — 10318-26-0.

Profile

Mitolactol is an antineoplastic which may act by alkylation, probably as epoxide metabolites including dianhydrogalactitol. It has been given by mouth in the treatment of metastatic breast and cervical carcinoma, although other drugs are usually preferred (see p.491 and p.492), and has also been tried in other malignant neoplasms, notably those of the brain (p.490).

In addition to myelosuppression, which is usually dose-limiting, and manifests chiefly as leucopenia and thrombocytopenia, adverse effects include gastrointestinal disturbances, skin rashes, grey pigmentation of the skin, transient disturbances of hepatic function, elevated blood-urea nitrogen (BUN), and hypersensitivity reactions. Blood counts should be taken regularly during treatment and mitolactol withdrawn if bone-marrow depression occurs.

Mitomycin (1850-a)

Mitomycin *(BAN, USAN, rINN).*
Mitomycin C; Mitomycine C; NSC-26980. 6-Amino-1,1a,2,8,8a,8b-hexahydro-8-hydroxymethyl-8a-methoxy-5-methylazirino[2',3':3,4]pyrrolo[1,2-a]indole-4,7-dione carbamate; (1S,2S,9S,9aR)-7-Amino-2,3,5,8,9,9a-hexahydro-9a-methoxy-6-methyl-5,8-dioxo-1,2-epimino-1-H-pyrrolo[1,2-a]indol-9-ylmethyl carbamate.
$C_{15}H_{18}N_4O_5 = 334.3$.
CAS — 50-07-7.
ATC — L01DC03.

Pharmacopoeias. In *Fr., Jpn,* and *US.*

An antineoplastic antibiotic produced by the growth of *Streptomyces caespitosus.*

Pharmacopoeial description

USP 25: A blue-violet crystalline powder. It has a potency of not less than 970 µg per mg. Slightly soluble in water; soluble in acetone, in butyl acetate, in cyclohexanone, and in methyl alcohol. A 0.5% suspension in water has a pH of 6.0 to 7.5. Store in airtight containers. Protect from light. Mitomycin may

be **incompatible** with drugs that are acid in solution—for a report of incompatibility with topotecan, see p.575.

Stability. Mitomycin undergoes degradation in acid solution,[1] and two studies[2,3] suggest that mitomycin is much less stable in glucose 5% injection than in sodium chloride 0.9%. These results have been queried by a manufacturer (*Bristol, USA*) whose results suggest that mitomycin is stable for 48 hours in glucose injection 5% at 25°,[4] and it is uncertain whether different manufacturers' formulations differ in stability, or, as has been suggested, that an unsuitable assay was used by the manufacturer to measure stability.[5]

1. Beijnen JH, Underberg WJM. Degradation of mitomycin C in acidic solution. *Int J Pharmaceutics* 1985; **24:** 219–29.
2. Benvenuto JA, *et al.* Stability and compatibility of antitumour agents in glass and plastic containers. *Am J Hosp Pharm* 1981; **38:** 1914–18.
3. Quebbeman EJ, *et al.* Stability of mitomycin admixtures. *Am J Hosp Pharm* 1985; **42:** 1750–4.
4. Keller JH. Stability of mitomycin admixtures. *Am J Hosp Pharm* 1986; **43:** 59,64.
5. Quebbeman EJ, Hoffman NE. Stability of mitomycin admixtures. *Am J Hosp Pharm* 1986; **43:** 64.

Adverse Effects, Treatment, and Precautions

For general discussions see Antineoplastics, p.476, p.479, and p.480.

The main adverse effect of mitomycin is delayed cumulative bone-marrow suppression. Profound leucopenia and thrombocytopenia occurs after about 4 weeks with recovery in about 8 to 10 weeks after a dose. Blood counts may not recover in about one-quarter of patients. Other serious adverse effects include renal damage and pulmonary reactions; a potentially fatal haemolytic-uraemic syndrome has been reported in some patients. The US manufacturer states that the degree of renal impairment does not appear to be related to dose or duration of therapy but some in the UK consider that the incidence of renal toxicity is greatly increased if the total cumulative dose exceeds 120 mg (see also Effects on the Kidneys, below). Gastrointestinal toxicity, dermatitis, alopecia, fever, malaise, and rarely cardiotoxicity may also occur. Local tissue necrosis, ulceration, and cellulitis may occur following extravasation.

Mitomycin is contra-indicated in patients with impaired renal function or coagulation disorders. Renal function should be tested before beginning treatment and after each course.

Effects on the bladder. Intravesical instillation of mitomycin after resection of superficial bladder tumours has led to the development of indolent asymptomatic ulcers at the resection site which may persist for months, and must be distinguished from persistent infiltrating bladder cancer.[1,2] Severe bladder contracture resulting in intolerable urinary frequency has also occurred.[3]

See also under Effects on the Skin, below.

1. Richards B, Tolley D. Benign ulcers after bladder instillation of mitomycin C. *Lancet* 1986; **i:** 45.
2. Hetherington JW, Whelan P. Persistent ulcers after bladder instillation of mitomycin C. *Lancet* 1986; **i:** 324.
3. Wajsman Z, *et al.* Severely contracted bladder following intravesical mitomycin C therapy. *J Urol (Baltimore)* 1983; **130:** 340–1.

Effects on the kidneys. A syndrome of thrombotic microangiopathy resembling the haemolytic-uraemic syndrome has been seen in patients receiving mitomycin,[1] either alone[2,3] or more frequently combined with other drugs,[1,4-6] particularly fluorouracil[4,6] or tamoxifen.[7] Symptoms of haemolysis and renal failure may be complemented by hypertension and cardiovascular problems, pulmonary oedema and hypertension, and neurological symptoms.[1] There is some uncertainty as to whether mitomycin dose is significant, but one study found that all of 25 cases they reported had received total doses of 70 mg or more.[3] Symptoms may be exacerbated if blood transfusions are given, sometimes fatally.[4] Plasma exchange has been suggested as possibly helpful,[5] although it may not relieve renal failure.[6] Captopril therapy may also be useful.[8]

1. Fields SM, Lindley CM. Thrombotic microangiopathy associated with chemotherapy: case report and review of the literature. *DICP Ann Pharmacother* 1989; **23:** 582–8.
2. Rumpf KW, *et al.* Mitomycin-induced haemolysis and renal failure. *Lancet* 1980; **ii:** 1037–8.
3. Cordonnier D, *et al.* La néphrotoxicité de la mitomycine (à propos de 25 observations): résultats d'une enquête multicentrique organisée par la société de néphrologie. *Nephrologie* 1985; **6:** 19–26.
4. Jones BG, *et al.* Intravascular haemolysis and renal impairment after blood transfusion in two patients on long-term 5-fluorouracil and mitomycin-C. *Lancet* 1980; **i:** 1275–7.
5. Karlin DA, Stroehlein JR. Rash, nephritis, hypertension, and haemolysis in a patient on 5-fluorouracil, doxorubicin, and mitomycin C. *Lancet* 1980; **ii:** 534–5.
6. Lempert KD. Haemolysis and renal impairment syndrome in patients on 5-fluorouracil and mitomycin-C. *Lancet* 1980; **ii:** 369–70.

7. Montes A, *et al.* A toxic interaction between mitomycin C and tamoxifen causing the haemolytic uraemic syndrome. *Eur J Cancer* 1993; **29A:** 1854–7.
8. Schiebe ME, *et al.* Mitomycin C-related hemolytic uremic syndrome in cancer patients. *Anticancer Drugs* 1998; **9:** 433–5.

Effects on the liver. Hepatic veno-occlusive disease developed in 6 of 29 patients given intensive mitomycin therapy and autologous bone-marrow transplantation.[1] The effect was manifest as abdominal pain, hepatomegaly, and ascites, and liver failure was progressive and fatal in 3. A further patient, who had no symptoms, was found to have veno-occlusive disease at post mortem.

1. Lazarus HM, *et al.* Veno-occlusive disease of the liver after high-dose mitomycin C therapy and autologous bone marrow transplantation. *Cancer* 1982; **49:** 1789–95.

Effects on respiratory function. Mitomycin-induced pulmonary toxicity has been reviewed.[1,2] There have been reports of toxicity at total dosages as low as 20 mg per m² of mitomycin,[2] although others report that the average cumulative dose associated with toxicity is 78 mg.[1] Premedication with corticosteroids may reduce the incidence of lung toxicity.[2]

See also Effects on the Lungs, p.478. For reference to the respiratory effects of mitomycin in combination with a vinca alkaloid see Interactions, Antineoplastics, under Vinblastine Sulfate, p.578.

1. Linette DC, *et al.* Mitomycin-induced pulmonary toxicity: case report and review of the literature. *Ann Pharmacother* 1992; **26:** 481–4.
2. Okuno SH, Frytak S. Mitomycin lung toxicity: acute and chronic phases. *Am J Clin Oncol* 1997; **20:** 282–4.

Effects on the skin. Severe eczematous symptoms in patients receiving intravesical mitomycin[1,2] appear to be due to a delayed hypersensitivity reaction,[2] which also appears to be responsible for the bladder irritation and cystitis which may follow intravesical mitomycin.[2]

1. Neild VS, *et al.* Dermatitis due to mitomycin bladder instillations. *J R Soc Med* 1984; **77:** 610–11.
2. Colver GB, *et al.* Dermatitis due to intravesical mitomycin C: a delayed-type hypersensitivity reaction? *Br J Dermatol* 1990; **122:** 217–24.

Interactions

Antineoplastics. Cardiotoxicity developed in 14 of 91 patients who received mitomycin therapy as second-line treatment for breast cancer after the failure of *doxorubicin*-containing regimens, compared with 3 of 89 similar patients whose second-line treatment did not include mitomycin.[1]

For reports of acute bronchospasm following injection of a *vinca alkaloid* in patients pretreated with mitomycin see Vinblastine Sulfate, p.578. For the increased risk of haemolytic-uraemic syndrome that may occur if mitomycin is given with *fluorouracil* or *tamoxifen* see under Effects on the Kidneys, above.

1. Buzdar AU, *et al.* Adriamycin and mitomycin C: possible synergistic cardiotoxicity. *Cancer Treat Rep* 1978; **62:** 1005–8.

Pharmacokinetics

Mitomycin disappears rapidly from the blood after intravenous injection with an initial (distribution) half-life of 17 minutes. It is widely distributed but does not appear to cross the blood-brain barrier. Mitomycin is metabolised mainly but not exclusively in the liver. The terminal half-life is about 50 minutes. Following normal doses about 10% of a dose is excreted unchanged in the urine; small amounts are also present in bile and faeces. With increasing doses metabolic pathways are saturated, and more drug is excreted unchanged in the urine.

Uses and Administration

Mitomycin is a highly toxic antibiotic with antineoplastic properties. It acts as an alkylating agent after activation *in vivo* and suppresses the synthesis of nucleic acids. It is a cell-cycle non-specific agent, but is most active in the late G_1 and early S phases.

Mitomycin is used, with other antineoplastic agents, in the treatment of many solid tumours including those of the bladder, breast, cervix, eye, liver, lung, stomach, and prostate as indicated by the cross-references given below. Mitomycin has been tried in various other neoplasms including those of the gastrointestinal tract, head and neck, pancreas, in melanoma, sarcomas, and in leukaemias.

Various dosage regimens have been tried. An initial dose of 10 to 20 mg per m² body-surface intravenously has been given; subsequent doses may be repeated at intervals of 6 to 8 weeks if blood counts permit, and should be reduced according to the previous haematological response. Another suggested regimen is 2 mg per m² daily for 5 days, repeated after 2 days.

Other regimens may be used, particularly in combination.

Doses are adjusted according to the effect on bone marrow and treatment should not be repeated until the leucocyte count is above at least 3000 per mm^3 and the platelet count above at least 75 000 per mm^3. The drug should not be given again if the nadir of the leucocyte count is below 2000 per mm^3. Dosage may need to be reduced when used in combination with other antineoplastics.

Mitomycin is also used as a bladder instillation: 10 to 40 mg is instilled one to three times a week for a total of 20 doses in the treatment of superficial bladder tumours. For the prevention of recurrent bladder tumours 20 mg may be instilled every 2 weeks, or 40 mg monthly or 3-monthly. Alternatively 4 to 10 mg may be instilled one to three times a week.

Mitomycin has been given by the intra-arterial route in the treatment of liver tumours, sometimes as an infusion of microcapsules designed to produce localised embolisation.

Malignant neoplasms. Mitomycin is used in the prevention of recurrent bladder cancer (p.490), in the palliative therapy of advanced breast cancer (p.491), in malignancies of the cervix (p.492), eye (p.493), gastrointestinal tract (p.493), liver (p.495), non-small-cell lung cancer (p.496), and has been tried in advanced prostatic cancer (see p.497).

Ocular disorders, non-malignant. GLAUCOMA. Mitomycin, like fluorouracil, is effective in improving the outcome of glaucoma filtering surgery in selected patients when used as an adjunct to prevent the formation of scar tissue (see p.1413). Fluorouracil is usually administered as a regimen of multiple injections but mitomycin given as a single intraoperative topical application in usual concentrations ranging from 0.2 to 0.5 mg per mL appears to be of similar efficacy.[1,2] A meta-analysis of 11 studies concluded that intra-operative mitomycin reduced the chances of failure in high-risk patients, and in those having their first trabeculectomy.[3] However it was noted that the nature of the data might have led to overestimation of the effect and that there was some evidence of an increased risk of cataract with mitomycin. Chronic hypotony, sometimes associated with maculopathy and irreversible visual loss, has been one of the most commonly reported adverse effects for mitomycin.

1. Skuta GL, et al. Intraoperative mitomycin versus postoperative 5-fluorouracil in high-risk glaucoma filtering surgery. Ophthalmology 1992; 99: 438–44.
2. Katz GJ, et al. Mitomycin C versus 5-fluorouracil in high-risk glaucoma filtering surgery: extended follow-up. Ophthalmology 1995; 102: 1263–9.
3. Wilkins M, et al. Intra-operative mitomycin C for glaucoma surgery (updated 30 November 2000). Available in The Cochrane Library. Issue 1. Oxford: Update Software; 2001.

PTERYGIUM. Pterygium is a degenerative condition of subconjunctival tissues that results in a vascularised overgrowth of the conjunctiva and cornea. It is cosmetically unappealing but does not usually require treatment. However, if it affects the pupillary area it can be treated surgically. Pterygium often recurs after removal. Methods used to prevent recurrence include radiotherapy or the use of eye drops containing mitomycin[1-4] or thiotepa.[5] Depigmentation of the eyelids may be a problem with topical thiotepa,[5] especially in darkly pigmented patients and most recent studies seem to have used mitomycin. Mitomycin has been applied topically to the surgical site,[3,6] or given as eye drops postoperatively.[1,2,4] The optimal concentration is uncertain; although 0.04% eye drops have been used there is some risk of adverse effects, which may be severe and sight-threatening,[7] and a 0.02% solution may be as effective, and better tolerated.[1,4,6,8] In one retrospective study,[9] intraoperative administration of 0.04% mitomycin was found to be more effective than β-irradiation in preventing recurrence after surgery. Batimastat is also under investigation for the prevention of pterygium recurrence.

1. Wong L. Ophthalmic mitomycin for preventing recurrent pterygium. Can J Hosp Pharm 1990; 43: 251–2.
2. Mahar PS, Nwokora GE. Role of mitomycin C in pterygium surgery. Br J Ophthalmol 1993; 77: 433–5.
3. Cano-Parra J, et al. Prospective trial of intraoperative mitomycin C in the treatment of primary pterygium. Br J Ophthalmol 1995; 79: 439–41.
4. Rachmiel R, et al. Results of treatment with topical mitomycin C 0.02% following excision of primary pterygium. Br J Ophthalmol 1995; 79: 233–6.
5. Meacham CT. Triethylene thiophosphoramide in the prevention of pterygium recurrence. Am J Ophthalmol 1962; 54: 751.
6. Mastropasqua L, et al. Long term results of intraoperative mitomycin C in the treatment of recurrent pterygium. Br J Ophthalmol 1996; 80: 288–91.
7. Rubinfeld RS, et al. Serious complications of topical mitomycin C after pterygium surgery. Ophthalmology 1992; 99: 1647–54.
8. Levartovsky S, Moskowitz Y. Application of mitomycin C 0.02% for 2 minutes at the end of pterygium surgery. Br J Ophthalmol 1998; 82: 97–100.
9. Amano S, et al. Comparative study of intraoperative mitomycin C and irradiation in pterygium surgery. Br J Ophthalmol 2000; 84: 618–21.

The symbol † denotes a preparation no longer actively marketed

Preparations

USP 25: Mitomycin for Injection.

Proprietary Preparations (details are given in Part 3)
Braz.: Mitocin; *Canad.:* Mutamycin; *Fin.:* Mitostat; Mutamycin; *Fr.:* Ametycine; *Ger.:* Ametycine; Mito-medac; *Mex.:* Mitocin-C; Mitolem; *Norw.:* Mutamycin; *Swed.:* Mutamycin; *Switz.:* Mutamycine; *USA:* Mutamycin.

Mitotane (1852-x)

Mitotane *(USAN, rINN)*.
CB-313; o,p'DDD; NSC-38721; WR-13045. 1,1-Dichloro-2-(2-chlorophenyl)-2-(4-chlorophenyl)ethane.
$C_{14}H_{10}Cl_4 = 320.0$.
CAS — 53-19-0.
Pharmacopoeias. In US.

Pharmacopoeial description

USP 25: A white crystalline powder with a slight aromatic odour. M.p. is between 75° and 81°. Practically insoluble in water; soluble in alcohol, in ether, in petroleum spirit, and in fixed oils and fats. Store in airtight containers. Protect from light.

Adverse Effects

Almost all patients given mitotane experience anorexia, nausea and vomiting, and sometimes diarrhoea, and about 40% suffer some central toxicity with dizziness, vertigo, sedation, lethargy, and mental depression. Permanent brain damage may develop with prolonged dosage. Ocular side-effects may occur including blurred vision, diplopia, lenticular opacities, and retinopathy. Other side-effects include hypersensitivity reactions, haematuria, albuminuria, skin rashes, fever, myalgia, haemorrhagic cystitis, flushing, hypertension, and orthostatic hypotension.

Precautions

Mitotane inhibits the adrenal cortex and adrenocortical insufficiency may develop during treatment; concomitant corticosteroid therapy is often required. In trauma or shock the drug should be temporarily withdrawn and corticosteroids should be given systemically. Mitotane should be given with care to patients with liver disease. Patients should not drive or operate machinery. Behavioural and neurological assessments should be carried out regularly in patients who have been receiving treatment for 2 years or more.

Interactions

Mitotane may induce hepatic microsomal enzymes and enhance the metabolism of some other drugs, including coumarin anticoagulants.

Spironolactone. Mitotane in a dose of up to 3 g daily in a 65-year-old patient with Cushing's syndrome appeared to be ineffective and did not produce the usual side-effects associated with mitotane while the patient was also receiving spironolactone.[1]

1. Wortsman J, Soler NG. Mitotane: spironolactone antagonism in Cushing's syndrome. JAMA 1977; 238: 2527.

Pharmacokinetics

Up to 40% of a dose of mitotane is absorbed from the gastrointestinal tract. After daily doses of 5 to 15 g, concentrations in the blood of 7 to 90 μg per mL of unchanged drug and 29 to 54 μg per mL of metabolite have been reported. Mitotane has been detected in the blood 6 to 9 weeks after stopping treatment. It is widely distributed and appears to be stored mainly in fatty tissues. It is metabolised in the liver and other tissues and excreted as metabolites in urine and bile. From 10 to 25% of a dose has been recovered in the urine as a water-soluble metabolite.

◊ Monitoring of mitotane and its major metabolite o,p'-DDE in 2 patients receiving mitotane in low doses for Cushing's disease demonstrated that there is a prolonged lag time in the plasma concentration changes in response to alterations in dosage,[1] presumably because of the lipophilicity of both compounds which leads to accumulation in adipose tissue.

1. Benecke R, et al. Plasma level monitoring of mitotane (o,p'-DDD) and its metabolite (o,p'-DDE) during long-term treatment of Cushing's disease with low doses. Eur J Clin Pharmacol 1991; 41: 259–61.

Uses and Administration

Mitotane is an antineoplastic with a selective inhibitory action on adrenal cortex activity. It may also modify peripheral steroid metabolism. It is given in the treatment of inoperable adrenocortical tumours and has also been used in patients with Cushing's syndrome (p.1272).

The usual initial dosage is 2 to 6 g daily by mouth in 3 or 4 divided doses, adjusted to the maximum tolerated dose which may range from 2 to 16 g daily.

◊ A retrospective study involving 105 patients with adrenocortical carcinoma found the prognosis to be generally poor with a 5-year survival of 22% among 88 patients followed up.[1] Surgical resection was the treatment of choice; mitotane treatment had no effect on survival although 8 patients had transient tumour regression and it was of some benefit in controlling adrenal hypersecretion. However, other workers have previously reported improved survival in patients with adrenocortical carcinoma in whom mitotane serum concentrations were above 14 μg per mL, and some[2] have suggested that the poor results with mitotane in the retrospective study may have been due to low serum-mitotane concentrations.

1. Luton J-P, et al. Clinical features of adrenocortical carcinoma, prognostic factors, and the effect of mitotane therapy. N Engl J Med 1990; 322: 1195–1201.
2. Haak HR, et al. Mitotane therapy of adrenocortical carcinoma. N Engl J Med 1990; 323: 758.

Preparations

USP 25: Mitotane Tablets.

Proprietary Preparations (details are given in Part 3)
Braz.: Lisodren; *Canad.:* Lysodren; *USA:* Lysodren.

Mitozantrone Hydrochloride (12967-s)

Mitozantrone Hydrochloride *(BANM)*.
Mitoxantrone Hydrochloride *(BANM, USAN, rINNM)*; CL-232315; DHAD; Dihydroxyanthracenedione Dihydrochloride; Mitoxantroni Hydrochloridum; NSC-301739. 1,4-Dihydroxy-5,8-bis[2-(2-hydroxyethylamino)ethylamino]anthraquinone dihydrochloride.
$C_{22}H_{28}N_4O_6,2HCl = 517.4$.
CAS — 65271-80-9 (mitozantrone [mitoxantrone]); 70476-82-3 (mitozantrone [mitoxantrone] hydrochloride).
Pharmacopoeias. In Eur. (see p.vi) and US.

Pharmacopoeial description

Ph. Eur.: A dark-blue, electrostatic, hygroscopic powder. Sparingly soluble in water; practically insoluble in acetone; slightly soluble in methyl alcohol. Store in airtight containers.
USP 25: A dark-blue powder. Sparingly soluble in water; practically insoluble in acetone, in acetonitrile, and in chloroform; slightly soluble in methyl alcohol. Store in airtight containers.

Adverse Effects, Treatment, and Precautions

As for Doxorubicin Hydrochloride, p.535. Mitozantrone [mitoxantrone] is reported to be better tolerated than doxorubicin. The nadir of the white blood cell count usually occurs about 10 days after a dose, with recovery by the 21st day. Elevation in liver enzyme values may occur; there are occasional reports of severe hepatic impairment in patients with leukaemia, in whom doses are generally higher and adverse effects of mitozantrone [mitoxantrone] may be more frequent and severe.

Transient blue-green coloration of the urine, and occasionally the sclerae, may occur. Tissue necrosis is rare following extravasation.

Severe neurotoxicity has resulted from erroneous intrathecal administration. Care is required in patients with pre-existing heart disease, or who have had prior anthracycline treatment or radiotherapy to the chest, as they are at increased risk of cardiotoxicity; regular examinations of cardiac function should be performed in such patients and in those who receive a total cumulative dose of mitozantrone [mitoxantrone] in excess of 160 mg per m^2 body-surface. Care is also required in patients with hepatic impairment.

Alopecia. Two patients receiving therapy with mitozantrone [mitoxantrone] developed selective alopecia of white but not of dark hair.[1]

1. Arlin ZA, et al. Selective alopecia with mitoxantrone. N Engl J Med 1984; 310: 1464.

Effects on the heart. Data from over 4000 patients treated with mitozantrone [mitoxantrone] included 172 reports of cardiac events, including 42 cases of congestive heart failure and 66 of decreased ejection fraction.[1] Prior treatment with an anthracycline increased the risk, and congestive heart failure seemed to be more likely in patients exposed to a cumulative mitozantrone [mitoxantrone] dose of 160 mg per m^2 body-surface or 100 mg per m^2 in those who had already received anthracyclines. In a further 78 patients,[2] clinical heart failure developed in 2 after cumulative doses of 174 and 243 per m^2. Four of 9 other patients who received mitozantrone [mitoxantrone] in doses above 100 mg per m^2 showed signs of cardiotoxicity, and a further patient who had previously received doxorubicin 313 mg per m^2 had a fall in stress ejection fraction after only 47 mg per m^2 of mitozantrone [mitoxantrone]. However, sinus bradycardia has also been reported[3] in 2 previously untreated patients after commencing continuous infusions of mitozantrone [mitoxantrone] 10 mg per m^2. For information on the cardiotoxicity of anthracyclines, to which mitozantrone [mitoxantrone] is structurally related, see under Adverse Effects and Treatment of Doxorubicin, p.535.

1. Crossley RJ. Clinical safety and tolerance of mitoxantrone. Sem in Oncol 1984; 11: (suppl 1): 54–8.
2. Stuart-Harris R, et al. Cardiotoxicity associated with mitoxantrone. Lancet 1984; ii: 219–20.
3. Benekli M, et al. Mitoxantrone-induced bradycardia. Ann Intern Med 1997; 126: 409.

Handling and disposal. *Urine and faeces* produced for up to 7 days after a dose of mitozantrone [mitoxantrone] should be handled wearing protective clothing.[1]

1. Harris J, Dodds LJ. Handling waste from patients receiving cytotoxic drugs. *Pharm J* 1985; **235:** 289–91.

Hypersensitivity. A report of 3 patients with allergic-type reactions to mitozantrone [mitoxantrone], including vasculitis, facial oedema and skin rashes, and in one, breathlessness, tachypnoea, cyanosis, and unrecordable pulse and blood pressure.[1] Allergic reactions to the drug appear to be rare.

1. Taylor WB, *et al.* Allergic reactions to mitoxantrone. *Lancet* 1986; **i:** 1439.

Pharmacokinetics

Following intravenous administration mitozantrone [mitoxantrone] is rapidly and extensively distributed to body tissues, and slowly excreted in urine and bile as unchanged drug and metabolites. The elimination half-life is reported to range from 5 to 18 days. Between 6 and 11% of a dose has been recovered from urine, and 13 to 25% in faeces, within 5 days of administration. It does not appear to cross the blood-brain barrier.

◊ References.

1. Ehninger G, *et al.* Pharmacokinetics and metabolism of mitoxantrone: a review. *Clin Pharmacokinet* 1990; **18:** 365–80.

Uses and Administration

Mitozantrone [mitoxantrone] is an antineoplastic structurally related to doxorubicin (p.534). Its mode of action has not been fully established but it inhibits topoisomerase II and causes DNA strand breakage, as well as intercalating with DNA. It is cell-cycle nonspecific but is most active against cells in the late S phase.

It is used in the treatment of advanced breast cancer (p.491), and of non-Hodgkin's lymphomas (p.487), alone or in combination with other agents. It may also be given to treat adult acute myeloid leukaemias (p.485), especially in relapse, and has been used in patients with hormone-refractory prostate cancer (p.497). Mitozantrone [mitoxantrone] has also been used in the treatment of ovarian and liver cancer.

In addition, mitozantrone [mitoxantrone] is used in the management of secondary progressive or relapsing multiple sclerosis (see below), to reduce neurological disability or the frequency of relapses.

In the treatment of breast cancer, prostate cancer, and lymphomas, mitozantrone [mitoxantrone] is given as the hydrochloride in an initial dose equivalent to 14 mg of base per m² body-surface, repeated every 3 weeks, by injecting a solution diluted in sodium chloride 0.9% or glucose 5% injection into a freely-running intravenous infusion of either, over at least 3 minutes. Subsequent doses may be adjusted according to the degree of myelosuppression produced. Initial dosage may need to be reduced to 12 mg per m² in debilitated patients or those who have had previous chemotherapy. Doses should also probably be reduced when mitozantrone [mitoxantrone] is given as part of a combination regimen: an initial dose of 10 to 12 mg per m² has been suggested.

In the treatment of patients with acute myeloid leukaemia a dose of 12 mg per m² daily for 5 days may be given to induce remission; alternatively a similar dose may be given for 3 days in association with cytarabine.

Cardiac examinations are recommended in all patients who receive a cumulative dose of mitozantrone [mitoxantrone] greater than 160 mg per m². Regular blood counts should be performed during treatment and courses should not be repeated until blood counts have recovered.

In the management of multiple sclerosis, the recommended dose is the equivalent of 12 mg of mitozantrone [mitoxantrone] per m² by intravenous infusion over 5 to 15 minutes. This dose may be given once every 3 months initially provided that neutrophil counts are above 1500 cells per mm³ and that left ventricular ejection fraction (LVEF) is greater than 50%. Blood counts should be monitored before each dose. LVEF should be evaluated before beginning mito-

zantrone [mitoxantrone] therapy and before all doses in patients who have received a cumulative dose in excess of 100 mg per m²; a total cumulative lifetime dose in excess of 140 mg per m² should be avoided. LVEF should also be measured if signs or symptoms of heart failure develop.

◊ References.

1. Faulds D, *et al.* Mitoxantrone: a review of its pharmacodynamic and pharmacokinetic properties, and therapeutic potential in the chemotherapy of cancer. *Drugs* 1991; **41:** 400–49.

Multiple sclerosis. Mitoxantrone [mitoxantrone] in intravenous doses ranging from 5 mg per m² every 3 months to 8 mg per m² every month has produced clinical benefit[1-3] in terms of reduced relapse rate and a slowing of disease progression in patients with multiple sclerosis (p.633). Benefit has also been demonstrated in combination with corticosteroids,[4] although the combination was not compared with mitoxantrone [mitoxantrone] alone. However, cardiotoxicity limits the dose that can be given.[1,4,5]

1. Millefiorini E, *et al.* Randomized placebo-controlled trial of mitoxantrone in relapsing-remitting multiple sclerosis: 24-month clinical and MRI results. *J Neurol* 1997; **244:** 153–9.
2. Hartung HP, Gonsett R. Mitoxantrone in progressive multiple sclerosis (MS): a placebo-controlled, randomized, observer-blind European phase III multicenter study - clinical results. *Multiple Sclerosis* 1998; **4:** 325.
3. Krapf H, *et al.* Mitoxantrone in progressive multiple sclerosis (MS): a placebo-controlled, randomised, observer-blind European phase III multicenter study - MRI results. *Multiple Sclerosis* 1998; **4:** 380.
4. Edan G, *et al.* Therapeutic effect of mitoxantrone combined with methylprednisolone in multiple sclerosis: a randomised multicentre study of active disease using MRI and clinical criteria. *J Neurol Neurosurg Psychiatry* 1997; **62:** 112–118.
5. Gonsette RE. Mitoxantrone immunotherapy in multiple sclerosis. *Multiple Sclerosis* 1996; **1:** 329–32.

Preparations

BP 2001: Mitoxantrone Intravenous Infusion;
USP 25: Mitoxantrone Injection.

Proprietary Preparations (details are given in Part 3)
Aust.: Novantron; **Austral.:** Novantrone; Onkotrone; **Belg.:** Novantrone; **Braz.:** Novantrone; **Canad.:** Novantrone; **Denm.:** Novantrone; **Fin.:** Novantrone; **Fr.:** Novantrone; **Ger.:** Novantron; Onkotrone; **Hong Kong:** Novantrone; **Irl.:** Novantrone; **Israel:** Novantrone; **Ital.:** Novantrone; **Mex.:** Mitroxone; Novantrone; **Neth.:** Novantrone; **Norw.:** Novantrone; **NZ:** Novantrone; **Port.:** Novantrone; **S.Afr.:** Novantrone; **Singapore:** Novantrone; **Spain:** Novantrone; Pralifan; **Swed.:** Novantrone; **Switz.:** Novantron; **Thai.:** Novantrone; **UK:** Novantrone; Onkotrone; **USA:** Novantrone.

Mizoribine (16900-f)

Mizoribine *(rINN).*

HE-69. 5-Hydroxy-1-β-D-ribofuranosylimidazole-4-carboxamide.

$C_9H_{13}N_3O_6 = 259.2.$
CAS — 50924-49-7.

Profile

Mizoribine is an oral immunosuppressant that has been used as an alternative to azathioprine.

◊ References.

1. Lee HA, *et al.* Mizoribine as an alternative to azathioprine in triple therapy immunosuppressant regimens in cadaveric renal transplantation: two successive studies. *Transplant Proc* 1995; **27:** 1050–1.
2. Tanabe K, *et al.* Long-term results in mizoribine-treated renal transplant recipients: a prospective, randomized trial of mizoribine and azathioprine under cyclosporine-based immunosuppression. *Transplant Proc* 1999; **31:** 2877–9.

Mopidamol (12975-s)

Mopidamol *(BAN, rINN).*

Ra-233. 2,2′,2″,2‴-(4-Piperidinopyrimido[5,4-d]pyrimidine-2,6-diyldinitrilo)tetraethanol.

$C_{19}H_{31}N_7O_4 = 421.5.$
CAS — 13665-88-8.

Profile

Mopidamol was formerly used as an antineoplastic. It is also a phosphodiesterase inhibitor which inhibits platelet aggregation.

Multialchilpeptide (10733-r)

CAS — 9076-25-9.

Profile

Multialchilpeptide is a complex of metamelfalan, an analogue of melphalan (p.551) with peptides. It has been used in the treatment of malignant neoplasms of the blood and lymphatic systems.

Preparations

Proprietary Preparations (details are given in Part 3)
Ital.: Peptichemio†.

Muromonab-CD3 (3278-f)

Muromonab-CD3 *(USAN, rINN).*
OKT3.
ATC — L04AA02.

A murine monoclonal antibody comprising a purified IgG₂ₐ immunoglobulin with a heavy chain having a molecular weight of about 50 000 Da and a light chain with a molecular weight of approximately 25 000 Da.

Adverse Effects, Treatment, and Precautions

An acute cytokine release syndrome ranging from fever, chills, gastrointestinal disturbances, myalgia, and tremor to dyspnoea, pulmonary oedema, collapse, and cardiac arrest has occurred, typically 30 to 60 minutes after the first few doses of muromonab-CD3 although risk persists for some 48 hours after a dose. Frequency and severity tend to decrease with successive doses, while prophylactic administration of corticosteroids may reduce initial adverse reactions (see Uses and Administration, below). Other reported effects include encephalopathy, cerebral oedema, and a syndrome resembling aseptic meningitis, with headache, fever, stiff neck, and photophobia; seizures have also occurred. Reversible impairment of renal function may also be seen.

Hypersensitivity reactions, including anaphylaxis, have occurred, and may be difficult to distinguish from the cytokine release syndrome.

As with other potent immunosuppressants, treatment with muromonab-CD3 may increase the risk of serious infections and the development of certain malignancies.

Muromonab-CD3 should not be given to patients with pre-existing fever, or in patients hypersensitive to products of murine origin. It should be avoided in patients with a history of seizures. Because fluid overload is associated with an increased risk of pulmonary oedema due to the cytokine release syndrome, muromonab-CD3 is contra-indicated in patients who have undergone a more than 3% weight gain in the week preceding therapy, or who have radiographic evidence of fluid overloading. Repeated courses of muromonab-CD3 may be less effective because of the development of antibodies to the drug. Paediatric patients may be at increased risk of serious adverse effects following muromonab-CD3 therapy.

Effects on the blood. THROMBOEMBOLISM. Intragraft thromboses developed in 9 of 93 consecutive kidney transplant recipients given high-dose muromonab-CD3 (10 mg daily) as part of their immunosuppressive regimen.[1] In one patient the thrombosis was in the renal artery, and in 3 in the renal vein; the remainder had thromboses in the glomerular capillaries and thrombotic microangiopathy similar to that of haemolytic-uraemic syndrome. The authors suggested that muromonab-CD3 has procoagulant effects, perhaps mediated by released tumour necrosis factor; these effects had also been seen in 3 patients receiving muromonab-CD3 at conventional doses (5 mg daily). Another group[2] has also reported an apparently increased incidence of acute vascular thrombosis in patients given muromonab-CD3 at conventional doses, but in the experience of others,[3] despite evidence of activation of coagulation by the drug, treatment of acute rejection with 5 mg daily was not associated with thromboembolic complications.

1. Abramowicz D, *et al.* Induction of thromboses within renal grafts by high-dose prophylactic OKT3. *Lancet* 1992; **339:** 777–8.
2. Gomez E, *et al.* Main graft vessels thromboses due to conventional-dose OKT3 in renal transplantation. *Lancet* 1992; **339:** 1612–13.
3. Raasveld MHM, *et al.* Thromboembolic complications and dose of monoclonal OKT3 antibody. *Lancet* 1992; **339:** 1363–4.

Effects on the ears. Bilateral sensorineural hearing loss has occurred following muromonab-CD3 therapy. In one case series, 5 out of 7 patients were affected, showing a mean hearing loss of 18dB.[1] Tinnitus may also occur[1,2]. Although symptoms are generally reversible,[1,2] one patient still showed a deficit in hearing after 6 months.[3]

1. Hartnick CJ, *et al.* Reversible sensorineural hearing loss following administration of muromonab-CD3 (OKT3) for cadaveric renal transplant immunosuppression. *Ann Otol Rhinol Laryngol* 1997; **106:** 45–7.
2. Hartnick CJ, *et al.* Reversible sensorineural hearing loss after renal transplant immunosuppression with OKT3 (muromonab-CD3). *Ann Otol Rhinol Laryngol* 1997; **106:** 640–2.
3. Michals M, *et al.* Hearing loss associated with muromonab-CD3 therapy. *Clin Pharm* 1988; **7:** 867–8.

Effects on the nervous system. A report of generalised seizures in 2 uraemic kidney-graft recipients following administration of muromonab-CD3.[1] Delayed graft function may result in the accumulation of uraemic toxins which combine with cytokines released by the immunosuppressant to produce the effects on the CNS.

1. Seifeldin RA, et al. Generalised seizures associated with the use of muromonab-CD3 in two patients after kidney transplantation. Ann Pharmacother 1997; 31: 586–9.

Uses and Administration

Muromonab-CD3 is a murine monoclonal antibody to the T3 (CD3) antigen of human T-lymphocytes, which is essential to antigen recognition and response; the antibody thus specifically blocks T-cell generation and function to exert an immunosuppressant effect without affecting the bone marrow.

It is used in the treatment of acute allograft rejection in organ transplant recipients, in doses of 5 mg daily by intravenous injection for 10 to 14 days. An initial dose of 2.5 mg daily is recommended in children weighing 30 kg or less, subsequently adjusted if necessary in increments of 2.5 mg according to response. The dose of any concomitant immunosuppressant therapy may need to be reduced. Patients should be monitored closely after the first few doses of muromonab-CD3 because of the risk of cytokine release syndrome and hypersensitivity reactions. The first dose may be preceded by intravenous administration of methylprednisolone sodium succinate, in a dose of 8 mg per kg, 1 to 4 hours before muromonab-CD3. Paracetamol and antihistamines may also be given concomitantly with muromonab-CD3 to reduce early reactions.

Muromonab-CD3 has also been given experimentally as part of regimens for the prophylaxis of graft rejection. For further details of the use of muromonab-CD3 in the treatment and prophylaxis of graft rejection see p.502, et seq.

◊ References.
1. Wilde MI, Goa KL. Muromonab CD3: a reappraisal of its pharmacology and use as prophylaxis of solid organ transplant rejection. Drugs 1996; 51: 865–94.
2. Burk ML, Matuszewski KA. Muromonab-CD3 and antithymocyte globulin in renal transplantation. Ann Pharmacother 1997; 31: 1370–7.
3. ten Berge IJM, et al. Guidelines for optimal use of muromonab CD3 in transplantation. BioDrugs 1999; 11: 277–84.
4. Flechner SM. A randomized prospective trial of low-dose OKT3 induction therapy to prevent rejection and minimize side effects in recipients of kidney transplants. Transplantation 2000; 69: 2374–81.

Preparations

Proprietary Preparations (details are given in Part 3)
Austral.: Orthoclone OKT3; *Belg.:* Orthoclone OKT3; *Braz.:* Anti CD3; *Canad.:* Orthoclone OKT3; *Fin.:* Orthoclone OKT3; *Fr.:* Orthoclone OKT3; *Ger.:* Orthoclone OKT3; *Hong Kong:* Orthoclone OKT3; *Israel:* Orthoclone OKT3; *Ital.:* Orthoclone OKT3; *Mex.:* Orthoclone OKT3; *Neth.:* Orthoclone OKT3; *Norw.:* Orthoclone OKT3; *NZ:* Orthoclone OKT3; *Swed.:* Orthoclone OKT3; *Switz.:* Orthoclone OKT3; *Thai.:* Orthoclone OKT3; *USA:* Orthoclone OKT3.

Mustine Hydrochloride (1853-r)

Mustine Hydrochloride (BANM).
Chlormethine Hydrochloride (BANM, rINNM); Chlorethazine Hydrochloride; HN2 (mustine [chlormethine]); Mechlorethamine Hydrochloride; Nitrogen Mustard (mustine [chlormethine]); NSC-762; WR-147650. Bis(2-chloroethyl)methylamine hydrochloride; 2,2'-Dichloro-N-methyldiethylamine hydrochloride.
$C_5H_{11}Cl_2N,HCl = 192.5$.
CAS — 51-75-2 (mustine [chlormethine]); 55-86-7 (mustine [chlormethine] hydrochloride).
Pharmacopoeias. In Br., Chin., Int., and US.

Solutions lose their activity very rapidly particularly at neutral or alkaline pH.

Pharmacopoeial description
BP 2001: A white or almost white, hygroscopic, vesicant, crystalline powder or mass. Very soluble in water. Store at a temperature of 8° to 15°.
USP 25: A white, hygroscopic, crystalline powder. A 0.2% solution in water has a pH of 3.0 to 5.0. Store in airtight containers. Protect from light.

◊ CAUTION. *Mustine [chlormethine] hydrochloride is a strong vesicant; avoid contact with skin and mucous membranes.*

Stability. A study using an assay specific for mustine [chlormethine][1] found that a 0.1% solution in Water for Injections or sodium chloride injection (0.9%) underwent a loss of approximately 10% when stored for 6 hours at room temperature, and of approximately 4 to 6% when stored for the same period at

4°; similar results were obtained whether the solution was stored in glass vials or plastic syringes. Solutions in 500 mL of sodium chloride or glucose (5%) injection and stored in PVC infusion bags were still less stable, with 15% and 10% degradation respectively after 6 hours at room temperature.

1. Kirk B. Stability of reconstituted Mustine Injection BP during storage. Br J Parenter Ther 1986; 7: 86–92.

Adverse Effects, Treatment, and Precautions

For general discussions see Antineoplastics, p.476, p.479, and p.480.

Mustine [chlormethine] hydrochloride is extremely toxic and its use is invariably accompanied by side-effects. Severe nausea and vomiting may commence within an hour of injection of the drug and last for some hours; antiemetics should be given before treatment. It causes varying degrees of bone-marrow depression depending on the dose. In heavily pretreated patients, or when the total dose for a single course exceeds 400 µg per kg body-weight, there is a risk of severe and possibly fatal depression with anaemia, lymphocytopenia, granulocytopenia, and thrombocytopenia with consequent haemorrhage. Depression of lymphocytes may be apparent within 24 hours of the administration of mustine [chlormethine] hydrochloride and maximum suppression of granulocytes and platelets occurs within 7 to 21 days; haematological recovery may be adequate after 4 weeks.

Tinnitus, vertigo, deafness, headache, drowsiness, and other neurological symptoms have been reported, as have episodes of jaundice. Skin reactions to mustine [chlormethine] hydrochloride include maculopapular rashes. There is a high incidence of hypersensitivity when topical preparations are used.

Mustine [chlormethine] hydrochloride has a powerful vesicant action on the skin and mucous membranes and great care must be taken to avoid contact with the eyes. Thrombophlebitis is a potential hazard of mustine [chlormethine] particularly if it is not sufficiently diluted. Extravasation of the injection causes severe irritation and even sloughing. If extravasation occurs during injection, the manufacturers suggest that the involved area should be infiltrated with an isotonic 4% solution of sodium thiosulfate, followed by the application of an ice compress intermittently for 6 to 12 hours, although the role of specific antidotes in antineoplastic extravasation is somewhat contentious (see p.480). A 1% lignocaine [lidocaine] solution may also be infiltrated.

Mustine [chlormethine] hydrochloride may produce temporary or permanent inhibition of fertility. There is some evidence of teratogenicity and carcinogenicity.

Effects on the nervous system. Severe immediate neurotoxicity developed in 14 of 21 evaluable patients who underwent bone-marrow transplantation after preparation with cytotoxic regimens including mustine [chlormethine] 0.3 to 2.0 mg per kg body-weight.[1] Symptoms, which developed a median of 4 days after treatment, included headache, hallucinations, confusion, convulsions, paraplegia, and tremor. Symptoms resolved in most, although in some they had not done so before their death. However, of the 13 patients who survived more than 60 days, 6, all of whom had earlier recovered from acute toxicity, developed a delayed neurotoxicity, beginning a median of 169 days after the first mustine [chlormethine] injection and characterised by symptoms including confusion, somnolence, personality change, dementia, focal motor seizures, and hydrocephalus. Patients older than 21 years, those who had received CNS irradiation, and those treated concomitantly with other cytotoxic agents were at increased risk of neurotoxicity.

1. Sullivan KM, et al. Immediate and delayed neurotoxicity after mechlorethamine preparation for bone marrow transplantation. Ann Intern Med 1982; 97: 182–9.

Handling and disposal. The manufacturers state that *unused injection* solutions of mustine [chlormethine] hydrochloride may be neutralised by mixing with an equal volume of a solution containing sodium thiosulfate 5% and sodium bicarbonate 5% and allowing to stand for 45 minutes. Equipment used in the preparation and administration of such solutions may be treated similarly. Alternatively a solution containing sodium carbonate 2.5% or sodium hydroxide in a mixture of industrial methylated spirit and water has been suggested for the decontamination of equipment.

Urine produced for up to 48 hours after a dose of mustine [chlormethine] should be handled wearing protective clothing.[1]

1. Harris J, Dodds LJ. Handling waste from patients receiving cytotoxic drugs. Pharm J 1985; 235: 289–91.

Pharmacokinetics

Following intravenous injection, mustine [chlormethine] is rapidly converted to a reactive ethyleneimmonium ion. It usually disappears from the blood in a few minutes. A very small proportion is excreted unchanged in the urine.

Uses and Administration

Mustine [chlormethine] belongs to the group of antineoplastic drugs described as alkylating agents. It also possesses weak immunosuppressant properties.

Mustine [chlormethine] hydrochloride is used in the treatment of advanced Hodgkin's disease (p.487), usually in conjunction with a vinca alkaloid, procarbazine, and prednisone or prednisolone (the MOPP regimen). Mustine [chlormethine] has also been tried in non-Hodgkin's lymphomas, notably mycosis fungoides (p.489), and some other malignancies including chronic leukaemias, tumours of the breast, ovary, and lung, and in polycythaemia vera. Mustine [chlormethine] has been used in the management of malignant effusions but is not the agent of choice.

In the MOPP regimen mustine [chlormethine] hydrochloride has been given in doses of 6 mg per m² body-surface. However, as a single agent, the usual dose of mustine [chlormethine] hydrochloride is 400 µg per kg body-weight, preferably as a single dose, although it may be divided into 2 or 4 equal doses on successive days. It is given by intravenous injection in a strength of 1 mg per mL in Water for Injections or sodium chloride 0.9%. Injection over 2 minutes into the tubing of a fast running intravenous infusion of sodium chloride 0.9% or glucose 5% may reduce the incidence of thrombophlebitis and the risk of extravasation.

The response should be assessed by the trend of the blood counts. Treatment with mustine [chlormethine] may be repeated when the bone-marrow function has recovered.

Intracavitary injections of 200 to 400 µg per kg have been given in the treatment of malignant, especially pleural, effusions. In mycosis fungoides with extensive skin involvement, very dilute solutions of mustine [chlormethine] (e.g. 200 µg per mL) have been applied topically.

Histiocytic syndromes. Dilute solutions of mustine [chlormethine] (200 µg per mL) have been applied topically for the cutaneous symptoms of Langerhans-cell histiocytosis (p.483).[1]

1. Sheehan MP, et al. Topical nitrogen mustard: an effective treatment for cutaneous Langerhans cell histiocytosis. J Pediatr 1991; 119: 317–21.

Preparations

BP 2001: Chlormethine Injection;
USP 25: Mechlorethamine Hydrochloride for Injection.

Proprietary Preparations (details are given in Part 3)
Aust.: Mustargen†; *Canad.:* Mustargen; *Fr.:* Caryolysine; *Israel:* Mustargen; *Switz.:* Mustargen; *USA:* Mustargen.

Mycophenolate Mofetil (11701-r)

Mycophenolate Mofetil (BANM, USAN).
Mycophenolate Morpholinoethyl; RS-61443; RS-61443-190 (mycophenolate mofetil hydrochloride). 2-Morpholinoethyl (E)-6-(4-hydroxy-6-methoxy-7-methyl-3-oxo-5-phthalanyl)-4-methyl-4-hexenoate.
$C_{23}H_{31}NO_7 = 433.5$.
CAS — 115007-34-6 (mycophenolate mofetil); 116680-01-4 (mycophenolate mofetil hydrochloride).

Adverse Effects, Treatment, and Precautions

For general discussions see Antineoplastics, p.476, p.479, and p.480.

Mycophenolate mofetil is associated with gastrointestinal disturbances, particularly diarrhoea; gastrointestinal haemorrhage and perforation has occurred. Leucopenia may develop; as with other immunosuppressants there is an increased risk of infection and certain malignancies in patients receiving mycophenolate mofetil. Other reported adverse effects include asthenia, fever, pain, headache, anaemia, thrombocytopenia, renal tubular necrosis, haematuria, hypertension, hyperglycaemia, disturbances of electrolytes and blood lipids, peripheral oedema, dyspnoea, cough, acne, dizziness, insomnia, and tremor. Hypersensitivity reactions have occurred. Mycophenolate is teratogenic in *animals*.

Mycophenolate mofetil should be given with care to patients with severe renal impairment or active disorders of the gastrointestinal tract.

Interactions

Mycophenolate mofetil may compete with other drugs that undergo active renal tubular secretion, resulting in increased concentrations of either drug. Concomitant administration with antacids, or to patients receiving colestyramine, may result in reduced absorption of mycophenolate.

Antacids. Although concomitant administration of mycophenolate mofetil and an antacid mixture (aluminium and magnesium hydroxides) or food both resulted in reductions in peak plasma concentrations of mycophenolic acid, the differences were small compared with interindividual variation, and were considered unlikely to be clinically significant.[1]

1. Bullingham R, *et al.* Effects of food and antacid on the pharmacokinetics of single doses of mycophenolate mofetil in rheumatoid arthritis patients. *Br J Clin Pharmacol* 1996; **41:** 513–16.

Immunosuppressants. Discontinuation of concomitant *ciclosporin* therapy was found to increase serum concentrations of mycophenolate mofetil in one study.[1]

1. Gregoor PJHS, *et al.* Effect of cyclosporine on mycophenolic acid trough levels in kidney transplant recipients. *Transplantation* 1999; **68:** 1603–6.

Iron. Absorption of mycophenolate mofetil following oral administration was markedly reduced by concomitant administration of iron preparations in a study in 7 healthy subjects:[1] mean peak serum concentrations of mycophenolate were reduced from 20.1 to 1.3 μg per mL.

1. Morii M, *et al.* Impairment of mycophenolate mofetil absorption by iron ion. *Clin Pharmacol Ther* 2000; **68:** 613–6.

Pharmacokinetics

Mycophenolate mofetil is rapidly and extensively absorbed from the gastrointestinal tract, and undergoes presystemic metabolism to active mycophenolic acid. It undergoes enterohepatic recirculation. Mycophenolic acid is metabolised by glucuronidation and excreted primarily in the urine; about 6% of a dose is recovered in faeces. Mycophenolic acid is 97% bound to plasma albumin. The half-life of mycophenolic acid after oral administration of mycophenolate is about 18 hours.

◊ Mycophenolate mofetil is rapidly de-esterified in the body to active mycophenolic acid which is subsequently excreted in the urine, mostly as the inactive glucuronide conjugate,[1] clearance being reduced in patients with impaired renal function. There is some evidence that the pharmacokinetics of mycophenolate mofetil alter with prolonged administration, resulting in reduction in trough plasma concentrations over time.[2] Patients with low mycophenolic acid concentrations may be at increased risk of transplant rejection.[3]

1. Shah J, *et al.* Pharmacokinetics of oral mycophenolate mofetil (MMF) and metabolites in renally impaired patients. *Clin Pharmacol Ther* 1995; **57:** 149.
2. Sanquer S, *et al.* Trough blood concentrations in long-term treatment with mycophenolate mofetil. *Lancet* 1998; **351:** 1557.
3. Van Gelder T, *et al.* A randomized double-blind, multicenter plasma concentration controlled study of the safety and efficacy of oral mycophenolate mofetil for the prevention of acute rejection after kidney transplantation. *Transplantation* 1999; **68:** 261–6.

Uses and Administration

Mycophenolic acid is an immunosuppressant derived from *Penicillium stoloniferum*. It is a reversible inhibitor of inosine monophosphate dehydrogenase and thus inhibits purine synthesis, with potent cytostatic effects on both T- and B-lymphocytes. It has been used mainly as the morpholinoethyl derivative, mycophenolate mofetil. It is given combined with other immunosuppressants, for the treatment and prevention of graft rejection, and has also been tried in various diseases with an auto-immune or immune-mediated inflammatory component. For mention of the use of mycophenolate mofetil in transplantation, see p.502 *et seq*.

In the prophylaxis of acute renal graft rejection mycophenolate mofetil is given by mouth in doses of 1 g twice daily; 1.5 g twice daily is recommended in the prophylaxis of cardiac graft rejection. For prevention of renal graft rejection in children and adolescents aged 2 to 18 years a dose of 600 mg per m² body-surface may be given by mouth twice daily, up to a maximum of 1 g twice daily, provided that body-surface area is at least 1.25 m².

In patients to whom oral therapy cannot initially be given, mycophenolate mofetil may be given for up to 14 days by intravenous infusion. Infusions are given as the hydrochloride salt, dissolved in glucose 5%, over 2 hours. Doses are described in terms of the base and are equivalent to those by mouth. For use in hepatic transplantation, the equivalent of 1 g twice daily is given for the first 4 days following transplantation, with subsequent conversion to 1.5 g twice daily by mouth as soon as it can be tolerated. Therapy should begin as soon as possible after transplantation, in combination with ciclosporin and corticosteroids. Patients should undergo regular blood counts; if neutropenia develops consideration should be given to interrupting mycophenolate therapy or reducing the dose.

◊ References.

1. European Mycophenolate Mofetil Cooperative Study Group. Placebo-controlled study of mycophenolate mofetil combined with cyclosporin and corticosteroids for prevention of acute rejection. *Lancet* 1995; **345:** 1321–5.
2. Fulton B, Markham A. Mycophenolate mofetil: a review of its pharmacodynamic and pharmacokinetic properties and clinical efficacy in renal transplantation. *Drugs* 1996; **51:** 278–98.
3. Simmons WD, *et al.* Preliminary risk-benefit assessment of mycophenolate mofetil in transplant rejection. *Drug Safety* 1997; **17:** 75–92.
4. Halloran P, *et al.* Mycophenolate mofetil in renal allograft recipients: a pooled efficacy analysis of three randomized, double-blind, clinical studies in prevention of rejection. *Transplantation* 1997; **63:** 39–47. Correction *ibid.*; 618.
5. Mathew TH. A blinded, long-term, randomized multicenter study of mycophenolate mofetil in cadaveric renal transplantation: results at three years. *Transplantation* 1998; **65:** 1450–4. Correction *ibid.*; **66:** 817.
6. Gruessner RW, *et al.* Mycophenolate mofetil in pancreas transplantation. *Transplantation* 1998; **66:** 318–23.
7. Kobashigawa J, *et al.* A randomized active-controlled trial of mycophenolate mofetil in heart transplant recipients. *Transplantation* 1998; **66:** 507–15.
8. Jain AB, *et al.* A prospective randomized trial of tacrolimus and prednisone versus tacrolimus, prednisone, and mycophenolate mofetil in primary adult liver transplant recipients: an interim report. *Transplantation* 1998; **66:** 1395–8.
9. Shapiro R, *et al.* A prospective, randomized trial of tacrolimus/prednisone versus tacrolimus/prednisone/mycophenolate mofetil in renal transplant recipients. *Transplantation* 1999; **67:** 411–15.
10. Furst DE. Leflunomide, mycophenolic acid and matrix metalloproteinase inhibitors. *Rheumatology* 1999; **38** (suppl 2): 14–18.

◊ Mycophenolate mofetil is being investigated in a number of conditions with an autoimmune component: these include IgA nephropathy (see Glomerular Kidney Disease, p.1051) and various vasculitic syndromes (see Polyarteritis Nodosa and Microscopic Polyangiitis, p.1056 and Wegener's Granulomatosis, p.1060). It has also been reported to be of benefit in refractory uveitis (p.1060).

Inflammatory bowel disease. Mycophenolate mofetil has been investigated as an alternative to azathioprine in Crohn's disease (p.1205). A randomised trial in 70 patients compared therapy with corticosteroids plus mycophenolate mofetil or azathioprine in patients with moderate or severe Crohn's disease. The authors concluded that the mycophenolate regimen produced a clinical response earlier than the azathioprine regimen, and that mycophenolate should be considered in patients allergic or unresponsive to azathioprine or mercaptopurine.[1] While some commentators and another case report supported the need for further investigation[2-4], others have questioned the long term safety and efficacy of this therapy.[5,6]

1. Neurath MF, *et al.* Randomised trial of mycophenolate mofetil versus azathioprine for treatment of chronic active Crohn's disease. *Gut* 1999; **44:** 625–8.
2. Florin THJ, *et al.* Treatment of steroid refractory inflammatory bowel disease (IBD) with mycophenolate mofetil (MMF). *Aust N Z J Med* 1998; **28:** 344–5.
3. Lowry PW, *et al.* Mycophenolate mofetil for Crohn's disease? *Lancet* 1999; **354:** 3–4.
4. Present DH. Is mycophenolate mofetil a new alternative in the treatment of inflammatory bowel disease? *Gut* 1999; **44:** 592–3.
5. Radford-Smith GL, *et al.* Mycophenolate mofetil in IBD patients. *Lancet* 1999; **354:** 1386–7.
6. Atherton JC. Mycophenolate mofetil for Crohn's disease. *Gut* 1999; **46:** 740–1.

Pemphigus and pemphigoid. Mycophenolate mofetil has been used successfully in the treatment of pemphigus and pemphigoid (p.1106), both in conjunction with prednisolone[1-4] and alone[5]. It may be of benefit in patients who cannot tolerate, or do not respond to, azathioprine.[6]

1. Böhm M, *et al.* Bullous pemphigoid treated with mycophenolate mofetil. *Lancet* 1997; **349:** 541.
2. Enk AH, Knop J. Treatment of pemphigus vulgaris with mycophenolate mofetil. *Lancet* 1997; **350:** 494.
3. Enk AH, Knop J. Mycophenolate is effective in the treatment of pemphigus vulgaris. *Arch Dermatol* 1999; **135:** 54–6.
4. Williams JV, *et al.* Use of mycophenolate mofetil in the treatment of paraneoplastic pemphigus. *Br J Dermatol* 2000; **142:** 506–8.
5. Bredlich R-O, *et al.* Mycophenolate mofetil monotherapy for pemphigus vulgaris. *Br J Dermatol* 1999; **141:** 934.
6. Stanley JR. Therapy of pemphigus vulgaris. *Arch Dermatol* 1999; **135:** 76–8.

Psoriasis. Mycophenolate mofetil has proved successful in some cases of psoriasis (p.1106) refractory to conventional therapies.[1-3]

1. Haufs MG, *et al.* Psoriasis vulgaris treated successfully with mycophenolate mofetil. *Br J Dermatol* 1998; **138:** 179–81.
2. Geilen CC, *et al.* Successful treatment of erythrodermic psoriasis with mycophenolate mofetil. *Br J Dermatol* 1998; **138:** 1101–2.
3. Grundmann-Kollmann M, *et al.* Treatment of chronic plaque-stage psoriasis and psoriatic arthritis with mycophenolate mofetil. *J Am Acad Dermatol* 2000; **42:** 835–7.

Preparations

Proprietary Preparations (details are given in Part 3)
Aust.: CellCept; *Austral.:* CellCept; *Belg.:* CellCept; *Canad.:* CellCept; *Denm.:* CellCept; *Fin.:* CellCept; *Fr.:* CellCept; *Ger.:* CellCept; *Hong Kong:* CellCept; *Irl.:* CellCept; *Israel:* CellCept; *Ital.:* CellCept; *Neth.:* CellCept; *Norw.:* CellCept; *NZ:* CellCept; *Port.:* CellCept; *S.Afr.:* CellCept; *Singapore:* CellCept; *Spain:* CellCept; *Swed.:* CellCept; *Switz.:* CellCept; *Thai.:* CellCept; *UK:* CellCept; *USA:* CellCept.

Nedaplatin (17044-g)

Nedaplatin (*rINN*).
cis-Diammine(glycolato-O^1,O^2)platinum.
$C_2H_8N_2O_3Pt = 303.2$.
CAS — 95734-82-0.

Profile

Nedaplatin is a platinum derivative with general properties similar to those of cisplatin (see p.525) although it may be associated with less nephrotoxicity. It is given by intravenous infusion over 1 hour or more, dissolved in at least 300 mL of an appropriate infusion solution, in doses of 80 to 100 mg per m² body-surface. Administration should be followed by infusion of at least 1 litre of fluid to ensure adequate hydration and reduce the risk of renal damage.

◊ References.

1. Adachi S, *et al.* A pilot study of nedaplatin and etoposide for recurrent gynecological malignancies. *Oncol Rep* 1998; **5:** 881–4.
2. Ito K, *et al.* A dose-finding study of nedaplatin and cyclophosphamide for patients with gynecological malignancies. *Jpn J Clin Oncol* 1999; **29:** 299–302.
3. Yoshioka T, *et al.* A new combination chemotherapy with cis-diammine-glycolatoplatinum (Nedaplatin) and 5-fluorouracil for advanced esophageal cancers. *Intern Med* 1999; **38:** 844–8.

Preparations

Proprietary Preparations (details are given in Part 3)
Jpn: Aqupla.

Nilutamide (2968-k)

Nilutamide (*BAN, USAN, rINN*).
RU-23908. 5,5-Dimethyl-3-(α,α,α-trifluoro-4-nitro-*m*-tolyl)-imidazolidine-2,4-dione.
$C_{12}H_{10}F_3N_3O_4 = 317.2$.
CAS — 63612-50-0.
ATC — L02BB02.

Adverse Effects and Precautions

As for Flutamide, p.542. Interstitial pneumonitis has occurred in patients receiving nilutamide, and the drug is contra-indicated in those with severe respiratory insufficiency. It should also not be given in severe hepatic impairment.

◊ Reversible visual disturbances have been associated with nilutamide.[1,2] Although some consider such visual disturbances to be mild and generally well tolerated,[3] others suggest that these, together with alcohol intolerance and, more seriously, effects on the lung, mean that other nonsteroidal anti-androgens should be preferred.[4]

1. Harnois C, *et al.* Ocular toxicity of Anandron in patients treated for prostatic cancer. *Br J Ophthalmol* 1986; **70:** 471–3.
2. Brisset JM, *et al.* Ocular toxicity of Anandron. *Br J Ophthalmol* 1987; **71:** 639.
3. Dijkman GA, *et al.* Comment: clinical experiences of visual disturbances with nilutamide. *Ann Pharmacother* 1997; **31:** 1550–1.
4. Dole EJ, Holdsworth MT. Comment: clinical experiences of visual disturbances with nilutamide. *Ann Pharmacother* 1997; **31:** 1551–2.

Interactions

Patients receiving nilutamide may exhibit intolerance to alcohol.

Uses and Administration

Nilutamide is a nonsteroidal anti-androgen which is used similarly to flutamide (p.542) in the treatment of prostatic carcinoma (p.497). It is given by mouth in usual doses of 300 mg daily, in patients who have undergone orchiectomy. Dosage may be reduced to 150 mg daily after 1 month. It has also been used in combination with a gonadorelin analogue.

◊ References.

1. Dole EJ, Holdsworth MT. Nilutamide: an antiandrogen for the treatment of prostate cancer. *Ann Pharmacother* 1997; **31:** 65–75.

Preparations

Proprietary Preparations (details are given in Part 3)
Austral.: Anandron; *Braz.:* Anandron; *Canad.:* Anandron; *Denm.:* Anandron; *Fin.:* Anandron; *Fr.:* Anandron; *Neth.:* Anandron; *Norw.:* Anandron; *Port.:* Anandron; *Swed.:* Anandron; *USA:* Nilandron.

Nimustine Hydrochloride (11478-q)

Nimustine Hydrochloride (*rINNM*).
ACNU; NSC-245382; Pimustine Hydrochloride. 3-[(4-Amino-2-methylpyrimidin-5-yl)methyl]-1-(2-chloroethyl)-1-nitrosourea hydrochloride.
$C_9H_{13}ClN_6O_2,HCl = 309.2$.
CAS — 42471-28-3 (nimustine); 55661-38-6 (nimustine hydrochloride).

Profile

Nimustine is a nitrosourea antineoplastic with actions and uses similar to those of carmustine (p.516). It is given as the hydrochloride in suggested doses of 2 to 3 mg per kg body-weight or 90 to 100 mg per m² body-surface as a single dose by slow intravenous administration, repeated at intervals of 4 to 6 weeks depending on haematological response. It may also be given intra-arterially. Solutions for injection must be freshly prepared and protected from light.

Preparations

Proprietary Preparations (details are given in Part 3)
Ger.: ACNU; *Jpn:* Nidran; *Neth.:* ACNU; *Switz.:* ACNU.

Nolatrexed (15981-p)

Nolatrexed (rINN).
AG-337 (nolatrexed dihydrochloride). 2-Amino-6-methyl-5-(4-pyridylthio)-4(3H)-quinazolinone.
$C_{14}H_{12}N_4OS$ = 284.3.
CAS — 147149-76-6 (nolatrexed); 152946-68-4 (nolatrexed dihydrochloride).

Profile

Nolatrexed is, like raltitrexed (p.567), a selective inhibitor of thymidylate synthase. It has been investigated as an antimetabolite antineoplastic.

◊ References.
1. Hughes AN, *et al.* Phase I studies with the nonclassical antifolate nolatrexed dihydrochloride (AG337, Thymitaq) administered orally for 5 days. *Clin Cancer Res* 1999; **5:** 111–8.
2. Stuart K, *et al.* A phase II trial of nolatrexed dihydrochloride in patients with advanced hepatocellular carcinoma. *Cancer* 1999; **86:** 410–4.

Oxaliplatin (2972-y)

Oxaliplatin (BAN, USAN, rINN).
JM-83; NSC-266046; l-OHP; RP-54780; SR-96669. [(1R,2R)-1,2-Cyclohexanediamine-N,N'][oxalato(2-)-O,O']platinum.
$C_8H_{14}N_2O_4Pt$ = 397.3.
CAS — 61825-94-3.
ATC — L01XA03.

Incompatibility. The manufacturers state that oxaliplatin should not be mixed with chloride-containing solutions (including sodium chloride) or alkaline drugs or solutions. It may degrade on contact with aluminium.

Adverse Effects and Precautions

The adverse affects of oxaliplatin are similar to those of cisplatin (p.525) but nausea and vomiting, and nephrotoxicity, seem to be less marked. Neurotoxicity can be dose-limiting. Peripheral neuropathy occurs in 85 to 95% of patients given oxaliplatin; pain, functional impairment, and loss of tendon reflexes may develop. Neurological examinations should be carried out at regular intervals during treatment and the dose should be reduced if symptoms are prolonged or severe. Oxaliplatin should not be given to patients with pre-existing sensory neuropathies, nor to those with severe renal impairment; renal function and toxicity should be carefully monitored in those with more moderate degrees of renal impairment.

Effects on the nervous system. Neurological toxicity is the principal dose-limiting adverse effect with oxaliplatin. The toxicity is biphasic:
- acute paraesthesias or dysaesthesias of the extremities, triggered or exacerbated by cold, are seen in 85 to 95% of patients within hours of infusion, but are normally mild and resolve within hours or days. Some patients also experience distressing laryngopharyngeal symptoms, such as difficulty in breathing or swallowing.
- with increasing cumulative dose, peripheral sensory symptoms increase in duration and intensity. Symptoms are sometimes associated with pain and cramps, and may progress to functional impairment (loss of fine sensorimotor coordination). Dosage reduction may be required, but in clinical practice the onset of functional impairment often occurs after the maximum response to therapy has been attained. Cumulative neurotoxicity is reversible in most cases, and about 80% of patients exhibit symptom regression within 4 to 6 months.

The incidence of neurotoxicity may be higher when oxaliplatin is given in combination with fluorouracil. There is some evidence that more prolonged infusion of oxaliplatin can reduce acute toxicity, particularly laryngopharyngeal symptoms. Antiepileptics such as carbamazepine or gabapentin have been investigated in the management of oxaliplatin-induced neurotoxicity.
References.
1. Extra JM, *et al.* Pharmacokinetics and safety profile of oxaliplatin. *Semin Oncol* 1998; **25** (suppl 5): 13–22.
2. Culy CR, *et al.* Oxaliplatin: a review of its pharmacological properties and clinical efficacy in metastatic colorectal cancer and its potential in other malignancies. *Drugs* 2000; **60:** 895–924.

Pharmacokinetics

Following intravenous administration, oxaliplatin is widely distributed throughout the body. It binds irre-

versibly to red blood cells, which can prolong the half-life of the drug. The mean terminal half-life is 273 hours.
Oxaliplatin is extensively metabolised to both inactive and active compounds and is predominantly excreted in the urine.

◊ References.
1. Lévi F, *et al.* Oxaliplatin: pharmacokinetics and chronopharmacological aspects. *Clin Pharmacokinet* 2000; **38:** 1–21.

Uses and Administration

Oxaliplatin is a platinum-containing complex similar to cisplatin (see p.525). It is given in combination with fluorouracil and folinic acid in the first-line treatment of metastatic colorectal cancer (p.493). The recommended dose is 85 mg per m^2 body-surface by intravenous infusion over 2 to 6 hours, dissolved in 250 to 500 mL of glucose 5%. The dose may be repeated at intervals of 2 weeks if toxicity permits, reduced according to tolerance. Oxaliplatin should always be administered before fluoropyrimidines.
Oxaliplatin is under investigation for the treatment of ovarian cancer.

◊ References.
1. Lévi FA, *et al.* Chronomodulated versus fixed-infusion-rate delivery of ambulatory chemotherapy with oxaliplatin, fluorouracil and folinic acid (leucovorin) in patients with colorectal cancer metastases: a randomized multi-institutional trial. *J Natl Cancer Inst* 1994; **86:** 1608–17.
2. Brienza S, *et al.* Oxaliplatin added to 5-fluorouracil-based therapy (5-Fu+/-FA) in the treatment of 5-Fu-pretreated patients with advanced colorectal carcinoma (ACRC): results from the European compassionate-use program. *Ann Oncol* 1999; **10:** 1311–16.
3. Lévi F, *et al.* Randomised multicentre trial of chronotherapy with oxaliplatin, fluorouracil, and folinic acid in metastatic colorectal cancer. *Lancet* 1997; **350:** 681–6.
4. Piccart MJ, *et al.* Oxaliplatin or paclitaxel in patients with platinum-pretreated advanced ovarian cancer: a randomized phase II study of the European Organization for Research and Treatment of Cancer Gynecology Group. *J Clin Oncol* 2000; **18:** 1193–1202.
5. Giacchetti S, *et al.* Phase III multicenter randomized trial of oxaliplatin added to chronomodulated fluorouracil-leucovorin as first-line treatment of metastatic colorectal cancer. *J Clin Oncol* 2000; **18:** 136–47.
6. Wiseman LR, *et al.* Oxaliplatin: a review of its use in the management of metastatic colorectal cancer. *Drugs Aging* 1999; **14:** 459–75.
7. Culy CR, *et al.* Oxaliplatin: a review of its pharmacological properties and clinical efficacy in metastatic colorectal cancer and its potential in other malignancies. *Drugs* 2000; **60:** 895–924.

Preparations

Proprietary Preparations (details are given in Part 3)
Austral.: Eloxatin; *Belg.:* Eloxatin; *Fr.:* Eloxatine; *Ger.:* Eloxatin; *Neth.:* Eloxatin; *Singapore:* Eloxatin; *Swed.:* Eloxatin; *Thai.:* Eloxatin; *UK:* Eloxatin.

Paclitaxel (2453-y)

Paclitaxel (BAN, USAN, rINN).
BMS-181339-01; NSC-125973; Taxol; Taxol A. (2S,5S,7S,10R,13S)-10,20-Bis(acetoxy)-2-benzoyloxy-1,7-dihydroxy-9-oxo-5,20-epoxytax-11-en-13-yl (3S)-3-benzoylamino-3-phenyl-D-lactate.
$C_{47}H_{51}NO_{14}$ = 853.9.
CAS — 33069-62-4.
ATC — L01CD01.

NOTE. Paclitaxel was formerly referred to as taxol, but the use of this name is now limited, as Taxol is a trademark.

Incompatibility. The vehicle for paclitaxel injection, which contains alcohol and polyethoxylated castor oil, was found to leach the plasticiser diethylhexyl phthalate from some plastic administration sets.[1,2] Consequently, the manufacturer recommends the use of non-PVC containers and administration sets. Paclitaxel was found to be compatible with doxorubicin for at least 24 hours, but microcrystalline precipitation of paclitaxel occurred after 3 to 5 days.[3] For mention of the incompatibility of paclitaxel and cisplatin see p.525.
1. Trissel LA, *et al.* Compatibility of paclitaxel injection vehicle with intravenous administration and extension sets. *Am J Hosp Pharm* 1994; **51:** 2804–10.
2. Mazzo DJ, *et al.* Compatibility of docetaxel and paclitaxel in intravenous solutions with polyvinyl chloride infusion materials. *Am J Health-Syst Pharm* 1997; **54:** 566–9.
3. Trissel LA, *et al.* Compatibility and stability of paclitaxel combined with doxorubicin hydrochloride in infusion solutions. *Ann Pharmacother* 1998; **32:** 1013–6.

Adverse Effects, Treatment, and Precautions

Paclitaxel produces severe dose-limiting bone marrow depression, the nadir of the white cell count usu-

ally occurring after about 11 days, with recovery usually by day 15 to 21 after a dose. Myelosuppression may be less frequent and less severe when infusions are given over 3 rather than 24 hours.
Peripheral neuropathy may also be severe, and occasionally dose-limiting. Hypersensitivity reactions, with flushing, rash, dyspnoea, hypotension, chest pain, and angioedema may occur, and patients receive initial premedication with corticosteroids, antihistamines, and histamine H_2-antagonists. Other adverse effects include alopecia, arthralgia and myalgia, gastrointestinal disturbances, mucositis, bradycardia and ECG changes, nail dystrophies, and elevation of liver enzyme values. Extravasation may result in tissue damage. Rare adverse events include hypertension, severe thrombotic events, myocardial infarction, severe cardiac conduction abnormalities, seizures, neuroencephalopathy, paralytic ileus, optic nerve disturbances, severe skin reactions, hepatic necrosis, and hepatic encephalopathy.
Paclitaxel is not recommended in patients with severely impaired hepatic function. The drug is formulated in polyethoxylated castor oil and should be avoided in patients hypersensitive to this substance. The formulation also contains alcohol, the CNS effects of which should be considered. Blood counts should be monitored frequently. Continuous cardiac monitoring should be performed in patients who have experienced previous significant conduction abnormalities while receiving paclitaxel.

Alcohol intoxication. Acute alcohol intoxication resulting from high-dose paclitaxel infusion has been reported;[1] it was calculated that the dose used (348 mg per m^2 body-surface) supplied 50 mL of alcohol, or the equivalent of about 3 drinks (half a bottle of wine).
1. Wilson DB, *et al.* Paclitaxel formulation as a cause of ethanol intoxication. *Ann Pharmacother* 1997; **31:** 873–5.

Effects on the eyes. Optic neuritis has occurred with paclitaxel. There is a report of glaucoma possibly related to the use of docetaxel and paclitaxel in a patient also receiving corticosteroids.[1]
1. Fabre-Guillevin E, *et al.* Taxane-induced glaucoma. *Lancet* 1999; **354:** 1181–2.

Effects on the heart. Infusion of paclitaxel has been associated with myocardial infarction,[1] sudden death[2] and symptoms suggestive of heart failure.[3] In another report sudden death 7 days after paclitaxel treatment raised the question of whether paclitaxel might have had a delayed effect.[4] There is some evidence of cellular damage to the myocardium of a patient with paclitaxel-associated cardiac symptoms.[3] The manufacturers note that severe cardiovascular events have been observed more frequently following the use of paclitaxel in patients with non-small cell lung cancer than in those with breast or ovarian carcinoma.
1. Rowinsky EK, *et al.* Cardiac disturbances during the administration of taxol. *J Clin Oncol* 1991; **9:** 1704–12.
2. Arbuck S, *et al.* A reassessment of cardiac toxicity associated with Taxol. *Proc Am Soc Clin Oncol* 1993; **12:** 138.
3. Jekunen A, *et al.* Paclitaxel-induced myocardial damage detected by electron microscopy. *Lancet* 1994; **343:** 727–8.
4. Alagaratnam TT. Sudden death 7 days after paclitaxel infusion for breast cancer. *Lancet* 1993; **342:** 1232–3.

Effects on the musculoskeletal system. Myalgia induced by paclitaxel and docetaxel was successfully treated with gabapentin in 2 patients.[1]
1. van Deventer H, Bernard S. Use of gabapentin to treat taxane-induced myalgias. *J Clin Oncol* 1999; **17:** 434–5.

Effects on the respiratory system. Acute bilateral interstitial pneumonitis has been reported rarely in patients receiving paclitaxel, despite premedication with corticosteroids and histamine antagonists.[1] Symptoms resolved on treatment with parenteral corticosteroids.
1. Khan A, *et al.* Paclitaxel-induced acute bilateral pneumonitis. *Ann Pharmacother* 1997; **31:** 1471–4.

Effects on the skin and nails. Nail changes, noted as pigmentation or discoloration of the nail-bed, may occur with paclitaxel. Onycholysis (separation of the nail from the nail-bed) has also been reported.[1]
1. Flory SM, *et al.* Onycholysis associated with weekly administration of paclitaxel. *Ann Pharmacother* 1999; **33:** 584–5.

Interactions

For a general outline of antineoplastic drug interactions, see p.481. Pretreatment with cisplatin may reduce the clearance of paclitaxel, resulting in increased toxicity, and when the 2 drugs are given in combination paclitaxel should be given first.

The symbol † denotes a preparation no longer actively marketed

Antineoplastics and immunosuppressants. For reference to enhanced cardiotoxicity when paclitaxel was given in association with *doxorubicin*, see p.535.

Pretreatment with *fluorouracil* has been reported to inhibit paclitaxel's cytotoxic action, possibly by preventing tumour cells from entering the G_2-M phases of the cell cycle.[1] The effect also occurred when the 2 drugs were given simultaneously, suggesting that combination therapy might not be appropriate.

Ciclosporin increased the oral absorption of paclitaxel, possibly by inhibiting the multidrug transporter P-glycoprotein in the gastrointestinal tract.[2]

1. Johnson KR, *et al*. 5-Fluorouracil interferes with paclitaxel cytotoxicity against human solid tumor cells. *Clin Cancer Res* 1997; **3:** 1739–45.
2. Meerum Terwogt JM, *et al*. Co-administration of cyclosporin enables oral therapy with paclitaxel. *Lancet* 1998; **352:** 285. Correction. *ibid.*: 824.

Pharmacokinetics

Following intravenous administration paclitaxel exhibits a biphasic decline in plasma concentrations, with a mean terminal half-life of anywhere between about 3 and 50 hours. The pharmacokinetics are nonlinear. The steady-state volume of distribution is reported to range from 200 to 700 litres per m^2, indicating extensive extravascular distribution, tissue binding, or both. Paclitaxel is 89% or more bound to plasma protein *in vitro*. The elimination of paclitaxel has not been fully elucidated; only about 1 to 12% of a dose is reported to be excreted in urine, as unchanged drug, indicating extensive non-renal clearance. Paclitaxel is metabolised in the liver, with the major metabolic pathway apparently mediated by the cytochrome P450 isoenzyme CYP2C8, although CYP3A4 may play a minor role. Metabolites are excreted in the faeces via the bile, the primary metabolite being 6α-hydroxypaclitaxel.

◊ References.

1. Wiernik PH, *et al*. Phase I clinical and pharmacokinetic study of Taxol. *Cancer Res* 1987; **47:** 2486–93.
2. Sonnichsen DS, Relling MV. Clinical pharmacokinetics of paclitaxel. *Clin Pharmacokinet* 1994; **27:** 256–69.
3. Walle T, *et al*. [³H]-Paclitaxel disposition and metabolism in cancer patients. *Clin Pharmacol Ther* 1995; **57:** 153.
4. Sonnichsen D, *et al*. Variability in human in vitro and in-vivo metabolism of paclitaxel. *Clin Pharmacol Ther* 1995; **57:** 193.

Uses and Administration

Paclitaxel is a taxane originally derived from the bark of the Pacific yew tree *Taxus brevifolia* (Taxaceae), and now obtained semisynthetically from a taxane precursor derived from the needles of the European yew, *Taxus baccata*. Its antineoplastic action arises from its induction of microtubule formation and stabilisation of microtubules, thereby disrupting normal cell division in the G_2 and M phases of the cell cycle. Paclitaxel is used for the primary treatment of advanced ovarian cancer (p.496) in combination with cisplatin or carboplatin, and for secondary treatment. It is also used for the primary adjuvant or second-line therapy of breast cancer (p.491), and, in combination with cisplatin or carboplatin, for the primary treatment of advanced non-small cell lung cancer (p.496). It may be used for the second-line treatment of AIDS-related Kaposi's sarcoma (p.501), and has been tried in a variety of other neoplasms including cancers of the head and neck, and relapsed germ-cell tumours.

The recommended dose for the primary treatment of ovarian cancer is 135 mg per m^2 body-surface infused over 24 hours, followed by cisplatin, and repeated at 3 week intervals. Alternatively 175 mg per m^2 may be infused over 3 hours, followed by cisplatin, every 3 weeks. For the secondary treatment of ovarian cancer, the suggested dose as a single agent is 135 or 175 mg per m^2 infused over 3 hours once every 3 weeks.

A dose of 175 mg per m^2 infused over 3 hours once every 3 weeks is recommended for the treatment of breast cancer; for adjuvant therapy 4 such courses may be given following sequentially to an anthracycline-based regimen. In non-small cell lung cancer, the recommended dose is 135 mg per m^2 over 24 hours or 175 mg per m^2 over 3 hours, followed by cisplatin, and repeated at 3-week intervals.

A dose of 135 mg per m^2 over 3 hours once every 3 weeks has been suggested for AIDS-related Kaposi's

sarcoma. Alternatively, 100 mg per m^2 over 3 hours every 2 weeks may be given, especially in patients with poor performance status.

Regular blood counts should be performed, and dosage should not be repeated until the neutrophil count is greater than 1500 per mm^3 (1000 per mm^3 in patients with AIDS) and the platelet count greater than 100 000 per mm^3. The dose should be reduced by 20% in subsequent courses in patients who experience severe neutropenia or peripheral neuropathy. Patients should be pretreated with corticosteroids, antihistamines, and histamine H_2-antagonists.

◊ References to paclitaxel, and to taxanes as a class.

1. Rowinsky EK, *et al*. Taxol: the first of the taxanes, an important new class of antitumor agents. *Semin Oncol* 1992; **19:** 646–62.
2. Gelmon K. The taxoids: paclitaxel and docetaxel. *Lancet* 1994; **344:** 1267–72.
3. Long HJ. Paclitaxel (Taxol): a novel anticancer chemotherapeutic drug. *Mayo Clin Proc* 1994; **69:** 341–5.
4. Spencer CM, Faulds D. Paclitaxel: a review of its pharmacodynamic and pharmacokinetic properties and therapeutic potential in the treatment of cancer. *Drugs* 1994; **48:** 794–847.
5. Rowinsky EK, Donehower RC. Paclitaxel (Taxol). *N Engl J Med* 1995; **332:** 1004–14. Correction. *ibid.*; **333:** 75.
6. Anonymous. Paclitaxel and docetaxel in breast and ovarian cancer. *Drug Ther Bull* 1997; **35:** 43–6.
7. Eisenhauer EA, Vermarken JB. The taxoids: comparative clinical pharmacology and therapeutic potential. *Drugs* 1998; **55:** 5–30.
8. Crown J O'Leary M. The taxanes: an update. *Lancet* 2000; **355:** 1176–8.

Administration. There has been considerable interest in evaluating the use of paclitaxel in reduced-dose *weekly* administration schedules. A variety of dosage regimens have been tried: most have found that doses of between 50 and about 100 mg per m^2 body-surface weekly, usually by infusion over 1 hour rather than a conventional 3-hour infusion, can be given with relatively modest toxicity. Although higher doses have been tried, neurotoxicity and myelosuppression become problematic and tend to limit dose intensity. A number of studies have addressed the combination of weekly paclitaxel with other antineoplastics, for example with trastuzumab in breast cancer, estramustine in prostate cancer, and in combination with platinum compounds or gemcitabine in other solid tumours such as those of the ovary or lung. Weekly paclitaxel is also under investigation in combination with radiotherapy in the management of lung cancer and glioblastoma multiforme.

References.

1. Seidman AD, *et al*. Dose-dense therapy with weekly 1-hour paclitaxel infusions in the treatment of metastatic breast cancer. *J Clin Oncol* 1998; **16:** 3353–61.
2. Fountzilas G, *et al*. Radiation and concomitant weekly administration of paclitaxel in patients with glioblastoma multiforme: a phase II study. *J Neurooncol* 1999; **45:** 159–65.
3. Markman M. Weekly paclitaxel in the management of ovarian cancer. *Semin Oncol* 2000; **27** (suppl 7): 37–40.
4. De Pas T, *et al*. Phase I and pharmacologic study of weekly gemcitabine and paclitaxel in chemo-naive patients with advanced non-small-cell lung cancer. *Ann Oncol* 2000; **11:** 821–7.
5. Langer CJ, *et al*. Paclitaxel by 1-h infusion in combination with carboplatin in advanced non-small cell lung carcinoma (NSCLC). *Eur J Cancer* 2000; **36:** 183–93.
6. Akerley W. Recent developments in weekly paclitaxel therapy in lung cancer. *Curr Oncol Rep* 2001; **3:** 165–9.
7. Haas N, *et al*. Phase I trial of weekly paclitaxel plus oral estramustine phosphate in patients with hormone-refractory prostate cancer. *Urology* 2001; **58:** 59–64.
8. Seidman AD, *et al*. Weekly trastuzumab and paclitaxel therapy for metastatic breast cancer with analysis of efficacy by HER2 immunophenotype and gene amplification. *J Clin Oncol* 2001; **19:** 2587–95.
9. Kouroussis C, *et al*. A dose-finding study of the weekly administration of paclitaxel in patients with advanced solid tumors. *Am J Clin Oncol* 2001; **24:** 404–7.

Preparations

Proprietary Preparations (details are given in Part 3)

Aust.: Taxol; **Austral.:** Anzatax; Taxol; **Belg.:** Taxol; **Braz.:** Taxol; **Canad.:** Taxol; **Denm.:** Taxol; **Fin.:** Taxol; **Fr.:** Taxol; **Ger.:** Taxol; **Hong Kong:** Anzatax; Taxol; **Irl.:** Taxol; **Israel:** Taxol; **Ital.:** Taxol; **Jpn:** Taxol; **Mex.:** Asotax; BrisTaxol; Praxel; **Neth.:** Taxol; **Norw.:** Taxol; **NZ:** Taxol; **Port.:** Taxol; **S.Afr.:** Taxol; Yewtaxan†; **Singapore:** Anzatax; Taxol; **Spain:** Taxol; **Swed.:** Taxol; **Switz.:** Taxol; **Thai.:** Anzatax; Taxol; **UK:** Taxol; **USA:** Onxol; Taxol.

Peldesine (17274-x)

Peldesine (USAN, pINN).

BCX-34; Peldesina; Peldésine. 2-Amino-3,5-dihydro-7-(3-pyridylmethyl)-4H-pyrrolo[3,2-d]pyrimidin-4-one.

$C_{12}H_{11}N_5O = 241.2$.

CAS — 133432-71-0.

Profile

Peldesine is an inhibitor of the enzyme purine nucleoside phosphorylase and is reported to suppress T-cell proliferation. It has been investigated in the management of cutaneous T-cell lymphomas, and has also been tried topically in psoriasis and some T-cell mediated eye disorders.

Pemetrexed Disodium (18590-k)

Pemetrexed Disodium (BANM, USAN, rINNM).

ALIMTA; LY-231514; MTA; Multi-targeted Antifolate. Disodium N-{p-[2-(2-amino-4,7-dihydro-4-oxo-1H-pyrrolo[2,3-d]pyrimidin-5-yl)ethyl]benzoyl}-L-glutamate.

$C_{20}H_{19}N_5Na_2O_6 = 471.4$.

CAS — 137281-23-3 (pemetrexed); 150399-23-8 (pemetrexed disodium).

Profile

Pemetrexed is a thymidylate synthase inhibitor under investigation as an antifolate antimetabolite in the treatment of lung, colon, and pancreatic cancer.

◊ References.

1. Miller KD, *et al*. Phase II study of the multitargeted antifolate LY231514 (ALIMTA, MTA, pemetrexed disodium) in patients with advanced pancreatic cancer. *Ann Oncol* 2000; **11:** 101–3.
2. John W, *et al*. Activity of multitargeted antifolate (pemetrexed disodium, LY231514) in patients with advanced colorectal carcinoma: results from a phase II study. *Cancer* 2000; **88:** 1807–13.
3. Manegold C, *et al*. Front-line treatment of advanced non-small-cell lung cancer with MTA (LY231514, pemetrexed disodium, ALIMTA) and cisplatin: a multicenter phase II trial. *Ann Oncol* 2000; **11:** 435–40.

Pentostatin (16946-y)

Pentostatin (BAN, USAN, rINN).

CI-825; Covidarabine; Co-vidarabine; Deoxycoformycin; 2′-Deoxycoformycin; NSC-218321; PD-81565. (R)-3-(2-Deoxy-β-D-*erythro*-pentofuranosyl)-3,6,7,8-tetrahydroimidazo[4,5-d][1,3]diazepin-8-ol; 1,2-Dideoxy-1-[(R)-3,6,7,8-tetrahydro-8-hydroxyimidazo[4,5-d][1,3]diazepin-3-yl]-D-*erythro*-pentofuranose.

$C_{11}H_{16}N_4O_4 = 268.3$.

CAS — 53910-25-1.

ATC — L01XX08.

Adverse Effects and Precautions

The most common adverse effects in patients receiving pentostatin include myelosuppression (and in particular suppression of CD4+ lymphocyte subset), headache, abdominal pain, fever and chills, gastrointestinal disturbances (notably diarrhoea and nausea and vomiting), hypersensitivity reactions, and hepatotoxicity. Central neurotoxicity may be manifest as tiredness, anxiety, depression, sleep disturbances, and paraesthesias: treatment should be withheld or discontinued in such patients. Impaired renal function and pulmonary toxicity (cough, dyspnoea, and pneumonia) may occur. Severe toxicity in early studies, affecting mainly the CNS, kidneys, and lungs, was associated with the use of doses higher than those currently recommended and produced some fatalities.

Other adverse effects reported with pentostatin include dry skin and rashes (sometimes severe and worsening with continued treatment), pruritus, conjunctivitis, alopecia, arthralgia and myalgia, peripheral oedema, thrombophlebitis, and cardiovascular disorders including arrhythmias, angina pectoris, and heart failure.

Pentostatin should not be given to patients with impaired renal function, or in active infection. It is teratogenic in *animals* and potentially genotoxic: men receiving pentostatin should not father children for 6 months after therapy.

Interactions

Pentostatin should not be given in association with fludarabine, as the combination may result in enhanced pulmonary toxicity. A similar increase in toxicity is expected when pentostatin is combined with vidarabine.

Use of pentostatin with carmustine, etoposide and high-dose cyclophosphamide, has produced acute pulmonary oedema and hypotension, leading to death. Pentostatin should therefore not be given in conjunction with high-dose cyclophosphamide.

Allopurinol. Fatal acute necrotising arteritis developed in a patient given pentostatin and allopurinol.[1] Although the hypersensitivity vasculitis may have been due to allopurinol alone there is circumstantial evidence to suggest that pentostatin may predispose patients to drug hypersensitivity and it may be wise to avoid this combination, and to observe pentostatin-treated patients closely for allergic manifestations.

1. Steinmetz JC, *et al*. Hypersensitivity vasculitis associated with 2-deoxycoformycin and allopurinol therapy. *Am J Med* 1989; **86:** 499.

Uses and Administration

Pentostatin is a potent inhibitor of the enzyme adenosine deaminase that probably exerts its cytotoxic actions through the interruption of normal purine metabolism and DNA synthesis. Lymphocytes are particularly sensitive to its actions.

Pentostatin is used in the treatment of hairy-cell leukaemia (see p.486), in usual doses of 4 mg per m^2 body-surface intravenously every other week. Hydration with 500 mL to 1 L of 5% glucose in 0.18% or 0.9% sodium chloride injection or equivalent is recommended before administration; a further 500 mL of the hydration solution should be infused once the drug has been given.

Pentostatin has been tried in some other lymphoid malignancies, including chronic lymphocytic leukaemia (see p.485), and in non-Hodgkin's lymphomas (see p.487).

◊ References.
1. Brogden RN, Sorkin EM. Pentostatin: a review of its pharmacodynamic and pharmacokinetic properties, and therapeutic potential in lymphoproliferative disorders. *Drugs* 1993; **46**: 652–77.

Preparations

Proprietary Preparations (details are given in Part 3)
Fr.: Nipent; *Ger.:* Nipent; *Ital.:* Nipent; *Port.:* Nipent; *Spain:* Nipent; *UK:* Nipent; *USA:* Nipent.

Peplomycin Sulfate (13092-v)

Peplomycin Sulfate (USAN, rINNM).
NK-631; Peplomycin Sulphate; Peplomycin Sulphate. N^1-{3-[(S)-(α-Methylbenzyl)amino]propyl}bleomycinamide sulphate.
$C_{61}H_{88}N_{18}O_{21}S_2,H_2SO_4 = 1571.7$.
CAS — 68247-85-8 (peplomycin); 70384-29-1 (peplomycin sulfate).
Pharmacopoeias. In Jpn.

Profile

Peplomycin is an antineoplastic derived from bleomycin (see p.511) and with similar properties. It has been given as the sulfate in the treatment of a variety of malignant neoplasms, including tumours of the head and neck, lung, prostate, and skin.

Preparations

Proprietary Preparations (details are given in Part 3)
Jpn: Pepleo†.

Pipobroman (1857-h)

Pipobroman (USAN, pINN).
A-8103; NSC-25154. 1,4-Bis(3-bromopropionyl)piperazine.
$C_{10}H_{16}Br_2N_2O_2 = 356.1$.
CAS — 54-91-1.
ATC — L01AX02.

Profile

Pipobroman is an antineoplastic which appears to act by alkylation. It may be used in the treatment of polycythaemia vera (p.486), in patients requiring myelosuppressive therapy, and in refractory chronic myeloid leukaemia (p.486).

The usual dose initially is 1 mg per kg body-weight by mouth daily, increased to 3 mg per kg, if necessary, according to the patient's response. Maintenance dosage is 100 to 200 µg per kg daily for polycythaemia vera.

The principal adverse effect is moderate bone-marrow depression, which may be delayed 4 weeks or more from initiation of treatment. Anaemia may be marked at higher doses and is usually accompanied by leucopenia. Thrombocytopenia and haemolysis have occurred. In the initial stages of treatment, white cell and platelet counts should be determined on alternate days and complete blood counts once or twice weekly. Doses should be discontinued if the white cell count is below 3000 per mm^3 or the platelet count below 150 000 per mm^3.

Preparations

Proprietary Preparations (details are given in Part 3)
Fr.: Vercyte; *Ital.:* Vercite.

Pirarubicin (2917-g)

Pirarubicin (rINN).
1609RB; Tepirubicin; THP-ADM; THP-doxorubicin. (8S,10S)-10-{[3-Amino-2,3,6-trideoxy-4-O-(2R-tetrahydro-2H-pyran-2-yl)-α-L-lyxo-hexopyranosyl]oxy}-8-glycoloyl-7,8,9,10-tetrahydro-6,8,11-trihydroxy-1-methoxy-5,12-naphthacenedione.
$C_{32}H_{37}NO_{12} = 627.6$.
CAS — 72496-41-4.
ATC — L01DB08.

Profile

Pirarubicin is an antineoplastic anthracycline antibiotic which is a structural analogue of doxorubicin (see p.534), and has similar properties. It is used in the management of breast cancer and has also been tried in other solid neoplasms, acute leukaemias and lymphomas.

Pirarubicin is formulated as the hydrochloride but doses are in terms of the base. A usual dose of 25 to 50 mg per m^2 body-surface every 3 to 4 weeks has been recommended in breast cancer, according to response, but other dosage regimens have been used. Doses may be given by intravenous injection over 5 to 10 minutes into a rapidly-flowing intravenous infusion. Patients should undergo regular blood counts and monitoring of cardiac function: at cumulative doses above 600 mg per m^2 ventricular ejection fraction should be checked before each course. Pirarubicin has also been given by the intra-arterial and intravesical routes.

Preparations

Proprietary Preparations (details are given in Part 3)
Aust.: Berirubin; *Fr.:* Theprubicine; *Jpn:* Therarubicin†.

Piritrexim Isetionate (18894-w)

Piritrexim Isetionate (rINNM).
BW-301U (piritrexim); NSC-351521; Piritrexim Isethionate (USAN). 2,4-Diamino-6-(2,5-dimethoxybenzyl)-5-methylpyrido[2,3-d]pyrimidine mono(2-hydroxyethanesulphonate).
$C_{17}H_{19}N_5O_2,C_2H_6O_4S = 451.5$.
CAS — 72732-56-0 (piritrexim); 79483-69-5 (piritrexim isetionate).

Profile

Piritrexim is a folate antagonist with general properties similar to those of methotrexate (see p.553) and which has been tried by mouth for its antineoplastic properties, and has also been used (as the isetionate) for the treatment of opportunistic infections in immunosuppressed patients. Myelosuppression, gastrointestinal disturbances, and hepatotoxicity have been reported.

Piritrexim isetionate has also been investigated for severe psoriasis.

◊ References.
1. Feun LG, et al. Phase II trial of piritrexim in metastatic melanoma using intermittent, low-dose administration. *J Clin Oncol* 1991; **9**: 464–7.
2. Perkins W, et al. Piritrexim in severe psoriasis. *Br J Dermatol* 1991; **125** (suppl 38): 26–7.
3. Guzzo C, et al. Treatment of psoriasis with piritrexim, a lipid-soluble folate antagonist. *Arch Dermatol* 1991; **127**: 511–14.
4. Perkins W, et al. A multicentre 12-week open study of a lipid-soluble folate antagonist, piritrexim in severe psoriasis. *Br J Dermatol* 1993; **129**: 584–9.

Piroxantrone Hydrochloride (6493-q)

Piroxantrone Hydrochloride (USAN, rINNM).
Anthrapyrazole Hydrochloride; CI-942; NSC-349174; Oxantrazole Hydrochloride; PD-111815 (piroxantrone). 5-[(3-Aminopropyl)amino]-7,10-dihydroxy-2-{2-[(2-hydroxyethyl)amino]ethyl}anthra[1,9-cd]pyrazol-6(2H)-one dihydrochloride.
$C_{21}H_{25}N_5O_4,2HCl = 484.4$.
CAS — 91441-23-5 (piroxantrone); 105118-12-5 (piroxantrone hydrochloride).

Profile

Piroxantrone like mitozantrone [mitoxantrone] (p.559) is a structural analogue of the anthracycline antibiotics. It has been investigated for its antineoplastic properties against various malignant neoplasms. Myelosuppression, which may be severe and cumulative, is dose-limiting.

◊ References.
1. Hantel A, et al. Phase I study and pharmacodynamics of piroxantrone (NSC 349174), a new anthrapyrazole. *Cancer Res* 1990; **50**: 3284–8.
2. Ames MM, et al. Phase I and clinical pharmacological evaluation of pirozantrone hydrochloride (oxantrazole). *Cancer Res* 1990; **50**: 3905–9.
3. Ingle JN, et al. Evaluation of piroxantrone in women with metastatic breast cancer and failure on nonanthracycline chemotherapy. *Cancer* 1994; **74**: 1733–8.

Plicamycin (1846-f)

Plicamycin (BAN, USAN, rINN).
A-2371; Aureolic Acid; Mithramycin; NSC-24559; PA-144.
$C_{52}H_{76}O_{24} = 1085.1$.
CAS — 18378-89-7.
ATC — L01DC02.
Pharmacopoeias. In US.

An antineoplastic antibiotic produced by the growth of *Streptomyces argillaceus, S. plicatus* and *S. tanashiensis*.

Pharmacopoeial description

USP 25: A yellow, odourless, hygroscopic, crystalline powder, with a potency of not less than 900 µg per mg, calculated on the dry basis. It loses not more than 8% of its weight when dried. Slightly soluble in water and in methyl alcohol; very slightly soluble in alcohol; freely soluble in ethyl acetate. A 0.05% solution in water has a pH of 4.5 to 5.5. Store at 2° to 8° in airtight containers. Protect from light.

Adsorption. Plicamycin is bound to cellulose filters used for inline filtration of intravenous infusions,[1] with more drug likely to be lost from glucose than from sodium chloride injection at the low concentrations of drug used in therapy.
1. Butler LD, et al. Effect of inline filtration on the potency of low-dose drugs. *Am J Hosp Pharm* 1980; **37**: 935–41.

Incompatibility. Plicamycin readily chelates divalent cations, especially iron. Admixture with trace element solutions should be avoided.[1]
1. D'Arcy PF. Reactions and interactions in handling anticancer drugs. *Drug Intell Clin Pharm* 1983; **17**: 532–8.

Adverse Effects, Treatment, and Precautions

For general discussions see Antineoplastics, p.476, p.479, and p.480.

The major adverse effect of plicamycin is a dose-related bleeding syndrome, manifest initially as epistaxis, which may progress to haematemesis and potentially fatal haemorrhage. Effects on clotting factors in the blood are thought to contribute

to this syndrome. Severe thrombocytopenia may also occur due to bone-marrow depression. Leucopenia is relatively uncommon.

Gastrointestinal effects are common during treatment with plicamycin. Other side-effects include fever, malaise, drowsiness, lethargy and weakness, headache, depression, skin rashes, facial flushing, and reduced serum concentrations of calcium, phosphorus, and potassium. There may also be reversible impairment of renal and hepatic function.

Extravasation of plicamycin solutions may cause local irritation, cellulitis, and phlebitis. Application of moderate heat to the site of extravasation may aid dispersal of plicamycin and minimise discomfort and local irritation.

Plicamycin should only be given with great care to patients with impaired hepatic or renal function. It should not be administered to patients with thrombocytopenia or depressed bone-marrow function, coagulation disorders, or increased susceptibility to bleeding for any cause.

◊ Although it is recommended that plicamycin is given as an intravenous infusion over 4 to 6 hours, on the grounds that more rapid administration is associated with increased severity of gastrointestinal toxicity, a search of the literature failed to find any evidence of improved tolerance or enhanced efficacy with infusion rather than bolus injection of plicamycin.[1]
1. Mutch RS, et al. Plicamycin: bolus or infusion? *DICP Ann Pharmacother* 1990; **24**: 885–6.

Effects on the kidneys. A report of reversible oliguria and deterioration of renal function occurring on 2 occasions in a patient given single doses of plicamycin.[1]
1. Benedetti RG, et al. Nephrotoxicity following single dose mithramycin therapy. *Am J Nephrol* 1983; **3**: 277–8.

Effects on the skin. Toxic epidermal necrolysis occurring in a 22-year-old man was attributed to treatment with plicamycin.[1]
1. Purpora D, et al. Toxic epidermal necrolysis after mithramycin. *N Engl J Med* 1978; **299**: 1412.

Local toxicity. Disodium edetate has been suggested as an antidote to local toxicity following extravasation of plicamycin.[1] However, there is a suggestion that the classification of plicamycin as a vesicant is inappropriate.[2]
1. MacCara ME. Extravasation: a hazard of intravenous therapy. *Drug Intell Clin Pharm* 1983; **17**: 713–17.
2. Loughner JE, Olek C. Comment; plicamycin infusion. *DICP Ann Pharmacother* 1991; **25**: 215.

Uses and Administration

Plicamycin is a highly toxic antibiotic with antineoplastic and hypocalcaemic properties. It may act by complexing with DNA in the presence of divalent cations and inhibiting synthesis of ribonucleic acid. Lowering of serum calcium concentrations has been suggested to result from antagonism of the effects of vitamin D and parathyroid hormone on osteoclasts.

Plicamycin is used in the symptomatic management of hypercalcaemia and hypercalciuria associated with malignancy if it cannot be managed by other means (see below). The usual dose is 25 µg per kg body-weight daily by slow intravenous infusion over 4 to 6 hours in a litre of glucose 5% or sodium chloride 0.9%, for 3 or 4 days if necessary. Further courses may be given at intervals of a week or more if required.

Plicamycin has also been used in the treatment of malignant neoplasms of the testis not susceptible to surgery or radiotherapy; however, other agents are preferred (p.499). The usual dose is 25 to 30 µg per kg daily by slow intravenous infusion for 8 to 10 doses. No more than 10 doses should be given and individual daily doses should not normally exceed 30 µg per kg, because of the increased risk of haemorrhage; however an alternative regimen employing up to 50 µg per kg on alternate days is reported to produce less toxicity. Courses may be repeated at monthly intervals.

Blood cell counts, bleeding time, prothrombin time, and hepatic and renal function should be determined frequently during treatment and for several days after, and treatment stopped if there is any sudden change.

Administration. The manufacturers recommend that plicamycin be given by infusion rather than bolus injection, as this is reportedly associated with fewer and less severe gastrointestinal adverse effects. For a suggestion that this distinction is unjustified, see under Adverse Effects, above.

Hypercalcaemia. Where treatment is required for hypercalcaemia it is aimed at increasing urinary excretion of calcium and maintaining adequate hydration. Drugs that inhibit bone resorption may also be employed if hypercalcaemia is severe, particularly when it is associated with malignancy (see p.1181). Although plicamycin is effective, it is highly toxic, and the bisphosphonates and calcitonins are generally preferred.

Paget's disease of bone. Plicamycin remains a second- or third-line drug in the therapy of Paget's disease of bone (p.746), reserved for patients refractory to other treatment. Nonetheless, occasional successes are reported: one patient with refractory Paget's disease had apparent cure of her symptoms after treatment with plicamycin 25 µg per kg body-weight daily for 15 doses, followed by 1500 µg weekly for about 2 months and every 2 weeks for 6 weeks.[1] She had remained asymptomatic for 18 years after treatment. However, similar regimens have been used in other patients without this degree of success.[1] Another patient, who was refractory to calcitonin and pamidronate therapy, showed a considerable improvement in pain relief and biochemical parameters when treated with 30 µg per kg plicamycin daily for 3 days.[2]

1. Ryan WG, et al. Apparent cure of Paget's disease of bone. Am J Med 1990; 89: 825–6.
2. Wimalawansa SJ. Dramatic response to plicamycin in a patient with severe Paget's disease refractory to calcitonin and pamidronate. Semin Arthritis Rheum 1994; 23: 267.

Preparations

USP 25: Plicamycin for Injection.

Proprietary Preparations (details are given in Part 3)
Fr.: Mithracine; **Neth.:** Mithracin†; **Norw.:** Mithracin; **USA:** Mithracin.

Porfimer Sodium (10687-p)

Porfimer Sodium (BAN, USAN, rINN).
CL-184116; Dihaematoporphyrin Ether.
CAS — 87806-31-3.
ATC — L01XD01.

Profile

Porfimer sodium is a haematoporphyrin derivative which reportedly accumulates in malignant tissue following administration, and is then activated by laser light to release oxygen radicals within malignant cells, producing cytotoxicity. It is used in the treatment of superficial bladder, lung, and oesophageal cancer, and has been investigated in some other neoplasms including tumours of gastrointestinal tract and cervix. Administration is by slow intravenous injection at a dose of 2 mg per kg body-weight. This is followed, 40 to 50 hours later, by activation using a laser tuned to a wavelength of 630 nm and delivered to the area of the tumour using a fibre optic guide. The tumour may subsequently be debrided surgically. A second laser treatment may be given 96 to 120 hours after the original injection. Prolonged photosensitivity, lasting several weeks, is likely in patients treated with porfimer sodium. Other reported adverse effects include local inflammation, constipation, abdominal pain, dysphagia, nausea and vomiting, tachycardia and atrial fibrillation, dyspnoea, pneumonia, pleural effusion, and anaemia.

Photodynamic therapy. Photodynamic therapy probably has the greatest potential of the various forms of light-activated treatment.[1] Photosensitising drugs are administered intravenously and are selectively retained by tumour cells. When exposed to the correct wavelength of light the drug produces toxic oxygen radicals which destroy cell membranes and therefore kill cells. Vascular damage and immune-mediated injury may also occur.[2,3] Tumour cells must have an adequate supply of oxygen to be sensitive to photodynamic therapy,[2] and as light penetration is usually limited, early or superficial malignant lesions respond best to therapy.[1,2] It has been tried in skin, gastrointestinal, head and neck, bladder, gynaecological, and various intraperitoneal malignancies[2-7] (for reference to the use of photodynamic therapy to relieve obstruction in advanced oesophageal cancer, see p.493). There is also an interesting report of cytotoxicity against leukaemic cells in vitro when exposure to porfimer sodium was combined with ultrasound.[6]

The main adverse effect of photosensitisers such as porfimer is photosensitivity lasting 4 to 8 weeks; patients should be advised to avoid sunlight during this period and therapy is best delayed until the darker winter months if possible.[1] Newer photosensitisers are being developed to show increased tissue penetration and less prolonged photosensitivity.[2] The natural haem precursor 5-aminolaevulinic acid (p.507) has the advantage that photosensitivity lasts only a few hours.

1. Bown SG. New techniques in laser therapy. BMJ 1998; 316: 754–7.
2. Hsi RA, et al. Photodynamic therapy in the treatment of cancer: current state of the art. Drugs 1999; 57: 725–34.
3. Ost D, et al. Photodynamic therapy in lung cancer. Oncology 2000; 14: 379–86.
4. Wilson JHP, et al. Photodynamic therapy for gastrointestinal tumors. Scand J Gastroenterol 1991; 26 (suppl 188): 20–5.
5. Abramson AL, et al. Clinical effects of photodynamic therapy on recurrent laryngeal papillomas. Arch Otolaryngol Head Neck Surg 1992; 118: 25–9.
6. Tachibana K, et al. Eliminating adult T-cell leukaemia cells with ultrasound. Lancet 1997; 349: 325.
7. Walther MM. The role of photodynamic therapy in the treatment of recurrent superficial bladder cancer. Urol Clin North Am 2000; 27: 163–70.

Preparations

Proprietary Preparations (details are given in Part 3)
Canad.: Photofrin; **UK:** Photofrin; **USA:** Photofrin.

Porfiromycin (6442-t)

Porfiromycin (BAN, USAN).
Methyl Mitomycin; NSC-56410; U-14743. 6-Amino-1,1a,2,8,8a,8b-hexahydro-8-(hydroxymethyl)-8a-methoxy-1,5-dimethylazirino[2',3':3,4]pyrrolo[1,2-a]-indole-4,7-dione carbamate ester.
$C_{16}H_{20}N_4O_5 = 348.4$.
CAS — 801-52-5.

Profile

Porfiromycin is an antibiotic antineoplastic structurally related to mitomycin (p.558). It is being studied as a radiosensitiser in the management of malignant neoplasms of the head and neck.

◊ References.
1. Haffty BG, et al. Bioreductive alkylating agent porfiromycin in combination with radiation therapy for the management of squamous cell carcinoma of the head and neck. Radiat Oncol Invest 1997; 5: 235–45.

Prednimustine (1859-b)

Prednimustine (USAN, rINN).
Leo-1031; NSC-134087. 11β,17,21-Trihydroxypregna-1,4-diene-3,20-dione 21-(4-{4-[bis(2-chloroethyl)amino]phenyl}butyrate).
$C_{35}H_{45}Cl_2NO_6 = 646.6$.
CAS — 29069-24-7.
ATC — L01AA08.

Profile

Prednimustine is the prednisolone ester of chlorambucil, (p.516) and has been given by mouth in the treatment of various malignant diseases.

Preparations

Proprietary Preparations (details are given in Part 3)
Swed.: Sterecyt†.

Procarbazine Hydrochloride (1860-x)

Procarbazine Hydrochloride (BANM, USAN, rINNM).
Ibenzmethyzin Hydrochloride; NSC-77213; Ro-4-6467/1. N-Isopropyl-α-(2-methylhydrazino)-p-toluamide hydrochloride.
$C_{12}H_{19}N_3O,HCl = 257.8$.
CAS — 671-16-9 (procarbazine); 366-70-1 (procarbazine hydrochloride).
Pharmacopoeias. In Chin., Int., Jpn, and US.

Procarbazine hydrochloride 116 mg is approximately equivalent to 100 mg of procarbazine.

Pharmacopoeial description
USP 25: Store in airtight containers. Protect from light.

Adverse Effects, Treatment, and Precautions

For general discussions see Antineoplastics, p.476, p.479, and p.480.

The most common adverse effects associated with procarbazine are gastrointestinal disturbances such as nausea and vomiting (although patients may soon become tolerant), and bone-marrow depression. Leucopenia and thrombocytopenia may be delayed with a nadir at about 4 weeks after a dose, and recovery usually within 6 weeks. Anaemia, haemolysis, and bleeding tendencies have been reported.

Neurotoxicity is also common, with central effects such as somnolence, depression, nervousness or confusion, headache, hallucinations, and dizziness, and peripheral neuropathies including paraesthesias and decreased reflexes. Lethargy, ataxia, and sleep disorders have also occurred, and tremors, convulsions, and coma have been reported.

Other side-effects reported include fever and myalgia, pulmonary fibrosis or pneumonitis, haematuria, urinary frequency, skin reactions including dermatitis, pruritus, and hyperpigmentation, tachycardia, orthostatic hypotension, ocular defects, infertility, and hepatic impairment.

Procarbazine is a carcinogen, mutagen, and teratogen.

Procarbazine should be used with caution in patients with impaired liver or kidney function, and is contra-indicated if impairment is severe. Care is also advisable in patients with phaeochromocytoma, epilepsy, or cardiovascular or cerebrovascular disease. Treatment should be interrupted if allergic skin reactions occur.

Handling and disposal. Urine produced for up to 48 hours after a dose of procarbazine should be handled wearing protective clothing.[1]

1. Harris J, Dodds LJ. Handling waste from patients receiving cytotoxic drugs. Pharm J 1985; 235: 289–91.

Interactions

For a general outline of antineoplastic drug interactions, see p.481. Procarbazine is a weak MAOI and the possibility of reactions with other drugs and food,

although very rare, must be borne in mind—for details of such reactions see p.305. Procarbazine may enhance the sedative effects of other CNS depressants. A disulfiram-like reaction has been reported with alcohol and the effects of antihypertensive agents may be enhanced.

Antiepileptics. Concomitant use of enzyme-inducing antiepileptics is associated with an increased risk of hypersensitivity reactions to procarbazine, possibly through a reactive intermediate generated by CYP3A isoform induction.[1] Non-enzyme-inducing antiepileptics might be more appropriate in patients with brain tumours in whom procarbazine therapy is anticipated.

1. Lehmann DF, et al. Anticonvulsant usage is associated with an increased risk of procarbazine hypersensitivity reactions in patients with brain tumors. Clin Pharmacol Ther 1997; 62: 225–9.

Pharmacokinetics

Procarbazine is readily absorbed from the gastrointestinal tract. It crosses the blood-brain barrier and diffuses into the cerebrospinal fluid. A plasma half-life of about 10 minutes has been reported. Procarbazine is rapidly metabolised (mainly in liver and kidneys) and only about 5% is excreted unchanged in the urine. The remainder is oxidised to N-isopropylterephthalamic acid and excreted in the urine, up to about 70% of a dose being excreted in 24 hours. Some of the drug is excreted as carbon dioxide and methane via the lungs. During oxidative breakdown in the body hydrogen peroxide is formed which may account for some of the drug's actions.

Uses and Administration

Procarbazine hydrochloride is an antineoplastic which appears to inhibit protein and nucleic acid synthesis and suppress mitosis. It is unrelated to the other antineoplastics and it may be effective when other drugs have become ineffective.

Its main use is the treatment of Hodgkin's disease (p.487) when it is usually given in association with other drugs such as mustine [chlormethine], vincristine, and prednisone (the MOPP regimen). Procarbazine has also been used in the treatment of other lymphomas (p.487) and in some other malignant neoplasms including tumours of the brain (p.490). Management of these conditions is discussed further in the introduction to this chapter as indicated by the cross-references given above.

Doses of procarbazine hydrochloride are calculated in terms of procarbazine. In many of the combination regimens it has been given to adults and children in doses of the equivalent of procarbazine 100 mg per m² body-surface on days 1 to 14 of each 4- or 6-week cycle. If used as a single agent a dose equivalent to 50 mg of procarbazine by mouth daily, increased by 50 mg daily to 250 to 300 mg daily in divided doses has been suggested in the UK, while in the USA the recommended regimen is 2 to 4 mg per kg body-weight daily for the first week, subsequently increased to 4 to 6 mg per kg, doses being given to the nearest 50 mg. These doses are continued until maximum response is achieved or leucopenia, thrombocytopenia, or other signs of toxicity ensue. Maintenance doses are usually 50 to 150 mg, or 1 to 2 mg per kg, daily, until a cumulative dose of at least 6 g has been given. In children, initial daily doses of the equivalent of 50 mg per m² have been suggested (some sources simply suggest a dose of 50 mg), increased to 100 mg per m² and then adjusted according to response.

The haematological status of the patient should be determined at least every 3 or 4 days and hepatic and renal function determined weekly.

Blood disorders, non-malignant. Combination chemotherapy with regimens including procarbazine has been employed in a few patients with refractory idiopathic thrombocytopenic purpura (p.1052), and has produced prolonged remission although in most cases of the disease such aggressive therapy is difficult to justify.

Preparations

USP 25: Procarbazine Hydrochloride Capsules.

Proprietary Preparations (details are given in Part 3)
Aust.: Natulan†; **Austral.:** Natulan; **Belg.:** Natulan†; **Braz.:** Natulanar; **Canad.:** Natulan†; **Fr.:** Natulan; **Ger.:** Natulan; **Israel:** Natulan; **Ital.:** Natulan; **Mex.:** Natulan; **Neth.:** Natulan; **Norw.:**

Natulan†; *NZ:* Natulan; *S.Afr.:* Natulan; *Spain:* Natulan; *Swed.:* Natulanar†; *Switz.:* Natulan†; *UK:* Natulan; *USA:* Matulane.

Raltitrexed (11782-z)

Raltitrexed *(BAN, USAN, rINN).*
ICI-D1694; ZD-1694. *N*-{5-[3,4-Dihydro-2-methyl-4-oxo-quinazolin-6-ylmethyl(methyl)amino]-2-thenoyl}-L-glutamic acid.
$C_{21}H_{22}N_4O_6S = 458.5$.
CAS — 112887-68-0.
ATC — L01BA03.

Adverse Effects, Treatment, and Precautions

Raltitrexed produces bone marrow depression, usually mild to moderate, with leucopenia, anaemia, and, less frequently, thrombocytopenia. The nadir of the white cell count usually occurs 7 to 14 days after a dose, with recovery by the third week. Gastrointestinal toxicity is also common, with nausea and vomiting, diarrhoea, and anorexia: mucositis may occur. Reversible increases in liver enzyme values have occurred. Other adverse effects include weakness and malaise, fever, pain, headache, skin rashes, arthralgia, muscle cramps, weight loss, peripheral oedema, alopecia, and conjunctivitis. The use of folinic acid 25 mg per m² every 6 hours intravenously has been suggested in patients who develop very severe toxicity.

Raltitrexed should be given with care to patients with hepatic impairment and should be avoided if impairment is severe. It should also be avoided in severe renal impairment and be given in reduced doses in moderate impairment. Care is also advisable in debilitated or elderly patients.

Raltitrexed is teratogenic; pregnancy should be avoided while either partner is receiving the drug and for at least 6 months after treatment. It may impair male fertility.

Toxicity. A large multicentre study comparing raltitrexed with fluorouracil plus folinic acid was suspended in 1999 due to an excess of deaths in the raltitrexed arm.[1] This decision has led to some controversy,[1-3] as in 11 of the 17 deaths in patients taking raltitrexed there was evidence that the dose had not been correctly adjusted to take account of renal function. In addition, and further confusing the issue, the incidence of reported serious adverse effects was lower in raltitrexed-treated patients than in controls.

1. Anonymous. Drug-company decision to end cancer trial. *Lancet* 1999; **354:** 1045.
2. Ford HER, Cunningham D. Safety of raltitrexed. *Lancet* 1999; **354:** 1824–5.
3. Kerr D. Safety of raltitrexed. *Lancet* 1999; **354:** 1825.

Interactions

Raltitrexed should not be given with folic or folinic acid which may impair its cytotoxic action. (For the deliberate use of folinic acid to counteract the effects of raltitrexed in patients with severe toxicity see above.)

Pharmacokinetics

Following intravenous administration raltitrexed exhibits triphasic pharmacokinetics, with an initial rapid decline from peak plasma concentrations followed by a slow terminal elimination phase. Raltitrexed is actively transported into cells and metabolised to active polyglutamate forms. The remainder of a dose is excreted unchanged, about 50% of a dose appearing in the urine, and about 15% in the faeces. The terminal elimination half-life is stated to be about 8 days. Clearance is markedly reduced in renal impairment.

◊ References.
1. Clarke SJ, *et al.* Clinical and preclinical pharmacokinetics of raltitrexed. *Clin Pharmacokinet* 2000; **39:** 429–43.

Uses and Administration

Raltitrexed is a folate analogue that is a potent and specific inhibitor of the enzyme thymidylate synthase, which is involved in the synthesis of DNA. It is used in the treatment of advanced colorectal cancer (p.493) and has also been tried in breast cancer (p.491) and other solid neoplasms.

The recommended initial dose in patients with normal renal function is 3 mg of raltitrexed per m² body-surface, given by intravenous infusion over 15 minutes. Subsequent doses, which should be reduced by up to 50% depending on the severity of initial toxicity, may be given at intervals of 3 weeks provided toxicity has resolved.

A full blood count should be performed before each dose and treatment withheld if the white cell count is below 4000 per mm³, the neutrophil count is below 2000 per mm³ or the platelet count less than 100 000 per mm³. Hepatic and renal function should also be tested. It is essential that doses be adjusted in renal impairment (creatinine clearance less than 65 mL per minute) as fatalities have been associated with the failure to make such adjustments (see under Adverse Effects, above). The dosage interval should be increased from 3 to 4 weeks and the dose adjusted on the basis of creatinine clearance (CC) as follows:

- CC of 55 to 65 mL per minute, 2.25 mg per m²
- CC of 25 to 54 mL per minute, 1.5 mg per m² (in some countries, adjustment of the dose to a percentage of the full dose equivalent to the value of the CC in mL per minute is suggested in this group, e.g. reduction to 30% in those with a CC of 30 mL per minute, or 40% if CC is 40 mL per minute)
- CC less than 25 mL per minute, treatment contra-indicated.

The symbol † denotes a preparation no longer actively marketed

---

◊ References.
1. Jackman AL, *et al.* ZD1694 (Tomudex): a new thymidylate synthase inhibitor with activity in colorectal cancer. *Eur J Cancer* 1995; **31A:** 1277–82.
2. Cunningham D, *et al.* Final results of a randomised trial comparing 'Tomudex' (raltitrexed) with 5-fluorouracil plus leucovorin in advanced colorectal cancer. *Ann Oncol* 1996; **7:** 961–5.
3. Cocconi G, *et al.* Open, randomized, multicenter trial of raltitrexed versus fluorouracil plus high-dose leucovorin in patients with advanced colorectal cancer. *J Clin Oncol* 1998; **16:** 2943–52.
4. Gunasekara NS, Faulds D. Raltitrexed: a review of its pharmacological properties and clinical efficacy in the management of advanced colorectal cancer. *Drugs* 1998; **55:** 423–35.
5. Cunningham D. Mature results from three large controlled studies with raltitrexed (Tomudex). *Br J Cancer* 1998; **77** (suppl 2): 15–21.

Preparations

Proprietary Preparations (details are given in Part 3)
Aust.: Tomudex; *Austral.:* Tomudex; *Belg.:* Tomudex; *Canad.:* Tomudex; *Fin.:* Tomudex; *Fr.:* Tomudex; *Irl.:* Tomudex; *Ital.:* Tomudex; *Neth.:* Tomudex; *Norw.:* Tomudex; *S.Afr.:* Tomudex; *Spain:* Tomudex; *Switz.:* Tomudex; *UK:* Tomudex.

Ranimustine (3170-w)

Ranimustine *(rINN).*
MCNU; NSC-0270516; Ranomustine. Methyl 6-[3-(2-chloroethyl)-3-nitrosoureido]-6-deoxy-α-D-glucopyranoside.
$C_{10}H_{18}ClN_3O_7 = 327.7$.
CAS — 58994-96-0.
ATC — L01AD07.

Profile

Ranimustine is a nitrosourea derivative with general properties similar to those of carmustine (see p.516). It is used intravenously in the treatment of malignant neoplasms in usual doses of 50 to 90 mg per m² body-surface every 6 to 8 weeks according to haematological response.

Preparations

Proprietary Preparations (details are given in Part 3)
Jpn: Cymerin.

Ranpirnase (10730-a)

Ranpirnase *(USAN, rINN).*
P-30 Protein.
CAS — 196488-72-9.

NOTE. P-30 protein has been incorrectly stated to contain ergotamine.

Profile

Ranpirnase is a ribonuclease reported to have antineoplastic properties. It is under investigation in the management of a variety of solid tumours, notably in advanced pancreatic cancer with variable results. It is also reported to have activity *in vitro* against HIV.

Razoxane (1861-r)

Razoxane *(BAN, rINN).*
ICI-59118; ICRF-159; NSC-129943. (±)-4,4′-Propylenebis(piperazine-2,6-dione).
$C_{11}H_{16}N_4O_4 = 268.3$.
CAS — 21416-87-5.

Profile

Razoxane is an antineoplastic with inhibitory activity during the pre-mitotic and early mitotic phases of cell growth (G₂-M). It enhances the effects of radiotherapy. It has been used in association with radiotherapy in the treatment of sarcomas, including Kaposi's sarcoma. Razoxane has also been tried in other malignant diseases including acute leukaemias and non-Hodgkin's lymphomas. However, it is no longer widely used. Razoxane was formerly used in psoriasis, but its carcinogenic properties militate against such use, as discussed below.

In the treatment of sarcomas it has generally been given by mouth in doses of 125 mg twice daily; higher doses have been given in the management of acute leukaemias and Kaposi's sarcoma. The peripheral blood count should be monitored during treatment.

The principal adverse effects of razoxane include bone-marrow depression, gastrointestinal disturbances, skin reactions, and alopecia. It may enhance the adverse effects of radiotherapy. Razoxane therapy has been associated with the development of secondary malignancies: it is contra-indicated in the treatment of non-malignant conditions.

Dexrazoxane (p.1006) is the (+)-enantiomer of razoxane. It is used to reduce anthracycline-induced cardiotoxicity.

Malignant neoplasms. References to the use of razoxane in association with radiotherapy.
1. Hellmann K, *et al.* Responses of liver metastases to radiotherapy and razoxane. *J R Soc Med* 1992; **85:** 136–8.
2. Rhomberg W, *et al.* Radiotherapy vs radiotherapy and razoxane in the treatment of soft tissue sarcomas: final results of a randomized study. *Int J Radiat Oncol Biol Phys* 1996; **36:** 1077–84.

Skin disorders, non-malignant. Razoxane was formerly used in the systemic treatment of psoriasis, and has been found to be extremely effective, with an initial response rate of 97% overall. It was found to be of use in all forms of cutaneous psoriasis and psoriatic arthropathy.[1] However, the development of acute myeloid leukaemias and other malignancies in patients given razoxane[2-5] has led to its being contra-indicated in non-malignant conditions.

For a discussion of psoriasis and its management, see p.1106.
1. Horton JJ, Wells RS. Razoxane: a review of 6 years' therapy in psoriasis. *Br J Dermatol* 1983; **109:** 669–73.
2. Horton JJ, *et al.* Epitheliomas in patients receiving razoxane therapy for psoriasis. *Br J Dermatol* 1983; **109:** 675–8.
3. Lakhani S, *et al.* Razoxane and leukaemia. *Lancet* 1984; **ii:** 288–9.
4. Caffrey EA, *et al.* Acute myeloid leukaemia after treatment with razoxane. *Br J Dermatol* 1985; **113:** 131–4.
5. Zuiable AG, *et al.* Razoxane and T-cell lymphoma. *Br J Dermatol* 1989; **121:** 149.

Preparations

Proprietary Preparations (details are given in Part 3)
UK: Razoxin.

Rituximab (17534-n)

Rituximab *(BAN, USAN, rINN).*
IDEC-102; IDEC-C2B8.
CAS — 174722-31-7.
ATC — L01XC02.

Adverse Effects, Treatment, and Precautions

Infusion of rituximab has been associated with a cytokine release syndrome of fever and rigors, usually within 2 hours of beginning therapy (see also below). Other reported symptoms include pruritus and rashes, dyspnoea, bronchospasm, angioedema, transient hypotension, and flushing. Severe cases may be associated with tumour lysis syndrome, respiratory failure, and death. Patients with an extensive tumour burden, pulmonary tumour infiltration or pulmonary insufficiency may be at increased risk of severe reactions and should be treated with caution and possibly a decreased initial infusion rate. Therapy should be interrupted in patients who develop severe symptoms and only resumed, at half the previous rate, once all signs and symptoms have resolved. Premedication with analgesics, antihistamines, and possibly corticosteroids is recommended in all patients before receiving rituximab. Thrombocytopenia, neutropenia, and anaemia have occurred in a few patients, as have exacerbation of angina pectoris and heart failure. Hypersensitivity reactions and skin rashes, including toxic epidermal necrolysis have also occurred.

Infusion-related reactions. By November 1998 there had been 74 cases of serious infusion-related reactions to rituximab reported worldwide, with 8 fatal cases.[1] An estimated 12 000 to 14 000 patients had been treated.

The reaction usually occurs within the first two hours of infusion and the underlying mechanism is believed to be a severe cytokine release syndrome, with some elements of tumour lysis syndrome.[1-3] In one series of cases tumour necrosis factor-α and interleukin-6 levels were found to peak 90 minutes after the onset of the infusion, and these elevated cytokine levels coincided with infusion-related symptoms.[2] The reaction is usually most marked after the first infusion and subsequent infusions are usually tolerated, emphasising that this is not a true hypersensitivity reaction.[4]

Patients with a high tumour burden (lesions over 10 cm in diameter or more than 500 000 circulating malignant cells per mm³), a history of pulmonary infiltration or insufficiency, or underlying cardiac disease are believed to be at greater risk of severe reactions.[1,2,4] The UK Committee on Safety of Medicines recommends that premedication with an analgesic and an antihistamine should always be given before rituximab, and corticosteroids should be considered.[1] However, serious or fatal reactions have occurred despite such premedication.[3,4] Alternative infusion schedules and/or combination therapy with chemotherapeutic drugs may be required to decrease the tumour burden before rituximab therapy.[2,4]

1. Committee on Safety of Medicines/Medicines Control Agency. Rituximab (MabThera): serious infusion-related adverse reactions. *Current Problems* 1999; **25:** 2–3.
2. Winkler U, *et al.* Cytokine-release syndrome in patients with B-cell chronic lymphocytic leukaemia and high lymphocyte counts after treatment with an anti-CD20 monoclonal antibody (rituximab, IDEC-C2B8). *Blood* 1999; **94:** 2217–24.
3. Lim L-C, *et al.* Fatal cytokine release syndrome with chimeric anti-CD20 monoclonal antibody rituximab in a 71-year-old patient with chronic lymphocytic leukaemia. *J Clin Oncol* 1999; **17:** 1962–3.
4. Byrd JC, *et al.* Rituximab therapy in hematologic malignancy patients with circulating blood tumor cells: association with increased infusion-related side effects and rapid blood tumor clearance. *J Clin Oncol* 1999; **17:** 791–5.

Uses and Administration

Rituximab is a chimeric monoclonal antibody to CD20 antigen used in the treatment of indolent low-grade non-Hodgkin's lymphoma (p.487). Recommended doses are 375 mg per m² body-surface by intravenous infusion once weekly, for 4 doses. The first infusion is given initially at a rate of 50 mg per hour; subsequently this may be increased in increments of 50 mg per hour every 30 minutes to a maximum of 400 mg per hour, if well tolerated. Subsequent doses may be begun at a rate of 100 mg per hour, and incremented to a maximum of 400 mg per hour. Combination with chemotherapy such as CHOP (cyclophosphamide, doxorubicin, vincristine, and prednisone) is being tried both for low-grade and high-grade lymphomas, and radiolabelled forms of rituximab have also been investigated.

◊ References.
1. Maloney DG, et al. IDEC-C2B8 (rituximab) anti-CD20 monoclonal antibody therapy in patients with relapsed low-grade non-Hodgkin's lymphoma. Blood 1997; 90: 2188–95.
2. Maloney DG, et al. IDEC-C2B8: results of a phase I multiple-dose trial in patients with relapsed non-Hodgkin's lymphoma. J Clin Oncol 1997; 15: 3266–74.
3. McLaughlin P, et al. Rituximab chimeric anti-CD20 monoclonal antibody therapy for relapsed indolent lymphoma: half of patients respond to a four-dose treatment program. J Clin Oncol 1998; 16: 2825–33.
4. Wood AM. Rituximab: an innovative therapy for non-Hodgkin's lymphoma. Am J Health-Syst Pharm 2001; 58: 215–32.

Preparations

Proprietary Preparations (details are given in Part 3)
Aust.: Mabthera; **Austral.:** Mabthera; **Belg.:** Mabthera; **Denm.:** Mabthera; **Fin.:** Mabthera; **Fr.:** Mabthera; **Ger.:** Mabthera; **Israel:** Mabthera; **Ital.:** Mabthera; **Mex.:** Mabthera; **Neth.:** Mabthera; **Norw.:** Mabthera; **NZ:** Mabthera; **Port.:** Mabthera; **S.Afr.:** Mabthera; **Singapore:** Mabthera; **Spain:** Mabthera; **Swed.:** Mabthera; **Switz.:** Mabthera; **Thai.:** Mabthera; **UK:** Mabthera; **USA:** Rituxan.

Rogletimide (15076-r)

Rogletimide (BAN, USAN, rINN).
Pyridoglutethimide. (±)-2-Ethyl-2-(4-pyridyl)glutarimide.
$C_{12}H_{14}N_2O_2 = 218.3$.
CAS — 121840-95-7.

Profile
Rogletimide is an inhibitor of the aromatase (oestrogen synthetase) system. It has been investigated in the treatment of breast cancer.

Roquinimex (2828-v)

Roquinimex (USAN, rINN).
FCF-89; LS-2616. 1,2-Dihydro-4-hydroxy-N,1-dimethyl-2-oxo-3-quinolinecarboxanilide.
$C_{18}H_{16}N_2O_3 = 308.3$.
CAS — 84088-42-6.
ATC — L03AX02.

Profile
Roquinimex is an immunomodulator which is reported to stimulate various immune functions including macrophage cytotoxicity. It has been investigated for its potential against various malignant neoplasms including as adjuvant therapy following bone marrow transplantation in acute leukaemia, to prolong the time to relapse. Roquinimex has also been investigated in various immune and auto-immune disorders including multiple sclerosis. However serious cardiovascular toxicity following roquinimex therapy has led to several trials being terminated.

◊ References.
1. Coutant R, et al. Low dose linomide in type I juvenile diabetes of recent onset: a randomised placebo-controlled double blind trial. Diabetologia 1998; 41: 1040–6.
2. Simonsson B, et al. Roquinimex (Linomide) vs placebo in AML after autologous bone marrow transplantation. Bone Marrow Transplant 2000; 25: 1121–7.
3. Tan IL, et al. Linomide in the treatment of multiple sclerosis: MRI results from prematurely terminated phase-III trials. Multiple Sclerosis 2000; 6: 99–104.
4. Noseworthy JH, et al. Linomide in relapsing and secondary progressive MS. Part 1: trial design and clinical results. Neurology 2000; 54: 1726–33.

Rubitecan (20424-n)

Rubitecan (USAN, rINN).
9-NC; 9-Nitrocamptothecin; RFS-2000. 9-Nitro-20(S)-camptothecin.
$C_{20}H_{15}N_3O_6 = 393.3$.
CAS — 91421-42-0.

Profile
Like irinotecan (p.549), rubitecan is a topoisomerase I inhibitor related to camptothecin. It is under investigation for its antineoplastic properties particularly in the treatment of pancreatic cancer.

Satraplatin (16686-s)

Satraplatin (USAN, rINN).
BMS-182751; BMY-45594; JM-216. (OC-6-43)-Bis(acetato)amminedichloro(cyclohexylamine)platinum.
$C_{10}H_{22}Cl_2N_2O_4Pt = 500.3$.
CAS — 129580-63-8.

Profile
Satraplatin is an analogue of cisplatin (p.525) with generally

similar properties, but which is well absorbed following oral administration. It is under investigation for its antineoplastic properties.

◊ References.
1. Weiss RB, Christian MC. New cisplatin analogues in development: a review. Drugs 1993; 46: 360–77.
2. McKeage MJ. Comparative adverse effect profiles of platinum drugs. Drug Safety 1995; 13: 228–44.
3. Fokkema E, et al. Phase II study of oral platinum drug JM216 as first-line treatment in patients with small-cell lung cancer. J Clin Oncol 1999; 17: 3822–7.

Sebriplatin (17110-d)

Sebriplatin (rINN).
CI-973; NK-121. (+)-cis-(1,1-Cyclobutanedicarboxylato)[(2R)-2-methyl-1,4-butanediamine-N,N']platinum.
$C_{11}H_{20}N_2O_4Pt = 439.4$.
CAS — 110172-45-7.

Profile
Sebriplatin is an analogue of cisplatin (p.525) with generally similar properties. It has been investigated in a variety of solid neoplasms and in the treatment of acute leukaemias.

◊ References.
1. Weiss RB, Christian MC. New cisplatin analogues in development: a review. Drugs 1993; 46: 360–77.
2. Kantarjian HM, et al. Evaluation of CI-973, a platinum analogue, in refractory or relapsed acute leukemia. Leukemia 1996; 10: 396–401.
3. Theriault RL, et al. A phase II study of CI-973 [SP-4-3(R)-1,1-cyclobutane-dicarboxylato (2-)] (2-methyl-1,4-butanediamine-N,N') platinum in patients with refractory advanced breast cancer. Cancer Chemother Pharmacol 1996; 38: 289–91.

Semustine (1863-d)

Semustine (USAN, rINN).
Methyl Lomustine; Methyl-CCNU; NSC-95441; WR-220076. 1-(2-Chloroethyl)-3-(4-methylcyclohexyl)-1-nitrosourea.
$C_{10}H_{18}ClN_3O_2 = 247.7$.
CAS — 13909-09-6.
ATC — L01AD03.

Adverse Effects, Treatment, and Precautions
As for Carmustine, p.516.

◊ Nephrotoxicity has been reported in patients receiving high cumulative doses of semustine. Severe renal damage was reported in 6 of 17 children given semustine after radiotherapy for brain tumours; all 6 children had received a total dose above 1.5 g per m^2 body-surface in contrast to those not so affected, who had received lower doses.[1] A decrease in kidney size was seen in 2 patients who had received lower cumulative doses. There had been no evidence during treatment that patients were losing renal function. Similarly others have reported an increased risk of renal abnormalities in patients given a cumulative dose of 1.4 g per m^2 or more.[2] Some 25% of patients given higher doses were so affected, while those given lower doses were not. Overall, however, the problem may not be particularly frequent: in one study it was considered that only 4 of 857 patients treated with semustine over 6 years might have had delayed renal insufficiency possibly related to semustine.[3]
1. Harmon WE, et al. Chronic renal failure in children treated with methyl-CCNU. N Engl J Med 1979; 300: 1200–3.
2. Micetich KC, et al. Nephrotoxicity of semustine (methyl-CCNU) in patients with malignant melanoma receiving adjuvant chemotherapy. Am J Med 1981; 71: 967–72.
3. Nichols WC, Moertel CG. Nephrotoxicity of methyl-CCNU. N Engl J Med 1979; 301: 1181.

Pharmacokinetics
Semustine is well absorbed from the gastrointestinal tract following oral doses, and is rapidly metabolised. The metabolites are reported to possess prolonged plasma half-lives, and cross the blood-brain barrier into the cerebrospinal fluid. It is excreted in urine as metabolites: up to 60% of a dose is excreted in this way within 48 hours. Small amounts may be excreted in faeces and via the lungs as carbon dioxide.

Uses and Administration
Semustine is a nitrosourea with actions and uses similar to those of carmustine (p.516) and lomustine (p.550).

Sirolimus (8273-e)

Sirolimus (BAN, USAN, rINN).
AY-22989; AY-022989; Rapamycin; Wy-090217. (3S,6R,7E,9R,10R,12R,14S,15E,17E,19E,21S,23S,26R,27R,34aS)-9,10,12,13,14,21,22,23,24,25,26,27,32,33,34,34a-Hexadecahydro-9,27-dihydroxy-3-{(1R)-2-[(1S,3R,4R)-4-hydroxy-3-methoxycyclohexyl]-1-methylethyl}-10,21-dimethoxy-6,8,12,14,20,26-hexamethyl-23,27-epoxy-3H-pyrido[2,1-c][1,4]oxaazacyclohentriacontine-1,5,11,28,29(4H,6H,31H)-pentone.
$C_{51}H_{79}NO_{13} = 914.2$.
CAS — 53123-88-9.
ATC — L04AA10.

Profile
Sirolimus is a macrolide compound obtained from Streptomyces hygroscopicus with potent immunosuppressant properties. It is used for the prevention of graft rejection in renal transplantation, and is being investigated for induction of remission in some auto-immune diseases. Sirolimus is given in conjunction with ciclosporin and corticosteroids as soon as possible after transplantation. A loading dose of 6 mg is given orally, followed by a maintenance dose of 2 mg daily, 4 hours after ciclosporin administration. In patients 13 years of age or more who weigh less than 40 kg a loading dose of 3 mg per m^2 body-surface, followed by initial maintenance doses of 1 mg per m^2, is recommended. The dose of sirolimus should be adjusted to obtain whole blood trough concentrations of 4 to 12 nanograms per mL, and the doses of ciclosporin and corticosteroids gradually reduced. After 2 to 3 months, ciclosporin should be gradually discontinued over 4 to 8 weeks, and the dose of sirolimus adjusted to obtain trough concentrations of 12 to 20 nanograms per mL. In patients in whom ciclosporin withdrawal is unsuccessful or cannot be attempted, sirolimus should not be used for more than 3 months after transplantation.

The most frequent adverse effects include gastrointestinal disturbances, tremor, acne, impaired renal function, hyperlipidaemia, peripheral oedema, headache, pain, asthenia, and hypertension.

Sirolimus has been shown to possess antifungal and antineoplastic properties. It is under investigation for gene regulation in gene therapy.

◊ References.
1. Vasquez EM. Sirolimus: a new agent for prevention of renal allograft rejection. Am J Health-Syst Pharm 2000; 57: 437–51.
2. Ferron GM, et al. Population pharmacokinetics of sirolimus in kidney transplant patients. Clin Pharmacol Ther 1997; 61: 416–28.
3. Kahan BD. Efficacy of sirolimus compared with azathioprine for reduction of acute renal allograft rejection: a randomised multicentre study. Lancet 2000; 356: 194–202.
4. Ingle GR, et al. Sirolimus: continuing the evolution of transplant immunosuppression. Ann Pharmacother 2000; 34: 1044–55.

Interactions. Trough concentrations of sirolimus, and area under the concentration-time curve (AUC) were significantly higher when sirolimus and ciclosporin were given together than when the 2 drugs were given 4 hours apart.[1]
1. Kaplan B, et al. The effects of relative timing of sirolimus and cyclosporine microemulsion formulation coadministration on the pharmacokinetics of each agent. Clin Pharmacol Ther 1998; 63: 48–53.

Use. PSORIASIS. Sirolimus has been investigated both systemically[1] and topically[2] in the treatment of psoriasis.
1. Reitamo S, et al. A double-blind study in patients with severe psoriasis to assess the clinical activity and safety of rapamycin (sirolimus) alone or in association with a reduced dose of cyclosporine. Br J Dermatol 1999; 141: 978–9.
2. Ormerod AD, et al. Penetration, safety and efficacy of the topical immunosuppressive sirolimus in psoriasis. Br J Dermatol 1999; 141: 975.

Preparations

Proprietary Preparations (details are given in Part 3)
UK: Rapamune; **USA:** Rapamune.

Sizofiran (1796-v)

Sizofiran (rINN).
Schizophyllan. Poly[3→(O-β-D-glucopyranosyl-(1→3)-O-[β-D-glucopyranosyl-(1→6)]-O-β-D-glucopyranosyl-(1→3)-O-β-D-glucopyranosyl)→1].
$(C_{24}H_{40}O_{20})_n$.
CAS — 9050-67-3.

Profile
Sizofiran is a polysaccharide obtained from cultures of the basidiomycete fungus Schizophyllum commune. It is reported to have antineoplastic and immunomodulating activity and is given in conjunction with radiotherapy in malignant neoplasms of the cervix (p.492). It is given by intramuscular injection in usual doses of 40 mg weekly. It has also been tried with chemotherapy or radiotherapy in other malignant neoplasms. Hypersensitivity reactions, including anaphylactoid shock, may occur.

◊ References.
1. Fujimoto S, et al. Clinical outcome of postoperative adjuvant immunochemotherapy with sizofiran for patients with resectable gastric cancer: a randomised controlled study. Eur J Cancer 1991; 27: 1114–18.
2. Shimizu Y, et al. Augmenting effect of sizofiran on the immunofunction of regional lymph nodes in cervical cancer. Cancer 1992; 69: 1188–94.
3. Kano Y, et al. Effect of sizofiran on regional lymph nodes in patients with head and neck cancer. Biotherapy 1996; 9: 257–62.

Preparations

Proprietary Preparations (details are given in Part 3)
Jpn: Sonifilan.

Sobuzoxane (5512-s)

Sobuzoxane (rINN).
MST-16. 4,4′-Ethylenebis[1-(hydroxymethyl)-2,6-piperazinedione] bis(isobutyl carbonate).
$C_{22}H_{34}N_4O_{10} = 514.5$.
CAS — 98631-95-9.

Profile

Sobuzoxane is an orally active inhibitor of topoisomerase II that has been used for its antineoplastic properties in the treatment of non-Hodgkin's lymphomas and adult T-cell leukaemia/lymphoma. Adverse effects include myelosuppression, bleeding tendency, renal and hepatic dysfunction, gastrointestinal disturbances, alopecia, headache, and fever.

Preparations

Proprietary Preparations (details are given in Part 3)
Jpn: Perazolin†.

Sodium Bromebrate (13243-b)

Sodium Bromebrate (BANM, rINN).
MBBA; NSC-104801; WR-149912. The sodium salt of (E)-3-p-anisoyl-3-bromoacrylic acid.
$C_{11}H_8BrNaO_4 = 307.1$.
CAS — 5711-40-0 (bromebric acid); 21739-91-3 (sodium bromebrate).

Profile

Sodium bromebrate is reported to possess antineoplastic properties and has been given in various gynaecological neoplasms.

Sparfosic Acid (16995-f)

Sparfosic Acid (rINN).
PALA. N-Phosphonoacetyl-L-aspartic acid.
$C_6H_{10}NO_8P = 255.1$.
CAS — 51321-79-0.

Sparfosate Sodium (12022-g)

Sparfosate Sodium (USAN, rINN).
CI-882; NSC-224131; PALA Disodium. The disodium salt of sparfosic acid.
$C_6H_8NNa_2O_8P = 299.1$.
CAS — 66569-27-5.

Adverse Effects and Precautions

Stomatitis, gastrointestinal disturbances, and effects on the skin have occurred. Central neurotoxicity has been reported, with seizures and encephalopathy.

Care should be taken to avoid extravasation.

◊ Transient hepatic abnormalities developed in 15 of 17 patients with a complete or partial response to combined therapy with sparfosic acid and fluorouracil,[1] comprising ascites (in 5), hyperbilirubinaemia (in 6), hypoalbuminaemia (in 12) and elevations of serum transaminase (in 7). Liver function abnormalities also developed in 12 of 27 patients who failed to respond to this regimen, but in most of these, changes were progressive. It is possible that some of these abnormalities could be related to the effects of the regimen on hepatic protein synthesis.

1. Kemeny N, *et al.* A new syndrome: ascites, hyperbilirubinemia, and hypoalbuminemia after biochemical modulation of fluorouracil with N-phosphonoacetyl-L-aspartate (PALA). *Ann Intern Med* 1991; **115:** 946–51.

Uses and Administration

Sparfosic acid is an antineoplastic agent that prevents the first step of pyrimidine biosynthesis by inhibition of the enzyme aspartate transcarbamylase. When combined with fluorouracil this depletion of cellular pyrimidines results in increased incorporation of the latter into nucleic acid, and increased inhibition of protein synthesis.

It has been tried with limited success in the management of various solid tumours, but is more frequently used in combination with other agents such as fluorouracil.

◊ References.
1. Fleming RA, *et al.* Phase I study of N-(phosphonacetyl)-L-aspartate with fluorouracil and with or without dipyridamole in patients with advanced cancer. *Clin Cancer Res* 1996; **2:** 1107–1114.
2. Nassim MA, *et al.* Effects of PALA on the pharmacokinetics of 5-fluorouracil. *Oncol Rep* 1998; **5:** 217–21.
3. Royce ME, *et al.* Sequential biochemical modulation of fluorouracil with folinic acid, N-phosphonacetyl-L-aspartic acid, and interferon alfa-2a in advanced colorectal cancer. *J Clin Oncol* 1999; **17:** 3276–82.

Streptozocin (1864-n)

Streptozocin (USAN, rINN).
NSC-85998; Streptozotocin; U-9889. 2-Deoxy-2-(3-methyl-3-nitrosoureido)-D-glucopyranose.
$C_8H_{15}N_3O_7 = 265.2$.
CAS — 18883-66-4.
ATC — L01AD04.

The manufacturers recommend that it be **stored** at 2° to 8° and protected from light.

Adverse Effects, Treatment, and Precautions

For general discussions see Antineoplastics, p.476, p.479, and p.480.

Cumulative nephrotoxicity is common with streptozocin and may be severe. Fatal irreversible renal failure has been reported. Intra-arterial administration may be associated with increased risk of nephrotoxicity.

Other adverse effects include severe nausea and vomiting and alterations in liver function or occasionally severe hepatotoxicity. Myelosuppression may occur but is rarely severe. Streptozocin may affect glucose metabolism. A diabetogenic effect has been reported; hypoglycaemia attributed to the release of insulin from damaged cells has also occurred.

Streptozocin is irritant to tissues and extravasation may lead to local ulceration and necrosis.

Streptozocin should be used with extreme care in patients with pre-existing renal impairment.

Handling and disposal. Methods for the destruction of streptozocin *waste* by reaction with hydrobromic acid in glacial acetic acid or by oxidation with a solution of potassium permanganate in sulfuric acid.[1] Residues produced by either method were free of mutagenic activity.

1. Castegnaro M, *et al.*, eds. Laboratory decontamination and destruction of carcinogens in laboratory wastes: some antineoplastic agents. *IARC Scientific Publications 73.* Lyon: WHO/International Agency for Research on Cancer, 1985.

Interactions

Streptozocin should not be given in association with other potentially nephrotoxic drugs. For increased doxorubicin toxicity when the latter was given with streptozocin see p.535.

Phenytoin. A suggestion that, since phenytoin appeared to protect the beta cells of the pancreas from the cytotoxic effects of streptozocin, its concomitant use with streptozocin should be avoided in patients being treated for pancreatic tumours.[1]

1. Koranyi L, Gero L. Influence of diphenylhydantoin on the effect of streptozotocin. *BMJ* 1979; **1:** 127.

Pharmacokinetics

Following intravenous administration streptozocin is rapidly cleared from the blood and distributed to body tissues, particularly the liver, kidneys, intestines, and pancreas. It is extensively metabolised, mainly in the liver and perhaps the kidney, and excreted principally in the urine as metabolites and a small amount of unchanged drug. Approximately 60 to 70% of an intravenous dose is excreted in urine within 24 hours. Some is also excreted via the lungs. Streptozocin itself does not cross the blood-brain barrier but its metabolites are found in the CSF.

Uses and Administration

Streptozocin is an antibiotic antineoplastic agent belonging to the nitrosoureas (see Carmustine, p.516) and is used, alone or in combination with other antineoplastic agents, mainly in the treatment of pancreatic endocrine (islet-cell) tumours (p.483). It has been tried in other tumours including exocrine pancreatic cancer and prostate cancer. It has been given by intravenous injection or infusion in doses of 1 g per m² body-surface weekly, increased if necessary after 2 weeks to up to 1.5 g per m². Alternatively doses of 500 mg per m² may be given daily for 5 days and repeated every 6 weeks.

Streptozocin has also been given by intra-arterial infusion (but see Adverse Effects above).

Full blood counts, and renal and hepatic function tests should be performed routinely during treatment; doses should be reduced or treatment withdrawn if renal toxicity occurs.

Preparations

Proprietary Preparations (details are given in Part 3)
Canad.: Zanosar; *Fr.:* Zanosar; *Israel:* Zanosar; *Neth.:* Zanosar†; *USA:* Zanosar.

Sulofenur (12231-z)

Sulofenur (BAN, USAN, rINN).
LY-186641. 1-(4-Chlorophenyl)-3-(indan-5-ylsulphonyl)urea.
$C_{16}H_{15}ClN_2O_3S = 350.8$.
CAS — 110311-27-8.

Profile

Sulofenur is a sulfonylurea derivative which has been investigated for its antineoplastic properties. Methaemoglobinaemia and haemolytic anaemia may be dose-limiting.

◊ References.
1. Hainsworth JD, *et al.* Phase I clinical study of N-[(4-chlorophenyl)amino]carbonyl-2,3-dihydro-1H-indene-5-sulfonamide (LY186641). *Cancer Res* 1989; **49:** 5217–20.
2. Mahjoubi M, *et al.* Phase II trial of LY 186641 in advanced renal cancer. *Invest New Drugs* 1993; **11:** 323–8.
3. Pratt CB, *et al.* A phase I study of sulofenur in refractory pediatric malignant solid tumors. *Invest New Drugs* 1995; **13:** 63–6.
4. Krarup-Hansen A, *et al.* Early clinical investigation of sulofenur with a daily schedule in advanced solid tumours. *Invest New Drugs* 1997; **15:** 147–51.

Tacrolimus (4992-w)

Tacrolimus (BAN, USAN, rINN).
FK-506; FR-900506.
(−)-(3S,4R,5S,8R,9E,12S,14S,15R,16S,18R,19R,26aS)-8-Allyl-5,6,8,11,12,13,14,15,16,17,18,19,24,25,26,26a-hexadecahydro-5,19-dihydroxy-3-{(E)-2-[(1R,3R,4R)-4-hydroxy-3-methoxycyclohexyl]-1-methylvinyl}-14,16,-dimethoxy-4,10,12,18-tetramethyl-15,19-epoxy-3H-pyrido[2,1-c][1,4]oxaazacyclotricosine-1,7,20,21(4H,23H)-tetrone monohydrate.
$C_{44}H_{69}NO_{12}, H_2O = 822.0$.
CAS — 104987-11-3 (anhydrous tacrolimus); 109581-93-3 (tacrolimus monohydrate).
ATC — L04AA05.

Adverse Effects and Precautions

Tacrolimus may produce nephrotoxicity and neurotoxicity. The most common adverse effects after systemic administration include tremor, headache, paraesthesias, nausea and diarrhoea, hypertension, leucocytosis, and impaired renal function. Disturbances of serum electrolytes, notably hyperkalaemia occur frequently. Other adverse effects include mood changes, sleep disturbances, confusion, dizziness, tinnitus, visual disturbances, and convulsions; disturbances of carbohydrate metabolism or frank diabetes mellitus; ECG changes and tachycardia, as well as hypertrophic cardiomyopathy (particularly in children); constipation, dyspepsia, and gastrointestinal haemorrhage; dyspnoea, asthma, pleural effusions; alopecia, hirsutism, skin rash and pruritus; and arthralgia or myalgia, spasm, leg cramps, peripheral oedema, liver dysfunction, and coagulation disorders. Topical administration of tacrolimus has been associated with local irritation and skin disorders including an increased incidence of herpes simplex and zoster infections; headache and 'flu-like' symptoms have also been reported.

Tacrolimus injection is formulated with polyethoxylated castor oil: anaphylactoid reactions have occurred, and appropriate means for their management should be available in patients given the injection. Use of tacrolimus should be avoided in patients hypersensitive to macrolides. Dosage reduction may be necessary in patients with hepatic impairment. Care is also required in patients with pre-existing renal impairment, and some sources consider that dosage reduction may prove advisable in such patients. Monitoring of blood concentrations of tacrolimus is recommended in all patients. Renal and hepatic function, blood pressure, serum glucose and electrolytes, and haematological and cardiac function, as well as visual function should be monitored regularly. As with other immunosuppressants, patients receiving tacrolimus are at increased risk of infection and malignancy. Tacrolimus may affect visual or neurological function, and patients so affected should not drive or operate dangerous machinery.

Effects on the blood. A report of severe anaemia due to selective depression of erythropoiesis in a patient given tacrolimus.[1] Anaemia resolved when tacrolimus was replaced with ciclosporin. More generalised bone marrow suppression has also been reported.[2]

1. Winkler M, *et al.* Anaemia associated with FK 506 immunosuppression. *Lancet* 1993; **341:** 1035–6.
2. de-la-Serna-Higuera C, *et al.* Tacrolimus-induced bone marrow suppression. *Lancet* 1997; **350:** 714–15.

Effects on carbohydrate metabolism. A retrospective study involving 52 patients given primary immunosuppression with tacrolimus and corticosteroids after liver transplantation found that 7 previously non-diabetic patients required temporary insulin therapy after transplantation.[1] Insulin requirements were not changed in 4 patients with pre-existing type 1 diabetes mellitus, although 3 patients with type 2 diabetes mellitus did experience a temporary need for insulin. The effects on blood glucose did not seem to depend on the dose of tacrolimus.

1. Tabasco-Minguillan J, *et al.* Insulin requirements after liver transplantation and FK-506 immunosuppression. *Transplantation* 1993; **56:** 862–7.

Effects on the cardiovascular system. Hypertrophic cardiomyopathy, and in some cases heart failure, has been described in paediatric patients receiving tacrolimus after organ grafting (small bowel or liver).[1] Symptoms largely resolved on discontinuation or dosage reduction. A similar case had been found *post mortem* in an adult,[2] and the UK Committee on Safety of Medicines[3] was aware of 29 reported cases worldwide as of July 1995. Echocardiographic monitoring of patients receiving

---

The symbol † denotes a preparation no longer actively marketed

tacrolimus has been recommended, with dose reduction or withdrawal in those who developed hypertrophic changes.[3] However, echocardiographic abnormalities may be quite common after orthotopic liver transplantation in adults, with no obvious relationship to the use of tacrolimus.[4]

Severe hypertension was documented in 5 out of 10 paediatric patients who received intravenous tacrolimus following renal transplant surgery. All patients responded to intravenous labetalol. By contrast none of 11 children who received ciclosporin at the same institution developed hypertension.[5]

1. Atkison P, et al. Hypertrophic cardiomyopathy associated with tacrolimus in paediatric transplant patients. Lancet 1995; 345: 894–6.
2. Natazuka T, et al. Immunosuppressive drugs and hypertrophic cardiomyopathy. Lancet 1995; 345: 1644.
3. Committee on Safety of Medicines/Medicines Control Agency. Tacrolimus (Prograf) and hypertrophic cardiomyopathy in transplant patients. Current Problems 1995; 21: 6.
4. Dollinger MM, et al. Cardiotoxicity in adult liver transplant recipients. Lancet 1995; 346: 507.
5. Booth CJ, et al. Intravenous tacrolimus may induce severe hypertension in renal transplant recipients. Arch Dis Child 1999; 80 (suppl 1): A27.

Effects on the kidney. A comparison in patients who had undergone liver transplantation suggested that nephrotoxicity was somewhat more of a problem in those receiving tacrolimus than in those given a ciclosporin-based regimen.[1] In particular intravenous administration of tacrolimus during the first week after transplantation was associated with acute renal failure in 4 of 20 patients. Furthermore, on follow-up for 1 year, glomerular filtration rate was somewhat lower in the tacrolimus-treated group.[1]

1. Porayko MK, et al. Nephrotoxic effects of primary immunosuppression with FK-506 and cyclosporine regimens after liver transplantation. Mayo Clin Proc 1994; 69: 105–11.

Effects on the nervous system. Severe peripheral neuropathy together with signs of cerebral dysfunction has been reported in 2 patients receiving tacrolimus.[1] Among other central effects, tacrolimus has also been associated with speech disorders, including severe dysarthria and mutism in 1 patient;[2] some degree of speech dysfunction, in the form of an apparent Norwegian accent, appeared to be permanent in this case.

1. Ayres RCS, et al. Peripheral neurotoxicity with tacrolimus. Lancet 1994; 343: 862–3.
2. Boeve BF, et al. Dysarthria and apraxia of speech associated with FK-506 (tacrolimus). Mayo Clin Proc 1996; 71: 969–72.

Effects on skeletal muscle. Severe acute rhabdomyolysis, leading to fatal acute renal failure, developed in an 18-month-old child given tacrolimus after bone-marrow transplantation.[1]

1. Hibi S, et al. Severe rhabdomyolysis associated with tacrolimus. Lancet 1995; 346: 702.

Hepatitis. For the suggestion that dosage requirements of tacrolimus may be reduced in children with hepatitis C see Administration, below.

Overdosage. A report[1] of 12 cases of acute overdose with tacrolimus described overdoses of up to 30 times the prescribed dose. Three patients were asymptomatic, while 7 showed mild transient renal and hepatic impairment, nausea, and mild hand tremors. One patient suffered renal failure, histoplasmosis and sepsis 48 hours after admission for the overdose. The outcome was unknown in one patient. All 8 symptomatic patients recovered when tacrolimus concentrations returned to normal. No specific treatment regimen has been recommended, but patients have been treated with gastric lavage, oral activated charcoal and phenytoin administration. The latter is used both to prevent seizures and to enhance tacrolimus metabolism by stimulation of cytochrome P450. Patients should be closely monitored for known signs and symptoms of tacrolimus toxicity.

1. Curran CF, et al. Acute overdoses of tacrolimus. Transplantation 1996; 62: 1376.

Interactions

Increased nephrotoxicity may result if tacrolimus is given with other potentially nephrotoxic drugs: concomitant use with ciclosporin should be avoided for this reason. Potassium-sparing diuretics should also be avoided in patients receiving tacrolimus.

Tacrolimus is metabolised by the cytochrome P450 isoenzyme CYP3A4, and drugs which inhibit this enzyme system, such as azole antifungals, bromocriptine, calcium-channel blockers, cimetidine, some corticosteroids, ciclosporin, danazol, HIV-protease inhibitors, macrolide antibacterials, and metoclopramide, may produce increased blood concentrations of tacrolimus if given concomitantly. Equally, inducers of this enzyme system (such as carbamazepine, phenobarbital, phenytoin, and rifampicin) may reduce blood concentrations of tacrolimus.

◊ A study[1] in vitro found that metabolism of tacrolimus by CYP3A in human liver microsomes was inhibited by bromocriptine, corticosterone, dexamethasone, ergotamine, erythromycin, ethinylestradiol, josamycin, ketoconazole, miconazole, midazolam, nifedipine, omeprazole, tamoxifen, troleandomycin, and verapamil. No effect on tacrolimus metabolism was

seen with aspirin, amphotericin B, captopril, cefotaxime, ciprofloxacin, diclofenac, diltiazem, doxycycline, frusemide [furosemide], glibenclamide, imipramine, lignocaine [lidocaine], paracetamol, prednisolone, progesterone, ranitidine, sulfamethoxazole, trimethoprim, or vancomycin.

1. Christians U, et al. Identification of drugs inhibiting the in vitro metabolism of tacrolimus by human liver microsomes. Br J Clin Pharmacol 1996; 41: 187–90.

Antibacterials. Increased concentrations of tacrolimus in plasma have been reported when erythromycin was given concomitantly;[1] the interaction was accompanied by some evidence of nephrotoxicity. A similar interaction has been reported between tacrolimus and clarithromycin.[2] For reference to the effects of macrolides on tacrolimus metabolism in vitro see above.

Concomitant treatment with rifampicin has been found to substantially decrease tacrolimus concentrations.[3,4] A pharmacokinetic study found that rifampicin induces metabolism of tacrolimus in both the liver and intestine, probably by induction of P450 CYP3A and P-glycoprotein.[5] Both metronidazole[6] and chloramphenicol[7] increased the blood concentrations of tacrolimus when given concurrently. This is probably due to inhibition of metabolism, and dosage reduction of the immunosuppressant may be necessary when either drug is given with tacrolimus.

Plasma concentrations of tacrolimus are also increased by quinupristin/dalfopristin.

1. Jensen C, et al. Interaction between tacrolimus and erythromycin. Lancet 1994; 344: 825.
2. Wolter K, et al. Interaction between FK 506 and clarithromycin in a renal transplant patient. Eur J Clin Pharmacol 1994; 47: 207–8.
3. Furlan V, et al. Interactions between FK506 and rifampicin or erythromycin in pediatric liver recipients. Transplantation 1995; 59: 1217–18.
4. Chenhsu R-Y, et al. Renal allograft dysfunction associated with rifampin-tacrolimus interaction. Ann Pharmacother 2000; 34: 27–31.
5. Hebert MF, et al. Effects of rifampin on tacrolimus pharmacokinetics in healthy volunteers. J Clin Pharmacol 1999; 39: 91–6.
6. Herzig K, Johnson DW. Marked elevation of blood cyclosporin and tacrolimus levels due to concurrent metronidazole therapy. Nephrol Dial Transplant 1999; 14: 521–3.
7. Schulman SL, et al. Interaction between tacrolimus and chloramphenicol in a renal transplant recipient. Transplantation 1998; 65: 1397–8.

Antiepileptics. For the effect of tacrolimus on phenytoin, see Phenytoin, p.360.

Antifungals. Elevated plasma-tacrolimus concentrations have been reported in patients given clotrimazole[1] or fluconazole[2] concomitantly; a reduction in the dose of tacrolimus was likely to be necessary if it were given with an azole antifungal. A study involving tacrolimus and ketoconazole suggested that an increase in the oral bioavailability of tacrolimus from a mean of 14 to 30% when given with the azole was probably due to decreased CYP3A4 metabolism in the gut wall, or improved absorption due to inhibition of P-glycoprotein mediated efflux, rather than an effect on hepatic metabolism.[3] Similarly, a 50% reduction in tacrolimus dosage was found to be necessary when the drug was given in combination with itraconazole.[4] It has been suggested that the interaction could be exploited to reduce the cost of immunosuppressant regimens.[5]

1. Mieles L, et al. Interaction between FK506 and clotrimazole in a liver transplant recipient. Transplantation 1991; 52: 1086–7.
2. Mañez R, et al. Fluconazole therapy in transplant recipients receiving FK506. Transplantation 1994; 57: 1521–3.
3. Floren LC, et al. Tacrolimus oral bioavailability doubles when coadministration of ketoconazole. Clin Pharmacol Ther 1997; 62: 41–9.
4. Capone D, et al. Effects of itraconazole on tacrolimus blood concentrations in a renal transplant recipient. Ann Pharmacother 1999; 33: 1124–5.
5. Kramer MR, et al. Dose adjustment and cost of itraconazole prophylaxis in lung transplant recipients receiving cyclosporine and tacrolimus (FK506). Transplant Proc 1997; 29: 2657–9.

Calcium-channel blockers. Dosage requirements for tacrolimus were substantially reduced in 22 liver graft recipients who also received nifedipine, compared with 28 patients who did not, in a 1-year retrospective study.[1]

1. Seifeldin RA, et al. Nifedipine interaction with tacrolimus in liver transplant recipients. Ann Pharmacother 1997; 31: 571–5.

Danazol. Nephrotoxicity and tremors associated with elevated concentrations of tacrolimus developed in a patient given danazol concomitantly with the immunosuppressant.[1] The effect might be due to inhibition of the metabolism of tacrolimus.

1. Shapiro R, et al. FK 506 interaction with danazol. Lancet 1993; 341: 1344–5.

Pharmacokinetics

Absorption of tacrolimus following oral administration is reported to be erratic. Oral bioavailability varies very widely, although a bioavailability of about 15 to 20% seems common. Following intravenous administration it is widely distributed to the tissues; in the blood, about 80% is bound to erythrocytes, and variations in red cell binding account for much of the variability in pharmacokinetics. The portion in plasma is approximately 99% bound to plasma proteins. Tacrolimus is extensively metabolised by the liver

and excreted, primarily in bile, almost entirely as metabolites. Some metabolism may occur in the gastrointestinal tract. Plasma elimination half-life has been reported to average 43 hours in healthy volunteers, and to range from about 12 to 16 hours in transplant patients.

◊ References.
1. Venkataramanan R, et al. Pharmacokinetics of FK 506: preclinical and clinical studies. Transplant Proc 1990; 22 (suppl 1): 52–6.
2. Lee C, et al. Pharmacokinetics of tacrolimus (FK506) in liver transplant patients. Clin Pharmacol Ther 1993; 53: 181.
3. Gruber SA, et al. Pharmacokinetics of FK506 after intravenous and oral administration in patients awaiting renal transplantation. J Clin Pharmacol 1994; 34: 859–64.
4. Gonschior A-K, et al. Measurement of blood concentrations of FK506 (tacrolimus) and its metabolites in seven liver graft patients after the first dose by hplc-MS and microparticle enzyme immunoassay (MEIA). Br J Clin Pharmacol 1994; 38: 567–71.
5. Jusko WJ, et al. Pharmacokinetics of tacrolimus in liver transplant patients. Clin Pharmacol Ther 1995; 57: 281–90.
6. Venkataramanan R, et al. Clinical pharmacokinetics of tacrolimus. Clin Pharmacokinet 1995; 29: 404–30.

Uses and Administration

Tacrolimus is a potent macrolide immunosuppressant derived from Streptomyces tsukubaensis, and has actions similar to those of ciclosporin (see p.523). It is used to prevent or reverse rejection in patients receiving organ transplants, as indicated by the cross-references given below, and has been tried in a few patients with refractory auto-immune or immune-mediated disorders. Tacrolimus is also applied topically in the management of moderate to severe atopic eczema.

For **transplantation**, the initial dose recommended in the UK for liver graft recipients is 100 to 200 µg per kg body-weight daily by mouth, in 2 divided doses. The initial oral dose in kidney transplant patients is 150 to 300 µg per kg daily in 2 divided doses. Administration should begin about 6 hours after completion of liver grafting and within 24 hours of a kidney transplant. If the patient's condition does not permit oral administration, therapy may be commenced intravenously, by continuous 24-hour infusion: suggested initial doses are 10 to 50 µg per kg daily for liver transplants and 50 to 100 µg per kg daily for kidney transplants. In the USA, initial oral doses in patients with liver grafts are 100 to 150 µg per kg daily, in 2 divided doses, and in kidney grafts 200 µg per kg daily, in 2 divided doses. The recommended starting dose of intravenous tacrolimus is 30 to 50 µg per kg daily.

Dosage should be adjusted according to whole-blood or plasma trough concentrations in individual patients: it is suggested that most patients can be satisfactorily maintained at whole-blood concentrations below 20 ng per mL. Children generally require doses 1.5 to 2 times greater than those recommended in adults to achieve the same blood concentrations.

For the treatment of **atopic eczema**, where conventional therapies are ineffective or unsuitable, tacrolimus may be applied twice daily as a 0.03 or 0.1% ointment. Treatment should be continued for 1 week after resolution of signs and symptoms of the disease.

◊ Reviews.
1. Hooks MA. Tacrolimus, a new immunosuppressant—a review of the literature. Ann Pharmacother 1994; 28: 501–11.
2. Winkler M, Christians U. A risk-benefit assessment of tacrolimus in transplantation. Drug Safety 1995; 12: 348–57.
3. Plosker GL, Foster RH. Tacrolimus: a further update of its pharmacology and therapeutic use in the management of organ transplantation. Drugs 2000; 59: 323–89.

◊ Experience with tacrolimus in applications other than transplantation is extremely limited; however, there are some reports of such use, including in focal glomerulosclerosis,[1] chronic active hepatitis,[2] atopic eczema,[3-5] psoriasis,[6] polymyositis,[7] pyoderma gangrenosum,[8,9] and scleroderma (see p.505). In addition to their use in atopic eczema,[10] topical formulations have been tried in lichen planus.[11]

1. McCauley J, et al. FK 506 in steroid-resistant focal sclerosing glomerulonephritis of childhood. Lancet 1990; 335: 674.
2. Van Thiel DH, et al. Tacrolimus: a potential new treatment for autoimmune chronic active hepatitis: results of an open-label preliminary trial. Am J Gastroenterol 1995; 90: 771–6.
3. Nakagawa H, et al. Tacrolimus ointment for atopic dermatitis. Lancet 1994; 344: 883.
4. Aoyama H, et al. Successful treatment of resistant facial lesions of atopic dermatitis with 0.1% FK506 ointment. Br J Dermatol 1995; 133: 494–6.
5. Ruzicka T, et al. A short-term trial of tacrolimus ointment for atopic dermatitis. N Engl J Med 1997; 337: 816–21.

6. European FK 506 Multicentre Psoriasis Study Group. Systemic tacrolimus (FK 506) is effective for the treatment of psoriasis in a double-blind, placebo-controlled study. *Arch Dermatol* 1996; **132:** 419–23.

7. Oddis CV, *et al.* Tacrolimus in refractory polymyositis with interstitial lung disease. *Lancet* 1999; **353:** 1762–3.

8. Abu-Elmagd K, *et al.* Resolution of severe pyoderma gangrenosum in a patient with streaking leukocyte factor disease after treatment with tacrolimus (FK 506). *Ann Intern Med* 1993; **119:** 595–8.

9. Schuppe H-C, *et al.* Topical tacrolimus for pyoderma gangrenosum. *Lancet* 1998; **351:** 832.

10. Boguniewicz M, *et al.* A randomized, vehicle-controlled trial of tacrolimus ointment for treatment or atopic dermatitis in children. *J Allergy Clin Immunol* 1998; **102:** 637–44.

11. Vente C, *et al.* Erosive mucosal lichen planus: response to topical treatment with tacrolimus. *Br J Dermatol* 1999; **140:** 338–42.

Administration. The mean dose of tacrolimus required to produce a standard trough concentration of 10 to 15 ng per mL was reported to be 96% higher in 7 black renal graft recipients than in 20 such patients of white or Asian descent.[1]

There is limited evidence that children with hepatitis C required on average one-third of the dose of tacrolimus needed by children without the virus.[2]

1. Andrews PA, *et al.* Racial variation in dosage requirements of tacrolimus. *Lancet* 1996; **348:** 1446.

2. Moreno M, *et al.* Monitoring of tacrolimus as rescue therapy in pediatric liver transplantation. *Ther Drug Monit* 1998; **20:** 376–9.

Organ and tissue transplantation. Tacrolimus has been used both for primary immunosuppression and for the control of graft rejection. Much of the initial experience with the drug was for liver grafts, (see p.504), but it is also employed in the transplantation of heart (p.503), kidney (p.503), lung (p.504), and other organs (p.504). It has also been tried for the prophylaxis of graft-versus-host disease following bone marrow transplantation (p.502).

A few selected references to the use of tacrolimus in transplantation are given below.

1. Jordan ML, *et al.* FK506 "rescue" for resistant rejection of renal allografts under primary cyclosporine immunosuppression. *Transplantation* 1994; **57:** 860–5.

2. European FK506 Multicentre Liver Study Group. Randomised trial comparing tacrolimus (FK506) and cyclosporin in prevention of liver allograft rejection. *Lancet* 1994; **344:** 423–8.

3. The US Multicenter FK506 Liver Study Group. A comparison of tacrolimus (FK506) and cyclosporine for immunosuppression in liver transplantation. *N Engl J Med* 1994; **331:** 1110–15.

4. Klein A. Tacrolimus rescue in liver transplant patients with refractory rejection or intolerance or malabsorption of cyclosporine. *Liver Transpl Surg* 1999; **5:** 502–8.

5. Gruessner RW. Tacrolimus in pancreas transplantation: a multicenter analysis. *Clin Transplant* 1997; **11:** 299–312.

6. Gruessner RWG, *et al.* Suggested guidelines for the use of tacrolimus in pancreas/kidney transplantation. *Clin Transplant* 1998; **12:** 260–2.

7. Reichart B, *et al.* European Multicenter Tacrolimus (FK506) Heart Pilot Study: one-year results. *J Heart Lung Transplant* 1998; **17:** 775–81.

8. Wiesner RH. A long-term comparison of tacrolimus (FK506) versus cyclosporine in liver transplantation: a report of the United States FK506 Study Group. *Transplantation* 1998; **66:** 493–9.

9. Taylor DO, *et al.* A randomized, multicenter comparison of tacrolimus and cyclosporine immunosuppressive regimens in cardiac transplantation: decreased hyperlipidemia and hypertension with tacrolimus. *J Heart Lung Transplant* 1999; **18:** 336–45.

Preparations

Proprietary Preparations (details are given in Part 3)
Aust.: Prograf; *Austral.:* Prograf; *Belg.:* Prograft; *Canad.:* Prograf; *Denm.:* Prograf; *Fin.:* Prograf; *Fr.:* Prograf; *Ger.:* Prograf; *Hong Kong:* Prograf; *Irl.:* Prograf; *Israel:* Prograf; *Ital.:* Prograf; *Jpn:* Prograf; *Mex.:* Prograf; *Norw.:* Prograf; *NZ:* Prograf; *Port.:* Prograf; *Singapore:* Prograf; *Spain:* Prograf; *Swed.:* Prograf; *Switz.:* Prograf; *Thai.:* Prograf; *UK:* Prograf; *USA:* Prograf; Protopic.

Tamoxifen Citrate   (1865-h)

Tamoxifen Citrate *(BANM, USAN, rINNM).*
ICI-46474; Tamoxifeni Citras. (Z)-2-[4-(1,2-Diphenylbut-1-enyl)phenoxy]ethyldimethylamine citrate.
$C_{26}H_{29}NO,C_6H_8O_7 = 563.6$.
CAS — 10540-29-1 (tamoxifen); 54965-24-1 (tamoxifen citrate).

Pharmacopoeias. In *Eur.* (see p.vi), *Int.,* and *US.*

Tamoxifen citrate 15.2 mg is approximately equivalent to 10 mg of tamoxifen.

Pharmacopoeial description

Ph. Eur.: A white or almost white, polymorphic, crystalline powder. Slightly soluble in water and in acetone; soluble in methyl alcohol.

USP 25: A white, fine, crystalline powder. Very slightly soluble in water, in alcohol, in acetone, and in chloroform; soluble in methyl alcohol. Protect from light.

Adverse Effects

The most frequent adverse effects of tamoxifen are hot flushes. Other adverse effects include fluid retention, nausea, gastrointestinal intolerance, vaginal bleeding or discharge, pruritus vulvae, rashes, and dry

skin. There have also been reports of dizziness, headache, depression, confusion, fatigue, and muscle cramps. There may be an increased tendency to thromboembolism, and pulmonary embolism has occurred. Tumour pain and flare may be a sign of response, but hypercalcaemia, sometimes severe, has developed in patients with bony metastases. Transient thrombocytopenia and leucopenia have been reported. Blurred vision and loss of visual acuity, corneal opacities, retinopathies, and cataracts have occurred rarely. Tamoxifen has been associated with increased liver enzymes, and rarely with cholestasis and hepatitis. Hypertriglyceridaemia has occurred. Uterine fibroids and endometrial changes including hyperplasia and polyps may occur, and an increased incidence of endometrial carcinoma has been reported. Suppression of menstruation may occur in premenopausal women and cystic ovarian swellings have occasionally occurred.

Carcinogenicity. Tamoxifen has a stimulant effect on the endometrium (probably by acting as a partial oestrogen agonist) and its use has been associated with the development of endometrial polyps[1] and endometriosis,[2] and an increased risk of endometrial cancer.[3-5] The risk, which increases with duration of therapy, is generally agreed to be modest, and the clinical benefit in women with breast cancer outweighs any increased risk of endometrial neoplasm.[6-9] Women taking tamoxifen to prevent breast cancer have been estimated to have a 2.53-fold greater risk of developing endometrial carcinoma than untreated women.[10] The risk may increase with more prolonged use and a case-control study has reported that long-term (over 2 years) users may have a worse prognosis if endometrial cancer develops, due to less favourable history and stage.[11] It has been recommended that women with breast cancer taking tamoxifen should be given annual gynaecological examinations, and any unusual symptoms, including abnormal bleeding or spotting should be investigated promptly.[12] Women taking tamoxifen for prophylaxis of breast cancer should be monitored carefully for endometrial hyperplasia. If atypical hyperplasia develops, tamoxifen should be discontinued while the condition is treated and a hysterectomy should be considered before tamoxifen is re-started.[12] However, up to 39% of postmenopausal women taking tamoxifen show endometrial changes and as these seldom progress to cancer, the value of routine endometrial biopsies has been questioned.[7,8,12] It has been suggested that colour doppler ultrasonography, which distinguishes vascularised lesions, such as polyps and carcinomas, from avascular atrophic lesions may be a useful and noninvasive diagnostic tool.[13] There is some evidence that a levonorgestrel-releasing intrauterine device can protect against the uterine changes induced by tamoxifen.[14]

Tamoxifen has been shown to form DNA adducts in *rat* livers, and there has been speculation that it may cause liver cancer in humans. However, there is considerable interspecies variation in the metabolism of tamoxifen and several large-scale clinical trials did not find an increase in liver carcinogenicity in humans.[9] There is also little evidence of an increased relative risk of other secondary malignancies such as gastrointestinal or ovarian cancers.[9]

1. Corley D, *et al.* Postmenopausal bleeding from unusual endometrial polyps in women on chronic tamoxifen therapy. *Obstet Gynecol* 1992; **79:** 111–16.

2. Cano A, *et al.* Tamoxifen and the uterus and endometrium. *Lancet* 1989; **i:** 376.

3. Fornander T, *et al.* Adjuvant tamoxifen in early breast cancer: occurrence of new primary cancers. *Lancet* 1989; **i:** 117–20.

4. Gusberg SB. Tamoxifen for breast cancer: associated endometrial cancer. *Cancer* 1990; **65:** 1463–4.

5. van Leeuwen FE, *et al.* Risk of endometrial cancer after tamoxifen treatment of breast cancer. *Lancet* 1994; **343:** 448–52.

6. Baum M, *et al.* Endometrial cancer during tamoxifen treatment. *Lancet* 1994; **343:** 1291.

7. Bissett D, *et al.* Gynaecological monitoring during tamoxifen therapy. *Lancet* 1994; **344:** 1244.

8. Neven P, Vergote I. Should tamoxifen users be screened for endometrial lesions? *Lancet* 1998; **351:** 155–7.

9. Stearns V, Gelmann EP. Does tamoxifen cause cancer in humans? *J Clin Oncol* 1998; **16:** 779–92.

10. Fisher B, *et al.* Tamoxifen for prevention of breast cancer: report of the National Surgical Adjuvant Breast and Bowel Project P-1 Study. *J Natl Cancer Inst* 1998; **90:** 1371–88.

11. Bergman L, *et al.* Risk and prognosis of endometrial cancer after tamoxifen for breast cancer. *Lancet* 2000; **356:** 881–7.

12. American College of Obstetrics and Gynaecologists. ACOG Committee Opinion: tamoxifen and endometrial cancer. *Int J Gynaecol Obstet* 1996; **53:** 197–9.

13. Aleem FA, Predanic M. Endometrial changes in patients on tamoxifen. *Lancet* 1995; **346:** 1292–3.

14. Gardner FJE, *et al.* Endometrial protection from tamoxifen-stimulated changes by a levonorgestrel-releasing intrauterine system: a randomised controlled trial. *Lancet* 2000; **356:** 1711–17.

Effects on the blood. Pancytopenia developed shortly after beginning tamoxifen therapy in an elderly woman, and persisted for some years;[1] the patient eventually developed very severe leucopenia and died of infection.

1. Miké V, *et al.* Fatal neutropenia associated with long-term tamoxifen therapy. *Lancet* 1994; **344:** 541–2.

Effects on blood lipids. Tamoxifen has been reported to have a generally favourable effect on serum lipid profiles.[1] However, some cases of increased serum triglycerides in women with pre-existing hypertriglyceridaemia have been reported. Pancreatitis has also resulted. It has been suggested that tamoxifen should be used with caution in patients with hypertriglyceridaemia.[2,3]

1. Love RR, *et al.* Effects of tamoxifen on cardiovascular risk factors in postmenopausal women. *Ann Intern Med* 1991; **115:** 860–4.

2. Kanel KT, *et al.* Delayed severe hypertriglyceridaemia from tamoxifen. *N Engl J Med* 1997; **337:** 281.

3. Colls BM, George PM. Severe hypertriglyceridaemia and hypercholesterolaemia associated with tamoxifen use. *Clin Oncol* 1998; **10:** 270–1.

Effects on the cardiovascular system. ISCHAEMIC HEART DISEASE. For discussion of whether the effects of tamoxifen on lipid profiles can alter the incidence of ischaemic heart disease, see Cardiovascular Disorders under Uses and Administration, below.

STROKE. An excess risk of stroke was seen in tamoxifen compared with placebo recipients (5 cases versus 1) in a study of adjuvant tamoxifen.[1] A non-statistically significant increase in stroke was seen in a study on the use of tamoxifen for breast cancer prevention (0.5 excess cases per 1000 women per year).[2]

1. Dignam JJ, Fisher B. Occurrence of stroke with tamoxifen in NSABP B-24. *Lancet* 2000; **355:** 848–9.

2. Fisher B, *et al.* Tamoxifen for prevention of breast cancer: report of the National Surgical Adjuvant Breast and Bowel Project P-1 study. *J Natl Cancer Inst* 1998; **90:** 1371–88.

THROMBOEMBOLISM. A case control study,[1] involving 25 cases of deep-vein thrombosis or pulmonary embolism among more than 10 000 women with breast cancer, suggested that current use of tamoxifen was associated with an estimated relative risk of developing idiopathic venous thromboembolism of 7.1 (95% confidence interval 1.5 to 33). Past use of tamoxifen was not associated with a materially increased risk. In a randomised placebo-controlled study, there was an increase in pulmonary emboli in women receiving tamoxifen for cancer prevention (excess of 0.46 cases per 1000 women per year).[2] The fatality rate from pulmonary emboli in tamoxifen recipients was about 17%. In this study, there was also a trend towards more deep-vein thrombosis in tamoxifen recipients.

1. Meier CR, Jick H. Tamoxifen and risk of idiopathic venous thromboembolism. *Br J Clin Pharmacol* 1998; **45:** 608–12.

2. Fisher B, *et al.* Tamoxifen for prevention of breast cancer: report of the National Surgical Adjuvant Breast and Bowel Project P-1 study. *J Natl Cancer Inst* 1998; **90:** 1371–88.

Effects on the eyes. Tamoxifen has been reported to be associated with decreased visual acuity, corneal opacities and cataract, and retinopathy. The latter is sometimes progressive although in most cases it has shown improvement once the drug was discontinued.[1] A prospective study in 63 patients receiving tamoxifen 20 mg daily found evidence of decreased visual acuity, macular oedema, and retinal opacities in 4, occurring after 10 to 35 months of therapy.[2] A small excess risk of developing cataracts (3.1 extra per year per 1000 women) and of requiring cataract surgery (1.7 per year per 1000 women) was found in women receiving tamoxifen for up to 5 years to reduce the risk of breast cancer when compared with women receiving placebo.[3] Studies *in vitro* have suggested that cataract formation may be due to inhibition of chloride channels in the lens by tamoxifen or its hydroxy metabolite.[4]

1. Mihm LM, Barton TL. Tamoxifen-induced ocular toxicity. *Ann Pharmacother* 1994; **28:** 740–2.

2. Pavlidis NA, *et al.* Clear evidence that long-term, low-dose tamoxifen treatment can induce ocular toxicity. *Cancer* 1992; **69:** 2961–4.

3. Fisher B, *et al.* Tamoxifen for prevention of breast cancer: report of the National Surgical Adjuvant Breast and Bowel Project P-1 study. *J Natl Cancer Inst* 1998; **90:** 1371–88.

4. Zhang JJ, *et al.* Tamoxifen blocks chloride channels: a possible mechanism for cataract formation. *J Clin Invest* 1994; **94:** 1690–7.

Effects on the genito-urinary system. A report of persistent nocturnal priapism in a man receiving tamoxifen 20 mg daily.[1] Symptoms abated within 24 hours of withdrawing the drug. Impotence has been reported in men receiving tamoxifen therapy, and has been attributed to a paradoxical oestrogenic effect.[2]

1. Fernando IN, Tobias JS. Priapism in patient on tamoxifen. *Lancet* 1989; **i:** 436.

2. Collinson MP, *et al.* Two case reports of tamoxifen as a cause of impotence in male subjects with carcinoma of the breast. *Breast* 1993; **2:** 48–9.

Effects on the liver. Cholestasis and increased liver enzyme values have been reported following administration of tamoxifen to a 75-year-old patient.[1] Enzyme activity rose again on rechallenge with tamoxifen. Fatal hepatocellular necrosis and agranulocytosis, possibly exacerbated by continuing to take the drug once jaundice developed, has also been reported;[2] the authors noted that 4 cases of hepatic failure (3 fatal) and 5 cases of hepatitis (1 fatal) had been reported to the UK Committee on Safety of Medicines. Patients taking tamoxifen may also develop steatohepatitis,[3-6] which must be distinguished from alcohol-induced liver disease. Steatohepatitis is reversible on withdrawal of tamoxifen.[3,5,6] Bezafibrate has been tried to prevent progression of steatohepatitis and permit continued tamoxifen treatment.[7]

The symbol † denotes a preparation no longer actively marketed

For a report of peliosis hepatis and liver haemorrhage in a patient receiving tamoxifen and warfarin, see under Interactions, below.

For reference to the development of liver cancer in *animals* given tamoxifen, see Carcinogenicity, above.

1. Blackburn AM, *et al.* Tamoxifen and liver damage. *BMJ* 1984; **289:** 288.
2. Ching CK, *et al.* Tamoxifen-associated hepatocellular damage and agranulocytosis. *Lancet* 1992; **339:** 940.
3. Pratt DS, *et al.* Tamoxifen-induced steatohepatitis. *Ann Intern Med* 1995; **123:** 236.
4. Van Hoof M, *et al.* Tamoxifen-induced steatohepatitis. *Ann Intern Med* 1996; **124:** 855–6.
5. Ogawa Y, *et al.* Tamoxifen-induced fatty liver in patients with breast cancer. *Lancet* 1998; **351:** 725.
6. Oien KA, *et al.* Cirrhosis with steatohepatitis after adjuvant tamoxifen. *Lancet* 1999; **353:** 36–7.
7. Saibara T, *et al.* Bezafibrate for tamoxifen-induced non-alcoholic steatohepatitis. *Lancet* 1999; **353:** 1802.

Effects on the ovaries. Ovarian cysts are relatively common as an adverse effect in women receiving adjuvant tamoxifen: a study[1] in 95 such women reported the development of ovarian cysts in 6 of 16 (37.5%) who were premenopausal and in 5 of 79 postmenopausal women (6.3%). In 2 of the premenopausal women the cysts were complex. Two women underwent laparotomy for persistent cysts that were found to be benign, and 1 for leiomyoma; the cysts in the other 8 women resolved after withdrawal of tamoxifen. A study of 142 breast cancer patients receiving tamoxifen found ovarian cysts in 24 patients after treatment. Cyst development was more common in premenopausal women, patients with high oestrogen levels, and patients who did not receive high-dose chemotherapy.[2] There is a little evidence that tamoxifen increases the risk of ovarian cancer (see Carcinogenicity, above).

1. Shushan A, *et al.* Ovarian cysts in premenopausal and postmenopausal tamoxifen-treated women with breast cancer. *Am J Obstet Gynecol* 1996; **174:** 141–4.
2. Mourits MJE, *et al.* Ovarian cysts in women receiving tamoxifen for breast cancer. *Br J Cancer* 1999; **79:** 1761–64.

Effects on the skin and hair. A report of purpuric leucocytoclastic vasculitis in a patient receiving tamoxifen.[1] Withdrawal of the drug resulted in complete clearance of the lesions within 2 weeks; on re-introduction purpura developed again within a few days. The results suggest that tamoxifen can produce immune-mediated vascular damage.

Another report concerned a patient with white hair who developed darkening and repigmentation of the hair after about 2½ years of tamoxifen therapy.[2] Alopecia has also been reported in women receiving tamoxifen,[3,4] and in older patients the follicle may not recover.[3]

1. Drago F, *et al.* Tamoxifen and purpuric vasculitis. *Ann Intern Med* 1990; **112:** 965–6.
2. Hampson JP, *et al.* Tamoxifen-induced hair colour change. *Br J Dermatol* 1995; **132:** 483–4.
3. Gateley CA, Bundred NJ. Alopecia and breast disease. *BMJ* 1997; **314:** 481.
4. Ayoub J-PM, *et al.* Tamoxifen-induced female androgenetic alopecia in a patient with breast cancer. *Ann Intern Med* 1997; **126:** 745–6.

Precautions

Tamoxifen should not be used for the prophylaxis of breast cancer in women with a history of thromboembolic events. When used to treat breast cancer in such women, the risks and benefits should be considered. Tamoxifen should not be given during pregnancy. Women treated with tamoxifen should have routine gynaecological monitoring, and any abnormal symptoms such as menstrual irregularities, abnormal vaginal bleeding or discharge, or pelvic pain should be investigated (see also under Carcinogenicity, above). Periodic complete blood counts and liver function tests have been suggested.

Porphyria. Tamoxifen has been associated with acute attacks of porphyria and is considered unsafe in porphyric patients.

Pregnancy and breast feeding. Ambiguous genitalia have been reported in an infant exposed to tamoxifen *in utero*, although no causal link was demonstrated.[1] Another infant was born with Goldenhar's syndrome (oculoauriculovertebral dysplasia) following exposure to tamoxifen throughout a 26-week pregnancy.[2] The mother had also taken cocaine and marijuana during the first 6 weeks of pregnancy, and a bone scan using technetium Tc99m medronate had been performed. The US manufacturer of tamoxifen (Zeneca USA) was aware of 50 pregnancies in patients taking tamoxifen, resulting in 19 normal births, 8 terminations, 13 unknown outcomes and 10 infants with fetal or neonatal abnormalities.[2]

Tamoxifen has also been used to stimulate ovulation in women with luteal phase dysfunction. In one study tamoxifen was given to 40 women, resulting in 14 pregnancies. Although 9 infants were born with no congenital abnormalities, there were 5 spontaneous abortions, which the authors felt was unacceptably high.[3] Another study, using lower doses of tamoxifen (in some cases sequentially with clomifene), reported 32 pregnancies and only 3 spontaneous abortions in 65 treated patients.[4]

Tamoxifen has been shown to inhibit lactation in 60 puerperal women.[5] The manufacturers recommend that it should not be given to lactating women.

1. Tewari K, *et al.* Ambiguous genitalia in infant exposed to tamoxifen in utero. *Lancet* 1997; **350:** 183.
2. Cullins SL, *et al.* Goldenhar's syndrome associated with tamoxifen given to the mother during gestation. *JAMA* 1994; **271:** 1905–6.
3. Ruiz-Velasco V, *et al.* Chemical inducers of ovulation: comparative results. *Int J Fertil* 1979; **24:** 61–64.
4. Wu CH. Less miscarriage in pregnancy following tamoxifen treatment of infertile patients with luteal phase dysfunction as compared to clomiphene treatment. *Early Pregnancy* 1997; **3:** 301–5.
5. Masala A, *et al.* Inhibition of lactation and inhibition of prolactin release after mechanical breast stimulation in puerperal women given tamoxifen or placebo. *Br J Obstet Gynaecol* 1978; **85:** 134–7.

Radiotherapy. Reports of radiation recall, with erythema at the site of previous radiotherapy, in patients receiving tamoxifen.[1,2]

1. Parry BR. Radiation recall induced by tamoxifen. *Lancet* 1992; **340:** 49.
2. Extermann M, *et al.* Radiation recall in a patient with breast cancer treated for tuberculosis. *Eur J Clin Pharmacol* 1995; **48:** 77–8.

Interactions

There is a risk of increased anticoagulant effect if tamoxifen is given concomitantly with coumarin anticoagulants. Conversely, concomitant use with cytotoxic drugs may increase the risk of thromboembolic events. Tamoxifen increases the dopaminergic effect of bromocriptine.

Allopurinol. For reference to exacerbation of hepatotoxicity when tamoxifen was given concurrently with allopurinol, see under Allopurinol, p.398.

Antibacterials. *Rifampicin* was found to decrease plasma concentrations of tamoxifen in 10 healthy subjects. This was thought to be due to induction of cytochrome P450 isoenzyme CYP3A4 by rifampicin.[1]

1. Kivistö KT, *et al.* Tamoxifen and toremifene concentrations in plasma are greatly decreased by rifampin. *Clin Pharmacol Ther* 1998; **64:** 648–54.

Anticoagulants. A potentially life-threatening interaction between tamoxifen and *warfarin*, with marked prolongation of prothrombin times, haematuria, and haematoma, has been reported in a number of cases.[1-3] It has been suggested that in addition to enhancement of the effects of warfarin, competition for the same metabolic enzyme systems might reduce the activity of tamoxifen against tumours,[2] but such a suggestion remains speculative.

Peliosis hepatis and fatal liver haemorrhage have been reported in a patient who was receiving tamoxifen with warfarin and a liothyronine-thyroxine [levothyroxine] preparation.[4]

1. Lodwick R, *et al.* Life threatening interaction between tamoxifen and warfarin. *BMJ* 1987; **295:** 1141.
2. Tenni P, *et al.* Life threatening interaction between tamoxifen and warfarin. *BMJ* 1989; **298:** 93.
3. Ritchie LD, Grant SMT. Tamoxifen-warfarin interaction: the Aberdeen hospitals drug file. *BMJ* 1989; **298:** 1253.
4. Loomis GN, *et al.* A case of peliosis hepatis in association with tamoxifen therapy. *Am J Clin Pathol* 1983; **80:** 881–3.

Antineoplastics. *Aminoglutethimide* reduces serum tamoxifen concentrations, possibly by increasing its metabolism. For mention of an increased risk of haemolytic-uraemic syndrome in patients who received therapy with tamoxifen and *mitomycin* see Effects on the Kidneys, under Mitomycin, p.558.

Immunosuppressants. For the results of a study *in vitro* suggesting that tamoxifen might inhibit the metabolism of tacrolimus, see under Interactions of Tacrolimus, p.570.

Neuromuscular blockers. For reference to prolonged neuromuscular blockade in a patient given atracurium while receiving tamoxifen, see p.1334.

Pharmacokinetics

Peak plasma concentrations of tamoxifen occur 4 to 7 hours after an oral dose. It is extensively protein bound. Plasma clearance is reported to be biphasic and the terminal half-life may be up to 7 days. It is extensively metabolised, the major serum metabolite being *N*-desmethyltamoxifen. Several of the metabolites are stated to have similar pharmacological activity to the parent compound. Tamoxifen is excreted slowly in the faeces, mainly as conjugates. Small amounts are excreted in urine. Tamoxifen appears to undergo enterohepatic circulation.

Uses and Administration

Tamoxifen is an oestrogen antagonist with actions similar to those of clomifene citrate (see p.1466). It may also inhibit the production or release of cellular growth factors and induce apoptosis. It is used as the citrate in the adjuvant endocrine therapy of early breast cancer and is also given for the palliative treatment of advanced disease and for prophylaxis in women at increased risk. It has been tried in some other malignancies including tumours of the ovary and in malignant melanoma. Tamoxifen citrate is also used to stimulate ovulation in women with anovulatory infertility. See also the cross-references below.

Tamoxifen is given by mouth as the citrate. Doses are calculated in terms of the base. In the treatment of breast cancer, usual doses are the equivalent of tamoxifen 20 mg daily, in 2 divided doses or as a single daily dose. Doses of up to 40 mg daily may be given but no additional benefit has been demonstrated. Adjuvant therapy is normally continued for up to 5 years, although the optimum duration is still uncertain (p.491). Tamoxifen may also be given to reduce breast cancer incidence in women at high risk of the disease. The recommended dose is 20 mg daily for 5 years.

In the treatment of anovulatory infertility the usual dose is the equivalent of tamoxifen 20 mg daily on days 2 to 5 of the menstrual cycle, increased if necessary in subsequent cycles up to 80 mg daily. In women with irregular menstruation the initial course may be begun on any day, and a second course begun at a higher dose after 45 days if there has been no response. If the patient responds with menstruation, subsequent courses may begin on day 2 of the cycle.

Tamoxifen methiodide and the isomer*z*-tamoxifen are reported to be under investigation.

◊ Reviews.

1. Osborne CK. Tamoxifen in the treatment of breast cancer. *N Engl J Med* 1998; **339:** 1609–18.
2. Mitlak BH, Cohen FJ. Selective estrogen receptor modulators: a look ahead. *Drugs* 1999; **57:** 653–63.

Breast disorders, non-malignant. GYNAECOMASTIA. Tamoxifen, usually in doses of 10 mg twice daily, has been reported to be effective[1-4] in relieving pain and swelling in men or pubertal boys with gynaecomastia (p.1470). Tamoxifen has been recommended as a drug of choice in patients requiring drug therapy, given for 3 months to see if a response occurs.[5]

1. Jefferys DB. Painful gynaecomastia treated with tamoxifen. *BMJ* 1979; **1:** 1119–20.
2. Hooper PD. Puberty gynaecomastia. *J R Coll Gen Pract* 1985; **35:** 142.
3. McDermott MT, *et al.* Tamoxifen therapy for painful idiopathic gynecomastia. *South Med J* 1990; **83:** 1283–5.
4. Ting AC, *et al.* Comparison of tamoxifen with danazol in the management of idiopathic gynecomastia. *Am Surg* 2000; **66:** 38–40.
5. Braunstein GD. Gynecomastia. *N Engl J Med* 1993; **328:** 490–5.

MASTALGIA. Tamoxifen 20 mg daily has been shown to be effective in patients with both cyclic and non-cyclic mastalgia,[1] and improvement has also been reported at a lower dose of 10 mg daily.[2] However, there is concern about the use of tamoxifen in otherwise healthy premenopausal women,[3-5] particularly since many patients relapse on withdrawal,[2] and it has been recommended[6,7] that tamoxifen be reserved for patients who fail to respond to other drugs (see p.1470).

1. Fentiman IS, *et al.* Double-blind controlled trial of tamoxifen therapy for mastalgia. *Lancet* 1986; **i:** 287–8.
2. Fentiman IS, *et al.* Studies of tamoxifen in women with mastalgia. *Br J Clin Pract* 1989; **43** (suppl 68): 34–6.
3. Anonymous. Tamoxifen for benign breast disease. *Lancet* 1986; **i:** 305.
4. Smallwood JA, Taylor I. Tamoxifen for mastalgia. *Lancet* 1986; **i:** 680–1.
5. Fentiman IS, *et al.* Tamoxifen for mastalgia. *Lancet* 1986; **i:** 681.
6. Gateley CA, Mansel RE. Management of the painful and nodular breast. *Br Med Bull* 1991; **47:** 284–94.
7. Anonymous. Cyclical breast pain: what works and what doesn't. *Drug Ther Bull* 1992; **30:** 1–3.

Cardiovascular disorders. Tamoxifen has been reported to have a generally favourable effect on lipid profiles (see Effects on Blood Lipids, under Adverse Effects, above) suggesting it may have cardiovascular benefits. A cohort study of adjuvant tamoxifen found that the drug reduced the incidence of myocardial infarction,[1] and a randomised study of the same therapy also showed a trend towards a decrease in mortality from coronary heart disease.[2] However, in a much larger breast cancer prevention trial, tamoxifen did not reduce the risk of and mortality from ischaemic heart disease, which did not differ between placebo and tamoxifen recipients.[3,4] This lack of difference was independent of pre-existing cardiovascular disease.[4]

1. McDonald CC, *et al.* Scottish Cancer Trials Breast Group. Cardiac and vascular morbidity in women receiving adjuvant tamoxifen for breast cancer in a randomised trial. *BMJ* 1995; **311:** 977–80.
2. Constantino JP, *et al.* Coronary heart disease mortality and adjuvant tamoxifen therapy. *J Natl Cancer Inst* 1997; **89:** 776–82.

3. Fisher B, *et al.* Tamoxifen for prevention of breast cancer: report of the National Surgical Adjuvant Breast and Bowel Project P-1 study. *J Natl Cancer Inst* 1998; **90:** 1371–88.

4. Reis SE, *et al.* Cardiovascular effects of tamoxifen in women with and without heart disease: breast cancer prevention trial. *J Natl Cancer Inst* 2001; **93:** 16–21.

Disorders related to the menstrual cycle. Apart from cyclic mastalgia (see above) tamoxifen has been used in a number of cases in which disorders were linked to the hormonal changes of the menstrual cycle, including menorrhagia due to myometrial hypertrophy,[1] an auto-immune dermatitis due to postovulatory rises in serum progesterone,[2,3] and premenstrual migraine.[4] However, tamoxifen was thought to be a cause of recurrent migraines in another patient, due to its action at oestrogen receptors.[5]

1. Fraser IS. Menorrhagia due to myometrial hypertrophy: treatment with tamoxifen. *Obstet Gynecol* 1987; **70:** 505–6.

2. Wojnarowska F, *et al.* Progesterone-induced erythema multiforme. *J R Soc Med* 1985; **78:** 407–8.

3. Stephens CJM, *et al.* Autoimmune progesterone dermatitis responding to tamoxifen. *Br J Dermatol* 1989; **121:** 135–7.

4. O'Dea JPK, Davis EH. Tamoxifen in the treatment of menstrual migraine. *Neurology* 1990; **40:** 1470–1.

5. Mathew P, Fung F. Recapitulation of menstrual migraine with tamoxifen. *Lancet* 1999; **353:** 467–8.

Infertility. Tamoxifen is reported to be as effective as clomifene in the treatment of anovulatory infertility (p.1275) in women,[1] and may be useful in women in whom abnormal cervical mucus acts as a barrier to spermatozoa.[2] In infertile men, however, results are reportedly contradictory, with some studies reporting increase in sperm density and improved pregnancy rates while others failed to demonstrate any effect.[3] A meta-analysis of 5 trials in men with oligo/asthenospermia showed that although anti-oestrogen therapy improved serum testosterone concentrations, there was no increase in the overall pregnancy rate.[4]

1. Messinis IE, Nillius SJ. Comparison between tamoxifen and clomiphene for induction of ovulation. *Acta Obstet Gynecol Scand* 1982; **61:** 377–9.

2. Roumen FJME, *et al.* Treatment of infertile women with a deficient postcoital test with two antiestrogens: clomiphene and tamoxifen. *Fertil Steril* 1984; **41:** 237–43.

3. Howards SS. Treatment of male infertility. *N Engl J Med* 1995; **312:** 312–17.

4. Vandekerckhove P, *et al.* Clomiphene or tamoxifen for idiopathic oligo/asthenospermia, (updated 28 May 2001). Available in The Cochrane Library; Issue 4. Oxford: Update Software; 2001.

Malignant neoplasms. For reference to the use of tamoxifen in malignant neoplasms of breast, ovary, and in cutaneous melanoma, see under Choice of Antineoplastic, p.491, p.496, and p.499. The most common use of tamoxifen is for the endocrine therapy of oestrogen-receptor positive or early or advanced breast cancer, where there seems to be a clear benefit. How long such therapy should be continued, however, remains uncertain although recent results suggest that continuing therapy beyond 5 years may not increase the overall benefit. Extension of tamoxifen use to the attempted prophylaxis of breast cancer, however, has proved controversial (see p.492). Nonetheless, evidence that tamoxifen can reduce short-term incidence of breast cancer in some women at increased risk has been seen, and tamoxifen has been approved for such use in the USA.

Despite some positive data, tamoxifen does not appear to be effective in the treatment of hepatocellular carcinoma (see p.495).

Osteoporosis. Tamoxifen has been reported to have favourable effects on bone mass,[1-3] but any general role in the prevention of osteoporosis (p.745) seems unlikely given concerns about the carcinogenicity of tamoxifen. The effects are reported to be comparable in magnitude to those of calcium supplementation, and less than those of oestrogens (see also p.1464) or bisphosphonates. It has been suggested that such an effect on bone would provide an additional benefit in women receiving tamoxifen for the prophylaxis of breast cancer,[4] although others dispute the benefits.[5]

1. Love RR, *et al.* Effects of tamoxifen on bone mineral density in postmenopausal women with breast cancer. *N Engl J Med* 1992; **326:** 852–6.

2. Love RR, *et al.* Effect of tamoxifen on lumbar spine bone mineral density in postmenopausal women after 5 years. *Arch Intern Med* 1994; **154:** 2585–8.

3. Grey AB, *et al.* The effect of the antiestrogen tamoxifen on bone mineral density in normal late postmenopausal women. *Am J Med* 1995; **99:** 636–41.

4. Powles TJ. The case for clinical trials of tamoxifen for prevention of breast cancer. *Lancet* 1992; **340:** 1145–7.

5. Fugh-Berman A, Epstein S. Tamoxifen: disease prevention or disease substitution? *Lancet* 1992; **340:** 1143–5.

Preparations

BP 2001: Tamoxifen Tablets;
USP 25: Tamoxifen Citrate Tablets.

Proprietary Preparations (details are given in Part 3)

Aust.: Ebefen; Kessar; Nolvadex; Tamax; Tamofen; Tamoplex; *Austral.:* Estroxyn; Genox; Kessar; Nolvadex; Noxitem†; Tamosin; Tamoxen; *Belg.:* Nolvadex; Tamizam; *Braz.:* Nolvadex; Tamofen; Tecnotax; *Canad.:* Apo-Tamox; Nolvadex; Tamofen; Tamone†; *Denm.:* Tamofen; *Fin.:* Nolvadex; Tadex; Tamexin; Tamofen; *Fr.:* Kessar; Nolvadex; Oncotam; Tamofene; *Ger.:* duratamoxifen†; Jenoxifen; Kessar; Nolvadex; Nourytam; Tamobeta; Tamofen; Tamokadin; Tamox; Tamoxasta; Tamoxigenat;

Tamoximerck; Tamoxistad; Zemide; Zitazonium†; *Hong Kong:* Apo-Tamox; Nolvadex; Tamifen; Tamofen; Zitazonium; *Irl.:* Clonoxifen; Nolgen; Nolvadex; Tamofen; Tamox; *Israel:* Nolvadex; Tamofen; Tamoplex; Tamoxen; Tamoxi; *Ital.:* Kessar; Ledertam; Nolvadex; *Mex.:* Bilem; Cryoxifeno; Kessar; Novaldex; Ralsifen-X; Tamofen; Tamoxan; Taxus; Tecnofen; *Neth.:* Nolvadex; *Norw.:* Nolvadex; Tamofen; *NZ:* Genox; Nolvadex; Tamofen; *Port.:* Nolvadex; Tamoxan; *S.Afr.:* Kessar; Neophedan; Nolvadex; Tamoplex; *Singapore:* Apo-Tamox; Nolvadex; Tamofen; Tamoplex; *Spain:* Nolvadex; Oxeprax; *Swed.:* Ledertam†; Nolvadex; Tamaxin†; *Switz.:* Kessar; Nolvadex; *Thai.:* Nolvadex; Novofen; Tamofen; Tamoplex; Tuosomin; Zitazonium; *UAE:* Tamophar; *UK:* Emblon; Fentamox†; Nolvadex; Oestrifen†; Soltamox; Tamofen; *USA:* Nolvadex.

Tegafur   (1866-m)

Tegafur *(BAN, USAN, rINN)*.

FT-207; Ftorafur; MJF-12264; NSC-148958; WR-220066. 5-Fluoro-1-(tetrahydro-2-furyl)uracil; 5-Fluoro-1-(tetrahydro-2-furyl)pyrimidine-2,4(1H,3H)-dione.

$C_8H_9FN_2O_3$ = 200.2.
CAS — 17902-23-7.
ATC — L01BC03.

Pharmacopoeias. In *Jpn.*

Adverse Effects, Treatment, and Precautions

As for Fluorouracil, p.540.

Bone-marrow depression may be less severe with tegafur but gastrointestinal toxicity is often dose-limiting and central neurotoxicity is more common.

Pharmacokinetics

Tegafur is well absorbed from the gastrointestinal tract after oral administration. Following an intravenous dose it is reported to have a prolonged plasma half-life of 6 to 16 hours, and to be slowly metabolised to fluorouracil. It crosses the blood-brain barrier and is found in the CSF.

Uses and Administration

Tegafur is an antineoplastic agent which appears to act by the release of fluorouracil (p.540) in the body. It has been used in the management of a variety of malignant neoplasms including those of the breast, gallbladder, gastrointestinal tract, head and neck, liver and pancreas. Tegafur is given by mouth in doses up to 1.8 g daily. It is often given in combination with uracil (UFT). A dose of 300 mg of tegafur per m² body-surface daily, combined with uracil 672 mg per m² daily, may be given in 3 divided doses by mouth, together with calcium folinate, in the management of metastatic colorectal cancer. Doses are given for a cycle of 28 days, followed by 7 days without treatment. The drugs should be taken 1 hour before or after meals, and doses modified according to toxicity. Doses of 1 to 3 g per m² body-surface daily for 5 days have been administered intravenously.

Administration. Tegafur is an orally active prodrug of fluorouracil. Although it has been administered as a single agent, it is more commonly given in combination with drugs that modify its bioavailability and toxicity.[1] These include drugs such as uracil and gimestat (5-chlorodihydropyrimidine, CDHP) which can increase fluorouracil concentrations by inhibition of dihydropyrimidine dehydrogenase, the enzyme responsible for its further catabolism,[1-3] and oxonic acid (otastat), which inhibits another enzyme, orotate pyrimidine phosphoribosyl transferase, thought to play a role in the gastrointestinal toxicity of fluorouracil and its prodrugs.[2]

UFT consists of tegafur and uracil in the optimal molar ratio 1:4.[1] It is available for the treatment of colorectal cancer (p.493)—for doses, see above. A preliminary analysis of a large trial comparing oral UFT and calcium folinate therapy with intravenous fluorouracil and calcium folinate found both regimens to be well tolerated with similar levels of toxicity.[4]

S-1 is a combination of tegafur, gimestat and the potassium salt of oxonic acid in the molar ratio 10:4:10. It has been tried in gastric and colorectal cancers,[2,3] and initial results have suggested comparable activity to fluorouracil and calcium folinate in induction regimens, but the incidence of diarrhoea and stomatitis was reduced.

1. Adjei AA. A review of the pharmacology and clinical activity of new chemotherapy agents for the treatment of colorectal cancer. *Br J Clin Pharmacol* 1999; **48:** 265–77.

2. Sakata Y, *et al.* Late phase II study of novel oral fluoropyrimidine anticancer drug S-1 (1 M tegafur-0.4 M gimestat-1 M otastat potassium) in advanced gastric cancer patients. *Eur J Cancer* 1998; **34:** 1715–20.

3. Sugimachi K, *et al.* An early phase II study of oral S-1, a newly developed 5-fluorouracil derivative for advanced and recurrent gastrointestinal cancers. *Oncology* 1999; **57:** 202–10.

4. Smith R, *et al.* UFT plus calcium folinate vs 5-FU plus calcium folinate in colon cancer. *Oncology (Huntingt)* 1999; **13** (suppl 3): 44–7.

Preparations

Proprietary Preparations (details are given in Part 3)

Aust.: Ftoralon†; *Hong Kong:* Ftoral; Futraful; *Israel:* Ftoral; *Ital.:* Citofur; *Jpn:* Futraful†; *Spain:* Utefos.

Multi-ingredient: *Hong Kong:* UFT; *Jpn:* UFT; *Mex.:* UFT; *Singapore:* UFT; *Spain:* UFT; *UK:* Uftoral.

Teloxantrone Hydrochloride   (14993-b)

Teloxantrone Hydrochloride *(USAN, rINNM)*.

DuP-937; Moxantrazole Hydrochloride; NSC-355644. 7,10-Dihydroxy-2-{2-[(2-hydroxyethyl)amino]ethyl}-5-{[2-(methylamino)ethyl]amino}anthra[1,9-*cd*]pyrazol-6(2*H*)-one dihydrochloride monohydrate.

$C_{21}H_{25}N_5O_4,2HCl,H_2O$ = 502.4.
CAS — 91441-48-4 (teloxantrone); 132937-88-3 (teloxantrone hydrochloride).

Profile

Teloxantrone is an anthrapyrazole derivative with structural similarities to mitozantrone [mitoxantrone] (see p.559). It has been investigated for its antineoplastic properties as the dihydrochloride.

Temoporfin   (17451-r)

Temoporfin *(BAN, USAN, rINN)*.

EF-9; mTHPC. 3,3',3'',3'''-(7,8-Dihydroporphyrin-5,10,15,20-tetrayl)tetraphenol; 7,8-Dihydro-5,10,15,20-tetrakis(3-hydroxyphenyl)porphyrin.

$C_{44}H_{32}N_4O_4$ = 680.7.
CAS — 122341-38-2.

Profile

Temoporfin is a porphyrin derivative under investigation as a photosensitiser in the photodynamic therapy of various superficial neoplasms. It is reported to require smaller light doses, and therefore shorter treatment times, than some other photosensitisers.

◊ References.

1. Dilkes MG, *et al.* Treatment of head and neck cancer with photodynamic therapy: results after one year. *J Laryngol Otol* 1995; **109:** 1072–6.

2. Savary JF, *et al.* Photodynamic therapy for early squamous cell carcinomas of the esophagus, bronchi, and mouth with m-tetra (hydroxyphenyl) chlorin. *Arch Otolaryngol Head Neck Surg* 1997; **123:** 162–8.

3. Wierrani F, *et al.* Clinical effect of meso-tetrahydroxyphenylchlorine based photodynamic therapy in recurrent carcinoma of the ovary: preliminary results. *Br J Obstet Gynaecol* 1997; **104:** 376–8.

4. Fan KF, *et al.* Photodynamic therapy using mTHPC for malignant disease in the oral cavity. *Int J Cancer* 1997; **73:** 25–32.

Preparations

Proprietary Preparations (details are given in Part 3)
UK: Foscan.

Temozolomide   (2543-z)

Temozolomide *(BAN, USAN, rINN)*.

CCRG-81045; M&B-39831; NSC-362856; Sch-52365. 3,4-Dihydro-3-methyl-4-oxoimidazo[5,1-*d*][1,2,3,5]tetrazine-8-carboxamide.

$C_6H_6N_6O_2$ = 194.2.
CAS — 85622-93-1.
ATC — L01AX03.

Adverse Effects, Treatment, and Precautions

For general discussions see Antineoplastics, p.476, p.479, and p.480. Myelosuppression is dose-limiting. The nadir of cell counts usually occurs 21 to 28 days after treatment, with recovery within the next 1 to 2 weeks. Patients over 70 years of age are thought to be more susceptible to severe myelosuppression. Other common adverse effects include gastrointestinal disturbances, headache, rashes, fever, and somnolence. Asthenia, dizziness, malaise, pain, pruritus, and paraesthesia have also been reported.

Pharmacokinetics

Temozolomide is rapidly and completely absorbed from the gastrointestinal tract, with peak plasma concentrations occurring 0.5 to 1.5 hours after a dose. Food reduces the rate and extent of absorption. It readily crosses the blood-brain barrier and can be detected in the CSF. The plasma elimination half-life is 1.8 hours. Temozolomide undergoes spontaneous hydrolysis to its active metabolite monomethyltriazenoimidazole carboxamide (MTIC), which is then further hydrolysed to active and inactive compounds. It is largely eliminated by the kidneys, about 5 to 10% as unchanged drug.

Uses and Administration

Temozolomide is a compound that is believed to act by spontaneous generation of the same active metabolite as dacarbazine (p.531), but can be given by mouth. It is used in the treatment of malignant gliomas (p.490) such as glioblastoma multiforme and anaplastic astrocytoma. It has also been investigated in malignant melanoma (below).

The usual dose for malignant gliomas in adults and children over 3 years of age is 200 mg per m² body-surface daily by mouth for 5 days, repeated every 28 days. In patients who have received previous courses of chemotherapy the dose should be reduced to 150 mg per m² for the first cycle of therapy, but may be increased for subsequent courses if there is no haematological toxicity.

The symbol † denotes a preparation no longer actively marketed

Malignant Neoplasms. References.

1. Newlands ES, *et al.* Temozolomide: a review of its discovery, chemical properties, pre-clinical development and clinical trials. *Cancer Treat Rev* 1997; **23**: 35–61.
2. Bower M, *et al.* Multicentre CRC phase II trial of temozolomide in recurrent or progressive high-grade glioma. *Cancer Chemother Pharmacol* 1997; **40**: 484–8.
3. Yung WKA, *et al.* Multicenter phase II trial of temozolomide in patients with anaplastic astrocytoma or anaplastic oligoastrocytoma at first relapse. *J Clin Oncol* 1999; **17**: 2762–71.
4. Estlin EJ, *et al.* Phase I study of temozolomide in paediatric patients with advanced cancer. *Br J Cancer* 1998; **78**: 652–61.

MELANOMA. Temozolomide has been investigated[1,2] as a treatment for advanced metastatic melanoma (p.499). A phase III trial compared the overall survival-time in 305 patients treated with either oral temozolomide or intravenous dacarbazine in standard doses for up to 12 cycles of therapy. Temozolomide was found to be at least equivalent to dacarbazine in these patients, and there were no major differences in adverse effects.[2] However, median survival-times were short in both groups (7.7 months and 6.4 months respectively).

1. Bleehen NM, *et al.* Cancer research campaign phase II trial of temozolomide in metastatic melanoma. *J Clin Oncol* 1995; **13**: 910–13.
2. Middleton MR, *et al.* Randomized phase III study of temozolomide versus dacarbazine in the treatment of patients with advanced metastatic malignant melanoma. *J Clin Oncol* 2000; **18**: 158–66.

Preparations

Proprietary Preparations (details are given in Part 3)
Aust.: Temodal; *Austral.:* Temodal; *Denm.:* Temodal; *Fin.:* Temodal; *Fr.:* Temodal; *Ger.:* Temodal; *Neth.:* Temodal; *NZ:* Temodal; *Port.:* Temodal; *S.Afr.:* Temoxol; *Spain:* Temodal; *Swed.:* Temodal; *UK:* Temodal; *USA:* Temodar.

Teniposide (1867-b)

Teniposide (BAN, USAN, rINN).

ETP; NSC-122819; VM-26. (5R,5aR,8aS,9R)-5,8,8a,9-Tetrahydro-5-(4-hydroxy-3,5-dimethoxyphenyl)-9-(4,6-O-thenylidene-β-D-glucopyranosyloxy)isobenzofuro[5,6-f][1,3]benzodioxol-6(5aH)-one.
$C_{32}H_{32}O_{13}S = 656.7$.
CAS — 29767-20-2.
ATC — L01CB02.

◊ Precipitation occurred repeatedly in preparations for infusion containing teniposide 0.2 mg per mL in either glucose 5% or sodium chloride 0.9% injection, although previously such preparations had been used uneventfully.[1] Dilution of teniposide solutions to 0.1 mg per mL or less reduced the frequency of the problem, which could not be attributed to a change in formulation and remained unexplained.

1. Strong DK, Morris LA. Precipitation of teniposide during infusion. *Am J Hosp Pharm* 1990; **47**: 512.

Adverse Effects, Treatment, and Precautions

As for Etoposide, p.538. There is some evidence that teniposide may be a more potent mutagen and carcinogen than etoposide.

Hypersensitivity. The development of haemolytic anaemia and acute renal failure with tubular necrosis has been reported in a patient who developed an antibody to teniposide.[1] Anaphylactic reactions occur, and may be severe;[2,3] the frequency may be as high as 13% in neuroblastoma patients.[2] Although it has been suggested that hypersensitivity reactions might be due to the polyethoxylated castor oil in the injection vehicle,[2] studies *in vitro* suggest that it is the drug rather than the vehicle which is responsible.[3]

1. Habibi B, *et al.* Immune hemolytic anemia and renal failure due to teniposide. *N Engl J Med* 1982; **306**: 1091–3.
2. Siddall SJ, *et al.* Anaphylactic reactions to teniposide. *Lancet* 1989; **i**: 394.
3. Carstensen H, *et al.* Teniposide-induced hypersensitivity reactions in children. *Lancet* 1989; **ii**: 55.

Interactions

For a general outline of antineoplastic drug interactions, see p.481.

Antiepileptics. Clearance of teniposide was markedly increased by concomitant treatment with *phenytoin* or *phenobarbital*; the resultant decrease in systemic exposure to the antineoplastic might reduce its efficacy, and increased dosage would be needed in patients receiving anticonvulsants to guarantee equivalent exposure.[1]

1. Baker DK, *et al.* Increased teniposide clearance with concomitant anticonvulsant therapy. *J Clin Oncol* 1992; **10**: 311–15.

Ciclosporin. Concomitant administration of ciclosporin with teniposide has been reported[1] to produce a decrease in the clearance of the latter, with increased terminal half-life, peak plasma concentrations, and toxicity.

1. Toffoli G, *et al.* Cyclosporin A as a multidrug-resistant modulator in patients with renal cell carcinoma treated with teniposide. *Br J Cancer* 1997; **75**: 715–21.

Uses and Administration

Teniposide is an antineoplastic agent with general properties similar to those of etoposide (p.538). It has been given alone or with other antineoplastic agents in the treatment of refractory acute lymphoblastic leukaemia (p.484). It has been tried in various solid tumours including neuroblastoma (p.500), and retinoblastoma (p.500).

A variety of dosage regimens have been used, ranging from 30 mg per m² body-surface every 5 days, to 180 mg per m² weekly, as a single agent. Doses of 165 mg per m² twice weekly for 8 or 9 doses with cytarabine, or up to 250 mg per m² weekly for 4 to 8 weeks with vincristine and prednisone have been given in the treatment of refractory acute lymphoblastic leukaemia. Teniposide is given by slow intravenous infusion over at least 30 to 60 minutes, as a solution of up to 1 mg teniposide per mL in sodium chloride 0.9% injection or glucose 5% injection.

Preparations

Proprietary Preparations (details are given in Part 3)
Aust.: Vumon; *Austral.:* Vumon; *Belg.:* Vumon; *Braz.:* Vumon; *Canad.:* Vumon; *Denm.:* Vumon†; *Fr.:* Vehem†; *Ger.:* VM 26; *Hong Kong:* Vumon; *Israel:* Vumon; *Ital.:* Vumon; *Mex.:* Vumon; *Neth.:* Vumon; *NZ:* Vumon; *S.Afr.:* Vumon; *Singapore:* Vumon; *Spain:* Vumon; *Swed.:* Vumon; *USA:* Vumon.

Testolactone (9107-v)

Testolactone (USAN, rINN).

1-Dehydrotestololactone; NSC-23759; SQ-9538. D-Homo-17a-oxaandrosta-1,4-diene-3,17-dione.
$C_{19}H_{24}O_3 = 300.4$.
CAS — 968-93-4.
Pharmacopoeias. In US.

Pharmacopoeial description

USP 25: A white to off-white, practically odourless, crystalline powder. Soluble 1 in 4050 of water; soluble in alcohol and in chloroform; slightly soluble in benzyl alcohol; insoluble in ether and in petroleum spirit. Store in airtight containers.

Profile

Testolactone is a derivative of testosterone (see p.1492). It is reported to be an aromatase inhibitor that reduces peripheral oestrogen synthesis but has no significant androgenic activity. It is used in the palliative treatment of advanced breast cancer in postmenopausal women (p.491).

The usual dose is 250 mg four times daily by mouth.

It should not be given to men with breast cancer.

Peripheral neuropathies have occurred in patients receiving testolactone; gastrointestinal disturbances, pain or oedema of the extremities, hypertension, rashes, and glossitis have also been reported.

Congenital adrenal hyperplasia. For mention of the use of testolactone with flutamide to block androgenic effects in congenital adrenal hyperplasia, see p.1049.

Precocious puberty. Encouraging results have been reported using testolactone in the treatment of 5 girls with precocious puberty (p.1277) due to the McCune-Albright syndrome.[1] Testolactone blocked the synthesis of oestrogens from androgens by virtue of its being an aromatase inhibitor. Long-term therapy (for up to 5 years) was associated with continued benefit in many patients; however, signs of puberty were not always completely suppressed, in some cases perhaps because of difficulties in maintaining the dosage regimen.[2] Encouraging results were also obtained using a combination of testolactone and spironolactone in the treatment of familial precocious puberty in boys, although neither agent was successful when used alone.[3] Again, signs of a diminished response to treatment occurred with longer-term therapy; in this case control was restored by addition of a gonadorelin analogue.[4]

1. Feuillan PP, *et al.* Treatment of precocious puberty in the McCune-Albright syndrome with the aromatase inhibitor testolactone. *N Engl J Med* 1986; **315**: 1115–19.
2. Feuillan PP, *et al.* Long term testolactone therapy for precocious puberty in girls with the McCune-Albright syndrome. *J Clin Endocrinol Metab* 1993; **77**: 647–51.
3. Laue L, *et al.* Treatment of familial male precocious puberty with spironolactone and testolactone. *N Engl J Med* 1989; **320**: 496–502.
4. Laue L, *et al.* Treatment of familial male precocious puberty with spironolactone, testolactone, and deslorelin. *J Clin Endocrinol Metab* 1993; **76**: 151–5.

Preparations

USP 25: Testolactone Tablets.

Proprietary Preparations (details are given in Part 3)
Ger.: Fludestrin; *USA:* Teslac.

Thiotepa (1869-g)

Thiotepa (BAN, rINN).

NSC-6396; TESPA; Thiophosphamide; Triethylenethiophosphoramide; TSPA; WR-45312. Phosphorothioic tri(ethyleneamide); Tris(aziridin-1-yl)phosphine sulphide.
$C_6H_{12}N_3PS = 189.2$.
CAS — 52-24-4.
ATC — L01AC01.
Pharmacopoeias. In Br., Chin., Fr., Jpn, and US.

Pharmacopoeial description

BP 2001: Fine white, odourless or almost odourless, crystalline flakes. M.p. 52° to 57°. Freely soluble in water, in alcohol, and in chloroform. Store at 2° to 8°. At higher temperatures it polymerises and becomes inactive.

USP 25: Fine white, crystalline flakes, having a faint odour. M.p. 52° to 57°. Soluble 1 in 13 of water, 1 in about 8 of alcohol, 1 in about 2 of chloroform, and 1 in about 4 of ether. Store at 2° to 8° in airtight containers. Protect from light.

Incompatibility. Lyophilised thiotepa 1 mg per mL in 5% glucose injection was incompatible when mixed with solutions of cisplatin or minocycline hydrochloride.

1. Trissel LA, Martinez JF. Compatibility of thiotepa (lyophilized) with selected drugs during simulated Y-site administration. *Am J Health-Syst Pharm* 1996; **53**: 1041–5.

Stability. A solution of a lyophilised thiotepa preparation 0.5 mg per mL in 5% glucose injection was considered to be stable (less than 10% loss of thiotepa) for 8 hours at both 4° and 23°.[1] After 24 hours losses ranged between about 10 and 17%. At a higher thiotepa concentration (5 mg per mL) thiotepa was stable for 3 days at 23° and 14 days at 4°. Another study found that solutions containing 1 or 3 mg of thiotepa per mL in 0.9% sodium chloride were stable for 24 hours at 25° and 48 hours at 8°, but solutions containing 0.5% thiotepa needed to be used immediately.[2]

1. Xu QA, *et al.* Stability of thiotepa (lyophilized) in 5% dextrose injection at 4 and 23°C. *Am J Health-Syst Pharm* 1996; **53**: 2728–30.
2. Murray KM, *et al.* Stability of thiotepa (lyophilized) in 0.9% sodium chloride injection. *Am J Health-Syst Pharm* 1997; **54**: 2588–91.

Adverse Effects, Treatment, and Precautions

For general discussions, see Antineoplastics, p.476, p.479, and p.480.

Bone-marrow depression may be delayed; the nadir of white cell and platelet counts may occur up to 30 days after therapy has been discontinued. Bone-marrow depression has been reported after intravesical as well as parenteral administration, and has occasionally been prolonged or fatal.

Gastrointestinal disturbances, fatigue, weakness, headache and dizziness, hypersensitivity reactions, blurred vision and conjunctivitis may occur. Amenorrhoea and impaired fertility have also been reported. Local irritation, and occasionally frank chemical or haemorrhagic cystitis may follow intravesical instillation. Depigmentation of periorbital skin has occurred following the use of thiotepa eye drops. As with other alkylating agents, thiotepa is potentially mutagenic, teratogenic, and carcinogenic.

Thiotepa should be given with extreme care, if at all, to patients with pre-existing impairment of hepatic, renal, or bone-marrow function.

Pharmacokinetics

The absorption of thiotepa from the gastrointestinal tract is incomplete and unreliable; variable absorption also occurs from intramuscular injection sites. Absorption through serous membranes such as the bladder and pleura occurs to some extent. Following intravenous administration it is rapidly cleared from plasma, with an elimination half-life of about 2.4 hours. It is extensively metabolised: triethylenephosphoramide (TEPA), the primary metabolite, and some of the other metabolites have cytotoxic activity and are eliminated more slowly than the parent compound. It is excreted in the urine: less than 2% of a dose is reported to be present as unchanged drug or its primary metabolite.

Uses and Administration

Thiotepa is an ethyleneimine compound whose antineoplastic effect is related to its alkylating action. It has generally been replaced by cyclophosphamide (p.529) or other drugs. It is not a vesicant and may be given by all parenteral routes, as well as directly into tumour masses.

Instillations of thiotepa may be used in the adjuvant treatment of superficial tumours of the bladder (p.490) and in the control of malignant effusions (p.489). It has been given parenterally in the palliative treatment of various solid tumours, including those of breast and ovary (p.491 and p.496). It has also been given intrathecally to patients with malignant meningeal disease, and has been used, in the form of eye drops, as an adjunct to the surgical removal of pterygium, to prevent recurrence (see p.559).

Thiotepa is given in a variety of dosage schedules. In general, initial doses to suit the individual patient are followed by maintenance doses given at intervals of one to 4 weeks. Blood counts are recommended before and during administration and should continue for at least 3 weeks after stopping therapy. Thiotepa should not be given if the white cell count falls below 3000 per mm³ or the platelet count below 150 000 per mm³ and treatment should be discontinued if the white cell count falls rapidly. Dosage should be reduced in patients with lesser degrees of leucopenia.

In the treatment of bladder cancer thiotepa in doses up to 60 mg may be instilled in 30 to 60 mL of sterile water into the bladder of a patient previously dehydrated for 8 to 12 hours, and retained if possible for 2 hours. The instillation may be repeated weekly for up to 4 weeks. Similar instillations have been given at intervals of 1 to 2 weeks, for up to 8 instillations in the prophylaxis of recurrence after surgical removal of bladder cancer. Single doses of 90 mg in 100 mL of sterile water have also been used prophylactically. For malignant effusions, suggested doses of up to 60 mg of thiotepa in 20 to 60 mL of sterile water may be instilled after aspiration; in the USA the usual recommended dose is 600 to 800 µg per kg body-weight, a dose similar to that suggested for injection directly into tumours. Thiotepa for local use may be mixed with solutions of procaine and adrenaline [epinephrine].

Intramuscular and intravenous dosage regimens vary considerably; several regimens have employed courses of 15 mg daily for 4 days. In the USA a suggested dose is 300 to 400 µg per kg given at 1- to 4-week intervals. A solution containing 1 mg per mL has been tried intrathecally in doses of up to 10 mg.

A 0.05% solution has been instilled as eye drops every 3 hours for up to 6 weeks following surgical removal of pterygium in order to reduce the likelihood of recurrence.

A dose of 60 mg weekly has been instilled into the urethra for the treatment of condylomata acuminata (genital warts). Topical application of thiotepa has also been used for condylomata.

Preparations

BP 2001: Thiotepa Injection;
USP 25: Thiotepa for Injection.

Proprietary Preparations (details are given in Part 3)
Belg.: Ledertepa; *Braz.:* Onco Tiotepa; *Ital.:* Thioplex; *Jpn:* Tespamin†; *Neth.:* Ledertepa; *Spain:* Onco Tiotepa; *USA:* Thioplex.

Tioguanine   (1868-v)

Tioguanine *(BAN, rINN)*.

NSC-752; 6-TG; Thioguanine *(USAN)*; 6-Thioguanine; WR-1141. 2-Aminopurine-6(1*H*)-thione; 2-Amino-6-mercaptopurine; 2-Aminopurine-6-thiol.

$C_5H_5N_5S = 167.2$.

CAS — 154-42-7 (anhydrous tioguanine); 5580-03-0 (tioguanine hemihydrate).

ATC — L01BB03.

Pharmacopoeias. In Br.
US permits anhydrous or hemihydrate.

Pharmacopoeial description

BP 2001: A pale yellow, odourless or almost odourless, crystalline powder. Practically insoluble in water, in alcohol, and in chloroform; dissolves in dilute solutions of alkali hydroxides.

USP 25: A pale yellow, odourless or practically odourless, crystalline powder. Insoluble in water and in chloroform; soluble 1 in 7700 of alcohol; freely soluble in dilute solutions of alkali hydroxides. Store in airtight containers.

Adverse Effects, Treatment, and Precautions

As for Mercaptopurine, p.552.

In some patients, gastrointestinal reactions are reported to be less frequent than with mercaptopurine. Normal doses of tioguanine may be employed when it is used with allopurinol.

Effects on the blood. For the view that it may be possible to predict those individuals likely to experience severe bone-marrow depression with tioguanine, see under Azathioprine, p.509.

Effects on the liver. There have been occasional reports of hepatic veno-occlusive disease attributed to tioguanine.[1,2]

1. Gill RA, *et al.* Hepatic veno-occlusive disease caused by 6-thioguanine. *Ann Intern Med* 1982; **96:** 58–60.
2. Krivoy N, *et al.* Reversible hepatic veno-occlusive disease and 6-thioguanine. *Ann Intern Med* 1982; **96:** 788.

Handling and disposal. For reference to a method for the destruction of tioguanine in wastes, see Mercaptopurine, p.552.

Pharmacokinetics

Tioguanine is incompletely and variably absorbed from the gastrointestinal tract; on average about 30% of a dose is absorbed following oral administration. It is rapidly activated in the body by intracellular conversion to its nucleotide, thioguanylic acid and its thioguanosine phosphate derivatives. With repeated doses increasing amounts of the nucleotide are incorporated into DNA. Very little unchanged tioguanine has been detected circulating in the blood but the half-

life of the nucleotide in the tissues is prolonged. Tioguanine is inactivated primarily by methylation to aminomethylthiopurine; small amounts are deaminated to thioxanthine, and may go on to be oxidised by xanthine oxidase to thiouric acid, but inactivation is essentially independent of xanthine oxidase and is not affected by inhibition of the enzyme.

It is excreted in the urine almost entirely as metabolites; only negligible amounts of tioguanine have been detected. Tioguanine does not appear to cross the blood-brain barrier to a significant extent; very little is found in cerebrospinal fluid after normal clinical doses. It crosses the placenta.

Uses and Administration

Tioguanine is an analogue of the naturally occurring purine, guanine, and is an antineoplastic with actions and uses similar to those of mercaptopurine (p.552). It appears to cause fewer gastrointestinal reactions but cross-resistance exists between it and mercaptopurine so that patients who do not respond to one are unlikely to respond to the other.

Tioguanine maybe given by mouth with other agents, usually cytarabine and an anthracycline, in the induction and maintenance of remissions in acute myeloid leukaemia (p.485) although there is some uncertainty about its value. It has also been used in other malignancies including acute lymphoblastic leukaemia (p.484) and chronic myeloid leukaemia.

Doses up to 200 mg per m² body-surface daily have been given for 5 to 20 days as part of a combined induction regimen. A dose of 2 to 2.5 mg per kg body-weight daily increased after 4 weeks, if there is no response or toxicity allows, to 3 mg per kg daily may be given to adults and children in those rare cases when single agent therapy is considered appropriate.

Blood counts should be made frequently, particularly during induction and when tioguanine is given with other antineoplastic agents. Therapy should be withdrawn at the first sign of severe bone-marrow depression.

It has been given intravenously as tioguanine sodium.

Psoriasis. A report of the use of tioguanine, in doses ranging from 20 mg twice weekly to 120 mg daily, in the management of patients with refractory psoriasis.[1] Dramatic improvement occurred in 14 of 18 patients, but a further 2 were unable to tolerate the drug. Myelosuppression was the principal toxic effect and it was suggested that thiopurine methyltransferase activity could be measured as a basis to determine initial dosage and the risk of toxicity. For the conventional management of psoriasis see p.1106.

1. Mason C, Krueger GG. Thioguanine for refractory psoriasis. *J Am Acad Dermatol* 2001; **44:** 67–72.

Preparations

BP 2001: Tioguanine Tablets;
USP 25: Thioguanine Tablets.

Proprietary Preparations (details are given in Part 3)
Austral.: Lanvis; *Belg.:* Lanvis; *Braz.:* Lanvis; *Canad.:* Lanvis; *Hong Kong:* Lanvis; *Irl.:* Lanvis; *Israel:* Lanvis; *Neth.:* Lanvis; *NZ:* Lanvis; *S.Afr.:* Lanvis; *Singapore:* Lanvis; *Swed.:* Lanvis; *Switz.:* Lanvis; *Thai.:* Lanvis; *UK:* Lanvis.

Tirapazamine   (17120-h)

Tirapazamine *(USAN, rINN)*.

Win-59075. 3-Amino-1,2,4-benzotriazine 1,4-dioxide.

$C_7H_6N_4O_2 = 178.1$.

CAS — 27314-97-2.

Profile

Tirapazamine is reported to be reduced in hypoxic cells to an active anion that causes DNA strand breaks. It is under investigation for its cytotoxic actions, alone or in combination with cisplatin or radiotherapy. Adverse effects reported with tirapazamine include nausea and vomiting, diarrhoea, skin rashes, muscle cramps and fatigue; myelosuppression is said to be rare.

◊ References.

1. Von Pawel J, *et al.* Tirapazamine plus cisplatin versus cisplatin in advanced non-small-cell lung cancer: a report of the international CATAPULT I study group. *J Clin Oncol* 2000; **18:** 1351–9.

Topotecan Hydrochloride   (15104-s)

Topotecan Hydrochloride *(BANM, USAN, pINNM)*.

SKF-104864A; SKFS-104864-A. (*S*)-10-Dimethylaminomethyl-4-ethyl-4,9-dihydroxy-1*H*-pyrano[3′,4′:6,7]indolizino[1,2*b*]quinoline-3,14(4*H*,12*H*)-dione hydrochloride.

$C_{23}H_{23}N_3O_5$,HCl = 457.9.

CAS — 123948-87-8 (topotecan); 119413-54-6 (topotecan hydrochloride).

Topotecan hydrochloride 1.09 mg is approximately equivalent to 1 mg of topotecan.

Incompatibility. Topotecan hydrochloride was found to degrade to 88.7% of its original concentration over 4 hours when mixed with ticarcillin sodium or potassium clavulanate. It was also found to be incompatible with dexamethasone sodium phosphate and fluorouracil.[1] When mixed with mitomycin solution an immediate colour change took place and concentrations of mitomycin fell by 15 to 20% over 4 hours. The pH of the mixtures remained constant at 3.3 to 3.5.

1. Mayron D, Gennaro AR. Stability and compatibility of topotecan hydrochloride with selected drugs. *Am J Health-Syst Pharm* 1999; **56:** 875–81.

Adverse Effects and Precautions

For general discussions, see Antineoplastics, p.476 and p.480. Neutropenia is common and is usually dose-limiting. The nadir of white cell count usually occurs about 9 to 12 days after a dose. Thrombocytopenia and anaemia are less frequent. Gastrointestinal disturbances are also common. Other adverse effects include fatigue and weakness, alopecia, malaise, and hyperbilirubinaemia.

Topotecan should be avoided in patients with pre-existing bone-marrow depression, and the manufacturers suggest that it should not be given in severe renal or hepatic impairment. Topotecan has been reported to produce fetal death and malformations in *animals*.

Pharmacokinetics

Topotecan is widely distributed following intravenous administration. It undergoes reversible hydrolysis of the lactone ring to the inactive hydroxy acid form; only small amounts are demethylated in the liver. A significant proportion of a dose is excreted in urine. Topotecan has a terminal half-life of 2 to 3 hours.

◊ References.

1. Herben VMM, *et al.* Clinical pharmacokinetics of topotecan. *Clin Pharmacokinet* 1996; **31:** 85–102.

Uses and Administration

Like irinotecan (p.549), topotecan is a semisynthetic derivative of the alkaloid camptothecin that exerts its antineoplastic activity by inhibition of topoisomerase I. It is used in the treatment of metastatic carcinoma of the ovary refractory to other therapy (see p.496) and in small cell lung cancer (p.496) refractory to standard therapy. Topotecan is also under investigation in the management of other malignancies.

Topotecan is given as the hydrochloride but doses are calculated in terms of the base. The recommended initial dose is the equivalent of topotecan 1.5 mg per m² body-surface, given by intravenous infusion over 30 minutes, on days 1 to 5 of a 21-day course. A minimum of 4 courses should be given, provided that blood counts and haemoglobin have recovered adequately.

If severe neutropenia occurs in any course the dose in the subsequent courses may be reduced by 0.25 mg per m², or a granulocyte colony-stimulating factor may be given from day 6 of the course once topotecan administration is complete. If severe toxicity recurs once the dose has been reduced to 1 mg per m² withdrawal of topotecan may be required. Dosage should also be reduced after severe thrombocytopenia, and in patients with impaired renal function: halving of the initial dose is recommended in those with a creatinine clearance between 20 and 39 mL per minute.

Oral formulations of topotecan are under investigation.

◊ References.

1. Macdonald D, *et al.* Phase II study of topotecan in patients with recurrent malignant glioma. *Ann Oncol* 1996; **7:** 205–7.

The symbol † denotes a preparation no longer actively marketed

2. Schiller JH, *et al.* Phase II study of topotecan in patients with extensive-stage small-cell carcinoma of the lung: an Eastern Co-operative Oncology Group Trial. *J Clin Oncol* 1996; **14:** 2345–52.
3. Beran M, *et al.* Topotecan, a topoisomerase I inhibitor, is active in the treatment of myelodysplastic syndrome and chronic mye-lomonocytic leukemia. *Blood* 1996; **88:** 2473–9.
4. Ardizzoni A, *et al.* Topotecan, a new active drug in the second-line treatment of small-cell lung cancer: a phase II study in pa-tients with refractory and sensitive disease. *J Clin Oncol* 1997; **15:** 2090–6.
5. ten Bokkel Huinink W, *et al.* Topotecan versus paclitaxel for the treatment of recurrent epithelial ovarian cancer. *J Clin Oncol* 1997; **15:** 2183–93.
6. Cersosimo RJ. Topotecan: a new topoisomerase I inhibiting an-tineoplastic agent. *Ann Pharmacother* 1998; **32:** 1332–43.
7. Estey EH. Topotecan for myelodysplastic syndromes. *Oncology (Huntingt)* 1998; **12:** 81–6.
8. von Pawel J, *et al.* Topotecan versus cyclophosphamide, doxoru-bicin, and vincristine for the treatment of recurrent small-cell lung cancer. *J Clin Oncol* 1999; **17:** 658–67.

Preparations

Proprietary Preparations (details are given in Part 3)
Aust.: Hycamtin; *Austral.:* Hycamtin; *Belg.:* Hycamtin; *Canad.:* Hycamtin; *Denm.:* Hycamtin; *Fin.:* Hycamtin; *Fr.:* Hycamtin; *Ger.:* Hycamtin; *Hong Kong:* Hycamtin; *Irl.:* Hycamtin; *Israel:* Hycamtin; *Ital.:* Hycamtin; *Neth.:* Hycamtin; *Norw.:* Hycamtin; *Port.:* Hycamtin; *S.Afr.:* Hycamtin; *Singapore:* Hycamtin; *Spain:* Hycamtin; *Swed.:* Hycamtin; *Switz.:* Hycamtin; *Thai.:* Hycamtin; *UK:* Hycamtin; *USA:* Hycamtin.

Toremifene (2830-f)

Toremifene (BAN, rINN).

FC-1157a (toremifene citrate). (Z)-2-[4-(4-Chloro-1,2-diphe-nylbut-1-enyl)phenoxy]ethyldimethylamine.
$C_{26}H_{28}ClNO = 406.0$.
CAS — 89778-26-7 (toremifene); 89778-27-8 (toremifene citrate).
ATC — L02BA02.

NOTE. Toremifene Citrate is *USAN*.

Adverse Effects and Precautions

As for Tamoxifen Citrate, p.571.

Use of toremifene is contra-indicated in patients with pre-exist-ing endometrial hyperplasia, or in those with severe cardiovas-cular disease or hepatic impairment.

Interactions

Toremifene is metabolised by cytochrome P450 isoenzyme CYP3A4, and potent enzyme-inducing drugs such as *pheny-toin*, *phenobarbital* and *carbamazepine*, might be expected to increase toremifene metabolism, thereby lowering the serum concentration. Conversely, azole antifungals and macrolide an-tibiotics may inhibit toremifene metabolism by inhibiting the isoenzyme.

Concomitant use of drugs that decrease renal calcium excre-tion, such as thiazide diuretics, may increase the incidence of hypercalcaemia.

Antibacterials. *Rifampicin* was found to decrease plasma concentrations of toremifene in 9 volunteers. This was thought to be due to induction of cytochrome P450 CYP3A4 by ri-fampicin.[1]

1. Kivistö KT, *et al.* Tamoxifen and toremifene concentrations in plasma are greatly decreased by rifampin. *Clin Pharmacol Ther* 1998; **64:** 648–54.

Uses and Administration

Toremifene is an anti-oestrogen with properties similar to those of tamoxifen (p.571), and is used similarly in the treatment of advanced breast cancer (p.491). It has also been investigated as an adjuvant for the treatment of lung tumours.

Toremifene is given by mouth as the citrate in doses equivalent to 60 mg of the base daily.

◊ References.

1. Wiseman LR, Goa KL. Toremifene: a review of its pharmacolog-ical properties and clinical efficacy in the management of ad-vanced breast cancer. *Drugs* 1997; **54:** 141–60.
2. Anonymous. Toremifene and letrozole for advanced breast can-cer. *Med Lett Drugs Ther* 1998; **40:** 43–5.
3. Holli K. Adjuvant trials of toremifene vs tamoxifen: the Europe-an experience. *Oncology (Huntingt)* 1998; **12** (suppl 5): 23–7.
4. Holli K, *et al.* Safety and efficacy results of a randomized trial comparing adjuvant toremifene and tamoxifen in postmenopau-sal patients with node-positive breast cancer. *J Clin Oncol* 2000; **18:** 3487–94.

Preparations

Proprietary Preparations (details are given in Part 3)
Aust.: Fareston; *Austral.:* Fareston; *Belg.:* Fareston; *Denm.:* Fare-ston†; *Fin.:* Fareston; *Fr.:* Fareston; *Ger.:* Fareston; *Irl.:* Fareston; *Ital.:* Fareston; *Mex.:* Fareston; *Neth.:* Fareston†; *NZ:* Fareston; *Port.:* Fareston; *S.Afr.:* Fareston; *Spain:* Fareston; *Swed.:* Fares-ton; *Switz.:* Fareston; *Thai.:* Fareston; *UK:* Fareston; *USA:* Fare-ston.

Trastuzumab (15020-v)

Trastuzumab (BAN, rINN).

HER-2 Monoclonal Antibody; rhuMAb HER2.
CAS — 180288-69-1.
ATC — L01XC03.

Adverse Effects, Treatment, and Precautions

Trastuzumab has been associated with fatal hypersensitivity re-actions, infusion reactions, and pulmonary events including acute respiratory distress syndrome. These usually occur after the first dose of trastuzumab and are more common in patients with reduced lung function. Use of trastuzumab is contra-indi-cated in patients with severe dyspnoea at rest. Cardiac dysfunc-tion and congestive heart failure may also occur and left ventricular function should be monitored before and during therapy. The risk of cardiotoxicity is increased if trastuzumab is given with or after doxorubicin (see p.535).

There is an increase in incidence of leucopenia and anaemia when trastuzumab is given with chemotherapy, but it rarely causes myelosuppression when given as a single agent. Diar-rhoea occurs in 25% of patients given trastuzumab. Other com-mon adverse effects include chills, fever, headache, arthralgia, myalgia, and rashes.

Uses and Administration

Trastuzumab is a monoclonal antibody directed against a cell surface protein produced by the HER2 gene, a growth-factor receptor which is overexpressed in about one-third of all breast cancers. Trastuzumab is used in the treatment of advanced breast cancer with such characteristics. The recommended dose, alone or in combination with paclitaxel, is 4 mg per kg body-weight initially, by intravenous infusion in 0.9% sodium chloride over 90 minutes. This may be followed by 2 mg per kg over 30 minutes at weekly intervals.

HER2 may also be overexpressed in other epithelial cancers, and trastuzumab is under investigation for use in non-small cell lung cancer, bladder, and ovarian malignancies.

◊ References.

1. Baselga J, *et al.* Phase II study of weekly intravenous recom-binant humanized anti-p185HER2 monoclonal antibody in pa-tients with HER2/neu-overexpressing metastatic breast cancer. *J Clin Oncol* 1996; **14:** 737–44.
2. Cobleigh MA, *et al.* Multinational study of the efficacy and safe-ty of humanized anti-HER2 monoclonal antibody in women who have HER2-overexpressing metastatic breast cancer that has pro-gressed after chemotherapy for metastatic disease. *J Clin Oncol* 1999; **17:** 2639–48.
3. Treish L, *et al.* Pharmacology and therapeutic use of trastuzumab in breast cancer. *Am J Health-Syst Pharm* 2000; **57:** 2063–79.
4. Agus DB, *et al.* HER-2/neu as a therapeutic target in non-small cell lung cancer, prostate cancer, and ovarian cancer. *Semin On-col* 2000; **27** (suppl 11): 53–63.
5. Seidman AD, *et al.* Weekly trastuzumab and paclitaxel therapy for metastatic breast cancer with analysis of efficacy by HER2 immunophenotype and gene amplification. *J Clin Oncol* 2001; **19:** 2587–95.
6. Eiermann W, *et al.* Trastuzumab combined with chemotherapy for the treatment of HER2-positive metastatic breast cancer: piv-otal trial data. *Ann Oncol* 2001; **12** (suppl 1): S57–S62.
7. Slamon DJ, *et al.* Use of chemotherapy plus a monoclonal anti-body against HER2 for metastatic breast cancer that overexpress-es HER2. *N Engl J Med* 2001; **344:** 783–92.

Preparations

Proprietary Preparations (details are given in Part 3)
Austral.: Herceptin; *Fr.:* Herceptin; *Irl.:* Herceptin; *Singapore:* Herceptin; *Switz.:* Herceptin; *UK:* Herceptin; *USA:* Herceptin.

Treosulfan (1871-d)

Treosulfan (BAN, rINN).

Dihydroxybusulphan; NSC-39069. L-Threitol 1,4-dimethane-sulphonate.
$C_6H_{14}O_8S_2 = 278.3$.
CAS — 299-75-2.
ATC — L01AB02.

Profile

Treosulfan is an antineoplastic agent related to busulfan (p.513), which is reported to act by alkylation after conversion *in vivo* to epoxide compounds. It is used palliatively or as an adjunct to surgery mainly in the treatment of ovarian cancer (p.496).

Treosulfan 1 g daily is given by mouth in 4 divided doses for 2 or 4 weeks followed by the same period without treatment. Al-ternatively 1.5 g daily in 3 divided doses may be given for 1 week, followed by 3 weeks without therapy. The cycle is then repeated, the dose being adjusted if necessary according to the effect on bone marrow. Lower doses should be used if treat-ment with other antineoplastic drugs or radiotherapy is being given concomitantly. Treosulfan may also be given intrave-nously in doses of 3 to 8 g per m² body-surface every one to three weeks. Doses larger than 3 g per m² should be given by infusion at a rate of 3 g per m² every 5 to 10 minutes. Doses up to 1.5 g per m² have been given intraperitoneally.

Regular blood counts should be made and treatment should be interrupted if the white-blood cell count is less than 3000 per mm³ or the platelet count below 100 000 per mm³. Because bone-marrow depression may be cumulative the interval be-tween blood counts should be reduced after the second course of treatment with treosulfan.

Preparations

Proprietary Preparations (details are given in Part 3)
Ger.: Ovastat.

Trimetrexate Glucuronate (19502-s)

Trimetrexate Glucuronate (BANM, USAN, rINNM).

CI-898 (trimetrexate); JB-11 (trimetrexate); NSC-352122; NSC-249008 (trimetrexate). 5-Methyl-6-(3,4,5-trimethoxy-anilinomethyl)quinazolin-2,4-diyldiamine mono-D-glucuronate.
$C_{19}H_{23}N_5O_3,C_6H_{10}O_7 = 563.6$.
CAS — 52128-35-5 (trimetrexate); 82952-64-5 (trimetrex-ate glucuronate).

Trimetrexate glucuronate 1.53 mg is approximately equivalent to 1 mg of trimetrexate.

Incompatibility. For reference to the incompatibility of tri-metrexate and foscarnet, see under Foscarnet Sodium, p.621. Trimetrexate should not be mixed with folinic acid or chloride ions, since precipitation occurs instantly.

Adverse Effects, Treatment, and Precau-tions

As for Methotrexate, p.553. Trimetrexate must be given in conjunction with folinic acid. Folinic acid therapy should be continued for 72 hours after the last dose of trimetrexate.

Interactions

Studies in *animals* suggest that cimetidine and imida-zole antifungal drugs such as clotrimazole and keto-conazole may inhibit trimetrexate metabolism, and there is a risk of possible interactions with all drugs that affect hepatic cytochrome P450 systems.

Uses and Administration

Trimetrexate is a dihydrofolate reductase inhibitor with general properties similar to those of methotrex-ate (p.556). It is used in the management of *Pneumo-cystis carinii* pneumonia in patients with AIDS where other therapy has proved ineffective (see also p.375). It has also been tried as an antineoplastic in the man-agement of various solid tumours.

Trimetrexate is given as the glucuronate, by intrave-nous infusion, over 60 to 90 minutes. A suggested schedule in *Pneumocystis carinii* pneumonia is 45 mg per m² daily for 21 days, in association with folinic acid rescue for 24 days. The dosage of trime-trexate and folinic acid should be adjusted according to the results of blood tests, which should be per-formed at least twice a week during therapy. Renal and hepatic function and haemoglobin values should also be monitored. It is recommended that treatment with zidovudine and other myelosuppressive drugs should be interrupted to allow full doses of trimetrex-ate to be given.

Doses of 8 mg per m² body-surface daily for 5 days at 3-week intervals, or 150 to 220 mg per m² every 28 days, have been given in the management of neoplas-tic disease, usually in combination with folinic acid rescue.

◊ Trimetrexate is a non-classical antifolate which is a potent inhibitor of dihydrofolate reductase but differs from methotrex-ate in two important aspects.[1] It is taken up avidly by most mammalian tumour cells by a process independent of the folate carrier system, and within the cell it does not undergo poly-glutamylation. In consequence, cell lines resistant to meth-otrexate may retain sensitivity to trimetrexate, particularly where resistance is due to polyglutamylation defects, uptake defects, or low level gene amplification. Only methotrexate re-sistant cells with altered dihydrofolate reductase have been shown to be insensitive to trimetrexate while those with high level amplification of the dihydrofolate reductase gene are par-tially cross resistant. A few cell lines have shown trimetrexate resistance of unknown cause.

1. Bertino JR. Folate antagonists: toward improving the therapeutic index and development of new analogs. *J Clin Pharmacol* 1990; **30:** 291–5.

◊ Further reviews.

1. Marshall JL, DeLap RJ. Clinical pharmacokinetics and pharma-cology of trimetrexate. *Clin Pharmacokinet* 1994; **26:** 190–200.
2. Fulton B, *et al.* Trimetrexate: a review of its pharmacodynamic and pharmacokinetic properties and therapeutic potential in the treatment of Pneumocystis carinii pneumonia. *Drugs* 1995; **49:** 563–76.

Preparations

Proprietary Preparations (details are given in Part 3)
Canad.: Neutrexin; *Denm.:* Neutrexin; *Fr.:* Neutrexin; *Hong Kong:* Neutrexin; *Irl.:* Neutrexin; *Ital.:* Neutrexin; *Spain:* Neu-trexin; *Swed.:* Neutrexin; *Thai.:* Neutrexin; *UK:* Neutrexin; *USA:* Neutrexin.

Trofosfamide (1875-b)

Trofosfamide (rINN).

A-4828; NSC-109723; Trilophosphamide; Trophosphamide; Z-4828. 3-(2-Chloroethyl)-2-[bis(2-chloroethyl)amino]tetrahydro-2H-1,3,2-oxazaphosphorine-2-oxide.

$C_9H_{18}Cl_3N_2O_2P = 323.6$.

CAS — 22089-22-1.
ATC — L01AA07.

Profile

Trofosfamide is a derivative of cyclophosphamide (see p.527) and has the same general properties. It is used in the treatment of a variety of malignant disorders in usual initial doses of 300 to 400 mg daily by mouth. Doses of 50 to 150 mg daily have been given for maintenance therapy.

Preparations

Proprietary Preparations (details are given in Part 3)
Aust.: Ixoten; *Ger.:* Ixoten; *Spain:* Genoxal Trofosfamida.

Tumour Necrosis Factor (1331-a)

TNF.

Tasonermin (9788-d)

Tasonermin (BAN, rINN).

TNFα-1a.

$C_{778}H_{1225}N_{215}O_{231}S_2 = 17350.5$.

CAS — 94948-59-1.

Profile

Tumour necrosis factor is a cytokine of which 2 forms have been identified with similar biological properties: TNFα or cachectin, which is produced predominantly by macrophages, and TNFβ or lymphotoxin, which is produced by lymphocytes. Various recombinant forms of TNFα, both human and mouse, are available: the names sonermin and sertenef have been used for such products.

The antitumour effects of tumour necrosis factor *in vitro* and in *animals* have prompted investigation of recombinant TNFα in the treatment of cancer either alone or in combination with other cytokines such as interleukin-2 or the interferons. Tasonermin is a recombinant TNFα used in combination with melphalan (p.551) for soft tissue sarcomas. It is administered by mild hyperthermic isolated limb perfusion at a total dose of 3 mg for upper limbs and 4 mg for lower limbs. Leakage of tasonermin into the systemic circulation should not exceed 10%, as severe toxicity may occur. Local adverse effects include skin reactions, oedema, and pain; less commonly, vascular thrombosis, onycholysis, or severe tissue damage have occurred. Systemic effects include fever, chills, nausea and vomiting, arrhythmias, hepatotoxicity, and infections. Shock or hypotension, neurological disorders, thrombocytopenia, leucopenia, acute renal failure, and hypersensitivity reactions have all been reported.

◊ References.

1. Meager A. 5th International congress on tumour necrosis factor and related cytokines: scientific advances and their medical applications. *Biologicals* 1994; **22:** 291–5.
2. Hieber U, Heim ME. Tumor necrosis factor for the treatment of malignancies. *Oncology* 1994; **51:** 142–53.
3. Bazzoni F, Beutler B. The tumor necrosis factor ligand and receptor families. *N Engl J Med* 1996; **334:** 1717–25.
4. Lejeune FJ. High dose recombinant tumour necrosis factor (rTNF alpha) administered by isolation perfusion for advanced tumours of the limbs: a model for biochemotherapy of cancer. *Eur J Cancer* 1995; **31A:** 1009–16.
5. Lienard D, et al. Isolated limb perfusion with tumour necrosis factor-alpha and melphalan with or without interferon-gamma for the treatment of in-transit melanoma metastases: a multicentre randomized phase II study. *Melanoma Res* 1999; **9:** 491–502.

Units. The first International Standard for human tumour necrosis factor α, which contained 40 000 international units per ampoule, was considered unsuitable for the assay of recombinant *mouse* tumour necrosis factor α, for human tumour necrosis factor β, or for preparations of tumour necrosis factor α of modified structure.[1]

1. WHO. WHO expert committee on biological standardisation: forty-second report. *WHO Tech Rep Ser 822* 1992.

Preparations

Proprietary Preparations (details are given in Part 3)
Neth.: Beromun†; *Spain:* Beromun; *Swed.:* Beromun.

Ubenimex (16531-y)

Ubenimex (rINN).

NK-421. (−)-N-[(2S,3R)-3-Amino-2-hydroxy-4-phenylbutyryl]-L-leucine.

$C_{16}H_{24}N_2O_4 = 308.4$.

CAS — 58970-76-6.

Profile

Ubenimex is a peptide derived from *Streptomyces olivoreticuli*. It is reported to have antineoplastic and immunostimulant properties. It has been used in the adjuvant treatment of acute myeloid leukaemia. Adverse effects include gastrointestinal

The symbol † denotes a preparation no longer actively marketed

---

and hepatic function disturbances, skin rashes, headache, and paraesthesias.

◊ Ubenimex has been tried as an adjuvant to tegafur and uracil in the treatment of bladder cancer.[1]

1. Uchibayashi T, et al. Adjuvant therapy with 5-fluoro-1-(2-tetrahydrofuryl)-2,4-(1H,3H)-pyrimidinedione (UFT) and Bestatin in patients with transitional cell carcinoma of the bladder—comparison between UFT therapy alone and UFT therapy in combination with Bestatin. *Int J Clin Pharmacol Ther* 1995; **33:** 465–8.

Preparations

Proprietary Preparations (details are given in Part 3)
Jpn: Bestatin†.

Uramustine (1876-v)

Uramustine (BAN, rINN).

NSC-34462; U-8344; Uracil Mustard (USAN). 5-Bis(2-chloroethylamino)uracil; 5-[Bis(2-chloroethyl)amino]pyrimidine-2,4(1H,3H)-dione.

$C_8H_{11}Cl_2N_3O_2 = 252.1$.

CAS — 66-75-1.

Profile

Uramustine is an antineoplastic agent derived from mustine [chlormethine] (see p.561) and has a similar mode of action but it has largely been replaced by more effective agents.

Valrubicin (20056-c)

Valrubicin (USAN, rINN).

AD-32; NSC-246131. (8S,10S)-8-Glycoloyl-7,8,9,10-tetrahydro-6,8,11-trihydroxy-1-methoxy-10-{[2,3,6-trideoxy-3-(2,2,2-trifluoroacetamido)-α-L-lyxo-hexopyranosyl]oxy}-5,12-naphthacenedione 8²-valerate.

$C_{34}H_{36}F_3NO_{13} = 723.6$.

CAS — 56124-62-0.
ATC — L01DB09.

Adverse Effects, Treatment, and Precautions

Increased urinary frequency and urgency, dysuria, bladder spasm and pain may follow intravesical administration of valrubicin due to local irritation of the bladder, and usually resolve within 1 to 7 days of treatment. Haematuria has occurred rarely but should be distinguished from drug-induced red coloration of the urine. Abdominal pain and nausea may occur.

Myelosuppression similar to that seen with other anthracyclines (see Adverse Effects of Doxorubicin, p.535) is possible if significant systemic exposure occurs. Therefore valrubicin should not be administered to patients with a perforated bladder or compromised bladder mucosa.

Because of the risk of metastasis cystectomy should be reconsidered for patients with carcinoma *in-situ* who do not respond completely to valrubicin treatment after three months.

Pharmacokinetics

Following intravesical administration valrubicin can penetrate the bladder wall but systemic absorption is low in patients who have an intact bladder mucosa. The drug is almost entirely excreted by voiding after the installation period.

Uses and Administration

Valrubicin is a semisynthetic analogue of the anthracycline doxorubicin (p.534). It is used for carcinoma *in situ* of the bladder (p.490) refractory to BCG vaccine, when surgery is contra-indicated, although only about 20% of such patients exhibit a complete response. The recommended dose is 800 mg given intravesically once a week for 6 weeks, as 75 mL of a solution diluted with sodium chloride 0.9%. The solution should be retained for 2 hours if possible before voiding.

◊ References.

1. Steinberg G, et al. Efficacy and safety of valrubicin for the treatment of Bacillus Calmette-Guerin refractory carcinoma in situ of the bladder. *J Urol (Baltimore)* 2000; **163:** 761–7.

Preparations

Proprietary Preparations (details are given in Part 3)
USA: Valstar.

Valspodar (9793-x)

Valspodar (BAN, USAN, rINN).

PSC-833; SDZ-PSC-833. Cyclo{[(2S,4R,6E)-4-methyl-2-(methylamino)-3-oxo-6-octenoyl]-L-valyl-N-methylglycyl-N-methyl-L-leucyl-L-valyl-N-methyl-L-leucyl-L-alanyl-D-alanyl-N-methyl-L-leucyl-N-methyl-L-leucyl-N-methyl-L-valyl}.

$C_{63}H_{111}N_{11}O_{12} = 1214.6$.

CAS — 121584-18-7.

Profile

Valspodar is an analogue of ciclosporin (p.518). It inhibits P-glycoprotein, which is associated with multidrug resistance. Valspodar is being investigated to restore sensitivity of resistant tumour cells to anticancer drugs, for example in the treatment of acute myeloid leukaemia.

Valspodar is an inhibitor of the cytochrome P450 isoenzyme CYP3A4, and may reduce the metabolism and clearance of other drugs given concomitantly.

◊ References.

1. Advani, R, et al. Treatment of poor prognosis AML patients using PSC833 (valspodar) plus mitoxantrone, etoposide, and cytarabine (PSC-MEC). *Adv Exp Med Biol* 1999; **457:** 47–56.
2. Sparreboom A, Nooter K. Does P-glycoprotein play a role in anticancer drug pharmacokinetics? *Drug Resist Updat* 2000; **3:** 357–63.
3. Kang MH, et al. The P-glycoprotein antagonist PSC 833 increases the plasma concentrations of 6alpha-hydroxypaclitaxel, a major metabolite of paclitaxel. *Clin Cancer Res* 2001; **7:** 1610–17.
4. Fracasso PM, et al. Phase II study of paclitaxel and valspodar (PSC 833) in refractory ovarian carcinoma: a gynecologic oncology group study. *J Clin Oncol* 2001; **19:** 2975–82.
5. Baekelandt M, et al. Phase I/II study of the multidrug-resistance modulator valspodar combined with cisplatin and doxorubicin in refractory ovarian cancer. *J Clin Oncol* 2001; **19:** 2983–93.

Verteporfin (14529-m)

Verteporfin (BAN, USAN, rINN).

Benzoporphyrin Derivative; BPD; CL-318952. trans-18-Ethenyl-4,4a-dihydro-3,4-bis(methoxycarbonyl)-4a,8,14,19-tetramethyl-23H,25H-benzo[b]porphine-9,13-dipropanoic acid monomethyl ester.

$C_{41}H_{42}N_4O_8 = 718.8$.

CAS — 129497-78-5.

Profile

Verteporfin is a photosensitiser used in the photodynamic therapy of age-related macular degeneration. Following intravenous administration verteporfin accumulates preferentially in the endothelial cells of actively growing blood vessels, including those in the retina. When activated by laser light it produces local vascular occlusion and this inhibits neovascularisation and reduces the decline in visual acuity. It is administered by intravenous infusion over 10 minutes at a dose of 6 mg per m² body-surface. This is followed 15 minutes after the start of the infusion by activation using a laser tuned to a wavelength of 689 nm and delivered to the eye via a fibre optic device and a slit lamp, together with a suitable contact lens.

Patients should not be exposed to direct sunlight for 2 to 5 days after treatment and care should be taken to avoid extravasation during injection of verteporfin, as this may lead to local burns. Verteporfin has also been investigated in the photodynamic therapy of a variety of other disorders, including malignant neoplasms.

Preparations

Proprietary Preparations (details are given in Part 3)
Austral.: Visudyne; *Fr.:* Visudyne; *UK:* Visudyne; *USA:* Visudyne.

Vinblastine Sulfate (1878-q)

Vinblastine Sulfate (USAN, rINNM).

29060-LE; NSC-49842; Sulfato de Vimblastina; Vinblastine Sulphate (BANM); Vinblastini Sulfas; Vincaleukoblastine Sulphate; VLB (vinblastine).

$C_{46}H_{58}N_4O_9,H_2SO_4 = 909.1$.

CAS — 865-21-4 (vinblastine); 143-67-9 (vinblastine sulfate).

Pharmacopoeias. In Chin., Eur. (see p.vi), Int., Jpn, and US.

The sulfate of an alkaloid, vincaleukoblastine, extracted from *Vinca rosea (Catharanthus roseus)* (Apocynaceae).

Pharmacopoeial description

Ph. Eur.: A white or slightly yellowish, very hygroscopic, crystalline powder. It loses not more than 15% of its weight on drying. Freely soluble in water; practically insoluble in alcohol and in ether. A 0.15% solution in water has a pH of 3.5 to 5.0. Store at a temperature not exceeding −20° in airtight glass containers. Protect from light.

USP 25: A white or slightly yellow, odourless, hygroscopic, amorphous or crystalline powder. It loses not more than 15% of its weight on drying. Freely soluble in water. A 0.15% solution in water has a pH of 3.5 to 5.0. Store at a temperature between −25° and −10° in airtight containers. Protect from light.

Stability. Between about 5 and 20% of active drug was lost from solution when a solution of vinblastine sulfate 3 µg per mL in 5% glucose injection was stored for 48 hours in a range of intravenous burette giving sets, the highest loss being from cellulose propionate sets and the lowest from one made from methacrylate butadiene styrene.[1] Similarly storage in polyvinyl chloride (PVC) tubing led to a 42 to 44% loss from solution whereas only about 6% was lost over the 48 hours in polybutadiene tubing. The losses appeared to be due to drug sorption, and were therefore greater from the tubing which had a greater surface-area-to-volume ratio than the burettes.

1. McElnay JC, et al. Stability of methotrexate and vinblastine in burette administration sets. *Int J Pharmaceutics* 1988; **47:** 239–47.

Adverse Effects, Treatment, and Precautions

For general discussions, see Antineoplastics, p.476, p.479, and p.480.

Bone-marrow depression, especially leucopenia, is the most common adverse effect with vinblastine and tends to be dose-limiting. Maximum depression occurs 5 to 10 days after administration with recovery in a further 7 to 14 days. Leucopenia may be more severe in patients with cachexia or extensive skin ulceration: vinblastine should not be used in elderly patients with these conditions. Gastrointestinal effects including stomatitis and gastrointestinal bleeding may occur; nausea and vomiting respond to treatment with antiemetics.

The vinca alkaloids can produce central and peripheral (including autonomic) neurotoxicity, although these effects are less frequent with vinblastine. Symptoms include malaise, dizziness, weakness, headache, depression, paraesthesia and numbness, loss of deep tendon reflexes, peripheral neuropathies, constipation and adynamic ileus, jaw pain, and convulsions. Damage to the eight cranial nerve may result in vestibular and auditory toxicity leading to nystagmus, vertigo, and partial or total deafness. A routine prophylactic regimen against constipation is recommended in patients receiving high doses of vinblastine. Overdosage has caused permanent damage to the central nervous system. Intrathecal administration of the vinca alkaloids is contra-indicated because of the likelihood of fatal neurotoxicity.

Other reported effects include skin reactions, alopecia, ischaemic cardiac toxicity, hypertension, dyspnoea and bronchospasm, and bone and tumour pain. A syndrome of inappropriate secretion of antidiuretic hormone has occurred at high doses, and may be relieved by fluid restriction and, if necessary, a suitable diuretic.

Vinblastine is irritant to the skin and mucous membranes and extravasation may cause necrosis, cellulitis, and sloughing. The application of warmth and local injection of hyaluronidase may be of benefit in relieving the effects of extravasation. Folinic acid has been suggested in overdosage, by analogy with vincristine.

Vinblastine should not be injected into an extremity with impaired circulation because of an increased risk of thrombosis. It should be given with caution and at reduced dosage to patients with hepatic impairment.

Administration error. *Intrathecal administration of vinca alkaloids, including vinblastine, results in ascending paralysis and death. For reference to the successful treatment of inadvertent intrathecal administration of vincristine, see p.579.*

Handling and disposal. A method for the destruction of vincristine or vinblastine *wastes* using sulfuric acid and potassium permanganate.[1] Residues produced by degradation of either drug by this method showed no mutagenicity *in vitro*.

Urine and faeces produced for up to 4 and 7 days respectively after a dose of vinblastine should be handled wearing protective clothing.[2]

1. Castegnaro M, *et al.*, eds. Laboratory decontamination and destruction of carcinogens in laboratory wastes: some antineoplastic agents. *IARC Scientific Publications 73* Lyon: WHO/International Agency for Research on Cancer, 1985.
2. Harris J, Dodds LJ. Handling waste from patients receiving cytotoxic drugs. *Pharm J* 1985; **235:** 289–91.

Porphyria. Vinblastine is considered to be unsafe in patients with porphyria because it has been shown to be porphyrinogenic in *in-vitro* systems, although there is conflicting evidence of porphyrinogenicity.

Interactions

For a general outline of antineoplastic drug interactions, see p.481. Concurrent administration of vinblastine with drugs that inhibit cytochromes of the CYP3A subfamily may result in decreased metabolism of vinblastine and increased toxicity.

Analgesics. A report of enhanced hepatotoxicity in patients treated with interferon alfa and vinblastine who were given *paracetamol*.[1]

1. Kellokumpu-Lehtinen P, *et al.* Hepatotoxicity of paracetamol in combination with interferon and vinblastine. *Lancet* 1989; **i:** 1143.

Antibacterials. There is a report of severe vinblastine toxicity in 3 patients who received vinblastine and ciclosporin with *erythromycin*.[1] Discontinuing erythromycin produced resolution of the adverse effects, which recurred following rechallenge with erythromycin in 1 patient.

1. Tobe SW, *et al.* Vinblastine and erythromycin: an unrecognised serious drug interaction. *Cancer Chemother Pharmacol* 1995; **35:** 188–90.

Antineoplastics. Acute bronchospastic reactions following injection of a vinca alkaloid have been reported, usually in patients who have also received *mitomycin*,[1] and presenting as acute respiratory distress, cyanosis, and dyspnoea, often with the development of pulmonary infiltrates and pneumonitis.[2,3] A number of fatalities due to respiratory complications have occurred. For reports of vascular toxicity and Raynauds syndrome associated with the use of vinca alkaloids with *bleomycin* and other drugs, see Effects on the Cardiovascular System, p.477.

1. Dyke RW. Acute bronchospasm after a vinca alkaloid in patients previously treated with mitomycin. *N Engl J Med* 1984; **310:** 389.
2. Konits PH, *et al.* Possible pulmonary toxicity secondary to vinblastine. *Cancer* 1982; **50:** 2771–4.
3. Ozols RF, *et al.* MVP (mitomycin, vinblastine, and progesterone): a second-line regimen in ovarian cancer with a high incidence of pulmonary toxicity. *Cancer Treat Rep* 1983; **67:** 721–2.

Interferons. Severe myelosuppression has occurred in patients receiving relatively high doses of vinblastine with interferon alfa-n1.

Pharmacokinetics

Vinblastine is not reliably absorbed from the gastrointestinal tract. Following intravenous administration it is rapidly cleared from the blood and distributed to tissues; it is reported to be concentrated in blood platelets. It is extensively protein bound. Vinblastine is metabolised in the liver, by cytochrome P450 isoenzymes of the CYP3A subfamily, to an active metabolite desacetylvinblastine, and is excreted in faeces via the bile, and in urine; some is excreted as unchanged drug. The terminal half-life is reported to be about 25 hours. It does not cross the blood-brain barrier in significant amounts.

Uses and Administration

Vinblastine sulfate is an antineoplastic agent which apparently acts by binding to the microtubular proteins of the spindle and arresting mitosis at the metaphase; it is thus specific for the M phase of the cell cycle. It also interferes with glutamate metabolism and possibly nucleic acid synthesis, and has some immunosuppressant activity. Significant cross-resistance with vincristine has not been reported although pleiotropic resistance may occur.

Vinblastine sulfate is used in the treatment of Hodgkin's disease and other lymphomas, usually with an alkylating agent such as cyclophosphamide or mustine [chlormethine], plus procarbazine and prednisone, or with doxorubicin, bleomycin, and dacarbazine (ABVD). It is also of use in the treatment of some inoperable malignant neoplasms including those of the breast, bladder, and kidney, and in non-small cell lung cancer, choriocarcinoma, and Kaposi's sarcoma; vinblastine has also been employed in the management of Langerhans-cell histiocytosis. It was formerly used with bleomycin and cisplatin (PVB) for testicular cancer, but other regimens are now preferred. The management of these conditions is discussed under Choice of Antineoplastic, as indicated by the cross-references given below.

Vinblastine sulfate is given by intravenous injection as a solution containing 1 mg per mL in sodium chloride 0.9%. Care should be taken to avoid extravasation and the injection may be given into a freely running infusion of sodium chloride injection if preferred. The usual dose is about 6 mg per m² body-surface, although doses of 400 μg per kg, divided over 2 consecutive days, may be given every 3 weeks in testicular cancer. One suggested dosage scheme is as follows: weekly injections starting with 3.7 mg per m² body-surface, raised by increments of 1.8 to 1.9 mg per m² to a maximum weekly dose of 18.5 mg per m², or until the white cell count has fallen to 3000 per mm³. Most patients respond to 5.5 to 7.4 mg per m² weekly. If a maintenance dose is required, it may be given every 7 days provided white cell counts permit (see below), and should be one increment smaller than the maximum dose that the patient is able to tolerate without serious leucopenia occurring.

Children may be given vinblastine sulfate in an initial dose of 2.5 mg per m² body-surface intravenously, increased by 1.25 mg per m² weekly to a usual maximum weekly dose of 7.5 mg per m². Doses of up to 12.5 mg per m² per week have been given.

White cell counts should be made before each injection and a repeat dose should never be given unless the count has risen to 4000 per mm³. A dosage reduction of 50% is advised in patients with moderately severe hepatic impairment (serum bilirubin above 3 mg per 100 mL).

Blood disorders, non-malignant. The vinca alkaloids vinblastine and vincristine have been used experimentally in the treatment of various auto-immune blood disorders such as idiopathic thrombocytopenic purpura, and auto-immune haemolytic anaemia (p.1052 and p.716 respectively). There are also reports of the haemolytic-uraemic syndrome/thrombotic thrombocytopenic purpura responding to treatment with intravenous injection of vincristine.[1,2] For further details on the treatment of thrombotic microangiopathies, see p.740. Vincristine has been given with normal immunoglobulin in the management of a patient with life-threatening thrombocytopenia due to *sarcoidosis*.[3]

1. Gutterman LA, *et al.* The hemolytic-uremic syndrome: recovery after treatment with vincristine. *Ann Intern Med* 1983; **98:** 612–13.
2. Wolf G, *et al.* Behandlung einer thrombotisch-thrombo-zytopenischen Purpura (Morbus Moschcowitz) mit Vincristine. *Dtsch Med Wochenschr* 1995; **120:** 442–6.
3. Larner AJ. Life threatening thrombocytopenia in sarcoidosis. *BMJ* 1990; **300:** 317–19.

Histiocytic syndromes. The value of systemic chemotherapy in patients with Langerhans-cell histiocytosis (p.483) is uncertain; however, it is certainly widely used in extensive disease, vinblastine being one of the drugs often employed.[1,2]

1. Ladisch S, *et al.* LCH-1: a randomized trial of etoposide vs vinblastine in disseminated Langerhans cell histiocytosis. *Med Pediatr Oncol* 1994; **23:** 107–10.
2. The French Langerhans' Cell Histiocytosis Study Group. A multicentre retrospective survey of Langerhans' cell histiocytosis: 348 cases observed between 1983 and 1993. *Arch Dis Child* 1996; **75:** 17–24.

Malignant neoplasms. Vinblastine plays an important role in the ABVD regimen in patients with Hodgkin's disease (see p.487). It also formed part of the effective, if toxic, PVB regimen used to treat testicular cancer, although other regimens tend now to be preferred, as mentioned on p.499. The vinca alkaloids are also active in gestational trophoblastic tumours (p.483), and vinblastine is also used in the therapy of invasive bladder cancer (p.490); it may be used in the adjuvant or palliative treatment of non-small-cell lung cancer (p.496) and in the palliative care of advanced breast cancer (p.491). It has been used in malignancies of the kidney (p.495). Vinca alkaloids are also used to treat Kaposi's sarcoma (p.501).

Preparations

BP 2001: Vinblastine Injection;
USP 25: Vinblastine Sulfate for Injection.

Proprietary Preparations (details are given in Part 3)
Aust.: Velbe; *Austral.:* Velbe; *Belg.:* Velbe; *Braz.:* Velban; *Canad.:* Velbe; *Denm.:* Velbe; *Fin.:* Velbe; *Fr.:* Velbe; *Ger.:* Cellblastin; Velbe; *Hong Kong:* Velbe; *Israel:* Blastovin; Velbe; *Ital.:* Velbe; *Mex.:* Lemblastine; Velbe; *Neth.:* Velbe; *Norw.:* Velbe; *Port.:* Solblastin; Velbe; *S.Afr.:* Periblastine†; *Swed.:* Velbe; *Switz.:* Velbe; *UK:* Velbe; *USA:* Alkaban†; Velban.

Vincristine Sulfate (1879-p)

Vincristine Sulfate *(USAN, rINNM)*.
Compound 37231; Leurocristine Sulphate; NSC-67574; 22-Oxovincaleukoblastine Sulphate; Sulfato de Vincristina; Vincristine Sulphate *(BANM)*; Vincristini Sulfas.
$C_{46}H_{56}N_4O_{10},H_2SO_4 = 923.0$.
CAS — 57-22-7 (vincristine); 2068-78-2 (vincristine sulfate).

Pharmacopoeias. In Chin., Eur. (see p.vi), Int., Jpn, Pol., and US.

The sulfate of an alkaloid, 22-oxovincaleukoblastine, obtained from *Vinca rosea (Catharanthus roseus)* (Apocynaceae).

Pharmacopoeial description
Ph. Eur.: A white or slightly yellowish, very hygroscopic, crystalline powder. It loses not more than 12% of its weight on drying. Freely soluble in water; slightly soluble in alcohol; practically insoluble in ether. A 0.1% solution in water has a pH of 3.5 to 4.5. Store at a temperature not exceeding −20° in airtight glass containers. Protect from light.

USP 25: A white to slightly yellow, odourless, hygroscopic, amorphous or crystalline powder. It loses not more than 12% of its weight on drying. Freely soluble in water; slightly soluble in alcohol; soluble in methyl alcohol. A 0.1% solution in water has a pH of 3.5 to 4.5. Store at a temperature between −25° and −20° in airtight containers. Protect from light.

Adverse Effects, Treatment, and Precautions

As for Vinblastine Sulfate, p.578.

Bone-marrow depression occurs less commonly than with vinblastine but neurological and neuromuscular effects are more severe with vincristine and are dose-limiting. Walking may be impaired and the neurological effects may not be reversed for several months after the drug is discontinued. Convulsions, often with hypertension, have occurred. Constipation is common and there may be abdominal pain. Urinary disturbances have occurred and alopecia is common.

Folinic acid has been given for the treatment of overdose: suggested doses are as much as 100 mg of folinic acid intravenously every 3 hours for 24 hours, then every 6 hours for at least 48 hours. However, this is unlikely to be of benefit in reversing neuromuscular toxicity. For mention of the use of glutamic acid in managing the usually fatal consequences of inadvertent intrathecal administration, see below.

Because severe constipation and impaction of faeces often occur with vincristine, laxatives or enemas may be necessary to ensure regular bowel function. Vincristine should be given with caution to patients with pre-existing neuromuscular disease and is contra-indicated in patients with the demyelinating form of Charcot-Marie-Tooth syndrome (see under Effects on the Nervous System, below). Doses may need to be adjusted in patients with hepatic impairment. Care should also be taken in elderly patients, who may be more susceptible to neurotoxicity.

Administration error. *Inadvertent intrathecal administration of vincristine results in ascending paralysis and death.*[1,2] However, in one case[3] treatment immediately following the error, and consisting of removal of contaminated spinal fluid and flushing with lactated Ringer's solution and fresh frozen plasma diluted in lactated Ringer's solution, plus intravenous and oral glutamic acid, was reported successful in stabilising neurological dysfunction and preventing death. The role of glutamic acid in this case is uncertain, but a study involving 84 patients found that the administration of glutamic acid 1.5 g daily by mouth in divided doses during a 6-week induction chemotherapy course decreased vincristine-induced neurotoxicity.[4]

1. Manelis J, et al. Accidental intrathecal vincristine administration: report of a case. J Neurol 1982; 228: 209–13.
2. Dyer C. Manslaughter convictions for making mistakes. BMJ 1991; 303: 1218.
3. Dyke RW. Treatment of inadvertent intrathecal injection of vincristine. N Engl J Med 1989; 321: 1270–1.
4. Jackson DV, et al. Amelioration of vincristine neurotoxicity by glutamic acid. Am J Med 1988; 84: 1016–22.

Effects on the nervous system. The neurotoxic effects of vincristine have been reviewed.[1] In its most typical form, neurotoxicity manifests as a mixed sensorimotor neuropathy of the distal type. The earliest symptoms are sensory changes in the form of paraesthesias, accompanied by impairment and ultimately loss of deep tendon reflexes. In more severe forms, impairment of motor function occurs with wrist drop and foot drop, ataxia and gait abnormalities, and occasionally progressive quadriparesis.

In contrast to these peripheral neuropathies which are usually associated with long-term usage there may be short-term autonomic neuropathy resulting in constipation and occasionally ileus, abdominal pain, atony of the urinary bladder (which may lead to urinary retention), postural hypotension, and rarely, impotence. There may be effects on the cranial nerves, resulting in ptosis, hoarseness (due to laryngeal nerve paralysis), or optic neuropathies. Effects on the CNS are rare, probably in part because of poor penetration into CSF, but include excessive release of antidiuretic hormone and consequent hyponatraemia.

Hallucinations have occurred[2] and effects on the special senses have been reported: both bilateral optic atrophy and blindness,[3] and profound neurological deafness (which was largely reversible on drug withdrawal)[4] have occurred. Convulsions associated with hypertension are another feature of vincristine toxicity.[5]

Toxicity is related to both the cumulative and the individual dose.[1] It usually begins in adults after receiving a total of 5 to 6 mg, and is significant by the time a cumulative dose of 15 to 20 mg is reached. If individual doses are low (less than 2 mg) or intervals between doses are longer than the usual week, patients can tolerate higher cumulative doses. Children tolerate vincristine better than adults, but the elderly are particularly prone to neurotoxicity. Patients with existing neurological disorders such as poliomyelitis or the Charcot-Marie-Tooth syndrome may be at increased risk of neurotoxicity.[6-9] It has been suggested that increased neurotoxicity may be associated with

the use of ready-to-use solutions rather than reconstituted lyophilised preparations but this has not been proved.[10-14]

There is no good treatment for the effects of vincristine on the nervous system: symptoms are largely reversible once administration is interrupted, and should be managed with appropriate symptomatic care.[1] However, there is some suggestion that glutamic acid may be of benefit in treating neurotoxicity—see above. For the use of dinoprost to alleviate ileus induced by vinca alkaloids, see p.1441.

1. Legha SS. Vincristine neurotoxicity: pathophysiology and management. Med Toxicol 1986; 1: 421–7.
2. Holland JF, et al. Vincristine treatment of advanced cancer: a cooperative study of 392 cases. Cancer Res 1973; 33: 1258–64.
3. Awidi AS. Blindness and vincristine. Ann Intern Med 1980; 93: 781.
4. Yousif H, et al. Partially reversible nerve deafness due to vincristine. Postgrad Med J 1990; 66: 688–9.
5. Ito S, et al. Seizures and hypertension complicating vincristine therapy in children. Clin Pharmacol Ther 1995; 57: 208.
6. Hogan-Dann CM, et al. Polyneuropathy following vincristine therapy in two patients with Charcot-Marie-Tooth syndrome. JAMA 1984; 252: 2862–3.
7. Miller BR. Neurotoxicity and vincristine. JAMA 1985; 253: 2045.
8. Chauncey TR, et al. Vincristine neurotoxicity. JAMA 1985; 254: 507.
9. Griffiths JD, et al. Vincristine neurotoxicity in Charcot-Marie-Tooth syndrome. Med J Aust 1985; 143: 305–6.
10. Arnold AM, et al. Acute vincristine neurotoxicity. Lancet 1985; i: 346.
11. Jalihal S, Roebuck N. Acute vincristine neurotoxicity. Lancet 1985; i: 637.
12. Davies CE, et al. Acute vincristine neurotoxicity. Lancet 1985; i: 637–8.
13. Warrier RP, Ducos R. Acute vincristine neurotoxicity. Lancet 1985; i: 980.
14. Gennery BA. Vincristine neurotoxicity. Lancet 1985; ii: 385.

Handling and disposal. For a method for the destruction of vincristine *wastes*, see under Vinblastine Sulfate, p.578.

Urine and faeces produced for up to 4 and 7 days respectively after a dose of vincristine should be handled wearing protective clothing.[1]

1. Harris J, Dodds LJ. Handling waste from patients receiving cytotoxic drugs. Pharm J 1985; 235: 289–91.

Porphyria. Vincristine is considered to be unsafe in patients with porphyria because it has been shown to be porphyrinogenic in *in-vitro* systems, although there is conflicting evidence of porphyrinogenicity.

Interactions

For a general outline of antineoplastic drug interactions, see p.481. Concurrent administration of vincristine with drugs that inhibit cytochromes of the CYP3A subfamily may result in decreased metabolism of vincristine and increased toxicity. If vincristine is used in combination with asparaginase it should be given 12 to 24 hours before the enzyme: administration of asparaginase with or before vincristine may reduce vincristine clearance and increase toxicity. For reports of vascular toxicity and Raynaud's syndrome associated with the concomitant use of vinca alkaloids with bleomycin and other drugs see Effects on the Cardiovascular System, p.477.

Antiepileptics. A pharmacokinetic study showed that systemic clearance of vincristine was 63% higher when it was administered with *phenytoin* or *carbamazepine*, two inducers of the cytochrome P450 isoenzyme CYP3A4. The clinical significance of this finding is unknown.[1]

1. Villikka K, et al. Cytochrome P450-inducing antiepileptics increase the clearance of vincristine in patients with brain tumours. Clin Pharmacol Ther 1999; 66: 589–93.

Antimicrobials. Toxicity has been reported to be increased in children who received *itraconazole* and nifedipine during leukaemia treatment involving vincristine.[1] Severe neurotoxicity has occurred when *isoniazid* was added to the regimen of a patient receiving vincristine.[2]

1. Murphy JA, et al. Vincristine toxicity in five children with acute lymphoblastic leukaemia. Lancet 1995; 346: 443.
2. Carrión C, et al. Possible vincristine-isoniazid interaction. Ann Pharmacother 1995; 29: 201.

Pharmacokinetics

Vincristine is not reliably absorbed from the gastrointestinal tract. After intravenous injection it disappears rapidly from the blood. It is extensively protein bound and is reported to be concentrated in blood platelets. It is metabolised in the liver and excreted primarily in the bile; about 70 to 80% of a dose is found in faeces, as unchanged drug and metabolites, while 10 to 20% appears in the urine. The terminal half-life is reported to be about 85 hours but may range from about 10 to 155 hours. Vincristine does not appear to cross the blood-brain barrier in significant amounts.

Uses and Administration

Vincristine sulfate is an antineoplastic agent which may act similarly to vinblastine (above) by arresting mitosis at the metaphase. Significant cross-resistance with vinblastine has not been reported although pleiotropic resistance may occur.

It is used principally in combination chemotherapy regimens for acute leukaemia and Hodgkin's disease and other lymphomas, including Burkitt's lymphoma. It may also be used in the treatment of Wilms' tumour, myeloma, neuroblastoma, in sarcomas including Kaposi's sarcoma and rhabdomyosarcoma and in tumours of the brain, breast, head and neck, and lung, among others. It has also been given in idiopathic thrombocytopenic purpura refractory to other agents. See also the cross-references given below.

Remissions are induced in acute lymphoblastic leukaemia with vincristine in association with prednisone alone or with an anthracycline or asparaginase or both. In Hodgkin's disease, vincristine may be given with mustine [chlormethine], procarbazine, and prednisone (MOPP), and similar regimens have been used in other lymphomas.

Vincristine sulfate is administered by intravenous injection, usually as a solution containing 1 mg per mL in sodium chloride 0.9%. Care should be taken to avoid extravasation and the injection may be given into a freely-running intravenous infusion of sodium chloride injection if preferred.

In acute leukaemia the usual weekly dose of vincristine sulfate for induction of remission in children is 2 mg per m² body-surface, or an initial dose of 50 µg per kg body-weight in those weighing 10 kg or less. Adults may be given about 1.4 mg per m² or 25 to 75 µg per kg weekly; a maximum weekly dose of 2 mg has been suggested (but see Administration, below). For other malignancies 25 µg per kg may be given weekly and reduced to 5 to 10 µg per kg for maintenance.

Blood counts should be carried out before giving each dose. A dose reduction of 50% is recommended in patients with moderately severe hepatic impairment (serum bilirubin above 3 mg per 100 mL).

A liposomal formulation of vincristine is under investigation.

Action. Results in vitro suggesting a selective action of vincristine against lymphocytes of patients with chronic lymphocytic leukaemia;[1] lymphocytes of healthy subjects were not so affected.

1. Vilpo J, et al. Selective toxicity of vincristine against chronic lymphocytic leukaemia in vitro. Lancet 1996; 347: 1491–2.

Administration. Although a maximum single dose of 2 mg is recommended for vincristine sulfate to reduce neurotoxicity, a review[1] has suggested that this guideline is overly rigid, since it does not take into account interindividual variations in pharmacokinetics and susceptibility to toxicity, which may be considerable. Furthermore the authors considered the evidence for effectiveness of this dosage limitation to be equivocal. They suggested beginning therapy at 1.4 mg per m² body-surface and adjusting subsequent doses according to toxicity.

1. McCune JS, Lindley C. Appropriateness of maximum-dose guidelines for vincristine. Am J Health-Syst Pharm 1997; 54: 1755–8.

Amyloidosis. For mention of regimens including vincristine used in the management of amyloidosis, see p.501.

Blood disorders, non-malignant. Vincristine may be employed in the treatment of refractory idiopathic thrombocytopenic purpura (p.1052), either by conventional injection or in the form of vincristine-loaded platelets, but results have been equivocal. Vincristine has also been used for life-threatening haemangioma (p.1052).

Malignant neoplasms. Vincristine is widely used in the treatment of malignant neoplasms. It is a fundamental part of potentially curative regimens for acute lymphoblastic leukaemia, Hodgkin's disease and aggressive non-Hodgkins lymphomas (see p.484, p.487 and p.487). It has also been used in chronic lymphocytic leukaemia (p.485) and in other non-Hodgkin's lymphomas including AIDS-related lymphoma (p.488), Burkitt's lymphoma (p.488) and mycosis fungoides (p.489). Other haematological malignancies in which it may be tried include multiple myeloma (p.489). Among the solid neoplasms, vincristine is used in regimens to treat gestational trophoblastic tumours (p.483), tumours of the brain (p.490), breast (p.491), head and neck (p.494), Wilms' tumour (p.495), small-cell lung cancer (p.496), and thymoma (p.499). It is also employed in regimens for neuroblastoma (p.500), retinoblasto-

The symbol † denotes a preparation no longer actively marketed

ma (p.500), and some sarcomas including sarcomas of bone, Kaposi's sarcoma, and rhabdomyosarcoma (see p.500, p.501, and p.501).

Preparations

BP 2001: Vincristine Injection;
USP 25: Vincristine Sulfate for Injection; Vincristine Sulfate Injection.

Proprietary Preparations (details are given in Part 3)

Aust.: Oncovin; *Austral.:* Oncovin; *Belg.:* Oncovin; *Braz.:* Oncovin; *Canad.:* Oncovin†; *Denm.:* Oncovin; *Fin.:* Oncovin; *Vincrin; Fr.:* Oncovin; *Ger.:* Cellcristin; Farmistin; *Irl.:* Oncovin; *Israel:* Oncovin; *Mex.:* Citomid RU; Filcrin; Oncovin; Vincasar; Vintec; *Neth.:* Oncovin†; *Norw.:* Oncovin; *NZ:* Oncovin; *Port.:* Faulcris; Oncovin; *S.Afr.:* Oncovin; Pericristine; *Spain:* Vincrisul; *Swed.:* Oncovin; *Switz.:* Oncovin; *UK:* Oncovin; *USA:* Oncovin; Vincasar PFS.

Vindesine Sulfate (1880-n)

Vindesine Sulfate (USAN, rINNM).

Compound 112531 (vindesine); Desacetyl Vinblastine Amide Sulfate; LY-099094; NSC-245467; Vindesine Sulphate (BANM); Vindesini Sulfas. 3-Carbamoyl-4-O-deacetyl-3-de(methoxycarbonyl)vincaleukoblastine.

$C_{43}H_{55}N_5O_7,H_2SO_4 = 852.0$.

CAS — 53643-48-4 (vindesine); 59917-39-4 (vindesine sulfate).

Pharmacopoeias. In Eur. (see p.vi).

Pharmacopoeial description

Ph. Eur.: A white or almost white, hygroscopic, amorphous substance. Freely soluble in water and in methyl alcohol; practically insoluble in cyclohexane. The pH of a 0.5% solution in water is 3.5 to 5.5. Store in airtight polypropylene containers with a polypropylene cap, at a temperature not exceeding −50°.

Adverse Effects, Treatment, and Precautions

As for Vinblastine Sulfate, p.578.

The main dose-limiting effect of vindesine is granulocytopenia with the nadir of the white cell count usually occurring 3 to 5 days after a dose, with recovery after a further 4 to 5 days. Although neurotoxicity occurs it may be less severe than that seen with vincristine (see p.579). Alopecia is the most common side-effect.

Folinic acid has been suggested for the treatment of overdosage by analogy with vincristine.

Vindesine should not be given by the intrathecal route, as this may produce fatal toxicity. Care should be taken if acute abdominal pain occurs: further administration may result in paralytic ileus.

Administration error. *Inadvertent intrathecal administration of vinca alkaloids results in ascending paralysis and death.* In a 10-year-old child who was accidentally given an intrathecal injection of vindesine, treatment with folinic acid and dexamethasone produced transient recovery but symptoms subsequently recurred and the patient died of progressive ascending paralysis.[1] The CNS showed changes at necropsy similar to those seen following intrathecal administration of vincristine. For reference to the treatment inadvertent intrathecal administration of vincristine, see p.579.

1. Robbins G. Accidental intrathecal injection of vindesine. *BMJ* 1985; **291:** 1094.

Interactions

As for Vinblastine Sulfate, p.578.

Pharmacokinetics

The pharmacokinetics of vindesine are similar to those of the other vinca alkaloids. After intravenous administration elimination from the blood is triphasic; the drug is rapidly distributed to body tissues. The terminal half-life is reported to be about 20 hours. It is metabolised primarily in the liver and excreted in bile and urine.

Uses and Administration

Vindesine sulfate is an antineoplastic agent derived from vinblastine (see p.577); like the other vinca alkaloids it causes mitotic arrest in metaphase by binding to microtubular protein. It has been tried in refractory malignant melanoma and in malignant neoplasms of the gastrointestinal tract, and lung. It has also been used in refractory acute lymphoblastic

or chronic myeloid leukaemias, and in malignant neoplasms of the breast. See all the cross references given below.

Vindesine sulfate is given weekly by intravenous injection as a solution containing 1 mg per mL in sodium chloride injection (0.9%). Care should be taken to avoid extravasation and it may be given into a fast-running infusion of sodium chloride, glucose (5%), or glucose-saline injection. The usual starting dose for adults is 3 mg per m² body-surface which may be raised by increments of 500 μg per m² weekly providing that the granulocyte count does not fall below 1500 per mm³, the platelet count does not fall below 100 000 per mm³, and acute abdominal pain is not experienced; weekly doses are usually between 3 and 4 mg per m². Children may be given 4 mg per m² initially, with weekly doses usually ranging between 4 and 5 mg per m². Blood counts should be made before each injection. It may be necessary to reduce initial doses in patients with significantly impaired hepatic function.

Malignant neoplasms. Vindesine has been tried in refractory metastatic melanoma (p.499), childhood acute lymphoblastic leukaemia (p.484) and chronic myeloid leukaemia in blastic crisis (p.486). It is also under investigation in lung cancer, particularly non-small cell lung cancer (p.496) and responses have been reported in oesophageal cancer (p.493) and advanced breast cancer (p.491).

Preparations

BP 2001: Vindesine Injection.

Proprietary Preparations (details are given in Part 3)

Aust.: Eldisin; *Austral.:* Eldisine; *Belg.:* Eldisine; *Canad.:* Eldisine; *Fin.:* Eldisine; *Fr.:* Eldisine; *Ger.:* Eldisine; *Hong Kong:* Eldisine; *Ital.:* Eldisine; *Neth.:* Eldisine; *Port.:* Gesidine; *S.Afr.:* Eldisine; *Spain:* Enison; *Swed.:* Eldisine; *Switz.:* Eldisine; *UK:* Eldisine.

Vinorelbine Tartrate (3773-j)

Vinorelbine Tartrate (BANM, USAN, rINNM).

Vinorelbine Ditartrate. 3′,4′-Didehydro-4′-deoxy-8′-norvincaleukoblastine ditartrate.

$C_{45}H_{54}N_4O_8,2C_4H_6O_6 = 1079.1$.

CAS — 71486-22-1 (vinorelbine); 125317-39-7 (vinorelbine tartrate).

Adverse Effects and Precautions

As for Vinblastine Sulfate, p.578. The nadir of the granulocyte count occurs 5 to 10 days after a dose with recovery usually after a further 7 to 14 days. The drug should be discontinued if moderate or severe neurotoxicity develops. Local pain and thrombophlebitis may be seen with repeated injection of vinorelbine.

Administration error. *Inadvertent intrathecal administration of vinca alkaloids results in ascending paralysis and death.* For reference to the treatment of inadvertent intrathecal administration of vincristine, see p.579.

Effects on the gastrointestinal tract. For reference to a report of vinorelbine possibly exacerbating ischaemic colitis in patients receiving docetaxel, see p.534.

Pharmacokinetics

As with the other vinca alkaloids, vinorelbine exhibits triphasic pharmacokinetics after intravenous injection, and has a terminal half-life of between about 28 and 44 hours. It is metabolised in the liver; deacetylvinorelbine has antineoplastic activity. Vinorelbine and its metabolites are excreted primarily in faeces via the bile but also in urine.

◊ References.

1. Levêque D, Jehl F. Clinical pharmacokinetics of vinorelbine. *Clin Pharmacokinet* 1996; **31:** 184–97.

Uses and Administration

Vinorelbine is a semisynthetic derivative of vinblastine (see p.578) with similar general properties. It is used as the tartrate in the treatment of advanced breast cancer and non-small cell lung cancers (see p.491 and p.496 respectively), and has been tried in other malignancies including lymphomas and tumours of ovary and prostate.

Vinorelbine is administered as the tartrate but doses are calculated in terms of vinorelbine. It is given by intravenous injection over 5 to 10 minutes, as a solution containing the equivalent of vinorelbine 1.5 to 3.0 mg per mL in glucose 5% or sodium chloride 0.9% injection, directly or into a freely-running intravenous infusion. It may also be given by intravenous infusion over 20 to 30 minutes after dilution in 125 mL of glucose 5% or sodium chloride 0.9%. The usual initial dose is the equivalent of vinorelbine 25 to 30 mg per m² body-surface weekly. In the UK, the manufacturers recommend that subsequent doses should be delayed until recovery if the neutrophil count falls below 2000 per mm³. In the USA it is suggested that subsequent doses should be halved if granulocyte counts fall to between 1000 and 1500 per mm³; treatment should be interrupted if counts are below 1000 per mm³ and discontinued if granulocytopenia persists for more than 2 weeks. Doses should also be reduced in hepatic impairment. In the UK a dose reduction of one-third has been suggested in patients with massive liver metastases (but see also below). In the USA, the manufacturers recommend that the dose of vinorelbine be reduced by 50% in patients with bilirubin values of 2.1 to 3.0 mg per 100 mL, and by 75% in those with bilirubin greater than 3.0 mg per 100 mL.

Oral use of vinorelbine has been studied.

◊ References.

1. Toso C, Lindley C. Vinorelbine: a novel vinca alkaloid. *Am J Health-Syst Pharm* 1995; **52:** 1287–1304.
2. Vokes EE, *et al.* Multicenter phase II study of weekly oral vinorelbine for stage IV non-small-cell lung cancer. *J Clin Oncol* 1995; **13:** 637–44.
3. Jones SF, Burris HA. Vinorelbine: a new antineoplastic drug for the treatment of non-small-cell lung cancer. *Ann Pharmacother* 1996; **30:** 501–6.
4. Rule S, *et al.* Vinorelbine in the treatment of lymphoma. *Hematol Oncol* 1998; **16:** 101–5.
5. Burger RA, *et al.* The P-glycoprotein antagonist PSC 833 increases the plasma concentrations of 6alpha-hydroxypaclitaxel, a major metabolite of paclitaxel. *Gynecol Oncol* 1999; **72:** 148–53.
6. Fields-Jones S, *et al.* Improvements in clinical benefit with vinorelbine in the treatment of hormone-refractory prostate cancer: a phase II trial. *Ann Oncol* 1999; **10:** 1307–10.
7. Gregory RK, Smith IE. Vinorelbine—a clinical review. *Br J Cancer* 2000; **82:** 1907–13.
8. Sarris AH, *et al.* Infusional vinorelbine in relapsed or refractory lymphomas. *Leuk Lymphoma* 2000; **39:** 291–9.
9. Sorensen P, *et al.* Phase II study of vinorelbine in the treatment of platinum-resistant ovarian carcinoma. *Gynecol Oncol* 2001; **81:** 58–62.
10. Oudard S, *et al.* Phase II study of vinorelbine in patients with androgen-independent prostate cancer. *Ann Oncol* 2001; **12:** 847–52.

Administration in hepatic impairment. Clearance of vinorelbine was markedly reduced in patients with diffuse liver metastases and hence severely altered hepatic function: a 50% dose reduction was probably appropriate in such patients even if hyperbilirubinaemia was not marked.[1] However, reduced doses were not necessary in patients with moderate liver involvement in whom liver function, as measured by lignocaine [lidocaine] metabolism, was not markedly reduced.

1. Robieux I, *et al.* Pharmacokinetics of vinorelbine in patients with liver metastases. *Clin Pharmacol Ther* 1996; **59:** 32–40.

Preparations

Proprietary Preparations (details are given in Part 3)

Aust.: Navelbine; *Austral.:* Navelbine; *Braz.:* Navelbine; *Canad.:* Navelbine; *Denm.:* Navelbine; *Fin.:* Navelbine; *Fr.:* Navelbine; *Ger.:* Navelbine; *Israel:* Navelbine; *Ital.:* Navelbine; *Mex.:* Navelbine; *Norw.:* Navelbine; *NZ:* Navelbine; *Port.:* Navelbine; *S.Afr.:* Navelbine; *Singapore:* Navelbine; *Spain:* Biovelbin†; Navelbine; *Swed.:* Navelbine; *Switz.:* Navelbine; *Thai.:* Navelbine; *UK:* Navelbine; *USA:* Navelbine.

Vorozole (15359-s)

Vorozole (BAN, USAN, rINN).

R-83842. (+)-6-[4-Chloro-α-(1,2,4-triazol-1-yl)benzyl]-1-methyl-1H-benzotriazole.

$C_{16}H_{13}ClN_6 = 324.8$.

CAS — 129731-10-8.
ATC — L02BG05.

Profile

Vorozole is a nonsteroidal inhibitor of the aromatase (oestrogen synthetase) system. It has been investigated in the treatment of breast cancer.

◊ References.

1. Goss PE, *et al.* Phase II study of vorozole (R83842), a new aromatase inhibitor, in postmenopausal women with advanced breast cancer in progression on tamoxifen. *Clin Cancer Res* 1995; **1:** 287–94.

2. Paridaens R, *et al.* Vorozole (Rivizor): an active and well tolerated new aromatase inhibitor for the treatment of advanced breast cancer patients with prior tamoxifen exposure. *Anticancer Drugs* 1998; **9:** 29–35.
3. Goss PE, *et al.* Randomized phase III trial comparing the new potent and selective third-generation aromatase inhibitor vorozole with megestrol acetate in postmenopausal advanced breast cancer patients. *J Clin Oncol* 1999; **17:** 52–63.

Zinostatin   (1881-h)

Zinostatin *(USAN, rINN)*.

Neocarzinostatin; NSC-157365 (formerly NSC-69856).

CAS — 9014-02-2.

An antineoplastic antibiotic obtained from *Streptomyces carzinostaticus.*

Profile
Zinostatin is an antibiotic with antineoplastic activity and has been used in the treatment of malignant neoplasms.

Zinostatin stimalamer (SMANCS), a conjugate of zinostatin with a styrene-maleic acid polymer, is used for the treatment of liver cancer.

Zolimomab Aritox   (9389-p)

Zolimomab Aritox *(USAN, rINN)*.

CD5 T-lymphocyte Immunotoxin; H65-RTA.

CAS — 141483-72-9.

Profile
Zolimomab aritox is a conjugate of a murine monoclonal antibody against the CD5 antigen of human lymphocytes with the A chain of ricin (see p.1658). It has been investigated in the prevention and treatment of graft-versus-host disease in patients receiving bone marrow transplants (p.502). Zolimomab aritox has also been investigated in the treatment of various auto-immune diseases, or diseases considered to have an immune component, including diabetes mellitus and rheumatoid arthritis.

◊ References.

1. Weisdorf D, *et al.* Combination graft-versus-host disease prophylaxis using immunotoxin (anti-CD5-RTA [Xomazyme-CD5]) plus methotrexate and cyclosporine or prednisone after unrelated donor marrow transplantation. *Bone Marrow Transplant* 1993; **12:** 531–6.
2. Stand V, *et al.* Effects of administration of an anti-CD5 plus immuno-conjugate in rheumatoid arthritis: results of two phase II studies. *Arthritis Rheum* 1993; **36:** 620–30.
3. Skyler JS, *et al.* Effects of an anti-CD5 immunoconjugate (CD5-plus) in recent onset type I diabetes mellitus: a preliminary investigation. *J Diabetes Complications* 1993; **7:** 224–32.
4. Olsen NJ, *et al.* A double-blind, placebo-controlled study of anti-CD5 immunoconjugate in patients with rheumatoid arthritis. *Arthritis Rheum* 1996; **39:** 1102–8.

Zorubicin Hydrochloride   (14032-n)

Zorubicin Hydrochloride *(USAN, rINNM)*.

NSC-164011; RP-22050 (zorubicin). Benzoic acid (2S-cis)-{1-[4-(3-amino-2,3,6-trideoxy-α-L-*lyxo*-hexopyranosyloxy)-1,2,3,4,6,11-hexahydro-2,5,12-trihydroxy-7-methoxy-6,11-dioxonaphthacen-2-yl]ethylidene}hydrazide hydrochloride.

$C_{34}H_{35}N_3O_{10}$,HCl = 682.1.

CAS — 54083-22-6 (zorubicin); 36508-71-1 (zorubicin hydrochloride).

Profile
Zorubicin is an anthracycline antibiotic with antineoplastic actions similar to those of doxorubicin (see p.534). It has been used as the hydrochloride in the treatment of acute leukaemias.

Antiprotozoals

The drugs described in this chapter are those used primarily in the treatment of parasitic protozoal infections. In addition to their use as antiprotozoals, metronidazole and related nitroimidazole derivatives are also important in the treatment of anaerobic bacterial infections. Some veterinary antiprotozoal drugs are included. Drugs used in the treatment of malaria are described in the Antimalarials chapter; some of these are also used in other protozoal infections.

The principal antiprotozoal drugs are listed in Table 1, below.

Choice of Antiprotozoal

Protozoal infections occur throughout the world and are a major cause of morbidity and mortality in some regions. The choice of treatment for the more important protozoal diseases in humans is discussed below.

Amoebic infections

The most common amoebic infection of man is amoebiasis caused by infection with the protozoan parasite *Entamoeba histolytica* and related species. Free-living amoebae can also cause disease in man, though these infections are rare. Infection with *Naegleria fowleri* results in primary amoebic meningoencephalitis, while infection with *Acanthamoeba* species or leptomyxid amoebae leads to granulomatous amoebic encephalitis. *Acanthamoeba* is also a cause of keratitis.

Acanthamoeba infections. ACANTHAMOEBA KERATITIS. *Acanthamoeba* keratitis is usually associated with the wearing of soft contact lenses. It is treated by prompt topical antiamoebic therapy, although an optimum regimen has yet to be determined. Surgery may be needed in severe cases. The antiseptic propamidine isetionate applied topically is a mainstay of treatment, and has been

Table 1. Classification of principal antiprotozoals.

Antimony compounds	*Nitrofurans*
Meglumine antimonate	Furazolidone
Sodium stibogluconate	Nifuratel
	Nifurtimox
Aromatic diamidines	
Pentamidine	*5-Nitroimidazoles*
	Metronidazole
Arsenicals, pentavalent	Nimorazole
Acetarsol	Ornidazole
Tryparsamide	Secnidazole
	Tinidazole
Arsenicals, trivalent	
Melarsoprol	*Miscellaneous*
	Atovaquone
Dichloroacetamides	Benznidazole
Diloxanide	Dehydroemetine
	Eflornithine
Halogenated hydroxyquinolines	Mepacrine
Diiodohydroxyquinoline	Suramin

used in various combinations with neomycin[1,2] or a neomycin-polymyxin-gramicidin preparation,[3,4] and/or a biguanide (usually polihexanide[2,5,6] but chlorhexidine[7] has also been proposed). Combinations of systemic itraconazole or ketoconazole with topical miconazole have also been tried with some success.[4,8] Hexamidine isetionate has been suggested[9] as an alternative to propamidine isetionate.

Acanthamoeba keratitis in contact lens wearers should be preventable by good lens hygiene (see Contact Lens Care, p.1129).

1. Wright P, *et al.* Acanthamoeba keratitis successfully treated medically. *Br J Ophthalmol* 1985; **69:** 778–82.
2. Varga JH, *et al.* Combined treatment of Acanthamoeba keratitis with propamidine, neomycin, and polyhexamethylene biguanide. *Am J Ophthalmol* 1993; **115:** 466–70.
3. Moore MB, McCulley JP. Acanthamoeba keratitis associated with contact lenses: six consecutive cases of successful management. *Br J Ophthalmol* 1989; **73:** 271–5.
4. Asbell PA, Torres MA. Therapeutic dilemmas in external ocular diseases. *Drugs* 1991; **42:** 606–15.
5. Illingworth CD, *et al.* Acanthamoeba keratitis: risk factors and outcome. *Br J Ophthalmol* 1995; **79:** 1078–82.
6. Elder MJ, Dart JKG. Chemotherapy for acanthamoeba keratitis. *Lancet* 1995; **345:** 791–2.
7. Seal DV, *et al.* Chlorhexidine or polyhexamethylene biguanide for acanthamoeba keratitis. *Lancet* 1995; **345:** 136.
8. Anonymous. Drugs for parasitic infections. *Med Lett Drugs Ther* 1998; **40:** 1–12.
9. Perrine D, *et al.* Amoebicidal efficiencies of various diamidines against two strains of Acanthamoeba polyphaga. *Antimicrob Agents Chemother* 1995; **39:** 339–42.

DISSEMINATED ACANTHAMOEBA INFECTION. Granulomatous amoebic encephalitis is caused by infection with free-living amoebae, usually *Acanthamoeba* spp. or sometimes leptomyxid amoebae. It is an opportunistic infection occurring mainly in debilitated or immunocompromised individuals. The protozoa spread to the CNS from pulmonary or skin lesions and produce focal neurological deficits that progress over days or weeks to a diffuse meningoencephalitis. The infection is usually fatal and most cases have been diagnosed postmortem so little is known about effective treatments.

Clinical responses to chemotherapy have been reported in a few patients[1,2] with disseminated infection, but no evidence of CNS involvement. Disseminated *Acanthamoeba* infection in an immunocompromised patient was successfully treated with intravenous pentamidine followed by maintenance therapy with oral itraconazole.[1] Skin lesions were treated topically with chlorhexidine and ketoconazole. Clinical improvement was reported in disseminated acanthamoebiasis in a patient with AIDS following treatment with intravenous pentamidine and oral flucytosine, and in an infant with HIV infection treated with fluconazole, flucytosine, and sulfadiazine.[2]

1. Slater CA, *et al.* Brief report: successful treatment of disseminated Acanthamoeba infection in an immunocompromised patient. *N Engl J Med* 1994; **331:** 85–7.
2. Murakawa GJ, *et al.* Disseminated Acanthamoeba in patients with AIDS: a report of five cases and a review of the literature. *Arch Dermatol* 1995; **131:** 1291–6.

Amoebiasis. The term amoebiasis is generally applied to infections with obligate parasitic species of amoeba, principally *Entamoeba histolytica.* Other parasitic species which occasionally cause human infections include *E. polecki* (primarily a parasite of pigs and reported mainly in Papua New Guinea) and *Dientamoeba fragilis* (often found in association with the helminth *Enterobius vermicularis* and now thought to be a trichomonad).

Transmission of *E. histolytica* is by the faeco-oral route and infection results from the ingestion of cysts, usually in contaminated food and drink. The cysts transform to trophozoites in the intestines and reproduction occurs by fission of the trophozoites. Further cysts develop and are excreted in the faeces. Amoebiasis occurs throughout the world. It is more prevalent and severe in the tropics and subtropics, but is more closely related to sanitation and socio-economic status than to climate. The majority of people infected with *E. histolytica* are asymptomatic cyst passers in whom trophozoites live as commensals in the large intestine. In others, the trophozoites invade the wall of the large intestine causing ulceration and may migrate to other tissues, especially the liver, where they continue to divide and destroy tissue. Factors increasing susceptibility to tissue invasion include malnutrition, immunosuppression, and pregnancy.

WHO has classified symptomatic amoebiasis into intestinal or extra-intestinal amoebiasis.[1] Intestinal amoebiasis comprises two main states, amoebic dysentery and non-dysenteric amoebic colitis; amoeboma, a localised

form of intestinal amoebiasis, and amoebic appendicitis may also occur. Hepatic amoebiasis, the most common form of extra-intestinal amoebic disease, may present as acute non-suppurative disease or as amoebic liver abscess. Amoebic infection is a less common cause of liver abscess than bacterial infection. Amoebiasis may also involve the skin, genito-urinary tract, or organs such as the lungs and brain.

Drugs used in the **treatment** of amoebiasis may be classified according to their site of action as follows:

- *luminal amoebicides* acting principally in the bowel lumen. These have included diloxanide furoate and other dichloroacetamide derivatives, diiodohydroxyquinoline and other halogenated hydroxyquinoline derivatives, and acetarsol and other arsenical derivatives. Diloxanide furoate is still widely used as the luminal amoebicide of choice. The arsenicals are toxic and are no longer used and, although some authorities still recommend diiodohydroxyquinoline, most oral preparations of halogenated hydroxyquinolines have been withdrawn since the association between clioquinol and subacute myelo-opticoneuropathy (SMON) was established. The antibiotics paromomycin and tetracycline have also been used.

- *tissue* or *systemic amoebicides* acting principally in the intestinal wall and liver. These have included the alkaloid emetine, and its synthetic derivative dehydroemetine, and the antimalarial chloroquine which acts principally in the liver.

- *mixed amoebicides* acting at all sites of infection, that is within the intestinal lumen and in the intestinal wall and other tissues. These have included metronidazole and other 5-nitroimidazole derivatives. However, because of their rapid absorption from the gastrointestinal tract, the nitroimidazoles are less effective against parasites in the lumen.

In non-endemic areas, patients with asymptomatic intestinal amoebiasis (cyst passers) are generally treated with a luminal amoebicide. The choice of drug is influenced by availability; diloxanide furoate is generally used in the UK while diiodohydroxyquinoline or paromomycin are used in the USA.[2] Invasive amoebiasis (amoebic dysentery; hepatic amoebiasis) requires treatment with a systemically absorbed amoebicide followed by a luminal amoebicide to eradicate any surviving organisms from the lumen of the large intestine and prevent relapse. Such treatment is generally with metronidazole or tinidazole followed by a luminal amoebicide. Other treatments that have been used in seriously ill patients are emetine or dehydroemetine, together with chloroquine in hepatic amoebiasis, followed by a luminal amoebicide.[3] Needle aspiration may be beneficial if there is a large liver abscess or if rupture of the abscess is imminent.[3] Tetracycline has been added to treatment regimens in severe amoebic dysentery.[3] In acute diarrhoea of any aetiology the priority is to maintain hydration by prevention or treatment of fluid and electrolyte depletion, especially in infants and the elderly. Oral rehydration therapy is discussed under Diarrhoea on p.1203.

Drugs suggested for the treatment of *Dientamoeba fragilis* infections include diiodohydroxyquinoline, paromomycin, or tetracycline.[2] Metronidazole has been suggested for *E. polecki* infections.[2]

1. WHO. Amoebiasis. *WHO Tech Rep Ser 421* 1969.
2. Anonymous. Drugs for parasitic infections. *Med Lett Drugs Ther* 1998; **40:** 1–12.
3. Anonymous. Protozoan intestinal infections. *WHO Drug Inf* 1988; **2:** 200–5.

Naegleria infections. PRIMARY AMOEBIC MENINGOENCEPHALITIS. Primary amoebic meningoencephalitis is usually caused by the free-living amoeba *Naegleria fowleri.* It occurs mainly in healthy children and young adults and is usually associated with swimming in warm fresh water. The protozoa invade the CNS directly through the nasal mucosa to produce a meningoencephalitis that is usually rapidly fatal. The few cases of successful treatment that have been reported[1-3] have all involved intravenous, and usually intrathecal, amphotericin B; some patients were also given oral rifampicin.

1. Anderson K, Jamieson A. Primary amoebic meningoencephalitis. *Lancet* 1972; **i:** 902–3.
2. Seidel JS, *et al.* Successful treatment of primary amebic meningoencephalitis. *N Engl J Med* 1982; **306:** 346–8.
3. Brown RL. Successful treatment of primary amebic meningoencephalitis. *Arch Intern Med* 1991; **151:** 1201–2.

Babesiosis

Babesiosis (piroplasmosis) is a rare infection caused by protozoa of the *Babesia* spp., which are transmitted to man by the bite of infected *Ixodes* ticks. Transmission by blood transfusion has also been reported.

Infections in North America are commonly due to *B. microti* and though often asymptomatic may produce prolonged severe illness with fever and haemolytic anaemia, particularly in patients who are asplenic, elderly, debilitated, or immunocompromised. Co-infection with *B. microti* and *Borrelia burgdorferi* (Lyme disease) has resulted in more severe symptoms. In Europe infections are principally caused by *B. divergens* or *B. bovis* and have only been described in asplenic persons, in most of whom the infection was rapidly fatal. Clinical features include severe haemolytic anaemia, jaundice, and renal failure.

There is no established specific treatment for babesiosis. For serious infections, supportive therapies include blood transfusion and haemodialysis. Exchange transfusions have been used to reduce parasitaemia. A combination of clindamycin and quinine has been used[1-3] for the treatment of *B. microti* infections. A prospective, randomised study[4] in 58 patients has suggested that azithromycin in combination with atovaquone may be equally effective as clindamycin and quinine. Azithromycin in combination with quinine has been reported to be effective in 2 patients who had not responded to quinine plus clindamycin.[5,6] In *B. divergens* infections, treatment is complicated by the rapid progression of the disease. A number of antiprotozoal and antimalarial drugs have been tried with limited success although a combination of pentamidine and co-trimoxazole was successful in a patient,[7] and a marked reduction in parasite load was seen in a patient treated with pentamidine in addition to exchange transfusions.[8] Pentamidine has also been reported to produce clinical improvement in patients with *B. microti* infection[9] but the efficacy and safety of pentamidine in this self-limiting disease has been questioned.[10]

1. Wittner M, *et al.* Successful chemotherapy of transfusion babesiosis. *Ann Intern Med* 1982; **96:** 601–4.
2. Anonymous. Clindamycin and quinine treatment for Babesia microti infections. *MMWR* 1983; **32:** 65–6,72.
3. Anonymous. Drugs for parasitic infections. *Med Lett Drugs Ther* 1998; **40:** 1–12.
4. Krause PJ, *et al.* Atovaquone and azithromycin for the treatment of babesiosis. *N Engl J Med* 2000; **343:** 1454–8.
5. Shaio MF, Yang KD. Response of babesiosis to a combined regimen of quinine and azithromycin. *Trans R Soc Trop Med Hyg* 1997; **91:** 214–15.
6. Shih C-M, Wang C-C. Ability of azithromycin in combination with quinine for the elimination of babesial infection in humans. *Am J Trop Med Hyg* 1998; **59:** 509–12.
7. Raoult D, *et al.* Babesiosis, pentamidine, and cotrimoxazole. *Ann Intern Med* 1987; **107:** 944.
8. Clarke CS, *et al.* Babesiosis: under-reporting or case-clustering? *Postgrad Med J* 1989; **65:** 591–3.
9. Francioli PB, *et al.* Response of babesiosis to pentamidine therapy. *Ann Intern Med* 1981; **94:** 326–30.
10. Teutsch SM, Juranek DD. Babesiosis. *Ann Intern Med* 1981; **95:** 241.

Balantidiasis

Infection with the ciliate protozoan *Balantidium coli* results from the ingestion of cysts, the commonest source of which is pigs.[1] Water-borne epidemics of balantidiasis have been reported. Most infections are asymptomatic and the organism lives in the large intestine as a luminal commensal, but those with symptomatic infections have diarrhoea. Colonic ulceration resulting in a severe dysenteric syndrome resembling amoebic dysentery may occur in some individuals, especially those who are malnourished. Treatment is with tetracycline; metronidazole or diiodohydroxyquinoline are alternatives.[1]

1. Anonymous. Drugs for parasitic infections. *Med Lett Drugs Ther* 1998; **40:** 1–12.

Blastocystis hominis infection

There is controversy over whether the protozoan parasite *Blastocystis hominis* is a pathogen or a harmless commensal of the intestinal tract. It has increasingly been reported both in immunocompetent and immunocompromised subjects,[1] with transmission probably by the faeco-oral route. Diarrhoea and other gastrointestinal symptoms have been ascribed to infection with the organism.

Treatment is with standard antiprotozoals, especially metronidazole, but with variable success. Co-trimoxazole was reported to have eliminated *B. hominis* from the stools of all but 1 of 47 otherwise healthy subjects with diarrhoea.[2]

1. Anonymous. Blastocystis hominis: commensal or pathogen? *Lancet* 1991; **337:** 521–2.
2. Schwartz E, Houston R. Effect of co-trimoxazole on stool recovery of Blastocystis hominis. *Lancet* 1992; **339:** 428–9.

Coccidiosis

Coccidiosis is a term sometimes applied to infections with protozoa of the order *Eucoccidiorida*. The predominant coccidian infections in man are caused by *Cryptosporidium* (below), *Cyclospora cayetanensis* (below), *Isospora* (below), *Plasmodium* (see Malaria, p.428), and *Toxoplasma* (below). Coccidian protozoa, primarily *Eimeria*, cause economically important infections in domesticated animals.

Cryptosporidiosis

Cryptosporidiosis is a gastrointestinal infection caused by species of the coccidian protozoan parasite *Cryptosporidium*. It has a worldwide distribution and occurs in many animal species as well as in man. Infection is acquired through ingestion, and perhaps inhalation, of oocysts. Infection in immunocompetent individuals usually causes a self-limiting diarrhoea lasting up to 2 weeks. In immunocompromised patients there may be profuse and persistent diarrhoea, profound weight loss, and severe abdominal pain, and the infection may be life-threatening. Cryptosporidiosis is increasingly recognised as a cause of diarrhoea in patients with AIDS. Other sites of infection include the respiratory and biliary tracts.

There is currently no consistently effective specific therapy and priority should be given to maintaining hydration by prevention or treatment of fluid and electrolyte depletion, especially in infants and the elderly. Oral rehydration therapy is discussed under Diarrhoea on p.1203. Responses to paromomycin have generally been favourable, although patient numbers are small.[1-8] There have also been reports indicating improvement in immunocompromised patients given azithromycin,[9,10] and combination therapy with paromomycin and azithromycin has produced some beneficial responses in patients with AIDS-related cryptosporidiosis.[11] Other treatments reported to have produced benefit include hyperimmune bovine colostrum,[12-15] eflornithine,[16] normal immunoglobulin with high cryptosporidium antibody titres,[17] or letrazuril,[18,19] but again the numbers of patients involved are small. Nitazoxanide may also be effective.[20] Responses to spiramycin have not been consistent.[21-23] Beneficial responses to octreotide have been reported in a few cases,[24,25] but a study in patients with refractory AIDS-related diarrhoea suggested that response was better in patients without identifiable pathogens.[26]

Clarithromycin and rifabutin may be useful for disease prophylaxis.[27]

1. Clezy K, *et al.* Paromomycin for the treatment of cryptosporidial diarrhoea in AIDS patients. *AIDS* 1991; **5:** 1146–7.
2. Armitage K, *et al.* Treatment of cryptosporidiosis with paromomycin: a report of five cases. *Arch Intern Med* 1992; **152:** 2497–9.
3. Danziger LH, *et al.* Treatment of cryptosporidial diarrhea in an AIDS patient with paromomycin. *Ann Pharmacother* 1993; **27:** 1460–2.
4. Fichtenbaum CJ, *et al.* Use of paromomycin for treatment of cryptosporidiosis in patients with AIDS. *Clin Infect Dis* 1993; **16:** 298–300.
5. White AC, *et al.* Paromomycin for cryptosporidiosis in AIDS: a prospective, double-blind trial. *J Infect Dis* 1994; **170:** 419–24.
6. Bissuel F, *et al.* Paromomycin: an effective treatment for cryptosporidial diarrhea in patients with AIDS. *Clin Infect Dis* 1994; **18:** 447–9.
7. Mohri H, *et al.* Case report: inhalation therapy of paromomycin is effective for respiratory infection and hypoxia by Cryptosporidium with AIDS. *Am J Med Sci* 1995; **309:** 60–2.
8. Flanigan TP, *et al.* Prospective trial of paromomycin for cryptosporidiosis in AIDS. *Am J Med* 1996; **100:** 370–2.
9. Vargas SL, *et al.* Azithromycin for treatment of severe Cryptosporidium diarrhea in two children with cancer. *J Pediatr* 1993; **123:** 154–6.
10. Bessette RE, Amsden GW. Treatment of non-HIV cryptosporidial diarrhea with azithromycin. *Ann Pharmacother* 1995; **29:** 991–3.
11. Smith NH, *et al.* Combination drug therapy for cryptosporidiosis in AIDS. *J Infect Dis* 1998; **178:** 900–903.
12. Tzipori S, *et al.* Remission of diarrhoea due to cryptosporidiosis in an immunodeficient child treated with hyperimmune bovine colostrum. *BMJ* 1986; **293:** 1276–7.
13. Tzipori S, *et al.* Chronic cryptosporidial diarrhoea and hyperimmune cow colostrum. *Lancet* 1987; **ii:** 344–5.
14. Nord J, *et al.* Treatment with bovine hyperimmune colostrum of cryptosporidial diarrhea in AIDS patients. *AIDS* 1990; **4:** 581–4.
15. Shield J, *et al.* Bovine colostrum immunoglobulin concentrate for cryptosporidiosis in AIDS. *Arch Dis Child* 1993; **69:** 451–3.
16. Rolston KVI, *et al.* Intestinal cryptosporidiosis treated with eflornithine: a prospective study among patients with AIDS. *J Acquir Immune Defic Syndr* 1989; **2:** 426–30.
17. Borowitz SM, Saulsbury FT. Treatment of chronic cryptosporidial infection with orally administered human serum immune globulin. *J Pediatr* 1991; **119:** 593–5.
18. Harris M, *et al.* A phase I study of letrazuril in AIDS-related cryptosporidiosis. *AIDS* 1994; **8:** 1109–13.
19. Loeb M, *et al.* Treatment with letrazuril of refractory cryptosporidial diarrhea complicating AIDS. *J Acquir Immune Defic Syndr Hum Retrovirol* 1995; **10:** 48–53.
20. Rossignol J-F, *et al.* A double-'blind' placebo-controlled study of nitazoxanide in the treatment of cryptosporidial diarrhoea in AIDS patients in Mexico. *Trans R Soc Trop Med Hyg* 1998; **92:** 663–6.
21. Portnoy D, *et al.* Treatment of intestinal cryptosporidiosis with spiramycin. *Ann Intern Med* 1984; **101:** 202–4.
22. Moskovitz BL, *et al.* Spiramycin therapy for cryptosporidial diarrhoea in immunocompromised patients. *J Antimicrob Chemother* 1988; **22** (suppl B): 189–91.
23. Wittenberg DF, *et al.* Spiramycin is not effective in treating cryptosporidium diarrhea in infants: results of a double-blind randomized trial. *J Infect Dis* 1989; **159:** 131–2.
24. Cook DJ, *et al.* Somatostatin treatment for cryptosporidial diarrhea in a patient with the acquired immunodeficiency syndrome (AIDS). *Ann Intern Med* 1988; **108:** 708–9.
25. Clotet B, *et al.* Efficacy of the somatostatin analogue (SMS-201-995), Sandostatin, for cryptosporidial diarrhea in patients with AIDS. *AIDS* 1989; **3:** 857–8.
26. Cello JP, *et al.* Effect of octreotide on refractory AIDS-associated diarrhea: a prospective, multicenter clinical trial. *Ann Intern Med* 1991; **115:** 705–10.
27. Holmberg SD, *et al.* Possible effectiveness of clarithromycin and rifabutin for cryptosporidiosis chemoprophylaxis in HIV disease. *JAMA* 1998; **279:** 384–6.

Cyclosporiasis

An organism originally described as cyanobacterium-like or coccidian-like bodies, but now identified as the coccidian protozoan *Cyclospora cayetanensis*, has been reported to be a cause of diarrhoea in both immunocompromised and immunocompetent patients. Infection results from ingestion of spores or oocysts in contaminated food or water. In immunocompetent patients, infection may be asymptomatic or cause a self-limiting diarrhoeal illness. Immunocompromised patients may develop severe or persistent symptoms. Beneficial responses have been reported with co-trimoxazole.[1-3]

1. Pape JW, *et al.* Cyclospora infection in adults infected with HIV: clinical manifestations, treatment, and prophylaxis. *Ann Intern Med* 1994; **121:** 654–7.
2. Hoge CW, *et al.* Placebo-controlled trial of co-trimoxazole for cyclospora infections among travellers and foreign residents in Nepal. *Lancet* 1995; **345:** 691–3. Correction. *ibid.*; 1060.
3. Verdier R-I, *et al.* Trimethoprim-sulfamethoxazole compared with ciprofloxacin for treatment and prophylaxis of Isospora belli and Cyclospora cayetanensis infection in HIV-infected patients: a randomized, controlled trial. *Ann Intern Med* 2000; **132:** 885–8.

Gastro-enteritis

Although bacteria and viruses are responsible for many cases of infective diarrhoea, protozoal infections are also recognised as a cause of diarrhoea, which can be severe especially in immunocompromised patients, including those with AIDS. In acute diarrhoea of any aetiology the priority is to maintain hydration by prevention or treatment of fluid and electrolyte depletion, especially in infants and the elderly. Oral rehydration is discussed under Diarrhoea on p.1203. Specific therapy with antiprotozoals may also be necessary to control enteric protozoal infections. For the management of the protozoal infections that are generally associated with diarrhoea, see under Amoebiasis (above), Balantidiasis (above), *Blastocystis hominis* infections (above), Cryptosporidiosis (above), Cyclosporiasis (above), Giardiasis (below), Isosporiasis (below), and Microsporidiosis (below).

References.

1. Guerrant RL, Bobak DA. Bacterial and protozoal gastroenteritis. *N Engl J Med* 1991; **325:** 327–40.
2. Goodgame RW. Diagnosis and treatment of gastrointestinal protozoal infections. *Curr Opin Infect Dis* 1996; **9:** 346–52.

Giardiasis

Infection with *Giardia intestinalis* (*G. lamblia*; *Lamblia intestinalis*) occurs throughout the world and is one of the commonest intestinal protozoal infections. Infection is acquired by oral ingestion of *Giardia* cysts, and transmission may be person-to-person or from contaminated drinking water or foodstuffs. Infected patients may have acute or chronic diarrhoea or they may be asymptomatic. In acute diarrhoea of any aetiology the priority is to maintain hydration by prevention or treatment of fluid and electrolyte depletion, especially in infants and the elderly. Oral rehydration is discussed under Diarrhoea on p.1203.

Treatment is with metronidazole or another nitroimidazole derivative such as tinidazole.[1] Albendazole, furazolidone, mebendazole, and mepacrine have all also been used but some of them may be less well tolerated than the nitroimidazoles. Paromomycin has also been suggested;[2] although it is less effective than other drugs, it is not absorbed systemically and may be a useful alternative during pregnancy. Treatment may sometimes need to be repeated, possibly due to resistance,[3,4] and drug combinations such as metronidazole with mepacrine have been reported to be of value in these cases.[3]

1. Zaat JOM, et al. Drugs for treating giardiasis (updated 29 November 2000). Available in The Cochrane Library; Issue 3. Oxford: Update Software; 2001.
2. Anonymous. Drugs for parasitic infections. Med Lett Drugs Ther 1998; 40: 1–12.
3. Farthing MJG. Giardia comes of age: progress in epidemiology, immunology and chemotherapy. J Antimicrob Chemother 1992; 30: 563–6.
4. Boreham PFL. Giardiasis and its control. Pharm J 1991; 247: 271–4.

Infections in immunocompromised patients

Patients with a defective immune system are at especial risk of infection. Primary immune deficiency is rare, whereas secondary deficiency is more common: immunosuppressive therapy, cancer and its treatment, HIV infection, and splenectomy may all cause neutropenia and impaired humoral and cellular immunity in varying degrees. The risk of infection is linked to the duration and severity of neutropenia. Most protozoal infections present in a more severe form in immunocompromised patients than in immunocompetent patients. Those of particular concern in patients with HIV infection include Cryptosporidiosis (above), Isosporiasis (below), Leishmaniasis (below), Microsporidiosis (below), and Toxoplasmosis (below).

References.

1. Canning EU. Protozoan infections. Trans R Soc Trop Med Hyg 1990; 84 (suppl 1): 19–24.
2. Wilson ME, et al. Infections in HIV-infected travelers: risks and prevention. Ann Intern Med 1991; 114: 582–92.
3. Sharpstone D, Gazzard B. Gastrointestinal manifestations of HIV infection. Lancet 1996; 348: 378–83.
4. Centers for Disease Control. 1999 USPHS/IDSA guidelines for the prevention of opportunistic infections in persons infected with human immunodeficiency virus. MMWR 1999; 48(RR-10): 1–66.

Isosporiasis

Isosporiasis is a coccidian protozoal infection of the gastrointestinal tract caused by Isospora belli. Oocysts are excreted in faeces and infection is acquired when sporulated oocysts are ingested. In immunocompetent individuals the infection is usually mild and self-limiting but in immunocompromised patients there may be severe, chronic gastro-enteritis. Treatment is usually with co-trimoxazole.[1-3] Pyrimethamine has been used successfully in individual patients with sulfonamide sensitivity.[4] In acute diarrhoea of any aetiology the priority is to maintain hydration by prevention or treatment of fluid and electrolyte depletion, especially in infants and the elderly. Oral rehydration therapy is discussed under Diarrhoea on p.1203.

Recurrence of infection is common and long-term suppressive treatment with either co-trimoxazole or pyrimethamine plus sulfadoxine has been recommended.[5]

1. WHO. WHO model prescribing information: drugs used in parasitic diseases. Geneva: WHO, 1995.
2. Anonymous. Drugs for parasitic infections. Med Lett Drugs Ther 1998; 40: 1–12.
3. Verdier R-I, et al. Trimethoprim-sulfamethoxazole compared with ciprofloxacin for treatment and prophylaxis of Isospora belli and Cyclospora cayetanensis infection in HIV-infected patients: a randomized, controlled trial. Ann Intern Med 2000; 132: 885–8.
4. Weiss LM, et al. Isospora belli infection: treatment with pyrimethamine. Ann Intern Med 1988; 109: 474–5.
5. Pape JW, et al. Treatment and prophylaxis of Isospora belli infection in patients with the acquired immunodeficiency syndrome. N Engl J Med 1989; 320: 1044–7.

Leishmaniasis

Leishmaniasis is caused by parasitic protozoa of the genus Leishmania. It occurs throughout Africa, the Middle East, Central Asia, and the Mediterranean (Old World leishmaniasis), and throughout Central and South America (New World leishmaniasis). In endemic areas there is generally a reservoir of disease in a mammalian host, often dogs or rodents. The usual vectors are sandflies of the genus Phlebotomus in the Old World and Lutzomyia in the New World. Leishmaniasis can be categorised as cutaneous, mucosal, and visceral and ranges from self-limiting, localised, cutaneous ulcers to widely disseminated progressive disease and involvement of the reticuloendothelial system. Incubation periods can be prolonged, with clinical features not appearing until several months or even years after the primary infection.

In endemic areas an integrated approach to controlling leishmaniasis involves case detection and treatment of patients, vector and animal reservoir control, environmental management to reduce suitable vector habitats, and personal protection against sandfly bites including the use of insect repellents and bednets.[1] Strategies aimed at controlling malaria are believed to have reduced leishmaniasis transmission dramatically.[1]

Visceral leishmaniasis of the Old World is mainly caused by L. donovani and L. infantum and of the New World by L. chagasi. The onset of the disease is gradual in residents of an endemic area but may present as an acute illness in non-immune visitors to the region. Many infections result in sub-clinical or self-limiting disease. Common symptoms are fever, malaise, shivering or chills, weight loss, anorexia, and discomfort in the left hypochondrium. Common clinical signs are non-tender splenomegaly with or without hepatomegaly, wasting, pallor of mucous membranes, anaemia, leucopenia, and lymphadenopathy. Continued deterioration can lead to potentially fatal secondary infection. Darkening of the skin of the face, hands, feet, and abdomen is common in endemic visceral leishmaniasis in India (kala-azar = black sickness). Rare complications can include severe acute haemolytic anaemia, acute renal damage, and severe mucosal haemorrhage. In recent years, visceral leishmaniasis has emerged as an opportunistic infection in patients with HIV or other conditions associated with reduced immunity, in whom it is particularly difficult to treat.

A small percentage of patients develop post-kala-azar dermal leishmaniasis following recovery from visceral leishmaniasis and such patients represent a human reservoir for the disease.

The pentavalent antimonials meglumine antimoniate and sodium stibogluconate are the traditional first-line drugs for the treatment of visceral leishmaniasis.[1-3] Patients relapsing after the initial course of treatment may be given a further course, but there is growing evidence that responsiveness to the antimonials is declining. Four regimens have been suggested for the first-line treatment of visceral leishmaniasis due to L. infantum in Mediterranean countries.[4] They are: pentavalent antimonials, pentavalent antimonials plus allopurinol, liposomal amphotericin B, and paromomycin alone or in combination with pentavalent antimonials. These regimens are also being evaluated in other regions and in patients with HIV infection.[5-14] Amphotericin B has also been tried successfully as a second-line drug in drug-resistant infections[15-18] and increasingly as a useful alternative first-line drug.[2,3] Lipid complex and other non-conventional forms of amphotericin B are better tolerated than conventional amphotericin B, and are likely to be preferred when the toxicity and duration of therapy with conventional forms would compromise patient compliance.[2] Pentamidine has also been used as a second-line drug but its usefulness as alternative first-line therapy is doubtful[19] due to its toxicity, increasing failure rates, and slow disease response. Nevertheless it has been tried as an adjunct to meglumine antimonate for first-line therapy[20] and alone for long-term secondary prophylaxis in patients with HIV infection.[21] In view of the toxicity of both first- and second-line drugs and the number of treatment failures the search for alternative therapies continues. Oral miltefosine has been shown to be effective[22] and appears to be of some promise. Beneficial responses to ketoconazole have also been reported in some patients[23,24] but unfavourable reports have also appeared.[25,26] Another line of investigation is to boost the immune response to the parasite by adding interferon gamma to conventional treatment, although results have been variable.[27-30]

Cutaneous leishmaniasis is caused by various species of Leishmania and a wide variety of clinical presentations is possible. A 'classical' lesion starts as a nodule at the site of inoculation. A crust develops centrally which may fall away exposing an ulcer which heals gradually. Satellite nodules at the edge of the lesion are common. Cutaneous leishmaniasis of the Old World is normally caused by L. tropica, L. major, or L. aethiopica, although cutaneous lesions due to L. infantum have been reported. Cutaneous leishmaniasis of the New World (American cutaneous leishmaniasis) is caused by numerous species and subspecies of Leishmania including L. braziliensis, L. mexicana, L. panamensis, and L. peruviana. In general, New World forms tend to be more severe and longer lasting than Old World forms. The disease ranges from single, self-healing lesions which are troublesome and unsightly but not a threat to life to multiple, deep, and destructive ulcers which cause considerable disfigurement and disability.

Diffuse cutaneous leishmaniasis occurs occasionally following infection with L. aethiopica or members of the L. mexicana complex and involves dissemination of the disease from the original site of infection to distant skin sites, typically the face and exterior surfaces of the limbs. The lesions resemble lepromatous leprosy, do not heal spontaneously, and are resistant to treatment.

Another variant is leishmaniasis recidivans which is a lupoid or tuberculoid form. This chronic disease often occurs as slowly progressive, destructive and disfiguring lesions on the face which are very resistant to most forms of therapy.

There is no established treatment for cutaneous leishmaniasis.[3] The decision to treat depends upon the site and extent of the lesions and the likelihood of dissemination. Small lesions, particularly in Old World cutaneous leishmaniasis, may be left untreated if they are not troublesome to the patient. Treatment for disfiguring or potentially disabling lesions may be local or systemic. Systemic treatment is required where there is a risk that the infecting organism may be one causing mucocutaneous leishmaniasis (see below) or where there is evidence of lymphatic spread or extensive local involvement. WHO[1] suggested that early noninflamed nodular lesions due to L. tropica, L. major, L. mexicana, L. panamensis, or L. peruviana may be treated with intralesional injections of mepacrine, sodium stibogluconate, or meglumine antimonate or removed by surgery and curettage. Beneficial responses have been reported with this therapy.[3,31,32] However, local infiltration of drugs can be difficult as well as painful. Surgical curettage may promote dissemination of the parasite.[33] Other local treatments include cryotherapy or, alternatively, application of heat to bring the temperature of the lesion to about 40° which may aid healing.[34] Topical treatment with paromomycin sulfate 15% plus methylbenzethonium chloride 5% or 12% has produced promising responses;[35,36] paromomycin 12 to 15% with urea 10% was better tolerated.[37] However, not all studies have shown beneficial responses.[38,39] Systemic treatment is similar to that used for visceral leishmaniasis[1,3,40,41] (see above). Treatment with topical paromomycin plus systemic meglumine antimonate was promising in patients with New World infections.[42] Cutaneous leishmaniasis due to L. aethiopica including diffuse cutaneous leishmaniasis does not generally respond to antimonials[1] although responses to antimonials in combination with paromomycin have been reported.[43] It may also be treated with pentamidine.[1,3] Other drugs tried in cutaneous leishmaniasis have included berberine derivatives,[44] itraconazole,[45-48] and ketoconazole.[49-52] Variable responses to allopurinol have been reported in patients with New World infections.[53-55] Dapsone was reported to be effective in a study in patients in India[56] but not in Colombia.[57] Among the non-specific therapies tried in cutaneous leishmaniasis, topical application of the nitric oxide donor S-nitroso-N-acetylpenicillamine (SNAP)[58] and intralesional injection of hypertonic sodium chloride solution[59] have produced beneficial responses. Immunomodulation using leishmania antigens mixed with BCG,[60,61] interferon gamma,[62,63] or interleukin-2[64] has produced encouraging results.

While there has been some work on vaccines against cutaneous leishmaniasis much more needs to be done. However, leishmanisation (deliberate infection with L. major) has been used as a last resort in some countries when other measures have failed.

Mucocutaneous leishmaniasis of the New World (espundia) is caused by L. braziliensis or L. panamensis. In mucocutaneous leishmaniasis the primary lesions do not heal spontaneously. Metastatic spread to the mucosa may occur during the presence of the primary lesion or up to 30 years later. The nasal mucosa is always affected. Ulceration and erosion progressively destroy the soft tissue and cartilage of the oronasal/pharyngeal cavity. Mutilation is severe and secondary bacterial infection is frequent and can be fatal. Mucocutaneous leishmaniasis responds poorly to treatment and relapses are common. Initial treatment is with pentavalent antimony;[3] failure to respond is an indication to use amphotericin B or pentamidine. Nifurtimox has been reported to be effective in some cases of mucocutaneous leishmaniasis.[1] Treatment with corticosteroids may be required to control severe inflammation. Mucosal disease in Old World leishmaniasis is much less common than visceral or cutaneous forms, but treatment with antimony compounds or ketoconazole has been described.[65]

1. WHO. Control of the leishmaniases. WHO Tech Rep Ser 793 1990.
2. Berman JD. Human leishmaniasis: clinical, diagnostic, and chemotherapeutic developments in the last 10 years. Clin Infect Dis 1997; 24: 684–703.
3. Herwaldt BL. Leishmaniasis. Lancet 1999; 354: 1191–9.

4. Gradoni L, *et al.* Treatment of Mediterranean visceral leishmaniasis. *Bull WHO* 1995; **73:** 191–7.
5. Mishra M, *et al.* Amphotericin versus sodium stibogluconate in first-line treatment of Indian Kala-azar. *Lancet* 1994; **344:** 1599–1600.
6. Dietze R, *et al.* Treatment of kala-azar in Brazil with Amphocil (amphotericin B cholesterol dispersion) for 5 days. *Trans R Soc Trop Med Hyg* 1995; **89:** 309–11.
7. Russo R, *et al.* Visceral leishmaniasis in HIV infected patients: treatment with high dose liposomal amphotericin B (AmBisome). *J Infect* 1996; **32:** 133–7.
8. Thakur CP, *et al.* Aminosidine plus sodium stibogluconate for the treatment of Indian kala-azar: a randomized dose-finding clinical trial. *Trans R Soc Trop Med Hyg* 1995; **89:** 219–23.
9. Scott JAG, *et al.* Aminosidine (paromomycin) in the treatment of leishmaniasis imported into the United Kingdom. *Trans R Soc Trop Med Hyg* 1992; **86:** 617–19.
10. Chunge CN, *et al.* Visceral leishmaniasis unresponsive to antimonial drugs III: successful treatment using a combination of sodium stibogluconate plus allopurinol. *Trans R Soc Trop Med Hyg* 1985; **79:** 715–18.
11. Dellamonica P, *et al.* Allopurinol for treatment of visceral leishmaniasis in patients with AIDS. *J Infect Dis* 1989; **160:** 904–5.
12. Laguna F, *et al.* Assessment of allopurinol plus meglumine antimoniate in the treatment of visceral leishmaniasis in patients infected with HIV. *J Infect* 1994; **28:** 255–9.
13. Sundar S, *et al.* Short-course, low-dose amphotericin B lipid complex therapy for visceral leishmaniasis unresponsive to antimony. *Ann Intern Med* 1997; **127:** 133–7.
14. Jha TK, *et al.* Randomised controlled trial of aminosidine (paromomycin) v sodium stibogluconate for treating visceral leishmaniasis in North Bihar, India. *BMJ* 1998; **316:** 1200–5.
15. Davidson RN, *et al.* Liposomal amphotericin B in drug-resistant visceral leishmaniasis. *Lancet* 1991; **337:** 1061–2.
16. Mishra M, *et al.* Amphotericin versus pentamidine in antimony-unresponsive kala-azar. *Lancet* 1992; **340:** 1256–7.
17. Jha TK, *et al.* Use of amphotericin B in drug-resistant cases of visceral leishmaniasis in North Bihar, India. *Am J Trop Med Hyg* 1995; **52:** 536–8.
18. Sundar S, Murray HW. Cure of antimony-unresponsive Indian visceral leishmaniasis with amphotericin B liquid complex. *J Infect Dis* 1996; **173:** 762–5.
19. Baily GG, Nandy A. Visceral leishmaniasis: more prevalent and more problematic. *J Infect* 1994; **29:** 241–7.
20. Özsoylu S. Treatment of kala azar. *Lancet* 1996; **347:** 1701.
21. Pérez-Molina JA, *et al.* Pentamidine isethionate as secondary prophylaxis against visceral leishmaniasis in HIV-positive patients. *AIDS* 1996; **10:** 237–8.
22. Jha TK, *et al.* Miltefosine, an oral agent, for the treatment of Indian visceral leishmaniasis. *N Engl J Med* 1999; **341:** 1795–1800.
23. Wali JP, *et al.* Ketoconazole in treatment of visceral leishmaniasis. *Lancet* 1990; **336:** 810–11.
24. Wali JP, *et al.* Ketoconazole in the treatment of antimony- and pentamidine-resistant kala-azar. *J Infect Dis* 1992; **166:** 215–16.
25. Sundar S, *et al.* Ketoconazole in visceral leishmaniasis. *Lancet* 1990; **336:** 1582–3.
26. Rashid JR, *et al.* The efficacy and safety of ketoconazole in visceral leishmaniasis. *East Afr Med J* 1994; **71:** 392–5.
27. Badaro R, *et al.* Treatment of visceral leishmaniasis with pentavalent antimony and interferon gamma. *N Engl J Med* 1990; **322:** 16–21.
28. Sundar S, *et al.* Successful treatment of refractory visceral leishmaniasis in India using antimony plus interferon-γ. *J Infect Dis* 1994; **170:** 659–62.
29. Sundar S, *et al.* Immunochemotherapy for a systemic intracellular infection: accelerated response using interferon-γ in visceral leishmaniasis. *J Infect Dis* 1995; **171:** 992–6.
30. Sundar S, *et al.* Response to interferon-γ plus pentavalent antimony in Indian visceral leishmaniasis. *J Infect Dis* 1997; **176:** 1117–19.
31. Alkhawajah AM, *et al.* Treatment of cutaneous leishmaniasis with antimony: intramuscular versus intralesional administration. *Ann Trop Med Parasitol* 1997; **91:** 899–905.
32. Aste N, *et al.* Intralesional treatment of cutaneous leishmaniasis with meglumine antimoniate. *Br J Dermatol* 1998; **138:** 370–1.
33. Moss JT, Wilson JP. Current treatment recommendations for leishmaniasis. *Ann Pharmacother* 1992; **26:** 1452–5.
34. Navin TR, *et al.* Placebo-controlled clinical trial of meglumine antimonate (Glucantime) vs localized controlled heat in the treatment of cutaneous leishmaniasis in Guatemala. *Am J Trop Med Hyg* 1990; **42:** 43–50.
35. El-On J, *et al.* Topical treatment of Old World cutaneous leishmaniasis caused by Leishmania major: a double-blind control study. *J Am Acad Dermatol* 1992; **27:** 227–31.
36. Krause G, Kroeger A. Topical treatment of American cutaneous leishmaniasis with paromomycin and methylbenzethonium chloride: a clinical study under field conditions in Ecuador. *Trans R Soc Trop Med Hyg* 1994; **88:** 92–4.
37. Bryceson ADM, *et al.* Treatment of Old World cutaneous leishmaniasis with aminosidine ointment: results of an open study in London. *Trans R Soc Trop Med Hyg* 1994; **88:** 226–8.
38. Ben Salah A, *et al.* A randomized, placebo-controlled trial in Tunisia treating cutaneous leishmaniasis with paromomycin ointment. *Am J Trop Med Hyg* 1995; **53:** 162–6.
39. Asilian A, *et al.* A randomized, placebo-controlled trial of a two week regimen of aminosidine (paromomycin) ointment for treatment of cutaneous leishmaniasis in Iran. *Am J Trop Med Hyg* 1995; **53:** 648–51.
40. Soto J, *et al.* Limited efficacy of injectable aminosidine as single-agent therapy for Colombian cutaneous leishmaniasis. *Trans R Soc Trop Med Hyg* 1994; **88:** 695–8.
41. Hepburn NC, *et al.* Aminosidine (paromomycin) versus sodium stibogluconate for the treatment of American Cutaneous leishmaniasis. *Trans R Soc Trop Med Hyg* 1994; **88:** 700–3.
42. Soto J, *et al.* Successful treatment of New World cutaneous leishmaniasis with a combination of topical paromomycin/methylbenzethonium chloride and injectable meglumine antimonate. *Clin Infect Dis* 1995; **20:** 47–51.
43. Teklemariam S, *et al.* Aminosidine and its combination with sodium stibogluconate in the treatment of diffuse cutaneous leishmaniasis caused by Leishmania aethiopica. *Trans R Soc Trop Med Hyg* 1994; **88:** 334–9.
44. Vennerstrom JL, *et al.* Berberine derivatives as antileishmanial drugs. *Antimicrob Agents Chemother* 1990; **34:** 918–21.
45. Albanese G, *et al.* Cutaneous leishmaniasis: treatment with itraconazole. *Arch Dermatol* 1989; **125:** 1540–2.
46. Pialoux G, *et al.* Cutaneous leishmaniasis in an AIDS patient: cure with itraconazole. *J Infect Dis* 1990; **162:** 1221–2.
47. Akuffo H, *et al.* The use of itraconazole in the treatment of leishmaniasis caused by Leishmania aethiopica. *Trans R Soc Trop Med Hyg* 1990; **84:** 532–4.
48. Dogra J, Saxena VN. Itraconazole and leishmaniasis: a randomised double-blind trial in cutaneous disease. *Int J Parasitol* 1996; **26:** 1413–15.
49. Dedet J-P, *et al.* Failure to cure Leishmania braziliensis guyanensis cutaneous leishmaniasis with oral ketoconazole. *Trans R Soc Trop Med Hyg* 1986; **80:** 176.
50. Weinrauch L, *et al.* Ketoconazole in cutaneous leishmaniasis. *Br J Dermatol* 1987; **117:** 666–7.
51. Saenz RE, *et al.* Efficacy of ketoconazole against Leishmania braziliensis panamensis cutaneous leishmaniasis. *Am J Med* 1990; **89:** 147–55.
52. Navin TR, *et al.* Placebo-controlled clinical trial of sodium stibogluconate (Pentostam) versus ketoconazole for treating cutaneous leishmaniasis in Guatemala. *J Infect Dis* 1992; **165:** 528–34.
53. Martinez S, Marr JJ. Allopurinol in the treatment of American cutaneous leishmaniasis. *N Engl J Med* 1992; **326:** 741–4.
54. Velez I, *et al.* Inefficacy of allopurinol as monotherapy for Colombian cutaneous leishmaniasis: a randomized, controlled trial. *Ann Intern Med* 1997; **126:** 232–6.
55. Martinez S, *et al.* Treatment of cutaneous leishmaniasis with allopurinol and stibogluconate. *Clin Infect Dis* 1997; **24:** 165–9.
56. Dogra J. A double-blind study on the efficacy of oral dapsone in cutaneous leishmaniasis. *Trans R Soc Trop Med Hyg* 1991; **85:** 212–13.
57. Osorio LE, *et al.* Treatment of cutaneous leishmaniasis in Colombia with dapsone. *Lancet* 1998; **351:** 498–9.
58. López-Jaramillo P, *et al.* Treatment of cutaneous leishmaniasis with nitric-oxide donor. *Lancet* 1998; **351:** 1176–7.
59. Sharquie KE. A new intralesional therapy of cutaneous leishmaniasis with hypertonic sodium chloride solution. *J Dermatol* 1995; **22:** 732–7.
60. Convit J, *et al.* Immunotherapy of localized, intermediate, and diffuse forms of American cutaneous leishmaniasis. *J Infect Dis* 1989; **160:** 104–15.
61. Sharifi I, *et al.* Randomised vaccine trial of single dose of killed Leishmania major plus BCG against anthroponotic cutaneous leishmaniasis in Bam, Iran. *Lancet* 1998; **351:** 1540–3.
62. Harms G, *et al.* A randomized trial comparing a pentavalent antimonial drug and recombinant interferon-γ in the local treatment of cutaneous leishmaniasis. *Trans R Soc Trop Med Hyg* 1991; **85:** 214–16.
63. Falcoff E, *et al.* Clinical healing of antimony-resistant cutaneous or mucocutaneous leishmaniasis following the combined administration of interferon-γ and pentavalent antimonial compounds. *Trans R Soc Trop Med Hyg* 1994; **88:** 95–7.
64. Akuffo H, *et al.* Administration of recombinant interleukin-2 reduces the local parasite load of patients with disseminated cutaneous leishmaniasis. *J Infect Dis* 1990; **161:** 775–80.
65. El-Hassan AM, *et al.* Sudanese mucosal leishmaniasis: epidemiology, clinical features, diagnosis, immune responses and treatment. *Trans R Soc Trop Med Hyg* 1995; **89:** 647–52.

Malaria

For a discussion of malaria, its prophylaxis and treatment, see p.428.

Microsporidiosis

Microsporidia are obligate intracellular spore-forming protozoal parasites. They were primarily regarded as a cause of disease in nonhuman species, but *Encephalitozoon*, *Enterocytozoon*, *Nosema*, *Pleistophora*, and *Septata* spp. are now recognised as human pathogens.[1,2] Transmission is believed to be predominantly faeco-oral although inhalation and direct inoculation also occur. Infections usually occur only in immunocompromised patients. Small bowel infection with *Enterocytozoon bieneusi* is being increasingly reported in AIDS patients as a cause of chronic diarrhoea and weight loss. Other manifestations of microsporidiosis in AIDS include keratoconjunctivitis, respiratory-tract infections, renal and urinary-tract infections, peritonitis, cholangitis, granulomatous hepatitis, and disseminated myositis.

There is no established effective treatment. Metronidazole has been reported to produce a transient symptomatic response in some patients[3] but not in those with severe diarrhoea.[4] Beneficial responses have been reported with albendazole[5-8] and atovaquone.[9] There has also been a report of a patient treated successfully with nitazoxanide.[10] Topical treatment of keratoconjunctivitis has been disappointing, although there are reports of individual patients responding to topical propamidine isetionate,[11] topical fumagillin,[12,13] or oral itraconazole plus topical antibacterials.[14]

1. Muscat I. Human microsporidiosis. *J Infect* 1990; **21:** 125–9.
2. Curry A, Canning EU. Human microsporidiosis. *J Infect* 1993; **27:** 229–36.
3. Schattenkerk JKME, *et al.* Clinical significance of small-intestinal microsporidiosis in HIV-1-infected individuals. *Lancet* 1991; **337:** 895–8.
4. Blanshard C, Gazzard BG. Microsporidiosis in HIV-1-infected individuals. *Lancet* 1991; **337:** 1488–9.
5. Blanshard C, *et al.* Treatment of intestinal microsporidiosis with albendazole in patients with AIDS. *AIDS* 1992; **6:** 311–13.
6. Dieterich DT, *et al.* Treatment with albendazole for intestinal disease due to Enterocytozoon bieneusi in patients with AIDS. *J Infect Dis* 1994; **169:** 178–82.
7. Franzen C, *et al.* Intestinal microsporidiosis with Septata intestinalis in a patient with AIDS—response to albendazole. *J Infect* 1995; **31:** 237–9.
8. Dore GJ, *et al.* Disseminated microsporidiosis due to Septata intestinalis in nine patients infected with the human immunodeficiency virus: response to therapy with albendazole. *Clin Infect Dis* 1995; **21:** 70–6.
9. Anwar-Bruni DM, *et al.* Atovaquone is effective treatment for the symptoms of gastrointestinal microsporidiosis in HIV-1-infected patients. *AIDS* 1995; **10:** 619–23.
10. Bicart-See A, *et al.* Successful treatment with nitazoxanide of Enterocytozoon bieneusi microsporidiosis in a patient with AIDS. *Antimicrob Agents Chemother* 2000; **44:** 167–8.
11. Metcalfe TW, *et al.* Microsporidial keratoconjunctivitis in a patient with AIDS. *Br J Ophthalmol* 1992; **76:** 177–8.
12. Diesenhouse MC, *et al.* Treatment of microsporidial keratoconjunctivitis with topical fumagillin. *Am J Ophthalmol* 1993; **115:** 293–8.
13. Garvey MJ, *et al.* Topical fumagillin in the treatment of microsporidial keratoconjunctivitis in AIDS. *Ann Pharmacother* 1995; **29:** 872–4.
14. Yee RW, *et al.* Resolution of microsporidial epithelial keratopathy in a patient with AIDS. *Ophthalmology* 1991; **98:** 196–201.

Pneumocystis carinii pneumonia

Although *Pneumocystis carinii* has been classified as a protozoan, current evidence suggests that it is probably a fungus. For the treatment of *Pneumocystis carinii* pneumonia, see p.375.

Toxoplasmosis

Toxoplasmosis is a zoonosis with a worldwide distribution caused by the protozoan parasite *Toxoplasma gondii*. There is a high incidence of *Toxoplasma* antibody, an indication of previous infection, in the general population although infection will have been diagnosed in few individuals. Sexual reproduction of *T. gondii* occurs in the gastrointestinal tract of cats. Soil becomes contaminated from excretion of oocysts in cat faeces. Other animals such as pigs and sheep may become infected by ingestion of these oocysts and act as intermediate hosts. In man, infection is acquired through contact with infected cat faeces or contaminated soil, or from eating raw or undercooked meat from infected animals. Ingested oocysts rapidly transform into trophozoites which multiply in tissue macrophages. The intracellular trophozoites disseminate in the blood stream and lymphatic system to reach the brain, heart, and lungs. As immunity develops the trophozoites form latent cystic aggregates (bradyzoites), mainly in the brain, heart, and skeletal muscle, and these are subject to reactivation throughout the life of the host.

Toxoplasma infection in immunocompetent individuals is usually asymptomatic and if symptomatic infection does occur it is usually self-limiting. Very rarely myocarditis or encephalitis may occur. Patients with impaired immunity may develop serious complications such as encephalitis, chorioretinitis, myocarditis, and pneumonitis. Toxoplasmic encephalitis is the most common presentation in patients with AIDS.

Congenital toxoplasmosis is not a problem in women who have *Toxoplasma* antibody before conception, but primary toxoplasmosis during early pregnancy is serious because of the risk of transplacental transmission which may result in fetal death or congenital toxoplasmosis. Primary infection during later pregnancy can also result in congenital infection, although this often only becomes symptomatic later in life. The sequelae in live-born infants with signs of infection are generally severe and include a potentially fatal syndrome in which hydrocephalus, hepatosplenomegaly with jaundice, mental retardation, and chorioretinitis may occur. Congenital disease that becomes clinically evident later in life is usually less severe, but it frequently results in ocular or neurological impairment. Infection in the pregnant woman is usually asymptomatic and antenatal screening programmes have been set up in some countries for the diagnosis of acute infections during pregnancy. However, the value and practicality of such schemes has been debated.[1-5] Ocular toxoplasmosis causes chorioretinitis and is often a result of congenital infection; patients may be asymptomatic until later in life.

Treatment. Toxoplasmosis in immunocompetent patients is not usually treated unless symptoms are severe. Currently there is no drug active against the cystic form, so any treatment is directed against the acute forms of the disease. Active toxoplasmosis in immunocompromised patients requires prompt treatment. Toxoplasmosis is normally treated with pyrimethamine together with sulfadiazine.[6] Folinic acid should also be given every third day during treatment to counteract the megaloblastic anaemia associated with these drugs. Treatment is ideally continued for several weeks after clinical cure. Indefinite, usually lifelong, maintenance therapy should be given to AIDS patients. Clindamycin plus pyrimethamine has been used as an alternative in patients unable to take the sulfonamide.[7-10] Other approaches for such patients are to give pyrimethamine alone[6] or to carry out sulfadiazine desensitisation.[11] Other drug regimens which have produced encouraging results in small numbers of AIDS patients with encephalitis include pyrimethamine with clarithromycin,[12] pyrimethamine with doxycycline,[13] atovaquone,[14,15] clindamycin with fluorouracil,[16] clarithromycin with minocycline,[17] co-trimoxazole,[18] and azithromycin with pyrimethamine.[19] Atovaquone has also been studied for long-term suppressive therapy.[15,20]

Pyrimethamine should not be used to treat primary toxoplasmosis during the first trimester of **pregnancy** in immunocompetent patients.[6] Spiramycin has been used throughout the first trimester but, although it reduces the risk of congenital transmission, it does not readily penetrate the cerebrospinal space and does not prevent toxoplasmic encephalitis in immunodeficient mothers. After the first trimester pyrimethamine may be given with sulfadiazine and folinic acid and, when there is evidence of placental or fetal infection, this treatment may be alternated with courses of spiramycin until term. In **neonates** without overt disease, but born to mothers known to have become infected during pregnancy, pyrimethamine together with sulfadiazine and folinic acid are given for the first 4 weeks with further courses of treatment if the infants are subsequently shown to be infected.[6] Some workers have suggested treatment for one year initially.[5,21] Alternating courses of pyrimethamine-sulfadiazine with spiramycin has been suggested as a means of reducing the risk of bone marrow suppression and has produced good results when given throughout the first year of life. Severely infected neonates are treated with daily pyrimethamine-sulfadiazine for 6 months after which alternating monthly courses of pyrimethamine-sulfadiazine and spiramycin for at least a further 6 months have been used.[6] A corticosteroid, usually prednisolone, is added for active chorioretinitis or CNS involvement.[6]

In immunocompetent individuals **ocular toxoplasmosis** is a self-limiting disease, and requires no treatment unless visual acuity is threatened or there is a large retinal lesion with marked vitritis.[22-24] All immunocompromised patients should be treated and prolonged treatment is necessary to prevent recrudescence. The optimum drug regimen is undecided. The most commonly used regimens are pyrimethamine with sulfadiazine or pyrimethamine with clindamycin (which is concentrated in the choroid). A beneficial response has been reported with clindamycin and corticosteroid therapy.[25] The role of corticosteroids is the subject of debate. They should never be used alone since fulminant cases may occur. Spiramycin is not indicated for ocular toxoplasmosis.

Prophylaxis. Primary prophylaxis against *T. gondii* infection has been investigated in AIDS patients and recipients of organ transplants. Clindamycin[26] alone was found to be too toxic. While some studies have suggested that pyrimethamine[26-28] alone was of value, increased mortality risk has been reported[29] and a controlled study has shown no benefit.[30] Co-trimoxazole, in regimens designed for *Pneumocystis carinii* pneumonia prophylaxis, appears to provide effective primary prophylaxis for toxoplasma encephalitis.[31] Alternatively, pyrimethamine plus dapsone may be effective[31,32] but in one study was not tolerated by 30% of patients.[33]

1. Anonymous. Antenatal screening for toxoplasmosis in the UK. *Lancet* 1990; **336:** 346–8. Correction. *ibid.*: 576.
2. Jeannel D, *et al.* What is known about the prevention of congenital toxoplasmosis? *Lancet* 1990; **336:** 359–61.
3. Ho-Yen DO, *et al.* Congenital toxoplasmosis and TORCH. *Lancet* 1990; **336:** 624.
4. Desmonts G. Preventing congenital toxoplasmosis. *Lancet* 1990; **336:** 1017–18.
5. Guerina NG, *et al.* Neonatal serologic screening and early treatment for congenital Toxoplasma gondii infection. *N Engl J Med* 1994; **330:** 1858–63.
6. WHO. *WHO model prescribing information: drugs used in parasitic diseases.* 2nd ed. Geneva: WHO, 1995.
7. Remington JS, Vilde JL. Clindamycin for toxoplasma encephalitis in AIDS. *Lancet* 1991; **338:** 1142–3.
8. Luft BJ, *et al.* Toxoplasmic encephalitis in patients with the acquired immunodeficiency syndrome. *N Engl J Med* 1993; **329:** 995–1000.
9. Dannemann B, *et al.* Treatment of toxoplasmic encephalitis in patients with AIDS: a randomized trial comparing pyrimethamine plus clindamycin to pyrimethamine plus sulfadiazine. *Ann Intern Med* 1992; **116:** 33–43.
10. Katlama C, *et al.* Pyrimethamine-clindamycin vs pyrimethamine-sulfadiazine as acute and long-term therapy for toxoplasmic encephalitis in patients with AIDS. *Clin Infect Dis* 1996; **22:** 268–75.
11. Tenant-Flowers M, *et al.* Sulphadiazine desensitization in patients with AIDS and cerebral toxoplasmosis. *AIDS* 1991; **5:** 311–15.
12. Fernandez-Martin J, *et al.* Pyrimethamine-clarithromycin combination for therapy of acute Toxoplasma encephalitis in patients with AIDS. *Antimicrob Agents Chemother* 1991; **35:** 2049–52.
13. Hagberg L, *et al.* Doxycycline and pyrimethamine for toxoplasmic encephalitis. *Scand J Infect Dis* 1993; **25:** 157–60.
14. Kovacs JA, *et al.* Efficacy of atovaquone in treatment of toxoplasmosis in patients with AIDS. *Lancet* 1992; **340:** 637–8.

15. Torres RA, *et al.* Atovaquone for salvage treatment and suppression of toxoplasmic encephalitis in patients with AIDS. *Clin Infect Dis* 1997; **24:** 422–9.
16. Dhiver C, *et al.* 5-Fluoro-uracil–clindamycin for treatment of cerebral toxoplasmosis. *AIDS* 1993; **7:** 143–4.
17. Lacassin F, *et al.* Clarithromycin-minocycline combination as salvage therapy for toxoplasmosis in patients infected with human immunodeficiency virus. *Antimicrob Agents Chemother* 1995; **39:** 276–7.
18. Torre D, *et al.* Randomized trial of trimethoprim-sulfamethoxazole versus pyrimethamine-sulfadiazine for therapy of toxoplasmic encephalitis in patients with AIDS. *Antimicrob Agents Chemother* 1998; **42:** 1346–9.
19. Saba J, *et al.* Pyrimethamine plus azithromycin for treatment of acute toxoplasmic encephalitis in patients with AIDS. *Eur J Clin Microbiol Infect Dis* 1993; **12:** 853–6.
20. Katlama C, *et al.* Atovaquone as long-term suppressive therapy for toxoplasmic encephalitis in patients with AIDS and multiple drug intolerance. *AIDS* 1996; **10:** 1107–12.
21. Roizen N, *et al.* Neurologic and developmental outcome in treated congenital toxoplasmosis. *Pediatrics* 1995; **95:** 11–20.
22. Rothova A. Ocular involvement in toxoplasmosis. *Br J Ophthalmol* 1993; **77:** 371–7.
23. Nussenblatt RB, Belfort R. Ocular toxoplasmosis: an old disease revisited. *JAMA* 1994; **271:** 304–7. Correction. *ibid.*; **272:** 356.
24. Hay J, Dutton GN. Toxoplasma and the eye. *BMJ* 1995; **310:** 1021–2.
25. Djurković-Djaković O, *et al.* Short-term effects of the clindamycin-steroid regimen in the treatment of ocular toxoplasmosis. *J Chemother* 1995; **7** (suppl 4): 199–201.
26. Jacobson MA, *et al.* Toxicity of clindamycin as prophylaxis for AIDS-associated toxoplasmic encephalitis. *Lancet* 1992; **339:** 333–4.
27. Wreghitt TG, *et al.* Efficacy of pyrimethamine for the prevention of donor-acquired Toxoplasma gondii infection in heart and heart-lung transplant recipients. *Transpl Int* 1992; **5:** 197–200.
28. Murphy K, *et al.* Pyrimethamine alone as long-term suppressive therapy in cerebral toxoplasmosis. *Am J Med* 1994; **96:** 95–6.
29. Jacobson MA, *et al.* Primary prophylaxis with pyrimethamine for toxoplasmic encephalitis in patients with advanced human immunodeficiency virus disease: results of a randomized trial. *J Infect Dis* 1994; **169:** 384–94.
30. Leport C, *et al.* Pyrimethamine for primary prophylaxis of toxoplasmic encephalitis in patients with human immunodeficiency virus infection: a double-blind, randomized trial. *J Infect Dis* 1996; **173:** 91–7.
31. Centers for Disease Control. 1997 USPHS/IDSA guidelines for the prevention of opportunistic infections in persons infected with human immunodeficiency virus. *MMWR* 1997; **46** (RR-12): 1–148.
32. Podzamczer D, *et al.* Intermittent trimethoprim-sulfamethoxazole compared with dapsone-pyrimethamine for the simultaneous primary prophylaxis of Pneumocystis pneumonia and toxoplasmosis in patients infected with HIV. *Ann Intern Med* 1995; **122:** 755–61.
33. Opravil M, *et al.* Once-weekly administration of dapsone/pyrimethamine vs aerosolized pentamidine as combined prophylaxis for Pneumocystis carinii pneumonia and toxoplasmic encephalitis in human immunodeficiency virus-infected patients. *Clin Infect Dis* 1995; **20:** 531–41.

Trichomoniasis

Trichomoniasis is caused by invasion of the genito-urinary tract with the protozoan *Trichomonas vaginalis*. Transmission is primarily sexual. Trichomoniasis is a common cause of vaginitis and vaginal discharge; some infected women are asymptomatic but should still be treated to prevent sexual transmission and symptomatic infection. Men are usually asymptomatic, although they may experience urethritis.

Treatment is usually with a nitroimidazole such as metronidazole when a single oral dose can be effective.[1-5] Sexual partners should be treated concomitantly. The incidence of treatment failures appears to be increasing and some at least have been due to metronidazole resistance. Patients who do not respond to single-dose treatment may be given a more intensive course of metronidazole for 5 to 7 days. Tinidazole has been widely used as an alternative to metronidazole, and may be effective in cases of metronidazole resistance.[6] A patient with metronidazole- and tinidazole-resistant infection was successfully treated with paromomycin.[7] Local application of paromomycin has also been tried in a small number of patients with moderate success.[8] Clotrimazole, administered intravaginally, has been suggested[1] for symptomatic relief during pregnancy, especially during the first trimester when metronidazole therapy is not recommended. However, clotrimazole is curative in only about 20% of patients and definitive treatment may be required later in pregnancy.

1. WHO. *WHO model prescribing information: drugs used in sexually transmitted diseases and HIV infection.* Geneva: WHO, 1995.
2. Centers for Disease Control. 1998 Guidelines for treatment of sexually transmitted diseases. *MMWR* 1998; **47** (RR-1): 74–5.
3. Association for Genitourinary Medicine/Medical Society for the Study of Venereal Diseases Clinical Effectiveness Group. National guideline for the management of Trichomonas vaginalis. Available at: http://www.mssvd.org.uk/ceg.htm (accessed 12/09/01).
4. Forna F, Gülmezoglu AM. Interventions for treating trichomoniasis in women (updated 7 December 2000). Available in The Cochrane Library; Issue 3. Oxford: Update Software; 2001.
5. WHO. Guidelines for the management of sexually transmitted infections. Geneva: WHO, 2001.

6. Hamed KA, Studemeister AE. Successful response to metronidazole-resistant trichomonal vaginitis to tinidazole: a case report. *Sex Transm Dis* 1992; **19:** 339–40.
7. Nyirjesy P, *et al.* Paromomycin for nitroimidazole-resistant trichomonosis. *Lancet* 1995; **346:** 1110.
8. Nyirjesy P, *et al.* Difficult-to-treat trichomoniasis: results with paromomycin cream. *Clin Infect Dis* 1998; **26:** 986–8.

African trypanosomiasis

African trypanosomiasis (sleeping sickness) is caused by subspecies of the protozoan *Trypanosoma brucei*, transmitted by the bite of infected tsetse flies (*Glossina* spp.). Gambian or West African sleeping sickness is caused by *T. brucei gambiense*, carried by riverine tsetse flies, and Rhodesian or East African sleeping sickness is caused by *T. brucei rhodesiense*, carried by savannah tsetse flies. Infection can follow blood transfusion and congenital trypanosomiasis has also occurred.

Although it has proven impractical to eliminate trypanosomiasis from endemic areas, the intensity of transmission can be reduced by detection and treatment of cases and vector control, including insecticide spraying of breeding sites and the use of insecticide-impregnated traps and screens.[1,2] Control of infection in domestic animals may also be beneficial.[1]

Trypanosomiasis can be divided into the early haematolymphatic stage (infection of the blood stream and lymph nodes) and the late or meningoencephalitic stage (infection of the CNS).[1] Trypanosomiasis due to *T. b. gambiense* develops slowly over several months or even years and the disease stages are relatively distinct. Infection with *T. b. rhodesiense* is more acute with a rapid onset of symptoms and indistinct disease stages and, if left untreated, will usually lead to death in a matter of weeks or months.

The haematolymphatic phase of African trypanosomiasis is treated with suramin or pentamidine. Pentamidine may be used for treatment of *T. b. gambiense* infections, but increasing resistance makes it unsuitable for *T. b. rhodesiense* infections; suramin is used for *T. b. rhodesiense* infections and for *T. b. gambiense* infections which are resistant to pentamidine. Combination therapy with pentamidine and suramin for *T. b. gambiense* infections has not been shown to reduce the incidence of relapse.[3] Eflornithine can also be effective in this phase of infection caused by *T. b. gambiense*; it is not very effective on its own against *T. b. rhodesiense*.[2]

Suramin and pentamidine penetrate the blood-brain barrier poorly and are only used in the meningoencephalitic stage as adjuncts before starting treatment with melarsoprol or eflornithine. Melarsoprol, which is effective against both *T. b. gambiense* and *T. b. rhodesiense*, is usually only given to treat the meningoencephalitic stage of the infection because it may produce potentially fatal encephalopathy. However, protection against this toxicity may be provided by prophylaxis with prednisolone.[4,5] Patients with *T. b. gambiense* infection may be treated more safely with eflornithine than melarsoprol on its own, although some consider that the cumbersome dosage schedule of eflornithine limits its use to those patients who relapse from melarsoprol.[6] Combination therapy with melarsoprol and eflornithine was reported to be effective in a patient who had not responded to either drug alone.[7] Eflornithine given in combination with suramin produced disappointing results in 6 patients with *T. b. rhodesiense*.[8]

Other alternative treatments to melarsoprol for *T. b. gambiense* infection include high doses of nifurtimox[9,10] or a combination of tryparsamide and suramin,[11] although tryparsamide is associated with a high risk of toxicity.

There is no established effective alternative treatment for melarsoprol-resistant *T. b. rhodesiense*, although suramin given in combination with high-dose metronidazole was successful in a patient.[12]

Patients should be seen every 6 months for a follow-up period of at least 2 years, to ascertain if treatment has been successful.

1. WHO. Control and surveillance of African trypanosomiasis. *WHO Tech Rep Ser* 881 1998.
2. WHO. *WHO model prescribing information: drugs used in parasitic diseases.* 2nd ed. Geneva: WHO, 1995.
3. Pépin J, Khonde N. Relapses following treatment of early-stage Trypanosoma brucei gambiense sleeping sickness with a combination of pentamidine and suramin. *Trans R Soc Trop Med Hyg* 1996; **90:** 183–6.
4. Pepin J, *et al.* Trial of prednisolone for prevention of melarsoprol-induced encephalopathy in gambiense sleeping sickness. *Lancet* 1989; **i:** 1246–50.
5. Pepin J, *et al.* Risk factors for encephalopathy and mortality during melarsoprol treatment of Trypanosoma brucei gambiense sleeping sickness. *Trans R Soc Trop Med Hyg* 1995; **89:** 92–7.

6. Milord F, *et al.* Efficacy and toxicity of eflornithine for treatment of Trypanosoma brucei gambiense sleeping sickness. *Lancet* 1992; **340:** 652–5.
7. Simarro PP, Asumu PN. Gambian trypanosomiasis and synergism between melarsoprol and eflornithine: first case report. *Trans R Soc Trop Med Hyg* 1996; **90:** 315.
8. Clerinx J, *et al.* Treatment of late stage rhodesiense trypanosomiasis using suramin and eflornithine: report of six cases. *Trans R Soc Trop Med Hyg* 1998; **92:** 449–50.
9. Pepin J, *et al.* An open clinical trial of nifurtimox for arseno-resistant Trypanosoma brucei gambiense sleeping sickness in central Zaire. *Trans R Soc Trop Med Hyg* 1989; **83:** 514–17.
10. Pepin J, *et al.* High-dose nifurtimox for arseno-resistant Trypanosoma brucei gambiense sleeping sickness: an open trial in central Zaire. *Trans R Soc Trop Med Hyg* 1992; **86:** 254–6.
11. Anonymous. Drugs for parasitic infections. *Med Lett Drugs Ther* 1998; **40:** 1–12.
12. Foulkes JR. Metronidazole and suramin combination in the treatment of arsenical refractory rhodesian sleeping sickness—a case study. *Trans R Soc Trop Med Hyg* 1996; **90:** 422.

American trypanosomiasis

South American trypanosomiasis (Chagas' disease) is caused by *Trypanosoma cruzi*, carried by reduviid or triatomine bugs which feed on human blood. Infected bugs defaecate on the human host while feeding and metacyclic trypanosomes are shed and enter the host via skin abrasions or by direct penetration of mucous membranes such as the conjunctiva. Transmission by blood transfusion is a growing problem. Congenital infection can also occur. Control measures include case detection and treatment, vector control by insecticide applications within domestic buildings, and screening of blood donors.

function, which may be a feature of visceral leishmaniasis, improved during treatment with sodium stibogluconate.

1. WHO. Control of the leishmaniases. *WHO Tech Rep Ser 793* 1990.
2. Ballou WR, *et al.* Safety and efficacy of high-dose sodium stibogluconate therapy of American cutaneous leishmaniasis. *Lancet* 1987; **ii:** 13–16.
3. Hepburn NC, *et al.* Hepatotoxicity of sodium stibogluconate in leishmaniasis. *Lancet* 1993; **342:** 238–9.
4. Misbahuddin M, *et al.* Stibogluconate for leishmaniasis. *Lancet* 1993; **342:** 804.

Effects on the musculoskeletal system. Arthralgia is common with pentavalent antimony compounds. It is usually dose-dependent[1] but a patient has been described who experienced symptoms early in treatment.[2] Palindromic arthropathy with effusion was associated with sodium stibogluconate treatment in a patient.[3]

1. Ballou WR, *et al.* Safety and efficacy of high-dose sodium stibogluconate therapy of American cutaneous leishmaniasis. *Lancet* 1987; **ii:** 13–16.
2. Castro C, *et al.* Severe arthralgia, not related to dose, associated with pentavalent antimonial therapy for mucosal leishmaniasis. *Trans R Soc Trop Med Hyg* 1990; **84:** 362.
3. Donovan KL, *et al.* Pancreatitis and palindromic arthropathy with effusions associated with sodium stibogluconate treatment in a renal transplant recipient. *J Infect* 1990; **21:** 107–10.

Effects on the nervous system. Peripheral neuropathy developed in a patient about 8 days after starting therapy with sodium stibogluconate.[1] The symptoms were generally reversible when treatment was stopped (after 17 days), although there was some slight persistent hypoaesthesia in the toes. An interaction with a single dose of amitriptyline, taken on the second day of stibogluconate therapy, seemed unlikely but could not be ruled out.

1. Brummitt CF, *et al.* Reversible peripheral neuropathy associated with sodium stibogluconate therapy for American cutaneous leishmaniasis. *Clin Infect Dis* 1996; **22:** 878–9.

Effects on the pancreas. Pancreatitis has been associated with sodium stibogluconate treatment.[1-3] Withdrawing treatment usually resulted in resolution of pancreatitis.

1. Donovan KL, *et al.* Pancreatitis and palindromic with effusions associated with sodium stibogluconate treatment in a renal transplant recipient. *J Infect* 1990; **21:** 107–10.
2. Gasser RA, *et al.* Pancreatitis induced by pentavalent antimonial agents during treatment of leishmaniasis. *Clin Infect Dis* 1994; **18:** 83–90.
3. Domingo P, *et al.* Treatment of Indian kala-azar with pentavalent antimony. *Lancet* 1995; **345:** 584–5.

Pharmacokinetics

The pentavalent antimony compounds are poorly absorbed from the gastrointestinal tract. After intravenous administration an initial distribution phase is followed by biexponential elimination by the kidneys. The elimination half-life of the initial phase is about 1.7 hours and that of the slow terminal phase is about 33 hours. The corresponding half-lives after intramuscular administration are 2 hours and 766 hours respectively. The slow elimination phase may reflect reduction to trivalent antimony. Accumulation occurs on daily administration and maximum tissue concentrations may not be reached for 7 days or more. Antimony has been detected in breast milk (see Breast Feeding in Precautions, above).

◊ References.
1. Rees PH, *et al.* Renal clearance of pentavalent antimony (sodium stibogluconate). *Lancet* 1980; **ii:** 226–9.
2. Chulay JD, *et al.* Pharmacokinetics of antimony during treatment of visceral leishmaniasis with sodium stibogluconate or meglumine antimoniate. *Trans R Soc Trop Med Hyg* 1988; **82:** 69–72.
3. Al Jaser M, *et al.* Pharmacokinetics of antimony in patients treated with sodium stibogluconate for cutaneous leishmaniasis. *Pharm Res* 1995; **12:** 113–16.

Uses and Administration

Pentavalent antimony, as sodium stibogluconate or meglumine antimonate, is the treatment of choice for all forms of leishmaniasis except *Leishmania aethiopica* infections.

Sodium stibogluconate is administered by intravenous or intramuscular injection as a solution containing the equivalent of 100 mg of pentavalent antimony per mL. Intravenous injections must be administered very slowly (over at least 5 minutes) and preferably through a fine needle to avoid thrombophlebitis; as with trivalent antimony compounds they should be discontinued immediately if coughing, vomiting, or substernal pain occurs. Meglumine antimonate is administered by deep intramuscular injection as a solution containing the equivalent of 85 mg of pentavalent antimony per mL. Doses are expressed in terms of the equivalent amount of pentavalent antimony. Local variations exist in treatment schedules but WHO recommends the following regimens.

In visceral leishmaniasis initial treatment is based on a daily injection of 20 mg of pentavalent antimony per kg body-weight to a maximum of 850 mg (but see below) for at least 20 days. The length of treatment varies from one endemic area to another, but is continued until no parasites are detected in consecutive splenic aspirates taken at 14-day intervals. Patients who relapse are re-treated at the same dose.

Early non-inflamed lesions of cutaneous leishmaniasis due to all forms of *Leishmania* except *L. aethiopica*, *L. amazonensis*, and *L. braziliensis* may be treated by infiltration with intralesional injections of 1 to 3 mL of sodium stibogluconate or meglumine antimonate (approximately 100 to 300 mg of pentavalent antimony), repeated once or twice if necessary at intervals of 1 to 2 days. Systemic therapy with 10 to 20 mg of pentavalent antimony per kg daily is given if the lesions are more severe and continued until a few days after clinical and parasitological cure is achieved. Cutaneous leishmaniasis due to *L. aethiopica* is not responsive to antimonials at conventional doses. In cutaneous leishmaniasis due to *L. braziliensis*, prolonged systemic treatment with 20 mg of pentavalent antimony per kg daily for a minimum of 4 weeks is indicated to prevent the later development of mucocutaneous leishmaniasis. Similar doses are required for diffuse cutaneous leishmaniasis due to *L. amazonensis* and are continued for several months after clinical improvement occurs.

In mucocutaneous leishmaniasis daily doses of 20 mg of pentavalent antimony per kg are given for a minimum of 4 weeks; if toxic effects develop or the response is poor, 10 to 15 mg per kg may be given every 12 hours. Relapses are well known and have generally been associated with inadequate or interrupted treatment; they are treated with the same drug given for at least twice as long as the original treatment. Only when that fails should alternative treatment be given.

Leishmaniasis. The main treatment for leishmaniasis (p.584) is a pentavalent antimony compound such as sodium stibogluconate. Higher doses of antimony compounds than those recommended by WHO (see above) have been tried in order to overcome the unresponsiveness of leishmaniasis to therapy. Drug-resistant strains of *Leishmania infantum* have been associated with unresponsiveness to treatment with meglumine antimonate.[1] It was suggested[2] that the use of suboptimal doses may be increasing the prevalence of drug-resistant strains of the parasite. The Centers for Disease Control (CDC) in the USA recommends the use of 20 mg per kg body-weight per day of pentavalent antimony without restriction to the 850-mg maximum daily dose.[3] At this dose the most common adverse effects are musculoskeletal disorders, elevated liver enzyme values, and T-wave changes on the ECG, and the CDC recommends that the ECG, blood chemistry, and blood count should be monitored throughout therapy if resources permit. Severe cardiotoxicity is rare at 20 mg per kg per day but fatal cardiac toxicity has been reported with doses of up to 60 mg per kg per day (see under Effects on the Heart, above). These findings notwithstanding, follow-up of patients with cutaneous *L. braziliensis* infections for up to 10 years suggested that low doses of antimony compounds (5 mg per kg body-weight daily for 30 days) could produce long-term cures.[4]

INTRALESIONAL ADMINISTRATION. Intralesional infiltration of 3 doses of sodium stibogluconate on alternate days or once weekly was more effective than daily treatment in a study of 96 patients in Saudi Arabia.[5] Local infiltration of meglumine antimonate in usual doses of 150 to 900 mg (maximum 1500 mg) once each week for up to 6 weeks produced microbiological and clinical cures in all of 45 patients in Italy with cutaneous leishmaniasis.[6]

1. Faraut-Gambarelli F, *et al.* In vitro and in vivo resistance of Leishmania infantum to meglumine antimoniate: a study of 37 strains collected from patients with visceral leishmaniasis. *Antimicrob Agents Chemother* 1997; **41:** 827–30.
2. Grogl M, *et al.* Drug resistance in leishmaniasis: its implication in systemic chemotherapy of cutaneous and mucocutaneous disease. *Am J Trop Med Hyg* 1992; **47:** 117–26.
3. Herwaldt BL, Berman JD. Recommendations for treating leishmaniasis with sodium stibogluconate (Pentostam) and review of pertinent clinical studies. *Am J Trop Med Hyg* 1992; **46:** 296–306.
4. Oliveira-Neto MP, *et al.* A low-dose antimony treatment in 159 patients with American cutaneous leishmaniasis: extensive follow-up studies (up to 10 years). *Am J Trop Med Hyg* 1997; **57:** 651–5.
5. Tallab TM, *et al.* Cutaneous leishmaniasis: schedules for intralesional treatment with sodium stibogluconate. *Int J Dermatol* 1996; **35:** 594–7.
6. Aste N, *et al.* Intralesional treatment of cutaneous leishmaniasis with meglumine antimoniate. *Br J Dermatol* 1998; **138:** 370–1.

PROPHYLAXIS. Sodium stibogluconate or meglumine antimonate given once a month provided effective secondary prophylaxis against visceral leishmaniasis in patients with HIV infection.[1]

1. Ribera E, *et al.* Prophylaxis of visceral leishmaniasis in human immunodeficiency virus-infected patients *Am J Med* 1996; **100:** 496–501.

Preparations

BP 2001: Sodium Stibogluconate Injection.

Proprietary Preparations (details are given in Part 3)
Braz.: Glucantime; *Fr.:* Glucantime; *Israel:* Pentostam; *Ital.:* Glucantim; *Spain:* Glucantime; *UK:* Pentostam.

Atovaquone (11117-v)

Atovaquone (BAN, USAN, rINN).

BW-A566C; BW-566C; BW-566C80; 566C; 566C80. 2-[*trans*-4-(4-Chlorophenyl)cyclohexyl]-3-hydroxy-1,4-naphthoquinone.

$C_{22}H_{19}O_3Cl = 366.8.$

CAS — 95233-18-4.
ATC — P01AX06.

Adverse Effects and Precautions

Adverse reactions to atovaquone include skin rashes, headache, fever, insomnia, and gastrointestinal effects such as nausea, diarrhoea, and vomiting. Raised liver enzyme values, hyponatraemia, and haematological disturbances such as anaemia and neutropenia may occur occasionally. Atovaquone should be avoided in patients with gastrointestinal disorders that may limit absorption of the drug.

Interactions

Concurrent administration of atovaquone with either metoclopramide, tetracycline, or rifampicin (and possibly also rifabutin) may result in decreases in plasma-atovaquone concentrations. Other drugs which have produced small reductions in plasma-atovaquone concentrations include aciclovir, antidiarrhoeals, benzodiazepines, cephalosporins, laxatives, opioids, and paracetamol.

Atovaquone is reported to decrease the metabolism of zidovudine resulting in moderate increases in zidovudine plasma concentrations. A decrease in the area under the time-concentration curve for didanosine has been reported when atovaquone is given concurrently. Small decreases in the plasma concentrations of co-trimoxazole have been noted in patients receiving atovaquone. There is a theoretical possibility that atovaquone could displace other highly protein-bound drugs from plasma-protein binding sites.

Pharmacokinetics

Atovaquone is poorly absorbed from the gastrointestinal tract following administration by mouth; bioavailability is especially poor in patients with AIDS. Bioavailability from commercial oral liquid formulations is better than from tablets and can be further improved by administration with food, particularly meals with a high fat content. Atovaquone is more than 99% bound to plasma proteins and has a long plasma half-life of between 60 and 70 hours, thought to be due to enterohepatic recycling. It is excreted almost exclusively in faeces as unchanged drug.

◊ References.
1. Hughes WT, *et al.* Safety and pharmacokinetics of 566C80, a hydroxynaphthoquinone with anti-Pneumocystis carinii activity: a phase I study in human immunodeficiency virus (HIV)-infected men. *J Infect Dis* 1991; **163:** 843–8.
2. Rolan PE, *et al.* Examination of some factors responsible for a food-induced increase in absorption of atovaquone. *Br J Clin Pharmacol* 1994; **37:** 13–20.
3. Dixon R, *et al.* Single-dose and steady-state pharmacokinetics of a novel microfluidized suspension of atovaquone in human immunodeficiency virus-seropositive patients. *Antimicrob Agents Chemother* 1996; **40:** 556–60.
4. Hussein Z, *et al.* Population pharmacokinetics of atovaquone in patients with acute malaria caused by Plasmodium falciparum. *Clin Pharmacol Ther* 1997; **61:** 518–30.
5. Rolan PE, *et al.* Disposition of atovaquone in humans. *Antimicrob Agents Chemother* 1997; **41:** 1319–21.

Uses and Administration

Atovaquone is a hydroxynaphthoquinone antiprotozoal that is also active against the fungus *Pneumocystis carinii*. It is used in the prophylaxis and treatment of *Pneumocystis carinii* pneumonia in patients unable to tolerate co-trimoxazole, and with proguanil in the prophylaxis and treatment of malaria.

In the treatment of mild to moderate *Pneumocystis carinii* pneumonia, atovaquone is given by mouth in a dose of 750 mg with food three times daily as tablets, or twice daily as a suspension, for 21 days. For prophylaxis 1500 mg is given once daily with food.

In the treatment of uncomplicated falciparum malaria, atovaquone is given in a dose of 1 g with proguanil hydrochloride 400 mg, given in combination as a single daily dose, for 3 days. Children weighing 11 to 20 kg may be given one-quarter the adult dose, those weighing 21 to 30 kg may be given half the adult dose, and those weighing 31 to 40 kg may be given three-quarters the adult dose.

For prophylaxis of falciparum malaria, atovaquone 250 mg is given once daily in combination with proguanil 100 mg.

◊ Reviews.
1. Haile LG, Flaherty JF. Atovaquone: a review. *Ann Pharmacother* 1993; **27:** 1488–94.
2. Artymowicz RJ, James VE. Atovaquone: a new antipneumocystis agent. *Clin Pharm* 1993; **12:** 563–70.
3. Spencer CM, Goa KL. Atovaquone: a review of its pharmacological properties and therapeutic efficacy in opportunistic infections. *Drugs* 1995; **50:** 176–96.

Babesiosis. In a prospective, randomised study[1] involving 58 patients with babesiosis, atovaquone in combination with azithromycin was found to be equivalent in efficacy to, and associated with fewer adverse effects than, standard therapy with quinine and clindamycin.
1. Krause PJ, *et al.* Atovaquone and azithromycin for the treatment of babesiosis. *N Engl J Med* 2000; **343:** 1454–8.

Malaria. Atovaquone with proguanil (Malarone) is used in the treatment and prophylaxis of uncomplicated malaria caused by *Plasmodium falciparum* (see p.428).

Atovaquone, a blood schizontocide, is associated with an unacceptably high rate of recrudescence when used alone[1,2] for *treatment* but is more successful in malaria when used with proguanil,[2,3] including that produced by multidrug-resistant strains.[4] Use of the combination to treat *P. ovale* and *P. malariae* malarias has also been studied.[5] Atovaquone with proguanil followed by primaquine may also be effective for the treatment of *P. vivax* malaria.[6]

The combination of atovaquone with proguanil has also been found to be useful for *prophylaxis* of falciparum malaria in both children[7] and adults[8] in endemic areas. Its use for prophylaxis in non-immune travellers has also been studied.[9]
1. Chiodini PL, *et al.* Evaluation of atovaquone in the treatment of patients with uncomplicated Plasmodium falciparum malaria. *J Antimicrob Chemother* 1995; **36:** 1073–5.
2. Looareesuwan S, *et al.* Clinical studies of atovaquone, alone or in combination with other antimalarial drugs, for treatment of acute uncomplicated malaria in Thailand. *Am J Trop Med Hyg* 1996; **54:** 62–6.
3. Radloff PD, *et al.* Atovaquone and proguanil for Plasmodium falciparum malaria. *Lancet* 1996; **347:** 1511–14.
4. Sabchareon A, *et al.* Efficacy and pharmacokinetics of atovaquone and proguanil in children with multidrug-resistant Plasmodium falciparum malaria. *Trans R Soc Trop Med Hyg* 1998; **92:** 201–6.
5. Radloff PD, *et al.* Atovaquone plus proguanil is an effective treatment for Plasmodium ovale and P. malariae malaria. *Trans R Soc Trop Med Hyg* 1996; **90:** 682.
6. Looareesuwan S, *et al.* Atovaquone and proguanil hydrochloride followed by primaquine for treatment of plasmodium vivax malaria in Thailand. *Trans R Soc Trop Med Hyg* 1999; **93:** 637–40.
7. Lell B, *et al.* Randomised placebo-controlled study of atovaquone plus proguanil for malaria prophylaxis in children. *Lancet* 1998; **351:** 709–13.
8. Shanks GD, *et al.* Efficacy and safety of atovaquone/proguanil as suppressive prophylaxis for Plasmodium falciparum malaria. *Clin Infect Dis* 1998; **27:** 494–9.
9. Høgh B, *et al.* Atovaquone-proguanil versus chloroquine-proguanil for malaria prophylaxis in non-immune travellers: a randomised, double-blind study. *Lancet* 2000; **356:** 1888–94.

Microsporidiosis. There is no established effective treatment for microsporidiosis (p.585). Beneficial responses were reported with atovaquone in a preliminary study.[1]
1. Anwar-Bruni DM, *et al.* Atovaquone is effective treatment for the symptoms of gastrointestinal microsporidiosis in HIV-1-infected patients. *AIDS* 1996; **10:** 619–23.

Pneumocystis carinii pneumonia. Atovaquone is one alternative to co-trimoxazole or pentamidine for the treatment of mild to moderate *Pneumocystis carinii* pneumonia (p.375). In open studies, a clinical response to atovaquone was reported in 78% of patients with mild to moderate disease and in 56% of patients with severe disease who were intolerant of, or who failed to respond to, both co-trimoxazole and pentamidine.[1] Comparative studies have shown atovaquone to be less effective than co-trimoxazole[2] and probably less effective than pentamidine,[3,4] but to produce fewer treatment-limiting adverse effects than either.

The symbol † denotes a preparation no longer actively marketed

For primary or secondary *prophylaxis*, atovaquone was as effective as dapsone[5] or inhaled pentamidine[6] in studies in patients intolerant of co-trimoxazole.
1. White A, *et al.* Clinical experience with atovaquone on a treatment investigational new drug protocol for Pneumocystis carinii pneumonia. *J Acquir Immune Defic Syndr Hum Retrovirol* 1995; **9:** 280–5.
2. Hughes W, *et al.* Comparison of atovaquone (566C80) with trimethoprim-sulfamethoxazole to treat Pneumocystis carinii pneumonia in patients with AIDS. *N Engl J Med* 1993; **328:** 1521–7.
3. Dohn MN, *et al.* Oral atovaquone compared with intravenous pentamidine for Pneumocystis carinii pneumonia in patients with AIDS. *Ann Intern Med* 1994; **121:** 174–80.
4. Lederman MM, van der Horst C. Atovaquone for Pneumocystis carinii pneumonia. *Ann Intern Med* 1995; **122:** 314.
5. El-Sadr WM, *et al.* Atovaquone compared with dapsone for the prevention of Pneumocystis carinii pneumonia in patients with HIV infection who cannot tolerate trimethoprim, sulfonamides, or both. *N Engl J Med* 1998; **339:** 1889–95.
6. Chan C, *et al.* Atovaquone suspension compared with aerosolized pentamidine for prevention of Pneumocystis carinii pneumonia in human immunodeficiency virus-infected subjects intolerant of trimethoprim or sulfonamides. *J Infect Dis* 1999; **180:** 369–76.

Toxoplasmosis. Atovaquone has produced encouraging results for treatment[1,2] or long-term suppression of toxoplasmosis (p.585) in patients with AIDS.[2,3]
1. Kovacs JA, *et al.* Efficacy of atovaquone in treatment of toxoplasmosis in patients with AIDS. *Lancet* 1992; **340:** 637–8.
2. Torres RA, *et al.* Atovaquone for salvage treatment and suppression of toxoplasmic encephalitis in patients with AIDS. *Clin Infect Dis* 1997; **24:** 422–9.
3. Katlama C, *et al.* Atovaquone as long-term suppressive therapy for toxoplasmic encephalitis in patients with AIDS and multiple drug intolerance. *AIDS* 1996; **10:** 1107–12.

Preparations

Proprietary Preparations (details are given in Part 3)
Aust.: Wellvone; *Austral.:* Wellvone; *Belg.:* Wellvone; *Canad.:* Mepron; *Denm.:* Wellvone; *Fr.:* Wellvone; *Ger.:* Wellvone; *Ital.:* Wellvone; *Neth.:* Wellvone; *S.Afr.:* Wellvone; *Swed.:* Wellvone; *Switz.:* Wellvone; *UK:* Wellvone; *USA:* Mepron.

Multi-ingredient: *Aust.:* Malarone; *Austral.:* Malarone; *Belg.:* Malarone; *Canad.:* Malarone; *Denm.:* Malarone; *Fr.:* Malarone; *Ger.:* Malarone; *Singapore:* Malarone; *Swed.:* Malarone; *Switz.:* Malarone; *UK:* Malarone; *USA:* Malarone.

Azanidazole (12411-t)

Azanidazole *(BAN, USAN, rINN)*.
F-4. 4-[(E)-2-(1-Methyl-5-nitroimidazol-2-yl)vinyl]pyrimidin-2-ylamine.
$C_{10}H_{10}N_6O_2 = 246.2$.
CAS — 62973-76-6.
ATC — G01AF13; P01AB04.

Profile
Azanidazole is a 5-nitroimidazole derivative similar to metronidazole (p.594) and is used in the treatment of trichomoniasis in usual doses of 200 mg twice daily by mouth or 250 mg once daily intravaginally.

Preparations
Proprietary Preparations (details are given in Part 3)
Ital.: Triclose.

Benznidazole (4756-r)

Benznidazole *(rINN)*.
Ro-7-1051. N-Benzyl-2-(2-nitroimidazol-1-yl)acetamide.
$C_{12}H_{12}N_4O_3 = 260.2$.
CAS — 22994-85-0.
ATC — P01CA02.

Adverse Effects
Nausea, vomiting, abdominal pain, peripheral neuropathy, blood dyscrasias, and severe skin reactions have been reported following the administration of benznidazole.

◊ A study[1] involving 20 patients with chronic American trypanosomiasis given benznidazole 5 mg per kg body-weight daily had to be stopped because of the high incidence of skin rashes and neurological symptoms.
1. Apt W, *et al.* Clinical trial of benznidazole and an immunopotentiator against Chagas disease in Chile. *Trans R Soc Trop Med Hyg* 1986; **80:** 1010.

Pharmacokinetics
Benznidazole is absorbed from the gastrointestinal tract following administration by mouth.

◊ Peak plasma concentrations of 2.22 to 2.81 µg per mL (average 2.54 µg per mL) of benznidazole were obtained in 6 healthy subjects 3 to 4 hours after administration of a single 100-mg dose of benznidazole by mouth.[1] The half-life of elimination ranged from 10.5 to 13.6 hours (average 12 hours). Benznidazole was about 44% bound to plasma proteins.
1. Raaflaub J, Ziegler WH. Single-dose pharmacokinetics of the trypanosomicide benznidazole in man. *Arzneimittelforschung* 1979; **29:** 1611–14.

Uses and Administration
Benznidazole is a 2-nitroimidazole derivative with antiprotozoal activity. It is of value in the treatment of South American trypanosomiasis (Chagas' disease) due to infection with *Trypanosoma cruzi*, especially the early acute stage of the disease.

Benznidazole has been given by mouth in a dose of 5 to 7 mg per kg body-weight daily in two divided doses usually for 60 days (but see below). Children have been given 10 mg per kg daily in two divided doses.

American trypanosomiasis. Available treatment for South American trypanosomiasis (p.587) is generally unsatisfactory, but benznidazole is of value especially in the acute phase. WHO[1] recommends that benznidazole should be given for 30 to 60 days but some in the USA[2] suggest courses of up to 90 days. Although treatment is usually confined to the acute phase of the disease, treatment during the early chronic phase was reported to be beneficial,[3] and long-term follow-up in patients who had received benznidazole has shown a reduction in cardiac complications and parasitaemia.[4]
1. WHO. Control of Chagas disease: report of a WHO expert committee. *WHO Tech Rep Ser 811* 1991.
2. Anonymous. Drugs for parasitic infections. *Med Lett Drugs Ther* 1998; **40:** 1–12.
3. de Andrade ALSS, *et al.* Randomised trial of efficacy of benznidazole in treatment of early Trypanosoma cruzi infection. *Lancet* 1996; **348:** 1407–13.
4. Viotti R, *et al.* Treatment of chronic Chagas' disease with benznidazole: clinical and serologic evolution of patients with long-term follow-up. *Am Heart J* 1994; **127:** 151–62.

Preparations
Proprietary Preparations (details are given in Part 3)
Arg.: Radanil; *Braz.:* Rochagan; *Ecuad.:* Ragonil.

Buparvaquone (18616-e)

Buparvaquone *(BAN, rINN)*.
BW-720C. trans-2-(4-tert-butylcyclohexylmethyl)-3-hydroxy-1,4-naphthoquinone.
$C_{21}H_{26}O_3 = 326.4$.
CAS — 88426-33-9.

Profile
Buparvaquone is an antiprotozoal used in veterinary practice for the treatment of theileriosis in cattle.

Carnidazole (4763-x)

Carnidazole *(BAN, USAN, pINN)*.
R-25831; R-28096 (carnidazole hydrochloride). O-Methyl [2-(2-methyl-5-nitroimidazol-1-yl)ethyl]thiocarbamate.
$C_8H_{12}N_4O_3S = 244.3$.
CAS — 42116-76-7.

Profile
Carnidazole is a 5-nitroimidazole derivative similar to metronidazole (p.594). It is used in veterinary practice for the control of trichomoniasis in pigeons.

Clazuril (2940-v)

Clazuril *(BAN, USAN, rINN)*.
R-62690. (±)-[2-Chloro-4-(4,5-dihydro-3,5-dioxo-as-triazin-2(3H)-yl)phenyl]-(p-chlorophenyl)acetonitrile.
$C_{17}H_{10}Cl_2N_4O_2 = 373.2$.
CAS — 101831-36-1.

Profile
Clazuril is an antiprotozoal used in veterinary practice for the control of coccidiosis in pigeons.

Clopidol (12589-f)

Clopidol *(BAN, USAN, rINN)*.
Clopindol; Meticlorpindol. 3,5-Dichloro-2,6-dimethylpyridin-4-ol.
$C_7H_7Cl_2NO = 192.0$.
CAS — 2971-90-6.

Profile
Clopidol is an antiprotozoal used in veterinary practice for the prevention of coccidiosis in poultry and rabbits either alone or in combination with methyl benzoquate (p.594).

Decoquinate (12626-e)

Decoquinate *(BAN, USAN, rINN)*.
HC-1528; M&B-15497. Ethyl 6-decyloxy-7-ethoxy-4-hydroxyquinoline-3-carboxylate.
$C_{24}H_{35}NO_5 = 417.5$.
CAS — 18507-89-6.
Pharmacopoeias. In BP(Vet). Also in US for veterinary use only.

Pharmacopoeial description

BP(Vet) 2001: A cream to buff-coloured, odourless or almost odourless, microcrystalline powder. Insoluble in water; practically insoluble in alcohol; very slightly soluble in chloroform and in ether.

USP 25: Store in airtight containers.

Profile
Decoquinate is an antiprotozoal used in veterinary practice for the control of coccidiosis in calves, sheep, and chickens. It is also used for toxoplasmosis in sheep.

Dehydroemetine Hydrochloride (4773-f)

Dehydroemetine Hydrochloride *(BANM, rINNM)*.

BT-436; 2,3-Dehydroemetine Hydrochloride; DHE; Ro-1-9334. 2,3-Didehydro-6′,7′,10,11-tetramethoxyemetan dihydrochloride; 3-Ethyl-1,6,7,11b-tetrahydro-9,10-dimethoxy-2-(1,2,3,4-tetrahydro-6,7-dimethoxy-1-isoquinolylmethyl)-4H-benzo[a]quinolizine dihydrochloride.

$C_{29}H_{38}N_2O_4,2HCl = 551.5$.

CAS — 4914-30-1 *(dehydroemetine)*; 2228-39-9 *(dehydroemetine hydrochloride)*.

NOTE. The name DHE has been used to denote a preparation of dihydroergotamine mesilate.

Pharmacopoeias. In Int.

Profile
Dehydroemetine, a synthetic derivative of emetine (p.591), is a tissue amoebicide with similar actions and uses, although probably of a lower toxicity.

Dehydroemetine should be avoided in patients with cardiac, renal, or neuromuscular disease and patients should be monitored for cardiac toxicity during treatment.

When used in the treatment of amoebiasis (p.582), dehydroemetine hydrochloride is given by intramuscular injection in a dose of 1 mg per kg body-weight daily, with no more than 60 mg daily, generally for up to 4 to 6 days (no more than 5 days in children). A dose of 0.5 mg per kg has been suggested for elderly or severely ill patients. At least 6 weeks should elapse before treatment is repeated. Following treatment with dehydroemetine, all patients should receive a luminal amoebicide to eliminate organisms from the colon. Patients with hepatic amoebiasis may be given supplementary treatment with chloroquine.

Liver fluke infections. Dehydroemetine has been given in the treatment of the liver fluke infection fascioliasis,[1] although the usual treatment is with bithionol (see p.93).
1. Farid Z, et al. Treatment of acute toxaemic fascioliasis. *Trans R Soc Trop Med Hyg* 1988; **82:** 299.

Diaveridine (12641-w)

Diaveridine *(BAN, USAN, rINN)*.

BW-49-210; NSC-408735. 5-Veratrylpyrimidine-2,4-diyldiamine.

$C_{13}H_{16}N_4O_2 = 260.3$.

CAS — 5355-16-8.

Pharmacopoeias. In Fr. for veterinary use.

Profile
Diaveridine is an antiprotozoal used in veterinary practice for the prevention of coccidiosis in poultry.

Diclazuril (2942-q)

Diclazuril *(BAN, USAN, rINN)*.

R-64433. (±)-4-Chlorophenyl[2,6-dichloro-4-(2,3,4,5-tetrahydro-3,5-dioxo-1,2,4-triazin-2-yl)phenyl]acetonitrile.

$C_{17}H_9Cl_3N_4O_2 = 407.6$.

CAS — 101831-37-2.

Profile
Diclazuril is an antiprotozoal that has been tried in AIDS patients for the management of diarrhoea associated with protozoal infection. It is used in veterinary medicine for the control of coccidiosis in lambs and poultry.

◊ References.
1. Kayembe K, et al. Diclazuril for Isospora belli infections in AIDS. *Lancet* 1989; **i:** 1397.
2. Connolly GM, et al. Diclazuril in the treatment of severe cryptosporidial diarrhoea in AIDS patients. *AIDS* 1990; **4:** 700–701.
3. Menichetti F, et al. Diclazuril for cryptosporidiosis in AIDS. *Am J Med* 1991; **90:** 271–2.
4. Limson-Pobre RNR, et al. Use of diclazuril for the treatment of isosporiasis in patients with AIDS. *Clin Infect Dis* 1995; **20:** 201–2.

Diiodohydroxyquinoline (4777-m)

Diiodohydroxyquinoline *(rINN)*.

Diiodohydroxyquin; Di-iodohydroxyquinoline *(BAN)*; Di-iodoxychinolinum; Diiodoxyquinoléine; Iodoquinol *(USAN)*. 5,7-Di-iodoquinolin-8-ol.

$C_9H_5I_2NO = 397.0$.

CAS — 83-73-8.

ATC — G01AC01.

Pharmacopoeias. In US.

Pharmacopoeial description
USP 25: A light yellowish to tan, microcrystalline powder, not readily wetted in water, odourless or has a faint odour. Practically insoluble in water; sparingly soluble in alcohol and in ether.

Adverse Effects
Major concerns have been expressed about the safety of the halogenated hydroxyquinolines since the recognition of severe neurotoxicity with clioquinol (p.190). In Japan, the epidemic development of subacute myelo-opticoneuropathy (SMON) in the 1960s was associated with the ingestion of normal or high doses of clioquinol for prolonged periods and the sale of clioquinol and related hydroxyquinolines was subsequently banned in Japan. Symptoms of subacute myelo-opticoneuropathy are principally those of peripheral neuropathy, including optic atrophy, and myelopathy. Abdominal pain and diarrhoea often precede neurological symptoms such as paraesthesias in the legs progressing to paraplegia in some patients and loss of visual acuity sometimes leading to blindness. Cerebral disturbances, including confusion and retrograde amnesia, have also been reported. Although many patients improved when clioquinol was withdrawn, others had residual disability.

It was suggested that the Japanese epidemic might have been due to genetic susceptibility, but a few similar cases of subacute myelo-opticoneuropathy have been reported from several other countries in association with clioquinol or related hydroxyquinoline derivatives, such as broxyquinoline or diiodohydroxyquinoline.

Diiodohydroxyquinoline has also been associated with gastrointestinal effects such as abdominal cramps, nausea, and diarrhoea. Adverse effects which may be attributable to the iodine content of diiodohydroxyquinoline include pruritus ani, skin eruptions, and enlargement of the thyroid gland. Fever, chills, headache, and vertigo have also occurred.

Precautions
Diiodohydroxyquinoline is contra-indicated in patients known to be hypersensitive to iodine or halogenated hydroxyquinolines and in those with impaired kidney or liver function. It should be used with caution in thyroid disease and may interfere with determinations of protein-bound iodine for up to 6 months in tests for thyroid function. Its use is best avoided in patients with neurological disorders. Long-term use should be avoided.

◊ The Committee on Drugs of the American Academy of Pediatrics[1] considered that there was a potential risk of toxicity to infants and children from clioquinol and diiodohydroxyquinoline applied topically. Since alternative effective preparations are available for dermatitis the Committee recommended that products containing either of these compounds should not be used.

Also WHO considered that the use of halogenated hydroxyquinolines for the treatment of acute diarrhoea or amoebiasis in children cannot be justified.[2] There is no evidence of their efficacy in acute diarrhoea and they have been associated with severe neurological effects. On the rare occasions when a luminal amoebicide is required other less toxic and more effective agents are available.
1. Kauffman RE, et al. Clioquinol (iodochlorhydroxyquin, Vioform) and iodoquinol (diiodohydroxyquin): blindness and neuropathy. *Pediatrics* 1990; **86:** 797–8.
2. WHO. The rational use of drugs in the management of acute diarrhoea in children. Geneva: WHO, 1990.

Pharmacokinetics
Diiodohydroxyquinoline is partly and irregularly absorbed from the gastrointestinal tract. Concern has been expressed about possible absorption following application to the skin (see under Precautions, above).

Uses and Administration
Diiodohydroxyquinoline, a halogenated hydroxyquinoline, is a luminal amoebicide acting principally in the bowel lumen and is used in the treatment of intestinal amoebiasis, although a less toxic amoebicide such as diloxanide furoate is usually preferred; children should not be treated with diiodohydroxyquinoline (see Precautions, above). It is given alone in the treatment of asymptomatic cyst passers and in conjunction with an amoebicide that acts in the tissues, such as metronidazole, in patients with invasive amoebiasis (p.582). The usual dosage in the treatment of amoebiasis is 630 or 650 mg three times daily by mouth for 20 days.

Diiodohydroxyquinoline has also been given in the treatment of *Dientamoeba fragilis* infections, in balantidiasis (p.583) as an alternative to tetracycline, and in *Blastocystis hominis* infections (p.583).

Diiodohydroxyquinoline was formerly used in the treatment of acrodermatitis enteropathica; it is reported to act by enhancing

---

zinc absorption and has now been superseded by oral zinc therapy.

Diiodohydroxyquinoline is claimed to have some antibacterial and antifungal activity and has been used topically (but see under Precautions, above).

Preparations
USP 25: Iodoquinol Tablets.

Proprietary Preparations (details are given in Part 3)
Canad.: Diodoquin; *Mex.:* Amabagyl; Antidifar; Carsuquin; Diameb; Diodolina; Diodoquin; Diyomex; Diyosul; Diyowil; Drioquilen; Entero-Diyod; Entodiba; Flanoquin; Versamiv; Yopin; *S.Afr.:* Floraquin†; *Thai.:* Dysetrin; *USA:* Sebaquin; Yodoxin.

Multi-ingredient: *Austral.:* Floraquin†; *Braz.:* Dexacloran; *Mex.:* Coralzul; Decadron Con Nistatina; Farmeban; Flagenase 400; Metodine; Metrodiyod; Norecil; *S.Afr.:* Vagarsol; Viocort; Viodor; *Thai.:* Coccila; Diolin; Disento; Floraquin; Gynoco; Mediocin; Nystin; Quinradon; Quinradon-N; Vagicin; *USA:* Vytone.

Diloxanide Furoate (4779-v)

Diloxanide Furoate *(BANM, rINNM)*.

4-(N-Methyl-2,2-dichloroacetamido)phenyl 2-furoate.

$C_{14}H_{11}Cl_2NO_4 = 328.1$.

CAS — 579-38-4 *(diloxanide)*; 3736-81-0 *(diloxanide furoate)*.

Pharmacopoeias. In Br., Int., and US.

Pharmacopoeial description
BP 2001: A white or almost white, odourless or almost odourless, crystalline powder. Very slightly soluble in water; slightly soluble in alcohol and in ether; freely soluble in chloroform. Protect from light.

USP 25: A white or almost white, crystalline powder. Very slightly soluble in water; slightly soluble in alcohol and in ether; freely soluble in chloroform. Protect from light.

Adverse Effects
Flatulence is the most common adverse effect during treatment with diloxanide furoate. Vomiting, pruritus, and urticaria may occasionally occur.

Pharmacokinetics
Diloxanide furoate is hydrolysed before absorption from the gastrointestinal tract. The resulting diloxanide is readily absorbed and excreted mainly in the urine as the glucuronide; less than 10% of a dose appears in the faeces.

Uses and Administration
Diloxanide furoate, a dichloroacetamide derivative, is a luminal amoebicide acting principally in the bowel lumen and is used in the treatment of intestinal amoebiasis (p.582). It is given alone in the treatment of asymptomatic cyst passers and in conjunction with an amoebicide that acts in the tissues, such as metronidazole, in patients with invasive amoebiasis.

Diloxanide furoate is administered by mouth in a dosage of 500 mg three times daily for 10 days; children weighing more than 25 kg may be given 20 mg per kg body-weight daily, in divided doses, for 10 days. The course of treatment may be repeated if necessary.

Preparations
BP 2001: Diloxanide Tablets.

Proprietary Preparations (details are given in Part 3)
Irl.: Furamide†; *Switz.:* Furamid; *UK:* Furamide†.

Multi-ingredient: *UK:* Entamizole.

Dimetridazole (12662-z)

Dimetridazole *(BAN, pINN)*.

1,2-Dimethyl-5-nitroimidazole.

$C_5H_7N_3O_2 = 141.1$.

CAS — 551-92-8.

Pharmacopoeias. In BP(Vet).

Fr. includes Dimetridazole and Dimetridazole Mesilate for veterinary use only.

Pharmacopoeial description
BP(Vet) 2001: An almost white to brownish-yellow, odourless or almost odourless powder which darkens on exposure to light. Slightly soluble in water; sparingly soluble in alcohol; freely soluble in chloroform; slightly soluble in ether. Protect from light.

Profile
Dimetridazole is a 5-nitroimidazole derivative similar to metronidazole. It is used in veterinary practice for the prevention and treatment of blackhead (histomoniasis) in turkeys and

other poultry, for the prevention of hexamitiasis and trichomoniasis in other birds, and for swine dysentery.

Diminazene Aceturate (4780-r)

Diminazene Aceturate (BANM, rINNM).

1,3-Bis(4-amidinophenyl)triazene bis(N-acetylglycinate).

$C_{22}H_{29}N_9O_6 = 515.5$.

CAS — 536-71-0 (diminazene); 908-54-3 (diminazene aceturate).

NOTE. Diminazene aceturate is often referred to by its veterinary proprietary name Berenil.

Profile

Diminazene aceturate, an aromatic diamidine derivative related to pentamidine, is an antiprotozoal that has been used in veterinary medicine in the treatment of trypanosomiasis and babesiosis. It has also been tried in human infections.

Dinitolmide (12665-a)

Dinitolmide (BAN, rINN).

Dinitrotoluamide; Methyldinitrobenzamide. 3,5-Dinitro-o-toluamide.

$C_8H_7N_3O_5 = 225.2$.

CAS — 148-01-6.

Pharmacopoeias. In BP(Vet).

Pharmacopoeial description

BP(Vet) 2001: A cream-coloured to light tan-coloured odourless or almost odourless powder. Practically insoluble in water; slightly soluble in alcohol, in chloroform, and in ether; soluble in acetone.

Profile

Dinitolmide is an antiprotozoal used in veterinary practice for the prevention of coccidiosis in poultry.

Eflornithine Hydrochloride (16604-j)

Eflornithine Hydrochloride (BANM, USAN, rINNM).

DFMO; α-Difluoromethylornithine Hydrochloride; MDL-71782; MDL-71782A; RMI-71782. 2-(Difluoromethyl)-DL-ornithine monohydrochloride monohydrate.

$C_6H_{12}F_2N_2O_2,HCl,H_2O = 236.6$.

CAS — 67037-37-0 (eflornithine); 96020-91-6 (eflornithine hydrochloride).

Adverse Effects and Precautions

Reported adverse effects with eflornithine include myelosuppression producing anaemia, leucopenia, and thrombocytopenia. Some patients have experienced hearing loss and alopecia. Gastrointestinal disturbances, especially diarrhoea, can be a problem with oral administration. Seizures have occurred in about 8% of patients given eflornithine but they may have been related to the disease rather than treatment.

Dosage should be reduced in patients with renal impairment.

Effects on the ears. A study in 58 patients[1] receiving eflornithine alone or in combination with interferon alfa for the treatment of metastatic melanoma demonstrated that hearing loss at multiple frequencies was related to the cumulative dose of eflornithine and was worse in patients with pre-existing hearing deficit.

1. Croghan MK, et al. Dose-related α-difluoromethylornithine ototoxicity. Am J Clin Oncol 1991; 14: 331–5.

Effects on the heart. Fatal cardiac arrest occurred in an AIDS patient with Pneumocystis carinii pneumonia during the intravenous infusion of eflornithine 100 mg per kg body-weight over 1 hour.[1] Sudden death after infusion of eflornithine had occurred in several other critically ill patients with AIDS.

1. Barbarash RA, et al. Alpha-difluoromethylornithine infusion and cardiac arrest. Ann Intern Med 1986; 105: 141–2.

Pharmacokinetics

Eflornithine hydrochloride is absorbed from the gastrointestinal tract. Following intravenous administration approximately 80% is excreted unchanged in the urine in 24 hours. The terminal elimination half-life is approximately 3 hours. It is distributed to the CSF.

◊ References.

1. Haegele KD, et al. Kinetics of α-difluoromethylornithine: an irreversible inhibitor of ornithine decarboxylase. Clin Pharmacol Ther 1981; 30: 210–17.
2. Milord F, et al. Eflornithine concentrations in serum and cerebrospinal fluid of 63 patients treated for Trypanosoma brucei gambiense sleeping sickness. Trans R Soc Trop Med Hyg 1993; 87: 473–7.

Uses and Administration

Eflornithine is an antiprotozoal that acts as an irreversible inhibitor of ornithine decarboxylase, the rate-limiting enzyme in polyamine biosynthesis; trypanosomes are more susceptible to the effects of eflornithine than are humans, probably because of their slower turnover of this enzyme.

Eflornithine is used in African trypanosomiasis due to Trypanosoma brucei gambiense. It is effective in the early and more importantly in the late stage of the disease when there is CNS involvement. Eflornithine also has activity against Pneumocystis carinii and there are several reports of it being effective in patients whose pneumonia due to this organism failed to respond to standard treatment such as co-trimoxazole or pentamidine.

It is administered as the hydrochloride intravenously or by mouth, though diarrhoea can be troublesome with the latter route. In the treatment of African trypanosomiasis the usual dose is 100 mg per kg body-weight every 6 hours by intravenous infusion for at least 14 days. Some clinicians then give 300 mg per kg per day by mouth for a further 3 to 4 weeks. Dosage should be reduced in patients with impaired renal function.

Eflornithine hydrochloride is also applied topically as a 13.9% cream for the reduction of unwanted facial hair in women.

Cryptosporidiosis. Eflornithine has been tried in the treatment of cryptosporidiosis (p.583) in AIDS patients.[1]

1. Rolston KVI, et al. Intestinal cryptosporidiosis treated with eflornithine: a prospective study among patients with AIDS. J Acquir Immune Defic Syndr 1989; 2: 426–30.

Malignant neoplasms. Eflornithine has antimetabolic activity and has been studied as a potential inhibitor of malignant disease. Palliative activity was reported in patients with recurrent gliomas[1] but eflornithine given in combination with interferon gamma had no therapeutic activity in patients with advanced renal cell carcinoma, malignant melanoma, or colorectal carcinoma.[2]

1. Levin VA, et al. Treatment of recurrent gliomas with eflornithine. J Natl Cancer Inst 1992; 84: 1432–7.
2. Zeller W, et al. Phase I-II study of interferon-γ and eflornithine (DFMO) in patients with advanced renal cell carcinoma, malignant melanoma and colorectal carcinoma. Oncol Rep 1996; 3: 447–51.

African trypanosomiasis. As discussed on p.586, eflornithine is effective in the treatment of Trypanosoma brucei gambiense infections, and is particularly valuable in providing an alternative to melarsoprol in meningoencephalitic disease. The cumbersome dosage schedule and relatively high cost may limit its use to patients who relapse after melarsoprol therapy.[1] Eflornithine 100 mg per kg body-weight intravenously every 6 hours for 7 days rather than the standard 14 days produced long-term responses in 42 of 47 patients who had previously relapsed following treatment with other regimens.[2] Similar positive results in relapsing cases were obtained with a short 7-day course in a multicentre randomised controlled study,[3] although this short course was inferior to the 14-day course for new cases and could not be recommended for them. A patient who had relapsed following treatment with melarsoprol and eflornithine given singly was cured when the drugs were given together.[4] Eflornithine is not effective when given alone in T. b. rhodesiense infections, and early reports of its use with suramin were not encouraging.[5]

1. Milord F, et al. Efficacy and toxicity of eflornithine for treatment of Trypanosoma brucei gambiense sleeping sickness. Lancet 1992; 340: 652–5.
2. Khonde N, et al. A seven days course of eflornithine for relapsing Trypanosoma brucei gambiense sleeping sickness. Trans R Soc Trop Med Hyg 1997; 91: 212–13.
3. Pepin J, et al. Short-course eflornithine in Gambian trypanosomiasis: a multicentre randomized controlled trial Bull WHO 2000; 78: 1284–95.
4. Simarro PP, Asumu PN. Gambian trypanosomiasis and synergism between melarsoprol and eflornithine: first case report. Trans R Soc Trop Med Hyg 1996; 90: 315.
5. Clerinx J, et al. Treatment of late stage rhodesiense trypanosomiasis using suramin and eflornithine: report of six cases. Trans R Soc Trop Med Hyg 1998; 92: 449–50.

Preparations

Proprietary Preparations (details are given in Part 3)

USA: Ornidyl; Vaniqa.

Emetine Hydrochloride (4782-d)

Emetine Hydrochloride (BANM).

Cloridrato de Emetina; Emet. Hydrochlor.; Emetine Dihydrochloride; Emetine Hydrochloride Heptahydrate; Emetini Chloridum; Emetini Hydrochloridum Heptahydricum; Ipecine Hydrochloride; Methylcephaëline Hydrochloride. 6′,7′,10,11-Tetramethoxyemetan dihydrochloride heptahydrate; (2S,3R,11bS)-3-Ethyl-1,3,4,6,7,11b-hexahydro-9,10-dimethoxy-2-[(1R)-1,2,3,4-tetrahydro-6,7-dimethoxy-1-isoquinolylmethyl]-2H-benzo[a]quinolizine dihydrochloride heptahydrate.

$C_{29}H_{40}N_2O_4,2HCl,7H_2O = 679.7$.

CAS — 483-18-1 (emetine); 316-42-7 (emetine hydrochloride, anhydrous); 7083-71-8 (emetine hydrochloride, hydrate); 79300-08-6 (emetine hydrochloride, heptahydrate).

Pharmacopoeias. In Eur. (see p.vi), which also has a monograph for Emetine Hydrochloride Pentahydrate; Int. permits the heptahydrate or pentahydrate in the same monograph. US has a monograph for the anhydrous salt.

Solutions are sterilised by heating in an autoclave.

Pharmacopoeial description

Ph. Eur.: A white or slightly yellow crystalline powder. Freely soluble in water and in alcohol. A 2% solution in water has a pH of 4.0 to 6.0. Protect from light.

USP 25: The hydrochloride of an alkaloid obtained from ipecacuanha, or prepared by methylation of cephaëline, or prepared synthetically. Anhydrous emetine hydrochloride is a white or slightly yellowish, odourless, crystalline powder. Freely soluble in water and in alcohol. Store in airtight containers. Protect from light.

Adverse Effects

Administration of emetine hydrochloride is commonly associated with aching, tenderness, stiffness, and weakness of the muscles in the area of the injection site; there may be necrosis and abscess formation. After injection diarrhoea and nausea and vomiting, sometimes accompanied by dizziness and headache, are common. There may be generalised muscle weakness and muscular pain, especially in the neck and limbs, and, more rarely, mild sensory disturbances. Eczematous, urticarial, and purpuric skin lesions have been reported.

Cardiovascular effects are considered the most serious and include precordial pain, dyspnoea, tachycardia, and hypotension. Changes in the ECG, particularly flattening or inversion of the T-wave and prolongation of the Q-T interval, occur in many patients. Emetine accumulates in the body and large doses or prolonged administration may cause lesions of the heart, gastrointestinal tract, kidneys, liver, and skeletal muscle. Severe acute degenerative myocarditis may occur and may give rise to sudden cardiac failure and death. In some patients cardiotoxic effects have appeared after the completion of treatment with therapeutic doses.

Emetine hydrochloride is very irritant and contact with mucous membranes should be avoided.

Precautions

Emetine is contra-indicated in cardiac, renal, or neuromuscular disease. Its use should be avoided during pregnancy and it should not be given to children, except in severe amoebic dysentery unresponsive to other drugs. It should be used with great caution in old or debilitated patients. Patients receiving emetine should be closely supervised; ECG monitoring is advisable during treatment.

Pharmacokinetics

After injection emetine hydrochloride is concentrated in the liver. Appreciable concentration occurs also in kidney, lung, and spleen. Excretion is slow and detectable concentrations may persist in urine 40 to 60 days after treatment has been discontinued.

Uses and Administration

Emetine, an alkaloid of ipecacuanha (p.1093), is a tissue amoebicide acting principally in the bowel wall and in the liver. It has been given by deep subcutaneous or intramuscular injection in the treatment of severe invasive amoebiasis (p.582) including hepatic amoebiasis in patients who do not respond to metronidazole although dehydroemetine has tended to replace it.

Emetine was formerly administered by mouth as emetine and bismuth iodide.

Preparations

USP 25: Emetine Hydrochloride Injection.

Proprietary Preparations (details are given in Part 3)

Multi-ingredient: Aust.: Spirbon; Canad.: Cophylac; Switz.: Ipeca; Sano Tuss.

Ethopabate (12705-w)

Ethopabate (BAN).

Methyl 4-acetamido-2-ethoxybenzoate.

$C_{12}H_{15}NO_4 = 237.3$.

CAS — 59-06-3.

Pharmacopoeias. In BP(Vet). Also in US for veterinary use only.

Pharmacopoeial description

BP(Vet) 2001: A white or pinkish-white powder. Very slightly soluble in water; sparingly soluble in alcohol; soluble in chloroform and in methyl alcohol; slightly soluble in ether.

USP 25: A white or pinkish-white, odourless or practically odourless, powder. Very slightly soluble in water; soluble in dehydrated alcohol, in acetone, in methyl alcohol, and in acetonitrile; slightly soluble in ether; sparingly soluble in dichloromethane, in dioxan, in ethyl acetate, and in isopropyl alcohol. Protect from light.

Profile

Ethopabate is an antiprotozoal used in veterinary practice, usually in conjunction with other drugs such as amprolium, for the control of coccidiosis in pigeons and in poultry.

Etofamide (4783-n)

Etofamide (rINN).

Ethychlordiphene; K-430. 2,2-Dichloro-N-(2-ethoxyethyl)-N-[4-(4-nitrophenoxy)benzyl]acetamide.

$C_{19}H_{20}Cl_2N_2O_5 = 427.3$.
CAS — 25287-60-9.
ATC — P01AC03.

Profile

Etofamide, a dichloroacetamide derivative, is a luminal amoebicide with actions and uses similar to those of diloxanide furoate (p.590).

Preparations

Proprietary Preparations (details are given in Part 3)
Braz.: Kitnos; **Mex.:** Kitnos.

Fumagillin (9454-n)

Fumagillin (BAN).

4-(1,2-Epoxy-1,6-dimethylhex-4-enyl)-5-methoxy-1-oxaspiro[2.5]oct-6-yl hydrogen deca-2,4,6,8-tetraenedioate.

$C_{26}H_{34}O_7 = 458.5$.
CAS — 23110-15-8.

Profile

Fumagillin is an alicyclic antibiotic produced by certain strains of *Aspergillus fumigatus*. It has activity against Microsporidia and is used in veterinary practice to control *Nosema apis* infection in honeybees. It has also been tried in humans in the topical treatment of microsporidial keratoconjunctivitis. It was formerly given by mouth in the treatment of intestinal amoebiasis, but produced an unacceptably high frequency of adverse effects. Analogues of fumagillin have been investigated for effects on angiogenesis in solid tumours.

Microsporidiosis. As discussed on p.585, topical treatment of microsporidial keratoconjunctivitis has been disappointing. There have been several reports of successful treatment in individual patients using fumagillin topically,[1-3] usually as a solution of bicyclohexylammonium fumagillin containing the equivalent of 70 mg of fumagillin per mL.

1. Rosberger DF, *et al.* Successful treatment of microsporidial keratoconjunctivitis with topical fumagillin in a patient with AIDS. *Cornea* 1993; **12:** 261–5.
2. Diesenhouse MC, *et al.* Treatment of microsporidial keratoconjunctivitis with topical fumagillin. *Am J Ophthalmol* 1993; **115:** 293–8.
3. Garvery MJ, *et al.* Topical fumagillin in the treatment of microsporidial keratoconjunctivitis in AIDS. *Ann Pharmacother* 1995; **29:** 872–4.

Furazolidone (4784-h)

Furazolidone (BAN, rINN).

Nifurazolidonum. 3-(5-Nitrofurfurylideneamino)-2-oxazolidone.

$C_8H_7N_3O_5 = 225.2$.
CAS — 67-45-8.
ATC — G01AX06.
Pharmacopoeias. In Br., Fr., It., and US.

Pharmacopoeial description

BP 2001: A yellow odourless or almost odourless crystalline powder. Very slightly soluble in water and in alcohol; slightly soluble in chloroform; practically insoluble in ether. The filtrate from a 1% suspension in water has a pH of 4.5 to 7.0. Protect from light.

USP 25: A yellow, odourless, crystalline powder. Practically insoluble in water, in alcohol, and in carbon tetrachloride. Store in airtight containers. Protect from light and avoid exposure to direct sunlight.

Adverse Effects

The most common adverse effects of furazolidone involve the gastrointestinal tract and include nausea and vomiting. Dizziness, drowsiness, headache, and a general malaise have also been reported.

Allergic reactions, most commonly skin reactions such as rashes or angioedema, may occur. There have been instances of acute pulmonary reactions, similar to those seen with the structurally related drug nitrofurantoin, and of hepatotoxicity.

Agranulocytosis has been reported rarely. Haemolytic anaemia may occur in patients with a deficiency of glucose-6-phosphate dehydrogenase given furazolidone.

Darkening of the urine has been attributed to the presence of metabolites.

Precautions

Furazolidone should be used with caution in those with glucose-6-phosphate dehydrogenase deficiency because of the risk of haemolytic anaemia. It should not be given to infants under 1 month of age since their enzyme systems are immature.

Interactions

A disulfiram-like reaction has been reported in patients taking alcohol while on furazolidone therapy; alcohol should be avoided during, and for a short period after, treatment with furazolidone.

Furazolidone is an MAOI and the cautions advised for these drugs regarding the concomitant administration of other drugs, especially indirect-acting sympathomimetic amines, and the consumption of food and drink containing tyramine, should be observed (see Phenelzine Sulfate, p.305). However, there appear to be no reports of hypertensive crises in patients receiving furazolidone and it has been suggested that, since furazolidone inhibits monoamine oxidase gradually over several days, the risks are small if treatment is limited to a 5-day course. Toxic psychosis has been reported in a patient receiving furazolidone and amitriptyline (see Antiprotozoals, under Interactions, p.277).

Pharmacokinetics

Although furazolidone has been considered to be largely unabsorbed when administered orally, the occurrence of systemic adverse effects and coloured metabolites in the urine suggest that this may not be the case. Rapid and extensive metabolism, possibly in the intestine, has been proposed.

Uses and Administration

Furazolidone is a nitrofuran derivative with antiprotozoal and antibacterial activity. It is active against the protozoan *Giardia intestinalis* (*Giardia lamblia*) and against a range of enteric bacteria *in vitro*, including staphylococci, enterococci, *Escherichia coli*, *Salmonella* spp., *Shigella* spp., and *Vibrio cholerae*. Furazolidone is bactericidal and appears to act by interfering with bacterial enzyme systems. Resistance is reported to be limited. It is used in the treatment of giardiasis (p.583) and cholera (p.122). It has been suggested for other bacterial gastrointestinal infections but antibacterial therapy is regarded as unnecessary in mild and self-limiting gastro-enteritis (see p.121).

Furazolidone is given by mouth in a dose of 100 mg four times daily; children may be given 1.25 mg per kg body-weight four times daily. It is usually given for 2 to 5 days, but may be given for up to 7 days in some patients, or for up to 10 days for giardiasis.

Peptic ulcer disease. Furazolidone is not one of the main antibacterials used in *Helicobacter pylori* eradication regimens for peptic ulceration (p.1208), but there are some studies suggesting its efficacy.[1-6]

1. Segura AM, *et al.* Furazolidone, amoxicillin, bismuth triple therapy for Helicobacter pylori infection. *Aliment Pharmacol Ther* 1997; **11:** 529–32.
2. Xiao S-D, *et al.* High cure rate of Helicobacter pylori infection using tripotassium dicitrato bismuthate, furazolidone and clarithromycin triple therapy for 1 week. *Aliment Pharmacol Ther* 1999; **13:** 311–15.
3. Liu W-Z, *et al.* Furazolidone-containing short-term triple therapies are effective in the treatment of Helicobacter pylori infection. *Aliment Pharmacol Ther* 1999; **13:** 317–22.
4. Dani R, *et al.* Omeprazole, clarithromycin and furazolidone for the eradication of Helicobacter pylori in patients with duodenal ulcer. *Aliment Pharmacol Ther* 1999; **13:** 1647–52.
5. Graham DY, *et al.* Furazolidone combination therapies for Helicobacter pylori infection in the United States. *Aliment Pharmacol Ther* 2000; **14:** 211–15.
6. Liu W-Z, *et al.* A new quadruple therapy for Helicobacter pylori using tripotassium dicitrate bismuthate, furazolidone, josamycin and famotidine. *Aliment Pharmacol Ther* 2000; **14:** 1519–22.

Preparations

USP 25: Furazolidone Oral Suspension; Furazolidone Tablets.

Proprietary Preparations (details are given in Part 3)
Braz.: Giarlam; **Ger.:** Nifuran; **Ital.:** Furoxone†; **Mex.:** Exofur; Furoxona; Fuxol; Novafur; Quimefuran; Salmocide; Seforman; **S.Afr.:** Furoxone†; **Thai.:** Furasian; Furion; **USA:** Furoxone.
Multi-ingredient: Braz.: Atapec; Colestase; Enterobion; Furazolin; Lisoquinol; Magnostase; Plasmocolit; Tratocoli; **Ital.:** Ginecofuran†; **Mex.:** Colfur; Coralzul; Dibapec Compuesto; Fuzotyl; Solfurol; **Spain:** Desinvag; **Thai.:** Attafur; Coccila; Di-Su-Frone; Difuran; Diolin; Disento; Disento PF; Furasian; Furopectin; Med-Kafuzone; Mediocin.

Halofuginone Hydrobromide (12813-j)

Halofuginone Hydrobromide (BANM, USAN, rINNM).

RU-19110. (±)-trans-7-Bromo-6-chloro-3-[3-(3-hydroxy-2-piperidyl)acetonyl]quinazolin-4(3H)-one hydrobromide.

$C_{16}H_{17}BrClN_3O_3,HBr = 495.6$.
CAS — 55837-20-2 (halofuginone); 64924-67-0 (halofuginone hydrobromide).

Profile

Halofuginone is an antiprotozoal used as the hydrobromide in veterinary practice for the prevention of coccidiosis in poultry and for the control of cryptosporidiosis in calves. It is also under investigation for use in neoplastic disease in humans and in the treatment of scleroderma.

Imidocarb Dipropionate (4983-s)

Imidocarb Dipropionate (BANM, rINNM).

4A65 (imidocarb hydrochloride). 1,3-Bis[3-(2-imidazolin-2-yl)phenyl]urea dipropionate; 3,3'-Di-2-imidazolin-2-ylcarbanilide dipropionate.

$C_{19}H_{20}N_6O,2C_3H_6O_2 = 496.6$.
CAS — 27885-92-3 (imidocarb); 55750-06-6 (imidocarb dipropionate); 5318-76-3 (imidocarb hydrochloride).

NOTE. Imidocarb Hydrochloride is USAN.

Profile

Imidocarb is an antiprotozoal used as the dipropionate in veterinary practice in the treatment of babesiosis in cattle. Imidocarb hydrochloride has also been used.

Isometamidium Chloride (7322-t)

Isometamidium Chloride (BAN, rINN).

Isometamidium. 8-[3-(m-Amidinophenyl)-2-triazeno]3-amino-5-ethyl-6-phenylphenanthridinium chloride.

$C_{28}H_{26}ClN_7 = 496.0$.
CAS — 34301-55-8.

Profile

Isometamidium is an antiprotozoal used as the chloride in veterinary practice for the control of trypanosomiasis.

Lasalocid Sodium (12890-b)

Lasalocid Sodium (BANM, rINNM).

Ro-02-2985 (lasalocid). Sodium 6-[(3R,4S,5S,7R)-7-{(2S,3S,5S)-5-ethyl-5-[(2R,5R,6S)-5-ethyltetrahydro-5-hydroxy-6-methyl-2H-pyran-2-yl]tetrahydro-3-methyl-2-furyl}-4-hydroxy-3,5-dimethyl-6-oxononyl]-2-hydroxy-m-toluate.

$C_{34}H_{53}NaO_8 = 612.8$.
CAS — 11054-70-9 (lasalocid); 25999-31-9 (lasalocid); 25999-20-6 (lasalocid sodium).

NOTE. Lasalocid is USAN.

An antibiotic produced by *Streptomyces lasaliensis*.

Profile

Lasalocid is an antiprotozoal used as the sodium salt in veterinary practice for the prevention of coccidiosis in poultry.

Letrazuril (11010-k)

Letrazuril (rINN).

(±)-[2,6-Dichloro-4-(4,5-dihydro-3,5-dioxo-as-triazin-2(3H)-yl)phenyl](p-fluorophenyl)acetonitrile.

$C_{17}H_9Cl_2FN_4O_2 = 391.2$.
CAS — 103337-74-2.

Profile

Letrazuril is an antiprotozoal that has been investigated in the treatment of cryptosporidiosis (p.583) in patients with AIDS.

Maduramicin (2749-g)

Maduramicin (BAN, USAN, rINN).

CL-273703; Maduramicin Ammonium. Ammonium (2R,3S,4S,5R,6S)-tetrahydro-2-hydroxy-6-{(R)-1-[(2S,5R,7S,8R,9S)-9-hydroxy-2,8-dimethyl-2-{(2S,2'R,3'S,5R,5'R)-octahydro-2-methyl-3'-[(2R,4S,5S,6S)-tetrahydro-4,5-dimethoxy-6-methyl-2H-pyran-2-yl]oxy}-5'-[(2S,5S,6S)-tetrahydro-6-hydroxy-3,5,6-trimethyl-2H-pyran-2-yl](2,2'-bifuran-5-yl)-1,6-dioxaspiro[4.5]dec-7-yl]ethyl}-4,5-dimethoxy-3-methyl-2H-pyran-2-acetate.

$C_{47}H_{80}O_{17},NH_3 = 934.2$.
CAS — 84878-61-5.

NOTE. The name maduramicin has also been used to denote the acid.

Profile

Maduramicin is an antiprotozoal used in veterinary practice for the prevention of coccidiosis in poultry.

Melarsomine (15288-w)

Melarsomine (rINN).

Bis(2-aminoethyl) p-[(4,6-diamino-s-triazin-2-yl)amino]dithiobenzenearsonite.

$C_{13}H_{21}AsN_8S_2 = 428.4$.
CAS — 128470-15-5.

Profile
Melarsomine is a trivalent arsenical derivative used in veterinary practice for the control of canine heartworm (dirofilariasis).

Melarsoprol (4788-g)

Melarsoprol (BAN, rINN).

Mel B; Melarsen Oxide-BAL; RP-3854. 2-[4-(4,6-Diamino-1,3,5-triazin-2-ylamino)phenyl]-1,3,2-dithiarsolan-4-ylmethanol.
$C_{12}H_{15}AsN_6OS_2 = 398.3$.
CAS — 494-79-1.
ATC — P01CD01.

Adverse Effects and Treatment
Adverse effects are common and may be severe during the treatment of African trypanosomiasis with melarsoprol. It may be difficult to distinguish between effects of the disease, Jarisch-Herxheimer reactions resulting from the trypanocidal activity of melarsoprol, and adverse effects of the drug itself attributed to its arsenic content or to hypersensitivity. For the adverse effects of arsenic and their treatment, see Arsenic Trioxide, p.1582.

A severe febrile reaction may occur after the first injection of melarsoprol, especially in patients with large numbers of trypanosomes in their blood. It is therefore common practice to give two or three injections of suramin or pentamidine before starting melarsoprol therapy.

The greatest risk is from reactive encephalopathy which occurs in about 10% of patients treated with melarsoprol and is usually seen between the end of the first 3- or 4-day course of injections and the start of the second course. Some have attributed it to a toxic effect of melarsoprol and others to a Jarisch-Herxheimer reaction resulting from the release of antigen from trypanosomes killed in the brain; a combination of drug toxicity and host immune responses may be responsible. Encephalopathy may be sudden in onset or develop slowly. Symptoms include fever, headache, tremor, slurring of speech, convulsions, and coma; death has occurred in up to 5% of patients treated with melarsoprol. Less commonly, haemorrhagic encephalopathy may occur. The prophylactic use of corticosteroids has been suggested during treatment courses of melarsoprol (see African Trypanosomiasis, below). Treatment of reactive encephalopathy has included the use of corticosteroids, hypertonic solutions to combat cerebral oedema, anticonvulsants such as diazepam, and subcutaneous adrenaline [epinephrine]; dimercaprol has been given on the assumption that encephalopathy resulted from arsenic poisoning, but has not generally been of benefit.

Hypersensitivity reactions to melarsoprol may occur during the second and subsequent courses of treatment. Desensitisation has been attempted by recommencing treatment with smaller and gradually increasing doses of melarsoprol; the concomitant administration of corticosteroids may help to control symptoms during this procedure. Some authorities consider that the use of small doses of melarsoprol may increase the risk of resistance.

Melarsoprol injection is very irritant and extravasation during intravenous administration should be avoided. Vomiting and abdominal colic may occur if it is injected too rapidly. Other adverse effects reported include agranulocytosis, hypertension, peripheral neuropathy, proteinuria, severe diarrhoea, myocardial damage, exfoliative dermatitis, and hepatic disturbances.

◊ References.
1. Pepin J, et al. Trial of prednisolone for prevention of melarsoprol-induced encephalopathy in gambiense sleeping sickness. Lancet 1989; i: 1246–50.
2. Pepin J, Milord F. African trypanosomiasis and drug-induced encephalopathy: risk factors and pathogenesis. Trans R Soc Trop Med Hyg 1991; 85: 222–4.
3. Pepin J, et al. Risk factors for encephalopathy and mortality during melarsoprol treatment of Trypanosoma brucei gambiense sleeping sickness. Trans R Soc Trop Med Hyg 1995; 89: 92–7.

The symbol † denotes a preparation no longer actively marketed

Precautions
Melarsoprol should not be administered during epidemics of influenza. Intercurrent infections such as malaria and pneumonia should be treated before melarsoprol is administered. Severe haemolytic reactions have been reported in patients with glucose-6-phosphate dehydrogenase deficiency. It may precipitate erythema nodosum when administered to patients with leprosy.

Patients should be in hospital when they are treated with melarsoprol and dosage decided after taking into account their general condition.

Treatment of pregnant women with trypanosomiasis should be deferred until after delivery. Pregnant women with meningoencephalitis may be treated with pentamidine (T. b. gambiense) or suramin (T. b. rhodesiense).

Pharmacokinetics
Melarsoprol is reported to be unreliably absorbed if given by mouth and is usually given by intravenous injection. A small amount penetrates to the CSF where it has a local trypanocidal action. It is rapidly metabolised and excreted in the faeces and urine so any prophylactic effect is short-lived.

Uses and Administration
Melarsoprol, a trivalent arsenical derivative, is a trypanocide which appears to act by inhibiting trypanosomal pyruvate kinase. It is effective in the treatment of all stages of African trypanosomiasis due to Trypanosoma brucei gambiense or T. brucei rhodesiense, but because of its toxicity its use is usually reserved for stages of the disease involving the CNS. Resistance has been reported to develop.

Patients undergoing therapy with melarsoprol should be treated in hospital. Melarsoprol is administered by intravenous injection as a 3.6% solution in propylene glycol. The injection should be given slowly, care being taken to prevent leakage into the surrounding tissues, and the patient should remain supine and fasting for several hours after the injection.

Treatment protocols vary, but in general melarsoprol is given in low doses initially, especially in children and debilitated patients, increased gradually to the maximum daily dose of 3.6 mg per kg body-weight. Doses are given daily for 3 or 4 days and the course repeated 2 or 3 times with an interval of at least 7 days between courses. Since massive destruction of parasites resulting in a Jarisch-Herxheimer reaction is particularly dangerous during treatment with melarsoprol, it may be preceded by several doses of suramin or pentamidine to induce the reaction beforehand.

Melarsonyl potassium is a water-soluble derivative of melarsoprol which was formerly used as an alternative to melarsoprol but was probably more toxic and less effective.

African trypanosomiasis. The treatment of African trypanosomiasis is discussed on p.586. Melarsoprol, which is effective against both Trypanosoma brucei gambiense and T. b. rhodesiense, is usually only given to treat the meningoencephalitic stage of the infection because it may produce potentially fatal encephalopathy. However, protection against this toxicity may be provided by prophylaxis with prednisolone.[1,2] Combination therapy with melarsoprol and eflornithine was reported to be effective in a patient who had not responded to either drug alone.[3] A comparative study[4] in 500 patients with second-stage infection with T.b gambiense found that a more concise dosage regimen of melarsoprol 2.2 mg per kg body-weight daily as a single course over 10 days, was similar in efficacy to standard regimens of 1.2 to 3.6 mg per kg daily for 3 or 4 days repeated twice over a 26-day period with 7-day intervals between series, although there was no difference between the regimens in the incidence of associated encephalopathy.

1. Pepin J, et al. Trial of prednisolone for prevention of melarsoprol-induced encephalopathy in gambiense sleeping sickness. Lancet 1989; i: 1246–50.
2. Pepin J, et al. Risk factors for encephalopathy and mortality during melarsoprol treatment of Trypanosoma brucei gambiense sleeping sickness. Trans R Soc Trop Med Hyg 1995; 89: 92–7.

3. Simarro PP, Asumu PN. Gambian trypanosomiasis and synergism between melarsoprol and eflornithine: first case report. Trans R Soc Trop Med Hyg 1996; 90: 315.
4. Burri C, et al. Efficacy of new, concise schedule for melarsoprol in treatment of sleeping sickness caused by Trypanosoma brucei gambiense: a randomised trial. Lancet 2000; 355: 1419–25.

Preparations
Proprietary Preparations (details are given in Part 3)
S.Afr.: Arsobal†.

Mepacrine Hydrochloride (1382-g)

Mepacrine Hydrochloride (BANM, rINNM).

Acrichinum; Acrinamine; Antimalarinae Chlorhydras; Chinacrina; Mepacrini Hydrochloridum; Quinacrine Hydrochloride. 6-Chloro-9-(4-diethylamino-1-methylbutylamino)-2-methoxyacridine dihydrochloride dihydrate.
$C_{23}H_{30}ClN_3O,2HCl,2H_2O = 508.9$.
CAS — 83-89-6 (mepacrine); 69-05-6 (anhydrous mepacrine dihydrochloride); 6151-30-0 (mepacrine dihydrochloride dihydrate).
Pharmacopoeias. In Aust. and It.

Adverse Effects
The most common adverse effects associated with mepacrine are dizziness, headache, and gastrointestinal disturbances such as nausea and vomiting. Reversible yellow discoloration of the skin and urine may occur during long-term administration or after large doses; blue/black discoloration of the palate and nails has also been reported. Doses such as those used in the treatment of giardiasis may occasionally cause transient acute toxic psychosis and CNS stimulation. Convulsions have been reported at high doses. Ocular toxicity similar to that seen with chloroquine (p.433) and chronic dermatoses, including severe exfoliative dermatitis and lichenoid eruptions, have also occurred after prolonged administration of mepacrine. Hepatotoxicity and aplastic anaemia occur rarely.

Effects on the nervous system. Two patients had convulsions a few hours after the intrapleural administration of mepacrine hydrochloride 400 mg for malignant effusions. One developed status epilepticus and died and the other was successfully treated with anticonvulsants.[1]
1. Borda I, Krant M. Convulsions following intrapleural administration of quinacrine hydrochloride. JAMA 1967; 201: 1049–50.

Precautions
Mepacrine should be used with caution in elderly patients or patients with a history of psychosis, or in the presence of hepatic disease. Mepacrine can cause exacerbation of psoriasis and should be avoided in psoriatic patients.

Porphyria. Mepacrine should be used with caution in patients with porphyria.

Interactions
Mepacrine has been reported to produce a mild disulfiram-like reaction (see p.1605) when taken with alcohol.

Theoretically, mepacrine may increase the plasma concentrations of primaquine resulting in a higher risk of toxicity, and it has been recommended that these drugs should not be used concomitantly.

Pharmacokinetics
Mepacrine is readily absorbed from the gastrointestinal tract and widely distributed throughout the body. It accumulates in body tissues, particularly the liver, and is liberated slowly. It is excreted slowly mainly in the urine, and is still detectable in the urine after 2 months. Mepacrine crosses the placenta.

Intrapleural administration. Peak plasma concentrations of mepacrine far above those associated with CNS effects were rapidly attained in 3 of 4 patients following intrapleural instillation of a solution of mepacrine hydrochloride and remained at these levels for several hours.[1]
1. Björkman S, et al. Pharmacokinetics of quinacrine after intrapleural instillation in rabbits and man. J Pharm Pharmacol 1989; 41: 160–73.

Uses and Administration
Mepacrine is a 9-aminoacridine antiprotozoal used as the hydrochloride mainly as an alternative to one of the nitroimidazoles in the treatment of giardiasis (p.583).

In giardiasis, mepacrine hydrochloride is given by mouth in doses of 100 mg three times daily after food for 5 to 7 days. A dose for children is 2 mg per kg body-weight given three times daily (maximum 300 mg daily).

Mepacrine hydrochloride has also been used locally in the treatment of some forms of cutaneous leishmaniasis, as a sterilisation technique for contraception, and in the management of malignant effusions. It was also formerly used to treat malaria. The mesilate was also formerly used.

Contraception. Sterilisation with intra-uterine mepacrine has been attempted as an irreversible method of contraception (p.1460). This technique produces occlusion of the fallopian tube and has been performed as an effective nonsurgical means of female sterilisation.[1] There has been speculation about the risk of cancer from this technique but there appeared to be no evidence to confirm such a risk.[2,3] However, the method remains controversial and some authorities[4] have recommended that a full evaluation of its safety and efficacy is still needed.

The Indian government has banned the use of mepacrine for sterilisation.

1. Hieu DT, *et al.* 31 781 Cases of non-surgical female sterilisation with quinacrine pellets in Vietnam. *Lancet* 1993; **342:** 213–17.
2. Anonymous. Death of a study: WHO, what, and why. *Lancet* 1994; **343:** 987–8.
3. Hieu DT. Quinacrine method of family planning. *Lancet* 1994; **343:** 1040.
4. Benagiano G. Sterilisation by quinacrine. *Lancet* 1994; **344:** 689.

Leishmaniasis. Mepacrine has been suggested for intralesional injection in the treatment of early noninflamed nodular lesions of cutaneous leishmaniasis (p.584) due to *Leishmania tropica, L. major, L. mexicana, L. panamensis,* or *L. peruviana.*[1] A suggested course of treatment is 3 intralesional injections of a 5% solution of mepacrine given at intervals of 3 to 5 days. However, local infiltration of drugs can be difficult and painful.

1. WHO. Control of the leishmaniases. *WHO Tech Rep Ser 793* 1990.

Malignant effusions. Intrapleural instillations of mepacrine hydrochloride or mesilate have been used as sclerosants in the management of malignant pleural effusions (p.489) and recurrent pneumothorax but the treatment is associated with pain and a high frequency of toxic effects.

Preparations

Proprietary Preparations (details are given in Part 3)
Multi-ingredient: *Aust.:* Acrisuxin; *Switz.:* Acrisuxin†.

Methyl Benzoquate (12946-b)

Methyl Benzoquate *(BAN)*.
Nequinate *(USAN, pINN)*; AY-20385; ICI-55052. Methyl 7-benzyloxy-6-butyl-1,4-dihydro-4-oxoquinoline-3-carboxylate.
$C_{22}H_{23}NO_4 = 365.4$.
CAS — 13997-19-8.

Profile
Methyl benzoquate is an antiprotozoal used in veterinary practice, in association with clopidol (p.589), for the prevention of coccidiosis in poultry.

Metronidazole (16893-c)

Metronidazole *(BAN, USAN, rINN)*.
Bayer-5360; Metronidazolum; NSC-50364; RP-8823; SC-10295. 2-(2-Methyl-5-nitroimidazol-1-yl)ethanol.
$C_6H_9N_3O_3 = 171.2$.
CAS — 443-48-1.
ATC — A01AB17; D06BX01; G01AF01; J01XD01; P01AB01.
Pharmacopoeias. In *Chin., Eur.* (see p.vi), *Int., Jpn, Pol.,* and *US.*

Pharmacopoeial description
Ph. Eur.: A white or yellowish, crystalline powder. Slightly soluble in water, in alcohol, in acetone, and in dichloromethane; very slightly soluble in ether. Protect from light.
USP 25: White to pale yellow, odourless crystals or crystalline powder. It darkens on exposure to light. Sparingly soluble in water and in alcohol; slightly soluble in chloroform and in ether. Protect from light.

Incompatibility. See below.

Metronidazole Benzoate (4757-f)

Metronidazole Benzoate *(BAN)*.
Benzoyl Metronidazole; RP-9712. 2-(2-Methyl-5-nitroimidazol-1-yl)ethyl benzoate.
$C_{13}H_{13}N_3O_4 = 275.3$.
CAS — 13182-89-3.
Pharmacopoeias. In *Eur.* (see p.vi).

Pharmacopoeial description
Ph. Eur.: White or slightly yellowish, crystalline powder or flakes. Practically insoluble in water; slightly soluble in alcohol; soluble in acetone; freely soluble in dichloromethane. Protect from light.

Metronidazole Hydrochloride (4751-c)

Metronidazole Hydrochloride *(BANM, USAN)*.
SC-32642.
$C_6H_9N_3O_3,HCl = 207.6$.
CAS — 69198-10-3.

Incompatibility. Solutions of metronidazole hydrochloride have a low pH, usually of less than 2.0, before dilution and neutralisation to produce a suitable solution for intravenous administration. These undiluted solutions react with aluminium in equipment such as needles to produce reddish-brown discoloration, and a precipitate has been reported with ready-to-use preparations of metronidazole hydrochloride, although this occurred after contact for 6 hours or more.[1,2]

Several studies have assessed the compatibility of antibacterial injections and other drugs when added to metronidazole solution for intravenous infusion.[3-7] Results have varied according

to the criteria applied and the preparations and conditions used. Physical incompatibilities due to the low pH of metronidazole injections appear to be more of a problem than chemical incompatibility. Regardless of these studies, it is generally recommended that other drugs should not be added to intravenous solutions of metronidazole or its hydrochloride. Specific information on the compatibility of individual formulations may be found in the manufacturers' literature.

1. Schell KH, Copeland JR. Metronidazole hydrochloride-aluminum interaction. *Am J Hosp Pharm* 1985; **42:** 1040, 1042.
2. Struthers BJ, Parr RJ. Clarifying the metronidazole hydrochloride-aluminum interaction. *Am J Hosp Pharm* 1985; **42:** 2660.
3. Bisaillon S, Sarrazin R. Compatibility of several antibiotics or hydrocortisone when added to metronidazole solution for intravenous infusion. *J Parenter Sci Technol* 1983; **37:** 129–32.
4. Gupta VD, Stewart KR. Chemical stabilities of hydrocortisone sodium succinate and several antibiotics when mixed with metronidazole injection for intravenous infusion. *J Parenter Sci Technol* 1985; **39:** 145–8.
5. Gupta VD, *et al.* Chemical stabilities of cefamandole nafate and metronidazole when mixed together for intravenous infusion. *J Clin Hosp Pharm* 1985; **10:** 379–83.
6. Barnes AR. Chemical stabilities of cefuroxime sodium and metronidazole in an admixture for intravenous infusion. *J Clin Pharm Ther* 1990; **15:** 187–96.
7. Nahata MC, *et al.* Stability of metronidazole and ceftizoxime sodium in ready-to-use metronidazole bags stored at 4 and 25° C. *Am J Health-Syst Pharm* 1996; **53:** 1046–8.

Adverse Effects

The adverse effects of metronidazole are generally dose-related. The most common are gastrointestinal disturbances, especially nausea and an unpleasant metallic taste. Vomiting, and diarrhoea or constipation may also occur. A furred tongue, glossitis, and stomatitis may be associated with an overgrowth of *Candida*. There have been rare reports of antibiotic-associated colitis associated with metronidazole, although it is also used in the treatment of this condition.

Weakness, dizziness, ataxia, headache, drowsiness, insomnia, and changes in mood or mental state such as depression or confusion have also been reported. Peripheral neuropathy, usually presenting as numbness or tingling in the extremities, and epileptiform seizures are serious adverse effects on the nervous system that have been associated with high doses of metronidazole or prolonged treatment.

Temporary moderate leucopenia and thrombocytopenia may occur in some patients receiving metronidazole. Skin rashes, urticaria, and pruritus occur occasionally and erythema multiforme, angioedema, and anaphylaxis have been reported rarely. Other side-effects include urethral discomfort and darkening of the urine. Raised liver enzyme values, cholestatic hepatitis, and jaundice have occasionally been reported. Thrombophlebitis may follow the intravenous administration of metronidazole.

Studies have shown metronidazole to be mutagenic in bacteria and carcinogenic in some *animals*.

Carcinogenicity and mutagenicity. Metronidazole is mutagenic in some strains of bacteria[1] and the urine of patients treated with metronidazole was found to be mutagenic in bacteria.[2] However, although increased chromosome aberrations were noted in patients following prolonged treatment with relatively high doses of metronidazole[3] no evidence of a cytogenic effect was found in a subsequent controlled study.[4] Tumours have been induced in *rats* and *mice* given metronidazole in chronic studies, but there was no appreciable increase in the incidence of cancer in a retrospective study of 771 patients given metronidazole for vaginal trichomoniasis[5] nor in another similar study of 2460 patients.[6] However, the first study[5] did show an excess of cases of lung cancer although all 4 were in women who were smokers. Subsequent follow-up[7] to 1984 covering a period of 15 to 25 years still showed an excess of lung cancer cases even after allowing for smoking status. However, the follow-up also continued to show no significant increase overall in cancer-related morbidity or mortality. Further follow-up[8] of the patients from the second study for 11 to 15 years to 1984 also showed no increase in the overall incidence of cancers nor did it confirm any increase in lung cancer.

Risks to the fetus are discussed under Pregnancy in Precautions, below.

1. Voogd CE, *et al.* The mutagenic action of nitroimidazoles I: metronidazole, nimorazole, dimetridazole and ronidazole. *Mutat Res* 1974; **26:** 483–90.
2. Speck WT, *et al.* Mutagenicity of metronidazole: presence of several active metabolites in human urine. *J Natl Cancer Inst* 1976; **56:** 283–4.
3. Mitelman F, *et al.* Chromosome aberrations and metronidazole. *Lancet* 1976; **ii:** 802.
4. Mitelman F, *et al.* No cytogenetic effect of metronidazole. *Lancet* 1980; **i:** 1249–50.
5. Beard CM, *et al.* Lack of evidence for cancer due to use of metronidazole. *N Engl J Med* 1979; **301:** 519–22.

6. Friedman GD. Cancer after metronidazole. *N Engl J Med* 1980; **302:** 519.
7. Beard CM, *et al.* Cancer after exposure to metronidazole. *Mayo Clin Proc* 1988; **63:** 147–53.
8. Friedman GD, Selby JV. Metronidazole and cancer. *JAMA* 1989; **261:** 866.

Effects on the blood. Adverse haematological effects associated with metronidazole therapy include a report of bone marrow aplasia, with leucopenia and markedly reduced erythropoiesis and granulopoiesis,[1] aplastic anaemia,[2] and the haemolytic-uraemic syndrome.[3]

1. White CM, *et al.* Bone marrow aplasia associated with metronidazole. *BMJ* 1980; **280:** 647.
2. Raman R, *et al.* Metronidazole induced aplastic anaemia. *Clinician* 1982; **46:** 464–8.
3. Powell HR, *et al.* Haemolytic-uraemic syndrome after treatment with metronidazole. *Med J Aust* 1988; **149:** 222–3.

Effects on the ears. A review of reports of ototoxicity notified to the Australian Adverse Drug Reactions Advisory Committee revealed a number of cases of deafness associated with the use of metronidazole.[1]

1. Anonymous. Drug-induced ototoxicity. *WHO Drug Inf* 1991; **5:** 12.

Effects on the eyes. Myopia which developed in a patient after 11 days of oral metronidazole for trichomoniasis had resolved 4 days after withdrawal of treatment but recurred when she resumed treatment.[1]

Retrobulbar or optic neuritis was reported in 7 patients receiving metronidazole.[2] Dosage varied from 0.75 to 1 g daily by mouth and duration of treatment from 7 days to a year. Abnormalities included defects in colour vision, decreased vision, and scotomas. Vision improved following withdrawal of metronidazole, although there was a residual deficit in 2 patients.

1. Grinbaum A, *et al.* Transient myopia following metronidazole treatment for Trichomonas vaginalis. *JAMA* 1992; **267:** 511–12.
2. Putnam D, *et al.* Metronidazole and optic neuritis. *Am J Ophthalmol* 1991; **112:** 737.

Effects on the gastrointestinal tract. ANTIBIOTIC-ASSOCIATED COLITIS. Reports of pseudomembranous colitis associated with the administration of metronidazole.

1. Thomson G, *et al.* Pseudomembranous colitis after treatment with metronidazole. *BMJ* 1981; **282:** 864–5.
2. Daly JJ, Chowdary KVS. Pseudomembranous colitis secondary to metronidazole. *Dig Dis Sci* 1983; **28:** 573–4.

Effects on the liver. Severely elevated liver enzyme values, consistent with a drug-induced hepatitis, occurred in a patient given metronidazole hydrochloride 500 mg every 6 hours intravenously for 4 days. He was also receiving cefapirin sodium and tobramycin sulfate.[1] A case of reversible hepatotoxicity caused by an overdose of metronidazole 12.5 g has also been reported.[2]

1. Appleby DH, Vogtland HD. Suspected metronidazole toxicity. *Clin Pharm* 1983; **2:** 373–4.
2. Lam S, Bank S. Hepatotoxicity caused by metronidazole overdose. *Ann Intern Med* 1995; **122:** 803.

Effects on the nervous system. EFFECTS ON MENTAL FUNCTION. Although metronidazole is sometimes used to reduce colonic flora in the treatment of hepatic encephalopathy, impaired metabolism of metronidazole in such patients can result in elevated plasma concentrations and consequent toxicity. Psychosis and manic behaviour was reported in one such patient during treatment for hepatic encephalopathy with metronidazole and lactulose, although plasma-metronidazole concentrations were not found to be elevated (24 µg per mL).[1] Symptoms resolved when metronidazole was discontinued. Acute psychosis has also been reported in a patient following a 5-day course of intravenous metronidazole 1 g daily for a gynaecological disorder.[2]

1. Uhl MD, Riely CA. Metronidazole in treating portosystemic encephalopathy. *Ann Intern Med* 1996; **124:** 455.
2. Schreiber W, Spernal J. Metronidazole-induced psychotic disorder. *Am J Psychiatry* 1997; **154:** 1170–1.

PERIPHERAL NEUROPATHY. Peripheral neuropathy has been reported in patients receiving prolonged treatment with metronidazole.[1-4] Discontinuation of metronidazole or reduction of the dose usually results in complete resolution or improvement of the neuropathy but in some patients it may persist despite these measures. For reports of retrobulbar or optic neuritis associated with metronidazole, see Effects on the Eyes, above.

1. Duffy LF, *et al.* Peripheral neuropathy in Crohn's disease patients treated with metronidazole. *Gastroenterology* 1985; **88:** 681–4.
2. Boyce EG, *et al.* Persistent metronidazole-induced peripheral neuropathy. *DICP Ann Pharmacother* 1990; **24:** 19–21.
3. Learned-Coughlin S. Peripheral neuropathy induced by metronidazole. *Ann Pharmacother* 1994; **28:** 536.
4. Dreger LM, *et al.* Intermittent-dose metronidazole-induced peripheral neuropathy. *Ann Pharmacother* 1998; **32:** 267–8.

Effects on the pancreas. A small number of cases of acute pancreatitis associated with metronidazole, in some cases recurrent on rechallenge, have been reported,[1-3] No cases were found in a retrospective study of about 6500 patients who had received metronidazole.[4]

1. Plotnick BH, *et al.* Metronidazole-induced pancreatitis. *Ann Intern Med* 1985; **103:** 891–2.
2. Sanford KA, *et al.* Metronidazole-associated pancreatitis. *Ann Intern Med* 1988; **109:** 756–7.
3. Sura ME, *et al.* Metronidazole-associated pancreatitis. *Ann Pharmacother* 2000; **34:** 1152–5.
4. Friedman GD, Selby JV. How often does metronidazole induce pancreatitis? *Gastroenterology* 1990; **98:** 1702–3.

Gynaecomastia. Gynaecomastia occurred in a 36-year-old man with ulcerative colitis after taking metronidazole for about a month.[1]

1. Fagan TC, et al. Metronidazole-induced gynecomastia. JAMA 1985; 254: 3217.

Hypersensitivity. A hypersensitivity reaction with chills, fever, generalised erythema, and a maculopapular rash developed after a single dose of metronidazole in a patient who had previously developed a rash during treatment with intravaginal metronidazole.[1]

1. Knowles S, et al. Metronidazole hypersensitivity. Ann Pharmacother 1994; 28: 325–6.

Precautions

Peripheral neuropathy, transient epileptiform seizures, and leucopenia have sometimes been associated with prolonged or intensive treatment with metronidazole (see Adverse Effects, above). Clinical and laboratory monitoring is advised in patients receiving metronidazole for more than 10 days. Doses should be reduced in patients with severe hepatic impairment.

It is suggested that the use of metronidazole should be avoided during pregnancy, and this caution applies especially to use during the first trimester and to the use of high-dose regimens (see also below). Some authorities consider that women taking metronidazole should not breast feed their babies (see also below).

Patients are advised not to drink alcoholic beverages while taking metronidazole (see Interactions, below).

Breast feeding. Metronidazole is distributed into breast milk giving it a bitter taste which may impair feeding.[1] The American Academy of Pediatrics considers that although the effects of metronidazole on breast-fed infants are unknown they may be of concern. It recommends that breast feeding should be discontinued for 12 to 24 hours when single-dose therapy is use;[2] no specific recommendations are given for long-term treatment.

1. Rubin PC. Prescribing in pregnancy: general principles. BMJ 1986; 293: 1415–17.
2. American Academy of Pediatrics, Committee on Drugs. The transfer of drugs and other chemicals into human milk. Pediatrics 2001; 108: 776–89.

Pregnancy. Metronidazole is mutagenic in bacteria and carcinogenic in rodents. It readily crosses the placenta to the fetus achieving similar concentrations in the placental cord and maternal plasma and its use in pregnancy is controversial. Meta-analyses of studies involving the use of metronidazole in the first trimester of pregnancy[1,2] concluded that there did not appear to be an increased risk of teratogenicity. However, in the USA the manufacturer considers metronidazole to be contraindicated during the first trimester in patients with trichomoniasis; use for trichomoniasis during the second and third trimesters may be acceptable. For other indications the risks and benefits of treatment with metronidazole should be weighed carefully, especially in the first trimester.

1. Burtin P, et al. Safety of metronidazole in pregnancy: a meta-analysis. Am J Obstet Gynecol 1995; 172: 525–9.
2. Caro-Patón T, et al. Is metronidazole teratogenic? A meta-analysis. Br J Clin Pharmacol 1997; 44: 179–82.

Interactions

When given with alcohol, metronidazole may provoke a disulfiram-like reaction in some patients. Acute psychoses or confusion have been associated with the use of metronidazole and disulfiram together.

Metronidazole is reported to impair the metabolism or excretion of several drugs including warfarin (p.996), phenytoin (p.361), lithium (p.295), and fluorouracil (p.541), with the consequent potential for an increased incidence of adverse effects. There is some evidence that phenytoin might accelerate the metabolism of metronidazole. Plasma concentrations of metronidazole are decreased by the concomitant administration of phenobarbital, with a consequent reduction in the effectiveness of metronidazole. Cimetidine has increased plasma concentrations of metronidazole and might increase the risk of neurological side-effects, see below. For references to some of these interactions, see below.

For incompatibilities between metronidazole and other drugs in solutions for injection, see above.

Alcohol. Metronidazole may provoke a disulfiram-like reaction in some individuals when given in conjunction with alcohol; reactions have occurred after the administration of pharmaceutical preparations formulated with alcohol, including injections, as well as after drinking alcohol.[1] Acute psychosis

or confusional state was reported in 6 of 29 alcoholic patients who were also receiving disulfiram.[2]

1. Edwards DL. et al. Disulfiram-like reaction associated with intravenous trimethoprim-sulfamethoxazole and metronidazole. Clin Pharm 1986; 5: 999–1000.
2. Rothstein E, Clancy DD. Toxicity of disulfiram combined with metronidazole. N Engl J Med 1969; 280: 1006–7.

Carbamazepine. For a report of a possible interaction between metronidazole and carbamazepine, see p.345.

Cimetidine. In a study in 6 healthy volunteers metronidazole plasma concentrations were increased by concurrent twice-daily administration of cimetidine. The effect was presumed to be due to inhibition of cytochrome P450 isoenzymes responsible for metronidazole metabolism.[1] However, cimetidine was not found to affect the pharmacokinetics of metronidazole in a study in patients with Crohn's disease[2] nor in a single-dose study in healthy subjects.[3]

1. Gugler R, Jansen JC. Interaction between cimetidine and metronidazole. N Engl J Med 1983; 309: 1518–19.
2. Eradiri O, et al. Interaction of metronidazole with cimetidine and phenobarbital in Crohn's disease. Clin Pharmacol Ther 1987; 41: 235.
3. Loft S, et al. Lack of effect of cimetidine on the pharmacokinetics and metabolism of a single oral dose of metronidazole. Eur J Clin Pharmacol 1988; 35: 65–8.

Disulfiram. For a report of acute psychosis or confusional state following metronidazole treatment in alcoholic patients receiving disulfiram, see under Alcohol, above.

Omeprazole. Although concentrations in plasma and saliva of metronidazole and its hydroxy metabolite were unaffected by concurrent administration of omeprazole in healthy volunteers, those in gastric juice were substantially lowered, possibly as a result of a reduction in transfer from the plasma.[1] However, this may be of limited clinical significance during treatment of Helicobacter pylori infections.

1. Jessa MJ, et al. The effect of omeprazole on the pharmacokinetics of metronidazole and hydroxymetronidazole in human plasma, saliva and gastric juice. Br J Clin Pharmacol 1997; 44: 245–53.

Phenobarbital. An increase in the rate of metabolism of metronidazole, resulting in treatment failure, was reported in a patient receiving concurrent treatment with phenobarbital.[1] In a retrospective survey of patients who had not responded to treatment with metronidazole, 80% were found to be receiving long-term phenobarbital therapy.[2] Subsequently it was found that up to three times the usual dose was required to produce a parasitological cure of giardiasis in such patients.

1. Mead PB, et al. Possible alteration of metronidazole metabolism by phenobarbital. N Engl J Med 1982; 306: 1490.
2. Gupte S. Phenobarbital and metabolism of metronidazole. N Engl J Med 1983; 308: 529.

Phenytoin. In addition to conflicting reports on the effects of metronidazole on the metabolism of phenytoin (p.361), increased metabolism of metronidazole was reported in a patient during treatment with phenytoin.[1]

1. Wheeler LA, et al. Use of high-pressure liquid chromatography to determine plasma levels of metronidazole and metabolites after intravenous administration. Antimicrob Agents Chemother 1978; 13: 205–9.

Antimicrobial Action

Metronidazole is active against several protozoa including Balantidium coli, Blastocystis hominis, Entamoeba histolytica, Giardia intestinalis (Giardia lamblia), and Trichomonas vaginalis. Most obligate anaerobic bacteria, including Bacteroides and Clostridium spp., are sensitive in vitro to metronidazole. It is bactericidal. Minimum inhibitory concentrations (MICs) for susceptible anaerobic bacteria generally range from 0.1 to 8 μg per mL. It also has activity against the facultative anaerobes Gardnerella vaginalis and Helicobacter pylori and against some spirochaetes. Resistance to metronidazole has been reported and cross-resistance to other nitroimidazoles, such as tinidazole, may occur.

◊ Metronidazole has well-established bactericidal activity against obligate anaerobic bacteria in vitro, including the Gram-negative organisms Bacteroides fragilis and other Bacteroides spp., Fusobacterium spp., and Veillonella spp., and the Gram-positive organisms Clostridium difficile, Cl. perfringens, and other Clostridium spp., Eubacterium spp., Peptococcus spp., and Peptostreptococcus spp.; Propionibacterium and Actinomyces spp. are often resistant.[1-6] It also has activity against the facultative anaerobe Gardnerella vaginalis, although its bactericidal effect is reported to be much slower than against obligate anaerobes,[7] against some strains of Campylobacter spp. including C. fetus subsp. jejuni,[8,9] and against Helicobacter pylori.[10,11]

The oxidative metabolites of metronidazole have antibacterial activity; MICs of the hydroxy metabolite against anaerobic bacteria are reported to be generally within one dilution of the parent compound whereas the acid metabolite is much less active.[12,13] The hydroxy metabolite has been reported to be con-

sistently more active than metronidazole against strains of G. vaginalis.[14,15]

The mode of action of metronidazole is not entirely clear, but is thought to involve reduction to an unstable intermediate which interacts with DNA, effectively preventing further replication.[16] A number of factors affect the sensitivity of micro-organisms to metronidazole in vitro. Anaerobic conditions are important for optimal activity. Interactions between micro-organisms and metronidazole have been described, including inhibition of Escherichia coli by metronidazole in the presence of B. fragilis and enhancement of the rate of killing of B. fragilis by metronidazole in the presence of E. coli.

Resistance to metronidazole has developed in sensitive species. Although no resistance among the B. fragilis group was observed over several years,[17,18] there have been occasional reports of resistance in this group[19-24] and in other Bacteroides spp.[25-27] now known as Prevotella spp. Nitroimidazole resistance in Helicobacter pylori has been increasing and may be associated with reduced response rates to anti-Helicobacter therapy for peptic ulcer disease in some populations (see Peptic Ulcer Disease under Uses, below).

1. Wüst J. Susceptibility of anaerobic bacteria to metronidazole, ornidazole, and tinidazole and routine susceptibility testing by standardized methods. Antimicrob Agents Chemother 1977; 11: 631–7.
2. Dubreuil L, et al. Susceptibility of anaerobic bacteria from several French hospitals to three major antibiotics. Antimicrob Agents Chemother 1984; 25: 764–6.
3. Hill GB, Ayers OM. Antimicrobial susceptibilities of anaerobic bacteria isolated from female genital tract infections. Antimicrob Agents Chemother 1985; 27: 324–31.
4. Chow AW, et al. In vitro susceptibility of Clostridium difficile to new β-lactam and quinolone antibiotics. Antimicrob Agents Chemother 1985; 28: 842–4.
5. Brazier JS, et al. Antibiotic susceptibility of clinical isolates of clostridia. J Antimicrob Chemother 1985; 15: 181–5.
6. Van der Auwera P, et al. Comparative serum bactericidal activity against test anaerobes in volunteers receiving imipenem, clindamycin, latamoxef and metronidazole. J Antimicrob Chemother 1987; 19: 205–10.
7. Ralph ED, Amatnieks YE. Metronidazole in treatment against Haemophilus vaginalis (Corynebacterium vaginale). Antimicrob Agents Chemother 1980; 18: 101–4.
8. Hof H, et al. Comparative in vitro activities of niridazole and metronidazole against anaerobic and microaerophilic bacteria. Antimicrob Agents Chemother 1982; 22: 332–3.
9. Freydière AM, et al. In vitro susceptibilities of 40 Campylobacter fetus subsp jejuni strains to niridazole and metronidazole. Antimicrob Agents Chemother 1984; 25: 145–6.
10. Marshall BJ, et al. Pyloric campylobacter infection and gastroduodenal disease. Med J Aust 1985; 142: 439–44.
11. Howden A, et al. In-vitro sensitivity of Campylobacter pyloridis to furazolidone. Lancet 1986; ii: 1035.
12. Haller I. In vitro activity of the two principal oxidative metabolites of metronidazole against Bacteroides fragilis and related species. Antimicrob Agents Chemother 1982; 22: 165–6.
13. O'Keefe JP, et al. Activity of metronidazole and its hydroxy and acid metabolites against clinical isolates of anaerobic bacteria. Antimicrob Agents Chemother 1982; 22: 426–30.
14. Ralph ED, Amatnieks YE. Relative susceptibilities of Gardnerella vaginalis (Haemophilus vaginalis), Neisseria gonorrhoeae, and Bacteroides fragilis to metronidazole and its two major metabolites. Sex Transm Dis 1980; 7: 157–60.
15. Shanker S, Munro R. Sensitivity of Gardnerella vaginalis to metabolites of metronidazole and tinidazole. Lancet 1982; i: 167.
16. Ingham HR, et al. Interactions between micro-organisms and metronidazole. J Antimicrob Chemother 1977; 10: 84–7.
17. Tally FP, et al. Susceptibility of the Bacteroides fragilis group in the United States in 1981. Antimicrob Agents Chemother 1983; 23: 536–40.
18. Tally FP, et al. Nationwide study of the susceptibility of the Bacteroides fragilis group in the United States. Antimicrob Agents Chemother 1985; 28: 675–7.
19. Ingham HR, et al. Bacteroides fragilis resistance to metronidazole after long-term therapy. Lancet 1978; i: 214.
20. Eme A, et al. Bacteroides fragilis resistant to metronidazole. J Antimicrob Chemother 1983; 12: 523–5.
21. Lamothe F, et al. Bacteroides fragilis resistant to both metronidazole and imipenem. J Antimicrob Chemother 1986; 18: 642–3.
22. Brogan O, et al. Bacteroides fragilis resistant to metronidazole, clindamycin and cefoxitin. J Antimicrob Chemother 1989; 23: 660–2.
23. Hickey MM, et al. Metronidazole resistant Bacteroides fragilis infection of a prosthetic hip joint. J Infect 1990; 20: 129–33.
24. Turner P, et al. Simultaneous resistance to metronidazole, coamoxiclav, and imipenem in clinical isolate of Bacteroides fragilis. Lancet 1995; 345: 1275–7.
25. Sprott MS, et al. Metronidazole-resistant anaerobes. Lancet 1983; i: 1220.
26. McWalter PW, Baird DR. Metronidazole-resistant anaerobes. Lancet 1983; i: 1220.
27. Sprott MS, Kearns AM. Metronidazole-resistant Bacteroides melaninogenicus. J Antimicrob Chemother 1988; 22: 951–2.

Pharmacokinetics

Metronidazole is readily absorbed following administration by mouth and bioavailability approaches 100%. Peak plasma concentrations of approximately 5 and 10 μg per mL are achieved, usually within 1 to 2 hours, after single doses of 250 and 500 mg respectively. Some accumulation occurs and consequently there are higher concentrations when multiple doses are given. Absorption may be delayed, but is not reduced overall by administration with food. Metronidazole benzoate given by mouth is hydrolysed in the

The symbol † denotes a preparation no longer actively marketed

gastrointestinal tract to release metronidazole, which in turn is then absorbed.

Following the intravenous administration of metronidazole, peak steady-state plasma concentrations of about 25 µg per mL with trough concentrations of about 18 µg per mL have been reported in patients given a loading dose of 15 mg per kg body-weight followed by 7.5 mg per kg every 6 hours. The bioavailability of metronidazole from rectal suppositories is 60 to 80%; peak plasma concentrations are half those achieved with equivalent oral doses and effective concentrations occur after about 5 to 12 hours. Absorption from vaginal pessaries has been reported to be poor with a bioavailability of about 20 to 25%; absorption is gradual producing peak plasma concentrations of about 2 µg per mL following a dose of 500 mg. An intravaginal gel formulation providing a dose of 37.5 mg metronidazole produced peak plasma concentrations of 0.3 µg per mL at 8 hours, with a bioavailability of 56%.

Metronidazole is widely distributed. It appears in most body tissues and fluids including bile, bone, breast milk, cerebral abscesses, CSF, liver and liver abscesses, saliva, seminal fluid, and vaginal secretions, and achieves concentrations similar to those in plasma. It also crosses the placenta and rapidly enters the fetal circulation. No more than 20% is bound to plasma proteins.

Metronidazole is metabolised in the liver by side-chain oxidation and glucuronide formation. The principal oxidative metabolites are 1-(2-hydroxyethyl)-2-hydroxymethyl-5-nitroimidazole (the hydroxy metabolite), which has antibacterial activity and is detected in plasma and urine, and 2-methyl-5-nitroimidazole-1-acetic acid (the acid metabolite), which has virtually no antibacterial activity and is often not detected in plasma, but is excreted in urine. Small amounts of reduced metabolites, acetamide and N-(2-hydroxyethyl)oxamic acid (HOA), have also been detected in urine and are probably formed by the intestinal flora.

The elimination half-life of metronidazole is about 8 hours; that of the hydroxy metabolite is slightly longer. The half-life of metronidazole is reported to be longer in neonates and in patients with severe hepatic impairment; that of the hydroxy metabolite is prolonged in patients with substantial renal impairment.

The majority of a dose of metronidazole is excreted in the urine, mainly as metabolites; a small amount appears in the faeces.

◊ References.
1. Cunningham FE, et al. Pharmacokinetics of intravaginal metronidazole gel. J Clin Pharmacol 1994; 34: 1060–5.
2. Lamp KC, et al. Pharmacokinetics and pharmacodynamics of the nitroimidazole antimicrobials. Clin Pharmacokinet 1999; 36: 353–73.

Hepatic impairment. There have been differing results from pharmacokinetic studies of the elimination of metronidazole in patients with hepatic impairment. No marked difference was reported[1] between patients with cirrhosis or hepatosplenic schistosomiasis given a single 500-mg oral dose of metronidazole when compared with healthy subjects which suggested that, in the absence of renal impairment, dosage adjustment was not needed in patients with hepatic impairment. However, others found[2] that elimination of metronidazole, administered intravenously, was considerably impaired in a study of 10 patients with alcoholic liver disease or chronic active hepatitis, 7 of whom had reduced creatinine clearance. Responding to the comment[3] that these differing results were probably due to impaired renal elimination, the authors suggested[4] that impaired elimination of metronidazole was due to impaired hepatic metabolism rather than decreased renal clearance; other studies have shown metronidazole clearance to be normal in renal impairment. They nevertheless agreed that reduction in the dosage of metronidazole is required only when hepatic function is very poor, particularly when renal function is impaired. A study in 10 severely ill patients with or without impaired hepatic and/or renal function[5] also suggested that hepatic function is a very important determinant of metronidazole elimination.

1. Daneshmend TK, et al. Disposition of oral metronidazole in hepatic cirrhosis and in hepatosplenic schistosomiasis. Gut 1982; 23: 807–13.
2. Farrell G, et al. Impaired elimination of metronidazole in decompensated chronic liver disease. BMJ 1983; 287: 1845.
3. Daneshmend TK, Roberts CJC. Impaired elimination of metronidazole in decompensated chronic liver disease. BMJ 1984; 288: 405.
4. Farrell G, et al. Impaired elimination of metronidazole in decompensated chronic liver disease. BMJ 1984; 288: 1009.
5. Ljungberg B, et al. Metronidazole: pharmacokinetic observations in severely ill patients. J Antimicrob Chemother 1984; 14: 275–83.

Infants and children. A single intravenous dose of 15 mg per kg body-weight has been suggested for neonates[1] which would produce therapeutic concentrations of metronidazole for around 24 hours in term neonates and 48 hours in preterm neonates. Renal and hepatic function is incompletely developed in newborn infants and consequently the elimination half-life of metronidazole is prolonged and has been reported to range from 25 to 109 hours.[1] Elimination half-life is inversely proportional to gestational age[1,2] and as the infant matures half-life is reduced to values closer to those in adults.[1,3]

1. Jager-Roman E, et al. Pharmacokinetics and tissue distribution of metronidazole in the newborn infant. J Pediatr 1982; 100: 651–4.
2. Hall P, et al. Intravenous metronidazole in the newborn. Arch Dis Child 1983; 58: 529–31.
3. Amon I, et al. Disposition kinetics of metronidazole in children. Eur J Clin Pharmacol 1983; 24: 113–19.

Renal impairment. Pharmacokinetic studies have indicated that doses of metronidazole need not be altered in patients with renal impairment,[1] although adjustments might be required in patients undergoing haemodialysis, since metronidazole and its hydroxy metabolite are efficiently cleared and extensively removed in such patients.[2] However, in another study[3] the amount of metronidazole and its hydroxy metabolite cleared was found to depend on the type of dialysis membrane used; the authors concluded that dosage supplementation may be needed only for seriously ill patients undergoing haemodialysis with a membrane having high metronidazole clearance.
Routine adjustment of dosage was not considered necessary in patients undergoing peritoneal dialysis.[4] However, the potential for metabolites to accumulate was noted in patients on continuous ambulatory peritoneal dialysis[5] and it was suggested that dosage reduction may be necessary if excessive concentrations of metabolites are found to be toxic.

1. Houghton GW, et al. Pharmacokinetics of metronidazole in patients with varying degrees of renal failure. Br J Clin Pharmacol 1985; 19: 203–9.
2. Somogyi A, et al. Disposition and removal of metronidazole in patients undergoing haemodialysis. Eur J Clin Pharmacol 1983; 25: 683–7.
3. Lau AH, et al. Hemodialysis clearance of metronidazole and its metabolites. Antimicrob Agents Chemother 1986; 29: 235–8.
4. Cassey JG, et al. Pharmacokinetics of metronidazole in patients undergoing peritoneal dialysis. Antimicrob Agents Chemother 1983; 24: 950–1.
5. Guay DR, et al. Pharmacokinetics of metronidazole in patients undergoing continuous ambulatory peritoneal dialysis. Antimicrob Agents Chemother 1984; 25: 306–10.

Uses and Administration

Metronidazole is a 5-nitroimidazole derivative with activity against anaerobic bacteria and protozoa (see Antimicrobial Action, above); it also has a radiosensitising effect on hypoxic tumour cells. Its mechanism of action is thought to involve interference with DNA by a metabolite in which the nitro group of metronidazole has been reduced.

Metronidazole is used in the treatment of susceptible protozoal infections such as amoebiasis, balantidiasis, Blastocystis hominis infections, giardiasis, and trichomoniasis; it has also been tried in leishmaniasis and microsporidiosis. For details of these infections and their treatment see under Choice of Antiprotozoal, p.582. Metronidazole is also used in the treatment and prophylaxis of anaerobic bacterial infections. Specific bacterial infections treated with metronidazole include bacterial vaginosis, acute necrotising ulcerative gingivitis, pelvic inflammatory disease, tetanus, and antibiotic-associated colitis. For details of these infections and their treatment see under Choice of Antibacterial, p.114.

It is used to eradicate Helicobacter pylori in peptic ulcer disease (in combination with other antimicrobials, and either bismuth compounds or proton pump inhibitors) and in the management of malodorous tumours and ulcers where there is anaerobic infection. It is also used in the treatment of rosacea and of dracunculiasis (guinea-worm infection) and has been given in the treatment of perianal Crohn's disease and hepatic encephalopathy. It has also been tried as an adjunct to the radiotherapy of malignant neoplasms. See below for these miscellaneous uses.

ADMINISTRATION AND DOSAGE. Metronidazole is administered by mouth in tablets or, as metronidazole benzoate, in oral suspension; the tablets are taken with or after food and the suspension at least 1 hour before food. Metronidazole is also given rectally in suppositories, applied topically as a cream or gel, or administered by intravenous infusion of metronidazole or metronidazole hydrochloride. Doses are expressed in terms of metronidazole base.

In **amoebiasis**, metronidazole acts as an amoebicide at all sites of infection with Entamoeba histolytica. Because of its rapid absorption it is probably less effective against parasites in the bowel lumen and is therefore used in conjunction with a luminal amoebicide such as diloxanide furoate or diiodohydroxyquinoline in the treatment of invasive amoebiasis. Metronidazole is given in doses of 400 to 800 mg three times daily by mouth for 5 to 10 days. Children aged 1 to 3 years may be given one-quarter, those aged 3 to 7 years one-third, and those aged 7 to 10 years one-half the adult dose; alternatively 35 to 50 mg per kg body-weight daily in divided doses has been used. An alternative adult dose is 1.5 to 2.5 g as a single dose daily for 2 or 3 days.

In **balantidiasis** and **Blastocystis hominis infection**, metronidazole has been given in doses similar to those used in amoebiasis.

In **giardiasis**, the usual dose of metronidazole is 2 g once daily by mouth for 3 successive days, or 400 mg three times daily for 5 days, or 500 mg twice daily for 7 to 10 days. Dosage for children is proportional, as for amoebiasis (above). An alternative schedule for children is 15 mg per kg daily in divided doses.

In **trichomoniasis**, metronidazole is given by mouth either as a single 2-g dose, as a 2-day course of 800 mg in the morning and 1.2 g in the evening, or as a 7-day course of 600 mg to 1 g daily in two or three divided doses. Sexual partners should be treated concomitantly. If treatment needs to be repeated, an interval of 4 to 6 weeks between courses has been recommended. Vaginal preparations containing metronidazole are available for the treatment of vaginal trichomoniasis in some countries. Children with trichomoniasis may be given a 7-day course of metronidazole by mouth as follows: 1 to 3 years, 50 mg three times daily; 3 to 7 years, 100 mg twice daily, and 7 to 10 years, 100 mg three times daily. An alternative children's dose is 15 mg per kg daily in divided doses for 7 days.

Bacterial vaginosis is treated similarly to vaginal trichomoniasis with which it may co-exist; metronidazole is usually given by mouth as a single 2-g dose or as a 5 to 7-day course of 400 or 500 mg twice daily. Alternatively it may be administered locally as 5 g of a 0.75% gel once or twice daily for 5 days.

In **acute necrotising ulcerative gingivitis**, metronidazole 200 mg three times daily is given by mouth for 3 days; similar doses are used in acute dental infections. A 25% dental gel has also been used as an adjunct to the treatment of chronic periodontal infections.

For the treatment of most **anaerobic bacterial infections**, metronidazole is given by mouth in an initial dose of 800 mg followed by 400 mg every 8 hours, usually for about 7 days. A regimen of 500 mg every 8 hours is alternatively used. When oral therapy is precluded metronidazole may be administered intravenously, 500 mg being infused as 100 mL of a 5 mg per mL solution at a rate of 5 mL per minute every 8 hours, or rectally as a 1-g suppository every 8 hours for 3 days, then every 12 hours; oral therapy should be substituted as soon as possible. Suppositories may be unsuitable for the initiation of therapy in serious infections because of the slower absorption of metronidazole. Children may be given 7.5 mg per kg every 8 hours by mouth, rectally, or by intravenous infusion. In the USA recommended adult doses of metronidazole are 7.5 mg per kg every 6 hours by mouth or 15 mg per kg by intravenous infusion followed by 7.5 mg per kg every 6 hours, doses being infused over 1 hour; by either route a total dose of 4 g in 24 hours should not be exceeded. In mixed anaerobic and aerobic infections metronidazole is given in association with the appropriate antibacterials.

For the **prevention of postoperative anaerobic bacterial infections**, especially in patients undergoing abdominal or gynaecological surgery, metronidazole is administered orally, intravenously, or rectally in doses similar to those used for the treatment of established infections, usually in combination with a beta-lactam or an aminoglycoside antibacterial. Various schedules have been employed. By mouth, 400 mg of metronidazole may be given every 8 hours in the 24 hours before surgery followed postoperatively by intravenous or rectal administration until oral therapy is possible. By intravenous infusion, 500 mg may be given shortly before operation and repeated every 8 hours, oral doses of 400 mg every 8 hours being substituted as soon as possible. By rectum, 1 g may be administered every 8 hours starting 2 hours before surgery. Children's prophylactic doses are as for treatment (above). In the USA the recommended schedule for adults undergoing colorectal surgery is metronidazole 15 mg per kg by intravenous infusion over 30 to 60 minutes, completed about 1 hour before surgery, followed by two further intravenous doses of 7.5 mg per kg infused at 6 and 12 hours after the initial dose.

In **peptic ulcer disease**, metronidazole is used in combination therapy to eradicate *Helicobacter pylori*. Typical regimens include metronidazole plus another antibacterial (clarithromycin or amoxicillin) given with either a proton pump inhibitor (omeprazole or lansoprazole) or with ranitidine bismuth citrate. The usual dose of metronidazole is 400 mg twice daily except when given in combination with omeprazole and amoxicillin, when metronidazole 400 mg three times daily is used. Treatment is continued for 1 week.

For **leg ulcers** and **pressure sores** infected with anaerobic bacteria, metronidazole 400 mg may be given three times daily by mouth for 7 days. Metronidazole is also applied topically as a 0.75% or 0.8% gel to reduce the odour associated with anaerobic infection in **fungating tumours**.

In the treatment of **rosacea** metronidazole is given by mouth or applied topically.

Administration in hepatic impairment. Since metronidazole is mainly metabolised by hepatic oxidation accumulation of metronidazole and its metabolites is likely in patients with severely impaired hepatic function. Metronidazole should therefore be administered with caution and at reduced doses to patients with severe hepatic impairment, and especially hepatic encephalopathy when adverse affects of metronidazole can add to the symptoms of the disease. One-third of the usual daily dose may be administered once daily in these patients. For patients with lesser degrees of hepatic impairment, pharmacokinetic studies have not produced consistent results (see under Pharmacokinetics, above) and no recommendations about dosage reduction have been made by the manufacturers.

Administration in renal impairment. The elimination of metronidazole is largely unchanged in patients with renal impairment although metabolites may accumulate in patients with end-stage renal disease on dialysis (see under Pharmacokinetics, above). Dosage reductions are therefore not usually recommended for patients with renal impairment, although, since both metronidazole and its metabolites are removed by haemodialysis, doses need to be administered immediately after haemodialysis.

Dracunculiasis. Metronidazole may be beneficial in the management of dracunculiasis (p.92). It provides symptomatic relief and is also thought to weaken the anchorage of the worms within subcutaneous tissue, thus allowing them to be removed more quickly.

Metronidazole has been given in a variety of dosage regimens including: 400 mg three times daily for 5 days;[1] 40 mg per kg body-weight daily in three divided doses, to a maximum daily dose of 2.4 g, for 3 days;[2] 400 mg daily for 10 to 20 days.[3] A dose of 250 mg three times daily for 10 days has also been recommended.[4]

1. Padonu KO. A controlled trial of metronidazole in the treatment of dracontiasis in Nigeria. *Am J Trop Med Hyg* 1973; **22:** 42–4.
2. Kale OO. A controlled field trial of the treatment of dracontiasis with metronidazole and niridazole. *Ann Trop Med Parasitol* 1974; **68:** 91–5.
3. Muller R. Guinea worm disease: epidemiology, control, and treatment. *Bull WHO* 1979; **57:** 683–9.
4. Anonymous. Drugs for parasitic infections. *Med Lett Drugs Ther* 1998; **40:** 1–12.

Hepatic encephalopathy. The treatment of hepatic encephalopathy is discussed on p.1205. It includes the administration of an antimicrobial such as metronidazole to reduce the intestinal flora.

The symbol † denotes a preparation no longer actively marketed

Inflammatory bowel disease. Metronidazole is used in the treatment of perineal Crohn's disease (see Inflammatory bowel disease, p.1205) and may also be used in colonic Crohn's disease, when it has been tried in combination with ciprofloxacin. It has also proved effective for the prevention of postsurgical recurrence. Duration of therapy is usually limited to 3 months.
References.
1. Bernstein LH, et al. Healing of perineal Crohn's disease with metronidazole. *Gastroenterology* 1980; **79:** 357–65.
2. Brandt LJ, et al. Metronidazole therapy for perineal Crohn's disease: a follow-up study. *Gastroenterology* 1982; **83:** 383–7.
3. Ursing B, et al. A comparative study of metronidazole and sulfasalazine for active Crohn's disease: the cooperative Crohn's disease study in Sweden. *Gastroenterology* 1982; **83:** 550–62.
4. Sutherland L, et al. Double blind, placebo controlled trial of metronidazole in Crohn's disease. *Gut* 1991; **32:** 1071–5.
5. Rutgeerts P, et al. Controlled trial of metronidazole treatment for prevention of Crohn's recurrence after ileal resection. *Gastroenterology* 1995; **108:** 1617–21.
6. Prantera C, et al. An antibiotic regimen for the treatment of active Crohn's disease: a randomized, controlled clinical trial of metronidazole plus ciprofloxacin. *Am J Gastroenterol* 1996; **91:** 328–32.

Metabolic disorders. There are case reports[1,2] of children with methylmalonic aciduria showing clinical improvement when given metronidazole which reduced the excretion of faecal propionate and urinary methylmalonate. Metronidazole is considered to act through its antimicrobial effect on gut anaerobes that are involved in propionate production; such propionate cannot be handled by these children who are deficient in the relevant enzyme.
1. Bain MD, et al. Contribution of gut bacterial metabolism to human metabolic disease. *Lancet* 1988; **i:** 1078–9.
2. Koletzko B, et al. Antibiotic therapy for improvement of metabolic control in methylmalonic aciduria. *J Pediatr* 1990; **117:** 99–101.

Mouth disorders and infections. Ciclosporin-induced gingival hyperplasia resolved in 4 patients following treatment with metronidazole.[1]
Metronidazole is considered to be effective for the treatment of acute necrotising ulcerative gingivitis and is an alternative to penicillin in other dental infections (see Mouth Infections, p.130).
1. Wong W, et al. Resolution of cyclosporin-induced gingival hypertrophy with metronidazole. *Lancet* 1994; **343:** 986.

Peptic ulcer disease. The use of metronidazole is well established in regimens for eradicating *Helicobacter pylori* (see Peptic Ulcer Disease p.1208). However, the emergence of metronidazole-resistant strains of *H. pylori* has been associated with an increased rate of treatment failures with some regimens.[1-4] Difficulties arise in assessing metronidazole resistance and in correlating *in-vitro* results with clinical response.[5] In populations in which the incidence of resistance is high, it may become necessary to use alternative regimens,[6] although some clinicians report that regimens containing metronidazole continue to produce adequate response rates.[7]
1. Buckley MJM, et al. Metronidazole resistance reduces efficacy of triple therapy and leads to secondary clarithromycin resistance. *Dig Dis Sci* 1997; **42:** 2111–15.
2. Lerang F, et al. Highly effective twice-daily triple therapies for Helicobacter pylori infection and peptic ulcer disease: does in vitro metronidazole resistance have any clinical relevance? *Am J Gastroenterol* 1997; **92:** 248–53.
3. Misiewicz JJ, et al. One week triple therapy for Helicobacter pylori: a multicentre comparative study. *Gut* 1997; **41:** 735–9.
4. van Zanten SV, et al. Adding once-daily omeprazole 20 mg to metronidazole/amoxicillin treatment for Helicobacter pylori gastritis: a randomized, double-blind trial showing the importance of metronidazole resistance. *Am J Gastroenterol* 1998; **93:** 5–10.
5. Goddard AF, Logan RPH. Antimicrobial resistance and Helicobacter pylori. *J Antimicrob Chemother* 1996; **37:** 639–43.
6. Fennerty MB. Should we abandon metronidazole containing Helicobacter pylori treatment regimens? The clinical relevance of metronidazole resistance. *Am J Gastroenterol* 1998; **93:** 2–3.
7. Walt RP. Metronidazole-resistance H pylori—of questionable clinical importance. *Lancet* 1996; **348:** 489–90.

Skin disorders. Metronidazole may be effective in the management of anaerobic skin infections associated with ulceration (p.140), including *pressure sores* and *fungating tumours*. Metronidazole 200 mg three times daily was reported to be successful in reducing the smell of fungating tumours.[1,2] Once-daily topical application of metronidazole has also proved effective. Treatment is supplemented by metronidazole irrigation for wound cleansing of large or deep cavities.[3,4]
In addition, several studies have indicated that metronidazole by mouth or applied topically is effective in the treatment of *rosacea* (p.1107). Metronidazole 200 mg twice daily by mouth was significantly better than placebo[5] and as effective as oxytetracycline by mouth.[6] Similarly, topical application of a 1% metronidazole cream was found to be better than placebo[7,8] and as effective as oxytetracycline by mouth.[9] A 0.75% metronidazole gel also proved effective when compared with placebo in patients with rosacea, although the telangiectatic component of the disease was not altered.[10]
1. Ashford RFU, et al. Metronidazole in smelly tumours. *Lancet* 1980; **i:** 874–5.
2. Ashford R, et al. Double-blind trial of metronidazole in malodorous ulcerating tumours. *Lancet* 1984; **i:** 1232–3.
3. Allwood MC, et al. Metronidazole topical gel. *Pharm J* 1986; **236:** 158.
4. Anonymous. Management of smelly tumours. *Lancet* 1990; **335:** 141–2.
5. Pye RJ, Burton JL. Treatment of rosacea by metronidazole. *Lancet* 1976; **i:** 1211–12.

6. Saihan EM, Burton JL. A double-blind trial of metronidazole versus oxytetracycline therapy for rosacea. *Br J Dermatol* 1980; **102:** 443–5.
7. Nielsen PG. Treatment of rosacea with 1% metronidazole cream. A double-blind study. *Br J Dermatol* 1983; **108:** 327–32.
8. Bitar A, et al. A double-blind randomised study of metronidazole (Flagyl®) 1% cream in the treatment of acne rosacea: a placebo-controlled study. *Drug Invest* 1990; **2:** 242–8.
9. Nielsen P. A double-blind study of 1% metronidazole cream versus systemic oxytetracycline therapy for rosacea. *Br J Dermatol* 1983; **109:** 63–5.
10. Aronson IK, et al. Evaluation of topical metronidazole gel in acne rosacea. *Drug Intell Clin Pharm* 1987; **21:** 346–51.

Surgical infection. Metronidazole and related nitroimidazoles are used in surgical infection prophylaxis (p.141) to reduce the rate of wound infection.

HAEMORRHOIDECTOMY. Prophylactic metronidazole reduced pain following haemorrhoidectomy in a small study.[1]
1. Carapeti EA, et al. Double-blind randomised controlled trial of effect of metronidazole on pain after day-case haemorrhoidectomy. *Lancet* 1998; **351:** 169–72.

African trypanosomiasis. Although there is no established alternative treatment for *Trypanosoma brucei rhodesiense* infections that are resistant to melarsoprol (see p.586), metronidazole and suramin were effective in 1 patient.[1]
1. Foulkes JR. Metronidazole and suramin combination in the treatment of arsenical refractory rhodesian sleeping sickness—a case study. *Trans R Soc Trop Med Hyg* 1996; **90:** 422.

Preparations

BP 2001: Metronidazole Gel; Metronidazole Intravenous Infusion; Metronidazole Suppositories; Metronidazole Tablets;
USP 25: Metronidazole Gel; Metronidazole Injection; Metronidazole Tablets.

Proprietary Preparations (details are given in Part 3)
Aust.: Acsacea; Anaerobex; Ariline†; Elyzol; Flagyl; Oeccozol; Trichex; *Austral.:* Flagyl; Metrogyl; Metronide; Metrozine†; Rozex; *Belg.:* Anaeromet; Flagyl; Pharmaflex; Rozex; *Braz.:* Flagyl; Metronix; Rozex; *Canad.:* Flagyl; Metrocream; Metrogel; NidaGel; Noritate; Novo-Nidazol; Trikacide†; *Denm.:* Elyzol; Flagyl; Metrogel; *Fin.:* Elyzol; Flagyl; Trikozol; *Fr.:* Elyzol; Flagyl; Rosiced; Rozacreme; Rozagel; Rozex; *Ger.:* Arilin; Clont; Elyzol; Flagyl; Fossyol; Metronid-Puren; Metronimerck; Metronour; Metront; Ulcolind Metro†; Vagimid; *Hong Kong:* Elyzol; Flagyl; Metrogyl; Metrozine; Noritate; Protogyl; Rozex; Trizole; *Irl.:* Anabact; Elyzol; Flagyl; Metrogel; Metronide; Metrotop; Rozex; *Israel:* Elyzol; Flagyl; Metrogyl; Rozex; Venogyl; Zadstat; *Ital.:* Deflamon; Elyzol; Flagyl; Pernyzol†; Rosased; Rozex; Vagilen; *Mex.:* Ameblin; Amiyodazol; Antral; Biomona; Biotazol; Cryozol; Dasmetrol; Dasolin; Dualizol; Elyzol; Epaq; Fagizol; Fartricon; Flagenase; Flaginazol; Flagyl; Fresenizol; Fusanidazol; Juaflor; Labitrix; Lagylan; Lamblit; Medizol; Meredazol; Metricom; Metrizol; Metrogel; Metronil; Metrosan; Mibazol; Niacel; Nidazol; Nidralon; Nidrozol; Nitromidagel; Ortrizol; Otrozol; Planizol; Proflag; Promibasol; Prozolin; Retofar; Selegil; Servizol; Solumidazol; Vatrix-S; Vertisal; *Neth.:* Flagyl; Metrogel; Rozex; *Norw.:* Elyzol; Flagyl; *NZ:* Flagyl; Rozex; Trichozole; *Port.:* Dumozol; Flagyl; Metroderme; Rodermil; *S.Afr.:* Acuzole†; Ambral; Anaerobyl†; Bemetrazole; Berazole†; Clinazole†; Dynametron; Flagyl; Medamet; Metagyl; Metazol; Metrazole†; Metrostat; Nabact†; Narobic; Nidatron†; Rozex; Trichazole; Urometron†; Zagyl; Zobacide; Zolerol; *Singapore:* Anabact; Elyzol; Flagyl; Metrozole; MND; Nizole; Protogyl; Rozex; Servizol; *Spain:* Amotein; Flagyl; Rozex; Tricowas B; *Swed.:* Elyzol; Flagyl; Rozex; *Switz.:* Arilin; Elyzol; Flagyl; Perilox; Rivozol; Rosalox; Rozex; Servizol†; *Thai.:* Anabact; Asiazole; Biogyl; Elyzol; Flagyl; Klion; Klont; Med-Tricocide; Medazyl; Mefiron; Menisole; Mepagyl; Mesolex; Metrazole; Metrocide; Metrogyl; Metrolex; Milanidazole; Servizol; Tricomed; Unimezol; Vagil; Vagyl; *UAE:* Negazole; *UK:* Anabact; Elyzol†; Flagyl; Metrogel; Metrolyl; Metrotop; Metrozol; Noritate; Norzol; Rozex; Vaginyl; Zadstat; Zidoval; Zyomet; *USA:* Flagyl; Metizol†; Metro; Metrocream; Metrogel; Metrogel Vaginal; Noritate; Protostat.

Multi-ingredient: *Aust.:* Helicocin†; *Austral.:* Helidac; Losec Helicopak; *Braz.:* Bio-Vagin; Colpanist; Colpatrin; Colpist MT; Colpistar; Colpistatin; Donnagel; Flagyl Nistatina; Fungimax; Ginestatin; Periodontil; Profargil; Sarcoton; Tricolpex; Trisdazol; Vagi Biotic; Vagimax; *Canad.:* Flagystatin; Losec 1-2-3 M; *Fin.:* Flagyl Comp; Helipak A; Helipak T; Losec Heliara; *Fr.:* Birodogyl; Rodogyl; *Irl.:* Flagyl Compak; *Ital.:* Meclon; *Mex.:* Flagenase 400; Flagystatin V; Madecassol C; Metodine; Metrodiyod; Norecil; Promibasol-Plus; Vagitrol-V; *NZ:* Helicosec; *Singapore:* Flagystatin; *Spain:* Blastoestimulina; Rhodogil; *UK:* Entamizole; Flagyl Compak; HeliMet; *USA:* Helidac.

Monensin Sodium (12973-q)

Monensin Sodium (*BANM, rINNM*).

Lilly-67314 (monensin). Sodium 4-{2-[2-ethyl-3′-methyl-5′-(tetrahydro-6-hydroxy-6-hydroxymethyl-3,5-dimethyl-2H-pyran-2-yl)perhydro-2,2′-bifuran-5-yl]-9-hydroxy-2,8-dimethyl-1,6-dioxaspiro[4.5]dec-7-yl}-3-methoxy-2-methylvalerate.
$C_{36}H_{61}NaO_{11} = 692.9$.
CAS — 17090-79-8 (monensin); 22373-78-0 (monensin sodium).

NOTE. Monensin is *USAN*.
Pharmacopoeias. US includes Monensin and Monensin Sodium for veterinary use only.

Pharmacopoeial description

USP 25: Monensin is a mixture of antibiotic substances produced by *Streptomyces cinnamonensis*. Monensin sodium is an off-white to tan crystalline powder. Slightly soluble in water; soluble in chloroform and in methyl alcohol; practically insoluble in petroleum spirit. Avoid moisture and excessive heat.

Profile
Monensin is an antiprotozoal used as the sodium salt in veterinary practice for the prevention of coccidiosis in poultry and as a growth promotor for cattle. It has also been used for toxoplasmosis in sheep.

Narasin (12016-p)
Narasin *(BAN, USAN, rINN)*.
Compound 79891; Lilly-79891. 2-(6-{5-[2-(5-Ethyltetrahydro-5-hydroxy-6-methylpyran-2-yl)-15-hydroxy-2,10,12-trimethyl-1,6,8-trioxadispiro[4.1.5.3]pentadec-13-en-9-yl]-2-hydroxy-1,3-dimethyl-4-oxoheptyl}tetrahydro-3,5-dimethylpyran-2-yl)butyric acid.
$C_{43}H_{72}O_{11} = 765.0$.
CAS — 55134-13-9.
Pharmacopoeias. In US for veterinary use only.

An antibiotic produced by *Streptomyces aureofaciens*.

Pharmacopoeial description
USP 25: A white to off-white crystalline powder. Soluble in water and in methyl alcohol.

Profile
Narasin is an antiprotozoal used in veterinary practice for the prevention of coccidiosis in poultry.

Nicarbazin (13007-z)
Nicarbazin *(BAN)*.
An equimolecular complex of 1,3-bis(4-nitrophenyl)urea ($C_{13}H_{10}N_4O_5$) and 4,6-dimethylpyrimidin-2-ol ($C_6H_8N_2O$).
$C_{19}H_{18}N_6O_6 = 426.4$.
CAS — 330-95-0.

Profile
Nicarbazin is an antiprotozoal used in veterinary practice for the prevention of coccidiosis in poultry.

Nifuratel (4789-q)
Nifuratel *(BAN, USAN, rINN)*.
Methylmercadone. 5-Methylthiomethyl-3-(5-nitrofurfurylideneamino)-2-oxazolidone.
$C_{10}H_{11}N_3O_5S = 285.3$.
CAS — 4936-47-4.
ATC — G01AX05.

Adverse Effects
Adverse effects associated with nifuratel include gastrointestinal disturbances, peripheral neuropathy, and thrombocytopenic purpura. Allergic reactions, hepatotoxicity, blood dyscrasias, and pulmonary reactions similar to those seen with the structurally related drug nitrofurantoin have been reported rarely. Haemolytic anaemia may occur in patients with a deficiency of glucose-6-phosphate dehydrogenase given nifuratel.

Hypersensitivity. A report of contact dermatitis after only one application of nifuratel ointment in a man whose wife was undergoing treatment with nifuratel vaginal pessaries.[1]

1. Bedello PG, *et al.* Contact dermatitis from nifuratel. *Contact Dermatitis* 1983; **9**: 166.

Precautions
Nifuratel should not be given to patients with renal impairment, neuropathies, or glucose-6-phosphate dehydrogenase deficiency.

Interactions
A disulfiram-like reaction may occur in patients taking alcohol while on nifuratel therapy.

Pharmacokinetics
When taken by mouth nifuratel is absorbed from the gastrointestinal tract. A metabolite, with activity against bacteria but not against trichomonads, is excreted in the urine.

Uses and Administration
Nifuratel is a nitrofuran derivative with a broad antimicrobial spectrum. It is active against the protozoan *Trichomonas vaginalis* and has an antibacterial spectrum similar to that of nitrofurantoin and some antifungal activity against *Candida albicans*. Although other drugs are preferred nifuratel has been used in the treatment of susceptible infections of the genitourinary tract in doses of 200 to 400 mg three times daily by mouth. It has also been administered vaginally.

Preparations
Proprietary Preparations (details are given in Part 3)
Aust.: Macmiror; *Ger.:* Inimur; *Hong Kong:* Macmiror; *Ital.:* Macmiror; *Mex.:* Macmiror; *Spain:* Macmiror†; *Switz.:* Macmiror†.

Multi-ingredient: *Fr.:* Mycomnes†; *Hong Kong:* Macmiror Complex; *Ital.:* Macmiror Complex; *Mex.:* Macmiror Complex V; *Port.:* Dafnegil; *Switz.:* Dafnegil†.

Nifursol (13015-z)
Nifursol *(BAN, USAN, pINN)*.
3,5-Dinitro-2'-(5-nitrofurfurylidene)salicylohydrazide.
$C_{12}H_7N_5O_9 = 365.2$.
CAS — 16915-70-1.

Profile
Nifursol is an antiprotozoal used in veterinary practice for the prevention of blackhead (histomoniasis) in poultry.

Nifurtimox (4790-d)
Nifurtimox *(BAN, rINN)*.
Bayer-2502. Tetrahydro-3-methyl-4-(5-nitrofurfurylideneamino)-1,4-thiazine 1,1-dioxide.
$C_{10}H_{13}N_3O_5S = 287.3$.
CAS — 23256-30-6.
ATC — P01CC01.
Pharmacopoeias. In Fr. and Int.

Adverse Effects
Adverse effects are common with nifurtimox and include gastrointestinal effects such as anorexia and loss of weight, abdominal pain, nausea and vomiting, and effects on the nervous system, especially peripheral neuropathy. Psychoses, CNS excitement, insomnia, drowsiness, headache, myalgia, arthralgia, dizziness, and convulsions have also been reported. Skin rashes and other allergic reactions may occur.

Mutagenesis. An increase in chromosomal aberrations has been observed in children given nifurtimox.[1]

1. Gorla NB, *et al.* Thirteenfold increase of chromosomal aberrations non-randomly distributed in chagasic children treated with nifurtimox. *Mutat Res* 1989; **224**: 263–7.

Pharmacokinetics
Nifurtimox is well absorbed and rapidly metabolised following administration by mouth.

◊ References.
1. Paulas C, *et al.* Pharmacokinetics of a nitrofuran compound, nifurtimox, in healthy volunteers. *Int J Clin Pharmacol Ther Toxicol* 1989; **27**: 454–7.
2. Gonzalez-Martin G, *et al.* The pharmacokinetics of nifurtimox in chronic renal failure. *Eur J Clin Pharmacol* 1992; **42**: 671–3.

Uses and Administration
Nifurtimox is a nitrofuran derivative with antiprotozoal activity. It is of value in the treatment of South American trypanosomiasis (Chagas' disease) due to infection by *Trypanosoma cruzi*, especially the early acute stage of the disease. In African trypanosomiasis it has some activity against *T. brucei gambiense*, the organism responsible for West African sleeping sickness.

Nifurtimox is given by mouth in divided doses. It is better tolerated by children than by adults. Treatment for South American trypanosomiasis is given for 60 to 120 days (but see below). Doses for adults are 8 to 10 mg per kg body-weight daily. Doses for children are: aged 1 to 10 years, 15 to 20 mg per kg daily for 90 days; aged 11 to 16 years, 12.5 to 15 mg per kg daily for 90 days.

Leishmaniasis. Mucocutaneous leishmaniasis of the New World (p.584) is usually treated with pentavalent antimony or, in those who do not respond, with amphotericin B or pentamidine. However, nifurtimox 10 mg per kg body-weight daily for a minimum of 4 weeks has been shown to be effective in cases of mucocutaneous leishmaniasis in Colombia and Brazil. Despite this, toxic effects with nifurtimox are common and its role as a second-line drug or in combination with pentavalent antimony has not been established.[1]

1. WHO. Control of the leishmaniases. *WHO Tech Rep Ser* 793, 1990.

African trypanosomiasis. Nifurtimox has been tried as an alternative to melarsoprol or eflornithine in the meningoencephalitic stage of *Trypanosoma brucei gambiense* infection (p.586) but higher doses than those used in South American trypanosomiasis are necessary. A good initial response was achieved[1] in 25 patients with nifurtimox 15 mg per kg body-weight daily for 60 days but 3 patients relapsed while still receiving nifurtimox and a further 12 of 19 patients who were followed up relapsed subsequently. An attempt to improve the response by increasing the daily dose even higher to 30 mg per

kg for 30 days[2] resulted in substantial toxicity and only a modest improvement in results with 9 of 25 patients relapsing.

1. Pepin J, *et al.* A clinical trial of nifurtimox for arseno-resistant Trypanosoma brucei gambiense sleeping sickness in central Zaire. *Trans R Soc Trop Med Hyg* 1989; **83**: 514–17.
2. Pépin J, *et al.* High-dose nifurtimox for arseno-resistant Trypanosoma brucei gambiense sleeping sickness: an open trial in central Zaire. *Trans R Soc Trop Med Hyg* 1992; **86**: 254–6.

American trypanosomiasis. The treatment of South American trypanosomiasis (p.587) is generally unsatisfactory, but nifurtimox is of value especially in the acute phase. However, there has been controversy over its ability to cure completely, that is to eradicate all parasites, in chronic disease.[1] Doses recommended by WHO[2] are 8 to 10 mg per kg body-weight daily in three divided doses for adults, and 15 to 20 mg per kg daily in four divided doses for children; however, up to 25 mg per kg daily has been used for the alleviation of acute meningoencephalitis.[3] WHO recommends that nifurtimox should be given for 60 to 90 days.[2,3] Some in the USA[4] suggest a 90- to 120-day regimen for adults but nifurtimox is not well tolerated and the experience of other workers[1] suggests that few patients may complete the full course. Doses of 8 to 25 mg per kg daily have been given for 30 days or more in the treatment of congenital infections.[3]

1. Gutteridge WE. Existing chemotherapy and its limitations. *Br Med Bull* 1985; **41**: 162–8.
2. WHO. WHO model prescribing information: drugs used in parasitic diseases. 2nd ed. Geneva: WHO, 1995.
3. WHO. Control of Chagas disease: report of a WHO expert committee. *WHO Tech Rep Ser* 811 1991.
4. Anonymous. Drugs for parasitic infections. *Med Lett Drugs Ther* 1998; **40**: 1–12.

Preparations
Proprietary Preparations (details are given in Part 3)
Ger.: Lampit†.

Nimorazole (4791-n)
Nimorazole *(BAN, rINN)*.
Nitrimidazine. 4-[2-(5-Nitroimidazol-1-yl)ethyl]morpholine.
$C_9H_{14}N_4O_3 = 226.2$.
CAS — 6506-37-2.
ATC — P01AB06.
Pharmacopoeias. In It.

Adverse Effects and Precautions
As for Metronidazole, p.594.

Pharmacokinetics
Nimorazole is readily absorbed from the gastrointestinal tract. Peak blood concentrations are achieved within 2 hours, and high concentrations are reported to occur in salivary and vaginal secretions. Trichomonicidal urinary concentrations are reported to persist for up to 48 hours after a dose. It is excreted in the urine together with 2 active metabolites. Unchanged drug and metabolites also appear in breast milk.

Uses and Administration
Nimorazole is a 5-nitroimidazole derivative. It has antimicrobial actions and uses similar to those of metronidazole (p.596).

In the treatment of trichomoniasis, the usual dose of nimorazole is 2 g by mouth as a single dose, with a main meal, repeated after about 1 month. Sexual partners should be treated concomitantly. In giardiasis or amoebiasis, nimorazole 1 g is given twice daily for 5 to 7 days; a dose for children is 15 to 30 mg per kg body-weight daily.

Preparations
Proprietary Preparations (details are given in Part 3)
Aust.: Naxogin; *Belg.:* Naxogin; *Braz.:* Naxogin; *Fr.:* Naxogyn; *Ger.:* Esclama; *Hong Kong:* Naxogin; *Mex.:* Naxogil; *S.Afr.:* Naxogin†; *Thai.:* Naxogin.

Multi-ingredient: *Braz.:* Floregin; Floregin Composto; Naxogin Composto.

Nitazoxanide (19580-d)
Nitazoxanide *(BAN, rINN)*.
N-(5-Nitro-2-thiazolyl)salicylamide acetate.
$C_{12}H_9N_3O_5S = 307.3$.
CAS — 55981-09-4.

Profile
Nitazoxanide is an antiprotozoal under investigation in the treatment of cryptosporidiosis in immunocompromised patients, including those with AIDS or HIV infection. It has also been used in helminth infections.

◊ References.
1. Doumbo O, *et al.* Nitazoxanide in the treatment of cryptosporidial diarrhea and other intestinal parasitic infections associated with acquired immunodeficiency syndrome in tropical Africa. *Am J Trop Med Hyg* 1997; **56**: 637–9.
2. Romero Cabello R, *et al.* Nitazoxanide for the treatment of intestinal protozoan and helminthic infections in Mexico. *Trans R Soc Trop Med Hyg* 1997; **91**: 701–3.
3. Rossignol J-F, *et al.* Successful treatment of human fascioliosis with nitazoxanide. *Trans R Soc Trop Med Hyg* 1998; **92**: 103–4.
4. Abaza H, *et al.* Nitazoxanide in the treatment of patients with intestinal protozoan and helminthic infections: a report on 546 patients in Egypt. *Curr Ther Res* 1998; **59**: 116–21.

5. Rossignol J-F, *et al.* A double-'blind' placebo-controlled study of nitazoxanide in the treatment of cryptosporidial diarrhoea in AIDS patients in Mexico. *Trans R Soc Trop Med Hyg* 1998; **92:** 663–6.
6. Megraud F, *et al.* Nitazoxanide, a potential drug for eradication of Helicobacter pylori with no cross-resistance to metronidazole. *Antimicrob Agents Chemother* 1998; **42:** 2836–40.
7. Bicart-See A, *et al.* Successful treatment with nitazoxanide of Enterocytozoon bieneusi microsporidiosis in a patient with AIDS. *Antimicrob Agents Chemother* 2000; **44:** 167–8.

Preparations

Proprietary Preparations (details are given in Part 3)
Mex.: Daxon.

Multi-ingredient: *Mex.:* Heliton.

Ornidazole   (4792-h)

Ornidazole *(USAN, rINN)*.
Ro-7-0207.   1-Chloro-3-(2-methyl-5-nitroimidazol-1-yl)propan-2-ol.
$C_7H_{10}ClN_3O_3 = 219.6$.
CAS — 16773-42-5.
ATC — G01AF06; J01XD03; P01AB03.

Adverse Effects and Precautions
As for Metronidazole, p.594.

Pharmacokinetics
Ornidazole is readily absorbed from the gastrointestinal tract and peak plasma concentrations of about 30 µg per mL have been achieved within 2 hours of a single dose of 1.5 g, falling to about 9 µg per mL after 24 hours and 2.5 µg per mL after 48 hours. After repeated oral doses of 500 mg every 12 hours, steady-state peak and trough concentrations are 14 and 6 µg per mL respectively. Ornidazole is also absorbed from the vagina and peak plasma concentrations of about 5 µg per mL have been reported 12 hours after the use of a 500-mg vaginal pessary.

The plasma elimination half-life of ornidazole is 12 to 14 hours. Less than 15% is bound to plasma proteins. It is widely distributed in body tissues and fluids, including the CSF.

Ornidazole is metabolised in the liver and is excreted in the urine, mainly as conjugates and metabolites, and to a lesser extent in the faeces. Biliary excretion may be important in the elimination of ornidazole and its metabolites.

◊ References.
1. Schwartz DE, Jeunet F. Comparative pharmacokinetic studies of ornidazole and metronidazole in man. *Chemotherapy* 1976; **22:** 19–29.
2. Matheson I, *et al.* Plasma levels after a single oral dose of 1.5 g ornidazole. *Br J Vener Dis* 1977; **53:** 236–9.
3. Schwartz DE, *et al.* Metabolic studies of ornidazole in the rat, in the dog and in man. *Xenobiotica* 1979; **9:** 571–81.
4. Turcant A, *et al.* Pharmacokinetics of ornidazole in neonates and infants after a single intravenous infusion. *Eur J Clin Pharmacol* 1987; **32:** 111–13.
5. Martin C, *et al.* Pharmacokinetics and tissue penetration of a single dose of ornidazole (1,000 milligrams intravenously) for antibiotic prophylaxis in colorectal surgery. *Antimicrob Agents Chemother* 1990; **34:** 1921–4.
6. Bourget P, *et al.* Disposition of ornidazole and its metabolites during pregnancy. *J Antimicrob Chemother* 1995; **35:** 691–6.

Hepatic impairment. The elimination of ornidazole following a single intravenous dose of 500 mg was impaired in 10 patients with severe liver cirrhosis when compared with 10 healthy subjects; mean half-lives were 21.9 hours and 14.1 hours respectively.[1] These results suggested that the interval between doses of ornidazole should be doubled in patients with marked hepatic impairment. The need for dose adjustment was confirmed in further studies of patients with other forms of liver disease.[2,3]

1. Taburet AM, *et al.* Pharmacokinetics of ornidazole in patients with severe liver cirrhosis. *Clin Pharmacol Ther* 1986; **40:** 359–64.
2. Bourget P, *et al.* Ornidazole pharmacokinetics in several hepatic diseases. *J Pharmacol Clin* 1988; **7:** 25–32.
3. Taburet AM, *et al.* Pharmacokinetics of ornidazole in patients with acute viral hepatitis, alcoholic cirrhosis, and extrahepatic cholestasis. *Clin Pharmacol Ther* 1989; **45:** 373–9.

Renal impairment. The half-life of ornidazole administered intravenously was not prolonged in a study in patients with advanced chronic renal failure, including those on continuous ambulatory peritoneal dialysis, although total plasma clearance was halved; modification of the usual dosage is not necessary in such patients. However, ornidazole was removed by haemodialysis and ornidazole should be given after the dialysis session rather than before.[1] In another study[2] the systemic availability and total body clearance of ornidazole were unaffected in

chronic renal failure; it was considered that an additional dose should be given before haemodialysis to compensate for removal during that procedure.

1. Merdjan H, *et al.* Pharmacokinetics of ornidazole in patients with renal insufficiency; influence of haemodialysis and peritoneal dialysis. *Br J Clin Pharmacol* 1985; **19:** 211–17.
2. Horber FF, *et al.* High haemodialysis clearance of ornidazole in the presence of a negligible renal clearance. *Eur J Clin Pharmacol* 1989; **36:** 389–93.

Uses and Administration
Ornidazole is a 5-nitroimidazole derivative. It has the antimicrobial actions of metronidazole and is used similarly (see p.596) in the treatment of susceptible protozoal infections and also in the treatment and prophylaxis of anaerobic bacterial infections.

It is administered by mouth in tablets after food, by vaginal pessary, or intravenously. When given intravenously, solutions of ornidazole should be diluted to 5 mg or less per mL and 100 or 200 mL infused over 15 to 30 minutes.

In amoebiasis, 0.5 g of ornidazole is given twice daily by mouth for 5 to 10 days; children are given 25 mg per kg body-weight daily as a single dose for 5 to 10 days. Patients with amoebic dysentery may be given 1.5 g as a single daily dose for 3 days; the children's dose is 40 mg per kg daily. In severe amoebic dysentery and amoebic liver abscess, ornidazole may be given by intravenous infusion in a dose of 0.5 to 1 g initially, followed by 0.5 g every 12 hours for 3 to 6 days; the children's dose is 20 to 30 mg per kg daily.

In giardiasis, 1 or 1.5 g of ornidazole is given by mouth as a single daily dose for 1 or 2 days; the children's dose is 30 or 40 mg per kg daily.

In trichomoniasis, a single dose of 1.5 g by mouth or 1 g by mouth together with 0.5 g vaginally is given; 5-day courses of ornidazole 0.5 g twice daily by mouth are also used. Sexual partners should be treated concomitantly. The children's dose is 25 mg per kg as a single dose by mouth.

For the treatment of anaerobic bacterial infections, ornidazole is given by intravenous infusion in an initial dose of 0.5 to 1 g, followed by 1 g daily as a single dose or in two divided doses for 5 to 10 days; oral therapy with 0.5 g every 12 hours should be substituted as soon as possible. Children may be given 10 mg per kg intravenously every 12 hours for 5 to 10 days.

For the prevention of postoperative anaerobic bacterial infections, 1 g is given by intravenous infusion about 30 minutes before surgery.

Administration in hepatic impairment. In view of the prolonged half-life and reduced clearance of ornidazole reported in patients with hepatic dysfunction (see above), the interval between doses should be doubled in patients with severe hepatic impairment.

Administration in renal impairment. The elimination of ornidazole is reported to be largely unaltered in patients with impaired renal function (see under Pharmacokinetics, above). Dosage adjustment is therefore usually unnecessary, although patients receiving haemodialysis should be given a supplemental dose equivalent to one-half of the usual dose before dialysis.

Preparations

Proprietary Preparations (details are given in Part 3)
Belg.: Tiberal; *Fr.:* Tiberal; *Israel:* Tiberal; *Ital.:* Tiberal; *Mex.:* Danubial; Tiberal; *NZ:* Tiberal; *Spain:* Tinerol; *Switz.:* Tiberal.

Paromomycin Sulfate   (123-h)

Paromomycin Sulfate *(rINNM)*.

Aminosidin Sulphate; Aminosidine Sulphate; Catenulin Sulphate; Crestomycin Sulphate; Estomycin Sulphate; Hydroxymycin Sulphate; Monomycin A Sulphate; Neomycin E Sulphate; Paromomycin Sulphate *(BANM)*; Paucimycin Sulphate. O-2,6-Diamino-2,6-dideoxy-β-L-idopyranosyl-(1→3)-O-β-D-ribofuranosyl-(1→5)-O-[2-amino-2-deoxy-α-D-glucopyranosyl-(1→4)]-2-deoxystreptamine sulphate.
$C_{23}H_{45}N_5O_{14},xH_2SO_4$.
CAS — 7542-37-2; 59-04-1 (both paromomycin); 1263-89-4 (paromomycin sulfate).

Pharmacopoeias. In Chin., Int., It., and US.

Pharmacopoeial description

USP 25: The sulfate salt of an antibiotic substance produced by the growth of *Streptomyces rimosus* var. *paromomycinus*, or a mixture of two or more such salts.

A creamy-white to light yellow, odourless or practically odourless, very hygroscopic powder. It loses not more than 5% of its weight on drying. Very soluble in water; insoluble in alcohol, in chloroform, and in ether. pH of a 3% solution in water is between 5.0 and 7.5. Store in airtight containers.

Adverse Effects, Treatment, and Precautions
As for Neomycin Sulfate, p.228.

Effects on the pancreas. Pancreatitis was associated with paromomycin administration during treatment of cryptosporidiosis in a patient with HIV infection.[1]

1. Tan WW, *et al.* Paromomycin-associated pancreatitis in HIV-related cryptosporidiosis. *Ann Pharmacother* 1995; **29:** 22–4.

Interactions
As for Neomycin Sulfate, p.228.

Antimicrobial Action
Paromomycin is active against various protozoa including *Leishmania* spp., *Entamoeba histolytica*, and *Cryptosporidium* spp. In addition, it has an antibacterial spectrum similar to that of neomycin (p.228). There is cross-resistance between paromomycin and kanamycin, framycetin, neomycin, and streptomycin.

Paromomycin also has anthelmintic properties against tapeworms.

Antimycobacterial activity. References.
1. Kanyok TP, *et al.* Activity of aminosidine (paromomycin) for Mycobacterium tuberculosis and Mycobacterium avium. *J Antimicrob Chemother* 1994; **33:** 323–7.
2. Piersimoni C, *et al.* Bacteriostatic and bactericidal activities of paromomycin against Mycobacterium avium complex isolates. *J Antimicrob Chemother* 1994; **34:** 421–4.
3. Kanyok TP, *et al.* In vivo activity of paromomycin against susceptible and multidrug-resistant Mycobacterium tuberculosis and M. avium complex strains. *Antimicrob Agents Chemother* 1994; **38:** 170–3.

Pharmacokinetics
Paromomycin is poorly absorbed from the gastrointestinal tract and most of the dose is eliminated unchanged in the faeces.

Parenteral administration. References.
1. Kanyok TP, *et al.* Pharmacokinetics of intramuscularly administered aminosidine in healthy subjects. *Antimicrob Agents Chemother* 1997; **41:** 982–6.

Uses and Administration
Paromomycin is an aminoglycoside antibiotic that has been administered by mouth as the sulfate in the treatment of intestinal protozoal infections, including amoebiasis, cryptosporidiosis, and giardiasis. It has also been tried parenterally for visceral, and topically for cutaneous, leishmaniasis. For details of these infections and their treatment, see under Choice of Antiprotozoal, p.582. It has also been used in the treatment of tapeworm infection, but it is not the treatment of choice. Similarly to neomycin (p.228), it has been used in the suppression of intestinal flora both preoperatively and in the management of hepatic encephalopathy.

In intestinal amoebiasis the dose for both adults and children is the equivalent of 25 to 35 mg of paromomycin per kg body-weight daily by mouth in 3 divided doses with meals for 5 to 10 days. Similar doses have been tried in cryptosporidiosis.

In taeniasis and other tapeworm infections, a dose of 4 g is given by mouth as a single dose or in divided doses over the course of one hour.

For hepatic encephalopathy, 4 g is given daily by mouth in divided doses at regular intervals for 5 to 6 days.

Preparations

USP 25: Paromomycin Sulfate Capsules; Paromomycin Sulfate Syrup.

Proprietary Preparations (details are given in Part 3)
Aust.: Humatin; *Belg.:* Gabbroral; *Canad.:* Humatin; *Ger.:* Humatin; *Hong Kong:* Gabbromicina; *Ital.:* Gabbroral; Humatin; *Spain:* Humatin; *Switz.:* Humatin; *USA:* Humatin.

The symbol † denotes a preparation no longer actively marketed

Pentamidine Isetionate (4794-b)

Pentamidine Isetionate (BANM, rINNM).

M&B-800; Pentamidine Diisetionate; Pentamidine Isethionate; Pentamidini Diisetionas; Pentamidini Isethionas. 4,4′-(Pentamethylenedioxy)dibenzamidine bis(2-hydroxyethanesulphonate).

$C_{19}H_{24}N_4O_2,2C_2H_6O_4S = 592.7$.

CAS — 100-33-4 (pentamidine); 140-64-7 (pentamidine isetionate).

ATC — P01CX01.

Pharmacopoeias. In Eur. (see p.vi) and Int.

Pentamidine isetionate 1.74 mg is approximately equivalent to 1 mg of pentamidine.

Pharmacopoeial description

Ph. Eur.: A white or almost white powder or colourless crystals; it is hygroscopic. Freely soluble in water; sparingly soluble in alcohol; practically insoluble in dichloromethane. A 5% solution in water has a pH of 4.5 to 6.5. Store in airtight containers.

Incompatibility. Immediate precipitation was observed when a solution of pentamidine isetionate 3 mg per mL in glucose 5% was mixed with each of 5 cephalosporin and 1 cephamycin injections.[1]

For reference to the incompatibility of pentamidine isetionate and foscarnet, see Foscarnet Sodium, p.621.

1. Lewis JD, El-Gendy A. Cephalosporin-pentamidine isethionate incompatibilities. Am J Health-Syst Pharm 1996; 53: 1461–2.

Pentamidine Mesilate (4793-m)

Pentamidine Mesilate (BANM, rINNM).

Pentamidine Dimethylsulphonate; Pentamidine Mesylate; Pentamidine Methanesulphonate; RP-2512. Pentamidine dimethanesulphonate.

$C_{19}H_{24}N_4O_2,2CH_3SO_3H = 532.6$.

CAS — 6823-79-6.

Pharmacopoeias. In Int.

Adverse Effects

Pentamidine is a toxic drug and adverse effects are frequent and sometimes severe following parenteral administration; fatalities have been reported. Impaired renal function is common, usually manifesting as mild and reversible raised blood urea nitrogen and serum creatinine concentrations, but acute renal failure can occur. Raised liver enzyme values and haematological disturbances such as leucopenia, anaemia, and occasionally thrombocytopenia, may occur. Hypoglycaemia, sometimes followed by hyperglycaemia and type 1 diabetes mellitus, is well documented; there have been occasional reports of acute pancreatitis.

The rapid intravenous injection of pentamidine has resulted in sudden hypotension and immediate reactions such as dizziness, headache, vomiting, breathlessness, tachycardia, and fainting. Hypotension may also occur when pentamidine is administered intramuscularly or by slow intravenous infusion. The intramuscular administration of pentamidine often causes pain, swelling, sterile abscess formation, and tissue necrosis at the site of injection. Similar damage can follow extravasation during intravenous administration.

Other adverse effects reported include hypocalcaemia, hyperkalaemia, skin rashes, the Stevens-Johnson syndrome, fever, flushing, gastrointestinal effects such as nausea, vomiting, and taste disturbances, confusion, hallucinations, and cardiac arrhythmias.

Pentamidine is not as toxic when administered by inhalation for the prophylaxis of *Pneumocystis carinii* pneumonia. The commonest adverse effects with this route are cough and bronchoconstriction and may be controlled by a bronchodilator. Inhalation may leave a bitter taste. Pneumothorax has been reported, but may be associated with *Pneumocystis carinii* infection. There have been rare reports of adverse effects such as those observed when pentamidine is given by injection.

◊ Adverse effects were observed in 46.8% of 404 patients given pentamidine parenterally for the treatment of *Pneumocystis carinii* pneumonia according to an analysis from the Center for Disease Control.[1] The reactions included impaired renal function (23.5% of patients), abnormal liver function (9.6%), hypoglycaemia (6.2%), haematological disturbances (4.2%), skin rashes (1.5%) and hypocalcaemia (1.2%). Local reactions at injection sites such as pain and abscess occurred in 18.3% and

immediate side-effects such as hypotension in 9.6%. **Nephrotoxicity** was often the most serious adverse reaction although it was impossible to attribute it solely to pentamidine. Severe renal impairment occurred in 15 patients and contributed materially to 12 of 14 ensuing deaths. However, elevation of blood urea nitrogen was usually relatively mild and reversible in those patients who had normal pretreatment renal function and had received no other nephrotoxic agents. Retrospective studies[2-4] suggest that adverse reactions, including nephrotoxicity, occur more commonly in patients with AIDS. In two such studies,[3,4] severe nephrotoxicity (increase in serum creatinine concentration of 0.5 mg per 100 mL) was reported in about 40% of patients. Analysis of risk factors suggested that the development of adverse reactions during parenteral administration is correlated with the total dose of pentamidine received and the duration of treatment,[3,4] but not with the initial degree of renal function.[3] There have been instances of renal failure occurring when pentamidine is inhaled as an aerosol for its local effect.[5,6]

An evaluation of pentamidine in the treatment of 82 patients with visceral leishmaniasis further illustrates its toxicity.[7] **Cardiotoxicity**, manifested by tachycardia, hypotension, and ECG changes of non-specific myocarditis, occurred in about 23% of patients. No hypoglycaemic reaction was noted, but 4 patients developed diabetes mellitus and 3 of them were found to be insulin-dependent. Other adverse reactions included gastrointestinal effects (anorexia, nausea, vomiting, abdominal pain, or diarrhoea) in about 78%; CNS effects (headache associated with flushing, delirium, or sensory disturbances resembling pins and needles) in about 24%; mild reversible albuminuria in about 7%; and allergic manifestations (generalised urticaria, itching, and conjunctival congestion) in about 5%. One patient had severe anaphylaxis.

As reported above[1,7] pentamidine can have a range of effects on **carbohydrate metabolism**. Four patients receiving pentamidine for *Pneumocystis carinii* pneumonia developed severe fasting hypoglycaemia followed later by hyperglycaemia and type 1 diabetes mellitus.[8] It has been suggested that pentamidine has a toxic effect on the β-cells of the pancreatic islets and can induce an early cytolytic release of insulin and hypoglycaemia, followed by β-cell destruction, insulin deficiency, and diabetes mellitus.[8,9] Once again AIDS patients appear to be highly susceptible, the incidence of hypoglycaemia due to pentamidine being higher in this group.[10] The action on the pancreas has led to fatal acute pancreatitis;[11-13] fatal hypoglycaemia has also been reported.[14] These reports[8-12,14] involved pentamidine administered by injection; there have also been reports of pancreatitis[15,16] and diabetes mellitus[17,18] occurring in patients given pentamidine by aerosol inhalation.

Hypotension is a problem with the **intravenous administration** of pentamidine, but can be reduced by infusing the dose over 60 minutes, when the incidence of hypotension appears to be similar to that with the intramuscular route.[19,20] Intravenous administration of pentamidine has also been associated with torsade de pointes.[21-23] It has been observed that renal toxicity is more common when pentamidine is given intramuscularly, rather than intravenously, to AIDS patients with diarrhoea, suggesting that fluid status might have an important role.[24]

Although there have been some reports of adverse reactions to inhaled pentamidine that are associated with the parenteral route, the main problem with the **inhalation route** is bronchoconstriction;[25] it can be prevented by giving a bronchodilator. Acute eosinophilic pneumonia has been reported with nebulised pentamidine administration in a patient.[26] Concern has been expressed at the risks to those who are with the patient at the time of inhalation and are exposed to nebulised pentamidine.[27-29]

1. Walzer PD, et al. Pneumocystis carinii pneumonia in the United States: epidemiologic, diagnostic and clinical features. Ann Intern Med 1974; 80: 83–93.
2. Lachaal M, Venuto RC. Nephrotoxicity and hyperkalemia in patients with acquired immunodeficiency syndrome treated with pentamidine. Am J Med 1989; 87: 260–3.
3. Briceland LL, Bailie GR. Pentamidine-associated nephrotoxicity and hyperkalemia in patients with AIDS. DICP Ann Pharmacother 1991; 25: 1171–4.
4. O'Brien JG, et al. A 5-year retrospective review of adverse drug reactions and their risk factors in human immunodeficiency virus-infected patients who were receiving intravenous pentamidine therapy for Pneumocystis carinii pneumonia. Clin Infect Dis 1997; 24: 854–9.
5. Miller RF, et al. Acute renal failure after nebulised pentamidine. Lancet 1989; i: 1271–2.
6. Chapelon C, et al. Renal insufficiency with nebulised pentamidine. Lancet 1989; ii: 1045–6.
7. Jha TK. Evaluation of diamidine compound (pentamidine isethionate) in the treatment of resistant cases of kala-azar occurring in North Bihar, India. Trans R Soc Trop Med Hyg 1983; 77: 167–70.
8. Bouchard P, et al. Diabetes mellitus following pentamidine-induced hypoglycemia in humans. Diabetes 1982; 31: 40–5.
9. Osei K, et al. Diabetogenic effect of pentamidine: in vitro and in vivo studies in a patient with malignant insulinoma. Am J Med 1984; 77: 41–6.
10. Stahl-Bayliss CM, et al. Pentamidine-induced hypoglycemia in patients with the acquired immune deficiency syndrome. Clin Pharmacol Ther 1986; 39: 271–5.
11. Salmeron S, et al. Pentamidine and pancreatitis. Ann Intern Med 1986; 105: 140–1.
12. Zuger A, et al. Pentamidine-associated fatal acute pancreatitis. JAMA 1986; 256: 2383–5.

13. Sauleda J, et al. Probable pentamidine-induced acute pancreatitis. Ann Pharmacother 1994; 28: 52–3.
14. Sattler FR, Waskin H. Pentamidine and fatal hypoglycemia. Ann Intern Med 1987; 107: 789–90.
15. Herer B, et al. Pancreatitis associated with pentamidine by aerosol. BMJ 1989; 298: 605.
16. Hart CC. Aerosolized pentamidine and pancreatitis. Ann Intern Med 1989; 111: 691.
17. Fisch A. Diabetes mellitus in a patient with AIDS after treatment with pentamidine aerosol. BMJ 1990; 301: 875.
18. Chen JP, et al. Diabetes after aerosolized pentamidine. Ann Intern Med 1991; 114: 913–14.
19. Navin TR, Fontaine RE. Intravenous versus intramuscular administration of pentamidine. N Engl J Med 1984; 311: 1701.
20. Helmick CG, Green JK. Pentamidine-associated hypotension and route of administration. Ann Intern Med 1985; 103: 480.
21. Harel Y, et al. Pentamidine-induced torsade de pointes. Pediatr Infect Dis J 1993; 12: 692–4.
22. Miller HC. Cardiac arrest after intravenous pentamidine in an infant. Pediatr Infect Dis J 1993; 12: 694–6.
23. Zanetti LAF, Oliphant CM. Pentamidine-induced torsade de pointes. Ann Pharmacother 1994; 28: 282–3.
24. Stehr-Green JK, Helmick CG. Pentamidine and renal toxicity. N Engl J Med 1985; 313: 694–5.
25. Smith DE, et al. Reversible bronchoconstriction with nebulised pentamidine. Lancet 1988; ii: 905.
26. Dupon M, et al. Acute eosinophilic pneumonia induced by inhaled pentamidine isethionate. BMJ 1993; 306: 109.
27. McDiarmid MA, Jacobson-Kram D. Aerosolised pentamidine and public health. Lancet 1989; ii: 863–4.
28. Thomas SHL, et al. Aerosolised pentamidine. Lancet 1989; ii: 1284.
29. Smaldone GC, et al. Detection of inhaled pentamidine in health care workers. N Engl J Med 1991; 325: 891–2.

Precautions

Pentamidine should be used under close supervision and great care is necessary if it is used in patients suffering from any condition likely to be exacerbated by its adverse effects. Patients should remain supine during administration and their blood pressure should be monitored. Kidney and liver function, blood-glucose concentrations, blood counts, and other parameters indicative of developing toxicity, such as serum-calcium concentrations and the ECG, should also be assessed regularly during courses of treatment with pentamidine.

Patients with a history of asthma or smoking may be at increased risk of cough and bronchospasm during inhalation of nebulised pentamidine. Symptoms may be controlled by administering a bronchodilator before giving pentamidine. Pentamidine solution should not be mixed with other drugs nor should a bronchodilator be administered in the same nebuliser. Extrapulmonary *P. carinii* infections may occur in patients receiving nebulised pentamidine and should be considered in patients with unexplained signs and symptoms. Precautions should be taken to minimise atmospheric pollution with pentamidine during nebulisation and to minimise exposure of medical personnel to pentamidine.

Interactions

The concomitant use of pentamidine with other nephrotoxic drugs such as amphotericin B or foscarnet should preferably be avoided. Extreme caution is also necessary if pentamidine is given with other drugs, such as foscarnet that can cause hypocalcaemia. There is an increased risk of ventricular arrhythmias if pentamidine is given with amiodarone or with levacetylmethadol.

Pharmacokinetics

Following intravenous administration of the isetionate, pentamidine is rapidly distributed to body tissues and this is followed by a prolonged elimination phase. Elimination half-lives of 6 hours following intravenous infusion and 9 hours following intramuscular injection have been cited, but probably represent an intermediate value, and terminal elimination half-lives of between several days and weeks have been reported. During repeated dosing accumulation is believed to occur, particularly in the liver and kidneys, and only small concentrations of pentamidine are found in the urine.

Distribution to the lung is relatively poor following administration by injection. Systemic absorption following inhalation is reported to result in peak plasma concentrations of between 5 and 10% of those observed after parenteral administration and there have been a few reports of systemic adverse effects. Particle or droplet size appears to be important in achieving adequate pulmonary distribution.

◊ References.
1. Waalkes TP, et al. Pentamidine: clinical pharmacologic correlations in man and mice. Clin Pharmacol Ther 1970; **11:** 505–12.
2. Bernard EM, et al. Use of a new bioassay to study pentamidine pharmacokinetics. J Infect Dis 1985; **152:** 750–4.
3. O'Doherty MJ, et al. Differences in relative efficiency of nebulisers for pentamidine administration. Lancet 1988; **ii:** 1283–6.
4. Simonds AK, et al. Aerosolised pentamidine. Lancet 1989; **i:** 221–2.
5. Baskin MI, et al. Regional deposition of aerosolized pentamidine: effects of body position and breathing pattern. Ann Intern Med 1990; **113:** 677–83.
6. Bronner U, et al. Pentamidine concentrations in plasma, whole blood and cerebrospinal fluid during treatment of Trypanosoma gambiense in Côte d'Ivoire. Trans R Soc Trop Med Hyg 1991; **85:** 608–11.
7. Lidman C, et al. Plasma pentamidine concentrations vary between individuals with Pneumocystis carinii pneumonia and the drug is actively secreted by the kidney. J Antimicrob Chemother 1994; **33:** 803–10.
8. Bronner U, et al. Pharmacokinetics and adverse reactions after a single dose of pentamidine in patients with Trypanosoma gambiense sleeping sickness. Br J Clin Pharmacol 1995; **39:** 289–95.
9. Conte JE, Golden JA. Intrapulmonary and systemic pharmacokinetics of aerosolized pentamidine used for prophylaxis of Pneumocystis carinii pneumonia in patients infected with the human immunodeficiency virus. J Clin Pharmacol 1995; **35:** 1166–73.

Renal impairment. In a study[1] of patients with normal renal function or on haemodialysis, renal clearance of pentamidine during the 24 hours after intravenous administration was 2.1% of the plasma clearance in those with normal renal function, suggesting that pentamidine elimination would be largely unaffected by renal impairment. In those with end-stage renal disease receiving haemodialysis the terminal elimination half-life following a single dose was prolonged to about 75 hours compared with 30 hours in the patients with normal renal function, but the volumes of distribution and area under the concentration-time curve were not significantly different. In patients with normal or mildly impaired renal function who had received between 12 and 21 doses the terminal elimination half-life after the final dose was about 12 days and pentamidine was still detectable in the plasma after 6 weeks. There was evidence of accumulation of pentamidine during repeated daily dosing.

1. Conte JE. Pharmacokinetics of intravenous pentamidine in patients with normal renal function or receiving hemodialysis. J Infect Dis 1991; **163:** 169–75.

Uses and Administration

Pentamidine, an aromatic diamidine derivative, is an antiprotozoal used in the treatment of the early stages of African trypanosomiasis, especially *Trypanosoma brucei gambiense* infections and in some forms of leishmaniasis. It is also used in the treatment and prophylaxis of pneumonia due to *Pneumocystis carinii*. It may act by several mechanisms including interference with protozoal DNA and folate transformation, and by inhibition of RNA and protein synthesis.

It has been given as the isetionate or mesilate salt, but pentamidine isetionate is the only form now available in most countries. There is considerable confusion in the literature regarding the dosage of pentamidine since it is often not clear whether doses are being expressed in terms of pentamidine base, the isetionate salt, or the mesilate salt. In general it would appear that when the isetionate is used doses are expressed in terms of pentamidine isetionate, individual doses usually being up to 4 mg per kg body-weight, whereas when the mesilate is used doses are expressed in terms of pentamidine base. Pentamidine isetionate 4 mg per kg is approximately equivalent to pentamidine base 2.3 mg per kg; pentamidine mesilate 3.6 mg per kg is approximately equivalent to pentamidine base 2.3 mg per kg.

Pentamidine isetionate is administered by deep intramuscular injection or by slow intravenous infusion over at least 60 minutes; direct intravenous injection must be avoided. Patients should be lying down during administration. The mesilate has usually been given intramuscularly.

In the treatment of early African trypanosomiasis due to *T. b. gambiense*, pentamidine isetionate 4 mg per kg may be given daily or on alternate days by intramuscular injection or intravenous infusion to a total of 7 to 10 doses. Pentamidine is not effective in trypanosomiasis with CNS involvement, but 2 injections of pentamidine may be given in late-stage *T. b. gambiense* infection before starting treatment with melarsoprol or eflornithine.

In the treatment of visceral leishmaniasis, and of mucocutaneous leishmaniasis due to *Leishmania braziliensis* or *L. aethiopica* that have not responded to antimonials, pentamidine isetionate 4 mg per kg may be given, preferably intramuscularly three times weekly, for 5 to 25 weeks or even longer. An alternative regimen in visceral leishmaniasis is to give 3 to 4 mg per kg on alternate days to a maximum of 10 injections; the course may need to be repeated. In cutaneous leishmaniasis due to *L. aethiopica* or *L. guyanensis*, pentamidine isetionate 3 to 4 mg per kg may be given, preferably intramuscularly once or twice weekly, until the condition resolves. A weekly dose of 3 to 4 mg per kg is also used for diffuse cutaneous leishmaniasis due to *L. aethiopica* and is given for at least 4 months.

In the treatment of *Pneumocystis carinii* pneumonia, pentamidine isetionate 4 mg per kg is given once daily for 14 days or longer by intramuscular injection or preferably slow intravenous infusion. Pentamidine isetionate is administered by inhalation through a nebuliser to prevent *P. carinii* pneumonia in HIV-positive patients in a dose of 300 mg once every 4 weeks; in those who cannot tolerate this dose 150 mg every 2 weeks may be used. It has also occasionally been used by this route for treating mild to moderate *P. carinii* infection in a dose of 600 mg daily for 3 weeks. Nebuliser design can affect the droplet size delivered and hence the amount of pentamidine reaching sites of action within the lungs. The optimal particle size is 1 to 2 microns. Precautions should be taken to minimise atmospheric pollution with pentamidine during nebulisation and to minimise exposure of medical personnel to pentamidine.

Administration in renal impairment. Since renal clearance accounts for only a small proportion of pentamidine elimination, dosage adjustment is not generally considered necessary for mild to moderate degrees of renal impairment. The UK manufacturer recommends dosage reductions in patients with *P. carinii* pneumonia who have a creatinine clearance of less than 10 mL per minute. In patients with life-threatening disease the recommended dose of 4 mg per kg daily should be given for 7 to 10 days and then on alternate days for the remainder of the 14-dose course. In less severe disease the suggested dose is 4 mg per kg on alternate days for 14 doses.

Amoebic infections. ACANTHAMOEBA INFECTIONS. Pentamidine was used to treat disseminated *Acanthamoeba* infection (p.582) without evidence of CNS involvement in 2 immunocompromised patients.[1,2] It is unlikely that pentamidine would be effective in infections involving the CNS.

1. Slater CA, et al. Brief report: successful treatment of disseminated Acanthamoeba infection in an immunocompromised patient. N Engl J Med 1994; **331:** 85–7.
2. Murakawa GJ, et al. Disseminated Acanthamoeba in patients with AIDS: a report of five cases and a review of the literature. Arch Dermatol 1995; **131:** 1291–6.

Babesiosis. Pentamidine has been tried for babesiosis (p.583), but while some patients were reported to have improved others had not and the value of pentamidine in this infection was considered to be doubtful.

References.
1. Teutsch SM, Juranek DD. Babesiosis. Ann Intern Med 1981; **95:** 241.
2. Francioli PB, et al. Response of babesiosis to pentamidine therapy. Ann Intern Med 1981; **94:** 326–30.
3. Raoult D, et al. Babesiosis, pentamidine, and cotrimoxazole. Ann Intern Med 1987; **107:** 944.
4. Clarke CS, et al. Babesiosis: under-reporting or case-clustering? Postgrad Med J 1989; **65:** 591–3.

Leishmaniasis. Pentamidine has been used in the treatment of visceral leishmaniasis (p.584) both alone and in combination with antimonials in patients who have failed to respond to antimonials alone.[1,2] It has also been tried for long-term secondary prophylaxis in patients with HIV infection.[3] Cutaneous leishmaniasis due to *L. guyanensis* is usually treated with pentamidine to reduce the risk of dissemination;[1] lesions due to *L. aethiopica* may also respond to pentamidine, but can be left to heal spontaneously since the risk of diffuse cutaneous involvement is small.[1] Diffuse cutaneous or mucocutaneous disease which is unresponsive to antimonials may respond to pentamidine, especially when due to *L. aethiopica*.[1]

1. WHO. WHO model prescribing information: drugs used in parasitic diseases. 2nd ed. Geneva: WHO, 1995.
2. Baily GG, Nandy A. Visceral leishmaniasis: more prevalent and more problematic. J Infect 1994; **29:** 241–7.
3. Pérez-Molina JA, et al. Pentamidine isethionate as secondary prophylaxis against visceral leishmaniasis in HIV-positive patients. AIDS 1996; **10:** 237–8.

Pneumocystis carinii pneumonia. In the treatment of *Pneumocystis carinii* pneumonia (p.375) intravenous pentamidine is generally reserved for patients who do not respond to, or cannot tolerate, co-trimoxazole.[1,2] Combination therapy with co-trimoxazole and pentamidine is no more effective than pentamidine alone in these patients and is potentially more toxic than either drug.[3] Inhaled pentamidine is occasionally suggested for mild to moderate infection but is now generally only used for prophylaxis. However, patients receiving inhaled pentamidine may be prone to extrapulmonary *Pneumocystis* infections.[4,5]

In both primary and secondary prophylaxis of *P. carinii* pneumonia in immunocompromised patients co-trimoxazole has been preferred to inhaled pentamidine. Comparative studies have shown that, in the short term, inhaled pentamidine has been less effective than co-trimoxazole[6,7] and no more effective than the other common prophylactic drug, dapsone.[8,9] In addition, both co-trimoxazole and dapsone (given with pyrimethamine) also provide protection against toxoplasmosis and, being given systemically, against extrapulmonary *P. carinii* infections. However, inhaled pentamidine is better tolerated than either of the alternatives, and studies have suggested that in the long term the efficacy of the three drugs is comparable,[10,11] at least in patients with CD4+ T lymphocyte counts of more than 100 per μL. Increasing the dose of pentamidine from 300 mg every four weeks to 300 mg every two weeks[12,13] or 600 mg every week[14] may improve efficacy further.

1. Anonymous. Prevention and treatment of Pneumocystis carinii pneumonia in patients infected with HIV. Drug Ther Bull 1994; **32:** 12–15.
2. Anonymous. Drugs for parasitic infections. Med Lett Drugs Ther 1998; **40:** 1–12.
3. PCP Therapy Project Group. Assessment of therapy for Pneumocystis carinii pneumonia. Am J Med 1984; **76:** 501–8.
4. Witt K, et al. Dissemination of Pneumocystis carinii in patients with AIDS. Scand J Infect Dis 1991; **23:** 691–5.
5. Sha BE, et al. Pneumocystis carinii choroiditis in patients with AIDS: clinical features, response to therapy, and outcome. J Acquir Immune Defic Syndr Hum Retrovirol 1992; **5:** 1051–8.
6. Schneider MME, et al. A controlled trial of aerosolized pentamidine or trimethoprim-sulfamethoxazole as primary prophylaxis against Pneumocystis carinii pneumonia in patients with human immunodeficiency virus infection. N Engl J Med 1992; **327:** 1836–41.
7. Hardy WD, et al. A controlled trial of trimethoprim-sulfamethoxazole or aerosolized pentamidine for secondary prophylaxis of Pneumocystis carinii pneumonia in patients with the acquired immunodeficiency syndrome. N Engl J Med 1992; **327:** 1842–8.
8. Girard P-M, et al. Dapsone-pyrimethamine compared with aerosolized pentamidine as primary prophylaxis against Pneumocystis carinii pneumonia and toxoplasmosis in HIV infection. N Engl J Med 1993; **328:** 1514–20.
9. Torres RA, et al. Randomized trial of dapsone and aerosolized pentamidine for the prophylaxis of Pneumocystis carinii pneumonia and toxoplasmic encephalitis. Am J Med 1993; **95:** 573–83.
10. Bozzette SA, et al. A randomized trial of three antipneumocystis agents in patients with advanced human immunodeficiency virus infection. N Engl J Med 1995; **332:** 693–9.
11. Rizzardi GP, et al. Risks and benefits of aerosolized pentamidine and cotrimoxazole in primary prophylaxis of Pneumocystis carinii pneumonia in HIV-1-infected patients: a two-year Italian multicentric randomized controlled trial. J Infect 1996; **32:** 123–31.
12. Kronawitter U, et al. Low incidence of Pneumocystis carinii pneumonia in HIV patients receiving 300 mg pentamidine aerosol every 2 weeks. Clin Invest 1992; **70:** 1089–91.
13. Rizzardi GP, et al. Better efficacy of twice-monthly than monthly aerosolised pentamidine for secondary prophylaxis of Pneumocystis carinii pneumonia in patients with AIDS: an Italian multicentric randomised controlled trial. J Infect 1995; **31:** 99–105.
14. Ong ELC, et al. Efficacy and effects on pulmonary function tests of weekly 600 mg aerosol pentamidine as prophylaxis against Pneumocystis carinii pneumonia. Infection 1992; **20:** 136–9.

African trypanosomiasis. Pentamidine is used for the haematolymphatic phase of African trypanosomiasis caused by *Trypanosoma brucei gambiense* (p.586), and as an adjunct to other treatment for the meningoencephalitic stage of the infection.[1] It is reported to be less effective against *T. b. rhodesiense* and in some areas resistance of *T. b. gambiense* to pentamidine is increasing.[2] Pentamidine has been used in combination with suramin for *T. b. gambiense* infections but this has not been shown to be clinically superior to pentamidine alone.[3]

1. WHO. Epidemiology and control of African trypanosomiasis. WHO Tech Rep Ser 739 1986.
2. WHO. WHO model prescribing information: drugs used in parasitic diseases. 2nd ed. Geneva: WHO, 1995.
3. Pépin J, Khonde N. Relapses following treatment of early-stage Trypanosoma brucei gambiense sleeping sickness with a combination of pentamidine and suramin. Trans R Soc Trop Med Hyg 1996; **90:** 183–6.

Preparations

BP 2001: Pentamidine Injection.

Proprietary Preparations (details are given in Part 3)
Aust.: Pentacarinat; *Austral.:* Pentacarinat†; *Belg.:* Pentacarinat; *Braz.:* Pentacarinat; *Canad.:* Pentacarinat; *Denm.:* Pentacarinat; *Fin.:* Pentacarinat; *Fr.:* Pentacarinat; *Ger.:* Pentacarinat; *Irl.:* Pentacarinat; *Israel:* Pentacarinat; *Ital.:* Pentacarinat; Pneumopent; *Mex.:* Pentam; *Neth.:* Pentacarinat; *Norw.:* Pentacarinat; *NZ:* Pentacarinat; *Port.:* Pentacarinat; Pentamina; *S.Afr.:* Pentacarinat; *Spain:* Pentacarinat; *Swed.:* Pentacarinat; *Switz.:* Pentacarinat; *Thai.:* Pentacarinat; *UK:* Pentacarinat; *USA:* NebuPent; Pentacarinat; Pentam.

The symbol † denotes a preparation no longer actively marketed

Propenidazole (3926-z)

Propenidazole (rINN).

Ethyl trans-α-acetyl-1-methyl-5-nitroimidazole-2-acrylate.

$C_{11}H_{13}N_3O_5 = 267.2$.

CAS — 76448-31-2.

ATC — G01AF14; P01AB05.

Profile

Propenidazole has been used for protozoal and fungal infections of the genito-urinary tract.

Robenidine Hydrochloride (13216-n)

Robenidine Hydrochloride (BANM, USAN, rINNM).

CL-78116; Robenzidene Hydrochloride. 1,3-Bis(4-chlorobenzylideneamino)guanidine hydrochloride.

$C_{15}H_{13}Cl_2N_5,HCl = 370.7$.

CAS — 25875-51-8 (robenidine); 25875-50-7 (robenidine hydrochloride).

Profile

Robenidine is an antiprotozoal used as the hydrochloride in veterinary practice for the prevention of coccidiosis in poultry and rabbits.

Ronidazole (13219-b)

Ronidazole (BAN, USAN, pINN).

(1-Methyl-5-nitroimidazol-2-yl)methyl carbamate.

$C_6H_8N_4O_4 = 200.2$.

CAS — 7681-76-7.

Pharmacopoeias. In BP(Vet).

Pharmacopoeial description

BP(Vet) 2001: A white to yellowish-brown, odourless or almost odourless powder. Slightly soluble in water, in alcohol, and in chloroform; very slightly soluble in ether. Protect from light.

Profile

Ronidazole is a 5-nitroimidazole antiprotozoal that is used in veterinary practice for the control of trichomoniasis in cage birds and pigeons. It has also been added to turkey feeding stuffs and has been used for the control of swine dysentery.

Salinomycin Sodium (12017-s)

Salinomycin Sodium (BANM, rINNM).

AHR-3096 (salinomycin); K-364 (salinomycin); K-748364A (salinomycin). Sodium (2R)-2-{(2R,5S,6R)-6-[(1S,2S,3S,5R)-5-{(2S,5S,7R,9S,10S,12R,15R)-2-[(2R,5R,6S)-5-ethyltetrahydro-5-hydroxy-6-methylpyran-2-yl]-15-hydroxy-2,10,12-trimethyl-1,6,8-trioxadispiro[4.1.5.3]pentadec-13-en-9-yl}-2-hydroxy-1,3-dimethyl-4-oxoheptyl]tetrahydro-5-methylpyran-2-yl}butyrate.

$C_{42}H_{69}NaO_{11} = 773.0$.

CAS — 53003-10-4 (salinomycin); 55721-31-8 (salinomycin sodium).

An antibiotic produced by Streptomyces albus.

Profile

Salinomycin is an antiprotozoal used as the sodium salt in veterinary practice for the prevention of coccidiosis in poultry and as a growth promotor in pigs.

Secnidazole (13227-b)

Secnidazole (BAN, rINN).

PM-185184; 14539-RP; RP-14539. 1-(2-Methyl-5-nitroimidazol-1-yl)propan-2-ol.

$C_7H_{11}N_3O_3 = 185.2$.

CAS — 3366-95-8.

ATC — P01AB07.

Profile

Secnidazole is a 5-nitroimidazole derivative with properties similar to those of metronidazole (p.594), apart from a much longer plasma half-life of about 20 hours. It is used in the treatment of amoebiasis, giardiasis, and trichomoniasis.

Secnidazole is given by mouth, usually as a single dose of 2 g in adults or 30 mg per kg body-weight in children. In invasive (hepatic) amoebiasis a dose of 1.5 g daily is given in single or divided doses for 5 days; children may be given 30 mg per kg body-weight daily.

◊ References.
1. Gillis JC, Wiseman LR. Secnidazole: a review of its antimicrobial activity, pharmacokinetic properties and therapeutic use in the management of protozoal infections and bacterial vaginosis. Drugs 1996; 51: 621–38.

Preparations

Proprietary Preparations (details are given in Part 3)
Braz.: Secni-Plus; Secnidal; **Fr.:** Flagentyl; **Mex.:** Minovag; Sabima; Secnidal; **Port.:** Flagentyl.
Multi-ingredient: Mex.: Sporasec.

Semduramicin (10424-p)

Semduramicin (BAN, USAN, rINN).

UK-61689; UK-61689-2 (semduramicin sodium). (2R,3S,4S,5R,6S)-Tetrahydro-2,4-dihydroxy-6-{(R)-1-[(2S,5R,7S,8R,9S)-9-hydroxy-2,8-dimethyl-2-{(2S,2′R,3′S,5′R)-octahydro-2-methyl-5′-[(2S,3S,5R,6S)-tetrahydro-6-hydroxy-3,5,6-trimethyl-2H-pyran-2-yl]-3′-[(2S, 5S, 6R)-tetrahydro-5-methoxy-6-methyl-2H-pyran-2-yloxy]-2,2′-bifuran-5-yl}-1,6-dioxaspiro[4.5]dec-7-yl]ethyl}-5-methoxy-3-methyl-2H-pyran-2-ylacetic acid.

$C_{45}H_{76}O_{16} = 873.1$.

CAS — 113378-31-7 (semduramicin); 119068-77-8 (semduramicin sodium).

NOTE. Semduramicin Sodium is also USAN.

Profile

Semduramicin is an antiprotozoal used in veterinary practice for the prevention of coccidiosis in poultry. It is also used as the sodium salt.

Suramin (4797-q)

Antrypol; Bayer-205; CI-1003; Fourneau-309; Naganinum; Naganol. The symmetrical 3″-urea of the sodium salt of 8-(3-benzamido-4-methylbenzamido)naphthalene-1,3,5-trisulphonic acid; Hexasodium 8,8′-{carbonylbis[imino-3,1-phenylenecarbonylimino(4-methyl-3,1-phenylene)carbonylimino]}bis(1,3,5-naphthalenetrisulfonate).

$C_{51}H_{34}N_6Na_6O_{23}S_6 = 1429.2$.

CAS — 145-63-1 (suramin); 129-46-4 (suramin sodium).

NOTE. The rINN is Suramin Sodium and the USAN is Suramin Hexasodium for this compound.

Pharmacopoeias. In Fr., Int., and It.

Adverse Effects

An immediate and potentially fatal reaction, with nausea, vomiting, shock, and loss of consciousness, may follow the injection of suramin in some patients and thus it is usual practice to give a small test dose before initiating treatment.

Abdominal pain, mouth ulceration, and skin reactions such as urticaria and pruritus may occur. The risk of hypersensitivity reactions is reported to be greater when onchocerciasis is present.

Later adverse effects include paraesthesia, hyperaesthesia of the palms and soles, skin eruptions, fever, polyuria, increased thirst, raised liver enzyme values, and effects on the eye including photophobia and lachrymation. Proteinuria is common; haematuria and casts in the urine may also occur. There have been occasional reports of adrenal insufficiency.

Effects on the blood. Thrombocytopenia has been reported in patients receiving suramin, generally during treatment for AIDS or cancer.[1-4] An immune-mediated mechanism has been proposed[3] although there is evidence that multiple mechanisms may be involved.[4] Other adverse effects on the blood include neutropenia,[1,5] anaemia,[1] deterioration of pre-existing lymphocytopenia,[1] and fatal myelosuppression.[5] Agranulocytosis and haemolytic anaemia have occurred rarely.
1. Levine AM, et al. Suramin antiviral therapy in the acquired immunodeficiency syndrome. Ann Intern Med 1986; 105: 32–7.
2. Arlt W, et al. Suramin in adrenocortical cancer: limited efficacy and serious toxicity. Clin Endocrinol (Oxf) 1994; 41: 299–307.
3. Seidman AD, et al. Immune-mediated thrombocytopenia secondary to suramin. Cancer 1993; 71: 851–4.
4. Tisdale JF, et al. Severe thrombocytopenia in patients treated with suramin: evidence for an immune mechanism in one. Am J Hematol 1996; 51: 152–7.
5. Rosen PJ, et al. Suramin in hormone-refractory metastatic prostate cancer: a drug with limited efficacy. J Clin Oncol 1996; 14: 1626–36.

Effects on the eyes. Late effects on the eyes associated with suramin include photophobia, lachrymation, and oedema. Keratopathy characterised by corneal deposits has been reported in patients receiving suramin. In a study of 114 patients receiving suramin for prostatic cancer, 13 developed corneal deposits similar to those reported with chloroquine therapy after 34 to 98 days of therapy.[1] Symptoms in 10 of the 13 included lachrymation and foreign body sensation. The remaining 3 patients were asymptomatic. Shifts in refractive error were also found. Keratopathy has also been reported in patients with AIDS receiving suramin.[2] In patients treated with suramin for ocular onchocerciasis the incidence of optic atrophy was higher

after 3 years than in untreated patients.[3] A prolonged inflammatory response to dying microfilariae in the optic nerve might be responsible, although a direct toxic or allergic effect could not be ruled out.
1. Hemady RK, et al. Ocular symptoms and signs associated with suramin sodium treatment for metastatic cancer of the prostate. Am J Ophthalmol 1996; 121: 291–6.
2. Teich SA, et al. Toxic keratopathy associated with suramin therapy. N Engl J Med 1986; 314: 1455–6.
3. Thylefors B, Rolland A. The risk of optic atrophy following suramin treatment of ocular onchocerciasis. Bull WHO 1979; 57: 479–80.

Effects on the kidneys. In addition to the proteinuria commonly seen during suramin therapy, there have been reports of individual cases of renal glycosuria[1] and of acute renal dysfunction.[2]
1. Awadzi K, et al. The chemotherapy of onchocerciasis XVIII: aspects of treatment with suramin. Trop Med Parasitol 1995; 46: 19–26.
2. Figg WD, et al. Acute renal toxicity associated with suramin in the treatment of prostate cancer. Cancer 1994; 74: 1612–14.

Effects on the nervous system. Neurological disorders reported in patients receiving suramin include paraesthesia and polyneuropathy. Severe polyneuropathy with generalised flaccid paralysis has generally been associated with serum-suramin concentrations greater than 350 µg per mL,[1,2] but motor neuropathy was reported in 8 patients with serum concentrations of 275 µg per mL.[3]
1. La Rocca RV, et al. Suramin-induced polyneuropathy. Neurology 1990; 40: 954–60.
2. Arlt W, et al. Suramin in adrenocortical cancer: limited efficacy and serious toxicity. Clin Endocrinol (Oxf) 1994; 41: 299–307.
3. Bitton RJ, et al. Pharmacologic variables associated with the development of neurologic toxicity in patients treated with suramin. J Clin Oncol 1995; 13: 2223–9.

Effects on the skin. Pruritus and urticaria may occur as hypersensitivity reactions to suramin. Late skin reactions include erythematous maculopapular rashes.[1] Severe reactions including erythema multiforme,[2] exfoliative dermatitis, and fatal toxic epidermal necrolysis[3,4] have been reported.
1. O'Donnell BP, et al. Suramin-induced skin reactions. Arch Dermatol 1992; 128: 75–9.
2. Katz SK, et al. Erythema multiforme induced by suramin. J Am Acad Dermatol 1995; 32: 292–3.
3. May E, Allolio B. Fatal toxic epidermal necrolysis during suramin therapy. Eur J Cancer 1991; 27: 1338.
4. Falkson G, Rapoport BL. Lethal toxic epidermal necrolysis during suramin treatment. Eur J Cancer 1992; 28A: 1294.

Precautions

Suramin should be administered under close medical supervision, and the general condition of patients improved as far as possible before treatment starts. Patients who experience a severe reaction after the first dose should never receive suramin again. It should not be used in elderly or infirm patients or in the presence of severe hepatic or renal disease. The urine should be tested before treatment starts and at weekly intervals during treatment; dosage should be reduced if moderate proteinuria develops and discontinued if it becomes severe or if casts appear in the urine.

Pregnancy. Suramin has been reported to be teratogenic in mice but not in rats.[1] WHO[2] recommends that when necessary suramin should be used in pregnant women with T. b. rhodesiense trypanosomiasis, even those with meningoencephalitic disease, because melarsoprol is contra-indicated; in onchocerciasis, suramin treatment should be delayed until after delivery.
1. Mercier-Parot L, Tuchmann-Duplessis H. Action abortive et tératogène d'un trypanocide, la suramine. C R Soc Biol 1973; 167: 1518–22.
2. WHO. WHO model prescribing information: drugs used in parasitic diseases. 2nd ed. Geneva: WHO, 1995.

Pharmacokinetics

Following intravenous injection, suramin becomes bound to plasma proteins and a low concentration in plasma is maintained for months. Unbound suramin is excreted in the urine. Penetration of suramin into the CSF appears to be poor.

◊ The clinical pharmacokinetics of suramin were studied in 4 patients with AIDS given 6.2 g intravenously over 5 weeks.[1] Suramin accumulated during treatment and plasma concentrations exceeded 100 µg per mL for several weeks. After the last dose the terminal half-life of suramin ranged from 44 to 54 days. At least 99.7% was bound to plasma proteins. Renal clearance accounted for most of the elimination of suramin from the body. There appeared to be little or no metabolism of suramin.
1. Collins JM, et al. Clinical pharmacokinetics of suramin in patients with HTLV-III/LAV infection. J Clin Pharmacol 1986; 26: 22–6.

Uses and Administration

Suramin is a trypanocide used in the treatment of African trypanosomiasis and as an anthelmintic in the treatment of onchocerciasis.

Suramin is administered by slow intravenous injection, usually as a 10% solution. Because of the danger of severe reactions it is advisable to give a test dose before initiating treatment.

In African trypanosomiasis suramin is used mainly for the early (haematolymphatic) stages of *Trypanosoma brucei rhodesiense* infection; pentamidine may be preferred for early-stage treatment of *T. b. gambiense* infection. Suramin is not used as sole therapy for late-stage infections with CNS involvement. Early-stage trypanosomiasis may be treated with a dose of 5 mg per kg body-weight of suramin on day 1, 10 mg per kg on day 3, then 20 mg per kg on days 5, 11, 17, 23, and 30. Other schedules consist of 5 doses of 1 g given over 3 weeks following a test dose of 100 to 200 mg. In late-stage *T. b. rhodesiense* infection 2 or 3 injections of suramin (5, 10, and 20 mg per kg respectively) are often given before starting treatment with melarsoprol. Combined therapy with suramin and tryparsamide has been used in late-stage *T. b. gambiense* infection; doses are suramin 10 mg per kg plus tryparsamide 30 mg per kg both given once every 5 days for 12 injections, repeated after another month if necessary.

Malignant neoplasms. Suramin is reported to have antineoplastic activity and has been studied in a number of malignant neoplasms, in particular hormone-resistant prostatic cancer (p.497). Hower, its clinical usefulness is hindered by dose-limiting toxicity and problems in developing a simple administration schedule.

References.

1. Stein CA, *et al.* Suramin: an anticancer drug with a unique mechanism of action. *J Clin Oncol* 1989; **7**: 499–508.
2. Kilbourn RG. Suramin: new therapeutic concepts for an old drug. *Cancer Bull* 1991; **43**: 265–7.
3. Rapoport BL, *et al.* Suramin in combination with mitomycin C in hormone-resistant prostate cancer: a phase II clinical study. *Ann Oncol* 1993; **4**: 567–73.
4. Woll PJ, *et al.* Suramin for breast and prostate cancer: a pilot study of intermittent short infusions without adaptive controls. *Ann Oncol* 1994; **5**: 597–600.
5. Arlt W, *et al.* Suramin in adrenocortical cancer: limited efficacy and serious toxicity. *Clin Endocrinol (Oxf)* 1994; **41**: 299–307.
6. Eisenberger MA, Reyno LM. Suramin. *Cancer Treat Rev* 1994; **20**: 259–73.
7. Rosen PJ, *et al.* Suramin in hormone-refractory metastatic prostate cancer: a drug with limited efficacy. *J Clin Oncol* 1996; **14**: 1626–36.

Onchocerciasis. Although suramin is the only drug in clinical use for onchocerciasis that is effective against adult worms, its use is restricted because of the frequency of associated complications and its intrinsic toxicity. Treatment of onchocerciasis (p.94) is currently based on continuous suppression of microfilariae by regular administration of ivermectin. WHO[1] advises that suramin should only be considered for the curative treatment of individuals in areas without transmission of onchocerciasis and of individuals leaving an endemic area, and for severe hyperreactive onchodermatitis where symptoms are not adequately controlled with ivermectin. WHO[2] also recommends that it should not be used to treat onchocerciasis in the elderly or infirm, in patients with severe liver or renal disease, in children aged less than 10 years, in totally blind patients (unless they require relief from intensely itchy lesions), in light to moderately infected people with no symptoms and whose eyes are not at risk, or in pregnant women (who should be treated after delivery).

A total dose of 66.7 mg per kg body-weight in six incremental weekly doses has been recommended.[1,2]

1. WHO. Onchocerciasis and its control: report of a WHO expert committee. *WHO Tech Rep Ser* 852 1995.
2. WHO. *WHO model prescribing information: drugs used in parasitic diseases.* 2nd ed. Geneva: WHO, 1995.

African trypanosomiasis. Suramin is used in the treatment of the early haematolymphatic phase of African trypanosomiasis (p.586) caused by *Trypanosoma brucei rhodesiense* and for *T. b. gambiense* infections which are resistant to pentamidine.[1] In some regions suramin is used in combination with pentamidine for *T. b. gambiense* infections but it has not been shown to be clinically superior to pentamidine alone.[2] Although suramin does not produce sufficient concentrations in the CNS to produce a cure in the meningoencephalitic phase,[3] it is used to reduce the number of trypanosomes in the blood and lymph before treatment with melarsoprol.[1] A combination of suramin with tryparsamide has been suggested as an alternative to melarsoprol or eflornithine in *T. b. gambiense* infections involving the CNS.[4] Case reports have suggested that suramin in combination with metronidazole[5] or eflornithine[6] could be useful in *T. b. rhodesiense* infections although response to suramin plus eflornithine was disappointing in a study involving 6 patients.[7]

1. WHO. *WHO model prescribing information: drugs used in parasitic diseases.* 2nd ed. Geneva: WHO, 1995.

The symbol † denotes a preparation no longer actively marketed

2. Pépin J, Khonde N. Relapses following treatment of early-stage Trypanosoma brucei gambiense sleeping sickness with a combination of pentamidine and suramin. *Trans R Soc Trop Med Hyg* 1996; **90**: 183–6.
3. Jennings FW. Suramin treatment of experimental Trypanosoma brucei infection of the central nervous system. *Trans R Soc Trop Med Hyg* 1995; **89**: 677.
4. Anonymous. Drugs for parasitic infections. *Med Lett Drugs Ther* 1998; **40**: 1–12.
5. Foulkes JR. Metronidazole and suramin combination in the treatment of arsenical refractory rhodesian sleeping sickness—a case study. *Trans R Soc Trop Med Hyg* 1996; **90**: 422.
6. Taelman H, *et al.* Combination treatment with suramin and eflornithine in late stage rhodesian trypanosomiasis: case report. *Trans R Soc Trop Med Hyg* 1996; **90**: 572–3.
7. Clerinx J, *et al.* Treatment of late stage rhodesiense trypanosomiasis using suramin and eflornithine: report of six cases. *Trans R Soc Trop Med Hyg* 1998; **92**: 449–50.

Preparations

Proprietary Preparations (details are given in Part 3)
Ger.: Germanin.

Teclozan   (4798-p)

Teclozan (USAN, rINN).
NSC-107433;   Win-13146.   NN'-p-Phenylenedimethyleneb-is[2,2-dichloro-N-(2-ethoxyethyl)acetamide].
$C_{20}H_{28}Cl_4N_2O_4 = 502.3$.
CAS — 5560-78-1.
ATC — P01AC04.

Profile
Teclozan, a dichloroacetamide derivative, is a luminal amoebicide with actions and uses similar to those of diloxanide furoate (p.590). It has been given by mouth in the treatment of intestinal amoebiasis.

Preparations

Proprietary Preparations (details are given in Part 3)
Braz.: Falmonox.

Tenonitrozole   (13318-q)

Tenonitrozole (rINN).
TC-109; Thenitrazole. N-(5-Nitrothiazol-2-yl)thiophene-2-carboxamide.
$C_8H_5N_3O_3S_2 = 255.3$.
CAS — 3810-35-3.
ATC — P01AX08.

Profile
Tenonitrozole is an antiprotozoal given in the treatment of trichomoniasis (p.586). It is also active against *Candida albicans*. It is given by mouth in a dose of 250 mg twice daily with meals, for 4 days.

Preparations

Proprietary Preparations (details are given in Part 3)
Fr.: Atrican.

Ternidazole   (13573-f)

Ternidazole (rINN).
2-Methyl-5-nitroimidazole-1-propanol.
$C_7H_{11}N_3O_3 = 185.2$.
CAS — 1077-93-6.

Profile
Ternidazole is a 5-nitroimidazole antiprotozoal with properties similar to those of metronidazole (p.594). It has been an ingredient of preparations used for the treatment of vaginitis.

Preparations

Proprietary Preparations (details are given in Part 3)
Multi-ingredient: *Fr.:* Tergynan†.

Tilbroquinol   (17008-h)

Tilbroquinol (pINN).
7-Bromo-5-methylquinolin-8-ol.
$C_{10}H_8BrNO = 238.1$.
CAS — 7175-09-9.
ATC — P01AA05.

Profile
Tilbroquinol is a halogenated hydroxyquinoline antiprotozoal with properties similar to those of diiodohydroxyquinoline (p.590). It has been used together with tiliquinol (below) in the treatment of intestinal infections including amoebiasis but less toxic drugs are preferred.

◊ A report of neurotoxicity, considered to be subacute myelo-opticoneuropathy, in a patient who had taken tilbroquinol together with tiliquinol for 4 years.[1] Hepatotoxicity has also been reported[2] with this combination.

1. Soffer M, *et al.* Oxyquinoline toxicity. *Lancet* 1983; **i**: 709.
2. Caroli-Bosc F-X, *et al.* Hépatite aiguë due à l'association de tiliquinol et tilbroquinol (Intétrix). *Gastroenterol Clin Biol* 1996; **20**: 605–6.

Preparations

Proprietary Preparations (details are given in Part 3)
Fr.: Intetrix P†.
Multi-ingredient: *Belg.:* Intetrix†; *Fr.:* Intetrix.

Tiliquinol   (17009-m)

Tiliquinol (rINN).
5-Methylquinolin-8-ol.
$C_{10}H_9NO = 159.2$.
CAS — 5541-67-3.

Profile
Tiliquinol has been used in conjunction with tilbroquinol (above) in the treatment of intestinal infections including amoebiasis but less toxic drugs are preferred.

Preparations

Proprietary Preparations (details are given in Part 3)
Multi-ingredient: *Belg.:* Intetrix†; *Fr.:* Intetrix.

Tinidazole   (4799-s)

Tinidazole (BAN, USAN, rINN).
CP-12574; Tinidazolum. 1-[2-(Ethylsulphonyl)ethyl]-2-methyl-5-nitroimidazole.
$C_8H_{13}N_3O_4S = 247.3$.
CAS — 19387-91-8.
ATC — J01XD02; P01AB02.
Pharmacopoeias. In Eur. (see p.vi), *Jpn, Pol.,* and *US.*

Pharmacopoeial description
Ph. Eur.: An almost white or pale yellow, crystalline powder. Practically insoluble in water; soluble in acetone and in dichloromethane; sparingly soluble in methyl alcohol. Protect from light.
USP 25: An almost white or pale yellow crystalline powder. Practically insoluble in water; soluble in acetone and in dichloromethane; sparingly soluble in methyl alcohol. Protect from light.

Adverse Effects and Precautions
As for Metronidazole, p.594.

Porphyria. Tinidazole is considered to be unsafe in patients with porphyria because it has been shown to be porphyrinogenic in *in-vitro* systems.

Pregnancy and breast feeding. Tinidazole readily crosses the placenta and is distributed into breast milk. The manufacturer recommends that tinidazole should not be given during the first trimester of pregnancy, since its effects on fetal development are unknown, and also that it should not be given to mothers who are breast feeding.

Shock. An acute severe toxic reaction, considered not to be allergic, occurred in a healthy subject shortly after the intravenous infusion of tinidazole 1.6 g over 80 minutes.[1] He fainted for about 10 seconds and low blood pressure, nausea, and tiredness persisted for several hours. Spasms in the left arm were also experienced but no generalised convulsions.

1. Aase S, *et al.* Severe toxic reaction to tinidazole. *Eur J Clin Pharmacol* 1983; **24**: 425–7.

Interactions
Tinidazole may, like metronidazole (p.595), produce a disulfiram-like reaction with alcohol.

Pharmacokinetics
The pharmacokinetics of tinidazole resemble those of metronidazole although the half-life is longer.

Tinidazole is almost completely absorbed following administration by mouth and, typically, a peak plasma concentration of about 40 µg per mL is achieved 2 hours after a single 2-g dose, falling to about 10 µg per mL at 24 hours and 2.5 µg per mL at 48 hours; concentrations above 8 µg per mL are maintained by daily maintenance doses of 1 g. Comparable concentrations are achieved with equivalent intravenous doses. The plasma elimination half-life of tinidazole is 12 to 14 hours.

Tinidazole is widely distributed and concentrations similar to those in plasma have been achieved in bile, breast milk, CSF, saliva, and a variety of body tissues; it crosses the placenta readily. Only 12% is reported to be bound to plasma proteins. An active hydroxy metabolite has been identified.

Unchanged drug and metabolites are excreted in the urine and, to a lesser extent, in the faeces.

◊ References.

1. Wood BA, *et al.* The pharmacokinetics, metabolism and tissue distribution of tinidazole. *J Antimicrob Chemother* 1982; **10** (suppl A): 43–57.
2. Karhunen M. Placental transfer of metronidazole and tinidazole in early human pregnancy after a single infusion. *Br J Clin Pharmacol* 1984; **18:** 254–7.
3. Evaldson GR, *et al.* Tinidazole milk excretion and pharmacokinetics in lactating women. *Br J Clin Pharmacol* 1985; **19:** 503–7.
4. Wood SG, *et al.* Pharmacokinetics and metabolism of ^{14}C-tinidazole in humans. *J Antimicrob Chemother* 1986; **17:** 801–9.

Renal impairment. Single-dose studies indicate that the pharmacokinetics of tinidazole in patients with chronic renal failure are not significantly different from those in healthy subjects and that no modification of tinidazole dosage is necessary. However, tinidazole is rapidly removed by haemodialysis.[1,2]

1. Flouvat BL, *et al.* Pharmacokinetics of tinidazole in chronic renal failure and in patients on haemodialysis. *Br J Clin Pharmacol* 1983; **15:** 735–41.
2. Robson RA, *et al.* Tinidazole pharmacokinetics in severe renal failure. *Clin Pharmacokinet* 1984; **9:** 88–94.

Uses and Administration

Tinidazole is a 5-nitroimidazole derivative. It has the antimicrobial actions of metronidazole and is used similarly (see p.596) in the treatment of susceptible protozoal infections and in the treatment and prophylaxis of anaerobic bacterial infections. It has also been used in regimens for the eradication of *Helicobacter pylori* in peptic ulcer disease.

Tinidazole is usually administered as a single daily dose by mouth with or after food; it is also given by intravenous infusion and as vaginal pessaries.

In invasive amoebiasis, tinidazole is administered, usually in conjunction with a luminal amoebicide, in a dose of 2 g as a single daily dose by mouth for 2 or 3 days; in hepatic amoebiasis, 1.5 to 2 g as a single daily dose may be given for 3 days or occasionally up to 6 days. Children are given 50 to 60 mg per kg body-weight daily for 3 or 5 days respectively.

A single dose of tinidazole 2 g is given by mouth in the treatment of giardiasis, trichomoniasis, and acute necrotising ulcerative gingivitis; 50 to 75 mg per kg as a single dose is given to children with giardiasis or trichomoniasis. It may sometimes be necessary to repeat this dose once. In trichomoniasis sexual partners should be treated concomitantly. In bacterial vaginosis, a single 2-g dose is usually given, although higher cure rates have been achieved with a 2-g dose on 2 successive days.

For the treatment of most anaerobic bacterial infections, tinidazole is given by mouth, usually for 5 or 6 days, in an initial dose of 2 g followed on subsequent days by 1 g daily or 500 mg twice daily. If oral therapy is not possible tinidazole may be administered intravenously, 800 mg being infused as 400 mL of a 2 mg per mL solution at a rate of 10 mL per minute; this initial dose is followed by 800 mg daily or 400 mg twice daily until oral therapy can be substituted. For the prevention of postoperative anaerobic bacterial infections, 2 g is given by mouth about 12 hours before surgery. Alternatively 1.6 g is given as a single intravenous infusion before surgery.

In regimens for the treatment of peptic ulcer disease, tinidazole 500 mg twice daily has been given with clarithromycin and omeprazole for 7 days.

Administration in renal impairment. The elimination of tinidazole is largely unchanged in patients with impaired renal function (see under Pharmacokinetics, above) and dosage adjustment is therefore not generally considered necessary. However tinidazole is removed by haemodialysis, and patients may need additional doses to compensate.

Preparations

Proprietary Preparations (details are given in Part 3)
Aust.: Fasigyn†; *Austral.:* Fasigyn; Simplotan; *Belg.:* Fasigyn; *Braz.:* Amplium; Fa-Cyl; Fasigyn; Ginosutin; Pletil; Trinizol; *Fr.:* Fasigyne†; *Ger.:* Simplotan; Sorquetan†; *Hong Kong:* Fasigyn; *Israel:* Fasigyn; Protocide; *Ital.:* Fasigin; Trimonase; *Mex.:* Amebysol; Ametricid; Estovyn-T; Fasigyn; Triseptil; *Neth.:* Fasigyn; *NZ:* Dyzole; *Port.:* Fasigyn; *S.Afr.:* Fasigyn; *Singapore:* Fasigyn; *Spain:* Tricolam; *Swed.:* Fasigyn; *Switz.:* Fasigyne; *Thai.:* Asiazole-TN; Fasigyn; Funida; Idazole; Sporinex; Tinazole; Tini; Tonid; Trichonas; Tricogyn; Tricozone; *UK:* Fasigyn.
Multi-ingredient: *Braz.:* Amplium-G; Cartrax; Colpolase; Fa-Cyl M; Gino Pletil; Ginometrim; Ginosutin M; Poliginax; Trinizol M; *Ital.:* Fasigin N; *Mex.:* Fasigyn VT; Mebeciclol.

Toltrazuril (18693-n)

Toltrazuril *(BAN, USAN, rINN)*.
Bay-Vi-9142. 1-Methyl-3-(4-{*p*-[(trifluoromethyl)thio]phenoxy}-*m*-tolyl)-s-triazine-2,4,6(1*H*,3*H*,5*H*)-trione.
$C_{18}H_{14}F_3N_3O_4S = 425.4$.
CAS — 69004-03-1.

Profile

Toltrazuril is an antiprotozoal used in veterinary practice for the treatment of coccidiosis in poultry and piglets.

Tryparsamide (6000-c)

Tryparsamide *(rINN)*.
Glyphenarsine; Tryparsam.; Tryparsone. Sodium hydrogen 4-(carbamoylmethylamino)phenylarsonate hemihydrate.
$C_8H_{10}AsN_2NaO_4,\frac{1}{2}H_2O = 305.1$.
CAS — 554-72-3 (anhydrous tryparsamide); 6159-29-1 (tryparsamide hemihydrate).

Profile

Tryparsamide, a pentavalent arsenical compound, is a trypanocide which penetrates into the CSF and has been used in combination with suramin in the treatment of late-stage African trypanosomiasis due to *Trypanosoma brucei gambiense*, as an alternative to melarsoprol or eflornithine (see p.586). However, because of its toxicity, especially the risk of blindness resulting from damage to the optic nerve, melarsoprol or eflornithine are preferred.

For the adverse effects of arsenic and their treatment, see Arsenic Trioxide, p.1582. Like melarsoprol, tryparsamide can cause encephalopathy.

Tryparsamide is administered in a dose of 30 mg per kg body-weight (to a maximum of 2 g), together with suramin 10 mg per kg, both given intravenously once every 5 days for 12 injections. Treatment may be repeated after one month.

Antivirals

The drugs described in this chapter are used in the treatment of viral infections; they may also be used to provide protection, usually for a brief period only, against infection. Treatment has to be started early in the infection for the drug to be effective and inhibit the replicating virus. There is little evidence that these compounds affect latent or nonreplicating viruses. They do not provide an alternative to available immunisation for the long-term prophylaxis of infection—for details of such treatment see the chapter on Vaccines, p.1529.

Choice of Antiviral
Antiviral drugs are effective for the treatment and prophylaxis of a range of viral infections as described below. Non-specific symptomatic and supportive treatments are also important in the management of viral infections. Those viral infections not amenable to antiviral drug therapy include mumps, poliomyelitis, rabies, and rubella.

Common cold
A cold is usually a mild, self-limiting respiratory infection with a range of viruses, the rhinoviruses and coronaviruses being most frequently involved. Symptoms include nasal discharge and obstruction, sneezing, sore throat, and cough; there is little or no fever. Occasionally there may be concurrent or subsequent bacterial infection of the upper respiratory tract.

The variety of causative agents makes vaccination an unlikely prospect. Not only are there different groups of viruses, but within the rhinoviruses, for example, there are many different serotypes.

Treatment of the common cold is symptomatic with analgesics, cough suppressants, and decongestants, and symptoms usually last for about a week whether or not treatment is taken. Antibacterial[1] and antiviral[2] therapy has consistently failed to show any benefit and antibacterials are indicated only if there is secondary bacterial infection. Treatment with very large doses of ascorbic acid has been widely used. Such treatment has been claimed to be beneficial in preventing and treating colds but a systematic review[3] has concluded that, although there has been evidence of benefit in published studies, it has generally been modest, and that long-term supplementation with vitamin C does not appear to prevent colds; there may be a slight reduction in duration of cold symptoms when it is used therapeutically. Other drugs[4] tried have included mast-cell stabilisers, interferon alfa-2b, and zinc lozenges. Intranasal interferons, tried for prophylaxis or treatment, have not fulfilled their early promise. Results of trials of zinc treatment have been inconclusive.[5] A soluble recombinant intercellular adhesion molecule 1 (ICAM-1), tremacamra, is also under investigation.

1. Arroll B, Kenealy T. Antibiotics for the common cold (updated 18 July 2001). Available in The Cochrane Library; Issue 4. Oxford: Update Software; 2001.

2. Jefferson TO, Tyrrell D. Antivirals for the common cold (updated 18 July 2001). Available in The Cochrane Library; Issue 4. Oxford: Update Software; 2001.
3. Douglas RM, et al. Vitamin C for preventing and treating the common cold (updated 18 July 2001). Available in The Cochrane Library; Issue 4. Oxford: Update Software; 2001.
4. Mossad SB. Treatment of the common cold. BMJ 1998; 317: 33–6.
5. Marshall I. Zinc for the common cold (updated 29 August 2001). Available in The Cochrane Library; Issue 4. Oxford: Update Software; 2001.

Encephalitis
Viral infections that may produce encephalitis include Epstein-Barr virus infections, herpes simplex infections, HIV infection, influenza, Lassa fever, measles, mumps, rubella, and varicella-zoster infections; the specific treatment of these infections, if any, is described under the appropriate heading. However, there is also a group of viruses known as encephalitis viruses that cause infections in which encephalitis is a major clinical feature.

They include:

- alphaviruses (previously arbovirus Group A) including Eastern, Western, and Venezuelan equine viruses transmitted by mosquitoes
- bunyaviruses including California encephalitis virus and La Crosse virus both transmitted by mosquitoes
- flaviviruses (previously arbovirus Group B) including Japanese encephalitis virus, St Louis encephalitis virus, Murray Valley encephalitis virus, Rocio virus, and West Nile virus all transmitted by mosquitoes and the tick-borne viruses of this group, louping ill virus, Powassan virus, and the Eastern and Western subtype viruses.

Encephalitis virus infections usually present with fever, headache, nausea, vomiting, and neck rigidity. Some infections progress to produce convulsions, confusion, coma, and sometimes death. Patients who recover may be left with some permanent neurological damage. There is generally no specific treatment for encephalitis virus infections and patients must be managed with vigorous supportive care. Control of mosquito and tick populations in endemic areas and minimising contact with these vectors are important means of preventing infections. Japanese encephalitis vaccine and tick-borne encephalitis vaccine are available for active immunisation of individuals at risk of infection and tick-borne encephalitis immunoglobulins are available in some countries for passive immunisation against infection.

Gastro-enteritis
Viral infections are an important cause of diarrhoea, especially in children and immunocompromised patients. Those causing diarrhoea and other gastrointestinal symptoms include adenovirus, astrovirus, calicivirus, rotavirus, Norwalk virus, and related small round structured virus infections. Cytomegalovirus is an important cause of diarrhoea in AIDS (see HIV-associated Wasting and Diarrhoea, below). Rotavirus infection is recognised as the commonest cause of endemic acute diarrhoea in childhood, and is associated with severe vomiting and fever. In acute diarrhoea of any aetiology the priority is to maintain hydration by prevention or treatment of fluid and electrolyte depletion, especially in infants and the elderly (see p.1203). Antivirals are not used in the management of viral diarrhoeas.[1-3] Several rotavirus vaccines are under development. Hyperimmune bovine colostrum in one study[4] reduced stool output and resulted in early recovery from illness and early clearance of viruses from stool.

1. Elliott EJ. Viral diarrhoeas in childhood. BMJ 1992; 305: 1111–12.
2. Kapikian AZ. Viral gastroenteritis. JAMA 1993; 269: 627–30.
3. Desselberger U. Rotavirus infections: guidelines for treatment and prevention. Drugs 1999; 58: 447–52.
4. Sarker SA, et al. Successful treatment of rotavirus diarrhea in children with immunoglobulin from immunized bovine colostrum. Pediatr Infect Dis J 1998; 17: 1149–54.

Haemorrhagic fevers
Viruses causing haemorrhagic fever form a diverse group from several viral families. They are usually transmitted via mosquitoes, ticks, or rodents.

The more important viruses responsible for haemorrhagic fevers in man include:

- alphaviruses (previously arbovirus Group A) causing Chikungunya, transmitted by mosquitoes
- arenaviruses causing Argentinian haemorrhagic fever, Bolivian haemorrhagic fever, and Lassa fever and transmitted by rodents

- Bunyaviridae causing Crimean Congo haemorrhagic fever, haemorrhagic fever with renal syndrome, and Rift Valley fever and transmitted by ticks, rodents and insectivores, and mosquitoes, respectively
- the filoviruses Ebola virus and Marburg virus
- flaviviruses (previously arbovirus Group B) causing dengue fever and yellow fever transmitted by mosquitoes, and Kyasanur forest fever and Omsk haemorrhagic fever transmitted by ticks.

As suggested by the name, fever and haemorrhage of varying severity are characteristics of these infections. Chills, headache, malaise, myalgia, and nausea usually occur and sometimes flushing and rashes. Severe vomiting, diarrhoea, and shock may occur in advanced infections. There is often some degree of renal or hepatic impairment and occasionally CNS involvement.

While ribavirin has been reported to reduce mortality in patients with Lassa fever, haemorrhagic fever with renal syndrome, and possibly Crimean Congo haemorrhagic fever, there is generally no specific antiviral treatment for haemorrhagic fever and patients must be managed symptomatically. Control of vector populations and prevention of vector contact have an important role to play (see p.1428). Guidelines for the prevention, control, and treatment of dengue and yellow fevers have been produced by WHO[1,2] and related organisations.[3] National guidelines exist in some countries.[4]

Rift Valley fever vaccine and yellow fever vaccine are available for active immunisation of individuals at risk of infection; dengue fever vaccines and haemorrhagic fever with renal syndrome vaccines are under development. Crimean Congo haemorrhagic fever immunoglobulins are available in some countries for passive immunisation against the disease.

1. WHO. Prevention and control of yellow fever in Africa. Geneva: WHO, 1986.
2. WHO. Prevention and control of dengue and dengue haemorrhagic fever: comprehensive guidelines. New Delhi: WHO, 1999.
3. Pan American Health Organization. Dengue and dengue hemorrhagic fever in the Americas: Guidelines for prevention and control. Washington, DC: PAHO, 1994.
4. Advisory Committee on Dangerous Pathogens. Management and control of viral haemorrhagic fevers. London: HMSO, 1996.

Hantavirus pulmonary syndrome
A number of hantaviruses related to the virus causing haemorrhagic fever with renal syndrome (see above) have been identified as the probable cause of an acute, severe respiratory illness which has been named hantavirus pulmonary syndrome. Its main symptoms are fever, myalgia, headache, and cough rapidly progressing to respiratory failure; the mortality rate may be about 50% and death is usually due to non-cardiogenic pulmonary oedema and acute respiratory distress syndrome. The virus is transmitted by rodents and the syndrome has mainly been described in the USA.

Treatment is primarily symptomatic including respiratory and circulatory support with the early use of cardiac inotropes being particularly important. Intravenous ribavirin has been tried but preliminary data have not indicated improved mortality. Guidelines for the management of hantavirus pulmonary syndrome have been produced in the USA.[1]

1. Pan American Health Organization. Hantavirus in the Americas: guidelines for diagnosis, treatment, prevention and control. Washington, DC: PAHO, 1999.

Hepatitis
Viral hepatitis refers to infection of the liver caused by a group of hepatitis viruses. Those so far identified are designated A, B, C, D, E, and G. Other viruses such as Epstein-Barr virus and yellow fever virus may be secondary causes of hepatitis and hepatitis may also be caused by nonviral infections, many drugs and chemicals, and alcoholism.

Hepatitis viruses are endemic throughout the world. Hepatitis A and E are spread via the faecal-oral route. Hepatitis B, C, and D, and probably also G are transmitted in blood and blood products and by sexual contact. Hepatitis B may also be transmitted by contact with infectious body fluids. Hepatitis C probably accounts for most cases of blood-transmitted hepatitis. Hepatitis D only occurs in the presence of hepatitis B since it requires multiplication of the hepatitis B virus for its own replication.

Acute viral hepatitis results in inflammation of the liver and hepatocellular necrosis but clinical presentation varies widely from subclinical asymptomatic illness to fulminant hepatic failure. Initial symptoms may include malaise, weakness, anorexia, nausea, vomiting, fever, and abdominal pain, followed after 3 to 10 days by jaundice. In some cases the condition may progress to fulminant hepatitis with hepatic encephalopathy, coma, and death. Recovery in patients who survive usually takes a few months but some patients will have residual liver damage. Also some patients infected with the B, C, or D virus may develop chronic hepatitis which may lead to hepatocellular carcinoma or cirrhosis.

Active immunisation of individuals at risk of infection is possible for hepatitis A and B with specific vaccines, or passive immunisation can be achieved using immunoglobulins.

The management of uncomplicated acute viral hepatitis is largely symptomatic. However, it has been suggested[1] that an *interferon* might prevent the progression of acute hepatitis C to the chronic stage and meta-analyses[2,3] also suggest that interferon treatment can promote more rapid resolution of viraemia and normalisation of aminotransferase. Additionally, improvements in liver function were reported in 4 patients with fulminant hepatitis A following treatment with interferon beta.[4] Chronic viral hepatitis has usually been treated with interferon alfa.[5-7] Guidelines have been produced in the UK for the management of hepatitis C.[8] Prolonged therapy for between 4 (hepatitis B) and 12 months (hepatitis C or D) is necessary, although long-term remission of disease is achieved in less than half of patients treated. Relapse is common and, in patients with hepatitis C especially, may be expected in half of responding patients on cessation of treatment.[6,9,10] Response rates may be determined by the level of viraemia and the genotype.[11] In view of these rather disappointing results and the as yet unproven effect on mortality, treatment has usually been reserved for high-risk patients and a number of other antiviral and immunomodulating drugs are either beginning to be used or are under investigation. In hepatitis B, responses to interferon alfa can be improved by pretreatment with prednisone[12,13] or prednisolone.[14,15] Recent studies[16] have shown once-weekly peginterferon alfa, a formulation of interferon alfa with monomethoxy polyethylene glycol, to be more effective than interferon alfa given three times weekly in patients with chronic hepatitis C, including those with cirrhosis or extensive fibrosis.[17] *Ribavirin* has also been shown to have some activity against hepatitis C although biochemical improvements are generally not sustained once treatment is stopped.[18,19] However, the use of ribavirin in combination with interferon alfa[20-25] (or beta[26]) is more effective than either drug alone with sustained responses having been recorded and some authorities now consider combination therapy to be the treatment of first choice.[8]

Several other nucleoside analogues are active against hepatitis B virus, the most widely used being *lamivudine*. It has been extensively studied and has produced promising responses, although relapse rates tend to be high once treatment is discontinued.[27-30] There is also a suggestion that lamivudine might prevent recurrence of hepatitis B infection in patients with chronic hepatitis B who undergo liver transplantation.[31]

Other drugs that have been tried as adjuncts to conventional therapy include thymosin α_1.[32,33]

1. Omata M, *et al.* Resolution of acute hepatitis C after therapy with natural beta interferon. *Lancet* 1991; **338**: 914–15.
2. Cammà C, *et al.* Interferon as treatment for acute hepatitis C: a meta-analysis. *Dig Dis Sci* 1996; **41**: 1248–55.
3. Quin JW. Interferon therapy for acute hepatitis C viral infection—a review by meta-analysis. *Aust N Z J Med* 1997; **27**: 611–18.
4. Yoshiba M, *et al.* Interferon for hepatitis A. *Lancet* 1994; **343**: 288–9.
5. Marwick C. Hepatitis C is focus of NIH consensus panel. *JAMA* 1997; **277**: 1268–9.
6. Hoofnagle JH, Di Bisceglie AM. The treatment of chronic viral hepatitis. *N Engl J Med* 1997; **336**: 347–56.
7. Centers for Disease Control. Recommendations for prevention and control of hepatitis C virus (HCV) infection and HCV-related chronic disease. *MMWR* 1998; **47** (RR-19): 1–39.
8. Booth JCL, *et al.*, Royal College of Physicians of London and the British Society of Gastroenterology. Clinical guidelines on the management of hepatitis C. *Gut* 2001; **49** (suppl 1): i1–i21.
9. van der Poel CL, *et al.* Hepatitis C virus six years on. *Lancet* 1994; **344**: 1475–9.
10. Dusheiko GM, *et al.* A rational approach to the management of hepatitis C infection. *BMJ* 1996; **312**: 357–64.
11. Main J. Hepatitis C: clinical aspects. *J Infect* 1995; **30**: 103–6.
12. Perrillo RP, *et al.* A randomized, controlled trial of interferon alfa-2b alone and after prednisone withdrawal for the treatment of chronic hepatitis B. *N Engl J Med* 1990; **323**: 295–301.
13. Fevery J, *et al.* Efficacy of interferon alfa-2b with or without prednisone withdrawal in the treatment of chronic viral hepatitis B: a prospective double-blind Belgian-Dutch study. *J Hepatol* 1990; **11**: S108–S112.
14. Krogsgaard K, *et al.* Prednisolone withdrawal therapy enhances the effect of human lymphoblastoid interferon in chronic hepatitis B. *J Hepatol* 1996; **25**: 803–13.
15. Lin S-M, *et al.* Long-term beneficial effect of interferon therapy in patients with chronic hepatitis B virus infection. *Hepatology* 1999; **29**: 971–5.
16. Zeuzem S, *et al.* Peginterferon alfa-2a in patients with chronic hepatitis C. *N Engl J Med* 2000; **343**: 1666–72.
17. Heathcote EJ, *et al.* Peginterferon alfa-2a in patients with chronic hepatitis C and cirrhosis. *N Engl J Med* 2000; **343**: 1673–80.
18. Reichard O, *et al.* Ribavirin treatment for chronic hepatitis C. *Lancet* 1991; **337**: 1058–61.
19. Di Bisceglie AM, *et al.* Ribavirin as therapy for chronic hepatitis C: a randomized, double-blind, placebo-controlled trial. *Ann Intern Med* 1995; **123**: 897–903.
20. Chemello L, *et al.* Response to ribavirin, to interferon and to a combination of both in patients with chronic hepatitis C and its relation to HCV genotypes. *J Hepatol* 1994; **21** (suppl): S12.
21. Braconier JH, *et al.* Combined alpha-interferon and ribavirin treatment in chronic hepatitis C: a pilot study. *Scand J Infect Dis* 1995; **27**: 325–9.
22. Reichard O, *et al.* Randomised, double-blind, placebo-controlled trial of interferon α-2b with and without ribavirin for chronic hepatitis C. *Lancet* 1998; **351**: 83–7.
23. Poynard T, *et al.* Randomised trial of interferon α2b plus ribavirin for 48 weeks or for 24 weeks versus interferon α2b plus placebo for 48 weeks for treatment of chronic infection with hepatitis C virus. *Lancet* 1998; **352**: 1426–32.
24. Davis GL, *et al.* Interferon alfa-2b alone or in combination with ribavirin for the treatment of relapse of chronic hepatitis C. *N Engl J Med* 1998; **339**: 1493–9.
25. McHutchison JG, *et al.* Interferon alfa-2b alone or in combination with ribavirin as initial treatment for chronic hepatitis C. *N Engl J Med* 1998; **339**: 1485–92.
26. Kakumu S, *et al.* A pilot study of ribavirin and interferon beta for the treatment of chronic hepatitis C. *Gastroenterology* 1993; **105**: 507–12.
27. Benhamou Y, *et al.* Efficacy of lamivudine on replication of hepatitis B virus in HIV-infected patients. *Lancet* 1995; **345**: 396–7.
28. Dienstag JL, *et al.* A preliminary trial of lamivudine for chronic hepatitis B infection. *N Engl J Med* 1995; **333**: 1657–61.
29. Lai C-L, *et al.* A one-year trial of lamivudine for chronic hepatitis B. *N Engl J Med* 1998; **339**: 61–8.
30. Dienstag JL, *et al.* Lamivudine as initial treatment for chronic hepatitis B in the United States. *N Engl J Med* 1999; **341**: 1256–63.
31. Perrillo RP, *et al.* A multicenter United States-Canadian trial to assess lamivudine monotherapy before and after liver transplantation for chronic hepatitis B. *Hepatology* 2001; **33**: 424–32.
32. Sherman KE, *et al.* Hepatitis C RNA response to combined therapy with thymosin alpha-1 and interferon. *Hepatology* 1994; **20**: 207A.
33. Chien R-N, *et al.* Efficacy of thymosin α-1 in patients with chronic hepatitis B: a randomized, controlled trial. *Hepatology* 1998; **27**: 1383–7.

Herpesvirus infections

Established herpesvirus pathogens discussed below include cytomegalovirus, Epstein-Barr virus, Herpesvirus simiae, herpes simplex virus, and varicella-zoster virus. Herpesviruses 6, 7, and 8 have also emerged as potential pathogens and have been associated with a variety of disorders including childhood febrile illnesses, various malignancies including Kaposi's sarcoma, and multiple sclerosis.

Cytomegalovirus infections. Cytomegaloviruses are members of the herpesvirus group, and are widely distributed in many animal species. Infection may occur through intra-uterine or perinatal transmission, by oral contact with the saliva of infected individuals, or by sexual transmission. Transmission by blood transfusion or by transplantation of infected tissue can also occur. After infection, viral DNA becomes incorporated into the host cells and persists for the life of the individual with occasional reactivation when infectious virions appear in the saliva and urine.

Most congenitally infected infants are asymptomatic, but some infants may present with intra-uterine growth retardation, jaundice, hepatosplenomegaly, encephalitis, and thrombocytopenia. Acquired infections generally do not cause clinical symptoms although they may occasionally present as infectious mononucleosis, lymphocytosis, or lymphadenopathy. The virus is a common cause of infection in the immunocompromised, particularly transplant recipients and patients with AIDS, when it commonly presents as cytomegalovirus retinitis or enteritis, and is a major cause of morbidity and mortality in these patients.

Specific **treatment** for cytomegalovirus infection is usually only given to immunocompromised patients, in whom the infection is often complicated by extensive tissue damage leading to target organ failure and secondary opportunistic infections. Relapses are likely to occur after treatment is stopped due to the latent nature of cytomegaloviruses. *Ganciclovir* is used in the treatment of severe cytomegalovirus infections in transplant recipients and patients with AIDS. However, ganciclovir may cause neutropenia and many AIDS patients receiving zidovudine cannot tolerate the combined haematological toxicity of these two drugs, hence the use of molgramostim to treat or prevent ganciclovir-induced neutropenia. Although less experience has been gained with *foscarnet* it appears to be an alternative to ganciclovir with similar

efficacy. It does not produce myelosuppression, but nephrotoxicity and electrolyte disturbances are common. The two drugs given in combination may be more effective than monotherapy with either. Other approaches to treatment have involved administration of ganciclovir in combination with *cytomegalovirus immunoglobulin* or *normal immunoglobulin*.

Cytomegalovirus retinitis is usually treated intravenously with ganciclovir or foscarnet,[1] this route having the advantage that extra-retinal and bilateral infections are also reduced. In AIDS patients, the initial induction treatment is generally followed by lifelong maintenance therapy, since ganciclovir and foscarnet both suppress rather than eliminate the virus.[2] However, some workers have expressed the view that maintenance therapy may be discontinued in patients who have received highly active antiretroviral therapy (HAART) with a resultant sufficient increase in their CD4+ count.[3-5] Oral ganciclovir is reported to be an effective and more convenient alternative to intravenous maintenance in selected patients. The oral prodrug of ganciclovir, valganciclovir, may be used for either induction or maintenance treatment as an alternative to intravenous administration. Despite maintenance treatment, recurrence is considered to be almost inevitable but it usually responds to an increase in dosage. Foscarnet therapy has been associated with improved survival in AIDS patients although it is often tolerated less well than ganciclovir and the need for long-term intravenous administration poses practical problems.

Cidofovir[6] is another alternative for the treatment of cytomegalovirus retinitis, and has the advantage of intermittent administration. However, long-term treatment may be limited by toxicity.

For patients unable to tolerate systemic therapy, administration of a modified-release intravitreal ganciclovir insert may be beneficial although the risk of increased bilateral and extra-ocular infection is not affected. Adjunctive treatment with oral ganciclovir has been tried to overcome this.[7] Intravitreal injection of the antisense oligonucleotide *fomivirsen* has also been used. Intra-ocular injection of cidofovir, foscarnet, or ganciclovir has been used but is now rarely employed because of the high incidence of complications associated with this technique.

Guidelines for the treatment of cytomegalovirus infections have been produced by the International AIDS Society in the USA.[8]

USA guidelines[9] for the **prevention** of opportunistic infections, including cytomegalovirus infection, in HIV-infected patients emphasise the importance of teaching patients to recognise early symptoms of cytomegalovirus retinitis. Ophthalmic screening is also sometimes used.

Primary prophylaxis of cytomegalovirus infection in high-risk patients, particularly transplant recipients, has been reported using intravenous *ganciclovir*,[10-12] *foscarnet*,[13] *valaciclovir*,[14] and *cytomegalovirus immunoglobulin*.[15] Oral ganciclovir may be useful for prophylaxis or pre-emptive therapy in selected transplant patients.[16] Conflicting results have been reported from studies of the efficacy of oral ganciclovir for primary prophylaxis in patients with HIV infection,[17,18] but it is recommended in the USA guidelines.[9]

Aciclovir with[19] or without[20,21] cytomegalovirus immunoglobulin has been successful in preventing infection in some transplant patients, but failure of prophylaxis has been reported,[22-24] and comparison of aciclovir with ganciclovir for prophylaxis in liver transplant recipients has found ganciclovir to be the more effective drug.[25] The USA guidelines[9] consider aciclovir and valaciclovir to be unsuitable for prophylaxis in patients with HIV infection although preliminary studies suggest that valaciclovir may be effective in these patients.[26] The efficacy of prophylaxis also varies with the organ transplanted.[27]

Cytomegalovirus vaccines are currently in development.

1. Jacobson MA. Treatment of cytomegalovirus retinitis in patients with the acquired immunodeficiency syndrome. *N Engl J Med* 1997; **337**: 105–14.
2. Dhillon B. The management of cytomegalovirus retinitis in AIDS. *Br J Ophthalmol* 1994; **78**: 66–9.
3. Whitcup SM. Cytomegalovirus retinitis in the era of highly active antiretroviral therapy. *JAMA* 2000; **283**: 653–7.
4. Jouan M, *et al.* Discontinuation of maintenance therapy for cytomegalovirus retinitis in HIV-infected patients receiving highly active antiretroviral therapy. *AIDS* 2001; **15**: 23–31.
5. Curi ALL, *et al.* Suspension of anticytomegalovirus maintenance therapy following immune recovery due to highly active antiretroviral therapy. *Br J Ophthalmol* 2001; **85**: 471–3.
6. Plosker GL, Noble S. Cidofovir: a review of its use in cytomegalovirus retinitis in patients with AIDS. *Drugs* 1999; **58**: 325–45.

7. Martin DF, *et al.* Oral ganciclovir for patients with cytomegalovirus retinitis treated with a ganciclovir implant. *N Engl J Med* 1999; **340:** 1063–70.
8. Whitley RJ, *et al.* Guidelines for the treatment of cytomegalovirus diseases in patients with AIDS in the era of potent antiretroviral therapy: recommendation of an international panel. *Arch Intern Med* 1998; **158:** 957–69.
9. Centers for Disease Control. 1999 USPHS/IDSA guidelines for the prevention of opportunistic infections in persons infected with human immunodeficiency virus. *MMWR* 1999; **48** (RR-10): 1–59.
10. Goodrich JM, *et al.* Ganciclovir prophylaxis to prevent cytomegalovirus disease after allogeneic marrow transplant. *Ann Intern Med* 1993; **118:** 173–8.
11. Winston DJ, *et al.* Ganciclovir prophylaxis of cytomegalovirus infection and disease in allogeneic bone marrow transplant recipients. *Ann Intern Med* 1993; **118:** 179–84.
12. Hibberd PL, *et al.* Preemptive ganciclovir therapy to prevent cytomegalovirus disease in cytomegalovirus antibody-positive renal transplant recipients: a randomized controlled trial. *Ann Intern Med* 1995; **123:** 18–26.
13. Reusser P, *et al.* Phase I-II trial of foscarnet for prevention of cytomegalovirus infection in autologous and allogeneic marrow transplant recipients. *J Infect Dis* 1992; **166:** 473–9.
14. Lowance D, *et al.* Valacyclovir for the prevention of cytomegalovirus disease after renal transplantation. *N Engl J Med* 1999; **340:** 1462–70.
15. Wittes JT, *et al.* Meta-analysis of CMVIG studies for the prevention and treatment of CMV infection in transplant patients. *Transplant Proc* 1996; **28** (suppl 2): 17–24.
16. Goodrich J, Khardori N. Cytomegalovirus: the taming of the beast? *Lancet* 1997; **350:** 1718–19.
17. Spector SA, *et al.* Oral ganciclovir for the prevention of cytomegalovirus disease in persons with AIDS. *N Engl J Med* 1996; **334:** 1491–7.
18. McCarthy M. Oral ganciclovir fails to prevent CMV in HIV trial. *Lancet* 1995; **346:** 895.
19. Eisenmann D, *et al.* Prevention of cytomegalovirus disease in heart transplant recipients by prophylaxis with cytomegalovirus hyperimmune globulin plus oral acyclovir. *Transplant Proc* 1990; **22:** 2322–3.
20. Balfour HH, *et al.* A randomized, placebo-controlled trial of oral acyclovir for the prevention of cytomegalovirus disease in recipients of renal allografts. *N Engl J Med* 1989; **320:** 1381–7.
21. Prentice HG, *et al.* Impact of long-term acyclovir on cytomegalovirus infection and survival after allogeneic bone marrow transplantation. *Lancet* 1994; **343:** 749–53.
22. Bailey TC, *et al.* Failure of high-dose oral acyclovir with or without immune globulin to prevent primary cytomegalovirus disease in recipients of solid organ transplants. *Am J Med* 1993; **95:** 273–8.
23. Singh N, *et al.* High-dose acyclovir compared with short-course pre-emptive ganciclovir therapy to prevent cytomegalovirus disease in liver transplant recipients: a randomized trial. *Ann Intern Med* 1994; **120:** 375–81.
24. Boeckh M, *et al.* Failure of high-dose acyclovir to prevent cytomegalovirus disease after autologous marrow transplantation. *J Infect Dis* 1995; **172:** 939–43.
25. Winston DJ, *et al.* Randomised comparison of ganciclovir and high-dose acyclovir for long-term cytomegalovirus prophylaxis in liver-transplant recipients. *Lancet* 1995; **346:** 69–74.
26. Feinberg JE, *et al.* A randomized, double-blind trial of valaciclovir prophylaxis for cytomegalovirus disease in patients with advanced human immunodeficiency virus infection. *J Infect Dis* 1998; **177:** 48–56.
27. Griffiths PD. Prophylaxis against CMV infection in transplant patients. *J Antimicrob Chemother* 1997; **39:** 299–301.

Epstein-Barr virus infections. Epstein-Barr virus (EBV) is a DNA virus of the herpesvirus group with a worldwide distribution. Following primary exposure the individual becomes a lifelong carrier of EBV, but associated disease only occurs if the normal immune mechanisms are compromised and the virus can be reactivated. EBV is the causative agent in infectious mononucleosis and is associated with several diseases including Burkitt's lymphoma, nasopharyngeal carcinoma, chronic interstitial pneumonitis in infants with AIDS, and oral hairy leukoplakia in AIDS patients. It may also be associated with Hodgkin's disease and with amyloidosis.

Infectious mononucleosis (glandular fever) is an acute, self-limiting, lymphoproliferative infection occurring mainly in adolescents and young adults, transmission usually being via close oral contact. Symptoms may last for several weeks and include sore throat, swelling of the neck, fever, sweating, chills, and anorexia. Lymphadenopathy and splenomegaly usually occur and some patients may experience hepatomegaly and jaundice. Most patients recover uneventfully with only supportive treatment although they may continue to be easily exhausted for some time. Complications may occur in a few patients and can be fatal. They include meningitis, encephalitis, seizures, hepatic necrosis, splenic rupture, haemolytic and aplastic anaemia, agranulocytosis, and thrombocytopenia. Very rarely the illness may become chronic, with symptoms persisting for years, and may result in death from lymphomatous disease.

There is no specific treatment for EBV infections. Aciclovir,[1-4] ganciclovir,[5,6] and interferons[3,7,8] are some of the drugs that have been reported to produce some clinical or immunological improvement, but this is usually reversible on stopping treatment. Corticosteroids may be useful in severe, prolonged, or complicated infections, although concern has been expressed that they might impair immunity and increase the risk of EBV-related tumours in later years.[9] Concurrent throat infection with streptococci should not be treated with amoxicillin or ampicillin since they may cause a maculopapular rash in patients with infectious mononucleosis.

1. Andersson J, *et al.* Effect of acyclovir on infectious mononucleosis: a double-blind, placebo-controlled study. *J Infect Dis* 1986; **153:** 283–90.
2. Yao QY, *et al.* The Epstein-Barr virus: host balance in acute infectious mononucleosis patients receiving acyclovir anti-viral therapy. *Int J Cancer* 1989; **43:** 61–6.
3. Drago F, *et al.* Epstein-Barr virus-related primary cutaneous amyloidosis: successful treatment with acyclovir and interferon-alpha. *Br J Dermatol* 1996; **134:** 170–4.
4. Tynell E, *et al.* Acyclovir and prednisolone treatment of acute infectious mononucleosis: a multicentre, double-blind, placebo-controlled study. *J Infect Dis* 1996; **174:** 324–31.
5. Ishida Y, *et al.* Ganciclovir for chronic active Epstein-Barr virus infection. *Lancet* 1993; **341:** 560–1.
6. Pirsch JD, *et al.* Treatment of severe Epstein-Barr virus-induced lymphoproliferative syndrome with ganciclovir: two cases after solid organ transplantation. *Am J Med* 1989; **86:** 241–4.
7. Cheeseman SH, *et al.* Epstein-Barr virus infection in renal transplant recipients: effects of antithymocyte globulin and interferon. *Ann Intern Med* 1980; **93:** 39–42.
8. Fujisaki T, *et al.* Gamma-interferon for severe chronic active Epstein-Barr virus. *Ann Intern Med* 1993; **118:** 474–5.
9. Sheagren JN. Corticosteroids for treatment of mononucleosis and aphthous stomatitis. *JAMA* 1986; **256:** 1051.

Herpes simplex infections. Herpes simplex virus (HSV, herpesvirus hominis) is distributed worldwide and is most often classified[1] into serotypes HSV-1 and HSV-2. Transmission is by direct contact with infected secretions, with HSV-1 being associated primarily with oral transmission and HSV-2 primarily with genital transmission. Symptomatic disease normally affects the skin or mucous membranes, when HSV replicates in the epithelium with subsequent lysis of infected cells and local inflammation to produce characteristic painful lesions. Viraemia occurs rarely, except in immunocompromised individuals in whom disseminated disease can develop.

HSV becomes latent within sensory nerve ganglia from where it can be reactivated by various triggers such as stress, bacterial infection, fever, irradiation (including sunlight), or menstruation. Reactivation leads to a prodromal period before the lesions emerge.

Primary infections are usually in the perioral, ocular, or genital areas, but infection may occur at any skin site if the skin is damaged or if the patient is immunocompromised. Anorectal lesions including herpes proctitis are especially prevalent in homosexual men with AIDS. Most primary HSV-1 infections are asymptomatic but may occasionally present as acute gingivostomatitis and pharyngitis. Infections commonly recur as *herpes labialis*, also known as fever blisters or cold sores. *Ocular herpes* is also generally caused by HSV-1, and infections range in severity from superficial conjunctivitis or dendritic keratitis to sight-threatening diseases of the inner eye such as iridocyclitis or herpetic disciform keratitis. *Genital herpes* is usually caused by HSV-2 and tends to be a more severe condition than other herpes simplex infections, especially in women. *Herpes encephalitis* and *neonatal herpes* are rare, but occasionally fatal, complications of herpes simplex infections.

MANAGEMENT. The most widely used antiviral for herpes simplex infections is aciclovir. In clinical practice, treatment of primary herpes simplex infections, while relieving symptoms and reducing the duration of viral shedding, does not prevent recurrences. Antiviral therapy is generally more effective for primary infections than for recurrences, and should be given as early as possible during the course of an active infection, preferably within 3 days of the onset of symptoms. Aciclovir may be administered topically, orally, or intravenously depending on the severity and nature of the infection. Resistance to aciclovir is emerging, mainly in immunocompromised patients.[2]

Assessment of antivirals with improved bioavailability or pharmacokinetic profiles which allow less frequent dosing and antivirals that are effective against aciclovir-resistant strains is continuing. Such drugs include the nucleoside analogues valaciclovir and cidofovir, and the immunomodulators interferon alfa and imiquimod.[3] Herpes simplex vaccines have also been tried but with generally disappointing results.

• **Herpes labialis** is a self-limiting disorder that rarely requires antiviral therapy. If it is used then such treatment should be started early in the prodromal phase. Topical preparations of antivirals, including aciclovir, penciclovir, and tromantadine, are used but there is conflicting evidence regarding their efficacy. Docosanol may be a further alternative. Oral aciclovir may suppress frequently recurrent herpes labialis,[4,5] and protect those at high risk of recurrence. However, for the majority of patients careful hygiene and, if necessary, symptomatic treatment with analgesics and the use of antiseptics such as povidone-iodine to reduce secondary infection will suffice; sunscreens may reduce the frequency of recurrences.

• **Ocular herpes simplex infections** usually require treatment with a suitable antiviral. Aciclovir is commonly applied as an ointment.[1] Trifluridine[1] and vidarabine are alternatives. Ganciclovir gel might be as effective as aciclovir.[6] The use of topical corticosteroids alone is contra-indicated for most forms of ocular herpes as they can increase disease severity, but a combination of a corticosteroid with an antiviral, such as prednisolone with aciclovir[7] or trifluridine[8] may be useful. Long-term treatment with oral aciclovir has been found to reduce the rate of recurrence of ocular herpes simplex disease.[9] Patients with intra-ocular infections require systemic treatment, usually with aciclovir. However, the addition of oral aciclovir to topical therapy with trifluridine and a corticosteroid was reported to be of no benefit in patients with stromal keratitis.[10] A systematic review[11] has concluded that the combination of an antiviral nucleoside and interferon appears to speed healing in patients with epithelial keratitis.

• **Genital herpes** is usually treated with systemic aciclovir; alternatives are famciclovir and valaciclovir.[12-14] Topical aciclovir has been used but it is less effective. As with other herpes simplex infections, therapy of the initial infection appears to have no effect on subsequent recurrences. In patients experiencing a recognisable prodrome, a 5-day course of oral aciclovir, famciclovir, or valaciclovir initiated by the patient may abort the recurrence or reduce its severity.[12] In patients who do not experience a prodrome or those with frequent recurrences, continuous suppressive therapy with aciclovir should be considered; there is less experience with famciclovir or valaciclovir.[12] Cidofovir gel has produced beneficial responses in mucocutaneous infections unresponsive to systemic aciclovir in patients with AIDS.[15] There is a risk of *neonatal herpes* in the infants of mothers with genital herpes infection. Prophylactic administration of aciclovir to the mother during late pregnancy is not routinely recommended[12] but may be indicated in HIV-infected mothers if recurrence is frequent.[16] Infants with evidence of neonatal herpes infection should be treated with systemic aciclovir.[12,14]

• **Severe or disseminated herpes simplex infections**, particularly those occurring in immunocompromised patients, usually require intravenous therapy. Aciclovir is used most commonly,[1] with foscarnet or cidofovir as alternatives for infections resistant to aciclovir.[12] Immunocompromised patients with frequent or disabling recurrences may benefit from prophylactic oral aciclovir or famciclovir administration.[16]

1. Whitley RJ, Roizman B. Herpes simplex virus infections. *Lancet* 2001; **357:** 1513–18.
2. Christophers J, *et al.* Survey of resistance of herpes simplex virus to aciclovir in Northwest England. *Antimicrob Agents Chemother* 1998; **42:** 868–72.
3. Cassady KA, Whitley RJ. New therapeutic approaches to the alphaherpesvirus infections. *J Antimicrob Chemother* 1997; **39:** 119–28.
4. Anonymous. Treatment of herpes simplex labialis. *Lancet* 1990; **335:** 1501–2.
5. Worrall G. Acyclovir in recurrent herpes labialis. *BMJ* 1996; **312:** 6.
6. Hoh HB, *et al.* Randomised trial of ganciclovir and acyclovir in the treatment of herpes simplex dendritic keratitis: a multicentre study. *Br J Ophthalmol* 1996; **80:** 140–3.
7. Collum LMT, *et al.* Acyclovir (Zovirax) in herpetic disciform keratitis. *Br J Ophthalmol* 1983; **67:** 115–18.
8. Wilhelmus KR, *et al.* Herpetic eye disease study: a controlled trial of topical corticosteroids for herpes simplex stromal keratitis. *Ophthalmology* 1994; **101:** 1883–96.
9. Herpetic Eye Disease Study Group. Acyclovir for the prevention of recurrent herpes simplex virus eye disease. *N Engl J Med* 1998; **339:** 300–6.
10. Barron BA, *et al.* Herpetic eye disease study: a controlled trial of oral acyclovir for herpes simplex stromal keratitis. *Ophthalmology* 1994; **101:** 1871–82.
11. Wilhelmus KR. Interventions for herpes simplex virus epithelial keratitis (updated 23 May 2001). Available in The Cochrane Library; Issue 4. Oxford: Update Software; 2001.
12. Centers for Disease Control. 1998 Guidelines for treatment of sexually transmitted diseases. *MMWR* 1998; **47:** 20–6.
13. Clinical Effectiveness Group (Association of Genitourinary Medicine and the Medical Society for the Study of Venereal Diseases). National guideline for the management of genital herpes. *Sex Transm Infect* 1999; **75** (suppl 1): S24–S28.
14. WHO. *Guidelines for the management of sexually transmitted infections.* Geneva: WHO, 2001
15. Lalezari J, *et al.* A randomized, double-blind, placebo-controlled trial of cidofovir gel for the treatment of acyclovir-unresponsive mucocutaneous herpes simplex virus infection in patients with AIDS. *J Infect Dis* 1997; **176:** 892–8.
16. Centers for Disease Control. 1999 USPHS/IDSA guidelines for the prevention of opportunistic infections in persons infected with human immunodeficiency virus. *MMWR* 1999; **48** (RR-10): 1–59.

Herpesvirus simiae infections. Herpesvirus simiae (monkey B virus, herpes B virus) is a herpesvirus that usually infects macaque monkeys, but may rarely be transmitted to man by laboratory accidents or bites or scratches from infected monkeys.

Initially there may be vesicles at the site of the bite or scratch. As the infection progresses there is increasing neurological involvement which can lead to encephalitis, coma, and death.

Aciclovir has been recommended for the prophylaxis and treatment of this infection. It should be started immediately an infection is suspected, usually intravenously for symptomatic infections or orally for those that are asymptomatic.[1] When treatment with intravenous aciclovir followed by ganciclovir was delayed in 2 patients until neurological symptoms had developed it was not successful.[2] Intravenous ganciclovir for one month followed by oral aciclovir has also been tried in a patient; he recovered from his meningitis.[3]

1. Wansbrough-Jones MH, *et al.* Prophylaxis against B virus infection. *BMJ* 1988; **297:** 909.
2. Holmes GP, *et al.* B virus (Herpesvirus simiae) infection in humans: epidemiologic investigation of a cluster. *Ann Intern Med* 1990; **112:** 833–9.
3. Scinicariello F, *et al.* Identification by PCR of meningitis caused by herpes B virus. *Lancet* 1993; **341:** 1660–1.

Varicella-zoster infections. Varicella-zoster virus (VZV) is a herpesvirus which causes chickenpox (varicella) and herpes zoster (zoster, shingles). The virus is easily transmitted, particularly by close contact with infected individuals.

Primary infection usually results in *chickenpox*, which presents with a characteristic generalised vesicular eruption, fever, and malaise. Chickenpox is commonly a benign disease of childhood of short duration. It can occur in adults when it can be severe, and is potentially fatal in immunocompromised patients: complications include secondary bacterial skin infections, pneumonia, and neurological disorders such as encephalitis and cerebral ataxia. Reye's syndrome, which is principally associated with viral infections in childhood, may also be a cause of encephalopathy in patients with chickenpox. Infection during early pregnancy may result rarely in fetal varicella syndrome while infection during late pregnancy may cause neonatal varicella after delivery.

Patients who recover from primary infections with varicella-zoster have lifelong immunity against chickenpox. However, a permanent latent infection of sensory nerve ganglia is established, and reactivation produces herpes zoster.

Herpes zoster is characterised by painful vesicular eruptions localised to a single dermatome of skin, and sometimes preceded by a prodromal phase with fever, malaise, and headache. Involvement of the trigeminal nerve can lead to sight-threatening ophthalmic herpes zoster. As with chickenpox, herpes zoster is more serious in immunocompromised patients and may be severe, prolonged, or disseminated. Chronic pain which persists after the rash has healed is termed postherpetic neuralgia (p.7) and occurs in about 10% of patients who have had herpes zoster.

Management of **chickenpox** in otherwise healthy patients is usually symptomatic using antipyretics, analgesics, and antipruritics. Antibacterials may be required for secondary infections. The value of antivirals in the treatment of chickenpox in such patients has been questioned,[1] and their use is not recommended for the treatment of uncomplicated chickenpox in otherwise healthy children.[2,3] However, oral aciclovir has been reported to reduce the duration and severity of symptoms when administered within 24 hours of onset of symptoms,[4-6] but not the incidence of chickenpox-associated complications.[4] It may be useful in immunocompromised patients or those who have developed complications. Intravenous therapy may be necessary in severe chickenpox. Recommendations for the use of aciclovir in children,[3] adults,[7] and during pregnancy[8] have been developed.

Transmission of chickenpox to household contacts is not prevented by administration of aciclovir to the primary case[4] but there is evidence to suggest that transmission can be suppressed by administering aciclovir to susceptible contacts during the incubation period.[9,10] Although the need for such prophylactic antiviral therapy has been questioned, especially in otherwise healthy children,[11] prophylaxis or early treatment may be useful for household contacts in whom the infection might prove to be more severe.[3,12,13]

Varicella-zoster immunoglobulins are used for the prevention of chickenpox in patients at high risk of develop-

ing complications such as the immunocompromised, neonates, and in susceptible pregnant women following significant exposure to chickenpox. There have been reports of severe chickenpox occurring in patients undergoing corticosteroid therapy and in the UK administration of varicella-zoster immunoglobulin is recommended in persons exposed to the virus who have received therapeutic doses of corticosteroids within the previous 3 months[14] (see also under Precautions for Corticosteroids, p.1043). Varicella-zoster vaccines are available in some countries.

The place of antivirals in the treatment of **herpes zoster** is well established and guidelines on management have been produced.[15] Antiviral treatment can reduce the severity and duration of acute pain, minimise complications and propagation of the rash, and reduce viral shedding.[15,16] Aciclovir may be given orally or intravenously, depending upon the severity of the infection. Oral famciclovir or valaciclovir are alternatives. Treatment should be initiated within 72 hours of the onset of the rash and is usually continued for 7 to 10 days. Amantadine has also been used in the acute phase. Nothing appears to be gained from extending the treatment period or from adding systemic corticosteroids[17] which are best avoided anyway in patients with acute infection since they can increase the risk of viral dissemination.[16] Immunocompromised patients or others at high risk of severe or disseminated varicella-zoster infections should receive intravenous aciclovir. Combined therapy with aciclovir and vidarabine may be considered in the severely immunocompromised.[16] Foscarnet may be of value in aciclovir-resistant varicella-zoster infections[18,19] although treatment failures have been reported.[20] Sorivudine has been reported to produce benefit in immunocompromised patients with recurrent cutaneously disseminated varicella-zoster infection refractory to aciclovir and to foscarnet,[21] and may be more effective than aciclovir.[22] Brivudine has displayed comparable efficacy to that of aciclovir.[23]

Ophthalmic herpes zoster may be treated with topical aciclovir, although concurrent treatment with systemic aciclovir may be needed for optimum results.[16,24] Oral famciclovir may have similar efficacy to oral aciclovir.[25] However, a study in 20 patients with AIDS suggested that ganciclovir given either alone or in combination with foscarnet was more effective than aciclovir in terms of preserving long-term visual acuity.[26] Topical corticosteroids are usually avoided during the acute phase of the infection, but may be needed if there is a substantial inflammatory component.

There has been controversy over the use of oral aciclovir to prevent postherpetic neuralgia and ocular complications. A meta-analysis suggested that treatment of herpes zoster with oral aciclovir within 72 hours of the onset of rash could reduce the incidence of residual pain at 6 months by 46% in immunocompetent adults.[27]

1. Anonymous. Controversy about chickenpox. *Lancet* 1992; **340:** 639–40.
2. Committee on Infectious Diseases. The use of oral acyclovir in otherwise healthy children with varicella. *Pediatrics* 1993; **91:** 674–6. Correction. *ibid.:* 858.
3. Tarlow MJ, Walters S. Chickenpox in childhood: a review prepared for the UK Advisory Group on Chickenpox on behalf of the British Society for the Study of Infection. *J Infect* 1998; **36** (suppl 1): 39–47.
4. Balfour HH, *et al.* Acyclovir treatment of varicella in otherwise healthy children. *J Pediatr* 1990; **116:** 633–9.
5. Feder HM. Treatment of adult chickenpox with oral acyclovir. *Arch Intern Med* 1990; **150:** 2061–5.
6. Balfour HH, *et al.* Acyclovir treatment of varicella in otherwise healthy adolescents. *J Pediatr* 1992; **120:** 627–33.
7. Wilkins EGL, *et al.* Management of chickenpox in the adult: a review prepared for the UK Advisory Group on Chickenpox on behalf of the British Society for the Study of Infection. *J Infect* 1998; **36** (suppl 1): 49–58.
8. Nathwani D, *et al.* Varicella infections in pregnancy and the newborn: a review prepared for the UK Advisory Group on Chickenpox on behalf of the British Society for the Study of Infection. *J Infect* 1998; **36** (suppl 1): 59–71.
9. Asano Y, *et al.* Postexposure prophylaxis of varicella in family contact by oral acyclovir. *Pediatrics* 1993; **92:** 219–22.
10. Suga S, *et al.* Effect of oral acyclovir against primary and secondary viraemia in incubation period of varicella. *Arch Dis Child* 1993; **69:** 639–42.
11. Conway SP. Effect of oral acyclovir against primary and secondary viraemia in incubation period of varicella: commentary. *Arch Dis Child* 1993; **69:** 642–3.
12. Ogilvie MM. Antiviral prophylaxis and treatment in chickenpox: a review prepared for the UK Advisory Group on Chickenpox on behalf of the British Society for the Study of Infection. *J Infect* 1998; **36:** (suppl 1): 31–8.
13. Lin TY, *et al.* Oral acyclovir prophylaxis of varicella after intimate contact. *Pediatr Infect Dis J* 1997; **16:** 1162–5.
14. Salisbury DM, Begg NT (eds), Joint Committee on Vaccination and Immunisation. *Immunisation against infectious disease.* London: HMSO, 1996.
15. BSSI Working Group. Guidelines for the management of shingles: report of a working group of the British Society for the Study of Infection (BSSI). *J Infect* 1995; **30:** 193–200.
16. Nikkels AF, Piérard GE. Recognition and treatment of shingles. *Drugs* 1994; **48:** 528–48.

17. Wood MJ, *et al.* A randomized trial of acyclovir for 7 days or 21 days with and without prednisolone for treatment of acute herpes zoster. *N Engl J Med* 1994; **330:** 896–900.
18. Safrin S, *et al.* Foscarnet therapy in five patients with AIDS and acyclovir-resistant varicella-zoster virus infection. *Ann Intern Med* 1991; **115:** 19–21.
19. Smith KJ. Acyclovir-resistant varicella zoster responsive to foscarnet. *Arch Dermatol* 1991; **127:** 1069–71.
20. Bendel AE, *et al.* Failure of foscarnet in disseminated herpes zoster. *Lancet* 1993; **341:** 1342.
21. Burdge DR, *et al.* Sorivudine (BV-ara-U) for the treatment of complicated refractory varicella zoster virus infection in HIV-infected patients. *AIDS* 1995; **9:** 610–2.
22. Gnann JW, *et al.* Sorivudine versus acyclovir for treatment of dermatomal herpes zoster in human immunodeficiency virus-infected patients: results from a randomized, controlled clinical trial. *Antimicrob Agents Chemother* 1998; **42:** 1139–45.
23. Wutzler P, *et al.* Oral brivudin vs intravenous acyclovir in the treatment of herpes zoster in immunocompromised patients: a randomized double-blind trial. *J Med Virol* 1995; **46:** 252–7.
24. Anonymous. Treatment of ocular herpes zoster. *Lancet* 1991; **338:** 1244–5.
25. Tyring S, *et al.* Famciclovir for ophthalmic zoster: a randomised acyclovir controlled study. *Br J Ophthalmol* 2001; **85:** 576–81.
26. Moorthy RS, *et al.* Management of varicella zoster virus retinitis in AIDS. *Br J Ophthalmol* 1997; **81:** 189–94.
27. Jackson JL, *et al.* The effect of treating herpes zoster with oral acyclovir in preventing postherpetic neuralgia: a meta-analysis. *Arch Intern Med* 1997; **157:** 909–12.

HIV infection and AIDS

The causative agent of AIDS (acquired immunodeficiency syndrome) is the human immunodeficiency virus (HIV; previously known as HTLV-III or LAV), a retrovirus transmitted by sexual contact, blood and blood products, the use of contaminated needles, or from mother to fetus. Two subtypes of HIV have been identified. The most common is HIV-1 which occurs worldwide. HIV-2 is found mainly in Africa and HIV-2 infection is associated with a slower progression to AIDS than HIV-1 infection.

HIV has a high affinity for the CD4 receptor on T lymphocytes and its major effect on the immune system is a progressive depletion of CD4+ T lymphocytes.[1] Although there is no rigid pattern in progression from HIV infection to AIDS, a typical course is as follows. Infection is followed by development of anti-HIV antibodies (seroconversion). During seroconversion the patient may remain asymptomatic or have transient symptoms including rash, sore throat, and lymphadenopathy. Despite the antibodies the infection progresses over a period of months to several years to persistent generalised lymphadenopathy (lymphadenopathy syndrome) or to a more serious collection of symptoms, sometimes known as AIDS-related complex (ARC), and including fatigue, weight loss, recurrent fever, diarrhoea, and persistent infections. AIDS is characterised by severe impairment of the immune system leading to the development of secondary infections particularly *Pneumocystis carinii* pneumonia, *Toxoplasma* encephalitis, oropharyngeal and oesophageal candidiasis, cryptococcal meningitis, cytomegalovirus retinitis, and tuberculosis, or to secondary neoplasms such as Kaposi's sarcoma, primary CNS lymphomas, invasive cervical cancer, and non-Hodgkin's lymphoma. Other complications are numerous and may include dementia and thrombocytopenia. Series of articles in *Lancet* 1996, *Med J Aust* 1995/96, and *J Antimicrob Chemother* 1996[2] have discussed various aspects of HIV infection and the associated disorders.

The revised definition of AIDS by the US Centers for Disease Control[1] (as all HIV-infected patients with a CD4+ T lymphocyte count of less than 200 per µL or less than 14% of the total lymphocyte count) has not generally been adopted outside the USA.[3] WHO has produced guidelines[4,5] for the diagnosis and treatment of HIV infection and related disorders which do not rely on the availability of advanced technological resources. Measurement of both the CD4+ T lymphocyte count and HIV RNA may be a more accurate surrogate marker for clinical outcome and is increasingly being used to assess prognosis before starting treatment and to monitor progress of the disease during treatment.[6]

In general, HIV infections eventually result in AIDS which appears to be invariably fatal. However, in a small proportion of patients the immune system stabilises after an initial decline in CD4+ count despite continued HIV infection.[7] Cases of clearance of HIV infection in neonates infected prenatally have been reported.[8] Variation in the genes for recently identified coreceptors necessary for HIV infection may be involved[9] and may offer new therapeutic targets.

Treatment. The following discussion relates to the use of antiretrovirals in HIV infection and AIDS. The treatment of secondary and opportunistic infections and other complications is covered under the relevant sections, below.

Treatment strategies for HIV infection have been changing rapidly with the advent of new antiretroviral drugs and improved timing of treatment. Indeed, as experience continues to be gained, guidelines for the treatment of HIV infection such as those published in the USA by the National Institutes of Health,[10,11] the International AIDS Society,[12] the Centers for Disease Control,[13] and the HIV/AIDS Treatment Information Service (ATIS),[14] and in the UK by the British HIV Association[15] will require frequent updating. Until recently monotherapy with zidovudine (or an alternative nucleoside reverse transcriptase inhibitor) was most commonly used, but combination therapy is now considered essential. The debate over whether to start treatment early in the course of the infection or to delay until the disease progresses continues.[16-18] However, in the USA treatment is being deferred to a later stage in the disease process than was formerly recommended in view of the adverse effects of current treatment regimens.[14] Treatment during the acute infection has also been advocated,[19] but a more conservative approach is being adopted in view of the lack of evidence of long-term benefits.[12]

The main drugs used in combination therapy are nucleoside reverse transcriptase inhibitors (such as zidovudine, abacavir, didanosine, lamivudine, stavudine, and zalcitabine), HIV-protease inhibitors (such as amprenavir, indinavir, lopinavir, nelfinavir, ritonavir, and saquinavir), and non-nucleoside reverse transcriptase inhibitors (such as delavirdine, efavirenz, and nevirapine). Those that inhibit reverse transcriptase act by preventing the spread of the virus to uninfected cells.[20,21] HIV-protease inhibitors act at a late stage of viral replication, preventing the maturation of the viral particle to an infective form.[22,23] Other drugs under investigation include transactivator gene (tat) inhibitors, integrase inhibitors,[24] TIBO derivatives,[25] and recombinant soluble CD4 (rs CD4). There are also strategies involving linking toxins to a CD4 carrier. Therapies aimed at modifying the immune response to HIV include the use of interleukin-2 (see p.548), normal immunoglobulins (see p.1553), and hyperimmune plasma products;[26] a number of vaccines are also being developed. The response to interferon therapy has generally been disappointing (see p.631). Gene therapies,[27,28] antisense oligonucleotides,[29] modified chemokines, and ribozymes[29,30] are at an early stage of development.

Monotherapy with zidovudine was generally considered to produce an improvement, albeit short-lived, in the incidence of opportunistic infections and in mortality in patients with ARC or AIDS (there might also be an improvement in some of the other features of AIDS such as dementia[31,32] and early studies produced promising results. For example, a placebo-controlled study[33] was terminated prematurely when the results at up to 24 weeks showed a significantly reduced mortality rate and incidence of opportunistic infections in the zidovudine group. Unfortunately, more recent studies have shown the benefits in AIDS and ARC patients to be limited to the first few months of treatment.[34] It has also been shown that while the death rate was reduced during the first year of zidovudine treatment,[35] after 2 years there was no difference between patients who did or did not receive zidovudine; beyond 2 years the death rate was higher in the zidovudine group.

Similarly, expectations that giving zidovudine monotherapy to patients in the early stages of HIV infection before symptoms developed might delay progression and reduce the mortality rate have not been fulfilled. Various studies in asymptomatic or mildly symptomatic patients showed that zidovudine started early could delay progression to ARC or AIDS within a follow-up period of about 2 years.[36-39] However, with the exception of the European-Australian Collaborative Group study[40] (which reported continued benefits at up to 3 years), the delay in disease progression has been transitory,[41,42] and in general no improvements in survival rates have been seen.[39,41,42] In addition, adverse effects of zidovudine may counterbalance any improvements in quality of life to be gained from a prolonged disease-free period.[43] Nevertheless, the successful reduction of vertical transmission from mother to child with zidovudine therapy (see under HIV Infection Prophylaxis, below) and findings that zidovudine given early in the primary infection might delay disease progression[44] suggest that early antiretroviral treatment may be beneficial.

The failure of monotherapy with antiretrovirals to produce sustained clinical benefits including improved survival is due, at least in part, to the selection of drug-resistant variants of HIV.[24,45] Resistance develops rapidly

during monotherapy and cross-resistance is reported between related drugs.

Combination therapy with antiretroviral drugs given early in the infection (a strategy analogous to the treatment of tuberculosis and other infectious diseases) aims to improve efficacy, minimise toxicity, and delay drug resistance. Results from the Delta study[46] and the US AIDS Clinical Trial Group 175 (ACTG 175) study,[47] showing combination therapy to be more effective than monotherapy in antiretroviral-naive patients, led to immediate changes in clinical practice. In patients who had not received antiretroviral therapy before, both studies showed substantial reductions in mortality at 30 months in patients treated with zidovudine plus either didanosine or zalcitabine compared with those receiving zidovudine alone.

The transience of the clinical benefit seen in most studies is attributable to the emergence of drug-resistant HIV variants, even during combination therapy. Combinations of three antiretrovirals, typically two nucleoside reverse transcriptase inhibitors plus either an HIV-protease inhibitor or a non-nucleoside reverse transcriptase inhibitor, referred to as highly active antiretroviral therapy (HAART), have produced reductions in viral loads, often to levels below the limits of detection associated with sustained improvements in disease progression.[48] It now appears that it is necessary to suppress viral replication to this extent in order to inhibit the emergence of resistant variants and consequent disease progression.[49] The decline in CD4+ count has been arrested or reversed in patients with AIDS on HAART therapy, even in the absence of profound suppression of viraemia,[50] and there is some evidence that immune function may be partially restored in the long term.[51] Declining morbidity and mortality among patients with HIV infection have been attributed to the introduction of more effective treatment regimens.[52-54]

Although HAART regimens are generally most effective in antiretroviral-naive patients, good responses can also be achieved in patients who have received previous treatment.[55] When a new regimen is started, drugs should be started simultaneously rather than sequentially.[56] Ideally, drug regimens should be changed entirely to drugs that have not been taken previously, or at least 2 drugs of a triple-drug regimen should be changed.[14]

Despite the ability of HAART regimens to maintain the viral loads at undetectable levels, clinical experience shows that viral load rapidly returns to pretreatment levels once treatment is stopped. The reason for this appears to be the persistence of the virus in a latent state or in compartments not accessible to antiretrovirals. At present it has not been possible to stop treatment in the majority of patients, although intermittent therapy may eventually be possible.[57] The continued effectiveness of any HAART regimen is dependent on compliance with treatment, since lapses in compliance can rapidly lead to the emergence of HIV variants resistant to one or more of the drugs being used and consequent disease progression. However, compliance is difficult to maintain due to the complexity of many regimens and to poor tolerability and long-term adverse effects of the drugs used. In addition, the cost of treatment is high and access to effective treatment in developing countries with high burdens of disease is of particular concern.[58] Recent interest in the use of hydroxyurea [hydroxycarbamide] in combination with conventional antiretrovirals may result in the development of regimens that are particularly useful in developing countries. Approaches being tried to overcome compliance problems include: the use of simplified dosage regimens using combined products or utilising pharmacokinetic interactions to reduce doses or extend the dosing interval;[48] the investigation of simplified maintenance regimens[48] (although preliminary results have been disappointing[59]); activating latent HIV-1 with immunostimulant treatment (for example interleukins, colony-stimulating factors, or antibodies to CD3) thereby making it susceptible to antiretrovirals;[60] and the development of new drugs with novel modes of action.

1. Anonymous. 1993 Revised classification system for HIV infection and expanded surveillance case definition for AIDS among adolescents and adults. *JAMA* 1993; **269:** 729–80.
2. Various. HIV infection. *J Antimicrob Chemother* 1996; **37** (suppl B): 1–198.
3. Ancelle Park RA. European AIDS definition. *Lancet* 1992; **339:** 671.
4. WHO. *Global programme on AIDS: guidelines for the clinical management of HIV infection in adults.* Geneva: WHO, 1991.
5. WHO. Safe and effective use of antiretroviral treatments in adults with particular reference to resource limited settings. Available at: http://www.who.int/HIV_AIDS/ WHO_HSI_2000.04_1.04/index.htm (accessed 11/09/01).

6. Saag MS. Use of HIV viral load in clinical practice: back to the future. *Ann Intern Med* 1997; **126:** 983–5.
7. Cao Y, *et al.* Virologic and immunologic characterization of long-term survivors of human immunodeficiency virus type 1 infection. *N Engl J Med* 1995; **332:** 201–8.
8. Bryson YJ, *et al.* Clearance of HIV infection in a perinatally infected infant. *N Engl J Med* 1995; **332:** 833–8.
9. Bradbury J. HIV-1-resistant individuals may lack HIV-1 coreceptor. *Lancet* 1996; **348:** 463. Correction. *ibid.*; 626.
10. NIH Panel. Guidelines for the use of antiretroviral agents in HIV-infected adults and adolescents. *Ann Intern Med* 1998; **128** (suppl): 1079–1100.
11. NIH Panel. Report of the NIH Panel to define principles of therapy of HIV infection. *Ann Intern Med* 1998; **128** (suppl): 1057–78.
12. Carpenter CCJ, *et al.* Antiretroviral therapy in adults: updated recommendations of the International AIDS Society—USA Panel. *JAMA* 2000; **283:** 381–90.
13. Centers for Disease Control. Guidelines for the use of antiretroviral agents in pediatric HIV infection. *MMWR* 1998; **47** (RR-4): 1–31.
14. HIV/AIDS Treatment Information Service. Guidelines for the use of antiretroviral agents in HIV-infected adults and adolescents. Available at: http://www.hivatis.org (accessed 11/09/01).
15. BHIVA Writing Committee. British HIV Association (BHIVA) guidelines for the treatment of HIV-infected adults with antiretroviral therapy. Available at: http://www.aidsmap.com/about/ bhiva/guidelines.pdf (accessed 11/09/01).
16. Walker BD, Basgoz N. Treat HIV-1 infection like other infections—treat it. *JAMA* 1998; **280:** 91–3.
17. Burman WJ, *et al.* The case for conservative management of early HIV disease. *JAMA* 1998; **280:** 93–5.
18. Levy JA. Caution: should we be treating HIV infection early? *Lancet* 1998; **352:** 982–3.
19. Kahn JO, Walker BD. Acute human immunodeficiency virus type 1 infection. *N Engl J Med* 1998; **339:** 33–9.
20. De Clercq E. HIV inhibitors targeted at the reverse transcriptase. *AIDS Res Hum Retroviruses* 1992; **8:** 119–34.
21. Sommadossi J-P. Nucleoside analogs: similarities and differences. *Clin Infect Dis* 1993; **16** (suppl 1): S7–S15.
22. Robins T, Plattner J. HIV protease inhibitors: their anti-HIV activity and potential role in treatment. *J Acquir Immune Defic Syndr* 1993; **6:** 162–70.
23. Deeks SG, *et al.* HIV-1 protease inhibitors: a review for clinicians. *JAMA* 1997; **277:** 145–53.
24. Anonymous. Update on AIDS. *WHO Drug Inf* 1995; **9:** 196–201.
25. Pauwels R, *et al.* New tetrahydroimidazo[4,5,1-jk][1,4]-benzodiazepin-2(1H)-one and -thione derivatives are potent inhibitors of human immunodeficiency virus type 1 replication and are synergistic with 2′,3′-dideoxynucleoside analogs. *Antimicrob Agents Chemother* 1994; **38:** 2863–70.
26. Levy J, *et al.* Passive hyperimmune plasma therapy in the treatment of acquired immunodeficiency syndrome: results of a 12-month multicenter double-blind controlled trial. *Blood* 1994; **84:** 2130–5.
27. Bridges SH, Sarver N. Gene therapy and immune restoration for HIV disease. *Lancet* 1995; **345:** 427–32.
28. Chen J-D, *et al.* Intra- and extracellular immunization against HIV-1 infection with lymphocytes transduced with an AAV vector expressing a human anti-gp120 antibody. *Hum Gene Ther* 1996; **7:** 1515–25.
29. Akhtar S, Rossi JJ. Anti-HIV therapy with antisense oligonucleotides and ribozymes: realistic approaches or expensive myths? *J Antimicrob Chemother* 1996; **38:** 159–65.
30. Rowe PM. Ribozymes enter clinical trials for HIV-1 treatment. *Lancet* 1996; **348:** 1302.
31. Portegies P, *et al.* Declining incidence of AIDS dementia complex after introduction of zidovudine treatment. *BMJ* 1989; **299:** 819–21. Correction. *ibid.*; 1141.
32. Schmitt FA, *et al.* Neuropsychological outcome of zidovudine (AZT) treatment of patients with AIDS and AIDS-related complex. *N Engl J Med* 1988; **319:** 1573–8.
33. Fischl MA, *et al.* The efficacy of azidothymidine (AZT) in the treatment of patients with AIDS and AIDS-related complex: a double-blind, placebo-controlled trial. *N Engl J Med* 1987; **317:** 185–91.
34. Dournon E, *et al.* Effects of zidovudine in 365 consecutive patients with AIDS or AIDS-related complex. *Lancet* 1988; **ii:** 1297–1302.
35. Lundgren JD, *et al.* Comparison of long-term prognosis of patients with AIDS treated and not treated with zidovudine. *JAMA* 1994; **271:** 1088–92.
36. Graham NMH, *et al.* The effects on survival of early treatment of human immunodeficiency virus infection. *N Engl J Med* 1992; **326:** 1037–42.
37. Fischl MA, *et al.* The safety and efficacy of zidovudine (AZT) in the treatment of subjects with mildly symptomatic human immunodeficiency virus type 1 (HIV) infection: a double-blind, placebo-controlled trial. *Ann Intern Med* 1990; **112:** 727–37.
38. Volberding PA, *et al.* Zidovudine in asymptomatic human immunodeficiency virus infection: a controlled trial in persons with fewer than 500 CD4-positive cells per cubic millimeter. *N Engl J Med* 1990; **322:** 941–9.
39. Hamilton JD, *et al.* A controlled trial of early versus late treatment with zidovudine in symptomatic human immunodeficiency virus infection. *N Engl J Med* 1992; **326:** 437–43.
40. Cooper DA, *et al.* Zidovudine in persons with asymptomatic HIV infection and CD4+ cell counts greater than 400 per cubic millimeter. *N Engl J Med* 1993; **329:** 297–303.
41. Concorde Coordinating Committee. Concorde: MRC/ANRS randomised double-blind controlled trial of immediate and deferred zidovudine in symptom-free HIV infection. *Lancet* 1994; **343:** 871–81.
42. Volberding PA, *et al.* The duration of zidovudine benefit in persons with asymptomatic HIV infection: prolonged evaluation of protocol 019 of the AIDS clinical trials group. *JAMA* 1994; **272:** 437–42.
43. Lenderking WR, *et al.* Evaluation of the quality of life associated with zidovudine treatment in asymptomatic human immunodeficiency virus infection. *N Engl J Med* 1994; **330:** 738–43.
44. Kinloch-de-Loës S, *et al.* A controlled trial of zidovudine in primary human immunodeficiency virus infection. *N Engl J Med* 1995; **333:** 408–13.
45. Moyle GJ. Use of viral resistance patterns to antiretroviral drugs in optimising selection of drug combinations and sequences. *Drugs* 1996; **52:** 168–85.

46. Delta Coordinating Committee. Delta: a randomised double-blind controlled trial comparing combination of zidovudine plus didanosine or zalcitabine with zidovudine alone in HIV-infected individuals. *Lancet* 1996; **348:** 283–91.
47. Hammer SM, *et al.* A trial comparing nucleoside monotherapy with combination therapy in HIV-infected adults with CD4 cell counts from 200 to 500 per cubic millimeter. *N Engl J Med* 1996; **335:** 1081–90.
48. Montaner JSG, *et al.* Antiretroviral treatment in 1998. *Lancet* 1998; **352:** 1919–22.
49. Raboud JM, *et al.* Suppression of plasma viral load below 20 copies/mL is required to achieve a long-term response to therapy. *AIDS* 1998; **12:** 1619–24.
50. Kaufmann D, *et al.* CD4-cell count in HIV-1-infected individuals remaining viraemic with highly active antiretroviral therapy (HAART). *Lancet* 1998; **351:** 723–4.
51. Graham BS. Infection with HIV-1. *BMJ* 1998; **317:** 1297–1301.
52. Palella FJ, *et al.* Declining morbidity and mortality among patients with advanced human immunodeficiency virus infection. *N Engl J Med* 1998; **338:** 853–60.
53. Detels R, *et al.* Effectiveness of potent antiretroviral therapy on time to AIDS and death in men with known HIV infection duration. *JAMA* 1998; **280:** 1497–1503.
54. Mocroft A, *et al.* Changing patterns of mortality across Europe in patients infected with HIV-1. *Lancet* 1998; **352:** 1725–30.
55. Ledergerber B, *et al.* Clinical progression and virological failure on highly active antiretroviral therapy in HIV-1 patients: a prospective cohort study. *Lancet* 1999; **353:** 863–8.
56. Gulick RM, *et al.* Simultaneous vs sequential initiation of therapy with indinavir, zidovudine, and lamivudine for HIV-1 infection: 100-week follow-up. *JAMA* 1998; **280:** 35–41.
57. Youle M. Is interruption of HIV therapy always harmful? *J Antimicrob Chemother* 2000; **45:** 137–8.
58. UK NGO AIDS Consortium Working Group on Access to Treatment for HIV in Developing Countries. Access to treatment for HIV in developing countries; statement from international seminar on access to treatment for HIV in developing countries, London, June 5 and 6, 1998. *Lancet* 1998; **352:** 1379–80.
59. Cooper DA, Emery S. Therapeutic strategies for HIV infection—time to think hard. *N Engl J Med* 1998; **339:** 1319–21.
60. Morris K. HAART and host: balancing the response to HIV-1. *Lancet* 1998; **352:** 1686.

HIV-associated infections. Patients with HIV infection and AIDS are at special risk of other infections as a consequence of their impaired cell-mediated immunity. The successful management of such patients depends as much on the prophylaxis and treatment of secondary and opportunistic infections as on the antiretroviral therapy aimed at the primary infection. There is growing concern that infections such as herpesviruses[1] and tuberculosis[2] may promote HIV replication and thereby accelerate the development of immunodeficiency. Some infections have particular significance in AIDS and are regarded as disease-defining events in patients testing positive for HIV.[3] They are: oesophageal candidiasis (p.372), cryptococcal meningitis (p.373), severe or recurrent pneumonia (p.135), and tuberculosis (p.143). Other common AIDS-related infections include mucosal candidiasis (p.372), coccidioidomycosis (p.373), cryptococcosis (p.373), herpesvirus infections (above), histoplasmosis (p.374), disseminated *Mycobacterium avium* complex infections (p.131), *Pneumocystis carinii* pneumonia (p.375), syphilis (p.141), and toxoplasmosis (p.585). Cytomegalovirus retinitis (above) is a common cause of blindness. Cryptosporidiosis (p.583) and microsporidiosis (p.585) have been identified as common causes of diarrhoea (see also below). Papovavirus infection can cause progressive multifocal leucoencephalopathy (see Infections in Immunocompromised Patients, below). Recommendations for both treatment[4,5] and infection prophylaxis in AIDS patients who have not previously contracted an opportunistic infection (primary prophylaxis) and following treatment of an infection (secondary prophylaxis) have been published.[6,7] Improvements in opportunistic infections have been reported in patients receiving combination antiretroviral therapy containing HIV-protease inhibitors.[8] Recovery of immune function in patients responding to intensive antiretroviral combination therapy may be sufficient to protect against some opportunistic infections.[9]

1. Wood MJ. Antivirals in the context of HIV disease. *J Antimicrob Chemother* 1996; **37** (suppl B): 97–112.
2. Goletti D, *et al.* Effect of Mycobacterium tuberculosis on HIV replication: role of immune activation. *J Immunol* 1996; **157:** 1271–8.
3. Harries AD, Maher D. *TB/HIV: a clinical manual.* Geneva: WHO, 1996.
4. British Society for Antimicrobial Chemotherapy Working Party. Antifungal chemotherapy in patients with acquired immunodeficiency syndrome. *Lancet* 1992; **340:** 648–51.
5. American Thoracic Society. Fungal infection in HIV-infected persons. *Am J Respir Crit Care Med* 1995; **152:** 816–22.
6. Mijch AM, Quin J. Recommendations for antimicrobial prophylaxis in HIV. *Med J Aust* 1996; **164:** 551.
7. Centers for Disease Control. 1999 USPHS/IDSA guidelines for the prevention of opportunistic infections in persons infected with human immunodeficiency virus. *MMWR* 1999; **48** (RR-10): 1–59.
8. Carr A, *et al.* Treatment of HIV-1-associated microsporidiosis and cryptosporidiosis with combination antiretroviral therapy. *Lancet* 1998; **351:** 256–61.
9. Powderly WG, *et al.* Recovery of the immune system with antiretroviral therapy: the end of opportunism? *JAMA* 1998; **280:** 72–7.

HIV-associated malignancies. There is an increased incidence of some malignancies in patients with the long-term immunodeficiency related to HIV infection. The malignancies most frequently associated with HIV infection are Kaposi's sarcoma (p.501), and non-Hodgkin's lymphoma and primary CNS lymphoma (see AIDS-related Lymphomas, p.488). In addition, invasive cervical cancer (p.492) may occur in a particularly aggressive form and this and Kaposi's sarcoma are classified as AIDS-defining events in patients testing positive for HIV. Other malignancies which may be associated with AIDS include Hodgkin's lymphoma (p.487) and, in some patient populations, tumours of the anus and rectum (see Malignant Neoplasms of the Gastrointestinal Tract p.493). Tumours may regress or the range of malignancies may change in patients responding to intensive antiretroviral combination therapy.

References.
1. Tirelli U, *et al.* Malignant tumours in patients with HIV infection. *BMJ* 1994; **308:** 1148–53.
2. Denton AS, Spittle MF. Management of malignancy in HIV infection. *J Antimicrob Chemother* 1996; **37** (suppl B): 121–33.
3. Milliken ST, *et al.* HIV-related lymphoma and other malignancies. *Med J Aust* 1996; **164:** 489–91.
4. Schulz TF, *et al.* HIV infection and neoplasia. *Lancet* 1996; **348:** 587–91.
5. Frisch M, *et al.* Association of cancer with AIDS-related immunosuppression in adults. *JAMA* 2001; **285:** 1736–45.
6. Little RF, *et al.* HIV-associated non-Hodgkin lymphoma: incidence, presentation, and prognosis. *JAMA* 2001; **285:** 1880–5.

HIV-associated neurological complications. Neurological complications of HIV infection can arise from opportunistic infections of the CNS, auto-immune disorders, HIV infection of the CNS, malignancies, and metabolic or drug toxicities.

AIDS dementia complex (HIV-1-associated cognitive/motor complex) and related transient neurological deficits occur mainly in patients with late HIV infection and severe immunodepression. It is thought to be due to HIV infection of the brain and there is evidence to suggest that antiretroviral therapy may have both prophylactic and therapeutic benefits. While most studies have used high-dose zidovudine, anecdotal reports suggest that intensive antiretroviral combination therapy may also be beneficial.

HIV headache is not well understood and occurs in late HIV infections. Headache can also be a symptom of meningitis.

Neuropathies may result from auto-immune mechanisms (for example idiopathic demyelinating neuropathies), cytomegalovirus infection, or HIV infection. One of the commonest is distal predominantly sensory polyneuropathy seen in the late stages of the disease. Effective antiretroviral combination therapy has produced improvement of neuropathies in some patients although toxicity caused by some antiretrovirals can produce similar symptoms.

Progressive multifocal leucoencephalopathy due to papovavirus infection is discussed under Infections in Immunocompromised Patients, below.

References.
1. Simpson DM, Tagliati M. Neurologic manifestations of HIV infection. *Ann Intern Med* 1994; **121:** 769–85. Correction. *ibid.* 1995; **122:** 317.
2. Wright EJ, *et al.* HIV-induced neurological disease. *Med J Aust* 1996; **164:** 414–17.
3. Price RW. Neurological complications of HIV infection. *Lancet* 1996; **348:** 445–52.
4. Brew BJ, Miller J. Human immunodeficiency virus type 1-related transient neurological deficits. *Am J Med* 1996; **101:** 257–61.
5. Melton ST, *et al.* Pharmacotherapy of HIV dementia. *Ann Pharmacother* 1997; **31:** 457–73.
6. Skolnick AA. Protease inhibitors may reverse AIDS dementia. *JAMA* 1998; **279:** 419.
7. Gendelman HE, *et al.* Suppression of inflammatory neurotoxins by highly active antiretroviral therapy in human immunodeficiency virus-associated dementia. *J Infect Dis* 1998; **178:** 1000–1007.
8. Markus R, Brew BJ. HIV-1 peripheral neuropathy and combination antiretroviral therapy. *Lancet* 1998; **352:** 1906–7.
9. Wulff EA, *et al.* HIV-associated peripheral neuropathy: epidemiology, pathophysiology and treatment. *Drugs* 2000; **59:** 1251–60.

HIV-associated wasting and diarrhoea. Diarrhoea and the wasting syndrome (with weight loss and cachexia) are major contributors to the morbidity and mortality of late HIV infection and AIDS, particularly in Africa where the syndrome has been termed 'slim disease'. Although the pathology is poorly understood, opportunistic infections, principally with Microsporidia and Cryptosporidia, cytomegalovirus, and *Mycobacterium avium-intracellulare*, are the most common causes of diarrhoea, while histopathological changes in the small bowel mucosa may also contribute. Malnutrition is thought to be a more likely cause of wasting than increased resting energy expenditure although nutritional supplementation is not consistently effective. Management of diarrhoea relies primarily on rehydration, antidiarrhoeal drugs, and antimicrobial treatment. If no causative pathogen is identified, elimination of common bacterial pathogens by empirical treatment with a fluoroquinolone such as ciprofloxacin has been suggested. Albendazole has also produced beneficial responses when given empirically. Details of specific management of the common infections are on p.583 (Cryptosporidiosis), p.606 (Cytomegalovirus Infections), p.585 (Microsporidiosis), and p.131 (Opportunistic Mycobacterial Infections). Other common microbial causes of diarrhoea are dealt with under Gastro-enteritis on p.121 (bacterial), p.583 (protozoal), and p.606 (viral). The use of antidiarrhoeals and rehydration techniques is discussed under Diarrhoea, p.1203. Antisecretory drugs such as octreotide have been tried with some success but are unlikely to have a wide role in the treatment of HIV-associated diarrhoea. Recombinant growth hormone has been suggested for cachectic patients who do not respond to nutritional supplementation. Other drugs tried in cachexia include megestrol and dronabinol (as appetite stimulants), the growth hormone mediator mecasermin, testosterone, and drugs that decrease cytokine production including oxpentifylline [pentoxifylline] and thalidomide.

References.
1. Von Roenn JH. Management of HIV-related bodyweight loss. *Drugs* 1994; **47:** 774–83.
2. Weinroth SE, *et al.* Wasting syndrome in AIDS: pathophysiologic mechanisms and therapeutic approaches. *Infect Agents Dis* 1995; **4:** 76–94.
3. DuPont HL, Marshall GD. HIV-associated diarrhoea and wasting. *Lancet* 1995; **346:** 352–6.
4. Grunfeld C. What causes wasting in AIDS? *N Engl J Med* 1995; **333:** 123–4.
5. Sharpstone D, Gazzard B. Gastrointestinal manifestations of HIV infection. *Lancet* 1996; **348:** 379–83.
6. Corcoran C, Grinspoon S. Treatments for wasting in patients with the acquired immunodeficiency syndrome. *N Engl J Med* 1999; **340:** 1740–50. Correction. *ibid.;* **341:** 776.
7. Nemechek PM, *et al.* Treatment guidelines for HIV-associated wasting. *Mayo Clin Proc* 2000; **75:** 386–94.

HIV infection prophylaxis

Despite remaining uncertainties over the efficacy and toxicity of prophylactic antiretroviral regimens following accidental exposure to HIV, they are becoming more widely accepted, particularly after **occupational exposure.**[1] Zidovudine has been commonly used, and has been reported[2] to reduce seroconversion after percutaneous exposure by 79%, but there are case reports of seroconversion,[3-6] including some where zidovudine was given within an hour of exposure.[5,6] The risk of seroconversion is estimated at about 0.3 to 0.4% following percutaneous contamination with HIV-infected blood[4,7,8] and considerably less for accidents involving contamination of intact skin or mucous membranes.[7,8] In view of short-term and potential long-term toxicity of antiretrovirals, chemoprophylaxis should only be offered to high-risk cases.[9] If chemoprophylaxis is given it should preferably be started as soon as possible after the accident. In the UK,[10] guidelines recommend that prophylaxis with a combination of zidovudine 200 mg three times daily (or 250 mg twice daily), lamivudine 150 mg twice daily, and indinavir 800 mg three times daily should be offered for 4 weeks following occupational percutaneous, mucous membrane, or broken skin site exposure to high-risk body fluids or tissues known to be, or strongly suspected of being, infected with HIV. Nelfinavir or saquinavir are considered suitable alternatives to indinavir to improve tolerability of the regimen. The US[7] guidelines recommend a two-drug regimen of zidovudine 600 mg daily in divided doses plus lamivudine 150 mg twice daily when there is a recognised risk of transmission, indinavir 800 mg every 8 hours or nelfinavir 750 mg three times daily being added for exposure with an increased risk for transmission. They also recommend that such treatment should continue for 4 weeks, if tolerated. Serious adverse effects have been reported following the use of regimens containing nevirapine.[11]

Hygienic measures and behavioural changes are the most effective methods of **reducing the spread of HIV infection in the general population.**[12,13] These include needle exchange schemes for intravenous drug abusers and the promotion of safe-sex practices. There is some evidence that heterosexual transmission may be inhibited if the infected partner is receiving zidovudine.[14] However transmission is only reduced by about 50%, and zidovudine treatment does not obviate the need for behavioural changes to reduce the risk of transmission. Prophylaxis following sexual exposure similar to that following occupational exposure has also been proposed,[15] although the disadvantages of antiretroviral prophylaxis in this setting may outweigh the advantages.[16,17] Vaccination against HIV infection is being investigated, but it is not clear yet if this is a feasible approach.

Measures aimed at **reducing vertical transmission** from mothers with HIV infection to their infants include perinatal chemotherapy and discouraging breast feeding. The Pediatric AIDS Clinical Trial Group protocol 076 (ACTG 076) study[18] of zidovudine therapy during pregnancy, labour, and given to the infant postpartum was stopped prematurely when good preliminary results were observed. Further analysis[19] of the results of ACTG 076 showed that the risk of vertical transmission was reduced regardless of the maternal viral load or CD4+ count. The protocol, which involved starting oral zidovudine at 14 to 34 weeks' gestation, giving the mother an intravenous dose at birth, and administering zidovudine to the infant for 6 weeks, has been widely adopted in the USA.[20,21] However, short-course oral therapy comprising less frequent doses given from 36 weeks' gestation, oral doses during labour and without treatment of the infant has also been shown to cut transmission,[22-24] and may be more appropriate for use in developing countries. There is also evidence that prophylactic zidovudine begun as late as the first 48 hours of life may still be of benefit in reducing vertical transmission.[25] Nevirapine given in single doses to the mother before delivery and to the neonate has also been shown to reduce transmission.[26] Maternal vitamin A deficiency has been identified as a risk factor for vertical transmission in Africa (see p.1384). Nutritional intervention and vaginal cleansing during labour could reduce vertical transmission in a region where zidovudine therapy is not readily available.

Other measures necessary to minimise the transmission of infection include the rigorous selection of blood donors, microbiological screening of the blood, and, where possible, heat treatment of blood products.

1. Henderson DK. Postexposure chemoprophylaxis for occupational exposures to the human immunodeficiency virus. *JAMA* 1999; **281**: 931–6.
2. Centers for Disease Control. Case-control study of HIV seroconversion in health-care workers after percutaneous exposure to HIV-infected blood—France, United Kingdom, and United States, January 1988–August 1994. *MMWR* 1995; **44**: 929–33.
3. Looke DFM, Grove DI. Failed prophylactic zidovudine after needlestick injury. *Lancet* 1990; **335**: 1280.
4. Tokars JI, *et al*. Surveillance of HIV infection and zidovudine use among health care workers after occupational exposure to HIV-infected blood. *Ann Intern Med* 1993; **118**: 913–19.
5. Lange JMA, *et al*. Failure of zidovudine prophylaxis after accidental exposure to HIV-1. *N Engl J Med* 1990; **322**: 1375–7.
6. Anonymous. HIV seroconversion after occupational exposure despite early prophylactic zidovudine therapy. *Lancet* 1993; **341**: 1077–8.
7. Centers for Disease Control. Public Health Service guidelines for the management of health-care worker exposures to HIV and recommendations for postexposure prophylaxis. *MMWR* 1998; **47** (RR-7): 1–33.
8. Jeffries DJ. Zidovudine after occupational exposure to HIV. *BMJ* 1991; **302**: 1349–51.
9. Easterbrook P, Ippolito G. Prophylaxis after occupational exposure to HIV. *BMJ* 1997; **315**: 557–8.
10. UK Health Departments. HIV post-exposure prophylaxis: guidance from the UK Chief Medical Officers' Expert Advisory Group on AIDS. London: Department of Health, 2000. Available at: www.doh.gov.uk/eaga/pepgu20fin.pdf (accessed 13/09/01).
11. Centers for Disease Control. Serious adverse events attributed to nevirapine regimens for postexposure prophylaxis after HIV exposure—worldwide, 1997-2000. *MMWR* 2001; **49**: 1153–6.
12. Coates TJ, *et al*. HIV prevention in developed countries. *Lancet* 1996; **348**: 1143–8.
13. d'Cruz-Grote D. Prevention of HIV infection in developing countries. *Lancet* 1996; **348**: 1071–4.
14. Musicco M, *et al*. Antiretroviral treatment of men infected with human immunodeficiency virus type 1 reduces the incidence of heterosexual transmission. *Arch Intern Med* 1994; **154**: 1971–6.
15. Katz MH, Gerberding JL. The care of persons with recent sexual exposure to HIV. *Ann Intern Med* 1998; **128**: 306–12.
16. Centers for Disease Control. Management of possible sexual, injecting-drug-use, or other nonoccupational exposure to HIV, including considerations related to antiretroviral therapy: Public Health Service statement. *MMWR* 1998; **47** (RR-17): 1–14.
17. Lurie P, *et al*. Postexposure prophylaxis after nonoccupational HIV exposure: clinical, ethical, and policy considerations. *JAMA* 1998; **280**: 1769–73.
18. Connor EM, *et al*. Reduction of maternal-infant transmission of human immunodeficiency virus type 1 with zidovudine treatment. *N Engl J Med* 1994; **331**: 1173–80.
19. Sperling RS, *et al*. Maternal viral load, zidovudine treatment, and the risk of transmission of human immunodeficiency virus type 1 from mother to infant. *N Engl J Med* 1996; **335**: 1621–9.
20. Centers for Disease Control. Public Health Service Task Force recommendations for the use of antiretroviral drugs in pregnant women infected with HIV-1 for maternal health and for reducing perinatal HIV-1 transmission in the United States. *MMWR* 1998; **47** (RR-2): 1–30.
21. Perinatal HIV Guidelines Working Group. Public health service task force recommendations for use of antiretroviral drugs in pregnant HIV-1-infected women for maternal health and interventions to reduce perinatal HIV-1 transmission in the United States. Available at: www.hivatis.org/guidelines/perinatal/May03_01/PerinatalMay04_01.pdf (accessed 13/09/01).
22. Shaffer N, *et al*. Short-course zidovudine for perinatal HIV-1 transmission in Bangkok, Thailand: a randomised controlled trial. *Lancet* 1999; **353**: 773–80.
23. Wiktor SZ, *et al*. Short-course oral zidovudine for prevention of mother-to-child transmission of HIV-1 in Abidjan, Côte d'Ivoire: a randomised trial. *Lancet* 1999; **353**: 781–5.
24. Dabis F, *et al*. 6-Month efficacy, tolerance, and acceptability of a short regimen of oral zidovudine to reduce vertical transmission of HIV in breastfed children in Côte d'Ivoire and Burkina Faso: a double-blind placebo-controlled multicentre trial. *Lancet* 1999; **353**: 786–92.
25. Wade NA, *et al*. Abbreviated regimens of zidovudine prophylaxis and perinatal transmission of the human immunodeficiency virus. *N Engl J Med* 1998; **339**: 1409–14.
26. Guay LA, *et al*. Intrapartum and neonatal single-dose nevirapine compared with zidovudine for prevention of mother-to-child transmission of HIV-1 in Kampala, Uganda: HIVNET 012 randomised trial. *Lancet* 1999; **354**: 795–802.

Infections in immunocompromised patients

Most viral infections present in a more severe form in immunocompromised patients than in immunocompetent patients. Among the viral infections that may be a particular problem in immunocompromised patients are hepatitis, herpesvirus infections (including cytomegalovirus and Epstein-Barr virus infections), measles, and respiratory syncytial virus infections. For further information and treatment of these infections, see under the individual diseases. For secondary infections occurring in HIV-infected patients, see above. The management of viral infections in transplant patients[1] and in neutropenic patients[2] has been reviewed.

Persistent infection with human **parvovirus B19** can cause red cell aplasia with resultant anaemia particularly in immunocompromised patients; treatment with high doses of immunoglobulin has been reported to be successful.[3]

Infection with a papovavirus (JC virus)[4,5] can cause **progressive multifocal leucoencephalopathy**. Although no treatment has been consistently successful,[4] prolonged survival has been reported in patients receiving interferon alfa[6] and in those receiving highly active antiretroviral therapy.[7-9]

1. Griffiths PD. Viral complications after transplantation. *J Antimicrob Chemother* 1995; **36** (suppl B): 91–106.
2. Wood MJ. Viral infections in neutropenia—current problems and chemotherapeutic control. *J Antimicrob Chemother* 1998; **41** (suppl D): 81–93.
3. Cohen B. Parvovirus B19: an expanding spectrum of disease. *BMJ* 1995; **311**: 1549–52.
4. Brink NS, Miller RF. Clinical presentation, diagnosis and therapy of progressive multifocal leukoencephalopathy. *J Infect* 1996; **32**: 97–102.
5. Greenlee JE. Progressive multifocal leukoencephalopathy—progress made and lessons relearned. *N Engl J Med* 1998; **338**: 1378–80.
6. Huang SS, *et al*. Survival prolongation in HIV-associated progressive multifocal leukoencephalopathy treated with alpha-interferon: an observational study. *J Neurovirol* 1998; **4**: 324–32.
7. Albrecht H, *et al*. Highly active antiretroviral therapy significantly improves the prognosis of patients with HIV-associated progressive multifocal leukoencephalopathy. *AIDS* 1998; **12**: 1149–54.
8. Elliot B, *et al*. 2.5 Year remission of AIDS-associated progressive multifocal leukoencephalopathy with combined antiretroviral therapy. *Lancet* 1997; **349**: 850.
9. Domingo P, *et al*. Remission of progressive multifocal leucoencephalopathy after antiretroviral therapy. *Lancet* 1997; **349**: 1554–5.

Influenza

Influenza is caused by RNA viruses of the family Orthomyxoviridae. Three types of influenza virus, A, B, and C, have been classified. Type A causes most infections in man; type B causes a similar though possibly milder infection than type A; type C causes only a mild infection. Epidemic influenza is usually caused by the type A influenza virus. Outbreaks of influenza due to the type A virus occur in most years while those due to the type B virus tend to occur at intervals of several years. Influenza viruses, especially influenza A, are antigenically labile with the principal surface antigens, haemagglutinin and neuraminidase, undergoing antigenic changes. Major changes (antigenic shifts) in these surface antigens of the influenza A virus occur periodically and are responsible for the emergence of the subtypes of virus which may cause pandemic influenza; more minor changes (antigenic drift) occur more frequently and are responsible for the annual epidemic outbreaks of influenza.

Influenza is transmitted from person to person in respiratory droplets. Infection with influenza A or B virus typically causes fever, chills, headache, malaise, myalgia, dry cough, nasal obstruction, and a dry or sore throat. Such infections are usually acute but self-limiting. Complications can occur though, and include primary viral pneumonia, secondary bacterial pneumonia, croup, exacerbation of asthma or chronic bronchitis, myositis, Reye's syndrome, and the toxic shock syndrome. Patients at high risk of complications include the elderly and those with heart and chronic chest disease.

Treatment of influenza is largely symptomatic and supportive. Amantadine and rimantadine have both been shown to reduce the duration of influenza A symptoms when given within 48 hours of the onset of symptoms and may be given to high-risk patients. Treatment and prophylaxis failures may be due to the rapid emergence of drug-resistant viruses. Oseltamivir and zanamivir, which inhibit viral neuraminidase, are active against both influenza A and B viruses, and are used for treatment. Response to ribavirin has generally been disappointing.

The most effective means of preventing influenza is with influenza vaccine adjusted to take account of current antigenic drifts and shifts and to provide protection against both influenza A and B. Amantadine and rimantadine are also effective at preventing influenza A but are not a substitute for vaccination unless the vaccine is contra-indicated. Prophylaxis with amantadine or rimantadine should be considered in addition to vaccination in individuals such as the immunosuppressed whose antibody response to the vaccine is likely to be incomplete, in persons vaccinated after an influenza outbreak has begun, and in residents and carers in institutions to prevent or abort outbreaks of influenza. To be fully effective chemoprophylaxis must be started as early as possible and be taken each day for the duration of influenza activity or until an adequate antibody response to vaccination has occurred. Neuraminidase inhibitors may also be useful for prophylaxis.

References.

1. Couch RB. Prevention and treatment of influenza. *N Engl J Med* 2000; **343**: 1778–87.
2. Jefferson T, *et al*. Neuraminidase inhibitors for preventing and treating influenza in healthy adults (updated 26 July 2001). Available in The Cochrane Library; Issue 4. Oxford: Update Software; 2001.
3. Jefferson TO, *et al*. Amantadine and rimantadine for preventing and treating influenza A in adults (updated 18 July 2001). Available in The Cochrane Library; Issue 4. Oxford: Update Software; 2001.

Measles

Measles is caused by an RNA virus of the family Paramyxoviridae. It is a highly contagious disease spread by direct contact with respiratory secretions of infected persons allowing the virus to invade the upper respiratory tract, nose, and possibly the conjunctivae. During the prodromal phase patients usually experience malaise, fever, conjunctivitis, cough, rhinitis, congestion, and later Koplik's spots on the buccal mucosa. An erythematous, maculopapular rash then develops starting on the face and spreading over the trunk and limbs. Immunocompromised patients are at special risk of respiratory and central complications. Recovery usually takes place during the week following the rash's appearance. However, potentially fatal complications may develop, especially in immunocompromised patients. There may be respiratory complications including giant cell pneumonia and bacterial and viral superinfections, and central complications including acute encephalitis, a progressive subacute encephalitis, and the more slowly progressive subacute sclerosing panencephalitis (SSPE) that may develop several years after the original measles infection.

Measles usually requires only symptomatic and supportive treatment.[1] Administration of vitamin A supplements to prevent complications from measles is well established in children in developing countries and may be beneficial in children in developed countries (see p.1383). The use of prophylactic antibacterials has not been supported by clinical trials.[2] There appears to be no good evidence for antiviral drugs being effective in the complications of measles.

Measles can be prevented by active immunisation with measles vaccine, and measles immunoglobulins may be used for passive immunisation against measles. Normal immunoglobulins may be used to prevent, or possibly modify, an attack of measles in those at risk of developing severe or fatal disease such as immunocompromised patients.

1. Hussey G. Managing measles. *BMJ* 1997; **314**: 316–17.
2. Shann F. Meta-analysis of trials of prophylactic antibiotics for children with measles: inadequate evidence. *BMJ* 1997; **314**: 334–7.

Respiratory syncytial virus infection

Respiratory syncytial virus (RSV) is an RNA virus of the family Paramyxoviridae. RSV infection is generally confined to the respiratory tract, occurs in young children, and is increasingly recognised as a common infection in the elderly. Acquired immunity is incomplete and of short duration and therefore re-infection is common. In young children the infection generally spreads to the lower respiratory-tract and may cause bronchiolitis and pneumonia which can be life-threatening. In older children and adults infection occurs as an upper respiratory-tract illness or tracheobronchitis. Severe or complicated infection is more common in children with underlying cardiac or pulmonary disease and in immunocompromised patients.

The management of RSV infection is largely supportive.[1-4] Supplementary oxygen is useful in patients with bronchiolitis. Measures to limit the spread of infection in hospitals and institutions through attention to good hygiene and control of cross-infection are important.[5-7] Ribavirin administered by aerosol has been shown to have beneficial effects in infants with lower respiratory-tract RSV infection, but trials lack sufficient power to provide reliable estimates of the effects and further study is needed.[8] The American Academy of Pediatrics has modified its recommendation[9] for use of ribavirin in the treatment of RSV infection in infants and children at high risk of developing severe or complicated disease to make ribavirin treatment discretionary.[10] Ribavirin is less frequently used in the UK and some[2] suggest its use be restricted to patients with RSV and cystic fibrosis, severe immunodeficiency, congenital heart disease and pulmonary hypertension, and patients with bronchopulmonary dysplasia and dependence on supplementary oxygen. Similarly, bronchodilators are reported to be more commonly used for RSV bronchiolitis in the USA than in the UK.[2] The difference in clinical management could result from differences in diagnostic criteria for bronchiolitis.[2,11] It has also been considered that the evidence of efficacy of bronchodilators in bronchiolitis is uncertain.[12] Corticosteroids are deemed to be of no value.[1,2,13-15]

Respiratory syncytial virus immunoglobulin or a human monoclonal antibody to RSV, palivizumab, is recommended in the USA for prophylaxis in infants and children at high risk of severe RSV infections, excepting those with cyanotic congenital heart disease.[16,17] RSV immunoglobulin has not, however, been found to be effective in the treatment of RSV infections.[18]

Vaccines to prevent RSV infection are currently under development.

1. Everard ML. Bronchiolitis: origins and optimal management. *Drugs* 1995; **49:** 885–96.
2. Rakshi K, Couriel JM. Management of acute bronchiolitis. *Arch Dis Child* 1994; **71:** 463–9.
3. Rodriguez WJ. Management strategies for respiratory syncytial virus infections in infants. *J Pediatr* 1999; **135:** S45–S50.
4. Simoes EAF. Respiratory syncytial virus infection. *Lancet* 1999; **354:** 847–52.
5. Madge P, et al. Prospective controlled study of four infection-control procedures to prevent nosocomial infection with respiratory syncytial virus. *Lancet* 1992; **340:** 1079–83.
6. O'Callaghan CA. Prevention of nosocomial respiratory syncytial virus infection. *Lancet* 1993; **341:** 182.
7. Madge P, et al. Prevention of nosocomial respiratory syncytial virus infection. *Lancet* 1993; **341:** 183.
8. Randolph AG, Wang EEL. Ribavirin for respiratory syncytial virus infection of the lower respiratory tract (updated 26 July 2001). Available in The Cochrane Library; Issue 4. Oxford: Update Software; 2001.
9. American Academy of Pediatrics, Committee on Infectious Diseases. Use of ribavirin in the treatment of respiratory syncytial virus infection. *Pediatrics* 1993; **92:** 501–4.
10. American Academy of Pediatrics, Committee on Infectious Diseases. Reassessment of the indications for ribavirin therapy in respiratory syncytial virus infections. *Pediatrics* 1996; **97:** 137–40.
11. Everard ML. Acute bronchiolitis—a perennial problem. *Lancet* 1996; **348:** 279–80.
12. Kellner JD, et al. Bronchodilators for bronchiolitis (updated 28 August 2001). Available in The Cochrane Library; Issue 4. Oxford: Update Software; 2001.
13. Isaacs D. Bronchiolitis. *BMJ* 1995; **310:** 4–5.
14. Roosevelt G, et al. Dexamethasone in bronchiolitis: a randomised controlled trial. *Lancet* 1996; **348:** 292–5.
15. Cade A, et al. Randomised placebo controlled trial of nebulised corticosteroids in acute respiratory syncytial viral bronchiolitis. *Arch Dis Child* 2000; **82:** 126–30.
16. Committee on Infectious Diseases, Committee on Fetus and Newborn American Academy of Pediatrics. Respiratory syncytial virus immune globulin intravenous: indications for use. *Pediatrics* 1997; **99:** 645–50.
17. Committee on Infectious Diseases and Committee on Fetus and Newborn, American Academy of Pediatrics. Prevention of respiratory syncytial virus infections: indications for the use of palivizumab and update on the use of RSV-IGIV. *Pediatrics* 1998; **102:** 1211–16.
18. Rodriguez WJ, et al. Respiratory syncytial virus (RSV) immune globulin intravenous therapy for RSV lower respiratory tract infection in infants and young children at high risk for severe RSV infections. *Pediatrics* 1997; **99:** 454–61.

Warts

Warts are caused by human papillomaviruses. The lesions present in several different forms and can affect any skin site although the hands, feet, and anogenital areas are most frequently affected. Anogenital warts are known as condylomata acuminata. Treatment generally relies on some form of local tissue destruction and is described on p.1108. Interferons have also been used (see p.632).

Abacavir (20325-r)

Abacavir *(BAN, rINN)*.

{(1S,4R)-4-[2-Amino-6-(cyclopropylamino)-9H-purin-9-yl]cyclopent-2-enyl}methanol.

$C_{14}H_{18}N_6O = 286.3$.

CAS — 136470-78-5.

ATC — J05AF06.

NOTE. The code 1592U89 has been applied to abacavir but is more properly reserved for abacavir sulfate.

Abacavir Succinate (9702-n)

Abacavir Succinate *(BANM, USAN, rINNM)*.

$C_{14}H_{18}N_6O,C_4H_6O_4 = 404.4$.

CAS — 168146-84-7.

NOTE. The code 1592U89 has been applied to abacavir succinate but is more properly reserved for abacavir sulfate.

Abacavir Sulfate (19949-k)

Abacavir Sulfate *(USAN, rINNM)*.

Abacavir Sulphate *(BANM)*; 1592U89.

$(C_{14}H_{18}N_6O)_2,H_2SO_4 = 670.7$.

CAS — 188062-50-2.

NOTE. The code 1592U89 and its abbreviated form, 1592, have also been applied to abacavir and abacavir succinate.

Adverse Effects

Severe hypersensitivity reactions, sometimes fatal, have occurred in approximately 4% of patients receiving abacavir, especially (but not exclusively) during the first 6 weeks of treatment, or during intermittent therapy. Symptoms of hypersensitivity commonly include fever, rash, cough, dyspnoea, lethargy, malaise, headache, myalgia, and gastrointestinal disturbances, particularly nausea and vomiting, diarrhoea, and abdominal pain. Caution is needed as hypersensitivity may be misdiagnosed as influenza, respiratory disease, or gastroenteritis. Other adverse effects associated with abacavir include pancreatitis and elevated blood glucose and triglyceride concentrations. There may be raised liver enzyme values. Lactic acidosis, sometimes fatal and usually associated with severe hepatomegaly and steatosis, has been reported in patients receiving nucleoside reverse transcriptase inhibitors (see Zidovudine, p.645).

Precautions

Abacavir should be discontinued immediately if symptoms associated with hypersensitivity occur and should *never be recommenced* in patients who have stopped therapy due to a hypersensitivity reaction. Patients should be closely monitored for signs of hypersensitivity during the first two months of treatment, although hypersensitivity reactions can occur at any time. Patients restarting therapy after an interruption are at particular risk even if they have not previously shown symptoms of hypersensitivity. Since intermittent therapy may increase the risk of hypersensitivity developing, patients should be advised of the importance of regular dosing.

Abacavir should not be used in patients with severe hepatic impairment, and should be used with caution in those with lesser degrees of impairment and those with risk factors for liver disease. Treatment should be discontinued if liver function deteriorates rapidly or if hepatomegaly or unexplained metabolic acidosis develop.

Interactions

Administration of abacavir with alcohol may result in decreased elimination of abacavir and consequent increases in the area under the plasma concentration-time curve.

Antiviral Action

Abacavir is converted intracellularly in stages to carbovir triphosphate (GR-90352; NSC-614846). This triphosphate halts the DNA synthesis of retroviruses, including HIV, through competitive inhibition of reverse transcriptase and incorporation into viral DNA.

◊ References.
1. Faletto MB, *et al.* Unique intracellular activation of the potent anti-human immunodeficiency virus agent 1592U89. *Antimicrob Agents Chemother* 1997; **41:** 1099–1107.

Pharmacokinetics

Abacavir is rapidly absorbed following oral administration with a bioavailability of about 80%. Absorption is not affected by food. Abacavir crosses the blood-brain barrier. It is about 50% bound to plasma proteins. The elimination half-life is about 1.5 hours following a single dose. Abacavir undergoes intracellular metabolism to the active antiviral metabolite carbovir triphosphate. Elimination is via hepatic metabolism primarily by alcohol dehydrogenase and by glucuronidation and the metabolites are excreted mainly in the urine. There is no significant metabolism by hepatic cytochrome P450 isoenzymes.

◊ References.
1. Kumar PN, *et al.* Safety and pharmacokinetics of abacavir (1592U89) following oral administration of escalating single doses in human immunodeficiency virus type 1-infected adults. *Antimicrob Agents Chemother* 1999; **43:** 603–8.
2. Hughes W, *et al.* Safety and single-dose pharmacokinetics of abacavir (1592U89) in human immunodeficiency virus type 1-infected children. *Antimicrob Agents Chemother* 1999; **43:** 609–15.
3. Wang LH, *et al.* Single-dose pharmacokinetics and safety of abacavir (1592U89), zidovudine, and lamivudine administered alone and in combination in adults with human immunodeficiency virus infection. *Antimicrob Agents Chemother* 1999; **43:** 1708–15.
4. McDowell JA, *et al.* Multiple-dose pharmacokinetics and pharmacodynamics of abacavir alone and in combination with zidovudine in human immunodeficiency virus-infected adults. *Antimicrob Agents Chemother* 2000; **44:** 2061–7.

Uses and Administration

Abacavir is a nucleoside reverse transcriptase inhibitor with antiretroviral activity against HIV. It is given by mouth as the sulfate in combination with other antiretrovirals in the treatment of HIV infection (p.608). The adult dose is the equivalent of 300 mg of abacavir twice daily. The dose for children over 3 months of age is 8 mg per kg body-weight twice daily up to a maximum of 600 mg daily.

◊ Reviews.
1. Hervey PS, Perry CM. Abacavir: a review of its clinical potential in patients with HIV infection. *Drugs* 2000; **60:** 447–79.

Preparations

Proprietary Preparations (details are given in Part 3)
Austral.: Ziagen; *Canad.:* Ziagen; *Denm.:* Ziagen; *Fin.:* Ziagen; *Fr.:* Ziagen; *Ger.:* Ziagen; *Israel:* Ziagen; *Ital.:* Ziagen; *Norw.:* Ziagen; *NZ:* Ziagen; *Port.:* Ziagen; *Singapore:* Ziagen; *Swed.:* Ziagen; *Switz.:* Ziagen; *UK:* Ziagen; *USA:* Ziagen.

Multi-ingredient: *UK:* Trizivir; *USA:* Trizivir.

Aciclovir (1682-a)

Aciclovir *(BAN, rINN)*.

Aciclovirum; Acycloguanosine; Acyclovir *(USAN)*; BW-248U. 9-[(2-Hydroxyethoxy)methyl]guanine; 2-Amino-1,9-dihydro-9-(2-hydroxyethoxymethyl)-6H-purin-6-one.

$C_8H_{11}N_5O_3 = 225.2$.

CAS — 59277-89-3.

ATC — D06BB03; J05AB01; S01AD03.

Pharmacopoeias. In *Eur.* (see p.vi) and *US*.

Pharmacopoeial description

Ph. Eur.: A white to almost white crystalline powder. Slightly soluble in water; very slightly soluble in alcohol; freely soluble in dimethyl sulfoxide; soluble in dilute solutions of alkali hydroxides and mineral acids.

USP 25: A white to off-white crystalline powder. Slightly soluble in water; insoluble in alcohol; soluble in dilute hydrochloric acid. Store in airtight containers.

Aciclovir Sodium (16177-e)

Aciclovir Sodium *(BANM, rINNM)*.

Acyclovir Sodium *(USAN)*.

$C_8H_{10}N_5NaO_3 = 247.2$.

CAS — 69657-51-8.

A white crystalline powder. **Soluble** more than 1 in 10 of water. Each g of aciclovir sodium represents 4.05 mmol of sodium.

Aciclovir sodium 1.1 g is approximately equivalent to 1 g of aciclovir.

Incompatibility. For references to the incompatibility of aciclovir and foscarnet, see Foscarnet Sodium, p.621.

Stability. References.
1. Zhang Y, *et al.* Stability of acyclovir sodium 1, 7, and 10 mg/mL in 5% dextrose injection and 0.9% sodium chloride injection. *Am J Health-Syst Pharm* 1998; **55:** 574–7.

Adverse Effects

Aciclovir is generally well tolerated. When administered intravenously as aciclovir sodium it may cause local reactions at the injection site with inflammation and phlebitis; these reactions may be associated with extravasation that leads rarely to ulceration. Renal impairment may occur in a few patients; it is usually reversible and is reported to respond to hydration and/or dosage reduction or withdrawal, but may progress to acute renal failure. The risk of renal toxicity is increased by conditions favouring deposition of aciclovir crystals in the tubules such as when the patient is poorly hydrated, has existing renal impairment, or when the drug is given at a high dosage or by rapid or bolus injection. Some patients receiving systemic aciclovir may experience transient increases in blood concentrations of urea and creatinine although this is more acute with intravenous administration.

Occasional adverse effects following systemic administration include increased serum bilirubin and liver enzymes, haematological changes, skin rashes (including erythema multiforme, Stevens-Johnson syndrome, and toxic epidermal necrolysis), fever, headache, dizziness, and gastrointestinal effects such as nausea, vomiting, and diarrhoea. Hepatitis and jaundice have been reported rarely. Neurological effects including lethargy, somnolence, confusion, hallucinations, agitation, tremors, psychosis, convulsions, and coma have been reported in a small number of patients, particularly in those receiving intravenous aciclovir and with predisposing factors such as renal impairment; these effects may be more marked in older patients. Thrombotic thrombocytopenic purpura and haemolytic uraemic syndrome, sometimes resulting in death, have occurred in immunocompromised patients receiving high parenteral doses of aciclovir. Accelerated diffuse hair loss has also been reported.

Topical application of aciclovir, especially to genital lesions, may sometimes produce transient stinging, burning, itching, or erythema. Eye ointments may occasionally produce transient stinging, superficial punctate keratopathy, blepharitis, or conjunctivitis.

◊ References.
1. Bean B, *et al.* Acyclovir therapy for acute herpes zoster. *Lancet* 1982; **ii:** 118–21.
2. Arndt KA. Adverse reactions to acyclovir: topical, oral, and intravenous. *J Am Acad Dermatol* 1988; **18:** 188–90.
3. Robbins MS, *et al.* Acyclovir pH—possible cause of extravasation tissue injury. *Ann Pharmacother* 1993; **27:** 238.

Effects on the blood. There has been no evidence of bone-marrow toxicity in patients given aciclovir following bone-marrow transplantation.[1,2] However, megaloblastic haematopoiesis has been observed in the bone marrow of 3 patients given aciclovir for suspected or proven herpes simplex encephalitis.[3] There has also been a report of inhibition of human peripheral blood lymphocytes in samples taken from healthy subjects given aciclovir.[4]
1. Serota FT, *et al.* Acyclovir treatment of herpes zoster infections: use in children undergoing bone marrow transplantation. *JAMA* 1982; **247:** 2132–5.
2. Gluckman E, *et al.* Oral acyclovir prophylactic treatment of herpes simplex infection after bone marrow transplantation. *J Antimicrob Chemother* 1983; **12** (suppl B): 161–7.
3. Amos RJ, Amess JAL. Megaloblastic haemopoiesis due to acyclovir. *Lancet* 1983; **i:** 242–3.
4. Tauris P, *et al.* Evaluation of the acyclovir-induced modulation of the plaque-forming cell response of human peripheral blood lymphocytes. *J Antimicrob Chemother* 1984; **13:** 71–7.

Effects on the kidneys. Transient renal impairment occurred in 2 adequately hydrated patients following aciclovir 10 mg per kg body-weight infused over 1 hour every 8 hours.[1] In another patient[2] severe acute renal failure occurred following administration of aciclovir 5 mg per kg over 90 minutes daily for 2 days. This reaction did not appear to be related to dosage or manner of administration, but may have been idiosyncratic or immunological.[2] Acute renal failure (with no evidence of crystals) and coma developed in 2 elderly patients receiving high dose oral therapy (800 mg five times daily) with aciclovir.[3,4]
1. Harrington MG, *et al.* Renal impairment and acyclovir. *Lancet* 1981; **ii:** 1281.

2. Giustina A, *et al.* Low-dose acyclovir and acute renal failure. *Ann Intern Med* 1988; **108:** 312.
3. Eck P, *et al.* Acute renal failure and coma after a high dose of oral acyclovir. *N Engl J Med* 1991; **325:** 1178.
4. Johnson GL, *et al.* Acute renal failure and neurotoxicity following oral acyclovir. *Ann Pharmacother* 1994; **28:** 460–3.

Effects on the nervous system. Of 143 patients given aciclovir by intravenous infusion in doses ranging from 0.75 to 3.6 g per m² body-surface daily for the treatment of herpesvirus infections following bone-marrow transplantation, 6 developed reversible neurological symptoms including tremor, agitation, nausea, lethargy, mild disorientation, autonomic instability, hemiparaesthesia, and slurred speech.[1] EEGs were diffusely abnormal in all 6. Symptoms improved in all patients on withdrawing aciclovir; reinstituting aciclovir in 2 produced a recurrence of symptoms. Concomitant therapy included irradiation and methotrexate intrathecally for all 6, interferon alfa for 3, and ciclosporin for 1.

There are individual case reports of neurological and, less frequently, psychiatric adverse effects in patients given intravenous aciclovir.[2-8] Neurological toxicity following oral aciclovir was possibly associated with elevated plasma concentrations in patients with end-stage renal disease.[9,10] The association between plasma-aciclovir concentrations and neurotoxicity has been difficult to establish because of a delay of 24 to 48 hours in the development of symptoms following a concentration peak.[11]
1. Wade JC, Meyers JD. Neurologic symptoms associated with parenteral acyclovir treatment after marrow transplantation. *Ann Intern Med* 1983; **98:** 921–5.
2. Vartian CV, Shlaes DM. Intravenous acyclovir and neurologic effects. *Ann Intern Med* 1983; **99:** 568.
3. Auwerx J, *et al.* Acyclovir and neurologic manifestations. *Ann Intern Med* 1983; **99:** 882–3.
4. Cohen SMZ, *et al.* Severe but reversible neurotoxicity from acyclovir. *Ann Intern Med* 1984; **100:** 920.
5. Tomson CR, *et al.* Psychiatric side-effects of acyclovir in patients with chronic renal failure. *Lancet* 1985; **ii:** 385–6.
6. Bataille P, *et al.* Psychiatric side-effects with acyclovir. *Lancet* 1985; **ii:** 724.
7. Sirota P, *et al.* Major depression with psychotic features associated with acyclovir therapy. *Drug Intell Clin Pharm* 1988; **22:** 306–8.
8. Revankar SG, *et al.* Delirium associated with acyclovir treatment in a patient with renal failure. *Clin Infect Dis* 1995; **21:** 435–6.
9. Swan SK, Bennett WM. Oral acyclovir and neurotoxicity. *Ann Intern Med* 1989; **111:** 188.
10. Mataix AL, *et al.* Oral acyclovir and neurologic adverse effects in endstage renal disease. *Ann Pharmacother* 1994; **28:** 961–2.
11. Haefeli WE, *et al.* Acyclovir-induced neurotoxicity: concentration-side effect relationship in acyclovir overdose. *Am J Med* 1993; **94:** 212–15.

Effects on the skin. A report of vesicular lesions associated with intravenous administration of aciclovir in a patient thought to have herpes simplex encephalitis.[1] Careful evaluation is necessary to differentiate the reaction from herpetic lesions.
1. Buck ML, *et al.* Vesicular eruptions following acyclovir administration. *Ann Pharmacother* 1993; **27:** 1458–9.

Vasculitis. Aciclovir has been associated with vasculitis. In one patient[1] it was one of many drugs given which may have caused a necrotising vasculitis. In another report an immunocompromised child with chickenpox given aciclovir by infusion developed a vasculitic rash which diminished on withdrawal of the drug.[2]
1. von Schulthess GK, Sauter C. Acyclovir and herpes zoster. *N Engl J Med* 1981; **305:** 1349.
2. Platt MPW, Eden OB. Vasculitis in association with chickenpox treatment in childhood acute lymphoblastic leukaemia. *Lancet* 1982; **ii:** 763–4.

Precautions

Aciclovir should be administered with caution to patients with renal impairment and doses should be adjusted according to creatinine clearance (see Administration in Renal Impairment, under Uses and Administration, below). Parenteral administration should be by slow intravenous infusion over one hour to avoid precipitation of aciclovir in the kidney; rapid or bolus injection should be avoided and adequate hydration maintained. The risk of renal impairment is increased by the concomitant use of other nephrotoxic drugs. Intravenous aciclovir should also be used with caution in patients with underlying neurological abnormalities, with significant hypoxia, or with serious hepatic or electrolyte abnormalities.

Breast feeding. The manufacturers report that aciclovir is distributed into breast milk following oral administration. A dose of 200 mg five times daily could expose a suckling infant to 300 µg per kg body-weight daily; caution is therefore recommended when treating nursing mothers.

Pregnancy. The incidence of congenital abnormality and spontaneous fetal loss did not appear to be greater among 312 cases of prenatal exposure to aciclovir than among the general population, and this data was supported by evidence from 145 further retrospective reports.[1]
1. Andrews EB, *et al.* Acyclovir in Pregnancy Registry: six years' experience. *Obstet Gynecol* 1992; **79:** 7–13.

Interactions

Probenecid is reported to block the renal clearance of aciclovir. The risk of renal impairment is increased by the concomitant use of other nephrotoxic drugs.

Antivirals. Combined therapy with *zidovudine* and aciclovir is not generally associated with additional toxicity.[1] However, there is a report[2] of a patient who had overwhelming fatigue when given aciclovir and zidovudine together; no such effect occurred when each drug was given alone.

The manufacturer of *interferon alfa-n1* has reported progressive renal failure in patients also given aciclovir.
1. Tartaglione TA, *et al.* Pharmacokinetic evaluations of low- and high-dose zidovudine plus high-dose acyclovir in patients with symptomatic human immunodeficiency virus infection. *Antimicrob Chemother* 1991; **35:** 2225–31.
2. Bach MC. Possible drug interaction during therapy with azidothymidine and acyclovir for AIDS. *N Engl J Med* 1987; **316:** 547.

Xanthines. For reference to evidence that aciclovir inhibits *theophylline* metabolism, resulting in accumulation, see p.781.

Antiviral Action

Aciclovir is active against herpes simplex virus type 1 and type 2 and against varicella-zoster virus. This activity is due to intracellular conversion of aciclovir by viral thymidine kinase to the monophosphate with subsequent conversion by cellular enzymes to the diphosphate and the active triphosphate. This active form inhibits viral DNA synthesis and replication by inhibiting the herpesvirus DNA polymerase enzyme as well as being incorporated into viral DNA. This process is highly selective for infected cells. Studies in *animals* and *in vitro* show various sensitivities but demonstrate that these viruses are inhibited by concentrations of aciclovir that are readily achieved clinically. Herpes simplex virus type 1 appears to be the most susceptible, then type 2, followed by varicella-zoster virus.

The Epstein-Barr virus and cytomegalovirus are also susceptible to aciclovir to a lesser extent. However, for cytomegalovirus it does not appear to be activated by thymidine kinase and may act via a different mechanism. Epstein-Barr virus may have reduced thymidine kinase activity but its DNA polymerase is very sensitive to inhibition by aciclovir triphosphate, which may account for the partial activity.

Aciclovir has no activity against latent viruses, but there is some evidence that it inhibits latent herpes simplex virus at an early stage of reactivation.

◊ Reviews of the antiviral activity of aciclovir.
1. Elion GB. Mechanism of action and selectivity of acyclovir. *Am J Med* 1982; **73** (suppl 1A): 7–13.
2. Elion GB. The biochemistry and mechanism of action of acyclovir. *J Antimicrob Chemother* 1983; **12** (suppl B): 9–17.
3. Collins P. The spectrum of antiviral activities of acyclovir in vitro and in vivo. *J Antimicrob Chemother* 1983; **12** (suppl B): 19–27.
4. Elion GB. Acyclovir: discovery, mechanism of action, and selectivity. *J Med Virol* 1993; **41** (suppl 1): 2–6.
5. Wagstaff AJ, *et al.* Aciclovir: a reappraisal of its antiviral activity, pharmacokinetic properties and therapeutic efficacy. *Drugs* 1994; **47:** 153–205.

Herpes simplex virus. In an in-vitro study using Vero cells, aciclovir was found to have a greater activity against herpes simplex virus (HSV) types 1 and 2 than idoxuridine, cytarabine, trifluridine, or vidarabine.[1] Another study[2] showed that for most cell lines aciclovir had lower potency than brivudine against HSV type 1.

Enhanced activity has been observed with human interferon and aciclovir against HSV types 1 and 2 in Vero cells.[3,4] This enhancement may be due to interferon-induced alterations in the nucleoside metabolism of infected cells.[5] An additive effect with aciclovir and vidarabine against HSV types 1 and 2 has also been reported.[6]
1. Collins P, Bauer DJ. The activity in vitro against herpes virus of 9-(2-hydroxyethoxymethyl)guanine (acycloguanosine), a new antiviral agent. *J Antimicrob Chemother* 1979; **5:** 431–6.
2. De Clercq E. Comparative efficacy of antiherpes drugs in different cell lines. *Antimicrob Agents Chemother* 1982; **21:** 661–3.
3. Stanwick TL, *et al.* Combined antiviral effect of interferon and acyclovir on herpes simplex virus types 1 and 2. *Antimicrob Agents Chemother* 1981; **19:** 672–4.
4. Hammer SM, *et al.* Alpha interferon and acyclovir treatment of herpes simplex virus in lymphoid cell cultures. *Antimicrob Agents Chemother* 1982; **21:** 634–40.
5. O'Brien WJ, *et al.* Nucleoside metabolism in herpes simplex virus-infected cells following treatment with interferon and acyclovir, a possible mechanism of synergistic antiviral activity. *Antimicrob Agents Chemother* 1990; **34:** 1178–82.
6. Schinazi RF, *et al.* Effect of combinations of acyclovir with vidarabine or its 5′-monophosphate on herpes simplex viruses in cell culture and in mice. *Antimicrob Agents Chemother* 1982; **22:** 499–507.

LATENT INFECTION. A study in vitro[1] in trigeminal ganglia cells of mice showed that aciclovir does not affect latent infections but could affect the latent virus during early stages of reactivation. Intermittent exposure in vitro of latently infected ganglia to aciclovir reduced the proportion of ganglia containing reactivatable herpes simplex virus. Another study in rabbits[2] showed that there was no evidence that aciclovir or brivudine given by mouth prevented the recurrence of viral shedding or clinical corneal disease in experimental herpes simplex keratitis; resistant viruses were not found in tears.

1. Klein RJ, et al. Effect of discontinuous acyclovir treatment on in vitro reactivation of herpes simplex virus from latently infected trigeminal ganglia. Antimicrob Agents Chemother 1983; 24: 129–31.
2. Kaufman HE, et al. Oral antiviral drugs in experimental herpes simplex keratitis. Antimicrob Agents Chemother 1983; 24: 888–91.

Herpesvirus 6. Human herpesvirus 6 was found to be comparatively resistant to aciclovir in vitro[1] with a concentration of approximately 100 μmol per mL needed to produce 50% viral inhibition. Other studies found this virus to be more susceptible to aciclovir.[2,3]

1. Russler SK, et al. Susceptibility of human herpesvirus 6 to acyclovir and ganciclovir. Lancet 1989; ii: 382.
2. Agut H, et al. Susceptibility of human herpesvirus 6 to acyclovir and ganciclovir. Lancet 1989; ii: 626.
3. Kikuta H, et al. Susceptibility of human herpesvirus 6 to acyclovir. Lancet 1989; ii: 861.

Resistance

Herpes simplex virus develops resistance to aciclovir in vitro and in vivo by selection of mutants deficient in thymidine kinase. Other mechanisms of resistance include altered substrate specificity of thymidine kinase and reduced sensitivity of viral DNA polymerase. Resistance has also been reported with varicella-zoster virus, probably by similar mechanisms.

Although occasional treatment failures have been reported, resistance has not yet emerged as a major problem in treating herpes simplex infections. This is partly because of the low incidence of resistant mutants in vivo and because viruses deficient in thymidine kinase generally appear to be of diminished virulence with reduced infectivity and latency. Viruses with altered thymidine kinase appear to be of normal or slightly diminished virulence and DNA polymerase mutants are of normal virulence, apart from apparently having a reduced neurological virulence. Resistant viruses are most likely to be a problem in patients with a suppressed immune response. AIDS patients may be particularly prone to aciclovir-resistant mucocutaneous herpes simplex virus infections.

Viruses resistant to aciclovir because of absence of thymidine kinase may be cross-resistant to other antivirals phosphorylated by this enzyme, such as brivudine, idoxuridine, and ganciclovir. Viruses resistant because of altered substrate specificity of thymidine kinase may display cross-resistance to brivudine; those with altered DNA polymerase sensitivity may be resistant to brivudine and vidarabine. However, those viruses with altered enzyme specificity or sensitivity tend to have variable cross-resistance patterns and may be relatively susceptible to the aforementioned antivirals.

◊ Reviews of the resistance of herpes simplex viruses to aciclovir[1-4] and cross-resistance to other antivirals.[2,4]

1. Field HJ. A perspective on resistance to acyclovir in herpes simplex virus. J Antimicrob Chemother 1983; 12 (suppl B): 129–35.
2. Crumpacker C. Resistance of herpes simplex virus to antiviral agents: is it clinically important? Drugs 1983; 26: 373–7.
3. Balfour HH. Resistance of herpes simplex to acyclovir. Ann Intern Med 1983; 98: 404–6.
4. Wagstaff AJ, et al. Aciclovir: a reappraisal of its antiviral activity, pharmacokinetic properties and therapeutic efficacy. Drugs 1994; 47: 153–205.

Resistance in human infections. Aciclovir resistance is still uncommon in clinical practice,[1] although more prevalent in immunocompromised patients. Most aciclovir-resistant herpes simplex and varicella zoster infections have been reported in immunocompromised patients receiving prolonged courses of aciclovir.[2-6] Aciclovir-resistant herpes simplex strains have generally been less virulent, but aggressive disease has been reported.[5,7,8] Recurrences in these patients may respond to increases in dosage of aciclovir,[9] but alternative antivirals may be required. Since resistance is commonly due to the emergence of strains deficient in thymidine kinase, they tend to retain sensitivity to foscarnet and vidarabine, drugs which do not depend on viral thymidine kinase for activation.[5,10,11] Aciclovir-resist-

ant varicella zoster infections have responded to increases in aciclovir dose[12] and to foscarnet.[13,14]

1. Christophers J, et al. Survey of resistance of herpes simplex virus to acyclovir in Northwest England. Antimicrob Agents Chemother 1998; 42: 868–72.
2. Christophers J, Sutton RNP. Characterisation of acyclovir-resistant and -sensitive clinical herpes simplex virus isolates from an immunocompromised patient. J Antimicrob Chemother 1987; 20: 389–98.
3. Erlich KS, et al. Acyclovir-resistant herpes simplex virus infections in patients with the acquired immunodeficiency syndrome. N Engl J Med 1989; 320: 293–6.
4. Englund JA, et al. Herpes simplex virus resistant to acyclovir: a study in a tertiary care center. Ann Intern Med 1990; 112: 416–22.
5. Ljungman P, et al. Acyclovir-resistant herpes simplex virus causing pneumonia after marrow transplantation. J Infect Dis 1990; 162: 244–8.
6. Jacobson MA, et al. Acyclovir-resistant varicella zoster virus infection after chronic oral acyclovir therapy in patients with the acquired immunodeficiency syndrome (AIDS). Ann Intern Med 1990; 112: 187–91.
7. Gateley A, et al. Herpes simplex virus type 2 meningoencephalitis resistant to acyclovir in a patient with AIDS. J Infect Dis 1990; 161: 711–15.
8. Sacks SL, et al. Progressive esophagitis from acyclovir resistant herpes simplex: clinical roles for DNA polymerase mutants and viral heterogeneity? Ann Intern Med 1989; 111: 893–9.
9. Modiano P, et al. Acyclovir-resistant chronic cutaneous herpes simplex in Wiskott-Aldrich syndrome. Br J Dermatol 1995; 133: 475–8.
10. Crumpacker CS, et al. Resistance to antiviral drugs of herpes simplex virus isolated from a patient treated with acyclovir. N Engl J Med 1982; 306: 343–6.
11. Chatis PA, et al. Successful treatment with foscarnet of an acyclovir-resistant mucocutaneous infection with herpes simplex virus in a patient with acquired immunodeficiency syndrome. N Engl J Med 1989; 320: 297–300.
12. Linnemann CC, et al. Emergence of acyclovir-resistant varicella zoster virus in an AIDS patient on prolonged acyclovir therapy. AIDS 1990; 4: 577–9.
13. Safrin S, et al. Foscarnet therapy in five patients with AIDS and acyclovir-resistant varicella-zoster virus infection. Ann Intern Med 1991; 115: 19–21.
14. Smith KJ, et al. Acyclovir-resistant varicella zoster responsive to foscarnet. Arch Dermatol 1991; 127: 1069–71.

Pharmacokinetics

The intravenous infusion of aciclovir as the sodium salt produces plasma-aciclovir concentrations that demonstrate a biphasic pattern. The infusion over one hour of a dose equivalent to 5 mg of aciclovir per kg body-weight in adults has produced steady-state plasma concentrations with a peak of 9.8 μg per mL and a trough of 0.7 μg per mL. Similar concentrations are achieved in children over 1 year following doses of 250 mg per m² body-surface; a dose of 10 mg per kg body-weight in neonates of up to 3 months of age has produced a peak plasma concentration of 13.8 μg per mL and a trough of 2.3 μg per mL.

Aciclovir is excreted through the kidney by both glomerular filtration and tubular secretion. The terminal or beta-phase half-life is reported to be about 2 to 3 hours for adults without renal impairment. In chronic renal failure this value is increased, and may be up to 19.5 hours in anuric patients. During haemodialysis the half-life is reduced to 5.7 hours, with 60% of a dose of aciclovir being removed in 6 hours. Most of a dose by intravenous infusion is excreted unchanged with only up to 14% appearing in the urine as the inactive metabolite 9-carboxymethoxymethylguanine. Faecal excretion may account for about 2% of a dose. There is wide distribution, including into the CSF where concentrations achieved are about 50% of those achieved in plasma. Protein binding is reported to range from 9 to 33%.

Prior administration of probenecid increases the half-life and the area under the plasma concentration-time curve of aciclovir.

About 15 to 30% of a dose of aciclovir given by mouth is considered to be absorbed from the gastrointestinal tract. A dose of 200 mg aciclovir every 4 hours by mouth is reported to produce maximum and minimum steady-state plasma concentrations of 0.7 and 0.4 μg per mL respectively; equivalent values following 400-mg doses are 1.2 and 0.6 μg per mL. Orally active prodrugs such as valaciclovir (p.643) have been developed to overcome this poor absorption.

Aciclovir crosses the placenta and is distributed into breast milk in concentrations approximately 3 times higher than those in maternal serum.

Absorption of aciclovir is usually slight following topical application to intact skin, although it may be increased by changes in formulation. Aciclovir is ab-

sorbed following application of a 3% ointment to the eye giving a relatively high concentration of 1.7 μg per mL in the aqueous humour but negligible amounts in the blood.

◊ The pharmacokinetics of aciclovir given intravenously as the sodium salt in single doses of 2.5, 5, 10, and 15 mg per kg body-weight as an infusion over 1 hour were studied in 13 patients with various malignant disorders.[1] The declining plasma concentration was considered to be well described by a two-compartment open model. At the end of the infusion the mean plasma-aciclovir concentrations were 4.52, 8.28, 14.6, and 22.7 μg per mL respectively. The mean terminal (beta) half-lives were 2.9, 2.8, 3.3, and 2.4 hours respectively. Total clearance was 239, 268, 321, and 394 mL per minute and the volumes of distribution at steady state were 44.1, 43.1, 55.9, and 53.4 litres per 1.73 m² body-surface respectively. Renal clearance amounted to 77.4% of total clearance and was about three times greater than the estimated creatinine clearance; 70.2% of total aciclovir was excreted in the urine over 72 hours. It was considered that elimination involved both tubular secretion and glomerular filtration. In another study,[2] probenecid 1 g given one hour before infusion of aciclovir in 3 patients given 5 mg per kg body-weight by intravenous infusion over one hour. Probenecid increased the mean terminal plasma half-life by 18% from 2.3 to 2.7 hours and the area under the plasma concentration-time curve by 40%. The mean 25-hour urinary excretion declined by 12.4% from 79.0 to 69.2% of the dose. Total body clearance declined by 29% from 300 to 213 mL/min per 1.73 m² body-surface; renal clearance declined by 32% but was still about twofold greater than the estimated creatinine clearance.

Further information on the pharmacokinetics of aciclovir can be obtained from the reviews listed below.[3-5]

1. Laskin OL, et al. Pharmacokinetics and tolerance of acyclovir, a new anti-herpesvirus agent, in humans. Antimicrob Agents Chemother 1982; 21: 393–8.
2. Laskin OL, et al. Effects of probenecid on the pharmacokinetics and elimination of acyclovir in humans. Antimicrob Agents Chemother 1982; 21: 804–7.
3. de Miranda P, Blum MR. Pharmacokinetics of acyclovir after intravenous and oral administration. J Antimicrob Chemother 1983; 12 (suppl B): 29–37.
4. Laskin OL. Clinical pharmacokinetics of acyclovir. Clin Pharmacokinet 1983; 8: 187–201.
5. Wagstaff AJ, et al. Aciclovir: a reappraisal of its antiviral activity, pharmacokinetic properties and therapeutic efficacy. Drugs 1994; 47: 153–205.

Distribution. Good intra-ocular penetration was achieved after the administration of aciclovir by mouth to 16 patients undergoing cataract extraction.[1] Patients received 5 doses of aciclovir 400 mg in the 24 hours before surgery and a mean concentration of aciclovir 3.26 μmol per litre (0.73 μg per mL) was found in aqueous humour removed during surgery. The mean concentration in plasma obtained at the same time was 8.74 μmol per litre (1.97 μg per mL). There was a significant correlation between plasma and aqueous humour concentrations.

Aciclovir 800 mg by mouth 3 times daily for 12 months was given to patients with multiple sclerosis.[2] In 3 patients the concentration of aciclovir in the CSF was 13 to 52% (mean 31%) of that in the blood, a value not as high as that found in earlier studies using short-term intravenous administration. Peak and trough CSF-aciclovir concentrations did not differ significantly and remained stable at 1, 4, 8, and 12 months at a level sufficient to inhibit clinically herpes simplex types 1 and 2 and varicella zoster viruses.

In another study,[3] patients seropositive for HIV given intravenous aciclovir 50 mg per kg once weekly as a 3-hour infusion with oral probenecid 1 g were found to have a meningeal penetration of aciclovir of 82%.

1. Hung SO, et al. Pharmacokinetics of oral acyclovir (Zovirax) in the eye. Br J Ophthalmol 1984; 68: 192–5.
2. Lycke J, et al. Acyclovir concentrations in serum and cerebrospinal fluid at steady state. J Antimicrob Chemother 1989; 24: 947–54.
3. Chavanet P, et al. Meningeal diffusion of high doses of acyclovir given with probenecid. J Antimicrob Chemother 1990; 26: 294–5.

Uses and Administration

Aciclovir is a synthetic purine nucleoside analogue structurally related to guanine. It is used mainly for the treatment of viral infections due to herpes simplex virus (types 1 and 2) and varicella-zoster virus (herpes zoster and chickenpox).

Herpes simplex infections including herpes keratitis, herpes labialis, and genital herpes respond to aciclovir given by the intravenous, oral, or topical route as soon as possible after symptoms appear. Both initial and recurrent infections can be successfully treated. Prolonged treatment can reduce the incidence of recurrence which is important in immunocompromised patients. However, when prolonged treatment is withdrawn infections may recur.

Aciclovir also improves the healing of herpes zoster lesions and reduces acute pain when given intravenously or by mouth; use to prevent postherpetic neuralgia is controversial. Beneficial effects may be more marked in immunocompromised patients.

ADMINISTRATION AND DOSAGE. Aciclovir is administered by *intravenous infusion* as the sodium salt over 1 hour. Solutions for infusion are usually prepared to give a concentration of 25 or 50 mg of aciclovir per mL; this must then be further diluted in a suitable infusion fluid such as water for injections or sodium chloride 0.9% to a final concentration not greater than about 5 mg per mL (0.5%). Alternatively a solution containing 25 mg per mL may be administered by injection using a controlled rate infusion pump, over 1 hour.

For herpes simplex infections in the immunocompromised, severe initial genital herpes, or varicella zoster infections the dose by the intravenous route is 5 mg per kg body-weight administered every 8 hours and recommended periods of treatment range from 5 to 7 days. A similar dose may be used for prophylaxis of herpes simplex infections in immunocompromised patients. A higher dose of 10 mg per kg every 8 hours is given in the treatment of herpes simplex encephalitis. This higher dose may also be required in varicella-zoster infections in immunocompromised patients. Herpes simplex encephalitis usually requires treatment for 10 days.

Oral doses of aciclovir vary according to indication. For treatment of primary herpes simplex infections, including genital herpes, the usual dose by mouth is 200 mg five times daily (usually every 4 hours while awake) for 5 to 10 days. Severely immunocompromised patients or those with impaired absorption may be given 400 mg five times daily for 5 days. For suppression of recurrent herpes simplex the dose by mouth is 800 mg daily in two to four divided doses; dosage reduction to 400 to 600 mg daily can be tried. Higher doses of 1 g daily have also been used. Therapy should be interrupted every 6 to 12 months for reassessment of the condition. For prophylaxis of herpes simplex in immunocompromised patients, the dose is 200 to 400 mg four times daily. Chronic suppressive treatment is not suitable for mild or infrequent recurrences of herpes simplex. In such cases episodic treatment of recurrences may be more beneficial; a dose of 200 mg five times daily (every 4 hours while awake) for 5 days has been recommended preferably initiated during the prodromal period. The usual oral dose for treatment of chickenpox is 800 mg of aciclovir four or five times daily for 5 to 7 days, while for herpes zoster 800 mg five times daily may be given for 7 to 10 days.

In herpes simplex infections of the skin, including genital herpes and herpes labialis, *topical treatment* with an ointment or cream containing aciclovir 5% may be applied 5 or 6 times daily every 3 or 4 hours for periods of 5 to 10 days. In herpes simplex keratitis a 3% eye ointment may be applied 5 times daily every 4 hours until 3 days after healing.

Doses should be reduced in *renal impairment* (see below).

Children's doses. In children the 8-hourly intravenous dose is best calculated by body-surface using 250 mg per m^2 for herpes simplex and varicella-zoster infections and 500 mg per m^2 for herpes simplex encephalitis. A suggested 8-hourly dose for infants and neonates is 10 mg per kg body-weight; treatment for neonatal herpes usually continues for 10 days. In the treatment of herpes simplex infections, and in the prophylaxis of herpes simplex infections in the immunocompromised, oral doses of aciclovir for children aged 2 years and over are as for adults. Children aged under 2 years are given half the adult dose. In the treatment of chickenpox, children over 2 years of age may be given 20 mg per kg body-weight, up to

a maximum of 800 mg, four times daily for 5 days. Alternatively, children aged 6 years and over may be given 800 mg four times daily, those aged 2 to 5 years may be given 400 mg four times daily, and those aged under 2 years may be given 200 mg four times daily.

◊ Reviews.
1. Dorsky DI, Crumpacker CS. Drugs five years later: acyclovir. *Ann Intern Med* 1987; **107:** 859–74.
2. Whitley RJ, Gnann JW. Acyclovir: a decade later. *N Engl J Med* 1992; **327:** 782–9. Correction. *ibid.* 1997; **337:** 1703.
3. Wagstaff AJ, *et al.* Aciclovir: a reappraisal of its antiviral activity, pharmacokinetic properties and therapeutic efficacy. *Drugs* 1994; **47:** 153–205.
4. Welsby PD. Acyclovir: is the honeymoon coming to an end? *J Infect* 1994; **28:** 121–9.

Administration in renal impairment. Doses of aciclovir should be reduced in renal impairment and the manufacturers have given the following guidance. For *intravenous* administration the interval between infusions may be increased to 12 hours when the creatinine clearance is between 25 and 50 mL per minute or to 24 hours when it is 10 to 25 mL per minute. When the creatinine clearance is less than 10 mL per minute, patients on peritoneal dialysis should receive half the usual appropriate dose given once every 24 hours. Patients on haemodialysis should receive half the usual dose every 24 hours plus an extra half-dose following haemodialysis. *Oral* doses of aciclovir may be reduced to the following: for patients with a creatinine clearance of less than 10 mL per minute, 200 mg every 12 hours for herpes simplex infections or 800 mg every 12 hours for varicella-zoster infections; for patients with a creatinine clearance of between 10 and 25 mL per minute the dose of aciclovir for varicella-zoster infections should be reduced to 800 mg three times daily at intervals of 6 to 8 hours.

Some references to the use of aciclovir in patients undergoing dialysis.
1. Burgess ED, Gill MJ. Intraperitoneal administration of acyclovir in patients receiving continuous ambulatory peritoneal dialysis. *J Clin Pharmacol* 1990; **30:** 997–1000.
2. Almond MK, *et al.* Avoiding acyclovir neurotoxicity in patients with chronic renal failure undergoing haemodialysis. *Nephron* 1995; **69:** 428–32.
3. Stathoulopoulou F, *et al.* Clinical pharmacokinetics of oral acyclovir in patients on continuous ambulatory peritoneal dialysis. *Nephron* 1996; **74:** 337–41.

Erythema multiforme. Recurrent erythema multiforme (p.1105) is a disorder that in some patients is associated with herpes simplex infection. In these patients a 5-day course of oral aciclovir at the start of the infection has been proposed, to prevent the subsequent skin lesions.[1] If this fails, a 6-month course of oral aciclovir may be tried, even if the association with herpes is not obvious. It should be noted, however, that erythema multiforme may occur as an adverse effect following systemic administration of aciclovir.
1. Schofield JK, *et al.* Recurrent erythema multiforme: clinical features and treatment in a large series of patients. *Br J Dermatol* 1993; **128:** 542–5.

Herpesvirus infections. Aciclovir is highly effective against replicating herpes simplex virus with lower activity against varicella zoster and herpesvirus simiae, slight activity against Epstein-Barr virus, and minimal activity against cytomegalovirus. Resistance is still uncommon in clinical practice (see Resistance in Human Infections above).

Aciclovir is widely used in *herpes simplex infections* (p.607).[1-10] It is still the main treatment and, although it does not prevent the development of latent infections, prophylactic administration of aciclovir can reduce the incidence and severity of recurrences. Treatment of *varicella-zoster infections* generally requires higher doses of aciclovir than those used for herpes simplex infections. Although its use in herpes zoster (p.608) is well established[11,12] its role in preventing postherpetic neuralgia is controversial. However, meta-analysis suggested that treatment of herpes zoster with aciclovir within 72 hours of the onset of rash could reduce the incidence of residual pain at 6 months by 46% in immunocompetent adults.[13] Aciclovir may be useful in *chickenpox* (p.608) where there are complications or the patient is immunosuppressed, but in otherwise healthy patients it is not worthwhile.[14-17] Also the value of using aciclovir to protect contacts of chickenpox is not clear and this use has been questioned.[14,18-20]

Aciclovir has also been tried in *Herpesvirus simiae infections* (see p.608).

Although aciclovir inhibits replication of *cytomegalovirus* (p.606) at high concentrations it is generally of no value in the treatment of acute infections and there have been conflicting reports of it preventing infection.[21-26] Various antivirals, including aciclovir,[27-29] have been tried in *Epstein-Barr virus infections* (see p.607), and, although some clinical improvements have been reported, any reductions in viral shedding were usually lost when treatment was stopped.
1. Whatley JD, Thin RN. Episodic acyclovir therapy to abort recurrent attacks of genital herpes simplex infection. *J Antimicrob Chemother* 1991; **27:** 677–81.
2. Kaplowitz LG, *et al.* Prolonged continuous acyclovir treatment of normal adults with frequently recurring genital herpes simplex virus infection. *JAMA* 1991; **265:** 747–51.

3. Whitley R, *et al.* A controlled trial comparing vidarabine with acyclovir in neonatal herpes simplex virus infection. *N Engl J Med* 1991; **324:** 444–9.
4. Rooney JF, *et al.* Oral acyclovir to suppress frequently recurrent herpes labialis: a double-blind, placebo-controlled trial. *Ann Intern Med* 1993; **118:** 268–72.
5. Goldberg LH. Long-term suppression of recurrent genital herpes with acyclovir: a 5-year benchmark. *Arch Dermatol* 1993; **129:** 582–7.
6. Barron BA, *et al.* Herpetic eye disease study: a controlled trial of oral acyclovir for herpes simplex stromal keratitis. *Ophthalmology* 1994; **101:** 1871–82.
7. Schirmer M, *et al.* Acyclovir in acute oligoarticular herpetic arthritis. *Lancet* 1995; **346:** 712–13.
8. Worrall G. Acyclovir in recurrent herpes labialis. *BMJ* 1996; **312:** 6.
9. Herpetic Eye Disease Study Group. Acyclovir for the prevention of recurrent herpes simplex virus eye disease. *N Engl J Med* 1998; **339:** 300–6.
10. Amir J, *et al.* Treatment of herpes simplex gingivostomatitis with aciclovir in children: a randomised double blind placebo controlled study. *BMJ* 1997; **314:** 1800–1803.
11. Anonymous. Treatment of ocular herpes zoster. *Lancet* 1991; **338:** 1244–5.
12. Nikkels AF, Piérard GE. Recognition and treatment of shingles. *Drugs* 1994; **48:** 528–48.
13. Jackson JL, *et al.* The effect of treating herpes zoster with oral acyclovir in preventing postherpetic neuralgia: a meta-analysis. *Arch Intern Med* 1997; **157:** 909–12.
14. Balfour HH, *et al.* Acyclovir treatment of varicella in otherwise healthy children. *J Pediatr* 1990; **116:** 633–9.
15. Feder HM. Treatment of adult chickenpox with oral acyclovir. *Arch Intern Med* 1990; **150:** 2061–5.
16. Balfour HH, *et al.* Acyclovir treatment of varicella in otherwise healthy adolescents. *J Pediatr* 1992; **120:** 627–33.
17. Committee on Infectious Diseases. The use of oral acyclovir in otherwise healthy children with varicella. *Pediatrics* 1993; **91:** 674–6. Correction. *ibid.:* 858.
18. Asano Y, *et al.* Postexposure prophylaxis of varicella in family contact by oral acyclovir. *Pediatrics* 1993; **92:** 219–22.
19. Suga S, *et al.* Effect of oral acyclovir against primary and secondary viraemia in incubation period of varicella. *Arch Dis Child* 1993; **69:** 639–42.
20. Conway SP. Effect of oral acyclovir against primary and secondary viraemia in incubation period of varicella: commentary. *Arch Dis Child* 1993; **69:** 642–3.
21. Balfour HH, *et al.* A randomized, placebo-controlled trial of oral acyclovir for the prevention of cytomegalovirus disease in recipients of renal allografts. *N Engl J Med* 1989; **320:** 1381–7.
22. Eisenmann D, *et al.* Prevention of cytomegalovirus disease in heart transplant recipients by prophylaxis with cytomegalovirus hyperimmune globulin plus oral acyclovir. *Transplant Proc* 1990; **22:** 2322–3.
23. Bailey TC, *et al.* Failure of high-dose oral acyclovir with or without immune globulin to prevent primary cytomegalovirus disease in recipients of solid organ transplants. *Am J Med* 1993; **95:** 273–8.
24. Prentice HG, *et al.* Impact of long-term acyclovir on cytomegalovirus infection and survival after allogeneic bone marrow transplantation. *Lancet* 1994; **343:** 749–53.
25. Singh N, *et al.* High-dose acyclovir compared with short-course preemptive ganciclovir therapy to prevent cytomegalovirus disease in liver transplant recipients: a randomized trial. *Ann Intern Med* 1994; **120:** 375–81.
26. Boeckh M, *et al.* Failure of high-dose acyclovir to prevent cytomegalovirus disease after autologous marrow transplantation. *J Infect Dis* 1995; **172:** 939–43.
27. Andersson J, *et al.* Effect of acyclovir on infectious mononucleosis: a double-blind, placebo-controlled study. *J Infect Dis* 1986; **153:** 283–90.
28. Yao QY, *et al.* The Epstein-Barr virus: host balance in acute infectious mononucleosis patients receiving acyclovir anti-viral therapy. *Int J Cancer* 1989; **43:** 61–6.
29. Tynell E, *et al.* Acyclovir and prednisolone treatment of acute infectious mononucleosis: a multicenter, double-blind, placebo-controlled study. *J Infect Dis* 1996; **174:** 324–31.

Preparations

BP 2001: Aciclovir Cream; Aciclovir Eye Ointment; Aciclovir Intravenous Infusion; Aciclovir Oral Suspension; Aciclovir Tablets; Dispersible Aciclovir Tablets;
USP 25: Acyclovir Capsules; Acyclovir for Injection; Acyclovir Ointment; Acyclovir Oral Suspension; Acyclovir Tablets.

Proprietary Preparations (details are given in Part 3)
Aust.: Aciclobene; Aciclotyrol; Activir; Nycovir; Simplex-Fieberblasen; Xorox; Zovirax; **Austral.:** Acihexal; Acyclo-V; Chemists Own Cold Sore; Lovir; Zolaten; Zovirax; Zyclir; **Belg.:** Zovirax; **Braz.:** Aviral; Zovirax; **Canad.:** Avirax; Zovirax; **Denm.:** Aciclodan; Geavir; Orivir; Zoviplus†; Zovir; **Fin.:** Aclovir; Acyclostad; Acyrax; Geavir; Herpolips; Zovirax; **Fr.:** Activir; Zovirax; **Ger.:** Aci-Sanorania†; Acic; Acic-Ophtal; Aciclobeta; Aciclostad; Acivir; Herpetad; Herpofug; Herpotern†; Herpoviric†; Mapox; Supraviran; Virax; Virupos; Viruseen; Virzin; Zoliparin; Zovirax; **Hong Kong:** Avorax; Vidaclovir; Zovirax; **Irl.:** Clonorax; Zovirax; **Israel:** Supra-Vir; Viroxy; Zovirax; **Ital.:** Aciclin; ACY; Acyvir; Alovir; Avirase; Avix; Avyclor; Avyplus; Avysal; Cevirin; Citivir; Cycloviran; Dravyr; Efriviral; Esavir; Herpesnil; Ipaviran; Ipsovir; Neviran; Rexan; Riduvir; Sifiviral; Zovirax; **Mex.:** Acifur; Akevir; Avirex; Cicloferon; Ciclor; Filivir; Herpilem; Isavir; Laciken; Opthavir; Virazone; Ziverone; Zovirax; **Neth.:** Previum†; Zovirax; **Norw.:** Geavir; Zovirax; **NZ:** Lovir; Viraban; Zolaten; Zovirax; **Port.:** Aciclosina; Cicloviral; Divicil; Faulviral; Hermixsofex†; Hermocil; Zov800; Zovirax; **S.Afr.:** Activir; Cyclivex; Lovire; Zovirax; **Singapore:** Avorax; Bearax; Cusiviral; Dravyr; Entir; Erlvirax; Lovir; Medovir; Vacrax; Zoral; **Spain:** Aciclostad; Cusiviral; Maynar; Milavir; Virbelte; Virherpes; Virmen; Zovirax; **Swed.:** Geavir; Zovir†; Zovirax; **Switz.:** Zovirax; **Thai.:** ACV; Acyvir; Clovin; Clovira; Colsor; Cyclorax; Entir; Herpenon; Medovir; Norum; Vilerm; Viraxy; Virogon; Viropox; Vivir; Zevin; Zocovin; Zovirax; **UAE:** Lovrak; **UK:** Herpetad; Soothelip; Virasorb; Virovir; Zovirax; **USA:** Zovirax.

The symbol † denotes a preparation no longer actively marketed

Adefovir (17807-w)

Adefovir (BAN, USAN, rINN).

GS-0393. {[2-(6-Amino-9H-purin-9-yl)ethoxy]methyl}phosphonic acid; 9-[2-(Phosphonomethoxy)ethyl]adenine.

$C_8H_{12}N_5O_4P = 273.2$.

CAS — 106941-25-7.

Adefovir Dipivoxil (17466-v)

Adefovir Dipivoxil (BANM, USAN, rINNM).

GS-0840. 9-[2-({Bis[(pivaloyloxy)methoxy]phosphinyl}methoxy)ethyl]adenine.

$C_{20}H_{32}N_5O_8P = 501.5$.

CAS — 142340-99-6.

Profile

Adefovir is a nucleoside reverse transcriptase inhibitor, structurally related to adenine, with antiviral activity. The oral prodrug adefovir dipivoxil is under investigation in the treatment of HIV infection and hepatitis B virus infection.

◊ References.
1. Noble S, Goa KL. Adefovir dipivoxil. Drugs 1999; 58: 479–87.
2. Kahn J, et al. Efficacy and safety of adefovir dipivoxil with antiretroviral therapy: a randomized controlled trial. JAMA 1999; 282: 2305–12.

Afovirsen (17400-w)

Afovirsen (rINN).

Isis-2105.

$C_{192}H_{250}N_{57}O_{107}P_{19}S_{19} = 6266.1$.

CAS — 151356-08-0.

NOTE. Afovirsen Sodium is USAN.

Profile

Afovirsen is an antisense oligonucleotide that has been investigated for the treatment of genital warts.

◊ References.
1. Crooke ST, et al. A pharmacokinetic evaluation of ¹⁴C-labeled afovirsen sodium in patients with genital warts. Clin Pharmacol Ther 1994; 56: 641–6.

Amprenavir (17909-c)

Amprenavir (BAN, USAN, rINN).

KVX-478; VX-478; 141W94. (3S)-Tetrahydro-3-furyl{(S)-α-[(1R)-1-hydroxy-2-(N¹-isobutylsulfanilamido)ethyl]phenethyl}carbamate.

$C_{25}H_{35}N_3O_6S = 505.6$.

CAS — 161814-49-9.

ATC — J05AE05.

Adverse Effects and Precautions

As for HIV-protease inhibitors in general (see Indinavir Sulfate, p.625). A possible association with Stevens-Johnson syndrome has been reported with amprenavir. Depressive or mood disorders have occurred in patients receiving amprenavir, and acute haemolytic anaemia has been reported.

Amprenavir should be permanently discontinued in patients who develop skin rashes with associated systemic or allergic symptoms or mucosal involvement. Amprenavir is a sulfonamide and should be used with caution in patients known to be allergic to sulfonamides. The oral solution and capsule formulations (Agenerase, Glaxo Wellcome, UK) also provide high daily doses of vitamin E (see p.1394); the oral solution has a high content of propylene glycol, present as an excipient, and appropriate precautions should be taken.

Interactions

Interactions involving HIV-protease inhibitors are discussed under Indinavir Sulfate, p.626. Amprenavir is reported to be both a substrate for, and inhibitor of, the cytochrome P450 isoenzyme CYP3A4 and may thus interact with drugs which are metabolised by, or which inhibit, this isoenzyme.

Antiviral Action

As for HIV-protease inhibitors in general (see Indinavir Sulfate, p.627). Mechanisms of resistance to amprenavir may differ sufficiently from those of other HIV-protease inhibitors to reduce the occurrence of cross-resistance between amprenavir and other HIV-protease inhibitors.

Pharmacokinetics

Amprenavir is absorbed from the gastrointestinal tract following oral administration. Absorption is impaired by ingestion with a high-fat meal. Bioavailability is approximately 14% lower from the oral solution formulation than from the capsule formulation (Agenerase, Glaxo Wellcome, UK). Peak plasma concentrations are attained 1 to 2 hours after a single dose. It is about 90% bound to plasma proteins. Amprenavir is metabolised by hepatic cytochrome P450 isoenzyme CYP3A4. It is excreted mainly in the faeces as metabolites. The plasma elimination half-life is 7.1 to 10.6 hours.

Uses and Administration

Amprenavir is a protease inhibitor with antiviral activity against HIV. It is used in combination with other antiretrovirals in the treatment of HIV infection (p.608).

Amprenavir is given by mouth as capsules (Agenerase, Glaxo Wellcome, UK) in an adult dose of 1.2 g twice daily or as an oral solution (Agenerase, Glaxo Wellcome, UK) in a dose of 17 mg per kg bodyweight three times daily (maximum daily dose 2.8 g). Children aged 4 to 12 years and patients under 50 kg body-weight may be given 20 mg per kg body-weight twice daily or 15 mg per kg three times daily to a maximum daily dose of 2.4 g as capsules or 22.5 mg per kg twice daily or 17 mg per kg three times daily as oral solution (maximum daily dose 2.8 g).

Doses should be reduced in patients with moderate to severe hepatic impairment.

◊ References.
1. Adkins JC, Faulds D. Amprenavir. Drugs 1998; 55: 837–42.
2. Sadler BM, et al. Safety and pharmacokinetics of amprenavir (141W94), a human immunodeficiency virus (HIV) type 1 protease inhibitor, following oral administration of single doses to HIV-infected adults. Antimicrob Agents Chemother 1999; 43: 1686–92.
3. Noble S, Goa KL. Amprenavir: a review of its clinical potential in patients with HIV infection. Drugs 2000; 60: 1383–1410.

Preparations

Proprietary Preparations (details are given in Part 3)
Fr.: Agenerase; Switz.: Agenerase; UK: Agenerase; USA: Agenerase.

Atevirdine (17287-h)

Atevirdine (rINN).

U-87201 (atevirdine); U-87201E (atevirdine mesilate). 1-[3-(Ethylamino)-2-pyridyl]-4-[(5-methoxyindol-2-yl)carbonyl]piperazine.

$C_{21}H_{25}N_5O_2 = 379.5$.

CAS — 136816-75-6 (atevirdine); 138540-32-6 (atevirdine mesilate).

NOTE. Atevirdine Mesilate is USAN.

Profile

Atevirdine is a non-nucleoside reverse transcriptase inhibitor under investigation for the treatment of HIV infection. Viral resistance emerges rapidly when atevirdine is given alone, and it would be likely to be used mainly in combination with nucleoside reverse transcriptase inhibitors.

◊ References.
1. Campbell TB, et al. Inhibition of human immunodeficiency virus type 1 replication in vitro by the bisheteroarylpiperazine atevirdine (U-87201E) in combination with zidovudine or didanosine. J Infect Dis 1993; 168: 318–26.
2. Morse GD, et al. Didanosine reduces atevirdine absorption in subjects with human immunodeficiency virus infections. Antimicrob Agents Chemother 1996; 40: 767–71.
3. Been-Tiktak AMM, et al. Safety, tolerance, and efficacy of atevirdine in asymptomatic human immunodeficiency virus-infected individuals. Antimicrob Agents Chemother 1996; 40: 2664–8.
4. Morse GD, et al. Concentration-targeted phase I trials of atevirdine mesylate in patients with HIV infection: dosage requirements and pharmacokinetic studies: the ACTG 187 and 199 study teams. Antiviral Res 2000; 45: 47–8.

Brivudine (12455-p)

Brivudine (rINN).

BVDU. (E)-5-(2-Bromovinyl)-2'-deoxyuridine.

$C_{11}H_{13}BrN_2O_5 = 333.1$.

CAS — 69304-47-8.

Profile

Brivudine is a nucleoside analogue effective in vitro against herpes simplex virus type 1 and varicella-zoster virus; other viruses including herpes simplex virus type 2 have been reported to be sensitive, but only at relatively high concentrations. The activity appears to be due, at least in part, to selective phosphorylation of brivudine by viral deoxythymidine kinase in preference to cellular kinases. There is the possibility of cross-resistance developing between brivudine and aciclovir because of some similar features in their mode of action (see p.614).

Brivudine is given by mouth in the treatment of herpes simplex (p.607) and herpes zoster (p.608) in a dose of 125 mg four times daily at intervals of 6 hours. It has also been used topically.

◊ References.
1. De Clercq E, et al. Oral (E)-5-(2-bromovinyl)-2'-deoxyuridine in severe herpes zoster. BMJ 1980; 281: 1178.
2. De Clercq E. The antiviral spectrum of (E)-5-(2-bromovinyl)-2'-deoxyuridine. J Antimicrob Chemother 1984; 14 (suppl A): 85–95.
3. Maudgal PC, et al. Efficacy of bromovinyldeoxyuridine in the treatment of herpes simplex virus and varicella-zoster virus eye infections. Antiviral Res 1984; 4: 281–91.
4. Wildiers J, De Clercq E. Oral (E)-5-(2-bromovinyl)-2'-deoxyuridine treatment of severe herpes zoster in cancer patients. Eur J Cancer Clin Oncol 1984; 20: 471–6.
5. van Bijsterveld OP, et al. Bromovinyldeoxyuridine and interferon in ulcerative herpetic keratitis: a double masked study. Br J Ophthalmol 1989; 73: 604–7.
6. Power WJ, et al. Randomised double-blind trial of bromovinyldeoxyuridine (BVDU) and trifluorothymidine (TFT) in dendritic corneal ulceration. Br J Ophthalmol 1991; 75: 649–51.
7. Wutzler P, et al. Oral brivudin vs intravenous acyclovir in the treatment of herpes zoster in immunocompromised patients: a randomized double-blind trial. J Med Virol 1995; 46: 252–7.

Preparations

Proprietary Preparations (details are given in Part 3)
Ger.: Helpin.

CD4 (10526-j)

Soluble CD4.

Profile

CD4 is a receptor on the cell membrane of helper T lymphocytes, macrophages, and related cells to which the gp120 glycoprotein of HIV binds with high affinity, thereby infecting the cell. Soluble CD4 produced by recombinant DNA technology has been tried in the treatment of AIDS and AIDS-related complex on the premise that excess CD4 in the blood will compete for HIV-binding and thus reduce HIV-binding to lymphocytes. It has been given parenterally.

◊ References.
1. Schooley RT, et al. Recombinant soluble CD4 therapy in patients with the acquired immunodeficiency syndrome (AIDS) and AIDS-related complex: a phase I–II escalating dosage trial. Ann Intern Med 1990; 112: 247–53.
2. Kahn JO, et al. The safety and pharmacokinetics of recombinant soluble CD4 (rCD4) in subjects with the acquired immunodeficiency syndrome (AIDS) and AIDS-related complex: a phase 1 study. Ann Intern Med 1990; 112: 254–61.
3. Daar ES, Ho DD. Relative resistance of primary HIV-1 isolates to neutralization by soluble CD4. Am J Med 1991; 90 (suppl 4A): 22–6S.
4. Schacker T, et al. Phase I study of high-dose, intravenous rsCD4 in subjects with advanced HIV-1 infection. J Acquir Immune Defic Syndr Hum Retrovirol 1995; 9: 145–52.

Cidofovir (15028-y)

Cidofovir (BAN, USAN, rINN).

GS-504; GS-0504; HPMPC. {[(S)-2-(4-Amino-2-oxo-1(2H)-pyrimidinyl)-1-(hydroxymethyl)ethoxy]methyl}phosphonic acid; 1-[(S)-3-Hydroxy-2-(phosphonomethoxy)propyl]-cytosine.

$C_8H_{14}N_3O_6P = 279.2$.

CAS — 113852-37-2 (anhydrous cidofovir); 149394-66-1 (anhydrous cidofovir or cidofovir dihydrate).

ATC — J05AB12.

Adverse Effects

The most serious dose-limiting adverse effect of cidofovir is nephrotoxicity, the incidence and severity of which can be reduced by concurrent administration of probenecid and by ensuring adequate hydration. There have been instances of acute renal failure occurring after only 1 or 2 doses, and some fatalities. Low plasma-bicarbonate concentrations and metabolic acidosis, sometimes associated with proximal tubule injury and renal wasting syndrome (including Fanconi's syndrome) or with liver dysfunction and pancreatitis, have been reported. Reversible neutropenia has also occurred. Other adverse effects include nausea and vomiting, fever, asthenia, skin rash, dyspnoea, alopecia, and ocular hypotony (decreased intraocular pressure). Iritis or uveitis has been reported.

Cidofovir is carcinogenic and embryotoxic in animals and may cause male infertility; for further details see Precautions, below.

Effects on the eyes. Ocular adverse effects associated with intravenous administration of cidofovir include iritis,[1] uveitis,[2] and ocular hypotony. While development of ocular hypotony is considered to warrant withdrawal of cidofovir,[2] uveitis or iritis alone may respond to topical corticosteroids and cycloplegics thus allowing antiviral therapy to be continued; no response or worsening of symptoms would necessitate discontinuation of cidofovir.

1. Tseng AL, *et al.* Iritis associated with intravenous cidofovir. *Ann Pharmacother* 1999; **33:** 167–71.
2. Ambati J, *et al.* Anterior uveitis associated with intravenous cidofovir use in patients with cytomegalovirus retinitis. *Br J Ophthalmol* 1999; **83:** 1153–8.

Effects on the kidneys. Dose-related nephrotoxicity is the most severe adverse effect of cidofovir and severe proteinuria has been reported in 13% of patients receiving it. There have been instances of acute renal failure occurring after only 1 or 2 doses, and some fatalities. Fanconi's syndrome associated with renal tubular damage has been reported in 2% of patients and, in one such patient, occurred on the third injection of cidofovir and resulted in irreversible renal impairment.[1] A case of nephrogenic diabetes insipidus occurring without premonitory laboratory abnormalities has also been reported in a patient receiving cidofovir.[2]

1. Vittecoq D, *et al.* Fanconi syndrome associated with cidofovir therapy. *Antimicrob Agents Chemother* 1997; **41:** 1846.
2. Schliefer K, *et al.* Nephrogenic diabetes insipidus in a patient taking cidofovir. *Lancet* 1997; **350:** 413–14. Correction. *ibid.;* 1558.

Precautions

Cidofovir is contra-indicated in patients with renal impairment. Renal function should be measured before each dose. In the UK it is recommended that treatment should be interrupted or discontinued if renal function deteriorates but in the USA reduction of the dosage is permitted for increases in serum creatinine up to 400 µg per dL above baseline. Patients should receive oral probenecid and prior intravenous hydration with each dose of cidofovir. Neutrophil counts should also be monitored and regular ophthalmological follow-up is recommended. Patients with diabetes mellitus are at increased risk of ocular hypotony. Cidofovir is carcinogenic and embryotoxic in *animals.* Cidofovir should not be administered during pregnancy and both sexes should use effective methods of contraception during treatment; in addition, women should use effective contraception for 1 month after the end of treatment and men for 3 months. There is also a possibility that cidofovir may cause male infertility.

Cidofovir should be administered intravenously only; direct intraocular injection has been associated with significant ocular hypotony and visual impairment and is contra-indicated.

Interactions

Additive nephrotoxicity may occur if cidofovir is given with other nephrotoxic drugs including aminoglycosides, amphotericin B, foscarnet, and intravenous pentamidine. Potentially nephrotoxic drugs should be discontinued at least 7 days before starting cidofovir. Probenecid, which is used with cidofovir, may alter the clearance of other drugs given concomitantly (see Interactions under Probenecid, p.402).

Patients with cytomegalovirus retinitis are at increased risk of adverse inflammatory effects if intravenous or intravitreal cidofovir is administered within 2 to 4 weeks of intravitreal fomivirsen.

Antiviral Action

Cidofovir undergoes intracellular phosphorylation by cellular kinases to the antiviral metabolite, cidofovir diphosphate, which acts as a competitive inhibitor of viral DNA polymerase. It is active against a range of herpesviruses including cytomegalovirus, and, since its activity is not reliant on viral enzymes, may retain activity against aciclovir- and foscarnet-resistant viruses. Cross-resistance has been noted with ganciclovir *in vitro.*

◊ References.
1. Moore MR, *et al.* Activity of (S)-1-(3-hydroxy-2-phosphonylmethoxypropyl) cytosine against human cytomegalovirus when administered as single-bolus dose and continuous infusion in in vitro cell culture perfusion system. *Antimicrob Agents Chemother* 1998; **38:** 2404–8.

The symbol † denotes a preparation no longer actively marketed

2. Polis MA, *et al.* Anticytomegaloviral activity and safety of cidofovir in patients with human immunodeficiency virus infection and cytomegalovirus viruria. *Antimicrob Agents Chemother* 1995; **39:** 882–6.
3. Cherrington JM, *et al.* In vitro antiviral susceptibilities of isolates from cytomegalovirus retinitis patients receiving first- or second-line cidofovir therapy: relationship to clinical outcome. *J Infect Dis* 1998; **178:** 1821–5.
4. Jabs DA, *et al.* Incidence of foscarnet resistance and cidofovir resistance in patients treated for cytomegalovirus retinitis. *Antimicrob Agents Chemother* 1998; **42:** 2240–4.

Pharmacokinetics

Following intravenous administration of cidofovir, serum concentrations decline with a reported terminal half-life of about 2.2 hours (the intracellular half-life of the active diphosphate may be up to 65 hours). Cidofovir is eliminated mainly by renal excretion, both by glomerular filtration and tubular secretion. Approximately 80 to 100% of a dose is recovered unchanged from the urine within 24 hours. Concomitant administration of probenecid may reduce the excretion of cidofovir to some extent by blocking tubular secretion, although 70 to 85% has still been reported to be excreted unchanged in the urine within 24 hours.

◊ References.
1. Cundy KC. Clinical pharmacokinetics of the antiviral nucleotide analogues cidofovir and adefovir. *Clin Pharmacokinet* 1999; **36:** 127–43.
2. Brody SR, *et al.* Pharmacokinetics of cidofovir in renal insufficiency and in continuous ambulatory peritoneal dialysis or high-flux hemodialysis. *Clin Pharmacol Ther* 1999; **65:** 21–8.

Uses and Administration

Cidofovir is a nucleoside analogue which is active against herpesviruses. It is used in the treatment of cytomegalovirus retinitis (p.606) in patients with AIDS, and is being investigated for herpes simplex infections.

In the treatment of cytomegalovirus retinitis, cidofovir is given in a dose of 5 mg per kg body-weight by intravenous infusion over 1 hour once a week for 2 consecutive weeks, then once every 2 weeks. Probenecid 2 g is given by mouth 3 hours before each dose of cidofovir and further doses of probenecid 1 g at 2 and 8 hours after completion of the infusion. To ensure adequate hydration 1 litre of sodium chloride 0.9% is administered by intravenous infusion over 1 to 2 hours immediately before each infusion of cidofovir; if the additional fluid load can be tolerated, a further 1 litre of sodium chloride 0.9% may be infused over 1 to 3 hours, starting at the same time as (or immediately after) the cidofovir infusion. In the UK it is recommended that cidofovir should be interrupted or discontinued if renal function deteriorates during treatment but in the USA a reduction in the maintenance dose from 5 to 3 mg per kg is permitted for increases of serum creatinine of up to 400 µg per dL above baseline.

Cidofovir has also been administered experimentally by intravitreal injection but the commercially available formulation is unsuitable for administration by this route and the manufacturers advise against it (see Precautions, above).

An orally active prodrug of cidofovir known as cyclic-HPMPC (GS-930) is under investigation.

◊ Reviews.
1. Lea AP, Bryson HM. Cidofovir. *Drugs* 1996; **52:** 225–30.
2. Kendle JB, Fan-Havard P. Cidofovir in the treatment of cytomegaloviral disease. *Ann Pharmacother* 1998; **32:** 1181–92.
3. Plosker GL, Noble S. Cidofovir: a review of its use in cytomegalovirus retinitis in patients with AIDS. *Drugs* 1999; **58:** 325–45.

Viral infections. In addition to its use in cytomegalovirus retinitis,[1-5] cidofovir has been studied in herpes simplex infections,[6-9] papillomavirus infections,[10-12] and molluscum contagiosum.[13,14]

1. Rahhal FM, *et al.* Treatment of cytomegalovirus retinitis with intravitreous cidofovir in patients with AIDS: a preliminary report. *Ann Intern Med* 1996; **125:** 98–103.
2. Studies of Ocular Complications of AIDS Research Group, AIDS Clinical Trials Group. Parenteral cidofovir for cytomegalovirus retinitis in patients with AIDS: the HPMPC peripheral cytomegalovirus retinitis trial: a randomized controlled trial. *Ann Intern Med* 1997; **126:** 264–74.
3. Lalezari JP, *et al.* Intravenous cidofovir for peripheral cytomegalovirus retinitis in patients with AIDS: a randomized, controlled trial. *Ann Intern Med* 1997; **126:** 257–63.
4. Lalezari JP, *et al.* Randomized, controlled study of the safety and efficacy of intravenous cidofovir for the treatment of relapsing cytomegalovirus retinitis in patients with AIDS. *J Acquir Immune Defic Syndr Hum Retrovirol* 1998; **17:** 339–44.

5. Berenguer J, *et al.* Intravenous cidofovir for compassionate use in AIDS patients with cytomegalovirus retinitis. *Clin Infect Dis* 2000; **30:** 182–4.
6. Snoeck R, *et al.* A new topical treatment for resistant herpes simplex infections. *N Engl J Med* 1993; **329:** 968–9.
7. Lalezari JP, *et al.* Treatment with intravenous (S)-1-[3-hydroxy-2-(phosphonylmethoxy)propyl]-cytosine of acyclovir-resistant mucocutaneous infection with herpes simplex virus in a patient with AIDS. *J Infect Dis* 1994; **170:** 570–2.
8. Lalezari J, *et al.* A randomized, double-blind, placebo-controlled trial of cidofovir gel for the treatment of acyclovir-unresponsive mucocutaneous herpes simplex virus infection in patients with AIDS. *J Infect Dis* 1997; **176:** 892–8.
9. Sacks SL, *et al.* A multicenter phase I/II dose escalation study of single-dose cidofovir gel for treatment of recurrent genital herpes. *Antimicrob Agents Chemother* 1998; **42:** 2996–9.
10. Snoeck R, *et al.* Treatment of anogenital papillomavirus infections with an acyclic nucleoside phosphonate analogue. *N Engl J Med* 1995; **333:** 943–4.
11. Davis MDP, *et al.* Large plantar wart caused by human papillomavirus-66 and resolution by topical cidofovir therapy. *J Am Acad Dermatol* 2000; **43:** 340–3.
12. Descamps V, *et al.* Topical cidofovir for bowenoid papulosis in an HIV-infected patient. *Br J Dermatol* 2001; **144:** 642–3.
13. Davies EG, *et al.* Topical cidofovir for severe molluscum contagiosum. *Lancet* 1999; **353:** 2042.
14. Toro JR, *et al.* Topical cidofovir: a novel treatment for recalcitrant molluscum contagiosum in children infected with human immunodeficiency virus 1. *Arch Dermatol* 2000; **136:** 983–5.

Preparations

Proprietary Preparations (details are given in Part 3)
Aust.: Vistide; *Austral.:* Vistide; *Belg.:* Vistide; *Fr.:* Vistide; *Ger.:* Vistide; *Ital.:* Vistide; *Port.:* Vistide; *Spain:* Vistide; *Switz.:* Vistide; *UK:* Vistide; *USA:* Vistide.

Delavirdine Mesilate (17191-k)

Delavirdine Mesilate (rINNM)

Delavirdine Mesylate (USAN); U-90152S. 1-[3-(Isopropylamino)-2-pyridyl]-4-[[(5-methanesulfonamidoindol-2-yl)carbonyl]-piperazine monomethanesulfonate.
$C_{22}H_{28}N_6O_3S,CH_4O_3S = 552.7.$
CAS — 136817-59-9 (delavirdine); 147221-93-0 (delavirdine mesilate).

Adverse Effects

The most common adverse effect of delavirdine is skin rash, usually occurring within the first 3 weeks of starting therapy and resolving in 3 to 14 days. Severe skin reactions including Stevens-Johnson syndrome have occurred. Additional adverse effects may include nausea and vomiting, diarrhoea, headache, and increased liver enzyme values.

Precautions

Delavirdine should be discontinued if a severe skin rash develops or if a rash is accompanied by fever, blistering, oral lesions, conjunctivitis, swelling, or muscle or joint aches. Delavirdine should be used with caution in patients with impaired hepatic function.

Interactions

Similarly to the HIV-protease inhibitors (see Indinavir, p.626), delavirdine is metabolised mainly by cytochrome P450 isoenzymes of the CYP3A family. Consequently it may compete with other drugs metabolised by this system, potentially resulting in toxic concentrations; co-administration of amfetamines, the non-sedating antihistamines astemizole and terfenadine, antiarrhythmics, the benzodiazepines alprazolam, midazolam, and triazolam, calcium-channel blockers, cisapride, ergot alkaloids, and sildenafil may be particularly hazardous. Alternatively, enzyme inducers such as rifabutin, rifampicin, and the antiepileptics carbamazepine, phenobarbital, and phenytoin, may decrease plasma concentrations of delavirdine. The absorption of delavirdine is reduced by drugs that raise gastric pH such as antacids and histamine H_2-receptor antagonists.

Antibacterials. Plasma concentrations of *dapsone* and *rifabutin* may be increased by delavirdine; *rifabutin* and *rifampicin*[1] may reduce delavirdine plasma concentrations and the use of either of these drugs with delavirdine is not recommended. Plasma concentrations of both delavirdine and *clarithromycin* may be increased by concurrent administration although this may not be clinically significant.

1. Borin MT, *et al.* Pharmacokinetic study of the interaction between rifampin and delavirdine mesylate. *Clin Pharmacol Ther* 1997; **61:** 544–53.

Antidepressants. Plasma concentrations of delavirdine may be increased by *fluoxetine.*

Antifungals. Plasma concentrations of delavirdine may be increased by *ketoconazole*.

Antivirals. Administration of delavirdine with *didanosine* may result in reduced plasma concentrations of both drugs[1] and they should be given at least 1 hour apart; plasma concentrations of HIV-protease inhibitors including *indinavir* and *saquinavir* may be increased by delavirdine (see Antivirals, under Interactions of Indinavir, p.626) and liver function should be monitored in patients receiving delavirdine and saquinavir.

1. Morse GD, *et al.* Single-dose pharmacokinetics of delavirdine mesylate and didanosine in patients with human immunodeficiency virus infection. *Antimicrob Agents Chemother* 1997; **41:** 169–74.

Pharmacokinetics

Delavirdine is rapidly absorbed following oral administration, peak plasma concentrations occurring after about 1 hour. It is about 98% bound to plasma proteins. Delavirdine is extensively metabolised by hepatic microsomal enzymes, principally by cytochrome P450 isoenzymes of the CYP3A family. It has been shown to reversibly inhibit P450 activity. Plasma half-life following the usual dosage has ranged from 2 to 11 hours. Delavirdine is excreted as metabolites in the urine and faeces. Less than 5% is excreted in the urine unchanged.

◊ **Reviews.**
1. Tran JQ, *et al.* Delavirdine: clinical pharmacokinetics and drug interactions. *Clin Pharmacokinet* 2001; **40:** 207–26.

Bioavailability. The manufacturers report that bioavailability of delavirdine tablets is about 85% of that from an oral solution following a single dose and that the bioavailability increases by about 20% if the tablets are dispersed in water before administration.

Uses and Administration

Delavirdine is a non-nucleoside reverse transcriptase inhibitor with activity against HIV-1. Viral resistance emerges rapidly when delavirdine is used alone, and it is therefore used in combination with other antiretroviral drugs in the treatment of HIV infection (p.608).

Delavirdine is given in a usual dose of 400 mg of delavirdine mesilate three times daily. Tablets may be dispersed in water before administration in order to increase bioavailability (see above).

◊ **Reviews.**
1. Scott LJ, Perry CM. Delavirdine: a review of its use in HIV infection. *Drugs* 2000; **60:** 1411–44.

Preparations

Proprietary Preparations (details are given in Part 3)
Austral.: Rescriptor; ***Canad.:*** Rescriptor; ***Mex.:*** Rescriptor; ***USA:*** Rescriptor.

Didanosine   (4889-e)

Didanosine *(BAN, USAN, rINN)*.
BMY-40900; DDI; ddI; ddIno; Dideoxyinosine; NSC-612049.
2′,3′-Dideoxyinosine.
$C_{10}H_{12}N_4O_3 = 236.2$.
CAS — 69655-05-6.
ATC — J05AF02.

Adverse Effects

The most common serious adverse effects of didanosine are peripheral neuropathy and potentially fatal pancreatitis. Abnormal liver function tests may occur and hepatitis or fatal liver failure has been reported rarely. Retinal depigmentation and optic neuritis have been reported in patients receiving high doses of didanosine. Other adverse effects include nausea, vomiting, and abdominal pain (which may also be symptoms of pancreatitis), diarrhoea, headache, hyperglycaemia, myalgia, rash, hypersensitivity reactions, and hyperuricaemia. Lactic acidosis, usually associated with severe hepatomegaly and steatosis, has been reported in patients receiving nucleoside reverse transcriptase inhibitors (see Zidovudine, p.645).

Effects on the blood. In general, haematological abnormalities are less common in patients taking didanosine than in those taking zidovudine. However, there have been reports of thrombocytopenia associated with didanosine.[1-3]

1. Butler KM, *et al.* Dideoxyinosine in children with symptomatic human immunodeficiency virus infection. *N Engl J Med* 1991; **324:** 137–44.

---

2. Lor E, Liu YQ. Didanosine-associated eosinophilia with acute thrombocytopenia. *Ann Pharmacother* 1993; **27:** 23–5.
3. Herranz P, *et al.* Cutaneous vasculitis associated with didanosine. *Lancet* 1994; **344:** 680.

Effects on the eyes. Retinal lesions with atrophy of the retinal pigment epithelium at the periphery of the retina was reported in 4 children receiving didanosine doses of 270 to 540 mg per m² body-surface per day.[1]

1. Whitcup SM, *et al.* Retinal lesions in children treated with dideoxyinosine. *N Engl J Med* 1992; **326:** 1226–7.

Effects on glucose metabolism. Hyperglycaemia, glucose intolerance, diabetes mellitus, and hyperosmolar nonketotic diabetic syndrome have been associated with didanosine administration.[1-3] The effect may be dose-related, and has been reported[4] in patients who subsequently developed pancreatitis (see Effects on the Pancreas, below). The manufacturer also reports cases of hypoglycaemia in patients taking didanosine.

1. Munshi MN, *et al.* Hyperosmolar nonketotic diabetic syndrome following treatment of human immunodeficiency virus infection with didanosine. *Diabetes Care* 1994; **17:** 316–17.
2. Jablonowski H, *et al.* A dose comparison study of didanosine in patients with very advanced HIV infection who are intolerant to or clinically deteriorate on zidovudine. *AIDS* 1995; **9:** 463–9.
3. Nguyen B-Y, *et al.* Five-year follow-up of a phase I study of didanosine in patients with advanced human immunodeficiency virus infection. *J Infect Dis* 1995; **171:** 1180–9.
4. Albrecht H, *et al.* Didanosine-induced disorders of glucose tolerance. *Ann Intern Med* 1993; **119:** 1050.

Effects on the liver. Fatal fulminant hepatic failure was reported[1] in a patient receiving didanosine. A further 14 cases had been noted by the manufacturer, and elevated liver enzymes had been recorded during clinical studies.[2-5]

1. Lai KK, *et al.* Fulminant hepatic failure associated with 2′,3′-dideoxyinosine (ddI). *Ann Intern Med* 1991; **115:** 283–4.
2. Dolin R, *et al.* Zidovudine compared with didanosine in patients with advanced HIV type 1 infection and little or no experience with zidovudine. *Arch Intern Med* 1995; **155:** 961–74.
3. Jablonowski H, *et al.* A dose comparison study of didanosine in patients with very advanced HIV infection who are intolerant to or clinically deteriorate on zidovudine. *AIDS* 1995; **9:** 463–9.
4. Alpha International Coordinating Committee. The Alpha trial: European/Australian randomized double-blind trial of two doses of didanosine in zidovudine-intolerant patients with symptomatic HIV disease. *AIDS* 1996; **10:** 867–80.
5. Gatell JM, *et al.* Switching from zidovudine to didanosine in patients with symptomatic HIV infection and disease progression. *J Acquir Immune Defic Syndr Hum Retrovirol* 1996; **12:** 249–58.

Effects on mental state. Recurrent mania associated with didanosine treatment has been reported in a patient.[1]

1. Brouillette MJ, *et al.* Didanosine-induced mania in HIV infection. *Am J Psychiatry* 1994; **151:** 1839–40.

Effects on metabolism. Hyperuricaemia has been reported to be a common adverse effect during clinical studies of didanosine.[1,2] Hypokalaemia occurred during didanosine therapy in 3 patients, 2 of whom had diarrhoea.[3] There has also been a report of hypertriglyceridaemia occurring on 2 occasions in a patient given didanosine;[4] it was suggested that this hyperlipidaemic effect might be a possible aetiological factor in the development of pancreatitis. For effects on glucose metabolism, see above.

1. Cooley TP, *et al.* Once-daily administration of 2′,3′-dideoxyinosine (ddI) in patients with the acquired immunodeficiency syndrome or AIDS-related complex: results of a phase I trial. *N Engl J Med* 1990; **322:** 1340–5.
2. Montaner JSG, *et al.* Didanosine compared with continued zidovudine therapy for HIV-infected patients with 200 to 500 CD4 cells/mm³: a double-blind, randomized, controlled trial. *Ann Intern Med* 1995; **123:** 561–71.
3. Katlama C, *et al.* Dideoxyinosine-associated hypokalaemia. *Lancet* 1991; **337:** 183.
4. Tal A, Dall L. Didanosine-induced hypertriglyceridemia. *Am J Med* 1993; **95:** 247.

Effects on the mouth. Xerostomia (dry mouth) may be a troublesome effect in patients receiving didanosine.[1,2]

1. Dodd CL, *et al.* Xerostomia associated with didanosine. *Lancet* 1992; **340:** 790.
2. Valentine C, *et al.* Xerostomia associated with didanosine. *Lancet* 1992; **340:** 1542.

Effects on the nervous system. Peripheral neuropathy is a well recognised adverse effect of didanosine and has been the subject of a review.[1]

1. Moyle GJ, Sadler M. Peripheral neuropathy with nucleoside antiretrovirals: risk factors, incidence and management. *Drug Safety* 1998; **19:** 481–94.

Effects on the pancreas. Pancreatitis is recognised as being the most serious adverse effect of didanosine and can be fatal.[1-3] It appears to be dose-related, occurring in up to 13% of patients receiving 750 mg of didanosine daily.[2,4] Pancreatitis can resolve if didanosine is withdrawn[5] and cautious reintroduction of didanosine has been possible in some patients.[6] Raised amylase concentrations[3] and glucose intolerance (see above) have been reported in patients who subsequently developed pancreatitis.

1. Bouvet E, *et al.* Fatal case of 2′,3′-dideoxyinosine-associated pancreatitis. *Lancet* 1990; **336:** 1515.
2. Kahn JO, *et al.* A controlled trial comparing continued zidovudine with didanosine in human immunodeficiency virus infection. *N Engl J Med* 1992; **327:** 581–7.
3. Dolin R, *et al.* Zidovudine compared with didanosine in patients with advanced HIV-type 1 infection and little or no previous experience with zidovudine. *Arch Intern Med* 1995; **155:** 961–74.
4. Jablonowski H, *et al.* A dose comparison study of didanosine in patients with very advanced HIV infection who are intolerant to or clinically deteriorate on zidovudine. *AIDS* 1995; **9:** 463–9.

---

5. Nguyen B-Y, *et al.* Five-year follow-up of a phase I study of didanosine in patients with advanced human immunodeficiency virus infection. *J Infect Dis* 1995; **171:** 1180–9.
6. Butler KM, *et al.* Pancreatitis in human immunodeficiency virus-infected children receiving dideoxyinosine. *Pediatrics* 1993; **91:** 747–51.

Effects on the skin. Didanosine has been implicated in a case of the Stevens-Johnson syndrome[1] and of cutaneous vasculitis.[2]

1. Parneix-Spake A, *et al.* Didanosine as probable cause of Stevens-Johnson syndrome. *Lancet* 1992; **340:** 857–8.
2. Herranz P, *et al.* Cutaneous vasculitis associated with didanosine. *Lancet* 1994; **344:** 680.

Precautions

Patients with a history of pancreatitis and those with increased triglyceride concentrations should be observed carefully for signs of pancreatitis during treatment with didanosine. Treatment with didanosine should be interrupted in all patients who develop abdominal pain, nausea, or vomiting, or in those with raised serum amylase or lipase, until pancreatitis has been excluded. Concomitant treatment with other drugs likely to cause pancreatitis or peripheral neuropathy (see Interactions, below) should be avoided if possible.

It may be necessary to interrupt didanosine treatment in patients who develop peripheral neuropathy; on recovery from peripheral neuropathy a reduced dose may be tolerated. Treatment should also be interrupted if uric acid concentrations are elevated.

Didanosine should be used with caution in patients with impaired renal or hepatic function, and dosage reduction may be necessary. Regular checks of liver function are recommended. If liver function deteriorates during treatment then didanosine should be withdrawn. Treatment with didanosine may be associated with lactic acidosis and should be discontinued if there is a rapid increase in aminotransferase concentrations, progressive hepatomegaly, or metabolic or lactic acidosis of unknown aetiology. Didanosine should be given with caution to patients with hepatomegaly or other risk factors for liver disease.

Children should be monitored for retinal lesions and didanosine withdrawn if they occur. Monitoring should also be considered in adults.

Interactions

Concurrent administration of didanosine with other drugs known to cause pancreatitis (for example intravenous pentamidine) or with drugs that may cause peripheral neuropathy (for example metronidazole, isoniazid, and vincristine) should be avoided. If co-administration is unavoidable, patients should be monitored carefully for these adverse effects.

An increase in the area under the plasma concentration-time curve for didanosine has been reported when allopurinol is given concurrently.

Since didanosine is generally taken in conjunction with an antacid (often included in the formulation), drugs which could be affected by an increased gastric pH (for example HIV-protease inhibitors, ketoconazole, fluoroquinolone antibacterials, and dapsone) should be given at least two hours before didanosine. Didanosine preparations containing magnesium or aluminium antacids should not be given with tetracyclines.

See also below for interactions with antivirals.

Antivirals. Plasma concentrations of didanosine are approximately doubled when *ganciclovir* is given concurrently.[1-3]

Changes in the pharmacokinetics of didanosine and *zidovudine* have occurred when these drugs are given together, but results of studies have not been consistent, and the effects have generally been of limited clinical significance. For further details, see under Interactions in Zidovudine, p.646.

Concurrent administration of didanosine and *delavirdine* resulted in reductions in the area under the concentration-time curve for both drugs in a single-dose study.[4] The manufacturer of delavirdine recommends that administration of these two drugs should be separated by at least 1 hour.

Absorption of some *HIV-protease inhibitors* may be reduced by the antacids in didanosine formulations and doses should be separated by at least 2 hours (see p.626).

1. Griffy KG. Pharmacokinetics of oral ganciclovir capsules in HIV-infected persons. *AIDS* 1996; **10** (suppl 4): S3–S6.

2. Jung D, et al. Effect of high-dose oral ganciclovir on didanosine disposition in human immunodeficiency virus (HIV)-positive patients. J Clin Pharmacol 1998; 38: 1057–62.
3. Cimoch PJ, et al. Pharmacokinetics of oral ganciclovir alone and in combination with zidovudine, didanosine, and probenecid in HIV-infected subjects. J Acquir Immune Defic Syndr Hum Retrovirol 1998; 17: 227–34.
4. Morse GD. Single-dose pharmacokinetics of delavirdine mesylate and didanosine in patients with human immunodeficiency virus infection. Antimicrob Agents Chemother 1997; 41: 169–74.

Antiviral Action

Didanosine is converted intracellularly to its active form dideoxyadenosine triphosphate. This triphosphate halts the DNA synthesis of retroviruses, including HIV, through competitive inhibition of reverse transcriptase and incorporation into viral DNA.

Didanosine-resistant strains of HIV emerge during didanosine therapy. Cross-resistance to other nucleoside reverse transcriptase inhibitors has been recognised.

Resistance. Evidence for the development of didanosine-resistant HIV was reported in 36 of 64 patients with advanced HIV infection within 24 weeks of switching from zidovudine to didanosine monotherapy.[1] Patients with the didanosine resistance mutation for HIV reverse transcriptase showed a greater decline in CD4+ T cell count and increase in viral burden than those without.

Multiple-drug resistant mutations have been identified in patients receiving long-term antiretroviral therapy with combinations containing didanosine.[2]

1. Kozal MJ, et al. Didanosine resistance in HIV-infected patients switched from zidovudine to didanosine monotherapy. Ann Intern Med 1994; 121: 263–8.
2. Kavlick MF, et al. Emergence of multi-dideoxynucleoside-resistant human immunodeficiency virus type 1 variants, viral sequence variation, and disease progression in patients receiving antiretroviral chemotherapy. J Infect Dis 1998; 98: 1506–13.

Pharmacokinetics

Didanosine is rapidly hydrolysed in the acid medium of the stomach and is therefore given by mouth with pH buffers or antacids. Bioavailability is reported to range from 20 to 40% depending on the formulation used; the bioavailability is substantially reduced by administration with or after food. Maximum plasma concentrations are achieved about 1 hour after oral administration. Binding to plasma proteins is reported to be less than 5%. The plasma elimination half-life is reported to be about 1.5 hours.

CSF concentrations of didanosine have been about 20% of those in plasma following intravenous infusion; it has been reported not to cross the blood brain barrier following oral administration.

Didanosine is metabolised intracellularly to the active antiviral metabolite dideoxyadenosine triphosphate. Renal clearance by glomerular filtration and active tubular secretion represents about 50% of total body clearance following intravenous administration. Urinary recovery following oral administration is about 20% of the dose. Didanosine is partially cleared by haemodialysis but not by peritoneal dialysis.

◊ References.

1. Balis FM, et al. Clinical pharmacology of 2′,3′-dideoxyinosine in human immunodeficiency virus-infected children. J Infect Dis 1992; 165: 99–104.
2. Morse GD. Comparative pharmacokinetics of antiviral nucleoside analogues. Clin Pharmacokinet 1993; 24: 101–23.
3. Mueller BU, et al. Clinical and pharmacokinetic evaluation of long-term therapy with didanosine in children with HIV infection. Pediatrics 1994; 94: 724–31.
4. Knupp CA, et al. Disposition of didanosine in HIV-seropositive patients with normal renal function or chronic renal failure: influence of hemodialysis and continuous ambulatory peritoneal dialysis. Clin Pharmacol Ther 1996; 60: 535–42.
5. Wintergerst U, et al. Lack of absorption of didanosine after rectal administration in human immunodeficiency virus-infected patients. Antimicrob Agents Chemother 1999; 43: 699–701.
6. Abreu T, et al. Bioavailability of once- and twice-daily regimens of didanosine in human immunodeficiency virus-infected children. Antimicrob Agents Chemother 2000; 44: 1375–6.

Pregnancy. Fetal blood concentrations of 14 and 19% of the maternal serum-didanosine concentrations have been reported.[1] There is evidence of extensive metabolism in the placenta.[2]

1. Pons JC, et al. Fetoplacental passage of 2′,3′-dideoxyinosine. Lancet 1991; 337: 732.
2. Dancis J, et al. Transfer and metabolism of dideoxyinosine by the perfused human placenta. J Acquir Immune Defic Syndr 1993; 6: 2–6.

Uses and Administration

Didanosine is a nucleoside reverse transcriptase inhibitor structurally related to inosine with activity against retroviruses including HIV. It is used in the treatment of HIV infection, usually in combination with other antiretrovirals.

Didanosine is administered by mouth, usually as buffered chewable/dispersible tablets, or enteric-coated tablets, or oral solution. The tablets have a bioavailability 20 to 25% greater than that of the solution. Doses should be taken at least 30 minutes before, or 2 hours after, a meal. The total daily dose may be given as either a single dose or as two divided doses, the choice being dependent upon both the formulation and the strength employed. Doses for adults are: greater than 60 kg body-weight, 400 mg (tablets) or 500 mg (oral solution) daily; under 60 kg body-weight, 250 mg (tablets) or 334 mg (oral solution) daily.

Children's doses are determined by body-surface: children over 3 months of age (or over 6 years with enteric-coated tablets) may be given 240 mg per m^2 body-surface daily, or 180 mg per m^2 daily when didanosine is given in combination with zidovudine.

Dosage reduction may be necessary in patients with renal or hepatic impairment.

◊ Reviews.

1. Shelton MJ, et al. Didanosine. Ann Pharmacother 1992; 26: 660–70.
2. Lipsky JJ. Zalcitabine and didanosine. Lancet 1993; 341: 30–2.
3. Perry CM, Noble S. Didanosine: an updated review of its use in HIV infection. Drugs 1999; 58: 1099–1135.

HIV infection and AIDS. Although formerly used as an alternative nucleoside reverse transcriptase inhibitor in patients with HIV infection who could not tolerate or no longer responded to zidovudine,[1-4] didanosine is now most commonly used in combinations of antiretroviral drugs. In patients who had not received antiretroviral treatment in the past, didanosine in combination with zidovudine delayed disease progression and reduced mortality compared to zidovudine alone.[5,6] In patients who had received previous antiretroviral treatment, the benefit was less marked[5-8] but responses were better than with zidovudine plus zalcitabine.[5,6] Didanosine is included in regimens, typically comprising two nucleoside reverse transcriptase inhibitors and either an HIV-protease inhibitor or a non-nucleoside reverse transcriptase inhibitor, which are capable of producing sustained suppression of viraemia (see p.608). Didanosine used in combination with hydroxyurea [hydroxycarbamide] has produced promising preliminary results (see p.545), and combinations including didanosine and interferons are also being investigated.[9] The use of doses of up to 750 mg didanosine daily has generally failed to produce better responses than conventional doses of up to 500 mg daily.[1,10,11] Reducing the dose to 200 mg daily has been tried but responses have been variable.[12,13] Although didanosine has been detected in the CNS following intravenous administration, a higher incidence of AIDS dementia complex was reported in patients with advanced disease receiving didanosine than in those receiving zidovudine.[14] However didanosine therapy reduced pathological changes in patients with less advanced CNS disease to a similar extent to zidovudine.[15]

1. Kahn JO, et al. A controlled trial comparing continued zidovudine with didanosine in human immunodeficiency virus infection. N Engl J Med 1992; 327: 581–7.
2. Spruance LS, et al. Didanosine compared with continuation of zidovudine in HIV-infected patients with signs of clinical deterioration while receiving zidovudine: a randomized, double-blind clinical trial. Ann Intern Med 1994; 120: 360–8.
3. Abrams DI, et al. A comparative trial of didanosine or zalcitabine after treatment with zidovudine in patients with human immunodeficiency virus infection. N Engl J Med 1994; 330: 657–62.
4. Montaner JSG, et al. Didanosine compared with continued zidovudine therapy for HIV-infected patients with 200 to 500 CD4 cells/mm³: a double-blind, randomized, controlled trial. Ann Intern Med 1995; 123: 561–71.
5. Delta Coordinating Committee. Delta: a randomised double-blind controlled trial comparing combinations of zidovudine plus didanosine or zalcitabine with zidovudine alone in HIV-infected individuals. Lancet 1996; 348: 283–91.
6. Hammer SM, et al. A trial comparing nucleoside monotherapy with combination therapy in HIV-infected adults with CD4 cell counts from 200 to 500 per cubic millimeter. N Engl J Med 1996; 335: 1081–90.
7. Graham NMH, et al. Survival in HIV-infected patients who have received zidovudine: comparison of combination therapy with sequential monotherapy and continued zidovudine monotherapy. Ann Intern Med 1996; 124: 1031–8.
8. D'Aquila RT, et al. Nevirapine, zidovudine, and didanosine compared with zidovudine and didanosine in patients with HIV-1 infection: a randomized, double-blind, placebo-controlled trial. Ann Intern Med 1996; 124: 1019–30.
9. Kovacs JA, et al. Combination therapy with didanosine and interferon-α in human immunodeficiency virus-infected patients: results of a phase I/II trial. J Infect Dis 1996; 173: 840–8.
10. Jablonowski H, et al. A dose comparison study of didanosine in patients with very advanced HIV infection who are intolerant to or clinically deteriorate on zidovudine. AIDS 1995; 9: 463–9.
11. Dolin R, et al. Zidovudine compared with didanosine in patients with advanced HIV type 1 infection and little or no previous experience with zidovudine. Arch Intern Med 1995; 155: 961–74.
12. Alpha International Coordinating Committee. The Alpha trial: European/Australian randomized double-blind trial of two doses of didanosine in zidovudine-intolerant patients with symptomatic HIV disease. AIDS 1996; 10: 867–80.
13. Gatell JM, et al. Switching from zidovudine to didanosine in patients with symptomatic HIV infection and disease progression. J Acquir Immune Defic Syndr Hum Retrovirol 1996; 12: 249–58.
14. Portegies P, et al. AIDS dementia complex and didanosine. Lancet 1994; 344: 759.
15. Chrétien F, et al. Protection of human immunodeficiency virus encephalitis by a switch from zidovudine to didanosine. Antimicrob Agents Chemother 1996; 40: 278.

Preparations

Proprietary Preparations (details are given in Part 3)
Aust.: Videx; Austral.: Videx; Belg.: Videx; Braz.: Videx; Canad.: Videx; Denm.: Videx; Fin.: Videx; Fr.: Videx; Ger.: Videx; Hong Kong: Videx; Irl.: Videx; Israel: Videx; Ital.: Videx; Mex.: Videx; Neth.: Videx; Norw.: Videx; NZ: Videx; Port.: Videx; S.Afr.: Videx; Singapore: Videx; Spain: Videx; Swed.: Videx; Switz.: Videx; Thai.: Videx; UK: Videx; USA: Videx.

Ditiocarb Sodium (1054-y)

Ditiocarb Sodium (rINN).

DDTC; Dithiocarb Sodium; DTC; Sodium Diethyldithiocarbamate.

$C_5H_{10}NNaS_2 = 171.3$.

CAS — 148-18-5.

Profile

Ditiocarb sodium is an immunomodulating drug that has been investigated in HIV infection. It is also a chelator that has been used in the destruction of cisplatin wastes and has been used in nickel carbonyl poisoning. Disulfiram is rapidly metabolised to ditiocarb; for its further metabolism, see p.1605.

◊ Reviews.

1. Renoux G. Immunopharmacologie et pharmacologie du diethyldithiocarbamate (DTC). J Pharmacol 1982; 13 (suppl 1): 95–134.

HIV infection and AIDS. Ditiocarb has been tried in patients with HIV infection and AIDS (p.608) with some success.[1-4] However, a study involving 1300 patients indicated a faster rate of progression to AIDS in patients receiving ditiocarb[5] and as a result of this another study, which had found no improvement in immune function, but evidence of haematological toxicity, was halted early.[6]

1. Lang J-M, et al. Immunomodulation with diethyldithiocarbamate in patients with AIDS-related complex. Lancet 1985; ii: 1066.
2. Lang J-M, et al. Randomised, double-blind, placebo-controlled trial of ditiocarb sodium ('Imuthiol') in human immunodeficiency virus infection. Lancet 1988; ii: 702–6.
3. Reisinger EC, et al. Inhibition of HIV progression by dithiocarb. Lancet 1990; 335: 679–82.
4. Hersh EM, et al. Ditiocarb sodium (diethyldithiocarbamate) therapy in patients with symptomatic HIV infection and AIDS: a randomized, double-blind, placebo-controlled, multicenter study. JAMA 1991; 265: 1538–44.
5. HIV87 Study Group. Multicenter, randomized, placebo-controlled study of ditiocarb (Imuthiol) in human immunodeficiency virus asymptomatic and minimally symptomatic patients. AIDS Res Hum Retroviruses 1993; 9: 83–9.
6. Shenep JL, et al. Decreased counts of blood neutrophils, monocytes, and platelets in human immunodeficiency virus-infected children and young adults treated with diethyldithiocarbamate. Antimicrob Agents Chemother 1994; 38: 1644–6.

Docosanol (15188-g)

Docosanol (USAN).

Behenyl Alcohol; n-Docosanol; Docosyl Alcohol; IK-2. 1-Docosanol.

$C_{22}H_{46}O = 326.6$.

CAS — 661-19-8.

Profile

Docosanol is an antiviral used topically five times daily as a 10% cream in the treatment of recurrent herpes simplex infections (p.607). Docosanol acts by inhibiting fusion between the cell plasma membrane and the herpes simplex virus, thereby preventing viral entry into cells and subsequent viral replication.

Preparations

Proprietary Preparations (details are given in Part 3)
USA: Abreva.

Edoxudine (12706-e)

Edoxudine (USAN, rINN).

EDU; Ethyl Deoxyuridine; EUDR; ORF-15817; RWJ-15817. 2′-Deoxy-5-ethyluridine.

$C_{11}H_{16}N_2O_5 = 256.3$.

CAS — 15176-29-1.

ATC — D06BB09.

Profile

Edoxudine is an antiviral used topically as a 1.2% gel in the treatment of mucocutaneous herpes simplex infections (p.607); it has also been used as a 3% cream and as a 0.3% ophthalmic preparation.

The symbol † denotes a preparation no longer actively marketed

Preparations

Efavirenz (3463-d)

Efavirenz *(BAN, rINN)*.

5B706; DMP-266; L-743; L-743726. (S)-6-Chloro-4-(cyclopropylethynyl)-1,4-dihydro-4-(trifluoromethyl)-2H-3,1-benzoxazin-2-one.

$C_{14}H_9ClF_3NO_2 = 315.7$.

CAS — 154598-52-4.

ATC — J05AG03.

Adverse Effects

The most common adverse effects associated with efavirenz are skin rashes and CNS disturbances. Mild rashes may resolve on continued treatment, but severe forms may occur and erythema multiforme and Stevens-Johnson syndrome have been reported occasionally. CNS symptoms include dizziness, headache, insomnia or somnolence, impaired concentration, and abnormal dreaming. Psychotic-like symptoms and severe acute depression have also been reported. Other adverse effects include nausea and diarrhoea, fatigue, and pancreatitis. Raised liver enzyme values have occurred, particularly in patients with viral hepatitis. Raised serum-cholesterol and -triglyceride concentrations have been reported.

Precautions

Efavirenz is contra-indicated in patients with severe hepatic impairment, and should be used with caution, and liver enzymes values monitored, in patients with mild to moderate liver disease. Efavirenz should be discontinued if a severe skin rash, associated with blistering, desquamation, mucosal involvement, or fever, develops. Monitoring of plasma-cholesterol concentrations may be considered during efavirenz treatment.

False-positive results in some urinary cannabinoid tests have been reported in subjects receiving efavirenz.

Interactions

Similarly to the HIV-protease inhibitors (see Indinavir, p.626), efavirenz is metabolised mainly by cytochrome P450 isoenzymes including CYP3A4. Consequently, it may compete with other drugs metabolised by this system, potentially resulting in mutually increased plasma concentrations and toxicity. Enzyme inducers may decrease plasma concentrations of efavirenz; efavirenz itself acts as an enzyme inducer and can reduce plasma concentrations of other drugs. Inhibition of some P450 isoenzymes has also been demonstrated *in vitro*.

Efavirenz can inhibit the metabolism of astemizole, terfenadine, cisapride, the benzodiazepines midazolam and triazolam, and ergot alkaloids, resulting in serious adverse effects and such combinations should be avoided.

Antibacterials. Plasma concentrations of efavirenz may be reduced by concurrent administration with *rifampicin* and may necessitate an increase in the dose of efavirenz. A similar interaction might be anticipated with *rifabutin*.

Administration of efavirenz with *clarithromycin* has resulted in a decrease in the plasma concentration of clarithromycin together with an increase in its active hydroxy metabolite. The combination has been associated with a high incidence of skin rashes.

Antivirals. For the effect of efavirenz on *HIV-protease inhibitors*, see p.626.

Grapefruit. The metabolism of efavirenz may be inhibited by concomitant ingestion of grapefruit juice.

Hormonal contraceptives. For the effect of efavirenz on *ethinylestradiol* concentrations, see p.1459.

Antiviral Action

Efavirenz acts by non-competitive inhibition of HIV reverse transcriptase.

Resistance to efavirenz and emergence of cross-resistance to other non-nucleoside reverse transcriptase inhibitors has been seen.

Pharmacokinetics

Efavirenz is absorbed following oral administration with peak plasma concentrations being achieved about 5 hours after the dose. Steady-state plasma concentrations are reached in 6 to 7 days following multiple dosing. Bioavailability is increased following a high-fat meal. Efavirenz is 99% bound to plasma proteins and is distributed into the CNS. It is metabolised principally by hepatic cytochrome P450 isoenzymes CYP3A4 and CYP2B6. Efavirenz acts as an enzyme inducer and induces its own metabolism resulting in a terminal half-life of 40 to 55 hours after multiple doses compared with 52 to 76 hours after a single dose. About 14 to 34% of a dose is excreted in the urine as metabolites, and 16 to 61% in the faeces.

Uses and Administration

Efavirenz is a non-nucleoside reverse transcriptase inhibitor with activity against HIV. It is used in the treatment of HIV infection (p.608) in combination with other antiretrovirals.

Efavirenz is administered by mouth in an adult dose of 600 mg once daily. Dosing at bedtime is recommended during the first 2 to 4 weeks of therapy to improve tolerability. Doses for children over the age of 3 years are based on body weight: children weighing 10 to 14 kg are given 200 mg once daily; those weighing 15 to 19 kg, 250 mg once daily; those weighing 20 to 24 kg, 300 mg once daily; those weighing 25 to 32.4 kg, 350 mg once daily; those weighing 32.5 to 39 kg, 400 mg once daily; and those weighing 40 kg or more, 600 mg once daily.

◊ References.
1. Adkins JC, Noble S. Efavirenz. *Drugs* 1998; **56:** 1055–64.
2. Gazzard BG. Efavirenz in the management of HIV infection. *Int J Clin Pract* 1999; **53:** 60–4.

Preparations

Emivirine (20328-n)

Emivirine *(rINN)*.

I-EBU; MKC-442. 6-Benzyl-1-(ethoxymethyl)-5-isopropyluracil.

$C_{17}H_{22}N_2O_3 = 302.4$.

CAS — 149950-60-7.

Profile

Emivirine is a non-nucleoside reverse transcriptase inhibitor under investigation for the treatment of HIV infection and AIDS.

Emtricitabine (20203-e)

Emtricitabine *(USAN, rINN)*.

BW-524W91; FTC; (–)-FTC; FTC-(–). 5-Fluoro-1-[(2R,5S)-2-(hydroxymethyl)-1,3-oxathiolan-5-yl]cytosine.

$C_8H_{10}FN_3O_3S = 247.2$.

CAS — 143491-57-0.

Profile

Emtricitabine is a nucleoside reverse transcriptase inhibitor under investigation for the treatment of HIV infection. It is also active against hepatitis B virus.

◊ References.
1. Molina J-M, *et al.* Once-daily combination therapy with emtricitabine, didanosine, and efavirenz in human immunodeficiency virus-infected patients. *J Infect Dis* 2000; **182:** 599–602.

Enfuvirtide (1743-z)

Enfuvirtide *(USAN)*.

DP-178; Pentafuside; T-20.

$C_{204}H_{301}N_{51}O_{64} = 4491.9$.

CAS — 159519-65-0.

Profile

Enfuvirtide is a synthetic 36-amino acid peptide that corresponds to residues 127–162 in the extracellular portion of the transmembrane segment (gp41) of the HIV envelope glycoprotein. It blocks HIV cell fusion and viral entry. It is under investigation for the treatment of HIV infection and AIDS.

◊ References.
1. Kilby JM, *et al.* Potent suppression of HIV-1 replication in humans by T-20, a peptide inhibitor of gp41-mediated virus entry. *Nature Med* 1998; **4:** 1302–7.
2. Nagashima KA, *et al.* Human immunodeficiency virus type 1 entry inhibitors PRO 542 and T-20 are potently synergistic in blocking virus-cell and cell-cell fusion. *J Infect Dis* 2001; **183:** 1121–5.
3. Zollner B, *et al.* Primary genotypic resistance of HIV-1 to the fusion inhibitor T-20 in long-term infected patients. *AIDS* 2001; **15:** 935–6.

Famciclovir (10521-s)

Famciclovir *(BAN, USAN, rINN)*.

BRL-42810. 2[2-(2-Amino-9H-purin-9-yl)ethyl]trimethylene diacetate.

$C_{14}H_{19}N_5O_4 = 321.3$.

CAS — 104227-87-4.

ATC — J05AB09; S01AD07.

Adverse Effects and Precautions

The most common adverse effects of famciclovir are headache and nausea. Other adverse effects include vomiting, dizziness, skin rash, confusion, and hallucinations. In addition, abdominal pain, fever, and, rarely, granulocytopenia and thrombocytopenia have been reported in immunocompromised patients receiving famciclovir.

Dosage should be reduced in patients with impaired renal function. Acute renal failure has been reported in patients with impaired renal function receiving inappropriately high doses of famciclovir.

◊ References.
1. Saltzman R, *et al.* Safety of famciclovir in patients with herpes zoster and genital herpes. *Antimicrob Agents Chemother* 1994; **38:** 2454–7.

Interactions

As for Penciclovir, p.638.

Antiviral Action

As for Penciclovir, p.638.

Pharmacokinetics

Famciclovir is rapidly absorbed following oral administration. Absorption is delayed but not reduced by administration with food. It is rapidly converted to penciclovir (see p.638), peak plasma concentrations occurring within about an hour of administration, and virtually no famciclovir is detectable in the plasma or urine. Bioavailability of penciclovir is reported to be 77%. Famciclovir is principally excreted in the urine (partly by renal tubular secretion) as penciclovir and its 6-deoxy precursor: elimination is reduced in patients with impaired renal function.

◊ References.
1. Pue MA, Benet LZ. Pharmacokinetics of famciclovir in man. *Antiviral Chem Chemother* 1993; **4** (suppl 1): 47–55.
2. Boike SC, *et al.* Pharmacokinetics of famciclovir in subjects with varying degrees of renal impairment. *Clin Pharmacol Ther* 1994; **55:** 418–26.
3. Boike SC, *et al.* Pharmacokinetics of famciclovir in subjects with chronic renal disease. *J Clin Pharmacol* 1994; **34:** 1199–1207.
4. Gill KS, Wood MJ. The clinical pharmacokinetics of famciclovir. *Clin Pharmacokinet* 1996; **31:** 1–8.

Uses and Administration

Famciclovir is a prodrug of the antiviral penciclovir (p.638). It is given by mouth in the treatment of herpes zoster (see Varicella-zoster Infections, p.608) and genital and mucocutaneous herpes (see Herpes Simplex Infections, p.607).

For herpes zoster, famciclovir is given in a dose of 250 mg three times daily, or 750 mg once daily, for 7 days (in the USA the recommended dose is 500 mg three times daily for 7 days); immunocompromised patients are given 500 mg three times daily for 10 days.

For first episodes of genital herpes, famciclovir is given in a dose of 250 mg three times daily for 5 days; immunocompromised patients are given 500 mg twice daily for 7 days. For acute treatment of recurrent episodes of genital herpes, 125 mg is given twice daily for 5 days; immunocompromised patients are given 500 mg twice daily for 7 days. For suppression of recurrent episodes of genital herpes, 250 mg is given twice daily; HIV patients may be given 500 mg twice daily. Such suppressive treatment is interrupted every 6 to 12 months in order to recognise possible changes in the natural history of the disease.

For acute treatment of recurrent mucocutaneous herpes in HIV-infected patients, 500 mg is given twice daily for 7 days.

Doses of famciclovir should be reduced in patients with renal impairment (see below).

◊ General references.
1. Vere Hodge RA. Famciclovir and penciclovir: the mode of action of famciclovir including its conversion to penciclovir. *Antiviral Chem Chemother* 1993; **4:** 67–84.
2. Perry CM, Wagstaff AJ. Famciclovir: a review of its pharmacological properties and therapeutic efficacy in herpesvirus infections. *Drugs* 1995; **50:** 396–415.

Administration in renal impairment. Doses of famciclovir need to be reduced in patients with impaired renal function. The UK manufacturer recommends the following doses based on creatinine clearance (CC):

Immunocompetent patients:
Herpes zoster or an initial episode of genital herpes
• for CC 30 to 59 mL per minute, 250 mg twice daily
• for CC 10 to 29 mL per minute, 250 mg once daily
Acute recurrent genital herpes, treatment
• for CC 30 to 59 mL per minute, no dosage adjustment necessary
• for CC 10 to 29 mL per minute, 125 mg once daily
Recurrent genital herpes, suppression
• for CC over 30 mL per minute, 250 mg twice daily
• for CC 10 to 29 mL per minute, 125 mg twice daily
Immunocompromised patients:
Herpes zoster
• for CC over 40 mL per minute, 500 mg three times daily
• for CC 30 to 39 mL per minute, 250 mg three times daily
• for CC 10 to 29 mL per minute, 125 mg three times daily
Herpes simplex infections
• for CC over 40 mL per minute, 500 mg twice daily
• for CC 30 to 39 mL per minute, 250 mg twice daily
• for CC 10 to 29 mL per minute, 125 mg twice daily

Patients on haemodialysis should be given doses of famciclovir immediately following dialysis.

Viral infections. Some studies of the use of famciclovir in herpes zoster[1-4] and genital herpes.[5-9]
1. Degreef H, et al. Famciclovir, a new oral antiherpes drug: results of the first controlled clinical study demonstrating its efficacy and safety in the treatment of uncomplicated herpes zoster in immunocompetent patients. *Int J Antimicrob Agents* 1994; **4:** 241–6.
2. Tyring S, et al. Famciclovir for the treatment of acute herpes zoster: effects on acute disease and postherpetic neuralgia: a randomized, double-blind, placebo-controlled trial. *Ann Intern Med* 1995; **123:** 89–96.
3. Klein JL, et al. Famciclovir in AIDS-related acute retinal necrosis. *AIDS* 1996; **10:** 1300–1.
4. Tyring S, et al. Famciclovir for ophthalmic zoster: a randomised aciclovir controlled study. *Br J Ophthalmol* 2001; **85:** 576–81.
5. Sacks SL, et al. Patient-initiated, twice daily oral famciclovir for early recurrent genital herpes: a randomized, double-blind multicenter trial. *JAMA* 1996; **276:** 44–9.
6. Mertz GJ, et al. Oral famciclovir for suppression of recurrent genital herpes simplex virus infection in women: a multicenter, double-blind, placebo-controlled trial. *Arch Intern Med* 1997; **157:** 343–9.
7. Schacker T, et al. Famciclovir for the suppression of symptomatic and asymptomatic herpes simplex virus reactivation in HIV-infected persons: a double-blind, placebo-controlled trial. *Ann Intern Med* 1998; **128:** 21–8.
8. Diaz-Mitoma F, et al. Oral famciclovir for the suppression of recurrent genital herpes: a randomized controlled trial. *JAMA* 1998; **280:** 887–92.
9. Chosidow O, et al. Famciclovir vs aciclovir in immunocompetent patients with recurrent genital herpes infections: a parallel-groups, randomized, double-blind clinical trial. *Br J Dermatol* 2001; **144:** 818–24.

Preparations

Proprietary Preparations (details are given in Part 3)
Aust.: Famvir; *Austral.:* Famvir; *Belg.:* Famvir; *Canad.:* Famvir; *Denm.:* Famvir; *Fin.:* Famvir; *Fr.:* Oravir; *Ger.:* Famvir; *Hong Kong:* Famvir; *Irl.:* Famvir; *Israel:* Famvir; *Neth.:* Famvir; *NZ:* Famvir; *S.Afr.:* Famvir; *Singapore:* Famvir; *Spain:* Famvir; *Swed.:* Famvir; *Switz.:* Famvir; *Thai.:* Famvir; *UK:* Famvir; *USA:* Famvir.

Fialuridine (19187-j)

Fialuridine (USAN, rINN).
FIAU; Fluoroiodoarauracil. 1-(2-Deoxy-2-fluoro-β-D-arabino-furanosyl)-5-iodouracil.
$C_9H_{10}FIN_2O_5 = 372.1$.
CAS — 69123-98-4.

Profile
Fialuridine is a synthetic nucleoside analogue structurally re-

lated to thymidine with activity against hepatitis B virus. Clinical studies were suspended after hepatic failure and lactic acidosis, including several fatalities, were associated with its use.

◊ References.
1. McKenzie R, et al. Hepatic failure and lactic acidosis due to fialuridine (FIAU), an investigational nucleoside analogue for chronic hepatitis B. *N Engl J Med* 1995; **333:** 1099–1105.
2. Honkoop P, et al. Mitochondrial injury: lessons from the fialuridine trial. *Drug Safety* 1997; **17:** 1–7.

Fomivirsen Sodium (20582-z)

Fomivirsen Sodium (BANM, USAN, rINNM).
Isis-2922.
$C_{204}H_{243}N_{63}Na_{20}O_{114}P_{20}S_{20} = 7122.0$.
CAS — 144245-52-3 (fomivirsen); 160369-77-7 (fomivirsen sodium).

Adverse Effects and Precautions
Adverse effects following intra-ocular administration of fomivirsen are confined to the treated eye. They include intra-ocular inflammation, transient increases in intra-ocular pressure, retinal detachments and oedema, and visual abnormalities. Other adverse effects associated with the intravitreal injection procedure include vitreal haemorrhage, endophthalmitis, uveitis, and cataract formation.
Patients should be monitored during treatment for changes in intra-ocular pressure and visual field.

Interactions
In order to reduce the risk of inflammation, intra-ocular administration of fomivirsen is not recommended within 2 to 4 weeks of intravenous or intravitreal cidofovir treatment.

Antiviral Action
Fomivirsen is an antisense oligonucleotide that inhibits human cytomegalovirus replication. It is active against strains of cytomegalovirus resistant to ganciclovir, foscarnet, and cidofovir. Resistance to fomivirsen has been induced *in vitro*, but cross-resistance to antivirals with other modes of action is unlikely.

Uses and Administration
Fomivirsen is an antisense oligonucleotide that is used as the sodium salt for the local treatment of cytomegalovirus retinitis (p.606) in patients with AIDS. A dose of 165 μg is given by intravitreal injection into the affected eye once each week for 3 weeks, then on alternate weeks thereafter. For previously treated disease, 330 μg may be injected into the affected eye; this dose is then repeated once after 2 weeks and then once every 4 weeks thereafter.

◊ Reviews.
1. Perry CM, Barman Balfour JA. Fomivirsen. *Drugs* 1999; **57:** 375–80.

Preparations

Proprietary Preparations (details are given in Part 3)
Denm.: Vitravene; *Fin.:* Vitravene; *Fr.:* Vitravene; *UK:* Vitravene; *USA:* Vitravene.

Foscarnet Sodium (16817-b)

Foscarnet Sodium (BAN, USAN, rINN).
A-29622; EHB-776 (anhydrous and hexahydrate); Foscarnetum Natricum Hexahydricum; Phosphonatoformate Trisodium; Phosphonoformate Trisodium. Trisodium phosphonatoformate hexahydrate.
$CNa_3O_5P,6H_2O = 300.0$.
CAS — 63585-09-1 (foscarnet sodium); 34156-56-4 (foscarnet sodium hexahydrate).
Pharmacopoeias. In Eur. (see p.vi).
Each g of foscarnet sodium represents about 15.6 mmol of sodium and about 5.2 mmol of phosphate.

Pharmacopoeial description
Ph. Eur.: A white crystalline powder. Soluble in water; practically insoluble in alcohol. A 2% solution in water has a pH of 9.0 to 11.0. Protect from light.

Incompatibility. Foscarnet sodium has been found to be visually incompatible with a number of commonly used injectable drugs including aciclovir sodium, ganciclovir, certain antibacterials, amphotericin B, pentamidine isetionate, and trimetrexate. The manufacturer also lists incompatibilities with glucose 30% solutions and solutions containing calcium along with a range of other drugs. It is therefore recommended that foscarnet should not be infused via an intravenous line with any other drugs.
References.
1. Lor E, Takagi J. Visual compatibility of foscarnet with other injectable drugs. *Am J Hosp Pharm* 1990; **47:** 157–9.
2. Baltz JK, et al. Visual compatibility of foscarnet with other injectable drugs during simulated Y-site administration. *Am J Hosp Pharm* 1990; **47:** 2075–7.

Adverse Effects and Treatment
Intravenous injection of foscarnet sodium may cause phlebitis at the site of injection. Foscarnet sodium can cause renal impairment which may be severe. Anae-

mia may be common and granulocytopenia and thrombocytopenia have been reported. Foscarnet sodium may cause hypocalcaemia and other electrolyte disturbances. Some patients may experience convulsions. Excretion of high concentrations in the urine can cause local irritation and genital ulceration. Other adverse effects reported include nausea, vomiting, and diarrhoea; malaise; fever; headache, fatigue, dizziness, paraesthesia, and tremor; mood disturbances; rash; abnormal liver function tests; blood pressure and ECG changes; and isolated reports of pancreatitis.

In cases of overdosage it is important to maintain hydration. Foscarnet elimination may be increased by haemodialysis.

Effects on the CNS. Convulsions may occur in up to 10% of AIDS patients receiving foscarnet and have been reported following overdoses. Contributing factors include underlying CNS pathology (HIV-related encephalopathy or other infections) and foscarnet-related electrolyte disturbances. However, seizures have been reported in patients without apparent risk factors.[1]
1. Lor E, Liu YQ. Neurologic sequelae associated with foscarnet therapy. *Ann Pharmacother* 1994; **28:** 1035–7.

Effects on electrolyte balance. Foscarnet chelates divalent metal ions and acute hypocalcaemia has been reported to occur in about 15% of patients receiving foscarnet. Other electrolyte disturbances include hypokalaemia and hypomagnesaemia (each in about 15%), hypophosphataemia (8%), and hyperphosphataemia (6%). The incidence of electrolyte disturbances is higher in patients receiving hydration. Hypocalcaemia may cause paraesthesias and, together with hypomagnesaemia and hypokalaemia, may predispose to seizures (see Effects on the CNS, above) and cardiovascular disturbances.
Administration of foscarnet in a liposomal formulation has been proposed to overcome the effects on electrolytes.[1]
1. Omar RF, et al. Liposomal encapsulation of foscarnet protects against hypocalcaemia induced by free foscarnet. *Antimicrob Agents Chemother* 1995; **39:** 1973–8.

Effects on the kidneys. The most serious common adverse effect of foscarnet sodium is nephrotoxicity. Clinically significant increases in serum-creatinine concentrations occur in about 30% of patients, and the incidence of nephrotoxicity tends to increase with increasing dose[1] and duration of therapy.[2] Foscarnet sodium is excreted unchanged in the urine and tubulo-interstitial lesions and deposition of crystals in the glomerular capillary lumen have been implicated.[3] Acute renal failure has occurred and haemodialysis has been reported to have reduced plasma-foscarnet concentrations in a patient.[4] The risk of nephrotoxicity can be minimised by ensuring adequate hydration, the use of intermittent dosing schedules,[5] and adjusting the dose according to serum-creatinine concentrations. Nephrogenic diabetes insipidus associated with foscarnet sodium has been reported.[6,7]
1. Jacobson MA, et al. A dose-ranging study of daily maintenance intravenous foscarnet therapy for cytomegalovirus retinitis in AIDS. *J Infect Dis* 1993; **168:** 444–8.
2. Gaub J, et al. The effect of foscarnet (phosphonoformate) on human immunodeficiency virus isolation, T-cell subsets and lymphocyte function in AIDS patients. *AIDS* 1987; **1:** 27–33.
3. Beaufils H, et al. Foscarnet and crystals in glomerular capillary lumens. *Lancet* 1990; **336:** 755.
4. Deray G, et al. Foscarnet-induced acute renal failure and effectiveness of haemodialysis. *Lancet* 1987; **1:** 216.
5. Deray G, et al. Prevention of foscarnet nephrotoxicity. *Ann Intern Med* 1990; **113:** 332.
6. Farese RV, et al. Nephrogenic diabetes insipidus associated with foscarnet treatment of cytomegalovirus retinitis. *Ann Intern Med* 1990; **112:** 955–6.
7. Conn J, et al. Nephrogenic diabetes insipidus associated with foscarnet—a case report. *J Antimicrob Chemother* 1996; **37:** 1180–1.

Effects on the skin and mucous membranes. A generalised pruritic macular rash was reported in a patient receiving foscarnet which subsided after the drug was withdrawn.[1]
There have been several reports of genital ulceration,[2-7] possibly related to local toxicity arising from high concentrations of foscarnet in the urine. Oral ulceration has occurred, usually in patients also presenting with genital ulceration during foscarnet treatment.[3-5] Uvular and oesophageal ulcerations have also been reported.[4,8]
1. Green ST, et al. Generalised cutaneous rash associated with foscarnet usage in AIDS. *J Infect* 1990; **21:** 227–8.
2. Van Der Pijl JW, et al. Foscarnet and penile ulceration. *Lancet* 1990; **335:** 286.
3. Gilquin J, et al. Genital and oral erosions induced by foscarnet. *Lancet* 1990; **335:** 287.
4. Féguex S, et al. Penile ulcerations with foscarnet. *Lancet* 1990; **335:** 547.
5. Moyle G, et al. Penile ulcerations with foscarnet. *Lancet* 1990; **335:** 547–8.
6. Lacey HB, et al. Vulval ulceration associated with foscarnet. *Genitourin Med* 1992; **68:** 182.
7. Caumes E, et al. Foscarnet-induced vulval erosion. *J Am Acad Dermatol* 1993; **28:** 799.
8. Saint-Marc T, et al. Uvula and oesophageal ulcerations with foscarnet. *Lancet* 1992; **340:** 970–1.

The symbol † denotes a preparation no longer actively marketed

Precautions

Foscarnet sodium should be used with caution in renal impairment and doses should be reduced if serum creatinine is raised. Serum-creatinine concentrations should be measured on alternate days throughout induction treatment; monitoring may be weekly during maintenance therapy. An adequate state of hydration must be maintained during therapy to prevent renal toxicity. Electrolytes, especially calcium and magnesium, should also be monitored and deficiencies corrected before starting foscarnet therapy.

Interactions

Foscarnet should not be given concurrently with other nephrotoxic drugs or with other drugs which can affect serum-calcium concentrations. Intravenous pentamidine can produce both of these effects and severe additive toxicity may result from its use in combination with foscarnet.

Ciprofloxacin. Tonic-clonic seizures associated with foscarnet administration in 2 patients receiving multiple antimicrobial drugs were thought to have been exacerbated by the concurrent administration of ciprofloxacin.[1]

1. Fan-Havard P, *et al.* Concurrent use of foscarnet and ciprofloxacin may increase the propensity for seizures. *Ann Pharmacother* 1994; **28:** 869–72.

Antiviral Action

Foscarnet inhibits replication of human herpesviruses including cytomegalovirus, herpes simplex virus types 1 and 2, herpesvirus 6 (see under Ganciclovir, p.623), Epstein-Barr virus, and varicella-zoster virus. Activity is also reported against hepatitis B virus and HIV. Foscarnet acts by inhibition of virus-specific DNA polymerases and reverse transcriptases: unlike the nucleoside reverse transcriptase inhibitors and ganciclovir, foscarnet does not require intracellular conversion to an active triphosphate.

◊ References.
1. Balfour HH, *et al.* Effect of foscarnet on quantities of cytomegalovirus and human immunodeficiency virus in blood of persons with AIDS. *Antimicrob Agents Chemother* 1996; **40:** 2721–6.
2. Jabs DA, *et al.* Incidence of foscarnet resistance and cidofovir resistance in patients treated for cytomegalovirus retinitis. *Antimicrob Agents Chemother* 1998; **42:** 2240–4.

Pharmacokinetics

The pharmacokinetics of foscarnet are complicated by the high incidence of renal impairment during therapy and by the deposition and subsequent gradual release of foscarnet from bone. Thus the estimation of half-life depends upon the duration of foscarnet therapy and the duration of the observation period. The plasma half-life in patients with normal renal function is in the order of 2 to 4 hours, but terminal half-lives in excess of 100 hours have been reported. Plasma protein binding is about 14 to 17%. Foscarnet crosses the blood-brain barrier in variable amounts; CSF concentrations ranging from zero to more than three times the plasma concentration have been reported. Foscarnet is mostly excreted unchanged in the urine.

◊ The pharmacokinetics of foscarnet [sodium] during and after continuous intravenous infusion (0.14 to 0.19 mg per kg body-weight per minute) were studied in 13 HIV-infected male patients with lymphadenopathy or AIDS-related complex.[1] During infusion there were wide inter- and intra-individual variations in plasma-foscarnet concentrations, which ranged from approximately 100 to 500 µmol per litre. There appeared to be a link between the degree of adverse effects experienced and plasma-foscarnet concentrations above 350 µmol per litre. Foscarnet was excreted mainly via the kidneys. It was thought that up to 20% of the cumulative intravenous dose may have been deposited in bone 7 days after the end of infusion.

A similar foscarnet pharmacokinetic study was performed in 8 AIDS patients with cytomegalovirus retinitis treated every 8 hours intermittently with 2-hour infusions.[2] This method of administration produced plasma concentrations high enough to exert an antiviral effect.

Penetration of foscarnet into the CSF is very variable. Lumbar puncture was performed in 5 patients[1] and foscarnet was found to be distributed into the CSF at concentrations of 13 to 68% of those in the plasma. Subsequent studies have shown that CSF concentrations of foscarnet would be virostatic in the majority of patients[3] attaining a mean concentration of about 25% of plasma concentration following a single infusion[3,4] and 66% under steady state conditions.[4] CSF concentrations ranged

from 0 to 340%[3] and 5 to 72%[4] of those in plasma. A correlation between the amount of foscarnet in the CSF and the inflammation of the meninges was found in one of the studies,[3] and with the HIV infection stage in another,[4] but neither reported a correlation with plasma concentration.

Evidence from a study of the effects of probenecid on foscarnet excretion[5] suggested that renal excretion was via glomerular filtration and not tubular excretion.

1. Sjövall J, *et al.* Pharmacokinetics of foscarnet and distribution to cerebrospinal fluid after intravenous infusion in patients with human immunodeficiency virus infection. *Antimicrob Agents Chemother* 1989; **33:** 1023–31.
2. Aweeka F, *et al.* Pharmacokinetics of intermittently administered intravenous foscarnet in the treatment of acquired immunodeficiency syndrome patients with serious cytomegalovirus retinitis. *Antimicrob Agents Chemother* 1989; **33:** 742–5.
3. Raffi F, *et al.* Penetration of foscarnet into cerebrospinal fluid of AIDS patients. *Antimicrob Agents Chemother* 1993; **37:** 1777–80.
4. Hengge UR, *et al.* Foscarnet penetrates the blood-brain barrier: rationale for therapy of cytomegalovirus encephalitis. *Antimicrob Agents Chemother* 1993; **37:** 1010–14.
5. Noormohamed FH, *et al.* Renal excretion and pharmacokinetics of foscarnet in HIV sero-positive patients: effect of probenecid pretreatment. *Br J Clin Pharmacol* 1997; **43:** 112–15.

Uses and Administration

Foscarnet sodium is a non-nucleoside pyrophosphate analogue active against herpesviruses. It is used mainly for the treatment of cytomegalovirus retinitis in AIDS patients and for aciclovir-resistant mucocutaneous herpes simplex virus infections in immunocompromised patients.

Foscarnet is administered by intravenous infusion. It is usually available as an infusion containing 24 mg of foscarnet sodium per mL. This may be administered via a central vein or diluted with glucose 5% or sodium chloride 0.9% to a concentration of 12 mg per mL and administered via a peripheral vein. Hydration with 0.5 to 1 litre of sodium chloride 0.9% or glucose 5% may be given with each infusion to reduce renal toxicity.

For the treatment of cytomegalovirus retinitis in adults with normal renal function a usual dose is 60 mg per kg body-weight infused over at least 1 hour every 8 hours or 90 mg per kg infused over 1½ to 2 hours every 12 hours for 2 to 3 weeks, followed by maintenance therapy with 60 mg per kg daily increasing to 90 to 120 mg per kg daily if tolerated. For the treatment of aciclovir-resistant mucocutaneous herpes simplex virus infections in adults with normal renal function, a dose of 40 mg per kg, infused over 1 hour, every 8 or 12 hours may be given for 2 to 3 weeks or until lesions have healed.

Doses should be reduced in patients with impaired renal function (see below).

◊ Reviews.
1. Chrisp P, Clissold SP. Foscarnet: a review of its antiviral activity, pharmacokinetic properties and therapeutic use in immunocompromised patients with cytomegalovirus retinitis. *Drugs* 1991; **41:** 104–29.
2. Wagstaff AJ, Bryson HM. Foscarnet: a reappraisal of its antiviral activity, pharmacokinetic properties and therapeutic use in immunocompromised patients with viral infections. *Drugs* 1994; **48:** 199–226.

Administration in renal impairment. For patients with varying degrees of renal impairment [based on creatinine clearance (CC)] the UK manufacturers of foscarnet sodium consider the following doses to be equivalent to the 60 mg per kg body-weight dose given to patients with normal renal function for the treatment of cytomegalovirus infection:

- for CC more than 1.6 mL per kg per minute, 60 mg per kg
- for CC 1.6 to 1.4 mL per kg per minute, 55 mg per kg
- for CC 1.4 to 1.2 mL per kg per minute, 49 mg per kg
- for CC 1.2 to 1.0 mL per kg per minute, 42 mg per kg
- for CC 1.0 to 0.8 mL per kg per minute, 35 mg per kg
- for CC 0.8 to 0.6 mL per kg per minute, 28 mg per kg
- for CC 0.6 to 0.4 mL per kg per minute, 21 mg per kg

Foscarnet is not recommended for patients with a CC of less than 0.4 mL per kg per minute.

They also suggest similar proportional reductions of the dose of 40 mg per kg used to treat herpes simplex infections in patients with normal renal function.

Cytomegalovirus infections. Foscarnet is used in the treatment of severe cytomegalovirus infections (p.606) in immunocompromised patients. It has been particularly useful instead of ganciclovir in patients with AIDS who require concurrent zidovudine therapy but are unable to tolerate ganciclovir (because of haematological toxicity) and appears to possess similar efficacy[1,2] (see also under Ganciclovir, p.624). It has also been tried in combination with ganciclovir in patients unresponsive to either drug alone.[3-6] One study[7] reported that a maintenance dose of 120 mg per kg body-weight of foscarnet daily was

more effective and no more toxic than 90 mg per kg per day in patients with cytomegalovirus retinitis, but long-term intravenous therapy is generally poorly tolerated.[2] Beneficial responses have been reported with intravitreal injections of foscarnet 1.2 mg every 48 hours for 4 doses[8] or 2.4 mg every 72 hours for 6 doses, then once weekly thereafter.[9]

Foscarnet has also been investigated for primary prophylaxis of cytomegalovirus infection in bone marrow transplant recipients at high risk of infection.[10,11]

1. Blanshard C, *et al.* Treatment of AIDS-associated gastrointestinal cytomegalovirus infection with foscarnet and ganciclovir: a randomised comparison. *J Infect Dis* 1995; **172:** 622–8.
2. Studies of Ocular Complications of AIDS Research Group, in collaboration with the AIDS Clinical Trials Group. Mortality in patients with the acquired immunodeficiency syndrome treated with either foscarnet or ganciclovir for cytomegalovirus retinitis. *N Engl J Med* 1992; **326:** 213–20.
3. Coker RJ, *et al.* Treatment of cytomegalovirus retinitis with ganciclovir and foscarnet. *Lancet* 1991; **338:** 574–5.
4. Enting R, *et al.* Ganciclovir/foscarnet for cytomegalovirus meningoencephalitis in AIDS. *Lancet* 1992; **340:** 559–60.
5. Dieterich DT, *et al.* Concurrent use of ganciclovir and foscarnet to treat cytomegalovirus infection in AIDS patients. *J Infect Dis* 1993; **167:** 1184–8.
6. Studies of Ocular Complications of AIDS Research Group, in Collaboration with the AIDS Clinical Trials Group. Combination foscarnet and ganciclovir therapy vs monotherapy for the treatment of relapsed cytomegalovirus retinitis in patients with AIDS: the Cytomegalovirus Retreatment Trial. *Arch Ophthalmol* 1996; **114:** 23–33.
7. Jacobson MA, *et al.* A dose-ranging study of daily maintenance intravenous foscarnet therapy for cytomegalovirus retinitis in AIDS. *J Infect Dis* 1993; **168:** 444–8.
8. Lieberman RM, *et al.* Efficacy of intravitreal foscarnet in a patient with AIDS. *N Engl J Med* 1994; **330:** 868–9.
9. Diaz-Llopis M, *et al.* High dose intravitreal foscarnet in the treatment of cytomegalovirus retinitis in AIDS. *Br J Ophthalmol* 1994; **78:** 120–4.
10. Reusser P, *et al.* Phase I-II trial of foscarnet for prevention of cytomegalovirus infection in autologous and allogeneic marrow transplant recipients. *J Infect Dis* 1992; **166:** 473–9.
11. Ippoliti C, *et al.* Foscarnet for prevention of cytomegalovirus infection in allogeneic marrow transplant recipients unable to receive ganciclovir. *Bone Marrow Transplant* 1997; **20:** 491–5.

Herpes simplex infections. Although foscarnet is effective in the treatment of herpes simplex infections it is usually reserved for severe infections, particularly in immunocompromised patients who have failed to respond to aciclovir (see p.607).[1-3] However, although the reason was not clear, herpes simplex infections were reported in 2 patients while receiving foscarnet for cytomegalovirus retinitis.[4]

1. Erlich KS, *et al.* Foscarnet therapy for severe acyclovir-resistant herpes simplex virus type-2 infections in patients with the acquired immunodeficiency syndrome (AIDS): an uncontrolled trial. *Ann Intern Med* 1989; **110:** 710–13.
2. Safrin S, *et al.* Foscarnet therapy for acyclovir-resistant mucocutaneous herpes simplex virus infection in 26 AIDS patients: preliminary data. *J Infect Dis* 1990; **161:** 1078–84.
3. Safrin S, *et al.* A controlled trial comparing foscarnet with vidarabine for acyclovir-resistant mucocutaneous herpes simplex in the acquired immunodeficiency syndrome. *N Engl J Med* 1991; **325:** 551–5.
4. Cotte L, *et al.* Herpes simplex virus infection during foscarnet therapy. *J Infect Dis* 1992; **166:** 447–8.

HIV infection and AIDS. A multicentre study[1] comparing foscarnet with ganciclovir for cytomegalovirus retinitis in patients with AIDS was prematurely terminated when patients in the foscarnet group showed improved survival compared with those given ganciclovir. Patients in the ganciclovir group received less concomitant antiretroviral therapy, in part because of additive toxicity, but it was considered that this alone was insufficient to explain the difference. Subsequent studies have supported these observations.[2-5] However, the toxicity of foscarnet at the doses necessary makes it unlikely to be used to treat HIV infection (p.608).

1. Studies of Ocular Complications of AIDS Research Group, in collaboration with the AIDS Clinical Trials Group. Mortality in patients with the acquired immunodeficiency syndrome treated with either foscarnet or ganciclovir for cytomegalovirus retinitis. *N Engl J Med* 1992; **326:** 213–20.
2. Reddy MM, *et al.* Effect of foscarnet therapy on human immunodeficiency virus p24 antigen levels in AIDS patients with cytomegalovirus retinitis. *J Infect Dis* 1992; **166:** 607–10.
3. Polis MA, *et al.* Increased survival of a cohort of patients with acquired immunodeficiency syndrome and cytomegalovirus retinitis who received sodium phosphonoformate (foscarnet). *Am J Med* 1993; **94:** 175–80.
4. Fletcher CV, *et al.* Foscarnet for suppression of human immunodeficiency virus replication. *Antimicrob Agents Chemother* 1994; **38:** 604–7.
5. Kaiser L, *et al.* Foscarnet decreases human immunodeficiency virus RNA. *J Infect Dis* 1995; **172:** 225–7.

Varicella-zoster infections. Although topical or systemic aciclovir is the usual treatment for ophthalmic herpes zoster (p.608), a study in 20 patients with AIDS suggested that ganciclovir alone or in combination with foscarnet was more effective than aciclovir in terms of preservation of long-term visual acuity.[1]

1. Moorthy RS, *et al.* Management of varicella zoster virus retinitis in AIDS. *Br J Ophthalmol* 1997; **81:** 189–94.

Preparations

BP 2001: Foscarnet Intravenous Infusion.

Proprietary Preparations (details are given in Part 3)
Aust.: Foscavir; **Austral.:** Foscavir; **Belg.:** Foscavir; **Denm.:** Foscovir; **Fin.:** Foscavir; **Fr.:** Foscavir; **Ger.:** Foscavir; Triapten; **Hong Kong:** Foscavir; **Israel:** Foscavir; **Ital.:** Foscavir; Virudin†; **Jpn:** Foscavir; **Neth.:** Foscavir; **Norw.:** Foscavir; **Port.:** Foscavir;

Spain: Foscavir; **Swed.:** Foscavir; **Switz.:** Foscavir; **Thai.:** Foscavir; **UK:** Foscavir; **USA:** Foscavir.

Ganciclovir (19746-g)

Ganciclovir (BAN, USAN, rINN).

BIOLF-62; BN-B759V; BW-759; BWB-759U; BW-759U; DH-PG; Dihydroxypropoxymethylguanine; 9-(1,3-Dihydroxy-2-propoxymethyl)guanine; 2′-NDG; 2′-Nor-2′-deoxyguanosine; RS-21592. 9-[2-Hydroxy-1-(hydroxymethyl)ethoxymethyl]guanine.

$C_9H_{13}N_5O_4 = 255.2$.

CAS — 82410-32-0.

ATC — J05AB06; S01AD09.

Ganciclovir Sodium (19084-q)

Ganciclovir Sodium (BANM, USAN, rINNM).

$C_9H_{12}N_5NaO_4 = 277.2$.

CAS — 107910-75-8.

Each g of ganciclovir sodium represents about 2.8 mmol of sodium.

Incompatibility. For reference to the incompatibility of ganciclovir and foscarnet, see Foscarnet Sodium, p.621.

Stability. Ganciclovir sodium solution in sodium chloride 0.9% was found to be stable when stored in polypropylene infusion-pump syringes for 12 hours at 25° and for 10 days at 4°.[1] Little variation was found in ganciclovir concentration following storage of a 2% solution at room temperature, 5°, and −8° for 10 to 24 days.[2]

1. Mulye NV, et al. Stability of ganciclovir sodium in an infusion-pump syringe. Am J Hosp Pharm 1994; **51:** 1348–9.
2. Morlet N, et al. High dose intravitreal ganciclovir for CMV retinitis: a shelf life and cost comparison study. Br J Ophthalmol 1995; **79:** 753–5.

Adverse Effects and Treatment

The most common adverse effects of intravenous ganciclovir are haematological and include neutropenia and thrombocytopenia; anaemia also occurs but less frequently. Neutropenia affects up to 40% of patients receiving ganciclovir intravenously, most commonly starting in the first or second week of ganciclovir treatment. It is usually reversible but may be prolonged or irreversible leading to potentially fatal infections. AIDS patients may be at a greater risk of neutropenia than other immunosuppressed patients. Thrombocytopenia occurs in about 20% of patients given ganciclovir intravenously. Those with iatrogenic immunosuppression may be more at risk of developing thrombocytopenia than AIDS patients. Other adverse effects occurring in patients given intravenous ganciclovir include fever, rash, and abnormal liver function tests. Irritation or phlebitis may occur at the site of injection due to the high pH. Less frequent adverse effects reported have included cardiovascular, CNS, gastrointestinal, metabolic, musculoskeletal, respiratory, urogenital, and cutaneous symptoms, and increased serum-creatinine and blood-urea nitrogen concentrations.

The most frequent adverse effects associated with orally administered ganciclovir include neutropenia, thrombocytopenia, anaemia, gastrointestinal disturbances, asthenia, headache, rash, pruritus, fever, abnormal liver function tests, pain, and infection.

Local adverse effects have been associated with the insertion of ocular implants containing ganciclovir.

Animal studies have suggested that there may be a risk of adverse testicular effects with temporary or permanent inhibition of spermatogenesis. Female fertility may also be affected. Such studies also suggest that ganciclovir is a potential mutagen, teratogen, and carcinogen.

Haemodialysis and hydration may be useful in reducing plasma concentrations of ganciclovir. Haematological adverse effects may be reversed in some patients by stopping treatment or reducing dosage; blood cell counts should return to normal within 3 to 7 days.

Colony-stimulating factors have been given with ganciclovir to limit its haematological toxicity.

◊ Molgramostim given intravenously at a dose of 5 µg per kg body-weight over a 4-hour period daily successfully treated

ganciclovir-induced neutropenia in a patient with cytomegalovirus retinitis and bone-marrow suppression.[1]

1. Russo CL, et al. Treatment of neutropenia associated with dyskeratosis congenita with granulocyte-macrophage colony-stimulating factor. Lancet 1990; **336:** 751–2.

Effects on mental function. Psychosis was associated with ganciclovir administration on 2 occasions in a patient.[1]

1. Hansen BA, et al. Ganciclovir-induced psychosis. N Engl J Med 1996; **335:** 1397.

Precautions

Ganciclovir should be administered with caution to patients with renal impairment and doses should be adjusted according to the serum-creatinine concentration (see Administration in Renal Impairment, below under Uses and Administration). It should not be given by rapid or bolus injection and adequate hydration should be maintained during intravenous infusion. It should be given with caution to patients with pre-existing cytopenias (low blood counts) or with a history of cytopenic reactions to drugs. Monitoring of white blood cell and platelet counts should be performed every 2 days or daily during the first 14 days of intravenous ganciclovir therapy and once weekly thereafter; ganciclovir should be withdrawn if the neutrophil count falls below 500 cells per µL and/or the platelet count falls below 25 000 cells per µL. Patients receiving oral ganciclovir should also be monitored regularly.

Ganciclovir is contra-indicated in pregnancy and in mothers who are breast feeding; contraception is recommended during ganciclovir treatment and, additionally for men, for 90 days thereafter.

Because of the risk of carcinogenicity and the high pH of the solution, contact with the skin and eyes should be avoided during the reconstitution of ganciclovir sodium injection.

Interactions

Zidovudine given concomitantly with ganciclovir may have an additive neutropenic effect and should not be given during intravenous ganciclovir induction therapy, although it has been given with caution during oral maintenance therapy. Probenecid and other drugs that inhibit renal tubular secretion and resorption may reduce the renal clearance of ganciclovir, and so increase its serum concentrations. Concomitant administration of intravenous ganciclovir and oral mycophenolate mofetil may result in increased plasma concentrations of both drugs due to competition for renal tubular secretion. Drugs that inhibit rapid cell division such as myelosuppressants may have additive toxic effects if given with ganciclovir. Convulsions have been reported when ganciclovir was given concomitantly with a combination of imipenem and cilastatin.

Antivirals. An additive neutropenic effect may occur if ganciclovir is given with *zidovudine* (see Zidovudine, p.646), there are reports of increased plasma concentrations of *didanosine* when given concurrently with ganciclovir (see p.618). There has also been a report[1] of decreased blood concentrations of ganciclovir when didanosine (200 mg every 12 hours) was given 2 hours before ganciclovir (1 g every 8 hours orally) but not when the two drugs were given at the same time. However, a later study[2] using twice the dose of ganciclovir found no effect irrespective of whether ganciclovir was administered 2 hours before or 2 hours after didanosine. The UK manufacturer also reports that decreased blood concentrations of ganciclovir have occurred when it is given orally 2 hours before didanosine.

When ganciclovir was given with *zalcitabine*, a 22% increase in the area under the concentration-time curve for ganciclovir was noted although it was believed that this did not necessitate any dosage modification.[3] No pharmacokinetic changes were reported when ganciclovir was given with *stavudine*.[3]

1. Cimoch PJ, et al. Pharmacokinetics of oral ganciclovir alone and in combination with zidovudine, didanosine, and probenecid in HIV-infected subjects. J Acquir Immune Defic Syndr Hum Retrovirol 1998; **17;** 227–34.
2. Jung D, et al. Effect of high-dose oral ganciclovir on didanosine disposition in human immunodeficiency virus (HIV)-positive patients. J Clin Pharmacol 1998; **38:** 1057–62.
3. Jung D, et al. The pharmacokinetics and safety profile of oral ganciclovir combined with zalcitabine or stavudine in asymptomatic HIV- and CMV-seropositive patients. J Clin Pharmacol 1999; **39;** 505–12.

Ciclosporin. Reversible acute unilateral or bilateral eye movement disorders typical of sixth cranial nerve palsies[1] occurred in 4 patients who received ciclosporin and ganciclovir following bone marrow transplantation.

1. Openshaw H, et al. Eye movement disorders in bone marrow transplant patients on cyclosporin and ganciclovir. Bone Marrow Transpl 1997; **19:** 503–5.

Antiviral Action

Ganciclovir inhibits replication of human herpesviruses *in vivo* and *in vitro*. It is active against cytomegalovirus, herpes simplex virus types 1 and 2, Epstein-Barr virus, varicella-zoster virus, and herpesvirus 6. This activity is due to intracellular conversion of ganciclovir by viral thymidine kinase (in herpes simplex and varicella-zoster infected cells) or possibly by cellular deoxyguanosine kinase (in Epstein-Barr infected cells) to ganciclovir monophosphate with subsequent cellular conversion to the diphosphate and the active triphosphate. The mechanism of phosphorylation in cells infected with cytomegalovirus has yet to be determined. Ganciclovir triphosphate inhibits viral DNA synthesis by inhibiting the viral DNA polymerase enzyme as well as being incorporated into the viral DNA. This process is selective for infected cells; the concentration of ganciclovir triphosphate is reported to be tenfold higher in cytomegalovirus-infected cells than in uninfected cells.

Ganciclovir has a similar spectrum of activity to aciclovir, herpes simplex virus types 1 and 2 being the most susceptible of the herpesviruses. However, cytomegalovirus is much more susceptible to ganciclovir than aciclovir.

Herpesvirus 6. Human herpesvirus 6 was susceptible to ganciclovir,[1-4] and foscarnet[2-4] *in vitro* but was relatively resistant to aciclovir,[1-4] brivudine,[4] and zidovudine.[3]

1. Russler SK, et al. Susceptibility of human herpesvirus 6 to aciclovir and ganciclovir. Lancet 1989; **ii:** 382.
2. Agut H, et al. Susceptibility of human herpesvirus 6 to acyclovir and ganciclovir. Lancet 1989; **ii:** 626.
3. Agut H, et al. In vitro sensitivity of human herpesvirus-6 to antiviral drugs. Res Virol 1989; **140:** 219–28.
4. Burns WH, Sandford GR. Susceptibility of human herpesvirus 6 to antivirals in vitro. J Infect Dis 1990; **162:** 634–7.

Resistance

Resistance to ganciclovir has been demonstrated *in vitro* in herpes simplex viruses, varicella-zoster virus, and cytomegalovirus. Possible mechanisms of resistance include a reduction in the phosphorylation of ganciclovir to the active form and reduced sensitivity of viral DNA polymerase. Resistance has also been reported in cytomegalovirus strains isolated from patients receiving ganciclovir for prolonged periods.

◊ The development of cytomegalovirus resistance to ganciclovir may be a factor in disease progression in patients receiving prolonged therapy with ganciclovir and the incidence of resistance is reported to increase with duration of therapy.[1] A ganciclovir-resistant isolate of cytomegalovirus has been detected in about 30% of 95 patients after 9 months of treatment and correlated with development of dissemination of infection to the contralateral eye.[2]

Ganciclovir-resistant cytomegalovirus has recently been reported[3] to be an important cause of late morbidity in seronegative patients who received cytomegalovirus-seropositive organ transplants; 5 of 67 seronegative recipients developed ganciclovir-resistant cytomegalovirus disease compared with none of 173 seropositive subjects.

1. Drew WL. Cytomegalovirus resistance to antiviral therapies. Am J Health-Syst Pharm 1996; **53** (suppl 2): S17–S23.
2. Jabs DA, et al. Cytomegalovirus retinitis and viral resistance: ganciclovir resistance. J Infect Dis 1998; **177:** 770–3.
3. Limaye AP, et al. Emergence of ganciclovir-resistant cytomegalovirus disease among recipients of solid-organ transplants. Lancet 2000; **356:** 645–9.

Pharmacokinetics

Ganciclovir is poorly absorbed from the gastrointestinal tract following oral administration and there is minimal systemic absorption after intravitreal injection. Bioavailability of oral ganciclovir is about 5%, and is increased by intake with food to 6 to 9%. Following intravenous administration as ganciclovir sodium it is widely distributed to body tissues and fluids including intra-ocular fluid and CSF. Binding to plasma proteins is reported to be 1 to 2%. Ganciclovir is excreted unchanged in the urine mainly by glomerular filtration and also active tubular secretion. The half-life is approximately 2.5 to 4.5 hours in patients with normal renal function following intravenous administration and about 4 to 5.7 hours after oral administration. In patients with renal impairment the renal clearance decreases and the half-life increases; a half-life of 28.5 hours has been reported when the serum-creatinine concentration was greater than 398 μmol per litre.

Haemodialysis has been reported to reduce ganciclovir plasma concentrations by about 50%.

◊ References.
1. Fletcher C, et al. Human pharmacokinetics of the antiviral drug DHPG. Clin Pharmacol Ther 1986; 40: 281–6.
2. Jacobson MA, et al. Human pharmacokinetics and tolerance of oral ganciclovir. Antimicrob Agents Chemother 1987; 31: 1251–4.
3. Rello J, et al. Effect of continuous arteriovenous hemodialysis on ganciclovir pharmacokinetics. DICP Ann Pharmacother 1990; 24: 544.
4. Morse GD, et al. Comparative pharmacokinetics of antiviral nucleoside analogues. Clin Pharmacokinet 1993; 24: 101–23.
5. Trang JM, et al. Linear single-dose pharmacokinetics of ganciclovir in newborns with congenital cytomegalovirus infections. Clin Pharmacol Ther 1993; 53: 15–21.
6. Combarnous F, et al. Pharmacokinetics of ganciclovir in a patient undergoing chronic haemodialysis. Eur J Clin Pharmacol 1994; 46: 379–81.
7. Arevalo JF, et al. Intravitreous and plasma concentrations of ganciclovir and foscarnet after intravenous therapy in patients with AIDS and cytomegalovirus retinitis. J Infect Dis 1995; 172: 951–6.
8. Morlet N, et al. High dose intravitreal ganciclovir injection provides a prolonged therapeutic intraocular concentration. Br J Ophthalmol 1996; 80: 214–16.
9. Lavelle J, et al. Effect of food on the relative bioavailability of oral ganciclovir. J Clin Pharmacol 1996; 36: 238–41.
10. Zhou X-J, et al. Population pharmacokinetics of ganciclovir in newborns with congenital cytomegalovirus infection. Antimicrob Agents Chemother 1996; 40: 2202–5.
11. Giffy KG. Pharmacokinetics of oral ganciclovir capsules in HIV-infected persons. AIDS 1996; 10 (suppl 4): S3–S6.
12. Jung D, et al. Steady-state relative bioavailability of three oral ganciclovir dosage regimens delivering 6,000 mg/day in patients with human immunodeficiency virus. J Clin Pharmacol 1998; 38: 1021–4.
13. Jung D, et al. Absolute bioavailability and dose proportionality of oral ganciclovir after ascending multiple doses in human immunodeficiency virus (HIV)-positive patients. J Clin Pharmacol 1998; 38: 1122–8.
14. Jung D, et al. Effect of food on high-dose oral ganciclovir disposition in HIV-positive subjects. J Clin Pharmacol 1999; 39: 161–5.
15. Snell GI, et al. Pharmacokinetic assessment of oral ganciclovir in lung transplant recipients with cystic fibrosis. J Antimicrob Chemother 2000; 45: 511–16.

Uses and Administration

Ganciclovir is a synthetic nucleoside analogue of guanine closely related to aciclovir, but with a greater activity against cytomegalovirus. It is used for the treatment and suppression of life- or sight-threatening cytomegalovirus infections in immunocompromised patients including those with AIDS and those with iatrogenic immunosuppression associated with organ transplantation or chemotherapy of neoplastic disease. It has also been used for superficial ocular herpes simplex infections and tried in Epstein-Barr virus and Herpesvirus simiae virus infections.

Ganciclovir is administered by intravenous infusion as the sodium salt over 1 hour. Solutions for infusion are usually prepared to give a concentration of 50 mg of ganciclovir per mL, then further diluted to contain not more than 10 mg per mL. Ganciclovir may also be given by mouth.

In **cytomegalovirus infections** the usual *initial* dose for *treatment* is 5 mg per kg body-weight by intravenous infusion every 12 hours for 14 to 21 days. This induction period may be followed by *maintenance* therapy to prevent recurrence or progression of the disease. The usual maintenance dosage is 5 mg per kg by intravenous infusion as a single daily dose for 7 days a week or 6 mg per kg daily for 5 days a week. If retinitis recurs or progresses a further induction course of ganciclovir may be given. AIDS patients who have received initial treatment with intravenous ganciclovir, and who have stable cytomegalovirus retinitis following at least 3 weeks of intravenous therapy, may be given ganciclovir orally in a dose of 3 g daily in 3 or 6 divided doses, with food.

For *prevention* of cytomegalovirus infection in immunocompromised patients, specifically those receiving immunosuppressive therapy following organ transplantation, ganciclovir may be given in an *initial* dose of 5 mg per kg by intravenous infusion every 12 hours for 7 to 14 days, followed by intravenous *mainte-*

nance therapy as above. Ganciclovir prophylaxis may be given orally in a dose of 1 g three times daily with food to immunocompromised patients including those with advanced HIV infection.

Doses should be reduced in renal impairment (see below).

Intravitreal implants providing controlled release of ganciclovir are available for those patients with cytomegalovirus retinitis who are unable to tolerate systemic therapy; the implants are designed to release ganciclovir over a period of 5 to 8 months.

Ganciclovir is used in some countries as a topical ophthalmic 0.15% gel for the treatment of superficial ocular **herpes simplex infections**.

◊ General references.
1. Faulds D, Heel RC. Ganciclovir: a review of its antiviral activity, pharmacokinetic properties and therapeutic efficacy in cytomegalovirus infections. Drugs 1990; 39: 597–638.
2. Markham A, Faulds D. Ganciclovir: an update of its therapeutic use in cytomegalovirus infection. Drugs 1994; 48: 455–84.
3. Crumpacker CS. Ganciclovir. N Engl J Med 1996; 335: 721–9.
4. McGavin JK, Goa KL. Ganciclovir: an update of its use in the prevention of cytomegalovirus infection and disease in transplant recipients. Drugs 2001; 61: 1153–83.

Administration in renal impairment. Doses of ganciclovir should be reduced in renal impairment. This may be done by reducing the dose and/or increasing the dosage interval according to creatinine clearance (CC). The following doses have been recommended by the manufacturer:
Intravenous dose:
• for CC of 70 mL per minute or more, 5 mg per kg body-weight every 12 hours for induction, followed by 5 mg per kg every 24 hours for maintenance
• for CC 50 to 69 mL per minute, 2.5 mg per kg every 12 hours for induction, 2.5 mg per kg every 24 hours for maintenance
• for CC 25 to 49 mL per minute, 2.5 mg per kg every 24 hours for induction, 1.25 mg per kg every 24 hours for maintenance
• for CC 10 to 24 mL per minute, 1.25 mg per kg every 24 hours for induction, 0.625 mg per kg every 24 hours for maintenance
• For dialysis patients a daily dose, on days when dialysis is performed, of 1.25 mg per kg for induction, or 0.625 mg per kg for maintenance, in each case given shortly after the end of dialysis has been recommended (in the USA, a maximum of 3 doses each week being recommended)
Oral dose:
• for CC of 70 mL per minute or more, 3000 mg daily in 3 or 6 divided doses
• for CC 50 to 69 mL per minute, 1500 mg daily
• for CC 25 to 49 mL per minute, 1000 mg daily
• for CC 10 to 24 mL per minute, 500 mg daily
• for CC less than 10 mL per minute, 500 mg three times a week, following haemodialysis.

Cytomegalovirus infections. Ganciclovir is used in both the treatment and prophylaxis of cytomegalovirus infections (p.606) in immunocompromised patients.

As with other herpesvirus infections, antiviral treatment tends to be suppressive rather than curative, and long-term maintenance therapy is necessary. Treatment in patients with AIDS is complicated by the additive haematological toxicity of ganciclovir and zidovudine. Clinical studies comparing ganciclovir with foscarnet for AIDS-related cytomegalovirus retinopathy have shown higher mortality rates in patients receiving ganciclovir than in those receiving foscarnet,[1,2] leading to the suggestion that foscarnet may possess intrinsic antiretroviral activity. However, an alternative explanation is that fewer patients receiving ganciclovir could tolerate full doses of zidovudine and were thus receiving suboptimal therapy. If it is possible to overcome the drug-induced neutropenia by giving colony-stimulating factors concomitantly (thus enabling the use of full therapeutic doses of zidovudine) ganciclovir may remain the preferred treatment for cytomegalovirus retinitis since foscarnet is less well tolerated. The use of ganciclovir in combination with cytomegalovirus immunoglobulins[3,4] or normal immunoglobulins,[5] or with foscarnet[6] may improve both efficacy and tolerance. An alternative is the use of intravitreal controlled-release ganciclovir implants[7-9] to avoid systemic adverse effects. Another development has been the introduction of oral preparations of ganciclovir for maintenance therapy.[10,11] Oral ganciclovir may be a useful adjunct to prevent systemic infection in patients treated with the intravitreal implants.[12] Cytomegalovirus infections at other sites in AIDS patients, including gastrointestinal and pulmonary infections, respond less well to ganciclovir than does retinitis.

Ganciclovir is also valuable for prophylaxis and early treatment of cytomegalovirus infections in transplant recipients.[13-17] For established infections, ganciclovir is reported to be more effective in solid organ transplant recipients than in bone marrow transplant recipients. Ganciclovir has also been

tried for prevention of cytomegalovirus infection in patients with AIDS, although results are conflicting.[18,19]

Treatment of congenital infections has a generally poor outcome. Prolonged treatment periods may improve the response, but the safety of extended treatment with ganciclovir in this age group has not been fully evaluated.
1. Studies of Ocular Complications of AIDS Research Group, in Collaboration with the AIDS Clinical Trials Group. Mortality in patients with the acquired immunodeficiency syndrome treated with either foscarnet or ganciclovir for cytomegalovirus retinitis. N Engl J Med 1992; 326: 213–20.
2. Polis MA, et al. Increases survival of a cohort of patients with acquired immunodeficiency syndrome and cytomegalovirus retinitis who received sodium phosphonoformate (foscarnet). Am J Med 1993; 94: 175–80.
3. D'Alessandro AM, et al. Successful treatment of severe cytomegalovirus infections with ganciclovir and CMV hyperimmune globulin in liver transplant recipients. Transplant Proc 1989; 21: 3560–1.
4. Salmela K, et al. Ganciclovir in the treatment of severe cytomegalovirus disease in liver transplant patients. Transplant Proc 1990; 22: 238–40.
5. Emanuel D, et al. Cytomegalovirus pneumonia after bone marrow transplantation successfully treated with the combination of ganciclovir and high-dose intravenous immune globulin. Ann Intern Med 1988; 109: 777–82.
6. Studies of Ocular Complications of AIDS Research Group, in Collaboration with the AIDS Clinical Trials Group. Combination foscarnet and ganciclovir therapy vs monotherapy for the treatment of relapsed cytomegalovirus retinitis in patients with AIDS: the Cytomegalovirus Retreatment Trial. Arch Ophthalmol 1996; 114: 23–33.
7. Anand R, et al. Control of cytomegalovirus retinitis using sustained release of intraocular gancyclovir. Arch Ophthalmol 1993; 111: 223–7.
8. Martin DF, et al. Treatment of cytomegalovirus retinitis with an intraocular sustained-release ganciclovir implant: a randomized controlled clinical trial. Arch Ophthalmol 1994; 112: 1531–9.
9. Musch DC, et al. Treatment of cytomegalovirus retinitis with a sustained-release ganciclovir implant. N Engl J Med 1997; 337: 83–90.
10. Oral Ganciclovir European and Australian Cooperative Study Group. Intravenous versus oral ganciclovir: European/Australian comparative study of efficacy and safety in the prevention of cytomegalovirus retinitis recurrence in patients with AIDS. AIDS 1995; 9: 471–7.
11. Drew WL, et al. Oral ganciclovir as maintenance treatment for cytomegalovirus retinitis in patients with AIDS. N Engl J Med 1995; 333: 615–20.
12. Martin DF, et al. Oral ganciclovir for patients with cytomegalovirus retinitis treated with a ganciclovir implant. N Engl J Med 1999; 340: 1063–70.
13. Goodrich JM, et al. Ganciclovir prophylaxis to prevent cytomegalovirus disease after allogeneic marrow transplant. Ann Intern Med 1993; 118: 173–8.
14. Winston DJ, et al. Ganciclovir prophylaxis of cytomegalovirus infection and disease in allogeneic bone marrow transplant recipients. Ann Intern Med 1993; 118: 179–84.
15. Hibberd PL, et al. Preemptive ganciclovir therapy to prevent cytomegalovirus disease in cytomegalovirus antibody-positive renal transplant recipients: a randomized controlled trial. Ann Intern Med 1995; 123: 18–26.
16. Winston DJ, et al. Randomised comparison of ganciclovir and high-dose acyclovir for long-term cytomegalovirus prophylaxis in liver-transplant recipients. Lancet 1995; 346: 69–74.
17. Gane E, et al. Randomised trial of efficacy and safety of oral ganciclovir in the prevention of cytomegalovirus disease in liver-transplant recipients. Lancet 1997; 350: 1729–33.
18. McCarthy M. Oral ganciclovir fails to prevent CMV in HIV trial. Lancet 1995; 346: 895.
19. Spector SA, et al. Oral ganciclovir for the prevention of cytomegalovirus disease in persons with AIDS. N Engl J Med 1996; 334: 1491–7.

Epstein-Barr virus infections. Ganciclovir has been reported to produce some improvement in patients with Epstein-Barr virus (EBV) infection, although no antiviral therapy is entirely satisfactory (p.607). Evidence of the efficacy of ganciclovir has been anecdotal, with eradication of EBV in an organ transplant recipient[1] and in a child who had relapsed after an initial response to interleukin-2 and splenectomy,[2] neither of whom had responded to aciclovir. However, it was ineffective in a second transplant recipient.[1]
1. Pirsch JD, et al. Treatment of severe Epstein-Barr virus-induced lymphoproliferative syndrome with ganciclovir: two cases after solid organ transplantation. Am J Med 1989; 86: 241–4.
2. Ishida Y, et al. Ganciclovir for chronic active Epstein-Barr virus infection. Lancet 1993; 341: 560–1.

Herpesvirus infections. In patients with herpes simplex keratitis, ganciclovir 0.15% gel was reported to be as effective as aciclovir 3% ointment,[1] the drug most commonly used in this infection (see Ocular Herpes Simplex Infections, p.607). Ganciclovir was also reported to produce beneficial responses in AIDS patients with ocular varicella zoster infections.[2]
1. Hoh HB, et al. Randomised trial of ganciclovir and acyclovir in the treatment of herpes simplex dendritic keratitis: a multicentre study. Br J Ophthalmol 1996; 80: 140–3.
2. Moorthy RS, et al. Management of varicella zoster virus retinitis in AIDS. Br J Ophthalmol 1997; 81: 189–94.

Preparations

Proprietary Preparations (details are given in Part 3)
Aust.: Cymevene; *Austral.:* Cymevene; Vitrasert; *Belg.:* Cymevene; *Canad.:* Cytovene; *Denm.:* Cymevene; *Fin.:* Cymevene; *Fr.:* Cymevan; Virgan; *Ger.:* Cymeven; *Hong Kong:* Cymevene; *Irl.:* Cymevene; *Israel:* Cymevene; *Ital.:* Citovirax; Cymevene; *Mex.:* Cymevene; *Neth.:* Cymevene; *Norw.:* Cymevene; *NZ:* Cymevene; *Port.:* Cymevene; *S.Afr.:* Cymevene; *Singapore:* Cymevene; *Spain:* Cymevene; *Swed.:* Cymevene; *Switz.:* Cymevene; *Thai.:* Cymevene; *UK:* Cymevene; Virgan; Vitrasert; *USA:* Cytovene; Vitrasert.

Ibacitabine (12854-d)

Ibacitabine (rINN).

Iododesoxycytidine. 2′-Deoxy-5-iodocytidine.

$C_9H_{12}IN_3O_4 = 353.1$.

CAS — 611-53-0.

ATC — D06BB08.

Profile

Ibacitabine is an antiviral used topically as a 1% gel in the treatment of mucocutaneous herpes simplex infections (p.607).

Preparations

Proprietary Preparations (details are given in Part 3)

Fr.: Cuterpes; **Hong Kong:** Cuterpes; **Ital.:** Herpes-Gel†.

Idoxuridine (1681-k)

Idoxuridine (BAN, USAN, rINN).

Allergan 211; GF-1115; Idoxuridina; IDU; 5-IDUR; 5-IUDR; NSC-39661; SKF-14287. 2′-Deoxy-5-iodouridine.

$C_9H_{11}IN_2O_5 = 354.1$.

CAS — 54-42-2.

ATC — D06BB01; J05AB02; S01AD01.

Pharmacopoeias. In Chin., Eur. (see p.vi), Jpn, and US.

Iodine vapour is liberated on heating. It has been reported that some decomposition products such as iodouracil are more toxic than idoxuridine and reduce its antiviral activity.

Pharmacopoeial description

Ph. Eur.: A white or almost white crystalline powder. M.p. about 180°, with decomposition. Slightly soluble in water and in alcohol; practically insoluble in ether; dissolves in dilute solutions of alkali hydroxides. A 0.1% solution in water has a pH of 5.5 to 6.5. Protect from light.

USP 25: A white, practically odourless, crystalline powder. Slightly soluble in water and in alcohol; practically insoluble in chloroform and in ether. Store in airtight containers. Protect from light.

Adverse Effects

Adverse effects which occur occasionally when idoxuridine is applied to the eyes include irritation, pain, conjunctivitis, oedema and inflammation of the eye or eyelids, photophobia, pruritus, and rarely, occlusion of the lachrymal duct. Hypersensitivity reactions may occur rarely. Prolonged use may damage the cornea.

Idoxuridine applied to the skin may produce irritation and hypersensitivity reactions. Excessive application of topical idoxuridine to the eyes or skin may cause punctate defects in the cornea or skin maceration.

Adverse effects after intravenous administration of idoxuridine have included bone-marrow depression and liver damage.

Idoxuridine is a potential carcinogen and teratogen.

Carcinogenicity. Squamous carcinoma in a patient was associated with topical idoxuridine treatment.[1] Reference is made to an earlier similar case.

1. Koppang HS, Aas E. Squamous carcinoma induced by topical idoxuridine therapy? Br J Dermatol 1983; 108: 501–3.

Precautions

Idoxuridine should be used with caution in conditions where there is deep ulceration involving the stromal layers of the cornea, as delayed healing has resulted in corneal perforation. Prolonged topical use should be avoided.

Idoxuridine's potential teratogenicity should be taken into account when treating pregnant patients or patients likely to become pregnant. Corticosteroids should be applied with caution in patients also receiving idoxuridine as they may accelerate the spread of viral infection. Boric acid preparations should not be applied to the eye in patients also receiving ocular preparations of idoxuridine as irritation ensues.

Antiviral Action

Following intracellular phosphorylation to the triphosphate, idoxuridine is incorporated into viral DNA instead of thymidine so inhibiting replication of the virus. Idoxuridine is also incorporated into mammalian DNA. Idoxuridine is active against herpes simplex and varicella zoster viruses. It has also been shown to inhibit vaccinia virus and cytomegalovirus.

Resistance to idoxuridine occurs in vitro and in vivo.

Pharmacokinetics

Penetration of idoxuridine into the cornea and skin is reported to be poor. Following systemic administration idoxuridine is rapidly metabolised to iodouracil, uracil, and iodide.

Uses and Administration

Idoxuridine is a pyrimidine nucleoside structurally related to thymidine. It has been used topically in the treatment of herpes simplex keratitis and cutaneous forms of herpes simplex (p.607) and herpes zoster (p.608), but has generally been superseded by other antivirals.

In the treatment of herpes simplex keratitis idoxuridine has been applied as a 0.1% ophthalmic solution.

Idoxuridine 5% in dimethyl sulfoxide (to aid absorption) can be painted onto the lesions of cutaneous herpes simplex and herpes zoster four times daily for 4 days.

The symbol † denotes a preparation no longer actively marketed

Preparations

BP 2001: Idoxuridine Eye Drops;

USP 25: Idoxuridine Ophthalmic Ointment; Idoxuridine Ophthalmic Solution.

Proprietary Preparations (details are given in Part 3)

Austral.: Herplex Liquifilm†; Herplex-D; Stoxil; **Belg.:** Virexen; **Canad.:** Herplex; **Fr.:** Iduviran; **Ger.:** Iducutit†; Ophtal; Virunguent; Zostrum; **Hong Kong:** Herpidu; Herplex; Oftalmolosa Cusi Virucida; Stoxil; **Irl.:** Zostrum; **Israel:** Virusan; **Ital.:** Iducher; Iduridin†; Idustatin; **Mex.:** Idina; **Norw.:** Iduridin†; **NZ:** Virasolve; **Port.:** Virexen†; Virunguent†; **S.Afr.:** Herplex-D†; **Singapore:** Stoxil; Virunguent; **Spain:** Antizona†; Virexen; **Switz.:** Iderpes; Virexen†; Virunguent; **Thai.:** Herpidu; **UK:** Herpid; Iduridin†; **USA:** Herplex†.

Multi-ingredient: Austral.: Virasolve; **Braz.:** Herpesine; **Ger.:** Virunguent P; **Hong Kong:** Virasolve; **Ital.:** Iducol; Idustatin†.

Imiquimod (11696-k)

Imiquimod (BAN, USAN, rINN).

R-837; S-26308. 4-Amino-1-isobutyl-1H-imidazo[4,5-c]quinoline.

$C_{14}H_{16}N_4 = 240.3$.

CAS — 99011-02-6.

ATC — D06BB10.

Adverse Effects

Adverse effects following topical application of imiquimod include local skin erosion, erythema, excoriation, flaking, and oedema. Skin reactions away from the site of application have been reported. Systemic effects following topical application include headache, influenza-like symptoms, and myalgia.

Hypotension has occurred after repeated ingestion.

Uses and Administration

Imiquimod is an immune response modifier used topically in the treatment of external genital and perianal warts. It is applied as a 5% cream three times each week for up to 16 weeks and is left on the skin for 6 to 10 hours.

◊ References.

1. Perry CM, Lamb HM. Topical imiquimod: a review of its use in genital warts. Drugs 1999; 58: 375–90.

Preparations

Proprietary Preparations (details are given in Part 3)

Austral.: Aldara; **Belg.:** Aldara; **Canad.:** Aldara; **Denm.:** Aldara; **Fin.:** Aldara; **Fr.:** Aldara; **Ger.:** Aldara; **Hong Kong:** Aldara; **Irl.:** Aldara; **Ital.:** Aldara; **Neth.:** Aldara; **Norw.:** Aldara; **NZ:** Aldara; **S.Afr.:** Aldara; **Singapore:** Aldara; **Spain:** Aldara; **Swed.:** Aldara; **Thai.:** Aldara; **UK:** Aldara; **USA:** Aldara.

Indinavir Sulfate (3883-x)

Indinavir Sulfate (USAN, pINNM).

Indinavir Sulfate (BANM); L-735524; MK-639; MK-0639. (αR,γS,2S)-α-Benzyl-2-(tert-butylcarbamoyl)-γ-hydroxy-N-[(1S,2R)-2-hydroxy-1-indanyl]-4-(3-pyridylmethyl)-1-piperazinevaleramide sulphate (1:1).

$C_{36}H_{47}N_5O_4,H_2SO_4 = 711.9$.

CAS — 150378-17-9 (indinavir); 157810-81-6 (indinavir sulfate).

Adverse Effects

The general spectrum of adverse effects associated with indinavir and other HIV-protease inhibitors commonly includes nausea, vomiting, and diarrhoea (which can be severe enough to cause dehydration with its potential for adverse renal effects). Other side-effects reported include taste disturbances, abdominal pain, anorexia, increased appetite, flatulence, asthenia, fatigue, sleep disturbances, headache, dizziness, paraesthesia, hypoaesthesia, myalgia, arthralgia, alopecia, pruritus, and renal insufficiency. Myositis and rhabdomyolysis have occurred. Skin rashes occur commonly and may occasionally be severe; a possible association with Stevens-Johnson syndrome and erythema multiforme has been reported for several HIV-protease inhibitors.

Lipodystrophy (redistribution of peripheral subcutaneous fat to the shoulders and abdomen) may occur.

Hyperglycaemia and an association with the onset or exacerbation of diabetes mellitus has also occurred in patients receiving HIV-protease inhibitors.

Allergic reactions (sometimes anaphylaxis) have been associated with several HIV-protease inhibitors including indinavir.

Effects on the blood associated with indinavir and other HIV-protease inhibitors are, notably, acute haemolytic anaemia and, generally, reduced neutrophil counts. Abnormal laboratory test results asso-

ciated with the administration of HIV-protease inhibitors have included raised liver enzymes and bilirubin (jaundice and hepatitis have occurred), raised creatine phosphokinase, and raised blood lipids (with rare cases of pancreatitis).

Nephrolithiasis, often with flank pain and occurring with or without haematuria, has been associated with indinavir. It is often resolved by withdrawal for one to three days and administration of fluids, but interstitial nephritis and acute renal failure have been reported.

There have been reports of ingrowing toenails and paronychia of the great toes associated with indinavir. Additional side-effects reported with indinavir include acid regurgitation, dyspepsia, dry mouth, dysuria, dry skin, and hyperpigmentation.

◊ Reviews.

1. Moyle GJ, Gazzard BG. A risk-benefit assessment of HIV protease inhibitors. Drug Safety 1999; 20: 299–321.

Effects on carbohydrate and lipid metabolism. HIV-protease inhibitors have been associated with a lipodystrophy syndrome characterised by peripheral fat wasting, central adiposity, hyperlipidaemia, and insulin resistance.[1]

A survey of 113 HIV-infected patients receiving HIV-protease inhibitors found lipodystrophy in 83% (severe in 11%) and impaired glucose tolerance in 23% (including diabetes mellitus in 7%) after a mean of 21 months of therapy.[2]

Hyperlipidaemia was identified in 41 of 124 patients receiving HIV-protease inhibitors, resulting in the development of angina pectoris in two.[3] There have been varying reports of the relative hyperlipidaemic effects of different HIV-protease inhibitors. Elevated lipid concentrations were found to be more frequent[4] or to have occurred more rapidly[2] in patients receiving ritonavir and/or saquinavir than in those receiving indinavir or nelfinavir. However, greater increases in lipid concentrations have been reported with indinavir than with saquinavir,[5] and increased abdominal girth was reported more frequently in patients taking indinavir than in those taking other HIV-protease inhibitors.[6] Treatment with lipid regulating drugs has been advocated[4] but concerns have been expressed over their safety in this patient group.[7]

Impaired glucose tolerance has been linked to reduction in insulin sensitivity[8] and has responded to treatment with sulfonylureas or insulin.[9]

1. Carr A, et al. Pathogenesis of HIV-1-protease inhibitor-associated peripheral lipodystrophy, hyperlipidaemia, and insulin resistance. Lancet 1998; 351: 1881–3.
2. Carr A, et al. Diagnosis, prediction, and natural course of HIV-1 protease-inhibitor-associated lipodystrophy, hyperlipidaemia, and diabetes mellitus: a cohort study. Lancet 1999; 353: 2093–9.
3. Henry K, et al. Severe premature coronary artery disease with protease inhibitors. Lancet 1998; 351: 1328.
4. Henry K, et al. Atorvastatin and gemfibrozil for protease-inhibitor-related lipid abnormalities. Lancet 1998; 352: 1031–2.
5. Segerer S, et al. Hyperlipidemia under treatment with proteinase inhibitors. Infection 1999; 27: 77–81.
6. De Luca A, et al. "Buffalo hump" in HIV-1 infection. Lancet 1998; 352: 320.
7. Wierzbicki AS, et al. Lipid lowering therapy in patients with HIV infection. Lancet 1998; 352: 1782.
8. Walli R, et al. Impaired glucose tolerance and protease inhibitors. Ann Intern Med 1998; 129: 837–8.
9. Dubé MP, et al. Protease inhibitor-associated hyperglycaemia. Lancet 1997; 350: 713–14.

Effects on the cardiovascular system. For adverse effects of HIV-protease inhibitors on carbohydrate and lipid metabolism that increase the risk of coronary vascular disease, see above.

Effects on the kidneys. Nephrolithiasis has been reported in about 10% of patients receiving indinavir, and the incidence may be higher in patients with haemophilia or hepatitis C infection.[1] Both asymptomatic[2] and symptomatic[3,4] crystalluria have been reported in patients receiving indinavir, with symptomatic urinary-tract disease in 8%. Indinavir has been identified as the major constituent of both urinary crystals[2] and calculi.[5] In addition there have been reports of acute interstitial nephritis associated with indinavir[6] and deterioration of renal function associated with both indinavir[7] and ritonavir.[8,9] Renal atrophy was associated with long-term treatment with indinavir.[10,11]

1. Brodie SB, et al. Variation in incidence of indinavir-associated nephrolithiasis among HIV-positive patients. AIDS 1998; 12: 2433–7.
2. Kopp JB, et al. Crystalluria and urinary tract abnormalities associated with indinavir. Ann Intern Med 1997; 127: 119–25.
3. Hachey DM, et al. Indinavir crystalluria in an HIV-positive man. Ann Pharmacother 2000; 34: 403.
4. Famularo G, et al. Symptomatic crystalluria associated with indinavir. Ann Pharmacother 2000; 34: 1414–18.
5. Daudon M, et al. Urinary stones in HIV-1-positive patients treated with indinavir. Lancet 1997; 349: 1294–5.
6. Marroni M, et al. Acute interstitial nephritis secondary to the administration of indinavir. Ann Pharmacother 1998; 32: 843–4.
7. Boubaker K, et al. Changes in renal function associated with indinavir. AIDS 1998; 12: F249–F254.
8. Duong M, et al. Renal failure after treatment with ritonavir. Lancet 1996; 348: 693–4.
9. Chugh S, et al. Ritonavir and renal failure. N Engl J Med 1997; 336: 138.

10. Hanabusa H, *et al.* Renal atrophy associated with long-term treatment with indinavir. *N Engl J Med* 1999; **340:** 392–3.
11. Cattelan AM, *et al.* Severe hypertension and renal atrophy associated with indinavir. *Clin Infect Dis* 2000; **30:** 619–21.

Effects on the liver. The use of indinavir, in combinations with other antiretroviral drugs, has been associated with the development of severe hepatitis.[1,2]

Hepatic failure was attributed to ritonavir in a patient receiving combination therapy for AIDS.[3]

1. Bräu N, *et al.* Severe hepatitis in three AIDS patients treated with indinavir. *Lancet* 1997; **349:** 924–5.
2. Matsuda J, *et al.* Severe hepatitis in patients with AIDS and haemophilia B treated with indinavir. *Lancet* 1997; **350:** 364.
3. Picard O, *et al.* Hepatotoxicity associated with ritonavir. *Ann Intern Med* 1998; **129:** 670–1.

Effects on the menstrual cycle. Irregular, prolonged, or heavy menstruation was reported[1] in 4 patients receiving ritonavir. Menstruation subsequently returned to normal in the 3 patients who were transferred to a different HIV-protease inhibitor.

1. Nielsen H. Hypermenorrhoea associated with ritonavir. *Lancet* 1999; **353:** 811–12.

Effects on mental state. Acute paranoid reactions were associated with saquinavir administration on two occasions in a patient.[1]

1. Finlayson JA, Laing RBS. Acute paranoid reaction to saquinavir. *Am J Health-Syst Pharm* 1998; **55:** 2016–17.

Effects on the pancreas. Pancreatitis was associated with administration of ritonavir and saquinavir in 1 patient,[1] and with ritonavir (other drugs unspecified) in 2 others,[2] and was believed to be secondary to hyperlipidaemia (see Effects on Carbohydrate and Lipid Metabolism, above).

1. McBride M, *et al.* Lipid lowering therapy in patients with HIV infection. *Lancet* 1998; **352:** 1782–3.
2. Di Perri G, *et al.* HIV-protease inhibitors. *N Engl J Med* 1998; **339:** 773–4.

Effects on sexual function. Sexual dysfunction has been reported in patients receiving combination antiretroviral therapy with HIV-protease inhibitors and reverse transcriptase inhibitors.[1,2]

1. Martínez E, *et al.* Sexual dysfunction with protease inhibitors. *Lancet* 1999; **353:** 810–11.
2. Colebunders R, *et al.* Sexual dysfunction with protease inhibitors. *Lancet* 1999; **353:** 1802.

Effects on the skin. Skin rashes have been reported in about 20% of patients receiving indinavir and in 3 to 5% of patients receiving nelfinavir or saquinavir. Rash is described as a frequent adverse effect of ritonavir. In patients taking indinavir who reported rashes,[1] the rash commonly appeared within 2 weeks of starting treatment, was frequently accompanied by pruritus, and was usually self-limiting, commonly resolving within 4 weeks.

Paronychia and pyogenic granuloma of the great toes has been reported in patients receiving indinavir.[2]

1. Gajewski LK, *et al.* Characterization of rash with indinavir in a national patient cohort. *Ann Pharmacother* 1999; **33:** 17–21.
2. Bouscarat F, *et al.* Paronychia and pyogenic granuloma of the great toes in patients treated with indinavir. *N Engl J Med* 1998; **338:** 1776–7.

Precautions

Indinavir and similar HIV-protease inhibitors are primarily metabolised in the liver which means that caution and possible dosage reduction are required in hepatic impairment; deterioration in hepatic function has been reported in patients with pre-existing hepatitis or hepatic impairment receiving HIV-protease inhibitors, and where the hepatic impairment is severe they should be avoided.

Although renal excretion is a relatively minor route of elimination, adequate hydration is recommended to reduce the risk of nephrolithiasis; monitoring is advised in the presence of renal impairment. Treatment may need to be temporarily interrupted or discontinued completely in patients developing nephrolithiasis.

Patients receiving HIV-protease inhibitors should be monitored for signs of lipodystrophy. Caution is needed in diabetic patients since HIV-protease inhibitors have been associated with hyperglycaemia and the onset or exacerbation of diabetes mellitus. Caution is also needed in patients with haemophilia who may experience increased bleeding. Treatment with HIV-protease inhibitors may need to be discontinued should acute haemolytic anaemia occur. Excessive diarrhoea may interfere with the absorption of HIV-protease inhibitors leading to subtherapeutic blood concentrations; resultant dehydration may also be a factor in renal damage.

Mycobacterial infections. Patients with a previously unsuspected *Mycobacterium avium* complex infection experienced a severe febrile syndrome with inflammatory lymphadenitis following initiation of indinavir treatment.[1] The reaction resolved with appropriate antimycobacterial therapy.

1. Race EM, *et al.* Focal mycobacterial lymphadenitis following initiation of protease-inhibitor therapy in patients with advanced HIV-1 disease. *Lancet* 1998; **351:** 252–5.

Pregnancy. A retrospective survey[1] involving 89 women who received protease inhibitors during pregnancy indicated that such drugs appeared generally safe.

1. Morris AB, *et al.* Multicenter review of protease inhibitors in 89 pregnancies. *J Acquir Immune Defic Syndr* 2000; **25:** 306–11.

Interactions

Indinavir and similar HIV-protease inhibitors are metabolised principally by cytochrome P450 isoenzymes of the CYP3A family. They consequently compete for the same metabolic pathways with a wide range of drugs that are metabolised similarly, often resulting in mutually increased plasma concentrations. The extent of such interactions depends on a number of factors, including the affinity of the relevant HIV-protease inhibitor for the various cytochrome P450 isoenzymes; in the case of indinavir, CYP3A4 is reported to be the only P450 isoenzyme that plays a major role. Where significant competition for metabolism does occur, the margin between therapeutic and toxic concentrations has a major role in determining the severity of the interaction. Thus, concurrent administration of a drug with a narrow therapeutic window, such as cisapride or terfenadine, is contra-indicated, whereas a drug with a wider therapeutic window, such as erythromycin, may only require dosage reduction at its highest dose level.

Conversely, a drug that is a significant inducer of microsomal enzymes, particularly isoenzymes of the CYP3A family, may reduce plasma concentrations of HIV-protease inhibitors. Thus, concurrent administration of a potent enzyme inducer, such as rifampicin, may reduce the plasma concentration of an HIV-protease inhibitor to a subtherapeutic level so that its concurrent administration is contra-indicated. Other well-known enzyme inducers, such as carbamazepine, phenobarbital, and phenytoin, also possibly reduce the plasma concentrations of HIV-protease inhibitors.

In turn, HIV-protease inhibitors may themselves induce metabolism and may reduce plasma concentrations of other drugs, such as theophylline and hormonal contraceptives.

The principal interactions that have been reported as a risk for one or more of the various HIV-protease inhibitors are listed below.

◊ References to interactions associated with HIV-protease inhibitors.

1. Eagling VA, *et al.* Differential inhibition of cytochrome P450 isoforms by the protease inhibitors, ritonavir, saquinavir and indinavir. *Br J Clin Pharmacol* 1997; **44:** 190–4.
2. von Moltke LL, *et al.* Protease inhibitors as inhibitors of human cytochromes P450: high risk associated with ritonavir. *J Clin Pharmacol* 1998; **38:** 106–11.
3. Malaty LI, Kuper JJ. Drug interactions of HIV protease inhibitors. *Drug Safety* 1999; **20:** 147–69.

Amfetamines. For mention of interactions, including a fatal serotonergic reaction, with *methylenedioxymethamfetamine* (Ecstasy) in patients receiving ritonavir, see p.1511.

Analgesics. Ritonavir and possibly other HIV-protease inhibitors produce complex and potentially serious interactions with some opioids (see p.68). Interactions between ritonavir and *dextropropoxyphene* (p.27) or *pethidine* (p.76) are considered to be especially hazardous.

Concomitant administration of ritonavir and *piroxicam* can result in potentially toxic concentrations of piroxicam (see p.79).

Antiarrhythmics. Concomitant administration of HIV-protease inhibitors and the antiarrhythmics *amiodarone, flecainide, propafenone,* or *quinidine* may result in potentially toxic plasma concentrations of these drugs with an increased risk of ventricular arrhythmias.

Antibacterials. Plasma concentrations of HIV-protease inhibitors may be reduced to subtherapeutic levels by concomitant administration of *rifabutin* or *rifampicin.* In addition, plasma concentrations of rifabutin may be increased, with a consequent risk of uveitis. In general, HIV-protease inhibitors should not be used together with rifampicin (p.244) and dosage modifications may be necessary if used with rifabutin; further information is given in Rifabutin under Interactions, p.242 and Uses, Tuberculosis, p.243.

HIV-protease inhibitors may inhibit the metabolism of *clarithromycin* (p.186).

Antidepressants. HIV-protease inhibitors may inhibit the metabolism of *desipramine* and other tricyclic antidepressants (p.277) and *fluoxetine* (p.287).

Plasma concentrations of HIV-protease inhibitors may be reduced by concurrent administration of *Hypericum* (St John's Wort) as a result of induction of cytochrome P450; concomitant use should be avoided.[1]

1. Piscitelli SC, *et al.* Indinavir concentrations and St John's wort. *Lancet* 2000; **355:** 547–8. Correction. *ibid.* 2001; **357:** 1210.

Antiepileptics. Reduced plasma concentrations of HIV-protease inhibitors may be anticipated if the enzyme inducers *carbamazepine, phenobarbital,* or *phenytoin* are given concurrently. In addition, carbamazepine concentrations have been reported to be increased by concurrent administration of ritonavir (p.345).

Antifungals. Plasma concentrations of HIV-protease inhibitors may be increased by concurrent administration of azole antifungals. The manufacturers recommend that the dose of indinavir should be reduced to 600 mg every 8 hours when given with *itraconazole* 200 mg twice daily. A dose reduction is not considered necessary by the UK manufacturer when indinavir is given with *ketoconazole,* but the US manufacturer recommends a reduction to indinavir 600 mg every 8 hours.

Conversely, plasma concentrations of ketoconazole are increased by concomitant administration of ritonavir.

Antihistamines. HIV-protease inhibitors inhibit the metabolism of non-sedating antihistamines such as *astemizole* and *terfenadine* resulting in increased plasma concentrations of these drugs and an increased risk of serious ventricular arrhythmias. Such combinations should be avoided.

Antipsychotics. Ritonavir and possibly other HIV-protease inhibitors may affect plasma concentrations of *clozapine* (p.673) and *pimozide* (p.700) resulting in increased toxicity. Concomitant use should be avoided.

Antivirals. HIV-protease inhibitors can inhibit metabolism of other drugs from the same class and increases in adverse effects have in particular resulted from concurrent administration of *saquinavir* and *ritonavir.* However, there have been suggestions that judicious administration of two of these drugs could be utilised to simplify dosage regimens and thereby improve compliance.[1] An increase in the plasma concentrations of both *indinavir* and *nelfinavir* occurs when the two drugs are co-administered. Ritonavir also appears to increase indinavir and nelfinavir plasma concentrations, and nelfinavir to increase saquinavir concentrations when given concomitantly.

Plasma concentrations of indinavir[2] and saquinavir may be reduced by concurrent administration of *nevirapine;* the manufacturers of indinavir recommend a dose increase of indinavir to 1 g every 8 hours be considered.

Plasma concentrations of indinavir[3] and saquinavir may be increased by *delavirdine;* the manufacturers of indinavir recommend a dose reduction of indinavir to 400 to 600 mg every 8 hours in patients receiving delavirdine concurrently and the manufacturers of saquinavir recommend that liver function should be monitored if saquinavir is given with delavirdine.

Plasma concentrations of indinavir and saquinavir are decreased when given with *efavirenz.* Increased doses of indinavir to 1 g every 8 hours are recommended when it is given in combination with efavirenz, but the use of saquinavir with efavirenz is not recommended unless saquinavir concentrations are increased by the addition of other antiretrovirals such as ritonavir. The use of efavirenz with ritonavir is associated with an increased frequency of adverse effects, presumably due to competitive inhibition of metabolism, and the manufacturer recommends that liver enzymes should be monitored in patients receiving this combination. Plasma concentrations of nelfinavir are increased when given with efavirenz, but the combination is usually well tolerated at standard doses.

Although there is no direct interaction between HIV-protease inhibitors and *didanosine,* the buffer included in the didanosine formulation can impair the absorption of indinavir; doses of nelfinavir or ritonavir, both of which should be given with food, should also be separated by at least 1 hour from didanosine doses, which should be given on an empty stomach.

For a report of reduced area under the plasma concentration-time curve for *zidovudine* in patients receiving ritonavir, see p.646.

1. Hsu A, *et al.* Pharmacokinetic interaction between ritonavir and indinavir in healthy volunteers. *Antimicrob Agents Chemother* 1998; **42:** 2784–91.
2. Murphy RL, *et al.* Antiviral effect and pharmacokinetic interaction between nevirapine and indinavir in persons infected with human immunodeficiency virus type 1. *J Infect Dis* 1999; **179:** 1116–23.
3. Ferry JJ, *et al.* Pharmacokinetic drug-drug interaction study of delavirdine and indinavir in healthy subjects. *J Acquir Immune Defic Syndr Hum Retrovirol* 1998; **18:** 252–9.

Benzodiazepines. For the effect of HIV-protease inhibitors on benzodiazepines, see Diazepam, p.678.

Ciclosporin. Mutual increases in the area under the plasma concentration-time curves for saquinavir and ciclosporin were reported in a kidney transplant recipient.[1] The resultant adverse effects subsided when doses of both drugs were reduced by half. Similar interactions with other HIV-protease inhibitors are possible.

1. Brinkman K, *et al.* Pharmacokinetic interaction between saquinavir and cyclosporine. *Ann Intern Med* 1998; **129:** 914–15.

Cisapride. For the effect of HIV-protease inhibitors on cisapride, see p.1220.

Corticosteroids. Corticosteroids, in particular *dexamethasone*, may induce the metabolism of HIV-protease inhibitors resulting in reduced plasma concentrations.

Ergot alkaloids. For reports of ergotism in patients receiving HIV-protease inhibitors and ergot alkaloids, see Ergotamine, p.452.

Grapefruit. The area under the plasma concentration-time curve for saquinavir was increased by 50% when administered with grapefruit juice.[1]

1. Kupferschmidt HHT, *et al.* Grapefruit juice enhances the bioavailability of the HIV protease inhibitor saquinavir in men. *Br J Clin Pharmacol* 1998; **45:** 355–9.

Hormonal contraceptives. For the effect of HIV-protease inhibitors on hormonal contraceptives, see p.1459.

Interleukin-2. Plasma concentrations of indinavir were increased during concurrent administration of interleukin-2.[1]

1. Piscitelli SC, *et al.* Alteration in indinavir clearance during interleukin-2 infusions in patients infected with the human immunodeficiency virus. *Pharmacotherapy* 1998; **18:** 1212–16.

Phenylpropanolamine. For a possible interaction between phenylpropanolamine and antiretrovirals including indinavir, see Stavudine, p.641.

Sildenafil. For the effect of HIV-protease inhibitors on sildenafil, including a report of fatal myocardial infarction following sildenafil in a patient receiving ritonavir and saquinavir, see p.1663.

Statins. HIV-protease inhibitors may inhibit the metabolism of statins metabolised by CYP3A4 isoenzymes resulting in an increased risk of myopathy. The use of indinavir with lovastatin or simvastatin should be avoided, and it should be given with caution in patients receiving atorvastatin or cerivastatin.

Tacrolimus. HIV-protease inhibitors may inhibit the metabolism of tacrolimus.

Theophylline. For a potential effect of ritonavir on theophylline, see p.781.

Warfarin. For the effect of HIV-protease inhibitors on warfarin, see p.996.

Antiviral Action
Indinavir and similar HIV-protease inhibitors are antiretrovirals that act by binding reversibly to HIV-protease thereby preventing cleavage of the viral precursor polyproteins. This results in the formation of immature viral particles incapable of infecting other cells. Viral resistance develops rapidly when HIV-protease inhibitors are given alone and therefore they are used in combination with other antiretrovirals. Cross-resistance between HIV-protease inhibitors may occur, but cross-resistance between HIV-protease inhibitors and reverse transcriptase inhibitors is considered unlikely.

Resistance. References.

1. Boden D, Markowitz M. Resistance to human immunodeficiency virus type 1 protease inhibitors. *Antimicrob Agents Chemother* 1998; **42:** 2775–83.

Pharmacokinetics
Indinavir is rapidly absorbed following oral administration producing peak plasma concentrations in 0.8 hours. Bioavailability is about 65% following a single dose. Absorption is reduced by administration with a meal high in calories, fat, and protein but is less affected by a light meal. At doses up to 800 mg, increases in plasma concentration are proportionally greater than increases in dose. Plasma protein binding is about 60%. Indinavir is reported to cross the blood-brain barrier into the CSF. It undergoes oxidative metabolism by cytochrome P450 isoenzyme CYP3A4 and glucuronidation. The elimination half-life is 1.8 hours. Less than 20% of the absorbed dose is excreted in the urine, about half of this as unchanged drug. The remainder is excreted in the faeces.

◊ References.

1. Ståhle L, *et al.* Indinavir in cerebrospinal fluid of HIV-1-infected patients. *Lancet* 1997; **350:** 1823.
2. Bernard L, *et al.* Indinavir concentrations in hair from patients receiving highly active antiretroviral therapy. *Lancet* 1998; **352:** 1757–8.
3. Wintergerst U, *et al.* Use of saliva specimens for monitoring indinavir therapy in human immunodeficiency virus-infected patients. *Antimicrob Agents Chemother* 2000; **44:** 2572–4.

4. Haas DW, *et al.* Steady-state pharmacokinetics of indinavir in cerebrospinal fluid and plasma among adults with human immunodeficiency virus type 1 infection. *Clin Pharmacol Ther* 2000; **68:** 367–74.
5. Burger DM, *et al.* Pharmacokinetics of the protease inhibitor indinavir in human immunodeficiency virus type 1-infected children. *Antimicrob Agents Chemother* 2001; **45:** 701–5.

Uses and Administration
Indinavir is a protease inhibitor with antiviral activity against HIV. It is used, in combination with nucleoside reverse transcriptase inhibitors, for the treatment of HIV infection (p.608).

Indinavir is given by mouth as the sulfate, but doses are expressed in terms of the base. It is given in an adult dose of 800 mg every 8 hours. It should be given either an hour before or two hours after meals, or with a light, low-fat meal. A reduction in dose to 600 mg every 8 hours is recommended for patients with mild to moderate hepatic insufficiency due to cirrhosis. Adequate hydration should be maintained. Treatment may have to be interrupted if acute episodes of nephrolithiasis occur. Children over 4 years of age may be given 500 mg per m² body-surface every 8 hours, the dose not to exceed the adult dose.

Indinavir has also been recommended as part of the chemoprophylactic regimen with zidovudine and lamivudine in patients at high risk of HIV infection following occupational percutaneous exposure (see p.610).

HIV infection and AIDS. Reviews on the use of indinavir and other HIV-protease inhibitors.

1. Moyle GJ, Barton SE. HIV-proteinase inhibitors in the management of HIV-infection. *J Antimicrob Chemother* 1996; **33:** 921–5.
2. Moyle G, Gazzard B. Current knowledge and future prospects for the use of HIV protease inhibitors. *Drugs* 1996; **51:** 701–12.
3. Barry M, *et al.* Protease inhibitors in patients with HIV disease: clinically important pharmacokinetic considerations. *Clin Pharmacokinet* 1997; **32:** 194–209.
4. Deeks SG, *et al.* HIV-1 protease inhibitors: a review for clinicians. *JAMA* 1997; **277:** 145–53.
5. Flexner C. HIV-protease inhibitors. *N Engl J Med* 1998; **338:** 1281–92.
6. Plosker GL, Noble S. Indinavir: a review of its use in the management of HIV infection. *Drugs* 1999; **58:** 1165–1203.

Other viral infections. Infection with HHV-8 (a virus associated with an increased risk of developing Kaposi's sarcoma) resolved in a patient when indinavir was added to combination therapy for HIV infection.[1] Regression of progressive multifocal leucoencephalopathy (the result of a papovavirus infection of the CNS) has been reported in 2 patients receiving combination antiretroviral therapy including indinavir for HIV infection.[2,3]

1. Rizzieri DA, *et al.* Clearance of HHV-8 from peripheral blood mononuclear cells with a protease inhibitor. *Lancet* 1997; **349:** 775–6.
2. Elliot B, *et al.* 2.5 Year remission of AIDS-associated progressive multifocal leukoencephalopathy with combined antiretroviral therapy. *Lancet* 1997; **349:** 850.
3. Domingo P, *et al.* Remission of progressive multifocal leucoencephalopathy after antiretroviral therapy. *Lancet* 1997; **349:** 1554–5.

Preparations

Proprietary Preparations (details are given in Part 3)

Aust.: Crixivan; *Austral.:* Crixivan; *Belg.:* Crixivan; *Canad.:* Crixivan; *Denm.:* Crixivan; *Fin.:* Crixivan; *Fr.:* Crixivan; *Ger.:* Crixivan; *Hong Kong:* Crixivan; *Irl.:* Crixivan; *Israel:* Crixivan; *Ital.:* Crixivan; *Jpn:* Crixivan; *Mex.:* Crixivan; *Neth.:* Crixivan; *Norw.:* Crixivan; *NZ:* Crixivan; *Port.:* Crixivan; *S.Afr.:* Crixivan; *Singapore:* Crixivan; *Spain:* Crixivan; *Swed.:* Crixivan; *Switz.:* Crixivan; *Thai.:* Crixivan; *UK:* Crixivan; *USA:* Crixivan.

Inosine Pranobex (12941-f)

Inosine Pranobex (BAN, rINNM).

Inosiplex; Isoprinosine; Methisoprinol; NP-113; NPT-10381. Inosine 2-hydroxypropyldimethylammonium 4-acetamidobenzoate (1:3).

$C_{10}H_{12}N_4O_5$:$C_{14}H_{22}N_2O_4$ (1:3) = 1115.2.

CAS — 36703-88-5.
ATC — J05AX05.

NOTE. Inosine pranobex has sometimes been expressed as inosine with dimepranol (*pINN*) ((±)-1-(dimethylamino)-2-propanol) and acedoben (*pINN*) (*p*-acetamidobenzoic acid). Dimepranol Acedoben is *USAN*.

Adverse Effects and Precautions
Some patients have experienced transient nausea and vomiting. Metabolism of the inosine content of inosine pranobex leads to increased serum and urine concentrations of uric acid; caution is therefore recommended in treating patients with impaired renal function, gout, or hyperuricaemia.

Antiviral Action
Inosine pranobex appears to owe its activity in viral infections more to its capacity to modify or stimulate cell-mediated immune processes than to a direct action on the virus.

◊ Inosine pranobex was found to have slight activity against some viruses *in vitro* and also some activity in *animals* infected with herpes simplex virus type 2 and influenza virus.[1] However, another study[2] showed it to lack activity in experimental model infections.

1. Chang T-W, Weinstein L. Antiviral activity of isoprinosine in vitro and in vivo. *Am J Med Sci* 1973; **265:** 143–6.
2. Glasgow LA, Galasso GJ. Isoprinosine: lack of antiviral activity in experimental model infections. *J Infect Dis* 1972; **126:** 162–9.

Pharmacokinetics
Inosine pranobex is reported to be rapidly absorbed following administration by mouth. It is also rapidly metabolised with a plasma half-life of 50 minutes, the inosine portion of the complex yielding uric acid; the other part of the complex undergoes oxidation and glucuronidation. The metabolites are excreted in the urine.

◊ References.

1. Nielsen P, Beckett AH. The metabolism and excretion in man of NN-dimethylamino-isopropanol and p-acetamido-benzoic acid after administration of isoprinosine. *J Pharm Pharmacol* 1981; **33:** 549–50.

Uses and Administration
Inosine pranobex has been used in the treatment of various viral infections. Preparations are available for use in herpes simplex, genital warts, and subacute sclerosing panencephalitis, although other treatments or measures are preferred. The dose in mucocutaneous herpes simplex is 1 g four times daily by mouth for 7 to 14 days. A dose of 1 g three times daily is given for 14 to 28 days as an adjunct to topical treatment for genital warts. In subacute sclerosing panencephalitis, the dose is 50 to 100 mg per kg body-weight daily in divided doses given every 4 hours.

◊ Reviews.

1. Campoli-Richards DM, *et al.* Inosine pranobex: a preliminary review of its pharmacodynamic and pharmacokinetic properties, and therapeutic efficacy. *Drugs* 1986; **32:** 383–424.

Herpes simplex infections. The usual antiviral used in the treatment of herpes simplex infections is aciclovir (see p.607), and it has been shown to be more effective than inosine pranobex for genital infections.[1,2] Inosine pranobex has also been tried in herpes labialis, but with equivocal results.[3-5]

1. Mindel A, *et al.* Treatment of first-attack genital herpes—aciclovir versus inosine pranobex. *Lancet* 1987; **i:** 1171–3.
2. Mindel A, *et al.* Suppression of frequently recurring genital herpes: acyclovir v inosine pranobex. *Genitourin Med* 1989; **65:** 103–5.
3. Galli M, *et al.* Inosiplex in recurrent herpes simplex infections. *Lancet* 1982; **ii:** 331–2.
4. Galli M, *et al.* Inosiplex in recurrent herpes simplex infections. *Lancet* 1982; **ii:** 926.
5. Kalimo KOK, *et al.* Failure of oral inosiplex treatment of recurrent herpes simplex virus infections. *Arch Dermatol* 1983; **119:** 463–7.

Subacute sclerosing panencephalitis. Inosine pranobex has been tried in the treatment of subacute sclerosing panencephalitis, a complication of measles (p.611), but the results of clinical studies have been equivocal.[1-8]

1. Streletz LJ, Cracco J. The effect of isoprinosine in subacute sclerosing panencephalitis (SSPE). *Ann Neurol* 1977; **1:** 183–4.
2. Huttenlocher PR, Mattson RH. Isoprinosine in subacute sclerosing panencephalitis. *Neurology* 1979; **29:** 763–71.
3. Silverberg R, *et al.* Inosiplex in the treatment of subacute sclerosing panencephalitis. *Arch Neurol* 1979; **36:** 374–5.
4. Haddad FS, Risk WS. Isoprinosine treatment in 18 patients with subacute sclerosing panencephalitis: a controlled study. *Ann Neurol* 1980; **7:** 185–8.
5. Jones CE, *et al.* Inosiplex therapy in subacute sclerosing panencephalitis: a multicentre, non-randomised study in 98 patients. *Lancet* 1982; **i:** 1034–7.
6. Anonymous. Inosiplex: antiviral, immunomodulator, or neither? *Lancet* 1982; **i:** 1052–4.
7. DuRant RH, *et al.* The influence of inosiplex treatment on the neurological disability of patients with subacute sclerosing panencephalitis. *J Pediatr* 1982; **101:** 288–93.
8. DuRant RH, Dyken PR. The effect of inosiplex on the survival of subacute sclerosing panencephalitis. *Neurology* 1983; **33:** 1053–5.

Preparations

Proprietary Preparations (details are given in Part 3)

Belg.: Isoprinosine; *Canad.:* Imunovir; *Fr.:* Isoprinosine; *Ger.:* delimmun; Isoprinosine; *Irl.:* Imunovir; Isoprinosine; *Ital.:* Avirin; Farviran; Isoprinosina†; Metivirol†; Stimuzim†; Virac†; Viralin; Virustop; Viruxan; *Mex.:* Isoprinosine; Pranosine; *NZ:* Imunovir; *Port.:* Isovir; *Spain:* Bodaril; *UK:* Imunovir.

The symbol † denotes a preparation no longer actively marketed

Interferon Alfa (11419-t)

Interferon Alfa *(BAN, rINN)*.

IFN-α; Interferon-α; Ro-22-8181 (interferon alfa-2a); Sch-30500 (interferon alfa-2b).

CAS — 74899-72-2 (interferon alfa); 76543-88-9 (interferon alfa-2a); 99210-65-8 (interferon alfa-2b); 118390-30-0 (interferon alfacon-1).

ATC — L03AB01 (natural); L03AB04 (2A); L03AB05 (2B); L03AB06 (N1).

NOTE. Interferon alfa was previously known as leucocyte interferon or lymphoblastoid interferon.
Interferon alfa-2a, alfa-2b, alfa-n1, and alfa-n3 are *USAN*.
Interferon alfacon-1 *(BAN, USAN, rINN)* is a recombinant non-naturally occurring alpha interferon.
Pharmacopoeias. Eur. (see p.vi) includes Interferon Alfa-2 Concentrated Solution.

Interferon alfa may be derived from leucocytes or lymphoblasts as well as through recombinant DNA technology. Sub-species of the human alfa gene may produce interferon alfa with protein variants or a mixture of proteins. The protein variants may be designated by a number (as in interferon alfa-2) which may be further qualified by a letter to indicate the amino-acid sequences at positions 23 and 34. Interferon alfa-2a has lysine at 23 and histidine at 34, interferon alfa-2b has arginine at 23 and histidine at 34, and interferon alfa-2c has arginine at both positions. In the case of a mixture of proteins an alphanumeric designation is given (as in interferon alfa-n1). Interferon alfacon-1 varies from interferon alfa-2 in 20 of 166 amino acids.

The name may be further elaborated on the label by approved sets of initials in parentheses to indicate the method of production: (rbe) indicates production from bacteria (*Escherichia coli*) genetically modified by recombinant DNA technology; (lns) indicates production from cultured lymphoblasts from the Namalwa cell line that have been stimulated by a Sendai virus; (bls) indicates production from leucocytes from human blood that have been stimulated by a Sendai virus.

Pharmacopoeial description

Ph. Eur.: Interferon Alfa-2 Concentrated Solution is produced by a method based on recombinant DNA technology using bacteria as host cells. It is a clear, colourless or slightly yellowish liquid. Store in airtight containers at a temperature of −20° or below. Protect from light.

◊ References to the nomenclature of interferon alfa.
1. Finter NB. The naming of cats—and alpha-interferons. *Lancet* 1996; **348:** 348–9.

Adverse Effects and Treatment

Most reports of the adverse effects of interferons have involved interferon alfa, but limited clinical experience suggests that interferons beta and gamma have similar adverse effects.

Interferons produce influenza-like symptoms with fever, chills, fatigue, headache, malaise, myalgia, and arthralgia. These symptoms tend to be dose-related, are most likely to occur at the start of treatment, and mostly respond to paracetamol (but for a possible interaction with paracetamol, see Interactions, below).

Other adverse effects include nausea, vomiting, diarrhoea, anorexia with weight loss, bone marrow depression, alopecia, rash, taste alteration and, rarely, epistaxis, cough, and pharyngitis. There may be signs of altered liver function and hepatitis has been reported. Renal failure and the nephrotic syndrome have occurred. Severe hypersensitivity reactions including anaphylaxis and bronchospasm have been reported rarely. Cardiovascular effects include hypotension or hypertension, arrhythmias, oedema, myocardial infarction, and stroke. High doses may cause electrolyte disturbances including decreased calcium concentrations. Hyperglycaemia and thyroid dysfunction have been reported as have pulmonary oedema and pneumonitis. EEG abnormalities and neurological symptoms including ataxia, paraesthesia, somnolence, dizziness, confusion, and rarely, convulsions and coma have been reported. Depression, anxiety, depersonalisation, or emotional lability may be severe. Visual disturbances and, rarely, ischaemic retinopathy may occur. Menstrual irregularities have been reported, particularly with interferon beta.

Subcutaneous injection may produce a reaction at the injection site. The reaction is reported frequently with interferon beta, which can produce severe reactions including local necrosis.

Nasal administration may produce mucosal irritation and damage.

◊ Reviews.
1. Vial T, Descotes J. Clinical toxicity of the interferons. *Drug Safety* 1994; **10:** 115–50.
2. Pardo M, *et al.* Risks and benefits of interferon-α in the treatment of hepatitis. *Drug Safety* 1995; **13:** 304–16.

Auto-immune disorders. For exacerbation or development of auto-immune disorders in patients receiving interferon, see under Precautions, below.

Effects on the blood. Restoration of bone-marrow function following marrow transplantation was delayed in 3 patients given a human interferon alfa preparation.[1] Laboratory results showed an inhibition of granulocyte colony growth by human leucocyte interferon alfa. It was considered that interferon alfa was contra-indicated in patients with severe bone-marrow insufficiency and should not be given to marrow transplant patients before the graft was fully functional. However, in another 5 patients recombinant interferon alfa did not affect bone-marrow transplants, although 3 patients experienced fever and chills, 4 experienced more than a 60% reduction in absolute peripheral granulocyte counts, and 4 had a 37 to 80% reduction in absolute platelet counts.[2] Lymphocytes were increased in all patients; blood counts returned to normal when interferon therapy stopped. Interferon alfa produced a decline in CD4+ T-lymphocytes resulting in opportunistic infections in 2 HIV-positive patients being treated for chronic hepatitis C.[3]

Other haematological effects reported to be associated with interferon alfa include immune haemolytic anaemia[4] and immune thrombocytopenia.[5,6] Haemorrhage occurred in a patient with immune thrombocytopenic purpura treated with interferon alfa,[7] and it was thought prudent to use interferons with caution, if at all, in this condition.[6,7] Bleeding associated with induction of factor VIII inhibitor has been reported in a patient receiving interferon alfa to enhance hydroxyurea therapy for chronic myeloid leukaemia.[8] Thrombosis associated with interferon alfa has also been reported.[9]

1. Nissen C, *et al.* Toxicity of human leucocyte interferon preparations in human bone-marrow cultures. *Lancet* 1977; **i:** 203–4.
2. Winston DJ, *et al.* Safety and tolerance of recombinant leukocyte A interferon in bone marrow transplant recipients. *Antimicrob Agents Chemother* 1983; **23:** 846–51.
3. Pesce A, *et al.* Opportunistic infections and CD4 lymphocytopenia with interferon treatment in HIV-1 infected patients. *Lancet* 1993; **341:** 1597.
4. Akard LP, *et al.* Alpha-interferon and immune hemolytic anemia. *Ann Intern Med* 1986; **105:** 306.
5. McLaughlin P, *et al.* Immune thrombocytopenia following α-interferon therapy in patients with cancer. *JAMA* 1985; **254:** 1353–4.
6. Färkkilä M, Iivanainen M. Thrombocytopenia and interferon. *BMJ* 1988; **296:** 642.
7. Matthey F, *et al.* Bleeding in immune thrombocytopenic purpura after alpha-interferon. *Lancet* 1990; **335:** 471–2.
8. English KE, *et al.* Acquired factor VIII inhibitor in a patient with chronic myelogenous leukaemia receiving interferon-alfa therapy. *Ann Pharmacother* 2000; **34:** 737–9.
9. Durand JM, *et al.* Thrombosis and recombinant interferon-α. *Am J Med* 1993; **95:** 115.

Effects on the cardiovascular system. There have been reports of cardiomyopathy[1,2] and of Raynaud's syndrome[3,4] associated with interferon alfa therapy.
1. Deyton LR, *et al.* Reversible cardiac dysfunction associated with interferon alfa therapy in AIDS patients with Kaposi's sarcoma. *N Engl J Med* 1989; **321:** 1246–9.
2. Sonnenblick M, *et al.* Reversible cardiomyopathy induced by interferon. *BMJ* 1990; **300:** 1174–5.
3. Roy V, Newland AC. Raynaud's phenomenon and cryoglobulinaemia associated with the use of recombinant human alpha-interferon. *Lancet* 1988; **i:** 944–5.
4. Bachmeyer C, *et al.* Raynaud's phenomenon and digital necrosis induced by interferon-alpha. *Br J Dermatol* 1996; **135:** 481–3.

Effects on the endocrine system. Both hypothyroidism[1,2] and hyperthyroidism[2,3] have been associated with interferon alfa therapy. Recombinant interferon gamma was reported not to affect thyroid function.[4] The development of type 1 diabetes has been associated with interferon alfa therapy.[5-8] Exacerbation of existing type 2 diabetes has also been reported.[9,10] Reversible hypopituitarism has been reported in a patient receiving interferon alfa.[11]

1. Fentiman IS, *et al.* Primary hypothyroidism associated with interferon therapy of breast cancer. *Lancet* 1985; **i:** 1166.
2. Burman P, *et al.* Autoimmune thyroid disease in interferon-treated patients. *Lancet* 1985; **ii:** 100–1.
3. Schultz M, *et al.* Induction of hyperthyroidism by interferon-α-2b. *Lancet* 1989; **i:** 1452.
4. Bhakri H, *et al.* Recombinant gamma interferon and autoimmune thyroid disease. *Lancet* 1985; **ii:** 457.
5. Fabris P, *et al.* Development of type 1 diabetes mellitus during interferon alfa therapy for chronic HCV hepatitis. *Lancet* 1992; **340:** 548.
6. Guerci A-P, *et al.* Onset of insulin-dependent diabetes mellitus after interferon-alfa therapy for hairy cell leukaemia. *Lancet* 1994; **343:** 1167–8.
7. Gori A, *et al.* Reversible diabetes in patient with AIDS-related Kaposi's sarcoma treated with interferon α-2a. *Lancet* 1995; **345:** 1438–9.
8. Murakami M, *et al.* Diabetes mellitus and interferon-α therapy. *Ann Intern Med* 1995; **123:** 318.
9. Campbell S, *et al.* Rapidly reversible increase in insulin requirement with interferon. *BMJ* 1996; **313:** 92.
10. Lopes EPA, *et al.* Exacerbation of type 2 diabetes mellitus during interferon-alfa therapy for chronic hepatitis B. *Lancet* 1994; **343:** 244. Correction. *ibid.:* 680.
11. Sakane N, *et al.* Reversible hypopituitarism after interferon-alfa therapy. *Lancet* 1995; **345:** 1305.

Effects on the eyes. Reports of interferon-associated retinopathy have been reviewed.[1]
In a study of 43 patients with chronic hepatitis receiving interferon alfa, retinopathy developed in 11 of 37 non-diabetic patients and in 3 of 6 diabetic patients after about 8 to 10 weeks of therapy.[2] None of the patients had had retinopathy before treatment; the condition was reversible in the non-diabetic patients on cessation of therapy. Visual acuity remained unchanged. Subconjunctival haemorrhage occurred in a further 3 of the non-diabetic patients. Severe irreversible loss of vision has been reported in a non-diabetic patient receiving interferon alfa.[3]
Pain in one eyeball leading to exophthalmos and complete visual loss has been reported in a patient receiving interferon alfa;[4] despite withdrawal of interferon and instigation of antibacterial and corticosteroid treatment, the eyeball subsequently ruptured necessitating ophthalmectomy.
1. Hayasaka S, *et al.* Interferon associated retinopathy. *Br J Ophthalmol* 1998; **82:** 323–5.
2. Hayasaka S, *et al.* Retinopathy and subconjunctival haemorrhage in patients with chronic viral hepatitis receiving interferon alfa. *Br J Ophthalmol* 1995; **79:** 150–2.
3. Lohmann CP, *et al.* Severe loss of vision during adjuvant interferon alfa-2b treatment for malignant melanoma. *Lancet* 1999; **353:** 1326.
4. Yamada H, *et al.* Acute onset of ocular complications with interferon. *Lancet* 1994; **343:** 914.

Effects on the gastrointestinal tract. There have been reports[1-3] of the onset of coeliac disease during treatment of hepatitis C with interferon alfa, in some cases in combination with ribavirin. Symptoms generally resolved after interferon was discontinued and a gluten-free diet instituted.
1. Bardella MT, *et al.* Celiac disease during interferon treatment. *Ann Intern Med* 1999; **131:** 157–8.
2. Cammarota G, *et al.* Onset of coeliac disease during treatment with interferon for chronic hepatitis C. *Lancet* 2000; **356:** 1494–5.
3. Bourlière M, *et al.* Onset of coeliac disease and interferon treatment. *Lancet* 2001; **357:** 803–4.

Effects on the hair. A report of marked greying of the hair in a patient beginning after 5 months of treatment with interferon alfa for metastatic malignant melanoma.[1] On completion of interferon therapy the hair regrowth returned to its normal colour. Reversible mild to moderate alopecia has been reported by the manufacturers.
1. Fleming CJ, MacKie RM. Alpha interferon-induced hair discolouration. *Br J Dermatol* 1996; **135:** 337–8.

Effects on hearing. Sensorineural hearing loss was reported in 18 of 49 patients and tinnitus in 14 of 49 patients receiving interferons.[1] The effects were more common in those receiving interferon beta than in those receiving interferon alfa, and resolved in all patients on discontinuation of therapy.
1. Kanda Y, *et al.* Sudden hearing loss associated with interferon. *Lancet* 1994; **343:** 1134–5.

Effects on the kidneys. In a double-blind parallel-group study all of 8 renal transplant patients given, in addition to routine immunosuppression, high doses of recombinant interferon alfa (36 million units intramuscularly three times a week for 6 weeks followed by twice weekly for a further 6 weeks) had early rejection episodes which were corticosteroid-resistant; 3 also had transient nephrotic syndrome.[1] All of 8 control patients, given human albumin and saline solution, also had early rejection episodes but only one was corticosteroid-resistant. These adverse effects on the transplant contrasted with the absence of adverse effects on kidney transplants reported by other workers[2] who gave lower doses of leucocyte interferon alfa for the prophylaxis of cytomegalovirus infections. There have been a number of other reports of nephrotic syndrome associated with interferon alfa;[3-5] in one patient this was secondary to membranoproliferative glomerulonephritis.[5]
1. Kramer P, *et al.* Recombinant leucocyte interferon A induces steroid-resistant acute vascular rejection episodes in renal transplant recipients. *Lancet* 1984; **i:** 989–90.
2. Hirsch MS, *et al.* Effects of interferon-alpha on cytomegalovirus reactivation syndromes in renal-transplant recipients. *N Engl J Med* 1983; **308:** 1489–93.
3. Averbuch SD, *et al.* Acute interstitial nephritis with the nephrotic syndrome following recombinant leukocyte A interferon therapy for mycosis fungoides. *N Engl J Med* 1984; **310:** 32–5.
4. Selby P, *et al.* Nephrotic syndrome during treatment with interferon. *BMJ* 1985; **290:** 1180.
5. Herrman J, Gabriel F. Membranoproliferative glomerulonephritis in a patient with hairy-cell leukemia treated with alpha-II interferon. *N Engl J Med* 1987; **316:** 112–13.

Effects on lipids. Reversible hypertriglyceridaemia has been associated with interferon alfa treatment for chronic hepatitis C.[1] Gemfibrozil reduced the hypertriglyceridaemia but lipid concentrations did not return to baseline values and interferon treatment had to be withdrawn. Reversible hypertriglyceridaemia has also occurred in patients given interferon alfa for malignant melanoma.[2]
1. Graessle D, *et al.* Alpha-interferon and reversible hypertriglyceridemia. *Ann Intern Med* 1993; **118:** 316–17.
2. Junghans V, Rünger TM. Hypertriglyceridaemia following adjuvant interferon-α treatment in two patients with malignant melanoma. *Br J Dermatol* 1999; **140:** 183–4.

Effects on the liver. Therapy with interferon alfa has been associated with cases of fatal liver failure,[1,2] sometimes in association with chronic hepatitis B and/or C infection.[3,4]
1. Durand JM, *et al.* Liver failure due to recombinant alpha interferon. *Lancet* 1991; **338:** 1268–9.

2. Wandl UB, *et al.* Liver failure due to recombinant alpha interferon for chronic myelogenous leukaemia. *Lancet* 1992; **339**: 123–4.

3. Marcellin P, *et al.* Fatal exacerbation of chronic hepatitis B induced by recombinant alpha-interferon. *Lancet* 1991; **338**: 828.

4. Janssen HLA, *et al.* Fatal hepatic decompensation associated with interferon alfa. *BMJ* 1993; **306**: 107–8.

Effects on the nervous system and mental state. Neurological effects reported in 10 women with advanced breast cancer treated for up to 12 weeks with recombinant interferon alfa in doses of 20 million units daily or 50 million units three times weekly included abnormal EEG patterns in all 10 patients, profound lethargy and somnolence in 6, confusion and dysphasia in 5, paraesthesia in 2, and an upper motor-neurone lesion of the legs in one.[1] These effects resolved when interferon alfa was withdrawn and all patients tolerated its reintroduction at a lower dose. Reversible EEG abnormalities were observed in a further 11 patients given interferon alfa in doses of 100 million units per m[2] body-surface daily for 7 days by continuous intravenous infusion,[2] in 3 patients given 5 to 10 million units per m[2] three times weekly by subcutaneous injection,[3] and in another patient given 4 million units per m[2] daily for 6 weeks.[4] Other adverse neurological effects reported with interferon alfa include neuropsychiatric changes,[5] neuralgic amyotrophy and polyradiculopathy,[6] seizures,[7,8] spastic diplegia (in infants),[9] and severe neuropathy.[10] Mania attributed to interferon-induced hypothyroidism has been described.[11] Some of these effects were observed with doses as low as 1.5 million units[7] or 3 million units daily.[5]

Psychiatric effects including depression and suicidal ideation have been associated with interferon alfa.[12-14] Preliminary findings suggest that patients who develop depression may have higher pretreatment depression scores in psychometric tests,[15] although a prospective study of 50 patients receiving interferon alfa found that patients with pre-existing mood or anxiety disorders were no more likely than controls to interrupt therapy.[16] SSRIs have been used successfully to both treat patients with interferon-associated depression, thus allowing therapy to be continued,[17,18] and to prevent its occurrence via pretreatment.[19]

1. Smedley H, *et al.* Neurological effects of recombinant human interferon. *BMJ* 1983; **286**: 262–4.

2. Rohatiner AZS, *et al.* Central nervous system toxicity of interferon. *Br J Cancer* 1983; **47**: 419–22.

3. Suter CC, *et al.* Electroencephalographic abnormalities in interferon encephalopathy: a preliminary report. *Mayo Clin Proc* 1984; **59**: 847–50.

4. Honigsberger L, *et al.* Neurological effects of recombinant human interferon. *BMJ* 1983; **286**: 719.

5. Adams F, *et al.* Neuropsychiatric manifestations of human leukocyte interferon therapy in patients with cancer. *JAMA* 1984; **252**: 938–41.

6. Bernsen PLJA, *et al.* Neuralgic amyotrophy and polyradiculopathy during interferon therapy. *Lancet* 1985; **i**: 50.

7. Janssen HLA, *et al.* Seizures associated with low-dose α-interferon. *Lancet* 1990; **336**: 1580.

8. Brouwers PJ, *et al.* Photosensitive seizures associated with interferon alpha-2a. *Ann Pharmacother* 1999; **33**: 113–14.

9. Barlow CF, *et al.* Spastic diplegia as a complication of interferon alfa-2a treatment of hemangiomas of infancy. *J Pediatr* 1998; **132**: 527–30.

10. Gastinne DA, *et al.* Severe neuropathy associated with low-dose recombinant interferon-alpha. *Am J Med* 1989; **87**: 116.

11. Kingsley D. Interferon-alpha induced 'tertiary mania'. *Hosp Med* 1999; **60**: 381–2.

12. Janssen HLA, *et al.* Suicide associated with alfa-interferon therapy for chronic viral hepatitis. *J Hepatol* 1994; **21**: 241–3.

13. Renault PF, *et al.* Psychiatric complications of long-term interferon alfa therapy. *Arch Intern Med* 1987; **147**: 1577–80.

14. Adverse Drug Reactions Advisory Committee (ADRAC). Depression with interferon. *Aust Adverse Drug React Bull* 1999; **18**: 6.

15. Capuron L, Ravaud A. Prediction of the depressive effects of interferon alfa therapy by the patient's initial affective state. *N Engl J Med* 1999; **340**: 1370.

16. Parinate CM, *et al.* Treatment with interferon-α in patients with chronic hepatitis and mood or anxiety disorders. *Lancet* 1999; **354**: 131–2.

17. Levenson JL, Fallon HJ. Fluoxetine treatment of depression caused by interferon-α. *Am J Gastroenterol* 1993; **88**: 760–1.

18. Schramm TM, *et al.* Sertraline treatment of interferon-alfa-induced depressive disorder. *Med J Aust* 2000; **173**: 359–61.

19. Musselman DL, *et al.* Paroxetine for the prevention of depression induced by high-dose interferon alfa. *N Engl J Med* 2001; **344**: 961–6.

Effects on the oral mucosa. Painful oral ulcers, necessitating withdrawal of interferon alfa therapy, have occurred in a patient treated for chronic hepatitis.[1] Oropharyngeal lichen planus was associated with interferon alfa in another patient.[2]

1. Qaseem T, *et al.* A case report of painful oral ulcerations associated with the use of alpha interferon in a patient with chronic hepatitis due to non-A non-B non-C virus. *Milit Med* 1993; **158**: 126–7.

2. Kütting B, *et al.* Oropharyngeal lichen planus associated with interferon-α treatment for mycosis fungoides: a rare side-effect in the therapy of cutaneous lymphomas. *Br J Dermatol* 1997; **137**: 836–7.

Effects on the respiratory system. Treatment with interferon alfa resulted in severe exacerbation of mild asthma in 2 patients with hepatitis C.[1]

1. Bini EJ, Weinshel EH. Severe exacerbation of asthma: a new side effect of interferon-α in patients with asthma and chronic hepatitis C. *Mayo Clin Proc* 1999; **74**: 367–70.

Effects on skeletal muscle. Myalgia is one of the influenza-like symptoms frequently associated with interferons. Fatal rhabdomyolysis and multiple organ failure was reported in a patient receiving high doses of interferon alfa.[1]

1. Reinhold U, *et al.* Fatal rhabdomyolysis and multiple organ failure associated with adjuvant high-dose interferon alfa in malignant melanoma. *Lancet* 1997; **349**: 540–1.

Effects on the skin. Exacerbation or development of psoriasis was reported in patients given recombinant interferon alfa.[1,2] However, no such effect was seen in 7 patients given interferon gamma.[3] Exacerbation of lichen planus has also been reported[4] during interferon alfa treatment (see also Effects on the Oral Mucosa, above). Cutaneous vascular lesions with punctate telangiectasias were noted in 18 of 44 patients treated with interferon alfa-2a; lesions did not appear at the injection site.[5] Severe necrotising cutaneous lesions were reported at injection sites in a patient receiving recombinant interferon beta-1b; the lesions healed when interferon alfa-n3 was substituted.[6] However, cutaneous necrosis has also been associated with interferon alfa.[7] Fatal paraneoplastic pemphigus developed in a patient receiving interferon alfa-2a.[8] Cutaneous sarcoidosis has also been reported.[9]

1. Quesada JR, Gutterman JU. Psoriasis and alpha-interferon. *Lancet* 1986; **i**: 1466–8.

2. Funk J, *et al.* Psoriasis induced by interferon-α. *Br J Dermatol* 1991; **125**: 463–5.

3. Schulze H-J, Mahrle G. Gamma interferon and psoriasis. *Lancet* 1986; **ii**: 926–7.

4. Protzer U, *et al.* Exacerbation of lichen planus during interferon alfa-2a therapy for chronic active hepatitis C. *Gastroenterology* 1993; **104**: 903–5.

5. Dreno B, *et al.* Alpha-interferon therapy and cutaneous vascular lesions. *Ann Intern Med* 1989; **111**: 95–6.

6. Sheremata WA, *et al.* Severe necrotizing cutaneous lesions complicating treatment with interferon beta-1b. *N Engl J Med* 1995; **332**: 1584.

7. Shinohara K. More on interferon-induced cutaneous necrosis. *N Engl J Med* 1995; **333**: 1222.

8. Kirsner RS, *et al.* Treatment with alpha interferon associated with the development of paraneoplastic pemphigus. *Br J Dermatol* 1995; **132**: 474–8.

9. Eberlein-König B, *et al.* Cutaneous sarcoid foreign body granulomas developing in sites of previous skin injury after systemic interferon-alpha treatment for chronic hepatitis C. *Br J Dermatol* 1999; **140**: 370–2.

Shock. Fatal non-cardiogenic shock occurred following the third dose of interferon alfa-2b in a patient with malignant melanoma.[1] There were similarities to a fatal reaction reported in another patient with malignant melanoma (see under Effects on Skeletal Muscle, above).

1. Carson JJ, *et al.* Fatality and interferon α for malignant melanoma. *Lancet* 1998; **352**: 1443–4.

Precautions

Interferons should be used with caution or avoided altogether in patients with depression or psychiatric disorders, epilepsy or other CNS diseases, severe renal or hepatic impairment, cardiac disorders, myelosuppression, poorly controlled thyroid dysfunction, pulmonary disease, diabetes mellitus, auto-immune diseases, coagulation disorders, or a history of these conditions. Patients with psoriasis have been reported to experience exacerbations during interferon alfa therapy.

Blood counts should be monitored, particularly in patients at high risk of myelosuppression (for example those with haematological malignancies). Assessment of cardiac function is advised before treatment is started. Patients receiving interferons who experience visual disturbances should receive an eye examination. A baseline ocular examination is recommended prior to treatment in patients predisposed to retinopathy such as those with diabetes mellitus or hypertension. Hepatic and renal function should be monitored during treatment with interferons. Interferon alfa should be discontinued in patients with chronic hepatitis who develop liver decompensation. Patients should receive adequate fluids to maintain hydration during treatment with interferon alfa.

Interferons may affect the ability to drive or operate machinery.

Antibodies may develop to exogenous interferon that reduce its activity.

Asthma. For a report of severe exacerbation of asthma in patients receiving interferon alfa, see Effects on the Respiratory System, above.

Auto-immune disorders. A number of disorders thought to have an auto-immune component have developed or been exacerbated during therapy with interferon alfa, including diabetes mellitus,[1] auto-immune hepatitis,[2,3] multiple sclerosis,[4,5] rheumatoid arthritis,[6] systemic lupus erythematosus,[7] and thyroid disease.[8]

For mention of a possible association between interferons and the occurrence of coeliac disease, see Effects on the Gastrointestinal Tract under Adverse Effects, above.

1. Fabris P, *et al.* Development of type 1 diabetes mellitus during interferon alfa therapy for chronic HCV hepatitis. *Lancet* 1992; **340**: 548.

2. Vento S, *et al.* Hazards of interferon therapy for HBV-seronegative chronic hepatitis. *Lancet* 1989; **ii**: 926.

3. Papo T, *et al.* Autoimmune chronic hepatitis exacerbated by alpha-interferon. *Ann Intern Med* 1992; **116**: 51–3.

4. Larrey D, *et al.* Exacerbation of multiple sclerosis after the administration of recombinant human interferon alfa. *JAMA* 1989; **261**: 2065.

5. Coyle JT. Multiple sclerosis and human interferon alfa. *JAMA* 1989; **262**: 2684.

6. Chazerain P, *et al.* Rheumatoid arthritis-like disease after alpha-interferon therapy. *Ann Intern Med* 1992; **116**: 427.

7. Tolaymat A, *et al.* Systemic lupus erythematosus in a child receiving long-term interferon therapy. *J Pediatr* 1992; **120**: 429–32.

8. Fernandez-Soto L, *et al.* Increased risk of autoimmune thyroid disease in hepatitis C vs hepatitis B before, during, and after discontinuing interferon therapy. *Arch Intern Med* 1998; **158**: 1445–8.

Psychiatric disorders. For comment on the incidence of adverse effects in patients with pre-existing mood or anxiety disorders, see Effects on the Nervous System and Mental State, above.

Interactions

Interactions involving interferons have not been fully evaluated, but it is known that they can inhibit hepatic oxidative metabolism and thus caution should be exercised during concomitant administration of drugs metabolised in this way. Drugs likely to exacerbate the effects of interferons, such as those with myelosuppressive activity, should also be used with caution.

See below for details of specific interactions.

ACE inhibitors. For a report of possible synergistic haematological toxicity in patients receiving interferon alfa and ACE inhibitors, see p.823.

Antineoplastics. The manufacturer of interferon alfa-n1 has reported occasional cases of severe cytopenia with or without bone marrow aplasia in patients with chronic myeloid leukaemia who received interferon alfa-n1 immediately following *busulfan*. Caution is advised if busulfan or *hydroxyurea [hydroxycarbamide]* are reintroduced in combination with interferon alfa-n1. Severe myelosuppression has been reported in patients receiving interferon alfa-n1 with relatively high doses of *vinblastine*.

For reduction in the area under the plasma concentration-time curve for *melphalan* in patients receiving interferon alfa, see Effects of Temperature, under Pharmacokinetics of Melphalan, p.551.

Antivirals. The manufacturer of interferon alfa-n1 has reported progressive renal failure in patients receiving interferon alfa-n1 and high doses of *aciclovir*.

For a report of synergistic bone-marrow toxicity with interferon alfa and *zidovudine*, see p.646.

Paracetamol. Three patients experienced increases in liver enzyme values when given paracetamol 1 g two or three times daily on three days each week to coincide with the days of administration of interferon alfa; vinblastine was also given every third week.[1] Paracetamol has also been found to enhance the antiviral effect of interferon alfa in healthy subjects.[2]

1. Kellokumpu-Lehtinen P, *et al.* Hepatotoxicity of paracetamol in combination with interferon and vinblastine. *Lancet* 1989; **i**: 1143.

2. Hendrix CW, *et al.* Modulation of α-interferon's antiviral and clinical effects by aspirin, acetaminophen, and prednisone in healthy volunteers. *Antiviral Res* 1995; **28**: 121–31.

Theophylline. For reference to reduced clearance of theophylline in patients receiving interferon alfa, see p.781.

Warfarin. For a report of potentiation of warfarin necessitating dosage reduction in a patient also receiving interferon alfa, see p.996.

Antiviral Action

Interferons are produced by virus-infected cells and confer protection on uninfected cells of the same species. They affect many cell functions demonstrating, in addition to their antiviral activity, antiproliferative and immunoregulatory properties; interferon gamma in particular is a potent macrophage-stimulating factor. These activities are considered to be interrelated. Following binding of interferons to a specific cell-surface protein, several enzyme systems appear to be activated to block viral and possibly cellular RNA development.

Studies have shown interferons to have benefit in infections with hepatitis B virus, hepatitis C virus, herpes simplex viruses, varicella-zoster virus, cytomegalovirus, rhinoviruses, and papillomaviruses.

Pharmacokinetics

Interferons are not absorbed from the gastrointestinal tract. More than 80% of a subcutaneous or intramuscular dose of interferon alfa is absorbed. Following intramuscular injection, interferon alfa produced by recombinant techniques or from cultured leucocytes produce similar plasma concentrations, usually reaching a peak within 4 to 8 hours. Half-lives of about 3 to 8 hours have been reported. Intravenous administration produces more rapid distribution and elimination. Interferon alfa does not readily cross the blood-brain barrier. Interferon alfa undergoes renal catabolism and negligible amounts of interferons are excreted in the urine.

Uses and Administration

The interferons have a range of activities. In addition to their action against viruses they are active against malignant neoplasms and have an immunomodulating effect. Several alfa-interferons are available: interferon alfa-2a (rbe), interferon alfa-2b (rbe), alfa-n1 (lns), alfa-n3 (bls), and alfacon-1 (rbe).

Alfa interferons are used in chronic hepatitis B (alfa-2a, alfa-2b, and alfa-n1) and chronic hepatitis C (alfa-2a, alfa-2b, alfa-n1, and alfacon-1); in several malignant neoplasms including AIDS-related Kaposi's sarcoma (alfa-2a and alfa-2b), hairy-cell leukaemia (alfa-2a, alfa-2b, and alfa-n1), chronic myeloid leukaemia (alfa-2a, alfa-2b, and alfa-n1), follicular lymphoma (alfa-2a and alfa-2b), cutaneous T-cell lymphoma (alfa-2a), carcinoid tumours (alfa-2b), melanoma (alfa-2a and alfa-2b), myeloma (alfa-2b), and renal cell carcinoma (alfa-2a); and in condylomata acuminata (alfa-2b and alfa-n3).

ADMINISTRATION AND DOSAGE. Dosage regimens are as follows.

- **Chronic active hepatitis B.** *Interferon alfa-2a* is given in a dose of 2.5 to 5 million units per m^2 body-surface three times weekly by subcutaneous injection for 4 to 6 months. *Interferon alfa-2b* is given in doses of 5 to 10 million units three times weekly for 4 to 6 months, or 5 million units daily for 4 months, by subcutaneous or intramuscular injection. *Interferon alfa-n1* is given either in doses of 10 to 15 million units (to a maximum of 7.5 million units per m^2) three times weekly for 12 weeks, or 5 to 10 million units (to a maximum of 5 million units per m^2) three times weekly for up to 6 months, by subcutaneous or intramuscular injection. An initial escalating dosing schedule, usually over 5 days, may improve tolerance.

- **Chronic hepatitis C.** *Interferon alfa-2a* is given in a dose of 3 to 4.5 million units three times weekly by subcutaneous or intramuscular injection for 6 months when it is used in combination with ribavirin. In patients unable to tolerate ribavirin, interferon alfa-2a monotherapy is given either in an initial dose of 3 to 6 million units three times weekly for 6 months followed by 3 million units three times weekly for an additional 6 months, or in a dose of 3 million units three times weekly for 12 months, by subcutaneous or intramuscular injection. *Interferon alfa-2b* is given in a dose of 3 million units three times weekly for 6 to 12 months in combination with ribavirin, or when given as monotherapy, for 12 to 18 months, or for up to 24 months, by subcutaneous or intramuscular injection. A formulation of interferon alfa-2b conjugated with monomethoxy polyethylene glycol (peginterferon alfa-2b) is available in some countries. It is given subcutaneously in a dose of 1.5 μg per kg body-weight once weekly for 6 to 12 months in combination with ribavirin, or in a dose of 0.5 or 1 μg per kg once weekly for 6 to 12 months when given as monotherapy. *Interferon alfa-n1* is given in a dose of 3 or 5 million units three times weekly for 48 weeks by subcutaneous or intramuscular injection. *Interferon alfacon-1* is given in a dose of 9 μg three times weekly by subcutaneous injection for 24 weeks followed by 15 μg three times weekly for 6 months if necessary.

- **AIDS-related Kaposi's sarcoma.** *Interferon alfa-2a* is usually given in an escalating dose of 3 million units daily for 3 days, 9 million units daily for 3 days, 18 million units daily for 3 days, and 36 million units daily, if tolerated, on days 10 to 84, by subcutaneous or intramuscular injection; thereafter the maximum tolerated dose (up to 36 million units) may be given three times weekly. *Interferon alfa-2b* is given in a dose of 30 million units per m^2 three times weekly, by subcutaneous or intramuscular injection.

- **Hairy-cell leukaemia.** *Interferon alfa-2a* is given in an initial dose of 3 million units daily for 16 to 24 weeks, then the same dose three times weekly, by subcutaneous or intramuscular injection. Treatment has continued for up to 20 months. *Interferon alfa-2b* is given in a dose of 2 million units per m^2 three times weekly by subcutaneous or intramuscular injection. *Interferon alfa-n1* is given in an initial dose of 3 million units daily by subcutaneous or intramuscular injection, commonly for 12 to 16 weeks, then the same dose three times weekly thereafter. Alternative doses of 2 million units per m^2 or 0.2 million units per m^2 of interferon alfa-n1 have also been tried. Treatment may continue for 6 months or more.

- **Chronic myeloid leukaemia.** *Interferon alfa-2a* is given by subcutaneous or intramuscular injection in an escalating dose of 3 million units daily for 3 days, 6 million units daily for 3 days, and 9 million units daily thereafter. Patients showing a response after 12 weeks should continue treatment until a complete haematological response is achieved or for a maximum of 18 months; those who achieve a complete haematological response should continue on 9 million units daily (or a minimum of 9 million units 3 times weekly) in order to achieve a cytogenetic response. *Interferon alfa-2b* is given in a dose of 4 to 5 million units per m^2 daily by subcutaneous injection, continuing at the maximum tolerated dose to maintain remission (usually 4 to 10 million units per m^2 daily). *Interferon alfa-n1* is given, once the white blood count has been controlled by cytotoxic chemotherapy, in a dose of 3 million units daily for three weeks by subcutaneous injection. The dose is then adjusted to maintain a suitable leucocyte count (typically about 20 million units per week). Doses of 3 or 6 million units (occasionally 9 million units) daily have been used to achieve initial control of the white blood cell count.

- **Follicular lymphoma.** *Interferon alfa-2a* is given as an adjunct to chemotherapy in a dose of 6 million units per m^2 daily by subcutaneous or intramuscular injection on days 22 to 26 of a 28-day chemotherapy cycle. *Interferon alfa-2b* is given as an adjunct to chemotherapy in a dose of 5 million units three times weekly by subcutaneous injection for 18 months.

- **Cutaneous T-cell lymphoma.** *Interferon alfa-2a* is given in an escalating dose of 3 million units daily for 3 days, then 9 million units daily for 3 days, and then 18 million units daily to complete 12 weeks of treatment, by subcutaneous or intramuscular injection. The maximum tolerated dose (but not exceeding 18 million units) is then given three times weekly for a minimum of 12 months in responding patients.

- **Carcinoid tumours.** *Interferon alfa-2b* is given in a dose of 3 to 9 million units (usually 5 million units) three times weekly by subcutaneous injection. In advanced disease, 5 million units may be given daily.

- **Melanoma.** *Interferon alfa-2a* is given in a dose of 3 million units three times weekly by subcutaneous or intramuscular injection for 18 months. Treatment should start no later than 6 weeks after surgery. *Interferon alfa-2b* is given in an initial dose of 20 million units per m^2 daily on 5 days each week for 4 weeks by intravenous infusion over 20 minutes, and then for maintenance 10 million units per m^2 three times weekly by subcutaneous injection for 48 weeks.

- **Multiple myeloma.** *Interferon alfa-2b* is given as maintenance treatment following chemotherapy induction at a dose of 3 million units per m^2 three times weekly by subcutaneous injection.

- **Renal cell carcinoma.** *Interferon alfa-2a* is given as an adjunct to cytotoxic chemotherapy in an escalating dose of 3 million units three times weekly for one week, then 9 million units three times weekly for one week, then 18 million units three times weekly thereafter for 3 to 12 months, by subcutaneous or intramuscular injection.

- **Condylomata acuminata.** *Interferon alfa-2b* is given in a dose of 1 million units injected into each lesion three times weekly for 3 weeks, and repeated after 12 to 16 weeks if necessary. No more than 5 lesions should be treated in each treatment course, but courses for additional lesions may run sequentially. *Interferon alfa-n3* is given in a dose of 0.25 million units per lesion twice weekly for up to 8 weeks, to a maximum of 2.5 million units in each session.

See below for further details of these as well as some other uses of alfa interferons.

◊ General reviews of interferons.

1. Baron S, *et al.* The interferons: mechanisms of action and clinical applications. *JAMA* 1991; **266:** 1375–83.
2. Finter NB, *et al.* The use of interferon-α in virus infections. *Drugs* 1991; **42:** 749–65.
3. Volz MA, Kirkpatrick CH. Interferons 1992: how much of the promise has been realised? *Drugs* 1992; **43:** 285–94.

4. Dorr RT. Interferon-α malignant and viral diseases: a review. *Drugs* 1993; **45:** 177–211.
5. Haria M, Benfield P. Interferon-α-2a: a review of its pharmacological properties and therapeutic use in the management of viral hepatitis. *Drugs* 1995; **50:** 873–96.

Age-related macular degeneration. In age-related macular degeneration (senile macular degeneration), a common cause of visual impairment in the elderly, there is a gradual and progressive deterioration of central vision usually affecting both eyes. Although some encouraging results[1-4] have been obtained with systemic interferon alfa-2a or alfa-2b for the treatment of choroidal neovascularisation considered unsuitable for laser therapy, adverse effects have been common and often severe and a randomised study in 481 patients showed no benefit after treatment for one year.[5]

1. Gillies MC, *et al.* Treatment of choroidal neovascularisation in age-related macular degeneration with interferon alfa-2a and alfa-2b. *Br J Ophthalmol* 1993; **77:** 759–65.
2. Kirkpatrick JNP, *et al.* Clinical experience with interferon alfa-2a for exudative age-related macular degeneration. *Br J Ophthalmol* 1993; **77:** 766–70.
3. Poliner LS, *et al.* Interferon alpha-2a for subfoveal neovascularization in age-related macular degeneration. *Ophthalmology* 1993; **100:** 1417–24.
4. Engler C, *et al.* Interferon alfa-2a modifies the course of subfoveal and juxtafoveal choroidal neovascularisation. *Br J Ophthalmol* 1994; **78:** 749–53.
5. Pharmacological Therapy for Macular Degeneration Study Group. Interferon alfa-2a in ineffective for patients with choroidal neovascularization secondary to age-related macular degeneration: results of a prospective randomized placebo-controlled clinical trial. *Arch Ophthalmol* 1997; **115:** 865–72.

Angiomatous disease. Encouraging responses were reported in 4 of 5 children treated with interferon alfa-2a for various angiomatous diseases.[1] Regression of haemangioma size by more than 50% was achieved in 11 of 18 infants and children given interferon alfa-2a for 1 to 5 months,[2] and in 11 of 19 children treated for at least 4 months.[3]

1. White CW, *et al.* Treatment of childhood angiomatous diseases with recombinant interferon alfa-2a. *J Pediatr* 1991; **118:** 59–66.
2. Deb G, *et al.* Treatment of hemangiomas of infants and babies with interferon alfa-2a: preliminary results. *Int J Pediatr Hematol/Oncol* 1996; **3:** 109–13.
3. Greinwald JH, *et al.* An update on the treatment of hemangiomas in children with interferon alfa-2a. *Arch Otolaryngol Head Neck Surg* 1999; **125:** 21–7.

Behçet's syndrome. Behçet's syndrome (p.1047) is usually managed with corticosteroids. Among many other drugs that have been tried, interferon alfa-2b was reported to produce beneficial responses in 3 patients with refractory ocular symptoms.[1] Encouraging results have also been obtained in other small studies of interferon alfa-2a.[2,3]

1. Feron EJ, *et al.* Interferon-α2b for refractory ocular Behçet's disease. *Lancet* 1994; **343:** 1428.
2. Azizlerli G, *et al.* Interferon alfa-2a in the treatment of Behçet's disease. *Dermatology* 1996; **192:** 239–41.
3. Kötter I, *et al.* Treatment of ocular symptoms of Behçet's disease with interferon α₂ₐ: a pilot study. *Br J Ophthalmol* 1998; **82:** 488–94.

Blood disorders. Interferon alfa may be used in the management of the myeloproliferative disorders *primary (essential) thrombocythaemia*[1] (p.486) and *polycythaemia vera*[1,2] (p.486). A study in patients with a variety of chronic myeloproliferative disorders suggested that interferon alfa-2b could also be useful in the management of *myeloid metaplasia*.[3]

Paradoxically, interferon alfa has also been tried in patients with HIV-associated *thrombocytopenia*[4] (see HIV Infection and AIDS, below).

Following case reports of interferon alfa producing improvements in patients with idiopathic *hypereosinophilic syndrome*[5,6] who had not responded to corticosteroids and hydroxyurea [hydroxycarbamide] 2 small studies have shown beneficial responses to interferon alfa alone[7] and in combination with hydroxyurea [hydroxycarbamide].[8]

See also under Malignant Neoplasms, below.

1. Elliott MA, Tefferi A. Interferon-alpha therapy in polycythemia vera and essential thrombocythemia. *Semin Thromb Hemost* 1997; **23:** 463–72.
2. Lengfelder E, *et al..* Interferon alpha in the treatment of polycythemia vera. *Ann Hematol* 2000; **79:** 103–9.
3. Gilbert HS. Long term treatment of *Cancer* 1998; **83:** 1205–13.
4. Marroni M, *et al.* Interferon-α is effective in the treatment of HIV-1-related, severe, zidovudine-resistant thrombocytopenia. *Ann Intern Med* 1994; **121:** 423–9.
5. Zielinski RM, Lawrence WD. Interferon-α for the hypereosinophilic syndrome. *Ann Intern Med* 1990; **113:** 716–18.
6. Busch FW, *et al.* Alpha-interferon for the hypereosinophilic syndrome. *Ann Intern Med* 1991; **114:** 338–9.
7. Butterfield JH, Gleich GJ. Interferon-α treatment of six patients with the idiopathic hypereosinophilic syndrome. *Ann Intern Med* 1994; **121:** 648–53.
8. Coutant G, *et al.* Traitement des syndromes hyperéosinophiliques à expression myeloproliferative par l'association hydroxyurée-interféron alpha. *Ann Med Interne (Paris)* 1993; **144:** 243–50.

Churg-Strauss syndrome. For a report that interferon alfa may be beneficial in Churg-Strauss syndrome, see p.1049.

Hepatitis. Interferon alfa is the main drug used in the treatment of chronic viral hepatitis (p.605). Interferon beta has also been used. Although the response and relapse rates following treatment of chronic hepatitis with interferon have been disappointing, prolonging treatment with higher doses (if tolerated) may be beneficial.[1-3] However, in an interim analysis of a study of 29 patients with AIDS and chronic hepatitis C, escalating doses of interferon alfa did not improve response rates.[4] A meta-analysis[5] has suggested that treatment with interferon alfa 3 million units three times weekly for at least 12 months had the best risk:benefit ratio for patients with chronic hepatitis C. Recent studies[6] have shown once-weekly peginterferon alfa, a formulation of interferon alfa with monomethoxy polyethylene glycol, to be more effective than interferon alfa given three times weekly in patients with chronic hepatitis C, including those with cirrhosis or extensive fibrosis.[7] The use of ribavirin in combination with interferon alfa[8-13] or beta[14] for the treatment of chronic hepatitis C is more effective than either drug alone with sustained responses having been recorded, and some authorities now consider combination therapy to be the treatment of first choice.[11-13]

In hepatitis B, responses to interferon alfa can be improved by pre-treatment with corticosteroids.[15-17]

Evidence of improved long-term outcomes following treatment is accumulating. Long-term follow-up of patients has demonstrated a lower incidence of hepatocellular carcinoma in patients who had received interferons than in untreated patients.[18-22] Risk reduction is apparently greatest in patients with chronic hepatitis C and without hepatitis B infection.[22]

Interferon alfa can produce benefit in some patients with chronic hepatitis D[23] or hepatitis G.[24]

Although antivirals are generally not required in uncomplicated acute hepatitis, treatment with interferons has been shown to produce more rapid resolution of viraemia[5,25,26] and may decrease the risk of chronic hepatitis developing.[27] Improvements in liver function were reported in 4 patients with fulminant hepatitis A treated with interferon beta.[28]

1. Reichard O, et al. Two-year biochemical, virological, and histological follow-up in patients with chronic hepatitis C responding in a sustained fashion to interferon alfa-2b treatment. Hepatology 1995; 21: 918–22.
2. Poynard T, et al. A comparison of three interferon alfa-2b regimens for the long-term treatment of chronic non-A, non-B hepatitis. N Engl J Med 1995; 332: 1457–62.
3. Degos F, et al. Reinforced regimen of interferon alfa-2a reduces the incidence of cirrhosis in patients with chronic hepatitis C: a multicentre randomised trial. J Hepatol 1998; 29: 224–32.
4. Soriano V, et al. A pilot study on the efficacy of escalating dosage of alpha-interferon for chronic hepatitis C in HIV-infected patients. J Infect 1997; 35: 225–30.
5. Poynard T, et al. Meta-analysis of interferon randomized trials in the treatment of viral hepatitis C: effects of dose and duration. Hepatology 1996; 24: 778–89.
6. Zeusen S, et al. Peginterferon alfa-2a in patients with chronic hepatitis C. N Engl J Med 2000; 343: 1666–72.
7. Heathcote EJ, et al. Peginterferon alfa-2a in patients with chronic hepatitis C and cirrhosis. N Engl J Med 2000; 343: 1673–80.
8. Chemello L, et al. Response to ribavirin, to interferon and to a combination of both in patients with chronic hepatitis C and its relation to HCV genotypes. J Hepatol 1994; 21: (suppl): S12.
9. Braconier JH, et al. Combined alpha-interferon and ribavirin treatment in chronic hepatitis C: a pilot study. Scand J Infect Dis 1995; 27: 325–9.
10. Reichard O, et al. Randomised, double-blind, placebo-controlled trial of interferon α-2b with and without ribavirin for chronic hepatitis C. Lancet 1998; 351: 83–7.
11. Poynard T, et al. Randomised trial of interferon α2b plus ribavirin for 48 weeks or for 24 weeks versus interferon α2b plus placebo for 48 weeks for treatment of chronic infection with hepatitis C virus. Lancet 1998; 352: 1426–32.
12. Davis GL, et al. Interferon alfa-2b alone or in combination with ribavirin for the treatment of relapse of chronic hepatitis C. N Engl J Med 1998; 339: 1493–9.
13. McHutchison JG, et al. Interferon alfa-2b alone or in combination with ribavirin as initial treatment for chronic hepatitis C. N Engl J Med 1998; 339: 1485–92.
14. Kakumu S, et al. A pilot study of ribavirin and interferon beta for the treatment of chronic hepatitis C. Gastroenterology 1993; 105: 507–12.
15. Perrillo RP, et al. A randomized, controlled trial of interferon alfa-2b alone and after prednisone withdrawal for the treatment of chronic hepatitis B. N Engl J Med 1990; 323: 295–301.
16. Fevery J, et al. Efficacy of interferon alfa-2b with or without prednisone withdrawal in the treatment for chronic viral hepatitis B: a prospective double-blind Belgian-Dutch study. J Hepatol 1991; 11: S108–S112.
17. Krogsgaard K, et al. Prednisolone withdrawal therapy enhances the effect of human lymphoblastoid interferon in chronic hepatitis B. J Hepatol 1996; 25: 803–13.
18. Nishiguchi S, et al. Randomised trial of effects of interferon-α on incidence of hepatocellular carcinoma in chronic active hepatitis C with cirrhosis. Lancet 1995; 346: 1051–5.
19. Kuwana K, et al. Risk factors and the effect of interferon therapy in the development of hepatocellular carcinoma: a multivariate analysis in 343 patients. J Gastroenterol Hepatol 1997; 12: 149–55.
20. Imai Y, et al. Relation of interferon therapy and hepatocellular carcinoma in patients with chronic hepatitis C. Ann Intern Med 1998; 129: 94–9.
21. Lin S-M, et al. Long-term beneficial effect of interferon therapy in patients with chronic hepatitis B virus infection. Hepatol 1999; 29: 971–5.
22. International Interferon-α Heptocellular Carcinoma Study Group. Effect of interferon-α on progression of cirrhosis to hepatocellular carcinoma: a retrospective cohort study. Lancet 1998; 351: 1535–9.
23. Farci P, et al. Treatment of chronic hepatitis D with interferon alfa-2a. N Engl J Med 1994; 330: 88–94.
24. Tanaka E, et al. Effect of hepatitis G virus infection on chronic hepatitis C. Ann Intern Med 1996; 125: 740–3.
25. Cammà C, et al. Interferon as treatment for acute hepatitis C: a meta-analysis. Dig Dis Sci 1996; 41: 1248–55.
26. Quin JW. Interferon therapy for acute hepatitis C viral infection—a review by meta-analysis. Aust N Z J Med 1997; 27: 611–18.
27. Omata M, et al. Resolution of acute hepatitis C after therapy with natural beta interferon. Lancet 1991; 338: 914–15.
28. Yoshiba M, et al. Interferon for hepatitis A. Lancet 1994; 343: 288–9.

Herpes simplex infections. Although herpes simplex infections are commonly treated with aciclovir (see p.607), beneficial responses to interferon alfa, applied topically, have been reported in genital herpes[1-4] and, in combination with trifluridine[5,6] or brivudine,[7] in herpes keratitis. A systematic review[8] of interventions for herpes simplex epithelial keratitis found that interferon monotherapy had a slightly beneficial effect on dendritic epithelial keratitis, but no more than that of other antiviral drugs, and concluded that the combination of an antiviral nucleoside and interferon seemed to speed healing.

Similarly, there are case reports of improvement in herpes labialis with interferon alfa in combination with trifluridine in 3 patients resistant to aciclovir, 2 of whom were also resistant to foscarnet.[9] Interferon beta has also been tried in a small number of patients for the treatment of labial and genital herpes.[10] However, in a comparative study[11] intramuscular interferon alfa was not superior to topical aciclovir either in treating first-episode genital herpes or in altering the frequency of recurrences.

1. Friedman-Kien AE, et al. Treatment of recurrent genital herpes with topical alpha interferon gel combined with nonoxynol 9. J Am Acad Dermatol 1986; 15: 989–94.
2. Sacks SL, et al. Randomized, double-blind, placebo-controlled, patient-initiated study of topical high- and low-dose interferon-α with nonoxynol-9 in the treatment of recurrent genital herpes. J Infect Dis 1990; 161: 692–8.
3. Shupack J, et al. Topical alpha-interferon in recurrent genital herpes simplex infection. Dermatologica 1990; 181: 134–8.
4. Syed TA, et al. Human leukocyte interferon-alpha in cream for the management of genital herpes in Asian women: a placebo-controlled, double-blind study. J Mol Med 1995; 73: 141–4.
5. de Koning EWJ, et al. Combination therapy for dendritic keratitis with human leucocyte interferon and trifluorothymidine. Br J Ophthalmol 1982; 66: 509–12.
6. Sundmacher R, et al. Combination therapy for dendritic keratitis: high-titer α-interferon and trifluridine. Arch Ophthalmol 1984; 102: 554–5.
7. van Bijsterveld OP, et al. Bromovinyldeoxyuridine and interferon treatment in ulcerative herpetic keratitis: a double masked study. Br J Ophthalmol 1989; 73: 604–7.
8. Wilhelmus KR. Interventions for herpes simplex virus epithelial keratitis (updated 23 May 2001). Available in The Cochrane Library; Issue 4. Oxford: Update Software; 2001.
9. Birch CJ, et al. Clinical effects and in vitro studies of trifluorothymidine combined with interferon-α for treatment of drug-resistant andsensitive herpes simplex virus infections. J Infect Dis 1992; 166: 108–12.
10. Glezerman M, et al. Placebo-controlled trial of topical interferon on labial and genital herpes. Lancet 1988; i: 150–2.
11. Levin MJ, et al. Comparison of intramuscular recombinant alpha interferon (rIFN-2A) with topical acyclovir for the treatment of first-episode herpes genitalis and prevention of recurrences. Antimicrob Agents Chemother 1989; 33: 649–52.

HIV infection and AIDS. The effects of interferons on the progression of AIDS (p.608) have been mixed.[1-5] Combinations of interferon alfa with antiretroviral reverse transcriptase inhibitors have produced variable responses,[6-10] with some investigators reporting enhanced[6,10] or synergistic[8] antiretroviral effects, though often at doses associated with a high incidence of adverse effects.

Interferons have been tried with some success in the management of Kaposi's sarcoma and mycobacterial infections in patients with AIDS (see below and under Interferon Gamma, p.634).

Promising results have been reported with interferon alfa in patients with HIV-associated thrombocytopenia,[11] although interferons have been reported to induce immune thrombocytopenia, and there has been a report of bleeding in a patient with idiopathic thrombocytopenic purpura (see Effects on the Blood under Adverse Effects, above).

1. Puppo F, et al. Low doses of alpha-interferon for the treatment of AIDS-related syndromes: a preliminary study. Int J Immunother 1988; 4: 165–8.
2. Brook MG, et al. Anti-HIV effects of alpha-interferon. Lancet 1989; i: 42.
3. Ellis ME, et al. An open study of interferon in HIV-antibody-positive men. AIDS 1989; 3: 851–3.
4. Lane HC, et al. Interferon-α in patients with asymptomatic human immunodeficiency virus (HIV) infection: a randomized placebo-controlled trial. Ann Intern Med 1990; 112: 805–11.
5. Frissen PHJ, et al. High-dose interferon-α2a exerts potent activity against human immunodeficiency virus type I not associated with antitumor activity in subjects with Kaposi's sarcoma. J Infect Dis 1997; 176: 811–14.
6. Berglund O, et al. Combined treatment of symptomatic human immunodeficiency virus type 1 infection with native interferon-α and zidovudine. J Infect Dis 1991; 163: 710–15.
7. Bissuel F, et al. Tolerance of a triple combination therapy with zidovudine, didanosine and interferon-α in seven HIV-infected patients. AIDS 1995; 9: 1285.
8. Mildvan D, et al. Synergy, activity and tolerability of zidovudine and interferon-alpha in patients with symptomatic HIV-1 infection: ACTG 068. Antiviral Ther 1996; 1: 77–88.
9. Kovacs JA, et al. Combination therapy with didanosine and interferon-α in human immunodeficiency virus-infected patients: results of a phase I/II trial. J Infect Dis 1996; 173: 840–8.
10. Fischl MA, et al. Safety and antiviral activity of combination therapy with zidovudine, zalcitabine, and two doses of interferon-α2a in patients with HIV: AIDS Clinical Trials Group Study 197. J Acquir Immune Defic Syndr Hum Retrovirol 1997; 16: 247–53.
11. Marroni M, et al. Interferon-α is effective in the treatment of HIV-1-related, severe, zidovudine-resistant thrombocytopenia. Ann Intern Med 1994; 121: 423–9.

PROGRESSIVE MULTIFOCAL LEUCOENCEPHALOPATHY. Beneficial responses were reported in patients with HIV-associated progressive multifocal leucoencephalopathy following treatment with interferon alfa.[1]

1. Huang SS, et al. Survival prolongation in HIV-associated progressive multifocal leukoencephalopathy treated with alpha-interferon: an observational study. J Neurovirol 1998; 4: 324–32.

Inflammatory bowel disease. Interferon alfa is one of many drugs that have been tried in inflammatory bowel disease (p.1205). A study[1] found that clinical remission was achieved in 26 of 28 patients with ulcerative colitis after 6 to 12 months of treatment with interferon alfa-2a. Partial remission was reported in 2 of 5 patients with Crohn's disease[2] who received interferon alfa, but in another study in 12 patients[3] interferon alfa was of no benefit.

1. Sümer N, Palabiyikoğlu M. Induction of remission by interferon-α in patients with chronic active ulcerative colitis. Eur J Gastroenterol Hepatol 1995; 7: 597–602.
2. Davidsen B, et al. Tolerability of interferon alfa-2b, a possible new treatment of active Crohn's disease. Aliment Pharmacol Ther 1995; 9: 75–9.
3. Gasché C, et al. Prospective evaluation of interferon-α in treatment of chronic active Crohn's disease. Dig Dis Sci 1995; 40: 800–4.

Kaposi's sarcoma. The various treatments used for Kaposi's sarcoma are discussed on p.501. Interferon alfa has been used in AIDS-related Kaposi's sarcoma[1-9] and in patients with the classical, nonepidemic form.[10-13] There have been several small studies of interferon alfa in patients with immunodeficiency- or AIDS-related Kaposi's sarcoma.[1-3] Results have been mixed. A review[8] concluded that the best responses to interferon alfa were achieved in asymptomatic patients with relatively high CD4+ T lymphocyte counts (200 cells per μL or better) and no prior opportunistic infections. However, the adverse effects which occur at the doses required limit the tolerability of long-term administration.

Interferons have also been tried in AIDS-related Kaposi's sarcoma in combination with other drugs including antineoplastics (with disappointing results)[9] and zidovudine (complete or partial tumour response and/or evidence of antiviral effects in some patients).[4-7] Low doses of interferons in combination with zidovudine have been used for AIDS-associated Kaposi's sarcoma.[9]

1. de Wit R, et al. Clinical and virological effects of high-dose recombinant interferon-α in disseminated AIDS-related Kaposi's sarcoma. Lancet 1988; ii: 1214–17.
2. Lane HC, et al. Anti-retroviral effects of interferon-α in AIDS-associated Kaposi's sarcoma. Lancet 1988; ii: 1218–22.
3. Sulis E, et al. Interferon administered intralesionally in skin and oral cavity lesions in heterosexual drug addicted patients with AIDS-related Kaposi's sarcoma. Eur J Cancer Clin Oncol 1989; 25: 759–61.
4. Kovacs JA, et al. Combined zidovudine and interferon-α therapy in patients with Kaposi sarcoma and the acquired immunodeficiency syndrome (AIDS). Ann Intern Med 1989; 111: 280–7.
5. Brockmeyer NH, et al. Regression of Kaposi's sarcoma and improvement of performance status by a combined interferon β and zidovudine therapy in AIDS patients. J Invest Dermatol 1989; 92: 776.
6. Edlin BR, et al. Interferon-alpha plus zidovudine in HIV infection. Lancet 1989; i: 156.
7. Krown SE, et al. Interferon-α with zidovudine: safety, tolerance, and clinical and virologic effects in patients with Kaposi sarcoma associated with the acquired immunodeficiency syndrome (AIDS). Ann Intern Med 1990; 112: 812–21.
8. Krown SE. Interferon and other biologic agents for the treatment of Kaposi's sarcoma. Hematol Oncol Clin North Am 1991; 5: 311–22.
9. Northfelt DW. Treatment of Kaposi's sarcoma: current guidelines and future perspectives. Drugs 1994; 48: 569–82.
10. Killeen RB, Marsh RD. α-Interferon for Kaposi's sarcoma in HIV-negative, non-homosexual man. Lancet 1991; 337: 309–10.
11. Trattner A, et al. The therapeutic effect of intralesional interferon in classical Kaposi's sarcoma. Br J Dermatol 1993; 129: 590–3.
12. Shimizu S, et al. Classic (non-AIDS-related) Kaposi's sarcoma in a Japanese patient, successfully treated with alpha-2b-interferon. Br J Dermatol 1995; 133: 332–4.
13. Deichmann M, et al. Non-human immunodeficiency virus Kaposi's sarcoma can be effectively treated with low-dose interferon-α despite the persistence of herpesvirus-8. Br J Dermatol 1998; 139: 1052–4.

Malignant neoplasms. Many reports have been published on the effects of interferons on various neoplasms; most have involved interferon alfa.

Interferons have become established in the treatment of a few malignant disorders, notably hairy-cell leukaemia (but see p.486), Kaposi's sarcoma (see above), and chronic myeloid leukaemia,[1-6] where interferon alfa may be regarded as the treatment of choice (p.486). Alfa interferons may improve the duration of remission in multiple myeloma,[7-9] but not necessarily survival.[9,10] Combination therapy including interferons has also been used in indolent low-grade non-Hodgkin's lymphoma (p.487) and interferon alfa has been used alone to maintain remission. In renal cell carcinoma (p.495) response to interferon alfa in combination with interleukin-2 has been promising, but toxicity high;[11,12] interferon alfa alone produces very modest benefit.[13] Beneficial responses have also been reported in a number of other neoplasms including melanoma (p.499); carcinoid tumours[14] (p.483); myelodysplasia; cutaneous T cell lymphomas including mycosis fungoides (p.489); and in one reported case of meningioma.[15] Interferons have been administered locally as an adjunct to surgery for superficial bladder tumours and intralesionally in basal cell carcinoma[16,17] and also for keloid scars.[18,19] Combination of interferon alfa with fluorouracil has been tried in inoperable colorectal cancer but does not appear to be more beneficial than fluorouracil alone.[20] Interferon alfa in combination with zidovudine has produced encouraging results in adult T-cell leukaemia-lymphoma.[21]

1. The Italian Cooperative Study Group on Chronic Myeloid Leukemia. Interferon alfa-2a as compared with conventional chemotherapy for the treatment of chronic myeloid leukemia. *N Engl J Med* 1994; **330:** 820–5.
2. Schofield JR, *et al.* Low doses of interferon-α are as effective as higher doses in inducing remissions and prolonging survival in chronic myeloid leukemia. *Ann Intern Med* 1994; **121:** 736–44.
3. Allan NC, *et al.* UK Medical Research Council randomised, multicentre trial of interferon-αnl for chronic myeloid leukaemia: improved survival irrespective of cytogenetic response. *Lancet* 1995; **345:** 1392–7.
4. Kantarjian HM, *et al.* Prolonged survival in chronic myelogenous leukemia after cytogenetic response to interferon-α therapy. *Ann Intern Med* 1995; **122:** 254–61.
5. Talpaz M, Kantarjian H. Low-dose interferon-α in chronic myeloid leukemia. *Ann Intern Med* 1995; **122:** 728.
6. Mahon F-X, *et al.* Response to IFNα in myelogenous leukaemia. *Lancet* 1996; **347:** 57–8.
7. Mandelli F, *et al.* Maintenance treatment with recombinant interferon alfa-2b in patients with multiple myeloma responding to conventional induction chemotherapy. *N Engl J Med* 1990; **322:** 1430–4.
8. Ludwig H, *et al.* Interferon-alpha for induction and maintenance in multiple myeloma: results of two multicenter randomized trials and summary of other studies. *Ann Oncol* 1995; **6:** 467–76.
9. Nordic Myeloma Study Group. Interferon-α2b added to melphalan-prednisone for initial and maintenance therapy in multiple myeloma: a randomized, controlled trial. *Ann Intern Med* 1996; **124:** 212–22.
10. Österborg A, *et al.* Natural interferon-α in combination with melphalan/prednisone versus melphalan/prednisone in the treatment of multiple myeloma stages II and III: a randomized study from the myeloma group of central Sweden. *Blood* 1993; **81:** 1428–34.
11. Besana C, *et al.* Treatment of advanced renal cell cancer with sequential intravenous recombinant interleukin-2 and subcutaneous α-interferon. *Eur J Cancer* 1994; **30A** 1292–8.
12. Négrier S, *et al.* Intensive regimen of cytokines with interleukin-2 and interferon alfa-2b in selected patients with metastatic renal carcinoma. *J Immunother* 1995; **17:** 62–8.
13. Medical Research Council Renal Cancer Collaborators. Interferon-α and survival in metastatic renal carcinoma: early results of a randomised controlled study. *Lancet* 1999; **353:** 14–17.
14. Öberg K, *et al.* Treatment of malignant carcinoid tumors: a randomized controlled study of streptozocin plus 5-FU and human leukocyte interferon. *Eur J Cancer Clin Oncol* 1989; **25:** 1475–9.
15. Wöber-Bingöl Ç, *et al.* Interferon-alfa-2b for meningioma. *Lancet* 1995; **345:** 331.
16. Pizarro A, Fonseca E. Treatment of basal cell carcinoma with intralesional interferon alpha-2b: evaluation of efficacy with emphasis on tumours located on "H" zone on face. *Eur J Dermatol* 1994; **4:** 287–90.
17. LeGrice P, *et al.* Treatment of basal cell carcinoma with intralesional interferon alpha-2A. *N Z Med J* 1995; **108:** 206–7.
18. Granstein RD, *et al.* A controlled trial of intralesional recombinant interferon-γ in the treatment of keloidal scarring. *Arch Dermatol* 1990; **126:** 1295–1302.
19. Larrabee WF, *et al.* Intralesional interferon gamma treatment for keloids and hypertrophic scars. *Arch Otolaryngol Head Neck Surg* 1990; **116:** 1159–62.
20. Makower D, Wadler S. Interferons as biomodulators of fluoropyrimidines in the treatment of colorectal cancer. *Semin Oncol* 1999; **26:** 663–71.
21. Gill PS, *et al.* Treatment of adult T-cell leukemia-lymphoma with a combination of interferon alfa and zidovudine. *N Engl J Med* 1995; **332:** 1744–8.

Mycobacterial infections. For the use of interferon alfa in mycobacterial infections, see Interferon Gamma, p.634.

Skin disorders. For the use of interferon alfa in skin disorders associated with raised IgE concentrations, see Interferon Gamma, p.634.

Warts. Various interferons by various routes have been tried in the treatment of anogenital warts (condylomata acuminata) (p.1108).

Intralesional injection has been used to ensure relatively high concentrations of interferon in the wart but the occurrence of systemic adverse effects demonstrates that there is absorption from this site. Complete responses were reported[1] in 36% of patients receiving intralesional interferon alfa-2b compared with 17% receiving placebo, and a corresponding overall reduction in the affected area of 62.4% compared with 1.2%. However, follow-up was not sufficiently long to comment on relapse rates. Another study[2] found similar responses using interferons alfa-2b, alfa-n1, or beta in patients with refractory warts, with complete responses in 47% of patients receiving intralesional interferons compared with 22% receiving placebo. A study[3] evaluating three different doses of intralesional interferon beta given three times weekly for three weeks reported complete responses in 63% of lesions injected with 1 million units compared with 38% of lesions injected with 33 000 units. Good responses have also been reported in patients with both refractory and recurrent warts treated with intralesional interferon alfa-n3.[4] Relapses were delayed and fewer warts recurred in patients who had received interferon rather than placebo. Intralesional interferon alfa-2b given in combination with podophyllum was more effective that podophyllum alone,[5] although about 66% of patients in each group subsequently relapsed.

Topical application of interferon alfa has also been reported to be more effective than podophyllotoxin.[6,7]

Theoretically, *systemic* administration should have advantages in controlling subclinical infections and reducing relapses. However, responses to subcutaneous interferon alfa have generally been disappointing[8-10] although responses comparable with cauterisation and a reduction in relapse rates with either subcutaneous or intramuscular interferon alfa-2b have been ob-

tained.[11] Information on the use of systemic interferons as an adjunct to conventional therapy is scarce but a study in 97 patients[12] with recurrent warts found no difference in either response or relapse rates in patients receiving cryotherapy with subcutaneous interferon alfa or cryotherapy alone. A study comparing subcutaneous interferon alfa, beta, and gamma in combination with cryotherapy found no significant difference in response rate, although patients receiving interferon beta or gamma developed new warts at a lower frequency.[13]

1. Eron LJ, *et al.* Interferon therapy for condylomata acuminata. *N Engl J Med* 1986; **315:** 1059–64.
2. Reichman RC, *et al.* Treatment of condyloma acuminatum with three different interferons administered intralesionally: a double-blind, placebo-controlled trial. *Ann Intern Med* 1988; **108:** 675–9.
3. Monsonego J, *et al.* Randomised double-blind trial of recombinant interferon-beta for condyloma acuminatum. *Genitourin Med* 1996; **72:** 111–14.
4. Friedman-Kien AE, *et al.* Natural interferon alfa for treatment of condylomata acuminata. *JAMA* 1988; **259:** 533–8.
5. Douglas JM, *et al.* A randomized trial of combination therapy with intralesional interferon α2b and podophyllin versus podophyllin alone for the therapy of anogenital warts. *J Infect Dis* 1990; **162:** 52–9.
6. Syed TA, *et al.* Human interferon-alpha versus podophyllotoxin in cream for the treatment of genital warts in males: a placebo-controlled, double-blind, comparative study. *Dermatology* 1995; **191:** 129–32.
7. Syed TA, *et al.* Management of genital warts in women with human leukocyte interferon-α vs podophyllotoxin in cream: a placebo-controlled, double-blind, comparative study. *J Mol Med* 1995; **73:** 255–8.
8. Reichman RC, *et al.* Treatment of condyloma acuminatum with three different interferon-α preparations administered parenterally: a double-blind, placebo-controlled trial. *J Infect Dis* 1990; **162:** 1270–6.
9. Condylomata International Collaborative Study Group. Recurrent condylomata acuminata treated with recombinant interferon alfa-2a: a multicenter double-blind placebo-controlled clinical trial. *JAMA* 1991; **265:** 2684–7.
10. Condylomata International Collaborative Study Group. Recurrent condylomata acuminata treated with recombinant interferon alpha-2a: a multicenter double-blind placebo-controlled clinical trial. *Acta Derm Venereol (Stockh)* 1993; **73:** 223–6.
11. Panici PB, *et al.* Randomized clinical trial comparing systemic interferon with diathermocoagulation in primary multiple and widespread anogenital condyloma. *Obstet Gynecol* 1989; **74:** 393–7.
12. Eron LJ, *et al.* Recurrence of condylomata acuminata following cryotherapy is not prevented by systemically administered interferon. *Genitourin Med* 1993; **69:** 91–3.
13. Bonnez W, *et al.* A randomized, double-blind, placebo-controlled trial of systemically administered interferon-α, -β, or -γ in combination with cryotherapy for the treatment of condyloma acuminatum. *J Infect Dis* 1995; **171:** 1081–9.

Preparations

Proprietary Preparations (details are given in Part 3)

Aust.: Berofor; Intron A; Roferon-A; Wellferon; **Austral.:** Intron A; Roferon-A; Wellferon; **Belg.:** Intron A; Roferon-A; **Braz.:** Inter IF; Intron A; Roferon-A; Wellferon; **Canad.:** Infergen; Intron A; Roferon-A; Wellferon; **Denm.:** Introna; Roceron-A; **Fin.:** Finnferon-Alpha; Introna; Roferon-A; Wellferon; **Fr.:** Introna; Laroferon; Roferon-A; Viraferon; **Ger.:** Cellferon†; Inferax; Intron A; Roferon-A; **Hong Kong:** Intron A; Roferon-A; Wellferon; **Irl.:** Introna; Roferon-A; ViraferonPeg; **Israel:** Intron A; Roferon-A; Wellferon; **Ital.:** Alfaferone; Alfater; Biaferone; Cilferon-A; Haimaferone; Humoferon; Infergen; Intron A; Isiferone; Roferon-A; Wellferon; **Jpn:** OIF; **Mex.:** Alferon; Altemol; Intron A; Roferon-A; Urifron; Viraferon; Wellferon; **Neth.:** Infergen; Intron A; Roferon-A; **Norw.:** Introna; Roceron; **NZ:** Intron A; Roferon-A; Wellferon; **Port.:** Intron A; Roferon-A; **S.Afr.:** Intron A; Roferon-A; **Singapore:** Intron A; Roferon-A; Wellferon; **Spain:** Intron A; Roferon-A; Viraferon†; Wellferon; **Swed.:** Interferon Alfanative; Introna; Roferon-A; Wellferon†; **Switz.:** Intron A; Roferon-A; Wellferon; **Thai.:** Bioferon; Introna; Roferon-A; Wellferon; **UK:** Introna; PegIntron; Roferon-A; Viraferon; ViraferonPeg; Wellferon†; **USA:** Alferon N; Infergen; Intron A; PegIntron; Roferon-A; Wellferon.

Multi-ingredient: **Austral.:** Rebetron; **Canad.:** Rebetron; **Switz.:** Intron A/Rebetol; **USA:** Rebetron.

Interferon Beta (11420-I)

Interferon Beta *(BAN, rINN).*

IFN-β; Interferon-β; SH-Y-579A (interferon beta-1b).

CAS — 74899-71-1 *(interferon beta);* 145258-61-3 *(interferon beta-1a);* 145155-23-3 *(interferon beta-1b);* 90598-63-3 *(interferon beta-1b).*

ATC — L03AB02 *(natural);* L03AB07 *(1A);* L03AB08 *(1B).*

NOTE. Interferon beta was previously known as fibroblast interferon.

Interferon beta-1a and Interferon beta-1b are both USAN.

Interferon beta may be derived from fibroblasts as well as through recombinant DNA technology. Sub-species of the human beta gene produce interferon beta with protein variants designated by a number (as in interferon beta-1). Interferon beta-1 is further qualified by a letter to indicate the amino-acid sequences at positions 1 and 17, and to indicate whether or not glycosylation is present. Interferon beta-1a has methionine at position 1 and cysteine at 17 and is glycosylated at position 80. Interferon beta-1b has serine at position 17 and is not glycosylated.

The name may be further elaborated on the label by approved sets of initials in parentheses to indicate the method of production: (rch) indicates production from genetically engineered

Chinese hamster ovary cells; (rbe) indicates production from bacteria (*Escherichia coli*) genetically modified by recombinant DNA technology.

Adverse Effects

As for interferons in general (see Interferon Alfa, p.628).

Severe local reactions at injection sites, including tissue necrosis, have been reported. Menstrual irregularities have been associated with interferon beta administration. Syncope and muscle hypotonia have been reported, usually early in a course of treatment.

Auto-immune disorders. Subacute cutaneous lupus erythematosus has been reported in a patient following administration of interferon beta.[1]

1. Nousari HC, *et al.* Subacute cutaneous lupus erythematosus associated with interferon beta-1a. *Lancet* 1998; **352:** 1825–6.

Effects on the cardiovascular system. Severe Raynaud's syndrome developed in a patient during treatment with interferon beta.[1] Symptoms subsided once interferon beta was stopped.

1. Linden D. Severe Raynaud's phenomenon associated with interferon-β treatment for multiple sclerosis. *Lancet* 1998; **352:** 878–9.

Effects on hearing. For a report of sensorineural hearing loss in patients receiving interferon beta, see Interferon Alfa, p.628.

Effects on the skin. For a report of severe necrotising cutaneous lesions at injection sites in a patient receiving interferon beta, see Interferon Alfa, p.629. See also Auto-immune Disorders, above for a report of cutaneous lupus erythematosus associated with interferon beta.

Precautions

As for interferons in general (see Interferon Alfa, p.629).

Interferon beta in high doses is fetotoxic and abortifacient in *primates* and should be avoided during pregnancy.

Interactions

As for interferons in general (see Interferon Alfa, p.629).

Antiviral Action

As for interferons in general (see Interferon Alfa, p.629).

Pharmacokinetics

Interferons are not absorbed from the gastrointestinal tract. About 50% of a subcutaneous or intramuscular dose of interferon beta is absorbed. For some formulations of interferon beta-1a, bioavailability and area under the plasma concentration-time curves are equivalent for subcutaneous and intramuscular administration, but for others, intramuscular administration produces higher values than subcutaneous administration. Peak serum concentrations of interferon beta-1a have been reported to be reached 3 hours after subcutaneous injection and between 5 and 15 hours after intramuscular injection, and those for beta-1b have been reported to be reached 1 to 8 hours after subcutaneous injection. The elimination half-life for interferon beta-1a is about 10 hours.

Uses and Administration

Interferon beta has antiviral and immunomodulating activities. It is mainly used in the management of multiple sclerosis, although its mode of action is unclear.

Interferon beta-1a is given in relapsing-remitting multiple sclerosis in a dose dependent upon the formulation used:

- *Avonex* (Biogen, UK) is given in a dose of 6 million units (30 μg) once weekly by intramuscular injection.

- *Rebif* (Serono, UK) is given in a dose, escalating over 4 weeks, to 12 million units (44 μg) three times weekly by subcutaneous injection, or to 6 million units (22 μg) three times weekly by subcutaneous injection in patients unable to tolerate the higher dose.

Interferon beta-1b is given in both relapsing-remitting and in secondary progressive multiple sclerosis in a dose of 8 million units (250 μg) on alternate days by subcutaneous injection.

◊ Reviews.
1. Goodkin DE. Interferon beta-1b. *Lancet* 1994; **344:** 1057–60.

Guillain-Barré syndrome. Rapid improvement in motor function was reported during administration of interferon beta-1a in a patient with Guillain-Barré syndrome associated with *Campylobacter jejuni* infection.[1] However, the relative contributions of interferon therapy and a course of plasma exchange which immediately preceded it could not be assessed.[2]

1. Créange A, *et al.* Treatment of Guillain-Barré syndrome with interferon-β. *Lancet* 1998; **352:** 368.
2. Sawaya RA. Interferon beta for Guillain-Barré syndrome. *Lancet* 1998; **352:** 1550–1.

Hepatitis. For mention of the use of interferon beta in chronic hepatitis, see Interferon Alfa, p.630.

Herpes simplex infections. For a report of the use of interferon beta in small numbers of patients for the treatment of labial and genital herpes, see Interferon Alfa, p.631.

Multiple sclerosis. Multiple sclerosis (MS) is characterised by patches of demyelination that can be scattered throughout the white matter of the CNS, but are usually localised in the brain stem, periventricular areas, the optic nerve, and the cervical spinal cord. The cause is unknown but may have an immunological basis. Symptoms may vary according to the areas affected but typically include weakness, paraesthesias, vision loss, incoordination, and bladder dysfunction. Most patients improve to some degree after the initial attack but the course and severity of the disease are unpredictable. The disease is classified according to the clinical course. In many patients the disease follows a relapsing-remitting course in which there are recurrent exacerbations followed by clinical improvement and relatively long periods of remission. The patients may subsequently develop progressive neurological deterioration, categorised as secondary progressive disease. About 10% of patients have gradual continuous deterioration, classified as primary progressive disease. In a few patients the disease is described as progressive relapsing when there is little or no improvement after each exacerbation and disability slowly increases.

The evaluation of therapy for any disease such as MS that has spontaneous remissions is difficult[1-8] and, until relatively recently, there has been little convincing evidence that any treatment affects the outcome of the disease. Despite the increasing use of disease-modifying treatment, **symptomatic treatment** aimed at the management of spasticity, pain, fatigue, and bladder dysfunction remains important. Baclofen, dantrolene, and diazepam are the usual drugs given for spasticity (see p.1322). There has also been a suggestion that the synthetic cannabinoid nabilone may improve spasticity.[9] Patients with MS can suffer from a number of different types of pain, including pain from spasticity, and therapy must be individualised for each specific pain syndrome[10] (see p.2). Pain, spasms, and spasticity have responded to gabapentin in preliminary studies.[11-14] Paraesthesia and dysaesthesia, which can be common, may respond to tricyclic antidepressants or antiepileptics. Amantadine may alleviate fatigue associated with MS.[15,16] Treatment of bladder dysfunction may include an alpha blocker such as phenoxybenzamine and appropriate parasympathomimetic or antimuscarinic therapy to control bladder contractions[1] (see Urinary Incontinence and Retention, p.459). Fampridine has been reported to produce improvement in walking, dexterity, and vision, possibly as a result of its potassium-channel blocking activity.[17-20] 3,4-Diaminopyridine has also been reported to produce beneficial symptomatic responses.[21]

A wide range of drugs with immunological actions has been tried in the **treatment** of MS itself with the aim of improving recovery from acute attacks, preventing or decreasing the number of relapses, and halting the progressive stage of the disease.

Corticosteroids are used for their immunomodulatory and anti-inflammatory effects in acute relapses. Corticosteroid therapy reduces the duration of the relapse and accelerates recovery, but it is not known whether it alters the course of the disease in the long term.[4,22] Methylprednisolone has superseded corticotropin and prednisolone as the drug of choice. Methylprednisolone is usually given intravenously in high doses (typically 1 g daily) for 3 to 5 days, sometimes followed by a tapering dose of oral prednisolone. Doses of up to 2 g daily have been tried.[23] In patients with acute optic neuritis (frequently the first manifestation of multiple sclerosis), methylprednisolone delayed the onset of other symptoms of multiple sclerosis[24] although the effect was not sustained beyond 2 years.[25] Beneficial responses have also been reported with oral methylprednisolone at doses including 500 mg once daily for 5 days followed by a tapering dose over 10 days[26] and 48 mg once daily for 7 days followed by a tapering dose over 14 days.[27]

In patients with primary progressive disease, the benefits of short-course methylprednisolone lasted no longer than 3 months[28] although in patients with secondary progressive disease, a preliminary study has suggested that progression may be delayed by intermittent high-dose methylprednisolone therapy.[29]

Interferon beta has become established for treatment of relapsing-remitting disease in selected patients, and is also used in secondary progressive disease. Many early studies using inter-

ferons were conducted before the immunomodulating effects of interferons were understood, but they did demonstrate that natural interferon beta could reduce exacerbations by inhibiting interferon gamma which in itself appeared to act as a disease activator. Natural interferon alfa alone was found to produce little or no benefit.[30] Subsequent studies in patients with relapsing-remitting disease have used recombinant interferon beta and patients treated with interferon *beta-1b* have obtained a reduction in the rate and severity of exacerbations;[31,32] there was also evidence from magnetic resonance imaging[33] of reduced disease activity and burden. Encouraging results have also been obtained in patients with secondary progressive disease.[34] Similar results in relapsing-remitting disease have been obtained with interferon *beta-1a*.[35-37] There may be some benefit from interferon beta in patients presenting with a first demyelinating event, or other manifestation of early disease, in terms of subsequent development of definitive disease.[38,39] However, the effect of interferon beta on the progression of disability remains to be determined. Concern has been expressed over the detection of neutralising antibodies against interferon in up to 36% of patients.[40,41]

Results of studies[42-44] with *glatiramer* have shown that it can reduce the number of relapses and may produce some improvements in neurological disability. These benefits are produced in a different way from those gained with interferon beta-1b leading to expectations of a study of treatment with both drugs.

Guidelines[45] have been produced by the Association of British Neurologists for the use of interferon beta and of glatiramer in selected patients.

Intermittent intravenous *normal immunoglobulins* might also be able to reduce the frequency of exacerbations and slow disease progression without producing troublesome adverse effects.[46,47]

Although some studies have shown modest benefits with *immunosuppressants*, the general conclusions of large controlled studies have tended to be that any slight benefits of existing therapies with immunosuppressants such as azathioprine, ciclosporin, or cyclophosphamide are outweighed by the toxicity of the doses required to have an effect.[48-54] However, it has been pointed out that in terms of relapse reduction azathioprine appeared to be as effective as newer treatments such as interferon beta.[55] Studies with cladribine suggested that it might provide some benefit at well-tolerated doses,[56,57] and low-dose methotrexate might also slow progression of chronic disease and provide a relatively non-toxic treatment option.[58] Mitozantrone [mitoxantrone] has also been studied[59-61] but its use may be limited by dose-related cardiotoxicity. Benefit has been reported with *roquinimex* (but see p.568).

Other immunological approaches evaluated have included the use of monoclonal antibodies such as CD4 antibodies, altered peptide ligands from myelin basic protein, and T-cell vaccination.[62] Combined total lymphoid irradiation with low-dose corticosteroid therapy has also been investigated and may slow progression of disease.[63]

A review of the relationship between *dietary fat* and MS concluded that the role of lipids remained to be proven.[64] Some studies found a reduction of severity and duration of relapse in patients taking linoleic acid supplements (as sunflower oil)[65] while another reported benefit in patients who limited their intake of dietary saturated fatty acids and supplemented their diet with polyunsaturated fatty acids.[66] Despite a lack of firm evidence many patients with MS practice dietary modification and take supplements of omega-6 group polyunsaturated acids, sunflower oil, evening primrose oil, fish oils, and omega-3 fatty acids.[64]

The use of *hyperbaric oxygen* therapy in MS was a matter of debate for many years. Some workers reported benefit, especially in bladder and bowel function or in cerebellar function.[67] Others were unable to substantiate any useful long-term effect[68] and a review of the current therapeutic options available in MS concluded that there was no convincing evidence that hyperbaric oxygen therapy was successful.[69]

1. Ebers GC. Treatment of multiple sclerosis. *Lancet* 1994; **343:** 275–9.
2. van Oosten BW, *et al.* Multiple sclerosis therapy: a practical guide. *Drugs* 1995; **49:** 200–12.
3. Weinstock-Guttman B, Cohen JA. Newer versus older treatments for relapsing-remitting multiple sclerosis. *Drug Safety* 1996; **14:** 121–30.
4. Rudick RA, *et al.* Management of multiple sclerosis. *N Engl J Med* 1997; **337:** 1604–11.
5. Weinstock-Guttman B, Jacobs LD. What is new in the treatment of multiple sclerosis? *Drugs* 2000; **59:** 401–10.
6. Pender MP. Multiple sclerosis. *Med J Aust* 2000; **172:** 556–62.
7. Polman CH, Vitdehaag BMJ. Drug treatment of multiple sclerosis. *BMJ* 2000; **321:** 490–4.
8. Noseworthy JH, *et al.* Multiple sclerosis. *N Engl J Med* 2000; **343:** 938–52.
9. Martyn CN, *et al.* Nabilone in the treatment of multiple sclerosis. *Lancet* 1995; **345:** 579.
10. Moulin DE. Pain syndromes in multiple sclerosis. *Neurology* 1988; **38:** 1830–4.
11. Mueller ME, *et al.* Gabapentin for relief of upper motor neuron symptoms in multiple sclerosis. *Arch Phys Med Rehabil* 1997; **78:** 521–4.
12. Samkoff LM, *et al.* Amelioration of refractory dysesthetic limb pain in multiple sclerosis by gabapentin. *Neurology* 1997; **49:** 304–5.
13. Solaro C, *et al.* An open-label trial of gabapentin treatment of paroxysmal symptoms in multiple sclerosis patients. *Neurology* 1998; **51:** 609–11.

14. Dunevsky A, Perel AB. Gabapentin for relief of spasticity associated with multiple sclerosis. *Am J Phys Med Rehabil* 1998; **77:** 451–4.
15. Kemp BA, Gora ML. Amantadine and fatigue of multiple sclerosis. *Ann Pharmacother* 1993; **27:** 893–5.
16. Krupp LB, *et al.* Fatigue therapy in multiple sclerosis: results of a double-blind, randomised, parallel trial of amantadine, pemoline, and placebo. *Neurology* 1995; **45:** 1956–61.
17. van Diemen HAM, *et al.* The effect of 4-aminopyridine on clinical signs in multiple sclerosis: a randomized, placebo-controlled, double-blind, cross-over study. *Ann Neurol* 1992; **32:** 123–30.
18. Van Diemen HAM, *et al.* 4-Aminopyridine in patients with multiple sclerosis: dosage and serum level related to efficacy and safety. *Clin Neuropharmacol* 1993; **16:** 195–204.
19. Bever CT, *et al.* The effects of 4-aminopyridine in multiple sclerosis patients: results of a randomised, placebo-controlled, double-blind, concentration-controlled, crossover trial. *Neurology* 1994; **44:** 1054–9.
20. Schwid SR, *et al.* Quantitative assessment of sustained-release 4-aminopyridine for symptomatic treatment of multiple sclerosis. *Neurology* 1997; **48:** 817–21.
21. Bever CT, *et al.* Treatment with oral 3,4 diaminopyridine improves leg strength in multiple sclerosis patients: results of a randomized, double-blind, placebo-controlled, crossover trial. *Neurology* 1996; **47:** 1457–62.
22. Filippini G, *et al.* Corticosteroids or ACTH for acute exacerbations in multiple sclerosis (updated 24 August 2001). Available in The Cochrane Library; Issue 4. Oxford: Update Software; 2001.
23. Oliveri RL, *et al.* Randomized trial comparing two different high doses of methylprednisolone in MS: a clinical and MRI study. *Neurology* 1998; **50:** 1833–6.
24. Beck RW, *et al.* The effect of corticosteroids for acute optic neuritis on the subsequent development of multiple sclerosis. *N Engl J Med* 1993; **329:** 1764–9.
25. Beck RW, *et al.* The optic neuritis treatment trial: three-year follow-up results. *Arch Ophthalmol* 1995; **113:** 136–7.
26. Sellebjerg F, *et al.* Double-blind, randomized, placebo-controlled study of oral, high-dose methylprednisolone in attacks of MS. *Neurology* 1998; **51:** 529–34.
27. Barnes D, *et al.* Randomised trial of oral and intravenous methylprednisolone in acute relapses of multiple sclerosis. *Lancet* 1997; **349:** 902–6.
28. Cazzato G, *et al.* Double-blind, placebo-controlled, randomized, crossover trial of high-dose methylprednisolone in patients with chronic progressive form of multiple sclerosis. *Eur Neurol* 1995; **35:** 193–8.
29. Goodkin DE, *et al.* A phase II study of IV methylprednisolone in secondary-progressive multiple sclerosis. *Neurology* 1998; **51:** 239–45.
30. Panitch HS. Interferons in multiple sclerosis: a review of the evidence. *Drugs* 1992; **44:** 946–62.
31. The IFNB Multiple Sclerosis Study Group. Interferon beta-1b is effective in relapsing-remitting multiple sclerosis I: clinical results of a multicenter, randomized, double-blind, placebo-controlled trial. *Neurology* 1993; **43:** 655–61.
32. The IFNB Multiple Sclerosis Study Group and the University of British Columbia MS/MRI Analysis Group. Interferon beta-1b in the treatment of multiple sclerosis: final outcome of the randomised controlled trial. *Neurology* 1995; **45:** 1277–85.
33. Paty DW. Interferon beta-1b is effective in relapsing-remitting multiple sclerosis II: MRI analysis results of a multicenter, randomized, double-blind, placebo-controlled trial. *Neurology* 1993; **43:** 662–7.
34. European Study Group on Interferon β-1b in Secondary Progressive MS. Placebo-controlled multicentre randomised trial of interferon β-1b in secondary progressive multiple sclerosis. *Lancet* 1998; **352:** 1491–7.
35. Jacobs LD, *et al.* Intramuscular interferon beta-1a for disease progression in relapsing multiple sclerosis. *Ann Neurol* 1996; **39:** 285–94.
36. Rudick RA, *et al.* Impact of interferon beta-1a on neurologic disability in relapsing multiple sclerosis. *Neurology* 1997; **49:** 358–63.
37. PRISMS Study Group. Randomised double-blind placebo-controlled study of interferon β-1a in relapsing/remitting multiple sclerosis. *Lancet* 1998; **352:** 1498–1504.
38. Jacobs LD, *et al.* Intramuscular interferon beta-1a therapy initiated during a first demyelinating event in multiple sclerosis. *N Engl J Med* 2000; **343:** 898–904.
39. Comi G, *et al.* Effect of early interferon treatment on conversion to definite multiple sclerosis: a randomised study. *Lancet* 2001; **357:** 1576–82.
40. Paty DW, *et al.* Guidelines for physicians with patients on IFNB-1b: the use of an assay for neutralizing antibodies (NAB). *Neurology* 1996; **47:** 865–6.
41. IFNB Multiple Sclerosis Study Group, University of British Columbia MS/MRI Analysis Group. Neutralizing antibodies during treatment of multiple sclerosis with interferon beta-1b: experience during the first three years. *Neurology* 1996; **47:** 889–94.
42. Johnson KP, *et al.* Copolymer 1 reduces relapse rate and improves disability in relapsing-remitting multiple sclerosis: results of a phase III multicenter, double-blind, placebo-controlled trial. *Neurology* 1995; **45:** 1268–76.
43. Johnson KP, *et al.* Extended use of glatiramer acetate (Copaxone) is well tolerated and maintains its clinical effect of multiple sclerosis relapse rate and degree of disability. *Neurology* 1998; **50:** 701–8.
44. Comi G, *et al.* European/Canadian multicenter, double-blind, randomized, placebo-controlled study of the effects of glatiramer acetate on magnetic resonance imaging-measured disease activity and burden in patients with relapsing multiple sclerosis. *Ann Neurol* 2001; **49:** 290–7.
45. Association of British Neurologists. Guidelines for the use of beta interferons and glatiramer acetate in multiple sclerosis. Available at: http://www.theabn.org/downloads/msdoc.pdf (accessed 16/10/01).
46. Achiron A, *et al.* Intravenous immunoglobulin treatment in multiple sclerosis. *Isr J Med Sci* 1995; **31:** 7–9.
47. Fazekas F, *et al.* Randomised placebo-controlled trial of monthly intravenous immunoglobulin therapy in relapsing-remitting multiple sclerosis. *Lancet* 1997; **349:** 589–93.
48. British and Dutch Multiple Sclerosis Azathioprine Trial Group. Double-masked trial of azathioprine in multiple sclerosis. *Lancet* 1988; **ii:** 179–83.
49. Ellison GW, *et al.* A placebo-controlled, randomized, double-masked, variable dosage, clinical trial of azathioprine with and without methylprednisolone in multiple sclerosis. *Neurology* 1989; **39:** 1018–26.

The symbol † denotes a preparation no longer actively marketed

50. Rudge P, *et al.* Randomised double blind controlled trial of cyclosporin in multiple sclerosis. *J Neurol Neurosurg Psychiatry* 1989; **52:** 559–65.
51. The Multiple Sclerosis Study Group. Efficacy and toxicity of cyclosporine in chronic progressive multiple sclerosis: a randomized, double-blinded, placebo-controlled clinical trial. *Ann Neurol* 1990; **27:** 591–605.
52. The Canadian Cooperative Multiple Sclerosis Study Group. The Canadian cooperative trial of cyclophosphamide and plasma exchange in progressive multiple sclerosis. *Lancet* 1991; **337:** 441–6.
53. Currier RD, *et al.* Cyclophosphamide and plasma exchange in multiple sclerosis. *Lancet* 1991; **337:** 1034.
54. Yudkin PL, *et al.* Overview of azathioprine treatment in multiple sclerosis. *Lancet* 1991; **338:** 1051–5.
55. Palace J, Rothwell P. New treatments and azathioprine in multiple sclerosis. *Lancet* 1997; **350:** 261.
56. Sipe JC, *et al.* Cladribine in treatment of chronic progressive multiple sclerosis. *Lancet* 1994; **344:** 9–13.
57. Romine JS, *et al.* A double-blind, placebo-controlled, randomized trial of cladribine in relapsing-remitting multiple sclerosis. *Proc Assoc Am Physicians* 1999; **111:** 35–44.
58. Goodkin DE, *et al.* Low-dose (7.5 mg) oral methotrexate reduces the rate of progression in chronic progressive multiple sclerosis. *Ann Neurol* 1995; **37:** 30–40.
59. Gonsette RE. Mitoxantrone immunotherapy in multiple sclerosis. *Multiple Sclerosis* 1996; **1:** 329–32.
60. Edan G, *et al.* Therapeutic effect of mitoxantrone combined with methylprednisolone in multiple sclerosis: a randomised multicentre study of active disease using MRI and clinical criteria. *J Neurol Neurosurg Psychiatry* 1997; **62:** 112–18.
61. Millefiorini E, *et al.* Randomized placebo-controlled trial of mitoxantrone in relapsing-remitting multiple sclerosis: 24-month clinical and MRI outcome. *J Neurol* 1997; **244:** 153–9.
62. Medaer R, *et al.* Depletion of myelin-basic-protein autoreactive T cells by T-cell vaccination: pilot trial in multiple sclerosis. *Lancet* 1995; **346:** 807–8.
63. Cook SD, *et al.* Combination total lymphoid irradiation and low-dose corticosteroid therapy for progressive multiple sclerosis. *Acta Neurol Scand* 1995; **91:** 22–7.
64. Anonymous. Lipids and multiple sclerosis. *Lancet* 1990; **336:** 25–6.
65. Millar JHD, *et al.* Double-blind trial of linoleate supplementation of the diet in multiple sclerosis. *BMJ* 1973; **1:** 765–8.
66. Swank RL, Dugan BB. Effect of low saturated fat diet in early and late cases of multiple sclerosis. *Lancet* 1990; **336:** 37–9.
67. James PB, Webster CJ. Long-term results of hyperbaric oxygen therapy in multiple sclerosis. *Lancet* 1989; **ii:** 327.
68. Kindwall EP, *et al.* Treatment of multiple sclerosis with hyperbaric oxygen: results of a national registry. *Arch Neurol* 1991; **48:** 195–9.
69. Webb HE. Multiple sclerosis: therapeutic pessimism. *BMJ* 1992; **304:** 1260–1.

Rheumatoid arthritis. Preliminary studies suggest that interferon beta may have a beneficial effect on rheumatoid arthritis[1] the conventional management of which is described on p.9.

1. Tak PP, *et al.* The effects of interferon beta treatment on arthritis. *Rheumatology* 1999; **38:** 362–9.

Warts. For the use of interferon beta in the management of warts, see Interferon Alfa, p.632.

Preparations

Proprietary Preparations (details are given in Part 3)

Aust.: Avonex; Betaferon; Rebif; *Austral.:* Avonex; Betaferon; Rebif; *Belg.:* Betaferon; Rebif; *Braz.:* Betaferon; Frone; *Canad.:* Avonex; Betaseron; Rebif; *Denm.:* Avonex; Betaferon; Rebif; *Fin.:* Avonex; Betaferon; Rebif; *Fr.:* Avonex; Betaferon; Rebif; *Ger.:* Avonex; Betaferon; Fiblaferon; Rebif; *Hong Kong:* Rebif; *Irl.:* Avonex; Betaferon; Rebif; *Israel:* Avonex; Betaferon; Rebif; *Ital.:* Avonex; Betaferon; Betantrone†; Betron R; Frone†; Naferon; Rebif; Serobif; *Jpn:* Feron; *Mex.:* Betaferon; Rebif; *Neth.:* Avonex; Betaferon; Rebif; *Norw.:* Avonex; Betaferon; Rebif; *NZ:* Avonex; Betaferon; Rebif; *Port.:* Avonex; Betaferon; Rebif; *S.Afr.:* Betaferon; *Singapore:* Betaferon; Rebif; *Spain:* Avonex; Betaferon; Frone; Rebif; *Swed.:* Avonex; Betaferon; Rebif; *Switz.:* Avonex; Betaferon; Rebif; *Thai.:* Rebif; *UK:* Avonex; Betaferon; Rebif; *USA:* Avonex; Betaseron.

Interferon Gamma (1683-t)

Interferon Gamma (BAN, rINN).

IFN-γ; Interferon-γ.

CAS — 98059-18-8 (interferon gamma-1a); 98059-61-1 (interferon gamma-1b).

ATC — L03AB03.

NOTE. Interferon gamma was previously known as immune interferon.

Interferon gamma-1b is *USAN* and was previously known as interferon gamma-2a.

Pharmacopoeias. Eur. (see p.vi) includes Interferon Gamma-1b Concentrated Solution.

Interferon gamma may be derived from immunologically stimulated T-lymphocytes (hence its former name of immune interferon) as well as through recombinant DNA technology. Similarly to interferon alfa, protein variants of interferon gamma are designated by a number and further qualified by a letter to indicate the amino-acid sequences at terminal positions 1 and 139. Interferon gamma-1a has at position 1 hydrogen, cysteine, tyrosine, and cysteine and at position 139 arginine, alanine, serine, glutamine, and a hydroxyl group. Interferon gamma-1b, formerly known as interferon gamma-2a, has at position 1 hydrogen and methionine and at position 139 a hydroxyl group. Interferon gamma derived through recombinant DNA technology is labelled (rbe).

Pharmacopoeial description

Ph. Eur.: Interferon Gamma-1b Concentrated Solution is a solution of the N-terminal methionyl form of interferon gamma. It is produced by a method based on recombinant DNA technology using bacteria as host cells. It is a clear, colourless or slightly yellowish liquid. The pH of the solution is 4.5 to 5.5. Store in airtight containers at a temperature of −70°. Protect from light.

Adverse Effects

As for interferons in general (see Interferon Alfa, p.628)

Precautions

As for interferons in general (see Interferon Alfa, p.629).

Interactions

As for interferons in general (see Interferon Alfa, p.629).

Antiviral Action

Interferons are produced by virus-infected cells and confer protection on uninfected cells of the same species. They affect many cell functions demonstrating, in addition to their antiviral activity, antiproliferative and immunomodulating properties. Interferon gamma in particular is a potent macrophage-stimulating factor.

Pharmacokinetics

Interferons are not absorbed from the gastrointestinal tract. Peak plasma concentrations of interferon gamma-1b occur about 4 hours after intramuscular injection and about 7 hours after subcutaneous injection. Half-lives of 38 minutes (intravenous administration), 2.9 hours (intramuscular administration), and 5.9 hours (subcutaneous administration) have been reported.

Uses and Administration

Interferon gamma has antiviral and immunomodulating effects. Interferon gamma-1b is used for its action as a macrophage-stimulating factor as an adjunct to antimicrobial therapy in chronic granulomatous disease. It is also used to delay time to disease progression in patients with severe malignant osteopetrosis.

Interferon gamma-1b is given in a dose of 50 μg per m² body-surface (1 million units per m²) three times weekly by subcutaneous injection. Patients with a body surface area less than 0.5 m² should receive 1.5 μg per kg body-weight three times weekly. Interferon gamma-n1 has also been used.

◊ Reviews.
1. Todd PA, Goa KL. Interferon gamma-1b: a review of its pharmacology and therapeutic potential in chronic granulomatous disease. *Drugs* 1992; **43:** 111–22.

Bacterial infections. In addition to its use to control infections in chronic granulomatous disease, interferon gamma was used with some success as an adjunct to antibacterials in a patient with Whipple's disease[1] but was of no benefit in a study in burn-related infections.[2] For the conventional management of these infections, see Whipple's Disease, p.147 and Skin Infections, p.140.

1. Schneider T, *et al.* Treatment of refractory Whipple disease with interferon-γ. *Ann Intern Med* 1998; **129:** 875–7.
2. Wasserman D, *et al.* Interferon-γ in the prevention of severe burn-related infections: a European phase III multicenter trial. *Crit Care Med* 1998; **26:** 434–9.

Chronic granulomatous disease. Interferon gamma reduces the incidence of infections in patients with chronic granulomatous disease[1-3] and is used as an adjunct to antimicrobial therapy in this condition.

1. The International Chronic Granulomatous Disease Cooperative Study Group. A controlled trial of interferon gamma to prevent infection in chronic granulomatous disease. *N Engl J Med* 1991; **324:** 509–16.
2. Bolinger AM, Taeubel MA. Recombinant interferon gamma for treatment of chronic granulomatous disease and other disorders. *Clin Pharm* 1992; **11:** 834–50.
3. Todd PA, Goa KL. Interferon gamma-1b: a review of its pharmacology and therapeutic potential in chronic granulomatous disease. *Drugs* 1992; **43:** 111–22.

Cryptogenic fibrosing alveolitis. In a preliminary study[1] in patients with cryptogenic fibrosing alveolitis who had not responded to treatment with corticosteroids or to other immunosuppressive therapy, lung capacity increased in 9 patients treated with interferon gamma-1b in combination with prednisolone for 12 months, but deteriorated in 9 who were

treated with prednisolone alone for the same period. The study was, however, criticised for its methodology and the statistical significance of its findings questioned.[2]

1. Ziesche R, *et al.* A preliminary study of long-term treatment with interferon gamma-1b and low-dose prednisolone in patients with idiopathic pulmonary fibrosis. *N Engl J Med* 1999; **341:** 1264–9.
2. King TE. Interferon gamma-1b for the treatment of idiopathic pulmonary fibrosis. *N Engl J Med* 2000; **342:** 974–5.

Juvenile osteopetrosis. Interferon gamma has been tried in the treatment of juvenile osteopetrosis (p.1053). A study[1] in 14 patients found that interferon gamma-1b increased bone resorption. In 11 who received this treatment for 18 months there was stabilisation or improvement in clinical condition and a reduction in the frequency of serious infection.

1. Key LL, *et al.* Long-term treatment of osteopetrosis with recombinant human interferon gamma. *N Engl J Med* 1995; **332:** 1594–9.

Leishmaniasis. Interferon gamma has been tried both systemically and locally as an adjunct to standard treatment of leishmaniasis (p.584) with encouraging results. A review[1] of the use of interferon gamma in non-viral infections concluded that interferon gamma was effective when combined with antimony compounds for treatment failures in visceral leishmaniasis and could enhance the response to initial therapy in untreated patients. However, the response to adjunctive interferon gamma was limited in patients with a high degree of resistance to antimony compounds.[2] For cutaneous infections, intralesional interferon gamma has been shown to be effective[3] but less so than intralesional antimony compounds.[4] Subcutaneous administration of interferon gamma with antimony given intravenously was no more effective than antimony alone when administered as a short course over 10 days.[5] However, encouraging responses have been reported in patients who have failed to respond to antimony compounds alone.[6]

1. Murray HW. Interferon-gamma and host antimicrobial defense: current and future clinical applications. *Am J Med* 1994; **97:** 459–67.
2. Sundar S, *et al.* Response to interon-γ plus pentavalent antimony in Indian visceral leishmaniasis. *J Infect Dis* 1997; **176:** 1117–19.
3. Harms G, *et al.* Effects of intradermal gamma-interferon in cutaneous leishmaniasis. *Lancet* 1989; **i:** 1287–92.
4. Harms G, *et al.* A randomized trial comparing a pentavalent antimonial drug and recombinant interferon-γ in the local treatment of cutaneous leishmaniasis. *Trans R Soc Trop Med Hyg* 1991; **85:** 214–16.
5. Arana BA, *et al.* Efficacy of a short course (10 days) of high-dose meglumine antimonate with or without interferon-γ in treating cutaneous leishmaniasis in Guatemala. *Clin Infect Dis* 1994; **18:** 381–4.
6. Falcoff E, *et al.* Clinical healing of antimony-resistant cutaneous or mucocutaneous leishmaniasis following the combined administration of interferon-γ and pentavalent antimonial compounds. *Trans R Soc Trop Med Hyg* 1994; **88:** 95–7.

Mycobacterial infections. Interferon alfa has been tried as an adjunct to conventional therapy in *multibacillary leprosy.*[1] Experience with interferons for *opportunistic mycobacterial infections* in patients with AIDS is limited. Interferon gamma given with antimycobacterials produced beneficial responses in 3 patients with *Mycobacterium avium* complex infections, but produced no response or only a transient response in 3 others who received interferon gamma alone.[2,3]

Beneficial responses have also been reported following use of interferon alfa[4] or gamma[5] as an adjunct to antimycobacterial therapy in HIV-negative patients with mycobacterial infections unresponsive to conventional therapy.

Inhaled interferon alfa[6] or gamma[7] may be a useful adjunct to conventional antimycobacterial treatment for *pulmonary tuberculosis.*

For discussion of these infections and their standard treatment, see under Leprosy, p.126, Opportunistic Mycobacterial Infections, p.131, and Tuberculosis, p.143.

1. Ganapati R, *et al.* A multicenter study of recombinant interferon-alpha2b in the treatment of multibacillary leprosy. *Int J Lepr* 1997; **65:** 495–7.
2. Squires KE, *et al.* Interferon-γ and Mycobacterium avium-intracellulare infection. *J Infect Dis* 1989; **159:** 599–600.
3. Squires KE, *et al.* Interferon-γ treatment for Mycobacterium avium-intracellulare complex bacillemia in patients with AIDS. *J Infect Dis* 1992; **166:** 686–7.
4. Maziarz RT, *et al.* Reversal of infection with Mycobacterium avium intracellulare by treatment with alpha-interferon in a patient with hairy cell leukemia. *Ann Intern Med* 1988; **109:** 292–4.
5. Holland SM, *et al.* Treatment of refractory disseminated nontuberculous mycobacterial infection with interferon gamma: a preliminary report. *N Engl J Med* 1994; **330:** 1348–55.
6. Giosuè S, *et al.* Effects of aerosolized interferon-α in patients with pulmonary tuberculosis. *Am J Respir Crit Care Med* 1998; **158:** 1156–62.
7. Condos R, *et al.* Treatment of multidrug-resistant pulmonary tuberculosis with interferon-γ via aerosol. *Lancet* 1997; **349:** 1513–15.

Skin disorders. Interferons have been tried in skin disorders in which IgE levels are raised. Subcutaneous interferon gamma improved *eczema* and reduced serum-IgE concentration in one patient, but the condition gradually returned within a week of stopping treatment.[1] In two studies[2,3] subcutaneous interferon gamma given to patients with severe atopic dermatitis and raised serum-IgE concentrations resulted in improvement of the skin condition; IgE concentrations were reduced in one study[2] but remained high in the other.[3] Subcutaneous interferon alfa, however, was unsuccessful in 2 patients with very severe atopic dermatitis; serum-IgE concentrations and severity of the skin condition remained unaffected.[4] Interferon alfa has been tried in subacute *cutaneous lupus erythematosus*[5,6] and *discoid lupus erythematosus*.[6] Although marked improvement generally occurred, the condition tended to recur within several weeks of stopping treatment. For discussion of the conventional treatment of eczema, see p.1105 and of lupus erythematosus, see Systemic Lupus Erythematosus, p.1059.

There have been reports[7,8] of the successful use of interferon alfa to control the symptoms of *urticaria* associated with mastocytosis (p.775).

Interferons have also been proposed for antifibrotic therapy in the management of diffuse *scleroderma* (see p.505). A multicentre study of interferon gamma in scleroderma[9] found that cutaneous symptoms might be improved but that treatment was associated with an unacceptable incidence of adverse effects. Interferon gamma has also been tried in *eosinophilic pustular folliculitis*.[10]

Interferons have also been used for the treatment of warts (see under Interferon Alfa, p.632).

1. Souillet G, *et al.* Alpha-interferon treatment of patient with hyper IgE syndrome. *Lancet* 1989; i: 1384.
2. Reinhold U, *et al.* Recombinant interferon-γ in severe atopic dermatitis. *Lancet* 1990; 335: 1282.
3. Boguniewicz M, *et al.* Recombinant gamma interferon in treatment of patients with atopic dermatitis and elevated IgE levels. *Am J Med* 1990; 88: 365–70.
4. MacKie RM. Interferon-α for atopic dermatitis. *Lancet* 1990; 335: 1282–3.
5. Nicolas J-F, Thivolet J. Interferon alfa therapy in severe unresponsive subacute cutaneous lupus erythematosus. *N Engl J Med* 1989; 321: 1550–1.
6. Thivolet J, *et al.* Recombinant interferon α2a is effective in the treatment of discoid and subacute cutaneous lupus erythematosus. *Br J Dermatol* 1990; 122: 405–9.
7. Kolde G, *et al.* Treatment of urticaria pigmentosa using interferon alpha. *Br J Dermatol* 1995; 133: 91–4.
8. Lippert U, Henz BM. Long-term effect of interferon alpha treatment in mastocytosis. *Br J Dermatol* 1996; 134: 1164–5.
9. Polisson RP, *et al.* A multicenter trial of recombinant human interferon gamma in patients with systemic sclerosis: effects on cutaneous fibrosis and interleukin 2 receptor levels. *J Rheumatol* 1996; 23: 654–8.
10. Fushimi M, *et al.* Eosinophilic pustular folliculitis effectively treated with recombinant interferon-γ: suppression of mRNA expression of interleukin 5 in peripheral blood mononuclear cells. *Br J Dermatol* 1996; 134: 766–72.

Preparations

Proprietary Preparations (details are given in Part 3)
Aust.: Imufor; Imukin; *Austral.:* Imukin; *Belg.:* Immukine; *Denm.:* Imukin; *Fin.:* Imukin; *Fr.:* Imukin; *Ger.:* Imukin; *Hong Kong:* Immukin; *Irl.:* Immukin; *Ital.:* Gammakine; Imukin; *Jpn:* Ogamma; *Neth.:* Immukine; *Norw.:* Imukin; *NZ:* Imukin; *Port.:* Imukin; *Spain:* Imukin; *Swed.:* Imukin; *Switz.:* Imukin; *UK:* Immukin; *USA:* Actimmune.

Lamivudine (15566-c)

Lamivudine *(BAN, USAN, rINN).*

3TC; (−)-2′-Deoxy-3′-thiacytidine; GR-109714X. (−)-1-[(2R,5S)-2-(Hydroxymethyl)-1,3-oxathiolan-5-yl]cytosine.
$C_8H_{11}N_3O_3S = 229.3$.
CAS — 131086-21-0; 134678-17-4.
ATC — J05AF05.

Adverse Effects

Adverse effects commonly associated with lamivudine include abdominal pain, nausea, vomiting, diarrhoea, headache, fever, rash, alopecia, malaise, insomnia, cough, nasal symptoms, musculoskeletal pain, and peripheral neuropathy. Pancreatitis has been reported rarely. Neutropenia and anaemia (usually when given in combination with zidovudine), thrombocytopenia, and increases in liver enzymes have occurred. Lactic acidosis, usually associated with severe hepatomegaly and steatosis, has been reported during treatment with nucleoside reverse transcriptase inhibitors (see Zidovudine, p.645).

Effects on the blood. Although anaemia associated with lamivudine usually occurs when it is used in combination with zidovudine, there has been a report[1] of severe anaemia in a 62-year-old HIV-infected man who received lamivudine in the absence of zidovudine.

1. Weitzel T, *et al.* Severe anaemia as a newly recognized side-effect caused by lamivudine. *AIDS* 1999; 13: 2309–11.

Effects on the hair. Hair loss was associated with lamivudine treatment in 5 patients.[1]

1. Fong IW. Hair loss associated with lamivudine. *Lancet* 1994; 344: 1702.

Effects on the nails. Paronychia was reported in 12 HIV-infected patients receiving lamivudine.[1] In a further report, 6 patients developed paronychia while receiving lamivudine in combination with indinavir.[2]

1. Zerboni R, *et al.* Lamivudine-induced paronychia. *Lancet* 1998; 351: 1256.
2. Tosti A, *et al.* Paronychia associated with antiretroviral therapy. *Br J Dermatol* 1999; 140: 1165–8.

The symbol † denotes a preparation no longer actively marketed

Effects on the nervous system. Exacerbation of peripheral neuropathy has been reported in a patient following substitution of lamivudine for zalcitabine.[1]

1. Cupler EJ, Dalakas MC. Exacerbation of peripheral neuropathy by lamivudine. *Lancet* 1995; 345: 460–1.

Hypersensitivity. Angioedema, urticaria, and anaphylactoid reaction occurred in a patient 30 minutes after receiving the first dose of lamivudine.[1]

1. Kainer MA, Mijch A. Anaphylactoid reaction, angioedema, and urticaria associated with lamivudine. *Lancet* 1996; 348: 1519.

Precautions

Lamivudine therapy should be stopped in patients who develop abdominal pain, nausea, or vomiting or with abnormal biochemical test results until pancreatitis has been excluded.

Treatment with lamivudine may be associated with lactic acidosis and should be discontinued if there is a rapid increase in aminotransferase concentrations, progressive hepatomegaly, or metabolic or lactic acidosis of unknown aetiology. Lamivudine should be used with caution in patients with hepatomegaly or other risk factors for hepatic disease. In patients with chronic hepatitis B, there is a risk of rebound hepatitis when lamivudine is discontinued, and liver function should be monitored in such patients. The possibility of HIV infection should be excluded before beginning lamivudine therapy for hepatitis B, since the lower doses used to treat the latter may permit the development of lamivudine-resistant strains of HIV.

Dosage reduction may be necessary in patients with impaired renal function (see below).

The manufacturers recommend that lamivudine should not be used during the first three months of pregnancy.

Interactions

The renal excretion of lamivudine may be inhibited by concomitant administration of other drugs mainly eliminated by active renal secretion, for example trimethoprim. Usual prophylactic doses of trimethoprim are unlikely to necessitate reductions in lamivudine dosage unless the patient has impaired renal function, but the co-administration of lamivudine with the high therapeutic doses of trimethoprim (as co-trimoxazole) used in *Pneumocystis carinii* pneumonia and toxoplasmosis should be avoided. Although there is usually no clinically significant interaction with zidovudine, severe anaemia has occasionally been reported in patients receiving lamivudine and zidovudine in combination (see Zidovudine, Interactions, p.646). Lamivudine may antagonise the antiviral action of zalcitabine and the two drugs should not be used in combination.

Phenylpropanolamine. For a possible interaction between phenylpropanolamine and antiretrovirals, see Stavudine, p.641.

Antiviral Action

Lamivudine is converted intracellularly in stages to the triphosphate. This triphosphate halts the DNA synthesis of retroviruses, including HIV, through competitive inhibition of reverse transcriptase and incorporation into viral DNA. Lamivudine is also active against hepatitis B virus. Resistance to lamivudine has been reported in isolates of HIV and hepatitis B virus.

◊ References.
1. Coates JAV, *et al.* (−)-2′-Deoxy-3′-thiacytidine is a potent, highly selective inhibitor of human immunodeficiency virus type 1 and type 2 replication in vitro. *Antimicrob Agents Chemother* 1992; 36: 733–9.
2. Bartholomew MM, *et al.* Hepatitis-B-virus resistance to lamivudine given for recurrent infection after orthotopic liver transplantation. *Lancet* 1997; 349: 20–2.
3. Honkoop P, *et al.* Lamivudine resistance in immunocompetent chronic hepatitis B: incidence and patterns. *J Hepatol* 1997; 26: 1393–5.
4. Conway B, *et al.* Primary lamivudine resistance in acute/early human immunodeficiency virus infection. *Clin Infect Dis* 1999; 28: 910–11.
5. Bessesen M, *et al.* Chronic active hepatitis B exacerbation in human immunodeficiency virus-infected patients following development of resistance to or withdrawal of lamivudine. *Clin Infect Dis* 1999; 28: 1032–5.

Microbiological interactions. The intracellular phosphorylation of lamivudine was increased by the addition of *hydroxyurea [hydroxycarbamide]* in an *in-vitro* study.[1]

Modest increases in *zidovudine* plasma concentrations may occur on concurrent administration of lamivudine, but are not usually clinically significant.

1. Palmer S, Cox S. Increased activation of the combination of 3′-azido-3′-deoxythymidine and 2′-deoxy-3′-thiacytidine in the presence of hydroxyurea. *Antimicrob Agents Chemother* 1997; 41: 460–4.

Pharmacokinetics

Lamivudine is rapidly absorbed following oral administration and peak plasma concentrations are achieved in about 1 hour. Absorption is delayed, but not reduced, by ingestion with food. Bioavailability is between 80 and 87%. Binding to plasma protein is reported to be less than 36%. Lamivudine crosses the blood-brain barrier with a ratio of CSF to serum concentrations of about 0.12. It crosses the placenta and is distributed into breast milk.

Lamivudine is metabolised intracellularly to the active antiviral triphosphate. Hepatic metabolism is low and it is cleared mainly unchanged by renal excretion. An elimination half-life of 5 to 7 hours has been reported following a single dose.

◊ References.
1. Mueller BU, *et al.* Serum and cerebrospinal fluid pharmacokinetics of intravenous and oral lamivudine in human immunodeficiency virus-infected children. *Antimicrob Agents Chemother* 1998; 42: 3187–92.
2. Johnson MA, *et al.* Clinical pharmacokinetics of lamivudine. *Clin Pharmacokinet* 1999; 36: 41–66.

Uses and Administration

Lamivudine is a nucleoside reverse transcriptase inhibitor structurally related to cytosine with activity against retroviruses including HIV. It is used, usually in combination with other antiretrovirals, in the treatment of HIV infection. It is also used for the treatment of chronic hepatitis B.

For HIV infection, the dose of lamivudine for adults is 150 mg by mouth twice daily. A dose for children aged between 3 months and 12 years is 4 mg per kg twice daily to a maximum of 150 mg twice daily.

For chronic hepatitis B the adult dose is 100 mg once daily by mouth; in patients with concomitant HIV and hepatitis B infection the dosage regimen appropriate for HIV should be used.

Reduction of dosage is recommended for patients with impaired renal function (see below).

◊ Reviews.
1. Perry CM, Faulds D. Lamivudine: a review of its antiviral activity, pharmacokinetic properties and therapeutic efficacy in the management of HIV infection. *Drugs* 1997; 53: 657–80.
2. Jarvis B, Faulds D. Lamivudine: a review of its therapeutic potential in chronic hepatitis B. *Drugs* 1999; 58: 101–41.

Administration in renal impairment. Dosage of lamivudine should be reduced in patients with moderate to severe renal impairment (creatinine clearance (CC) below 50 mL per minute).

Doses employed in adults for the treatment of HIV infection are:
• for CC 30 to 50 mL per minute, 150 mg for the first dose then 150 mg once daily
• for CC 15 to 30 mL per minute, 150 mg for the first dose then 100 mg once daily.
• for CC 5 to 15 mL per minute, 150 mg for the first dose then 50 mg once daily
• for CC less than 5 mL per minute, 50 mg for the first dose then 25 mg once daily.

Lamivudine is not recommended for HIV infection in patients undergoing dialysis.

Doses employed in adults for the treatment of chronic hepatitis B infection are:
• for CC 30 to 50 mL per minute, 100 mg for the first dose then 50 mg once daily
• for CC 15 to 30 mL per minute, 100 mg for the first dose then 25 mg once daily
• for CC 5 to 15 mL per minute, 35 mg for the first dose then 15 mg once daily
• for CC less than 5 mL per minute, 35 mg for the first dose then 10 mg once daily.

Lamivudine may be given to patients for chronic hepatitis B who are undergoing haemodialysis; no further dose adjustment other than in accordance with creatinine clearance is required. It is not recommended in patients undergoing peritoneal dialysis.

It is recommended that doses in children with renal impairment be reduced according to creatinine clearance by the same proportions as in adults.

Hepatitis. Lamivudine is one of the more promising antivirals being used as an alternative to interferon alfa in the treatment of chronic hepatitis B (p.605).[1,2] In a preliminary study, lamivudine 100 or 300 mg daily reduced hepatitis B virus DNA to low or undetectable levels.[3] In a 1-year double-blind study involving about 350 patients with chronic hepatitis B, lamivudine 100 mg daily was associated with substantial histological improvement in many patients; a dose of 25 mg daily was less effective.[4] Relapses have been reported once treatment with lamivudine is stopped, and a case of reactivation of hepatitis B infection has been observed.[5] Lamivudine may also be effective in preventing re-infection with hepatitis B in patients who have received liver transplants,[6,7] and beneficial responses have been seen in transplant patients with acute hepatitis B infection treated with lamivudine 100 mg daily for prolonged periods.[8]

1. Dienstag JL, et al. Lamivudine as initial treatment for chronic hepatitis B in the United States. N Engl J Med 1999; 341: 1256–63.
2. Hagmeyer KO, Pan Y-Y. Role of lamivudine in the treatment of chronic hepatitis B virus infection. Ann Pharmacother 1999; 33: 1104–12.
3. Dienstag JL, et al. A preliminary trial of lamivudine for chronic hepatitis B infection. N Engl J Med 1995; 333: 1657–61.
4. Lai C-L, et al. A one-year trial of lamivudine for chronic hepatitis B. N Engl J Med 1998; 339: 61–8.
5. Honkoop P, et al. Hepatitis B reactivation after lamivudine. Lancet 1995; 346: 1156–7.
6. Grellier L, et al. Lamivudine prophylaxis against reinfection in liver transplantation for hepatitis B cirrhosis. Lancet 1996; 348: 1212–15. Correction. ibid. 1997; 349: 364.
7. Perrillo RP, et al. A multicenter United States-Canadian trial to assess lamivudine monotherapy before and after liver transplantation for chronic hepatitis B. Hepatology 2001; 33: 424–32.
8. Andreone P, et al. Lamivudine treatment for acute hepatitis B after liver transplantation. J Hepatol 1998; 29: 985–9.

HIV infection and AIDS. Lamivudine is a potent inhibitor of HIV-1 and HIV-2 in vitro, including variants resistant to zidovudine.[1] Resistance emerges rapidly when lamivudine is given alone to patients with HIV infections,[2] although sustained responses have been reported despite the emergence of resistance.[3] Combination therapy with lamivudine delays, and may even reverse, the emergence of zidovudine resistance and produces a sustained synergistic antiretroviral effect,[4] but HIV strains resistant to both lamivudine and zidovudine may arise.[5] As discussed on p.608, combination therapy, typically with two nucleoside reverse transcriptase inhibitors and either a non-nucleoside reverse transcriptase inhibitor or an HIV-protease inhibitor, is standard therapy for HIV infection. Treatment with lamivudine plus zidovudine has produced better responses than either drug alone in antiretroviral-naive patients,[6,7] and has produced additional responses in antiretroviral-experienced patients,[8,9] with little additional toxicity. The addition of lamivudine to existing antiretroviral therapy was reported to slow the progression of the disease and improve survival,[10] and treatment with lamivudine, indinavir, and nevirapine produced beneficial responses in patients who had previously failed on combined nucleoside analogue therapy.[11] Clinically useful CNS concentrations of lamivudine were achieved in patients with HIV infection given combination therapy with lamivudine and zidovudine or stavudine.[12]

Lamivudine is also used in prophylactic regimens following occupational exposure to HIV infection (see p.610) and has been tried for reducing vertical transmission from mother to neonate.[13]

1. Anonymous. Lamivudine: impressive benefits in combination with zidovudine. WHO Drug Inf 1996; 10: 5–7.
2. Wainberg MA, et al. Development of HIV-1 resistance to (–)2′-deoxy-3′-thiacytidine in patients with AIDS or advanced AIDS-related complex. AIDS 1995; 9: 351–7.
3. Ingrand D, et al. Phase I/II study of 3TC in HIV-positive, asymptomatic or mild AIDS-related complex patients: sustained reduction in viral markers. AIDS 1995; 9: 1323–9.
4. Larder BA, et al. Potential mechanism for sustained antiretroviral efficacy of AZT-3TC combination therapy. Science 1995; 269: 696–9.
5. Miller V, et al. Dual resistance to zidovudine and lamivudine in patients treated with zidovudine-lamivudine combination therapy: association with therapeutic failure. J Infect Dis 1998; 177: 1521–32.
6. Eron JJ, et al. Treatment with lamivudine, zidovudine, or both in HIV-positive patients with 200 to 500 CD4+ cells per cubic millimeter. N Engl J Med 1995; 333: 1662–9.
7. Katlama C, et al. Safety and efficacy of lamivudine-zidovudine combination therapy in antiretroviral-naive patients: a randomized controlled comparison with zidovudine monotherapy. JAMA 1996; 276: 118–25.
8. Staszewski S, et al. Safety and efficacy of lamivudine-zidovudine combination therapy in zidovudine-experienced patients: a randomized controlled comparison with zidovudine monotherapy. JAMA 1996; 276: 111–17.
9. Bartlett JA, et al. Lamivudine plus zidovudine compared with zalcitabine plus zidovudine in patients with HIV infection: a randomized, double-blind, placebo-controlled trial. Ann Intern Med 1996; 125: 161–72.
10. CAESAR Coordinating Committee. Randomised trial of addition of lamivudine or lamivudine plus loviride to zidovudine-containing regimens for patients with HIV-1 infection: the CAESAR trial. Lancet 1997; 349: 1413–21.
11. Harris M, et al. A pilot study of nevirapine, indinavir, and lamivudine among patients with advanced human immunodeficiency virus disease who have had failure of combination nucleoside therapy. J Infect Dis 1998; 177: 1514–20.
12. Foudraine NA, et al. Cerebrospinal-fluid HIV-1 RNA and drug concentrations after treatment with lamivudine plus zidovudine or stavudine. Lancet 1998; 351: 1547–51.
13. Mandelbrot L, et al. Lamivudine-zidovudine combination for prevention of maternal-infant transmission of HIV-1. JAMA 2001; 285: 2083–93.

Preparations

Proprietary Preparations (details are given in Part 3)
Aust.: Epivir; *Austral.:* 3TC; Zeffix; *Belg.:* Epivir; Zeffix; *Canad.:* 3TC; Heptovir; *Denm.:* Epivir; Zeffix; *Fin.:* Epivir; Zeffix; *Fr.:* Epivir; Zeffix; *Ger.:* Epivir; Zeffix; *Hong Kong:* 3TC; Zeffix; *Irl.:* Zeffix; *Israel:* Epivir; *Ital.:* Epivir; Zeffix; *Jpn:* Epivir; *Mex.:* 3TC; *Neth.:* Epivir; *Norw.:* Epivir; *NZ:* Zeffix; *Port.:* Epivir; Zeffix; *S.Afr.:* 3TC; *Singapore:* Epivir; *Spain:* Epivir; *Swed.:* Epivir; Zeffix; *Switz.:* 3TC; Zeffix; *Thai.:* Epivir; Zeffix; *UK:* Epivir; Zeffix; *USA:* Epivir.

Multi-ingredient: *Aust.:* Combivir; *Austral.:* Combivir; *Belg.:* Combivir; *Canad.:* Combivir; *Denm.:* Combivir; *Fin.:* Combivir; *Fr.:* Combivir; *Ger.:* Combivir; *Hong Kong:* Combivir; *Irl.:* Combivir; *Israel:* Combivir; *Ital.:* Combivir; *Mex.:* Combivir; *Neth.:* Combivir; *NZ:* Combivir; *Port.:* Combivir; *S.Afr.:* Retrovir/3TC Post-HIV Exposure; *Singapore:* Combivir; *Spain:* Combivir; *Swed.:* Combivir; *Switz.:* Combivir; *Thai.:* Combid; *UK:* Combivir; Trizivir; *USA:* Combivir; Trizivir.

Lobucavir (17834-y)

Lobucavir (USAN, rINN).
BMS-180194; SQ-34514. 9-[(1R,2R,3S)-2,3-Bis(hydroxymethyl)cyclobutyl]guanine.
$C_{11}H_{15}N_5O_3 = 265.3$.
CAS — 127759-89-1.

Profile

Lobucavir is a nucleoside analogue with antiviral activity that has been studied for the treatment of herpesvirus and hepatitis B infections. Clinical studies were suspended in 1999 following observation of possible carcinogenicity in *rodents*.

Lopinavir (20215-z)

Lopinavir (BAN, USAN, rINN).
A-157378.0; ABT-378. (αS)-Tetrahydro-N-((αS)-α-{(2S,3S)-2-hydroxy-4-phenyl-3-[2-(2,6-xylyloxy)acetamido]butyl}phenethyl)-α-isopropyl-2-oxo-1(2H)-pyrimidineacetamide.
$C_{37}H_{48}N_4O_5 = 628.8$.
CAS — 192725-17-0.

Adverse Effects and Precautions

As for HIV-protease inhibitors in general (see Indinavir Sulfate, p.625). Lopinavir has been associated with increases in serum cholesterol and triglycerides, and cases of pancreatitis have been reported. It should be discontinued if symptoms of pancreatitis occur.

The oral solution (*Kaletra, Abbott, UK*) has a high content of alcohol and propylene glycol, present as excipients, and appropriate precautions should be taken.

Interactions

Interactions involving HIV-protease inhibitors are discussed under Indinavir Sulfate, p.626.

Antiviral Action

As for HIV-protease inhibitors in general (see Indinavir Sulfate, p.627).

Uses and Administration

Lopinavir is a protease inhibitor with antiviral activity against HIV. It is used, in combination with other antiretrovirals, in the treatment of HIV infection (p.608). It is given with low-dose ritonavir, which acts as a pharmacokinetic enhancer. The dose in adults is lopinavir 400 mg (with ritonavir 100 mg) twice daily with food. Children over 2 years of age may be given lopinavir 230 mg (with ritonavir 57.5 mg) per m² body-surface twice daily, up to a maximum of lopinavir 400 mg twice daily.

◊ Reviews.
1. Hurst M, Faulds D. Lopinavir. Drugs 2000; 60: 1371–9.

Preparations

Proprietary Preparations (details are given in Part 3)
Multi-ingredient: *UK:* Kaletra; *USA:* Kaletra.

Loviride (17434-x)

Loviride (BAN, USAN, rINN).
R-89439. (±)-2-(6-Acetyl-m-toluidino)-2-(2,6-dichlorophenyl)acetamide; N²-(6-Acetyl-m-tolyl)-DL-2-(2,6-dichlorophenyl)glycinamide.
$C_{17}H_{16}Cl_2N_2O_2 = 351.2$.
CAS — 147362-57-0.

Profile

Loviride is a non-nucleoside reverse transcriptase inhibitor under investigation for the treatment of HIV infection. Viral resistance emerges rapidly when loviride is given alone, and it would be likely to be used mainly in combination with nucleoside reverse transcriptase inhibitors.

◊ References.
1. CAESAR Coordinating Committee. Randomised trial of addition of lamivudine or lamivudine plus loviride to zidovudine-containing regimens for patients with HIV-1 infection: the CAESAR trial. Lancet 1997; 349: 1413–21.
2. Miller V, et al. Patterns of resistance and cross-resistance to human immunodeficiency virus type 1 reverse transcriptase inhibitors in patients treated with the nonnucleoside reverse transcriptase inhibitor loviride. Antimicrob Agents Chemother 1998; 42: 3123–9.
3. Gatell J, et al. AVANTI 1: randomized, double-blind trial to evaluate the efficacy and safety of zidovudine plus lamivudine versus zidovudine plus lamivudine plus loviride in HIV-infected antiretroviral-naive patients: AVANTI Study Group. Antiviral Ther 1999; 4: 79–86.

Moroxydine Hydrochloride (12979-y)

Moroxydine Hydrochloride (BANM, rINNM).
Abitilguanide Hydrochloride; ABOB. 1-(Morpholinoformimidoyl)guanidine hydrochloride.
$C_6H_{13}N_5O,HCl = 207.7$.
CAS — 3731-59-7 (moroxydine); 3160-91-6 (moroxydine hydrochloride).

Profile

Moroxydine hydrochloride has been given by mouth in the treatment of herpes simplex and varicella-zoster infections. It has also been used topically. It is included as an ingredient in preparations for the treatment of cold and influenza symptoms.

Preparations

Proprietary Preparations (details are given in Part 3)
Hong Kong: Virustat.
Multi-ingredient: *Hong Kong:* Virulex Forte; *S.Afr.:* Corenza C; Virobis.

Nelfinavir Mesilate (17721-b)

Nelfinavir Mesilate (BANM, rINNM).
AG-1343 (nelfinavir or nelfinavir mesilate); Nelfinavir Mesylate (USAN). 3S[2(2S*,3S*),3α,4aβ,8aβ]-N-(1,1-Dimethylethyl)decahydro-2-2-hydroxy-3-[(3-hydroxy-2-methylbenzoyl)amino]-4-(phenylthio)butyl-3-isoquinolinecarboxamide monomethanesulphonate; (3S,4aS,8aS)-N-tert-Butyldecahydro-2-[(2R,3R)-3-(3-hydroxy-o-toluamido)-2-hydroxy-4-(phenylthio)butyl]isoquinoline-3-carboxamide monomethanesulphonate.
$C_{32}H_{45}N_3O_4S,CH_4O_3S = 663.9$.
CAS — 159989-64-7 (nelfinavir); 159989-65-8 (nelfinavir mesilate).

NOTE. Nelfinavir should not be confused with nevirapine (p.637).

Adverse Effects and Precautions

As for HIV-protease inhibitors in general (see Indinavir Sulfate, p.625).

Interactions

Interactions involving HIV-protease inhibitors are discussed under Indinavir Sulfate, p.626. Nelfinavir is reported to be metabolised in part by cytochrome P450 isoenzymes of the CYP3A family and to be unlikely to inhibit other cytochrome P450 isoforms at therapeutic concentrations.

Antiviral Action

As for HIV-protease inhibitors in general (see Indinavir Sulfate, p.627). Mechanisms of resistance to nelfinavir may differ sufficiently from those to other HIV-protease inhibitors to reduce the occurrence of cross-resistance between nelfinavir and other HIV-protease inhibitors.

Resistance. References.
1. Patick AK, et al. Genotypic and phenotypic characterization of human immunodeficiency virus type 1 variants isolated from patients treated with the protease inhibitor nelfinavir. Antimicrob Agents Chemother 1998; 42: 2637–44.

Pharmacokinetics

Nelfinavir is absorbed from the gastrointestinal tract and peak plasma concentrations occur in 2 to 4 hours. Absorption is enhanced by administration with food. Nelfinavir is extensively bound to plasma proteins (98%). It is distributed into breast milk. Nelfinavir is metabolised by oxidation by cytochrome P450 isoenzymes including CYP3A. The major oxidative metabolite has *in-vitro* antiviral activity equal to that of nelfinavir. The terminal half-life is 3.5 to 5 hours. Nelfinavir is excreted in the faeces mainly as metabolites. Only about 1 to 2% is excreted in the urine.

Uses and Administration
Nelfinavir is a protease inhibitor with antiviral activity against HIV. It is used, in combination with nucleoside reverse transcriptase inhibitors, for the treatment of HIV infection (p.608).

Nelfinavir is given by mouth as the mesilate, but doses are expressed in terms of the base. It is given in an adult dose of 1.25 g twice daily or 0.75 g three times daily with food. Children aged 2 to 13 years may be given 20 to 30 mg per kg body-weight three times daily.

◊ Reviews.
1. Perry C, Benfield P. Nelfinavir. *Drugs* 1997; **54:** 81–7.
2. Pai VB, Nahata MC. Nelfinavir mesylate: a protease inhibitor. *Ann Pharmacother* 1999; **33:** 325–39.
3. Bardsley-Elliot A, Plosker GL. Nelfinavir: an update on its use in HIV infection. *Drugs* 2000; **59:** 581–620.

Preparations
Proprietary Preparations (details are given in Part 3)
Aust.: Viracept; *Austral.:* Viracept; *Belg.:* Viracept; *Canad.:* Viracept; *Denm.:* Viracept; *Fin.:* Viracept; *Fr.:* Viracept; *Ger.:* Viracept; *Israel:* Viracept; *Ital.:* Viracept; *Jpn:* Viracept; *Neth.:* Viracept; *Norw.:* Viracept; *NZ:* Viracept; *Port.:* Viracept; *S.Afr.:* Viracept; *Singapore:* Viracept; *Spain:* Viracept; *Swed.:* Viracept; *Switz.:* Viracept; *Thai.:* Viracept; *UK:* Viracept; *USA:* Viracept.

Netivudine (14532-r)
Netivudine (BAN, rINN).
BW-882C; BW-882C87; 882C; 882C87. 1-β-D-Arabinofuranosyl-5-prop-1-ynyluracil.
$C_{12}H_{14}N_2O_6 = 282.2$.
CAS — 84558-93-0.

Profile
Netivudine is a synthetic nucleoside analogue structurally related to thymidine, with activity against varicella-zoster virus. It is being studied for the treatment of herpes zoster, although concerns have been expressed over its toxicity following long-term administration to *rodents*.

◊ References.
1. Easterbrook P, Wood MJ. Successors to acyclovir. *J Antimicrob Chemother* 1994; **34:** 307–11.
2. Peck RW, *et al.* Pharmacokinetics and tolerability of single oral doses of 882C87, a potent, new anti-varicella-zoster virus agent, in healthy volunteers. *Antimicrob Agents Chemother* 1995; **39:** 20–7.
3. Peck RW, *et al.* The bioavailability and disposition of 1-(β-D-arabinofuranosyl)-5-(1-propynyl)uracil (882C87), a potent, new anti-varicella zoster virus agent. *Br J Clin Pharmacol* 1995; **39:** 143–9.
4. Peck RW, *et al.* Multiple dose netivudine, a potent anti-varicella zoster virus agent, in healthy elderly volunteers and patients with shingles. *J Antimicrob Chemother* 1996; **37:** 583–97.
5. Fillastre JP, *et al.* Pharmacokinetics of netivudine, a potent anti-varicella zoster virus drug, in patients with renal impairment. *J Antimicrob Chemother* 1996; **37:** 965–74.
6. Söltz-Szöts J, *et al.* A randomised controlled trial of acyclovir versus netivudine for treatment of herpes zoster. *J Antimicrob Chemother* 1998; **41:** 549–56.

Nevirapine (14530-t)
Nevirapine (BAN, USAN, rINN).
BI-RG-587; BIRG-0587. 11-Cyclopropyl-5,11-dihydro-4-methyl-6H-dipyrido[3,2-b:2′,3′-e]-[1,4]diazepin-6-one.
$C_{15}H_{14}N_4O = 266.3$.
CAS — 129618-40-2.
ATC — J05AG01.

NOTE. Nevirapine should not be confused with nelfinavir (p.636).

Adverse Effects
The most common adverse effect of nevirapine is skin rash, usually occurring within the first 6 weeks of starting therapy. Severe and life-threatening skin reactions (with some fatalities) have occurred, including Stevens-Johnson syndrome and, more rarely, toxic epidermal necrolysis. Hypersensitivity reactions including angioedema, urticaria, and anaphylaxis have been reported. Abnormalities in liver function tests are also common, and severe hepatitis and hepatic necrosis, occasionally fatal, have occurred. Other

common adverse effects include nausea, vomiting, diarrhoea, abdominal pain, fatigue, fever, drowsiness, myalgia, and headache. Granulocytopenia has occurred and has been observed more commonly in children than in adults.

Effects on the liver. References.
1. Cattelan AM, *et al.* Severe hepatic failure related to nevirapine treatment. *Clin Infect Dis* 1999; **29:** 455–6.
2. Clarke S, *et al.* Late onset hepatitis and prolonged deterioration in hepatic function associated with nevirapine therapy. *Int J STD AIDS* 2000; **11:** 336–7.
3. Prakash M, *et al.* Jaundice and hepatocellular damage associated with nevirapine therapy. *Am J Gastroenterol* 2001; **96:** 1571–4.
4. Martinez E, *et al.* Hepatotoxicity in HIV-1-infected patients receiving nevirapine-containing antiretroviral therapy. *AIDS* 2001; **15:** 1261–8.
5. Committee on Safety of Medicines/Medicines Control Agency. Nevirapine (Viramune): serious adverse reactions when used in HIV post exposure prophylaxis. *Current Problems* 2001; **27:** 13.

Effects on the skin. References.
1. Warren KJ, *et al.* Nevirapine-associated Stevens-Johnson syndrome. *Lancet* 1998; **351:** 567.
2. Barner A, Myers M. Nevirapine and rashes. *Lancet* 1998; **351:** 1133.
3. Wetterwald E, *et al.* Nevirapine-induced overlap Stevens-Johnson syndrome/toxic epidermal necrolysis. *Br J Dermatol* 1999; **140:** 980–2.
4. Committee on Safety of Medicines/Medicines Control Agency. Nevirapine (Viramune): serious adverse reactions when used in HIV post exposure prophylaxis. *Current Problems* 2001; **27:** 13.

Precautions
Patients receiving nevirapine should be closely monitored for adverse skin reactions during the first 8 weeks of treatment. Nevirapine should be permanently discontinued if a severe skin rash develops or if a rash is accompanied by fever, blistering, oral lesions, conjunctivitis, swelling, muscle or joint aches, or general malaise. Dose escalation should not be attempted in patients developing any rash during the first 14 days of treatment until the rash has resolved.

Liver function should be monitored every 2 weeks during the first 2 months of treatment, again at 3 months, and every 3 to 6 months thereafter; treatment should be interrupted if moderate or severe abnormalities occur; nevirapine may be restarted at the initial dose if liver function returns to normal, but should be permanently discontinued if abnormalities recur or if abnormalities in liver function are accompanied by symptoms suggestive of a hypersensitivity reaction. Nevirapine should be used with caution in patients with renal or hepatic insufficiency and not at all in those with renal or hepatic failure.

Interactions
Similarly to the HIV-protease inhibitors (see Indinavir, p.626), nevirapine is metabolised mainly by cytochrome P450 isoenzymes of the CYP3A family. Consequently it may compete with other drugs metabolised by this system, possibly resulting in mutually increased plasma concentrations. Alternatively enzyme inducers may decrease plasma concentrations of nevirapine; nevirapine itself acts as a mild to moderate enzyme inducer and may thus reduce plasma concentrations of other drugs.

Antibacterials. Plasma concentrations of nevirapine may be decreased by *rifabutin* and *rifampicin*, probably as a result of enzyme induction.

Antifungals. Concurrent administration of nevirapine and *ketoconazole* may result in reduction in the plasma concentration of ketoconazole and increase in that of nevirapine. The manufacturers recommend that this combination should be avoided.

Antivirals. For the effect of nevirapine on *indinavir* and *saquinavir*, see p.626.

Hormonal contraceptives. The manufacturers suggest that nevirapine may decrease the plasma concentrations of hormonal contraceptives. Although the clinical significance of this potential interaction is unknown they advise the use of alternative contraceptive methods.

Methadone. Nevirapine may induce the metabolism of methadone (p.54) resulting in reduced plasma-methadone concentrations.

Pharmacokinetics
Nevirapine is readily absorbed following oral administration and absorption is not affected by food. Bioavailability is greater than 90%. Peak plasma concen-

trations occur 4 hours after a single dose. Nevirapine is about 60% bound to plasma proteins. Concentrations in the CSF are about 45% of those in plasma. Nevirapine crosses the placenta and is distributed into breast milk. It is extensively metabolised by hepatic microsomal enzymes, principally by cytochrome P450 isoenzymes of the CYP3A family. Autoinduction of these enzymes results in a 1.5- to 2-fold increase in apparent oral clearance after 2 to 4 weeks' administration of usual doses, and a decrease in terminal half-life from 45 hours to 25 to 30 hours over the same period. In children, half-life at steady state varies with age, being 32 hours in children less than 1 year of age, 21 hours in children aged 1 to 4 years, 18 hours in children aged 4 to 8 years, and 28 hours in children over 8 years. Apparent clearance, adjusted for body-weight, also varies with age, that in children under 8 years being approximately twice that in adults. Nevirapine is mainly excreted in the urine as glucuronide conjugates of the hydroxylated metabolites.

◊ References.
1. Cheeseman SH, *et al.* Pharmacokinetics of nevirapine: initial single-rising-dose study in humans. *Antimicrob Agents Chemother* 1993; **37:** 178–82.
2. Zhou X-J, *et al.* Population pharmacokinetics of nevirapine, zidovudine, and didanosine in human immunodeficiency virus-infected patients. *Antimicrob Agents Chemother* 1999; **43:** 121–8.
3. Mirochnick M, *et al.* Nevirapine: pharmacokinetic considerations in children and pregnant women. *Clin Pharmacokinet* 2000; **39:** 281–93.

Uses and Administration
Nevirapine is a non-nucleoside reverse transcriptase inhibitor with activity against HIV-1. It is used in the treatment of HIV infection (p.608). Viral resistance emerges rapidly when nevirapine is used alone, and it is used in combination with other antiretrovirals.

Nevirapine is given in an adult dose of 200 mg once daily for the first 14 days, then increased to 200 mg twice daily provided that no rash is present (see Precautions, above). Children aged 2 months to 8 years may be given 4 mg per kg body-weight once daily for 14 days, then, if no rash is present, 7 mg per kg twice daily; those aged 8 to 16 years may be given 4 mg per kg once daily for 14 days, then 4 mg per kg twice daily thereafter. A total dose of 400 mg daily should not be exceeded.

If treatment is interrupted for more than 7 days, it should be reintroduced using the lower dose for the first 14 days as for new treatment.

◊ References.
1. Havlir D, *et al.* A pilot study to evaluate the development of resistance to nevirapine in asymptomatic human immunodeficiency virus-infected patients with CD4 cell counts of >500/mm³: AIDS Clinical Trials Group Protocol 208. *J Infect Dis* 1995; **172:** 1379–83.
2. Carr A, *et al.* A controlled trial of nevirapine plus zidovudine versus zidovudine alone in p24 antigenaemic HIV-infected patients. *AIDS* 1996; **10:** 635–41.
3. D'Aquila RT, *et al.* Nevirapine, zidovudine, and didanosine compared with zidovudine and didanosine in patients with HIV-1 infection: a randomized, double-blind, placebo-controlled trial. *Ann Intern Med* 1996; **124:** 1019–30.
4. Harris M, *et al.* A pilot study of nevirapine, indinavir, and lamivudine among patients with advanced human immunodeficiency virus disease who have had failure of combination nucleoside therapy. *J Infect Dis* 1998; **177:** 1514–20.
5. Floridia M, *et al.* A randomized, double-blind trial on the use of a triple combination including nevirapine, a nonnucleoside reverse transcriptase HIV inhibitor, in antiretroviral-naive patients with advanced disease. *J Acquir Immune Defic Syndr Hum Retrovirol* 1999; **20:** 11–19.
6. Guay LA, *et al.* Intrapartum and neonatal single-dose nevirapine compared with zidovudine for prevention of mother-to-child transmission of HIV-1 in Kampala, Uganda: HIVNET 012 randomised trial. *Lancet* 1999; **354:** 795–802.
7. Bardsley-Elliot A, Perry CM. Nevirapine: a review of its use in the prevention and treatment of paediatric HIV infection. *Paediatr Drugs* 2000; **2:** 373–407.

Preparations
Proprietary Preparations (details are given in Part 3)
Aust.: Viramune; *Austral.:* Viramune; *Belg.:* Viramune; *Canad.:* Viramune; *Denm.:* Viramune; *Fin.:* Viramune; *Fr.:* Viramune; *Ger.:* Viramune; *Hong Kong:* Viramune; *Irl.:* Viramune; *Ital.:* Viramune; *Jpn:* Viramune; *Mex.:* Viramune; *Neth.:* Viramune; *Norw.:* Viramune; *NZ:* Viramune; *Port.:* Viramune; *S.Afr.:* Viramune; *Singapore:* Viramune; *Spain:* Viramune; *Swed.:* Viramune; *Switz.:* Viramune; *Thai.:* Viramune; *UK:* Viramune; *USA:* Viramune.

The symbol † denotes a preparation no longer actively marketed

Oseltamivir Phosphate (20273-h)

Oseltamivir Phosphate (USAN, rINNM).
GS-4104/002; Ro-64-0796/002. Ethyl (3R,4R,5S)-4-acetamido-5-amino-3-(1-ethylpropoxy)-1-cyclohexene-1-carboxylate phosphate (1:1).
$C_{16}H_{28}N_2O_4,H_3PO_4 = 410.4$.
CAS — 196618-13-0 (oseltamivir); 204255-11-8 (oseltamivir phosphate).

Adverse Effects

The most commonly reported adverse effects associated with oseltamivir are nausea and vomiting, bronchitis, insomnia, and vertigo. Diarrhoea, dizziness, headache, cough, and fatigue may occur, but many adverse effects may be difficult to distinguish from the symptoms of influenza. Other adverse effects occurring less commonly have included unstable angina, anaemia, pseudomembranous colitis, pneumonia, pyrexia, and peritonsillar abscess.

Precautions

Oseltamivir should be given with caution, and dosage reduced, in patients with moderate to severe renal impairment.

Pharmacokinetics

Oseltamivir is readily absorbed from the gastrointestinal tract following oral administration and is extensively metabolised in the liver to the active entity, oseltamivir carboxylate. At least 75% of an oral dose reaches the systemic circulation as the carboxylate. Binding to plasma proteins is about 3% for the carboxylate and 42% for the parent drug. Oseltamivir has a plasma half-life of 1 to 3 hours. The carboxylate is not metabolised further and is eliminated primarily in the urine.

Uses and Administration

Oseltamivir is an oral prodrug of oseltamivir carboxylate, an inhibitor of the enzyme neuraminidase (sialidase), which has a role in the infectivity and replication of influenza A and B viruses. It is used for the treatment and prevention of influenza A and B. For treatment, oseltamivir is given as the phosphate in an adult dose of 75 mg twice daily for 5 days, beginning as soon as possible (within 48 hours) after the onset of symptoms.

For the prevention of influenza, the dose of oseltamivir is 75 mg once daily for at least 7 days; therapy should begin within 48 hours of exposure.

Dosage should be reduced in patients with moderate to severe renal impairment; the dose in adult patients with a creatinine clearance below 30 mL per minute should be 75 mg once daily for treatment, or 75 mg on alternate days for prevention.

Doses in children over 1 year for the treatment of influenza are, according to body-weight: over 40 kg body-weight, the adult dose; 23 to 40 kg, 60 mg twice daily; 15 to 23 kg, 45 mg twice daily; less than 15 kg, 30 mg twice daily.

◊ Reviews.
1. McClellan K, Perry CM. Oseltamivir: a review of its use in influenza. Drugs 2001; 61: 263–83.
2. Gubareva LV, et al. Influenza virus neuraminidase inhibitors. Lancet 2000; 355: 827–35.
3. Jefferson T, et al. Neuraminidase inhibitors for preventing and treating influenza in healthy adults (updated 26 July 2001). Available in The Cochrane Library; Issue 4. Oxford: Update Software; 2001.

Preparations

Proprietary Preparations (details are given in Part 3)
Austral.: Tamiflu; *USA:* Tamiflu.

Penciclovir (3035-m)

Penciclovir (BAN, USAN, rINN).
BRL-39123 (penciclovir); BRL-39123-D (penciclovir sodium). 9-[4-Hydroxy-3-(hydroxymethyl)butyl]guanine.
$C_{10}H_{15}N_5O_3 = 253.3$.
CAS — 39809-25-1 (penciclovir); 97845-62-0 (penciclovir sodium).
ATC — D06BB06; J05AB13.

Adverse Effects and Precautions

Penciclovir applied topically may cause transient stinging, burning, and numbness.

For the effects of systemic administration, see Famciclovir, p.620.

Interactions

Plasma concentrations of penciclovir may be increased in patients receiving *probenecid* concomitantly.

Antiviral Action

Penciclovir has antiviral activity similar to that of aciclovir (p.613). It is active in vitro and in vivo against herpes simplex virus types 1 and 2 and against varicella-zoster virus. This activity is due to intracellular conversion by virus-induced thymidine kinase into penciclovir triphosphate, which inhibits replication of viral DNA and persists in infected cells for more than 12 hours. It also has activity against Epstein-Barr virus and hepatitis B virus.

◊ References.
1. Weinberg A, et al. In vitro activities of penciclovir and acyclovir against herpes simplex virus types 1 and 2. Antimicrob Agents Chemother 1992; 36: 2037–8.
2. Vere-Hodge RA. Famciclovir and penciclovir: the mode of action of famciclovir including its conversion to penciclovir. Antiviral Chem Chemother 1993; 4: 67–84.
3. Boyd MR, et al. Penciclovir: a review of its spectrum of activity, selectivity, and cross-resistance pattern. Antiviral Chem Chemother 1993; 4 (suppl 1): 3–11.
4. Bacon TH, Boyd MR. Activity of penciclovir against Epstein-Barr virus. Antimicrob Agents Chemother 1995; 39: 1599–1602.

Pharmacokinetics

Penciclovir is poorly absorbed from the gastrointestinal tract. For systemic use it is usually administered orally as the prodrug famciclovir which is rapidly converted to penciclovir, producing peak plasma concentrations proportional to the dose (over the range 125 to 750 mg) after 45 minutes to 1 hour. The plasma elimination half-life is approximately 2 hours. The intracellular half-life of the active triphosphate metabolite is more prolonged. Penciclovir is less than 20% bound to plasma proteins. Penciclovir is mainly excreted unchanged in the urine.

◊ References.
1. Fowles SE, et al. The tolerance to and pharmacokinetics of penciclovir (BRL39123A), a novel antiherpes agent, administered by intravenous infusion to healthy subjects. Eur J Clin Pharmacol 1992; 43: 513–16.
2. Pue MA, et al. Linear pharmacokinetics of penciclovir following administration of single oral doses of famciclovir 125, 250, 500 and 750 mg to healthy volunteers. J Antimicrob Chemother 1994; 33: 119–27.

Uses and Administration

Penciclovir is a nucleoside analogue structurally related to guanine, which is active against herpesviruses. It is applied topically as a 1% cream every 2 hours during waking hours for 4 days in the treatment of herpes labialis (see Herpes Simplex Infections, p.607).

For systemic use, penciclovir is administered by mouth as the prodrug famciclovir (see p.620). Intravenous administration of penciclovir is being investigated.

◊ References.
1. Spruance SL, et al. Penciclovir cream for the treatment of herpes simplex labialis: a randomized, multicenter, double-blind, placebo-controlled trial. JAMA 1997; 277: 1374–9.
2. Lazarus HM, et al. Intravenous penciclovir for treatment of herpes simplex infections in immunocompromised patients: results of a multicenter, acyclovir-controlled trial. Antimicrob Agents Chemother 1999; 43: 1192–7.

Preparations

Proprietary Preparations (details are given in Part 3)
Aust.: Famvir; *Austral.:* Vectavir; *Belg.:* Vectavir; *Denm.:* Vectavir; *Fin.:* Vectavir; *Fr.:* Denavir; *Ger.:* Vectavir; *Hong Kong:* Vectavir; *Israel:* Vectavir; *Ital.:* Vectavir; *Neth.:* Famvir; *Norw.:* Vectavir; *NZ:* Vectavir; *Spain:* Vectavir; *Swed.:* Vectavir; *Switz.:* Famvir; *UK:* Vectavir; *USA:* Denavir.

Peptide T (3160-p)

D-Ala-peptide-T-amide.

Profile

Peptide T is an octapeptide segment of the envelope glycoprotein of HIV. It has been investigated for the treatment of HIV

infection and HIV-associated neurological disorders. Peptide T has also been tried in the treatment of psoriasis.

◊ References.
1. Wetterberg L, et al. Peptide T in treatment of AIDS. Lancet 1987; i: 159.
2. Bridge TP, et al. Improvement in AIDS patients on peptide T. Lancet 1989; ii: 226–7.
3. Poizot-Martin I, et al. Are CD4 antibodies and peptide T new treatments for psoriasis? Lancet 1991; 337: 1477.
4. Farbar EM, et al. Peptide T improves psoriasis when infused into lesions in nanogram amounts. J Am Acad Dermatol 1991; 25: 658–64.
5. Delfino M, et al. Peptide T in the treatment of severe psoriasis. Acta Derm Venereol (Stockh) 1992; 72: 68–9.
6. Simpson DM, et al. Peptide T in the treatment of painful distal neuropathy associated with AIDS: results of a placebo-controlled trial. Neurology 1996; 47: 1254–9.
7. Heseltine PN, et al. Randomized double-blind controlled trial of peptide T for HIV-associated cognitive impairment. Arch Neurol 1998; 55: 41–51.
8. Gulliver WP, et al. Peptide T—a novel neuro peptide analog for the treatment of psoriasis. Br J Dermatol 1999; 141: 980.

Pirodavir (14650-b)

Pirodavir (BAN, USAN, rINN).
R-77975. Ethyl 4-{2-[1-(6-methylpyridazin-3-yl)-4-piperidyl]ethoxy}benzoate.
$C_{21}H_{27}N_3O_3 = 369.5$.
CAS — 124436-59-5.

Profile

Pirodavir is an antiviral reported to be active against rhinoviruses. It has been investigated for the treatment of the common cold.

◊ References.
1. Hayden FG, et al. Intranasal pirodavir (R77, 975) treatment of rhinovirus colds. Antimicrob Agents Chemother 1995; 39: 290–4.

Pleconaril (3662-q)

Pleconaril (USAN, rINN).
VP-63843; Win-63843. 3-{4-[3-(3-Methyl-5-isoxazolyl)propoxy]-3,5-xylyl}-5-(trifluoromethyl)-1,2,4-oxadizole.
$C_{18}H_{18}F_3N_3O_3 = 381.3$.
CAS — 153168-05-9.

Profile

Pleconaril is an oral antiviral with activity against a range of picornaviruses. It is under investigation for the treatment of viral meningitis, upper respiratory-tract viral infections including the common cold, and other enteroviral infections.

◊ References.
1. Abdel-Rahman SM, Kearns GL. Single-dose pharmacokinetics of a pleconaril (VP63843) oral solution and effect of food. Antimicrob Agents Chemother 1998; 42: 2706–9.
2. Abdel-Rahman SM, Kearns GL. Single oral dose escalation pharmacokinetics of pleconaril (VP63843) capsules in adults. J Clin Pharmacol 1999; 39: 613–18.
3. Kearns GL, et al. Single-dose pharmacokinetics of a pleconaril (VP63843) oral solution in children and adolescents. Antimicrob Agents Chemother 1999; 43: 634–8.
4. Rogers JM, et al. Pleconaril: a broad spectrum antipicornaviral agent. Adv Exp Med Biol 1999; 458: 69–76.
5. Schmugge M, et al. Chronic enteroviral meningo-encephalitis in X-linked agammaglobulinaemia: favourable response to anti-enteroviral treatment. Eur J Pediatr 1999; 158: 1010–11.
6. Kearns GL, et al. Single dose pharmacokinetics of pleconaril in neonates. Pediatr Infect Dis J 2000; 19: 833–9.
7. Nowak-Wegrzyn A, et al. Successful treatment of enterovirus infection with the use of pleconaril in 2 infants with severe combined immunodeficiency. Clin Infect Dis 2001; 32: E13–E14.
8. Rotbart HA, Webster AD. Treatment of potentially life-threatening enterovirus infections with pleconaril. Clin Infect Dis 2001; 32: 228–35.

Poly I.poly C12U (3322-w)

Poly(I):poly(C_{12},U).

Profile

Poly I.poly C12U is a synthetic mismatched polymer of double-stranded RNA with antiviral and immunomodulatory activity. It is under investigation in the treatment of AIDS and HIV infection, and also in renal cell carcinoma, chronic fatigue syndrome, invasive melanoma, and hepatitis B and C.

For a reference to the enhancement by poly I.poly C12U of zidovudine's anti-HIV activity in vitro, see Microbiological Interactions under Antiviral Action of Zidovudine, p.647.

◊ References.
1. Carter WA, et al. Clinical, immunological, and virological effects of Ampligen, a mismatched double-stranded RNA, in patients with AIDS or AIDS-related complex. Lancet 1987; i: 1286–92.
2. Strayer DR, et al. A controlled clinical trial with a specifically configured RNA drug, poly(I).poly(C12U), in chronic fatigue syndrome. Clin Infect Dis 1994; 18 (suppl 1): S88–S95.
3. Thompson KA, et al. Results of a double-blind placebo-controlled study of the double-stranded RNA drug polyI:polyC12U in the treatment of HIV infection. Eur J Clin Microbiol Infect Dis 1996; 15: 580–7.

Propagermanium (14652-g)

Propagermanium (rINN).

A polymer obtained from 3-(trihydroxygermyl)propionic acid. $(C_3H_5GeO_{3.5})_n$.

Profile

Propagermanium is an immunomodulator which has been used in chronic hepatitis B infections. Acute exacerbation of hepatitis, including some fatalities, has been reported in patients receiving propagermanium.

Preparations

Proprietary Preparations (details are given in Part 3)

Jpn: Serocion†.

Resiquimod (20638-z)

Resiquimod (rINN).

R-848.   4-Amino-2-(ethoxymethyl)-α,α-dimethyl-1H-imidazo[4,5-c]quinoline-1-ethanol.
$C_{17}H_{22}N_4O_2 = 314.4$.
CAS — 144875-48-9.

Profile

Resiquimod is an immune response modifier under investigation for the topical treatment of genital herpes.

◊ References.

1. Spruance SL, *et al.* Application of a topical immune response modifier, resiquimod gel, to modify the recurrence rate of recurrent genital herpes: a pilot study. *J Infect Dis* 2001; **184:** 196–200.

Ribavirin (1685-r)

Ribavirin (USAN, rINN).

ICN-1229; Tribavirin (BAN). 1-β-D-Ribofuranosyl-1H-1,2,4-triazole-3-carboxamide.
$C_8H_{12}N_4O_5 = 244.2$.
CAS — 36791-04-5.
ATC — J05AB04.

Pharmacopoeias. In *Br.* and *US.*

Pharmacopoeial description

BP 2001: A white crystalline powder. Freely soluble in water; slightly soluble in alcohol. Protect from light.

USP 25: A white crystalline powder. Freely soluble in water; slightly soluble in dehydrated alcohol. Store in airtight containers.

Adverse Effects

When given *by inhalation* ribavirin has sometimes led to deterioration in pulmonary function, bacterial pneumonia, and pneumothorax, to adverse effects on the cardiovascular system (including a fall in blood pressure and cardiac arrest), and, rarely, to anaemia and reticulocytosis. Conjunctivitis and skin rash have also occurred. Precipitation of inhaled ribavirin and consequent accumulation of fluid in the tubing has occurred in ventilating equipment being used during the period of treatment.

Patients receiving ribavirin *by mouth* have experienced haemolytic anaemia, sometimes with associated increased serum concentrations of bilirubin and uric acid. Other effects that have been reported include reticulocytosis, anorexia, dyspepsia, nausea, dizziness, insomnia, irritability, dyspnoea, pharyngitis, skin rashes, and pruritus.

◊ Report of damage to a nurse's soft contact lenses following intermittent occupational exposure to ribavirin over a period of 1 month.[1]

1. Diamond SA, Dupuis LL. Contact lens damage due to ribavirin exposure. *DICP Ann Pharmacother* 1989; **23:** 428–9.

Precautions

SPECIFIC CAUTIONS FOR ORAL TREATMENT. Ribavirin should not be administered by mouth to patients with pre-existing medical conditions that could be exacerbated by ribavirin-induced haemolysis including unstable cardiac disease or haemoglobinopathies (thalassaemia or sickle-cell anaemia). Blood cell counts and chemistry should be measured at the start of treatment, after 2 and 4 weeks of treatment, and periodically thereafter. Patients with renal impairment and a creatinine clearance of less than 50 mL per minute should not receive oral ribavirin. It should be avoided in patients with severe hepatic impairment

The symbol † denotes a preparation no longer actively marketed

or decompensated cirrhosis of the liver. The potential for development of gout should be considered in predisposed patients.

Ribavirin has been reported to be teratogenic in *animals* and is contra-indicated in pregnancy or in those who may become pregnant. Pregnancy should also be avoided in partners of male patients taking ribavirin orally. The UK manufacturer recommends that effective contraception should be used for 4 months after the end of treatment in women and 7 months after the end of treatment in men. Male patients whose partner is pregnant should use a condom to minimise vaginal exposure to ribavirin.

SPECIFIC CAUTIONS FOR INHALED TREATMENT. Standard supportive respiratory and fluid management should be maintained during aerosol treatment with ribavirin and electrolytes should be monitored closely. Administration equipment should be monitored for precipitation of ribavirin. Precautions should be taken to minimise atmospheric pollution with ribavirin during aerosol administration. Pregnant women and those planning pregnancy should avoid exposure to the aerosol.

Antiviral Action

Ribavirin inhibits a wide variety of viruses *in vitro* and in *animal* models. However, this activity has not necessarily correlated with activity against human infections. Ribavirin is phosphorylated but its mode of action is still unclear; it may act at several sites, including cellular enzymes, to interfere with viral nucleic acid synthesis. The mono- and triphosphate derivatives are believed to be responsible for the antiviral activity of the compound. Susceptible DNA viruses include herpesviruses, adenoviruses, and poxviruses. Susceptible RNA viruses include Lassa virus, members of the bunyaviridae group, influenza, parainfluenza, measles, mumps, and respiratory syncytial viruses, and human immunodeficiency virus (HIV).

Microbiological interactions. Ribavirin and *zidovudine* inhibited each others' antiviral activity *in vitro*.[1]

1. Vogt MW, *et al.* Ribavirin antagonizes the effect of azidothymidine on HIV replication. *Science* 1987; **235:** 1376–9.

Pharmacokinetics

Ribavirin is rapidly absorbed following oral administration and peak blood concentrations have been reported within 1 to 2 hours. Bioavailability following oral administration is about 50% as a result of first-pass metabolism. Steady-state plasma concentrations are achieved after about 4 weeks with twice-daily oral doses. Ribavirin is also absorbed from the respiratory tract following inhalation. Ribavirin crosses the blood-brain barrier and at steady state concentrations in the CSF are 70% or more of those in the plasma. Accumulation occurs in the red blood cells and ribavirin is detectable in sperm. Ribavirin undergoes phosphorylation by cellular enzymes to the mono-, di-, and triphosphate derivatives. Distribution and elimination is triphasic. The β-phase half-life is about 2 hours, and the terminal elimination half-life is reported to be 20 to 50 hours depending on the sampling time. Ribavirin is mainly excreted in the urine as unchanged drug and metabolites. Insignificant amounts of the drug are removed by haemodialysis. Ribavirin is still detectable in the plasma for up to 4 weeks after cessation of therapy.

◊ References.

1. Crumpacker C, *et al.* Ribavirin enters cerebrospinal fluid. *Lancet* 1986; **ii:** 45–6.
2. Laskin OL, *et al.* Ribavirin disposition in high-risk patients for acquired immunodeficiency syndrome. *Clin Pharmacol Ther* 1987; **41:** 546–55.
3. Roberts RB, *et al.* Ribavirin pharmacodynamics in high-risk patients for acquired immunodeficiency syndrome. *Clin Pharmacol Ther* 1987; **42:** 365–73.
4. Paroni R, *et al.* Pharmacokinetics of ribavirin and urinary excretion of the major metabolite 1,2,4-triazole-3-carboxamide in normal volunteers. *Int J Clin Pharmacol Ther Toxicol* 1989; **27:** 302–7.

5. Kramer TH, *et al.* Hemodialysis clearance of intravenously administered ribavirin. *Antimicrob Agents Chemother* 1990; **34:** 489–90.
6. Connor E, *et al.* Safety, tolerance, and pharmacokinetics of systemic ribavirin in children with human immunodeficiency virus infection. *Antimicrob Agents Chemother* 1993; **37:** 532–9.
7. Glue P, *et al.* The single dose pharmacokinetics of ribavirin in subjects with chronic liver disease. *Br J Clin Pharmacol* 2000; **49:** 417–21.

Uses and Administration

Ribavirin is a synthetic nucleoside analogue structurally related to guanine. It is administered by aerosol in the treatment of respiratory syncytial virus infections (p.612); this route appears to give better results than the oral route although its efficacy by any route is questionable. It is used in combination with interferon alfa-2b (or peginterferon alfa-2b) in the treatment of chronic hepatitis C unresponsive to interferon alone (p.605). Ribavirin has been tried in haemorrhagic fever with renal syndrome and in other types of haemorrhagic fever including Lassa fever.

Preparations of ribavirin are available for aerosol administration to infants and children with *severe respiratory syncytial virus infections* via a small particle aerosol generator. Solutions containing 20 mg per mL are used; over a 12- to 18-hour period 300 mL, representing 6 g of ribavirin, are delivered by aerosol at an average concentration of 190 μg per litre of air. Treatment is for 3 to 7 days.

For the treatment of *chronic hepatitis C* refractory to interferon alone, ribavirin is given daily by mouth in doses determined according to body-weight. In the UK, the dose of ribavirin is 400 mg twice daily, in the morning and evening, for patients up to 65 kg body-weight; 400 mg in the morning and 600 mg in the evening for those between 65 and 85 kg; and 600 mg twice daily, in the morning and evening, for those over 85 kg. In the USA, the dose is 400 mg (in patients up to 75 kg) or 600 mg (in patients over 75 kg) in the morning, and 600 mg in the evening (regardless of body-weight). Treatment is continued for at least 6 months, in combination with interferon alfa-2b 3 million units by subcutaneous injection 3 times weekly or peginterferon alfa-2b 1.5 μg per kg per week. Dose reductions of ribavirin may be necessary in patients who develop low haemoglobin concentrations.

Encephalitis. A beneficial response to ribavirin was reported in a child with severe La Crosse encephalitis.[1] Ribavirin was given intravenously in a dose of 25 mg per kg body-weight over the first 24 hours and then reduced to 15 mg per kg daily for a further 9 days.

1. McJunkin JE, *et al.* Treatment of severe La Crosse encephalitis with intravenous ribavirin following diagnosis by brain biopsy. *Pediatrics* 1997; **99:** 261–7.

Haemorrhagic fevers. The treatment of haemorrhagic fevers (p.605) is primarily symptomatic. However, ribavirin has been reported to reduce mortality in patients with Lassa fever,[1] haemorrhagic fever with renal syndrome,[2] and possibly Crimean-Congo haemorrhagic fever[3] and Bolivian haemorrhagic fever.[4] Ribavirin has also been tried in the related hantavirus pulmonary syndrome,[5,6] but preliminary results did not indicate an improvement in mortality.[7]

For treatment of *Lassa fever*, ribavirin has been given intravenously in a dose of 2 g initially, then 1 g every 6 hours for 4 days, then 500 mg every 8 hours for 6 days.[1] Treatment is most effective if instituted within 6 days of the onset of fever. Experience has shown that rigors may occur if the drug is given as a bolus injection, but that this can be overcome by giving it as an infusion over 30 minutes.[8] For prophylaxis, a dose of ribavirin 600 mg by mouth 4 times daily for 10 days has been suggested for adults,[9] although this was considered to be excessive by other commentators[10] who suggested that oral doses of 1 g daily (following an intravenous loading dose for those in whom the start of prophylaxis is delayed) might be suitable.

1. McCormick JB, *et al.* Lassa fever: effective therapy with ribavirin. *N Engl J Med* 1986; **314:** 20–6.
2. Huggins JW, *et al.* Prospective, double-blind, concurrent, placebo-controlled clinical trial of intravenous ribavirin therapy of hemorrhagic fever with renal syndrome. *J Infect Dis* 1991; **164:** 1119–27.
3. Fisher-Hoch SP, *et al.* Crimean Congo-haemorrhagic fever treated with oral ribavirin. *Lancet* 1995; **346:** 472–5.
4. Kilgore PE, *et al.* Treatment of Bolivian hemorrhagic fever with intravenous ribavirin. *Clin Infect Dis* 1997; **24:** 718–22.
5. Anonymous. Hantavirus pulmonary syndrome—northeastern United States, 1994. *JAMA* 1994; **272:** 997–8.
6. Prochoda K, *et al.* Hantavirus-associated acute respiratory failure. *N Engl J Med* 1993; **329:** 1744.

7. Khan AS, *et al.* Hantavirus pulmonary syndrome. *Lancet* 1996; **347:** 739–41.
8. Fisher-Hoch SP, *et al.* Unexpected adverse reactions during a clinical trial in rural West Africa. *Antiviral Res* 1992; **19:** 139–47.
9. Holmes GP, *et al.* Lassa fever in the United States: investigation of a case and new guidelines for management. *N Engl J Med* 1990; **323:** 1120–23.
10. Johnson KM, Monath TP. Imported Lassa fever—reexamining the algorithms. *N Engl J Med* 1990; **323:** 1139–41.

Preparations

BP 2000: Tribavirin Solution for Nebulisation;
BP 2001: Ribavirin Nebuliser Solution;
USP 25: Ribavirin for Inhalation Solution.

Proprietary Preparations (details are given in Part 3)

Aust.: Rebetol; **Austral.:** Virazide; **Belg.:** Virazole; **Canad.:** Virazole; **Denm.:** Rebetol; **Fin.:** Rebetol; **Fr.:** Rebetol; **Ger.:** Rebetol; Virazole; **Hong Kong:** Virazole; **Irl.:** Rebetol; **Ital.:** Rebetol; Viramid†; **Mex.:** Vilona; Virazide; **Neth.:** Rebetol; Virazole†; **Port.:** Rebetol; **Singapore:** Virazole; **Spain:** Rebetol; Virazid; **Swed.:** Rebetol; Virazole; **UK:** Rebetol; Virazole; **USA:** Virazole.

Multi-ingredient: *Austral.:* Rebetron; *Canad.:* Rebetron; *Switz.:* Intron A/Rebetol; *USA:* Rebetron.

Rimantadine Hydrochloride (1686-f)

Rimantadine Hydrochloride (*BANM, USAN, rINNM*).
EXP-126. (*RS*)-1-(Adamantan-1-yl)ethylamine hydrochloride; α-Methyl-1-adamantanemethylamine hydrochloride.
$C_{12}H_{21}N,HCl = 215.8$.
CAS — 13392-28-4 (rimantadine); 1501-84-4 (rimantadine hydrochloride).

Adverse Effects and Precautions

The incidence and severity of adverse effects associated with rimantadine appear to be low. Those reported include gastrointestinal disturbances such as nausea, vomiting, and anorexia and CNS effects such as headache, insomnia, nervousness, lightheadedness, and concentration difficulties. It should be given with caution to patients with epilepsy. Doses are reduced in severe renal or hepatic impairment; reduced doses are also used in the elderly.

◊ A review[1] of clinical studies in healthy subjects concluded that rimantadine and amantadine were equally effective for prevention and treatment of influenza A, but rimantadine was significantly better tolerated than amantadine at usual doses.

In a study to evaluate the safety of long-term rimantadine hydrochloride for elderly, chronically ill individuals during an influenza A epidemic,[2] a significantly greater proportion of patients taking rimantadine developed anxiety and/or nausea compared with those taking placebo. There was also a significantly greater number of days in which anxiety, nausea, confusion, depression, or vomiting were reported. Most of these side-effects lasted less than 9 days and were seldom severe except in 2 patients who withdrew from the study because of insomnia, anxiety, or both and a third who suffered a generalised convulsion. In a larger study[3] the incidence of these symptoms was similar in treatment and placebo groups.

Observations of seizures in 2 patients receiving influenza prophylaxis with rimantadine hydrochloride emphasised that chronically ill and elderly patients prone to seizures (especially those who may have had antiepileptic therapy withdrawn) may be at risk of developing seizures.[4] A precautionary measure of reducing the rimantadine hydrochloride dosage to 100 mg daily together with temporary re-introduction of antiepileptics was suggested.

1. Jefferson TO, *et al.* Amantadine and rimantadine for preventing and treating influenza A in adults (updated 18 July 2001). Available in The Cochrane Library; Issue 4. Oxford: Update Software; 2001.
2. Patriarca PA, *et al.* Safety of prolonged administration of rimantadine hydrochloride in the prophylaxis of influenza A virus infections in nursing homes. *Antimicrob Agents Chemother* 1984; **26:** 101–3.
3. Monto AS, *et al.* Safety and efficacy of long-term use of rimantadine for prophylaxis of type A influenza in nursing homes. *Antimicrob Agents Chemother* 1995; **39:** 2224–8.
4. Bentley DW, *et al.* Rimantadine and seizures. *Ann Intern Med* 1989; **110:** 323–4.

Antiviral Action

Rimantadine inhibits influenza A viruses, probably at an early stage of replication.

Resistance to rimantadine can be induced in influenza A virus *in vitro* and *in vivo* although resistance in clinical isolates is reported to occur infrequently. Transmission of rimantadine-resistant influenza A virus has been found among household contacts, and young children treated for established influenza A infection may excrete resistant virus within a week of beginning treatment.

◊ References to rimantadine resistance in influenza A virus.

1. Hall CB, *et al.* Children with influenza A infection: treatment with rimantadine. *Pediatrics* 1987; **80:** 275–82.
2. Belshe RB, *et al.* Genetic basis of resistance to rimantadine emerging during treatment of influenza virus infection. *J Virol* 1988; **62:** 1508–12.
3. Belshe RB, *et al.* Resistance of influenza A virus to amantadine and rimantadine: results of one decade of surveillance. *J Infect Dis* 1989; **159:** 430–5.
4. Hayden FG, *et al.* Emergence and apparent transmission of rimantadine-resistant influenza A virus in families. *N Engl J Med* 1989; **321:** 1696–1702.
5. Ziegler T, *et al.* Low incidence of rimantadine resistance in field isolates of influenza A viruses. *J Infect Dis* 1999; **180:** 935–9.

Pharmacokinetics

Rimantadine hydrochloride is well, but slowly, absorbed from the gastrointestinal tract. Maximum plasma concentrations are reached 3 to 6 hours after administration. It has a long plasma half-life; reported figures range from 24 to 36 hours. Protein binding of rimantadine is about 40%. The elimination half-life following a single dose is 13 to 65 hours in healthy subjects. It is extensively metabolised with less than 25% of a dose being excreted unchanged in the urine; about 75% is excreted as hydroxylated metabolites over 72 hours. In severe renal or hepatic impairment the half-life approximately doubles, necessitating a dosage reduction.

◊ References.

1. Wills RJ, *et al.* Rimantadine pharmacokinetics after single and multiple doses. *Antimicrob Agents Chemother* 1987; **31:** 826–8.
2. Anderson EL, *et al.* Pharmacokinetics of a single dose of rimantadine in young adults and children. *Antimicrob Agents Chemother* 1987; **31:** 1140–2.

Uses and Administration

Rimantadine hydrochloride is used similarly to amantadine hydrochloride (p.1161) in the prophylaxis and treatment of influenza A infections (p.611). It is given in usual adult doses of 200 mg daily by mouth in divided doses. Children may be given 5 mg per kg body-weight daily, up to a maximum of 150 mg. In elderly patients and in those with severe renal or hepatic impairment the usual daily dose is 100 mg.

◊ Reviews.

1. Jefferson TO, *et al.* Amantadine and rimantadine for preventing and treating influenza A in adults (updated 18 July 2001). Available in The Cochrane Library; Issue 4. Oxford: Update Software; 2001.

Preparations

Proprietary Preparations (details are given in Part 3)
Israel: Flumadine; *USA:* Flumadine.

Ritonavir (17872-t)

Ritonavir (*BAN, USAN, rINN*).
A-84538; Abbott-84538; ABJ-538. 5-Thiazolylmethyl {(αS)-α-[(1S,3S)-1-hydroxy-3-((2S)-2-{3-[(2-isopropyl-4-thiazolyl)methyl]-3-methylureido}-3-methylbutyramido)-4-phenylbutyl]phenethyl}carbamate; N¹-[(1S,3S,4S)-1-Benzyl-3-hydroxy-5-phenyl-4-(1,3-thiazol-5-ylmethoxycarbonylamino)pentyl]-N²-{[(2-isopropyl-1,3-thiazol-4-yl)methyl](methyl)carbamoyl}-L-valinamide.
$C_{37}H_{48}N_6O_5S_2 = 720.9$.
CAS — 155213-67-5.
ATC — J05AE03.

Adverse Effects and Precautions

As for HIV-protease inhibitors in general (see Indinavir Sulfate, p.625). Vasodilatation has been commonly associated with ritonavir, and syncope and orthostatic hypotension have been reported. Pancreatitis has occurred in patients receiving ritonavir, and has been associated with hypertriglyceridaemia. Additional adverse effects reported with ritonavir include dyspepsia, dry mouth, ulceration of the oral mucosa, throat irritation and cough, hyperaesthesia, seizures, anxiety, sweating, and fever. Allergic reactions, rarely anaphylaxis, have been associated with ritonavir. There may be increases in uric acid concentrations and decreased free and total thyroxine concentrations. Neutrophil counts may be reduced or increased.

Ritonavir treatment should be discontinued in patients developing pancreatitis.

Interactions

Interactions involving HIV-protease inhibitors are discussed under Indinavir Sulfate, p.626. Ritonavir is reported to have a high affinity for several cytochrome P450 isoenzymes with the following ranked order:

$$CYP3A > CYP2D6 > CYP2C9$$

Oral liquid formulations of ritonavir currently contain alcohol and concurrent administration with disulfiram or metronidazole should be avoided.

Antiviral Action

As for HIV-protease inhibitors in general (see Indinavir Sulfate, p.627).

Pharmacokinetics

Ritonavir is absorbed following oral administration and peak plasma concentrations occur in about 2 to 4 hours. Absorption is enhanced when ritonavir is taken with food, and is dose-related. Protein binding is reported to be about 98% and penetration into the CNS is minimal. Ritonavir is extensively metabolised in the liver principally by cytochrome P450 isoenzymes CYP3A and CYP2D6. The major metabolite has antiviral activity, but concentrations in plasma are low. Ritonavir is mainly excreted in the faeces, with a half-life of 3 to 5 hours.

◊ References.

1. Hsu A, *et al.* Multiple-dose pharmacokinetics of ritonavir in human immunodeficiency virus-infected subjects. *Antimicrob Agents Chemother* 1997; **41:** 898–905.

Uses and Administration

Ritonavir is a protease inhibitor with antiviral activity against HIV (see Antiviral Action, under Indinavir, p.627). It is used in combination with other antiretrovirals for the treatment of HIV infection (p.608).

Ritonavir is given by mouth in an adult dose of 600 mg twice daily with food. In order to minimise nausea, ritonavir may be started at a dose of 300 mg twice daily and gradually increased over a period of up to 14 days by 100 mg twice daily to a total of 600 mg twice daily. Children over the age of 2 years may be given an initial dose of ritonavir of 250 mg per m^2 body-surface twice daily increasing by 50 mg per m^2 twice daily at 2- or 3-day intervals up to 350 to 400 mg per m^2 twice daily, but not exceeding 600 mg twice daily.

◊ Reviews.

1. Lea AP, Faulds D. Ritonavir. *Drugs* 1996; **52:** 541–6.
2. Hsu A, *et al.* Ritonavir: clinical pharmacokinetics and interactions with other anti-HIV agents. *Clin Pharmacokinet* 1998; **35:** 275–91.

Administration. Adjusting the dosage regimen for ritonavir from 600 mg twice daily to 300 mg every 6 hours improved tolerability in two patients who would otherwise have discontinued the drug.[1]

1. Merry C, *et al.* Improved tolerability of ritonavir derived from pharmacokinetic principles. *Br J Clin Pharmacol* 1996; **42:** 787.

Molluscum contagiosum. Intractable molluscum contagiosum, a viral skin infection, resolved when a patient was given ritonavir for treatment of HIV infection.[1]

1. Hicks CB, *et al.* Resolution of intractable molluscum contagiosum in a human immunodeficiency virus-infected patient after institution of antiretroviral therapy with ritonavir. *Clin Infect Dis* 1997; **24:** 1023–5.

Preparations

Proprietary Preparations (details are given in Part 3)
Austral.: Norvir; *Belg.:* Norvir; *Canad.:* Norvir; *Denm.:* Norvir; *Fin.:* Norvir; *Fr.:* Norvir; *Ger.:* Norvir; *Hong Kong:* Norvir; *Israel:* Norvir; *Ital.:* Norvir; *Jpn:* Norvir; *Mex.:* Norvir; *Neth.:* Norvir; *Norw.:* Norvir; *NZ:* Norvir; *Port.:* Norvir; *S.Afr.:* Norvir; *Spain:* Norvir; *Swed.:* Norvir; *Switz.:* Norvir; *Thai.:* Norvir; *UK:* Norvir; *USA:* Norvir.

Multi-ingredient: *UK:* Kaletra; *USA:* Kaletra.

Saquinavir (13846-p)

Saquinavir (BAN, USAN, rINN).

Ro-31-8959. N^1-{(1S,2R)-1-Benzyl-3-[(3S,4aS,8aS)-3-(tert-butylcarbamoyl)perhydroisoquinolin-2-yl]-2-hydroxypropyl}-N^2-(2-quinolylcarbonyl)-L-aspartamide; (S)-N-[(αS)-α-{(1R)-2-[(3S,4aS,8aS)-3-(tert-Butylcarbamoyl)octahydro-2(1H)-isoquinolyl]-1-hydroxyethyl}phenethyl]-2-quinaldamidosuccinamide.

$C_{38}H_{50}N_6O_5 = 670.8$.

CAS — 127779-20-8.

ATC — J05AE01.

Saquinavir Mesilate (17244-j)

Saquinavir Mesilate (BANM, rINNM).

Ro-31-8959/003; Saquinavir Mesylate (USAN). Saquinavir methanesulfonate.

$C_{38}H_{50}N_6O_5,CH_4O_3S = 766.9$.

CAS — 149845-06-7.

Pharmacopoeias. In US.

Pharmacopoeial description

USP 25: Store in airtight containers.

Adverse Effects and Precautions

As for HIV-protease inhibitors in general (see Indinavir Sulfate, p.625). Stevens-Johnson syndrome, nephrolithiasis, and pancreatitis (in some cases fatal) have possibly been associated with saquinavir. Additional adverse effects reported with saquinavir include ulceration of the oral mucosa, depression, seizures, and peripheral neuropathy. Allergic reactions have been associated with saquinavir. Acute haemolytic anaemia has occurred.

Bioavailability of some formulations of saquinavir is reported to be low owing to a combination of incomplete absorption and extensive first-pass metabolism; it may therefore be particularly susceptible to malabsorption (e.g. in the presence of diarrhoea).

Interactions

Interactions involving HIV-protease inhibitors are discussed under Indinavir Sulfate, p.626.

Saquinavir is reported to be metabolised by the cytochrome P450 system, with the specific isoenzyme CYP3A4 responsible for more than 90% of the hepatic metabolism.

Antiviral Action

As for HIV-protease inhibitors in general (see Indinavir Sulfate, p.627). HIV isolates resistant to saquinavir are reported to show cross-resistance to at least one other HIV-protease inhibitor in a proportion of patients.

Resistance. References.
1. Ives KJ, et al. Emergence of resistant variants of HIV in vivo during monotherapy with the proteinase inhibitor saquinavir. J Antimicrob Chemother 1997; 39: 771–9.

Pharmacokinetics

Saquinavir is absorbed to a limited extent (about 30%) following oral administration of saquinavir mesilate and undergoes extensive first-pass hepatic metabolism, resulting in a bioavailability of 4% when taken with food. Bioavailability is greater from a soft gelatin capsule formulation of saquinavir base in a suitable vehicle (Fortovase, Roche, UK) than from the hard capsule formulation (Invirase, Roche, UK). Bioavailability is substantially less when saquinavir is taken in the fasting state. Plasma concentrations are reported to be higher in HIV-infected patients than in healthy subjects. Saquinavir is about 98% bound to plasma proteins and extensively distributed into the tissues, although CNS concentrations are reported to be negligible. It is rapidly metabolised by the cytochrome P450 system (specifically the isoenzyme CYP3A4) to a number of inactive monohydroxylated and dihydroxylated compounds. It is excreted predominantly in the faeces with a reported terminal elimination half-life of 13.2 hours.

◊ References.
1. Regazzi MB, et al. Pharmacokinetic variability and strategy for therapeutic drug monitoring of saquinavir (SQV) in HIV-1 infected individuals. Br J Clin Pharmacol 1999; 47: 379–82.

Uses and Administration

Saquinavir is a protease inhibitor with antiviral activity against HIV (see Antiviral Action, under Indinavir, p.627). It is used, in combination with other antiretrovirals, for the treatment of HIV infection (p.608).

Saquinavir is given by mouth as the mesilate (Invirase, Roche, UK), but doses are expressed in terms of the base. It is given in an adult dose of 600 mg three times daily after meals. Despite the greater bioavailability of saquinavir base formulated as soft gelatin capsules, this formulation (Fortovase, Roche, UK) is nevertheless given in a higher dose of 1200 mg three times daily after meals.

◊ Reviews.
1. Noble S, Faulds D. Saquinavir: a review of its pharmacology and clinical potential in the management of HIV infection. Drugs 1996; 52: 93–112.
2. Moyle G. Saquinavir in the management of HIV infection. Br J Hosp Med 1997; 57: 560–4.
3. Vella S, Floridia M. Saquinavir: clinical pharmacology and efficacy. Clin Pharmacokinet 1998; 34: 189–201.

Administration. A soft gelatin capsule formulation of saquinavir has been developed to overcome some of the problems associated with the low bioavailability of the conventional formulation.[1]
1. Figgitt DP, Plosker GL. Saquinavir soft-gel capsule: an updated review of its use in the management of HIV infection. Drugs 2000; 60: 481–516.

Preparations

USP 25: Saquinavir Capsules.

Proprietary Preparations (details are given in Part 3)

Aust.: Fortovase; Invirase; Austral.: Fortovase; Invirase; Belg.: Fortovase; Invirase; Canad.: Fortovase; Invirase; Denm.: Fortovase; Invirase; Fin.: Fortovase; Invirase; Fr.: Fortovase; Invirase; Ger.: Fortovase; Invirase; Hong Kong: Invirase; Irl.: Invirase; Israel: Invirase; Ital.: Fortovase; Invirase; Jpn.: Invirase; Mex.: Invirase; Neth.: Fortovase; Invirase; Norw.: Invirase; NZ: Fortovase; Invirase; Port.: Fortovase; Invirase†; S.Afr.: Invirase; Singapore: Invirase; Spain: Fortovase; Invirase; Swed.: Fortovase; Invirase; Switz.: Fortovase; Invirase; Thai.: Fortovase; Invirase; UK: Fortovase; Invirase; USA: Fortovase; Invirase.

Sorivudine (18871-m)

Sorivudine (BAN, USAN, rINN).

Bravavir; Bromovinylarauracil; Brovavir; BV-araU; BVAU; SQ-32756; YN-72. (E)-1-β-D-Arabinofuranosyl-5-(2-bromovinyl)uracil.

$C_{11}H_{13}BrN_2O_6 = 349.1$.

CAS — 77181-69-2.

Profile

Sorivudine is a synthetic thymidine derivative with antiviral activity against varicella-zoster virus. It has been investigated for the treatment of herpes zoster but has been withdrawn from the market in Japan following deaths in patients receiving fluorouracil concomitantly.

◊ References.
1. Yawata M. Deaths due to drug interaction. Lancet 1993; 342: 1166.
2. Diasio RB. Sorivudine and 5-fluorouracil: a clinically significant drug-drug interaction due to inhibition of dihydropyrimidine dehydrogenase. Br J Clin Pharmacol 1998; 46: 1–4.

Stavudine (15405-f)

Stavudine (BAN, USAN, pINN).

BMY-27857; d4T. 1-(2,3-Dideoxy-β-D-glycero-pent-2-enofuranosyl)thymine.

$C_{10}H_{12}N_2O_4 = 224.2$.

CAS — 3056-17-5.

ATC — J05AF04.

Adverse Effects

Stavudine produces dose-related peripheral neuropathy. Raised liver enzyme concentrations may also occur during treatment. Pancreatitis has been reported and fatalities have occurred.

Other adverse effects noted in patients taking stavudine have included asthenia, chest pain, hypersensitivity reactions, and an influenza-like syndrome; dizziness, headache, and insomnia; abdominal pain, anorexia, constipation, diarrhoea, nausea, and vomiting; neutropenia and thrombocytopenia; arthralgia and myalgia; mood changes; dyspnoea; pruritus and rashes; and lymphadenopathy and neoplasms.

Lactic acidosis, usually associated with severe hepatomegaly and steatosis, has been associated with

treatment with nucleoside reverse transcriptase inhibitors (see Zidovudine, p.645).

Effects on the nervous system. Peripheral neuropathy is a well recognised adverse effect of stavudine and has been the subject of a review.[1]
1. Moyle GJ, Sadler M. Peripheral neuropathy with nucleoside antiretrovirals: risk factors, incidence and management. Drug Safety 1998; 19: 481–94.

Gynaecomastia. Bilateral gynaecomastia was associated with stavudine administration in a patient with HIV infection who was also receiving lamivudine and co-trimoxazole.[1] Symptoms resolved when stavudine was discontinued. Four further cases of gynaecomastia were reported in HIV-infected patients receiving highly active antiretroviral therapy (HAART) regimens all involving stavudine.[2]
1. Melbourne KM, et al. Gynecomastia with stavudine treatment in an HIV-positive patient. Ann Pharmacother 1998; 32: 1108.
2. Manfredi R, et al. Gynecomastia associated with highly active antiretroviral therapy. Ann Pharmacother 2001; 35: 438–9.

Precautions

Stavudine should be used with caution in patients with a history of peripheral neuropathy and treatment suspended if peripheral neuropathy develops; if symptoms resolve on withdrawal stavudine may be resumed at half the previous dose. Treatment with stavudine may be associated with lactic acidosis and should be discontinued if there is a rapid increase in aminotransferase concentrations, progressive hepatomegaly, or metabolic or lactic acidosis of unknown aetiology. Stavudine should be given with caution to patients with hepatomegaly or other risk factors for liver disease. Patients with a history of pancreatitis should also be observed carefully for signs of pancreatitis during treatment with stavudine. Concomitant treatment with other drugs likely to cause peripheral neuropathy or pancreatitis (see Interactions, below) should be avoided if possible. Stavudine should be used with caution and doses reduced in patients with renal impairment.

Interactions

The intracellular activation of stavudine and hence its antiviral effect may be inhibited by zidovudine and doxorubicin.

Concurrent administration of stavudine with other drugs known to cause pancreatitis (e.g. intravenous pentamidine) or peripheral neuropathy (e.g. metronidazole, isoniazid, and vincristine) should be avoided if possible.

Antivirals. References to in-vivo antagonism of the antiretroviral effect of stavudine and zidovudine when used in combination.[1]
1. Havlir DV, et al. In vivo antagonism with zidovudine plus stavudine combination therapy. J Infect Dis 2000; 182: 321–5.

Phenylpropanolamine. Hypertensive crisis associated with administration of phenylpropanolamine and clemastine occurred in a patient receiving HIV prophylaxis with indinavir, lamivudine, and stavudine. The most likely cause was an interaction between phenylpropanolamine and stavudine, although interactions with the other antiretrovirals could not be ruled out.
1. Khurana V, et al. Hypertensive crisis secondary to phenylpropanolamine interacting with triple-drug therapy for HIV prophylaxis. Am J Med 1999; 106: 118–19.

Antiviral Action

Stavudine is converted intracellularly in stages to the triphosphate. This triphosphate halts the DNA synthesis of retroviruses, including HIV, through competitive inhibition of reverse transcriptase and incorporation into viral DNA. Stavudine-resistant strains of HIV have been identified and cross-resistance to other nucleoside reverse transcriptase inhibitors may occur.

Pharmacokinetics

Stavudine is absorbed rapidly following oral administration producing peak plasma concentrations within 1 hour and with a reported bioavailability of about 86%. Administration with food delays but does not reduce absorption. Stavudine crosses the blood-brain barrier producing a CSF:plasma ratio of about 0.4 after 4 hours. Binding to plasma proteins is negligible. Stavudine is metabolised intracellularly to the active antiviral triphosphate. The elimination half-life is re-

The symbol † denotes a preparation no longer actively marketed

ported to be about 1 to 1.5 hours following single or multiple doses. The intracellular half-life of stavudine triphosphate has been estimated to be 3.5 hours *in vitro*. About 40% of a dose is excreted in the urine at between 6 and 24 hours after administration by active tubular secretion and glomerular filtration. Stavudine is removed by haemodialysis.

◊ References.
1. Rana KZ, Dudley MN. Clinical pharmacokinetics of stavudine. *Clin Pharmacokinet* 1997; **33:** 276–84.
2. Kaul S, *et al.* Effect of food on bioavailability of stavudine in subjects with human immunodeficiency virus infection. *Antimicrob Agents Chemother* 1998; **42:** 2295–8.
3. Grasela DM, *et al.* Pharmacokinetics of single-dose oral stavudine in subjects with renal impairment and in subjects requiring hemodialysis. *Antimicrob Agents Chemother* 2000; **44:** 2149–53.

Uses and Administration

Stavudine is a nucleoside reverse transcriptase inhibitor related to thymidine with activity against retroviruses including HIV. It is used in the treatment of HIV infection, usually in combination with other antiretrovirals. However, use in combination with zidovudine is not recommended (see Interactions, above). Doses of stavudine are 40 mg every 12 hours by mouth for patients weighing 60 kg or more or 30 mg every 12 hours for patients weighing less than 60 kg. The dose in children over 3 months of age and weighing less than 30 kg is 1 mg per kg body-weight every 12 hours; children weighing more than 30 kg are given the adult dose.

Dosage reduction is recommended for patients with renal impairment; in patients with a creatinine clearance of 26 to 50 mL per minute, the dose is 20 mg every 12 hours (those weighing 60 kg or more) or 15 mg every 12 hours (those weighing less than 60 kg); for creatinine clearance below 25 mL per minute, the dose is 20 mg every 24 hours (those weighing 60 kg or more) or 15 mg every 24 hours (those weighing less than 60 kg).

◊ Reviews.
1. Hurst M, Noble S. Stavudine: an update of its use in the treatment of HIV infection. *Drugs* 1999; **58:** 919–49.

Preparations

Proprietary Preparations (details are given in Part 3)
Aust.: Zerit; *Austral.:* Zerit; *Belg.:* Zerit; *Braz.:* Zeritavir; *Canad.:* Zerit; *Denm.:* Zerit; *Fin.:* Zerit; *Fr.:* Zerit; *Ger.:* Zerit; *Hong Kong:* Zerit; *Irl.:* Zerit; *Israel:* Zerit; *Ital.:* Zerit; *Jpn:* Zerit; *Mex.:* Zerit; *Neth.:* Zerit; *Norw.:* Zerit; *NZ:* Zerit; *Port.:* Zerit; *S.Afr.:* Zerit; *Singapore:* Zerit; *Spain:* Zerit; *Swed.:* Zerit; *Switz.:* Zerit; *Thai.:* Zerit; *UK:* Zerit; *USA:* Zerit.

Talviraline (5671-n)

Talviraline (rINN).
HBY-097. Isopropyl (2S)-3,4-dihydro-7-methoxy-2-[(methylthio)methyl]-3-thioxo-1(2H)-quinoxalinecarboxylate.
$C_{15}H_{20}N_2O_3S_2 = 340.5$.
CAS — 169312-27-0.

Profile

Talviraline is a quinoxaline non-nucleoside reverse transcriptase inhibitor that has been investigated for the treatment of HIV infection.

Tenofovir (7211-l)

Tenofovir (BAN, USAN, rINN).
GS-1278; PMPA; (R)-PMPA. 9-[(R)-2-(Phosphonomethoxy)propyl]adenine monohydrate; {[(R)-2-(6-Amino-9H-purin-9-yl)-1-methylethoxy]methyl}phosphonic acid monohydrate.
$C_9H_{14}N_5O_4P,H_2O = 305.2$.
CAS — 147127-20-6 (anhydrous tenofovir); 206184-49-8 (tenofovir monohydrate).

Tenofovir Disoproxil Fumarate (20549-j)

Tenofovir Disoproxil Fumarate (BANM, USAN, rINNM).
GS-4331/05. 9-{(R)-2-[[Bis[[(isopropoxycarbonyl)oxy]methoxy]phosphinyl]methoxy]propyl}adenine fumarate (1:1).
$C_{19}H_{30}N_5O_{10}P,C_4H_4O_4 = 635.5$.
CAS — 202138-50-9.

Profile

Tenofovir is a nucleoside reverse transcriptase inhibitor used, in combination with other antiretrovirals, for the treatment of HIV infection. It is given by mouth in a dose of 300 mg of the disoproxil fumarate ester once daily with food. The base is given intravenously.

Lactic acidosis, sometimes fatal and usually associated with severe hepatomegaly and steatosis, has been reported in patients

receiving nucleoside reverse transcriptase inhibitors (see Zidovudine, p.645).

◊ References.
1. Deeks SG, *et al.* Safety, pharmacokinetics, and antiretroviral activity of intravenous 9-[2-(R)-(phosphonomethoxy)propyl]adenine, a novel anti-human immunodeficiency virus (HIV) therapy, in HIV-infected adults. *Antimicrob Agents Chemother* 1998; **42:** 2380–4.

Preparations

Proprietary Preparations (details are given in Part 3)
USA: Viread.

Tipranavir (20234-a)

Tipranavir (rINN).
PNU-140690; U-140690. 3'-{(1R)-1-[(6R)-5,6-Dihydro-4-hydroxy-2-oxo-6-phenethyl-6-propyl-2H-pyran-3-yl]propyl}-5-(trifluoromethyl)-2-pyridinesulfonanilide.
$C_{31}H_{33}F_3N_2O_5S = 602.7$.
CAS — 174484-41-4 (tipranavir); 191150-83-1 (tipranavir disodium).

NOTE. Tipranavir Disodium is *USAN.*

Profile

Tipranavir is an HIV-protease inhibitor under investigation, in combination with other antiretrovirals, for the treatment of HIV infection.

Tremacamra (20099-b)

Tremacamra (USAN, rINN).
BIRR-004; 1-453-Glycoprotein ICAM-1 (human reduced). 1-453-Glycoprotein ICAM-1 (human reduced).
CAS — 155576-45-7.

Profile

Tremacamra is a recombinant soluble intercellular adhesion molecule 1 (ICAM-1) under investigation for the treatment of the common cold.

◊ References.
1. Turner RB, *et al.* Efficacy of tremacamra, a soluble intercellular adhesion molecule 1, for experimental rhinovirus infection: a randomized clinical trial. *JAMA* 1999; **281:** 1797–1804.

Trichosanthin (2467-t)

Compound Q; GLQ-223 (a purified form of trichosanthin).
CAS — 60318-52-7 (trichosanthins); 116899-30-0 (Trichosanthes kirilowii); 160185-58-0 (Trichosanthes kirilowii root); 120947-28-6 (GLQ-223).

Profile

Trichosanthin is a polypeptide extracted from the tuber of the Chinese cucumber, *Trichosanthes kirilowii* (Cucurbitaceae). It is under investigation in the treatment of HIV infection and is used in China as an abortifacient.

◊ Trichosanthin has been given to patients with AIDS, AIDS-related complex, or HIV infection.[1,2] It has generally been given by intravenous injection. In one study[1] it was also given by intramuscular injection but that route was abandoned due to the occurrence of pain and necrosis at the injection site. A common adverse effect on intravenous administration was a flu-like syndrome with headache, myalgias, fever, and arthralgia and was generally mild to moderate,[3] although neurological effects progressing to coma with fatalities have been reported.[1,2] Improvements in surrogate markers for HIV infection have been reported including increases in CD4+ T lymphocyte counts in patients with moderate disease[3] and in patients failing to respond to reverse transcriptase inhibitors.[4]
1. Byers VS, *et al.* A phase I/II study of trichosanthin treatment of HIV disease. *AIDS* 1990; **4:** 1189–96.
2. Kahn JO, *et al.* The safety and pharmacokinetics of GLQ223 in subjects with AIDS and AIDS-related complex: a phase I study. *AIDS* 1990; **4:** 1197–1204.
3. Kahn JO, *et al.* Safety, activity, and pharmacokinetics of GLQ223 in patients with AIDS and AIDS-related complex. *Antimicrob Agents Chemother* 1994; **38:** 260–7.
4. Byers VS, *et al.* A phase II study of effect of addition of trichosanthin to zidovudine in patients with HIV disease and failing antiretroviral agents. *AIDS Res Hum Retroviruses* 1994; **10:** 413–20.

Trifluridine (1688-n)

Trifluridine (USAN, rINN).
F_3TDR; F_3T; NSC-75520; Trifluorothymidine. ααα-Trifluorothymidine; 2'-Deoxy-5-trifluoromethyluridine.
$C_{10}H_{11}F_3N_2O_5 = 296.2$.
CAS — 70-00-8.
ATC — S01AD02.
Pharmacopoeias. In *US.*

Pharmacopoeial description

USP 25: A white, odourless powder, appearing under the microscope as rod-like crystals. Store in airtight containers. Protect from light.

Adverse Effects

Adverse effects occurring after the use of trifluridine in the eyes are similar to those for idoxuridine (p.625) but have been reported to occur less frequently.

◊ References.
1. Udell IJ. Trifluridine-associated conjunctival cicatrization. *Am J Ophthalmol* 1985; **99:** 363–4.

Antiviral Action

Trifluridine acts similarly to idoxuridine to interfere with viral DNA synthesis following phosphorylation. It is reported to be active against herpes simplex viruses, some adenoviruses, vaccinia viruses, and cytomegalovirus. Like idoxuridine it is incorporated into mammalian DNA.

Pharmacokinetics

Trifluridine is absorbed through the cornea following ocular administration and penetration may be increased in the presence of damage or inflammation. Systemic absorption does not appear to follow ocular administration.

Uses and Administration

Trifluridine is a pyrimidine nucleoside structurally related to thymidine. It is used in the treatment of primary keratoconjunctivitis and recurrent epithelial keratitis due to herpes simplex viruses. One drop of a 1% ophthalmic solution is instilled into the eye every 2 hours up to a maximum of 9 times daily until complete re-epithelialisation has occurred. Treatment is then reduced to one drop every 4 hours to a minimum of 5 drops daily for a further 7 days.

◊ Reviews.
1. Heidelberger C, King DH. Trifluorothymidine. *Pharmacol Ther* 1979; **6:** 427–42.
2. Carmine AA, *et al.* Trifluridine: a review of its antiviral activity and therapeutic use in the topical treatment of viral eye infections. *Drugs* 1982; **23:** 329–53.

Herpes simplex infections. Trifluridine may be used as an alternative to topical aciclovir in ocular herpes simplex infections (p.607). It has been used in combination with a corticosteroid for herpes simplex stromal keratitis.[1]

Trifluridine produced varied improvement when applied topically in combination with interferon alfa in 3 AIDS patients with mucocutaneous herpes unresponsive to aciclovir (and to foscarnet in 2).[2] A pilot study in AIDS patients indicated that topical trifluridine alone might be of benefit for aciclovir-resistant mucocutaneous herpes simplex.[3]
1. Wilhelmus KR, *et al.* Herpetic eye disease study: a controlled trial of topical corticosteroids for herpes simplex stromal keratitis. *Ophthalmology* 1994; **101:** 1883–96.
2. Birch CJ, *et al.* Clinical effects and in vitro studies of trifluorothymidine combined with interferon-α for treatment of drug-resistant and -sensitive herpes simplex virus infections. *J Infect Dis* 1992; **166:** 108–12.
3. Kessler HA, *et al.* Pilot study of topical trifluridine for the treatment of acyclovir-resistant mucocutaneous herpes simplex disease in patients with AIDS (ACTG 172). *J Acquir Immune Defic Syndr Hum Retrovirol* 1996; **12:** 147–52.

Preparations

Proprietary Preparations (details are given in Part 3)
Belg.: TFT Ophtiole; *Braz.:* Zost; *Canad.:* Viroptic; *Fr.:* Triherpine; Virophta; *Ger.:* TFT; Triflumann; *Hong Kong:* Bephen; Triherpine; *Ital.:* Triherpine; *Neth.:* TFT Ophtiole; *Port.:* Adrocil; Viridin; *S.Afr.:* TFT; *Spain:* Viromidin; *Switz.:* Triherpine; *Thai.:* Triherpine; *USA:* Viroptic.

Tromantadine Hydrochloride (1689-h)

Tromantadine Hydrochloride (rINNM).
D-41. N-1-Adamantyl-2-(2-dimethylaminoethoxy)acetamide hydrochloride; 2-(2-Dimethylaminoethoxy)-N-(tricyclo[3.3.1.1^{3,7}]dec-1-yl)acetamide hydrochloride.
$C_{16}H_{28}N_2O_2,HCl = 316.9$.
CAS — 53783-83-8 (tromantadine); 41544-24-5 (tromantadine hydrochloride).

Adverse Effects

Contact dermatitis has been reported following the topical use of tromantadine hydrochloride.

◊ References.
1. Fanta D, Mischer P. Contact dermatitis from tromantadine hydrochloride. *Contact Dermatitis* 1976; **2:** 282–4.
2. Lembo G, *et al.* Allergic dermatitis from Viruserol ointment probably due to tromantadine hydrochloride. *Contact Dermatitis* 1984; **10:** 317.
3. Jauregui I, *et al.* Allergic contact dermatitis from tromantadine. *J Investig Allergol Clin Immunol* 1997; **7:** 260–1.

Uses and Administration

Tromantadine hydrochloride is a derivative of amantadine (p.1161) used for its antiviral activity. It is applied at a concentration of 1% in the treatment of herpes simplex infections of the skin and mucous membranes and of herpes zoster.

Preparations

Proprietary Preparations (details are given in Part 3)
Aust.: Viru-Merz; *Belg.:* Viru-Merz; *Braz.:* Herpex; *Denm.:* Viru-Merz†; *Ger.:* Viru-Merz; *Hong Kong:* Viru-Merz; *Israel:* Viru-Merz; *Ital.:* Viruserol; *Mex.:* Viru-Serol; *Neth.:* Viru-Merz; *Port.:* Viru-Merz; *Singapore:* Viru-Merz; *Spain:* Viru-Serol; *Switz.:* Viru-Merz Serol.

Valaciclovir Hydrochloride (17334-c)

Valaciclovir Hydrochloride (BANM, rINNM).
256U87 (valaciclovir); Valacyclovir Hydrochloride (USAN). L-Valine, ester with 9-[(2-hydroxyethoxy)methyl]guanine hydrochloride.
$C_{13}H_{20}N_6O_4$,HCl = 360.8.
CAS — 124832-26-4 (valaciclovir); 124832-27-5 (valaciclovir hydrochloride);.

Valaciclovir hydrochloride 1.11 g is approximately equivalent to 1 g of valaciclovir.

Adverse Effects and Precautions
As for Aciclovir, p.613.

Interactions
As for Aciclovir, p.613.

Antiviral Action
As for Aciclovir, p.613.

Pharmacokinetics
Valaciclovir is readily absorbed from the gastrointestinal tract following oral administration, and is rapidly converted to aciclovir and valine by first-pass intestinal and/or hepatic metabolism. The bioavailability of aciclovir following valaciclovir administration is reported to be 54% and peak plasma concentrations of aciclovir are achieved after 1.5 hours. Valaciclovir is eliminated principally as aciclovir and its metabolite 9-carboxymethoxymethylguanine (see p.614); less than 1% of a dose of valaciclovir is excreted unchanged in the urine.

◊ References.
1. Weller S, et al. Pharmacokinetics of the acyclovir pro-drug valaciclovir after escalating single- and multiple-dose administration to normal volunteers. Clin Pharmacol Ther 1993; 54: 595–605.
2. Rolan P. Pharmacokinetics of new antiherpetic agents. Clin Pharmacokinet 1995; 29: 333–40.
3. Soul-Lawton J, et al. Absolute bioavailability and metabolic disposition of valaciclovir, the L-valyl ester of acyclovir, following oral administration to humans. Antimicrob Agents Chemother 1995; 39: 2759–64.
4. Wang LH, et al. Pharmacokinetics and safety of multiple-dose valaciclovir in geriatric volunteers with and without concomitant diuretic therapy. Antimicrob Agents Chemother 1996; 40: 80–5.
5. Steingrimsdottir H, et al. Bioavailability of aciclovir after oral administration of aciclovir and its prodrug valaciclovir to patients with leukopenia after chemotherapy. Antimicrob Agents Chemother 2000; 44: 207–9.

Uses and Administration
Valaciclovir is a prodrug of the antiviral aciclovir (p.614) that is used in the treatment of herpes zoster (p.608) and herpes simplex infections (p.607) of the skin and mucous membranes, including genital herpes. It is given by mouth as the hydrochloride; doses are expressed in terms of valaciclovir. Treatment should be started as soon as symptoms occur.

For herpes zoster the dose is 1 g three times daily for 7 days. For treatment of herpes simplex infections, 500 mg is given twice daily for 5 days for recurrent episodes or for up to 10 days for a first episode; in the USA the recommended dose for a first episode of genital herpes is 1 g twice daily for 10 days. For the suppression of herpes simplex infection a dose of 500 mg daily, as a single dose or in 2 divided doses, is recommended; in the USA a dose of 1 g once daily is recommended for suppression of recurrent genital herpes. A dose of 500 mg twice daily may be used in immunocompromised patients.

Doses of valaciclovir may need to be reduced in patients with impaired renal function. The following dosage reductions are suggested by the UK manufacturer: for herpes zoster in patients with a creatinine clearance (CC) of 15 to 30 mL per minute, 1 g twice daily and for those with a CC of less than 15 mL per minute, 1 g daily; for treatment of herpes simplex infections in patients with a CC of 15 to 30 mL per minute, no modification, but for those with a CC of less than 15 mL per minute, 500 mg daily. For the suppression of herpes simplex, usual doses are halved in patients with a CC below 15 mL per minute, to 250 mg once daily in immunocompetent and 500 mg once daily in immunocompromised patients. For pa-

tients undergoing haemodialysis, doses are as for patients with a CC of less than 15 mL per minute and should be administered after haemodialysis.

◊ Reviews.
1. Ormrod D, et al. Valaciclovir: a review of its long term utility in the management of genital herpes simplex virus and cytomegalovirus infections. Drugs 2000; 59: 839–63.
2. Ormrod D, Goa K. Valaciclovir: a review of its use in the management of herpes zoster. Drugs 2000; 59: 1317–40.

Preparations
Proprietary Preparations (details are given in Part 3)
Aust.: Valtrex; Austral.: Valtrex; Belg.: Zelitrex; Canad.: Valtrex; Denm.: Zelitrex; Fin.: Valavir; Valtrex; Fr.: Zelitrex; Ger.: Valtrex; Hong Kong: Valtrex; Irl.: Valtrex; Israel: Valtrex; Ital.: Talavir; Zelitrex; Mex.: Rapivir; Neth.: Zelitrex; Norw.: Valtrex; S.Afr.: Zelitrex; Singapore: Valtrex; Spain: Valherpes; Valpridol; Valtrex; Virval; Swed.: Valtrex; Switz.: Valtrex; Thai.: Valtrex; UK: Valtrex; USA: Valtrex.

Valganciclovir Hydrochloride (20277-g)

Valganciclovir Hydrochloride (USAN, rINNM).
Ro-107-9070/194; RS-079070-194. L-Valine, ester with 9-{[2-hydroxy-1-(hydroxymethyl)-ethoxy]methyl} guanine hydrochloride.
$C_{14}H_{22}N_6O_5$,HCl = 390.8.
CAS — 175865-60-8 (valganciclovir); 175865-59-5 (valganciclovir hydrochloride).

Adverse Effects, Treatment, and Precautions
As for Ganciclovir, p.623.

Interactions
As for Ganciclovir, p.623.

Antiviral Action
As for Ganciclovir, p.623.

Pharmacokinetics
Valganciclovir is well absorbed from the gastrointestinal tract following oral administration and is rapidly converted to ganciclovir by first-pass intestinal and/or hepatic metabolism. The bioavailability of ganciclovir following valganciclovir administration is reported to be approximately 60% and peak plasma concentrations of ganciclovir are achieved between 1 and 3 hours after administration. Valganciclovir is eliminated in the urine as ganciclovir (see p.623).

◊ References.
1. Brown F, et al. Pharmacokinetics of valganciclovir and ganciclovir following multiple oral dosages of valganciclovir in HIV- and CMV-seropositive volunteers. Clin Pharmacokinet 1999; 37: 167–76.
2. Jung D, Dorr A. Single-dose pharmacokinetics of valganciclovir in HIV- and CMV-seropositive subjects. J Clin Pharmacol 1999; 39: 800–4.
3. Pescovitz MD, et al. Valganciclovir results in improved oral absorption of ganciclovir in liver transplant recipients. Antimicrob Agents Chemother 2000; 44: 2811–15.

Uses and Administration
Valganciclovir is a prodrug of the antiviral ganciclovir (p.624) that is used for the treatment of cytomegalovirus retinitis in patients with AIDS. It is given by mouth with food as the hydrochloride; doses are expressed in terms of valganciclovir. For induction in patients with active cytomegalovirus retinitis, the dose is 900 mg twice daily for 21 days. For maintenance following induction, or in patients with inactive cytomegalovirus retinitis, the dose is 900 mg daily.

Doses of valganciclovir may need to be reduced according to creatinine clearance (CC) in patients with impaired renal function. For patients with a CC of 40 to 59 mL per minute, the dose is 450 mg twice daily for induction and 450 mg daily for maintenance; for CC 25 to 39 mL per minute, 450 mg daily for induction and 450 mg every two days for maintenance; for CC 10 to 24 mL per minute, 450 mg every two days for induction and 450 mg twice weekly for maintenance. Valganciclovir should not be given to patients undergoing haemodialysis.

◊ Reviews.
1. Curran M, Noble S. Valganciclovir. Drugs 2001; 61: 1145–50.

Preparations
Proprietary Preparations (details are given in Part 3)
USA: Valcyte.

Vidarabine (17027-v)

Vidarabine (BAN, USAN, rINN).
Adenine Arabinoside; Ara-A; CI-673. 9-β-D-Arabinofuranosyladenine monohydrate.
$C_{10}H_{13}N_5O_4$,H_2O = 285.3.
CAS — 5536-17-4 (anhydrous vidarabine); 24356-66-9 (vidarabine monohydrate).
ATC — J05AB03; S01AD06.
Pharmacopoeias. In US.

A purine nucleoside obtained from Streptomyces antibioticus.
Pharmacopoeial description
USP 25: A white to off-white powder. Very slightly soluble in water; slightly soluble in dimethylformamide. Store in airtight containers.

Vidarabine Phosphate (1690-a)

Vidarabine Phosphate (BANM, USAN, rINNM).
Ara-AMP; Arabinosyladenine Monophosphate; CI-808; Vidarabine 5′-Monophosphate. 9-β-D-Arabinofuranosyladenine 5′-(dihydrogen phosphate).
$C_{10}H_{14}N_5O_7P$ = 347.2.
CAS — 29984-33-6 (vidarabine phosphate); 71002-10-3 (vidarabine sodium phosphate).

Adverse Effects
Adverse effects which may occur when vidarabine is applied to the eyes include irritation, pain, superficial punctate keratitis, photophobia, lachrymation, and occlusion of the lachrymal duct.

Vidarabine has been reported to be teratogenic, carcinogenic, and mutagenic in some species of animals.

Antiviral Action
Vidarabine appears to act by interfering in the early stages of viral DNA synthesis, but several mechanisms may be involved. It is phosphorylated intracellularly to the triphosphate which inhibits among other enzymes viral DNA polymerase; it may also be incorporated into the viral DNA.

Following administration, vidarabine is rapidly converted to hypoxanthine arabinoside which also appears to interfere with viral DNA synthesis but is reported to have less antiviral activity than the parent compound.

The activity of vidarabine in vitro and in vivo is limited to DNA viruses such as herpes simplex virus types 1 and 2, varicella-zoster virus, cytomegalovirus, and Epstein-Barr and vaccinia viruses; with few exceptions it does not inhibit RNA viruses.

Pharmacokinetics
Systemic absorption does not occur following application of vidarabine to the eye; trace amounts of its principal metabolite hypoxanthine arabinoside (arabinosyl hypoxanthine), and vidarabine, if the cornea is damaged, may be found in the aqueous humour.

Uses and Administration
Vidarabine is a purine nucleoside that has been used in the treatment of herpes simplex and varicella-zoster infections although aciclovir is generally preferred.

Vidarabine is administered topically in the treatment of herpes simplex keratitis and keratoconjunctivitis as a 3% ophthalmic ointment and can be used when there has been no response to treatment with other antivirals or when ocular toxicity or hypersensitivity to other drugs has occurred. The ointment is applied 5 times daily every 3 hours until corneal re-epithelialisation has occurred, then twice daily for a further 7 days to prevent recurrence. If there is no improvement within 7 days after the start of therapy, or if complete healing has not occurred within 21 days, other forms of therapy should be considered.

Vidarabine was formerly used intravenously in the treatment of severe and disseminated herpes simplex infections and herpes zoster but aciclovir is preferred.

Herpes simplex infections. Although vidarabine has been shown to be moderately effective in the treatment of disseminated herpes simplex infections, aciclovir or foscarnet are preferred (see p.607) and vidarabine is now only used topically for the treatment of herpes simplex infections. Topically applied vidarabine was reported to be as effective as idoxuridine[1,2] or trifluridine[3,4] in early studies in herpes keratitis. Responses to topical vidarabine in genital herpes[5] and herpes labialis[6] have generally been disappointing.

1. Pavan-Langston D. Clinical evaluation of adenine arabinoside and idoxuridine in the treatment of ocular herpes simplex. Am J Ophthalmol 1975; 80: 495–502.
2. Pavan-Langston D, Buchanan RA. Vidarabine therapy of simple and IDU-complicated herpetic keratitis. Trans Am Acad Ophthalmol Otolaryngol 1976; 81: 813–25.
3. Travers JP, Patterson A. A controlled trial of adenine arabinoside and trifluorothymidine in herpetic keratitis. J Int Med Res 1978; 6: 102–4.
4. van Bijsterveld OP, Post H. Trifluorothymidine versus adenine arabinoside in the treatment of herpes simplex keratitis. Br J Ophthalmol 1980; 64: 33–6.
5. Eron LJ, et al. Topically applied vidarabine sodium phosphate in genital herpes infection. J Antimicrob Chemother 1988; 21: 801–5.
6. Spruance SL, et al. Ineffectiveness of topical adenine arabinoside 5′-monophosphate in the treatment of recurrent herpes simplex labialis. N Engl J Med 1979; 300: 1180–4.

Preparations
USP 25: Vidarabine Ophthalmic Ointment.

Proprietary Preparations (details are given in Part 3)
Austral.: Vira-A†; Fr.: Vira-MP; Jpn: Arasena-A†; NZ: Vira-A; USA: Vira-A.

The symbol † denotes a preparation no longer actively marketed

Zalcitabine (1731-e)

Zalcitabine (BAN, USAN, rINN).

DDC; ddC; ddCyd; Dideoxycytidine; NSC-606170; Ro-24-2027; Ro-24-2027/000. 2',3'-Dideoxycytidine.
$C_9H_{13}N_3O_3 = 211.2$.
CAS — 7481-89-2.
ATC — J05AF03.
Pharmacopoeias. In US.

Pharmacopoeial description

USP 25: A white to off-white, crystalline powder. Soluble in water and in methyl alcohol; sparingly soluble in alcohol, in acetonitrile, in chloroform, and in dichloromethane; slightly soluble in cyclohexane. Store in airtight containers. Protect from light.

◊ CAUTION. Avoid exposure to the skin and inhalation of zalcitabine powder.

Adverse Effects

The most serious adverse effects of zalcitabine are peripheral neuropathy which can affect up to one third of patients and pancreatitis which is rare, affecting less than 1% of patients, but which can be fatal. Other severe adverse effects include oral and oesophageal ulceration, hypersensitivity reactions, cardiomyopathy and heart failure, lactic acidosis and severe hepatomegaly with steatosis (both potentially life-threatening), and hepatic failure.

Other adverse effects noted in patients taking zalcitabine have included asthenia, chest pain, fatigue, and fever; dizziness, headache, and insomnia; abdominal pain, anorexia, constipation, diarrhoea, dysphagia, nausea, and vomiting; anaemia, leucopenia, neutropenia, and thrombocytopenia; raised liver enzyme values; arthralgia and myalgia; mood changes; dyspnoea and pharyngitis; alopecia, pruritus, and rashes; hearing and visual disturbances; hyperuricaemia; and renal disorders.

Effects on the nervous system. Peripheral neuropathy is a well recognised adverse effect of zalcitabine and has been the subject of a review.[1]

1. Moyle GJ, Sadler M. Peripheral neuropathy with nucleoside antiretrovirals: risk factors, incidence and management. Drug Safety 1998; 19: 481–94.

Precautions

Zalcitabine should be interrupted or discontinued if peripheral neuropathy develops. Neuropathy is usually slowly reversible if treatment is stopped promptly but may be irreversible if treatment is continued after symptoms develop. Zalcitabine should be avoided in patients who already have peripheral neuropathy. It should be used with caution in patients at risk of developing peripheral neuropathy (especially those with a low CD4+ cell count) and in those receiving other drugs that may cause peripheral neuropathy (see Interactions, below).

Treatment should be interrupted in patients who develop abdominal pain, nausea, or vomiting or with abnormal biochemical test results until pancreatitis has been excluded. Zalcitabine should be discontinued permanently if pancreatitis develops. Patients with a history of pancreatitis or of raised serum amylase should be monitored closely. Zalcitabine should not be administered with other drugs known to cause pancreatitis (see Interactions, below).

Zalcitabine should be used with caution in patients with impaired hepatic function and treatment interrupted or discontinued if hepatic function deteriorates or there are signs of hepatic damage or unexplained lactic acidosis. It should be used with caution in patients with impaired renal function, and dosage reductions may be necessary. It should also be used with caution in patients with cardiomyopathy or heart failure.

Complete blood count and biochemical tests should be carried out before treatment starts and at regular intervals throughout therapy.

Interactions

Zalcitabine should not be administered with other drugs known to cause pancreatitis (for example intravenous pentamidine). Caution is necessary when zal-

citabine is given with other drugs that may cause peripheral neuropathy such as other nucleoside reverse transcriptase inhibitors, metronidazole, isoniazid (the clearance of which may also be affected—see p.217), and vincristine.

The absorption of zalcitabine is reduced by about 25% when administered concurrently with aluminium- or magnesium-containing antacids.

The administration of either cimetidine, probenecid, or trimethoprim can reduce the renal excretion of zalcitabine, resulting in elevated plasma concentrations. Renal excretion of zalcitabine may also be reduced by concurrent administration of amphotericin B, aminoglycosides, or foscarnet, potentially increasing its toxicity.

The antiviral action of zalcitabine may be antagonised by lamivudine and the two drugs should not be used in combination.

Antiviral Action

Zalcitabine is converted intracellularly in stages to the triphosphate. This triphosphate halts the DNA synthesis of retroviruses, including HIV, through competitive inhibition of reverse transcriptase and incorporation into viral DNA.

The emergence of zalcitabine-resistant strains of HIV has been reported.

◊ References.
1. Jeffries DJ. The antiviral activity of dideoxycytidine. J Antimicrob Chemother 1989; 23 (suppl A): 29–34.

Pharmacokinetics

Zalcitabine is absorbed from the gastrointestinal tract with a bioavailability of greater than 80%. The rate of absorption is reduced by administration with food. Peak plasma concentrations in the fasting state are achieved within about 1 hour. Zalcitabine crosses the blood-brain barrier producing CSF concentrations ranging from 9 to 37% of those in plasma. Binding to plasma proteins is negligible. The plasma elimination half-life is about 2 hours.

Zalcitabine is metabolised intracellularly to the active antiviral triphosphate. It does not appear to undergo any substantial hepatic metabolism and is excreted mainly in the urine, in part by active tubular secretion.

◊ References.
1. Morse GD, et al. Comparative pharmacokinetics of antiviral nucleoside analogues. Clin Pharmacokinet 1993; 24: 101–23.
2. Devineni D, Gallo JM. Zalcitabine: clinical pharmacokinetics and efficacy. Clin Pharmacokinet 1995; 28: 351–60.
3. Chadwick EG, et al. Phase I evaluation of zalcitabine administered to human immunodeficiency virus-infected children. J Infect Dis 1995; 172: 1475–9.
4. Bazunga M, et al. The effects of renal impairment on the pharmacokinetics of zalcitabine. J Clin Pharmacol 1998; 38: 28–33.

Uses and Administration

Zalcitabine is a nucleoside reverse transcriptase inhibitor derived from cytidine with activity against retroviruses including HIV. It is used in the treatment of HIV infection, usually in combination with other antiretrovirals.

Zalcitabine is given by mouth in a dose of 750 µg every 8 hours. Doses for patients with impaired renal function are: creatinine clearance 10 to 40 mL per minute, 750 µg every 12 hours; creatinine clearance less than 10 mL per minute, 750 µg every 24 hours.

◊ Reviews.
1. Whittington R, Brodgen RN. Zalcitabine: a review of its pharmacology and clinical potential in acquired immunodeficiency syndrome (AIDS). Drugs 1992; 44: 656–83.
2. Lipsky JJ. Zalcitabine and didanosine. Lancet 1993; 341: 30–2.
3. Shelton MJ, et al. Zalcitabine. Ann Pharmacother 1993; 27: 480–9.
4. Adkins JC, et al. Zalcitabine: an update of its pharmacodynamic and pharmacokinetic properties and clinical efficacy in the management of HIV infection. Drugs 1997; 53: 1054–80.

HIV infection and AIDS. Zalcitabine has been used as an alternative antiretroviral to treat HIV infection in patients intolerant of or unresponsive to zidovudine, although it has not been shown to have any great advantage over zidovudine in patients with advanced disease[1,2] and may be less well tolerated.[3] Alternating schedules of zalcitabine and zidovudine[4-6] were tried in an attempt to minimise the toxicities of both drugs. In patients who had ceased to respond to zidovudine, zalcitabine was reported to produce a response similar to that with didanosine.[7]

Zalcitabine is now generally used together with other antiretrovirals, usually another nucleoside reverse transcriptase inhibitor and either an HIV-protease inhibitor or a non-nucleoside reverse transcriptase inhibitor. Combination therapy with zalcitabine and zidovudine was superior to zidovudine alone in delaying disease progression and in prolonging life in patients who had not previously received antiretroviral therapy.[8,9] Combination therapy has been less successful in patients who have previously received zidovudine than in zidovudine-naive patients,[10] and zalcitabine with zidovudine was reported to be less effective than combinations of zidovudine with didanosine[8,9] or lamivudine.[11] Preliminary studies of zalcitabine with zidovudine and the HIV-protease inhibitor saquinavir have shown favourable responses.[12]

For a general discussion on the management of HIV infection and AIDS, see p.608.

1. Fischl MA, et al. Zalcitabine compared with zidovudine in patients with advanced HIV-1 infection who received previous zidovudine therapy. Ann Intern Med 1993; 118: 762–9.
2. Fischl MA, et al. Combination and monotherapy with zidovudine and zalcitabine in patients with advanced HIV disease. Ann Intern Med 1995; 122: 24–32.
3. Bozzette SA, et al. Health status and function with zidovudine or zalcitabine as initial therapy for AIDS: a randomized controlled trial. JAMA 1995; 273: 295–301.
4. Yarchoan R, et al. Phase I studies of 2',3'-dideoxycytidine in severe human immunodeficiency virus infection as a single agent and alternating with zidovudine (AZT). Lancet 1988; i: 76–81.
5. Pizzo PA, et al. Dideoxycytidine alone and in an alternating schedule with zidovudine in children with symptomatic human immunodeficiency virus infection. J Pediatr 1990; 117: 799–808.
6. Skowron G, et al. Alternating and intermittent regimens of zidovudine and dideoxycytidine in patients with AIDS or AIDS-related complex. Ann Intern Med 1993; 118: 321–30.
7. Abrams DI, et al. A comparative trial of didanosine or zalcitabine after treatment with zidovudine in patients with human immunodeficiency virus infection. N Engl J Med 1994; 330: 657–62.
8. Delta Coordinating Committee. Delta: a randomised double-blind controlled trial comparing combinations of zidovudine plus didanosine or zalcitabine with zidovudine alone in HIV-infected individuals. Lancet 1996; 348: 283–91.
9. Hammer SM, et al. A trial comparing nucleoside monotherapy with combination therapy in HIV-infected adults with CD4 cell counts from 200 to 500 per cubic millimeter. N Engl J Med 1996; 335: 1081–90.
10. Saravolatz LD, et al. Zidovudine alone or in combination with didanosine or zalcitabine in HIV-infected patients with the acquired immunodeficiency syndrome or fewer than 200 CD4 cells per cubic millimeter. N Engl J Med 1996; 335: 1099–1106.
11. Bartlett JA, et al. Lamivudine plus zidovudine compared with zalcitabine plus zidovudine in patients with HIV infection: a randomized, double-blind, placebo-controlled trial. Ann Intern Med 1996; 125: 161–72.
12. Collier AC, et al. Treatment of human immunodeficiency virus infection with saquinavir, zidovudine, and zalcitabine. N Engl J Med 1996; 334: 1011–17.

Preparations

USP 25: Zalcitabine Tablets.

Proprietary Preparations (details are given in Part 3)
Aust.: Hivid; Austral.: Hivid; Belg.: Hivid; Braz.: Hivid; Canad.: Hivid; Denm.: Hivid; Fin.: Hivid; Fr.: Hivid; Ger.: Hivid; Hong Kong: Hivid; Irl.: Hivid; Israel: Hivid; Ital.: Hivid; Jpn: Hivid; Mex.: Hivid; Neth.: Hivid; Norw.: Hivid; NZ: Hivid; Port.: Hivid; S.Afr.: Hivid; Singapore: Hivid; Spain: Hivid; Swed.: Hivid; Switz.: Hivid; Thai.: Hivid; UK: Hivid; USA: Hivid.

Zanamivir (17658-y)

Zanamivir (BAN, USAN, rINN).

GG-167; GR-121167X; 4-Guanidino-2,4-dideoxy-2,3-dehydro-N-acetylneuraminic Acid. 5-Acetamido-2,6-anhydro-3,4,5-trideoxy-4-guanidino-D-glycero-D-galacto-non-2-enonic acid.
$C_{12}H_{20}N_4O_7 = 332.3$.
CAS — 139110-80-8.
ATC — J05AH01.

Adverse Effects

Inhaled zanamivir has generally been well tolerated. Acute bronchospasm and/or decline in respiratory function, with some fatalities, has been reported rarely in patients with a previous history of respiratory disease and very rarely in those with no such previous history. Other effects which have been noted include nasal symptoms, headache, gastrointestinal symptoms, cough, and bronchitis, but they may be difficult to distinguish from the symptoms of influenza. There have also been rare reports of hypersensitivity reactions, including oropharyngeal oedema and severe skin rashes, in association with zanamivir.

Precautions

Zanamivir should be used with caution in patients with chronic respiratory diseases as they may be at increased risk of bronchospasm; if zanamivir administration is considered appropriate, patients with asthma or chronic obstructive pulmonary disease should have a fast-acting bronchodilator available during treatment. Patients on maintenance therapy with inhaled bronchodilators should administer the bronchodilator before zanamivir administration. Patients experiencing bronchospasm should be advised to discontinue zanamivir and seek medical evaluation.

Antiviral Action

Zanamivir inhibits the viral surface enzyme neuraminidase (sialidase) which is essential for the release of newly formed viral particles from infected cells, and may facilitate access of virus through mucus to the cell surface. Zanamivir is active against influenza A and B virus replication.

Resistance. References.
1. Gubareva LV, et al. Evidence for zanamivir resistance in an immunocompromised child infected with influenza B virus. *J Infect Dis* 1998; **178:** 1257–62.
2. McKimm-Breschkin JL. Resistance of influenza viruses to neuraminidase inhibitors—a review. *Antiviral Res* 2000; **47:** 1–17.

Pharmacokinetics

Zanamivir is poorly absorbed following oral administration with a bioavailability of about 2%. About 10 to 20% of the inhaled dose is absorbed producing peak serum concentrations at about 1 to 2 hours. The remainder is deposited in the oropharynx and eliminated via the gastrointestinal tract. The absorbed portion is excreted unchanged in the urine with a serum half-life of 2.6 to 5 hours.

◊ References.
1. Aoki FY, Hayden FG (eds). The pharmacokinetics of zanamivir: a new inhaled antiviral for influenza. *Clin Pharmacokinet* 1999; **36** (suppl 1): 1–58.

Uses and Administration

Zanamivir is a neuraminidase inhibitor used for the treatment of influenza A and B (p.611).

It is administered by inhalation in a dose of 10 mg twice daily for 5 days, starting as soon as possible (within 48 hours) after the onset of symptoms.

It is also under investigation for prophylaxis of influenza.

◊ Reviews.
1. Waghorn SL, Goa KL. Zanamivir. *Drugs* 1998; **55:** 721–5.
2. Freund B, et al. Zanamivir: a review of clinical safety. *Drug Safety* 1999; **21:** 267–81.
3. Dunn CJ, Goa KL. Zanamivir: a review of its use in influenza. *Drugs* 1999; **58:** 761–84.
4. Gubareva LV, et al. Influenza virus neuraminidase inhibitors. *Lancet* 2000; **355:** 827–35.
5. Jefferson T, et al. Neuraminidase inhibitors for preventing and treating influenza in healthy adults (updated 26 July 2001). Available in The Cochrane Library; Issue 4. Oxford: Update Software; 2001.

Influenza. Randomised, placebo-controlled studies in healthy subjects[1] have shown intranasal zanamivir to be well tolerated and effective for prophylaxis of experimental influenza A. Early administration (within 32 hours of inoculation with the virus) reduced the occurrence of fever, peak viral titres, and the duration of viral shedding by 3 days.[1] Delayed administration (beginning 50 hours after inoculation) produced rapid decline in viral titres and subsequent reduction of the duration of viral shedding by 1 day, but had no effect on symptoms.[1] Inhaled zanamivir has also been shown to be therapeutically active in acute, uncomplicated, naturally occurring influenza.[2,3] In patients presenting within 48 hours of the onset of symptoms in whom influenza was confirmed, the duration of major symptoms was reduced by about 1 day by zanamivir.[2] Analysis of the intention-to-treat population showed a smaller benefit, however, due to the inclusion of patients subsequently shown to have non-influenza respiratory illnesses. Treatment was most effective in patients who began treatment within 30 hours of the onset of symptoms, and in those with fever, and was equally effective against influenza A and B. Similar results were obtained in a study of patients recruited within 36 hours of the onset of symptoms.[3] The main disadvantages of zanamivir include the need to begin treatment soon after the onset of symptoms and difficulties in administering the drug to the very young and very old.[4,5]

1. Hayden FG, et al. Safety and efficacy of the neuraminidase inhibitor GG167 in experimental human influenza. *JAMA* 1996; **275:** 295–9.
2. Hayden FG, et al. Efficacy and safety of the neuraminidase inhibitor zanamivir in the treatment of influenzavirus infection. *N Engl J Med* 1997; **337:** 874–80.
3. The MIST (Management of Influenza in the Southern Hemisphere Trialists) Study Group. Randomised trial of efficacy and safety of inhaled zanamivir in treatment of influenza A and B virus infections. *Lancet* 1998; **352:** 1877–81. Corrections. *ibid.* 1999; **353:** 504 and 1104.

4. Read RC. Treating influenza with zanamivir. *Lancet* 1998; **352:** 1872–3.
5. Nguyen-Van-Tam JS. Zanamivir for influenza: a public health perspective. *BMJ* 1999; **319:** 655–6.

Preparations

Proprietary Preparations (details are given in Part 3)
Austral.: Relenza; *Belg.:* Relenza; *Denm.:* Relenza; *Fin.:* Relenza; *Fr.:* Relenza; *Ger.:* Relenza; *Irl.:* Relenza; *Ital.:* Relenza; *Neth.:* Relenza; *Norw.:* Relenza; *NZ:* Relenza; *Port.:* Relenza; *Singapore:* Relenza; *Spain:* Relenza; *Swed.:* Relenza; *Switz.:* Relenza; *UK:* Relenza; *USA:* Relenza.

Zidovudine   (18797-s)

Zidovudine (BAN, USAN, rINN).

Azidodeoxythymidine; Azidothymidine; AZT; BW-A509U; BW-509U; Compound-S; Zidovudinum. 3′-Azido-3′-deoxythymidine.
$C_{10}H_{13}N_5O_4 = 267.2$.
CAS — 30516-87-1.
ATC — J05AF01.

NOTE. The abbreviation AZT has also been used for azathioprine.
Pharmacopoeias. In *Eur.* (see p.vi) and *US*.

Pharmacopoeial description
Ph. Eur.: A white to brownish powder. It shows polymorphism. Sparingly soluble in water; soluble in dehydrated alcohol. Protect from light.
USP 25: A white to yellowish powder. Exhibits polymorphism. Sparingly soluble in water; freely soluble in alcohol. Store in airtight containers. Protect from light.

Adverse Effects

The commonest serious adverse effects reported with zidovudine are anaemia and leucopenia, mainly neutropenia, occurring within a few weeks of starting treatment. This haematological toxicity occurs most commonly in those with pre-existing haematological abnormalities and is usually reversed by interrupting treatment or reducing dosage but it can be severe enough to require blood transfusion.

Other frequently reported adverse effects include asthenia, fever, and malaise; dizziness, headache, insomnia, myopathy, and paraesthesia; abdominal pain, anorexia, dyspepsia, diarrhoea, nausea, and vomiting; myalgia; and rashes. Lactic acidosis and severe hepatomegaly with steatosis have been reported as rare, but potentially fatal, occurrences in patients taking zidovudine. Pancreatitis, convulsions, and pigmentation of nails, skin, and oral mucosa have occurred.

Zidovudine is reported to be carcinogenic in *mice* and *rats*.

◊ Adverse effects with zidovudine tend to be dose-related and reversible. The more advanced the state of the disease being treated, the greater the risk of zidovudine toxicity.

Some references to the incidence and range of adverse effects are given below.
1. Richman DD, et al. The toxicity of azidothymidine (AZT) in the treatment of patients with AIDS and AIDS-related complex: a double-blind, placebo-controlled trial. *N Engl J Med* 1987; **317:** 192–7.
2. Gelmon K, et al. Nature, time course and dose dependence of zidovudine-related side effects: results from the Multicenter Canadian Azidothymidine Trial. *AIDS* 1989; **3:** 555–61.
3. Fischl MA, et al. The safety and efficacy of zidovudine (AZT) in the treatment of subjects with mildly symptomatic human immunodeficiency virus type 1 (HIV) infection: a double-blind, placebo-controlled trial. *Ann Intern Med* 1990; **112:** 727–37.
4. McKinney RE, et al. Safety and tolerance of intermittent intravenous and oral zidovudine therapy in human immunodeficiency virus-infected pediatric patients. *J Pediatr* 1990; **116:** 640–7.
5. Koch MA, et al. Toxic effects of zidovudine in asymptomatic human immunodeficiency-virus-infected individuals with CD4+ cell counts of 0.5×10⁹/L or less: detailed and updated results from protocol 019 of the AIDS Clinical Trials Group. *Arch Intern Med* 1992; **152:** 2286–92.

Effects on the blood. Adverse haematological effects reported with zidovudine may be severe and include anaemia with erythroid aplasia or hypoplasia, and neutropenia.[1-5] Although these effects may be reversed by stopping treatment,[5] they may persist for weeks after zidovudine has been withdrawn[2,3] and blood transfusions may be required in some patients.[1-4] A study indicated that zidovudine-induced neutropenia only significantly increased the risk of bacterial infection in patients whose polymorphonuclear cell count fell below 500 per μL.[6] The effects of zidovudine on the platelet count are considered to be complex, but patients with thrombocytopenia appeared not to be at risk during treatment.[7]

Recombinant erythropoietin has been used in an attempt to reduce blood-transfusion requirements in zidovudine-induced anaemia,[8,9] although the proportion of patients who derive ben-

efit may be limited and some have reported it to have no effect.[10] Similarly granulocyte-macrophage colony-stimulating factor has been reported to improve the neutrophil count in some but not all patients.[11]
1. Forester G. Profound cytopenia secondary to azidothymidine. *N Engl J Med* 1987; **317:** 772.
2. Gill PS, et al. Azidothymidine associated with bone marrow failure in the acquired immunodeficiency syndrome (AIDS). *Ann Intern Med* 1987; **107:** 502–5.
3. Mir N, Costello C. Zidovudine and bone marrow. *Lancet* 1988; **ii:** 1195–6.
4. Walker RE, et al. Anemia and erythropoiesis in patients with the acquired immunodeficiency syndrome (AIDS) and Kaposi sarcoma treated with zidovudine. *Ann Intern Med* 1988; **108:** 372–6.
5. Cohen H, et al. Reversible zidovudine-induced pure red-cell aplasia. *AIDS* 1989; **3:** 177–8.
6. Shaunak S, Bartlett JA. Zidovudine-induced neutropenia: are we too cautious? *Lancet* 1989; **ii:** 91–2.
7. Flegg PJ, et al. Effect of zidovudine on platelet count. *BMJ* 1989; **298:** 1074–5.
8. Fischl M, et al. Recombinant human erythropoietin for patients with AIDS treated with zidovudine. *N Engl J Med* 1990; **322:** 1488–93.
9. Henry DH, et al. Recombinant human erythropoietin in the treatment of anemia associated with human immunodeficiency virus (HIV) infection and zidovudine therapy: overview of four clinical trials. *Ann Intern Med* 1992; **117:** 739–48.
10. Shepp DH, et al. Erythropoietin for zidovudine-induced anemia. *N Engl J Med* 1990; **323:** 1069–70.
11. Hewitt RG, et al. Pharmacokinetics and pharmacodynamics of granulocyte-macrophage colony-stimulating factor and zidovudine in patients with AIDS and severe AIDS-related complex. *Antimicrob Agents Chemother* 1993; **37:** 512–22.

Effects on the CNS. Reports of adverse effects on the CNS associated with zidovudine include mania,[1,2] seizures[3,4] (following an overdose in one patient[5]), psychogenic panic,[6] and Wernicke's encephalopathy,[7] mostly involving one or two patients in each case. CNS toxicity, thought to be zidovudine-related, contributed to the death of an AIDS patient.[8]

For reports of neurological symptoms associated with mitochondrial dysfunction in infants whose mothers received perinatal zidovudine, see Effects on Mitochondria, below.
1. Maxwell S, et al. Manic syndrome associated with zidovudine treatment. *JAMA* 1988; **259:** 3406–7.
2. Wright JM, et al. Zidovudine-related mania. *Med J Aust* 1989; **150:** 339–40.
3. Harris PJ, Caceres CA. Azidothymidine in the treatment of AIDS. *N Engl J Med* 1988; **318:** 250.
4. D'Silva M, et al. Seizure associated with zidovudine. *Lancet* 1995; **346:** 452.
5. Routy JP, et al. Seizure after zidovudine overdose. *Lancet* 1989; **i:** 384–5.
6. Levitt AJ, Lippert GP. Psychogenic panic after zidovudine therapy—the therapeutic benefit of an N of 1 trial. *Can Med Assoc J* 1990; **142:** 341–2.
7. Davtyan DG, Vinters HV. Wernicke's encephalopathy in AIDS patient treated with zidovudine. *Lancet* 1987; **i:** 919–20.
8. Hagler DN, Frame PT. Azidothymidine neurotoxicity. *Lancet* 1986; **ii:** 1392–3.

Effects on the liver. The development of acute cholestatic hepatitis necessitated the withdrawal of zidovudine in a patient who was later unable to tolerate its re-institution.[1] Zidovudine also had to be withdrawn in 3 patients after abnormal liver-function values occurred;[2] it was reinstated in 2 patients without further liver changes. Reversible increases in liver enzymes and rashes were also reported in 2 patients receiving prophylaxis with zidovudine and zalcitabine following exposure to HIV.[3] There has been a report of iron deposition in the liver of patients receiving blood transfusions for zidovudine-related anaemia.[4]

Fatal hepatic dysfunction associated with steatosis in the liver was reported in 6 patients with HIV infection, who were either receiving zidovudine or had previously done so.[5] Five of these 6 patients also developed metabolic acidosis. Cases of fatal lactic acidosis and hepatic failure have been reported in patients receiving zidovudine and other nucleoside analogues.[6]
1. Dubin G, Braffman MN. Zidovudine-induced hepatotoxicity. *Ann Intern Med* 1989; **110:** 85–6.
2. Melamed AJ, et al. Possible zidovudine-induced hepatotoxicity. *JAMA* 1987; **258:** 2063.
3. Henry K, et al. Hepatotoxicity and rash associated with zidovudine and zalcitabine chemoprophylaxis. *Ann Intern Med* 1996; **124:** 855.
4. Lindley R, et al. Iron deposition in liver in zidovudine-related transfusion-dependent anaemia. *Lancet* 1989; **ii:** 681.
5. Freiman JP, et al. Hepatomegaly with severe steatosis in HIV-seropositive patients. *AIDS* 1993; **7:** 379–85.
6. Sundar K, et al. Zidovudine-induced fatal lactic acidosis and hepatic failure in patients with acquired immunodeficiency syndrome: report of two patients and review of the literature. *Crit Care Med* 1997; **25:** 1425–30.

Effects on the metabolism. Lactic acidosis, sometimes in association with myopathy[1] or hepatotoxicity (see above), has been reported following zidovudine treatment. However, lactic acidosis with no apparent cause[2] has also been reported in 7 patients with HIV infection: 4 patients were receiving zidovudine, 1 ganciclovir, and 1 clofazimine. The disorder in these patients resembled Reye's syndrome and it was not clear whether the acidosis was induced by zidovudine or the HIV infection.

Lactic acidosis associated with nucleoside reverse transcriptase inhibitors responded to treatment with riboflavin in 4 patients.[3,4]
1. Gopinath R, et al. Chronic lactic acidosis in a patient with acquired immunodeficiency syndrome and mitochondrial myopathy: biochemical studies. *J Am Soc Nephrol* 1992; **3:** 1212–19.

The symbol † denotes a preparation no longer actively marketed

2. Chattha G, *et al.* Lactic acidosis complicating the acquired immunodeficiency syndrome. *Ann Intern Med* 1993; **118:** 37–9.
3. Fouty B, *et al.* Riboflavin to treat nucleoside analogue-induced lactic acidosis. *Lancet* 1998; **352:** 291–2.
4. Luzzati R, *et al.* Riboflavine and severe lactic acidosis. *Lancet* 1999; **353:** 901–2.

Effects on mitochondria. Concern has been expressed[1] over the effects of nucleoside reverse transcriptase inhibitors on mitochondria following reports in France[2] of mitochondrial dysfunction in 8 infants whose mothers had received zidovudine alone, or combined zidovudine and lamivudine, to prevent vertical transmission of HIV infection during pregnancy. The effects manifested themselves as severe demyelinating neurological disorder in 2 of the 8, both of whom died after about one year of life. Three other infants experienced seizures, 1 with severe cardiomyopathy and 1 with spastic diplegia, while the remaining 3 were asymptomatic. None were infected with HIV. A study[3] involving echocardiograms performed from birth to 5 years of age in 382 infants without HIV infection (36 with zidovudine exposure) and 58 infants with HIV infection (12 with zidovudine exposure), all of whom were born to HIV-infected women, found, however, that there was no evidence of abnormality in left ventricular structure or function associated with perinatal zidovudine. While it was considered that further assessment of this toxicity was required, it was emphasised that current recommendations for zidovudine monotherapy during pregnancy should be maintained.[1,2]

1. Committee on Safety of Medicines. Antiretroviral drugs in pregnancy and mitochondrial cytopathy in infants. *Current Problems* 1999; **25:** 15.
2. Blanche S, *et al.* Persistent mitochondrial dysfunction and perinatal exposure to antiretroviral nucleoside analogues. *Lancet* 1999; **354:** 1084–9.
3. Lipshultz SE, *et al.* Absence of cardiac toxicity of zidovudine in infants. *N Engl J Med* 2000; **343:** 759–66.

Effects on the musculoskeletal system. Myalgia can occur in patients taking zidovudine; so too can other adverse muscle effects although it has sometimes been difficult to determine whether the effects were caused by the drug or the underlying HIV infection.[1-4] Zidovudine-induced myopathy has been considered to be a distinct condition characterised by the presence of abnormal mitochondria in muscle-biopsy specimens;[2] this view is supported by the fact that the myopathy readily responded to the withdrawal of zidovudine or to treatment with corticosteroids or other anti-inflammatory drugs.[1-3] For further discussion of the effects of zidovudine on mitochondria, see above.

Arthralgia involving the knees, elbows, ankles, and wrists has been reported in a patient receiving zidovudine.[5]

1. Gertner E, *et al.* Zidovudine-associated myopathy. *Am J Med* 1989; **86:** 814–18.
2. Dalakas MC, *et al.* Mitochondrial myopathy caused by long-term zidovudine therapy. *N Engl J Med* 1990; **322:** 1098–1105.
3. Till M, MacDonell KB. Myopathy with human immunodeficiency virus type 1 (HIV-1) infection: HIV-1 or zidovudine? *Ann Intern Med* 1990; **113:** 492–4.
4. Simpson DM, *et al.* Myopathies associated with human immunodeficiency virus and zidovudine: can their effects be distinguished? *Neurology* 1993; **43:** 971–6.
5. Murphy D, *et al.* Zidovudine related arthropathy. *BMJ* 1994; **309:** 97.

Effects on the nails. Bluish or brownish discoloration of fingernails and/or toenails has been reported in a number of patients receiving zidovudine.[1-5] Dark-skinned patients appear to be most commonly affected.[2,4] Occasionally the abnormal pigmentation also involves the skin.[3,5] It has been pointed out that discoloration of nails has occurred in HIV-infected patients without exposure to zidovudine.[6]

1. Furth PA, Kazakis AM. Nail pigmentation changes associated with azidothymidine (zidovudine). *N Engl J Med* 1987; **107:** 350.
2. Vaiopoulos G, *et al.* Nail pigmentation and azidothymidine. *Ann Intern Med* 1988; **108:** 777.
3. Merenich JA, *et al.* Azidothymidine-induced hyperpigmentation mimicking primary adrenal insufficiency. *Am J Med* 1989; **86:** 469–70.
4. Don PC, *et al.* Nail dyschromia associated with zidovudine. *Ann Intern Med* 1990; **112:** 145–6.
5. Bendick C, *et al.* Azidothymidine-induced hyperpigmentation of skin and nails. *Arch Dermatol* 1989; **125:** 1285–6.
6. Chandrasekar PH. Nail discoloration and human immunodeficiency virus infection. *Am J Med* 1989; **86:** 506–7.

Precautions

Zidovudine should be used with care in patients with anaemia or bone-marrow suppression. The incidence of neutropenia is greater in patients with low vitamin B_{12} concentrations. Dosage adjustments may be necessary and it has been recommended that it should not be used if the neutrophil count or haemoglobin value is abnormally low. Care is also required in the elderly and in patients with reduced kidney or liver function who may require reductions in dose. Patients with risk factors for liver disease should be monitored during treatment. Zidovudine treatment should be stopped if there is a rapid increase in aminotransferase concentrations, progressive hepatomegaly, or metabolic or lactic acidosis of unknown aetiology. It should not be given to neonates with hyperbilirubinaemia requiring treatment other than phototherapy or with markedly increased aminotransferase concentrations.

Because of the haematological toxicity of zidovudine it is recommended that, in patients with advanced symptomatic HIV disease taking oral zidovudine, blood tests should be carried out at least every 2 weeks for the first 3 months of treatment and at least monthly thereafter; blood tests should be performed at least every week in those receiving intravenous zidovudine. In patients with early HIV infection blood tests may be performed less frequently (e.g. every 1 to 3 months).

Interference with laboratory tests. Raised urinary thymine concentrations in neonates, due to maternal zidovudine treatment, could produce erroneous results in screening tests for inborn errors of metabolism.[1]

1. Sewell AC. Zidovudine and confusion in urinary metabolic screening. *Lancet* 1998; **352:** 1227.

Pregnancy. Administration of zidovudine to pregnant women with HIV infection from 14 weeks of gestation until delivery, and subsequently to the neonate, has been shown to reduce vertical transmission of the infection (see Uses and Administration, below). However, studies have shown that zidovudine can be fetotoxic in *animals* when given early in pregnancy, and the long-term consequences for the infant are as yet unknown although no adverse effects were seen in a group of infants followed for up to 5.6 years.[1] The manufacturer therefore recommends that zidovudine should not generally be administered before 14 weeks of gestation.

1. Culnane M, *et al.* Lack of long-term effects of in utero exposure to zidovudine among uninfected children born to HIV-infected women. *JAMA* 1999; **281:** 151–7.

Interactions

Care should be taken during concomitant therapy with zidovudine and drugs that are myelosuppressive or nephrotoxic. Drugs that undergo glucuronidation may delay the metabolism of zidovudine but few of these appear to produce clinically important increases in zidovudine plasma concentrations. Increased toxicity and decreased antiretroviral activity has been reported when zidovudine is given with some other antiviral drugs, and pharmacokinetic interactions have been reported with a number of anti-infective drugs used commonly in patients with HIV infection. See below for further details of interactions.

Analgesics. There may be an increased risk of haematotoxicity during concomitant use of zidovudine and *NSAIDs*.

Decreased zidovudine clearance[1] and increased area under the zidovudine plasma concentration-time curve[2] has been observed in patients receiving *methadone*.

Severe hepatotoxicity has occurred in a patient taking zidovudine and co-trimoxazole following *paracetamol* administration.[3] However, neither short-term[4] nor long-term[5] studies (the latter also in an individual patient) have shown any alteration of zidovudine elimination in patients taking zidovudine and paracetamol.

1. Burger DM, *et al.* Pharmacokinetic variability of zidovudine in HIV-infected individuals: subgroup analysis and drug interactions. *AIDS* 1994; **8:** 1683–9.
2. Schwartz EL, *et al.* Pharmacokinetic interactions of zidovudine and methadone in intravenous drug-using patients with HIV infection. *J Acquir Immune Defic Syndr* 1992; **5:** 619–26.
3. Shriner K, Goetz MB. Severe hepatotoxicity in a patient receiving both acetaminophen and zidovudine. *Am J Med* 1992; **93:** 94–6.
4. Sattler FR, *et al.* Acetaminophen does not impair clearance of zidovudine. *Ann Intern Med* 1991; **114:** 937–40.
5. Burger DM, *et al.* Pharmacokinetics of zidovudine and acetaminophen in a patient on chronic acetaminophen therapy. *Ann Pharmacother* 1994; **28:** 327–30.

Antibacterials. Studies have indicated that the absorption of zidovudine could be reduced by concurrent administration of *clarithromycin*.[1] The manufacturers of clarithromycin recommend administering zidovudine and clarithromycin 1 to 2 hours apart since this has been shown to have no overall effect on the bioavailability of zidovudine.[2] Administration of *rifampicin* to patients taking zidovudine has been reported to reduce the area under the plasma concentration-time curve of zidovudine, probably by inducing glucuronidation and amination.[3,4] *Rifabutin* has not been shown to have a marked effect on zidovudine clearance.[5] *Trimethoprim* has been reported[6,7] to decrease the renal clearance of zidovudine by up to 60% with a consequent increase in plasma concentrations, although it was only thought likely to be of clinical significance in patients with impaired liver function.[7]

For a report of reduced *pyrazinamide* concentrations in patients receiving zidovudine, see p.240.

1. Polis MA, *et al.* Clarithromycin lowers plasma zidovudine levels in persons with human immunodeficiency virus infection. *Antimicrob Agents Chemother* 1997; **41:** 1709–14.
2. Vance E, *et al.* Pharmacokinetics of clarithromycin and zidovudine in patients with AIDS. *Antimicrob Agents Chemother* 1995; **39:** 1355–60.

3. Burger DM, *et al.* Pharmacokinetic interaction between rifampin and zidovudine. *Antimicrob Agents Chemother* 1993; **37:** 1426–31.
4. Gallicano KD, *et al.* Induction of zidovudine glucuronidation and amination pathways by rifampicin in HIV-infected patients. *Br J Clin Pharmacol* 1999; **48:** 168–79.
5. Narang PK, Sale M. Population based assessment of rifabutin effect on zidovudine disposition in AIDS patients. *Clin Pharmacol Ther* 1993; **53:** 219.
6. Chatton JY, *et al.* Trimethoprim, alone or in combination with sulphamethoxazole, decreases the renal excretion of zidovudine and its glucuronide. *Br J Clin Pharmacol* 1992; **34:** 551–4.
7. Lee BL, *et al.* Zidovudine, trimethoprim, and dapsone pharmacokinetic interactions in patients with human immunodeficiency virus infection. *Antimicrob Agents Chemother* 1996; **40:** 1231–6.

Antiepileptics. Administration of *valproic acid* to 6 patients receiving zidovudine produced increases in plasma-zidovudine concentrations and the area under the plasma concentration-time curve.[1] The evidence suggested that this was due to reduced glucuronidation of zidovudine. Zidovudine may possibly reduce or increase plasma concentrations of *phenytoin*.

1. Lertora JJL, *et al.* Pharmacokinetic interaction between zidovudine and valproic acid in patients infected with human immunodeficiency virus. *Clin Pharmacol Ther* 1994; **56:** 272–8.

Antifungals. Administration of *fluconazole* in combination with zidovudine produced higher serum-zidovudine concentrations, increases in the area under the serum concentration-time curve and prolonged terminal half-life compared with zidovudine alone in a study in 12 patients.[1] Studies *in vitro* suggested that fluconazole could inhibit the glucuronidation of zidovudine; inhibition was also seen with *amphotericin B*, *ketoconazole*, and *miconazole*, but not with *flucytosine* or *itraconazole*.[2]

1. Sahai J, *et al.* Effect of fluconazole on zidovudine pharmacokinetics in patients infected with human immunodeficiency virus. *J Infect Dis* 1994; **169:** 103–7.
2. Sampol E, *et al.* Comparative effects of antifungal agents on zidovudine glucuronidation by human liver microsomes. *Br J Clin Pharmacol* 1995; **40:** 83–6.

Antivirals. Studies *in vitro* showed that ribavirin and zidovudine inhibited each other's anti-HIV activity[1] and the manufacturer recommends that this combination should be avoided. The manufacturer also recommends that the combination of zidovudine and *stavudine* should be avoided since similar antagonism has been shown *in vivo*.[2] *Interferon alfa* and zidovudine had a synergistic cytotoxicity to bone-marrow progenitor cells.[3] Severe haematological toxicity occurred when zidovudine was added to *ganciclovir* therapy in AIDS patients with cytomegalovirus retinitis, necessitating substantial dosage reductions or withdrawal of zidovudine in the majority of patients;[4,5] this additive toxicity with ganciclovir may be one reason why patients receiving zidovudine and ganciclovir do less well than those receiving zidovudine and foscarnet. Combined therapy with zidovudine and *aciclovir* is not generally associated with additional toxicity[6] but severe fatigue and lethargy were reported in a patient receiving aciclovir with zidovudine; this did not occur when either drug was given alone.[7] Evidence of a pharmacokinetic interaction between zidovudine and *didanosine* has been conflicting, with reports of no effect,[8] increased,[9] and decreased[10] plasma concentrations of zidovudine. Small reductions in didanosine plasma concentrations have been reported in patients also receiving zidovudine.[11] However, all changes have generally been small and are likely to be of limited clinical significance. Exposure to zidovudine (as measured by peak plasma concentrations and area under the concentration-time curve) was reduced in HIV patients given *ritonavir* concomitantly, whereas the pharmacokinetics of ritonavir were not affected by zidovudine;[12] the clinical relevance of this was not known. Modest increases in plasma-zidovudine concentrations occur on concurrent administration with *lamivudine*. Although this interaction is usually clinically insignificant, profound anaemia has been reported rarely in patients receiving this combination.[13,14]

For the enhanced *in-vitro* antiviral activity of zidovudine in combination with other antivirals, see Microbiological Interactions under Antiviral Action, below.

1. Vogt MW, *et al.* Ribavirin antagonizes the effect of azidothymidine on HIV replication. *Science* 1987; **235:** 1376–9.
2. Havlir DV, *et al.* In vivo antagonism with zidovudine plus stavudine combination therapy. *J Infect Dis* 2000; **182:** 321–5.
3. Berman E, *et al.* Synergistic cytotoxic effect of azidothymidine and recombinant interferon alpha on normal human bone marrow progenitor cells. *Blood* 1989; **74:** 1281–6.
4. Millar AB, *et al.* Treatment of cytomegalovirus retinitis with zidovudine and ganciclovir in patients with AIDS: outcome and toxicity. *Genitourin Med* 1990; **66:** 156–8.
5. Hochster H, *et al.* Toxicity of combined ganciclovir and zidovudine for cytomegalovirus disease associated with AIDS: an AIDS Clinical Trials Group study. *Ann Intern Med* 1990; **113:** 111–17.
6. Tartaglione TA, *et al.* Pharmacokinetic evaluations of low- and high-dose zidovudine plus high-dose acyclovir in patients with symptomatic human immunodeficiency virus infection. *Antimicrob Agents Chemother* 1991; **35:** 2225–31.
7. Bach MC. Possible drug interaction during therapy with azidothymidine and acyclovir for AIDS. *N Engl J Med* 1987; **316:** 547.
8. Collier AC, *et al.* Combination therapy with zidovudine and didanosine compared with zidovudine alone in HIV-1 infection. *Ann Intern Med* 1993; **119:** 786–93.
9. Barry M, *et al.* Pharmacokinetics of zidovudine and dideoxyinosine alone and in combination in patients with the acquired immunodeficiency syndrome. *Br J Clin Pharmacol* 1994; **37:** 421–6.
10. Burger DM, *et al.* Pharmacokinetic interaction study of zidovudine and didanosine. *J Drug Dev* 1994; **6:** 187–94.

11. Gibb D, *et al.* Pharmacokinetics of zidovudine and dideoxyinosine alone and in combination in children with HIV infection. *Br J Clin Pharmacol* 1995; **39:** 527–30.

12. Cato A, *et al.* Multidose pharmacokinetics of ritonavir and zidovudine in human immunodeficiency virus-infected patients. *Antimicrob Agents Chemother* 1998; **42:** 1788–93.

13. Hester EK, Peacock JE. Profound and unanticipated anemia with lamivudine-zidovudine combination therapy in zidovudine-experienced patients with HIV infection. *AIDS* 1998; **12:** 439–40.

14. Tseng A, *et al.* Precipitous declines in hemoglobin levels associated with combination zidovudine and lamivudine therapy. *Clin Infect Dis* 1998; **27:** 908–9.

Atovaquone. Administration of atovaquone in combination with zidovudine produced moderate increases in the zidovudine plasma concentration and area under the plasma concentration-time curve, probably by inhibition of glucuronidation.[1]

1. Lee BL, *et al.* Atovaquone inhibits the glucuronidation and increases the plasma concentrations of zidovudine. *Clin Pharmacol Ther* 1996; **59:** 14–21.

Probenecid. Administration of probenecid with zidovudine results in increased plasma concentrations and area under the plasma concentration-time curve of zidovudine, probably due to inhibition of glucuronidation;[1] tubular secretion of the glucuronide metabolite is also reduced. A high incidence of adverse effects has been reported in some patients receiving this combination.[2]

1. de Miranda P, *et al.* Alteration of zidovudine pharmacokinetics by probenecid in patients with AIDS or AIDS-related complex. *Clin Pharmacol Ther* 1989; **46:** 494–500.

2. Petty BG, *et al.* Zidovudine with probenecid: a warning. *Lancet* 1990; **335:** 1044–5.

Antiviral Action

Zidovudine is converted intracellularly in stages to the triphosphate via thymidine kinase and other kinases. This triphosphate halts the DNA synthesis of retroviruses, including HIV, through competitive inhibition of reverse transcriptase and incorporation into viral DNA. It has also been shown to possess activity against Epstein-Barr virus and Gram-negative bacteria *in vitro.*

Zidovudine-resistant strains of HIV emerge rapidly during zidovudine therapy and are responsible for the lack of benefit with long-term monotherapy. Cross-resistance to other nucleoside reverse transcriptase inhibitors has been recognised.

Microbiological interactions. The anti-HIV activity of zidovudine has been enhanced *in vitro* by a number of drugs including dextran sulfate,[1] granulocyte-macrophage colony-stimulating factor,[2,3] hydroxyurea [hydroxycarbamide],[4] foscarnet,[5,6] poly I.poly C12U,[7] carbovir,[8] castanospermine,[9] zalcitabine,[10] and didanosine.[11] Antiviral synergy was demonstrated against HIV *in vitro* with a combination of zidovudine, soluble CD4, and interferon alfa.[12] Interferon alfa also enhanced the activity of zidovudine in cells acutely and persistently infected with HIV.[13] Zidovudine blocked the HIV replication-enhancing effect of tumour necrosis factor.[14]

For a report of zidovudine and ribavirin mutually inhibiting each other's antiviral activity *in vitro*, and reports of increased toxicity of some antiviral combinations, see Antivirals, under Interactions, above.

1. Ueno R, Kuno S. Dextran sulphate, a potent anti-HIV agent in vitro having synergism with zidovudine. *Lancet* 1987; **i:** 1379.

2. Hammer SM, Gillis JM. Synergistic activity of granulocyte-macrophage colony-stimulating factor and 3′-azido-3′-deoxythymidine against human immunodeficiency virus in vitro. *Antimicrob Agents Chemother* 1987; **31:** 1046–50.

3. Perno C-F, *et al.* Replication of human immunodeficiency virus in monocytes: granulocyte/macrophage colony-stimulating factor (GM-CSF) potentiates viral production yet enhances the antiviral effect mediated by 3′-azido-2′3′-dideoxythymidine (AZT) and other dideoxynucleoside congeners of thymidine. *J Exp Med* 1989; **169:** 933–51.

4. Palmer S, Cox S. Increased activity of the combination of 3′-azido-3′-deoxythymidine and 2′-deoxy-3′-thiacytidine in the presence of hydroxyurea. *Antimicrob Agents Chemother* 1997; **41:** 460–4.

5. Eriksson BFH, Schinazi RF. Combinations of 3′-azido-3′-deoxythymidine (zidovudine) and phosphonoformate (foscarnet) against human immunodeficiency virus type 1 and cytomegalovirus replication in vitro. *Antimicrob Agents Chemother* 1989; **33:** 663–9.

6. Koshida R, *et al.* Inhibition of human immunodeficiency virus in vitro by combination of 3′-azido-3′-deoxythymidine and foscarnet. *Antimicrob Agents Chemother* 1989; **33:** 778–80.

7. Mitchell WM, *et al.* Mismatched double-stranded RNA (ampligen) reduces concentration of zidovudine (azidothymidine) required for in-vitro inhibition of human immunodeficiency virus. *Lancet* 1987; **i:** 890–2.

8. Smith MS, *et al.* Evaluation of synergy between carbovir and 3′-azido-2′3′-dideoxythymidine for inhibition of human immunodeficiency virus type 1. *Antimicrob Agents Chemother* 1993; **37:** 144–7.

9. Johnson VA, *et al.* Synergistic inhibition of human immunodeficiency virus type 1 and type 2 replication in vitro by castanospermine and 3′-azido-3′-deoxythymidine. *Antimicrob Agents Chemother* 1989; **33:** 53–7.

10. Spector SA, *et al.* Human immunodeficiency virus inhibition is prolonged by 3′-azido-3′-deoxythymidine alternating with 2′,3′-dideoxycytidine compared with 3′-azido-3′-deoxythymidine alone. *Antimicrob Agents Chemother* 1989; **33:** 920–3.

11. Dornsife RE, *et al.* Anti-human immunodeficiency virus synergism by zidovudine (3′-azidothymidine) and didanosine (dideoxyinosine) contrasts with their additive inhibition of normal human marrow progenitor cells. *Antimicrob Agents Chemother* 1991; **35:** 322–8.

12. Johnson VA, *et al.* Three-drug synergistic inhibition of HIV-1 replication in vitro by zidovudine, recombinant soluble CD4, and recombinant interferon-alpha A. *J Infect Dis* 1990; **161:** 1059–67.

13. Pincus SH, Wehrly K. AZT demonstrates anti-HIV-1 activity in persistently infected cell lines: implications for combination chemotherapy and immunotherapy. *J Infect Dis* 1990; **162:** 1233–8.

14. Michihiko S, *et al.* Augmentation of in-vitro HIV replication in peripheral blood mononuclear cells of AIDS and ARC patients by tumour necrosis factor. *Lancet* 1989; **i:** 1206–7.

Resistance. The emergence of zidovudine-resistant HIV strains in patients receiving long-term therapy with zidovudine has been recognised since 1989.[1,2] The emergence of drug resistance is associated with the duration[3] of treatment with zidovudine, but not the dose,[4] and is attributed to a high frequency of mutations in the HIV reverse transcriptase gene.[3,5] Development of high-level resistance to zidovudine in patients with advanced HIV infection is associated with rapid disease progression and death.[6] Primary infection with zidovudine-resistant HIV strains has been recorded,[7] as has zidovudine resistance in patients receiving other nucleoside reverse transcriptase inhibitors,[8,9] although it is possible that these patients had unrecorded exposure to zidovudine.[8] Emerging resistance to zidovudine is believed to be a factor in the loss of effect of long-term therapy. Cross-resistance with other reverse transcriptase inhibitors has been recorded and, although the use of zidovudine in combination with lamivudine has been reported to delay or reverse the emergence of some mutations conferring zidovudine resistance, dual resistance to zidovudine and lamivudine has occurred.[10] Analysis of the Delta trial[11] found no delay in the emergence of zidovudine resistance when used in combinations with didanosine or zalcitabine, although circulating concentrations of resistant virus were lower during combination therapy and antiviral activity was apparently not impaired. Nevertheless, it could be anticipated that the use of zidovudine in combination with other antiretrovirals, and particularly the highly active regimens which suppress viral replication to a high degree, could delay the emergence of resistance. The clinical response of patients with previous exposure to a number of regimens could be compromised by the presence of multidrug resistance.[12,13]

1. Larder BA, *et al.* HIV with reduced sensitivity to zidovudine (AZT) isolated during prolonged therapy. *Science* 1989; **243:** 1731–4.

2. Rooke R, *et al.* Isolation of drug-resistant variants of HIV-1 from patients on long-term zidovudine therapy. *AIDS* 1989; **3:** 411–15.

3. Japour AJ, *et al.* Prevalence and clinical significance of zidovudine resistance mutations in human immunodeficiency virus isolated from patients after long-term zidovudine treatment. *J Infect Dis* 1995; **171:** 1172–9.

4. Richman DD, *et al.* Effect of stage of disease and drug dose on zidovudine susceptibilities of isolates of human immunodeficiency virus. *J Acquir Immune Defic Syndr* 1990; **3:** 743–6.

5. Loveday C, *et al.* HIV-1 RNA serum-load and resistant viral genotypes during early zidovudine therapy. *Lancet* 1995; **345:** 820–4.

6. D'Aquila RT, *et al.* Zidovudine resistance and HIV-1 disease progression during antiretroviral therapy. *Ann Intern Med* 1995; **122:** 401–8.

7. Erice A, *et al.* Brief report: primary infection with zidovudine-resistant human immunodeficiency virus type 1. *N Engl J Med* 1993; **328:** 1163–5.

8. Lin P-F, *et al.* Genotypic and phenotypic analysis of human immunodeficiency virus type 1 isolates from patients on prolonged stavudine therapy. *J Infect Dis* 1994; **170:** 1157–64.

9. Demeter LM, *et al.* Development of zidovudine resistance mutations in patients receiving prolonged didanosine monotherapy. *J Infect Dis* 1995; **172:** 1480–5.

10. Miller V, *et al.* Dual resistance to zidovudine and lamivudine in patients treated with zidovudine-lamivudine combination therapy: association with therapy failure. *J Infect Dis* 1998; **177:** 1521–32.

11. Brun-Vézinet F, *et al.* HIV-1 viral load, phenotype, and resistance in a subset of drug-naive participants from the Delta trial. *Lancet* 1997; **350:** 983–90.

12. Kavlick MF, *et al.* Emergence of multi-dideoxynucleoside-resistant human immunodeficiency virus type 1 variants, viral sequence variation, and disease progression in patients receiving antiretroviral chemotherapy. *J Infect Dis* 1998; **177:** 1506–13.

13. Shafer RW, *et al.* Multiple concurrent reverse transcriptase and protease mutations and multidrug resistance of HIV-1 isolates from heavily treated patients. *Ann Intern Med* 1998; **128:** 906–11.

Pharmacokinetics

Zidovudine is rapidly absorbed from the gastrointestinal tract and undergoes first-pass hepatic metabolism with a bioavailability of about 60 to 70%. Peak plasma concentrations occur after about 1 hour. Absorption is delayed by administration with food, but bioavailability is probably unaffected. Zidovudine crosses the blood-brain barrier producing CSF to plasma ratios of about 0.5. It crosses the placenta and is distributed into breast milk. Plasma protein binding is reported to be 34 to 38%. The plasma half-life is about 1 hour.

Zidovudine is metabolised intracellularly to the antiviral triphosphate. It is also metabolised in the liver mainly to the inactive glucuronide and is excreted in the urine as unchanged drug and metabolite.

◊ Reviews.

1. Acosta EP, *et al.* Clinical pharmacokinetics of zidovudine: an update. *Clin Pharmacokinet* 1996; **30:** 251–62.

Bioavailability. Absorption of oral zidovudine was delayed or reduced when the dose was taken with a meal compared with when taken after an overnight fast.[1-3] It was suggested that to achieve high peak plasma concentrations of zidovudine, it should be taken on an empty stomach. The bioavailability in HIV-positive patients is reported to be erratic[4,5] but not greatly reduced by diarrhoea.[5]

1. Unadkat JD, *et al.* Pharmacokinetics of oral zidovudine (azidothymidine) in patients with AIDS when administered with and without a high-fat meal. *AIDS* 1990; **4:** 229–32.

2. Lotterer E, *et al.* Decreased and variable systemic availability of zidovudine in patients with AIDS if administered with a meal. *Eur J Clin Pharmacol* 1991; **40:** 305–8.

3. Ruhnke M, *et al.* Effects of standard breakfast on pharmacokinetics of oral zidovudine in patients with AIDS. *Antimicrob Agents Chemother* 1993; **37:** 2153–8.

4. Macnab KA, *et al.* Erratic zidovudine bioavailability in HIV seropositive patients. *J Antimicrob Chemother* 1993; **31:** 421–8.

5. Zorza G, *et al.* Absorption of zidovudine in patients with diarrhoea. *Eur J Clin Pharmacol* 1993; **44:** 501–3.

Neonates. The pharmacokinetics of zidovudine in infants more than 14 days old are reported to be similar to those in adults. Following maternal administration the half-life of zidovudine in 7 neonates has been reported to be extended to a mean of 13 hours.[1] In infants receiving zidovudine, those under 14 days of age had lower total clearance, longer terminal half-life (about 3 hours), and higher bioavailability than older infants.[2] Zidovudine clearance was low and the half-life prolonged to about 7 hours in premature infants.[3]

1. O'Sullivan MJ, *et al.* The pharmacokinetics and safety of zidovudine in the third trimester of pregnancy for women infected with human immunodeficiency virus and their infants: phase 1 Acquired Immunodeficiency Syndrome Clinical Trials Group Study (protocol 082). *Am J Obstet Gynecol* 1993; **168:** 1510–16.

2. Boucher FD, *et al.* Phase 1 evaluation of zidovudine administered to infants exposed at birth to the human immunodeficiency virus. *J Pediatr* 1993; **122:** 137–44.

3. Mirochnick M, *et al.* Zidovudine pharmacokinetics in premature infants exposed to human immunodeficiency virus. *Antimicrob Agents Chemother* 1998; **42:** 808–12.

Pregnancy. In a study in 3 pregnant women with HIV infection,[1] the area under the concentration-time curve for zidovudine was reduced and the clearance of an oral dose increased during pregnancy when compared with up to 4 weeks postpartum. These results differed from those reported from another study which reported no differences during or after pregnancy.[2] This latter study, however, used values obtained no later than 48 hours postpartum for comparison, at which time it is unlikely that physiological functions would have returned to the non-pregnant state. Zidovudine and its glucuronide metabolite cross the placenta reaching concentrations in the fetal blood similar to those in maternal blood.[3,4] However, concentrations of zidovudine in the fetal CNS have been reported to be below those required to exert an anti-HIV effect.[5]

1. Watts DH, *et al.* Pharmacokinetic disposition of zidovudine during pregnancy. *J Infect Dis* 1991; **163:** 226–32.

2. O'Sullivan MJ, *et al.* The pharmacokinetics and safety of zidovudine in the third trimester of pregnancy for women infected with human immunodeficiency virus and their infants: phase 1 Acquired Immunodeficiency Syndrome Clinical Trials Group Study (protocol 082). *Am J Obstet Gynecol* 1993; **168:** 1510–16.

3. Gillet JY, *et al.* Fetoplacental passage of zidovudine. *Lancet* 1989; **ii:** 269–70.

4. Chavanet P, *et al.* Perinatal pharmacokinetics of zidovudine. *N Engl J Med* 1989; **321:** 1548–9.

5. Lyman WD, *et al.* Zidovudine concentrations in human fetal tissue: implications for perinatal AIDS. *Lancet* 1990; **335:** 1280–1.

Uses and Administration

Zidovudine is a nucleoside reverse transcriptase inhibitor structurally related to thymidine. It has activity against retroviruses including HIV and is used in the management of HIV infection. Zidovudine is usually given in combination with other antiretrovirals to symptomatic and selected asymptomatic patients. It is used alone to prevent vertical transmission from mother to infant.

Zidovudine is given by mouth in *adult* doses of 500 to 600 mg daily in divided doses. Higher doses may be required for neurological disease. Zidovudine may be given by intravenous infusion of a solution containing 2 to 4 mg per mL over 1 hour for short-term management of patients unable to take it by mouth. The adult dose is 1 to 2 mg per kg body-weight every 4 hours (equivalent to an oral dose of 1.5 to 3 mg per kg every 4 hours).

The oral dose for *children* over 3 months of age is 360 to 480 mg per m^2 body-surface daily in 3 or 4 divided doses, although doses of up to 720 mg per m^2 daily (180 mg per m^2 every 6 hours) are used and may be necessary for neurological disease. The dose should not exceed 200 mg every 6 hours. Intravenous doses of 80 to 160 mg per m² have been given every 6 hours. An intravenous dose of 120 mg per m² every 6 hours is approximately equivalent to an oral dose of 180 mg per m² every 6 hours.

For the *prevention of maternal-fetal HIV transmission*, zidovudine may be given after the fourteenth week of pregnancy until the beginning of labour in a dose of 100 mg five times daily by mouth. During labour and delivery, zidovudine is given by intravenous infusion in a dose of 2 mg per kg over 1 hour, then 1 mg per kg per hour until the umbilical cord is clamped. When a caesarean section is planned the intravenous infusion is started 4 hours before the operation. The newborn infant is given 2 mg per kg orally every 6 hours starting within 12 hours after birth and continuing for 6 weeks. Low-dose regimens are being assessed (see HIV Infection Prophylaxis, below). Neonates unable to receive oral doses are given 1.5 mg per kg by intravenous infusion over 30 minutes every 6 hours.

Blood tests should be carried out regularly as described under Precautions, above. If the white cell count or haemoglobin level fall, the dose should be reduced or, alternatively, treatment interrupted briefly, until there is evidence of recovery. Treatment should be discontinued if toxicity is severe and cautiously reintroduced once the bone marrow has recovered. Dosage adjustments may also be necessary in patients with renal or hepatic impairment.

◊ Reviews.
1. Wilde MI, Langtry HD. Zidovudine: an update of its pharmacodynamic and pharmacokinetic properties, and therapeutic efficacy. *Drugs* 1993; **46:** 515–78.

Administration and dosage. A number of studies have been performed to determine the optimal dosage regimen of zidovudine and as a result there has been a general trend to use lower doses for both prophylaxis and treatment of HIV infection and AIDS. Doses studied in patients with AIDS have ranged from 400 to 1500 mg daily in a variety of divided-dose regimens.[1,2] These studies found that low-dose regimens were as effective as higher doses in terms of prolongation of survival and were better tolerated. Similar results were found in patients with AIDS-related complex[3] and asymptomatic HIV infection,[4] and it was concluded that doses above 400 to 600 mg daily[5,6] offered no clinical advantage.

Although zidovudine should ideally be administered every 4 hours owing to its short half-life, patients have been reported to take it in three or even two daily doses,[7] and there is preliminary evidence that efficacy is unaffected.[8] HAART regimens have typically used zidovudine in doses of 200 mg three times daily. Modified-release formulations are under development which may allow less frequent dosing while maintaining zidovudine plasma concentrations.

1. Fischl MA, *et al.* A randomized controlled trial of a reduced daily dose of zidovudine in patients with the acquired immunodeficiency syndrome. *N Engl J Med* 1990; **323:** 1009–14.
2. Nordic Medical Research Councils' HIV Therapy Group. Double blind dose-response study of zidovudine in AIDS and advanced HIV infection. *BMJ* 1992; **304:** 13–17.
3. Collier AC, *et al.* A pilot study of low-dose zidovudine in human immunodeficiency virus infection. *N Engl J Med* 1990; **323:** 1015–21.
4. Volberding PA, *et al.* Zidovudine in asymptomatic human immunodeficiency virus infection: a controlled trial in persons with fewer than 500 CD4-positive cells per cubic millimeter. *N Engl J Med* 1990; **322:** 941–9.
5. Gøtzshe PC. Zidovudine dosage. *BMJ* 1993; **307:** 682–3.
6. McLeod GX, Hammer SM. Zidovudine: five years later. *Ann Intern Med* 1992; **117:** 487–501.
7. Clumeck N. Current use of anti-HIV drugs in AIDS. *J Antimicrob Chemother* 1993; **32** (suppl A): 133–8.
8. Shepp DH, *et al.* A comparative trial of zidovudine administered every four versus every twelve hours for the treatment of advanced HIV disease. *J Acquir Immune Defic Syndr Hum Retrovirol* 1997; **15:** 283–8.

HIV infection and AIDS. As discussed on p.608, the use of antiretroviral drugs in HIV infection has changed following studies which indicated that combination therapy could improve response. Monotherapy with zidovudine reduced the incidence of opportunistic infections and mortality in patients with AIDS or ARC. Benefit might also be seen in other features of AIDS such as dementia (see HIV-associated Neurological Complications, below). Unfortunately such benefit was found to be transient[1-4] and treatment during the early stages of HIV infection, while delaying disease progression,[5-10] failed to produce improvements in long-term outcome or the quality of life;[7,10-12] in addition there are concerns about resistance.[13,14]

Therapy with a combination of zidovudine and other antiretroviral drugs might improve efficacy, minimise toxicity, and delay drug resistance. Results from the Delta study[15] and the US AIDS Clinical Trial Group 175 (ACTG 175) study[16] showed combination therapy to be more effective than monotherapy in antiretroviral-naive patients and led to immediate changes in clinical practice. In patients who had not received zidovudine before, both studies showed substantial reductions in mortality at 30 months in patients treated with zidovudine plus either didanosine or zalcitabine compared with those receiving zidovudine alone. Triple therapy with zidovudine combined with another nucleoside reverse transcriptase inhibitor and either an HIV-protease inhibitor or a non-nucleoside reverse transcriptase inhibitor (HAART regimens) have been found to reduce viral loads more effectively than monotherapy or two-drug combination therapy[17-19] and such regimens are currently regarded as standard.

1. Fischl MA, *et al.* The efficacy of azidothymidine (AZT) in the treatment of patients with AIDS and AIDS-related complex: a double-blind, placebo-controlled trial. *N Engl J Med* 1987; **317:** 185–91.
2. Dournon E, *et al.* Effects of zidovudine in 365 consecutive patients with AIDS or AIDS-related complex. *Lancet* 1988; **ii:** 1297–1302.
3. Lundgren JD, *et al.* Comparison of long-term prognosis of patients with AIDS treated and not treated with zidovudine. *JAMA* 1994; **271:** 1088–92.
4. Kinloch-de Loës S, Perneger TV. Primary HIV infection: follow-up of patients initially randomized to zidovudine or placebo. *J Infect* 1997; **35:** 111–16.
5. Fischl MA, *et al.* The safety and efficacy of zidovudine (AZT) in the treatment of subjects with mildly symptomatic human immunodeficiency virus type 1 (HIV) infection: a double-blind, placebo-controlled trial. *Ann Intern Med* 1990; **112:** 727–37.
6. Volberding PA, *et al.* Zidovudine in asymptomatic human immunodeficiency virus infection: a controlled trial in persons with fewer than 500 CD4-positive cells per cubic millimeter. *N Engl J Med* 1990; **322:** 941–9.
7. Hamilton JD, *et al.* A controlled trial of early versus late treatment with zidovudine in symptomatic human immunodeficiency virus infection. *N Engl J Med* 1992; **326:** 437–43.
8. Graham NMH, *et al.* The effects on survival of early treatment of human immunodeficiency virus infection. *N Engl J Med* 1992; **326:** 1037–42.
9. Cooper DA, *et al.* Zidovudine in persons with asymptomatic HIV infection and CD4+ cell counts greater than 400 per cubic millimeter. *N Engl J Med* 1993; **329:** 297–303.
10. Concorde Coordinating Committee. Concorde: MRC/ANRS randomised double-blind controlled trial of immediate and deferred zidovudine in symptom-free HIV infection. *Lancet* 1994; **343:** 871–81.
11. Volberding PA, *et al.* The duration of zidovudine benefit in persons with asymptomatic HIV infection: prolonged evaluation of protocol 019 of the AIDS clinical trials group. *JAMA* 1994; **272:** 437–42.
12. Lenderking WR, *et al.* Evaluation of the quality of life associated with zidovudine treatment in asymptomatic human immunodeficiency virus infection *N Engl J Med* 1994; **330:** 738–43.
13. Ogino MT, *et al.* Development and significance of zidovudine resistance in children infected with human immunodeficiency virus. *J Pediatr* 1993; **123:** 1–8.
14. Husson RN, *et al.* High-level resistance to zidovudine but not to zalcitabine or didanosine in human immunodeficiency virus from children receiving antiretroviral therapy. *J Pediatr* 1993; **123:** 9–16.
15. Delta Coordinating Committee. Delta: a randomised double-blind controlled trial comparing combinations of zidovudine plus didanosine or zalcitabine with zidovudine alone in HIV-infected individuals. *Lancet* 1996; **348:** 283–91.
16. Hammer SM, *et al.* A trial comparing nucleoside monotherapy with combination therapy in HIV-infected adults with CD4 cell counts from 200 to 500 per cubic millimeter. *N Engl J Med* 1996; **335:** 1081–90.
17. Hammer SM, *et al.* A controlled trial of two nucleoside analogues plus indinavir in persons with human immunodeficiency virus infection and CD4 cell counts of 200 per cubic millimeter or less. *N Engl J Med* 1997; **337:** 725–33.
18. Gulick RM, *et al.* Treatment with indinavir, zidovudine, and lamivudine in adults with human immunodeficiency virus infection and prior antiretroviral therapy. *N Engl J Med* 1997; **337:** 734–9.
19. Montaner JSG, *et al.* A randomized, double-blind trial comparing combinations of nevirapine, didanosine, and zidovudine for HIV-infected patients: the INCAS trial. *JAMA* 1998; **279:** 930–7.

HIV-associated malignancies. As discussed on p.501, zidovudine in combination with interferons has been advocated for the management of Kaposi's sarcoma in HIV-infected patients with a CD4+ count of 200 cells per μL or above.[1-5]

In patients with AIDS-associated non-Hodgkin's lymphoma, zidovudine in combination with interferon alfa[6] and with methotrexate[7] has been reported to produce beneficial responses in small numbers of patients.

1. Brockmeyer NH, *et al.* Regression of Kaposi's sarcoma and improvement of performance status by a combined interferon β and zidovudine therapy in AIDS patients. *J Invest Dermatol* 1989; **92:** 776.
2. Edlin BR, *et al.* Interferon-alpha plus zidovudine in HIV infection. *Lancet* 1989; **i:** 156.
3. Northfelt DW. Treatment of Kaposi's sarcoma: current guidelines and future perspectives. *Drugs* 1994; **48:** 569–82.
4. Kovacs JA, *et al.* Combined zidovudine and interferon-α therapy in patients with Kaposi sarcoma and the acquired immunodeficiency syndrome (AIDS). *Ann Intern Med* 1989; **111:** 280–7.
5. Krown SE, *et al.* Interferon-α with zidovudine: safety, tolerance, and clinical and virologic effects in patients with Kaposi sarcoma associated with the acquired immunodeficiency syndrome (AIDS). *Ann Intern Med* 1990; **112:** 812–21.
6. Harrington WJ, *et al.* Azothymidine and interferon-α are active in AIDS-associated small non-cleaved cell lymphoma but not large-cell lymphoma. *Lancet* 1996; **348:** 283–91.
7. Tosi P, *et al.* 3′-Azido-3′-deoxythymidine + methotrexate as a novel antineoplastic combination in the treatment of human immunodeficiency virus-related non-Hodgkin's lymphomas. *Blood* 1997; **89:** 419–25.

HIV-associated neurological complications. Dementia is one of the complications associated with HIV infection and AIDS (see p.610). In a retrospective study of AIDS patients it was noted that the incidence of dementia fell after the institution of zidovudine therapy.[1] Despite criticisms of this study,[2] others have also noted an improvement in dementia and other AIDS-related neurological disorders with zidovudine.[3-7] The improvement was sustained for up to 18 months in one patient.[3] Zidovudine given intrathecally for AIDS-related dementia produced improvement in 3 patients, with minimal toxicity,[8] but no improvement was observed in a further patient given zidovudine intrathecally and intravenously.[9]

1. Portegies P, *et al.* Declining incidence of AIDS dementia complex after introduction of zidovudine treatment. *BMJ* 1989; **299:** 819–21. Correction. *ibid.*; 1141.
2. Morriss R, House A. Zidovudine in AIDS dementia complex. *BMJ* 1989; **299:** 1218.
3. Yarchoan R, *et al.* Long-term administration of 3′-azido-2′,3′-dideoxythymidine to patients with AIDS-related neurological disease. *Ann Neurol* 1988; **23** (suppl): S82–7.
4. Schmitt FA, *et al.* Neuropsychological outcome of zidovudine (AZT) treatment of patients with AIDS and AIDS-related complex. *N Engl J Med* 1988; **319:** 1573–8.
5. Conway B, *et al.* Human immunodeficiency virus-associated progressive multifocal leukoencephalopathy: apparent response to 3′-azido-3′-deoxythymidine. *Rev Infect Dis* 1990; **12:** 479–82.
6. Chiesi A, *et al.* Epidemiology of AIDS dementia complex in Europe. *J Acquir Immune Defic Syndr Hum Retrovirol* 1996; **11:** 39–44.
7. Evers S, *et al.* Impact of antiretroviral treatment on AIDS dementia: a longitudinal prospective event-related potential study. *J Acquir Immune Defic Syndr Hum Retrovirol* 1998; **17:** 143–8.
8. Routy JP, *et al.* Intrathecal zidovudine for AIDS dementia. *Lancet* 1990; **336:** 248.
9. Lucht F, *et al.* Intrathecal zidovudine for AIDS dementia. *Lancet* 1990; **336:** 813.

HIV infection prophylaxis. Antiretroviral drugs are becoming more widely accepted for chemoprophylaxis after exposure to HIV infection. Zidovudine is commonly used in combination with other antiretroviral drugs, such as lamivudine and an HIV-protease inhibitor, after occupational exposure with a high risk of infection. For suggested regimens, see p.610.

Zidovudine has also been shown to be of value in reducing vertical transmission from mother to infant.[1] A typical dosage regimen is given under Uses and Administration, above, but the effectiveness of lower doses is being assessed in developing countries. Short-course regimens have typically involved starting zidovudine 300 mg twice daily by mouth at 36 to 38 weeks' gestation, and giving, during labour, either 300 mg every 3 hours,[2,3] or 500 or 600 mg as a single dose.[4] In the latter study, treatment was continued for a further week postpartum,[4] but no treatment was given to the infants in any of these studies. Although the reductions in transmission rates were lower than those achieved with the high-dose regimen, they were nevertheless regarded as useful in the populations studied.[5] Abbreviated regimens, even begun as late as the first 48 hours of life, do seem still to be of benefit.[6]

1. Sperling RS, *et al.* Maternal viral load, zidovudine treatment, and the risk of transmission of human immunodeficiency virus type 1 from mother to infant. *N Engl J Med* 1996; **335:** 1621–9.
2. Shaffer N, *et al.* Short-course zidovudine for perinatal HIV-1 transmission in Bangkok, Thailand: a randomised controlled trial. *Lancet* 1999; **353:** 773–80.
3. Wiktor SZ, *et al.* Short-course oral zidovudine for prevention of mother-to-child transmission of HIV-1 in Abidjan, Côte d'Ivoire: a randomised trial. *Lancet* 1999; **353:** 781–5.
4. Dabis F, *et al.* 6-Month efficacy, tolerance, and acceptability of a short regimen of oral zidovudine to reduce vertical transmission of HIV in breastfed children in Côte d'Ivoire and Burkina Faso: a double-blind placebo-controlled multicentre trial. *Lancet* 1999; **353:** 786–92.
5. Mofenson LM. Short-course zidovudine for prevention of perinatal infection. *Lancet* 1999; **353:** 766–7.
6. Wade NA, *et al.* Abbreviated regimens of zidovudine prophylaxis and perinatal transmission of the human immunodeficiency virus. *N Engl J Med* 1998; **339:** 1409–14.

Preparations

USP 25: Zidovudine Capsules; Zidovudine Injection; Zidovudine Oral Solution.

Proprietary Preparations (details are given in Part 3)

Aust.: Retrovir; *Austral.:* Retrovir; *Belg.:* Retrovir; *Braz.:* Retrovir; Virustat; *Canad.:* Novo-AZT; Retrovir; *Denm.:* Retrovir; *Fin.:* Retrovir; *Fr.:* Retrovir; *Ger.:* Retrovir; *Hong Kong:* Retrovir; *Irl.:* Retrovir; *Israel:* Retrovir; *Ital.:* Retrovir; *Mex.:* Dipedyne; Isadol; Novavir; Retrovir; Serovidina; Zidovir; *Neth.:* Retrovir; *Norw.:* Retrovir; *NZ:* Retrovir; *Port.:* Retrovir; *S.Afr.:* Retrovir; *Singapore:* Retrovir; *Spain:* Retrovir; *Swed.:* Retrovir; *Switz.:* Retrovir; *Thai.:* Retrovir; T-ZA; T.O.Vir; *UK:* Retrovir; *USA:* Retrovir.

Multi-ingredient: *Aust.:* Combivir; *Austral.:* Combivir; *Belg.:* Combivir; *Canad.:* Combivir; *Denm.:* Combivir; *Fin.:* Combivir; *Fr.:* Combivir; *Ger.:* Combivir; *Hong Kong:* Combivir; *Irl.:* Combivir; *Israel:* Combivir; *Ital.:* Combivir; *Mex.:* Combivir; *Neth.:* Combivir; *NZ:* Combivir; *Port.:* Combivir; *S.Afr.:* Retrovir/3TC Post-HIV Exposure; *Singapore:* Combivir; *Spain:* Combivir; *Swed.:* Combivir; *Switz.:* Combivir; *Thai.:* Combid; *UK:* Combivir; Trizivir; *USA:* Combivir; Trizivir.

Anxiolytic Sedatives Hypnotics and Antipsychotics

The drugs in this chapter include anxiolytic sedatives, formerly called minor tranquillisers, which have been used in the management of anxiety disorders; drugs used to produce sleep (hypnotics); and drugs used in the treatment of psychoses (antipsychotics, formerly called major tranquillisers). The term neuroleptic is sometimes used to describe those antipsychotics that have effects on the extrapyramidal system. The difference in action between anxiolytics and hypnotics is mainly one of degree and the same drug or group of drugs can have both effects, larger doses being necessary to produce a state of sleep.

The benzodiazepines (typified by Diazepam, p.674) replaced the barbiturates (typified by Amobarbital, p.655) and related sedatives as the major group of drugs used as anxiolytics and hypnotics. Some benzodiazepines are also used for their muscle relaxant and anticonvulsant properties. Newer anxiolytics include buspirone (p.657), a drug which affects serotonin neurotransmission.

The classical antipsychotics (typified by Chlorpromazine, p.660) include the butyrophenones, the diphenylbutylpiperidines, the indole derivatives, the phenothiazines, and the thioxanthenes. Some newer antipsychotics such as clozapine (p.671), risperidone (p.704), olanzapine (p.696), quetiapine (p.703), and amisulpride (p.655) are often referred to as atypical antipsychotics because of their reduced tendency to cause the extrapyramidal effects typical of classical antipsychotics.

◊ General references.
1. WHO. Evaluation of methods for the treatment of mental disorders. *WHO Tech Rep Ser 812* 1991.

Anxiety disorders

Anxiety is an emotional condition characterised by feelings such as apprehension and fear accompanied by physical symptoms such as tachycardia, increased respiration, sweating, and tremor. It can be a normal emotion but when it is severe and disabling it becomes pathological.

Anxiety disorders are difficult to define and various classifications exist. In **acute stress disorder** anxiety is associated with a recent extremely stressful event such as bereavement, and is likely to resolve within a few weeks, whereas in **generalised anxiety disorders** there is persistent pervasive anxiety usually lasting 6 months or more. Symptoms include motor tension, autonomic hyperactivity, irritability, and loss of concentration.

The first step in the management of anxiety that cannot be attributed to an underlying disease is the use of psychological treatments. Such therapy can be effective in most types of anxiety. If unsuccessful, short-term treatment with a benzodiazepine may be considered. Although benzodiazepines can exert an effect very rapidly, possibly even after the first dose, their use is limited by serious problems of dependence (see under Diazepam, p.675). Tolerance may develop to the anxiolytic effects of benzodiazepines although this appears to be less likely than tolerance to the psychomotor effects. There do not

appear to be clear advantages for any one benzodiazepine in the treatment of anxiety disorders.

Buspirone, an azaspirodecanedione, appears to have broadly similar efficacy to the benzodiazepines but a slower onset of action. It is reported to lack euphoriant effect, and may cause less sedation and dependence than the benzodiazepines. Its efficacy is reduced in patients who have had previous extensive use of benzodiazepines.[1,2]

Other drugs used as alternatives to the benzodiazepines for the treatment of anxiety disorders include the tricyclic antidepressants.[2,3] Some consider them preferable to benzodiazepines for the treatment of generalised anxiety disorders;[1,4] they are particularly appropriate when medium or long-term therapy is necessary or when depression is also present. It may be several weeks before their effects are apparent, therefore combined therapy with benzodiazepines may be required initially. SSRIs have been used as alternatives to the tricyclics although they have been less well studied in the treatment of generalised anxiety disorders.[3] The noradrenaline and serotonin reuptake inhibitor venlafaxine may also be used.

Beta blockers may be useful for the control of the physical symptoms of anxiety.[5] There is little evidence to support the efficacy of antihistamines such as hydroxyzine in anxious patients,[1] and the use of antihistamines solely for their sedative effect in anxiety is not considered appropriate. Antipsychotics have been used by some in severe anxiety for their sedative effects; long-term use should be avoided because of the risk of tardive dyskinesia.

Anxiety may be present with other disorders such as depression in **mixed anxiety and depressive disorders** the management of which is discussed under Depression on p.271.

1. Lader M. Treatment of anxiety. *BMJ* 1994; **309**: 321–4.
2. Nutt DJ. The psychopharmacology of anxiety. *Br J Hosp Med* 1996; **55**: 187–91.
3. Feighner JP. Overview of antidepressants currently used to treat anxiety disorders. *J Clin Psychiatry* 1999; **60** (suppl 22): 18–22.
4. Lader M, *et al.* Royal College of Psychiatrists. Guidelines for the management of patients with generalised anxiety. *Psychiatr Bull* 1992; **16**: 560–5.
5. Anonymous. Drugs for depression and anxiety. *Med Lett Drugs Ther* 1999; **41**: 33–8.

Obsessive-compulsive disorder. Obsessive-compulsive disorder is associated with intrusive, recurrent, obsessional thoughts and/or repetitive compulsive behaviour (e.g. hand washing) performed in a ritualistic manner. A combination of pharmacological, behavioural, and psychosocial methods appears to have the most successful long-term outcome in the treatment of obsessive-compulsive disorder.[1] Drug therapy is based on antidepressants which inhibit reuptake of serotonin.[2-5] These include clomipramine and the SSRIs. There is some evidence that clomipramine is more effective than the SSRIs but its adverse effects are more problematic.[5] It may take 4 to 6 weeks before any response is obtained and up to about 12 weeks to achieve an optimal effect.[4,6] If one serotonin reuptake inhibitor fails then another can be tried.[2,4,5] About 40 to 60% of patients do not respond to these drugs and of those who do, many do not experience complete remission.[5] The optimum duration of treatment in responders remains to be determined. Some suggest therapy for at least a year or longer[1,6,7] but many patients relapse when drug therapy is withdrawn and prolonged therapy may be necessary. It has been suggested that patients may be maintained on reduced dosage.[8] Gradual withdrawal over several months may be more successful if patients are also receiving behavioural therapy.[1] Drugs such as buspirone, pindolol, and some antipsychotics have also been tried as adjuncts when patients are refractory to serotonin reuptake inhibitors and behavioural therapy but results have been variable.[1,4,5,7] Benzodiazepines have been tried as alternatives to serotonin reuptake inhibitors but they are unsuitable because of the problems associated with prolonged therapy.[7]

1. Rasmussen SA, *et al.* Current issues in the pharmacologic management of obsessive compulsive disorder. *J Clin Psychiatry* 1993; **54** (suppl): 4–9.
2. Anonymous. Drugs for depression and anxiety. *Med Lett Drugs Ther* 1999; **41**: 33–8.
3. Piccinelli M, *et al.* Efficacy of drug treatment in obsessive-compulsive disorder: a meta-analytic review. *Br J Psychiatry* 1995; **166**: 424–43.
4. Carpenter LL, *et al.* A risk-benefit assessment of drugs used in the management of obsessive-compulsive disorder. *Drug Safety* 1996; **15**: 116–34.

5. Goodman WK. Obsessive-compulsive disorder: diagnosis and treatment. *J Clin Psychiatry* 1999; **60** (suppl 18): 27–32.
6. March JS, *et al.* Expert Consensus Guideline Series: treatment of obsessive-compulsive disorder. *J Clin Psychiatry* 1997; **58** (suppl 4): 1–73.
7. Zohar J, *et al.* Current concepts in the pharmacological treatment of obsessive-compulsive disorder. *Drugs* 1992; **43**: 210–18.
8. Mundo E, *et al.* Long-term pharmacotherapy of obsessive-compulsive disorder: a double-blind controlled study. *J Clin Psychopharmacol* 1997; **17**: 4–10.

Panic attacks. Panic attacks are severe, sudden, unexpected, recurrent exacerbations of anxiety. During an attack there is a feeling of fear, terror, and impending doom or even death accompanied by autonomic symptoms. If behavioural or cognitive therapy fails in the management of panic disorders drug therapy can then be tried, but it may need to be prolonged as there is a high rate of relapse on discontinuation.[1] Antidepressants are the drugs of choice in the treatment of panic disorder.[2] Tricyclic antidepressants or SSRIs can reduce the frequency of attacks and can often prevent them completely.[3-5] Efficacy is broadly comparable, although SSRIs may be associated with a lower incidence of serious adverse effects.[6,7] MAOIs such as phenelzine are also effective but dietary restrictions and serious adverse effects limit their use to patients unresponsive to tricyclics and SSRIs.[5,6] Other antidepressants are being evaluated in panic attacks. It may take several weeks before the effects of antidepressants are seen and initially there may be an increase in anxiety and the frequency of panic attacks. Benzodiazepines are sometimes used as adjuncts until antidepressants exert their full effect.[5-7] Short courses of benzodiazepines may also be of use in patients who cannot tolerate, or are refractory to, antidepressants,[3] but any benefit may be outweighed by the risk of dependence.[4] There is little evidence to support the use of beta blockers, but they may control physical symptoms. Other drugs that might produce beneficial effects in some patients include valproate[3,5,7] and possibly clonidine.[8]

1. Michels R, Marzuk PM. Progress in psychiatry. *N Engl J Med* 1993; **329**: 628–38.
2. Anonymous. Drugs for depression and anxiety. *Med Lett Drugs Ther* 1999; **41**: 33–8.
3. Johnson MR, *et al.* Panic disorder: pathophysiology and drug treatment. *Drugs* 1995; **49**: 328–44.
4. Anonymous. Stopping panic attacks. *Drug Ther Bull* 1997; **35**: 58–62.
5. Bennett JA, *et al.* A risk-benefit assessment of pharmacological treatments for panic disorder. *Drug Safety* 1998; **18**: 419–30.
6. American Psychiatric Association. Practice guideline for the treatment of patients with panic disorder. *Am J Psychiatry* 1998; **155** (suppl): 1–34.
7. Ballenger JC, *et al.* Consensus statement on panic disorder from the International Consensus Group on Depression and Anxiety. *J Clin Psychiatry* 1998; **59** (suppl 8): 47–54.
8. Puzantian T, Hart LL. Clonidine in panic disorder. *Ann Pharmacother* 1993; **27**: 1351–3.

Phobic disorders. Phobic disorders consist of an irrational or exaggerated fear of, and a wish to avoid, specific objects, activities, or situations. As there is a strong link between **agoraphobia** and panic attacks (see above) it is treated similarly. Simple or specific phobias are usually unresponsive to pharmacotherapy and respond better to behaviour therapy. SSRIs, and particularly paroxetine, are considered to be the first choice for the treatment of social anxiety disorders.[1-3] MAOIs such as phenelzine are also effective in social phobias and can improve anticipatory anxiety and functional disability;[4-8] however, as in panic attacks, their use is limited. Results with moclobemide have been variable.[1-3] The benzodiazepine clonazepam has also been reported to be of some benefit,[1,3,5,6,9,10] although benzodiazepines should be used with caution because of the risk of dependence and abuse. Beta blockers may help to reduce the physical symptoms in performance-related anxiety.[3,4,6,8,9]

1. Ballenger JC, *et al.* Consensus statement on social anxiety disorder from the International Consensus Group on Depression and Anxiety. *J Clin Psychiatry* 1998; **59** (suppl 17): 54–60.
2. Liebowitz MR. Update on the diagnosis and treatment of social anxiety disorder. *J Clin Psychiatry* 1999; **60** (suppl 18): 22–6.
3. Sareen J, Stein M. A review of the epidemiology and approaches to the treatment of social anxiety disorder. *Drugs* 2000; **59**: 497–509.
4. Michels R, Marzuk PM. Progress in psychiatry. *N Engl J Med* 1993; **329**: 628–38.
5. Liebowitz MR. Pharmacotherapy of social phobia. *J Clin Psychiatry* 1993; **54** (suppl): 31–5.
6. den Boer JA. Social phobia: epidemiology, recognition, and treatment. *BMJ* 1997; **315**: 796–800.
7. Hale AS. Anxiety. *BMJ* 1997; **314**: 1886–9.
8. Anonymous. Drugs for depression and anxiety. *Med Lett Drugs Ther* 1999; **41**: 33–8.
9. Healy D. Social phobia in primary care. *Prim Care Psychiatry* 1995; **1**: 31–8.
10. Stein MB. How shy is too shy? *Lancet* 1996; **347**: 1131–2.

Post-traumatic stress disorder. In post-traumatic stress disorder anxiety is precipitated by recall of a traumatic experience. Patients may also suffer from negative symptoms such as avoidance, alienation, emotional numbness, and social withdrawal. The main treatment is psychotherapy.[1-3] Drug therapy is largely aimed at accompanying symptoms of anxiety or depression.[1,4] SSRIs are the treatment of choice for most of the symptoms of post-traumatic stress disorder.[3] Tricyclic antidepressants, or in refractory patients MAOIs, may be used as alternatives to SSRIs to help reduce traumatic recollections and nightmares and to repress flashbacks.[2,3] Negative symptoms are usually resistant to pharmacotherapy. A minimum of 8 weeks of treatment is considered necessary to judge the efficacy of treatment.[2] Antiepileptics such as carbamazepine and valproate appear to improve symptoms of hyper-reactivity, violent behaviour, and angry outbursts but only a small number of patients have been studied. Benzodiazepines may be helpful for short-term management of anxiety and sleep disturbances, (although some studies have failed to show benefit[4]), but must be used with caution because of the risk of dependence and abuse.[3]

1. Michels R, Marzuk PM. Progress in psychiatry. *N Engl J Med* 1993; **329:** 628–38.
2. McIvor RJ, Turner SW. Drug treatment in post-traumatic stress disorder. *Br J Hosp Med* 1995; **53:** 501–6.
3. Foa EB, *et al.* Treatment of posttraumatic stress disorder. *J Clin Psychiatry* 1999; **60** (suppl 16): 1–75.
4. Stein DJ, *et al.* Pharmacotherapy for posttraumatic stress disorder (updated 14 December 2000). Available in The Cochrane Library; Issue 4. Oxford: Update Software; 2001.

Extrapyramidal disorders
Extrapyramidal disorders are movement disorders involving the brain's motor systems outside the pyramidal tract. They are usually characterised by akinesia (a loss of movement) or bradykinesia (abnormal slowness of movement) accompanied by an increase in muscle tone (typified by parkinsonism, p.1160); or by dyskinesias (abnormal involuntary movements), often accompanied by a reduction in muscle tone (see below for some examples). Drug-induced extrapyramidal disorders are discussed under Chlorpromazine, p.662.

Ballism. Ballism, sometimes called hemiballism or hemiballismus because it is usually unilateral, consists of involuntary flinging movements of the upper extremities and most often results from acute vascular infarction or haemorrhage of the subthalamic nucleus. It often improves spontaneously but dopamine-blocking antipsychotics such as haloperidol or dopamine-depleting drugs such as tetrabenazine may be needed to control severe symptoms. Surgery may be necessary in severe cases.

Chorea. Chorea is characterised by brief involuntary muscle contractions and an inability to sustain voluntary contractions. It may be related to neurological abnormalities in the caudate nucleus and putamen of the striatum as well as other basal ganglia structures. Overactivity of dopaminergic nigrostriatal pathways and depletion of gamma-aminobutyric acid (GABA) and acetylcholine may also play a part. Chorea may be an adverse effect of some drugs, including antipsychotics, levodopa, and oral contraceptives; it may also be a symptom of an underlying disorder such as systemic lupus erythematosus.

Huntington's chorea (Huntington's disease, progressive hereditary chorea) is a hereditary autosomal dominant disease characterised by chorea, behavioural disturbances, and a progressive decline in cognitive function culminating in dementia and death. The identification of a gene marker for Huntington's chorea now makes it possible to identify carriers of the abnormal gene. Symptoms usually appear in mid-life, with death following after about 15 years, although there are also juvenile-onset forms. Westphal variant, a form commonest in children, tends to be characterised more by rigidity than by chorea.

Sydenham's chorea (St Vitus' dance; Chorea Minor) is an acute, usually self-limiting, disorder with an auto-immune basis, characterised by chorea and behavioural disturbances. It commonly occurs about 6 months after rheumatic fever but is now rare since the incidence of rheumatic fever has declined. It may also arise during pregnancy (chorea gravidarum).

Treatment of chorea is symptomatic only and does not alter the progressive decline of Huntington's chorea; Sydenham's chorea resolves spontaneously within weeks or months but antibiotic prophylaxis to prevent recurrence of rheumatic fever (p.138) has been recommended. Other forms of chorea may resolve with treatment of the underlying disorder or withdrawal of any causative drug.

Tetrabenazine has been used effectively in chorea, although not all patients respond, and it may produce depression. The mode of action is thought to involve depletion of striatal dopamine. Reserpine, which has a similar action and effects, has also been used.

Phenothiazines such as chlorpromazine and fluphenazine have dopamine-receptor blocking activity and have also been used to treat chorea. Other antipsychotics with a similar mode of action that have been used include haloperidol, pimozide, sulpiride, and tiapride. Adverse effects such as tardive dyskinesias may limit the use of antipsychotics, and doses should be kept as low as possible; attempts to control choreiform movements completely are not recommended. In addition to improving chorea, antipsychotics may also be of value in controlling the behavioural symptoms associated with Huntington's chorea; anxiolytics and antidepressants may also be of use.

Carbamazepine and lamotrigine have been tried with some degree of success in a limited number of patients. The use of drugs to increase GABA activity has been of little value. Implantation of human and porcine fetal neural cells is being studied.

References.
1. Marsden CD. Basal ganglia disease. *Lancet* 1982; **ii:** 1141–6.
2. Kremer B, *et al.* A worldwide study of the Huntington's disease mutation: the sensitivity and specificity of measuring CAG repeats. *N Engl J Med* 1994; **330:** 1401–6.
3. Furtado S, Suchowersky O. Huntington's disease: recent advances in diagnosis and management. *Can J Neurol Sci* 1995; **22:** 5–12.
4. Quinn N, Schrag A. Huntington's disease and other choreas. *J Neurol* 1998; **245:** 709–16.

Tics. Tics may manifest as sudden, involuntary, brief, isolated, repetitive movements which may be simple (e.g. eye blinking, nose twitching, or head jerking) or complex (e.g. touching, jumping, or kicking); they may also be sensory in nature or may present in a vocal or phonic way and may range from simple clearing of the throat to more complex symptoms such as echolalia (involuntary repetition of others speech) or coprolalia (involuntary and inappropriate swearing). Symptoms can usually be suppressed voluntarily and may increase with stress and decrease with distraction. Some tics persist during sleep. The most common cause is **Tourette's syndrome** (Gilles de la Tourette's syndrome), in which behavioural disturbances accompany the tics. It is mainly a genetic disorder with an onset during childhood but may also be precipitated by various substances (e.g. antipsychotics), trauma, streptococcal infection, or viral encephalitis.

Most patients' symptoms wax and wane and behavioural therapy and reassurance may be sufficient to resolve mild tics. Drug treatment may be necessary when tics are severe enough to cause discomfort or embarrassment. Dopamine blockers, usually pimozide or haloperidol, often decrease the frequency and severity of tics and may improve any accompanying behavioural disturbances. Superiority of either drug in terms of efficacy or adverse effects has not been clearly demonstrated. It is usually recommended that doses are titrated to as low as possible bearing in mind that optimum treatment does not necessarily lead to the complete control of symptoms. The risk of developing serious adverse effects such as tardive dyskinesia with these drugs should be balanced against the perceived benefits of treatment. Medication can often be discontinued after a few years. Alternative drugs may be required for those unresponsive to or intolerant of haloperidol or pimozide. Other drugs that are also used in the management of tics and/or behavioural aspects of Tourette's syndrome include clonidine and sulpiride; in some patients clonidine may be used initially in preference to haloperidol or pimozide due to its relative lack of serious side-effects. Baclofen, botulinum toxin, clonazepam, fluphenazine, levodopa, pergolide, risperidone, and tiapride have also been tried. Nicotine has been reported to produce benefit when used alone or with haloperidol in patients whose symptoms were not satisfactorily controlled with haloperidol.

For drugs used in the treatment of comorbid disorders commonly associated with Tourette's syndrome, such as obsessive-compulsive disorder and attention deficit hyperactivity disorder, see above and p.1505, respectively.

References.
1. Sandor P. Clinical management of Tourette's syndrome and associated disorders. *Can J Psychiatry* 1995; **40:** 577–83.
2. Peterson BS. Considerations of natural history and pathophysiology in the psychopharmacology of Tourette's syndrome. *J Clin Psychiatry* 1996; **57** (suppl 9): 24–34.
3. Robertson MM, Stern JS. Gilles de la Tourette syndrome. *Br J Hosp Med* 1997; **58:** 253–6.

4. Kurlan R. Treatment of tics. *Neurol Clin North Am* 1997; **15:** 403–9.
5. Peterson BS, Cohen DJ. The treatment of Tourette's syndrome: multimodal, developmental intervention. *J Clin Psychiatry* 1998; **59** (suppl 1): 62–74.

Hypochondriasis
Hypochondriasis (hypochondriacal neurosis) is a morbid preoccupation with one's health characterised by a fear or belief that normal bodily sensations are indicative of serious disease. It persists despite medical reassurance and management is difficult. If hypochondriasis is associated with a psychiatric disorder, treatment is aimed at the primary condition.

Pimozide is used in the management of hypochondriacal psychoses such as delusions of parasitic infestation or sexually transmitted disease. The SSRIs are an alternative to pimozide.

References.
1. Lyell A. Delusions of parasitosis. *Br J Dermatol* 1983; **108:** 485–99.
2. Hamann K, Avnstorp C. Delusions of infestation treated by pimozide: a double-blind crossover clinical study. *Acta Derm Venereol (Stockh)* 1982; **62:** 55–8.
3. Goldmeier D. Psychological and sexual problems. In: Adler MW, ed. *ABC of sexually transmitted diseases.* 4th ed. London: BMJ Publishing Group, 1999; 63–5.
4. Fallon BA, *et al.* The pharmacotherapy of hypochondriasis. *Psychopharmacol Bull* 1996; **32:** 607–11.
5. Perkins RJ. SSRI antidepressants are effective for treating delusional hypochondriasis. *Med J Aust* 1999; **170:** 140–1.

Psychoses
Psychoses and psychotic disorders are terms that have been used to describe a collection of severe psychiatric disorders in which the patient has disordered thinking and loses contact with reality due to delusions and/or hallucinations. There may be accompanying mood or behavioural disturbances. *Organic psychoses* arise from organic brain disease produced by toxic insults, metabolic disturbances, infections, or structural abnormalities and may be acute (delirium) or chronic (dementia) in nature.

Disturbed behaviour. Drug therapy is sometimes indicated for the immediate control of severely disturbed, agitated, or violent behaviour associated with a variety of conditions such as toxic delirium, brain damage, mania (see Bipolar Disorder, p.271), or other psychotic disorders. Antipsychotics and benzodiazepines, either alone or in combination, are commonly used for disturbed behaviour. There is little agreement on the best antipsychotic for these indications, selection depending mainly on the condition of the patient and the adverse effect profile of the drug. The high-potency butyrophenone haloperidol is commonly used for **acutely disturbed behaviour.** Benzodiazepines such as diazepam and lorazepam are valuable sedatives for the disturbed or delirious patient. A combination of haloperidol and lorazepam allows the use of lower doses of each drug.

Other drugs that have had some success in the control of symptoms such as agitation, aggression, rage, or violent behaviour include beta blockers, lithium, carbamazepine, and valproate. Buspirone and antidepressants such as the SSRIs and trazodone may also be useful.

Antipsychotics appear to be modestly effective for the control of disturbed behaviour associated with chronic conditions such as senile **dementia** or Alzheimer's disease (p.1412). However, antipsychotics can themselves precipitate confusion or exacerbate dementia and may hasten cognitive decline, increase the risk of falls, incontinence, and drowsiness, and interfere with the performance of motor skills. Elderly patients with dementia, especially Lewy-body dementia, are reported to be highly susceptible to the extrapyramidal adverse effects of antipsychotics and the reaction can be life-threatening. Antipsychotics are used only after careful consideration of the causes of disturbed behaviour and the benefits and risks of antipsychotic treatment. Very low doses are given at first and increased gradually according to clinical response and development of side-effects; the necessity for continued use is reviewed periodically. Again, there is no agreement over the choice of antipsychotic. Atypical antipsychotics may be less likely to produce extrapyramidal symptoms but any advantage remains to be determined. The sedative drug, clomethiazole, may be a useful alternative to antipsychotics for the control of agitated behaviour in elderly patients, generally causing fewer side-effects; respiratory depression, excessive sedation, and dependence may, however, be a problem. Benzodiazepines are not generally indicated for the management of elderly demented patients because of the risks of dependence with continued use, disinhibiting effects, and the special problems of these drugs in old people (see the Elderly, under Diazepam, p.676). They are not as effective as antipsychotics in reducing behavioural problems, but may be useful in short courses for the management of severe anxiety disorders, or given as required for patients who only have rare episodes of agitation.

The use of antipsychotics in the control of **disturbed behaviour in children** is controversial and can probably be justified only in severe cases resistant to other therapy. Autistic and mentally retarded children are among those who may require antipsychotics on a short-term basis. Some suggest the use of high-potency antipsychotics such as haloperidol on the grounds that they are less likely to cause sedation or impair arousal, cognitive function, and learning; others have favoured a drug such as thioridazine which carries a lower risk of dystonic reactions, but thioridazine is no longer recommended for use in children because of cardiotoxic risks. The tendency of antipsychotics to lower the seizure threshold is an important consideration in autistic children who are at a higher than normal risk of seizure disorders.

Antipsychotics and benzodiazepines have been used to control the symptoms of **drug-induced delirium**. Psychosis in patients with Parkinson's disease may be particularly difficult to treat, since the extrapyramidal effects of classical antipsychotics can exacerbate the movement disorder; benefit has been reported with the atypical antipsychotic clozapine (which must be used with caution because of the risk of agranulocytosis) but results with other atypical antipsychotics such as risperidone and olanzapine have been mixed; quetiapine appears to be reasonably well tolerated.

Benzodiazepines are favoured for palliative treatment of agitation and restlessness in patients with **terminal restlessness** since antipsychotics may exacerbate the existing tendency to myoclonus and convulsions in these patients and may not produce adequate sedation in the terminal phase.

Paraphilias and other **deviant sexual behaviour** are rare in women so treatment is focussed largely towards men; it consists mainly of psychotherapy and the use of libido-suppressing drugs such as the anti-androgens. The use of such pharmacotherapy is controversial and involves not only medical but legal issues. Drugs used for their anti-androgenic action include cyproterone and medroxyprogesterone. Gonadorelin analogues have also been tried for suppression of libido. Medroxyprogesterone has also been used for the control of intrusive disinhibited sexual behaviour in elderly men with dementia. There have been some case reports of fluoxetine being used with some success in the control of fantasies associated with various paraphilias. The butyrophenone antipsychotic benperidol is used in some countries for the management of sexual deviations but its value is not established. In general few well-controlled blinded studies have been conducted into the pharmacological treatment of sexual offenders and there is no evidence that drug treatment reduces the recidivism rate.

References.
1. Schneider LS, et al. A metaanalysis of controlled trials of neuroleptic treatment in dementia. *J Am Geriatr Soc* 1990; **38:** 553–63.
2. Anonymous. Management of behavioural emergencies. *Drug Ther Bull* 1991; **29:** 62–4. Correction. *ibid.;* 80.
3. Fish DN. Treatment of delirium in the critically ill patient. *Clin Pharm* 1991; **10:** 456–66.
4. Druckenbrod RW, et al. As-needed dosing of antipsychotic drugs: limitations and guidelines for use in the elderly agitated patient. *Ann Pharmacother* 1993; **27:** 645–8.
5. Richer M, Crismon ML. Pharmacotherapy of sexual offenders. *Ann Pharmacother* 1993; **27:** 316–19.
6. Yeager BF, et al. Management of the behavioral manifestations of dementia. *Arch Intern Med* 1995; **155:** 250–60.
7. Carter GL, et al. Drug-induced delirium: incidence, management and prevention. *Drug Safety* 1996; **15:** 291–301.
8. Pabis DJ, Stanislav SW. Pharmacotherapy of aggressive behaviour. *Ann Pharmacother* 1996; **30:** 278–87.
9. Connor DF, Steingard RJ. A clinical approach to the pharmacotherapy of aggression in children and adolescents. *Ann N Y Acad Sci* 1996; **794:** 290–307.
10. American Psychiatric Association. Practice guideline for the treatment of patients with Alzheimer's disease and other dementias of late life. *Am J Psychiatry* 1997; **154** (suppl): 1–39.
11. McShane R, et al. Do neuroleptic drugs hasten cognitive decline in dementia: prospective study with necropsy follow up. *BMJ* 1997; **314:** 266–70.
12. Burke AL. Palliative care: an update on "terminal restlessness". *Med J Aust* 1997; **166:** 39–42.
13. Fava M. Psychopharmacologic treatment of pathologic aggression. *Psychiatr Clin North Am* 1997; **20:** 427–51.
14. Bradford JMW. Treatment of men with paraphilia. *N Engl J Med* 1998; **338:** 464–5.
15. Alexopoulos GS, et al. Treatment of agitation in older persons with dementia. *Postgrad Med* 1998; Apr (suppl): 1–88.
16. American Psychiatric Association. Practice guideline for the treatment of patients with delirium. *Am J Psychiatry* 1999; **156** (suppl): 1–20.
17. Davies T. Management of the acutely disturbed patient. *Prescribers' J* 1999; **39:** 129–35.
18. Ballard C, O'Brien J. Treating behavioural and psychological signs in Alzheimer's disease. *BMJ* 1999; **319:** 138–9.
19. Friedman JH, Factor SA. Atypical antipsychotics in the treatment of drug-induced psychosis in Parkinson's disease. *Mov Disord* 2000; **15:** 201–11.

Mania. Mania usually occurs as part of bipolar disorder (manic depression). The treatment of acute attacks of mania including mention of the role of antipsychotics is described under Bipolar Disorder, p.271.

Schizophrenia. Schizophrenia is a complex disorder associated with a high morbidity; it may be a group of related syndromes rather than a single disorder. Schizophrenia begins most commonly in adolescence and many patients develop a chronic illness with repeated relapses. The predominant clinical features of acute schizophrenia syndrome can be divided into psychotic features such as delusions and hallucinations, and disorganised features involving speech, thought, and behaviour (together often known as 'positive' symptoms). The main features of the chronic syndrome are apathy, lack of drive, and social withdrawal (so-called 'negative' symptoms). Positive symptoms tend to respond better to drug therapy than negative symptoms. The pathophysiological mechanism of schizophrenia is unclear. Since classical antipsychotics used in the treatment of schizophrenia block dopamine D_2 receptors in the midbrain it has been suggested that dopaminergic system overactivity may be involved. However, the efficacy of atypical antipsychotics such as clozapine (see below), which is a relatively weak dopamine D_2 inhibitor, has raised the possibility that an imbalance of other neurotransmitters such as serotonin may also be involved (see also Action, under Chlorpromazine, p.666).

The **treatment** of schizophrenia consists mainly of a combination of social therapy and antipsychotics. Drug treatment needs to be started promptly for best outcome, and involves a choice between classical antipsychotics such as chlorpromazine or haloperidol, and the atypical antipsychotics such as clozapine and risperidone.

There is little difference in the efficacy of classical antipsychotics. Clozapine appears to be more effective than classical antipsychotics in the management of both positive and negative symptoms, although adverse effects limit its use (see below). Comparative studies have shown that other atypical antipsychotics are at least as effective on positive symptoms as the classical antipsychotics, although claims of greater effects on negative symptoms remain to be proven.

Classical antipsychotics are associated with anti-adrenergic, antimuscarinic, extrapyramidal, and sedative effects. The frequency and pattern of these vary between the different groups of antipsychotics (see p.660). Sedative and antimuscarinic effects usually diminish with continued use, although sedative effects may be useful for behavioural control in acute illness. However, extrapyramidal effects are particularly troublesome with classical antipsychotics. Some, such as thioridazine, are also restricted by the risk of cardiotoxicity.

In comparison, extrapyramidal disorders appear to be less of a problem with the atypical antipsychotics, although they may have other troublesome side-effects. In particular, the use of clozapine is restricted because it can cause potentially fatal agranulocytosis.

Consequently, choice of therapy depends on the risk of adverse effects, any past treatment, and, unfortunately, cost. Classical antipsychotics are still widely used. The diversity of their preparations (tablets, oral liquids, injections, and depot injections) and lower cost also offer advantages over the atypical antipsychotics. Atypical antipsychotic therapy (with the exception of clozapine) may be more appropriate in patients intolerant of previous therapy with classical antipsychotics, particularly for those at a high risk of extrapyramidal effects. Their use in patients experiencing a first schizophrenic episode is also recommended by some physicians.

There is great interindividual variation in response to antipsychotics, and choosing the most appropriate one may require a trial of antipsychotics from different chemical groups and careful adjustment of dosage. The Royal College of Psychiatrists in the UK has issued advice for those considering the use of higher than normally recommended doses of antipsychotics (see under Adminstration in the Uses and Administration of Chlorpromazine, p.666). However, in recent years there has been a trend in favour of lower doses of antipsychotics, often with adjunctive benzodiazepines (see below). The use of more

than one antipsychotic at the same time is not recommended.

About 30% of patients may have little or no response to classical antipsychotics while many others have only a partial response. Such **resistant schizophrenia** may be due to poor patient compliance, which is a major problem in schizophrenic patients; lack of compliance may be a result of adverse effects (see below for possible treatments) or because the patient experiences a relapse while on medication and is unable to maintain treatment. A patient should not be considered resistant to therapy until at least 2 different antipsychotics have each been given for an adequate trial period. If other drugs are still ineffective clozapine may be tried; it should be given for at least 3 months before resorting to measures such as ECT or the use of adjunctive drugs (see below).

Following the initial control of schizophrenia with antipsychotics relapse rates are high in those who stop treatment, therefore maintenance therapy is probably warranted. Some recommend the use of lower doses of antipsychotics during maintenance to reduce adverse effects, although this may increase the risk of relapse. The decision to withdraw an antipsychotic completely in a stabilised patient is complex and depends on the number of previous psychotic episodes. In some cases maintenance therapy may need to be indefinite. Regular injections of long-acting depot antipsychotics are sometimes used for maintenance therapy especially if compliance is a problem. They are particularly useful for patients living in the community, and may also be advantageous for those who respond poorly to therapy because of increased first-pass metabolism or intestinal malabsorption. Concern over the possibility of increased extrapyramidal effects and other adverse effects with depot antipsychotics has not been substantiated.

Adjunctive drugs have been used in schizophrenia either to augment antipsychotic therapy or reduce their adverse effects. The short-term addition of a benzodiazepine to the initial treatment of acute episodes of schizophrenia can provide a useful extra sedative and anxiolytic effect. It may also allow a smaller dose of antipsychotic to be used and thereby reduce the likelihood of extrapyramidal effects.

The use of antimuscarinics for the treatment or prophylaxis of antipsychotic-induced extrapyramidal side-effects is controversial (see Extrapyramidal Disorders on p.662). They are particularly effective in the management of acute dystonic reactions but efficacy in parkinsonism may be minimal and little benefit has been demonstrated in akathisia. Fears that the long-term use of antimuscarinics increases the risk of tardive dyskinesia appear to be unfounded, although they may worsen the condition and should be discontinued if it develops. However, the side-effects of antimuscarinics may be troublesome and may be additive with the antimuscarinic actions of the antipsychotic. Antimuscarinics also have euphoric effects. Routine administration of prophylactic antimuscarinics is therefore not indicated with the possible exception of short-term use in patients at high risk of developing dystonias, or in patients with a previous history of drug-induced dystonias. Antimuscarinics may be given on a short-term basis to treat dystonias.

Addition of lithium to antipsychotic treatment may be worthwhile in some patients who fail to respond to an antipsychotic alone, although there is the danger of an interaction (see p.295).

The value of treatment of depressive symptoms of schizophrenia with antidepressants is not established but the addition of antidepressants such as the tricyclics is considered worth a trial for depression occurring during the recovery phase after an acute episode of psychosis.

Carbamazepine has produced modest benefit in some patients with refractory schizophrenia, the main effect being a reduction in accompanying symptoms such as excitement, impulsivity, and aggression, but concomitant administration of carbamazepine and haloperidol has also resulted in reduced haloperidol concentrations and clinical deterioration in a few patients. Valproate has also been tried.

Propranolol in high doses has been reported to be beneficial in refractory schizophrenia but several controlled studies of adjunctive use have found slight or no benefit. However, it may be of use as an adjunct in patients who develop akathisia unresponsive to antimuscarinics.

References.
1. Davis JM, et al. Depot antipsychotic drugs: place in therapy. *Drugs* 1994; **47:** 741–73.

2. Johns CA, Thompson JW. Adjunctive treatments in schizophrenia: pharmacotherapies and electroconvulsive therapy. *Schizophr Bull* 1995; **21:** 607–19.
3. Fleischhacker WW, Hummer M. Drug treatment of schizophrenia in the 1990s: achievements and future possibilities in optimising outcomes. *Drugs* 1997; **53:** 915–29.
4. Buckley PF. New dimensions in the pharmacologic treatment of schizophrenia and related psychoses. *J Clin Pharmacol* 1997; **37:** 363–78. Correction. *ibid.* 1998; **38:** 27.
5. American Academy of Child and Adolescent Psychiatry. Practice parameters for the assessment and treatment of children and adolescents with schizophrenia. *J Am Acad Child Adolesc Psychiatry* 1997; **36** (suppl): 177S–193S.
6. American Psychiatric Association. Practice guideline for the treatment of patients with schizophrenia. *Am J Psychiatry* 1997; **154** (suppl): 1–63.
7. McGrath J, Emmerson WB. Treatment of schizophrenia. *BMJ* 1999; **319:** 1045–8.
8. Campbell M, *et al*. The use of atypical antipsychotics in the management of schizophrenia. *Br J Clin Pharmacol* 1999; **47:** 13–22.
9. Pearsall R, *et al*. A new algorithm for treating schizophrenia. *Psychopharmacol Bull* 1998; **34:** 349–53.
10. Frankenburg FR. Choices in antipsychotic therapy in schizophrenia. *Harv Rev Psychiatry* 1999; **6:** 241–9.
11. Kane JM. Management strategies for the treatment of schizophrenia. *J Clin Psychiatry* 1999; **60** (suppl. 12): 13–17.
12. Kane JM. Pharmacologic treatment of schizophrenia. *Biol Psychiatry* 1999; **46:** 1396–1408.

Sedation

Since sedatives reduce excitement and anxiety, they may be used before or during various medical procedures to alleviate fear and produce a state of calmness in the patient. The optimum degree of sedation required depends on the particular procedure. A practical aim for situations requiring **conscious sedation**, for example in *dentistry*, may be the reduction or abolition of physiological and psychological responses to the stress without loss of consciousness, cooperation, or protective reflexes. A greater degree of sedation may be required for patients in *intensive care* and some consider that patients should be maintained asleep but easily rousable. The difference between sedatives and hypnotics is mainly dose related. The same drug or group of drugs can have both effects, larger doses being necessary for a hypnotic effect, that is to produce a state of sleep.

The use of sedatives in premedication for anaesthesia is discussed on p.1256.

Dental sedation. Intravenous midazolam has largely superseded diazepam for sedation in dental procedures. Although benzodiazepines have no analgesic activity, concomitant use of analgesics is rarely required. However, midazolam needs to be given slowly in small increments as its sedative end-point is reached much more abruptly than with diazepam. Midazolam has a rapid onset of action and produces good anterograde amnesia, but the response in children may be poor. Full recovery can take several hours. Concurrent administration of benzodiazepines such as midazolam with opioid analgesics to supplement sedation and provide postoperative analgesia is not recommended because of the possibility of respiratory depression.

Nitrous oxide is a powerful analgesic and sedative, well tolerated by children, and relatively safe and simple to use, although there is some concern over its long-term effect on dental staff. It also requires a certain amount of patient cooperation.

Oral sedatives may also be used to provide dental sedation and are particularly useful to ensure that the patient has a restful night prior to the procedure. Those drugs used include the benzodiazepines diazepam, nitrazepam, and temazepam, and the antihistamines promethazine and trimeprazine [alimemazine]. Temazepam is preferred when it is important to minimise any residual effects.

Endoscopy. The practice of giving sedation routinely before endoscopy varies widely between and within countries. It is unclear whether sedation improves patient comfort and the ease of performing the procedure; there may be a failure to distinguish between the need for sedation and the need for analgesia in such procedures. Ultimately the acceptability of unsedated endoscopy differs from patient to patient and procedure to procedure, and it may be appropriate to offer patients the choice of having sedation or not.

Benzodiazepines are commonly used for intravenous sedation during endoscopy. Midazolam is generally preferred to diazepam because of its shorter duration of action. Since hypoventilation and oxygen desaturation may occur with benzodiazepines and the procedure itself can lower oxygen saturation, some recommend the administration of prophylactic nasal oxygen in conjunction with oxygen saturation monitoring.

Opioid analgesics such as morphine and pethidine have also been given but they have largely been replaced by the newer shorter-acting opioids, for example fentanyl, which have faster recovery times. Combination of a benzodiazepine with an opioid analgesic is not advocated in the UK because of the increased risk of cardiorespiratory effects. However, in the USA, benzodiazepines have often been given with opioids, including pethidine, since such combinations may reduce gagging and increase patient tolerance.

The intravenous anaesthetic propofol has also been used for sedation as an alternative to, or in combination with, midazolam. However the risk of adverse effects may limit its use and require the presence of an anaesthetist.

The use of topical anaesthetics such as lignocaine [lidocaine] should probably be reserved for those who prefer to undergo endoscopy without sedation as topical anaesthesia appears to serve little useful function in patients premedicated with benzodiazepines or opioids. There appears to be no practical difference between individual topical anaesthetics. Sprays are safer and may be more effective than lozenges, but even when using a spray it is difficult to anaesthetise the oropharyngeal region effectively.

References.

1. Arrowsmith JB, *et al*. Results from the American Society for Gastrointestinal Endoscopy/US Food and Drug Administration collaborative study on complication rates and drug use during gastrointestinal endoscopy. *Gastrointest Endosc* 1991; **37:** 421–7.
2. The Royal College of Surgeons of England Commission on the Provision of Surgical Services. *Report of the working party on guidelines for sedation by non-anaesthetists.* London: Royal College of Surgeons, 1993.
3. Williams TJ. Sedation in fibreoptic bronchoscopy. *BMJ* 1995; **310:** 872.
4. Sutherland FWH. Sedation in fibreoptic bronchoscopy. *BMJ* 1995; **310:** 872.
5. Charlton JE. Monitoring and supplemental oxygen during endoscopy. *BMJ* 1995; **310:** 886–7.
6. Ristikankare M, *et al*.. Is routinely given conscious sedation of benefit during colonoscopy? *Gastrointest Endosc* 1999; **49:** 566–72.
7. Davis DE, *et al*. Topical pharyngeal anesthesia does not improve upper gastrointestinal endoscopy in conscious sedated patients. *Am J Gastroenterol* 1999; **94:** 1853–6.
8. Bell GD. Premedication, preparation, and surveillance. *Endoscopy* 2000; **32:** 92–100.
9. Zuccaro G. Sedation and sedationless endoscopy. *Gastrointest Endosc Clin N Am* 2000; **10:** 1–20.

Intensive care. Most patients in an intensive care unit require analgesia, sedation, or both during at least part of their stay. The required level of sedation may vary but, in general, many consider patients should be maintained asleep but easily rousable. Most sedatives and analgesics are given parenterally. Continuous intravenous infusion avoids the peaks and troughs of analgesia and sedation associated with intermittent intramuscular or intravenous administration, but to what extent it improves patient outcomes is unclear: sedation produced in this way may prolong the need for mechanical ventilation.

Opioid analgesics, which have both sedative and analgesic properties, are commonly administered for sedation and are appropriate for any patient in whom pain is anticipated, although special care is required in those not artificially ventilated. The antitussive action of the opioids may also help ventilated patients to tolerate a tracheal tube. Morphine is a suitable opioid in many situations in intensive care but has a slow onset of action. If prolonged sedation is required analgesia can be obtained by a loading dose followed by a continuous infusion. Fentanyl has a short duration of action after single doses as a result of redistribution in the body. However, following repeated administration it is not a short-acting drug and therefore offers little advantage over morphine. Alfentanil has a short duration of action and has provided satisfactory sedation in patients requiring overnight sedation but does not appear to offer any advantage over other opioids. In some patients, elimination and duration of action have been prolonged. It may be suitable for use at the start and end of prolonged periods of sedation to produce a rapid effect and to decrease the risk of prolonged respiratory depression respectively.

Not all patients require sedatives if sufficient analgesia is achieved, particularly after the first 24 to 48 hours, but most will require a balanced combination of analgesics and sedatives to relieve pain and anxiety. It is inappropriate to use high doses of opioids to achieve deep sedation and it is also inappropriate to use sedatives alone for patients who are in pain.

Benzodiazepines induce sleep and reduce anxiety and muscle tone. Although they produce profound amnesia, they often fail to achieve satisfactory sedation; doses that do achieve sedation often interfere with verbal contact with the patient. All benzodiazepines tend to produce cardiovascular and respiratory depression and care is required if they are used with opioids. Midazolam has a rapid onset and short duration of action and has largely replaced diazepam as the benzodiazepine of choice for sedation. However, the half-life of midazolam can be substantially increased when given as a continuous intravenous infusion for long-term sedation in patients in intensive care. Lorazepam has also been used.

Flumazenil is a specific benzodiazepine antagonist and some suggest that it may be of use to assist the return of spontaneous respiration and consciousness in patients receiving benzodiazepines. Multiple doses may be required as it has a short duration of action.

Propofol is used successfully for sedation in adults in intensive care, and weaning times in propofol-sedated patients on mechanical ventilation have been demonstrated to be shorter than those seen with midazolam. However, propofol is not recommended for use in children because of adverse effects (see p.1265).

Ketamine has also been investigated for sedation in the intensive care setting and appears to be effective; it may be given in combination with a benzodiazepine.

Sedation and analgesia for **children** in intensive care is a subject of debate. Many of the regimens used appear to be similar to those used in adults or modifications of existing regimens for paediatric sedation. Drugs commonly used include midazolam and opioids such as fentanyl or morphine. However, there has been some concern over a report of encephalopathy associated with the prolonged use of midazolam with fentanyl for sedation in infants under intensive care (see under Effects on the Nervous System, p.676). As mentioned above, propofol is not recommended for children in intensive care.

References.

1. Wolf AR. Neonatal sedation: more art than science. *Lancet* 1994; **344:** 628–9.
2. Barker DP, Rutter N. Neonatal sedation. *Lancet* 1994; **344:** 1362.
3. Wagner BKJ, O'Hara DA. Pharmacokinetics and pharmacodynamics of sedatives and analgesics in the treatment of agitated critically ill patients. *Clin Pharmacokinet* 1997; **33:** 426–53.
4. Lerch C, Park GR. Sedation and analgesia. *Br Med Bull* 1999; **55:** 76–95.
5. Bennett NR. Paediatric intensive care. *Br J Anaesth* 1999; **83:** 139–56.
6. Ostermann ME, *et al*. Sedation in the intensive care unit: a systematic review. *JAMA* 2000; **283:** 1451–9.

Sleep disorders

The exact function of sleep is uncertain but it is believed to be involved in energy conservation and total body restoration and recuperation. Initially there is a period of light sleep (stages 1 and 2) followed by deep sleep (stages 3 and 4); this latter period is also known as slow-wave sleep. After stage 4, which occurs about 90 minutes after first falling asleep, there is a period of rapid-eye-movement (REM) sleep during which most dreams occur and EEG traces show high frequency waves. During a period of sleep there are several cycles of stages 1 to 4 followed by REM sleep, with periods of non-REM sleep becoming shorter and periods of REM sleep longer. It is the slow-wave sleep that is considered to be the more restorative. Most healthy adults sleep for single periods of between 7 to 9 hours a day. In old age there is less slow-wave sleep and sleep becomes more fragmented.

Sleep disorders include insomnia (see below), hypersomnia such as narcolepsy, p.1505, in which the timing, length, and quality of sleep is altered, and the parasomnias (see below) in which abnormal events occur during sleep.

Insomnia. Insomnia[1-8] is the inability to achieve or maintain sleep and is the most common of the sleep disorders. It often leaves sufferers feeling unrefreshed by sleep and may lead to impaired daytime performance.

- Transient insomnia may occur in those who normally sleep well and may be due to an alteration in the conditions that surround sleep, for example noise, or to an unusual pattern of rest as in shift work or travelling between time zones. It may also be associated with acute disorders.

- Short-term insomnia is often related to an emotional problem or more serious medical illness such as acute pain and may recur.

- Chronic insomnia may be attributed to an underlying psychiatric disorder, especially depression, to alcohol or drug abuse, to excessive caffeine intake, or to daytime cat napping, or physical causes such as pain, pruritus, or dyspnoea.

Management of insomnia requires resolution of any stressful precipitant or identification and treatment of any underlying causes, with an emphasis on non-pharmacological measures such as counselling, behavioural therapy, development of relaxation techniques, and avoidance of stimulant substances. Hypnotic drugs should ideally be reserved for short courses in the acutely distressed patient; they should be avoided in the elderly, and their use is rarely justified in children. Generally, hypnotics should be given at the lowest effective dose for as short a period as possible. In transient insomnia one or two doses of a short-acting hypnotic may be indicated, whereas in short-term insomnia intermittent doses of a short-acting hypnotic given for no more than 3 weeks may be appropriate. Routine use of hypnotics is undesirable. Tolerance can develop rapidly with continuous use and withdrawal following long-term use can lead to rebound insomnia and a withdrawal syndrome.

Benzodiazepines are generally regarded as the hypnotics of choice. They hasten sleep onset, decrease nocturnal awakenings, increase total sleeping time, and often impart a sense of deep and refreshing sleep. Slow-wave sleep and REM sleep are, however, reduced and the extra sleeping time is largely made up of relatively light sleep. A short-acting benzodiazepine such as temazepam is generally used when residual sedation is undesirable, if falling asleep is a problem, or, when necessary, in elderly patients. Longer-acting benzodiazepines such as nitrazepam are indicated when early waking is a problem and possibly when an anxiolytic effect is needed during the day or when some impairment of psychomotor function is acceptable.

Because of the hazard of dependence with benzodiazepines (see p.675), the UK Committee on Safety of Medicines (CSM)[9] has issued certain recommendations: they should be used to treat insomnia only when it is severe, disabling, or subjecting the individual to extreme distress; they should be given in the lowest dose which controls symptoms (if possible, intermittently); they should not be continued beyond 4 weeks; and they should be withdrawn by gradual tapering of the dose to zero. Subsequently, the EU Committee on Proprietary Medicinal Products (EU CPMP) has recommended that the treatment period should be limited to 2 weeks when brotizolam, midazolam, or triazolam are used.[10]

Tolerance to the hypnotic effects of benzodiazepines develops rapidly, with sleep latency and pattern returning to pretreatment levels within a few weeks of starting treatment.

A number of other drugs have been used as alternatives to the benzodiazepines. Zaleplon, zopiclone, and zolpidem act on the same receptors or receptor subtypes as the benzodiazepines although structurally they are unrelated. Their short duration of action makes them more suitable for patients who have trouble falling asleep. The EU CPMP has recommended that treatment with zolpidem should be limited to a maximum of 4 weeks.[10] It remains to be proven whether these drugs offer any advantages over the benzodiazepines. Indeed, the CSM considers that zopiclone has the same potential for adverse psychiatric reactions, including dependence, as benzodiazepines.[11]

The use of cloral hydrate and its derivatives as hypnotics is now very limited. They have been used as alternatives to benzodiazepines in the elderly, although there is no convincing evidence of any special value in these patients. They used to be considered useful hypnotics for children but such use is rarely justified.

Clomethiazole has also been used as an alternative to benzodiazepines in the elderly. Nasal and conjunctival irritation may be troublesome, and the danger of overdosage and risk of dependence should be considered.

Some antihistamines have hypnotic properties and a number, including diphenhydramine, doxylamine, promethazine, and trimeprazine [alimemazine], are marketed for insomnia. They may cause troublesome antimuscarinic effects and those with longer half-lives may cause hangover effects. Promethazine is also popular for use in children, but such use is not usually justified.

Barbiturates are no longer recommended as hypnotics because of their adverse effects. The CSM[12] has advised that barbiturates should only be used for insomnia that is severe and intractable when there are compelling reasons to, and then only in patients already taking barbiturates. It was also advised that attempts should be made to wean patients off barbiturate hypnotics. Similarly, compounds such as ethchlorvynol, glutethimide, and methaqualone are not recommended.

Alcohol is not recommended because it has a short weak hypnotic action, and rebound excitation can result in early morning insomnia. Its diuretic effects can interrupt sleep and chronic use can lead to rapid development of tolerance and addiction.

Tryptophan, sometimes in the form of dietary supplements, has enjoyed some popularity in the treatment of insomnia. Its efficacy is difficult to substantiate and, since the publication of reports linking tryptophan with the eosinophilic-myalgia syndrome, preparations indicated for insomnia have been withdrawn from the market in many countries.

Melatonin, a hormone believed to be involved in the maintenance of circadian rhythms, may be useful in the treatment of insomnias such as those due to jet lag[13] or other disorders (where it might act by resetting the body clock), and in the elderly. However, evidence for a direct hypnotic effect is less conclusive; its sleep-inducing properties are usually only seen after very high, supraphysiological concentrations have been attained.[7,8]

1. National Medical Advisory Committee. The management of anxiety and insomnia. A report by the National Medical Advisory Committee. Edinburgh: HMSO 1994.
2. Mendelson WB, Jain B. An assessment of short-acting hypnotics. *Drug Safety* 1995; **13:** 257–70.
3. NIH Technology Assessment Panel. Integration of behavioral and relaxation approaches into the treatment of chronic pain and insomnia. *JAMA* 1996; **276:** 313–18.
4. Anonymous. Hypnotic drugs. *Med Lett Drugs Ther* 1996; **38:** 59–61.
5. Kupfer DJ, Reynolds CF. Management of insomnia. *N Engl J Med* 1997; **336:** 341–6.
6. Ashton CH. Management of insomnia. *Prescribers' J* 1997; **37:** 1–10.
7. Wagner J, *et al.* Beyond benzodiazepines: alternative pharmacologic agents for the treatment of insomnia. *Ann Pharmacother* 1998; **32:** 680–91.
8. Nishino S, Mignot E. Drug treatment of patients with insomnia and excessive daytime sleepiness: pharmacokinetic considerations. *Clin Pharmacokinet* 1999; **37:** 305–30.
9. Committee on Safety of Medicines. Benzodiazepines, dependence and withdrawal symptoms. *Current Problems 21* 1988.
10. Anonymous. Short-acting hypnotics: a comparative assessment. *WHO Drug Inf* 1993; **7:** 125–6.
11. Committee on Safety of Medicines. Zopiclone (Zimovane) and neuro-psychiatric reactions. *Current Problems 30* 1990.
12. Committee on Safety of Medicines/Medicines Control Agency. Barbiturate hypnotics: avoid wherever possible. *Current Problems* 1996; **22:** 7.
13. Herxheimer A, Petrie KJ. Melatonin for the prevention and treatment of jet lag (updated 11 May 2001). Available in The Cochrane Library; Issue 4. Oxford: Update Software; 2001.

Parasomnias. Parasomnias are motor or autonomic disturbances that occur during sleep or are exaggerated by sleep. Some of the main parasomnias include nightmares, night terrors, sleepwalking (somnambulism), restless legs syndrome, periodic movements in sleep, nocturnal enuresis (p.459), bruxism (teeth grinding), head banging, and aggression during sleep. Parasomnias are common but rarely require treatment with drugs other than the symptomatic treatment of sleep-related medical problems. The management of some parasomnias is discussed briefly below.

The **restless legs syndrome** is characterised by an unpleasant creeping sensation deep in the legs with an irresistible urge to move them. The disorder is intermittent and begins during relaxation in the evenings and in bed. The aetiology of this condition is obscure and treatment has been largely empirical. Although there have been reports of efficacy with a wide range of treatments, few have been well studied. Levodopa, dopamine agonists such as bromocriptine, cabergoline, pergolide, pramipexole, and ropinirole, some opioids, clonazepam, carbamazepine, and clonidine are amongst those drugs shown in controlled studies to produce beneficial effects. Many patients with restless legs syndrome exhibit **periodic limb movements in sleep**, characterised by repetitive periodic leg and foot jerking during sleep. Treatments tried are similar to those for the restless legs syndrome; clonazepam and levodopa are amongst the drugs shown to be of benefit.

Some **other parasomnias** have responded to treatment with benzodiazepines. These include bruxism, head banging, aggression during sleep, night terrors, and sleep walking.

References.
1. Parkes JD. The parasomnias. *Lancet* 1986; **ii:** 1021–5.
2. Kales A, *et al.* Sleep disorders: insomnia, sleepwalking, night terrors, nightmares, and enuresis. *Ann Intern Med* 1987; **106:** 582–92.
3. Krueger BR. Restless leg syndrome and periodic movements of sleep. *Mayo Clin Proc* 1990; **65:** 999–1006.
4. Montplaisir J, *et al.* The treatment of the restless leg syndrome with or without periodic leg movements in sleep. *Sleep* 1992; **15:** 391–5.
5. Silber MH. Restless legs syndrome. *Mayo Clin Proc* 1997; **72:** 261–4.
6. Collado-Seidel V, *et al.* Aetiology and treatment of restless legs syndrome. *CNS Drugs* 1999; **12:** 9–20.

7. Hening W, *et al.* The treatment of restless legs syndrome and periodic limb movement disorder. *Sleep* 1999; **22:** 970–99.
8. Weimerskirch PR, Ernst ME. Newer dopamine agonists in the treatment of restless legs syndrome. *Ann Pharmacother* 2001; **35:** 627–30.

Abecarnil (9339-r)

Abecarnil (rINN).

ZK-112119. Isopropyl 6-(benzyloxy)-4-(methoxymethyl)-9H-pyrido(3,4-b)indole-3-carboxylate.

$C_{24}H_{24}N_2O_4 = 404.5$.

CAS — 111841-85-1.

Profile

Abecarnil is a beta-carboline compound reported to be a partial agonist at benzodiazepine receptors. It is being studied for its anxiolytic and anticonvulsant actions in anxiety disorders and alcohol withdrawal syndrome.

◊ References.
1. Krause W, *et al.* Pharmacokinetics and acute toleration of the β-carboline derivative abecarnil in man. *Arzneimittelforschung* 1990; **40:** 529–32.
2. Karara AH, *et al.* Pharmacokinetics of abecarnil in patients with renal insufficiency. *Clin Pharmacol Ther* 1996; **59:** 520–8.
3. Lydiard RB, *et al.* Abecarnil Work Group. A double-blind evaluation of the safety and efficacy of abecarnil, alprazolam, and placebo in outpatients with generalized anxiety disorder. *J Clin Psychiatry* 1997; **58** (suppl 11): 11–18.
4. Pollack MH, *et al.* Abecarnil for the treatment of generalized anxiety disorder: a placebo-controlled comparison of two dosage ranges of abecarnil and buspirone. *J Clin Psychiatry* 1997; **58** (suppl 11): 19–23.
5. Anton RF, *et al.* A double-blind comparison of abecarnil and diazepam in the treatment of uncomplicated alcohol withdrawal. *Psychopharmacology (Berl)* 1997; **131:** 123–9.
6. Rickels K, *et al.* A double-blind, placebo-controlled trial of abecarnil and diazepam in the treatment of patients with generalized anxiety disorder. *J Clin Psychopharmacol* 2000; **20:** 12–8.

Acamprosate Calcium (10919-p)

Acamprosate Calcium (BANM, rINNM).

Acamprosatum Calcium. The calcium salt of 3-acetamido-1-propanesulphonic acid.

$C_{10}H_{20}CaN_2O_8S_2 = 400.5$.

CAS — 77337-76-9 (acamprosate); 77337-73-6 (acamprosate calcium).

Pharmacopoeias. In Eur. (see p.vi).

Pharmacopoeial description

Ph. Eur.: A white powder. Freely soluble in water; practically insoluble in alcohol and in dichloromethane. A 5% solution in water has a pH of 5.5 to 7.0.

Adverse Effects

The main adverse effect of acamprosate is a dosage-related diarrhoea; nausea, vomiting, and abdominal pain occur less frequently. Other adverse effects have included pruritus, and occasionally a maculopapular rash; bullous skin reactions have occurred rarely. Depression and fluctuations in libido have also been reported.

Effects on the skin. A case of erythema multiforme in a woman with cirrhosis of the liver has been attributed to use of acamprosate[1] although both the diagnosis and any association with acamprosate has been seriously challenged.[2]
1. Fortier-Beaulieu M, *et al.* Possible association of erythema multiforme with acamprosate. *Lancet* 1992; **339:** 991.
2. Potgieter AS, Opsomer L. Acamprosate as cause of erythema multiforme contested. *Lancet* 1992; **340:** 856–7.

Precautions

Acamprosate is contra-indicated in patients with renal or severe hepatic impairment.

Renal impairment. It is considered[1] likely that accumulation of acamprosate would occur with prolonged administration of therapeutic doses to patients with renal impairment. It has been reported that the mean maximum concentration of acamprosate after a single 666-mg dose was 813 nanograms per mL in 12 patients with moderate or severe renal impairment compared with 198 nanograms per mL in 6 healthy subjects; values for the plasma elimination half-life were 47 and 18 hours respectively.
1. Wilde MI, Wagstaff AJ. Acamprosate: a review of its pharmacology and clinical potential in the management of alcohol dependence after detoxification. *Drugs* 1997; **53:** 1038–53.

Pharmacokinetics

Absorption of acamprosate from the gastrointestinal tract is slow but sustained and is subject to considerable interindividual variation. Steady-state concentrations are achieved after 7 days' administration. Bioavailability is reduced by administration with food. Acamprosate is not protein bound and although it is hydrophilic it is reported to cross the blood-brain barrier. Acamprosate does not appear to be metabolised and is excreted unchanged in the urine. The apparent half-life after oral administration has been reported to be 13 hours.

◊ References.
1. Saivin S, *et al.* Clinical pharmacokinetics of acamprosate. *Clin Pharmacokinet* 1998; **35:** 331–45.

Uses and Administration

Acamprosate has a chemical structure similar to that of gamma-aminobutyric acid (GABA) (p.1613). It is given by mouth as the calcium salt to prevent relapse in alcoholics who have been weaned off alcohol. The usual dose for patients weighing 60 kg or more is 666 mg of acamprosate calcium given three times daily; for patients less than 60 kg a dose of 666 mg may be given at breakfast followed by 333 mg at midday and 333 mg at night. Treatment should be started as soon as possible after alcohol withdrawal and maintained, even if the patient relapses, for the recommended period of 1 year.

Alcohol dependence. Acamprosate is considered to be of use as an adjunct to psychotherapy in maintaining abstinence after alcohol withdrawal in patients with alcohol dependence (p.1131). Reviews[1,2] of placebo-controlled studies conclude that acamprosate helps to prevent relapse and increase the number of drink-free days during a 1-year course of treatment and possibly for up to one year thereafter. Efficacy appears to be dose related but its effects in promoting abstinence may wane during treatment. Use with disulfiram may improve results but published data on concomitant use is relatively limited. Several mechanisms have been proposed to account for acamprosate's action including inhibition of neuronal hyperexcitability by antagonising excitatory amino acids such as glutamate.

1. Wilde MI, Wagstaff AJ. Acamprosate: a review of its pharmacology and clinical potential in the management of alcohol dependence after detoxification. *Drugs* 1997; **53:** 1038–53.
2. Anonymous. Acamprosate for alcohol dependence? *Drug Ther Bull* 1997; **35:** 70–2.

Preparations

Proprietary Preparations (details are given in Part 3)
Aust.: Campral; *Austral.:* Campral; *Belg.:* Campral; *Denm.:* Campral; *Fr.:* Aotal; *Ger.:* Campral; *Irl.:* Campral; *Neth.:* Campral; *Norw.:* Campral; *Port.:* Campral; *Singapore:* Campral; *Spain:* Campral; Zulex; *Swed.:* Campral; *Switz.:* Campral; *UK:* Campral.

Acepromazine   (18320-a)

Acepromazine (*BAN, rINN*).

10-(3-Dimethylaminopropyl)phenothiazin-2-yl methyl ketone.
$C_{19}H_{22}N_2OS = 326.5$.
CAS — 61-00-7.
ATC — N05AA04.

Acepromazine Maleate   (7001-h)

Acepromazine Maleate (*BANM, USAN, rINNM*).

Acetylpromazine Maleate. 10-(3-Dimethylaminopropyl)phenothiazin-2-yl methyl ketone hydrogen maleate.
$C_{19}H_{22}N_2OS,C_4H_4O_4 = 442.5$.
CAS — 3598-37-6.
Pharmacopoeias. In US for veterinary use only. Also in BP(Vet).

Acepromazine maleate 13.5 mg is approximately equivalent to 10 mg of acepromazine.

Pharmacopoeial description

BP(Vet) 2001: A yellow odourless or almost odourless crystalline powder. Soluble in water and in alcohol; freely soluble in chloroform; slightly soluble in ether. A 1% solution in water has a pH of 4.0 to 4.5.
USP 25: pH of a 1% solution is between 4.0 and 5.5. Protect from light.

Profile

Acepromazine is a phenothiazine with general properties similar to those of chlorpromazine (p.660). It has been given by mouth as the maleate in the treatment of anxiety disorders, hiccups, and nausea and vomiting; doses (expressed as the base) of up to 60 mg daily in divided doses have been given. Acepromazine, as the base, has also been given in preparations for the management of insomnia.

Preparations

Proprietary Preparations (details are given in Part 3)
Denm.: Plegicil.
Multi-ingredient: *Fr.:* Noctran.

Aceprometazine   (12302-j)

Aceprometazine (*rINN*).

16-64 CB. 10-(2-Dimethylaminopropyl)phenothiazin-2-yl methyl ketone.
$C_{19}H_{22}N_2OS = 326.5$.
CAS — 13461-01-3.

Profile

Aceprometazine is a phenothiazine with general properties similar to those of chlorpromazine (p.660). It is available usually as the maleate in preparations for the management of insomnia.

Preparations

Proprietary Preparations (details are given in Part 3)
Multi-ingredient: *Fr.:* Mepronizine; Noctran.

Adinazolam Mesilate   (12327-d)

Adinazolam Mesilate (*BANM, rINNM*).

Adinazolam Mesylate (*USAN*); U-41123 (adinazolam); U-41123F (adinazolam mesilate). 8-Chloro-1-(dimethylaminomethyl)-6-phenyl-4*H*-1,2,4-triazolo[4,3-*a*][1,4]benzodiazepine methanesulphonate.
$C_{19}H_{18}CIN_5,CH_4O_3S = 447.9$.
CAS — 37115-32-5 (adinazolam); 57938-82-6 (adinazolam mesilate).

Profile

Adinazolam is a short-acting benzodiazepine structurally related to alprazolam (p.654) and is reported to have similar properties. It has been studied in the short-term management of anxiety disorders and depression. It is also reported to exert a uricosuric effect.

◊ References.
1. Fleishaker JC, *et al.* Clinical pharmacology of adinazolam and N-desmethyladinazolam mesylate after single oral doses of each compound in healthy volunteers. *Clin Pharmacol Ther* 1990; **48:** 652–64.
2. Davidson JRT, *et al.* Adinazolam sustained-release treatment of panic disorder: a double-blind study. *J Clin Psychopharmacol* 1994; **14:** 255–63.
3. Golden PL, *et al.* Effect of probenecid on the pharmacokinetics and pharmacodynamics of adinazolam in humans. *Clin Pharmacol Ther* 1994; **56:** 133–41.
4. Carter CS, *et al.* Adinazolam-SR in panic disorder with agoraphobia: relationship of daily dose to efficacy. *J Clin Psychiatry* 1995; **56:** 202–10.

Allobarbital   (4003-m)

Allobarbital (*USAN, rINN*).

Allobarbitone; Diallylbarbitone; Diallylbarbituric Acid; Diallylmalonylurea; Diallymalum; NSC-9324. 5,5-Diallylbarbituric acid.
$C_{10}H_{12}N_2O_3 = 208.2$.
CAS — 52-43-7.
ATC — N05CA21.
Pharmacopoeias. In Aust.

Profile

Allobarbital is a barbiturate with general properties similar to those of amobarbital (p.655). It was formerly used in combination preparations for the treatment of sleep disorders and pain but barbiturates are no longer considered appropriate for such purposes.

Alpidem   (1676-x)

Alpidem (*BAN, USAN, rINN*).

SL-80.0342-00. 2-(6-Chloro-2-*p*-chlorophenylimidazo[1,2-*a*]pyridin-3-yl)-*N,N*-dipropylacetamide.
$C_{21}H_{23}Cl_2N_3O = 404.3$.
CAS — 82626-01-5.

Profile

Alpidem is an imidazopyridine derivative that was given by mouth for its anxiolytic properties but it was withdrawn from the market following reports of hepatic dysfunction.

Alprazolam   (7003-b)

Alprazolam (*BAN, USAN, rINN*).

Alprazolamum; U-31889. 8-Chloro-1-methyl-6-phenyl-4*H*-1,2,4-triazolo[4,3-*a*][1,4]benzodiazepine.
$C_{17}H_{13}CIN_4 = 308.8$.
CAS — 28981-97-7 (alprazolam).
ATC — N05BA12.
Pharmacopoeias. In Eur. (see p.vi) and US.

Pharmacopoeial description

Ph. Eur.: A white crystalline powder. It exhibits polymorphism. Practically insoluble in water; sparingly soluble in alcohol and in acetone; freely soluble in dichloromethane. Protect from light.
USP 25: A white to off-white crystalline powder. Insoluble in water; soluble in alcohol; sparingly soluble in acetone; freely soluble in chloroform; slightly soluble in ethyl acetate.

◊ CAUTION. *Care should be taken to prevent inhaling particles of alprazolam and exposing the skin to it.*

Dependence and Withdrawal

As for Diazepam, p.675. Dependence may be a particular problem at the high doses used in the treatment of panic attacks.

Adverse Effects and Treatment

As for Diazepam, p.675.

Effects on the liver. Abnormal liver enzyme values occurred on 2 occasions when alprazolam was added to the treatment regimen of a patient receiving phenelzine for depression.[1] It was not possible to say if this was due to alprazolam alone or a synergistic effect with phenelzine.
1. Roy-Byrne P, *et al.* Alprazolam-related hepatotoxicity. *Lancet* 1983; **ii:** 786–7.

Effects on the skin. A report of a patient with alprazolam-induced photosensitivity confirmed on rechallenge.[1]
1. Kanwar AJ, *et al.* Photosensitivity due to alprazolam. *Dermatologica* 1990; **181:** 75.

Precautions

As for Diazepam, p.676.

Abuse. Report of the abuse of alprazolam by patients receiving methadone maintenance therapy for opioid dependence.[1] Ingestion of high doses of alprazolam after taking methadone produced a 'high' without pronounced sedation. Alprazolam was also being reportedly abused by nonopioid-drug abusers. The usual urine toxicology screens for benzodiazepines often give false-negative results for alprazolam because of the extremely low concentrations of metabolites excreted, making abuse difficult to detect. A subsequent review[2] considered that the literature did not support the widely held belief that alprazolam had a greater liability for abuse than other benzodiazepines, but the possibility could not be discounted.
1. Weddington WW, Carney AC. Alprazolam abuse during methadone maintenance therapy. *JAMA* 1987; **257:** 3363.
2. Rush CR, *et al.* Abuse liability of alprazolam relative to other commonly used benzodiazepines: a review. *Neurosci Biobehav Rev* 1993; **17:** 277–85.

Hepatic impairment. Alprazolam 1 mg by mouth was absorbed more slowly in 17 patients with alcoholic cirrhosis but no ascites than in 17 healthy subjects;[1] the peak alprazolam concentrations in the 2 groups were achieved at a mean of 3.34 hours and 1.47 hours respectively, and the mean elimination half-lives were 19.7 hours and 11.4 hours. However, there were no significant differences in the maximum plasma concentrations achieved. The results indicate that alprazolam, in common with other benzodiazepines which undergo oxidative metabolism, would accumulate to a greater extent in patients with alcoholic liver disease than in healthy subjects; the daily dose of alprazolam may need to be reduced by half in this population.
1. Juhl RP, *et al.* Alprazolam pharmacokinetics in alcoholic liver disease. *J Clin Pharmacol* 1984; **24:** 113–19.

Porphyria. Alprazolam is considered to be unsafe in patients with porphyria because it has been shown to be porphyrinogenic in *in-vitro* systems.

Interactions

As for Diazepam, p.677.

Pharmacokinetics

Alprazolam is well absorbed from the gastrointestinal tract following oral administration, with peak plasma concentrations being achieved within 1 to 2 hours of a dose. The mean plasma half-life is 11 to 15 hours. Alprazolam is 70 to 80% bound to plasma protein. It is metabolised in the liver primarily to α-hydroxyalprazolam, which is reported to be approximately half as active as the parent compound, and to an inactive benzophenone; plasma concentrations of metabolites are very low; it is excreted in urine as unchanged drug and metabolites.

◊ References.
1. Greenblatt DJ, Wright CE. Clinical pharmacokinetics of alprazolam: therapeutic implications. *Clin Pharmacokinet* 1993; **24:** 453–71.
2. Wright CE, *et al.* Pharmacokinetics and psychomotor performance of alprazolam: concentration-effect relationship. *J Clin Pharmacol* 1997; **37:** 321–9.
3. Kaplan GB, *et al.* Single-dose pharmacokinetics and pharmacodynamics of alprazolam in elderly and young subjects. *J Clin Pharmacol* 1998; **38:** 14–21.

Distribution into breast milk. From a study[1] of the distribution of alprazolam into breast milk in 8 lactating women it was estimated that the average daily dose of alprazolam ingested by a breast-fed infant would range from 0.3 to 5 μg per kg body-weight or about 3% of a maternal dose.
1. Oo CY, *et al.* Pharmacokinetics in lactating women: prediction of alprazolam transfer into milk. *Br J Clin Pharmacol* 1995; **40:** 231–6.

Uses and Administration

Alprazolam is a short-acting benzodiazepine with general properties similar to those of diazepam (p.680). It is used in the short-term treatment of anxiety disorders in doses of 0.25 to 0.5 mg three times daily by mouth, increased where necessary to a total daily dose of 3 or 4 mg. In elderly or debilitated patients and in those with advanced liver disease, an initial dose of 0.25 mg two or three times daily has been suggested.

Doses of up to 10 mg of alprazolam daily have been used in the treatment of panic attacks.

Anxiety disorders. The management of anxiety disorders, including the use of benzodiazepines, is discussed on p.649. References.

1. Cross-National Collaborative Panic Study, Second Phase Investigators. Drug treatment of panic disorder: comparative efficacy of alprazolam, imipramine, and placebo. *Br J Psychiatry* 1992; **160:** 191–202.
2. Lepola UM, *et al.* Three-year follow-up of patients with panic disorder after short-term treatment with alprazolam and imipramine. *Int Clin Psychopharmacol* 1993; **8:** 115–18.
3. Pollack MH, *et al.* Long-term outcome after acute treatment with alprazolam or clonazepam for panic disorder. *J Clin Psychopharmacol* 1993; **13:** 257–63.
4. Woodman CL, *et al.* Predictors of response to alprazolam and placebo in patients with panic disorder. *J Affect Disord* 1994; **30:** 5–13.

Depression. Although they may be useful for associated anxiety, benzodiazepines are not usually considered appropriate for treatment of depression (p.271); however, some drugs such as alprazolam have been tried for this indication.[1]

1. Kravitz HM, *et al.* Alprazolam and depression: a review of risks and benefits. *J Clin Psychiatry* 1993; **54:** (suppl.): 78–84.

Premenstrual syndrome. Alprazolam has been reported[1-3] to have produced a marginal to good response in the premenstrual syndrome (p.1475) but others have not found it to be of benefit,[4] and the role of benzodiazepines is limited by their adverse effects. If benzodiazepines are selected it is recommended that in order to reduce the risk of dependence and withdrawal symptoms they should be carefully restricted to the luteal phase in selected patients.[5] Withdrawal symptoms may be more severe after short-acting drugs such as alprazolam. Antidepressant drugs such as SSRIs may be preferred.

1. Smith S, *et al.* Treatment of premenstrual syndrome with alprazolam: results of a double-blind, placebo-controlled, randomized crossover clinical trial. *Obstet Gynecol* 1987; **70:** 37–43.
2. Harrison WM, *et al.* Treatment of premenstrual dysphoria with alprazolam: a controlled study. *Arch Gen Psychiatry* 1990; **47:** 270–5.
3. Freeman EW, *et al.* A double-blind trial of oral progesterone, alprazolam, and placebo in treatment of severe premenstrual syndrome. *JAMA* 1995; **274:** 51–7.
4. Evans SM, *et al.* Mood and performance changes in women with premenstrual dysphoric disorder: acute effects of alprazolam. *Neuropsychopharmacology* 1998; **19:** 499–516.
5. Mortola JF. A risk-benefit appraisal of drugs used in the management of premenstrual syndrome. *Drug Safety* 1994; **10:** 160–9.

Preparations

USP 25: Alprazolam Tablets.

Proprietary Preparations (details are given in Part 3)
Aust.: Xanor; *Austral.:* Kalma; Ralozam; Xanax; *Belg.:* Alpraz; Xanax; *Braz.:* Frontal; *Canad.:* Apo-Alpraz; Novo-Alprazol; Nu-Alpraz; Xanax; *Denm.:* Alprox; Tafil; *Fin.:* Alprox; Xanor; *Fr.:* Xanax; *Ger.:* Cassadan; Esparon; Tafil; Xanax; *Hong Kong:* Xanax; *Irl.:* Alprox; Calmax; Gerax; Xanax; *Israel:* Alpralid; Alprox; Apox; Xanagis; Xanax; *Ital.:* Frontal; Mialin; Valeans; Xanax; *Mex.:* Tafil; *Neth.:* Xanax; *Norw.:* Xanor; *NZ:* Xanax; *Port.:* Alpronax†; Pazolam; Prazam; Unilan; Xanax; *S.Afr.:* Alzam; Anxirid; Azor; Drimpam; Panix; Xanolam; Xanor; Zopax; *Singapore:* Alzolam; Apo-Alpraz; Dizolam; Xanax; Zacetin; *Spain:* Trankimazin; *Swed.:* Alpralid†; Xanor; *Switz.:* Xanax; *Thai.:* Alcelam; Alnax; Anpress; Dizolam; Pharnax; Siampraxol; Xanax; Xiemed; *UK:* Xanax; *USA:* Xanax.

Amisulpride (1759-d)

Amisulpride (BAN, rINN).

Amisulpridum; DAN-216. 4-Amino-N-[(1-ethyl-2-pyrrolidinyl)methyl]-5-(ethylsulphonyl)-2-methoxybenzamide; (RS)-4-Amino-N-[(1-ethylpyrrolidin-2-yl)methyl]-5-(ethylsulfonyl)-o-anisamide.
$C_{17}H_{27}N_3O_4S = 369.5$.
CAS — 71675-85-9.
ATC — N05AL05.

Pharmacopoeias. In Eur. (see p.vi).

Pharmacopoeial description

Ph. Eur.: A white or almost white crystalline powder. Practically insoluble in water; sparingly soluble in dehydrated alcohol; freely soluble in dichloromethane.

Adverse Effects, Treatment, and Precautions

As for Sulpiride, p.706.

Overdosage. The effects of overdosage of amisulpride in 2 patients have been reported.[1] The first patient had taken about 3 g of amisulpride and an unknown amount of dothiepin [dosulepin] and was found to have had a blood-amisulpride concentration of 9.63 μg per mL. Generalised convulsions, which resolved spontaneously, were followed by coma, motor restlessness, tachycardia, and slight prolongation of the QT interval. The patient was treated with gastric lavage and had recovered within 48 hours. The second patient, who had been found dead, had a blood-amisulpride concentration of 41.7 μg per mL.

1. Tracqui A, *et al.* Amisulpride poisoning: a report on two cases. *Hum Exp Toxicol* 1995; **14:** 294–8.

The symbol † denotes a preparation no longer actively marketed

Interactions

As for Chlorpromazine, p.664.

Pharmacokinetics

Amisulpride is absorbed from the gastrointestinal tract but bioavailability is reported to be only about 43 to 48%. An initial peak in plasma concentration has been reported to occur one hour after oral administration and a second higher one after 3 to 4 hours. Plasma protein binding is reported to be low. Metabolism is limited, with most of a dose appearing in the urine and faeces as unchanged drug. The terminal elimination half-life is about 12 hours.

Uses and Administration

Amisulpride is a substituted benzamide atypical antipsychotic with general properties similar to those of sulpiride (p.706). It is reported to have a high affinity for dopamine D_2 and D_3 receptors. Amisulpride is used mainly in the management of psychoses such as schizophrenia (p.651) but has also been tried in depression (p.271).

For acute psychotic episodes daily doses of between 400 and 800 mg may be given by mouth in 2 divided doses, increased if necessary to 1200 mg daily. For patients with predominantly negative symptoms daily doses between 50 and 300 mg are recommended. Daily doses of up to 300 mg may be administered once daily. For patients with renal impairment the dose should be reduced to half the normal dose for patients with a creatinine clearance (CC) of between 30 and 60 mL per minute and to one-third in patients with a CC between 10 and 30 mL per minute. Amisulpride has also been given by intramuscular injection in doses of 400 mg daily.

◊ References.

1. Boyer P, *et al.* Treatment of negative symptoms in schizophrenia with amisulpride. *Br J Psychiatry* 1995; **166:** 68–72.
2. Möller H-J, *et al.* Improvement of acute exacerbations of schizophrenia with amisulpride: a comparison with haloperidol. *Psychopharmacology (Berl)* 1997; **132:** 396–401.
3. Loo H, *et al.* Amisulpride versus placebo in the medium-term treatment of the negative symptoms of schizophrenia. *Br J Psychiatry* 1997; **170:** 18–22.
4. Lecrubier Y, *et al.* Amisulpride Study Group. Amisulpride versus imipramine and placebo in dysthymia and major depression. *J Affect Disord* 1997; **43:** 95–103.
5. Smeraldi E. Amisulpride versus fluoxetine in patients with dysthymia or major depression in partial remission: a double-blind, comparative study. *J Affect Disord* 1998; **48:** 47–56.
6. Boyer P, *et al.* Amisulpride versus amineptine and placebo for the treatment of dysthymia. *Neuropsychobiology* 1999; **39:** 25–32.

Preparations

Proprietary Preparations (details are given in Part 3)
Aust.: Deniban†; *Braz.:* Socian; *Fr.:* Solian; *Ger.:* Solian; *Irl.:* Solian; *Ital.:* Deniban; Sulamid; *Port.:* Amitrex; Socian; *Singapore:* Solian; *Switz.:* Solian; *UK:* Solian.

Amobarbital (4005-v)

Amobarbital (BAN, rINN).

Amobarbitalum; Amylobarbitone; Pentymalum. 5-Ethyl-5-isopentylbarbituric acid.
$C_{11}H_{18}N_2O_3 = 226.3$.
CAS — 57-43-2.
ATC — N05CA02.

Pharmacopoeias. In Chin., Eur. (see p.vi), and Jpn.

Pharmacopoeial description

Ph. Eur.: A white crystalline powder. Very slightly soluble in water; freely soluble in alcohol and in ether; soluble in dichloromethane. Forms water-soluble compounds with alkali hydroxides and carbonates and with ammonia.

Amobarbital Sodium (4006-g)

Amobarbital Sodium (BANM, rINNM).

Amobarbitalum Natricum; Amylobarbitone Sodium; Barbamylum; Pentymalnatrium; Sodium Amobarbital; Soluble Amylobarbitone. Sodium 5-ethyl-5-isopentylbarbiturate.
$C_{11}H_{17}N_2NaO_3 = 248.3$.
CAS — 64-43-7.

Pharmacopoeias. In Chin., Eur. (see p.vi), and US.
Jpn includes Amobarbital Sodium for Injection.

Amobarbital may be precipitated from preparations containing amobarbital sodium, depending on the concentration and pH. Amobarbital sodium has, therefore, been reported to be incompatible with many other drugs, particularly acids and acidic salts.

Pharmacopoeial description

Ph. Eur.: A white, hygroscopic, granular powder. Very soluble in carbon dioxide-free water (a small fraction may be insoluble); freely soluble in alcohol; practically insoluble in ether. A 10% solution in water has a pH of not more than 11.0. Store in airtight containers.

USP 25: A white, odourless, hygroscopic, friable, granular powder. Very soluble in water; soluble in alcohol; practically insoluble in chloroform and in ether. Solutions decompose on standing; decomposition is accelerated by heat. pH of a 10% solution in water is not more than 11.0. Store in airtight containers.

Dependence and Withdrawal

The development of dependence is a high risk with amobarbital and other barbiturates and may occur after regular use even in therapeutic doses for short periods. Barbiturates should not therefore be discontinued abruptly, but should be withdrawn by gradual reduction of the dose over a period of days or weeks. A long-acting barbiturate such as phenobarbital may be substituted for a short- or intermediate-acting one, followed by gradual reduction of the phenobarbital dose.

Withdrawal symptoms are similar to those of alcohol withdrawal and are characterised after several hours by apprehension and weakness, followed by anxiety, headache, dizziness, irritability, tremors, nausea and vomiting, abdominal cramps, insomnia, distortion in visual perception, muscle twitching, and tachycardia. Orthostatic hypotension and convulsions may develop after a day or two, sometimes leading to status epilepticus. Hallucinations and delirium tremens may develop after several days followed by coma before the symptoms disappear or death occurs.

Adverse Effects

Drowsiness, sedation, and ataxia are the most frequent adverse effects of amobarbital and other barbiturates and are a consequence of dose-related CNS depression. Other adverse effects include respiratory depression, headache, gastrointestinal disturbances, skin reactions, confusion, and memory defects. Paradoxical excitement and irritability may occur, particularly in children, the elderly, and patients in acute pain. Hypersensitivity reactions occur rarely and include skin rashes (erythema multiforme and exfoliative dermatitis, sometimes fatal, have been reported), hepatitis and cholestasis, and photosensitivity. Blood disorders, including megaloblastic anaemia after chronic use of barbiturates, have also occurred occasionally.

Neonatal intoxication, drug dependence, and symptoms resembling vitamin-K deficiency have been reported in infants born to mothers who received barbiturates during pregnancy. Congenital malformations have been reported in children of women who took barbiturates during pregnancy, but the causal role is a matter of some debate.

Nystagmus, miosis, slurred speech, and ataxia may occur with excessive doses of barbiturates. The toxic effects of overdosage result from profound central depression and include coma, respiratory and cardiovascular depression, with hypotension and shock leading to renal failure and death. Hypothermia may occur with subsequent pyrexia on recovery. Erythematous or haemorrhagic blisters reportedly occur in about 6% of patients, but are not characteristic solely of barbiturate poisoning.

Solutions of the sodium salts of barbiturates are extremely alkaline, and necrosis has followed subcutaneous injection. Intravenous injection may be hazardous; hypotension, shock, laryngospasm, and apnoea have occurred particularly after rapid administration. Gangrene has resulted from intra-arterial injection into an extremity.

Overdosage. A detailed review of drug-induced stupor and coma, including that caused by barbiturates.[1]

1. Ashton CH, *et al.* Drug-induced stupor and coma: some physical signs and their pharmacological basis. *Adverse Drug React Acute Poisoning Rev* 1989; **8:** 1–59.

Treatment of Adverse Effects

Following an overdose of a barbiturate endotracheal intubation may be necessary if the patient is unconscious. Administration of activated charcoal by mouth or nasogastric tube is advocated in patients who have ingested more than 25 mg per kg bodyweight within 1 hour of treatment. Patients should be managed with intensive supportive therapy, with particular attention being paid to the maintenance of cardiovascular, respiratory, and renal functions, and to the maintenance of the electrolyte balance. Charcoal haemoperfusion can be life-saving in the most severe cases and should be considered if there is no improvement after 24 hours of supportive care. The value of other measures aimed at the active removal of barbiturates is questionable.

Precautions

Amobarbital and other barbiturates are best avoided in elderly and debilitated patients, in young adults, in children, and in those with depression.

Amobarbital is contra-indicated in patients with pulmonary insufficiency, sleep apnoea, pre-existing CNS depression or coma, and severe hepatic impairment, and should be given with caution to those with renal insufficiency. Barbiturates given to patients in pain may provoke a paradoxical excitatory reaction, unless an analgesic is given concomitantly. With continued administration, tolerance develops to the sedative or hypnotic effects of the barbiturates to a greater extent than to their lethal effects. Barbiturates may cause drowsiness which may persist the next day; affected patients should not drive or operate machinery.

See under Adverse Effects, above, for the hazards of administration of barbiturates during pregnancy. Small amounts of barbiturates are distributed into breast milk; they should not, therefore, be given to nursing mothers.

Dependence readily develops after use of barbiturates with a **withdrawal syndrome** on abrupt discontinuation (see under Dependence and Withdrawal, above).

Barbiturates are abused for their euphoriant effects.

Porphyria. Barbiturates including amobarbital have been associated with acute attacks of porphyria and are considered unsafe in porphyric patients.

Interactions
Sedation or respiratory depression may be enhanced by drugs with CNS-depressant properties; in particular alcohol should be avoided. Barbiturates generally induce liver enzymes, and thus increase the rate of metabolism (and decrease the activity) of many other drugs as well as endogenous substances. Continued use may result in induction of their own metabolism. MAOIs may prolong the CNS depressant effects of some barbiturates, probably by inhibition of their metabolism. However, MAOIs, like other antidepressants, also reduce the convulsive threshold and thereby antagonise the anticonvulsant action of barbiturates.

For some further interactions involving barbiturates, see under Phenobarbital, p.355.

Pharmacokinetics
Amobarbital is readily absorbed from the gastrointestinal tract. It is about 60% bound to plasma proteins. It has a half-life of about 20 to 25 hours which is considerably extended in neonates. It crosses the placenta and small amounts are distributed into breast milk. Amobarbital is metabolised in the liver; up to about 50% is excreted in the urine as 3'-hydroxyamylobarbital and up to about 30% as N-hydroxyamylobarbital, less than 1% appearing unchanged; up to about 5% is excreted in the faeces.

Uses and Administration
Amobarbital is a barbiturate that has been used as a hypnotic and sedative. Its use can no longer be recommended because of its adverse effects and risk of dependence, although continued use may occasionally be considered necessary for severe intractable insomnia (p.652) in patients already taking it. The usual dose by mouth at bedtime was 100 to 200 mg of the base or 60 to 200 mg of the sodium salt. A more rapid onset of effect was obtained with the sodium salt.

Barbiturates with a longer action such as phenobarbital (p.355) are still used in epilepsy and those with a shorter action such as methohexital (p.1263) or thiopental (p.1269) for anaesthesia.

Cerebrovascular disorders. For reference to the use of barbiturate-induced coma in the management of patients with cerebral ischaemia, see p.1270.

Epilepsy. Amobarbital is used for specialised procedures in expert epilepsy centres only. It is given by deep intramuscular or slow intravenous injection as the sodium salt.

Preparations
USP 25: Amobarbital Sodium for Injection; Secobarbital Sodium and Amobarbital Sodium Capsules.

Proprietary Preparations (details are given in Part 3)
Austral.: Amytal; Neur-Amyl; *Canad.:* Amytal; *Irl.:* Amytal; *UK:* Amytal; *USA:* Amytal.
Multi-ingredient: *Belg.:* Bellanox†; *Canad.:* Tuinal†; *Irl.:* Tuinal†; *S.Afr.:* Amesec†; Daral†; Fabasma†; Medikasma†; Panasma†; Repasma†; *Thai.:* Ama; *UK:* Tuinal; *USA:* Tuinal.

Amperozide (18810-y)
Amperozide *(BAN, rINN)*.
FG-5606. 4-[4,4-Bis(4-fluorophenyl)butyl]-N-ethylpiperazine-1-carboxamide.
$C_{23}H_{29}F_2N_3O = 401.5$.
CAS — 75558-90-6 (amperozide); 75529-73-6 (amperozide hydrochloride).

Profile
Amperozide is an antipsychotic used in veterinary medicine.

Aprobarbital (4007-q)
Aprobarbital *(rINN)*.
Allylisopropylmalonylurea; Allypropymal; Aprobarbitone. 5-Allyl-5-isopropylbarbituric acid.
$C_{10}H_{14}N_2O_3 = 210.2$.
CAS — 77-02-1.
ATC — N05CA05.

Profile
Aprobarbital is a barbiturate with general properties similar to those of amobarbital (p.655). It has been given by mouth for insomnia (p.652) in doses of 40 to 160 mg at night and as a sedative in usual doses of 40 mg three times daily, but barbitu-

rates are no longer considered appropriate for such purposes. Aprobarbital sodium was also formerly used.

Preparations
Proprietary Preparations (details are given in Part 3)
USA: Alurate†.

Azaperone (12412-x)
Azaperone *(BAN, USAN, rINN)*.
Azaperonum; R-1929. 4'-Fluoro-4-[4-(2-pyridyl)piperazin-1-yl]butyrophenone.
$C_{19}H_{22}FN_3O = 327.4$.
CAS — 1649-18-9.
Pharmacopoeias. In Eur. (see p.vi) and US for veterinary use only.

Pharmacopoeial description
Ph. Eur.: A white or almost white powder. It exhibits polymorphism. Practically insoluble in water; soluble in alcohol; freely soluble in acetone and in dichloromethane. Protect from light.
USP 25: M.p. 92° to 95°. Protect from light.

Profile
Azaperone is a butyrophenone antipsychotic used as a tranquilliser in veterinary practice.

Barbital (4009-s)
Barbital *(BAN, rINN)*.
Barbitalum; Barbitone; Diemalum; Diethylmalonylurea. 5,5-Diethylbarbituric acid.
$C_8H_{12}N_2O_3 = 184.2$.
CAS — 57-44-3.
ATC — N05CA04.
Pharmacopoeias. In Eur. (see p.vi), Jpn, and Pol.

Pharmacopoeial description
Ph. Eur.: A white, crystalline powder or colourless crystals. Slightly soluble in water; soluble in boiling water, in alcohol, and in ether. It forms water-soluble compounds with alkali hydroxides and carbonates and with ammonia.

Barbital Sodium (4010-h)
Barbital Sodium *(BANM, rINN)*.
Barbitalum Natricum; Barbitone Sodium; Diemalnatrium; Soluble Barbitone. Sodium 5,5-diethylbarbiturate.
$C_8H_{11}N_2NaO_3 = 206.2$.
CAS — 144-02-5.
Pharmacopoeias. In Aust., Pol., and Swiss.

Profile
Barbital is a barbiturate with general properties similar to those of amobarbital (p.655). It was formerly used for its hypnotic and sedative properties.

Preparations
Proprietary Preparations (details are given in Part 3)
Mex.: Neurinase.

Benperidol (7006-q)
Benperidol *(BAN, USAN, rINN)*.
Benperidolum; Benzperidol; CB-8089; McN-JR-4584; R-4584. 1-{1-[3-(4-Fluorobenzoyl)propyl]-4-piperidyl}benzimidazolin-2-one.
$C_{22}H_{24}FN_3O_2 = 381.4$.
CAS — 2062-84-2.
ATC — N05AD07.
Pharmacopoeias. In Eur. (see p.vi).

Pharmacopoeial description
Ph. Eur.: A white or almost white powder. It exhibits polymorphism. Practically insoluble in water; slightly soluble in alcohol; soluble in dichloromethane; freely soluble in dimethylformamide. Protect from light.

Profile
Benperidol is a butyrophenone with general properties similar to those of haloperidol (p.686). Doses of 0.25 to 1.5 mg daily in divided doses are given by mouth in the management of deviant sexual behaviour. Elderly or debilitated patients may require reduced doses of benperidol.

In some countries benperidol is given by mouth or parenterally for the treatment of psychotic conditions (p.650).

Pharmacokinetics. References.
1. Furlanut M, *et al.* Pharmacokinetics of benperidol in volunteers after oral administration. *Int J Clin Pharmacol Res* 1988; **8:** 13–16.

Deviant sexual behaviour. Results of a double-blind placebo-controlled crossover study demonstrated no difference between the effect of benperidol 1.25 mg daily, chlorpromazine 125 mg daily, or placebo, on sexual drive and arousal in 12 paedophilic sexual offenders, except for a lower frequency of sexual thoughts with benperidol.[1] The effects of benperidol are unlikely to be sufficient to control severe forms of antisocial

sexually deviant behaviour. The management of deviant sexual behaviour is discussed under Disturbed Behaviour on p.650.
1. Tennent G, *et al.* The control of deviant sexual behaviour by drugs: a double-blind controlled study of benperidol, chlorpromazine, and placebo. *Arch Sex Behav* 1974; **3:** 261–71.

Preparations
Proprietary Preparations (details are given in Part 3)
Belg.: Frenactil; *Ger.:* Glianimon; *Irl.:* Anquil; *Neth.:* Frenactil; *UK:* Anquil.

Bentazepam (12429-g)
Bentazepam *(USAN, rINN)*.
CI-718; QM-6008. 1,3,6,7,8,9-Hexahydro-5-phenyl-2H-[1]benzothieno[2,3-e]-1,4-diazepin-2-one.
$C_{17}H_{16}N_2OS = 296.4$.
CAS — 29462-18-8.

Profile
Bentazepam is a benzodiazepine with general properties similar to those of diazepam (p.674). It has been given by mouth in the short-term treatment of anxiety disorders and insomnia.

Effects on the liver. Severe chronic active hepatitis has been reported in a 65-year-old man who had received long-term treatment with bentazepam.[1]
1. Andrade RJ, *et al.* Bentazepam-associated chronic liver disease. *Lancet* 1994; **343:** 860.

Preparations
Proprietary Preparations (details are given in Part 3)
Spain: Tiadipona.

Brallobarbital (5149-g)
Brallobarbital *(rINN)*.
UCB-5033. 5-Allyl-5-(2-bromoallyl)barbituric acid.
$C_{10}H_{11}BrN_2O_3 = 287.1$.
CAS — 561-86-4.

Profile
Brallobarbital is a barbiturate with general properties similar to those of amobarbital (p.655). It has been used in preparations for the management of insomnia but barbiturates are no longer considered appropriate for such a purpose. Brallobarbital calcium has been used similarly.

Preparations
Proprietary Preparations (details are given in Part 3)
Multi-ingredient: *Belg.:* Bellanox†; Vesparax†; *Neth.:* Vesparax; *Port.:* Vesparax†; *S.Afr.:* Vesparax†; *Spain:* Somatarax.

Bromazepam (7008-s)
Bromazepam *(BAN, USAN, rINN)*.
Bromazepamum; Ro-5-3350. 7-Bromo-1,3-dihydro-5-(2-pyridyl)-1,4-benzodiazepin-2-one.
$C_{14}H_{10}BrN_3O = 316.2$.
CAS — 1812-30-2.
ATC — N05BA08.
Pharmacopoeias. In Eur. (see p.vi) and Jpn.

Pharmacopoeial description
Ph. Eur.: A white or yellowish crystalline powder. Practically insoluble in water; sparingly soluble in alcohol and in dichloromethane. Protect from light.

Dependence and Withdrawal
As for Diazepam, p.675.

Adverse Effects, Treatment, and Precautions
As for Diazepam, p.675.

Interactions
As for Diazepam, p.677.

Pharmacokinetics
Bromazepam is well absorbed from the gastrointestinal tract following oral administration and peak plasma concentrations are achieved within 1 to 4 hours. It is highly bound to plasma proteins. Reported values for the mean plasma elimination half-life have ranged from about 12 to 32 hours. It is excreted mainly in the urine in the form of inactive conjugated metabolites.

◊ References.
1. Kaplan SA, *et al.* Biopharmaceutical and clinical pharmacokinetic profile of bromazepam. *J Pharmacokinet Biopharm* 1976; **4:** 1–16.
2. Ochs HR, *et al.* Bromazepam pharmacokinetics: influence of age, gender, oral contraceptives, cimetidine, and propranolol. *Clin Pharmacol Ther* 1987; **41:** 562–70.

Uses and Administration
Bromazepam is a benzodiazepine with general properties similar to those of diazepam (p.680). It is used in the short-term treatment of anxiety disorders (p.649) occurring alone or associated with insomnia. A usual dose for anxiety is 3 to 18 mg daily in divided doses by mouth. Higher doses up to 60 mg daily have occasionally been given to hospitalised patients. Doses

should be reduced by at least half in elderly patients and in those with hepatic or renal impairment.

◊ References.
1. Erb T, *et al.* Preoperative anxiolysis with minimal sedation in elderly patients: bromazepam or clorazepate-dipotassium? *Acta Anaesthesiol Scand* 1998; **42:** 97–101.

Preparations

Proprietary Preparations (details are given in Part 3)
Aust.: Lexotanil; **Austral.:** Lexotan; **Belg.:** Bromidem; Lexotan; **Braz.:** Brozepax; Calmex; Deptran; Lexotan; Nervium; Somalium; **Canad.:** Lectopam; **Denm.:** Bromam; Lexotan; **Fr.:** Anxyrex; Lexomil; Quietiline; **Ger.:** Bromazanil; Bromazep; durazanil; Gityl; Lexostad; Lexotanil; neo OPT; Normoc; **Hong Kong:** Akamon; Lexilium; Lexotan; **Irl.:** Lexotan; **Israel:** Lenitin; **Ital.:** Compendium; Lexotan; **Mex.:** Lexotanil; **Neth.:** Lexotanil; **Port.:** Bromalex; Lexotan; Ultramidol; **S.Afr.:** Brazepam; Bromaze; Brozam; Lexotan; **Singapore:** Lexotan; **Spain:** Lexatin; **Switz.:** Lexotanil; **Thai.:** Lexotan; **UK:** Lexotan.

Multi-ingredient: **Braz.:** Bromopirin; Sulpan; **Ital.:** Lexil.

Bromisoval   (4013-v)

Bromisoval *(rINN)*.

Bromisovalerylurea; Bromisovalum; Bromvalerylurea; Bromvaletone; Bromylum. *N*-(2-Bromo-3-methylbutyryl)urea.
$C_6H_{11}BrN_2O_2 = 223.1$.
CAS — 496-67-3.
ATC — N05CM03.

Pharmacopoeias. In Aust., Jpn, and Neth.

Profile
Bromisoval has actions and uses similar to those of carbromal (p.659).

Bromperidol   (7009-w)

Bromperidol *(BAN, USAN, rINN)*.

Bromperidolum; R-11333. 4-[4-(*p*-Bromophenyl)-4-hydroxypiperidino]-4′-fluorobutyrophenone.
$C_{21}H_{23}BrFNO_2 = 420.3$.
CAS — 10457-90-6.
ATC — N05AD06.

Pharmacopoeias. In Eur. (see p.vi).

Pharmacopoeial description
Ph. Eur.: A white or almost white powder. Practically insoluble in water; slightly soluble in alcohol; sparingly soluble in dichloromethane and in methyl alcohol. Protect from light.

Bromperidol Decanoate   (16551-k)

Bromperidol Decanoate *(BANM, USAN, rINNM)*.

Bromperidoli Decanoas; R-46541.
$C_{31}H_{41}BrFNO_3 = 574.6$.
CAS — 75067-66-2.

Pharmacopoeias. In Eur. (see p.vi).

Pharmacopoeial description
Ph. Eur.: A white or almost white powder. Practically insoluble in water; soluble in alcohol; very soluble in dichloromethane. It melts at about 60°. Store at a temperature below 25°. Protect from light.

Profile
Bromperidol is a butyrophenone with general properties similar to those of haloperidol (p.686). It is given in the treatment of schizophrenia (p.651) and other psychoses. Some bromperidol preparations are prepared with the aid of lactic acid and may be stated to contain bromperidol lactate. However, doses are expressed in terms of the equivalent amount of bromperidol. A usual dose is 1 to 15 mg daily by mouth, although up to 80 mg daily has been given. Elderly patients may require reduced doses of bromperidol. Bromperidol may also be administered by intramuscular or intravenous injection.

The long-acting decanoate ester may be used for patients requiring long-term therapy with bromperidol. A usual dose, given by deep intramuscular injection, is the equivalent of up to 300 mg of bromperidol every 4 weeks.

◊ References.[1-5] A systematic review[5] suggested that depot bromperidol had some benefits in schizophrenia but was less effective than haloperidol or fluphenazine.

1. Benfield P, *et al.* Bromperidol: a preliminary review of its pharmacodynamic and pharmacokinetic properties, and therapeutic efficacy in psychoses. *Drugs* 1988; **35:** 670–84.
2. McLaren S, *et al.* Positive and negative symptoms, depression and social disability in chronic schizophrenia: a comparative trial of bromperidol and fluphenazine decanoates. *Int J Clin Psychopharmacol* 1992; **7:** 67–72.
3. Yamagami S, *et al.* A single-blind comparison of bromperidol and sulpiride in hospitalized schizophrenics. *Acta Psychiatr Belg* 1993; **93:** 236–44.
4. Yasui N, *et al.* Prolactin response to bromperidol treatment in schizophrenic patients. *Pharmacol Toxicol* 1998; **82:** 153–6.
5. Quraishi S, *et al.* Depot bromperidol decanoate for schizophrenia (updated 30 August 2000). Available in The Cochrane Library; Issue 4. Oxford: Update Software; 2001.

Preparations

Proprietary Preparations (details are given in Part 3)
Belg.: Impromen; **Denm.:** Bromidol†; **Ger.:** Impromen; Tesoprel; **Ital.:** Impromen; **Neth.:** Impromen; **Thai.:** Impromen.

Brotizolam   (12458-e)

Brotizolam *(BAN, USAN, rINN)*.

We-941; We-941-BS. 2-Bromo-4-(2-chlorophenyl)-9-methyl-6*H*-thieno[3,2-*f*][1,2,4]triazolo[4,3-*a*][1,4]diazepine.
$C_{15}H_{10}BrClN_4S = 393.7$.
CAS — 57801-81-7.
ATC — N05CD09.

Profile
Brotizolam is a short-acting benzodiazepine with general properties similar to those of diazepam (p.674). It is given by mouth for the short-term (up to 2 weeks) management of insomnia (p.652) in usual doses of 250 µg at night. The suggested dose for elderly and debilitated patients is 125 µg.

Abuse. Reference to abuse of brotizolam in Germany and Hong Kong.[1]
1. WHO. WHO expert committee on drug dependence: twenty-ninth report. *WHO Tech Rep Ser 856* 1995.

Pharmacokinetics. References.
1. Bechtel WD. Pharmacokinetics and metabolism of brotizolam in humans. *Br J Clin Pharmacol* 1983; **16:** 279S–283S.
2. Jochemsen R, *et al.* Pharmacokinetics of brotizolam in healthy subjects following intravenous and oral administration. *Br J Clin Pharmacol* 1983; **16:** 285S–290S.

Preparations

Proprietary Preparations (details are given in Part 3)
Aust.: Lendorm; **Belg.:** Lendormin; **Denm.:** Lendorm; **Ger.:** Lendormin; **Israel:** Bondormin; **Ital.:** Lendormin; Nimbisan†; **Jpn:** Lendormin†; **Mex.:** Lindormin; **Neth.:** Lendormin; **Port.:** Lendormin; **S.Afr.:** Lendormin; **Spain:** Sintonal; **Switz.:** Lendormine.

Buspirone Hydrochloride   (12471-p)

Buspirone Hydrochloride *(BANM, USAN, rINNM)*.

MJ-9022-1.   8-[4-(4-Pyrimidin-2-ylpiperazin-1-yl)butyl]-8-azaspiro[4.5]decane-7,9-dione hydrochloride.
$C_{21}H_{31}N_5O_2,HCl = 422.0$.
CAS — 36505-84-7 (buspirone); 33386-08-2 (buspirone hydrochloride).

Pharmacopoeias. In US.

Pharmacopoeial description
USP 25: A white crystalline powder. Very soluble in water; sparingly soluble in alcohol and in acetonitrile; freely soluble in dichloromethane and in methyl alcohol; very slightly soluble in ethyl acetate; practically insoluble in hexanes. Store in airtight containers at a temperature between 15° and 30°. Protect from light.

Dependence and Adverse Effects
Dizziness, nausea, headache, nervousness, light-headedness, excitement, paraesthesias, sleep disturbances, chest pain, tinnitus, sore throat, and nasal congestion are amongst the most frequent adverse effects reported following the use of buspirone hydrochloride. Other adverse effects have included tachycardia, palpitations, drowsiness, confusion, dry mouth, fatigue, and sweating. A syndrome of restlessness appearing shortly after the start of treatment has been reported in a small number of patients given buspirone. Buspirone is reported to produce less sedation, and to have a lower potential for dependence, than the benzodiazepines.

◊ Mild acute hypertension and panic were reported on two occasions after the addition of single 10-mg doses of buspirone to therapy with tricyclic antidepressants in a 40-year-old man with panic disorder. Adrenergic or serotonin dysfunction were postulated as possible mechanisms for the reaction.[1,2] Psychotic reactions associated with buspirone treatment have also been reported in a few patients.[3] There have also been isolated reports of mania.[4]
1. Chignon JM, Lepine JP. Panic and hypertension associated with single dose of buspirone. *Lancet* 1989; **ii:** 46–7.
2. Norman TR, Judd FK. Panic attacks, buspirone, and serotonin function. *Lancet* 1989; **ii:** 615.
3. Friedman R. Possible induction of psychosis by buspirone. *Am J Psychiatry* 1991; **148:** 1606.
4. Price WA, Bielefeld M. Buspirone-induced mania. *J Clin Psychopharmacol* 1989; **9:** 150–1.

Extrapyramidal disorders. There have been isolated reports of exacerbation or precipitation of movement disorders[1-4] associated with the use of buspirone. However, buspirone has also been reported to have been of benefit in some patients with tardive dyskinesia (see under Uses and Administration, below).
1. Hammerstad JP, *et al.* Buspirone in Parkinson's disease. *Clin Neuropharmacol* 1986; **9:** 556–60.

---

2. Ritchie EC, *et al.* Acute generalized myoclonus following buspirone administration. *J Clin Psychiatry* 1988; **49:** 242–3.
3. Strauss A. Oral dyskinesia associated with buspirone use in an elderly woman. *J Clin Psychiatry* 1988; **49:** 322–3.
4. LeWitt PA, *et al.* Persistent movement disorders induced by buspirone. *Mov Disord* 1993; **8:** 331–4.

Precautions
Buspirone hydrochloride should be used with caution in patients with renal or hepatic disease and is contra-indicated if the disease is severe. Buspirone should preferably be avoided during pregnancy and breast feeding. It should not be used in patients with epilepsy or a history of such disorders. It does not exhibit cross-tolerance with benzodiazepines or other common sedatives or hypnotics and will not block symptoms of their withdrawal; they should, therefore, be gradually withdrawn before commencing treatment with buspirone. Buspirone may impair the patient's ability to drive or operate machinery.

Diagnosis and testing. Buspirone may interfere with diagnostic assays of urinary catecholamines.[1]
1. Cook FJ, *et al.* Effect of buspirone on urinary catecholamine assays. *N Engl J Med* 1995; **332:** 401.

Hepatic impairment. Caution has been advised when using buspirone in patients with liver disease. The mean peak plasma-buspirone concentration after a dose by mouth was about 16 times higher in cirrhotic patients than in controls[1] and the elimination half-life was prolonged about twofold. A secondary peak concentration was seen in some subjects, occurring between 4 and 24 hours after a dose in the cirrhotics and after between 2 and 8 hours in controls. Data from a multiple-dose study[2] suggested that there was accumulation of buspirone and its metabolite 1-(2-pyrimidinyl)-piperazine in hepatic impairment, but that plasma concentrations appeared to reach steady state after 3 days regardless of the state of liver function. The area under the curve and mean peak concentration for buspirone were both higher in patients with hepatic impairment than in healthy subjects, but there were no significant differences for its metabolites. Specific dosing recommendations could not be made for patients with hepatic impairment because of the high intra- and inter-subject variations in plasma-buspirone concentrations.
1. Dalhoff K, *et al.* Buspirone pharmacokinetics in patients with cirrhosis. *Br J Clin Pharmacol* 1987; **24:** 547–50.
2. Barbhaiya RH, *et al.* Disposition kinetics of buspirone in patients with renal or hepatic impairment after administration of single and multiple doses. *Eur J Clin Pharmacol* 1994; **46:** 41–7.

Renal impairment. As for hepatic impairment (above) caution is advised when giving buspirone to patients with renal impairment.[1,2] There is evidence of accumulation of buspirone and its metabolite following repeated administration but plasma concentrations appeared to reach steady state after 3 days regardless of the state of renal function. At steady state both the area under the curve and maximum concentrations for buspirone and its metabolite were greater in patients with renal failure than in healthy subjects. The metabolite, but not the parent drug, was removed by haemodialysis. Specific dosing recommendations could not be made for patients with renal impairment because of the high intra- and inter-subject variations in buspirone plasma concentrations following repeated administration.
1. Caccia S, *et al.* Clinical pharmacokinetics of oral buspirone in patients with impaired renal function. *Clin Pharmacokinet* 1988; **14:** 171–7.
2. Barbhaiya RH, *et al.* Disposition kinetics of buspirone in patients with renal or hepatic impairment after administration of single and multiple doses. *Eur J Clin Pharmacol* 1994; **46:** 41–7.

Interactions
The sedative effects of buspirone are enhanced by the simultaneous administration of alcohol or other CNS depressants. Because of reports of increased blood pressure in patients receiving buspirone hydrochloride with an MAOI, the manufacturers of buspirone recommend that it should not be given with a MAOI. The metabolism of buspirone is mediated by the cytochrome P450 isoenzyme CYP3A4 and therefore there is the potential for interactions between buspirone and other drugs that inhibit or act as a substrate for this enzyme. The dose of buspirone may need to be reduced during concomitant administration of potent inhibitors of CYP3A4. Plasma concentrations of buspirone may be reduced by enzyme-inducing drugs such as rifampicin.

Antibacterials. Pretreatment with *erythromycin* in healthy subjects given buspirone resulted in mild to moderate side-effects associated with increased plasma concentrations of buspirone.[1]

Pretreatment with *rifampicin* greatly reduced plasma concentrations of buspirone in healthy subjects.[2] A reduced anxiolytic effect could be expected if buspirone is used with rifampicin or

---

other potent inducers of the cytochrome P450 isoenzyme CYP3A4.

1. Kivistö KT, *et al.* Plasma buspirone concentrations are greatly increased by erythromycin and itraconazole. *Clin Pharmacol Ther* 1997; **62**: 348–54.
2. Lamberg TS, *et al.* Concentrations and effects of buspirone are considerably reduced by rifampicin. *Br J Clin Pharmacol* 1998; **45**: 381–5.

Antidepressants. Concomitant administration of buspirone and *nefazodone* can raise plasma concentrations of buspirone. The UK manufacturer of nefazodone recommends that the initial dose of buspirone be lowered to 2.5 mg and subsequent dose adjustments of either drug should be based on tolerance and clinical response. A possible serotonin syndrome (p.304) has been reported[1] in one patient following concomitant administration of buspirone and *fluoxetine*.

1. Manos GH. Possible serotonin syndrome associated with buspirone added to fluoxetine. *Ann Pharmacother* 2000; **34**: 871–4.

Antifungals. Pretreatment with *itraconazole* in healthy subjects given buspirone resulted in mild to moderate side-effects associated with increased plasma concentrations of buspirone.[1]

1. Kivistö KT, *et al.* Plasma buspirone concentrations are greatly increased by erythromycin and itraconazole. *Clin Pharmacol Ther* 1997; **62**: 348–54.

Antipsychotics. For the effect of buspirone on serum concentrations of *haloperidol*, see under Chlorpromazine, p.665. For a report of potentially fatal gastrointestinal bleeding and marked hyperglycaemia following concomitant administration of buspirone and *clozapine*, see under Clozapine, p.673.

Calcium-channel blockers. Increases in buspirone plasma concentrations have been seen in healthy subjects pretreated with *diltiazem* or *verapamil*.[1]

1. Lamberg TS, *et al.* Effects of verapamil and diltiazem on the pharmacokinetics and pharmacodynamics of buspirone. *Clin Pharmacol Ther* 1998; **63**: 640–5.

Grapefruit. Grapefruit juice increased the plasma concentrations of buspirone in healthy subjects.[1]

1. Lilja JJ, *et al.* Grapefruit juice substantially increases plasma concentrations of buspirone. *Clin Pharmacol Ther* 1998; **64**: 655–60.

Pharmacokinetics

Buspirone hydrochloride is rapidly absorbed from the gastrointestinal tract reaching peak plasma concentrations within 40 to 90 minutes after administration by mouth. Systemic bioavailability is low because of extensive first-pass metabolism, but may be increased on administration with food as this delays absorption from the gastrointestinal tract and thereby reduces presystemic clearance. Buspirone is about 95% bound to plasma proteins. Metabolism in the liver is extensive; hydroxylation yields several inactive metabolites and oxidative dealkylation produces 1-(2-pyrimidinyl)-piperazine which is reported to be about 25% as potent as the parent drug in one model of anxiolytic activity. The elimination half-life of buspirone is usually about 2 to 4 hours but half-lives of up to 11 hours have been reported. Buspirone is excreted mainly as metabolites in the urine, and also in the faeces.

◊ References.
1. Mahmood I, Sahajwalla C. Clinical pharmacokinetics and pharmacodynamics of buspirone, an anxiolytic drug. *Clin Pharmacokinet* 1999; **36**: 277–87.

Uses and Administration

Buspirone hydrochloride is an azaspirodecanedione anxiolytic. It is reported to be largely lacking in sedative, anticonvulsant, and muscle relaxant actions.

Buspirone hydrochloride is given, in initial doses of 5 mg two or three times daily, in the short-term management of anxiety disorders. The dose may be increased in increments of 5 mg at 2- to 3-day intervals if required. The recommended maximum daily dose, to be administered in divided doses, is 45 mg in the UK and 60 mg in the USA.

◊ General reviews.
1. Fulton B, Brogden RN. Buspirone: an updated review of its clinical pharmacology and therapeutic applications. *CNS Drugs* 1997; **7**: 68–88.
2. Apter JT, Allen LA. Buspirone: future directions. *J Clin Psychopharmacol* 1999; **19**: 86–93.

Action. Buspirone has dopaminergic, noradrenergic, and serotonin-modulating properties[1] and its anxiolytic effects appear to be related to its action on serotonin (5-hydroxytryptamine, 5-HT) neurotransmission. Buspirone, and the related drugs gepirone (p.686) and ipsapirone (p.688), are partial agonists at 5-HT$_{1A}$ receptors.[1,2] While such drugs may inhibit serotonin neurotransmission (most likely via 5-HT$_{1A}$ autoreceptor stimulation), they may also have postsynaptic 5-HT$_{1A}$ agonist activity and thus facilitate serotonin neurotransmission.[1] To compli-

cate matters further, 5-HT$_{1A}$ partial agonists have demonstrated both anxiolytic and anxiogenic properties in *animal* models of anxiety. Clinical studies have, however, shown that buspirone is effective in the treatment of generalised anxiety.[1,2]

Clinical studies with buspirone and gepirone suggest that 5-HT$_{1A}$ partial agonists may be useful in the treatment of depression, possibly by downregulation of either 5-HT$_{1A}$ or 5-HT$_2$ receptors or both.[1] There is some suggestion that buspirone has an anti-aggressive action in humans; it is unclear whether this is mediated via dopaminergic or serotonergic mechanisms.

Buspirone also has characteristics of both a dopamine agonist and antagonist; this may result in stimulation of both growth hormone and prolactin secretion.[3]

1. Glitz DA, Pohl R. 5-HT$_{1A}$ partial agonists: what is their future? *Drugs* 1991; **41**: 11–18.
2. Marsden CA. The pharmacology of new anxiolytics acting on 5-HT neurones. *Postgrad Med J* 1990; **66** (suppl 2): S2–S6.
3. Meltzer HY, *et al.* The effect of buspirone on prolactin and growth hormone secretion in man. *Arch Gen Psychiatry* 1983; **40**: 1099–1102.

Anxiety disorders. Buspirone has been shown to be as effective as the benzodiazepines in the short-term treatment of generalised anxiety disorder (p.649) and to be less likely to cause sedation or psychomotor and cognitive impairment. It also appears to have a lower propensity for interaction with alcohol and a lower risk of abuse and dependence. However, its usefulness may be limited by a relatively slow response to treatment, which some commentators consider may take up to 2 to 4 weeks to appear. Its efficacy may be reduced in patients who have recently taken benzodiazepines. It appears to be ineffective in panic disorders and convincing evidence of efficacy in other anxiety disorders is lacking.

References.
1. Caven P. Drugs in focus: 5. buspirone. *Prescribers' J* 1992; **32**: 200–204.
2. Deakin JFW. A review of clinical efficacy of 5-HT$_{1A}$ agonists in anxiety and depression. *J Psychopharmacol* 1993; **7**: 283–9.
3. Pecknold JC. A risk-benefit assessment of buspirone in the treatment of anxiety disorders. *Drug Safety* 1997; **16**: 118–32.
4. Fulton B, Brogden RN. Buspirone: an updated review of its clinical pharmacology and therapeutic applications. *CNS Drugs* 1997; **7**: 68–88.

Bruxism. SSRI-induced bruxism has been successfully controlled by adjunctive therapy with buspirone.[1,2]

1. Romanelli F, *et al.* Possible paroxetine-induced bruxism. *Ann Pharmacother* 1996; **30**: 1246–7.
2. Bostwick JM, Jaffee MS. Buspirone as an antidote to SSRI-induced bruxism in 4 cases. *J Clin Psychiatry* 1999; **60**: 857–60.

Cerebellar ataxias. In general the management of cerebellar ataxias is mainly supportive; buspirone has improved some symptoms of ataxia in a small study of patients with cerebellar cortical activity.[1]

1. Trouillas P, *et al.* Buspirone, a 5-hydroxytryptamine$_{1A}$ agonist, is active in cerebellar ataxia: results of a double-blind drug placebo study in patients with cerebellar cortical atrophy. *Arch Neurol* 1997; **54**: 749–52.

Depression. Buspirone has been investigated for augmentation of therapy with antidepressants with serotonin reuptake inhibiting activity in patients with refractory depression (p.271), but results have been variable.

References.
1. Fischer P, *et al.* Weak antidepressant response after buspirone augmentation of serotonin reuptake inhibitors in refractory severe depression. *Int Clin Psychopharmacol* 1998; **13**: 83–6.
2. Dimitriou EC, Dimitriou CE. Buspirone augmentation of antidepressant therapy. *J Clin Psychopharmacol* 1998; **18**: 465–9.
3. Landen M, *et al.* A randomized, double-blind, placebo-controlled trial of buspirone in combination with an SSRI in patients with treatment-refractory depression. *J Clin Psychiatry* 1998; **59**: 664–8.

Disturbed behaviour. Buspirone has been tried in various disorders for the control of symptoms such as agitation, aggression, and disruptive behaviour (see Disturbed Behaviour, p.650) but evidence of efficacy is limited. Nonetheless, in the management of dementia, some[1] consider that it might be worth trying in nonpsychotic patients with disturbed behaviour, especially those with mild symptoms or those intolerant or unresponsive to antipsychotics.

1. American Psychiatric Association. Practice guideline for the treatment of patients with Alzheimer's disease and other dementias of late life. *Am J Psychiatry* 1997; **154** (suppl): 1–39.

Extrapyramidal disorders. Although there have been reports[1,2] that buspirone may improve symptoms of drug-induced dyskinesia (p.662), drugs with dopaminergic actions have mostly exacerbated symptoms and there are a few reports of extrapyramidal disorders with buspirone (see under Adverse Effects, above).

1. Moss LE, *et al.* Buspirone in the treatment of tardive dyskinesia. *J Clin Psychopharmacol* 1993; **13**: 204–9.
2. Bonifati V, *et al.* Buspirone in levodopa-induced dyskinesias. *Clin Neuropharmacol* 1994; **17**: 73–82.

Substance dependence. ALCOHOL. Despite an early study[1] suggesting that buspirone could reduce alcohol craving in alcohol dependent patients, later studies[2–4] have overall failed to confirm that buspirone improves abstinence or reduces alcohol consumption. Although some studies[3,5] have found that buspirone may improve certain psychopathological symptoms in these patients, others[4] have found no such benefit; a meta-analysis[6] of 5 studies favoured the former interpretation.

The management of alcohol withdrawal and abstinence is discussed on p.1131.

1. Bruno F. Buspirone in the treatment of alcoholic patients. *Psychopathology* 1989; **22** (suppl 1): 49–59.
2. George DT, *et al.* Buspirone does not promote long term abstinence in alcoholics. *Clin Pharmacol Ther* 1995; **57**: 161.
3. Malec E, *et al.* Buspirone in the treatment of alcohol dependence: a placebo-controlled trial. *Alcohol Clin Exp Res* 1996; **20**: 307–12.
4. Malcolm R, *et al.* A placebo-controlled trial of buspirone in anxious inpatient alcoholics. *Alcohol Clin Exp Res* 1992; **16**: 1007–13.
5. Kranzler HR, *et al.* Buspirone treatment of anxious alcoholics: a placebo-controlled trial. *Arch Gen Psychiatry* 1994; **51**: 720–31.
6. Malec TS, *et al.* Efficacy of buspirone in alcohol dependence: a review. *Alcohol Clin Exp Res* 1996; **20**: 853–8.

NICOTINE. Buspirone has produced conflicting results[1-5] in the management of smoking cessation (p.1642). Although some studies suggest that in the short-term buspirone can increase the numbers of patients who are able to cease smoking, it does not necessarily decrease withdrawal symptoms.

1. West R, *et al.* Effect of buspirone on cigarette withdrawal symptoms and short-term abstinence rates in a smokers clinic. *Psychopharmacology (Berl)* 1991; **104**: 91–6.
2. Hilleman DE, *et al.* Effect of buspirone on withdrawal symptoms associated with smoking cessation. *Arch Intern Med* 1992; **152**: 350–2.
3. Hilleman DE, *et al.* Comparison of fixed-dose transdermal nicotine, tapered-dose transdermal nicotine, and buspirone in smoking cessation. *J Clin Pharmacol* 1994; **34**: 222–4.
4. Schneider NG, *et al.* Efficacy of buspirone in smoking cessation: a placebo-controlled trial. *Clin Pharmacol Ther* 1996; **60**: 568–76.
5. Farid P, Abate MA. Buspirone use for smoking cessation. *Ann Pharmacother* 1998; **32**: 1362–4.

Tourette's syndrome. Report[1] of a 42-year-old patient with Tourette's syndrome (p.650) refractory to antipsychotics who had a 70% reduction in tic severity during treatment with buspirone 30 mg daily. Worsening of symptoms was noted during the period in which buspirone was discontinued.

1. Dursun SM, *et al.* Buspirone treatment of Tourette's syndrome. *Lancet* 1995; **345**: 1366–7.

Preparations

USP 25: Buspirone Hydrochloride Tablets.

Proprietary Preparations (details are given in Part 3)
Aust.: Buspar; *Austral.:* Buspar; *Belg.:* Buspar; *Braz.:* Buspanil; Buspar; Buspiril; Seduspar; *Canad.:* Buspar; Buspirex; Bustab; *Denm.:* Buspar; Stesiron; *Fin.:* Buspar; Stesiron; *Fr.:* Buspar; *Ger.:* Bespar; Busp; *Hong Kong:* Buspar; *Irl.:* Buspar; *Israel:* Buspirol; Sorbon; *Ital.:* Axoren; Buspar; Buspimen; *Mex.:* Buspar; Neurosine; *Neth.:* Buspar; *Norw.:* Buspar; Stesiron; *NZ:* Biron; Buspar; *Port.:* Ansiten; Busansil; Buscalma; Buspar; Establix†; Itagil; *S.Afr.:* Buspar; Pasrin; *Singapore:* Buspar; *Spain:* Buspar; Buspisal†; Effiplen; Narol; *Swed.:* Buspar; *Switz.:* Buspar; *Thai.:* Anxiolan; Barpil; *UK:* Buspar; *USA:* Buspar.

Butalbital   (4014-g)

Butalbital *(USAN, rINN)*.

Alisobumalum; Allylbarbital; Allylbarbituric Acid; Itobarbital; Tetrallobarbital. 5-Allyl-5-isobutylbarbituric acid.

$C_{11}H_{16}N_2O_3 = 224.3$.
CAS — 77-26-9.

NOTE. The name Butalbital has also been applied to talbutal, the *S*-butyl analogue, which was formerly used as a hypnotic and sedative.

Compounded preparations of butalbital may be represented by the following names:

• Co-bucafAPAP *(USP 25)*—butalbital, paracetamol, and caffeine.

Pharmacopoeias. In *US*.

Pharmacopoeial description

USP 25: A white odourless crystalline powder. Slightly soluble in cold water; soluble in boiling water; freely soluble in alcohol, in chloroform, and in ether; soluble in solutions of fixed alkalis and alkali carbonates. A saturated solution is acid to litmus.

Profile

Butalbital is a barbiturate with general properties similar to those of amobarbital (p.655). It has been used mainly in combination with analgesics in the treatment of occasional tension-type headaches (p.450), but other treatments are generally preferred.

Preparations

USP 25: Butalbital and Aspirin Tablets; Butalbital, Acetaminophen, and Caffeine Capsules; Butalbital, Acetaminophen, and Caffeine Tablets; Butalbital, Aspirin, and Caffeine Capsules; Butalbital, Aspirin, and Caffeine Tablets; Butalbital, Aspirin, Caffeine, and Codeine Phosphate Capsules.

Proprietary Preparations (details are given in Part 3)
Multi-ingredient: *Canad.:* Fiorinal; Fiorinal C; Tecnal; Tecnal C; Trianal; Trianal C; *Denm.:* Gynergen Comp; *Ital.:* Optalidon; *Norw.:* Cafergot Comp; *S.Afr.:* Cafergot-PB; *Spain:* Cafergot-PB; *Switz.:* Cafergot-PB; *USA:* Amaphen with Codeine; Amphen†; Anolor; Anoquan†; Arcet†; Axocet; Axotal†; B-A-C; Bucet†; Bupap; Endolor; Esgic; Esgic-Plus; Femcet†; Fiorgen PF†; Fioricet; Fioricet with Codeine; Fiorinal; Fiorinal with Codeine; Fiorpap†; Fiortal with Codeine; Fiortal†; Isocet†; Isollyl Improved†; Lanorinal†; Margesic; Marnal†; Marten-Tab; Medi-

gesic; Pacaps; Phrenilin; Prominol; Pyridium Plus; Repan; Repan CF; Sedapap; Tencet; Tencon; Triad; Triaprin†; Two-Dyne†.

Butobarbital (4015-q)

Butobarbital (BAN).

Butethal; Butobarbitalum; Butobarbitone. 5-Butyl-5-ethylbarbituric acid.

$C_{10}H_{16}N_2O_3 = 212.2$.
CAS — 77-28-1.
ATC — N05CA03.

NOTE. Butobarbital should be distinguished from Butabarbital, which is Secbutabarbital (p.705).

Pharmacopoeias. In Aust., Belg., Fr., It., Neth., and Port.

Dependence and Withdrawal
As for Amobarbital, p.655.

Adverse Effects, Treatment, and Precautions
As for Amobarbital, p.655.

Interactions
As for Amobarbital, p.656.

Antibacterials. Results suggesting that metronidazole alters the metabolism of butobarbital when taken concomitantly.[1]

1. Al Sharifi MA, et al. The effect of anti-amoebic drug therapy on the metabolism of butobarbitone. J Pharm Pharmacol 1982; 34: 126–7.

Pharmacokinetics
Butobarbital is metabolised in the liver mainly by hydroxylation; small amounts are excreted in the urine as unchanged drug. It has been reported to have a half-life of about 40 to 55 hours and to be about 26% bound to plasma proteins.

Uses and Administration
Butobarbital is a barbiturate with general properties similar to those of amobarbital (p.656). Its use can no longer be recommended because of the risk of its adverse effects and of dependence, although continued use may occasionally be considered necessary for severe intractable insomnia (p.652) in patients already taking it. It is given by mouth in usual doses of 100 to 200 mg at night.

Preparations
Proprietary Preparations (details are given in Part 3)
Austral.: Soneryl†; UK: Soneryl.
Multi-ingredient: Fr.: Hypnasmine; Thai.: Belloid.

Calcium Bromolactobionate (12504-n)

Calcium bromide lactobionate hexahydrate.

$Ca(C_{12}H_{21}O_{12})_2,CaBr_2,6H_2O = 1062.6$.
CAS — 33659-28-8 (anhydrous calcium bromolactobionate).

Profile
Calcium bromolactobionate has sedative properties and has been given by mouth and intravenous injection in the treatment of insomnia and nervous disorders. The use of bromides is generally deprecated.

◊ Bromide intoxication has been reported[1] in a patient following overdosage with calcium bromolactobionate tablets.

1. Danel VC, et al. Bromide intoxication and pseudohyperchloremia. Ann Pharmacother 2001; 35: 386–7.

Preparations
Proprietary Preparations (details are given in Part 3)
Fr.: Calcibronat; Ital.: Calcibronat; Mex.: Calcibronat.
Multi-ingredient: Fr.: Assagix†.

Camazepam (7012-v)

Camazepam (rINN).

SB-5833. 7-Chloro-2,3-dihydro-1-methyl-2-oxo-5-phenyl-1H-1,4-benzodiazepin-3-yl dimethylcarbamate.

$C_{19}H_{18}ClN_3O_3 = 371.8$.
CAS — 36104-80-0.
ATC — N05BA15.

Profile
Camazepam is a benzodiazepine with general properties similar to those of diazepam (p.674). It has been given by mouth for the short-term treatment of anxiety disorders and insomnia.

Preparations
Proprietary Preparations (details are given in Part 3)
Spain: Albego†.

Captodiame Hydrochloride (7013-g)

Captodiame Hydrochloride (BANM, pINNM).

Captodiamine Hydrochloride. 2-(4-Butylthiobenzhydrylthio)ethyldimethylamine hydrochloride.

$C_{21}H_{29}NS_2,HCl = 396.1$.
CAS — 486-17-9 (captodiame); 904-04-1 (captodiame hydrochloride).

Profile
Captodiame hydrochloride has been given in doses of 50 mg three times daily by mouth for the treatment of anxiety disorders (p.649).

Preparations
Proprietary Preparations (details are given in Part 3)
Fr.: Covatine.

Carbromal (4018-w)

Carbromal (BAN, rINN).

Bromodiethylacetylurea; Karbromal. N-(2-Bromo-2-ethylbutyryl)urea.

$C_7H_{13}BrN_2O_2 = 237.1$.
CAS — 77-65-6.
ATC — N05CM04.

Pharmacopoeias. In Aust. and Belg.

Profile
Carbromal is a bromureide with general properties similar to those of the barbiturates (see Amobarbital, p.655). It was formerly used for its hypnotic and sedative properties. Chronic use of carbromal could result in bromide accumulation and symptoms resembling bromism (see Bromides, p.1587). The use of bromides is generally deprecated.

Porphyria. Carbromal has been associated with acute attacks of porphyria and is considered unsafe in porphyric patients.

Carpipramine Hydrochloride (7015-p)

Carpipramine Hydrochloride (rINNM).

PZ-1511. 1-[3-(10,11-Dihydro-5H-dibenz[b,f]azepin-5-yl)propyl]-4-piperidinopiperidine-4-carboxamide dihydrochloride monohydrate.

$C_{28}H_{38}N_4O,2HCl,H_2O = 537.6$.
CAS — 5942-95-0 (carpipramine); 7075-03-8 (anhydrous carpipramine hydrochloride).

Profile
Carpipramine is structurally related both to imipramine (p.291) and to butyrophenones such as haloperidol (p.686). It has been used in the management of anxiety disorders (p.649) and psychoses such as schizophrenia (p.651). Carpipramine is given as the hydrochloride in a usual dose equivalent to 50 mg of the base three times daily by mouth, with a range of 50 to 400 mg daily.

Porphyria. Carpipramine is considered to be unsafe in patients with porphyria although there is conflicting experimental evidence of porphyrinogenicity.

Preparations
Proprietary Preparations (details are given in Part 3)
Fr.: Prazinil.

Chlordiazepoxide (7017-w)

Chlordiazepoxide (BAN, rINN).

Chlordiazepoxidum; Methaminodiazepoxide. 7-Chloro-2-methylamino-5-phenyl-3H-1,4-benzodiazepine 4-oxide.

$C_{16}H_{14}ClN_3O = 299.8$.
CAS — 58-25-3.
ATC — N05BA02.

Pharmacopoeias. In Chin., Eur. (see p.vi), Jpn, Pol., and US.

Chlordiazepoxide 1 mg is approximately equivalent to 1.1 mg of chlordiazepoxide hydrochloride.

Chlordiazepoxide or chlordiazepoxide hydrochloride is reported to be incompatible with benzquinamide hydrochloride and with pentazocine lactate.

Pharmacopoeial description
Ph. Eur.: An almost white or light yellow, crystalline powder. Practically insoluble in water; sparingly soluble in alcohol; slightly soluble in ether. Protect from light.

USP 25: A yellow, practically odourless, crystalline powder. Insoluble in water; soluble 1 in 50 of alcohol, 1 in 6250 of chloroform, and 1 in 130 of ether. Store in airtight containers. Protect from light.

Chlordiazepoxide Hydrochloride (7018-e)

Chlordiazepoxide Hydrochloride (BANM, USAN, rINNM).

Chlordiazepoxidi Hydrochloridum; Methaminodiazepoxide Hydrochloride; NSC-115748; Ro-5-0690.

$C_{16}H_{14}ClN_3O,HCl = 336.2$.
CAS — 438-41-5.

Pharmacopoeias. In Eur. (see p.vi), Pol., and US.

For incompatibilities of chlordiazepoxide hydrochloride see under Chlordiazepoxide, above.

Pharmacopoeial description
Ph. Eur.: A white or slightly yellow crystalline powder. Soluble in water; sparingly soluble in alcohol; practically insoluble in ether. Protect from light.

USP 25: A white or practically white, odourless, crystalline powder. Soluble in water; sparingly soluble in alcohol; insoluble in petroleum spirit. Store in airtight containers. Protect from light.

Dependence and Withdrawal
As for Diazepam, p.675.

◊ For the purpose of withdrawal regimens, 15 mg of chlordiazepoxide is considered roughly equivalent to 5 mg of diazepam.

Adverse Effects, Treatment, and Precautions
As for Diazepam, p.675.

Hepatic impairment. A report of progressive drowsiness beginning after 20 days of administration of chlordiazepoxide to a woman with cirrhosis and hepatitis.[1] One week after discontinuing the drug, the patient could not be roused and full consciousness was not regained for another week. Accumulation of active metabolites of chlordiazepoxide may have been responsible for the prolonged stupor.

1. Barton K, et al. Chlordiazepoxide metabolite accumulation in liver disease. Med Toxicol 1989; 4: 73–6.

Porphyria. Chlordiazepoxide has been associated with acute attacks of porphyria and is considered unsafe in porphyric patients.

Interactions
As for Diazepam, p.677.

Pharmacokinetics
Absorption of chlordiazepoxide is almost complete after oral administration; peak plasma concentrations are achieved after 1 to 2 hours. Absorption after intramuscular injection may be slow and erratic depending on the site of injection. Chlordiazepoxide is about 96% bound to plasma proteins. Reported values for the elimination half-life of chlordiazepoxide have ranged from about 5 to 30 hours, but its main active metabolite desmethyldiazepam (nordazepam, p.696) has a half-life of several days. Other pharmacologically active metabolites of chlordiazepoxide include desmethylchlordiazepoxide, demoxepam, and oxazepam (p.697). Chlordiazepoxide passes into the CSF and breast milk, and crosses the placenta. Unchanged drug and metabolites are excreted in the urine, mainly as conjugated metabolites.

◊ References.
1. Greenblatt DJ, et al. Clinical pharmacokinetics of chlordiazepoxide. Clin Pharmacokinet 1978; 3: 381–94.

Uses and Administration
Chlordiazepoxide is a benzodiazepine with general properties similar to those of diazepam (p.680). It is used in the short-term treatment of anxiety disorders (p.649) and insomnia (p.652). Chlordiazepoxide is also used in muscle spasm (p.1322), in alcohol withdrawal syndromes (p.1131), and for premedication (p.1256).

Chlordiazepoxide is administered by mouth as the hydrochloride or the base; the doses given refer equally to both. It may also be administered by deep intramuscular or slow intravenous injection as the hydrochloride. Preparations formulated for intramuscular use are stated to be unsuitable for intravenous administration due to the formation of air bubbles in the solvent.

Elderly and debilitated patients should be given one-half or less of the usual adult dose.

The usual dose by mouth for the treatment of anxiety is up to 30 mg daily in divided doses; in severe conditions up to 100 mg daily has been given. For acute or severe anxiety an initial dose of 50 to 100 mg of the hydrochloride has been given by injection, followed if necessary by 25 to 50 mg three or four times daily.

For relief of muscle spasm a dose of 10 to 30 mg daily by mouth in divided doses is recommended, and 10 to 30 mg by mouth may be given before retiring for insomnia associated with anxiety.

For the control of the acute symptoms of alcohol withdrawal chlordiazepoxide or chlordiazepoxide hydrochloride may be given by mouth in a dose of 25 to 100 mg repeated as needed up to a maximum of

---

The symbol † denotes a preparation no longer actively marketed

300 mg daily. For severe symptoms treatment may be initiated by injection of 50 to 100 mg, repeated if necessary after 2 to 4 hours.

Chlordiazepoxide hydrochloride has also been given for anaesthetic **premedication** in a dose of 50 to 100 mg intramuscularly one hour before surgery.

Preparations

BP 2001: Chlordiazepoxide Capsules; Chlordiazepoxide Hydrochloride Tablets;
USP 25: Chlordiazepoxide and Amitriptyline Hydrochloride Tablets; Chlordiazepoxide Hydrochloride and Clidinium Bromide Capsules; Chlordiazepoxide Hydrochloride Capsules; Chlordiazepoxide Hydrochloride for Injection; Chlordiazepoxide Tablets.

Proprietary Preparations (details are given in Part 3)
Braz.: Psicosedin; Tensil; *Canad.:* Novo-Poxide; *Denm.:* Klopoxid; Risolid; *Fin.:* Risolid; *Ger.:* Librium; Multum; Radepur; *Hong Kong:* Librium; *Irl.:* Librium; *Israel:* Servium; *Ital.:* Librium; Psicofar†; Reliberan; Seren Vita†; *Mex.:* Kalmocaps; *Neth.:* Librium†; *NZ:* Novapam; *Port.:* Paxium; *S.Afr.:* Librium; *Singapore:* Benpine; *Spain:* Huberplex; Omnalio; *Thai.:* Benpine; Epoxide; *UK:* Librium; Tropium; *USA:* Libritabs; Librium; Mitran; Reposans.

Multi-ingredient: *Aust.:* Librax†; Limbitrol; Pantrop; *Belg.:* Librax†; Limbitrol†; *Braz.:* Limbitrol; Menostress; Menotensil; *Canad.:* Apo-Chlorax; Corium†; Librax; *Fin.:* Librax; Limbitrol; *Fr.:* Librax; *Ger.:* Limbatril; *Hong Kong:* Bralix; Librax; *Israel:* Librax; Nirvaxal; *Ital.:* Diapatol; Librax; Limbitryl; Sedans; *Neth.:* Limbitrol†; *Port.:* Gabil†; Librax; *S.Afr.:* Librax; Limbitrol; *Singapore:* Apo-Chlorax; Chlobax; Librax; Medocalum; *Spain:* Psico Blocan; Relaxedans†; *Swed.:* Librax†; *Switz.:* Librax; Limbitrol; *Thai.:* Kenspa; Liblan; Librax; Pobrax; Tumax; *USA:* Clindex; Librax; Lidox†; Limbitrol; Menrium†.

Chlormezanone (7019-l)

Chlormezanone (BAN, rINN).
Chlormethazanone; Chlormezanonum. 2-(4-Chlorophenyl)-3-methylperhydro-1,3-thiazin-4-one 1,1-dioxide.
$C_{11}H_{12}CINO_3S = 273.7$.
CAS — 80-77-3.
ATC — M03BB02.

Profile

Chlormezanone has been used in the treatment of anxiety disorders (p.649) and insomnia (p.652), but was withdrawn from use in many countries following reports of serious skin reactions (see below). It was also used in conditions associated with painful muscle spasm (p.1322), often in compound preparations with analgesics; its mechanism of action is not clear but is probably related to its sedative effect.

Effects on the skin. Chlormezanone was responsible for 5 of 86 cases of fixed drug eruption detected in a Finnish hospital from 1971 to 1981.[1] In the period from 1981 to 1985 chlormezanone was responsible for 1 out of 77 such eruptions.[2] In a case control study[3] comparing drug use in 245 patients hospitalised because of toxic epidermal necrolysis or Stevens-Johnson syndrome and 1147 controls, 13 patients and one control were found to have taken chlormezanone. From these figures a high crude relative risk of 62 was calculated; the excess risk was estimated to be 1.7 cases per million users per week.

1. Kauppinen K, Stubb S. Fixed eruptions: causative drugs and challenge tests. *Br J Dermatol* 1985; **112:** 575–8.
2. Stubb S, *et al.* Fixed drug eruptions: 77 cases from 1981 to 1985. *Br J Dermatol* 1989; **120:** 583.
3. Roujeau J-C, *et al.* Medication use and the risk of Stevens-Johnson syndrome or toxic epidermal necrolysis. *N Engl J Med* 1995; **333:** 1600–7.

Porphyria. Chlormezanone has been associated with acute attacks of porphyria and is considered unsafe in porphyric patients.

Preparations

Proprietary Preparations (details are given in Part 3)
Aust.: Trancopal†; *Belg.:* Lyseen New†; *Neth.:* Trancopal†; *Swed.:* Trancopal†; *Switz.:* Trancopal†; *USA:* Trancopal†.

Multi-ingredient: *Aust.:* Trancopal compositum†; *Braz.:* Besaprin; Beserol; *S.Afr.:* Arcanaflex†; Besenol†; Betaflex†; Lobak†; Myoflex†; Rexachlor†; Spasmoflex†; *Singapore:* Relexic; *Spain:* Lumbaxol Para†; *Switz.:* Trancopal compositum†.

Chlorproethazine Hydrochloride (7020-v)

Chlorproethazine Hydrochloride (rINNM).
RP-4909 (chlorproethazine). 3-(2-Chlorophenothiazin-10-yl)-NN-diethylpropylamine hydrochloride.
$C_{19}H_{23}CIN_2S,HCl = 383.4$.
CAS — 84-01-5 (chlorproethazine); 4611-02-3 (chlorproethazine hydrochloride).

Profile

Chlorproethazine is a phenothiazine derivative differing chemically from chlorpromazine by the substitution of a diethyl for a dimethyl group. It has general properties similar to those of chlorpromazine (below) but has been used mainly as a muscle relaxant in the management of muscle spasm (p.1322). Although exposure of the skin to phenothiazines has been associated with sensitivity reactions, chlorproethazine hydrochloride

has been applied topically in an ointment, with the warning to avoid direct exposure to sunlight. It has also been given by mouth or by intramuscular or slow intravenous injection.

Preparations

Proprietary Preparations (details are given in Part 3)
Fr.: Neuriplege.

Multi-ingredient: *Fr.:* Neuriplege†.

Chlorpromazine (7021-g)

Chlorpromazine (BAN, rINN).
3-(2-Chlorophenothiazin-10-yl)propyldimethylamine.
$C_{17}H_{19}CIN_2S = 318.9$.
CAS — 50-53-3.
ATC — N05AA01.
Pharmacopoeias. In Br. and US.

Chlorpromazine 100 mg is approximately equivalent to 111 mg of chlorpromazine hydrochloride.

Pharmacopoeial description

BP 2001: A white or creamy-white powder or waxy solid; odourless or almost odourless. M.p. 56° to 58°. Practically insoluble in water; freely soluble in alcohol and in ether; very soluble in chloroform. Protect from light.

USP 25: A white crystalline solid with an amine-like odour. It darkens on prolonged exposure to light. Practically insoluble in water; soluble 1 in 3 of alcohol, 1 in 2 of chloroform, 1 in 3 of ether, and 1 in 2 of benzene; freely soluble in dilute mineral acids; practically insoluble in dilute alkali hydroxides. Store in airtight containers. Protect from light.

Chlorpromazine Embonate (7022-q)

Chlorpromazine Embonate (BANM, rINNM).
Chlorpromazine Pamoate. Chlorpromazine 4,4′-methylenebis(3-hydroxy-2-naphthoate).
$(C_{17}H_{19}CIN_2S)_2,C_{23}H_{16}O_6 = 1026.1$.
Chlorpromazine hydrochloride 100 mg is approximately equivalent to 144 mg of chlorpromazine embonate.

Chlorpromazine Hydrochloride (7023-p)

Chlorpromazine Hydrochloride (BANM, rINNM).
Aminazine; Chlorpromazini Hydrochloridum.
$C_{17}H_{19}CIN_2S,HCl = 355.3$.
CAS — 69-09-0.
Pharmacopoeias. In *Chin.*, *Eur.* (see p.vi), *Int.*, *Jpn*, *Pol.*, and *US*.

Incompatibility has been reported between chlorpromazine hydrochloride injection and several other compounds; precipitation of chlorpromazine base from solution is particularly likely if the final pH is increased. Compounds reported to be incompatible with chlorpromazine hydrochloride include aminophylline, amphotericin B, aztreonam, some barbiturates, chloramphenicol sodium succinate, chlorothiazide sodium, cimetidine hydrochloride, dimenhydrinate, heparin sodium, morphine sulfate (when preserved with chlorocresol), some penicillins, ranitidine hydrochloride, and remifentanil.

For a warning about incompatibility between chlorpromazine solution (Thorazine) and carbamazepine suspension (Tegretol), see p.342.

Pharmacopoeial description

Ph. Eur.: A white or almost white crystalline powder. It decomposes on exposure to air and light. Very soluble in water; freely soluble in alcohol; practically insoluble in ether. A freshly prepared 10% solution in water has a pH of 3.5 to 4.5. Store in airtight containers. Protect from light.

USP 25: A white or slightly creamy-white odourless crystalline powder. It darkens on prolonged exposure to light. Soluble 1 in 1 of water, 1 in 1.5 of alcohol, and 1 in 1.5 of chloroform; insoluble in ether and in benzene. Store in airtight containers. Protect from light.

◊ CAUTION. *Owing to the risk of contact sensitisation health workers should avoid direct contact with chlorpromazine; tablets should not be crushed and solutions should be handled with care.*

Dilution. Solutions containing 2.5% of chlorpromazine hydrochloride could be diluted to 100 mL with 0.9% sodium chloride solution provided the pH of the saline solution was such that the pH of the dilution did not exceed the critical range of pH 6.7 to 6.8.[1] With saline of pH 7.0 or 7.2, the final solution had a pH of 6.4.

1. D'Arcy PF, Thompson KM. Stability of chlorpromazine hydrochloride added to intravenous infusion fluids. *Pharm J* 1973; **210:** 28.

Sorption. There was a 41% loss of chlorpromazine hydrochloride from solution when infused for 7 hours via a plastic infusion set (cellulose propionate burette with polyvinyl chloride tubing), and a 79% loss after infusion for 1 hour from a glass syringe through silastic tubing.[1] Loss was negligible after infusion for 1 hour from a system comprising a glass syringe with polyethylene tubing.

1. Kowaluk EA, *et al.* Interactions between drugs and intravenous delivery systems. *Am J Hosp Pharm* 1982; **39:** 460–7.

Adverse Effects

Chlorpromazine generally produces less central depression than the barbiturates or benzodiazepines, and tolerance to its initial sedative effects develops fairly quickly in most patients. It has antimuscarinic properties and may cause adverse effects such as dry mouth, constipation, difficulty with micturition, blurred vision, and mydriasis. Tachycardia, ECG changes (particularly Q- and T-wave abnormalities), and, rarely, cardiac arrhythmias may occur and hypotension (usually orthostatic) is common. Other adverse effects include delirium, agitation and, rarely, catatonic-like states, insomnia or drowsiness, nightmares, depression, miosis, EEG changes and convulsions, nasal congestion, minor abnormalities in liver function tests, inhibition of ejaculation, impotence, and priapism.

Hypersensitivity reactions include urticaria, exfoliative dermatitis, erythema multiforme, and contact sensitivity. A syndrome resembling systemic lupus erythematosus has been reported. Jaundice has occurred, and probably has an immunological origin. Prolonged therapy may lead to deposition of pigment in the skin, or more frequently the eyes; corneal and lens opacities have been observed. Pigmentary retinopathy has occurred only rarely with chlorpromazine. Photosensitivity reactions are more common with chlorpromazine than with other antipsychotics.

Various haematological disorders, including haemolytic anaemia, aplastic anaemia, thrombocytopenic purpura, leucocytosis, and a potentially fatal agranulocytosis have occasionally been reported; they may be manifestations of a hypersensitivity reaction. Most cases of agranulocytosis have occurred within 4 to 10 weeks of starting treatment, and symptoms such as sore throat or fever should be watched for and white cell counts instituted should they appear. Mild leucopenia has been stated to occur in up to 30% of patients on prolonged high dosage.

Extrapyramidal dysfunction and resultant disorders include acute dystonia, a parkinsonism-like syndrome, and akathisia; late effects include tardive dyskinesia and perioral tremor. The neuroleptic malignant syndrome may also occur.

Chlorpromazine alters endocrine and metabolic functions. Patients have experienced amenorrhoea, galactorrhoea, gynaecomastia, weight gain, and hyperglycaemia and altered glucose tolerance. Body temperature regulation is impaired and may result in hypo- or hyperthermia depending on environment.

There have been isolated reports of sudden death with chlorpromazine; possible causes include cardiac arrhythmias or aspiration and asphyxia due to suppression of the cough and gag reflexes.

Pain and irritation at the injection site may occur on injection. Nodule formation may occur after intramuscular administration.

Phenothiazines do not cause dependence of the type encountered with barbiturates or benzodiazepines. However, withdrawal symptoms have been seen following the abrupt withdrawal from patients receiving prolonged and/or high-dose maintenance therapy.

Although the adverse effects of other phenothiazines are broadly similar in nature to those of chlorpromazine, their frequency and pattern tend to fall into 3 groups:

• group 1 (e.g. chlorpromazine, methotrimeprazine [levomepromazine], and promazine) are generally characterised by pronounced sedative effects and moderate antimuscarinic and extrapyramidal effects

• group 2 (e.g. pericyazine, pipotiazine, and thioridazine) are generally characterised by moderate sedative effects, marked antimuscarinic effects, and fewer extrapyramidal effects than groups 1 or 3

- group 3 (e.g. fluphenazine, perphenazine, prochlorperazine, and trifluoperazine) are generally characterised by fewer sedative and antimuscarinic effects but more pronounced extrapyramidal effects than groups 1 or 2

Classical antipsychotics of other chemical groups tend to resemble the phenothiazines of group 3. They include the butyrophenones (e.g. benperidol, droperidol, and haloperidol); diphenylbutylpiperidines (e.g. pimozide); thioxanthenes (flupentixol and zuclopenthixol); substituted benzamides (e.g. sulpiride); oxypertine; and loxapine.

Carcinogenicity. See Effects on Endocrine Function, below.

Convulsions. Treatment with antipsychotics can result in EEG abnormalities and lowered seizure threshold.[1,2] Seizures can be induced particularly in patients with a history of epilepsy or drug-induced seizures, abnormal EEG, previous electroconvulsive therapy, or pre-existing CNS abnormalities. The risk appears to be greatest at the start of antipsychotic therapy, or with high doses, or abrupt increases of dose, or with the use of more than one antipsychotic. The incidence of antipsychotic-induced convulsions is, however, probably less than 1%.

Phenothiazines with an aliphatic side-chain such as chlorpromazine, promazine, and trifluoperazine appear to present a higher risk than those with a piperazine or piperidine moiety. Despite conflicting evidence, haloperidol appears to carry a relatively low risk of seizures. In general, the epileptic potential has been correlated with the propensity of the antipsychotic to cause sedation. The following drugs have been suggested when antipsychotic therapy is considered necessary in patients at risk of seizures or being treated for epilepsy: fluphenazine, haloperidol, molindone, and pimozide. Antipsychotic dosage should be increased slowly and the possibility of interactions with antiepileptic therapy considered (see under Interactions, below).

The atypical antipsychotic clozapine appears to be associated with a particularly high risk of seizures (see p.671).

1. Cold JA, *et al.* Seizure activity associated with antipsychotic therapy. *DICP Ann Pharmacother* 1990; **24:** 601–6. Correction. *ibid.*; 1012.
2. Zaccara G, *et al.* Clinical features, pathogenesis and management of drug-induced seizures. *Drug Safety* 1990; **5:** 109–51.

Effects on the blood. The UK Committee on Safety of Medicines provided data on the reports it had received between July 1963 and January 1993 on agranulocytosis and neutropenia.[1] Several groups of drugs were commonly implicated, among them phenothiazines for which there were 87 reports of agranulocytosis (42 fatal) and 33 of neutropenia (22 fatal). The most frequently implicated phenothiazines were chlorpromazine with 51 reports of agranulocytosis (26 fatal) and 12 of neutropenia (2 fatal) and thioridazine with 20 reports of agranulocytosis (9 fatal) and 10 of neutropenia (0 fatal).

1. Committee on Safety of Medicines/Medicines Control Agency. Drug-induced neutropenia and agranulocytosis. *Current Problems* 1993; **19:** 10–11.

Effects on body-weight. Most antipsychotic drugs are associated with weight gain. A meta-analysis[1] found evidence of weight gain in patients receiving both classical (chlorpromazine, fluphenazine, haloperidol, loxapine, perphenazine, thioridazine, tiotixene, or trifluoperazine) and atypical (clozapine, olanzapine, quetiapine, risperidone, sertindole, and ziprasidone) antipsychotics. Two drugs, molindone and pimozide, appeared in contrast to be associated with weight loss, although in the case of pimozide this could not be confirmed statistically. Placebo treatment was also associated with weight loss.

1. Allison DB, *et al.* Antipsychotic-induced weight gain: a comprehensive research synthesis. *Am J Psychiatry* 1999; **156:** 1686–96.

Effects on the cardiovascular system. Orthostatic hypotension is a common problem in patients taking psychotropic drugs and is particularly pronounced with low-potency antipsychotics.[1] T-wave changes have also been reported with low-potency antipsychotics; they are usually benign and reversible, and subject to diurnal fluctuations. Low-potency antipsychotics, particularly *thioridazine* and *mesoridazine*, and the high-potency drug *pimozide*, prolong the QT interval in a similar manner to class I antiarrhythmics such as quinidine or procainamide; their use is therefore contra-indicated in patients taking such antiarrhythmics. Droperidol, another high-potency drug, has also been reported to prolong the QT interval.[2] Thioridazine is most frequently discussed in case reports of psychotropic drug-induced torsade de pointes, which has led to restrictions on its use (see Precautions and Uses and Administration of Thioridazine, p.708); *chlorpromazine* and *pimozide* have also been implicated. Torsade de pointes has also been reported following overdosage[3-5] with, or high intravenous[6] doses of, the high-potency antipsychotic *haloperidol*. There are also isolated reports of cardiac arrhythmias following attempts at rapid control with high doses of haloperidol.[7,8] *Melperone*, a butyrophenone antipsychotic related to haloperidol, has been reported to have class III electrophysiologic and antiarrhythmic activity.[9,10]

Results from a case-control study[11] have suggested that use of classical antipsychotics may be associated with an increased risk of idiopathic venous thromboembolism. The risk was most pronounced during the first 3 months of treatment, and was higher for low potency than high potency antipsychotics. This study did not examine the risk of venous thromboembolism with atypical antipsychotics, but see under Clozapine, p.672.

1. DiGiacomo J. Cardiovascular effects of psychotropic drugs. *Cardiovasc Rev Rep* 1989; **10:** 31–2, 39–41, and 47.
2. Reilly JG, *et al.* QTc-interval abnormalities and psychotropic drug therapy in psychiatric patients. *Lancet* 2000; **355:** 1048–52.
3. Zee-Cheng C-S, *et al.* Haloperidol and torsades de pointes. *Ann Intern Med* 1985; **102:** 418.
4. Henderson RA, *et al.* Life-threatening ventricular arrhythmia (torsades de pointes) after haloperidol overdose. *Hum Exp Toxicol* 1991; **10:** 59–62.
5. Wilt JL, *et al.* Torsade de pointes associated with the use of intravenous haloperidol. *Ann Intern Med* 1993; **119:** 391–4.
6. O'Brien JM, *et al.* Haloperidol-induced torsade de pointes. *Ann Pharmacother* 1999; **33:** 1046–50.
7. Mehta D, *et al.* Cardiac arrhythmia and haloperidol. *Am J Psychiatry* 1979; **136:** 1468–9.
8. Bett JHN, Holt GW. Malignant ventricular tachyarrhythmia and haloperidol. *BMJ* 1983; **287:** 1264.
9. Møgelvang JC, *et al.* Antiarrhythmic properties of a neuroleptic butyrophenone, melperone, in acute myocardial infarction. *Acta Med Scand* 1980; **208:** 61–4.
10. Hui WKK, *et al.* Melperone: electrophysiologic and antiarrhythmic activity in humans. *J Cardiovasc Pharmacol* 1990; **15:** 144–9.
11. Zornberg GL, Jick H. Antipsychotic drug use and risk of first-time idiopathic venous thromboembolism: a case-control study. *Lancet* 2000; **356:** 1219–23.

Effects on endocrine function. Antipsychotics can alter the secretion of prolactin, growth hormone, and thyrotrophin from the anterior pituitary[1] via their ability to block central dopamine-D_2 receptors. Therapeutic doses of antipsychotics increase serum-prolactin concentrations; this effect occurs at lower doses and after shorter latent periods than the antipsychotic effects. However, raised prolactin concentrations have not always been observed after long-term use, suggesting that tolerance may develop to the hyperprolactinaemic effect. Serum prolactin declines to normal values within 2 to 4 days of stopping oral antipsychotic therapy.

Although long-term antipsychotic treatment increases the incidence of mammary tumours in the *rat*, studies[2,3] have found little or no evidence that chronic use in humans alters the risk of breast cancer among women with schizophrenia. Fears about pituitary abnormalities, including pituitary tumours,[4] might develop in patients on long-term phenothiazine therapy have not been confirmed.[5,6]

Antipsychotics can in some circumstances reduce both basal and stimulated growth-hormone secretion but attempts to use them to treat dysfunctions in growth-hormone regulation have not been successful.[1] Although a number of clinical studies show that acute administration of antipsychotics increased both basal and stimulated thyrotrophin secretion, the majority of studies find either no change or only a small increase in thyrotrophin secretion following long-term use.

One small study has suggested that thioridazine may be more likely than other antipsychotics to decrease serum concentrations of testosterone or luteinising hormone in men.[7] However, concentrations were within the normal range in most patients taking antipsychotics.[7]

See also Effects on Fluid and Electrolyte Homoeostasis, below and Effects on Sexual Function, below.

1. Gunnet JW, Moore KE. Neuroleptics and neuroendocrine function. *Ann Rev Pharmacol Toxicol* 1988; **28:** 347–66.
2. Mortensen PB. The incidence of cancer in schizophrenic patients. *J Epidemiol Community Health* 1989; **43:** 43–7.
3. Mortensen PB. The occurrence of cancer in first admitted schizophrenic patients. *Schizophr Res* 1994; **12:** 185–94.
4. Asplund K, *et al.* Phenothiazine drugs and pituitary tumors. *Ann Intern Med* 1982; **96:** 533.
5. Rosenblatt S, *et al.* Chronic phenothiazine therapy does not increase sellar size. *Lancet* 1978; **ii:** 319–20.
6. Lilford VA, *et al.* Long-term phenothiazine treatment does not cause pituitary tumours. *Br J Psychiatry* 1984; **144:** 421–4.
7. Brown WA, *et al.* Differential effects of neuroleptic agents on the pituitary-gonadal axis in men. *Arch Gen Psychiatry* 1981; **38:** 1270–2.

Effects on the eyes. Phenothiazines may induce a pigmentary retinopathy which is dependent on both the dose and the duration of treatment.[1] Those phenothiazine derivatives with piperidine side-chains such as thioridazine have a higher risk of inducing retinal toxicity than other phenothiazine derivatives, with relatively few cases reported for those with aliphatic side-chains such as chlorpromazine; the piperazine group does not appear to exert direct ocular toxicity.[2] The retinopathy may present acutely, (sudden loss of vision associated with retinal oedema and hyperaemia of the optic disc), or chronically, (a fine pigment scatter appearing in the central area of the fundus, extending peripherally but sparing the macula). Chronic paracentral and pericentral scotomas may be found. Although pigmentary disturbances may progress after withdrawal of thioridazine, they are not always paralleled by deterioration in visual function; nonetheless, some cases have led to progressive chorioretinopathy.[3] The critical ocular toxic dose of thioridazine is reported to be 800 mg daily and the UK manufacturers recommend that a daily dose of 600 mg should not usually be exceeded. However, there is a report[4] of pigmentary retinopathy in a patient who received long-term thioridazine in daily doses not exceeding 400 mg; the total dose was 752 g.

Pigmentation may also occur in the cornea, lens, and conjunctiva following administration of phenothiazines. It may occur in association with pigmentary changes in the skin and is dose-related. In a study of 100 Malaysian patients, ocular pigmentation was observed in slightly more than half of those who had received a total dose of chlorpromazine of 100 to 299 g and in 13 of 15 who had received 300 to 599 g.[5] All those who had received more than 600 g of chlorpromazine or thioridazine had ocular pigmentation. Cataract formation, mainly of an anterior polar variety, has been observed rarely, mainly in patients on chlorpromazine. It does not appear to be dose-related.[2]

A patient who had received fortnightly injections of fluphenazine for 10 years to an estimated total dose of 3.25 g, developed bilateral maculopathy following unprotected exposure of less than 2-minute's duration to a welding arc.[6] It was postulated that accumulation of phenothiazine in the retinal epithelium sensitised the patient to photic damage.

1. Spiteri MA, James DG. Adverse ocular reactions to drugs. *Postgrad Med J* 1983; **59:** 343–9.
2. Crombie AL. Drugs causing eye problems. *Prescribers' J* 1981; **21:** 222–7.
3. Marmor MF. Is thioridazine retinopathy progressive? Relationship of pigmentary changes to visual function. *Br J Ophthalmol* 1990; **74:** 739–42.
4. Lam RW, Remick RA. Pigmentary retinopathy associated with low-dose thioridazine treatment. *Can Med Assoc J* 1985; **132:** 737.
5. Ngen CC, Singh P. Long-term phenothiazine administration and the eye in 100 Malaysians. *Br J Psychiatry* 1988; **152:** 278–81.
6. Power WJ, *et al.* Welding arc maculopathy and fluphenazine. *Br J Ophthalmol* 1991; **75:** 433–5.

Effects on fluid and electrolyte homoeostasis. There have been occasional reports of water intoxication in patients taking antipsychotics. A review[1] of hyponatraemia and the syndrome of inappropriate antidiuretic hormone secretion associated with psychotropics summarised 20 such reports for antipsychotics in the literature. The drugs implicated were thioridazine (8 patients), 3 reports with haloperidol, 2 each for chlorpromazine, trifluoperazine, and fluphenazine, and 1 each with flupentixol, tiotixene, and clozapine. The majority of reports did not permit clear conclusions and, particularly in the cases of prolonged treatment, the role of the medication was unclear. However, at least 3 of the cases were well documented and supported the view that antipsychotics could cause hyponatraemia.

One report not considered by the above review described water retention and peripheral oedema associated with chlorpromazine.[2] A small controlled study[3] found that 5 of 10 evaluated patients receiving haloperidol decanoate had impaired fluid homoeostasis.

1. Spigset O, Hedenmalm K. Hyponatraemia and the syndrome of inappropriate antidiuretic hormone secretion (SIADH) induced by psychotropic drugs. *Drug Safety* 1995; **12:** 209–25.
2. Witz L, *et al.* Chlorpromazine induced fluid retention masquerading as idiopathic oedema. *BMJ* 1987; **294:** 807–8.
3. Rider JM, *et al.* Water handling in patients receiving haloperidol decanoate. *Ann Pharmacother* 1995; **29:** 663–6.

Effects on lipid metabolism. There are scant data implicating phenothiazines as a cause of elevated cholesterol and decreased high-density lipoprotein concentrations.[1] The possibility of such effects should nevertheless be considered in dyslipidaemic patients treated with these drugs.

1. Henkin Y, *et al.* Secondary dyslipidemia: inadvertent effects of drugs in clinical practice. *JAMA* 1992; **267:** 961–8.

Effects on the liver. Chlorpromazine and other phenothiazines may cause hepatocanalicular cholestasis often with hepatocyte damage suggestive of immunological liver injury.[1] Only a small number of patients taking the drug are affected and the onset is usually in the first 4 weeks of therapy. The drug or one of its metabolites may induce alteration in the liver-cell membrane so that it becomes antigenic; there is also good evidence for direct hepatotoxicity related to the production of free drug radical. There may be an individual idiosyncrasy in the metabolism of chlorpromazine and in the production of these radicals. One study has suggested that patients who have poor sulfoxidation status combined with unimpaired hydroxylation capacity may be most likely to develop jaundice with chlorpromazine.[2]

A preliminary study[3] showing a high incidence of gallstones in psychiatric inpatients in Japan found a correlation between the presence of gallstones and the duration of illness and use of antipsychotics. It was speculated that gallstones could be a consequence of phenothiazine-induced cholestasis.

1. Sherlock S. The spectrum of hepatotoxicity due to drugs. *Lancet* 1986; **ii:** 440–4.
2. Watson RGP, *et al.* A proposed mechanism for chlorpromazine jaundice—defective hepatic sulphoxidation combined with rapid hydroxylation. *J Hepatol* 1988; **7:** 72–8.
3. Fukuzako H, *et al.* Ultrasonography detected a higher incidence of gallstones in psychiatric inpatients. *Acta Psychiatr Scand* 1991; **84:** 83–5.

Effects on sexual function. The phenothiazines can cause both impotence and ejaculatory dysfunction.[1] Thioridazine has been frequently implicated, and in an early report 60% of 57 male patients taking the drug reported sexual dysfunction compared with 25% of 64 men taking other antipsychotics.[2] There are also several reports of priapism with phenothiazines;[1,3,4] alpha-adrenoceptor blocking properties of these compounds may be partly responsible. Male sexual dysfunction, including priapism, has been reported only rarely with other antipsychotics

The symbol † denotes a preparation no longer actively marketed

such as the butyrophenones, diphenylbutylpiperidines, and thioxanthenes.[5] Priapism has also been reported with clozapine.[6] The effects of antipsychotics on female sexual function are less well studied. Orgasmic dysfunction has been reported with thioridazine, trifluoperazine, and fluphenazine.[7]

The effects of hyperprolactinaemia (see Effects on Endocrine Function, above) on sexual function are described on p.1274.

1. Beeley L. Drug-induced sexual dysfunction and infertility. *Adverse Drug React Acute Poisoning Rev* 1984; **3:** 23–42.
2. Kotin J, *et al.* Thioridazine and sexual dysfunction. *Am J Psychiatry* 1976; **133:** 82–5.
3. Baños JE, *et al.* Drug-induced priapism: its aetiology, incidence and treatment. *Med Toxicol* 1989; **4:** 46–58.
4. Chan J, *et al.* Perphenazine-induced priapism. *DICP Ann Pharmacother* 1990; **24:** 246–9.
5. Fabian J-L. Psychotropic medications and priapism. *Am J Psychiatry* 1993; **150:** 349–50.
6. Patel AG, *et al.* Priapism associated with psychotropic drugs. *Br J Hosp Med* 1996; **55:** 315–19.
7. Segraves RT. Psychiatric drugs and inhibited female orgasm. *J Sex Marital Ther* 1988; **14:** 202–7.

Effects on the skin. DEPOT INJECTION. Of 217 patients who received a combined total of 2354 depot antipsychotic injections 42 (19.4%) had local problems at the site of injection; 18 (8.3%) experienced chronic complications and 30 (13.8%) acute reactions.[1] Acute problems reported included 31 episodes of unusual pain, 21 of bleeding or haematoma, 19 of clinically important leakage of drug from injection site, 11 of acute inflammatory indurations, and 2 of transient nodules. Complications were more common in patients receiving concentrated preparations, higher doses, weekly injections, haloperidol decanoate or zuclopenthixol decanoate, and injection volumes greater than 1 mL and in those treated for more than 5 years. Chronic reactions were more common in patients aged over 50 years.

1. Hay J. Complications at site of injection of depot neuroleptics. *BMJ* 1995; **311:** 421.

PHOTOSENSITIVITY. Testing in 7 subjects taking chlorpromazine revealed that photosensitivity reactions manifested primarily as immediate erythema and that sensitivity was primarily to light in the long ultraviolet (UVA) and visible wavebands. Sensitivity to UVB was normal.[1]

The incidence of photosensitivity reactions to chlorpromazine has been given as 3%. However, a higher incidence of 16-25% has also been reported.[2]

See also Effects on the Eyes, above.

1. Ferguson J, *et al.* Further clinical and investigative studies of chlorpromazine phototoxicity. *Br J Dermatol* 1986; **115** (suppl 30): 35.
2. Harth Y, Rapoport M. Photosensitivity associated with antipsychotics, antidepressants and anxiolytics. *Drug Safety* 1996; **14:** 252–9.

PIGMENTATION. The pigment found in the skin of patients treated with chlorpromazine was considered[1] to be a chlorpromazine-melanin polymer formed in a light-catalysed anaerobic reaction. Hydrogen chloride liberated during the reaction could account for the skin irritation. Intracutaneous injection of a preparation of the polymer into 2 volunteers produced a bluish-purple discoloration which faded in 3 days.

1. Huang CL, Sands FL. Effect of ultraviolet irradiation on chlorpromazine II: anaerobic condition. *J Pharm Sci* 1967; **56:** 259–64.

Extrapyramidal disorders. Antipsychotics and a number of other drugs, including antiemetics such as metoclopramide and some antidepressants, can produce a range of dyskinesias or involuntary movement disorders involving the extrapyramidal motor system, including parkinsonism, akathisia, acute dystonia, and chronic tardive dyskinesia.[1-4] Such reactions are a major problem in the clinical management of patients receiving antipsychotics. Reactions of this type can occur with any antipsychotic, but (excluding tardive dyskinesia) are particularly prominent during treatment with high-potency drugs such as the tricyclic piperazines and butyrophenones. Clozapine carries a low risk of extrapyramidal effects and is therefore described as an atypical antipsychotic. Other atypical antipsychotics include risperidone, olanzapine, quetiapine, and amisulpride. The incidence of tardive dyskinesia does appear to be minimal with clozapine, although there is less evidence for other atypical antipsychotics (but see also below).

Of 2811 patients studied[5] in the first few months of therapy with prochlorperazine (a drug with a high propensity to cause extrapyramidal reactions), 57 reported adverse effects, 16 of which involved the extrapyramidal system. There were 4 dystonic-dyskinesic reactions (an incidence of 1 in 464 and 1 in 707 for patients aged under and over 30 years respectively), 9 reports of parkinsonism (under 60 years, 1 in 1555; over 60 years, 1 in 159), and 3 reports of akathisia (1 in 562).

One explanation of extrapyramidal disorders is an imbalance between dopaminergic and cholinergic systems in the brain. However, this simple model fails to explain the co-existence of a variety of extrapyramidal effects, and several alternative mechanisms have been proposed.[2,6] Hypotheses based on interactions between different dopamine receptor types may help to explain the decreased tendency of some antipsychotic drugs to induce these reactions (see Action under Uses and Administration, below).

Akathisia is a condition of mental and motor restlessness in which there is an urge to move about constantly and an inability to sit or stand still. It is the most common motor side-effect of

treatment with antipsychotics.[7] Acute akathisia is dose-dependent, usually develops within a few days of beginning treatment or following a rapid increase in dose, and usually improves if the drug is stopped or the dose reduced. *Antimuscarinics* appear to provide only limited benefit, although success may be more likely in patients with concomitant parkinsonism. A low dose of a *beta blocker* such as *propranolol* or a *benzodiazepine* may be helpful. Improvement has also been reported with *clonidine* and *amantadine* but the usefulness of these drugs may be limited by side-effects or development of tolerance respectively. The tardive form, like tardive dyskinesia (see below) which appears after several months of treatment, does not respond to antimuscarinics, and is difficult to treat.

Acute **dystonic reactions**, which mainly affect the muscles of the face, neck, and trunk and include jaw clenching (trismus), torticollis, and oculogyric crisis are reported to occur in up to 10% of patients taking antipsychotics. Laryngeal dystonia is rare, but potentially fatal.[8] Dystonias usually occur within the first few days of treatment or after a dosage increase but may also develop on withdrawal. They are transitory, and are most common in children and young adults. Dystonic reactions may be controlled by the administration of *antimuscarinics* or *antihistamines* such as *diphenhydramine* or *promethazine*.[9] *Benzodiazepines* such as *diazepam* can also be used. Prophylactic administration of antimuscarinics can prevent the development of dystonias, but routine use is not recommended as not all patients require them and tardive dyskinesia may be unmasked or worsened (see below); such a strategy should probably be reserved for short-term use in those at high risk of developing dystonic reactions, such as young adults starting treatment with high-potency antipsychotics or in patients with a previous history of drug-induced dystonias.[10,11] Some patients may develop tardive dystonia. A range of drugs has been tried in this condition but without consistent benefit.[12]

Parkinsonism, often indistinguishable from idiopathic Parkinson's disease (p.1160), may develop during therapy with antipsychotics, usually after the first few weeks or months of treatment. It is generally stated to be more common in adults and the elderly, although a retrospective study with haloperidol found an inverse relationship between drug-induced parkinsonism and age.[13] This parkinsonism is generally reversible on drug withdrawal or dose reduction, and may sometimes disappear gradually despite continued drug therapy. *Antimuscarinic* drugs are used to suppress the symptoms of parkinsonism.[14] However, they are often minimally effective and commonly cause adverse effects. Routine use for prophylaxis is not recommended because of the risk of unmasking or exacerbating tardive dyskinesia (see below). *Amantadine* is an alternative to the antimuscarinics.[14]

The central feature of **tardive dyskinesia** is orofacial dyskinesia characterised by protrusion of the tongue ('fly catching'), lipsmacking, sucking, lateral chewing, and pouting of the lips and cheeks. The trunk and limbs also become involved with choreiform movements such as repetitive 'piano-playing' hand movements, shoulder shrugging, foot tapping, or rocking movements. The prevalence of tardive dyskinesia among those receiving antipsychotics varies widely but up to 60% of patients may develop symptoms. In most cases the condition is mild and not progressive and tends to wax and wane. Although tardive dyskinesia usually develops after many years of antipsychotic therapy no clear correlation has been shown between development of the condition and the length of drug treatment or the type and class of drug. However, administration of *clozapine* does not appear to be associated with development of the condition and in some cases has resulted in improvement of established tardive dyskinesia (see Schizophrenia under Clozapine, p.674). Whether other atypical antipsychotics also have a lower incidence of tardive dyskinesia remains to be established, although there are some data to suggest that this may be the case.[15,16] Symptoms of tardive dyskinesia often develop after discontinuation of the antipsychotic or after dose reduction. Risk factors include old age, female sex, affective disorder, schizophrenia characterised by negative symptoms, and organic brain damage.

Suggested causes of tardive dyskinesia include dopaminergic overactivity, imbalance between dopaminergic and cholinergic activity, supersensitivity of postsynaptic dopamine receptors, presynaptic catecholaminergic hyperfunction, and alterations of the gamma-aminobutyric acid (GABA) system. This had led to trials with antidopaminergics, noradrenergic antagonists, cholinergic drugs, and GABAergic drugs as well as attempts to reverse postsynaptic supersensitivity with dopamine. Although many drugs have been tried in the treatment of tardive dyskinesia there have been relatively few double-blind studies. Reviews of tardive dyskinesia[15,17-19] have concluded that there appeared to be no reliable or safe treatment. Overall, standard antipsychotics appeared to be the most effective in masking symptoms of tardive dyskinesia but tolerance may develop and a worsening of the underlying pathophysiology by antipsychotics had to be assumed on theoretical grounds. Other drugs with antidopaminergic actions which were probably of comparable efficacy included *reserpine, oxypertine, tetrabenazine,* and *metirosine.* The next most effective drugs were considered to be noradrenergic antagonists such as *clonidine.* Some encouraging results had also been obtained with GABAergic drugs such as the *benzodiazepines, baclofen, progabide, valproate,* and

vigabatrin, although a systematic review[20] of studies of some GABAergic drugs found the evidence unconvincing. However, the efficacy of cholinergics could not be confirmed. Dopaminergics and antimuscarinics mostly exacerbated symptoms but others[11] had commented that there was no convincing evidence that long-term administration of antimuscarinics increased the risk of developing the condition. Other drugs whose value is unclear include *vitamin E,* although one study[21] found favourable results, and some calcium-channel blockers.[22]

In view of the unsatisfactory management of tardive dyskinesia, emphasis is placed on its prevention. Antipsychotics should be prescribed only when clearly indicated, should be given in the minimum dose, and continued only when there is evidence of benefit. Although drug holidays have been suggested for reducing the risk of tardive dyskinesia, the limited evidence indicates that interruptions in drug treatment may increase the risk of both persistent dyskinesia and psychotic relapse. Increasing the dose of antipsychotic generally improves the condition, but only temporarily. Options in the management of tardive dyskinesia include withdrawal of antimuscarinic therapy, and either withdrawal of the antipsychotic or reduction of the dosage to the minimum required or transfer to an atypical antipsychotic. Success is most likely in younger patients. Stopping the drug usually worsens the condition although symptoms often diminish or disappear over a period of weeks or sometimes a year or so. During withdrawal drugs such as *diazepam* or *clonazepam* may be given to alleviate symptoms. Although standard antipsychotics are effective their routine use to suppress symptoms is not recommended but they may be required for acute distressing or life-threatening reactions or in chronic tardive dyskinesia unresponsive to other treatment. In extremely severe resistant cases some have used an antipsychotic with *valproate* or *carbamazepine* or *reserpine* with *metirosine.*

1. Committee on Safety of Medicines/Medicines Control Agency. Drug-induced extrapyramidal reactions. *Current Problems* 1994; **20:** 15–16.
2. Ebadi M, Srinivasan SK. Pathogenesis, prevention, and treatment of neuroleptic-induced movement disorders. *Pharmacol Rev* 1995; **47:** 575–604.
3. Holloman LC, Marder SR. Management of acute extrapyramidal effects induced by antipsychotic drugs. *Am J Health-Syst Pharm* 1997; **54:** 2461–77.
4. Jiménez-Jiménez FJ, *et al.* Drug-induced movement disorders. *Drug Safety* 1997; **16:** 180–204.
5. Bateman DN, *et al.* Extrapyramidal reactions to metoclopramide and prochlorperazine. *Q J Med* 1989; **71:** 307–11.
6. Ereshefsky L, *et al.* Pathophysiologic basis for schizophrenia and the efficacy of antipsychotics. *Clin Pharm* 1990; **9:** 682–707.
7. Miller CH, Fleischhacker WW. Managing antipsychotic-induced acute and chronic akathisia. *Drug Safety* 2000; **22:** 73–81.
8. Koek RJ, Pi EH. Acute laryngeal dystonic reactions to neuroleptics. *Psychosomatics* 1989; **30:** 359–64.
9. van Harten PN, *et al.* Acute dystonia induced by drug treatment. *BMJ* 1999; **319:** 623–6.
10. WHO. Prophylactic use of anticholinergics in patients on long-term neuroleptic treatment: a consensus statement. *Br J Psychiatry* 1990; **156:** 412.
11. Barnes TRE. Comment on the WHO consensus statement. *Br J Psychiatry* 1990; **156:** 413–14.
12. Raja M. Managing antipsychotic-induced acute and tardive dystonia. *Drug Safety* 1998; **19:** 57–72.
13. Moleman P, *et al.* Relationship between age and incidence of parkinsonism in psychiatric patients treated with haloperidol. *Am J Psychiatry* 1986; **143:** 232–4.
14. Mamo DC, *et al.* Managing antipsychotic-induced parkinsonism. *Drug Safety* 1999; **20:** 269–75.
15. Casey DE. Tardive dyskinesia and atypical antipsychotic drugs. *Schizophr Res* 1999; **35** (suppl): S61–S66.
16. Kane JM. Tardive dyskinesia in affective disorders. *J Clin Psychiatry* 1999; **60** (suppl 5): 43–7.
17. Haag H, *et al.,* eds. Tardive Dyskinesia. *WHO Expert Series on Biological Psychiatry Volume 1.* Seattle: Hogrefe & Huber, 1992.
18. Egan MF, *et al.* Treatment of tardive dyskinesia. *Schizophr Bull* 1997; **23:** 583–609.
19. Najib J. Tardive dyskinesia: a review and current treatment options. *Am J Ther* 1999; **6:** 51–60.
20. Soares KVS, *et al.* Gamma-aminobutyric acid agonists for neuroleptic-induced tardive dyskinesia (updated 28 February 2001). Available in The Cochrane Library; Issue 4. Oxford: Update Software; 2001.
21. Adler LA, *et al.* Long-term treatment effects of vitamin E for tardive dyskinesia. *Biol Psychiatry* 1998; **43:** 868–72.
22. Soares KVS, McGrath JJ. Calcium channel blockers for neuroleptic-induced tardive dyskinesia (updated 9 May 2001). Available in The Cochrane Library; Issue 4. Oxford: Update Software; 2001.

Neuroleptic malignant syndrome. The neuroleptic malignant syndrome (NMS) is a potentially fatal reaction to a number of drugs including antipsychotics and dopamine antagonists such as metoclopramide. The clinical features of the classic syndrome are usually considered to include hyperthermia, severe extrapyramidal symptoms including muscular rigidity, autonomic dysfunction, and altered levels of consciousness. Skeletal muscle damage may occur and resulting myoglobinuria may lead to renal failure. However, there appear to be no universal criteria for the diagnosis of the syndrome. Some believe the classic syndrome to be the extreme of a range of effects associated with antipsychotics and have introduced the concept of milder variants or incomplete forms. Others consider it to be a rare idiosyncratic reaction and suggest that the term neuroleptic malignant syndrome should be reserved for the full blown reaction. Consequently estimates of the incidence vary greatly and recent estimates have ranged from 0.02 to 2.5%. The mortality rate has been substantial; although it has decreased over the years with improved diagnosis and management this may also be due to the detection and inclusion of the milder or incomplete variants. Possible risk factors include dehydration, pre-existing organic brain disease, and a history of a previous episode; young males have also been reported to be particularly susceptible.

The pathogenesis of NMS is still unclear. Blockade of dopaminergic receptors in the corpus striatum is thought to cause muscular contraction and rigidity generating heat while blockade of dopaminergic receptors in the hypothalamus leads to impaired heat dissipation. Peripheral mechanisms such as vasomotor paralysis may also play a role. Also a syndrome resembling NMS has been seen following withdrawal of treatment with dopamine agonists such as levodopa (see p.1171). Symptoms develop rapidly over 24 to 72 hours and may occur days to months after initiation of antipsychotic medication or increase in dosage, but no consistent correlation with dosage or duration of therapy has been found. Symptoms may last for up to 14 days after cessation of oral antipsychotics, or for up to 4 weeks after cessation of depot preparations. All antipsychotics are capable of inducing the condition; depot preparations may, however, be associated with prolonged recovery from the syndrome if it develops, and hence a higher mortality rate. Concomitant administration of lithium carbonate or antimuscarinics may increase the likelihood of developing the syndrome.

Antipsychotic medication should be withdrawn immediately the diagnosis of the classic syndrome is made, followed by symptomatic and supportive therapy including cooling measures, correction of dehydration, and treatment of cardiovascular, respiratory, and renal complications. Whether antipsychotics should be withdrawn from patients with mild attacks and how they should be managed is a matter of debate. The efficacy of specific drug therapy remains to be proven and justification for use is based mainly on case reports. *Dantrolene* was first used because of its effectiveness in malignant hyperthermia. It has a direct action on skeletal muscle and may be particularly effective for the reversal of hyperthermia of muscle origin. In contrast, dopaminergic agonists may resolve hyperthermia of central origin, restoring dopaminergic transmission and hence alleviating extrapyramidal symptoms. There have been isolated reports of success with *amantadine* and *levodopa* but *bromocriptine* is generally preferred. Any underlying psychosis may, however, be aggravated by dopaminergic drugs. In view of the differing modes of action of dantrolene and dopaminergics a combination of the two might be useful but any advantage remains to be demonstrated. *Antimuscarinics* are generally considered to be of little use and may aggravate the associated hyperthermia. *Benzodiazepines* may be used for sedation in agitated patients and may be of use against concomitant catatonia. Electroconvulsive therapy may be an alternative in refractory cases of NMS or when catatonic symptoms are present. Reintroduction of antipsychotic therapy may be possible but is not always successful and extreme caution is advised. It has been recommended that a gap of at least 5 to 14 days should be left after resolution of the symptoms before attempting re-introduction.

References.
1. Wells AJ, *et al.* Neuroleptic rechallenge after neuroleptic malignant syndrome: case report and literature review. *Drug Intell Clin Pharm* 1988; **22:** 475–80.
2. Bristow MF, Kohen D. How "malignant" is the neuroleptic malignant syndrome? *BMJ* 1993; **307:** 1223–4.
3. Kornhuber J, Weller M. Neuroleptic malignant syndrome. *Curr Opin Neurol* 1994; **7:** 353–7.
4. Velamoor VR, *et al.* Management of suspected neuroleptic malignant syndrome. *Can J Psychiatry* 1995; **40:** 545–50.
5. Ebadi M, Srinivasan SK. Pathogenesis, prevention, and treatment of neuroleptic-induced movement disorders. *Pharmacol Rev* 1995; **47:** 575–604.
6. Bristow MF, Kohen D. Neuroleptic malignant syndrome. *Br J Hosp Med* 1996; **55:** 517–20.
7. Velamoor VR. Neuroleptic malignant syndrome: recognition, prevention and management. *Drug Safety* 1998; **19:** 73–82.
8. Adnet P, *et al.* Neuroleptic malignant syndrome. *Br J Anaesth* 2000; **85:** 129–35.

Withdrawal. Abrupt discontinuation of an antipsychotic may be accompanied by withdrawal symptoms, the most common of which are nausea, vomiting, anorexia, diarrhoea, rhinorrhoea, sweating, myalgias, paraesthesias, insomnia, restlessness, anxiety, and agitation.[1] Patients may also experience vertigo, alternate feelings of warmth and coldness, and tremor. Symptoms generally begin within 1 to 4 days of withdrawal and abate within 7 to 14 days. They are more severe and frequent when antimuscarinics are discontinued simultaneously.

1. Dilsaver SC. Withdrawal phenomena associated with antidepressant and antipsychotic agents. *Drug Safety* 1994; **10:** 103–14.

Treatment of Adverse Effects

Following an overdose of chlorpromazine patients should be managed with intensive symptomatic and supportive therapy. Activated charcoal should be given by mouth if a substantial amount of the phenothiazine has been taken within 1 hour, provided that the airway can be protected; emptying the stomach by gastric lavage has sometimes been recommended. Dialysis is of little or no value in poisoning by phenothiazines.

Hypotension should be corrected by raising the patient's legs, or in severe cases by intravascular volume expansion. If a vasoconstrictor is considered necessary in the management of phenothiazine-induced hypotension the use of adrenaline [epinephrine] or other sympathomimetics with high beta-adrenergic agonist properties should be avoided since the alpha-blocking effects of phenothiazines may impair the usual alpha-mediated vasoconstriction of these drugs, resulting in unopposed beta-adrenergic stimulation and increased hypotension.

The treatment of neuroleptic malignant syndrome and the difficulties of treating extrapyramidal side-effects, especially tardive dyskinesia, are discussed above.

Precautions

Chlorpromazine and other phenothiazines are contraindicated in patients with pre-existing CNS depression or coma, bone-marrow suppression, phaeochromocytoma, or prolactin-dependent tumours. They should be used with caution or not at all in patients with impaired liver, kidney, cardiovascular, cerebrovascular, and respiratory function and in those with angle-closure glaucoma, a history of jaundice, parkinsonism, diabetes mellitus, hypothyroidism, myasthenia gravis, paralytic ileus, prostatic hyperplasia, or urinary retention. Care is required in patients with epilepsy or a history of seizures as phenothiazines may lower the seizure threshold. Debilitated patients may be more prone to the adverse effects of phenothiazines as may the elderly, especially those with dementia.

The sedative effects of phenothiazines are most marked during the first few days of administration; affected patients should not drive or operate machinery.

Phenothiazine effects on the vomiting centre may mask the symptoms of overdosage of other drugs, or of disorders such as gastrointestinal obstruction. Administration at extremes of temperature may be hazardous since body temperature regulation is impaired by phenothiazines.

Regular eye examinations are advisable for patients receiving long-term phenothiazine therapy and avoidance of undue exposure to direct sunlight is recommended. Phenothiazines should be used with caution in the presence of acute infection or leucopenia. Blood counts are advised if the patient develops an unexplained infection or fever.

Phenothiazines are generally not recommended late in pregnancy; such use may be associated with intoxication of the neonate. Chlorpromazine may prolong labour and should be withheld until the cervix is dilated 3 to 4 cm. For other possible risks of phenothiazine administration during pregnancy, see below.

Patients should remain supine for at least 30 minutes after parenteral administration of chlorpromazine; blood pressure should be monitored.

Abrupt withdrawal of phenothiazine therapy is best avoided.

AIDS. Isolated reports[1,2] have suggested that patients with AIDS may be particularly susceptible to antipsychotic-induced extrapyramidal effects.

1. Hollander H, *et al.* Extrapyramidal symptoms in AIDS patients given low-dose metoclopramide or chlorpromazine. *Lancet* 1985; **ii:** 1186.
2. Edelstein H, Knight RT. Severe parkinsonism in two AIDS patients taking prochlorperazine. *Lancet* 1987; **ii:** 341–2.

Asthma. Findings of a retrospective case-control study[1] appeared to indicate that asthmatic patients who receive antipsychotics were at an increased risk of death or near death from asthma.

1. Joseph KS, *et al.* Increased morbidity and mortality related to asthma among asthmatic patients who use major tranquillisers. *BMJ* 1996; **312:** 79–82.

Children. Few phenothiazines are recommended for use in children; in particular there have been concerns about the use of phenothiazine derivatives in infants (see Sudden Infant Death Syndrome, p.423). For reference to the wide use of chlorpromazine in infants suffering neonatal abstinence syndrome see Substance Dependence, Opioids, under Uses and Administration, below.

References.
1. Dyer KS, Woolf AD. Use of phenothiazines as sedatives in children: what are the risks? *Drug Safety* 1999; **21:** 81–90.

The elderly. The risk of *hip fracture* has been reported to be increased in elderly patients given antipsychotics. A large case-control study in patients over 65 found that current users of antipsychotics had a twofold increase in the risk of hip fractures.[1] The effect was dose-related and the increased risk was similar for chlorpromazine, haloperidol, and thioridazine. It was suggested that antipsychotic-induced sedation or orthostatic hypotension could increase the risk of falls in elderly persons. A study in 12 schizophrenic patients receiving antipsychotics plus other drugs such as antimuscarinics or benzodiazepines has suggested that long-term treatment with antipsychotics may decrease bone mineralisation.[2] A later study suggested that any increased risk of falls might be due to an effect of antipsychotics on balance as thioridazine was found to increase sway in elderly but not young subjects.[3] A meta-analysis of forty studies[4] concluded that there was a small, but consistent, association between the use of most classes of psychotropic drugs, including antipsychotics, and falls. However, the evidence from these studies was based solely on observational data, with minimal adjustment for confounders, dosage, or duration of therapy.

There is some evidence[5,6] to suggest that the use of antipsychotics to manage behavioural complications of *dementia* may increase the rate of cognitive decline. Elderly patients with dementia, especially Lewy-body dementia, are reported to be highly susceptible to the extrapyramidal adverse effects of antipsychotic drugs,[7,8] and the reaction can be extremely serious, even fatal. If these drugs are to be used in elderly patients with dementia, then very low doses should be employed, and special care should be taken if the dementia is suspected to be of the Lewy-body type since sudden life-threatening deterioration may occur.[9] Depot preparations should not be used and since dopamine D$_2$ receptors may be involved, it has been suggested that consideration could be given to using an antipsychotic such as clozapine that does not principally antagonise those receptors,[8] although it too is not without its problems.

For further discussion of the problems associated with the use of antipsychotics in disturbed behaviour in the elderly, see p.650.

1. Ray WA, *et al.* Psychotropic drug use and the risk of hip fracture. *N Engl J Med* 1987; **316:** 363–9.
2. Higuchi T, *et al.* Certain neuroleptics reduce bone mineralization in schizophrenic patients. *Neuropsychobiology* 1987; **18:** 185–8.
3. Liu Y, *et al.* Comparative clinical effects of thioridazine (THD) on fall risk in young and elderly subjects. *Clin Pharmacol Ther* 1995; **57:** 200.
4. Leipzig RM, *et al.* Drugs and falls in older people: a systematic review and meta-analysis: I. Psychotropic drugs. *J Am Geriatr Soc* 1999; **47:** 30–9.
5. McShane R, *et al.* Do neuroleptic drugs hasten cognitive decline in dementia? Prospective study with necropsy follow up. *BMJ* 1997; **314:** 266–70.
6. Holmes C, *et al.* Do neuroleptic drugs hasten cognitive decline in dementia? Carriers of apolipoprotein E ε4 allele seem particularly susceptible to their effects. *BMJ* 1997; **314:** 1411.
7. McKeith I, *et al.* Neuroleptic sensitivity in patients with senile dementia of Lewy body type. *BMJ* 1992; **305:** 673–8.
8. Piggott MA, *et al.* DRD2 Ser311/Cys311 polymorphism in schizophrenia. *Lancet* 1994; **343:** 1044–5. Correction. *ibid.*; 1170. [Title: Dopamine D2 receptors in demented patients with severe neuroleptic sensitivity.]
9. Committee on Safety of Medicines/Medicines Control Agency. Neuroleptic sensitivity in patients with dementia. *Current Problems* 1994; **20:** 6.

Epilepsy. See Convulsions under Adverse Effects, above.

Folic acid deficiency. Concentrations of folate in serum and erythrocytes were reduced in 15 patients receiving long-term treatment with chlorpromazine or thioridazine.[1] All the patients showed significant induction of hepatic microsomal enzymes. It was suggested that folate deficiency due to the induction of microsomal enzymes might subsequently limit enzyme induction and hence reduce drug metabolism, which could lead to symptoms of toxicity in patients apparently stabilised for a number of years. The dietary intake of patients on long-term treatment with enzyme-inducing drugs might be inadequate.

1. Labadarios D, *et al.* The effects of chronic drug administration on hepatic enzyme induction and folate metabolism. *Br J Clin Pharmacol* 1978; **5:** 167–73.

Hypoparathyroidism. There have been rare reports[1,2] of acute dystonic reactions associated with the use of phenothiazines in patients with untreated hypoparathyroidism. Caution was recommended in giving phenothiazine derivatives to patients with hypoparathyroidism and it was suggested that any acute reaction to such a drug should prompt investigation for some form of latent tetany.

1. Schaaf M, Payne CA. Dystonic reactions to prochlorperazine in hypoparathyroidism. *N Engl J Med* 1966; **275:** 991–5.
2. Gur H, *et al.* Acute dystonic reaction to methotrimeprazine in hypoparathyroidism. *Ann Pharmacother* 1996; **30:** 957–9.

Pregnancy and breast feeding. A review[1] of the use of phenothiazines in pregnancy and during breast feeding concluded that there was no clear evidence that these drugs caused a significant increase in fetal malformations. Nevertheless it was considered advisable that if pregnant patients required such treatment, then a single phenothiazine should be used and that it should be one of the established drugs. Use during labour could be effective in controlling nausea and vomiting, but the effects of interactions should be considered, as should the possibility of lethargy and extrapyramidal effects in the neonate due to slow elimination. It was also considered that there were no major problems related to use during breast feeding.

Another review[2] considered that the criteria for the selection of an antipsychotic for use in pregnant women did not differ from that used in nonpregnant women. It was also concluded that the benefits of continuing antipsychotic treatment at the minimum effective dose would usually outweigh any risks to the fetus.

1. McElhatton PR. The use of phenothiazines during pregnancy and lactation. *Reprod Toxicol* 1992; **6:** 475–90.
2. Trixler M, Tényi T. Antipsychotic use in pregnancy: what are the best treatment options? *Drug Safety* 1997; **16:** 403–10.

Renal impairment. Phenothiazine-induced toxic psychosis occurred in 4 patients with chronic renal failure who had been given chlorpromazine.[1]

1. McAllister CJ, *et al.* Toxic psychosis induced by phenothiazine administration in patients with chronic renal failure. *Clin Nephrol* 1978; **10:** 191–5.

Interactions

The most common interactions encountered with phenothiazines are those resulting from concomitant administration of drugs with similar pharmacological actions. When given with other drugs that produce orthostatic hypotension dosage adjustments may be necessary. However, it should be noted that phenothiazines have been reported to reduce the antihypertensive action of guanethidine and other adrenergic neurone blockers. As many phenothiazines possess antimuscarinic actions they may potentiate the adverse effects of other drugs with antimuscarinic actions, including tricyclic antidepressants and the antimuscarinic antiparkinsonian drugs that may be given to treat phenothiazine-induced extrapyramidal effects. In theory, antipsychotics with dopamine-blocking activity and dopaminergic drugs such as those used to treat parkinsonism may be mutually antagonistic. Concomitant administration of metoclopramide may increase the risk of antipsychotic-induced extrapyramidal effects.

There is an increased risk of arrhythmias when antipsychotics are used with drugs which prolong the QT interval including certain antiarrhythmics, antihistamines, antimalarials, and cisapride; the co-administration of diuretics that cause electrolyte imbalance particularly hypokalaemia may also have the same effect. There is also an increased risk of arrhythmia when tricyclic antidepressants are used with antipsychotics which prolong the QT interval. Because of an increased risk of seizures the US manufacturers recommend discontinuation of chlorpromazine before the use of metrizamide for radiographic procedures. Symptoms of CNS depression may be enhanced by other drugs with CNS-depressant properties including alcohol, general anaesthetics, hypnotics, anxiolytics, and opioids.

◊ Most interactions with antipsychotics are as a result of additive pharmacological effects.[1] Since tolerance develops to many of these side-effects, interactions are likely to be most important in the early stages of combination therapy.

1. Livingston MG. Interactions that matter: 11 antipsychotic drugs. *Prescribers' J* 1987; **27** (Dec): 26–9.

Alcohol. Akathisia and dystonia occurred after consumption of alcohol by patients taking antipsychotics.[1] Alcohol might lower the threshold of resistance to neurotoxic side-effects.

1. Lutz EG. Neuroleptic-induced akathisia and dystonia triggered by alcohol. *JAMA* 1976; **236:** 2422–3.

Antacids. Studies in 6 patients showed that chlorpromazine plasma concentrations were significantly lower after administration of chlorpromazine with an aluminium hydroxide and magnesium trisilicate antacid gel (Gelusil) than after chlorpromazine alone.[1] *In-vitro* studies indicated that chlorpromazine was highly bound to the gel.

1. Fann WE, *et al.* Chlorpromazine: effects of antacids on its gastrointestinal absorption. *J Clin Pharmacol* 1973; **13:** 388–90.

Antiarrhythmics. There is an increased risk of arrhythmias when antipsychotics are given with other drugs which prolong the QT interval. It has been recommended that the concomitant use of pimozide, sertindole, or thioridazine with antiarrhythmics (especially amiodarone, disopyramide, procainamide, and quinidine) should be avoided. Concomitant use of haloperidol and amiodarone is also not recommended. A study[1] in healthy subjects has suggested that quinidine might increase plasma concentrations of haloperidol.

1. Young D, *et al.* Effect of quinidine on the interconversion kinetics between haloperidol and reduced haloperidol in humans: implications for the involvement of cytochrome P450IID6. *Eur J Clin Pharmacol* 1993; **44:** 433–8.

Antibacterials. Seven schizophrenic patients whose antitubercular therapy included *rifampicin* (in addition to isoniazid, and in some cases also ethambutol) had lower serum concentrations of haloperidol compared with tuberculotic schizophrenic patients receiving no antimycobacterials and with non-tuberculotic schizophrenics.[1] Pharmacokinetic studies involving some of these patients indicated accelerated haloperidol clearance in the presence of rifampicin. Abnormally high serum-haloperidol concentrations were observed in 3 of 18 patients treated with *isoniazid* alone.

Black galactorrhoea occurred in a patient receiving concomitant therapy with *minocycline*, perphenazine, amitriptyline hydrochloride, and diphenhydramine hydrochloride.[2] Simultaneous occurrence of phenothiazine-induced galactorrhoea and tetracycline-induced pigmentation was considered responsible.

Sudden cardiac deaths have been reported[3] in patients given *clarithromycin* and pimozide. The manufacturer of pimozide has recommended that pimozide should not be used with macrolide antibacterials.

1. Takeda M, *et al.* Serum haloperidol levels of schizophrenics receiving treatment for tuberculosis. *Clin Neuropharmacol* 1986; **9:** 386–97.
2. Basler RSW, Lynch PJ. Black galactorrhea as a consequence of minocycline and phenothiazine therapy. *Arch Dermatol* 1985; **121:** 417–18.
3. Flockhart DA, *et al.* A metabolic interaction between clarithromycin and pimozide may result in cardiac toxicity. *Clin Pharmacol Ther* 1996; **59:** 189.

Anticoagulants. For reference to the effects of some antipsychotics on the activity of anticoagulants, see under Warfarin, p.996.

Antidepressants. Interactions between antipsychotics and *tricyclic antidepressants* are generally of two forms: either additive pharmacological effects such as antimuscarinic effects or hypotension, or pharmacokinetic interactions. Although not commonly reported in the literature additive antimuscarinic activity may be a significant risk especially in the elderly. Careful drug selection might help to prevent the development of serious adverse effects. Mutual inhibition of liver enzymes concerned with the metabolism of both the antipsychotic and the tricyclic antidepressant might result in increased plasma concentrations of either drug. In one study[1] addition of nortriptyline to chlorpromazine therapy produced an increase in plasma concentrations of chlorpromazine but this resulted in a paradoxical increase in agitation and tension.

There is an increased risk of arrhythmias when tricyclic antidepressants are given with other drugs which prolong the QT interval. It has been recommended that the concomitant use of pimozide, sertindole, or thioridazine with tricyclic antidepressants should be avoided.

Increased serum concentrations of haloperidol have occurred in patients given haloperidol with *fluoxetine*,[2] *fluvoxamine*,[3] or *nefazodone*. Isolated reports[4-9] of extrapyramidal symptoms, psychoneuromotor syndrome, stupor, bradycardia, and urinary retention associated with concomitant use of fluoxetine and antipsychotics (including the atypical antipsychotic risperidone[10]) suggest that fluoxetine might exacerbate the adverse effects of antipsychotics or produce additive toxicity. Similar CNS effects have been noted in volunteers given perphenazine and *paroxetine*.[11] There has also been an isolated report of a patient who complained of amenorrhoea and galactorrhoea after fluvoxamine was added to loxapine therapy.[12] Significant increases in the plasma concentrations of thioridazine have occurred after concurrent administration with fluvoxamine.[13] Plasma concentrations of olanzapine have been reported to be doubled by concomitant use of fluvoxamine but not *sertraline*.[14]

Combinations of antipsychotics and lithium should be used with care. Lithium can reduce plasma-chlorpromazine concentrations and there is a report of ventricular fibrillation on withdrawal of lithium from concomitant therapy with chlorpromazine. Chlorpromazine has also been reported to enhance the excretion of lithium. Neurotoxic or extrapyramidal symptoms have been reported rarely in patients taking antipsychotics and lithium; these may be atypical cases of lithium toxicity or neuroleptic malignant syndrome. The above issues are discussed in detail, and references given, on p.295.

A patient on long-term trifluoperazine treatment developed neuroleptic malignant syndrome after the concomitant administration of a single dose of *venlafaxine*.[15] The authors noted that the manufacturers of venlafaxine have received a small number of similar reports after introduction of venlafaxine in patients receiving antipsychotics (risperidone, olanzapine, or molindone).

There have been occasional reports of sexual disinhibition in patients taking *tryptophan* with phenothiazines.

1. Loga S, *et al.* Interaction of chlorpromazine and nortriptyline in patients with schizophrenia. *Clin Pharmacokinet* 1981; **6:** 454–62.
2. Goff DC, *et al.* Elevation of plasma concentrations of haloperidol after the addition of fluoxetine. *Am J Psychiatry* 1991; **148:** 790–2.
3. Daniel DG, *et al.* Coadministration of fluvoxamine increases serum concentrations of haloperidol. *J Clin Psychopharmacol* 1994; **14:** 340–3.
4. Tate JL. Extrapyramidal symptoms in a patient taking haloperidol and fluoxetine. *Am J Psychiatry* 1989; **146:** 399–400.
5. Ahmed I, *et al.* Possible interaction between fluoxetine and pimozide causing sinus bradycardia. *Can J Psychiatry* 1993; **38:** 62–3.
6. Ketai R. Interaction between fluoxetine and neuroleptics. *Am J Psychiatry* 1993; **150:** 836–7.
7. Hansen-Grant S, *et al.* Fluoxetine-pimozide interaction. *Am J Psychiatry* 1993; **150:** 1751–2.

8. D'Souza DC, *et al.* Precipitation of a psychoneuromotor syndrome by fluoxetine in a haloperidol-treated schizophrenic patient. *J Clin Psychopharmacol* 1994; **14:** 361–3.
9. Benazzi F. Urinary retention with fluoxetine-haloperidol combination in a young patient. *Can J Psychiatry* 1996; **41:** 606–7.
10. Brown ES. Extrapyramidal side effects with low-dose risperidone. *Can J Psychiatry* 1997; **42:** 325–6.
11. Özdemir V, *et al.* Paroxetine potentiates the central nervous system side effects of perphenazine: contribution of cytochrome P4502D6 inhibition in vivo. *Clin Pharmacol Ther* 1997; **62:** 334–47.
12. Jeffries J, *et al.* Amenorrhea and galactorrhea associated with fluvoxamine in a loxapine-treated patient. *J Clin Psychopharmacol* 1992; **12:** 296–7.
13. Carrillo JA, *et al.* Pharmacokinetic interaction of fluvoxamine and thioridazine in schizophrenic patients. *J Clin Psychopharmacol* 1999; **19:** 494–9.
14. Weigmann H, *et al.* Fluvoxamine but not sertraline inhibits the metabolism of olanzapine: evidence from a therapeutic drug monitoring service. *Ther Drug Monit* 2001; **23:** 410–13.
15. Nimmagadda SR, *et al.* Neuroleptic malignant syndrome after venlafaxine. *Lancet* 2000; **354:** 289–90.

Antidiabetic drugs. Since chlorpromazine may cause hyperglycaemia or impair glucose tolerance the dose of oral hypoglycaemics or of insulin may need to be increased in diabetics.

Antiepileptics. *Carbamazepine, phenobarbital,* and *phenytoin* are potent enzyme inducers and concomitant administration may decrease plasma concentrations of antipsychotics or their active metabolites.[1-5] The clinical effect of any interaction has not been consistent; worsening, improvement, or no change in psychotic symptoms have all been noted. Delirium has been reported in one patient given haloperidol and carbamazepine.[6] One case report[7] has suggested that phenytoin might also exacerbate antipsychotic-induced dyskinesia. Care should be taken when withdrawing enzyme-inducing antiepileptics as this may result in a rise in antipsychotic serum concentrations.[8]

The effect of antipsychotics on antiepileptic concentrations is discussed on p.345 (carbamazepine) and p.361 (phenytoin). It should also be remembered that antipsychotics may lower the seizure threshold.

1. Loga S, *et al.* Interactions of orphenadrine and phenobarbitone with chlorpromazine: plasma concentrations and effects in man. *Br J Clin Pharmacol* 1975; **2:** 197–208.
2. Linnoila M, *et al.* Effect of anticonvulsants on plasma haloperidol and thioridazine levels. *Am J Psychiatry* 1980; **137:** 819–21.
3. Jann MW, *et al.* Effects of carbamazepine on plasma haloperidol levels. *J Clin Psychopharmacol* 1985; **5:** 106–9.
4. Arana GW, *et al.* Does carbamazepine-induced reduction of plasma haloperidol levels worsen psychotic symptoms? *Am J Psychiatry* 1986; **143:** 650–1.
5. Ereshefsky L, *et al.* Thiothixene pharmacokinetic interactions: a study of hepatic enzyme inducers, clearance inhibitors, and demographic variables. *J Clin Psychopharmacol* 1991; **11:** 296–301.
6. Kanter GL, *et al.* Case report of a possible interaction between neuroleptics and carbamazepine. *Am J Psychiatry* 1984; **141:** 1101–2.
7. DeVeaugh-Geiss J. Aggravation of tardive dyskinesia by phenytoin. *N Engl J Med* 1978; **298:** 457–8.
8. Jann MW, *et al.* Clinical implications of increased antipsychotic plasma concentrations upon anticonvulsant cessation. *Psychiatry Res* 1989; **28:** 153–9.

Antihistamines. For the effect of a preparation containing chlorpheniramine [chlorphenamine] maleate and phenylpropanolamine hydrochloride on thioridazine, see Sympathomimetics (below). There is an increased risk of arrhythmias when antipsychotics are given with other drugs which prolong the QT interval. It has been recommended that the concomitant use of pimozide, sertindole, or thioridazine with antihistamines such as astemizole or terfenadine should be avoided.

Antihypertensives. For discussion of the interaction between phenothiazines and drugs with hypotensive properties, see Interactions, above. For a report of chlorpromazine enhancing the hyperglycaemic effect of diazoxide, see p.868. For reports of hypertension or dementia in patients given methyldopa and antipsychotics, see p.929.

Antimalarials. Pretreatment with single doses of chloroquine sulfate, amodiaquine hydrochloride, or sulfadoxine with pyrimethamine increased the plasma concentrations of chlorpromazine and 7-hydroxychlorpromazine, but not of chlorpromazine sulfoxide, in schizophrenic patients maintained on chlorpromazine.[1] The raised plasma concentrations appeared to be associated with a greater level of sedation.

There is an increased risk of arrhythmias when antipsychotics are given with other drugs which prolong the QT interval. It has been recommended that the concomitant use of antipsychotics, and pimozide in particular, with antimalarials such as halofantrine, mefloquine, or quinine should be avoided. For the possible effects of the use of quinidine with antipsychotics see Antiarrhythmics, above.

1. Makanjuola ROA, *et al.* Effects of antimalarial agents on plasma levels of chlorpromazine and its metabolites in schizophrenic patients. *Trop Geogr Med* 1988; **40:** 31–3.

Antimigraine drugs. A report[1] of a patient receiving loxapine who had a dystonic reaction within 15 minutes of subcutaneous administration of *sumatriptan* suggests that these two drugs might interact or potentiate each other's adverse effects. However, the patient had a previous history of dystonic reactions associated with haloperidol and was receiving benzatropine prophylactically. Furthermore, the dose of loxapine had been increased 2 days before the event and this may have predisposed the patient to dystonia.

1. Garcia G, *et al.* Dystonic reaction associated with sumatriptan. *Ann Pharmacother* 1994; **28:** 1199.

Antiparkinsonian drugs. Antiparkinsonian drugs are sometimes given with antipsychotics for the management of antipsychotic-induced side-effects including extrapyramidal disorders (see under Adverse Effects, above). Theoretically, dopaminergics such as *levodopa* and *bromocriptine* might induce or exacerbate psychotic symptoms. A study in 18 subjects and review of the literature suggested that bromocriptine can be used safely in patients at risk of psychotic illness provided they are clinically stable and maintained on antipsychotics.[1] Conversely, antipsychotics might antagonise the effects of dopaminergics; diminished therapeutic effects of levodopa have been noted with several antipsychotics (see p.1171) and thioridazine has been reported to oppose the prolactin-lowering action of bromocriptine (see p.1166).

Additive antimuscarinic side-effects are obviously a risk when antimuscarinic antiparkinsonian drugs are given with antipsychotics. Although these are generally mild, serious reactions have occurred. *Benzhexol [trihexyphenidyl]*[2] and *orphenadrine*[3] have both been reported to decrease plasma concentrations of chlorpromazine, possibly by interfering with absorption from the gastrointestinal tract. Reports suggesting that antimuscarinics may antagonise the antipsychotic effects of antipsychotics at the neurotransmitter level require substantiating.

1. Perovich RM, *et al.* The behavioral toxicity of bromocriptine in patients with psychiatric illness. *J Clin Psychopharmacol* 1989; **9:** 417–22.
2. Rivera-Calimlim L, *et al.* Effects of mode of management on plasma chlorpromazine in psychiatric patients. *Clin Pharmacol Ther* 1973; **14:** 978–86.
3. Loga S, *et al.* Interactions of orphenadrine and phenobarbitone with chlorpromazine: plasma concentrations and effects in man. *Br J Clin Pharmacol* 1975; **2:** 197–208.

Antipsychotics. Elevated plasma levels of haloperidol were reported[1] in a patient being treated for schizophrenia when *chlorpromazine* or *clozapine* were also given.

1. Allen SA. Effect of chlorpromazine and clozapine on plasma concentrations of haloperidol in a patient with schizophrenia. *J Clin Pharmacol* 2000; **40:** 1296–7.

Antivirals. *Ritonavir* may increase the plasma concentration of some antipsychotics. The increases expected for pimozide were considered by the manufacturer of ritonavir to be large enough to recommend that these drugs should not be used together. The UK prescribing information for ritonavir gives a similar warning with respect to clozapine (but see p.673 for evidence to the contrary). Other antipsychotics predicted to have increases include haloperidol, perphenazine, risperidone, and thioridazine and it was recommended that monitoring of drug concentrations and/or adverse effects were required when used with ritonavir.

Beta blockers. When given together, chlorpromazine and propranolol may mutually inhibit the liver metabolism of the other drug. *Propranolol* has been reported to increase plasma concentrations of chlorpromazine[1] and thioridazine,[2,3] and *pindolol* to increase plasma-thioridazine concentrations.[4] Neither beta blocker tested had a significant effect on haloperidol concentrations,[3,4] although there is a report of severe hypotension or cardiopulmonary arrest occurring on 3 occasions in a schizophrenic patient given haloperidol and propranolol concomitantly.[5] The clinical significance of antipsychotic-beta blocker interactions is unclear.

For the effect of chlorpromazine on propranolol, see under Beta Blockers, p.847.

There is an increased risk of arrhythmias when antipsychotics are given with other drugs which prolong the QT interval. The concomitant use of antipsychotics, and pimozide in particular, with *sotalol* should be avoided.

1. Peet M, *et al.* Pharmacokinetic interaction between propranolol and chlorpromazine in schizophrenic patients. *Lancet* 1980; **ii:** 978.
2. Silver JM, *et al.* Elevation of thioridazine plasma levels by propranolol. *Am J Psychiatry* 1986; **143:** 1290–2.
3. Greendyke RM, Kanter DR. Plasma propranolol levels and their effect on plasma thioridazine and haloperidol concentrations. *J Clin Psychopharmacol* 1987; **7:** 178–82.
4. Greendyke RM, Gulya A. Effect of pindolol administration on serum levels of thioridazine, haloperidol, phenytoin, and phenobarbital. *J Clin Psychiatry* 1988; **49:** 105–7.
5. Alexander HE, *et al.* Hypotension and cardiopulmonary arrest associated with concurrent haloperidol and propranolol therapy. *JAMA* 1984; **252:** 87–8.

Buspirone. The manufacturers have reported that concomitant administration of haloperidol and buspirone has resulted in increased serum haloperidol concentrations. However, while some[1] found the mean rise in serum-haloperidol concentrations to be 26%, that observed by others[2] was not statistically significant.

1. Goff DC, *et al.* An open trial of buspirone added to neuroleptics in schizophrenic patients. *J Clin Psychopharmacol* 1991; **11:** 193–7.
2. Huang HF, *et al.* Lack of pharmacokinetic interaction between buspirone and haloperidol in patients with schizophrenia. *J Clin Pharmacol* 1996; **36:** 963–9.

Cimetidine. Despite expectations that cimetidine might reduce the metabolism of chlorpromazine, mean steady-state plasma concentrations of chlorpromazine fell rather than rose

in 8 patients given cimetidine for 7 days in addition to regular chlorpromazine therapy.[1] The explanation was probably that cimetidine interfered with chlorpromazine absorption. Excessive sedation, necessitating a reduction in chlorpromazine dosage, has been reported[2] after addition of cimetidine to the drug therapy of 2 chronic schizophrenics.

1. Howes CA, *et al.* Reduced steady-state plasma concentrations of chlorpromazine and indomethacin in patients receiving cimetidine. *Eur J Clin Pharmacol* 1983; **24:** 99–102.
2. Byrne A, O'Shea B. Adverse interaction between cimetidine and chlorpromazine in two cases of chronic schizophrenia. *Br J Psychiatry* 1989; **155:** 413–15.

Cocaine. The risk of antipsychotic-induced dystonic reactions may be increased in cocaine abusers. Dystonia occurred in 6 of 7 cocaine abusers treated with haloperidol.[1]

1. Kumor K, *et al.* Haloperidol-induced dystonia in cocaine addicts. *Lancet* 1986; **ii:** 1341–2.

Desferrioxamine. Loss of consciousness lasting 48 to 72 hours occurred in 2 patients given prochlorperazine during desferrioxamine therapy.[1] Prochlorperazine may enhance the removal of transition metals from brain cells by desferrioxamine.

1. Blake DR, *et al.* Cerebral and ocular toxicity induced by desferrioxamine. *Q J Med* 1985; **56:** 345–55.

Disulfiram. A psychotic patient, previously maintained with plasma-perphenazine concentrations of 2 to 3 nanomoles per mL on a dose of 8 mg twice daily by mouth, was readmitted with subtherapeutic plasma-perphenazine concentrations of less than 1 nanomole per mL, despite unchanged dosage, following concomitant disulfiram therapy.[1] The concentration of the sulfoxide metabolite of perphenazine was much increased. Following a change from oral to intramuscular perphenazine therapy there was a substantial clinical improvement associated with a return to therapeutic plasma concentrations of perphenazine and a fall in concentration of the metabolite. Disulfiram appears to greatly enhance biotransformation of perphenazine given by mouth to inactive metabolites, but parenteral administration avoids the 'first-pass' effect in the liver.

1. Hansen LB, Larsen N-E. Metabolic interaction between perphenazine and disulfiram. *Lancet* 1982; **ii:** 1472.

General anaesthetics. A schizophrenic patient without a history of epilepsy who was receiving chlorpromazine by mouth and flupentixol depot injection had a convulsive seizure when given *enflurane* anaesthesia.[1]

1. Vohra SB. Convulsions after enflurane in a schizophrenic patient receiving neuroleptics. *Can J Anaesth* 1994; **41:** 420–2.

Naltrexone. Two patients maintained on thioridazine experienced intense sleepiness and lethargy after receiving 2 doses of naltrexone.[1]

1. Maany I, *et al.* Interaction between thioridazine and naltrexone. *Am J Psychiatry* 1987; **144:** 966.

NSAIDs. A report of severe drowsiness and confusion in patients given haloperidol with *indometacin*.[1]

1. Bird HA, *et al.* Drowsiness due to haloperidol/indomethacin in combination. *Lancet* 1983; **i:** 830–1.

Opioid analgesics. For reference to the effects of phenothiazines on *pethidine*, see p.76.

Piperazine. Caution has been advised when giving piperazine to patients receiving phenothiazines because of the possibility that piperazine might enhance their adverse effects. There has been an isolated report[1] of convulsions associated with the use of chlorpromazine in a child who had received piperazine several days earlier. Subsequent *animal*[1-3] studies produced conflicting evidence for an interaction but one worker[3] concluded that an interaction would only be clinically significant when high concentrations of piperazine were reached in the body.

1. Boulos BM, Davis LE. Hazard of simultaneous administration of phenothiazine and piperazine. *N Engl J Med* 1969; **280:** 1245–6.
2. Armbrecht BH. Reaction between piperazine and chlorpromazine. *N Engl J Med* 1970; **282:** 1490–1.
3. Sturman G. Interaction between piperazine and chlorpromazine. *Br J Pharmacol* 1974; **50:** 153–5.

Sympathomimetics. For reference to the possible interaction between phenothiazines and *adrenaline [epinephrine]*, see Treatment of Adverse Effects, above.

A 27-year-old woman with schizophrenia and T-wave abnormality of the heart,[1] receiving thioridazine 100 mg daily with procyclidine 2.5 mg twice daily, died from ventricular fibrillation within 2 hours of taking a single dose of a preparation reported to contain chlorpheniramine [chlorphenamine] maleate 4 mg with *phenylpropanolamine hydrochloride* 50 mg (Contac C), concurrently with thioridazine.

1. Chouinard G, *et al.* Death attributed to ventricular arrhythmia induced by thioridazine in combination with a single Contac C capsule. *Can Med Assoc J* 1978; **119:** 729–31.

Tobacco smoking. Smoking has been shown to decrease the incidence of chlorpromazine-induced sedation[1,2] and orthostatic hypotension.[2] Studies indicate that the clearance of chlorpromazine,[3] fluphenazine,[4] tiotixene,[5] and haloperidol[6] may be increased in patients who smoke. It has been suggested that some of the components of smoke may act as liver-enzyme inducers. The clinical significance of this effect is unclear but the possible need to use increased doses in smokers should be borne in mind.

1. Swett C. Drowsiness due to chlorpromazine in relation to cigarette smoking: a report from the Boston Collaborative Drug Surveillance Program. *Arch Gen Psychiatry* 1974; **31:** 211–13.
2. Pantuck EJ, *et al.* Cigarette smoking and chlorpromazine disposition and actions. *Clin Pharmacol Ther* 1982; **31:** 533–8.
3. Chetty M, *et al.* Smoking and body weight influence the clearance of chlorpromazine. *Eur J Clin Pharmacol* 1994; **46:** 523–6.
4. Ereshefsky L, *et al.* Effects of smoking on fluphenazine clearance in psychiatric inpatients. *Biol Psychiatry* 1985; **20:** 329–32.
5. Ereshefsky L, *et al.* Thiothixene pharmacokinetic interactions: a study of hepatic enzyme inducers, clearance inhibitors, and demographic variables. *J Clin Psychopharmacol* 1991; **11:** 296–301.
6. Jann MW, *et al.* Effects of smoking on haloperidol and reduced haloperidol plasma concentrations and haloperidol clearance. *Psychopharmacology (Berl)* 1986; **90:** 468–70.

Vitamins. Administration of ascorbic acid, for vitamin C deficiency, to a patient receiving fluphenazine for bipolar disorder was associated with a fall in serum concentrations of fluphenazine and a deterioration of behaviour.[1]

1. Dysken MW, *et al.* Drug interaction between ascorbic acid and fluphenazine. *JAMA* 1979; **241:** 2008.

Xanthine-containing beverages. Studies *in vitro* have shown precipitation of some antipsychotics from solution by addition of coffee and tea.[1,2] However, in a study of 16 patients taking antipsychotics no correlation could be found between plasma-antipsychotic concentrations or behaviour and tea or coffee consumption.[3]

1. Kulhanek F, *et al.* Precipitation of antipsychotic drugs in interaction with coffee or tea. *Lancet* 1979; **ii:** 1130.
2. Lasswell WL, *et al.* In vitro interaction of neuroleptics and tricyclic antidepressants with coffee, tea, and gallotannic acid. *J Pharm Sci* 1984; **73:** 1056–8.
3. Bowen S, *et al.* Effect of coffee and tea on blood levels and efficacy of antipsychotic drugs. *Lancet* 1981; **i:** 1217–18.

Pharmacokinetics

Chlorpromazine is readily, although sometimes erratically, absorbed from the gastrointestinal tract; peak plasma concentrations are attained 2 to 4 hours after ingestion. It is subject to considerable first-pass metabolism in the gut wall and is also extensively metabolised in the liver and is excreted in the urine and bile in the form of numerous active and inactive metabolites; there is some evidence of enterohepatic recycling. Owing to the first-pass effect, plasma concentrations following oral administration are much lower than those following intramuscular administration. Moreover, there is very wide intersubject variation in plasma concentrations of chlorpromazine; no simple correlation has been found between plasma concentrations of chlorpromazine and its metabolites, and their therapeutic effect (see Administration under Uses and Administration, below). Paths of metabolism of chlorpromazine include hydroxylation and conjugation with glucuronic acid, *N*-oxidation, oxidation of a sulfur atom, and dealkylation. Although the plasma half-life of chlorpromazine itself has been reported to be about 30 hours, elimination of the metabolites may be very prolonged. There is limited evidence that chlorpromazine induces its own metabolism.

Chlorpromazine is about 95 to 98% bound to plasma proteins. It is widely distributed in the body and crosses the blood-brain barrier to achieve higher concentrations in the brain than in the plasma. Chlorpromazine and its metabolites also cross the placental barrier and are distributed into breast milk.

◊ References.
1. Rivera-Calimlim L, *et al.* Plasma chlorpromazine concentrations in children with behavioral disorders and mental illness. *Clin Pharmacol Ther* 1979; **26:** 114–21.
2. Furlanut M, *et al.* Chlorpromazine disposition in relation to age in children. *Clin Pharmacokinet* 1990; **18:** 329–31.
3. Caccia S, Garattini S. Formation of active metabolites of psychotropic drugs: an updated review of their significance. *Clin Pharmacokinet* 1990; **18:** 434–59.
4. Yeung PK-F, *et al.* Pharmacokinetics of chlorpromazine and key metabolites. *Eur J Clin Pharmacol* 1993; **45:** 563–9.

Uses and Administration

Chlorpromazine is a phenothiazine antipsychotic. It has a wide range of activity arising from its depressant actions on the CNS and its alpha-adrenergic blocking and antimuscarinic activities. Chlorpromazine is a dopamine inhibitor and stimulates the release of prolactin. The turnover of dopamine in the brain is also increased. There is some evidence that the antagonism of central dopaminergic function, especially at the D_2-dopaminergic receptor, is related to therapeutic effect in psychotic conditions. Chlorpromazine possesses sedative properties but patients usually develop tolerance rapidly to the sedation. It has antiemetic, serotonin-blocking, and weak antihistaminic properties and slight ganglion-blocking activity. It inhibits the heat-regulating centre so that the patient tends to acquire the temperature of the surroundings (poikilothermy). Chlorpromazine can relax skeletal muscle.

Chlorpromazine is widely used in the management of psychotic conditions. It is used in acute and chronic schizophrenia (p.651) and reduces acute mania, as in bipolar disorder (p.271). It is used to control severely disturbed, agitated, or violent behaviour (p.650) and is sometimes given in other psychiatric conditions and as an adjunct for the short-term treatment of severe anxiety (but see also p.649).

Chlorpromazine is an antiemetic and is used to control some forms of nausea and vomiting (p.1206); it is ineffective in motion sickness.

Chlorpromazine is effective in the alleviation of intractable hiccup (below).

Chlorpromazine has been given to reduce pre-operative anxiety.

Chlorpromazine has also been used as an adjunct in the treatment of tetanus (p.142 and p.1332) and to control symptoms in acute intermittent porphyria (p.1011).

Chlorpromazine is administered as the hydrochloride by mouth or injection, as the embonate by mouth in doses equivalent to those of the hydrochloride, and as the base rectally by suppository.

Dosage varies both with the individual and with the purpose for which the drug is being used. In most patients with psychiatric conditions oral treatment may be used from the start, typically commencing with a dosage of 25 mg of the hydrochloride, or its equivalent as the embonate, three times daily and increasing as necessary; daily doses of 75 mg may be given as a single dose at night. In some patients doses of 10 mg three times daily may be adequate. Maintenance doses, when required, usually range from 25 to 100 mg three times daily, although psychotic patients may require daily doses of up to 1 g or more. Doses of 10 to 25 mg every 4 to 6 hours are recommended for control of nausea and vomiting.

For parenteral use, deep intramuscular injection is preferable, but diluted solutions have sometimes been given by slow intravenous infusion for indications such as tetanus, severe intractable hiccup, or nausea and vomiting associated with surgery. Subcutaneous injection is contra-indicated. After injection of chlorpromazine, patients should remain in the supine position for at least 30 minutes. The usual dose by intramuscular injection is 25 to 50 mg repeated every 6 to 8 hours if required.

If intractable hiccup does not respond to 25 to 50 mg three or four times daily by mouth for 2 to 3 days then 25 to 50 mg may be administered intramuscularly; if this fails 25 to 50 mg in 500 to 1000 mL of 0.9% sodium chloride intravenous infusion should be given by slow intravenous infusion, with the patient supine and careful monitoring of the blood pressure.

If the oral and parenteral routes are not suitable chlorpromazine may be administered rectally as suppositories containing 100 mg of chlorpromazine base; this is stated to have an effect comparable with 40 to 50 mg of the hydrochloride by mouth or 20 to 25 mg intramuscularly. Up to 4 suppositories may be given in 24 hours.

Initial doses of chlorpromazine of one-third to one-half the normal adult dose have been recommended for elderly or debilitated patients; doses should be increased more gradually.

Children aged 1 to 12 years may be given chlorpromazine hydrochloride in a dose of 500 µg per kg body-weight every 4 to 6 hours by mouth or every 6 to 8 hours by intramuscular injection, but for psychiatric indications the oral dose for children aged over 5 years is usually one-third to one-half the adult dose. Daily doses should not normally exceed 40 mg of chlorpromazine hydrochloride for children aged 1 to 5 years or 75 mg for children over 5 years of age. Suppositories containing 25 mg of chlorpromazine base are available in some countries for use in children.

Action. The therapeutic effects of antipsychotics appear to be mediated, at least in part, by interference with dopamine transmission in the brain. Chlorpromazine, thioridazine, and thioxanthene derivatives have relatively equal affinity for D_1 or D_2 receptors, although their metabolites tend to be more potent as D_2 blockers.[1] Butyrophenones and diphenylbutylpiperidines are relatively selective for D_2 receptors, and the substituted benzamides such as sulpiride and remoxipride are highly D_2-specific. Clozapine is a relatively weak inhibitor of D_2 receptors but its actions are complex and it has a high affinity for a number of different receptors including serotonin$_2$ (5-HT$_2$) receptors.[2] Risperidone has a high affinity both for 5-HT$_2$ and D_2 receptors.[2]

The traditional hypothesis of the action of antipsychotics has been that blockade of D_2 receptors in the limbic and cortical regions is responsible for the antipsychotic effects, and that extrapyramidal motor side-effects result from blockade of D_2 receptors in the striatum (a typical motor region of the basal ganglia).[3] Modification of prolactin secretion results from blockade of D_2 receptors in the anterior pituitary. However, this hypothesis cannot satisfactorily account for the pharmacological profiles of atypical antipsychotics such as clozapine, remoxipride, risperidone, and sulpiride. Their mode of action or reasons for their relative lack of extrapyramidal effects still remain largely unclear.[2]

Unlike phenothiazines and butyrophenones, the diphenylbutylpiperidines are potent calcium antagonists. This action may explain the ability of this group of drugs to relieve the negative symptoms of schizophrenia.[4]

Division of antipsychotics into low- and high-potency drugs is discussed under Administration, below. For reference to the actions of antipsychotics on neuroendocrine function, see Effects on Endocrine Function under Adverse Effects, above.

1. Ereshefsky L, *et al.* Pathophysiologic basis for schizophrenia and the efficacy of antipsychotics. *Clin Pharm* 1990; **9:** 682–707.
2. Kerwin RW. The new atypical antipsychotics: a lack of extrapyramidal side-effects and new routes in schizophrenia research. *Br J Psychiatry* 1994; **164:** 141–8.
3. Anonymous. Now we understand antipsychotics? *Lancet* 1990; **336:** 1222–3.
4. Snyder SH. Drug and neurotransmitter receptors: new perspectives with clinical relevance. *JAMA* 1989; **261:** 3126–9.

Administration. The traditional antipsychotics are often divided into:

- **low-potency** drugs (phenothiazines with an aliphatic or piperidine side-chain or thioxanthenes with an aliphatic side-chain)
- **high-potency** drugs (butyrophenones, diphenylbutylpiperidines, and phenothiazines or thioxanthenes with a piperazine side-chain)

At doses with equipotent antipsychotic activity, the low-potency drugs are more prone to cause sedation and antimuscarinic or α-adrenergic-blocking effects than the high-potency drugs. However, they are associated with a lower incidence of extrapyramidal effects, with the exception of tardive dyskinesia which is likely to occur to the same extent with all conventional antipsychotics.

Equivalent doses of antipsychotics quoted in the literature have varied considerably. In the UK the following daily doses of oral antipsychotics have been suggested to have approximately equipotent antipsychotic activity for doses up to the maximum licensed doses:

- chlorpromazine hydrochloride 100 mg
- clozapine 50 mg
- haloperidol 2 to 3 mg
- loxapine 10 to 20 mg
- pimozide 2 mg
- risperidone 0.5 to 1 mg
- sulpiride 200 mg
- thioridazine 100 mg
- trifluoperazine 5 mg.

In specialist psychiatric units where very high doses are required the equivalent dose of haloperidol might be up to 10 mg. It should be noted that all patients receiving pimozide require an annual ECG and all those receiving more than 16 mg of pimozide daily require periodic ECGs (see p.699).

Suggested equipotent doses of intramuscular depot antipsychotics are:

- flupentixol decanoate 40 mg every 2 weeks
- fluphenazine decanoate 25 mg every 2 weeks
- haloperidol (as the decanoate) 100 mg every 4 weeks
- pipotiazine palmitate 50 mg every 4 weeks
- zuclopenthixol decanoate 200 mg every 2 weeks.

It has been noted[1] that *high doses* of antipsychotics (greater than the equivalent of 600 mg of chlorpromazine daily) are generally not necessary for the treatment (both initial and maintenance) of psychotic disorders, and may be associated with an increased risk of side-effects as well as with a diminished clinical response. However, if high doses of antipsychotics have to be used, then doses should be increased gradually and with caution and under the supervision of a specialist with facilities for emergency resuscitation available. The Royal College of Psychiatrists in the UK has issued advice for those considering the use of high doses of antipsychotics.[2]

- When patients have failed to respond to recommended doses of two different antipsychotics the diagnosis, patient compliance, and the duration of treatment already given should be reviewed before increasing the dose
- Alternative approaches to treatment including the use of adjuvant therapy and newer antipsychotics such as clozapine should also be considered
- Contra-indications to high-dose therapy such as cardiac disease and hepatic and renal impairment and other risk factors such as obesity and old age should be borne in mind
- An ECG should be carried out to exclude QT prolongation and repeated every 1 to 3 months while the dose remains high. The dose should be reduced if a prolonged QT interval develops
- Regular checks on pulse, blood pressure, temperature, and hydration are also advised
- If possible dosage should be increased gradually at intervals of at least one week
- The use of high-dose therapy should be considered as a limited course. The patient should be reviewed regularly and the dose reduced back to accepted levels after 3 months if there has been no improvement

The existence of a *therapeutic range* (or therapeutic window) has not been demonstrated for most antipsychotics (with the possible exception of haloperidol[3]), and plasma concentrations of these drugs must be interpreted with caution.[1,3] Many factors make it difficult to establish a meaningful correlation between dose, plasma concentrations, and clinical improvement. These include incomplete absorption, first-pass effect, enzyme induction, the presence of active and inactive metabolites, ethnic group, smoking, and factors occurring at the receptor level.[3]

1. Baldessarini RJ, *et al.* Significance of neuroleptic dose and plasma level in the pharmacological treatment of psychoses. *Arch Gen Psychiatry* 1988; **45:** 79–91.
2. The Royal College of Psychiatrists. Consensus statement on the use of high dose antipsychotic medication. *Council Report CR26* London: Royal College of Psychiatrists, October 1993. Also in: Thompson C. Royal College of Psychiatrists' Consensus Panel. The use of high-dose antipsychotic medication. *Br J Psychiatry* 1994; **164:** 448–58.
3. Sramek JJ, *et al.* Neuroleptic plasma concentrations and clinical response: in search of a therapeutic window. *Drug Intell Clin Pharm* 1988; **22:** 373–80.

Administration in children. For reference to the use of lytic cocktails containing chlorpromazine, promethazine, and pethidine and the view that alternatives should be considered in children, see under Pethidine, p.76.

Bipolar disorder. Patients with bipolar disorder (p.271) suffering from acute mania with coexisting psychotic features, agitation, or disruptive behaviour are usually treated with antipsychotics as they produce rapid control of symptoms. Typical drugs used include chlorpromazine, droperidol, or haloperidol.

Chorea. For a discussion of the management of various choreas, including mention of the use of phenothiazines such as chlorpromazine, see p.650.

Dyspnoea. It has been shown that in healthy subjects an oral dose of 25 mg of chlorpromazine hydrochloride can reduce exercise-induced breathlessness without affecting ventilation or causing sedation.[1] Some workers[2] have reported that chlorpromazine relieves air hunger in patients with advanced cancer and dyspnoea (p.69) unresponsive to other measures and, if required, can be used to sedate dying patients who have unrelieved distress. It is recommended that initial doses be small; 12.5 mg by slow intravenous injection or 25 mg by suppository may be given.

1. O'Neill PA, *et al.* Chlorpromazine—a specific effect on breathlessness? *Br J Clin Pharmacol* 1985; **19:** 793–7.
2. Walsh D. Dyspnoea in advanced cancer. *Lancet* 1993; **342:** 450–1.

Dystonia. Antipsychotics such as phenothiazines, haloperidol, or pimozide are sometimes useful in the treatment of idiopathic dystonia (p.1173) in patients who have failed to respond to other drugs.[1] However, they often act non-specifically, damping down excessive movements by causing a degree of drug-induced parkinsonism and there is the risk of adding drug-induced extrapyramidal disorders to the dystonia being treated (see Extrapyramidal Disorders under Adverse Effects, above).

1. Marsden CD, Quinn NP. The dystonias. *BMJ* 1990; **300:** 139–44.

Eclampsia and pre-eclampsia. Drug combinations known as lytic cocktails have been used in many countries for the management of pre-eclampsia and imminent eclampsia. The cocktail has usually consisted of a combination of chlorpromazine, pethidine, and/or promethazine. However, phenothiazines are not generally recommended late in pregnancy and other treatments are preferred for hypertension (see Hypertension in Pregnancy, under Hypertension, p.802); the management of eclampsia, which is the convulsive phase, is discussed on p.341.

Headache. The phenothiazines chlorpromazine and prochlorperazine have been used in migraine to control severe nausea and vomiting unresponsive to antiemetics such as metoclopramide and domperidone (see p.449). Parenteral phenothiazines may also relieve the pain of severe migraine attacks unresponsive to parenteral dihydroergotamine or sumatriptan. Some phenothiazines have also been tried in the management of other types of headache including cluster headache (p.449) and tension-type headache (p.450).

References.
1. Caviness VS, O'Brien P. Cluster headache: response to chlorpromazine. *Headache* 1980; **20:** 128–31.
2. Lane PL, *et al.* Comparative efficacy of chlorpromazine and meperidine with dimenhydrinate in migraine headache. *Ann Emerg Med* 1989; **18:** 360–5.
3. Jones J, *et al.* Randomized double-blind trial of intravenous prochlorperazine for the treatment of acute headache. *JAMA* 1989; **261:** 1174–6.
4. Bell R, *et al.* A comparative trial of three agents in the treatment of acute migraine headache. *Ann Emerg Med* 1990; **19:** 1079–82.
5. Stiell IG, *et al.* Methotrimeprazine versus meperidine and dimenhydrinate in the treatment of severe migraine: a randomized, controlled trial. *Ann Emerg Med* 1991; **20:** 1201–5.
6. Jones EB, *et al.* Safety and efficacy of rectal prochlorperazine for the treatment of migraine in the emergency department. *Ann Emerg Med* 1994; **24:** 237–41.
7. Coppola M, *et al.* Randomized, placebo-controlled evaluation of prochlorperazine versus metoclopramide for emergency department treatment of migraine headache. *Ann Emerg Med* 1995; **26:** 541–6.

Hiccup. A hiccup is an involuntary spasmodic contraction of the diaphragm which causes a sudden inspiration of air which is then checked abruptly by closure of the glottis. Hiccups often have a simple cause such as gastric distension and usually resolve spontaneously or respond to simple measures. Intractable hiccups may stem from a serious underlying cause such as brain disorders, metabolic or endocrine disturbances, CNS infections, and oesophageal or other gastrointestinal disorders. Other precipitants include anaesthesia or drug therapy.

Treatment of intractable hiccups should initially be aimed at controlling or removing the underlying cause including the relief of gastric distension or oesophageal obstruction.[1-4] Measures which raise carbon dioxide pressure such as breath holding, rebreathing, or alteration of normal respiratory rhythm can be effective. Stimulation of the pharynx can also interrupt hiccups and may explain the action of a host of remedies such as sipping iced water, gargling, and swallowing granulated sugar. Many drugs have been tried in the treatment of hiccups but evidence of efficacy is largely from anecdotal reports or uncontrolled studies. However, the following treatment protocol[5] has been formulated for intractable hiccups from a review of the early literature and the authors' experience:

- correct any metabolic abnormality, then granulated sugar should be swallowed dry; if this is successful the sugar should be repeated if hiccups recur
- if not effective, pass nasogastric tube, decompress stomach, then irritate pharynx; if successful, repeat if hiccups recur
- if stimulation is unsuccessful, give chlorpromazine 25 to 50 mg intravenously; repeat up to 3 times if necessary; if parenteral therapy is effective maintain on chlorpromazine by mouth for 10 days (some manufacturers recommend the use of oral therapy first and if symptoms persist for 2 to 3 days they then recommend one dose by the intramuscular route followed if necessary by a slow intravenous infusion of a dilute solution—see under Uses and Administration, above)
- if hiccups are not controlled by chlorpromazine give metoclopramide 10 mg intravenously and if successful maintain on metoclopramide by mouth for 10 days
- if metoclopramide is not effective give quinidine 200 mg by mouth 4 times daily
- if this fails consider left phrenic nerve block and crush.

In later discussions[1,3] chlorpromazine still emerged as the most consistently effective drug treatment; metoclopramide appeared to be an acceptable second choice and nifedipine an appropriate third choice,[3] although haloperidol has also been considered to be of value.[1,4] Other phenothiazine drugs which have been used for intractable hiccup include perphenazine and promazine. It was also considered that clonazepam, carbamazepine, phenytoin, and valproic acid might be of value, especially in neurogenic hiccups.[1] Further reports had described some beneficial results with amitriptyline, amantadine, and baclofen.

Other methods which have been used in the treatment of hiccups include swallowing a solution of lignocaine [lidocaine].

1. Howard RS. Persistent hiccups: if excluding or treating any underlying pathology fails try chlorpromazine. *BMJ* 1992; **305:** 1237–8.
2. Rousseau P. Hiccups. *South Med J* 1995; **88:** 175–81.
3. Friedman NL. Hiccups: a treatment review. *Pharmacotherapy* 1996; **16:** 986–95.
4. WHO. Hiccup. In: *Symptom relief in terminal illness.* Geneva: WHO, 1998.
5. Williamson BWA, Macintyre IMC. Management of intractable hiccup. *BMJ* 1977; **2:** 501–3.

Lesch-Nyhan syndrome. The Lesch-Nyhan syndrome is an inherited disorder caused by a complete deficiency of hypoxanthine-guanine phosphoribosyl transferase, an enzyme involved in purine metabolism. It is characterised by hyperuricaemia, spasticity, choreoathetosis, self-mutilation, and mental retardation. The hyperuricaemia (see p.397) can be controlled by drugs such as allopurinol but there appears to be no effective treatment for the neurological deficits. It has been suggested that the behavioural problems might be associated with alterations in the brain's dopamine system. There have been rare reports of improvement in self-mutilation in patients given anti-

psychotics or antiepileptics such as carbamazepine and gabapentin.

References.
1. Nyhan WL, Wong DF. New approaches to understanding Lesch-Nyhan disease. *N Engl J Med* 1996; **334:** 1602–4.

Migraine. See under Headache, above.

Nausea and vomiting. Many antipsychotics, with the notable exception of thioridazine, have antiemetic properties and have been used in the prevention and treatment of nausea and vomiting (p.1206) arising from a variety of causes such as radiation sickness, malignancy, and emesis caused by drugs, including antineoplastics and opioid analgesics. Reference to the risk to the fetus of antiemetic therapy with phenothiazines during pregnancy can be found under Precautions, above.

Schizophrenia. Classical antipsychotics such as chlorpromazine, haloperidol, and thioridazine have been the traditional drug treatment of choice for patients with schizophrenia (p.651); however, with the advent of the atypical antipsychotics such as clozapine and risperidone there has been much debate over which should be used as first-line therapy. There is little difference in efficacy between the classical antipsychotics, but thioridazine is now restricted to second-line treatment of schizophrenia because of the risk of cardiotoxicity.

Substance dependence. ALCOHOL. For advice against the use of antipsychotics for alcohol withdrawal, see p.1131.

OPIOIDS. In a discussion of neonatal abstinence syndrome (p.67), it was observed in 1986 that, although opioids, diazepam, and phenobarbital were widely used in the USA for the management of this condition, chlorpromazine had tended to be the preferred treatment in the UK.[1] This was still true as late as 1996, although practice varied widely.[2] The following dosage schedule has been suggested: chlorpromazine is initiated with a loading dose of 3 mg per kg body-weight, followed by a total maintenance dose of 3 mg per kg by mouth daily, divided in 4 or 6 doses. This dose may be increased by 3 mg per kg daily if withdrawal symptoms are particularly severe. Once stabilised a reduction in the dose of chlorpromazine by 2 mg per kg every third day is attempted. Complications of phenothiazine usage have been notably absent, although rarely seizures may occur.

1. Rivers RPA. Neonatal opiate withdrawal. *Arch Dis Child* 1986; **61:** 1236–9.
2. Morrison CL, Siney C. A survey of the management of neonatal opiate withdrawal in England and Wales. *Eur J Pediatr* 1996; **155:** 323–6.

Taste disorders. Disturbances of the sense of taste may be broadly divided into either loss or distortion of taste. Loss of taste may be either complete (ageusia) or partial (hypogeusia). Distortion of taste (dysgeusia) may occur as aliageusia in which stimuli such as food or drink produce an inappropriate taste or as phantogeusia in which an unpleasant taste is not associated with an external stimuli and is sometimes referred to as a gustatory hallucination. Taste disturbances have many causes including infections, metabolic or nutritional disturbances, radiation, CNS disorders, neoplasms, drug therapy, or may occur as a consequence of normal aging.[1] Management primarily consists of treatment of any underlying disorder. Withdrawal of offending drug therapy is commonly associated with resolution but occasionally effects persist and may require treatment.[2] Zinc or vitamin therapy has been used but there is insufficient evidence to indicate efficacy[1,3] for taste disturbances secondary to drug therapy or medical conditions that do not involve low zinc or vitamin concentrations. Phantogeusia might be linked to excessive activity of dopaminergic receptors as it has been reported[4] to respond to short-term treatment with small doses of drugs such as haloperidol or pimozide.

1. Schiffman SS. Taste and smell losses in normal aging and disease. *JAMA* 1997; **278:** 1357–62.
2. Henkin RI. Drug-induced taste and smell disorders: incidence, mechanisms and management related primarily to treatment of sensory receptor dysfunction. *Drug Safety* 1994; **11:** 318–77.
3. Heyneman CA. Zinc deficiency and taste disorders. *Ann Pharmacother* 1996; **30:** 186–7.
4. Henkin RI. Salty and bitter taste. *JAMA* 1991; **265:** 2253.

Preparations

BP 2001: Chlorpromazine Injection; Chlorpromazine Oral Solution; Chlorpromazine Suppositories; Chlorpromazine Tablets;
USP 25: Chlorpromazine Hydrochloride Injection; Chlorpromazine Hydrochloride Oral Concentrate; Chlorpromazine Hydrochloride Syrup; Chlorpromazine Hydrochloride Tablets; Chlorpromazine Suppositories.

Proprietary Preparations (details are given in Part 3)
Aust.: Largactil; *Austral.:* Largactil; *Belg.:* Largactil†; *Braz.:* Amplictil; *Canad.:* Chlorpromanyl; Largactil; *Denm.:* Largactil; *Fin.:* Klorproman; *Fr.:* Largactil; *Ger.:* Propaphenin; *Hong Kong:* Largactil; *Irl.:* Clonazine; Largactil; *Israel:* Taroctyl; *Ital.:* Largactil; Prozin; *Mex.:* Largactil; *Neth.:* Largactil; *Norw.:* Largactil; *NZ:* Largactil; *Port.:* Largactil; Largatrex; *S.Afr.:* Largactil; *Singapore:* Matcine; *Spain:* Largactil; *Swed.:* Hibernal; *Switz.:* Chlorazin; Largactil†; *Thai.:* Chlorpromed; Matcine; Prozine; *UK:* Chloractil; Largactil; *USA:* Ormazine†; Thorazine.

Multi-ingredient: *Spain:* Diminex Balsamico†; Largatrex; *Thai.:* Ama.

Chlorprothixene (7024-s)

Chlorprothixene *(BAN, USAN, rINN).*
N-714; Ro-4-0403. (Z)-3-(2-Chlorothioxanthen-9-ylidene)-NN-dimethylpropylamine.
$C_{18}H_{18}ClNS = 315.9.$
CAS — 113-59-7.
ATC — N05AF03.

Chlorprothixene Hydrochloride (18327-h)

Chlorprothixene Hydrochloride *(BANM, rINNM).*
Chlorprothixeni Hydrochloridum.
$C_{18}H_{19}Cl_2NS = 352.3.$
Pharmacopoeias. In *Eur.* (see p.vi).

Pharmacopoeial description

Ph. Eur.: A white or almost white, crystalline powder. Soluble in water and in alcohol; slightly soluble in dichloromethane. A 1% solution in water has a pH of 4.4 to 5.2. Protect from light.

Chlorprothixene Mesilate (17494-s)

Chlorprothixene Mesilate *(BANM, rINNM).*
Chlorprothixene Mesylate; Chlorprothixenium Mesylicum.
$C_{19}H_{22}ClNO_3S_2,H_2O = 430.0.$

Adverse Effects, Treatment, and Precautions
As for Chlorpromazine, p.660.

Effects on the liver. A 59-year-old man receiving chlorprothixene (for the second time) for acute mania developed severe obstructive jaundice within a few days; he was also taking chlorpropamide, digoxin, and diuretics.[1] Chlorprothixene was considered the most likely cause of the jaundice, though chlorpropamide could not be excluded.

1. Ruddock DGS, Hoenig J. Chlorprothixene and obstructive jaundice. *BMJ* 1973; **1:** 231.

Interactions
As for Chlorpromazine, p.664.

Pharmacokinetics

Distribution into breast milk. Chlorprothixene and its sulfoxide metabolite were concentrated in the breast milk of 2 mothers receiving chlorprothixene 200 mg daily but it was calculated that the amount supplied to the nursing infant was only 0.1% of the maternal dose per kg body-weight.[1]

1. Matheson I, *et al.* Presence of chlorprothixene and its metabolites in breast milk. *Eur J Clin Pharmacol* 1984; **27:** 611–13.

Metabolism. Studies on the metabolism of chlorprothixene in *animals* and man.[1] In addition to the major metabolite chlorprothixene-sulfoxide, 2 further urinary metabolites were identified, namely N-desmethylchlorprothixene-sulfoxide and chlorprothixene-sulfoxide-N-oxide.

1. Raaflaub J. Zum Metabolismus des Chlorprothixen. *Arzneimittelforschung* 1967; **17:** 1393–5.

Uses and Administration

Chlorprothixene is a thioxanthene antipsychotic with general properties similar to those of the phenothiazine, chlorpromazine (p.665). It is used mainly in the treatment of psychoses (p.650). Some preparations of chlorprothixene are prepared with the aid of hydrochloric and/or lactic acid and may be stated to contain chlorprothixene hydrochloride or chlorprothixene lactate. Chlorprothixene acetate, chlorprothixene mesilate, and chlorprothixene citrate have also been used. Doses are usually expressed in terms of the equivalent amount of chlorprothixene. A usual initial dose by mouth for the treatment of psychoses is 15 to 50 mg three or four times daily, increased according to response; doses of up to 600 mg or more daily have been given in severe or resistant conditions. It may also be given intramuscularly in doses of 25 to 100 mg up to four times daily. Chlorprothixene should be used in reduced dosage for elderly or debilitated patients.

Preparations

Proprietary Preparations (details are given in Part 3)
Aust.: Truxal; Truxaletten; *Denm.:* Truxal; *Fin.:* Cloxan; Truxal; *Ger.:* Truxal; *Israel:* Truquil; *Neth.:* Truxal; *Norw.:* Truxal; *Swed.:* Truxal; *Switz.:* Truxal; Truxaletten.

Cinolazepam (9402-l)

Cinolazepam *(rINN).*
OX-373. 7-Chloro-5-(2-fluorophenyl)-2,3-dihydro-3-hydroxy-2-oxo-1H-1,4-benzodiazepine-1-propionitrile.
$C_{18}H_{13}ClFN_3O_2 = 357.8.$
CAS — 75696-02-5.
ATC — N05CD13.

Profile
Cinolazepam is a benzodiazepine derivative with general properties similar to those of diazepam (p.674).

Preparations

Proprietary Preparations (details are given in Part 3)
Aust.: Gerodorm.

The symbol † denotes a preparation no longer actively marketed

Clobazam (7025-w)

Clobazam (BAN, USAN, rINN).

H-4723; HR-376; LM-2717. 7-Chloro-1,5-dihydro-1-methyl-5-phenyl-1,5-benzodiazepine-2,4(3H)-dione.

$C_{16}H_{13}CIN_2O_2 = 300.7$.

CAS — 22316-47-8.

ATC — N05BA09.

Pharmacopoeias. In Br.

Pharmacopoeial description

BP 2001: A white crystalline powder. Very slightly soluble in water; soluble in alcohol and in methyl alcohol. A 1% suspension in water has a pH of 5.5 to 7.5.

Dependence and Withdrawal

As for Diazepam, p.675.

Adverse Effects, Treatment, and Precautions

As for Diazepam, p.675.

Effects on menstruation. Occasionally the use of clobazam before menstruation for catamenial epilepsy appeared to delay the period.[1]

1. Feely M. Prescribing anticonvulsant drugs 3: clonazepam and clobazam. *Prescribers' J* 1989; **29:** 111–15.

Effects on the skin. Report[1] of toxic epidermal necrolysis which developed in light-exposed areas in a patient being treated with clobazam.

1. Redondo P, *et al.* Photo-induced toxic epidermal necrolysis caused by clobazam. *Br J Dermatol* 1996; **135:** 999–1002.

Porphyria. Clobazam is considered to be unsafe in patients with porphyria although there is conflicting evidence of porphyrinogenicity.

Interactions

As for Diazepam, p.677.

Pharmacokinetics

Clobazam is well absorbed from the gastrointestinal tract and peak plasma concentrations have been reached 1 to 4 hours after oral administration. It is about 85% bound to plasma proteins. Clobazam is highly lipophilic and rapidly crosses the blood-brain barrier. It is metabolised in the liver by demethylation and hydroxylation but unlike the 1,4-benzodiazepines such as diazepam, clobazam, a 1,5-benzodiazepine, is hydroxylated at the 4-position rather than the 3-position (see also Metabolism, under Diazepam, p.680). Clobazam is excreted unchanged and as metabolites mainly in the urine. Mean half-lives of 18 hours and 42 hours have been reported for clobazam and its main active metabolite N-desmethylclobazam, respectively.

◊ References.

1. Greenblatt DJ, *et al.* Clinical pharmacokinetics of the newer benzodiazepines. *Clin Pharmacokinet* 1983; **8:** 233–52.
2. Ochs HR, *et al.* Single and multiple dose kinetics of clobazam, and clinical effects during multiple dosage. *Eur J Clin Pharmacol* 1984; **26:** 499–503.

Uses and Administration

Clobazam is a long-acting 1,5-benzodiazepine with uses similar to those of diazepam (a 1,4-benzodiazepine; see p.680). The usual dose for the short-term treatment of anxiety (p.649) is 20 to 30 mg daily given in divided doses or as a single dose at night; in severe conditions up to 60 mg daily has been given. Similar daily doses have been given as adjunctive therapy in the management of epilepsy.

Doses of 10 to 20 mg daily have been suggested in elderly or debilitated patients; in children aged 3 years or over not more than half the recommended adult dose may be given.

Epilepsy. Benzodiazepines are sometimes employed in the management of epilepsy (p.338), but their long-term use is limited by problems of sedation, dependence, and tolerance to the antiepileptic effects.

Clobazam, along with clonazepam, is one of the benzodiazepines most commonly used as an oral antiepileptic. Sedation appears to be less of a problem with clobazam than with clonazepam, and this advantage may make it more appropriate as adjunctive therapy for adults.[1] Clobazam is active against partial and generalised seizures in epilepsy of widely differing aetiology in patients of all ages but is usually only indicated for adjunctive therapy. Intermittent therapy with clobazam has been used successfully in women with catamenial epilepsy (seizures associated with menstruation). Short-term therapy may also be useful for patients whose epileptic attacks occur in clusters or as cover for special events. Clobazam has also been tried with some success in children with refractory epilepsy.[2,3]

1. Feely M. Prescribing anticonvulsant drugs 3: clonazepam and clobazam. *Prescribers' J* 1989; **29:** 111–15.
2. Munn R, Farrell K. Open study of clobazam in refractory epilepsy. *Pediatr Neurol* 1993; **9:** 465–9.
3. Sheth RD, *et al.* Clobazam for intractable pediatric epilepsy. *J Child Neurol* 1995; **10:** 205–8.

Phantom limb pain. There has been a mention[1] of the complete relief of phantom limb pain (p.7) refractory to other therapy in an elderly patient given clobazam 10 mg three times daily.

1. Rice-Oxley CP. The limited list: clobazam for phantom limb pain. *BMJ* 1986; **293:** 1309.

Preparations

BP 2001: Clobazam Capsules.

Proprietary Preparations (details are given in Part 3)
Aust.: Frisium; *Austral.:* Frisium; *Belg.:* Frisium; *Braz.:* Frisium; Urbanil; *Canad.:* Frisium; *Denm.:* Frisium; *Fin.:* Frisium; *Fr.:* Urbanyl; *Ger.:* Frisium; *Hong Kong:* Frisium; *Irl.:* Frisium; *Israel:* Frisium; *Ital.:* Frisium; *Mex.:* Frisium; Urbadan; *Neth.:* Frisium; Urbadan†; *NZ:* Frisium; *Port.:* Castilium; Urbanil; *S.Afr.:* Urbanol; *Singapore:* Frisium; *Spain:* Clarmyl†; Noiafren; *Switz.:* Urbanyl; *Thai.:* Frisium; *UK:* Frisium.

Clocapramine Hydrochloride (12582-z)

Clocapramine Hydrochloride (rINNM).

Chlorcarpipramine Hydrochloride; Y-4153. 1'-[3-(3-Chloro-10,11-dihydro-5H-dibenz[b,f]azepin-5-yl)propyl][1,4'-bipiperidine]-4'-carboxamide dihydrochloride monohydrate.

$C_{28}H_{37}CIN_4O,2HCl,H_2O = 572.0$.

CAS — 47739-98-0 (clocapramine); 28058-62-0 (clocapramine hydrochloride).

Pharmacopoeias. In Jpn.

Profile

Clocapramine is a chlorinated derivative of carpipramine (p.659). The hydrochloride has been given by mouth in the treatment of schizophrenia.

◊ References.

1. Yamagami S. A crossover study of clocapramine and haloperidol in chronic schizophrenia. *J Int Med Res* 1985; **13:** 301–10.
2. Yamagami S, *et al.* A single-blind study of clocapramine and sulpiride in hospitalized chronic schizophrenic patients. *Drugs Exp Clin Res* 1988; **14:** 707–13.

Clomethiazole (18200-w)

Clomethiazole (BAN, rINN).

Chlormethiazole. 5-(2-Chloroethyl)-4-methyl-1,3-thiazole.

$C_6H_8CINS = 161.7$.

CAS — 533-45-9.

ATC — N05CM02.

Pharmacopoeias. In Br.

Pharmacopoeial description

BP 2001: A colourless to slightly yellowish-brown liquid with a characteristic odour. Slightly soluble in water; miscible with alcohol, with chloroform, and with ether. A 0.5% solution in water has a pH of 5.5 to 7.0. Store at a temperature of 2° to 8°.

Clomethiazole Edisilate (4024-p)

Clomethiazole Edisilate (BANM, rINNM).

Chlormethiazole Edisylate; Chlormethiazole Ethanedisulphonate. 5-(2-Chloroethyl)-4-methylthiazole ethane-1,2-disulphonate.

$(C_6H_8CINS)_2,C_2H_6O_6S_2 = 513.5$.

CAS — 1867-58-9.

Pharmacopoeias. In Br. and Pol.

Pharmacopoeial description

BP 2001: A white crystalline powder with a characteristic odour. Freely soluble in water; soluble in alcohol; practically insoluble in ether.

Incompatibility. Several studies have demonstrated that clomethiazole edisilate may permeate through or be sorbed onto plastics used in intravenous infusion bags or giving sets.[1-4] The drug may also react with and soften the plastic.[1] The UK manufacturers of clomethiazole edisilate have suggested that thrombophlebitis, fever, and headache reported in young children during prolonged infusions may have been due to reaction with plastic giving sets and silastic cannulae, and recommend the use of a motor-driven glass syringe in preference to a plastic drip set in small children. If a plastic drip set is used in older patients it should be changed at least every 24 hours. In all cases, teflon intravenous cannulas should be used.

1. Lingam S, *et al.* Problems with intravenous chlormethiazole (Hemineurin) in status epilepticus. *BMJ* 1980; **280:** 155–6.
2. Tsuei SE, *et al.* Sorption of chlormethiazole by intravenous infusion giving sets. *Eur J Clin Pharmacol* 1980; **18:** 333–8.
3. Kowaluk EA, *et al.* Dynamics of chlormethiazole edisylate interaction with plastic infusion systems. *J Pharm Sci* 1984; **73:** 43–7.
4. Lee MG. Sorption of four drugs to polyvinyl chloride and polybutadiene intravenous administration sets. *Am J Hosp Pharm* 1986; **43:** 1945–50.

Dependence and Withdrawal

Dependence may develop, particularly with prolonged use of higher than recommended doses of clomethiazole. Features of dependence and withdrawal are similar to those of barbiturates (see Amobarbital, p.655).

Adverse Effects and Treatment

Clomethiazole may produce nasal congestion and irritation, sneezing, and conjunctival irritation sometimes associated with a headache. Nasopharyngeal or bronchial secretions may be increased. Skin rashes and urticaria have also occurred and in rare cases bullous eruptions have been reported. Gastrointestinal disturbances including nausea and vomiting, have been reported following oral administration. Reversible increases in liver enzyme values and blood-bilirubin concentrations have also been noted. Clomethiazole may cause excessive drowsiness particularly in high doses; paradoxical excitation or confusion may occur rarely. Anaphylaxis has been reported rarely with clomethiazole. Tachycardia and a transient fall in blood pressure, related to the rate of infusion, may follow intravenous dosage, and rapid infusion has resulted in hypotension and apnoea. Phlebitis or thrombophlebitis may occur after intravenous infusion.

Excessive doses may produce coma, respiratory depression, hypotension, and hypothermia; pneumonia may follow increased respiratory secretion. Treatment is as for barbiturate overdose (see Amobarbital, p.655).

Effects on the heart. Cardiac arrest in 2 chronic alcoholics might have been associated with clomethiazole infusion.[1]

1. McInnes GT, *et al.* Cardiac arrest following chlormethiazole infusion in chronic alcoholics. *Postgrad Med J* 1980; **56:** 742–3.

Overdosage. A report of clomethiazole poisoning on 16 occasions in 13 patients, some of whom had also taken other drugs and alcohol.[1] There was increased salivation on 7 occasions; otherwise the clinical features were those of barbiturate poisoning. The highest plasma-clomethiazole concentration was 36 µg per mL, with the highest value in a conscious patient 11.5 µg per mL. All the patients survived following intensive supportive treatment as for barbiturate poisoning.

1. Illingworth RN, *et al.* Severe poisoning with chlormethiazole. *BMJ* 1979; **2:** 902–3.

Parotitis. Acute bilateral parotitis has been reported in a patient given clomethiazole.[1] The swelling disappeared after withdrawal of clomethiazole and recurred on rechallenge.

1. Bosch X, *et al.* Parotitis induced by chlormethiazole. *BMJ* 1994; **309:** 1620.

Precautions

Clomethiazole is contra-indicated in patients with acute pulmonary insufficiency, and should be given with care to patients with chronic pulmonary insufficiency, or renal, liver, cerebral, or cardiac disease. When given parenterally, close supervision is necessary and facilities to maintain the airway should be at hand. Paradoxical worsening of epilepsy may occur in the Lennox Gastaut syndrome.

Clomethiazole may cause drowsiness which may persist the next day, affected patients should not drive or operate machinery.

Administration. Facilities for intubation and resuscitation must be available when clomethiazole is given intravenously and care should be taken to ensure that the patient's airway is maintained since there is a risk of mechanical obstruction during deep sedation. With intravenous administration it is important to adjust the dosage to the patient's response. With too high a rate of infusion sleep induced with clomethiazole may lapse into deep unconsciousness and patients must be kept under close and constant observation. Rapid infusion may cause transient apnoea and hypotension, and special care is needed in patients susceptible to cerebral or cardiac complications, including the elderly. With prolonged infusion there is a risk of electrolyte imbalance due to the water load involved with the glucose vehicle. Recovery can be considerably delayed after prolonged infusion.

Pregnancy. There have been reports of neonates being adversely affected by clomethiazole given to their mothers for toxaemia of pregnancy.[1,2] Effects included sedation, hypotonia, and apnoea. In one report[1] it was suggested that the effects might have been due to a synergistic interaction between clomethiazole and diazoxide as these drugs were given to most of the mothers with affected infants.

1. Johnson GT. Adverse neonatal reaction to maternal administration of intravenous chlormethiazole and diazoxide. *BMJ* 1976; 1: 943.
2. Wood C, Renou P. Sleepy and hypotonic neonates. *Med J Aust* 1978; 2: 73.

Interactions

The sedative effects of clomethiazole are enhanced by the simultaneous administration of CNS depressants such as alcohol, barbiturates, other hypnotics and sedatives, and antipsychotics.

Alcohol. Comment on the dangers of concomitant ingestion of clomethiazole and alcohol.[1] Although clomethiazole is a popular choice for the treatment of alcohol withdrawal symptoms (p.1131), if it is given long-term, patients readily transfer dependency to it; if they also continue to abuse alcohol this may lead to severe self-poisoning with deep coma and potentially fatal respiratory depression.

1. McInnes GT. Chlormethiazole and alcohol: a lethal cocktail. *BMJ* 1987; 294: 592.

Beta blockers. Sinus bradycardia developed in an 84-year-old woman taking *propranolol* for hypertension 3 hours after she took a second dose of clomethiazole 192 mg.[1] Her pulse rate increased on discontinuation of propranolol and clomethiazole and later stabilised when she took propranolol with haloperidol.

1. Adverse Drug Reactions Advisory Committee (Australia). *Med J Aust* 1979; 2: 553.

Diazoxide. For a report of severe adverse reactions in neonates born to mothers given clomethiazole and diazoxide, see Pregnancy under Precautions, above.

Histamine H$_2$-antagonists. A study of the pharmacokinetics of clomethiazole edisilate 1 g by mouth in 8 healthy subjects, before and after administration of *cimetidine* 1 g daily for 1 week, demonstrated that mean clearance of clomethiazole was reduced to 69% of its original value by cimetidine therapy.[1] This was associated with an increase in the mean peak plasma concentration of the hypnotic from 2.664 to 4.507 μg per mL and an increase in the mean elimination half-life from 2.33 to 3.63 hours. After the original dose of clomethiazole subjects slept for 30 to 60 minutes, whereas following cimetidine treatment, most slept for at least 2 hours.

Ranitidine did not significantly affect the pharmacokinetics of clomethiazole in a study in 7 healthy subjects.[2]

1. Shaw G, *et al.* Cimetidine impairs the elimination of chlormethiazole. *Eur J Clin Pharmacol* 1981; 21: 83–5.
2. Mashford ML, *et al.* Ranitidine does not affect chlormethiazole or indocyanine green disposition. *Clin Pharmacol Ther* 1983; 34: 231–3.

Pharmacokinetics

Clomethiazole is rapidly absorbed from the gastrointestinal tract, peak plasma concentrations appearing about 15 to 90 minutes after oral administration depending on the formulation used. It is widely distributed in the body and is reported to be 65% bound to plasma proteins. Clomethiazole is extensively metabolised, probably by first-pass metabolism in the liver with only small amounts appearing unchanged in the urine. The elimination half-life has been reported to be about 4 hours but this may be increased to 8 hours or longer in the elderly or in patients with hepatic impairment. Clomethiazole crosses the placenta and has been detected in breast milk.

Hepatic impairment. Studies in 8 patients with advanced cirrhosis of the liver and in 6 healthy men showed that the amount of unmetabolised clomethiazole reaching the circulation after an oral dose was about 10 times higher in the patients than in the controls.[1] Low concentrations in the controls were related to extensive first-pass metabolism in the liver.

1. Pentikäinen PJ, *et al.* Pharmacokinetics of chlormethiazole in healthy volunteers and patients with cirrhosis of the liver. *Eur J Clin Pharmacol* 1980; 17: 275–84.

Uses and Administration

Clomethiazole is a hypnotic and sedative with anticonvulsant effects. It is used in disturbed behaviour (p.650) such as agitation and restlessness, particularly of geriatric patients, in the short-term management of severe insomnia (p.652) in the elderly, and in the treatment of acute alcohol withdrawal symptoms (p.1131). It is one of the drugs used for the control of status epilepticus (p.341), usually to prevent recurrence of seizures once they have been brought under control with a benzodiazepine. It has been used for the initial control of impending or actual eclampsia (p.341) but magnesium sulfate is generally the preferred treatment now. It was also used as a sedative in

regional anaesthesia but is no longer used for this purpose in the UK.

Clomethiazole as Heminevrin (*AstraZeneca*) is commonly used as capsules containing 192 mg of clomethiazole base, as syrup containing 250 mg of the edisilate in 5 mL, or as a 0.8% intravenous infusion of the edisilate; tablets containing 500 mg of the edisilate have been available in some countries. As a result of differences in the bioavailability of these preparations, 500 mg of the edisilate in the tablets is considered therapeutically equivalent to 192 mg of the base in the capsules, but it is also equivalent to only 250 mg (5 mL) of the edisilate in the syrup, i.e. one tablet or one capsule or 5 mL of syrup are all equivalent in their effects.

When clomethiazole edisilate is administered by intravenous infusion, a loading dose is generally given to produce the desired effect, followed by a maintenance infusion. The precise dose will vary from patient to patient and close supervision is essential to avoid overdosage (see also Administration, above). Rapid reversal of sedative effects usually occurs after stopping the infusion, but recovery may be considerably delayed after large and prolonged dosage. See under Incompatibility, above, for reference to the incompatibility of clomethiazole with plastic infusion bags and administration sets.

The usual hypnotic dose of clomethiazole for **insomnia** is 1 or 2 capsules (192 or 384 mg of the base) or the equivalent. For **daytime sedation** 1 capsule (192 mg of the base), or the equivalent dose as one of the other dosage forms, may be given 3 times daily.

Various clomethiazole regimens have been suggested for the treatment of **alcohol withdrawal**, usually starting with 9 to 12 capsules, or the equivalent, divided into 3 or 4 doses, on the first day, and gradually reducing the dosage over the following 5 days. Treatment should be carried out in hospital or in specialist centres, and administration for longer than 9 days is not recommended because of the risk of dependence (see above).

For acute alcohol withdrawal symptoms, including delirium tremens, when oral therapy is insufficiently rapid or not practicable, an infusion of clomethiazole edisilate 0.8% is given at an initial rate of 3.0 to 7.5 mL per minute until shallow sleep is induced from which the patient can easily be awakened, and reduced thereafter to a usual rate of 0.5 to 1.0 mL per minute to maintain shallow sleep and adequate spontaneous respiration. Urgent deep sedation is obtained with an initial infusion of 40 to 100 mL given over 3 to 5 minutes and then reduced to a maintenance rate as before.

In **status epilepticus**, an infusion of 5 to 15 mL per minute of the 0.8% solution up to a total of 40 to 100 mL will usually stop convulsions; thereafter a slower maintenance infusion may be required depending on the patient's response (usual rate 0.5 to 1.0 mL per minute). In the management of status epilepticus in children the 0.8% solution is given at a suggested initial infusion rate of 0.01 mL per kg body-weight per minute, adjusted upwards according to response until seizures are abolished or drowsiness occurs. The dose is then gradually reduced once seizures have been absent for about 2 days.

For impending **eclampsia** an initial infusion of clomethiazole edisilate 0.8% solution at the rate of 0.5 to 0.75 mL per minute during labour has been suggested with a maintenance rate of 0.5 mL per minute for 12 hours following delivery. Clomethiazole edisilate 0.8% solution is also used to control or prevent the recurrence of eclamptic seizures. While seizures are occurring an infusion of 5 to 10 mL per minute is given until the seizures stop and then decreased to a maintenance rate of 0.5 to 1.0 mL per minute, adjusted according to response. If the infusion is started while a patient is not having a seizure clomethiazole edisilate is given at an initial infusion rate of 3 to 5 mL per minute until deep sedation is obtained; maintenance rates are then as before.

Porphyria. Clomethiazole is one of the drugs that has been used for seizure prophylaxis in patients with porphyria (p.342) who continue to experience convulsions while in remission.

Stroke. Clomethiazole has been studied[1] as a neuroprotective drug in the acute management of patients with stroke, but no beneficial effect on long-term outcome was demonstrated.

1. Wahlgren NG, *et al.* CLASS Study Group. Clomethiazole Acute Stroke Study (CLASS): results of a randomized, controlled trial of clomethiazole versus placebo in 1360 acute stroke patients. *Stroke* 1999; 30: 21–8.

Substance dependence. For a discussion of the management of *opioid* withdrawal symptoms, including mention of the use of clomethiazole, see p.66.

Preparations

BP 2001: Clomethiazole Capsules; Clomethiazole Intravenous Infusion; Clomethiazole Oral Solution.

Proprietary Preparations (details are given in Part 3)
Aust.: Heminevrin; *Austral.:* Heminevrin; *Belg.:* Distraneurine; *Denm.:* Heminevrin; *Fin.:* Heminevrin; *Ger.:* Distraneurin; *Hong Kong:* Heminevrin; *Irl.:* Heminevrin; *Neth.:* Distraneurine; *Norw.:* Heminevrin; *NZ:* Heminevrin; *S.Afr.:* Heminevrin; *Spain:* Distraneurine; *Swed.:* Heminevrin; *Switz.:* Distraneurin; *UK:* Heminevrin.

Cloral Betaine (4019-e)

Cloral Betaine (BAN, rINN).

Chloral Betaine (USAN); Compound 5107. An adduct of chloral hydrate and betaine.

$C_7H_{12}Cl_3NO_3,H_2O = 282.5$.
CAS — 2218-68-0.

Profile

Cloral betaine rapidly dissociates in the stomach to release cloral hydrate and has actions and uses similar to those of cloral hydrate (below). It is given by mouth in the short-term management of insomnia (p.652), as tablets containing 707 mg (approximately equivalent to 414 mg of cloral hydrate). The usual hypnotic dose is one or two tablets taken at night with water or milk. The maximum daily dose is five tablets (equivalent to about 2 g of cloral hydrate). A reduction in dosage may be appropriate in frail elderly patients or in those with hepatic impairment.

Preparations

Proprietary Preparations (details are given in Part 3)
UK: Welldorm.

Cloral Hydrate (4020-b)

Chloral Hydrate (BAN); Chlorali Hydras. 2,2,2-Trichloroethane-1,1-diol.

$C_2H_3Cl_3O_2 = 165.4$.
CAS — 302-17-0.
ATC — N05CC01.

Pharmacopoeias. In Chin., Eur. (see p.vi), Jpn, Pol., and US.

Incompatible with alkalis, alkaline earths, alkali carbonates, soluble barbiturates, borax, tannin, iodides, oxidising agents, permanganates, and alcohol (cloral alcoholate may crystallise out). It forms a liquid mixture when triturated with many organic compounds, such as camphor, menthol, phenazone, phenol, thymol, and quinine salts.

Pharmacopoeial description

Ph. Eur.: Colourless, transparent crystals. Very soluble in water; freely soluble in alcohol. A 10% solution in water has a pH of 3.5 to 5.5. Store in airtight containers.

USP 25: Colourless, transparent, or white crystals having an aromatic, penetrating, and slightly acrid odour. It volatilises slowly on exposure to air and melts at about 55°. Soluble 1 in 0.25 of water, 1 in 1.3 of alcohol, 1 in 2 of chloroform, and 1 in 1.5 of ether; very soluble in olive oil. Store in airtight containers.

Dependence and Withdrawal, Adverse Effects, and Treatment

Cloral hydrate has an unpleasant taste and is corrosive to skin and mucous membranes unless well diluted. The most frequent adverse effect is gastric irritation; abdominal distension and flatulence may also occur. CNS effects such as drowsiness, light-headedness, ataxia, headache, and paradoxical excitement, hallucinations, nightmares, delirium, and confusion (sometimes with paranoia) occur occasionally. Hypersensitivity reactions include skin rashes (erythema multiforme and Stevens-Johnson syndrome have been reported with the related compound triclofos). Ketonuria may occur.

The effects of acute overdosage resemble acute barbiturate intoxication (see Amobarbital, p.655 and below), and are managed similarly. In addition the irritant effect may cause initial vomiting, and gastric necrosis leading to strictures. Cardiac arrhythmias have been reported. Jaundice may follow liver damage, and albuminuria may follow kidney damage.

Tolerance may develop and dependence may occur. Features of dependence and withdrawal are similar to those of barbiturates (see Amobarbital, p.655).

The symbol † denotes a preparation no longer actively marketed

◊ In a drug surveillance programme,[1] side-effects of cloral hydrate, which were reversible, occurred in 2.3% of 1130 patients evaluated and included gastrointestinal symptoms (10 patients), CNS depression in 20, and skin rash in 5. In 1 patient the prothrombin time was increased; in 1 patient hepatic encephalopathy seemed to worsen; and bradycardia developed in 1 patient. In another such programme, side-effects occurred in approximately 2% of 5435 patients who received cloral hydrate.[2] Three reactions were described as life-threatening.

1. Shapiro S, et al. Clinical effects of hypnotics II: an epidemiologic study. JAMA 1969; 209: 2016–20.
2. Miller RR, Greenblatt DJ. Clinical effects of chloral hydrate in hospitalized medical patients. J Clin Pharmacol 1979; 19: 669–74.

Carcinogenicity. Cloral hydrate has been widely used as a sedative, especially in children. Concern over warnings that cloral hydrate was carcinogenic in rodents[1] has prompted some experts, including the American Academy of Pediatrics, to review the relative risks of the medical use of this drug.[2,3] The original warnings appear to have been based, in part, on the assumption that cloral hydrate was a reactive metabolite of trichloroethylene and was responsible for its carcinogenicity, but there is evidence to suggest that the carcinogenicity of trichloroethylene is due to a reactive intermediate epoxide metabolite. Studies in vitro indicate that choral hydrate can damage chromosomes in some mammalian test systems but there have been no studies of the carcinogenicity of cloral hydrate in humans. Some long-term studies in mice have linked cloral hydrate with the development of hepatic adenomas or carcinomas. However, it was noted that cloral hydrate was not the only sedative that had been shown to be a carcinogen in experimental animals. The American Academy of Pediatrics considered cloral hydrate to be an effective sedative with a low incidence of acute toxicity when given short-term as recommended and, although the information on carcinogenicity was of concern, it was not sufficient to justify the risk associated with the use of less familiar sedatives. There was no evidence in infants or children demonstrating that any of the available alternatives were safer or more effective. However, the use of repetitive dosing with cloral hydrate to maintain prolonged sedation in neonates and other children was of concern because of the potential for accumulation of drug metabolites and resultant toxicity.

1. Smith MT. Chloral hydrate warning. Science 1990; 250: 359.
2. Steinberg AD. Should chloral hydrate be banned? Pediatrics 1993; 92: 442–6.
3. American Academy of Pediatrics Committee on Drugs and Committee on Environmental Health. Use of chloral hydrate for sedation in children. Pediatrics 1993; 92: 471–3.

Effects on the CNS. Report[1] of a 2-year-old child who experienced the first of 2 seizures 60 minutes after receiving cloral hydrate 70 mg per kg body-weight for sedation.

1. Muñoz M, et al. Seizures caused by chloral hydrate sedative doses. J Pediatr 1997; 131: 787–8.

Hyperbilirubinaemia. Small retrospective studies[1] have suggested that prolonged administration of cloral hydrate in neonates may be associated with the development of hyperbilirubinaemia. This may possibly be related to the prolonged half-life of the metabolite trichloroethanol in neonates.

1. Lambert GH, et al. Direct hyperbilirubinemia associated with chloral hydrate administration in the newborn. Pediatrics 1990; 86: 277–81.

Overdosage. The general management of poisoning with cloral hydrate resembles that for barbiturates (see, p.655). Activated charcoal has been recommended if more than 2 g has been taken by an adult within 1 hour of treatment, or 30 mg per kg body-weight in a child, provided the airway can be protected. Gastric lavage may be considered before giving charcoal in serious cases. Of 76 cases of cloral hydrate poisoning reported to the UK National Poisons Information Service, 47 were severe.[1] Of 39 adults, 12 had cardiac arrhythmias including 5 with cardiac arrest. Antiarrhythmic drugs were recommended unless obviously contra-indicated. Haemoperfusion through charcoal or haemodialysis was recommended for patients in profound coma. Cardiac arrhythmias and CNS depression were also major features of 12 cases of cloral hydrate overdosage reported from Australia.[2] Lignocaine [lidocaine] was not always successful in controlling arrhythmias, but propranolol was successful in all 7 patients in whom it was used. It was noted that resistant arrhythmias, particularly ventricular fibrillation, ventricular tachycardia, and supraventricular tachycardia, were the usual cause of death in patients who had taken an overdosage of cloral hydrate. Although there had been no controlled studies of antiarrhythmic therapy in overdosage with cloral hydrate, the successful use of beta blockers appeared to be a recurring feature in reports in the literature.

Administration of flumazenil produced an increased level of consciousness, pupillary dilatation, and return of respiratory rate and blood pressure towards normal in a patient who had taken an overdosage of cloral hydrate.[3]

1. Wiseman HM, Hampel G. Cardiac arrhythmias due to chloral hydrate poisoning. BMJ 1978; 2: 960.
2. Graham SR, et al. Overdose with chloral hydrate: a pharmacological and therapeutic review. Med J Aust 1988; 149: 686–8.
3. Donovan KL, Fisher DJ. Reversal of chloral hydrate overdose with flumazenil. BMJ 1989; 298: 1253.

Precautions

Cloral hydrate should not be used in patients with marked hepatic or renal impairment or severe cardiac disease, and oral administration is best avoided in the presence of gastritis. As with all sedatives, it should be used with caution in those with respiratory insufficiency.

Cloral hydrate may cause drowsiness which may persist the next day; affected patients should not drive or operate machinery. Prolonged administration and abrupt withdrawal of cloral hydrate should be avoided to prevent precipitation of withdrawal symptoms. Repeated administration in infants and children may lead to accumulation of metabolites and thereby increase the risk of adverse effects. Use is best avoided during pregnancy. Cloral hydrate is distributed into breast milk and may lead to sedation in breast-fed infants.

Cloral hydrate may interfere with tests for urinary glucose or 17-hydroxycorticosteroids.

Neonates. The half-life of trichloroethanol, an active metabolite of cloral hydrate, is prolonged in neonates;[1] values of up to 66 hours have been reported in some studies. Short-term sedation in the neonate with single oral doses of 25 to 50 mg per kg body-weight of cloral hydrate is considered[1] to be probably relatively safe, but repeated administration carries the risk of accumulation of metabolites which may result in serious toxicity. Toxic reactions may occur even after the drug has been discontinued since the metabolites may accumulate for several days.

1. Jacqz-Aigrain E, Burtin P. Clinical pharmacokinetics of sedatives in neonates. Clin Pharmacokinet 1996; 31: 423–43.

Obstructive sleep apnoea. Children with obstructive sleep apnoea could be at risk from life-threatening respiratory obstruction if cloral hydrate is used for sedation. Details of 2 such children who suffered respiratory failure following sedation with cloral hydrate for lung function studies have been reported.

1. Biban P, et al. Adverse effect of chloral hydrate in two young children with obstructive sleep apnea. Pediatrics 1993; 92: 461–3.

Porphyria. The UK manufacturer recommends that cloral hydrate should not be used in patients with porphyria, although some authorities consider it safe; caution would seem appropriate.

Interactions

The sedative effects of cloral hydrate are enhanced by the simultaneous administration of depressants of the CNS such as alcohol (the 'Mickey Finn' of detective fiction), barbiturates, and other sedatives.

Cloral hydrate may enhance the effects of coumarin anticoagulants (see Warfarin, p.996). A hypermetabolic state, apparently due to displacement of thyroid hormones from their binding proteins, has been reported in patients given an intravenous dose of frusemide [furosemide] subsequent to cloral hydrate.

Pharmacokinetics

Cloral hydrate is rapidly absorbed from the gastrointestinal tract and starts to act within 30 minutes of oral administration. It is widely distributed throughout the body. It is rapidly metabolised to trichloroethanol and trichloroacetic acid (p.1674) in the erythrocytes, liver, and other tissues. It is excreted partly in the urine as trichloroethanol and its glucuronide (urochloralic acid) and as trichloroacetic acid. Some is also excreted in the bile.

Trichloroethanol is the active metabolite, and passes into the CSF, into breast milk, and across the placenta. The half-life of trichloroethanol in plasma is reported to range from about 7 to 11 hours but is considerably prolonged in the neonate. Trichloroacetic acid has a plasma half-life of several days.

Uses and Administration

Cloral hydrate is a hypnotic and sedative with properties similar to those of the barbiturates. It is used in the short-term management of insomnia (p.652) and has been used as a sedative for premedication (p.1256). In the USA it has been widely used for sedation of children before diagnostic, dental, or medical procedures (but see under Carcinogenicity above).

Externally, cloral hydrate has a rubefacient action and has been employed as a counter-irritant.

Cloral hydrate is administered by mouth as an oral liquid or as gelatin capsules with cloral hydrate dissolved in a suitable vehicle. It has also been dissolved in a bland fixed oil and given by enema or as suppositories.

It should not be given as tablets because of the risk of damage to the mucous membrane of the alimentary tract.

The usual hypnotic dose by mouth is 0.5 to 2 g given as a single dose at night; as a sedative 250 mg can be given three times daily to a maximum daily dose of 2 g. Oral dosage forms should be taken well diluted or with plenty of water or milk. Children may be given 30 to 50 mg per kg body-weight to a maximum single dose of 1 g as a hypnotic. A suggested sedative dose for premedication in children is 25 to 50 mg per kg to a maximum single dose of 1 g.

A reduction in dosage may be appropriate in frail elderly patients or in those with hepatic impairment.

Derivatives of cloral hydrate, such as cloral betaine (above), chloralose (p.1429), and dichloralphenazone (p.682), which break down in the body to yield cloral hydrate, have been used similarly.

◊ References.
1. McCarver-May DG, et al. Comparison of chloral hydrate and midazolam for sedation of neonates for neuroimaging studies. J Pediatr 1996; 128: 573–6.
2. Napoli KL, et al. Safety and efficacy of chloral hydrate sedation in children undergoing echocardiography. J Pediatr 1996; 129: 287–91.

Preparations

USP 25: Chloral Hydrate Capsules; Chloral Hydrate Syrup.

Proprietary Preparations (details are given in Part 3)
Aust.: Chloraldurat; *Ger.:* Chloraldurat; *Neth.:* Chloraldurat†; *Switz.:* Chloraldurat; Medianox; *UK:* Noctec†; Welldorm; *USA:* Aquachloral.

Multi-ingredient: *Belg.:* Babygencal; Dentophar; Syntholt†; *Canad.:* Analgesic Balm†; *Fr.:* Bain de Bouche Lipha; Dolodent; Lini-Bombe†; Pipiol; Sirop Teyssedre; Synthol; *Ger.:* Leukona-Sedativ-Bad; *Spain:* Dentol Topico; *Switz.:* Nervifene.

Clorazepic Acid (17899-q)

Clorazepic Acid (BAN).

7-Chloro-2,3-dihydro-2,2-dihydroxy-5-phenyl-1H-1,4-benzodiazepine-3-carboxylic acid.

$C_{16}H_{11}ClN_2O_3 = 314.7$.
CAS — 23887-31-2.

Clorazepate Monopotassium (7029-j)

Clorazepate Monopotassium (USAN).

Abbott-39083; 4311-CB. Potassium 7-chloro-2,3-dihydro-2-oxo-5-phenyl-1H-1,4-benzodiazepine-3-carboxylate.

$C_{16}H_{10}ClKN_2O_3 = 352.8$.
CAS — 5991-71-9.

Dipotassium Clorazepate (7030-q)

Dipotassium Clorazepate (BANM, rINN).

Abbott-35616; AH-3232; 4306-CB; Clorazepate Dipotassium (USAN); Dikalii Clorazepas; Potassium Clorazepate. Compound of Potassium 7-chloro-2,3-dihydro-2-oxo-5-phenyl-1H-1,4-benzodiazepine-3-carboxylate with potassium hydroxide.

$C_{16}H_{11}ClK_2N_2O_4 = 408.9$.
CAS — 57109-90-7.
ATC — N05BA05.
Pharmacopoeias. In Eur. (see p.vi) and US.

Pharmacopoeial description

Ph. Eur.: A white or light yellow, crystalline powder. Solutions in water and in alcohol are unstable and should be used immediately. Freely soluble or very soluble in water; very slightly soluble in alcohol; practically insoluble in dichloromethane. Store in airtight containers. Protect from light.

USP 25: A light yellow, crystalline powder which darkens on exposure to light. Soluble in water but, upon standing, may precipitate from the solution; slightly soluble in alcohol and in isopropyl alcohol; practically insoluble in acetone, in chloroform, in dichloromethane, in ether, and in benzene. Store under nitrogen in airtight containers. Protect from light.

Dependence and Withdrawal

As for Diazepam, p.675.

Adverse Effects, Treatment, and Precautions

As for Diazepam, p.675.

Effects on the liver. A report of jaundice and hepatic necrosis associated with clorazepate administration.[1]

1. Parker JLW. Potassium clorazepate (Tranxene)-induced jaundice. Postgrad Med J 1979; 55: 908–910.

Effects on the nervous system. For reference to extrapyramidal disorders associated with administration of clorazepate, see Diazepam, p.675.

Porphyria. Clorazepate has been associated with acute attacks of porphyria and is considered unsafe in porphyric patients.

Interactions

As for Diazepam, p.677.

Pharmacokinetics

Clorazepate is decarboxylated rapidly at the low pH in the stomach to form desmethyldiazepam (nordazepam, see p.696), which is quickly absorbed.

◊ References.
1. Ochs HR, et al. Comparative single-dose kinetics of oxazolam, prazepam, and clorazepate: three precursors of desmethyldiazepam. J Clin Pharmacol 1984; 24: 446–51.
2. Bertler Å, et al. Intramuscular bioavailability of chlorazepate as compared to diazepam. Eur J Clin Pharmacol 1985; 28: 229–30.

Uses and Administration

Clorazepate is a long-acting benzodiazepine with general properties similar to those of diazepam (p.680). It is mainly used in the short-term treatment of anxiety disorders (p.649), as an adjunct in the management of epilepsy, and in the alcohol withdrawal syndrome (p.1131).

Dipotassium clorazepate is usually given by mouth but preparations for intravenous or intramuscular administration are also available in some countries. In the UK, a usual dose of 15 mg of dipotassium clorazepate by mouth is given as a single dose at night for the treatment of anxiety; alternatively a dose of 7.5 mg may be given up to three times daily. In the USA rather higher doses have been recommended; 15 to 60 mg of dipotassium clorazepate may be given daily, in divided doses or as a single dose at night. Up to 90 mg has been given daily in divided doses in the management of epilepsy or the alcohol withdrawal syndrome. Children aged between 9 and 12 years may be given a maximum of 60 mg daily in the management of epilepsy.

Reduced doses should be given in elderly or debilitated patients.

Preparations

USP 25: Clorazepate Dipotassium Tablets.

Proprietary Preparations (details are given in Part 3)
Aust.: Tranxilium; *Austral.:* Tranxene†; *Belg.:* Tranxene; Uni-Tranxene; *Braz.:* Tranxilene; *Canad.:* Novo-Clopate; Tranxene; *Denm.:* Tranxen†; *Fr.:* Tranxene; *Ger.:* Tranxilium; *Hong Kong:* Tranxene; *Irl.:* Tranxene; *Israel:* Tranxal; *Ital.:* Transene; *Mex.:* Tranxene; *Neth.:* Tranxene; *Port.:* Medipax; Tranxene; *S.Afr.:* Tranxene; *Singapore:* Tranxene; *Spain:* Dorken; Nansius; Tranxilium; *Switz.:* Tranxilium; *Thai.:* Cloraxene; Diposef; Dipot; Flulium; Polizep; Sanor; Serene; Trancap; Tranclor; Trancon; Tranxene; Zetran; *UK:* Tranxene; *USA:* Gen-Xene; Tranxene.

Multi-ingredient: *Fr.:* Noctran.

Clotiapine (7031-p)

Clotiapine *(BAN, rINN)*.

Clothiapine *(USAN)*; HF-2159. 2-Chloro-11-(4-methylpiperazin-1-yl)dibenzo[b,f][1,4]thiazepine.
$C_{18}H_{18}ClN_3S = 343.9$.
CAS — 2058-52-8.
ATC — N05AX09.

Profile

Clotiapine is a dibenzothiazepine antipsychotic with general properties similar to those of the phenothiazines (see Chlorpromazine, p.660). It is used in a variety of psychiatric disorders including schizophrenia (p.651), mania (see Bipolar Disorder, p.271), and anxiety (p.649). It is given by mouth in doses of 10 to 200 mg daily in divided doses; doses of up to 360 mg daily have been given in severe or resistant psychoses. It may also be given by slow intravenous or deep intramuscular injection.

◊ A systematic review[1] found that good evidence to support the use of clotiapine over other treatments in acute psychotic illness was lacking.

1. Carpenter S, Berk M. Clotiapine for acute psychotic illnesses (updated 28 February 2001). Available in The Cochrane Library; Issue 4. Oxford: Update Software; 2001.

Preparations

Proprietary Preparations (details are given in Part 3)
Belg.: Etumine; *Israel:* Etumin/Entumin; *Ital.:* Entumin; *S.Afr.:* Etomine; *Spain:* Etumina; *Switz.:* Entumine.

Clotiazepam (12592-k)

Clotiazepam *(rINN)*.

Y-6047. 5-(2-Chlorophenyl)-7-ethyl-1,3-dihydro-1-methyl-2H-thieno[2,3-e]-1,4-diazepin-2-one.
$C_{16}H_{15}ClN_2OS = 318.8$.
CAS — 33671-46-4.
ATC — N05BA21.
Pharmacopoeias. In Jpn.

Profile

Clotiazepam is a short-acting thienodiazepine with general properties similar to those of diazepam (p.674). A usual daily dose for the short-term management of anxiety disorders (p.649) is 5 to 15 mg by mouth given in divided doses but up to 60 mg daily has been used. For insomnia (p.652) up to 20 mg has been given as a single dose at night.

◊ References.

1. Jibiki I, *et al.* Beneficial effect of high-dose clotiazepam on intractable auditory hallucinations in chronic schizophrenic patients. *Eur J Clin Pharmacol* 1994; **46**: 367–9.

Effects on the liver. Development of hepatitis in a 65-year-old woman was attributed to clotiazepam begun 7 months earlier.[1] The patient took triazolam and lorazepam without any apparent effect on the liver, and it was speculated that the hepatotoxic effect of clotiazepam was related to the thiophene ring present in the chemical structure.

1. Habersetzer F, *et al.* Clotiazepam-induced acute hepatitis. *J Hepatol* 1989; **9**: 256–9.

Porphyria. Clotiazepam is considered to be unsafe in patients with porphyria because it has been shown to be porphyrinogenic in *in-vitro* systems.

Preparations

Proprietary Preparations (details are given in Part 3)
Belg.: Clozan; *Fr.:* Veratran; *Ger.:* Trecalmo†; *Ital.:* Rizen; Tienor; *Jpn:* Rize; *Spain:* Distensan.

Cloxazolam (7032-s)

Cloxazolam *(rINN)*.

CS-370. 10-Chloro-11b-(2-chlorophenyl)-2,3,7,11b-tetrahydro-oxazolo[3,2-d][1,4]benzodiazepin-6(5H)-one.
$C_{17}H_{14}Cl_2N_2O_2 = 349.2$.
CAS — 24166-13-0.
ATC — N05BA22.
Pharmacopoeias. In Jpn.

Profile

Cloxazolam is a long-acting benzodiazepine with general properties similar to those of diazepam (p.674). It is given by mouth in doses of up to 12 mg daily in divided doses for the short-term treatment of anxiety disorders (p.649). A dose of 100 µg per kg body-weight may be used for premedication (p.1256).

Preparations

Proprietary Preparations (details are given in Part 3)
Aust.: Olcadil†; *Belg.:* Akton; *Braz.:* Elum; Olcadil; *Hong Kong:* Sepazon; *Jpn:* Sepazon†; *Port.:* Cloxam; Olcadil; *Switz.:* Lubalix.

Clozapine (12595-x)

Clozapine *(BAN, USAN, rINN)*.

Clozapinum; HF-1854. 8-Chloro-11-(4-methylpiperazin-1-yl)-5H-dibenzo[b,e][1,4]diazepine.
$C_{18}H_{19}ClN_4 = 326.8$.
CAS — 5786-21-0.
ATC — N05AH02.
Pharmacopoeias. In Eur. (see p.vi).

Pharmacopoeial description

Ph. Eur.: A yellow crystalline powder. Practically insoluble in water; soluble in alcohol; freely soluble in dichloromethane. It dissolves in dilute acetic acid.

Stability. A suspension of clozapine 100 mg in 5 mL, made by crushing clozapine tablets and suspending the powder in a syrup-based mixture containing carboxymethylcellulose preserved with methyl hydroxybenzoate and propyl hydroxybenzoate (Guy's Hospital paediatric base formula), was considered to be stable for at least 18 days after preparation.[1]

1. Ramuth S, *et al.* A liquid clozapine preparation for oral administration in hospital. *Pharm J* 1996; **257**: 190–1.

Adverse Effects and Treatment

As for Chlorpromazine, p.660 but antimuscarinic effects may be more pronounced.

Clozapine can cause reversible neutropenia which may progress to a potentially fatal agranulocytosis; strict monitoring of white blood cell counts is essential (see Precautions, below). Eosinophilia may also occur.

Extrapyramidal disorders, including tardive dyskinesia appear to be rare with clozapine. Clozapine has little effect on prolactin secretion. Clozapine appears to carry a greater epileptic potential than chlorpromazine but a comparable risk of cardiovascular effects such as tachycardia and orthostatic hypotension. In rare cases circulatory collapse with cardiac and respiratory arrest has occurred. Hypertension and isolated cases of myocarditis or pericarditis have also been reported.

Additional side-effects of clozapine include dizziness, hypersalivation (particularly at night), headache, nausea, vomiting, constipation (which, in a few cases, has led to gastrointestinal obstruction and paralytic ileus), anxiety, confusion, fatigue, and transient fever which must be distinguished from the signs of impending agranulocytosis. There have also been rare reports of dysphagia, parotid gland enlargement, thromboembolism, acute pancreatitis, hepatitis and cholestatic jaundice, and very rarely fulminant hepatic necrosis. Isolated cases of acute interstitial nephritis have been reported. Abnormalities of glucose homoeostasis occur uncommonly; severe hyperglycaemia, sometimes leading to ketoacidosis, has been reported. Many of the adverse effects of clozapine are most common at the beginning of therapy and may be minimised by gradual increase in dosage.

Convulsions. As with other antipsychotics (see Chlorpromazine, p.661), clozapine can lower the seizure threshold and cause EEG abnormalities, although treatment with clozapine appears to be associated with a higher frequency of seizures. A review[1] of 1418 patients treated with clozapine in the USA between 1972 and 1988 found that 41 had experienced generalized tonic-clonic seizures. It was considered that the risk of clo-

zapine-induced seizures was dose-related. The seizure frequency was calculated to be 1% at a dose less than 300 mg daily, 2.7% at 300 to 599 mg daily, and 4.4% with a dosage of 600 mg or more daily. Six of the patients had been taking other drugs reported to lower the seizure threshold. Therapy with clozapine was continued in 31 of the 41 patients by reducing the total daily dose of clozapine; antiepileptic drug therapy was initiated in about half of the patients. The UK Committee on Safety of Medicines[2] considered that although the epileptogenic effect of clozapine was claimed to be dose-related, the metabolism and plasma concentrations of clozapine were highly variable and data from 8 cases reported to the Committee suggest that convulsions may possibly be related to high plasma concentrations in susceptible individuals. A low initial dosage followed by careful increases according to response and downward titration thereafter to a maintenance dose was recommended to avoid convulsions in susceptible individuals.

1. Devinsky O, *et al.* Clozapine-related seizures. *Neurology* 1991; **41**: 369–71.
2. Committee on Safety of Medicines. Convulsions may occur in patients receiving clozapine (Clozaril®, Sandoz). *Current Problems 31* 1991.

Effects on the blood. Clozapine can cause reversible neutropenia which, if the drug is not withdrawn immediately, may progress to a potentially fatal **agranulocytosis**. Particular concern over this side-effect dates from 1975 when 17 cases of neutropenia or agranulocytosis, 8 of them fatal, were reported in Finland;[1] the calculated incidence[2] of agranulocytosis or severe granulocytopenia during this Finnish epidemic was 7.1 per 1000. These reports led to the withdrawal of clozapine in some countries or to restrictions in its use and intense haematological monitoring in others. Following studies demonstrating the efficacy of clozapine in severely ill schizophrenic patients unresponsive to adequate therapy with standard antipsychotics, the drug became available in the UK and USA in 1990 with strict procedures for monitoring of white blood cell counts. The UK Committee on Safety of Medicines provided data on the reports it had received between July 1963 and January 1993 on agranulocytosis and neutropenia.[3] Clozapine was one of the individual drugs most frequently implicated with 14 reports of agranulocytosis (one fatal) and 119 of neutropenia (none fatal). Various estimates of the **incidence** of clozapine-associated agranulocytosis have been made; analysis of data from 11 555 patients who had received clozapine in the USA[4] showed a cumulative incidence of agranulocytosis of 8.0 per 1000 at 1 year and 9.1 per 1000 at 1½ years with the risk being increased in elderly patients. The majority of cases of agranulocytosis occurred within 3 months of the start of treatment with the risk peaking in the third month. The manufacturers report a lower incidence of agranulocytosis of 4.8 per 1000 patients for the first 6 months[5] and an annual rate of 0.8 per 1000 patients during the next 2.5 years. These figures were based on data on 56 000 patients in the USA who had received clozapine up to the end of March 1993. Analysis of data[6] on 6316 patients registered in the UK and Ireland between January 1990 and July 1994 to receive (although not necessarily given) clozapine produced a cumulative incidence of agranulocytosis of 0.7% during the first year and 0.8% over the whole study period. Most cases of agranulocytosis and neutropenia occurred during the first 6 to 18 weeks of treatment. The incidence of agranulocytosis (0.07%) and neutropenia (0.7%) seen during the second year of therapy was of the same order of magnitude noted for some phenothiazine antipsychotics.

These data[6] and comparable data from the USA[7] were considered to indicate that mandatory haematological monitoring (see Precautions, below) helped to reduce the risks of clozapine-induced neutropenia and agranulocytosis and associated deaths.

The mechanism for clozapine-induced agranulocytosis is unclear and may be the result of direct toxicity or an immune response.[8,9] **Predisposing factors** for development of agranulocytosis have not been identified, apart from a possible excess of cases in female patients and an increased risk with increasing age. Furthermore, both agranulocytosis and neutropenia do not appear to be dose-related effects with clozapine. A postulated higher incidence of agranulocytosis in patients of Jewish background may be related to genetic factors.[10] Africans and Afro-Caribbeans appear to be at increased risk of developing neutropenia[6] and it has been noted[11] that many patients from these ethnic groups are currently already excluded from treatment with clozapine because their normal white blood cell and neutrophil counts are below the recommended range for treatment (see Precautions, below).

Evidence would suggest that development of clozapine-induced leucopenia or granulocytopenia precludes **retreatment** with clozapine at any future date; in one series of 9 patients retreated all again developed leucopenia or agranulocytosis.[12] In the USA patients who have had clozapine withdrawn because of moderate leucopenia (judged to be when counts fall to 2000 to 3000 per mm³) are considered eligible for a return to clozapine treatment when this count returns to normal; such patients are considered to have a five- or sixfold greater risk of agranulocytosis.[5]

1. Idänpään-Heikkilä J, *et al.* Agranulocytosis during treatment with clozapine. *Eur J Clin Pharmacol* 1977; **11**: 193–8.
2. Anderman B, Griffith RW. Clozapine-induced agranulocytosis: a situation report up to August 1976. *Eur J Clin Pharmacol* 1977; **11**: 199–201.

The symbol † denotes a preparation no longer actively marketed

3. Committee on Safety of Medicines/Medicines Control Agency. Drug-induced neutropenia and agranulocytosis. *Current Problems* 1993; **19:** 10–11.

4. Alvir JMJ, *et al.* Clozapine-induced agranulocytosis: incidence and risk factors in the United States. *N Engl J Med* 1993; **329:** 162–7.

5. Finkel MJ, Arellano F. White-blood-cell monitoring and clozapine. *Lancet* 1995; **346:** 849.

6. Atkin K, *et al.* Neutropenia and agranulocytosis in patients receiving clozapine in the UK and Ireland. *Br J Psychiatry* 1996; **169:** 483–8.

7. Honigfeld G, *et al.* Reducing clozapine-related morbidity and mortality: 5 years experience with the Clozaril National Registry. *J Clin Psychiatry* 1998; **59** (suppl 3): 3–7.

8. Gerson SL, *et al.* Polypharmacy in fatal clozapine-associated agranulocytosis. *Lancet* 1991; **338:** 262–3.

9. Hoffbrand AV, *et al.* Mechanisms of clozapine-induced agranulocytosis. *Drug Safety* 1992; **7** (suppl 1): 1–60.

10. Lieberman JA, *et al.* HLA-B38, DR4, DQw3 and clozapine-induced agranulocytosis in Jewish patients with schizophrenia. *Arch Gen Psychiatry* 1990; **47:** 945–8.

11. Fisher N, Baigent B. Treatment with clozapine: black patients' low white cell counts currently mean that they cannot be treated. *BMJ* 1996; **313:** 1262.

12. Safferman AZ, *et al.* Rechallenge in clozapine-induced agranulocytosis. *Lancet* 1992; **339:** 1296–7.

Effects on the cardiovascular system. The UK Committee on Safety of Medicines (CSM)[1] issued a warning in November 1993 of the risk of myocarditis with clozapine. Three patients who died while taking clozapine had evidence of myocarditis. The CSM had also received one other report of myocarditis and one of cardiomyopathy associated with clozapine. The Australian Adverse Drug Reactions Advisory Committee (ADRAC) subsequently reported[2] another 5 cases of clozapine-associated myocarditis in November 1994. A later report[3] from Australia identified 15 cases of myocarditis, including 5 fatalities, between January 1993 and March 1999 (these figures were established using both data from ADRAC and the Australian manufacturers). Between September 1989 and December 1999 the FDA in the USA had received reports of 28 cases of myocarditis (18 fatal) and 41 of cardiomyopathy (10 fatal) temporally associated with clozapine use.[4] A review[5] by the pharmacovigilance authorities in New Zealand stated that by November 1999 the manufacturers Novartis had analysed 125 reports of myocarditis received worldwide including 35 fatalities; 53% had occurred during the first month of treatment but about 5% occurred more than 2 years after starting treatment. As myocarditis can be difficult to diagnose and confirmation is not always possible, the CSM recommended that if there was a high clinical suspicion of myocarditis, antipsychotic medication should be stopped. Presenting features might include heart failure, arrhythmia, or symptoms mimicking myocardial infarction or pericarditis.

There is also evidence that clozapine may be associated with fatal thromboembolism. The Swedish Adverse Reactions Advisory Committee had received reports[6] on 6 cases (5 fatal) of pulmonary embolism and 6 of venous thrombosis associated with clozapine treatment as of March 2000. The effect seemed to occur mainly in the first 3 months of treatment, and the majority of the cases involved men. However, analysis of data[7] from Germany and Switzerland suggests that the incidence of clozapine-associated thromboembolism is no different from that in psychiatric patients treated with classical antipsychotics or no psychotics at all (see also under Chlorpromazine, p.661).

Some studies[8] have suggested that serious cardiovascular effects might occur more frequently and might be more severe in healthy subjects than in patients with schizophrenia. The manufacturers had requested that for the purpose of pharmacokinetic studies, clozapine should not be given to healthy subjects.

There have been isolated reports[9,10] of paradoxical hypertension in patients receiving clozapine. Concomitant administration of atenolol has controlled the hypertension and allowed therapy with clozapine to be continued.

A small preliminary study[11] has suggested that serum triglyceride concentrations may be higher in patients taking clozapine than in those treated with conventional antipsychotics.

For further details of effects of clozapine on the cardiovascular system, see Benzodiazepines under Interactions, below.

1. Committee on Safety of Medicines/Medicines Control Agency. Myocarditis with antipsychotics: recent cases with clozapine (Clozaril). *Current Problems* 1993; **19:** 9–10.

2. Adverse Drug Reactions Advisory Committee. Clozapine and myocarditis. *Aust Adverse Drug React Bull* 1994; **13** (Nov): 14–15.

3. Kilian JG, *et al.* Myocarditis and cardiomyopathy associated with clozapine. *Lancet* 1999; **354:** 1841–5.

4. La Grenada L, *et al.* Myocarditis and cardiomyopathy associated with clozapine use in the United States. *N Engl J Med* 2001; **345:** 224–5.

5. New Zealand Medicines and Medical Devices Safety Authority. Potentially fatal complications of clozapine therapy: myocarditis, venous thromboembolism and constipation. Available at: http://www.medsafe.govt.nz/profs/puarticles/cloz1.htm (accessed 13/11/2001).

6. Hägg S, *et al.* Association of venous thromboembolism and clozapine. *Lancet* 2000; **355:** 1155–6.

7. Wolstein J, *et al.* Antipsychotic drugs and venous thromboembolism. *Lancet* 2000; **356:** 252.

8. Pokorny R, *et al.* Normal volunteers should not be used for bioavailability or bioequivalence studies of clozapine. *Pharm Res* 1994; **11:** 1211.

9. Gupta S. Paradoxical hypertension associated with clozapine. *Am J Psychiatry* 1994; **151:** 148.

10. Ennis LM, Parker RM. Paradoxical hypertension associated with clozapine. *Med J Aust* 1997; **166:** 278.

11. Ghaeli P, Dufresne RL. Serum triglyceride levels in patients treated with clozapine. *Am J Health-Syst Pharm* 1996; **53:** 2079–81.

Effects on fluid and electrolyte homoeostasis. Hyponatraemia has been reported to be associated with clozapine,[1] as with other antipsychotics (p.661). It was emphasised that hyponatraemia should be excluded as a possible trigger when considering the epileptogenic potential of clozapine.

1. Ogilvie AD, Croy MF. Clozapine and hyponatraemia. *Lancet* 1992; **340:** 672.

Effects on the gastrointestinal tract. The UK Committee on Safety of Medicines had received 20 reports of serious gastrointestinal reactions resembling obstruction associated with clozapine treatment as of March 1999, of which 3 were fatal.[1] These reactions were thought to be due to the antimuscarinic actions of clozapine and, therefore, more likely to occur when clozapine was taken together with other drugs with antimuscarinic actions such as tricyclic antidepressants, some antiparkinsonian drugs, and other antipsychotics; care was also warranted in those patients with a history of colonic disease or previous bowel surgery. It was also important to recognise and treat constipation in patients receiving clozapine to prevent the development of more serious complications such as obstruction and paralytic ileus.

1. Committee on Safety of Medicines/Medicines Control Agency. Clozapine (Clozaril) and gastrointestinal obstruction. *Current Problems* 1999; **25:** 5.

Effects on the kidneys. Acute interstitial nephritis developed in a 38-year-old woman after 11 days of treatment with clozapine 250 mg daily;[1] she recovered after stopping clozapine.

1. Elias TJ, *et al.* Clozapine-induced acute interstitial nephritis. *Lancet* 1999; **354:** 1180–1.

Effects on the pancreas. There have been isolated reports of pancreatitis associated with clozapine.[1,2] Pancreatitis has also been reported[3] following overdosage with clozapine.

1. Martin A. Acute pancreatitis associated with clozapine use. *Am J Psychiatry* 1992; **149:** 714.

2. Frankenburg FR, Kando J. Eosinophilia, clozapine, and pancreatitis. *Lancet* 1992; **340:** 251.

3. Jubert P, *et al.* Clozapine-related pancreatitis. *Ann Intern Med* 1994; **121:** 722–3.

Hypersalivation. Hypersalivation has been reported[1] to occur in up to 54% of patients receiving clozapine. The pathophysiology for this effect is unclear, but proposed mechanisms include action at muscarinic (M_3 and M_4) receptors, blockade of α_2-adrenoceptors, or distortion of the swallowing reflex. Management strategies have included chewing gum to increase frequency of swallowing or reduction of clozapine dosage in stabilised patients; antimuscarinics or α_2-agonists have been tried when other methods have failed. However, antimuscarinics could potentially exacerbate the antimuscarinic adverse effects of clozapine, and intranasal administration of ipratropium bromide has been tried as an alternative with beneficial results in one small uncontrolled study.[2]

1. Davydov L, Botts SR. Clozapine-induced hypersalivation. *Ann Pharmacother* 2000; **34:** 662–5.

2. Calderon J, *et al.* Potential use of ipatropium [sic] bromide for the treatment of clozapine-induced hypersalivation: a preliminary report. *Int Clin Psychopharmacol* 2000; **15:** 49–52.

Neuroleptic malignant syndrome. A review of the literature[1] suggested that clozapine may produce fewer extrapyramidal effects and a lower rise in creatine kinase concentrations than classical antipsychotics. The incidence of neuroleptic malignant syndrome with clozapine appeared to be similar to that with classical antipsychotics;[1] however, its presentation may differ, with fever and rigidity less frequent, and possibly less severe, but diaphoresis more common.[2]

1. Sachdev P, *et al.* Clozapine-induced neuroleptic malignant syndrome: a review and report of new cases. *J Clin Psychopharmacol* 1995; **15:** 365–71.

2. Karagianis JL, *et al.* Clozapine-associated neuroleptic malignant syndrome: two new cases and a review of the literature. *Ann Pharmacother* 1999; **33:** 623–30. Correction. *ibid.*; 1011.

Withdrawal. A report[1] of 3 patients who experienced delirium with psychotic symptoms shortly after discontinuation of clozapine. One of the patients had developed symptoms within 24 hours despite gradual withdrawal of clozapine over a 2-week period. All the patients responded rapidly to resumption of low doses of clozapine.

1. Stanilla JK, *et al.* Clozapine withdrawal resulting in delirium with psychosis: a report of three cases. *J Clin Psychiatry* 1997; **58:** 252–5.

Precautions

As for Chlorpromazine, p.663.

Clozapine should not be given to patients with uncontrolled epilepsy, alcoholic or toxic psychoses, drug intoxication, or a history of circulatory collapse. It is contra-indicated in patients with bone-marrow suppression, myeloproliferative disorders, or any abnormalities of white blood cell count or differential blood count. It is also contra-indicated in patients with a history of drug-induced neutropenia or agranulocytosis. It should not be used concurrently with

drugs which carry a high risk of bone-marrow suppression (see Interactions, below). Clozapine is contra-indicated in patients with severe renal impairment; caution is required in mild to moderate renal impairment. It should be used with caution in hepatic impairment and avoided in symptomatic or progressive liver disease or hepatic failure. Clozapine should not be used in severe heart failure.

A white blood cell count and a differential blood count must be performed before starting clozapine therapy and regularly throughout treatment. Treatment should not be started if the white blood cell count is less than 3500 per mm³ or if there is an abnormal differential count. In the UK, monitoring is performed at weekly intervals for the first 18 weeks and then at least every 2 weeks for the first year of treatment; if the neutrophil count has remained stable during that period then monitoring can be changed to every 4 weeks. In the USA blood counts are monitored weekly for the first 6 months and then every 2 weeks thereafter. Monitoring should continue for 4 weeks after discontinuation. Clozapine should be withdrawn immediately if the white blood cell count falls below 3000 per mm³ and/or the absolute neutrophil count drops below 1500 per mm³. Repeat blood counts and more intense monitoring are required for counts just above these values. Patients or their carers should report the development of any infection or signs such as fever, sore throat, or flu-like symptoms which suggest infection.

Patients who develop tachycardia at rest, dyspnoea, or signs or symptoms of heart failure should be investigated immediately and clozapine treatment discontinued if a diagnosis of myocarditis is confirmed.

Because of an increased risk of collapse due to hypotension associated with initial titration of dosage of clozapine it is recommended that treatment be initiated under close medical supervision. On planned withdrawal the dose of clozapine should be reduced gradually over at least a 1- to 2-week period in order to avoid the risk of rebound psychosis. If abrupt withdrawal is necessary (see above) then patients should be observed carefully.

Interactions

As for Chlorpromazine, p.664.

Clozapine may enhance the central effects of MAOIs.

Clozapine should not be used concurrently with drugs which carry a high risk of bone-marrow suppression including carbamazepine, co-trimoxazole, chloramphenicol, penicillamine, sulfonamides, antineoplastics, or pyrazolone analgesics such as azapropazone. Long-acting depot antipsychotics should not be used with clozapine as they cannot be withdrawn rapidly should neutropenia occur.

Concomitant use of phenytoin or other enzyme-inducing drugs may accelerate the metabolism of clozapine and reduce its plasma concentrations. The metabolism of clozapine is mediated mainly by the cytochrome P450 isoenzyme CYP1A2. Concomitant use of drugs which inhibit or act as a substrate to this isoenzyme may affect plasma concentrations of clozapine.

◊ References.

1. Taylor D. Pharmacokinetic interactions involving clozapine. *Br J Psychiatry* 1997; **171:** 109–12.

Antibacterials. A patient with schizophrenia controlled with clozapine therapy had a tonic-clonic seizure 7 days after starting treatment with *erythromycin*.[1] It appeared that erythromycin had inhibited the metabolism of clozapine and raised its serum concentrations. Increased drowsiness and hypersalivation have been seen in a patient receiving clozapine and *ampicillin*; he recovered when ampicillin was replaced with doxycycline.[2] Co-administration of clozapine and *rifampicin* has resulted in decreased clozapine concentrations with consequent return of paranoid thoughts in a patient with a complicated history of schizophrenia.[3] An improvement was seen after rifampicin was substituted with ciprofloxacin. The interaction was thought to be due to the induction of cytochrome P450 isoenzymes, particularly CYP1A2, by rifampicin, resulting in the accelerated metabolism of clozapine.

1. Funderburg LG, *et al.* Seizure following addition of erythromycin to clozapine treatment. *Am J Psychiatry* 1994; **151:** 1840–1.

2. Csík V, Molnár J. Possible adverse interaction between clozapine and ampicillin in an adolescent with schizophrenia. *J Child Adolesc Psychopharmacol* 1994; **4:** 123–8.
3. Joos AAB, *et al.* Pharmacokinetic interaction of clozapine and rifampicin in a forensic patient with atypical mycobacterial infection. *J Clin Psychopharmacol* 1998; **18:** 83–5.

Antidepressants. Rises in serum concentrations of clozapine have been found in patients receiving clozapine after addition of *fluoxetine*[1] or *fluvoxamine*[2] to therapy. Increased serum concentrations of clozapine have also been reported when *paroxetine* or *sertraline* was added to therapy.[3] A possible serotonin syndrome (p.304) has been reported[4] in a patient receiving clomipramine after clozapine was gradually withdrawn from the treatment regimen, although the symptoms were also similar to those of clozapine withdrawal. There has been an isolated report[5] of a patient who developed myoclonic jerks 79 days after fluoxetine was added to treatment with clozapine and lorazepam, although some[6] doubt whether the effects were entirely due to an interaction. Giving clozapine with *lithium* may increase the risk of neuroleptic malignant syndrome. For reference to neurological reactions in patients receiving *lithium* concomitantly with clozapine, see p.295.

1. Centorrino F, *et al.* Serum concentrations of clozapine and its major metabolites: effects of cotreatment with fluoxetine or valproate. *Am J Psychiatry* 1994; **151:** 123–5.
2. Jerling M, *et al.* Fluvoxamine inhibition and carbamazepine induction of the metabolism of clozapine: evidence from a therapeutic drug monitoring service. *Ther Drug Monit* 1994; **16:** 368–74.
3. Centorrino F, *et al.* Serum levels of clozapine and norclozapine in patients treated with selective serotonin reuptake inhibitors. *Am J Psychiatry* 1996; **153:** 820–2.
4. Zerjav-Lacombe S, Dewan V. Possible serotonin syndrome associated with clomipramine after withdrawal of clozapine. *Ann Pharmacother* 2001; **35:** 180–2.
5. Kingsbury SJ, Puckett KM. Effects of fluoxetine on serum clozapine levels. *Am J Psychiatry* 1995; **152:** 473.
6. Baldessarini RJ, *et al.* Effects of fluoxetine on serum clozapine levels. *Am J Psychiatry* 1995; **152:** 473–4.

Antiepileptics. Concomitant use of *phenytoin* or other *enzyme-inducing antiepileptics* may accelerate the metabolism of clozapine and reduce its plasma concentrations. Studies have found that addition of *sodium valproate* to clozapine therapy may increase[1] or decrease[2] plasma concentrations of clozapine. Although no increase in clozapine-related adverse effects or loss of control of psychotic symptoms were reported in these studies there has been a report[3] of a patient who experienced sedation, confusion, slurring of speech and other functional impairment after valproate was given with clozapine.

See also under Benzodiazepines, below.

1. Centorrino F, *et al.* Serum concentrations of clozapine and its major metabolites: effects of cotreatment with fluoxetine or valproate. *Am J Psychiatry* 1994; **151:** 123–5.
2. Finley P, Warner D. Potential impact of valproic acid therapy on clozapine disposition. *Biol Psychiatry* 1994; **36:** 487–8.
3. Costello LE, Suppes T. A clinically significant interaction between clozapine and valproate. *J Clin Psychopharmacol* 1995; **15:** 139–41.

Antipsychotics. Adding *risperidone* in a patient with schizoaffective disorder partially controlled by clozapine produced clinical improvement but was associated with a 74% rise in serum-clozapine concentrations over a 2-week period.[1] Although no adverse effects had occurred in this patient the potential for serious adverse effects with elevated clozapine concentrations required caution if these drugs were used together. Neuroleptic malignant syndrome associated with concomitant use of clozapine and *haloperidol* has been reported.[2] See also under Chlorpromazine, p.665.

1. Tyson SC, *et al.* Pharmacokinetic interaction between risperidone and clozapine. *Am J Psychiatry* 1995; **152:** 1401–2.
2. Garcia G, *et al.* Neuroleptic malignant syndrome with antidepressant/antipsychotic drug combination. *Ann Pharmacother* 2001; **35:** 784–5.

Antivirals. Although the UK manufacturers of *ritonavir* state that it may increase plasma concentrations of clozapine with a resultant increase in the risk of toxicity, there is evidence to suggest that, in fact, ritonavir may decrease the plasma concentrations of clozapine.[1] Ritonavir has been noted to induce the cytochrome P450 isoenzyme CYP1A2 and hence, as clozapine is primarily metabolised via this isoenzyme, an acceleration of the metabolism of clozapine would be expected. US prescribing information has been amended accordingly.

1. Penzak SR, *et al.* Comment: significant interactions with new antiretrovirals and psychotropic drugs. *Ann Pharmacother* 1999; **33:** 1372–3.

Benzodiazepines. Concern has been expressed over reports of cardiorespiratory collapse in patients taking both clozapine and benzodiazepines.[1,2] In response, the manufacturers of clozapine outlined[3] similar cases reported to them in the USA. Of 7 cases of respiratory arrest or depression only 2 involved recent use of a benzodiazepine; among 26 cases of orthostatic hypotension with syncope reported during the first year the drug was marketed, only 8 included recent benzodiazepine use. The manufacturers concluded that an increased risk of such reactions in patients taking both drugs simultaneously was possible but not established, and advised caution when initiating clozapine therapy in patients taking benzodiazepines.

Hypersalivation associated with clozapine and benzodiazepines may be exacerbated when these drugs are used together. One patient[4] experienced increased hypersalivation, salivary thickening, and distension of the parotid glands when clon-

azepam was added to treatment with clozapine. Adverse effects reported in 5 other patients given clozapine and benzodiazepines together included hypersalivation, sedation, ataxia, and symptoms of delirium.[5,6]

1. Sassim N, Grohmann R. Adverse drug reactions with clozapine and simultaneous application of benzodiazepines. *Pharmacopsychiatry* 1988; **21:** 306–7.
2. Friedman LJ, *et al.* Clozapine—a novel antipsychotic agent. *N Engl J Med* 1991; **325:** 518.
3. Finkel MJ, Schwimmer JL. Clozapine—a novel antipsychotic agent. *N Engl J Med* 1991; **325:** 518–19.
4. Martin SD. Drug-induced parotid swelling. *Br J Hosp Med* 1993; **50:** 426.
5. Cobb CD, *et al.* Possible interaction between clozapine and lorazepam. *Am J Psychiatry* 1991; **148:** 1606–7.
6. Jackson CW, *et al.* Delirium associated with clozapine and benzodiazepine combinations. *Ann Clin Psychiatry* 1995; **7:** 139–41.

Buspirone. Potentially fatal gastrointestinal bleeding, accompanied by severe acidosis and hyperglycaemia, developed in a patient given buspirone in addition to clozapine.[1] The patient had previously been receiving clozapine for over a year without adverse effect, and was subsequently maintained on clozapine alone without a recurrence of symptoms.

1. Good MI. Lethal interaction of clozapine and buspirone? *Am J Psychiatry* 1997; **154:** 1472–3.

Histamine H₂-antagonists. A patient stabilised on clozapine developed increased serum clozapine concentrations and signs of clozapine toxicity after starting treatment with *cimetidine*.[1] Cimetidine was withdrawn and ranitidine substituted without recurrence of toxicity.

1. Szymanski S, *et al.* A case report of cimetidine-induced clozapine toxicity. *J Clin Psychiatry* 1991; **52:** 21–2.

Xanthines. *Caffeine* may inhibit the metabolism of clozapine.[1,2] Care should be taken before stopping or starting caffeine-containing beverages in patients stabilised on clozapine treatment.

1. Carrillo JA, *et al.* Effects of caffeine withdrawal from the diet on the metabolism of clozapine in schizophrenic patients. *J Clin Psychopharmacol* 1998; **18:** 311–16.
2. Hägg S, *et al.* Effect of caffeine on clozapine pharmacokinetics in healthy volunteers. *Br J Clin Pharmacol* 2000; **49:** 59–63.

Pharmacokinetics

Although clozapine is well absorbed from the gastrointestinal tract, its bioavailability is limited to about 50% by first-pass metabolism. Peak plasma concentrations are achieved an average of about 2.5 hours after administration by mouth. Clozapine is about 95% bound to plasma proteins and has a mean terminal elimination half-life of approximately 12 hours at steady state. It is almost completely metabolised; routes of metabolism include *N*-demethylation, hydroxylation, and *N*-oxidation. The metabolism of clozapine is mediated mainly by the cytochrome P450 isoenzyme CYP1A2. Metabolites and trace amounts of unchanged drug are excreted mainly in the urine and also in the faeces. There is wide interindividual variation in plasma concentrations of clozapine and no simple correlation has been found between plasma concentrations and therapeutic effect.

◊ References.

1. Jann MW, *et al.* Pharmacokinetics and pharmacodynamics of clozapine. *Clin Pharmacokinet* 1993; **24:** 161–76.
2. Lin S-K, *et al.* Disposition of clozapine and desmethylclozapine in schizophrenic patients. *J Clin Pharmacol* 1994; **34:** 318–24.
3. Freeman DJ, Oyewumi LK. Will routine therapeutic drug monitoring have a place in clozapine therapy? *Clin Pharmacokinet* 1997; **32:** 93–100.
4. Olesen OV. Therapeutic drug monitoring of clozapine treatment: therapeutic threshold value for serum clozapine concentrations. *Clin Pharmacokinet* 1998; **34:** 497–502.
5. Guitton C, *et al.* Clozapine and metabolite concentrations during treatment of patients with chronic schizophrenia. *J Clin Pharmacol* 1999; **39:** 721–8.

Uses and Administration

Clozapine is a dibenzodiazepine derivative described as an atypical antipsychotic. It has relatively weak dopamine receptor-blocking activity at D₁, D₂, D₃, and D₅ receptors but has a high affinity for the D₄ receptor. It causes only a minimal increase in prolactin secretion. Clozapine possesses alpha-adrenergic blocking, antimuscarinic, antihistamine, antiserotonergic, and sedative properties.

Clozapine is used for the management of schizophrenia; because of the risk of agranulocytosis, it is reserved for patients who fail to respond to, or who experience severe extrapyramidal side-effects with, classical antipsychotics. Clozapine use must be accompanied by strict procedures for the monitoring of white blood cell counts (see Precautions, above).

To minimise the incidence of adverse effects, clozapine therapy should be introduced gradually, beginning with low doses and increasing according to response. The usual dose by mouth is 12.5 mg once or twice on the first day followed by 25 mg once or twice on the second day. Thereafter the daily dosage may be increased gradually in increments of 25 to 50 mg to achieve a daily dose of up to 300 mg within 14 to 21 days; subsequent increments of 50 to 100 mg may be made once or twice weekly. Most patients respond to 200 to 450 mg daily; a daily dosage of 900 mg should not be exceeded. The total daily dose is given in divided doses; a larger proportion may be given at night. Once a therapeutic response has been obtained, a gradual reduction of dosage to a maintenance dose of 150 to 300 mg daily may be possible. Daily maintenance doses of 200 mg or less may be given as a single dose in the evening. If clozapine is to be withdrawn this should be done gradually over a 1- to 2-week period. However, immediate discontinuation with careful observation is essential if neutropenia develops (see Precautions, above).

Elderly patients may require lower doses of clozapine and it is recommended that treatment should be initiated with a dose of 12.5 mg on the first day and that subsequent dose increments should be restricted to 25 mg per day.

Patients with a history of epilepsy and those suffering from cardiovascular, renal, or hepatic disorders should receive a dose of 12.5 mg on the first day and subsequent dosage increases should be made slowly and in small increments. If seizures occur treatment should be suspended for 24 hours and resumed at a lower dose.

For patients who are restarting treatment after an interval of more than 2 days 12.5 mg may be given once or twice on the first day. If that dose is well tolerated it may be possible to increase the dosage more quickly than on initiation. However, patients who previously experienced respiratory or cardiac arrest with initial dosing should be re-titrated with extreme caution after even 24 hours discontinuation.

It is recommended that therapy with classical antipsychotics should be withdrawn gradually before treatment with clozapine is started.

Clozapine has also been given by intramuscular injection.

◊ References.

1. Fitton A, Heel RC. Clozapine: a review of its pharmacological properties, and therapeutic use in schizophrenia. *Drugs* 1990; **40:** 722–47.
2. Anonymous. Clozapine and loxapine for schizophrenia. *Drug Ther Bull* 1991; **29:** 41–2. Correction. *ibid.*; 52.
3. Baldessarini RJ, Frankenburg FR. Clozapine: a novel antipsychotic agent. *N Engl J Med* 1991; **324:** 746–54.
4. Hirsch SR, Puri BK. Clozapine: progress in treating refractory schizophrenia. *BMJ* 1993; **306:** 1427–8.
5. Taylor D. Clozapine—five years on. *Pharm J* 1995; **254:** 260–3.
6. Kerwin RW. Clozapine: back to the future for schizophrenia research. *Lancet* 1995; **345:** 1063–4.

Action. Antipsychotics are thought to work through inhibition of dopamine D₂-receptors (see p.666), but this hypothesis fails to explain the activity of the atypical antipsychotics such as clozapine. How clozapine produces its antipsychotic activity is not clear; it has a high affinity for a number of different receptors.[1]

1. Kerwin RW. The new atypical antipsychotics: a lack of extrapyramidal side-effects and new routes in schizophrenia research. *Br J Psychiatry* 1994; **164:** 141–8.

Disturbed behaviour. For mention that atypical antipsychotics such as clozapine might be more appropriate than classical antipsychotics for elderly patients with dementia, see the Elderly in Precautions for Chlorpromazine, p.663. For further discussion of the management of disturbed behaviour, see p.650.

Parkinsonism. Clozapine appears to be of potential use as an alternative to classical antipsychotics for the treatment of psychosis in patients with Parkinson's disease (p.1160). Some neurologists even consider clozapine to be the antipsychotic of choice in these patients although this remains to be determined. A review[1] in 1994 considered that there was little evidence to support clozapine as first choice given the quality of the available studies and the need for extensive monitoring. However a more recent double-blind, placebo-controlled study[2] demonstrated that low-dose clozapine treatment (up to 50 mg daily) significantly improved drug-induced psychosis without worsening parkinsonism. Adverse effects noted in this study were generally mild although in the clozapine group of 30 patients, there was one report of leucopenia. Adverse effects reported from other individuals have also included a patient with parkinsonism who experienced worsening of psychotic symptoms when her dose of clozapine was increased,[3] and the sudden return of psychosis in another patient with parkinsonism whose psychosis was successfully treated with clozapine for 5 years.[4]

1. Pfeiffer C, Wagner ML. Clozapine therapy for Parkinson's disease and other movement disorders. *Am J Hosp Pharm* 1994; **51:** 3047–53.
2. The Parkinson Study Group. Low-dose clozapine for the treatment of drug-induced psychosis in Parkinson's disease. *N Engl J Med* 1999; **340:** 757–63.
3. Auzou P, *et al.* Worsening of psychotic symptoms by clozapine in Parkinson's disease. *Lancet* 1994; **344:** 955.
4. Greene P. Clozapine therapeutic plunge in patient with Parkinson's disease. *Lancet* 1995; **345:** 1172–3.

Schizophrenia. Clozapine is an effective antipsychotic for the management of schizophrenia (p.651) but its use is limited by its blood toxicity. Its effectiveness and superiority over classical antipsychotics was demonstrated by Kane *et al.* in a multicentre study.[1] Patients refractory to at least 3 different antipsychotics and who failed to improve after a single-blind trial of haloperidol, were randomised, double-blind, to treatment for 6 weeks with either clozapine, up to 900 mg daily, or chlorpromazine hydrochloride up to 1800 mg daily with benzatropine mesilate up to 6 mg daily. Of the 267 patients included in the evaluation, 5 of 141 (4%) improved with chlorpromazine and benzatropine, and 38 of 126 (30%) improved with clozapine. Clozapine was superior to chlorpromazine in the treatment of negative as well as positive symptoms. Reviews[2,3] of clozapine indicate that these findings have been well replicated both in subsequent studies and in clinical practice. It is, however, unclear for how long clozapine should initially be tried: although one study[4] identified new responses up to 12 months after initiation of therapy others have indicated that if improvement was not seen within the first 6 to 24 weeks, it was unlikely to occur.[2,5]

Clozapine has shown consistent clinical benefit in schizophrenic patients with persistent aggressive or violent behaviour.[2] Whether this is due to a sedative effect, a specific antiaggressive action, or just reflects an overall improvement in psychosis remains to be determined.

Clozapine also appears to reduce suicide risk in patients with refractory chronic schizophrenia.[6] The reported suicide rate of 0.05% per year in 6300 patients in the UK given clozapine since 1990 was considered to be tenfold less than expected.[7]

Clozapine has been advocated for use in schizophrenic patients with moderate to severe tardive dyskinesia. It is still unclear whether clozapine can itself cause tardive dyskinesia but some patients with established tardive dyskinesia have experienced improvement in their symptoms when using clozapine.[8,9]

1. Kane J, *et al.* Clozapine for the treatment-resistant schizophrenic: a double-blind comparison with chlorpromazine. *Arch Gen Psychiatry* 1988; **45:** 789–96.
2. Buckley PF. New dimensions in the pharmacologic treatment of schizophrenia and related psychoses. *J Clin Pharmacol* 1997; **37:** 363–78. Correction. *ibid.* 1998; **38:** 27.
3. Wahlbeck K, *et al.* Clozapine versus typical neuroleptic medication for schizophrenia (dated 29 March 2001). Available in The Cochrane Library; Issue 4. Oxford: Update Software; 2001.
4. Meltzer HY, *et al.* A prospective study of clozapine in treatment-resistant schizophrenic patients I: preliminary report. *Psychopharmacology (Berl)* 1989; **99:** S68–S72.
5. Conley RR, *et al.* Time to clozapine response in a standardized trial. *Am J Psychiatry* 1997; **154:** 1243–7.
6. Meltzer HY, Okayli G. Reduction of suicidality during clozapine treatment of neuroleptic-resistant schizophrenia: impact on risk-benefit assessment. *Am J Psychiatry* 1995; **152:** 183–90.
7. Kerwin RW. Clozapine: back to the future for schizophrenia research. *Lancet* 1995; **345:** 1063–4.
8. Tamminga CA, *et al.* Clozapine in tardive dyskinesia: observations from human and animal model studies. *J Clin Psychiatry* 1994; **55** (suppl B): 102–106.
9. Nair C, *et al.* Dose-related effects of clozapine on tardive dyskinesia among "treatment-refractory" patients with schizophrenia. *Biol Psychiatry* 1996; **39:** 529–30.

Preparations

Proprietary Preparations (details are given in Part 3)
Aust.: Leponex; **Austral.:** Clopine; Clozaril; **Belg.:** Leponex; **Braz.:** Leponex; **Canad.:** Clozaril; **Denm.:** Leponex; **Fin.:** Froidir; **Fr.:** Leponex; **Ger.:** Elcrit; Leponex; **Hong Kong:** Clozaril; **Irl.:** Clozaril; **Israel:** Leponex; **Ital.:** Leponex; **Mex.:** Clopsine; Leponex; **Neth.:** Leponex; **NZ:** Clozaril; **Port.:** Leponex; **S.Afr.:** Leponex; **Singapore:** Clozaril; **Spain:** Leponex; **Swed.:** Leponex; **Switz.:** Leponex; **Thai.:** Clozaril; **UK:** Clozaril; **USA:** Clozaril.

Cyamemazine (7033-w)

Cyamemazine (rINN).

Cyamepromazine; RP-7204. 10-(3-Dimethylamino-2-methylpropyl)phenothiazine-2-carbonitrile.
$C_{19}H_{21}N_3S = 323.5$.
CAS — 3546-03-0.
ATC — N05AA06.

Profile

Cyamemazine is a phenothiazine with general properties similar to those of chlorpromazine (p.660). It is available as a preparation for the management of a variety of psychiatric disorders including anxiety disorders (p.649) and aggressive behaviour (p.650).

Cyamemazine has been given by mouth as the base or the tartrate and by injection as the base. Doses (expressed in terms of the equivalent amount of cyamemazine) have ranged from 25 to 600 mg daily by mouth, depending on the individual and the condition being treated; the daily dosage is given in 2 or 3 divided doses with the larger amount at night. Doses given by intramuscular injection have ranged from 25 to 200 mg daily. Cyamemazine should be given in reduced dosage to elderly patients; the parenteral route is not recommended for the elderly.

Preparations

Proprietary Preparations (details are given in Part 3)
Fr.: Tercian; **Port.:** Tercian.

Cyclobarbital (4025-s)

Cyclobarbital (BAN, rINN).

Ciclobarbital; Cyclobarbitalum; Cyclobarbitone; Ethylhexabital; Hexemalum. 5-(Cyclohex-1-enyl)-5-ethylbarbituric acid.
$C_{12}H_{16}N_2O_3 = 236.3$.
CAS — 52-31-3.
ATC — N05CA10.

NOTE. The name ciclobarbital has sometimes been applied to hexobarbital.

Pharmacopoeias. In Aust.

Cyclobarbital Calcium (4026-w)

Cyclobarbital Calcium (BANM, rINNM).

Ciclobarbital Calcium; Cyclobarbitalum Calcicum; Cyclobarbitone Calcium; Hexemalcalcium. Calcium 5-(cyclohex-1-enyl)-5-ethylbarbiturate.
$(C_{12}H_{15}N_2O_3)_2Ca = 510.6$.
CAS — 5897-20-1.

Pharmacopoeias. In Aust., Belg., Fr., It., Neth., Pol., and Port.

Profile

Cyclobarbital is a barbiturate with general properties similar to those of amobarbital (p.655). The calcium salt has been used as a hypnotic.

Preparations

Proprietary Preparations (details are given in Part 3)
Multi-ingredient: Belg.: Domidorm†.

Delorazepam (12552-s)

Delorazepam (pINN).

Chlordesmethyldiazepam; Clordesmethyldiazepam. 7-Chloro-5-(2-chlorophenyl)-1,3-dihydro-2H-1,4-benzodiazepin-2-one.
$C_{15}H_{10}Cl_2N_2O = 305.2$.
CAS — 2894-67-9.

Profile

Delorazepam is a long-acting benzodiazepine with general properties similar to those of diazepam (p.674). It has been used in the short-term treatment of anxiety disorders (p.649) in doses of 0.5 to 2 mg given two or three times daily by mouth. A dose of 0.5 to 2 mg has been used at night for insomnia (p.652). It has also been given by intramuscular injection for premedication, for anxiety disorders, and in the management of epilepsy.

Administration in hepatic or renal impairment. The pharmacokinetics of total delorazepam were unchanged in patients with renal failure undergoing haemodialysis compared with controls.[1] However, the apparent volume of distribution of unbound drug was smaller and the clearance slower. The volume of distribution and clearance of unchanged drug was also reduced in patients with liver disease[2] and delorazepam should therefore be used with caution in patients with hepatic impairment.

1. Sennesael J, *et al.* Pharmacokinetics of intravenous and oral chlordesmethyldiazepam in patients on regular haemodialysis. *Eur J Clin Pharmacol* 1991; **41:** 65–8.
2. Bareggi SR, *et al.* Effects of liver disease on the pharmacokinetics of intravenous and oral chlordesmethyldiazepam. *Eur J Clin Pharmacol* 1995; **48:** 265–8.

Preparations

Proprietary Preparations (details are given in Part 3)
Ital.: En.

Detomidine Hydrochloride (18627-j)

Detomidine Hydrochloride (BAN, USAN, rINNM).

Demotidini Hydrochloridum; MPV-253-AII. 4-(2,3-Dimethylbenzyl)imidazole monohydrochloride.
$C_{12}H_{14}N_2,HCl = 222.7$.
CAS — 90038-01-0 (detomidine hydrochloride); 76631-46-4 (detomidine).

Pharmacopoeias. In Eur. (see p.vi) for veterinary use only.

Pharmacopoeial description

Ph. Eur.: A white or almost white, hygroscopic, crystalline powder. Soluble in water; freely soluble in alcohol; practically insoluble in acetone; very slightly soluble in dichloromethane. Protect from moisture.

Profile

Detomidine is an α_2-adrenoceptor agonist with sedative, muscle relaxant, and analgesic properties. It is used as the hydrochloride in veterinary medicine.

Dexmedetomidine Hydrochloride (20689-m)

Dexmedetomidine Hydrochloride (BANM, USAN, rINNM).
MPV-1440 (dexmedetomidine). (S)-4-[1-(2,3-Xylyl)ethyl]imidazole hydrochloride.
$C_{13}H_{16}N_2,HCl = 236.7$.
CAS — 113775-47-6 (dexmedetomidine); 145108-58-3 (dexmedetomidine hydrochloride).

Adverse Effects and Precautions

The most frequently observed adverse effect with dexmedetomidine is hypotension. Other common adverse effects include hypertension, nausea and vomiting, bradycardia, tachycardia, fever, hypoxia, and anaemia. Patients should be continuously monitored during administration. Dexmedetomidine should be used with caution in patients with advanced heart block, or hepatic or renal impairment, or in the elderly.

Pharmacokinetics

Dexmedetomidine is approximately 94% protein bound, but this has been reported to be significantly decreased in patients with hepatic impairment. Dexmedetomidine is almost completely metabolised by direct glucuronidation or by isoenzymes of the cytochrome P450 system. It is excreted mainly as metabolites in the urine and faeces. The terminal elimination half-life is approximately 2 hours.

Uses and Administration

Dexmedetomidine is a selective alpha$_2$-adrenergic receptor agonist with anxiolytic, analgesic, and sedative properties. It is used as the hydrochloride for the sedation of mechanically ventilated patients in intensive care.

Dexmedetomidine hydrochloride is administered in 0.9% sodium chloride by intravenous infusion in a loading dose of 1 µg per kg body-weight over 10 minutes, followed by a maintenance infusion of 0.2 to 0.7 µg per kg per hour for up to 24 hours. Reduced doses may be necessary in patients with hepatic or renal impairment, or in the elderly.

The racemate, medetomidine (p.690), is used as the hydrochloride in veterinary medicine.

◊ References.
1. Peden CJ, Prys-Roberts C. Dexmedetomidine—a powerful new adjunct to anaesthesia? *Br J Anaesth* 1992; **68:** 123–5.
2. Scheinin H, *et al.* Pharmacodynamics and pharmacokinetics of intramuscular dexmedetomidine. *Clin Pharmacol Ther* 1992; **52:** 537–46.
3. Aho M, *et al.* Comparison of dexmedetomidine and midazolam sedation and antagonism of dexmedetomidine with atipamezole. *J Clin Anesth* 1993; **5:** 194–203.
4. Kivistö KT, *et al.* Pharmacokinetics and pharmacodynamics of transdermal dexmedetomidine. *Eur J Clin Pharmacol* 1994; **46:** 345–9.
5. Venn RM, *et al.* Preliminary UK experience of dexmedetomidine, a novel agent for postoperative sedation in the intensive care unit. *Anaesthesia* 1999; **54:** 1136–42.
6. Bhana N, *et al.* Dexmedetomidine. *Drugs* 2000; **59:** 263–8.

Preparations

Proprietary Preparations (details are given in Part 3)
USA: Precedex.

Diazepam (7036-y)

Diazepam (BAN, USAN, rINN).

Diazepamum; LA-III; NSC-77518; Ro-5-2807; Wy-3467. 7-Chloro-1,3-dihydro-1-methyl-5-phenyl-2H-1,4-benzodiazepin-2-one.
$C_{16}H_{13}ClN_2O = 284.7$.
CAS — 439-14-5.
ATC — N05BA01.

Pharmacopoeias. In Chin., Eur. (see p.vi), Int., Jpn, Pol., and US.

Pharmacopoeial description

Ph. Eur.: A white or almost white, crystalline powder. Very slightly soluble in water; soluble in alcohol. Protect from light.

USP 25: An off-white to yellow, practically odourless, crystalline powder. Soluble 1 in 333 of water, 1 in 16 of alcohol, 1 in 2 of chloroform, and 1 in 39 of ether. Store in airtight containers. Protect from light.

Dilution. Great care should be observed on dilution of diazepam injections for administration by infusion because of problems of precipitation. The manufacturer's directions should be followed regarding diluent and concentration of diazepam and all solutions should be freshly prepared.

Incompatibility. Incompatibility has been reported between diazepam and several other drugs. Manufacturers of diazepam injection (Roche and others) have advised against its admixture with other drugs.

Sorption. Substantial adsorption of diazepam onto some plastics may cause problems when administering the drug by continuous intravenous infusion. More than 50% of diazepam in solution may be adsorbed onto the walls of PVC infusion bags and their use should, therefore, be avoided. Administration sets should contain the minimum amount of polyvinyl chloride tubing and should not contain a cellulose propionate volume-control chamber. Suitable materials for infusion containers, syringes, and administration sets when administering diazepam include glass, polyolefin, polypropylene, and polyethylene.

References.
1. Cloyd JC, et al. Availability of diazepam from plastic containers. Am J Hosp Pharm 1980; 37: 492–6.
2. Parker WA, MacCara ME. Compatibility of diazepam with intravenous fluid containers and administration sets. Am J Hosp Pharm 1980; 37: 496–500.
3. Kowaluk EA, et al. Interactions between drugs and intravenous delivery systems. Am J Hosp Pharm 1982; 39: 460–7.
4. Kowaluk EA, et al. Factors affecting the availability of diazepam stored in plastic bags and administered through intravenous sets. Am J Hosp Pharm 1983; 40: 417–23.
5. Martens HJ, et al. Sorption of various drugs in polyvinyl chloride, glass, and polyethylene-lined infusion containers. Am J Hosp Pharm 1990; 47: 369–73.

Dependence and Withdrawal

The development of dependence is common after regular use of diazepam or other benzodiazepines, even in therapeutic doses for short periods. Dependence is particularly likely in patients with a history of alcohol or drug abuse and in patients with marked personality disorders. Benzodiazepines should not therefore be discontinued abruptly after regular use for even a few weeks, but should be withdrawn by gradual reduction of the dose; the time needed for withdrawal can vary from about 4 weeks to a year or more. The extent to which tolerance occurs has been debated but appears to involve psychomotor performance more often than anxiolytic effects. Drug-seeking behaviour is uncommon with therapeutic doses of benzodiazepines. High doses of diazepam and other benzodiazepines, injected intravenously, have been abused for their euphoriant effects.

Benzodiazepine withdrawal syndrome. Development of dependence to benzodiazepines cannot be predicted but risk factors include high dosage, regular continuous use, the use of benzodiazepines with a short half-life, use in patients with dependent personality characteristics or a history of drug or alcohol dependence, and the development of tolerance.

The mechanism of benzodiazepine dependence is unclear. One possible mechanism is a relative deficiency of functional gamma-aminobutyric acid (GABA) activity resulting from down-regulation of GABA receptors.

Symptoms of benzodiazepine withdrawal include anxiety, depression, impaired concentration, insomnia, headache, dizziness, tinnitus, loss of appetite, tremor, perspiration, irritability, perceptual disturbances such as hypersensitivity to physical, visual, and auditory stimuli and abnormal taste, nausea, vomiting, abdominal cramps, palpitations, mild systolic hypertension, tachycardia, and orthostatic hypotension. Rare and more serious symptoms include muscle twitching, confusional or paranoid psychosis, convulsions, hallucinations, and a state resembling delirium tremens. Broken sleep with vivid dreams and increased REM sleep may persist for some weeks after withdrawal of benzodiazepines.

Symptoms typical of withdrawal have been observed despite continued use of benzodiazepines and have been attributed either to the development of tolerance or, as in the case of very short-acting drugs such as triazolam, to rapid benzodiazepine elimination. Pseudowithdrawal has been reported in patients who believed incorrectly that their dose of benzodiazepine was being reduced. Benzodiazepine withdrawal syndrome can theoretically be distinguished from these reactions and from rebound phenomena (return of original symptoms at greater than pretreatment severity) by the differing time course. A withdrawal syndrome is characterised by its onset, by the development of new symptoms, and by a peak in intensity followed by resolution. Onset of withdrawal symptoms depends on the half-life of the drug and its active metabolites. Symptoms can begin within a few hours after withdrawal of a short-acting benzodiazepine, but may not develop for up to 3 weeks after stopping a longer-acting benzodiazepine. Resolution of symptoms may take several days or months. The dependence induced by short- and long-acting benzodiazepines appears to be qualitatively similar although withdrawal symptoms may be more severe with short-acting benzodiazepines. Rebound effects are also more likely with short-acting benzodiazepines. Rebound and withdrawal symptoms develop particularly rapidly with the very short-acting drug triazolam.

With increased awareness of the problems of benzodiazepine dependence, emphasis has been placed on prevention by proper use and careful patient selection. For example, the UK Committee on Safety of Medicines has recommended that benzodiazepines should be reserved for the short-term relief (2 to 4 weeks only) of anxiety that is severe, disabling, or subjecting the individual to unacceptable distress and is occurring alone or in association with insomnia or short-term psychosomatic, organic, or psychotic illness. These recommendations are similar to those of the UK Royal College of Psychiatrists.

The symbol † denotes a preparation no longer actively marketed

Withdrawal from long-term benzodiazepine use should generally be encouraged. The patient should have professional and family support and behavioural therapy may be helpful. Withdrawal in a specialist centre may be required for some patients. Since abrupt withdrawal of benzodiazepines may result in severe withdrawal symptoms dosage should be tapered. The British National Formulary considers that benzodiazepines can be withdrawn in steps of about one-eighth of the daily dose every fortnight (range one-tenth to one-quarter). There are no comparative studies of the efficacy of various withdrawal schedules and in practice the protocol should be titrated against the response of the patient. Clinicians often favour transferring the patient to an equivalent dose of diazepam given at night and the following approximate dosage equivalents to diazepam 5 mg have been recommended in the UK:

- chlordiazepoxide 15 mg
- loprazolam 0.5 to 1 mg
- lorazepam 500 µg
- lormetazepam 0.5 to 1 mg
- nitrazepam 5 mg
- oxazepam 15 mg
- temazepam 10 mg.

The daily dosage of diazepam can then be reduced in steps of 0.5 to 2.5 mg at fortnightly intervals. If troublesome abstinence effects occur the dose should be held level for a longer period before further reduction; increased dosage should be avoided if possible. It is better to reduce too slowly than too quickly. Time required for withdrawal can vary from about 4 weeks to a year or longer. In many cases the rate of withdrawal is best decided by the patient.

Adjuvant therapy should generally be avoided although a beta blocker may be given for prominent sympathetic overactivity and an antidepressant for clinical depression. Antipsychotic drugs may aggravate symptoms.

Symptoms gradually improve after withdrawal but postwithdrawal syndromes lasting for several weeks or months have been described. Continued support may be required for the first year after withdrawal to prevent relapse.

References.
1. Committee on Safety of Medicines. Benzodiazepines, dependence and withdrawal symptoms. Current Problems 21 1988.
2. Royal College of Psychiatrists. Benzodiazepines and dependence: a college statement. Bull R Coll Psychiatrists 1988; 12: 107–8.
3. Marriott S, Tyrer P. Benzodiazepine dependence: avoidance and withdrawal. Drug Safety 1993; 9: 93–103.
4. Pétursson H. The benzodiazepine withdrawal syndrome. Addiction 1994; 89: 1455–59.
5. Ashton H. The treatment of benzodiazepine dependence. Addiction 1994; 89: 1535–41.
6. DoH. Drug misuse and dependence: guidelines on clinical management. London: The Stationery Office, 1999.

Adverse Effects

Drowsiness, sedation, muscle weakness, and ataxia are the most frequent adverse effects of diazepam use. They generally decrease on continued administration and are a consequence of CNS depression. Less frequent effects include vertigo, headache, confusion, depression (but see Effects on Mental Function, below), slurred speech or dysarthria, changes in libido, tremor, visual disturbances, urinary retention or incontinence, gastrointestinal disturbances, changes in salivation, and amnesia. Some patients may experience a paradoxical excitation which may lead to hostility, aggression, and disinhibition. Jaundice, blood disorders, and hypersensitivity reactions have been reported rarely. Respiratory depression and hypotension occasionally occur with high dosage and parenteral administration.

Pain and thrombophlebitis may occur with some intravenous formulations of diazepam; raised liver enzyme values have occurred.

Overdosage can produce CNS depression and coma or paradoxical excitation. However, fatalities are rare when taken alone.

Use of diazepam in the first trimester of pregnancy has occasionally been associated with congenital malformations in the infant but no clear relationship has been established. This topic is reviewed under Pregnancy and Breast Feeding, below. Administration of diazepam in late pregnancy has been associated with intoxication of the neonate.

Carcinogenicity. The International Agency for Research on Cancer concluded[1] that there was sufficient evidence from human studies that diazepam did not produce breast cancer, and that there was inadequate data to support its potential carcinogenicity at other sites. For most other benzodiazepines the lack of human studies meant that the carcinogenic risk to humans was not classifiable. However, there appeared to be sufficient

evidence of carcinogenicity in animal studies for oxazepam to be classified as possibly carcinogenic in humans.
1. IARC/WHO. Some pharmaceutical drugs. IARC monographs on the evaluation of carcinogenic risks to humans volume 66 1996.

Effects on body temperature. Studies in healthy subjects[1,2] indicate that benzodiazepines can reduce body temperature. After a single dose of diazepam 10 mg by mouth in 11 subjects, body temperature on exposure to cold fell to a mean of 36.93° compared with 37.08° on exposure without the drug.[1] An 86-year-old woman developed hypothermia[3] after administration of nitrazepam 5 mg. After recovery she was mistakenly given another 5-mg dose of nitrazepam and again developed hypothermia.

Hypothermia has been reported in the neonates of mothers given benzodiazepines during the late stages of pregnancy.
1. Martin SM. The effect of diazepam on body temperature change in humans during cold exposure. J Clin Pharmacol 1985; 25: 611–13.
2. Matsukawa T, et al. I.M. midazolam as premedication produces a concentration-dependent decrease in core temperature in male volunteers. Br J Anaesth 1997; 78: 396–9.
3. Impallomeni M, Ezzat R. Hypothermia associated with nitrazepam administration. BMJ 1976; 1: 223–4.

Effects on endocrine function. Galactorrhoea with normal serum-prolactin concentrations has been noted in 4 women taking benzodiazepines.[1] Gynaecomastia has been reported in a man taking up to 140 mg diazepam daily[2] and in 5 men taking diazepam in doses of up to 30 mg daily.[3] Serum-oestradiol concentrations were raised in the latter group. However, raised plasma-testosterone concentrations have also been observed in men taking diazepam 10 to 20 mg daily for 2 weeks.[4]
1. Kleinberg DL, et al. Galactorrhea: a study of 235 cases, including 48 with pituitary tumors. N Engl J Med 1977; 296: 589–600.
2. Moerck HJ, Magelund G. Gynaecomastia and diazepam abuse. Lancet 1979; i: 1344–5.
3. Bergman D, et al. Increased oestradiol in diazepam related gynaecomastia. Lancet 1981; ii: 1225–6.
4. Argüelles AE, Rosner J. Diazepam and plasma-testosterone levels. Lancet 1975; ii: 607.

Effects on the eyes. Brown opacification of the lens occurred in a married couple who took diazepam 5 mg or more daily by mouth over several years.[1]
1. Pau H. Braune scheibenförmige Einlagerungen in die Linse nach Langzeitgabe von Diazepam (Valium). Klin Monatsbl Augenheilkd 1985; 187: 219–20.

Effects on the liver. Reports of cholestatic jaundice[1] in one patient and focal hepatic necrosis with intracellular cholestasis[2] in another associated with the use of diazepam.
1. Jick H, et al. Drug-induced liver disease. J Clin Pharmacol 1981; 21: 359–64.
2. Tedesco FJ, Mills LR. Diazepam (Valium) hepatitis. Dig Dis Sci 1982; 27: 470–2.

Effects on mental function. The effects of benzodiazepines on psychomotor performance in laboratory tests[1] are not easily extrapolated to the clinical situation.

Concern has been expressed over the possible effects of long-term benzodiazepine use on the brain. A detailed study[2] found that performance of tasks involving visual-spatial ability and sustained attention was poor in patients taking high doses of benzodiazepines for long periods of time. There was no evidence of impairment in global measures of intellectual functioning such as memory, flexibility, and simple reaction time. The authors could draw no conclusions about the effect of benzodiazepine withdrawal on these changes. A study of 17 long-term users of benzodiazepines has indicated a dose-dependent increase in cerebral ventricle size.[3]

Sexual fantasies have been reported in women sedated with intravenous diazepam or midazolam.[4] These appear to be dose-related.[5]

The view that benzodiazepines can cause depression, albeit infrequently, has been queried.[6]

Adverse effects of alprazolam on behaviour have also been reviewed.[7]
1. Woods JH, et al. Abuse liability of benzodiazepines. Pharmacol Rev 1987; 39: 251–413.
2. Golombok S, et al. Cognitive impairment in long-term benzodiazepine users. Psychol Med 1988; 18: 365–74.
3. Schmauss C, Krieg J-C. Enlargement of cerebrospinal fluid spaces in long-term benzodiazepine abusers. Psychol Med 1987; 17: 869–73.
4. Dundee JW. Fantasies during benzodiazepine sedation in women. Br J Clin Pharmacol 1990; 30: 311P.
5. Brahams D. Benzodiazepine sedation and allegations of sexual assault. Lancet 1989; i: 1339–40.
6. Patten SB, Love EJ. Drug-induced depression: incidence, avoidance and management. Drug Safety 1994; 10: 203–19.
7. Cole JO, Kando JC. Adverse behavioral events reported in patients taking alprazolam and other benzodiazepines. J Clin Psychiatry 1993; 54 (suppl): 49–61.

Effects on the nervous system. There are a few isolated reports of extrapyramidal symptoms in patients taking benzodiazepines.[1-4] Benzodiazepines have been used to treat such symptoms induced by antipsychotics (see Chlorpromazine, p.662).
1. Rosenbaum AH, De La Fuente JR. Benzodiazepines and tardive dyskinesia. Lancet 1979; ii: 900.
2. Sandyk R. Orofacial dyskinesias associated with lorazepam therapy. Clin Pharm 1986; 5: 419–21.

3. Stolarek IH, Ford MJ. Acute dystonia induced by midazolam and abolished by flumazenil. *BMJ* 1990; **300:** 614.

4. Joseph AB, Wroblewski BA. Paradoxical akathisia caused by clonazepam, clorazepate and lorazepam in patients with traumatic encephalopathy and seizure disorders: a subtype of benzodiazepine-induced disinhibition? *Behav Neurol* 1993; **6:** 221–3.

ENCEPHALOPATHY. Prolonged use of midazolam with fentanyl has been associated with encephalopathy in infants sedated under intensive care.[1]

1. Bergman I, *et al.* Reversible neurologic abnormalities associated with prolonged intravenous midazolam and fentanyl administration. *J Pediatr* 1991; **119:** 644–9.

Effects on sexual function. Benzodiazepines have no direct effects on erection or ejaculation but their sedative effect may reduce sexual arousal and lead to impotence in some patients. Conversely sexual performance may be improved when it is impaired by anxiety.[1] Increased libido and orgasmic function has been reported in 2 women after withdrawal of long-term benzodiazepine use.[2]

1. Beeley L. Drug-induced sexual dysfunction and infertility. *Adverse Drug React Acute Poisoning Rev* 1984; **3:** 23–42.

2. Nutt D, *et al.* Increased sexual function in benzodiazepine withdrawal. *Lancet* 1986; **ii:** 1101–2.

Effects on skeletal muscle. In a report[1] of 2 patients who developed rhabdomyolysis secondary to hyponatraemia it was suggested that the use of benzodiazepines might have contributed to the rhabdomyolysis. Of 8 reported cases of rhabdomyolysis associated with hyponatraemia, 5 had received benzodiazepines.

1. Fernández-Real JM, *et al.* Hyponatremia and benzodiazepines result in rhabdomyolysis. *Ann Pharmacother* 1994; **28:** 1200–1.

Effects on the skin. Analysis by the Boston Collaborative Drug Surveillance Program of data on 15 438 patients hospitalised between 1975 and 1982 detected 2 allergic skin reactions attributed to diazepam among 4707 recipients of the drug.[1] A reaction rate of 0.4 per 1000 recipients was calculated from these figures.

1. Bigby M, *et al.* Drug-induced cutaneous reactions. *JAMA* 1986; **256:** 3358–63.

Hypersensitivity. Hypersensitivity reactions including anaphylaxis are very rare following administration of diazepam. Reactions have been attributed to the polyethoxylated castor oil (p.1347) vehicle used for some parenteral formulations.[1] There is also a report of a type I hypersensitivity reaction to a lipid emulsion formulation of diazepam.[2]

See also under Effects on the Skin, above.

1. Hüttel MS, *et al.* Complement-mediated reactions to diazepam with Cremophor as solvent (Stesolid MR). *Br J Anaesth* 1980; **52:** 77–9.

2. Deardon DJ, Bird GLA. Acute (type 1) hypersensitivity to iv Diazemuls. *Br J Anaesth* 1987; **59:** 391.

Local reactions. Ischaemia and gangrene have been reported after accidental intra-arterial injection of diazepam.[1,2] Clinical signs may not occur until several days after the event. Pain and thrombophlebitis after intravenous administration may be similarly delayed. Local reactions after intravenous injection have been attributed to the vehicle, and have been observed more often when diazepam is given as a solution in propylene glycol than in polyethoxylated castor oil.[3] An emulsion of diazepam in soya oil and water has been associated with a lower incidence of local reactions.[3] Pain and phlebitis may also be caused by precipitation of diazepam at the site of infusion.[4] Arterial spasm experienced by a patient given diazepam intravenously was probably due to pressure from a cuff on the arm being inflated causing extravasation of diazepam out of the vein and into the radial artery.[5]

Local irritation has also been observed after rectal administration of diazepam.[6]

For a report of the exacerbation of diazepam-induced thrombophlebitis by penicillamine, see below.

1. Gould JDM, Lingam S. Hazards of intra-arterial diazepam. *BMJ* 1977; **2:** 298–9.

2. Rees M, Dormandy J. Accidental intra-arterial injection of diazepam. *BMJ* 1980; **281:** 289–90.

3. Olesen AS, Hüttel MS. Local reactions to iv diazepam in three different formulations. *Br J Anaesth* 1980; **52:** 609–11.

4. Hussey EK, *et al.* Correlation of delayed peak concentration with infusion-site irritation following diazepam administration. *DICP Ann Pharmacother* 1990; **24:** 678–80.

5. Ng Wing Tin L, *et al.* Arterial spasm after administration of diazepam. *Br J Anaesth* 1994; **72:** 139.

6. Hansen HC, *et al.* Local irritation after administration of diazepam in a rectal solution. *Br J Anaesth* 1989; **63:** 287–9.

Overdosage. Impairment of consciousness is fairly rapid in poisoning by benzodiazepines.[1] Deep coma or other manifestations of severe depression of brainstem vital functions are rare; more common is a sleep-like state from which the patient can be temporarily roused by appropriate stimuli. There is usually little or no respiratory depression, and cardiac rate and rhythm remain normal in the absence of anoxia or severe hypotension. Since tolerance to benzodiazepines develops rapidly, consciousness is often regained when concentrations of drug in the blood are higher than those which induced coma. Anxiety and insomnia can occur during recovery from acute overdosage, while a full-blown withdrawal syndrome, possibly with major convulsions, can occur in patients who have previously been chronic users.

During the years 1980 to 1989, 1576 fatal poisonings in Britain were attributed to benzodiazepines.[2] Of these, 891 were linked to overdosage with benzodiazepines alone and another 591 to overdosage combined with alcohol. A comparison of these mortality statistics with prescribing data for the same period, to calculate a toxicity index of deaths per million prescriptions, suggested that there were differences between the relative toxicities of individual benzodiazepines in overdosage. A later study of another 303 cases of benzodiazepine poisoning[3] supported these findings of differences in toxicity as well as pointing to the relative safety of the benzodiazepines in overdosage.

1. Ashton CH, *et al.* Drug-induced stupor and coma: some physical signs and their pharmacological basis. *Adverse Drug React Acute Poisoning Rev* 1989; **8:** 1–59.

2. Serfaty M, Masterton G. Fatal poisonings attributed to benzodiazepines in Britain during the 1980s. *Br J Psychiatry* 1993; **163:** 386–93.

3. Buckley NA, *et al.* Relative toxicity of benzodiazepines in overdose. *BMJ* 1995; **310:** 219–21.

Treatment of Adverse Effects

The treatment of benzodiazepine overdosage is generally symptomatic and supportive. Activated charcoal may be given to those patients who have taken more than 1 mg per kg body-weight of diazepam (or its equivalent) and who present within 1 hour. Gastric lavage is generally not advocated in overdoses of benzodiazepines alone. The specific benzodiazepine antagonist, flumazenil, is rarely required; if used expert advice is essential since serious adverse effects may occur in patients dependent on benzodiazepines (see p.1009). It should be used with extreme caution, if at all, in multiple drug overdoses or for the differential diagnosis of unclear cases of overdose.

Precautions

Diazepam should be avoided in patients with pre-existing CNS depression or coma, respiratory depression, acute pulmonary insufficiency, or sleep apnoea, and used with care in those with chronic pulmonary insufficiency. Diazepam should be given with care to elderly or debilitated patients who may be more prone to adverse effects. Caution is required in patients with muscle weakness, or impaired liver or kidney function; its use should be avoided in severe hepatic impairment. The sedative effects of diazepam are most marked during the first few days of administration; affected patients should not drive or operate machinery (see also Driving, below). Monitoring of cardiorespiratory function is generally recommended when benzodiazepines are used for deep sedation.

Diazepam is not appropriate for the treatment of chronic psychosis or for phobic or obsessional states. Diazepam-induced disinhibition may precipitate suicide or aggressive behaviour and it should not, therefore, be used alone to treat depression or anxiety associated with depression; it should also be used with care in patients with personality disorders. Caution is required in patients with organic brain changes particularly arteriosclerosis. In cases of bereavement, psychological adjustment may be inhibited by diazepam.

Many manufacturers of diazepam and other benzodiazepines advise against their use in patients with glaucoma, but the rationale for this contra-indication is unclear.

For warnings on benzodiazepines during pregnancy and breast feeding, see below.

Dependence characterised by a withdrawal syndrome may develop after regular use of diazepam, even in therapeutic doses for short periods (see above); because of its dependence liability, diazepam should be used with caution in patients with a history of alcohol or drug addiction.

Since hypotension and apnoea may occur when diazepam is given intravenously it has been recommended that this route should only be used when facilities for reversing respiratory depression with mechanical ventilation are available. Patients should remain supine and under medical supervision for at least one hour after intravenous injection. Intravenous infusion is best undertaken in specialist centres with intensive care facilities where close and constant supervision can be undertaken.

Administration. INTRAVENOUS. A warning[1] that prolonged use of high-dose intravenous infusions of diazepam preparations containing benzyl alcohol can result in benzyl alcohol poisoning.

1. López-Herce J, *et al.* Benzyl alcohol poisoning following diazepam intravenous infusion. *Ann Pharmacother* 1995; **29:** 632.

Cardiovascular disorders. See under Respiratory System Disorders, below.

Driving. Most benzodiazepines can adversely affect parameters of driving performance in healthy subjects.[1] It is not entirely clear to what extent benzodiazepines contribute to the risk of driving accidents. A large case-control study[2] in elderly drivers suggested that the risk of accidents was increased in those who took longer-acting benzodiazepines. Another study[3] suggested that, for users of benzodiazepines or zopiclone as a group, the increased risk was greatest in younger drivers and was increased by alcohol consumption. Patients affected by drowsiness while taking benzodiazepines should not drive or operate machinery. Drowsiness often becomes less troublesome with continued use of these drugs.

1. Woods JH, *et al.* Abuse liability of benzodiazepines. *Pharmacol Rev* 1987; **39:** 251–413.

2. Hemmelgarn B, *et al.* Benzodiazepine use and the risk of motor vehicle crash in the elderly. *JAMA* 1997; **278:** 27–31.

3. Barbone F, *et al.* Association of road-traffic accidents with benzodiazepine use. *Lancet* 1998; **352:** 1331–6.

The elderly. Old age may alter the distribution, elimination, and clearance of benzodiazepines.[1,2] Metabolic clearance of benzodiazepines metabolised principally by oxidation appears to be reduced but not clearance of those biotransformed by glucuronide conjugation or nitroreduction. Prolonged half-life in the elderly may be a result of such a decrease in clearance or of an increase in the volume of distribution. The clinical consequence of these changes depends on factors such as dosage schedule and extent of first-pass extraction by the liver.

Irrespective of pharmacokinetic changes, the elderly may exhibit increased sensitivity to acute doses of benzodiazepines.[1-3] Impairment of memory, cognitive function, and psychomotor performance and behaviour disinhibition may be more common than with younger patients.[4] Long-term use commonly exacerbates underlying dementia in elderly patients.[4]

The upshot of the pharmacokinetic and pharmacodynamic changes of benzodiazepines in the elderly is that adverse effects may be more frequent in these patients and lower doses are commonly required. An epidemiological study of persons 65 years and older found an increased rate of hip fracture among current users of long-acting benzodiazepines (*chlordiazepoxide, clorazepate, diazepam,* and *flurazepam*), but not among users of short-acting drugs (*alprazolam, bromazepam, lorazepam, oxazepam,* and *triazolam*).[5] However, a case-control study[6] of patients with falls leading to femur fractures suggested that the most important factor in increasing risk was the dose of benzodiazepine. However, another case-control study[7] found no correlation between hip fracture and benzodiazepines either as a group or according to half-life or to characterisation as an anxiolytic or a hypnotic; there might, however, be an increase in risk with lorazepam. There was also an increased risk associated with use of two or more benzodiazepines. Nonetheless, if administration of a benzodiazepine is considered necessary in elderly patients, a short-acting drug is to be preferred. It should also be remembered that the elderly are at increased risk of sleep-related breathing disorders, such as sleep apnoea and the use of hypnotics such as benzodiazepines should be avoided in these patients (see Respiratory System Disorders, below).

1. Greenblatt DJ, *et al.* Implications of altered drug disposition in elderly: studies of benzodiazepines. *J Clin Pharmacol* 1989; **29:** 866–72.

2. Greenblatt DJ, *et al.* Clinical pharmacokinetics of anxiolytics and hypnotics in the elderly: therapeutic considerations. *Clin Pharmacokinet* 1991; **21:** 165–77 and 262–73.

3. Swift CG. Pharmacodynamics: changes in homeostatic mechanisms, receptor and target organ sensitivity in the elderly. *Br Med Bull* 1990; **46:** 36–52.

4. Juergens SM. Problems with benzodiazepines in elderly patients. *Mayo Clin Proc* 1993; **68:** 818–20.

5. Ray WA, *et al.* Benzodiazepines of long and short elimination half-life and the risk of hip fracture. *JAMA* 1989; **262:** 3303–7.

6. Herings RMC, *et al.* Benzodiazepines and the risk of falling leading to femur fractures: dosage more important than elimination half-life. *Arch Intern Med* 1995; **155:** 1801–7.

7. Pierfitte C, *et al.* Benzodiazepines and hip fractures in elderly people: case-control study. *BMJ* 2001; **322:** 704–8.

Gout. A 40-year-old Chinese man with a history of gout had acute attacks on 5 occasions after taking nitrazepam 10 mg;[1] attacks were also precipitated by diazepam 5 mg, chlordiazepoxide 15 mg, and by methaqualone with diphenhydramine.

1. Leng CO. Drug-precipitated acute attacks of gout. *BMJ* 1975; **2:** 561.

Hangover effects. Long-acting benzodiazepines accumulate in the body to a greater extent than ones with a shorter half-life. Although this might be expected to increase the frequency of daytime sedation and impairment of performance (so-called hangover effects) after a hypnotic dose, such a straightforward relationship has not always been observed in practice.[1]

Anterograde amnesia is more common with short-acting drugs such as triazolam; 'traveller's amnesia' has been used to describe amnesia in persons taking benzodiazepines for sleep disturbances resulting from jet lag.[2]

1. Greenblatt DJ, et al. Neurochemical and pharmacokinetic correlates of the clinical action of benzodiazepine hypnotic drugs. *Am J Med* 1990; **88** (suppl 3A): 18S–24S.
2. Meyboom RHB. Benzodiazepines and pilot error. *BMJ* 1991; **302:** 1274–5.

Hepatic impairment. Studies of the pharmacokinetics of diazepam in patients with liver disorders suggest that oxidative metabolism is impaired resulting in a prolonged half-life and reduced clearance.[1-3] A reduction in dosage was generally required.

1. Branch RA, et al. Intravenous administration of diazepam in patients with chronic liver disease. *Gut* 1976; **17:** 975–83.
2. Klotz U, et al. Disposition of diazepam and its major metabolite desmethyldiazepam in patients with liver disease. *Clin Pharmacol Ther* 1977; **21:** 430–6.
3. Ochs HR, et al. Repeated diazepam dosing in cirrhotic patients: cumulation and sedation. *Clin Pharmacol Ther* 1983; **33:** 471–6.

High-altitude disorders. Sleep may be impaired at high altitude due to frequent arousals associated with pronounced oxygen desaturation and periodic breathing. Traditional advice has been that sedatives should not be given at high altitude.[1] Caution may also be warranted at moderate altitudes especially in non-acclimatised climbers.[2] It has been argued that since diazepam, and possibly other sedatives, blunt the hypoxic ventilatory response, sleep hypoxaemia might be exacerbated. A recent small study[3] has suggested that small doses of a short-acting benzodiazepine, such as temazepam, might actually improve the subjective quality of sleep and reduce episodes of arterial desaturation without changing mean oxygen saturation. However the possibility of an interaction between acetazolamide taken for prophylaxis or treatment of acute mountain sickness and the benzodiazepine should be borne in mind; ventilatory depression in a mountain climber with acute mountain sickness was considered to be due to the potentiation of triazolam by acetazolamide.[4]

1. Sutton JR, et al. Insomnia, sedation, and high altitude cerebral oedema. *Lancet* 1979; **i:** 165.
2. Röggla G, et al. Effect of temazepam on ventilatory response at moderate altitude. *BMJ* 2000; **320:** 56.
3. Dubowitz G. Effect of temazepam on oxygen saturation and sleep quality at high altitude: randomised placebo controlled crossover trial. *BMJ* 1998; **316:** 587–9.
4. Masuyama S, et al. 'Ondine's curse': side effect of acetazolamide? *Am J Med* 1989; **86:** 637.

Nervous system disorders. Benzodiazepines can reduce cerebral perfusion pressure and blood oxygenation to an extent that results in irreversible neurological damage in patients with head injuries. Consequently, they should be administered with great care to such patients.[1,2] Their use should be avoided for the control of seizures in patients with head injuries or other acute neurological lesions as these patients can be managed effectively with phenytoin.

1. Eldridge PR, Punt JAG. Risks associated with giving benzodiazepines to patients with acute neurological injuries. *BMJ* 1990; **300:** 1189–90.
2. Papazian L, et al. Effect of bolus doses of midazolam on intracranial pressure and cerebral perfusion pressure in patients with severe head injury. *Br J Anaesth* 1993; **71:** 267–71.

EPILEPSY. There have been rare reports of benzodiazepines producing paradoxical exacerbation of seizures in patients with epilepsy.[1,2]

1. Prior PF, et al. Intravenous diazepam. *Lancet* 1971; **2:** 434–5.
2. Tassinari CA, et al. A paradoxical effect: status epilepticus induced by benzodiazepines (Valium and Mogadon). *Electroencephalogr Clin Neurophysiol* 1971; **31:** 182.

Porphyria. Diazepam has been associated with acute attacks of porphyria and is considered unsafe in porphyric patients. Intravenous diazepam has been used successfully, however, to control status epilepticus occurring after the acute porphyric attack. For a discussion of the management of seizures associated with acute porphyric attacks, see p.342.

Pregnancy and breast feeding. Benzodiazepines have been widely used in pregnant patients.[1] Use of benzodiazepines in the *third trimester* and during *labour* seems to be associated with some infants with neonatal withdrawal symptoms or the floppy infant syndrome. Also a small number exposed *in utero* to benzodiazepines have shown slow development in the early years but by 4 years of age most had developed normally, and for those that had not it was not possible to prove a cause-effect relationship with benzodiazepine exposure. In a meta-analysis[2] of live births following benzodiazepine use during the *first trimester* of pregnancy, pooled data from cohort studies showed no apparent association between benzodiazepine use and the risk of major malformations or oral cleft alone. There was, however, a small but significantly increased risk of oral cleft according to data from case-control studies. Although benzodiazepines did not appear to be a major human teratogen, use of ultrasonography was advised to rule out visible forms of cleft lip. The UK Committee on Safety of Medicines (CSM) has recommended[3] that women of child-bearing potential prescribed benzodiazepines should be advised to contact the physician regarding discontinuation of the drug if they intend to become, or suspect they are, pregnant.

In one reviewer's opinion[1] the limited distribution into breast milk did not constitute a hazard to the breast-fed infant but the infant should be monitored for sedation and the inability to suckle. Another group has also reported a low incidence of toxicity and adverse effects in the breast-fed infants of mothers taking psychotropic drugs including benzodiazepines.[4] However, the American Academy of Pediatrics Committee considered that benzodiazepine use by nursing mothers for long periods was a cause for concern,[5] and the CSM has recommended[3] that benzodiazepines should not be given to lactating mothers. It has been suggested[6] that if a benzodiazepine must be used during breast feeding it would be preferable to use a short-acting drug with minimal distribution into breast milk and inactive metabolites; oxazepam, lorazepam, alprazolam, or midazolam might be suitable.

1. McElhatton PR. The effects of benzodiazepine use during pregnancy and lactation. *Reprod Toxicol* 1994; **8:** 461–75.
2. Dolovich LR, et al. Benzodiazepine use in pregnancy and major malformations or oral cleft: meta-analysis of cohort and case-control studies. *BMJ* 1998; **317:** 839–43.
3. Committee on Safety of Medicines/Medicines Control Agency. Reminder: avoid benzodiazepines in pregnancy and lactation. *Current Problems* 1997; **23:** 10.
4. Birnbaum CS, et al. Serum concentrations of antidepressants and benzodiazepines in nursing infants: a case series. Abstract: *Pediatrics* 1999; **104:** 104. Full version: http://www.pediatrics.org/cgi/content/full/104/1/e11
5. American Academy of Pediatrics Committee on Drugs. The transfer of drugs and other chemicals into human milk. *Pediatrics* 2001; **108:** 776–89.
6. Chisholm CA, Kuller JA. A guide to the safety of CNS-active agents during breastfeeding. *Drug Safety* 1997; **17:** 127–42.

Renal impairment. Although plasma protein binding of diazepam was reduced in 8 patients with advanced renal failure, the clearance of unbound drug after a single intravenous dose was not significantly changed.[1]

See also under Flurazepam, p.685.

1. Ochs HR, et al. Diazepam kinetics in patients with renal insufficiency or hyperthyroidism. *Br J Clin Pharmacol* 1981; **12:** 829–32.

Respiratory system disorders. Benzodiazepines may affect the control of ventilation during sleep and may worsen sleep apnoea or other sleep-related breathing disorders especially in patients with chronic obstructive pulmonary disease or cardiac failure.[1] Risk factors for sleep apnoea, which often goes undiagnosed, include old age, obesity, male sex, postmenopausal status in women, and a history of heavy snoring. Although benzodiazepines may reduce sleep fragmentation, their long-term use may result in conversion from partial to complete obstructive sleep apnoea in heavy snorers or in short repetitive central sleep apnoea in patients with recent myocardial infarction.

1. Guilleminault C. Benzodiazepines, breathing, and sleep. *Am J Med* 1990; **88** (suppl 3A): 25S–28S.

Interactions

Enhanced sedation or respiratory and cardiovascular depression may occur if diazepam or other benzodiazepines are given with other drugs that have CNS-depressant properties; these include alcohol, antidepressants, antihistamines, antipsychotics, general anaesthetics, other hypnotics or sedatives, and opioid analgesics. The sedative effect of benzodiazepines may also be enhanced by cisapride. Adverse effects may also be produced by concomitant administration with drugs which interfere with the metabolism of benzodiazepines. Drugs which have been reported to alter the pharmacokinetics of benzodiazepines are discussed in detail below but few of these interactions are likely to be of clinical significance. Benzodiazepines such as diazepam which are metabolised primarily by hepatic microsomal oxidation may be more susceptible to pharmacokinetic changes than those eliminated primarily by glucuronide conjugation.

Analgesics. The peak plasma concentration of oxazepam was significantly decreased during treatment with *diflunisal* in 6 healthy subjects, while the renal clearance of the glucuronide metabolite was reduced and its mean elimination half-life increased from 10 to 13 hours.[1] Diflunisal also displaced oxazepam from plasma protein binding sites *in vitro*. *Aspirin* shortened the time to induce anaesthesia with midazolam in 78 patients also possibly due to competition for plasma protein binding sites.[2] *Paracetamol* produced no significant change in plasma concentrations of diazepam or its major metabolite and only marginal changes in urine concentrations in 4 healthy subjects.[3]

Benzodiazepines such as diazepam, lorazepam, and midazolam may be used with opioid analgesics in anaesthetic or analgesic regimens. An additive sedative effect is to be expected[4] but there are also reports of severe respiratory depression with midazolam and *fentanyl*[5] or sudden hypotension with midazolam and fentanyl[6] or *sufentanil*.[7] The clearance of midazolam appears to be reduced by fentanyl,[8] possibly as a result of competitive inhibition of metabolism by the cytochrome P450 isoenzyme CYP3A. Careful monitoring is therefore required during concomitant administration of midazolam with these opioids and the dose of both drugs may need to be reduced. Synergistic potentiation of the induction of anaesthesia has been reported between midazolam and fentanyl,[9] but one study has suggested that midazolam can diminish the analgesic effects of sufentanil.[10] Pretreatment with *morphine* or *pethidine* has decreased the rate of oral absorption of diazepam. This has been attributed to the effect of opioid analgesics on gastrointestinal motility.[11]

Dextropropoxyphene prolonged the half-life and reduced the clearance of alprazolam but not diazepam or lorazepam in healthy subjects.[12]

1. Van Hecken AM, et al. The influence of diflunisal on the pharmacokinetics of oxazepam. *Br J Clin Pharmacol* 1985; **20:** 225–34.
2. Dundee JW, et al. Aspirin and probenecid pretreatment influences the potency of thiopentone and the onset of action of midazolam. *Anesthesiol* 1986; **3:** 247–51.
3. Mulley BA, et al. Interactions between diazepam and paracetamol. *J Clin Pharm* 1978; **3:** 25–35.
4. Tverskoy M, et al. Midazolam-morphine sedative interaction in patients. *Anesth Analg* 1989; **68:** 282–5.
5. Yaster M, et al. Midazolam-fentanyl intravenous sedation in children: case report of respiratory arrest. *Pediatrics* 1990; **86:** 463–7.
6. Burtin P, et al. Hypotension with midazolam and fentanyl in the newborn. *Lancet* 1991; **337:** 1545–6.
7. West JM, et al. Sudden hypotension associated with midazolam and sufentanil. *Anesth Analg* 1987; **66:** 693–4.
8. Hase I, et al. I.V. fentanyl decreases the clearance of midazolam. *Br J Anaesth* 1997; **79:** 740–3.
9. Ben-Shlomo I, et al. Midazolam acts synergistically with fentanyl for induction of anaesthesia. *Br J Anaesth* 1990; **64:** 45–7.
10. Luger TJ, Morawetz RF. Clinical evidence for a midazolam-sufentanil interaction in patients with major trauma. *Clin Pharmacol Ther* 1991; **49:** 133.
11. Gamble JAS, et al. Some pharmacological factors influencing the absorption of diazepam following oral administration. *Br J Anaesth* 1976; **48:** 1181–5.
12. Abernethy DR, et al. Interaction of propoxyphene with diazepam, alprazolam and lorazepam. *Br J Clin Pharmacol* 1985; **19:** 51–7.

Antiarrhythmics. An interaction between clonazepam and existing therapy with amiodarone was suspected in a 78-year-old man who experienced symptoms of benzodiazepine toxicity 2 months after starting with clonazepam 0.5 mg given at bedtime for restless leg syndrome;[1] symptoms resolved on withdrawal of clonazepam.

1. Witt DM, et al. Amiodarone-clonazepam interaction. *Ann Pharmacother* 1993; **27:** 1463–4.

Antibacterials. Both *erythromycin*[1] and *troleandomycin*[2] have been reported to inhibit the hepatic metabolism of triazolam in healthy subjects. Peak plasma-triazolam concentrations were increased, half-life prolonged, and clearance reduced. Troleandomycin prolonged the psychomotor impairment and amnesia produced by triazolam.[2] Loss of consciousness following erythromycin infusion in a child premedicated with midazolam was attributed to a similar interaction,[3] and increases in peak plasma concentrations of midazolam with profound and prolonged sedation have been reported following administration of erythromycin.[4] Use of midazolam with erythromycin should be avoided or the dose of midazolam reduced by 50 to 75%. The clearance of midazolam is also reduced by *clarithromycin*, with an approximate doubling of the benzodiazepine's oral bioavailability.[5] The manufacturers of *quinupristin/dalfopristin* state that it too may increase plasma concentrations of midazolam. *Roxithromycin* has been reported[6] to have some effects on the pharmacokinetics and pharmacodynamics of midazolam but these changes were not thought clinically relevant. However, it was recommended that as a precaution the lowest possible effective dose of midazolam should be used when given with roxithromycin. In another study[7] *azithromycin* did not appear to have any effect on the metabolism or psychomotor effects of midazolam.

There is an isolated report of significant rises in steady-state blood-midazolam concentration coinciding with administration of *ciprofloxacin*.[8] Also ciprofloxacin has been reported to reduce diazepam clearance and prolong its terminal half-life,[9] although psychometric tests did not show any changes in diazepam's pharmacodynamics. However, ciprofloxacin appears to have no effect on the pharmacokinetics or pharmacodynamics of temazepam.[10]

Isoniazid has been reported to increase the half-life of a single dose of diazepam[11] and triazolam[12] but not of oxazepam[12] in healthy subjects. In contrast, *rifampicin* has decreased the half-life of diazepam[13] and midazolam,[14] and more or less abolishes the effects of triazolam,[15] while *ethambutol* has no effect on diazepam pharmacokinetics.[11] In patients receiving therapy for tuberculosis with a combination of isoniazid, rifampicin, and ethambutol the half-life of a single diazepam dose was shortened and its clearance increased.[11] Thus the enzyme-inducing effect of rifampicin appears to predominate over the enzyme-inhibiting effect of isoniazid.

1. Phillips JP, et al. A pharmacokinetic drug interaction between erythromycin and triazolam. *J Clin Psychopharmacol* 1986; **6:** 297–9.
2. Warot D, et al. Troleandomycin-triazolam interaction in healthy volunteers: pharmacokinetic and psychometric evaluation. *Eur J Clin Pharmacol* 1987; **32:** 389–93.
3. Hiller A, et al. Unconsciousness associated with midazolam and erythromycin. *Br J Anaesth* 1990; **65:** 826–8.
4. Olkkola KT, et al. A potentially hazardous interaction between erythromycin and midazolam. *Clin Pharmacol Ther* 1993; **53:** 298–305.
5. Gorski JC, et al. The contribution of intestinal and hepatic CYP3A to the interaction between midazolam and clarithromycin. *Clin Pharmacol Ther* 1998; **64:** 133–43.

6. Backman JT, *et al.* A pharmacokinetic interaction between roxithromycin and midazolam. *Eur J Clin Pharmacol* 1994; **46**: 551–5.

7. Mattila MJ, *et al.* Azithromycin does not alter the effects of oral midazolam on human performance. *Eur J Clin Pharmacol* 1994; **47**: 49–52.

8. Orko R, *et al.* Intravenous infusion of midazolam, propofol and vecuronium in a patient with severe tetanus. *Acta Anaesthesiol Scand* 1988; **32**: 590–2.

9. Kamali F, *et al.* The influence of steady-state ciprofloxacin on the pharmacokinetics and pharmacodynamics of a single dose of diazepam in healthy volunteers. *Eur J Clin Pharmacol* 1993; **44**: 365–7.

10. Kamali F, *et al.* The influence of ciprofloxacin on the pharmacokinetics and pharmacodynamics of a single dose of temazepam in the young and elderly. *J Clin Pharm Ther* 1994; **19**: 105–9.

11. Ochs HR, *et al.* Diazepam interaction with antituberculous drugs. *Clin Pharmacol Ther* 1981; **29**: 671–8.

12. Ochs HR, *et al.* Differential effect of isoniazid on triazolam oxidation and oxazepam conjugation. *Br J Clin Pharmacol* 1983; **16**: 743–6.

13. Brockmeyer N, *et al.* The metabolism of diazepam following different enzyme inducing agents. *Br J Clin Pharmacol* 1985; **19**: 544P.

14. Backman JT, *et al.* Rifampin drastically reduces plasma concentrations and effects of oral midazolam. *Clin Pharmacol Ther* 1996; **59**: 7–13.

15. Villikka K, *et al.* Triazolam is ineffective in patients taking rifampicin. *Clin Pharmacol Ther* 1997; **61**: 8–14.

Anticoagulants. Plasma binding of diazepam and desmethyldiazepam was reduced, and free concentrations increased, immediately following *heparin* intravenously.[1]

Benzodiazepines do not usually interact with oral anticoagulants although there have been rare reports of altered anticoagulant activity.

1. Routledge PA, *et al.* Diazepam and N-desmethyldiazepam redistribution after heparin. *Clin Pharmacol Ther* 1980; **27**: 528–32.

Antidepressants. It has been recommended that the dosage of alprazolam should be reduced when given with *fluvoxamine*, as concomitant use has resulted in doubling of plasma-alprazolam concentrations.[1] Since plasma concentrations of bromazepam[2] and of diazepam[3] also appear to be affected by fluvoxamine, it has been suggested that patients taking fluvoxamine who require a benzodiazepine should preferentially receive one such as lorazepam which has a different metabolic pathway.[3] Small studies suggest that *fluoxetine* can also increase plasma concentrations of alprazolam.[4,5] Fluoxetine appears to have a similar effect on diazepam but plasma concentrations of diazepam's active metabolite desmethyldiazepam are reduced and it is considered that the overall effect is likely to be minor.[6] The potential for a clinically significant interaction with *sertraline*, *paroxetine*, or *citalopram* is considered to be less.[7]

The manufacturers in the USA have reported that alprazolam may increase the steady-state plasma concentrations of *imipramine* and *desipramine*, although the clinical significance of such changes is unknown. For a suggestion that benzodiazepines may increase the oxidation of *amineptine* to a toxic metabolite, see under Effects on the Liver in Adverse Effects of Amitriptyline, p.274.

Concomitant administration of *nefazodone* has been reported to result in raised concentrations of alprazolam and triazolam, increased sedation, and impairment of psychomotor performance.[8,9] Nefazodone may inhibit the oxidative metabolism of alprazolam and triazolam. Raised concentrations of midazolam have similarly been seen when given by mouth with nefazodone.[10] No interaction was reported with lorazepam which is primarily eliminated by conjugation.

For reference to an isolated report of hypothermia after administration of diazepam and *lithium*, see p.295.

There have been occasional reports of sexual disinhibition in patients taking *tryptophan* with benzodiazepines.

1. Fleishaker JC, Hulst LK. A pharmacokinetic and pharmacodynamic evaluation of the combined administration of alprazolam and fluvoxamine. *Eur J Clin Pharmacol* 1994; **46**: 35–9.

2. Van Harten J, *et al.* Influence of multiple-dose administration of fluvoxamine on the pharmacokinetics of the benzodiazepines bromazepam and lorazepam: a randomized crossover study. *Eur Neuropsychopharmacol* 1992; **2**: 381.

3. Perucca E, *et al.* Inhibition of diazepam metabolism by fluvoxamine: a pharmacokinetic study in normal volunteers. *Clin Pharmacol Ther* 1994; **56**: 471–6.

4. Lasher TA, *et al.* Pharmacokinetic pharmacodynamic evaluation of the combined administration of alprazolam and fluoxetine. *Psychopharmacology (Berl)* 1991; **104**: 323–7.

5. Greenblatt DJ, *et al.* Fluoxetine impairs clearance of alprazolam but not of clonazepam. *Clin Pharmacol Ther* 1992; **52**: 479–86.

6. Lemberger L, *et al.* The effect of fluoxetine on the pharmacokinetics and psychomotor responses of diazepam. *Clin Pharmacol Ther* 1988; **43**: 412–19.

7. Sproule BA, *et al.* Selective serotonin reuptake inhibitors and CNS drug interactions: a critical review of the evidence. *Clin Pharmacokinet* 1997; **33**: 454–71.

8. Greene DS, *et al.* Coadministration of nefazodone (NEF) and benzodiazepines I: pharmacokinetic assessment. *Clin Pharmacol Ther* 1994; **55**: 141.

9. Kroboth P, *et al.* Coadministration of nefazodone and benzodiazepines II: pharmacodynamic assessment. *Clin Pharmacol Ther* 1994; **55**: 142.

10. Lam YWF, *et al.* Effect of antidepressants and ketoconazole on oral midazolam pharmacokinetics. *Clin Pharmacol Ther* 1998; **63**: 229.

Antiepileptics. *Carbamazepine*, *phenobarbital*, and *phenytoin* are all inducers of hepatic drug-metabolising enzymes. Therefore, in patients receiving long-term therapy with these drugs the metabolism of benzodiazepines may be enhanced.

For oral midazolam the effects of carbamazepine or phenytoin may be sufficient to virtually abolish the effects of a standard dose, with a more than 90% reduction in peak serum concentrations of the benzodiazepine.[1] Interactions between benzodiazepines and these antiepileptics are further discussed on p.345 (carbamazepine) and p.361 (phenytoin). Results from a study[2] involving 66 children and adults receiving clobazam as adjunctive therapy for epilepsy showed a significant increase in clobazam clearance, leading to accumulation of its principle active metabolite N-desmethyl-clobazam, in the 16 patients also taking *felbamate*.

Sodium valproate has been reported to displace diazepam from plasma-protein binding sites.[3] Sporadic reports exist of adverse effects when valproate is given with clonazepam[4,5] with the development of drowsiness and, more seriously, absence status epilepticus, but the existence of an interaction is considered to be unproven.[6] Drowsiness has also been reported when valproate was given with nitrazepam.[7] Concomitant administration of valproate semisodium and lorazepam has resulted in raised concentrations of lorazepam due to inhibition of glucuronidation of lorazepam.[8]

1. Backman JT, *et al.* Concentrations and effects of oral midazolam are greatly reduced in patients treated with carbamazepine or phenytoin. *Epilepsia* 1996; **37**: 253–7.

2. Contin M, *et al.* Effect of felbamate on clobazam and its metabolite kinetics in patients with epilepsy. *Ther Drug Monit* 1999; **21**: 604–8.

3. Dhillon S, Richens A. Valproic acid and diazepam interaction in vivo. *Br J Clin Pharmacol* 1982; **13**: 553–60.

4. Watson WA. Interaction between clonazepam and sodium valproate. *N Engl J Med* 1979; **300**: 678.

5. Browne TR. Interaction between clonazepam and sodium valproate. *N Engl J Med* 1979; **300**: 679.

6. Levy RH, Koch KM. Drug interactions with valproic acid. *Drugs* 1982; **24**: 543–56.

7. Jeavons PM, *et al.* Treatment of generalized epilepsies of childhood and adolescence with sodium valproate (Epilim). *Dev Med Child Neurol* 1977; **19**: 9–25.

8. Samara EE, *et al.* Effect of valproate on the pharmacokinetics and pharmacodynamics of lorazepam. *J Clin Pharmacol* 1997; **37**: 442–50.

Antifungals. Both a single dose and multiple doses of *ketoconazole* decreased the clearance of a single intravenous injection of chlordiazepoxide.[1] Studies[2-4] have shown that ketoconazole and *itraconazole* can produce marked pharmacokinetic interactions with midazolam or triazolam and greatly increase the intensity and duration of action of these benzodiazepines. The area under the plasma concentration-time curve for midazolam was increased by 15 times by ketoconazole and by 10 times by itraconazole while peak plasma concentrations of midazolam were increased fourfold and threefold respectively.[2] The area under the curve for triazolam was increased by 22 times by ketoconazole and by 27 times by itraconazole;[3] peak plasma concentrations of triazolam were increased about threefold by both antifungals. One study[5] indicated that the risk of interaction persists for several days after cessation of itraconazole therapy. It is recommended that the concomitant use of these antifungals and benzodiazepines should be avoided or that the dose of the benzodiazepine should be greatly reduced. A similar but less pronounced interaction occurs between *fluconazole* and midazolam[6] or triazolam;[7] nonetheless the dosage of the benzodiazepine should be reduced during concomitant use.

1. Brown MW, *et al.* Effect of ketoconazole on hepatic oxidative drug metabolism. *Clin Pharmacol Ther* 1985; **37**: 290–7.

2. Olkkola KT, *et al.* Midazolam should be avoided in patients receiving the systemic antimycotics ketoconazole or itraconazole. *Clin Pharmacol Ther* 1994; **55**: 481–5.

3. Varhe A, *et al.* Oral triazolam is potentially hazardous to patients receiving systemic antimycotics ketoconazole or itraconazole. *Clin Pharmacol Ther* 1994; **56**: 601–7.

4. Greenblatt DJ, *et al.* Interaction of triazolam and ketoconazole. *Lancet* 1995; **345**: 191.

5. Neuvonen PJ, *et al.* The effect of ingestion time interval on the interaction between itraconazole and triazolam. *Clin Pharmacol Ther* 1996; **60**: 326–31.

6. Ahonen J, *et al.* Effect of route of administration of fluconazole on the interaction between fluconazole and midazolam. *Eur J Clin Pharmacol* 1997; **51**: 415–19.

7. Varhe A, *et al.* Effect of fluconazole dose on the extent of fluconazole-triazolam interaction. *Br J Clin Pharmacol* 1996; **42**: 465–70.

Antihistamines. A suggestion[1] that a reduction in temazepam metabolism caused by *diphenhydramine* may have contributed to perinatal death after ingestion of these drugs by the mother.

1. Kargas GA, *et al.* Perinatal mortality due to interaction of diphenhydramine and temazepam. *N Engl J Med* 1985; **313**: 1417–18.

Antivirals. The non-nucleoside reverse transcriptase inhibitors *delavirdine* and *efavirenz*, and HIV-protease inhibitors such as *indinavir*, *nelfinavir*, *ritonavir*,[1] and *saquinavir*[2] may inhibit the hepatic microsomal systems involved in the metabolism of some benzodiazepines. (Prolonged administration of protease inhibitors may also *induce* these metabolic systems; interactions may therefore be complex and difficult to predict.) Concomitant administration requires monitoring with dosage adjustments for the benzodiazepine or else should be avoided. Benzodiazepines which should **not** be used concomitantly with

HIV-protease inhibitors include alprazolam, clorazepate, diazepam, estazolam, flurazepam, midazolam, and triazolam.

1. Greenblatt DJ, *et al.* Extensive impairment of triazolam and alprazolam clearance by short-term low-dose ritonavir: the clinical dilemma of concurrent inhibition and induction *J Clin Psychopharmacol* 1999; **19**: 293–6.

2. Palkama VJ, *et al.* Effect of saquinavir on the pharmacokinetics and pharmacodynamics of oral and intravenous midazolam. *Clin Pharmacol Ther* 1999; **66**: 33–9.

Beta blockers. A clear pattern of interactions between benzodiazepines and beta blockers has not emerged. *Propranolol* may inhibit the metabolism of diazepam[1,2] and bromazepam,[3] and *metoprolol* may inhibit the metabolism of diazepam[1,4] or bromazepam[5] to some extent, although in many cases the effect on pharmacokinetics and pharmacodynamics is unlikely to be of clinical significance. No significant pharmacokinetic interaction has been observed between propranolol and alprazolam,[2] lorazepam,[2] or oxazepam,[6] although the rate of alprazolam absorption may be decreased.[2] Similarly no pharmacokinetic interaction has been observed between *atenolol* and diazepam,[1] *labetalol* and oxazepam,[6] or metoprolol and lorazepam.[5]

1. Hawksworth G, *et al.* Diazepam/β-adrenoceptor antagonist interactions. *Br J Clin Pharmacol* 1984; **17**: 69S–76S.

2. Ochs HR, *et al.* Propranolol interactions with diazepam, lorazepam, and alprazolam. *Clin Pharmacol Ther* 1984; **36**: 451–5.

3. Ochs HR, *et al.* Bromazepam pharmacokinetics: influence of age, gender, oral contraceptives, cimetidine, and propranolol. *Clin Pharmacol Ther* 1987; **41**: 562–70.

4. Klotz U, Reimann IW. Pharmacokinetic and pharmacodynamic interaction study of diazepam and metoprolol. *Eur J Clin Pharmacol* 1984; **26**: 223–6.

5. Scott AK, *et al.* Interaction of metoprolol with lorazepam and bromazepam. *Eur J Clin Pharmacol* 1991; **40**: 405–9.

6. Sonne J, *et al.* Single dose pharmacokinetics and pharmacodynamics of oral oxazepam during concomitant administration of propranolol and labetalol. *Br J Clin Pharmacol* 1990; **29**: 33–7.

Calcium-channel blockers. Peak plasma concentrations of midazolam were doubled and the elimination half-life of midazolam prolonged when midazolam was given to healthy subjects receiving *diltiazem* or *verapamil*.[1] A similar interaction has been demonstrated between diltiazem and triazolam.[2,3] Concomitant use should be avoided or the dose of these benzodiazepines reduced.

1. Backman JT, *et al.* Dose of midazolam should be reduced during diltiazem and verapamil treatments. *Br J Clin Pharmacol* 1994; **37**: 221–5.

2. Varhe A, *et al.* Diltiazem enhances the effects of triazolam by inhibiting its metabolism. *Clin Pharmacol Ther* 1996; **59**: 369–75.

3. Kosuge K, *et al.* Enhanced effect of triazolam with diltiazem. *Br J Clin Pharmacol* 1997; **43**: 367–72.

Ciclosporin. *In-vitro* studies suggested that ciclosporin could inhibit the metabolism of midazolam.[1] However, bloodciclosporin concentrations in patients given ciclosporin to prevent graft rejection were considered too low to result in such an interaction.

1. Li G, *et al.* Is cyclosporin A an inhibitor of drug metabolism? *Br J Clin Pharmacol* 1990; **30**: 71–7.

Clonidine. Anxiety was reduced and sedation was enhanced when *clonidine* was given with flunitrazepam for premedication.[1]

1. Kulka PJ, *et al.* Sedative and anxiolytic interactions of clonidine and benzodiazepines. *Br J Anaesth* 1994; **72** (suppl 1): 81.

Clozapine. For reports of cardiorespiratory collapse and other adverse effects in patients taking benzodiazepines and clozapine, see p.673.

Corticosteroids. The metabolism of midazolam was increased in chronic users of *glucocorticoids*,[1] perhaps due to the induction of cytochrome P450 isoenzyme CYP3A4, or of enzymes responsible for glucuronidation. The changes were not considered clinically relevant if midazolam was given intravenously, but might be so if it were given by mouth.

1. Nakajima M, *et al.* Effects of chronic administration of glucocorticoid on midazolam pharmacokinetics in humans. *Ther Drug Monit* 1999; **21**: 507–13.

Digoxin. For the effects of alprazolam and diazepam on digoxin pharmacokinetics, see p.872.

Disulfiram. Evidence from healthy and alcoholic subjects suggests that chronic treatment with disulfiram can inhibit the metabolism of chlordiazepoxide and diazepam leading to a prolonged half-life and reduced clearance; there was little effect on the disposition of oxazepam.[1] No significant pharmacokinetic interaction was observed between disulfiram and alprazolam in alcoholic patients.[2] Temazepam toxicity, attributed to concomitant administration of disulfiram and temazepam, has been reported.[3]

See also under Disulfiram, p.1605.

1. MacLeod SM, *et al.* Interaction of disulfiram with benzodiazepines. *Clin Pharmacol Ther* 1978; **24**: 583–9.

2. Diquet B, *et al.* Lack of interaction between disulfiram and alprazolam in alcoholic patients. *Eur J Clin Pharmacol* 1990; **38**: 157–60.

3. Hardman M, *et al.* Temazepam toxicity precipitated by disulfiram. *Lancet* 1994; **344**: 1231–2.

Gastrointestinal drugs. *Antacids* have variable effects on the absorption of benzodiazepines[1-6] but any resulting interaction is unlikely to be of major clinical significance.

Several studies, usually involving single doses of diazepam given to healthy subjects, have demonstrated that *cimetidine* can inhibit the hepatic metabolism of diazepam.[7-10] The clearance of diazepam has generally been decreased and the half-life prolonged. Some studies have also demonstrated impaired metabolic clearance of the major metabolite, desmethyldiazepam (nordazepam). Cimetidine has also been reported to inhibit the metabolism of other benzodiazepines (generally those metabolised by oxidation) including adinazolam,[11] alprazolam,[12,13] bromazepam,[14] chlordiazepoxide,[15] clobazam,[16,17] flurazepam,[18] midazolam,[19] nitrazepam,[20] and triazolam.[12,13] Cimetidine does not appear to inhibit the hepatic metabolism of lorazepam,[18] oxazepam,[18] or temazepam.[21] The clinical significance of these interactions between cimetidine and benzodiazepines remains dubious, and little effect on cognitive function or degree of sedation has been shown.

Most studies have failed to demonstrate an effect of *ranitidine* on the hepatic metabolism of diazepam,[22-25] although one study[26] reported an increase in the bioavailability of a single dose of midazolam given by mouth, and considered that an effect on hepatic clearance was more likely than an effect on absorption. These results were consistent with those of another study which demonstrated an enhanced sedative effect of midazolam in patients pretreated with ranitidine.[27] Ranitidine has been reported to have no effect on the pharmacokinetics of lorazepam[23] or on the sedative effect of temazepam[27] but has increased the bioavailability of triazolam.[28]

Famotidine[10] or *nizatidine*[25] do not appear to inhibit the hepatic metabolism of diazepam.

Oral diazepam was absorbed more rapidly after the intravenous administration of *metoclopramide*.[29] Enhanced motility of the gastrointestinal tract was implicated. *Cisapride* may also accelerate the absorption of diazepam.[30]

Studies of continuous *omeprazole* administration on the pharmacokinetics of a single intravenous dose of diazepam in healthy subjects indicate inhibition of diazepam metabolism in a similar manner to cimetidine.[31,32] Omeprazole decreases the clearance and prolongs the elimination half-life of diazepam; in addition both the formation and elimination of desmethyldiazepam appear to be decreased. The effects may be greater in rapid than in slow metabolisers of omeprazole[33] and vary between ethnic groups.[34] The clinical significance of the interaction remains to be established. *Lansoprazole*[35] and *pantoprazole*[36] have been reported not to affect the pharmacokinetics of diazepam.

1. Nair SG, *et al.* The influence of three antacids on the absorption and clinical action of oral diazepam. *Br J Anaesth* 1976; **48:** 1175–80.
2. Greenblatt DJ, *et al.* Influence of magnesium and aluminum hydroxide mixture on chlordiazepoxide absorption. *Clin Pharmacol Ther* 1976; **19:** 234–9.
3. Chun AHC, *et al.* Effect of antacids on absorption of clorazepate. *Clin Pharmacol Ther* 1977; **22:** 329–35.
4. Shader RI, *et al.* Impaired absorption of desmethyldiazepam from clorazepate by magnesium aluminum hydroxide. *Clin Pharmacol Ther* 1978; **24:** 308–15.
5. Greenblatt DJ, *et al.* Diazepam absorption: effect of antacids and food. *Clin Pharmacol Ther* 1978; **24:** 600–9.
6. Shader RI, *et al.* Steady-state plasma desmethyldiazepam during long-term clorazepate use: effect of antacids. *Clin Pharmacol Ther* 1982; **31:** 180–3.
7. Klotz U, Reimann I. Delayed clearance of diazepam due to cimetidine. *N Engl J Med* 1980; **302:** 1012–14.
8. Gough PA, *et al.* Influence of cimetidine on oral diazepam elimination with measurement of subsequent cognitive change. *Br J Clin Pharmacol* 1982; **14:** 739–42.
9. Greenblatt DJ, *et al.* Clinical importance of the interaction of diazepam and cimetidine. *N Engl J Med* 1984; **310:** 1639–43.
10. Locniskar A, *et al.* Interaction of diazepam with famotidine and cimetidine, two H₂-receptor antagonists. *J Clin Pharmacol* 1986; **26:** 299–303.
11. Hulhoven R, *et al.* Influence of repeated administration of cimetidine on the pharmacokinetics and pharmacodynamics of adinazolam in healthy subjects. *Eur J Clin Pharmacol* 1988; **35:** 59–64.
12. Abernethy DR, *et al.* Interaction of cimetidine with the triazolobenzodiazepines alprazolam and triazolam. *Psychopharmacology (Berl)* 1983; **80:** 275–8.
13. Pourbaix S, *et al.* Pharmacokinetic consequences of long term coadministration of cimetidine and triazolobenzodiazepines, alprazolam and triazolam, in healthy subjects. *Int J Clin Pharmacol Ther Toxicol* 1985; **23:** 447–51.
14. Ochs HR, *et al.* Bromazepam pharmacokinetics: influence of age, gender, oral contraceptives, cimetidine, and propranolol. *Clin Pharmacol Ther* 1987; **41:** 562–70.
15. Desmond PV, *et al.* Cimetidine impairs elimination of chlordiazepoxide (Librium) in man. *Ann Intern Med* 1980; **93:** 266–8.
16. Grigoleit H-G, *et al.* Pharmacokinetic aspects of the interaction between clobazam and cimetidine. *Eur J Clin Pharmacol* 1983; **25:** 139–42.
17. Pullar T, *et al.* The effect of cimetidine on the single dose pharmacokinetics of oral clobazam and N-desmethylclobazam. *Br J Clin Pharmacol* 1987; **23:** 317–21.
18. Greenblatt DJ, *et al.* Interaction of cimetidine with oxazepam, lorazepam, and flurazepam. *J Clin Pharmacol* 1984; **24:** 187–93.
19. Sanders LD, *et al.* Interaction of H2-receptor antagonists and benzodiazepine sedation: a double-blind placebo-controlled investigation of the effects of cimetidine and ranitidine on recovery after intravenous midazolam. *Anaesthesia* 1993; **48:** 286–92.
20. Ochs HR, *et al.* Cimetidine impairs nitrazepam clearance. *Clin Pharmacol Ther* 1983; **34:** 227–30.
21. Greenblatt DJ, *et al.* Noninteraction of temazepam and cimetidine. *J Pharm Sci* 1984; **73:** 399–401.
22. Klotz U, *et al.* Effect of ranitidine on the steady state pharmacokinetics of diazepam. *Eur J Clin Pharmacol* 1983; **24:** 357–60.

23. Abernethy DR, *et al.* Ranitidine does not impair oxidative or conjugative metabolism: noninteraction with antipyrine, diazepam, and lorazepam. *Clin Pharmacol Ther* 1984; **35:** 188–92.
24. Fee JPH, *et al.* Diazepam disposition following cimetidine or ranitidine. *Br J Clin Pharmacol* 1984; **17:** 617P–18P.
25. Klotz U, *et al.* Nocturnal doses of ranitidine and nizatidine do not affect the disposition of diazepam. *J Clin Pharmacol* 1987; **27:** 210–12.
26. Fee JPH, *et al.* Cimetidine and ranitidine increase midazolam bioavailability. *Clin Pharmacol Ther* 1987; **41:** 80–4.
27. Wilson CM, *et al.* Effect of pretreatment with ranitidine on the hypnotic action of single doses of midazolam, temazepam and zopiclone. *Br J Anaesth* 1986; **58:** 483–6.
28. Vanderveen RP, *et al.* Effect of ranitidine on the disposition of orally and intravenously administered triazolam. *Clin Pharm* 1991; **10:** 539–43.
29. Gamble JAS, *et al.* Some pharmacological factors influencing the absorption of diazepam following oral administration. *Br J Anaesth* 1976; **48:** 1181–5.
30. Bateman DN. The action of cisapride on gastric emptying and the pharmacokinetics of oral diazepam. *Eur J Clin Pharmacol* 1986; **30:** 205–8.
31. Gugler R, Jensen JC. Omeprazole inhibits elimination of diazepam. *Lancet* 1984; **i:** 969.
32. Andersson T, *et al.* Effect of omeprazole and cimetidine on plasma diazepam levels. *Eur J Clin Pharmacol* 1990; **39:** 51–4.
33. Andersson T, *et al.* Effect of omeprazole treatment on diazepam plasma levels in slow versus normal rapid metabolizers of omeprazole. *Clin Pharmacol Ther* 1990; **47:** 79–85.
34. Caraco Y, *et al.* Interethnic difference in omeprazole's inhibition of diazepam metabolism. *Clin Pharmacol Ther* 1995; **58:** 62–72.
35. Lefebvre RA, *et al.* Influence of lansoprazole treatment on diazepam plasma concentrations. *Clin Pharmacol Ther* 1992; **52:** 458–63.
36. Gugler R, *et al.* Lack of pharmacokinetic interaction of pantoprazole with diazepam in man. *Br J Clin Pharmacol* 1996; **42:** 249–52.

General anaesthetics. A synergistic interaction has been demonstrated for the hypnotic effects of midazolam and thiopental.[1] Although midazolam failed to produce anaesthesia at the doses used, the drug caused a twofold increase in the anaesthetic potency of thiopental. Similar synergistic interactions have been observed between midazolam and both *methohexital*[2] and *propofol*.[3,4] The interaction between midazolam and propofol could not be explained solely by alteration in free-plasma concentration of either drug,[5] although a later study[6] does suggest that propofol reduces the clearance of midazolam via its inhibitory effects on the metabolism of midazolam by the cytochrome P450 isoenzyme CYP3A4. Midazolam has also been reported to be able to produce a marked reduction in the concentration of halothane required for anaesthesia.[7]

1. Short TG, *et al.* Hypnotic and anaesthetic action of thiopentone and midazolam alone and in combination. *Br J Anaesth* 1991; **66:** 13–19.
2. Tverskoy M, *et al.* Midazolam acts synergistically with methohexitone for induction of anaesthesia. *Br J Anaesth* 1989; **63:** 109–12.
3. McClune S, *et al.* Synergistic interaction between midazolam and propofol. *Br J Anaesth* 1992; **69:** 240–5.
4. Short TG, Chui PT. Propofol and midazolam act synergistically in combination. *Br J Anaesth* 1991; **67:** 539–45.
5. Teh J, *et al.* Pharmacokinetic interactions between midazolam and propofol: an infusion study. *Br J Anaesth* 1994; **72:** 62–5.
6. Hamaoka N, *et al.* Propofol decreases the clearance of midazolam by inhibiting CYP3A4: an in vivo and in vitro study. *Clin Pharmacol Ther* 1999; **66:** 110–7.
7. Inagaki Y, *et al.* Anesthetic interaction between midazolam and halothane in humans. *Anesth Analg* 1993; **76:** 613–7.

Grapefruit juice. Grapefruit juice has been reported to be able to increase the bioavailability of oral midazolam[1] or triazolam[2] and to raise peak plasma concentrations. However, these results have been contradicted by another study,[3] which found no evidence for an interaction.

1. Kupferschmidt HHT, *et al.* Interaction between grapefruit juice and midazolam in humans. *Clin Pharmacol Ther* 1995; **58:** 20–8.
2. Hukkinen SK, *et al.* Plasma concentrations of triazolam are increased by concomitant ingestion of grapefruit juice. *Clin Pharmacol Ther* 1995; **58:** 127–31.
3. Vanakoski J, *et al.* Grapefruit juice does not enhance the effects of midazolam and triazolam in man. *Eur J Clin Pharmacol* 1996; **50:** 501–8.

Kava. A patient whose medication included alprazolam, cimetidine, and terazosin became lethargic and disoriented after starting to take kava.[1] An interaction between kava and the benzodiazepine was suspected.

1. Almeida JC, Grimsley EW. Coma from the health food store: interaction between kava and alprazolam. *Ann Intern Med* 1996; **125:** 940–1.

Levodopa. For reference to the effects of benzodiazepines on levodopa, see p.1172.

Neuromuscular blockers. For reference to the effect of diazepam on neuromuscular blockade, see p.1334.

Oral contraceptives. Some studies with alprazolam,[1] chlordiazepoxide,[2] and diazepam[3] have supported suggestions that oral contraceptives may inhibit the biotransformation of benzodiazepines metabolised by oxidation, although no significant pharmacokinetic alterations have been observed with clotiazepam,[4] or triazolam.[1] The biotransformation of benzodiazepines metabolised by conjugation, such as lorazepam, oxazepam, or temazepam, may be enhanced[1,2] or unchanged.[5] No consistent correlation has been observed between the above pharmacokinetic changes and clinical effects. It has been observed[6] that psychomotor impairment due to oral diazepam

was greater during the menstrual pause than during the 21-daily oral contraceptive cycle. This may have been due to an effect of oral contraceptives on diazepam absorption. Another study[7] noted that women taking oral contraceptives appeared to be more sensitive to psychomotor impairment following single oral doses of alprazolam, lorazepam, or triazolam, than controls. The effects of temazepam were minimal in both groups. Alterations in sedative or amnesic effect could not be established with any certainty.

1. Stoehr GP, *et al.* Effect of oral contraceptives on triazolam, temazepam, alprazolam, and lorazepam kinetics. *Clin Pharmacol Ther* 1984; **36:** 683–90.
2. Patwardhan RV, *et al.* Differential effects of oral contraceptive steroids on the metabolism of benzodiazepines. *Hepatology* 1983; **3:** 248–53.
3. Abernethy DR, *et al.* Impairment of diazepam metabolism by low-dose estrogen-containing oral-contraceptive steroids. *N Engl J Med* 1982; **306:** 791–2.
4. Ochs HR, *et al.* Disposition of clotiazepam: influence of age, sex, oral contraceptives, cimetidine, isoniazid and ethanol. *Eur J Clin Pharmacol* 1984; **26:** 55–9.
5. Abernethy DR, *et al.* Lorazepam and oxazepam kinetics in women on low-dose oral contraceptives. *Clin Pharmacol Ther* 1983; **33:** 628–32.
6. Ellinwood EH, *et al.* Effects of oral contraceptives on diazepam-induced psychomotor impairment. *Clin Pharmacol Ther* 1984; **35:** 360–6.
7. Kroboth PD, *et al.* Pharmacodynamic evaluation of the benzodiazepine-oral contraceptive interaction. *Clin Pharmacol Ther* 1985; **38:** 525–32.

Penicillamine. Phlebitis associated with intravenous diazepam resolved with local heat but recurred on two separate occasions after oral penicillamine.[1]

1. Brandstetter RD, *et al.* Exacerbation of intravenous diazepam-induced phlebitis by oral penicillamine. *BMJ* 1981; **283:** 525.

Probenecid. Probenecid increased the half-life of intravenous lorazepam in 9 healthy subjects.[1] Probenecid was considered to impair glucuronide formation selectively and thus the clearance of drugs like lorazepam. Probenecid has also shortened the time to induce anaesthesia with midazolam in 46 patients.[2] The effect was considered to be due to competition for plasma protein binding sites. It has been suggested that the initial dose of adinazolam should be reduced and subsequent dosage monitored when it is administered with probenecid.[3] A study[3] in 16 subjects had indicated that probenecid could potentiate the psychomotor effects of adinazolam. This appeared to be mainly due to inhibition of the renal clearance of N-desmethyladinazolam. Probenecid has also been reported[4] to reduce the clearance of nitrazepam but not of temazepam.

1. Abernethy DR, *et al.* Probenecid inhibition of acetaminophen and lorazepam glucuronidation. *Clin Pharmacol Ther* 1984; **35:** 224.
2. Dundee JW, *et al.* Aspirin and probenecid pretreatment influences the potency of thiopentone and the onset of action of midazolam. *Eur J Anaesthesiol* 1986; **3:** 247–51.
3. Golden PL, *et al.* Effects of probenecid on the pharmacokinetics and pharmacodynamics of adinazolam in humans. *Clin Pharmacol Ther* 1994; **56:** 133–41.
4. Brockmeyer NH, *et al.* Comparative effects of rifampin and/or probenecid on the pharmacokinetics of temazepam and nitrazepam. *Int J Clin Pharmacol Ther Toxicol* 1990; **28:** 387–93.

Smooth muscle relaxants. Intracavernosal *papaverine* produced prolonged erection in 2 patients who had been given intravenous diazepam as an anxiolytic before the papaverine.[1]

1. Vale JA, *et al.* Papaverine, benzodiazepines, and prolonged erections. *Lancet* 1991; **337:** 1552.

Tobacco smoking. The Boston Collaborative Drug Surveillance Program reported drowsiness as a side-effect of diazepam or chlordiazepoxide less frequently in smokers than non-smokers.[1] Pharmacokinetic studies have, however, been divided between those indicating that smoking induces the hepatic metabolism of benzodiazepines and those showing no effect on benzodiazepine pharmacokinetics.[2] Hence, diminished end-organ responsiveness may in part account for the observed clinical effects. Concomitant consumption of large amounts of xanthine-containing beverages may decrease any enzyme-inducing effects of smoking.[3]

1. Boston Collaborative Drug Surveillance Program, Boston University Medical Center. Clinical depression of the central nervous system due to diazepam and chlordiazepoxide in relation to cigarette smoking and age. *N Engl J Med* 1973; **288:** 277–80.
2. Miller LG. Cigarettes and drug therapy: pharmacokinetic and pharmacodynamic considerations. *Clin Pharm* 1990; **9:** 125–35.
3. Downing RW, Rickels K. Coffee consumption, cigarette smoking and reporting of drowsiness in anxious patients treated with benzodiazepines or placebo. *Acta Psychiatr Scand* 1981; **64:** 398–408.

Xanthines. There are reports of *aminophylline* given intravenously reversing the sedation from intravenous diazepam,[1-3] although not always completely[2] nor as effectively as flumazenil.[4] Blockade of adenosine receptors by aminophylline has been postulated as the mechanism of this interaction.[3,5]

Xanthine-containing beverages may be expected to decrease the incidence of benzodiazepine-induced drowsiness because of their CNS-stimulating effects and their ability to induce hepatic drug-metabolising enzymes. However, decreased drowsiness has only sometimes been observed and the actions of xanthines may themselves be decreased by concomitant heavy tobacco smoking.[6,7]

1. Arvidsson SB, *et al.* Aminophylline antagonises diazepam sedation. *Lancet* 1982; **ii:** 1467.
2. Kleindienst G, Usinger P. Diazepam sedation is not antagonised completely by aminophylline. *Lancet* 1984; **i:** 113.

3. Niemand D, et al. Aminophylline inhibition of diazepam sedation: is adenosine blockade of GABA-receptors the mechanism? Lancet 1984; i: 463–4.
4. Sibai AN, et al. Comparison of flumazenil with aminophylline to antagonise midazolam in elderly patients. Br J Anaesth 1991; 66: 591–5.
5. Henauer SA, et al. Theophylline antagonises diazepam-induced psychomotor impairment. Eur J Clin Pharmacol 1983; 25: 743–7.
6. Downing RW, Rickels K. Coffee consumption, cigarette smoking and reporting of drowsiness in anxious patients treated with benzodiazepines or placebo. Acta Psychiatr Scand 1981; 64: 398–408.
7. Ghoneim MM, et al. Pharmacokinetic and pharmacodynamic interactions between caffeine and diazepam. J Clin Psychopharmacol 1986; 6: 75–80.

Pharmacokinetics

Diazepam is readily and completely absorbed from the gastrointestinal tract, peak plasma concentrations occurring within about 30 to 90 minutes of oral administration. Diazepam is rapidly absorbed after administration as a rectal solution; peak plasma concentrations are achieved after about 10 to 30 minutes but are lower than those after intravenous administration. Absorption may be erratic following intramuscular administration and lower peak plasma concentrations may be obtained compared with those following oral administration. Diazepam is highly lipid soluble and crosses the blood-brain barrier; it acts promptly on the brain, and its initial effects decrease rapidly as it is redistributed into fat depots and tissues.

Diazepam has a biphasic half-life with an initial rapid distribution phase followed by a prolonged terminal elimination phase of 1 or 2 days; its action is further prolonged by the even longer half-life of 2 to 5 days of its principal active metabolite, desmethyldiazepam (nordazepam). Diazepam and desmethyldiazepam accumulate on repeated administration and the relative proportion of desmethyldiazepam in the body increases on long-term administration. No simple correlation has been found between plasma concentrations of diazepam or its metabolites and their therapeutic effect.

Diazepam is extensively metabolised in the liver and, in addition to desmethyldiazepam, its active metabolites include oxazepam, and temazepam. It is excreted in the urine, mainly in the form of free or conjugated metabolites. Diazepam is 98 to 99% bound to plasma proteins.

The plasma elimination half-life of diazepam and/or its metabolites is prolonged in neonates, in the elderly, and in patients with liver disease. In addition to crossing the blood-brain barrier, diazepam and its metabolites also cross the placental barrier and are distributed into breast milk.

◊ Reviews.
1. Bailey L, et al. Clinical pharmacokinetics of benzodiazepines. J Clin Pharmacol 1994; 34: 804–11.

◊ For reference to the altered pharmacokinetics of diazepam in patients with impaired liver and kidney function and in the elderly, see under Precautions, above.

Absorption and plasma concentrations. CHRONIC ORAL ADMINISTRATION. In 36 patients who had received diazepam 2 to 30 mg daily for periods from one month to 10 years, plasma-diazepam concentrations were directly related to dose and inversely related to age.[1] There was a close association between the plasma concentrations of diazepam and its metabolite desmethyldiazepam and both concentrations were independent of the duration of therapy. Plasma-diazepam concentration ranges were 0.02 to 1.01 µg per mL, and plasma-desmethyldiazepam concentration ranges were 0.055 to 1.765 µg per mL. Another similar study[2] reached the same general conclusions.

1. Rutherford DM, et al. Plasma concentrations of diazepam and desmethyldiazepam during chronic diazepam therapy. Br J Clin Pharmacol 1978; 6: 69–73.
2. Greenblatt DJ, et al. Plasma diazepam and desmethyldiazepam concentrations during long-term diazepam therapy. Br J Clin Pharmacol 1981; 1: 35–40.

RECTAL. In 6 adults given diazepam 10 mg by mouth or as a solution (Valium injection) by rectum, mean bioavailability was 76 and 81%, respectively compared with the same dose by intravenous injection.[1] Bioavailability was lower with suppositories than with the solution given rectally. Studies support the use of rectal solution rather than suppositories in children.[2,3]

1. Dhillon S, et al. Bioavailability of diazepam after intravenous, oral and rectal administration in adult epileptic patients. Br J Clin Pharmacol 1982; 13: 427–32.
2. Dhillon S, et al. Rectal absorption of diazepam in epileptic children. Arch Dis Child 1982; 57: 264–7.
3. Sonander H, et al. Effects of the rectal administration of diazepam. Br J Anaesth 1985; 57: 578–80.

Distribution into breast milk. Studies measuring concentrations of diazepam and desmethyldiazepam transferred from mother to infant via breast milk.[1,2]
See also under Precautions, above.

1. Erkkola R, Kanto J. Diazepam and breast-feeding. Lancet 1972; i: 1235–6.
2. Brandt R. Passage of diazepam and desmethyldiazepam into breast milk. Arzneimittelforschung 1976; 26: 454–7.

Metabolism. Most benzodiazepines are highly lipophilic compounds requiring biotransformation before excretion from the body, and many form active metabolites that affect the duration of action. The benzodiazepines may be classified as long-, intermediate-, or short-acting compounds.[1]

• **Long-acting** benzodiazepines are either N_1-desalkyl derivatives (delorazepam and nordazepam) or are oxidised in the liver to N_1-desalkyl derivatives (benzodiazepines so oxidised include chlordiazepoxide, clobazam, clorazepate, cloxazolam, diazepam, flurazepam, halazepam, ketazolam, medazepam, oxazolam, pinazepam, prazepam, and quazepam). Clorazepate and prazepam may be considered as prodrugs since the metabolite is the expected active principle. Both parent drug and metabolites contribute to the activity of the other long-acting drugs. Further biotransformation of N_1-desalkylated metabolites proceeds much more slowly than for the parent drug, and they therefore accumulate in the body after a few days of treatment. The rate-limiting step of their metabolism (with the exception of the 1,5-derivatives) is C3-hydroxylation to the pharmacologically active oxazepam or its 2'-halogenated analogues.

• **Intermediate-acting** benzodiazepines are 7-nitrobenzodiazepines such as clonazepam, flunitrazepam, and nitrazepam which are metabolised by nitroreduction with no important known active metabolites. The metabolites of long- and intermediate-acting benzodiazepines require conjugation before excretion in the urine.

• **Short-acting** benzodiazepines include the C3-hydroxylated benzodiazepines such as lorazepam, lormetazepam, oxazepam, and temazepam which undergo rapid conjugation with glucuronic acid to water-soluble inactive metabolites that are excreted in the urine, and drugs such as alprazolam, brotizolam, estazolam, etizolam, midazolam, tofisopam, and triazolam which require oxidation involving aliphatic hydroxylation before subsequent conjugation. Although these hydroxylated metabolites may retain pharmacological activity, they are unlikely to contribute significantly to the clinical activity because of their negligible plasma concentrations and rapid inactivation by glucuronidation.

Drug-metabolising capacity is influenced by many factors including genetics, age, sex, endocrine and nutritional status, smoking, disease, and concurrent drug therapy. This results in wide interindividual variation in both parent drug concentrations and metabolite-to-parent drug ratios.

1. Caccia S, Garattini S. Formation of active metabolites of psychotropic drugs: an updated review of their significance. Clin Pharmacokinet 1990; 18: 434–59.

Pregnancy. Passage of diazepam across the placenta depends in part on the relative degrees of protein binding in mother and fetus, which in turn is influenced by factors such as stage of pregnancy and plasma concentrations of free fatty acids in mother and fetus.[1-6] Adverse effects may persist in the neonate for several days after birth because of immature drug-metabolising enzymes. Competition between diazepam and bilirubin for protein binding sites could result in hyperbilirubinaemia in the neonate.[7]

See also under Precautions, above.

1. Lee JN, et al. Serum protein binding of diazepam in maternal and foetal serum during pregnancy. Br J Clin Pharmacol 1982; 14: 551–4.
2. Kuhnz W, Nau H. Differences in in vitro binding of diazepam and N-desmethyldiazepam to maternal and fetal plasma proteins at birth: relation to free fatty acid concentration and other parameters. Clin Pharmacol Ther 1983; 34: 220–6.
3. Kanto J, et al. Accumulation of diazepam and N-desmethyldiazepam in the fetal blood during the labour. Ann Clin Res 1973; 5: 375–9.
4. Nau H, et al. Decreased serum protein binding of diazepam and its major metabolite in the neonate during the first postnatal week related to increased free fatty acid levels. Br J Clin Pharmacol 1984; 17: 92–8.
5. Ridd MJ, et al. The disposition and placental transfer of diazepam in cesarean section. Clin Pharmacol Ther 1989; 45: 506–12.
6. Idänpään-Heikkilä J, et al. Placental transfer and fetal metabolism of diazepam-C14 in early human pregnancy. Clin Pharmacol Ther 1971; 12: 363.
7. Notarianni LJ. Plasma protein binding of drugs in pregnancy and in neonates. Clin Pharmacokinet 1990; 18: 20–36.

Uses and Administration

Diazepam is a long-acting benzodiazepine with anticonvulsant, anxiolytic, sedative, muscle relaxant, and amnestic properties. Its actions are mediated by enhancement of the activity of gamma-aminobutyric acid (GABA), a major inhibitory neurotransmitter in the brain. It is used in the short-term treatment of severe anxiety disorders (p.649), as a hypnotic in the short-term management of insomnia (p.652), as a sedative (p.652) and premedicant (p.1256), as an anticonvulsant (particularly in the management of status epilepticus and febrile convulsions), in the control of muscle spasm, and in the management of withdrawal symptoms (see the references below).

Diazepam is **administered** orally, rectally, and parenterally with the risk of dependence very much influencing the dose and duration of treatment. Doses should be the lowest that can control symptoms and courses of treatment should be short, not normally exceeding 4 weeks, with diazepam being withdrawn gradually (see above). Elderly and debilitated patients should be given not more than one-half the usual adult dose. Dosage reduction may also be required in patients with liver or kidney dysfunction.

Oral administration is appropriate for many indications and modified-release formulations are available in some countries. Rectal administration may be by suppository or rectal solution or gel. Diazepam is also given by deep intramuscular or slow intravenous injection, although absorption following intramuscular injection may be erratic and provides lower blood concentrations than those following oral administration. Intravenous injection should be carried out slowly into a large vein of the antecubital fossa at a recommended rate of no more than 1 mL of a 0.5% solution (5 mg) per minute. It is advisable to keep the patient in the supine position and under medical supervision for at least an hour after administration. Diazepam may be administered by continuous intravenous infusion; because of the risk of precipitation of diazepam, solutions should be freshly prepared following the manufacturer's directions regarding diluent and concentration of diazepam. Diazepam is substantially adsorbed onto some plastics (see under Sorption, above). Facilities for resuscitation should always be available when diazepam is given intravenously.

Diazepam may be given for **severe anxiety** in oral doses of 2 mg three times daily to a maximum of 30 mg daily. A wider dose range of 4 to 40 mg daily in divided doses is used in the USA with children over 6 months of age receiving up to 10 mg daily. Diazepam may be given as a rectal solution in a dose of 500 µg per kg body-weight repeated after 12 hours if necessary or as suppositories in a dose of 10 to 30 mg. Diazepam may sometimes have to be given by intramuscular or intravenous injection when a dose of up to 10 mg may be given, repeated if necessary after 4 hours.

The benzodiazepines have a limited role in **insomnia** and diazepam is used for the short-term management of insomnia associated with anxiety in a dose of 5 to 15 mg by mouth at bedtime. Doses of 1 to 5 mg at bedtime have been used in children to control **night terrors** and **sleepwalking**.

Diazepam may be given for **premedication** before general anaesthesia or to provide sedative cover for minor surgical or investigative procedures. Doses by mouth are in the range of 5 to 20 mg; a dose of 10 mg as a rectal solution may also be suitable. When given by intravenous injection the dose is usually 100 to 200 µg per kg body-weight. Some regard the perioperative use of diazepam in children undesirable since its effect and onset of action are unreliable and paradoxical effects may occur. Diazepam may also be given for **sedation** during minor surgical and medical procedures; doses of 10 to 20 mg, given by intravenous injection over 2 to 4 minutes are recommended.

Diazepam is used in a variety of **seizures**. It is given by mouth as an adjunct in some types of epilepsy; for this purpose, 2 to 60 mg may be given daily in divided doses. A rectal gel formulation is also available for adjunctive use in the management of episodes of increased seizure activity in patients with refractory epilepsy; doses range from 200 to 500 µg per kg, depending on age, repeated after 4 to 12 hours if necessary. For febrile convulsions, status epilepticus, and convulsions due to poisoning, administration of a rectal solution may be appropriate; suppositories are not suitable because absorption is too slow. Recommended doses for the rectal solution differ. Some recommend a dose of 500 μg per kg body-weight for adults and children over 10 kg, repeated every 12 hours if necessary, but if convulsions are not controlled by the first dose the use of other anticonvulsive measures is recommended. Others recommend a dose of 10 mg for adults and children over 3 years of age and 5 mg for children 1 to 3 years of age. Alternatively diazepam may be given *intravenously* to adults in a dose of 10 to 20 mg given at a rate of 5 mg per minute and repeated if necessary after 30 to 60 minutes. Other schedules involve administering smaller amounts more frequently or giving diazepam *intramuscularly*, though again absorption may be too slow. Once the seizures have been controlled, a slow intravenous infusion providing up to 3 mg per kg over 24 hours has been administered to protect against recurrence. Doses by intravenous or intramuscular injection in children are within the range of 200 to 300 μg per kg; alternatively 1 mg may be given for each year of age.

Diazepam may be given *by mouth* in daily divided doses of 2 to 15 mg to alleviate **muscle spasm**. The dose may be increased in severe spastic disorders, such as cerebral palsy, to up to 60 mg daily in adults or up to 40 mg daily in children. If given by intramuscular or slow intravenous *injection* the dose is 10 mg repeated if necessary after 4 hours. Larger doses are used in tetanus in adults and children with 100 to 300 μg per kg body-weight being given every 1 to 4 hours by intravenous injection. Alternatively 3 to 10 mg per kg may be given over 24 hours by continuous intravenous infusion or by nasoduodenal tube using a suitable liquid oral dose form. Diazepam may also be given by the rectal route as a *rectal solution* in a dose of 500 μg per kg body-weight for adults and children over 10 kg in weight, repeated every 12 hours if necessary.

Symptoms of the **alcohol withdrawal syndrome** may be controlled by diazepam given *by mouth* in a dose of 5 to 20 mg, repeated if required after 2 to 4 hours; another approach is to give 10 mg three or four times on the first day reducing to 5 mg three or four times daily as required. Diazepam may need to be given *by injection* if the symptoms are severe and if delirium tremens has developed; 10 to 20 mg by intramuscular or intravenous injection may be adequate, although some patients may require higher doses.

◊ Reviews.
1. Ashton H. Guidelines for the rational use of benzodiazepines: when and what to use. *Drugs* 1994; **48:** 25–40.

Action. Gamma-aminobutyric acid (GABA) is the major inhibitory neurotransmitter in the brain. GABA's functions within the CNS include involvement in sleep induction and the control of neuronal excitability, epilepsy, anxiety, memory, and hypnosis.[1] Two subtypes of GABA receptors have been identified: A and B. Benzodiazepines interact with GABA$_A$ receptors to produce their sedative, hypnotic, anxiolytic, anticonvulsant, and antinociceptive effects. The GABA$_A$ receptors within the CNS are composed of different subunits, 4 of which have been described: α, β, γ, and δ. These subunits combine to form macromolecular complexes which include a chloride ion channel and regions to which GABA and benzodiazepines bind, as well as binding sites for other substances. The different types of subunit comprising the GABA$_A$ receptor determine its activity. The presence of a γ subunit confers benzodiazepine sensitivity and it is the type of α subunit(s) present that determines whether the benzodiazepine activity is mainly anxiolytic or mainly sedative. Two types of benzodiazepine receptor are suggested: type I, found throughout the brain and in large concentrations in the cerebellum and type II found mainly in the cerebral cortex, spinal cord, and hippocampus. It is the benzodiazepine type I receptors that are thought to be responsible for the anxiolytic actions of benzodiazepines. The possibility of different types of GABA receptor associated with different functions remains to be fully exploited with the development of a benzodiazepine specially selected for its anxiolytic effect and lacking sedative and muscle relaxant activity. The 1–5 benzodiazepines such as clobazam are examples of compounds possessing a certain degree of selectivity, being less sedating, although having muscle relaxant activity.
1. Goodchild CS. GABA receptors and benzodiazepines. *Br J Anaesth* 1993; **71:** 127–33.

Cardiac arrhythmias. Although not considered to be an antiarrhythmic, diazepam has been tried with good effect in treating the cardiotoxicity of chloroquine poisoning (see p.433).

However, diazepam has been reported to possess both antiarrhythmic and pro-arrhythmic properties, possibly depending on the dose.[1]
1. Kumagai K, *et al.* Antiarrhythmic and proarrhythmic properties of diazepam demonstrated by electrophysiological study in humans. *Clin Cardiol* 1991; **14:** 397–401.

Chloroquine poisoning. For reference to the possible use of diazepam to decrease the cardiotoxic effects of chloroquine, see p.433.

Conversion and dissociative disorders. Conversion and dissociative disorders (formerly known as hysteria) are characterised by physical symptoms that occur in the absence of organic disease. Medication has no part to play in the treatment of these disorders unless they are secondary to conditions such as depression or anxiety disorders requiring treatment in their own right.

There have been suggestions that sedatives such as diazepam or midazolam may be used to confirm the diagnosis of hysterical paralysis.[1,2] The test tends to exacerbate organic disease while psychiatric dysfunction may improve.
1. Ellis SJ. Diazepam as a truth drug. *Lancet* 1990; **336:** 752–3.
2. Keating JJ, *et al.* Hysterical paralysis. *Lancet* 1990; **336:** 1506–7.

Disturbed behaviour. For a discussion of the management of behaviour disturbances associated with various psychotic disorders, and the value of benzodiazepines, see p.650. Benzodiazepines are considered to be useful in palliative care for the relief of terminal restlessness. Midazolam is often used although other benzodiazepines such as diazepam have also been tried.[1] A suggested dose for diazepam is 5 to 10 mg given slowly as a rectal solution and repeated every 8 to 12 hours.
1. Burke AL. Palliative care: an update on "terminal restlessness." *Med J Aust* 1997; **166:** 39–42.

Dyspnoea. Despite the hazards of administration to patients with any form of respiratory depression or pulmonary insufficiency (see under Precautions, above) benzodiazepines such as diazepam have been tried in the treatment of dyspnoea (p.69), in the belief that reduction of an elevated respiratory drive may alleviate respiratory distress. However, benefits have not been confirmed. Benzodiazepines may be of use in patients with advanced cancer who have rapid shallow respiration. A daily dose of 5 to 10 mg has been suggested for diazepam.

Eclampsia and pre-eclampsia. Diazepam has been used for the initial control of impending or actual eclampsia (p.341), but magnesium sulfate is now generally the preferred treatment.

Epilepsy and other convulsive disorders. Some benzodiazepines such as diazepam are used for the control of status epilepticus (p.341), including status epilepticus in patients with porphyria (p.342—but see also under Porphyria in Precautions, above), and for febrile convulsions (p.341); diazepam has also been used in eclampsia (see above) and for neonatal seizures (p.342). Benzodiazepines such as clobazam and clonazepam may be employed in the management of epilepsy (p.338), but their long-term use is limited by problems of sedation, dependence, and tolerance to the antiepileptic effects. Diazepam has been used as an adjunct in the management of some types of epilepsy including myoclonus.

References.
1. Rosman NP, *et al.* A controlled trial of diazepam administered during febrile illnesses to prevent recurrence of febrile seizures. *N Engl J Med* 1993; **329:** 79–84.
2. Somerville ER, Antony JH. Position statement on the use of rectal diazepam in epilepsy. *Med J Aust* 1995; **163:** 268–9.
3. Uhari M, *et al.* Effect of acetaminophen and low intermittent doses of diazepam on prevention of recurrences of febrile seizures. *J Pediatr* 1995; **126:** 991–5.
4. Akinbi MS, Welty TE. Benzodiazepines in the home treatment of acute seizures. *Ann Pharmacother* 1999; **33:** 99–102.
5. Rey E, *et al.* Pharmacokinetic optimisation of benzodiazepine therapy for acute seizures: focus on delivery routes. *Clin Pharmacokinet* 1999; **36:** 409–24.

Extrapyramidal disorders. For reference to the use of benzodiazepines in the treatment of antipsychotic-induced extrapyramidal disorders, see Chlorpromazine, p.662.

Irritable bowel syndrome. Although some benzodiazepines have been used in the management of irritable bowel syndrome (p.1206) there is no evidence to support their use in this condition.

Mania. Benzodiazepines have been used as short-term adjuncts in the initial control of manic episodes in patients with bipolar disorder (p.271) until lithium has achieved its full effect.

Muscle spasm. Diazepam and other benzodiazepines may be used for the relief of muscle spasm (p.1322) of various aetiologies including that secondary to muscle or joint inflammation or trauma, such as in acute **low back pain** (p.6), or resulting from **spasticity** (p.1322), **dystonias** (p.1173), **stiff-man syndrome** (see below), **cerebral palsy**, **poisoning**, or **tetanus** (p.1332). High doses are often required and treatment may be limited by adverse effects or by risk of dependence.

STIFF-MAN SYNDROME. Stiff-man syndrome is a rare condition characterised by painful intermittent spasms and rigidity of the axial and limb muscles. Its exact cause is unknown but there is some evidence to implicate autoantibodies against one of the enzymes involved in the synthesis of the neurotransmitter gam-

ma-aminobutyric acid. It is frequently associated with auto-immune diseases and type 1 diabetes mellitus. Patients typically respond to benzodiazepines and this may be of use in the differential diagnosis of the syndrome. Diazepam has been the mainstay of treatment but clonazepam may also be of use, especially in familial startle disease, a rare congenital form of stiff-man syndrome. Although rigidity and spasms in stiff-man syndrome are not completely resolved by diazepam the degree of improvement can be sufficient to restore the functional level to near normal. However, large doses are often required and sedation might be a limiting factor in some patients. Other drugs which have been used when diazepam is ineffective or poorly tolerated include baclofen or sodium valproate but benefit may be less evident. There have been isolated anecdotal reports of improvement with vigabatrin. Although corticosteroids may be of benefit, the chronic nature of the disorder and the high incidence of type 1 diabetes mellitus make their use undesirable. Other attempts at immunomodulation such as plasmapheresis have yielded variable results and evidence of the efficacy of immunoglobulins is largely limited to anecdotal reports and uncontrolled studies.

References.
1. Toro C, *et al.* Stiff-man syndrome. *Semin Neurol* 1994; **14:** 154–8.
2. Gerhardt CL. Stiff-man syndrome revisited. *South Med J* 1995; **88:** 805–808.
3. Stayer C, Meinck H-M. Stiff-man syndrome: an overview. *Neurologia* 1998; **13:** 83–8.
4. Levy LM, *et al.* The stiff-person syndrome - an autoimmune disorder affecting neurotransmission of γ-aminobutyric acid. *Ann Intern Med* 1999; **131:** 522–30.

Nausea and vomiting. Benzodiazepines, particularly lorazepam, are used as adjuncts in the management of nausea and vomiting induced by cancer chemotherapy (p.1206), particularly anticipatory emesis.

Parasomnias. Parasomnias (p.653) rarely require treatment other than the symptomatic treatment of sleep-related medical problems. A number of parasomnias such as restless leg syndrome, sleepwalking, and night terrors have been reported to respond to benzodiazepines. Although the muscle relaxant and anxiolytic action of a benzodiazepine can be helpful in bruxism (teeth grinding) it has been recommended that they should only be prescribed on a short-term basis during the acute phase.

References.
1. Schenck CH, Mahowald MW. Long-term, nightly benzodiazepine treatment of injurious parasomnias and other disorders of disrupted nocturnal sleep in 170 adults. *Am J Med* 1996; **100:** 333–7.

Premenstrual syndrome. For mention of the limited role of benzodiazepines in the management of premenstrual syndrome, see p.1475.

Schizophrenia. Benzodiazepines may be useful adjuncts to antipsychotics in the initial management of schizophrenia (p.651).

Substance dependence. The benzodiazepines are used in the management of symptoms of *alcohol* withdrawal (p.1131), of *opioid* withdrawal (p.66), and of *cocaine* withdrawal (p.1310).

Vertigo. Although intravenous diazepam has been used to abort acute attacks of vertigo of peripheral origin (p.408), it can prolong compensation and recovery from vestibular lesions.[1]
1. Rascol O, *et al.* Antivertigo medications and drug-induced vertigo: a pharmacological review. *Drugs* 1995; **50:** 777–91.

Preparations

BP 2001: Diazepam Injection; Diazepam Oral Solution; Diazepam Rectal Solution; Diazepam Tablets;
USP 25: Diazepam Capsules; Diazepam Extended-release Capsules; Diazepam Injection; Diazepam Tablets.

Proprietary Preparations (details are given in Part 3)
Aust.: Gewacalm; Psychopax; Stesolid; Umbrium; Valium; *Austral.:* Antenex; Diazemuls; Ducene; Valium; *Belg.:* Valium; *Braz.:* Ansilive; Calmociteno; Diazelong; Dienpax; Kiatrium; Noan; Pazolini; Somaplus; Valium; *Canad.:* Diazemuls; Novo-Dipam†; Valium; Vivol; *Denm.:* Apozepam; Hexalid; Stesolid; Valaxona; Valium; Fin.: Diapam; Medipam; Stesolid; *Fr.:* Novazem; Valium; *Ger.:* Diazep; Faustan; Lamra; Stesolid; Tranquase; Valiquid; Valium; Valocordin-Diazepam; *Hong Kong:* Diazemuls; Kratium; *Irl.:* Anxicalm; Diazemuls; Stesolid; Valium; *Israel:* Assival; Diaz; Disopam; Stesolid; Valium; *Ital.:* Aliseum; Ansiolin; Diazemuls; Eridan†; Micronoan; Noan; Tranquirit; Valium; Vatran; *Mex.:* Alboral; Arzepam; Benzyme; Diapanil; Diatex; Farmin; Freudal; Impepas; Laxyl; Nerolid; Onapan; Ortopsique; Paxate; Prizem; Rayne; Relasan; Relazepam; Sediver; Seredyn; Tandial; Valium; Vanzor; Zepan; Zeprat; *Neth.:* Valium; *Norw.:* Stesolid; Valium; Vival; *NZ:* D-Pam; Diazemuls; Propam; Stesolid; *Port.:* Bialzepam; Metamidol; Stesolid; Unisedil; Valium; *S.Afr.:* Benzopin; Betapam; Calmpose; Diaquel; Doval; Dynapam†; Ethipam†; Pax; Scriptopam†; Valium; *Singapore:* Diapine; Stesolid; Valium; *Spain:* Aneurol; Aspaserine B6 Tranq; Calmaven†; Complutine; Diaceplex; Diaceplex Simple†; Dicepin B6†; Drenian; Gobanal; Pacium; Podium; Sico Relax; Stesolid; Valium; Vincosedan; *Swed.:* Apozepam; Stesolid; Valium†; *Switz.:* Paceum; Psychopax; Stesolid; Valium; *Thai.:* Diapam; Diapine; Dizan; Dizepam; Sipam; Stesolid; V Day Zepam; Valenium; Valium; Zopam; *UK:* Dialar; Diazemuls; Rimapam; Stesolid; Tensium; Valclair; Valium; *USA:* Dizac†; Valium.

Multi-ingredient: *Aust.:* Acordin†; Betamed; Harmomed; *Braz.:* Dialudon; Dobesix; Fastium; Moderine; Nofagus; *Fin.:* Gastrodyn comp; Nitrapamil; Relapamil; Vertipam; *Ital.:* Gamibetal Plus; Spasen Somatico; Spasmeridan; Spasmomen Somatico;

The symbol † denotes a preparation no longer actively marketed

Valpinax; Valtrax; *Mex.:* Adepsique; Esbelcaps; Numencil; *Port.:* Gamibetal Compositum; *Spain:* Ansium; Edym Sedante†; Pertranquil; Tepazepan; Tropargal; *USA:* Emergent-Ez.

Dichloralphenazone (4028-l)

Dichloralphenazone *(BAN)*.
$C_{15}H_{18}Cl_6N_2O_5 = 519.0$.
CAS — 480-30-8.
ATC — N05CC04.
Pharmacopoeias. In US.

In aqueous solution it dissociates into cloral hydrate and phenazone.

Pharmacopoeial description

USP 25: A white microcrystalline powder with a slight odour characteristic of cloral hydrate. Freely soluble in water, in alcohol, and in chloroform; soluble in dilute acids. It is decomposed by dilute alkalis liberating chloroform.

Profile

Dichloralphenazone dissociates on administration to form cloral hydrate and phenazone. It has the general properties of cloral hydrate (p.669), although it is less likely to cause gastric irritation after administration by mouth. Phenazone-induced skin eruptions may, however, occur (see p.77). Dichloralphenazone is used in some countries in combination preparations mainly for the treatment of tension and vascular headaches.

Porphyria. Dichloralphenazone has been associated with acute attacks of porphyria and is considered unsafe in porphyric patients.

Preparations

USP 25: Isometheptene Mucate, Dichloralphenazone, and Acetaminophen Capsules.

Proprietary Preparations (details are given in Part 3)

Multi-ingredient: *USA:* Duradrin; Isocom; Isopap; Midchlor†; Midrin; Migratine.

Difebarbamate (13412-v)

Difebarbamate *(rINN)*.
1,3-Bis(3-butoxy-2-hydroxypropyl)-5-ethyl-5-phenylbarbituric acid dicarbamate ester.
$C_{28}H_{42}N_4O_9 = 578.7$.
CAS — 15687-09-9.

Profile

Difebarbamate is a barbiturate with general properties similar to those of amobarbital (p.655). Tetrabamate, a complex of difebarbamate, febarbamate, and phenobarbital has been used in the management of anxiety disorders. However, barbiturates are not considered appropriate in the management of these conditions.

Preparations

Proprietary Preparations (details are given in Part 3)

Multi-ingredient: *Fr.:* Atrium†; *Switz.:* Atrium†.

Dixyrazine (7037-j)

UCB-3412.   2-(2-{4-[2-Methyl-3-(phenothiazin-10-yl)propyl]piperazin-1-yl}ethoxy)ethanol.
$C_{24}H_{33}N_3O_2S = 427.6$.
CAS — 2470-73-7.
ATC — N05AB01.

Profile

Dixyrazine is a phenothiazine with general properties similar to those of chlorpromazine (p.660). It has a piperazine side-chain. It is given by mouth for its antipsychotic, antiemetic, and sedative properties in doses ranging from 20 to 75 mg daily. Dixyrazine has also been given by injection.

◊ References.
1. Larsson S, *et al.* Premedication with intramuscular dixyrazine (Esucos®): a controlled double-blind comparison with morphine-scopolamine and placebo. *Acta Anaesthesiol Scand* 1988; **32:** 131–4.
2. Karlsson E, *et al.* The effects of prophylactic dixyrazine on postoperative vomiting after two different anaesthetic methods for squint surgery in children. *Acta Anaesthesiol Scand* 1993; **37:** 45–8.
3. Oikkonen M, *et al.* Dixyrazine premedication for cataract surgery: a comparison with diazepam. *Acta Anaesthesiol Scand* 1994; **38:** 214–17.
4. Feet PO, Götestam KG. Increased antipanic efficacy in combined treatment with clomipramine and dixyrazine. *Acta Psychiatr Scand* 1994; **89:** 230–4.
5. Oikkonen M, *et al.* CSF concentrations and clinical effects following intravenous dixyrazine premedication. *Eur J Clin Pharmacol* 1995; **47:** 445–7.

Porphyria. Dixyrazine is considered to be unsafe in patients with porphyria because it has been shown to be porphyrinogenic in *animals.*

Preparations

Proprietary Preparations (details are given in Part 3)
Aust.: Esucos; *Belg.:* Esucos; *Denm.:* Esucos; *Fin.:* Esucos; *Ital.:* Esucos; *Norw.:* Esucos; *Swed.:* Esucos.

Multi-ingredient: *Spain:* Vertigum†.

Droperidol (7038-z)

Droperidol *(BAN, USAN, rINN)*.
Droperidolum; McN-JR-4749; R-4749. 1-{1-[3-(4-Fluorobenzoyl)propyl]-1,2,3,6-tetrahydro-4-pyridyl}-benzimidazolin-2-one.
$C_{22}H_{22}FN_3O_2 = 379.4$.
CAS — 548-73-2.
ATC — N01AX01; N05AD08.
Pharmacopoeias. In Eur. (see p.vi), Jpn, and US.

Pharmacopoeial description

Ph. Eur.: A white or almost white powder. It exhibits polymorphism. Practically insoluble in water; sparingly soluble in alcohol; freely soluble in dichloromethane and in dimethylformamide. Protect from light.

USP 25: A white to light tan amorphous or microcrystalline powder. Practically insoluble in water; soluble 1 in 140 of alcohol, 1 in 4 of chloroform, and 1 in 500 of ether. Store under nitrogen in airtight containers at a temperature of 8° to 15°. Protect from light.

Adverse Effects, Treatment, and Precautions

As for Chlorpromazine, p.660. There is an increased risk of cardiotoxicity and prolongation of the QT interval (see p.661). Droperidol should not be used in patients at risk of arrhythmias, including those with impairment of cardiac function, hypokalaemia or other electrolyte imbalance, or with pre-existing QT prolongation.

Uses and Administration

Droperidol is a butyrophenone with general properties similar to those of haloperidol (p.687). The duration of action of droperidol has been reported to last about 2 to 4 hours although alteration of alertness may last 12 hours or longer. Droperidol has been given by mouth or by injection as a premedicant (p.1256), as an adjunct in anaesthesia, as an antiemetic, and for the control of agitated patients in acute psychoses (see Disturbed Behaviour, p.650) and in mania (see Bipolar Disorder, p.271). It has also been used in conjunction with an opioid analgesic such as fentanyl citrate to maintain patients in a state of neuroleptanalgesia (p.1256) in which they are calm and indifferent to the surroundings and able to cooperate with the surgeon. The longer duration of action of droperidol must be kept in mind when using it in association with such opioid analgesics. One of the manufacturers of droperidol (*Janssen-Cilag*) voluntarily withdrew it from the market worldwide in March 2001 following reports of QT prolongation, serious ventricular arrhythmias, or sudden death in association with its use.

Droperidol should be used in reduced dosage in elderly or debilitated patients. In general half the initial dose in adults has been recommended.

Preparations

BP 2001: Droperidol Injection; Droperidol Tablets;
USP 25: Droperidol Injection.

Proprietary Preparations (details are given in Part 3)
Aust.: Dehydrobenzperidol†; *Austral.:* Droleptan†; *Belg.:* Dehydrobenzperidol†; *Canad.:* Inapsine†; *Denm.:* Dehydrobenzperidol†; *Fin.:* Dehydrobenzperidol; *Fr.:* Droleptan; *Ger.:* Dehydrobenzperidol†; *Hong Kong:* Dehydrobenzperidol†; *Ital.:* Sintodian†; *Mex.:* Dehydrobenzperidol†; *Neth.:* Dehydrobenzperidol†; *Norw.:* Dridol†; *NZ:* Droleptan†; *S.Afr.:* Inapsin†; Paxical; *Spain:* Dehidrobenzperidol; *Swed.:* Dridol†; *Switz.:* Dehydrobenzperidol†; *Thai.:* Dehydrobenzperidol†; *UK:* Droleptan†; *USA:* Inapsine†.

Multi-ingredient: *Aust.:* Thalamonal†; *Belg.:* Thalamonal†; *Braz.:* Inoval†; *Ger.:* Thalamonal†; *Ital.:* Leptofen; *Neth.:* Thalamonal†; *USA:* Innovar†.

Eltoprazine (3678-z)

Eltoprazine *(rINN)*.
DU-28853. 1-(1,4-Benzodioxan-5-yl)piperazine.
$C_{12}H_{16}N_2O_2 = 220.3$.
CAS — 98224-03-4.

Profile

Eltoprazine is a serotonin agonist with a selective action at the 5-HT$_{1AB}$ receptors that is reported to inhibit aggression without causing sedation or motor impairment. It has been investigated in the treatment of behaviour disorders.

◊ References.
1. Verhoeven WMA, *et al.* Eltoprazine in mentally retarded self-injuring patients. *Lancet* 1992; **340:** 1037–8.
2. Tiihonen J, *et al.* Eltoprazine for aggression in schizophrenia and mental retardation. *Lancet* 1993; **341:** 307.
3. Kohen D. Eltoprazine for aggression in mental handicap. *Lancet* 1993; **341:** 628–9.

Estazolam (4030-g)

Estazolam *(USAN, rINN)*.
Abbott-47631; D-40TA. 8-Chloro-6-phenyl-4*H*-1,2,4-triazolo[4,3-*a*]-1,4-benzodiazepine.
$C_{16}H_{11}ClN_4 = 294.7$.
CAS — 29975-16-4.
ATC — N05CD04.
Pharmacopoeias. In Chin. and Jpn.

Dependence and Withdrawal

As for Diazepam, p.675.

Adverse Effects, Treatment, and Precautions

As for Diazepam, p.675.

Interactions

As for Diazepam, p.677.

Pharmacokinetics

Peak plasma concentrations of estazolam are reached on average within 2 hours of administration by mouth. A high proportion of estazolam is protein bound (about 93%). Reported mean elimination half-lives have generally been in the range of 10 to 24 hours. Estazolam is extensively metabolised, mainly to 4-hydroxyestazolam and 1-oxoestazolam which are considered inactive. These metabolites are excreted, either free or conjugated, in the urine with small amounts detected in the faeces. Only a small proportion of a dose is excreted as unchanged drug.

Uses and Administration

Estazolam is a short-acting benzodiazepine with general properties similar to those of diazepam (p.680). It is given by mouth as a hypnotic in the short-term management of insomnia (p.652) in usual doses of 1 to 2 mg at night. Small or debilitated elderly patients may be given an initial dose of 0.5 mg.

Preparations

Proprietary Preparations (details are given in Part 3)
Braz.: Noctal; *Denm.:* Domnamid; *Fr.:* Nuctalon; *Ital.:* Esilgan; *Jpn:* Eurodin; *Mex.:* Tasedan; *Port.:* Kainever; *USA:* Prosom.

Ethchlorvynol (4031-q)

Ethchlorvynol *(BAN, rINN)*.
β-Chlorovinyl Ethyl Ethynyl Carbinol; *E*-Ethchlorvynol. 1-Chloro-3-ethylpent-1-en-4-yn-3-ol.
$C_7H_9ClO = 144.6$.
CAS — 113-18-8.
ATC — N05CM08.
Pharmacopoeias. In US.

Pharmacopoeial description

USP 25: A colourless to yellow, slightly viscous liquid having a characteristic pungent odour. It darkens on exposure to air and light. Immiscible with water; miscible with most organic solvents. Store in airtight containers of glass or polyethylene, using polyethylene-lined closures. Protect from light.

Dependence and Withdrawal

Prolonged use of ethchlorvynol may lead to dependence similar to that with barbiturates (see Amobarbital, p.655).

Adverse Effects

Side-effects of ethchlorvynol include gastrointestinal disturbances, dizziness, headache, unwanted sedation and other symptoms of CNS depression such as ataxia, facial numbness, blurred vision, and hypotension. Hypersensitivity reactions include skin rashes, urticaria, and occasionally, thrombocytopenia and cholestatic jaundice. Idiosyncratic reactions include excitement, severe muscular weakness, and syncope without marked hypotension.

Acute overdosage is characterised by prolonged deep coma, respiratory depression, hypothermia, hypotension, and relative bradycardia. Pancytopenia and nystagmus have occurred. Pulmonary oedema has followed abuse by intravenous injection.

Treatment of Adverse Effects

Treatment is as for barbiturate overdose (see Amobarbital, p.655). Haemoperfusion may be of value in the treatment of severe poisoning with ethchlorvynol.

Precautions

Ethchlorvynol should be used with caution in patients with hepatic or renal impairment or with mental depression, in patients with severe uncontrolled pain, and, as with all sedatives, in those with impaired respiratory function. It may cause drowsiness; affected patients should not drive or operate machinery.

Excessively rapid absorption of ethchlorvynol in some patients has been reported to produce giddiness and ataxia; this may be reduced by administration with food.

Porphyria. Ethchlorvynol has been associated with acute attacks of porphyria and is considered unsafe in porphyric patients.

Interactions

The effect of ethchlorvynol may be enhanced by alcohol, barbiturates, and other CNS depressants. It has been reported to decrease the effects of coumarin anticoagulants.

Tricyclic antidepressants. The US manufacturers state that transient delirium has been reported with the concomitant use of ethchlorvynol and amitriptyline but details of such an interaction do not appear to have been published in the literature.

Pharmacokinetics
Ethchlorvynol is readily absorbed from the gastrointestinal tract, peak plasma concentrations usually occurring within 2 hours of ingestion. It is widely distributed in body tissues and is extensively metabolised in the liver, and possibly to some extent in the kidneys. It has a biphasic plasma half-life with a rapid initial phase and a terminal phase reported to last from 10 to 20 hours. Ethchlorvynol is excreted mainly in the urine as metabolites and their conjugates. Ethchlorvynol crosses the placenta.

Uses and Administration
Ethchlorvynol is a hypnotic and sedative with some anticonvulsant and muscle relaxant properties. It is given by mouth for the short-term management of insomnia (p.652); use for periods greater than one week are not recommended. Ethchlorvynol has, however, been largely superseded by other drugs. The usual hypnotic dose is 500 mg at night but doses ranging from 200 mg to 1 g have been given. Administration with food has been recommended—see Precautions, above.

Preparations
USP 25: Ethchlorvynol Capsules.

Proprietary Preparations (details are given in Part 3)
USA: Placidyl.

Ethyl Loflazepate (15319-n)
Ethyl Loflazepate *(rINN)*.
CM-6912. Ethyl 7-chloro-5-(2-fluorophenyl)-2,3-dihydro-2-oxo-1*H*-1,4-benzodiazepine-3-carboxylate.
$C_{18}H_{14}ClFN_2O_3 = 360.8$.
CAS — 29177-84-2.
ATC — N05BA18.

Profile
Ethyl loflazepate is a long-acting benzodiazepine derivative with general properties similar to those of diazepam (p.674). It is used in the short-term treatment of anxiety disorders (p.649) in usual doses of 1 to 3 mg daily by mouth in a single dose or in divided doses.

Preparations
Proprietary Preparations (details are given in Part 3)
Belg.: Victan; *Fr.:* Victan; *Jpn:* Meilax; *Mex.:* Victan; *Port.:* Victan; *Thai.:* Victan.

Etifoxine Hydrochloride (19158-s)
Etifoxine Hydrochloride *(BANM, rINNM)*.
Etifoxin Hydrochloride; Hoe-36801. 6-Chloro-4-methyl-4-phenyl-3,1-benzoxazin-2-yl(ethyl)amine hydrochloride.
$C_{17}H_{17}ClN_2O,HCl = 337.2$.
CAS — 21715-46-8 (etifoxine); 56776-32-0 (etifoxine hydrochloride).

Profile
Etifoxine hydrochloride is an anxiolytic (p.649) given by mouth in usual doses of 150 or 200 mg daily for up to 30 days.

Preparations
Proprietary Preparations (details are given in Part 3)
Fr.: Stresam.

Etizolam (16639-h)
Etizolam *(rINN)*.
AHR-3219; Y-7131. 4-(2-Chlorophenyl)-2-ethyl-9-methyl-6*H*-thieno[3,2-*f*]-s-triazolo[4,3-*a*][1,4]diazepine.
$C_{17}H_{15}ClN_4S = 342.8$.
CAS — 40054-69-1.
ATC — N05BA19.

Profile
Etizolam is a short-acting benzodiazepine derivative with general properties similar to those of diazepam (p.674). It is given by mouth for the short-term treatment of insomnia (p.652) and anxiety disorders (p.649) in doses of up to 3 mg daily in divided doses or as a single dose at night.

Preparations
Proprietary Preparations (details are given in Part 3)
Ital.: Depas; Pasaden; *Jpn:* Depas.

Etodroxizine (12718-z)
Etodroxizine *(rINN)*.
2-{2-[2-(4-*p*-Chlorobenzhydrylpiperazin-1-yl)ethoxy]ethoxy}ethanol.
$C_{23}H_{31}ClN_2O_3 = 419.0$.
CAS — 17692-34-1.

Profile
Etodroxizine was formerly used as the base or the maleate as a hypnotic and for the relief of hypersensitivity disorders.

Febarbamate (12728-k)
Febarbamate *(rINN)*.
Go-560. 1-(3-Butoxy-2-carbamoyloxypropyl)-5-ethyl-5-phenylbarbituric acid.
$C_{20}H_{27}N_3O_6 = 405.4$.
CAS — 13246-02-1.
ATC — M03BA05.

Profile
Febarbamate is a barbiturate with general properties similar to those of amobarbital (p.655). It has been used in the management of anxiety, insomnia, and alcohol withdrawal symptoms. However, barbiturates are no longer considered appropriate in the management of these conditions.

Tetrabamate, a complex of febarbamate, difebarbamate, and phenobarbital has been used similarly.

Preparations
Proprietary Preparations (details are given in Part 3)
Spain: G Tril†.
Multi-ingredient: *Fr.:* Atrium†; *Switz.:* Atrium†.

Fluanisone (7040-s)
Fluanisone *(BAN, rINN)*.
Haloanisone; MD-2028; R-2028; R-2167. 4'-Fluoro-4-[4-(2-methoxyphenyl)piperazin-1-yl]butyrophenone.
$C_{21}H_{25}FN_2O_2 = 356.4$.
CAS — 1480-19-9.
ATC — N05AD09.
Pharmacopoeias. In BP(Vet).

Pharmacopoeial description
BP(Vet) 2001: White or almost white to buff-coloured, odourless or almost odourless crystals or powder. It exhibits polymorphism. M.p. 72° to 76°. Practically insoluble in water; freely soluble in alcohol, in chloroform, in ether, and in dilute solutions of organic acids. Protect from light.

Profile
Fluanisone is a butyrophenone with general properties similar to those of haloperidol (p.686). It has been used in the management of agitated states in psychiatric patients and as anaesthetic premedication.

Fluanisone is used in veterinary medicine for neuroleptanalgesia.

Fludiazepam (16810-x)
Fludiazepam *(rINN)*.
ID-540. 7-Chloro-5-(2-fluorophenyl)-1,3-dihydro-1-methyl-2*H*-1,4-benzodiazepin-2-one.
$C_{16}H_{12}ClFN_2O = 302.7$.
CAS — 3900-31-0.
ATC — N05BA17.
Pharmacopoeias. In Jpn.

Profile
Fludiazepam is a short-acting benzodiazepine with general properties similar to those of diazepam (p.674). It has been used in the short-term treatment of anxiety disorders.

Preparations
Proprietary Preparations (details are given in Part 3)
Jpn: Erispan†.

Flunitrazepam (4034-w)
Flunitrazepam *(BAN, USAN, rINN)*.
Flunitrazepamum; Ro-5-4200. 5-(2-Fluorophenyl)-1,3-dihydro-1-methyl-7-nitro-1,4-benzodiazepin-2-one.
$C_{16}H_{12}FN_3O_3 = 313.3$.
CAS — 1622-62-4.
ATC — N05CD03.
Pharmacopoeias. In Eur. (see p.vi) and Jpn.

Pharmacopoeial description
Ph. Eur.: A white or yellowish crystalline powder. Practically insoluble in water; slightly soluble in alcohol and in ether; soluble in acetone. Protect from light.

Dependence and Withdrawal
As for Diazepam, p.675.

Adverse Effects, Treatment, and Precautions
As for Diazepam, p.675.

Abuse. A WHO review[1] concluded that flunitrazepam had a moderate abuse potential which might be higher than that of other benzodiazepines. It was reported that there was current evidence of widespread abuse of flunitrazepam among drug abusers, particularly among those who used opioids or cocaine.

Flunitrazepam has also been misused as a sedative in sexual assaults[2] or so called 'date rapes'.

1. WHO expert committee on drug dependence: twenty-ninth report. *WHO Tech Rep Ser 856* 1995.
2. Simmons MM, Cupp MJ. Use and abuse of flunitrazepam. *Ann Pharmacother* 1998; **32:** 117–19.

Local reactions. Of 43 patients given a single intravenous dose of flunitrazepam 1 to 2 mg, two had local thrombosis 7 to 10 days later.[1] The incidence was lower than in those given diazepam [in solution]. However, there was little difference in the incidence of local reactions after intravenous administration of flunitrazepam and diazepam in another study.[2]

1. Hegarty JE, Dundee JW. Sequelae after the intravenous injection of three benzodiazepines—diazepam, lorazepam, and flunitrazepam. *BMJ* 1977; **2:** 1384–5.
2. Mikkelsen H, *et al.* Local reactions after iv injections of diazepam, flunitrazepam and isotonic saline. *Br J Anaesth* 1980; **52:** 817–19.

Porphyria. Flunitrazepam has been associated with acute attacks of porphyria and is considered unsafe in porphyric patients.

Interactions
As for Diazepam, p.677.

Pharmacokinetics
Flunitrazepam is readily absorbed from the gastrointestinal tract. About 77 to 80% is bound to plasma proteins. It is extensively metabolised in the liver and excreted mainly in the urine as metabolites (free or conjugated). Its principal metabolites are 7-aminoflunitrazepam and *N*-desmethylflunitrazepam; *N*-desmethylflunitrazepam is reported to be pharmacologically active. The elimination half-life of flunitrazepam is reported to be between 16 and 35 hours. Flunitrazepam crosses the placental barrier and is distributed into breast milk.

◊ References.
1. Davis PJ, Cook DR. Clinical pharmacokinetics of the newer intravenous anaesthetic agents. *Clin Pharmacokinet* 1986; **11:** 18–35.
2. Pariente-Khayat A, *et al.* Pharmacokinetics and tolerance of flunitrazepam in neonates and in infants. *Clin Pharmacol Ther* 1999; **66:** 136–9.

Pregnancy and breast feeding. Concentrations of flunitrazepam in umbilical-vein and umbilical-artery plasma were close to those in maternal venous plasma about 11 to 15 hours after administration of flunitrazepam 1 mg to 14 pregnant women; concentrations in amniotic fluid were lower still.[1] Concentrations in breast milk the morning after a single evening 2-mg dose were considered to be too low to produce clinical effects in breast-fed infants, although accumulation in the milk might occur after repeated administration.[1]

1. Kanto J, *et al.* Placental transfer and breast milk levels of flunitrazepam. *Curr Ther Res* 1979; **26:** 539–46.

Uses and Administration
Flunitrazepam is a short-acting benzodiazepine with general properties similar to those of diazepam (p.680). It is used in the short-term management of insomnia (p.652), as a premedicant in surgical procedures, and for induction of anaesthesia (p.1256). A usual dose for insomnia is 0.5 to 1 mg by mouth at night; up to 2 mg may be given if necessary. In elderly or debilitated patients the initial dose should not exceed 0.5 mg at night; up to 1 mg may be given if necessary. A dose of 1 to 2 mg (0.015 to 0.030 mg per kg body-weight) has been given intramuscularly or by mouth for premedication or by slow intravenous injection for induction of general anaesthesia.

Preparations
Proprietary Preparations (details are given in Part 3)
Aust.: Rohypnol; Somnubene; *Austral.:* Hypnodorm; Rohypnol; *Belg.:* Rohypnol; *Braz.:* Fluserin; Rohypnol; *Denm.:* Flunipam; Rohypnol; Ronal; *Fr.:* Narcozep; Rohypnol; *Ger.:* Flunimerck; Fluninoc; Rohypnol; *Hong Kong:* Absint; Rohypnol; *Irl.:* Rohypnol; *Israel:* Hypnodorm; Rohypnol; *Ital.:* Darkene; Rohypnol; Valsera; *Mex.:* Rohypnol; *Neth.:* Rohypnol; *Norw.:* Flunipam; Flutraz†; Rohypnol; *Port.:* Rohypnol; Sedex†; *S.Afr.:* Hypnor; Insom†; Rohypnol; *Spain:* Rohypnol; *Swed.:* Flupam†; Fluscand; Rohypnol; *Switz.:* Rohypnol; *Thai.:* Rohypnol; *UK:* Rohypnol.

The symbol † denotes a preparation no longer actively marketed

Flupentixol Decanoate (7044-y)

Flupentixol Decanoate (BANM, rINNM).

Flupenthixol Decanoate; (Z)-Flupentixol Decanoate; cis-Flu-penthixol Decanoate. (Z)-2-{4-[3-(2-Trifluoromethylthioxan-then-9-ylidene)propyl]piperazin-1-yl}ethyl decanoate.

$C_{33}H_{43}F_3N_2O_2S = 588.8$.

CAS — 2709-56-0 (flupentixol); 30909-51-4 (flupentixol decanoate).

Pharmacopoeias. In Br.

Pharmacopoeial description

BP 2001: A yellow viscous oil. Very slightly soluble in water; soluble in alcohol; freely soluble in chloroform and in ether. Store at a temperature below −15° and protect from light.

Flupentixol Hydrochloride (7045-j)

Flupentixol Hydrochloride (BANM, rINNM).

Flupenthixol Dihydrochloride; Flupenthixol Hydrochloride; Flu-pentixoli Dihydrochloridum; LC-44 (flupentixol); N-7009 (flu-pentixol). 2-{4-[3-(2-Trifluoromethylthioxanthen-9-yli-dene)propyl]piperazin-1-yl}ethanol dihydrochloride.

$C_{23}H_{25}F_3N_2OS,2HCl = 507.4$.

CAS — 2413-38-9.

Pharmacopoeias. In Eur. (see p.vi).

Pharmacopoeial description

Ph. Eur.: A white or almost white powder. Very soluble in wa-ter; soluble in alcohol; practically insoluble in dichloromethane. A 1% solution in water has a pH of 2.0 to 3.0. Protect from light.

Stability. References.

1. Enever RP, et al. Flupenthixol dihydrochloride decomposition in aqueous solution. *J Pharm Sci* 1979; **68:** 169–71.
2. Li Wan Po A, Irwin WJ. The photochemical stability of cis- and trans-isomers of tricyclic neuroleptic drugs. *J Pharm Pharmacol* 1980; **32:** 25–9.

Adverse Effects and Treatment

As for Chlorpromazine, p.660. Flupentixol is less likely to cause sedation, but extrapyramidal disorders are more frequent.

Sudden death. A report of sudden death in 3 patients who had received depot injections of flupentixol decanoate.[1]

1. Turbott J, Smeeton WMI. Sudden death and flupentixol de-canoate. *Aust N Z J Psychiatry* 1984; **18:** 91–4.

Precautions

As for Chlorpromazine, p.663. Flupentixol is not rec-ommended in states of excitement or overactivity, in-cluding mania.

Porphyria. Flupentixol is considered to be unsafe in patients with porphyria because it has been shown to be porphyrinogen-ic in *animals*.

Interactions

As for Chlorpromazine, p.664.

Pharmacokinetics

Flupentixol is readily absorbed from the gastrointes-tinal tract and is probably subject to first-pass metab-olism in the gut wall. It is also extensively metabo-lised in the liver and is excreted in the urine and faeces in the form of numerous metabolites; there is evidence of enterohepatic recycling. Owing to the first-pass effect, plasma concentrations following oral administration are much lower than those following estimated equivalent doses of the intramuscular depot preparation. Moreover, there is very wide intersubject variation in plasma concentrations of flupentixol, but, in practice, no simple correlation has been found be-tween plasma concentrations of flupentixol and its metabolites, and the therapeutic effect. Paths of me-tabolism of flupentixol include sulfoxidation, side-chain N-dealkylation, and glucuronic acid conjuga-tion. It is widely distributed in the body, and crosses the blood-brain barrier. Flupentixol crosses the pla-cental barrier and small amounts have been detected in breast milk.

The decanoate ester of flupentixol is very slowly ab-sorbed from the site of intramuscular injection and is therefore suitable for depot injection. It is gradually released into the blood stream where it is rapidly hy-drolysed to flupentixol.

Uses and Administration

Flupentixol is a thioxanthene antipsychotic with gen-eral properties similar to those of the phenothiazine, chlorpromazine (p.665). It has a piperazine side-chain. Flupentixol is used mainly in the treatment of schizophrenia (p.651) and other psychoses. Unlike chlorpromazine, a certain activating effect has been ascribed to flupentixol and, accordingly, it is not indi-cated in overactive, including manic, patients. Flu-pentixol has also been used for its antidepressant properties.

Flupentixol is administered as the hydrochloride by mouth or as the longer-acting decanoate ester by deep intramuscular injection.

The usual initial dose of the hydrochloride for the treatment of **psychoses** is the equivalent of 3 to 9 mg of flupentixol twice daily adjusted according to the response; the maximum recommended dose is a total of 18 mg daily. The initial dose in elderly and debili-tated patients may need to be reduced to a quarter or a half of the normal starting dose. The long-acting de-canoate preparation available in the UK contains flu-pentixol as the cis(Z)-isomer (see Action, below) and doses are expressed in terms of the amount of cis(Z)-flupentixol decanoate. It should be given by deep in-tramuscular injection in an initial test dose of 20 mg, as 1 mL of a 2% oily solution. Then after at least 7 days and according to the patient's response, this may be followed by doses of 20 to 40 mg at intervals of 2 to 4 weeks. Shorter dosage intervals or greater amounts may be required according to the patient's response. The initial dose in elderly and debilitated patients may need to be reduced to a quarter or a half of the normal starting dose. If doses greater than 40 mg are considered necessary they should be divid-ed between 2 separate injection sites. Another means of reducing the volume of fluid to be injected in pa-tients requiring high-dose therapy with flupentixol decanoate is to give an injection containing 100 or 200 mg of the decanoate per mL (10 or 20%). The usual maintenance dose is between 50 mg every 4 weeks and 300 mg every 2 weeks but doses of up to 400 mg weekly have been given in severe or resistant conditions.

Flupentixol has also been given as the hydrochloride, by mouth, for the treatment of mild to moderate **de-pression**, with or without anxiety. The usual initial dose, expressed in terms of the equivalent amount of flupentixol, is 1 mg (0.5 mg in the elderly) daily, in-creased after 1 week to 2 mg (1 mg in the elderly) and then to a maximum of 3 mg (2 mg in the elderly) dai-ly. Doses above 2 mg (1 mg in the elderly) should be given in 2 divided doses. The last dose of the day should be given no later than 4 p.m. and if no effect has been noted within 1 week of administration of the maximum dose, the treatment should be withdrawn.

Action. Patients with acute schizophrenic illnesses taking α-flupentixol [(Z)-flupentixol or cis-flupentixol] improved more after 3 weeks than patients who were taking equal doses of β-flupentixol [(E)-flupentixol or trans-flupentixol] or a placebo.[1] The α-isomer had more effect on the positive symptoms of the disease; this difference was less apparent for the negative symptoms. The difference in activity between the isomers was attributed to the greater dopamine-receptor blocking activity of the α-isomer rather than to differences in distribution.[2]

1. Johnstone EC, et al. Mechanism of the antipsychotic effect in the treatment of acute schizophrenia. *Lancet* 1978; **i:** 848–51.
2. Crow TJ, Johnstone EC. Mechanism of action of neuroleptic drugs. *Lancet* 1978; **i:** 1050.

Depression. Small studies[1,2] comparing flupentixol with standard drugs for treatment of depression (p.271) suggest that it may be of benefit.

1. Hamilton BA, et al. Flupenthixol and fluvoxamine in mild to moderate depression: a comparison in general practice. *Pharma-therapeutica* 1989; **5:** 292–7.
2. Dwivedi VS, et al. Depression in general practice: a comparison of flupenthixol dihydrochloride and dothiepin hydrochloride. *Curr Med Res Opin* 1990; **12:** 191–7.

Substance dependence. Depot flupentixol decanoate has produced some promising results as an aid in reducing *cocaine* usage (see Withdrawal, p.1310).

References.

1. Gawin FH, et al. Flupentixol-induced aversion to crack cocaine. *N Engl J Med* 1996; **334:** 1340–1.

Preparations

BP 2001: Flupentixol Injection.

Proprietary Preparations (details are given in Part 3)

Aust.: Fluanxol; **Austral.:** Fluanxol; **Belg.:** Fluanxol; **Canad.:** Fluanxol; **Denm.:** Fluanxol; **Fin.:** Fluanxol; **Fr.:** Fluanxol; **Ger.:** Fluanxol; **Hong Kong:** Fluanxol; **Irl.:** Depixol; Fluanxol; **Israel:** Fluanxol; **Mex.:** Fluanxol; **Neth.:** Fluanxol; **Norw.:** Fluanxol; **NZ:** Depixol; **Port.:** Fluanxol; **S.Afr.:** Fluanxol; **Singapore:** Fluanxol; **Swed.:** Fluanxol; **Switz.:** Fluanxol; **Thai.:** Fluanxol; **UK:** Depixol; Fluanxol.

Multi-ingredient: **Aust.:** Deanxit; **Belg.:** Deanxit; **Hong Kong:** Deanxit; **Ital.:** Deanxit; **Singapore:** Deanxit; **Spain:** Deanxit; **Switz.:** Deanxit; **Thai.:** Deanxit.

Fluphenazine (17391-h)

Fluphenazine (BAN, rINN).

2-{4-[3-(2-Trifluoromethylphenothiazin-10-yl)propyl]piper-azin-1-yl}ethanol.

$C_{22}H_{26}F_3N_3OS = 437.5$.

CAS — 69-23-8.

ATC — N05AB02.

Fluphenazine Decanoate (7046-z)

Fluphenazine Decanoate (BANM, rINNM).

Fluphenazini Decanoas.

$C_{32}H_{44}F_3N_3O_2S = 591.8$.

CAS — 5002-47-1.

Pharmacopoeias. In Chin., Eur. (see p.vi), Int., and US.

Fluphenazine decanoate 12.5 mg is approximately equivalent to 10.75 mg of fluphenazine hydrochloride.

Pharmacopoeial description

Ph. Eur.: A pale yellow viscous liquid or a yellow solid. Prac-tically insoluble in water; very soluble in dehydrated alcohol, in dichloromethane, and in ether; freely soluble in methyl alco-hol. Protect from light.

USP 25: Store in airtight containers. Protect from light.

Fluphenazine Enantate (7047-c)

Fluphenazine Enantate (BANM, rINNM).

Fluphenazine Enanthate; Fluphenazine Heptanoate; Fluphenazi-ni Enantas.

$C_{29}H_{38}F_3N_3O_2S = 549.7$.

CAS — 2746-81-8.

Pharmacopoeias. In Eur. (see p.vi), Int., Jpn, and US.

Fluphenazine enantate 12.5 mg is approximately equivalent to 11.6 mg of fluphenazine hydrochloride.

Pharmacopoeial description

Ph. Eur.: A pale yellow viscous liquid or a yellow solid. Prac-tically insoluble in water; very soluble in dehydrated alcohol, in dichloromethane, and in ether; freely soluble in methyl alco-hol. Protect from light.

USP 25: A pale yellow to yellow-orange, clear to slightly tur-bid, viscous liquid having a characteristic odour. Insoluble in water; soluble 1 in less than 1 of alcohol and of chloroform and 1 in 2 of ether. Stable in air at room temperature but unstable in strong light. Store in airtight containers. Protect from light.

Fluphenazine Hydrochloride (7048-k)

Fluphenazine Hydrochloride (BANM, rINNM).

Fluphenazini Hydrochloridum.

$C_{22}H_{26}F_3N_3OS,2HCl = 510.4$.

CAS — 146-56-5.

Pharmacopoeias. In Chin., Eur. (see p.vi), Int., Pol., and US.

Pharmacopoeial description

Ph. Eur.: A white or almost white, crystalline powder. Freely soluble in water; slightly soluble in alcohol and in dichlo-romethane; practically insoluble in ether. Protect from light.

USP 25: A white or nearly white, odourless crystalline powder. Soluble 1 in 1.4 of water and 1 in 6.7 of alcohol; slightly solu-ble in acetone and in chloroform; practically insoluble in ether and in benzene. Store in airtight containers. Protect from light.

Adverse Effects and Treatment

As for Chlorpromazine, p.660. Fluphenazine is less likely to cause sedation, hypotension, or antimus-carinic effects but is associated with a higher inci-dence of extrapyramidal effects.

◊ A significant incidence of akinesia, involuntary movement, autonomic disturbances, and drowsiness may occur in the first few hours following injection of fluphenazine decanoate and in the first 2 days following injection of fluphenazine enantate.[1]

1. Curry SH, et al. Unwanted effects of fluphenazine enanthate and decanoate. *Lancet* 1979; **i:** 331–2.

Convulsions. For mention of fluphenazine as one of the antip-sychotics suitable for patients at risk of seizures, see p.661.

Effects on the liver. A patient given 3 injections of a depot antipsychotic containing fluphenazine decanoate over a 2-week period developed jaundice 17 days after the first dose.[1] The patient developed indicators of severe liver toxicity, with extreme hyperbilirubinaemia and raised liver enzyme values, and remained very ill for the next 4 months. The patient showed cross-sensitivity to haloperidol but not to flupentixol.

See also under Chlorpromazine, p.661.

1. Kennedy P. Liver cross-sensitivity to antipsychotic drugs. *Br J Psychiatry* 1983; **143:** 312.

Overdosage. A patient who took about 30 fluphenazine hydrochloride 2.5-mg tablets was treated with gastric lavage.[1] Twenty hours after hospital admission he experienced difficulty in breathing due to spasm of the respiratory muscles; other very severe extrapyramidal side-effects were also present. Muscle spasm was controlled by diazepam.

There were few ill-effects in a patient given intramuscular fluphenazine decanoate 50 mg every 4 hours, instead of the intended 4 weeks, to a total of 1050 mg.[2] About three weeks after the period of overdosage the patient had some degree of hypothermia and tachycardia, and after a further week parkinsonian signs appeared. No specific treatment was given.

1. Ladhani FM. Severe extrapyramidal manifestations following fluphenazine overdose. *Med J Aust* 1974; **2:** 26.
2. Cheung HK, Yu ECS. Effect of 1050 mg fluphenazine decanoate given intramuscularly over six days. *BMJ* 1983; **286:** 1016–17.

Precautions

As for Chlorpromazine, p.663. Fluphenazine may exacerbate depression; depot injections are therefore contra-indicated in severely depressed patients.

Pregnancy. Nasal congestion with severe rhinorrhoea, respiratory distress, vomiting, and extrapyramidal symptoms occurred in a neonate delivered to a mother who had received fluphenazine hydrochloride 10 to 20 mg daily throughout pregnancy.[1] Respiratory symptoms appeared to respond to pseudoephedrine.

1. Nath SP, *et al.* Severe rhinorrhea and respiratory distress in a neonate exposed to fluphenazine hydrochloride prenatally. *Ann Pharmacother* 1996; **30:** 35–7.

Interactions

As for Chlorpromazine, p.664.

Pharmacokinetics

Fluphenazine hydrochloride is absorbed following oral administration, and has a reported plasma half-life of 14.7 hours after doses by mouth. Fluphenazine decanoate and fluphenazine enantate are very slowly absorbed from the site of subcutaneous or intramuscular injection. They both gradually release fluphenazine into the body and are therefore suitable for use as depot injections.

◊ The plasma half-life of fluphenazine after a single dose was 14.7 hours in 1 patient given the hydrochloride by mouth and 14.9 and 15.3 hours in 2 patients given the hydrochloride by intramuscular injection.[1] The half-life was 3.6 and 3.7 days in 2 patients given the enantate intramuscularly and 9.6 and 6.8 days in 2 patients given the decanoate intramuscularly. Peak plasma-fluphenazine concentrations occurred earlier in patients given fluphenazine decanoate compared with those who received the enantate. Fluphenazine sulfoxide and 7-hydroxyfluphenazine were identified in the urine and faeces.

1. Curry SH, *et al.* Kinetics of fluphenazine after fluphenazine dihydrochloride, enanthate and decanoate administration to man. *Br J Clin Pharmacol* 1979; **7:** 325–31.

◊ Further references to the pharmacokinetics of fluphenazine.

1. Wistedt B, *et al.* Slow decline of plasma drug and prolactin levels after discontinuation of chronic treatment with depot neuroleptics. *Lancet* 1981; **i:** 1163.
2. Midha KK, *et al.* Kinetics of oral fluphenazine disposition in humans by GC-MS. *Eur J Clin Pharmacol* 1983; **25:** 709–11.
3. Marder SR, *et al.* Plasma levels of parent drug and metabolites in patients receiving oral and depot fluphenazine. *Psychopharmacol Bull* 1989; **25:** 479–82.

Uses and Administration

Fluphenazine is a phenothiazine with general properties similar to those of chlorpromazine (p.665). It has a piperazine side-chain. Fluphenazine is used in the treatment of a variety of psychiatric disorders including schizophrenia (p.651), mania (see Bipolar Disorder, p.271), severe anxiety (p.649), and behavioural disturbances (p.650). Fluphenazine is administered as the hydrochloride usually by mouth or sometimes by intramuscular injection; longer-acting decanoate or enantate esters of fluphenazine are given by intramuscular or sometimes subcutaneous injection.

The usual initial dose of the hydrochloride for the treatment of schizophrenia, mania, and other **psychoses** is 2.5 to 10 mg daily in two or three divided doses *by mouth*; the dose is then increased according to response up to a usual maximum of 20 mg daily (10 mg daily in the elderly), although higher doses have oc-

The symbol † denotes a preparation no longer actively marketed

casionally been given. Dosage may subsequently be reduced to a usual maintenance dose of 1 to 5 mg daily. Treatment is sometimes started with an initial *intramuscular* injection of 1.25 mg of the hydrochloride adjusted thereafter according to response. The usual initial intramuscular daily dose is 2.5 to 10 mg given in divided doses every 6 to 8 hours. In general the required parenteral doses of fluphenazine hydrochloride have been found to be approximately one-third to one-half of those given by mouth.

The long-acting decanoate or enantate esters of fluphenazine are usually given by deep intramuscular injection and are used mainly for the *maintenance* treatment of patients with schizophrenia or other chronic psychoses. The onset of action is usually within 1 to 3 days of injection and significant effects on psychosis are usually evident within 2 to 4 days. An initial dose of fluphenazine decanoate or enantate 12.5 mg (6.25 mg in the elderly) is given intramuscularly to assess the extrapyramidal effects. Subsequent adjustments in the amounts and the dosage interval should be made according to the patient's response; the amounts required may range from 12.5 to 100 mg and the intervals required may range from 2 weeks to 5 or 6 weeks. Lower doses may be possible in some patients (see Schizophrenia, below). If doses greater than 50 mg are considered necessary cautious increments should be made in steps of 12.5 mg.

Fluphenazine hydrochloride has also been given *by mouth* in doses of 1 mg twice daily, increased if necessary to 2 mg twice daily, for the short-term adjunctive management of severe **anxiety** or **behavioural disturbances**.

Chorea. For a discussion of the management of various choreas, including mention of the use of phenothiazines such as fluphenazine, see p.650.

References.

1. Terrence CF. Fluphenazine decanoate is the treatment of chorea: a double-blind study. *Curr Ther Res* 1976; **20:** 177–83.

Schizophrenia. References[1-3] to fluphenazine decanoate in schizophrenia (p.651) indicating that low doses (10 mg or less every 2 weeks) may be effective in some patients. Administration of standard doses at greater intervals (6 weeks) has also been investigated.[4] A systematic review of the use of depot fluphenazine in schizophrenia considered the evidence to be very limited.[5]

1. Kane JM, *et al.* Low-dose neuroleptic treatment of outpatient schizophrenics: I preliminary results for relapse rates. *Arch Gen Psychiatry* 1983; **40:** 893–6.
2. Marder SR, *et al.* Low- and conventional-dose maintenance therapy with fluphenazine decanoate: two-year outcome. *Arch Gen Psychiatry* 1987; **44:** 581–21.
3. Hogarty GE, *et al.* Dose of fluphenazine, familial expressed emotion, and outcome in schizophrenia: results of a two-year controlled study. *Arch Gen Psychiatry* 1988; **45:** 797–805.
4. Carpenter WT, *et al.* Comparative effectiveness of fluphenazine decanoate injections every 2 weeks versus every 6 weeks. *Am J Psychiatry* 1999; **156:** 412–18.
5. Adams CE, Eisenbruch M. Depot fluphenazine for schizophrenia (updated 28 February 2001). Available in The Cochrane Library; Issue 4. Oxford: Update Software; 2001.

Tourette's syndrome. Fluphenazine has been tried[1] as an alternative to standard dopamine antagonists such as haloperidol or pimozide in the symptomatic management of Tourette's syndrome (p.650).

1. Singer HS, *et al.* Haloperidol, fluphenazine and clonidine in tourette syndrome: controversies in treatment. *Pediatr Neurosci* 1985–86; **12:** 71–4.

Preparations

BP 2001: Fluphenazine Decanoate Injection; Fluphenazine Tablets;
USP 25: Fluphenazine Decanoate Injection; Fluphenazine Enanthate Injection; Fluphenazine Hydrochloride Elixir; Fluphenazine Hydrochloride Injection; Fluphenazine Hydrochloride Oral Solution; Fluphenazine Hydrochloride Tablets.

Proprietary Preparations (details are given in Part 3)
Aust.: Dapotum; *Austral.:* Anatensol; Modecate; *Belg.:* Sevinol; *Braz.:* Anatensol; Flufenan; *Canad.:* Modecate; Moditen; *Denm.:* Pacinol; Siqualone; *Fin.:* Pacinol; Siqualone; *Fr.:* Modecate; Moditen; *Ger.:* Dapotum; Lyogen; Lyorodin; Omca; *Hong Kong:* Modecate; *Irl.:* Modecate; Moditen†; *Israel:* Fludecate; Modecate; Sediten; Selecten; *Ital.:* Anatensol; Moditen Depot; *Mex.:* Siqualine; *Neth.:* Anatensol; *Norw.:* Siqualone; *NZ:* Modecate; *Port.:* Anatensol; Cenilene; Phenazin; *S.Afr.:* Decafen†; Fludecate; Modecate; Modecate Acutum†; *Singapore:* Modecate; *Spain:* Modecate; *Swed.:* Pacinol; Siqualone; *Switz.:* Dapotum; *Thai.:* Deca; Fluzine; Modecate; Phenazine; Potensone; *UK:* Decazate†; Modecate; Moditen; *USA:* Permitil; Prolixin.

Multi-ingredient: *Fr.:* Motival†; *Hong Kong:* Motival; *Irl.:* Motipress†; Motival; *Ital.:* Dominans; *S.Afr.:* Mendrome†; Motival; *Thai.:* Motival; *UK:* Motipress; Motival.

Flurazepam (11384-n)

Flurazepam (BAN, rINN).
7-Chloro-1-(2-diethylaminoethyl)-5-(2-fluorophenyl)-1,3-dihydro-1,4-benzodiazepin-2-one.
$C_{21}H_{23}ClFN_3O = 387.9$.
CAS — 17617-23-1.
ATC — N05CD01.
Pharmacopoeias. In Jpn.

Flurazepam Monohydrochloride (4035-e)

Flurazepam Monohydrochloride (BANM, rINNM).
Flurazepami Monohydrochloridum.
$C_{21}H_{23}ClFN_3O,HCl = 424.3$.
CAS — 36105-20-1.
Pharmacopoeias. In Eur. (see p.vi) and Jpn.

Flurazepam monohydrochloride 32.8 mg is approximately equivalent to 30 mg of flurazepam.

Pharmacopoeial description
Ph. Eur.: A white or almost white crystalline powder. Very soluble in water; freely soluble in alcohol; practically insoluble in ether. A 5% solution in water has a pH of 5.0 to 6.0. Protect from light.

Flurazepam Dihydrochloride (4036-l)

Flurazepam Dihydrochloride (BANM, rINNM).
Flurazepam Hydrochloride (USAN); NSC-78559; Ro-5-6901.
$C_{21}H_{23}ClFN_3O,2HCl = 460.8$.
CAS — 1172-18-5.
Pharmacopoeias. In US.

Flurazepam dihydrochloride 30 mg is approximately equivalent to 25.3 mg of flurazepam.

Pharmacopoeial description
USP 25: An off-white to yellow crystalline powder. Is odourless or has a slight odour. Soluble 1 in 2 of water, 1 in 4 of alcohol, 1 in 90 of chloroform, 1 in 3 of methyl alcohol, 1 in 69 of isopropyl alcohol, 1 in 5000 of ether and of petroleum spirit, and 1 in 2500 of benzene. A solution in water is acid to litmus. Store in airtight containers. Protect from light.

Dependence and Withdrawal

As for Diazepam, p.675.

Adverse Effects, Treatment, and Precautions

As for Diazepam, p.675.

Effects on the liver. Reports of cholestatic jaundice following the use of flurazepam.[1,2]

1. Fang MH, *et al.* Cholestatic jaundice associated with flurazepam hydrochloride. *Ann Intern Med* 1978; **89:** 363–4.
2. Reynolds R, *et al.* Cholestatic jaundice induced by flurazepam hydrochloride. *Can Med Assoc J* 1981; **124:** 893–4.

Effects on taste. Flurazepam had been reported to cause dysgeusia.[1]

1. Willoughby JMT. Drug-induced abnormalities of taste sensation. *Adverse Drug React Bull* 1983 (June): 368–71.

Porphyria. Flurazepam has been associated with acute attacks of porphyria and is considered unsafe in porphyric patients.

Renal impairment. Five patients on maintenance haemodialysis developed encephalopathy attributed to flurazepam and diazepam.[1]

1. Taclob L, Needle M. Drug-induced encephalopathy in patients on maintenance haemodialysis. *Lancet* 1976; **ii:** 704–5.

Interactions

As for Diazepam, p.677.

Pharmacokinetics

Flurazepam is readily absorbed from the gastrointestinal tract. It undergoes extensive first-pass metabolism and is excreted in the urine, chiefly as conjugated metabolites. The major active metabolite is *N*-desalkylflurazepam, which is reported to have a half-life ranging from 47 to 100 hours or more.

Metabolism. The metabolism of flurazepam was studied in 4 healthy male subjects given 30 mg daily for 2 weeks.[1] A hydroxyethyl metabolite was present in the blood shortly after administration. The *N*-desalkyl metabolite, the major metabolite in the blood, had a half-life ranging from 47 to 100 hours. Steady-state concentrations were reached after 7 to 10 days and were about 5 to 6 times greater than those observed on day 1. Results from a study in 3 patients indicated that some metabolism of flurazepam may occur in the small bowel mucosa.[2]

1. Kaplan SA, *et al.* Blood level profile in man following chronic oral administration of flurazepam hydrochloride. *J Pharm Sci* 1973; **62:** 1932–5.
2. Mahon WA, *et al.* Metabolism of flurazepam by the small intestine. *Clin Pharmacol Ther* 1977; **22:** 228–33.

Uses and Administration

Flurazepam is a long-acting benzodiazepine with general properties similar to those of diazepam (p.680). It is used as a hypnotic in the short-term management of insomnia (p.652). In the USA flurazepam is given in doses of 15 to 30 mg of the dihydrochloride by mouth at night. In the UK it is given as the monohydrochloride in doses equivalent to 15 to 30 mg of flurazepam at night. A maximum initial dose of 15 mg has been suggested in the UK and the USA for elderly or debilitated patients.

Preparations

BP 2001: Flurazepam Capsules;
USP 25: Flurazepam Hydrochloride Capsules.

Proprietary Preparations (details are given in Part 3)
Belg.: Staurodorm; **Braz.:** Dalmadorm; **Canad.:** Dalmane; Novo-Flupam†; Somnol; **Ger.:** Dalmadorm; Staurodorm Neu; **Hong Kong:** Dalmadorm; **Irl.:** Dalmane; **Ital.:** Dalmadorm; Felison; Flunox; Remdue; Valdorm; **Neth.:** Dalmadorm†; **Port.:** Dalmadorm; Morfex; **S.Afr.:** Dalmadorm; **Singapore:** Dalmadorm; **Spain:** Dormodor; **Switz.:** Dalmadorm; **Thai.:** Dalmadorm; **UK:** Dalmane; **USA:** Dalmane.

Fluspirilene (7049-a)

Fluspirilene (BAN, USAN, rINN).

McN-JR-6218; R-6218. 8-[4,4-Bis(4-fluorophenyl)butyl]-1-phenyl-1,3,8-triazaspiro[4.5]decan-4-one.
$C_{29}H_{31}F_2N_3O = 475.6$.
CAS — 1841-19-6.
ATC — N05AG01.

Profile

Fluspirilene is a diphenylbutylpiperidine antipsychotic and has general properties similar to those of the phenothiazine, chlorpromazine (p.660). It is less likely to cause sedation. Fluspirilene has been given by deep intramuscular injection for the treatment of schizophrenia (p.651). A usual initial dose is up to 2 mg weekly by deep intramuscular injection, increased according to the patient's response. The usual maintenance dose is 2 to 10 mg weekly.

Adverse effects. References.
1. McCreadie RG, et al. Probable toxic necrosis after prolonged fluspirilene administration. BMJ 1979; 1: 523–4.

Preparations

Proprietary Preparations (details are given in Part 3)
Belg.: Imap; **Canad.:** Imap†; **Ger.:** Fluspi; Imap; kivat; **Irl.:** Redeptin; **Israel:** Imap; **Neth.:** Imap; **Norw.:** Imap†; **Switz.:** Imap†.

Flutoprazepam (19191-w)

Flutoprazepam (rINN).

KB-509. 7-Chloro-1-(cyclopropylmethyl)-5-(2-fluorophenyl)-1,3-dihydro-2H-1,4-benzodiazepin-2-one.
$C_{19}H_{16}ClFN_2O = 342.8$.
CAS — 25967-29-7.

Profile

Flutoprazepam is a benzodiazepine with general properties similar to those of diazepam (p.674).

Gepirone Hydrochloride (19247-w)

Gepirone Hydrochloride (USAN, rINNM).

BMY-13805-1; MJ-13805-1. 3,3-Dimethyl-N-{4-[4-(2-pyrimidinyl)-1-piperazinyl]butyl}glutarimide hydrochloride.
$C_{19}H_{29}N_5O_2,HCl = 395.9$.
CAS — 83928-76-1 (gepirone); 83928-66-9 (gepirone hydrochloride).

Profile

Gepirone is structurally related to buspirone (p.657). It is being investigated as the hydrochloride for the treatment of anxiety disorders and depression.

Action. Gepirone is a partial agonist at serotonin (hydroxytryptamine, 5-HT) receptors of the 5-HT$_{1A}$ subtype. For reference to the actions and potential uses of such drugs, see Buspirone, p.658.

References.
1. Feiger AD. A double-blind comparison of gepirone extended release, imipramine, and placebo in the treatment of outpatient major depression. Psychopharmacol Bull 1996; 32: 659–65.
2. Rickels K, et al. Gepirone and diazepam in generalized anxiety disorder: a placebo-controlled trial. J Clin Psychopharmacol 1997; 17: 272–7.

Glutethimide (4037-y)

Glutethimide (BAN, rINN).

Glutethimidum; Glutetimide. 2-Ethyl-2-phenylglutarimide; 3-Ethyl-3-phenylpiperidine-2,6-dione.
$C_{13}H_{15}NO_2 = 217.3$.
CAS — 77-21-4.
ATC — N05CE01.

Dependence and Withdrawal

As for the barbiturates (see Amobarbital, p.655).

Adverse Effects and Treatment

Side-effects of glutethimide include nausea, headache, blurred vision, unwanted sedation and other CNS effects such as ataxia, impaired memory, and paradoxical excitement, and occasional skin rashes. Acute hypersensitivity reactions, blood disorders, and exfoliative dermatitis have been reported in rare instances.

Overdosage with glutethimide produces symptoms similar to those of barbiturate overdosage; respiratory depression is usually less severe, and circulatory failure more severe than with the barbiturates (see Amobarbital, p.655). There are considerable fluctuations in the depth of coma and wakefulness. Antimuscarinic effects such as mydriasis, dryness of the mouth, paralytic ileus, and urinary bladder atony often occur. Treatment is as for barbiturate overdose (see Amobarbital, p.655). Irregular absorption and storage in fat depots may complicate treatment.

Precautions

Glutethimide should be used with care in patients with renal impairment and, as with all sedatives, in patients with impaired respiratory function. Because of its antimuscarinic actions it should be given with great care to patients with conditions such as angle-closure glaucoma, prostatic hyperplasia or urinary tract obstruction, pyloroduodenal obstruction, or cardiac arrhythmias.

Glutethimide may cause drowsiness; affected patients should not drive or operate machinery.

Abuse. A warning of the hazards associated with the abuse of glutethimide in a combination with codeine termed 'loads'.[1]
1. Sramek JJ, Khajawall A. "Loads". N Engl J Med 1981; 305: 231.

Porphyria. Glutethimide has been associated with acute attacks of porphyria and is considered unsafe in porphyric patients.

Interactions

The sedative effects of glutethimide are enhanced by the simultaneous administration of CNS depressants such as alcohol, barbiturates, and other sedatives; absorption of glutethimide is also markedly enhanced by concomitant administration of alcohol. Glutethimide induces microsomal hepatic enzymes, and it can thus cause increased metabolism of coumarin anticoagulants and other drugs, with reduced effect. Chronic administration of glutethimide may also enhance vitamin D metabolism.

Pharmacokinetics

Glutethimide is irregularly absorbed from the gastrointestinal tract and extensively metabolised in the liver. It has a biphasic plasma half-life; half-lives of up to 22 hours have been reported for the terminal phase. Glutethimide is excreted in urine, almost entirely as metabolites, with less than 2% of unchanged drug. Up to 2% of a dose has been reported to be present in the faeces. Glutethimide is reported to be about 50% bound to plasma proteins. It is highly lipid-soluble and may be stored in adipose tissue. It crosses the placental barrier and traces are found in breast milk.

Uses and Administration

Glutethimide is a piperidinedione hypnotic and sedative. It has been given by mouth for the short-term management of insomnia (p.652) in usual doses of 250 to 500 mg at night but has been superseded by other drugs.

Halazepam (7050-e)

Halazepam (BAN, USAN, rINN).

Sch-12041. 7-Chloro-1,3-dihydro-5-phenyl-1-(2,2,2-trifluoroethyl)-1,4-benzodiazepin-2-one.
$C_{17}H_{12}ClF_3N_2O = 352.7$.
CAS — 23092-17-3.
ATC — N05BA13.

Profile

Halazepam is a benzodiazepine with general properties similar to those of diazepam (p.674). It has been given by mouth for the short-term treatment of anxiety disorders (p.649).

Preparations

Proprietary Preparations (details are given in Part 3)
Ital.: Paxipam; **Port.:** Pacinone; **Spain:** Alapryl.

Haloperidol (18332-f)

Haloperidol (BAN, USAN, rINN).

Aloperidolo; Haloperidolum; McN-JR-1625; R-1625. 4-[4-(4-Chlorophenyl)-4-hydroxypiperidino]-4'-fluorobutyrophenone.
$C_{21}H_{23}ClFNO_2 = 375.9$.
CAS — 52-86-8.
ATC — N05AD01.

Pharmacopoeias. In Chin., Eur. (see p.vi), Int., Jpn, Pol., and US.

Pharmacopoeial description

Ph. Eur.: A white or almost white powder. Practically insoluble in water; slightly soluble in alcohol, in dichloromethane, and in methyl alcohol. Protect from light.

USP 25: A white to faintly yellowish amorphous or microcrystalline powder. Practically insoluble in water; soluble 1 in 60 of alcohol, 1 in 15 of chloroform, and 1 in 200 of ether. A saturated solution is neutral to litmus. Store in airtight containers. Protect from light.

Dilution. See Incompatibility, below.

Incompatibility. Formation of a precipitate was observed after dilution of haloperidol (as the lactate) in sodium chloride 0.9% injection when the final haloperidol concentration was 1.0 mg per mL or higher.[1] Undiluted haloperidol (5 mg per mL) injection has been reported to be incompatible with heparin sodium (diluted in sodium chloride 0.9% or glucose 5% injection),[2] sodium nitroprusside (diluted in glucose 5%),[1] cefmetazole sodium,[3] and diphenhydramine.[4] A mixture of equal volumes of sargramostim 10 µg per mL and haloperidol (as the lactate) 0.2 mg per mL resulted in a precipitate at 4 hours.[5]
1. Outman WR, Monolakis J. Visual compatibility of haloperidol lactate with 0.9% sodium chloride injection or injectable critical-care drugs during simulated Y-site injection. Am J Hosp Pharm 1991; 48: 1539–41.
2. Solomon DA, Nasinnyk KK. Compatibility of haloperidol lactate and heparin sodium. Am J Hosp Pharm 1982; 39: 843–4.
3. Hutchings SR, et al. Compatibility of cefmetazole sodium with commonly used drugs during Y-site delivery. Am J Health-Syst Pharm 1996; 53: 2185–8.
4. Ukhun IA. Compatibility of haloperidol and diphenhydramine in a hypodermic syringe. Ann Pharmacother 1995; 29: 1168–9.
5. Trissel LA, et al. Visual compatibility of sargramostim with selected antineoplastic agents, anti-infectives, or other drugs during simulated Y-site injection. Am J Hosp Pharm 1992; 49: 402–6.

Stability. Mention that a combination of the stabilisers benzyl alcohol and vanillin could protect haloperidol from photodegradation.[1]
1. Thoma K, Klimek R. Photostabilisation of drugs in dosage forms without protection from packaging materials. Int J Pharmaceutics 1991; 67: 169–75.

Haloperidol Decanoate (7051-l)

Haloperidol Decanoate (BANM, USAN, rINNM).

Haloperidoli Decanoas; R-13672.
$C_{31}H_{41}ClFNO_3 = 530.1$.
CAS — 74050-97-8.
Pharmacopoeias. In Eur. (see p.vi).

Pharmacopoeial description

Ph. Eur.: A white or almost white powder. It melts at about 42°. Practically insoluble in water; very soluble in alcohol, in dichloromethane, and in methyl alcohol. Store at a temperature below 25°. Protect from light.

Adverse Effects and Treatment

As for Chlorpromazine, p.660. Haloperidol is less likely to cause sedation, hypotension, or antimuscarinic effects, but is associated with a higher incidence of extrapyramidal effects.

Convulsions. For mention of haloperidol as one of the antipsychotics suitable for patients at risk of seizures, see p.661.

Effects on the liver. Liver dysfunction with jaundice and eosinophilia developed in a 15-year-old male 4 weeks after administration of haloperidol and benzatropine mesilate.[1] This treatment was discontinued 2 weeks later but some symptoms lasted for 28 months. The reaction was suggestive of a drug-induced hypersensitivity reaction and haloperidol was the most likely cause. Haloperidol-induced liver injury was considered to be rare.
1. Dincsoy HP, Saelinger DA. Haloperidol-induced chronic cholestatic liver disease. Gastroenterology 1982; 83: 694–700.

Overdosage. Symptoms of haloperidol overdose in children have ranged from the expected, such as drowsiness, restlessness, confusion, marked extrapyramidal symptoms, and hypothermia,[1,2] to unexpected reactions such as bradycardia (possibly secondary to hypothermia)[1] and an episode of severe, delayed hypertension.[3]

Torsade de pointes has followed overdosage in adults (for references, see Effects on the Cardiovascular System under Chlorpromazine, p.661).
1. Scialli JVK, Thornton WE. Toxic reactions from a haloperidol overdose in two children: thermal and cardiac manifestations. JAMA 1978; 239: 48–9.

2. Sinaniotis CA, *et al.* Acute haloperidol poisoning in children. *J Pediatr* 1978; **93**: 1038–9.
3. Cummingham DG, Challapalli M. Hypertension in acute haloperidol poisoning. *J Pediatr* 1979; **95**: 489–90.

Retroperitoneal fibrosis. Obstructive uropathy was noted in a 45-year-old woman who had received haloperidol 5 to 15 mg daily for 8 years.[1] Benzatropine was also taken during that time, and in the previous 5 years she had taken chlorpromazine and fluphenazine. A diagnosis of retroperitoneal fibrosis was made and was tentatively associated with long-term antipsychotic therapy.

1. Jeffries JJ, *et al.* Retroperitoneal fibrosis and haloperidol. *Am J Psychiatry* 1982; **139**: 1524–5.

Toxic encephalopathy. A report[1] of possible toxic encephalopathy following the use of high intravenous doses of haloperidol. The patient, who had a history of bipolar disorder and cerebrovascular accident, had been given increasing intravenous doses of haloperidol (up to 270 mg daily) to control post-surgical agitation. The encephalopathy had resolved 8 days after discontinuation of haloperidol.

1. Maxa JL, *et al.* Possible toxic encephalopathy following high-dose intravenous haloperidol. *Ann Pharmacother* 1997; **31**: 736–7.

Precautions

As for Chlorpromazine, p.663.

Severe dystonic reactions have followed the use of haloperidol, particularly in children and adolescents. It should therefore be used with extreme care in children. Haloperidol may also cause severe extrapyramidal reactions in patients with hyperthyroidism.

Porphyria. Haloperidol is considered to be unsafe in patients with porphyria although there is conflicting experimental evidence of porphyrinogenicity.

Interactions

As for Chlorpromazine, p.664.

Haloperidol must be used with extreme caution in patients receiving lithium; an encephalopathic syndrome has been reported following their concomitant use (see p.295).

Pharmacokinetics

Haloperidol is readily absorbed from the gastrointestinal tract. It is metabolised in the liver and is excreted in the urine and, via the bile, in the faeces; there is evidence of enterohepatic recycling. Owing to first-pass metabolism in the liver, plasma concentrations following oral administration are lower than those following intramuscular administration. Moreover, there is wide intersubject variation in plasma concentrations of haloperidol, but, in practice, no strong correlation has been found between plasma concentrations of haloperidol and its therapeutic effect. Paths of metabolism of haloperidol include oxidative *N*-dealkylation and reduction of the ketone group to form an alcohol known as reduced haloperidol. Haloperidol has been reported to have a plasma elimination half-life ranging from about 12 to 38 hours after oral administration. Haloperidol is about 92% bound to plasma proteins. It is widely distributed in the body and crosses the blood-brain barrier. Haloperidol is distributed into breast milk.

The decanoate ester of haloperidol is very slowly absorbed from the site of injection and is therefore suitable for depot injection. It is gradually released into the blood stream where it is rapidly hydrolysed to haloperidol.

◊ References.
1. Kudo S, Ishizaki T. Pharmacokinetics of haloperidol: an update. *Clin Pharmacokinet* 1999 **37**: 435–56.

◊ The clinical significance of the reduced metabolite of haloperidol has been much debated.[1,2] Its activity appears to be substantially less than that of the parent drug but there is some evidence for re-oxidation of reduced haloperidol to haloperidol.[1-3] Some studies suggest that nonresponders to haloperidol have elevated ratios of reduced haloperidol to haloperidol in the plasma, although other workers have reported contrary findings.[2] Pyridinium metabolites resulting from oxidation of haloperidol have been detected in the urine and there is concern that they may be neurotoxic in a manner similar to MPTP (p.1160), a compound which can induce irreversible parkinsonism.[4]

Measurement of concentrations of haloperidol or reduced haloperidol in scalp hair has been suggested as a useful means of monitoring compliance.[5,6] Evidence for the existence of any re-

lationship between plasma concentrations of haloperidol and therapeutic effect in schizophrenia has been discussed.[7]

1. Sramek JJ, *et al.* Neuroleptic plasma concentrations and clinical response: in search of a therapeutic window. *Drug Intell Clin Pharm* 1988; **22**: 373–80.
2. Froemming JS, *et al.* Pharmacokinetics of haloperidol. *Clin Pharmacokinet* 1989; **17**: 396–423.
3. Chakraborty BS, *et al.* Interconversion between haloperidol and reduced haloperidol in healthy volunteers. *Eur J Clin Pharmacol* 1989; **37**: 45–8.
4. Eyles DW, *et al.* Quantitative analysis of two pyridinium metabolites of haloperidol in patients with schizophrenia. *Clin Pharmacol Ther* 1994; **56**: 512–20.
5. Uematsu T, *et al.* Human scalp hair as evidence of individual dosage history of haloperidol: method and retrospective study. *Eur J Clin Pharmacol* 1989; **37**: 239–44.
6. Matsuno H, *et al.* The measurement of haloperidol and reduced haloperidol in hair as an index of dosage history. *Br J Clin Pharmacol* 1990; **29**: 187–94.
7. Ulrich S, *et al.* The relationship between serum concentration and therapeutic effect of haloperidol in patients with acute schizophrenia. *Clin Pharmacokinet* 1998; **34**: 227–63.

Uses and Administration

Haloperidol is a butyrophenone with general properties similar to those of the phenothiazine, chlorpromazine (p.665). It is an antipsychotic with actions most closely resembling those of phenothiazines with a piperazine side-chain.

Haloperidol is used in the treatment of various psychoses including schizophrenia (p.651) and mania (see Bipolar Disorder, p.271), and in behaviour disturbances (p.650), in Tourette's syndrome and severe tics (p.650), in intractable hiccups (p.667), and in severe anxiety (p.649). Haloperidol has also been used for its antiemetic effect in the management of nausea and vomiting of various causes (p.1206).

Haloperidol is usually given by mouth or injection as the base or intramuscularly as the long-acting decanoate ester. Some haloperidol preparations are prepared with the aid of lactic acid and may be stated to contain haloperidol lactate. Doses are expressed in terms of the equivalent amount of haloperidol. It should be used in reduced dosage in elderly or debilitated patients; doses at the lower end of the scale are also advised for adolescents.

The usual initial dose *by mouth* for the treatment of **psychoses** and associated behaviour disorders is 0.5 to 5 mg twice or three times daily. In severe or resistant psychoses doses of up to 100 mg daily may be required; rarely doses above 100 mg daily have been used. The dose should be reduced gradually according to response. Maintenance doses as low as 3 to 10 mg daily may be sufficient. A suitable initial dose for children by mouth is 25 to 50 µg per kg bodyweight daily in two divided doses, increased cautiously, if necessary; a maximum daily dose of 10 mg has been recommended in the UK but in the USA the suggested maximum daily dose is 150 µg per kg as the manufacturer has stated that there is little evidence of behaviour improvement with daily doses of more than 6 mg.

For the control of acute psychotic conditions haloperidol may be given *intramuscularly* in doses of 2 to 10 mg; subsequent doses may be given hourly until symptoms are controlled although dosage intervals of 4 to 8 hours may be adequate. Up to 30 mg intramuscularly has been used for the initial emergency control of very severely disturbed patients, although some manufacturers recommend an initial maximum dose of no more than 18 mg. The *intravenous* route may also be used.

In patients already stabilised on an oral dose of haloperidol and requiring long-term therapy the long-acting decanoate ester may be given by *deep intramuscular* injection. The usual initial dose is the equivalent of 10 to 20 times the total daily dose of haloperidol by mouth, up to a maximum of 100 mg; if more than 100 mg is required for an initial dose the excess should be given after 3 to 7 days. Subsequent doses, usually given every 4 weeks, may be increased to up to 300 mg or more, according to the patient's requirements, both dose and dose interval being adjusted as required.

In the management of **nausea and vomiting** haloperidol has been given in usual doses of 0.5 to 2 mg

daily by *intramuscular* injection. In palliative care haloperidol 1.5 mg may be given *by mouth* once or twice daily or by *subcutaneous* infusion (via a syringe driver) in doses of 2.5 to 10 mg over 24 hours.

A starting dose of 0.5 to 1.5 mg three times daily *by mouth* has been suggested for the management of **Tourette's syndrome** and severe **tics**. Up to about 10 mg daily may be needed in Tourette's syndrome, although requirements vary considerably and the dose must be very carefully adjusted to obtain the optimum response.

For intractable **hiccups** a suggested dose is 1.5 mg given three times daily *by mouth* adjusted according to response; alternatively 3 to 15 mg may be given daily by intramuscular or intravenous *injection* in divided doses.

A dose of 0.5 mg twice daily *by mouth* has been used as adjunctive treatment in the short-term management of severe **anxiety disorders**.

In palliative care, haloperidol has been given in a dose of 1 to 3 mg every 8 hours *by mouth* for the treatment of **restlessness and confusion**. It may also be given as a *subcutaneous* infusion in a dose of 5 to 15 mg over 24 hours.

Ballism. Dopamine-blocking antipsychotics such as haloperidol may sometimes be needed for the management of patients with ballism (p.650) when symptoms are severe.

Chorea. For a discussion of the management of various choreas, including mention of the use of haloperidol, see p.650.

Dystonia. Antipsychotics such as phenothiazines, haloperidol, or pimozide are sometimes useful in the treatment of idiopathic dystonia (p.1173) in patients who have failed to respond to other drugs. However, they often act non-specifically and there is the risk of adding drug-induced extrapyramidal disorders to the dystonia being treated (see Extrapyramidal Disorders under Adverse Effects of Chlorpromazine, p.662).

Sneezing. Report[1] of a patient whose intractable sneezing was controlled by haloperidol given in doses of up to 5 mg twice daily. Symptoms recurred when treatment was stopped after 5 weeks but responded again to 5 mg three times daily. On gradual reduction of dosage over 6 months the patient experienced no recurrence and had remained symptom-free after 6 months without medication.

1. Davison K. Pharmacological treatment for intractable sneezing. *BMJ* 1982; **284**: 1163–4.

Stuttering. Stuttering (stammering) is a disorder which affects the fluency of speech. Developmental stuttering usually occurs in early childhood and is more common in boys than girls. While stuttering may cease in some children after only a few months it may become a chronic condition in others. Stuttering which starts during adulthood is rarer and may be the result of a neurological insult. It should also be remembered that stuttering may be drug induced. While stuttering may be greatly improved with intensive speech training the effectiveness of other forms of management such as hypnosis, psychotherapy, counselling, and drug therapy has been largely unconvincing.[1] Although many drugs have been used to treat stuttering a review of the literature[2] indicated that there were few adequate studies of their efficacy. Haloperidol was considered to be the most well studied drug and its efficacy had been demonstrated by several double-blind placebo-controlled studies. However, most patients needed to continue taking haloperidol to maintain improvement but few did so because of its adverse effects. Double-blind studies have on the whole failed to confirm reports of benefit for drugs such as bethanechol, beta blockers, and calcium-channel blockers although isolated patients may have marked improvement. Other drugs which are being studied and which might be of benefit include clomipramine.

1. Andrews G, *et al.* Stuttering. *JAMA* 1988; **260**: 1445.
2. Brady JP, *et al.* The pharmacology of stuttering: a critical review. *Am J Psychiatry* 1991; **148**: 1309–16.

Taste disorders. For reference to the use of haloperidol in the treatment of taste disorders, see Chlorpromazine, p.667.

Tourette's syndrome. Many patients with Tourette's syndrome (p.650) do not require medication but when treatment is needed dopamine antagonists such as the antipsychotics haloperidol or pimozide are most commonly used. They often decrease the frequency and severity of tics and may improve any accompanying behavioural disturbances. However, superiority of either drug in terms of efficacy or adverse effects has not been clearly demonstrated.[1,2] Because of the potential for acute and long-term adverse effects it is usually recommended that doses are titrated to be as low as possible; the aim of treatment is not necessarily to control symptoms completely. Medication can often be discontinued after a few years.

1. Shapiro E, *et al.* Controlled study of haloperidol, pimozide, and placebo for the treatment of Gilles de la Tourette's syndrome. *Arch Gen Psychiatry* 1989; **46:** 722–30.
2. Sallee FR, *et al.* Relative efficacy of haloperidol and pimozide in children and adolescents with Tourette's disorder. *Am J Psychiatry* 1997; **154:** 1057–62.

Preparations

BP 2001: Haloperidol Capsules; Haloperidol Injection; Haloperidol Oral Solution; Haloperidol Tablets; Strong Haloperidol Oral Solution;
USP 25: Haloperidol Injection; Haloperidol Oral Solution; Haloperidol Tablets.

Proprietary Preparations (details are given in Part 3)
Aust.: Haldol; *Austral.:* Haldol; Serenace; *Belg.:* Haldol; *Braz.:* Haldol; *Canad.:* Haldol; Novo-Peridol; Peridol; *Denm.:* Serenase; *Fin.:* Serenase; *Fr.:* Haldol; *Ger.:* Buteridol; Haldol; Haloneural; Haloper; Sigaperidol; *Hong Kong:* Haldol; Serenace; *Irl.:* Haldol; Serenace; *Israel:* Haldol; Haloper; Pericate; Peridor; *Ital.:* Bioperidolo; Haldol; Serenase; *Mex.:* Haldol; Haloperil; Kepsidol; Pulsit; *Neth.:* Haldol; *Norw.:* Haldol; *NZ:* Haldol; Serenace; *Port.:* Serenelfi; *S.Afr.:* Cereen; Serenace; *Singapore:* Serenace; *Swed.:* Haldol; *Switz.:* Haldol; Sigaperidol; *Thai.:* H-Tab; Haldol; Halo-P; Halomed; Halopol; Haricon; Haridol; Perida; Polyhadol; Senorm; Serenace; Tensidol; *UK:* Dozic; Haldol; Serenace; *USA:* Haldol.

Multi-ingredient: *Aust.:* Vesalium; *Belg.:* Vesalium†; *Fr.:* Vesadol.

Haloxazolam (19283-j)

Haloxazolam *(rINN)*.

10-Bromo-11b-(2-fluorophenyl)-2,3,7,11b-tetrahydrooxazolo[3,2-*d*][1,4]benzodiazepin-6(5*H*)-one.
$C_{17}H_{14}BrFN_2O_2 = 377.2$.
CAS — 59128-97-1.

Pharmacopoeias. In *Jpn.*

Profile
Haloxazolam is a benzodiazepine with general properties similar to those of diazepam (p.674). It has been given by mouth as a hypnotic in the short-term management of insomnia.

Preparations

Proprietary Preparations (details are given in Part 3)
Jpn: Somelin†.

Hexapropymate (4039-z)

Hexapropymate *(BAN, rINN)*.

L-2103; Propinylcyclohexanol Carbamate. 1-(Prop-2-ynyl)cyclohexyl carbamate.
$C_{10}H_{15}NO_2 = 181.2$.
CAS — 358-52-1.
ATC — N05CM10.

Profile
Hexapropymate is a carbamate derivative formerly used as a hypnotic.

Porphyria. Hexapropymate is considered to be unsafe in patients with porphyria because it has been shown to be porphyrinogenic in *in-vitro* systems.

Hexobarbital (4040-p)

Hexobarbital *(BAN, rINN)*.

Enhexymalum; Enimal; Hexobarbitalum; Hexobarbitone; Methexenyl; Methyl-cyclohexenylmethyl-barbitursäure; Methylhexabarbital. 5-(Cyclohex-1-enyl)-1,5-dimethylbarbituric acid.
$C_{12}H_{16}N_2O_3 = 236.3$.
CAS — 56-29-1.
ATC — N01AF02; N05CA16.

NOTE. The name ciclobarbital (see Cyclobarbital, p.674) has sometimes been applied to hexobarbital.

Pharmacopoeias. In *Eur.* (see p.vi).

Pharmacopoeial description

Ph. Eur.: A white crystalline powder. Very slightly soluble in water; sparingly soluble in alcohol and in ether. Forms water-soluble compounds with alkali hydroxides and carbonates and with ammonia.

Hexobarbital Sodium (4041-s)

Hexobarbital Sodium *(BANM, rINNM)*.

Enhexymalnatrium; Hexenalum; Hexobarbitalum Natricum; Hexobarbitone Sodium; Sodium Hexobarbital; Soluble Hexobarbitone. Sodium 5-(cyclohex-1-enyl)-1,5-dimethylbarbiturate.
$C_{12}H_{15}N_2NaO_3 = 258.2$.
CAS — 50-09-9.
Pharmacopoeias. In *Aust.* and *Pol.*

Profile
Hexobarbital is a barbiturate with the general properties of amobarbital (p.655). It has been used as a hypnotic and sedative but barbiturates are no longer considered appropriate for such purposes.

Homofenazine Hydrochloride (7052-y)

Homofenazine Hydrochloride *(rINNM)*.

D-775 (homofenazine); HFZ (homofenazine). 2-{Hexahydro-4-[3-(2-trifluoromethylphenothiazin-10-yl)propyl]-1,4-diazepin-1-yl}ethanol dihydrochloride.
$C_{23}H_{28}F_3N_3OS,2HCl = 524.5$.
CAS — 3833-99-6 (homofenazine); 1256-01-5 (homofenazine hydrochloride).

Profile
Homofenazine hydrochloride is a phenothiazine with general properties similar to those of chlorpromazine (p.660). It has been used in the management of neuropsychiatric disorders.

Preparations

Proprietary Preparations (details are given in Part 3)
Multi-ingredient: *Aust.:* Pelvichthol†.

Ipsapirone Hydrochloride (19356-z)

Ipsapirone Hydrochloride *(BANM, USAN, rINNM)*.

Bay-q-7821; TVX-Q-7821. 2-[4-(4-Pyrimidin-2-ylpiperazin-1-yl)butyl]-1,2-benzothiazol-3(2*H*)-one 1,1-dioxide hydrochloride.
$C_{19}H_{23}N_5O_3S,HCl = 437.9$.
CAS — 95847-70-4 (ipsapirone); 92589-98-5 (ipsapirone hydrochloride).

Profile
Ipsapirone is structurally related to buspirone (p.657). It is under investigation as the hydrochloride for the treatment of anxiety disorders and depression.

◊ Ipsapirone is a partial agonist at serotonin (hydroxytryptamine, 5-HT) receptors of the 5-HT$_{1A}$ subtype. For reference to the actions and potential uses of such drugs, see Buspirone, p.658.

References.
1. Cutler NR, *et al.* A double-blind, placebo-controlled study comparing the efficacy and safety of ipsapirone versus lorazepam in patients with generalized anxiety disorder: a prospective multicenter trial. *J Clin Psychopharmacol* 1993; **13:** 429–37.
2. Fuhr U, *et al.* Absorption of ipsapirone along the human gastrointestinal tract. *Br J Clin Pharmacol* 1994; **38:** 83–6.
3. Mandos LA, *et al.* Placebo-controlled comparison of the clinical effects of rapid discontinuation of ipsapirone and lorazepam after 8 weeks of treatment for generalized anxiety disorder. *Int Clin Psychopharmacol* 1995; **10:** 251–6.
4. Lapierre YD, *et al.* A Canadian multicenter study of three fixed doses of controlled-release ipsapirone in outpatients with moderate to severe major depression. *J Clin Psychopharmacol* 1998; **18:** 268–73.

Ketazolam (7055-c)

Ketazolam *(BAN, USAN, rINN)*.

U-28774. 11-Chloro-8,12b-dihydro-2,8-dimethyl-12b-phenyl-4*H*-[1,3]oxazino[3,2-*d*][1,4]benzodiazepine-4,7(6*H*)-dione.
$C_{20}H_{17}ClN_2O_3 = 368.8$.
CAS — 27223-35-4.
ATC — N05BA10.

Profile
Ketazolam is a long-acting benzodiazepine with general properties similar to those of diazepam (p.674). It is given by mouth in the short-term treatment of anxiety (p.649) in usual doses of 15 to 60 mg daily, either in divided doses or as a single dose at night.

◊ References.
1. Angelini G, *et al.* Ketazolam, a new long-acting benzodiazepine, in the treatment of anxious patients: a multicenter study of 2,056 patients. *Curr Ther Res* 1989; **45:** 294–304.

Preparations

Proprietary Preparations (details are given in Part 3)
Belg.: Solatran; Unakalm; *Ital.:* Anseren; *Neth.:* Unakalm; *Port.:* Unakalm; *S.Afr.:* Solatran; *Spain:* Marcen; Sedotime; *Switz.:* Solatran†.

Loprazolam Mesilate (18341-d)

Loprazolam Mesilate *(BANM, rINNM)*.

HR-158; Loprazolam Mesylate; Loprazolam Methanesulphonate; RU-31158. 6-(2-Chlorophenyl)-2,4-dihydro-2-(4-methylpiperazin-1-ylmethylene)-8-nitroimidazo[1,2-*a*][1,4]benzodiazepin-1-one methanesulphonate monohydrate.
$C_{23}H_{21}ClN_6O_3,CH_4O_3S,H_2O = 579.0$.
CAS — 61197-73-7 (loprazolam); 70111-54-5 (anhydrous loprazolam mesilate).
Pharmacopoeias. In *Br.*

Pharmacopoeial description

BP 2001: A yellow crystalline powder. Slightly soluble in water, in alcohol, and in chloroform; very slightly soluble in ether.

Dependence and Withdrawal
As for Diazepam, p.675.

◊ For the purpose of withdrawal regimens, 0.5 to 1 mg of loprazolam is considered roughly equivalent to 5 mg of diazepam.

Adverse Effects, Treatment, and Precautions
As for Diazepam, p.675.

Porphyria. Loprazolam is considered to be unsafe in patients with porphyria because it has been shown to be porphyrinogenic in *in-vitro* systems.

Interactions
As for Diazepam, p.677.

Pharmacokinetics

◊ After oral administration, peak plasma concentrations of loprazolam are achieved in about 1 to 2 hours.[1] The elimination half-life has varied from 4 to 15 hours and appears to be prolonged in elderly patients to some extent. Loprazolam is reported to be about 80% bound to plasma proteins and has been detected in breast milk. The major pathway of metabolism in humans is *N*-oxidation of the piperazine ring. Loprazolam and its metabolites are excreted in the urine and faeces. In some studies, a secondary peak in plasma-loprazolam concentrations has been observed; this could be a result of enterohepatic recycling.

1. Garzone PD, Kroboth PD. Pharmacokinetics of the newer benzodiazepines. *Clin Pharmacokinet* 1989; **16:** 337–64.

Uses and Administration
Loprazolam is an intermediate-acting benzodiazepine with general properties similar to those of diazepam (p.680).

Loprazolam mesilate is usually used for its hypnotic properties in the short-term management of insomnia (p.652), in usual doses equivalent to 1 mg of loprazolam at night. Dosage may be increased to up to 2 mg if necessary. A starting dose of 0.5 mg increased to a maximum of 1 mg may be appropriate for elderly or debilitated patients.

Preparations

BP 2001: Loprazolam Tablets.

Proprietary Preparations (details are given in Part 3)
Belg.: Dormonoct; *Fr.:* Havlane; *Ger.:* Sonin; *Irl.:* Dormonoct†; *Neth.:* Dormonoct; *Port.:* Dormonoct; *S.Afr.:* Dormonoct; *Spain:* Somnovit; *UK:* Dormonoct.

Lorazepam (7060-y)

Lorazepam *(BAN, USAN, rINN)*.

Lorazepamum; Wy-4036. 7-Chloro-5-(2-chlorophenyl)-1,3-dihydro-3-hydroxy-1,4-benzodiazepin-2-one.
$C_{15}H_{10}Cl_2N_2O_2 = 321.2$.
CAS — 846-49-1.
ATC — N05BA06.
Pharmacopoeias. In *Eur.* (see p.vi), *Jpn*, and *US.*

Pharmacopoeial description

Ph. Eur.: A white or almost white, crystalline powder. It exhibits polymorphism. Practically insoluble in water; sparingly soluble in alcohol; sparingly or slightly soluble in dichloromethane. Store in airtight containers. Protect from light.

USP 25: A white or practically white, practically odourless powder. Insoluble in water; sparingly soluble in alcohol; slightly soluble in chloroform. Store in airtight containers. Protect from light.

Incompatibility. Visual incompatibility has been noted with lorazepam and sargramostim[1] or aztreonam.[2]

1. Trissel LA, *et al.* Visual compatibility of sargramostim with selected antineoplastic agents, anti-infectives, or other drugs during simulated Y-site injection. *Am J Hosp Pharm* 1992; **49:** 402–6.
2. Trissel LA, Martinez JF. Compatibility of aztreonam with selected drugs during simulated Y-site administration. *Am J Health-Syst Pharm* 1995; **52:** 1086–90.

Solubility. The solubility of lorazepam in fluids for intravenous administration (water, glucose injection, lactated Ringer's injection, and sodium chloride injection) was greatest in glucose injection (5%) at 62 µg per mL and lowest in sodium chloride injection (0.9%) at 27 µg per mL;[1] these differences in solubility appeared to be pH related. Commercial injections are reported to contain polyethylene glycol in propylene glycol to overcome this poor solubility. However, precipitation has been noted[2] in solutions prepared by dilution of lorazepam injection with sodium chloride injection (0.9%) to a concentration of 500 µg per mL. One group of workers[3] have reported that they had overcome such problems with precipitation by using glucose injection (5%) as a diluent and by avoiding final concentrations of lorazepam between 0.08 mg per mL and 1 mg per mL. It was suggested that the propylene glycol in the mixture might account for the unusual concentration effect. Such recommendations have been adopted by another group[4] although they observed that precipitation occurred if a formulation of lorazepam containing 4 mg per mL was used to prepare the injection; no precipitation was noted when a formulation containing 2 mg per mL was used. The group also commented that, in the USA, the manufacturers of lorazepam injection advise that admixtures should be prepared with the 2 mg per mL formulation only.

1. Newton DW, *et al.* Lorazepam solubility in and sorption from intravenous admixture solutions. *Am J Hosp Pharm* 1983; **40:** 424–7.
2. Boullata JI, *et al.* Precipitation of lorazepam infusion. *Ann Pharmacother* 1996; **30:** 1037–8.
3. Volles DF, *et al.* More on usability of lorazepam admixtures for continuous infusion. *Am J Health-Syst Pharm* 1996; **53:** 2753–4.
4. Levanda M. Noticeable difference in admixtures prepared from lorazepam 2 and 4 mg/ml. *Am J Health-Syst Pharm* 1998; **55:** 2305.

Sorption. Significant loss of lorazepam has been reported from solutions stored in PVC[1] or polypropylene[2] giving equipment; polyolefin[3] or glass[4] equipment appears to be more suitable.

1. Hoey LL, *et al.* Lorazepam stability in parenteral solutions for continuous intravenous administration. *Ann Pharmacother* 1996; **30:** 343–6.
2. Stiles ML, *et al.* Stability of deferoxamine mesylate, floxuridine, fluorouracil, hydromorphone hydrochloride, lorazepam, and midazolam hydrochloride in polypropylene infusion-pump syringes. *Am J Health-Syst Pharm* 1996; **53:** 1583–8.
3. Trissel LA, Pearson SD. Storage of lorazepam in three injectable solutions in polyvinyl chloride and polyolefin bags. *Am J Hosp Pharm* 1994; **51:** 368–72.
4. Martens HJ, *et al.* Sorption of various drugs in polyvinyl chloride, glass, and polyethylene-lined infusion containers. *Am J Hosp Pharm* 1990; **47:** 369–73.

Dependence and Withdrawal

As for Diazepam, p.675.

◊ For the purpose of withdrawal regimens, 0.5 mg of lorazepam may be considered roughly equivalent to 5 mg of diazepam.

Adverse Effects, Treatment, and Precautions

As for Diazepam, p.675. Pain and a sensation of burning have occurred following injection of lorazepam.

◊ There have been reports of toxicity, presumed to be due to polyethylene glycol[1] or propylene glycol,[2] following prolonged parenteral administration of lorazepam; polyethylene glycol in propylene glycol is included as a solubiliser in lorazepam solutions. Diarrhoea in an infant given large enteral doses of lorazepam or diazepam solutions may have been due to the combined osmotic effect of polyethylene glycol and propylene glycol in these preparations.[3]

1. Laine GA, *et al.* Polyethylene glycol nephrotoxicity secondary to prolonged high-dose intravenous lorazepam. *Ann Pharmacother* 1995; **29:** 1110–4.
2. Seay RE, *et al.* Possible toxicity from propylene glycol in lorazepam infusion. *Ann Pharmacother* 1997; **31:** 647–8. Woycik CL, Walker PC. Correction and comment: possible toxicity from propylene glycol in injectable drug preparations. *ibid.*: 1413.
3. Marshall JD, *et al.* Diarrhea associated with enteral benzodiazepine solutions. *J Pediatr* 1995; **126:** 657–9.

Effects on the blood. A case of pancytopenia associated with oral lorazepam was reported[1] in 1988; only 5 instances of thrombocytopenia and none of leucopenia had been reported to the UK Committee on Safety of Medicines or the UK manufacturers over the previous 13 years.

1. El-Sayed S, Symonds RP. Lorazepam induced pancytopenia. *BMJ* 1988; **296:** 1332.

Effects on fluid and electrolyte homoeostasis. Inappropriate secretion of antidiuretic hormone related to ingestion of lorazepam was considered to be the cause of hyponatraemia in an 81-year-old woman.[1]

1. Engel WR, Grau A. Inappropriate secretion of antidiuretic hormone associated with lorazepam. *BMJ* 1988; **297:** 858.

Effects on the nervous system. For reference to extrapyramidal disorders associated with administration of lorazepam, see Diazepam, p.675.

The elderly. For discussion of the need for reduced dosage of benzodiazepines in elderly patients, including mention of lorazepam, see Diazepam, p.676.

Hepatic impairment. Lorazepam is contra-indicated in severe hepatic impairment; patients with mild to moderate impairment may require reduced doses. Although the elimination half-life of lorazepam was increased in 13 patients with alcoholic cirrhosis compared with 11 control subjects, this was not associated with an impairment in systemic plasma clearance.[1] With the exception of a modest decrease in the extent of plasma protein binding, acute viral hepatitis had no effect on the disposition kinetics of lorazepam.

1. Kraus JW, *et al.* Effects of aging and liver disease on disposition of lorazepam. *Clin Pharmacol Ther* 1978; **24:** 411–19.

Local reactions. Of 40 patients given a single intravenous dose of lorazepam 4 mg three had local thrombosis 2 to 3 days later and 6 had local thrombosis 7 to 10 days later.[1] The incidence was lower than in those given diazepam [in solution].

1. Hegarty JE, Dundee JW. Sequelae after the intravenous injection of three benzodiazepines—diazepam, lorazepam, and flunitrazepam. *BMJ* 1977; **2:** 1384–5.

Interactions

As for Diazepam, p.677.

The symbol † denotes a preparation no longer actively marketed

Pharmacokinetics

Lorazepam is readily absorbed from the gastrointestinal tract following oral administration, with a bioavailability of about 90%; peak plasma concentrations are reported to occur about 2 hours after an oral dose. The absorption profile after intramuscular injection is similar to that after administration by mouth.

Lorazepam is about 85% bound to plasma protein. It crosses the blood-brain barrier and the placenta; it is also distributed into breast milk. Lorazepam is metabolised in the liver to the inactive glucuronide, and excreted in urine. The elimination half-life has been reported to range from about 10 to 20 hours.

◊ References.
1. Greenblatt DJ. Clinical pharmacokinetics of oxazepam and lorazepam. *Clin Pharmacokinet* 1981; **6:** 89–105.

Children. References to the pharmacokinetics of lorazepam in children.
1. Relling MV, *et al.* Lorazepam pharmacodynamics and pharmacokinetics in children. *J Pediatr* 1989; **114:** 641–6.

Neonates. References to slow elimination of lorazepam by neonates.
1. Cummings AJ, Whitelaw AGL. A study of conjugation and drug elimination in the human neonate. *Br J Clin Pharmacol* 1981; **12:** 511–15.
2. McDermott CA, *et al.* Pharmacokinetics of lorazepam in critically ill neonates with seizures. *J Pediatr* 1992; **120:** 479–83.
3. Reiter PD, Stiles AD. Lorazepam toxicity in a premature infant. *Ann Pharmacother* 1993; **27:** 727–9.

Distribution. Evidence that lorazepam undergoes enterohepatic recirculation with possible first-pass metabolism.[1]
1. Herman RJ, *et al.* Disposition of lorazepam in human beings: enterohepatic recirculation and first-pass effect. *Clin Pharmacol Ther* 1989; **46:** 18–25.

BREAST MILK. Free lorazepam concentrations in the breast milk of 4 lactating mothers who had received lorazepam 3.5 mg by mouth as premedication, ranged from 8 to 9 nanograms per mL four hours after the dose.[1] This represented about 15 to 26% of the concentration in plasma, and was probably sufficiently low to cause no adverse effects in breast-fed infants.
1. Summerfield RJ, Nielsen MS. Excretion of lorazepam into breast milk. *Br J Anaesth* 1985; **57:** 1042–3.

CNS. In a study involving 6 healthy subjects, peak plasma-lorazepam concentrations were reached 5 minutes after the end of a one-minute intravenous injection.[1] CNS effects, as measured by EEG activity, did not reach a maximum until 30 minutes after injection; they declined to baseline values slowly over 5 to 8 hours in a similar manner to plasma concentrations. In contrast, CNS effects of diazepam were maximal immediately after the injection. They also declined more rapidly than lorazepam, but again in a similar way to plasma concentrations. Studies in *mice* suggested that the slow onset of action of lorazepam that has been reported by some is at least partly explained by a delay in passage from systemic blood into brain tissue.
1. Greenblatt DJ, *et al.* Kinetic and dynamic study of intravenous lorazepam; comparison with intravenous diazepam. *J Pharmacol Exp Ther* 1989; **250:** 134–40.

Uses and Administration

Lorazepam is a short-acting benzodiazepine with general properties similar to those of diazepam (p.680). It is used in the short-term treatment of anxiety disorders (p.649), as a hypnotic in the short-term management of insomnia (p.652), and as an anticonvulsant in the management of status epilepticus (p.341). When used in the treatment of status epilepticus lorazepam has a prolonged antiepileptic action. It is also used for its sedative and amnestic properties in premedication and in antiemetic regimens for the control of nausea and vomiting associated with cancer chemotherapy (p.1206).

Lorazepam is usually given by mouth or by injection as the base although the pivalate is available for oral administration in some countries. Sublingual tablets are used in some countries in doses similar to those for standard tablets. The intramuscular route is usually only used when oral or intravenous administration is not possible. Injections should usually be diluted before administration; intravenous injections should be given at a rate of not more than 2 mg per minute into a large vein. Lorazepam should be given in reduced dosage to elderly or debilitated patients; one-half the usual adult dose, or less, may be sufficient.

The usual dose of lorazepam by mouth for the treatment of **anxiety disorders** is 1 to 6 mg daily in 2 or 3 divided doses with the largest dose taken at night; up to 10 mg daily has been given. A dose of 25 to 30 µg

per kg body-weight may be given by injection every 6 hours for acute anxiety. A single oral dose of 1 to 4 mg at bedtime may be given for **insomnia** associated with anxiety.

For **premedication** adults may be given a dose of 2 to 3 mg by mouth the night before the operation followed if necessary the next morning by a smaller dose. Alternatively, 2 to 4 mg may be given 1 to 2 hours before an operation. A dose of 50 µg per kg may be administered 30 to 45 minutes before the operation if given intravenously or 1 to 1½ hours before if given intramuscularly.

In the management of **status epilepticus** 4 mg may be given as a single intravenous dose; a dose of 2 mg has been suggested for children.

A dose of 1 to 2 mg of lorazepam by mouth given with dexamethasone before chemotherapy has been suggested for prevention of acute symptoms in patients at increased risk of antineoplastic-induced **emesis**.

Disturbed behaviour. For a discussion of the management of behaviour disturbances associated with various psychotic disorders and the value of benzodiazepines, see p.650.
References.
1. Bieniek SA, *et al.* A double-blind study of lorazepam versus the combination of haloperidol and lorazepam in managing agitation. *Pharmacotherapy* 1998; **18:** 57–62.

Premedication and sedation. Lorazepam is used as a premedicant (p.1256) and as a sedative for therapeutic and investigative procedures such as dental treatment (p.652) and endoscopy (p.652), and also in intensive care (p.652).
References.
1. Maltais F, *et al.* A randomized, double-blind, placebo-controlled study of lorazepam as premedication for bronchoscopy. *Chest* 1996; **109:** 1195–8.

Substance dependence. Lorazepam has been used in the management of symptoms of alcohol withdrawal (p.1131).
References.
1. D'Onofrio G, *et al.* Lorazepam for the prevention of recurrent seizures related to alcohol. *N Engl J Med* 1999; **340:** 915–9.

Preparations

BP 2001: Lorazepam Injection; Lorazepam Tablets;
USP 25: Lorazepam Injection; Lorazepam Oral Concentrate; Lorazepam Tablets.

Proprietary Preparations (details are given in Part 3)

Aust.: Ergocalm; Merlit; Temesta; *Austral.:* Ativan; *Belg.:* Loridem; Serenase; Temesta; Vigiten; *Braz.:* Anosedil; Calmogenol; Lorax; Lorium; Max-Pax; Mesmerin; *Canad.:* Ativan; Novo-Lorazem; Nu-Loraz; *Denm.:* Lorabenz; Temesta; *Fin.:* Temesta; *Fr.:* Equitam; Temesta; *Ger.:* duralozam; Laubeel; Pro Dorm†; Punktyl; Somagerol; Tavor; Tolid; *Hong Kong:* Ativan; Lorivan; *Irl.:* Ativan; *Israel:* Lorivan; *Ital.:* Control; Lorans; Quait†; Tavor; *Mex.:* Ativan; Sinestron; Tem. . . Nz Temesta; *NZ:* Ativan; Lorapam; Lorzem; *Port.:* Ansilor; Lorenin; Lorsedal; *S.Afr.:* Ativan; TranQil†; Tranqipam; *Singapore:* Ativan; Lorans; *Spain:* Divial†; Donix; Idalprem; Orfidal; Piralone†; Placinoral; Sedicepan; Sedizepan†; *Swed.:* Temesta; *Switz.:* Lorasifar; Temesta; *Thai.:* Anta; Anxira; Ativan; Lora; Loramed; Lorapam; Lorazene; Lorazep; Ora; *UK:* Ativan; *USA:* Ativan.

Multi-ingredient: *Aust.:* Somnium; *Switz.:* Somnium.

Lormetazepam (4077-r)

Lormetazepam *(BAN, USAN, rINN)*.

Wy-4082. (RS)-7-Chloro-5-(2-chlorophenyl)-1,3-dihydro-3-hydroxy-1-methyl-1,4-benzodiazepin-2-one.

$C_{16}H_{12}Cl_2N_2O_2 = 335.2$.

CAS — 848-75-9.
ATC — N05CD06.

Pharmacopoeias. In Br.

Pharmacopoeial description

BP 2001: A white crystalline powder. Practically insoluble in water; soluble in alcohol and in methyl alcohol. Protect from light.

Dependence and Withdrawal

As for Diazepam, p.675.

◊ For the purpose of withdrawal regimens, 0.5 to 1 mg of lormetazepam is considered roughly equivalent to 5 mg of diazepam.

Adverse Effects, Treatment, and Precautions

As for Diazepam, p.675.

Interactions

As for Diazepam, p.677.

Pharmacokinetics

Lormetazepam is rapidly absorbed from the gastrointestinal tract and metabolised to the inactive glucuronide. The terminal half-life is reported to be about 11 hours.

◊ A brief review of the pharmacokinetics of lormetazepam.[1]

1. Greenblatt DJ, *et al.* Clinical pharmacokinetics of the newer benzodiazepines. *Clin Pharmacokinet* 1983; **8**: 233–52.

Uses and Administration

Lormetazepam is a short-acting benzodiazepine with general properties similar to those of diazepam (p.680). It is mainly used as a hypnotic in the short-term management of insomnia (p.652) in usual doses of 0.5 to 1.5 mg by mouth at night. A dose of 500 µg is recommended for elderly or debilitated patients. Lormetazepam is also used in some countries for premedication (p.1256).

Preparations

BP 2001: Lormetazepam Tablets.

Proprietary Preparations (details are given in Part 3)
Aust.: Noctamid; *Belg.:* Loramet; Noctamid; Octonox; Stilaze; *Denm.:* Pronoctan; *Fr.:* Noctamide; *Ger.:* Ergocalm; Loretam; Noctamid; *Hong Kong:* Loramet; *Irl.:* Loramet; Noctamid; *Ital.:* Minias; *Neth.:* Loramet; Noctamid; *NZ:* Noctamid; *Port.:* Noctamid; *S.Afr.:* Loramet; Noctamid; *Singapore:* Loramet; *Spain:* Aldosomnil; Loramet; Noctamid; Sedobrina†; *Switz.:* Loramet; Noctamid; *Thai.:* Loramet.

Loxapine (7061-j)

Loxapine (BAN, USAN, rINN).
CL-62362; Oxilapine; SUM-3170. 2-Chloro-11-(4-methylpiperazin-1-yl)dibenz[b,f][1,4]oxazepine.
$C_{18}H_{18}ClN_3O = 327.8$.
CAS — 1977-10-2.
ATC — N05AH01.

Loxapine Hydrochloride (3843-l)

Loxapine Hydrochloride (BANM, rINNM).
$C_{18}H_{18}ClN_3O,HCl = 364.3$.

Loxapine hydrochloride 28 mg is approximately equivalent to 25 mg of loxapine.

Loxapine Succinate (7062-z)

Loxapine Succinate (BANM, USAN, rINNM).
CL-71563.
$C_{18}H_{18}ClN_3O,C_4H_6O_4 = 445.9$.
CAS — 27833-64-3.
Pharmacopoeias. In *US*.

Loxapine succinate 34 mg is equivalent to 25 mg of loxapine.

Pharmacopoeial description

USP 25: A white to yellowish, odourless, crystalline powder. Store in airtight containers.

Adverse Effects, Treatment, and Precautions

As for Chlorpromazine, p.660.

Other side-effects reported include nausea and vomiting, seborrhoea, dyspnoea, ptosis, headache, paraesthesia, flush, weight gain or loss, and polydipsia.

Abuse. A report of 3 cases of loxapine succinate abuse.[1]

1. Sperry L, *et al.* Loxapine abuse. *N Engl J Med* 1984; **310**: 598.

Effects on carbohydrate metabolism. Reversible nonketotic hyperglycaemia, coma, and delirium, developed in a patient receiving loxapine 150 mg daily in addition to lithium therapy.[1] Symptoms improved following discontinuation of loxapine, but subsequently recurred when the patient was given amoxapine. The causative agent may have been 7-hydroxyamoxapine, a common metabolite of both amoxapine and loxapine.

1. Tollefson G, Lesar T. Nonketotic hyperglycemia associated with loxapine and amoxapine: case report. *J Clin Psychiatry* 1983; **44**: 347–8.

Mania. A patient, initially diagnosed as suffering from schizophrenia, developed manic symptoms after receiving loxapine.[1] The diagnosis was revised to schizoaffective disorder but it was suspected that loxapine had a role in the emergence of the affective symptoms. As loxapine shares common metabolites with the antidepressant amoxapine it was suggested that an antidepressant effect might have been instrumental in the production of manic symptoms.

1. Gojer JAC. Possible manic side-effects of loxapine. *Can J Psychiatry* 1992; **37**: 669–70.

Overdosage. An 8-year-old child was treated with activated charcoal within 30 minutes of being given 375 mg of loxapine by accident.[1] The child became drowsy and was asleep but arousable one hour after ingestion. The degree of sedation appeared to reach peak after 3.75 hours and the child was discharged about 20 hours postingestion.

1. Tarricone NW. Loxitane overdose. *Pediatrics* 1998; **101**: 496.

Porphyria. Loxapine is considered to be unsafe in patients with porphyria because it has been shown to be porphyrinogenic in *in-vitro* systems.

Interactions

As for Chlorpromazine, p.664.

Pharmacokinetics

Loxapine is readily absorbed from the gastrointestinal tract. It is very rapidly and extensively metabolised and there is evidence for a first-pass effect. It is mainly excreted in the urine, in the form of its conjugated metabolites, with smaller amounts appearing in the faeces as unconjugated metabolites; a substantial proportion of a dose is excreted in the first 24 hours. The major metabolites of loxapine are the active 7- and 8-hydroxyloxapine, which are conjugated to the glucuronide or sulfate; other metabolites include hydroxyloxapine-*N*-oxide, loxapine-*N*-oxide, and hydroxydesmethylloxapine (hydroxyamoxapine). Loxapine is widely distributed and *animal* studies have indicated that it crosses the placenta and is distributed into breast milk.

Uses and Administration

Loxapine is a dibenzoxazepine with general properties similar to those of the phenothiazine, chlorpromazine (p.665). It is given by mouth as the hydrochloride or the succinate and by intramuscular injection as the hydrochloride in the treatment of psychoses, but doses are expressed in terms of the base.

The usual dose by mouth is 20 to 50 mg daily initially, in 2 divided doses, increased according to requirements over the next 7 to 10 days to 60 to 100 mg daily or more in 2 to 4 divided doses; the maximum recommended dose is 250 mg daily. Maintenance doses are usually in the range of 20 to 100 mg daily. For the control of acute conditions it is given by intramuscular injection in doses of 12.5 to 50 mg at intervals of 4 to 6 hours or longer.

Reduced dosage may be required in elderly patients.

Disturbed behaviour. For a discussion of the use and limitations of antipsychotics such as loxapine in patients with disturbed behaviour, see p.650.

References.
1. Carlyle W, *et al.* Aggression in the demented patient: a double-blind study of loxapine versus haloperidol. *Int J Clin Psychopharmacol* 1993; **8**: 103–8.

Schizophrenia. A brief review of loxapine[1] concluded that suggestions that loxapine was particularly effective in patients with paranoid schizophrenia (p.651) had not been confirmed. A subsequent systematic review considered that the limited evidence did not indicate a clear difference in its effects from other antipsychotics.[2]

1. Anonymous. Clozapine and loxapine for schizophrenia. *Drug Ther Bull* 1991; **29**: 41–2.
2. Fenton M, *et al.* Loxapine for schizophrenia (updated 26 January 2001). Available in The Cochrane Library; Issue 4. Oxford: Update Software; 2001.

Preparations

USP 25: Loxapine Capsules.

Proprietary Preparations (details are given in Part 3)
Belg.: Loxapac†; *Canad.:* Loxapac; *Denm.:* Loxapac; *Fr.:* Loxapac; *Irl.:* Loxapac; *NZ:* Loxapac; *Spain:* Desconex; *UK:* Loxapac; *USA:* Loxitane.

Magnesium Aspartate Hydrobromide (11439-d)

Magnesium L-aspartate hydrobromide trihydrate.

Profile

Magnesium aspartate hydrobromide has been used as a sedative but the use of bromides is generally deprecated.

Preparations

Proprietary Preparations (details are given in Part 3)
Ger.: Vernelan.

Medazepam (7064-k)

Medazepam (BAN, rINN).
Ro-5-4556 (medazepam hydrochloride). 7-Chloro-2,3-dihydro-1-methyl-5-phenyl-1*H*-1,4-benzodiazepine.
$C_{16}H_{15}ClN_2 = 270.8$.
CAS — 2898-12-6 (medazepam); 2898-11-5 (medazepam hydrochloride).
ATC — N05BA03.

NOTE. Medazepam Hydrochloride is *USAN*.
Pharmacopoeias. In *Jpn*.

Profile

Medazepam is a long-acting benzodiazepine with properties similar to those of diazepam (p.674). It is given by mouth for the short-term treatment of anxiety disorders (p.649) and disturbed behaviour (p.650).

A usual dose is 10 to 20 mg daily in divided doses; in severe conditions up to 60 mg daily has been given. Reduced doses should be given in elderly or debilitated patients.

Preparations

Proprietary Preparations (details are given in Part 3)
Ger.: Rudotel; *Neth.:* Nobrium†.

Multi-ingredient: *Ital.:* Debrum; *Spain:* Nobritol.

Medetomidine Hydrochloride (2813-r)

Medetomidine Hydrochloride (BANM, USAN, rINNM).
MPV-785. (±)-4-[1-(2,3-Xylyl)ethyl]imidazole monohydrochloride.
$C_{13}H_{16}N_2,HCl = 236.7$.
CAS — 86347-15-1 (medetomidine hydrochloride); 86347-14-0 (medetomidine).

Profile

Medetomidine is an α_2-adrenoceptor agonist with sedative, muscle relaxant, and analgesic properties. It is used as the hydrochloride in veterinary medicine.

Dexmedetomidine (p.674) is used as the hydrochloride in intensive care.

Melperone Hydrochloride (7150-z)

Melperone Hydrochloride (BANM, rINNM).
FG-5111; Flubuperone Hydrochloride; Methylperone Hydrochloride. 4′-Fluoro-4-(4-methylpiperidino)butyrophenone hydrochloride.
$C_{16}H_{22}FNO,HCl = 299.8$.
CAS — 3575-80-2 (melperone); 1622-79-3 (melperone hydrochloride).

Profile

Melperone is a butyrophenone with general properties similar to those of haloperidol (p.686). It is given as the hydrochloride by mouth or by intramuscular injection for the management of psychoses such as schizophrenia (p.651) and in disturbed behaviour (p.650); doses are expressed as the hydrochloride. A usual dose by mouth is up to 400 mg daily in divided doses. In acute conditions it may be given intramuscularly in doses of 25 to 100 mg repeated to a usual maximum of 200 mg daily.

Cardiac arrhythmias. Melperone has been reported to have class III electrophysiologic and antiarrhythmic activity[1,2] but its clinical use as an antiarrhythmic would be limited by a high incidence of adverse effects.[2] For a discussion of the cardiovascular effects of antipsychotics in general, see under Chlorpromazine, p.661.

1. Møgelvang JC, *et al.* Antiarrhythmic properties of a neuroleptic butyrophenone, melperone, in acute myocardial infarction. *Acta Med Scand* 1980; **208**: 61–4.
2. Hui WKK, *et al.* Melperone: electrophysiologic and antiarrhythmic activity in humans. *J Cardiovasc Pharmacol* 1990; **15**: 144–9.

Pharmacokinetics. References.
1. Köppel C, *et al.* Gas chromatographic-mass spectrometric study of urinary metabolism of melperone. *J Chromatogr Biomed Appl* 1988; **427**: 144–50.

Preparations

Proprietary Preparations (details are given in Part 3)
Aust.: Buronil; Neuril; *Belg.:* Buronil; *Denm.:* Buronil; *Fin.:* Buronil; Melpax; *Ger.:* Eunerpan; Harmosin; Mel-Puren; Melneurin; Melperomerck; *Norw.:* Buronil; *Port.:* Bunil; *Swed.:* Buronil.

Mephenoxalone (7065-a)

Mephenoxalone (rINN).
AHR-233; Methoxadone; OM-518. 5-(2-Methoxyphenoxymethyl)oxazolidin-2-one.
$C_{11}H_{13}NO_4 = 223.2$.
CAS — 70-07-5.
ATC — N05BX01.

Profile

Mephenoxalone has actions similar to those of meprobamate (below). It has been given by mouth in a dose of 400 mg three times daily as a muscle relaxant in the treatment of muscle spasm (p.1322). It has also been given for the treatment of anxiety.

Preparations

Proprietary Preparations (details are given in Part 3)
Neth.: Dorsiflex; *Switz.:* Control†.

Multi-ingredient: *Switz.:* Dorsilon†.

Meprobamate (7066-t)

Meprobamate (BAN, rINN).

Meprobamatum; Meprotanum. 2-Methyl-2-propyltrimethylene dicarbamate.

$C_9H_{18}N_2O_4 = 218.3$.

CAS — 57-53-4.

ATC — N05BC01.

Pharmacopoeias. In Chin., Eur. (see p.vi), and US.

Pharmacopoeial description

Ph. Eur.: A white or almost white, crystalline or amorphous powder. Slightly soluble in water and in ether; freely soluble in alcohol.

USP 25: A white powder having a characteristic odour. Slightly soluble in water; freely soluble in alcohol and in acetone; practically insoluble or insoluble in ether. Store in airtight containers.

Dependence and Withdrawal

As for the barbiturates (see Amobarbital, p.655).

Adverse Effects and Treatment

Drowsiness is the most frequent side-effect of meprobamate. Other effects include nausea, vomiting, diarrhoea, paraesthesia, weakness, and CNS effects such as headache, paradoxical excitement, dizziness, ataxia, and disturbances of vision. There may be hypotension, tachycardia, and cardiac arrhythmias. Hypersensitivity reactions occur occasionally. These may be limited to skin rashes, urticaria, and purpura or may be more severe with angioedema, bronchospasm, or anuria. Erythema multiforme or Stevens-Johnson syndrome, and exfoliative or bullous dermatitis have been reported.

Blood disorders including agranulocytosis, eosinophilia, leucopenia, thrombocytopenia, and aplastic anaemia have occasionally been reported.

Overdosage with meprobamate produces symptoms similar to those of barbiturate overdosage (see Amobarbital, p.655), and is managed similarly.

Overdosage. Two children aged 2 and 2.5 years recovered with conservative management alone following overdosage of meprobamate with bendrofluazide [bendroflumethiazide] despite measured plasma-meprobamate concentrations of 170 and 158 μg per mL respectively.[1] Although recommendations advise that haemoperfusion should be considered at plasma-meprobamate concentrations above 100 μg per mL, the authors considered that experience with adults suggested haemoperfusion should normally only be considered at plasma concentrations above 200 μg per mL.

1. Dennison J, et al. Meprobamate overdosage. Hum Toxicol 1985; **4:** 215–17.

Precautions

Meprobamate should be used with caution in patients with impaired hepatic or renal function, depression, muscle weakness, and, as with all sedatives, in patients with impaired respiratory function. Meprobamate should be given with care to elderly or debilitated patients. Meprobamate may induce seizures in patients with a history of epilepsy.

Meprobamate may cause drowsiness; affected patients should not drive or operate machinery.

The use of meprobamate should be avoided in breast feeding mothers as concentrations in milk may exceed maternal plasma concentrations fourfold and may cause drowsiness in the infant.

Porphyria. Meprobamate has been associated with acute attacks of porphyria and is considered unsafe in porphyric patients.

Pregnancy. Studies on the use of meprobamate during pregnancy.

1. Milkovich L, van den Berg BJ. Effects of prenatal meprobamate and chlordiazepoxide hydrochloride on human embryonic and fetal development. N Engl J Med 1974; **291:** 1268–71.
2. Crombie DL, et al. Fetal effects of tranquilizers in pregnancy. N Engl J Med 1975; **293:** 198–9.
3. Hartz SC, et al. Antenatal exposure to meprobamate and chlordiazepoxide in relation to malformations, mental development, and childhood mortality. N Engl J Med 1975; **292:** 726–8.

Interactions

The sedative effects of meprobamate are enhanced by CNS depressants including alcohol. Meprobamate is capable of inducing hepatic microsomal enzyme systems involved in drug metabolism: the metabolism of other drugs may be enhanced if given concurrently.

Pharmacokinetics

Meprobamate is readily absorbed from the gastrointestinal tract and peak plasma concentrations occur 1 to 3 hours after ingestion. Meprobamate is widely distributed. It is extensively metabolised in the liver and is excreted in the urine mainly as an inactive hydroxylated metabolite and its glucuronide conjugate. About 10% of a dose is excreted unchanged. Meprobamate has a half-life reported to range from about 6 to 17 hours, although this may be prolonged after chronic administration.

It diffuses across the placenta and appears in breast milk at concentrations of up to 4 times those in the maternal plasma.

Uses and Administration

Meprobamate is a carbamate with hypnotic, sedative, and some muscle relaxant properties, although in therapeutic doses its sedative effect rather than a direct action may be responsible for muscle relaxation. It has been used in the short-term treatment of anxiety disorders (p.649) and also for the short-term management of insomnia (p.652) but has largely been superseded by other drugs. Meprobamate has sometimes been used, alone or in combination with an analgesic, in the management of muscle spasm (p.1322) and painful musculoskeletal disorders but such use is no longer considered appropriate.

The usual anxiolytic dose is 400 mg by mouth three or four times daily to a maximum of 2.4 g daily. In elderly patients, no more than half the usual adult dose has been suggested.

Preparations

USP 25: Meprobamate Oral Suspension; Meprobamate Tablets.

Proprietary Preparations (details are given in Part 3)
Aust.: Cyrpon; Epikur; Microbamat; Miltaun; Pertranquil; *Austral.:* Equanil†; *Belg.:* Pertranquil; Procalmadiol†; Reposo-Mono; Sanobamat†; *Canad.:* Equanil; Novo-Mepro†; *Fr.:* Equanil; Norgagil†; Novalm†; *Ger.:* Visano N; Visano-mini N; *Israel:* Mepro; *Ital.:* Quanil; *S.Afr.:* Equanil; *Spain:* Dapaz; Oasil Simes†; *Swed.:* Restenil†; *Switz.:* Meprodil; *UK:* Equanil†; Meprate; *USA:* Equanil; MB-Tab†; Meprospan†; Miltown; Neuramate.

Multi-ingredient: *Belg.:* Spasmosedine†; *Canad.:* 282 Mep; Equagesic†; *Fin.:* Anervan; Crampiton; Potentol; *Fr.:* Kaologeais; Meprorinine; Palpipax; Precyclan; *Norw.:* Anervan; *Port.:* Vitasma; *S.Afr.:* Acugesil†; Antipyn Forte; Ban Pain; Briscopyn†; Dimiprol†; Dynapayne; Equagesic†; Go-Pain; Maxadol Forte; Megapyn; Meprogesic; Mepromol; Nopyn; Noralget; Painagon; Painrite†; Pynmed; Salterpyn; Scriptogesic†; Spectrapain Forte; Stilpane; Stopayne; Supragesic; Synaleve; Tenston; Trinagesic; Vacudol Forte; Xeramax; Xerogesic; *Swed.:* Anervan; *UK:* Equagesic; Paxidal; *USA:* Epromate†; Equagesic; Equazine M†; Micrainin; PMB†.

Mesoridazine Besilate (7067-x)

Mesoridazine Besilate (BANM, rINNM).

Mesoridazine Benzenesulphonate; Mesoridazine Besylate; Mesuridazine Benzenesulphonate; NC-123 (mesoridazine); TPS-23 (mesoridazine). 10-[2-(1-Methyl-2-piperidyl)ethyl]-2-(methylsulphinyl)phenothiazine benzenesulphonate.

$C_{21}H_{26}N_2OS_2,C_6H_6O_3S = 544.7$.

CAS — 5588-33-0 (mesoridazine); 32672-69-8 (mesoridazine besilate).

NOTE. Mesoridazine is USAN.

Pharmacopoeias. In US.

Pharmacopoeial description

USP 25: A white to pale yellowish powder having not more than a faint odour. Soluble 1 in 1 of water, 1 in 11 of alcohol, 1 in 3 of chloroform, and 1 in 6300 of ether; freely soluble in methyl alcohol. pH of a freshly prepared 1 in 100 solution is between 4.2 and 5.7. Store in airtight containers. Protect from light.

Adverse Effects, Treatment, and Precautions

As for Chlorpromazine, p.660. Mesoridazine has been shown to prolong the QT interval in a dose-related manner which increases the risk of life-threatening arrhythmias such as torsade de pointes and sudden death; consequently its use has been restricted. Details of these restrictions are given under Precautions of Thioridazine, the parent drug of mesoridazine (see p.708).

For all patients starting mesoridazine it is recommended that a baseline ECG and potassium screening are performed. These tests should also be repeated periodically, especially during periods of dosage adjustment.

Interactions

As for Chlorpromazine, p.664. Concomitant use of mesoridazine with other drugs known to prolong the QT interval is contra-indicated.

Pharmacokinetics

Mesoridazine is a metabolite of thioridazine (p.708).

Uses and Administration

Mesoridazine is a phenothiazine with general properties similar to those of chlorpromazine (p.665). It has a piperidine side-chain and is a metabolite of thioridazine (p.708).

The use of mesoridazine is restricted to the treatment of schizophrenia (p.651) in patients who fail to show an adequate response to treatment with other antipsychotics. Its use in other psychiatric disorders was abandoned after it was felt that there was an unacceptable balance of risks and benefits as a result of its cardiotoxic potential.

For all patients starting mesoridazine it is recommended that a baseline ECG and potassium screening are performed. These tests should also be repeated periodically, especially during periods of dosage adjustment. Mesoridazine is usually given as the besilate but the doses are expressed in terms of the base.

The usual initial dose for the treatment of schizophrenia is 50 mg three times daily by mouth; doses may be adjusted to 100 to 400 mg daily according to response.

Mesoridazine may be given intramuscularly in an initial dose of 25 mg repeated after 30 to 60 minutes if necessary; up to 200 mg daily has been given.

Preparations

USP 25: Mesoridazine Besylate Injection; Mesoridazine Besylate Oral Solution; Mesoridazine Besylate Tablets.

Proprietary Preparations (details are given in Part 3)
Canad.: Serentil; *USA:* Serentil.

Metaclazepam Hydrochloride (19474-r)

Metaclazepam Hydrochloride (rINNM).

Brometazepam Hydrochloride; Ka-2547 (metaclazepam); KC-2547 (metaclazepam). 7-Bromo-5-(2-chlorophenyl)-2,3-dihydro-2-(methoxymethyl)-1-methyl-1H-1,4-benzodiazepine hydrochloride.

$C_{18}H_{18}BrClN_2O,HCl = 430.2$.

CAS — 65517-27-3 (metaclazepam).

Profile

Metaclazepam is a short-acting benzodiazepine with general properties similar to those of diazepam (p.674). It has been given by mouth as the hydrochloride for the short-term treatment of anxiety disorders.

Preparations

Proprietary Preparations (details are given in Part 3)
Ger.: Talis†.

Methaqualone (4045-y)

Methaqualone (BAN, USAN, rINN).

CI-705; CN-38703; Methachalonum; Methaqualonum; QZ-2; R-148; TR-495. 2-Methyl-3-o-tolylquinazolin-4-(3H)-one.

$C_{16}H_{14}N_2O = 250.3$.

CAS — 72-44-6 (methaqualone); 340-56-7 (methaqualone hydrochloride).

ATC — N05CM01.

Pharmacopoeias. In Eur. (see p.vi).

Pharmacopoeial description

Ph. Eur.: A white or almost white, crystalline powder. Very slightly soluble in water; soluble in alcohol; sparingly soluble in ether; dissolves in dilute sulfuric acid. Protect from light.

Profile

Methaqualone is a quinazoline derivative with hypnotic and sedative properties. It has been given by mouth in the short-term management of insomnia but the use of methaqualone for this purpose is no longer considered appropriate. It was also given with diphenhydramine for an enhanced effect.

Methaqualone has been withdrawn from the market in many countries because of problems with abuse.

Adverse effects and symptoms of overdosage are similar to those of barbiturates (see Amobarbital, p.655) although cardiac and respiratory depression reportedly occur less frequently.

Preparations

Proprietary Preparations (details are given in Part 3)
Spain: Pallidan†.

Multi-ingredient: *Switz.:* Toquilone compositum.

Methotrimeprazine (7068-r)

Methotrimeprazine (BAN, USAN).

Levomepromazine (BAN, rINN); CL-36467; CL-39743; RP-7044; SKF-5116. (−)-NN-Dimethyl-3-(2-methoxyphenothiazin-10-yl)-2-methylpropylamine; 3-(2-Methoxyphenothiazin-10-yl)-2-methylpropyldimethylamine.

$C_{19}H_{24}N_2OS = 328.5$.

CAS — 60-99-1.

ATC — N05AA02.

Pharmacopoeias. In US. Also in BP(Vet).

Pharmacopoeial description

BP(Vet) 2001: A white or slightly cream-coloured odourless or almost odourless crystalline powder. Practically insoluble in water; slightly soluble in alcohol; freely soluble in chloroform and in ether. Protect from light.

USP 25: A fine white, practically odourless, crystalline powder. Soluble 1 in 10 of water, of alcohol, and of methyl alcohol, and 1 in 2 of chloroform; freely soluble in ether; sparingly soluble in alcohol at 25° but freely soluble in boiling alcohol. Protect from light.

Methotrimeprazine Hydrochloride (7069-f)

Methotrimeprazine Hydrochloride (BANM).

Levomepromazine Hydrochloride (BANM, rINNM); Levomepromazini Hydrochloridum.

$C_{19}H_{24}N_2OS,HCl = 364.9$.

CAS — 4185-80-2.

Pharmacopoeias. In Eur. (see p.vi).

Methotrimeprazine [levomepromazine] hydrochloride 1.11 g is approximately equivalent to 1 g of methotrimeprazine [levomepromazine].

Methotrimeprazine [levomepromazine] hydrochloride is reported to be incompatible with alkaline solutions.

Pharmacopoeial description

Ph. Eur.: A white or very slightly yellow, slightly hygroscopic crystalline powder. It deteriorates on exposure to air and light. Freely soluble in water and in alcohol; practically insoluble in ether. Store in airtight containers. Protect from light.

Methotrimeprazine Maleate (7070-z)

Methotrimeprazine Maleate (BANM).
Levomepromazine Maleate (BANM, rINNM); Levomepromazini Maleas; Methotrimeprazine Hydrogen Maleate.
$C_{19}H_{24}N_2OS,C_4H_4O_4 = 444.5$.
CAS — 7104-38-3.
Pharmacopoeias. In Eur. (see p.vi), Jpn, and Pol.

Methotrimeprazine [levomepromazine] maleate 1.35 g is approximately equivalent to 1 g of methotrimeprazine [levomepromazine].

Pharmacopoeial description

Ph. Eur.: A white or slightly yellowish crystalline powder. It deteriorates when exposed to air and light. Slightly soluble in water and in alcohol; sparingly soluble in dichloromethane; practically insoluble in ether. The supernatant of a 2% dispersion in water has a pH of 3.5 to 5.5. Protect from light.

Adverse Effects, Treatment, and Precautions

As for Chlorpromazine, p.660, although it may be more sedating. See also the sedating antihistamines, p.404.

Methotrimeprazine [levomepromazine] may cause severe postural hypotension therefore patients receiving large initial doses, patients over 50 years of age, or those receiving injections, should be recumbent. Children are very susceptible to the hypotensive and sedative effects of methotrimeprazine [levomepromazine].

Interactions

As for Chlorpromazine, p.664.

Antidepressants. Although MAOIs have been used with phenothiazines without untoward effects the concomitant use of methotrimeprazine [levomepromazine] and MAOIs should probably be avoided as this combination has been implicated in 2 fatalities.[1,2]

1. Barsa JA, Saunders JC. A comparative study of tranylcypromine and pargyline. Psychopharmacologia 1964; 6: 295–8.
2. McQueen EG. New Zealand committee on adverse drug reactions: fourteenth annual report 1979. N Z Med J 1980; 91: 226–9.

Pharmacokinetics

◊ In a study involving a total of 5 psychiatric patients peak plasma concentrations of methotrimeprazine [levomepromazine] were noted 1 to 4 hours after administration by mouth and 30 to 90 minutes after injection into the gluteal muscle.[1] About 50% of orally administered drug reached the systemic circulation. Although the metabolite methotrimeprazine sulfoxide could not be detected after a single intramuscular injection it was found in concentrations higher than unmetabolised methotrimeprazine after single and multiple oral dosage, both substances reaching a steady state in the plasma within 7 days of starting multiple dose oral therapy. Fluctuations in plasma concentration during multiple dose oral therapy indicated that until the correlation between acute side-effects and peak plasma concentration of methotrimeprazine had been further studied the total daily dose should be divided into 2 or 3 portions when larger doses of methotrimeprazine were given by mouth.

1. Dahl SG. Pharmacokinetics of methotrimeprazine after single and multiple doses. Clin Pharmacol Ther 1976; 19: 435–42.

Half-life. In 8 psychiatric patients given methotrimeprazine [levomepromazine] 50 to 350 mg daily the plasma half-life showed wide variation, from 16.5 to 77.8 hours, and did not correlate with the dose given.[1]

1. Dahl SG, et al. Pharmacokinetics and relative bioavailability of levomepromazine after repeated administration of tablets and syrup. Eur J Clin Pharmacol 1977; 11: 305–310.

Uses and Administration

Methotrimeprazine [levomepromazine] is a phenothiazine with pharmacological activity similar to that of both chlorpromazine (p.665) and promethazine (p.424). It has antihistaminic actions (p.404) together with CNS effects resembling those of chlorpromazine. It is also reported to have analgesic activity. It is used in the treatment of various psychoses including schizophrenia (p.651), as an analgesic for moderate to severe pain usually in non-ambulatory patients, and for premedication (p.1256). It is also used for the control of symptoms such as restlessness, agitation, and vomiting and as an adjunct to opioid analgesia in terminally ill patients.

Methotrimeprazine [levomepromazine] is also used in veterinary medicine.

Methotrimeprazine [levomepromazine] is given by mouth as the maleate or by injection as the hydrochloride; the embonate has also been used. Care is required in elderly patients because of the risk of severe hypotension; if methotrimeprazine [levomepromazine] is given to such patients reduced doses may be necessary.

The usual initial dose of methotrimeprazine [levomepromazine] maleate for the treatment of **schizophrenia** is 25 to 50 mg by mouth; the daily dosage is usually divided into 3 portions with a larger portion taken at night. Doses of 100 to 200 mg have been given to non-ambulant patients increased gradually up to 1 g daily if necessary. Children are very susceptible to the hypotensive and sedative effects of methotrimeprazine [levomepromazine]: a suggested dose for a 10-year-old is 12.5 to 25 mg of the maleate daily in divided doses by mouth; a dose of 37.5 mg daily should not be exceeded. For the management of **nausea and vomiting** in palliative care methotrimeprazine [levomepromazine] maleate 12.5 to 25 mg may be given by mouth where first-line antiemetics have proved inadequate.

As an adjunct to analgesics in the management of severe terminal **pain**, methotrimeprazine [levomepromazine] maleate is given by mouth in a dose of 12.5 to 50 mg every 4 to 8 hours. Alternatively 12.5 to 25 mg of methotrimeprazine [levomepromazine] hydrochloride may be given intramuscularly every 6 or 8 hours but patients should remain in bed for at least the first few doses; doses of up to 50 mg have been given for severe agitation. Methotrimeprazine [levomepromazine] hydrochloride may also be given intravenously in similar doses following dilution with an equal volume of sodium chloride 0.9% injection. Alternatively it may be given, suitably diluted with sodium chloride 0.9% injection, by continuous subcutaneous infusion via a syringe driver, in doses ranging from a total of 25 to 200 mg daily although lower doses of 5 to 25 mg daily may also be effective against nausea and vomiting and produce less sedation. Experience with parenteral administration of methotrimeprazine [levomepromazine] hydrochloride in children is limited but a dose of 0.35 to 3 mg per kg body-weight daily has been suggested.

A dose of 10 to 20 mg of methotrimeprazine [levomepromazine] hydrochloride given intramuscularly every 4 to 6 hours adjusted as required has been used for the control of acute pain. If used for postoperative analgesia an initial intramuscular dose of 2.5 to 7.5 mg has been given.

Methotrimeprazine [levomepromazine] hydrochloride has also been given as a **premedicant** in doses ranging from 2 to 20 mg administered intramuscularly 45 minutes to 3 hours prior to surgical procedures.

Pain. As methotrimeprazine [levomepromazine] appears to possess intrinsic analgesic activity in addition to its antiemetic and antipsychotic actions it has been used for the symptomatic control of restlessness and vomiting and as an adjunct to opioid analgesics in pain control (p.2) in terminally ill patients.

References.

1. Oliver DJ. The use of methotrimeprazine in terminal care. Br J Clin Pract 1985; 39: 339–40.
2. Patt RB, et al. The neuroleptics as adjuvant analgesics. J Pain Symptom Manage 1994; 9: 446–53.
3. O'Neill J, Fountain A. Levomepromazine (methotrimeprazine) and the last 48 hours. Hosp Med 1999; 60: 564–7.
4. Skinner J, Skinner A. Levomepromazine for nausea and vomiting in advanced cancer. Hosp Med 1999; 60: 568–70.

HEADACHE. Similarly to chlorpromazine (p.666) and prochlorperazine (p.702), methotrimeprazine [levomepromazine][1] has been effective in relieving the pain of severe migraine attacks.

1. Stiell IG, et al. Methotrimeprazine versus meperidine and dimenhydrinate in the treatment of severe migraine: a randomized, controlled trial. Ann Emerg Med 1991; 20: 1201–5.

Preparations

USP 25: Methotrimeprazine Injection.

Proprietary Preparations (details are given in Part 3)
Aust.: Nozinan; **Belg.:** Nozinan; **Braz.:** Levozine; Neozine; **Canad.:** Novo-Meprazine; Nozinan; **Denm.:** Nozinan; **Fin.:** Levozin; **Fr.:** Nozinan; **Ger.:** Levium; Neurocil; Tisercin†; **Irl.:** Nozinan; **Israel:** Nozinane; Nozinan; **Ital.:** Nozinan; **Mex.:** Levocina; Sinogan; **Neth.:** Nozinan; **Norw.:** Nozinan; **NZ:** Nozinan; **Port.:** Nozinan; **Spain:** Sinogan; **Swed.:** Nozinan; **Switz.:** Minozinan†; Nozinan; **UK:** Nozinan; **USA:** Levoprome.

Methylpentynol (4048-c)

Methylpentynol (BAN, rINN).
Meparfynol; Methylparafynol. 3-Methylpent-1-yn-3-ol.
$C_6H_{10}O = 98.14$.
CAS — 77-75-8.
ATC — N05CM15.

Profile

Methylpentynol is a hypnotic and sedative. It has been given by mouth as a hypnotic in the short-term management of insomnia.

Preparations

Proprietary Preparations (details are given in Part 3)
Switz.: Oblivon†.

Mexazolam (16895-a)

Mexazolam (rINN).
CS-386; Methylcloxazolam. 10-Chloro-11b-(2-chlorophenyl)-2,3,7,11b-tetrahydro-3-methyloxazolo[3,2-d][1,4]benzodiazepin-6(5H)-one.
$C_{18}H_{16}Cl_2N_2O_2 = 363.2$.
CAS — 31868-18-5.

Profile

Mexazolam is a benzodiazepine with general properties similar to those of diazepam (p.674). It has been given by mouth for its anxiolytic and sedative properties.

Preparations

Proprietary Preparations (details are given in Part 3)
Jpn: Melex†; **Port.:** Sedoxil.

Midazolam (13499-v)

Midazolam (BAN, rINN).
Midazolamum; Ro-21-3971. 8-Chloro-6-(2-fluorophenyl)-1-methyl-4H-imidazo[1,5-a][1,4]benzodiazepine.
$C_{18}H_{13}ClFN_3 = 325.8$.
CAS — 59467-70-8.
ATC — N05CD08.
Pharmacopoeias. In Eur. (see p.vi).

Pharmacopoeial description

Ph. Eur.: A white or yellowish crystalline powder. Practically insoluble in water; freely soluble in alcohol and in acetone; soluble in methyl alcohol. Protect from light.

Midazolam Hydrochloride (12958-p)

Midazolam Hydrochloride (BANM, USAN, rINNM).
Ro-21-3981/003.
$C_{18}H_{13}ClFN_3,HCl = 362.2$.
CAS — 59467-96-8.

Incompatibility. The visual compatibility of midazolam hydrochloride with a range of drugs was studied over a period of 4 hours.[1] A white precipitate was formed immediately with dimenhydrinate, pentobarbital sodium, perphenazine, prochlorperazine edisilate, and ranitidine hydrochloride. Similar incompatibility has been reported[2,3] with frusemide [furosemide], thiopental, and parenteral nutrition solutions. Other workers[4] have reported that a precipitate is formed with midazolam hydrochloride if the resultant mixture has a pH of 5 or more.

1. Forman JK, Souney PF. Visual compatibility of midazolam hydrochloride with common preoperative injectable medications. Am J Hosp Pharm 1987; 44: 2298–9.
2. Chiu MF, Schwartz ML. Visual compatibility of injectable drugs used in the intensive care unit. Am J Health-Syst Pharm 1997; 54: 64–5.
3. Trissel LA, et al. Compatibility of parenteral nutrient solutions with selected drugs during simulated Y-site administration. Am J Health-Syst Pharm 1997; 54: 1295–300.
4. Swart EL, et al. Compatibility of midazolam hydrochloride and lorazepam with selected drugs during simulated Y-site administration. Am J Health-Syst Pharm 1995; 52: 2020–2.

Stability. The manufacturers have stated that solutions of midazolam hydrochloride in sodium chloride 0.9% or glucose 5% are stable at room temperature for up to 24 hours. However, one group of workers[1] has reported that similar solutions containing midazolam hydrochloride equivalent to 0.5 mg per mL of the base were stable for 36 days when stored in glass bottles at temperatures of 4 to 6°, 24 to 26°, and 39 to 41°. Other workers[2] found that a solution containing midazolam hydrochloride equivalent to 1 mg per mL of the base in sodium chloride 0.9% was stable for at least 10 days when stored in PVC bags. The manufacturer advises against admixture with Compound Sodium Lactate Intravenous Infusion (Hartmann's solution) as the potency of midazolam is reduced.

1. Pramar YV, *et al.* Stability of midazolam hydrochloride in syringes and i.v. fluids. *Am J Health-Syst Pharm* 1997; **54**: 913–15.
2. McMullin ST, *et al.* Stability of midazolam hydrochloride in polyvinyl chloride bags under fluorescent light. *Am J Health-Syst Pharm* 1995; **52**: 2018–20.

Midazolam Maleate (15125-j)

Midazolam Maleate *(BANM, USAN, rINNM)*.
Ro-21-3981/001.
$C_{18}H_{13}ClFN_3,C_4H_4O_4 = 441.8$.
CAS — 59467-94-6.

Dependence and Withdrawal

As for Diazepam, p.675.

◊ Details have been reported[1] of 2 children who developed withdrawal symptoms following discontinuation of midazolam, which had been used for sedation during mechanical ventilation.

1. van Engelen BGM, *et al.* Benzodiazepine withdrawal reaction in two children following discontinuation of sedation with midazolam. *Ann Pharmacother* 1993; **27**: 579–81.

Adverse Effects, Treatment, and Precautions

As for Diazepam, p.675. There have been reports of life-threatening adverse respiratory and cardiovascular events occurring after administration of midazolam; when giving midazolam the precautions given below should be observed to lessen the risk of such reactions. Pain, tenderness, and thrombophlebitis have occurred following injection of midazolam. Hiccups have been reported.

◊ There has been concern over reports of death due to respiratory depression, hypotension, or cardiac arrest in patients given intravenous midazolam for conscious sedation.[1] Within about 6 months of its introduction in the USA in May 1986, 13 fatalities due to cardiorespiratory depression had been reported, although higher doses were used initially than in the UK. By January 1988, 66 deaths had been reported, although in November 1987 the adult dosage recommendation had been reduced to 70 µg per kg body-weight and to 50 µg per kg for elderly patients. Fatalities have also occurred in the UK [where the dose is 70 µg per kg, reduced in the elderly], 4 deaths having been reported to the UK Committee on Safety of Medicines by November 1987.
While it appears that midazolam and diazepam produce very similar degrees of hypoventilation and oxygen desaturation when used in equivalent doses,[2] the sedative end-point does appear to be reached more abruptly with midazolam.[3]
Facilities for resuscitation should always be available when intravenous midazolam is used, and respiratory and cardiac function monitored continuously. The dose of midazolam should be carefully titrated against the response of the patient and the manufacturer's recommendations concerning speed of administration be observed. Particular care, including a reduction in midazolam dosage, is required in patients also receiving opioid analgesics, in the elderly and children, and in patients with compromised cardiorespiratory function. Similar warnings apply to the use of oral midazolam where it is available.
The availability of the benzodiazepine antagonist, flumazenil, should not be an encouragement to use larger doses of midazolam.[1]
Since endoscopy of the upper gastrointestinal tract can itself reduce oxygen saturation, some workers have advocated the prophylactic administration of nasal oxygen during this procedure for those patients at particular risk as outlined above.

1. Anonymous. Midazolam—is antagonism justified? *Lancet* 1988; **ii**: 140–2.
2. Bell GD. Review article: premedication and intravenous sedation for upper gastrointestinal endoscopy. *Aliment Pharmacol Ther* 1990; **4**: 103–22.
3. Ryder W, Wright PA. Dental sedation: a review. *Br Dent J* 1988; **165**: 207–16.

Children. Administration of an intravenous bolus injection of midazolam to children already receiving intravenous morphine after cardiac surgery produced an undesirable transient fall in cardiac output.[1] It was suggested that for patients already receiving other drugs which provide sedation the use of midazolam in the early postoperative period should be limited to a continuous infusion. Similarly, it has been recommended[2] that bolus intravenous administration of midazolam should be avoided in neonates due to the occurrence of hypotension.
The initial dosage of midazolam used for continuous intravenous sedation may need to be reduced in critically ill children under 3 years of age since the plasma clearance of midazolam appears to be reduced in these patients.[3]

1. Shekerdemian L, *et al.* Cardiovascular effects of intravenous midazolam after open heart surgery. *Arch Dis Child* 1997; **76**: 57–61.
2. Jacqz-Aigrain E, Burtin P. Clinical pharmacokinetics of sedatives in neonates. *Clin Pharmacokinet* 1996; **31**: 423–43.
3. Hughes J, *et al.* Steady-state plasma concentrations of midazolam in critically ill infants and children. *Ann Pharmacother* 1996; **30**: 27–30.

Effects on mental function. For discussion of the adverse effects of benzodiazepines on mental function, including reports of sexual fantasies in women sedated with intravenous midazolam, see Diazepam, p.675.

Effects on the nervous system. For reference to acute dystonia associated with administration of midazolam, see Diazepam, p.675.

ENCEPHALOPATHY. For a report of prolonged use of midazolam with fentanyl being associated with encephalopathy in infants sedated under intensive care, see Diazepam, p.676.

MYOCLONUS. Myoclonic twitching of all four limbs was noted[1] in 6 of 102 neonates who received a continuous intravenous infusion of midazolam at a rate of 30 to 60 µg per kg bodyweight per hour. Myoclonus ceased a few hours after discontinuing the infusion and never recurred. No ictal activity was detected in EEGs recorded during the myoclonus.

1. Magny JF, *et al.* Midazolam and myoclonus in neonate. *Eur J Pediatr* 1994; **153**: 389–90.

The elderly. Sedation with midazolam in elderly volunteers was achieved at approximately half the dose necessary to produce comparable effects in younger subjects.[1] Pharmacodynamic differences due to age suggested an increase in sensitivity of the CNS to midazolam in the elderly subjects.

1. Albrecht S, *et al.* The effect of age on the pharmacokinetics and pharmacodynamics of midazolam. *Clin Pharmacol Ther* 1999; **65**: 630–9.

Hepatic impairment. For the precautions to be observed in patients with impaired liver function, see under Pharmacokinetics, below.

Renal impairment. Five patients with severe renal impairment experienced prolonged sedation when given midazolam; this was attributed to accumulation of conjugated metabolites.[1]

1. Bauer TM, *et al.* Prolonged sedation due to accumulation of conjugated metabolites of midazolam. *Lancet* 1995; **346**: 145–7.

Interactions

As for Diazepam, p.677.

Pharmacokinetics

Absorption of midazolam is rapid, peak plasma concentrations being achieved within 20 to 60 minutes of administration depending on the route. Extensive first-pass metabolism results in a low systemic bioavailability after oral administration. Bioavailability is higher, but variable, after intramuscular injection; figures of more than 90% are often cited.

Midazolam is lipophilic at physiological pH. It crosses the placenta and is distributed into breast milk (but see below). Midazolam is about 96% bound to plasma proteins.

Midazolam usually has a short elimination half-life of about 2 hours although half-lives longer than 7 hours have been reported in some patients. The half-life of midazolam is prolonged in neonates, in the elderly, and in patients with liver disorders.

Midazolam is metabolised in the liver. The major metabolite, 1-hydroxymethylmidazolam, is less active than midazolam; its half-life is similar to that of midazolam. Midazolam metabolites are excreted in the urine, mainly as glucuronide conjugates.

◊ Reviews.

1. Garzone PD, Kroboth PD. Pharmacokinetics of the newer benzodiazepines. *Clin Pharmacokinet* 1989; **16**: 337–64.

Children. A study of the pharmacokinetics of midazolam in children.[1] Bioavailability of a dose of 0.15 mg per kg bodyweight was 100, 87, 27, and 18% after administration by the intravenous, intramuscular, oral, and rectal routes respectively. The oral bioavailability was reduced to 16 and 15% after increasing the dose to 0.45 and 1 mg per kg respectively. There was bioequivalence between the 0.15 mg per kg intramuscular dose and the 0.45 mg per kg oral dose from 45 to 120 minutes after administration. Absorption from the rectal route gave lower serum-midazolam concentrations than the oral route at the 0.15 mg per kg dose.
Midazolam appears to be absorbed rapidly when given by the intranasal route to children with mean maximum plasma concentrations being achieved within about 12 minutes;[2–4] values of 30% and 55% have been reported for the bioavailability[3,4] but methods to optimise nasal delivery have resulted in higher bioavailability in studies in adults (see below). A study comparing intranasal, intravenous, and rectal administration of midazolam to children found that plasma concentrations from 45 minutes after intranasal and intravenous administration were similar; those following rectal administration were consistently less than after these other 2 routes.[2] Possible reasons suggested by the authors for this included the effect that the wide interindividual variations in rectal pH may have had on the absorption of midazolam.

Another study has investigated the relationship between intravenous dose and plasma-midazolam concentrations in children.[5]
See also Children under Precautions, above.

1. Payne K, *et al.* The pharmacokinetics of midazolam in paediatric patients. *Eur J Clin Pharmacol* 1989; **37**: 267–72.
2. Malinovsky J-M, *et al.* Plasma concentrations of midazolam after iv, nasal or rectal administration in children. *Br J Anaesth* 1993; **70**: 617–20.
3. Rey E, *et al.* Pharmacokinetics of midazolam in children: comparative study of intranasal and intravenous administration. *Eur J Clin Pharmacol* 1991; **41**: 355–7.
4. Kauffman RE, *et al.* Intranasal absorption of midazolam. *Clin Pharmacol Ther* 1995; **57**: 209.
5. Tolia V, *et al.* Pharmacokinetic and pharmacodynamic study of midazolam in children during esophagogastroduodenoscopy. *J Pediatr* 1991; **119**: 467–71.

NEONATES. References to the pharmacokinetics of midazolam in neonates. See also Children under Precautions, above.

1. Jacqz-Aigrain E, *et al.* Pharmacokinetics of midazolam in critically ill neonates. *Eur J Clin Pharmacol* 1990; **39**: 191–2.
2. Jacqz-Aigrain E, *et al.* Pharmacokinetics of midazolam during continuous infusion in critically ill neonates. *Eur J Clin Pharmacol* 1992; **42**: 329–32.
3. Burtin P, *et al.* Population pharmacokinetics of midazolam in neonates. *Clin Pharmacol Ther* 1994; **56**: 615–25.
4. Jacqz-Aigrain E, Burtin P. Clinical pharmacokinetics of sedatives in neonates. *Clin Pharmacokinet* 1996; **31**: 423–43.
5. Harte GJ, *et al.* Haemodynamic responses and population pharmacokinetics of midazolam following administration to ventilated, preterm neonates. *J Paediatr Child Health* 1997 **33**: 335–8.
6. Lee TC, *et al.* Population pharmacokinetic modeling in very premature infants receiving midazolam during mechanical ventilation: midazolam neonatal pharmacokinetics. *Anesthesiology* 1999; **90**: 451–7.

Distribution into breast milk. Midazolam could not be detected in breast milk from 11 mothers the morning after either the first or the fifth nightly 15-mg dose by mouth.[1] Additional study of 2 mothers found that midazolam and its hydroxy-metabolite disappeared rapidly from milk with undetectable concentrations at 4 hours. The mean milk to plasma ratio for midazolam was 0.15 in 6 paired samples.

1. Matheson I, *et al.* Midazolam and nitrazepam in the maternity ward: milk concentrations and clinical effects. *Br J Clin Pharmacol* 1990; **30**: 787–93.

Half-life. Data collected from seven studies involving 90 participants has suggested that the prolonged midazolam half-lives reported in a small number of patients are secondary to increases in the volume of distribution and not a result of alterations in clearance and metabolism.[1] Prolongation of the half-life of midazolam has been reported[2] in 2 patients following sustained infusion for status epilepticus.

1. Wills RJ, *et al.* Increased volume of distribution prolongs midazolam half-life. *Br J Clin Pharmacol* 1990; **29**: 269–72.
2. Naritoku DK, Sinha S. Prolongation of midazolam half-life after sustained infusion for status epilepticus. *Neurology* 2000 **54**: 1366–8.

Intranasal administration. Plasma concentrations of midazolam sufficient to induce conscious sedation are rapidly attained following intranasal administration.[1] Although bioavailability of up to 55% had previously been obtained in children following intranasal administration (see above) slow administration and other methods to optimise nasal delivery had resulted in a bioavailability of 83% in adults.[2] Similar techniques should be developed for use in children.

1. Burstein AH, *et al.* Pharmacokinetics and pharmacodynamics of midazolam after intranasal administration. *J Clin Pharmacol* 1997; **37**: 711–18.
2. Björkman S, *et al.* Pharmacokinetics of midazolam given as an intranasal spray to adult surgical patients. *Br J Anaesth* 1997; **79**: 575–80.

Liver disorders. The pharmacokinetics of midazolam in patients with advanced cirrhosis of the liver were characterised by an increase in oral systemic bioavailability[1] and by a decrease in clearance with consequent prolongation of elimination half-life.[1,2] Dosage may need to be reduced. Metabolism of midazolam has been demonstrated, however, in the anhepatic period of liver transplantation indicating extrahepatic metabolism (see below).

1. Pentikäinen PJ, *et al.* Pharmacokinetics of midazolam following intravenous and oral administration in patients with chronic liver disease and in healthy subjects. *J Clin Pharmacol* 1989; **29**: 272–7.
2. MacGilchrist AJ, *et al.* Pharmacokinetics and pharmacodynamics of intravenous midazolam in patients with severe alcoholic cirrhosis. *Gut* 1986; **27**: 190–5.

Metabolism. For a discussion of the metabolism of benzodiazepines, see Diazepam, p.680. Midazolam appears to be metabolised by at least 3 different cytochrome P450 isoenzymes which are found in the liver and in the kidney.[1] Variations in the activity of these enzymes might account for some of the interindividual differences in pharmacokinetics and pharmacodynamics seen with midazolam.[2] However, a study[3] in patients undergoing liver transplantation has indicated that the small intestine is a significant site for the first-pass metabolism of midazolam, metabolism presumably being catalysed by the cytochrome P450 isoenzyme CYP3A4 found in intestinal mucosa.

1. Wandel C, *et al.* Midazolam is metabolized by at least three different cytochrome P450 enzymes. *Br J Anaesth* 1994; **73**: 658–61.

2. Lown KS, *et al.* The erythromycin breath test predicts the clearance of midazolam. *Clin Pharmacol Ther* 1995; **57:** 16–24.
3. Paine MF, *et al.* First-pass metabolism of midazolam by the human intestine. *Clin Pharmacol Ther* 1996; **60:** 14–24.

Sublingual administration. High bioavailability (approximately 75%) and reliable plasma concentrations have been achieved following sublingual administration of midazolam.[1]

1. Schwagmeier R, *et al.* Midazolam pharmacokinetics following intravenous and buccal administration. *Br J Clin Pharmacol* 1998; **46:** 203–6.

Uses and Administration

Midazolam is a short-acting benzodiazepine with general properties similar to those of diazepam (p.680), except that it has a more potent amnestic action. It is mainly used for premedication and sedation and for induction of general anaesthesia. When midazolam is used as a premedicant or for conscious sedation, onset of sedation occurs at about 15 minutes after intramuscular injection reaching a peak at 30 to 60 minutes, and within 3 to 5 minutes after intravenous injection. When given intravenously as an anaesthetic induction agent, anaesthesia is induced in about 2 to 2.5 minutes. Onset of action is more rapid when premedication with an opioid analgesic has been given. Since the sedative end-point is reached abruptly with midazolam, dosage must be titrated carefully against the response of the patient; lower doses of midazolam are required when it is used in conjunction with opioid analgesics. Respiratory and cardiac function should be monitored continuously, and facilities for resuscitation should always be available. It is advisable to keep the patient supine during intravenous administration and throughout the procedure. The doses given below are, except where specified, the usual adult doses: midazolam should be given in reduced doses to elderly or debilitated patients.

Midazolam is used as the hydrochloride for oral, parenteral, and rectal administration; the maleate may also be given orally. All doses are given in terms of the base.

Midazolam may be given for premedication before general anaesthesia or to provide sedation for minor surgical or investigative procedures. A usual total **sedative** dose for dental and minor surgical and other procedures ranges from 2.5 to 7.5 mg (about 70 µg per kg body-weight) *intravenously*; an initial dose of 2 mg over 30 seconds has been suggested, with further incremental doses of 0.5 to 1 mg at intervals of 2 minutes if required until the desired end-point is reached. In the USA a suggested initial dose of up to 2.5 mg is given intravenously over at least 2 minutes and repeated if necessary after an additional 2 or more minutes to a maximum total dose of 5 mg. Sedation in children aged 6 months and over may be achieved with *oral* midazolam hydrochloride. A single dose of 250 to 500 µg per kg, up to a maximum of 20 mg, is recommended although younger patients (6 months to less than 6 years) may require up to 1 mg per kg.

Midazolam is given *intramuscularly* as a **premedicant** about 30 to 60 minutes before surgery. The usual dose is about 5 mg; doses range from 70 to 100 µg per kg. Children may be premedicated with *oral* midazolam in similar doses to those used for sedation (see above). The *rectal* route is used for premedication in some countries.

The usual dose of midazolam for **induction of anaesthesia** (p.1256) is about 200 µg per kg by slow *intravenous injection* in premedicated patients and at least 300 µg per kg in those who have not received a premedicant. In the USA further incremental doses of midazolam of approximately 25% of the induction dose have been given as a component of the regimens used for the maintenance of anaesthesia during short surgical procedures. A dose of 150 µg per kg has been recommended for the induction of anaesthesia in children over 7 years of age.

Patients in **intensive care** who require continuous sedation (p.652) can be given midazolam by *intravenous infusion*. An initial loading dose of 30 to 300 µg per kg may be given by intravenous infusion over 5 minutes to induce sedation; in the USA a lower dose

of 10 to 50 µg per kg is recommended. The maintenance dose required varies considerably but a dose of between 20 and 200 µg per kg per hour has been suggested. The loading dose should be reduced or omitted, and the maintenance dose reduced, for patients with hypovolaemia, vasoconstriction, or hypothermia. The need for continuous administration should be reassessed on a daily basis to reduce the risk of accumulation and prolonged recovery. Sedation can also be achieved by giving intermittent *intravenous bolus injections* of midazolam; doses of 1 to 2 mg may be given, and repeated, until the desired level of sedation has been reached. Abrupt withdrawal should be avoided after prolonged administration.

Midazolam maleate is also given *by mouth* for the short-term management of **insomnia**; the usual dose is the equivalent of midazolam 7.5 to 15 mg at night.

◊ References.
1. Blumer JL. Clinical pharmacology of midazolam in infants and children. *Clin Pharmacokinet* 1998; **35:** 37–47.
2. Marshall J, *et al.* Pediatric pharmacodynamics of midazolam oral syrup. *J Clin Pharmacol* 2000; **40:** 578–89.

Administration. The rectal,[1] intranasal,[1-5] and sublingual[1,6] routes have all been proposed as alternatives to parenteral administration of midazolam.

One group of workers reported that intranasal midazolam caused intense burning, irritation, and lachrymation on instillation into the nares and they now use a nasal spray containing lignocaine [lidocaine] before administering midazolam to children.[7] The use of midazolam spray intranasally in adults would be impractical and uncomfortable because of the large volume required. It has therefore been tried as a nebulised solution.[8]
1. Wong L, McQueen KD. Midazolam routes of administration. *DICP Ann Pharmacother* 1991; **25:** 476–7.
2. Theroux MC, *et al.* Efficacy of intranasal midazolam in facilitating suturing of lacerations in preschool children in the emergency department. *Pediatrics* 1993; **91:** 624–7.
3. Louon A, *et al.* Sedation with nasal ketamine and midazolam for cryotherapy in retinopathy of prematurity. *Br J Ophthalmol* 1993; **77:** 529–30.
4. Bates BA, *et al.* A comparison of intranasal sufentanil and midazolam to intramuscular meperidine, promethazine, and chlorpromazine for conscious sedation in children. *Ann Emerg Med* 1994; **24:** 646–51.
5. Ljungman G, *et al.* Midazolam nasal spray reduces procedural anxiety in children. *Pediatrics* 2000; **105:** 73–8.
6. Karl HW, *et al.* Transmucosal administration of midazolam for premedication of pediatric patients: comparison of the nasal and sublingual routes. *Anesthesiology* 1993; **78:** 885–91.
7. Lugo RA, *et al.* Complication of intranasal midazolam. *Pediatrics* 1993; **92:** 638.
8. Hodgson PE, *et al.* Administration of nebulized intranasal midazolam to healthy adult volunteers: a pilot study. *Br J Anaesth* 1994; **73:** 719P.

INTRATHECAL. See Pain, below.

Conversion and dissociative disorders. For reference to the use of midazolam in the diagnosis of conversion disorders, such as hysterical paralysis, see p.681.

Dyspnoea. Midazolam has been suggested[1] as an alternative to chlorpromazine in patients with advanced cancer and intractable dyspnoea (p.69) to relieve air hunger and to sedate dying patients who have unrelieved distress. Suggested[2] initial doses are 2.5 to 5 mg subcutaneously or 10 mg administered by infusion over a period of 24 hours, increased as necessary.
1. Walsh D. Dyspnoea in advanced cancer. *Lancet* 1993; **342:** 450–1.
2. Davis CL. ABC of palliative care: breathlessness, cough, and other respiratory problems. *BMJ* 1997; **315:** 931–4.

Hiccup. A protocol for the management of intractable hiccups may be found under Chlorpromazine, p.667. Midazolam given intravenously or subcutaneously has been reported[1] to have been effective in 2 patients with metastatic cancer who had hiccups unresponsive to conventional treatment. However, it has been noted[1,2] that benzodiazepines such as midazolam may exacerbate or precipitate hiccups.
1. Wilcock A, Twycross R. Midazolam for intractable hiccup. *J Pain Symptom Manage* 1996; **12:** 59–61.
2. Rousseau P. Hiccups. *South Med J* 1995; **88:** 175–81.

Insomnia. For discussion of the management of insomnia including limitations on the use of benzodiazepines and a recommendation that the period of treatment with midazolam should be limited to 2 weeks, see p.652.

References.
1. Monti JM, *et al.* The effect of midazolam on transient insomnia. *Eur J Clin Pharmacol* 1993; **44:** 525–7.

Pain. The conventional use of benzodiazepines in pain management is as muscle relaxants to relieve pain associated with skeletal muscle spasm (see under Choice of Analgesic, p.2). Midazolam has been studied[1-4] for use as an intrathecal analgesic but efficacy has been inconsistent.
1. Cripps TP, Goodchild CS. Intrathecal midazolam and the stress response to upper abdominal surgery. *Clin J Pain* 1988; **4:** 125–8.
2. Serrao JM, *et al.* Intrathecal midazolam for the treatment of chronic mechanical low back pain: a controlled comparison with epidural steroid in a pilot study. *Pain* 1992; **48:** 5–12.
3. Baaijens PFJ, *et al.* Intrathecal midazolam for the treatment of chronic mechanical low back pain: a randomized double-blind placebo-controlled study. *Br J Anaesth* 1995; **74** (suppl 1): 143.
4. Valentine JMJ, *et al.* The effect of intrathecal midazolam on post-operative pain. *Eur J Anaesthesiol* 1996; **13:** 589–93.

Premedication and sedation. Midazolam is used as a premedicant (p.1256) and as a sedative for therapeutic and investigative procedures such as dental treatment (p.652) and endoscopy (see below). It is also used to provide continuous sedation in patients in intensive care (p.652) although a systematic review has raised concerns about such use in neonates.

References.
1. Sandler ES, *et al.* Midazolam versus fentanyl as premedication for painful procedures in children with cancer. *Pediatrics* 1992; **89:** 631–4.
2. Stenhammar L, *et al.* Intravenous midazolam in small bowel biopsy. *Arch Dis Child* 1994; **71:** 558.
3. Jacqz-Aigrain E, *et al.* Placebo-controlled trial of midazolam sedation in mechanically ventilated newborn babies. *Lancet* 1994; **344:** 646–50.
4. Mitchell V, *et al.* Comparison of midazolam with trimeprazine as an oral premedicant for paediatric anaesthesia. *Br J Anaesth* 1995; **74** (suppl 1): 94–5.
5. McCarver-May DG, *et al.* Comparison of chloral hydrate and midazolam for sedation of neonates for neuroimaging studies. *J Pediatr* 1996; **128:** 573–6.
6. Zedie N, *et al.* Comparison of intranasal midazolam and sufentanil premedication in pediatric outpatients. *Clin Pharmacol Ther* 1996; **59:** 341–8.
7. Ng E, *et al.* Intravenous midazolam infusion for sedation of infants in the neonatal intensive care unit (updated 16 August 2001). Available in The Cochrane Library; Issue 4. Oxford: Update Software; 2001.

ENDOSCOPY. Intravenous benzodiazepines such as diazepam or midazolam are often the preferred drugs for sedation in patients undergoing endoscopy (p.652). They are sometimes used in conjunction with opioid analgesics for sedation.[1]

A reduced dose of midazolam was required for endoscopy when it was given as a bolus intravenous injection rather than as a slow intravenous titration. A study in 788 patients undergoing endoscopy found that a mean dose of 4.65 mg of midazolam given as a bolus intravenous injection was safe and effective in patients under 70 years of age whereas a mean dose of 1.89 mg was sufficient for patients over 70 years of age.[2] Furthermore, topical pharyngeal anaesthesia was not required with these doses of midazolam.
1. Bahal-O'Mara N, *et al.* Sedation with meperidine and midazolam in pediatric patients undergoing endoscopy. *Eur J Clin Pharmacol* 1994; **47:** 319–23.
2. Smith MR, *et al.* Small bolus injections of intravenous midazolam for upper gastrointestinal endoscopy: a study of 788 consecutive cases. *Br J Clin Pharmacol* 1993; **36:** 573–8.

Status epilepticus. Benzodiazepines such as diazepam or lorazepam given parenterally are often tried first to control status epilepticus (p.341). Midazolam has been used as an alternative.[1] It may be of value when intravenous access is difficult as effective concentrations of midazolam can be obtained after intramuscular injection.[2,3] Intravenous midazolam has been used in some centres[4] for status epilepticus refractory to diazepam, lorazepam, or phenytoin but reviews of the literature[5] reveal that evidence of efficacy is limited mainly to uncontrolled studies and anecdotal reports. The use of intranasal[6,7] or buccal[8] midazolam for the management of seizures is being studied.
1. Hanley DF, *et al.* Use of midazolam in the treatment of refractory status epilepticus. *Clin Ther* 1998; **20:** 1093–1105.
2. Bauer J, Elger CE. Management of status epilepticus in adults. *CNS Drugs* 1994; **1:** 26–44.
3. Towne AR, DeLorenzo RJ. Use of intramuscular midazolam for status epilepticus. *J Emerg Med* 1999; **17:** 323–8.
4. Bebin M, Bleck TP. New anticonvulsant drugs: focus on flunarizine, fosphenytoin, midazolam and stiripentol. *Drugs* 1994; **48:** 153–71.
5. Denzel D, Burstein AH. Midazolam in refractory status epilepticus. *Ann Pharmacother* 1996; **30:** 1481–3.
6. Wallace SJ. Nasal benzodiazepines for management of acute childhood seizures? *Lancet* 1997; **349:** 222.
7. Lahat E, *et al.* Intranasal midazolam for childhood seizures. *Lancet* 1998; **352:** 620.
8. Scott RC, *et al.* Buccal midazolam and rectal diazepam for treatment of prolonged seizures in childhood and adolescence: a randomised trial. *Lancet* 1999; **353:** 623–6.

Preparations

BP 2001: Midazolam Injection.

Proprietary Preparations (details are given in Part 3)
Aust.: Dormicum; *Austral.:* Hypnovel; *Belg.:* Dormicum; *Braz.:* Dormonid; *Canad.:* Versed; *Denm.:* Dormicum; *Fin.:* Dormicum; *Fr.:* Hypnovel; *Ger.:* Dormicum; *Hong Kong:* Dormicum; *Irl.:* Hypnovel; *Israel:* Dormicum; Midolam; *Ital.:* Ipnovel; *Mex.:* Dormicum; *Neth.:* Dormicum; *Norw.:* Dormicum; *NZ:* Hypnovel; *Port.:* Dormicum; *S.Afr.:* Dormicum; *Singapore:* Dormicum; *Spain:* Dormicum; *Swed.:* Dormicum; *Switz.:* Dormicum; *Thai.:* Dormicum; *UK:* Hypnovel; *USA:* Versed.

Molindone Hydrochloride (7072-k)

Molindone Hydrochloride (BANM, USAN, rINNM).

EN-1733A. 3-Ethyl-1,5,6,7-tetrahydro-2-methyl-5-(morpholinomethyl)indol-4-one hydrochloride.

$C_{16}H_{24}N_2O_2,HCl = 312.8$.

CAS — 7416-34-4 (molindone); 15622-65-8 (molindone hydrochloride).

Pharmacopoeias. In US.

Pharmacopoeial description

USP 25: pH of a 1% solution in water is between 4.0 and 5.0. Store in airtight containers. Protect from light.

Adverse Effects, Treatment, and Precautions

As for Chlorpromazine, p.660. Molindone hydrochloride is less likely to cause hypotension than chlorpromazine and extrapyramidal effects may be frequent but less severe. The incidence of sedation is intermediate between that of chlorpromazine and of phenothiazines with a piperazine side-chain. Weight gain or loss may occur, but weight loss appears to be more prominent (see p.661).

Convulsions. For mention of molindone as one of the antipsychotics suitable for patients at risk of seizures, see p.661.

Effects on the liver. A report of hepatotoxicity, associated with a flu-like syndrome, in a patient given molindone.[1] Symptoms and liver-enzyme values returned to normal on discontinuation of the drug and recurred on rechallenge with low doses. The effect was probably due to a hypersensitivity reaction.

1. Bhatia SC, *et al.* Molindone and hepatotoxicity. *Drug Intell Clin Pharm* 1985; **19**: 744–6.

Interactions

As for Chlorpromazine, p.664.

Pharmacokinetics

Molindone is readily absorbed from the gastrointestinal tract, peak concentrations of unchanged molindone being obtained within about 1.5 hours of administration. It is rapidly and extensively metabolised and a large number of metabolites have been identified. It is excreted in the urine and faeces almost entirely in the form of its metabolites. The pharmacological effect from a single dose by mouth is reported to last for 24 to 36 hours.

◊ References.

1. Zetin M, *et al.* Bioavailability of oral and intramuscular molindone hydrochloride in schizophrenic patients. *Clin Ther* 1985; **7**: 169–75.

Uses and Administration

Molindone is an indole derivative with general properties similar to those of the phenothiazine, chlorpromazine (p.665). It is given as the hydrochloride by mouth for the treatment of psychoses including schizophrenia (p.651).

The usual dose of molindone hydrochloride by mouth is 50 to 75 mg daily initially, increased in 3 or 4 days to 100 mg daily; in severe or resistant conditions doses of up to 225 mg daily may be required. The maintenance dosage can range from 15 to 225 mg daily according to severity of symptoms. The daily dosage is usually divided into 3 or 4 portions.

Molindone should be given in reduced dosage to elderly or debilitated patients.

◊ A systematic review[1] found that molindone appeared to be effective in mental illness but evidence of differences from other classical antipsychotics was lacking.

1. Bagnall A-M, *et al.* Molindone for schizophrenia and severe mental illness (updated 21 June 2000). Available in The Cochrane Library; Issue 4. Oxford: Update Software; 2001.

Preparations

USP 25: Molindone Hydrochloride Tablets.

Proprietary Preparations (details are given in Part 3)
Hong Kong: Moban; *USA:* Moban.

Moperone Hydrochloride (7073-a)

Moperone Hydrochloride *(rINNM)*.

Methylperidol Hydrochloride; R-1658 (moperone). 4′-Fluoro-4-(4-hydroxy-4-*p*-tolylpiperidino)butyrophenone hydrochloride.

$C_{22}H_{26}FNO_2,HCl = 391.9$.
CAS — 1050-79-9 (moperone); 3871-82-7 (moperone hydrochloride).

Profile

Moperone is a butyrophenone with general properties similar to those of haloperidol (p.686). It has been given by mouth for the treatment of psychoses.

Preparations

Proprietary Preparations (details are given in Part 3)
Switz.: Luvatren†.

Mosapramine (15295-s)

Mosapramine *(rINN)*.

Clospipramine; Y-516. (±)-1′-[3-(3-Chloro-10,11-dihydro-5*H*-dibenz[*b,f*]azepin-5-yl)propyl]hexahydrospiro[imidazo[1,2-*a*]pyridine-3(2*H*),4′-piperidin]-2-one.

$C_{28}H_{35}CIN_4O = 479.1$.
CAS — 89419-40-9.
ATC — N05AX10.

Profile

Mosapramine is an antipsychotic under investigation for the treatment of schizophrenia.

The symbol † denotes a preparation no longer actively marketed

---

◊ References.

1. Ishigooka J, *et al.* Pilot study of plasma concentrations of mosapramine, a new iminodibenzyl antipsychotic agent, after multiple oral administration in schizophrenic patients. *Curr Ther Res* 1994; **55**: 331–42.
2. Takahashi N, *et al.* Comparison of risperidone and mosapramine addition to neuroleptic treatment in chronic schizophrenia. *Neuropsychobiology* 1999; **39**: 81–5.

Nemonapride (10985-a)

Nemonapride *(rINN)*.

(±)-*cis*-N-(1-Benzyl-2-methyl-3-pyrrolidinyl)-5-chloro-4-(methylamino)-*o*-anisamide.

$C_{21}H_{26}CIN_3O_2 = 387.9$.
CAS — 93664-94-9.

Profile

Nemonapride is a substituted benzamide antipsychotic with general properties similar to those of sulpiride (p.706). It is given by mouth in the treatment of schizophrenia in usual doses of 9 to 36 mg daily in divided doses; up to 60 mg daily may be given if necessary.

◊ References.

1. Satoh K, *et al.* Effects of nemonapride on positive and negative symptoms of schizophrenia. *Int Clin Psychopharmacol* 1996; **11**: 279–81.

Preparations

Proprietary Preparations (details are given in Part 3)
Jpn: Emilace.

Nimetazepam (13018-a)

Nimetazepam *(rINN)*.

Menifazepam; S-1530. 1,3-Dihydro-1-methyl-7-nitro-5-phenyl-1,4-benzodiazepin-2-one.

$C_{16}H_{13}N_3O_3 = 295.3$.
CAS — 2011-67-8.

Profile

Nimetazepam is a benzodiazepine with the general properties of diazepam (p.674). It has been given by mouth for the short-term management of insomnia.

Preparations

Proprietary Preparations (details are given in Part 3)
Jpn: Erimin†.

Nitrazepam (4054-j)

Nitrazepam *(BAN, USAN, rINN)*.

Nitrazepamum; NSC-58775; Ro-4-5360; Ro-5-3059. 1,3-Dihydro-7-nitro-5-phenyl-2*H*-1,4-benzodiazepin-2-one.

$C_{15}H_{11}N_3O_3 = 281.3$.
CAS — 146-22-5.
ATC — N05CD02.

Pharmacopoeias. In *Chin., Eur.* (see p.vi), *Int., Jpn,* and *Pol.*

Pharmacopoeial description

Ph. Eur.: A yellow, crystalline powder. Practically insoluble in water; slightly soluble in alcohol and in ether. Protect from light.

Dependence and Withdrawal

As for Diazepam, p.675.

◊ For the purpose of withdrawal regimens, 5 mg of nitrazepam may be considered roughly equivalent to 5 mg of diazepam.

Adverse Effects, Treatment, and Precautions

As for Diazepam, p.675.

Effects on the digestive system. Two children given nitrazepam as part of their antiepileptic therapy developed drooling, eating difficulty, and aspiration pneumonia; symptoms improved in one patient when the dosage of nitrazepam was reduced.[1] Manometric studies indicated that the onset of normal cricopharyngeal relaxation in swallowing was delayed in these patients until after hypopharyngeal contraction, resulting in impaired swallowing and spillover of material into the trachea. Other workers[2] have found similar effects on swallowing and cricopharyngeal relaxation in children given nitrazepam. The deaths of six epileptic children under 5 years of age who were treated with nitrazepam have been reported.[3] Three of the deaths were unexpected, and in view of the previous reports of swallowing difficulties and aspiration, it was recommended that the use of nitrazepam in young children be restricted to those in whom seizure control fails to improve with other antiepileptics. Another study[4] also found an apparently increased risk of death, especially in young patients with intractable epilepsy, associated with nitrazepam therapy.

1. Wyllie E. *et al.* The mechanism of nitrazepam-induced drooling and aspiration. *N Engl J Med* 1986; **314**: 35–8.

---

2. Lim HCN, *et al.* Nitrazepam-induced cricopharyngeal dysphagia, abnormal esophageal peristalsis and associated bronchospasm: probable cause of nitrazepam-related sudden death. *Brain Dev* 1992; **14**: 309–14.
3. Murphy JV, *et al.* Deaths in young children receiving nitrazepam. *J Pediatr* 1987; **111**: 145–7.
4. Rintahaka PJ, *et al.* Incidence of death in patients with intractable epilepsy during nitrazepam treatment. *Epilepsia* 1999; **40**: 492–6.

Porphyria. Nitrazepam has been associated with acute attacks of porphyria and is considered unsafe in porphyric patients.

Interactions

As for Diazepam, p.677.

Pharmacokinetics

Nitrazepam is fairly readily absorbed from the gastrointestinal tract, although there is some individual variation. It is extensively bound to plasma proteins. It crosses the blood-brain and the placental barriers and traces are found in breast milk. Nitrazepam is metabolised in the liver, mainly by nitroreduction followed by acetylation; none of the metabolites possess significant activity. It is excreted in the urine in the form of its metabolites (free or conjugated) with only small amounts of a dose appearing unchanged. Up to about 20% of an oral dose is found in the faeces. Mean elimination half-lives of 24 to 30 hours have been reported.

Distribution into breast milk. A mean milk-to-plasma ratio of 0.27 was obtained after administration of nitrazepam 5 mg for 5 nights to 9 puerperal women.[1] The degree of nitrazepam accumulation in milk over the study period was similar to that in plasma.

1. Matheson I, *et al.* Midazolam and nitrazepam in the maternity ward: milk concentrations and clinical effects. *Br J Clin Pharmacol* 1990; **30**: 787–93.

Hepatic impairment. A study of the pharmacokinetics of intravenous nitrazepam in 12 patients with cirrhosis of the liver compared with 9 healthy subjects aged 22 to 49 years and 8 healthy elderly subjects aged 67 to 76 years.[1] The mean elimination half-life of nitrazepam was 26 hours in young and 38 hours in elderly subjects, the difference, which was not significant, being chiefly due to the greater volume of distribution in elderly subjects. Although there was also no significant difference between young and elderly subjects in percentage of unbound nitrazepam (13.0 and 13.9% respectively) there was a substantially higher unbound fraction in the patients with cirrhosis, the mean value being 18.9%, and clearance of unbound nitrazepam was reduced relative to healthy subjects.

1. Jochemsen R, *et al.* Effect of age and liver cirrhosis on the pharmacokinetics of nitrazepam. *Br J Clin Pharmacol* 1983; **15**: 295–302.

Metabolism. Although the acetylation of the reduced metabolite of nitrazepam has been reported to be controlled by acetylator phenotype,[1] Swift *et al.*[2] observed no significant differences between either half-life or residual effects of nitrazepam in slow and fast acetylators.

1. Karim AKMB, Price Evans DA. Polymorphic acetylation of nitrazepam. *J Med Genet* 1976; **13**: 17–19.
2. Swift CG, *et al.* Acetylator phenotype, nitrazepam plasma concentrations and residual effects. *Br J Clin Pharmacol* 1980; **9**: 312P–313P.

Uses and Administration

Nitrazepam is an intermediate-acting benzodiazepine with general properties similar to those of diazepam (p.680). It is used as a hypnotic in the short-term management of insomnia (p.652) and is reported to act in 30 to 60 minutes to produce sleep lasting for 6 to 8 hours. Nitrazepam has also been used in epilepsy, notably for infantile spasms (as for example in West's syndrome).

The usual dose for insomnia is 5 mg at night, although 10 mg may be required in some patients. Elderly or debilitated patients should not be given more than half of the normal adult dose.

Epilepsy. Benzodiazepines are sometimes employed in the management of epilepsy (p.338), but their long-term use is limited by problems of sedation, dependence, and tolerance to the antiepileptic effects. Nitrazepam has perhaps been most useful in the treatment of infantile spasms (as for example in West's syndrome) and the so-called infantile myoclonic seizures. Doses of 125 µg per kg body-weight twice daily, increased gradually to 250 to 500 µg per kg twice daily have been suggested. There has been concern, however, over swallowing difficulties with subsequent aspiration and reports of unexpected death associated with the use of nitrazepam in young children (see Effects on the Digestive System under Adverse Effects, above).

Preparations

BP 2001: Nitrazepam Oral Suspension; Nitrazepam Tablets.

Proprietary Preparations (details are given in Part 3)
Aust.: Mogadon; *Austral.:* Alodorm; Mogadon; *Belg.:* Mogadon; *Braz.:* Nitrazepan; Nitrazepol; Sonebon; Sonotrat; *Canad.:* Mogadon; Nitrazadon; *Denm.:* Apodorm; Dumolid; Mogadon; Pacisyn; *Fin.:* Insomin; *Fr.:* Nitrazepam; *Ger.:* Dormalon; Dormo-Puren; Eatan N; Imeson; Mogadan; Nitrazep†; Novanox; Rade-dorm; *Hong Kong:* Mogadon; *Irl.:* Mogadon; Somnite; *Israel:* Numbon; *Ital.:* Mogadon; *Neth.:* Mogadon†; *Norw.:* Apodorm; Mogadon; *NZ:* Insoma; Nitrados; *S.Afr.:* Arem; Mogadon; Ormo-don; Paxadorm; Protraz†; Somnipar; *Singapore:* Dima; Nitrados; *Spain:* Nitrazepam†; Pelson†; Serenade†; *Swed.:* Apodorm; Moga-don; *Switz.:* Mogadon; *UK:* Mogadon; Remnos; Somnite; Uni-somnia†.

Nordazepam (7035-I)

Nordazepam (rINN).

A-101; Demethyldiazepam; Desmethyldiazepam; *N*-Desmeth-yldiazepam; Nordiazepam; Ro-5-2180. 7-Chloro-1,3-dihydro-5-phenyl-2*H*-1,4-benzodiazepin-2-one.

$C_{15}H_{11}ClN_2O = 270.7$.
CAS — 1088-11-5.
ATC — N05BA16.

Profile

Nordazepam is a long-acting benzodiazepine with the general properties of diazepam (p.674). It is the principal active metab-olite of a number of benzodiazepines and has a half-life of 2 to 5 days. It is given by mouth in doses of up to 15 mg daily for the short-term treatment of anxiety disorders (p.649) and in-somnia (p.652).

Porphyria. Nordazepam is considered to be unsafe in patients with porphyria because it has been shown to be porphyrinogen-ic in *animals* or *in-vitro* systems.

Preparations

Proprietary Preparations (details are given in Part 3)
Aust.: Stilny†; *Belg.:* Calmday; *Fr.:* Nordaz; *Ger.:* Tranxilium N; *Ital.:* Madar; *Neth.:* Calmday; *Port.:* Sopax; *Singapore:* Nordaz; *Switz.:* Vegesan.

Olanzapine (16785-I)

Olanzapine (BAN, USAN, rINN).

LY-170053.   2-Methyl-4-(4-methyl-1-piperazinyl)-10*H*-thieno[2,3-b][1,5]benzodiazepine.
$C_{17}H_{20}N_4S = 312.4$.
CAS — 132539-06-1.
ATC — N05AH03.

Stability. A suspension of olanzapine 1 mg in 1 mL, made by crushing olanzapine tablets and suspending the powder in a syrup-based mixture containing carboxymethylcellulose pre-served with methyl hydroxybenzoate and propyl hydroxyben-zoate (Guy's Hospital paediatric base formula) was considered to be stable for 2 weeks when stored in a refrigerator.[1]

1. Harvey EJ, *et al.* The preparation and stability of a liquid olanza-pine preparation for oral administration in hospitals. *Pharm J* 2000; **265:** 275–6.

Adverse Effects, Treatment, and Precautions

As for Chlorpromazine, p.660. The most frequent ad-verse effects with olanzapine are somnolence, dizzi-ness, and weight gain; increased appetite, oedema, or-thostatic hypotension, and mild transient antimuscarinic effects are also relatively common. Olanzapine has been associated with a low incidence of extrapyramidal symptoms including tardive dyski-nesia; extrapyramidal symptoms may be more likely at high doses. Hyperprolactinaemia may occur but is usually asymptomatic. Abnormalities of glucose ho-moeostasis occur uncommonly; severe hyperglycae-mia, or exacerbation of pre-existing diabetes, some-times leading to ketoacidosis or coma, has been reported.

Patients receiving olanzapine intramuscularly should be closely observed for 2 to 4 hours for hypotension, bradyarrhythmia, and hypoventilation.

◊ References.
1. Beasley CM, *et al.* Safety of olanzapine. *J Clin Psychiatry* 1997; **58** (suppl 10): 13–17.

Convulsions. A 31-year-old woman with a complicated medi-cal history suffered three generalised tonic-clonic seizures af-ter 13 days' therapy with olanzapine.[1] She recovered after treatment with phenytoin.

1. Lee JW, *et al.* Seizure associated with olanzapine. *Ann Pharma-cother* 1999; **33:** 554–6.

Effects on the blood. Agranulocytosis developed in a 27-year-old man about 9 days after starting treatment with olanza-pine.[1] Although he had received clozapine up to 5 months pre-viously his blood values were normal prior to olanzapine treat-ment. Neutropenia has also been reported in a 31-year-old woman who was being treated with olanzapine;[2] she had previ-ously developed clozapine-induced neutropenia. The authors recommended that neutrophil counts should be monitored dur-ing treatment with olanzapine in those patients who have a his-tory of neutropenia with clozapine therapy. Olanzapine has also apparently delayed recovery of granulocyte counts in patients with clozapine-induced granulocytopenia who were switched to olanzapine before blood counts had returned to the normal range.[3]

1. Naumann R, *et al.* Olanzapine-induced agranulocytosis. *Lancet* 1999; **354:** 566–7.
2. Benedetti F, *et al.* Olanzapine-induced neutropenia after clozap-ine-induced neutropenia. *Lancet* 1999; **354:** 567.
3. Flynn SW, *et al.* Prolongation of clozapine-induced granulocyto-penia associated with olanzapine. *J Clin Psychopharmacol* 1997; **17:** 494–5.

Effects on sexual function. Priapism has been reported[1] in a patient receiving olanzapine therapy.

1. Deirmenjian JM, *et al.* Olanzapine-induced reversible priapism: a case report. *J Clin Psychopharmacol* 1998; **18:** 351–3.

Extrapyramidal disorders. A report of 2 isolated cases of tardive dyskinesia associated with olanzapine treatment.[1]

1. Herrán A, Vázquez-Barquero JL. Tardive dyskinesia associated with olanzapine. *Ann Intern Med* 1999; **131:** 72.

Mania. Mania has been reported following treatment with olanzapine.[1,2]

1. Lindenmayer J-P, Klebanov R. Olanzapine-induced manic-like syndrome. *J Clin Psychiatry* 1998; **59:** 318–19.
2. Fitz-Gerald MJ, *et al.* Olanzapine-induced mania. *Am J Psychia-try* 1999; **156:** 1114.

Neuroleptic malignant syndrome. Cases of neuroleptic malignant syndrome associated with olanzapine therapy.[1,2]

1. Filice GA, *et al.* Neuroleptic malignant syndrome associated with olanzapine. *Ann Pharmacother* 1998; **32:** 1158–9.
2. Nyfort-Hansen K, Alderman CP. Possible neuroleptic malignant syndrome associated with olanzapine. *Ann Pharmacother* 2000; **34:** 667.

Overdosage. A 2½-year-old boy was found sleeping and dif-ficult to arouse after taking either one or two 7.5-mg olanzapine tablets.[1] His reported symptoms included agitation, aggressive behaviour, miosis, hypersalivation, tachycardia, and ataxia; he recovered after 24 hours.

1. Yip L, *et al.* Olanzapine toxicity in a toddler. *Pediatrics* 1998; **102:** 1494.

Parkinsonism. Worsening of motor function has been reported[1-4] in patients with parkinsonism following olanzapine administration.

1. Graham JM, *et al.* Olanzapine in the treatment of hallucinosis in idiopathic Parkinson's disease: a cautionary note. *J Neurol Neu-rosurg Psychiatry* 1998 **65:** 774–7.
2. Molho ES, Factor SA. Worsening of motor features of parkinson-ism with olanzapine. *Mov Disord* 1999; **14:** 1014–16.
3. Goetz CG, *et al.* Olanzapine and clozapine: comparative effects on motor function in hallucinating PD patients. *Neurology* 2000; **55:** 789–94.
4. Manson AJ, *et al.* Low-dose olanzapine for levodopa induced dyskinesias. *Neurology* 2000; **55:** 795–9.

Interactions

As for Chlorpromazine, p.664. The metabolism of olanzapine is mediated to some extent by the cyto-chrome P450 isoenzyme CYP1A2. Concomitant ad-ministration of drugs which inhibit or act as a sub-strate to this isoenzyme may affect plasma concentrations of olanzapine.

The clearance of olanzapine is increased by tobacco smoking.

Pharmacokinetics

Olanzapine is well absorbed from the gastrointestinal tract but undergoes considerable first-pass metabo-lism. Peak plasma concentrations are achieved about 5 to 8 hours after oral administration. Olanzapine is about 93% bound to plasma proteins. It is extensively metabolised in the liver primarily by direct glucuroni-dation and by oxidation mediated through the cyto-chrome P450 isoenzymes CYP1A2 and to a lesser ex-tent CYP2D6. The two major metabolites 10-*N*-glucuronide and 4′-*N*-desmethyl olanzapine appear to be inactive. About 57% of a dose is excreted in the urine, mainly as metabolites and about 30% appears in the faeces. The plasma elimination half-life has been variously reported to be about 30 to 38 hours; half-lives tend to be longer in female than in male pa-tients.

◊ References.
1. Callaghan JT, *et al.* Olanzapine: pharmacokinetic and pharmaco-dynamic profile. *Clin Pharmacokinet* 1999; **37:** 177–93.

Uses and Administration

Olanzapine is a thienobenzodiazepine atypical antip-sychotic. It has affinity for various dopamine, serot-onin, and muscarinic receptors, as well as histamine-H_1 and adrenergic ($α_1$) receptors.

Olanzapine is used for the management of schizo-phrenia and for the short-term treatment of mania as-sociated with bipolar disorder.

A usual initial dose for **schizophrenia** is 10 mg daily as a single dose *by mouth*; thereafter dosage adjust-ments of 5 mg daily may be made according to re-sponse at intervals of not less than one week to within the range of 5 to 20 mg daily. It is recommended that doses of 15 mg or more daily should be given only after clinical reassessment.

Metabolism might be slower in female, elderly, or non-smoking patients; if more than one of these fac-tors is present a lower initial dose and a more gradual dose escalation should be considered. A starting dose of 5 mg daily by mouth may be necessary for patients with renal impairment; for patients with moderate he-patic insufficiency the starting dose should be 5 mg daily, and only increased with caution.

For the rapid control of agitation and disturbed behav-iour in patients with schizophrenia olanzapine may be given *intramuscularly* in an initial dose of 5 to 10 mg, followed by 5 to 10 mg as required after 2 hours. Not more than three injections should be given in any 24-hour period and the maximum daily dose, including olanzapine given by mouth, should not exceed 20 mg. Parenteral administration may be used for up to a maximum of 3 days but transfer to oral therapy should be initiated as soon as possible. The intramus-cular dose should be reduced by half in the elderly. An initial dose of 5 mg should be considered for pa-tients with renal or hepatic impairment; for patients with moderate hepatic insufficiency the starting dose should only be increased with caution.

For the treatment of **acute manic episodes** a recom-mended initial dose is 10 or 15 mg daily by mouth; dosage adjustments of 5 mg daily may subsequently be made at intervals of not less than 24 hours if nec-essary to within the range 5 to 20 mg daily, for 3 to 4 weeks. As in schizophrenia, a lower initial dose and more cautious dose escalation may be appropriate in patients in whom metabolism is liable to be reduced or sensitivity increased.

Bipolar disorder. Olanzapine is of benefit for the treatment of mania, with or without psychosis, in patients with bipolar disorder (p.271). However, there have been individual case re-ports of olanzapine-induced mania (see above).

References.
1. Tohen M, *et al.* Olanzapine HGEH Study Group. Olanzapine ver-sus placebo in the treatment of acute mania. *Am J Psychiatry* 1999; **156:** 702–9.

Parkinsonism. Olanzapine is associated with a relatively low incidence of extrapyramidal disorders and is therefore being studied[1] for use in the treatment of psychosis in patients with Parkinson's disease (see Disturbed Behaviour, p.650). Howev-er, there have been a number of reports of exacerbation of the movement disorder (see above).

1. Wolters EC, *et al.* Olanzapine in the treatment of dopaminomi-metic psychosis in patients with Parkinson's disease. *Neurology* 1996; **47:** 1085–7.

Schizophrenia. Studies suggest that olanzapine is as effective as haloperidol against positive symptoms of schizophrenia (p.651) and more effective against negative symptoms in the short-term and possibly in the long-term,[1-5] although a system-atic review considered the evidence equivocal.[6] Quality of life has also been judged to be greater in patients treated with olan-zapine.[7] In comparative studies, extrapyramidal symptoms have been less frequent with olanzapine than haloperidol and fewer patients have discontinued treatment with olanzapine. There are few published comparisons with other atypical anti-psychotics, but one study[8] has suggested that response of neg-ative symptoms might be greater than with risperidone; pa-tients in this study were also more likely to maintain their initial response with olanzapine and less likely to experience extrapy-ramidal effects, although risperidone had been given in doses higher than usually used clinically. Olanzapine's efficacy in the treatment of patients with refractory schizophrenia remains to be determined.

1. Beasley CM, *et al.* Olanzapine HGAD Study Group. Olanzapine versus placebo and haloperidol: acute phase results of the North American double-blind olanzapine trial. *Neuropsychopharma-cology* 1996; **14:** 111–23.

2. Beasley C, *et al.* Olanzapine versus haloperidol: long-term results of the multi-center international trial. *Eur Neuropsychopharmacol* 1996; **6** (suppl 3): 59.
3. Beasley CM, *et al.* Olanzapine versus haloperidol: acute phase results of the international double-blind olanzapine trial. *Eur Neuropsychopharmacol* 1997; **7**: 125–37.
4. Tollefson GD, *et al.* Olanzapine versus haloperidol in the treatment of schizophrenia and schizoaffective and schizophreniform disorders: results of an international collaborative trial. *Am J Psychiatry* 1997; **154**: 457–65.
5. Bhana N, *et al.* Olanzapine: an updated review of its use in the management of schizophrenia. *Drugs* 2001; **61**: 111–61.
6. Duggan L, *et al.* Olanzapine for schizophrenia (updated 16 March 2001). Available in The Cochrane Library; Issue 4. Oxford: Update Software; 2001.
7. Hamilton SH, *et al.* Olanzapine versus placebo and haloperidol: quality of life and efficacy results of the North American double-blind trial. *Neuropsychopharmacology* 1998; **18**: 41–9.
8. Tran PV, *et al.* Double-blind comparison of olanzapine versus risperidone in the treatment of schizophrenia and other psychotic disorders. *J Clin Psychopharmacol* 1997; **17**: 407–18.

Preparations

Proprietary Preparations (details are given in Part 3)
Aust.: Zyprexa; *Austral.:* Zyprexa; *Belg.:* Zyprexa; *Canad.:* Zyprexa; *Denm.:* Zyprexa; *Fin.:* Zyprexa; *Fr.:* Zyprexa; *Ger.:* Zyprexa; *Hong Kong:* Zyprexa; *Irl.:* Zyprexa; *Israel:* Zyprexa; *Mex.:* Zyprexa; *Neth.:* Zyprexa; *Norw.:* Zyprexa; *NZ:* Zyprexa; *Port.:* Zyprexa; *S.Afr.:* Zyprexa; *Singapore:* Zyprexa; *Spain:* Zyprexa; *Swed.:* Zyprexa; *Switz.:* Zyprexa; *Thai.:* Zyprexa; *UK:* Zyprexa; *USA:* Zyprexa.

Oxazepam (7076-r)

Oxazepam (BAN, USAN, rINN).

Oxazepamum; Wy-3498. 7-Chloro-1,3-dihydro-3-hydroxy-5-phenyl-1,4-benzodiazepin-2-one.

$C_{15}H_{11}ClN_2O_2 = 286.7$.

CAS — 604-75-1.

ATC — N05BA04.

Pharmacopoeias. In Eur. (see p.vi), Pol., and US.

Pharmacopoeial description

Ph. Eur.: A white or almost white crystalline powder. Practically insoluble in water; slightly soluble in alcohol and in dichloromethane. Protect from light.

USP 25: A creamy-white to pale yellow, practically odourless powder. Practically insoluble in water; soluble 1 in 220 of alcohol, 1 in 270 of chloroform, and 1 in 2200 of ether. pH of a 2% suspension in water is between 4.8 and 7.0.

Dependence and Withdrawal

As for Diazepam, p.675.

◊ For the purpose of withdrawal regimens, 15 mg of oxazepam is considered roughly equivalent to 5 mg of diazepam.

Adverse Effects, Treatment, and Precautions

As for Diazepam, p.675.

Hepatic impairment. All benzodiazepines should be used with caution in patients with hepatic impairment, but short acting ones such as oxazepam may be preferred.

Seven patients with acute viral hepatitis, 6 with cirrhosis of the liver, and 16 age-matched healthy control subjects received a single dose of oxazepam 15 or 45 mg by mouth.[1] Urinary excretion rates and plasma elimination patterns were unaltered in patients with acute and chronic parenchymal liver disease. Oxazepam 15 mg was also administered three times daily by mouth for 2 weeks to 2 healthy subjects and to 2 patients with cirrhosis and did not appear to accumulate in any of the four.

1. Shull HJ, *et al.* Normal disposition of oxazepam in acute viral hepatitis and cirrhosis. *Ann Intern Med* 1976; **84**: 420–5.

Porphyria. Oxazepam is considered to be unsafe in patients with porphyria although there is conflicting experimental evidence of porphyrinogenicity.

Renal impairment. Pharmacokinetic studies suggesting that, in general, the dosage of oxazepam does not need adjusting in patients with renal impairment.[1-3]

1. Murray TG, *et al.* Renal disease, age, and oxazepam kinetics. *Clin Pharmacol Ther* 1981; **30**: 805–9.
2. Busch U, *et al.* Pharmacokinetics of oxazepam following multiple administration in volunteers and patients with chronic renal disease. *Arzneimittelforschung* 1981; **31**: 1507–11.
3. Greenblatt DJ, *et al.* Multiple-dose kinetics and dialyzability of oxazepam in renal insufficiency. *Nephron* 1983; **34**: 234–8.

Thyroid disorders. There was a reduction in half-life and an increase in the apparent oral clearance of oxazepam in 7 hyperthyroid patients.[1] In 6 hypothyroid patients there was no overall change in oxazepam elimination, although 5 of the 6 complained of drowsiness despite a relatively low dose (15 mg).

1. Scott AK, *et al.* Oxazepam pharmacokinetics in thyroid disease. *Br J Clin Pharmacol* 1984; **17**: 49–53.

Interactions

As for Diazepam, p.677.

The symbol † denotes a preparation no longer actively marketed

Pharmacokinetics

Oxazepam is well absorbed from the gastrointestinal tract and reaches peak plasma concentrations about 2 to 3 hours after ingestion. It crosses the placenta and has been detected in breast milk. Oxazepam is extensively bound to plasma proteins and has been reported to have an elimination half-life ranging from about 4 to 15 hours. It is largely metabolised to the inactive glucuronide which is excreted in the urine.

Pregnancy. A study on the placental passage of oxazepam and its metabolism in 12 women given a single dose of oxazepam 25 mg during labour.[1] Oxazepam was readily absorbed and peak plasma concentrations were in the same range as those reported in healthy males and non-pregnant females given the same dose, although the plasma half-life (range 5.3 to 7.8 hours in 8 subjects studied) was shorter than that reported for non-pregnant subjects. Oxazepam was detected in the umbilical vein of all 12 patients with the ratio between umbilical to maternal vein concentration of oxazepam reaching a value of about 1.35 and remaining constant beyond a dose-delivery time of 3 hours. All of the babies had a normal Apgar score value. The oxazepam plasma half-life in the newborns was about 3 to 4 times that in the mothers, although in 3 the plasma concentration of oxazepam conjugate rose during the first 6 to 10 hours after delivery indicating the ability of the neonate to conjugate oxazepam.

1. Tomson G, *et al.* Placental passage of oxazepam and its metabolism in mother and newborn. *Clin Pharmacol Ther* 1979; **25**: 74–81.

Uses and Administration

Oxazepam is a short-acting benzodiazepine with general properties similar to those of diazepam (p.680). It is used in the short-term management of anxiety disorders (p.649) and insomnia (p.652) associated with anxiety. Oxazepam is also used for the control of symptoms associated with alcohol withdrawal (p.1131). Oxazepam is usually administered as the base but the hemisuccinate has been used in some multi-ingredient preparations.

The usual dose of oxazepam for the treatment of anxiety or for control of symptoms of alcohol withdrawal is 15 to 30 mg three or four times daily by mouth. A suggested initial dose for elderly or debilitated patients is 10 mg three times daily increased if necessary up to 10 to 20 mg three or four times daily. Oxazepam 15 to 25 mg may be given one hour before retiring for the treatment of insomnia associated with anxiety; up to 50 mg may occasionally be necessary.

Preparations

BP 2001: Oxazepam Tablets;
USP 25: Oxazepam Capsules; Oxazepam Tablets.

Proprietary Preparations (details are given in Part 3)
Aust.: Adumbran; Anxiolit; Oxahexal; Praxiten; *Austral.:* Alepam; Murelax; Serepax; *Belg.:* Seresta; Tranquo; *Canad.:* Novoxapam†; Serax; *Denm.:* Alopam; Oxabenz; Oxapax; Serepax; *Fin.:* Alopam; Opamox; Oxamin; Oxepam; *Fr.:* Seresta; *Ger.:* Adumbran; Azutranquil; durazepam; Mirfudorm; Noctazepam; oxa; Praxiten; Sigacalm; Uskan; *Israel:* Vaben; *Ital.:* Limbial; Oxapam; Serpax; *Neth.:* Seresta; *Norw.:* Alopam; Sobril; *NZ:* Benzotran; Ox-Pam; Serepax; *Port.:* Serenal; *S.Afr.:* Medopam†; Noripam; Oxaline; Purata; Serepax; *Spain:* Adumbran; *Swed.:* Alopam†; Oxascand; Serepax†; Sobril; *Switz.:* Anxiolit; Seresta; Uskan†; *USA:* Serax.

Multi-ingredient: *Aust.:* Anxiolit plus; *Fin.:* Spasmo-Oxepam; *Ital.:* Persumbrax†; *Port.:* Sedioton†; *Spain:* Novo Aerofil Sedante; Suxidina.

Oxazolam (7077-f)

Oxazolam (rINN).

Oxazolazepam. 10-Chloro-2,3,7,11b-tetrahydro-2-methyl-11b-phenyloxazolo[3,2-d][1,4]benzodiazepin-6(5H)-one.

$C_{18}H_{17}ClN_2O_2 = 328.8$.

CAS — 24143-17-7.

Pharmacopoeias. In Jpn.

Profile

Oxazolam is a long-acting benzodiazepine with general properties similar to those of diazepam (p.674). It has been given by mouth for the short-term treatment of anxiety disorders.

Oxazolam has also been used as a premedicant in general anaesthesia.

Preparations

Proprietary Preparations (details are given in Part 3)
Hong Kong: Serebon; *Jpn:* Serenal†.

Oxypertine (7078-d)

Oxypertine (BAN, USAN, rINN).

Win-18501-2. 5,6-Dimethoxy-2-methyl-3-[2-(4-phenylpiperazin-1-yl)ethyl]indole.

$C_{23}H_{29}N_3O_2 = 379.5$.

CAS — 153-87-7 (oxypertine); 40523-01-1 (oxypertine hydrochloride).

ATC — N05AE01.

Adverse Effects, Treatment, and Precautions

As for Chlorpromazine, p.660. It is claimed to cause fewer sedative, antimuscarinic, and, possibly, extrapyramidal effects although its sedative effects may increase with high doses. In low doses oxypertine may produce agitation and hyperactivity. Photophobia may occur occasionally.

Interactions

As for Chlorpromazine, p.664.

The manufacturers have recommended that since oxypertine has been observed in *animal* studies to release small amounts of catecholamines it should be avoided in patients taking MAOIs.

Uses and Administration

Oxypertine is an indole derivative with general properties similar to those of the phenothiazine, chlorpromazine (p.665). It is used in the treatment of various psychoses including schizophrenia (p.651), mania (see Bipolar Disorder, p.271), and disturbed behaviour (p.650), and in the short-term, adjunctive management of severe anxiety (p.649). Oxypertine is given by mouth in the treatment of psychoses and associated disorders initially in doses of 80 to 120 mg daily in divided doses adjusted according to response up to a maximum of 300 mg daily.

Doses of 10 mg three or four times daily have been used as adjunctive treatment in the short-term management of severe anxiety disorders. The maximum recommended dose is 60 mg daily.

Oxypertine should be given in reduced dosage to elderly patients.

Paraldehyde (4055-z)

Paracetaldehyde; Paraldehydum. The trimer of acetaldehyde; 2,4,6-Trimethyl-1,3,5-trioxane.

$(C_2H_4O)_3 = 132.2$.

CAS — 123-63-7.

ATC — N05CC05.

Pharmacopoeias. In Eur. (see p.vi) and US.

Because of its solvent action upon rubber, polystyrene, and styrene-acrylonitrile copolymer, paraldehyde should not be administered in plastic syringes made with these materials.

At low temperature it solidifies to form a crystalline mass. If it solidifies, the whole should be liquefied before use.

Pharmacopoeial description

Ph. Eur.: A colourless or slightly yellow, transparent liquid. It solidifies on cooling to form a crystalline mass. It may contain a suitable amount of an antioxidant. Relative density 0.991 to 0.996. F.p. is 10° to 13°; not more than 10% distils below 123° and not less than 95% below 126°. Soluble in water but less soluble in boiling water; miscible with alcohol, with ether, and with volatile oils. Store in small well-filled airtight containers at a temperature of 8° to 15°. Protect from light.

USP 25: A colourless transparent liquid with a strong characteristic, but not unpleasant or pungent, odour. It is subject to oxidation to form acetic acid. It may contain a suitable stabiliser. Specific gravity is about 0.99. It has a congealing temperature of not lower than 11° and distils completely between 120° and 126°.

Soluble 1 in 10 of water v/v, but only 1 in 17 of boiling water v/v; miscible with alcohol, with chloroform, with ether, and with volatile oils. Store in well-filled airtight containers of not more the 30 mL at a temperature not exceeding 25°. Protect from light. It must not be used more than 24 hours after opening the container.

◊ CAUTION. *Paraldehyde decomposes on storage, particularly after the container has been opened. The administration of partly decomposed paraldehyde is dangerous. It must not be used if it has a brownish colour or a sharp penetrating odour of acetic acid.*

Incompatibility. An evaluation of the compatibility of paraldehyde with plastic syringes and needle hubs concluded that, if possible, all-glass syringes should be used with paraldehyde.[1] Needles with plastic hubs could be used. Polypropylene syringes with rubber-tipped plastic plungers (Plastipak), or glass syringes with natural rubber-tipped plastic plungers (Glaspak) were acceptable only for the immediate administration or measurement of paraldehyde doses.

1. Johnson CE, Vigoreaux JA. Compatibility of paraldehyde with plastic syringes and needle hubs. *Am J Hosp Pharm* 1984; **41**: 306–8.

Dependence and Withdrawal

Prolonged use of paraldehyde may lead to dependence, especially in alcoholics. Features of dependence and withdrawal are similar to those of barbiturates (see Amobarbital, p.655).

Adverse Effects and Treatment

Paraldehyde decomposes on storage and deaths from corrosive poisoning have followed the use of such material. Paraldehyde has an unpleasant taste and imparts a smell to the breath; it may cause skin rashes.

Oral and rectal administration of paraldehyde may cause gastric or rectal irritation. Intramuscular administration is painful and associated with tissue necrosis, sterile abscesses, and nerve damage. Intravenous administration is extremely hazardous since it may cause pulmonary oedema and haemorrhage, hypotension and cardiac dilatation, and circulatory collapse; thrombophlebitis is also associated with intravenous use.

Overdosage results in rapid laboured breathing owing to damage to the lungs and to acidosis. Nausea and vomiting may follow an overdose by mouth. Respiratory depression and coma as well as hepatic and renal damage may occur. Treatment is as for barbiturate overdose (see Amobarbital, p.655).

Precautions

Paraldehyde should not be given to patients with gastric disorders and it should be used with caution, if at all, in patients with bronchopulmonary disease or hepatic impairment. It should not be given rectally in the presence of colitis. Old paraldehyde must never be used.

Paraldehyde must be well diluted before oral or rectal administration; if it is deemed essential to give paraldehyde intravenously it must be well diluted and given very slowly with extreme caution (see also Adverse Effects, above and Uses, below). Intramuscular injections may be given undiluted but care should be taken to avoid nerve damage. Plastic syringes should be avoided (see Incompatibility, above).

Interactions

The sedative effects of paraldehyde are enhanced by simultaneous administration of CNS depressants such as alcohol, barbiturates, and other sedatives. A few case reports suggest that disulfiram may enhance the toxicity of paraldehyde.

Pharmacokinetics

Paraldehyde is generally absorbed readily, although absorption is reported to be slower after rectal than after oral or intramuscular administration. It is widely distributed and has a reported half-life of 4 to 10 hours. About 80% of a dose is metabolised in the liver probably to acetaldehyde, which is oxidised by aldehyde dehydrogenase to acetic acid. Unmetabolised drug is largely excreted unchanged through the lungs; only small amounts appear in the urine. It crosses the placental barrier and is distributed into breast milk.

Uses and Administration

Paraldehyde is a hypnotic and sedative with antiepileptic effects. However, because of the hazards associated with its administration, its tendency to react with plastic, and the risks associated with its deterioration, it has largely been superseded by other drugs. It is still occasionally used to control status epilepticus (p.341) resistant to conventional treatment. Given rectally or intramuscularly it causes little respiratory depression and is therefore useful where facilities for resuscitation are poor. A usual dose for adults is 10 to 20 mL administered rectally as a 10% solution in sodium chloride 0.9% solution or diluted with 1 or 2 parts of oil. Doses of 5 to 10 mL are also occasionally given intramuscularly up to a maximum of 20 mL daily with not more than 5 mL being given at any one site. Recommended doses rectally or intramuscularly in children are: up to 3 months, 0.5 mL; 3 to 6 months, 1 mL; 6 to 12 months, 1.5 mL; 1 to 2 years, 2 mL; 3 to 5 years, 3 to 4 mL; 6 to 12 years, 5 to 6 mL.

Paraldehyde has been given by slow intravenous infusion in specialist centres with intensive care facilities but this method of administration is not usually recommended; it must be diluted to a 4% solution in sodium chloride 0.9% before administration.

Paraldehyde has been given by mouth; it should always be well diluted to avoid gastric irritation.

Preparations

BP 2001: Paraldehyde Injection.

Proprietary Preparations (details are given in Part 3)
USA: Paral.

Penfluridol (7080-k)

Penfluridol (BAN, USAN, rINN).

McN-JR-16341; R-16341. 4-(4-Chloro-3-trifluoromethylphenyl)-1-[3-(p,p'-difluorobenzhydryl)propyl]piperidin-4-ol.
$C_{28}H_{27}ClF_5NO = 524.0$.
CAS — 26864-56-2.
ATC — N05AG03.
Pharmacopoeias. In Chin.

Adverse Effects, Treatment, and Precautions

As for Chlorpromazine, p.660.

Interactions

As for Chlorpromazine, p.664.

Pharmacokinetics

Although penfluridol is absorbed from the gastrointestinal tract, peak plasma concentrations are not achieved until about 12 hours after a dose by mouth. The initial peak plasma concentration is followed by a rapid decrease over the next 36 hours, probably due to tissue redistribution, followed by a slower decline over the next 120 hours. Penfluridol, according-ly, has a very long duration of action possibly partly related to its storage in, and slow release from, adipose tissue.

There is evidence of enterohepatic recycling, and penfluridol is excreted mainly as the N-dealkylated metabolite in the faeces and urine.

Uses and Administration

Penfluridol is a diphenylbutylpiperidine antipsychotic and shares the general properties of the phenothiazine, chlorpromazine (p.660). Following administration by mouth it has a prolonged duration of action which lasts for about a week. It is used in the treatment of various psychoses including schizophrenia (p.651).

The usual dose of penfluridol for the treatment of chronic psychoses is 20 to 60 mg weekly by mouth. Doses of up to 250 mg once a week may be required in severe or resistant conditions.

Preparations

Proprietary Preparations (details are given in Part 3)
Aust.: Semap; *Belg.:* Semap; *Braz.:* Semap; *Denm.:* Semap; *Fr.:* Semap; *Israel:* Semap; *Mex.:* Semap; *Neth.:* Semap; *Switz.:* Semap.

Pentobarbital (4056-c)

Pentobarbital (BAN, rINN).

Aethaminalum; Mebubarbital; Mebumal; Pentobarbitalum; Pentobarbitone. 5-Ethyl-5-(1-methylbutyl)barbituric acid.
$C_{11}H_{18}N_2O_3 = 226.3$.
CAS — 76-74-4.
ATC — N05CA01.
Pharmacopoeias. In Eur. (see p.vi) and US.

Pharmacopoeial description

Ph. Eur.: Colourless crystals or a white crystalline powder. Very slightly soluble in water; freely soluble in dehydrated alcohol and in ether; It forms water-soluble compounds with alkali hydroxides and carbonates, and with ammonia.

USP 25: A white or practically white, practically odourless, fine powder. Very slightly soluble in water and in carbon tetrachloride; soluble 1 in 4.5 of alcohol, 1 in 4 of chloroform, and 1 in 10 of ether; very soluble in acetone and in methyl alcohol; soluble in benzene. Store in airtight containers.

Pentobarbital Calcium (4057-k)

Pentobarbital Calcium (BANM, rINNM).

Pentobarbitone Calcium. Calcium 5-ethyl-5-(1-methylbutyl)barbiturate.
$(C_{11}H_{17}N_2O_3)_2Ca = 490.6$.

Pentobarbital Sodium (4058-a)

Pentobarbital Sodium (BANM, rINNM).

Aethaminalum-Natrium; Ethaminal Sodium; Mebumalnatrium; Pentobarbitalum Natricum; Pentobarbitone Sodium; Sodium Pentobarbital; Soluble Pentobarbitone. Sodium 5-ethyl-5-(1-methylbutyl)barbiturate.
$C_{11}H_{17}N_2NaO_3 = 248.3$.
CAS — 57-33-0.
Pharmacopoeias. In Eur. (see p.vi) and US.

Pentobarbital may be precipitated from preparations containing pentobarbital sodium, depending on the concentration and pH. Pentobarbital sodium has, therefore, been reported to be incompatible with many other drugs particularly acids and acidic salts.

Pharmacopoeial description

Ph. Eur.: A white, hygroscopic, crystalline powder. Very soluble in water. A 10% solution in water has a pH of 9.6 to 11.0 when freshly prepared. Store in airtight containers.

USP 25: White, crystalline granules or white powder. Is odourless or has a slight characteristic odour. Very soluble in water; freely soluble in alcohol; practically insoluble in ether. pH of a 10% solution in water is between 9.8 and 11.0. Solutions decompose on standing, the decomposition being accelerated at higher temperatures. Store in airtight containers.

Dependence and Withdrawal

As for Amobarbital, p.655.

Adverse Effects, Treatment, and Precautions

As for Amobarbital, p.655.

Interactions

As for Amobarbital, p.656.

Pharmacokinetics

Following oral or rectal administration pentobarbital is well absorbed from the gastrointestinal tract, and is reported to be approximately 60 to 70% bound to plasma protein. The elimination half-life appears to be dose dependent and reported values have ranged from 15 to 50 hours. It is metabolised in the liver, mainly by hydroxylation, and excreted in the urine mainly as metabolites.

Uses and Administration

Pentobarbital is a barbiturate that has been used as a hypnotic and sedative. It has general properties and uses similar to those of amobarbital (p.656). It has been used as a sedative and in the short-term management of insomnia (p.652) but barbiturates are not considered appropriate for such purposes. Pentobarbital sodium, administered by mouth or by deep intramuscular or slow intravenous injection, has been used for premedication in anaesthetic procedures (p.1256) but the use of barbiturates for pre-operative sedation has been replaced by other drugs. Pentobarbital is usually administered as the sodium salt although pentobarbital and its calcium salt have also been used.

A usual dose of pentobarbital sodium given at night for insomnia is 100 mg by mouth or up to 200 mg rectally. A dose of 20 mg of the sodium salt has been given by mouth 3 or 4 times daily as a sedative; alternatively, 30 mg has been given rectally 2 to 4 times daily.

Cerebrovascular disorders. For reference to the use of barbiturate-induced coma in the management of patients with cerebral ischaemia, see p.1270. See also p.811 for reference to the use of barbiturates in the management of raised intracranial pressure.

Status epilepticus. Anaesthesia in conjunction with assisted ventilation may be instituted to control refractory tonic-clonic status epilepticus (p.341). A short-acting barbiturate such as thiopental is usually used, but pentobarbital has been used similarly.

Preparations

BP 2001: Pentobarbital Tablets;
USP 25: Pentobarbital Elixir; Pentobarbital Sodium Capsules; Pentobarbital Sodium Injection.

Proprietary Preparations (details are given in Part 3)
Braz.: Hypnol; *Canad.:* Nembutal; Nova Rectal†; *USA:* Nembutal.

Multi-ingredient: *Canad.:* Cafergot-PB; *USA:* Cafatine-PB.

Perazine Dimalonate (7081-a)

P-725 (perazine); Pemazine Dimalonate. 10-[3-(4-Methylpiperazin-1-yl)propyl]phenothiazine dimalonate.
$C_{20}H_{25}N_3S,2C_3H_4O_4 = 547.6$.
CAS — 84-97-9 (perazine); 14777-25-4 (perazine dimalonate).
Pharmacopoeias. In Pol.

Profile

Perazine dimalonate is a phenothiazine with general properties similar to those of chlorpromazine (p.660). It has a piperazine side-chain. It is given by mouth for the treatment of psychotic conditions in usual doses equivalent to 25 to 600 mg of the base daily; up to 1000 mg daily has been given in resistant cases. It may also be given intramuscularly.

Adverse effects. A report of 5 patients receiving perazine dimalonate who developed acute axonal neuropathies of superficial nerve fibres after exposure to sunlight.[1]

1. Roelcke U, *et al.* Acute neuropathy in perazine-treated patients after sun exposure. *Lancet* 1992; **340:** 729–30.

Preparations

Proprietary Preparations (details are given in Part 3)
Ger.: Taxilan; *Neth.:* Taxilan†.

Pericyazine (7082-t)

Pericyazine (BAN).

Periciazine (pINN); Propericiazine; RP-8909; SKF-20716. 10-[3-(4-Hydroxypiperidino)propyl]phenothiazine-2-carbonitrile; 1-[3-(2-Cyanophenothiazin-10-yl)propyl]piperidin-4-ol.
$C_{21}H_{23}N_3OS = 365.5$.
CAS — 2622-26-6.
ATC — N05AC01.

Adverse Effects, Treatment, and Precautions

As for Chlorpromazine, p.660. Sedation and orthostatic hypotension may be marked.

Interactions

As for Chlorpromazine, p.664.

Uses and Administration

Pericyazine is a phenothiazine with general properties similar to those of chlorpromazine (p.665). It has a piperidine side-chain. It is used in the treatment of various psychoses including schizophrenia (p.651) and disturbed behaviour (p.650), and in the short-term management of severe anxiety (p.649).

Pericyazine is usually given as the base but the mesilate and tartrate have also been used.

The usual dose by mouth for the treatment of severe anxiety, agitation, aggression, or impulsive behaviour is 15 to 30 mg daily given in 2 portions, the larger amount in the evening. In schizophrenia and severe psychoses initial doses of 75 mg daily may be given in divided doses, increased if necessary, at weekly intervals by steps of 25 mg, to up to 300 mg daily. It has also been given by intramuscular injection.

A recommended initial daily dose by mouth in children over one year of age is 500 µg for a child of 10 kg body-weight; for heavier children this initial dose may be increased by 1 mg for each additional 5 kg of body-weight, to a maximum total of 10 mg daily. Thereafter the dose may be gradually increased according to response but the daily maintenance dose should not exceed twice the initial dose.

Elderly subjects should be given reduced doses: a recommended initial dose is 5 to 10 mg daily for anxiety or behaviour disorders and 15 to 30 mg daily for schizophrenia or psychosis, both in divided doses.

Preparations

Proprietary Preparations (details are given in Part 3)
Aust.: Neuleptil; **Austral.:** Neulactil; **Belg.:** Neuleptil†; **Braz.:** Neuleptil; **Canad.:** Neulactil; **Denm.:** Neulactil; **Fin.:** Neulactil; **Fr.:** Neuleptil; **Hong Kong:** Neulactil; **Irl.:** Neulactil; **Israel:** Neuleptil; **Ital.:** Neuleptil; **Neth.:** Neuleptil; **Norw.:** Neulactil†; **NZ:** Neulactil; **S.Afr.:** Neulactil; **Spain:** Nemactil; **Swed.:** Neulactil†; **Switz.:** Neuleptil†; **UK:** Neulactil.

Perospirone (17642-v)

Perospirone (rINN).

cis-N-{4-[4-(1,2-Benzisothiazol-3-yl)-1-piperazinyl]butyl}-1,2-cyclohexanedicarboximide.

$C_{23}H_{30}N_4O_2S = 426.6$.

CAS — 150915-41-6.

Profile

Perospirone is an atypical antipsychotic used in the treatment of schizophrenia.

◊ References.
1. Onrust SV, McClellan K. Perospirone. *CNS Drugs.* 2001; **15:** 329–37

Perphenazine (7084-r)

Perphenazine (BAN, rINN).

Perphenazinum. 2-{4-[3-(2-Chlorophenothiazin-10-yl)propyl]piperazin-1-yl}ethanol.

$C_{21}H_{26}ClN_3OS = 404.0$.

CAS — 58-39-9.

ATC — N05AB03.

Pharmacopoeias. In Chin., Eur. (see p.vi), Jpn, Pol., and US. Jpn also includes the maleate.

Pharmacopoeial description

Ph. Eur.: A white or yellowish-white crystalline powder. Practically insoluble in water; soluble in alcohol; freely soluble in dichloromethane; sparingly soluble in ether; dissolves in dilute solutions of hydrochloric acid. Protect from light.

USP 25: A white to creamy-white odourless powder. M.p. 94° to 100°. Practically insoluble in water; soluble 1 in 7 of alcohol and 1 in 13 of acetone; freely soluble in chloroform. Store in airtight containers. Protect from light.

Incompatibility. Perphenazine has been reported to be incompatible with cefoperazone sodium[1] and with midazolam hydrochloride (see p.692).
1. Gasca M, *et al.* Visual compatibility of perphenazine with various antimicrobials during simulated Y-site injection. *Am J Hosp Pharm* 1987; **44:** 574–5.

Perphenazine Decanoate (15578-x)

Perphenazine Decanoate (BANM, rINNM).

2-{4-[3-(2-Chlorophenothiazin-10-yl)propyl]piperazin-1-yl}ethyl decanoate.

$C_{31}H_{44}ClN_3O_2S = 558.2$.

Perphenazine decanoate 108.2 mg is approximately equivalent to 78.3 mg of perphenazine.

Perphenazine Enantate (18340-f)

Perphenazine Enantate (BANM, rINNM).

Perphenazine Enanthate; Perphenazine Heptanoate. 2-{4-[3-(2-Chlorophenothiazin-10-yl)propyl]piperazin-1-yl}ethyl heptanoate.

$C_{28}H_{38}ClN_3O_2S = 516.1$.

CAS — 17528-28-8.

Perphenazine enantate 100 mg is approximately equivalent to 78.3 mg of perphenazine.

Adverse Effects, Treatment, and Precautions

As for Chlorpromazine, p.660. Perphenazine has been associated with a lower frequency of sedation, but a higher incidence of extrapyramidal symptoms.

Interactions

As for Chlorpromazine, p.664.

Pharmacokinetics

Perphenazine is well absorbed following oral administration and undergoes some first-pass metabolism, resulting in a relative bioavailability of about 60 to 80%. Perphenazine decanoate and perphenazine enantate are slowly absorbed from the site of intra-muscular injection. They gradually release perphenazine into the body and are therefore suitable for use as depot injections.

◊ Perphenazine 5 or 6 mg administered intravenously had a plasma half-life from 8.4 to 12.3 hours in a study of 4 schizophrenic patients and 4 healthy subjects.[1] Considerable fluctuations in plasma-perphenazine concentrations were observed 3 to 5 hours after administration before the exponential elimination phase. A dose of 6 mg by mouth in 4 healthy subjects failed to produce a detectable plasma concentration and only low plasma concentrations of its sulfoxide metabolite could be detected; this was attributed to a marked first-pass effect. Systemic availability was variable and poor in 4 schizophrenic patients given perphenazine 12 mg three times daily. However, it was considered that oral therapy should be on an 8-hour dosage regimen. Intramuscular injection of perphenazine enantate 50 or 100 mg every 2 weeks gave plasma-perphenazine concentrations similar to those after continuous oral administration but with a high initial absorption within 2 to 3 days associated with the most serious neurological and sedative side-effects.
1. Hansen CE, *et al.* Clinical pharmacokinetic studies of perphenazine. *Br J Clin Pharmacol* 1976; **3:** 915–23.

Distribution into breast milk. The distribution of perphenazine into breast milk was studied[1] in a mother who was receiving perphenazine 24 mg daily, later reduced to 16 mg daily, by mouth. Breast feeding was started after 1 week and it was estimated that a breast-fed infant would ingest about 0.1% of a maternal dose. Treatment with perphenazine lasted for 3.5 months and during this period the child thrived normally and no drug-induced symptoms were seen.
1. Olesen OV, *et al.* Perphenazine in breast milk and serum. *Am J Psychiatry* 1990; **147:** 1378–9.

Metabolism. In a study in 12 healthy subjects there was a clear difference in the disposition of a single oral dose of perphenazine between poor and extensive hydroxylators of debrisoquine.[1]
1. Dahl-Puustinen M-L, *et al.* Disposition of perphenazine is related to polymorphic debrisoquin hydroxylation in human beings. *Clin Pharmacol Ther* 1989; **46:** 78–81.

Uses and Administration

Perphenazine is a phenothiazine with general properties similar to those of chlorpromazine (p.665). It has a piperazine side-chain. It is used in the treatment of various psychoses including schizophrenia (p.651) and mania (see Bipolar Disorder, p.271) as well as disturbed behaviour (p.650) and in the short-term, adjunctive management of severe anxiety (p.649). Perphenazine is also used for the management of postoperative or chemotherapy-induced nausea and vomiting (p.1206) and for the treatment of intractable hiccup (p.667).

Perphenazine is usually given as the base by mouth or sometimes by intramuscular or intravenous injection. Long-acting decanoate or enantate esters of perphenazine, available in some countries, are given by intramuscular injection.

The usual initial dose for the treatment of schizophrenia, mania, and other psychoses is 4 to 8 mg three times daily by mouth. The dose is adjusted according to response up to a usual maximum of 24 mg daily although up to 64 mg daily has occasionally been used in hospitalised patients. Similar doses have been used for the management of severe agitated or violent behaviour or in severe anxiety. Perphenazine has sometimes been used in combination with tricyclic antidepressants such as amitriptyline in the treatment of anxiety with depression.

For the control of nausea and vomiting the usual dose by mouth is 4 mg three times daily but up to 8 mg three times daily may be required.

Perphenazine may be given by intramuscular injection for control of acute psychotic symptoms or for severe nausea and vomiting. An initial dose of 5 or 10 mg is followed, if necessary, by 5 mg every 6 hours to a maximum of 15 to 30 mg daily.

Perphenazine, diluted to a concentration of 0.5 mg per mL in sodium chloride 0.9% solution, is occasionally given by intravenous injection in divided doses, not more than 1 mg being administered every 1 to 2 minutes or by continuous infusion at a rate not greater than 1 mg per minute; the maximum intravenous dose is 5 mg. The intravenous route of administration is usually reserved for the control of severe vomiting or intractable hiccup.

The long-acting decanoate or enantate esters of perphenazine are administered by deep intramuscular injection in doses ranging from approximately 50 to 300 mg of ester given at intervals of 2 to 4 weeks.

Elderly subjects should be given reduced doses of perphenazine or its esters but it should be noted that perphenazine is not indicated for the management of agitation and restlessness in the elderly.

Preparations

BP 2001: Perphenazine Tablets;

USP 25: Perphenazine and Amitriptyline Hydrochloride Tablets; Perphenazine Injection; Perphenazine Oral Solution; Perphenazine Syrup; Perphenazine Tablets.

Proprietary Preparations (details are given in Part 3)
Aust.: Decentan; **Belg.:** Trilafon; **Canad.:** Trilafon; **Denm.:** Trilafon; **Fin.:** Peratsin; **Fr.:** Trilifan; **Ger.:** Decentan; **Irl.:** Fentazin†; **Israel:** Perphenan; **Ital.:** Trilafon; **Mex.:** Leptopsique; Trilafon; Zerfenazin; **Neth.:** Trilafon; **Norw.:** Trilafon; **S.Afr.:** Trilafon; **Spain:** Decentan; **Swed.:** Trilafon; **Switz.:** Trilafon; **Thai.:** Conazine; Pernamed; Pernazine; Perzine; Porazine; **UK:** Fentazin; **USA:** Trilafon.

Multi-ingredient: **Austral.:** Mutabon D†; **Canad.:** Elavil Plus; Etrafon; PMS-Levazine†; Triavil; **Fin.:** Pertriptyl; **Irl.:** Triptafen†; **Ital.:** Mutabon; **Mex.:** Adepsique; **Port.:** Mutabon; **S.Afr.:** Etrafon; **Spain:** Mutabase; **Thai.:** Anxipress-D; Neuragon; **UK:** Triptafen; **USA:** Etrafon; Triavil.

Phenprobamate (7086-d)

Phenprobamate (BAN, rINN).

MH-532; Proformiphen. 3-Phenylpropyl carbamate.

$C_{10}H_{13}NO_2 = 179.2$.

CAS — 673-31-4.

ATC — M03BA01.

Profile

Phenprobamate is a carbamate with general properties similar to those of meprobamate (p.691). It has been used for its anxiolytic and muscle relaxant actions.

Preparations

Proprietary Preparations (details are given in Part 3)
Multi-ingredient: **Switz.:** Dolo-Prolixan†.

Pimozide (7087-n)

Pimozide (BAN, USAN, rINN).

McN-JR-6238; Pimozidum; R-6238. 1-{1-[4,4-Bis(4-fluorophenyl)butyl]-4-piperidyl}benzimidazolin-2-one; 1-{1-[3-(4,4'-Difluorobenzhydryl)propyl]-4-piperidyl}benzimidazolin-2-one.

$C_{28}H_{29}F_2N_3O = 461.5$.

CAS — 2062-78-4.

ATC — N05AG02.

Pharmacopoeias. In Eur. (see p.vi), Pol., and US.

Pharmacopoeial description

Ph. Eur.: A white or almost white powder. Practically insoluble in water; slightly soluble in alcohol; soluble in dichloromethane; sparingly soluble in methyl alcohol. Protect from light.

USP 25: A white crystalline powder. Insoluble in water; soluble 1 in 1000 of alcohol, of ether, and of methyl alcohol, 1 in 100 of acetone, 1 in 10 of chloroform, and 1 in more than 1000 of 0.1N hydrochloric acid. Store in airtight containers. Protect from light.

Adverse Effects, Treatment, and Precautions

As for Chlorpromazine, p.660.

Extrapyramidal symptoms may be more common than those associated with chlorpromazine, whereas pimozide may be less likely to cause sedation, hypotension, or antimuscarinic effects.

In view of reports of ventricular arrhythmias and other ECG abnormalities such as prolongation of the QT interval and T-wave changes associated with the use of pimozide, an ECG should be performed prior to treatment and repeated annually or earlier if indicated. In the UK, periodic assessment of cardiac function is recommended for patients receiving more than 16 mg daily. If repolarisation changes appear or arrhythmias develop, the need for continuing treatment with pimozide should be reviewed; at the very least dose reduction and close supervision are advised. Pimozide is contra-indicated in patients with pre-existing prolongation of the QT interval and in patients with a history of cardiac arrhythmias. Electrolyte disturbances such as hypokalaemia in patients receiving pimozide may lead to cardiotoxicity.

The symbol † denotes a preparation no longer actively marketed

Effects on the cardiovascular system. The UK Committee on Safety of Medicines (CSM) has received reports of ventricular arrhythmias and other ECG abnormalities such as prolongation of the QT interval and T-wave changes associated with the use of pimozide.[1,2] In August 1990 they had received 13 reports of sudden unexpected death since 1971; many of these patients had no evidence of pre-existing cardiac disease, and 7 were aged between 17 and 30 years of age. Five of the 13 were also taking other antipsychotics. In ten cases, the dose of pimozide was greater than 20 mg daily, and in many of the patients for whom information was available the dose had been increased rapidly, possibly resulting in substantial tissue accumulation. By February 1995 the CSM had received a total of 40 reports (16 fatal) of serious cardiac reactions most of which involved arrhythmias.

See also under Chlorpromazine, p.661.

1. Committee on Safety of Medicines. Cardiotoxic effects of pimozide. *Current Problems* 29 1990.
2. Committee on Safety of Medicines/Medicines Control Agency. Cardiac arrhythmias with pimozide (Orap). *Current Problems* 1995; **21**: 2.

Interactions

As for Chlorpromazine, p.664. The risk of arrhythmias with pimozide may be increased by other drugs which prolong the QT interval including some antiarrhythmics, tricyclic antidepressants, the antihistamines terfenadine and astemizole, antimalarials, and cisapride; concomitant use should be avoided. Concomitant use should also be avoided with drugs which induce electrolyte disturbances such as diuretics. The concomitant use of drugs that inhibit the cytochrome P450 isoenzyme CYP3A4 is contra-indicated; the resultant decrease in the metabolism of pimozide may lead to increased plasma concentrations and hence greater risk of cardiac arrhythmias. CYP3A4 inhibitors include the macrolide antibacterials such as clarithromycin, erythromycin, and troleandomycin; the azole antifungals including itraconazole and ketoconazole; the HIV-protease inhibitors ritonavir, saquinavir, indinavir, and nelfinavir; nefazodone, and zileuton. The metabolism of pimozide may also be inhibited by grapefruit juice and concomitant use should be avoided.

Antibacterials. Two sudden deaths have occurred in patients on high-dose pimozide treatment following the co-administration of *clarithromycin*. In a study[1] in healthy volunteers elevated pimozide plasma concentrations were recorded after pretreatment with clarithromycin.

1. Desta Z, *et al.* Effect of clarithromycin on the pharmacokinetics and pharmacodynamics of pimozide in healthy poor and extensive metabolisers of cytochrome P450 2D6 (CYP2D6). *Clin Pharmacol Ther* 1999; **65**: 10–20.

Pharmacokinetics

Following oral administration, more than half of a dose of pimozide is reported to be absorbed. It undergoes significant first-pass metabolism. Peak plasma concentrations have been reported after 4 to 12 hours and there is a considerable interindividual variation in the concentrations achieved. Pimozide is metabolised in the liver mainly by N-dealkylation and excreted in the urine and faeces, both unchanged and in the form of metabolites. Metabolism is mediated mainly by the cytochrome P450 isoenzyme CYP3A4 and to a lesser extent by CYP2D6. Pimozide has a long terminal half-life generally considered to be approximately 55 hours, although half-lives of up to 150 hours have been noted in some patients.

Uses and Administration

Pimozide is a member of the diphenylbutylpiperidine group of antipsychotics, which are structurally similar to the butyrophenones. It is a long-acting antipsychotic with general properties similar to those of the phenothiazine, chlorpromazine (p.665), although it also has some calcium-blocking activity. Pimozide is given by mouth in the management of psychoses including schizophrenia, paranoid states, and monosymptomatic hypochondria (p.650) and in Tourette's syndrome. An ECG should be performed in all patients before starting treatment with pimozide (see Adverse Effects, Treatment, and Precautions, above).

For **schizophrenia**, treatment is usually initiated with a dose of 2 mg daily adjusted thereafter according to response in increments of 2 to 4 mg at intervals of not less than one week. A maximum daily dose of 20 mg

should not be exceeded. It is usually given as a single daily dose.

In **monosymptomatic hypochondria** and **paranoid psychoses** the initial dose is 4 mg daily adjusted as above to a maximum daily dose of 16 mg.

For the treatment of **Tourette's syndrome** an initial dose of 1 to 2 mg daily is recommended, increased to a maximum of 10 mg daily, or 200 µg per kg body-weight, daily.

Pimozide treatment should be begun at half the standard dosage in elderly patients.

Chorea. Antipsychotics such as pimozide have some action against choreiform movements (p.650) as well as being of use to control the behavioural disturbances of Huntington's chorea.

References.

1. Shannon KM, Fenichel GM. Pimozide treatment of Sydenham's chorea. *Neurology* 1990; **40**: 186.

Dystonia. Antipsychotics such as phenothiazines, haloperidol, or pimozide are sometimes useful in the treatment of idiopathic dystonia (p.1173) in patients who have failed to respond to other drugs.[1] In very severe dystonia combination therapy may be required. Pimozide in gradually increasing doses up to 12 mg daily with tetrabenazine and benzhexol [trihexyphenidyl] is sometimes effective. However, antipsychotics often act non-specifically and there is the risk of adding drug-induced extrapyramidal disorders to the dystonia being treated (see Extrapyramidal Disorders under Adverse Effects of Chlorpromazine, p.662).

1. Marsden CD, Quinn NP. The dystonias. *BMJ* 1990; **300**: 139–44.

Schizophrenia. A meta-analysis[1] concluded that pimozide appears to be of similar efficacy to other classical antipsychotics in the treatment of schizophrenia (p.651). However, there was no evidence that pimozide was particularly useful for those with delusional disorders or with predominantly negative symptoms.

1. Sultana A, McMonagle T. Pimozide for schizophrenia or related psychoses (updated 21 November 2000). Available in The Cochrane Library; Issue 4. Oxford: Update Software; 2001.

Taste disorders. For reference to the use of pimozide in the treatment of taste disorders, see Chlorpromazine, p.667.

Tourette's syndrome. Tourette's syndrome (p.650) is a disorder characterised by motor and vocal tics and behavioural disturbances. Many patients with Tourette's syndrome do not require medication but when treatment is needed dopamine antagonists such as the antipsychotics haloperidol or pimozide[1,2] are most commonly used. They often decrease the frequency and severity of tics and may improve any accompanying behavioural disturbances. However, superiority of either drug in terms of efficacy or adverse effects has not been clearly demonstrated. Because of the potential for acute and long-term adverse effects it is usually recommended that doses are titrated to as low as possible; the aim of treatment is not necessarily to control symptoms completely. Medication can often be discontinued after a few years.

1. Shapiro E, *et al.* Controlled study of haloperidol, pimozide, and placebo for the treatment of Gilles de la Tourette's syndrome. *Arch Gen Psychiatry* 1989; **46**: 722–30.
2. Sallee FR, *et al.* Relative efficacy of haloperidol and pimozide in children and adolescents with Tourette's disorder. *Am J Psychiatry* 1997; **154**: 1057–62.

Preparations

BP 2001: Pimozide Tablets;
USP 25: Pimozide Tablets.

Proprietary Preparations (details are given in Part 3)
Aust.: Orap; *Austral.:* Orap; *Belg.:* Orap; *Braz.:* Orap; *Canad.:* Orap; *Denm.:* Orap; *Fr.:* Orap; *Ger.:* Antalon†; Orap; *Hong Kong:* Orap; *Irl.:* Orap; *Israel:* Orap; *Ital.:* Orap; *Neth.:* Orap; *Norw.:* Orap; *NZ:* Orap; *S.Afr.:* Orap; *Singapore:* Orap; *Spain:* Orap; *Swed.:* Orap†; *Switz.:* Orap; *Thai.:* Orap; Pizide; *UK:* Orap; *USA:* Orap.

Pinazepam (7088-h)

Pinazepam *(rINN)*.

7-Chloro-1,3-dihydro-5-phenyl-1-(prop-2-ynyl)-2H-1,4-benzodiazepin-2-one.

$C_{18}H_{13}ClN_2O = 308.8$.
CAS — 52463-83-9.
ATC — N05BA14.

Profile

Pinazepam is a long-acting benzodiazepine with general properties similar to those of diazepam (p.674). It is given by mouth in doses of 5 to 20 mg daily in divided doses for the short-term treatment of anxiety disorders (p.649) and insomnia (p.652).

Preparations

Proprietary Preparations (details are given in Part 3)
Hong Kong: Domar; *Ital.:* Domar; *Singapore:* Domar; *Spain:* Duna; *Thai.:* Domar.

Pipamperone Hydrochloride (7090-t)

Pipamperone Hydrochloride *(BANM, rINNM)*.

Floropipamide Hydrochloride; R-3345 (pipamperone). 1-[3-(4-Fluorobenzoyl)propyl]-4-piperidinopiperidine-4-carboxamide dihydrochloride.

$C_{21}H_{30}FN_3O_2,2HCl = 448.4$.
CAS — 1893-33-0 (pipamperone); 2448-68-2 (pipamperone hydrochloride).

NOTE. Pipamperone is *USAN*.

Pipamperone hydrochloride 1.2 mg is approximately equivalent to 1 mg of pipamperone.

Profile

Pipamperone is a butyrophenone with general properties similar to those of haloperidol (p.686). It is given by mouth as the hydrochloride for the treatment of psychoses. Starting doses equivalent to 20 mg of the base have been given daily, increased gradually thereafter according to response; doses of 360 mg or more have been given daily in divided doses.

Preparations

Proprietary Preparations (details are given in Part 3)
Belg.: Dipiperon; *Denm.:* Dipiperon; *Fr.:* Dipiperon; *Ger.:* Dipiperon; *Ital.:* Piperonil; *Neth.:* Dipiperon; *Switz.:* Dipiperon.

Piperacetazine (7091-x)

Piperacetazine *(USAN, rINN)*.

PC-1421. 10-{3-[4-(2-Hydroxyethyl)piperidino]propyl}phenothiazin-2-yl methyl ketone.

$C_{24}H_{30}N_2O_2S = 410.6$.
CAS — 3819-00-9.

Profile

Piperacetazine is a phenothiazine antipsychotic used as a sedative in veterinary medicine.

Pipotiazine (7092-r)

Pipotiazine *(BAN, rINN)*.

Pipothiazine; RP-19366. 10-{3-[4-(2-Hydroxyethyl)piperidino]propyl}-NN-dimethylphenothiazine-2-sulphonamide; 2-{4-[3-(2-Dimethylsulphamoylphenothiazin-10-yl)propyl]piperazin-1-yl}ethanol.

$C_{24}H_{33}N_3O_3S_2 = 475.7$.
CAS — 39860-99-6.
ATC — N05AC04.

Pipotiazine Palmitate (7093-f)

Pipotiazine Palmitate *(BANM, USAN, rINNM)*.

IL-19552; Pipothiazine Palmitate; RP-19552.

$C_{40}H_{63}N_3O_4S_2 = 714.1$.
CAS — 37517-26-3.

Adverse Effects, Treatment, and Precautions

As for Chlorpromazine, p.660.

◊ Manic symptoms developed in a schizophrenic patient following administration of pipotiazine palmitate. Symptoms recurred on subsequent rechallenge.[1] The possible mania-inducing or antidepressant effects of pipotiazine should be investigated further.

1. Singh AN, Maguire J. Pipothiazine palmitate induced mania. *BMJ* 1984; **289**: 734.

Pharmacokinetics

Pipotiazine palmitate is very slowly absorbed from the site of intramuscular injection. It gradually releases pipotiazine into the body and is therefore suitable for use as a depot injection.

Uses and Administration

Pipotiazine is a phenothiazine with general properties similar to those of chlorpromazine (p.665). It has a piperidine side-chain. It is used in the treatment of schizophrenia (p.651) and other psychoses.

A usual oral dose of pipotiazine for the treatment of psychoses is 10 to 20 mg daily in a single dose; in severe psychoses higher doses have been given for brief periods. In acute conditions treatment has sometimes been started with intramuscular injections.

The long-acting palmitate ester of pipotiazine is given by deep intramuscular injection. An initial test dose of 25 mg is followed by a further 25 to 50 mg after 4 to 7 days. The dosage is then adjusted in increments of 25 to 50 mg according to response at intervals of 4 weeks. Usual maintenance doses of 50 to 100 mg are given at average intervals of 4 weeks; the maximum recommended dose is 200 mg.

Pipotiazine should be given in reduced dosage to elderly patients; a starting dose of 5 to 10 mg has been suggested for pipotiazine palmitate intramuscular injections.

Schizophrenia. A systematic review[1] concluded that depot pipotiazine palmitate appeared to be no different in terms of efficacy or adverse effects to other antipsychotics given orally or by depot injection.

1. Quraishi S, David A. Depot pipothiazine palmitate and undecylenate for schizophrenia (updated 30 May 2001). Available in The Cochrane Library; Issue 4. Oxford: Update Software; 2001.

Preparations

Proprietary Preparations (details are given in Part 3)
Belg.: Piportil; **Braz.:** Piportil; **Canad.:** Piportil L4; **Fr.:** Piportil; **Hong Kong:** Piportil; **Irl.:** Piportil; **Mex.:** Piportil L4; **Neth.:** Piportil; **NZ:** Piportil; **S.Afr.:** Piportil†; **Singapore:** Piportil; **Spain:** Lonseren; **Switz.:** Piportil†; **UK:** Piportil.

Prazepam   (7095-n)

Prazepam (BAN, USAN, rINN).

Prazepamum; W-4020. 7-Chloro-1-(cyclopropylmethyl)-1,3-dihydro-5-phenyl-2H-1,4-benzodiazepin-2-one.
$C_{19}H_{17}ClN_2O = 324.8$.
CAS — 2955-38-6.
ATC — N05BA11.
Pharmacopoeias. In Eur. (see p.vi) and Jpn.

Pharmacopoeial description

Ph. Eur.: A white to almost white crystalline powder. Practically insoluble in water; sparingly soluble in dehydrated alcohol; freely soluble in dichloromethane. Protect from light.

Dependence and Withdrawal
As for Diazepam, p.675.

Adverse Effects, Treatment, and Precautions
As for Diazepam, p.675.

Porphyria. Prazepam is considered to be unsafe in patients with porphyria because it has been shown to be porphyrinogenic in *in-vitro* systems.

Interactions
As for Diazepam, p.677.

Pharmacokinetics
After oral administration, prazepam undergoes extensive first-pass metabolism in the liver to oxazepam (p.697) and desmethyldiazepam (nordazepam, p.696). Desmethyldiazepam is largely responsible for the pharmacological activity of prazepam. Peak plasma concentrations of desmethyldiazepam are reached within about 6 hours after oral administration of prazepam although considerable individual variation has been reported.

◊ References.
1. Ochs HR, *et al.* Comparative single-dose kinetics of oxazolam, prazepam, and clorazepate: three precursors of desmethyldiazepam. *J Clin Pharmacol* 1984; **24:** 446–51.

Distribution into breast milk. The ratio of desmethyldiazepam in plasma to that in breast milk of 5 lactating women given prazepam 20 mg three times daily for 3 days was 9.6 from measurements 12 hours after the last dose.[1] It was estimated that a breast-fed infant of a mother on continuous prazepam therapy would ingest the equivalent of about 4% of the daily maternal dose.
1. Brodie RR, *et al.* Concentrations of N-descyclopropylmethylprazepam in whole-blood, plasma, and milk after administration of prazepam to humans. *Biopharm Drug Dispos* 1981; **2:** 59–68.

Uses and Administration
Prazepam is a long-acting benzodiazepine with general properties similar to those of diazepam (p.680). The usual dose by mouth for the short-term treatment of anxiety disorders (p.649) is 30 mg daily as a single nightly dose or in divided doses; in severe conditions up to 60 mg daily has been given. In elderly or debilitated patients, treatment should be initiated with a daily dose of 10 to 15 mg.

Preparations

Proprietary Preparations (details are given in Part 3)
Aust.: Demetrin; **Belg.:** Lysanxia; **Fr.:** Lysanxia; **Ger.:** Demetrin; Mono Demetrin; **Irl.:** Centrax; **Ital.:** Prazene; Trepidan; **Neth.:** Reapam; **Port.:** Demetrin; **S.Afr.:** Demetrin; **Switz.:** Demetrin; **Thai.:** Pozapam; Prasepine; **UK:** Centrax.

Prochlorperazine   (7096-h)

Prochlorperazine (BAN, rINN).

Chlormeprazine; Prochlorpemazine. 2-Chloro-10-[3-(4-methylpiperazin-1-yl)propyl]phenothiazine.
$C_{20}H_{24}ClN_3S = 373.9$.
CAS — 58-38-8.
ATC — N05AB04.
Pharmacopoeias. In US.

Pharmacopoeial description

USP 25: A clear, pale yellow, viscous liquid, sensitive to light. Very slightly soluble in water; freely soluble in alcohol, in chloroform, and in ether. Store in airtight containers. Protect from light.

Prochlorperazine Edisilate   (7097-m)

Prochlorperazine Edisilate (BANM, rINNM).

Chlormeprazine Edisylate; Prochlorpemazine Edisylate; Prochlorperazine Edisylate; Prochlorperazine Ethanedisulphonate. Prochlorperazine ethane-1,2-disulphonate.
$C_{20}H_{24}ClN_3S, C_2H_6O_6S_2 = 564.1$.
CAS — 1257-78-9.
Pharmacopoeias. In US.

The symbol † denotes a preparation no longer actively marketed

---

Prochlorperazine edisilate 7.5 mg is approximately equivalent to 5 mg of prochlorperazine.

Pharmacopoeial description

USP 25: A white to very light yellow odourless crystalline powder. Soluble 1 in 2 of water and 1 in 1500 of alcohol; insoluble in chloroform and in ether. Solutions in water are acid to litmus. Store in airtight containers. Protect from light.

Incompatibility. See under Prochlorperazine Mesilate, below.

Prochlorperazine Maleate   (7098-b)

Prochlorperazine Maleate (BANM, rINNM).

Chlormeprazine Maleate; Prochlorpemazine Maleate; Prochlorperazine Dihydrogen Maleate; Prochlorperazine Dimaleate; Prochlorperazini Maleas.
$C_{20}H_{24}ClN_3S, 2C_4H_4O_4 = 606.1$.
CAS — 84-02-6.
Pharmacopoeias. In Eur. (see p.vi), Jpn, Pol., and US.

Prochlorperazine maleate 8 mg is approximately equivalent to 5 mg of prochlorperazine.

Pharmacopoeial description

Ph. Eur.: A white or pale yellow, crystalline powder. Very slightly soluble in water and in alcohol; practically insoluble in ether. A freshly prepared saturated solution in water has a pH of 3.0 to 4.0. Protect from light.

USP 25: A white or pale yellow, practically odourless, crystalline powder. Practically insoluble in water; soluble 1 in 1200 of alcohol; slightly soluble in warm chloroform. Its saturated solution is acid to litmus. Store in airtight containers. Protect from light.

Prochlorperazine Mesilate   (7099-v)

Prochlorperazine Mesilate (BANM, rINNM).

Chlormeprazine Mesylate; Prochlorpemazine Mesylate; Prochlorperazine Dimethanesulphonate; Prochlorperazine Mesylate; Prochlorperazine Methanesulphonate; Prochlorperazini Mesylas.
$C_{20}H_{24}ClN_3S, 2CH_3SO_3H = 566.2$.
CAS — 5132-55-8.
Pharmacopoeias. In Br.

Prochlorperazine mesilate 7.6 mg is approximately equivalent to 5 mg of prochlorperazine.

Pharmacopoeial description

BP 2001: A white or almost white, odourless or almost odourless powder. Very soluble in water; sparingly soluble in alcohol; slightly soluble in chloroform; practically insoluble in ether. A 2% solution in water has a pH of 2.0 to 3.0. Protect from light.

Incompatibility. Incompatibility has been reported between the edisilate or mesilate salts of prochlorperazine and several other compounds: these include aminophylline, amphotericin B, ampicillin sodium, aztreonam, some barbiturates, benzylpenicillin salts, calcium gluconate, cefalotin sodium, cefmetazole sodium, chloramphenicol sodium succinate, chlorothiazide sodium, dimenhydrinate, heparin sodium, hydrocortisone sodium succinate, midazolam hydrochloride, and some sulfonamides. Incompatibility between prochlorperazine edisilate and morphine sulfate has been attributed to phenol present in some formulations of the opioid.[1,2] Incompatibility has been reported on dilution of prochlorperazine edisilate injection with sodium chloride injection containing methyl hydroxybenzoate and propyl hydroxybenzoate as preservatives.[3] The problem did not occur with unpreserved sodium chloride or when benzyl alcohol was used as preservative. Prochlorperazine mesilate syrup has been reported to be incompatible with magnesium trisilicate mixture.[4]

1. Stevenson JG, Patriarca C. Incompatibility of morphine sulfate and prochlorperazine edisylate in syringes. *Am J Hosp Pharm* 1985; **42:** 2651.
2. Zuber DEL. Compatibility of morphine sulfate injection and prochlorperazine edisylate injection. *Am J Hosp Pharm* 1987; **44:** 67.
3. Jett S, *et al.* Prochlorperazine edisylate incompatibility. *Am J Hosp Pharm* 1983; **40:** 210.
4. Greig JR. Stemetil syrup and magnesium trisilicate. *Pharm J* 1986; **237:** 504.

Adverse Effects, Treatment, and Precautions

As for Chlorpromazine, p.660. Prochlorperazine may cause less sedation and fewer antimuscarinic effects but extrapyramidal effects may be more frequent.

Severe dystonic reactions have followed the use of prochlorperazine, particularly in children and adolescents. It should therefore be used with extreme care in children.

Transient numbness of the gum and tongue has occurred after the use of buccal tablets of prochlorperazine maleate.

Effects on the cardiovascular system. Hypertension has been reported[1] in some patients given prochlorperazine intrave-

---

nously for prophylaxis of cisplatin-induced nausea and vomiting.

1. Roche H, *et al.* Hypertension and intravenous antidopaminergic drugs. *N Engl J Med* 1985; **312:** 1125–6.

Effects on the mouth. Reports of ulceration and soreness of the lip and tongue associated with administration of prochlorperazine maleate oral tablets.[1,2] The erosive cheilitis resolved after withdrawal of prochlorperazine and recurred on rechallenge.

1. Duxbury AJ, *et al.* Erosive cheilitis related to prochlorperazine maleate. *Br Dent J* 1982; **153:** 271–2.
2. Reilly GD, Wood ML. Prochlorperazine—an unusual cause of lip ulceration. *Acta Derm Venereol (Stockh)* 1984; **64:** 270–1.

Interactions
As for Chlorpromazine, p.664.

Pharmacokinetics

◊ A study of the pharmacokinetics of prochlorperazine in 8 healthy subjects following doses of 6.25 and 12.5 mg intravenously, and 25 mg by mouth.[1] There was a marked interindividual variation in pharmacokinetics following intravenous administration but no evidence of dose-dependent pharmacokinetics; mean terminal half-lives were 6.8 hours for the higher and 6.9 hours for the lower dose. The apparent volume of distribution was very high and plasma clearance values were apparently greater than liver plasma flow, suggesting that the liver may not be the only site of metabolism. After oral administration prochlorperazine concentrations were detectable in only 4 of the 8 subjects due in part to a low bioavailability but also to the lack of sensitivity of the high-pressure liquid chromatographic assay used. The time to peak plasma concentration varied from 1.5 to 5 hours, and the peak concentrations varied from 1.6 to 7.6 ng per mL. Bioavailability was estimated to range from 0 to 16%. A low bioavailability due to high first-pass metabolism would be expected because of the high plasma clearance of prochlorperazine.

1. Taylor WB, Bateman DN. Preliminary studies of the pharmacokinetics and pharmacodynamics of prochlorperazine in healthy volunteers. *Br J Clin Pharmacol* 1987; **23:** 137–42.

Buccal administration. Comparative studies of the bioavailability of buccal and oral prochlorperazine maleate.[1] Both single- and multiple-dose studies indicated that bioavailability was greater after buccal administration. Doses of 3 mg twice daily by the buccal route and 5 mg three times daily by mouth produced similar steady-state plasma-prochlorperazine concentrations.

1. Hessell PG, *et al.* A comparison of the availability of prochlorperazine following im buccal and oral administration. *Int J Pharmaceutics* 1989; **52:** 159–64.

Uses and Administration

Prochlorperazine is a phenothiazine antipsychotic with general properties similar to those of chlorpromazine (p.665). It has a piperazine side-chain. Prochlorperazine and its salts are widely used in the prevention and treatment of nausea and vomiting (p.1206) including that associated with migraine or drug-induced emesis. They are also used for the short-term symptomatic relief of vertigo (p.408) as occurs in Ménière's disease (p.407) or labyrinthitis and in the management of schizophrenia (p.651), mania (see Bipolar Disorder, p.271), and other psychoses. Prochlorperazine has been used as an adjunct in the short-term management of severe anxiety (p.649).

Prochlorperazine base is generally administered by the rectal route and prochlorperazine maleate by the oral or buccal routes, while prochlorperazine edisilate and mesilate are given orally or parenterally.

Depending on the country or the manufacturer, doses of prochlorperazine are expressed either as the base or the salt. Most doses in the UK, including the rectal doses, are expressed in terms of the maleate or mesilate, while most doses in the USA are expressed in terms of the base. As a result there is a disparity in the dosage recommendations for these countries, with the doses in the USA tending to be higher.

Reduced dosage may be required in elderly patients.

Doses of 5 to 10 mg of the maleate or mesilate (or, in the USA, the equivalent of 5 mg of the base) up to 3 or 4 times daily have been used for short-term adjunctive management of **severe anxiety disorders**. A modified-release preparation may be given in doses similar to those used in nausea and vomiting.

For **nausea and vomiting** doses are as follows:

• in the UK, the usual dose *by mouth* for prevention is 5 to 10 mg of the maleate or mesilate (roughly equivalent to about 3 to 6.5 mg of the base) two or three times daily. Similar doses may be given by the *rectal* route

- for the treatment of nausea and vomiting recommended UK doses are 20 mg of the maleate or mesilate *by mouth*, 12.5 mg of the mesilate by deep *intramuscular* injection, or the equivalent of prochlorperazine maleate 25 mg *rectally* as suppositories; further doses, preferably by mouth, are given if necessary. The recommended *buccal* dose of prochlorperazine maleate for the management of nausea and vomiting is 3 to 6 mg twice daily

- in the USA the dose *by mouth* for the control of nausea and vomiting is the equivalent of 5 to 10 mg of the base (as edisilate or maleate) given 3 or 4 times daily; alternatively the equivalent of 10 mg of the base twice daily or 15 mg daily of the base (both as the maleate) may be taken as modified-release capsules. The recommended *intramuscular* dosage is the equivalent of 5 to 10 mg of the base (as edisilate) given every 3 to 4 hours if necessary, up to a total of 40 mg of the base daily. The *rectal* dose is 25 mg of the base given twice daily. In the management of severe nausea and vomiting the equivalent of 2.5 to 10 mg of prochlorperazine (as the edisilate) may be given by slow *intravenous* injection or infusion at a rate not exceeding 5 mg per minute; doses should not exceed 40 mg per day.

For treatment of **psychoses** the following doses have been given:

- in the UK, prochlorperazine maleate or mesilate may be given *by mouth* in a dose of 12.5 mg twice daily for 7 days adjusted gradually to 75 to 100 mg daily according to response; some patients may be maintained on doses of 25 to 50 mg daily. The equivalent of prochlorperazine maleate 25 mg two or three times daily may be given by the *rectal* route or 12.5 to 25 mg of the mesilate two or three times daily by deep *intramuscular* injection

- in the USA prochlorperazine is given as the maleate or edisilate in usual initial doses equivalent to 5 to 10 mg of the base 3 or 4 times daily *by mouth* adjusted according to response up to a maximum of 150 mg of base daily. In severe disturbances it may be given by deep *intramuscular* injection as the edisilate in doses equivalent to 10 to 20 mg of base and repeated every 2 to 6 hours if necessary.

There are similar discrepancies with **children's doses;** owing to the risk of severe extrapyramidal reactions, prochlorperazine should be administered with extreme caution in children: in particular it is not recommended for those weighing less than 10 kg or below 1 year of age. Where the use of prochlorperazine in children is unavoidable, UK sources have suggested that 250 μg of the maleate or mesilate per kg body-weight, may be given two or three times daily by mouth for the prevention and treatment of nausea and vomiting; the intramuscular or rectal routes are considered unsuitable. In contrast, in the USA oral, rectal, and intramuscular routes have all been advocated. The usual oral or rectal antiemetic dose ranges up to 7.5 mg of the base or its equivalent daily in children weighing 10 to 13 kg; in children 14 to 17 kg, up to 10 mg daily; from 18 to 39 kg, up to 15 mg daily. Higher doses have been given for psychoses. The suggested intramuscular dose for children in the USA is the equivalent of about 130 μg of base per kg given as a single deep intramuscular injection of the edisilate.

Prochlorperazine is also used in the UK in the treatment of **vertigo** including that due to Ménière's disease. It is given *by mouth* in doses of 15 to 30 mg of the maleate or mesilate daily in divided doses; after several weeks the dose may be gradually reduced to 5 to 10 mg daily. The recommended *buccal* dose of prochlorperazine maleate for the treatment of vertigo due to Ménière's disease is 3 to 6 mg twice daily.

Headache. The phenothiazines chlorpromazine and prochlorperazine have been used in migraine to control severe nausea and vomiting unresponsive to antiemetics such as metoclopra-

mide and domperidone (see p.449). Parenteral phenothiazines may also relieve the pain of severe migraine attacks unresponsive to parenteral dihydroergotamine or sumatriptan. In comparative studies[1,2] prochlorperazine appears to have been more effective in relieving migraine headache and nausea and vomiting than metoclopramide when these drugs were given parenterally. Prochlorperazine was shown to be effective in aborting intractable migraine in children in a small uncontrolled study.[3]

For further references to the use of phenothiazines in the management of headache including migraine, see under Chlorpromazine, p.666.

1. Coppola M, *et al.* Randomized, placebo-controlled evaluation of prochlorperazine versus metoclopramide for emergency department treatment of migraine headache. *Ann Emerg Med* 1995; **26:** 541–6.
2. Jones J, *et al.* Intramuscular prochlorperazine versus metoclopramide as single-agent therapy for the treatment of acute migraine headache. *Am J Emerg Med* 1996; **14:** 262–4.
3. Kabbouche MA, *et al.* Tolerability and effectiveness of prochlorperazine for intractable migraine in children. *Pediatrics* 2001; **107:** 767. Full version: http://www.pediatrics.org/cgi/content/full/107/4/e62

Preparations

BP 2001: Prochlorperazine Buccal Tablets; Prochlorperazine Injection; Prochlorperazine Oral Solution; Prochlorperazine Tablets; **USP 25:** Prochlorperazine Edisylate Injection; Prochlorperazine Maleate Tablets; Prochlorperazine Oral Solution; Prochlorperazine Suppositories.

Proprietary Preparations (details are given in Part 3)
Austral.: Stemetil; Stemzine; **Canad.:** Nu-Prochlor; Stemetil; **Denm.:** Stemetil; **Fin.:** Stemetil; **Hong Kong:** Dhaperazine; Stella; Stemetil; **Irl.:** Buccastem; Stemetil; **Ital.:** Stemetil; **Neth.:** Stemetil; **Norw.:** Stemetil; **NZ:** Antinaus; Buccastem; Stemetil; **S.Afr.:** Mitil; Scripto-Metic; Stemetil; **Singapore:** Dhaperazine; Stemetil; **Swed.:** Stemetil; **Thai.:** Proclozine; Stemetil; **UK:** Buccastem; Proziere; Stemetil; **USA:** Compazine; Compro.

Multi-ingredient: *Ital.:* Difmetre.

Prolonium Bromide   (14253-j)

(2-Hydroxytrimethylene)bis(trimethylammonium bromide).
$C_9H_{24}Br_2N_2O = 336.1$.

NOTE. Prolonium Iodide is *rINNM.*

Profile
Prolonium bromide was formerly used for its hypnotic and sedative properties.

Prolonium iodide (p.1525) has been used as a source of iodine as part of the treatment of thyroid storm and for the pre-operative management of hyperthyroidism.

Promazine Embonate   (7100-v)

Promazine Embonate (BANM, rINNM).
Promazine Pamoate.
$(C_{17}H_{20}N_2S)_2,C_{23}H_{16}O_6 = 957.2$.
CAS — 58-40-2 (promazine).

Promazine embonate 1.5 g is approximately equivalent to 1 g of promazine hydrochloride.

Promazine Hydrochloride   (7101-g)

Promazine Hydrochloride (BANM, rINNM).
Promazini Hydrochloridum; Propazinum. NN-Dimethyl-3-phenothiazin-10-ylpropylammonium chloride.
$C_{17}H_{20}N_2S,HCl = 320.9$.
CAS — 53-60-1.
Pharmacopoeias. In Eur. (see p.vi), Pol., and US.

Incompatibility has been reported between promazine hydrochloride and several other compounds: these include aminophylline, some barbiturates, benzylpenicillin potassium, chloramphenicol sodium succinate, chlortetracycline, chlorothiazide sodium, dimenhydrinate, heparin, hydrocortisone sodium succinate, nafcillin sodium, phenytoin sodium, prednisolone sodium phosphate, and sodium bicarbonate.

Pharmacopoeial description
Ph. Eur.: A white or almost white, slightly hygroscopic, crystalline powder. Very soluble in water, in alcohol, and in dichloromethane. A freshly prepared 5% solution in water has a pH of 4.2 to 5.2. Protect from light.

USP 25: A white or slightly yellow, practically odourless, crystalline powder. It oxidises upon prolonged exposure to air and acquires a pink or blue colour. Soluble 1 in 3 of water; freely soluble in chloroform. pH of a 1 in 20 solution is between 4.2 and 5.2. Store in airtight containers. Protect from light.

Sorption. A study[1] of drug loss from intravenous delivery systems reported an 11% loss of promazine hydrochloride from solution when infused for 7 hours via a plastic infusion set, and a 59% loss after infusion for one hour from a glass syringe through silastic tubing. Loss was negligible after infusion for one hour from a system comprising a glass syringe with polyethylene tubing.

1. Kowaluk EA, *et al.* Interactions between drugs and intravenous delivery systems. *Am J Hosp Pharm* 1982; **39:** 460–7.

Stability. A study of the stability of promazine diluted to a 0.1% infusion in sodium chloride solution (0.9%) or glucose (5%) found that solutions in glucose (5%) remained stable for up to 6 days at 4°, and at room temperature, provided they were stored in the dark.[1] However, with saline as the diluent deterioration of the promazine was observed 24 hours after preparation, even when stored in the dark, and after 8 hours when exposed to light. Temperature had no effect on degradation rate.

1. Tebbett IR, *et al.* Stability of promazine as an intravenous infusion. *Pharm J* 1986; **237:** 172–4.

Adverse Effects, Treatment, and Precautions
As for Chlorpromazine, p.660.

Pregnancy and the neonate. An increased incidence of neonatal jaundice coincided with the increased use of promazine.[1] A decrease in the incidence of jaundice was noted 3 months after the total withdrawal of the drug from the hospital although restriction of its use during labour had no impact.

1. John E. Promazine and neonatal hyperbilirubinaemia. *Med J Aust* 1975; **2:** 342–4.

Interactions
As for Chlorpromazine, p.664.

Uses and Administration
Promazine is a phenothiazine with general properties similar to those of chlorpromazine (p.665). It has relatively weak antipsychotic activity and is not generally used for the management of psychoses. It is mainly used for the short-term management of agitated or disturbed behaviour (p.650). It has also been given for the alleviation of nausea and vomiting (p.1206) and relief of intractable hiccup (p.667). Promazine is given by mouth or intramuscularly as the hydrochloride. It is also given as the embonate by mouth, in doses equivalent to those of the hydrochloride. Promazine hydrochloride has also been given by slow intravenous injection, in concentrations not exceeding 25 mg per mL.

For the treatment of agitated behaviour, promazine is given in doses of 100 to 200 mg of the hydrochloride four times daily by mouth or 50 mg by intramuscular injection repeated if necessary after 6 to 8 hours. It has also been given by slow intravenous injection for severely agitated hospitalised patients in doses similar to those given by the intramuscular route.

A dose of 25 to 50 mg by intramuscular injection has been given for the control of nausea and vomiting; it has also been given by mouth for this indication. For intractable hiccup 25 to 50 mg is given by intramuscular injection 3 or 4 times daily.

Promazine should be given in reduced dosage to elderly or debilitated subjects; 25 mg by mouth of the hydrochloride initially, increasing, if necessary, to 50 mg four times daily has been suggested for the control of agitation and restlessness; for intramuscular injection a dose of 25 mg may be sufficient.

Preparations
BP 2001: Promazine Injection; Promazine Oral Suspension; Promazine Tablets;
USP 25: Promazine Hydrochloride Injection; Promazine Hydrochloride Oral Solution; Promazine Hydrochloride Syrup; Promazine Hydrochloride Tablets.

Proprietary Preparations (details are given in Part 3)
Austral.: Sparine†; **Belg.:** Prazine; **Denm.:** Sparine; **Fin.:** Sparine; **Ger.:** Protactyl; Sinophenin; **Irl.:** Sparine; **Ital.:** Talofen; **S.Afr.:** Sparine†; **Switz.:** Prazine; **UK:** Sparine; **USA:** Prozine; Sparine†.

Propionylpromazine   (16727-h)

Dipropimazine; Propiopromazine.
CAS — 3568-24-9.

Profile
Propionylpromazine is a phenothiazine antipsychotic used for sedation and premedication in veterinary medicine.

Prothipendyl Hydrochloride   (7102-q)

Prothipendyl Hydrochloride (BANM, rINNM).
D-206; Phrenotropin. NN-Dimethyl-3-(pyrido[3,2-b][1,4]benzothiazin-10-yl)propylamine hydrochloride monohydrate.
$C_{16}H_{19}N_3S,HCl,H_2O = 339.9$.
CAS — 303-69-5 (prothipendyl); 1225-65-6 (anhydrous prothipendyl hydrochloride).

Profile
Prothipendyl is an azaphenothiazine with general properties similar to those of chlorpromazine (p.660). It is given by mouth as the hydrochloride in doses of 40 to 80 mg two to four times daily for the treatment of psychoses and agitation, and as an adjunct to analgesics in the treatment of severe pain. Prothipendyl hydrochloride may also be given by injection.

Preparations
Proprietary Preparations (details are given in Part 3)
Aust.: Dominal; **Belg.:** Dominal; **Ger.:** Dominal.
Multi-ingredient: Belg.: Domidorm†.

Proxibarbal (4064-c)
Proxibarbal (rINN).
HH-184; Proxibarbital. 5-Allyl-5-(2-hydroxypropyl)barbituric acid.
$C_{10}H_{14}N_2O_4 = 226.2$.
CAS — 2537-29-3.
ATC — N05CA22.
Pharmacopoeias. In Pol.

Profile
Proxibarbal is a barbiturate with general properties similar to those of amobarbital (p.655). It has been given by mouth as a sedative in the management of anxiety disorders. It has also been used in the treatment of headache. However, barbiturates are not considered appropriate in the management of these conditions. Proxibarbal has been associated with severe hypersensitivity-induced thrombocytopenia.

Preparations
Proprietary Preparations (details are given in Part 3)
Fr.: Centralgol†.

Pyrithyldione (4065-k)
Pyrithyldione (rINN).
Didropyridinum; NU-903. 3,3-Diethylpyridine-2,4(1H,3H)-dione.
$C_9H_{13}NO_2 = 167.2$.
CAS — 77-04-3.
ATC — N05CE03.

Profile
Pyrithyldione has been given in preparations with diphenhydramine in the short-term management of insomnia but there have been reports of agranulocytosis associated with the use of this combination.

Preparations
Proprietary Preparations (details are given in Part 3)
Multi-ingredient: Belg.: Dormen.

Quazepam (13196-y)
Quazepam (BAN, USAN, rINN).
Sch-16134. 7-Chloro-5-(2-fluorophenyl)-1,3-dihydro-1-(2,2,2-trifluoroethyl)-1,4-benzodiazepine-2-thione.
$C_{17}H_{11}ClF_4N_2S = 386.8$.
CAS — 36735-22-5.
ATC — N05CD10.
Pharmacopoeias. In US.

Off-white to yellowish powder.
Pharmacopoeial description
USP 25: Off-white to yellowish powder.

Dependence and Withdrawal
As for Diazepam, p.675.

Adverse Effects, Treatment, and Precautions
As for Diazepam, p.675.

Interactions
As for Diazepam, p.677.

Pharmacokinetics
Quazepam is readily absorbed from the gastrointestinal tract after administration by mouth, peak plasma concentrations being reached in about 2 hours. It is metabolised extensively in the liver. The principal active metabolites are 2-oxoquazepam and N-desalkyl-2-oxoquazepam (N-desalkylflurazepam) which have elimination half-lives of about 39 and 73 hours respectively compared with a half-life of 39 hours for quazepam. Further hydroxylation occurs and quazepam is excreted in urine and faeces mainly as conjugated metabolites.

Quazepam and its two active metabolites are more than 95% bound to plasma proteins. Quazepam and its metabolites have been detected in breast milk.

Uses and Administration
Quazepam is a long-acting benzodiazepine with general properties similar to those of diazepam (p.680). It is given by mouth as a hypnotic in the short-term management of insomnia (p.652), in an initial dose of 15 mg at night; in elderly or debilitated patients and some other patients this can be reduced to 7.5 mg.

The symbol † denotes a preparation no longer actively marketed

Preparations
USP 25: Quazepam Tablets.
Proprietary Preparations (details are given in Part 3)
Ital.: Quazium; **Port.:** Prosedar; **S.Afr.:** Dorme†; **Spain:** Quiedorm; **USA:** Doral.

Quetiapine Fumarate (17253-z)
Quetiapine Fumarate (BANM, USAN, pINNM).
ICI-204636; ZD-5077; ZM-204636. 2-[2-(4-Dibenzo[b,f][1,4]thiazepin-11-yl-1-piperazinyl)ethoxy]ethanol fumarate (2:1) salt.
$(C_{21}H_{25}N_3O_2S)_2, C_4H_4O_4 = 883.1$.
CAS — 111974-69-7 (quetiapine); 111974-72-2 (quetiapine fumarate).

Adverse Effects and Treatment
As for Chlorpromazine, p.660. The most frequent adverse effect with quetiapine has been somnolence. Quetiapine has been associated with a low incidence of extrapyramidal symptoms. Rises in prolactin concentrations may be less than with chlorpromazine. Other adverse effects have included mild asthenia, anxiety, dizziness, myalgia, rhinitis, dyspepsia, rises in plasma-triglyceride and cholesterol concentrations, and reduced plasma-thyroid hormone concentrations. There have been rare reports of priapism or peripheral oedema. Asymptomatic changes in the lens of the eye have occurred in patients during long-term treatment with quetiapine; cataracts have developed in dogs during chronic dosing studies.

Hyperventilation. A report of hyperventilation and respiratory alkalosis associated with quetiapine administration.[1]
1. Shelton PS, et al. Hyperventilation associated with quetiapine. Ann Pharmacother 2000; 34: 335–7.

Overdosage. Hypotension, tachycardia, and somnolence were the main clinical events observed in a patient who had ingested an overdose of 3 g of quetiapine.[1] Tachycardia of an unexpectedly long duration was also noted. Management was symptomatic, including maintenance of fluids. Asymptomatic prolongation of the QT interval was observed in another patient who had ingested a 2 g overdose of quetiapine.[2] Her treatment regimen also included risperidone, and the authors warned that considerable QT interval prolongation may occur when patients overdose on quetiapine while taking therapeutic doses of risperidone.
1. Beelen AP, et al. Asymptomatic QTc prolongation associated with quetiapine fumarate overdose in a patient being treated with risperidone. Hum Exp Toxicol 2001; 20: 215–19.
2. Pollak PT, Zbuk K. Quetiapine fumarate overdose: clinical and pharmacokinetic lessons from extreme conditions. Clin Pharmacol Ther 2000; 68: 92–7.

Precautions
As for Chlorpromazine, p.663. In the USA it is recommended that patients should have an eye examination to detect cataract formation before starting therapy with quetiapine and every 6 months during treatment.

Interactions
As for Chlorpromazine, p.664. The clearance of quetiapine is increased by concomitant administration with thioridazine.

CYP3A4 is the main isoenzyme responsible for cytochrome P450 mediated metabolism of quetiapine and caution is advised when quetiapine is administered with potent inhibitors of CYP3A4 such as erythromycin, fluconazole, itraconazole, and ketoconazole. Phenytoin and thioridazine have been reported to increase the clearance of quetiapine.

Antipsychotics. For a report of asymptomatic QT prolongation associated with quetiapine in a patient also receiving risperidone, see under Overdosage, above.

Pharmacokinetics
Quetiapine is well absorbed following oral administration and widely distributed throughout the body. It is about 83% bound to plasma proteins. Quetiapine is extensively metabolised in the liver by sulfoxidation mediated mainly by the cytochrome P450 isoenzyme CYP3A4 and by oxidation. It is excreted mainly as inactive metabolites, about 73% of a dose appearing in the urine and about 20% in the faeces. The elimi-

nation half-life has been reported to be about 6 to 7 hours.

◊ References.
1. DeVane CL, Nemeroff CB. Clinical pharmacokinetics of quetiapine: an atypical antipsychotic. Clin Pharmacokinet 2001; 40: 509–22.

Uses and Administration
Quetiapine fumarate is a dibenzothiazepine atypical antipsychotic. It is reported to have affinity for serotonin (5-HT$_2$), dopamine (D$_2$), histaminergic (H$_1$), and adrenergic (α_1 and α_2) receptors.

Quetiapine fumarate is given by mouth in the treatment of schizophrenia. The usual initial dose is the equivalent of 25 mg of the base twice daily on day one, 50 mg twice daily on day two, 100 mg twice daily on day three, and 150 mg twice daily on day four. The dosage is then adjusted according to response to a usual range of 300 to 450 mg daily given in 2 divided doses, although 150 mg daily may be adequate for some patients. The maximum recommended dose is 750 mg daily. Quetiapine should be given in reduced doses to the elderly or patients with impaired hepatic or renal function; a recommended starting dose is 25 mg daily increased in steps of 25 to 50 mg daily according to response.

Quetiapine is under investigation in the treatment of bipolar disorder.

Parkinsonism. Quetiapine has been tried as an antipsychotic in patients with parkinsonism (see under Disturbed Behaviour, p.650).

Schizophrenia. A meta-analysis[1] noted that although the short-term benefits of quetiapine for positive and negative symptoms of schizophrenia appeared comparable with classical antipsychotics, and the incidence of extrapyramidal effects was low (equivalent to placebo), conclusions were necessarily limited by high drop-out rates in the studies considered.
1. Srisurapanont M, et al. Quetiapine for schizophrenia (updated 30 May 2001). Available in The Cochrane Library; Issue 4. Oxford: Update Software; 2001.

Preparations
Proprietary Preparations (details are given in Part 3)
Austral.: Seroquel; **Canad.:** Seroquel; **Fin.:** Seroquel; **Hong Kong:** Seroquel; **Irl.:** Seroquel; **Ital.:** Seroquel; **Mex.:** Seroquel; **NZ:** Seroquel; **S.Afr.:** Seroquel; **Singapore:** Seroquel; **Thai.:** Seroquel; **UK:** Seroquel; **USA:** Seroquel.

Raclopride (2420-b)
Raclopride (BAN, rINN).
A-40664 (raclopride tartrate); FLA-870. (S)-3,5-Dichloro-N-(1-ethylpyrrolidin-2-ylmethyl)-2-hydroxy-6-methoxybenzamide.
$C_{15}H_{20}Cl_2N_2O_3 = 347.2$.
CAS — 84225-95-6 (raclopride); 98185-20-7 (raclopride tartrate).

Profile
Raclopride is a substituted benzamide related to sulpiride (p.706). It has been investigated for the treatment of psychoses. Since it binds selectively and with high affinity to D$_2$ dopaminergic receptors raclopride labelled with carbon-11 has been tried as a tracer in computerised tomographic studies of neurological disorders associated with dysfunction of brain D$_2$ dopaminergic receptors.

Remoxipride Hydrochloride (497-s)
Remoxipride Hydrochloride (BANM, USAN, rINNM).
A-33547 (remoxipride); FLA-731 (remoxipride). (S)-3-Bromo-N-(1-ethylpyrrolidin-2-ylmethyl)-2,6-dimethoxybenzamide hydrochloride monohydrate.
$C_{16}H_{23}BrN_2O_3,HCl,H_2O = 425.7$.
CAS — 80125-14-0 (remoxipride); 73220-03-8 (anhydrous remoxipride hydrochloride); 117591-79-4 (remoxipride hydrochloride monohydrate).
NOTE. Remoxipride is USAN.

Profile
Remoxipride is a substituted benzamide with general properties similar to those of sulpiride (p.706). It is described as an atypical antipsychotic. Remoxipride has been given by mouth or intramuscularly for the treatment of schizophrenia and other psychoses but was withdrawn by the manufacturer following reports of aplastic anaemia associated with its use. However, it remained available from the manufacturer for the compassionate treatment of psychoses in individual patients intolerant of other antipsychotics.

Effects on the blood. By November 1993 the UK Committee on Safety of Medicines had received 8 reports (5 in the UK) of aplastic anaemia associated with remoxipride treatment.[1] The

UK patients, one of whom died, had received a dose of 150 to 600 mg daily for between 3 and 8 months. The committee recommended that treatment with remoxipride should only be initiated by psychiatrists in patients who are intolerant of other antipsychotics. They also recommended that it should not be given to patients with a history of blood disorders and that blood counts should be determined before treatment, every week for the first 6 months of treatment, and monthly thereafter. Patients or their carers should be advised to seek immediate medical attention if bruising, bleeding, fever, or a sore throat develops during treatment. Treatment should be stopped immediately if there is any evidence of a blood disorder.

1. Committee on Safety of Medicines/Medicines Control Agency. Stop press: remoxipride (Roxiam)-aplastic anaemia. *Current Problems* 1993; **19**: 9.

Preparations

Proprietary Preparations (details are given in Part 3)
Aust.: Roxiam†.

Risperidone (5648-h)

Risperidone *(BAN, USAN, rINN).*

R-64766; Risperidonum. 3-{2-[4-(6-Fluoro-1,2-benzisoxazol-3-yl)piperidino]ethyl}-6,7,8,9-tetrahydro-2-methylpyrido[1,2-a]pyrimidin-4-one.

$C_{23}H_{27}FN_4O_2 = 410.5.$
CAS — 106266-06-2.
ATC — N05AX08.

Pharmacopoeias. In Eur. (see p.vi).

Pharmacopoeial description

Ph. Eur.: A white or almost white powder. It exhibits polymorphism. Practically insoluble in water; sparingly soluble in alcohol; freely soluble in dichloromethane; dissolves in dilute acid solutions. Protect from light.

Adverse Effects, Treatment, and Precautions

As for Chlorpromazine, p.660. Risperidone is reported to be less likely to cause sedation or extrapyramidal effects (see also Uses and Administration, below) but agitation may occur more frequently. Dyspepsia, nausea, abdominal pain, anxiety, concentration difficulties, headache, dizziness, fatigue, and rhinitis have also been reported. In addition to orthostatic hypotension, hypertension has been reported infrequently.

Effects on the liver. A report of 2 cases of hepatotoxicity associated with risperidone.[1] An idiosyncratic reaction to risperidone was suspected in another patient who developed hepatotoxicity after receiving only 2 doses of risperidone.[2]

1. Fuller MA, *et al.* Risperidone-associated hepatotoxicity. *J Clin Psychopharmacol* 1996; **16**: 84–5.
2. Phillips EJ, *et al.* Rapid onset of risperidone-induced hepatotoxicity. *Ann Pharmacother* 1998; **32**: 843.

Effects on the skin. A patient developed facial and periorbital oedema 2 weeks after her dose of risperidone reached 6 mg daily.[1] The oedema subsided when the dose was halved but recurred shortly after it was again increased to 6 mg. She had previously had a similar reaction to lithium and there was also a family history of angioedema.

1. Cooney C, Nagy A. Angio-oedema associated with risperidone. *BMJ* 1995; **311**: 1204.

Extrapyramidal disorders. In reports of 3 cases of tardive dystonia associated with risperidone therapy,[1,2] onset ranged from 3 to 8 months after starting the drug. Dyskinesia has also been reported 5 days after the withdrawal of risperidone and citalopram.[3]

1. Vercueil L, Foucher J. Risperidone-induced tardive dystonia and psychosis. *Lancet* 1999; **353**: 981.
2. Krebs MO, Olie JP. Tardive dystonia induced by risperidone. *Can J Psychiatry* 1999; **44**: 507–508.
3. Miller LJ. Withdrawal-emergent dyskinesia in a patient taking risperidone/citalopram. *Ann Pharmacother* 2000; **34**: 269.

Mania. There has been a report[1] that all of 6 patients with bipolar schizoaffective disorder displayed the onset of, or an increase in, manic symptoms shortly after initiation of treatment with risperidone. Symptoms resolved in some patients without the use of mood-stabilising drugs but others required the addition of valproate to treatment. It was considered that it was more likely that risperidone precipitated or exacerbated symptoms of mania rather than this being a coincidental worsening of the patients' symptoms. Since this report, additional cases[2] of risperidone-induced mania have been published.

1. Dwight MM, *et al.* Antidepressant activity and mania associated with risperidone treatment of schizoaffective disorder. *Lancet* 1994; **344**: 554–5.
2. Zolezzi M, Badr MG. Risperidone-induced mania. *Ann Pharmacother* 1999; **33**: 380–1.

Neuroleptic malignant syndrome. Neuroleptic malignant syndrome (p.662) has occasionally been associated with risperidone.[1-3]

1. Sharma R, *et al.* Risperidone-induced neuroleptic malignant syndrome. *Ann Pharmacother* 1996; **30**: 775–8.

2. Tarsy D. Risperidone and neuroleptic malignant syndrome. *JAMA* 1996; **275**: 446.
3. Reeves RR, *et al.* Neuroleptic malignant syndrome during a change from haloperidol to risperidone. *Ann Pharmacother* 2001; **35**: 698–701.

Overdosage. A 3½-year-old child developed extrapyramidal symptoms after accidental ingestion of a single 4-mg tablet of risperidone.[1] The child was initially treated with gastric lavage, activated charcoal, and sorbitol; extrapyramidal symptoms responded to treatment with diphenhydramine and the child recovered completely. The need to monitor for and treat hypotension following overdosage with risperidone was highlighted in a report[2] of a 15-year-old girl who took 40 mg of risperidone.

1. Cheslik TA, Erramouspe J. Extrapyramidal symptoms following accidental ingestion of risperidone in a child. *Ann Pharmacother* 1996; **30**: 360–3.
2. Himstreet JE, Daya M. Hypotension and orthostasis following a risperidone overdose. *Ann Pharmacother* 1998; **32**: 267.

Interactions

As for Chlorpromazine, p.664.

Antipsychotics. For a report suggesting that risperidone might increase plasma concentrations of *clozapine*, see p.673. For a report of asymptomatic QT prolongation associated with *quetiapine* in a patient also receiving risperidone, see under Overdosage of Quetiapine, p.703.

Pharmacokinetics

Risperidone is readily absorbed after oral doses, peak plasma concentrations being reached within 1 to 2 hours. It is extensively metabolised in the liver by hydroxylation to its main active metabolite, 9-hydroxyrisperidone; oxidative *N*-dealkylation is a minor metabolic pathway. Hydroxylation is mediated by the cytochrome P450 isoenzyme CYP2D6 and is the subject of genetic polymorphism. Excretion is mainly in the urine and to a lesser extent, in the faeces. Risperidone and 9-hydroxyrisperidone are about 88% and 77% bound to plasma proteins, respectively.

Metabolism. Although the hydroxylation of risperidone is subject to genetic polymorphism, the pharmacokinetics and effects of the active antipsychotic fraction (risperidone plus 9-hydroxyrisperidone) have been reported to vary little between extensive and poor metabolisers.[1] A mean value of 19.5 hours has been reported for the terminal elimination half-life of the active fraction following oral administration of risperidone.[1]

1. Huang M-L, *et al.* Pharmacokinetics of the novel antipsychotic agent risperidone and the prolactin response in healthy subjects. *Clin Pharmacol Ther* 1993; **54**: 257–68.

Uses and Administration

Risperidone is a benzisoxazole antipsychotic, reported to be an antagonist at dopamine D_2 and serotonin (5-HT$_2$), adrenergic (α_1 and α_2), and histamine (H$_1$) receptors. It is described as an atypical antipsychotic. It is given by mouth for the treatment of schizophrenia and other psychoses.

Risperidone may be given in 1 or 2 divided doses daily. The usual initial daily dose of risperidone is 2 mg; this may be increased to 4 mg daily on the second day, and subsequently adjusted further as required in increments or decrements of 1 or 2 mg daily, generally at intervals of not less than one week, although other titration regimens have been employed. Most patients benefit from doses of 4 to 6 mg daily. Extrapyramidal symptoms may be more likely with doses above 10 mg daily; the US manufacturer does not recommend daily doses above 6 mg if divided into 2 doses, although higher doses are permitted if given as a single dose. The maximum recommended dose is 16 mg daily.

An initial dose of 0.5 mg twice daily slowly increased in steps of 0.5 mg twice daily if necessary to a dose of 1 to 2 mg twice daily is recommended for the elderly and for patients with renal or hepatic impairment.

Action. Risperidone is described as an atypical antipsychotic but although it has a lower propensity to produce parkinsonism, dystonias and akathisias have been reported.[1] (See also Extrapyramidal Disorders, above.) The traditional hypothesis is that antipsychotics work through inhibition of dopamine D_2 receptors and that extrapyramidal motor side-effects result from blockade of D_2 receptors in the striatum (see p.666). Like clozapine, risperidone has a high affinity for 5-HT$_2$ receptors and like haloperidol it has a high affinity for dopamine D_2 receptors. Risperidone also binds to alpha-adrenergic and histamine H_1 sites. It is unclear whether risperidone's antipsychotic effect is due to activity at dopamine D_2 receptors or at another site. It

has been suggested[1] that other potent effects of risperidone may be counterbalancing the D_2 activity to produce its atypicality.

1. Kerwin RW. The new atypical antipsychotics: a lack of extrapyramidal side-effects and new routes in schizophrenia research. *Br J Psychiatry* 1994; **164**: 141–8.

AIDS. Risperidone has been used successfully to control AIDS-related psychosis in 4 patients who also had manic symptoms.[1] No extrapyramidal symptoms were reported during treatment. For reports suggesting that risperidone can induce or exacerbate manic symptoms in patients with schizoaffective disorders, see under Mania in Adverse Effects, above.

1. Singh AN, Catalan J. Risperidone in HIV-related manic psychosis. *Lancet* 1994; **344**: 1029–30.

Anxiety disorders. Although there have been anecdotal reports[1,2] of improvement following the addition of risperidone to treatment in patients with obsessive-compulsive disorder refractory to conventional treatment there has also been a report[3] of a patient whose obsessive-compulsive behaviour recurred when he was treated with risperidone for tardive dyskinesia.

1. Jacobsen FM. Risperidone in the treatment of affective illness and obsessive-compulsive disorder. *J Clin Psychiatry* 1995; **56**: 423–9.
2. McDougle CJ, *et al.* Risperidone addition in fluvoxamine-refractory obsessive-compulsive disorder: three cases. *J Clin Psychiatry* 1995; **56**: 526–8.
3. Remington G, Adams M. Risperidone and obsessive-compulsive symptoms. *J Clin Psychopharmacol* 1994; **14**: 358–9.

Dementia. Risperidone has been used for the management of behavioural disturbances[1,2] in patients with dementia (p.650). Although there have been anecdotal reports[3] of efficacy in patients with Lewy-body dementia, other reports[4] suggest that these patients are likely to be just as sensitive to risperidone as to standard antipsychotics (see the Elderly in Precautions for Chlorpromazine, p.663).

1. DeDeyn PP, *et al.* A randomized trial of risperidone, placebo, and haloperidol for behavioral symptoms of dementia. *Neurology* 1999; **53**: 946–55.
2. Falsetti AE. Risperidone for control of agitation in dementia patients. *Am J Health-Syst Pharm* 2000; **57**: 862–70.
3. Allen RL, *et al.* Risperidone for psychotic and behavioural symptoms in Lewy body dementia. *Lancet* 1995; **346**: 185.
4. McKeith IG, *et al.* Neuroleptic sensitivity to risperidone in Lewy body dementia. *Lancet* 1995; **346**: 699.

Dystonias. Antipsychotics are sometimes useful in the treatment of idiopathic dystonia (p.1173) in patients who have failed to respond to treatment with levodopa or antimuscarinics, but with classic antipsychotics there is the risk of adding drug-induced extrapyramidal effects to the dystonia. Risperidone has been reported to be of benefit in 5 patients with idiopathic segmental dystonia partly insensitive to haloperidol.[1]

1. Zuddas A, Cianchetti C. Efficacy of risperidone in idiopathic segmental dystonia. *Lancet* 1996; **347**: 127–8.

Parkinsonism. There have been conflicting reports of the use of risperidone as an antipsychotic in a small number of patients with Parkinson's disease (see also Disturbed Behaviour, p.650). While some have found that risperidone ameliorated levodopa-induced hallucinations without worsening of extrapyramidal symptoms,[1,2] in other patients with Parkinson's disease given risperidone substantial worsening of symptoms has occurred.[2,3]

1. Meco G, *et al.* Risperidone for hallucinations in levodopa-treated Parkinson's disease patients. *Lancet* 1994; **343**: 1370–1.
2. Leopold NA. Risperidone treatment of drug-induced psychosis in patients with parkinsonism. *Mov Disord* 2000; **15**: 301–4.
3. Ford B, *et al.* Risperidone in Parkinson's disease. *Lancet* 1994; **344**: 681.

Schizophrenia. Risperidone is claimed to produce a relatively low incidence of extrapyramidal effects and to have efficacy against both positive and negative symptoms of schizophrenia. Most studies have compared risperidone with haloperidol but, of these, some of the major studies[1-3] have been criticised for potential methodological flaws[4,5] and it is difficult to determine any difference in efficacy including effect on negative symptoms. A systematic review[6] suggested that risperidone's benefits over haloperidol or other classical antipsychotics were marginal; although it did appear to reduce the risk of extrapyramidal effects compared with haloperidol, the latter produces a relatively high incidence of such effects. Furthermore, the risk of extrapyramidal effects with risperidone appears to be dose dependent;[7] although similar to that for placebo overall, at doses of more than 10 mg it appears to approach that associated with haloperidol. In the few comparative studies with other atypical antipsychotics risperidone has appeared to be of similar efficacy to clozapine.[8] However, another systematic review[9] concluded that such equivalence with clozapine cannot be assumed. For a comparative study with olanzapine, see p.696. There is insufficient evidence to indicate whether risperidone is effective for treatment-resistant or poorly responsive patients.

1. Chouinard G, *et al.* A Canadian multicenter placebo-controlled study of fixed doses of risperidone and haloperidol in the treatment of chronic schizophrenic patients. *J Clin Psychopharmacol* 1993; **13**: 25–40.
2. Marder SR, Meibach RC. Risperidone in the treatment of schizophrenia. *Am J Psychiatry* 1994; **151**: 825–35.
3. Peuskens J, *et al.* Risperidone Study Group. Risperidone in the treatment of patients with chronic schizophrenia: a multi-national, multi-centre, double-blind, parallel-group study versus haloperidol. *Br J Psychiatry* 1995; **166**: 712–26.

4. Livingston MG. Risperidone. *Lancet* 1994; **343:** 457–60.
5. Musser WS, Kirisci L. Critique of the Canadian multicenter placebo-controlled study of risperidone and haloperidol. *J Clin Psychopharmacol* 1995; **15:** 226–8.
6. Kennedy E, *et al.* Risperidone versus typical antipsychotic medication for schizophrenia (updated 12 February 2001). Available in The Cochrane Library; Issue 4. Oxford: Update Software; 2001.
7. Owens DGC. Extrapyramidal side effects and tolerability of risperidone: a review. *J Clin Psychiatry* 1994; **55** (suppl 5): 29–35.
8. Klieser E, *et al.* Randomized, double-blind, controlled trial of risperidone versus clozapine in patients with chronic schizophrenia. *J Clin Psychopharmacol* 1995; **15** (suppl 1): 45S–51S.
9. Gilbody SM, *et al.* Risperidone versus other atypical antipsychotic medication for schizophrenia (updated 12 February 2001). Available in The Cochrane Library; Issue 4. Oxford: Update Software; 2001.

Tourette's syndrome. When treatment is required for tics and behavioural disturbances in Tourette's syndrome (p.650) haloperidol or pimozide are commonly used but risperidone has also been tried.[1,2]

1. Bruun RD, Budman CL. Risperidone as a treatment for Tourette's syndrome. *J Clin Psychiatry* 1996; **57:** 29–31.
2. Bruggeman R, *et al.* Risperidone versus pimozide in Tourette's disorder: a comparative double-blind parallel-group study. *J Clin Psychiatry* 2001; **62:** 50–6.

Preparations

Proprietary Preparations (details are given in Part 3)
Aust.: Belivon; Risperdal; Rispolin†; *Austral.:* Risperdal; *Belg.:* Risperdal; *Braz.:* Risperdal; *Canad.:* Risperdal; *Denm.:* Risperdal; *Fin.:* Risperdal; *Fr.:* Risperdal; *Ger.:* Risperdal; *Hong Kong:* Risperdal; *Irl.:* Risperdal; *Israel:* Risperdal; *Ital.:* Belivon; Risperdal; *Jpn:* Risperdal; *Mex.:* Risperdal; *Neth.:* Risperdal; *Norw.:* Risperdal; *NZ:* Risperdal; *Port.:* Risperdal; *S.Afr.:* Risperdal; *Singapore:* Risperdal; *Spain:* Risperdal; *Swed.:* Risperdal; *Switz.:* Risperdal; *Thai.:* Risperdal; *UK:* Risperdal; *USA:* Risperdal.

Ritanserin   (18677-n)

Ritanserin (*BAN, USAN, rINN*).

R-55667.   6-{2-[4-(4,4′-Difluorobenzhydrylidene)piperidino]ethyl}-7-methyl[1,3]thiazolo[3,2-*a*]pyrimidin-5-one.

$C_{27}H_{25}F_2N_3OS = 477.6$.
CAS — 87051-43-2.

Profile

Ritanserin is a serotonin antagonist which has been studied in a variety of disorders including anxiety disorders, depression, and schizophrenia. It is reported to have little sedative action.

Action. Ritanserin is a relatively selective antagonist at serotonin (5-hydroxytryptamine, 5-HT) receptors of the 5-HT$_2$ subtype, although it also has appreciable affinity for 5-HT$_{1C}$ receptors.[1] Unlike ketanserin (p.917), it does not block α$_1$-adrenergic receptors. Ritanserin has anxiolytic activity; it also hastens the onset of slow-wave sleep although sleep may be impaired on withdrawal.

Ritanserin may interfere with platelet function[2,3] and has been reported to have no significant effect on blood pressure, blood flow, or heart rate in patients with hypertension.[2,4] Features characteristic of class III antiarrhythmic activity have also been noted.[2]

1. Marsden CA. The pharmacology of new anxiolytics acting on 5-HT neurones. *Postgrad Med J* 1990; **66** (suppl 2): S2–S6.
2. Stott DJ, *et al.* The effects of the 5HT$_2$ antagonist ritanserin on blood pressure and serotonin-induced platelet aggregation in patients with untreated essential hypertension. *Eur J Clin Pharmacol* 1988; **35:** 123–9.
3. Wagner B, *et al.* Effect of ritanserin, a 5-hydroxytryptamine$_2$-receptor antagonist, on platelet function and thrombin generation at the site of plug formation in vivo. *Clin Pharmacol Ther* 1990; **48:** 419–23.
4. Chau NP, *et al.* Comparative haemodynamic effects of ketanserin and ritanserin in the proximal and distal upper limb circulations of hypertensive patients. *Eur J Clin Pharmacol* 1989; **37:** 215–20.

Schizophrenia. Ritanserin has produced some beneficial effects[1,2] when tried in small numbers of patients with schizophrenia (p.651).

1. Duinkerke SJ, *et al.* Ritanserin, a selective 5-HT$_{2/1C}$ antagonist, and negative symptoms in schizophrenia: a placebo-controlled double-blind trial. *Br J Psychiatry* 1993; **163:** 451–5.
2. Wiesel F-A, *et al.* An open clinical and biochemical study of ritanserin in acute patients with schizophrenia. *Psychopharmacology (Berl)* 1994; **114:** 31–8.

Substance dependence. Despite some encouraging preliminary data[1] suggesting that ritanserin might influence the desire to drink alcohol, subsequent studies[2] have failed to support a role for ritanserin in reducing alcohol intake in patients with *alcohol* dependence (p.1131).

1. Meert TF. Ritanserin and alcohol abuse and dependence. *Alcohol Alcohol* 1994; **2** (suppl): 523–30.
2. Johnson BA, *et al.* Ritanserin Study Group. Ritanserin in the treatment of alcohol dependence—a multi-center clinical trial. *Psychopharmacology (Berl)* 1996; **128:** 206–15.

Romifidine   (5670-d)

Romifidine (*BAN, rINN*).

STH-2130. 2-Bromo-6-fluoro-*N*-(1-imidazolin-2-yl)aniline.

$C_9H_9BrFN_3 = 258.1$.
CAS — 65896-16-4.

Profile

Romifidine is an α$_2$-adrenoceptor agonist with sedative, muscle relaxant, and analgesic properties and is used in veterinary medicine.

Secbutabarbital   (4068-x)

Secbutabarbital (*rINN*).

Butabarbital; Butabarbitone; Secbutobarbital (*BAN*); Secbutobarbitone. 5-sec-Butyl-5-ethylbarbituric acid.

$C_{10}H_{16}N_2O_3 = 212.2$.
CAS — 125-40-6.

NOTE. Butabarbital should be distinguished from Butobarbital (p.659).

Pharmacopoeias. In US.

Pharmacopoeial description

USP 25: A white, odourless, crystalline powder. Very slightly soluble in water; soluble in alcohol, in chloroform, in ether, and in aqueous solutions of alkali hydroxides and carbonates. Store in airtight containers.

Secbutabarbital Sodium   (4069-r)

Secbutabarbital Sodium (*rINNM*).

Butabarbital Sodium; Secbutabarbital Sodium (*BANM*); Secbutobarbitone Sodium; Secumalnatrium; Sodium Butabarbital. Sodium 5-sec-butyl-5-ethylbarbiturate.

$C_{10}H_{15}N_2NaO_3 = 234.2$.
CAS — 143-81-7.

Pharmacopoeias. In US.

Pharmacopoeial description

USP 25: A white powder. Soluble 1 in 2 of water, 1 in 7 of alcohol, and 1 in 7000 of chloroform; practically insoluble in absolute ether. pH of a 10% solution in water is between 10.0 and 11.2. Store in airtight containers.

Profile

Secbutabarbital is a barbiturate with general properties similar to those of amobarbital (p.655). It was used as a hypnotic and sedative although barbiturates are no longer considered appropriate for such purposes. For the short-term management of insomnia (p.652) it was usually given as the sodium salt in doses of 50 to 100 mg by mouth at night; as a sedative 15 to 30 mg has been given 3 or 4 times daily. Secbutabarbital base has been given.

Preparations

USP 25: Butabarbital Sodium Elixir; Butabarbital Sodium Tablets.

Proprietary Preparations (details are given in Part 3)
Canad.: Butisol†; *USA:* Butisol.

Multi-ingredient: *USA:* Butibel.

Secobarbital   (4066-a)

Secobarbital (*rINN*).

Meballymal; Quinalbarbitone; Secobarbitalum; Secobarbitone. 5-Allyl-5-(1-methylbutyl)barbituric acid.

$C_{12}H_{18}N_2O_3 = 238.3$.
CAS — 76-73-3.
ATC — N05CA06.

Pharmacopoeias. In US.

Pharmacopoeial description

USP 25: A white amorphous or crystalline odourless powder. Very slightly soluble in water; freely soluble in alcohol, in ether, and in solutions of fixed alkali hydroxides and carbonates; soluble in chloroform; soluble 1 in 8.5 of 0.5N sodium hydroxide. A saturated solution in water has a pH of about 5.6. Store in airtight containers.

Secobarbital Sodium   (4067-t)

Secobarbital Sodium (*BAN, rINNM*).

Meballymalnatrium; Quinalbarbitone Sodium; Secobarbitalum Natricum; Secobarbitone Sodium. Sodium 5-allyl-5-(1-methylbutyl)barbiturate.

$C_{12}H_{17}N_2NaO_3 = 260.3$.
CAS — 309-43-3.

Pharmacopoeias. In Aust., Belg., Chin., Fr., It., Neth., Port., Swiss, and US.

Secobarbital may be precipitated from preparations containing secobarbital sodium depending on the concentration and pH. Secobarbital sodium has, therefore, been reported to be **incompatible** with many other drugs, particularly acids and acidic salts.

Pharmacopoeial description

USP 25: A white odourless hygroscopic powder. Very soluble in water; soluble in alcohol; practically insoluble in ether. pH

of a 10% solution in water is between 9.7 and 10.5. Solutions decompose on standing, heat accelerating the decomposition. Store in airtight containers.

Dependence and Withdrawal

As for Amobarbital, p.655.

Adverse Effects, Treatment, and Precautions

As for Amobarbital, p.655.

◊ Exposure to secobarbital sodium among 6 workers in the pharmaceutical industry resulted in absorption of substantial amounts of the drug, with blood concentrations approaching those expected after a therapeutic dose.[1] There continued to be evidence of absorption, despite protective masks to reduce inhalation, and it appeared that substantial absorption was taking place through the skin.

1. Baxter PJ, *et al.* Exposure to quinalbarbitone sodium in pharmaceutical workers. *BMJ* 1986; **292:** 660–1.

Porphyria. Secobarbital has been associated with acute attacks of porphyria and is considered unsafe in porphyric patients.

Interactions

As for Amobarbital, p.656.

Pharmacokinetics

Secobarbital is well absorbed from the gastrointestinal tract following oral doses and is reported to be about 46 to 70% bound to plasma proteins. The mean elimination half-life is reported to be 28 hours. It is metabolised in the liver, mainly by hydroxylation, and excreted in urine as metabolites and a small amount of unchanged drug.

Uses and Administration

Secobarbital is a barbiturate that has been used as a hypnotic and sedative. It has general properties similar to those of amobarbital (p.656). As a hypnotic in the short-term management of insomnia (p.652) it was usually given by mouth in a dose of 100 mg of the sodium salt at night, but barbiturates are no longer considered appropriate for such use.

Secobarbital sodium has also been given by mouth or by intramuscular or intravenous injection for premedication in anaesthetic procedures (p.1256) but the use of barbiturates for preoperative sedation has been replaced by other drugs.

Preparations

USP 25: Secobarbital Elixir; Secobarbital Sodium and Amobarbital Sodium Capsules; Secobarbital Sodium Capsules; Secobarbital Sodium for Injection; Secobarbital Sodium Injection.

Proprietary Preparations (details are given in Part 3)
Canad.: Seconal†; *Irl.:* Seconal†; *S.Afr.:* Seconal†; *UK:* Seconal; *USA:* Seconal.

Multi-ingredient: *Belg.:* Bellanox†; Vesparax†; *Canad.:* Tuinal†; *Irl.:* Tuinal†; *Neth.:* Vesparax; *Port.:* Vesparax†; *S.Afr.:* Vesparax†; *Spain:* Somatarax; *UK:* Tuinal; *USA:* Tuinal.

Sertindole   (11056-p)

Sertindole (*BAN, USAN, rINN*).

Lu-23-174. 1-(2-{4-[5-Chloro-1-(*p*-fluorophenyl)indol-3-yl]piperidino}ethyl)-2-imidazolidinone.

$C_{24}H_{26}ClFN_4O = 440.9$.
CAS — 106516-24-9.
ATC — N05AE03.

Adverse Effects, Treatment, and Precautions

As for Chlorpromazine, p.660. Sertindole is associated with a low incidence of extrapyramidal symptoms and does not appear to cause sedation. Prolactin elevation may be less frequent. Other adverse effects have included peripheral oedema, rhinitis, dyspnoea, and paraesthesia.

Marketing of sertindole was suspended in the UK in December 1998, and subsequently in a number of other countries, because of cardiac arrhythmias and sudden cardiac deaths associated with its use. However it has remained available on a named-patient basis and its suspension from European markets was lifted in 2001. Since sertindole has been associated with prolongation of the QT interval, usually during the first 3 to 6 weeks of treatment, it was recommended that patients should have an ECG before the start of therapy and periodically during treatment. Patients with pre-existing prolongation of the QT interval should not be given sertindole and sertindole should be discontinued if such prolongation occurs during treatment.

Sertindole should not be given to patients with uncorrected hypokalaemia or hypomagnesaemia. It was also recommended that blood pressure should be monitored during dose titration and in early maintenance therapy.

Effects on the cardiovascular system. The manufacturer has stated that in clinical studies prolongation of the QT interval had been seen in 24 of 1446 (1.66%) patients given sertindole. The effect did not correlate with plasma concentrations of sertindole and/or its metabolites. In evidence presented to the FDA it was reported that as of 1st June 1996 there had been 27 deaths, 16 due to adverse cardiac events, among the 2194 patients given sertindole in clinical studies.[1] By the end of November 1998, the UK Committee on Safety of Medicines (CSM) was aware of 36 suspected adverse drug reactions with a fatal outcome, 9 of which originated in the UK.[2] In addition there had been 13 reports of serious but non-fatal cardiac arrhythmias in the UK. Although not all the fatalities were related to sudden cardiac events, the CSM considered that, given the number of serious arrhythmias and sudden cardiac deaths, the risk-benefit ratio of sertindole was no longer favourable.

1. Barnett AA. Safety concerns over antipsychotic drug, sertindole. *Lancet* 1996; **348:** 256.
2. Committee on Safety of Medicines/Medicines Control Agency. Suspension of availability of sertindole (Serdolect). *Current Problems* 1999; **25:** 1.

Interactions
As for Chlorpromazine, p.664. The risk of arrhythmias with sertindole may be increased by other drugs which prolong the QT interval and concomitant use should be avoided. Concomitant use should also be avoided with drugs which produce electrolyte disturbances.

Sertindole is extensively metabolised by the cytochrome P450 isoenzymes CYP2D6 and CYP3A. Ketoconazole and itraconazole are potent inhibitors of CYP3A and their use with sertindole is contra-indicated. Minor increases in sertindole plasma concentrations have been noted in patients also given macrolide antibacterials or calcium-channel blockers which also inhibit CYP3A. Fluoxetine and paroxetine, potent inhibitors of CYP2D6, have increased plasma concentrations of sertindole by a factor of 2 to 3 and lower maintenance doses of sertindole may be required during concomitant treatment.

Pharmacokinetics
Sertindole is slowly absorbed with peak concentrations occurring about 10 hours after oral administration. It is about 99.5% bound to plasma proteins and readily crosses the placenta. Sertindole is extensively metabolised in the liver by the cytochrome P450 isoenzymes CYP2D6 and CYP3A. There is moderate intersubject variation in the pharmacokinetics of sertindole due to polymorphism in the isoenzyme CYP2D6. Poor metabolisers, deficient in this isoenzyme, may have plasma concentrations of sertindole 2 to 3 times higher than other patients. The two major metabolites identified, dehydrosertindole and norsertindole, appear to be inactive. Sertindole and its metabolites are excreted slowly, mainly in the faeces with a minor amount appearing in the urine. The mean terminal half-life is about 3 days.

Uses and Administration
Sertindole is an atypical antipsychotic that is an antagonist at central dopamine (D_2), serotonin (5-HT$_2$), and adrenergic (α_1) receptors. It was used in the treatment of schizophrenia (p.651) but marketing was suspended (see Adverse Effects, above); it is currently available on a named-patient basis for those already stabilised on the drug in whom other antipsychotics are inappropriate.

Sertindole was given by mouth in an initial dose of 4 mg daily, increased gradually by 4 mg every 4 or 5 days to a usual maintenance dose of 12 to 20 mg given once daily. The maximum dose was 24 mg daily. Slower dose titration and lower maintenance doses are advisable for the elderly and patients with hepatic impairment.

Preparations
Proprietary Preparations (details are given in Part 3)
Aust.: Serdolect; **Denm.:** Serdolect†; **Ger.:** Serdolect; **Irl.:** Serdolect†; **Neth.:** Serdolect†; **Norw.:** Serdolect; **Switz.:** Serdolect; **UK:** Serdolect†.

Sulpiride (7107-l)

Sulpiride (BAN, USAN, rINN).

Sulpiridum. *N*-(1-Ethylpyrrolidin-2-ylmethyl)-2-methoxy-5-sulphamoylbenzamide.

$C_{15}H_{23}N_3O_4S = 341.4$.

CAS — 15676-16-1 (sulpiride); 23672-07-3 (levosulpiride).

ATC — N05AL01.

NOTE. Levosulpiride is *pINN*.

Pharmacopoeias. In Eur. (see p.vi) and Jpn.

Pharmacopoeial description
Ph. Eur.: A white or almost white crystalline powder. Practically insoluble in water; slightly soluble in alcohol and in dichloromethane; sparingly soluble in methyl alcohol. It dissolves in dilute solutions of mineral acids and in alkali hydroxides.

Adverse Effects, Treatment, and Precautions
As for Chlorpromazine, p.660.

Sleep disturbances, overstimulation, and agitation may occur. Extrapyramidal effects appear to occur as frequently as for chlorpromazine but have usually been mild. Whether sulpiride is less likely to cause tardive dyskinesia remains to be established. Sulpiride is less likely to cause sedation than chlorpromazine and antimuscarinic effects are minimal. Cardiovascular effects such as hypotension are generally rare although they may occur with overdosage.

Sulpiride should be given with care to manic or hypomanic patients in whom it may exacerbate symptoms.

Sulpiride may be distributed into breast milk in relatively large amounts and some recommend that its use should be avoided in mothers wishing to breast feed.

Effects on the cardiovascular system. Sulpiride 100 mg by mouth caused an attack of hypertension in 6 of 26 hypertensive patients; in 4 it induced a rise in urinary excretion of vanillylmandelic acid and catecholamines.[1] A transient rise in blood pressure and catecholamines after administration of sulpiride occurred in 3 patients who were found to have a phaeochromocytoma; another patient probably had a phaeochromocytoma. The means by which sulpiride provoked hypertension were not known but appeared to be due to a noradrenergic effect. Sulpiride should be avoided during the treatment of phaeochromocytoma, and prescribed with great care in hypertensive patients.

1. Corvol P, *et al.* Poussées hypertensives déclenchées par le sulpiride. *Sem Hop Paris* 1974; **50:** 1265–9.

Porphyria. Sulpiride is considered to be unsafe in patients with porphyria because it has been shown to be porphyrinogenic in *animals*.

Renal impairment. For the precautions to be observed in patients with impaired renal function, see under Uses and Administration, below.

Interactions
As for Chlorpromazine, p.664

Gastrointestinal drugs. Giving sulpiride with therapeutic doses of *sucralfate* or an *antacid* containing aluminium and magnesium hydroxides to 6 healthy subjects reduced the mean oral bioavailability of sulpiride by 40 and 32% respectively.[1] When sulpiride was given 2 hours after the antacid or sucralfate (each in 2 subjects), the reduction in bioavailability was about 25%. This interaction was expected to be clinically significant, and it was recommended that sulpiride should be given before, rather than with or after, sucralfate or antacids.

1. Gouda MW, *et al.* Effect of sucralfate and antacids on the bioavailability of sulpiride in humans. *Int J Pharmaceutics* 1984; **22:** 257–63.

Pharmacokinetics
Sulpiride is slowly absorbed from the gastrointestinal tract; bioavailability is low and subject to interindividual variation. It is rapidly distributed to the tissues but passage across the blood-brain barrier is poor. Sulpiride is less than 40% bound to plasma proteins and is reported to have a plasma half-life of about 6 to 9 hours. It is excreted in the urine and faeces, chiefly as unchanged drug. Sulpiride is distributed into breast milk.

◊ References.
1. Wiesel F-A, *et al.* The pharmacokinetics of intravenous and oral sulpiride in healthy human subjects. *Eur J Clin Pharmacol* 1980; **17:** 385–91.
2. Bressolle F, *et al.* Sulpiride pharmacokinetics in humans after intramuscular administration at three dose levels. *J Pharm Sci* 1984; **73:** 1128–36.
3. Bressolle F, *et al.* Absolute bioavailability, rate of absorption, and dose proportionality of sulpiride in humans. *J Pharm Sci* 1992; **81:** 26–32.

Distribution into breast milk. On the fifth day after starting administration of D-sulpiride, DL-sulpiride, or L-sulpiride in a dose of 50 mg twice daily, mean concentrations of sulpiride in breast milk were 840 nanograms, 850 nanograms, and 810 nanograms per mL respectively.[1]

1. Polatti F. Sulpiride isomers and milk secretion in puerperium. *Clin Exp Obstet Gynecol* 1982; **9:** 144–7.

Uses and Administration
Sulpiride is a substituted benzamide antipsychotic which is reported to be a selective antagonist of central dopamine (D_2, D_3, and D_4) receptors. It is also claimed to have mood elevating properties.

Sulpiride is mainly used in the treatment of psychoses such as schizophrenia. It has also been given in the management of Tourette's syndrome, anxiety disorders (p.649), vertigo (p.408), and benign peptic ulceration. Levosulpiride, the L-isomer of sulpiride, has been used similarly to sulpiride.

In the treatment of schizophrenia initial doses of 200 to 400 mg of sulpiride are given twice daily by mouth, increased if necessary up to a maximum of 1.2 g twice daily in patients with mainly positive symptoms or up to a total of 800 mg daily in patients with predominantly negative symptoms. Sulpiride is also given in some countries by intramuscular injection, in doses ranging from 200 to 800 mg daily. A daily dose of 3 to 5 mg per kg body-weight may be

given by mouth to children over 14 years of age. Lower initial doses have been recommended in elderly patients, subsequently adjusted as required. Dosage adjustment is also advised in patients with renal impairment (see below).

◊ Reviews.
1. Caley CF, Weber SS. Sulpiride: an antipsychotic with selective dopaminergic antagonist properties. *Ann Pharmacother* 1995; **29:** 152–60.
2. Mauri MC, *et al.* A risk-benefit assessment of sulpiride in the treatment of schizophrenia. *Drug Safety* 1996; **14:** 288–98.

Administration in renal impairment. A single intravenous dose of sulpiride 100 mg was administered to 6 healthy subjects with normal renal function (creatinine clearance greater than 90 mL per minute) and to three groups of 6 patients each with creatinine clearances (CC) in the ranges 30 to 60, 10 to 30, and less than 10 mL per minute.[1] There was a progressive diminution in the rate of elimination and an increase in half-life with decreasing renal function. The mean plasma elimination half-lives were 5.90, 11.02, 19.27, and 25.96 hours in the four groups respectively. In the UK it has been recommended that the dose be reduced to two-thirds of the normal amount in patients with CC of 30 to 60 mL per minute, to half the normal dose where CC is 10 to 30 mL per minute, and to one-third where CC is less than 10 mL per minute; alternatively the dosage interval can be prolonged by a factor of 1.5, 2, and 3 respectively. However, the *British National Formulary* suggests that sulpiride should be avoided if possible in moderate renal impairment.

1. Bressolle F, *et al.* Pharmacokinetics of sulpiride after intravenous administration in patients with impaired renal function. *Clin Pharmacokinet* 1989; **17:** 367–73.

Chorea. Antipsychotics have some action against choreiform movements (p.650) as well as being of use to control the behavioural disturbances of Huntington's chorea. Although sulpiride was found to have produced an overall reduction in abnormal movements in 11 patients with Huntington's chorea when compared with placebo in a double-blind study[1] there was generally no accompanying functional improvement and patients with mild disease tended to worsen when taking sulpiride.

1. Quinn N, Marsden CD. A double blind trial of sulpiride in Huntington's disease and tardive dyskinesia. *J Neurol Neurosurg Psychiatry* 1984; **47:** 844–7.

Gastrointestinal disorders. Although sulpiride is used in some countries as an adjunct in the treatment of peptic ulcer disease (p.1208) it is not among the more usual drugs used for this indication. Efficacy has also been claimed for sulpiride or levosulpiride in a variety of other gastrointestinal disorders, including irritable colon (p.1206), gastrointestinal motility disorders (p.1202), and nausea and vomiting (p.1206), but again they are not among the drugs usually considered for use in these conditions.

Lactation. Drug therapy has been used occasionally to stimulate lactation in breast-feeding mothers, although mechanical stimulation of the nipple remains the primary method. Dopamine antagonists such as sulpiride can produce modest increases in breast milk production[1-3] although metoclopramide has been more widely used (see p.1276). However, there is concern about the adverse effects of these drugs. As sulpiride appears in breast milk in relatively large amounts and may be associated with adverse effects in the infant it has been recommended that it should not be used to enhance milk production.[4]

1. Aono T, *et al.* Effect of sulpiride on poor puerperal lactation. *Am J Obstet Gynecol* 1982; **143:** 927–32.
2. Ylikorkala O, *et al.* Sulpiride improves inadequate lactation. *BMJ* 1982; **285:** 249–51.
3. Ylikorkala O, *et al.* Treatment of inadequate lactation with oral sulpiride and buccal oxytocin. *Obstet Gynecol* 1984; **63:** 57–60.
4. Pons G, *et al.* Excretion of psychoactive drugs into breast milk: pharmacokinetic principles and recommendations. *Clin Pharmacokinet* 1994; **27:** 270–89.

Schizophrenia. A meta-analysis[1] of studies of the use of sulpiride for schizophrenia (p.651) or serious mental illness concluded that while sulpiride might be as effective as the classical antipsychotics for schizophrenia, evidence of its value for treating negative symptoms was lacking. It appeared to produce fewer adverse effects than the classical antipsychotics. Comparisons with the atypical antipsychotic drugs were lacking.

1. Soares BGO, *et al.* Sulpiride for schizophrenia (updated 16 March 2001). Available in The Cochrane Library; Issue 4. Oxford: Update Software; 2001.

Tourette's syndrome. When treatment is needed for tics and behavioural disturbances in Tourette's syndrome (p.650) dopamine antagonists such as the antipsychotics haloperidol or pimozide are most commonly used but sulpiride has also been tried.[1]

1. Robertson MM, *et al.* Management of Gilles de la Tourette syndrome using sulpiride. *Clin Neuropharmacol* 1990; **13:** 229–35.

Preparations
BP 2001: Sulpiride Tablets.

Proprietary Preparations (details are given in Part 3)
Aust.: Dogmatil; Meresa; **Belg.:** Dogmatil; **Braz.:** Dogmatil; Equilid; **Denm.:** Dogmatil; Sulpril; **Fin.:** Suprium; **Fr.:** Aiglonyl; Dogmatil; Synedil; **Ger.:** Arminol; Desisulpid; Dogmatil; Intrasil; Meresa; neogama; neogama D novo; Sulp; Sulpivert; Vertigo-Meresa; vertigo-neogama; **Hong Kong:** Dogmatil; Sulpiren; **Irl.:**

Dolmatil; *Israel:* Modal; *Ital.:* Championyl; Dobren; Equilid; Levobren; Levopraid; Normum†; Quiridil†; *Mex.:* Dogmatil; Ekilid; Pontiride; *Neth.:* Dogmatil; *Port.:* Dogmatil; Lisopride; *S.Afr.:* Depex; Eglonyl; Espiride; *Singapore:* Dogmatil; *Spain:* Digton; Dogmatil; Guastil; Leboptide; Psicocen; Tepavil; *Switz.:* Dogmatil; *UK:* Dolmatil; Sulparex†; Sulpitil; Sulpor.

Multi-ingredient: *Braz.:* Bromopirin; Sulpan; *Mex.:* Numencial; *Spain:* Ansium; Roter Complex†; Sirodina; Tepazepan.

Sultopride Hydrochloride (7108-y)

Sultopride Hydrochloride (rINNM).

LIN-1418. *N*-(1-Ethylpyrrolidin-2-ylmethyl)-5-ethylsulphonyl-2-methoxybenzamide hydrochloride.

$C_{17}H_{26}N_2O_4S,HCl = 390.9$.

CAS — 53583-79-2 (sultopride); 23694-17-9 (sultopride hydrochloride).

Profile
Sultopride is a substituted benzamide with general properties similar to those of sulpiride (above). It is used in the emergency management of agitation in psychotic or aggressive patients (see Disturbed Behaviour, p.650) and in psychoses such as schizophrenia (p.651). It is given as the hydrochloride but doses are expressed in terms of the base. For acute agitation it may be given in doses of 400 to 800 mg daily by mouth or intramuscularly. In psychoses daily doses of 400 to 1600 mg have been given by mouth or intramuscularly. For chronically aggressive patients, maintenance doses of sultopride 400 to 600 mg daily may be given.

Ventricular arrhythmias, including torsade de pointes, have been reported. It has been recommended that sultopride should not be used in patients with bradycardia.

Porphyria. Sultopride is considered to be unsafe in patients with porphyria because it has been shown to be porphyrinogenic in *in-vitro* systems.

Preparations
Proprietary Preparations (details are given in Part 3)
Belg.: Barnetil; *Fr.:* Barnetil; *Ital.:* Barnotil; *Port.:* Barnetil†.

Suriclone (13291-I)

Suriclone (BAN, rINN).

31264-RP; RP-31264. (*RS*)-6-(7-Chloro-1,8-naphthyridin-2-yl)-2,3,6,7-tetrahydro-7-oxo-5*H*-[1,4]dithi-ino[2,3-c]pyrrol-5-yl 4-methylpiperazine-1-carboxylate.

$C_{20}H_{20}ClN_5O_3S_2 = 478.0$.

CAS — 53813-83-5.

Profile
Suriclone is a cyclopyrrolone structurally related to zopiclone (p.713) and reported to possess similar properties. It has been investigated as an anxiolytic.

◊ References.
1. Saletu B, *et al.* Sleep laboratory studies on single dose effects of suriclone. *Br J Clin Pharmacol* 1990; **30:** 703–10.
2. Ansseau M, *et al.* Controlled comparison of the efficacy and safety of four doses of suriclone, diazepam, and placebo in generalized anxiety disorder. *Psychopharmacology (Berl)* 1991; **104:** 439–443.
3. Saletu B, *et al.* Pharmacokinetic and -dynamic studies with a new anxiolytic, suriclone, utilizing EEG mapping and psychometry. *Br J Clin Pharmacol* 1994; **37:** 154–56.

Tandospirone Citrate (10442-w)

Tandospirone Citrate (BANM, USAN, rINNM).

Metanopirone Citrate; SM-3997 (tandospirone); SM-3997 (tandospirone citrate). (1*R*,2*S*,3*R*,4*S*)-*N*-{4-[4-(2-Pyrimidinyl)-1-piperazinyl]butyl}-2,3-norbornanedicarboximide citrate.

$C_{21}H_{29}N_5O_2,C_6H_8O_7 = 575.6$.

CAS — 87760-53-0 (tandospirone); 112457-95-1 (tandospirone citrate).

Profile
Tandospirone, a partial agonist at serotonin (5-HT) receptors of the 5-HT$_{1A}$ subtype, is an anxiolytic structurally related to buspirone (p.657). It is given by mouth as the citrate in usual doses of 30 mg daily in divided doses.

◊ References.
1. Sumiyoshi T, *et al.* The effect of tandospirone, a serotonin(1A) agonist, on memory function in schizophrenia. *Biol Psychiatry* 2001; **49:** 861–8.

Preparations
Proprietary Preparations (details are given in Part 3)
Jpn: Sediel.

Temazepam (4072-c)

Temazepam (BAN, USAN, rINN).

ER-115; 3-Hydroxydiazepam; K-3917; Ro-5-5345; Temazepamum; Wy-3917. 7-Chloro-1,3-dihydro-3-hydroxy-1-methyl-5-phenyl-1,4-benzodiazepin-2-one.

$C_{16}H_{13}ClN_2O_2 = 300.7$.

CAS — 846-50-4.

ATC — N05CD07.

Pharmacopoeias. In Eur. (see p.vi), Pol., and US.

Pharmacopoeial description

Ph. Eur.: A white or almost white crystalline powder. Practically insoluble in water; sparingly soluble in alcohol; freely soluble in dichloromethane. Protect from light

USP 25: A white or nearly white crystalline powder. Very slightly soluble in water; sparingly soluble in alcohol. Protect from light.

Dependence and Withdrawal
As for Diazepam, p.675.

◊ For the purpose of withdrawal regimens, 10 mg of temazepam may be considered roughly equivalent to 5 mg of diazepam.

Adverse Effects, Treatment, and Precautions
As for Diazepam, p.675.

Abuse. Liquid-filled temazepam capsules (known on the street as 'eggs') were widely abused on the illicit drugs market, the liquid gel lending itself to intravenous administration.[1] This formulation was, therefore, replaced in the UK by tablets and semi-solid gel-filled capsules. The manufacturer of one such capsule formulation considers that the gel is difficult to inject even after heating or diluting in various solvents.[2] In spite of this there is evidence of abuse of these capsules[3] and there are reports of ischaemia, in some cases necessitating amputation.[4,5] The contents have also been subject to intra-arterial abuse.[6,7] The tablets may also be liable to abuse; there has been a report of death following intravenous injection of a solution containing crushed temazepam tablets.[8] The manufacturers of a temazepam elixir consider that, because of its viscosity and its low strength relative to the liquid in the capsules, it has a low potential for intravenous abuse.[9] Nonetheless, there have been reports[3] of some drug abusers injecting large quantities of diluted elixir.

1. Farrell M, Strang J. Misuse of temazepam. *BMJ* 1988; **297:** 1402.
2. Launchbury AP. Temazepam abuse. *Pharm J* 1990; **244:** 749.
3. Ruben SM, Morrison CL. Temazepam misuse in a group of injecting drug users. *Br J Addict* 1992; **87:** 1387–92.
4. Blair SD, *et al.* Leg ischaemia secondary to non-medical injection of temazepam. *Lancet* 1991; **338:** 1393–4.
5. Fox R, *et al.* Misuse of temazepam. *BMJ* 1992; **305:** 253.
6. Scott RN, *et al.* Intra-arterial temazepam. *BMJ* 1992; **304:** 1630.
7. Adiseshiah M, *et al.* Intra-arterial temazepam. *BMJ* 1992; **304:** 1630.
8. Vella EJ, Edwards CW. Death from pulmonary microembolization after intravenous injection of temazepam. *BMJ* 1993; **307:** 26.
9. Drake J, Ballard R. Misuse of temazepam. *BMJ* 1988; **297:** 1402.

Effects on the skin. Generalised lichenoid drug eruption that had persisted for 5 months in an elderly patient receiving therapy including temazepam resolved within 10 days of discontinuing the benzodiazepine.[1]

1. Norris P, Sounex TS. Generalised lichenoid drug eruption associated with temazepam. *BMJ* 1986; **293:** 510.

Hepatic impairment. All benzodiazepines should be used with caution in patients with hepatic impairment, and the manufacturers in the UK advise that temazepam should be avoided in severe cases. However, short-acting benzodiazepines such as temazepam may pose less risk in patients with hepatic impairment; in a study of 15 patients with cirrhosis and 16 healthy subjects, liver disease had no significant effect on the pharmacokinetic parameters or pattern of elimination of temazepam.[1]

1. Ghabrial H, *et al.* The effects of age and chronic liver disease on the elimination of temazepam. *Eur J Clin Pharmacol* 1986; **30:** 93–7.

Interactions
As for Diazepam, p.677.

Pharmacokinetics
Temazepam is fairly readily absorbed from the gastrointestinal tract, although the exact rate of absorption depends on the formulation. It is about 96% bound to plasma protein. Mean elimination half-lives of about 8 to 15 hours or longer have been reported. It is excreted mainly in the urine in the form of its inactive glucuronide conjugate together with small amounts of the demethylated derivative, oxazepam, also in conjugated form.

◊ The elimination half-life was significantly longer at 16.8 hours among 17 women given temazepam 30 mg compared

with 12.3 hours among 15 men.[1] The total clearance was also lower among women. After correction for differences in protein binding, unbound clearance was still lower in women than men but there was no significant effect of age on this parameter. Time to peak plasma concentration and volume of distribution were not affected by the age or sex of the subjects.

1. Divoll M, *et al.* Effect of age and gender on disposition of temazepam. *J Pharm Sci* 1981; **70:** 1104–7.

Absorption and plasma concentration. Various oral temazepam formulations have been available worldwide. These included powder-filled hard gelatin capsules, liquid-filled soft gelatin capsules, semi-solid gel-filled soft gelatin capsules, and an elixir. There has been considerable debate over the comparative absorption profiles of temazepam from these formulations which have, in some cases, been modified over the years. It should be noted that pharmacokinetic studies of temazepam do not always clearly state the formulation used.

Temazepam 30 mg was given as a premedicant to 80 patients undergoing surgery in the form of capsules [type not stated] or elixir.[1] Mean peak plasma concentrations of about 800 nanograms per mL occurred 30 minutes after administration of either formulation although there was wide interindividual variation in plasma concentrations. The evidence corresponded with previous suggestions that a plasma concentration of about 250 nanograms or more per mL was required to ensure sedation. The presence or absence of anxiety did not influence the absorption of the preparations.

1. Hosie HE, Nimmo WS. Temazepam absorption in patients before surgery. *Br J Anaesth* 1991; **66:** 20–4.

Distribution. BREAST MILK. Temazepam was detected in breast milk in only one of 10 lactating mothers given temazepam as a bedtime sedative;[1] temazepam was given in a dose of 10 to 20 mg and milk concentrations were measured about 15 hours after a dose. The authors considered that breast-fed neonates would receive negligible amounts of temazepam.

1. Lebedevs TH, *et al.* Excretion of temazepam in breast milk. *Br J Clin Pharmacol* 1992; **33:** 204–6.

CSF. A study in 13 male patients demonstrating a correlation between the unbound concentration of temazepam in plasma and the amount of temazepam detected in CSF.[1] The mean CSF to total plasma temazepam concentration ratio was 5.2.

1. Badcock NR. Plasma and cerebrospinal fluid concentrations of temazepam following oral drug administration. *Eur J Clin Pharmacol* 1990; **38:** 153–5.

Metabolism. References.

1. Locniskar A, Greenblatt DJ. Oxidative versus conjugative biotransformation of temazepam. *Biopharm Drug Dispos* 1990; **11:** 499–506.

Uses and Administration
Temazepam is a short-acting benzodiazepine with general properties similar to those of diazepam (p.680). It is used as a hypnotic in the short-term management of insomnia (p.652) and for premedication before surgical or investigative procedures (p.1256).

A usual dose for insomnia is 10 to 20 mg by mouth at night; exceptionally, doses up to 40 mg may be required. For premedication the usual dose is 20 to 40 mg by mouth given half to one hour beforehand. The *British National Formulary* states that children may be given 1 mg per kg body-weight for premedication, to a maximum total dose of 30 mg.

Temazepam should be given in reduced dosage to elderly or debilitated patients; one-half the usual adult dose, or less, may be sufficient.

Administration. For reference to the various formulations of oral temazepam that have been used, see Abuse under Adverse Effects, Treatment, and Precautions, above.

Administration in the elderly. In one small study[1] a dose of temazepam of 7.5 mg was found to be adequate for the short-term management of insomnia in elderly patients.

1. Vgontzas AN, *et al.* Temazepam 7.5 mg: effects on sleep in elderly insomniacs. *Eur J Clin Pharmacol* 1994; **46:** 209–13.

Preparations
BP 2001: Temazepam Oral Solution; Temazepam Tablets; **USP 25:** Temazepam Capsules.

Proprietary Preparations (details are given in Part 3)
Aust.: Levanxol; Remestan; *Austral.:* Euhypnos; Nocturne; Nomapam†; Normison; Temaze; Temtabs; *Belg.:* Euhypnos; Levanxol; Normison; Temador†; *Canad.:* Restoril; *Denm.:* Normison; *Fin.:* Normison; Tenox; *Fr.:* Normison; *Ger.:* Neodorm SP†; Norkotral Tema; Planum; Pronervon T; Remestan; temazep; *Irl.:* Euhypnos; Normison; Nortem; Temazine†; Tenox; *Ital.:* Euipnos; Normison; *Neth.:* Normison; NZ: Euhypnos; Normison; Somapam; *Port.:* Normison; *S.Afr.:* Euhypnos†; Levanxol†; Normison; Z-Pam†; *Switz.:* Normison; Planum†; *Thai.:* Euhypnos; *UK:* Euhypnos; Normison; *USA:* Restoril.

The symbol † denotes a preparation no longer actively marketed

Tetrazepam (13314-m)

Tetrazepam (BAN, pINN).

CB-4261; Tetrazepamum. 7-Chloro-5-(cyclohex-1-enyl)-1,3-dihydro-1-methyl-2H-1,4-benzodiazepin-2-one.
$C_{16}H_{17}ClN_2O = 288.8$.
CAS — 10379-14-3.
ATC — M03BX07.

Pharmacopoeias. In Eur. (see p.vi).

Pharmacopoeial description

Ph. Eur.: A light yellow or yellow crystalline powder. Practically insoluble in water; soluble in acetonitrile; freely soluble in dichloromethane. Protect from light.

Profile

Tetrazepam is a benzodiazepine with general properties similar to those of diazepam (p.674). It is used for its muscle relaxant properties in the treatment of muscle spasm (p.1322). The usual initial dose is 25 to 50 mg by mouth increased, if necessary, to 150 mg or more daily.

Pharmacokinetics. References.
1. Bun H, et al. Plasma levels and pharmacokinetics of single and multiple dose of tetrazepam in healthy volunteers. Arzneimittelforschung 1987; 37: 199–202.

Porphyria. Tetrazepam is considered to be unsafe in patients with porphyria because it has been shown to be porphyrinogenic in in-vitro systems.

Preparations

Proprietary Preparations (details are given in Part 3)
Aust.: Myolastan; **Belg.:** Myolastan; **Fr.:** Megavix; Myolastan; Panos; **Ger.:** Mobiforton; Musapam; Musaril; Muskelat; Myospasmal; Rilex; Tepam; Tethexal; Tetra-saar; Tetramdura; Tetrazep; **Mex.:** Miolastan; **Spain:** Myolastan.

Thioproperazine Mesilate (7113-w)

Thioproperazine Mesilate (BANM, rINNM).

RP-7843; SKF-5883; Thioproperazine Dimethanesulphonate; Thioproperazine Mesylate; Thioproperazine Methanesulphonate. NN-Dimethyl-10-[3-(4-methylpiperazin-1-yl)propyl]phenothiazine-2-sulphonamide dimethanesulphonate.
$C_{22}H_{30}N_4O_2S_2,2CH_4O_3S = 638.8$.
CAS — 316-81-4 (thioproperazine); 2347-80-0 (thioproperazine mesilate).

Pharmacopoeias. In Fr.

Profile

Thioproperazine is a phenothiazine with general properties similar to those of chlorpromazine (p.660). It has a piperazine side-chain. It is used in the treatment of schizophrenia (p.651), mania (see Bipolar Disorder, p.271), and other psychoses. Thioproperazine is given as the mesilate in initial doses of the equivalent of 5 mg of thioproperazine daily, increased as necessary; the usual effective dosage is 30 to 40 mg daily. In severe or resistant cases doses of 90 mg or more daily have been given.

Preparations

Proprietary Preparations (details are given in Part 3)
Belg.: Majeptil; **Canad.:** Majeptil; **Fr.:** Majeptil; **Mex.:** Majeptil; **Spain:** Majeptil.

Thioridazine (7114-e)

Thioridazine (BAN, USAN, rINN).

Thioridazinum; TP-21. 10-[2-(1-Methyl-2-piperidyl)ethyl]-2-methylthiophenothiazine.
$C_{21}H_{26}N_2S_2 = 370.6$.
CAS — 50-52-2.
ATC — N05AC02.

Pharmacopoeias. In Eur. (see p.vi) and US.

Thioridazine 100 mg is approximately equivalent to 110 mg of thioridazine hydrochloride.

Pharmacopoeial description

Ph. Eur.: A white or almost white powder. Practically insoluble in water; soluble in alcohol; very soluble in dichloromethane; freely soluble in methyl alcohol. Protect from light.

USP 25: A white to slightly yellow crystalline or micronised powder; odourless or having a faint odour. Practically insoluble in water; freely soluble in dehydrated alcohol and in ether; very soluble in chloroform. Protect from light.

Thioridazine Hydrochloride (7115-l)

Thioridazine Hydrochloride (BANM, rINNM).

Thioridazini Hydrochloridum.
$C_{21}H_{26}N_2S_2,HCl = 407.0$.
CAS — 130-61-0.

Pharmacopoeias. In Eur. (see p.vi), Jpn, Pol., and US.

Pharmacopoeial description

Ph. Eur.: A white or almost white, crystalline powder. Freely soluble in water and in methyl alcohol; soluble in alcohol; practically insoluble in ether. A 1% solution in water has a pH of 4.2 to 5.2. Protect from light.

USP 25: A white to slightly yellow granular powder having a slight odour. Freely soluble in water, in chloroform, and in methyl alcohol; insoluble in ether. pH of a 1% solution in water is between 4.2 and 5.2. Store in airtight containers. Protect from light.

Incompatibility. For a warning about incompatibility between thioridazine hydrochloride solution (Mellaril) and carbamazepine suspension (Tegretol), see p.342.

Adverse Effects and Treatment

As for Chlorpromazine, p.660.

Thioridazine has been associated with a higher incidence of antimuscarinic effects, but lower incidence of extrapyramidal symptoms than chlorpromazine. It may also be less sedating. However, it is more likely to induce hypotension and there is an increased risk of cardiotoxicity and dose-related prolongation of the QT interval. Because of this and the consequent danger of life-threatening arrhythmias such as torsade de pointes and sudden death, its use is restricted (see Precautions and Uses and Administration, below). Sexual dysfunction also appears to be more frequent with thioridazine.

Pigmentary retinopathy characterised by diminution of visual acuity, brownish colouring of vision, and impairment of night vision has been observed particularly in patients taking large doses.

Effects on the cardiovascular system. Between 1964 and 2001, the UK Committee on Safety of Medicines received 42 reports of suspected heart rate and rhythm disorders associated with thioridazine.[1] There were 21 fatalities reported out of 39 cases where the outcome was known.

See also under Chlorpromazine, p.661.
1. Committee on Safety of Medicines/Medicines Control Agency. QT interval prolongation with antipsychotics. Current Problems 2001; 27: 4.

Hypersensitivity. Pruritus and erythematous rash on the genitals of a woman following sexual intercourse were found to be due to thioridazine present in the seminal fluid of her husband, who was receiving 100 mg daily at night.[1]
1. Sell MB. Sensitization to thioridazine through sexual intercourse. Am J Psychiatry 1985; 142: 271–2.

Overdosage. Rhabdomyolysis has been reported in a patient after overdosage with thioridazine.[1] Twenty-four hours after taking 9.4 g of thioridazine the patient presented with difficulty in moving and speaking. On examination he had swelling and tenderness over his upper arms, thighs, and calves. Ataxia and transient dysarthria were attributed to generalised muscle weakness. Other effects were consistent with antimuscarinic effects of thioridazine. He had no signs of neuroleptic malignant syndrome but his urine contained myoglobin. The patient was treated with gastric lavage, activated charcoal, and rehydration. Serum biochemistry returned to normal over one week and the muscle tenderness and weakness disappeared.
1. Nankivell BJ, et al. Rhabdomyolysis induced by thioridazine. BMJ 1994; 309: 378.

Precautions

As for Chlorpromazine, p.663. Thioridazine should not be used in patients with clinically significant cardiac disorders, uncorrected hypokalaemia or other electrolyte imbalance, or with known or suspected QT prolongation or a history of ventricular arrhythmias including torsade de pointes. Use is also contraindicated in patients known to have reduced activity of the cytochrome P450 isoenzyme CYP2D6, which is responsible for thioridazine metabolism. The concomitant administration of drugs liable to interfere with the metabolism of thioridazine, of other drugs known to prolong the QT interval, and of drugs likely to cause electrolyte imbalance should also be avoided (see under Interactions, below).

For all patients starting thioridazine it is recommended that a baseline ECG and electrolyte screening are performed. An ECG should also be repeated before each dose increase, one week after the maximum therapeutic dose has been reached, and at 6-monthly intervals in those who continue treatment. Serum electrolyte concentrations should also be monitored periodically during treatment and any imbalance corrected.

Porphyria. Thioridazine has been associated with acute attacks of porphyria and is considered unsafe in porphyric patients.

Interactions

As for Chlorpromazine, p.664. The metabolism of thioridazine is mediated by the cytochrome P450 isoenzyme CYP2D6; thioridazine itself is also an inhibitor of CYP2D6. Therefore there is the potential for interactions between thioridazine and other drugs that inhibit or act as a substrate for this enzyme; such drugs should not be given concomitantly with thioridazine. Some examples include antiarrhythmics, certain antidepressants including the SSRIs and tricyclics, certain antipsychotics, beta blockers, HIV-protease inhibitors, and opiates. Concomitant administration with other drugs known to prolong the QT interval such as class IA and class III antiarrhythmics, tricyclic antidepressants, and some antipsychotics should also be avoided as should the co-administration of those drugs known to cause electrolyte imbalance.

Pharmacokinetics

The pharmacokinetics of thioridazine appear to be generally similar to those of chlorpromazine (p.665). Thioridazine is metabolised by the cytochrome P450 isoenzyme CYP2D6. The

principal active metabolite of thioridazine is mesoridazine (p.691); the metabolite, sulforidazine, also has some activity. Thioridazine and its active metabolites are reported to be highly bound to plasma proteins. The plasma half-life of thioridazine has been estimated to range from about 6 to over 40 hours.

◊ References.
1. Mårtensson E, Roos B-E. Serum levels of thioridazine in psychiatric patients and healthy volunteers. Eur J Clin Pharmacol 1973; 6: 181–6.
2. Axelsson R, Mårtensson E. Serum concentration and elimination from serum of thioridazine in psychiatric patients. Curr Ther Res 1976; 19: 242–65.

Metabolism. In 10 psychiatric patients stabilised on thioridazine, therapy was replaced by equipotent doses of the side-chain sulfoxide (mesoridazine) and side-chain sulfone (sulforidazine) metabolites of thioridazine.[1] Both metabolites were shown to have an antipsychotic effect, the dose of each required being about two-thirds that of thioridazine. The serum half-lives were thioridazine 21 hours, mesoridazine 16 hours, and sulforidazine 13 hours. Apathy, depression, and restlessness gradually developed during treatment with the 2 metabolites and they could not be used for any length of time. Extrapyramidal symptoms, hypersalivation, and drowsiness were more common with the metabolites; 2 patients had epileptic seizures, and one receiving sulforidazine developed probable cholestatic jaundice.

There is some evidence that the metabolism of thioridazine is influenced by debrisoquine hydroxylation phenotype.[2] A single-dose study in 19 healthy male subjects demonstrated slower formation of mesoridazine, and hence higher serum-thioridazine concentrations in poor debrisoquine hydroxylators compared with extensive hydroxylators. Formation of thioridazine ring-sulfoxide appeared to be compensatorily increased in slow hydroxylators.
1. Axelsson R. On the serum concentrations and antipsychotic effects of thioridazine, thioridazine side-chain sulfoxide and thioridazine side-chain sulfone, in chronic psychotic patients. Curr Ther Res 1977; 21: 587–605.
2. von Bahr C, et al. Plasma levels of thioridazine and metabolites are influenced by the debrisoquin hydroxylation phenotype. Clin Pharmacol Ther 1991; 49: 234–40.

Uses and Administration

Thioridazine is a phenothiazine with general properties similar to those of chlorpromazine (p.665). It has a piperidine side-chain and, unlike chlorpromazine, has little antiemetic activity.

The use of thioridazine is restricted to the treatment of schizophrenia (p.651) in patients who fail to show an adequate response to treatment with other antipsychotics. Its use in other psychiatric disorders was abandoned after it was felt that there was an unacceptable balance of risks and benefits as a result of its cardiotoxic potential.

For all patients starting thioridazine it is recommended that a baseline ECG and electrolyte screening are performed. An ECG should also be repeated before each dose increase, one week after the maximum therapeutic dose has been reached, and at 6-monthly intervals in those who continue treatment. Serum electrolyte concentrations should also be monitored periodically during treatment and any imbalance corrected.

Thioridazine is administered by mouth as the hydrochloride or the base, but doses are normally given in terms of the hydrochloride. In the UK, oral suspensions contain 25 mg of thioridazine base (approximately equivalent to 27.5 mg of thioridazine hydrochloride) per unit dosage, or 100 mg of thioridazine base (approximately equivalent to 110 mg of thioridazine hydrochloride) per unit dosage, whereas other oral liquid preparations contain 27.5 mg of thioridazine hydrochloride per unit dosage and the tablets contain 10, 25, 50 or 100 mg of thioridazine hydrochloride.

In the treatment of schizophrenia thioridazine should be initiated at the lowest recommended dose and slowly titrated upwards. A usual dosage range for outpatients is 50 to 300 mg of the hydrochloride daily, which may be given in divided doses. In the UK the maximum licensed dose is 600 mg daily in hospitalised patients but up to 800 mg daily is permitted in the USA; such doses should be reduced once effective control is achieved. It is recommended that increases in doses should be no more than 100 mg weekly.

Thioridazine should be given in lower initial doses to patients with a low body-mass or those with hepatic or renal impairment; dosage increases should also be more gradual.

In those patients who require withdrawal of thioridazine, the dose should be gradually reduced over 1 to 2 weeks to avoid symptoms such as gastrointestinal disorders, dizziness, anxiety, and insomnia that are sometimes seen after abrupt discontinuation of high-dose or long-term treatment.

Preparations

BP 2001: Thioridazine Oral Solution; Thioridazine Oral Suspension; Thioridazine Tablets;
USP 25: Thioridazine Hydrochloride Oral Solution; Thioridazine Hydrochloride Tablets; Thioridazine Oral Suspension.

Proprietary Preparations (details are given in Part 3)
Aust.: Melleretten; Melleril; **Austral.:** Aldazine; Melleril; **Belg.:** Melleril; **Braz.:** Melleril; **Canad.:** Mellaril; Novo-Ridazine†; **Denm.:** Melleril; **Fin.:** Melleril; Orsanil; **Fr.:** Melleril; **Ger.:** Melleril; Melleretten; **Hong Kong:** Melleril; **Irl.:** Melleril; Melzine; Thiozine; **Israel:** Melleril; Ridazin; **Ital.:** Mellerette; Melleril; **Mex.:** Melleril; **Neth.:** Melleretten; Melleril; **Norw.:** Melleril; **NZ:**

Aldazine; Melleril; *Port.:* Melleril; *S.Afr.:* Melleril; Ridazine†; *Spain:* Meleril; *Swed.:* Mallorol; *Switz.:* Mellerettes; Melleril; *Thai.:* Calmaril; Dazine; Ridazine; Thiomed; Thiosia; *UK:* Melleril; Rideril; *USA:* Mellaril.

Multi-ingredient: *Ital.:* Visergil; *Spain:* Visergil.

Tiapride Hydrochloride (13339-I)

Tiapride Hydrochloride *(BAN, rINNM).*
FLO-1347; Tiapridi Hydrochloridum. *N*-(2-Diethylaminoethyl)-2-methoxy-5-methylsulphonylbenzamide hydrochloride.
$C_{15}H_{24}N_2O_4S,HCl = 364.9$.
CAS — 51012-32-9 *(tiapride)*; 51012-33-0 *(tiapride hydrochloride)*.
Pharmacopoeias. In *Eur.* (see p.vi).

Pharmacopoeial description

Ph. Eur.: A white or almost white crystalline powder. Very soluble in water; slightly soluble in dehydrated alcohol; soluble in methyl alcohol. A 5% solution in water has a pH of 4.0 to 6.0.

Adverse Effects, Treatment, and Precautions

As for Chlorpromazine, p.660.

Interactions

As for Chlorpromazine, p.664.

Pharmacokinetics

Tiapride is rapidly absorbed following oral administration and excreted largely unchanged in the urine. The plasma half-life is reported to range from 3 to 4 hours.

◊ A study of the steady-state pharmacokinetics of tiapride in 5 elderly patients with tardive dyskinesia, and in 2 patients with Huntington's chorea.[1] All patients received tiapride 100 mg three times daily by mouth for 7 days. The mean peak plasma concentration of tiapride was 1.47 µg per mL, achieved a mean of 1.4 hours after dosing, and the mean elimination half-life was 3.8 hours. These values did not differ significantly from those previously reported in younger healthy subjects, although renal clearance was slightly lower in these patients. About half of the dose of tiapride was excreted unchanged by the kidney; a metabolite, probably *N*-monodesethyltiapride was detected in the urine but its identity was not confirmed.

1. Roos RAC, *et al.* Pharmacokinetics of tiapride in patients with tardive dyskinesia and Huntington's disease. *Eur J Clin Pharmacol* 1986; **31:** 191–4.

Uses and Administration

Tiapride is a substituted benzamide with general properties similar to those of sulpiride (p.706).

It is usually given as the hydrochloride in the management of behaviour disorders and to treat dyskinesias; doses are expressed in terms of the equivalent amount of tiapride. Doses of 200 to 400 mg daily by mouth are usually given, although higher daily doses have been used, in particular in the management of dyskinesias. Tiapride hydrochloride has also been given by intramuscular or intravenous injection.

Disturbed behaviour. For a discussion of the management of disturbed behaviour including limitations on the use of antipsychotics, see p.650.
References.
1. Gutzmann H, *et al.* Measuring the efficacy of psychopharmacological treatment of psychomotoric restlessness in dementia: clinical evaluation of tiapride. *Pharmacopsychiatry* 1997; **30:** 6–11.

Extrapyramidal disorders. For reference to the use of tiapride in suppressing the adverse effects of levodopa on respiration, see p.1170.

Tiapride has been tried in the treatment of antipsychotic-induced tardive dyskinesia (p.662), but as with all antipsychotics improvement may only be short-term.

Tiapride has also been tried in the treatment of Tourette's syndrome (p.650).

CHOREA. Antipsychotics have some action against choreiform movements as well as being of use to control the behavioural disturbances of Huntington's chorea. For a discussion of the management of various choreas, see p.650.
References to the use of tiapride.
1. Roos RAC, *et al.* Tiapride in the treatment of Huntington's chorea. *Acta Neurol Scand* 1982; **65:** 45–50.
2. Deroover J, *et al.* Tiapride versus placebo: a double-blind comparative study in the management of Huntington's chorea. *Curr Med Res Opin* 1984; **9:** 329–38.

Substance dependence. A review[1] concluded that the role of tiapride in acute *alcohol* withdrawal (p.1131) is likely to be limited as patients at risk of severe reactions would still require adjunct therapy for the control of hallucinations and seizures. Following detoxification tiapride may help to alleviate distress, improve abstinence and drinking behaviour, and facilitate reintegration within society.[2] However, the potential risk of tardive dyskinesias (at the dosage used (300 mg daily) still needed to be evaluated and patients would require medical supervision.[1]

1. Peters DH, Faulds D. Tiapride: a review of its pharmacology and therapeutic potential in the management of alcohol dependence syndrome. *Drugs* 1994; **47:** 1010–32.
2. Shaw GK, *et al.* Tiapride in the prevention of relapse in recently detoxified alcoholics. *Br J Psychiatry* 1994; **165:** 515–23.

The symbol † denotes a preparation no longer actively marketed

Preparations

Proprietary Preparations (details are given in Part 3)
Aust.: Delpral; *Belg.:* Tiapridal; *Braz.:* Tiapridal; *Fr.:* Clemental; Equilium; Tiapridal; *Ger.:* Tiapridex; *Hong Kong:* Tiapridal; *Israel:* Doparid; *Ital.:* Italprid; Luxoben†; Sereprile; *Neth.:* Tiapridal; *Port.:* Normagit†; Tiapridal; *Singapore:* Tiapridal; *Spain:* Tiapridal; *Switz.:* Tiapridal.

Timiperone (17010-t)

Timiperone *(rINN).*
DD-3480. 4′-Fluoro-4-[4-(2-thioxo-1-benzimidazolinyl)piperidino]butyrophenone.
$C_{22}H_{24}FN_3OS = 397.5$.
CAS — 57648-21-2.

Profile

Timiperone is a butyrophenone with general properties similar to those of haloperidol (p.686). It has been used by mouth in the treatment of schizophrenia. Timiperone has also been given by injection.

Tiotixene (7116-y)

Tiotixene *(BAN, rINN).*
NSC-108165; P-4657B; Thiothixene *(USAN).* *(Z)-NN*-Dimethyl-9-[3-(4-methylpiperazin-1-yl)propylidene]thioxanthene-2-sulphonamide.
$C_{23}H_{29}N_3O_2S_2 = 443.6$.
CAS — 5591-45-7; 3313-26-6 *(tiotixene Z-isomer).*
ATC — N05AF04.
Pharmacopoeias. In *US.*

Tiotixene 1 mg is approximately equivalent to 1.25 mg of tiotixene hydrochloride (dihydrate) or to 1.16 mg of the anhydrous hydrochloride.

Pharmacopoeial description

USP 25: White to tan, practically odourless, crystals. Practically insoluble in water; soluble 1 in 110 of dehydrated alcohol, 1 in 2 of chloroform, and 1 in 120 of ether; slightly soluble in acetone and in methyl alcohol. Store in airtight containers. Protect from light.

Tiotixene Hydrochloride (7117-j)

Tiotixene Hydrochloride *(BANM, rINNM).*
CP-12252-1; Thiothixene Hydrochloride *(USAN).*
$C_{23}H_{29}N_3O_2S_2,2HCl,2H_2O = 552.6$.
CAS — 58513-59-0 *(anhydrous tiotixene hydrochloride);* 49746-04-5 *(anhydrous tiotixene hydrochloride, Z-isomer);* 22189-31-7 *(tiotixene hydrochloride dihydrate);* 49746-09-0 *(tiotixene hydrochloride dihydrate, Z-isomer).*
Pharmacopoeias. In *US,* which permits both the dihydrate and the anhydrous form ($C_{23}H_{29}N_3O_2S_2,2HCl = 516.5$).

Pharmacopoeial description

USP 25: A white or practically white crystalline powder having a slight odour. Soluble 1 in 8 of water, 1 in 270 of dehydrated alcohol, and 1 in 280 of chloroform; practically insoluble in acetone, in ether, and in benzene. Store in airtight containers. Protect from light.

Stability. A combination of the stabilisers hydroxyquinoline sulfate and vanillin could protect tiotixene from photodegradation.[1]

1. Thoma K, Klimek R. Photostabilization of drugs in dosage forms without protection from packaging materials. *Int J Pharmaceutics* 1991; **67:** 169–75.

Adverse Effects, Treatment, and Precautions

As for Chlorpromazine, p.660. Tiotixene is less likely to cause sedation but extrapyramidal disorders are more frequent.

Interactions

As for Chlorpromazine, p.664.

Pharmacokinetics

◊ In 15 adequately controlled schizophrenic patients receiving tiotixene 15 to 60 mg daily in 2, 3, or 4 divided doses by mouth, plasma concentrations were found to be in the relatively narrow range of 10 to 22.5 nanograms per mL 126 to 150 minutes after the last daily dose despite the fourfold difference in dosage.[1] Investigations in a further 5 patients indicated that peak plasma concentrations were obtained about 1 to 3 hours after a dose, indicating rapid absorption with an absorption half-time of about 30 minutes. There was an early plasma half-life of about 210 minutes and a late half-life of about 34 hours; resurgence of drug concentrations in some subjects might have been due to enterohepatic recycling.

1. Hobbs DC, *et al.* Pharmacokinetics of thiothixene in man. *Clin Pharmacol Ther* 1974; **16:** 473–8.

Metabolism. A study[1] indicating that tiotixene may induce its own metabolism.

1. Bergling R, *et al.* Plasma levels and clinical effects of thioridazine and thiothixene. *J Clin Pharmacol* 1975; **15:** 178–86.

Uses and Administration

Tiotixene is a thioxanthene antipsychotic with general properties similar to those of the phenothiazine, chlorpromazine (p.665). It has a piperazine side-chain. It is used in the treat-

ment of various psychoses including schizophrenia (p.651). Tiotixene is given by mouth as the base or hydrochloride and sometimes intramuscularly as the hydrochloride. Doses are expressed in terms of the base.

The usual initial dose is 2 mg three times daily by mouth (or 5 mg twice daily in more severe conditions) gradually increasing to 20 to 30 mg daily if necessary; once-daily dosage may be adequate. In severe or resistant psychoses doses of up to 60 mg daily may be given. The usual initial intramuscular dose is 4 mg two to four times daily increased if necessary to a maximum of 30 mg daily.

Tiotixene should be given in reduced dosage to elderly patients.

Preparations

USP 25: Thiothixene Capsules; Thiothixene Hydrochloride for Injection; Thiothixene Hydrochloride Injection; Thiothixene Hydrochloride Oral Solution.
Proprietary Preparations (details are given in Part 3)
Austral.: Navane; *Braz.:* Navane; *Canad.:* Navane; *Hong Kong:* Navane; *Neth.:* Navane; *NZ:* Thixit; *Thai.:* Navane; *USA:* Navane.

Tofisopam (7118-z)

Tofisopam *(rINN).*
EGYT-341; Tofizopam. 1-(3,4-Dimethoxyphenyl)-5-ethyl-7,8-dimethoxy-4-methyl-5*H*-2,3-benzodiazepine.
$C_{22}H_{26}N_2O_4 = 382.5$.
CAS — 22345-47-7.
ATC — N05BA23.
Pharmacopoeias. In *Jpn.*

Profile

Tofisopam is a 2,3-benzodiazepine related structurally to the 1,4-benzodiazepines such as diazepam (p.674) and sharing some of the same actions. It is reported, however, to be largely lacking in the sedative, anticonvulsant, and muscle relaxant properties of the conventional benzodiazepines. Tofisopam has been given by mouth in the short-term treatment of anxiety disorders.

Preparations

Proprietary Preparations (details are given in Part 3)
Hung.: Grandaxin; *Thai.:* Grandaxin.

Triazolam (4073-k)

Triazolam *(BAN, USAN, rINN).*
Clorazolam; U-33030. 8-Chloro-6-(2-chlorophenyl)-1-methyl-4*H*-[1,2,4]triazolo[4,3-*a*][1,4]benzodiazepine.
$C_{17}H_{12}Cl_2N_4 = 343.2$.
CAS — 28911-01-5.
ATC — N05CD05.
Pharmacopoeias. In *US.*

Pharmacopoeial description

USP 25: A white to off-white, practically odourless, crystalline powder. Practically insoluble in water and in ether; soluble 1 in 1000 of alcohol, 1 in 25 of chloroform, and 1 in 600 of 0.1N hydrochloric acid.

Dependence and Withdrawal

As for Diazepam, p.675.

Adverse Effects and Treatment

As for Diazepam, p.675.

Effects on the liver. A 44-year-old man developed severe pruritus with jaundice which subsequently proved fatal. Liver histology showed intense cholestasis. Triazolam was considered to be the most likely precipitant.[1]

1. Cobden I, *et al.* Fatal intrahepatic cholestasis associated with triazolam. *Postgrad Med J* 1981; **57:** 730–1.

Effects on mental function. The effects of triazolam on mental function have been controversial since van der Kroef first described in 1979 a range of symptoms including anxiety, amnesia, depersonalisation and derealisation, depression, paranoia, and severe suicidal tendencies that he had observed in 25 patients and attributed to the administration of triazolam.[1] This led to suspension of triazolam in the Netherlands (re-approved in 1990) and removal of the 1-mg tablet from other markets. Continued reporting of similar symptoms of cognitive impairment with triazolam resulted in discontinuation of the 500-µg dosage form in several countries in 1987 and 1988 and in a gradual reduction of recommended dosage from 1 mg at night down to 125 to 250 µg at night. Triazolam was withdrawn from the UK[2] and some other markets in 1991. Opinion still remains divided over the adverse effects of triazolam, the main issues being its propensity to cause side-effects relative to other benzodiazepines and whether its risk-benefit ratio is acceptable to justify its continued use.[3,4]

Others[5] have reviewed spontaneous adverse effects reported to the FDA in the USA for triazolam, temazepam, and flurazepam. Daytime sedation was noted with all three, but triazolam caused more agitation, confusion, hallucinations, and amnesia. Such effects occurred frequently with the 250-µg dose as well as with the 500-µg dose. Similar results were obtained after analysis of reports for triazolam and temazepam in the first 7 years of marketing, although the possibility that selection factors were producing higher reporting rates for triazolam could not be entirely excluded.[6] One study[7] gave triazolam 500 µg, lormetazepam 2 mg, or placebo, to groups of 40 patients for 25 nights and observed the greatest frequency of daytime anxiety, panic, derealisation, and paranoia with triazolam. Another[8] found a greater total number of reports of memory impairment or amnesia after nightly administration of triazolam 500 µg compared with temazepam 30 mg. Triazolam also impaired delayed, but not immediate, memory recall. Similar cases of memory impairment occurring with triazolam at doses of 125 and 250 µg have reportedly been submitted to the UK Committee on Safety of Medicines.[2] The emergence of daytime symptoms after more than a few days' treatment with triazolam could be attributed to rebound or withdrawal phenomena occurring as a result of rapid elimination of the drug. As regards the risk-benefit ratio of triazolam some workers have questioned the hypnotic efficacy of the drug at a dose of 250 µg and consider that reduction of the dose has decreased efficacy more than side-effects.[3]

In defence of triazolam, the FDA and the manufacturers (Upjohn) have considered epidemiological studies which, unlike the FDA spontaneous reporting scheme, have been unable to demonstrate a substantial difference in its adverse effects compared with other benzodiazepines except, perhaps, in the incidence of amnesia.[9] Retrospective studies[10,11] claiming similar findings have been the subject of criticism.[12-14] Other workers have cited studies indicating benefit of triazolam 250 µg for the treatment of insomnia.[15] A review by the US Institute of Medicine found that triazolam was safe when given in a dose of 250 µg daily for 7 to 10 days but called for studies of lower doses and of long-term use.[16]

1. Van der Kroef C. Reactions to triazolam. *Lancet* 1979; **ii**: 526.
2. Anonymous. The sudden withdrawal of triazolam—reasons and consequences. *Drug Ther Bull* 1991; **29**: 89–90.
3. O'Donovan MC, McGuffin P. Short acting benzodiazepines. *BMJ* 1993; **306**: 945–6.
4. Ghaeli P, *et al.* Triazolam treatment controversy. *Ann Pharmacother* 1994; **28**: 1038–40.
5. Bixler EO, *et al.* Adverse reactions to benzodiazepine hypnotics: spontaneous reporting system. *Pharmacology* 1987; **35**: 286–300.
6. Wysowski DK, Barash D. Adverse behavioral reactions attributed to triazolam in the Food and Drug Administration's spontaneous reporting system. *Arch Intern Med* 1991; **151**: 2003–8.
7. Adam K, Oswald I. Can a rapidly-eliminated hypnotic cause daytime anxiety? *Pharmacopsychiatry* 1989; **22**: 115–19.
8. Bixler EO, *et al.* Next-day memory impairment with triazolam use. *Lancet* 1991; **337**: 827–31.
9. Drucker RF, MacLeod N. Benzodiazepines. *Pharm J* 1989; **243**: 508.
10. Hindmarch I, *et al.* Adverse events after triazolam substitution. *Lancet* 1993; **341**: 55.
11. Rothschild AJ, *et al.* Triazolam and disinhibition. *Lancet* 1993; **341**: 186.
12. Hawley CJ, *et al.* Adverse events after triazolam substitution. *Lancet* 1993; **341**: 567.
13. Vela-Bueno A. Adverse events after triazolam substitution. *Lancet* 1993; **341**: 567.
14. Kales A, *et al.* Adverse events after triazolam substitution. *Lancet* 1993; **341**: 567–8.
15. Gillin JC, Byerley WF. Diagnosis and management of insomnia. *N Engl J Med* 1990; **323**: 487.
16. Ault A. FDA advisers find no major Halcion dangers. *Lancet* 1997; **350**: 1760.

Precautions

As for Diazepam, p.676.

Hepatic impairment. Cirrhosis decreased the apparent oral clearance of triazolam to an extent depending on the severity of the liver disease.[1] An initial dose of 125 µg was suggested for patients with severe liver dysfunction. It was suggested that the relative lack of effect that mild to moderate cirrhosis had on the metabolism of oral triazolam might be due to some first-pass metabolism occurring in the intestinal wall.[2]

1. Kroboth PD, *et al.* Nighttime dosing of triazolam in patients with liver disease and normal subjects: kinetics and daytime effects. *J Clin Pharmacol* 1987; **27**: 555–60.
2. Robin DW, *et al.* Triazolam in cirrhosis: pharmacokinetics and pharmacodynamics. *Clin Pharmacol Ther* 1993; **54**: 630–7.

Renal impairment. Peak plasma-triazolam concentrations were lower in 11 dialysis patients compared with 11 controls.[1] It was postulated that a relatively high basal gastric acid secretion in dialysis patients could result in hydrolysis and opening of the ring structure of triazolam effectively reducing its systemic availability. Administration of an antacid could reverse this effect. Renal failure had no other effect on the pharmacokinetics of triazolam which could probably be administered in usual doses.

1. Kroboth PD, *et al.* Effects of end stage renal disease and aluminium hydroxide on triazolam pharmacokinetics. *Br J Clin Pharmacol* 1985; **19**: 839–42.

Interactions

As for Diazepam, p.677.

Pharmacokinetics

Triazolam is rapidly and nearly completely absorbed from the gastrointestinal tract, peak plasma concentrations being achieved within 2 hours of administra-

---

tion by mouth. Triazolam has a plasma elimination half-life ranging from 1.5 to 5.5 hours. It is reported to be about 89% bound to plasma proteins. Hydroxylation of triazolam in the liver is mediated by the cytochrome P450 isoenzyme CYP3A4. Triazolam is excreted in the urine mainly in the form of its conjugated metabolites with only small amounts appearing unchanged.

◊ Reviews of the pharmacokinetics of triazolam.

1. Garzone PD, Kroboth PD. Pharmacokinetics of the newer benzodiazepines. *Clin Pharmacokinet* 1989; **16**: 337–64.

Uses and Administration

Triazolam is a short-acting benzodiazepine with general properties similar to those of diazepam (p.680). It is used as a hypnotic in the short-term management of insomnia (p.652) in doses of 125 to 250 µg at night for no more than 2 weeks; doses of up to 500 µg at night have been used for resistant cases but these may be associated with an increased risk of severe adverse effects (see Effects on Mental Function, above). Initial doses of 125 µg at night have been suggested for elderly or debilitated subjects, increased up to a maximum of 250 µg only if necessary.

Preparations

USP 25: Triazolam Tablets.

Proprietary Preparations (details are given in Part 3)

Aust.: Halcion; *Austral.:* Halcion; *Belg.:* Halcion; *Canad.:* Apo-Triazo; Halcion; Novo-Triolam†; *Denm.:* Halcion; Rilamir; *Fin.:* Halcion; *Fr.:* Halcion; *Ger.:* Halcion; *Hong Kong:* Halcion; *Irl.:* Halcion; Trilam; *Israel:* Halcion; *Ital.:* Halcion; Songar; *Mex.:* Halcion; *Neth.:* Halcion; *NZ:* Halcion; Hypam; Trycam; *Port.:* Halcion; *S.Afr.:* Halcion; *Singapore:* Somese; *Spain:* Halcion; *Swed.:* Halcion; *Switz.:* Halcion; *Thai.:* Halcion; *USA:* Halcion.

Triclofos Sodium (4074-a)

Triclofos Sodium (BANM, USAN, rINNM).

Sch-10159; Sodium Triclofos. Sodium 2,2,2-trichloroethyl hydrogen orthophosphate.

$C_2H_3Cl_3NaO_4P = 251.4$.

CAS — 306-52-5 (triclofos); 7246-20-0 (triclofos sodium).

Pharmacopoeias. In *Br.* and *Jpn.*

Pharmacopoeial description

BP 2001: A white or almost white, odourless or almost odourless, hygroscopic powder. Freely soluble in water; slightly soluble in alcohol; practically insoluble in ether. A 2% solution in water has a pH of 3.0 to 4.5.

Dependence and Withdrawal, Adverse Effects, Treatment, and Precautions

As for Cloral Hydrate, p.669 but causes fewer gastrointestinal disturbances.

Triclofos sodium is not corrosive to skin and mucous membranes.

Interactions

As for Cloral Hydrate, p.670.

Pharmacokinetics

Triclofos sodium is rapidly hydrolysed to trichloroethanol, peak serum concentrations being achieved within about one hour after oral administration. For the pharmacokinetics of trichloroethanol, see Cloral Hydrate, p.670.

Uses and Administration

Triclofos sodium has hypnotic and sedative actions similar to those of cloral hydrate (p.670) but it is more palatable and causes less gastric irritation. It is given by mouth in the short-term management of insomnia (p.652).

The usual adult dose as a hypnotic is 1 g (therapeutically equivalent to about 600 mg of cloral hydrate) at night, but up to 2 g may be necessary in some patients. A suggested hypnotic dose for children up to 1 year of age is 25 to 30 mg per kg body-weight; children aged 1 to 5 years may be given single doses of 250 to 500 mg, and children aged 6 to 12 years may be given single doses of 0.5 to 1 g.

Preparations

BP 2001: Triclofos Oral Solution.

Proprietary Preparations (details are given in Part 3)

Irl.: Tricloryl; *Israel:* Triclonam.

Trifluoperazine Hydrochloride

(7120-s)

Trifluoperazine Hydrochloride (BANM, rINNM).

Trifluoperazini Hydrochloridum; Triphthazinum. 10-[3-(4-Methylpiperazin-1-yl)propyl]-2-trifluoromethylphenothiazine dihydrochloride.

$C_{21}H_{24}F_3N_3S,2HCl = 480.4$.

CAS — 117-89-5 (trifluoperazine); 440-17-5 (trifluoperazine hydrochloride).

Pharmacopoeias. In *Chin., Eur.* (see p.vi), *Pol.*, and *US.*

Trifluoperazine 1 mg is approximately equivalent to 1.2 mg of trifluoperazine hydrochloride.

Pharmacopoeial description

Ph. Eur.: A white to pale yellow, hygroscopic, crystalline powder. Freely soluble in water; soluble in alcohol; practically insoluble in ether. A 10% solution in water has a pH of 1.6 to 2.5. Protect from light.

USP 25: A white to pale yellow, practically odourless, crystalline powder. Soluble 1 in 3.5 of water, 1 in 11 of alcohol, and 1 in 100 of chloroform; insoluble in ether and in benzene. pH of a 1 in 20 solution is between 1.7 and 2.6. Store in airtight containers. Protect from light.

Adverse Effects, Treatment, and Precautions

As for Chlorpromazine, p.660. Trifluoperazine is less likely to cause sedation, hypotension, hypothermia, or antimuscarinic effects but is associated with a higher incidence of extrapyramidal effects particularly when the daily dose exceeds 6 mg.

Interactions

As for Chlorpromazine, p.664.

Pharmacokinetics

◊ A study of the pharmacokinetics of trifluoperazine as a single 5-mg dose by mouth in 5 healthy subjects.[1] Peak plasma concentrations of trifluoperazine were reached from 1.5 to 4.5 hours after ingestion and varied widely between subjects, ranging from 0.53 to 3.09 nanograms per mL. Elimination of trifluoperazine was multiphasic; the mean elimination half-life was estimated to be 5.1 hours over the period from 4.5 to 12 hours after ingestion, while the mean apparent terminal elimination half-life was estimated to be 12.5 hours.

1. Midha KK, *et al.* Kinetics of oral trifluoperazine disposition in man. *Br J Clin Pharmacol* 1983; **15**: 380–2.

Uses and Administration

Trifluoperazine is a phenothiazine antipsychotic with general properties similar to those of chlorpromazine (p.665). It has a piperazine side-chain.

Trifluoperazine is used in the treatment of a variety of psychiatric disorders including schizophrenia (p.651), severe anxiety (p.649), and disturbed behaviour (p.650). It is also used for the control of nausea and vomiting (p.1206).

Trifluoperazine is given as the hydrochloride but its doses are expressed in terms of the base. A modified-release preparation is also available; the total daily dosage, as given below, may be administered in a single dose by mouth. Trifluoperazine should be given in reduced dosage to elderly or debilitated patients.

The usual initial dose for the treatment of schizophrenia and other **psychoses** is 2 to 5 mg twice daily *by mouth*, gradually increased to a usual range of 15 to 20 mg daily; in severe or resistant psychoses daily doses of 40 mg or more have been given. For the control of acute psychotic symptoms it may be given by deep *intramuscular* injection in a dose of 1 to 2 mg, repeated if necessary at intervals of not less than every 4 hours; more than 6 mg daily is rarely required. The initial dose for use in *children* is up to 5 mg daily by mouth in divided doses adjusted according to age, body-weight, and response, or 1 mg given once or twice daily by intramuscular injection.

For the control of **nausea and vomiting** the usual adult dose *by mouth* is 1 or 2 mg twice daily; up to 6 mg daily may be given in divided doses. *Children* aged 3 to 5 years may be given up to 1 mg daily in divided doses; this may be increased to a maximum of 4 mg daily in children aged 6 to 12 years.

When used as an adjunct in the short-term management of **severe anxiety disorders** doses are similar to those used for the control of nausea and vomiting.

Preparations

BP 2001: Trifluoperazine Tablets;
USP 25: Trifluoperazine Hydrochloride Injection; Trifluoperazine Hydrochloride Syrup; Trifluoperazine Hydrochloride Tablets.
Proprietary Preparations (details are given in Part 3)
Aust.: Jatroneural; *Austral.:* Stelazine; *Braz.:* Stelazine; *Canad.:* Novo-Flurazine†; Stelazine; Terfluzine†; *Fr.:* Terfluzine†; *Ger.:* Jatroneural†; *Irl.:* Stelazine; *Israel:* Terfluzine; *Ital.:* Modalina; *Mex.:* Flupazine; Stelazine; *Neth.:* Terfluzine; *NZ:* Stelazine; *S.Afr.:* Stelazine; *Spain:* Eskazine; *Thai.:* Triplex; *UK:* Stelazine; *USA:* Stelazine.
Multi-ingredient: *Aust.:* Stelabid†; *Braz.:* Stelapar; *Canad.:* Stelabid; *Irl.:* Parstelin; Stelabid; *Ital.:* Parmodalin; *Mex.:* Stelabid; *S.Afr.:* Stelabid†; *UK:* Parstelin†.

Trifluperidol (7121-w)

Trifluperidol *(BAN, USAN, rINN).*
McN-JR-2498; R-2498. 4′-Fluoro-4-[4-hydroxy-4-(3-trifluoromethylphenyl)piperidino]butyrophenone.
$C_{22}H_{23}F_4NO_2 = 409.4$.
CAS — 749-13-3.
ATC — N05AD02.

Trifluperidol Hydrochloride (7122-e)

Trifluperidol Hydrochloride *(BANM, rINNM).*
$C_{22}H_{23}F_4NO_2,HCl = 445.9$.
CAS — 2062-77-3.

Profile
Trifluperidol is a butyrophenone with general properties similar to those of haloperidol (p.686), and has been used as the hydrochloride in the treatment of psychoses including schizophrenia (p.651).

Preparations
Proprietary Preparations (details are given in Part 3)
Fr.: Triperidol†; *Ger.:* Triperidol†.

Triflupromazine (7041-w)

Triflupromazine *(BAN, rINN).*
Fluopromazine. NN-Dimethyl-3-(2-trifluoromethylphenothiazin-10-yl)propylamine.
$C_{18}H_{19}F_3N_2S = 352.4$.
CAS — 146-54-3.
ATC — N05AA05.
Pharmacopoeias. In US.

Pharmacopoeial description
USP 25: A light amber viscous oily liquid which crystallises into large irregular crystals during prolonged storage. Practically insoluble in water. Store in airtight containers. Protect from light.

Triflupromazine Hydrochloride (7042-e)

Triflupromazine Hydrochloride *(BANM, rINNM).*
Fluopromazine Hydrochloride.
$C_{18}H_{19}F_3N_2S,HCl = 388.9$.
CAS — 1098-60-8.
Pharmacopoeias. In US.

Pharmacopoeial description
USP 25: A white to pale tan crystalline powder having a slight characteristic odour. Soluble 1 in less than 1 of water and of alcohol and 1 in 1.7 of chloroform; soluble in acetone; insoluble in ether. Store in glass containers. Protect from light.

Profile
Triflupromazine hydrochloride is a phenothiazine with general properties similar to those of chlorpromazine (p.660). It is used mainly in the management of psychoses (p.650) and the control of nausea and vomiting (p.1206). Triflupromazine hydrochloride is usually given by injection but in some countries preparations are available for administration by mouth or by rectal suppository.

In the management of psychosis, the usual dose is 60 to 150 mg daily by intramuscular injection. For the control of nausea and vomiting 5 to 15 mg is given intramuscularly and repeated after 4 hours if necessary up to a maximum of 60 mg daily; a dose of 1 mg to a maximum total daily dose of 3 mg may be given intravenously.

A suggested intramuscular dose for children over 2½ years of age is 200 to 250 µg per kg body-weight daily up to a maximum of 10 mg daily.

Reduced doses should be used in elderly or debilitated patients.

Preparations
USP 25: Triflupromazine Hydrochloride Injection; Triflupromazine Hydrochloride Tablets; Triflupromazine Oral Solution.
Proprietary Preparations (details are given in Part 3)
Aust.: Psyquil; *Ger.:* Psyquil; *Neth.:* Siquil†; *USA:* Vesprin.

Valnoctamide (7125-j)

Valnoctamide *(USAN, rINN).*
McN-X-181; NSC-32363. 2-Ethyl-3-methylvaleramide.
$C_8H_{17}NO = 143.2$.
CAS — 4171-13-5.
ATC — N05CM13.

Profile
Valnoctamide, an isomer of valpromide (p.366), has been given by mouth in the treatment of anxiety disorders.

◊ References.
1. Bialer M, *et al.* Pharmacokinetics of a valpromide isomer, valnoctamide, in healthy subjects. *Eur J Clin Pharmacol* 1990; **38:** 289–91.
2. Barel S, *et al.* Stereoselective pharmacokinetic analysis of valnoctamide in healthy subjects and in patients with epilepsy. *Clin Pharmacol Ther* 1997; **61:** 442–9.

Interactions. For a discussion of the potential interaction between carbamazepine and valnoctamide, see Antiepileptics, p.344.

Preparations
Proprietary Preparations (details are given in Part 3)
Ital.: Nirvanil†.

Veralipride (17026-b)

Veralipride *(rINN).*
N-[(1-Allyl-2-pyrrolidinyl)methyl]-5-sulphamoyl-2-veratramide.
$C_{17}H_{25}N_3O_5S = 383.5$.
CAS — 66644-81-3.
ATC — N05AL06.

Profile
Veralipride is a substituted benzamide antipsychotic. It has been used in the treatment of cardiovascular and psychological symptoms associated with the menopause; the usual dose by mouth is 100 mg daily for 20 days repeated at intervals of 7 to 10 days.

Menopausal disorders. Hormone replacement therapy (HRT) with oestrogens is the mainstay of treatment for acute symptoms associated with the menopause (see p.1464). When HRT is considered to be unsuitable a variety of other drugs including veralipride have been tried.[1]
1. Young RL, *et al.* Management of menopause when estrogen cannot be used. *Drugs* 1990; **40:** 220–30.

Porphyria. Veralipride is considered to be unsafe in patients with porphyria because it has been shown to be porphyrinogenic in *in-vitro* systems.

Preparations
Proprietary Preparations (details are given in Part 3)
Belg.: Agreal; *Braz.:* Agreal; *Fr.:* Agreal; *Hong Kong:* Agreal; *Ital.:* Agradil; Veralipril; *Mex.:* Aclimafel; Veraligral; *Port.:* Agreal; *Spain:* Agreal; Faltium.

Vinylbital (4076-x)

Vinylbital *(BAN, rINN).*
Butyvinal; JD-96; Vinylbitone; Vinymalum. 5-(1-Methylbutyl)-5-vinylbarbituric acid.
$C_{11}H_{16}N_2O_3 = 224.3$.
CAS — 2430-49-1.
ATC — N05CA08.

Profile
Vinylbital is a barbiturate with general properties similar to those of amobarbital (p.655). It was used as a hypnotic but barbiturates are no longer considered appropriate for such use.

Zaleplon (17862-k)

Zaleplon *(BAN, USAN, rINN).*
CL-284846; L-846; LJC-10846; ZAL-846. 3′-(3-Cyanopyrazolo[1,5-a]pyrimidin-7-yl)-N-ethylacetanilide.
$C_{17}H_{15}N_5O = 305.3$.
CAS — 151319-34-5.
ATC — N05CF03.

Dependence and Withdrawal
As for Diazepam, p.675.

Adverse Effects, Treatment, and Precautions
As for Diazepam, p.675. Zaleplon should be used with caution and in reduced doses in patients with hepatic impairment, and should be avoided where this is severe.

Abuse. In a controlled study in healthy patients with a history of drug abuse, zaleplon was shown to have a comparable abuse potential to that of the benzodiazepine, triazolam.[1]
1. Rush CR, *et al.* Zaleplon and triazolam in humans: acute behavioral effects and abuse potential. *Psychopharmacology (Berl)* 1999; **145:** 39–51.

Interactions
As for Diazepam, p.677. Zaleplon is primarily metabolised by aldehyde oxidase and concurrent administration with inhibitors of this enzyme, such as cimetidine, may result in increased plasma concentrations of zaleplon (see Uses and Administra-

---

tion, below). Zaleplon is also partly metabolised by the cytochrome P450 isoenzyme CYP3A4 and consequently caution is advised when zaleplon is co-administered with drugs that are substrates for, or potent inhibitors of, this isoenzyme.
Concomitant administration of rifampicin or other potent enzyme-inducing drugs may accelerate the metabolism of zaleplon and reduce its plasma concentrations.

Pharmacokinetics
Zaleplon is rapidly absorbed from the gastrointestinal tract with peak plasma concentrations reached in about one hour. A heavy meal or one with a high-fat content delays absorption and reduces peak concentrations. Bioavailability is about 30% due to significant first-pass hepatic metabolism. Zaleplon is metabolised primarily by aldehyde oxidase to form 5-oxo-zaleplon and, to a lesser extent, by the cytochrome P450 isoenzyme CYP3A4 to desethylzaleplon, which is further metabolised by aldehyde oxidase to 5-oxo-desethylzaleplon. The plasma-elimination half-life of zaleplon is approximately 1 hour. About 70% of a dose is excreted in the urine as these inactive metabolites or their glucuronides; less than 1% is excreted unchanged. About 17% of a dose is eliminated in the faeces, mainly as 5-oxo-zaleplon. Zaleplon is distributed into breast milk.

◊ References.
1. Greenblatt DJ, *et al.* Comparative kinetics and dynamics of zaleplon, zolpidem, and placebo. *Clin Pharmacol Ther* 1998; **64:** 553–61.
2. Drover D, *et al.* Pharmacokinetics, pharmacodynamics, and relative pharmacokinetic/pharmacodynamic profiles of zaleplon and zolpidem. *Clin Ther* 2000; **22:** 1443–61.

Distribution into breast milk. Zaleplon was detected in the breast milk of 5 lactating women who had been given a 10-mg dose.[1] The milk-to-plasma concentration ratio for zaleplon was approximately 0.5.
1. Darwish M, *et al.* Rapid disappearance of zaleplon from breast milk after oral administration to lactating women. *J Clin Pharmacol* 1999; **39:** 670–4.

Uses and Administration
Zaleplon is a pyrazolopyrimidine which is reported to have similar sedative properties to the benzodiazepines (see Diazepam, p.680). It is used as a hypnotic in the short-term management of insomnia (p.652). Zaleplon has a rapid onset and short duration of action. The usual dose is 10 mg at bedtime although the US manufacturer notes that occasional patients may require 20 mg. Elderly or debilitated patients and those with mild to moderate hepatic impairment should be given 5 mg. It is also recommended that the dose of zaleplon should be reduced to 5 mg in patients taking cimetidine concomitantly.

◊ Zaleplon is a pyrazolopyrimidine hypnotic. Although not related structurally to the benzodiazepines it appears to act by binding selectively to the benzodiazepine type I receptor (BZ1- or ω1-receptors) on the GABA subtype A complex. Zaleplon reduces sleep latency but has little effect on sleep duration; it is rapidly absorbed and eliminated and consequently residual effects the next day are said to be minimal. These characteristics make it best suited for the treatment of patients with insomnia who have difficulty falling asleep; zaleplon can either be taken at bedtime or during the night if a patient has trouble falling back to sleep, provided they are assured of at least 4 hours uninterrupted sleep.
References.
1. Anonymous. Zaleplon for insomnia. *Med Lett Drugs Ther* 1999; **41:** 93–4.
2. Danjou P, *et al.* A comparison of the residual effects of zaleplon and zolpidem following administration 5 to 2 h before awakening. *Br J Clin Pharmacol* 1999; **48:** 367–74.
3. Elie R, *et al.* Sleep latency is shortened during 4 weeks of treatment with zaleplon, a novel nonbenzodiazepine hypnotic. *J Clin Psychiatry* 1999; **60:** 536–44.
4. Dooley M, Plosker GL. Zaleplon: a review of its use in the treatment of insomnia. *Drugs* 2000; **60:** 413–45

Preparations
Proprietary Preparations (details are given in Part 3)
Belg.: Sonata; *Denm.:* Sonata; *Fin.:* Sonata; *Ger.:* Sonata; *Irl.:* Sonata; *Ital.:* Sonata; *Swed.:* Sonata; *Switz.:* Sonata; *UK:* Sonata; *USA:* Sonata.

Ziprasidone (17144-w)

Ziprasidone *(BAN, rINN).*
CP-88059 (ziprasidone hydrochloride); CP-88059/27 (ziprasidone mesilate). 5-{2-[4-(1,2-Benzisothiazol-3-yl)-1-piperazinyl]ethyl}-6-chloro-2-indolinone.
$C_{21}H_{21}ClN_4OS = 412.9$.
CAS — 146939-27-7 (ziprasidone); 138982-67-9 (ziprasidone hydrochloride); 199191-69-0 (ziprasidone mesilate).
ATC — N05AE04.

NOTE. Ziprasidone Hydrochloride and Ziprasidone Mesilate are *USAN*.

Adverse Effects, Treatment, and Precautions
As for Chlorpromazine, p.660.

Ziprasidone has been associated with dose-related prolongation of the QT interval. Because of this and the consequent danger of life-threatening arrhythmias such as torsade de pointes and sudden death, its use is contra-indicated in patients with a known history of QT prolongation or cardiac arrhythmias, with

---

The symbol † denotes a preparation no longer actively marketed

recent acute myocardial infarction, or with decompensated heart failure. The concomitant administration of drugs liable to interfere with the metabolism of ziprasidone, of other drugs known to prolong the QT interval, and of drugs likely to cause electrolyte imbalance should also be avoided (see under Interactions, below).

For all patients starting ziprasidone, it is recommended that baseline serum potassium and magnesium screening should be performed. Serum electrolytes should be monitored in patients who commence diuretic therapy during ziprasidone treatment. Patients who present during ziprasidone treatment with symptoms that might indicate torsade de pointes (e.g. dizziness, palpitations, or syncope) should be further evaluated.

Interactions
Concomitant administration of ziprasidone with other drugs known to prolong the QT interval such as *dofetilide, moxifloxacin, pimozide, quinidine, sotalol, sparfloxacin*, and *thioridazine* is contra-indicated.

The metabolism of ziprasidone is mediated by the cytochrome P450 isoenzyme CYP3A4. Therefore, there is the potential for interactions between ziprasidone and other drugs that inhibit or act as a substrate for this enzyme, and such drugs should not be given concomitantly. Ziprasidone may enhance the effects of certain antihypertensives, and it may antagonise the effects of levodopa and dopamine antagonists.

Pharmacokinetics
Ziprasidone is well absorbed following oral administration with peak plasma concentrations being reached after 6 to 8 hours. The presence of food may double the absorption. Plasma protein binding is about 99%. Ziprasidone is extensively metabolised by aldehyde oxidase (approximately 66% of the original dose) and by the cytochrome P450 isoenzyme CYP3A4. The terminal elimination half-life has been reported to be about 7 hours. Ziprasidone is excreted predominantly as metabolites in the faeces (66%) and urine (20%); less than 5% appears as unchanged drug.

◊ References.
1. Various. The pharmacokinetics of ziprasidone. *Br J Clin Pharmacol* 2000; **49** (suppl 1): 1S–76S.

Uses and Administration
Ziprasidone is an atypical antipsychotic used for the treatment of schizophrenia (p.651). Like other atypical antipsychotics it appears to be associated with a low incidence of extrapyramidal adverse effects. It is reported to have affinity for serotonin (5-HT$_2$) and dopamine (D$_2$) receptors. Ziprasidone is given as the hydrochloride by mouth in an initial dose of 20 mg twice daily with food. Doses may be increased if necessary at intervals of not less than 2 days up to 80 mg twice daily. For maintenance, doses as low as 20 mg twice daily may be effective.

Psychoses. A meta-analysis[1] of the effectiveness and safety of ziprasidone in patients with schizophrenia found that from the limited data available ziprasidone was as effective as haloperidol; it was less likely to provoke extrapyramidal disorders but appeared to cause more nausea and vomiting, and pain at the site of injection. Comparisons with other atypical antipsychotics were lacking. A comparative study[2] of intramuscular ziprasidone compared with intramuscular haloperidol also demonstrated a favourable outcome in patients with acute psychoses.

1. Bagnall A-M, *et al.* Ziprasidone for schizophrenia and severe mental illness (updated 16 March 2001). Available in The Cochrane Library; Issue 4. Oxford: Update Software; 2001.
2. Brook S, *et al.* Intramuscular ziprasidone compared with intramuscular haloperidol in the treatment of acute psychosis. *J Clin Psychiatry* 2000; **61**: 933–41.

Preparations
Proprietary Preparations (details are given in Part 3)
Swed.: Zeldox†; *USA*: Geodon.

Zolazepam Hydrochloride (18695-m)
Zolazepam Hydrochloride (*BANM, USAN, rINNM*).
CI-716. 4-(o-Fluorophenyl)-6,8-dihydro-1,3,8-trimethylpyrazolo[3,4-e][1,4]diazepin-7(1H)-one monohydrochloride.
$C_{15}H_{15}FN_4O$,HCl = 322.8.
CAS — 31352-82-6 (*zolazepam*); 33754-49-3 (*zolazepam hydrochloride*).
Pharmacopoeias. In *US* for veterinary use only.

Pharmacopoeial description
USP 25: A white to off-white crystalline powder. Freely soluble in water and in 0.1N hydrochloric acid; slightly soluble in chloroform; practically insoluble in ether; soluble in methyl alcohol. pH of a 10% solution in water is between 1.5 and 3.5. Store in airtight containers.

Profile
Zolazepam hydrochloride is a benzodiazepine with general properties similar to those of diazepam (p.680). It is used with tiletamine (p.1270) for general anaesthesia in veterinary medicine.

Zolpidem Tartrate (1667-t)
Zolpidem Tartrate (*BANM, USAN, rINNM*).
SL-80.0750 (zolpidem); SL-80.0750-23N; Zolpidemi Tartras.
N,N-Dimethyl-2-(6-methyl-2-p-tolylimidazo[1,2-a]pyridin-3-yl)acetamide hemitartrate.
$(C_{19}H_{21}N_3O)_2,C_4H_6O_6$ = 764.9.
CAS — 82626-48-0 (*zolpidem*); 99294-93-6 (*zolpidem tartrate*).
Pharmacopoeias. In *Eur.* (see p.vi).

Pharmacopoeial description
Ph. Eur.: A white or almost white hygroscopic crystalline powder. Slightly soluble in water; practically insoluble in dichloromethane; sparingly soluble in methyl alcohol. Store in airtight containers. Protect from light.

Dependence and Withdrawal
As for Diazepam, p.675.

◊ A 37-year-old male suffered a generalised tonic-clonic seizure after zolpidem was abruptly stopped.[1] He had himself escalated the dose from 10 mg to 130 mg daily over 2 months. The patient recovered after being started on a benzodiazepine dosage tapering programme. Symptoms attributed to daytime abstinence following excessive night-time doses have been reported[2] in 2 patients and included anxiety, tremor, sweating, nausea, gastric and abdominal pain, swallowing difficulties, tachycardia, and tachypnoea. The patients had increased their doses because of the development of tolerance to the hypnotic effect but had begun to experience muscle twitches and myoclonic jerks.

1. Gilbert DL, Staats PS. Seizure after withdrawal from supratherapeutic doses of zolpidem tartrate, a selective omega I benzodiazepine receptor agonist. *J Pain Symptom Manage* 1997; **14**: 118–20.
2. Cavallaro R, *et al.* Tolerance and withdrawal with zolpidem. *Lancet* 1993; **342**: 374–5.

Adverse Effects, Treatment, and Precautions
As for Diazepam, p.675.

◊ Reviews.
1. Darcourt G, *et al.* The safety and tolerability of zolpidem—an update. *J Psychopharmacol* 1999; **13**: 81–93.

Abuse. Chronic abuse has been reported in a patient with depression who obtained a stimulant effect when taking large doses of zolpidem.[1] Tolerance also developed. See also under Dependence and Withdrawal, above.

1. Gericke CA, Ludolph AC. Chronic abuse of zolpidem. *JAMA* 1994; **272**: 1721–2.

Effects on the liver. Hepatitis developed on two separate occasions in a 53-year-old woman following the use of zolpidem for insomnia.[1]

1. Karsenti D, *et al.* Hepatotoxicity associated with zolpidem treatment. *BMJ* 1999; **318**: 1179.

Effects on mental function. Psychotic reactions, which may not subsequently be recalled, have been reported in patients taking therapeutic doses of zolpidem.[1,2]

1. Ansseau M, *et al.* Psychotic reactions to zolpidem. *Lancet* 1992; **339**: 809.
2. Iruela LM, *et al.* Zolpidem-induced macropsia in anorexic woman. *Lancet* 1993; **342**: 443–4.

Overdosage. A retrospective analysis of 344 cases of acute overdosage with zolpidem reported to the Paris Poison Center and the manufacturers Synthelabo has been published.[1] For those patients whose details were available the ingested dose had ranged from 10 to 1400 mg. Drowsiness which occurred in 89 patients was the most common adverse effect reported. Adverse effects also considered to be associated with zolpidem overdosage included coma in 4 patients and vomiting in 7. Recovery was usually rapid when overdosage involved only zolpidem. It was recommended that patients who had ingested more than 100 mg of zolpidem should undergo gastric lavage and should be monitored for at least 12 hours. (UK authorities make similar recommendations; activated charcoal may also be considered, and should be employed in children who have ingested more than 5 mg.) Although it has been shown that flumazenil[2] can effectively antagonise the CNS effects of zolpidem the authors of this analysis[1] found that in general it was not required.

1. Garnier R, *et al.* Acute zolpidem poisoning—analysis of 344 cases. *J Toxicol Clin Toxicol* 1994; **32**: 391–404.
2. Patat A, *et al.* Flumazenil antagonizes the central effects of zolpidem, an imidazopyridine hypnotic. *Clin Pharmacol Ther* 1994; **56**: 430–6.

Interactions
As for Diazepam, p.677.

Antidepressants. A 16-year-old girl who had been taking *paroxetine* 20 mg daily for 3 days began to hallucinate and became disorientated one hour after taking zolpidem 10 mg at night. The delirium cleared spontaneously 4 hours later without treatment.[1] When questioned, at least one other of the author's patients receiving this combination reported transient visual hallucinations. Other isolated cases of visual hallucinations have been reported in patients taking zolpidem concomitantly

with antidepressants including *bupropion, desipramine, fluoxetine, sertraline*, and *venlafaxine*.[2]

1. Katz SE. Possible paroxetine-zolpidem interaction. *Am J Psychiatry* 1995; **152**: 1689.
2. Elko CJ, *et al.* Zolpidem-associated hallucinations and serotonin reuptake inhibition: a possible interaction. *J Toxicol Clin Toxicol* 1998; **36**: 195–203.

Antifungals. Use of *ketoconazole* with zolpidem has resulted in increased plasma concentrations, and an enhanced sedative effect, of zolpidem, albeit only modest.[1] The co-administration of zolpidem and *fluconazole*[1] or *itraconazole*[1,2] has resulted in small but non-significant changes in the pharmacokinetics and sedative effects of zolpidem.

1. Greenblatt DJ, *et al.* Kinetic and dynamic interaction study of zolpidem with ketoconazole, itraconazole, and fluconazole. *Clin Pharmacol Ther* 1998; **64**: 661–71.
2. Luurila H, *et al.* Effect of itraconazole on the pharmacokinetics and pharmacodynamics of zolpidem. *Eur J Clin Pharmacol* 1998; **54**: 163–6.

Antivirals. HIV-protease inhibitors such as *ritonavir* may increase plasma concentrations of zolpidem with a risk of extreme sedation and respiratory depression; concomitant administration is not recommended.

Rifampicin. Rifampicin reduced the hypnotic effect of zolpidem in a study in 8 healthy female subjects.[1] The area under the curve for zolpidem was reduced by 73% after administration of rifampicin and the peak plasma concentration by 58%. The elimination half-life of zolpidem was reduced from 2.5 to 1.6 hours. Similar effects could be expected with other potent inducers of the cytochrome P450 isoenzyme CYP3A4 such as carbamazepine and phenytoin.

1. Villikka K, *et al.* Rifampin reduces plasma concentrations and effects of zolpidem. *Clin Pharmacol Ther* 1997; **62**: 629–34.

Pharmacokinetics
Zolpidem is rapidly absorbed from the gastrointestinal tract, peak plasma concentrations being reached within 3 hours. Zolpidem undergoes first-pass metabolism and an absolute bioavailability of about 70% has been reported. Zolpidem has an elimination half-life of about 2.5 hours and is approximately 92% bound to plasma proteins. It is metabolised primarily by the cytochrome P450 isoenzyme CYP3A4; the inactive metabolites of zolpidem are excreted in the urine and faeces. Zolpidem is distributed into breast milk.

◊ References.
1. Salvà P, Costa J. Clinical pharmacokinetics and pharmacodynamics of zolpidem: therapeutic implications. *Clin Pharmacokinet* 1995; **29**: 142–53.
2. von Moltke LL, *et al.* Zolpidem metabolism in vitro: responsible cytochromes, chemical inhibitors, and vivo correlations. *Br J Clin Pharmacol* 1999; **48**: 89–97.
3. Drover D, *et al.* Pharmacokinetics, pharmacodynamics, and relative pharmacokinetic/pharmacodynamic profiles of zaleplon and zolpidem. *Clin Ther* 2000; **22**: 1443–61.

Distribution into breast milk. In 5 lactating women given a 20-mg dose of zolpidem, the amount of drug excreted in breast milk after 3 hours ranged between 0.76 and 3.88 µg, which represented 0.004 to 0.019% of the administered dose.[1] No detectable (below 0.5 nanograms per mL) zolpidem was found in subsequent milk samples.

1. Pons G, *et al.* Zolpidem excretion in breast milk. *Eur J Clin Pharmacol* 1989; **37**: 245–8.

Uses and Administration
Zolpidem tartrate is an imidazopyridine which is reported to have similar sedative properties to the benzodiazepines (see Diazepam, p.680), but minimal anxiolytic, muscle relaxant, and anticonvulsant properties. It has a rapid onset and short duration of action, and is used as a hypnotic in the short-term management of insomnia (p.652). The usual dose by mouth is 10 mg taken immediately before retiring. In elderly or debilitated patients or patients with hepatic impairment, treatment should be initiated with a dose of 5 mg at night.

◊ Zolpidem is an imidazopyridine with strong sedative actions, but only minor anxiolytic, muscle relaxant, or anticonvulsant properties. Some degree of amnesia has been reported. Zolpidem appears to act by binding to the benzodiazepine receptor component of the GABA receptor complex. It has, however, a selective affinity for the subtype of benzodiazepine receptors prevalent in the cerebellum (BZ1- or ω$_1$-receptors) as opposed to those more commonly found in the spinal cord (BZ2- or ω$_2$-receptors) or in the peripheral tissues (BZ3- or ω$_3$-receptors). Zolpidem has a rapid onset and short duration of hypnotic action and at usual doses decreases time to sleep onset and increases duration of sleep with little apparent effect on sleep stages. Reviews agree that clinical studies have shown zolpidem to have hypnotic activity superior to placebo and generally similar to comparative benzodiazepines. Although it does not appear to produce rebound insomnia to any great extent, there appears to be little evidence that zolpidem offers any advantage over short-acting benzodiazepines in terms of residual effects the next day, or its potential to induce tolerance or withdrawal symptoms or dependence (see also under Dependence and Withdrawal, above).

References.
1. Langtry HD, Benfield P. Zolpidem: a review of its pharmacodynamic and pharmacokinetic properties and therapeutic potential. *Drugs* 1990; **40:** 291–313.
2. Lobo BL, Greene WL. Zolpidem: distinct from triazolam? *Ann Pharmacother* 1997; **31:** 625–32.
3. Nowell PD, *et al.* Benzodiazepines and zolpidem for chronic insomnia: a meta-analysis of treatment efficacy. *JAMA* 1997; **278:** 2170–7.
4. Holm KJ, Goa KL. Zolpidem: an update of its pharmacology, therapeutic efficacy and tolerability in the treatment of insomnia. *Drugs* 2000; **59:** 865–89.

Catatonia. Anecdotal reports[1,2] suggesting that zolpidem may be a useful test in the diagnosis of catatonia.
1. Thomas P, *et al.* Test for catatonia with zolpidem. *Lancet* 1997; **349:** 702.
2. Zaw ZF, Bates GDL. Replication of zolpidem test for catatonia in an adolescent. *Lancet* 1997; **349:** 1914.

Parkinsonism. Although preliminary findings[1] in 10 patients suggested that zolpidem might improve symptoms of Parkinson's disease concern has been expressed[2] over the risk of falls associated with zolpidem-induced drowsiness and the serious consequences for these patients. Benefit has also been reported[3] in the treatment of antipsychotic-induced parkinsonism in one patient with symptoms of repetitive persistent gross tremors of the hands.
1. Daniele A, *et al.* Zolpidem in Parkinson's disease. *Lancet* 1997; **349:** 1222–3.
2. Lavoisy J, Marsac J. Zolpidem in Parkinson's disease. *Lancet* 1997; **350:** 74.
3. Farver DK, Khan MH. Zolpidem for antipsychotic-induced parkinsonism. *Ann Pharmacother* 2001; **35:** 435–7.

Preparations

Proprietary Preparations (details are given in Part 3)
Aust.: Ivadal; Stilnox†; *Austral.:* Stilnox; *Belg.:* Stilnoct; *Braz.:* Stilnox; *Denm.:* Stilnoct; *Fin.:* Stilnoct; *Fr.:* Ivadal†; *Ger.:* Bikalm; Stilnox; *Hong Kong:* Stilnox; *Irl.:* Stilnoct; *Israel:* Stilnox; *Ital.:* Ivadal†; *Niotal; Nottem; Stilnox; *Neth.:* Stilnoct; *Norw.:* Stilnoct; *Port.:* Cymerion; Stilnox; *S.Afr.:* Stilnox; *Singapore:* Stilnox; *Spain:* Cedrol; Dalparan; Stilnox; *Swed.:* Stilnoct; *Switz.:* Stilnox; *UK:* Stilnoct; *USA:* Ambien.

Zopiclone   (14031-d)

Zopiclone *(BAN, rINN)*.

27267-RP; Zopiclonum. 6-(5-Chloro-2-pyridyl)-6,7-dihydro-7-oxo-5H-pyrrolo[3,4-b]pyrazin-5-yl 4-methylpiperazine-1-carboxylate.

$C_{17}H_{17}ClN_6O_3 = 388.8$.
CAS — 43200-80-2.
ATC — N05CF01.

Pharmacopoeias. In Eur. (see p.vi).

Pharmacopoeial description

Ph. Eur.: A white or slightly yellowish powder. Practically insoluble in water and in alcohol; sparingly soluble in acetone; freely soluble in dichloromethane. It dissolves in dilute mineral acids. Protect from light.

Dependence and Withdrawal

As for Diazepam, p.675.

◊ Reports[1,2] of zopiclone dependence and associated withdrawal symptoms on dosage reduction or cessation of use.
1. Jones IR, Sullivan G. Physical dependence on zopiclone: case reports. *BMJ* 1998; **316:** 117.
2. Sikdar S. Physical dependence on zopiclone. *BMJ* 1998; **317:** 146.

Adverse Effects, Treatment, and Precautions

As for Diazepam, p.675. A bitter or metallic taste in the mouth has been reported with zopiclone.

Treatment of overdose is largely supportive. Activated charcoal may be given orally within one hour of ingestion of more than 150 mg zopiclone by adults, or 1.5 mg per kg body-weight by children. Alternatively gastric lavage may be considered in adults if they present within 1 hour of a potentially life-threatening overdose. Flumazenil has been used in cases of severe CNS depression.

◊ In a French postmarketing survey[1] of 20 513 patients treated with zopiclone the most commonly reported adverse events were bitter taste (3.6%), dry mouth (1.6%), difficulty arising in the morning (1.3%), sleepiness (0.5%), nausea (0.5%) and nightmares (0.5%). The UK Committee on Safety of Medicines (CSM)[2] had received 122 reports of adverse reactions to zopiclone over a period of about one year since the product's introduction in November 1989. A fifth of these were neuropsychiatric reactions, a proportion similar to that found with other

hypnotics. Many of these reactions were potentially serious and involved hallucinations (3 auditory and 2 visual), amnesia (4) and behavioural disturbances (10, including 3 cases of aggression). Most reactions started immediately or shortly after the first dose and improved rapidly on stopping the drug. Three patients had difficulty in stopping treatment, 2 because of withdrawal symptoms and one due to repeated rebound insomnia. The CSM considered that, although differing structurally from the benzodiazepines, zopiclone has the same potential for adverse psychiatric reactions, including dependence. As with the benzodiazepines it should be reserved for patients with severe sleep disturbance and its duration of use limited to 28 days; also care should be taken in the elderly, those who have a history of previous psychiatric illness, or who are prone to drug abuse.
1. Allain H, *et al.* Postmarketing surveillance of zopiclone in insomnia: analysis of 20,513 cases. *Sleep* 1991; **14:** 408–13.
2. Committee on Safety of Medicines. Zopiclone (Zimovane) and neuro-psychiatric reactions. *Current Problems 30* 1990.

Administration. Results in 9 healthy subjects given zopiclone indicated a significant delay in onset of action when the drug was taken in the supine, as opposed to the standing, position; this was associated with a prolongation of more than 20 minutes in the lag time before absorption began.[1] In order to obtain a rapid and complete hypnotic effect from zopiclone the tablet should be swallowed in the standing position.
1. Channer KS, *et al.* The effect of posture at the time of administration on the central depressant effects of the new hypnotic zopiclone. *Br J Clin Pharmacol* 1984; **18:** 879–86.

Driving. For reference to the increased risk of road-traffic accidents for drivers taking zopiclone, see p.676.

Hepatic impairment. Zopiclone was given in a dose of 7.5 mg to 7 cirrhotic patients and 8 healthy subjects; a further 2 cirrhotic patients received 3.75 mg.[1] Mean peak plasma concentrations were similar in healthy subjects and those with hepatic impairment following equivalent doses but time to peak plasma concentration was 4 hours in the latter as compared with 2 hours in the healthy subjects. Elimination was greatly prolonged in cirrhotic patients, in whom the mean plasma half-life was 8.53 compared with 3.50 hours. The CNS-depressant effects of zopiclone were delayed in the cirrhotic patients in a way consistent with the pharmacokinetic changes. There was also some evidence of an increased response in these patients. The authors recommended caution when administering zopiclone to patients with severe hepatic disease; the manufacturers contra-indicate the use of zopiclone in such patients.
1. Parker G, Roberts CJC. Plasma concentrations and central nervous system effects of the new hypnotic agent zopiclone in patients with chronic liver disease. *Br J Clin Pharmacol* 1983; **16:** 259–65.

Overdosage. Consciousness was rapidly regained after intravenous flumazenil administration in a patient who had taken an overdosage of zopiclone.[1] Fatalities following zopiclone overdose have been reported.[2,3]
1. Ahmad Z, *et al.* Diagnostic utility of flumazenil in coma with suspected poisoning. *BMJ* 1991; **302:** 292.
2. Boniface PJ, Russell SGG. Two cases of fatal zopiclone overdose. *J Anal Toxicol* 1996; **20:** 131–3.
3. Meatherall RC. Zopiclone fatality in a hospitalized patient. *J Forensic Sci* 1997; **42:** 340–3.

Interactions

As for Diazepam, p.677. Concomitant administration of rifampicin or other potent inducers of the cytochrome P450 isoenzyme CYP3A4, such as carbamazepine or phenytoin, is likely to reduce the effects of zopiclone.

Antibacterials. In a study in healthy subjects *erythromycin* increased the rate of absorption of zopiclone and prolonged its elimination.[1] In a study[2] in 8 healthy subjects concomitant administration of *rifampicin* was associated with an 82% reduction in the area under the curve for zopiclone. The peak plasma concentration of zopiclone was reduced from 76.9 to 22.5 nanograms per mL and the elimination half-life from 3.8 to 2.3 hours.
1. Aranko K, *et al.* The effect of erythromycin on the pharmacokinetics and pharmacodynamics of zopiclone. *Br J Clin Pharmacol* 1994; **37:** 363–7.
2. Villikka K, *et al.* Concentrations and effects of zopiclone are greatly reduced by rifampicin. *Br J Clin Pharmacol* 1997; **43:** 471–4.

Pharmacokinetics

Zopiclone is rapidly absorbed and widely distributed following administration by mouth. It has an elimination half-life of 3.5 to 6.5 hours and is reported to be about 45 to 80% bound to plasma proteins. Zopiclone is extensively metabolised in the liver; the 2 major metabolites, the less active zopiclone N-oxide and the inactive N-desmethylzopiclone, are excreted mainly in the urine. About 50% of a dose is converted by decarboxylation to inactive metabolites, which are partly eliminated via the lungs as carbon dioxide. Only about 5% of a dose appears unchanged in the urine and about 16% appears in the faeces. Excretion

of zopiclone in the saliva may explain reports of a bitter taste. It is also distributed into breast milk.

◊ Reviews.
1. Fernandez C, *et al.* Clinical pharmacokinetics of zopiclone. *Clin Pharmacokinet* 1995; **29:** 431–41.

Distribution into breast milk. Zopiclone was distributed into breast milk in 12 lactating women in concentrations approximately half those in plasma.[1] The calculated dose that would be received by a neonate was 1.5 µg per kg body-weight, corresponding to 1.2% of the maternal dose.
1. Matheson I, *et al.* The excretion of zopiclone into breast milk. *Br J Clin Pharmacol* 1990; **30:** 267–71.

Uses and Administration

Zopiclone is a cyclopyrrolone which is reported to have similar sedative, anxiolytic, muscle relaxant, amnestic, and anticonvulsant properties to those of the benzodiazepines (see Diazepam, p.680). Like diazepam, its actions are mediated by enhancement of the activity of aminobutyric acid (GABA) in the brain. Zopiclone is reported to bind to the benzodiazepine receptor component of the GABA receptor complex but at a different site to the benzodiazepines. It has a short duration of action.

Zopiclone is used as a hypnotic in the short-term management of insomnia (p.652). The usual dose is 7.5 mg by mouth before retiring. In elderly patients and in those with renal insufficiency or mild to moderate hepatic insufficiency, treatment should be initiated with a dose of 3.75 mg before retiring.

◊ Zopiclone has a similar pharmacological and pharmacokinetic profile to the short-acting benzodiazepines. It is claimed to initiate sleep rapidly, without reduction of rapid-eye-movement (REM) sleep, and then sustain it with preservation of normal slow-wave sleep. It is generally considered to be as effective as a hypnotic as the benzodiazepines.[1,2] Rebound insomnia has occurred but does not appear to be common. Residual effects the next day may be less pronounced after zopiclone than after short-acting benzodiazepines but there appears to be little evidence that zopiclone offers any clinical advantage in terms of its potential to induce tolerance, withdrawal symptoms, or dependence. For recommendations of the UK Committee on Safety of Medicines concerning its use as a hypnotic, see under Adverse Effects, Treatment, and Precautions, above.
1. Noble S, *et al.* Zopiclone: an update of its pharmacology, clinical efficacy and tolerability in the treatment of insomnia. *Drugs* 1998; **55:** 277–302.
2. Hajak G. A comparative assessment of the risks and benefits of zopiclone: a review of 15 years' clinical experience. *Drug Safety* 1999; **21:** 457–69.

Preparations

Proprietary Preparations (details are given in Part 3)
Aust.: Imovane; *Austral.:* Imovane; *Belg.:* Imovane; *Braz.:* Imovane; Serenex; *Canad.:* Imovane; Rhovane; *Denm.:* Imoclone; Imovane; Imozop; *Fin.:* Imovane; Zopinox; *Fr.:* Imovane; Noctirex; *Ger.:* espa-dorm; Optidorm; Somnosan; Ximovan; *Hong Kong:* Imovane; *Irl.:* Zilese; Zimoclone; Zimovane; Zopitan; Zorclone; *Israel:* Imovane; Nocturno; *Ital.:* Imovane; *Mex.:* Imovane; *Neth.:* Imovane; *Norw.:* Imovane; *NZ:* Imovane; Zo-Tab; *S.Afr.:* Alchera; Imovane; Zopimed; *Singapore:* Imovane; *Spain:* Datolan; Limovan; Siaten; *Swed.:* Imovane; *Switz.:* Imovane; *UK:* Zileze; Zimovane.

Zotepine   (2479-d)

Zotepine *(BAN, rINN)*.

2-[(8-Chlorodibenzo[b,f]-thiepin-10-yl)oxy]-N,N-dimethylethylamine.

$C_{18}H_{18}ClNOS = 331.9$.
CAS — 26615-21-4.

Adverse Effects, Treatment, and Precautions

As for Chlorpromazine, p.660.

Zotepine is contra-indicated in patients with a personal or close family history of epilepsy. It has uricosuric properties and should not be given to patients with acute gout or a history of nephrolithiasis. Since zotepine can prolong the QT interval it is recommended that an ECG is performed before starting treatment. Patients with pre-existing prolongation of the QT interval should not be given zotepine. A reduced dosage is recommended in the elderly or in those with renal or hepatic impairment. Weekly monitoring of liver function is recommended for at least the first 3 months of therapy in patients with hepatic impairment.

Interactions

As for Chlorpromazine, p.664.

The risk of arrhythmias with zotepine may be increased by use with other drugs that prolong the QT interval or cause hypokalaemia. Concomitant administration of zotepine with fluoxetine or diazepam may lead to increased plasma concentrations of zotepine.

The symbol † denotes a preparation no longer actively marketed

Pharmacokinetics

Zotepine is absorbed from the gastrointestinal tract and peak plasma concentrations have been achieved 2 to 3 hours after oral administration. It undergoes extensive first-pass metabolism to the equipotent metabolite norzotepine and inactive metabolites. CYP1A2 and CYP3A4 are the major cytochrome P450 isoenzymes involved in the metabolism of zotepine. Protein binding of zotepine and norzotepine is 97%. Zotepine is excreted mainly in the urine and faeces as metabolites and has an elimination half-life of about 14 hours.

Uses and Administration

Zotepine is an atypical antipsychotic that is an antagonist at central dopamine (D_1 and D_2) receptors; it also binds to serotonin (5-HT_2), adrenergic (α_1), and histamine (H_1) receptors and inhibits noradrenaline reuptake. It is given by mouth in the treatment of schizophrenia (p.651) in an initial dose of 25 mg three times daily increased at intervals of 4 days according to response to a maximum dose of 100 mg three times daily. There is an appreciable increase in the incidence of seizures at total daily doses above the recommended maximum of 300 mg. For elderly patients or those with renal or hepatic insufficiency the recommended starting dose is 25 mg given twice daily increased gradually up to a maximum of 75 mg twice daily.

Schizophrenia. A systematic review[1] of short-term studies of zotepine for schizophrenia concluded tentatively that it was as effective as classical antipsychotics and might be of benefit in patients with negative symptoms; in addition it seemed less likely to provoke extrapyramidal disorders. Comparisons with atypical antipsychotics were too scanty for a meaningful comparison to be drawn.

1. Fenton M, et al. Zotepine for schizophrenia (updated 21 November 2000). Available in The Cochrane Library; Issue 4. Oxford: Update Software; 2001.

Preparations

Proprietary Preparations (details are given in Part 3)
Aust.: Nipolept; *Ger.:* Nipolept; *Jpn:* Lodopin; *UK:* Zoleptil.

Zuclopenthixol (12014-g)

Zuclopenthixol (BAN, rINN).

AY-62021 (clopenthixol); Z-Clopenthixol; cis-Clopenthixol; α-Clopenthixol; N-746 (clopenthixol); NSC-64087 (clopenthixol). (Z)-2-{4-[3-(2-Chloro-10H-dibenzo[b,e]thiin-10-ylidene)propyl]piperazin-1-yl}ethanol.

$C_{22}H_{25}ClN_2OS = 401.0$.

CAS — 53772-83-1 (zuclopenthixol); 982-24-1 (clopenthixol).

ATC — N05AF05.

NOTE. Clopenthixol (the racemic mixture) is *BAN* and *USAN*.

Zuclopenthixol Acetate (14093-j)

Zuclopenthixol Acetate (BANM, rINNM).

$C_{24}H_{27}ClN_2O_2S = 443.0$.

CAS — 85721-05-7.

Pharmacopoeias. In *Br.*

Pharmacopoeial description

BP 2001: A yellowish, viscous oil. Very slightly soluble in water; very soluble in alcohol, in dichloromethane, and in ether. Store at a temperature not exceeding −20°. Protect from light.

Zuclopenthixol Decanoate (7027-l)

Zuclopenthixol Decanoate (BANM, rINNM).

Zuclopenthixoli Decanoas.

$C_{32}H_{43}ClN_2O_2S = 555.2$.

CAS — 64053-00-5.

Pharmacopoeias. In *Eur.* (see p.vi).

Pharmacopoeial description

Ph. Eur.: A yellow viscous oily liquid. Very slightly soluble in water; very soluble in alcohol and in dichloromethane. Store under an inert gas in airtight containers at a temperature not exceeding −20°. Protect from light.

Zuclopenthixol Hydrochloride (7028-y)

Zuclopenthixol Hydrochloride (BANM, rINNM).

Zuclopenthixol dihydrochloride.

$C_{22}H_{25}ClN_2OS,2HCl = 473.9$.

CAS — 633-59-0.

Pharmacopoeias. In *Br.*

Zuclopenthixol hydrochloride 11.8 mg is approximately equivalent to 10 mg of zuclopenthixol.

Pharmacopoeial description

BP 2001: An off-white granular powder. Very soluble in water; sparingly soluble in alcohol; slightly soluble in chloroform; very slightly soluble in ether. A 1% solution in water has a pH of 2.0 to 3.0. Protect from light.

Stability. References.

1. Li Wan Po A, Irwin WJ. The photochemical stability of cis- and trans-isomers of tricyclic neuroleptic drugs. *J Pharm Pharmacol* 1980; 32: 25–9.

Adverse Effects, Treatment, and Precautions

As for Chlorpromazine, p.660. Zuclopenthixol is less likely to cause sedation. It should not be used in apathetic or withdrawn states.

Porphyria. Zuclopenthixol is considered to be unsafe in patients with porphyria because it has been shown to be porphyrinogenic in *animals*.

Interactions

As for Chlorpromazine, p.664.

Pharmacokinetics

Zuclopenthixol is absorbed following oral administration with peak plasma concentrations occurring 3 to 6 hours after a dose. The biological half-life is reported to be about 1 day. Small amounts of drug or metabolites cross the placenta and are distributed into breast milk. Following intramuscular injection the acetate and decanoate esters of zuclopenthixol are hydrolysed to release zuclopenthixol. Zuclopenthixol acetate has a relatively quick onset of action after injection, and has a duration of action of 2 to 3 days; it is, therefore, useful for the control of acute psychotic symptoms while avoiding repeated injections. The decanoate has a much longer duration of action and is a suitable depot preparation for maintenance treatment.

Metabolism. Determination of metaboliser phenotype with regard to cytochrome P450 isoenzyme CYP2D6 appeared to be of limited value in patients receiving zuclopenthixol as interindividual variation appeared to be the main factor affecting dose to serum concentration ratios.[1]

1. Linnet K, Wiborg O. Influence of Cyp2d6 genetic polymorphism on ratios of steady-state serum concentration to dose of the neuroleptic zuclopenthixol. *Ther Drug Monit* 1996; 18: 629–34.

Uses and Administration

Zuclopenthixol is a thioxanthene of high potency with general properties similar to the phenothiazine, chlorpromazine (p.665). It has a piperazine sidechain.

Zuclopenthixol is used for the treatment of schizophrenia (p.651), mania (see Bipolar Disorder, p.271), and other psychoses. It may be particularly suitable for agitated or aggressive patients who may become over-excited with flupentixol. Zuclopenthixol hydrochloride is usually administered by mouth with doses expressed in terms of the base. Zuclopenthixol acetate and zuclopenthixol decanoate are given by deep intramuscular injection; doses are expressed in terms of the ester. The acetate ester has an onset of action shortly after injection and a duration of action of 2 to 3 days; it is used for the initial treatment of acute psychoses and for exacerbations of chronic psychoses. The longer-acting decanoate ester is used for the maintenance treatment of chronic psychoses.

The usual initial oral dose of the hydrochloride for the treatment of psychoses is the equivalent of 20 to 30 mg of the base daily in divided doses; in severe or resistant schizophrenia up to 150 mg daily has been given. The usual maintenance dose is 20 to 50 mg daily. Zuclopenthixol hydrochloride has also been given intramuscularly.

The usual dose of zuclopenthixol acetate is 50 to 150 mg by deep intramuscular injection repeated, if necessary, after 2 or 3 days. Some patients may need an additional injection between 1 and 2 days after the first dose. Zuclopenthixol acetate is not intended for maintenance treatment; not more than four injections should be given in a course of treatment and the total dose should not exceed 400 mg. When maintenance therapy is required, zuclopenthixol hydrochloride by mouth may be introduced 2 to 3 days after the last injection of zuclopenthixol acetate, or intramuscular injections of the decanoate (see below) commenced with the last injection of the acetate.

The long-acting decanoate should be given by deep intramuscular injection; treatment is usually initiated with a test dose of 100 mg. This may be followed after at least one week by a dose of 200 to 500 mg or more, repeated at intervals of 1 to 4 weeks, and adjusted according to response. Injection volumes greater than 2 mL should be divided between 2 separate injection sites. The maximum recommended dose of zuclopenthixol decanoate is 600 mg per week.

Elderly or debilitated patients should be given reduced doses of zuclopenthixol. The manufacturers recommend that for the acetate ester, half the normal recommended dose be used for patients with hepatic impairment; a dosage reduction is considered to be unnecessary in patients with renal impairment but where there is renal failure half the normal dosage is recommended.

Schizophrenia. A systematic review[1] comparing zuclopenthixol decanoate with other depot antipsychotic preparations considered that although it may induce more adverse effects, limited data might offer advantages such as lower relapse rates and increased acceptability in the treatment of schizophrenia (p.651) and similar serious mental illnesses. A similar review of the use of zuclopenthixol acetate in the management of acute psychiatric illness found, however, that evidence of additional benefit over other antipsychotics was lacking.[2]

1. Coutinho E, et al. Zuclopenthixol decanoate for schizophrenia and other serious mental illnesses (updated 28 February 2001). Available in The Cochrane Library; Issue 4. Oxford: Update Software, 2001.
2. Fenton M, et al. Zuclopenthixol acetate in the treatment of acute schizophrenia and similar serious mental illnesses (updated 30 May 2001). Available in The Cochrane Library; Issue 4. Oxford: Update Software; 2001.

Preparations

BP 2001: Zuclopenthixol Acetate Injection; Zuclopenthixol Decanoate Injection; Zuclopenthixol Tablets.

Proprietary Preparations (details are given in Part 3)
Aust.: Cisordinol; *Austral.:* Clopixol; *Belg.:* Clopixol; *Canad.:* Clopixol; *Denm.:* Cisordinol; *Fin.:* Cisordinol; *Fr.:* Clopixol; *Ger.:* Ciatyl-Z; *Hong Kong:* Clopixol; *Irl.:* Clopixol; *Israel:* Clopixol; *Ital.:* Clopixol; Sordinol†; *Mex.:* Clopixol; *Neth.:* Cisordinol; *Norw.:* Cisordinol; *NZ:* Clopixol; *Port.:* Cisordinol; *S.Afr.:* Clopixol; *Singapore:* Clopixol; *Spain:* Cisordinol; Clopixol; *Swed.:* Cisordinol; *Switz.:* Clopixol; *Thai.:* Clopixol; *UK:* Clopixol.

Blood Products Plasma Expanders and Haemostatics

This chapter describes the management of blood disorders including anaemias, haemorrhagic disorders, and neutropenia. It covers blood, blood products and substitutes, and colloid plasma expanders; crystalloid plasma expanders are generally solutions of sodium chloride (p.1196) or glucose (p.1364) or both. Also included in the chapter are haemostatic drugs and erythropoietin and other colony-stimulating factors.

Anaemias

Anaemia is usually understood to mean a lowering of haemoglobin concentration, red cell count, or packed cell volume to below 'normal' values, but the criteria for normality are difficult to establish. WHO's suggested definition of anaemia in populations living at around sea level is a haemoglobin concentration below 13 g per 100 mL in adult men and below 12 g per 100 mL in women; children would be considered anaemic below 12 g per 100 mL if aged 6 to 14 years, or below 11 g per 100 mL if aged 6 months to 6 years. However, because of individual variation, some apparently normal individuals have blood haemoglobin concentrations below these values, while others may be above these values and still be effectively anaemic.

Reduction in overall haemoglobin concentrations may be due just to fewer red cells with the cells retaining normal amounts of haemoglobin (normochromic anaemia), or the amount of haemoglobin in the cells may be reduced (hypochromic anaemia). Red cells themselves may be reduced in size (microcytic), enlarged (macrocytic), or normal in size (normocytic).

The immediate cause of anaemia may be decreased red cell production (due to defective proliferation and/or maturation of red cells from their precursors in bone marrow), increased red cell destruction (i.e. haemolysis), or loss of red cells from the circulation due to haemorrhage, either occult or overt. These conditions may occur due to underlying disease, nutritional deficiency, congenital disorders, or toxicity due to drugs or other substances and the cause must always be sought before an appropriate treatment can be determined.

The symptoms of anaemia are as variable as its causes but may include fatigue, pallor, dyspnoea, palpitations, headache, faintness or lightheadedness, tinnitus, anorexia and gastrointestinal disturbances, and loss of libido; tachycardia, heart failure, and retinal haemorrhage may occur in severe anaemia.

The treatment of anaemia depends upon its type and cause. Some of the principal types are classified in Table 1, below, and their management is discussed in more detail under the relevant headings. Sickle-cell disease and β-thalassaemia are discussed under Haemoglobinopathies.

Aplastic anaemia

Aplastic anaemia is characterised by pancytopenia and hypoplasia of the bone marrow, with less than 25% of the marrow occupied by haematopoietic cells but without evident fibrosis or malignant infiltration. It is relatively rare, although it may be somewhat more common in the Far East, is predominantly seen in younger adults, and is slightly more frequent in men than women. Some forms, such as Fanconi's anaemia, are inherited but most are acquired from various causes, including the effects of cytotoxic drugs or radiation, idiosyncratic reactions to other drugs, viral infections such as hepatitis C, or auto-immune reactions. In about 50% of cases aplastic anaemia is classified as idiopathic. All cell lines are affected and patients consequently develop thrombocytopenia and neutropenia as well as anaemia, and symptoms include bleeding syndromes and infections as well as typical symptoms of anaemia.

Although spontaneous recovery has occurred, untreated aplastic anaemia is usually fatal. Management may be divided into supportive care and attempts to restore bone-marrow function and has been the subject of guidelines and reviews.[1-3]

Supportive care. Supportive care involves the prevention and treatment of infection (see Infections in Immunocompromised Patients, p.125), the control of haemorrhage with platelet concentrates, and where necessary, infusions of red blood cells (with platelets to prevent haemorrhage) for anaemia. Transfusions should be minimised in candidates for bone-marrow transplant (see below).

Restoration of bone-marrow function. In patients aged under 40 years with severe disease and with a suitable HLA-matched donor, bone-marrow transplantation has been considered the treatment of choice. Ideally this should be performed early before the patient has received too many transfusions, which increase the risk of rejection, and before infection develops. Transfusion of cord blood from an HLA-identical sibling can also produce permanent engraftment, and may be associated with less acute graft-versus-host disease than bone-marrow transplantation.[1]

In patients unsuitable for bone-marrow transplantation, or where a suitable donor is not available, treatment with immunosuppressants may be tried. About 50% of patients are reported to respond to a course of equine antilymphocyte or antithymocyte immunoglobulin, although response may be slow; if there is no sign of response after about 4 months a second course (usually of a rabbit-derived product) may produce benefit in some.[4] Ciclosporin may be of benefit in nonresponders to antilymphocyte immunoglobulins;[4,5] combined immunosuppression with antilymphocyte immunoglobulins, methylprednisolone, and ciclosporin produces better response rates than regimens without ciclosporin,[6] but the combined regimen has not yet been shown to produce improved survival.[1] Androgens may also be added to a second course of immunosuppressants.[1] Good response rates have been reported from combined regimens including a granulocyte colony-stimulating factor.[7] Cyclophosphamide is commonly used in preparation for bone-marrow transplantation and complete remission has also been reported with high-dose cyclophosphamide alone.[8] However, a randomised trial[9] of high-dose cyclophosphamide plus ciclosporin compared with conventional immunosuppression was stopped early when a higher mortality was observed in those receiving cyclophosphamide.

Overall, the results of immunosuppression seem to be comparable to those of bone-marrow transplantation, except perhaps in children,[4] who generally respond less well to immunosuppressants. Responses are often partial, but this may be sufficient to free the patient from dependency on transfusions and intensive antibacterial cover, and is considered well worth achieving. Some groups have preferred immunosuppression for initial therapy even in patients suitable for transplantation, reserving the transplant for salvage in nonresponders or relapse.[10] Such an approach has been reported to result in a 5-year survival of some 80%, but there is concern that patients treated with immunosuppression retain some underlying defect in marrow function, as many patients subsequently develop leukaemias or myelodysplasias.[11,12]

In moderate disease, or where immunosuppression fails, a trial of an anabolic steroid such as oxymetholone may be considered, although responses are likely to be disappointing.[4] Other drugs that have been tried include normal immunoglobulins, although it has been suggested that responses are uncommon.[11] The availability of recombinant haematopoietic growth factors has led to trials of colony-stimulating factors in a few patients,[13-15] but although some responses have occurred during therapy there is no evidence of sustained remission. The use of colony-stimulating factors alone has been criticised[16] on the grounds that such treatment delays bone-marrow transplantation or immunosuppressive therapy and thus reduces the chance of a successful outcome. They may, however, have a role in conjunction with immunosuppressive therapy (see above).

1. Bacigalupo A. Guidelines for the treatment of severe aplastic anemia. *Haematologica* 1994; **79:** 438–44.
2. Young NS. Aplastic anaemia. *Lancet* 1995; **346:** 228–32.
3. Marsh JCW, Gordon-Smith EC. Treatment options in severe aplastic anaemia. *Lancet* 1998; **351:** 1830–1.
4. Webb DKH, *et al.* Acquired aplastic anaemia: still a serious disease. *Arch Dis Child* 1991; **66:** 858–61.
5. Werner EJ, *et al.* Immunosuppressive therapy versus bone marrow transplantation for children with aplastic anemia. *Pediatrics* 1989; **83:** 61–5.

Table 1. Types of anaemias.

Classification	Anaemia	Mean cell volume	Haemoglobin	Associated with
Microcytic	Iron-deficiency anaemia	Decreased (or normal in early stages)	Hypochromic	Blood loss, malabsorption, inadequate iron intake
	Hereditary sideroblastic anaemia	Decreased	Hypochromic	
	Thalassaemias	Decreased	Hypochromic	
Macrocytic	Megaloblastic anaemia	Increased	Normochromic	Vitamin B$_{12}$ deficiency, folate deficiency (including drug induced)
	Acquired sideroblastic anaemia	Increased	Hypochromic	Alcoholism, drug or other toxicity
Normocytic	Normocytic-normochromic anaemia	Normal	Normochromic	Anaemia of chronic disorders, bone-marrow disorders (including aplastic anaemia), malignancy, renal failure, endocrine disorders, prematurity
Haemolytic	Haemolytic anaemia	Increased		Immune disorders, drug toxicity, hereditary disorders
	Sickle-cell anaemia			

6. Frickhofen N, *et al.* Treatment of aplastic anemia with antilymphocyte globulin and methylprednisolone with or without cyclosporine. *N Engl J Med* 1991; **324:** 1297–1304.
7. Bacigalupo A, *et al.* Antilymphocyte globulin, cyclosporin, and granulocyte colony-stimulating factor in patients with acquired severe aplastic anemia (SAA): a pilot study of the EBMT SAA Working Party. *Blood* 1995; **85:** 1348–53.
8. Brodsky RA, *et al.* Complete remission in severe aplastic anemia after high-dose cyclophosphamide without bone marrow transplantation. *Blood* 1996; **87:** 491–4.
9. Tisdale JF, *et al.* High-dose cyclophosphamide in severe aplastic anaemia: a randomised trial. *Lancet* 2000; **356:** 1554–9.
10. Crump M, *et al.* Treatment of adults with severe aplastic anemia: primary therapy with antithymocyte globulin (ATG) and rescue of ATG failures with bone marrow transplantation. *Am J Med* 1992; **92:** 596–602.
11. Moore MAS, Castro-Malaspina H. Immunosuppression in aplastic anemia—postponing the inevitable? *N Engl J Med* 1991; **324:** 1358–60.
12. Socié G, *et al.* Malignant tumors occurring after treatment of aplastic anemia. *N Engl J Med* 1993; **329:** 1152–7.
13. Vadhan-Raj S, *et al.* Stimulation of myelopoiesis in patients with aplastic anemia by recombinant human granulocyte-macrophage colony-stimulating factor. *N Engl J Med* 1988; **319:** 1628–34.
14. Kurzrock R, *et al.* Very low doses of GM-CSF administered alone or with erythropoietin in aplastic anemia. *Am J Med* 1992; **93:** 41–8.
15. Geissler K, *et al.* Effect of interleukin-3 on responsiveness to granulocyte-colony-stimulating factor in severe aplastic anemia. *Ann Intern Med* 1992; **117:** 223–5.
16. Marsh JCW, *et al.* Haemopoietic growth factors in aplastic anaemia: a cautionary note. *Lancet* 1994; **344:** 172–3.

Haemolytic anaemia

The normal life span of an erythrocyte is about 120 days; a haemolytic state is defined as a reduction in this mean life span due to premature destruction of red cells, either intravascularly, or more commonly after sequestration by the spleen or liver. Healthy bone marrow can compensate for even quite severe haemolysis by increased erythropoiesis; however, if the red cell survival-time is less than 15 days, or if the bone marrow is abnormal, or there is a deficiency of folate, iron, or other necessary nutrients, then compensation will be inadequate and haemolytic anaemia will result. In addition to typical symptoms of anaemia (above) patients frequently exhibit jaundice and splenomegaly, while the increased erythropoiesis results in reticulocytosis (elevated counts of immature red cells).

Haemolytic anaemias may be either congenital or acquired. The congenital disorders include those due to membrane defects in the erythrocyte such as spherocytosis or elliptocytosis; those due to enzyme defects (including the various forms of glucose-6-phosphate dehydrogenase deficiency); and those due to haemoglobin defects (haemoglobinopathies) including sickle-cell disease and β-thalassaemia (below).

The acquired haemolytic anaemias arise from numerous causes but may be divided into immune and non-immune types. The immune types include some drug-induced haemolytic anaemias (including those produced by penicillins, rifampicin, and methyldopa); auto-immune haemolytic anaemia (further classified into warm or cold depending on the temperature at which the red cell antibodies are most active); and haemolytic disease of the newborn (see p.1532). The non-immune types include haemolysis due to infections such as malaria; chemically-induced haemolysis (due to a direct effect on the red cell rather than an immunologically-mediated one, and including the effects of toxins such as copper and arsenic as well as some snake venoms, and drugs such as amphotericin B, dapsone, and sulfasalazine); and the effects of mechanical trauma.

Treatment of haemolytic anaemia depends on the underlying cause, although general supportive measures (bed rest, transfusion if haemodynamic abnormalities make it necessary, and supplementation with folate) will be similar in all poorly-compensated patients. Well compensated haemolysis may require no treatment at all, though clearly elucidation and, where possible, removal of the cause is desirable.

Hereditary haemolytic disorders such as spherocytosis mostly respond well to splenectomy, although milder forms may not require treatment. In patients with glucose-6-phosphate dehydrogenase deficiency, treatment consists essentially of avoidance of drugs or foodstuffs likely to provoke haemolysis.

Acquired haemolytic anaemia is best treated by identification and where possible elimination of any underlying cause. Most drug-induced haemolytic anaemias respond rapidly to discontinuation of the offending substance.

Auto-immune haemolytic anaemias require treatment aimed at maintaining the patient and controlling haemolysis. Although treatment may need to be prolonged, in many patients with idiopathic disease antibodies eventually disappear or decrease to insignificant titres after

months or years. The auto-immune haemolytic anaemias may be secondary to other disorders including leukaemias, lymphomas, and systemic lupus erythematosus; correction of the underlying disease often results in marked improvement of accompanying haemolysis.

In patients with warm auto-immune haemolytic anaemia initial treatment is with corticosteroids. A typical initial dose is prednisone or prednisolone 80 mg by mouth daily; higher doses are rarely required. The initial dose may be reduced over 2 to 4 weeks to 20 mg daily; thereafter, the dose may be decreased more slowly and cautiously to the minimum necessary to control symptoms. If oral therapy is inappropriate hydrocortisone has been given intravenously. If symptoms do not respond to tolerable doses of corticosteroids splenectomy should be considered. Alternative approaches include the use of vinblastine- or vincristine-loaded platelets,[1] or intravenous infusions of high-dose normal immunoglobulin.[2,3] Immunosuppressants such as azathioprine may be considered in patients refractory to other therapy; responses are reportedly variable, but they sometimes permit reduction of corticosteroid maintenance doses. Transfusion is problematic in these patients because of the difficulty in establishing compatibility between patient and donor.[4,5] Nonetheless, transfusion may be life-saving in acute disease, and the least incompatible blood should be used.

In patients with cold auto-immune haemolytic anaemias such as cold haemagglutinin disease it is additionally important to keep the patient warm. Corticosteroids and splenectomy are generally of no benefit in these patients (although there may be a responsive subgroup[6]), but treatment with chlorambucil 2 to 4 mg daily by mouth may produce a response. Blood transfusion should be avoided if possible, and if given it should be preferably via a warming coil and infused slowly.

1. Ahn YS, *et al.* Treatment of autoimmune hemolytic anemia with vinca-loaded platelets. *JAMA* 1983; **249:** 2189–94.
2. Mitchell CA, *et al.* High dose intravenous gammaglobulin in Coombs positive hemolytic anemia. *Aust N Z J Med* 1987; **17:** 290–4.
3. Blanchette VS, *et al.* Role of intravenous immunoglobulin G in autoimmune hematologic disorders. *Semin Hematol* 1992; **29:** 72–82.
4. Salama A, *et al.* Red blood cell transfusion in warm-type autoimmune haemolytic anaemia. *Lancet* 1992; **340:** 1515–17.
5. Garratty G, Petz LD. Transfusing patients with autoimmune haemolytic anaemia. *Lancet* 1993; **341:** 1220.
6. Silberstein LE, *et al.* Cold hemagglutinin disease associated with IgG cold-reactive antibody. *Ann Intern Med* 1987; **106:** 238–42.

Iron-deficiency anaemia

The iron content of the body is normally kept constant by regulation of the amount absorbed to balance the amount lost. If loss is increased, and/or intake inadequate, a negative iron-balance may lead by degrees to depletion of body iron stores, iron deficiency, and eventually to anaemia. Iron requirements are increased during infancy, puberty, pregnancy, and during menstruation, and iron-deficiency anaemias are most common in women and children; the most common cause in adult males and postmenopausal women is blood loss, usually from the gastrointestinal tract.

Iron deficiency usually results in a microcytic, hypochromic anaemia, but the diagnosis of iron deficiency should be confirmed, if there is any doubt, by measurement of serum ferritin or total iron binding capacity (transferrin). Iron therapy can begin once deficiency is confirmed, but the underlying cause of the deficiency should still be sought and treated.

Treatment. The prevention and control of iron-deficiency anaemias has been reviewed.[1-3] Almost all iron-deficiency anaemias respond readily to treatment with iron. The treatment of choice is oral administration of a ferrous salt (ferrous iron is better absorbed than ferric iron). Many iron compounds have been used for this purpose, but do not offer any real advantage over the simple ferrous fumarate, gluconate, or sulfate salts. The usual adult dose is sufficient of these salts to supply about 100 to 200 mg of elemental iron daily (for the elemental iron content of various iron salts, see p.1368). A rise in haemoglobin concentration of about 0.1 g or more per 100 mL daily is considered a positive response. Haemoglobin response is greatest in the first few weeks of therapy and is proportional to the severity of the original anaemia. Once haemoglobin concentrations have risen to the normal range, iron therapy should be continued for a further 3 months to aid replenishment of iron stores.

Oral iron has been given with agents such as ascorbic acid which enhances iron absorption significantly if given in large enough doses, but such combinations may increase the incidence of adverse effects. Modified-release

preparations have been used in patients intolerant of ordinary formulations of iron but some consider them therapeutically ineffective.

Failure to respond to oral iron after about 3 weeks of therapy may be indicative of non-compliance, continued blood loss with inadequate replacement of iron, malabsorption, wrong diagnosis, or other complicating factors, and the treatment should be reassessed.

Parenteral iron therapy is rarely indicated, may produce severe adverse effects, and should be reserved for patients who are genuinely intolerant of oral iron, persistently non-compliant, who have gastrointestinal disorders exacerbated by oral iron therapy, continuing blood loss too severe for oral treatment to provide sufficient iron, or for those unable to absorb iron adequately from the gastrointestinal tract. The most common parenteral forms are iron sorbitol (given intramuscularly), iron sucrose (given intravenously), and iron dextran (given intravenously, in which case the complete iron requirement may be given as a single infusion, or intramuscularly).

Exceptionally, in patients with profound anaemia, blood transfusion may be necessary to restore dangerously low concentrations of haemoglobin. This may be the case, for example, in elderly patients with long-standing iron deficiency leading to heart failure. However, transfusion should always be avoided if possible.

Prophylaxis. Prophylaxis may be desirable in some groups at risk of iron deficiency and consequent anaemia, and may include therapy with oral iron supplements, measures to improve dietary iron intake, fortification of food staples, or control of infection.

Therapy with prophylactic iron supplements is justifiable in pregnancy where there are risk factors for deficiency, but the practice of universal supplementation is less widespread than formerly, and some authorities consider that it should be reserved for documented deficiency.[4-6] The US Preventive Services Task Force has reviewed the subject of iron supplementation during pregnancy,[7] and concluded that there was insufficient evidence for or against routine supplementation.[8]

Iron supplementation is accepted in menorrhagia, after gastrectomy, and in the management of low birth-weight infants such as the premature. Iron deficiency in infants and children may result in developmental delay,[9-12] reversible with iron supplements,[13] and WHO has suggested supplementation in pre-school children;[1] however, this does not seem to be the practice in developed countries, although there is some suggestion that screening would be valuable to identify iron-deficient children in this age group.[12,14,15]

The usual prophylactic dose in adults is sufficient of a ferrous salt to provide about 60 to 120 mg of elemental iron daily. Doses of around 1 mg per kg body-weight of elemental iron daily have been suggested for prophylaxis in children.

Dietary measures, such as addition of vitamin-C-rich foods, or other enhancers of iron absorption including iron in the form of haem (found in meat or fish) to the diet, and control of parasitic infections such as hookworm (which are responsible for considerable occult blood loss), are particularly important for the general community in developing countries. Fortification of food staples poses technical problems as iron salts react with food components and may produce rancidity or other undesirable changes on storage. Nonetheless, wheat flour, bread, and milk products are often so fortified, and consideration has been given to fortification of salt, sugar, rice, and fish sauce.

1. De Maeyer EM, *et al. Preventing and controlling iron deficiency anaemia through primary health care: a guide for health administrators and programme managers.* Geneva: WHO, 1989.
2. Chipping P. Management of iron deficiency anaemia. *Prescribers' J* 1990; **30:** 65–71.
3. Frewin R, *et al.* ABC of clinical haematology. Iron deficiency anaemia. *BMJ* 1997; **314:** 360–3.
4. Hibbard BM. Iron and folate supplements during pregnancy: supplementation is valuable only in selected patients. *BMJ* 1988; **297:** 1324 and 1326.
5. Horn E. Iron and folate supplements during pregnancy: supplementing everyone treats those at risk and is cost effective. *BMJ* 1988; **297:** 1325 and 1327.
6. Chamberlain G. Medical problems in pregnancy—II. *BMJ* 1991; **302:** 1327–30.
7. US Preventive Services Task Force. Routine iron supplementation during pregnancy: review article. *JAMA* 1993; **270:** 2848–54.
8. US Preventive Services Task Force. Routine iron supplementation during pregnancy: policy statement. *JAMA* 1993; **270:** 2846–8.
9. Walter T, *et al.* Iron deficiency anemia: adverse effects on infant psychomotor development. *Pediatrics* 1989; **84:** 7–17.
10. Filer LJ. Iron needs during rapid growth and mental development. *J Pediatr* 1990; **117:** S143–6.
11. Lozoff B, *et al.* Long-term developmental outcome of infants with iron deficiency. *N Engl J Med* 1991; **325:** 687–94.

12. Booth IW, Aukett MA. Iron deficiency anaemia in infancy and early childhood. *Arch Dis Child* 1997; **76:** 549–54.
13. Idjradinata P, Pollitt E. Reversal of developmental delays in iron-deficient anaemic infants treated with iron. *Lancet* 1993; **341:** 1–4.
14. James J, *et al*. Preventing iron deficiency in preschool children by implementing an educational and screening programme in an inner city practice. *BMJ* 1989; **299:** 838–40.
15. James J, *et al*. Treatment of iron deficiency anaemia with iron in children. *Lancet* 1993; **341:** 572.

Megaloblastic anaemia

The megaloblastic anaemias are characterised by macrocytosis (an increased mean cell volume) and the production of distinctive morphological changes and abnormal maturation in developing haematopoietic cells in the bone marrow: white cell and platelet lines are affected as well as erythroid precursors, and in severe cases anaemia may be associated with leucopenia and thrombocytopenia. Megaloblastic anaemia is a consequence of impaired DNA biosynthesis in the bone marrow, usually due to a deficiency of vitamin B_{12} (cobalamins) or folate, both of which are essential for this process. Although the haematological symptoms of B_{12} deficiency and folate deficiency are similar it is important to distinguish between them since the use of folate alone in B_{12}-deficient megaloblastic anaemia may improve haematological symptoms without preventing aggravation of accompanying neurological symptoms, and may lead to severe nervous system sequelae such as subacute combined degeneration of the spinal cord. Where it is desirable to commence therapy immediately, combined treatment for both deficiencies may be started once suitable samples have been taken to permit diagnosis of the deficiency, and the patient converted to the appropriate treatment once the cause of the anaemia is known.

Vitamin B_{12} deficiency anaemia. Vitamin B_{12} deficiency and its associated symptoms may be due to malabsorption (including following gastrectomy), dietary deficiency (mainly in strict vegetarians), competition with intestinal bacteria or parasites, or to the effect of drugs such as nitrous oxide. In populations of northern European origin pernicious anaemia, in which atrophy of the gastric mucosa results in a lack of the intrinsic factor essential for B_{12} absorption, is the most frequent cause. Owing to large body stores of the vitamin it may take several years for signs of deficiency to manifest once the defect in absorption occurs.

In addition to megaloblastic anaemia, vitamin B_{12} deficiency may result in neurological damage, including peripheral neuropathy and effects on mental function ranging from mild neurosis to dementia.

TREATMENT. The treatment is with vitamin B_{12}, almost always by the intramuscular or sometimes the deep subcutaneous route since in most patients absorption from the gastrointestinal tract is inadequate. Hydroxocobalamin is generally preferred to cyanocobalamin since it need be given less often. Regimens may vary, but hydroxocobalamin 1 mg every few days for 6 to 8 doses will restore normal body stores of the vitamin. The haematological response to therapy is rapid, with improvement in most parameters and symptoms beginning within 48 hours. Neurological abnormalities may take much longer to respond, and may not do so completely.

PROPHYLAXIS. Where the defect in B_{12} handling is irreversible, as in pernicious anaemia, maintenance therapy must continue for life to prevent a recurrence of the deficiency. Therapy must also be given prophylactically after total gastrectomy or total ileal resection, or where gastrointestinal surgery is shown to have impaired absorption of the vitamin. Typically, injection of hydroxocobalamin 1 mg every 2 to 3 months is used. In patients in whom injection is not possible, 1 mg may be given daily by mouth, since a few micrograms may be absorbed by passive diffusion. In patients whose diet supplies inadequate B_{12}, deficiency may be prevented, in the absence of other causes, by much lower oral doses given as a supplement; up to 0.15 mg (150 µg) of cyanocobalamin daily has been recommended.

Folate-deficiency anaemia. Deficiency of folate may be due to inadequate diet, or malabsorption syndromes (as in coeliac disease or sprue), to increased utilisation (as in pregnancy, one of the most common causes of megaloblastic anaemia, or the increased haematopoiesis of haemolytic syndromes), to increased urinary loss or loss due to haemodialysis, or to an adverse effect of alcohol, antiepileptics, or other drugs.

The clinical features of folate-deficient megaloblastic anaemia are similar to those of disease due to vitamin-B_{12} deficiency except that the accompanying severe neu-

ropathy does not occur, and deficiency may develop much more rapidly. Deficiency may also be associated with neural tube defects (p.1362) if it occurs in pregnancy.

TREATMENT. Once folate deficiency has been established the usual treatment in the UK is folic acid 5 mg by mouth daily. Lower doses of 0.25 to 1.0 mg are suggested in the USA. It is customary to continue therapy for at least 4 months, the time necessary for complete red cell replacement. In patients with malabsorption, therapy may require higher doses, up to 15 mg of folic acid daily. As in B_{12}-deficiency anaemia, the response to therapy is rapid.

PROPHYLAXIS. Long-term maintenance is rarely needed, except in a few patients in whom the underlying cause of folate deficiency cannot be treated (for example in some severe haemolytic syndromes). Doses of 5 mg daily or even weekly have been suggested for prophylaxis in patients undergoing dialysis or with chronic haemolytic states, depending on the diet and rate of haemolysis; a dose of 0.4 mg daily is recommended in the USA.

For primary prophylaxis of megaloblastic anaemia in pregnancy, folic acid is given in the UK in usual doses of 0.2 to 0.5 mg daily, often in combination with a ferrous salt for prophylaxis of iron deficiency. In the USA, doses of up to, but not more than, 1 mg daily are suggested.

Drugs which act as inhibitors of dihydrofolate reductase, such as methotrexate, may produce severe megaloblastic anaemia which cannot be reversed by therapy with folic acid. The adverse effects of such drugs may be largely prevented or reversed by therapy with folinic acid, which can be incorporated into folate metabolism without the need for reduction by the inhibited enzyme. For details of such 'folinic acid rescue', see under Folinic Acid, p.1363.

General references.

1. Hoffbrand V, Provan D. ABC of clinical haematology: macrocytic anaemias. *BMJ* 1997; **314:** 430–33.
2. Wickramasinghe SN. Folate and vitamin B_{12} deficiency and supplementation. *Prescribers' J* 1997; **37:** 88–95.

Normocytic-normochromic anaemia

Anaemias in which red cell size and cellular haemoglobin are not significantly different from normal (normocytic-normochromic anaemias) form a substantial proportion of all cases. Such anaemias are usually secondary to another disease and include the anaemia of chronic disorders (associated with chronic infection such as tuberculosis, malignancy, inflammatory disorders such as inflammatory bowel disease, polymyalgia rheumatica, rheumatoid arthritis, and systemic lupus erythematosus), anaemia of renal failure, anaemia of prematurity, anaemia associated with endocrine disorders such as hypothyroidism or hypopituitarism, and anaemias associated with primary bone-marrow failure (including aplastic anaemia, above, pure red cell aplasia, marrow fibrosis or infiltration as in myelodysplasia or leukaemia, and marrow failure associated with AIDS). Iron-deficiency anaemia, which is usually classified as microcytic and hypochromic may in fact be neither, particularly in the early stages, and should be differentiated from anaemia of chronic disease. The latter is also accompanied by changes in iron metabolism, notably sequestration of iron in reticuloendothelial cells: plasma iron is low but in contrast to iron deficiency the total iron binding capacity is reduced and serum ferritin is often increased.

The **treatment** of most of these anaemias is essentially that of the underlying disease. Blood transfusion has been given when anaemia is severe. In patients with anaemia of renal failure, which is due at least in part to decreased erythropoietin production by the damaged kidney, regular subcutaneous or intravenous injection of recombinant human erythropoietins (epoetin alfa or epoetin beta) can completely reverse the anaemia. Epoetins may also have a role in anaemia of prematurity and some drug-induced anaemias, and have been investigated in patients with the anaemia of chronic disease and some other normocytic-normochromic anaemias.

Sideroblastic anaemia

The sideroblastic anaemias are characterised by a population of hypochromic red cells in the presence of increased serum-iron concentrations, and abnormal erythroid precursors, known as ring sideroblasts, in the bone marrow. They are associated with abnormalities in porphyrin biosynthesis leading to diminished production of haem, and increased cellular iron uptake. Sideroblastic anaemias may be of various types, and are classified as acquired or hereditary.

Acquired sideroblastic anaemia. Acquired sideroblastic anaemia may either be idiopathic, or secondary to either a drug or toxin (such as alcohol, isoniazid, chloramphenicol, or lead) or to a disease (including hypothyroidism, rheumatoid arthritis, haemolytic or megaloblastic anaemias, leukaemias, and lymphomas). The treatment of the secondary forms is essentially the treatment of the underlying disease or removal of the precipitating cause. The anaemia is usually mild and often macrocytic.

Patients with idiopathic disease usually have only mild anaemia, and most require no treatment. Although rarely suffering from vitamin B_6 deficiency a few patients will respond at least partially to high doses of pyridoxine by mouth, up to 400 mg daily, and a trial is considered worthwhile in all patients. If patients become symptomatic, transfusion may be required, but should be kept to a minimum because of the problems of iron overload. All patients with sideroblastic anaemia must have their serum-iron and -ferritin concentrations regularly monitored, and be given desferrioxamine by regular bolus injection when there is evidence of iron overload.

Hereditary sideroblastic anaemia. The hereditary forms of the disease appear to be sex-linked, and almost always manifest themselves in males. The anaemia may be more severe than in acquired sideroblastic anaemia, and is usually microcytic.

A trial of pyridoxine, as in the acquired form, is considered worthwhile as some forms are responsive, but in many cases there is no benefit. Some patients develop gradually increasing iron loads, and may eventually develop haemosiderosis; to prevent this, regular venesection or the use of desferrioxamine are indicated if there is evidence of iron accumulation.

Haemoglobinopathies

Haemoglobinopathies are clinical abnormalities due to altered structure, function, or production of haemoglobin. Human haemoglobins are tetramers, constructed of 4 globin chains each enfolding an iron-containing haem moiety: two of these globins are of the 'α-like' types (globins α or ζ) and two are 'non-α' (types β, γ, δ, or ε). The normal major adult haemoglobin, haemoglobin A, comprises two α and two β chains, while the predominant fetal haemoglobin, haemoglobin F (also present in minute amounts in normal adults), is composed of two α and two γ globins. The erythroblast inherits two genes for the production of α globin and one for β globin production from each parent, and a mutation in a single α gene will therefore affect only 25% of the haemoglobin produced, whereas a single β mutation will affect 50%: the β-haemoglobinopathies, due to defective β globin production, are therefore more likely to produce symptoms, and the most widespread forms are the β-thalassaemias and sickle-cell disease, which are discussed below.

Sickle-cell disease

Sickle-cell disease is a haemoglobinopathy (above) in which a structural abnormality in the β globin chain results in the formation of an abnormal haemoglobin, haemoglobin S, that polymerises in the deoxygenated state, making the red cell less flexible and, when present in sufficient amounts, deforming it into a sickle shape. Normal haemoglobins may be incorporated into the polymer although some, such as fetal haemoglobin (haemoglobin F), do not participate and if present in sufficient amounts reduce sickling.

The heterozygous form, sickle-cell trait, is generally asymptomatic except in conditions of extreme anoxia, although characteristic abnormalities of renal function (inadequate concentration of the urine) may be present. As with thalassaemia trait (below) it is more common in populations of tropical origin, and has been postulated to offer a degree of protection against malaria. In the homozygous form a varying degree of haemolytic anaemia is present, accompanied by increased erythropoiesis. In addition to shortened survival, the decreased flexibility of the deformed erythrocytes can lead to occlusion of the microvasculature, and sickle-cell crisis. The latter may manifest as excruciating pain due to infarction of the blood supply to the bones, or infarction of other organs including lung, liver, kidney, penis (leading to priapism), and brain (stroke). An acute chest syndrome occurs in many patients, and may be fatal. It is a form of acute lung injury associated with infarction, fat embolism, and infection, and may progress to acute respiratory distress syndrome. Occasionally a large proportion of red cell mass may become trapped in spleen or liver (sequestration crisis) with death due to gross anaemia. Chronic complications include skin ulceration, renal failure, retinal detachment, and increased susceptibility to infection.

Treatment of sickle-cell disease is essentially symptomatic.[1,2] Young children should receive prophylactic penicillin and pneumococcal vaccine, to reduce the risk of infection (see Spleen Disorders, p.140). Infection should be treated early, and folate supplementation given if necessary since the increased erythropoiesis resulting from chronic haemolysis may increase folate requirements.

Sickle-cell crisis requires hospitalisation, with the use of large volumes of intravenous fluids for dehydration, analgesia including opioids for pain (see p.7), and treatment of any concurrent infection. Oxygen should be given if the patient is hypoxaemic. Where crisis affects a vital organ with life-threatening or potentially disabling consequences partial exchange transfusion should be carried out promptly, as no other therapy exists. Where rapid enlargement of spleen or liver indicates a sequestration crisis, transfusion is also important to avoid fatal anaemia.

Maintenance transfusion is rarely indicated, although it may be given to patients who have already had a stroke; measures to avoid iron overload such as phlebotomy or desferrioxamine chelation are necessary in patients receiving regular transfusions. Prophylactic transfusions in children at high risk has been reported[3] to reduce the incidence of first stroke but the risks and benefits of treatment must be carefully considered.

Research into specific therapy for sickling has produced some promising results.[4] Because haemoglobin F is known to protect against sickling, considerable interest has centred on attempts to stimulate fetal haemoglobin production. Most studies have used hydroxyurea [hydroxycarbamide]. Initial trials showed some elevation in mean fetal haemoglobin concentrations, but responses were very variable. However, a subsequent randomised controlled study in 299 patients[5] reported that therapy with hydroxyurea [hydroxycarbamide] caused a 44% reduction in the median annual rate of painful crises. The beneficial effects did not become evident for several months. Beneficial effects have also been reported in initial studies in children.[6,7] However, the potential toxicity of long-term therapy with hydroxyurea [hydroxycarbamide] (especially in children) remains a concern. Use of hydroxyurea [hydroxycarbamide] with erythropoietin has been reported to increase fetal haemoglobin concentrations further in one study,[8] although not in another using a different dosage regimen.[9] A short-chain fatty acid, butyric acid, which has a low order of toxicity, has been reported to stimulate fetal haemoglobin in patients with sickle-cell disease when given by infusion as arginine butyrate.[10]

As in thalassaemia (below), bone-marrow transplantation is potentially curative in a small minority of patients, but the indications for transplantation are much less well established, and its use and benefits remain a matter for debate.[11-13]

1. Davies SC, Oni L. Management of patients with sickle cell disease. *BMJ* 1997; **315:** 656–60.
2. Steinberg MH. Management of sickle cell disease. *N Engl J Med* 1999; **340:** 1021–30.
3. Adams RJ, *et al.* Prevention of a first stroke by transfusions in children with sickle cell anemia and abnormal results on transcranial doppler ultrasonography. *N Engl J Med* 1998; **339:** 5–11.
4. Bunn HF. Pathogenesis and treatment of sickle cell disease. *N Engl J Med* 1997; **337:** 762–9.
5. Charache S, *et al.* Effect of hydroxyurea on the frequency of painful crises in sickle cell anemia. *N Engl J Med* 1995; **332:** 1317–22.
6. Scott JP, *et al.* Hydroxyurea therapy in children severely affected with sickle cell disease. *J Pediatr* 1996; **128:** 820–8.
7. Ferster A, *et al.* Hydroxyurea for treatment of severe sickle cell anemia: a pediatric clinical trial. *Blood* 1996; **88:** 1960–4.
8. Rodgers GP, *et al.* Augmentation by erythropoietin of the fetal-hemoglobin response to hydroxyurea in sickle cell disease. *N Engl J Med* 1993; **328:** 73–80.
9. Goldberg MA, *et al.* Treatment of sickle cell anemia with hydroxyurea and erythropoietin. *N Engl J Med* 1990; **323:** 366–72.
10. Perrine SP, *et al.* A short-term trial of butyrate to stimulate fetal-globin-gene expression in the β-globin disorders. *N Engl J Med* 1993; **328:** 81–6.
11. Vermylen C, Cornu G, Roberts IAG. Bone marrow transplant for sickle cell disease—an update. *Arch Dis Child* 1996; **75:** 3–6.
12. Walters MC, *et al.* Bone marrow transplantation for sickle cell disease. *N Engl J Med* 1996; **335:** 369–76.
13. Platt OS, Guinan EC. Bone marrow transplantation in sickle cell anemia—the dilemma of choice. *N Engl J Med* 1996; **335:** 426–8.

β-Thalassaemia

β-Thalassaemia is a haemoglobinopathy (above) that is due to a deficiency in β globin production accompanied by normal production of α globin chains that, in the absence of sufficient partner chains, are insoluble and precipitate out in erythrocytes and erythroid precursors as large cellular inclusions. These interfere with red cell maturation resulting in ineffective haematopoiesis, retard the passage of red cells from the bone marrow, and create a tendency for those red cells which do mature to be trapped and destroyed in the spleen. The condition is therefore characterised by a hypochromic, microcytic anaemia accompanied by haemolysis. In the heterozygous form, where only one of the β globin genes is affected (known as thalassaemia trait or thalassaemia minor) the anaemia is mild and clinically insignificant. There is some evidence that patients with this form of the disease experience a degree of protection from malaria, which may account for the more frequent distribution of the trait in the populations of areas such as the Mediterranean, parts of Africa, and Asia.

The more severe forms of the disease (known as thalassaemia intermedia if haemoglobin levels are high enough not to require regular transfusion, or thalassaemia major in transfusion-dependent patients) occur in homozygous patients who inherit a defective β globin gene from both parents. Severe anaemia develops in the first year of life as fetal haemoglobin production (which does not involve a β globin) is replaced by the production of adult haemoglobin. The anaemia stimulates erythropoietin production, and if not corrected massive proliferation of red cell precursors develops within, and eventually beyond, the bone marrow, resulting in recurrent bone fractures, deformity of the skull due to expansion of the marrow spaces, and compression of vital structures such as the spinal cord with consequent paresis. Other symptoms include splenomegaly and hypersplenism (resulting in neutropenia and thrombocytopenia), increased susceptibility to infection, and hypermetabolism which may lead to folate deficiency because of the increased folate requirement. If untreated, death in patients with thalassaemia major usually occurs by the 2nd or 3rd year.

Treatment. The mainstay of treatment for severe β-thalassaemia has been regular blood transfusion to correct the anaemia. Transfusions should be begun as early as possible in life once it is clear that anaemia is severe enough to warrant them. Transfusion of washed or frozen red cells every 6 to 8 weeks is usually required, to maintain haemoglobin values of between 9 and 14 g per 100 mL; a sudden increase in transfusion requirements is a sign of hypersplenism, which may be an indication for splenectomy although this should be avoided if possible below the age of 5 because of the increased risk of infection. For a discussion of antibacterial prophylaxis in splenectomised patients, see Spleen Disorders, p.140.

If anaemia is corrected by transfusion, growth and development proceed fairly normally in thalassaemic children. However, because the body lacks a mechanism for the excretion of excess iron repeated transfusion invariably results in iron overload (p.1005), leading eventually to haemochromatosis. The consequences of haemochromatosis include mild liver dysfunction, endocrine dysfunction (failure of the adolescent growth spurt, hypogonadism, sometimes diabetes and hypothyroidism), and particularly heart disease (pericarditis, heart failure, and arrhythmias). If unchecked, the iron build-up usually leads to death (mainly through heart failure or arrhythmia) by the time patients reach their mid-20s. The accumulation of iron can be retarded by the use of the chelator desferrioxamine. This has been shown to improve survival in thalassaemic children given regular systemic therapy,[1-3] the greatest increase in iron excretion being seen in patients given the drug by continuous subcutaneous infusion rather than intramuscular bolus. There is some suggestion that intensive desferrioxamine therapy can improve impaired organ function,[4-7] but it is considered preferable to begin chelation therapy as early as possible (in practice usually at 2 to 3 years of age) to try to prevent organ damage developing in the first place. Better iron excretion is achieved if patients are given ascorbic acid 100 to 200 mg daily in addition to desferrioxamine (but see under Interactions for Desferrioxamine, p.1004). Patients with thalassaemia may have increased folate requirements and folate supplementation may also be necessary. Although it is not yet certain how much chelation therapy will prolong survival the fact that a nearly normal iron balance can be achieved long term[4] seems hopeful. Deferiprone has been used as an oral alternative to des-

ferrioxamine,[8,9] but may not be effective in the longer term;[10] it may have a role in patients for whom desferrioxamine therapy is unsuitable.

In addition to the essentially symptomatic treatment of thalassaemia a very few patients may be candidates for bone-marrow transplantation where suitable facilities and compatible donors exist; if transplantation is carried out before organ damage is marked, successfully transplanted patients are apparently cured and can lead a normal life.[11-13] Gene therapy is also under investigation.

An alternative approach using hydroxyurea [hydroxycarbamide] in an attempt to stimulate fetal haemoglobin production and 'mop up' some of the excess α globin chains has been tried experimentally but results have been mixed. Results of an initial study in patients given butyric acid (as an arginine butyrate infusion) for the same purpose appeared more promising[14] although a subsequent study failed to show any benefit.[15]

1. Zurlo MG, *et al.* Survival and causes of death in thalassaemia major. *Lancet* 1989; **ii:** 27–30.
2. Ehlers KH, *et al.* Prolonged survival in patients with beta-thalassaemia major treated with deferoxamine. *J Pediatr* 1991; **118:** 540–5.
3. Olivieri NF, *et al.* Survival in medically treated patients with homozygous β-thalassaemia. *N Engl J Med* 1994; **331:** 574–8.
4. Hoffbrand AV, *et al.* Improvement in iron status and liver function in patients with transfusional iron overload with long-term subcutaneous desferrioxamine. *Lancet* 1979; **i:** 947–9.
5. Freeman AP, *et al.* Early left ventricular dysfunction and chelation therapy in thalassemia major. *Ann Intern Med* 1983; **99:** 450–4.
6. Marcus RE, *et al.* Desferrioxamine to improve cardiac function in iron-overloaded patients with thalassaemia major. *Lancet* 1984; **i:** 392–3.
7. Maurer HS, *et al.* A prospective evaluation of iron chelation therapy in children with severe β-thalassemia: a six-year study. *Am J Dis Child* 1988; **142:** 287–92.
8. Olivieri NF, *et al.* Iron-chelation therapy with oral deferiprone in patients with thalassemia major. *N Engl J Med* 1995; **332:** 918–22.
9. Nathan DG. An orally active iron chelator. *N Engl J Med* 1995; **332:** 953–4.
10. Olivieri NF, *et al.* Long-term safety and effectiveness of iron-chelation therapy with deferiprone for thalassemia major. *N Engl J Med* 1998; **339:** 417–23.
11. Lucarelli G. Bone marrow transplantation for severe thalassaemia 1: the view from Pesaro. *Br J Haematol* 1991; **78:** 300–1.
12. Weatherall DJ. Bone marrow transplantation for severe thalassaemia 2: to be or not to be. *Br J Haematol* 1991; **78:** 301–3.
13. Lucarelli G, *et al.* Marrow transplantation in patients with thalassemia responsive to iron chelation therapy. *N Engl J Med* 1993; **329:** 840–4.
14. Perrine SP, *et al.* A short-term trial of butyrate to stimulate fetal-globin-gene expression in the β-globin disorders. *N Engl J Med* 1993; **328:** 81–6.
15. Sher GD, *et al.* Extended therapy with intravenous arginine butyrate in patients with β-hemoglobinopathies. *N Engl J Med* 1995; **332:** 1606–10.

Haemostasis and Fibrinolysis

Haemostasis is the physiological response that occurs when blood vessels are damaged. It results in coagulation (formation of a blood clot) and thus arrests bleeding. The initial response is the formation of a plug of platelets which adhere both to the injured tissue and to each other. The vessel injury together with factors released by the platelets trigger a series of reactions (the coagulation 'cascade') mediated by proteins circulating in the plasma (blood clotting factors). This results in formation of an insoluble fibrin clot that reinforces the initial platelet plug. Regulatory mechanisms come into operation to prevent widespread coagulation. Lysis of the clot (fibrinolysis) then occurs when wound healing and tissue repair are underway.

Platelet aggregation. Platelets usually circulate in plasma in an inactive form. Contact with damaged endothelium causes them to become activated and to adhere to the site of injury. This adhesion is partly mediated by binding of von Willebrand factor, a plasma protein that also acts as a carrier for factor VIII, to a glycoprotein (termed GPIb) on the platelet membrane surface. Substances are secreted by the activated platelets which cause further platelet aggregation (adenosine diphosphate and thromboxane A$_2$) and vasoconstriction (serotonin and thromboxane A$_2$). Thromboxane A$_2$ secreted by platelets is derived from arachidonic acid. The enzyme cyclo-oxygenase is required for the synthesis of thromboxane A$_2$ and this enzyme is inhibited by the **antiplatelet drugs** aspirin and sulfinpyrazone. Aspirin binds irreversibly to the enzyme and therefore the antiplatelet effect lasts for the lifetime of the platelet. Sulfinpyrazone is a reversible inhibitor of the enzyme. Platelet aggregation involves interaction of fibrinogen with a receptor, glycoprotein IIb/IIIa, on the platelet surface. Antiplatelet drugs such as abciximab act by blocking this receptor. In addition to their action in forming the initial haemostatic plug, platelets are also involved in coagulation by providing a surface on which interactions between clotting factors take place, resulting in more efficient coagulation.

Coagulation. The series of reactions that results in formation of a fibrin clot may be conveniently considered as two pathways, the *intrinsic* pathway (initiated within the blood) and the *extrinsic* pathway (initiated by substances extraneous to the blood). While this distinction is useful for understanding *in-vitro* coagulation and is the basis for tests that are specific for each pathway (see below), the mechanism of *in-vivo* coagulation is not so segregated and factors appearing in one pathway are also necessary for reactions in the other pathway. The intrinsic and extrinsic pathways of coagulation and the *in-vivo* pathways are discussed further below and are represented in summary form in Figure 1, p.720 and Figure 2, p.721 respectively. Factors circulate in the blood in an inactive form and are activated by cleavage of peptide bonds. The numerals attached to the factors reflect the order in which they were discovered and not their importance or position in the chain of reaction. The letter 'a' after a factor name or number denotes the activated form. Factors involved in blood coagulation are listed in Table 2, below. Once the coagulation cascade is initiated, activated factors act in positive feedback mechanisms to amplify the activation steps thus producing rapid coagulation. Cofactors are necessary as they increase the speed of the reactions. Other components necessary for coagulation are calcium ions and a membrane surface. Calcium ions are required for nearly all the reactions. Many of the activation steps, notably those involving factors VII, IX, and X, take place on a membrane surface provided by tissue factor or platelets. Factors bind to phospholipids on the membrane surface.

The *extrinsic* pathway is initiated when *tissue factor* (factor III) is released from damaged tissue. This forms a complex with *factor VII* and factor VIIa and directly activates *factor X*. The *intrinsic* pathway is initiated when blood comes into contact with a negatively charged surface. *Factor XII* interacts with high molecular weight kininogen (Fitzgerald factor) and prekallikrein (Fletcher factor) to produce *kallikrein* which activates factor XII. The active factor XIIa then activates *factor XI* which in turn activates *factor IX*. Factor IXa, together with activated *factor VIII* (VIIIa) as a cofactor, converts *factor X* to factor Xa. The extrinsic and intrinsic pathways therefore converge with the activation of factor X. Factor Xa, together with activated *factor V* (Va) as a cofactor, converts prothrombin to thrombin with the subsequent formation of a *fibrin* gel which is stabilised by *factor XIIIa* to form a stable clot.

The dependence on calcium ions of many steps in the coagulation cascade allows coagulation *in vitro* to be blocked by the addition of calcium chelators, such as sodium citrate, to collected blood. When collected blood is tested for coagulation function, addition of calcium ions allows clotting to proceed. Tests of coagulation function include activated partial thromboplastin time (APTT), which is a measure of the activity of the intrinsic system, prothrombin time (PT), a measure of the activity of the extrinsic system, and thrombin clotting time, which measures the conversion of fibrinogen to fibrin.

The factors involved in initiating the *in-vitro* intrinsic pathway, that is prekallikrein, factor XII, and possibly factor XI, are probably not important in *in-vivo* blood coagulation as deficiency of any of these factors is not associated with a serious bleeding disorder. The important step in initiating the clotting cascade *in vivo* is release of *tissue factor* (factor III) from damaged tissue. As has already been mentioned, tissue factor forms a complex with *factor VII* and factor VIIa which activates *factor X*. Factor Xa activates *prothrombin* resulting in formation of a *fibrin clot* which occurs as described above under the *in-vitro* systems. To enhance coagulation, various positive feedback mechanisms and other clotting factors operate to increase production of activated factors VII and X. For example, formation of factor VIIa is amplified by factor VIIa itself and by factor Xa. Formation of factor Xa is amplified by factor IXa produced by the action of thrombin on factor XI.

Regulation of coagulation. The process of blood coagulation is regulated to ensure that it remains localised at the site of injury and does not result in more widespread clotting. This is achieved by dilution of clotting factors in flowing blood, by rapid hepatic clearance of many activated factors or products, and by natural anticoagulant mechanisms which include antithrombin III, protein C, and protein S (see Figure 2, p.721). *Antithrombin III* inhibits the serine protease clotting factors, that is, thrombin, IXa, Xa, XIa, and XIIa. Antithrombin III is activated by binding to glycosaminoglycans, such as heparan glycosaminoglycan and dermatan sulfate, present in vascular endothelium. Heparin and low-molecular-weight heparins act as **anticoagulants** by binding antithrombin III at a specific binding site and enhancing its inhibitory effect on the serine protease clotting factors. At therapeutic doses of heparin the factors inhibited are thrombin and factor Xa. Low-dose heparin, such as that given for the prophylaxis of thromboembolism, inhibits factor Xa. Very high doses of heparin have a direct inhibitory effect on antithrombin III. Heparinoids which lack the specific binding site for antithrombin III do not have the anticoagulant properties of heparin. Low-molecular-weight heparins have a higher ratio of anti-factor-Xa to antithrombin activity than heparin and therefore mainly inhibit factor Xa.

Proteins C and S are both vitamin K-dependent plasma proteins. Protein C circulates in plasma in an inactive form. It is activated by contact with thrombin that is bound to thrombomodulin, a receptor located on the surface of endothelial cells. Activated protein C inhibits factors Va and VIIIa and therefore slows blood clotting. Protein S acts as a cofactor in this inhibition.

Vitamin K is essential for the activities of factors II, VII, IX, and X. It is also essential for the activity of proteins C and S. These factors contain glutamic acid residues that undergo carboxylation in the liver, a reaction requiring reduced vitamin K as a cofactor. This carboxylation step allows the factors to bind calcium, a reaction necessary for their function in the clotting cascade. Deficiency of vitamin K or the use of **oral anticoagulants** (which are vitamin K antagonists) therefore impairs the function of these clotting factors. Oral anticoagulants have no effect on circulating clotting factors and thus the time required before the anticoagulant effect is seen depends on the individual clearance rate of the factor.

Fibrinolysis is the mechanism of clot dissolution. It is mediated by *plasminogen* which circulates in plasma in an inactive form; conversion to its active form, *fibrinolysin (plasmin)*, occurs when plasminogen binds to fibrin in the presence of a *plasminogen activator* (see Figure 2, p.721). Fibrinolysin, a *proteolytic enzyme,* digests fibrin clots and hydrolyses other proteins, including factors II, V, VIII, and XII. As fibrin is lysed, fibrinolysin is released which is inhibited by α_2-antiplasmin to prevent a systemic lytic state developing. There are two types of plasminogen activator, *tissue plasminogen activator* (tPA) which originates from the endothelium, and *urokinase*, which is activated from prourokinase. Activators of prourokinase include fibrinolysin. Tissue plasminogen activator binds to fibrin and thus activates plasminogen bound to fibrin much more rapidly than circulating plasminogen; therefore the fibrinolytic action of tissue plasminogen activator is fibrin specific. Urokinase

Table 2. Proteins involved in blood coagulation and in fibrinolysis.

	Proteins	Synonyms
Blood coagulation	Factor I	Fibrinogen
	Factor II*	Prothrombin
	Factor III	Tissue thromboplastin; tissue factor
	Factor IV	Calcium ion
	Factor V	Ac-globulin; labile factor; proaccelerin
	Factor VI (unassigned)	
	Factor VII*	Proconvertin; SPCA; stable factor
	Factor VIII	Antihaemophilic factor; AHF
	Factor IX*	Christmas factor; plasma thromboplastin component; PTC
	Factor X*	Stuart factor; Stuart-Prower factor
	Factor XI	Plasma thromboplastin antecedent; PTA
	Factor XII	Hageman factor
	Factor XIII	Fibrin stabilising factor; FSF
	von Willebrand factor	Factor VIII-related antigen; vWF
	High molecular weight kininogen	HMWK; Fitzgerald factor
	Prekallikrein	Fletcher factor
Fibrinolysis	Plasminogen	
	Prourokinase	
	Tissue plasminogen activator	tPA
	Antithrombin III	Major antithrombin; AT-III; Heparin cofactor
	Protein C*	Autoprothrombin
	Protein S*	
	α_2-Antiplasmin	

* denotes vitamin K-dependent factor

Figure 1. Simplified representation of *in-vitro* coagulation.

does not bind to fibrin, and therefore its fibrinolytic action is not fibrin specific, although it is activated by fibrinolysin that is bound to fibrin. *In vivo*, fibrinolysis is almost entirely due to the activity of tissue plasminogen activator. The two types of plasminogen activator with their different modes of action provide the basis for the specificity of **thrombolytics** (the so-called 'clot specific' effect) which act by promoting the conversion of plasminogen to fibrinolysin. The tissue plasminogen activators alteplase and duteplase are fibrin-specific thrombolytics, and streptokinase and urokinase are fibrin-nonspecific. The **antifibrinolytic drugs** aminocaproic acid and tranexamic acid act primarily by blocking the binding of plasminogen and fibrinolysin to fibrin thereby preventing the breakdown of fibrin clots. Aprotinin, an inhibitor of proteolytic enzymes, acts as a **haemostatic** by inhibiting the action of fibrinolysin and therefore preventing the breakdown of fibrin clots. Other drugs acting as haemostatics include batroxobin, which is reported to promote the production of fibrin from fibrinogen and etamsylate which has a stabilising effect on the capillary wall. Drugs such as oxidised cellulose, calcium alginate, collagen, and gelatin act by providing a physical meshwork within which clotting can occur. Adrenaline [epinephrine], adrenalone, and noradrenaline [norepinephrine] produce haemostasis by causing vasoconstriction. Drugs with astringent properties such as alum, ferric chloride, silver nitrate, and trichloroacetic acid are also used for haemostasis. The use of haemostatics may be considered when bleeding cannot be controlled by direct measures

such as the application of pressure, suture or ligation, or electrocoagulation.

Dysfunction of the haemostatic mechanisms or the systems regulating haemostasis produces haemorrhagic (below) or thromboembolic (p.816) disorders.

◊ General references.

1. Furie B, Furie BC. Molecular and cellular biology of blood coagulation. *N Engl J Med* 1992; **326**: 800–806.
2. Dahlbäck B. Blood coagulation. *Lancet* 2000; **355**: 1627–32.

Disseminated intravascular coagulation

Disseminated intravascular coagulation (DIC) is an acute or chronic syndrome resulting from an underlying condition that causes pathological stimulation of coagulation at some point in the coagulation pathway (above); thrombin generation triggered by uncontrolled tissue factor is probably the predominant factor in most cases. Causes include obstetric emergencies (placental abruption, eclampsia), infection (notably Gram-negative septicaemia), neoplasms, trauma (head injury, burns), venomous snake bites, transfusion of incompatible blood, liver disease, and various vascular causes.

Stimulation of coagulation leads to microvascular thrombosis that produces widespread tissue ischaemia and may lead to ischaemia of major organs. Simultaneously, secondary activation of the fibrinolytic system and consumption of coagulation factors produces bleeding, which is often the predominant manifestation. Symptoms are therefore very variable and include those of bleeding, such as spontaneous bruising, prolonged bleeding from intravenous puncture sites, and gastrointestinal and pulmonary haemorrhage, and those of thrombosis, such as acute renal failure, venous thromboembolism, skin necrosis, liver failure, cerebral infarction, acute res-

piratory distress, and coma. Some cases may be asymptomatic.

Treatment of DIC is aimed primarily at the underlying cause since the condition will not resolve until the underlying trigger is removed. Recovery is often fairly rapid once treatment is instituted. Supportive therapy to ensure adequate hydration and tissue oxygenation is also vital. These measures may be sufficient in patients with asymptomatic DIC. Most patients with symptomatic DIC also require administration of plasma and other blood components including platelets and cryoprecipitate as necessary to replace coagulation factors and arrest bleeding. Heparin has been used in the management of DIC with the aim of switching off the coagulatory mechanisms. Although benefit has been shown with some underlying causes, heparin may worsen bleeding and its use in DIC is considered by some to be controversial. Where bleeding is the main clinical problem, heparin should only be given if replacement of coagulation factors fails to stop the bleeding. Where the risk of bleeding is relatively minor and thrombosis predominates, heparin may be appropriate. Other measures that have been tried in limited numbers of patients include administration of a low-molecular-weight heparin, a thrombin inhibitor such as antithrombin III, and protein C.

General references.

1. Rubin RN, Colman RW. Disseminated intravascular coagulation: approach to treatment. *Drugs* 1992; **44**: 963–71.
2. Baglin T. Disseminated intravascular coagulation: diagnosis and treatment. *BMJ* 1996; **312**: 683–7.
3. Frewin R, *et al.* ABC of clinical haematology. Haematological emergencies. *BMJ* 1997; **314**: 1333–6.
4. de Jonge E, *et al.* Current drug treatment strategies for disseminated intravascular coagulation. *Drugs* 1998; **55**: 767–77.
5. Levi M, ten Cate H. Disseminated intravascular coagulation. *N Engl J Med* 1999; **341**: 586–92.

Figure 2. Simplified representation of *in-vivo* coagulation and fibrinolysis

Haemorrhagic disorders

Haemorrhage is bleeding from any part of the vascular system. The mechanisms responsible for haemostasis and its control, that is, platelet aggregation, blood coagulation, and fibrinolysis, are described under Haemostasis and Fibrinolysis, above. Dysfunction of any of these systems may produce a haemorrhagic disorder, as discussed below. The dysfunction may be an inherited disorder or it may be acquired as a result of disease or a medical or surgical procedure.

Inherited haemorrhagic disorders. Inherited disorders which lead to abnormal bleeding include platelet and vascular disorders, and disturbances in clotting factors.

Inherited *platelet disorders* are rare; they include

• Bernard-Soulier syndrome (a lack of platelet GPIb receptor)
• thrombasthenia (defective glycoproteins IIb and IIIa)
• storage pool disease (lack of platelet ADP)

Disorders of *vascular function* include

• hereditary telangiectasia

The most common inherited haemorrhagic disorders are due to absent, reduced, or malfunctioning *clotting factors*. The most important are

• **haemophilia A**
• **haemophilia B**
• **von Willebrand's disease**

Hereditary deficiency of all the clotting factors (other than calcium and thromboplastin) has been described although the incidence and clinical significance varies.

Haemophilia A (classical haemophilia, factor VIII deficiency) is the most common of the serious hereditary bleeding disorders. It is an X-linked recessive disorder and therefore with rare exceptions males are affected and females are carriers. The condition is due to deficiency of factor VIII; severity of bleeding is related to the residual factor level. The condition is severe when there is no detectable factor VIII activity, moderate when the factor VIII concentration is 2 to 5% of normal, and mild when the factor concentration is greater than 5%. Clots are slow to form and break up easily, and bleeding following trauma or surgery may continue for days or weeks. In moderate and severe haemophilia A bleeding may occur into major joints producing long-term joint destruction, a major cause of morbidity in haemophilia. Other frequent sites of bleeding are large muscles and renal and intestinal tracts. CNS haemorrhage may also occur, especially after trauma.

Treatment of bleeding episodes depends on the severity of the haemophilia.[1-4] Patients with mild haemophilia may be satisfactorily treated with desmopressin, which produces an increase in factor VIII and von Willebrand factor. Desmopressin also stimulates release of plasminogen activator, and an antifibrinolytic, such as tranexamic acid, may be given at the same time to inhibit the enhanced fibrinolytic activity. Desmopressin is usually given intravenously; it can be given intranasally, but the factor VIII response is less predictable than with the injection.[5]

Desmopressin is ineffective in patients with more severe haemophilia A, and treatment of bleeding episodes in these patients requires replacement with a factor VIII preparation. The amount of factor given depends on the severity of bleeding.

In addition to use of factor VIII to treat bleeding episodes, it may also be given prophylactically in situations where haemorrhage may be anticipated, for example following trauma, and before surgery. Patients with haemophilia should also not be given intramuscular injections (because of potential muscle damage and bleeding into muscle) unless they are given during a period when the patient is covered by replacement factor. Dental extraction and other oral surgical procedures are examples of situations that may be followed by bleeding lasting days and weeks. Oral secretions which can cause clot lysis contribute to this bleeding. Patients undergoing dental or oral surgery should be given factor VIII and an antifibrinolytic, usually tranexamic acid, before the procedure. The antifibrinolytic should be continued for five days following the procedure. Fibrin glue[6] and topical aminocaproic acid[7] or tranexamic acid[8] are methods that have also been used.

An alternative method of management has been practised in Sweden since 1958 where continuous prophylaxis with factor VIII is given to patients with severe haemophilia with the aim of preventing arthropathy. Therapy is started at 1 to 2 years of age and the factor VIII concentration is maintained at a level of at least 1% of normal. Patients who began receiving prophylaxis before the age of 2 have had almost no bleeding episodes and joints have remained normal for up to 11 years of follow-up.[9,10] This approach has subsequently been adopted in a number of other countries.

There are various factor VIII preparations available that vary in activity and source.[11] Most products were previously derived from pooled donor plasma and were associated with transmission of viruses including HIV (leading to the subsequent development of AIDS), hepatitis B, and other hepatitis viruses. The introduction of products treated with heat or chemicals together with efforts to screen the donor material from which factor VIII is obtained seem to have overcome problems with transmission of HIV and hepatitis B, although there is concern that non-lipid-enveloped viruses such as human parvovirus B19 and hepatitis A may still be transmitted. It is recommended that patients not already immune should be vaccinated against hepatitis A and B. Factor VIII produced by recombinant DNA technology may avoid the dangers of possible viral transmission (but see under Factor VIII, Transmission of Infections, p.734) and is therefore the factor VIII preparation of choice. There are some reports[12,13] that high-purity factor VIII preparations slow the decline in CD4 count in HIV-positive patients, although the evidence is conflicting.[14]

A complication of replacement therapy in haemophilia is the development of antibodies to factor VIII. Antibodies are more likely to develop in young patients with severe haemophilia, but on rare occasions can also arise in patients with mild haemophilia. An incidence of 10 to 15% is frequently cited, although prospective studies are lacking and it has been suggested that this is an underestimate.[15]

A number of strategies have been developed to overcome the resulting resistance to treatment.[1-3,16] Continued treatment with factor VIII may produce a clinical response and a decline in antibody titre in patients with a low antibody titre. Porcine factor VIII may be useful at least in the short term, although with longer use antibodies to the porcine material can develop in turn. Other strategies to reverse inhibition are the use of factor VIII inhibitor bypassing fraction; the use of recombinant factor VIIa which bypasses the factor VIII-dependent step in the coagulation cascade; routine infusion of small doses of factor VIII; and concurrent administration of factor VIII, intravenous normal immunoglobulin, and cyclophosphamide.[16] Immunosuppressive therapy (cyclophosphamide, vincristine, prednisone) with factor VIII has been found to eliminate factor VIII inhibitor in 11 of 12 non-haemophilic patients but only transiently in 1 of 5 haemophilic patients.[17] In patients with a severe haemorrhage or those undergoing surgery plasmapheresis can be used to reduce antibody concentrations. The use of tissue factor and factor Xa is also being studied.[2]

A future development that may provide a clinical cure for haemophilia is gene therapy.[18,19] Gene therapy for haemophilia A and B is being investigated and successful treatment has been carried out in an *animal* model with conversion to less severe haemophilia.

Haemophilia B (Christmas disease, factor IX deficiency) is less common than haemophilia A. The condition is due to deficiency of factor IX. The clinical features are identical to haemophilia A. Treatment follows the same principles as haemophilia A, bleeding episodes being treated with factor IX replacement.[1,2] Mild or moderate disease may be treated with fresh frozen plasma. Factor IX preparations derived from plasma, however, contain other clotting factors in addition to factor IX (such as the activated factors IX, X, and XII) and are therefore potentially associated with thromboembolic complications (mainly in patients with liver disease). Antifibrinolytic drugs, which may sometimes be used concurrently, increase the risk of thromboembolism further, and should be used with care. Highly purified factor IX preparations have been developed which do not contain other clotting factors and therefore may be expected to avoid this risk of thromboembolism. It has been suggested that these preparations should be used when very large amounts of replacement factor are required, or the risk of thrombotic complications is otherwise high.[2,4] Recently, a recombinant factor IX has been introduced.

Inhibitors to factor IX can be produced although the incidence is lower than the inhibition seen in haemophilia A. As in patients with haemophilia A, vaccination against hepatitis A and hepatitis B is recommended for all haemophiliacs not already immune.

As mentioned under haemophilia A, gene therapy is under investigation as a possible clinical cure.

von Willebrand's disease is due to deficiency of von Willebrand factor, a plasma protein which stimulates platelet aggregation and acts as a carrier for factor VIII, protecting it from premature destruction. Deficiency therefore slows clotting by reducing the platelet response to injury and reducing levels of factor VIII. There are many different types, and severity ranges from severe haemorrhagic disease to asymptomatic disease. Bleeding episodes in patients with mild to moderate forms of the disease may be managed with desmopressin, which increases levels of von Willebrand factor and factor VIII.[1,2,20,21] However, some forms of von Willebrand's disease do not respond to desmopressin therapy and in these patients, and in those with more severe disease, factor VIII concentrates are used; the very highly purified factor VIII preparations or recombinant forms should not be used as they do not contain appreciable amounts of von Willebrand factor and are thus ineffective. Cryoprecipitate (obtained from a very small donor pool to reduce the risk of transmission of infection) may also be used. Antifibrinolytic drugs may be used in open bleeding and in dental or oral surgery as for haemophilia A. A recombinant activated factor VII preparation has been developed that may also be used.

OTHER INHERITED DISORDERS. *Factor XI deficiency* is quite common in Jews of eastern European origin. Spontaneous bleeding is rare. Bleeding following trauma or surgery is generally mild and infusion of fresh frozen plasma is usually sufficient to maintain haemostasis. A factor XI concentrate is available.

Inherited deficiencies of other clotting factors are rare. Concentrates of factors II, VII, and X are available. Fresh frozen plasma or cryoprecipitate may be used in factor XIII deficiency.

Acquired haemorrhagic disorders. Bleeding disorders sometimes arise due to disturbances in either clotting factors or platelets or to vascular wall defects occurring as a result of a disease or a medical or surgical procedure. Disturbances and defects may also be drug induced. In some conditions, including renal and liver disease, cardiopulmonary bypass procedures, or following massive blood transfusion, disturbances in many of the homoeostatic mechanisms occur simultaneously producing complex haemorrhagic disorders, sometimes referred to as complex acquired coagulopathies.

One of the commoner causes of haemorrhagic disorder caused by **disturbance of clotting factors** is overdose with heparin, oral anticoagulants, or thrombolytics. Heparin overdose is rarely accompanied by serious haemorrhage. Stopping treatment is usually sufficient; protamine sulfate, which reverses the action of heparin, may be given. Bleeding in patients on oral anticoagulants is more difficult to control as the patient remains anticoagulated for several days after treatment is stopped. Local measures may be sufficient, although in life-threatening haemorrhage administration of phytomenadione (vitamin K₁), a concentrate of factors II, VII, IX, and X, or fresh frozen plasma may be necessary (see Treatment of Adverse Effects under Warfarin Sodium, p.993). Overdose with a thrombolytic, such as streptokinase or urokinase, may be managed with an antifibrinolytic drug (for example aminocaproic acid or tranexamic acid), aprotinin, and packed red blood cells.

Deficiencies in clotting factors may occur in several diseases. Disorders producing a deficiency of vitamin K will lead to reduced levels of clotting factors (see also under Haemostasis and Fibrinolysis, above). Vitamin K deficiency due to impaired absorption, metabolism, or synthesis may occur in small bowel disease, biliary obstruction, or liver disease. Vitamin K deficiency in neonates produces haemorrhagic disease of the newborn (p.1397). Vitamin K deficiency is treated by administration of vitamin K, although this is not always effective in patients with liver diseases. Rarely, deficiencies in clotting factors may be caused by the development of antibodies against a particular factor; factor VIII is the factor most frequently affected.

Disturbances in platelet function can give rise to a haemorrhagic disorder.[22] Sometimes the bleeding disorder is due to abnormally functioning platelets, such as occurs in renal failure or following the administration of some drugs (for example, aspirin and high doses of beta-lactam antibiotics). More often the bleeding disorder is due to a reduction is the number of platelets, that is, **thrombocytopenia**. Thrombocytopenia may occur in a

wide range of disorders and can result from decreased production, increased destruction, or abnormal splenic sequestration of platelets. Decreased platelet production may occur in bone marrow diseases such as leukaemias and aplastic anaemia, chronic alcohol toxicity, and some viral illnesses. Decreased platelet production also occurs following bone-marrow transplantation. Some drugs, for example thiazide diuretics and many antineoplastics, also reduce platelet production. Increased destruction of platelets occurs in many disorders including idiopathic thrombocytopenic purpura (p.1052), neonatal alloimmune thrombocytopenia, sepsis, disseminated intravascular coagulation (above), and thrombotic thrombocytopenic purpura and haemolytic uraemic syndrome (see Thrombotic Microangiopathies, p.740). Many drugs also cause increased platelet destruction; they include aminosalicylic acid, cimetidine, digitalis, frusemide [furosemide], heparin, methyldopa, paracetamol, and sulfonamides. Thrombocytopenia as a result of abnormal splenic sequestration may occur in hypersplenism from any cause. Thrombocytopenia also occurs in a few very rare congenital abnormalities such as Fanconi's anaemia and the Wiskott-Aldrich syndrome.

In thrombocytopenia, the severity of bleeding depends on the platelet count; clotting is impaired following surgery or trauma and spontaneous bleeding may occasionally occur when the platelet count is less than 50×10^9 per litre. Treatment is management of the underlying disorder where appropriate or discontinuation of therapy with the offending drug. If surgery is contemplated or haemorrhage occurs and the platelet count is less than 50×10^9 per litre or a platelet abnormality is manifested by a prolonged bleeding time, platelet transfusion may be given. Patients requiring long-term treatment may develop antibodies to HLA with repeated transfusions from random donors, which results in impaired responsiveness to subsequent transfusion; these patients should receive platelets obtained from a single donor for each transfusion. When thrombocytopenia is a result of increased platelet destruction, the condition is usually refractory to platelet transfusion. Interleukin-11 (oprelvekin) has recently been introduced for the treatment of thrombocytopenia. Other haematopoietic growth factors under investigation include interleukin-3 and -6, and thrombopoietin.

Complex acquired coagulopathies can arise in many surgical settings, such as cardiopulmonary bypass procedures and liver transplantation, as well as in association with, or following, infection, massive blood transfusion, prolonged hypotension, and renal failure.

In renal failure the bleeding tendency is related to the degree and duration of uraemia. The bleeding defect is the result of platelet dysfunction and clotting factor deficiencies. There may also be mild thrombocytopenia. Correction of anaemia and dialysis seems to improve the bleeding disorder. If bleeding occurs desmopressin and conjugated oestrogens may be used. Cryoprecipitate and platelet transfusions may be necessary in life-threatening haemorrhage.

In liver disease the haemorrhagic disorder is a result of impaired synthesis of clotting factors, thrombocytopenia, and impaired clearance of activated clotting factors. Desmopressin has been used to control bleeding episodes. Patients undergoing liver transplantation frequently develop a bleeding disorder as a result of the procedure itself as well as from the existing haemostatic defect. Small studies on the use of aprotinin in liver transplant patients have generally shown reductions in blood loss.

Various drugs including desmopressin, epoprostenol, tranexamic acid, aminocaproic acid, aprotinin, and nafamostat have been investigated for their effect on blood loss in patients undergoing surgery. Most of the investigations have been in surgery which involves cardiopulmonary bypass, a procedure that may be complicated by a postperfusion syndrome which includes impairment of haemostasis and pulmonary dysfunction. Aprotinin is the only agent that has shown a consistent effect in decreasing perioperative blood loss,[23] perhaps due to preservation of platelet function mediated by inhibition of fibrinolysin. Desmopressin may be effective in those patients with excessive bleeding after cardiac surgery.[24]

1. WHO/World Federation of Haemophilia. Prevention and control of haemophilia: memorandum from a joint WHO/WFH meeting. *Bull WHO* 1991; **69:** 17–26.
2. Seremetis SV, Aledort LM. Congenital bleeding disorders: rational treatment options. *Drugs* 1993; **45:** 541–7.
3. Hoyer LW. Haemophilia A. *N Engl J Med* 1994; **330:** 38–47.
4. Berntorp E, *et al.* Modern treatment of haemophilia. *Bull WHO* 1995; **73:** 691–701.

5. Rose EH, Aledort LM. Nasal spray desmopressin (DDAVP) for mild hemophilia A and von Willebrand disease. *Ann Intern Med* 1991; **114**: 563–8.
6. Baudo F, *et al.* Management of oral bleeding in haemophilic patients. *Lancet* 1988; **ii**: 1082.
7. Casdorph DL. Topical aminocaproic acid in hemophiliac patients undergoing dental extraction. *DICP Ann Pharmacother* 1990; **24**: 160–1.
8. Sindet-Pedersen S, *et al.* Management of oral bleeding in haemophilic patients. *Lancet* 1988; **ii**: 566.
9. Nilsson IM, *et al.* Twenty-five years' experience of prophylactic treatment in severe haemophilia A and B. *J Intern Med* 1992; **232**: 25–32.
10. Aledort LM. Prophylaxis: the next haemophilia treatment. *J Intern Med* 1992; **232**: 1–2.
11. United Kingdom Haemophilia Centre Directors Organisation Executive Committee. Guidelines on therapeutic products to treat haemophilia and other hereditary coagulation disorders. *Haemophilia* 1997; **3**: 63–77.
12. Hilgartner MW, *et al.* Purity of factor VIII concentrates and serial CD4 counts. *Lancet* 1993; **341**: 1373–4.
13. Seremetis SV, *et al.* Three-year randomised study of high-purity or intermediate-purity factor VIII concentrates in symptom-free HIV-seropositive haemophiliacs: effects on immune status. *Lancet* 1993; **342**: 700–703.
14. Schwarz HP, *et al.* High-purity factor concentrates in prevention of AIDS. *Lancet* 1994; **343**: 478–9.
15. Ehrenforth S, *et al.* Incidence of development of factor VIII and factor IX inhibitors in haemophiliacs. *Lancet* 1992; **339**: 594–8.
16. Anonymous. Anti-factor-VIII inhibitors in haemophilia. *Lancet* 1989; **ii**: 363–4.
17. Lian EC-Y, *et al.* Combination immunosuppressive therapy after factor VIII infusion for acquired factor VIII inhibitor. *Ann Intern Med* 1989; **110**: 774–8.
18. Lozier JN, Brinkhous KM. Gene therapy and the hemophilias. *JAMA* 1994; **271**: 47–51.
19. Brownlee GG. Prospects for gene therapy for haemophilia A and B. *Br Med Bull* 1995; **51**: 91–105.
20. Scott JP, Montgomery RR. Therapy of von Willebrand disease. *Semin Thromb Hemost* 1993; **19**: 37–47.
21. Castaman G, Rodeghiero F. Current management of von Willebrand's disease. *Drugs* 1995; **50**: 602–14.
22. Liesner RJ, Machin SJ. ABC of clinical haematology: platelet disorders. *BMJ* 1997; **314**: 809–12.
23. Royston D. Perioperative bleeding. *Lancet* 1993; **341**: 1629.
24. Cattaneo M, Mannucci PM. Desmopressin and blood loss after cardiac surgery. *Lancet* 1993; **342**: 812.

Neonatal intraventricular haemorrhage

Intraventricular haemorrhage, also referred to as periventricular or periventricular-intraventricular haemorrhage, is bleeding from vessels in or around the ventricles of the brain. It is the major cause of death in very low birthweight neonates and affects up to 60% of neonates weighing less than 1500 g. Intraventricular haemorrhage is rare in neonates over 32 weeks' gestation, since the vessels which bleed involute early in the third trimester. Intraventricular haemorrhage usually develops within the first 3 days of life. The haemorrhage may be graded from 1 to 4 according to severity, the higher numbered grades being the most severe and most likely to produce the long-term consequences of impaired motor and mental function. The aetiology is probably multifactorial and may include fluctuations in cerebral blood flow due to failure of autoregulatory mechanisms and tissue damage caused by oxygen free-radicals.

Once intraventricular haemorrhage has occurred **treatment** is supportive and includes correction of anaemia, hypotension, and acidaemia, and management of raised intracranial pressure. As intraventricular haemorrhage is a major risk factor for impaired motor and mental development **prevention** is very important. Numerous interventions aim to reduce its incidence and include prevention of premature births, avoidance of hypercapnia, correction of major haemodynamic disturbances, and correction of coagulation abnormalities. Various drugs have also been tried including corticosteroids, etamsylate, indometacin, pancuronium, phenobarbital, vitamin E, and vitamin K. Some of these drugs have been administered to the mother antenatally since the development of intraventricular haemorrhage may be related to perinatal events.

Administration of corticosteroids to pregnant women at risk of preterm delivery is recommended to prevent neonatal respiratory distress syndrome (p.1055) and may also reduce the incidence of intraventricular haemorrhage.[1] A review of data from 12 controlled studies involving antenatal corticosteroid administration (primarily to prevent respiratory distress syndrome)[2] suggested that the risk of intraventricular haemorrhage was also reduced but this was based on limited data. Further studies[3,4] have supported this finding, although none has involved randomised administration of corticosteroids. The mechanism for the beneficial effect of corticosteroids is not clear but avoidance of neonatal hypotension has been suggested.[3]

Etamsylate limits capillary bleeding through its action on hyaluronic acid and initial studies showed a reduction in intraventricular haemorrhage. A subsequent study[5]

showed little evidence of benefit on short-term follow-up, although confidence intervals were wide. The results of long-term follow-up are awaited.

Indometacin may reduce cerebral blood flow as a result of vasoconstriction, reduce oxygen free-radical damage, and accelerate maturation of blood vessels around the ventricles. Early studies produced conflicting results but a later larger multicentre study[6] showed a reduction in both incidence and severity although there was an unusually large number of neonates with severe intraventricular haemorrhage in the control group.[7] A concern with the use of indometacin is the possibility that it may produce cerebral ischaemia due to its vasoconstrictor action and therefore increase the risk of developmental handicaps.[7] A review[8] of studies of prophylactic indometacin concluded that more studies of possible adverse effects and long-term outcome are needed before indometacin can be recommended for routine use. However, follow-up of the infants included in the multicentre study at the ages of 3 years[9] and 4.5 years[10] reported no adverse effects on cognitive or motor development.

Pancuronium abolishes non-synchronous respiration and therefore stabilises both cerebral and arterial blood flow velocity and some studies have shown a reduction in intraventricular haemorrhage in mechanically ventilated neonates (p.1332). However, other studies have produced conflicting results.

Phenobarbital was also suggested to act by stabilising fluctuations in cerebral blood flow, and studies of administration to neonates show similarly inconsistent results with many failing to show any benefit. Initial studies of antenatal phenobarbital were more promising with a decrease in severity of haemorrhage being reported.[11] However, a larger randomised study[12] in 610 women failed to show any effect of antenatal phenobarbital on incidence or severity of intraventricular haemorrhage. A concern with the use of phenobarbital in the perinatal period is that it may lower Apgar scores and produce respiratory depression.

Vitamin E protects polyunsaturated fatty acids and thus membranes from oxidation. As oxygen free-radical damage may contribute to the development of intraventricular haemorrhage, vitamin E may have a role in its prevention. Results have been conflicting. Some studies have shown a reduction in incidence of intraventricular haemorrhage and a review of studies suggested vitamin E may be useful in the smallest, most susceptible neonates.[13] However, larger studies and studies to assess long-term outcome are needed.

The activity of vitamin K-dependent coagulation factors is reduced in neonates and thus antenatal administration of vitamin K to mothers has been tried as a means of preventing intraventricular haemorrhage. However, results of studies have not been promising. Most trials have been too small to produce conclusive results and a larger randomised controlled study[14] in 139 mothers failed to find any benefit from vitamin K prophylaxis.

Plasma volume expansion using fresh frozen plasma or a plasma substitute has also been thought to reduce intraventricular haemorrhage by stabilising the circulation, but a prospective multicentre study found no evidence of reduction in haemorrhage[15] or subsequent death and disability[16] following the use of plasma or gelatin as volume expanders.

1. NIH Consensus Development Panel. Effect of corticosteroids for fetal maturation on perinatal outcomes. *JAMA* 1995; **273**: 413–18.
2. Crowley P, *et al.* The effect of corticosteroid administration before preterm delivery: an overview of the evidence from controlled trials. *Br J Obstet Gynaecol* 1990; **97**: 11–25.
3. Garland JS, *et al.* Effect of maternal glucocorticoid exposure on risk of severe intraventricular haemorrhage in surfactant-treated preterm infants. *J Pediatr* 1995; **126**: 272–9.
4. Ment LR, *et al.* Antenatal steroids, delivery mode, and intraventricular haemorrhage in preterm infants. *Am J Obstet Gynecol* 1995; **172**: 795–800.
5. The EC Ethamsylate Trial Group. The EC randomised controlled trial of prophylactic ethamsylate for very preterm neonates: early mortality and morbidity. *Arch Dis Child* 1994; **70**: F201–F205.
6. Ment LR, *et al.* Low-dose indomethacin and prevention of intraventricular haemorrhage: a multicenter randomized trial. *Pediatrics* 1994; **93**: 543–50.
7. Volpe JJ. Brain injury caused by intraventricular hemorrhage: is indomethacin the silver bullet for prevention? *Pediatrics* 1994; **93**: 673–6.
8. Fowlie PW. Prophylactic indomethacin: systematic review and meta-analysis. *Arch Dis Child* 1996; **74**: F81–F87.
9. Ment LR, *et al.* Neurodevelopment outcome at 36 months' corrected age of preterm infants in the multicenter indomethacin intraventricular hemorrhage prevention trial. *Pediatrics* 1996; **98**: 714–18.
10. Ment LR, *et al.* Outcome of children in the indomethacin intraventricular hemorrhage prevention trial. *Pediatrics* 2000; **105**: 485–91.
11. Barnes ER, Thompson DF. Antenatal phenobarbital to prevent or minimize intraventricular hemorrhage in the low-birthweight neonate. *Ann Pharmacother* 1993; **27**: 49–52.
12. Shankaran S, *et al.* The effect of antenatal phenobarbital therapy on neonatal intracranial hemorrhage in preterm infants. *N Engl J Med* 1997; **337**: 466–71.
13. Poland RL. Vitamin E for prevention of perinatal intracranial hemorrhage. *Pediatrics* 1990; **85**: 865–7.
14. Thorp JA, *et al.* Antepartum vitamin K and phenobarbital for preventing intraventricular hemorrhage in the premature newborn: a randomized, double-blind, placebo-controlled trial. *Obstet Gynecol* 1994; **83**: 70–6.
15. The Northern Neonatal Nursing Initiative Trial Group. A randomized trial comparing the effect of prophylactic intravenous fresh frozen plasma, gelatin or glucose on early mortality and morbidity in preterm babies. *Eur J Pediatr* 1996; **155**: 580–8.
16. Northern Neonatal Nursing Initiative Trial Group. Randomized trial of prophylactic early fresh-frozen plasma or gelatin or glucose in preterm babies: outcome at 2 years. *Lancet* 1996; **348**: 229–32.

Neutropenia

A circulating neutrophil count below 1.5×10^9 per litre is usually regarded as abnormal and neutrophil counts below 0.5×10^9 per litre are associated with increased risk of infections. Neutropenia may be a result of reduced production, increased peripheral destruction, or increased peripheral pooling of neutrophils, and can be inherited or acquired.

Inherited forms of neutropenia are rare and include congenital agranulocytosis (Kostmann's syndrome: severe persistent neutropenia with frequent and severe infections that start in infancy) and cyclic neutropenia (fluctuating periods of neutropenia accompanied by fever, mouth ulceration, and serious infection).

Granulocyte colony-stimulating factors have been shown to reduce the incidence of severe infections and have improved substantially the quality of life of patients with congenital neutropenias although there are some concerns over their safety. Before the development of colony-stimulating factors various treatments including plasma, glucocorticoids, androgens, and lithium were tried in patients with severe congenital neutropenias with the aim of stimulating neutrophil production. However, none was particularly effective.

There are many causes of **acquired** neutropenia. Drugs are a common cause, either by direct toxicity to the bone marrow, or by immune-mediated marrow suppression or peripheral destruction. Drugs that cause dose-related direct toxicity include cytotoxic and immunosuppressive drugs, flucytosine, ganciclovir, and zidovudine. Drugs that appear to cause neutropenia by immune-mediated mechanisms include sulfur-containing drugs (such as captopril, co-trimoxazole, and some antithyroid drugs), clozapine, penicillins, and cephalosporins. Patients with drug-induced neutropenia usually present with fever of sudden onset, sore throat, mouth ulcers, headache, and malaise. This condition is also known as **agranulocytosis**. Other causes of acquired neutropenia include serious bacterial and viral infections and radiotherapy, neoplasms that invade bone marrow, and some auto-immune disorders.

The management of acquired neutropenia includes the treatment of any contributory condition. Drug-induced neutropenia is usually managed by withdrawal of the offending drug. In idiosyncratic reactions readministration of the implicated drug should be avoided, since abrupt neutropenia will usually be precipitated. Administration of colony-stimulating factors can be used to manage drug-induced neutropenia.

In all neutropenic patients onset of fever is indicative of serious infection and is treated immediately with empirical antibacterial therapy as described on p.125.

◊ General references.

1. Anonymous. Drug-induced agranulocytosis. *Drug Ther Bull* 1997; **35**: 49–52.
2. Provan D, O'Connell S. Management of the neutropenic patient. *Prescribers' J* 1999; **39**: 144–53.

Albumin (1215-j)

ATC — B05AA01.

Pharmacopoeial description

Ph. Eur.: Human Albumin Solution (Albumini Humani Solutio; Albumin Solution (BP 2001); Albumin; Human Albumin) is an aqueous solution of protein obtained from the plasma of healthy donors; the plasma is tested for the absence of hepatitis B surface antigen and antibodies against HIV-1 and HIV-2 and hepatitis C virus. It is prepared as a concentrated solution containing 15 to 25% of total protein or as an isotonic solution containing 3.5 to 5% of total protein; not less than 95% of the total protein is albumin. A suitable stabiliser, such as sodium octanoate or *N*-acetyltryptophan or a combination of the two, may be added but no antimicrobial preservative is added. It contains not more than 160 mmol of sodium per litre and not more than 200 µg of aluminium per litre. The solution is sterilised by filtration and distributed aseptically into containers which are sealed to prevent contamination and maintained at 59° to 61° for not less than 10 hours. Finally, the containers are incubated for not less than 14 days at 30° to 32° or for not less than 4 weeks at 20° to 25° and examined visually for signs of microbial contamination. It should be protected from light.

A clear, almost colourless, yellow, amber, or green slightly viscous liquid. A solution in sodium chloride 0.9% containing 1% protein has a pH of 6.7 to 7.3.

USP 25: Albumin Human is a sterile, nonpyrogenic, preparation of serum albumin obtained by fractionating material (blood, plasma, serum, or placentas) from healthy human donors, the source material being tested for the absence of hepatitis B surface antigen. It is made by a process that yields a product that is safe for intravenous use. It contains 4, 5, 20, or 25% of serum albumin and not less than 96% of the total protein is albumin. It may contain sodium acetyltryptophanate with or without sodium caprylate as a stabilising agent; it contains no added antimicrobial agent. It contains 130 to 160 mmol of sodium per litre. It is a practically odourless, moderately viscous, clear, brownish fluid.

Adverse Effects and Precautions

Adverse reactions to albumin infusion occur rarely and include nausea and vomiting, increased salivation, and febrile reactions. Allergic reactions, including severe anaphylactic shock, are possible. Rapid increases in circulatory volume can cause vascular overload, haemodilution, and pulmonary oedema. Solutions containing albumin 20% or 25% are hyperosmotic and draw fluid from the extravascular compartment. Heating to about 60° in the presence of a stabiliser during preparation has reduced the risk of transmitting some viral infections.

Infusion of albumin solutions is contra-indicated in patients with severe anaemia or heart failure. They should be given with caution to patients with hypertension or low cardiac reserve. Dehydrated patients may require additional fluids. Injured or postoperative patients should be observed carefully following the administration of albumin as the rise in blood pressure may result in bleeding from previously undetected sites.

◊ Volume expansion with albumin (a colloid) has been widely used in critically ill patients, although its use has never been formally tested in large controlled studies. A systematic review based on available studies up to March 1998 (relatively small, old trials that recorded only a small number of deaths) suggested that albumin was of no benefit in critically ill patients with hypovolaemia, burns, or hypoalbuminaemia, and that it might be linked to increased mortality.[1] The authors of the review stressed that these results should be treated with caution but nevertheless called for an urgent reconsideration of the use of albumin in critically ill patients. The review was severely criticised[2] and while it was recognised that albumin has probably been overused in the past it was considered that more studies were required to define the effect of albumin on mortality.[3-5] An update[6] to the review, however, including some more recent studies, came to the same conclusions as the original review. On a broader level, debate continues about the relative merits and risks of such colloid solutions, compared with those of crystalloids such as glucose or sodium chloride solutions, in the management of hypovolaemia and shock (p.813).

1. Cochrane Injuries Group Albumin Reviewers. Human albumin administration in critically ill patients: systematic review of randomised controlled trials. *BMJ* 1998; **317:** 235–40.
2. Various. Human albumin administration in critically ill patients. *BMJ* 1998; **317:** 882–6. [Letters.]
3. Tomlin M. Albumin usage in the critically ill. *Pharm J* 1998; **261:** 193.
4. McClelland B. Albumin: don't confuse us with the facts. *BMJ* 1998; **317:** 829–30.

5. Committee on Safety of Medicines/Medicines Control Agency. The safety of human albumin. *Current Problems* 1999; **25:** 11.
6. The Albumin Reviewers. Human albumin solution for resuscitation and volume expansion in critically ill patients (updated 28 August 2001). Available in The Cochrane Library; Issue 4. Oxford: Update Software; 2001.

Aluminium toxicity. Albumin solutions may contain appreciable amounts of aluminium. Marked increases in plasma aluminium concentrations have been demonstrated in patients receiving large volumes by infusion and accumulation of aluminium may occur in patients with impaired renal function.[1-3] In the UK albumin solutions with an aluminium content of less than 200 µg per litre are available for use in patients undergoing dialysis and premature infants.

1. Milliner DS, *et al.* Inadvertent aluminum administration during plasma exchange due to aluminum contamination of albumin-replacement solutions. *N Engl J Med* 1985; **312:** 165–7.
2. Maher ER, *et al.* Accumulation of aluminium in chronic renal failure due to administration of albumin replacement solutions. *BMJ* 1986; **292:** 306.
3. Maharaj D, *et al.* Aluminium bone disease in patients receiving plasma exchange with contaminated albumin. *BMJ* 1987; **295:** 693–6.

Dilution. If concentrated albumin solutions are diluted before administration, a suitable solution such as sodium chloride 0.9% or glucose 5% must be used. Albumin 25% that was erroneously diluted with water to produce a hypo-osmolar albumin 5% solution has produced severe haemolysis and renal failure in patients undergoing plasmapheresis,[1,2] including a fatality in one patient.[3]

1. Steinmuller DR. A dangerous error in the dilution of 25 percent albumin. *N Engl J Med* 1998; **338:** 1226.
2. Pierce LR, *et al.* Hemolysis and renal failure associated with use of sterile water for injection to dilute 25% human albumin solution. *Am J Health-Syst Pharm* 1998; **55:** 1057,1062, 1070.
3. Anonymous. Hemolysis associated with 25% human albumin diluted with sterile water—United States, 1994–1998. *MMWR* 1999; **48:** 157–9.

Transmission of infections. There has been concern that albumin preparations may carry a potential risk of transmission of viral and subviral particles, notably Creutzfeldt-Jakob disease. In 1993, *Pasteur-Mérieux* (one of the largest producers of blood products) withdrew all products containing albumin derived from placental blood[1] due to uncertainty regarding the adequacy of screening procedures for placentas as a source. It was considered that the agent responsible for Creutzfeldt-Jakob disease might be contained in placentas from women who have been treated with growth hormone derived from cadaver pituitaries. More recently, the production of blood products (including albumin) using plasma from UK donors has been phased out due to the possible risk of transmission of Creutzfeldt-Jakob disease.

1. Anonymous. Placental-derived albumin preparations withdrawn. *WHO Drug Inf* 1994; **8:** 29–30.

Uses and Administration

Albumin is the major protein involved in maintaining colloid osmotic pressure in the blood. It also binds a number of endogenous and exogenous substances including bilirubin, steroid hormones, and many, mainly acidic, drugs.

Albumin solutions are used for plasma volume replacement and to restore colloid osmotic pressure. They have been used in conditions such as burns, severe acute albumin loss, and acute hypovolaemic shock (p.813). They are also used as an exchange fluid in therapeutic plasmapheresis. Concentrated albumin solutions are used in neonatal hyperbilirubinaemia associated with haemolytic disease of the newborn (p.1532). They have also been suggested for short-term management of hypoproteinaemia in hepatic disease and in diuretic-resistant patients with nephrotic syndrome but are of little value in chronic hypoproteinaemias. Albumin preparations labelled with technetium-99m are used as radiopharmaceuticals in heart and lung scanning (p.1451) and air-filled albumin microspheres are available for enhancing cardiac ultrasound imaging.

Albumin solutions are usually available as 4.5% or 5% solutions, which are iso-osmotic with plasma, and as 20% or 25% solutions which, being hyperosmotic with respect to plasma, cause a movement of fluid from the extravascular to the intravascular compartment. These concentrated solutions may be used undiluted or may be diluted with a suitable solution, commonly sodium chloride 0.9% or glucose 5%. Adequate hydration should be maintained in patients receiving hyperosmotic solutions of albumin.

The amount of albumin solution administered will depend upon the clinical condition of the patient and the response to treatment. The following doses have been suggested: in acute hypovolaemic shock an initial

dose of 25 g of albumin for adults (for example, 500 mL of a 5% solution or 100 mL of a 25% solution) and up to about 1 g per kg body-weight for children; in hypoproteinaemia a maximum daily dose of 2 g per kg; and in neonatal hyperbilirubinaemia a dose of 1 g per kg before exchange transfusion (albumin, in a dose of 1.5 to 2.5 g per 100 mL of blood, may also be added to the exchange transfusion).

A suggested rate of infusion is 1 to 2 mL per minute (5% solution) or 1 mL per minute (25% solution) although high rates may be needed in the treatment of shock.

Albumin solutions should not be used for parenteral nutrition.

◊ References.

1. Erstad BL, *et al.* The use of albumin in clinical practice. *Arch Intern Med* 1991; **151:** 901–11.
2. Tomlin M. Albumin usage on intensive care. *Pharm J* 1997; **259:** 856–9. Comment including corrections—Dash C, *et al. ibid.* 1998; **260:** 88–9.
3. McClelland DBL. Human albumin solutions. In Contreras M, ed. *ABC of transfusion.* 3rd ed. London: BMJ Books, 1998: 45–8.

Preparations

Ph. Eur.: Human Albumin Solution;
USP 25: Albumin Human.

Proprietary Preparations (details are given in Part 3)
Austral.: Albumex; NSA†; *Belg.:* Albuman†; *Canad.:* Plasbumin; *Ger.:* Humanalbin; *Hong Kong:* Albutein; Biseko; Buminate; Plasbumin; Zenalb; *Irl.:* Albuminar; *Israel:* Albuminar; Plasbumin; *Ital.:* Albital; Albuman; Albutein; Endalbumin†; Haimalbumin; Seralbuman†; *Mex.:* Albumyn; Biomina; Probi-Albumin; Seralbumin; Vanderbumin; *Norw.:* Infosan†; *NZ:* Albumex; *S.Afr.:* Albusol; *Singapore:* Albutein; Buminate; Plasbumin; Zenalb; *Spain:* Plasbumin; *Swed.:* Albuminar†; Infoson†; *Switz.:* Albuman; *Thai.:* Albuman; Albutein; Buminate; Zenalb; *UK:* Alba; Albuminar†; Albutein; Zenalb; *USA:* Albumarc; Albuminar; Albunex†; Albutein; Buminate; Plasbumin.

Multi-ingredient: *Denm.:* Tisseel Duo Quick; *Swed.:* Tisseel Duo Quick.

Aminaphthone (12357-g)

Aminaftone; Aminaphtone; Aminonaphthone. 2-Hydroxy-3-methylnaphtho-1,4-hydroquinone 2-(4-aminobenzoate); 3-Methylnaphthalene-1,2,4-triol 2-(4-aminobenzoate).

$C_{18}H_{15}NO_4 = 309.3.$
CAS — 14748-94-8.

Profile

Aminaphthone is a haemostatic. Daily doses of 150 to 225 mg by mouth have been employed.

Preparations

Proprietary Preparations (details are given in Part 3)
Braz.: Capilarema; *Ital.:* Capilarema; *Port.:* Capilarema; *Spain:* Capilarema.

Aminocaproic Acid (1712-p)

Aminocaproic Acid *(BAN, USAN, rINN).*

Acidum Aminocaproicum; CL-10304; CY-116; EACA; Epsilon Aminocaproic Acid; JD-177; NSC-26154. 6-Aminohexanoic acid.

$C_6H_{13}NO_2 = 131.2.$
CAS — 60-32-2.
ATC — B02AA01.
Pharmacopoeias. In Eur. (see p.vi), Pol., and US.

Pharmacopoeial description

Ph. Eur.: A white, crystalline powder or colourless crystals. Freely soluble in water; slightly soluble in alcohol; practically insoluble in ether. A 20% solution in water has a pH of 7.5 to 8.0.

USP 25: A fine, white, odourless or practically odourless, crystalline powder. Soluble 1 in 3 of water and 1 in 450 of methyl alcohol; slightly soluble in alcohol; practically insoluble in chloroform and in ether; freely soluble in acids and in alkalis. Its solutions are neutral to litmus. Store in airtight containers.

Adverse Effects

Adverse effects associated with the administration of aminocaproic acid include dose-related gastrointestinal disturbances, dizziness, tinnitus, headache, nasal and conjunctival congestion, and skin rashes. Aminocaproic acid may cause muscle damage. This has usually occurred with high doses given for prolonged periods; renal failure may develop. Thrombotic complications have been reported, although they are usually a consequence of inappropriate use. If aminocaproic acid is given by rapid intravenous administration it can produce hypotension, bradycardia, and arrhythmias. There have been reports of a few patients suffering from convulsions, dry ejaculation, or cardiac and hepatic damage.

Effects on the blood. Very high doses of aminocaproic acid (36 g or more daily) have been given intravenously in the management of subarachnoid haemorrhage. One study[1] reported rebleeding and excessive intra-operative bleeding in patients with subarachnoid haemorrhage receiving aminocaproic acid and suggested that this was due to an antiplatelet effect of the aminocaproic acid. However, a comment on this report[2] pointed out that any antiplatelet effect was independent of its antifibrinolytic action and that this effect could only aggravate rebleeding, if it occurs, rather than initiating it.

1. Glick R, *et al.* High dose ε-aminocaproic acid prolongs the bleeding time and increases rebleeding and intraoperative hemorrhage in patients with subarachnoid hemorrhage. *Neurosurgery* 1981; **9:** 398–401.
2. Kassell NF. Comment. *Neurosurgery* 1981; **9:** 401.

Effects on the muscles. There have been a number of cases of reversible myopathy reported with aminocaproic acid,[1-4] associated with daily doses ranging from 10 to 49 g and treatment durations of about one to three months. In some patients myoglobinuria or acute tubular necrosis also occurred. Suggested mechanisms for the reaction have included a direct dose-related effect on the muscle fibre[2] or a defect in aerobic energy provision induced by aminocaproic acid.[3]

1. Brown JA, *et al.* Myopathy induced by epsilon-aminocaproic acid. *J Neurosurg* 1982; **57:** 130–4.
2. Vanneste JAL, van Wijngaarden GK. Epsilon-aminocaproic acid myopathy. *Eur Neurol* 1982; **21:** 242–8.
3. Van Renterghem D, *et al.* Epsilon amino caproic acid myopathy: additional features. *Clin Neurol Neurosurg* 1984; **86:** 153–7.
4. Seymour BD, Rubinger M. Rhabdomyolysis induced by epsilon-aminocaproic acid. *Ann Pharmacother* 1997; **31:** 56–8.

Precautions

As for Tranexamic Acid, p.742.

The range of adverse effects that have been noted with aminocaproic acid indicates that caution is required in patients with renal or cardiac disorders. Should treatment be prolonged, it is advisable to monitor creatine phosphokinase values for signs of muscle damage.

Renal impairment. High anion gap metabolic acidosis developed in a 65-year-old woman with sepsis and acute renal failure who received aminocaproic acid for a haemorrhagic coagulopathy.[1] The acidosis improved temporarily following haemodialysis and resolved after discontinuation of aminocaproic acid and systemic alkalinisation. Although the dose of aminocaproic acid had been reduced due to her renal impairment, it was suggested that more conservative dosing and close monitoring may be indicated in such patients.

1. Budris WA, *et al.* High anion gap metabolic acidosis associated with aminocaproic acid. *Ann Pharmacother* 1999; **33:** 308–11.

Pharmacokinetics

Aminocaproic acid is readily absorbed when given by mouth and peak plasma concentrations are reached within 2 hours. It is widely distributed and is rapidly excreted in the urine, mainly unchanged, with a terminal elimination half-life of approximately 2 hours.

Uses and Administration

Aminocaproic acid is an antifibrinolytic used similarly to tranexamic acid (p.742) in the treatment and prophylaxis of haemorrhage associated with excessive fibrinolysis. It has also been used in the prophylaxis of hereditary angioedema (p.743).

A plasma concentration of about 130 μg per mL is considered to be necessary for effective inhibition of fibrinolysis and the recommended dosage schedules are aimed at producing and maintaining this concentration for as long as is necessary. For the treatment and prophylaxis of haemorrhage, aminocaproic acid may be given by mouth in an initial dose of 4 to 5 g, followed by 1 to 1.25 g every hour. Alternatively, the same dose may be given intravenously as a 2% solution; the initial dose (4 to 5 g) should be given over one hour followed by a continuous infusion of 1 g per hour. Up to 8 hours of treatment is often sufficient. Should treatment need to be extended, then the maximum dose over 24 hours should not normally exceed 24 g. Care is required when aminocaproic acid is used in patients with renal impairment and dosage should be reduced.

The symbol † denotes a preparation no longer actively marketed

Preparations

USP 25: Aminocaproic Acid Injection; Aminocaproic Acid Syrup; Aminocaproic Acid Tablets.

Proprietary Preparations (details are given in Part 3)
Austral.: Amicar; *Braz.:* Ipsilon; *Canad.:* Amicar; *Fr.:* Hexalense; *Ital.:* Caprolisin; *Mex.:* Amicar; *NZ:* Amicar; *Port.:* Epsicaprom; *S.Afr.:* Amicar; *Spain:* Caproamin; *USA:* Amicar.
Multi-ingredient: *Braz.:* Eaca Balsamico; Expectovac; Ginurovac; *Spain:* Caprofides Hemostatico.

Aminomethylbenzoic Acid (1713-s)

PAMBA. 4-Aminomethylbenzoic acid.
$C_8H_9NO_2 = 151.2$.
CAS — 56-91-7.
ATC — B02AA03.
Pharmacopoeias. In *Chin.* which specifies the monohydrate.

Profile

Aminomethylbenzoic acid is an antifibrinolytic with actions and uses similar to those of tranexamic acid (p.742). It is given by mouth, by intramuscular injection, or intravenously by slow injection or infusion.

Preparations

Proprietary Preparations (details are given in Part 3)
Aust.: Gumbix; *Ger.:* Gumbix; Pamba.

Antithrombin III (1216-z)

Antithrombin III (BAN, rINN).
Antithrombin III Human; AT-III; Heparin Cofactor; Heparin Cofactor I; Major Antithrombin.
CAS — 52014-67-2.
ATC — B01AB02.

Pharmacopoeial description

Ph. Eur.: Human Antithrombin III Concentrate (Antithrombinum III Humanum Densatum; Antithrombin III Concentrate (BP 2001)) is a preparation of a glycoprotein fraction obtained from human plasma that inactivates thrombin in the presence of an excess of heparin. The plasma is obtained from healthy donors and is tested for the absence of hepatitis B surface antigen and antibodies against HIV-1 and HIV-2 and hepatitis C virus. The method of preparation includes a step or steps that have been shown to remove or to inactivate known agents of infection. The antithrombin III concentrate is passed through a bacteria-retentive filter, distributed into sterile containers, and immediately frozen. The preparation is freeze-dried and the containers sealed under vacuum or in an atmosphere of inert gas. No antimicrobial preservative is added but a suitable stabiliser (such as albumin) may be added. When reconstituted in the volume of solvent stated on the label, the resulting solution contains not less than 25 units of antithrombin III per mL.
A white, friable solid or powder. Protect from light.

Units

The potency of antithrombin III is expressed in international units and preparations may be assayed using the first International Standard for antithrombin III concentrate (1990).

Uses and Administration

Antithrombin III is a protein in plasma; it is the major endogenous inhibitor of thrombin and other activated clotting factors including factors IX, X, XI, and XII (p.718), and is the cofactor through which heparin (p.904) exerts its effect. Genetic and acquired deficiency of antithrombin III occurs and is associated with susceptibility to thromboembolic disorders.

Antithrombin III is administered intravenously in the management of acute thrombotic episodes and for prophylaxis during surgery and pregnancy in patients with antithrombin III deficiency. The aim of therapy is to restore plasma-antithrombin III concentrations to at least 80% of normal. The dose, frequency of administration, and duration of therapy are individualised for each patient taking into account the patient's pretreatment concentration and presence of active coagulation. A usual initial dose is about 30 to 50 international units per kg body-weight.

A recombinant human antithrombin III preparation is being developed.

◊ Reviews of antithrombin III.
1. Rosenberg RD, ed. Role of antithrombin III in coagulation disorders: state-of-the-art review. *Am J Med* 1989; **87** (3B): 1S–67S.
2. Harper PL. The clinical use of antithrombin concentrate in septicaemia. *Br J Hosp Med* 1994; **52:** 571–4.

Preparations

Ph. Eur.: Human Antithrombin III Concentrate.

Proprietary Preparations (details are given in Part 3)
Aust.: Atenativ; Athimbin P; Kybernin P; Thrombhibin; *Austral.:* Thrombotrol-VF; *Canad.:* Thrombate; *Denm.:* Atenativ; *Fin.:* Atenativ; *Fr.:* Aclotine; *Ger.:* AT III; Atenativ; Kybernin P; *Hong Kong:* Thrombate; *Ital.:* Anbin; Kybernin P; *Neth.:* Atenativ; *Norw.:* Atenativ; *NZ:* Thrombotrol; *Spain:* Atenativ; Kybernin P; *Swed.:* Atenativ; *Switz.:* Atenativ; Kybernin; *UK:* Kybernin P†; *USA:* ATnativ†; Thrombate; Thrombate III.

Aprotinin (1714-w)

Aprotinin (BAN, USAN, rINN).
Aprotininum; Bayer A-128; Riker 52G; RP-9921.
CAS — 9087-70-1.
ATC — B02AB01.
Pharmacopoeias. In *Chin.* and *Eur.* (see p.vi).

A single-chain polypeptide derived from bovine tissues consisting of 58 amino-acid residues and having a molecular weight of about 6500.

Aprotinin is reported to be incompatible with corticosteroids, heparin, tetracyclines, and nutrient solutions containing amino acids or fat emulsions.

Pharmacopoeial description

Ph. Eur.: Aprotinin is a polypeptide consisting of 58 amino acids that inhibits the activity of several proteolytic enzymes such as chymotrypsin, kallikrein, fibrinolysin, and trypsin. It contains not less than 3 Ph. Eur. units per mg calculated with reference to the dried substance. An almost white, hygroscopic powder. Soluble in water and in isotonic solutions; practically insoluble in organic solvents. Store in airtight containers. Protect from light.

Aprotinin Concentrated Solution is a solution of aprotinin containing not less than 15 Ph. Eur. units per mL. A clear colourless solution. Store in airtight containers. Protect from light.

Units

The potency of aprotinin is expressed in terms of kallikrein (kallidinogenase) inactivator units (KIU) or of trypsin inactivation (Ph. Eur. units). One KIU is contained in 140 nanograms of aprotinin. One Ph. Eur. unit is approximately equivalent to 1800 KIU.

Potency has also been expressed in terms of fibrinolysin (plasmin) inactivation (antiplasmin units).

Adverse Effects and Precautions

Aprotinin is usually well tolerated. Side-effects that have been observed include bronchospasm, gastrointestinal disturbances, skin rashes, and tachycardia; most of these effects are considered to be hypersensitivity reactions. Anaphylaxis has occasionally occurred as has local thrombophlebitis.

◊ Aprotinin has been used to reverse resistance to subcutaneous insulin. After one year's successful treatment of a diabetic patient with aprotinin and insulin given subcutaneously,[1] loss of effect from the aprotinin was accompanied by development of lipohypertrophy; this was not seen during prior or subsequent use of insulin alone. On continuing treatment glomerulonephritis was detected. It was suggested that development of antibodies against aprotinin might explain these effects.
1. Boag F, *et al.* Lipohypertrophy and glomerulonephritis after the use of aprotinin in an insulin-dependent diabetic. *N Engl J Med* 1985; **312:** 245–6.

Disseminated intravascular coagulation. Disseminated intravascular coagulation resulting in death has been reported in a patient following the use of intraoperative autotransfusion and aprotinin during surgery.[1] Activation of the clotting system occurs during autotransfusion although this usually causes no systemic adverse effects. While there were other possible causes, it was suggested that aprotinin could have contributed to deposition of fibrin microthrombi in the microvasculature and prevented subsequent fibrinolysis.
1. Milne AA, *et al.* Disseminated intravascular coagulation after aortic aneurysm repair, intraoperative salvage autotransfusion, and aprotinin. *Lancet* 1994; **344:** 470–1.

Effects on coagulation tests. In patients receiving heparin, administration of aprotinin may prolong the activated clotting time when measured by some methods, but this may not represent increased anticoagulation. It has been recommended that an alternative to the activated clotting time be used to monitor heparin therapy when aprotinin is administered concurrently.

It should also be noted that aprotinin injection and heparin injection are pharmaceutically incompatible.

Effects on the respiratory system. Acute respiratory distress syndrome developed in a 24-year-old male two hours after the start of an intravenous infusion of aprotinin for bleeding following tonsillectomy.[1] Mechanical ventilation was required for 4 days.

1. Vucicevic Z, Suskovic T. Acute respiratory distress syndrome after aprotinin infusion. *Ann Pharmacother* 1997; **31:** 429–32.

Hypersensitivity. Acute allergic reactions were noted[1] in 2 of 136 courses of aprotinin; one patient experienced acute anaphylaxis, the other an acute urticarial reaction. Such patients might be detected by challenging their reactivity using aprotinin eye drops as an alternative to intradermal testing. However, a severe anaphylactic reaction occurred[2] in a patient after the intravenous administration of aprotinin despite negative ocular sensitivity tests. Repeat administration of aprotinin (2 months after the initial dose) has produced anaphylactic shock in a 3-year-old boy.[3] In a study[4] of 248 re-exposures to aprotinin in 240 patients undergoing cardiac surgery, there were 7 cases of anaphylactic reactions ranging from mild to severe with a higher incidence of reactions occurring in those patients re-exposed within 6 months of the previous dose. It has been suggested that re-exposure should be avoided for at least 6 months,[4] that a test dose be used in all patients,[4] and that histamine H_1- and H_2-antagonists should be given before re-exposure to aprotinin to ameliorate severe anaphylactic reactions.[4,5]

1. Freeman JG, *et al.* Serial use of aprotinin and incidence of allergic reactions. *Curr Med Res Opin* 1983; **8:** 559–61.
2. LaFerla GA, Murray WR. Anaphylactic reaction to aprotinin despite negative ocular sensitivity tests. *BMJ* 1984; **289:** 1176–7.
3. Wüthrich B, *et al.* IgE-mediated anaphylactic reaction to aprotinin during anaesthesia. *Lancet* 1992; **340:** 173–4.
4. Dietrich W, *et al.* Prevalence of anaphylactic reactions to aprotinin: analysis of two hundred forty-eight reexposures to aprotinin in heart operations. *J Thorac Cardiovasc Surg* 1997; **113:** 194–201.
5. Lamparter-Schummert B, *et al.* Aprotinin re-exposure in patients undergoing repeat cardiac surgery: effect of prophylaxis with H1- and H2-receptor antagonists. *Br J Anaesth* 1995; **74** (suppl 2): 3.

Interactions

◊ For comment on the use of aprotinin with heparin, see under Effects on Coagulation Tests, above.

For potentiation of the activity of neuromuscular blockers by aprotinin, see p.1334.

Pharmacokinetics

Aprotinin, being a polypeptide, is inactivated in the gastrointestinal tract. Following intravenous administration, it is excreted in the urine as inactive degradation products. The terminal elimination half-life is about 7 to 10 hours.

Renal impairment. The terminal elimination half-life of aprotinin was reported as 13.3 and 14.9 hours, respectively, in two patients with chronic renal impairment given aprotinin by intravenous infusion over 30 minutes.[1]

1. Müller FO, *et al.* Pharmacokinetics of aprotinin in two patients with chronic renal impairment. *Br J Clin Pharmacol* 1996; **41:** 619–20.

Uses and Administration

Aprotinin is a haemostatic. It is an inhibitor of proteolytic enzymes including chymotrypsin, kallikrein (kallidinogenase), fibrinolysin (plasmin), and trypsin.

Aprotinin is used in the treatment of haemorrhage associated with raised plasma concentrations of fibrinolysin. It is also used to reduce blood loss and transfusion requirements in patients at high risk of major blood loss during and following open-heart surgery with extracorporeal circulation. Aprotinin has been tried in the management of pancreatitis (p.1646) because of the postulated role of proteolytic enzymes in this condition. Aprotinin is applied topically as a component of fibrin glues (p.735).

In the treatment of haemorrhage, 500 000 to 1 000 000 KIU of aprotinin are given by slow intravenous injection or infusion at a maximum rate of 100 000 KIU per minute with the patient in the supine position. This may be followed by 200 000 KIU every hour until the haemorrhage is controlled.

In open-heart surgery, an intravenous loading dose of 2 000 000 KIU is given after induction of anaesthesia but before incision, or re-opening of the wound. It is recommended that because of the risk of hypersensitivity reactions the first 50 000 KIU of the loading dose should be administered over several minutes, the remainder being given over 20 minutes. Alternatively, a test dose of 10 000 KIU may be given at least 10 minutes before the loading dose. The loading dose is followed by a continuous infusion of 500 000 KIU per hour until skin closure at the end of the operation. An additional dose of 2 000 000 KIU is added to the prime volume of the oxygenator. In patients with sep-

tic endocarditis, a dose of 3 000 000 KIU is added to the prime volume of the oxygenator and the continuous infusion may be continued into the early postoperative period.

Haemorrhagic disorders. Aprotinin is indicated in the treatment of life-threatening haemorrhage caused by raised plasma concentrations of fibrinolysin. It is used alone, or with tranexamic acid or aminocaproic acid, in the treatment of severe bleeding arising from overdosage with thrombolytics.

It is also used to reduce blood loss in patients undergoing surgery, including that involving cardiopulmonary bypass.[1-3] (See also Complex Acquired Coagulopathies under Haemorrhagic Disorders, p.721.)

Cardiac surgery may be complicated by a postperfusion syndrome which includes impairment of haemostasis and pulmonary dysfunction. This syndrome has been interpreted as a 'whole-body inflammatory response'. The beneficial effect of aprotinin on haemostasis during cardiopulmonary bypass has been attributed, not to an antifibrinolytic action, but to a preservation of platelet function, possibly mediated by inhibition of fibrinolysin.[2-7] Administration of aprotinin has reduced blood loss and transfusion requirements in patients undergoing both primary and repeat cardiac surgery.[1,8,9] The usual dosage regimen is given under Uses and Administration, above. In addition, 500 000 KIU may be added to each litre of whole blood given during the operation.[4,5]

A slightly different dosage regimen has been used in a group of patients undergoing heart-valve replacement for infective endocarditis.[10] Other workers have investigated the use of reduced dosage regimens omitting the loading dose, including the administration of aprotinin in the priming volume alone.[11-15]

Encouraging reductions in blood loss have been obtained in some patients undergoing liver transplantation,[16,17] peripheral vascular surgery,[18] orthopaedic surgery,[19] and lung transplantation,[20] but it has been advised that until risks such as postoperative thromboembolic disease and loss of graft patency have been investigated aprotinin should be used with caution.[21]

Aprotinin has been tried with a low-dose regimen of tranexamic acid in the prevention of rebleeding in patients with subarachnoid haemorrhage[22] (p.813). Results suggested a reduced risk of rebleeding, without the increased incidence of ischaemic complications observed after treatment with conventional doses of tranexamic acid alone.

Aprotinin is a component of fibrin glues (p.735), also known as fibrin sealants or tissue glues, that are applied topically in the control of bleeding or as a suture system. The other components of these glues include fibrinogen, factor XIII, and other plasma proteins, mixed with calcium and thrombin immediately prior to use.

1. Davis R, Whittington R. Aprotinin: a review of its pharmacology and therapeutic efficacy in reducing blood loss associated with cardiac surgery. *Drugs* 1995; **49:** 954–83.
2. Robert S, *et al.* Aprotinin. *Ann Pharmacother* 1996; **30:** 372–80.
3. Dobkowski WB, Murkin JM. A risk-benefit assessment of aprotinin in cardiac surgical procedures. *Drug Safety* 1998; **18:** 21–41.
4. van Oeveren W, *et al.* Effects of aprotinin on hemostatic mechanisms during cardiopulmonary bypass. *Ann Thorac Surg* 1987; **44:** 640–5.
5. Royston D, *et al.* Effect of aprotinin on need for blood transfusion after repeat open-heart surgery. *Lancet* 1987; **ii:** 1289–91.
6. Anonymous. Can drugs reduce surgical blood loss? *Lancet* 1988; **i:** 155–6.
7. van Oeveren W, *et al.* Platelet preservation by aprotinin during cardiopulmonary bypass. *Lancet* 1988; **i:** 644.
8. Bidstrup BP, *et al.* Aprotinin therapy in cardiac operations: a report on use in 41 cardiac centers in the United Kingdom. *Ann Thorac Surg* 1993; **55:** 971–6.
9. Laupacis A, Fergusson D. Drugs to minimize perioperative blood loss in cardiac surgery: meta-analyses using perioperative blood transfusion as the outcome. *Anesth Analg* 1997; **85:** 1258–67.
10. Bidstrup BP, *et al.* Effect of aprotinin on need for blood transfusion in patients with septic endocarditis having open-heart surgery. *Lancet* 1988; **i:** 366–7.
11. Locatelli A, *et al.* Aprotinin in cardiac surgery. *Lancet* 1991; **338:** 254.
12. Carrel T, *et al.* Low-dose aprotinin for reduction of blood loss after cardiopulmonary bypass. *Lancet* 1991; **337:** 673.
13. Vandenvelde C, *et al.* Low-dose aprotinin for reduction of blood loss after cardiopulmonary bypass. *Lancet* 1991; **337:** 1157–8.
14. Bailey CR, Wielogorski AK. Randomised placebo controlled double blind study of two low dose aprotinin regimens in cardiac surgery. *Br Heart J* 1994; **71:** 349–53.
15. Levy JH, *et al.* A multicenter, double-blind, placebo-controlled trial of aprotinin for reducing blood loss and the requirement for donor-blood transfusion in patients undergoing repeat coronary artery bypass graftings. *Circulation* 1995; **92:** 2236–44.
16. Neuhaus P, *et al.* Effect of aprotinin on intraoperative bleeding and fibrinolysis in liver transplantation. *Lancet* 1989; **i:** 924–5.
17. Mallett SV, *et al.* Aprotinin and reduction of blood loss and transfusion requirements in orthotopic liver transplantation. *Lancet* 1990; **336:** 886–7.
18. Thompson JF, *et al.* Aprotinin in peripheral vascular surgery. *Lancet* 1990; **335:** 911.
19. Janssens M, *et al.* High-dose aprotinin reduces blood loss in patients undergoing total hip replacement surgery. *Anesthesiology* 1994; **80:** 23–9.
20. Jaquiss RDB, *et al.* Use of aprotinin in pediatric lung transplantation. *J Heart Lung Transplant* 1995; **14:** 302–7.
21. Hunt BJ, Yacoub M. Aprotinin and cardiac surgery. *BMJ* 1991; **303:** 660–1.
22. Spallone A, *et al.* Low-dose tranexamic acid combined with aprotinin in the pre-operative management of ruptured intracranial aneurysms. *Neurochirurgia (Stuttg)* 1987; **30:** 172–6.

Preparations

BP 2001: Aprotinin Injection;
Ph. Eur.: Fibrin Sealant Kit.

Proprietary Preparations (details are given in Part 3)
Aust.: Pantinol; Trasylol; *Austral.:* Trasylol; *Belg.:* Iniprol†; Trasylol; *Canad.:* Trasylol; *Denm.:* Trasylol; *Fin.:* Trasylol; *Fr.:* Antagosan; Trasylol; *Ger.:* Antagosan; Trasylol; *Hong Kong:* Trasylol; *Israel:* Protosol; *Ital.:* Antagosan†; Fase†; Kir Richter†; Trasylol†; *Mex.:* Protinin; Trasylol; *Neth.:* Trasylol; *NZ:* Trasylol; *S.Afr.:* Midran†; Trasylol; *Singapore:* Trasylol; *Swed.:* Trasylol; *Switz.:* Trasylol; *Thai.:* Trasylol; *UK:* Trasylol; *USA:* Trasylol.

Multi-ingredient: *Aust.:* Beriplast; TachoComb; Tissucol; Tissucol Duo Quick; *Belg.:* Tissucol; *Braz.:* Tissucol; *Canad.:* Tisseel; *Denm.:* Tisseel Duo Quick; *Fin.:* Beriplast; Tisseel Duo Quick; *Fr.:* Beriplast; Biocol; *Ger.:* Beriplast; TachoComb; Tissucol Duo S; Tissucol Fibrinkleber tiefgefroren†; Tissucol-Kit; *Hong Kong:* Beriplast; TachoComb; Tisseel; *Irl.:* Tisseel; *Israel:* Beriplast P; Tisseel; *Ital.:* Tissucol; *Mex.:* Beriplast P; Tisseel; *Spain:* Tissucol; *Swed.:* Tisseel Duo Quick; *Switz.:* Tissucol; Tissucol Duo S; *Thai.:* TachoComb; *UK:* Tisseel.

Batroxobin (12419-b)

Batroxobin (rINN).

CAS — 9039-61-6 (batroxobin); 9001-13-2 (haemocoagulase).
ATC — B02BX03.

Batroxobin is an enzyme obtained from the venom of the viper *Bothrops atrox*. It has also been obtained from *Bothrops moojeni* and a similar preparation is derived from *Bothrops jararaca*. The name haemocoagulase (hemocoagulase) is used for a preparation of batroxobin with a factor-X activator.

Profile

Batroxobin is reported to act on fibrinogen to produce a fibrin monomer that can be converted by thrombin to a fibrin clot. It is used both as a haemostatic and, in larger doses, to induce a hypofibrinogen state in the management of thromboembolic disorders. When used as a haemostatic it is usually given with a factor-X activator; such a combined preparation is known as haemocoagulase. Batroxobin may be administered parenterally or by local application.

Preparations

Proprietary Preparations (details are given in Part 3)
Aust.: Defibrase; Reptilase; *Fr.:* Reptilase; *Ital.:* Botropase; Reptilase†; *Port.:* Reptilase; *Spain:* Reptilase.

Blood (1212-e)

Pharmacopoeial description

USP 25: Whole Blood (ACD Whole Blood; CPD Whole Blood; CPDA-1 Whole Blood; Heparin Whole Blood) is blood from suitable human donors that has been collected under rigid aseptic precautions. It contains acid citrate dextrose, citrate phosphate dextrose, citrate phosphate dextrose with adenine, or heparin sodium as an anticoagulant. It may consist of blood from which the antihaemophilic factor has been removed, in which case it is termed 'Modified'. It should be stored in hermetically-sealed sterile containers at 1° to 6° (with a range of not more than 2°) except during transport when the temperature may be 1° to 10°. The expiration date is not later than 48 hours after withdrawal (heparin anticoagulant), not later than 21 days after withdrawal (acid citrate dextrose or citrate phosphate dextrose), or not later than 35 days after withdrawal (citrate phosphate dextrose with adenine).

It is a deep red, opaque liquid from which the corpuscles readily settle upon standing for 24 to 48 hours, leaving a clear, yellowish or pinkish supernatant layer of plasma.

Adverse Effects

The rapid transfusion of large volumes of whole blood may overload the circulation and cause pulmonary oedema. Repeated transfusions of blood, as in thalassaemia, may lead to iron overload. Transfusion of very large volumes of citrated blood can lead to hypocalcaemia which is not usually a problem unless there is impaired liver function or hypothermia. Hyperkalaemia may occur but on its own is rarely clinically significant. Hypothermia may result from rapid transfusion of large volumes of cooled blood and may, in combination with hypocalcaemia, hyperkalaemia, and resultant acidosis, lead to cardiac toxicity. Disseminated intravascular coagulation may also occur in patients receiving large-volume transfusions.

The transfusion of incompatible blood causes haemolysis, possibly with renal failure. Pyrexia, rigors, and urticaria may be due to antibodies towards a number of blood components. Severe allergic reactions and anaphylaxis may occur.

Transmission of infections. The use of blood, blood components, or blood products has been associated with the transmission of viruses, most notably transmission of the hepatitis B virus and HIV; other reports of transmission include cytomegalovirus, hepatitis C and possibly other hepatitis viruses, HTLV-I and -II, and the agent causing Creutzfeldt-Jakob disease. Transmission of bacterial and parasitic diseases is also possible including syphilis, Chagas' disease, and malaria.

The main methods of minimising the risk of transmission of infection are by rigorous selection of blood donors and by microbiological screening tests. Contamination during collection and processing is minimised by using closed systems and by strict aseptic technique. Some organisms cannot survive storage under refrigeration, for example staphylococci, while others, like malaria parasites, can survive storage in blood at 4° for at least a week. Treatment of blood products with heat or chemicals can inactivate some organisms including some viruses, in particular HIV-I, but blood and blood components cannot be treated in either of these ways. Patients receiving multiple transfusions of pooled plasma products are at increased risk of contracting infections and can be offered immunological protection, for example hepatitis B vaccine.

◊ Reviews.
1. Donaldson MDJ, et al. Massive blood transfusion. *Br J Anaesth* 1992; **69:** 621–30.
2. Contreras M, Mollison PL. Immunological complications of transfusion. In: Contreras M, ed. *ABC of transfusion.* 3rd ed. London: BMJ Books, 1998: 53–7.
3. Barbara JAJ, Contreras M. Infectious complications of blood transfusion: bacteria and parasites. In: Contreras M. ed. *ABC of transfusion.* 3rd ed. London: BMJ Books, 1998: 58–61.
4. Barbara JAJ, Contreras M. Infectious complications of blood transfusion: viruses. In: Contreras M. ed. *ABC of transfusion.* 3rd ed. London: BMJ Books, 1998: 62–6.
5. McClelland DBL, ed. *Handbook of transfusion medicine: Blood Transfusion Services of the United Kingdom.* 3rd ed. London: The Stationery Office, 2001.

Creutzfeldt-Jakob disease. While there is no proof that transmission of Creutzfeldt-Jakob disease by blood or blood products has occurred,[1] it is recognised that there is a need for further assessment of the potential risk of transmission of new variant Creutzfeldt-Jakob disease by such products.[2] As precautionary measures, production of blood products using plasma from UK donors has been phased out and in some countries (including the UK) leucocytes are removed from donated blood (a procedure that early evidence suggests may remove infectivity).

Concern at the risk of transmitting Creutzfeldt-Jakob disease by albumin prepared from placental blood has lead to restriction on this source of albumin (see p.724).
1. Wilson K, et al. Risk of acquiring Creutzfeldt-Jakob disease from blood transfusions: systematic review of case-control studies. *BMJ* 2000; **321:** 17–19.
2. Barbara J, Flanagan P. Blood transfusion risk: protecting against the unknown. *BMJ* 1998; **316:** 717–18.

Effects on leucocytes. A study of 50 patients in an intensive care unit found that 45 of them developed leucocytosis following transfusion of packed red blood cells.[1] The leucocytosis, which was accounted for by neutrophils, occurred immediately after transfusion and persisted for 12 hours.
1. Fenwick JC, et al. Blood transfusion as a cause of leucocytosis in critically ill patients. *Lancet* 1994; **344:** 855–6.

Effects on the lungs. A rare but life-threatening complication of transfusion of blood or other plasma-containing products is acute lung injury.[1] The symptoms, which usually develop 1 to 6 hours after the start of infusion, are those of acute respiratory distress syndrome but usually resolve within about 2 to 4 days with vigorous supportive therapy. The presence of HLA-specific antileucocyte antibodies in plasma from multiparous female donors appears to play a role in initiating the reaction.
1. Popovsky MA, et al. Transfusion-related acute lung injury: a neglected, serious complication of hemotherapy. *Transfusion* 1992; **32:** 589–92.

Graft-versus-host disease. Acute graft-versus-host disease (p.502) has been reported in both immunocompromised and apparently immunocompetent patients following blood transfusion.[1-4] The reaction can be severe and fatal. Symptoms include fever, rash, hepatomegaly and abnormal liver function tests, diarrhoea, and pronounced pancytopenia. Infusion of products containing viable lymphocytes appears to be responsible and patients considered to be at risk may be given products depleted of viable lymphocytes by irradiation. Risk factors are incompletely defined. High-risk groups include bone marrow transplant recipients, patients with congenital immunodeficiencies, and possibly also premature infants undergoing exchange transfusions and patients receiving intensive chemotherapy for Hodgkin's disease. Immunocompetent patients who share an HLA haplotype with HLA-homozygous blood donors also appear to be at increased risk. A study in Japan[5] found that fresh and consanguineous blood transfusion was a major risk factor and that others were cardiovascular surgery, cancer, and being male.
1. Anonymous. Transfusions and graft-versus-host disease. *Lancet* 1989; **i:** 529–30.
2. Anderson KC, Weinstein HJ. Transfusion-associated graft-versus-host disease. *N Engl J Med* 1990; **323:** 315–21.
3. Webb DKH. Irradiation in the prevention of transfusion associated graft-versus-host disease. *Arch Dis Child* 1995; **73:** 388–9.
4. Williamson LM. Transfusion associated graft versus host disease and its prevention. *Heart* 1998; **80:** 211–12.
5. Takahashi K, et al. Analysis of risk factors for post-transfusion graft-versus-host disease in Japan. *Lancet* 1994; **343:** 700–2.

Malignant neoplasms. Blood transfusion is reported to have immunosuppressant effects, and several retrospective studies have suggested that perioperative blood transfusion in patients undergoing surgical resection of their tumours may be associated with an increased rate of tumour recurrence and decreased long-term survival.[1-5] This has been supported by experimental *animal* data.[6] However, the association has not been found in other studies[7,8] and at present there is insufficient data from prospective studies on which to base clinical recommendations.

Blood transfusions have also been associated with increased risk of non-Hodgkin's lymphoma in some studies, although it has been pointed out[9] that confounding factors could account for both the positive and negative associations that have been reported.
1. Burrows L, Tartter P. Effect of blood transfusions on colonic malignancy recurrence rate. *Lancet* 1982; **ii:** 662.
2. Blumberg N, et al. Relation between recurrence of cancer of the colon and blood transfusion. *BMJ* 1985; **290:** 1037–9.
3. Blumberg N, et al. Association between transfusion of whole blood and recurrence of cancer. *BMJ* 1986; **293:** 530–3.
4. Jackson RM, Rice DH. Blood transfusions and recurrence in head and neck cancer. *Ann Otol Rhinol Laryngol* 1989; **98:** 171–3.
5. Blumberg N, et al. The relationship of blood transfusion, tumor staging, and cancer recurrence. *Transfusion* 1990; **30:** 291–4.
6. Waymack JP, Chance WT. Effect of blood transfusions on immune function: IV effect on tumor growth. *J Surg Oncol* 1988; **39:** 159–64.
7. Blair SD, Janvrin SB. Relation between cancer of the colon and blood transfusion. *BMJ* 1985; **290:** 1516–17.
8. Frankish PD, et al. Relation between cancer of the colon and blood transfusion. *BMJ* 1985; **290:** 1827.
9. Alexander FE. Blood transfusion and risk of non-Hodgkin lymphoma. *Lancet* 1997; **350:** 1414–15.

Precautions

Whole blood should generally not be transfused unless the ABO and Rh groups of the patient's and the donor's blood have been verified and a compatibility check made between the patient's serum and the donor's red cells (see under Blood Groups, below).

The Rh group of the recipient should always be determined and ideally all patients should be transfused with blood of homologous Rh groups.

To reduce the possibility of cardiac arrest from cardiac hypothermia when large volumes are used or the blood is transfused rapidly, and to minimise postoperative shivering, stored blood should be carefully warmed to about 37° before transfusion.

Whole blood should not be given to patients with chronic anaemia who have a normal or elevated plasma volume.

Drugs should *not* be added to blood.

Transfusion of blood from donors who have recently been receiving drug treatment may be hazardous to the recipient.

◊ Suggested guidelines[1] for accepting blood from donors who have been receiving drugs.
1. Ferner RE, et al. Drugs in donated blood. *Lancet* 1989; **ii:** 93–4.

Blood groups. The chief blood group systems are the ABO system and the Rhesus system.

In simple terms red blood cells carry on their surface genetically determined antigens. A person with antigen A, B, A plus B, or neither is classified as group A, B, AB, or O respectively. Such persons will have, in their serum, antibodies to B, A, neither, or both respectively—anti-B (β), anti-A (α), or anti-B plus anti-A (α + β). Administration of blood containing red cells from a person of group A to a person with anti-A results in agglutination or possibly haemolysis. For the determination of the ABO group the agglutinogens of the red cells and the agglutinins of the serum are determined by testing against known standards.

In the Rhesus system many persons carry an antigen (Rh-positive) which stimulates antibody formation in Rh-negative persons; subsequent exposure to Rh-positive blood causes haemolysis.

Many variants of these systems, and other systems, are recognised.

Uses and Administration

Blood is a complex fluid with many functions including the maintenance of hydration of the tissues, maintenance of body temperature, and the transport within the body of gases, ions, nutrients, hormones, enzymes, antibodies, waste products of metabolism, and drugs.

The main components of blood are plasma, red blood cells (erythrocytes), white blood cells (leucocytes), and platelets. The leucocytes are classified according to their morphological appearance into granulocytes, lymphocytes, and monocytes. The granulocytes are further classified as neutrophils, eosinophils, and basophils, according to the characteristics of their granules. The term polymorphonuclear leucocytes can be applied to granulocytes in general but applies in particular to neutrophils. Serum is the fluid which remains once blood or plasma has clotted; it is in effect plasma with fibrinogen removed.

Whole blood is used as a source of red cell concentrates, clotting factors, platelets, plasma and plasma fractions, and immunoglobulins, each of which has specific indications for use. Because of the risks involved in transfusing whole blood and the need for economy in its use, the appropriate blood component should be used whenever possible.

Whole blood may be used where replacement of plasma proteins as well as red blood cells is needed, for example following acute blood loss during surgery and severe haemorrhage. It may also be used to supplement the circulation during cardiac bypass surgery.

The amount of whole blood transfused and the rate at which it is given depend upon the patient's age and general condition, upon the state of their circulatory system, and upon the therapeutic indication for transfusion.

The expression 'unit of blood' generally represents a volume of about 510 mL, including anticoagulant. For blood preparations a unit generally refers to the quantity of a blood component obtained from 1 unit of whole blood. Specific units of activity are used for some blood components.

The haemoglobin concentration of the blood of the average adult is raised by about 1 g per 100 mL by the transfusion of 1 unit of whole blood.

◊ Reviews of uses of blood and blood components.
1. Donaldson MDJ, et al. Massive blood transfusion. *Br J Anaesth* 1992; **69:** 621–30.
2. British Committee for Standards in Haematology Blood Transfusion Task Force. Guidelines for administration of blood products: transfusion of infants and neonates. *Transfus Med* 1994; **4:** 63–9.
3. Contreras M, ed. *ABC of transfusion.* 3rd ed. London: BMJ Books, 1998.
4. Goodnough LT, et al. Transfusion medicine: blood transfusion. *N Engl J Med* 1999; **340:** 438–47.
5. McClelland DBL, ed. *Handbook of transfusion medicine: Blood Transfusion Services of the United Kingdom.* 3rd ed. London: The Stationery Office, 2001.

Autologous blood transfusion. Reviews and guidelines regarding autologous blood transfusion, the procedure of a patient acting as his own blood donor, the blood usually being collected shortly before elective surgery or salvaged during the surgical procedure.
1. The National Blood Resource Education Program Expert Panel. The use of autologous blood. *JAMA* 1990; **263:** 414–17.
2. British Committee for Standards in Haematology Blood Transfusion Task Force. Guidelines for autologous transfusion I: preoperative autologous donation. *Transfus Med* 1993; **3:** 307–16.
3. British Committee for Standards in Haematology Blood Transfusion Task Force. Guidelines for autologous transfusion II: perioperative haemodilution and cell salvage. *Br J Anaesth* 1997; **78:** 768–71.
4. Gillon J, Thomas DW. Autologous transfusion. In: Contreras M, ed. *ABC of transfusion.* 3rd ed. London: BMJ Books, 1998: 23–8.
5. Goodnough LT, et al. Transfusion medicine: blood conservation. *N Engl J Med* 1999; **340:** 525–33.
6. McClelland DBL, ed. *Handbook of transfusion medicine: Blood Transfusion Services of the United Kingdom.* 3rd ed. London: The Stationery Office, 2001.

Preparations

USP 25: Whole Blood.

Calcium Alginate (1715-e)

E404.
CAS — 9005-35-0.
ATC — B02BC08.

The calcium salt of alginic acid, a polyuronic acid composed of residues of D-mannuronic and L-guluronic acids. It may be obtained from seaweeds, mainly species of *Laminaria*.

Profile

Calcium alginate is used as an absorbable haemostatic and for the promotion of wound healing (p.1108); it is also used in the form of a mixed calcium-sodium salt of alginic acid as a fibre made into a dressing or packing material. Calcium ions in the calcium alginate fibres are exchanged for sodium ions in the blood and exudate to form a hydrophilic gel.

Alginic acid and its calcium and sodium salts are widely used in the food industry.

◊ References.
1. Thomas S, Tucker CA. Sorbsan in the management of leg ulcers. *Pharm J* 1989; 243: 706–9.
2. Anonymous. Scalpel and seaweed, nurse. *Lancet* 1990; 336: 914.
3. Henderson NJ, *et al.* A randomised trial of calcium alginate swabs to control blood loss in 3–5-year-old children. *Br Dent J* 1998; 184: 187–90. Correction. *ibid.*; 526.

Preparations

Proprietary Preparations (details are given in Part 3)
Austral.: Hydroheal Algin; Kaltostat; Sorbsan; *Fr.:* Algosteril; Coalgan; Sorbalgon; Sorbsan; Stop Hemo; Trophiderm†; *Ger.:* Algosteril; *Irl.:* Algosteril; *Ital.:* Algosteril; Cutinova Alginate; Kaltostat; Sorbsan; *S.Afr.:* Kaltostat; *Switz.:* Stop Hemo†; *UK:* Algistat†; Algosteril; Comfeel Seasorb; Kaltostat; Sorbsan; Stop Hemo†; *USA:* Kaltostat†.

Multi-ingredient: *Austral.:* Kaltocarb†; *Fr.:* Comfeel Seasorb; Melgisorb; *Israel:* Kaltocarb; Kaltostat; *Port.:* Carboflex; Kaltostat; *UK:* Comfeel Plus; Kaltocarb†.

Carbazochrome (1716-I)

Carbazochrome *(rINN)*.
Adrenochrome Monosemicarbazone. 3-Hydroxy-1-methyl-5,6-indolinedione semicarbazone.
$C_{10}H_{12}N_4O_3 = 236.2$.
CAS — 69-81-8 *(carbazochrome)*; 13051-01-9 *(carbazochrome salicylate)*; 51460-26-5 *(carbazochrome sodium sulfonate)*.
ATC — B02BX02.
Pharmacopoeias. Jpn includes Carbazochrome Sodium Sulfonate $(C_{10}H_{11}N_4NaO_5S,3H_2O = 376.3)$.

Profile

Carbazochrome, an oxidation product of adrenaline [epinephrine], has been given as a haemostatic by mouth and by injection; it appears to be given as the dihydrate. It has also been used as the salicylate and the sodium sulfonate.

Preparations

Proprietary Preparations (details are given in Part 3)
Braz.: Adrenoplasma; Adrenoxil; *Ger.:* Adrenoxyl; *Hong Kong:* Adona; Adrezon; *Ital.:* Adona; *Jpn:* Adona; *Port.:* Adrenoxil; *Thai.:* Neo-Hesna.

Multi-ingredient: *Ital.:* Fleboside; *Mex.:* Hemosin-K; *Spain:* Cromoxin K; Flebeside; Perfus Multivitaminico; Quercetol Hemostatico; Quercetol K†.

Oxidised Cellulose (1719-z)

Cellulosic Acid; Oxidized Cellulose.
CAS — 9032-53-5.
ATC — B02BC02.
Pharmacopoeias. In It. and US.
US also includes Oxidized Regenerated Cellulose.

A sterile polyanhydroglucuronic acid, prepared by the oxidation of a suitable form of cellulose.

Pharmacopoeial description

USP 25: Oxidized Cellulose contains not less than 16% and not more than 24% of carboxyl groups, calculated on the dried basis. It is a slightly off-white gauze or lint with a slight, charred odour. Insoluble in water and in acids; soluble in dilute alkalis. Store at a temperature not exceeding 8°. Protect from direct sunlight.

Oxidized Regenerated Cellulose contains 18 to 24% of carboxyl groups calculated on the dried basis. It is a slightly off-white knit fabric, with a slight odour. Insoluble in water and in dilute acids; soluble in dilute alkalis. Store at a temperature between 15° and 30°. Protect from direct sunlight.

Adverse Effects and Precautions

Foreign body reactions may occur after the use of oxidised cellulose or oxidised regenerated cellulose. Headache, burning, and stinging have been reported and sneezing has been noted after use in epistaxis. Oxidised cellulose swells on contact with a bleeding surface; this could result in tissue necrosis, nerve damage, obstruction, or vascular stenosis if packed closely, especially into bony cavities, or if wrapped tightly around blood vessels. To minimise such complications the removal of excess material should be considered after haemostasis is achieved, and oxidised cellulose should always be removed after use near the spinal cord or optic nerve. Oxidised cellulose should not be used in packing or implantation in fractures since it may interfere with bone regeneration or cause cyst formation. It should not be used as a surface dressing, except for immediate control of haemorrhage, as it inhibits epithelialisation.

Oxidised cellulose should be used as the dry material as moistening will reduce its ability to absorb blood. Silver nitrate or other escharotic chemicals should not be applied prior to use as cauterisation might inhibit absorption of oxidised cellulose. Thrombin is inactivated by the low pH of oxidised cellulose; it is recommended that oxidised cellulose should not be impregnated with other haemostatics or antibacterial agents.

Uses and Administration

Oxidised cellulose and oxidised regenerated cellulose are absorbable haemostatics (p.718). When applied to a bleeding surface, they swell to form a gelatinous mass which aids in the formation of a clot. It is gradually absorbed by the tissues, usually within 2 to 7 days. Complete absorption of large amounts of such material may take 6 weeks or more. These materials also have a weak bactericidal action. They are employed in surgery as adjuncts in the control of moderate bleeding where suturing or ligation is impracticable or ineffective; they should not be used to control haemorrhage from large arteries. The gauze, lint, or knitted material should be laid on the bleeding surface or held firmly against the tissues until haemostasis is achieved; removal should then be considered (see Adverse Effects and Precautions, above). Oxidised cellulose should be used as the dry material as moistening will reduce its ability to absorb blood.

Preparations

Proprietary Preparations (details are given in Part 3)
Fr.: Interceed†; Surgicel; *Ger.:* Interceed†; Tabotamp†; *Ital.:* Tabotamp†; *UK:* Interceed; Oxycel; Surgicel; *USA:* Interceed (TC7)†; Oxycel; Surgicel.

Multi-ingredient: *UK:* Seal-On.

Darbepoetin Alfa (20270-f)

Darbepoetin Alfa *(BAN, USAN)*.
NESP; Novel Erythropoiesis Stimulating Protein. 30-L-Asparagine-32-L-threonine-87-L-valine-88-L-asparagine-90-L-threonineerythropoietin (human).
CAS — 209810-58-2.

Profile

Darbepoetin alfa is an analogue of the endogenous protein hormone erythropoietin with similar properties to the epoetins (p.730). It is used in the management of anaemia associated with chronic renal failure (p.717). Darbepoetin alfa is given by subcutaneous or intravenous injection in an initial dose of 0.45 μg per kg body-weight once weekly, as a single injection. The dose should be adjusted at intervals of not less than 4 weeks, according to response, until the target haemoglobin concentration is achieved. Maintenance doses may be given once every 1 or 2 weeks.

Preparations

Proprietary Preparations (details are given in Part 3)
Austral.: Aranesp; *UK:* Aranesp; *USA:* Aranesp.

Dextran 1 (14124-v)

Dextran 1 *(BAN, rINN)*.
Dextranum 1.
CAS — 9004-54-0 *(dextran)*.
Pharmacopoeias. Eur. (see p.vi) describes Dextran 1 for Injection.

Pharmacopoeial description

Ph. Eur.: Dextran 1 for Injection is a low-molecular-weight fraction of dextran, consisting of a mixture of isomalto-oligosaccharides. It is obtained by hydrolysis and fractionation of dextrans produced by fermentation of sucrose using a certain strain or substrains of *Leuconostoc mesenteroides*. The average relative molecular mass is about 1000.

A white or almost white, hygroscopic powder. Very soluble in water; very slightly soluble in alcohol.

Uses and Administration

Dextran 1 is used to prevent severe anaphylactic reactions to infusions of dextran. It is reported to occupy the binding sites of dextran-reactive antibodies and so prevent the formation of large immune complexes with higher molecular weight dextrans.

Dextran 1 is given in usual doses of 20 mL of a solution containing 150 mg per mL by intravenous injection about 1 to 2 minutes before the infusion of the higher molecular weight dextran; the interval should not exceed 15 minutes. A suggested dose for children is 0.3 mL per kg body-weight. The dose of dextran 1 should be repeated if further infusions of dextran are required more than 48 hours after the initial dose.

◊ Two large multicentre studies (involving about 29 200 and 34 950 patients) have suggested that dextran 1 prevented anaphylactic reactions by hapten inhibition in a dose-dependent way.[1,2] It did not reduce the incidence of mild reactions, which are not generally mediated by antibodies. Another large study[3] comparing the effects of giving dextran 1 either 2 minutes before injection of dextran 40 or 70 or mixed with the injection, was discontinued after the occurrence of 2 severe reactions in the admixture group. A comparison[4] of severe anaphylactic reactions to dextran infusion during the period 1983 to 1992 (when prophylaxis with dextran 1 was used) with reactions reported during the period 1975 to 1979 (no prophylaxis) found that the use of dextran 1 was associated with a 35-fold reduction in severe anaphylactic reactions to dextran infusion.

There were 21, 20, and 2 adverse reactions to dextran 1 in the first 3 studies respectively, including nausea, skin reactions, bradycardia, and hypotension. Apart from one patient, reactions to dextran 1 were mild and were considered to be of minor clinical importance. In the fourth study, side-effects to dextran 1 were reported in approximately one case per 100 000 doses.

1. Ljungström K-G, *et al.* Prevention of dextran-induced anaphylactic reactions by hapten inhibition I: a Scandinavian multicenter study on the effects of 10 mL dextran 1, 15% administered before dextran 70 or dextran 40. *Acta Chir Scand* 1983; 149: 341–8.
2. Renck H, *et al.* Prevention of dextran-induced anaphylactic reactions by hapten inhibition III: Scandinavian multicenter study on the effects of 20 mL dextran 1, 15% administered before dextran 70 or dextran 40. *Acta Chir Scand* 1983; 149: 355–60.
3. Renck H, *et al.* Prevention of dextran-induced anaphylactic reactions by hapten inhibition II: a comparison of the effects of 20 mL dextran 1, 15% administered either admixed to or before dextran 70 or dextran 40. *Acta Chir Scand* 1983; 149: 349–53.
4. Ljungström K-G. Hapten inhibition of dextran reactions. Ten years' experience with dextran 1. *Br J Anaesth* 1995; 74 (suppl 1): 127.

Preparations

Proprietary Preparations (details are given in Part 3)
Aust.: Praedex; Promit; *Austral.:* Promit; *Denm.:* Promiten; *Fr.:* Promit; *Ger.:* Promit; *Norw.:* Promiten; *S.Afr.:* Promit; *Swed.:* Promiten; *Switz.:* Promit; *USA:* Promit.

Dextran 40 (251-w)

Dextran 40 *(BAN, USAN, rINN)*.
Dextranum 40; LMD; LMWD; Low-molecular-weight Dextran; LVD.
CAS — 9004-54-0 *(dextran)*.
Pharmacopoeias. In Chin., Jpn, Pol., and US.
Eur. (see p.vi) and Jpn describe Dextran 40 for Injection.

Incompatibilities may arise from the slightly acid pH of dextran 40 preparations.

Pharmacopoeial description

Ph. Eur.: Dextran 40 for Injection is a mixture of polysaccharides, principally of the α-1,6-glucan type, obtained by hydrolysis and fractionation of dextrans produced by fermentation of sucrose using a certain strain or substrains of *Leuconostoc mesenteroides*. The average relative molecular mass is about 40 000.

A white or almost white powder. Very soluble in water; very slightly soluble in alcohol; slightly soluble in ether.

USP 25: Dextran 40 is derived by controlled hydrolysis and fractionation of polysaccharides elaborated by the fermentative action of certain strains of *Leuconostoc mesenteroides* on a sucrose substrate. It is a glucose polymer in which the linkages between glucose units are almost entirely of the α-1:6 type. Its weight average molecular weight is in the 35 000 to 45 000 range. A 10% solution in water has a pH of 4.5 to 7.0.

Adverse Effects, Treatment, and Precautions

As for Dextran 70, p.729.

Rapid renal excretion of dextran 40 in patients with reduced urine flow can result in high urinary concentrations which increase urinary viscosity and may cause oliguria or acute renal failure. Therefore, infusions of dextran 40 are contra-indicated in renal disease with oliguria; should anuria or oliguria occur during treatment dextran 40 should be withdrawn. Dehydration should preferably be corrected before administration of dextran 40. Dextran 40 can cause capillary oozing of wound surfaces.

Effects on the kidneys. Acute renal failure has been associated with dextran 40[1-3] and less frequently with dextran 70.[4-5] The mechanism of the effect is still unclear[2-5] but low-molecular-weight dextran has been cited[1] as a common cause of drug-induced acute renal failure. Dextran should be withheld if the urine output falls during administration and diuresis induced with diuretics and a high fluid intake. Plasmapheresis has been used successfully to remove dextran from the circulation.[2]

1. Feest TG. Low molecular weight dextran: a continuing cause of acute renal failure. *BMJ* 1976; **2**: 1300.
2. Moran M, Kapsner C. Acute renal failure associated with elevated plasma oncotic pressure. *N Engl J Med* 1987; **317**: 150–3.
3. Druml W, *et al.* Dextran-40, acute renal failure, and elevated plasma oncotic pressure. *N Engl J Med* 1988; **318**: 252–3.
4. Stein HD. Dextran-40, acute renal failure, and elevated plasma oncotic pressure. *N Engl J Med* 1988; **318**: 253.
5. Moran M, Kapsner C. Dextran-40, acute renal failure, and elevated plasma oncotic pressure. *N Engl J Med* 1988; **318**: 253–4.

Effects on the lungs. In a study[1] of 45 women undergoing gynaecological surgery, 25 received 400 to 500 mL of a 10% solution of dextran 40 intraperitoneally for prevention of adhesions. After 5 to 7 days, 12 of the dextran group and none of the controls had a pleural effusion visible on chest X-ray. The effusions were small to moderate, asymptomatic, and resolved without treatment.

1. Adoni A, *et al.* Postoperative pleural effusion caused by dextran. *Int J Gynaecol Obstet* 1980; **18**: 243–74.

Hypersensitivity. For reports of anaphylactic reactions associated with administration of dextran 40, see Dextran 70, below, and Dextran 1, above.

Pharmacokinetics
After intravenous infusion of dextran 40, about 70% is excreted unchanged in the urine within 24 hours. The dextran not excreted is slowly metabolised to glucose. A small amount is excreted into the gastrointestinal tract and eliminated in the faeces.

Uses and Administration
Dextran 40 is a plasma volume expander used in the management of hypovolaemic shock (p.813). As a 10% solution, dextran 40 exerts a slightly higher colloidal osmotic pressure than plasma proteins and thus produces a greater expansion of plasma volume than dextrans of a higher molecular weight, although the expansion may have a shorter duration because of more rapid renal excretion. Dextran 40 also reduces blood viscosity and inhibits sludging or aggregation of red blood cells. It is used in the prophylaxis and treatment of postoperative thromboembolic disorders, in conditions where improved circulatory flow is required, and as a priming solution during extracorporeal circulation.

Dextran 40 is given by intravenous infusion as a 10% solution in sodium chloride 0.9% or glucose 5%. Doses depend on the clinical condition of the patient.

In shock, a maximum of 20 mL per kg body-weight during the first 24 hours has been recommended; the first 10 mL per kg may be given by rapid intravenous infusion. Doses of up to 10 mL per kg may be given daily thereafter for up to 5 days. Dehydration should preferably be corrected before dextran 40 is administered.

In the treatment of thromboembolic disorders a suggested regimen is 500 to 1000 mL over 4 to 6 hours on the first day, then 500 mL over 4 to 6 hours on the next and subsequent alternate days for not more than 10 days.

For prophylaxis of postoperative thromboembolic disorders, 500 mL over 4 to 6 hours may be given during or at the end of surgery and the dose repeated on the next day; treatment may be continued in high risk patients on alternate days for up to 10 days.

Infants may be given up to 5 mL per kg body-weight and children up to 10 mL per kg.

A dose of 10 to 20 mL per kg has been added to extracorporeal perfusion fluids.

Dextran 40 is also an ingredient of artificial tears.

Venous thromboembolism. Dextran 40 is only one of a variety of drugs that have been used for the prophylaxis of venous thromboembolism (p.817) resulting from surgical operations. In hip replacement surgery[1] warfarin and dextran 40 gave similar protection whereas in general surgery[2] heparin was better than dextran 40 in preventing deep-vein thrombosis. Dextran 40 was considerably less effective than a combination of antithrombin III and heparin in total knee arthroplasty.[3]

1. Harris WH, *et al.* Prevention of venous thromboembolism following total hip replacement: warfarin vs dextran 40. *JAMA* 1972; **220**: 1319–22.
2. Gruber UF, *et al.* Prevention of postoperative thromboembolism by dextran 40, low doses of heparin, or xantinol nicotinate. *Lancet* 1977; **i**: 207–10.
3. Francis CW, *et al.* Prevention of venous thrombosis after total knee arthroplasty: comparison of antithrombin III and low-dose heparin with dextran. *J Bone Joint Surg Am* 1990; **72-A**; 976–82.

Preparations
BP 2001: Dextran 40 Intravenous Infusion;
USP 25: Dextran 40 in Dextrose Injection; Dextran 40 in Sodium Chloride Injection.

Proprietary Preparations (details are given in Part 3)
Aust.: Elorheo; Laevodex; Onkovertin N; Rheofusin; Rheomacrodex; *Austral.:* Rheomacrodex; *Braz.:* Isodex; Rheomacrodex; *Canad.:* Gentran 40; Rheomacrodex†; *Denm.:* Rheomacrodex; *Fr.:* Plasmacair†; Rheomacrodex; *Ger.:* Infukoll M 40; Longasteril 40; Onkovertin N; Rheomacrodex; Thomaedex 40; *Israel:* Rheomacrodex; *Ital.:* Eudextran; Plander R; Solplex 40; *Mex.:* Rheomacrodex; *Norw.:* Rheomacrodex; *Port.:* Neodextril 40; *S.Afr.:* Rheomacrodex; *Spain:* Rheomacrodex; *Swed.:* Perfadex;

Rheomacrodex; *Switz.:* Rheomacrodex; *UK:* Gentran 40; Rheomacrodex†; *USA:* Gentran 40; Rheomacrodex.

Multi-ingredient: *Canad.:* Ocutears†; *Port.:* Bas-Dextrano.

Dextran 60 (16294-c)

Pharmacopoeias. Eur. (see p.vi) describes Dextran 60 for Injection.

Incompatibilities may arise from the slightly acid pH of dextran 60 preparations.

Pharmacopoeial description
Ph. Eur.: Dextran 60 for Injection is a mixture of polysaccharides, principally of the α-1,6-glucan type, obtained by hydrolysis and fractionation of dextrans produced by fermentation of sucrose using a certain strain or substrains of *Leuconostoc mesenteroides*. The average relative molecular mass is about 60 000.

A white or almost white powder. Very soluble in water; very slightly soluble in alcohol; slightly soluble in ether.

Profile
Dextran 60 is a plasma volume expander with actions and uses similar to those of dextran 70 (below). It is given by intravenous infusion as a 3% or 6% solution in sodium chloride 0.9% or a mixture of electrolytes.

Dextran 60 is also used topically for dry eyes.

Preparations
Proprietary Preparations (details are given in Part 3)
Aust.: Laevodex; Macrodex; Onkovertin; *Fr.:* Dialens†; Hemodex; *Ger.:* Macrodex; Onkovertin†; Thomaedex 60; *Norw.:* Plasmodex; *Swed.:* Plasmodex; *Switz.:* Dialens.

Dextran 70 (252-e)

Dextran 70 (BAN, USAN, rINN).
Dextranum 70; Polyglucin (dextran).
CAS — 9004-54-0 (dextran).

Pharmacopoeias. In *Chin., Jpn, Pol.,* and *US.*
Eur. (see p.vi) and *Jpn* describe Dextran 70 for Injection.

Incompatibilities may arise from the slightly acid pH of dextran 70 preparations.

Crystals may form in solutions of dextran if they are stored at low temperatures. These may be redissolved by warming for a short time.

Pharmacopoeial description
Ph. Eur.: Dextran 70 for Injection is a mixture of polysaccharides, principally of the α-1,6-glucan type, obtained by hydrolysis and fractionation of dextrans produced by fermentation of sucrose using a certain strain or substrains of *Leuconostoc mesenteroides*. The average relative molecular mass is about 70 000.

A white or almost white powder. Very soluble in water; very slightly soluble in alcohol; slightly soluble in ether.

USP 25: Dextran 70 is derived by controlled hydrolysis and fractionation of polysaccharides elaborated by the fermentative action of certain appropriate strains of *Leuconostoc mesenteroides* on a sucrose substrate. It is a glucose polymer in which the linkages between glucose units are almost entirely of the α-1:6 type. Its weight average molecular weight is in the 63 000 to 77 000 range. A 6% solution in water has a pH of 4.5 to 7.0.

Adverse Effects and Treatment
Infusions of dextrans may occasionally produce hypersensitivity reactions such as fever, nasal congestion, joint pains, urticaria, hypotension, and bronchospasm. Severe anaphylactic reactions occur rarely and may be fatal. Dextran-reactive antibodies may arise in response to dietary or bacterial polysaccharides in patients who have not previously received dextran. Nausea and vomiting have also been reported. These reactions are treated symptomatically after withdrawal of the dextran.

Dextran 1 (p.728) may be used to block the formation of dextran-reactive antibodies and hence the hypersensitivity reactions.

Effects on the blood. Disseminated intravascular coagulation and acute respiratory distress syndrome developed following hysteroscopy during which 1200 mL of dextran 70 was used to dilate the uterus.[1] The large volume used was considered to have contributed to the reaction by increasing the systemic absorption of the dextran solution.

1. Jedeikin R, *et al.* Disseminated intravascular coagulopathy and adult respiratory distress syndrome: life-threatening complications of hysteroscopy. *Am J Obstet Gynecol* 1990; **162**: 44–5.

Effects on the kidneys. For a report of acute renal failure associated with use of dextran 70, see Dextran 40, above.

Hypersensitivity. In a retrospective study of allergic reactions to dextran 40 and dextran 70 reported in Sweden from 1970 to 1979,[1] there were 478 reports of reactions, 458 of

which were considered to be due to dextran, out of 1 365 266 infusions given. There was a male to female ratio of 1.5 to 1 for all reactions and a ratio of 3 to 1 for the most severe reactions. The mean age of the patients was higher in those with severe reactions. Of the 28 fatal reactions, 27 occurred within 5 minutes of the start of the infusion and 25 when less than 25 mL had been infused. Three of the fatal reactions occurred after a test dose of only 0.5 to 1.0 mL and it was strongly recommended that such test doses should not be used.

An anaphylactic reaction has also been reported[2] more than 75 minutes after intraperitoneal instillation. After successful symptomatic treatment symptoms recurred 20 minutes later, due to slow absorption of dextran from the peritoneal cavity. No further reaction occurred after removal of 200 mL of intraperitoneal fluid by culdocentesis.

Anaphylactoid reactions after BCG vaccination have been attributed to hypersensitivity to dextran in the formulation.[3,4]

The use of dextran 1 for the prevention of hypersensitivity reactions is discussed under that monograph (p.728).

1. Ljungström K-G, *et al.* Adverse reactions to dextran in Sweden 1970–1979. *Acta Chir Scand* 1983; **149**: 253–62.
2. Borten M, *et al.* Recurrent anaphylactic reaction to intraperitoneal dextran 75 used for prevention of postsurgical adhesions. *Obstet Gynecol* 1983; **61**: 755–7.
3. Rudin C, *et al.* Anaphylactoid reaction to BCG vaccination. *Lancet* 1991; **337**: 377.
4. Pönnighaus JM, *et al.* Hypersensitivity to dextran in BCG vaccine. *Lancet* 1991; **337**: 1039.

Precautions
Dextran infusions produce a progressive dilution of oxygen-carrying capacity, coagulation factors, and plasma proteins and may overload the circulation. They are therefore contra-indicated in patients with severe heart failure, bleeding disorders such as hypofibrinogenaemia or thrombocytopenia, or renal failure and should be administered with caution to patients with impaired renal function, haemorrhage, chronic liver disease, or those at risk of developing pulmonary oedema or heart failure. Central venous pressure should be monitored during the initial period of infusion to detect fluid overload. Also patients should be watched closely during the early part of the infusion period, and the infusion stopped immediately if signs of anaphylactic reactions appear. Infusions should also be stopped if there are signs of oliguria or renal failure. The haematocrit should not be allowed to fall below 30% and all patients should be observed for early signs of bleeding complications. The bleeding time may be increased especially in patients receiving large volumes of dextrans. Deficiency of coagulation factors should be corrected and fluid and electrolyte balance maintained. Dehydration should be corrected before or at least during dextran infusions, in order to maintain an adequate urine flow.

The anticoagulant effect of heparin may be enhanced by dextran.

The higher molecular weight dextrans may interfere with blood grouping and cross-matching of blood, while the lower molecular weight dextrans may interfere with some methods. Therefore, whenever possible, a sample of blood should be collected before giving the dextran infusion and kept frozen in case such tests become necessary.

The presence of dextran may interfere with the determination of glucose, bilirubin, or protein in blood or urine.

Pharmacokinetics
After intravenous infusion dextrans with a molecular weight of less than 50 000 are excreted unchanged by the kidney. Dextrans with a molecular weight greater than 50 000 are slowly metabolised to glucose. Small amounts of dextrans are excreted into the gastrointestinal tract and eliminated in the faeces.

About 50% of dextran 70 is excreted unchanged in the urine within 24 hours.

Uses and Administration
Dextran 70 is a plasma volume expander used in the management of hypovolaemic shock (p.813). As a 6% solution dextran 70 exerts a colloidal osmotic pressure similar to that of plasma proteins and thus produces less expansion of plasma volume than dextrans of a lower molecular weight, although the expansion may have a longer duration because of less

rapid renal excretion. Dextran 70 also reduces blood viscosity and inhibits sludging or aggregation of red blood cells. It is used in the prophylaxis of postoperative thromboembolic disorders (p.817).

Dextran 70 is given by intravenous infusion as a 6% solution in sodium chloride 0.9% or glucose 5%.

Doses depend on the severity of the plasma loss and on the degree of haemoconcentration.

In shock, the usual initial dose for rapid expansion of plasma volume is 500 to 1000 mL infused at a rate of 20 to 40 mL per minute. A suggested maximum dose is 20 mL per kg body-weight during the first 24-hour period and 10 mL per kg per day thereafter; treatment should not continue for longer than 3 days. Patients may also require administration of blood, coagulation factors, and electrolytes.

For the prophylaxis of pulmonary embolism or venous thrombosis in moderate- to high-risk patients undergoing surgery, a dose of 500 to 1000 mL may be given over 4 to 6 hours either during or immediately after surgery. A dose of 500 mL should be given on the next day and in high-risk patients on subsequent alternate days for up to 2 weeks after the operation.

A 32% solution of dextran 70 has been instilled into the uterus in a dose of 50 to 100 mL as a rinsing and dilatation fluid to aid hysteroscopy.

Dextran 70 is also an ingredient of artificial tears.

Preparations

BP 2001: Dextran 70 Intravenous Infusion;
USP 25: Dextran 70 in Dextrose Injection; Dextran 70 in Sodium Chloride Injection.

Proprietary Preparations (details are given in Part 3)
Austral.: Hyskon; Macrodex†; *Canad.:* Gentran 70; Hyskon†; Macrodex†; *Denm.:* Macrodex; RescueFlow; *Ger.:* Hyskon†; Longasteril 70; *Israel:* Macrodex; *Ital.:* Plander; Solplex 70; *Mex.:* Macrodex; *Norw.:* Macrodex; *Port.:* Neodextril 70; *S.Afr.:* Macrodex; *Spain:* Macrodex; *Swed.:* Hyskon†; Macrodex; RescueFlow; *Switz.:* Macrodex; *UK:* Gentran 70; Hyskon; Macrodex; RescueFlow; *USA:* Gentran 70; Hyskon; Macrodex.

Multi-ingredient: *Austral.:* Bion Tears; Poly-Tears; Tears Naturale; Visine Advanced Relief; *Belg.:* Alcon Adequad; Lacrystat; Tears Naturale; *Canad.:* Aquasite; Bion Tears; Tears Naturale; *Denm.:* Dacriosol; *Ger.:* Isopto Naturale; *Irl.:* Tears Naturale; *Israel:* Tears Naturale; *Ital.:* Dacriosol; *Neth.:* Duratears†; *NZ:* Poly-Tears; Tears Naturale; *Port.:* Tears Naturale; *S.Afr.:* Tears Naturale; *Singapore:* Bion Tears; Dacrolux; Tears Naturale; *Spain:* Dacrolux; Tears Humectante; *Swed.:* Bion Tears; Tears Naturale; *Switz.:* Tears Naturale; *Thai.:* Tears Naturale; *UK:* Tears Naturale; *USA:* Advanced Relief Visine; Aquasite; Bion Tears; Lacri-Tears; LubriTears; Moisture Drops; Nature's Tears; Ocucoat; Tears Naturale; Tears Renewed.

Dextran 75 (14125-g)

Dextran 75 *(BAN, USAN, rINN)*.
Dextranum 75.
CAS — 9004-54-0 (dextran).

Dextran 75 consists of dextrans (glucose polymers) of weight average molecular weight about 75 000 that are derived from the dextrans produced by the fermentation of sucrose by means of a certain strain of *Leuconostoc mesenteroides*.

Profile
Dextran 75 is a plasma volume expander with actions and uses similar to dextran 70 (p.729). It is given by intravenous infusion as a 6% solution in sodium chloride 0.9% or glucose 5%.

Preparations

Proprietary Preparations (details are given in Part 3)
USA: Gentran 75†.

Dextran 110 (253-l)

Dextran 110 *(BAN, rINN)*.
Dextranum 110.
CAS — 9004-54-0 (dextran).
Pharmacopoeias. Br. describes Dextran 110 Intravenous Infusion.

Pharmacopoeial description
BP 2001: Dextran 110 Intravenous Infusion is a sterile solution of dextrans of weight average molecular weight about 110 000, derived from dextrans produced by the fermentation of sucrose using a certain strain of *Leuconostoc mesenteroides*. The dextrans are polymers of glucose in which the linkages between the glucose units are almost entirely of the α-1,6 type.
An almost colourless, slightly viscous solution.

Profile
Dextran 110 is a plasma volume expander with actions and uses similar to dextran 70 (p.729). It has been given by intravenous infusion as a 6% solution.

Epoetins (16635-r)

BI-71.052 (epoetin gamma); BM-06.019 (epoetin beta); EPO (epoetin alfa); EPOCH (epoetin beta).
CAS — 113427-24-0 (epoetin alfa); 122312-54-3 (epoetin beta); 130455-76-4 (epoetin gamma).

Pharmacopoeias. Eur. (see p.vi) includes Erythropoietin Concentrated Solution.

Erythropoietin is a glycosylated protein hormone and a haematopoietic growth factor produced primarily in the kidneys. Erythropoietin for clinical use is produced by recombinant DNA technology and the name epoetin is often applied to such material. **Epoetin alfa** *(BAN, USAN, rINN)*, **epoetin beta** *(BAN, USAN, rINN)*, and **epoetin gamma** *(BAN, rINN)* are recombinant human erythropoietins derived from a cloned human erythropoietin gene. All have the same 165 amino acid sequence but differ in the glycosylation pattern.

Pharmacopoeial description
Ph. Eur.: Erythropoietin Concentrated Solution is a clear or slightly turbid colourless solution, containing 0.05 to 1% of glycoproteins indistinguishable from naturally occurring human erythropoietin in terms of amino acid sequence and glycosylation pattern. It has a potency of not less than 100 000 units per mg of active substance. Store in airtight containers below −20° and avoid repeated freezing and thawing.

Stability. Proprietary preparations of recombinant human erythropoietin contain albumin or amino acids for stability. Administration to neonates may necessitate making very dilute solutions. A study of the stability of epoetin alfa in various intravenous fluids[1] found that a minimum of 0.05% protein was required to prevent loss of drug from solutions containing epoetin alfa 0.1 units per mL. In another study,[2] 0.0125% albumin was sufficient to prevent loss of drug from a solution containing epoetin alfa 100 units per mL.
1. Ohls RK, Christensen RD. Stability of human recombinant epoetin alfa in commonly used neonatal intravenous solutions. *Ann Pharmacother* 1996; **30:** 466–8.
2. Widness JA, Schmidt RL. Comment: epoetin alfa loss with NaCl 0.9% dilution. *Ann Pharmacother* 1996; **30:** 1501–2.

Adverse Effects
Headache, hypertension, and seizures have been reported in patients treated with recombinant human erythropoietin particularly in those with poor renal function. These adverse effects are probably associated with haemodynamic changes produced by the increase in haematocrit. In patients with normal or low blood pressure there have been isolated reports of hypertensive crisis with encephalopathy-like symptoms, including headache and confusion, and generalised seizures. Other adverse effects include thrombosis at vascular access sites and clotting in the dialyser, transient increases in the platelet count, flu-like symptoms including chills and myalgia, hyperkalaemia, and skin rashes. There have been rare reports of anaphylactoid reactions. Pure red cell aplasia has been reported rarely in patients with chronic renal failure after months to years of treatment with epoetin alfa; most patients have been found to have antibodies to epoetins.

◊ General references.
1. Macdougall IC. Adverse reactions profile: erythropoietin in chronic renal failure. *Prescribers' J* 1992; **32:** 40–4.

Effects on the blood. Changes in rheological properties of the blood following recombinant human erythropoietin therapy were attributed to high red cell aggregation, possibly due to hyperfibrinogenaemia.[1] The increased viscosity could have contributed to an early kidney graft thrombosis in 1 patient[2] and a delay in the onset of graft function in 7 others.[3] Pre-operative haemodilution was suggested as a possible solution.[3]
1. Koppensteiner R, *et al.* Changes in determinants of blood rheology during treatment with haemodialysis and recombinant human erythropoietin. *BMJ* 1990; **300:** 1626–7.
2. Zaoui P, *et al.* Early thrombosis in kidney grafted into patient treated with erythropoietin. *Lancet* 1988; **ii:** 956.
3. Wahlberg J, *et al.* Haemodilution in renal transplantation in patients on erythropoietin. *Lancet* 1988; **ii:** 1418.

Effects on electrolytes. Hyperkalaemia and hyperphosphataemia may occur in patients receiving recombinant human erythropoietin. However, hypophosphataemia has also been reported in cirrhotic patients given erythropoietin prior to autologous blood donation.[1]
1. Kajikawa M, *et al.* Recombinant human erythropoietin and hypophosphatemia in patients with cirrhosis. *Lancet* 1993; **341:** 503–4.

Effects on mental function. Visual hallucinations occurred in 4 patients during treatment with recombinant human erythropoietin, stopped when treatment was withdrawn, and re-occurred in 2 patients when erythropoietin was reinstituted.[1] Commenting on these and a further 7 cases,[2] the manufacturers considered the reaction to be extremely rare and that the contribution of concurrent medication could not be discounted. In two groups of dialysis patients treated with recombinant human erythropoietin, 15 of 134 and 2 of 103 experienced visual hallucinations.[3] Increasing age appeared to be a risk factor.
1. Steinberg H. Erythropoietin and visual hallucinations. *N Engl J Med* 1991; **325:** 285.
2. Stead RB. Erythropoietin and visual hallucinations. *N Engl J Med* 1991; **325:** 285.
3. Steinberg H, *et al.* Erythropoietin and visual hallucinations in patients on dialysis. *Psychosomatics* 1996; **37:** 556–63.

Effects on the skin. Skin rashes may occur during treatment with recombinant human erythropoietin.
Pseudoporphyria cutanea tarda, a photosensitivity disorder, has been reported in 2 children undergoing peritoneal dialysis and receiving erythropoietin.[1] However, it was pointed out that this disorder has occurred in adults undergoing dialysis and the children were also receiving other potentially photosensitising drugs.
1. Harvey E, *et al.* Pseudoporphyria cutanea tarda: two case reports on children receiving peritoneal dialysis and erythropoietin therapy. *J Pediatr* 1992; **121:** 749–52.

Effects on the spleen. Aggravation of splenomegaly was reported in 2 patients with myeloproliferative disorders following administration of recombinant human erythropoietin.[1] Splenic infarction has been reported in a patient with aplastic anaemia treated with erythropoietin.[2]
1. Iki S, *et al.* Adverse effect of erythropoietin in myeloproliferative disorders. *Lancet* 1991; **337:** 187–8.
2. Imashuku S, *et al.* Splenic infarction after erythropoietin therapy. *Lancet* 1993; **342:** 182–3.

Effects of subcutaneous injection. More pain at the injection site was experienced by patients given subcutaneous injections of epoetin alfa than in those given epoetin beta.[1,2] It was suggested that different excipients in the two formulations could be responsible.[1,2]
1. Frenken LAM, *et al.* Assessment of pain after subcutaneous injection of erythropoietin in patients receiving haemodialysis. *BMJ* 1991; **303:** 288.
2. Lui SF, *et al.* Pain after subcutaneous injection of erythropoietin. *BMJ* 1991; **303:** 856.

Treatment of adverse effects. Venesection successfully reduced the blood pressure in 4 patients with life-threatening hypertension unresponsive to antihypertensive therapy associated with recombinant human erythropoietin treatment.[1]
1. Fahal IH, *et al.* Phlebotomy for erythropoietin-associated malignant hypertension. *Lancet* 1991; **337:** 1227.

Precautions
Recombinant human erythropoietin should be used with caution in patients with hypertension, a history of seizures, thrombocytosis, chronic hepatic impairment, ischaemic vascular disease, or in patients with malignant tumours. Hypertension should be well controlled before treatment is started and the blood pressure monitored during treatment.

Response to recombinant human erythropoietin may be diminished by iron deficiency, infection or inflammatory disorders, haemolysis, or aluminium intoxication. Anaemia due to folic acid and vitamin B_{12} deficiencies should also be excluded, since these may also reduce the response. Patients developing sudden lack of efficacy should be investigated. If pure red cell aplasia is diagnosed treatment should be discontinued and testing for epoetin antibodies considered; patients should not be transferred to another epoetin.

Patients undergoing dialysis may require increased doses of heparin in view of the increase in packed cell volume.

Platelet counts and serum-potassium concentrations should be monitored regularly.

Dosage must be carefully controlled to avoid too fast an increase in haematocrit and recommended haematocrit levels should not be exceeded due to the increased risk of thrombotic events.

◊ A study[1] involving 1233 patients undergoing haemodialysis and suffering from heart failure or ischaemic heart disease found that erythropoietin in doses sufficient to increase haematocrit to 42% (within the normal range) was associated with lack of benefit and a trend towards increased mortality when compared with administration in doses sufficient to maintain a lower haematocrit of around 30%. However, these results are difficult to interpret, since within each group, increased haematocrit was associated with lower mortality, despite the between-group differences. The possibility that intravenous iron supplementation might have contributed to these adverse results was considered, but commentators suggested that until further data was available aiming for a haematocrit of 33 to 36%, and using intravenous iron supplementation where necessary, was still appropriate.[2]

1. Besarab A, *et al.* The effects of normal as compared with low hematocrit values in patients with cardiac disease who are receiving hemodialysis and epoetin. *N Engl J Med* 1998; **339:** 584–90.
2. Adamson JW, Eschbach JW. Erythropoietin for end-stage renal disease. *N Engl J Med* 1998; **339:** 625–7.

Abuse. Comments on the dangers of the abuse of recombinant human erythropoietin by athletes as an alternative to 'blood doping'.[1-4] Haematocrit may continue to rise for several days after administration of recombinant human erythropoietin, possibly reaching dangerously high levels. Lack of medical supervision and fluid loss during endurance events increase the risk of serious adverse consequences of changes in blood viscosity produced by such misuse.

1. Scott WC. The abuse of erythropoietin to enhance athletic performance. *JAMA* 1990; **264:** 1660.
2. Adamson JW, Vapnek D. Recombinant erythropoietin to improve athletic performance. *N Engl J Med* 1991; **324:** 698–9.
3. Kennedy M. Drugs and athletes—an update. *Adverse Drug React Bull* 1994; **169:** 639–42.
4. MacAuley D. Drugs in sport. *BMJ* 1996; **313:** 211–15.

Resistance. Many factors may contribute to a poor response to recombinant human erythropoietin (see above). A study in patients with anaemia of end-stage renal disease[1] found that inadequate dialysis was associated with a reduced response to erythropoietin treatment. Antibodies to recombinant human erythropoietin have also been reported.[2] Delayed clinical response to recombinant human erythropoietin in a patient[3] could have been due to an inherited subclinical pyruvate kinase deficiency.

1. Ifudu O, *et al.* The intensity of hemodialysis and the response to erythropoietin in patients with end-stage renal disease. *N Engl J Med* 1996; **334:** 420–5.
2. Peces R, *et al.* Antibodies against recombinant human erythropoietin in a patient with erythropoietin-resistant anemia. *N Engl J Med* 1996; **335:** 523–4.
3. Zachée P, *et al.* Pyruvate kinase deficiency and delayed clinical response to recombinant human erythropoietin treatment. *Lancet* 1989; **i:** 1327–8.

Pharmacokinetics

Epoetin alfa and epoetin beta exhibit some differences in their pharmacokinetics, possibly due to differences in glycosylation and in the formulation of the commercial preparations.

Epoetin alfa is slowly and incompletely absorbed following subcutaneous injection, and a bioavailability of about 10 to 50% relative to intravenous administration has been reported. Peak concentrations following epoetin alfa intravenously are attained within 15 minutes, and within 4 to 24 hours following subcutaneous injection.

The elimination half-life of epoetin alfa following intravenous administration has been reported to be 4 to 16 hours in patients with chronic renal failure; the half-life is generally less in patients with normal renal function. An estimated elimination half-life of about 24 hours has been reported for epoetin alfa given subcutaneously.

Epoetin beta is similarly slowly and incompletely absorbed after subcutaneous injection, and its absolute bioavailability has been reported to be 23 to 42%. Peak serum concentrations are attained within 12 to 28 hours of subcutaneous administration. An elimination half-life of 4 to 12 hours has been reported following intravenous administration and a terminal half-life of 13 to 28 hours following subcutaneous administration.

◊ References.

1. Macdougall IC, *et al.* Clinical pharmacokinetics of epoetin (recombinant human erythropoietin). *Clin Pharmacokinet* 1991; **20:** 99–113.
2. Halstenson CE, *et al.* Comparative pharmacokinetics and pharmacodynamics of epoetin alfa and epoetin beta. *Clin Pharmacol Ther* 1991; **50:** 702–12.
3. Gladziwa U, *et al.* Pharmacokinetics of epoetin (recombinant human erythropoietin) after long term therapy in patients undergoing haemodialysis and haemofiltration. *Clin Pharmacokinet* 1993; **25:** 145–53.
4. Montini G, *et al.* Pharmacokinetics and hematologic response to subcutaneous administration of recombinant human erythropoietin in children undergoing long-term peritoneal dialysis: a multicenter study. *J Pediatr* 1993; **122:** 297–302.
5. Brown MS, *et al.* Single-dose pharmacokinetics of recombinant human erythropoietin in preterm infants after intravenous and subcutaneous administration. *J Pediatr* 1993; **122:** 655–7.

Uses and Administration

Erythropoietin is a glycosylated protein hormone and a haematopoietic growth factor. It is secreted primarily by the kidneys, although a small amount is pro-

duced in extrarenal sites such as the liver. Erythropoietin regulates erythropoiesis by stimulating the differentiation and proliferation of erythroid precursors, stimulating the release of reticulocytes into the circulation, and stimulating the synthesis of cellular haemoglobin. The release of erythropoietin is promoted by hypoxia or anaemia, and up to 1000 times the normal serum-erythropoietin concentration may be reached under these conditions; this response may be impaired in some disease states such as chronic renal failure. The haematological response to erythropoietin is reduced if there is an inadequate supply of iron.

Epoetin alfa and epoetin beta are recombinant human erythropoietins available for clinical use that have the same pharmacological actions as endogenous erythropoietin. They are used in the management of anaemia associated with chronic renal failure in dialysis and predialysis patients; they may reduce or obviate the need for blood transfusions in these patients. They are also used in the management of chemotherapy-induced anaemia in patients with non-myeloid malignant disease. Epoetin alfa is used in zidovudine-related anaemia in HIV-positive patients. Epoetin beta is used in the management of anaemia of prematurity. Recombinant human erythropoietin is also being evaluated in the management of other types of normocytic-normochromic anaemias, including that associated with inflammatory disorders such as rheumatoid arthritis. In all patients, iron status should be monitored and supplementation provided if necessary.

Epoetin alfa and epoetin beta may also be used in patients with moderate anaemia (but no iron deficiency) before elective surgery to increase the yield of blood collected for autologous blood transfusion. Epoetin alfa may also be used in such patients to reduce the need for allogeneic blood transfusion.

In the management of **anaemia of chronic renal failure** epoetin alfa or epoetin beta may be given subcutaneously or intravenously. The aim of treatment is to increase the haemoglobin concentration to 10 to 12 g per 100 mL or to increase the haematocrit to 30 to 36%. The rate of rise in haemoglobin should be gradual to minimise side-effects such as hypertension; a rate not exceeding 2 g per 100 mL per month is suggested.

Epoetin alfa may be given subcutaneously or by intravenous injection over at least 1 minute; slow intravenous injection over 5 minutes may be used in patients who experience flu-like symptoms as side-effects. In predialysis and haemodialysis patients, a recommended initial dose of epoetin alfa is 50 international units per kg body-weight three times weekly; a higher initial dose of 50 to 100 units per kg three times weekly has been suggested in the USA. Doses may be increased at 4-week intervals in increments of 25 units per kg three times weekly until the target is reached. In patients on peritoneal dialysis an initial dose of 50 units per kg given subcutaneously twice weekly is recommended. Once the target is reached doses may need to be adjusted, and even decreased, for maintenance therapy.

The usual total weekly maintenance dose of epoetin alfa in predialysis patients is 50 to 100 units per kg given in three divided doses, and in haemodialysis patients it is about 75 to 300 units per kg given in three divided doses. In predialysis patients a total weekly dose of 600 units per kg should not be exceeded. In patients on peritoneal dialysis, the usual total weekly maintenance dose is 50 to 100 units per kg given subcutaneously in two divided doses.

In children, epoetin alfa may be given intravenously to those on haemodialysis at an initial dose of 50 units per kg three times weekly. The dose may be increased at 4-week intervals in increments of 25 units per kg three times weekly until a target haemoglobin concentration of 9.5 to 11 g per 100 mL is reached; the usual total weekly maintenance dose given in three divided doses is: 225 to 450 units per kg for those

weighing less than 10 kg; 180 to 450 units per kg for those weighing 10 to 30 kg; and 90 to 300 units per kg for those weighing over 30 kg.

Epoetin beta is used similarly in the management of anaemia of chronic renal failure in dialysis and predialysis patients. It may be given subcutaneously, by intravenous injection over 2 minutes, or by intravenous infusion. The following dosages may be used in adults and children. For subcutaneous injection the initial dose is 60 units per kg once weekly for 4 weeks; alternatively, the total weekly dose may be given in daily doses or three times a week. For intravenous injection the initial dose is 40 units per kg three times weekly for 4 weeks. The dose may then be increased to 80 units per kg three times weekly. Thereafter the dose of epoetin beta may be increased at 4-week intervals (if the increase in haemoglobin concentration is less than 1 g per 100 mL per month) in increments of 20 units per kg three times weekly for intravenous administration or 60 units per kg per week for subcutaneous administration until a target haemoglobin concentration of 10 to 12 g per 100 mL is reached. A total weekly dose of 720 units per kg of epoetin beta should not be exceeded. For maintenance, the dose is halved initially and then adjusted every 1 to 2 weeks according to response.

In patients with **non-myeloid malignant disease** receiving chemotherapy, epoetin alfa or epoetin beta may be given by subcutaneous injection in an initial dose of 150 units per kg three times weekly. The dose may be increased after 4 or 8 weeks, if necessary, to 300 units per kg three times weekly. If the response is still inadequate after 4 weeks at this higher dose, treatment should be discontinued. As an alternative regimen, the total weekly dose of epoetin beta may be divided into 7 daily doses.

To increase the yield of **autologous blood**, epoetin alfa or epoetin beta may be used in conjunction with iron supplementation. The dose depends on the volume of blood required for collection and on factors such as the patient's whole blood volume and haematocrit. Suggested regimens are: epoetin alfa 600 units per kg given intravenously twice weekly starting 3 weeks before surgery; or up to 800 units per kg of epoetin beta intravenously, or up to 600 units per kg subcutaneously, twice weekly for 4 weeks before surgery. To reduce the need for allogeneic blood transfusion epoetin alfa may be given in a dose of 600 units per kg subcutaneously once weekly starting 3 weeks before surgery or 300 units per kg subcutaneously daily starting 10 days before surgery.

In **HIV-positive patients** on zidovudine therapy, epoetin alfa may be beneficial if the endogenous serum-erythropoietin concentration is 500 milliunits or less per mL. Epoetin alfa is given by subcutaneous or intravenous injection in an initial dose of 100 units per kg three times weekly for 8 weeks. The dose may then be increased every 4 to 8 weeks by 50 to 100 units per kg three times weekly according to response. However, patients are unlikely to benefit from doses above 300 units per kg three times weekly if lower doses have failed to elicit a satisfactory response.

In the management of **anaemia of prematurity** epoetin beta is given subcutaneously in a dose of 250 units per kg three times weekly. Treatment should be started as early as possible and continued for six weeks.

◊ General references.

1. Markham A, Bryson HM. Epoetin alfa: a review of its pharmacodynamic and pharmacokinetic properties and therapeutic use in nonrenal applications. *Drugs* 1995; **49:** 232–54.
2. Dunn CJ, Markham A. Epoetin beta: a review of its pharmacological properties and clinical use in the management of anaemia associated with chronic renal failure. *Drugs* 1996; **51:** 299–318.
3. Beguin Y. A risk-benefit assessment of epoetin in the management of anaemia associated with cancer. *Drug Safety* 1998; **19:** 269–82.

Administration to neonates. Recombinant human erythropoietin may be given to neonates for anaemia of prematurity. It is usually administered by subcutaneous injection. Administration by intravenous infusion in total parenteral nutrition solutions produced satisfactory results in a group of 20 neonates.[1]

For a warning about diluting recombinant human erythropoietin solutions, see under Stability, above.

1. Ohls RK, *et al.* Pharmacokinetics and effectiveness of recombinant erythropoietin administered to preterm infants by continuous infusion in total parenteral nutrition solution. *J Pediatr* 1996; **128:** 518–23.

Anaemias. Epoetins are used in normocytic-normochromic anaemias (p.717) associated with low endogenous erythropoietin concentrations.

Clinical studies have shown the effectiveness of epoetins in correcting the anaemia of end-stage renal disease in patients maintained by haemodialysis,[1,2] and they are also effective in anaemia in predialysis patients. Although several factors contribute to the aetiology of the anaemia, including blood loss associated with dialysis, the main cause is inadequate production of erythropoietin in the kidney. Consistently good results have been obtained with epoetins not only for correction of anaemia but also for quality of life and exercise capacity[3,4] and for improvements in haemostatic[5] and cardiorespiratory function.[6] Guidelines have been introduced for their use in chronic renal failure.[7]

Over 90% of patients with renal anaemia respond to treatment with epoetins.[8] Many factors may contribute to a poor response (see Precautions, above) and the patient should always be investigated and the cause corrected where possible.[8,9]

Epoetins may be administered intravenously or subcutaneously. Epoetin given subcutaneously produces lower but more sustained plasma concentrations and comparative studies have shown that total weekly maintenance doses are reduced by between 23% and 52% with subcutaneous rather than intravenous administration.[10,11] The subcutaneous route is thus preferred especially in patients not on haemodialysis. The frequency of administration may also be important in maximising the response to treatment;[12] daily subcutaneous administration has been reported to give a better response than the same total weekly dose given two or three times a week.[2] Intraperitoneal administration has also been investigated.[13]

Epoetins are also used to treat anaemias from other causes. Epoetins may be used for zidovudine-induced anaemia in AIDS patients, in chemotherapy-induced anaemia in patients with non-myeloid malignant disease, and in anaemia of prematurity.[14-22] Epoetins have a potential application for other anaemias associated with impaired or insufficient erythropoietin production, such as anaemias in infants with bronchopulmonary dysplasia[23,24] and infants with haemolytic disease of the newborn,[25,26] postpartum anaemia,[27,28] and in arthritis[29-31] and inflammatory bowel disease.[32-34]

1. Winearls C. Treatment of anaemia in renal failure. *Prescribers' J* 1992; **3:** 238–44.
2. De Marchi S, *et al.* Erythropoietin and the anemia of chronic diseases. *Clin Exp Rheumatol* 1993; **11:** 429–44.
3. Canadian Erythropoietin Study Group. Association between recombinant human erythropoietin and quality of life and exercise capacity of patients receiving haemodialysis. *BMJ* 1990; **300:** 573–8.
4. Evans RW, *et al.* The quality of life of hemodialysis recipients treated with recombinant human erythropoietin. *JAMA* 1990; **263:** 825–30.
5. Moia M, *et al.* Improvement in the haemostatic defect of uraemia after treatment with recombinant human erythropoietin. *Lancet* 1987; **ii:** 1227–9.
6. Macdougall IC, *et al.* Long-term cardiorespiratory effects of amelioration of renal anaemia by erythropoietin. *Lancet* 1990; **335:** 489–93. Correction. *ibid.*; 614.
7. National Kidney Foundation. NKF-DOQI clinical practice guidelines for the treatment of anemia of chronic renal failure. *Am J Kidney Dis* 1997; **30** (suppl 3): S192–S240.
8. Macdougall IC. Poor response to erythropoietin. *BMJ* 1995; **310:** 1424–5.
9. Koury MJ. Investigating erythropoietin resistance. *N Engl J Med* 1993; **328:** 205–6.
10. Zachée P. Controversies in selection of epoetin dosages: issues and answers. *Drugs* 1995; **49:** 536–47.
11. Kaufman JS, *et al.* Subcutaneous compared with intravenous epoetin in patients receiving hemodialysis. *N Engl J Med* 1998; **339:** 578–83.
12. Abraham PA, *et al.* Controversies in determination of epoetin (recombinant human erythropoietin) dosages. *Clin Pharmacokinet* 1992; **22:** 409–15.
13. Taylor CA, *et al.* Clinical pharmacokinetics during continuous ambulatory peritoneal dialysis. *Clin Pharmacokinet* 1996; **31:** 293–308.
14. Bechensteen AG, *et al.* Erythropoietin, protein, and iron supplementation and the prevention of anaemia of prematurity. *Arch Dis Child* 1993; **69:** 19–23.
15. Maier RF, *et al.* The effect of epoetin beta (recombinant human erythropoietin) on the need for transfusion in very-low-birth-weight infants. *N Engl J Med* 1994; **330:** 1173–8.
16. Strauss RG. Erythropoietin and neonatal anemia. *N Engl J Med* 1994; **330:** 1227–8.
17. Shannon KM, *et al.* Recombinant human erythropoietin stimulates erythropoiesis and reduces erythrocyte transfusions in very low birth weight preterm infants. *Pediatrics* 1995; **95:** 1–8.
18. Wilimas JA, Crist WM. Erythropoietin—not yet a standard treatment for anemia of prematurity. *Pediatrics* 1995; **95:** 9–10.
19. Wandstrat TL, Kaplan B. Use of erythropoietin in premature neonates: controversies and the future. *Ann Pharmacother* 1995; **29:** 166–73.
20. Williamson P, *et al.* Blood transfusions and human recombinant erythropoietin in premature newborn infants. *Arch Dis Child* 1996; **75:** F65–F68.
21. Strauss RG. Recombinant erythropoietin for the anaemia of prematurity: still a promise, not a panacea. *J Pediatr* 1997; **131:** 653–5.
22. Ohls RK, *et al.* The effect of erythropoietin on the transfusion requirements of preterm infants weighing 750 grams or less: a randomized, double-blind, placebo-controlled study. *J Pediatr* 1997; **131:** 661–5.
23. Ohls RK, *et al.* A randomized, double-blind, placebo-controlled trial of recombinant erythropoietin in treatment of the anemia of bronchopulmonary dysplasia. *J Pediatr* 1993; **123:** 996–1000.
24. Al-Kharfy T, *et al.* Erythropoietin therapy in neonates at risk of having bronchopulmonary dysplasia and requiring multiple transfusions. *J Pediatr* 1996; **129:** 89–96.
25. Ohls RK, *et al.* Recombinant erythropoietin as treatment for the late hyporegenerative anemia of Rh hemolytic disease. *Pediatrics* 1992; **90:** 678–80.
26. Scaradavou A, *et al.* Suppression of erythropoiesis by intrauterine transfusions in hemolytic disease of the newborn: use of erythropoietin to treat the late anemia. *J Pediatr* 1993; **123:** 279–84.
27. Huch A, *et al.* Recombinant human erythropoietin in the treatment of postpartum anemia. *Obstet Gynecol* 1992; **80:** 127–31.
28. Breymann C, *et al.* Use of recombinant human erythropoietin in combination with parenteral iron in the treatment of postpartum anaemia. *Eur J Clin Invest* 1996; **26:** 123–30.
29. Pincus T, *et al.* Multicenter study of recombinant human erythropoietin in correction of anemia in rheumatoid arthritis. *Am J Med* 1990; **89:** 161–8.
30. Murphy EA, *et al.* Study of erythropoietin in treatment of anaemia in patients with rheumatoid arthritis. *BMJ* 1994; **309:** 1337–8.
31. Peeters HRM, *et al.* Effect of recombinant human erythropoietin on anaemia and disease activity in patients with rheumatoid arthritis and anaemia of chronic disease: a randomised placebo controlled double blind 52 weeks clinical trial. *Ann Rheum Dis* 1996; **55:** 739–44.
32. Schreiber S, *et al.* Recombinant erythropoietin for the treatment of anemia in inflammatory bowel disease. *N Engl J Med* 1996; **334:** 619–23.
33. Gasché C, *et al.* Intravenous iron and erythropoietin for anemia associated with Crohn disease: a randomized, controlled trial. *Ann Intern Med* 1997; **126:** 782–7.
34. Dohil R, *et al.* Recombinant human erythropoietin for treatment of anemia for chronic disease in children with Crohn's disease. *J Pediatr* 1998; **132:** 155–9.

Surgery. Concern over the safety of blood transfusions and the need to conserve blood supplies has led to interest in methods of reducing blood use in surgery. Recombinant human erythropoietin has been used to increase the number of units harvested for autologous transfusion[1-4] and to reduce transfusion requirements.[4-6] It has also been used as an alternative to blood transfusions.[7,8]

1. Goodnough LT, *et al.* Increased preoperative collection of autologous blood with recombinant human erythropoietin therapy. *N Engl J Med* 1989; **321:** 1163–8.
2. Graf H, *et al.* Recombinant human erythropoietin as adjuvant treatment for autologous blood donation. *BMJ* 1990; **300:** 1627–8.
3. Tasaki T, *et al.* Recombinant human erythropoietin for autologous blood donation: effects on perioperative red-blood-cell and serum erythropoietin production. *Lancet* 1992; **339:** 773–5.
4. Goodnough LT. The role of recombinant growth factors in transfusion medicine. *Br J Anaesth* 1993; **70:** 80–6.
5. Canadian Orthopedic Perioperative Erythropoietin Study Group. Effectiveness of perioperative recombinant human erythropoietin in elective hip replacement. *Lancet* 1993; **341:** 1227–32.
6. Biesma DH, *et al.* Lower homologous blood requirement in autologous blood donors after treatment with recombinant human erythropoietin. *Lancet* 1994; **344:** 367–70.
7. Green D, Handley E. Erythropoietin for anemia in Jehovah's Witnesses. *Ann Intern Med* 1990; **113:** 720–1.
8. Busuttil D, Copplestone A. Management of blood loss in Jehovah's Witnesses. *BMJ* 1995; **311:** 1115–16.

Preparations

Proprietary Preparations (details are given in Part 3)
Aust.: Culat; Erypo; NeoRecormon; Recormon; **Austral.:** Eprex; **Belg.:** Eprex; NeoRecormon; Recormon†; **Braz.:** Hemax-Eritron; **Canad.:** Eprex; **Denm.:** Eprex; NeoRecormon; Recormon†; **Fin.:** Eprex; NeoRecormon; **Fr.:** Eprex; NeoRecormon; Recormon†; **Ger.:** Erypo; NeoRecormon; Recormon†; **Hong Kong:** Eprex; Recormon; **Irl.:** Eprex; NeoRecormon; Recormon; **Israel:** Eprex; Recormon; **Ital.:** Epoxitin; Eprex; Eritrogen†; Globuren; NeoRecormon; **Jpn:** Epogin; Espo; **Mex.:** Bioyetin; Epomax; Eprex; Recormon; **Neth.:** Eprex; Recormon†; **Norw.:** Eprex; NeoRecormon; Recormon†; **NZ:** Eprex; Recormon; **Port.:** NeoRecormon; Recormon†; **S.Afr.:** Eprex; Recormon; Repotin; **Singapore:** Eprex; Recormon; **Spain:** Epopen; Eprex; Erantin†; NeoRecormon; **Swed.:** Eprex; NeoRecormon; **Switz.:** Eprex; NeoRecormon; Recormon; **Thai.:** Eprex; Hemax; Recormon; **UAE:** Epotin; **UK:** Eprex; NeoRecormon; Recormon†; **USA:** Epogen; Procrit.

Etamsylate (1720-p)

Etamsylate (*BAN, rINN*).

Cyclonamine; E-141; Etamsylatum; Ethamsylate (*USAN*); MD-141. Diethylammonium 2,5-dihydroxybenzenesulphonate.

$C_{10}H_{17}NO_5S = 263.3.$

CAS — 2624-44-4.

ATC — B02BX01.

Pharmacopoeias. In *Chin., Eur.* (see p.vi), and *Pol.*

Pharmacopoeial description

Ph. Eur.: A white or almost white, crystalline powder. It shows polymorphism. Very soluble in water; soluble in dehydrated alcohol; practically insoluble in dichloromethane; freely soluble in methyl alcohol. A 10% solution in water has a pH of 4.5 to 5.6. Store in airtight containers. Protect from light.

Adverse Effects and Precautions

Nausea, headache, and skin rash have occurred after administration of etamsylate. Transient hypotension has been reported following intravenous injection.

Porphyria. Etamsylate is considered to be unsafe in patients with porphyria because it has been shown to be porphyrinogenic in *animals*.

Pharmacokinetics

Etamsylate is absorbed from the gastrointestinal tract. It is excreted unchanged, mainly in the urine. Etamsylate is distributed into breast milk.

Uses and Administration

Etamsylate is a haemostatic that appears to maintain the stability of the capillary wall and correct abnormal platelet adhesion. It is given for the prophylaxis and control of haemorrhages from small blood vessels.

For short-term blood loss in menorrhagia a dose of 500 mg is given by mouth four times daily during menstruation. For the prophylaxis and treatment of periventricular haemorrhage in low birth-weight neonates 12.5 mg per kg body-weight is given by intramuscular or intravenous injection every 6 hours. For the control of haemorrhage following surgery etamsylate may be given to adults by mouth, or by intramuscular or intravenous injection in a dose of 250 to 500 mg; this dose may be repeated every 4 to 6 hours as necessary.

Menorrhagia. When administered during menstruation to women with idiopathic menorrhagia (p.1490), etamsylate was as effective as mefenamic acid in reducing uterine blood loss in 1 study,[1] but was ineffective in another.[2] A review, which included published and unpublished results from these and 2 earlier studies, reported that etamsylate produced about a 10 to 15% reduction in menstrual blood loss.[3]

1. Chamberlain G, *et al.* A comparative study of ethamsylate and mefenamic acid in dysfunctional uterine bleeding. *Br J Obstet Gynaecol* 1991; **98:** 707–11.
2. Bonnar J, Sheppard BL. Treatment of menorrhagia during menstruation: randomised controlled trial of ethamsylate, mefenamic acid, and tranexamic acid. *BMJ* 1996; **313:** 579–82.
3. Coulter A, *et al.* Treating menorrhagia in primary care: an overview of drug trials and a survey of prescribing practice. *Int J Technol Assess Health Care* 1995; **11:** 456–71.

Neonatal intraventricular haemorrhage. Etamsylate is one of several drugs that have been tried in the prevention of intraventricular haemorrhage in very low birth-weight infants (p.723). In a multicentre, placebo-controlled, double-blind study,[1] etamsylate was given in an initial dose of 12.5 mg per kg body-weight intravenously or intramuscularly within 1 hour of delivery, followed by the same dose intravenously every 6 hours for 4 days to a total dose of 200 mg per kg. Of 330 infants who had had no evidence of haemorrhage soon after delivery, the subsequent incidence of haemorrhage in the 162 who received etamsylate was reduced, particularly the more extensive grades when compared with the 168 who received placebo. Of a further 30 infants with evidence of periventricular haemorrhage before treatment, 21 were given etamsylate and 9 placebo; treatment with etamsylate limited the extension of bleeding. There was also a reduction in patent ductus arteriosus in the treated infants. However, a more recent study using the same dosage regimen,[2] showed little benefit on short-term follow-up. It was considered that the study size may have been too small and the drug administered too late; the initial dose was given within four hours of birth whereas, in the previous study, treatment was started within one hour of birth. The results of long-term follow-up are awaited.

1. Benson JWT, *et al.* Multicentre trial of ethamsylate for prevention of periventricular haemorrhage in low birthweight infants. *Lancet* 1986; **ii:** 1297–1300.
2. The EC Ethamsylate Trial Group. The EC randomised controlled trial of prophylactic ethamsylate for very preterm neonates: early mortality and morbidity. *Arch Dis Child* 1994; **70:** F201–F205.

Preparations

Proprietary Preparations (details are given in Part 3)
Belg.: Dicynone; **Braz.:** Dicinone; **Fr.:** Dicynone; **Ger.:** Altodor; **Irl.:** Dicynene; **Ital.:** Dicynone; Eselin; **Singapore:** Dicynone; **Spain:** Dicinone; Hemo 141; **Switz.:** Dicynone; **UK:** Dicynene.

Etherified Starches (255-j)

HES; Hydroxyethyl Starch. 2-Hydroxyethyl ether starch.
CAS — 9005-27-0.

NOTE. The names hetastarch (*BAN, USAN*) and pentastarch (*BAN, USAN*) are in use for etherified starches with specified degrees of etherification.

Etherified starches are starches that are composed of more than 90% of amylopectin and that have been etherified to varying extents. In hetastarch an average of 7 to 8 of the hydroxy groups in each 10 D-glucopyranose units of starch polymer have been converted into OCH_2CH_2OH groups, whereas in pentastarch an average of 4 to 5 of the hydroxy groups in each 10 D-glucopyranose units of the starch polymer have been converted to OCH_2CH_2OH groups. Etherified starches also vary in terms of average molecular weight and the position of etherification within the glucopyranose unit.

Incompatibilities. Hetastarch is incompatible with many compounds including a number of injectable antibacterials. References.

1. Wohlford JG, Fowler MD. Visual compatibility of hetastarch with injectable critical-care drugs. *Am J Hosp Pharm* 1989; **46:** 995–6.
2. Wohlford JG, *et al.* More information on the visual compatibility of hetastarch with injectable critical-care drugs. *Am J Hosp Pharm* 1990; **47:** 297–8.

Adverse Effects and Precautions
Hypersensitivity reactions including anaphylactic reactions have occurred after infusion of etherified starches.

Precautions that should be observed with plasma expanders are described under Dextran 70, p.729, and these should be considered when etherified starches are used. There does not appear to be any interference with blood grouping and cross-matching of blood.

Effects on the blood. Use of plasma expanders causes dilution of clotting factors and may also have direct effects on coagulation. Coagulopathy and haemorrhage has been reported in neurosurgical patients,[1,2] in a patient with coagulation defects,[3] and in a Jehovah's Witness[4] in whom large volumes of hetastarch solution were used during major orthopaedic surgery. It was suggested that hetastarch should probably be avoided in neurosurgical patients in whom the prevention of intracranial haemorrhage is critical, and in patients with a pre-existing bleeding disorder.

1. Syrington BE. Hetastarch and bleeding complications. *Ann Intern Med* 1986; **105:** 627–8.
2. Damon L, *et al.* Intracranial bleeding during treatment with hydroxyethyl starch. *N Engl J Med* 1987; **317:** 964–5.
3. Abramson N. Plasma expanders and bleeding. *Ann Intern Med* 1988; **108:** 307.
4. Lockwood DNJ, *et al.* A severe coagulopathy following volume replacement with hydroxyethyl starch in a Jehovah's Witness. *Anaesthesia* 1988; **43:** 391–3.

Effects on the kidneys. Osmotic-nephrosis-like lesions found at biopsy in some transplanted kidneys have been attributed to use of solutions of etherified starches in the donor patient.[1] Such use has also been reported to impair immediate graft function.[2] However, another study[3] found no association between the use of these solutions in the donor patient and osmotic-nephrosis-like lesions or delayed graft function.

1. Legendre CH, *et al.* Hydroxyethylstarch and osmotic-nephrosis-like lesions in kidney transplantation. *Lancet* 1993; **342:** 248–9.
2. Cittanova ML, *et al.* Effect of hydroxyethylstarch in brain-dead kidney donors on renal function in kidney-transplant recipients. *Lancet* 1996; **348:** 1620–22.
3. Coronel B, *et al.* Hydroxyethylstarch and renal function in kidney transplant recipients. *Lancet* 1997; **349:** 884.

Effects on the skin. Pruritus has been reported after infusion of etherified starches. A review[1] indicated that severe pruritus developed in 32% of patients and occurred, usually on the trunk, 3 days to 15 weeks after administration; the mean duration was nearly 9 weeks. Prolonged pruritus lasting more than 2 years has been reported.[2] The reaction is dose dependent and usually refractory to treatment. There are individual reports of response to capsaicin.[3] Etherified starches have been shown to accumulate in the skin and other tissues but are eliminated over time.[4] Marked and persistent periocular swelling developed in a patient following 15 daily infusions of hetastarch.[5] Abnormal accumulation of hetastarch was found in the periocular tissues.

1. Gall H, *et al.* Persistierender pruritus nach hydroxyäthylstärke-infusionen. *Hautarzt* 1993; **44:** 713–16.
2. Cox NH, Popple AW. Persistent erythema and pruritus, with a confluent histiocytic skin infiltrate, following the use of a hydroxyethylstarch plasma expander. *Br J Dermatol* 1996; **134:** 353–7.
3. Szeimies R-M, *et al.* Successful treatment of hydroxyethyl starch-induced pruritus with topical capsaicin. *Br J Dermatol* 1994; **131:** 380–2.
4. Sirtl C, *et al.* Tissue deposits of hydroxyethyl starch (HES): dose-dependent and time-related. *Br J Anaesth* 1999; **82:** 510–15.
5. Kiehl P, *et al.* Decreased activity of acid α-glucosidase in a patient with persistent periocular swelling after infusions of hydroxyethyl starch. *Br J Dermatol* 1998; **138:** 672–77.

Pharmacokinetics
Etherified starches consist of mixtures of molecules with a range of molecular weights and with varying degrees of etherification. After intravenous infusion the molecules with a molecular weight of less than 50 000 are readily excreted unchanged by the kidney; larger molecules are metabolised and eliminated more slowly. The rate of metabolism depends upon the size of the molecule and the degree and position of etherification, with a high molecular weight, high degree of etherification, and etherification predominantly at the C2 position leading to a slower rate of metabolism and hence a longer duration of action. About 33% of a dose of high-molecular-weight heta-

The symbol † denotes a preparation no longer actively marketed

starch (weight average molecular weight 450 000) and about 70% of a dose of medium-molecular-weight pentastarch (weight average molecular weight 250 000) is excreted in the urine in 24 hours.

◊ References.

1. Mishler JM, *et al.* Changes in the molecular composition of circulating hydroxyethyl starch following consecutive daily infusions in man. *Br J Clin Pharmacol* 1979; **7:** 505–9.
2. Mishler JM, *et al.* Post-transfusion survival of hydroxyethyl starch 450/0.70 in man: a long-term study. *J Clin Pathol* 1980; **33:** 155–9.
3. Yacobi A, *et al.* Pharmacokinetics of hydroxyethyl starch in normal subjects. *J Clin Pharmacol* 1982; **22:** 206–12.

Uses and Administration
Etherified starches are plasma volume expanders used in the management of hypovolaemic shock (p.813). Those most commonly used include high-molecular-weight hetastarch (weight average molecular weight 450 000 to 480 000) and medium-molecular-weight pentastarch (weight average molecular weight 200 000 to 250 000). Other etherified starches that are used include low-molecular-weight pentastarch and medium-molecular-weight hexastarch, which has a degree of etherification between that of pentastarch and hetastarch. A higher molecular weight hetastarch is also available. Iso-oncotic solutions of etherified starches, for example, 6% hetastarch or 6% medium-molecular-weight pentastarch, exert a similar colloidal osmotic pressure to human albumin, and when given by intravenous infusion produce an expansion of plasma volume slightly in excess of the infused volume. Hyperoncotic solutions, for example 10% medium-molecular-weight pentastarch, produce an expansion of plasma volume of about 1.5 times the infused volume. The duration of effect depends on the characteristics of the starch used; for 6% hetastarch the effect lasts for 24 to 36 hours.

Etherified starches are given intravenously as solutions in sodium chloride 0.9% or other electrolytes; concentrations used are usually 6 or 10%, although 3% solutions are also available for some. The dose and rate of infusion depend on the amount of fluid lost and degree of haemoconcentration; usual doses are in the range of 500 to 2500 mL daily, depending on the preparation used, and the infusion rate may be up to about 20 mL per kg body-weight per hour if necessary.

Hetastarch and pentastarch increase the erythrocyte sedimentation rate when added to whole blood. They are therefore used in leucopheresis procedures to increase the yield of granulocytes. Doses of 250 to 700 mL may be added to venous blood in the ratio 1 part to at least 8 parts of whole blood in such procedures. Up to 2 such procedures per week and a total of 7 to 10 have been reported to be safe.

Hetastarch has also been used in extracorporeal perfusion fluids.

◊ References.

1. Treib J, *et al.* An international view of hydroxyethyl starches. *Intensive Care Med* 1999; **25:** 258–68.

Administration in children. A 6% solution of a low-molecular-weight etherified starch (average molecular weight 200 000) was considered effective and safe when compared with human albumin in the management of volume replacement in children under 3 years of age undergoing cardiac surgery.[1]

1. Boldt J, *et al.* Volume replacement with hydroxyethyl starch solutions in children. *Br J Anaesth* 1993; **70:** 661–5.

Stroke. Haemodilution with pentastarch has been tried in patients with acute ischaemic stroke (p.813) in an attempt to improve reperfusion of the brain by lowering blood viscosity. However, one study was terminated early when an excess mortality was noted in the haemodilution group.[1] The early fatalities occurred almost exclusively in patients with severe strokes; cerebral oedema was the main cause of death within one week of the onset of symptoms. Among the survivors neurological recovery was better among those who received haemodilution.

1. Hemodilution in Stroke Study Group. Hypervolemic hemodilution treatment of stroke: results of a randomized multicenter trial using pentastarch. *Stroke* 1989; **20:** 317–23.

Preparations
Proprietary Preparations (details are given in Part 3)
Aust.: Elohast; Expafusin; Expahes; HAES; Hyperhes; Isohes; Osmohes; Plasmasteril; Varihes; *Belg.:* Elohaes†; HAES-steril†; Plasmasteril†; *Braz.:* Plasmasteril; *Canad.:* Pentaspan; *Denm.:*

HAES-steril; *Fin.:* HAES-steril; Hemohes; Plasmafusin; *Fr.:* Elohes; Heafusine; Hesteril; *Ger.:* Expafusin; Haemofusin; HAES-Rheopond; HAES-steril; Hemohes; Infukoll HES; Plasmafusin HES; Plasmasteril; Rheohes; Serag-HAES; Voluven; *Israel:* HAES-steril; *Ital.:* HAES-steril; *Jpn:* Hespander; *Mex.:* HAES-steril; Pentastan; *Norw.:* HAES-steril; *NZ:* Pentaspan; *Port.:* HAES-steril; Voluven; *S.Afr.:* HAES-steril; *Singapore:* HAES-steril; Hemohes; *Spain:* Elohes; Expafusin; HAES Esteril; *Swed.:* HAES-steril; Hemohes; *Switz.:* Elohast; Expahes; HAES-steril; Hemohes; Isohes; Plasmasteril; Varihes; *Thai.:* HAES-steril; Hespander; *UK:* Elohaes; HAES-steril; Hemohes; Hespan; Pentaspan; Voluven; *USA:* Hespan; Pentaspan.

Multi-ingredient: *Norw.:* Hemohes.

Factor VII (10819-b)

Proconvertin; SPCA; Stable Factor.
ATC — B02BD08.

NOTE. The name Eptacog Alfa (Activated) *(BAN, rINN)* is in use for a recombinant factor VIIa.

Pharmacopoeial description

Ph. Eur.: Human Coagulation Factor VII (Factor VII Coagulationis Humanus; Dried Factor VII Fraction (BP 2001)) is a plasma protein fraction that contains the single-chain glycoprotein factor VII and may also contain small amounts of the activated form, the two-chain derivative factor VIIa, as well as coagulation factors II, IX, and X, and protein C and protein S. It is prepared from human plasma obtained from blood from healthy donors; the plasma is tested for the absence of hepatitis B surface antigen and antibodies against HIV-1 and HIV-2 and hepatitis C virus. The method of preparation is designed to minimise activation of any coagulation factor and includes a step or steps that have been shown to remove or inactivate known agents of infection. The factor VII fraction is dissolved in a suitable liquid, passed through a bacteria-retentive filter, distributed aseptically into the final containers, and immediately frozen. The preparation is freeze-dried and the containers sealed under vacuum or under an inert gas. Heparin, antithrombin, and other auxiliary substances such as a stabiliser may be added. No antimicrobial preservative is added. The specific activity is not less than 2 international units of factor VII per mg of protein before the addition of any protein stabiliser. When reconstituted as stated on the label the resulting solution contains not less than 15 international units per mL.

A white, pale yellow, green, or blue powder or friable solid. Protect from light.

Units
The potency of factor VIIa (activated factor VII) is expressed in international units and preparations may be assayed using the first International Standard for blood coagulation factor VIIa concentrate (1993).

Adverse Effects and Precautions
Administration of factor VIIa (activated factor VII) may be associated with minor skin reactions, fever, headache, and changes in blood pressure. Factor VIIa should be used with caution in patients with conditions associated with circulating tissue factor, such as advanced atherosclerosis, crush injury, or septicaemia, since there is a risk of precipitating thrombosis or disseminated intravascular coagulation.

Uses and Administration
Factor VII may be used as replacement therapy in patients with rare genetic deficiencies of factor VII.

Factor VIIa (activated factor VII) is used to treat bleeding episodes and to prevent bleeding associated with surgery in patients with haemophilia A or haemophilia B (p.721) who have developed antibodies to factor VIII or factor IX, respectively. It may also be useful in patients with von Willebrand's disease. Factor VIIa is given by intravenous injection in an initial dose of 4500 units per kg body-weight. Subsequent doses of 3000 to 6000 units per kg may be given, the dose and frequency of administration depending on the type and severity of haemorrhage.

Preparations
Ph. Eur.: Human Coagulation Factor VII.

Proprietary Preparations (details are given in Part 3)
Aust.: NovoSeven; *Austral.:* NovoSeven; *Denm.:* NovoSeven; *Fin.:* NovoSeven; *Fr.:* Acset†; NovoSeven; *Ger.:* NovoSeven; *Irl.:* NovoSeven†; *Israel:* NovoSeven; *Ital.:* NovoSeven; Provertin-UM TIM 3; *Neth.:* NovoSeven; *Norw.:* NovoSeven; *NZ:* NovoSeven; *S.Afr.:* NovoSeven; *Spain:* NovoSeven; *Swed.:* NovoSeven; *Switz.:* NovoSeven; *UK:* NovoSeven; *USA:* NovoSeven.

Multi-ingredient: *Spain:* Hemofactor HT.

Factor VIII (1225-c)

AHF; Antihaemophilic Factor.

NOTE. The names Moroctocog Alfa *(BAN, rINN)* and Octocog Alfa *(BAN, rINN)* are in use for recombinant factor VIII.

Factor VIII is prepared from human plasma as described below. It may also be prepared using recombinant DNA technology.

Pharmacopoeial description

Ph. Eur.: Human Coagulation Factor VIII (Factor VIII Coagulationis Humanus; Dried Factor VIII Fraction (BP 2001); Dried Human Antihaemophilic Fraction) is a plasma protein fraction that contains the glycoprotein coagulation factor VIII together with varying amounts of von Willebrand factor, depending on the method of preparation. It is prepared from human plasma obtained from blood from healthy donors; the plasma is tested for the absence of hepatitis B surface antigen and antibodies against HIV-1 and HIV-2 and hepatitis C virus. The method of preparation includes a step or steps that have been shown to remove or inactivate known agents of infection. The factor VIII fraction is dissolved in an appropriate liquid, passed through a bacteria-retentive filter, distributed aseptically into the final containers, and immediately frozen. The preparation is freeze-dried and the containers sealed under vacuum or under an inert gas. Auxiliary substances such as a stabiliser may be added. No antimicrobial preservative is added. The specific activity is not less than 1 international unit of factor VIII:C per mg of total protein before the addition of any protein stabiliser. When reconstituted as stated on the label the resulting solution contains not less than 20 international units of factor VI-II:C per mL.

A white or pale yellow powder or friable solid. Protect from light.

USP 25: Antihemophilic Factor is a sterile freeze-dried powder containing the factor VIII fraction prepared from units of human venous plasma that have been tested for the absence of hepatitis B surface antigen, obtained from whole-blood donors and pooled; it may contain heparin sodium or sodium citrate. It contains not less than 100 units per g of protein. Unless otherwise specified it should be stored at 2° to 8° in hermetically-sealed containers. It should be used within 4 hours of reconstitution and should be administered with equipment that includes a filter.

A white or yellowish powder. On reconstitution it is opalescent with a slight blue tinge or is a yellowish liquid.

Cryoprecipitated Antihemophilic Factor is a sterile frozen concentrate of human antihaemophilic factor prepared from the cryoprecipitate, rich in factor VIII, of human venous plasma obtained from suitable whole-blood donors from a single unit of plasma derived from whole blood or by plasmapheresis, collected and processed in a closed system. It contains no preservative. It has an average potency of not less than 80 units per container. It should be stored at or below −18° in hermetically-sealed containers. It should be thawed to 20° to 37° before use; this liquid should be stored at room temperature and used within 6 hours of thawing; it should also be used within 4 hours of opening the container and administered with equipment that includes a filter.

A yellowish frozen solid. On thawing it becomes a very viscous, yellow, gummy liquid.

Units

The potency of factor VIII is expressed in international units and preparations may be assayed using the fifth International Standard for blood coagulation factor VIII:C concentrate, human (1994).

Adverse Effects and Precautions

Allergic reactions may sometimes follow the use of factor VIII preparations and chills, urticaria, and fever experienced by some patients may be allergic manifestations. Headache may occur. There is the possibility of intravascular haemolysis in patients with blood groups A, B, or AB receiving high doses or frequently repeated doses of factor VIII preparations due to the content of blood group isoagglutinins; also massive doses of some preparations may produce hyperfibrinogenaemia. Such risks should be reduced with more highly purified preparations.

Factor VIII preparations have been associated with the transmission of some viral infections, including hepatitis B and C, and more notably transmission of HIV. Strenuous efforts are now undertaken to screen the donor material from which factor VIII material is obtained and new methods of manufacture have also been introduced with the aim of inactivating any viruses present. Vaccination against hepatitis B is recommended for patients not already immune. Recombinant preparations are also available.

Some patients develop antibodies to factor VIII and, although large doses of preparations of both factor

VIII and factor IX or porcine or highly purified factor VIII concentrates may be effective in the management of such patients, some patients remain resistant to treatment.

Effects on blood platelets. Thrombocytopenia was associated with administration of porcine factor VIII concentrate in 2 patients.[1] Platelet aggregation was noted in addition in one patient. Platelet counts improved when treatment with factor VIII was withdrawn.

1. Green D, Tuite GF. Declining platelet counts and platelet aggregation during porcine VIII:C infusions. *Am J Med* 1989; **86:** 222–4.

Transmission of infections. Treatment with heat or chemicals together with efforts to screen the donor material from which factor VIII and other clotting factors are obtained seem to have overcome problems with transmission of HIV and hepatitis B and C, although there is concern that non-lipid-enveloped viruses, such as human parvovirus B19 and hepatitis A, may still be transmitted. A solvent-detergent-treated factor VIII product[1-4] and a similar factor IX product[4] have been associated with reports of hepatitis A in patients with haemophilia and vaccination against hepatitis A has been recommended for patients treated with these factor preparations. Plasma-derived factor VIII preparations or recombinant preparations containing added albumin may carry a risk of transmission of Creutzfeldt-Jakob disease (see under Blood, p.727). It has been pointed out[5] that, since recombinant factor VIII is prepared from mammalian cell lines, there is a theoretical risk of transmission of infection with recombinant preparations.

1. Prowse C. Hepatitis A virus infection: no conclusive link to factor VIII. *BMJ* 1993; **307:** 561–2.
2. Thomas DP. Viral contamination of blood products. *Lancet* 1994; **343:** 1583–4.
3. Colvin BT. Viral contamination of blood products. *Lancet* 1994; **344:** 405.
4. Anonymous. Hepatitis A among persons with hemophilia who received clotting factor concentrate—United States, September-December 1995. *JAMA* 1996; **275:** 427–8.
5. Foster PR, *et al.* Hepatitis C and haemophilia. *BMJ* 1995; **311:** 754–5.

Pharmacokinetics

◊ References.

1. Messori A, *et al.* Clinical pharmacokinetics of factor VIII in patients with classic haemophilia. *Clin Pharmacokinet* 1987; **13:** 365–80.
2. Björkman S, *et al.* Pharmacokinetics of factor VIII in humans: obtaining clinically relevant data from comparative studies. *Clin Pharmacokinet* 1992; **22:** 385–95.

Uses and Administration

Factor VIII is used as replacement therapy in patients with haemophilia A (p.721), a genetic deficiency of factor VIII.

Preparations of factor VIII are used to control bleeding episodes in the treatment of patients with haemophilia A and to prevent bleeding episodes in such patients undergoing dental and surgical procedures. They may also be used for long-term prophylaxis in patients with severe haemophilia A.

Preparations of factor VIII are given by slow intravenous infusion. The dosage of factor VIII should be determined for each patient and will vary with the circumstances involving bleeding or type of surgery to be performed. In adults, a dose of 1 unit per kg body-weight has been reported to raise the plasma concentration of factor VIII by about 2% (of normal). A suggested formula to calculate, approximately, the dose required for a given effect is:

$$\text{units} = \text{wt (kg)} \times 0.5 \times \% \text{ desired increase (of normal)}$$

Recommended doses vary depending on the preparation used, but the following have been suggested: for mild to moderate haemorrhage the plasma concentration of factor VIII should be raised to 20 to 30% of normal, usually achieved with a single dose of 10 to 15 units per kg body-weight; for more serious haemorrhage or minor surgery it should be raised to 30 to 50% of normal, achieved with a usual initial dose of 15 to 25 units per kg followed by 10 to 15 units per kg every 8 to 12 hours if required; and for severe haemorrhage or major surgery an increase to 80 to 100% of normal may be necessary, achieved with a usual initial dose of 40 to 50 units per kg followed by 20 to 25 units per kg every 8 to 12 hours.

In patients with inhibitory antibodies to human factor VIII, a porcine factor VIII preparation may be used in doses of 25 to 100 units per kg depending upon the severity of the haemorrhage.

Cryoprecipitate is an alternative source of clotting factors and contains factor VIII, factor XIII, von Willebrand's factor, fibrinogen, and fibronectin. Some factor VIII concentrates also contain von Willebrand's factor and these preparations or cryoprecipitate may be used in the management of von Willebrand's disease. Commercial very highly purified and recombinant factor VIII preparations do not contain appreciable amounts of von Willebrand's factor and are thus ineffective.

Administration. Surgical prophylaxis or significant haemorrhage in patients with haemophilia A is usually managed with injections of factor VIII given intravenously every 8 to 12 hours. Continuous intravenous infusion prevents wide fluctuations in factor VIII plasma concentrations and has been used successfully following major surgery in patients with haemophilia.[1-3]

1. Bona RD, *et al.* The use of continuous infusion of factor concentrates in the treatment of hemophilia. *Am J Hematol* 1989; **32:** 8–13.
2. Martinowitz U, *et al.* Adjusted dose continuous infusion of factor VIII in patients with haemophilia A. *Br J Haematol* 1992; **82:** 729–34.
3. Hawkins TE, *et al.* Treatment of haemophilia A by continuous factor VIII infusion. *Aust N Z J Med* 1995; **25:** 37–9.

Preparations

Ph. Eur.: Human Coagulation Factor VIII;
USP 25: Antihemophilic Factor; Cryoprecipitated Antihemophilic Factor.

Proprietary Preparations (details are given in Part 3)
Aust.: Beriate; Helixate; Immunate; Koate†; Kogenate; Kryobulin s-TIM 3†; Monoclate-P; ReFacto; *Austral.:* AHF; Kogenate; Recombinate; *Belg.:* Kogenate; Recombinate; ReFacto; *Braz.:* Emoclot DI; Kryobulin; Monoclate-P; Vueffe; *Canad.:* Koate-HP†; Kogenate; Recombinate; *Denm.:* Bioclate; Haemate; Helixate; Kogenate; Monoclate-P; Nordiate; Recombinate; ReFacto; *Fin.:* Amofil; Helixate; Recombinate; ReFacto; *Fr.:* Helixate; Hemofil M†; Kogenate; Monoclate-P; Recombinate; ReFacto; *Ger.:* Beriate P; Bioclate; Fanhdi; Haemate; Haemoctin SDH; Helixate; Hemofil; Immunate STIM; Kogenate; Monoclate-P; Octanate; Octavi†; Profilate; Recombinate; ReFacto; *Hong Kong:* Alphanate; Hemofil M; Koate-HP; *Irl.:* Kogenate; Monoclate-P; *Israel:* Haemate P; Hyate:C; Koate-HP; Monoclate-P; Omrixate; Profilate; *Ital.:* Alphanate; Beriate P; Emoclot DI; Fanhdi; Haemate; Helixate; Hemofil M; Immunate STIM; Koate-HS†; Kogenate; Kryobulin TIM 3-I†; Recombinate; ReFacto; Uman-Cry DI; Vueffe; *Jpn:* Recombinate; *Mex.:* Koate-HP; Monoclate-P; *Neth.:* Haemate; Helixate; Kogenate; ReFacto; *Norw.:* Kogenate; Octavi; Octonativ-M; *NZ:* AHF; Kogenate; Recombinate; *Port.:* Haemoctin SDH; Hemofil M†; Kogenate; Recombinate†; ReFacto; *S.Afr.:* Haemosolvate; *Singapore:* Alphanate; Haemoctin SDH; Hemofil M; Koate-HP; *Spain:* Beriate P; Bioclate†; Criostat SD 2†; Fanhdi; Haemate; Helixate; Hemofil M; Kogenate; Kryobulin TIM 3†; Monoclate-P; Recombinate; ReFacto; *Swed.:* Beriate P; Haemate; Helixate; Hemofil M; Immunate; Kogenate; Monoclate-P; Octonativ-M; Recombinate; ReFacto; *Switz.:* Haemate HS; Helixate; Hyate:C; Immunate STIM plus; Kogenate; Kryobuline S-TIM 3†; Premofil M; Recombinate; *Thai.:* Alphanate; Alpha VIII†; *UK:* Alphanate; Beriate P; Bioclate; Fanhdi; Haemate P; Helixate; Hemofil HT; Hemofil M; Hyate:C; Kogenate; Monoclate-P; Recombinate; ReFacto; Replenate; *USA:* Alphanate; Bioclate; Helixate; Hemofil M; Humate-P; Hyate:C; Koate-DVI; Koate-HP†; Kogenate; Monarc-M; Monoclate-P; Profilate HP, OSD†; Recombinate; ReFacto.

Multi-ingredient: *Fr.:* Innobrand.

Factor VIII Inhibitor Bypassing Fraction (19165-p)

Activated Prothrombin Complex Concentrate; Anti-inhibitor Coagulant Complex.

Preparations with factor VIII inhibitor bypassing activity are prepared from human plasma.

Adverse Effects and Precautions

Allergic reactions may follow the administration of preparations having factor VIII inhibitor bypassing activity. Rapid infusion may cause headache, flushing, and changes in blood pressure and pulse rate.

It should not be given if disseminated intravascular coagulation is suspected or if there are signs of fibrinolysis. It should be used with caution in patients with liver disease.

As with other plasma-derived products, there is a risk of transmission of infection.

Uses and Administration

Preparations with factor VIII inhibitor bypassing activity are used in patients with haemophilia A (p.721) who have antibodies to factor VIII and in patients with acquired antibodies to factor VIII. The dose is administered intravenously and depends on the preparation used.

Preparations

Proprietary Preparations (details are given in Part 3)
Aust.: Feiba S-TIM 4; *Belg.:* Autoplex T†; Feiba; *Braz.:* Feiba; *Canad.:* Feiba; *Denm.:* Feiba; *Fin.:* Feiba; *Fr.:* Feiba; *Ger.:* Autoplex; Feiba S-TIM 4; *Hong Kong:* Feiba TIM 4; *Israel:* Anti-Inhibitor Coagulant Complex (Autoplex T); Feiba TIM 4; *Ital.:* Feiba; *S.Afr.:* Feiba TIM 4; *Singapore:* Autoplex T; *Spain:* Auto-

plex T†; Feiba TIM 4; *Swed.:* Autoplex; Feiba; *Switz.:* Feiba; *UK:* Anti-inhibitor Coagulant Complex; Autoplex; Feiba; *USA:* Autoplex T; Feiba.

Factor IX (1227-a)

Christmas Factor; Plasma Thromboplastin Component; PTC.
CAS — 181054-95-5 (nonacog alfa).
ATC — B02BD09.

NOTE. The name Nonacog Alfa *(BAN, rINN, USAN)* is in use for recombinant factor IX.

Factor IX is prepared from human plasma as described below. It may also be prepared using recombinant DNA technology.

Pharmacopoeial description

Ph. Eur.: Human Coagulation Factor IX (Factor IX Coagulationis Humanus; Dried Factor IX Fraction (BP 2001)) is a plasma protein fraction containing coagulation factor IX, prepared by a method that effectively separates it from other prothrombin complex factors (factors II, VII, and X). It is prepared from human plasma obtained from healthy donors; the plasma is tested for the absence of hepatitis B surface antigen and antibodies against HIV-1 and HIV-2 and hepatitis C virus. The method of preparation is designed to maintain functional integrity of factor IX, to minimise activation of any coagulation factor, and includes a step or steps that have been shown to remove or inactivate known agents of infection. The factor IX fraction is dissolved in a suitable liquid, passed through a bacteria-retentive filter, distributed aseptically into the final containers, and immediately frozen. The preparation is freeze-dried and the containers are sealed under vacuum or under an inert gas. Heparin, antithrombin, or other auxiliary substances such as a stabiliser may be included. No antimicrobial preservative is added. The specific activity is not less than 50 international units of factor IX per mg of total protein before the addition of any protein stabiliser. The dried product is a white or pale yellow powder or friable solid and should be protected from light. When reconstituted as stated on the label the resulting solution contains not less than 20 international units per mL.

Human Prothrombin Complex (Ph. Eur.) (Prothrombinum Multiplex Humanum; Dried Prothrombin Complex (BP 2001)) contains factor IX together with variable amounts of coagulation factors II, VII, and X. It is prepared by fractionation of human plasma obtained from blood from healthy donors; the plasma is tested for the absence of hepatitis B surface antigen and antibodies against HIV-1 and HIV-2 and hepatitis C virus. The method of preparation is designed in particular to minimise thrombogenicity and includes a step or steps that have been shown to remove or inactivate known agents of infection. The prothrombin complex fraction is dissolved in a suitable liquid, sterilised by filtration, distributed aseptically into final containers, and immediately frozen. The preparation is freeze-dried and the containers are sealed under vacuum or under an inert gas. No antimicrobial preservative is added. Heparin, antithrombin, and other auxiliary substances such as a stabiliser may be added. The potency of the preparation is not less than 0.6 international units of factor IX per mg of total protein before the addition of any protein stabiliser. The dried product is a white or slightly coloured, very hygroscopic, powder or friable solid and should be protected from light. When reconstituted as stated on the label the resulting solution contains not less than 20 international units per mL.

USP 25: Factor IX Complex is a sterile freeze-dried powder consisting of partially purified factor IX fraction, as well as concentrated factor II, VII, and X fractions of venous plasma obtained from healthy human donors. It contains no preservatives. It should be stored at 2° to 8° in hermetically-sealed containers. It should be used within 4 hours after reconstitution and administered with equipment that includes a filter.

Units

The activity of factor IX is expressed in terms of international units and preparations may be assayed using the second International Standard for blood coagulation factor IX concentrate (1994).

Adverse Effects and Precautions

Allergic reactions may follow the administration of factor IX preparations and there may be chills, fever, and urticaria. Other adverse effects include nausea and vomiting, headache, and flushing particularly following rapid administration. Intravascular coagulation and thrombosis have been reported, mainly in patients with liver disease, and factor IX should be used with care in patients at risk of thromboembolism or disseminated intravascular coagulation. The risk should be less with more highly purified preparations.

As with other plasma derivatives there is a possibility of transmitting viral infection, although selection of donors and heat or chemical treatments of products

The symbol † denotes a preparation no longer actively marketed

are used to minimise the risk. Vaccination against hepatitis B is recommended for patients not already immune.

Antibodies to Factor IX may develop rarely.

Effects on blood coagulation. Some factor IX preparations derived from plasma contain other clotting factors in addition to factor IX (such as the activated factors IX, X and XII) and administration of these preparations has the potential to produce thromboembolic complications. Reports of thrombosis[1] and intravascular coagulation[2,3] have generally been associated with the use of these factor IX preparations in patients with liver disease, although there has been a report[4] of deep-vein thrombosis in a patient with normal hepatic function who had been given factor IX postoperatively. Highly purified factor IX preparations which do not contain other clotting factors may be expected to avoid this risk of thromboembolism.

1. Blatt PM, *et al.* Thrombogenic materials in prothrombin complex concentrates. *Ann Intern Med* 1974; **81:** 766–70.
2. Gazzard BG, *et al.* Coagulation factor concentrate in the treatment of the haemorrhagic diathesis of fulminant hepatic failure. *Gut* 1974; **15:** 993–8.
3. Cederbaum AI, *et al.* Intravascular coagulation with use of human prothrombin complex concentrates. *Ann Intern Med* 1976; **84:** 683–7.
4. Machin SJ, Miller BR. Thrombosis and factor-IX concentrates. *Lancet* 1978; **i:** 1367.

Effects on the heart. Myocardial infarction has occurred in patients receiving factor IX concentrates[1-3] and may be associated with the large doses employed.[4]

1. Fuerth JH, Mahrer P. Myocardial infarction after factor IX therapy. *JAMA* 1981; **245:** 1455–6.
2. Schimpf K, *et al.* Myocardial infarction complicating activated prothrombin complex concentrate substitution in patient with haemophilia A. *Lancet* 1982; **ii:** 1043.
3. Gruppo RA, *et al.* Fatal myocardial necrosis associated with prothrombin-complex-concentrate therapy in hemophilia A. *N Engl J Med* 1983; **309:** 242–3.
4. Lusher JM. Myocardial necrosis after therapy with prothrombin-complex concentrate. *N Engl J Med* 1984; **310:** 464.

Transmission of infections. For a report of hepatitis A in a patient receiving a solvent-detergent-treated factor IX preparation, see under Adverse Effects and Precautions of Factor VIII, p.734.

Uses and Administration

Factor IX is used as replacement therapy in patients with haemophilia B (Christmas disease), a genetic deficiency of factor IX (p.721).

There are two forms of factor IX preparation derived from plasma; one is of high purity, the other is rich in other clotting factors. A recombinant factor IX preparation is also available. Preparations that contain other factors as well as factor IX may sometimes be useful for the treatment of bleeding due to deficiencies of factors II, VII, and X, as well as IX, and in the preparation of such patients for surgery; they may also be used for immediate reversal of coumarin anticoagulants and in the management of patients with haemophilia A who have antibodies to factor VIII.

Factor IX is given by slow intravenous infusion. In patients with factor IX deficiency the dosage should be determined for each patient and will vary with the preparation used and the circumstances of bleeding or type of surgery to be performed. Suggested target factor IX concentrations vary considerably.

Preparations

Ph. Eur.: Human Coagulation Factor IX; Human Prothrombin Complex;
USP 25: Factor IX Complex.

Proprietary Preparations (details are given in Part 3)
Aust.: Bebulin S-TIM 4†; Benefix; Beriplex; Immunine; Prothromplex S-TIM 4; *Austral.:* Benefix; Monofix-VF; *Belg.:* Benefix; *Braz.:* Bebulin; Mononine; Prothromplex-T; *Canad.:* Immunine; *Denm.:* Benefix; Immunine; Mononine; *Fin.:* Bemofil; *Fr.:* Benefix; Kaskadil; Mononine; Octanate†; Benefix; Berinin; Beriplex PN; Immunine STIM; Mononine; Octanine; PPSB Konzentrat S-TIM; Prothrombinkomplex BaWu; Prothromplex S-TIM 4†; *Hong Kong:* Konyne 80; Proplex T; *Irl.:* Mononine; *Israel:* Konyne; Monofine; Proplex; *Ital.:* Aimafix; Alphanine; Bebulin TIM 3†; Benefix; Immunine STIM; Mononine; Protromplex TIM 3; Uman-Complex; *Mex.:* Berinin P; Konyne 80; *Neth.:* Mononine; Norw.:* Nanotiv; Octanyne; *NZ:* Monofix; Prothrombinex; *S.Afr.:* Bebulin TIM 4†; Haemosolvex; Prothromplex-T TIM 4; *Singapore:* Alphanine; Profilnine; Proplex T; Replenine; *Spain:* Bebulin TIM 4; Benefix; Immunine; Mononine; Proplex T†; *Swed.:* Benefix; Immunine; Mononine; Nanotiv; *Switz.:* Benefix; Berinin HS; Immunine STIM plus; Prothromplex Total S-TIM 4; *Thai.:* Profilnine; *UK:* Alphanine; Benefix; Beriplex PN; Mononine; Proplex; Prothromplex; Replenine; *USA:* Alphanine; Bebulin VH; Benefix; Konyne 80†; Mononine; Profilnine; Proplex T.

Multi-ingredient: *Spain:* Hemofactor HT.

Factor XIII (1228-t)

Fibrin-stabilising Factor; FSF.

Profile

Factor XIII is used as replacement therapy in patients with a genetic deficiency of factor XIII. Dosage of factor XIII is based on the degree of deficiency and the condition of the patient. For prophylaxis of haemorrhage approximately 10 units per kg body-weight may be given intravenously every 4 weeks. For pre-operative use, a dose of up to 35 units per kg may be given immediately before the operation and followed by approximately 10 units per kg daily for 5 days or until the wound is healed. For the treatment of severe bleeding episodes 10 to 20 units per kg should be given daily.

Cryoprecipitate is also used as a source of factor XIII.

Factor XIII is also a component of fibrin glues (see Fibrin, p.735).

Inflammatory bowel disease. Some patients with inflammatory bowel disease may be deficient in factor XIII, possibly due to increased intestinal blood loss seen in severe ulcerative colitis or increased mucosal deposition of factor XIII in Crohn's disease. Factor XIII concentrate given intravenously has produced beneficial results in 12 patients with active ulcerative colitis resistant to conventional therapy with corticosteroids and mesalazine[1] and has also been associated with healing of intractable fistulae in 3 of 4 patients with Crohn's disease.[2]

1. Lorenz R, *et al.* Factor XIII substitution in ulcerative colitis. *Lancet* 1995; **345:** 449–50.
2. Oshitani N, *et al.* Treatment of Crohn's disease fistulas with co-agulation factor XIII. *Lancet* 1996; **347:** 119–20.

Preparations

Ph. Eur.: Fibrin Sealant Kit.

Proprietary Preparations (details are given in Part 3)
Aust.: Fibrogammin; *Ger.:* Fibrogammin; *Israel:* Fibrogammin P; *UK:* Fibrogammin P.

Multi-ingredient: *Aust.:* Beriplast; Tissucol; Tissucol Duo Quick; *Canad.:* Tisseel; *Denm.:* Tisseel Duo Quick; *Fin.:* Beriplast; Tisseel Duo Quick; *Fr.:* Beriplast; Biocol; *Ger.:* Beriplast; Tissucol Duo S; Tissucol Fibrinkleber tiefgefroren†; Tissucol-Kit; *Hong Kong:* Beriplast; Tisseel; *Irl.:* Tisseel; *Israel:* Tisseel; *Mex.:* Beriplast P; *Spain:* Tissucol; *Swed.:* Tisseel Duo Quick; *Switz.:* Tissucol; Tissucol Duo S; *UK:* Tisseel.

Fibrin (1229-x)

Pharmacopoeial description

Ph. Eur.: Fibrin Sealant Kit (Fibrini Glutinum) is composed of two components, a fibrinogen concentrate containing human fibrinogen and human factor XIII, and a human thrombin preparation. The kit may also contain other ingredients, such as human fibronectin, aprotinin, and human albumin. The human constituents are obtained from plasma for fractionation and the method of preparation includes a step or steps that have been shown to remove or inactivate known agents of infection. The constituents are passed through a bacteria-retentive filter and distributed aseptically into sterile containers. Containers of freeze-dried components are sealed under vacuum or filled with oxygen-free nitrogen or other suitable inert gas before sealing. No antimicrobial preservative is added. When thawed or reconstituted in the volume of solvent stated on the label, the fibrinogen concentrate contains not less than 60 g per litre of clottable protein and not less than 10 international units of factor XIII per mL; the activity of the thrombin preparation varies over a wide range (approximately 4 to 500 international units per mL). Protect from light.

Uses and Administration

Fibrin glue is prepared by mixing solutions containing fibrinogen, factor XIII, and often other clotting components with thrombin and calcium ions usually, with the addition of aprotinin to inhibit fibrinolysis. It is used as a haemostatic to control haemorrhage during surgical procedures or as a spray to bleeding surfaces.

A dry artificial sponge of human fibrin, prepared by clotting with human thrombin a foam of a solution of human fibrinogen and known as human fibrin foam, has been used similarly.

◊ Reviews.

1. Dunn CJ, Goa KL. Fibrin sealant: a review of its use in surgery and endoscopy. *Drugs* 1999; **58:** 863–86.

Adverse effects. Fatal neurotoxicity has been reported[1] following the use of a fibrin sealant during neurosurgical procedures. The toxicity may have been due to the presence of tranexamic acid as a stabiliser in the formulation, and such formulations should not be used in surgical operations where contact with the CSF or dura mater could occur.[2]

1. Committee on Safety of Medicines/Medicines Control Agency. Quixil human surgical sealant: reports of fatal reactions. *Current Problems* 1999; **25:** 19.
2. Committee on Safety of Medicines/Medicines Control Agency. Quixil human surgical sealant: update on fatal neurotoxic reactions. *Current Problems* 2000; **26:** 10.

Preparations

Ph. Eur.: Fibrin Sealant Kit.

Proprietary Preparations (details are given in Part 3)
Braz.: Fibrinol; *Ital.:* Hemofibrine Spugna†; Zimospuma†.

Multi-ingredient: *Aust.:* Tissucol; Tissucol Duo Quick; *Belg.:* Tissucol; *Braz.:* Tissucol; *Canad.:* Tisseel; *Denm.:* Tisseel Duo Quick; *Fin.:* Beriplast; Tisseel Duo Quick; *Fr.:* Biocol; Tissucol; *Ger.:* Beriplast; Tissucol Duo S; Tissucol Fibrinkleber tiefgefroren†; Tissucol-Kit; *Hong Kong:* Tisseel; *Irl.:* Tisseel; *Israel:* Beriplast P; Tisseel; *Ital.:* Tissucol; *Mex.:* Beriplast P; *Spain:* Tissucol; *Swed.:* Tisseel Duo Quick; *Switz.:* Tissucol; Tissucol Duo S; *UK:* Tisseel.

Fibrinogen (1230-y)

Factor I.

Pharmacopoeial description

Ph. Eur.: Human Fibrinogen (Fibrinogenum Humanum; Dried Fibrinogen (BP 2001)) contains the soluble constituent of human plasma that is transformed to fibrin on addition of thrombin. It is obtained from plasma by fractionation and the method of preparation includes a step or steps that have been shown to remove or inactivate known agents of infection. Stabilisers, including protein such as human albumin, salts, and buffers may be added. No antimicrobial preservative is added. When dissolved in the volume of solvent stated on the label, the solution contains not less than 10 g per litre of fibrinogen.

A white or pale yellow powder or friable solid. Protect from light.

Profile

Fibrinogen has been used to control haemorrhage associated with low blood-fibrinogen concentration in afibrinogenaemia or hypofibrinogenaemia but the use of plasma or cryoprecipitate is usually preferred. It has also been used in disseminated intravascular coagulation (p.720). Fibrinogen is a component of fibrin glue (see Fibrin, above).

Fibrinogen labelled with radionuclides has also been used in diagnostic procedures.

Preparations

Ph. Eur.: Fibrin Sealant Kit; Human Fibrinogen.

Proprietary Preparations (details are given in Part 3)
Aust.: Haemocomplettan; *Ger.:* Haemocomplettan; *Ital.:* Fibrinomer†; Uman-Fibrin†; *Switz.:* Haemocomplettan; *UK:* Haemocomplettan P.

Multi-ingredient: *Aust.:* Beriplast; TachoComb; Tissucol; Tissucol Duo Quick; *Braz.:* Tissucol; *Canad.:* Tisseel; *Denm.:* Tisseel Duo Quick; *Fin.:* Beriplast; Tisseel Duo Quick; *Fr.:* Biocol; Tissucol; *Ger.:* Beriplast; Tisseel Duo Quick; Tissucol Duo S; Tissucol Fibrinkleber tiefgefroren†; Tissucol-Kit; *Hong Kong:* Beriplast; TachoComb; Tisseel; *Israel:* Beriplast P; Tisseel; *Mex.:* Beriplast P; *Spain:* Tissucol; *Swed.:* Tisseel Duo Quick; *Switz.:* Tissucol; Tissucol Duo S; *Thai.:* TachoComb; *UK:* Tisseel.

Filgrastim (14677-z)

Filgrastim (BAN, USAN, rINN).

r-metHuG-CSF. A recombinant human granulocyte colony-stimulating factor.

CAS — 121181-53-1.
ATC — L03AA02.

Solutions of filgrastim must not be diluted with sodium chloride solutions as precipitation will occur. Solutions of filgrastim may be adsorbed onto glass or plastic materials, therefore they should not be diluted below the recommended minimum concentration (2 μg per mL). When albumin must be added to give a final concentration of 2 mg per mL to solutions that are diluted to concentrations below 15 μg of filgrastim per mL.

Incompatibilities. References.
1. Trissel LA, Martinez JF. Compatibility of filgrastim with selected drugs during simulated Y-site administration. *Am J Hosp Pharm* 1994; **51:** 1907–13.

Adverse Effects

The main adverse effects of granulocyte colony-stimulating factors such as filgrastim during short-term treatment are musculoskeletal pain and dysuria. Hypersensitivity reactions have been reported rarely. In patients receiving long-term treatment the most frequent adverse effects are bone pain and musculoskeletal pain. Other side-effects include splenic enlargement, thrombocytopenia, anaemia, epistaxis, headache, diarrhoea, and cutaneous vasculitis. There have been reports of pulmonary infiltrates leading to respiratory failure or acute respiratory distress syndrome.

Preparations of filgrastim may contain sorbitol as an excipient; care is advisable in patients with hereditary fructose intolerance.

Colony-stimulating factors are fetotoxic in *animal* studies.

◊ General references.
1. Vial T, Descotes J. Clinical toxicity of cytokines used as haemopoietic growth factors. *Drug Safety* 1995; **13:** 371–406.

Disseminated intravascular coagulation. Long-term treatment with granulocyte colony-stimulating factor in a 7-year-old boy with HIV infection and zidovudine-induced neutropenia produced evidence of disseminated intravascular coagulation on 2 occasions.[1]

1. Mueller BU, *et al.* Disseminated intravascular coagulation associated with granulocyte colony-stimulating factor therapy in a child with human immunodeficiency virus infection. *J Pediatr* 1995; **126:** 749–52.

Effects on the bones. Bone mineral loss and osteoporosis have been reported in children with severe congenital neutropenia receiving granulocyte colony-stimulating factor for long periods.[1,2] However, the role of granulocyte colony-stimulating factor in producing this effect is uncertain since bone mineral loss may be a feature of the underlying disease.

1. Bishop NJ, *et al.* Osteoporosis in severe congenital neutropenia treated with granulocyte colony-stimulating factor. *Br J Haematol* 1995; **89:** 927–8.
2. Yakisan E, *et al.* High incidence of significant bone loss in patients with severe congenital neutropenia (Kostmann's syndrome). *J Pediatr* 1997; **131:** 592–7.

Effects on the eyes. Subretinal haemorrhage resulting in irreversible loss of vision in one eye occurred in a 4-year-old girl who received filgrastim and nartogramostim for chemotherapy-induced neutropenia and for mobilising peripheral blood stem cells.[1] It was postulated that the colony-stimulating factor reactivated a primary ocular inflammation probably caused by an infection.

1. Matsumura T, *et al.* Subretinal haemorrhage after granulocyte colony-stimulating factor. *Lancet* 1997; **350:** 336. Correction. *ibid.;* 1406.

Effects on the lungs. There have been reports of exacerbation of chemotherapy-induced pulmonary toxicity in patients receiving granulocyte colony-stimulating factor in conjunction with bleomycin[1,2] and cyclophosphamide.[3] The patients were also receiving other antineoplastics. However, analysis of 2 randomised controlled studies failed to show increased pulmonary toxicity when granulocyte colony-stimulating factor was added to bleomycin therapy[4,5] and it has been suggested[5] that confounding factors, including the use of other antineoplastics, may account for the increased pulmonary toxicity.

1. Matthews JH. Pulmonary toxicity of ABVD chemotherapy and G-CSF in Hodgkin's disease: possible synergy. *Lancet* 1993; **342:** 988.
2. Dirix LY, *et al.* Pulmonary toxicity and bleomycin. *Lancet* 1994; **344:** 56.
3. van Woensel JBM, *et al.* Acute respiratory insufficiency during doxorubicin, cyclophosphamide, and G-CSF therapy. *Lancet* 1994; **344:** 759–60.
4. Bastion Y, *et al.* Possible toxicity with the association of G-CSF and bleomycin. *Lancet* 1994; **343:** 1221–2.
5. Bastion Y, Coiffier B. Pulmonary toxicity of bleomycin: is G-CSF a risk factor? *Lancet* 1994; **344:** 474.

Effects on the skin. Skin reactions may occur in patients given colony-stimulating factors. In a study in women with inflammatory breast cancer, a pruritic skin reaction developed at the subcutaneous injection site in all 7 given granulocyte-macrophage colony-stimulating factor.[1] Exacerbation of psoriasis[2] and precipitation or exacerbation of neutrophilic dermatoses including Sweet's syndrome,[3,4] pyoderma gangrenosum,[5] and neutrophilic eccrine hidradenitis[6] have been reported following administration of granulocyte colony-stimulating factor.

1. Steger GG, *et al.* Cutaneous reactions to GM-CSF in inflammatory breast cancer. *N Engl J Med* 1992; **327:** 286.
2. Kavanaugh A. Flare of psoriasis and psoriatic arthritis following treatment with granulocyte colony-stimulating factor. *Am J Med* 1996; **101:** 567.
3. Petit T, *et al.* Lymphoedema-area-restricted Sweet syndrome during G-CSF treatment. *Lancet* 1996; **347:** 690.
4. Garty BZ, *et al.* Sweet syndrome associated with G-CSF treatment in a child with glycogen storage disease type Ib. *Pediatrics* 1996; **97:** 401–3.
5. Johnson ML, Grimwood RE. Leukocyte colony-stimulating factors: a review of associated neutrophilic dermatoses and vasculitides. *Arch Dermatol* 1994; **130:** 77–81.
6. Bachmeyer C, *et al.* Neutrophilic eccrine hidradenitis induced by granulocyte colony-stimulating factor. *Br J Dermatol* 1998; **139:** 354–5.

Effects on the thyroid. Reversible thyroid dysfunction has been reported in patients with pre-existing thyroid antibodies during treatment with granulocyte-macrophage colony-stimulating factor,[1] but not with granulocyte colony-stimulating factor.[2] However, clinical hypothyroidism has been reported in a patient with no history of thyroid dysfunction or thyroid antibodies during treatment with granulocyte colony-stimulating factor.[3]

1. Hoekman K, *et al.* Reversible thyroid dysfunction during treatment with GM-CSF. *Lancet* 1991; **338:** 541–2.
2. van Hoef MEHM, Howell A. Risk of thyroid dysfunction during treatment with G-CSF. *Lancet* 1992; **340:** 1169–70.
3. de Luis DA, Romero E. Reversible thyroid dysfunction with filgrastim. *Lancet* 1996; **348:** 1595–6.

Inflammatory disorders. Reactivation of various inflammatory disorders including rheumatoid arthritis[1] and pseudogout[2,3] has been reported following administration of granulocyte colony-stimulating factors. For further reports of

reactivation of sites of inflammation, see under Effects on the Eyes and Effects on the Skin, above.

1. Vildarsson B, *et al.* Reactivation of rheumatoid arthritis and development of leukocytoclastic vasculitis in a patient receiving granulocyte colony-stimulating factor for Felty's syndrome. *Am J Med* 1995; **98:** 589–91.
2. Sandor V, *et al.* Exacerbation of pseudogout by granulocyte colony-stimulating factor. *Ann Intern Med* 1996; **125:** 781.
3. Teramoto S, *et al.* Increased synovial interleukin-8 and interleukin-6 levels in pseudogout associated with granulocyte colony-stimulating factor. *Ann Intern Med* 1998; **129:** 424–5.

Precautions

Since granulocyte colony-stimulating factors such as filgrastim can promote growth of myeloid cells *in vitro* their use in myeloid malignancies has been contraindicated, although recently colony-stimulating factors have been used in some patients with myeloid diseases without stimulation of malignant cells. However, caution is required when they are used in patients with any pre-malignant or malignant myeloid condition. They should not be used from 24 hours before until 24 hours after cytotoxic chemotherapy due to the sensitivity of rapidly dividing myeloid cells.

The complete blood count should be monitored regularly during therapy with granulocyte colony-stimulating factors. Treatment should be withdrawn in patients who develop signs of pulmonary infiltrates. Bone density should be monitored in patients with osteoporosis who are receiving long-term treatment with filgrastim.

Uses and Administration

Filgrastim is a granulocyte colony-stimulating factor that acts as a haematopoietic growth factor stimulating the development of granulocytes. It is used to treat or prevent neutropenia in patients receiving myelosuppressive cancer chemotherapy and to reduce the period of neutropenia in patients undergoing bone-marrow transplantation (p.480). It is also used to mobilise peripheral blood progenitor cells for use as an alternative to bone marrow transplantation, in the management of chronic neutropenia (congenital, cyclic, or idiopathic), and for persistent neutropenia in patients with advanced HIV infection.

Filgrastim may be given intravenously or subcutaneously. Doses may be expressed in μg or in units; 10 μg is equivalent to 1 million units.

As an adjunct to antineoplastic therapy, filgrastim is given in a dose of 5 μg per kg body-weight daily starting not less than 24 hours after the last dose of antineoplastic. It can be given as a single daily subcutaneous injection, as a continuous intravenous or subcutaneous infusion, or as a daily intravenous infusion over 15 to 30 minutes. Treatment is continued until the neutrophil count has stabilised within the normal range which may take up to 14 days or more.

The initial dose following bone-marrow transplantation is 10 μg per kg daily, adjusted according to response. This may be given by intravenous infusion over 30 minutes, intravenous infusion over 4 hours, or by continuous intravenous or subcutaneous infusion over 24 hours.

For mobilisation of peripheral blood progenitor cells, a dose of 10 μg per kg daily of filgrastim may be given subcutaneously as a single daily injection or by continuous infusion; if given after myelosuppressive chemotherapy this dose is halved to 5 μg per kg daily by subcutaneous injection.

In patients with congenital neutropenia the recommended initial dose is 12 μg per kg daily and in patients with idiopathic or cyclic neutropenia the recommended initial dose is 5 μg per kg daily. In these forms of neutropenia the dose is given subcutaneously in single or divided doses and should be adjusted according to response.

In patients with HIV infection and persistent neutropenia the initial dose is 1 μg per kg daily by subcutaneous injection. The dose may be titrated up to a maximum of 4 μg per kg daily until a normal neutrophil count is achieved and then adjusted for maintenance according to response. Maintenance doses of 300 μg daily on 1 to 7 days a week have been used.

The doses described above for patients receiving antineoplastic therapy and for chronic neutropenias may also be given to children.

◊ Colony-stimulating factors or haematopoietic growth factors are naturally occurring glycoprotein growth factors (cytokines) that promote the proliferation and differentiation of haematopoietic precursors. Many colony-stimulating factors have been identified that stimulate development of different cell lines. These include: erythropoietin (p.730); granulocyte colony-stimulating factors; granulocyte-macrophage colony-stimulating factors such as molgramostim (p.738); thrombopoietin (p.742); interleukin-3 (p.738); and oprelvekin (interleukin-11) (p.739). Other factors under investigation include macrophage colony-stimulating factors and ancestim (stem cell factor).

◊ References.
1. Frampton JE, et al. Filgrastim: a review of its pharmacological properties and therapeutic efficacy in neutropenia. Drugs 1994; 48: 731–60.
2. American Society of Clinical Oncology. Recommendations for the use of hematopoietic colony-stimulating factors: evidence-based, clinical practice guidelines. J Clin Oncol 1994; 12: 2471–2508.
3. American Society of Clinical Oncology. Update of recommendations for the use of hematopoietic colony-stimulating factors: evidence-based clinical practice guidelines. J Clin Oncol 1996; 14: 1957–60.
4. Nemunaitis J. A comparative review of colony-stimulating factors. Drugs 1997; 54: 709–29.
5. Ozer H, et al. 2000 Update of recommendations for the use of hematopoietic colony-stimulating factors: evidence-based, clinical practice guidelines. J Clin Oncol 2000; 18: 3558–85.

Aplastic anaemia. Colony-stimulating factors, including granulocyte colony-stimulating factors, have been tried in a few patients with aplastic anaemia (p.715).

Infections. It has been suggested[1] that colony-stimulating factors may be useful as adjuncts to antibacterial or antifungal therapy in patients with severe infections and defects in phagocytic cell function. Such defects may occur in patients with diabetes mellitus or AIDS. Addition of granulocyte colony-stimulating factor to conventional therapy improved clinical outcome of foot infection in a small study in diabetic patients[2] and 3 of 4 patients with AIDS and resistant oral candidiasis responded to treatment with granulocyte-macrophage colony-stimulating factor.[3] A controlled study in 258 patients with advanced HIV infection found that prophylactic administration of granulocyte colony-stimulating factor reduced the incidence of severe neutropenia and also suggested that the incidence and duration of bacterial infections was reduced.[4]

Granulocyte colony-stimulating factors have also been tried as an adjunct to conventional therapy in chronic viral hepatitis.[5]

1. Khwaja A, Linch DC. Haemopoietic growth factors in the treatment of infection in non-neutropenic patients. J Antimicrob Chemother 1994; 33: 679–83.
2. Gough A, et al. Randomised placebo-controlled trial of granulocyte-colony stimulating factor in diabetic foot infection. Lancet 1997; 350: 855–9.
3. Capetti A, et al. Employment of recombinant human granulocyte-macrophage colony stimulating factor in oesophageal candidiasis in AIDS patients. AIDS 1995; 9: 1378–9.
4. Kuritzkes DP, et al. Filgrastim prevents severe neutropenia and reduces infective morbidity in patients with advanced HIV infection: results of a randomized, multicenter, controlled trial. AIDS 1998; 12: 65–74.
5. Pardo M, et al. Treatment of chronic hepatitis C with cirrhosis with recombinant human granulocyte colony-stimulating factor plus recombinant interferon-alpha. J Med Virol 1995; 45: 439–44.

Neutropenia. Granulocyte colony-stimulating factors are used in the management of neutropenia (p.723). They are used to treat or prevent antineoplastic-induced neutropenia and have also been tried in patients with neutropenia induced by a wide range of other drugs.[1-6] They may be used for long-term treatment in patients with chronic neutropenias.[7] Short-term administration has been tried in a few preterm neonates with neutropenia and severe infections and increases in neutrophil counts have been reported in some,[8,9] though not in others.[10] There has also been a preliminary report that prophylaxis with filgrastim may reduce the incidence of sepsis in critically-ill neonates with neutropenia.[11] Granulocyte colony-stimulating factors have also been tried with mixed results in neonates with the rare condition of alloimmune neutropenia.[12-14]

1. Gerson SL, et al. Granulocyte colony-stimulating factor for clozapine-induced agranulocytosis. Lancet 1992; 340: 1097.
2. Wyatt S, et al. Filgrastim for mesalazine-associated neutropenia. Lancet 1993; 341: 1476.
3. Teitelbaum AH, et al. Filgrastim (r-met HuG-CSF) reversal of drug-induced agranulocytosis. Am J Med 1993; 95: 245–6.
4. Geibig CB, Marks LW. Treatment of clozapine- and molindone-induced agranulocytosis with granulocyte colony-stimulating factor. Ann Pharmacother 1993; 27: 1190–2.
5. Chia HM, et al. Filgrastim for low-dose, captopril-induced agranulocytosis. Lancet 1993; 342: 304.
6. Gales BJ, Gales MA. Granulocyte-colony stimulating factor for sulfasalazine-induced agranulocytosis. Ann Pharmacother 1993; 27: 1052–4.
7. Bonilla MA, et al. Long-term safety of treatment with recombinant human granulocyte colony-stimulating factor (r-metHuG-CSF) in patients with severe congenital neutropenias. Br J Haematol 1994; 88: 723–30.
8. Bedford Russell AR, et al. Granulocyte colony stimulating factor treatment for neonatal neutropenia. Arch Dis Child 1995; 72: F53–F54.

The symbol † denotes a preparation no longer actively marketed

9. Carr R, Modi N. Haemopoietic colony stimulating factors for preterm neonates. Arch Dis Child 1997; 76: F128–F133.
10. Schibler KR, et al. A randomized, placebo-controlled trial of granulocyte colony-stimulating factor administration to newborn infants with neutropenia and clinical signs of early-onset sepsis. Pediatrics 1998; 102: 6–13.
11. Kocherlakota P, La Gamma EF. Preliminary report: rhG-CSF may reduce the incidence of neonatal sepsis in prolonged preeclampsia-associated neutropenia. Pediatrics 1998; 102: 1107–11.
12. Gilmore MM, et al. Treatment of alloimmune neonatal neutropenia with granulocyte colony-stimulating factor. J Pediatr 1994; 125: 948–51.
13. Bedu A, et al. Failure of granulocyte colony-stimulating factor in alloimmune neonatal neutropenia. J Pediatr 1995; 127: 508.
14. Rodwell RL, et al. Granulocyte colony stimulating factor treatment for alloimmune neonatal neutropenia. Arch Dis Child 1996; 75: F57–F58.

Preparations

Proprietary Preparations (details are given in Part 3)
Aust.: Neupogen; *Austral.:* Neupogen; *Belg.:* Neupogen; *Braz.:* Granulokine; *Canad.:* Neupogen; *Denm.:* Neupogen; *Fin.:* Neupogen; *Fr.:* Neupogen; *Ger.:* Neupogen; *Hong Kong:* Neupogen; *Irl.:* Neupogen; *Israel:* Neupogen; *Ital.:* Granulokine; Neupogen; *Jpn:* Gran; *Mex.:* Neupogen; *Neth.:* Neupogen; *Norw.:* Neupogen; *NZ:* Neupogen; *Port.:* Neupogen; *S.Afr.:* Neupogen; *Singapore:* Neupogen; *Spain:* Granulokine; Neupogen; *Swed.:* Neupogen; *Switz.:* Neupogen; *Thai.:* Neupogen; *UK:* Neupogen; *USA:* Neupogen.

Gelatin   (5425-w)

Gelatina.

Pharmacopoeias. In Chin., Eur. (see p.vi), Int., Jpn, and Pol. Also in USNF.

Gelatins are usually graded by jelly strength, expressed as 'Bloom strength' or 'Bloom rating'.

The gelatin described in some pharmacopoeias is not necessarily suitable for preparations for parenteral use or for other special purposes.

Pharmacopoeial description

Ph. Eur.: Gelatin is a purified protein obtained either by partial acid hydrolysis (type A) or by partial alkaline hydrolysis (type B) of animal collagen or it may be a mixture of types A and B. It is not necessarily suitable for preparations for parenteral use or for other special purposes.

Light amber to faintly yellow translucent sheets, shreds, powder, or granules.

Gelatin swells in cold water and on heating it gives a colloidal solution which on subsequent cooling forms a more or less firm gel. It is practically insoluble in common organic solvents. A 1% solution in water at about 55° has a pH of 3.8 to 7.6. Store in airtight containers.

USNF 20: Gelatin is obtained by the partial hydrolysis of collagen derived from the skin, white connective tissue, and bones of animals. Gelatin derived from an acid-treated precursor is known as Type A, and gelatin derived from an alkali-treated precursor is known as Type B.

Faintly yellow or amber sheets, flakes, or shreds, or a coarse to fine powder, the colour varying in depth according to the particle size. A solution has a slight, characteristic, bouillon-like odour. It is stable in air when dry, but is subject to microbial decomposition when moist or in solution. Gelatin swells and softens when immersed in cold water, gradually absorbing 5 to 10 times its weight of water. Soluble in hot water, in 6N acetic acid, and in a hot mixture of glycerol and water; insoluble in alcohol, in chloroform, in ether, and in fixed and volatile oils.

Incompatibilities. A white precipitate was formed immediately when vancomycin injection was administered through a giving set containing modified fluid gelatin solution.[1]

1. Taylor A, Hornbrey P. Incompatibility of vancomycin and gelatin plasma expanders. Pharm J 1991; 246: 466.

Adverse Effects

Hypersensitivity reactions including anaphylactic reactions have occurred after the infusion of gelatin or its derivatives. Rapid infusion of gelatin derivatives may directly stimulate the release of histamine and other vasoactive substances.

For adverse reactions associated with the topical use of gelatin, see Haemostasis under Uses and Administration, below.

Effects on the kidneys. Acute renal failure developed in a patient undergoing aortobifemoral graft surgery who received modified fluid gelatin, blood transfusion, and diuretics following a fall in urine output.[1,2] The conclusion that gelatin was the most likely cause of the renal failure was contested[3-5] on the basis of previous experience and other major contributory factors such as diminished intravascular volume and reduced organ perfusion.

1. Hussain SF, Drew PJT. Acute renal failure after infusion of gelatins. BMJ 1989; 299: 1137–8.

2. Drew PJT, Hussain SF. Acute renal failure after infusion of gelatin. BMJ 1989; 299: 1400. Correction. ibid.; 1531.
3. Frazer RS, Macmillan RR. Acute renal failure after infusion of gelatin. BMJ 1989; 299: 1399.
4. Fawcett WJ. Acute renal failure after infusion of gelatin. BMJ 1989; 299: 1399.
5. Wilkins RG. Acute renal failure after infusion of gelatin. BMJ 1989; 299: 1399–1400.

Hypersensitivity. Ten severe anaphylactoid reactions to an infusion of a modified fluid gelatin were reported over a period of 3 years.[1] Some hypersensitivity reactions associated with vaccine administration in children have also been attributed to the use of gelatin as an excipient.[2]

For reports of fatal reactions in asthmatic patients following administration of gelatin derivatives, see Polygeline, p.741.

1. Blanloeil Y, et al. Accidents anaphylactoïdes sévères après perfusion d'une gélatine fluide modifiée en solution équilibrée Therapie 1983; 38: 519–21.
2. Kumagai T, et al. Gelatin-specific humoral and cellular immune responses in children with immediate- and nonimmediate-type reactions to live measles, mumps, rubella, and varicella vaccines. J Allergy Clin Immunol 1997; 100: 130–4.

Precautions

Precautions that should be observed with plasma expanders are described under Dextran 70, p.729, and these should be considered when gelatin and gelatin derivatives are used for this purpose. There does not appear to be any interference with blood grouping and cross-matching of blood.

Pharmacokinetics

Following infusion of modified fluid gelatin (succinylated gelatin), 75% of the dose is excreted in the urine in 24 hours. The half-life is about 4 hours.

Uses and Administration

Gelatin is a protein that has both clinical and pharmaceutical uses.

Gelatin is used as a haemostatic in surgical procedures as an absorbable film or sponge and can absorb many times its weight of blood. It is also employed as a plasma volume expander similarly to the dextrans in hypovolaemic shock (p.813). A 4% solution of a modified fluid gelatin (succinylated gelatin) has been infused in doses of 500 to 1000 mL. It may also be used in the form of a gelatin-derived polymer, see Polygeline, p.741.

Gelatin rods may be employed to temporarily block tear outflow in the diagnosis of dry eye (p.1498).

Gelatin is used in the preparation of pastes, pastilles, suppositories, tablets, and hard and soft capsule shells. It is also used for the microencapsulation of drugs and other industrial materials. It has been used as a vehicle for injections; Pitkin's Menstruum, which consists of gelatin, glucose, and acetic acid, has been used in a modified form for heparin while hydrolysed gelatin has been used for corticotropin. Gelatin is an ingredient of preparations used for the protection of stoma and lesions.

Haemostasis. Gelatin acts as a haemostatic (p.718) by providing a physical meshwork within which clotting can occur.

Gelatin powder may be applied dry to wound beds and may be most useful when mixed with saline or thrombin and applied to bone. Gelatin sponge can be applied dry or soaked in saline or thrombin solutions. When applied to skin wounds the gelatin liquefies within 2 to 5 days; when implanted into tissues it is absorbed within 4 to 6 weeks. Adverse reactions include an increased incidence of infection, compression of surrounding tissue due to fluid absorption, granuloma formation, and fibrosis. Generally, gelatin sponges cause little tissue reaction and can be applied to bone, dura, and pleural tissue.

References.
1. Larson PO. Topical hemostatic agents for dermatologic surgery. J Dermatol Surg Oncol 1988; 14: 623–32.

Neonatal intraventricular haemorrhage. Plasma volume expansion in preterm neonates has been thought to help prevent neonatal intraventricular haemorrhage (p.723). However, a study using plasma or gelatin as plasma volume expanders,[1,2] found no evidence of a decreased risk of such haemorrhage or subsequent death or disability.

1. The Northern Neonatal Nursing Initiative Trial Group. A randomized trial comparing the effect of prophylactic intravenous fresh frozen plasma, gelatin or glucose on early mortality and morbidity in preterm babies. Eur J Pediatr 1996; 155: 580–8.
2. Northern Neonatal Nursing Initiative Trial Group. Randomised trial of prophylactic early fresh-frozen plasma or gelatin or glucose in preterm babies: outcome at 2 years. Lancet 1996; 348: 229–32.

Preparations

USP 25: Absorbable Gelatin Film; Absorbable Gelatin Sponge.

Proprietary Preparations (details are given in Part 3)
Aust.: Gelofusin; Spongostan†; **Austral.:** Gelfilm; Gelfoam; Gelofusine; **Belg.:** Gelfoam; Gelofusine; Geloplasma†; Willspon†; **Braz.:** Hisocel; **Canad.:** Gelfilm; Gelfoam; **Fin.:** Gelofusine; **Fr.:** Epiphane; Gel-Phan; Gelodiet; Gelofusine; Hydrocoll; Orangel; **Ger.:** Gelafundin; Gelafusal-N in Ringeracetat; Gelaspon; Gelastypt; stypro; Thomaegelin; **Hong Kong:** Gelafundin; Gelfilm; Gelfoam; Gelofusine; **Israel:** Gelfoam; **Ital.:** Cutanplast; Eufusin; Spongostan†; **Neth.:** Gelfilm; Gelfoam; Geloplasma†; Willspon; **NZ:** Gelfilm; Gelfoam; **Port.:** Epiphane 7; Gelafundina; **S.Afr.:** Gelofusine; Spongostan†; **Singapore:** Gelfoam; Gelofusine; **Spain:** Espongostan†; Geloplasma; **Switz.:** Gelfoam†; Physiogel; **Thai.:** Gelafundin; Gelofusine; **UK:** Geloflex; Gelofusine; **USA:** Gelfilm; Gelfoam.

Multi-ingredient: Aust.: Gelacet; **Austral.:** Orabase; Orahesive; Stomahesive; **Canad.:** Orabase; Orahesive; **Fr.:** Gelogastrine†; Plasmagel; Plasmion; Rectopanbiline; **Ger.:** Gelacet N; Gerontamin; **Irl.:** Orabase; **Israel:** Orabase; **Ital.:** Solecin; **NZ:** Stomahesive; **Port.:** Combiderm; Varihesive; **Switz.:** Gelacet; Varihesive Hydroactive†; **UK:** Orabase; Orahesive; Stomahesive; Varihesive†; **USA:** Dome-Paste.

Haemoglobin (12812-y)

Profile

Haemoglobin has the property of reversible oxygenation and is the respiratory pigment of blood. Solutions of haemoglobin or modified haemoglobin are being investigated as blood substitutes.

◊ The structure of haemoglobin gives a non-linear oxygen dissociation curve; almost maximum oxygen saturation occurs in normal arterial blood without the need for oxygen-enriched air. Thus the use of haemoglobin solutions for emergency use appears logical. Initial *animal* experiments with haemoglobin from haemolysed erythrocytes resulted in serious renal damage but haemoglobin is not itself nephrotoxic and the development of stroma-free haemoglobin solutions reduced this toxicity. However, once released from the erythrocytes, haemoglobin loses its ability to hold 2,3-diphosphoglycerate, which is essential for the delivery of oxygen, and haemoglobin, being a small molecule, is rapidly excreted by the kidneys. Various methods have been tried to overcome these problems; addition of pyridoxine 5-phosphate and formation of crosslinked haemoglobin restore the oxygen affinity to that of whole blood and polymerisation or microencapsulation in a lipid membrane extend the half-life. Polymerisation has the added advantages that this process is virucidal and also lowers the osmolality of the solution permitting higher concentrations to be used. There are, however, reservations concerning haemoglobin solutions as blood substitutes; blood itself must be available for their production, although expired blood may be employed and there is also concern about impairment of immune mechanisms. The development of recombinant human haemoglobin may overcome these problems and may allow further modification of the haemoglobin molecule.

References.
1. Anonymous. Blood substitutes: has the right solution been found? *Lancet* 1986; **i:** 717–18.
2. Urbaniak SJ. Artificial blood. *BMJ* 1991; **303:** 1348–50.
3. Jones JA. Red blood cell substitutes: current status. *Br J Anaesth* 1995; **74:** 697–703.
4. Mallick A, Bodenham AR. Modified haemoglobins as oxygen-transporting blood substitutes. *Br J Hosp Med* 1996; **55:** 443–8.
5. Lowe KC. Red cell substitutes. In: Contreras M, ed. *ABC of transfusion.* 3rd ed. London: BMJ Books, 1998: 71–5.

Preparations

Proprietary Preparations (details are given in Part 3)
Multi-ingredient: Belg.: Aperop; Vitathion†.

Interleukin-3 (16855-w)

Profile

Interleukin-3 (IL-3) is a cytokine that acts as a colony-stimulating factor. It is under investigation in the management of myelosuppression associated with cancer chemotherapy and following bone marrow transplantation. A fusion molecule with granulocyte-macrophage colony-stimulating factor, known as milodistim (PIXY-321), is also under investigation.

Lenograstim (15280-h)

Lenograstim (BAN, USAN, rINN).
rG-CSF. A recombinant human granulocyte colony-stimulating factor.
CAS — 135968-09-1.
ATC — L03AA10.

Solutions of colony-stimulating factors may be adsorbed onto glass or plastic materials. Solutions of lenograstim should not be diluted below the minimum recommended concentration for the formulation used.

Adverse Effects and Precautions

As for Filgrastim, p.736.

Uses and Administration

Lenograstim is a granulocyte colony-stimulating factor with actions and uses similar to those of filgrastim (p.736). It is used to treat or prevent neutropenia in patients receiving myelosuppressive cancer chemotherapy and to reduce the period of neutropenia in patients undergoing bone-marrow transplantation (p.480). It is also used to mobilise peripheral blood progenitor cells for use as an alternative to bone-marrow transplantation.

Lenograstim may be given in a dose of 150 µg (19.2 million international units) per m² body-surface daily to patients following bone-marrow transplantation and also to patients established on antineoplastic therapy; in post-transplant patients it is given by intravenous infusion over 30 minutes or by subcutaneous injection, and in patients on antineoplastics it is given subcutaneously. Treatment is given until the neutrophil count has stabilised within the normal range, but a maximum treatment period of 28 consecutive days should not be exceeded.

For mobilisation of peripheral blood progenitor cells after cytotoxic chemotherapy a dose of 150 µg (19.2 million international units) per m² daily may be administered by subcutaneous injection starting the day after completion of chemotherapy. When used alone, or in healthy donors, a dose of 10 µg (1.28 million international units) per kg body-weight daily is given subcutaneously for 4 to 6 days.

◊ References.
1. Frampton JE, et al. Lenograstim: a review of its pharmacological properties and therapeutic efficacy in neutropenia and related clinical settings. *Drugs* 1995; **49:** 767–93.
2. Dunn CJ, Goa KL. Lenograstim: an update of its pharmacological properties and use in chemotherapy-induced neutropenia and related clinical settings. *Drugs* 2000; **59:** 681–717.

Preparations

Proprietary Preparations (details are given in Part 3)
Aust.: Granocyte; **Austral.:** Granocyte; **Belg.:** Granocyte; **Denm.:** Granocyte; **Fin.:** Granocyte; **Fr.:** Granocyte; **Ger.:** Granocyte; **Irl.:** Granocyte; **Israel:** Granocyte; **Ital.:** Myelostim; **Jpn:** Neutrogin; **Neth.:** Granocyte; **Norw.:** Granocyte; **NZ:** Granocyte; **Port.:** Granocyte; **S.Afr.:** Granocyte; **Singapore:** Granocyte; **Spain:** Euprotin; Granocyte; **Swed.:** Granocyte; **Switz.:** Granocyte; **Thai.:** Granocyte; **UK:** Granocyte.

Leucocytes (1244-t)

Preparations of leucocytes contain granulocytes with a variable content of red blood cells, lymphocytes, and platelets. Depending on the method of collection they may also contain dextran or hetastarch.

Adverse Effects and Precautions

Leucocyte transfusions may cause severe transfusion reactions and fever. As with other blood products, there is a risk of transmission of infection. Severe lung reactions including fluid overload with pulmonary oedema are a particular problem in patients with active pulmonary infections.

Red blood cell compatibility testing is necessary because of the content of red blood cells. Graft-versus-host disease may occur in immunosuppressed recipients, and may be avoided by irradiating the product before administration.

Uses and Administration

Transfusion of leucocytes has been used in patients with severe granulocytopenia and infection which has not been controlled by treatment with appropriate antimicrobials for 48 to 72 hours. Transfusion of 1×10^{10} granulocytes once or twice daily has been suggested as an effective dose. Daily transfusions for at least 3 to 4 days are usually advised. Hydrocortisone and chlorpheniramine [chlorphenamine] may be given intravenously before transfusion to reduce the severity of adverse reactions.

◊ References.
1. Brozović B, et al. Platelet and granulocyte transfusions. In: Contreras M, ed. *ABC of transfusion.* 3rd ed. London: BMJ Books, 1998: 17–22.

Preparations

Proprietary Preparations (details are given in Part 3)
Ger.: LeukoNorm.

Metacresolsulfonic Acid-Formaldehyde (1723-e)

m-Cresolsulphonic acid-formaldehyde condensation product; Dicresulene polymer; Metacresulphonic Acid-Formaldehyde; Polycresulfonate. Dihydroxydimethyldiphenylmethanedisulphonic acid polymer; Methylenebis(hydroxytoluenesulphonic acid) polymer.
$(C_{15}H_{16}O_8S_2)_n$.
CAS — 9011-02-3.

Profile

Preparations of metacresolsulfonic acid-formaldehyde are highly acidic and are used as topical haemostatics and antiseptics. There are a number of vaginal preparations.

Preparations

Proprietary Preparations (details are given in Part 3)
Belg.: Lotagen†; **Denm.:** Nelex†; **Fin.:** Nelex; **Fr.:** Negatol; **Ger.:** Albothyl; **Hong Kong:** Albothyl; **Ital.:** Negatol; **Mex.:** Albothyl; **Port.:** Nelex; **S.Afr.:** Nelex; **Singapore:** Albothyl; **Spain:** Negatol; **Swed.:** Nelex†; **Switz.:** Negatol; Negatol Dental; **Thai.:** Albothyl.

Molgramostim (15057-a)

Molgramostim (BAN, USAN, rINN).
Sch-39300. A recombinant human granulocyte-macrophage colony-stimulating factor; Colony-stimulating factor 2 (human clone pHG25 protein moiety reduced).
CAS — 99283-10-0.
ATC — L03AA03.

Solutions of molgramostim may be adsorbed onto glass and plastic materials and therefore should not be diluted below the recommended minimum concentration of 7 µg per mL.

Adverse Effects

Granulocyte-macrophage colony-stimulating factors such as molgramostim may cause transient hypotension and flushing, bone pain and musculoskeletal pain, fever and chills, dyspnoea, rash, fatigue, and gastrointestinal effects. Antibodies have been detected. Anaphylactic reactions, pleural and pericardial effusion, and cardiac rhythm abnormalities have been reported rarely.

Colony-stimulating factors are fetotoxic in *animal* studies.

◊ General references.
1. Vial T, Descotes J. Clinical toxicity of cytokines used as haemopoietic growth factors. *Drug Safety* 1995; **13:** 371–406.

Antibodies. Antibodies have been reported in patients following administration of granulocyte-macrophage colony-stimulating factors produced in yeast[1] or in *Escherichia coli.*[2] Such factors are nonglycosylated or only partially glycosylated. A study[2] in 20 nonimmunocompromised patients given *E. coli*-derived granulocyte-macrophage colony-stimulating factors found that antibodies that were associated with reduced biological effectiveness developed in 95% of the patients. Only 1 of 8 immunocompromised patients given the colony-stimulating factor developed antibodies.
1. Gribben JG, et al. Development of antibodies to unprotected glycosylation sites on recombinant human GM-CSF. *Lancet* 1990; **335:** 434–7.
2. Ragnhammar P, et al. Induction of anti-recombinant human granulocyte-macrophage colony-stimulating factor (Escherichia coli-derived) antibodies and clinical effects in nonimmunocompromised patients. *Blood* 1994; **84:** 4078–87.

Effects on the skin. See under Filgrastim, p.736.

Effects on the thyroid. See under Filgrastim, p.736.

Hypoalbuminaemia. In a series of 9 patients given prolonged treatment with granulocyte-macrophage colony-stimulating factor for myelodysplasia or aplastic anaemia, 4 developed hypoalbuminaemia that was symptomatic in 2 of the patients.[1]
1. Kaczmarski RS, Mufti GJ. Hypoalbuminaemia after prolonged treatment with recombinant granulocyte macrophage colony stimulating factor. *BMJ* 1990; **301:** 1312–13.

Precautions

Since granulocyte-macrophage colony-stimulating factors such as molgramostim can promote growth of myeloid cells *in vitro* their use in myeloid malignancies has been contra-indicated, although recently colony-stimulating factors have been used in some patients with myeloid diseases without stimulation of malignant cells. However, caution is required when they are used in patients with any pre-malignant or malignant myeloid condition. They should not be used from 24 hours before until 24 hours after cytotoxic chemotherapy or radiotherapy due to the sensitivity of rapidly dividing myeloid cells.

Granulocyte-macrophage colony-stimulating factors should be used with caution in patients with pulmonary disease as they may be predisposed to dyspnoea. Treatment should be withdrawn in patients who develop signs of pulmonary infiltrates. Caution is also necessary in patients with fluid retention or heart failure as fluid retention may be aggravated.

The complete blood count should be monitored regularly during therapy.

Uses and Administration

Molgramostim is a granulocyte-macrophage colony-stimulating factor (GM-CSF) that acts as a haematopoietic growth factor stimulating the development of white blood cells, particularly granulocytes, macrophages, and monocytes. It is used to treat or prevent neutropenia in patients receiving myelosuppressive cancer chemotherapy and to reduce the period of neutropenia in patients undergoing bone marrow transplantation (p.480). It is also used to reduce ganciclovir-induced neutropenia (p.623).

As an adjunct to antineoplastic therapy, molgramostim is given by subcutaneous injection, starting 24 hours after the last dose of antineoplastic, in a dose of 5 to 10 µg (60 000 to 110 000 international units) per kg body-weight daily. Treatment should be continued for 7 to 10 days.

Following bone marrow transplantation, molgramostim may be given by intravenous infusion over 4 to 6 hours in a dose of 10 µg (110 000 international units) per kg daily. Treatment should be initiated the day after bone marrow transplantation and continued for up to 30 days depending on the neutrophil count.

For the management of ganciclovir-induced neutropenia, molgramostim may be given by subcutaneous injection in a dose of 5 µg (60 000 international units) per kg daily. After 5 doses have been given the dose of molgramostim should be adjusted according to the neutrophil count.

The maximum dose for any indication should not exceed 10 µg (110 000 international units) per kg daily.

Granulocyte colony-stimulating factors such as filgrastim (p.736) are also used. Macrophage colony-stimulating factors such as mirimostim are under investigation.

◊ General references.
1. American Society of Clinical Oncology. Recommendations for the use of hematopoietic colony-stimulating factors: evidence-based, clinical practice guidelines. *J Clin Oncol* 1994; **12:** 2471–2508.
2. American Society of Clinical Oncology. Update of recommendations for the use of hematopoietic colony-stimulating factors: evidence-based clinical practice guidelines. *J Clin Oncol* 1996; **14:** 1957–60.
3. Nemunaitis J. A comparative review of colony-stimulating factors. *Drugs* 1997; **54:** 709–29.
4. Ozer H, *et al.* 2000 Update of recommendations for the use of hematopoietic colony-stimulating factors: evidence-based, clinical practice guidelines. *J Clin Oncol* 2000; **18:** 3558–85.

Aplastic anaemia. Colony-stimulating factors, including granulocyte-macrophage colony-stimulating factors, have been tried in a few patients with aplastic anaemia (p.715).

Infections. See under Filgrastim, p.737.

Wounds and ulcers. Molgramostim modifies several mechanisms involved in wound healing and is being investigated in non-healing wounds and ulcers. It has been tried as an incubation solution for skin grafts,[1] and by perilesional injection[2,3] and topical application.[4]
1. Pojda Z, Struzyna J. Treatment of non-healing ulcers with rhGM-CSF and skin grafts. *Lancet* 1994; **343:** 1100.
2. Marques da Costa R, *et al.* Quick healing of leg ulcers after molgramostim. *Lancet* 1994; **344:** 481–2.
3. Wheeler DJ, Brodie GN. GM-CSF and wound healing. *Med J Aust* 1998; **168:** 580.
4. Pieters RC, *et al.* Molgramostim to treat SS-sickle cell leg ulcers. *Lancet* 1995; **345:** 528.

Preparations

Proprietary Preparations (details are given in Part 3)
Aust.: Leucomax; *Belg.:* Leucomax; *Braz.:* Leucomax; *Denm.:* Leucomax; *Fin.:* Leucomax; *Fr.:* Leucomax; *Ger.:* Leucomax; *Hong Kong:* Leucomax; *Irl.:* Leucomax; *Ital.:* Leucomax; *Mielogen; Mex.:* Gramal; Leucomax; *Neth.:* Leucomax; *Norw.:* Leucomax; *NZ:* Leucomax; *Port.:* Leucomax; *S.Afr.:* Leucomax; *Singapore:* Leucomax; *Spain:* Leucomax; *Swed.:* Leucomax; *Switz.:* Leucomax; *Thai.:* Leucomax; *UK:* Leucomax.

Naftazone (1724-I)
Naftazone (*BAN, rINN*).
1,2-Naphthoquinone 2-semicarbazone.
$C_{11}H_9N_3O_2 = 215.2$.
CAS — 15687-37-3.

Profile
Naftazone is a haemostatic used in venous insufficiency and in capillary haemorrhage. It is given by mouth in doses of up to 30 mg daily. It was formerly given by injection.

Preparations
Proprietary Preparations (details are given in Part 3)
Belg.: Mediaven; *Fr.:* Etioven; *Spain:* Metorene; *Switz.:* Mediaven.

Nartograstim (15909-d)
Nartograstim (*rINN*).
A recombinant human granulocyte colony-stimulating factor; *N*-L-Methionyl-1-L-alanine-3-L-threonine-4-L-tyrosine-5-L-arginine-17-L-serine colony-stimulating factor (human clone 1034).
CAS — 134088-74-7.

Profile
Nartograstim is a granulocyte colony-stimulating factor with properties similar to those of filgrastim (p.736). It has been given by intravenous or subcutaneous injection in the management of neutropenia.

Preparations
Proprietary Preparations (details are given in Part 3)
Jpn: Neu-Up†.

Oprelvekin (9779-f)
Oprelvekin (*USAN, rINN*).
$C_{854}H_{1411}N_{253}O_{235}S_2 = 19047.0$.
CAS — 145941-26-0.
ATC — L03AC02.

Adverse Effects and Precautions
Fluid retention may occur producing oedema and dyspnoea; caution is required when giving oprelvekin to patients with a history or signs of heart failure. Fluid balance and electrolytes should be monitored in patients receiving long-term diuretic therapy. Transient atrial arrhythmias have occasionally been reported. Other adverse effects include exfoliative dermatitis, mild blurred vision, and conjunctival injection.
Fetotoxicity has been reported in *animals.*

Uses and Administration
Oprelvekin, a recombinant human interleukin-11, is a platelet growth factor that stimulates the proliferation and maturation of megakaryocytes and thus increases the production of platelets. Oprelvekin is given by subcutaneous injection in a dose of 50 µg per kg body-weight daily to prevent severe antineoplastic-induced thrombocytopenia in patients with non-myeloid malignancies.

◊ References.
1. Tepler I, *et al.* A randomized placebo-controlled trial of recombinant human interleukin-11 in cancer patients with severe thrombocytopenia due to chemotherapy. *Blood* 1996; **87:** 3607–14.
2. Isaacs C, *et al.* Randomized placebo-controlled study of recombinant human interleukin-11 to prevent chemotherapy-induced thrombocytopenia in patients with breast cancer receiving dose-intensive cyclophosphamide and doxorubicin. *J Clin Oncol* 1997; **15:** 3368–77.

Preparations
Proprietary Preparations (details are given in Part 3)
USA: Neumega.

Oxypolygelatin (5446-z)

Profile
Oxypolygelatin is a polymer derived from gelatin (p.737). It is used as a 5.5% solution as a plasma volume expander. There have been reports of anaphylaxis.

Preparations
Proprietary Preparations (details are given in Part 3)
Aust.: Gelifundol; *Ger.:* Gelifundol; *Hong Kong:* Gelifundol; *S.Afr.:* Gelifundol; *Switz.:* Gelifundol†; *Thai.:* Gelifundol.

Plasma (1245-x)

Pharmacopoeial description
Ph. Eur.: Human Plasma for Fractionation (Plasma Humanum ad Separationem; Plasma for Fractionation (BP 2001)) is the liquid part of human blood remaining after separation of the cellular elements from whole blood or collected in an apheresis procedure; it is intended for the manufacture of plasma-derived products. It is obtained from healthy donors and is tested for the absence of hepatitis B surface antigen and antibodies against HIV-1 and HIV-2 and hepatitis C virus.

A light yellow to green, clear or slightly turbid liquid, without visible signs of haemolysis. Frozen plasma should be stored at or below −20°; it may still be used for fractionation if a temperature of −20° is exceeded on at most one occasion for not more than 72 hours and if the plasma is at all times maintained at a temperature of −5° or lower.

Human Plasma (Pooled and Treated for Virus Inactivation) (Plasma Humanum Collectum Deinde Conditum ad Viros Exstinguendos) is a frozen or freeze-dried, sterile, non-pyrogenic preparation obtained from human plasma derived from donors belonging to the same ABO blood group. The plasma used complies with the requirements for Human Plasma for Fractionation (above). The method of preparation is designed to minimise activation of any coagulation factor and includes a step or steps that have been shown to inactivate known agents of infection.

The frozen preparation, after thawing, is a clear or slightly opalescent liquid free from solid and gelatinous particles. The freeze-dried preparation is an almost white or slightly yellow powder or friable solid.

Adverse Effects and Precautions
As for Blood, p.726, though with a low risk of transmitting cell-associated viruses. However, the production of blood products using plasma from UK donors has been phased out due to the possible risk of transmission of Creutzfeldt-Jakob disease.

Uses and Administration
Fresh frozen plasma contains useful amounts of clotting factors. It should be reserved for patients with proven abnormalities in blood coagulation (see Haemorrhagic Disorders, p.721). Indications include congenital deficiencies in clotting factors for which specific concentrates are unavailable, severe multiple clotting factor deficiencies for example in patients with liver disease, rapid reversal of the action of coumarin anticoagulants, and disseminated intravascular coagulation. It may be used following massive blood transfusion when there is evidence of coagulation deficiency but its value for routine prophylaxis against abnormal bleeding tendencies in patients receiving massive blood transfusions is contentious except where clotting abnormalities have been confirmed. It has also been used in the treatment of thrombotic thrombocytopenic purpura and as a source of plasma proteins.

The amount of fresh frozen plasma transfused depends on the required level of clotting factors. A unit of fresh frozen plasma refers to the quantity of plasma obtained from 1 unit of whole blood; this generally represents a volume of about 250 mL, including anticoagulant.

Fresh frozen plasma should not be used as a volume expander or as a nutritional source.

Therapeutic plasma exchange or plasmapheresis (see below) are used in a wide variety of disorders.

Plasma is used for the production of various blood products including albumin, antithrombin III, blood clotting factors, immunoglobulins, and platelets. Other preparations include cryoprecipitate depleted plasma from which approximately half the fibrinogen, factor VIII, and fibronectin has been removed, and single donor plasma which is not frozen. A solvent-detergent-treated plasma preparation is available.

◊ References.
1. British Committee for Standards in Haematology, Working Party of the Blood Transfusion Task Force. Guidelines for the use of fresh frozen plasma. *Transfus Med* 1992; **2:** 57–63.
2. Fresh-frozen Plasma, Cryoprecipitate, and Platelets Administration Practice Guidelines Development Task Force of the College of American Pathologists. Practice parameter for the use of fresh-frozen plasma, cryoprecipitate, and platelets. *JAMA* 1994; **271:** 777–81.
3. Cohen H, *et al.* Plasma, plasma products, and indications for their use. In: Contreras M, ed. *ABC of transfusion.* 3rd ed. London: BMJ Books, 1998: 40–44.

Hereditary angioedema. For a mention of fresh frozen plasma being used in hereditary angioedema, see p.743.

Neonatal intraventricular haemorrhage. Plasma volume expansion in preterm neonates has been thought to help prevent neonatal intraventricular haemorrhage (p.723). However, a study using plasma or gelatin as plasma volume expanders,[1,2]

---

found no evidence of a decreased risk of such haemorrhage or subsequent death or disability.

1. The Northern Neonatal Nursing Initiative Trial Group. A randomized trial comparing the effect of prophylactic intravenous fresh frozen plasma, gelatin or glucose on early mortality and morbidity in preterm babies. *Eur J Pediatr* 1996; **155**: 580–8.
2. Northern Neonatal Nursing Initiative Trial Group. Randomised trial of prophylactic early fresh-frozen plasma or gelatin or glucose in preterm babies: outcome at 2 years. *Lancet* 1996; **348**: 229–32.

Plasma exchange. Therapeutic plasma exchange or plasmapheresis are procedures in which plasma is selectively removed from the body while the cellular constituents of blood are retained. They have been tried in a number of disorders, including many with an immunological basis, when conventional treatment has not been successful. The aim is removal or reduction of those constituents of plasma causing or aggravating a disease or replacement of deficient plasma factors if the deficiency is the cause of the disorder. Although the two terms are commonly used synonymously, plasmapheresis generally involves the removal of small volumes of plasma, whereas plasma exchange removes larger volumes which must be replaced with a suitable fluid. Volume and frequency of plasma exchange is determined by the pathophysiology of the undesirable plasma constituent. For example, removal of antibody usually requires exchange of 1.5 times the estimated plasma volume (3 to 4 litres) repeated daily or on alternate days until the desired reduction is obtained. The replacement fluid used depends on the volume and the condition being treated; albumin solutions, plasma expanders, or sodium chloride 0.9% are frequently used, whereas in conditions where there is deficiency of a plasma factor replacement of blood components such as immunoglobulins may be required. Fresh frozen plasma has been used as a replacement fluid but is associated with a high incidence of adverse effects and is generally reserved for the management of thrombotic thrombocytopenic purpura. Technological developments, such as the use of specific adsorbents and the use of multiple filters with different pore sizes, may enable removal of only the desired constituent and avoid removal and subsequent replacement of total plasma.

References.

1. Urbaniak SJ, Robinson EA. Therapeutic apheresis. In: Contreras M, ed. *ABC of transfusion*. 3rd ed. London: BMJ Books, 1998: 67–70.

Thrombotic microangiopathies. Thrombotic thrombocytopenic purpura and haemolytic-uraemic syndrome are both syndromes characterised by intravascular platelet clumping.[1,2] Thrombocytopenia also occurs and fragmentation of erythrocytes, partly caused by the red cells passing through areas of the microvasculature occluded by the platelet aggregation, leads to microvascular haemolytic anaemia. In **thrombotic thrombocytopenic purpura** (TTP) the platelet aggregation is extensive and obstructs the vessels of various organs producing ischaemia or even infarction. The CNS, notably the brain, is often the area predominantly affected although some degree of renal involvement may occur in over 50% of cases. It is an uncommon disorder; adult women, in whom the condition presents as a chronic relapsing illness, are slightly more frequently affected.

In **haemolytic-uraemic syndrome** (HUS) the platelet aggregation is relatively less widespread and less severe and mainly affects the renal microvasculature although extra-renal manifestations may also occur. The primary consequences of HUS are hypertension and acute renal insufficiency or ultimately, if untreated, renal failure. Most cases of HUS occur in early childhood and follow a diarrhoeal illness caused by *Shigella dysenteriae* or *Escherichia coli*. However, the condition is becoming increasingly recognised in adults, particularly the elderly. Some cases may be drug induced. With appropriate symptomatic therapy HUS is typically a self-limiting disease with spontaneous recovery although fatalities have been known.

The **management** of both syndromes follows similar lines. In HUS, or TTP with renal symptoms, special attention needs to be directed towards the prevention of renal failure. If hypovolaemia has occurred due to preceding diarrhoeal illness it should be corrected,[2] and as oliguria is common crystalloids and frusemide [furosemide] intravenously should be given to induce a diuresis. This will usually maintain renal function and, if performed early enough, avoid the need for dialysis;[2,3] if renal failure is already established haemodialysis will need to be started. Severe anaemia requires blood transfusion.[2] Hypertension can usually be controlled by conventional means.[2]

Specific therapies for both conditions include the administration of fresh frozen plasma.[2,4] The mechanism of action is unclear, as is the optimum dose although amounts in the region of 1 litre daily are suggested. An alternative to direct infusion of plasma is plasma exchange (plasmapheresis), using fresh frozen plasma as the replacement fluid. A comparison of plasma infusion with plasma exchange[5] found no difference in outcome when similar plasma volumes were delivered. Plasma exchange may be the preferred method in patients with impaired renal function and fluid overload, and in oliguric patients with HUS may be the only way of administering enough plasma.

Antiplatelet therapy and corticosteroids are often given, although neither has been adequately investigated and antiplatelets such as ticlopidine and clopidogrel have been reported to cause TTP (see p.981). Improved outcome with antiplatelet drugs has been noted in patients with TTP but not in those with

HUS;[2] however, the failures in the latter case may have been due to late administration. Some reports have described improved outcome in both syndromes with corticosteroids.[6] However, a randomised, double-blind trial[7] in children with HUS failed to show any difference between oral corticosteroids and placebo in terms of haematological or neurological recovery, although renal function appeared to improve more rapidly in those receiving corticosteroids.

Other drugs may also be used. Administration of epoprostenol may be tried[2] in order to inhibit platelet-endothelial interactions and to help promote diuresis but again has not been subject to controlled studies; anecdotal evidence presents both favourable[8,9] and negative[10,11] results. Alteplase has been used successfully in one patient with HUS.[12] Improved outcome has been reported with vincristine[13,14] as part of the overall management strategy. Normal immunoglobulin has been of benefit in HUS[15] but mixed results have been reported in TTP.[4] In chronic relapsing forms of the disorder immunosuppressants may be tried.[2] Splenectomy may also be considered.[4]

1. Moake JL. Haemolytic-uraemic syndrome: basic science. *Lancet* 1994; **343**: 393–7.
2. Neild GH. Haemolytic-uraemic syndrome in practice. *Lancet* 1994; **343**: 398–401. Correction. *ibid.*; 552.
3. Rousseau E, *et al.* Decreased necessity for dialysis with loop diuretic therapy in hemolytic uremic syndrome. *Clin Nephrol* 1990; **34**: 22–5.
4. Gillis S. The thrombocytopenic purpuras: recognition and management. *Drugs* 1996; **51**: 942–53.
5. Novitzky N, *et al.* The treatment of thrombotic thrombocytopenic purpura: plasma infusion or exchange? *Br J Haematol* 1994; **87**: 317–20.
6. Bell WR, *et al.* Improved survival in thrombotic thrombocytopenic purpura-hemolytic uremic syndrome: clinical experience in 108 patients. *N Engl J Med* 1991; **325**: 398–403.
7. Perez N, *et al.* Steroids in the hemolytic uremic syndrome. *Pediatr Nephrol* 1998; **12**: 101–4.
8. Fitzgerald GA, *et al.* Intravenous prostacyclin in thrombotic thrombocytopenic purpura. *Ann Intern Med* 1981; **95**: 319–22.
9. Payton CD, *et al.* Successful treatment of thrombotic thrombocytopenic purpura by epoprostenol infusion. *Lancet* 1985; **i**: 927–8.
10. Budd GT, *et al.* Prostacyclin therapy of thrombotic thrombocytopenic purpura. *Lancet* 1980; **ii**: 915.
11. Johnson JE, *et al.* Ineffective epoprostenol therapy for thrombotic thrombocytopenic purpura. *JAMA* 1983; **250**: 3089–91.
12. Kruez W, *et al.* Successful treatment of haemolytic-uraemic syndrome with recombinant tissue-type plasminogen activator. *Lancet* 1993; **341**: 1665–6.
13. Gutterman LA, *et al.* The hemolytic-uremic syndrome: recovery after treatment with vincristine. *Ann Intern Med* 1983; **98**: 612–13.
14. Wolf G, *et al.* Behandlung einer thrombotisch-thrombo-zytopenischen purpura (morbus Moschcowitz) mit vincristin. *Dtsch Med Wochenschr* 1995; **120**: 442–6.
15. Sheth KJ, *et al.* High-dose intravenous gamma globulin infusions in hemolytic-uremic syndrome: a preliminary report. *Am J Dis Child* 1990; **144**: 268–70.

Preparations

Proprietary Preparations (details are given in Part 3)
Aust.: Octaplas; *Ger.:* Octaplas; *Switz.:* Octaplas; *UK:* Octaplas.

Plasma Protein Fraction (1248-d)

Pharmacopoeial description

USP 25: Plasma Protein Fraction is a sterile preparation of serum albumin and globulin obtained by fractionating material (blood, plasma, or serum) from healthy human donors, the source material being tested for the absence of hepatitis B surface antigen. It contains 5% of protein; not less than 83% of the total protein is albumin; not more than 17% is alpha and beta globulins; not more than 1% has the electrophoretic properties of gamma globulin. It contains sodium acetyltryptophanate with or without sodium caprylate as a stabilising agent but no antimicrobial preservative. It contains 130 to 160 mmol of sodium per litre, and not more than 2 mmol of potassium per litre. A solution in 0.15M sodium chloride containing 1% protein has a pH between 6.7 and 7.3. It should be used within 4 hours of opening the container.

Uses and Administration

Plasma protein fraction consists mainly of albumin with a small proportion of globulins; it does not contain blood-clotting factors. It has properties and uses similar to those of other albumin solutions (p.724). It is given intravenously as a solution containing 4 to 5% of total protein. The amount of plasma protein fraction administered will depend upon the clinical condition of the patient. For most indications an initial infusion of up to 500 mL for adults has been suggested at a rate not normally exceeding 10 mL per minute. Patients with normal blood volume may require slower rates of administration to prevent excessive volume expansion. In hypoproteinaemia administration of 1 to 1.5 litres of a 5% solution will provide 50 to 75 g of protein. A suggested dose in infants and small children for shock with dehydration is up to 33 mL per kg body-weight given at a rate of up to 5 to 10 mL per minute.

As with other albumin solutions, plasma protein fraction should not be used for parenteral nutrition.

Preparations

USP 25: Plasma Protein Fraction.

Proprietary Preparations (details are given in Part 3)
Aust.: Biseko; *Canad.:* Plasmanate†; *Ger.:* Biseko; Tecelac; *Hong Kong:* Plasmanate; Protenate; *Israel:* Plasmanate; *Ital.:* Haimaserum†; Plasmaviral; PPS; Uman-Serum; *S.Afr.:* Bioplasma FDP;

Singapore: Plasmanate; *Thai.:* Biseko; *USA:* Plasma-Plex; Plasmanate; Protenate.

Multi-ingredient: *Belg.:* Tissucol; *Fin.:* Tisseel Duo Quick; *Ger.:* Tissucol Duo S; Tissucol Fibrinkleber tiefgefroren†; Tissucol-Kit; *Ital.:* Tissucol; *Swed.:* Tisseel Duo Quick; *Switz.:* Tissucol Duo S.

Platelets (1221-l)

Pharmacopoeial description

USP 25: Platelet Concentrate contains the platelets taken from plasma obtained, in a single procedure, by whole blood collection, plasmapheresis, or plateletpheresis from a single suitable human donor. The platelets are suspended in a specified volume (20 to 30 mL, or 30 to 50 mL) of the original plasma. The suspension contains not less than 5.5×10^{10} platelets per unit in not less than 75% of the units tested. It should be stored in hermetically-sealed sterile containers at 20° to 24° (30 to 50 mL volume), or at 1° to 6° (20 to 30 mL volume) except during transport when the temperature may be 1° to 10°. The expiration time is not more than 72 hours from the time of collection of the source material. Continuous gentle agitation must be maintained if stored at 20° to 24°. The suspension must be used within 4 hours of opening the container and should be administered with equipment that contains a filter.

Adverse Effects and Precautions

Transmission of infection has been associated with the transfusion of blood products including platelets (p.726). Since platelets are stored at room temperature there is increased risk of bacterial infection following transfusion. Transfusion reactions including fever and urticaria are not uncommon. Recipients of multiple transfusions of platelet concentrates from random donors may develop antibodies to HLA which result in impaired responsiveness to subsequent transfusions. Use of leucodepleted platelet concentrates reduces the incidence of transfusion reactions and of HLA sensitisation. Platelet concentrates prepared from RhD-positive donors should generally not be given to RhD-negative women of child-bearing potential. Ideally platelet concentrates should also be ABO-compatible with the recipient.

ABO compatibility. A discussion[1] of ABO incompatibility and platelet transfusions concluded that, while ABO compatibility is desirable, it is better to transfuse incompatible platelets than none at all. However, acute haemolysis has occurred[2] after transfusion of platelet concentrate with high-titre anti-A. Increased use of single-donor, machine-harvested material from panels of regular platelet donors should make screening for high-titre isoagglutinins more practical.[1]

1. Anonymous. ABO incompatibility and platelet transfusion. *Lancet* 1990; **335**: 142–3.
2. Murphy MF, *et al.* Acute haemolysis after ABO-incompatible platelet transfusion. *Lancet* 1990; **335**: 974–5.

HLA antibodies. Platelets obtained from single donors have been used in patients receiving multiple transfusions of platelet concentrates to reduce the formation of antibodies to HLA. Leucocyte-depleted platelets and UVB-irradiated platelets have also been tried. A study[1] in 530 patients found that the incidence of platelet refractoriness was reduced from 13% in those patients receiving pooled platelet concentrates to 3% and 5% of those receiving leucocyte-depleted and UVB-irradiated platelets, respectively.

1. The Trial to Reduce Alloimmunization to Platelets Study Group. Leukocyte reduction and ultraviolet B irradiation of platelets to prevent alloimmunization and refractoriness to platelet transfusions. *N Engl J Med* 1997; **337**: 1861–9.

Uses and Administration

Blood platelets assist in the haemostatic process (p.718) by aggregation to form a platelet thrombus and by releasing factors involved in initiating coagulation.

Transfusions of platelet concentrates are given to patients with thrombocytopenic haemorrhage (see p.721). They are also given prophylactically to reduce the frequency of haemorrhage in thrombocytopenia associated with the chemotherapy of neoplastic disease.

◊ References.

1. Fresh-frozen Plasma, Cryoprecipitate, and Platelets Administration Practice Guidelines Development Task Force of the College of American Pathologists. Practice parameter for the use of fresh-frozen plasma, cryoprecipitate, and platelets. *JAMA* 1994; **271**: 777–81.
2. Brozović B, *et al.* Platelet and granulocyte transfusions. In: Contreras M, ed. *ABC of transfusion*. 3rd ed. London: BMJ Books, 1998: 17–22.
3. Schiffer CA, *et al.* Platelet transfusion for patients with cancer: clinical practice guidelines of the American Society of Clinical Oncology. *J Clin Oncol* 2001; **19**: 1519–38.

Preparations

USP 25: Platelet Concentrate.

Polygeline (5449-a)

Polygeline (BAN, pINN).

Polygelinum.

CAS — 9015-56-9.

Polygeline is a polymer prepared by cross-linking polypeptides derived from denatured gelatin with a di-isocyanate to form urea bridges.

Intravenous preparations of polygeline contain calcium ions and are incompatible with citrated blood.

Adverse Effects

As for Gelatin, p.737.

Hypersensitivity. Fatal reactions following polygeline infusion have been reported in 2 patients with bronchial asthma.[1,2] In both cases, the patients were undergoing epidural analgesia with bupivacaine. Polygeline was administered to correct hypotension which had not responded to infusion of crystalloids. Both patients developed refractory bronchospasm and cardiac arrhythmias and died despite intensive resuscitation attempts. One patient also developed focal seizures.[2]

The manufacturer recommends that prophylaxis with histamine H_1- or H_2-antagonists should be given to patients with known allergic conditions such as asthma. Similar advice has been offered[3] for patients undergoing anaesthesia and receiving polygeline following findings of an increased incidence of severe histamine-related reactions in such patients.

1. Freeman MK. Fatal reaction to haemaccel. *Anaesthesia* 1979; **34:** 341–3.
2. Barratt S, Purcell GJ. Refractory bronchospasm following "Haemaccel" infusion and bupivacaine epidural anaesthesia. *Anaesth Intensive Care* 1988; **16:** 208–11.
3. Lorenz W, *et al.* Incidence and clinical importance of perioperative histamine release: randomised study of volume loading and antihistamines after induction of anaesthesia. *Lancet* 1994; **343:** 933–40.

Precautions

Precautions that should be observed with plasma expanders are described under Dextran 70, p.729, and these should be considered when polygeline is used for this purpose.

Polygeline preparations contain calcium ions and therefore should be used with caution in patients being treated with cardiac glycosides.

Renal impairment. In a study[1] in 52 patients with normal or impaired renal function given 500 mL of polygeline 3.5% about 50% of the dose was excreted in the urine within 48 hours in those with normal renal function. Excretion was not impaired in those with a glomerular filtration rate (GFR) of 31 to 90 mL per minute, slightly reduced in those with a GFR of 11 to 30 mL, reduced to 27% in 48 hours in those with a GFR of 2 to 10 mL, and to 9.3% in 48 hours in those with a GFR of 0.5 to 2 mL. The mean half-life of the elimination phase was 505 minutes in those with adequate renal function, increasing to 985 minutes in those with end-stage renal failure. Polygeline 500 mL of 3.5% solution could be given twice weekly for 1 to 2 months even in patients with total anuria.

1. Köhler H, *et al.* Elimination of hexamethylene diisocyanate cross-linked polypeptides in patients with normal or impaired renal function. *Eur J Clin Pharmacol* 1978; **14:** 405–12.

Pharmacokinetics

Like gelatin, polygeline is excreted mainly in the urine. The half-life is about 5 hours.

Uses and Administration

Polygeline is a plasma volume expander used as a 3.5% solution with electrolytes in the management of hypovolaemic shock (p.813). The rate of infusion depends on the condition of the patient and does not normally exceed 500 mL in 60 minutes although it may be greater in emergencies. Initial doses for hypovolaemic shock usually consist of 500 to 1000 mL; up to 1500 mL of blood loss can be replaced by polygeline alone. Patients losing greater volumes of blood will require blood transfusion as well as plasma expanders.

Polygeline is also used in extracorporeal perfusion fluids, as a perfusion fluid for isolated organs, as fluid replacement in plasma exchange, and as a carrier solution for insulin. For plasma exchange, up to 2 litres of polygeline may be given as sole replacement fluid.

The symbol † denotes a preparation no longer actively marketed

Preparations

Proprietary Preparations (details are given in Part 3)
Aust.: Haemaccel; *Austral.:* Haemaccel; *Belg.:* Haemaccel; *Braz.:* Haemaccel; *Denm.:* Haemaccel; *Fin.:* Haemaccel; *Fr.:* Haemaccel; *Ger.:* Haemaccel; *Hong Kong:* Haemaccel; *Irl.:* Haemaccel; *Israel:* Haemaccel; *Ital.:* Emagel; Gelplex; *Mex.:* Haemaccel; *Neth.:* Haemaccel; *Norw.:* Haemaccel; *NZ:* Haemaccel; *Port.:* Haemaccel; *S.Afr.:* Haemaccel; *Singapore:* Haemaccel; *Spain:* Hemoce; *Swed.:* Haemaccel; *Switz.:* Haemaccel; *Thai.:* Haemaccel; *UK:* Haemaccel.

Protein C (247-j)

Profile

Protein C is an endogenous inhibitor of blood coagulation. A preparation of protein C purified from human plasma is used in the management of thromboembolic disorders in patients with congenital deficiency of protein C. It is given by intravenous injection in an initial dose of 60 to 80 international units per kg body-weight, adjusted according to response.

Drotrecogin alfa is a recombinant activated protein C that is used in the management of severe sepsis. It is given by intravenous infusion in a dose of 24 µg per kg body-weight per hour for 96 hours.

◊ References.

1. Rintala E, *et al.* Protein C in the treatment of coagulopathy in meningococcal disease. *Lancet* 1996; **347:** 1767.
2. Smith OP, *et al.* Use of protein-C concentrate, heparin, and haemodiafiltration in meningococcus-induced purpura fulminans. *Lancet* 1997; **350:** 1590–3.
3. Bernard GR, *et al.* Efficacy and safety of recombinant human activated protein C for severe sepsis. *N Engl J Med* 2001; **344:** 699–709.

Preparations

Proprietary Preparations (details are given in Part 3)
UK: Ceprotin; *USA:* Xigris.

Red Blood Cells (1218-k)

Pharmacopoeial description

USP 25: Red Blood Cells is the remaining red blood cells of whole human blood from suitable donors, from which plasma has been removed. It is prepared not later than 21 days after the blood has been withdrawn except that the period may be 35 days if the anticoagulant used was acid citrate dextrose adenine solution. If intended for extended manufacturer's storage at or below −65° it contains a portion of the plasma sufficient to ensure cell preservation, or a cryophylactic substance. It should be stored in hermetically-sealed sterile containers; store if unfrozen at 1° to 6° (with a range of not more than 2°) except during transport when the temperature may be 1° to 10°. The expiration date of unfrozen Red Blood Cells is not later than that of the whole human blood from which it is derived if plasma has not been removed, unless the hermetic seal is broken, in which case it should be used within 24 hours. The expiration date of frozen Red Blood Cells is not later than 3 years after the date of collection of the source blood when stored at or below −65° and not later than 24 hours after removal from −65° provided that it is then stored at the temperature for unfrozen Red Blood Cells. Red Blood Cells should be administered using equipment incorporating a filter.

Dark red in colour when packed and may show a slight creamy layer on the surface and a small supernatant layer of yellow or opalescent plasma.

Adverse Effects and Precautions

As for Blood, p.726.

◊ Patients with sickle-cell anaemia frequently require repeated transfusions of red blood cells. Alloimmunisation is a common problem in these patients. Alloantibodies were detected in 32 of 107 black patients with sickle-cell anaemia who had received red cell transfusions compared with 1 of 19 non black patients who had received transfusions for other chronic anaemias.[1] The incidence of antibody formation was related to the number of transfusions received. An analysis of the red cell phenotypes suggested that the high rate of alloimmunisation among patients with sickle-cell anaemia could be due to racial differences between donors and recipients.

1. Vichinsky EP, *et al.* Alloimmunization in sickle cell anemia and transfusion of racially unmatched blood. *N Engl J Med* 1990; **322:** 1617–21.

Uses and Administration

Transfusions of red blood cells are given for the treatment of severe anaemia without hypovolaemia (p.715).

Red blood cells are also used for exchange transfusion in babies with haemolytic disease of the newborn (p.1532). Red cells may be used with volume expanders for acute blood loss of less than half of the blood volume; if more than half of the blood volume has been lost, whole blood should be used.

Other red blood cell products are available. Concentrated red cells in an optimal additive solution containing sodium chloride, adenine, glucose, and mannitol has reduced viscosity and an extended shelf-life. Leucocyte-depleted red cells may be used in patients who have developed antibodies to previous transfusions or in whom development of antibodies is undesirable. Frozen, thawed, and washed red cell concentrates in which plasma proteins are removed in addition to leucocytes and platelets may be used in patients with rare antibodies.

◊ References.

1. Flanagan P. Red cell transfusions including autologous transfusion. *Prescribers' J* 1992; **32:** 15–21.
2. Welch HG, *et al.* Prudent strategies for elective red blood cell transfusion. *Ann Intern Med* 1992; **116:** 393–402.
3. American College of Physicians. Practice strategies for elective red blood cell transfusion. *Ann Intern Med* 1992; **116:** 403–6.
4. Royal College of Physicians of Edinburgh. Consensus statement on red cell transfusion. *Br J Anaesth* 1994; **73:** 857–9.
5. Davies SC, Williamson LM. Transfusion of red cells. In: Contreras M, ed. *ABC of transfusion.* 3rd ed. London: BMJ Books, 1998: 10–16.

Preparations

USP 25: Red Blood Cells.

Sargramostim (14745-e)

Sargramostim (BAN, USAN, rINN).

BI-61.012; rhu GM-CSF. A recombinant human granulocyte-macrophage colony-stimulating factor; 23-L-Leucinecolony-stimulating factor 2 (human clone pHG$_{25}$ protein moiety).

CAS — 123774-72-1.

ATC — L03AA09.

Pharmacopoeias. In US.

Albumin must be added to give a final concentration of 1 mg per mL to solutions for injection that are diluted to concentrations below 10 µg of sargramostim per mL to prevent adsorption to glass or plastic materials.

Pharmacopoeial description

USP 25: Sargramostim is a highly purified glycosylated protein consisting of 127 amino acids, produced by recombinant DNA synthesis in yeast culture. Store in sealed containers at a temperature of −20° or below.

Adverse Effects and Precautions

As for Molgramostim, p.738.

Uses and Administration

Sargramostim is a granulocyte-macrophage colony-stimulating factor with actions and uses similar to those of molgramostim (p.739). It is used to treat or prevent neutropenia in patients receiving myelosuppressive cancer chemotherapy and to reduce the period of neutropenia in patients undergoing bone marrow transplantation (p.480). It is also used to mobilise autologous peripheral blood progenitor cells for an alternative to bone marrow transplantation.

As an adjunct to antineoplastic therapy, sargramostim is given by intravenous infusion over 4 hours in a dose of 250 µg per m^2 body-surface daily for up to 42 days as required.

Following bone marrow transplantation, sargramostim may be given in a dose of 250 µg per m^2 daily by intravenous infusion over 2 hours. The dose may be increased to 500 µg per m^2 daily if engraftment is delayed.

For mobilisation of peripheral blood progenitor cells a dose of 250 µg per m^2 daily is given by continuous intravenous infusion over 24 hours or by subcutaneous injection.

Preparations

USP 25: Sargramostim for Injection.

Proprietary Preparations (details are given in Part 3)
Aust.: Interberin†; *USA:* Leukine.

Thrombin (1250-k)

Factor IIa.

CAS — 9002-04-4.

ATC — B02BC06; B02BD30.

Pharmacopoeial description

USP 25: Thrombin is a sterile, freeze-dried powder derived from bovine plasma containing the protein substance prepared from prothrombin through interaction with added thromboplastin in the presence of calcium. It is capable, without the addition of other substances, of causing the clotting of whole blood, plasma, or a solution of fibrinogen. It should be stored at 2° to 8°. Once reconstituted, solutions should be used within a few hours of preparation. The label should state that the prepared solution should not be injected into or otherwise allowed to enter large blood vessels.

A white to greyish, amorphous substance dried from the frozen state.

Adverse Effects and Precautions

Hypersensitivity reactions, including anaphylaxis, have occurred rarely. Thrombin solutions must not be injected into blood vessels.

Effects on the blood. Repeated exposure to thrombin preparations of bovine origin has led to the development of antibodies to bovine thrombin and factor V with cross-reactivity, in some cases, to human factors.[1-3] The presence of inhibitors to human factors may produce bleeding abnormalities and interfere with clotting measurements.

1. Rapaport SI, et al. Clinical significance of antibodies to bovine and human thrombin and factor V after surgical use of bovine thrombin. Am J Clin Pathol 1992; **97:** 84–91.
2. Bänninger H, et al. Fibrin glue in surgery: frequent development of inhibitors of bovine thrombin and human factor V. Br J Haematol 1993; **85:** 528–32.
3. Ortel TL, et al. Topical thrombin and acquired coagulation factor inhibitors: clinical spectrum and laboratory diagnosis. Am J Hematol 1994; **45:** 128–35.

Uses and Administration

Thrombin is a protein substance produced *in vivo* from prothrombin that converts soluble fibrinogen into insoluble fibrin thus producing coagulation.

Thrombin of either human or bovine origin is applied topically to control bleeding from capillaries and small venules. It is applied directly to the bleeding surface either as a solution or dry powder. It may also be used in conjunction with absorbable gelatin sponge during surgical procedures.

Thrombin is a component of fibrin glue (p.735).

Preparations

Ph. Eur.: Fibrin Sealant Kit;
USP 25: Thrombin.

Proprietary Preparations (details are given in Part 3)
Austral.: Thrombinar†; Thrombostat; *Canad.:* Thrombostat; *Ger.:* Thrombocoll†; *Ital.:* Zimotrombina†; *NZ:* Thrombostat; *S.Afr.:* Tisseel; *Singapore:* Thrombostat; *USA:* Thrombinar; Thrombogen; Thrombostat.

Multi-ingredient: *Aust.:* Beriplast; TachoComb; Tissucol; Tissucol Duo Quick; *Belg.:* Tissucol; *Braz.:* Tissucol; *Canad.:* Tisseel; *Denm.:* Tisseel Duo Quick; *Fin.:* Beriplast; Tisseel Duo Quick; *Fr.:* Beriplast; Biocol; *Ger.:* Beriplast; TachoComb; Tissucol Duo S; Tissucol Fibrinkleber tiefgefroren†; Tissucol-Kit; *Hong Kong:* Beriplast; TachoComb; Tisseel; *Irl.:* Tisseel; *Israel:* Beriplast P; Tisseel; *Ital.:* Tissucol; *Mex.:* Beriplast P; *Spain:* Tissucol; *Swed.:* Tisseel Duo Quick; *Switz.:* Tissucol; Tissucol Duo S; *Thai.:* TachoComb; *UK:* Tisseel.

Thromboplastin (1251-a)

Cytozyme; Thrombokinase.

Profile

Tissue thromboplastin (tissue factor; factor III) is a membrane glycoprotein that is released from damaged tissue and initiates coagulation. The term thromboplastin may also be applied to other related substances with similar activity. Commercial preparations may contain tissue extracts comprising a variety of such substances.

Preparations of thromboplastin have been used as haemostatics.

A preparation of thromboplastin derived from rabbit brain is employed in the determination of the prothrombin time for the control of anticoagulant therapy (for further details see under Warfarin Sodium, p.998).

Preparations

Proprietary Preparations (details are given in Part 3)
Multi-ingredient: *Braz.:* Claudemor; *Port.:* Claudemor.

Thrombopoietin (17553-b)

Profile

Thrombopoietin is a naturally occurring colony-stimulating factor that regulates thrombopoiesis. Recombinant thrombopoietin is under investigation for the management of thrombocytopenia in patients receiving myelosuppressive chemotherapy. A form of recombinant thrombopoietin conjugated with polyethylene glycol (pegacaristim, PEG-megakaryocyte growth and development factor, PEG-MGDF) has also been investigated.

◊ References.

1. Basser RL, et al. Thrombopoietic effects of pegylated recombinant human megakaryocyte growth and development factor (PEG-rHuMGDF) in patients with advanced cancer. Lancet 1996; **348:** 1279–81.

2. Fanucchi M, et al. Effects of polyethylene glycol-conjugated recombinant human megakaryocyte growth and development factor on platelet counts after chemotherapy for lung cancer. N Engl J Med 1997; **336:** 404–9.
3. Vadhan-Raj S, et al. Stimulation of megakaryocyte and platelet production by a single dose of recombinant human thrombopoietin in patients with cancer. Ann Intern Med 1997; **126:** 673–81.
4. Kaushansky K. Thrombopoietin: platelets on demand? Ann Intern Med 1997; **126:** 731–3.
5. Kaushansky K. Thrombopoietin. N Engl J Med 1998; **339:** 746–54.

Tranexamic Acid (1726-j)

Tranexamic Acid (BAN, USAN, rINN).
Acidum Tranexamicum; AMCA; trans-AMCHA; CL-65336. trans-4-(Aminomethyl)cyclohexanecarboxylic acid.
$C_8H_{15}NO_2 = 157.2$.
CAS — 1197-18-8.
ATC — B02AA02.
Pharmacopoeias. In Chin., Eur. (see p.vi), and Jpn.

Solutions of tranexamic acid are incompatible with benzylpenicillin.

Pharmacopoeial description

Ph. Eur.: A white crystalline powder. Freely soluble in water and in glacial acetic acid; practically insoluble in alcohol and in acetone. A 5% solution in water has a pH of 7.0 to 8.0.

Adverse Effects

Tranexamic acid appears to be well tolerated. It can produce dose-related gastrointestinal disturbances. Hypotension has occurred, particularly after rapid intravenous administration. Thrombotic complications have been reported in patients receiving tranexamic acid, but these are usually a consequence of its inappropriate use (see under Precautions, below).

Manufacturers of tranexamic acid report that there have been a few instances of transient disturbance of colour vision associated with its use.

◊ A patient undergoing regular peritoneal dialysis for Epstein's syndrome developed ligneous conjunctivitis, gingival hyperplasia, and peritoneal protein loss associated with the use of tranexamic acid.[1]

1. Diamond JP, et al. Tranexamic acid-associated ligneous conjunctivitis with gingival and peritoneal lesions. Br J Ophthalmol 1991; **75:** 753–4.

Effects on the skin. A widespread, patchy rash with associated blisters, considered on skin biopsy to be a fixed-drug eruption, occurred in a 33-year-old woman.[1] Tranexamic acid, which she had taken for 8 years and which had been well tolerated, was identified as the causative agent. Desensitisation was unsuccessful. Tranexamic acid was also suspected as being the cause of a fixed-drug eruption in a 36-year-old woman.[2] Pruritic, vesicle-bullous lesions appeared within a few hours of commencing treatment with tranexamic acid and the lesions resolved completely 3 days after discontinuing therapy even though other drug treatment was continued.

1. Kavanagh GM, et al. Tranexamic acid (Cyklokapron®)-induced fixed-drug eruption. Br J Dermatol 1993; **128:** 229–30.
2. Carrión-Carrión C, et al. Bullous eruption induced by tranexamic acid. Ann Pharmacother 1994; **28:** 1305–6.

Precautions

Tranexamic acid should not be used in patients with active intravascular clotting because of the risk of thrombosis. Patients with a predisposition to thrombosis are also at risk if given antifibrinolytic therapy. Haemorrhage due to disseminated intravascular coagulation should therefore not be treated with antifibrinolytic compounds unless the condition is predominantly due to disturbances in fibrinolytic mechanisms; tranexamic acid has been used when the latter conditions are met, but with careful monitoring and anticoagulant cover.

Lysis of existing extravascular clots may be inhibited in patients receiving tranexamic acid. Clots in the renal system can lead to intrarenal obstruction, so caution is required in the treatment of patients with haematuria. Doses of tranexamic acid should be reduced in patients with renal impairment (see Uses and Administration, below). The manufacturers recommend that regular eye examinations and liver function tests should be performed if tranexamic acid is used long term.

Some studies have suggested that tranexamic acid when given to patients following a subarachnoid haemorrhage increases the incidence of cerebral is-

chaemic complications (see Haemorrhagic Disorders under Uses, below).

Rapid intravenous administration may be associated with adverse effects (see above).

Interactions

Drugs with actions on haemostasis should be given with caution to patients on antifibrinolytic therapy. The potential for thrombus formation may be increased by oestrogens, for example, or the action of the antifibrinolytic antagonised by compounds such as thrombolytics.

Pharmacokinetics

Tranexamic acid is absorbed from the gastrointestinal tract with peak plasma concentrations occurring after about 3 hours. Bioavailability is about 30 to 50%. Tranexamic acid is widely distributed throughout the body and has very low protein binding. It diffuses across the placenta and is distributed into breast milk. Tranexamic acid has a plasma elimination half-life of about 2 hours. It is excreted in the urine mainly as unchanged drug.

◊ References.

1. Andersson L, et al. Role of urokinase and tissue activator in sustaining bleeding and the management thereof with EACA and AMCA. Ann N Y Acad Sci 1968; **146:** 642–56.
2. Kullander S, Nilsson IM. Human placental transfer of an antifibrinolytic agent (AMCA). Acta Obstet Gynecol Scand 1970; **49:** 241–2.
3. Pilbrant Å, et al. Pharmacokinetics and bioavailability of tranexamic acid. Eur J Clin Pharmacol 1981; **20:** 65–72.

Uses and Administration

Tranexamic acid is an antifibrinolytic drug which inhibits breakdown of fibrin clots. It acts primarily by blocking the binding of plasminogen and fibrinolysin to fibrin; direct inhibition of fibrinolysin occurs only to a limited degree. Tranexamic acid is used in the treatment and prophylaxis of haemorrhage associated with excessive fibrinolysis. It is also used in the prophylaxis of hereditary angioedema.

Tranexamic acid is given by mouth and by slow intravenous injection or continuous infusion. Administration by injection is usually changed to oral administration after a few days. Alternatively, an initial intravenous injection may be followed by continuous infusion. Oral doses are 1 to 1.5 g (or 15 to 25 mg per kg body-weight) 2 to 4 times daily. When given by slow intravenous injection doses are 0.5 to 1 g (or 10 to 15 mg per kg) 3 times daily. Tranexamic acid is administered by continuous infusion at a rate of 25 to 50 mg per kg daily. These doses are used in the short term for haemorrhage. Tranexamic acid is given for prolonged periods in hereditary angioedema in doses of 1 to 1.5 g by mouth 2 or 3 times daily.

Children may be given doses of 25 mg per kg by mouth or 10 mg per kg intravenously usually administered 2 or 3 times daily.

Reduced doses recommended by the UK manufacturer for patients with renal impairment and having serum-creatinine concentrations of 120 to 250, 250 to 500, and greater than 500 µmol per litre are: oral doses of 25 mg per kg twice daily, 25 mg per kg once daily, and 12.5 mg per kg once daily, respectively; intravenous doses of 10 mg per kg twice daily, 10 mg per kg once daily, and 5 mg per kg once daily, respectively.

Solutions of tranexamic acid have been applied topically, for example as a bladder irrigation or mouthwash.

Haemorrhagic disorders. Tranexamic acid, aminocaproic acid, and aminomethylbenzoic acid are structurally related synthetic antifibrinolytic drugs that block the binding of plasminogen and fibrinolysin to fibrin, thereby preventing dissolution of the haemostatic plug. Tranexamic acid is also a direct, but weak, inhibitor of fibrinolysin.[1,2] A plasma concentration of tranexamic acid of 5 to 10 µg per mL has been considered necessary for effective inhibition of fibrinolysis.[1]

Antifibrinolytics are used to control haemorrhage that is considered to be caused by excessive fibrinolysis. Antifibrinolytic therapy may also be indicated in the prevention of rebleeding in some haemorrhagic conditions, the rationale being to retard dissolution of the haemostatic plug formed in response to vascular injury.[1,2]

In haemorrhage caused by a congenital or acquired deficiency of blood coagulation factors (p.721), haemostatic drugs have a secondary role and may be useful in reducing requirements of factor concentrates.[2] The most established use of antifibrinolytics in these conditions is in the prophylaxis of bleeding after dental procedures in haemophiliacs.[1,2] A standard regimen is the intravenous administration of tranexamic acid 10 mg per kg body-weight given pre-operatively with factor VIII or factor IX. Tranexamic acid is continued postoperatively in a dose of 25 mg per kg 3 or 4 times daily by mouth for up to 8 days. Some workers have found that local treatment with a 4.8% solution of tranexamic acid as a mouthwash is a useful addition to systemic therapy.[3] A similar approach using tranexamic acid mouthwashes has been used to reduce the risk of bleeding after oral surgery in patients on anticoagulant therapy.[4] Tranexamic acid may prove beneficial in patients with other congenital bleeding disorders such as α_2-antiplasmin deficiency.[5,6] Aminocaproic acid has been tried in a few patients with hereditary haemorrhagic telangiectasia with mixed results.[7,8] Benefit from treatment with aminocaproic acid or tranexamic acid has been reported in coagulopathies associated with thrombocytopenia[9,10] and acute promyelocytic leukaemia.[11]

Tranexamic acid and aminocaproic acid have each been used in an attempt to prevent rebleeding in patients with subarachnoid haemorrhage (p.813), particularly if surgery is to be delayed. However, while rebleeding may be reduced, there can be an increase in the incidence of cerebral ischaemic complications resulting in little overall improvement in outcome.[1] Paradoxically, rebleeding has been noted in patients given high doses of aminocaproic acid after subarachnoid haemorrhage (see Adverse Effects, Effects on the Blood, under Aminocaproic Acid, p.725). Possible methods of overcoming the ischaemic complications have included the administration of drugs such as nimodipine[12] or nicardipine[13] or the use of aprotinin with a low-dose regimen of tranexamic acid.[14]

Tranexamic acid has been used to control haemorrhage of gastrointestinal origin. In a meta-analysis[15] of 6 studies, involving a total of 1267 patients given tranexamic acid for acute upper gastrointestinal haemorrhage, treatment with tranexamic acid was associated with a 20 to 30% decrease in the rate of rebleeding, a 30 to 40% decrease in the need for surgery, and a 40% decrease in mortality. However, the validity of the results of one study included in the analysis has been disputed.[16,17] The management of bleeding associated with peptic ulcer disease and varices is discussed on p.1208 and p.1637, respectively.

Tranexamic acid or aminocaproic acid have been suggested to control bleeding in many other conditions. These include haemorrhage after surgical or other procedures including prostatectomy, bladder surgery, and cervical conisation, perioperative blood loss in cardiac surgery, and other conditions associated with excessive fibrinolysis such as menorrhagia (see below), epistaxis, and placental abruption.

1. Verstraete M. Clinical application of inhibitors of fibrinolysis. *Drugs* 1985; **29**: 236–61.
2. Verstraete M. Haemostatic drugs. In: Bloom AL, Thomas DP, eds. *Haemostasis and thrombosis*. 2nd ed. London: Churchill Livingstone, 1987: 607–17.

3. Sindet-Pedersen S, *et al.* Management of oral bleeding in haemophilic patients. *Lancet* 1988; **ii**: 566.
4. Sindet-Pedersen S, *et al.* Hemostatic effect of tranexamic acid mouthwash in anticoagulant-treated patients undergoing oral surgery. *N Engl J Med* 1989; **320**: 840–3.
5. Koie K, *et al.* α_2-Plasmin-inhibitor deficiency (Miyasato disease). *Lancet* 1978; **ii**: 1334–6.
6. Kettle P, Mayne EE. A bleeding disorder due to deficiency of α_2-antiplasmin. *J Clin Pathol* 1985; **38**: 428–9.
7. Saba HI, *et al.* Brief report: treatment of bleeding in hereditary hemorrhagic telangiectasia with aminocaproic acid. *N Engl J Med* 1994; **330**: 1789–90.
8. Korzenik JR, *et al.* Treatment of bleeding in hereditary hemorrhagic telangiectasia with aminocaproic acid. *N Engl J Med* 1994; **331**: 1236.
9. Warrell RP, Kempin SJ. Treatment of severe coagulopathy in the Kasabach-Merritt syndrome with aminocaproic acid and cryoprecipitate. *N Engl J Med* 1985; **313**: 309–12.
10. Poon M-C, *et al.* Epsilon-aminocaproic acid in the reversal of consumptive coagulopathy with platelet sequestration in a vascular malformation of Klippel-Trenaunay syndrome. *Am J Med* 1989; **87**: 211–13.
11. Avvisati G, *et al.* Tranexamic acid for control of haemorrhage in acute promyelocytic leukaemia. *Lancet* 1989; **ii**: 122–4.
12. van Gijn J. Subarachnoid haemorrhage. *Lancet* 1992; **339**: 653–5.
13. Beck DW, *et al.* Combination of aminocaproic acid and nicardipine in treatment of aneurysmal subarachnoid hemorrhage. *Stroke* 1988; **19**: 63–7.
14. Spallone A, *et al.* Low-dose tranexamic acid combined with aprotinin in the pre-operative management of ruptured intracranial aneurysms. *Neurochirurgia (Stuttg)* 1987; **30**: 172–6.
15. Henry DA, O'Connell DL. Effects of fibrinolytic inhibitors on mortality from upper gastrointestinal haemorrhage. *BMJ* 1989; **298**: 1142–6.
16. Brown C, Rees WDW. Drug treatment for acute upper gastrointestinal bleeding. *BMJ* 1992; **304**: 135–6.
17. Barer D. Drug treatment for acute upper gastrointestinal bleeding. *BMJ* 1992; **304**: 383.

Hereditary angioedema. Hereditary angioedema, formerly known as hereditary angioneurotic oedema, is a rare autosomal dominant disease caused by either a deficiency of complement C1 esterase inhibitor or, more rarely, a lack of functioning inhibitor.[1,2] The disease presents as episodic attacks of oedema, usually of the extremities and face, and often involving the gastrointestinal mucosa producing abdominal pain. A non-pruritic rash may also occur. A few patients develop life-threatening laryngeal oedema. Attacks generally last about 1 to 3 days and may occur as frequently as weekly or there may be years between attacks. The first attack may occur at any age although initial presentation in childhood is most common. Trauma, especially dental surgery, illness, and emotional stress may provoke an attack although often there is no precipitating factor.

Treatment of the acute attack is essentially supportive. If laryngeal oedema is present adrenaline [epinephrine], antihistamines, and corticosteroids may be given (as for Anaphylactic Shock, p.832) even though patients with hereditary angioedema often fail to respond adequately to them. The mainstay of treatment of an acute attack is replacement therapy with complement C1 esterase inhibitor. Fresh frozen plasma has been used although there is a risk of initially exacerbating the oedema due to the presence of other complements in the plasma. Tracheostomy or tracheal intubation may be necessary.

Once the acute attack has subsided most patients will not require further treatment, but those who experience life-threatening attacks, repeated episodes of swelling around the face or neck, or incapacitating attacks require long-term prophylactic therapy. A synthetic androgen (danazol or stanozolol) or an antifibrinolytic (aminocaproic acid or tranexamic acid) is effective for long-term prophylaxis. Danazol and stanozolol raise serum concentrations of C1 esterase inhibitor possibly by enhancing its synthesis in the liver. Aminocaproic acid and tranexamic acid may act by inhibiting fibrinolysin activation. A synthetic androgen is often preferred, with an antifibrinolytic being reserved for patients refractory to, or intolerant of, androgens. An antifibrinolytic may be preferred in premenopausal women. A combination of an androgen and an antifibrinolytic may be used. These drugs may also be used for short-term prophylaxis in situations expected to provoke an attack, such as surgery involving the head, neck, or respiratory tract. Prophylaxis should be started a few days before the procedure. Fresh frozen plasma has also been used in situations likely to precipitate an attack.

1. Sim TC, Grant JA. Hereditary angioedema: its diagnostic and management perspectives. *Am J Med* 1990; **88**: 656–64.
2. Orphan NA, Kolski GB. Angioedema and C1 inhibitor deficiency. *Ann Allergy* 1992; **69**: 167–72.

Menorrhagia. Tranexamic acid is used in women with menorrhagia (p.1490) who do not require contraception or hormonal therapy. It reduces uterine blood loss in such women when used during menstruation.[1-3] A comparative trial[1] found tranexamic acid to be more effective than the NSAID mefenamic acid, a commonly used treatment for the condition. It is also more effective than cyclical norethisterone[2] (although less so than a progesterone-releasing intra-uterine device[3]). A review,[4] which included these and some earlier studies, reported that tranexamic acid reduces menstrual blood loss by about 46%.

1. Bonnar J, Sheppard BL. Treatment of menorrhagia during menstruation: randomised controlled trial of ethamsylate, mefenamic acid, and tranexamic acid. *BMJ* 1996; **313**: 579–82.
2. Preston JT, *et al.* Comparative study of tranexamic acid and norethisterone in the treatment of ovulatory menorrhagia. *Br J Obstet Gynaecol* 1995; **102**: 401–406.
3. Milsom I, *et al.* A comparison of flurbiprofen, tranexamic acid, and a levonorgestrel-releasing intrauterine contraceptive device in the treatment of idiopathic menorrhagia. *Am J Obstet Gynecol* 1991; **164**: 879–83.
4. Coulter A, *et al.* Treating menorrhagia in primary care: an overview of drug trials and a survey of prescribing practice. *Int J Technol Assess Health Care* 1995; **11**: 456–71.

Preparations

BP 2001: Tranexamic Acid Injection; Tranexamic Acid Tablets.

Proprietary Preparations (details are given in Part 3)
Aust.: Cyklokapron; *Austral.:* Cyklokapron; *Belg.:* Exacyl†; *Braz.:* Transamin; *Canad.:* Cyklokapron; *Denm.:* Cyklokapron; *Fin.:* Caprilon; Cyklokapron; *Fr.:* Exacyl; Spotof; *Ger.:* Anvitoff; Cyklokapron; Ugurol; *Hong Kong:* Cyklokapron; Transamin; *Irl.:* Cyklokapron; *Israel:* Hexakapron; *Ital.:* Tranex; Ugurol; *Jpn:* Transamin; *Neth.:* Cyklokapron; *Norw.:* Cyklokapron; *NZ:* Cyklokapron; *S.Afr.:* Cyklokapron; *Singapore:* Cyklokapron; *Spain:* Amchafibrin; *Swed.:* Cyklo-F; Cyklokapron; *Switz.:* Anvitoff; Cyklokapron; *Thai.:* Transamin; *UK:* Cyklokapron; *USA:* Cyklokapron.

Bone Modulating Drugs

The processes of bone turnover, and the regulation of body calcium, are intimately connected. The concentration of calcium in plasma is normally kept within a narrow range (p.1180) by regulation of the absorption and excretion of calcium, and also by modulation of the normal resorption and formation of bone and hence the movement of calcium to and from the skeletal reservoir. The endogenous substances, parathyroid hormone, calcitonin, and vitamin D, are involved in the regulation of calcium homoeostasis.

Calcitonins and the bisphosphonates inhibit bone resorption and thus have a hypocalcaemic effect. They are therefore used in the treatment of conditions associated with increased bone resorption, such as osteoporosis and Paget's disease of bone, and in the management of hypercalcaemia, especially that associated with malignancy (p.1181). Bisphosphonates have a high affinity for bone and radioactively labelled bisphosphonates are used as bone scanning agents. Gallium nitrate also inhibits bone resorption, and is used for Paget's disease of bone and hypercalcaemia of malignancy.

Parathyroid hormone, which has a hypercalcaemic effect, is under investigation to promote bone formation. It was formerly used in the differential diagnosis of hypoparathyroidism and pseudohypoparathyroidism, but has been replaced by teriparatide, the synthetic 1-34 amino-acid fragment of human parathyroid hormone.

The inorganic fluoride salts, which can promote bone formation when given in appropriate doses, are discussed in the chapter on Nutritional Agents (see Sodium Fluoride, p.1375).

Bone and Bone Disease

The skeleton acts as mechanical support and protection to softer tissues and organs. It is also important in electrolyte homoeostasis, acting as a reservoir of certain ions and minerals such as calcium, phosphorus, and magnesium.

Bone has two components: an organic matrix, called **osteoid**, consisting mainly of collagen, and a mineral phase deposited through that matrix; the latter, comprising about 70% of the skeletal mass, is composed chiefly of hydroxyapatite (a complex crystalline salt of calcium and phosphate). Two structural forms are known in mature bone, namely cortical (lamellar) bone, which has a dense, continuous structure, and trabecular (cancellous) bone, which has a 'spongy' structure of linked plates and is associated with high bone turnover and growth. The peripheral or appendicular parts of the skeleton are predominantly cortical bone, while the axial or central parts, such as the spine and pelvis, contain substantial amounts of trabecular bone.

Bone is a dynamic tissue: once new bone has been laid down it is subject to a continual process of formation and resorption called **remodelling**. Remodelling takes place along bone surfaces and is carried out by bone cells (osteoclasts and osteoblasts) that originate in the marrow and share common origins with blood cells. Stimulated by physical or chemical signals, **osteoclasts** dig a cavity into the bone (bone resorption); they are then replaced by **osteoblasts** that synthesise new osteoid to fill the cavity (bone formation) and

may help to promote its subsequent mineralisation. The actions of these two types of bone cell are closely linked, and agents that suppress resorption ultimately decrease bone formation too. However, at any given time there is a deficit in potential bone mass, the **remodelling space**, which represents sites of bone resorption that have not yet been filled in. Any stimulus that affects bone turnover by altering the recruitment of osteoblasts and osteoclasts to remodelling will result in an increase or decrease in the remodelling space, until a new steady state is achieved, and this will be seen as a decrease or increase in bone mass.

Bone also contains **osteocytes**, which are cells derived from osteoblasts thought to be involved in the movement of minerals.

Bone cells are controlled by systemic hormones including parathyroid hormone, 1,25-dihydroxycholecalciferol (calcitriol), and calcitonin and local regulators such as bone morphogenetic proteins and interleukin-1; vitamin K is also thought to have a role, and bone cells are affected by other hormones including corticosteroids and sex hormones.

Bone diseases may be due to defects in the production of osteoid or its mineralisation, or to an imbalance in resorption and formation of bone.

Ectopic ossification

Ectopic ossification (heterotopic ossification) is a condition in which mature bone develops in non-skeletal tissues, commonly the connective tissue of muscles. It occurs following local trauma, for example after joint dislocation or surgery such as total hip replacement, and also after neurological damage such as severe head or spinal cord injuries. Ectopic bone formation usually starts about 2 weeks after the injury, though symptoms which include localised pain, swelling, and restriction of movement, may not appear for 8 to 10 weeks. A congenital form of ectopic ossification, myositis ossificans progressiva, also occurs but is rare.

Ectopic ossification should be distinguished from the calcification of soft tissue which may occur in connective-tissue disorders or in parathyroid disorders due to high circulating concentrations of calcium and or phosphate; in these conditions calcification occurs without bone formation.

Treatment of established ectopic bone is limited to surgical resection. Patients at high risk of ectopic bone formation should therefore receive prophylaxis with radiotherapy, physiotherapy, or drug therapy. While prophylaxis does not always prevent the development of ectopic ossification, it can decrease its occurrence and severity. Prophylactic measures should be begun as early as possible and for orthopaedic surgery may be started before the operation. Prophylaxis is also required if mature ectopic bone is to be surgically excised in order to minimise the rate of recurrence. NSAIDs appear to significantly reduce the incidence of ectopic bone formation,[1-4] possibly by inhibiting the synthesis of osteoactive prostaglandins. Studies suggest that NSAID prophylaxis is of similar effectiveness to radiotherapy.[5-8] Bisphosphonates that inhibit the mineralisation of the deposited bone, such as etidronate, have also been used[9,10] but they do not prevent the formation of the osteoid matrix. Also when etidronate is discontinued, some mineralisation can occur, resulting in delayed ectopic ossification, though it is usually less severe.

1. Schmidt SA, *et al.* The use of indomethacin to prevent the formation of heterotopic bone after total hip replacement: a randomized, double-blind clinical trial. *J Bone Joint Surg Am* 1988; **70A:** 834–8.
2. Pagnani MJ, *et al.* Effect of aspirin on heterotopic ossification after total hip arthroplasty in men who have osteoarthrosis. *J Bone Joint Surg Am* 1991; **73A:** 924–9.
3. Knelles D, *et al.* Prevention of heterotopic ossification after total hip replacement: a prospective, randomised study using acetylsalicylic acid, indomethacin and fractional or single-dose irradiation. *J Bone Joint Surg Br* 1997; **79B:** 596–602.
4. Neal B, *et al.* Non-steroidal anti-inflammatory drugs for preventing heterotopic bone formation after hip arthroplasty (updated 30 November 2000). Available in The Cochrane Library; Issue 1. Oxford: Update Software; 2001.
5. Moore KD, *et al.* Indomethacin versus radiation therapy for prophylaxis against heterotopic ossification in acetabular fractures: a randomised, prospective study. *J Bone Joint Surg Br* 1998; **80:** 259–63.
6. Kölbl O, *et al.* Preoperative irradiation versus the use of nonsteroidal anti-inflammatory drugs for prevention of heterotopic ossification following total hip replacement: the results of a randomized trial. *Int J Radiat Oncol Biol Phys* 1998; **42:** 397–401.
7. Sell S, *et al.* The suppression of heterotopic ossifications: radiation versus NSAID therapy-a prospective study. *J Arthroplasty* 1998; **13:** 854–9.
8. Kienapfel H, *et al.* Prevention of heterotopic bone formation after total hip arthroplasty: a prospective randomised study comparing postoperative radiation therapy with indomethacin medication. *Arch Orthop Trauma Surg* 1999; **119:** 296–302.
9. Finerman GAM, Stover SL. Heterotopic ossification following hip replacement or spinal cord injury: two clinical studies with EHDP. *Metab Bone Dis Relat Res* 1981; **4 & 5:** 337–42.
10. Banovac K, *et al.* Intravenous disodium etidronate therapy in spinal cord injury patients with heterotopic ossification. *Paraplegia* 1993; **31:** 660–6.

Malignant neoplasms of the bone

The bisphosphonates and calcitonins are used to control the hypercalcaemia that often accompanies malignant disease (p.1181). Bisphosphonates are also used in metastatic bone disease (p.490) to control bone pain and to reduce skeletal complications such as fractures. Evidence of the ability of bisphosphonates to prevent the development of bone metastases is conflicting.

Osteogenesis imperfecta

Osteogenesis imperfecta (brittle bone syndrome) is a heterogeneous congenital disorder of connective tissue characterised by bone fragility, osteopenia, short stature, joint laxity, teeth defects, and hearing abnormalities. It may be classified into 4 forms, which vary in clinical severity.

Orthopaedic treatment and physical activity programmes form the basis of therapy: at present there is no accepted drug therapy. Beneficial effects have been reported with calcitonins,[1,2] bisphosphonates,[3-5] and growth hormone.[6,7] Bisphosphonates may also be useful for associated immobilisation hypercalcaemia.[8] Bone-marrow transplantation and the potential of antisense gene therapy are being investigated.[7]

1. Castells S, *et al.* Therapy of osteogenesis imperfecta with synthetic salmon calcitonin. *J Pediatr* 1979; **95:** 807–11.
2. Nishi Y, *et al.* Effect of long-term calcitonin therapy by injection and nasal spray on the incidence of fractures in osteogenesis imperfecta. *J Pediatr* 1992; **121:** 477–80.
3. Bembi B, *et al.* Intravenous pamidronate treatment in osteogenesis imperfecta. *J Pediatr* 1997; **131:** 622–5.
4. Shaw NJ. Bisphosphonates in osteogenesis imperfecta. *Arch Dis Child* 1997; **77:** 92–3.
5. Glorieux FH, *et al.* Cyclic administration of pamidronate in children with severe osteogenesis imperfecta. *N Engl J Med* 1998; **339:** 947–52.
6. Antoniazzi F, *et al.* Growth hormone treatment in osteogenesis imperfecta with quantitative defect of type I collagen synthesis. *J Pediatr* 1996; **129:** 432–9.
7. Marini JC, Gerber NL. Osteogenesis imperfecta: rehabilitation and prospects for gene therapy. *JAMA* 1997; **277:** 746–50.
8. Williams CJC, *et al.* Hypercalcaemia in osteogenesis imperfecta treated with pamidronate. *Arch Dis Child* 1997; **76:** 169–70.

Osteomalacia

Osteomalacia occurs when there is impaired mineralisation of the bone matrix resulting in 'soft' bones. Patients usually present with bone pain and muscle weakness and may have subclinical fractures. **Rickets** refers to defective mineralisation of growing bone and is therefore restricted to children; it is associated with retarded growth, skeletal deformities, teeth defects, and muscle hypotonia.

Inadequate bone mineralisation is usually caused by vitamin D deficiency or its abnormal metabolism, but may also be due to phosphate depletion, calcium deficiency, or a primary disorder of bone matrix such as hypophosphatasia in which a deficiency of alkaline phosphatase results in an increase in pyrophosphate, an inhibitor of bone mineralisation. Some drugs including various antiepileptics (p.358), etidronate, and aluminium salts, can interfere with bone mineralisation and cause osteomalacia. Osteomalacia also occurs in renal osteodystrophy associated with chronic renal failure (see below).

Several hereditary disorders are associated with the development of rickets including vitamin D-pseudodeficiency rickets (vitamin D-dependent rickets), in which there is impaired synthesis of 1,25-dihydroxycholecalciferol (Type I) or receptor resistance to 1,25-dihydroxycholecalciferol (Type II), and X-linked hypophosphataemic rickets.[1]

Treatment of osteomalacia and rickets is primarily aimed at correcting any underlying deficiency. Vitamin D substances, calcium, or phosphate supplements can be given by mouth as appropriate but doses require careful individual adjustment to maintain calcium and phosphate concentrations within normal limits. A variety of forms or analogues of vitamin D are available. For the treatment of simple vitamin D deficiency colecalciferol or ergocalciferol are generally preferred. If malabsorption is suspected, larger doses or parenteral administration may be necessary, but where large doses are required it may be preferable to use one of the more potent forms of vitamin D such as calcitriol. Simple calcium deficiency may be a more important cause of rickets than vitamin D deficiency in some populations. A study in African children with rickets found that their calcium intake was low and that they responded better to calcium supplementation, with or without vitamin D, than to vitamin D alone.[2]

Type I vitamin D-pseudodeficiency rickets requires replacement therapy with calcitriol. In Type II disease, resistance to calcitriol treatment may be so extreme that only very large supplements of calcium may be effective.[1,3] X-linked hypophosphataemic rickets is considered to be best treated with combined phosphate supplementation and calcitriol.[1,4] There has also been some interest in the use of growth hormone in children with hypophosphataemic rickets.[5] A form of hypophosphataemic rickets, rickets of prematurity (p.1194), may occur in small, premature infants fed exclusively on breast milk, and phosphate supplementation with concomitant calcium and vitamin D has been suggested in such cases.

1. Glorieux FH. Rickets, the continuing challenge. *N Engl J Med* 1991; **325:** 1875–7.
2. Thacher TD, *et al.* A comparison of calcium, vitamin D, or both for nutritional rickets in Nigerian children. *N Engl J Med* 1999; **341:** 563–8.
3. Hochberg Z, *et al.* Calcium therapy for calcitriol-resistant rickets. *J Pediatr* 1992; **121:** 803–8.
4. Verge CF, *et al.* Effects of therapy in X-linked hypophosphatemic rickets. *N Engl J Med* 1991; **325:** 1843–8.
5. Shaw NJ, *et al.* Growth hormone and hypophosphataemic rickets. *Arch Dis Child* 1995; **72:** 543–4.

Osteoporosis

Osteoporosis is a disease characterised by low bone mass and microarchitectural deterioration of bone tissue, leading to enhanced bone fragility and risk of fracture,[1] particularly of the long bones (distal forearm and neck of the femur) and the vertebrae. Although bone formation outstrips resorption in youth, accumulated small deficits from remodelling (see Bone and Bone Disease, above) result in a gradual loss of bone mass after the third decade. Primary osteoporosis is therefore usually an age-related disease. It can affect both sexes, though women are at greater risk because bone loss is accelerated, to a variable degree, after the menopause. Osteoporosis can also be secondary to diseases such as thyrotoxicosis, hypogonadism, Cushing's syndrome, hypoparathyroidism, and rheumatoid arthritis, or to drugs such as corticosteroids (p.1040), gonadorelin analogues (p.1284), and heparin (p.903). Also, immobility, especially in younger patients, can result in osteoblastic failure with an increase in osteoclastic resorption and the development of osteoporosis. Other risk factors for osteoporosis include smoking, high alcohol intake, physical inactivity, thin body type, early menopause, and a family history of osteoporosis.[2,3]

Patients are usually asymptomatic until fractures occur, and up to half of vertebral fractures may also be asymptomatic. Fractures may result in pain, deformity (kyphosis, loss of height), and disability. Currently, the most reliable method of assessing osteoporosis and fracture risk is measurement of bone mass density (BMD), usually by dual energy X-ray absorptiometry.[1] WHO have defined osteoporosis as a BMD 2.5 standard deviations or more below the young adult mean, and severe osteoporosis (established osteoporosis) as this BMD in the presence of one or more fragility fractures.[1,4] There is no universally agreed policy on screening for osteoporosis,[5] but measurement of BMD should be considered in those thought to be at risk of osteoporosis if the result is likely to affect treatment decisions.[3,4] Different approaches to the management of osteoporosis have been suggested, including changes in life-style, interventions to reduce falls, the use of drugs to decrease bone resorption such as calcium, oestrogens, calcitonins, and bisphosphonates, and the administration of drugs to stimulate bone formation, such as sodium fluoride.[3,6-13] Because bone remodelling is a coupled process decreases in resorption ultimately reduce the rate of bone formation, and antiresorptive drugs can therefore only produce modest increases in bone mass. Trials with such drugs must be sufficiently prolonged to determine whether an increase

in bone mass represents more than just a constriction in the remodelling space.[14] Moreover, experience with fluoride indicates that increases in BMD do not always equate to decreases in fracture risk. Thus, there is also a need to show that drugs decrease fracture rate; currently there are few trials with fracture rates as primary endpoints. In addition, the optimum timing and duration of drug therapy to optimise the benefits on bone and minimise the risks is not known, particularly for the prevention of primary osteoporosis.

Prevention is the most effective method of dealing with osteoporosis as once bone mass has decreased it is difficult to replace. Optimising peak bone mass is therefore important; regular moderate weight-bearing exercise and adequate dietary calcium during growth[15,16] have been advocated. After the third decade of life, interventions should be aimed at reducing the rate of bone loss. This includes life-style modifications such as avoiding smoking,[17] moderation of alcohol intake, improving diet to ensure an adequate calcium and vitamin D intake (see under Human Requirements, p.1189 and p.1392), and regular weight-bearing exercise.[18,19] Secondary causes of osteoporosis should be identified and treated as appropriate.[3] Antiresorptive drugs may be considered.

In *postmenopausal women*, HRT (p.1464) slows or eliminates postmenopausal bone loss at all skeletal sites. Many observational studies and a few randomised trials have shown that this reduces the risk of fractures. Efficacy is dependent on dose, but the duration of therapy for maximum benefit is unknown. It has been suggested that HRT may need to be continued indefinitely, since there is evidence that the risk of fracture returns to baseline after 10 or more years without HRT. However, the potential value of long-term HRT must be balanced against the potential risks, particularly breast cancer. It is generally considered that HRT is indicated in women with risk factors for osteoporosis. In women with no risk factors for osteoporosis and without menopausal symptoms, use of HRT is more controversial. In these women it may be appropriate to start HRT several years after the menopause.

Alternatives to HRT for the prevention of postmenopausal osteoporosis include tibolone and raloxifene as well as the bisphosphonates alendronate, etidronate, and risedronate. There is good evidence that these drugs prevent loss of bone mineral density in postmenopausal women. However, as yet there is little experience of the long-term use of these drugs (beyond 2 to 5 years). In postmenopausal women, the effects of calcium supplementation (about 1 g of calcium daily by mouth) have been conflicting; some studies have reported a reduction in bone loss[20-22] but others have found calcium supplements to be of little benefit.[23] However, a subsequent meta-analysis[24] found that increasing calcium intake by diet or supplements potentiated the effect of oestrogens and calcitonins on bone, confirming that an adequate intake of calcium is important when antiresorptive drugs are being used.

The use of calcitonins as prophylactic drugs has been limited by the necessity for parenteral administration. However, intranasal spray formulations of salcatonin have been developed and oral formulations are under investigation.

Other drugs that have been reported to have favourable effects on bone mass in postmenopausal women include thiazide diuretics, tamoxifen, intermittent teriparatide, diclofenac,[25] and potassium bicarbonate. However, their role, if any, in the prevention of osteoporosis has not yet been determined.

Treatment. In patients with osteoporosis with or without fragility fractures (established osteoporosis), treatment involves supportive therapy and interventions to prevent further bone loss and reduce the risk of fractures.[3,4,6-13] Supportive therapy in the acute phase of a fracture includes pain relief, physiotherapy, and appropriate orthopaedic management of fracture of long bones; surgery is required for the majority of hip fractures.[11] Life-style modifications and drugs to prevent further bone loss and fractures are similar to those outlined above. In the elderly, interventions to reduce the risk of falls may be important,[26] and measures to protect the patient should falls occur may also be considered.[27]

In *postmenopausal women* with established osteoporosis, HRT increases bone mass and reduces the incidence of fractures. Alternatively, a bisphosphonate such as alendronate or etidronate may be used. Both of these drugs have been shown to increase bone mass and decrease fracture rate in established osteoporosis. Combined therapy with HRT and a bisphosphonate is also being investigated.[28] Improvements in bone mass and fracture rate

have also been shown with raloxifene. Calcitonins may also have a role. It has been suggested that, in particular, the analgesic effects of calcitonins may be advantageous in patients with acute pain due to osteoporotic fractures. Studies using the vitamin D substance calcitriol for the treatment of osteoporosis have produced conflicting results; although some have reported an increase in spinal bone density[29] and a reduction in the rate of new vertebral fractures,[30] others have found no significant effects.[31]

Vitamin D supplements have shown beneficial effects in the elderly, and it is considered that they may have a particular role in frail or housebound individuals, who are at high risk of vitamin D deficiency and resulting hyperparathyroidism.[10,11,13]

Postmenopausal osteoporosis has also been treated with drugs that promote bone formation. Fluoride stimulates osteoblasts and increases the density of trabecular bone and has been administered as sodium fluoride or sodium monofluorophosphate. However, increases in BMD with fluoride have not always resulted in decreased fracture rate, and may even be associated with increased bone fragility; thus, the role of fluoride remains unclear.[4,10,12,13,32] Anabolic steroids have been tried but have considerable adverse effects. Other drugs that have been investigated for postmenopausal osteoporosis include teriparatide, mecasermin, and ipriflavone.

There is less evidence to guide decisions on the management of osteoporosis in men[33-35] than in postmenopausal women. In hypogonadal men with osteoporosis, testosterone replacement therapy should be used.[35] In eugonadal men, there are concerns regarding the potential long-term adverse effects of exogenous testosterone. Therefore, in men with idiopathic osteoporosis, bisphosphonates may be the treatment of choice.[35] Calcium and vitamin D supplements did not affect the rate of bone mineral loss in healthy men with adequate diets.[36] However, there is some evidence that, as for women, elderly men may benefit from vitamin D supplements and calcium.[37] Other drugs that have been reported to have favourable effects on BMD in men include thiazides[38] and parathyroid hormone.[39]

1. WHO. Assessment of fracture risk and its application to screening for postmenopausal osteoporosis. *WHO Tech Rep Ser 843* 1994.
2. Dempster DW, Lindsay R. Pathogenesis of osteoporosis. *Lancet* 1993; **341:** 797–801.
3. Peel N, Eastell R. Osteoporosis. *BMJ* 1995; **310:** 989–92.
4. Kanis JA, *et al.* Guidelines for diagnosis and management of osteoporosis. *Osteoporosis Int* 1997; **7:** 390–406.
5. Fogelman I. Screening for osteoporosis. *BMJ* 1999; **319:** 1148–9.
6. Riggs BL, Melton LJ. The prevention and treatment of osteoporosis. *N Engl J Med* 1992; **327:** 620–7.
7. Lindsay R. Prevention and treatment of osteoporosis. *Lancet* 1993; **341:** 801–5.
8. Conference Report. Consensus Development Conference: diagnosis, prophylaxis, and treatment of osteoporosis. *Am J Med* 1993; **94:** 646–50.
9. Khosla S, Riggs BL. Treatment options for osteoporosis. *Mayo Clin Proc* 1995; **70:** 978–82.
10. Anonymous. Managing osteoporosis. *Drug Ther Bull* 1996; **34:** 45–8.
11. Compston JE. Osteoporosis: management of established disease. *Prescribers' J* 1997; **37:** 119–24.
12. Gibaldi M. Prevention and treatment of osteoporosis: does the future belong to hormone replacement therapy? *J Clin Pharmacol* 1997; **37:** 1087–99.
13. Eastell R. Treatment of postmenopausal osteoporosis. *N Engl J Med* 1998; **338:** 736–46.
14. Heaney RP. Interpreting trials of bone-active agents. *Am J Med* 1995; **98:** 329–30.
15. Johnston CC, *et al.* Calcium supplementation and increases in bone mineral density in children. *N Engl J Med* 1992; **327:** 82–7.
16. Lloyd T, *et al.* Calcium supplementation and bone mineral density in adolescent girls. *JAMA* 1993; **270:** 841–4.
17. Law MR, Hackshaw AK. A meta-analysis of cigarette smoking, bone mineral density and risk of hip fracture: recognition of a major effect. *BMJ* 1997; **315:** 841–6.
18. Nelson ME, *et al.* Effects of high intensity strength training on multiple risk factors for osteoporotic fractures: a randomized controlled trial. *JAMA* 1994; **272:** 1909–14.
19. Gregg EW, *et al.* Physical activity and osteoporotic fracture risk in older women. *Ann Intern Med* 1998; **129:** 81–8.
20. Reid IR, *et al.* Effect of calcium supplementation on bone loss in postmenopausal women. *N Engl J Med* 1993; **328:** 460–4. Correction. *ibid.*; **329:** 1281.
21. Aloia JF, *et al.* Calcium supplementation with and without hormone replacement therapy to prevent postmenopausal bone loss. *Ann Intern Med* 1994; **120:** 97–103.
22. Reid IR, *et al.* Long-term effects of calcium supplementation on bone loss and fractures in postmenopausal women: a randomized controlled trial. *Am J Med* 1995; **98:** 331–5.
23. Riis B, *et al.* Does calcium supplementation prevent postmenopausal bone loss? *N Engl J Med* 1987; **316:** 173–7.
24. Nieves JW, *et al.* Calcium potentiates the effects of estrogen and calcitonin on bone mass: review and analysis. *Am J Clin Nutr* 1998; **67:** 18–24.
25. Bell NH, *et al.* Diclofenac sodium inhibits bone resorption in postmenopausal women. *Am J Med* 1994; **96:** 349–53.
26. Dargent-Molina P, *et al.* Fall-related factors and risk of hip fracture: the EPIDOS prospective study. *Lancet* 1996; **348:** 145–9.
27. Lauritzen JB, *et al.* Effect of external hip protectors on hip fractures. *Lancet* 1993; **341:** 11–13.

28. Altkorn D, Vokes T. Treatment of postmenopausal osteoporosis. *JAMA* 2001; **285**: 1415–18.
29. Gallagher JC, Goldgar D. Treatment of postmenopausal osteoporosis with high doses of synthetic calcitriol: a randomized controlled study. *Ann Intern Med* 1990; **113**: 649–55.
30. Tilyard MW, *et al.* Treatment of postmenopausal osteoporosis with calcitriol or calcium. *N Engl J Med* 1992; **326**: 357–62.
31. Ott SM, Chesnut CH. Calcitriol treatment is not effective in postmenopausal osteoporosis. *Ann Intern Med* 1989; **110**: 267–74.
32. Haguenauer D, *et al.* Fluoride for treating postmenopausal osteoporosis (updated 30 November 2000). Available in The Cochrane Library; Issue 3. Oxford: Update Software; 2001.
33. Anderson DC. Osteoporosis in men. *BMJ* 1992; **305**: 489–90.
34. Seeman E. The dilemma of osteoporosis in men. *Am J Med* 1995; **98** (suppl 2A): 76S–88S.
35. Eastell R, *et al.* Management of male osteoporosis: report of the UK Consensus Group. *Q J Med* 1998; **91**: 71–92.
36. Orwoll ES, *et al.* The rate of bone mineral loss in normal men and the effects of calcium and cholecalciferol supplementation. *Ann Intern Med* 1990; **112**: 29–34.
37. Dawson-Hughes B, *et al.* Effect of calcium and vitamin D supplementation on bone density in men and women 65 years of age and older. *N Engl J Med* 1997; **337**: 670–6.
38. Wasnich R, *et al.* Effect of thiazide on rates of bone mineral loss: a longitudinal study. *BMJ* 1990; **301**: 1303–5. Correction. *ibid.* 1991; **302**: 218.
39. Slovik DM, *et al.* Restoration of spinal bone in osteoporotic men by treatment with human parathyroid hormone (1–34) and 1,25-dihydroxyvitamin D. *J Bone Miner Res* 1986; **1**: 377–81.

Paget's disease of bone

Paget's disease of bone (osteitis deformans) is characterised by excessive and disorganised bone resorption and formation. It may affect one or more bones, usually the cranium, spine, clavicles, pelvis, or long bones, but in most patients the majority of the skeleton is uninvolved. Paget's disease occurs in about 3 to 4% of the population over 40 years of age and its frequency increases with age. Patients are often asymptomatic, but some present with musculoskeletal and bone pain, or with bone weakness and deformity that can result in fractures. Other complications include hearing loss, nerve compression (especially of the spinal cord), and, in severe disease, heart failure due to increased skeletal vascularity.

Patients who are asymptomatic and in whom the sites of disease are associated with little or no risk of complications do not require any treatment. Bone or joint pain may be treated with NSAIDs or paracetamol. Therapy with drugs that reduce bone resorption,[1-3] such as the calcitonins and bisphosphonates, is indicated if bone pain is persistent or to prevent further progression of the disease, especially if complications such as spinal-cord compression are present or there is a risk of such complications. Such treatment is suppressive and while osteolytic lesions may be healed, the underlying disorder is not cured. Drug therapy is guided by monitoring biochemical improvement in disease activity.

Bisphosphonates give symptomatic relief and heal osteolytic lesions. In contrast to the short-lived effects of calcitonins, which generally need to be given continuously to suppress disease activity,[3] disease activity may be reduced for several months, or years, after bisphosphonate therapy has ceased; therefore, bisphosphonates have largely superseded the calcitonins.[2,4] Initial experience was with etidronate, which has the advantage that it may be given by mouth, but unfortunately it impairs bone mineralisation and can cause osteomalacia especially with high doses or prolonged use. Bisphosphonates that have less effect on bone mineralisation, such as oral alendronate or tiludronate and intravenous pamidronate are also effective in Paget's disease of bone and may be preferred.[3,4]

Concomitant administration of a calcitonin with a bisphosphonate has been reported to induce a better response than either drug given alone,[5] but some workers consider that such combinations should be reserved for patients only partially responsive to a single drug.[1] Others suggest that a calcitonin may be useful in the first few weeks of bisphosphonate therapy for more rapid relief of bone pain.[3] When administered consecutively, results have been conflicting.[6,7]

Plicamycin, a cytotoxic antibiotic with particular activity against osteoclasts, is highly effective in the treatment of Paget's disease of bone when given daily by intravenous infusion for 5 to 10 days. However, it is associated with severe toxicity and is therefore now avoided or reserved for patients refractory to other drugs.[3,8]

Studies with gallium nitrate,[9] another inhibitor of bone resorption, have indicated beneficial effects in the treatment of Paget's disease of bone.

In selected patients, orthopaedic surgery such as hip replacement or correction of a bone deformity may be appropriate. A calcitonin or bisphosphonate is usually given 1 to 3 months before surgery in order to reduce bone vascularity (thus minimising blood loss during the operation) and also to prevent development of postoperative hypercalcaemia of immobilisation.

1. Gennari C, *et al.* Management of osteoporosis and Paget's disease: an appraisal of the risks and benefits of drug treatment. *Drug Safety* 1994; **11**: 179–95.
2. Hosking D, *et al.* Paget's disease of bone: diagnosis and management. *BMJ* 1996; **312**: 491–4.
3. Delmas PD, Meunier PJ. The management of Paget's disease of bone. *N Engl J Med* 1997; **336**: 558–66.
4. Roux C, Dougados M. Treatment of patients with Paget's disease of bone. *Drugs* 1999; **58**: 823–30.
5. O'Donoghue DJ, Hosking DJ. Biochemical response to combination of disodium etidronate with calcitonin in Paget's disease. *Bone* 1987; **8**: 219–25.
6. Perry HM, *et al.* Alternate calcitonin and etidronate disodium therapy for Paget's bone disease. *Arch Intern Med* 1984; **144**: 929–33.
7. Rico H, *et al.* Biochemical assessment of acute and chronic treatment of Paget's bone disease with calcitonin and calcium with and without biphosphonate. *Bone* 1988; **9**: 63–6.
8. Ryan WG, *et al.* Apparent cure of Paget's disease of bone. *Am J Med* 1990; **89**: 825–6.
9. Bockman RS, *et al.* A multicenter trial of low dose gallium nitrate in patients with advanced Paget's disease of bone. *J Clin Endocrinol Metab* 1995; **80**: 595–602.

Renal osteodystrophy

Renal osteodystrophy is a complex condition associated with chronic renal failure (p.1185) which involves the development of osteitis fibrosa (hyperparathyroid bone disease) and osteomalacia.[1,2] Osteosclerosis, osteoporosis, and adynamic bone disease (suppression of remodelling) may also occur.[3]

Vitamin D is metabolised in the kidney to its most active form, 1,25-dihydroxycholecalciferol. In renal disease a reduction in the synthesis of this metabolite results in reduced intestinal absorption of calcium, and thus hypocalcaemia. In addition, a reduction in the renal excretion of phosphate leads to hyperphosphataemia, which exacerbates these changes and increases the risk of soft tissue and vascular calcification.

The result is inadequate bone mineralisation with the development of osteomalacia (see above) and excessive production of parathyroid hormone, resulting in secondary hyperparathyroidism (see below). Hyperparathyroidism increases bone turnover and leads to osteitis fibrosa, a condition characterised by an abundance of osteoclasts, osteoblasts, and osteocytes, and the deposition of fibrous tissue in the bone marrow.

In patients with chronic renal failure on dialysis, the accumulation of aluminium from either the dialysis water supply or from the use of aluminium-containing phosphate binders may also have adverse effects on bone (see Aluminium Hydroxide, p.1210) and is associated with the development of osteomalacia and adynamic bone disease.

Most patients are asymptomatic at presentation and **treatment** is aimed at controlling the plasma concentrations of calcium, phosphate, and parathyroid hormone.[2] Severe hyperphosphataemia should be corrected first to reduce the risk of metastatic calcification which may be aggravated by the use of vitamin D compounds which increase calcium absorption.

Hyperphosphataemia is initially controlled with a low-phosphate diet but many patients, especially those on dialysis, also need an oral phosphate binder to complex with dietary phosphate in the gastrointestinal tract and reduce its absorption.[2,4]

Calcium salts such as the carbonate or acetate are effective phosphate binders[5,6] and have been found to suppress hyperparathyroidism. Calcium salts also raise plasma-calcium concentrations and reduce acidosis but hypercalcaemia can occur;[7,8] the use of dialysis fluids with a lower calcium content has been suggested for these patients.[2,9]

Alternatively, aluminium hydroxide may be given but relatively large doses are required and as mentioned above, aluminium accumulation can lead to osteomalacia and adynamic bone disease in patients with impaired renal function. Long-term use is not generally recommended,[2] and alternative drugs are probably preferable.

Vitamin D compounds that do not require renal hydroxylation such as calcitriol (1,25-dihydroxycholecalciferol) or its synthetic analogue, alfacalcidol, are the drugs of choice for correcting the *hypocalcaemia* and also contribute to the control of *secondary hyperparathyroidism*;[2] calcium supplements may also occasionally be required. Newer vitamin D analogues for secondary hyperparathyroidism related to chronic renal failure include doxercalciferol, paricalcitol, and falecalcitriol. Administration of alfacalcidol in the early stages of renal failure, before dialysis is required, has been reported to improve subclinical bone disease.[10] Calcitriol or its analogues are given by mouth; the dose is adjusted according to response but must be carefully monitored as the dose required for adequate suppression of parathyroid hormone secretion may be close to that which causes hypercalcaemia. It has also been recommended that a close watch should be kept on renal function since deterioration may be accelerated by calcitriol, an effect that may be independent of any induced hypercalcaemia.[11]

Patients unresponsive to drug treatment or who develop hypercalcaemia (which may itself accelerate the decline in renal function) may require sub-total parathyroidectomy.[1,2] Alternatively, the administration of calcitriol as intermittent intravenous infusions (3 times a week during haemodialysis) has been reported to be effective in reducing plasma concentrations of parathyroid hormone and ameliorating osteitis fibrosa in some patients with moderate to severe secondary hyperparathyroidism due to chronic renal failure who had failed to respond adequately to oral calcitriol.[12]

Patients with *adynamic bone disease* related to aluminium retention require removal of aluminium from the body; desferrioxamine has been used to mobilise aluminium before haemodialysis.[13] Use of aluminium-containing phosphate binders is clearly undesirable in such patients, and it has also been suggested that vitamin D compounds should not be given because they decrease the proliferation of osteoblasts.[3]

1. Malluche HH, Faugere M-C. Renal osteodystrophy. *N Engl J Med* 1989; **321**: 317–19.
2. Gower P. Prevention of bone disease in chronic renal failure. *Prescribers' J* 1992; **32**: 245–51.
3. Hruska KA, Teitelbaum SL. Renal osteodystrophy. *N Engl J Med* 1995; **333**: 166–74.
4. Coburn JW, Salusky IB. Control of serum phosphorus in uremia. *N Engl J Med* 1989; **320**: 1140–42.
5. Mak RHK, *et al.* Suppression of secondary hyperparathyroidism in children with chronic renal failure by high dose phosphate binders: calcium carbonate versus aluminium hydroxide. *BMJ* 1985; **291**: 623–7.
6. Slatopolsky E, *et al.* Calcium carbonate as a phosphate binder in patients with chronic renal failure undergoing dialysis. *N Engl J Med* 1986; **315**: 157–61.
7. Stein HD, *et al.* Calcium carbonate as a phosphate binder. *N Engl J Med* 1987; **316**: 109–10.
8. Raine AEG, Oliver DO. Management of hyperphosphataemia in renal dialysis patients. *Lancet* 1987; **i**: 633–4.
9. Slatopolsky E, *et al.* Calcium carbonate as a phosphate binder. *N Engl J Med* 1987; **316**: 110.
10. Hamdy NAT, *et al.* Effect of alfacalcidol on natural course of renal bone disease in mild to moderate renal failure. *BMJ* 1995; **310**: 358–63.
11. Chan JCM, *et al.* A prospective, double-blind study of growth failure in children with chronic renal insufficiency and the effectiveness of treatment with calcitriol versus dihydrotachysterol. *J Pediatr* 1994; **124**: 520–8.
12. Andress DL, *et al.* Intravenous calcitriol in the treatment of refractory osteitis fibrosa of chronic renal failure. *N Engl J Med* 1989; **321**: 274–9.
13. McCarthy JT, *et al.* Clinical experience with desferrioxamine in dialysis patients with aluminium toxicity. *Q J Med* 1990; **74**: 257–76.

Rickets

See Osteomalacia, above.

Parathyroid Disorders

Parathyroid hormone, secreted by the parathyroid gland, maintains concentrations of ionised calcium in extracellular fluid within normal limits. It acts directly on the kidney to enhance renal reabsorption of calcium, to increase phosphate excretion, and to promote the conversion of vitamin D to its active metabolite, 1,25-dihydroxycholecalciferol, which in turn, enhances calcium absorption from the gastrointestinal tract. Parathyroid hormone also acts on bone, to accelerate bone resorption and the release of calcium and phosphate into the extracellular fluid. Secretion of parathyroid hormone is primarily regulated by the extracellular concentration of ionised calcium; hypocalcaemia stimulates secretion whereas hypercalcaemia has an inhibitory effect. 1,25-Dihydroxycholecalciferol can also suppress parathyroid hormone secretion.

Disorders of parathyroid hormone secretion cause a disruption of calcium homoeostasis and in the long-term, may result in bone disease.

Hyperparathyroidism

Primary hyperparathyroidism is a disorder of parathyroid hormone hypersecretion usually caused by adenomas or hyperplasia of the parathyroid glands. Patients are commonly asymptomatic but may have signs of hypercalcaemia (p.1181); nephrolithiasis may also be present. Secondary hyperparathyroidism occurs in response to hypocalcaemia as in chronic renal failure (p.1185) and if prolonged may progress to autonomous hypersecretion by the parathyroid gland (tertiary hyperparathyroidism).

Severe hypercalcaemia requires immediate treatment, but is rare in primary hyperparathyroidism. In the long-term, the treatment of choice for primary and tertiary hyperparathyroidism is usually surgical parathyroidectomy;[1-3] in patients with asymptomatic primary hyperparathyroidism no therapy may be necessary,[1] but the precise indications for surgery have been subject to debate.[3] The treatment of secondary hyperparathyroidism is usually aimed at the underlying cause of the hypocalcaemia; for example, for the treatment of secondary hyperparathyroidism associated with chronic renal disease, see Renal Osteodystrophy, above.

Drug treatment plays only a modest role in primary hyperparathyroidism. Oral phosphate supplements have been given in the short-term to alleviate hypercalciuria and hypercalcaemia. Bisphosphonates can be used in the acute management of hypercalcaemia, but seem to be of little benefit in the long-term treatment of hyperparathyroidism.[4] Oestrogens have been reported to reduce the rate of bone turnover and perhaps plasma-concentrations of calcium in postmenopausal women with primary hyperparathyroidism.[3,5,6] Calcium receptor agonists (calcimimetics) are under development for hyperparathyroidism.[7] Use of parathyroid hormone peptides to induce autoantibodies against parathyroid hormone resulted in improvement in hypercalcaemia in a woman with parathyroid carcinoma.[8]

1. Consensus Development Conference Panel. Diagnosis and management of asymptomatic primary hyperparathyroidism: consensus development conference statement. *Ann Intern Med* 1991; 114: 593–7.
2. Scott-Coombes DM, Lynn JA. Surgical treatment of parathyroid disease. *Br J Hosp Med* 1997; 57: 488–91.
3. Marx SJ. Hyperparathyroid and hypoparathyroid disorders. *N Engl J Med* 2000; 343: 1863–75. Correction. *ibid.*; 344: 696.
4. Al Zahrani A, Levine MA. Primary hyperparathyroidism. *Lancet* 1997; 349: 1233–8.
5. Marcus R, *et al.* Conjugated estrogens in the treatment of postmenopausal women with hyperparathyroidism. *Ann Intern Med* 1984; 100: 633–40.
6. Selby PL, Peacock M. Ethinyl estradiol and norethindrone in the treatment of primary hyperparathyroidism in postmenopausal women. *N Engl J Med* 1986; 314: 1481–5.
7. Silverberg SJ, *et al.* Short-term inhibition of parathyroid hormone secretion by a calcium-receptor agonist in patients with primary hyperparathyroidism. *N Engl J Med* 1997; 337: 1506–10.
8. Bradwell AR, *et al.* Control of hypercalcaemia of parathyroid carcinoma by immunisation. *Lancet* 1999; 353: 370–3.

Hypoparathyroidism

Hypoparathyroidism occurs when there is a deficiency of parathyroid hormone secretion due to lack of parathyroid gland development or destruction of the gland, for example by auto-immune disease or surgical removal.[1] Other factors that may lead to a deficiency in parathyroid hormone include hypomagnesaemia and parathyroid adenomas. Where the deficiency results from resistance to parathyroid hormone the condition is termed pseudohypoparathyroidism. Parathyroid hormone, as teriparatide, is used in the differential diagnosis of hypoparathyroidism and pseudohypoparathyroidism. Hypoparathyroidism leads to hypocalcaemia and hyperphosphataemia, though in some patients these may not become significant until there is an increased calcium demand as in pregnancy.

Treatment is aimed at correcting the hypocalcaemia (p.1181); in patients with hypocalcaemic tetany the parenteral administration of calcium salts may be necessary. In the long-term, treatment is usually with oral vitamin D compounds which increase the intestinal absorption of calcium; calcium supplements may be required if dietary calcium is inadequate. Calcium concentrations and renal function require careful monitoring, especially since the lack of parathyroid hormone results in an increase in the renal excretion of calcium and the risk of nephrolithiasis. Beneficial effects on plasma-calcium concentrations have been reported following the use of thiazide diuretics to reduce the urinary excretion of calcium.[2,3] However, these effects tended to be modest and thiazide diuretics have not been found to be effective in all patients with hypoparathyroidism;[4] adverse effects such as metabolic alkalosis may also be a problem.[5]

Teriparatide also has potential in the treatment of hypoparathyroidism. In one study,[6] it maintained serum calcium in the normal range and decreased urine calcium excretion. Good results have been reported following transplantation of parathyroid cells depleted of antigenbearing cells in a few patients with postsurgical hypopar-

athyroidism.[7,8] It was considered that this might prove a promising technique in the future.

1. Marx SJ. Hyperparathyroid and hypoparathyroid disorders. *N Engl J Med* 2000; 343: 1863–75. Correction. *ibid.*; 344: 696.
2. Porter RH, *et al.* Treatment of hypoparathyroid patients with chlorthalidone. *N Engl J Med* 1978; 298: 577–81.
3. Newman GH, *et al.* Effect of bendrofluazide on calcium reabsorption in hypoparathyroidism. *Eur J Clin Pharmacol* 1984; 27: 41–6.
4. Gertner JM, Genel M. Chlorthalidone for hypoparathyroidism. *N Engl J Med* 1978; 298: 1478.
5. Barzel US. Chlorthalidone for hypoparathyroidism. *N Engl J Med* 1978; 298: 1478.
6. Winer KK, *et al.* Synthetic human parathyroid hormone 1-34 vs calcitriol and calcium in the treatment of hypoparathyroidism: results of a short-term randomized crossover trial. *JAMA* 1996; 276: 631–6.
7. Decker GAG, *et al.* Allotransplantation of parathyroid cells. *Lancet* 1995; 345: 124. Correction. *ibid.*; 464.
8. Hasse C, *et al.* Parathyroid allotransplantation without immunosuppression. *Lancet* 1997; 350: 1296–7.

Alendronic Acid (4537-w)

Alendronic Acid *(BAN, rINN)*.
AHButBP; Aminohydroxybutylidene Diphosphonic Acid. 4-Amino-1-hydroxybutane-1,1-diylbis(phosphonic acid).
$C_4H_{13}NO_7P_2 = 249.1$.
CAS — 66376-36-1.
ATC — M05BA04.

Alendronate Sodium (19721-x)

Alendronate Sodium *(BANM, USAN, rINNM)*.
G-704650; L-670452; MK-0217; MK-217; Monosodium alendronate; Natrii Alendronas. Sodium trihydrogen (4-amino-1-hydroxybutylidene)diphosphonate trihydrate.
$C_4H_{12}NNaO_7P_2,3H_2O = 325.1$.
CAS — 121268-17-5.
Pharmacopoeias. In Eur. (see p.vi).

Alendronate sodium 1.3 mg is approximately equivalent to 1 mg of alendronic acid.

Pharmacopoeial description

Ph. Eur.: A white or almost white crystalline powder. Soluble in water; practically insoluble in dichloromethane; very slightly soluble in methyl alcohol. A 1% solution in water has a pH of 4.0 to 5.0.

Adverse Effects and Precautions

As for the bisphosphonates in general, p.748. Gastrointestinal symptoms such as abdominal pain, dyspepsia, diarrhoea or constipation are the most frequent adverse effects. Severe oesophageal reactions such as oesophagitis, erosions, and ulceration have occurred (see below); patients should be advised to stop taking the tablets and seek medical attention if they develop symptoms such as dysphagia, new or worsening heartburn, pain on swallowing, or retrosternal pain. Peptic ulceration has been reported.

Alendronate should not be given to patients with abnormalities of the oesophagus or other factors that might delay oesophageal emptying, or those unable to stand or sit upright for at least 30 minutes. It should be used with caution in patients with upper gastrointestinal abnormalities. *To minimise the risk of oesophageal reactions, patients should be instructed to swallow alendronate tablets whole with plenty of water (not less than 200 mL), in an upright position (standing or sitting). Tablets should be taken on rising for the day, on an empty stomach, at least 30 minutes before breakfast and any other oral medication; patients should remain upright after taking the tablets, and should not lie down before eating the first meal of the day. Alendronate should not be taken at bedtime, or before getting up for the day.* Hypocalcaemia should be corrected before starting alendronate therapy.

Effects on the oesophagus. Between September 1995 and March 1996 the UK Committee on Safety of Medicines (CSM) had received 10 reports of adverse effects on the oesophagus in patients receiving alendronate sodium.[1] Of these, 4 were of oesophageal reflux, 4 of oesophagitis, and 2 of oesophageal ulceration. As of March 1996, worldwide an estimated 475 000 patients had received alendronate and 199 patients had oesophageal reactions reported to the manufacturer, of which 51 were serious or severe.[2] Endoscopic findings included erosions, ulcerations, exudative inflammation, and thickening of the oesophagus. Bleeding was rare, and oesophageal perforation was not reported. Most oesophageal reactions occurred within 1 week to 2 months of starting alendronate therapy. Recovery occurred when alendronate was stopped; however, it

was considered important that patients be followed up for the possible development of strictures.[2] In about 60% of the cases where the information was available, alendronate had not been taken in accordance with the precautions for use (see above).

The CSM subsequently noted[3] that it had continued to receive reports of reactions; by July 1998 there had been 97 reports in the UK, in 1 case associated with a fatality. It was estimated that 1 to 2% of patients might experience oesophageal reactions even when following the precautions for use. Some have reported a much higher incidence of unacceptable upper gastrointestinal symptoms in clinical practice.[4] However, a large placebo-controlled trial of alendronate did not find any increase in upper gastrointestinal events in patients taking alendronate.[5]

1. Committee on Safety of Medicines/Medicines Control Agency. Oesophageal reactions with alendronate sodium (Fosamax). *Current Problems* 1996; 22: 5.
2. de Groen PC, *et al.* Esophagitis associated with the use of alendronate. *N Engl J Med* 1996; 335: 1016–21.
3. Committee on Safety of Medicines/Medicines Control Agency. Reminder: severe oesophageal reactions with alendronate sodium (Fosamax). *Current Problems* 1998; 24: 13.
4. Kelly R, Taggart H. Incidence of gastrointestinal side effects due to alendronate is high in clinical practice. *BMJ* 1997; 315: 1235.
5. Bauer DC, *et al.* Upper gastrointestinal tract safety profile of alendronate: the fracture intervention trial. *Arch Intern Med* 2000; 160: 517–25.

Interactions

As for the bisphosphonates in general, p.748.

Pharmacokinetics

Like other bisphosphonates, alendronate is poorly absorbed following oral administration. Absorption is decreased by food, especially by products containing calcium or other polyvalent cations. Bioavailability is about 0.4% when administered half an hour before food, reduced from 0.7% in the fasting state; absorption is negligible when taken up to 2 hours after a meal. About half of the absorbed portion is excreted in the urine; the remainder is sequestered to bone for a prolonged period. Bisphosphonates do not appear to be metabolised.

◊ References.

1. Gertz BJ, *et al.* Studies of the oral bioavailability of alendronate. *Clin Pharmacol Ther* 1995; 58: 288–98.

Uses and Administration

Alendronate is an aminobisphosphonate with general properties similar to those of the other bisphosphonates (p.749). It is a potent inhibitor of bone resorption and is used as the sodium salt in osteoporosis and Paget's disease of bone. It has also been given in the treatment of bone metastases and hypercalcaemia of malignancy.

Alendronate sodium is given by mouth, and the specific instructions for its administration (see Adverse Effects and Precautions, above) should be followed to minimise adverse effects and permit adequate absorption. Doses are expressed in terms of alendronic acid. The usual dosage for the treatment of osteoporosis in men and women is 10 mg daily. Postmenopausal women may be given 5 mg daily for prophylaxis. Alendronic acid may also be given once weekly to postmenopausal women in a dose of 70 mg for treatment of osteoporosis, or 35 mg for prophylaxis. Alendronate is used for the treatment and prevention of corticosteroid-induced osteoporosis in a dose of 5 mg daily; postmenopausal women who do not receive HRT should be given 10 mg daily. In adults with Paget's disease of bone the usual dose is 40 mg daily for 6 months; treatment may be repeated if necessary after an interval of a further 6 months.

Alendronic acid has also been given by intravenous infusion.

Malignant neoplasms of the bone. Bisphosphonates are of benefit in some patients with metastatic bone disease (p.490). An open study with alendronate given intravenously suggested that it might be useful in such circumstances,[1] while a randomised dose-response study[2] found that single intravenous doses of alendronate 5 mg or more effectively lowered serum-calcium concentrations in patients with hypercalcaemia of malignancy.

1. Attardo-Parrinello G, *et al.* Effects of a new aminodiphosphonate (aminohydroxybutylidene diphosphonate) in patients with osteolytic lesions from metastases and myelomatosis: comparison with dichloromethylene diphosphonate. *Arch Intern Med* 1987; 147: 1629–33.
2. Nussbaum SR, *et al.* Dose-response study of alendronate sodium for the treatment of cancer-associated hypercalcemia. *J Clin Oncol* 1993; 11: 1618–23.

Osteoporosis. The use of alendronate for the prevention and treatment of osteoporosis (p.745) has been reviewed.[1] In randomised controlled trials of up to 3 years duration, alendronate increased bone mass density of the spine, hip, and total body in postmenopausal women with osteoporosis,[2-4] those with osteoporosis and existing vertebral fractures,[5,6] and those without osteoporosis.[7,8] In postmenopausal women without osteoporosis, alendronate increased bone mass density, but not quite to the same extent as HRT.[7,9] Continuous therapy with alendronate for 4 years was more effective than 2 years of active therapy followed by placebo for 2 years.[9] Where incidence of vertebral fracture was the primary end-point, alendronate reduced the incidence of new vertebral and nonvertebral fractures in women with prior fractures.[5,6,10] In women without prior fractures, alendronate reduced the incidence of clinical fractures in those with osteoporosis,[10,11] but not in those with higher bone mass density.[11] Alendronate is also used in men with osteoporosis; in a 2-year randomised trial it was found to increase bone mineral density and help prevent vertebral fractures.[12]

Alendronate also increases bone mass density in men and women receiving oral corticosteroids at doses equivalent to at least 7.5 mg prednisone daily.[13]

1. Sharpe M, et al. Alendronate: an update of its use in osteoporosis. *Drugs* 2001; **61:** 999–1039.
2. Chesnut CH, et al. Alendronate treatment of the postmenopausal osteoporotic woman: effect of multiple dosages on bone mass and bone remodeling. *Am J Med* 1995; **99:** 144–52.
3. Liberman UA, et al. Effect of oral alendronate on bone mineral density and the incidence of fractures in postmenopausal osteoporosis. *N Engl J Med* 1995; **333:** 1437–43.
4. Tucci JR, et al. Effect of three years of oral alendronate treatment in postmenopausal women with osteoporosis. *Am J Med* 1996; **101:** 488–501.
5. Black DM, et al. Randomised trial of effect of alendronate on risk of fracture in women with existing vertebral fractures. *Lancet* 1996; **348:** 1535–41.
6. Ensrud KE, et al. Treatment with alendronate prevents fractures in women at highest risk: results from the Fracture Intervention Trial. *Arch Intern Med* 1997; **157:** 2617–24.
7. Hosking D, et al. Prevention of bone loss with alendronate in postmenopausal women under 60 years of age. *N Engl J Med* 1998; **338:** 485–92.
8. McClung M, et al. Alendronate prevents postmenopausal bone loss in women without osteoporosis: a double-blind, randomized, controlled trial. *Ann Intern Med* 1998; **128:** 253–61.
9. Ravn P, et al. Alendronate and estrogen-progestin in the long-term prevention of bone loss: four-year results from the early postmenopausal intervention cohort study: a randomized, controlled trial. *Ann Intern Med* 1999; **131:** 935–42.
10. Black DM, et al. Fracture risk reduction with alendronate in women with osteoporosis: the fracture intervention trial. *J Clin Endocrinol Metab* 2000; **85:** 4118–24.
11. Cummings SR, et al. Effect of alendronate on risk of fracture in women with low bone density but without vertebral fractures: results from the Fracture Intervention Trial. *JAMA* 1998; **280:** 2077–82.
12. Orwoll E, et al. Alendronate for the treatment of osteoporosis in men. *N Engl J Med* 2000; **343:** 604–10.
13. Saag KG, et al. Alendronate for the prevention and treatment of glucocorticoid-induced osteoporosis. *N Engl J Med* 1998; **339:** 292–9.

Paget's disease of bone. Bisphosphonates may be indicated to control the excessive and disorganised resorption and formation of bone that occurs in Paget's disease of bone (p.746). References.

1. Adami S, et al. Effects of two oral doses of alendronate in the treatment of Paget's disease of bone. *Bone* 1994; **15:** 415–17.
2. Reid LR, et al. Biochemical and radiologic improvement in Paget's disease of bone treated with alendronate: a randomized, placebo-controlled trial. *Am J Med* 1996; **101:** 341–8.
3. Siris E, et al. Comparative study of alendronate versus etidronate for the treatment of Paget's disease of bone. *J Clin Endocrinol Metab* 1996; **81:** 961–7.

Preparations

Proprietary Preparations (details are given in Part 3)
Aust.: Fosamax; *Austral.:* Fosamax; *Belg.:* Fosamax; *Braz.:* Endronax; Fosamax; *Canad.:* Fosamax; *Denm.:* Fosamax; *Fin.:* Fosamax; *Fr.:* Fosamax; *Ger.:* Fosamax; *Hong Kong:* Fosamax; *Irl.:* Fosamax; *Israel:* Fosalan; *Ital.:* Adronat; Alendros; Dronal; Fosamax; *Jpn:* Onclast; *Mex.:* Fosamax; *Neth.:* Fosamax; *Norw.:* Fosamax; *NZ:* Fosamax; *Port.:* Adronat; Fosamax; *S.Afr.:* Fosamax; *Singapore:* Fosamax; *Spain:* Fosamax; *Swed.:* Fosamax; *Switz.:* Fosamax; *Thai.:* Fosamax; *UK:* Fosamax; *USA:* Fosamax.

Bisphosphonates (3267-t)

Biphosphonates; Diphosphonates.

Bisphosphonates are analogues of pyrophosphate, in which the central oxygen atom is replaced by a carbon atom with two further substituents—see Figure 1, below. Like pyrophosphate they have a strong affinity for bone. The bisphosphonates are used chiefly for their antiresorptive and hypocalcaemic properties (see Uses and Administration, below).

Adverse Effects, Treatment, and Precautions

Bisphosphonates may cause gastrointestinal disturbances including abdominal pain, nausea and vomiting, and diarrhoea or constipation. Existing gastrointestinal problems may be exacerbated, and oral bisphosphonates should generally be given with care or avoided if acute upper gastrointestinal inflammation is present. Abdominal pain may be more frequent with aminobisphosphonates such as alendronate and oesophagitis has occurred.

Disturbances in serum electrolytes may occur, most commonly hypocalcaemia and hypophosphataemia. Bisphosphonates may cause musculoskeletal pain and headache. Hypersensitivity reactions have occurred rarely; angioedema, rashes, and pruritus have been reported. Other rare adverse effects include blood disorders such as leucopenia and disturbances in liver enzyme values.

Transient fever and influenza-like symptoms are common with infusions of ibandronate and pamidronate. There may be local reactions, including thrombophlebitis, following parenteral administration.

Impairment of renal function has been reported with bisphosphonates, particularly when given parenterally. As a result their use should generally be avoided in patients with moderate to severe renal insufficiency and they should be used with care in those with lesser degrees of renal impairment.

Etidronate interferes with bone mineralisation, especially at higher doses, which can result in osteomalacia and an increased incidence of fracture. Etidronate should be discontinued if a fracture occurs, until healing is complete. It has also been associated with a flare in bone pain in some patients with Paget's disease. Impaired mineralisation is much less marked at usual doses of other bisphosphonates.

Overdosage with bisphosphonates would be likely to result in symptoms of hypocalcaemia; if necessary, parenteral infusion of a calcium salt could be given. Administration of milk or antacids, to bind the bisphosphonate and minimise absorption, has been suggested for oral overdosage.

There is no clinical experience with bisphosphonates in pregnancy and they are generally contra-indicated; bisphosphonates have been associated with skeletal abnormalities in the fetus when given to pregnant *animals*.

◊ Reviews.

1. Adami S, Zamberlan N. Adverse effects of bisphosphonates: a comparative review. *Drug Safety* 1996; **14:** 158–70.

Effects on the eyes. There have been a few reports of ocular effects associated with aminobisphosphonates. Although adverse ocular reactions to bisphosphonates appeared to be rare, the manufacturers were aware of 23 cases up to September 1993 which were possibly associated with the drug.[1] The reactions included anterior uveitis in 7 patients and unilateral episcleritis or scleritis in 3. In one previously reported case,[2] bilateral iritis was associated with risedronate and subsequently pamidronate in a patient who had earlier received etidronate without ill-effect.

1. Macarol V, Fraunfelder FT. Pamidronate disodium and possible ocular adverse drug reactions. *Am J Ophthalmol* 1994; **118:** 220–4.
2. Siris ES. Bisphosphonates and iritis. *Lancet* 1993; **341:** 436–7.

Effects on the kidneys. Renal failure was associated with the intravenous administration of etidronate to 2 patients with hypercalcaemia of malignancy.[1] One had been given a high dose (1 g) by short intravenous infusion on two successive days and the other had an elevated serum-creatinine concentration before administration. A third patient given clodronate also developed renal failure but had a slightly raised serum-creatinine concentration before administration. Kanis *et al.*[2] commented that with smaller doses of bisphosphonates (up to 300 mg daily) by intravenous infusion over 2 to 3 hours they had not seen renal impairment in more than 40 patients treated with disodium etidronate or disodium clodronate. They noted a trend towards raised creatinine concentrations which was reversed when etidronate infusions were discontinued. Hasling *et al.*[3] found increased serum-creatinine concentrations after the first infusion of etidronate when compared with placebo, but not after subsequent infusions.

1. Bounameaux HM, et al. Renal failure associated with intravenous diphosphonates. *Lancet* 1983; **i:** 471.
2. Kanis JA, et al. Effects of intravenous diphosphonates on renal function. *Lancet* 1983; **i:** 1328.
3. Hasling C, et al. Etidronate disodium for treating hypercalcaemia of malignancy: a double blind placebo-controlled study. *Eur J Clin Invest* 1986; **16:** 433–7.

Effects on the respiratory system. Bronchospasm has been induced by bisphosphonates in 2 patients who were aspirin-sensitive asthmatics. The first patient complained of shortness of breath and wheezing 10 minutes after the start of an infusion of clodronate while the second developed similar symptoms 2 days after the start of cyclical therapy with etidronate by mouth. Oral rechallenge in both patients resulted in a fall in the forced expiratory values at 1 second.[1] The reaction in these 2 patients was not considered to be immune-mediated.

1. Rolla G, et al. Bisphosphonate-induced bronchoconstriction in aspirin-sensitive asthma. *Lancet* 1994; **343:** 426–7.

Hypersensitivity. Bisphosphonates may rarely cause hypersensitivity reactions such as angioedema, urticaria, and pruritus. Published reports include a severe allergic reaction to sodium medronate in the form of a radiopharmaceutical,[1] and mild skin rashes in two patients given pamidronate by mouth.[2] There has also been a report of erythroderma with lesions of the mucous membranes being associated with clodronate administration in one patient,[3] and severe epidermal necrosis may have been associated with tiludronate in another.[4] A possibly drug-related rash has also been reported in a patient receiving alendronate.[5] Two patients experiencing cutaneous reactions to pamidronate or clodronate were able to continue oral clodronate after desensitisation.[6]

1. Elliott AT, et al. Severe reaction to diphosphonate: implications for treatment of Paget's disease. *BMJ* 1988; **297:** 592–3.
2. Mautalen CA, et al. Side effects of disodium aminohydroxypropylidenediphosphonate (APD) during treatment of bone diseases. *BMJ* 1984; **288:** 828–9.
3. Pajus I, et al. Erythroderma after clodronate treatment. *BMJ* 1993; **307:** 484.
4. Roux C, et al. Long-lasting dermatological lesions after tiludronate therapy. *Calcif Tissue Int* 1992; **50:** 378–80.
5. Chesnut CH, et al. Alendronate treatment of the postmenopausal osteoporotic woman: effect of multiple dosages on bone mass and bone remodeling. *Am J Med* 1995; **99:** 144–52.
6. Phillips EJ, et al. Allergic reactions to bisphosphonates: a report of three cases and an approach to management. *J Clin Pharmacol* 1998; **38:** 842–86.

Interactions

The bisphosphonates are not well absorbed from the gastrointestinal tract, and administration with food further impairs their absorption.

Compounds containing aluminium, calcium, iron, or magnesium, including antacids and mineral supplements and some osmotic laxatives, can also impair the absorption of bisphosphonates given by mouth.

Figure 1. Comparative structures of the bisphosphonates.

Pyrophosphate

Generic structure of a bisphosphonate

R_1	R_2	Name
$C_3H_6.NH_2$	OH	Alendronic Acid
Cl	Cl	Clodronic Acid
CH_3	OH	Etidronic Acid
$C_2H_4.NCH_3.C_5H_{11}$	OH	Ibandronic Acid
$C_7H_{13}.NH$	H	Incadronic Acid
H	H	Medronic Acid
$C_5H_{10}.NH_2$	OH	Neridronic Acid
H	OH	Oxidronic Acid
$C_2H_4.NH_2$	OH	Pamidronic Acid
$CH_2.C_5H_4N$	OH	Risedronic Acid
$S.C_6H_4Cl$	H	Tiludronic Acid
$CH_2.C_3H_3N_2$	OH	Zoledronic Acid

It has been suggested that the administration of certain bisphosphonates with NSAIDs may result in an increased incidence of gastrointestinal or renal adverse effects.

There may be additive hypocalcaemic effects with aminoglycosides.

Aminoglycosides. A report of a patient who developed persisting severe hypocalcaemia after treatment with clodronate and *netilmicin*. Bisphosphonates and aminoglycosides can induce hypocalcaemia by different mechanisms and care should be taken when administering them simultaneously.[1]

1. Pedersen-Bjergaard U, Myhre J. Severe hypocalcaemia after treatment with diphosphonate and aminoglycoside. *BMJ* 1991; **302:** 295. Correction. *ibid.*; 791.

Pharmacokinetics

The bisphosphonates are poorly absorbed following oral administration, with bioavailabilities in the fasting state ranging from about 0.7% (alendronate; risedronate) to up to 6% (etidronate; tiludronate). Absorption is reduced by food, especially by products containing calcium or other polyvalent cations. They have a high affinity for bone, with about 50% of an absorbed dose bound to ossified tissues and retained in the body for prolonged periods. Excretion is in the urine, as unchanged drug; they do not appear to be metabolised.

Uses and Administration

The bisphosphonates inhibit bone resorption and thus have a hypocalcaemic effect. They are pyrophosphate analogues which have a high affinity for the hydroxyapatite of bone, and which inhibit bone resorption by osteoclasts; because of the coupling of resorption and formation this results in an overall reduction in remodelling and bone turnover (see Bone and Bone Disease, p.744). Their antiresorptive potency varies widely. The bisphosphonates also inhibit the formation and dissolution of hydroxyapatite crystals and thus have the potential to interfere with bone mineralisation. The degree to which the bisphosphonates inhibit mineralisation in clinical practice varies; disodium etidronate is the most potent inhibitor of those now in general clinical use.

Because bone resorption increases plasma-calcium concentrations, the bisphosphonates are used as adjuncts to the treatment of severe hypercalcaemia, especially when associated with malignancy. They are also used in disorders associated with excessive bone resorption and turnover, such as Paget's disease of bone and osteoporosis, as well as in the management of bone metastases. Etidronate has been used in the prevention and treatment of ectopic ossification.

Because of the affinity of bisphosphonates for bone, complexes labelled with radioactive technetium-99m (see p.1451) have been used diagnostically as bone scanning agents.

Bisphosphonates have been given by intravenous infusion or by mouth. In the latter case food should be avoided for a suitable period before and after administration, especially products with a high calcium content such as milk.

◊ References.
1. Compston JE. The therapeutic use of bisphosphonates. *BMJ* 1994; **309:** 711–15.
2. Rosen CJ, Kessenich CR. Comparative clinical pharmacology and therapeutic use of bisphosphonates in metabolic bone diseases. *Drugs* 1996; **51:** 537–51.
3. Brown DL, Robbins R. Developments in the therapeutic applications of bisphosphonates. *J Clin Pharmacol* 1999; **39:** 651–60.
4. Shoemaker LR. Expanding role of bisphosphonate therapy in children. *J Pediatr* 1999; **134:** 264–7.
5. Hillner BE, *et al.* American Society of Clinical Oncology guideline on the role of bisphosphonates in breast cancer. *J Clin Oncol* 2000; **18:** 1378–91.
6. Homik J, *et al.* Bisphosphonates for steroid induced osteoporosis (updated 9 May 2001). Available in The Cochrane Library; Issue 3. Oxford: Update Software; 2001.

Ectopic ossification. The only treatment for established ectopic ossification (p.744) is surgery, but drugs have been used for prophylaxis or prevention of recurrence. Bisphosphonates that are potent inhibitors of mineralisation such as etidronate have been advocated for this purpose, but they do not prevent the formation of the osteoid matrix and delayed mineralisation may occur once they are withdrawn.

The symbol † denotes a preparation no longer actively marketed

Hypercalcaemia. In patients with severe symptomatic hypercalcaemia restoration and maintenance of adequate hydration and urine flow is essential, and helps to reduce plasma-calcium concentrations by promoting calcium diuresis. In hypercalcaemia of malignancy (p.1181) therapy with inhibitors of bone resorption such as the bisphosphonates may also be considered, and some have suggested that pamidronate is the drug of choice for this purpose. Although sustained, the action of bisphosphonates is not particularly rapid; they may be combined with a calcitonin where both rapid and prolonged diminution of plasma-calcium concentration is desired.

Hyperparathyroidism. Bisphosphonates have been used to inhibit bone resorption in the treatment of hypercalcaemia associated with hyperparathyroidism (p.746), but seem to be of little benefit for long-term treatment.

Malignant neoplasms of the bone. There is good evidence that some bisphosphonates are of benefit in patients with metastatic bone disease (p.490) not only to control bone pain and to manage the attendant hypercalcaemia, but also to reduce skeletal complications such as fractures. There is also much interest in the use of bisphosphonates to prevent the development of bone metastases; however, preliminary evidence of their efficacy is conflicting. Specific references may be found under the individual drugs.

Osteogenesis imperfecta. Bisphosphonates have been tried in osteogenesis imperfecta (p.744), but orthopaedic treatment and physical activity programmes form the basis of therapy.

Osteoporosis. Bisphosphonates are used in the prevention and treatment of postmenopausal and corticosteroid-induced osteoporosis (p.745). Both alendronate and etidronate have been shown to be effective in terms of effect on bone mass density. There is less evidence for a consequent reduction in fracture rates, although this has been shown for alendronate in postmenopausal osteoporosis (see p.748). Alendronate is given continuously, whereas etidronate is given intermittently, alternating with a calcium supplement; both drugs are administered orally. Although there is less evidence for their efficacy in men with idiopathic osteoporosis, some consider bisphosphonates are the preferred treatment for this condition.

Paget's disease of bone. Paget's disease of bone (p.746) is characterised by excessive and disorganised bone resorption and formation. Not all patients require treatment, and pain can be managed in some with NSAIDs or paracetamol. Bisphosphonates may be indicated if bone pain is persistent or to prevent further progression of the disease particularly if there is a risk of complications.

Reflex sympathetic dystrophy. Osteoporosis is one of the features of reflex sympathetic dystrophy (see under Sympathetic Pain Syndromes, p.8) and preliminary data indicate that bisphosphonates may be of benefit in controlling associated pain in some patients.[1]

1. Schott GD. Bisphosphonates for pain relief in reflex sympathetic dystrophy? *Lancet* 1997; **350:** 1117. Correction. *ibid.* 1998; **351:** 682.

Calcitonins (12106-w)

Calcitonin (Human) (11091-e)

Calcitonin-human; Human Calcitonin.
$C_{151}H_{226}N_{40}O_{45}S_3,3HCl = 3527.2$.
ATC — H05BA03 (Human Synthetic).
Pharmacopoeias. In Swiss.

A synthetic polypeptide comprising 32 amino acids in the same linear sequence as in naturally occurring human calcitonin.

Calcitonin (Pork) (8053-f)

Calcitonin (Pork) (BANM).
CAS — 12321-44-7.
ATC — H05BA02 (Pork Natural).

NOTE. The synonym thyrocalcitonin and the CAS number 9007-12-9 have been used for calcitonin that is often of pork origin.
Pharmacopoeias. In It.

A polypeptide hormone obtained from pork thyroid.

Elcatonin (19126-n)

Elcatonin (rINN).
[Aminosuberic Acid 1,7]-eel Calcitonin; [Asu^{1,7}]-E-CT; Carbocalcitonin. 1-Butyric acid-7-(L-2-aminobutyric acid)-26-L-aspartic acid-27-L-valine-29-L-alaninecalcitonin (salmon).
$C_{148}H_{244}N_{42}O_{47} = 3363.8$.
CAS — 60731-46-6.
ATC — H05BA04.
Pharmacopoeias. In Jpn.

A synthetic analogue of eel calcitonin.

Salcatonin (8054-d)

Salcatonin (BAN).
Calcitonin (Salmon) (BAN); Calcitonin-salmon; Calcitoninum Salmonis; Salmon Calcitonin; SCT-1.
$C_{145}H_{240}N_{44}O_{48}S_2 = 3431.9$.
CAS — 47931-85-1.
ATC — H05BA01 (Salmon Synthetic).

NOTE. There may be some confusion between the terms Salcatonin and Calcitonin (Salmon) (Salmon Calcitonin; Calcitonin-salmon) although in practice these names appear to be used for the same substance.
The Ph. Eur. defines Calcitonin (Salmon) as a synthetic polypeptide having the structure of salmon calcitonin I.
Calcitonin (Salmon)/Salcatonin (BAN) is defined as a *component* of natural salmon calcitonin. The BP 2001 defines Calcitonin (Salmon)/Salcatonin as a synthetic polypeptide having the structure determined for salmon calcitonin I.
In the USA, Calcitonin (USAN) includes calcitonin (human) and calcitonin (salmon). Salcatonin is there understood to be a synthetic polypeptide structurally similar to natural salmon calcitonin (Calcitonin Salmon (Synthesis)). The US manufacturers use Calcitonin-salmon for a synthetic polypeptide with the same structure as calcitonin of salmon origin.
Pharmacopoeias. In Eur. (see p.vi).

Like some other peptide drugs, calcitonin may be adsorbed onto the plastic of intravenous giving sets; it has been suggested that solutions for intravenous infusion should contain some protein to prevent the sorption and consequent loss of potency (see under Administration, below).

Pharmacopoeial description

Ph. Eur.: A white or almost white powder. Freely soluble in water. Store at 2° to 8°. If the substance is sterile store in a sterile, airtight, tamper-proof container. Protect from light.

Units

0.8 units of calcitonin, porcine, are contained in one ampoule of the second International Standard Preparation (1991).

128 units of calcitonin, salmon, are contained in approximately 20 µg of freeze-dried purified synthetic salmon calcitonin, with mannitol 2 mg in one ampoule of the second International Standard Preparation (1989).

17.5 units of calcitonin, human, are contained in one ampoule of the second International Standard Preparation (1991).

There is also a first International Standard Preparation (1989) of elcatonin.

Potency of calcitonins is estimated by comparing the hypocalcaemic effect, in *rats*, with that of the standard preparation, and is expressed in international or MRC units which are considered to be equivalent. One manufacturer states that 100 international units by this assay is equivalent to 1 mg of porcine or human calcitonin, and to 25 µg of salmon calcitonin although other, slightly different, equivalencies have been cited for other preparations. However, although 1 unit of pork calcitonin, 1 unit of salmon calcitonin, and 1 unit of human calcitonin should give the same response in humans this is not necessarily the case. Clinically, doses of pork and salmon calcitonin are expressed in units whereas those of human calcitonin can be expressed by weight, probably a reflection of its purity. Doses of calcitonin considered approximately equivalent in practice are 80 units of pork calcitonin, 50 units of salmon calcitonin, and 0.5 mg of human calcitonin (see Uses and Administration, below).

Adverse Effects, Treatment, and Precautions

Calcitonins may cause nausea, vomiting, diarrhoea, dizziness, flushing, and tingling of the hands. These reactions are dose dependent, usually transient, and occur more often with intravenous administration. Other adverse effects have included skin rash, an unpleasant taste, abdominal pain, urinary frequency, and tremor. A diabetogenic effect has been reported rarely. Inflammatory reactions at the injection site have been reported with some calcitonins, and rhinitis and other local reactions have been reported with nasal formulations. Transient hypocalcaemia may occur after injections of calcitonin.

Calcitonins should be given with care to patients with renal impairment (see below) or heart failure. If children receive calcitonin it should preferably be for short periods and bone growth should be monitored.

Circulating antibodies may develop after several months of use but resistance does not necessarily follow (see also below). In patients with a history of allergy, a skin test has been advised prior to administration as hypersensitivity reactions, including anaphylaxis, have occurred.

Calcitonin has inhibited lactation in *animals*.

Nausea and vomiting may be reduced by administration at bedtime or by prior administration of an antiemetic.

Calcitonin (pork) may contain trace amounts of thyroid hormones, but clinical effects are unlikely in most patients.

Antibody formation. Long-term treatment with heterologous calcitonins may lead to the formation of neutralising antibodies. This appears to be common in patients given pork or to a lesser extent salmon calcitonin. Human calcitonin is less immunogenic than pork or salmon, but a study[1] has also detected antibodies to human calcitonin in 1 of 33 women with postmenopausal osteoporosis after 6 months of therapy.

The degree to which such antibodies affect therapeutic activity is uncertain. Some studies have suggested a significant loss of therapeutic activity in patients who developed neutralising antibodies to salmon calcitonin,[2] or a restoration in activity following a switch from salmon to human calcitonin in such patients;[3] equally, others have presented evidence that the activity of salmon calcitonin was not reduced by the development of antibodies to the drug.[4]

1. Grauer A, *et al.* Formation of neutralizing antibodies after treatment with human calcitonin. *Am J Med* 1993; **95**: 439–42.
2. Grauer A, *et al.* In vitro detection of neutralizing antibodies after treatment of Paget's disease of bone with nasal salmon calcitonin. *J Bone Miner Res* 1990; **5**: 387–91.
3. Muff R, *et al.* Efficacy of intranasal human calcitonin in patients with Paget's disease refractory to salmon calcitonin. *Am J Med* 1990; **89**: 181–4.
4. Reginster JY, *et al.* Influence of specific anti-salmon calcitonin antibodies on biological effectiveness of nasal salmon calcitonin in Paget's disease of bone. *Scand J Rheumatol* 1990; **19**: 83–6.

Effect on glucose metabolism. A single subcutaneous injection of salmon calcitonin has been reported to increase blood-glucose concentrations,[1] but long-term treatment with calcitonins was considered unlikely to cause diabetes.[2] Nevertheless, deterioration in diabetic control has been noted in a patient given calcitonin (pork)[3] and postprandial release of insulin was abolished by intravenous salmon calcitonin in 8 patients with duodenal ulcers.[4]

1. Gattereau A, *et al.* Hyperglycaemic effect of synthetic salmon calcitonin. *Lancet* 1977; **ii**: 1076–7.
2. Evans IMA, *et al.* Hyperglycaemic effect of synthetic salmon calcitonin. *Lancet* 1978; **i**: 280.
3. Thomas DW, *et al.* Deterioration in diabetic control during calcitonin therapy. *Med J Aust* 1979; **2**: 699–70.
4. Jonderko K. Effect of calcitonin on gastric emptying in patients with an active duodenal ulcer. *Gut* 1989; **30**: 430–5.

Gynaecomastia. A 62-year-old man developed painful gynaecomastia on two occasions following treatment with salcatonin administered by subcutaneous injection.[1]

1. Vankrunkelsven PJ, Thijs MM. Salcatonin and gynaecomastia. *Lancet* 1994; **344**: 482.

Renal impairment. Calcitonins are metabolised mainly in the kidneys and pharmacokinetic studies (see below) have indicated that the dosage of calcitonins may need to be reduced in patients with renal insufficiency, but there have been no specific guidelines.

Interactions

There is a theoretical possibility that dosage adjustments may be required in patients receiving cardiac glycosides who are given injections of calcitonin, because of the effects of the latter on serum calcium.

Pharmacokinetics

Calcitonins are rapidly inactivated when given by mouth. After injection, calcitonins are quickly metabolised, primarily in the kidneys but also in blood and peripheral tissues. The inactive metabolites and a small proportion of unchanged drug are excreted in the urine. The half-life of human calcitonin is stated to be 60 minutes and that of salmon calcitonin about 70 to 90 minutes.

Calcitonins are also absorbed through the nasal and rectal mucosa. Although figures have varied widely, about 3% of a nasally administered dose of salmon calcitonin is reported to be bioavailable compared with the same dose administered by intramuscular injection, with peak plasma concentrations occurring

after about 30 to 40 minutes compared with 15 to 25 minutes after the parenteral dose.

◊ Following the subcutaneous injection of 19.9 μg of synthetic salmon-calcitonin in 16 healthy subjects,[1] absorption was rapid with an absorption half-life of 23.4 minutes. The maximum mean plasma concentration was 384 picograms per mL at 60 minutes after which excretion was fairly rapid with an elimination half-life of 87 minutes. These results and those from previously reported investigations of salmon, human, and porcine calcitonin could not easily be compared, especially since different assay methods had been used. Nevertheless it was concluded that bioavailability from subcutaneous and intramuscular injection sites was good; that dosage may need to be adjusted in renal insufficiency because of low metabolic clearance rate; and that the higher potency of salcatonin is due to higher intrinsic activity at the receptor site rather than to pharmacokinetic differences. The US manufacturers have cited a half-life of 1.02 hours after a single subcutaneous injection of human calcitonin 500 μg. The plasma elimination half-life of elcatonin was about 4.8 hours following intramuscular injection in healthy subjects.[2]

Calcitonins are absorbed following intranasal or rectal administration. Peak plasma concentrations of salmon calcitonin were achieved 20 to 60 minutes after administration by nasal spray in doses ranging from 200 to 400 units.[3] In another study[4] salmon calcitonin 200 units, repeated once after 3 hours, was given by nasal spray or suppository to healthy subjects. Absorption was prompt and the total amount absorbed was similar with either route. However, whereas intranasal administration produced low peaks with salcatonin still detectable in the blood after 3 to 5 hours, rectal administration produced peak plasma concentrations about 6 to 8 times higher than intranasal administration but salcatonin was undetectable within 2 hours; plasma concentrations were lower than those found after injection. Another group of workers[5] found human calcitonin to be poorly absorbed when given intranasally to healthy subjects. Absorption from nasal powder or spray solutions was improved by the presence of the surfactants dihydrofusinate or glycocholate.

Investigations carried out in 4 osteoporotic patients[6] suggested that the rectal administration of salcatonin could provide 65% of the bioavailability of intramuscular administration.

1. Nüesch E, Schmidt R. Comparative pharmacokinetics of calcitonins. In: Pecile A, ed. *Calcitonin international congress series no. 540.* Amsterdam: Excerpta Medica, 1980: 352–64.
2. Sergre G, *et al.* Pharmacokinetics of carbocalcitonin in humans. *Clin Trials J* 1986; **23** (suppl 1): 23–8.
3. Kurose H, *et al.* Intranasal absorption of salmon calcitonin. *Calcif Tissue Int* 1987; **41**: 249–51.
4. Buclin T, *et al.* The effect of rectal and nasal administration of salmon calcitonin in normal subjects. *Calcif Tissue Int* 1987; **41**: 252–8.
5. Pontiroli AE, *et al.* Nasal administration of glucagon and human calcitonin to healthy subjects: a comparison of powders and spray solutions and of different enhancing agents. *Eur J Clin Pharmacol* 1989; **37**: 427–30.
6. Gennari C, *et al.* Pharmacodynamic activity of synthetic salmon calcitonin in osteoporotic patients: comparison between rectal and intramuscular administration: pilot study. *Curr Ther Res* 1993; **53**: 301–8.

Uses and Administration

Calcitonin is a hormone produced by mammalian thyroid parafollicular cells or the ultimobranchial gland in non-mammalian vertebrates. In man its secretion and biosynthesis are regulated by the plasma-calcium concentration. It has a hypocalcaemic action that is due primarily to inhibition of osteoclastic bone resorption; of less importance is a direct effect on the kidneys resulting in increased urinary excretion of calcium and phosphorus. Calcitonin contains 32 amino acids; the sequence varies according to the species. Naturally occurring porcine calcitonin, synthetic salmon calcitonin (salcatonin), and synthetic human calcitonin are in clinical use; salcatonin is the most potent. Elcatonin, a synthetic derivative of eel calcitonin, is available in some countries.

Calcitonins are used in the treatment of diseases characterised by high bone turnover such as Paget's disease of bone. They are also given as an adjunct in the treatment of severe hypercalcaemia, especially that associated with malignancy. Some calcitonins are used in the management of osteoporosis, and osteolysis and bone pain due to malignancies of bone.

Calcitonins are generally given by subcutaneous or intramuscular injection; some have been given intranasally, rectally, or by intravenous infusion.

In **Paget's disease of bone** the usual dose range for calcitonin (pork) by subcutaneous or intramuscular injection is 80 units three times weekly to 160 units daily in single or divided doses; patients with bone pain or nerve compression syndromes may be given

80 or 160 units daily for 3 to 6 months. For salcatonin the range is 50 units three times weekly to 100 units daily in single or divided doses by subcutaneous or intramuscular injection. Human calcitonin is usually given by subcutaneous or intramuscular injection in a dose range of 0.5 mg two or three times weekly to 0.5 mg daily; severe cases may require up to 1 mg daily.

As an adjunct to the treatment of **hypercalcaemia**, calcitonins have a rapid effect which is greatest in patients with an increased bone turnover. Calcitonin (pork) may be given in a dose of 4 units per kg bodyweight daily by intramuscular or subcutaneous injection according to the patient's needs. In severe hypercalcaemia larger doses of calcitonin may be more conveniently administered as the more potent salcatonin. Salcatonin may be given by subcutaneous or intramuscular injection in a dose of 5 to 10 units per kg daily in one or two divided doses or up to 400 units every 6 or 8 hours. Doses greater than 8 units per kg every 6 hours are considered to have no additional benefit. In the emergency treatment of hypercalcaemic crisis, salcatonin has also been given intravenously: a suggested dose is 5 to 10 units per kg daily, diluted in 500 mL of sodium chloride 0.9% and given by slow intravenous infusion over at least 6 hours (see also under Administration below for the problems of intravenous administration). Human calcitonin has also been given intravenously for acute hypercalcaemia.

Salcatonin is used in the treatment of **postmenopausal osteoporosis** in a dose of 100 units daily or every other day by subcutaneous or intramuscular injection, or 200 units daily intranasally by nasal spray, alternating nostrils each day. Supplementary calcium (equivalent to at least 600 mg of elemental calcium daily) and, if necessary, vitamin D (400 units daily) should also be given.

Salcatonin has also been used for the control of **bone pain due to malignant neoplasms**. The usual dose by intramuscular or subcutaneous injection is 200 units every 6 hours or 400 units every 12 hours for up to 48 hours. The treatment course may be repeated as appropriate.

Oral formulations of salcatonin are being studied.

Administration. Calcitonins have poor oral bioavailability and administration is usually by subcutaneous or intramuscular injection. To improve patient acceptability, especially in diseases requiring long-term drug therapy such as osteoporosis or Paget's disease of bone, alternative methods of administration have been investigated.

Salcatonin has proved effective when given intranasally in usual doses of 50 to 200 units daily (for references, see Osteoporosis below), and intranasal products for osteoporosis are available. Suppositories containing 300 units of salcatonin have been used in the management of hypercalcaemia, one suppository being administered three times daily (total daily dose of 900 units).[1,2] Daily doses of 100 units of salcatonin by suppository have been tried in postmenopausal osteoporosis[3] and in patients with bone pain.[4]

Calcitonins have been given by intravenous infusion, but this is rarely necessary and may cause more side-effects. If intravenous administration is essential, it has been suggested[5] that some protein must be present in the solution to prevent adsorption onto the plastic of the giving set. However, in practice this does not seem to be the case; in the UK, manufacturer's recommendations are for dilution with normal saline, while acknowledging that such dilution results in a loss of potency, and dosage is adjusted accordingly. Presumably dilution with a protein-containing solution would allow lower doses to be used. The manufacturers do specify that solutions for infusion should be prepared immediately before use and that glass or hard plastic containers should not be used.

1. Thiébaud D, *et al.* Effectiveness of salmon calcitonin administered as suppositories in tumor-induced hypercalcemia. *Am J Med* 1987; **82**: 745–50.
2. Thiébaud D, *et al.* Fast and effective treatment of malignant hypercalcaemia: combination of suppositories of calcitonin and a single infusion of 3-amino 1-hydroxypropylidene-1-bisphosphonate. *Arch Intern Med* 1990; **150**: 2125–8.
3. Gonnelli S, *et al.* Effect of rectal salmon calcitonin treatment on bone mass and bone turnover in patients with established postmenopausal osteoporosis: a 1-year crossover study. *Curr Ther Res* 1993; **54**: 458–65.
4. Mannarini M, *et al.* Analgesic effect of salmon calcitonin suppositories in patients with bone pain. *Curr Ther Res* 1994; **55**: 1079–83.
5. Stevenson JC. Current management of malignant hypercalcaemia. *Drugs* 1988; **36**: 229–38.

Hypercalcaemia. Calcitonins can be used in the management of moderate to severe symptomatic hypercalcaemia (p.1181) in addition to rehydration and diuresis. Because of their rapid effect, they may be particularly useful in life-threatening hypercalcaemia. However, although they have a rapid effect it is usually short-lived; calcitonins are therefore generally given as an adjunct with other therapy such as a bisphosphonate.

References.
1. Ralston SH, *et al.* Treatment of cancer associated hypercalcaemia with combined aminohydroxypropylidene diphosphonate and calcitonin. *BMJ* 1986; **292:** 1549–50.
2. Thiébaud D, *et al.* Effectiveness of salmon calcitonin administered as suppositories in tumor-induced hypercalcemia. *Am J Med* 1987; **82:** 745–50.
3. Thiébaud D, *et al.* Fast and effective treatment of malignant hypercalcemia: combination of suppositories of calcitonin and a single infusion as 3-amino 1-hydroxypropylidene-1-bisphosphonate. *Arch Intern Med* 1990; **150:** 2125–8.
4. Kaul S, Sockalosky JJ. Human synthetic calcitonin therapy for hypercalcemia of immobilization. *J Pediatr* 1995; **126:** 825–7.

Malignant neoplasms of the bone. Calcitonins may be useful adjuvants in the treatment of malignant disease involving the bone (p.490), not only to correct hypercalcaemia of malignancy, but also to relieve bone pain and osteolysis. The analgesic properties of calcitonins (see Pain, below) may play some part in this, although relief of bone pain has also been seen with bisphosphonates, suggesting that if such actions are of significance, they are not the sole reason for pain relief.

References.
1. Roth A, Kolarić K. Analgetic activity of calcitonin in patients with painful osteolytic metastases of breast cancer. *Oncology* 1986; **43:** 283–7.
2. Blomqvist C, *et al.* Evaluation of salmon calcitonin treatment in bone metastases from breast cancer—a controlled trial. *Bone* 1988; **9:** 45–51.
3. Gennari C, *et al.* Salmon calcitonin treatment in bone metastases. *Curr Ther Res* 1989; **45:** 804–12.

Osteogenesis imperfecta. There have been reports[1,2] of beneficial effects with calcitonins in the treatment of osteogenesis imperfecta (p.744).
1. Castells S, *et al.* Therapy of osteogenesis imperfecta with synthetic salmon calcitonin. *J Pediatr* 1979; **95:** 807–11.
2. Nishi Y, *et al.* Effect of long-term calcitonin therapy by injection and nasal spray on incidence of fractures in osteogenesis imperfecta. *J Pediatr* 1992; **121:** 477–80.

Osteoporosis. Calcitonins are used in the prevention and treatment of osteoporosis (p.745). In postmenopausal osteoporosis they are usually second-line agents. However, they may be particularly useful in women with high-turnover osteoporosis, and in those with bone pain due to vertebral crush fractures. References to the use of calcitonins for postmenopausal osteoporosis[1-10] and corticosteroid-induced osteoporosis[11-15] are given below.
1. Reginster JY, *et al.* 1-Year controlled randomised trial of prevention of early postmenopausal bone loss by intranasal calcitonin. *Lancet* 1987; **ii:** 1481–3.
2. MacIntyre I, *et al.* Calcitonin for prevention of postmenopausal bone loss. *Lancet* 1988; **i:** 900–2.
3. Pun KK, Chan LWL. Analgesic effect of intranasal salmon calcitonin in the treatment of osteoporotic vertebral fractures. *Clin Ther* 1989; **11:** 205–9.
4. Overgaard K, *et al.* Effect of salcatonin given intranasally on early postmenopausal bone loss. *BMJ* 1989; **299:** 477–9.
5. Overgaard K, *et al.* Discontinuous calcitonin treatment of established osteoporosis—effects of withdrawal of treatment. *Am J Med* 1990; **89:** 1–6.
6. Overgaard K, *et al.* Effect of salcatonin given intranasally on bone mass and fracture rates in established osteoporosis: a dose response study. *BMJ* 1992; **305:** 556–61.
7. Reginster JY, *et al.* A 5-year controlled randomized study of prevention of postmenopausal trabecular bone loss with nasal salmon calcitonin and calcium. *Eur J Clin Invest* 1994; **24:** 565–9.
8. Reginster JY, *et al.* A double-blind, placebo-controlled, dose-finding trial of intermittent nasal salmon calcitonin for prevention of postmenopausal lumbar spine bone loss. *Am J Med* 1995; **98:** 452–8.
9. Downs RW, *et al.* Comparison of alendronate and intranasal calcitonin for treatment of osteoporosis in postmenopausal women. *J Clin Endocrinol Metab* 2000; **85:** 1783–8.
10. Chesnut CH, *et al.* A randomized trial of nasal spray salmon calcitonin in postmenopausal women with established osteoporosis: the prevent recurrence of osteoporotic fractures study. *Am J Med* 2000; **109:** 267–76.
11. Ringe J-D, Welzel D. Salmon calcitonin in the therapy of corticoid-induced osteoporosis. *Eur J Clin Pharmacol* 1987; **33:** 35–9.
12. Rizzato G, *et al.* Administration of salmon calcitonin nasal spray for long-term treatment of corticosteroid-induced osteoporosis, a preliminary report. *Curr Ther Res* 1989; **45:** 761–6.
13. Nishioka T, *et al.* Nasal administration of salmon calcitonin for prevention of glucocorticoid-induced osteoporosis in children with nephrosis. *J Pediatr* 1991; **118:** 703–7.
14. Adachi JD, *et al.* Salmon calcitonin nasal spray in the prevention of corticosteroid-induced osteoporosis. *Br J Rheumatol* 1997; **36:** 255–9.
15. Cranney A, *et al.* Calcitonin for preventing and treating corticosteroid-induced osteoporosis (updated 30 August 2000). Available in The Cochrane Library; Issue 3. Oxford: Update Software; 2001.

Paget's disease of bone. Patients with Paget's disease of bone (p.746) may require no treatment or just analgesics alone, but calcitonins may be indicated if bone pain is persistent and to prevent further progression of the disease. However, the bisphosphonates have largely superseded the calcitonins in this

role. References to the use of calcitonins for Paget's disease of bone are given below.
1. Nagant de Deuxchaisnes C, *et al.* New modes of administration of salmon calcitonin in Paget's disease. *Clin Orthop* 1987; **217:** 56–71.
2. Muff R, *et al.* Efficacy of intranasal human calcitonin in patients with Paget's disease refractory to salmon calcitonin. *Am J Med* 1990; **89:** 181–4.

Pain. In addition to bone pain associated with malignancy and with bone disorders such as Paget's disease, calcitonins may also have other analgesic properties.[1] Beneficial results have been seen in various painful syndromes.[2-5]
1. Fraioli F, *et al.* Subarachnoid injection of salmon calcitonin induces analgesia in man. *Eur J Pharmacol* 1982; **78:** 381–2.
2. Ricevuti G. Effects of human calcitonin on pain in the treatment of Tietze's syndrome. *Clin Ther* 1985; **7:** 669–73.
3. Patti F, *et al.* Calcitonin and migraine. *Headache* 1986; **26:** 172–4.
4. Micieli G, *et al.* Effectiveness of salmon calcitonin nasal spray preparation in migraine treatment. *Headache* 1988; **28:** 196–200.
5. Mannerini M, *et al.* Analgesic effect of salmon calcitonin suppositories in patients with bone pain. *Curr Ther Res* 1994; **55:** 1079–83.

Preparations

BP 2001: Calcitonin (Salmon) Injection.

Proprietary Preparations (details are given in Part 3)
Aust.: Calcitonin; Casalm; Cibacalcin; Elcimen; Ucecal; *Austral.:* Calcitare†; Calsynar; Cibacalcin†; Miacalcic; *Belg.:* Calsynar; Cibacalcine†; Miacalcic; *Braz.:* Acticalcin; Calsynar; Cibacalcina; Miacalcic; Staporos; Turbocalcin; *Canad.:* Calcimar; Caltine; Miacalcin; *Denm.:* Miacalcic; *Fin.:* Miacalcic; *Fr.:* Cadens; Calcitar†; Calsyn; Cibacalcine; Miacalcic; *Ger.:* Azucalcit; Calci; Calcimonta; Calsynar; Calsynar Lyo†; Casalm; Cibacalcin; Karil; Osteos; Ostostabil; *Hong Kong:* Calsynar; Miacalcic; Osteocalcin; Osteostabil; *Irl.:* Calcitare†; Calsynar; *Israel:* Calsynar; Cibacalcin; Miacalcic; Salco; *Ital.:* Aima-Calcin†; Biocalcin; Calciben; Calcinil; Calciosint; Calcioton; Calcitar†; Calcitonina; Calco; Carbicalcin; Catonin; Cibacalcin; Ipocalcin; Isi-Calcin†; Miacalcic; Miadenil; Osteocalcin; Osteotonina; Osteovis; Porostenina†; Quosten; Rulicalcin; Salmocalcin†; Salmofar; Sical; Sintocalcin†; Stalcin†; Steocin; Tonocalcin; Turbocalcin; *Jpn:* Calcitoran; Elcitonin†; Mex.: Endocal; Miacalcic; Oseum; Serocalcin; Tonocalcin; *Neth.:* Calsynar†; Cibacalcin†; *Norw.:* Miacalcic; *NZ:* Miacalcic; *Port.:* Bionocalcin†; Calcimon; Calogen; Calsyn; Cibacalcina†; Miacalcic; Osseocalcina†; Ostosalm†; Salcat; Tonocaltin; *S.Afr.:* Miacalcic; *Singapore:* Calco; Menocal; Miacalcic; Osteocalcin; *Spain:* Bionocalcin; Calogen; Calsynar; Carbicalcin; Cibacalcina; Diatin; Kalsimin; Miacalcic; Oseototal; Osteobion; Sical; Tonocaltin; Ucecal; *Swed.:* Cibacalcin; Miacalcic; *Switz.:* Cibacalcine†; Miacalcic; *Thai.:* Calco; Miacalcic; Osteocalcin; Ostostabil; Tonocalcin; *UK:* Calcitare†; Calsynar; Forcaltonin; Miacalcic; *USA:* Calcimar; Miacalcin; Osteocalcin.

Clodronic Acid (3273-k)

Clodronic Acid *(BAN, USAN, rINN).*
(Dichloromethylene)diphosphonic acid.
$CH_4Cl_2O_6P_2 = 244.9$.
CAS — 10596-23-3.
ATC — M05BA02.

Disodium Clodronate (12673-a)

BM-06.011; Cl_2MBP; Cl_2MDP; Clodronate Disodium; Clodronate Sodium; Dichloromethane Diphosphonate Disodium; Dichloromethylene Diphosphonate Disodium; Sodium Clodronate *(BANM).* Disodium (dichloromethylene)diphosphonate tetrahydrate.
$CH_2Cl_2Na_2O_6P_2,4H_2O = 360.9$.
CAS — 22560-50-5.

124.9 mg of disodium clodronate tetrahydrate is approximately equivalent to 100 mg of anhydrous substance.

Adverse Effects and Precautions

As for the bisphosphonates in general, p.748. Gastrointestinal symptoms following oral dosage may be reduced by giving the drug in divided doses rather than as a single daily dose. Reversible increases in liver enzyme values and moderate leucopenia have been seen in a few patients. Monitoring of hepatic and renal function and white cell counts is advised. Disodium clodronate has precipitated bronchospasm, even in patients with no history of asthma. Transient proteinuria has been reported immediately after intravenous infusion.

Effects on the respiratory system. For a report of bronchospasm in an aspirin-sensitive asthmatic, induced by an infusion of clodronate, see p.748.

Hypersensitivity. Allergic reactions to bisphosphonates are rare. For published reports of cutaneous reactions associated with clodronate administration, see p.748.

Renal impairment. For mention of renal failure developing in a patient with slightly raised serum-creatinine concentrations who subsequently received an intravenous infusion of clodronate, see Effects on the Kidneys, p.748. The manufacturers recommend that *intravenous* infusion of clodronate should

be avoided in patients with moderate to severe renal impairment (serum creatinine greater than 440 μmol (50 mg) per litre) and that the *oral* dosage form should be avoided in patients with a creatinine clearance below 10 mL per minute and the dosage halved in patients with creatinine clearance between 10 and 30 mL per minute.

Interactions

As for the bisphosphonates in general, p.748.

Aminoglycosides. A report of a patient who developed persisting severe hypocalcaemia after treatment with clodronate and *netilmicin*. Bisphosphonates and aminoglycosides can induce hypocalcaemia by different mechanisms and care should be taken when administering them simultaneously.[1]
1. Pedersen-Bjergaard U, Myhre J. Severe hypocalcaemia after treatment with diphosphonate and aminoglycoside. *BMJ* 1991; **302:** 295. Correction. *ibid.;* 791.

Pharmacokinetics

Disodium clodronate is poorly absorbed from the gastrointestinal tract and absorption is reduced by food, especially products containing calcium or other polyvalent cations; bioavailability is only 1 to 4%. Following absorption or intravenous administration it is cleared rapidly from the blood with a reported plasma half-life of only about 2 hours, but has a high affinity for bone. Over 70% of an intravenous dose is excreted unchanged in the urine within 24 hours the remainder being sequestered in bone tissue. Disodium clodronate is not metabolised.

◊ References.
1. Conrad KA, Lee SM. Clodronate kinetics and dynamics. *Clin Pharmacol Ther* 1981; **30:** 114–20.
2. Yakatan GJ, *et al.* Clodronate kinetics and bioavailability. *Clin Pharmacol Ther* 1982; **31:** 402–10.

Bioavailability. Enhanced bioavailability tablets of disodium clodronate are available in some countries, the licensed dose of which is 35% less than the dose of the standard formulation (see below). However, an open, randomised, crossover study in 88 volunteers found that a 1040-mg dose of the new formulation provided only 52% of the bioavailable dose of 1600 mg of the standard capsule formulation.[1]
1. Lapham G, *et al.* Bioavailability of two clodronate formulations. *Br J Hosp Med* 1996; **56:** 231–3.

Uses and Administration

Clodronate is a bisphosphonate with general properties similar to those of the other bisphosphonates (p.749). It inhibits bone resorption, but appears to have less effect on bone mineralisation than etidronate at comparable doses.

Disodium clodronate is used as an adjunct in the treatment of severe hypercalcaemia, especially when associated with malignancy. In addition, it is used in the treatment of osteolytic bone metastases.

It is administered by slow intravenous infusion or by mouth, as a single daily dose or in 2 divided doses; food should be avoided for at least 1 hour before or after oral administration. Doses are expressed in terms of the anhydrous substance. Disodium clodronate is available in capsules of 400 mg and standard tablets of 800 mg. Tablets of disodium clodronate 520 mg are also available in some countries, and have a greater bioavailability than the capsules or standard tablets; one such tablet of disodium clodronate 520 mg is approximately equivalent to two capsules each containing disodium clodronate 400 mg or one 800-mg standard tablet (but see Bioavailability, above).

In the management of osteolytic lesions, hypercalcaemia, and bone pain associated with skeletal metastases in patients with breast cancer or multiple myeloma, disodium clodronate 1.6 g daily has been given by mouth as capsules or standard tablets, and may be increased if necessary to a maximum of 3.2 g daily. Alternatively a dose of 1.04 g daily, increased if necessary up to 2.08 g daily, may be given as enhanced bioavailability tablets.

In hypercalcaemia of malignancy disodium clodronate is given by intravenous infusion over not less than 2 hours as a dose of 300 mg daily on successive days until normocalcaemia is achieved; duration of treatment should not exceed 10 days. Alternatively, it may be given as a single intravenous infusion of 1.5 g in 500 mL of infusion solution administered over a period of 4 hours. Once serum-calcium concentrations have been reduced to an acceptable level, maintenance therapy may be given by mouth in similar doses to those used for initial oral treatment of metastases.

◊ General references.
1. Plosker GL, Goa KL. Clodronate: a review of its pharmacological properties and therapeutic efficacy in resorptive bone disease. *Drugs* 1994; **47:** 945–82.

Hypercalcaemia. Treatment with bisphosphonates may be considered in patients with moderate to severe symptomatic hypercalcaemia of malignancy (p.1181) in addition to rehydration and diuresis.

References.
1. Urwin GH, *et al.* Treatment of the hypercalcaemia of malignancy with intravenous clodronate. *Bone* 1987; **8** (suppl 1): S43–S51.
2. Ralston SH, *et al.* Comparison of three intravenous bisphosphonates in cancer-associated hypercalcaemia. *Lancet* 1989; **ii:** 1180–2.
3. Rostom AY. Clodronate as outpatient treatment for hypercalcaemia. *Lancet* 1990; **336:** 1390.
4. O'Rourke NP, *et al.* Effective treatment of malignant hypercalcaemia with a single intravenous infusion of clodronate. *Br J Cancer* 1993; **67:** 560–3.

Hyperparathyroidism. Bisphosphonates have been used to inhibit bone resorption in the treatment of hypercalcaemia associated with hyperparathyroidism (p.746) but seem to be of little benefit for long-term treatment.

References.
1. Shane E, *et al.* Effects of dichloromethylene diphosphonate on serum and urinary calcium in primary hyperparathyroidism. *Ann Intern Med* 1981; **95:** 23–7.
2. Douglas DL, *et al.* Drug treatment of primary hyperparathyroidism: use of clodronate disodium. *BMJ* 1983; **286:** 587–90.
3. Hamdy NAT, *et al.* Clodronate in the medical management of hyperparathyroidism. *Bone* 1987; **8** (suppl 1): S69–77.

Malignant neoplasms of the bone. Bisphosphonates are of benefit in some patients with metastatic bone disease (p.490).

References.
1. Elomaa I, *et al.* Treatment of skeletal disease in breast cancer: a controlled clodronate trial. *Bone* 1987; **8** (suppl 1): S53–56.
2. Lahtinen R, *et al.* Randomised, placebo-controlled multicentre trial of clodronate in multiple myeloma. *Lancet* 1992; **340:** 1049–52. Correction. *ibid.*; 1420.
3. Diel IJ, *et al.* Reduction in new metastases in breast cancer with adjuvant clodronate treatment. *N Engl J Med* 1998; **339:** 357–63.
4. Kristensen B, *et al.* Oral clodronate in breast cancer patients with bone metastases: a randomized study. *J Intern Med* 1999; **246:** 67–74.

Paget's disease of bone. Patients with Paget's disease of bone (p.746) may require no treatment or just analgesics, but bisphosphonates may be indicated if bone pain is persistent or to prevent further progression of the disease.

References.
1. Yates AJP, *et al.* Intravenous clodronate in the treatment and re-treatment of Paget's disease of bone. *Lancet* 1985; **i:** 1474–7.
2. Gray RES, *et al.* Duration of effect of oral diphosphonate therapy in Paget's disease of bone. *Q J Med* 1987; **64:** 755–67.

Preparations

Proprietary Preparations (details are given in Part 3)
Aust.: Ascredar; Bonefos; Lodronat; Lytos†; **Austral.:** Bonefos; **Belg.:** Bonefos; Ostac; **Braz.:** Bonefos; Ostac; **Canad.:** Bonefos; Ostac; **Denm.:** Bonefos; Loron†; **Fin.:** Bonefos; **Fr.:** Clastoban; Lytos; **Ger.:** Bonefos; Ostac; **Hong Kong:** Ostac; **Irl.:** Bonefos; Loron; **Israel:** Bonefos; Ostac; **Ital.:** Clasteon; Clody; Difosfonal; Niklod; Ossiten; **Neth.:** Bonefos; Ostac; **Norw.:** Bonefos; Ostac; **NZ:** Ostac; **Port.:** Bonefos; Ostac; **S.Afr.:** Ostac; **Singapore:** Bonefos; Ostac; **Spain:** Bonefos; Hemocalcin; Mebonat; **Swed.:** Bonefos; Ostac; **Switz.:** Bonefos; Ostac; **Thai.:** Bonefos; **UK:** Bonefos; Loron.

Etidronic Acid   (3274-a)

Etidronic Acid *(BAN, USAN, rINN)*.
1-Hydroxyethylidenedi(phosphonic acid).
$C_2H_8O_7P_2 = 206.0$.
CAS — 2809-21-4.
ATC — M05BA01.

Disodium Etidronate   (12674-t)

Disodium Etidronate *(BANM)*.
EHDP; Etidronate Disodium *(USAN)*. Disodium dihydrogen (1-hydroxyethylidene)diphosphonate.
$C_2H_6Na_2O_7P_2 = 250.0$.
CAS — 7414-83-7.

NOTE. Other etidronic acid sodium salts are designated as etidronate monosodium, etidronate trisodium, and etidronate tetrasodium. The name sodium etidronate is used only where the salt cannot be identified more precisely.
Pharmacopoeias. In US.

Pharmacopoeial description
USP 25: Store in airtight containers. pH of a 1% solution in water is between 4.2 and 5.2.

Adverse Effects and Precautions

As for the bisphosphonates in general, p.748. Unlike the newer bisphosphonates etidronate produces marked impairment of bone mineralisation at high therapeutic doses. An increase in bone pain may occur in patients with Paget's disease. Impairment of bone mineralisation may result in osteomalacia and fractures have been reported. Etidronate should be discontinued if a fracture occurs until healing is complete. Hyperphosphataemia may occur, usually at high doses, but generally resolves 2 to 4 weeks after therapy. There have been reports of paraesthesias and peripheral neuropathy. Transient loss or alteration of taste has been reported mainly during and after intravenous infusion.

Effects on the gastrointestinal tract. Oral etidronate was not associated with an increased incidence of upper gastrointestinal problems in a retrospective cohort study.[1] There was also no evidence of an increased incidence of gastrointestinal effects when given with NSAIDs or corticosteroids.

1. van Staa T, *et al.* Upper gastrointestinal adverse events and cyclical etidronate. *Am J Med* 1997; **103:** 462–7.

Effects on the respiratory system. For a report of bronchospasm induced by etidronate in an aspirin-sensitive asthmatic, see p.748.

Hypersensitivity. Allergic reactions to bisphosphonates do occur but appear to be rare (see p.748).

Renal impairment. Bisphosphonates are excreted by the kidneys, thus caution is advised in patients with impaired renal function. When given by intravenous infusion for the treatment of hypercalcaemia of malignancy they have been reported to affect renal function adversely; hypercalcaemia or malignancy may also have contributed. For reports of renal failure associated with etidronate administration see Effects on the Kidneys, p.748.

The manufacturers have recommended that disodium etidronate should not be given *intravenously* to patients with serum-creatinine concentrations greater than 440 μmol (50 mg) per litre, and that doses may need to be reduced in patients with serum creatinine concentrations between 220 and 440 μmol (25 to 50 mg) per litre. Reduced *oral* doses are similarly recommended in mild renal impairment, and avoidance in moderate to severe impairment.

Interactions

As for the bisphosphonates in general, p.748.

◊ For a lack of apparent interaction between cyclical etidronate and corticosteroids or NSAIDs see under Effects on the Gastrointestinal Tract, above.

Pharmacokinetics

Following administration by mouth, absorption is variable and appears to be dose dependent. At usual dosage ranges about 1 to 6% of a dose of disodium etidronate is absorbed. Absorption is reduced by food, especially by products containing calcium or other polyvalent cations. Disodium etidronate is rapidly cleared from the blood and has been reported to have a plasma half-life of 1 to 6 hours. It is not metabolised. About 50% is excreted in the urine within 24 hours, the remainder being chemically adsorbed on bone and slowly eliminated. The half-life of disodium etidronate in bone exceeds 90 days. Unabsorbed disodium etidronate appears in the faeces.

Uses and Administration

Etidronate is a bisphosphonate with general properties similar to those of the other bisphosphonates (p.749). It inhibits the growth and dissolution of hydroxyapatite crystals in bone and may also directly impair osteoclast activity. It diminishes bone resorption and thus reduces bone turnover.

Disodium etidronate is used as an adjunct in the treatment of severe hypercalcaemia, especially when associated with malignancy. It is also given in bone disorders in which excessive bone resorption is a problem, such as Paget's disease of bone and osteoporosis. In addition, it may be used for the prevention and treatment of ectopic (heterotopic) ossification and the management of malignancies of bone. A chelate of etidronate with radioactive techne-

tium-99m (p.1451) is used diagnostically as a bone scanning agent.

Disodium etidronate is administered by intravenous infusion over at least 2 hours, or by mouth, usually as a single daily dose. Food should be avoided for 2 hours before and after oral administration.

In the treatment of **Paget's disease**, disodium etidronate is given by mouth in a usual initial dose of 5 mg per kg body-weight daily for not more than 6 months. Doses above 10 mg per kg daily should be reserved for severe disease and should not be given for more than 3 months at a time. The maximum dose is 20 mg per kg daily. The response to disodium etidronate may be slow in onset and may continue for several months after cessation of therapy. Therefore, further treatment should only be given after a drug-free interval of at least 3 months and after evidence of relapse; it should not be continued for more than the duration of the initial treatment.

In the treatment of **hypercalcaemia of malignancy** the recommended dose of disodium etidronate by slow intravenous infusion is 7.5 mg per kg body-weight daily for 3 successive days, although infusions may be continued for up to 7 days if necessary. This daily dose should be diluted in at least 250 mL of 0.9% sodium chloride and infused over at least 2 hours. There should be at least a 7-day interval between courses of treatment. Once serum-calcium concentrations have been reduced to an acceptable level, maintenance therapy with disodium etidronate 20 mg per kg daily by mouth for 30 days may be started on the day following the last intravenous dose; treatment may be extended to a maximum of 90 days.

For the prevention and treatment of **ectopic ossification** complicating hip replacement disodium etidronate has been given by mouth in a dose of 20 mg per kg daily for one month before and 3 months after the operation. For ectopic ossification due to spinal cord injury it has been given in a dose of 20 mg per kg daily for 2 weeks followed by 10 mg per kg daily for 10 weeks.

For the treatment of **osteoporosis**, the prevention of bone loss in postmenopausal women, and the prevention and treatment of corticosteroid-induced osteoporosis, etidronate is given in an intermittent or cyclical regimen with a calcium salt; disodium etidronate 400 mg is given by mouth daily for 14 days followed by the equivalent of 500 mg of elemental calcium by mouth for 76 days. Treatment has continued for 3 years in most patients; the optimum duration of treatment has not been established.

Ectopic ossification. Bisphosphonates that inhibit bone mineralisation such as disodium etidronate have been used to prevent ectopic ossification (p.744).[1,2]

1. Finerman GAM, Stover SL. Heterotopic ossification following hip replacement or spinal cord injury: two clinical studies with EHDP. *Metab Bone Dis Relat Res* 1981; **4 & 5:** 337–42.
2. Banovac K, *et al.* Intravenous disodium etidronate therapy in spinal cord injury patients with heterotopic ossification. *Paraplegia* 1993; **31:** 660–6.

Hypercalcaemia. Treatment with bisphosphonates may be considered in patients with moderate to severe symptomatic hypercalcaemia of malignancy (p.1181) in addition to rehydration and diuresis.

References.
1. Hasling C, *et al.* Etidronate disodium for treating hypercalcaemia of malignancy: a double blind, placebo-controlled study. *Eur J Clin Invest* 1986; **16:** 433–7.
2. Ringenberg QS, Ritch PS. Efficacy of oral administration of etidronate disodium in maintaining normal serum calcium levels in previously hypercalcemic cancer patients. *Clin Ther* 1987; **9:** 318–25.
3. Ralston SH, *et al.* Comparison of three intravenous bisphosphonates in cancer-associated hypercalcaemia. *Lancet* 1989; **ii:** 1180–2.
4. Singer FR, *et al.* Treatment of hypercalcaemia of malignancy with intravenous etidronate: a controlled, multicenter study. *Arch Intern Med* 1991; **151:** 471–6.

Hyperparathyroidism. Bisphosphonates have been used to inhibit bone resorption in the treatment of hypercalcaemia associated with hyperparathyroidism (p.746) but seem to be of little benefit in long-term treatment.

References.
1. Licata AA, O'Hanlon E. Treatment of hyperparathyroidism with etidronate disodium. *JAMA* 1983; **249:** 2063–4.

Malignant neoplasms of the bone. Bisphosphonates are of benefit in some patients with metastatic bone disease (p.490).
References.
1. Carey PO, Lippert MC. Treatment of painful prostatic bone metastases with oral etidronate disodium. *Urology* 1988; **32:** 403–7.
2. Smith JA. Palliation of painful bone metastases from prostate cancer using sodium etidronate: results of a randomized, prospective, double-blind, placebo-controlled study. *J Urol (Baltimore)* 1989; **141:** 85–7.

Osteoporosis. Bisphosphonates are used in the prevention and treatment of osteoporosis (p.745). For the treatment of postmenopausal osteoporosis, disodium etidronate is given in an intermittent or cyclical regimen;[1-4] additive effects with oestrogen have been described.[5,6] Similar cyclical regimens are used in the prevention of early postmenopausal bone loss.[7,8] Etidronate is also effective in both men and women for the prevention and treatment of corticosteroid-induced osteoporosis.[9-11] There is some interest in the use of etidronate to treat idiopathic vertebral osteoporosis in men.[12]

1. Storm T, *et al.* Effect of intermittent cyclical etidronate therapy on bone mass and fracture rate in women with postmenopausal osteoporosis. *N Engl J Med* 1990; **322:** 1265–71.
2. Watts NB, *et al.* Intermittent cyclical etidronate treatment of postmenopausal osteoporosis. *N Engl J Med* 1990; **323:** 73–9.
3. Harris ST, *et al.* Four-year study of intermittent cyclic etidronate treatment of postmenopausal osteoporosis: three years of blinded therapy followed by one year of open therapy. *Am J Med* 1993; **95:** 557–67.
4. Miller PD, *et al.* Cyclical etidronate in the treatment of postmenopausal osteoporosis: efficacy and safety after seven years of treatment. *Am J Med* 1997; **103:** 468–76.
5. Wimalawansa SJ. Combined therapy with estrogen and etidronate has an additive effect on bone mineral density in the hip and vertebrae: four-year randomized study. *Am J Med* 1995; **99:** 36–42.
6. Wimalawansa SJ. A four-year randomized controlled trial of hormone replacement and bisphosphonate, alone or in combination, in women with postmenopausal osteoporosis. *Am J Med* 1998; **104:** 219–26.
7. Herd RJM, *et al.* The prevention of early postmenopausal bone loss by cyclical etidronate therapy: a 2-year, double-blind, placebo-controlled study. *Am J Med* 1997; **103:** 92–9.
8. Meunier PJ, *et al.* Prevention of early postmenopausal bone loss with cyclical etidronate therapy. *J Clin Endocrinol Metab* 1997; **82:** 2784–91.
9. Struys A, *et al.* Cyclical etidronate reverses bone loss of the spine and proximal femur in patients with established corticosteroid-induced osteoporosis. *Am J Med* 1995; **99:** 235–42.
10. Adachi JD, *et al.* Intermittent etidronate therapy to prevent corticosteroid-induced osteoporosis. *N Engl J Med* 1997; **337:** 382–7.
11. Pitt P, *et al.* A double blind placebo controlled study to determine the effects of intermittent cyclical etidronate on bone mineral density in patients on long term oral corticosteroid treatment. *Thorax* 1998; **53:** 351–6.
12. Anderson FH, *et al.* Effect of intermittent cyclical disodium etidronate therapy on bone mineral density in men with vertebral fractures. *Age Ageing* 1997; **26:** 359–65.

Paget's disease of bone. Patients with Paget's disease of bone (p.746) may require no treatment or just analgesics, but bisphosphonates may be indicated if bone pain is persistent or to prevent further progression of the disease.
References.
1. Johnston CC, *et al.* Review of fracture experience during treatment of Paget's disease of bone with etidronate disodium (EHDP). *Clin Orthop* 1983; **172:** 186–94.
2. Preston CJ, *et al.* Effective short term treatment of Paget's disease with oral etidronate. *BMJ* 1986; **292:** 79–80.
3. Gibbs CJ, *et al.* Osteomalacia in Paget's disease treated with short term, high dose sodium etidronate. *BMJ* 1986; **292:** 1227–9.
4. Perry HM, *et al.* Alternate calcitonin and etidronate disodium therapy for Paget's bone disease. *Arch Intern Med* 1984; **144:** 929–33.

Preparations

USP 25: Etidronate Disodium Tablets.

Proprietary Preparations (details are given in Part 3)
Aust.: Didronel; *Austral.:* Didronel; *Belg.:* Didronel; Osteodidronel; *Canad.:* Didronel; *Denm.:* Didronate; *Fin.:* Didronate; *Fr.:* Didronel; *Ger.:* Didronel; Diphos; *Hong Kong:* Didronel; *Irl.:* Didronel; *Israel:* Didronel; *Ital.:* Etidron; *Neth.:* Didronel†; *Norw.:* Didronate; *NZ:* Didronel; *Port.:* Didronel; *S.Afr.:* Didronel†; *Singapore:* Difosen; *Spain:* Osteum; *Swed.:* Didronate; *Switz.:* Didronel; *UK:* Didronel; *USA:* Didronel.

Multi-ingredient: *Austral.:* Didrocal; *Canad.:* Didrocal; *Denm.:* Didronate Calcium; *Fin.:* Didronate + Calcium; *Irl.:* Didronel PMO; *Ital.:* Didro-Kit†; *Neth.:* Didrokit; *Norw.:* Didronate + Calsium; *Swed.:* Didronate + Calcium; *UK:* Didronel PMO.

Gallium Nitrate (12780-r)

Gallium Nitrate *(USAN).*
NSC-15200; WR-135675.
$Ga(NO_3)_3,9H_2O = 417.9$.
CAS — 13494-90-1 *(anhydrous gallium nitrate)*; 135886-70-3 *(gallium nitrate nonahydrate).*

Adverse Effects, Treatment, and Precautions

Gallium nitrate may produce serious nephrotoxicity, especially when given as a brief intravenous infusion; administration by continuous infusion, with adequate hydration, may reduce the incidence of renal damage. Serum creatinine should be monitored during therapy and treatment discontinued if it exceeds

25 mg per litre. Gallium nitrate should be given with great care and in reduced doses, if at all, to patients with existing renal dysfunction.

Gastrointestinal disturbances, rashes, metallic taste, visual and auditory disturbances, anaemia, hypophosphataemia, and hypocalcaemia have also been reported.

◊ Although it has been suggested, given the chemical similarity of gallium to aluminium, that repeated administration, particularly in the presence of renal impairment, might lead to severe neurotoxicity,[1] studies in *rats* do not provide any evidence of central neurological abnormalities.[2]

1. Altmann P, Cunningham J. Hazards of gallium for the treatment of Paget's disease of bone. *Lancet* 1990; **335:** 477.
2. Matkovic V, *et al.* Hazards of gallium for Paget's disease of bone. *Lancet* 1990; **335:** 1099.

Uses and Administration

Gallium nitrate is an inorganic metallic salt with hypocalcaemic properties. It acts to decrease bone resorption by osteoclasts, with a lesser and probably indirect increase in bone formation, and a consequent decline in serum calcium.

Gallium nitrate is used in the treatment of hypercalcaemia associated with malignant neoplasms and has been investigated in other disorders associated with abnormally enhanced bone turnover, such as Paget's disease of bone. For the treatment of hypercalcaemia of malignancy doses of 100 to 200 mg per m² body-surface may be given daily for up to 5 days, diluted in 1 litre of sodium chloride 0.9% or glucose 5% injection and infused intravenously over 24 hours. Treatment may be repeated after 2 to 4 weeks, if necessary. Adequate hydration before and during treatment is essential: a urinary output of at least 2 litres daily should be maintained, and renal function should be regularly monitored.

Gallium nitrate has been tried, with limited benefit, as an antineoplastic in the management of lymphomas and some solid neoplasms.

Hypercalcaemia. References to the use of gallium nitrate in hypercalcaemia of malignancy (p.1181).

1. Warrell RP, *et al.* Gallium nitrate for treatment of refractory hypercalcemia from parathyroid carcinoma. *Ann Intern Med* 1987; **107:** 683–6.
2. Warrell RP, *et al.* Gallium nitrate for acute treatment of cancer-related hypercalcemia: a randomized, double-blind comparison to calcitonin. *Ann Intern Med* 1988; **108:** 669–74.
3. Warrell RP, *et al.* A randomized double-blind study of gallium nitrate compared with etidronate for acute control of cancer-related hypercalcemia. *J Clin Oncol* 1991; **9:** 1467–75.

Paget's disease of bone. Beneficial results[1] were reported when gallium nitrate was given subcutaneously in doses of 0.25 or 0.5 mg per kg body-weight daily for 14 days to patients with advanced Paget's disease of bone (p.746). In this pilot multicentre study 14 days of gallium nitrate injections were followed by 4 weeks off medication and the cycle repeated once.

1. Bockman RS, *et al.* A multicenter trial of low dose gallium nitrate in patients with advanced Paget's disease of bone. *J Clin Endocrinol Metab* 1995; **80:** 595–602.

Preparations

Proprietary Preparations (details are given in Part 3)
USA: Ganite†.

Ibandronic Acid (17608-m)

Ibandronic Acid *(BAN, rINN).*
BM-21.0955. [1-Hydroxy-3-(methylpentylamino)propylidene]diphosphonic acid.
$C_9H_{23}NO_7P_2 = 319.2$.
CAS — 114084-78-5.
ATC — M05BA06.

Sodium Ibandronate (17801-b)

Sodium Ibandronate *(BANM, rINNM).*
Ibandronate Sodium *(USAN).*
$C_9H_{22}NNaO_7P_2,H_2O = 359.2$.
CAS — 138926-19-9.

Profile

Ibandronate is an aminobisphosphonate (p.748) which is a potent inhibitor of bone resorption. It is used as the sodium salt in hypercalcaemia of malignancy and is under investigation in various disorders of increased bone turnover.

Sodium ibandronate is administered by intravenous infusion over 2 hours. The dose is expressed in terms of ibandronic acid. For hypercalcaemia of malignancy, a single dose of the equivalent of 2 to 4 mg ibandronic acid is usually administered, up to a maximum of 6 mg. An oral formulation has been investigated.

The most common adverse effect is fever and influenza-like symptoms.

◊ General references.
1. Dooley M, Balfour JA. Ibandronate. *Drugs* 1999; **57:** 101–108.

Hypercalcaemia. Treatment with bisphosphonates may be considered in patients with moderate to severe symptomatic

hypercalcaemia of malignancy (p.1181) in addition to rehydration and diuresis.
References.
1. Pecherstorfer M, *et al.* Randomized phase II trial comparing different doses of the bisphosphonate ibandronate in the treatment of hypercalcaemia of malignancy. *J Clin Oncol* 1996; **14:** 268–76.
2. Ralston SH, *et al.* Dose-response study of ibandronate in the treatment of cancer-associated hypercalcaemia. *Br J Cancer* 1997; **75:** 295–300.

Osteoporosis. Bisphosphonates may be used for the prevention and treatment of osteoporosis (p.745).
References.
1. Ravn P, *et al.* The effect on bone mass and bone markers of different doses of ibandronate: a new bisphosphonate for the prevention and treatment of postmenopausal osteoporosis: a 1-year randomized, double-blind, placebo-controlled dose-finding study. *Bone* 1996; **19:** 527–33.
2. Thiébaud D, *et al.* Three monthly intravenous injections of ibandronate in the treatment of postmenopausal osteoporosis. *Am J Med* 1997; **103:** 298–307.

Preparations

Proprietary Preparations (details are given in Part 3)
Aust.: Bondronat; *Denm.:* Bondronat; *Fin.:* Bondronat; *Fr.:* Bondronat; *Ger.:* Bondronat; *Spain:* Bondronat; *Swed.:* Bondronat; *Switz.:* Bondronat; *Thai.:* Bondronat.

Imidazole Oxoglurate (3906-e)

Imidazole Cetoglutarate; Imidazole α-Ketoglutarate; Imidazole 2-Oxoglutarate.

Profile

Imidazole oxoglurate was used in the treatment of bone disorders and disorders of calcium metabolism; it was also used for its reported effects on platelet aggregation in the treatment of thrombotic disorders.

Preparations

Proprietary Preparations (details are given in Part 3)
Spain: Retencal†.

Incadronic Acid (17397-p)

Incadronic Acid *(rINN).*
Cimadronic Acid; YM-175. [(Cycloheptylamino)methylene]diphosphonic acid.
$C_8H_{19}NO_6P_2 = 287.2$.
CAS — 124351-85-5.

Disodium Incadronate (20336-n)

Disodium Incadronate *(rINNM).*
Disodium [(cycloheptylamino)methylene]diphosphonate.
$C_8H_{17}NNa_2O_6P_2 = 331.2$.
CAS — 138330-18-4.

Profile

Incadronic acid is an aminobisphosphonate (p.748) which is a potent inhibitor of bone resorption. It is given by intravenous infusion as disodium incadronate for hypercalcaemia of malignancy in a dose of 10 mg over 2 to 4 hours; if necessary this dose may be repeated at intervals of no less than 1 week. An oral formulation is under investigation for osteoporosis.

◊ References.
1. Usui T, *et al.* Pharmacokinetics of incadronate, a new bisphosphonate, in healthy volunteers and patients with malignancy-associated hypercalcemia. *Int J Clin Pharmacol Ther* 1997; **35:** 239–44.

Preparations

Proprietary Preparations (details are given in Part 3)
Jpn: Bisphonal.

Ipriflavone (7310-z)

Ipriflavone *(rINN).*
FL-113. 7-Isopropoxyisoflavone.
$C_{18}H_{16}O_3 = 280.3$.
CAS — 35212-22-7.
ATC — M05BX01.

Profile

Ipriflavone is a synthetic isoflavonoid that inhibits resorption of bone and is available in some countries for the treatment of osteoporosis (p.745). It is given by mouth in a dose of 200 mg three times daily.

◊ References.[1-4] Despite earlier favourable reports, a prospective randomised controlled study in postmenopausal women with low bone mass failed to show prevention of bone loss or improvements in markers of bone metabolism with ipriflavone.[4] There was also a significant incidence of lymphopenia with the drug.

1. Agnusdei D, *et al.* Metabolic and clinical effects of ipriflavone in established post-menopausal osteoporosis. *Drugs Exp Clin Res* 1989; **15:** 97–104.
2. Hyodo T, *et al.* A study of the effects of ipriflavone administration on hemodialysis patients with renal osteodystrophy: preliminary report. *Nephron* 1991; **58:** 114–15.

---

3. Agnusdei D, *et al.* Effects of ipriflavone on bone mass and bone remodeling in patients with established postmenopausal osteoporosis. *Curr Ther Res* 1992; **51**: 82–91.
4. Alexandersen P, *et al.* Ipriflavone in the treatment of postmenopausal osteoporosis: a randomized controlled trial. *JAMA* 2001; **285**: 1482–8.

Preparations

Proprietary Preparations (details are given in Part 3)
Ital.: Iprosten; Osteofix; **Jpn**: Osten.

Multi-ingredient: *UK*: Osteopro.

Medronic Acid (3279-d)

Medronic Acid *(BAN, USAN, pINN)*.
Methylenebis(phosphonic acid).
$CH_6O_3P_2 = 176.0$.
CAS — 1984-15-2.

Disodium Medronate (9425-t)

Disodium Medronate *(BANM)*.

Disodium Methylene Diphosphonate; MDP; Medronate Disodium *(USAN)*. Disodium dihydrogen methylenediphosphonate.
$CH_4Na_2O_6P_2 = 220.0$.
CAS — 25681-89-4.

Profile
Medronate is a bisphosphonate with general properties similar to those of the other bisphosphonates (p.748). Like other members of the class it has a strong affinity for bone, and a complex of disodium medronate and stannous chloride or fluoride labelled with radioactive technetium-99m (p.1451) is used diagnostically as a bone scanning agent; it is given intravenously.

Hypersensitivity. For reference to a severe allergic reaction attributed to the sodium medronate component of a radiopharmaceutical, see under Adverse Effects and Precautions of Bisphosphonates, p.748.

Neridronic Acid (4536-s)

Neridronic Acid *(rINN)*.

AHDP; AHHexBP; Aminohexane Diphosphonate. (6-Amino-1-hydroxyhexylidene)diphosphonic acid.
$C_6H_{17}NO_7P_2 = 277.1$.
CAS — 79778-41-9.

Profile
Neridronic acid is an aminobisphosphonate with similar properties to those of the bisphosphonates in general (p.748). It inhibits bone resorption and has been given intravenously or by mouth as a neridronate salt in the treatment of malignant hypercalcaemia and diseases associated with excessive bone turnover such as Paget's disease of bone.

◊ Bisphosphonates are widely used in the treatment of Paget's disease of bone (p.746) and hypercalcaemia of malignancy (p.1181).
References.
1. Delmas PD, *et al.* Beneficial effects of aminohexane diphosphonate in patients with Paget's disease of bone resistant to sodium etidronate. *Am J Med* 1987; **83**: 276–82.
2. O'Rourke NP, *et al.* Treatment of malignant hypercalcaemia with aminohexane bisphosphonate (neridronate). *Br J Cancer* 1994; **69**: 914–17.
3. Filipponi P, *et al.* Paget's disease of bone: benefits of neridronate as a first treatment and in cases of relapse after clodronate. *Bone* 1998; **23**: 543–8.

Oxidronic Acid (3280-c)

Oxidronic Acid *(BAN, USAN, pINN)*.

(Hydroxymethylene)diphosphonic acid.
$CH_6O_7P_2 = 192.0$.
CAS — 15468-10-7.

Disodium Oxidronate (2544-c)

HMDP; Oxidronate Disodium; Oxidronate Sodium; Sodium Oxidronate *(BANM)*. Disodium (hydroxymethylene)diphosphonate.
$CH_4Na_2O_7P_2 = 236.0$.
CAS — 14255-61-9.

Profile
Oxidronate is a bisphosphonate with general properties similar to those of the other bisphosphonates (p.748). Like other members of the class it has a strong affinity for bone, and a chelate of oxidronate with radioactive technetium-99m (p.1451) is used diagnostically as a bone scanning agent; it is given intravenously.

Pamidronic Acid (3392-n)

Pamidronic Acid *(BAN, rINN)*.

Aminohydroxypropylidenebisphosphonate; APD. 3-Amino-1-hydroxypropylidenebis(phosphonic acid).
$C_3H_{11}NO_7P_2 = 235.1$.
CAS — 40391-99-9.
ATC — M05BA03.

Disodium Pamidronate (12672-k)

Disodium Pamidronate *(BANM)*.

Aminohydroxypropylidenebisphosphonate Disodium; CGP-23339A; CGP-23339AE; Disodium Aminohydroxypropylidenediphosphonate; Pamidronate Disodium *(USAN)*. Disodium 3-amino-1-hydroxypropylidenebisphosphonate pentahydrate.
$C_3H_9NNa_2O_7P_2,5H_2O = 369.1$.
CAS — 109552-15-0 *(disodium pamidronate pentahydrate)*; 57248-88-1 *(anhydrous disodium pamidronate)*.
Pharmacopoeias. In *Br.*

Pharmacopoeial description
BP 2001: A white crystalline powder. Soluble in water and in 2M sodium hydroxide; sparingly soluble in 0.1M hydrochloric acid; practically insoluble in organic solvents. A 1% solution in water has a pH of 7.8 to 8.8.

Adverse Effects and Precautions
As for the bisphosphonates in general, p.748.

Fever and influenza-like symptoms (sometimes accompanied by malaise, rigors, fatigue, and flushes) are common during treatment with disodium pamidronate but generally resolve spontaneously. Severe local reactions and thrombophlebitis have followed administration as a bolus injection. Rare CNS effects include agitation, confusion, dizziness, somnolence, and insomnia. Seizures have been precipitated in a few patients. In addition to hypocalcaemia and hypophosphataemia (which are common), hypomagnesaemia, and rarely hypernatraemia, and hyperkalaemia or hypokalaemia have occurred. Hypotension and hypertension have been reported.

Pamidronate should be used with caution in those with cardiac disease because of the potential for fluid overload and in those who have had thyroid surgery because of the increased risk of hypocalcaemia. Serum electrolytes, calcium and phosphate should be monitored during therapy. Patients should be warned against driving or operating machinery after treatment if somnolence or dizziness occur. Pamidronate should not be administered by bolus injection.

Effects on the eyes. Although adverse ocular reactions to pamidronate appeared to be rare, the manufacturers were aware of 23 cases up to September 1993 which were possibly associated with the drug.[1] The reactions included anterior uveitis in 7 patients and unilateral episcleritis or scleritis in 3 (see also under Bisphosphonates, p.748).
1. Macarol V, Fraunfelder FT. Pamidronate disodium and possible ocular adverse drug reactions. *Am J Ophthalmol* 1994; **118**: 220–4.

Effects on the gastrointestinal tract. The tolerability of pamidronate administered *by mouth* may depend to some extent on the particular formulation. Gastrointestinal disturbances (in 21.8%) and haematological abnormalities (in 9.4%) were the predominant side-effects associated with oral pamidronate in an open study of elderly patients.[1] Oesophagitis, noted earlier[2] in 4 of 49 patients given a different formulation, was not reported in this study.[1]
1. Spivacow FR, *et al.* Tolerability of oral pamidronate in elderly patients with osteoporosis and other metabolic bone diseases. *Curr Ther Res* 1996; **57**: 123–30.
2. Lufkin EG, *et al.* Pamidronate: an unrecognised problem in gastrointestinal tolerability. *Osteoporosis Int* 1994; **4**: 320–2.

Hypersensitivity. Allergic reactions to bisphosphonates are rare. Rash and pruritus occasionally follow pamidronate infusion. Mild skin rashes have also been reported in some patients taking pamidronate by mouth (see also under Bisphosphonates, p.748).

Musculoskeletal effects. Although pamidronate appears to be a less potent inhibitor of bone mineralisation than etidronate, mineralisation defects of bone have been reported in patients with Paget's disease of bone receiving pamidronate.[1] The resultant osteomalacia was not associated with any adverse clinical effects. Acute pseudogout occurred in a woman treated with pamidronate for acute hypercalcaemia, possibly due to deposition of calcium in the joints.[2] Severe bone pain occurred in more patients than expected when pamidronate was used for low bone density in cystic fibrosis;[3] an increase in proinflammatory cytokines was postulated as a mechanism for this effect.[4]
1. Adamson BB, *et al.* Mineralisation defects with pamidronate therapy for Paget's disease. *Lancet* 1993; **342**: 1459–60.

2. Malnick SDH *et al.* Acute pseudogout as a complication of pamidronate. *Ann Pharmacother* 1997; **31**: 499–500.
3. Haworth CS, *et al.* Severe bone pain after intravenous pamidronate in adult patients with cystic fibrosis. *Lancet* 1998; **352**: 1753–4.
4. Teramoto S, *et al.* Increased cytokines and pamidronate-induced bone pain in adults with cystic fibrosis. *Lancet* 1999; **353**: 750.

Renal impairment. Like other bisphosphonates (see Effects on the Kidneys, p.748), pamidronate may cause adverse renal effects. The manufacturer notes there have been isolated cases of haematuria, acute renal failure, and deterioration of pre-existing renal disease. Therefore, it is recommended that renal function be monitored during long-term pamidronate therapy, especially in patients with pre-existing renal disease or a predisposition to renal impairment.

Pharmacokinetic studies suggest that no dosage reduction is required in patients with renal impairment.[1] However, the UK manufacturer currently recommends that the rate of infusion be reduced to a maximum of 20 mg per hour in patients with established or suspected renal impairment.
1. Berenson JR, *et al.* Pharmacokinetics of pamidronate disodium in patients with cancer with normal or impaired renal function. *J Clin Pharmacol* 1997; **37**: 285–90.

Interactions
As for the bisphosphonates in general, p.748.

Pharmacokinetics
After intravenous administration of disodium pamidronate, about 20 to 55% of the dose is excreted in the urine unchanged within 72 hours, while the remainder is mainly adsorbed onto bone and only very slowly eliminated. Renal clearance is slower in patients with severe renal impairment and infusion rates may need to be reduced (see above).

Disodium pamidronate is poorly absorbed (about 1 to 3%) from the gastrointestinal tract.

Uses and Administration
Pamidronate is an aminobisphosphonate with general properties similar to those of the other bisphosphonates (p.749). It inhibits bone resorption, but appears to have less effect on bone mineralisation than etidronate at comparable doses.

Disodium pamidronate is used as an adjunct in the treatment of severe hypercalcaemia, especially when associated with malignancy. It is also used in the treatment of osteolytic lesions and bone pain in multiple myeloma or bone metastases associated with breast cancer. It may also be of benefit in bone disorders associated with excessive bone resorption, including Paget's disease of bone.

Disodium pamidronate is administered by slow intravenous infusion. The UK manufacturer recommends infusion at a rate not exceeding 60 mg per hour (or not exceeding 20 mg per hour in patients with established or suspected renal impairment) and at a concentration not exceeding 60 mg per 250 mL of sodium chloride 0.9%. In the USA, the recommended concentration of infusion and its rate of administration vary depending on the indication.

In **hypercalcaemia of malignancy** disodium pamidronate is given by slow intravenous infusion in a total dose of 15 to 90 mg according to the initial plasma-calcium concentration. In the UK, the total dose is given as a single infusion or in divided doses over 2 to 4 days. In the USA, the total dose is given as a single infusion, doses of 60 mg being given over at least 4 hours, and 90 mg over 24 hours. Plasma-calcium concentrations generally start declining 24 to 48 hours after administration of pamidronate with normalisation within 3 to 7 days. Treatment may be repeated if normocalcaemia is not achieved within this time or if hypercalcaemia recurs.

In patients with **osteolytic lesions and bone pain** of multiple myeloma or bone metastases associated with breast cancer, disodium pamidronate may be given in doses of 90 mg by intravenous infusion every 3 to 4 weeks.

In the treatment of **Paget's disease** the dosage regimen in the UK is 30 mg by slow infusion once a week for 6 weeks (total dose 180 mg), or 30 mg in the first week then 60 mg every other week for 6 weeks (total dose 210 mg). These courses may be repeated every 6 months, and the total dose increased if necessary up to a maximum of 360 mg. Alternatively, the dose used in the USA is 30 mg by infusion over 4 hours, repeated on consecutive days to a total dose of 90 mg. This course is repeated when clinically indicated.

Disodium pamidronate has also been given by mouth.

◊ General references.
1. Fitton A, McTavish D. Pamidronate: a review of its pharmacological properties and therapeutic efficacy in resorptive bone disease. *Drugs* 1991; **41**: 289–318. Correction. *ibid.* 1992; **43**: 145.
2. Anonymous. Pamidronate. *Med Lett Drugs Ther* 1992; **34**: 1–2.
3. Kellihan MJ, Mangino PD. Pamidronate. *Ann Pharmacother* 1992; **26**: 1262–9.

Gaucher disease. Treatment with oral disodium pamidronate in doses of 600 mg daily in adults,[1] and 150 to 300 mg daily in children,[2] or intravenous disodium pamidronate in doses of 45 mg every 3 weeks,[3] has been reported to improve bone lesions of Gaucher disease (p.1575) in a few patients.
1. Harinck HIJ, *et al.* Regression of bone lesions in Gaucher's disease during treatment with aminohydroxypropylidene bisphosphonate. *Lancet* 1984; **i**: 513.
2. Samuel R, *et al.* Aminohydroxy propylidine bisphosphonate (APD) treatment improves the clinical skeletal manifestations of Gaucher's disease. *Pediatrics* 1994; **94**: 385–9.
3. Ciana G, *et al.* Short-term effects of pamidronate in patients with Gaucher's disease and severe skeletal involvement. *N Engl J Med* 1997; **337**: 712.

Hypercalcaemia. In patients with moderate to severe symptomatic hypercalcaemia of malignancy (p.1181) treatment with bisphosphonates may be considered in addition to rehydration and diuresis.

References.
1. Thiébaud D, *et al.* Oral versus intravenous AHP,BP (APD) in the treatment of hypercalcemia of malignancy. *Bone* 1986; **7**: 247–53.
2. Morton AR, *et al.* Single dose versus daily intravenous aminohydroxypropylidene biphosphonate (APD) for the hypercalcaemia of malignancy. *BMJ* 1988; **296**: 811–14.
3. Ralston SH, *et al.* Comparison of three intravenous bisphosphonates in cancer-associated hypercalcaemia. *Lancet* 1989; **ii**: 1180–2.
4. Nussbaum SR, *et al.* Single-dose intravenous therapy with pamidronate for the treatment of hypercalcaemia of malignancy: comparison of 30-, 60-, and 90-mg dosages. *Am J Med* 1993; **95**: 297–304.
5. Kutluk MT, *et al.* Childhood cancer and hypercalcemia: report of a case treated with pamidronate. *J Pediatr* 1997; **130**: 828–31.

Malignant neoplasms of the bone. Bisphosphonates are of benefit in some patients with metastatic bone disease (p.490).

References.
1. Pelger RCM, *et al.* Short-term metabolic effects of pamidronate in patients with prostatic carcinoma and bone metastases. *Lancet* 1989; **ii**: 865.
2. Man Z, *et al.* Use of pamidronate for multiple myeloma osteolytic lesions. *Lancet* 1990; **335**: 663.
3. van Holten-Verzantvoort AT, *et al.* Palliative pamidronate treatment in patients with bone metastases from breast cancer. *J Clin Oncol* 1993; **11**: 491–8.
4. Berenson JR, *et al.* Efficacy of pamidronate in reducing skeletal events in patients with advanced multiple myeloma. *N Engl J Med* 1996; **334**: 488–93.
5. Conte PF, *et al.* Delayed progression of bone metastases with pamidronate therapy in breast cancer patients: a randomized, multicenter phase III trial. *Ann Oncol* 1994; **5** (suppl 7): 41S–44S.
6. Hortobagyi GN, *et al.* Efficacy of pamidronate in reducing skeletal complications in patients with breast cancer and lytic bone metastases. *N Engl J Med* 1996; **335**: 1785–91.
7. Theriault RL, *et al.* Pamidronate reduces skeletal morbidity in women with advanced breast cancer and lytic bone lesions: a randomized, placebo-controlled trial. *J Clin Oncol* 1999; **17**: 846–54.
8. Lipton A, *et al.* Pamidronate prevents skeletal complications and is effective palliative treatment in women with breast carcinoma and osteolytic bone metastases: long term follow-up of two randomized, placebo-controlled trials. *Cancer* 2000; **88**: 1082–90.

Osteogenesis imperfecta. Pamidronate has produced some benefit in children with osteogenesis imperfecta (p.744).

Paget's disease of bone. Patients with Paget's disease of bone (p.746) may require no treatment or just analgesics, but bisphosphonates may be indicated if bone pain is persistent or to prevent further progression of the disease. References to the use of disodium pamidronate in Paget's disease are given below.[1-5] Bisphosphonates have also been given in other bone diseases with a similar pathology, particularly increased osteoclastic resorption. For example, pamidronate has had beneficial effects in patients with fibrous dysplasia of bone, a rare congenital disease leading to osteolytic lesions.[6]
1. Mautalen CA, *et al.* Efficacy of the bisphosphonate APD in the control of Paget's bone disease. *Bone* 1985; **6**: 429–32.
2. Cantrill JA, *et al.* Low dose intravenous 3-amino-1-hydroxypropylidene-1,1-bisphosphonate (APD) for the treatment of Paget's disease of bone. *Ann Rheum Dis* 1986; **45**: 1012–18.
3. Harinck HIJ, *et al.* Paget's disease of bone: early and late responses to three different modes of treatment with aminohydroxypropylidene bisphosphonate (APD). *BMJ* 1987; **295**: 1301–5.
4. Drake S, *et al.* Pamidronate sodium and calcitonin-resistant Paget's disease: immediate response in a patient. *Arch Intern Med* 1989; **149**: 401–3.
5. Crisp AJ. Pamidronate for Paget's disease of the bone. *Br J Hosp Med* 1995; **53**: 66–8.
6. Liens D, *et al.* Long-term effects of intravenous pamidronate in fibrous dysplasia of bone. *Lancet* 1994; **343**: 953–4.

The symbol † denotes a preparation no longer actively marketed

Rheumatoid arthritis. Intravenous[1] and oral[2] administration of pamidronate has reportedly produced some modification of disease in a few patients with rheumatoid arthritis (p.9). Continuous oral pamidronate therapy was shown to be effective in preserving and increasing bone mass in a 3-year randomised controlled trial involving 105 patients with rheumatoid arthritis.[3]
1. Eggelmeijer F, *et al.* Clinical and biochemical response to single infusion of pamidronate in patients with active rheumatoid arthritis: a double blind placebo controlled study. *J Rheumatol* 1994; **21**: 2016–20.
2. Maccagno A, *et al.* Double blind radiological assessment of continuous oral pamidronic acid in patients with rheumatoid arthritis. *Scand J Rheumatol* 1994; **23**: 211–14.
3. Eggelmeijer F, *et al.* Increased bone mass with pamidronate treatment in rheumatoid arthritis: results of a three-year randomized, double-blind trial. *Arthritis Rheum* 1996; **39**: 396–402.

Preparations

BP 2001: Disodium Pamidronate Intravenous Infusion.

Proprietary Preparations (details are given in Part 3)
Aust.: Aredia; *Austral.:* Aredia; *Belg.:* Aredia; *Braz.:* Aredia; *Canad.:* Aredia; *Denm.:* Aredia; *Fin.:* Aredia; *Fr.:* Aredia; *Ger.:* Aredia; *Hong Kong:* Aredia; *Irl.:* Aredia; *Israel:* Aredia; *Ital.:* Aredia; *Neth.:* Aredia; *Norw.:* Aredia; *NZ:* Aredia; *Port.:* Aredia; *S.Afr.:* Aredia; *Singapore:* Aredia; *Spain:* Aredia; *Swed.:* Aredia; *Switz.:* Aredia; *Thai.:* Aredia; *UK:* Aredia; *USA:* Aredia.

Parathyroid Hormone (8051-x)

Parathyrin; PTH.
CAS — 9002-64-6.

Profile
Parathyroid hormone is a single-chain polypeptide isolated from the parathyroid glands. It contains 84 amino acids and in man the first (N-terminal) 34 appear to be responsible for the hormonal activity. The amino-acid sequence varies according to the source.

Endogenous parathyroid hormone is involved in the maintenance of plasma-calcium concentrations having a hypercalcaemic effect through its actions on bone, kidney, and indirectly on the gastrointestinal tract (see also under Parathyroid Disorders, p.746).

Exogenous parathyroid hormone was formerly used in acute hypoparathyroidism with tetany. It has also been used in the differential diagnosis of hypoparathyroidism and pseudohypoparathyroidism.

Synthetic preparations of the first 34 amino acids of human and bovine parathyroid hormones (PTH 1-34; teriparatide) are now used for diagnostic purposes, and are under investigation for the treatment of osteoporosis (see Teriparatide Acetate, p.755).

Risedronic Acid (10591-d)

Risedronic Acid *(BAN, rINN)*.
[1-Hydroxy-2-(3-pyridinyl)ethylidene]diphosphonic acid.
$C_7H_{11}NO_7P_2 = 283.1$.
CAS — 105462-24-6.

Risedronate Sodium (3406-j)

Risedronate Sodium *(BANM, USAN, rINNM)*.
Monosodium Risedronate; NE-58095; Sodium Risedronate. Sodium trihydrogen [1-hydroxy-2-(3-pyridyl)ethylidene]diphosphonate.
$C_7H_{10}NNaO_7P_2 = 305.1$.
CAS — 115436-72-1.

Adverse Effects and Precautions
As for the bisphosphonates in general, p.748. The most frequent adverse effects are arthralgia and gastrointestinal disturbances. *To minimise the risk of gastrointestinal effects patients should be instructed to swallow risedronate tablets with plenty of water (at least 200 mL), in an upright position (standing or sitting). Tablets should be taken on rising for the day, on an empty stomach, at least 30 minutes before breakfast and any other oral medication; if taken at any other time food and drink should be avoided for at least 2 hours before or after risedronate. Tablets should not be taken at bedtime or before rising. Patients should remain upright after taking the tablets, and should not lie down for at least 30 minutes.* Hypocalcaemia should be corrected before beginning risedronate therapy.

Effects on the eyes. For a reported case of bilateral iritis associated with risedronate, see under Bisphosphonates, p.748.

Interactions
As for the bisphosphonates in general, p.748.

Pharmacokinetics
Like other bisphosphonates, risedronate is poorly absorbed after oral administration. Absorption is reduced by food, especially by products containing calcium or other polyvalent cations. The mean bioavailability is 0.63% in the fasting state, and is reduced by 30% when administered 1 hour before breakfast, and by 55% when administered half an hour before breakfast. Unabsorbed drug is eliminated unchanged in the faeces. Risedronate is not metabolised, and 50% of the absorbed dose is excreted unchanged in the urine within 24 hours. The remainder of the absorbed dose is apparently sequestered to bone for a prolonged period.

Absorption. Absorption of a single dose of risedronate was comparable when given 0.5 to 1 hour before breakfast or 2 hours after an evening meal in a study in healthy subjects.[1]
1. Mitchell DY, *et al.* The effect of dosing regimen on the pharmacokinetics of risedronate. *Br J Clin Pharmacol* 1999; **48**: 536–42.

Uses and Administration
Risedronate is an aminobisphosphonate with similar properties to those of the bisphosphonates in general (p.749). It inhibits bone resorption and is used as the sodium salt in Paget's disease of bone and for prevention and treatment of postmenopausal or corticosteroid-induced osteoporosis.

Risedronate sodium is given by mouth, and the specific instructions for its administration (see above) should be followed to minimise gastrointestinal adverse effects and permit adequate absorption. The recommended dosage for Paget's disease of bone is 30 mg once daily for 2 months. Treatment may be repeated if necessary after an interval of a further 2 months. The recommended dosage for the treatment or prevention of osteoporosis is 5 mg daily.

◊ Some references to the use of risedronate for osteolysis in malignant disease (p.490), for Paget's disease of bone (p.746), for primary hyperparathyroidism (p.746), and for the prevention of postmenopausal osteoporosis (p.745).
1. Roux C, *et al.* Biologic, histologic and densitometric effects of oral risedronate on bone in patients with multiple myeloma. *Bone* 1994; **15**: 41–9.
2. Brown JP, *et al.* Risedronate in Paget's disease: preliminary results of a multicenter study. *Semin Arthritis Rheum* 1994; **23**: 272.
3. Reasner CA, *et al.* Acute changes in calcium homeostasis during treatment of primary hyperparathyroidism with risedronate. *J Clin Endocrinol Metab* 1993; **77**: 1067–71.
4. Delmas PD, *et al.* Bisphosphonate risedronate prevents bone loss in women with artificial menopause due to chemotherapy of breast cancer: a double-blind, placebo-controlled study. *J Clin Oncol* 1997; **15**: 955–62.
5. Mortensen L, *et al.* Risedronate increases bone mass in early postmenopausal population: two years of treatment plus one year of follow-up. *J Clin Endocrinol Metab* 1998; **83**: 396–402.
6. Fogelman I, *et al.* Risedronate reverses bone loss in postmenopausal women with low bone mass: results from a multinational, double-blind, placebo-controlled trial. *J Clin Endocrinol Metab* 2000; **85**: 1895–1900.
7. Crandall C. Risedronate: a clinical review. *Arch Intern Med* 2001; **161**: 353–60.
8. McClung MR, *et al.* Effect of risedronate on the risk of hip fracture in elderly women. *N Engl J Med* 2001; **344**: 333–40.
9. Harris ST, *et al.* Effect of combined risedronate and hormone replacement therapies on bone mineral density in postmenopausal women. *J Clin Endocrinol Metab* 2001; **86**: 1890–7.
10. Dunn CJ, Goa KL. Risedronate: a review of its pharmacological properties and clinical use in resorptive bone disease. *Drugs* 2001; **61**: 685–712.

Preparations

Proprietary Preparations (details are given in Part 3)
Austral.: Actonel; *Fin.:* Optinate; *Fr.:* Actonel; *Irl.:* Actonel; *Swed.:* Optinate; *UK:* Actonel; *USA:* Actonel.

Teriparatide Acetate (3640-n)

Teriparatide Acetate *(USAN, rINNM)*.
hPTH 1-34 (teriparatide); LY-333334 (teriparatide).
$C_{181}H_{291}N_{55}O_{51}S_2, xH_2O, yC_2H_4O_2$.
CAS — 52232-67-4 (teriparatide); 99294-94-7 (teriparatide acetate).

Units
The potency of teriparatide acetate is expressed in terms of units of human parathyroid hormone activity.

The first International Reference Preparation (1981) of parathyroid hormone, human, for immunoassay contains 0.1 unit in approximately 100 ng of freeze-dried purified hormone.

Adverse Effects
Gastrointestinal disturbances, a metallic taste, tingling of the extremities, and pain at the site of injection have occasionally been associated with the intravenous infusion of teriparatide acetate. It is a peptide and the possibility of systemic hypersen-

sitivity reactions should be borne in mind. Hypercalcaemia may develop.

Uses and Administration
Teriparatide is a synthetic polypeptide that consists of the 1-34 amino-acid biologically active N-terminal region of human parathyroid hormone (p.755). Teriparatide acetate has been given by intravenous infusion in the differential diagnosis of hypoparathyroidism and pseudohypoparathyroidism.

Teriparatide is under investigation as a potential stimulant of bone formation in patients with osteoporosis (see below).

Hypoparathyroidism. Hypoparathyroidism is characterised by a deficiency in endogenous parathyroid hormone, whereas pseudohypoparathyroidism is characterised by resistance to the effects of parathyroid hormone (see p.747). Teriparatide acetate is used *diagnostically* to distinguish between these 2 conditions.[1] A synthetic 1-38 fragment of human parathyroid hormone (1-38 hPTH) has been used similarly.[2] Teriparatide has also been used to *treat* hypoparathyroidism.[3,4]

1. Mallette LE. Synthetic human parathyroid hormone 1-34 fragment for diagnostic testing. *Ann Intern Med* 1988; **109:** 800–4.
2. Kruse K, Kracht U. A simplified diagnostic test in hypoparathyroidism and pseudohypoparathyroidism type I with synthetic 1-38 fragment of human parathyroid hormone. *Eur J Pediatr* 1987; **146:** 373–7.
3. Winer KK, et al. Synthetic human parathyroid hormone 1-34 vs calcitriol and calcium in the treatment of hypoparathyroidism. *JAMA* 1996; **276:** 631–6.
4. Winer KK, et al. A randomized, cross-over trial of once-daily versus twice-daily parathyroid hormone 1-34 in treatment of hypoparathyroidism. *J Clin Endocrinol Metab* 1998; **83:** 3480–6.

Osteoporosis. Parathyroid hormone is capable of stimulating both formation and resorption of bone; at low doses the former effect predominates and may avoid the development of hypercalcaemia. These different actions appear to be modulated by different signalling pathways in the osteoblast, and there is much interest in developing a hormone fragment or analogue which would stimulate bone formation but not resorption.[1] Parathyroid hormone appears to have less effect on cortical than trabecular bone, suggesting that, although it may be helpful in preventing vertebral fractures, its impact on fractures of the proximal femur may be more limited. However, combination with an antiresorptive agent such as oestrogen or a bisphosphonate, the currently preferred treatments for osteoporosis (p.745), might protect other parts of the skeleton. References[2-10] to the use of teriparatide and other synthetic parathyroid hormone fragments in osteoporosis are given below.

1. Bonn D. Parathyroid hormone for osteoporosis. *Lancet* 1996; **347:** 50.
2. Slovik DM, et al. Restoration of spinal bone in osteoporotic men by treatment with human parathyroid hormone (1-34) and 1,25-dihydroxyvitamin D. *J Bone Miner Res* 1986; **1:** 377–81.
3. Rittinghaus EF, et al. Increase of vertebral density in osteoporosis: combination therapy with 1-38 hPTH and calcitonin nasal spray. *Acta Endocrinol (Copenh)* 1988; **117** (suppl 287): 167–8.
4. Reeve J, et al. Treatment of osteoporosis with human parathyroid peptide and observations on effect of sodium fluoride. *BMJ* 1990; **301:** 314–18. Correction. *ibid.;* 477.
5. Finkelstein JS, et al. Parathyroid hormone for the prevention of bone loss induced by estrogen deficiency. *N Engl J Med* 1994; **331:** 1618–23.
6. Hodsman AB, et al. A randomized controlled trial to compare the efficacy of cyclical parathyroid hormone versus cyclical parathyroid hormone and sequential calcitonin to improve bone mass in postmenopausal women with osteoporosis. *J Clin Endocrinol Metab* 1997; **82:** 620–8.
7. Lindsay R, et al. Randomised controlled study of effect of parathyroid hormone on vertebral-bone mass and fracture incidence among postmenopausal women on oestrogen with osteoporosis. *Lancet* 1997; **350:** 550–5.
8. Finkelstein JS, et al. Prevention of estrogen deficiency-related bone loss with human parathyroid hormone-(1-34): a randomized controlled trial. *JAMA* 1998; **280:** 1067–73.
9. Lane NE, et al. Parathyroid hormone treatment can reverse corticosteroid-induced osteoporosis. *J Clin Invest* 1998; **102:** 1627–33.
10. Neer RM, et al. Effect of parathyroid hormone (1-34) on fractures and bone mineral density in postmenopausal women with osteoporosis. *N Engl J Med* 2001; **344:** 1434–41.

Tiludronic Acid (10451-e)

Tiludronic Acid *(BAN, rINN)*.

ME-3737; SR-41319. {[(p-Chlorophenyl)thio]methylene}diphosphonic acid.

$C_7H_9ClO_6P_2S = 318.6$.

CAS — 89987-06-4.

ATC — M05BA05.

Tiludronate Sodium (17782-k)

Tiludronate Sodium *(BANM, rINNM)*.

Disodium Tiludronate; SR-41319B; Tiludronate Disodium *(USAN)*. Disodium dihydrogen {[(p-chlorophenyl)thio]methylene}diphosphonate hemihydrate.

$C_7H_7ClNa_2O_6P_2S, \frac{1}{2}H_2O = 371.6$.

CAS — 149845-07-8 *(anhydrous tiludronate sodium); 155453-10-4 (tiludronate sodium hemihydrate)*.

Adverse Effects and Precautions
As for the bisphosphonates in general, p.748.

Effects on the skin. As with other bisphosphonates, tiludronate has been associated with rash and pruritus. For reference to a case of massive epidermal necrosis possibly associated with tiludronate, see Hypersensitivity, under Bisphosphonates, p.748.

Interactions
As for the bisphosphonates in general, p.748. Indometacin may increase the bioavailability of tiludronate two to fourfold if taken concomitantly; diclofenac does not appear to have this effect. Aspirin may decrease the bioavailability of tiludronate by 50%.

Pharmacokinetics
Like other bisphosphonates tiludronate is poorly absorbed following oral administration. Absorption is reduced by food, especially by products containing calcium or other polyvalent cations. Following oral administration the bioavailability of tiludronate is about 6% in the fasting state, and is reduced by about 90% when administered within 2 hours of food. About half of the absorbed portion of tiludronate is bound to bone, and only very slowly excreted; the remainder is excreted unchanged in the urine.

Uses and Administration
Tiludronate is a bisphosphonate with similar properties to those of the bisphosphonates in general (p.749). It inhibits bone resorption and is used for Paget's disease of bone and has been tried in postmenopausal osteoporosis.

It is given by mouth as tiludronate sodium, but doses are expressed in terms of the equivalent amount of tiludronic acid. To ensure adequate absorption doses should be taken, together with plenty of water (at least 200 mL), at least 2 hours before or after meals. In Paget's disease of bone the usual dose is 400 mg once daily for 3 months, and this may be repeated if necessary after an interval of at least 3 months.

◊ Some references to the use of tiludronate in Paget's disease of bone (p.746), and for the management of osteoporosis (p.745).

1. Chesnut CH. Tiludronate: development as an osteoporosis therapy. *Bone* 1995; **17** (suppl 5): 517S–19S.
2. McClung MR, et al. Tiludronate therapy for Paget's disease of bone. *Bone* 1995; **17** (suppl 5): 493S–6S.
3. Roux C, et al. Comparative prospective, double-blind, multicenter study of the efficacy of tiludronate and etidronate in the treatment of Paget's disease of bone. *Arthritis Rheum* 1995; **38:** 851–8.
4. Anonymous. Tiludronate for Paget's disease of bone. *Med Lett Drugs Ther* 1997; **39:** 65–6.
5. Fraser WD, et al. A double-blind, multicentre, placebo-controlled study of tiludronate in Paget's disease of bone. *Postgrad Med J* 1997; **73:** 496–502.

Preparations
Proprietary Preparations (details are given in Part 3)
Aust.: Skelid†; *Austral.:* Skelid; *Belg.:* Skelid; *Fin.:* Skelid; *Fr.:* Skelid; *Ger.:* Skelid; *Neth.:* Skelid; *Spain:* Skelid; *Swed.:* Skelid; *Switz.:* Skelid; *UK:* Skelid; *USA:* Skelid.

Zoledronic Acid (17610-x)

Zoledronic Acid *(BAN, USAN, rINN)*.

CGP-42446. (1-Hydroxy-2-imidazol-1-ylethylidene)diphosphonic acid.

$C_5H_{10}N_2O_7P_2 = 272.1$.

CAS — 118072-93-8 *(anhydrous zoledronic acid); 165800-06-6 (zoledronic acid monohydrate)*.

Zoledronate Disodium (19851-q)

Zoledronate Disodium *(BANM, USAN, rINNM)*.

CGP-42446A. Disodium dihydrogen (1-hydroxy-2-imidazol-1-ylethylidene)diphosphonate tetrahydrate.

$C_5H_8N_2O_7P_2, 4H_2O = 388.1$.

CAS — 165800-07-7.

Zoledronate Trisodium (19852-p)

Zoledronate Trisodium *(BANM, USAN, rINNM)*.

CGP-42446B. Trisodium hydrogen (1-hydroxy-2-imidazol-1-ylethylidene)diphosphonate hydrate (5:2).

$C_5H_7N_2Na_3O_7P_2, 2\frac{1}{2}H_2O = 383.1$.

CAS — 165800-08-8.

Profile
Zoledronate is an aminobisphosphonate (p.748) which is a potent inhibitor of bone resorption. It is used for hypercalcaemia of malignancy, in a single dose of 4 mg administered by intravenous infusion over 15 minutes. The treatment may be repeated if necessary after at least 7 days at a dose of 8 mg. In the USA, however, it is stated that individual doses should not exceed 4 mg, because of the increased risk of adverse renal effects, including renal failure, reported in patients who have received doses of 8 mg. It is also under investigation for various other disorders of increased bone turnover such as Paget's disease of bone and osteoporosis, and for malignancies of bone.

◊ References.

1. Arden-Cordone M, et al. Antiresorptive effect of a single infusion of microgram quantities of zoledronate in Paget's disease of bone. *Calcif Tissue Int* 1997; **60:** 415–18.
2. Body JJ, et al. A dose-finding study of zoledronate in hypercalcemic cancer patients. *J Bone Miner Res* 1999; **14:** 1557–61.
3. Buckler H, et al. Single infusion of zoledronate in Paget's disease of bone: a placebo-controlled, dose-ranging study. *Bone* 1999; **24** (suppl): 81S–85S.
4. Major P, et al. Zoledronic acid is superior to pamidronate in the treatment of hypercalcemia of malignancy: a pooled analysis of two randomised, controlled clinical trials. *J Clin Oncol* 2001; **19:** 558–67.

Preparations
Proprietary Preparations (details are given in Part 3)
Austral.: Zometa; *UK:* Zometa; *USA:* Zometa.

Bronchodilators and Anti-asthma Drugs

This chapter includes many of those drugs used for their bronchodilator or anti-inflammatory properties in the management of reversible airways obstruction, as in asthma and some patients with chronic obstructive pulmonary disease.

The main bronchodilators discussed in this chapter are the sympathomimetic beta agonists (stimulants of beta-adrenoceptors), and the xanthines, primarily theophylline. The antimuscarinic bronchodilators ipratropium and oxitropium are also included. The major class of anti-inflammatory drugs, the corticosteroids, are discussed separately, on p.1039; other drugs considered to act on the processes of airway inflammation and which are included in this section include sodium cromoglicate and its analogues, and the various drugs that act on leukotriene synthesis and receptor binding, on platelet-activating factor (PAF), or on other aspects of the inflammatory cascade.

Anti-asthma Drug Groups

Antimuscarinics. The parasympathetic nervous system plays a role in the regulation of bronchomotor tone, and antimuscarinic drugs have bronchodilator properties. The quaternary ammonium compounds ipratropium bromide (p.766) and oxitropium bromide (p.769) are the main antimuscarinic (anticholinergic) bronchodilators in current use; as well as reduced CNS effects they have less effect on mucociliary clearance than drugs such as atropine, which can produce accumulation of viscid lower airway secretions and a risk of mucus plugging in these patients. An antimuscarinic may be the bronchodilator of choice in the management of chronic obstructive pulmonary disease. In patients with chronic asthma they are usually reserved for addition to the therapy of those who cannot be managed with beta agonists and corticosteroids, and are used in life-threatening acute asthma exacerbations.

Beta agonists. The sympathetic nervous system plays a role in the regulation of bronchomotor tone and beta$_2$-adrenoceptors in bronchial smooth muscle produce bronchodilatation when stimulated. This makes short-acting selective agonists of beta$_2$-adrenoceptors (beta$_2$ agonists; beta$_2$ stimulants), of which salbutamol (p.770) is the paradigmatic example, first-line drugs for the relief of asthma symptoms. They are also widely employed in the management of chronic obstructive pulmonary disease, although antimuscarinic bronchodilators may be preferred or used in addition. Long-acting beta$_2$ agonists are used in patients also requiring anti-inflammatory therapy; their role is less clearly established.

Corticosteroids. Corticosteroids are widely employed for their anti-inflammatory (glucocorticoid) properties in the management of asthma, and may be beneficial in some patients with chronic obstructive pulmonary disease. Because of the potential adverse effects associated with prolonged systemic corticosteroid therapy, inhalation of corticosteroids with reduced systemic activity is widely employed; oral corticosteroids are preferably only employed in short courses, and at relatively low doses, to gain control of the disease. The actions and uses of the corticosteroids are discussed in much greater detail in the section beginning on p.1039.

Leukotriene inhibitors and antagonists. Leukotrienes appear to play an important role in the inflammatory process of asthma, and a number of drugs may modify or inhibit this action. Leukotriene synthesis may be prevented by blockade of the enzyme 5-lipoxygenase with inhibitors such as zileuton (p.786); indirect inhibition by targeting 5-lipoxygenase activating protein (FLAP) is also under investigation. Alternatively, leukotriene antagonists such as zafirlukast (p.785) may be used to block specific receptors (usually those of leukotriene D$_4$) and prevent their activation. The role of such anti-leukotriene drugs in the prophylactic management of asthma is not yet clearly established.

Mast cell stabilisers. The role of the mast cell in initiating an inflammatory cascade has long been recognised as important, and the best established of the mast cell stabilisers are sodium cromoglicate (p.774) and nedocromil sodium (p.768). These compounds inhibit mast cell degranulation in response to antigens or other stimuli, and hence prevent the release of histamine, leukotrienes, and other inflammatory mediators. They are generally well tolerated and guidelines for the treatment of asthma mention their use for prophylactic therapy as an alternative, or a supplement, to corticosteroids, particularly in children. However, it is generally felt that the corticosteroids are more effective.

Xanthines. Xanthines are drugs with complex actions which include, in varying degrees, relaxation of bronchial smooth muscle and relief of bronchospasm, as well as stimulant effects on respiration. Theophylline (p.777) and its derivatives have long been used for their bronchodilator properties in the man-

agement of asthma and chronic obstructive pulmonary disease, but the narrow therapeutic range and the propensity for interactions with other drugs make theophylline a difficult drug to use, and it tends to be reserved for combination therapy in patients who cannot be managed with other bronchodilators (such as the beta$_2$ agonists) alone.

Management of Reversible Airways Obstruction

Asthma

Asthma is a chronic inflammatory disease in which the patient suffers episodes of reversible airways obstruction due to bronchial hyperresponsiveness; in a few patients, inflammation may lead to irreversible obstruction. It is a common disorder occurring in up to 5% of the adult population and perhaps up to 10% of children. Fatalities can occur and mortality rates are reported to be increasing.[1]

The aetiology of asthma is poorly understood, but resistance to airflow is increased by a number of factors, including contraction of the airway smooth muscle, the presence of excessive secretions within the airway lumen, and shedding and thickening of the airway epithelium.[2] Asthma may be described as extrinsic when it is associated with exposure to a specific allergen such as pollen or house-dust mite, or to a non-specific stimulus such as a chemical irritant or exercise. It may be described as intrinsic when no external precipitating factor is identifiable.

The principal symptom of asthma is dyspnoea (breathlessness). Wheezing, cough, and chest tightness are often present[1,3] and these symptoms are often worse at night.[1,3,4] In an acute attack, the respiratory rate is rapid and tachycardia is common. The peak expiratory flow (PEF), maximal mid-expiratory flow (MMEF), and forced expiratory volume in the first second (FEV$_1$) are all decreased in asthma, and in a severe asthmatic attack the PEF and FEV$_1$ are generally less than 50% of predicted values with a MMEF of 10 to 30% of predicted value. Life-threatening features include exhaustion, cyanosis, bradycardia, hypotension, confusion, and coma.[3]

Management of asthma. As asthma is a chronic disease, management involves prophylactic measures to reduce inflammation and airway resistance and to maintain airflow, as well as specific regimens for the treatment of acute attacks. Measurements of lung function play an important part in determining treatment and patients are encouraged to monitor their own disease by using a simple peak flow meter to measure PEF and adjust their therapy accordingly.

The standard drugs employed in the management of asthma are the beta$_2$ agonists and corticosteroids.[1,3,5-7] Therapy is preferably administered by inhalation to deliver the drugs to the desired site of action. This permits smaller dosages than would be required with oral administration, with a consequent reduction in side-effects. Spacer devices can be fitted to some metered-dose inhalers to act as reservoirs for the drug to make it easier for the patient (especially if a child) to inhale each dose correctly. There is a general trend towards the use of metered-dose inhalers with spacer devices rather than nebulisers,[5] although the choice of spacer and the method of use may substantially affect drug delivery.[8,9] A large volume spacer device is recommended for the inhalation of high doses of corticosteroids to reduce oropharyngeal deposition and systemic absorption.[3]

Beta$_2$ agonists relax the bronchial smooth muscle to produce bronchodilatation by selectively stimulating beta$_2$-adrenergic receptors. Short-acting beta$_2$ agonists such as salbutamol or terbutaline are the initial drugs of choice for acute bronchospasm; if inhaled, they can have an almost immediate bronchodilating effect. The epidemics of increased asthma mortality associated with inhaled beta agonists (see under Fenoterol, p.765) receded some time ago and since then the way in which these compounds are used has changed. Doses have fallen and selective agonists are preferred (nonselective beta agonists such as isoprenaline no longer have a role), and there has been a change from regular administration to administration as required. Regular administration of beta$_2$ agonists is mainly restricted to 'long-acting' beta$_2$ agonists such as salmeterol xinafoate in patients also requiring anti-inflammatory prophylactic treatment;[3,5,10] a 'short-acting' beta$_2$ agonist should still be used as required.

Corticosteroids are used for their anti-inflammatory properties and to reduce bronchial hyperresponsiveness; they must be taken regularly to achieve maximum benefit. Corticosteroid therapy is recommended both for acute attacks and chronic asthma prophylaxis. Although the use of corticosteroids for the treatment of acute asthma attacks has been questioned,[11] meta-analysis suggests that they do speed the resolution of exacerbations and reduce the rate of relapse.[12,13]

In addition, *xanthines* such as aminophylline or theophylline, and *antimuscarinics* such as ipratropium bromide or oxitropium bromide may be given for their bronchodilating properties; there is disagreement concerning xanthine administration in addition to bronchodilating therapy with beta$_2$ agonists for the management of acute severe asthma (see below). *Cromoglicate or nedocromil* may be used as an alternative to corticosteroids for the prophylaxis of less severe asthma or in conjunction with other therapy. *Anti-leukotrienes*[14,15] such as zafirlukast and zileuton are now available as another alternative or adjunct to inhaled corticosteroids.

Chronic asthma. Advice for patients with chronic asthma includes avoidance of smoking, of allergens such as pollen, and of bronchoconstricting drugs such as beta blockers. Patients who have had asthma induced by aspirin and NSAIDs should also avoid these drugs. Skin testing to determine allergen sensitivity may be advisable. US guidelines[6] suggest consideration of immunotherapy to desensitise patients with poorly controlled disease unavoidably exposed to a precipitating allergen, but evidence of benefit from this approach is ambiguous, particularly for multiple allergen immunotherapy, and the potential adverse effects make it controversial (see under Hyposensitisation, p.1576). UK guidelines[3] do not recommend immunotherapy for asthma management.[3] Gastro-oesophageal reflux has been suggested as another exacerbating factor, but this has been disputed[16] and a review of acid suppressive therapy concluded this did not benefit asthma in most patients.[17]

Drug therapy for chronic asthma is managed by a stepwise approach depending on the severity of the disease at presentation and its subsequent progression. Guidelines have been issued in the UK by the British Thoracic Society,[3] and subsequently updated;[5] guidelines in the USA have also been recently re-issued and are broadly similar.[6] These guidelines provide for a progressive approach, but now emphasise the importance of obtaining initial control, with the early use of anti-inflammatory drugs, and subsequently 'stepping-down' therapy as far as possible. Treatment strategies for the management of asthma in infants and young children are similar to those outlined for adults and older children though some modifications are usually made.[3,5,6] Some, but not all, authorities prefer to employ cromoglicate or nedocromil before trying low-dose inhaled corticosteroids in mild asthma in children; current guidelines permit initiation of prophylactic therapy with either option.[5,6] Specially adapted or modified inhalation devices are available to enable children to achieve a correct technique when using inhaled drug therapy,[3,5] but alternative routes of delivery such as oral administration or nebulisation may be necessary for some infants and small children.[18]

The recommendations for **adults and children over 5 years of age** with chronic asthma are as follows.

- Patients requiring only occasional relief from symptoms may be adequately managed with an inhaled short-acting beta$_2$ agonist such as salbutamol or terbutaline taken when needed, provided this is not more than once daily (Step 1; mild intermittent asthma).

- If the beta$_2$ agonist is required more than once daily then regular inhalation of a corticosteroid such as beclometasone dipropionate or budesonide (100 to 400 µg twice daily) or fluticasone (50 to 200 µg twice daily) should be added. *Alternatively* cromoglicate or nedocromil could be started with a change to inhaled corticosteroids if this fails to provide control (Step 2; mild persistent asthma).

At this stage, US guidelines permit consideration of sustained-release oral theophylline, or in patients over 12 years of age, the use of zafirlukast or zileuton.

- If adequate control is not achieved, the inhaled corticosteroid dose can be increased to 800 to 2000 µg of beclometasone or budesonide, or 400 to 1000 µg of fluticasone, daily given via a large volume spacer.

Alternatively, inhaled corticosteroids at lower doses may be supplemented by a long-acting inhaled beta₂ agonist such as salmeterol xinafoate (Step 3; moderate persistent asthma).

At this stage there are slight differences of emphasis between US and UK guidelines. *In the USA*, modified-release oral theophylline or a modified-release oral beta₂ agonist preparation may be considered as an alternative to an inhaled long-acting beta₂ agonist, and if necessary such long-acting bronchodilators may be combined with high-dose inhaled corticosteroids. *In the UK*, although oral theophylline and cromoglicate or nedocromil may be added to lower doses of inhaled corticosteroids, combination of the latter at high doses with regular bronchodilators is considered as the next step:

- treatment with high-dose inhaled corticosteroids and inhaled beta₂ agonists is supplemented with one or more of the following bronchodilating drugs: inhaled long-acting beta₂ agonists, modified-release oral theophylline, inhaled antimuscarinics, oral modified-release beta₂ agonists, and high doses of inhaled bronchodilators; cromoglicate or nedocromil may also be given (UK Step 4).
- If further control is needed, then a corticosteroid such as prednisolone may also be given by mouth in single daily doses (UK Step 5; US Step 4; severe persistent asthma).

A short 'rescue' course of oral prednisolone 30 to 60 mg may also be needed at any time and at any step for an acute exacerbation.

Treatment should be reviewed every 3 to 6 months and if the asthma is adequately controlled a stepwise reduction in treatment may be possible.

The UK recommendations[5] for the management of chronic asthma in **children under 5 years of age** are as follows. Treatment should be started at the step most appropriate to the initial severity.

- Step 1 involves the use of a short-acting beta₂ agonist as required, but not more than once daily.
- Should that not provide control, then cromoglicate may be added in a dose of 20 mg three or four times daily as an inhaled powder or 10 mg three times daily via a metered dose inhaler if a large volume spacer is used. *Alternatively*, or if there is no control after 4 to 6 weeks cromoglicate may be replaced by inhaled beclometasone or budesonide in doses up to 400 μg daily, or fluticasone up to 200 μg daily (Step 2).

The dose of inhaled corticosteroid may be doubled initially for stabilisation, or a short course of prednisolone may be added at a dose of 1 to 2 mg per kg body-weight daily for those under 1 year of age and 20 mg daily for those aged 1 to 5 years, for five days. (Recent evidence[19] suggests that lower doses of prednisolone [0.5 mg per kg daily] may be as effective.)

- If further control is necessary, then the dose of inhaled beclometasone or budesonide is increased to 800 μg daily, or that of fluticasone to 500 μg daily, given via a large volume spacer. *In addition* a short course of prednisolone should be considered, as should the addition of an inhaled long-acting beta₂ agonist twice daily or modified-release oral theophylline (Step 3).
- Further increasing the inhaled corticosteroid dose is then recommended; again a short course of prednisolone should be considered, as should the addition of an inhaled long-acting beta₂ agonist or modified-release oral theophylline. Addition of a nebulised beta₂ agonist should also be considered (Step 4).

Treatment should be regularly reviewed and reduced in a stepwise manner if asthma is well controlled.

Acute severe asthma (status asthmaticus). An acute attack of severe asthma is potentially life-threatening and treatment should be instituted as soon as possible. UK guidelines provide guidance on the assessment and initial treatment of exacerbations of asthma in general practice and in the accident and emergency department. Acute severe attacks require admission to hospital, and the guidelines suggest the following regimen for the hospital management of **adults**.[3,5]

- Initially, oxygen should be given at the highest concentration available (40 to 60%) with a high flow rate.
- High doses of inhaled beta₂ agonists, such as salbutamol 5 mg or terbutaline 10 mg, should be administered via a nebuliser with oxygen or compressed air, or if neither of these is available, by multiple actuations of a metered-dose inhaler into a large spacer device.
- High doses of systemic corticosteroids are also required: for example, prednisolone 30 to 60 mg by

mouth or hydrocortisone 200 mg intravenously, or both.

- If life-threatening features are present, ipratropium bromide (0.5 mg) can be added to the nebuliser and aminophylline (250 mg over 20 minutes) or a beta₂ agonist (salbutamol or terbutaline 250 μg over 10 minutes) may be given intravenously. However, aminophylline should not be given to patients already taking oral theophylline.
- Subsequently, oxygen therapy should be continued as should corticosteroid treatment (prednisolone 30 to 60 mg daily by mouth or hydrocortisone 200 mg every 6 hours intravenously).
- Nebulised beta₂ agonists may be given every 4 hours, but if the patient's condition has not improved after 15 to 30 minutes, the nebulised beta₂ agonist should be given more frequently (up to every 15 minutes) and ipratropium bromide (0.5 mg every 6 hours) added.
- If progress is still unsatisfactory, then an infusion of aminophylline (0.5 to 0.9 mg per kg body-weight per hour, monitoring blood concentrations if continued for more than 24 hours), salbutamol (5 μg per minute), or terbutaline (1.5 to 5.0 μg per minute) may be required.
- Patients who deteriorate further with drowsiness, unconsciousness, or respiratory arrest need intermittent positive-pressure ventilation.

Once lung function is stabilised the patient can be discharged taking oral prednisolone, inhaled corticosteroids, inhaled or nebulised beta₂ agonists as required, and oral theophylline, long-acting beta₂ agonists, or inhaled ipratropium bromide as necessary.

UK guidelines suggest the following regimen for **children**.

- Immediate treatment involves the administration of oxygen, nebulised beta₂ agonists, and oral prednisolone (1 to 2 mg per kg daily, to a maximum of 20 mg daily in children aged 1 to 5 years, or 40 mg daily in those aged 5 to 15 years).
- If life-threatening features are present, nebulised ipratropium bromide (0.125 to 0.25 mg), intravenous hydrocortisone (100 mg every 6 hours), and intravenous aminophylline (5 mg per kg over 20 minutes then 1 mg per kg per hour) can be given. Aminophylline should not be used before hospital admission or in children already receiving oral theophylline.

Subsequent management follows a similar routine to that in adults.[5] (Although the guidelines do not suggest the use of intravenous beta₂ agonists in children, a subsequent study[20] has suggested that intravenous salbutamol may be of benefit.)

In the USA guidelines for acute severe asthma are slightly different.[6] Although subcutaneous adrenaline [epinephrine] or terbutaline has been employed in the management of acute severe asthma, the guidelines now suggest that the parenteral use of beta₂ agonists is an unproven treatment. Moreover, in contrast to the UK the intravenous administration of xanthines is not recommended. In compiling the UK guidelines the British Thoracic Society has taken the view that although most patients on maximal doses of nebulised beta₂ agonists derive no additional benefit from intravenous aminophylline, some could obtain more rapid and effective bronchodilatation; intravenous aminophylline was therefore recommended for patients with severe or unresponsive acute asthma attacks;[3] a subsequent trial in children supports this.[21] In contrast, the most recent US guidelines issued by the National Asthma Education and Prevention Program do not recommend the use of xanthines as they are considered to offer no benefit over the optimal use of inhaled beta₂ agonists.[6] In consequence, in the US guidelines patients whose asthma cannot be managed with oxygen, inhaled beta₂ agonists and antimuscarinics, and systemic corticosteroids are suggested as candidates for intubation and mechanical ventilation. The UK guidelines acknowledge that not all studies have demonstrated additional benefit with the use of ipratropium; a subsequent meta-analysis[22] and further large trial[23] concluded that the addition of multiple doses of nebulised antimuscarinics to beta agonists was effective in reducing hospital admissions in children and adolescents with severe exacerbations. In a study in children specifically with mild to moderate asthma exacerbation, there was no additional benefit from the addition of nebulised ipratropium.[24] A further meta-analysis indicated that ipratropium also provides modest benefits in lung function in adults with acute asthma exacerbation.[25]

Investigational therapy. A number of other therapeutic approaches for the management of asthma are currently under investigation.[26] Immunomodulators such as methotrexate, ciclosporin, and gold have been used for their anti-inflammatory, immunosuppressant, and corticosteroid-sparing properties: their use must be balanced against their potentially serious adverse effects and they are therefore reserved for individual patients with chronic severe asthma dependent on systemic corticosteroid therapy.[27]

Interestingly, frusemide [furosemide] administered by oral inhalation has been found to protect against bronchoconstriction induced by exercise[28] and external stimuli,[29,30] but was not effective in improving bronchial hyperresponsiveness in a 4-week study;[31] any clinical application has yet to be determined.[26]

Results of clinical studies of intravenous magnesium in acute asthma have been conflicting; a meta-analysis concluded that its routine use was not justified, but that it may benefit some patients with severe exacerbations.[32] There has been some interest in heparin given by inhalation,[26,33] and nebulised lignocaine [lidocaine] may be of some benefit;[26,34] intravenous lignocaine [lidocaine] or oral mexiletine have been shown to block reflex bronchoconstriction.[35]

At a molecular level, bronchodilatation involves an increase in intracellular cyclic adenosine monophosphate (cAMP) and a reduction in the cytosolic calcium ion concentration. Selective phosphodiesterase inhibitors have been used to inhibit the breakdown of cAMP and are being investigated.[26] Potassium channel activators such as cromakalim[36] have also been investigated. Other studies have concentrated on antagonising the various mediators of asthma using platelet-activating factor (PAF) antagonists, thromboxane inhibitors, neurokinin antagonists, and mast cell tryptase inhibitors.[26] Anti-IgE therapies, such as the monoclonal antibody omalizumab,[37] are being studied in allergen-induced asthma.

In patients with acute severe asthma, in whom respiratory muscle fatigue can lead to ventilatory failure, use of helium-oxygen mixture, which has a lower density than air and can reduce turbulent flow and respiratory work, may be beneficial.[38]

Pregnancy. It is particularly important that asthma should be well controlled during pregnancy; where this is achieved asthma has no important effects on pregnancy, labour, or the fetus.

Inhalation has particular advantages as a means of drug administration during pregnancy because the therapeutic action can be achieved without the need for plasma drug concentrations liable to have a pharmacological effect on the fetus.

Severe exacerbations can have an adverse effect on pregnancy and should be treated promptly with conventional therapy, including oral or parenteral administration of corticosteroids and nebulisation of a selective beta₂ agonist. UK authorities advise that prednisolone is the preferred corticosteroid for oral use since very little of the drug reaches the fetus.

1. McFadden ER, Gilbert IA. Asthma. *N Engl J Med* 1992; **327**: 1928–37. Correction. *ibid.* 1993; **328**: 1640–1.
2. Barnes PJ. Pathophysiology of asthma. *Br J Clin Pharmacol* 1996; **42**: 3–10.
3. British Thoracic Society, *et al.* Guidelines on the management of asthma. *Thorax* 1993; **48** (suppl): S1–S24. Correction. *ibid.* 1994; **49**: 386. (Summary published in *BMJ* 1993; **306**: 776–82. Correction. *ibid.* 307: 1054.)
4. Catterall JR, Shapiro CM. Nocturnal asthma. *BMJ* 1993; **306**: 1189–92.
5. British Thoracic Society, *et al.* The British guidelines on asthma management: 1995 review and position statement. *Thorax* 1997; **52** (suppl 1): S1–S21. Comment. *ibid.*; 932.
6. National Asthma Education and Prevention Program. *Expert Panel Report 2: guidelines for the diagnosis and management of asthma.* Bethesda: National Heart, Lung, and Blood Institute, 1997.
7. Lipworth BJ. Modern drug treatment of chronic asthma. *BMJ* 1999; **318**: 380–4.
8. Bisgaard H. Drug delivery from inhaler devices. *BMJ* 1996; **313**: 895–6. Correction. *ibid.* 1997; **314**: 990.
9. O'Callaghan C, Barry P. Spacer devices in the treatment of asthma. *BMJ* 1997; **314**: 1061–2.
10. Boulet L-P. Long- versus short-acting β₂-agonists: implications for drug therapy. *Drugs* 1994; **47**: 207–22.
11. McFadden ER, Hejal R. Asthma. *Lancet* 1995; **345**: 1215–20.
12. Rowe BH, *et al.* Effectiveness of steroid therapy in acute exacerbations of asthma: a meta-analysis. *Am J Emerg Med* 1992; **10**: 301–10.
13. Rowe BH, *et al.* Corticosteroids for preventing relapse following acute exacerbations of asthma (updated 30 July 2001). Available in The Cochrane Library; Issue 4. Oxford: Update Software; 2001.
14. Drazen JM, *et al.* Treatment of asthma with drugs modifying the leukotriene pathway. *N Engl J Med* 1999; **340**: 197–206. Correction. *ibid.*; 663.
15. Lipworth BJ. Leukotriene-receptor antagonists. *Lancet* 1999; **353**: 57–62.

16. Field SK. A critical review of the studies of the effects of simulated or real gastroesophageal reflux on pulmonary function in asthmatic adults. *Chest* 1999; **115:** 848–56.
17. Gibson PG, *et al.* Gastro-oesophageal reflux treatment for asthma in adults and children (updated 30 July 2001). Available in the Cochrane Library; Issue 4. Oxford: Update Software; 2001.
18. Warner JO, *et al.* Asthma: a follow up statement from an international paediatric asthma consensus group. *Arch Dis Child* 1992; **67:** 240–8.
19. Langton Hewer S, *et al.* Prednisolone in acute childhood asthma: clinical responses to three dosages. *Respir Med* 1998; **92:** 541–6.
20. Browne GJ, *et al.* Randomised trial of intravenous salbutamol in early management of acute severe asthma in children. *Lancet* 1997; **349:** 301–5.
21. Yung M, South M. Randomised controlled trial of aminophylline for severe acute asthma. *Arch Dis Child* 1998; **79:** 405–10.
22. Plotnick LH, Ducharme FM. Should inhaled anticholinergics be added to β_2 agonists for treating acute childhood and adolescent asthma? A systematic review. *BMJ* 1998; **317:** 971–7.
23. Qureshi F, *et al.* Effect of nebulized ipratropium on the hospitalization rates of children with asthma. *N Engl J Med* 1998; **339:** 1030–5.
24. Ducharme FM, Davis GM. Randomized controlled trial of ipratropium bromide and frequent low doses of salbutamol in the management of mild and moderate acute pediatric asthma. *J Pediatr* 1998; **133:** 479–85.
25. Stoodley RG, *et al.* The role of ipratropium bromide in the emergency management of acute asthma exacerbation: a metaanalysis of randomized clinical trials. *Ann Emerg Med* 1999; **34:** 8–18.
26. Floreani AA, Rennard SI. Experimental treatments for asthma. *Curr Opin Pulm Med* 1997; **3:** 30–41.
27. Kon OM, Barnes N. Immunosuppressive treatment in asthma. *Br J Hosp Med* 1997; **57:** 383–6.
28. Munyard P, *et al.* Inhaled frusemide and exercise-induced bronchoconstriction in children with asthma. *Thorax* 1995; **50:** 677–9.
29. Bianco S, *et al.* Protective effect of inhaled furosemide on allergen-induced early and late asthmatic reactions. *N Engl J Med* 1989; **321:** 1069–73.
30. Seidenberg J, *et al.* Inhaled frusemide against cold air induced bronchoconstriction in asthmatic children. *Arch Dis Child* 1992; **67:** 214–17.
31. Yates DH, *et al.* Effect of acute and chronic inhaled furosemide on bronchial hyperresponsiveness in mild asthma. *Am J Respir Crit Care Med* 1995; **152:** 2173–5.
32. Rowe BH, *et al.* Magnesium sulfate for treating exacerbations of acute asthma in the emergency department (updated 30 July 2001). Available in The Cochrane Library; Issue 4. Oxford: Update Software; 2001.
33. Diamant Z, *et al.* Effect of inhaled heparin on allergen-induced early and late asthmatic responses in patients with atopic asthma. *Am J Respir Crit Care Med* 1996; **153:** 1790–5.
34. Hunt LW, *et al.* Effect of nebulized lidocaine on severe glucocorticoid-dependent asthma. *Mayo Clin Proc* 1996; **71:** 361–8.
35. Groeben H, *et al.* Intravenous lidocaine and oral mexiletine block reflex bronchoconstriction in asthmatic subjects. *Am J Respir Crit Care Med* 1996; **154:** 885–8.
36. Williams AJ, *et al.* Attenuation of nocturnal asthma by cromakalim. *Lancet* 1990; **336:** 334–6.
37. Easthope S, Jarvis B. Omalizumab. *Drugs* 2001; **61:** 253–60.
38. Kudukis TM, *et al.* Inhaled helium-oxygen revisited: effect of inhaled helium-oxygen during the treatment of status asthmaticus in children. *J Pediatr* 1997; **130:** 217–24.

Chronic obstructive pulmonary disease

Chronic obstructive pulmonary disease (COPD, chronic obstructive lung disease, chronic obstructive airways disease) covers a range of disorders of progressive airflow limitation including chronic bronchitis and emphysema. Unlike asthma, the obstruction of airflow, indicated by an abnormal decline in the forced expiratory volume in one second (FEV_1), is more or less continuous and largely irreversible. Chronic obstructive pulmonary disease is a common disorder, frequently associated with cigarette smoking; infections, environmental pollution, and occupational dust exposure may also have an aetiological role.

In *chronic bronchitis* there is enlargement of the mucous glands and an increase in the number of goblet cells within the bronchial mucosa which leads to an increase in mucus production and thickening of the bronchial wall. Patients suffer from a chronic productive cough with excessive sputum production. They may also experience dyspnoea, bronchospasm, and frequent respiratory-tract infections. In severe cases (chronic obstructive bronchitis, small airways disease), irreversible narrowing of the airways leads to a disabling condition in which there is cyanosis, hypoxia, hypercapnia, and right-sided heart failure (cor pulmonale, see below); such patients have been described as 'blue bloaters'.

Emphysema is an abnormal permanent enlargement of air spaces distal to the terminal bronchioles accompanied by destruction of the alveolar wall and without obvious fibrosis. There is excessive airway collapse upon expiration and irreversible airways obstruction. Dyspnoea is a prominent symptom; a productive cough, wheezing, recurrent respiratory infection, and a marked loss of weight may also be noted. Patients may hyperventilate to maintain oxygen levels in the blood and have been called 'pink puffers' in contrast to the 'blue bloaters' of the classic bronchitic presentation. Rarely, emphysema can be caused by a hereditary deficiency of alpha$_1$ antitrypsin (alpha$_1$-proteinase inhibitor), see p.1577.

Patients with severe COPD can develop *cor pulmonale* (heart disease secondary to disease of the lungs and respiratory system) with pulmonary hypertension, right ventricular hypertrophy, and right heart failure.[1] Cor pulmonale is more often associated with chronic bronchitis than with emphysema.

Management of COPD. Although there is less consensus than for asthma, guidelines for the treatment of COPD have been issued in a number of countries.[2-6] The most important therapeutic intervention is encouraging those patients who smoke to stop; psychological support and adjunctive drug therapy may be required (see Smoking Cessation, p.1642). Prevention of respiratory infection should be considered, and influenza and pneumococcal vaccination are recommended,[3,6-8] although the value of pneumococcal vaccination in these patients has not been unequivocally established.[6,7]

Drug treatment is primarily symptomatic and palliative using bronchodilators, corticosteroids, and oxygen therapy. Purulent sputum indicates a respiratory infection (see under Exacerbations, below).

First-line drug therapy for the treatment of COPD consists of bronchodilators to alleviate bronchospasm and any reversible component of the airways obstruction. Either an inhaled *antimuscarinic*, such as ipratropium bromide, or a short-acting *beta$_2$ agonist*, is suggested as the initial bronchodilator.[2-6] UK guidelines recommend beginning with a beta$_2$ agonist, because of their more rapid action,[5] but there is some suggestion that antimuscarinics are slightly more effective than beta$_2$ agonists in this group of patients.[3,7] Patients vary in their responsiveness and a beta$_2$ agonist should be tried in those who do not respond well to an antimuscarinic, and vice versa.[4] Some patients benefit further from combined therapy;[2,5,9] US guidelines suggest addition of an inhaled short-acting beta$_2$ agonist to ipratropium, on an 'as needed' basis.[3] The role of longer-acting beta$_2$ agonists such as salmeterol has yet to be clearly established, but some consider that they may have a role in maintenance, particularly in the prevention of nocturnal symptoms.[6] A *xanthine* such as theophylline by mouth may also be considered and has been given in addition to inhaled agents.[2-6,9] Theophylline has been reported to improve respiratory muscle function in patients with COPD and may have positive cardiac inotropic effects which could be of value in cor pulmonale.

Meta-analysis suggests that only about 10% of COPD patients receiving optimal bronchodilator therapy exhibit a substantial further response to oral *corticosteroids*.[10] It is recommended that patients requiring frequent bronchodilator therapy should receive a trial of prednisolone 30 to 40 mg daily by mouth for 2 weeks; an increase in FEV_1 of more than 15% from baseline is considered evidence of responsiveness.[5,6] In patients showing an objective response, guidelines suggest the continued use of corticosteroids, preferably by the inhaled route[5] as this is associated with fewer adverse effects. One 6-month study[11] has reported a trend towards a reduction in exacerbations of COPD with inhaled corticosteroid therapy. However, whether corticosteroids improve the long-term outcome of COPD remains to be confirmed. An analysis[12] of data from 3 small studies suggested that inhaled corticosteroids may reduce the decline in FEV_1. However, recent evidence from larger studies in patients without significant bronchodilator[13] or corticosteroid[14,15] responsiveness suggests that standard- or high-dose inhaled corticosteroids have limited benefits in terms of decline in FEV_1, and alternative treatments are needed.[16]

In patients with severe COPD and persistent hypoxaemia, supplemental *oxygen* provided on an almost continuous long-term basis at home has been found to improve survival and alleviate complications such as cor pulmonale, polycythaemia and neuropsychological impairment.[17,18] Guidelines recommend the institution of oxygen therapy in patients whose resting PaO_2 is less than 55 mmHg (about 7.3 kPa), or whose arterial oxygen saturation is less than about 90%.[2,3,5,6] Non-invasive nocturnal ventilation (via a mask) may be of benefit in some patients.[7,19] Lung transplantation (p.504) may be considered in a small number of patients with end-stage disease.[5] In patients with severe emphysema and marked air trapping, lung volume reduction surgery is being investigated.[5]

The use of *mucolytics* or *expectorants* is controversial,[2,6] although meta-analysis has suggested a modest benefit in reducing exacerbations,[20] and some guidelines allow for their use.[6] Initially promising results with dornase alfa have not been borne out in later study.[8] Improved pulmo-

nary function has been reported in patients given aerosolised surfactant.[21]

Investigational approaches to COPD include blocking various mediators of the inflammatory processes with, for example, inhibitors of phosphodiesterase, neutrophil elastase, and matrix metalloproteinases.[22]

Exacerbations. Patients with COPD frequently suffer acute exacerbations of their symptoms, and may require hospitalisation. Treatment options include maximal bronchodilators, antibacterials, systemic corticosteroids, and oxygen as necessary, together with appropriate management of any associated cardiovascular disorder.[5,23,24] Systemic corticosteroids are widely used, despite limited evidence of clinical benefit. Studies[25,26] of severe acute exacerbation requiring hospitalisation have found systemic corticosteroids to improve lung function and reduce the length of hospital stay. However, the most effective dose and duration of treatment is yet to be established, although one study[25] found that a 2-week course was as effective as a longer course of 8 weeks. There is also no evidence of long-term benefit.[25,26] The use of *antibacterials* for acute exacerbations has long been controversial, but meta-analysis suggests that a modest benefit exists,[27] mainly in patients with more severe disease (see also Bronchitis, p.116). Guidelines recommend their use on an empirical basis where signs of infection are present;[4,5,23] it has been suggested that in patients with only mild exacerbations they can be withheld until the patient deteriorates or fails to improve.[6] The use of prophylactic antibacterial cover for those with recurrent acute exacerbations is even more controversial, but US guidelines have suggested that prolonged courses of antibacterials may be appropriate, particularly in winter.[3] Oxygen therapy is required in patients with hypoxia; the goal is to maintain oxygen saturation above 90% but prevent increasing CO_2 retention. Relatively low oxygen concentrations (beginning at about 25%) are advised in these generally hypercapnic patients, as high concentrations may impair ventilation and respiratory drive.[3,5] *Respiratory stimulants* such as doxapram are of limited use but may be considered in the short term for certain patients.[5] Despite intensive therapy, some patients progress to respiratory muscle fatigue and require ventilatory support.

1. Palevsky HI, Fishman AP. Chronic cor pulmonale: etiology and management. *JAMA* 1990; **263:** 2347–53.
2. Canadian Thoracic Society Workshop Group. Guidelines for the assessment and management of chronic obstructive pulmonary disease. *Can Med Assoc J* 1992; **147:** 420–8.
3. American Thoracic Society. Standards for the diagnosis and care of patients with chronic obstructive pulmonary disease. *Am J Respir Crit Care Med* 1995; **152** (suppl): S77–S120.
4. Siafakas NM, *et al.* ERS consensus statement: optimal assessment and management of chronic obstructive pulmonary disease (COPD). *Eur Respir J* 1995; **8:** 1398–1420.
5. British Thoracic Society. BTS Guidelines for the management of chronic obstructive pulmonary disease. *Thorax* 1997; **52** (suppl 5): S1–S28.
6. Leuenberger P, *et al.* Management 1997 of chronic obstructive pulmonary disease. *Schweiz Med Wochenschr* 1997; **127:** 766–82.
7. Chapman KR. Therapeutic approaches to chronic obstructive pulmonary disease: an emerging consensus. *Am J Med* 1996; **100** (suppl 1A): 5S–10S.
8. Fiel SB. Chronic obstructive pulmonary disease: mortality and mortality reduction. *Drugs* 1996; **52** (suppl 2): 55–61.
9. Karpel JP, *et al.* A comparison of inhaled ipratropium, oral theophylline plus inhaled beta-agonist, and the combination of all three in patients with COPD. *Chest* 1994; **105:** 1089–94.
10. Callahan CM, *et al.* Oral corticosteroid therapy for patients with stable chronic obstructive pulmonary disease. *Ann Intern Med* 1991; **114:** 216–23.
11. Paggiaro PL, *et al.* Multicentre randomised placebo-controlled trial of inhaled fluticasone propionate in patients with chronic obstructive pulmonary disease. *Lancet* 1998; **351:** 773–80. Correction. *ibid.*; 1968.
12. van Grunsven PM, *et al.* Long term effects of inhaled corticosteroids in chronic obstructive pulmonary disease: a meta-analysis. *Thorax* 1999; **54:** 7–14.
13. Pauwels RA, *et al.* Long-term treatment with inhaled budesonide in persons with mild chronic obstructive pulmonary disease who continue smoking. *N Engl J Med* 1999; **340:** 1948–53.
14. Bourbeau J, *et al.* Randomised controlled trial of inhaled corticosteroids in patients with chronic obstructive pulmonary disease. *Thorax* 1998; **53:** 477–82.
15. Vestbo J, *et al.* Long-term effect of inhaled budesonide in mild and moderate chronic obstructive pulmonary disease: a randomised controlled trial. *Lancet* 1999; **353:** 1819–23.
16. Bruge PS. EUROSCOP, ISOLDE and the Copenhagen City Lung Study. *Thorax* 1999; **54:** 287–8.
17. Medical Research Council Working Party. Long-term domiciliary oxygen therapy in chronic hypoxic cor pulmonale complicating chronic bronchitis and emphysema. *Lancet* 1981; **i:** 681–6.
18. Nocturnal Oxygen Therapy Trial Group. Continuous or nocturnal oxygen therapy in hypoxemic chronic obstructive lung disease: a clinical trial. *Ann Intern Med* 1980; **93:** 391–8.
19. Elliott MW. Non-invasive ventilation in chronic obstructive pulmonary disease. *Br J Hosp Med* 1997; **57:** 83–6.
20. Poole PJ, Black PN. Mucolytic agents for chronic bronchitis (updated 30 July 2001). Available in The Cochrane Library; Issue 4. Oxford: Update Software; 2001.

21. Anzueto A, *et al.* Effects of aerosolized surfactant in patients with stable chronic bronchitis: a prospective randomized controlled trial. *JAMA* 1997; **278:** 1426–31.
22. Barnes PJ. New therapies for chronic obstructive pulmonary disease. *Thorax* 1998; **53:** 137–47.
23. Snow V, *et al.* Evidence base for management of acute exacerbations of chronic obstructive pulmonary disease. *Ann Intern Med* 2001; **134:** 595–9.
24. Madison JM, Irwin RS. Chronic obstructive pulmonary disease. *Lancet* 1998; **352:** 467–73.
25. Niewoehner DE, *et al.*. Effect of systemic glucocorticoids on exacerbations of chronic obstructive pulmonary disease. *N Engl J Med* 1999; **340:** 1941–7.
26. Davies L, *et al.* Oral corticosteroids in patients admitted to hospital with exacerbations of chronic obstructive pulmonary disease: a prospective randomised controlled trial. *Lancet* 1999; **354:** 456–60.
27. Saint S, *et al.* Antibiotics in chronic obstructive pulmonary disease exacerbations: a meta-analysis. *JAMA* 1995; **273:** 957–60.

Aminophylline (3873-a)

Aminophylline *(BAN, pINN)*.

Aminofilina; Aminophyllin; Euphyllinum; Metaphyllin; Theophyllaminum; Theophylline and Ethylenediamine; Theophylline Ethylenediamine Compound; Theophyllinum et Ethylenediaminum. A mixture of theophylline and ethylenediamine (2:1), its composition approximately corresponding to the formula below.

$(C_7H_8N_4O_2)_2, C_2H_4(NH_2)_2 = 420.4$.
CAS — 317-34-0 (anhydrous aminophylline).
ATC — R03DA05.

Pharmacopoeias. In *Eur.* (see p.vi), *Int.*, and *US*. Some pharmacopoeias include anhydrous and hydrated aminophylline in one monograph. Some pharmacopoeias do not specify the hydration state.

Solutions should not be allowed to come into contact with metals.

Pharmacopoeial description

Ph. Eur.: Theophylline-ethylenediamine contains 84.0 to 87.4% of anhydrous theophylline and 13.5 to 15.0% of anhydrous ethylenediamine. A white or slightly yellowish powder, sometimes granular. Freely soluble in water (the solution becomes cloudy through absorption of carbon dioxide); practically insoluble in dehydrated alcohol. Store in airtight containers. Protect from light.

USP 25: Aminophylline is anhydrous or contains not more than two molecules of water of hydration. It contains not less than 84.0 and not more than 87.4% of anhydrous theophylline. It consists of white or slightly yellowish granules or powder, having a slight ammoniacal odour. Upon exposure to air it gradually loses ethylenediamine and absorbs carbon dioxide with the liberation of theophylline. One g dissolves in 25 mL of water to give a clear solution; 1 g dissolved in 5 mL of water crystallises upon standing, but redissolves when a small amount of ethylenediamine is added; insoluble in alcohol and in ether. Its solutions are alkaline to litmus. Store in airtight containers.

Aminophylline Hydrate (628-b)

Aminophylline Hydrate *(BANM, pINNM)*.

$(C_7H_8N_4O_2)_2, C_2H_4(NH_2)_2, 2H_2O = 456.5$.
CAS — 49746-06-7 (aminophylline dihydrate).

Pharmacopoeias. In *Chin.*, *Eur.* (see p.vi), *Jpn*, *Pol.*, and *US*. Some pharmacopoeias include anhydrous and hydrated aminophylline in one monograph. Some pharmacopoeias do not specify the hydration state.

Aminophylline hydrate 1.09 mg is approximately equivalent to 1 mg of aminophylline.

Solutions should not be allowed to come into contact with metals.

Pharmacopoeial description

Ph. Eur.: Theophylline-ethylenediamine hydrate contains 84.0 to 87.4% of anhydrous theophylline and 13.5 to 15.0% of anhydrous ethylenediamine. A white or slightly yellowish powder, sometimes granular. Freely soluble in water (the solution becomes cloudy through absorption of carbon dioxide); practically insoluble in dehydrated alcohol. Store in well-filled airtight containers. Protect from light.

USP 25: Aminophylline is anhydrous or contains not more than two molecules of water of hydration. It contains not less than 84.0 and not more than 87.4% of anhydrous theophylline. It consists of white or slightly yellowish granules or powder, having a slight ammoniacal odour. Upon exposure to air it gradually loses ethylenediamine and absorbs carbon dioxide with the liberation of theophylline. One g dissolves in 25 mL of water to give a clear solution; 1 g dissolved in 5 mL of water crystallises upon standing, but redissolves when a small amount of ethylenediamine is added; insoluble in alcohol and in ether. Its solutions are alkaline to litmus. Store in airtight containers.

Incompatibility. Solutions of aminophylline are alkaline and if the pH falls below 8, crystals of theophylline will deposit.[1] Drugs known to be unstable in alkaline solutions, or that would

lower the pH below the critical value, should not be mixed with aminophylline.

1. Edward M. pH—an important factor in the compatibility of additives in intravenous therapy. *Am J Hosp Pharm* 1967; **24:** 440–9.

Adverse Effects, Treatment, and Precautions

As for Theophylline, p.777. Hypersensitivity has been associated with the ethylenediamine content.

Porphyria. Aminophylline is considered to be unsafe in patients with porphyria because it has been shown to be porphyrinogenic in *animals* or *in-vitro* systems.

Interactions

As for Theophylline, p.779.

Pharmacokinetics

Aminophylline, a complex of theophylline with ethylenediamine, readily liberates theophylline in the body. The pharmacokinetics of theophylline are discussed on p.782.

◊ Studies in healthy subjects suggested that ethylenediamine does not affect the pharmacokinetics of theophylline after oral or intravenous administration.[1,2]

1. Aslaksen A, *et al.* Comparative pharmacokinetics of theophylline and aminophylline in man. *Br J Clin Pharmacol* 1981; **11:** 269–73.
2. Caldwell J, *et al.* Theophylline pharmacokinetics after intravenous infusion with ethylenediamine or sodium glycinate. *Br J Clin Pharmacol* 1986; **22:** 351–5.

Uses and Administration

Aminophylline has the actions and uses of theophylline (see p.783) and is used similarly as a bronchodilator in the management of asthma (p.757) and chronic obstructive pulmonary disease (p.759). Aminophylline is also used to relieve apnoea in neonates. It was formerly used in heart failure, and may occasionally have a role in patients with this condition who are also suffering from obstructive airways disease. Aminophylline is usually preferred to theophylline when greater solubility in water is required, particularly in intravenous formulations.

Aminophylline may be given in the anhydrous form or as the hydrate, and doses may be expressed as either. The USP 25 specifies that aminophylline preparations should be labelled with respect to their anhydrous *theophylline* content. As the pharmacokinetics of theophylline are affected by a number of factors including age, smoking, disease, diet, and drug interactions, the dose of aminophylline must be carefully individualised and serum-theophylline concentrations monitored (see under Uses and Administration of Theophylline, p.783).

In the management of **acute severe bronchospasm**, aminophylline may be administered intravenously by slow injection or infusion. To reduce adverse effects, the rate of intravenous administration of aminophylline should not exceed 25 mg per minute. In patients who have not been taking aminophylline, theophylline, or other xanthine-containing medication, 250 to 500 mg of aminophylline (25 mg per mL) may be given by slow intravenous injection over 20 minutes. When administered by infusion, a suggested loading dose is 5 mg per kg ideal (lean) body-weight given over 20 to 30 minutes, followed by a maintenance dose of 0.5 mg per kg per hour. Older patients and those with cor pulmonale, heart failure, or liver disease may require lower maintenance doses; smokers often need higher maintenance doses. A loading dose may not be considered necessary unless the patient's condition is deteriorating. Children (also not currently on xanthine medication) may be given the same loading dose per kg as adults; suggested maintenance doses are 1 mg per kg per hour for children aged 6 months to 9 years and 0.8 mg per kg per hour for children aged 10 to 16 years. Some authorities suggest that the maintenance doses should be slightly higher for the first 12 hours of the infusion in both adults and children.

Intravenous aminophylline is best avoided in patients already taking theophylline, aminophylline, or other xanthine-containing medication but, if considered

necessary, the serum-theophylline concentration should first be assessed and the initial loading dose should be calculated on the basis that each 0.6 mg per kg of aminophylline (equivalent to 0.5 mg per kg theophylline) will increase serum theophylline concentration by 1 µg per mL.

In the treatment of **acute bronchospasm** that does not require intravenous therapy, aminophylline has been given by mouth in conventional dosage forms; modified-release preparations are not suitable. Doses used have generally ranged from 100 to 300 mg three or four times daily after food.

In the management of **chronic bronchospasm** aminophylline may be given by mouth as conventional or as modified-release preparations. The modified-release products are generally preferred and a usual dose is aminophylline hydrate 225 to 450 mg twice daily by mouth. Therapy should be initiated with the lower dose and increased as appropriate. Retitration of the dosage is required if the patient is changed from one modified-release preparation to another as the bioavailability of modified-release aminophylline preparations may vary. Children (over 3 years) have been given modified-release aminophylline hydrate in doses of 12 mg per kg body-weight daily, increased after 1 week to 24 mg per kg daily, in 2 divided doses.

Intramuscular administration of aminophylline causes intense local pain and is not recommended.

Aminophylline has also been used as the hydrochloride.

Administration. RECTAL ADMINISTRATION. Absorption from aminophylline suppositories is erratic and this dose form has been associated with toxicity, hence the warnings that suppositories should not be used especially in children. In the UK suppositories are no longer readily available and one hospital wishing to use the rectal route for apnoea in premature infants (see Neonatal Apnoea, p.784) achieved therapeutic plasma-theophylline concentrations with a specially formulated rectal gel.[1]

1. Cooney S, *et al.* Rectal aminophylline gel in treatment of apnoea in premature newborn babies. *Lancet* 1991; **337:** 1351.

Methotrexate neurotoxicity. For reference to the use of aminophylline or theophylline to relieve the acute neurotoxicity of methotrexate, see p.554.

Reduction of body fat. Discussion of the cosmetic use of aminophylline cream to remove fat ('cellulite') from the thighs.[1] Concern has been raised about the potential for topical sensitisation with this use.[2]

1. Dickinson BI, Gora-Harper ML. Aminophylline for cellulite removal. *Ann Pharmacother* 1996; **30:** 292–3.
2. Simon PA. Comment: aminophylline-containing cream. *Ann Pharmacother* 1996; **30:** 1341.

Preparations

BP 2001: Aminophylline Injection; Aminophylline Tablets;
USP 25: Aminophylline Delayed-release Tablets; Aminophylline Rectal Solution; Aminophylline Injection; Aminophylline Oral Solution; Aminophylline Suppositories; Aminophylline Tablets.

Proprietary Preparations (details are given in Part 3)
Aust.: Euphyllin; Mundiphyllin; *Braz.:* Asmodrin; Eufilin; *Canad.:* Phyllocontin; *Denm.:* Teofylamin; *Fin.:* Aminocont; Theophyllaminum; *Fr.:* Planphylline†; *Ger.:* Afonilum†; Phyllotemp; *Hong Kong:* Phyllocontin; *Irl.:* Clonofilin; Phyllocontin; *Israel:* Elixophyllin; *Ital.:* Aminomal; Euphyllina; Tefamin; *Mex.:* Drafilyn Z; *Neth.:* Euphyllin; *Port.:* Filotempo; *S.Afr.:* Peterphyllin; Phyllocontin; *Switz.:* Aminomal; Escophylline; Euphyllin; Phyllotemp; *UK:* Amnivent; Norphyllin SR; Pecram†; Phyllocontin; *USA:* Phyllocontin†; Truphylline.

Multi-ingredient: *Aust.:* Asthma-Hilfe; Euphyllin-Calcium†; Limptar; Myocardon; *Braz.:* Alergo Filinal; Alergotox; Alergotox Expectorante; Dispneitrat; Teodrin; *Ger.:* Limptar; *Hong Kong:* Asmeton; *Port.:* Anti-Asmatico; Fluidin Antiasmatico; *S.Afr.:* Amesec†; Daral†; Diphenamill; Efcod†; Fabasma†; Lotussin Expectorant; Medikasma†; Panasma†; Repasma†; *Spain:* Angiosedante; Lasa Antiasmatico†; *Switz.:* Limptar†; *Thai.:* Asmeton; *USA:* Emergent-Ez; Mudrane; Mudrane GG; Mudrane GG-2.

Amlexanox (2893-j)

Amlexanox *(BAN, USAN, rINN)*.

AA-673; Amoxanox; CHX-3673. 2-Amino-7-isopropyl-5-oxo-5*H*-[1]benzopyrano[2,3-b]pyridine-3-carboxylic acid.
$C_{16}H_{14}N_2O_4 = 298.3$.
CAS — 68302-57-8.
ATC — R03DX01.

Profile

Amlexanox has a stabilising action on mast cells resembling that of sodium cromoglicate (p.774) and is also a leukotriene inhibitor. It is administered by mouth in the management of asthma (p.757) and for allergic rhinitis (p.407); a dose of 25 or 50 mg three times daily has been suggested. Amlexanox is also given as a metered-dose nasal spray for allergic rhinitis.

Amlexanox is also applied as a 5% oral paste four times daily in the management of aphthous ulcers (p.1206).

Preparations

Proprietary Preparations (details are given in Part 3)
Jpn: Solfa; *USA:* Aphthasol.

Apafant (3658-e)

Apafant (USAN, rINN).
WEB-2086; WEB-2086-BS. 4-{3-[4-(o-Chlorophenyl)-9-methyl-6H-thieno[3,2-f]-s-triazolo[4,3-a][1,4]diazepin-2-yl]propionyl}morpholine.
$C_{22}H_{22}ClN_5O_2S = 456.0.$
CAS — 105219-56-5.

Profile
Apafant is a platelet-activating factor antagonist that has been investigated for the prophylactic management of asthma. It has been tried in other conditions, including acute pancreatitis.

◊ References.
1. Brecht HM, et al. Pharmacodynamics, pharmacokinetics and safety profile of the new platelet-activating factor antagonist apafant in man. Arzneimittelforschung 1991; 41: 51–9.

Asthma. In a study involving 106 patients with stable atopic asthma, apafant 40 mg by mouth three times daily was no more effective than placebo in reducing the requirement for inhaled corticosteroids.[1] It was concluded that these negative results, at a dose known to produce active concentrations in the airways, cast doubt upon the role of platelet-activating factor in the pathogenesis of asthma (p.757).
1. Spence DPS, et al. The effect of the orally active platelet-activating factor antagonist WEB 2086 in the treatment of asthma. Am J Respir Crit Care Med 1994; 149: 1142–8.

Bambuterol Hydrochloride (18825-x)

Bambuterol Hydrochloride (BANM, rINNM).
KWD-2183. (RS)-5-(2-tert-Butylamino-1-hydroxyethyl)-m-phenylene bis(dimethylcarbamate) hydrochloride.
$C_{18}H_{29}N_3O_5,HCl = 403.9.$
CAS — 81732-65-2 (bambuterol); 81732-46-9 (bambuterol monohydrochloride).
Pharmacopoeias. In Eur. (see p.vi).

Pharmacopoeial description
Ph. Eur.: A white or almost white crystalline powder. It exhibits polymorphism. Freely soluble in water; soluble in alcohol.

Adverse Effects and Precautions
As for Salbutamol, p.770. Bambuterol is not recommended for patients with severe hepatic impairment as its metabolism would be unpredictable. It is unsuitable for the relief of acute bronchospasm or in patients with unstable respiratory disease.

Effects on the heart. A prescription event monitoring study found an excess risk of non-fatal heart failure in elderly patients receiving bambuterol, particularly in the first month of treatment.[1] See also under Salbutamol, p.771.
1. Martin RM, et al. Risk of non-fatal cardiac failure and ischaemic heart disease with long acting β_2 agonists. Thorax 1998; 53: 558–62.

Interactions
As for Salbutamol, p.771. Bambuterol inhibits plasma cholinesterases and can prolong the action of drugs such as suxamethonium (see Sympathomimetics, under Suxamethonium, p.1342) that are inactivated by these enzymes.

Pharmacokinetics
Nearly 20% of a dose of bambuterol is absorbed from the gastrointestinal tract following oral administration. It is slowly metabolised in the body to its active metabolite, terbutaline; peak terbutaline concentrations are reported to occur about 4 to 7 hours after a dose of bambuterol as tablets. The slow rate at which metabolism occurs determines the prolonged duration of action of bambuterol of at least 24 hours. Hydrolysis of bambuterol to terbutaline and carbamic acid leads to inhibition of plasma-cholinesterase activity that can be correlated with plasma concentrations of terbutaline. For the metabolism and excretion of terbutaline, see p.776.

◊ References.
1. Sitar DS. Clinical pharmacokinetics of bambuterol. Clin Pharmacokinet 1996; 31: 246–56.
2. Nyberg L, et al. Pharmacokinetics of bambuterol in healthy subjects. Br J Clin Pharmacol 1998; 45: 471–8.
3. Bang U, et al. Pharmacokinetics of bambuterol in subjects homozygous for the atypical gene for plasma cholinesterase. Br J Clin Pharmacol 1998; 45: 479–84.

Uses and Administration
Bambuterol is an inactive prodrug of terbutaline (p.776), a direct-acting sympathomimetic with predominantly beta-adrenergic activity and a selective action on beta$_2$ receptors (a beta$_2$ agonist). It has similar actions to those of salbutamol (p.772) except that it has a more prolonged duration of action (at least 24 hours). Bambuterol hydrochloride is used as a long-acting bronchodilator for persistent reversible airways obstruction in conditions such as asthma (p.757). The usual dose is 10 to 20 mg by mouth once daily at bedtime; starting doses should be halved in patients with moderate or severe renal impairment.

The symbol † denotes a preparation no longer actively marketed

◊ References.
1. Fugleholm AM, et al. Therapeutic equivalence between bambuterol, 10 mg once daily, and terbutaline controlled release, 5 mg twice daily, in mild to moderate asthma. Eur Respir J 1993; 6: 1474–8.
2. Gunn SD, et al. Comparison of the efficacy, tolerability and patient acceptability of once-daily bambuterol tablets against twice-daily controlled release salbutamol in nocturnal asthma. Eur J Clin Pharmacol 1995; 48: 23–8.

Preparations
Proprietary Preparations (details are given in Part 3)
Aust.: Bambec; *Denm.:* Bambec; *Fr.:* Oxeol; *Ger.:* Bambec; *Hong Kong:* Bambec; *Ital.:* Bambec; *Norw.:* Bambec; *NZ:* Bambec; *Singapore:* Bambec; *Spain:* Bambec; *Swed.:* Bambec; *Switz.:* Bambec; *Thai.:* Bambec; *UK:* Bambec.

Bamifylline Hydrochloride (629-v)

Bamifylline Hydrochloride (BANM, USAN, rINNM).
AC-3810; BAX-2739Z; CB-8102. 8-Benzyl-7-[2-(N-ethyl-N-2-hydroxyethylamino)ethyl]theophylline hydrochloride.
$C_{20}H_{27}N_5O_3,HCl = 421.9.$
CAS — 2016-63-9 (bamifylline); 20684-06-4 (bamifylline hydrochloride).

Profile
Bamifylline hydrochloride is a xanthine derivative (see Theophylline, p.777) which is used for its bronchodilator properties in reversible airways obstruction. It is given by mouth in usual doses of 600 or 900 mg daily. It is also given rectally as suppositories, and by slow intravenous infusion.

Preparations
Proprietary Preparations (details are given in Part 3)
Belg.: Trentadil; *Braz.:* Bamifix; *Fr.:* Trentadil; *Ital.:* Airest; Bamifix; Bamixol; Briofil.

Bitolterol Mesilate (12447-p)

Bitolterol Mesilate (BANM, rINNM).
Bitolterol Mesylate (USAN). Win-32784. 4-[2-(tert-Butylamino)-1-hydroxyethyl]-o-phenylene di-p-toluate methanesulphonate.
$C_{28}H_{31}NO_5,CH_4O_3S = 557.7.$
CAS — 30392-40-6 (bitolterol); 30392-41-7 (bitolterol mesilate).

Profile
Bitolterol is an inactive prodrug which is hydrolysed in the body to colterol, a direct-acting sympathomimetic with predominantly beta-adrenergic activity and a selective action on beta$_2$ receptors (a beta$_2$ agonist). It has similar properties to those of salbutamol (p.770).

It is used as a bronchodilator in the management of diseases with reversible airways obstruction such as asthma (p.757) or in some patients with chronic obstructive pulmonary disease (p.759); administration by inhalation results in the rapid onset of bronchodilatation (2 to 4 minutes) with a duration of action of 5 or more hours.

Bitolterol is given by inhalation via a metered-dose aerosol supplying 370 μg of bitolterol mesilate per inhalation. For the relief of bronchospasm the usual adult dose is 2 inhalations (740 μg) followed by a third inhalation (370 μg) if required. For the prevention of bronchospasm the usual adult dose is 2 inhalations (740 μg) every 8 hours. Maximum doses have been stated to be 3 inhalations (1110 μg) every 6 hours or 2 inhalations (740 μg) every 4 hours. In patients with asthma, as-required beta agonist therapy is preferable to regular use. An increased need for, or decreased duration of effect of, bitolterol indicates deterioration of asthma control and the need for review of therapy.

Alternatively, a 0.2% inhalation solution of bitolterol mesilate may be given by nebulisation.

Preparations
Proprietary Preparations (details are given in Part 3)
Ital.: Asmalene; *USA:* Tornalate.

Broxaterol (18872-b)

Broxaterol (rINN).
Z-1170. (±)-3-Bromo-α-[(tert-butylamino)methyl]-5-isoxazolemethanol.
$C_9H_{15}BrN_2O_2 = 263.1.$
CAS — 76596-57-1.

Profile
Broxaterol is a direct-acting sympathomimetic with predominantly selective beta-adrenergic activity on beta$_2$ receptors (a beta$_2$ agonist). It has similar properties to those of salbutamol (p.770). It has been investigated as a bronchodilator by mouth and by inhalation.

◊ References.
1. Casali L, et al. A comparison of the bronchodilator effects of broxaterol and salbutamol. Int J Clin Pharmacol Ther Toxicol 1988; 26: 93–7.

2. Robuschi M, et al. Dose-response curve of the bronchodilating effect of broxaterol inhaled by patients with reversible airway obstruction. Curr Ther Res 1988; 43: 725–33.
3. Ziment I. Broxaterol: therapeutic trials and safety profile. Respiration 1989; 55 (suppl 2): 28–40.
4. Robuschi M, et al. The protective effect of transdermal broxaterol on exercise-induced bronchoconstriction. Eur J Clin Pharmacol 1995; 47: 465–6.

Bufylline (630-r)

Bufylline (BAN).
Ambuphylline (USAN); Theophylline-aminoisobutanol. 2-Amino-2-methylpropan-1-ol theophyllinate.
$C_{11}H_{19}N_5O_3 = 269.3.$
CAS — 5634-34-4.
ATC — R03DA10.

Profile
Bufylline is a theophylline derivative (p.777), which has been used for its bronchodilator effects as an ingredient of preparations promoted for coughs and other respiratory-tract disorders. The ethiodide has also been used.

Preparations
Proprietary Preparations (details are given in Part 3)
Multi-ingredient: *Braz.:* Bronco-Ped; Broncolex; EMS Expectorante; Revenil; Reveníl Dospan; Reveníl Expectorante; *S.Afr.:* Nethaprin Dospan; Nethaprin Expectorant.

Caffeine (621-x)

Caffeine (BAN).
Anhydrous Caffeine; Caféine; Coffeinum; Guaranine; Methyltheobromine; Théine. 1,3,7-Trimethylpurine-2,6(3H,1H)-dione; 1,3,7-Trimethylxanthine; 7-Methyltheophylline.
$C_8H_{10}N_4O_2 = 194.2.$
CAS — 58-08-2.
ATC — N06BC01.

NOTE. Compounded preparations of caffeine may be represented by the following names:
• Co-bucafAPAP (USP 25)—butalbital, paracetamol, and caffeine.
Pharmacopoeias. In Eur. (see p.vi), Int., Jpn, Pol., and US. Some pharmacopoeias include caffeine and caffeine hydrate under one monograph.

Pharmacopoeial description
Ph. Eur.: A white crystalline powder or silky white crystals. It sublimes readily. Sparingly soluble in water; freely soluble in boiling water; slightly soluble in dehydrated alcohol and in ether. It dissolves in concentrated solutions of alkali benzoates or salicylates.
USP 25: Caffeine is anhydrous or contains one molecule of water of hydration. An odourless white powder or white, glistening needles, usually matted together. The hydrate is efflorescent in air. The hydrate is soluble 1 in 50 of water, 1 in 75 of alcohol, 1 in 6 of chloroform, and 1 in 600 of ether. The hydrate should be stored in airtight containers.

Caffeine Citrate (626-h)

Caffeine Citrate (BANM).
Citrated Caffeine; Coffeinum Citricum.
$C_8H_{10}N_4O_2,C_6H_8O_7 = 386.3.$
CAS — 69-22-7.
Pharmacopoeias. In Aust.

Caffeine Hydrate (622-r)

Caffeine Hydrate (BANM).
Caffeine Monohydrate; Coffeinum Monohydricum.
$C_8H_{10}N_4O_2,H_2O = 212.2.$
CAS — 5743-12-4.
Pharmacopoeias. In Chin., Eur. (see p.vi), Int., Jpn, Pol., and US. Some pharmacopoeias include caffeine and caffeine hydrate under one monograph.

Pharmacopoeial description
Ph. Eur.: A white crystalline powder or silky white crystals. It sublimes readily. Sparingly soluble in water; freely soluble in boiling water; slightly soluble in dehydrated alcohol and in ether. It dissolves in concentrated solutions of alkali benzoates or salicylates.
USP 25: Caffeine is anhydrous or contains one molecule of water of hydration. An odourless white powder or white, glistening needles, usually matted together. The hydrate is efflorescent in air. The hydrate is soluble 1 in 50 of water, 1 in 75 of alcohol, 1 in 6 of chloroform, and 1 in 600 of ether. The hydrate should be stored in airtight containers.

Stability. References to the stability of caffeine and caffeine citrate.
1. Eisenberg MG, Kang N. Stability of citrated caffeine solutions for injectable and enteral use. Am J Hosp Pharm 1984; 41: 2405–6.
2. Nahata MC, et al. Stability of caffeine injection in intravenous admixtures and parenteral nutrition solutions. DICP Ann Pharmacother 1989; 23: 466–7.

3. Hopkin C, et al. Stability study of caffeine citrate. Br J Pharm Pract 1990; 12: 133.
4. Donnelly RF, Tirona RG. Stability of citrated caffeine injectable solution in glass vials. Am J Hosp Pharm 1994; 51: 512–14.

Adverse Effects, Treatment, and Precautions

As for Theophylline, p.777.

Prolonged high intake of caffeine may lead to tolerance of some of the pharmacological actions and physical signs of withdrawal including irritability, lethargy, and headache may occur if intake is discontinued abruptly.

◊ General references.
1. Wills S. Drugs and substance misuse: caffeine. Pharm J 1994; 252: 822–4.
2. Fredholm BB, et al. Actions of caffeine in the brain with special reference to factors that contribute to its widespread use. Pharmacol Rev 1999; 51: 83–133.

Effects on the heart. For a discussion of the effects of caffeine-containing beverages on cardiovascular risk factors, see p.1681.

Effects on mental function. A report of 6 cases of excessive daytime sleepiness associated with high caffeine intake.[1]
1. Regestein QR. Pathologic sleepiness induced by caffeine. Am J Med 1989; 87: 586–8.

Overdosage. Reports and reviews of caffeine toxicity.
1. Kulkarni PB, Dorand RD. Caffeine toxicity in a neonate. Pediatrics 1979; 64: 254–5.
2. Banner W, Czajka PA. Acute caffeine overdose in the neonate. Am J Dis Child 1980; 134: 495–8.
3. Zimmerman PM, et al. Caffeine intoxication: a near fatality. Ann Emerg Med 1985; 14: 1227–9.
4. Dalvi RR. Acute and chronic toxicity of caffeine: a review. Vet Hum Toxicol 1986; 28: 144–50.
5. Rivenes SM, et al. Intentional caffeine poisoning in an infant. Pediatrics 1997; 99: 736–8.

Pregnancy. In the USA, the FDA has advised pregnant women to limit their intake of caffeine and caffeine-containing beverages to a minimum, but this recommendation was based largely on animal studies and the effect of caffeine on the human fetus and fetal loss during pregnancy is controversial.[1] Although some studies found no evidence that moderate caffeine use increased the risk of spontaneous abortion,[2,3] others have reported conflicting results.[4,5] There is some evidence for an effect on fetal growth, but again it is not clear that this applies generally: a prospective population-based study in the UK found that a decreased birth-weight with increased caffeine intake was only significant in smokers.[6] The authors of this study concurred that a reduction in caffeine intake during pregnancy would be prudent, together with stopping smoking. An association between high maternal caffeine intake during pregnancy and an increased risk of the sudden infant death syndrome has also been reported,[7] although another study found no such association.[8]
1. Eskenazi B. Caffeine during pregnancy: grounds for concern? JAMA 1993; 270: 2973–4.
2. Mills JL, et al. Moderate caffeine use and the risk of spontaneous abortion and intrauterine growth retardation. JAMA 1993; 269: 593–7.
3. Klebanoff MA, et al. Maternal serum paraxanthine, a caffeine metabolite, and the risk of spontaneous abortion. N Engl J Med 1999; 341: 1639–44.
4. Infante-Rivard C, et al. Fetal loss associated with caffeine intake before and during pregnancy. JAMA 1993; 270: 2940–3.
5. Cnattingius S, et al. Caffeine intake and the risk of first-trimester spontaneous abortion. N Engl J Med 2000; 343: 1839–45.
6. Cook DG, et al. Relation of caffeine intake and blood caffeine concentrations during pregnancy to fetal growth: prospective population based study. BMJ 1996; 313: 1358–62.
7. Ford RPK, et al. Heavy caffeine intake in pregnancy and sudden infant death syndrome. Arch Dis Child 1998; 78: 9–13.
8. Alm B, et al. Caffeine and alcohol as risk factors for sudden infant death syndrome. Arch Dis Child 1999; 81: 107–11.

Sport. The International Olympic Committee has banned the use of large amounts of caffeine by athletes but smaller amounts, compatible with a moderate intake of coffee or soft drinks, are permitted.[1] The concentration of caffeine in the urine should not exceed 12 μg per mL.[2] However, because of the marked interindividual variation in urine-caffeine concentrations, even a modest caffeine intake equivalent to 3 to 6 cups of coffee daily, may give a urine concentration in excess of the permissible limit.[3]
1. Anonymous. Drugs in the Olympics. Med Lett Drugs Ther 1984; 26: 65–6.
2. MacAuley D. Drugs in sport. BMJ 1996; 313: 211–15.
3. Birkett DJ, Miners JO. Caffeine renal clearance and urine caffeine concentrations during steady state dosing: implications for monitoring caffeine intake during sports events. Br J Clin Pharmacol 1991; 31: 405–8.

Withdrawal. Headache is a recognised symptom of caffeine withdrawal and even subjects who drink moderate amounts of coffee can develop headaches lasting 1 to 6 days when switched to a decaffeinated brand.[1] It has also been suggested that postoperative headache could be attributed to caffeine withdrawal as fasting patients are required to abstain from drinking tea or coffee before surgical procedures. Several studies[2-4] have found a positive association between postoperative headache and daily caffeine consumption, although there have also been negative findings.[5] A prospective study suggest-

ed that prophylactic intravenous administration of caffeine on the day of surgery reduced the likelihood of postoperative headache in patients at risk of caffeine withdrawal.[6]
1. van Dusseldorp M, Katan MB. Headache caused by caffeine withdrawal among moderate coffee drinkers switched from ordinary to decaffeinated coffee: a 12 week double blind trial. BMJ 1990; 300: 1558–9.
2. Galletly DC, et al. Does caffeine withdrawal contribute to postanaesthetic morbidity? Lancet 1989; i: 1335.
3. Weber JG, et al. Perioperative ingestion of caffeine and postoperative headache. Mayo Clin Proc 1993; 68: 842–5.
4. Nikolajsen L, et al. Effect of previous frequency of headache, duration of fasting and caffeine abstinence on perioperative headache. Br J Anaesth 1994; 72: 295–7.
5. Verhoeff FH, Millar JM. Does caffeine contribute to postoperative morbidity? Lancet 1990; 336: 632.
6. Weber JG, et al. Prophylactic intravenous administration of caffeine and recovery after ambulatory surgical procedures. Mayo Clin Proc 1997; 72: 621–6.

Interactions

Like theophylline (see p.779) caffeine undergoes extensive metabolism by hepatic microsomal cytochrome P450, and is subject to numerous interactions with other drugs and substances which enhance or reduce its metabolic clearance.

Alcohol. In a study of 8 healthy subjects given alcohol by mouth in a dose of 2.2 mL per kg body-weight, caffeine 150 mg by mouth did not antagonise the central effects of alcohol and, instead, a synergistic interaction occurred which further increased reaction time. The common practice of drinking coffee after drinking alcohol in order to sober up is not supported by these results.[1] Another study[2] found that some antagonism of the central effects of alcohol was produced by caffeine, although there was no reversal of subjective sensations of drunkenness; however, the dose of caffeine in this study (400 mg) was considerably higher.
1. Oborne DJ, Rogers Y. Interactions of alcohol and caffeine on human reaction time. Aviat Space Environ Med 1983; 54: 528–34.
2. Azcona O, et al. Evaluation of the central effects of alcohol and caffeine interaction. Br J Clin Pharmacol 1995; 40: 393–400.

Antiarrhythmics. In 7 healthy subjects and 5 patients with cardiac arrhythmias, mexiletine in a single dose of 200 mg or a dose of 600 mg daily respectively, reduced the elimination of caffeine by 30 to 50%.[1] Lignocaine [lidocaine], flecainide, and tocainide had no effect on caffeine elimination in healthy subjects.[1]
1. Joeres R, Richter E. Mexiletine and caffeine elimination. N Engl J Med 1987; 317: 117.

Antibacterials. Caffeine elimination half-life has been reported to be increased and clearance decreased by the concomitant administration of ciprofloxacin,[1-3] enoxacin,[2,3] and pipemidic acid,[2,3] whereas lomefloxacin,[4] norfloxacin,[2,3] and ofloxacin[2,3] had little or no effect on these parameters. Enoxacin had the greatest inhibitory effect on caffeine clearance.[2,3]
1. Healy DP, et al. Interaction between oral ciprofloxacin and caffeine in normal volunteers. Antimicrob Agents Chemother 1989; 33: 474–8.
2. Harder S, et al. Ciprofloxacin-caffeine: a drug interaction established using in vivo and in vitro investigations. Am J Med 1989; 87 (suppl 5A): 89–91S.
3. Barnett G, et al. Pharmacokinetic determination of relative potency of quinolone inhibition of caffeine disposition. Eur J Clin Pharmacol 1990; 39: 63–9.
4. Healy DP, et al. Lack of interaction between lomefloxacin and caffeine in normal volunteers. Antimicrob Agents Chemother 1991; 35: 660–4.

Antiepileptics. The mean clearance of caffeine was increased and its half-life decreased in epileptic patients taking phenytoin compared with healthy controls, resulting in lower plasma-caffeine concentrations. Treatment with carbamazepine or valproic acid had no effect on the pharmacokinetics of caffeine.[1]
1. Wietholtz H, et al. Effects of phenytoin, carbamazepine, and valproic acid on caffeine metabolism. Eur J Clin Pharmacol 1989; 36: 401–6.

Antifungals. In a single-dose study in healthy subjects, terbinafine 500 mg by mouth decreased the clearance and increased the elimination half-life of caffeine 3 mg per kg body-weight given intravenously. Ketoconazole 400 mg by mouth did not prolong the elimination of caffeine to a significant extent.[1]
1. Wahlländer A, Paumgartner G. Effect of ketoconazole and terbinafine on the pharmacokinetics of caffeine in healthy volunteers. Eur J Clin Pharmacol 1989; 37: 279–83.

Antigout drugs. In a study in 2 healthy subjects, the plasma half-life of caffeine was essentially unchanged by 7 days' treatment with allopurinol 300 mg or 600 mg daily by mouth. However, allopurinol caused a specific, dose-dependent inhibition of the conversion of 1-methylxanthine to 1-methyluric acid.[1]
1. Grant DM, et al. Effect of allopurinol on caffeine disposition in man. Br J Clin Pharmacol 1986; 21: 454–8.

Gastrointestinal drugs. Cimetidine 1 g daily by mouth reduced the systemic clearance of caffeine and prolonged its elimination half-life in 5 healthy subjects. Although the steady-state plasma-caffeine concentration would increase by approximately 70%, it was thought unlikely that this would produce adverse clinical effects.[1] However, in contrast a study in 11 children given cimetidine in doses of 11 to 36 mg per kg body-

weight daily for gastritis found no evidence that it altered the metabolism of a dose of ^{13}C-labelled caffeine.[2]
1. Broughton LJ, Rogers HJ. Decreased systemic clearance of caffeine due to cimetidine. Br J Clin Pharmacol 1981; 12: 155–9.
2. Parker AC, et al. Lack of inhibitory effect of cimetidine on caffeine metabolism in children using the caffeine breath test. Br J Clin Pharmacol 1997; 43: 467–70.

Lithium. For mention of the effect of caffeine on serum-lithium concentrations, see Xanthines, p.296.

Oral contraceptives. The clearance of caffeine has been reported to be reduced and its elimination half-life increased in women taking oral contraceptives.[1-3] This interaction was thought to be due to impairment of hepatic metabolism of caffeine by sex hormones and could result in increased accumulation of caffeine.
1. Patwardhan RV, et al. Impaired elimination of caffeine by oral contraceptive steroids. J Lab Clin Med 1980; 95: 603–8.
2. Abernethy DR, Todd EL. Impairment of caffeine clearance by chronic use of low-dose oestrogen-containing oral contraceptives. Eur J Clin Pharmacol 1985; 28: 425–8.
3. Balogh A, et al. Influence of ethinylestradiol-containing combination oral contraceptives with gestodene or levonorgestrel on caffeine elimination. Eur J Clin Pharmacol 1995; 48: 161–6.

Sympathomimetics. Administration of caffeine 400 mg with phenylpropanolamine 75 mg, both given orally as modified-release preparations, produced greater plasma-caffeine concentrations in healthy subjects than administration of caffeine alone. Greater increases in blood pressure and more reports of physical side-effects occurred after the combination than after either drug alone.[1]
1. Lake CR, et al. Phenylpropanolamine increases plasma caffeine levels. Clin Pharmacol Ther 1990; 47: 675–85.

Theophylline. For the effect of caffeine on the metabolism and elimination of theophylline, see p.781.

Pharmacokinetics

Caffeine is absorbed readily after oral administration and is widely distributed throughout the body. It is also absorbed through the skin. Absorption following rectal administration by suppository may be slow and erratic. Absorption following intramuscular injection may be slower than after oral administration. Caffeine passes readily into the CNS and into saliva; low concentrations are also present in breast milk. Caffeine crosses the placenta.

In adults, caffeine is metabolised almost completely in the liver via oxidation, demethylation, and acetylation, and is excreted in the urine as 1-methyluric acid, 1-methylxanthine, 7-methylxanthine, 1,7-dimethylxanthine (paraxanthine), 5-acetylamino-6-formylamino-3-methyluracil (AFMU), and other metabolites with only about 1% unchanged. Neonates have a greatly reduced capacity to metabolise caffeine and it is largely excreted unchanged in the urine until hepatic metabolism becomes significantly developed, usually by about 6 months of age. Elimination half-lives are approximately 3 to 7 hours in adults but may be in excess of 100 hours in neonates.

Breast feeding. Studies examining the transfer of caffeine into breast milk after doses of 35 to 336 mg of caffeine by mouth have recorded peak maternal plasma concentrations of 2.4 to 4.7 μg per mL, peak maternal saliva concentrations of 1.2 to 9.2 μg per mL, and peak breast-milk concentrations of 1.4 to 7.2 μg per mL. At these concentrations in breast milk, the calculated daily caffeine ingestion by breast-fed infants ranged from 1.3 to 3.1 mg, which was not thought to present a hazard, although irritability and a poor sleeping pattern have been reported.[1-4]
1. Tyrala EE, Dodson WE. Caffeine secretion into breast milk. Arch Dis Child 1979; 54: 787–800.
2. Hildebrandt R, et al. Transfer of caffeine to breast milk. Br J Clin Pharmacol 1983; 15: 612P.
3. Sagraves R, et al. Pharmacokinetics of caffeine in human breast milk after a single oral dose of caffeine. Drug Intell Clin Pharm 1984; 18: 507.
4. Berlin CM, et al. Disposition of dietary caffeine in milk, saliva, and plasma of lactating women. Pediatrics 1984; 73: 59–63.

Metabolism and excretion. The metabolism of caffeine has been shown to be dose dependent[1,2] with clearance decreasing as the dose is increased suggesting saturable metabolism. Four- to fivefold differences in plasma half-lives of caffeine are common among healthy people. The plasma half-life of caffeine is decreased by smoking[3] and by exercise,[4] and is increased by liver disease such as cirrhosis and viral hepatitis,[3,5] and in pregnancy.[3] The plasma half-life of caffeine is not affected by old age[6] or obesity.[7] Drug interactions also affect the pharmacokinetics of caffeine (see above).
1. Cheng WSC, et al. Dose-dependent pharmacokinetics of caffeine in humans: relevance as a test of quantitative liver function. Clin Pharmacol Ther 1990; 47: 516–24.
2. Denaro CP, et al. Dose-dependency of caffeine metabolism with repeated dosing. Clin Pharmacol Ther 1990; 48: 277–85.

3. Kalow W. Variability of caffeine metabolism in humans. *Arznei-mittelforschung* 1985; **35**: 319–24.
4. Collomp K, *et al.* Effects of moderate exercise on the pharma-cokinetics of caffeine. *Eur J Clin Pharmacol* 1991; **40**: 279–82.
5. Scott NR, *et al.* The pharmacokinetics of caffeine and its dimeth-ylxanthine metabolites in patients with chronic liver disease. *Br J Clin Pharmacol* 1989; **27**: 205–13.
6. Blanchard J, Sawers SJA. Comparative pharmacokinetics of caf-feine in young and elderly men. *J Pharmacokinet Biopharm* 1983; **11**: 109–26.
7. Abernethy DR, *et al.* Caffeine disposition in obesity. *Br J Clin Pharmacol* 1985; **20**: 61–6.

Uses and Administration

Caffeine is a methylxanthine which, like theophylline (p.783), inhibits the enzyme phosphodiesterase and has an antagonistic effect at central adenosine recep-tors. It is a stimulant of the CNS, particularly the higher centres, and it can produce a condition of wakefulness and increased mental activity. It may also stimulate the respiratory centre, increasing the rate and depth of respiration. Its bronchodilating properties are weaker than those of theophylline. Caf-feine facilitates the performance of muscular work and increases the total work which can be performed by a muscle. The diuretic action of caffeine is weaker than that of theophylline.

Caffeine is used as a mild CNS stimulant in usual dos-es of 50 to 100 mg by mouth, although doses of up to 200 mg may be used. A total dose of 1 g daily should not be exceeded. It is also frequently included in oral analgesic preparations with aspirin, paracetamol, or codeine in unit doses of about 15 to 65 mg but its clin-ical benefit is debated (see Pain, below). It is some-times given with ergotamine in preparations for the treatment of migraine, usually in unit doses of 100 mg. Caffeine citrate has been used similarly.

Caffeine is also used in the short-term treatment of neonatal apnoea of prematurity (p.784). An initial dose for caffeine citrate is 20 mg per kg body-weight (equivalent to 10 mg per kg caffeine), followed by a maintenance dose of caffeine citrate 5 mg per kg daily. These doses are given either orally or by intra-venous infusion. Serum concentrations of caffeine should be measured before starting treatment in infants who have already been treated with theophyl-line (which is metabolised to caffeine in infants) or whose mothers consumed caffeine before delivery; serious toxicity has been associated with serum con-centrations greater than 50 μg per mL.

Caffeine and sodium benzoate and caffeine and sodi-um salicylate are readily soluble in water and have been used for the administration of caffeine by injec-tion. Caffeine and sodium iodide (iodocaffeine) was formerly used in a similar manner.

Beverages of coffee, tea, and cola provide active dos-es of caffeine (see p.1681).

◊ General references.
1. Sawynok J. Pharmacological rationale for the clinical use of caf-feine. *Drugs* 1995; **49**: 37–50.

Asthma. Caffeine's bronchodilating activity is about 40% that of theophylline[1] and doses of 5 or 10 mg per kg body-weight by mouth have been shown to produce an effect.[2,3] Because of its weak action other xanthines are generally recommended in asthma (p.757), but it may need to be avoided before tests of lung function.[4]
1. Gong H, *et al.* Bronchodilator effects of caffeine in coffee: a dose-response study of asthmatic subjects. *Chest* 1986; **89**: 335–42.
2. Becker AB, *et al.* The bronchodilator effects and pharmacokinet-ics of caffeine in asthma. *N Engl J Med* 1984; **310**: 743–6.
3. Bukowskyj M, Nakatsu K. The bronchodilator effect of caffeine in adult asthmatics. *Am Rev Respir Dis* 1987; **135**: 173–5.
4. Bara AI, Barley EA. Caffeine for asthma (updated 30 July 2001). Available in The Cochrane Library; Issue 4. Oxford: Update Software; 2001.

Diagnosis and testing. Caffeine excretion assessed by meas-uring its urinary metabolites or by the exhalation of labelled CO_2 in breath following administration of ^{13}C- or ^{14}C-labelled caffeine has been used to develop liver function tests and to determine the activity of specific enzymes such as xanthine ox-idase, P450 cytochromes, and polymorphic N-acetyltrans-ferase.[1]

Caffeine administered orally has been used to assess acetylator status by determining the metabolic ratio of the metabolites 5-acetylamino-6-formylamino-1-methyluracil (AFMU) to 1-methylxanthine in urine,[2] but some have questioned its value.[3]
1. Kalow W, Tang B-K. The use of caffeine for enzyme assays: a critical appraisal. *Clin Pharmacol Ther* 1993; **53**: 503–14.

2. Hildebrand M, Seifert W. Determination of acetylator phenotype in caucasians with caffeine. *Eur J Clin Pharmacol* 1989; **37**: 525–6.
3. Notarianni LJ, *et al.* Caffeine as a metabolic probe: NAT2 phe-notyping. *Br J Clin Pharmacol* 1996; **41**: 169–73.

ECT. In patients whose seizure duration is declining despite maximal ECT stimulation, pretreatment with high-dose intra-venous caffeine increases seizure duration without affecting seizure threshold. Theophylline has been used similarly, see p.779.
References.
1. Hinkle PE, *et al.* Use of caffeine to lengthen seizures in ECT. *Am J Psychiatry* 1987; **144**: 1143–8.
2. Coffey CE, *et al.* Caffeine augmentation of ECT. *Am J Psychia-try* 1990; **147**: 579–85.
3. Kelsey MC, Grossberg GT. Safety and efficacy of caffeine-aug-mented ECT in elderly depressives: a retrospective study. *J Ger-iatr Psychiatry Neurol* 1995; **8**: 168–72.

Hypoglycaemia. A single dose of caffeine 250 mg proved beneficial in augmenting warning symptoms and physiological responses to experimentally-induced hypoglycaemia in diabet-ic patients,[1] and was suggested as a potentially useful treatment for diabetics who have difficulty in recognising the onset of hy-poglycaemia (p.318).
1. Debrah K, *et al.* Effect of caffeine on recognition of and physio-logical responses to hypoglycaemia in insulin-dependent diabe-tes. *Lancet* 1996; **347**: 19–24.

Orthostatic hypotension. Caffeine has been of benefit in the treatment of orthostatic hypotension (p.1070) due to auto-nomic failure in some patients, especially for postprandial hy-potension.[1-3] However, efficacy has only been demonstrated in mild cases and it is usually ineffective in severe cases.[4]
1. Onrot J, *et al.* Hemodynamic and humoral effects of caffeine in autonomic failure. *N Engl J Med* 1985; **313**: 549–54.
2. Hoeldtke RD, *et al.* Treatment of orthostatic hypotension with dihydroergotamine and caffeine. *Ann Intern Med* 1986; **105**: 168–73.
3. Tonkin AL. Postural hypotension. *Med J Aust* 1995; **162**: 436–8.
4. Mathias CJ. Orthostatic hypotension. *Prescribers' J* 1995; **35**: 124–32.

Pain. Caffeine has been widely used in analgesic preparations to enhance the effects of both non-opioid and opioid analgesics but is of debatable benefit (see under Choice of Analgesic, p.2). Some investigators have failed to show that caffeine offers any benefit[1,2] but others have shown that the adjuvant use of caf-feine can increase analgesic activity.[3-7] A meta-analysis of 10 studies comparing paracetamol plus caffeine with paracetamol alone in women with postpartum uterine cramp found any ben-efit of the combination to be minimal.[8]

Whether caffeine enhances the gastrointestinal absorption of ergotamine is not clear.

In the UK it is generally recommended that caffeine-containing analgesic preparations should not be used not only because of doubts about caffeine enhancing the analgesic effect but be-cause it can add to gastrointestinal adverse effects and in large doses can itself cause headache.
1. Winter L, *et al.* A double-blind, comparative evaluation of aceta-minophen, caffeine, and the combination of acetaminophen and caffeine in outpatients with post-operative oral surgery pain. *Curr Ther Res* 1983; **33**: 115–22.
2. Sawynok J. Pharmacological rationale for the clinical use of caf-feine. *Drugs* 1995; **49**: 37–50.
3. Laska EM, *et al.* Caffeine as an analgesic adjuvant. *JAMA* 1984; **251**: 1711–18.
4. Rubin A, Winter L. A double-blind randomized study of an aspi-rin/caffeine combination versus acetaminophen/aspirin combi-nation versus acetaminophen versus placebo in patients with moderate to severe post-partum pain. *J Int Med Res* 1984; **12**: 338–45.
5. Schachtel BP, *et al.* Caffeine as an analgesic adjuvant: a double-blind study comparing aspirin with caffeine to aspirin and place-bo in patients with sore throat. *Arch Intern Med* 1991; **151**: 733–7.
6. Migliardi JR, *et al.* Caffeine as an analgesic adjuvant in tension headache. *Clin Pharmacol Ther* 1994; **56**: 576–86.
7. Kraetsch HG, *et al.* Analgesic effects of propyphenazone in com-parison to its combination with caffeine. *Eur J Clin Pharmacol* 1996; **49**: 377–82.
8. Zhang WY, Li Wan Po A. Analgesic efficacy of paracetamol and its combination with codeine and caffeine in surgical pain—a meta-analysis. *J Clin Pharm Ther* 1996; **21**: 261–82.

POST-DURAL PUNCTURE HEADACHE. Intravenous caffeine sodium benzoate may relieve post-dural puncture headache (p.1303) which persists despite conservative therapy.

Preparations

BP 2001: Aspirin and Caffeine Tablets;
USP 25: Acetaminophen and Caffeine Tablets; Acetaminophen, Aspirin, and Caffeine Tablets; Butalbital, Acetaminophen, and Caffeine Capsules; Butalbital, Acetaminophen, and Caffeine Tab-lets; Butalbital, Aspirin, and Caffeine Capsules; Butalbital, Aspi-rin, and Caffeine Tablets; Butalbital, Aspirin, Caffeine, and Co-deine Phosphate Capsules; Caffeine and Sodium Benzoate Injection; Ergotamine Tartrate and Caffeine Suppositories; Ergot-amine Tartrate and Caffeine Tablets; Propoxyphene Hydrochlo-ride, Aspirin, and Caffeine Capsules.

Proprietary Preparations (details are given in Part 3)
Aust.: Coffekapton; **Austral.:** No Doz; **Braz.:** Cefaldina; **Canad.:** Wake-Up Tablets; **Fin.:** Cofi-Tabs; **Fr.:** Percutafeine; **Ger.:** Auton-ic†; Percoffedrinol N; **S.Afr.:** Doxypol; Universal Concentration Tablets†; **Spain:** Durvitan; Prolert; **UK:** Pro-Plus; **USA:** Cafcit;

Caffedrine; Enerjets; Keep Alert; NoDoz; Quick Pep†; Spray-n-Wake†; Stay Alert; Tirend†; Vivarin.

Multi-ingredient: numerous preparations are listed in Part 3.

Choline Theophyllinate   (631-f)

Choline Theophyllinate (BAN, rINN).
Oxtriphylline; Theophylline Cholinate.
$C_{12}H_{21}N_5O_3 = 283.3$.
CAS — 4499-40-5.
ATC — R03DA02.
Pharmacopoeias. In *Br., Chin.,* and *US.*

Choline theophyllinate 1.57 mg is approximately equivalent in theophylline content to 1 mg of anhydrous theophylline.

Pharmacopoeial description
BP 2001: A white crystalline powder, odourless or with a faint amine-like odour. It contains between 41.9% and 43.6% of choline and between 61.7% and 65.5% of theophylline, each calculated with reference to the dried substance. Very soluble in water; soluble in alcohol; very slightly soluble in chloroform and in ether. Store at a temperature not exceeding 25°. Protect from light.

USP 25: A white crystalline powder, having an amine-like odour. It contains not less than 61.7% and not more than 65.5% of anhydrous theophylline. Soluble 1 in 1 of water; freely sol-uble in alcohol; very slightly soluble in chloroform. A 1% so-lution in water has a pH of about 10.3. Store in airtight contain-ers.

Profile
Choline theophyllinate is a theophylline salt which liberates theophylline (p.777) in the body. It is used as a bronchodilator for reversible airways obstruction. The usual maintenance dos-age for adults is 0.8 to 1.2 g daily by mouth, in 3 or 4 divided doses, preferably after food to reduce gastrointestinal side-ef-fects. Low doses (0.2 to 0.4 g daily) should be given initially and gradually increased according to clinical response and se-rum-theophylline concentrations (see Uses and Administration of Theophylline, p.783). A suggested maintenance dosage for children aged 5 to 9 years is 200 to 400 mg in 4 divided doses, and for children aged 10 to 14 years, 400 to 800 mg daily in 4 divided doses. Children under 5 years of age may receive 24 to 36 mg per kg body-weight daily in 3 divided doses.

Preparations
BP 2001: Choline Theophyllinate Tablets;
USP 25: Oxtriphylline Delayed-release Tablets; Oxtriphylline Ex-tended-release Tablets; Oxtriphylline Oral Solution; Oxtriphylline Tablets.

Proprietary Preparations (details are given in Part 3)
Austral.: Brondecon Elixir; **Canad.:** Choledyl; Novo-Triphyl†; Rouphylline; **Ger.:** Euspirax; **Hong Kong:** Rouphylline; **Irl.:** Choledyl; **Norw.:** Teovent; **S.Afr.:** Choledyl†; **Swed.:** Teovent; **UK:** Choledyl†; **USA:** Choledyl.

Multi-ingredient: **Austral.:** Brondecon Expectorant; **Canad.:** Choledyl Expectorant; **NZ:** Broncelix; Brondecon; Pharmacycare Expectorant; **Port.:** Vitasma; **Spain:** Dimayon†; Tilfilin†.

Clenbuterol Hydrochloride   (2047-f)

Clenbuterol Hydrochloride (BANM, rINNM).
NAB-365 (clenbuterol). 1-(4-Amino-3,5-dichlorophenyl)-2-*tert*-butylaminoethanol hydrochloride.
$C_{12}H_{18}Cl_2N_2O,HCl = 313.7$.
CAS — 37148-27-9 (clenbuterol); 21898-19-1 (clenbuterol hydrochloride).

NOTE. Clenbuterol has been referred to as angel dust; this name has also been used to describe illicit phencyclidine.

Profile
Clenbuterol hydrochloride is a direct-acting sympathomimetic with predominantly beta-adrenergic activity and a selective ac-tion on $beta_2$ receptors (a $beta_2$ agonist). It has properties simi-lar to those of salbutamol (p.770). It is used as a bronchodilator in the management of reversible airways obstruction, as in asth-ma (p.757) and in certain patients with chronic obstructive pul-monary disease (p.759). A usual dose is 20 μg twice daily by mouth; doses of up to 40 μg twice daily have occasionally been employed. Clenbuterol hydrochloride is also given by inhala-tion in usual doses of 20 μg three times daily. In patients with asthma, as-required beta agonist therapy is preferable to regular use. An increased need for, or decreased duration of effect of, clenbuterol indicates deterioration of asthma control and the need for review of therapy.

Abuse. Clenbuterol has been used illicitly in animal feeds in an attempt to promote weight gain and to increase muscle to lipid mass. Adverse effects typical of sympathomimetic activi-ty have been attributed to such misuse both in farmers perpe-trating such acts[1] and in innocent persons consuming meat products from affected animals.[2-4] Clenbuterol has been abused by sportsmen for its anabolic effects,[5] although it is doubtful that it leads to enhanced performance.[6]
1. Dawson P. β Agonists put meat in the limelight again. *BMJ* 1990; **301**: 1238–9.
2. Martínez-Navarro JF. Food poisoning related to consumption of illicit β-agonist in liver. *Lancet* 1990; **336**: 1311.

3. Maistro S, *et al.* Beta blockers to prevent clenbuterol poisoning. *Lancet* 1995; **346:** 180.
4. Brambilla G, *et al.* Food poisoning following consumption of clenbuterol-treated veal in Italy. *JAMA* 1997; **278:** 635.
5. Anonymous. Muscling in on clenbuterol. *Lancet* 1992; **340:** 403.
6. Spann C, Winter ME. Effect of clenbuterol on athletic performance. *Ann Pharmacother* 1995; **29:** 75–7.

Preparations

Proprietary Preparations (details are given in Part 3)
Aust.: Spiropent; *Braz.:* Ventilan; *Ger.:* Contraspasmin; Spiropent; *Hong Kong:* Clenasma; *Ital.:* Broncodil†; Clenasma; Contrasmina; Monores; Prontovent; Spiropent; *Mex.:* Novegam; Spiropent; *Port.:* Broncoterol; *Spain:* Spiropent; Ventolase.

Multi-ingredient: *Aust.:* Mucospas; *Ger.:* Spasmo-Mucosolvan; *Mex.:* Brogal Compuesto; Broxofar Compuesto; Broxol Plus; Mucosolvan Compositum; Mucovibrol C; Septacin Ex; *Port.:* Clembroxol; Mucospas; Ventoliber.

Diprophylline (633-n)

Diprophylline (BAN, rINN).

Dihydroxypropyltheophyllinum; Diprophyllinum; Dyphylline; Glyphyllinum; Hyphylline. 7-(2,3-Dihydroxypropyl)-1,3-dimethylxanthine; 7-(2,3-Dihydroxypropyl)theophylline.

$C_{10}H_{14}N_4O_4 = 254.2$.
CAS — 479-18-5.
ATC — R03DA01.

Pharmacopoeias. In Chin., Eur. (see p.vi), Pol., and US.

Pharmacopoeial description

Ph. Eur.: A white crystalline powder. Freely soluble in water; slightly soluble in alcohol. Protect from light.

USP 25: A white, odourless, amorphous or crystalline solid. Freely soluble in water; sparingly soluble in alcohol and in chloroform; practically insoluble in ether. A 1% solution in water has a pH of 5.0 to 7.5. Store in airtight containers.

Adverse Effects, Treatment, and Precautions
As for Theophylline, p.777. Diprophylline is primarily excreted unchanged in the urine and should therefore be used with caution in patients with renal impairment. However, unlike theophylline, plasma concentrations of diprophylline are not greatly affected by changes in liver function or hepatic enzyme activity such as those produced by smoking, age, and heart failure.

Interactions
Since diprophylline does not undergo metabolism by hepatic microsomal cytochrome P450 it does not exhibit the numerous interactions seen with theophylline (p.779). However, the possibility of synergistic effects should be borne in mind if it is prescribed concomitantly with other xanthines.

Probenecid. Probenecid has been reported to decrease the clearance of diprophylline thus prolonging its half-life.[1-3]

1. May DC, Jarboe CH. Inhibition of clearance of dyphylline by probenecid. *N Engl J Med* 1981; **304:** 791.
2. May DC, Jarboe CH. Effect of probenecid on dyphylline elimination. *Clin Pharmacol Ther* 1983; **33:** 822–5.
3. Acara M, *et al.* Probenecid inhibition of the renal excretion of dyphylline in chicken, rat and man. *J Pharm Pharmacol* 1987; **39:** 526–30.

Pharmacokinetics
Diprophylline is rapidly absorbed from the gastrointestinal tract and from the site of intramuscular injections. Diprophylline does not liberate theophylline in the body and is largely excreted unchanged in the urine with an elimination half-life of approximately 2 hours.

Breast feeding. In a study of 20 lactating women given diprophylline by intramuscular injection,[1] diprophylline was found to concentrate in breast milk, with a milk to serum concentration ratio of approximately 2. However, it was felt that the quantity of diprophylline a breast-feeding infant would ingest was unlikely to produce any pharmacological action unless the child was very sensitive.

1. Jarboe CH, *et al.* Dyphylline elimination kinetics in lactating women: blood to milk transfer. *J Clin Pharmacol* 1981; **21:** 405–10.

Uses and Administration
Diprophylline is a theophylline derivative which is used similarly to theophylline (p.783) as a bronchodilator in reversible airways obstruction.

The usual dose of diprophylline by mouth is up to 15 mg per kg body-weight every 6 hours. It has also been given intramuscularly. Diprophylline is also an ingredient of preparations that have been promoted for coughs.

◊ Improvements in measurements of lung function after diprophylline in doses of 15 and 20 mg per kg body-weight by mouth were only one-third to one-half those obtained after theophylline 6 mg per kg by mouth.[1]

1. Furukawa CT, *et al.* Diphylline versus theophylline: a double-blind comparative evaluation. *J Clin Pharmacol* 1983; **23:** 414–18.

Preparations

USP 25: Dyphylline and Guaifenesin Elixir; Dyphylline and Guaifenesin Tablets; Dyphylline Elixir; Dyphylline Injection; Dyphylline Tablets.

Proprietary Preparations (details are given in Part 3)
Aust.: Austrophyllin; Isophyllen; Neothyllin†; *Ger.:* Asthmolysin†; *Ital.:* Katasma; *Port.:* Neufil; *USA:* Dilor; Dyflex†; Dylix; Lufyllin; Neothylline†.

Multi-ingredient: *Aust.:* Laevostrophan compositum; *Fr.:* Ozothine a la Diprophylline; *Ger.:* Neobiphyllin-Clys†; Neobiphyllin†; Ozothin; *Israel:* Philinal; *Ital.:* Cort-Inal; *Spain:* Alergical Expect; Bronsal; Difilina Asmorax†; Novofilin; *Switz.:* Astho-Med; Brosol; Neo-Biphyllin†; *UK:* Noradran; *USA:* Dilor-G; Dy-G; Dyflex-G; Dyline GG; Dyphylline-GG; Lufyllin-EPG; Lufyllin-GG; Panfil G.

Doxofylline (1737-k)

Doxofylline (USAN, rINN).

ABC 12/3. 7-(1,3-Dioxolan-2-ylmethyl)theophylline.

$C_{11}H_{14}N_4O_4 = 266.3$.
CAS — 69975-86-6.
ATC — R03DA11.

Profile
Doxofylline is a theophylline derivative (p.777) which is used as a bronchodilator in reversible airways obstruction. It is given by mouth in doses of up to 1200 mg daily. It may also be given by slow intravenous injection.

Preparations

Proprietary Preparations (details are given in Part 3)
Ital.: Ansimar.

Eformoterol Fumarate (19193-l)

Eformoterol Fumarate (BANM).

Formoterol Fumarate (BANM, USAN, rINNM); BD-40A; CGP-25827A; YM-08316. (±)-2′-Hydroxy-5′-[(RS)-1-hydroxy-2-{[(RS)-p-methoxy-α-methylphenethyl]amino}ethyl]formanilide fumarate.

$(C_{19}H_{24}N_2O_4)_2, C_4H_4O_4 = 804.9$.
CAS — 73573-87-2 (eformoterol [formoterol]); 43229-80-7 (eformoterol [formoterol] fumarate).

Pharmacopoeias. In Jpn.

Adverse Effects and Precautions
As for Salbutamol, p.770. Inhalation of eformoterol [formoterol] may be associated with paradoxical bronchospasm.

Long-acting beta$_2$ agonists such as eformoterol [formoterol] are not appropriate for the treatment of acute bronchospasm.

Conjunctival irritation and eyelid oedema have been reported in isolated cases.

Tolerance. Regular use of eformoterol [formoterol] produced bronchodilator desensitisation,[1] and tachyphylaxis to bronchoprotection against methacholine,[2] effects that have been noted with other long-acting beta$_2$ agonists (see Salmeterol, p.773) and short-acting beta$_2$ agonists (see Salbutamol, p.771).

1. Newnham DM, *et al.* Bronchodilator subsensitivity after chronic dosing with eformoterol in patients with asthma. *Am J Med* 1994; **97:** 29–37.
2. Lipworth B, *et al.* Effects of treatment with formoterol on bronchoprotection against methacholine. *Am J Med* 1998; **104:** 431–8.

Interactions
As for Salbutamol, p.771.

Pharmacokinetics
Inhaled eformoterol [formoterol] is rapidly absorbed. It is largely metabolised by glucuronidation and O-demethylation, with about 10% being excreted as unchanged drug. The terminal elimination half-life after inhalation is estimated to be 8 hours.

Uses and Administration
Eformoterol [formoterol] is a direct-acting sympathomimetic with predominantly beta-adrenoceptor stimulant activity specific to beta$_2$ receptors (a beta$_2$ agonist). It has properties similar to those of salbutamol (p.772), but like salmeterol (p.773) it has a prolonged duration of action of up to 12 hours; it is therefore not considered suitable for the symptomatic relief of acute attacks of bronchospasm. It is used when the regular administration of a long-acting beta$_2$ agonist is required for management of reversible airways ob-

struction, as in chronic asthma (p.757) or in some patients with chronic obstructive pulmonary disease (p.759).

Eformoterol [formoterol] is given as the fumarate. A usual dose for adults and children aged 5 years or older is 12 µg of eformoterol [formoterol] fumarate twice daily by inhalation from a metered-dose aerosol or inhalational capsules, increased to 24 µg twice daily in severe disease. Usual doses from a metered-dose dry powder inhaler are 6 or 12 µg once or twice daily, increased to 24 µg twice daily in severe disease. Treatment should be reassessed if this proves inadequate; in the UK, some preparations are licensed for additional short-term symptom relief, but such use is contrary to current asthma guidelines (see p.757). Doses of 80 µg have been given twice daily by mouth.

◊ References.

1. Faulds D, *et al.* Formoterol: a review of its pharmacological properties and therapeutic potential in reversible obstructive airways disease. *Drugs* 1991; **42:** 115–37.
2. van Noord JA, *et al.* Salmeterol versus formoterol in patients with moderately severe asthma: onset and duration of action. *Eur Respir J* 1996; **9:** 1684–8.
3. van der Molen T, *et al.* Effects of the long acting β agonist formoterol on asthma control in asthmatic patients using inhaled corticosteroids. *Thorax* 1996; **52:** 535–9.
4. Pauwels RA, *et al.* Effect of inhaled formoterol and budesonide on exacerbations of asthma. *N Engl J Med* 1997; **337:** 1405–11. Correction. *ibid.* 1998; **338:** 139.
5. Bartow RA, Brogden RN. Formoterol: an update of its pharmacological properties and therapeutic efficacy in the management of asthma. *Drugs* 1998; **55:** 303–22.

Preparations

Proprietary Preparations (details are given in Part 3)
Aust.: Oxis; *Austral.:* Foradile; Oxis; *Belg.:* Foradil; Oxis; *Canad.:* Foradil; Oxeze; *Denm.:* Foradil; Oxis; *Fin.:* Foradil; Oxis; *Fr.:* Foradil; *Ger.:* Foradil; Oxis; *Hong Kong:* Foradil; *Irl.:* Oxis; *Israel:* Foradil; *Ital.:* Eolus; Foradil; *Jpn:* Atock; *Mex.:* Foradil; Oxis; *Neth.:* Foradil; Oxis; *Norw.:* Foradil; Oxis; *NZ:* Oxis; *Port.:* Foradil; Oxis; *S.Afr.:* Foradil; Oxis; *Singapore:* Foradil; Oxis; *Spain:* Broncoral; Foradil; Neblik; Oxis; *Swed.:* Foradil; Oxis; *Switz.:* Foradil; Oxis; *Thai.:* Oxis; *UK:* Foradil; Oxis; *USA:* Foradil.

Multi-ingredient: *UK:* Symbicort.

Enprofylline (16624-a)

Enprofylline (USAN, rINN).

D-4028; 3-Propylxanthine. 3,7-Dihydro-3-propyl-1H-purine-2,6-dione.

$C_8H_{10}N_4O_2 = 194.2$.
CAS — 41078-02-8.

Profile
Enprofylline is a theophylline derivative (p.777) that has been investigated for its bronchodilating properties in reversible airways obstruction.

◊ Enprofylline differs from theophylline in that it has no adenosine-antagonist activity, undergoes little hepatic metabolism,[1] and appears to have little CNS stimulant effect.[2] Enprofylline demonstrated effective bronchodilatation in clinical trials at comparable doses to theophylline,[3,4] but appeared to cause more headache and nausea than theophylline.[3] Elevation in liver enzyme values, and unpredictable blood concentrations have also been reported.[4]

1. Lunell E, Borgå O. Pharmacokinetics of enprofylline in healthy elderly subjects. *Eur J Clin Pharmacol* 1987; **32:** 67–70.
2. Tiplady B, *et al.* A comparison of the CNS effects of enprofylline and theophylline in healthy subjects assessed by performance testing and subjective measures. *Br J Clin Pharmacol* 1990; **30:** 55–61.
3. Arnold JD, *et al.* Comparative assessment of enprofylline and theophylline for chronic obstructive airways disease in the elderly. *Respir Med* 1990; **84:** 211–15.
4. Chapman KR, *et al.* Long-term xanthine therapy of asthma: enprofylline and theophylline compared. *Chest* 1994; **106:** 1407–13.

Etamiphylline Camsilate (634-h)

Etamiphylline Camsilate (BANM, rINNM).

Diétamiphylline Camphosulfonate; Etamiphylline Camsylate; Etamiphyllin Camsylate. 7-(2-Diethylaminoethyl)-1,3-dimethylxanthine camphor-10-sulphonate; 7-(2-Diethylaminoethyl)theophylline camphor-10-sulphonate.

$C_{23}H_{37}N_5O_6S = 511.6$.
CAS — 314-35-2 (etamiphylline); 19326-29-5 (etamiphylline camsilate).

Pharmacopoeias. In Br.

Pharmacopoeial description

BP 2001: A white or almost white powder with a faint camphoraceous odour. Very soluble in water; soluble in alcohol and in chloroform; very slightly soluble in ether. A 10% solution in water has a pH of 3.9 to 5.4.

Profile

Etamiphylline camsilate is a derivative of theophylline (p.777) and has been used as a bronchodilator in reversible airways obstruction. Etamiphylline does not liberate theophylline in the body.

Etamiphylline and its dehydrocholate, hydrochloride, and methiodide salts have also been used.

Preparations

BP 2001: Etamiphylline Injection; Etamiphylline Suppositories.
Proprietary Preparations (details are given in Part 3)
Spain: Solufilina; Solufilina Simple.
Multi-ingredient: *Aust.:* Longtussin†; *Spain:* Solufilina Sedante†.

Etofylline (635-m)

Etofylline (BAN, rINN).

Aethophyllinum; Etofyllinum; Hydroxyaethyltheophyllinum; Hydroxyéthylthéophylline; Oxyethylline. 7-(2-Hydroxyethyl)-1,3-dimethylxanthine; 3,7-Dihydro-7-(2-hydroxyethyl)-1,3-dimethyl-1H-purine-2,6-dione; 7-(2-Hydroxyethyl)theophylline.

$C_9H_{12}N_4O_3 = 224.2$.
CAS — 519-37-9.
Pharmacopoeias. In Eur. (see p.vi).

Pharmacopoeial description

Ph. Eur.: A white crystalline powder. Soluble in water; slightly soluble in alcohol. Protect from light.

Profile

Etofylline is a derivative of theophylline (p.777) that is an ingredient of preparations promoted for various respiratory and cardiovascular disorders. It does not liberate theophylline in the body.

Etofylline nicotinate has also been used.

Preparations

Proprietary Preparations (details are given in Part 3)
S.Afr.: Theostat†.

Multi-ingredient: *Aust.:* Alpha-Apoplectal†; Apoplectal; Coroverlan†; Instenon; Peripherin†; Perphyllon; *Braz.:* Geri-Kan H3; *Ger.:* Coroverlan; Eucebral-N†; *Hong Kong:* Instenon; *S.Afr.:* Actophlem; Alcophyllex; D-Tussin†; Dilinct; Solphyllex; Solphyllin; Theophen; Theophen Comp; *Spain:* Flebo Stop; Vasperdil†; *Switz.:* Theo-Talusin†; *Thai.:* Instenon.

Fenoterol Hydrobromide (2063-f)

Fenoterol Hydrobromide (BANM, rINNM).

Fenoteroli Hydrobromidum; TH-1165a. 1-(3,5-Dihydroxyphenyl)-2-(4-hydroxy-α-methylphenethylamino)ethanol hydrobromide.

$C_{17}H_{21}NO_4,HBr = 384.3$.
CAS — 13392-18-2 (fenoterol); 1944-12-3 (fenoterol hydrobromide).

NOTE. Fenoterol is USAN.
Pharmacopoeias. In Eur. (see p.vi) and Pol.

Pharmacopoeial description

Ph. Eur.: A white crystalline powder. Soluble in water and in alcohol; practically insoluble in ether. A 4% solution in water has a pH of 4.2 to 5.2. Protect from light.

Adverse Effects and Precautions

As for Salbutamol, p.770.

Increased mortality. Since the introduction of metered-dose aerosols of beta agonists there have been two reported epidemics of increased morbidity and mortality in asthmatic patients associated with their use. The first occurred in the 1960s and was linked with the use of high-dose isoprenaline inhalers.[1] The use of isoprenaline was subsequently largely discontinued in favour of more selective beta₂ agonists.

The second epidemic occurred in New Zealand in the late 1970s and 1980s and was associated with the use of fenoterol.[1-5] When use of fenoterol fell in New Zealand, so too did the asthma mortality rate.[5] Heavy or regular use of fenoterol was implicated.[6,7] Fenoterol was also implicated in increased asthma morbidity and mortality in a study in Canada,[7] as was salbutamol, and results from Japan also suggested a relation between asthma deaths and excessive use of beta agonists, particularly fenoterol.[8] However, an analysis of the New Zealand deaths could not identify such a risk with beta agonists other than fenoterol.[5]

There is still debate about this second epidemic. The individual case control studies, including the one from Canada,[7] showed an increased morbidity and mortality in patients taking fenoterol, but a meta-analysis of the accumulated data to 1992 suggested that the increase in mortality in the patients taking beta₂ agonists was slight and only significant when administration was by nebulisation.[9] Also a working party of the UK Committee on Safety of Medicines considered[10] that a causal link be-

The symbol † denotes a preparation no longer actively marketed

tween asthma mortality and beta-agonist use could neither be confirmed nor refuted.

Not surprisingly there are different views on the cause of the increased asthma mortality. The cardiotoxicity of the beta agonist might have to be considered, although evidence for such an effect is felt by some to be slight.[11] The severity of the asthma might have been a factor in two different ways. One hypothesis is that patients used more fenoterol because they had severe asthma and were already at increased risk of dying.[12] Another proposes that heavy beta-agonist use led to an increase in asthma severity[13] which could be explained by a down regulation of beta receptors.[14]

This may appear to be only of historical interest since mortality rates have fallen and current recommendations for the use of short-acting beta₂ agonists, which are generally more selective than fenoterol, are for them to be taken as required rather than on a regular basis; indeed increasing use of such drugs is seen as an indication to amend the treatment schedule. Moreover, the dose of fenoterol has been reduced in recent years. However, controversy over regular use of beta₂ agonists continues to be fed by conflicting studies of their benefit.[15,16] It is possible that some benefit exists in more severe disease, and current recommendations for asthma treatment do permit the regular use of long-acting beta₂ agonists in severe chronic asthma. It is not clear to what extent the same concerns, particularly of down-regulation of beta receptors, apply to such therapy (see Tolerance, under Salmeterol, p.773).

1. Pearce N, *et al.* Beta agonists and asthma mortality: déjà vu. *Clin Exp Allergy* 1991; **21:** 401–10.
2. Crane J, *et al.* Prescribed fenoterol and death from asthma in New Zealand, 1981-83: case-control study. *Lancet* 1989; **i:** 917–22.
3. Pearce N, *et al.* Case-control study of prescribed fenoterol and death from asthma in New Zealand, 1977–81. *Thorax* 1990; **45:** 170–5.
4. Grainger J, *et al.* Prescribed fenoterol and death from asthma in New Zealand, 1981–7: a further case-control study. *Thorax* 1991; **46:** 105–111.
5. Pearce N, *et al.* End of the New Zealand asthma mortality epidemic. *Lancet* 1995; **345:** 41–4.
6. Sears MR, *et al.* Regular inhaled beta-agonist treatment in bronchial asthma. *Lancet* 1990; **336:** 1391–6.
7. Spitzer WO, *et al.* The use of β-agonists and the risk of death and near death from asthma. *N Engl J Med* 1992; **326:** 501–6.
8. Beasley R, *et al.* β-agonist therapy and asthma mortality in Japan. *Lancet* 1998; **351:** 1406–7.
9. Mullen M, *et al.* The association between β-agonist use and death from asthma: a meta-analytic integration of case control studies. *JAMA* 1993; **270:** 1842–5.
10. Committee on Safety of Medicines. Beta-agonist use in asthma: report from the CSM Working Party. *Current Problems 33* 1992.
11. Sears MR, Taylor DR. The β₂-agonist controversy: observations, explanations and relationship to asthma epidemiology. *Drug Safety* 1994; **11:** 259–83.
12. Fuller RW. Use of β₂ agonists in asthma: much ado about nothing? *BMJ* 1994; **309:** 795–6.
13. Sears MR. Asthma deaths in New Zealand. *Lancet* 1995; **345:** 655–6.
14. Tattersfield AE. Use of β₂ agonists in asthma: much ado about nothing? *BMJ* 1994; **309:** 794–5.
15. Chapman KR, *et al.* Regular vs as-needed inhaled salbutamol in asthma control. *Lancet* 1994; **343:** 1379–82.
16. Drazen JM, *et al.* Comparison of regularly scheduled with as-needed use of albuterol in mild asthma. *N Engl J Med* 1996; **335:** 841–7.

Pulmonary oedema. Pulmonary oedema has occurred in women given beta agonists, including fenoterol,[1] for premature labour. The risk factors, the most important of which is fluid overload, are discussed under Precautions for Salbutamol, on p.771.

1. Hawker F. Pulmonary oedema associated with β₂-sympathomimetic treatment of premature labour. *Anaesth Intensive Care* 1984; **12:** 143–51.

Interactions

As for Salbutamol, p.771.

Pharmacokinetics

Fenoterol is incompletely absorbed from the gastrointestinal tract and is also subject to extensive first-pass metabolism by sulfate conjugation. It is excreted in the urine and bile almost entirely as the inactive sulfate conjugate.

◊ References.
1. Rominger KL, Pollmann W. Vergleichende Pharmakokinetik von Fenoterol-Hydrobromid bei Ratte, Hund und Mensch. *Arzneimittelforschung* 1972; **22:** 1190–6.
2. Hildebrandt R, *et al.* Pharmacokinetics of fenoterol in pregnant and nonpregnant women. *Eur J Clin Pharmacol* 1993; **45:** 275–7.

Uses and Administration

Fenoterol is a direct-acting sympathomimetic with beta-adrenoceptor stimulant activity largely selective for beta₂ receptors (a beta₂ agonist). It has actions and uses similar to those of salbutamol (p.772) and is used as a bronchodilator in the management of reversible airways obstruction, as occurs in asthma (p.757) and in some patients with chronic obstructive pulmonary disease (p.759). Following inhalation, fenoterol acts

rapidly (2 to 3 minutes) and has a duration of action of about 6 to 8 hours.

In the management of **reversible airways obstruction**, fenoterol hydrobromide may be administered by inhalation in a dose of 1 or 2 inhalations of 100 µg up to 3 or 4 times daily; children over the age of 6 years will only normally require one inhalation (100 µg) up to 3 times daily. If symptoms are not adequately controlled with this low-dose inhaler then a high-dose inhaler administering 200 µg per inhalation has been employed in adults; 2 inhalations of 200 µg may be given up to 3 times daily. The dose should not exceed 400 µg every six hours or 1.6 mg in a 24-hour period; this high-dose inhaler is not recommended for children under 16 years of age. Current asthma guidelines recommend that inhaled short-acting beta₂ agonists such as fenoterol be used on an 'as-required', not regular, basis. In those patients requiring more than occasional use of fenoterol, anti-inflammatory therapy is also needed. An increased requirement for, or decreased duration of effect of, fenoterol indicates deterioration of asthma control and the need for increased anti-inflammatory therapy.

Fenoterol hydrobromide may be given as a nebulised solution; the usual dose for inhalation by this route is 200 to 400 µg, up to a maximum of 1.6 mg daily.

Fenoterol hydrobromide has also been used similarly to salbutamol in the management of **premature labour** (see p.773). A suggested dose, by intravenous infusion, has been 0.5 to 3 µg per minute, continued until contractions are suppressed, and followed by oral administration of 5 mg every 3 to 6 hours.

Preparations

BP 2001: Fenoterol Pressurised Inhalation.

Proprietary Preparations (details are given in Part 3)
Aust.: Berotec; *Austral.:* Berotec; *Belg.:* Berotec; *Braz.:* Berotec; *Canad.:* Berotec; *Denm.:* Berotec; *Fin.:* Berotec; *Fr.:* Berotec; *Ger.:* Berotec; Partusisten; *Hong Kong:* Berotec; *Irl.:* Berotec; *Ital.:* Dosberotec; *Mex.:* Berotec; Partusisten; *Neth.:* Berotec; Partusisten; *Norw.:* Berotec; *NZ:* Berotec; *Port.:* Berotec; *S.Afr.:* Berotec; Fensol†; *Singapore:* Berotec; *Spain:* Berotec; *Swed.:* Berotec; *Switz.:* Berotec; Partusisten†; *Thai.:* Berotec; *UK:* Berotec†.

Multi-ingredient: *Aust.:* Arelcant; Berodual; Berodualin; Ditec; *Belg.:* Duovent; *Braz.:* Duovent; Fymnal; *Canad.:* Duovent; *Denm.:* Berodual; *Fin.:* Atrovent Comp; *Fr.:* Bronchodual; *Ger.:* Berodual; Berodue solvens†; Ditec; *Hong Kong:* Berodual; *Irl.:* Duovent; *Ital.:* Duovent; Iprafen; *Neth.:* Berodual; *NZ:* Duovent; *Port.:* Berodual; *S.Afr.:* Atrovent Beta; Duovent; *Singapore:* Berodual; Duovent; *Spain:* Berodual; Crismol; *Switz.:* Berodual; *Thai.:* Berodual; *UK:* Duovent.

Fenspiride Hydrochloride (12746-t)

Fenspiride Hydrochloride (USAN, rINNM).

Decaspiride; JP-428; NAT-333; NDR-5998A. 8-Phenethyl-1-oxa-3,8-diazaspiro[4.5]decan-2-one hydrochloride.

$C_{15}H_{20}N_2O_2,HCl = 296.8$.
CAS — 5053-06-5 (fenspiride); 5053-08-7 (fenspiride hydrochloride).

Profile

Fenspiride is reported to have bronchodilator and anti-inflammatory properties. It is given as the hydrochloride in asthma (p.757) and other respiratory disorders in usual doses of 160 to 240 mg daily by mouth in divided doses before meals. It has also been administered rectally and by intramuscular or intravenous injection.

Preparations

Proprietary Preparations (details are given in Part 3)
Belg.: Pneumorel†; *Fr.:* Pneumorel; *Hong Kong:* Pneumorel; *Ital.:* Espiran†; Fenspir; Fluiden; Pneumorel; *Port.:* Fenspin; Pneumorel.

Heptaminol Acephyllinate (636-b)

Acéfyllinate d'Heptaminol; Acefyllinum Heptaminolum; Heptaminol Theophylline Ethanoate; Heptaminol Theophylline-7-acetate. The 6-amino-2-methylheptan-2-ol salt of theophyllin-7-ylacetic acid .

$C_8H_{19}NO,C_9H_{10}N_4O_4 = 383.4$.
CAS — 5152-72-7; 10075-18-0.
Pharmacopoeias. In Fr.

Profile

Heptaminol acephyllinate is a derivative of theophylline (p.777) that has been used for its bronchodilator and cardiovascular effects.

Preparations

Proprietary Preparations (details are given in Part 3)

Multi-ingredient: *Braz.:* Sureptil; *Fr.:* Sureptil; *Spain:* Clinadil Compositum; Diclamina.

Hexoprenaline Hydrochloride (2065-n)

Hexoprenaline Hydrochloride (*BANM, rINNM*).

ST-1512. *N,N'*-Hexamethylenebis[4-(2-amino-1-hydroxyethyl)pyrocatechol] dihydrochloride; *N,N'*-Hexamethylenebis[2-amino-1-(3,4-dihydroxyphenyl)ethanol] dihydrochloride.

$C_{22}H_{32}N_2O_6,2HCl = 493.4$.

CAS — 3215-70-1 (hexoprenaline); 4323-43-7 (hexoprenaline dihydrochloride).

Hexoprenaline Sulfate (2066-h)

Hexoprenaline Sulfate (*USAN, rINNM*).

Hexoprenaline Sulphate (*BANM*). (±)-α,α'-[Hexamethylenebis(iminomethylene)]-bis[3,4-dihydroxybenzyl alcohol] sulfate (1:1).

$C_{22}H_{32}N_2O_6,H_2SO_4 = 518.6$.

CAS — 32266-10-7.

Profile

Hexoprenaline is a direct-acting sympathomimetic with predominantly beta-adrenergic activity selective to beta$_2$ receptors (a beta$_2$ agonist). It has properties similar to those of salbutamol (p.770) and is used as a bronchodilator in the treatment of reversible airways obstruction as occurs with asthma (p.757) and in some patients with chronic obstructive pulmonary disease (p.759). It has sometimes been used similarly to salbutamol in the management of premature labour (p.773).

Hexoprenaline is usually given as the hydrochloride or sulfate.

For bronchodilatation, usual doses of the salts are 0.5 to 1 mg three times daily by mouth or 200 to 400 µg by inhalation three to four times daily. In patients with asthma, as-required beta agonist therapy is preferable to regular use. An increased need for, or decreased duration of effect of, hexoprenaline indicates deterioration of asthma control and the need for review of therapy. Hexoprenaline salts have also been given parenterally.

In the management of premature labour an intravenous infusion of hexoprenaline sulfate can be given at an initial rate of about 0.1 to 0.3 µg per minute. Infusion may be preceded by slow intravenous injection of 10 µg as a loading dose over 5 to 10 minutes.

Preparations

Proprietary Preparations (details are given in Part 3)

Aust.: Gynipral; Ipradol; *Hong Kong:* Ipradol; *S.Afr.:* Ipradol; *Spain:* Ipradol†; *Switz.:* Gynipral; *Thai.:* Ipradol.

Ibudilast (19376-t)

Ibudilast (*rINN*).

KC-404. 1-(2-Isopropylpyrazolo[1,5-a]pyridin-3-yl)-2-methyl-1-propanone.

$C_{14}H_{18}N_2O = 230.3$.

CAS — 50847-11-5.

ATC — R03DX04.

Profile

Ibudilast is an orally active leukotriene antagonist and platelet-activating factor antagonist. It is administered by mouth in the management of asthma (p.757) in a dose of 10 mg twice daily.

Ibudilast has also been promoted for a variety of cerebrovascular disorders in doses of 10 mg three times daily.

Preparations

Proprietary Preparations (details are given in Part 3)

Jpn: Ketas.

Ipratropium Bromide (386-h)

Ipratropium Bromide (*BAN, USAN, rINN*).

Ipratropii Bromidum; Sch-1000; Sch-1000-Br-monohydrate. (1R,3r,5S,8r)-8-Isopropyl-3-[(±)-tropoyloxy]tropanium bromide monohydrate.

$C_{20}H_{30}BrNO_3,H_2O = 430.4$.

CAS — 22254-24-6 (anhydrous ipratropium bromide); 66985-17-9 (ipratropium bromide monohydrate).

ATC — R01AX03; R03BB01.

Pharmacopoeias. In Eur. (see p.vi) and Jpn.

Pharmacopoeial description

Ph. Eur.: White or almost white crystalline powder. Soluble in water; slightly soluble in alcohol; freely soluble in methyl alcohol. The pH of a 1% solution in water is 5.0 to 7.5.

Stability. In a study[1] of the stability of admixtures of ipratropium and salbutamol nebuliser solutions equal ratio mixtures were found to retain more than 90% of their initial concentra-

tions after storage for 5 days at 4° or 22° in the dark or at 22° under continuous fluorescent lighting.

1. Jacobson GA, Peterson GM. Stability of ipratropium bromide and salbutamol nebuliser solution admixtures. *Int J Pharm Pract* 1995; **3:** 169–73.

Adverse Effects and Precautions

Ipratropium and other inhaled antimuscarinic bronchodilators may occasionally cause dry mouth, and rarely constipation and urinary retention. They should be used with care in prostatic hyperplasia. Acute angle-closure glaucoma has been reported with *nebulised* ipratropium; the mist or solution should not be allowed to enter the eyes, particularly in patients susceptible to glaucoma. As with other bronchodilators, paradoxical bronchospasm has occurred.

Intranasal ipratropium has been associated with nasal dryness and epistaxis.

For details of the adverse effects of, and precautions for, antimuscarinics in general, see Atropine, p.461.

Buccal ulceration. A report[1] of inflammation and ulceration of the buccal mucosa associated with the use of an ipratropium bromide inhaler.

1. Spencer PA. Buccal ulceration with ipratropium bromide. *BMJ* 1986; **292:** 380.

Effects on the eyes. Although short-term studies in patients with angle-closure glaucoma and normal subjects indicate that inhalation of ipratropium alone has no effect on intra-ocular pressure, accommodation, or pupil diameter[1,2] there has been a report[3] of a patient with a history of glaucoma who developed angle-closure glaucoma after receiving ipratropium using a metered dose inhaler and nebulised salbutamol together. Angle-closure glaucoma,[4-6] pupillary dilatation,[6,7] and anisocoria[8] have been reported in patients receiving *nebulised* ipratropium, usually with salbutamol, through a poorly fitting face mask. The antimuscarinic effects of ipratropium can lead to impaired drainage of aqueous humour in the eyes of patients predisposed to angle-closure glaucoma; co-administration of salbutamol may intensify this problem by increasing the production of aqueous humour.[5] Studies[9,10] suggest that patients with a history of angle-closure glaucoma might be at an increased risk of developing glaucoma when nebulised ipratropium and salbutamol are used together.

1. Scheufler G. Ophthalmotonometry, pupil diameter and visual accommodation following repeated administration of Sch 1000 MDI in patients with glaucoma. *Postgrad Med J* 1975; **51** (suppl 7): 132.
2. Thumm HW. Ophthalmic effects of high doses of Sch 1000 MDI in healthy volunteers and patients with glaucoma. *Postgrad Med J* 1975; **51** (suppl 7): 132–3.
3. Hall SK. Acute angle-closure glaucoma as a complication of combined β-agonist and ipratropium bromide therapy in the emergency department. *Ann Emerg Med* 1994; **23:** 884–7.
4. Packe GE, *et al.* Nebulised ipratropium bromide and salbutamol causing closed-angle glaucoma. *Lancet* 1984; **ii:** 691.
5. Shah P, *et al.* Acute angle closure glaucoma associated with nebulised ipratropium bromide and salbutamol. *BMJ* 1992; **304:** 40–1.
6. Mulpeter KM, *et al.* Ocular hazards of nebulized bronchodilators. *Postgrad Med J* 1992; **68:** 132–3.
7. Roberts TE, Pearson DJ. Wide eyed and breathless. *BMJ* 1989; **299:** 1348.
8. Lust K, Livingstone I. Nebulizer-induced anisocoria. *Ann Intern Med* 1998; **128:** 327.
9. Watson WTA, *et al.* Effect of nebulized ipratropium bromide on intraocular pressures in children. *Chest* 1994; **105:** 1439–41.
10. Kalra L, Bone MF. The effect of nebulized bronchodilator therapy on intraocular pressures in patients with glaucoma. *Chest* 1988; **93:** 739–41.

Effects on the gastrointestinal tract. Paralytic ileus developed shortly after initiation of ipratropium therapy in 2 patients, apparently due to the inadvertent swallowing of the drug during inhalation.[1,2] Both patients also had other predisposing factors for paralytic ileus (cystic fibrosis,[1] spastic diplegia[2]).

1. Mulherin D, FitzGerald MX. Meconium ileus equivalent in association with nebulised ipratropium bromide in cystic fibrosis. *Lancet* 1990; **355:** 552.
2. Markus HS. Paralytic ileus associated with ipratropium. *Lancet* 1990; **355:** 1224.

Effects on the respiratory tract. Antimuscarinics typically inhibit mucociliary clearance and inhibit secretions of the nose, mouth, pharynx, and bronchi. However, inhaled ipratropium bromide has virtually no effect on sputum viscosity or volume and, in contrast to atropine, it does not affect mucociliary function in the respiratory tract.[1,2]

1. Gross NJ. Ipratropium bromide. *N Engl J Med* 1988; **319:** 486–94.
2. Mann KV, *et al.* Use of ipratropium bromide in obstructive lung disease. *Clin Pharm* 1988; **7:** 670–80.

BRONCHOSPASM. Paradoxical bronchoconstriction occurring after the use of ipratropium was reported in 3 patients.[1] The authors of a further report[2] of paradoxical bronchoconstriction following nebulisation therapy with salbutamol and ipratropium suggested that this adverse effect may have been caused by benzalkonium chloride present in the nebuliser solutions. Nebuliser solutions of ipratropium in some countries contain benzalkonium chloride as a preservative. Solutions available in the UK are preservative-free but the manufacturers still recom-

mend that the first doses of ipratropium nebuliser solution should be inhaled under medical supervision.

1. Connolly CK. Adverse reaction to ipratropium bromide. *BMJ* 1982; **285:** 934–5.
2. Boucher M, *et al.* Possible associations of benzalkonium chloride in nebulizer solutions with respiratory arrest. *Ann Pharmacother* 1992; **26:** 772–4.

Effects on the urinary tract. Treatment with nebulised ipratropium bromide has resulted in urinary retention in elderly men especially those with prostatic hyperplasia.[1,2]

1. Lozewicz S. Bladder outflow obstruction induced by ipratropium bromide. *Postgrad Med J* 1989; **65:** 260–1.
2. Pras E, *et al.* Urinary retention associated with ipratropium bromide. *DICP Ann Pharmacother* 1991; **25:** 939–40.

Increased mortality. A case-control study found an unexpected association between death and treatment with ipratropium, which was not explained by co-morbidity due to chronic obstructive airways disease.[1] A later retrospective cohort study[2] of elderly patients found no increase in all-cause mortality associated with the use of ipratropium for chronic obstructive pulmonary disease. In patients with asthma there was a slight increase in the risk of death, but this may have been due to the confounding effect of disease severity.

1. Guite HF, *et al.* Risk factors for death from asthma, chronic obstructive pulmonary disease, and cardiovascular death after a hospital admission for asthma. *Thorax* 1999; **54:** 301–7.
2. Sin DD, Tu JV. Lack of association between ipratropium bromide and mortality in elderly patients with chronic obstructive airway disease. *Thorax* 2000; **55:** 194–7.

Interactions

For interactions associated with antimuscarinics in general, see Atropine, p.461. However, these interactions are not usually seen with antimuscarinics, such as ipratropium, given by inhalation.

Salbutamol. For reference to nebulised salbutamol exacerbating the adverse effects of nebulised ipratropium in patients predisposed to angle-closure glaucoma, see under Effects on the Eyes, above.

Pharmacokinetics

Following inhalation, only a small amount of ipratropium reaches the systemic circulation. Some ipratropium is inadvertently swallowed but it is poorly absorbed from the gastrointestinal tract. Ipratropium and its metabolites are eliminated in the urine and faeces.

◊ References.

1. Ensing K, *et al.* Pharmacokinetics of ipratropium bromide after single dose inhalation and oral and intravenous administration. *Eur J Clin Pharmacol* 1989; **36:** 189–94.

Uses and Administration

Ipratropium bromide is a quaternary ammonium antimuscarinic (p.757). It is used by inhalation as a bronchodilator in the treatment of reversible airways obstruction, as in asthma (p.757) and in some patients with chronic obstructive pulmonary disease (p.759).

In the UK the dose of ipratropium bromide from the metered-dose aerosol is expressed in terms of the amount of drug released from the valve into the mouthpiece (20 µg) whereas in the USA it is expressed in terms of the dose emitted from the mouthpiece (18 µg); recommended doses therefore appear lower in the USA. For **reversible airways obstruction,** the usual UK dose by inhalation from a metered-dose aerosol is 20 or 40 µg three or four times daily; single doses of up to 80 µg may be required. Comparable doses are used in the USA, but it is recommended that the daily dose should not exceed 216 µg (12 inhalations). In children aged 6 to 12 years the usual dose is 20 or 40 µg three times daily, and below 6 years the usual dose is 20 µg three times daily. Dry powder inhalation capsules are also available for use in adults, the usual dose being 40 µg three or four times daily.

Ipratropium bromide may also be administered by inhalation as a nebulised solution in doses of 100 to 500 µg up to 4 times daily. In children aged 3 to 14 years the usual dose by nebuliser is 100 to 500 µg up to 3 times daily. Doses of 62.5 to 250 µg up to 3 times daily have been given to children 1 month to 3 years of age.

Ipratropium bromide, given intranasally, is also used in the management of rhinorrhoea associated with **rhinitis.** A dose of 42 µg is administered into each nostril by metered-dose nasal spray 2 or 3 times daily. In the USA, doses of 84 µg may be given into each nostril 3 or 4 times daily when rhinorrhoea is associated with the common cold.

Rhinitis. Ipratropium bromide is used intranasally for the treatment of rhinorrhoea in allergic and non-allergic rhinitis (p.407). It has also relieved rhinorrhoea and sneezing associated with the common cold.

References.
1. Georgitis JW, *et al.* Ipratropium bromide nasal spray in non-allergic rhinitis: efficacy, nasal cytological response and patient evaluation on quality of life. *Clin Exp Allergy* 1994; **24:** 1049–55.
2. Hayden FG, *et al.* Effectiveness and safety of intranasal ipratropium bromide in common colds: a randomized, double-blind, placebo-controlled trial. *Ann Intern Med* 1996; **125:** 89–97.
3. Dockhorn R, *et al.* Ipratropium bromide nasal spray 0.03% and beclomethasone nasal spray alone and in combination for the treatment of rhinorrhoea in perennial rhinitis. *Ann Allergy Asthma Immunol* 1999; **82:** 349–59.

Preparations

BP 2001: Ipratropium Pressurised Inhalation.

Proprietary Preparations (details are given in Part 3)
Aust.: Atronase; Atrovent; Itrop; *Austral.:* Apoven; Atrovent; Ipratrin; Ipravent; *Belg.:* Atronase; Atrovent; *Braz.:* Atrovent; *Canad.:* Apo-Ipravent; Atrovent; Novo-Ipramide; *Denm.:* Atrovent; *Fin.:* Atrovent; *Fr.:* Atrovent; *Ger.:* Atrovent; Itrop; *Hong Kong:* Atrovent; *Irl.:* Atrovent; Rinatec; *Israel:* Aerovent; Apovent; *Ital.:* Atem; Atrovent; Rinovagos; *Mex.:* Atrovent; *Neth.:* Atrovent; *Norw.:* Atrovent; Respontin; *NZ:* Atrovent; *Port.:* Atrovent; *S.Afr.:* Atronase†; Atrovent; Ipvent; *Singapore:* Atrovent; *Spain:* Atrovent; Disne Asmol†; Narilet†; *Swed.:* Atrovent; *Switz.:* Atrovent; Rhinovent; *Thai.:* Atrovent; *UK:* Atrovent; Respontin; Rinatec; Tropiovent; *USA:* Atrovent.

Multi-ingredient: *Aust.:* Arelcant; Berodual; Berodualin; Combivent; Di-Promal; *Austral.:* Combivent; *Belg.:* Combivent; Duovent; *Braz.:* Duovent; *Canad.:* Combivent; Duovent; *Denm.:* Berodual; Combivent; *Fin.:* Berodual; Atrovent Comp; *Fr.:* Bronchodual; Combivent; *Ger.:* Berodual; *Hong Kong:* Berodual; Combivent; *Irl.:* Combivent; Duovent; *Ital.:* Breva; Duovent; Iprafen; *Mex.:* Combivent; *Neth.:* Berodual; Combivent†; *NZ:* Combivent; Duovent; *Port.:* Berodual; Combivent; *S.Afr.:* Atrovent Beta; Combivent; Duovent; *Singapore:* Berodual; Combivent; Duovent; *Spain:* Berodual; Combivent; Crismol; *Swed.:* Combivent; *Switz.:* Berodual; Dospir; *Thai.:* Berodual; Combivent; *UK:* Combivent; Duovent; *USA:* Combivent; DuoNeb.

Isoetarine Hydrochloride (2070-r)

Isoetarine Hydrochloride *(BANM, rINNM).*

Etyprenaline Hydrochloride; Isoetharine Hydrochloride; *N*-Isopropylethylnoradrenaline Hydrochloride. 1-(3,4-Dihydroxyphenyl)-2-isopropylaminobutan-1-ol hydrochloride.
$C_{13}H_{21}NO_3,HCl = 275.8.$
CAS — 530-08-5 (isoetarine); 50-96-4 (isoetarine hydrochloride); 2576-92-3 (isoetarine hydrochloride).
NOTE. Isoetharine is *USAN.*
Pharmacopoeias. In US.

Pharmacopoeial description

USP 25: A white to off-white, odourless, crystalline solid. Soluble in water; sparingly soluble in alcohol; practically insoluble in ether. A 1% solution in water has a pH of 4.0 to 5.6. Store in airtight containers.

Isoetarine Mesilate (2071-f)

Isoetarine Mesilate *(BANM, rINNM).*

Isoetharine Mesylate; Isoetharine Methanesulphonate; *N*-Isopropylethylnoradrenaline Mesylate; Win-3406 (isoetarine).
$C_{13}H_{21}NO_3,CH_4O_3S = 335.4.$
CAS — 7279-75-6.
NOTE. Isoetharine is *USAN.*
Pharmacopoeias. In US.

Pharmacopoeial description

USP 25: White or practically white, odourless, crystals. Freely soluble in water; soluble in alcohol; practically insoluble in acetone and in ether. A 1% solution in water has a pH of 4.5 to 5.5. Store in airtight containers.

Profile

Isoetarine is a sympathomimetic with predominantly beta-adrenergic activity. It has actions similar to those of salbutamol (p.770) but is less selective for beta$_2$ adrenoceptors (for the actions of a non-selective beta agonist see Isoprenaline, p.914). Isoetarine has been used as a bronchodilator in the management of reversible airways obstruction.

Isoetarine is given by inhalation, as a nebulised solution of the hydrochloride in strengths up to 0.25%; a 1% solution can be administered by a hand nebuliser. It has also been given as an aerosol inhalation of the mesilate.

Preparations

USP 25: Isoetharine Inalation Solution; Isoetharine Mesylate Inhalation Aerosol.

Proprietary Preparations (details are given in Part 3)
USA: Beta-2†; Bronkometer†; Bronkosol†.

The symbol † denotes a preparation no longer actively marketed

---

Ketotifen Fumarate (7724-j)

Ketotifen Fumarate *(BANM, USAN, rINNM).*

HC-20511 (ketotifen); Ketotifen Hydrogen Fumarate; Ketotifeni Hydrogenofumaras. 4-(1-Methylpiperidin-4-ylidene)-4*H*-benzo[4,5]cyclohepta-[1,2-*b*]thiophen-10(9*H*)-one hydrogen fumarate.
$C_{19}H_{19}NOS,C_4H_4O_4 = 425.5.$
CAS — 34580-13-7 (ketotifen); 34580-14-8 (ketotifen fumarate).
Pharmacopoeias. In Eur. (see p.vi).

Ketotifen fumarate 1.38 mg is approximately equivalent to 1 mg of ketotifen.

Pharmacopoeial description

Ph. Eur.: A white to brownish-yellow, fine crystalline powder. Sparingly soluble in water; very slightly soluble in acetonitrile; slightly soluble in methyl alcohol.

Adverse Effects and Precautions

As for the antihistamines in general, p.404; drowsiness may be a problem, and dry mouth and dizziness may occur. Increased appetite and weight gain, and CNS stimulation, have been reported. Cystitis has occurred rarely, and isolated cases of severe skin reactions have been reported.

For precautions to be observed in asthmatic patients, see Sodium Cromoglicate, p.774. Exacerbation of asthma has been reported; existing anti-asthma treatment should be continued for at least 2 weeks after starting ketotifen therapy. It should not be used for the treatment of acute asthma attacks.

Overdosage. Overdoses of ketotifen in doses stated to range from 10 to 120 mg occurred in 8 patients.[1] Symptoms included drowsiness, confusion, dyspnoea, bradycardia or tachycardia, disorientation, and convulsions. Gastric lavage was performed in 6 patients, and all 8 recovered within 12 hours after supportive treatment.

In an overview of 21 cases of overdosage (including those reported above) the manufacturers stated that no serious signs or symptoms had been reported with doses below 20 mg, and there had been no fatalities.[2] The most serious effects reported had included unconsciousness, convulsions, bradycardia and tachycardia, and a severe hypotensive reaction. Management is essentially supportive and symptomatic.

1. Jefferys DB, Volans GN. Ketotifen overdose: surveillance of the toxicity of a new drug. *BMJ* 1981; **282:** 1755–6.
2. Le Blaye I, *et al.* Acute ketotifen overdosage: a review of present clinical experience. *Drug Safety* 1992; **7:** 387–92.

Interactions

A reversible fall in the platelet count has been observed in a few patients receiving ketotifen concomitantly with oral antidiabetics and it has been suggested that this combination should therefore be avoided. Since ketotifen has the properties of the antihistamines, it may potentiate the effects of other CNS depressant drugs such as alcohol, antihistamines, hypnotics, and sedatives. For the interactions of antihistamines in general, see p.406.

Pharmacokinetics

Ketotifen fumarate is almost completely absorbed from the gastrointestinal tract following oral administration, but bioavailability is reported to be only about 50% due to hepatic first-pass metabolism. Peak plasma concentrations occur 2 to 4 hours after a dose by mouth. It is mainly excreted in the urine as inactive metabolites with a small amount of unchanged drug; the terminal elimination half-life is about 21 hours.

Uses and Administration

Ketotifen has the properties of the antihistamines (p.406) in addition to a stabilising action on mast cells analogous to that of sodium cromoglicate (p.775). It is given orally as the fumarate in the prophylactic management of asthma, when it may take several weeks to exert its full effect; it should not be used to treat acute asthma attacks. Ketotifen is also used in the treatment of allergic conditions such as rhinitis (p.407) and conjunctivitis (p.406).

Ketotifen fumarate is taken by mouth in doses equivalent to 1 mg of ketotifen twice daily with food, increased if necessary to 2 mg twice daily; 0.5 to 1 mg at night may be preferable for the first few days of treatment if drowsiness is likely to be a problem. Children over 2 or 3 years may be given the equivalent of 1 mg of ketotifen twice daily. A dose equivalent to 0.5 mg twice daily has been suggested for children between 6 months and 3 years of age.

Ketotifen fumarate has also been applied topically, as eye drops equivalent to 0.025% ketotifen.

Action. It has been suggested that the anti-allergic action of ketotifen was independent of its antihistaminic properties.[1] This might be due to its effect on responses to platelet-activating factor (PAF).[2] However, the significance of PAF in the pathogenesis of asthma has been questioned.

1. Greenwood C. The pharmacology of ketotifen. *Chest* 1982; **82** (suppl): 45S–5S.
2. Morley J, *et al.* Effects of ketotifen upon responses to platelet activating factor: a basis for asthma prophylaxis. *Ann Allergy* 1986; **56:** 335–40.

Asthma. Results of studies on the effectiveness of ketotifen in the treatment of asthma (p.757) have been conflicting; although some have found it effective in reducing symptoms[1-4] and in enabling a reduction in concomitant anti-asthmatic drug thera-

py,[2,4] others have reported no significant benefits.[5,6] A study in children described as 'preasthmatic' (that is, being at high risk of developing asthma) suggested that long-term therapy with ketotifen decreased the risk of asthma onset.[7]

Although doubts exist about the efficacy of ketotifen in the management of chronic asthma, guidelines by the British Thoracic Society suggest that it may be of some help in very young children intolerant of other drugs.[8]

1. Paterson JW, *et al.* Evaluation of ketotifen (HC-20-511) in bronchial asthma. *Eur J Clin Pharmacol* 1983; **25:** 187–93.
2. Tinkelman DG, *et al.* A multicenter trial of the prophylactic effect of ketotifen, theophylline, and placebo in atopic asthma. *J Allergy Clin Immunol* 1985; **76:** 487–97.
3. Miraglia Del Giudice M, *et al.* Study of the efficacy of ketotifen treatment in asthmatic children under 3 years of age. *Curr Ther Res* 1986; **40:** 685–93.
4. Rackham A, *et al.* A Canadian multicenter study with Zaditen (ketotifen) in the treatment of bronchial asthma in children aged 5 to 17 years. *J Allergy Clin Immunol* 1989; **84:** 286–96.
5. White MP, *et al.* Ketotifen in the young asthmatic—a double-blind placebo-controlled trial. *J Int Med Res* 1988; **16:** 107–13.
6. Volovitz B, *et al.* Efficacy and safety of ketotifen in young children with asthma. *J Allergy Clin Immunol* 1988; **81:** 526–30.
7. Bustos GJ, *et al.* Prevention of asthma with ketotifen in preasthmatic children: a three-year follow-up study. *Clin Exp Allergy* 1995; **25:** 568–73.
8. British Thoracic Society, *et al.* The British guidelines on asthma management: 1995 review and position statement. *Thorax* 1997; **52** (suppl 1): S1–S21.

Preparations

Proprietary Preparations (details are given in Part 3)
Aust.: Zaditen; *Belg.:* Zaditen; *Braz.:* Asdron; Asmalergin; Asmax; Asmen; Broncoten; Nemesil; Profilasmin-Ped; Zaditen; *Canad.:* Zaditen; *Fr.:* Zaditen; *Ger.:* Airvitess; Astifat; Ketof; Padiatifen; Zaditen; Zatofug; *Hong Kong:* Asmafen; Zaditen; *Irl.:* Zaditen; *Israel:* Profiten; Zaditen; *Ital.:* Zaditen; *Jpn:* Zaditen†; *Mex.:* Asmaral-K; Fin-A; Hidroazer; Kasmal; Nemodine; Nomotec; Saluket-H1; Ventisol; Waytifeno; Zaditen; *Neth.:* Zaditen; *NZ:* Asmafen; *Port.:* Cipanfeno; Quefeno; Zaditen; *S.Afr.:* Zaditen; Zetofen; *Singapore:* Asmafen; Denerel; Dhatifen; Erliten; Zaditen; *Spain:* Ketasma; Zasten; *Switz.:* Zaditen; *Thai.:* Asmanoc; Denerel; Ibis; Katifen; Kenefen; Keten; Ketifen; Keto; Ketofen; Ketotab; Medkofen; Medotifen; Politifen; Servitifen; Sykofen; Xidanef; Zadino; Zaditen; *UAE:* Asmafort; *UK:* Zaditen; *USA:* Zaditor.

Levosalbutamol Hydrochloride (20160-c)

Levosalbutamol Hydrochloride *(rINNM).*

Levalbuterol Hydrochloride *(USAN).* (R)-α[1]-[(*tert*-Butylamino)methyl]-4-hydroxy-*m*-xylene-α,α′-diol hydrochloride.
$C_{13}H_{21}NO_3,HCl = 275.8.$
CAS — 34391-04-3 (levosalbutamol); 50293-90-8 (levosalbutamol hydrochloride).

Adverse Effects and Precautions

As for Salbutamol, p.770.

◊ Beta-adrenergic adverse effects (e.g. nervousness and increased heart rate) appeared less frequent with nebulised levosalbutamol 0.63 mg than with racemic salbutamol 2.5 mg.[1] There is preliminary evidence that the increased airway hyper-responsiveness occasionally seen with long-term racemic salbutamol (see Tolerance, p.771) may be due to the S(+)-enantiomer, and therefore might not occur with levosalbutamol.[2]

1. Nelson HS, *et al.* Improved bronchodilation with levalbuterol compared with racemic albuterol in patients with asthma. *J Allergy Clin Immunol* 1998; **102:** 943–52.
2. Perrin-Fayolle M. Salbutamol in the treatment of asthma. *Lancet* 1995; **346:** 1101.

Interactions

As for Salbutamol, p.771.

Pharmacokinetics

There is some systemic absorption of inhaled levosalbutamol. It appears to be stereochemically stable *in vivo* and not metabolised to S(+)-salbutamol. After a single dose levosalbutamol has a half-life of 3.3 hours.

Metabolism. There is evidence that levosalbutamol is metabolised faster than S(+)-salbutamol.

References.
1. Boulton DW, Fawcett JP. Enantioselective disposition of salbutamol in man following oral and intravenous administration. *Br J Clin Pharmacol* 1996; **41:** 35–40.
2. Lipworth BJ, *et al.* Pharmacokinetics and extrapulmonary β$_2$ adrenoceptor activity of nebulised racemic salbutamol and its R and S isomers in healthy volunteers. *Thorax* 1997; **52:** 849–52.
3. Gumbhir-Shah K, *et al.* Pharmacokinetic and pharmacodynamic characteristics and safety of inhaled albuterol enantiomers in healthy volunteers. *J Clin Pharmacol* 1998; **38:** 1096–1106.
4. Boulton DW, Fawcett JP. The pharmacokinetics of levosalbutamol: what are the clinical implications? *Clin Pharmacokinet* 2001; **40:** 23–40.

Uses and Administration

Levosalbutamol, the R(−)-enantiomer of salbutamol (p.770), may be used as an alternative to racemic salbutamol for the management of asthma (p.757). It is administered as the hydrochloride but doses are expressed in terms of the base. Usual doses of 0.63 mg are inhaled three times daily as a nebulised solution, increased if necessary to 1.25 mg three times daily.

◊ References.
1. Nelson HS, *et al.* Improved bronchodilation with levalbuterol compared with racemic albuterol in patients with asthma. *J Allergy Clin Immunol* 1998; **102:** 943–52.

2. Jenne JW. The debate on S-enantiomers of β-agonists: tempest in a teapot or gathering storm? *J Allergy Clin Immunol* 1998; **102**: 893–5.
3. Gawchick SM, *et al.* The safety and efficacy of nebulized leval-buterol compared with racemic albuterol and placebo in the treatment of asthma in pediatric patients. *J Allergy Clin Immunol* 1999; **103**: 615–21.
4. Anonymous. Levalbuterol for asthma. *Med Lett Drugs Ther* 1999; **41**: 51–3.

Action. *In vitro,* levosalbutamol had slightly higher affinity than racemic salbutamol for beta$_1$ and beta$_2$ adrenoceptors.[1] The $S(+)$-enantiomer had low affinity for these receptors. All 3 were mildly selective for beta$_2$ adrenoceptors.

1. Penn RB, *et al.* Comparison of R-, S-, and RS-albuterol interaction with human β$_1$- and β$_2$-adrenergic receptors. *Clin Rev Allergy Immunol* 1996; **14**: 37–45.

Preparations

Proprietary Preparations (details are given in Part 3)
USA: Xopenex.

Lodoxamide Trometamol (12899-y)

Lodoxamide Trometamol (*BANM, rINNM*).
Lodoxamide Tromethamine (*USAN*); U-42585 (lodoxamide); U-42718 (lodoxamide ethyl); U-42585E (lodoxamide trometamol). *N,N'*-(2-Chloro-5-cyano-*m*-phenylene)dioxamic acid compound with trometamol.
$C_{11}H_6ClN_3O_6,2C_4H_{11}NO_3 = 553.9$.
CAS — 53882-12-5 (lodoxamide); 53882-13-6 (lodoxamide ethyl); 63610-09-3 (lodoxamide trometamol).

NOTE. Lodoxamide Ethyl is also *USAN.*

Adverse Effects

The application of lodoxamide eye drops may cause local irritation. Reported effects include burning or stinging, and itching. Flushing and dizziness have also been reported.

Uses and Administration

Lodoxamide has a stabilising action on mast cells resembling that of sodium cromoglicate (p.774). It has been given by mouth, generally as the ethyl ester, or by aerosol inhalation, generally as the trometamol salt, in studies of its prophylactic effect in the treatment of asthma, but has not proved to be of benefit.

Lodoxamide trometamol has, however, been found to be effective when employed as eye drops for allergic conjunctivitis (p.406), particularly vernal keratoconjunctivitis; a concentration equivalent to 0.1% of lodoxamide is used, one or two drops usually being instilled into the eye four times daily.

Conjunctivitis. Lodoxamide is an effective treatment for vernal keratoconjunctivitis.[1,2] There is some evidence that it may be more effective than sodium cromoglicate for this purpose (see p.776).

1. Anonymous. Lodoxamide for vernal keratoconjunctivitis. *Med Lett Drugs Ther* 1994; **36**: 26.
2. Lee S, Allard TRFK. Lodoxamide in vernal keratoconjunctivitis. *Ann Pharmacother* 1996; **30**: 535–7.

Preparations

Proprietary Preparations (details are given in Part 3)
Austral.: Lomide; *Belg.:* Alomide; *Braz.:* Alomide; *Canad.:* Alomide; *Denm.:* Alomide; *Fin.:* Alomide; *Fr.:* Alomide; *Ger.:* Alomide; InfectoTop; *Hong Kong:* Alomide; *Irl.:* Alomide†; *Israel:* Alomide; *Ital.:* Alomide; *Mex.:* Alomide; *Norw.:* Alomide; *NZ:* Lomide; *Port.:* Alomide; *S.Afr.:* Alomide; *Singapore:* Alomide; *Spain:* Alomide; *Switz.:* Alomide; *Thai.:* Alomide; *UK:* Alomide; *USA:* Alomide.

Montelukast Sodium (17380-f)

Montelukast Sodium (*BANM, USAN, rINNM*).
MK-476. Sodium 1-[({(R)-*m*-[(E)-2-(7-chloro-2-quinolyl)-vinyl]-α-[o-(1-hydroxy-1-methylethyl)phenethyl]-benzyl}thio)methyl] cyclopropaneacetate.
$C_{35}H_{35}ClNNaO_3S = 608.2$.
CAS — 158966-92-8 (montelukast); 151767-02-1 (montelukast sodium).

Montelukast sodium 10.37 mg is equivalent to montelukast 10 mg.

Adverse Effects and Precautions

As for Zafirlukast, p.785.

◊ Suspected adverse effects reported to the UK Committee on Safety of Medicines following the launch of montelukast included oedema, agitation and restlessness, allergy including anaphylaxis, angioedema, and urticaria, chest pain, tremor, dry mouth, vertigo, and arthralgia.[1] Further suspected effects included nightmares, sedation, palpitations, and increased sweating.[2]

1. Committee on Safety of Medicines/Medicines Control Agency. Leukotriene antagonists: a new class of asthma treatment. *Current Problems* 1998; **24**: 14.
2. Committee on Safety of Medicines/Medicines Control Agency. Leukotriene receptor antagonists: update on adverse reaction profiles. *Current Problems* 1999; **25**: 14.

Churg-Strauss syndrome. Churg-Strauss syndrome has been reported in association with montelukast.[1,2] For discussion of the unresolved role of leukotriene antagonists in this disorder and precautions to be observed, see under Zafirlukast, p.785.

1. Franco J, Artés MJ. Pulmonary eosinophilia associated with montelukast. *Thorax* 1999; **54**: 558–60.
2. Tuggey JM, Hosker HSR. Churg-Strauss syndrome associated with montelukast therapy. *Thorax* 2000; **55**: 805–6.

Hepatic and renal impairment. Although there is some evidence of effects on the liver in patients receiving montelukast, and although it is largely eliminated by hepatic metabolism, montelukast (unlike zafirlukast) is not considered by its UK manufacturer to be contra-indicated in hepatic impairment, and no dose adjustment is considered necessary in mild to moderate hepatic impairment.

No dosage adjustment is anticipated to be necessary in patients with renal impairment.

Interactions

The manufacturer recommends clinical monitoring when potent hepatic enzyme inducers such as phenytoin, phenobarbital, or rifampicin are given with montelukast.

Phenobarbital. Peak serum concentrations after a single dose of montelukast 10 mg were reduced by 20% in 14 healthy subjects who took phenobarbital 100 mg daily for 14 days, and area under the serum concentration-time curve was reduced by 38%. However, it was not thought that montelukast doses would need adjustment if given with phenobarbital.[1]

1. Holland S, *et al.* Metabolism of montelukast (M) is increased by multiple doses of phenobarbital (P). *Clin Pharmacol Ther* 1998; **63**: 231.

Pharmacokinetics

Peak plasma concentrations of montelukast are achieved in 2 to 4 hours after oral administration. The mean oral bioavailability is 64%. Montelukast is more than 99% bound to plasma proteins. It is extensively metabolised in the liver by cytochrome P450 isoenzymes CYP3A4, CYP2A6, and CYP2C9, and is excreted principally in the faeces via the bile. Metabolism was reduced and the elimination half-life prolonged in patients with mild to moderate hepatic impairment.

Uses and Administration

Montelukast is a selective leukotriene receptor antagonist with actions and uses similar to those of zafirlukast (p.786) although it is reported to have a longer duration of action. It is used as the sodium salt in the management of chronic asthma (p.757), in doses equivalent to 10 mg of montelukast once daily at bedtime; children aged 6 to 14 years may be given the equivalent of 5 mg at bedtime and children aged 2 to 5 years may be given 4 mg. It should not be used to treat an acute asthma attack.

Asthma. Montelukast produced modest improvements compared with placebo in chronic asthma and exercise-induced asthma in both adults[1,2] and children.[3,4] It was not as effective as low-dose inhaled beclometasone in 1 study,[5] but did permit reduction in the dose of concomitant inhaled corticosteroid in another.[6] Montelukast has been reviewed,[7-9] and further general references for leukotriene antagonists can be found under Zafirlukast, p.786.

1. Leff JA, *et al.* Montelukast, a leukotriene-receptor antagonist, for the treatment of mild asthma and exercise-induced bronchoconstriction. *N Engl J Med* 1998; **339**: 147–52.
2. Reiss TF, *et al.* Montelukast, a once-daily leukotriene receptor antagonist, in the treatment of chronic asthma: a multicenter, randomized, double-blind trial. *Arch Intern Med* 1998; **158**: 1213–20.
3. Knorr B, *et al.* Montelukast for chronic asthma in 6- to 14-year-old children: a randomized, double-blind trial. *JAMA* 1998; **279**: 1181–6.
4. Kemp JP, *et al.* Montelukast once daily inhibits exercise-induced bronchoconstriction in 6- to 14-year-old children with asthma. *J Pediatr* 1998; **133**: 424–8.
5. Malmstrom K, *et al.* Oral montelukast, inhaled beclomethasone, and placebo for chronic asthma: a randomized, controlled trial. *Ann Intern Med* 1999; **130**: 487–95.
6. Löfdahl C-G, *et al.* Randomised, placebo controlled trial of effect of a leukotriene receptor antagonist, montelukast, on tapering inhaled corticosteroids in asthma. *BMJ* 1999; **319**: 87–90.
7. Anonymous. Montelukast for persistent asthma. *Med Lett Drugs Ther* 1998; **40**: 71–3.
8. Anonymous. Montelukast and zafirlukast in asthma. *Drug Ther Bull* 1998; **36**: 65–8.
9. Jarvis B, Markham A. Montelukast: a review of its therapeutic potential in persistent asthma. *Drugs* 2000; **59**: 891–928.

Preparations

Proprietary Preparations (details are given in Part 3)
Aust.: Singulair; *Austral.:* Singulair; *Belg.:* Singulair; *Canad.:* Singulair; *Denm.:* Singulair; *Fin.:* Singulair; *Fr.:* Singulair; *Ger.:* Singulair; *Hong Kong:* Singulair; *Irl.:* Singulair; *Israel:* Singulair; *Ital.:* Lukasm; Montegen; Singulair; *Mex.:* Singulair; *Neth.:* Singulair; *Norw.:* Singulair; *NZ:* Singulair; *Port.:* Singulair; *S.Afr.:* Singulair; *Singapore:* Singulair; *Spain:* Singulair; *Swed.:* Singulair; *Switz.:* Singulair; *Thai.:* Singulair; *UK:* Singulair; *USA:* Singulair.

Nedocromil Sodium (18666-r)

Nedocromil Sodium (*BANM, USAN, rINNM*).
FPL-59002 (nedocromil); FPL-59002KC (nedocromil calcium); FPL-59002KP (nedocromil sodium). Disodium 9-ethyl-6,9-dihydro-4,6-dioxo-10-propyl-4H-pyrano[3,2-g]quinoline-2,8-dicarboxylate.
$C_{19}H_{15}NNa_2O_7 = 415.3$.
CAS — 69049-73-6 (nedocromil); 69049-74-7 (nedocromil sodium); 101626-68-0 (nedocromil calcium).

NOTE. Nedocromil Calcium is also *USAN.*

Adverse Effects and Precautions

Inhaled nedocromil sodium may cause headache, nausea, abdominal discomfort (mild and transient), and a bitter taste. Increased bronchospasm has occurred in a few patients. Eye drops may cause transient burning and stinging.

It should not be used for the treatment of acute asthma attacks. The general cautions described under sodium cromoglicate (see p.774) also apply.

◊ A review[1] of nedocromil sodium commented that adverse effects were infrequent, mild, and short-lived. The most common effect appeared to be an unpleasant or bitter taste which was experienced by 12 to 13% of patients, although less than 1% of patients discontinued treatment because of it. Other adverse effects included cough (in 7%), headache (6%), sore throat (5.7%), nausea (4%), and vomiting (1.7%).

1. Brogden RN, Sorkin EM. Nedocromil sodium: an updated review of its pharmacological properties and therapeutic efficacy in asthma. *Drugs* 1993; **45**: 693–715.

Pharmacokinetics

Nedocromil sodium is poorly absorbed from the gastrointestinal tract. About 5% of the inhaled dose is absorbed from the lungs and is excreted unchanged in the urine and bile. The half-life is stated to range from about 1.5 to 3.3 hours.

◊ The extent of absorption or bioavailability of nedocromil sodium after inhalation in healthy subjects was 7 to 9% of the dose, including 2 to 3% oral absorption and 5 to 6% absorption from the respiratory tract.[1] Following inhalation of nedocromil sodium 4 mg the mean peak plasma concentration was 3.3 nanograms per mL in healthy subjects and 2.8 nanograms per mL in asthmatic patients, with peak values being reached at approximately 20 and 40 minutes respectively. The mean total urinary excretion after 24 hours following a single dose was 5.4% of the dose in healthy subjects and 2.3% in asthmatics.

1. Neale MG, *et al.* The pharmacokinetics of nedocromil sodium, a new drug for the treatment of reversible obstructive airways disease, in human volunteers and patients with reversible obstructive airways disease. *Br J Clin Pharmacol* 1987; **24**: 493–501.

Uses and Administration

Nedocromil sodium has a stabilising action on mast cells resembling that of sodium cromoglicate (p.775) and is used similarly in the management of chronic asthma. It should not be used to treat an acute attack of asthma.

For **asthma,** nedocromil sodium is given by metered-dose aerosol inhalation. The usual dose is 4 mg inhaled four times daily which may be decreased to 4 mg twice daily once control of symptoms is achieved. Clinical improvement usually occurs within 2 to 4 weeks of beginning therapy.

Nedocromil sodium is also used topically in the treatment of **allergic conjunctivitis** and allergic **rhinitis.** For allergic conjunctivitis it is given as a 2% solution, being instilled into each eye twice daily. This may be increased to 4 times daily if necessary, which is the usual dose in vernal keratoconjunctivitis. In allergic rhinitis nedocromil sodium is used as a 1% nasal spray: one spray is given into each nostril 4 times daily.

◊ General references.
1. Brogden RN, Sorkin EM. Nedocromil sodium: an updated review of its pharmacological properties and therapeutic efficacy in asthma. *Drugs* 1993; **45:** 693–715.
2. Parish RC, Miller LJ. Nedocromil sodium. *Ann Pharmacother* 1993; **27:** 599–606.

Asthma. Nedocromil sodium is generally considered to be an alternative to sodium cromoglicate in the management of asthma (p.757). Nedocromil has been shown to improve symptoms and reduce bronchodilator intake in adults[1] and children[2] with chronic asthma and it may be used before exercise to reduce exercise-induced bronchoconstriction.[3]
1. Edwards AM, Stevens MT. The clinical efficacy of inhaled nedocromil sodium (Tilade) in the treatment of asthma. *Eur Respir J* 1993; **6:** 35–41.
2. Armenio L, *et al.* Double blind, placebo controlled study of nedocromil sodium in asthma. *Arch Dis Child* 1993; **68:** 193–7.
3. Spooner CH, *et al.* Nedocromil sodium for preventing exercise-induced bronchoconstriction (updated 25 February 1999). Available in The Cochrane Library; Issue 4. Oxford: Update Software; 1999.

Cough. For references indicating a positive response to sodium cromoglicate but not to nedocromil sodium in the management of cough induced by ACE inhibitor therapy, see Cough, p.775.

Rhinitis and conjunctivitis. Nedocromil has been employed in the management of allergic rhinitis (p.407) and conjunctivitis (p.406). There is some evidence that nedocromil may be more effective than cromoglicate in the management of vernal keratoconjunctivitis (see p.776), but is less effective than fluorometholone.[1]
1. Tabbara KF, Al-Kharashi SA. Efficacy of nedocromil 2% versus fluorometholone 0.1%: a randomised, double masked trial comparing the effects on severe vernal keratoconjunctivitis. *Br J Ophthalmol* 1999; **83:** 180–4.

Preparations

Proprietary Preparations (details are given in Part 3)
Aust.: Tilade; Tilarin; Tilavist; *Austral.:* Tilade; *Braz.:* Tilade; *Canad.:* Mireze; Tilade; *Denm.:* Tilade; Tilavist; *Fin.:* Tilade; Tilarin; Tilavist; *Fr.:* Tilade; Tilavist; *Ger.:* Halamid; Irtan; Tilade; *Hong Kong:* Tilade; *Irl.:* Tilade; Tilavist; *Israel:* Tilade; Tilavist; *Ital.:* Kovilen; Kovinal; Tilade; Tilarin; Tilavist; *Mex.:* Irtan; Tilaire; *Neth.:* Tilade; Tilavist; *Norw.:* Tilavist; *NZ:* Tilade; Tilarin; Tilavist; *Port.:* Tilavist; *S.Afr.:* Tilade; *Singapore:* Tilavist; *Spain:* Brionil; Cetimil; Ildor†; Tilad; Tilavist; *Swed.:* Tilavist; *Switz.:* Tilade; Tilarin; Tilavist; *UK:* Rapitil; Tilade; Tilarin†; *USA:* Alocril; Tilade.

Multi-ingredient: *Ital.:* Zarent.

Omalizumab (290-k)

Omalizumab (BAN, pINN).
rhuMab-E25.
CAS — 242138-07-4.

Profile
Omalizumab is a recombinant humanised anti-IgE monoclonal antibody. It is under investigation in the prophylactic management of allergic asthma and seasonal allergic rhinitis.

◊ References.
1. Milgrom H, *et al.* Treatment of allergic asthma with monoclonal anti-IgE antibody. *N Engl J Med* 1999; **341:** 1966–73.
2. Easthope S, Jarvis B. Omalizumab. *Drugs* 2001; **61:** 253–60.
3. Milgrom H, *et al.* Treatment of childhood asthma with anti-immunoglobulin E antibody (omalizumab). *Pediatrics* 2001; **108:** 462–3. Full version: http://www.pediatrics.org/cgi/content/full/108/2/e36
4. Busse W, *et al.* Omalizumab, anti-IgE recombinant humanized monoclonal antibody, for the treatment of severe allergic asthma. *J Allergy Clin Immunol* 2001; **108:** 184–90.
5. Boushey HA. Experiences with monoclonal antibody therapy for allergic asthma. *J Allergy Clin Immunol* 2001; **108** (suppl 2): S77–S83.
6. Casale TB. Experience with monoclonal antibodies in allergic mediated disease: seasonal allergic rhinitis. *J Allergy Clin Immunol* 2001; **108** (suppl 2): S84–S88.

Orciprenaline Sulfate (2091-m)

Orciprenaline Sulfate (rINNM).
Metaproterenol Sulfate (USAN); Metaproterenol Sulphate; Orciprenaline Sulphate (BANM); Orciprenalini Sulfas; Th-152. 1-(3,5-Dihydroxyphenyl)-2-isopropylaminoethanol sulphate; N-Isopropyl-N(β,3,5-trihydroxyphenethyl)ammonium sulphate.
$(C_{11}H_{17}NO_3)_2,H_2SO_4$ = 520.6.
CAS — 586-06-1 (orciprenaline); 5874-97-5 (orciprenaline sulfate).

Pharmacopoeias. In *Eur.* (see p.vi), *Jpn, Pol.*, and *US.*

Pharmacopoeial description

Ph. Eur.: A white, slightly hygroscopic, crystalline powder. Freely soluble in water and in alcohol; practically insoluble in dichloromethane and in ether. A 10% solution in water has a pH of 4.0 to 5.5. Protect from light.

The symbol † denotes a preparation no longer actively marketed

---

USP 25: A white to off-white crystalline powder. Freely soluble in water. A 10% solution in water has a pH of 4.0 to 5.5. Store in airtight containers. Protect from light.

Adverse Effects and Precautions
As for Salbutamol, p.770. Adverse effects are more common because of the non-selective beta agonist effect of orciprenaline. For the adverse effects and precautions pertaining to a non-selective beta agonist see Isoprenaline Sulfate, p.914.

Interactions
As for Salbutamol, p.771.

Pharmacokinetics
Following oral administration orciprenaline is absorbed from the gastrointestinal tract and undergoes extensive first-pass metabolism in the liver; about 40% of an oral dose is reported to reach the circulation unchanged. It is excreted in the urine primarily as metabolites.

Uses and Administration
Orciprenaline sulfate is a direct-acting sympathomimetic with predominantly beta-adrenoceptor stimulant activity. It has actions and uses similar to those of salbutamol (p.772) but is less selective for beta$_2$ receptors.

Orciprenaline sulfate is used as a bronchodilator in the management of reversible airways obstruction, as in asthma (p.757) and in some patients with chronic obstructive pulmonary disease (p.759). However, more selective beta$_2$ agonists such as salbutamol or terbutaline are now preferred. Following inhalation, the onset of action is usually within 5 to 30 minutes and can last up to 6 hours, though there is wide variation.

A typical adult dose for the relief of acute **bronchospasm** has been 1 or 2 inhalations of orciprenaline sulfate 750 µg from a metered-dose aerosol, repeated if required after not less than 30 minutes, up to a maximum of 12 inhalations (9 mg) in 24 hours. A suggested maximum dose within a 24-hour period for children is: under 6 years, up to 4 inhalations; 6 to 12 years, up to 8 inhalations. In patients with asthma, 'as-required' beta agonist therapy is preferable to regular use. An increased need for, or decreased duration of effect of, orciprenaline indicates deterioration of asthma control and the need for review of therapy.

Orciprenaline sulfate has also been inhaled in 5% solution from a hand nebuliser, the usual adult dose being 10 inhalations. If the solution is used with any other nebulising device such as an intermittent positive pressure breathing (IPPB) apparatus the adult dose is 0.2 to 0.3 mL of a 5% solution diluted up to about 2.5 mL with sterile water or physiological saline (i.e. dilution to a 0.4 to 0.6% solution) administered not more often than every 4 hours. Unit-dose vials containing a prediluted solution of orciprenaline sulfate 0.4% and 0.6% are also available for nebulisation by an IPPB device.

In the chronic management of reversible airways obstruction, orciprenaline sulfate has been given by mouth in a usual adult dose of 20 mg three or four times daily.

Orciprenaline sulfate has also been used similarly to isoprenaline (see p.915) for its cardiovascular effects in the treatment of **bradycardia** of various types, notably in AV heart block and sinus bradycardia. In such cases doses of up to 240 mg daily by mouth in divided doses, or 0.25 to 0.5 mg by slow intravenous injection have been given; orciprenaline sulfate may also be given by intravenous infusion, or intramuscular or subcutaneous injection.

Preparations

BP 2001: Orciprenaline Tablets;
USP 25: Metaproterenol Sulfate Inhalation Aerosol; Metaproterenol Sulfate Inhalation Solution; Metaproterenol Sulfate Syrup; Metaproterenol Sulfate Tablets.

Proprietary Preparations (details are given in Part 3)
Aust.: Alupent; *Austral.:* Alupent; *Belg.:* Alupent†; *Canad.:* Alupent; *Fr.:* Alupent†; *Ger.:* Alupent; *Irl.:* Alupent; *Ital.:* Alupent; *Mex.:* Alupent; *Neth.:* Alupent†; *NZ:* Alupent; *S.Afr.:* Alupent; *Spain:* Alupent; *Switz.:* Alupent†; *Thai.:* Alupent; *UK:* Alupent; *USA:* Alupent; Metaprel†; Prometa†.

Multi-ingredient: *Braz.:* Bisolvon Complex; *Irl.:* Alupent Expectorant; *S.Afr.:* Adco-Linctopent; Benylin Chesty; Bisolvon Linctus DA; Bronkese Compound; Flemeze; Silomat DA; *Swed.:* Silomat Compositum†; *Thai.:* Silomat Compositum; *UAE:* Orcinol.

Oxitropium Bromide (13065-h)

Oxitropium Bromide (BAN, rINN).
Ba-253. 6,7-Epoxy-8-ethyl-3-[(S)-tropoyloxy]tropanium bromide; (3s,6R,7S,8r)-8-Ethyl-3-[(S)-tropoyloxy]-6,7-epoxytropanium bromide.
$C_{19}H_{26}BrNO_4$ = 412.3.
CAS — 30286-75-0.
ATC — R03BB02.

Profile
Oxitropium bromide is a quaternary ammonium antimuscarinic with actions similar to those of ipratropium bromide (p.766), to which it is structurally related. It is used as a bronchodilator in the treatment of reversible airways obstruction. Doses of 200 µg by inhalation from a metered-dose aerosol are given 2 or 3 times daily. *Animal* studies have shown reproductive tox-

---

icity with high doses of oxitropium, hence the manufacturer's recommendation that it should not be used during pregnancy.

Administration and dosage. Oxitropium bromide is usually administered by inhalation from an aerosol (see above). The optimal dosage of oxitropium bromide given as a nebulised solution in studies of patients with chronic obstructive pulmonary disease has been reported[1] to be in the range of 1000 to 2000 µg.
1. Stappaerts I, *et al.* Dose-response study of oxitropium bromide inhaled as a nebulised solution. *Eur J Clin Pharmacol* 1994; **46:** 305–7.

Preparations

Proprietary Preparations (details are given in Part 3)
Aust.: Oxivent†; *Belg.:* Oxivent; *Denm.:* Oxivent†; *Fin.:* Ventox; *Fr.:* Tersigat; *Ger.:* Ventilat; *Irl.:* Oxivent; *Ital.:* Oxivent; *UK:* Oxivent.

Pemirolast Potassium (11030-r)

Pemirolast Potassium (USAN, rINNM).
BMY-26517. Potassium 9-methyl-3-(1H-tetrazol-5-yl)-4H-pyrido[1,2-a]-pyrimidin-4-one.
$C_{10}H_7KN_6O$ = 266.3.
CAS — 69372-19-6 (pemirolast); 100299-08-9 (pemirolast potassium).

Profile
Pemirolast potassium has mast cell stabilising properties like sodium cromoglicate (p.774) and may also be a leukotriene inhibitor. It has been used in the treatment of chronic asthma (p.757) and in the prophylaxis of allergic rhinitis (p.407) and conjunctivitis (p.406). For asthma, the usual dose used for adults is 10 mg orally twice daily after food. Children aged 1 to 4 years are given 2.5 mg twice daily, and those aged 5 to 10 years are given 5 mg twice daily. For allergic rhinitis, these doses for adults and children are halved. Pemirolast potassium 0.1% ophthalmic solution is used 4 times daily in the prophylactic management of allergic conjunctivitis. Pemirolast potassium has no bronchodilator properties and should not be used for the treatment of acute asthma attacks.

◊ References.
1. Tinkelman DG, Berkowitz RB. A pilot study of pemirolast in patients with seasonal allergic rhinitis. *Ann Allergy* 1991; **66:** 162–5.
2. Hasegawa T, *et al.* Kinetic interaction between theophylline and a newly developed anti-allergic drug, pemirolast potassium. *Eur J Clin Pharmacol* 1994; **46:** 55–8.
3. Anonymous. New drugs for allergic conjunctivitis. *Med Lett Drugs Ther* 2000; **42:** 39–40.

Preparations

Proprietary Preparations (details are given in Part 3)
Jpn: Alegysal; *USA:* Alamast.

Pirbuterol Acetate (3776-k)

Pirbuterol Acetate (BANM, USAN, rINNM).
CP-24314-14. 2-tert-Butylamino-1-(5-hydroxy-6-hydroxymethyl-2-pyridyl)ethanol acetate.
$C_{12}H_{20}N_2O_3,C_2H_4O_2$ = 300.4.
CAS — 38677-81-5 (pirbuterol); 65652-44-0 (pirbuterol acetate).

Pirbuterol Hydrochloride (13127-d)

Pirbuterol Hydrochloride (BANM, USAN, rINNM).
CP-24314-1; Pyrbuterol Hydrochloride. 2-tert-Butylamino-1-(5-hydroxy-6-hydroxymethyl-2-pyridyl)ethanol dihydrochloride.
$C_{12}H_{20}N_2O_3,2HCl$ = 313.2.
CAS — 38029-10-6.

Profile
Pirbuterol is a direct-acting sympathomimetic with predominantly beta-adrenoceptor stimulant activity and a selective action on beta$_2$ receptors (a beta$_2$ agonist). It has properties similar to those of salbutamol (p.770).

Pirbuterol is used for its bronchodilating properties. It is given as the acetate in the management of reversible airways obstruction, as in asthma (p.757) and in some patients with chronic obstructive pulmonary disease (p.759). Following inhalation, pirbuterol exerts an effect within 10 minutes which is reported to last at least 5 hours.

Pirbuterol is given by inhalation as the acetate via a metered-dose aerosol in a usual dose equivalent to pirbuterol 200 to 400 µg (1 to 2 inhalations) as required but not more often than every four hours. In patients with asthma, 'as-required' beta agonist therapy is preferable to regular use. An increased need for, or decreased duration of effect of, pirbuterol indicates deterioration of asthma control and the need for review of therapy.

Pirbuterol has also been given by mouth as the hydrochloride.

Preparations

Proprietary Preparations (details are given in Part 3)
Aust.: Exirel; *Belg.:* Spirolair; *Canad.:* Maxair†; *Fr.:* Maxair; *Ger.:* Zeisin; *Switz.:* Maxair; *UK:* Exirel†; *USA:* Maxair.

Pranlukast (16795-j)

Pranlukast (BAN, rINN).

ONO-1078. N-[4-Oxo-2-(1H-tetrazol-5-yl)-4H-1-benzopyran-8-yl]-p-(4-phenylbutoxy)benzamide.

$C_{27}H_{23}N_5O_4 = 481.5$.

CAS — 103177-37-3.

ATC — R03DC02.

Profile

Pranlukast is a selective antagonist of the leukotriene D_4 receptor with similar properties to zafirlukast (p.785). It is used in the management of asthma (p.757) at a usual dose of 225 mg of the hydrate twice daily.

◊ References.

1. Tamaoki J, et al. Leukotriene antagonist prevents exacerbation of asthma during reduction of high-dose inhaled corticosteroid. Am J Respir Crit Care Med 1997; 155: 1235–40.
2. Barnes NC, et al. Pranlukast, a novel leukotriene receptor antagonist: results of the first European, placebo-controlled, multicentre clinical study in asthma. Thorax 1997; 52: 523–7.
3. Grossman J, et al. Results of the first US double-blind, placebo-controlled, multicenter clinical study in asthma with pranlukast, a novel leukotriene receptor antagonist. J Asthma 1997; 34: 321–8.
4. Kinoshita M, et al. Churg-Strauss syndrome after corticosteroid withdrawal in an asthmatic patient treated with pranlukast. J Allergy Clin Immunol 1999; 103: 534–5.

Preparations

Proprietary Preparations (details are given in Part 3)

Jpn: Onon.

Procaterol Hydrochloride (13171-b)

Procaterol Hydrochloride (BANM, USAN, rINNM).

CI-888; OPC-2009. (±)-erythro-8-Hydroxy-5-(1-hydroxy-2-isopropylaminobutyl)quinolin-2(1H)-one hydrochloride; (±)-8-Hydroxy-5-[(1R*,2S*)-1-hydroxy-2-isopropylaminobutyl]-2-quinolone hydrochloride.

$C_{16}H_{22}N_2O_3,HCl = 326.8$.

CAS — 72332-33-3 (procaterol); 59828-07-8 (procaterol hydrochloride).

NOTE. The commercial substance is the hemihydrate $(C_{16}H_{22}N_2O_3,HCl,\frac{1}{2}H_2O = 335.8)$.

Pharmacopoeias. In Jpn.

Profile

Procaterol hydrochloride is a direct-acting sympathomimetic with predominantly beta-adrenoceptor stimulant activity selective to beta$_2$ receptors (a beta$_2$ agonist). It has properties similar to those of salbutamol (p.770) and it is used as a bronchodilator in the management of reversible airways obstruction, as in asthma (p.757) or in some patients with chronic obstructive pulmonary disease (p.759). Administration by oral inhalation produces an effect within 5 minutes and the effect can last up to 8 hours.

To relieve acute bronchospasm, 10 to 20 µg of procaterol hydrochloride is given by inhalation from a metered-dose aerosol up to 3 times daily. In patients with asthma, 'as-required' beta agonist therapy is preferable to regular use. An increased need for, or decreased duration of effect of, procaterol indicates deterioration of asthma control and the need for review of therapy. An inhalation solution containing 100 µg per mL has been given via a nebuliser in usual doses of 30 to 50 µg. Procaterol hydrochloride can also be given by mouth in doses of 50 µg once or twice daily.

Preparations

Proprietary Preparations (details are given in Part 3)

Hong Kong: Meptin; *Ital.:* Procadil; Propulm; *Jpn:* Meptin; *Port.:* Onsudil; *S.Afr.:* Normalin†; *Singapore:* Meptin; *Spain:* Onsukil; Promaxol; *Thai.:* Caterol; Meptin.

Proxyphylline (640-d)

Proxyphylline (BAN, rINN).

Proxyphyllinum. 7-(2-Hydroxypropyl)-1,3-dimethylxanthine; (RS)-1,3-Dimethyl-7-(2-hydroxypropyl)purine-2,6(3H,1H)-dione; 7-(2-Hydroxypropyl)theophylline.

$C_{10}H_{14}N_4O_3 = 238.2$.

CAS — 603-00-9.

ATC — R03DA03.

Pharmacopoeias. In Eur. (see p.vi).

Pharmacopoeial description

Ph. Eur.: A white crystalline powder. Very soluble in water; soluble in alcohol. Protect from light.

Profile

Proxyphylline is a derivative of theophylline (p.777) which is used as a bronchodilator and for its cardiovascular properties. Proxyphylline is readily absorbed from the gastrointestinal tract and it does not liberate theophylline in the body.

Preparations

Proprietary Preparations (details are given in Part 3)

Denm.: Neofyllin†; *Mex.:* Purofilina.

Multi-ingredient: *Aust.:* Asthma Efeum; Omega; *Braz.:* Santussal; *Ger.:* Antihypertonicum S; Neobiphyllin-Clys†; Neobiphyllin†; *Spain:* Novofilin; *Switz.:* Neo-Biphyllin†.

Pyridofylline (641-n)

Pyridofylline (rINN).

Pyridophylline; Pyridoxine O-(Theophyllin-7-ylethyl)sulphate. 3-Hydroxy-4,5-bis(hydroxymethyl)-2-methylpyridine 2-(theophyllin-7-yl)ethyl sulphate.

$C_{17}H_{23}N_5O_9S = 473.5$.

CAS — 53403-97-7.

Profile

Pyridofylline is a derivative of theophylline (p.777) that has been used as an ingredient of preparations promoted for respiratory-tract disorders.

Preparations

Proprietary Preparations (details are given in Part 3)

Multi-ingredient: *Spain:* Aletor Compositum†.

Repirinast (2921-h)

Repirinast (USAN, rINN).

MY-5116. Isopentyl 5,6-dihydro-7,8-dimethyl-4,5-dioxo-4H-pyrano[3,2-c]quinoline-2-carboxylate.

$C_{20}H_{21}NO_5 = 355.4$.

CAS — 73080-51-0.

Profile

Repirinast is an orally active anti-allergic with a stabilising action on mast cells resembling that of sodium cromoglicate (p.774). It has been given by mouth in the management of asthma (p.757).

◊ References.

1. Takagi K, et al. Lack of effect of repirinast on the pharmacokinetics of theophylline in asthmatic patients. Eur J Clin Pharmacol 1989; 37: 301–3.
2. Patel PC, et al. The effect of repirinast on airway responsiveness to methacholine and allergen. J Allergy Clin Immunol 1992; 90: 782–8.

Preparations

Proprietary Preparations (details are given in Part 3)

Jpn: Romet.

Reproterol Hydrochloride (2101-l)

Reproterol Hydrochloride (BANM, USAN, rINNM).

D-1959 (reproterol); W-2946M. 7-{3-[(3,5,β-Trihydroxyphenethyl)amino]propyl}theophylline hydrochloride.

$C_{18}H_{23}N_5O_5,HCl = 425.9$.

CAS — 54063-54-6 (reproterol); 13055-82-8 (reproterol hydrochloride).

Profile

Reproterol is a direct-acting sympathomimetic with predominantly beta-adrenergic activity and a selective action on beta$_2$ receptors (a beta$_2$ agonist). It has properties similar to those of salbutamol (p.770).

Reproterol hydrochloride is used as a bronchodilator in the management of reversible airways obstruction, as in asthma (p.757) and in some patients with chronic obstructive pulmonary disease (p.759).

For the relief of acute attacks of bronchospasm the usual dose of reproterol hydrochloride is 1 or 2 inhalations of 500 µg from a metered-dose aerosol repeated every 3 to 6 hours as required. For children of 6 to 12 years of age the suggested dose is one inhalation of 500 µg every 3 to 6 hours. In patients with asthma, 'as-required' beta agonist therapy is preferable to regular use. An increased need for, or decreased duration of effect of, reproterol indicates deterioration of asthma control and the need for review of therapy. It has also been given by mouth (adult doses are 10 to 20 mg three times daily), and by slow intravenous injection.

Preparations

Proprietary Preparations (details are given in Part 3)

Aust.: Bronchospasmin; *Ger.:* Bronchospasmin; *Ital.:* Broncospasmine; *Spain:* Broncospasmin†; *Switz.:* Bronchospasmine; *UK:* Bronchodil†.

Multi-ingredient: *Aust.:* Aarane; Allergospasmin; *Ger.:* Aarane N; Allergospasmin; *Switz.:* Aarane; Allergospasmine.

Rimiterol Hydrobromide (2102-y)

Rimiterol Hydrobromide (BANM, USAN, rINNM).

R-798; WG-253. erythro-3,4-Dihydroxy-α-(2-piperidyl)benzyl alcohol hydrobromide; erythro-(3,4-Dihydroxyphenyl)(2-piperidyl)methanol hydrobromide.

$C_{12}H_{17}NO_3,HBr = 304.2$.

CAS — 32953-89-2 (rimiterol); 31842-61-2 (rimiterol hydrobromide).

Profile

Rimiterol is a direct-acting sympathomimetic with predominantly beta-adrenergic activity and a selective action on beta$_2$ receptors (a beta$_2$ agonist). It has properties similar to those of salbutamol (p.770).

Rimiterol hydrobromide has been used as a bronchodilator for reversible airways obstruction, as in asthma (p.757) and in certain patients with chronic obstructive pulmonary disease (p.759). The usual dose is 1 to 3 inhalations of 200 µg from a metered-dose aerosol as required. This treatment dose should not be repeated in less than 30 minutes. No more than 8 treatments should be taken in any 24-hour period. In patients with asthma, 'as-required' beta agonist therapy is preferable to regular use. An increased need for, or decreased duration of effect of, rimiterol indicates deterioration of asthma control and the need for review of therapy.

Preparations

Proprietary Preparations (details are given in Part 3)

Belg.: Pulmadil†; *Denm.:* Pulmadil†; *Neth.:* Pulmadil†; *S.Afr.:* Pulmadil†; *UK:* Pulmadil†.

Salbutamol (2104-z)

Salbutamol (BAN, rINN).

AH-3365; Albuterol (USAN); Salbutamolum; Sch-13949W. 2-tert-Butylamino-1-(4-hydroxy-3-hydroxymethylphenyl)ethanol.

$C_{13}H_{21}NO_3 = 239.3$.

CAS — 18559-94-9.

ATC — R03AC02; R03CC02.

Pharmacopoeias. In Eur. (see p.vi), Int., and US.

Pharmacopoeial description

Ph. Eur.: A white or almost white, crystalline powder. Sparingly soluble in water; soluble in alcohol; slightly soluble in ether. Protect from light.

USP 25: A white crystalline powder. Sparingly soluble in water; soluble in alcohol. Protect from light.

Salbutamol Sulfate (2105-c)

Salbutamol Sulfate (rINNM).

Albuterol Sulfate (USAN); Salbutamol Hemisulphate; Salbutamol Sulphate (BANM); Salbutamoli Sulfas.

$(C_{13}H_{21}NO_3)_2,H_2SO_4 = 576.7$.

CAS — 51022-70-9.

Pharmacopoeias. In Chin., Eur. (see p.vi), Int., Jpn, Pol., and US.

Salbutamol sulfate 1.2 mg is approximately equivalent to 1 mg of salbutamol.

Pharmacopoeial description

Ph. Eur.: A white or almost white crystalline powder. Freely soluble in water; slightly soluble in alcohol and in ether; very slightly soluble in dichloromethane. Protect from light.

USP 25: A white or practically white powder. Freely soluble in water; slightly soluble in alcohol, in chloroform, and in ether. Protect from light.

Stability. For mention of the stability of a 1:1 mixture of salbutamol and ipratropium nebuliser solutions, see under Ipratropium, p.766.

Adverse Effects

Salbutamol and other beta agonists may cause fine tremor of skeletal muscle (particularly the hands), palpitations, tachycardia, nervous tension, headaches, peripheral vasodilatation, and rarely muscle cramps. Inhalation causes fewer side-effects than systemic administration, and the more selective beta$_2$ agonists cause fewer side-effects than less selective beta agonists. Potentially serious hypokalaemia has been reported after large doses. Hypersensitivity reactions have occurred, including paradoxical bronchospasm, angioedema, urticaria, hypotension, and collapse.

The high doses of salbutamol used intravenously to delay premature labour have additionally been associated with nausea and vomiting, and with severe adverse cardiac and metabolic effects and pulmonary oedema.

For details of the adverse effects of sympathomimetics in general, including distinction between alpha, beta$_1$, and beta$_2$ agonist effects, see under Adrenaline, p.829.

Effects on electrolytes and metabolism. Salbutamol, in common with other beta$_2$-agonists, may cause *hypokalaemia* and *hyperglycaemia*. These effects are related to the dose and route of salbutamol employed; hypokalaemia is more common after parenteral and nebulised administration. Hypokalaemia may be potentiated by concomitant therapy with corticosteroids, diuretics, or xanthines, and by hypoxia; potassium concentrations should therefore be monitored in severe asthma.

Effects on the eyes. It has been suggested that salbutamol and to a greater extent ritodrine may contribute to retinopathy in the premature infant when used for premature labour.[1]

For reports of glaucoma precipitated by the combined administration of ipratropium bromide and salbutamol via a nebuliser, see Ipratropium Bromide, p.766.

1. Michie CA, *et al.* Do maternal β-sympathomimetics influence the development of retinopathy in the premature infant? *Arch Dis Child* 1994; **71:** F149.

Effects on the heart. The main adverse cardiac effect of salbutamol is tachycardia due to increased sympathetic effects on the cardiovascular system. Such tachycardia is dose dependent and is more common after systemic than inhaled therapy. It has been suggested that the increased metabolic demand produced by tachycardia, especially following oral beta$_2$ agonists, might predispose to heart failure or angina in some older patients.[1]

The decreased vagal (parasympathetic) stimulation, and consequently increased sympathetic dominance of cardiac function, together with a tendency to decreased baroreflex sensitivity, that may occur with beta$_2$ agonist inhalation are similar to the risk factors which predispose to ventricular tachyarrhythmias.[2] Hypokalaemia (see under Effects on Electrolytes and Metabolism above) induced by salbutamol may also lead to arrhythmias. The manufacturers note that cardiac arrhythmias, including atrial fibrillation, supraventricular tachycardia, and extrasystoles, have been reported with beta$_2$ agonists, usually in susceptible patients. See also Pregnancy, below.

1. Jenne JW. Can oral β$_2$ agonists cause heart failure? *Lancet* 1998; **352:** 1081–2.
2. Jartti T, *et al.* The acute effects of inhaled salbutamol on the beat-to-beat variability of heart rate and blood pressure assessed by spectral analysis. *Br J Clin Pharmacol* 1997; **43:** 421–8.

Effects on mental function. Visual hallucinations lasting for an hour have been reported[1] following administration of nebulised salbutamol to an elderly patient. At the time of the report the manufacturers were aware of 3 cases of hallucinations in children given oral salbutamol but no such reaction had been previously reported in adults given recommended doses.

1. Khanna PB, Davies R. Hallucinations associated with the administration of salbutamol via a nebuliser. *BMJ* 1991; **292:** 1430.

Effects on the respiratory system. Paradoxical bronchoconstriction has occasionally been reported following bronchodilating therapy. With nebuliser solutions, it has been suggested that the preservatives present could be responsible (see also under Ipratropium, p.766), or that the pH may contribute if non-neutral. In addition, regular use of beta$_2$ agonists such as salbutamol (as opposed to use on an as-needed basis) has been shown to increase airway hyperresponsiveness to various stimuli and to lead to the possible development of tolerance to the bronchoprotective effect (see below).

The increased risk of pulmonary oedema associated with salbutamol is mentioned under Pulmonary Oedema, below.

Increased mortality. The increased incidence of morbidity and mortality that occurred in asthmatic patients mainly involved fenoterol, but salbutamol has been implicated.[1] The debate on the relevance of beta agonist therapy to this increased morbidity and mortality is discussed under Fenoterol on p.765.

1. Spitzer WO, *et al.* The use of β-agonists and the risk of death or near death from asthma. *N Engl J Med* 1992; **326:** 501–6.

Overdosage. Reports of overdosage with salbutamol[1-4] have generally only described the features that may be expected such as tachycardia, CNS stimulation, tremor, hypokalaemia, and hyperglycaemia. Symptomatic treatment of the adverse effects has proved successful. The plasma-potassium concentration and pulse rate have been found to correlate with the plasma concentration of salbutamol.[5]

1. Morrison GW, Farebrother MJB. Overdose of salbutamol. *Lancet* 1973; **ii:** 681.
2. O'Brien IAD, *et al.* Hypokalaemia due to salbutamol overdosage. *BMJ* 1981; **282:** 1515–16.
3. Prior JG, *et al.* Self-poisoning with oral salbutamol. *BMJ* 1981; **282:** 1932.
4. Connell JMC, *et al.* Metabolic consequences of salbutamol poisoning reversed by propranolol. *BMJ* 1982; **285:** 779.
5. Lewis LD, *et al.* A study of self poisoning with oral salbutamol—laboratory and clinical features. *Hum Exp Toxicol* 1993; **12:** 397–401. Correction. *ibid.* 1994; **13:** 371.

Pregnancy. Most adverse effects associated with salbutamol in pregnancy relate to the cardiovascular and metabolic effects of the very high doses given by intravenous infusion in attempts to delay premature labour (see also under Pulmonary Oedema, below). Thus myocardial ischaemia on stopping an infusion[1] and unifocal ventricular ectopics associated with the hypokalaemic response to intravenous salbutamol[2] have been reported. A further report concerned congestive heart failure in a hypertensive woman.[3] Metabolic acidosis following salbutamol infusions in diabetic women has also been reported.[4,5]

1. Whitehead MI, *et al.* Myocardial ischaemia after withdrawal of salbutamol for pre-term labour. *Lancet* 1979; **ii:** 904.
2. Chew WC, Lew LC. Ventricular ectopics after salbutamol infusion for preterm labour. *Lancet* 1979; **ii:** 1383–4.
3. Whitehead MI, *et al.* Acute congestive cardiac failure in a hypertensive woman receiving salbutamol for premature labour. *BMJ* 1980; **280:** 1221–2.
4. Chapman MG. Salbutamol-induced acidosis in pregnant diabetics. *BMJ* 1979; **1:** 639–40.
5. Thomas DJB, *et al.* Salbutamol-induced diabetic ketoacidosis. *BMJ* 1977; **2:** 438.

The symbol † denotes a preparation no longer actively marketed

Pulmonary oedema. Pulmonary oedema has occurred in women given beta$_2$ agonists, including salbutamol,[1,2] for premature labour. The risk factors, the most important of which is fluid overload, are discussed under Precautions, below.

1. Hawker F. Pulmonary oedema associated with β$_2$-sympathomimetic treatment of premature labour. *Anaesth Intensive Care* 1984; **12:** 143–51.
2. Pisani RJ, Rosenow EC. Pulmonary edema associated with tocolytic therapy. *Ann Intern Med* 1989; **110:** 714–18.

Tolerance. Some studies suggest that regular inhalation of a short-acting beta$_2$ agonist, although it continues to produce bronchodilatation, increases airway hyperresponsiveness and may reduce the protective effect against bronchoconstriction provoked by stimuli such as bradykinin, methacholine, or allergen.[1-5] Such tolerance is considered another argument against regular use of short-acting drugs.[1] Reduced bronchoprotective effects have also been demonstrated with long-acting beta$_2$ agonists (see Salmeterol, p.773). There is some evidence that for salbutamol the effect may be due to the $S(+)$-enantiomer,[6] which unlike the $R(-)$-enantiomer does not possess bronchodilating activity: stereoselective metabolism (see under Pharmacokinetics, below) means that regular use of the racemate could lead to accumulation of the S-enantiomer, which provides a possible mechanism for the effect.

1. Cockcroft DW, *et al.* Regular inhaled salbutamol and airway responsiveness to allergen. *Lancet* 1993; **342:** 833–7.
2. O'Connor BJ, *et al.* Tolerance to the nonbronchodilator effects of inhaled β$_2$-agonists in asthma. *N Engl J Med* 1992; **327:** 1204–8.
3. Cockcroft DW, *et al.* Regular use of inhaled albuterol and the allergen-induced late asthmatic response. *J Allergy Clin Immunol* 1995; **96:** 44–9.
4. Inman MD, O'Byrne PM. The effect of regular inhaled albuterol on exercise-induced bronchoconstriction. *Am Respir Crit Care Med* 1996; **153:** 65–9.
5. Crowther SD, *et al.* Varied effects of regular salbutamol on airway responsiveness to inhaled spasmogens. *Lancet* 1997; **350:** 1450.
6. Perrin-Fayolle M. Salbutamol in the treatment of asthma. *Lancet* 1995; **346:** 1101.

Precautions

Salbutamol and other beta agonists should be given with caution in hyperthyroidism, myocardial insufficiency, arrhythmias, susceptibility to QT-interval prolongation, hypertension, and diabetes mellitus (especially on intravenous administration—blood glucose should be monitored since ketoacidosis has been reported).

In *severe asthma* particular caution is also required to avoid inducing hypokalaemia as this effect may be potentiated by hypoxia or by concomitant administration of other anti-asthma drugs (see Interactions, below); plasma-potassium concentrations should be monitored.

Beta$_2$ agonists such as salbutamol are not appropriate for use alone in the treatment of more than mild asthma (see under Asthma, p.757). Increasing need for, or decreased duration of effect of, inhaled salbutamol and other short-acting beta$_2$ agonists indicates deterioration of asthma control and the likely requirement for increased anti-inflammatory therapy.

In *women being treated for premature labour* the risk of pulmonary oedema means that the patient's state of hydration and cardiac and respiratory function should be monitored very carefully; the volume of infusion fluid should be kept to the minimum (normally using glucose 5% as the diluent), and beta$_2$-agonist therapy should be discontinued immediately and diuretic therapy instituted if signs of pulmonary oedema develop. Other risk factors for pulmonary oedema include multiple pregnancy and cardiac disease, which is a specific contra-indication; where cardiac disease is suspected assessment by a physician experienced in cardiology is needed. Eclampsia and severe pre-eclampsia are also contra-indications, with special care needed in mild to moderate pre-eclampsia. Other contra-indications include intra-uterine infection, intra-uterine fetal death, antepartum haemorrhage (which requires immediate delivery), placenta praevia, and cord compression; beta$_2$ agonists should not be used for threatened miscarriage. See also Uses and Administration, below.

For details of the precautions to be observed with sympathomimetics in general, see Adrenaline, p.830.

Abuse. Salbutamol inhalers have been subject to abuse, particularly by children and young adults.[1-5] This has occurred in both asthmatic and non-asthmatic individuals and has been thought to be for the effect of sympathetic stimulation and for the effect of the fluorocarbon propellants. The introduction of

fluorocarbon-free inhalers should reduce the latter motivation, although not the former.

1. Brennan PO. Inhaled salbutamol: a new form of drug abuse? *Lancet* 1983; **ii:** 1030–1.
2. Thompson PJ, *et al.* Addiction to aerosol treatment: the asthmatic alternative to glue sniffing. *BMJ* 1983; **287:** 1515–16.
3. Brennan PO. Addiction to aerosol treatment. *BMJ* 1983; **287:** 1877.
4. Wickramasinghe H, Liebeschuetz HJ. Addiction to aerosol treatment. *BMJ* 1983; **287:** 1877.
5. O'Callaghan C, Milner AD. Aerosol treatment abuse. *Arch Dis Child* 1988; **63:** 70.

Interactions

Concomitant administration of salbutamol and other beta$_2$ agonists with corticosteroids, diuretics, or xanthines increases the risk of hypokalaemia, and monitoring of potassium concentrations is recommended in severe asthma, where such combination therapy is the rule (see also Effects on Electrolytes and Metabolism, above). For an outline of interactions associated with sympathomimetics in general, see Adrenaline, p.830.

Antidepressants. For an apparent interaction between terbutaline and *toloxatone*, a reversible inhibitor of monoamine oxidase type A (RIMA) see Sympathomimetics, p.300.

Beta$_2$ agonists. Patients receiving *salmeterol* may require salbutamol to control an acute attack of bronchospasm. One study indicated that the effects might be additive,[1] but another demonstrated that patients receiving salmeterol had reduced sensitivity to salbutamol and might need higher doses of the latter for acute relief.[2]

1. Smyth ET, *et al.* Interaction and dose equivalence of salbutamol and salmeterol in patients with asthma. *BMJ* 1993; **306:** 543–5.
2. Grove A, Lipworth BJ. Bronchodilator subsensitivity to salbutamol after twice daily salmeterol in asthmatic patients. *Lancet* 1995; **346:** 201–6.

Cardiac glycosides. Hypokalaemia produced by beta$_2$ agonists may result in an increased susceptibility to digitalis-induced arrhythmias although salbutamol intravenously and by mouth can also decrease serum concentrations of *digoxin* (see Beta$_2$ Agonists, p.872).

Corticosteroids. Corticosteroids and beta$_2$ agonists may both produce falls in plasma potassium concentrations; there is evidence that such falls can be exacerbated by concomitant administration.[1] The possibility of enhanced hyperglycaemic effects from such a combination should also be borne in mind.

1. Taylor DR, *et al.* Interaction between corticosteroid and beta-agonist drugs: biochemical and cardiovascular effects in normal subjects. *Chest* 1992; **102:** 519–24.

Diuretics. Hypokalaemia is known to be a possible side-effect during treatment with beta$_2$ agonists such as salbutamol or terbutaline, and this may be enhanced during concomitant diuretic therapy;[1,2] in addition the arrhythmogenic potential of this interaction may be clinically important in patients with ischaemic heart disease.[1]

1. Lipworth BJ, *et al.* Prior treatment with diuretic augments the hypokalemic and electrocardiographic effects of inhaled albuterol. *Am J Med* 1989; **86:** 653–7.
2. Newnham DM, *et al.* The effects of frusemide and triamterene on the hypokalaemic and electrocardiographic responses to inhaled terbutaline. *Br J Clin Pharmacol* 1991; **32:** 630–2.

Neuromuscular blockers. Salbutamol given intravenously has been reported to enhance the neuromuscular blockade produced by *pancuronium* and by *vecuronium* (see Sympathomimetics, p.1335).

Xanthines. An enhanced hypokalaemic effect may occur during coadministration of salbutamol with *theophylline*.[1,2] See also under Terbutaline, p.776 and Sympathomimetics, under Theophylline, p.1327 for the potentiation of other effects.

1. Whyte KF, *et al.* Salbutamol induced hypokalaemia: the effect of theophylline alone and in combination with adrenaline. *Br J Clin Pharmacol* 1988; **25:** 571–8.
2. Kolski GB, *et al.* Hypokalemia and respiratory arrest in an infant with status asthmaticus. *J Pediatr* 1988; **112:** 304–7.

Pharmacokinetics

Salbutamol is readily absorbed from the gastrointestinal tract. It is subject to first-pass metabolism in the liver and possibly in the gut wall; the main metabolite is an inactive sulfate conjugate. Salbutamol is rapidly excreted in the urine as metabolites and unchanged drug; there is some excretion in the faeces. Salbutamol does not appear to be metabolised in the lung, therefore its ultimate metabolism and excretion following inhalation depends upon the delivery method used, which determines the proportion of inhaled salbutamol relative to the proportion inadvertently swallowed. It has been suggested that the majority of an inhaled dose is swallowed and absorbed from the gut.

The plasma half-life of salbutamol has been estimated to range from 4 to 6 hours.

◊ General references.
1. Walker SR, et al. The clinical pharmacology of oral and inhaled salbutamol. Clin Pharmacol Ther 1972; 13: 861–7.
2. Hetzel MR, Clark TJH. Comparison of intravenous and aerosol salbutamol. BMJ 1976; 2: 919.
3. Lin C, et al. Isolation and identification of the major metabolite of albuterol in human urine. Drug Metab Dispos 1977; 5: 234–8.
4. Morgan DJ, et al. Pharmacokinetics of intravenous and oral salbutamol and its sulphate conjugate. Br J Clin Pharmacol 1986; 22: 587–93.
5. Lipworth BJ, et al. Single dose and steady-state pharmacokinetics of 4 mg and 8 mg oral salbutamol controlled-release in patients with bronchial asthma. Eur J Clin Pharmacol 1989; 37: 49–52.
6. Rey E, et al. Pharmacokinetics of intravenous salbutamol in renal insufficiency and its biological effects. Eur J Clin Pharmacol 1989; 37: 387–9.
7. Hindle M, Chrystyn H. Determination of the relative bioavailability of salbutamol to the lung following inhalation. Br J Clin Pharmacol 1992; 34: 311–15.
8. Milliez JM, et al. Pharmacokinetics of salbutamol in the pregnant woman after subcutaneous administration with a portable pump. Obstet Gynecol 1992; 80: 182–5.

Stereoselectivity. The R(−)-enantiomer of salbutamol (levosalbutamol—p.767) is preferentially metabolised and is therefore cleared from the body more rapidly than the S(+)-enantiomer, which lacks bronchodilator activity but may be implicated in some of the adverse effects of salbutamol (see Tolerance, under Adverse Effects, above).

References.
1. Boulton DW, Fawcett JP. Enantioselective disposition of salbutamol in man following oral and intravenous administration. Br J Clin Pharmacol 1996; 41: 35–40.
2. Boulton DW, et al. Transplacental distribution of salbutamol enantiomers at Caesarian section. Br J Clin Pharmacol 1997; 44: 587–90.
3. Lipworth BJ, et al. Pharmacokinetics and extrapulmonary β₂ adrenoceptor activity of nebulised racemic salbutamol and its R and S isomers in healthy volunteers. Thorax 1997; 52: 849–52.

Uses and Administration

Salbutamol is a direct-acting sympathomimetic with predominantly beta-adrenergic activity and a selective action on beta₂ receptors (a beta₂ agonist—p.757). This results in its bronchodilating action being more prominent than its effect on the heart.

Salbutamol and salbutamol sulfate are used as bronchodilators in the management of reversible airways obstruction, as in asthma and in some patients with chronic obstructive pulmonary disease. Salbutamol also decreases uterine contractility and may be given as the sulfate to arrest premature labour (below).

Administration by inhalation results in the rapid onset (within 5 to 15 minutes) of bronchodilatation which lasts for about 3 to 6 hours. Following administration by mouth, the onset of action is within 30 minutes, with a peak effect between 2 to 3 hours after the dose, and a duration of action of up to 8 hours; modified-release preparations that have a longer duration of action are available.

Salbutamol is used as the base or sulfate in aerosol inhalers and as the sulfate in other preparations. The dosage is expressed in terms of salbutamol base.

For the relief of **acute bronchospasm**, 1 or 2 inhalations of salbutamol 100 µg may be given from a conventional *metered-dose aerosol* as required, up to every 4 to 6 hours or 3 or 4 times daily. Two inhalations (1 or 2 in children) may also be given just prior to exertion for the prophylaxis of exercise-induced bronchospasm. (In the USA these inhalations may be expressed as supplying 100 µg, the amount delivered *into* the mouthpiece, or 90 µg, the amount delivered *from* the mouthpiece.) Current asthma guidelines (see p.757) recommend that inhaled short-acting beta₂ agonists such as salbutamol be used on an as-required, not regular, basis. In those patients requiring more than occasional use of salbutamol, anti-inflammatory therapy is also needed. An increased requirement for, or decreased duration of effect of, salbutamol indicates deterioration of asthma control and the need for increased anti-inflammatory therapy. Salbutamol sulfate is now available in chlorofluorocarbon (CFC)-free aerosols. Doses for these aerosols (expressed in terms of salbutamol) are the same as for conventional aerosols.

Salbutamol may also be inhaled as the sulfate from *inhalation capsules* or *discs* containing powder for inhalation, particularly by patients who experience difficulty in using aerosol formulations. Owing to differences in the relative bioavailability to the lungs

between these dry powder systems and the inhalation aerosol a 200-µg dose (expressed in terms of salbutamol) from an inhalation capsule or disc is approximately equivalent in activity to a 100-µg dose from a conventional aerosol and the recommended doses are therefore usually twice those suggested for the aerosol.

When inhalation is ineffective, salbutamol may be given *by mouth* in a dose of 2 to 4 mg three or four times daily as the sulfate; some patients may require doses of up to 8 mg three or four times daily, but such increased doses are unlikely to be tolerated or to provide much extra benefit. Elderly patients should be given the lower doses initially. A dose of 1 to 2 mg three or four times daily is recommended for children aged 2 to 6 years or 2 mg three or four times daily for older children. Modified-release preparations are also available; a usual adult dose is 8 mg twice daily.

In more severe or unresponsive bronchospasm salbutamol sulfate may be given intermittently via a *nebuliser* in adults and children in doses of 2.5 to 5 mg of salbutamol repeated up to 4 times daily; more frequent administration may be required (see Acute Severe Asthma, under Asthma, p.757). Single-dose units of 0.1% or 0.2%, or a concentrated solution of salbutamol 0.5%, are available for this method of administration. Continuous administration via a nebuliser is also possible, usually at a rate of 1 to 2 mg of salbutamol per hour as a 0.005 to 0.01% solution in sodium chloride 0.9%. The efficacy of nebulised salbutamol in infants under 18 months of age is uncertain. Patients with asthma may require supplemental oxygen.

In emergency situations where delivery via a nebuliser is not available, 2 inhalations of salbutamol 100 µg can be repeated 10 to 20 times by multiple actuations of a metered-dose inhaler, preferably into a large spacer device.

In the management of a severe attack of bronchospasm a slow *intravenous injection* of salbutamol 250 µg as a solution containing 50 µg per mL as the sulfate may be required; alternatively salbutamol may be given by intravenous infusion of a solution containing 5 mg in 500 mL (10 µg per mL) at a usual rate of 3 to 20 µg per minute according to the patient's need; higher dosages have been used in patients with respiratory failure.

Salbutamol sulfate can also be given for bronchospasm by *subcutaneous* or *intramuscular* injection in doses of salbutamol 500 µg every 4 hours as required.

For the arrest of uncomplicated **premature labour** between 24 and 33 weeks of gestation salbutamol sulfate is given by *intravenous infusion* preferably with the aid of a syringe pump when the concentration should be 200 µg of salbutamol per mL, glucose 5% having been used for dilution. If no syringe pump is available then the infusion should be with a more dilute solution of 20 µg per mL in glucose 5%. The same dose is employed as with the syringe pump. The recommended initial rate of infusion is 10 µg per minute increased at intervals of 10 minutes until there is a response; the rate is then increased slowly until contractions cease. The usual effective dose is 10 to 45 µg per minute. The infusion should be maintained at the rate at which contractions cease for one hour, then reduced by decrements of 50% at intervals of 6 hours. Prolonged therapy should be avoided as the risks to the mother (see Precautions, above) increase after 48 hours, and furthermore myometrial response is reduced.

The maternal pulse should be monitored throughout the infusion and the rate adjusted to avoid a maternal heart rate of more than 140 beats per minute. A close watch should also be kept on the patient's state of hydration since fluid overload is considered to be a key risk factor for pulmonary oedema.

Salbutamol may subsequently be given *by mouth* in a dose of 4 mg three or four times daily but such usage is not recommended by the *British National Formu-

lary, given the problems with prolonged therapy already mentioned.

Administration. Beta₂ agonists are used extensively in the management of reversible airways obstruction. A common, effective, and convenient method of administration is by a pressurised aerosol inhaler. With this route of administration relief is provided rapidly and fewer systemic side-effects are likely to occur than with oral administration. It is important that patients using conventional inhalers employ the correct technique which involves coordinating actuation of the aerosol with inhalation. If patients have difficulty with correct technique, alternatives are available. Breath-actuated aerosol inhalers may be used. Spacing devices may be used with inhalers. These are added on to the inhaler and reduce the velocity of the aerosol; also more propellant may evaporate before inhalation allowing a greater proportion of the drug to reach the lungs, and coordination of actuation of the aerosol and inhalation is less important. Inhalers of dry powder are also available and are actuated by the patient's inspiration and thus avoid entirely the need for coordination of actuation and inhalation; however, inhalation of the dry powder has occasionally caused irritation of the throat or coughing.

The oral route can be employed although generally a form of inhaled therapy as described above is preferable. A variety of formulations intended for oral administration is commercially available, including modified-release formulations. Nebulisation is an alternative method of delivery and this may be used in the management of severe acute attacks as may parenteral therapy.

Chlorofluorocarbon (CFC) propellants in pressurised aerosol inhalers are being replaced by hydrofluoroalkane (HFA) propellants. Conventional and breath-actuated HFA preparations are available. HFA aerosols may feel and taste different to CFC aerosols.

Asthma. Short-acting beta₂ agonists such as salbutamol form the initial therapy of chronic as well as acute asthma (p.757). High doses are used in acute asthma, but current recommendations for chronic asthma are for low doses to be inhaled as required rather than regularly. Should patients with mild asthma find that more than one dose is required daily, then that should be a sign for additional treatment with anti-inflammatory drugs. Increasing need for, or decreased effect of, short-acting beta₂ agonists indicates deteriorating asthma and the requirement for stepping up therapy. It has been reported that regular salbutamol provided better control than taking it as required,[1] but others have not found this to be the case;[2] any benefit might be proportional to the severity of disease,[3] and whether regular use of short-acting beta₂ agonists helps patients with severe asthma requires more study.[4] In one placebo-controlled study,[5] patients with stable asthma receiving regular high doses of a short-acting inhaled beta₂ agonist were able to reduce the dose considerably with no change in asthma control, lending support to the recommendation for 'as-required' rather than regular use of these drugs. The discussion under Fenoterol on p.765 on the increased mortality that has been observed in asthma patients and the connection with asthma therapy includes a view that regular administration might have contributed to the increased mortality.

1. Chapman KR, et al. Regular vs as-needed inhaled salbutamol in asthma control. Lancet 1994; 343: 1379–82.
2. Drazen JM, et al. Comparison of regularly scheduled with as-needed use of albuterol in mild asthma. N Engl J Med 1996; 335: 841–7.
3. O'Byrne PM, Kerstjens HAM. Inhaled β₂-agonists in the treatment of asthma. N Engl J Med 1996; 335: 886–8.
4. Anonymous. Using β₂-stimulants in asthma. Drug Ther Bull 1997; 35: 1–4.
5. Harrison TW, et al. Randomised placebo controlled trial of β agonist dose reduction in asthma. Thorax 1999; 54: 98–102.

Bronchiolitis. Acute bronchiolitis (inflammation of the bronchioles associated with viral respiratory-tract infection, usually due to respiratory syncytial virus—see p.612) is a poorly defined respiratory condition seen in children. The diagnostic criteria, and the usual management, vary considerably from country to country. Beta₂ agonists such as salbutamol are widely prescribed in the USA, but not in the UK, and attempts to establish their benefits have produced conflicting results.[1] Modest benefit (but no difference in hospital admission rate) has been reported from a meta-analysis of bronchodilator therapy in general,[2] but a meta-analysis of beta₂ agonist therapy in bronchiolitis did not show it to be effective.[3] Comparative studies have suggested that nebulised adrenaline [epinephrine] is more effective than salbutamol,[4,5] and a study in hospitalised children found no benefit from nebulised salbutamol in terms of improved oxygenation or length of hospital stay.[6]

1. Everard ML. Acute bronchiolitis—a perennial problem. Lancet 1996; 348: 279–80.
2. Kellner JD, et al. Bronchodilators for bronchiolitis (updated 28 August 2001). Available in The Cochrane Library; Issue 4. Oxford: Update Software; 2001.
3. Flores G, Horwitz RI. Efficacy of β₂-agonists in bronchiolitis: a reappraisal and meta-analysis. Pediatrics 1997; 100: 233–9.
4. Reijonen T, et al. The clinical efficacy of nebulized racemic epinephrine and albuterol in acute bronchiolitis. Arch Pediatr Adolesc Med 1995; 149: 686–92.
5. Menon K, et al. A randomized trial comparing the efficacy of epinephrine with salbutamol in the treatment of acute bronchiolitis. J Pediatr 1995; 126: 1004–7.
6. Dobson JV, et al. The use of albuterol in hospitalized infants with bronchiolitis. Pediatrics 1998; 101: 361–8.

Chronic obstructive pulmonary disease. Salbutamol and other beta₂ agonist bronchodilators form part of the first-line treatment of chronic obstructive pulmonary disease, although, as discussed on p.759, there is some evidence that an inhaled quaternary ammonium antimuscarinic, such as ipratropium bromide, may have slight advantages compared with a beta₂ agonist.

Cough. For a study indicating that inhaled salbutamol was ineffective in the treatment of children with recurrent cough, see under Beclometasone, p.1062.

Hyperkalaemia. Salbutamol can lower plasma-potassium concentrations by promoting intracellular uptake,[1,2] and this effect has been used in treating mild hyperkalaemia (p.1182) associated with chronic disorders such as renal failure[3,4] and hyperkalaemic periodic paralysis.[5] However, such use is controversial: the effects of salbutamol may be inconsistent[6] and some clinicians prefer to avoid the use of beta₂ agonists because of fears that large doses may induce cardiac arrhythmias.[7]

1. Bushe C. Salbutamol for hyperkalaemia. *Lancet* 1983; **ii**: 797.
2. Anonymous. Hyperkalaemia—silent and deadly. *Lancet* 1989; **i**: 1240.
3. Allon M, *et al.* Nebulized albuterol for acute hyperkalemia in patients on hemodialysis. *Ann Intern Med* 1989; **110**: 426–9.
4. McClure RJ, *et al.* Treatment of hyperkalaemia using intravenous and nebulised salbutamol. *Arch Dis Child* 1994; **70**: 126–8.
5. Wang P, Clausen T. Treatment of attacks in hyperkalaemic familial periodic paralysis by inhalation of salbutamol. *Lancet* 1976; **i**: 221–3.
6. Wong S-L, Maltz HC. Albuterol for the treatment of hyperkalemia. *Ann Pharmacother* 1999; **33**: 103–6.
7. Halperin ML, Kamel KS. Potassium. *Lancet* 1998; **352**: 135–40.

Lymphangioleiomyomatosis. Inhaled beta₂ agonists are often helpful in treating the reversible component of airway obstruction in women with pulmonary lymphangioleiomyomatosis, and a trial of treatment is warranted.[1,2] For mention of the use of medroxyprogesterone in this rare disease, see Respiratory Disorders, p.1481.

1. Johnson S. Lymphangioleiomyomatosis: clinical features, management and basic mechanisms. *Thorax* 1999; **54**: 254–64.
2. Johnson SR, Tattersfield AE. Clinical experience of lymphangioleiomyomatosis in the UK. *Thorax* 2000; **55**: 1052–7.

Premature labour. Premature (preterm labour) is the onset of labour before the expected date, resulting in delivery of an immature infant. Conventionally the definition includes women giving birth before 37 weeks gestation but in practice most problems arise with births before 32 weeks or when the baby's birth-weight is less than 1.5 kg.[1] Risk factors for premature labour include infection, premature rupture of the membranes, cervical incompetence, and multiple pregnancy. There are few proven measures to prevent premature labour, but cervical cerclage may be used for cervical incompetence, and treatment of infections is being investigated.[1,2] In women with premature rupture of the membranes who have not gone into spontaneous labour there is some evidence that antibacterial therapy may be effective in delaying delivery and improving outcomes (see Premature Labour, p.137).

A diagnosis of premature labour is not always easy to make and evidence of cervical change should usually be present in addition to uterine activity.[2,3] Once a diagnosis has been established, a decision must be made as to whether to postpone delivery by the use of drugs that inhibit uterine contractions (tocolysis). It may not be considered appropriate to stop labour in some women. However, in patients of less than about 28 to 32 weeks gestation without complications, attempts to postpone delivery are usually worth trying, if only in the short-term, to allow emergency treatment such as corticosteroids to be given to the mother to enhance the maturation of the fetal respiratory system (see Neonatal Respiratory Distress Syndrome, p.1055) and to enable the patient to be transferred to a specialised unit for preterm delivery.[1-4] Tocolysis is rarely considered necessary after 34 weeks gestation, provided adequate neonatal support facilities are available.[2,3]

The commonest tocolytics are the beta-adrenoceptor agonists, which relax the smooth muscle of the uterus by stimulation of beta₂-adrenoceptors.[2,3] Nonselective agonists, for example orciprenaline and isoxsuprine, have been replaced by more selective beta₂ agonists such as ritodrine and salbutamol.[2,3] These can postpone labour for a few days and the preferred route for starting treatment is intravenous infusion.[3] Oral maintenance therapy with beta₂ agonists after successful treatment of an episode of acute premature labour produces no further benefit.[5] There is little evidence that beta₂ agonists significantly reduce perinatal mortality rates.[6] The patient may experience adverse cardiovascular and metabolic effects and, in particular, pulmonary oedema has been reported in some women given beta₂ agonists intravenously to suppress labour (see above). It is therefore essential that the patient's heart rate and state of hydration are carefully monitored throughout administration. In the event of caesarean section beta blockers may be needed to combat an increased tendency to uterine bleeding.

Magnesium salts have been given intravenously and by mouth as tocolytics, though their precise mode of action is unclear.[3] An intravenous infusion of magnesium sulfate can be given for the initial suppression of uterine contractions and is considered to have similar efficacy to treatment with a beta₂-agonist.[7,8] It has, however, been suggested that tocolytic use of magnesium may be associated with increased paediatric mortality—see

p.1192. Plasma-magnesium concentrations should be monitored during therapy.[3]

Prostaglandins have a role in the induction of labour as mediators of uterine contractions and cervical softening and dilatation. Cyclo-oxygenase (prostaglandin-synthetase) inhibitors such as indometacin may therefore be given by mouth or rectally to inhibit premature labour.[2,3] Although this treatment is as effective as ritodrine,[9,10] a number of adverse effects on the fetus have been reported, such as constriction of the ductus arteriosus and consequent pulmonary hypertension, bronchopulmonary dysplasia, oligohydramnios (a deficiency in amniotic fluid volume), and fatal renal toxicity. A retrospective study suggested that antenatal indometacin therapy for premature labour increased the risk of prematurity-related complications,[11] but some consider the benefits to outweigh the potential risks.[12] Indometacin is therefore generally reserved as a second-line drug or given in conjunction with intravenous tocolytic therapy for an additive effect.[3] Sulindac, a cyclo-oxygenase inhibitor which seems to have little placental transfer, may reduce the incidence of fetal side-effects.[13] More recently it has been suggested that the enzyme isoform cyclo-oxygenase-2 is associated with labour, while cyclo-oxygenase-1 is responsible for constant prostaglandin synthesis in body tissues. The selective cyclo-oxygenase-2 inhibitor nimesulide is under investigation for its potential in the prevention of premature labour.[14]

Atosiban is a peptide analogue of oxytocin with oxytocin antagonist properties. A pooled analysis[15] of three trials found atosiban to be as effective as beta agonists in the management of premature labour, with fewer maternal cardiovascular adverse effects.

Other tocolytics under investigation are the calcium-channel blockers. These suppress the influx of calcium ions across the cell membrane resulting in a reduction in the intracellular concentration of free calcium which inhibits smooth muscle contraction.[3] Initial studies with nifedipine administered by mouth or sublingually have been promising; it appears to be as effective as a beta₂ agonist in suppressing premature labour and may have fewer adverse effects.[16] Similar results have been reported with nicardipine.[17] Application of patches of the nitric oxide donor glyceryl trinitrate to the abdomen to produce uterine relaxation is reported to be as effective as ritodrine treatment.[18]

1. Goldenberg RL, Rouse DJ. Prevention of premature birth. *N Engl J Med* 1998; **339**: 313–20.
2. Steer P, Flint C. Preterm labour and premature rupture of membranes. *BMJ* 1999; **318**: 1059–62.
3. Johnson P. Suppression of preterm labour: current concepts. *Drugs* 1993; **45**: 684–92.
4. Report of a Joint Working Group of the British Association of Perinatal Medicine and the Research Unit of the Royal College of Physicians. Development of audit measures and guidelines for good practice in the management of neonatal respiratory distress syndrome. *Arch Dis Child* 1992; **67**: 1221–7.
5. Macones GA, *et al.* Efficacy of oral beta-agonist maintenance therapy in preterm labor: a meta-analysis. *Obstet Gynecol* 1995; **85**: 313–17.
6. The Canadian Preterm Labor Investigators Group. Treatment of preterm labor with the beta-adrenergic agonist ritodrine. *N Engl J Med* 1992; **327**: 308–12.
7. Wilkins IA, *et al.* Efficacy and side effects of magnesium sulfate and ritodrine as tocolytic agents. *Am J Obstet Gynecol* 1988; **159**: 685–9.
8. Ridgway LE, *et al.* A prospective randomized comparison of oral terbutaline and magnesium oxide for the maintenance of tocolysis. *Am J Obstet Gynecol* 1990; **163**: 879–82.
9. Morales WJ, *et al.* Efficacy and safety of indomethacin versus ritodrine in the management of preterm labor: a randomized study. *Obstet Gynecol* 1989; **74**: 567–72.
10. Besinger RE, *et al.* Randomized comparative trial of indomethacin and ritodrine for the long-term treatment of preterm labor. *Am J Obstet Gynecol* 1991; **164**: 981–8.
11. Norton ME, *et al.* Neonatal complications after the administration of indomethacin for preterm labor. *N Engl J Med* 1993; **329**: 1602–7.
12. Macones GA, Robinson CA. Is there justification for using indomethacin in preterm labor? An analysis of neonatal risks and benefits. *Am J Obstet Gynecol* 1997; **177**: 819–24.
13. Carlan SJ, *et al.* Randomized comparative trial of indomethacin and sulindac for the treatment of refractory preterm labor. *Obstet Gynecol* 1992; **79**: 223–8.
14. Sawdy R, *et al.* Use of cyclo-oxygenase type-2-selective nonsteroidal anti-inflammatory agent to prevent preterm delivery. *Lancet* 1997; **350**: 265–6.
15. The Worldwide Atosiban versus Beta-agonists Study Group. Effectiveness and safety of the oxytocin antagonist atosiban versus beta-adrenergic agonists in the treatment of preterm labour. *Br J Obstet Gynaecol* 2001; **108**: 133–42.
16. Ray JG. Meta-analysis of nifedipine versus beta-sympathomimetic agents for tocolysis during preterm labour. *J Soc Obstet Gynaecol Can* 1998; **20**: 259–69.
17. Jannet D, *et al.* Nicardipine versus salbutamol in the treatment of premature labor: a prospective randomized study. *Eur J Obstet Gynecol Reprod Biol* 1997; **73**: 11–16.
18. Lees CC, *et al.* Glyceryl trinitrate and ritodrine in tocolysis: an international multicenter randomized study. *Obstet Gynecol* 1999; **94**: 403–8.

Proctalgia fugax. Inhalation of salbutamol from a metered-dose inhaler at the beginning of an attack has been shown to reduce the duration of pain in patients with proctalgia fugax.[1]

1. Eckardt VF, *et al.* Treatment of proctalgia fugax with salbutamol inhalation. *Am J Gastroenterol* 1996; **91**: 686–9.

Preparations

BP 2001: Salbutamol Injection; Salbutamol Nebuliser Solution; Salbutamol Oral Solution; Salbutamol Pressurised Inhalation; Salbutamol Tablets;
USP 25: Albuterol Tablets.

Proprietary Preparations (details are given in Part 3)
Aust.: Astec†; Buventol; Epaq; Sultanol; Zaperin; *Austral.:* Airomir; Asmol; Epaq; Respax; Respolin; Ventolin; *Belg.:* Airomir; Ventolin; *Braz.:* Aero-Clenil; Aerolin; Aerotrat; Asmaliv; Broncodil; Broncolin; Broncosedol; Pneumolat; Salbutalin; Suxar; *Canad.:* Apo-Salvent; Asmavent; Novo-Salmol; Ventodisk; Ventolin; *Denm.:* Airomir; Buventol; Salbulin†; Salbutard; Salbuvent; Ventoline; Volmax; *Fin.:* Airomir; Buventol; Salbuvent; Ventoline; *Fr.:* Airomir; Asmasal; Buventol; Salbumol; Spreor; Ventodisks; Ventoline; *Ger.:* Aerolind; Apsomol; Arubendol; Asthma-Spray; Asthmalitan; Broncho Fertiginhalat; Broncho Inhalat; Bronchospray Novo; Cyclocaps; Epaq; Loftan; Padiamol; Pentamol; Salbu; Salbuhexal; Salbulair; Salbupp; Salmundin; Salvent; Sultanol; Volmac; *Hong Kong:* Apo-Salvent; Buto Asma; Respax; Respolin; Salmol; Ventodisks; Ventolin; Volmax; Zenmolin; *Irl.:* Aerolin; Airomir; Asmasal; Gerivent; Salamol; Salomol; Steri-Neb Salamol; Ventamol; Ventodisks; Ventolin; *Israel:* Aerolin; Ventolin; Volmax; *Ital.:* Aerotec; Broncovaleas; Salbufax; Salbutard; Ventolin; Volmax; *Mex.:* Anebron; Assal; Biorenyn; Brodil; Butotal; Cobamol; Inspiryl; Salbulin; Salbutalan; Ventolin; Volmax; *Neth.:* Aerolin; Airomir; Ventolin; Volmax; *Norw.:* Airomir; Buventol; Inspiryl; Salbuvent; Ventoline; *NZ:* Airomir; Asmol; Respax; Respolin; Salbuvent; Ventodisk; Ventolin; Volmax; *Port.:* Ventilan; *S.Afr.:* Abbutamol†; Airomir; Asthavent; Breatheze†; Bronchospray†; Salbulin; Veneze; Ventimax; Ventodisk; Ventolin; Viavent†; Volmax; *Singapore:* Airomir; Butahale; Buventol; Medolin; Respolin; Sabutol; Salmol; Ventolin; Volmax; *Spain:* Aldobronquial; Buto Asma; Dipulmin; Emican; Respiroma; Ventadur; Ventolin; *Swed.:* Airomir; Buventol; Inspiryl; Ventoline; *Switz.:* Airomir; Butohaler†; Butovent; Buventol; Ecovent; Servitamol†; Ventodisk; Ventolin; Volmax; *Thai.:* Airomir; Asmasal; Asthmolin; Butamol; Butovent; Buventol; Medolin; Respolin; Salbusian; Salbutac; Salmol; Saltamol; Servitamol; Venterol; Ventodisk; Ventolin; Violin; Volmax; *UAE:* Butalin; *UK:* Aerolin; Airomir; Asmasal; Asmaven; Kentamol; Libetist; Maxivent; Rimasal; Salamol; Salapin; Salbulin; Ventmax; Ventodisks; Ventolin; Volmax; *USA:* Accuneb; Airet; Proventil; Ventolin; Volmax.

Multi-ingredient: *Aust.:* Combivent; Di-Promal; Duospirel†; Vertide; *Austral.:* Combivent; *Belg.:* Combivent; *Braz.:* Aeroflux Edulito; Aerotide; Clenil Compositum; Pneumolat Expectorante; *Canad.:* Combivent; *Denm.:* Combivent; *Fin.:* Atrodual; Redol Comp; *Fr.:* Combivent; *Hong Kong:* Combivent; Ventide; Ventolin Expectorant; *Irl.:* Combivent; *Ital.:* Breva; Clenil Compositum; Plenaer; Ventolin Espettorante; Ventolin Flogo; Zarent; *Mex.:* Aerocrom; Aeroflux; Combivent; Ventide; *Neth.:* Combivent†; *NZ:* Combivent; Ventide; *Port.:* Combivent; Propavente; *S.Afr.:* Combivent; *Singapore:* Clenil Compositum; Combivent; Ventide; *Spain:* Butosol; Combivent; *Swed.:* Combivent; *Switz.:* Dospir; *Thai.:* Almasal; Asmasal Expectorant; Clenil Compositum; Combivent; Royalin; Salceryl; Salmol Expectorant; Theosal; Ventide; Ventolin Expectorant; *UK:* Aerocrom; Combivent; Ventide; *USA:* Combivent; DuoNeb.

Salmeterol Xinafoate (18680-t)

Salmeterol Xinafoate *(BANM, USAN, rINNM).*

GR-33343G; Salmeterol Xinafoate; Salmeterol 1-Hydroxy-2-naphthoate. *(RS)*-5-{1-Hydroxy-2-[6-(4-phenylbutoxy)hexylamino]ethyl}salicyl alcohol 1-hydroxy-2-naphthoate.
$C_{25}H_{37}NO_4, C_{11}H_8O_3 = 603.7$.

CAS — 89365-50-4 (salmeterol); 94749-08-3 (salmeterol xinafoate).

Adverse Effects and Precautions

As for Salbutamol, p.770. Inhalation of salmeterol may be associated with paradoxical bronchospasm.

Long-acting beta₂ agonists such as salmeterol are not appropriate for the treatment of acute bronchospasm or for patients whose asthma is deteriorating.

Effects on the respiratory system. Transient paradoxical bronchoconstriction with breathlessness, wheeze, or cough has been reported in 6 asthmatic patients following inhalation of salmeterol from a metered-dose aerosol but not after inhalation of the dry powder formulation by diskhaler.[1] The fluorocarbon propellants in the metered-dose aerosol were suspected as the irritants causing bronchoconstriction.

1. Wilkinson JRW, *et al.* Paradoxical bronchoconstriction in asthmatic patients after salmeterol by metered dose inhaler. *BMJ* 1992; **305**: 931–2.

Effects on the skin. A case has been reported in which an urticarial rash was demonstrated to be associated with inhaled salmeterol and in which the propellant as a cause was excluded. Although many urticarial reactions and a variety of rashes had been attributed to beta-agonist therapy their reproducibility had not always been documented.[1]

1. Hatton MQF, *et al.* Salmeterol rash. *Lancet* 1991; **337**: 1169–70.

Tolerance. As with short-acting beta₂ agonists (see Salbutamol, p.771), there is evidence that regular use of long-acting beta₂ agonists such as salmeterol produces tachyphylaxis to their protective effect against bronchoconstriction, as provoked by stimuli such as allergen, methacholine, or exercise.[1-4] The authors of a study of the long-term effect of salmeterol on exercise-induced asthma concluded that the decreased bronchoprotective effect over time was due to a decrease in duration of action (to less than 9 hours) rather than tachyphylaxis,[5] but this interpretation was criticised.[6,7] Whatever the mechanism, the reduced bronchoprotective effect is perhaps more of a concern with long-acting beta$_2$ agonists, since, unlike the short-acting beta$_2$ agonists, their use on a regular basis is recommended.[8] There is little evidence at present that symptomatic relief is significantly reduced by regular use of beta$_2$ agonists, or that patients using salmeterol are at increased risk of death[9,10] or severe (near fatal) attacks,[11] despite a suggestion that receptor downregulation induced by regular salmeterol might mean that patients required higher doses of inhaled salbutamol to attain relief from an acute asthma attack[12,13] (see also Beta$_2$ Agonists, under Interactions of Salbutamol, p.771).

1. Cheung D, et al. Long-term effects of a long-acting β$_2$-adrenoceptor agonist, salmeterol, on airway hyperresponsiveness in patients with mild asthma. N Engl J Med 1992; 327: 1198–1203.
2. Bhagat R, et al. Rapid onset of tolerance to the bronchoprotective effect of salmeterol. Chest 1995; 108: 1235–9.
3. Booth H, et al. Salmeterol tachyphylaxis in steroid treated asthmatic subjects. Thorax 1996; 51: 1100–4.
4. Simons FER, et al. Tolerance to the bronchoprotective effect of salmeterol in adolescents with exercise-induced asthma using concurrent inhaled glucocorticoid treatment. Pediatrics 1997; 99: 655–9.
5. Nelson JA, et al. Effect of long-term salmeterol treatment on exercise-induced asthma. N Engl J Med 1998; 339: 141–6.
6. Aziz I, Lipworth BJ. Exercise-induced asthma. N Engl J Med 1998; 339: 1783.
7. Dickey BF, Adachi R. Exercise-induced asthma. N Engl J Med 1998; 339: 1783–4.
8. Abisheganaden J, Bonshey HA. Long-acting inhaled β$_2$-agonists and the loss of "bronchoprotective" efficacy. Am J Med 1998; 104: 494–7.
9. Castle W, et al. Serevent nationwide surveillance study: comparison of salmeterol with salbutamol in asthmatic patients who require regular bronchodilator treatment. BMJ 1993; 306: 1034–7.
10. Mann RD, et al. Salmeterol: a study by prescription-event monitoring in a UK cohort of 15,407 patients. J Clin Epidemiol 1996; 49: 247–50.
11. Williams C, et al. Case-control study of salmeterol and nearfatal attacks of asthma. Thorax 1998; 53: 7–13.
12. Lipworth B, Grove A. Bronchodilation subsensitivity to salbutamol after salmeterol. Lancet 1995; 346: 968–9.
13. Lipworth BJ. Airway subsensitivity with long-acting β$_2$-agonists: is there cause for concern? Drug Safety 1997; 16: 295–308.

Interactions

As for Salbutamol, p.771.

◊ For a study suggesting a decreased effect of salbutamol in patients receiving salmeterol, as well as a report of additive effects, see Beta$_2$ Agonists under Interactions of Salbutamol, p.771.

Pharmacokinetics

The manufacturers report that at therapeutic inhalation doses plasma concentrations of salmeterol are negligible.

Uses and Administration

Salmeterol is a direct-acting sympathomimetic with beta-adrenoceptor stimulant activity and a selective action on beta$_2$ receptors (a beta$_2$ agonist). When given by oral inhalation, salmeterol acts as a bronchodilator. The onset of action is about 10 to 20 minutes but the full effect may not be apparent until after regular administration of several doses. Unlike short-acting beta$_2$ agonists (see Salbutamol, p.772), salmeterol is therefore not suitable for the symptomatic relief of an acute attack of bronchospasm. However, it is long-acting with a duration of action of about 12 hours and is indicated where the regular administration of a long-acting beta$_2$ agonist is required for persistent reversible airways obstruction, as in chronic asthma or in some patients with chronic obstructive pulmonary disease. It may be useful in protecting against nocturnal and exercise-induced asthma attacks. Short-acting beta$_2$ agonists (on an as-required basis) and regular anti-inflammatory therapy should continue to be used.

Salmeterol is employed in the form of the xinafoate; doses are expressed in terms of the equivalent amount of salmeterol.

The usual dose is two inhalations of salmeterol 25 μg twice daily from a metered-dose aerosol; if necessary, up to 100 μg may be inhaled twice daily. Alternatively, a dry powder inhalation of 50 μg, or if necessary 100 μg, twice daily may be used. Children of 4 years and over may be given 50 μg of salmeterol twice daily by inhalation.

◊ Reviews.
1. Brogden RN, Faulds D. Salmeterol xinafoate: a review of its pharmacological properties and therapeutic potential in reversible obstructive airways disease. Drugs 1991; 42: 895–912.
2. Meyer JM, et al. Salmeterol: a novel, long-acting beta$_2$-agonist. Ann Pharmacother 1993; 27: 1478–87.
3. Bennett J, Tattersfield A. Drugs in focus: 15. Salmeterol. Prescribers' J 1995; 35: 84–8.
4. Adkins JC, McTavish D. Salmeterol: a review of its pharmacological properties and clinical efficacy in the management of children with asthma. Drugs 1997; 54: 331–54.

Asthma. Salmeterol is a long-acting beta$_2$ agonist (duration of action about 12 hours). Guidelines on the management of asthma, see p.757, generally recommend that the use of salmeterol be reserved for patients with chronic asthma who have already progressed to inhaled corticosteroids; it is not a substitute for corticosteroids. Increasing data suggest that, apart from in severe exacerbations, adding a long-acting beta$_2$ agonist to standard dose inhaled corticosteroid therapy may be more effective than doubling the dose of corticosteroid. Salmeterol may also be useful in controlling persistent nocturnal asthma or preventing exercise-induced attacks. There is some evidence that after prolonged use, duration of protection against exercise-induced bronchoconstriction is reduced (see Tolerance, above).

References.
1. Twentyman OP, et al. Protection against allergen-induced asthma by salmeterol. Lancet 1990; 336: 1338–42.
2. Fitzpatrick MF, et al. Salmeterol in nocturnal asthma: a double blind, placebo controlled trial of a long acting inhaled β$_2$ agonist. BMJ 1990; 301: 1365–8.
3. Pearlman DS, et al. A comparison of salmeterol with albuterol in the treatment of mild-to-moderate asthma. N Engl J Med 1992; 327: 1420–5.
4. Green CP, Price JF. Prevention of exercise induced asthma by inhaled salmeterol xinafoate. Arch Dis Child 1992; 67: 1014–17.
5. Smyth ET, et al. Interaction and dose equivalence of salbutamol and salmeterol in patients with asthma. BMJ 1993; 306: 543–5.
6. D'Alonzo GE, et al. Salmeterol xinafoate as maintenance therapy compared with albuterol in patients with asthma. JAMA 1994; 271: 1412–16.
7. Greening AP, et al. Added salmeterol versus higher-dose corticosteroid in asthma patients with symptoms on existing inhaled corticosteroid. Lancet 1994; 344: 219–24.
8. Woolcock A, et al. Comparison of addition of salmeterol to inhaled steroids with doubling of the dose of inhaled steroids. Am J Respir Crit Care Med 1996; 153: 1481–8.
9. Wilding P, et al. Effect of long term treatment with salmeterol on asthma control: a double blind, randomised crossover study. BMJ 1997; 314: 1441–6.
10. Simons FER, et al. A comparison of beclomethasone, salmeterol, and placebo in children with asthma. N Engl J Med 1997; 337: 1659–65.
11. van Noord JA, et al. Addition of salmeterol versus doubling the dose of fluticasone propionate in patients with mild to moderate asthma. Thorax 1999; 54: 207–12.

Chronic obstructive pulmonary disease. Short-acting beta$_2$ agonists are used as bronchodilators in patients with chronic obstructive pulmonary disease (see p.759), although there is some evidence to suggest that an antimuscarinic might be preferable. However the role, if any, of long-acting beta$_2$ agonists such as salmeterol, remains to be clearly established. Improvement in lung function and symptoms has been seen in such patients following regular treatment with inhaled salmeterol,[1,2] and some consider that long-acting beta$_2$ agonists may have a role in maintenance, particularly for nocturnal symptoms.[3]
1. Boyd G, et al. An evaluation of salmeterol in the treatment of chronic obstructive pulmonary disease (COPD). Eur Respir J 1997; 10: 815–21.
2. Mahler DA, et al. Efficacy of salmeterol xinafoate in the treatment of COPD. Chest 1999; 115: 957–65.
3. Leuenberger P, et al. Management 1997 of chronic obstructive pulmonary disease. Schweiz Med Wochenschr 1997; 127: 766–82.

Preparations

Proprietary Preparations (details are given in Part 3)
Aust.: Serevent; **Austral.:** Optrol; Serevent; **Belg.:** Serevent; **Braz.:** Serevent; **Canad.:** Serevent; **Denm.:** Serevent; **Fin.:** Serevent; **Fr.:** Serevent; **Ger.:** Aeromax; Serevent; **Hong Kong:** Serevent; **Irl.:** Serevent; **Israel:** Arial; Salmetedur; Serevent; **Ital.:** Arial; Salmetedur; Serevent; **Mex.:** Serevent; **Neth.:** Serevent; **Norw.:** Serevent; **NZ:** Serevent; **Port.:** Dilamax; Serevent; Ultrabeta; **S.Afr.:** Serevent; **Singapore:** Serevent; **Spain:** Beglan; Betamican; Inaspir; Serevent; **Swed.:** Serevent; **Switz.:** Serevent; **Thai.:** Serevent; **UK:** Serevent; **USA:** Serevent.

Multi-ingredient: Aust.: Seretide; **Austral.:** Seretide; **Canad.:** Advair; **Denm.:** Seretide; **Fin.:** Seretide; **Irl.:** Seretide; **Neth.:** Seretide; **Norw.:** Seretide; **Port.:** Seretaide; **Singapore:** Seretide; **Swed.:** Seretide; **Switz.:** Seretide; **UK:** Seretide; **USA:** Advair.

Seratrodast (17446-n)

Seratrodast (USAN, rINN).

A-73001; AA-2414; Abbott-73001; ABT-001. (±)-2,4,5-Trimethyl-3,6-dioxo-ζ-phenyl-1,4-cyclohexadiene-1-heptanoic acid.
$C_{22}H_{26}O_4 = 354.4$.
CAS — 112665-43-7; 103186-19-2.

Profile

Seratrodast is a thromboxane A$_2$ antagonist that is reported to reduce airway hyperresponsiveness. It is given by mouth in the prophylactic management of asthma (p.757), in single doses of 80 mg in the evening after food.

Adverse effects include gastrointestinal disturbances, drowsiness, headache, palpitations, and hepatitis. Hepatic function should be monitored and the drug should be withdrawn if hypersensitivity reactions such as rashes and pruritus occur, or if there is elevation of liver enzyme values. Seratrodast should be used with care in patients with pre-existing hepatic impairment. It is not suitable for the treatment of an acute asthmatic attack.

◊ References.
1. Tamaoki J, et al. Effect of a thromboxane A$_2$ antagonist on sputum production and its physicochemical properties in patients with mild to moderate asthma. Chest 2000; 118: 73–9.

Preparations

Proprietary Preparations (details are given in Part 3)
Jpn: Bronica.

Sodium Cromoglicate (7721-e)

Sodium Cromoglicate (BANM, rINNM).

Cromolyn Sodium (USAN); Disodium Cromoglycate; FPL-670; Natrii Cromoglicas; Sodium Cromoglycate. Disodium 4,4′-dioxo-5,5′-(2-hydroxytrimethylenedioxy)di(4H-chromene-2-carboxylate).
$C_{23}H_{14}Na_2O_{11} = 512.3$.
CAS — 16110-51-3 (cromoglycic acid); 15826-37-6 (sodium cromoglicate).
Pharmacopoeias. In Chin., Eur. (see p.vi), Int., Jpn, and US.

Pharmacopoeial description

Ph. Eur.: A white or almost white, hygroscopic, crystalline powder. Soluble in water; practically insoluble in alcohol and in ether. Store in airtight containers. Protect from light.

USP 25: A white, odourless, hygroscopic, crystalline powder. Soluble in water; insoluble in alcohol and in chloroform. Store in airtight containers.

Adverse Effects

Inhalation of sodium cromoglicate may cause transient bronchospasm, wheezing, cough, nasal congestion, and irritation of the throat. Nausea, headache, dizziness, an unpleasant taste, and joint pain and swelling have been reported. Other reactions, which have sometimes occurred after treatment for several weeks or months, include aggravation of existing asthma, urticaria, rashes, pulmonary infiltrates with eosinophilia, dysuria, and urinary frequency. Severe reactions such as marked bronchospasm, laryngeal oedema, angioedema, and anaphylaxis have been reported rarely; these have sometimes been referred to as pseudo-allergic.

Intranasal use of sodium cromoglicate may cause transient irritation of the nasal mucosa, sneezing, and occasionally epistaxis. Nausea, skin rashes, and joint pains have occurred when it is taken by mouth. Transient burning and stinging have occasionally been reported following use of sodium cromoglicate eye drops.

Formulation. Some of the adverse effects reported with sodium cromoglicate may be due to its formulation: there is a view that some of the irritant effects reported on inhalation may be due to the use of dry powder inhalers. It has also been suggested that in some patients receiving sodium cromoglicate via a nebuliser, hypotonicity of the nebuliser solution may induce bronchospasm,[1] although others consider this debatable.[2]
1. Chin TW, Nussbaum E. Detrimental effect of hypotonic cromolyn sodium. J Pediatr 1992; 120: 641–3.
2. Rachelefsky GS, et al. Detrimental effects of hypotonic cromolyn sodium. J Pediatr 1992; 121: 992.

Precautions

Sodium cromoglicate has no role in the treatment of acute asthmatic attacks. Withdrawal of sodium cromoglicate may lead to recurrence of the symptoms of asthma. Should withdrawal be necessary it has been suggested that the dose be reduced gradually over a period of one week; patients in whom sodium cromoglicate therapy has permitted a reduction of corticosteroid dosage may require restoration of full steroid cover.

Systemic corticosteroid therapy that has been reduced or discontinued in asthmatic patients may need to be reinstated if symptoms increase, during periods of stress such as infection, illness, trauma, or severe antigen challenge, or where airways obstruction impairs inhalation of sodium cromoglicate.

◊ Nausea, bloating, abdominal cramps, and flatulence developed in a 24-year-old lactase-deficient woman 2 hours after the use of Intal (sodium cromoglicate) via a turbo-haler for exercise-induced asthma.[1] These symptoms recurred on rechallenge and were attributed to ingestion of lactose contained within the Intal capsules.

1. Brandstetter RD, et al. Lactose intolerance associated with Intal capsules. N Engl J Med 1986; 315: 1613–14.

Pharmacokinetics

Sodium cromoglicate is poorly absorbed from the gastrointestinal tract, with a reported bioavailability of only 1%. It has been reported that following inhalation as a fine powder only 8 to 10% of a dose is deposited in the lungs from where it is rapidly absorbed and excreted unchanged in the urine and bile. Less than 7% of an intranasal dose appears to be absorbed. The majority of an inhaled or an intranasal dose is swallowed and excreted unchanged in the faeces. Approximately 0.03% of an ophthalmic dose is reported to be absorbed. The elimination half-life has been reported to be about 20 to 60 minutes following intravenous administration, but the elimination half-life following oral administration or inhalation is longer, being stated to be about 80 minutes.

◊ A study[1] in patients with exercise-induced asthma concluded that plasma concentration of cromoglicate was almost certainly not related directly to protective effect, although another study in asthmatic children given sodium cromoglicate by dry-powder inhalation, found both blood concentration and clinical response to be correlated with inhalation technique.[2]

1. Patel KR, et al. Plasma concentrations of sodium cromoglicate given by nebulisation and metered dose inhalers in patients with exercise-induced asthma: relationship to protective effect. Br J Clin Pharmacol 1986; 21: 231–3.
2. Yahav Y, et al. Sodium cromoglycate in asthma: correlation between response and serum concentrations. Arch Dis Child 1988; 63: 592–7.

Uses and Administration

Sodium cromoglicate is used for the prevention of allergic reactions. Although its precise mode of action remains uncertain, it is believed to act primarily by preventing release of mediators of inflammation from sensitised mast cells through stabilisation of mast-cell membranes. It has no intrinsic antihistaminic action and has generally been considered to possess no bronchodilator activity.

Sodium cromoglicate can prevent the asthmatic response to a variety of allergic and non-allergic stimuli. It is used in the management of chronic asthma that cannot be managed with inhaled beta$_2$ agonists alone; it is not used for acute attacks of asthma.

Sodium cromoglicate is also used in the prophylaxis and treatment of seasonal and perennial allergic rhinitis and allergic conditions of the eye including acute and chronic allergic conjunctivitis and vernal keratoconjunctivitis. It has been given by mouth for the prevention of food allergies, in conjunction with dietary restriction, and is also used in the treatment of mastocytosis.

It is important that the regular administration of sodium cromoglicate is maintained both in the prophylactic control of asthma and in the management of other allergic conditions. Beneficial effects may take several weeks to become established.

In the prophylaxis of **asthma**, sodium cromoglicate is administered by inhalation either as a dry powder, or as a nebulised solution, or from a metered aerosol. The usual dose as dry powder or nebulised solution is 20 mg by inhalation 4 times daily increased, if necessary, to 6 or, for the powder, even to 8 times daily. Once the asthma has been stabilised it may be possible to reduce the dosage. The usual dose by aerosol in the UK is 10 mg four times daily, increased to 6 to 8 times daily if necessary; it may be possible to reduce the dosage to 5 mg four times daily once the asthma has been stabilised. Additional doses as the aerosol or dry powder may be taken before exercise. Doses are administered from metered aerosols providing units of 5 mg. However, aerosols providing units of about 1 mg are also available in some countries and doses of about 2 mg four times daily have been used. The adequacy of this low dosage has been questioned (see

The symbol † denotes a preparation no longer actively marketed

under Administration, below) and in the UK the manufacturers have discontinued the 1-mg aerosol.

Inhalation of sodium cromoglicate may cause bronchospasm; separate inhalation of a beta$_2$ agonist such as salbutamol a few minutes beforehand should prevent this. Use of a combination product containing a beta$_2$ agonist is not recommended as this is liable to be used inappropriately for relief of bronchospasm rather than for its prophylactic effect.

For the prophylaxis of **allergic rhinitis**, approximately 2.5 or 5 mg as a 2 or 4% solution is administered as a spray into each nostril up to 6 times daily. Prophylactic treatment for seasonal allergic rhinitis should begin 2 to 3 weeks before exposure to the offending allergen and should continue throughout the season. In **allergic conjunctivitis** sodium cromoglicate is applied as drops of 2 or 4%, or as a 4% eye ointment; eye drops are generally applied 4 to 6 times daily and eye ointment is applied 2 to 3 times daily.

In **food allergy** and in **mastocytosis**, sodium cromoglicate may be given by mouth in doses of 200 mg four times daily before meals; children over 2 years may be given 100 mg four times daily. If satisfactory control is not achieved within 2 to 3 weeks the dosage may be doubled, but should not exceed 40 mg per kg body-weight daily; a reduction in dosage may be possible once symptoms have been controlled.

Action. Sodium cromoglicate has a range of actions at cellular level. It is known as a mast-cell stabiliser and such an action inhibits the release of histamine and other inflammatory mediators from sensitised mast cells. Other actions that have been reported include a direct effect on airway nerves[1,2] and antagonism of substance P,[3] which lay up with its inhibition of the effects of platelet activating factor (PAF).[4,5] However, sodium cromoglicate is viewed clinically as an anti-inflammatory, and it is still the view, at least of the manufacturers, that sodium cromoglicate's activity in asthma is due to mast-cell stabilisation.[6]

There have been a few reports[7-9] of sodium cromoglicate producing bronchodilatation. However, in practice other drugs with accepted bronchodilating activity are used for this effect in asthma treatment schedules, see p.757.

1. Barnes PJ. Asthma as an axon reflex. Lancet 1986; i: 242–5.
2. Dixon M, et al. The effects of sodium cromoglycate on lung irritant receptors and left ventricular cardiac receptors in the anaesthetized dog. Br J Pharmacol 1979; 67: 569–74.
3. Page C. Sodium cromoglycate, a tachykinin antagonist? Lancet 1994; 343: 70.
4. Morley J, et al. The platelet in asthma. Lancet 1984; ii: 1142–4.
5. Morley J. PAF and airway hyperreactivity: prospects for novel prophylactic anti-asthma drugs. In: PAF, Platelets, and Asthma. Basel, Birkhäuser Verlag, 1987: 87–95.
6. Edwards AM, Norris AA. Cromoglycate and asthma. Lancet 1994; 343: 426.
7. Horn CR, et al. Bronchodilator effect of disodium cromoglycate administered as a dry powder in exercise induced asthma. Br J Clin Pharmacol 1984; 18: 798–801.
8. Weiner P, et al. Bronchodilating effect of cromolyn sodium in asthmatic patients at rest and following exercise. Ann Allergy 1984; 53: 186–8.
9. Yuksel B, Greenough A. Bronchodilator effect of nebulized sodium cromoglycate in children born prematurely. Eur Respir J 1993; 6: 387–90.

Administration. The effectiveness of sodium cromoglicate 2 mg four times daily by metered-dose aerosol inhaler has been reported by a number of controlled studies in adults and children with asthma.[1-5] However, although sodium cromoglicate 2 mg by inhalation from a metered-dose aerosol was reported[6] to be as effective as 20 mg inhaled as powder, the tenfold difference in dosage has been questioned,[7] and others have reported contrary results.[8,9] It has been suggested that an aerosol supplying 5 mg per metered dose (currently favoured in the UK, see above) would be preferable.[10] In a comparison of single-dose pretreatment from metered-dose inhalers, sodium cromoglicate 10 mg (2 × 5 mg puffs) was as effective as beclometasone dipropionate 200 µg in inhibiting bronchial responsiveness to histamine.[11]

Care is required if inhaled sodium cromoglicate is given via a spacer device; evidence suggests that these may greatly influence the amount of drug delivered, reducing it to one-third of the dose delivered by inhaler actuation in some cases.[12]

1. Geller-Bernstein C, Levin S. Sodium cromoglycate pressurised aerosol in childhood asthma. Curr Ther Res 1983; 34: 345–9.
2. Wheatley D. Sodium cromoglycate in aerosol form in regular users of bronchodilator drugs. Curr Med Res Opin 1983; 8: 333–7.
3. Rubin AE, et al. The treatment of asthma in adults using sodium cromoglycate pressurized aerosol: a double-blind controlled trial. Curr Med Res Opin 1983; 8: 553–8.
4. Blumenthal MN, et al. A multicenter evaluation of the clinical benefits of cromolyn sodium aerosol by metered-dose inhaler in the treatment of asthma. J Allergy Clin Immunol 1988; 81: 681–7.
5. Selcow JE, et al. Clinical benefits of cromolyn sodium aerosol (MDI) in the treatment of asthma in children. Ann Allergy 1989; 62: 195–9.

6. Latimer KM, et al. Inhibition by sodium cromoglycate of bronchoconstriction stimulated by respiratory heat loss: comparison of pressurised aerosol and powder. Thorax 1984; 39: 277–81.
7. Anonymous. Sodium cromoglycate aerosol. Drug Ther Bull 1982; 20: 27.
8. Robson RA, et al. Sodium cromoglycate: spincaps or metered dose aerosol. Br J Clin Pharmacol 1981; 11: 383–4.
9. Bar-Yishay E, et al. Duration of action of sodium cromoglycate on exercise induced asthma: comparison of 2 formulations. Arch Dis Child 1983; 58: 624–7.
10. Tullett WM, et al. Dose-response effect of sodium cromoglycate pressurised aerosol in exercise induced asthma. Thorax 1985; 40: 41–4.
11. Cockcroft DW, Murdock KY. Comparative effects of inhaled salbutamol, sodium cromoglycate, and beclomethasone dipropionate on allergen-induced early asthmatic responses, late asthmatic responses, and increased bronchial responsiveness to histamine. J Allergy Clin Immunol 1987; 79: 734–40.
12. Barry PW, O'Callaghan C. Inhalational drug delivery from seven different spacer devices. Thorax 1996; 51: 835–40.

Asthma. Sodium cromoglicate is used as a prophylactic agent in the management of chronic asthma (p.757), but in practice inhaled corticosteroids are generally preferred if the condition cannot be managed with occasional use of an inhaled beta$_2$ agonist alone, when regular prophylactic treatment is therefore considered to be indicated. Even in children, in whom cromoglicate has tended to be more widely used, the trend appears to be towards greater use of inhaled corticosteroids. However, guidelines still specify the use of cromoglicate or nedocromil as a valid alternative to inhaled corticosteroids in some circumstances.

Response to treatment with nebulised sodium cromoglicate was found to be age-related in a study of children under 2 years of age with recurrent wheezy bronchitis and a history of allergic symptoms.[1] It was effective in children of 12 to 24 months of age but not in those below 12 months. Similarly, nebulised sodium cromoglicate was no more effective than placebo in the treatment of a group of 31 infants with persistent wheezing aged under 1 year,[2] and long-term inhalation therapy was ineffective in children aged 1 to 4 years.[3]

1. Geller-Bernstein C, Levin S. Nebulised sodium cromoglycate in the treatment of wheezy bronchitis in infants and young children. Respiration 1982; 43: 294–8.
2. Furfaro S, et al. Efficacy of cromoglycate in persistently wheezing infants. Arch Dis Child 1994; 71: 331–4.
3. Tasche MJA, et al. Randomised placebo-controlled trial of inhaled sodium cromoglicate in 1-4-year-old children with moderate asthma. Lancet 1997; 350: 1060–4. Correction. ibid. 1998; 351: 376.

Cogan's syndrome. Sodium cromoglicate eye drops improved blurred vision in a patient with Cogan's syndrome (p.1049) of 18 years' duration.[1] Sodium cromoglicate capsules [by mouth] also reduced the frequency of fever attacks in this patient.

1. Carter F, Nabarro J. Cromoglycate for Cogan's syndrome. Lancet 1987; i: 858.

Cough. Sodium cromoglicate has been used with modest success by aerosol inhalation to suppress the cough associated with ACE inhibitor therapy (p.820) in some patients.[1,2] However, inhalation of nedocromil sodium was not helpful in the treatment of ACE inhibitor induced cough in 6 diabetic patients.[3]

1. Keogh A. Sodium cromoglycate prophylaxis for angiotensin-converting enzyme inhibitor cough. Lancet 1993; 341: 560.
2. Hargreaves MR, Benson MK. Inhaled sodium cromoglycate in angiotensin-converting enzyme inhibitor cough. Lancet 1995; 345: 13–16.
3. Puolijoki H, Rekiaro M. Lack of effect of nedocromil sodium in ACE-inhibitor-induced cough. Lancet 1995; 345: 394.

Food allergy. Oral sodium cromoglicate has been used in the prophylaxis of food allergy reactions (p.406). However, efficacy has not been unequivocally established.

Mastocytosis. Mastocytosis is a condition characterised by abnormal proliferation of mast cells and their accumulation in body tissues.[1] It occurs in cutaneous or systemic forms, the former most often manifesting as urticaria pigmentosa, the latter involving diverse organs and tissues including the bones, liver, spleen, lymph nodes, haematopoietic system, gastrointestinal tract, and also the skin.

Treatment is aimed at relieving symptoms and does not alter the course of the disease. A combination of H$_1$ and H$_2$-antagonist antihistamines is widely used to control cutaneous and gastrointestinal symptoms, while antimuscarinics may be useful for diarrhoea.[1] Patients should carry adrenaline [epinephrine] for self-injection in the event of severe attacks.

Sodium cromoglicate has been tried in systemic mastocytosis in doses of 100 to 200 mg four times daily by mouth, generally with favourable results.[2-4] In a comparative study in 6 patients sodium cromoglicate 200 mg four times daily was indistinguishable from chlorpheniramine [chlorphenamine] 4 mg plus cimetidine 300 mg four times daily in relieving overall symptoms of systemic mastocytosis.[4] However, individual symptoms responded to varying degrees. A much higher dose of sodium cromoglicate of 100 mg per kg body-weight daily by mouth in divided doses was used with some success in a 5-year-old boy with systemic mastocytosis after lower doses had proved ineffective.[3] Responses to interferon alfa have been reported.[5,6]

1. Golkar L, Bernhard JD. Mastocytosis. Lancet 1997; 349: 1379–85.
2. Soter NA, et al. Oral disodium cromoglycate in the treatment of systemic mastocytosis. N Engl J Med 1979; 301: 465–9.

3. Businco L, *et al.* Systemic mastocytosis in a 5-year-old child: successful treatment with disodium cromoglycate. *Clin Allergy* 1984; **14**: 147–52.
4. Frieri M, *et al.* Comparison of the therapeutic efficacy of cromolyn sodium with that of combined chlorpheniramine and cimetidine in systemic mastocytosis. *Am J Med* 1985; **78**: 9–14.
5. Kolde G, *et al.* Treatment of urticaria pigmentosa using interferon alpha. *Br J Dermatol* 1995; **133**: 91–4.
6. Lippert U, Henz BM. Long-term effect of interferon alpha treatment in mastocytosis. *Br J Dermatol* 1996; **134**: 1164–5.

Rhinitis and conjunctivitis. Many drugs, including sodium cromoglicate, are employed in the management of allergic rhinitis (p.407) and conjunctivitis (p.406). There is some evidence that nedocromil[1] or lodoxamide[2] may be more effective than cromoglicate in the management of vernal keratoconjunctivitis.

1. El Hennawi M. A double-blind placebo controlled group comparative study of ophthalmic sodium cromoglycate and nedocromil sodium in the treatment of vernal keratoconjunctivitis. *Br J Ophthalmol* 1994; **78**: 365–9.
2. Leonardi A, *et al.* Effect of lodoxamide and disodium cromoglycate on tear eosinophil cationic protein in vernal keratoconjunctivitis. *Br J Ophthalmol* 1997; **81**: 23–6.

Preparations

BP 2001: Sodium Cromoglicate Eye Drops; Sodium Cromoglicate Powder for Inhalation;
USP 25: Cromolyn Sodium Inhalation Powder; Cromolyn Sodium Inhalation Solution; Cromolyn Sodium Nasal Solution; Cromolyn Sodium Ophthalmic Solution.

Proprietary Preparations (details are given in Part 3)
Aust.: Acromax; Allercrom; Cromal; Cromoglin; Intal; Lomusol; Opticrom; Pulmosin; Vividrin; *Austral.:* Cromese; Intal; Opticrom; Rynacrom; *Belg.:* Lomudal; Lomusol; Opticrom; Vividrin; *Braz.:* Cromoberg; Intal; Maxicrom; Opticrom; Rilan; *Canad.:* Apo-Cromolyn; Cromolyn; Intal; Nalcrom; Novo-Cromolyn; Opticrom; Rynacrom†; Solu-Crom; Vistacrom†; *Denm.:* Hexacroman; Lecrolyn; Lomudal; *Fin.:* Glinor; Lecrolyn; Lomudal; *Fr.:* Cromabak; Cromoptic; Intercron; Lomudal; Lomusol; Nalcron; Ophtacalm; Opticron; *Ger.:* Acecromol; Allergo-COMOD; Allergocrom; Colimune; Crom-Ophtal; Cromo; Cromo Pur; Cromoglicin; Cromohexal; Cromol; Cromolind; Cromolyn; Cromopp; Diffusyl; Dispacromil; DNCG; duracroman; Flenid; Flui-DNCG; Gelodrin; Intal; Logomed Heuschnupfen-Spray†; Lomupren; Opticrom; Otriven H; Padiacrom; Pentacrom; Pentatop; Prothanon cromo; Pulbil; Vividrin; *Hong Kong:* Cromabak; Cusicrom; Intal; Opticrom; Rynacrom M; Stadaglicin; *Irl.:* Cromogen; Hay-Crom; Intal; Nalcrom; Opticrom; Rynacrom; Steri-Neb Cromogen; Vividrin; *Israel:* Cromogen; Cromoptic; Cromunal; Cronase; Lomudal; Nalcrom; Opticrom; Vicrom; *Ital.:* Acticrom; Cromantal†; Cromosan; Cronacol†; Frenal; Frenal Rinologico; Gaster; Gastrofrenal; Glicacil†; Lomudal; Lomuspray; Nalcrom; Sificrom; *Mex.:* Alercrom; Cusicrom; Intal; Maxicrom; Opticrom; Rynacrom; *Mon.:* Allergodose; Cromedil; *Neth.:* Allergocrom†; Lomudal; Lomusol; Nalcrom; Opticrom; Prevalin†; Vividrin; *Norw.:* Lecrolyn; Lomudal; *NZ:* Intal; Nalcrom; Opticrom; Optrex Hayfever Allergy; Rynacrom; Vicrom; *Port.:* Croglina; Cromex; Cusicrom†; Fenolip; Intal; Opticrom; Rynacrom; *S.Afr.:* Cromal; Cromogen†; Cromohexal; Hay-Crom†; Kiddicrom†; Lomudal; Nalcrom; Opticrom; Rynacrom; Vistacrom; Vividrin; *Singapore:* Cromabak; Cusicrom; Intal; Opticrom; Rynacrom; Sificrom; Stadaglicin; Vividrin; *Spain:* Alergocrom; Cromo Asma; Cusicrom; Farmacrom; Frenal; Gastrofrenal†; Intal; Nalcrom†; Nebulasma; Nebulcrom; Oralcrom; Poledin; Primover; Rinilyn; Rinofrenal; Vividrin; *Swed.:* Lecrolyn; Lomudal; Pollyferm; Rinil; *Switz.:* Cromodyn; Cromosol Ophta; Cromosol UD; Glicinal; Lomudal; Lomusol; Nalcrom; Opticrom; Vividrin; *Thai.:* Ifiral; Intal; Lecrolyn; Opticrom; Rynacrom; Stadaglicin; Vividrin; *UK:* Brol-eze; Clariteyes; Cromogen; Hay-Crom; Hayfever Eye Drops; Intal; Nalcrom; Opticrom; Optrex Hayfever Allergy Eye Drops; Pollenase Allergy; Rynacrom; Vividrin; Viz-On; *USA:* Crolom; Gastrocrom; Intal; Nasalcrom; Opticrom.

Multi-ingredient: *Aust.:* Aarane; Allergospasmin; Ditec; Lomusol comp†; *Belg.:* Lomusol plus Xylometazoline; *Denm.:* Kombicrom; *Ger.:* Aarane N; Allergospasmin; Ditec; Lomupren compositum; Vividrin comp; *Hong Kong:* Rynacrom Compound; *Irl.:* Rynacrom Compound; *Ital.:* Cromozil; Rinofrenal; Visuglican; *Mex.:* Cromosil; *Port.:* Rinoglin; Rynacrom Compound; *Singapore:* Rynacrom Compound; *Spain:* Cromoftol†; Frenal Compositum; Rinofrenal Plus; *Switz.:* Aarane; Allergospasmine; Lomusol-X; *Thai.:* Rynacrom Compound; *UK:* Aerocrom; Resiston One†; Rynacrom Allergy; Rynacrom Compound.

Suplatast Tosilate (11884-r)

Suplatast Tosilate (rINN).
IPD-1151T; Suplatast Tosylate; Suplatastum Tosilas. (±)-(2-{[p-(3-Ethoxy-2-hydroxypropoxy)phenyl]carbamoyl}ethyl)dimethylsulphonium p-toluenesulphonate; (3-{[4-(3-Ethoxy-2-hydroxypropoxy)phenyl]amino}-3-oxopropyl)dimethylsulphonium p-toluenesulphonate.
$C_{23}H_{33}NO_7S_2 = 499.6$.
CAS — 94055-76-2.

Profile

Suplatast tosilate is an anti-allergic given by mouth in the prophylactic management of asthma and other allergic conditions.

◊ References.

1. Sano Y, *et al.* Anti-inflammatory effect of suplatast tosilate on mild asthma. *Chest* 1997; **112**: 862–3.
2. Nihei Y, *et al.* Suplatast tosilate (IPD), a new immunoregulator, is effective in vitiligo treatment. *J Dermatol* 1998; **25**: 250–5.
3. Tamaoki J, *et al.* Effect of suplatast tosilate, a Th2 cytokine inhibitor, on steroid-dependent asthma: a double-blind randomised study. *Lancet* 2000; **356**: 273–8.

Terbutaline Sulfate (2107-a)

Terbutaline Sulfate (USAN, rINNM).
KWD-2019; Terbutaline Sulphate (BANM); Terbutalini Sulfas. 2-*tert*-Butylamino-1-(3,5-dihydroxyphenyl)ethanol sulphate. $(C_{12}H_{19}NO_3)_2,H_2SO_4 = 548.6$.
CAS — 23031-25-6 (terbutaline); 23031-32-5 (terbutaline sulfate).
Pharmacopoeias. In *Eur.* (see p.vi), *Jpn*, and *US*.

Pharmacopoeial description
Ph. Eur.: A white or almost white crystalline powder. It exhibits polymorphism. Freely soluble in water; slightly soluble in alcohol.
USP 25: A white to grey-white crystalline powder; odourless or has a faint odour of acetic acid. Soluble in water and in 0.1N hydrochloric acid; insoluble in chloroform; slightly soluble in methyl alcohol. Store at 15° to 30°. Protect from light.

Adverse Effects and Precautions

As for Salbutamol, p.770.

Overdosage. An overdose of terbutaline due to transcutaneous absorption has been reported following inappropriate topical application to skin infected with tinea.[1] Transcutaneous absorption should be considered especially when children with facial eczema or dermatitis are given terbutaline via a nebuliser and mask.

1. Ingrams GJ, Morgan FB. Transcutaneous overdose of terbutaline. *BMJ* 1993; **307**: 484.

Pulmonary oedema. Pulmonary oedema has occurred in women given beta$_2$ agonists, including terbutaline, for premature labour.[1] The risk factors, the most important of which is fluid overload, are discussed under Precautions for Salbutamol, p.771.

1. Hawker F. Pulmonary oedema associated with β$_2$-sympathomimetic treatment of premature labour. *Anaesth Intensive Care* 1984; **12**: 143–51.

Tolerance. As with other beta$_2$ agonists (see p.771) there is some evidence[1] that tolerance may develop to terbutaline when it is used regularly.

1. O'Connor BJ, *et al.* Tolerance to the nonbronchodilator effects of inhaled β$_2$-agonists in asthma. *N Engl J Med* 1992; **327**: 1204–8.

Tooth erosion. The pH of some inhaled powder formulations of anti-inflammatory and bronchodilator drugs (including terbutaline) was found to be below 5.5, and it was suggested that this might contribute to the dissolution of enamel surfaces of teeth.[1]

1. O'Sullivan EA, Curzon MEJ. Drug treatments for asthma may cause erosive tooth damage. *BMJ* 1998; **317**: 820.

Interactions

As for Salbutamol, p.771.

Xanthines. The metabolic and cardiovascular responses to terbutaline infusion were significantly enhanced following administration of *theophylline* in a study in 7 healthy subjects; in particular the fall in serum potassium was greater when both drugs were given.[1] Careful monitoring of serum potassium is recommended in severe asthma where theophylline and beta$_2$-agonists may be given together.
Terbutaline conversely has an effect on theophylline. Terbutaline can reduce serum-theophylline concentrations by increasing its systemic clearance. This may, or may not, have clinical implications, as improved clinical scores have still occurred with combined therapy despite the theophylline concentration being lower than when used alone; if respiratory symptoms persist, an increase in dosage may be contemplated while monitoring theophylline side-effects and concentration.[2]

1. Smith SR, Kendall MJ. Potentiation of the adverse effects of intravenous terbutaline by oral theophylline. *Br J Clin Pharmacol* 1986; **21**: 451–3.
2. Garty M, *et al.* Increased theophylline clearance in asthmatic patients due to terbutaline. *Eur J Clin Pharmacol* 1989; **36**: 25–8.

Pharmacokinetics

Terbutaline is variably absorbed from the gastrointestinal tract and about 60% of the absorbed dose undergoes first-pass metabolism by sulfate (and some glucuronide) conjugation in the liver and the gut wall. It is accordingly excreted in the urine partly as the inactive conjugates and partly as unchanged terbutaline, the ratio depending upon the route of administration. The half-life is reported to be about 3 to 4 hours. There is some placental transfer. Traces are distributed into breast milk.

Stereoselectivity. Terbutaline, like many other sympathomimetics, exists in two stereoisometric forms but only the (−)-enantiomer of terbutaline is pharmacologically active. Pharmacokinetic studies have been conducted on the two enantiomers and on the racemate.
The oral bioavailability of (−)-terbutaline was 14.8% which was similar to that of the racemate; the bioavailability of (+)-terbutaline was much lower at 7.5%. The difference in bioavailability between the two enantiomers was mainly due to a difference in absorption (about 75% and 50% respectively) although a small difference in subsequent first-pass metabolism also occurred, with the (+)-isomer undergoing slightly more metabolism. It appeared that the (+)-isomer governed the elimination behaviour, both first-pass metabolism and renal clearance, of the racemate whereas the (−)-isomer determined the absorption.[1]
Other studies have also demonstrated stereoselective sulfate conjugation of terbutaline with sulfation of the (+)-enantiomer being double that of the (−)-enantiomer.[2] The primary site of terbutaline sulfation for both enantiomers appears to be in the gut and is significantly correlated with the activity of catechol sulfotransferase.[3]

1. Borgström L, *et al.* Pharmacokinetic evaluation in man of terbutaline given as separate enantiomers and as the racemate. *Br J Clin Pharmacol* 1989; **27**: 49–56.
2. Walle T, Walle UK. Stereoselective sulphate conjugation of racemic terbutaline by human liver cytosol. *Br J Clin Pharmacol* 1990; **30**: 127–33.
3. Pacifici GM, *et al.* (+) and (−) terbutaline are sulphated at a higher rate in human intestine than in the liver. *Eur J Clin Pharmacol* 1993; **45**: 483–7.

Uses and Administration

Terbutaline sulfate is a direct-acting sympathomimetic with predominantly beta-adrenergic activity and a selective action on beta$_2$ receptors (a beta$_2$ agonist). It has actions and uses similar to those of salbutamol (p.772).

Terbutaline is given as the sulfate for its bronchodilating properties in reversible airways obstruction, as occurs in asthma (p.757) and in some patients with chronic obstructive pulmonary disease (p.759). It also decreases uterine contractility and may be used to arrest premature labour (p.773).

After inhalation, the bronchodilating effect of terbutaline usually begins within 5 minutes and lasts for about 3 to 4 hours. The onset of action following oral administration is about 30 minutes and its duration is up to 8 hours; the maximum effect occurs 2 to 3 hours after the dose.

To relieve **acute bronchospasm** in adults and children, 1 or 2 inhalations of terbutaline sulfate 250 µg can be taken as required from a *metered-dose aerosol* every 4 to 6 hours, to a maximum of 8 inhalations in 24 hours. (In the USA, these inhalations may be expressed as supplying 250 µg, the amount delivered into the mouthpiece, or 200 µg, the amount delivered from the mouthpiece.) Current asthma guidelines (see p.757) recommend that inhaled short-acting beta$_2$ agonists such as terbutaline be used on an 'as-required', not regular, basis. In those patients requiring more than occasional use of terbutaline, anti-inflammatory therapy is also needed. An increased requirement for, or decreased duration of effect of, terbutaline indicates deterioration of asthma control and the need for increased anti-inflammatory therapy. A breath-actuated metered-dose *powder inhaler* delivering 500 µg of terbutaline sulfate per inhalation is also available. One inhalation of 500 µg is taken when required up to a maximum of 4 inhalations in 24 hours.

When inhalation is ineffective, terbutaline sulfate may be given *by mouth*; for adults the usual initial dose is 2.5 or 3 mg three times daily increased to 5 mg three times daily as necessary. Children's doses may be calculated on the basis of body-weight; a dose of 75 µg per kg three times daily is suggested. A usual dose in children over 7 years of age is 2.5 mg two or three times daily. Modified-release tablets are also available; the usual adult dose is 7.5 mg twice daily.

Severe or unresponsive bronchospasm may require the administration of terbutaline sulfate intermittently via a *nebuliser*. A usual dose is 2 to 5 mg for children and 5 to 10 mg for adults inhaled 2 to 4 times daily. Single-dose units or a suitable dilution of a concentrated solution containing terbutaline sulfate 1% are used for this purpose. For continuous administration, a suitable adult dose is 1 to 2 mg of terbutaline sulfate per hour given as a 0.01% nebuliser solution in sodium chloride 0.9%.

In emergency situations, where delivery via a nebuliser is not available, 2 inhalations of terbutaline sulfate 250 µg can be repeated 10 to 20 times by multiple actuations of a metered-dose inhaler, preferably into a large spacer device. In children over 5 years of age, inhalation from a metered-dose inhaler has been as effective as the same dose given by nebulisation.

In the treatment of severe forms of bronchospasm, terbutaline sulfate may be given by subcutaneous, intramuscular, or slow intravenous *injection*; a dose of 250 to 500 µg may be given up to four times daily. A suggested dose by injection for children over 2 years of age is 10 µg per kg body-weight to a maximum total dose of 300 µg. Terbutaline sulfate may also be given by *intravenous infusion*, as a solution containing 3 to 5 µg per mL at a rate of 0.5 to 1 mL per minute for adults.

Terbutaline sulfate is also used to arrest uncomplicated **premature labour** between 24 and 33 weeks of gestation. It is given by *intravenous infusion* in glucose 5%, preferably by syringe pump when the concentration is 100 µg per mL. If no syringe pump is available then the concentration of the infusion should be 10 µg per mL. The recommended initial rate of infusion is 5 µg per minute increased by 2.5 µg per minute at intervals of 20 minutes until contractions stop. Usually, a rate of up to 10 µg per minute is sufficient; rates in excess of 20 µg per minute should not be used and if that maximum rate does not delay labour then the infusion should be stopped. The maternal pulse should be monitored throughout the infusion which should be adjusted to avoid a maternal heart rate of more than 135 to 140 beats per minute. A close watch should also be kept on the patient's state of hydration since fluid overload is considered to be a key risk factor for pulmonary oedema. Once contractions have ceased and the infusion has been given for one hour, the dose may be decreased by 2.5 µg per minute at 20-minute intervals to the lowest maintenance dose that produces continued suppression of contractions. After a further 12 hours, *oral* maintenance therapy with 5 mg three times daily may be started. However, such usage is not recommended by the *British National Formulary* as the risks to the mother (see Precautions under Salbutamol, p.771) increase after 48 hours, and furthermore myometrial response is reduced. *Subcutaneous* doses of 250 µg four times daily have been given for a few days before oral treatment was commenced.

Hypoglycaemia. Administration of terbutaline 5 mg by mouth at night reduced the risk of nocturnal hypoglycaemia in a study in patients with type 1 diabetes.[1]

1. Saleh TY, Cryer PE. Alanine and terbutaline in the prevention of nocturnal hypoglycemia in IDDM. *Diabetes Care* 1997; **20:** 1231–6.

Systemic capillary leak syndrome. Systemic capillary leak syndrome is a rare disorder marked by shifts of plasma from the intravascular to the extracellular space, and is often fatal. Acute attacks are treated with intravenous fluid resuscitation, but there is some anecdotal evidence that treatment with terbutaline combined with aminophylline or theophylline, both by mouth, may be useful in preventing further attacks.[1-3] Infusion of epoprostenol has also been used in acute management.[4]

1. Droder RM, *et al.* Control of systemic capillary leak syndrome with aminophylline and terbutaline. *Am J Med* 1992; **92:** 523–6.
2. Amoura Z, *et al.* Systemic capillary leak syndrome: report on 13 patients with special focus on course and treatment. *Am J Med* 1997; **103:** 514–19.
3. Tahirkheli NK, Greipp PR. Treatment of the systemic capillary leak syndrome with terbutaline and theophylline: a case series. *Ann Intern Med* 1999; **130:** 905–9.
4. Fellows IW, *et al.* Epoprostenol in systemic capillary leak syndrome. *Lancet* 1988; **ii:** 1143.

Urticaria. Patients with various types of urticaria unresponsive to conventional therapy with antihistamines (see p.1107) have obtained benefit from treatment with a combination of terbutaline and ketotifen; the urticarias have included chronic idiopathic urticaria,[1] dermographism,[1] and cold urticaria.[1,2] Terbutaline on its own was relatively ineffective and the mechanism of the combination was believed to be due to a stabilising effect on mast cells.[1]

1. Saihan EM. Ketotifen and terbutaline in urticaria. *Br J Dermatol* 1981; **104:** 205–6.
2. Edge JA, Osborne JP. Terbutaline and ketotifen in cold urticaria in a child. *J R Soc Med* 1989; **82:** 439–40.

Preparations

BP 2001: Terbutaline Tablets;
USP 25: Terbutaline Sulfate Inhalation Aerosol; Terbutaline Sulfate Injection; Terbutaline Sulfate Tablets.

Proprietary Preparations (details are given in Part 3)
Aust.: Bricanyl; **Austral.:** Bricanyl; **Belg.:** Bricanyl; **Braz.:** Bricanyl; **Canad.:** Bricanyl; **Denm.:** Bricanyl; **Fin.:** Bricanyl; **Fr.:** Bricanyl; **Ger.:** Aerodur; Aritabendol; Asthma-Kranit Mono; Asthmaprotect; Bricanyl; Butaliret; Butalitab; Contimit; Terbul;

Terbuturmant; **Hong Kong:** Ataline; Bricanyl; Dhatalin; **Irl.:** Bricanyl; **Israel:** Bricalin; Terbulin; **Ital.:** Bricanyl; **Mex.:** Bricanyl; Taziken; Terbuken; **Neth.:** Bricanyl; **Norw.:** Bricanyl; **NZ:** Bricanyl; **Port.:** Bricanyl; **S.Afr.:** Bricanyl; **Singapore:** Ataline; Bricanyl; Butylin; Tolbin; **Spain:** Tedipulmo; Terbasmin; **Swed.:** Bricanyl; **Switz.:** Bricanyl; **Thai.:** Asmaline; Asthamsian; Ataline; Bricanyl; Broncholine; Bucaril; Med-Broncodil; Proasma-T; Sulterline; Terbron; Terbulin; Terbuno; Vacanyl; **UK:** Bricanyl; Monovent; **USA:** Brethaire†; Brethine; Bricanyl.

Multi-ingredient: Aust.: Bricanyl comp; Eudur†; **Braz.:** Bricanyl Composto; Broncasmin Composto; **Ger.:** Bricanyl comp; Eudur†; **Hong Kong:** Bricanyl Expectorant; **Irl.:** Bricanyl Expectorant; **Mex.:** Bricanyl EX; **S.Afr.:** Bronchoped; **Spain:** Terbasmin Expectorante; **Thai.:** Bricanyl Expectorant; Med-Broncodil Expectorant; Terbosil; Terbron Expectorant; Terbulin Expectorant.

Theobromine (643-m)

Theobromine (*BAN*).

Santheose; Theobrominum. 3,7-Dihydro-3,7-dimethylpurine-2,6(1H)-dione; 3,7-Dimethylxanthine.
$C_7H_8N_4O_2 = 180.2$.
CAS — 83-67-0.
ATC — C03BD01; R03DA07.
Pharmacopoeias. In *Eur.* (see p.vi) and *Pol.*

Pharmacopoeial description

Ph. Eur.: A white powder. Very slightly soluble in water and in dehydrated alcohol; practically insoluble in ether; slightly soluble in ammonia. It dissolves in dilute solutions of alkali hydroxides and in mineral acids.

Profile

Theobromine has the general properties of the other xanthines (see Theophylline, p.777). It has a weaker activity than theophylline or caffeine and has practically no stimulant effect on the CNS. Large doses can cause nausea and vomiting. Theobromine has been used for its bronchodilating properties and in the treatment of cardiovascular disorders. Theobromine and calcium salicylate (theosalicin), theobromine and sodium acetate, and theobromine and sodium salicylate (themisalum, theobromsal) have all been used similarly to theobromine.

Theobromine is the chief xanthine in the beverage cocoa (p.1681). It is also present in chocolate and in small amounts in tea. Theobroma oil may contain up to 2% theobromine.

Preparations

Proprietary Preparations (details are given in Part 3)

Multi-ingredient: Aust.: Asthma-Hilfe; Theo-Lanicor†; **Braz.:** Urodonal; **Ger.:** Angiocardyl N†; Eupond†; **Spain:** Propyre T.

Theophylline (647-q)

Theophylline (*BAN*).

Anhydrous Theophylline; Teofillina; Theophyllinum. 3,7-Dihydro-1,3-dimethylpurine-2,6(1H)-dione; 1,3-Dimethylxanthine.
$C_7H_8N_4O_2 = 180.2$.
CAS — 58-55-9.
ATC — R03DA04.
Pharmacopoeias. In *Eur.* (see p.vi), *Jpn, Pol.,* and *US.* Some pharmacopoeias include anhydrous and hydrated theophylline in one monograph.

Pharmacopoeial description

Ph. Eur.: A white crystalline powder. Slightly soluble in water; sparingly soluble in dehydrated alcohol. It dissolves in solutions of alkali hydroxides, in ammonia, and in mineral acids.

USP 25: Theophylline contains one molecule of water of hydration or is anhydrous. It is a white, odourless, crystalline powder. Slightly soluble in water, more soluble in hot water; sparingly soluble in alcohol, in chloroform, and in ether; freely soluble in solutions of alkali hydroxides and in ammonia.

Theophylline Hydrate (648-p)

Theophylline Hydrate (*BANM*).

Theophylline Monohydrate; Theophyllinum Monohydricum.
$C_7H_8N_4O_2,H_2O = 198.2$.
CAS — 5967-84-0.

Pharmacopoeias. In *Chin., Eur.* (see p.vi), *Pol.,* and *US.* Some pharmacopoeias include anhydrous and hydrated theophylline in one monograph.

Theophylline hydrate 1.1 mg is approximately equivalent to 1 mg of theophylline.

Pharmacopoeial description

Ph. Eur.: A white crystalline powder. Slightly soluble in water; sparingly soluble in dehydrated alcohol. It dissolves in solutions of alkali hydroxides, in ammonia, and in mineral acids.

USP 25: Theophylline contains one molecule of water of hydration or is anhydrous. It is a white, odourless, crystalline powder. Slightly soluble in water, more soluble in hot water; sparingly soluble in alcohol, in chloroform, and in ether; freely soluble in solutions of alkali hydroxides and in ammonia.

Stability. Alcohol-free theophylline liquid repackaged in clear or amber polypropylene oral syringes could be stored at room temperature under continuous fluorescent lighting for at least 180 days without significant change in the concentration of theophylline.[1] However, it was recommended that solutions be protected from light because of the potential for discoloration.

1. Johnson CE, Drabik BT. Stability of alcohol-free theophylline liquid repackaged in plastic oral syringes. *Am J Hosp Pharm* 1989; **46:** 980–1.

Adverse Effects

The side-effects commonly encountered with theophylline and xanthine derivatives irrespective of the route of administration, are gastrointestinal irritation and stimulation of the CNS. Serum concentrations of theophylline greater than 20 µg per mL (110 µmol per litre) are associated with an increased risk of adverse effects (but see below).

Theophylline may cause nausea, vomiting, abdominal pain, diarrhoea, gastro-oesophageal reflux, and other gastrointestinal disturbances, insomnia, headache, anxiety, restlessness, dizziness, tremor, and palpitations. Overdosage may also lead to agitation, diuresis and repeated vomiting (sometimes haematemesis) and consequent dehydration, cardiac arrhythmias including tachycardia, hypotension, electrolyte disturbances including profound hypokalaemia, hyperglycaemia, metabolic acidosis, convulsions, and death. Severe toxicity may not be preceded by milder symptoms. Convulsions, cardiac arrhythmias, and hypotension may follow intravenous injection, particularly if the injection is too rapid, and sudden deaths have been reported; the drug is too irritant for intramuscular use. Proctitis may follow repeated administration of suppositories.

◊ Adverse effects are uncommon at serum-theophylline concentrations of 5 to 10 µg per mL but begin to become more frequent at 15 µg per mL or above, and are greatly increased in frequency and severity at concentrations greater than 20 µg per mL.[1-3] The severity of toxicity is generally correlated with age, underlying disease, and serum-theophylline concentration, but a distinction has been made between acute and chronic theophylline intoxication; symptoms appear to occur at a lower theophylline concentration in chronic toxicity than following acute ingestion of large amounts.[1,2,4] Young infants and the elderly (over 60 years) appear to be at particular risk from chronic intoxication with theophylline.[5,6] Common clinical manifestations of theophylline toxicity following overdosage of aminophylline or theophylline include nausea, vomiting, diarrhoea, agitation, tremor, hypertonicity, hyperventilation, supraventricular and ventricular arrhythmias, hypotension, and seizures. Metabolic disturbances such as hypokalaemia, hyperglycaemia, hypophosphataemia, hypercalcaemia, metabolic acidosis, and respiratory alkalosis often occur.[1-3] Other toxic effects reported include dementia,[7] toxic psychosis,[8] symptoms of acute pancreatitis,[9] rhabdomyolysis[10-12] with associated renal failure,[10] and acute compartment syndrome.[13]

Serious toxic symptoms may not be preceded by minor symptoms. In acute intoxication with sustained-release preparations the onset of major toxic symptoms may be delayed for up to 24 hours[1] and prolonged monitoring of such patients is required. Patients have recovered despite serum-theophylline concentrations in excess of 200 µg per mL[11,13] but fatalities have occurred with much lower serum concentrations.[9,14,15] Mortality in severe poisoning may be as high as 10%.

1. Dawson AH, Whyte IM. The assessment and treatment of theophylline poisoning. *Med J Aust* 1989; **151:** 689–93.
2. Minton NA, Henry JA. Acute and chronic human toxicity of theophylline. *Hum Exp Toxicol* 1996; **15:** 471–81.
3. Hardy CC, Smith J. Adverse reactions profile: theophylline and aminophylline. *Prescribers' J* 1997; **37:** 96–101.
4. Olson KR, *et al.* Theophylline overdose: acute single ingestion versus chronic repeated overmedication. *Am J Emerg Med* 1985; **3:** 386–94.
5. Shannon M, Lovejoy FH. Effect of acute versus chronic intoxication on clinical features of theophylline poisoning in children. *J Pediatr* 1992; **121:** 125–30.
6. Shannon M. Predictors of major toxicity after theophylline overdose. *Ann Intern Med* 1993; **119:** 1161–7.
7. Drummond I. Aminophylline toxicity in the elderly. *BMJ* 1982; **285:** 779–80.
8. Wasser WG, *et al.* Theophylline madness. *Ann Intern Med* 1981; **95:** 191.
9. Burgan THS, *et al.* Fatal overdose of theophylline simulating acute pancreatitis. *BMJ* 1982; **284:** 939–40.
10. Macdonald JB, *et al.* Rhabdomyolysis and acute renal failure after theophylline overdose. *Lancet* 1985; **i:** 932–3.
11. Rumpf KW, *et al.* Rhabdomyolysis after theophylline overdose. *Lancet* 1985; **i:** 1451–2.
12. Modi KB, *et al.* Theophylline poisoning and rhabdomyolysis. *Lancet* 1985; **ii:** 160–1.
13. Lloyd DM, *et al.* Acute compartment syndrome secondary to theophylline overdose. *Lancet* 1990; **ii:** 312.
14. Whyte KF, Addis GJ. Toxicity of salbutamol and theophylline together. *Lancet* 1983; **ii:** 618–19.
15. Davies RJ, Hawkey CJ. Fatal theophylline toxicity precipitated by in situ pulmonary artery thrombosis. *Postgrad Med J* 1989; **65:** 49–50.

Effects on carbohydrate metabolism. Hyperglycaemia is a frequent feature of theophylline intoxication, and is thought to be secondary to theophylline-induced adrenal catecholamine release.[1,2] Whether the effects on blood glucose are significant at more modest serum concentrations of theophylline is unclear, although in 29 preterm infants, mean plasma-glucose concentrations were significantly higher after treatment with intravenous aminophylline and oral theophylline than in those not treated. Two of 15 treated infants developed clinically significant hyperglycaemia and glycosuria. It was recommended that plasma-glucose concentrations be monitored in preterm infants receiving theophylline.[3]

1. Kearney TE, et al. Theophylline toxicity and the beta-adrenergic system. Ann Intern Med 1985; 102: 766–9.
2. Shannon M. Hypokalemia, hyperglycemia and plasma catecholamine activity after severe theophylline intoxication. J Toxicol Clin Toxicol 1994; 32: 41–7.
3. Srinivasan G, et al. Plasma glucose changes in preterm infants during oral theophylline therapy. J Pediatr 1983; 103: 473–6.

Effects on electrolytes. Hypokalaemia is a common metabolic disturbance in theophylline intoxication, but it has also been reported[1] in patients with plasma-theophylline concentrations within the therapeutic range. It is considered to be secondary to theophylline-induced adrenal catecholamine release, with cellular influx of potassium ions.[2] It is recommended[1] that plasma-potassium is monitored during intravenous theophylline therapy particularly if other drugs predisposing to hypokalaemia are also administered (see also Interactions, below). Hypophosphataemia[1,3] and hyponatraemia[1] can also occur at therapeutic plasma-theophylline concentrations. Hypomagnesaemia[4] and hypercalcaemia[5] have occurred in theophylline overdose.

1. Zantvoort FA, et al. Theophylline and serum electrolytes. Ann Intern Med 1986; 104: 134–5.
2. Minton NA, Henry JA. Acute and chronic human toxicity of theophylline. Hum Exp Toxicol 1996; 15: 471–81.
3. Laaban J-P, et al. Hypophosphatemia complicating management of acute severe asthma. Ann Intern Med 1990; 112: 68–9.
4. Hall KW, et al. Metabolic abnormalities associated with intentional theophylline overdose. Ann Intern Med 1984; 101: 457–62.
5. McPherson ML, et al. Theophylline-induced hypercalcemia. Ann Intern Med 1986; 105: 52–4.

Effects on the heart. ARRHYTHMIAS. Theophylline or aminophylline can precipitate sinus tachycardia and supraventricular and ventricular premature contractions at therapeutic serum-theophylline concentrations[1] and in overdose.[2,3] Multifocal atrial tachycardia has also been associated with both theophylline overdose[2] and serum-theophylline concentrations within the generally accepted therapeutic range of 10 to 20 µg per mL.[4] Combined administration of theophylline with beta-adrenoceptor stimulants by mouth is associated with a significant increase in the mean heart rate.[5,6]

1. Josephson GW, et al. Cardiac dysrhythmias during the treatment of acute asthma: a comparison of two treatment regimens by a double blind protocol. Chest 1980; 78: 429–35.
2. Greenberg A, et al. Severe theophylline toxicity: role of conservative measures, antiarrhythmic agents, and charcoal hemoperfusion. Am J Med 1984; 76: 854–60.
3. Minton NA, Henry JA. Acute and chronic human toxicity of theophylline. Hum Exp Toxicol 1996; 15: 471–81.
4. Levine JH, et al. Multifocal atrial tachycardia: a toxic effect of theophylline. Lancet 1985; i: 12–14.
5. Coleman JJ, et al. Cardiac arrhythmias during the combined use of β-adrenergic agonist drugs and theophylline. Chest 1986; 90: 45–51.
6. Conradson T-B, et al. Arrhythmogenicity from combined bronchodilator therapy in patients with obstructive lung disease and concomitant ischemic heart disease. Chest 1987; 91: 5–9.

Effects on the kidneys. For a report of rhabdomyolysis-induced acute renal failure occurring after aminophylline overdose, see the general discussion on toxicity, above.

Effects on mental function. As mentioned in the general discussion on toxicity above, theophylline toxicity has been associated with reports of dementia and toxic psychosis, as well as the more common adverse effects of anxiety and restlessness.

LEARNING AND BEHAVIOUR PROBLEMS. Several small studies[1-3] have suggested that theophylline may be associated with learning and behaviour problems in children, especially those with a low IQ. However, the FDA has concluded[4] that such studies provide insufficient evidence to support an adverse effect of theophylline on learning behaviour or school performance. Other studies have found no marked behavioural side-effects that could be attributed to theophylline.[5,6] Additionally, academic achievement generally appeared to be unaffected by either asthma or by treatment with appropriate doses of theophylline.[7]

1. Furukawa CT, et al. Learning and behaviour problems associated with theophylline therapy. Lancet 1984; i: 621.
2. Springer C, et al. Clinical, physiologic, and psychologic comparison of treatment by cromolyn or theophylline in childhood asthma. J Allergy Clin Immunol 1985; 76: 64–9.
3. Schlieper A, et al. Effect of therapeutic plasma concentrations of theophylline on behavior, cognitive processing, and affect in children with asthma. J Pediatr 1991; 118: 449–55.
4. Anonymous. Theophylline and school performance. FDA Drug Bull 1988; 18: 32–3.
5. Bender B, Milgrom H. Theophylline-induced behavior change in children: an objective evaluation of parents' perceptions. JAMA 1992; 267: 2621–4.
6. Bender BG, et al. Neuropsychological behavioral changes in asthmatic children treated with beclomethasone dipropionate versus theophylline. Pediatrics 1998; 101: 355–60.
7. Lindgren S, et al. Does asthma or treatment with theophylline limit children's academic performance? N Engl J Med 1992; 327: 926–30.

Effects on the nervous system. CONVULSIONS. The risk of convulsions with acute theophylline toxicity is low at serum theophylline concentrations less than 60 µg per mL;[1] seizures are most likely in patients with peak concentrations above 100 µg per mL.[2] However, the risk of seizures is much greater after chronic overdosage;[1,2] seizure activity has been reported at serum concentrations just above or even within the therapeutic range.[3] Elderly patients or those with previous brain injury or neurological disease may be at increased risk,[2-4] although some have questioned the association.[1] The outcome of seizures appears to be variable: death and severe neurological deficit have occurred,[2,3] but other series have recorded recovery without serious morbidity.[4]

1. Paloucek FP, Rodvold KA. Evaluation of theophylline overdoses and toxicities. Ann Emerg Med 1988; 17: 135–44.
2. Olson KR, et al. Theophylline overdose: acute single ingestion versus chronic repeated overmedication. Am J Emerg Med 1985; 3: 386–94.
3. Bahls FH, et al. Theophylline-associated seizures with "therapeutic" or low toxic serum concentrations: risk factors for serious outcome in adults. Neurology 1991; 41: 1309–12.
4. Covelli HD, et al. Predisposing factors to apparent theophylline-induced seizures. Ann Allergy 1985; 54: 411–15.

Effects on the skin. For reports of cutaneous reactions to theophylline and aminophylline, see under Hypersensitivity, below.

Effects on the urinary tract. Although diuresis is more commonly seen, urinary retention has been reported in male patients during therapy with aminophylline[1] or theophylline.[2]

1. Owens GR, Tannenbaum R. Theophylline-induced urinary retention. Ann Intern Med 1981; 94: 212–13.
2. Prakash M, Washburne JD. Theophylline and urinary retention. Ann Intern Med 1981; 94: 823.

Hypersensitivity. Hypersensitivity reactions have been reported following oral or intravenous administration of aminophylline. Reactions include erythematous rash with pruritus,[1,2] erythroderma,[2] and exfoliative dermatitis.[3] Aminophylline can produce both type I (immediate) and type IV (delayed) hypersensitivity reactions, the latter being due to the ethylenediamine component and can be confirmed by skin patch tests.[1-3] If hypersensitivity to ethylenediamine is confirmed it is recommended that aminophylline is avoided and treatment continued with theophylline or another theophylline salt.[1,3,4] Hypersensitivity reactions to theophylline have been reported rarely but type I reactions have occurred.[4] An erythematous, maculopapular rash has been reported[5] during treatment with a modified-release theophylline preparation which did not occur when another modified-release theophylline product was given.

1. Hardy C, et al. Allergy to aminophylline. BMJ 1983; 286: 2051–2.
2. Mohsenifar Z, et al. Two cases of allergy to aminophylline. Ann Allergy 1982; 49: 281–2.
3. Nierenberg DW, Glazener FS. Aminophylline-induced exfoliative dermatitis: cause and implications. West J Med 1982; 137: 328–31.
4. Gibb WRG. Delayed-type hypersensitivity to theophylline/aminophylline. Lancet 1985; i: 49.
5. Mendel S, et al. Dermatologic reaction to a sustained-release theophylline product. Clin Pharm 1985; 4: 334–5.

Hyperuricaemia. In a study of 112 asthmatic patients receiving modified-release theophylline 200 to 400 mg 12-hourly, there was a significant correlation of serum-uric-acid concentrations and serum-theophylline concentrations.[1] Gout has been reported in a woman receiving theophylline and aminophylline;[2] her serum-uric acid concentration was increased while receiving the xanthines, but subsequently fell when they were discontinued, and rose again when treatment was resumed.

1. Morita Y, et al. Theophylline increases serum uric acid levels. J Allergy Clin Immunol 1984; 74: 707–12.
2. Toda K, et al. Gout due to xanthine derivatives. Br J Rheumatol 1997; 36: 1131–2.

Necrotising enterocolitis. Although there have been reports of necrotising enterocolitis in neonates associated with oral theophylline and aminophylline administration,[1,2] a study of 275 infants concluded that theophylline did not significantly contribute to its development.[3] It has been suggested that the high osmolality of liquid feeds and drugs including oral theophylline preparations may be involved in the aetiology of necrotising enterocolitis.[4]

1. Robinson MJ, et al. Xanthines and necrotising enterocolitis. Arch Dis Child 1980; 55: 494–5.
2. Williams AJ. Xanthines and necrotising enterocolitis. Arch Dis Child 1980; 55: 973–4.
3. Davis JM, et al. Role of theophylline in pathogenesis of necrotizing enterocolitis. J Pediatr 1986; 109: 344–7.
4. Watkinson M, et al. Hyperosmolar preparations for neonates. Pharm J 1987; 241: 488.

Withdrawal syndromes. Episodes of apnoea beginning 28 hours after birth and increasing in frequency and severity over the next 4 days occurred in a neonate whose mother had taken aminophylline and theophylline throughout pregnancy. Measurement of serum-theophylline concentration showed the increasing apnoea was coincident with falling theophylline concentration and administration of theophylline to the infant resulted in resolution of apnoea; treatment was discontinued after 4 months.[1]

Worsening asthma control may occur when theophylline is withdrawn; there is some evidence of a rebound deterioration in lung function due to the development of tolerance.[2]

1. Horowitz DA, et al. Apnea associated with theophylline withdrawal in a term neonate. Am J Dis Child 1982; 136: 73–4.
2. Bennett JA, et al. The airway effects of stopping regular oral theophylline in patients with asthma. Br J Clin Pharmacol 1998; 45: 402–4.

Treatment of Adverse Effects

After theophylline or aminophylline overdosage by mouth the stomach may be emptied by lavage if within 2 hours of the overdose. Elimination may be enhanced by repeated oral doses of activated charcoal regardless of the route of theophylline overdose (see below). An osmotic laxative may also be considered, especially if modified-release preparations have been taken. Treatment is symptomatic and supportive. Serum-theophylline concentrations should be monitored and if modified-release preparations have been taken monitoring should be prolonged. Metabolic abnormalities, particularly hypokalaemia, should be corrected; hypokalaemia may be so severe as to require intravenous infusion of potassium under ECG monitoring. In the non-asthmatic patient extreme tachycardia, hypokalaemia, and hyperglycaemia may be reversed by a non-selective beta blocker (see also below). Isolated convulsions may be controlled by the intravenous administration of diazepam or a barbiturate; phenytoin may not be effective. In the most refractory cases general anaesthesia, and neuromuscular blockade, together with ventilation, may be required. Ventricular arrhythmias in a patient who is having convulsions may be best treated with disopyramide rather than lignocaine [lidocaine] or mexiletine since the latter may exacerbate convulsions.

Charcoal haemoperfusion or haemodialysis may be required.

◊ Reviews.

1. Dawson AH, Whyte IM. The assessment and treatment of theophylline poisoning. Med J Aust 1989; 151: 689–93.
2. Skinner MH. Adverse reactions and interactions with theophylline. Drug Safety 1990; 5: 275–85.
3. Minton NA, Henry JA. Treatment of theophylline overdose. Am J Emerg Med 1996; 14: 606–12.

Activated charcoal. Multiple-dose oral activated charcoal (p.1000) is considered the cornerstone of treatment for theophylline and xanthine poisoning. It reduces the absorption of orally administered theophylline, and also enhances the elimination of theophylline from the body even after absorption or intravenous xanthine administration. Aggressive antiemetic therapy may be required to allow administration and retention of activated charcoal, since theophylline toxicity causes protracted vomiting. A cathartic such as sorbitol may be given with the activated charcoal to aid elimination of theophylline, but can cause fluid and electrolyte disturbances. The use of gastric lavage before oral activated charcoal administration may not be better than activated charcoal alone after oral theophylline overdose.

References.

1. Neuvonen PJ, et al. Comparison of activated charcoal and ipecac syrup in prevention of drug absorption. Eur J Clin Pharmacol 1983; 24: 557–62.
2. Berlinger WG, et al. Enhancement of theophylline clearance by oral activated charcoal. Clin Pharmacol Ther 1983; 33: 351–4.
3. Mahutte CK, et al. Increased serum theophylline clearance with orally administered activated charcoal. Am Rev Respir Dis 1983; 128: 820–2.
4. Park GD, et al. Effects of size and frequency of oral doses of charcoal on theophylline clearance. Clin Pharmacol Ther 1983; 34: 663–6.
5. Goldberg MJ, et al. The effect of sorbitol and activated charcoal on serum theophylline concentrations after slow-release theophylline. Clin Pharmacol Ther 1987; 41: 108–11.
6. Al-Shareef AH, et al. The effects of charcoal and sorbitol (alone and in combination) on plasma theophylline concentrations after a sustained-release formulation. Hum Exp Toxicol 1990; 9: 179–82.
7. Minton NA, et al. Prevention of drug absorption in simulated theophylline overdose. Hum Exp Toxicol 1995; 14: 170–4.

Beta blockers. During the infusion of propranolol in 2 patients with hyperglycaemia, hypokalaemia, tachycardia, and hypotension following theophylline overdose, plasma glucose fell, plasma potassium increased, the pulse rate fell, and blood pressure rose. Beta-adrenergic blockade may be of benefit in the management of the metabolic changes of theophylline poisoning, especially in the non-asthmatic patient.[1,2] However, in asthmatic patients, beta blockers should be reserved for those with severe hypokalaemia or cardiac arrhythmias when mechanical ventilation is available as beta blockers can cause bronchoconstriction.[1,2] Propranolol reduces the clearance of theophylline (see under Interactions, below) and it has been suggested that a non-interacting beta blocker may be more appropriate.[3] Esmolol has been used successfully to manage cardiovascular symptoms of overdosage.[4]

1. Kearney TE, et al. Theophylline toxicity and the beta-adrenergic system. Ann Intern Med 1985; 102: 766–9.
2. Amin DN, Henry JA. Propranolol administration in theophylline overdose. Lancet 1985; i: 520–1.
3. Farrar KT, Dunn AM. Beta-blockers in treatment of theophylline overdose. Lancet 1985; i: 983.
4. Seneff M, et al. Acute theophylline toxicity and the use of esmolol to reverse cardiovascular instability. Ann Emerg Med 1990; 19: 671–3.

Endoscopy. Absorption is delayed following overdosage with modified-release oral preparations of aminophylline or theophylline and may be further prolonged by the formation of tablet aggregates, or bezoars, in the stomach.[1-3] Of 11 patients admitted with overdosage, one vomited a bezoar, 2 had bezoars removed at gastroscopy, and in one a bezoar was found at necropsy.[3] If bezoar formation occurs gastric lavage and activated charcoal will have little if any effect and the patient may appear to stabilise before experiencing increasing serum-theophylline concentration and clinical deterioration;[1,2] fatalities have been reported.[1] Endoscopy should be considered in cases of modified-release theophylline overdosage in which clinical signs and serial concentration measurements suggest continuing drug absorption.[2]

1. Coupe M. Self-poisoning with sustained-release aminophylline: a mechanism for observed secondary rise in serum theophylline. Hum Toxicol 1986; 5: 341–2.
2. Cereda J-M, et al. Endoscopic removal of pharmacobezoar of slow release theophylline. BMJ 1986; 293: 1143.
3. Smith WDF. Endoscopic removal of a pharmacobezoar of slow release theophylline. BMJ 1987; 294: 125.

Haemodialysis and haemoperfusion. Extracorporeal theophylline removal techniques following overdosage of aminophylline or theophylline have been reviewed.[1] Neither peritoneal dialysis nor exchange transfusion produced a significant increase in the total body clearance of theophylline, whereas haemodialysis could be expected to double clearance, and haemoperfusion results in four- to sixfold increases in clearance. Charcoal haemoperfusion should be considered if the plasma-theophylline concentration exceeds 100 μg per mL in an acute intoxication, or 60 μg per mL in chronic overdose (40 μg per mL if there is significant respiratory or heart failure, or liver disease) though plasma concentrations alone should not determine its use (see under Adverse Effects, above). If there is intractable vomiting, arrhythmias, or seizures charcoal haemoperfusion should be commenced without delay. In most patients a 4-hour haemoperfusion allows significant clinical improvement, but treatment should continue until plasma concentrations are below 15 μg per mL. Plasma concentrations should be followed at least every 4 hours for the first 12 hours post-perfusion, as rebound increases have been noted on terminating perfusion. Haemodialysis may rarely be an alternative if haemoperfusion is not available, or in series with haemoperfusion if significant rhabdomyolysis is present.

1. Heath A, Knudsen K. Role of extracorporeal drug removal in acute theophylline poisoning: a review. Med Toxicol 1987; 2: 294–308.

Precautions

Theophylline or aminophylline should be given with caution to patients with peptic ulceration, hyperthyroidism, hypertension, cardiac arrhythmias or other cardiovascular disease, or epilepsy, as these conditions may be exacerbated. They should also be given with caution to patients with heart failure, hepatic dysfunction or chronic alcoholism, acute febrile illness, and to neonates and the elderly, since in all of these circumstances theophylline clearance may be decreased, resulting in increases in serum-theophylline concentrations and serum half-life. Conversely, smoking increases theophylline clearance. Many drugs interact with theophylline; for details see Interactions, below.

Intravenous injections of theophylline or aminophylline must be administered very slowly to prevent dangerous CNS and cardiovascular side-effects resulting from the direct stimulant effect.

Dosage requirements of theophylline vary widely between subjects; in view of the many factors affecting theophylline pharmacokinetics, serum concentration monitoring is necessary to ensure concentrations are within the therapeutic range.

Patients should not be transferred from one modified-release theophylline or aminophylline preparation to another without clinical assessment and the measurement of serum-theophylline concentrations because of bioavailability differences.

Acute febrile illness. A reduction in theophylline clearance has been noted in patients presenting with acute respiratory illness[1] and appears to be associated with the severity of the underlying pulmonary disease and the rate of change in the patient's condition.[2] Caution has been advised in administering theophylline to patients with chronic obstructive pulmonary disease with acute exacerbations of a concomitant respiratory illness such as pneumonia since these patients appear most likely to exhibit altered theophylline metabolism.[2] Similarly, a decrease in theophylline clearance and an increase in the incidence of adverse effects has been reported during acute viral infections such as influenza in children receiving theophylline therapy for chronic asthma.[3,4] Influenza vaccination has also been reported to reduce theophylline clearance (see Interactions, below). The mechanism by which theophylline metabolism is reduced in these patients may be related to increased interferon production during the acute febrile response. A dosage reduction of one half has been recommended[5] in children receiving chronic theophylline therapy who are febrile for more than 24 hours. Further dose adjustments should be based on serum-theophylline concentrations until the patients have recovered from their acute illness and are restabilised on their usual dosage. However, conflicting results have been reported and in one controlled study respiratory syncytial virus infection was found to have no significant effect on theophylline disposition in children.[6]

1. Vozeh S, et al. Changes in theophylline clearance during acute illness. JAMA 1978; 240: 1882–4.
2. Richer M, Lam YWF. Hypoxia, arterial pH and theophylline disposition. Clin Pharmacokinet 1993; 25: 283–99.
3. Chang KC, et al. Altered theophylline pharmacokinetics during acute respiratory viral illness. Lancet 1978; i: 1132–3.
4. Kraemer MJ, et al. Altered theophylline clearance during an influenza B outbreak. Pediatrics 1982; 69: 476–80.
5. American Academy of Pediatrics Committee on Drugs. Precautions concerning the use of theophylline. Pediatrics 1992; 89: 781–3.
6. Muslow HA, et al. Lack of effect of respiratory syncytial virus infection on theophylline disposition in children. J Pediatr 1992; 121: 466–71.

Age. For the effects of age on the metabolism and excretion of theophylline see under Pharmacokinetics, below. Dosage regimens for infants are discussed under Administration in Infants, in Uses and Administration, below.

ECT. Patients receiving theophylline are at risk of prolonged seizures during ECT, and status epilepticus has been reported.[1,2] The ability of theophylline to prolong seizures has led to it being used as an adjunct in ECT.[3] Caffeine has been used similarly, see p.763.

1. Peters SG, et al. Status epilepticus as a complication of concurrent electroconvulsive and theophylline therapy. Mayo Clin Proc 1984; 59: 568–70.
2. Rasmussen KG, Zorumski CF. Electroconvulsive therapy in patients taking theophylline. J Clin Psychiatry 1993; 54: 427–31.
3. Leentjens AFG, et al. Facilitation of ECT by intravenous administration of theophylline. Convuls Ther 1996; 12: 232–7.

Porphyria. Theophylline has been associated with acute attacks of porphyria and is considered unsafe in porphyric patients.

Pregnancy and breast feeding. It has been recommended[1] that serum-theophylline concentrations are measured at monthly intervals throughout pregnancy and 1 and 4 weeks after delivery since the pharmacokinetics of theophylline may be altered. An increase in the volume of distribution of theophylline, a decrease in plasma-protein binding, and a continuing decrease in clearance throughout pregnancy have been noted in some patients, especially during the later part of pregnancy,[2-4] but other studies have noted an increase in theophylline clearance during pregnancy.[1,5] Some studies have found that after delivery there is a return of clearance values to those existing before pregnancy,[2] while others have not.[4]

In a study of 12 neonates whose mothers received various theophylline preparations throughout their pregnancies[6] maternal, cord, and neonatal heelstick theophylline concentrations were not notably different, and ranged from 2.3 to 19.6 μg per mL. Transient jitteriness was seen in 2 neonates and tachycardia in one, at cord theophylline concentrations of 11.7 to 17 μg per mL. There were no instances of vomiting, seizure, arrhythmias, diarrhoea, or feeding disturbances, which had been reported previously.

Toxic concentrations of theophylline are unlikely in breast-fed infants whose mothers are given appropriate doses of theophylline;[7] less than 1% of the total theophylline eliminated by breast-feeding women was found in breast milk.

1. Rubin PC. Prescribing in pregnancy: general principles. BMJ 1986; 293: 1415–17.
2. Carter BL, et al. Theophylline clearance during pregnancy. Obstet Gynecol 1986; 68: 555–9.
3. Frederiksen MC, et al. Theophylline pharmacokinetics in pregnancy. Clin Pharmacol Ther 1986; 40: 321–8.
4. Gardner MJ, et al. Longitudinal effects of pregnancy on the pharmacokinetics of theophylline. Eur J Clin Pharmacol 1987; 31: 289–95.
5. Romero R, et al. Pharmacokinetics of intravenous theophylline in pregnant patients at term. Am J Perinatol 1983; 1: 31–5.
6. Labovitz E, Spector S. Placental theophylline transfer in pregnant asthmatics. JAMA 1982; 247: 786–8.
7. Stec GP, et al. Kinetics of theophylline transfer to breast milk. Clin Pharmacol Ther 1980; 28: 404–8.

Renal impairment. Theophylline is eliminated mainly by hepatic metabolism and usual doses of aminophylline or theophylline can be given to patients with renal impairment. In patients undergoing haemodialysis the clearance of theophylline is increased and its elimination half-life reduced; mean values of 84.8 and 83 mL per minute and 2.5 and 2.3 hours respective-ly have been reported.[1,2] Haemodialysis removes up to 40% of a dose of theophylline.[1] Peritoneal dialysis has little effect on the pharmacokinetics of theophylline removing about 3.2% of a dose.[1]

1. Lee C-SC, et al. Comparative pharmacokinetics of theophylline in peritoneal dialysis and hemodialysis. J Clin Pharmacol 1983; 23: 274–80.
2. Anderson JR, et al. Effects of hemodialysis on theophylline kinetics. J Clin Pharmacol 1983; 23: 428–32.

Smoking. Certain components of tobacco smoke, notably aromatic hydrocarbons, induce hepatic drug-metabolising enzymes and cigarette smoking has been reported[1-3] to increase theophylline clearance and shorten its elimination half-life. The effect of smoking may override factors that tend to decrease theophylline clearance, such as old age.[4] The duration of enzyme induction after stopping smoking is uncertain; theophylline clearance decreased by 38% after one week of abstinence from smoking in one study,[5] while others have found changes in clearance persisting for at least 3 months.[1] Tobacco chewing has also been reported to increase theophylline clearance,[6] but nicotine chewing gum appears to have no effect.[5]

1. Hunt SN, et al. Effect of smoking on theophylline disposition. Clin Pharmacol Ther 1976; 19: 546–51.
2. Jusko WJ, et al. Enhanced biotransformation of theophylline in marihuana and tobacco smokers. Clin Pharmacol Ther 1978; 24: 406–10.
3. Grygiel JJ, Birkett DJ. Cigarette smoking and theophylline clearance and metabolism. Clin Pharmacol Ther 1981; 30: 491–6.
4. Cusack B, et al. Theophylline kinetics in relation to age: the importance of smoking. Br J Clin Pharmacol 1980; 10: 109–14.
5. Lee BL, et al. Cigarette abstinence, nicotine gum, and theophylline disposition. Ann Intern Med 1987; 106: 553–5.
6. Rockwood R, Henann N. Smokeless tobacco and theophylline clearance. Drug Intell Clin Pharm 1986; 20: 624–5.

Interactions

The toxic effects of theophylline, aminophylline, and other xanthines are additive. Concomitant use with other xanthine medications should therefore be avoided; if intravenous aminophylline is to be given for acute bronchospasm in patients who have been taking maintenance theophylline therapy, serum-theophylline concentrations should be measured first and the initial dose reduced as appropriate (see Uses and Administration, below).

Theophylline clearance may be reduced by interaction with other drugs including allopurinol, some antiarrhythmics, cimetidine, disulfiram, fluvoxamine, interferon alfa, macrolide antibacterials and quinolones, oral contraceptives, tiabendazole, and viloxazine, necessitating dosage reduction. Phenytoin and some other anticonvulsants, ritonavir, rifampicin, and sulfinpyrazone may increase theophylline clearance, necessitating an increase in dose or dosing frequency.

Xanthines can potentiate hypokalaemia caused by hypoxia or associated with the administration of beta$_2$-adrenoceptor stimulants (beta$_2$ agonists), corticosteroids, and diuretics. There is a risk of synergistic toxicity if theophylline is given concomitantly with halothane or ketamine, and it may antagonise the effects of adenosine and of competitive neuromuscular blockers; lithium elimination may be enhanced with a consequent loss of effect. The interaction between theophylline and beta blockers is complex (see below) but concomitant administration tends to be avoided on pharmacological grounds since beta blockers produce bronchospasm.

◊ Theophylline is metabolised by several hepatic cytochrome P450 isoenzymes, of which the most important seems to be CYP1A2.[1] Numerous drugs affect the metabolic clearance of theophylline and aminophylline,[2] but the variability in theophylline pharmacokinetics makes the clinical significance of these interactions difficult to predict. Giving theophylline with drugs that inhibit its metabolism should be avoided but, if unavoidable, the dose of theophylline should be halved and subsequently adjusted based on serum-theophylline monitoring.[3] Even when introducing medication for which no interaction is suspected, a check on the serum-theophylline concentration within 24 hours of beginning the new drug has been advised.[3] Theophylline reduces liver plasma flow[4] and may therefore prolong the half-life and increase steady-state levels of hepatically eliminated drugs but it is claimed to have no effect on antipyrine clearance.[5]

1. Ha HR, et al. Metabolism of theophylline by cDNA-expressed human cytochromes P-450. Br J Clin Pharmacol 1995; 39: 321–6.
2. Upton RA. Pharmacokinetic interactions between theophylline and other medication. Clin Pharmacokinet 1991; 20: 66–80 (part I) and 135–50 (part II).
3. American Academy of Pediatrics Committee on Drugs. Precautions concerning the use of theophylline. Pediatrics 1992; 89: 781–3.

4. Onrot J, *et al.* Reduction of liver plasma flow by caffeine and theophylline. *Clin Pharmacol Ther* 1986; **40:** 506–10.
5. Døssing M, *et al.* Effect of theophylline and salbutamol on hepatic drug metabolism. *Hum Toxicol* 1989; **8:** 225–8.

Antiarrhythmics. An increase in serum-theophylline concentration from 93.2 to 194.2 μmol per litre with symptoms of tachycardia, nervousness, and tremors occurred in a patient 9 days after starting *amiodarone* therapy.[1] Elevated theophylline concentrations and/or decreased clearance have also been reported following addition of *mexiletine* to theophylline therapy.[2-6] Amiodarone and mexiletine probably interact with theophylline through inhibition of its hepatic metabolism. *Tocainide* has also been found to impair theophylline metabolism resulting in a reduction in theophylline clearance but the effect was substantially smaller than that of mexiletine.[7] In one patient stabilised on theophylline therapy, an increase in the plasma-theophylline concentration with subsequent toxicity was noted following the initiation of treatment with *propafenone*.[8] See also under Calcium-channel Blockers, below.

1. Soto J, *et al.* Possible theophylline-amiodarone interaction. *DICP Ann Pharmacother* 1990; **24:** 1115.
2. Stanley R, *et al.* Mexiletine-theophylline interaction. *Am J Med* 1989; **86:** 733–4.
3. Ueno K, *et al.* Interaction between theophylline and mexiletine. *DICP Ann Pharmacother* 1990; **24:** 471–2.
4. Hurwitz A, *et al.* Mexiletine effects on theophylline disposition. *Clin Pharmacol Ther* 1991; **50:** 299–307.
5. Loi C-M, *et al.* Inhibition of theophylline metabolism by mexiletine in young male and female nonsmokers. *Clin Pharmacol Ther* 1991; **49:** 571–80.
6. Ueno K, *et al.* Mechanism of interaction between theophylline and mexiletine. *DICP Ann Pharmacother* 1991; **25:** 727–30.
7. Loi C-M, *et al.* The effect of tocainide on theophylline metabolism. *Br J Clin Pharmacol* 1993; **35:** 437–40.
8. Lee BL, Dohrmann ML. Theophylline toxicity after propafenone treatment: evidence for drug interaction. *Clin Pharmacol Ther* 1992; **51:** 353–5.

Antibacterials. IMIPENEM. Seizures have been reported in three patients receiving theophylline who were given imipenem,[1] although serum concentrations of theophylline were not affected.

1. Semel JD, Allen N. Seizures in patients simultaneously receiving theophylline and imipenem or ciprofloxacin or metronidazole. *South Med J* 1991; **84:** 465–8.

ISONIAZID. Isoniazid inhibits oxidative enzymes in the liver and has been found to impair the elimination of theophylline. Both clearance and volume of distribution of theophylline were reduced with an increase in serum-theophylline concentrations in healthy subjects after 14 days' pretreatment with isoniazid[1] and theophylline toxicity has been reported[2] in a patient one month after adding theophylline to isoniazid therapy.

1. Samigun, *et al.* Lowering of theophylline clearance by isoniazid in slow and rapid acetylators. *Br J Clin Pharmacol* 1990; **29:** 570–3.
2. Torrent J, *et al.* Theophylline-isoniazid interaction. *DICP Ann Pharmacother* 1989; **23:** 143–5.

MACROLIDES. There are conflicting reports of the effect of *erythromycin* on the pharmacokinetics of theophylline. Significant decreases in the clearance of theophylline and prolonged elimination half-life have been reported[1-3] but other studies have found no interaction.[4,5] It has also been noted that the serum concentrations and bioavailability of erythromycin may be reduced by theophylline.[6,7] The clearance of theophylline is also markedly decreased by the concomitant administration of *troleandomycin*,[8-10] but there have been reports that for clinical purposes the pharmacokinetics of theophylline do not seem to be significantly altered by *dirithromycin*,[11,12] *josamycin*,[9,13] *midecamycin*,[10,14,15] *rokitamycin*,[16] *roxithromycin*,[17] or *spiramycin*.[18] *Clarithromycin* also seems unlikely to have a significant effect in most patients, but in a few theophylline dosage may need to be adjusted.[19,20]

1. Zarowitz BJM, *et al.* Effect of erythromycin base on theophylline kinetics. *Clin Pharmacol Ther* 1981; **29:** 601–5.
2. Renton KW, *et al.* Depression of theophylline elimination by erythromycin. *Clin Pharmacol Ther* 1981; **30:** 422–6.
3. May DC, *et al.* The effects of erythromycin on theophylline elimination in normal males. *J Clin Pharmacol* 1982; **22:** 125–30.
4. Maddux MS, *et al.* The effect of erythromycin on theophylline pharmacokinetics at steady state. *Chest* 1982; **81:** 563–5.
5. Hildebrandt R, *et al.* Lack of clinically important interaction between erythromycin and theophylline. *Eur J Clin Pharmacol* 1984; **26:** 485–9.
6. Iliopoulou A, *et al.* Pharmacokinetic interaction between theophylline and erythromycin. *Br J Clin Pharmacol* 1982; **14:** 495–9.
7. Paulsen O, *et al.* The interaction of erythromycin with theophylline. *Eur J Clin Pharmacol* 1987; **32:** 493–8.
8. Weinberger M, *et al.* Inhibition of theophylline clearance by troleandomycin. *J Allergy Clin Immunol* 1977; **59:** 228–31.
9. Brazier JL, *et al.* Retard d'élimination de la théophylline dû à la troléandomycine: absence d'effet de la josamycine. *Therapie* 1980; **35:** 545–9.
10. Lavarenne J, *et al.* Influence d'un nouveau macrolide, la midécamycine, sur les taux sanguins de théophylline. *Therapie* 1981; **36:** 451–6.
11. Bachmann K, *et al.* Changes in the steady-state pharmacokinetics of theophylline during treatment with dirithromycin. *J Clin Pharmacol* 1990; **30:** 1001–5.
12. Bachmann K, *et al.* Steady-state pharmacokinetics of theophylline in COPD patients treated with dirithromycin. *J Clin Pharmacol* 1993; **33:** 861–5.
13. Ruff F, *et al.* Macrolide et théophylline: absence d'interaction josamycine-théophylline. *Nouv Presse Med* 1981; **10:** 175.
14. Principi N, *et al.* Effect of miocamycin on theophylline kinetics in children. *Eur J Clin Pharmacol* 1987; **31:** 701–4.

15. Couet W, *et al.* Lack of effect of ponsinomycin on the plasma pharmacokinetics of theophylline. *Eur J Clin Pharmacol* 1989; **37:** 101–4.
16. Ishioka T. Effect of a new macrolide antibiotic, 3″-O-propionyl-leucomycin A₅ (rokitamycin) on serum concentrations of theophylline and digoxin in the elderly. *Acta Ther* 1987; **13:** 17–24.
17. Saint-Salvi B, *et al.* A study of the interaction of roxithromycin with theophylline and carbamazine. *J Antimicrob Chemother* 1987; **20** (suppl B): 121–9.
18. Debruyne D, *et al.* Spiramycin has no effect on serum theophylline in asthmatic patients. *Eur J Clin Pharmacol* 1986; **30:** 505–7.
19. Bachand RT. Comparative study of clarithromycin and ampicillin in the treatment of patients with acute bacterial exacerbations of chronic bronchitis. *J Antimicrob Chemother* 1991; **27** (suppl A): 91–100.
20. Gillum JG, *et al.* Effect of combination therapy with ciprofloxacin and clarithromycin on theophylline pharmacokinetics in healthy volunteers. *Antimicrob Agents Chemother* 1996; **40:** 1715–16.

QUINOLONES. The fluoroquinolone antibacterials vary in their ability to interact with theophylline. *Enoxacin* shows the strongest interaction and has been reported[1] to cause serious nausea and vomiting, tachycardia, and headaches, associated with unexpectedly high plasma-theophylline concentrations in patients with respiratory-tract infections. Studies,[2-5] mainly in healthy subjects, have found that enoxacin decreases theophylline clearance by up to 74%[3] with an increase in the elimination half-life and serum-theophylline concentration. A 50% decrease in theophylline clearance has been reported with *grepafloxacin*.[6]

Ciprofloxacin[2,7-9] and *pefloxacin*[2] interact with theophylline to a lesser extent than enoxacin, decreasing theophylline clearance by about 30%. Eight clinically important interactions between ciprofloxacin and theophylline had been reported to the UK Committee on Safety of Medicines[10] including 1 death. A ciprofloxacin-induced seizure has been reported[11] which may have been due to the combined inhibitory effects of the 2 drugs on GABA binding. It has been recommended that ciprofloxacin should not be used in patients treated with theophylline.[10] *Norfloxacin*[4,12-14] and *ofloxacin*[4,12,15] have been reported to have minor effects on the pharmacokinetics of theophylline. Although their effects were usually considered not to be clinically significant, the US FDA had received 9 reports of theophylline toxicity associated with concomitant norfloxacin administration, including 1 death.[16] *Fleroxacin*,[17] *flumequine*,[18] *lomefloxacin*,[9,19,20] *moxifloxacin*,[21] and *rufloxacin*[22] have been reported to have no significant effect on the pharmacokinetics of theophylline in small studies in healthy subjects.

The mechanism of interaction involves a reduction in the metabolic clearance of theophylline due to inhibition of hepatic microsomal enzymes. However, the exact mechanism is unknown and it is difficult to predict which patients will be at risk. Extreme caution should be used when giving quinolones in conjunction with theophylline, particularly in the elderly[16] and it may be advisable to prescribe a non-interacting fluoroquinolone, although theophylline concentrations should still be monitored.

Of the non-fluorinated quinolones, *nalidixic acid*[2] has been reported not to affect theophylline clearance whereas *pipemidic acid* has markedly inhibited theophylline clearance.[20]

1. Wijnands WJA, *et al.* Enoxacin raises plasma theophylline concentrations. *Lancet* 1984; **ii:** 108–9.
2. Wijnands WJA, *et al.* The influence of quinolone derivatives on theophylline clearance. *Br J Clin Pharmacol* 1986; **22:** 677–83.
3. Beckmann J, *et al.* Enoxacin—a potent inhibitor of theophylline metabolism. *Eur J Clin Pharmacol* 1987; **33:** 227–30.
4. Sano M, *et al.* Inhibitory effect of enoxacin, ofloxacin and norfloxacin on renal excretion of theophylline in humans. *Eur J Clin Pharmacol* 1989; **36:** 323–4.
5. Koup JR, *et al.* Theophylline dosage adjustment during enoxacin coadministration. *Antimicrob Agents Chemother* 1990; **34:** 803–7.
6. Efthymiopoulos C, *et al.* Theophylline and warfarin interaction studies with grepafloxacin. *Clin Pharmacokinet* 1997; **33** (suppl 1): 39–46.
7. Nix DE, *et al.* Effect of multiple dose oral ciprofloxacin on the pharmacokinetics of theophylline and indocyanine green. *J Antimicrob Chemother* 1987; **19:** 263–9.
8. Schwartz J, *et al.* Impact of ciprofloxacin on theophylline clearance and steady-state concentrations in serum. *Antimicrob Agents Chemother* 1988; **32:** 75–7.
9. Robson RA. Comparative effects of ciprofloxacin and lomefloxacin on the oxidative metabolism of theophylline. *Br J Clin Pharmacol* 1990; **29:** 491–3.
10. Bem JL, Mann RD. Danger of interaction between ciprofloxacin and theophylline. *BMJ* 1988; **296:** 1131.
11. Karki SD, *et al.* Seizure with ciprofloxacin and theophylline combined therapy. *DICP Ann Pharmacother* 1990; **24:** 595–6.
12. Sano M, *et al.* Comparative pharmacokinetics of theophylline following two fluoroquinolones co-administration. *Eur J Clin Pharmacol* 1987; **32:** 431–2.
13. Ho G, *et al.* Evaluation of the effect of norfloxacin on the pharmacokinetics of theophylline. *Clin Pharmacol Ther* 1988; **44:** 35–8.
14. Davis RL, *et al.* Effect of norfloxacin on theophylline metabolism. *Antimicrob Agents Chemother* 1989; **33:** 212–14.
15. Gregoire SL, *et al.* Inhibition of theophylline clearance by coadministered ofloxacin without alteration of theophylline effects. *Antimicrob Agents Chemother* 1987; **31:** 375–8.
16. Grasela TH, Dreis MW. An evaluation of the quinolone-theophylline interaction using the Food and Drug Administration spontaneous reporting system. *Arch Intern Med* 1992; **152:** 617–21.
17. Parent M, *et al.* Safety of fleroxacin coadministered with theophylline to young and elderly volunteers. *Antimicrob Agents Chemother* 1990; **34:** 1249–53.
18. Lacarelle B, *et al.* The quinolone, flumequine, has no effect on theophylline pharmacokinetics. *Eur J Clin Pharmacol* 1994; **46:** 477–8.

19. LeBel M, *et al.* Influence of lomefloxacin on the pharmacokinetics of theophylline. *Antimicrob Agents Chemother* 1990; **34:** 1254–6.
20. Staib AH, *et al.* Interaction of quinolones with the theophylline metabolism in man: investigations with lomefloxacin and pipemidic acid. *Int J Clin Pharmacol Ther Toxicol* 1989; **27:** 289–93.
21. Stass H, Kubitza D. Lack of pharmacokinetic interaction between moxifloxacin, a novel 8-methoxyfluoroquinolone, and theophylline. *Clin Pharmacokinet* 2001; **40** (suppl 1): 63–70.
22. Kinzig-Schippers M, *et al.* Absence of effect of rufloxacin on theophylline pharmacokinetics in steady state. *Antimicrob Agents Chemother* 1998; **42:** 2359–64.

RIFAMPICIN. Rifampicin induces hepatic oxidative enzymes and a dose of 600 mg daily by mouth for 6 to 14 days has been shown to increase mean plasma-theophylline clearance by 25 to 82% due to enhancement of hepatic theophylline metabolism. This increase in clearance is sufficient to require dosage adjustment in some patients,[1-4] including children.[5]

1. Straughn AB, *et al.* Effect of rifampin on theophylline disposition. *Ther Drug Monit* 1984; **6:** 153–6.
2. Robson RA, *et al.* Theophylline-rifampicin interaction: non-selective induction of theophylline metabolic pathways. *Br J Clin Pharmacol* 1984; **18:** 445–8.
3. Boyce EG, *et al.* The effect of rifampin on theophylline kinetics. *J Clin Pharmacol* 1986; **26:** 696–9.
4. Adebayo GE, *et al.* Attenuation of rifampicin-induced theophylline metabolism by diltiazem/rifampicin coadministration in healthy volunteers. *Eur J Clin Pharmacol* 1989; **37:** 127–31.
5. Brocks DR, *et al.* Theophylline-rifampin interaction in a pediatric patient. *Clin Pharm* 1986; **5:** 602–4.

TETRACYCLINES. *Tetracycline* weakly inhibited theophylline clearance after 5 days of therapy in 5 non-smoking adults with chronic obstructive airways disease[1] and theophylline toxicity has been reported[2] in a patient given a 10-day course of tetracycline during theophylline therapy. *Doxycycline* has been reported not to have any significant effect on theophylline pharmacokinetics in healthy subjects.[3]

1. Gotz VP, Ryerson GG. Evaluation of tetracycline on theophylline disposition in patients with chronic obstructive airways disease. *Drug Intell Clin Pharm* 1986; **20:** 694–7.
2. McCormack JP, *et al.* Theophylline toxicity induced by tetracycline. *Clin Pharm* 1990; **9:** 546–9.
3. Jonkman JHG, *et al.* No influence of doxycycline on theophylline pharmacokinetics. *Ther Drug Monit* 1985; **7:** 92–4.

Antidepressants. Significantly reduced clearance and increased plasma concentrations of theophylline have been reported when given with *viloxazine*.[1,2] The dosage of theophylline should be decreased and its plasma concentrations monitored when viloxazine is also prescribed.[2] The interaction probably involves competition between the two drugs for hepatic microsomal enzymes.

Fluvoxamine has also been associated with a significant reduction in theophylline clearance[3] and theophylline toxicity has been described in patients when fluvoxamine was added to their therapy.[4,5] This interaction which is due to potent liver enzyme inhibition[6] has been the subject of a warning by the UK Committee on Safety of Medicines[7] in which they issued the standard advice of avoiding the two drugs if at all possible and, where they could not be avoided, of giving half the dose of theophylline and monitoring plasma concentrations.

Hypericum may have decreased theophylline concentrations, leading to a need for increased theophylline dosage in one case report.[8]

For a mention of the effect of theophylline on the renal clearance of *lithium*, see Xanthines, under Interactions of Lithium, p.296.

1. Thomson AH, *et al.* Theophylline toxicity following coadministration of viloxazine. *Ther Drug Monit* 1988; **10:** 359–60.
2. Perault MC, *et al.* A study of the interaction of viloxazine with theophylline. *Ther Drug Monit* 1989; **11:** 520–2.
3. Donaldson KM, *et al.* The effect [of] fluvoxamine at steady state on the pharmacokinetics of theophylline after a single dose in healthy male volunteers. *Br J Clin Pharmacol* 1994; **37:** 492P.
4. Sperber AD. Toxic interaction between fluvoxamine and sustained release theophylline in an 11-year-old boy. *Drug Safety* 1991; **6:** 460–2.
5. Thomson AH, *et al.* Interaction between fluvoxamine and theophylline. *Pharm J* 1992; **249:** 137.
6. Rasmussen BB, *et al.* Selective serotonin reuptake inhibitors and theophylline metabolism in human liver microsomes: potent inhibition by fluvoxamine. *Br J Clin Pharmacol* 1995; **39:** 151–9.
7. Committee on Safety of Medicines/Medicines Control Agency. Fluvoxamine increases plasma theophylline levels. *Current Problems* 1994; **20:** 12.
8. Nebel A, *et al.* Potential metabolic interaction between St John's wort and theophylline. *Ann Pharmacother* 1999; **33:** 502.

Antiepileptics. *Phenytoin* markedly decreases the elimination half-life and increases the clearance of theophylline, probably due to hepatic enzyme induction, at therapeutic serum-phenytoin concentrations,[1-3] at subtherapeutic phenytoin concentrations,[2,4] and even in heavy smokers.[2] A preliminary report suggested that the serum concentration of phenytoin may be decreased simultaneously,[5] perhaps due to enzyme induction by theophylline[5] or reduced phenytoin absorption.[6] The interaction between phenytoin and theophylline has been reported to occur within 5 to 14 days of commencing concomitant therapy, and theophylline clearance has increased by up to 350%, and reductions in serum half-life have ranged from 25 to 70% of initial values.[3,4]

Carbamazepine has also been observed to increase theophylline elimination. In one patient, theophylline serum half-life was decreased by approximately 24 to 60%, and clearance was increased by about 35 to 100% when carbamazepine was given concomitantly.[2] In an 11-year-old girl theophylline-serum half-life was almost halved with loss of asthma control after 3 weeks of concurrent carbamazepine therapy.[7] In turn, theophylline has been reported to reduce the half-life of carbamazepine—see p.345.

Although *phenobarbital* was not found to have a significant effect on the pharmacokinetics of a single dose of theophylline given intravenously,[8] enhanced theophylline clearance has been seen in patients after longer periods of treatment with phenobarbital.[9,10] The magnitude of the changes in theophylline elimination appears to be smaller with phenobarbital than phenytoin. *Pentobarbital* in high doses has also been reported to increase theophylline metabolism.[11] A more recent study[12] has also shown that therapeutic doses of pentobarbital (100 mg daily) increase plasma clearance of theophylline by a mean of 40%, although this was subject to marked interindividual variations. Renal clearance was not affected, suggesting hepatic enzyme induction as the probable mechanism.

1. Marquis J-F, *et al.* Phenytoin-theophylline interaction. *N Engl J Med* 1982; **307:** 1189–90.
2. Reed RC, Schwartz HJ. Phenytoin-theophylline-quinidine interaction. *N Engl J Med* 1983; **308:** 724–5.
3. Sklar SJ, Wagner JC. Enhanced theophylline clearance secondary to phenytoin therapy. *Drug Intell Clin Pharm* 1985; **19:** 34–6.
4. Miller M, *et al.* Influence of phenytoin on theophylline clearance. *Clin Pharmacol Ther* 1984; **35:** 666–9.
5. Taylor JW, *et al.* The interaction of phenytoin and theophylline. *Drug Intell Clin Pharm* 1980; **14:** 638.
6. Hendeles L, *et al.* Decreased oral phenytoin absorption following concurrent theophylline administration. *J Allergy Clin Immunol* 1979; **63:** 156.
7. Rosenberry KR, *et al.* Reduced theophylline half-life induced by carbamazepine therapy. *J Pediatr* 1983; **102:** 472–4.
8. Piafsky KM, *et al.* Effect of phenobarbital on the disposition of intravenous theophylline. *Clin Pharmacol Ther* 1977; **22:** 336–9.
9. Jusko WJ, *et al.* Factors affecting theophylline clearances: age, tobacco, marijuana, cirrhosis, congestive heart failure, obesity, oral contraceptives, benzodiazepines, barbiturates, and ethanol. *J Pharm Sci* 1979; **68:** 1358–66.
10. Saccar CL, *et al.* The effect of phenobarbital on theophylline disposition in children with asthma. *J Allergy Clin Immunol* 1985; **75:** 716–19.
11. Gibson GA, *et al.* Influence of high-dose phenobarbital on theophylline pharmacokinetics: a case report. *Ther Drug Monit* 1985; **7:** 181–4.
12. Dahlqvist R, *et al.* Induction of theophylline metabolism by pentobarbital. *Ther Drug Monit* 1989; **11:** 408–10.

Antifungals. There have been reports that *ketoconazole* does not appear significantly to alter the pharmacokinetics of theophylline.[1,2] The manufacturer of *fluconazole* has, however, stated that plasma clearance of theophylline may be decreased by fluconazole. A 16% reduction in theophylline clearance has been reported[3] following oral fluconazole administration but fluconazole was considered to have only a minor inhibitory effect on theophylline metabolism and theophylline disposition was not significantly affected. A similar degree of inhibition has been seen in theophylline metabolism when *terbinafine* was given concomitantly.[4]

1. Brown MW, *et al.* Effect of ketoconazole on hepatic oxidative drug metabolism. *Clin Pharmacol Ther* 1985; **37:** 290–7.
2. Heusner JJ, *et al.* Effect of chronically administered ketoconazole on the elimination of theophylline in man. *Drug Intell Clin Pharm* 1987; **21:** 514–17.
3. Konishi H, *et al.* Effect of fluconazole on theophylline disposition in humans. *Eur J Clin Pharmacol* 1994; **46:** 309–12.
4. Trépanier EF, *et al.* Effect of terbinafine on theophylline pharmacokinetics in healthy volunteers. *Antimicrob Agents Chemother* 1998; **42:** 695–7.

Antigout drugs. *Allopurinol* 300 mg by mouth daily for 7 days was found to have no effect on the pharmacokinetics of theophylline following a single intravenous dose of aminophylline[1,2] or following theophylline given by mouth to steady state.[1] However, allopurinol 600 mg by mouth daily for 28 days has been found to inhibit the metabolism of theophylline,[3] increasing the mean half-life by 25% after 14 days and 29% after 28 days and there has been a report of allopurinol increasing peak plasma-theophylline concentrations by 38% in one patient within 2 days of concomitant administration.[4]

Probenecid has been reported[5] to have no effect on the hepatic metabolism or total body clearance of theophylline in a single-dose study in healthy subjects.

Sulfinpyrazone 800 mg daily for 7 days increased the total plasma clearance of theophylline by 22% in healthy subjects due to selective induction of certain cytochrome P450 isoenzymes.[6]

1. Grygiel JJ, *et al.* Effects of allopurinol on theophylline metabolism and clearance. *Clin Pharmacol Ther* 1979; **26:** 660–7.
2. Vozeh S, *et al.* Influence of allopurinol on theophylline disposition in adults. *Clin Pharmacol Ther* 1980; **27:** 194–7.
3. Manfredi RL, Vesell ES. Inhibition of theophylline metabolism by long-term allopurinol administration. *Clin Pharmacol Ther* 1981; **29:** 224–9.
4. Barry M, *et al.* Allopurinol influences aminophenazone elimination. *Clin Pharmacokinet* 1990; **19:** 167–9.
5. Chen TWD, Patton TF. Effect of probenecid on the pharmacokinetics of aminophylline. *Drug Intell Clin Pharm* 1983; **17:** 465–6.
6. Birkett DJ, *et al.* Evidence for a dual action of sulphinpyrazone on drug metabolism in man: theophylline-sulphinpyrazone interaction. *Br J Clin Pharmacol* 1983; **15:** 567–9.

Antineoplastics. There has been a report of increased clearance of theophylline in 3 patients receiving *aminoglutethimide*.[1]

For reference to a possible interaction between theophylline and *lomustine*, see Lomustine, p.550.

1. Lønning PE, *et al.* Effect of aminoglutethimide on antipyrine, theophylline, and digitoxin disposition in breast cancer. *Clin Pharmacol Ther* 1984; **36:** 796–802.

Antivirals. A single injection of recombinant human *interferon alfa* reduced theophylline clearance by 33 to 81% in 8 of 9 subjects, resulting in a 1.5 to sixfold increase in the theophylline elimination half-life.[1] Injection of interferon alfa once daily for 3 days in 11 healthy subjects also reduced theophylline clearance and increased elimination half-life,[2] but the magnitude of the changes were of a similar order to normal intra-individual variation and the interaction was considered of minor clinical significance.

The manufacturers of *ritonavir* state that it substantially increases the clearance of theophylline; theophylline dosage may need to be increased to maintain efficacy.

There is evidence[3] that *aciclovir* inhibits theophylline metabolism, resulting in accumulation.

1. Williams SJ, *et al.* Inhibition of theophylline metabolism by interferon. *Lancet* 1987; **ii:** 939–41.
2. Jonkman JHG, *et al.* Effects of α-interferon on theophylline pharmacokinetics and metabolism. *Br J Clin Pharmacol* 1989; **27:** 795–802.
3. Maeda Y, *et al.* Inhibition of theophylline metabolism by aciclovir. *Biol Pharm Bull* 1996; **19:** 1591–5.

Benzodiazepines. For reference to the antagonism of benzodiazepine sedation by aminophylline, see Xanthines, under Interactions of Diazepam, p.679.

Beta blockers. *Propranolol* reduced theophylline clearance by 36% in healthy subjects given aminophylline intravenously. *Metoprolol* did not reduce clearance in the group as a whole, but a reduction was noted in some smokers whose theophylline clearance was initially high.[1] Propranolol is thought to exert a dose-dependent selective inhibitory effect on the separate cytochrome P450 isoenzymes involved in theophylline demethylation and 8-hydroxylation.[2] The less lipophilic beta blockers *atenolol*[3,4] and *nadolol*[4] had no significant effect on the pharmacokinetics of theophylline.

In general, however, beta blockers should be avoided in patients taking theophylline as they can dangerously exacerbate bronchospasm in patients with a history of asthma or chronic obstructive pulmonary disease.

1. Conrad KA, Nyman DW. Effects of metoprolol and propranolol on theophylline elimination. *Clin Pharmacol Ther* 1980; **28:** 463–7.
2. Miners JO, *et al.* Selectivity and dose-dependency of the inhibitory effect of propranolol on theophylline metabolism in man. *Br J Clin Pharmacol* 1985; **20:** 219–23.
3. Cerasa LA, *et al.* Lack of effect of atenolol on the pharmacokinetics of theophylline. *Br J Clin Pharmacol* 1988; **26:** 800–2.
4. Corsi CM, *et al.* Lack of effect of atenolol and nadolol on the metabolism of theophylline. *Br J Clin Pharmacol* 1990; **29:** 265–8.

Caffeine. Abstention from dietary methylxanthines by healthy subjects has resulted in faster elimination of theophylline.[1] While the addition of extra caffeine to the diet has been reported not to alter theophylline disposition,[2] some studies in healthy subjects have indicated that the ingestion of moderate amounts of caffeine (120 to 900 mg daily), which could be consumed by drinking several cups of coffee a day, can have a pronounced influence on the pharmacokinetics of theophylline.[3,4] In these latter studies the mean theophylline clearance was reduced by 23% and 29% with a corresponding increase in the elimination half-lives.

1. Monks TJ, *et al.* Influence of methylxanthine-containing foods on theophylline metabolism and kinetics. *Clin Pharmacol Ther* 1979; **26:** 513–24.
2. Monks TJ, *et al.* The effect of increased caffeine intake on the metabolism and pharmacokinetics of theophylline in man. *Biopharm Drug Dispos* 1981; **2:** 31–7.
3. Jonkman JHG, *et al.* The influence of caffeine on the steady-state pharmacokinetics of theophylline. *Clin Pharmacol Ther* 1991; **49:** 248–55.
4. Sato J, *et al.* Influence of usual intake of dietary caffeine on single-dose kinetics of theophylline in healthy human subjects. *Eur J Clin Pharmacol* 1993; **44:** 295–8.

Calcium-channel blockers. *Verapamil* has been reported[1] to decrease the clearance of theophylline by a mean of 14% in healthy subjects and although this was not considered to be clinically significant, symptoms of theophylline toxicity, associated with near doubling of the serum-theophylline concentration have occurred in a 76-year-old woman taking theophylline after 6 days of therapy with verapamil.[2] Studies in healthy subjects and asthmatic patients have produced conflicting results of the effect of *nifedipine* on the pharmacokinetics of theophylline. Reduced clearance[1] and an increase in the volume of distribution[3,4] of theophylline have been reported and both decreased[4] and increased[5] serum-theophylline concentrations; theophylline toxicity has been reported.[6,7] However, most studies have concluded that the effects of nifedipine are unlikely to be of clinical importance.[1,4,5,8]

Diltiazem has been reported[5] to cause an increase in serum-theophylline concentration and *felodipine*[9] a decrease in serum-theophylline concentration; neither of these effects were considered to be clinically significant.

1. Robson RA, *et al.* Selective inhibitory effects of nifedipine and verapamil on oxidative metabolism: effects on theophylline. *Br J Clin Pharmacol* 1988; **25:** 397–400.
2. Burnakis TG, *et al.* Increased serum theophylline concentrations secondary to oral verapamil. *Clin Pharm* 1983; **2:** 458–61.

3. Jackson SHD, *et al.* The interaction between iv theophylline and chronic oral dosing with slow release nifedipine in volunteers. *Br J Clin Pharmacol* 1986; **21:** 389–92.
4. Adebayo GI, Mabadeje AFB. Effect of nifedipine on antipyrine and theophylline disposition. *Biopharm Drug Dispos* 1990; **11:** 157–64.
5. Smith SR, *et al.* The influence of nifedipine and diltiazem on serum theophylline concentration-time profiles. *J Clin Pharm Ther* 1989; **14:** 403–8.
6. Parrillo SJ, Venditto M. Elevated theophylline blood levels from institution of nifedipine therapy. *Ann Emerg Med* 1984; **13:** 216–17.
7. Harrod CS. Theophylline toxicity and nifedipine. *Ann Intern Med* 1987; **106:** 480.
8. Spedini C, Lombardi C. Long-term treatment with oral nifedipine plus theophylline in the management of chronic bronchial asthma. *Eur J Clin Pharmacol* 1986; **31:** 105–6.
9. Bratel T, *et al.* Felodipine reduces the absorption of theophylline in man. *Eur J Clin Pharmacol* 1989; **36:** 481–5.

Cannabis. A search of the literature[1] revealed 2 studies, both published in the 1970s, that showed that marijuana smoking increased the clearance of theophylline.

1. Brown D. Influence on theophylline clearance. *Pharm J* 1994; **253:** 595.

Corticosteroids. In 3 patients with acute severe asthma given aminophylline intravenously, serum-theophylline concentrations rose rapidly from the therapeutic range to between 40 and 50 µg per mL when *hydrocortisone* was given intravenously.[1] In studies in healthy subjects, no significant changes in serum-theophylline concentrations were noted after the concomitant administration of hydrocortisone, methylprednisolone,[2] or prednisone[3] although there was a trend towards increased theophylline clearance during corticosteroid therapy.[2,3] In preterm neonates, exposure to *betamethasone in utero* stimulated the hepatic metabolism of theophylline,[4,5] but did not affect dosage requirements.

The possibility that adverse effects such as hypokalaemia may be potentiated by concomitant administration of theophylline and corticosteroids should be borne in mind.

1. Buchanan N, *et al.* Asthma—a possible interaction between hydrocortisone and theophylline. *S Afr Med J* 1979; **56:** 1147–8.
2. Leavengood DC, *et al.* The effect of corticosteroids on theophylline metabolism. *Ann Allergy* 1983; **50:** 249–51.
3. Anderson JL, *et al.* Potential pharmacokinetic interaction between theophylline and prednisone. *Clin Pharm* 1984; **3:** 187–9.
4. Jager-Roman E, *et al.* Increased theophylline metabolism in premature infants after prenatal betamethasone administration. *Dev Pharmacol Ther* 1982; **5:** 127–35.
5. Baird-Lambert J, *et al.* Theophylline metabolism in preterm neonates during the first weeks of life. *Dev Pharmacol Ther* 1984; **7:** 239–44.

Disulfiram. In a study involving 20 recovering alcoholic patients, disulfiram decreased the plasma clearance and prolonged the elimination half-life of theophylline in a dose-dependent manner when administered concomitantly.[1] It was concluded that disulfiram exerts a dose-dependent inhibitory effect on the hepatic metabolism of theophylline and that, in order to minimise the risk of toxicity, the dosage of theophylline may need to be reduced by up to 50% during co-administration.

1. Loi C-M, *et al.* Dose-dependent inhibition of theophylline metabolism by disulfiram in recovering alcoholics. *Clin Pharmacol Ther* 1989; **45:** 476–86.

Diuretics. Although increased mean serum-theophylline concentrations were noted in 10 patients receiving continuous intravenous aminophylline infusions after intravenous injection of *frusemide [furosemide]*,[1] in 8 patients with chronic stable asthma, mean peak serum-theophylline concentrations were reduced from 12.14 µg per mL with placebo to 7.16 µg per mL when frusemide [furosemide] was given. Reduced concentrations were noted for up to 6 hours after frusemide [furosemide] administration.[2] Decreased theophylline concentrations were also noted in 4 neonates receiving oral or intravenous theophylline when given frusemide [furosemide].[3] Serum-theophylline concentrations returned to normal when frusemide [furosemide] and theophylline were given more than 2 hours apart.

The possibility that adverse effects such as hypokalaemia may be potentiated by concomitant administration of theophylline and diuretics should be borne in mind.

1. Conlon PF, *et al.* Effect of intravenous furosemide on serum theophylline concentration. *Am J Hosp Pharm* 1981; **38:** 1345–7.
2. Carpentiere G, *et al.* Furosemide and theophylline. *Ann Intern Med* 1985; **103:** 567.
3. Toback JW, Gilman ME. Theophylline-furosemide inactivation. *Pediatrics* 1983; **71:** 140–1.

Gastrointestinal drugs. Oral administration of *antacids* does not appear to affect the total absorption of theophylline from the gut.[1-5] However, some studies have shown a reduction in the rate of absorption from both immediate-[1] and modified-release theophylline preparations[2] following administration of antacids. Also an increase in peak serum-theophylline concentrations has been noted with certain modified-release formulations.[3]

Cimetidine inhibits the oxidative metabolism of theophylline reducing its clearance by 20 to 35% and prolonging its serum half-life;[6-8] toxic effects have been reported.[6] It has been recommended that the dose of aminophylline should be reduced by about one-third if cimetidine is used concomitantly.[6] This inhibition of theophylline metabolism may be enhanced by liver disease,[9] but there is wide interindividual variation. The reduction in clearance may be greater in smokers.[10] Studies have suggested that *ranitidine* does not significantly inhibit theophylline metabolism,[11-14] even at very high doses.[15] However, there have been occasional reports of theophylline toxicity after concomitant ranitidine therapy.[16-18] *Famotidine*[19] has also been reported to not alter theophylline disposition but one small study found a significant decrease in theophylline clearance in some patients with chronic obstructive pulmonary disease.[20]

Omeprazole, lansoprazole, and *pantoprazole* generally have insignificant or no effect on theophylline clearance.[21,22] A modest increase in theophylline clearance in CYP2C19 poor metabolisers receiving omeprazole was not considered clinically relevant.[23]

1. Arnold LA, *et al.* Effect of an antacid on gastrointestinal absorption of theophylline. *Am J Hosp Pharm* 1979; 36: 1059–62.
2. Shargel L, *et al.* Effect of antacid on bioavailability of theophylline from rapid and timed-release drug products. *J Pharm Sci* 1981; 70: 599–602.
3. Darzentas LJ, *et al.* Effect of antacid on bioavailability of a sustained-release theophylline preparation. *Drug Intell Clin Pharm* 1983; 17: 555–7.
4. Myhre KI, Walstad RA. The influence of antacid on the absorption of two different sustained-release formulations of theophylline. *Br J Clin Pharmacol* 1983; 15: 683–7.
5. Muir JF, *et al.* Lack of effect of magnesium-aluminium hydroxide on the absorption of theophylline given as a pH-dependent sustained-release preparation. *Eur J Clin Pharmacol* 1993; 44: 85–8.
6. Bauman JH, *et al.* Cimetidine-theophylline interaction: report of four patients. *Ann Allergy* 1982; 48: 100–2.
7. Vestal RE, *et al.* Cimetidine inhibits theophylline clearance in patients with chronic obstructive pulmonary disease: a study using stable isotope methodology during multiple oral dose administration. *Br J Clin Pharmacol* 1983; 15: 411–18.
8. Roberts RK, *et al.* Cimetidine-theophylline interaction in patients with chronic obstructive airways disease. *Med J Aust* 1984; 140: 279–80.
9. Gugler R, *et al.* The inhibition of drug metabolism by cimetidine in patients with liver cirrhosis. *Klin Wochenschr* 1984; 62: 1126–31.
10. Grygiel JJ, *et al.* Differential effects of cimetidine on theophylline metabolic pathways. *Eur J Clin Pharmacol* 1984; 26: 335–40.
11. Breen KJ, *et al.* Effects of cimetidine and ranitidine on hepatic drug metabolism. *Clin Pharmacol Ther* 1982; 31: 297–300.
12. Segger JS, *et al.* No evidence for interaction between ranitidine and theophylline. *Arch Intern Med* 1987; 147: 179–80.
13. Adebayo GI. Effects of equimolar doses of cimetidine and ranitidine on theophylline elimination. *Biopharm Drug Dispos* 1989; 10: 77–85.
14. Boehning W. Effect of cimetidine and ranitidine on plasma theophylline in patients with chronic obstructive airways disease treated with theophylline and corticosteroids. *Eur J Clin Pharmacol* 1990; 38: 43–5.
15. Kelly HW, *et al.* Ranitidine at very large doses does not inhibit theophylline elimination. *Clin Pharmacol Ther* 1986; 39: 577–81.
16. Fernandes E, Melewicz FM. Ranitidine and theophylline. *Ann Intern Med* 1984; 100: 459.
17. Gardner ME, Sikorski GW. Ranitidine and theophylline. *Ann Intern Med* 1985; 102: 559.
18. Hegman GW, Gilbert RP. Ranitidine-theophylline interaction—fact or fiction? *DICP Ann Pharmacother* 1991; 25: 21–5.
19. Chremos AN, *et al.* Famotidine does not interfere with the disposition of theophylline in man: comparison to cimetidine. *Clin Pharmacol Ther* 1986; 39: 187.
20. Dal Negro R, *et al.* Famotidine and theophylline pharmacokinetics: an unexpected cimetidine-like interaction in patients with chronic obstructive pulmonary disease. *Clin Pharmacokinet* 1993; 24: 255–8.
21. Kokufu T, *et al.* Effects of lansoprazole on pharmacokinetics and metabolism of theophylline. *Eur J Clin Pharmacol* 1995; 48: 391–5.
22. Dilger K, *et al.* Lack of drug interaction between omeprazole, lansoprazole, pantoprazole and theophylline. *Br J Clin Pharmacol* 1999; 48: 438–44.
23. Cavuto NJ, *et al.* Effect of omeprazole on theophylline clearance in poor metabolizers of omeprazole. *Clin Pharmacol Ther* 1995; 57: 215.

General anaesthetics. There have been several reports[1,2] of increased cardiotoxicity when patients taking theophylline were anaesthetised with *halothane.* There was also an early report of seizures and tachycardia attributed to an interaction between theophylline and *ketamine.*[3]

1. Barton MD. Anesthetic problems with aspirin-intolerant patients. *Anesth Analg* 1975; 54: 376–80.
2. Richards W, *et al.* Cardiac arrest associated with halothane anesthesia in a patient receiving theophylline. *Ann Allergy* 1988; 61: 83–4.
3. Hirschman CA, *et al.* Ketamine-aminophylline-induced decrease in seizure threshold. *Anesthesiology* 1982; 56: 464–7.

Leukotriene inhibitors and antagonists. *Zileuton* prolongs the half-life and reduces the clearance of theophylline;[1] dosage of theophylline should be reduced to avoid toxicity when both drugs are given together, and plasma-theophylline concentrations should be monitored. Use of *zafirlukast* with theophylline decreased zafirlukast plasma concentrations but had no effect on theophylline plasma concentrations in clinical trials. However, toxic serum-theophylline concentrations occurred in one patient when zafirlukast was added to therapy, and reduced on rechallenge.[2]

1. Granneman GR, *et al.* Effect of zileuton on theophylline pharmacokinetics. *Clin Pharmacokinet* 1995; 29 (suppl 2): 77–83.
2. Katial RK, *et al.* A drug interaction between zafirlukast and theophylline. *Arch Intern Med* 1998; 158: 1713–15.

Neuromuscular blockers. For reference to resistance to neuromuscular block with pancuronium in patients receiving aminophylline, see p.1335.

Oral contraceptives. Oral contraceptives have been reported to decrease the clearance of theophylline by about 30%, and serum concentrations may be increased,[1-3] due to the inhibitory effects of oral contraceptives on hepatic P450 isoenzymes.

1. Tornatore KM, *et al.* Effect of chronic oral contraceptive steroids on theophylline disposition. *Eur J Clin Pharmacol* 1982; 23: 129–34.
2. Gardner MJ, *et al.* Effects of tobacco smoking and oral contraceptive use on theophylline disposition. *Br J Clin Pharmacol* 1983; 16: 271–80.
3. Roberts RK, *et al.* Oral contraceptive steroids impair the elimination of theophylline. *J Lab Clin Med* 1983; 101: 821–5.

Sympathomimetics. The effect of beta-adrenoceptor agonists on the pharmacokinetics of theophylline is unclear. Whereas some studies have found that concomitant use of *orciprenaline*[1] or *terbutaline*[2] had no effect on theophylline disposition, others have shown an increase in theophylline clearance following the concurrent use of *isoprenaline*[3,4] or *terbutaline.*[5,6]

Concurrent use of theophylline with beta-adrenoceptor agonists can potentiate adverse effects including hypokalaemia,[7,8] hyperglycaemia,[7] tachycardia,[7,8] hypertension,[7] and tremor.[9] Of 9 patients reported to the UK Committee on Safety of Medicines with hypokalaemia during such combined therapy, 4 had clinical sequelae of cardiorespiratory arrest, intestinal pseudo-obstruction, or confusion. Monitoring of serum-potassium concentrations was recommended in patients with severe asthma receiving concomitant treatment with beta-adrenoceptor agonists and xanthine derivatives.[10]

The possibility of an interaction with *phenylpropanolamine* should also be borne in mind, as it has been shown to reduce the clearance of theophylline significantly.[11]

1. Conrad KA, Woodworth JR. Orciprenaline does not alter theophylline elimination. *Br J Clin Pharmacol* 1981; 12: 756–7.
2. Snidow J, *et al.* Acute effects of short-term subcutaneous terbutaline on theophylline disposition. *Eur J Clin Pharmacol* 1987; 32: 191–3.
3. Hemstreet MP, *et al.* Effect of intravenous isoproterenol on theophylline kinetics. *J Allergy Clin Immunol* 1982; 69: 360–4.
4. Griffith JA, Kozloski GD. Isoproterenol-theophylline interaction: possible potentiation by other drugs. *Clin Pharm* 1990; 9: 54–7.
5. Danziger Y, *et al.* Reduction of serum theophylline levels by terbutaline in children with asthma. *Clin Pharmacol Ther* 1985; 37: 469–71.
6. Garty M, *et al.* Increased theophylline clearance in asthmatic patients due to terbutaline. *Eur J Clin Pharmacol* 1989; 36: 25–8.
7. Smith SR, Kendall MJ. Potentiation of the adverse effects of intravenous terbutaline by oral theophylline. *Br J Clin Pharmacol* 1986; 21: 451–3.
8. Whyte KF, *et al.* Salbutamol induced hypokalaemia: the effect of theophylline alone and in combination with adrenaline. *Br J Clin Pharmacol* 1988; 25: 571–8.
9. van der Vet APH, *et al.* Pharmacodynamics (lungfunction tests, tremor measurements and cAMP determinations) of a single dose of 0.5 mg terbutaline subcutaneously during sustained-release theophylline medication in patients with asthmatic bronchitis. *Int J Clin Pharmacol Ther Toxicol* 1986; 24: 569–73.
10. Committee on Safety of Medicines. β₂ agonists, xanthines and hypokalaemia. *Current Problems* 28 1990.
11. Wilson HA. Phenylpropanolamine significantly reduces the clearance of theophylline. *Am Rev Respir Dis* 1991; 143: A629.

Tacrine. Results of a study in healthy subjects indicated that tacrine reduced theophylline clearance by about 50% and increased plasma-theophylline concentrations. Competitive inhibition by tacrine of theophylline metabolism was proposed.[1]

1. deVries TM, *et al.* Effect of multiple-dose tacrine administration on single-dose pharmacokinetics of digoxin, diazepam, and theophylline. *Pharm Res* 1993; 10 (suppl): S333.

Tiabendazole. Tiabendazole has been reported[1,2] to increase serum-theophylline concentrations and to decrease theophylline clearance. It has been recommended[2] that theophylline dosage should be reduced by 50% when tiabendazole therapy is initiated.

1. Sugar AM, *et al.* Possible thiabendazole-induced theophylline toxicity. *Am Rev Respir Dis* 1980; 122: 501–3.
2. Lew G, *et al.* Theophylline-thiabendazole drug interaction. *Clin Pharm* 1989; 8: 225–7.

Ticlopidine. Theophylline elimination half-life was increased and plasma clearance was decreased in 10 healthy subjects after the use of ticlopidine 500 mg daily by mouth for 10 days.[1]

1. Colli A, *et al.* Ticlopidine-theophylline interaction. *Clin Pharmacol Ther* 1987; 41: 358–62.

Vaccines. Transient inhibition of the hepatic metabolism of theophylline, possibly secondary to interferon production, resulting in increased theophylline serum half-life and concentration has been reported after BCG vaccination[1] and influenza vaccination.[2,3] Other studies have not been able to confirm the interaction with influenza vaccine.[4-7] The differing findings are probably due to differences in vaccine; modern purified subvirion vaccines which do not induce interferon production do not appear to alter theophylline metabolism.[8,9]

1. Gray JD, *et al.* Depression of theophylline elimination following BCG vaccination. *Br J Clin Pharmacol* 1983; 16: 735–7.
2. Renton KW, *et al.* Decreased elimination of theophylline after influenza vaccination. *Can Med Assoc J* 1980; 123: 288–90.
3. Walker S, *et al.* Serum theophylline levels after influenza vaccination. *Can Med Assoc J* 1981; 125: 243–4.
4. Goldstein RS, *et al.* Decreased elimination of theophylline after influenza vaccination. *Can Med Assoc J* 1982; 126: 470.
5. Fischer RG, *et al.* Influence of trivalent influenza vaccine on serum theophylline levels. *Can Med Assoc J* 1982; 126: 1312–13.
6. Britton L, Ruben FL. Serum theophylline levels after influenza vaccination. *Can Med Assoc J* 1982; 126: 1375.
7. Patriarca PA, *et al.* Influenza vaccination and warfarin or theophylline toxicity in nursing-home residents. *N Engl J Med* 1983; 308: 1601–2.
8. Stults BM, Hashisaki PA. Influenza vaccination and theophylline pharmacokinetics in patients with chronic obstructive lung disease. *West J Med* 1983; 139: 651–4.
9. Winstanley PA, *et al.* Lack of effect of highly purified subunit influenza vaccination on theophylline metabolism. *Br J Clin Pharmacol* 1985; 20: 47–53.

Pharmacokinetics

Theophylline is rapidly and completely absorbed from liquid preparations, capsules, and uncoated tablets; the rate, but not the extent, of absorption is decreased by food and food may also affect theophylline clearance. Modified-release preparations of theophylline can usually provide adequate plasma concentrations when given every 12 hours. However, there is a considerable variability in their absorption characteristics and in the effect of food. It is generally recommended that if a patient is transferred from one such preparation to another then the dose should be re-titrated. Peak serum-theophylline concentrations occur 1 to 2 hours after ingestion of liquid preparations, capsules, and uncoated tablets, and generally about 4 hours after ingestion of modified-release preparations. Rectal absorption is rapid from enemas, but may be slow and erratic from suppositories. Absorption following intramuscular injection is slow and incomplete.

Theophylline is approximately 40% bound to plasma proteins, but in neonates, or adults with liver disease, binding is reduced. Optimum therapeutic serum concentrations are generally considered to range from 10 to 20 µg per mL (55 to 110 µmol per litre) although some consider a lower range appropriate (see Therapeutic Drug Monitoring, below).

Theophylline is metabolised in the liver to 1,3-dimethyluric acid, 1-methyluric acid (via the intermediate 1-methylxanthine), and 3-methylxanthine. Demethylation to 3-methylxanthine (and possibly to 1-methylxanthine) is catalysed by the cytochrome P450 isoenzyme CYP1A2; hydroxylation to 1-methyluric acid is catalysed by CYP2E1 and CYP3A3. The metabolites are excreted in the urine. In adults, about 10% of a dose of theophylline is excreted unchanged in the urine, but in neonates around 50% is excreted unchanged, and a large proportion is excreted as caffeine. Considerable interindividual differences in the rate of hepatic metabolism of theophylline result in large variations in clearance, serum concentrations, and half-lives. Hepatic metabolism is further affected by factors such as age, smoking, disease, diet, and drug interactions. The serum half-life of theophylline in an otherwise healthy, non-smoking asthmatic adult is 6 to 12 hours, in children 1 to 5 hours, in cigarette smokers 4 to 5 hours, and in neonates and premature infants 10 to 45 hours. The serum half-life of theophylline may be increased in the elderly and in patients with heart failure or liver disease.

Theophylline crosses the placenta; it also enters breast milk.

Absorption. FOOD. The effect of food on the absorption of theophylline from modified-release formulations of theophylline and its derivatives has been reviewed.[1] Substantial but variable effects have been reported but it is difficult to predict whether a particular modified-release theophylline formulation will be affected. Some formulations are not affected by the presence of food but for others increases or decreases in the rate and/or extent of absorption have been reported. The composition and fluid content of the food appears to be important and a rapid release of theophylline ('dose-dumping') has occurred with some formulations following a meal, especially one with a high fat content.

A diet high in protein and low in carbohydrate has been reported to increase theophylline clearance, and a low-protein, high-carbohydrate diet to decrease theophylline clearance.[2-6] The consumption of methylxanthines, particularly caffeine, in the diet may decrease theophylline clearance (see under Interactions, above).

1. Jonkman JHG. Food interactions with sustained-release theophylline preparations: a review. *Clin Pharmacokinet* 1989; 16: 162–79.
2. Kappas A, *et al.* Influence of dietary protein and carbohydrate on antipyrine and theophylline metabolism in man. *Clin Pharmacol Ther* 1976; 20: 643–53.

3. Feldman CH, *et al.* Effect of dietary protein and carbohydrate on theophylline metabolism in children. *Pediatrics* 1980; **66**: 956–62.
4. Feldman CH, *et al.* Interaction between nutrition and theophylline metabolism in children. *Ther Drug Monit* 1982; **4**: 69–76.
5. Juan D, *et al.* Effects of dietary protein on theophylline pharmacokinetics and caffeine and aminopyrine breath tests. *Clin Pharmacol Ther* 1986; **40**: 187–94.
6. Juan D, *et al.* Impairment of theophylline clearance by a hypocaloric low-protein diet in chronic obstructive pulmonary disease. *Ther Drug Monit* 1990; **12**: 111–14.

Metabolism and excretion. AGE. From approximately one year of age until adolescence, children have a rapid theophylline clearance.[1] Premature infants and those under one year of age have a slower clearance[2,3] due to immature metabolic pathways.[3-5] In neonates the capacity of hepatic cytochrome P450 enzymes is much reduced compared with older children and adults, and *N*-demethylation and oxidation reactions play a minor role in the metabolism of theophylline.[4-6] Neonates are, however, capable of methylating theophylline at the N7 position to form caffeine which is present at about one-third the concentration of theophylline at steady state.[5,6] The proportion of theophylline excreted unchanged is also increased in premature neonates and decreases with age as hepatic enzyme systems develop.[6] More rapid clearance on the first day of life in premature neonates has been reported.[7]

Some studies have demonstrated a progressive decline in clearance throughout adult years[8] whereas others have not.[9] Similarly, some studies have found a decreased clearance in the elderly[10,11] but others have found no significant change.[12,13]

1. Zaske DE, *et al.* Oral aminophylline therapy: increased dosage requirements in children. *JAMA* 1977; **237**: 1453–5.
2. Aranda JV, *et al.* Pharmacokinetic aspects of theophylline in premature newborns. *N Engl J Med* 1976; **295**: 413–16.
3. Kraus DM, *et al.* Alterations in theophylline metabolism during the first year of life. *Clin Pharmacol Ther* 1993; **54**: 351–9.
4. Grygiel JJ, Birkett DJ. Effect of age on patterns of theophylline metabolism. *Clin Pharmacol Ther* 1980; **28**: 456–62.
5. Tserng K-Y, *et al.* Theophylline metabolism in premature infants. *Clin Pharmacol Ther* 1981; **29**: 594–600.
6. Tserng K-Y, *et al.* Developmental aspects of theophylline metabolism in premature infants. *Clin Pharmacol Ther* 1983; **33**: 522–8.
7. Stile IL, *et al.* Pharmacokinetics of theophylline in premature infants on the first day of life. *Clin Ther* 1986; **8**: 336–41.
8. Randolph WC, *et al.* The effect of age on theophylline clearance in normal subjects. *Br J Clin Pharmacol* 1982; **22**: 603–5.
9. Wiffen JK, *et al.* Does theophylline clearance alter within the adult age range? *Br J Clin Pharmacol* 1984; **17**: 219P.
10. Antal EJ, *et al.* Theophylline pharmacokinetics in advanced age. *Br J Clin Pharmacol* 1981; **12**: 637–45.
11. Jackson SHD, *et al.* The relationship between theophylline clearance and age in adult life. *Eur J Clin Pharmacol* 1989; **36**: 29–34.
12. Bauer LA, Blouin RA. Influence of age on theophylline clearance in patients with chronic obstructive pulmonary disease. *Clin Pharmacokinet* 1981; **6**: 469–74.
13. Fox RW, *et al.* Theophylline kinetics in a geriatric group. *Clin Pharmacol Ther* 1983; **34**: 60–7.

ELIMINATION KINETICS. There is evidence that the elimination of theophylline is dose-dependent and that at high serum concentrations, a small change in dose of a theophylline preparation could cause a disproportionate increase in serum-theophylline concentration, due to a reduction in clearance.[1-3] However, it is not clear that this effect is clinically significant when serum-theophylline concentrations are within the therapeutic range.[4-8] It has also been suggested that repeated oral dosing of theophylline might result in a decrease of clearance compared with pre-treatment values.[9]

1. Weinberger M, Ginchansky E. Dose-dependent kinetics of theophylline disposition in asthmatic children. *J Pediatr* 1977; **91**: 820–4.
2. Tang-Liu DD-S, *et al.* Nonlinear theophylline elimination. *Clin Pharmacol Ther* 1982; **31**: 358–69.
3. Butcher MA, *et al.* Dose-dependent pharmacokinetics with single daily dose slow release theophylline in patients with chronic lung disease. *Br J Clin Pharmacol* 1982; **13**: 241–3.
4. Koëter GH, *et al.* Pharmacokinetics of sustained release theophylline in low and high multidose regimens. *Br J Clin Pharmacol* 1981; **12**: 647–51.
5. Rovei V, *et al.* Pharmacokinetics of theophylline: a dose-range study. *Br J Clin Pharmacol* 1982; **14**: 769–78.
6. Gundert-Remy U, *et al.* Non-linear elimination processes of theophylline. *Eur J Clin Pharmacol* 1983; **24**: 71–8.
7. Brown PJ, *et al.* Lack of dose dependent kinetics of theophylline. *Eur J Clin Pharmacol* 1983; **24**: 525–7.
8. Milavetz G, *et al.* Dose dependency for absorption and elimination rates of theophylline: implications for studies of bioavailability. *Pharmacotherapy* 1984; **4**: 216–20.
9. Efthimiou H, *et al.* Influence of chronic dosing on theophylline clearance. *Br J Clin Pharmacol* 1984; **17**: 525–30.

GENDER. A higher theophylline clearance and shorter elimination half-life has been reported in healthy premenopausal women than in healthy men, probably due to sex-related differences in hepatic metabolism.[1] Changes in the pharmacokinetics of theophylline in women have also been reported according to the stage of the menstrual cycle.[2,3]

1. Nafziger AN, Bertino JS. Sex-related differences in theophylline pharmacokinetics. *Eur J Clin Pharmacol* 1989; **37**: 97–100.
2. Bruguerolle B, *et al.* Influence of the menstrual cycle on theophylline pharmacokinetics in asthmatics. *Eur J Clin Pharmacol* 1990; **39**: 59–61.
3. Nagata K, *et al.* Increased theophylline metabolism in the menstrual phase of healthy women. *J Allergy Clin Immunol* 1997; **100**: 39–43.

Pregnancy and breast feeding. For mention of the pharmacokinetics of theophylline during pregnancy and breast feeding, see under Precautions, above.

Protein binding. Albumin is the major plasma binding protein for theophylline, binding is pH-dependent, and the percentage of theophylline bound at physiological pH is reported to range from about 35 to 45%.[1,2] Some studies have found the plasma protein binding of theophylline to be concentration dependent,[3] but others have not confirmed this.[1,4] Protein binding has been reported to be slightly but significantly higher in patients with bronchial asthma than in healthy controls.[5] Reduced protein binding occurs in patients with hypoalbuminaemia;[6,7] it has also been found in obese subjects[8] possibly due to elevated concentrations of free fatty acids which can displace theophylline from binding sites.

1. Buss D, *et al.* Determinants of the plasma protein binding of theophylline in health. *Br J Clin Pharmacol* 1983; **15**: 399–405.
2. Brørs O, *et al.* Binding of theophylline in human serum determined by ultrafiltration and equilibrium dialysis. *Br J Clin Pharmacol* 1983; **15**: 393–7.
3. Gundert-Remy U, Hildebrandt R. Binding of theophylline and its metabolites to human plasma proteins. *Br J Clin Pharmacol* 1983; **15**: 573–4.
4. Buss DC, *et al.* Protein binding of theophylline. *Br J Clin Pharmacol* 1985; **19**: 529–31.
5. Trnavská Z. Theophylline protein binding. *Arzneimittelforschung* 1990; **40**: 166–9.
6. Leopold D, *et al.* The ex vivo plasma protein binding of theophylline in renal disease. *Br J Clin Pharmacol* 1985; **19**: 823–5.
7. Connelly TJ, *et al.* Characterization of theophylline binding to serum proteins in pregnant and nonpregnant women. *Clin Pharmacol Ther* 1990; **47**: 68–72.
8. Shum L, Jusko WJ. Effects of obesity and ancillary variables (dialysis time, drug, albumin, and fatty acid concentrations) on theophylline serum protein binding. *Biopharm Drug Dispos* 1989; **10**: 549–62.

Therapeutic drug monitoring. Dosage requirements of theophylline preparations vary widely between subjects and even vary with time in individuals, since serum-theophylline concentrations are influenced by a number of factors including disease states, concurrent medication, diet, smoking, and age. Serious toxicity is related to serum concentration and may not be preceded by minor symptoms. For these reasons it is recommended that serum-theophylline concentrations should be monitored if theophylline is to be used safely. The generally accepted optimal serum concentration is between 10 and 20 μg per mL,[1-3] but this should be regarded as a guide and not a rigid barrier and clinical decisions should never be based solely on the serum concentration.[1] The therapeutic range in the treatment of neonatal apnoea is usually considered to be 5 to 15 μg per mL although some babies may respond at lower concentrations.[4] Some now consider that this is a more appropriate range in asthma (except perhaps acute severe asthma).[5] It has been suggested that pulmonary function tests provide a better guide in long-term therapy with theophylline.[6]

Serum-theophylline concentrations were originally measured by spectrophotometry but this is subject to considerable interference from other drugs. High performance liquid chromatography is now the method of choice when extreme accuracy is important and the enzyme multiplied immunoassay technique (EMIT) has become popular because of its rapidity and adaptability to processing large batches.[2] Devices are also available which provide serum-theophylline measurements within several minutes using monoclonal antibody technology.[2,7]

The use of salivary concentrations for monitoring theophylline dosage requirements has been tried, because it is noninvasive, but poor correlations between salivary- and serum-theophylline concentrations mean it has not gained general usage.

1. Hampson JP. The theophylline "therapeutic window"—fact or fallacy? *Pharm J* 1988; **241**: 722–4.
2. Bierman CW, Williams PV. Therapeutic monitoring of theophylline: rationale and current status. *Clin Pharmacokinet* 1989; **17**: 377–84.
3. Holford N, *et al.* Theophylline target concentration in severe airways obstruction—10 or 20 mg/L. A randomised concentration-controlled trial. *Clin Pharmacokinet* 1993; **25**: 495–505.
4. Edwards C. Theophylline and caffeine. *Pharm J* 1986; **237**: 128–9.
5. Hardy CC, Smith J. Adverse reactions profile: theophylline and aminophylline. *Prescribers' J* 1997; **37**: 96–101.
6. Ashutosh K, *et al.* Use of serum theophylline level as a guide to optimum therapy in patients with chronic obstructive lung disease. *J Clin Pharmacol* 1990; **30**: 324–9.
7. Clifton GD, *et al.* Accuracy and time requirements for use of three rapid theophylline assay methods. *Clin Pharm* 1988; **7**: 462–6.

Uses and Administration

Theophylline is a xanthine (p.757) and relaxes bronchial smooth muscle, relieves bronchospasm, and has a stimulant effect on respiration. It stimulates the myocardium and CNS, decreases peripheral resistance and venous pressure, and causes diuresis. It is still not clear how theophylline exerts these effects. Inhibition of phosphodiesterase with a resulting increase in intracellular cyclic adenosine monophosphate (cyclic AMP) occurs, and may play a role. Other proposed mechanisms of action include adenosine receptor antagonism, prostaglandin antagonism, and effects on intracellular calcium.

Theophylline is used as a bronchodilator in the management of reversible airways obstruction, such as in asthma. Although selective beta₂ adrenoceptor stimulants (beta₂ agonists) such as salbutamol are generally the preferred bronchodilators for initial treatment, theophylline is commonly used as an adjunct to beta₂ agonist and corticosteroid therapy in patients requiring an additional bronchodilating effect. Some patients with chronic obstructive pulmonary disease can also exhibit a beneficial response to theophylline therapy. Theophylline is also used to relieve apnoea in neonates. It was formerly used in the treatment of heart failure, and may occasionally have a role in patients with this condition who are also suffering from asthma and bronchitis.

Theophylline may be given in the anhydrous form or as the hydrate. Doses of theophylline are usually expressed as anhydrous theophylline.

The pharmacokinetics of theophylline may be altered by a number of factors including age, smoking, disease, diet, and drug interactions (see above under Precautions, Interactions, and Pharmacokinetics). Theophylline doses should therefore be adjusted for each individual patient according to clinical response, adverse effects, and serum-theophylline concentrations. Optimum therapeutic serum concentrations of theophylline are traditionally considered to range from 10 to 20 μg per mL (55 to 110 μmol per litre) and toxic effects are more common above 20 μg per mL. A range of 5 to 15 μg per mL may be effective, and associated with fewer adverse effects. For long-term administration, once a maintenance dose has been established, monitoring of serum-theophylline concentrations at 6- to 12-monthly intervals has been recommended.

In the management of **acute severe bronchospasm**, theophylline may be given by *intravenous infusion*, though usually aminophylline is preferred (see p.760). (Anhydrous theophylline 1 mg is approximately equivalent to 1.17 mg anhydrous aminophylline or 1.27 mg aminophylline hydrate.) In patients not currently receiving theophylline, aminophylline, or other xanthine-containing medications, a suggested loading dose of 4 to 5 mg per kg body-weight may be given by intravenous infusion over 20 to 30 minutes followed by a suggested maintenance dose of 0.4 mg per kg per hour. Lower doses should be used in the elderly and those with cor pulmonale, heart failure, or liver disease; smokers may require a higher maintenance dose. Dosage should be calculated in terms of lean or ideal body-weight. Some authorities do not consider a loading dose is necessary unless the patient's condition is deteriorating.

Suggested doses for children (not taking theophylline or other xanthine medication) are theophylline 4 to 5 mg per kg by intravenous infusion over 20 to 30 minutes, followed by maintenance doses of: in children 1 to 9 years, 0.8 mg per kg per hour; in children over 9 years, 0.6 to 0.7 mg per kg per hour.

Intravenous theophylline therapy is best avoided in patients already taking theophylline, aminophylline, or other xanthine-containing medication but, if considered necessary, serum-theophylline concentrations should be monitored and the initial dose should be calculated on the basis that each 0.5 mg of theophylline per kg of lean body-weight will result in an increase of serum theophylline concentration of 1 μg per mL.

In the treatment of **acute bronchospasm** which has not required intravenous therapy, theophylline has been given *by mouth* in conventional dosage forms; modified-release preparations are not suitable. In the USA, one suggested oral regimen for adults and children not currently taking theophylline or xanthine-containing products is 5 mg per kg, to produce an average peak serum concentration of 10 μg per mL, and followed by appropriate oral maintenance doses. These are given every 6 to 8 hours in adults, and every 4 to 6 hours in children. Doses should again be reduced in the elderly and those with cor pulmonale, heart failure, or liver disease; smokers may require a higher maintenance dose.

In the long-term management of **chronic broncho-spasm**, theophylline may be given *by mouth* in doses ranging from 300 to 1000 mg daily in divided doses as conventional tablets, capsules, liquid preparations, or modified-release preparations.

For conventional dosage forms the divided doses are generally given every 6 to 8 hours. However, modi-fied-release preparations are more commonly used as they reduce adverse effects and the need for frequent dosing, especially in patients with a rapid theophyl-line clearance. A usual dose of modified-release theo-phylline is 175 to 500 mg every 12 hours, though the bioavailability of different modified-release theo-phylline preparations may not be comparable and retitration of dosage is required if the patient is changed from one modified-release preparation to an-other.

Initially, low doses of theophylline should be given and they should be gradually adjusted according to clinical response and serum-theophylline measure-ments. In the USA a preferred approach to initial dos-age titration, in adults and children weighing over 45 kg, may be to begin with 300 mg daily, in divided doses, for 3 days; if well tolerated to increase the total daily dose to 400 mg for 3 days, and then 600 mg for a further 3 days, before titrating to a final dose based on serum-theophylline concentrations.

The total dose of some modified-release preparations may be given as a single daily dose, for example, in the evening if nocturnal symptoms and early morning wheezing are a problem.

In the UK, suggested oral doses for children weighing 20 to 35 kg (about 6 to 12 years old) are approximate-ly half the adult dose; dosage recommendations for children aged 2 to 6 years are scarce and inconsistent, but one manufacturer recommends approximately quarter the adult dose; use for chronic bronchospasm in children under 2 years is not recommended. In the USA, suggested daily doses in children weighing less than 45 kg and 1 year of age or older are 12 to 14 mg per kg (maximum 300 mg) for 3 days initially, in-creased, if well tolerated, to 16 mg per kg (maximum 400 mg) for 3 days, and then up to 20 mg per kg (maximum 600 mg), before titrating to a final dose based on serum-theophylline concentrations.

Intramuscular injection and administration by sup-pository are not recommended due to severe local ir-ritation and slow unreliable absorption.

Theophylline is an ingredient of some preparations promoted for coughs.

There are topical cosmetic preparations containing theophylline derivatives, particularly aminophylline, that have been promoted for the local reduction of body fat (p.760).

Theophylline monoethanolamine (theophylline olamine), theophylline calcium salicylate, theophyl-line and sodium acetate (theophylline sodium ace-tate), theophylline sodium glycinate (theophylline so-dium aminoacetate), theophylline calcium glycinate, and theophylline glycinate have all been used similar-ly to theophylline.

◊ General references.
1. Vasallo R, Lipsky JJ. Theophylline: recent advances in the un-derstanding of its mode of action and uses in clinical practice. *Mayo Clin Proc* 1998; **73:** 346–54.

Administration. Various methods have been proposed for es-timating theophylline pharmacokinetic parameters to enable optimisation of initial dosage but none should be substituted for the subsequent determination of serum-theophylline concen-trations and clearance at steady state.[1-3]

It was noted in 1997 that dosage requirements for theophylline had declined relative to those of historical controls, apparently due to a downward shift in theophylline clearance in the US population (perhaps due to environmental changes, such as a decrease in exposure to tobacco smoke).[4] It was suggested that earlier dosage guidelines for theophylline needed to be revised in the light of these data, so that the initial dose did not exceed 300 mg daily by mouth—for an approach to initial dosage titra-tion consonant with this view, see Uses and Administration, above.

1. Erdman SM, *et al.* An updated comparison of drug dosing meth-ods part II: theophylline. *Clin Pharmacokinet* 1991; **20:** 280–92.

2. Hogue SL, Phelps SJ. Evaluation of three theophylline dosing equations for use in infants up to one year of age. *J Pediatr* 1993; **123:** 651–6.
3. Lee TC, *et al.* Theophylline population pharmacokinetics from routine monitoring data in very premature infants with apnoea. *Br J Clin Pharmacol* 1996; **41:** 191–200.
4. Asmus MJ, *et al.* Apparent decrease in population clearance of theophylline: implications for dosage. *Clin Pharmacol Ther* 1997; **62:** 483–9.

ADMINISTRATION IN INFANTS. Theophylline clearance is reduced in premature neonates and infants under one year of age due to an immature hepatic microsomal enzyme system (see under Metabolism and Excretion in Pharmacokinetics, above). Post-conceptional age may have a slight influence on theophylline clearance but postnatal age is thought to be more significant.[1]
Theophylline dosage guidelines for infants under one year of age were suggested by the FDA in 1985,[2] but a number of cli-nicians considered that higher doses might be necessary.[1,3,4] Subsequent guidelines for oral theophylline,[5] issued in 1995, suggested a modified regimen: premature infants should re-ceive initial doses of 1 mg per kg body-weight every 12 hours if less than 24 days postnatal age, or 1.5 mg per kg every 12 hours if more than 24 days; in full-term infants initial daily dos-age (to be given in 3 or 4 divided doses) could be calculated on the basis of the equation:

$$\text{Daily dose (mg per kg)} = (0.2 \times \text{age in weeks}) + 5.0$$

Subsequent dosage should be adjusted based on steady-state serum theophylline concentrations, which might take as long as 5 days to be achieved in premature neonates if a loading dose is not used.[5] The recommended serum concentrations were 5 to 10 µg per mL in neonates and 10 to 15 µg per mL in older in-fants. If a loading dose is considered necessary, 5 mg per kg (or 1 mg per kg for each 2 µg per mL increase in serum-theophyl-line concentration in those already receiving theophylline) has been suggested.

Other equations and models of population pharmacokinetics have been proposed for the calculation of appropriate theophyl-line doses in neonates.[6-8]

1. Gilman JT, Gal P. Inadequacy of FDA dosing guidelines for theo-phylline use in neonates. *Drug Intell Clin Pharm* 1986; **20:** 481–4.
2. Anonymous. Use of theophylline in infants. *FDA Drug Bull* 1985; **15:** 16–17.
3. Murphy JE, *et al.* New FDA guidelines for theophylline dosing in infants. *Clin Pharm* 1986; **5:** 16.
4. Kriter KE, Blanchard J. Management of apnea in infants. *Clin Pharm* 1989; **8:** 577–87.
5. Hendeles L, *et al.* Revised FDA labeling guideline for theophyl-line oral dosage forms. *Pharmacotherapy* 1995; **15:** 409–27.
6. Hogue SL, Phelps SJ. Evaluation of three theophylline dosing equations for use in infants up to one year of age. *J Pediatr* 1993; **123:** 651–6.
7. Lee TC, *et al.* Theophylline population pharmacokinetics from routine monitoring data in very premature infants with apnoea. *Br J Clin Pharmacol* 1996; **41:** 191–200.
8. Gagnon AJ. Aminophylline dosing in the treatment of apnea of prematurity—a commentary. *Pharmacotherapy* 1996; **16:** 317–18.

Asthma. Theophylline and its derivatives may be used in the treatment of chronic asthma (p.757) as an adjunct to beta$_2$ ago-nists and corticosteroid therapy when an additional bronchodi-lator is indicated. Modified-release preparations can be useful in the control of nocturnal asthma.
Evidence suggests[1,2] that adding low-dose oral theophylline to inhaled corticosteroids is as effective as increasing the dose of corticosteroid in patients with moderate asthma and persistent symptoms.

The use of xanthines in acute asthma attacks is more controver-sial. UK guidelines permit the use of intravenous aminophyl-line in patients with severe or unresponsive acute asthma, whereas US guidelines do not consider xanthines have any ben-efit over the optimal use of beta agonists and consequently do not recommend their use (see p.757).

1. Evans DJ, *et al.* A comparison of low-dose inhaled budesonide plus theophylline and high-dose inhaled budesonide for moder-ate asthma. *N Engl J Med* 1997; **337:** 1412–18.
2. Ukena D, *et al.* Comparison of addition of theophylline to in-haled steroid with doubling of the dose of inhaled steroid in asth-ma. *Eur Respir J* 1997; **10:** 2754–60.

Cardiac arrhythmias. Theophylline has been tried in vari-ous bradyarrhythmias, usually when other treatment has failed.[1-5]

1. Viskin S, *et al.* Aminophylline for bradyasystolic cardiac arrest refractory to atropine and epinephrine. *Ann Intern Med* 1993; **118:** 279–81.
2. Sra JS, *et al.* Comparison of cardiac pacing with drug therapy in the treatment of neurocardiogenic (vasovagal) syncope with bradycardia or asystole. *N Engl J Med* 1993; **328:** 1085–90.
3. Bertolet BD, *et al.* Theophylline for the treatment of atrioven-tricular block after myocardial infarction. *Ann Intern Med* 1995; **123:** 509–11.
4. Alboni P, *et al.* Effects of permanent pacemaker and oral theo-phylline in sick sinus syndrome: the THEOPACE study: a rand-omized controlled trial. *Circulation* 1997; **96:** 260–6.
5. Ling CA, Crouch MA. Theophylline for chronic symptomatic bradycardia in the elderly. *Ann Pharmacother* 1998; **32:** 837–9.

Cheyne-Stokes respiration. Oral theophylline considera-bly reduced Cheyne-Stokes respiration (periodic breathing) and episodes of central apnoea in a study in 15 patients with stable heart failure and left ventricular systolic dysfunction.[1] This was associated with an improvement in arterial-oxygen saturation during sleep. There was no significant change in car-

diac function, although pulmonary function did improve. Theophylline was also effective in one patient with Cheyne-Stokes respiration possibly related to diabetic autonomic neuropathy.[2]

1. Javaheri S, *et al.* Effect of theophylline on sleep-disordered breathing in heart failure. *N Engl J Med* 1996; **335:** 562–7.
2. Pesek CA, *et al.* Theophylline therapy for near-fatal Cheyne-Stokes respiration: a case report. *Ann Intern Med* 1999; **130:** 427–30.

Chronic obstructive pulmonary disease. In the treatment of chronic obstructive pulmonary disease (p.759), the bron-chodilators of first choice are usually either an antimuscarinic such as ipratropium bromide, or a beta$_2$ agonist such as salbuta-mol, given by inhalation. However the addition of a xanthine such as theophylline, administered by mouth, may be of value in some patients to maximise respiratory function and for its positive cardiac inotropic effects.

ECT. For mention of the use of theophylline as an adjunct to electroconvulsive therapy, see under Precautions, above.

Erythrocytosis. Erythrocytosis (secondary polycythaemia) is an absolute increase in red cell mass that may occur as a result of tissue hypoxia, as in chronic obstructive airways disease, or excessive erythropoietin production, as in some renal tumours or after renal transplant. Post-transplantation erythrocytosis is usually self-limiting but weekly phlebotomy may be required to avoid thromboembolic complications. Theophylline 8 mg per kg body-weight daily by mouth has been shown to reduce haematocrit, red cell mass, and serum-erythropoietin concen-trations in post-transplantation erythrocytosis,[1,2] being benefi-cial in up to 60% of patients.[2] However, there is evidence that an ACE inhibitor (p.824) may be more effective than theophyl-line for this purpose.[3] Theophylline treatment may also reduce erythrocytosis associated with chronic obstructive pulmonary disease.[4]

1. Bakris GL, *et al.* Effects of theophylline on erythropoietin pro-duction in normal subjects and in patients with erythrocytosis after renal transplantation. *N Engl J Med* 1990; **323:** 86–90.
2. Ilan Y, *et al.* Erythrocytosis after renal transplantation: the re-sponse to theophylline treatment. *Transplantation* 1994; **57:** 661–4.
3. Ok E, *et al.* Comparison of the effects of enalapril and theophyl-line on polycythemia after renal transplantation. *Transplantation* 1995; **59:** 1623–45.
4. Oren R, *et al.* Effect of theophylline on erythrocytosis in chronic obstructive pulmonary disease. *Arch Intern Med* 1997; **157:** 1474–8.

Methotrexate neurotoxicity. For reference to the use of aminophylline or theophylline to relieve the acute neurotoxici-ty of methotrexate, see p.554.

Neonatal apnoea. Apnoea of infancy has been defined as cessation of breathing either lasting 20 seconds or more or as-sociated with bradycardia, cyanosis, pallor, and marked hypot-onia, for which no specific cause can be identified.[1] Premature infants (less than 37 weeks' gestation) can exhibit periodic breathing with pathological apnoea (apnoea of prematurity); this usually resolves as the infant approaches term and the neu-rological systems controlling ventilation mature.[1,2]

The management of neonatal apnoea for which no underlying disorder can be found may involve supportive measures such as water beds and cardiorespiratory monitoring, or in some cases, drug therapy.

Administration of either caffeine (as the citrate) or theophylline has been found to reduce the number and severity of apnoeic episodes within 24 to 48 hours in premature infants;[3-6] it is im-portant to rule out any underlying seizure disorder before be-ginning such therapy. Caffeine has a wider therapeutic index and fewer peripheral adverse effects than theophylline, and a longer half-life enabling once-daily administration, and is therefore preferred.[1,6] It may be effective in some children unresponsive to theophylline.[5] Administration by the oral route is generally preferred.[1] Appropriate serum concentrations have been considered to be 5 to 15 µg per mL for theophylline (see also under Administration in Infants, above) and 8 to 20 µg per mL for caffeine.[1] High doses of caffeine (to produce a desired serum concentration of 26 to 40 µg per mL) have been used to obtain a faster response (within 8 hours) without apparent side-effects.[5] During the first year of life, the elimination half-life of both caffeine and theophylline decreases significantly as the in-fant matures; regular monitoring of serum concentrations and constant dosage adjustments are therefore required.[1]

As the patient gets older or becomes asymptomatic (for at least 4 to 8 weeks), xanthine therapy can be withdrawn on a trial basis to see if apnoea will recur.

In infants with apnoea that does not respond to xanthine thera-py, treatment with doxapram may be considered.[1,2] Doxapram is as effective as theophylline, and may also be of benefit as an addition to xanthine therapy[7,8] but must be administered by continuous intravenous infusion and blood pressure must be monitored for signs of hypertension.[2] Adverse effects such as irritability and convulsions may also be a problem.[2]

1. Kriter KE, Blanchard J. Management of apnea in infants. *Clin Pharm* 1989; **8:** 577–87.
2. Ruggins NR. Pathophysiology of apnoea in preterm infants. *Arch Dis Child* 1991; **66:** 70–73.
3. Murat I, *et al.* The efficacy of caffeine in the treatment of recur-rent idiopathic apnea in premature infants. *J Pediatr* 1981; **99:** 984–9.

4. Autret E, *et al.* Comparaison de deux doses d'entretien différentes de caféine dans le traitment des apnées du prématuré. *Therapie* 1985; **40:** 235–9.

5. Scanlon JEM, *et al.* Caffeine or theophylline for neonatal apnoea? *Arch Dis Child* 1992; **67:** 425–8.

6. Henderson-Smart DJ, Steer P. Methylxanthine treatment for apnea in preterm infants (updated 23 August 2001). Available in The Cochrane Library; Issue 4. Oxford: Update Software; 2001.

7. Eyal F, *et al.* Aminophylline versus doxapram in idiopathic apnea of prematurity: a double-blind controlled study. *Pediatrics* 1985; **75:** 709–13.

8. Peliowski A, Finer NN. A blinded, randomized, placebo-controlled trial to compare theophylline and doxapram for the treatment of apnea of prematurity. *J Pediatr* 1990; **116:** 648–53.

Preparations

USP 25: Theophylline and Guaifenesin Capsules; Theophylline and Guaifenesin Oral Solution; Theophylline Capsules; Theophylline Extended-release Capsules; Theophylline in Dextrose Injection; Theophylline Sodium Glycinate Elixir; Theophylline Sodium Glycinate Tablets; Theophylline Tablets; Theophylline, Ephedrine Hydrochloride, and Phenobarbital Tablets.

Proprietary Preparations (details are given in Part 3)
Aust.: Aerodyne; Euphyllin; Pulmidur; Respicur; Theohexal; Theoplus; Theospirex; Unifyl; *Austral.:* Austyn; Nuelin; Theo-Dur; *Belg.:* Euphyllin; Theo-Dur; Theolair; Theophyllard; Xanthium; *Braz.:* Bronquiasma; Codrinan; Talofilina; Teolong; *Canad.:* Apo-Theo; Novo-Theophyl; Pulmophylline†; Quibron-T; Slo-Bid; Theo-Dur; Theo-SR†; Theochron; Theolair; Uniphyl; *Denm.:* Nuelin; Pulmo-Timelets; Theo-Dur; UniXan; Uno-Lin; *Fin.:* Euphyllin; Nuelin; Retafyllin; Theo-Dur; Theofol; *Fr.:* Dilatrane; Euphylline; Pneumogeine; Theolair; Theostat; Xanthium; *Ger.:* Aerobin; Afonilum; Afonilum novo; afpred-THEO; Bronchoparat; Bronchoretard; Contiphyllin; Cronasma; Ditenate N; duraphyllin; Etheophyl†; Euphyllin†; Euphylong; Flui-Theophylline†; Myocardon N†; Perasthman N; Pulmidur; Pulmo-Timelets; Solosin; theo; Theolair; Theophyllard†; Tromphyllin; Unilair; Uniphyllin; *Hong Kong:* Apo-Theo; Euphylong; Nuelin; Phenedrine; Slo-Bid; Theo-Dur; Theovent; Uniphyl; *Irl.:* Lasma; Nuelin; ProVent†; Slo-Phyllin; Theo-Dur; Theolan; Uniphyllin Continus; Zepholin; *Israel:* Asthma T; Glyphyllin; Theotard; Theotrim; *Ital.:* Aminomal; Diffumal; Euphyllina; Frivent; Paidomal; Respicur; Tefamin; Teobid; Teonova†; Theo-24; Theo-Dur; Theolair; Uni-Dur; *Jpn:* Theolong; *Mex.:* Elixofilina; Slo-Bid; Teolong; Uni-Dur; *Mon.:* Tedralan; *Neth.:* Euphylong; Pediaphyllin PL†; Theo₂†; Theolin; Unilair†; *Norw.:* Euphyllin†; Nuelin; Theo-Dur; *NZ:* Nuelin; Theo-Dur; *Port.:* Eufilina; Theo₂†; Teovent; Unicontin; *S.Afr.:* Alcophyllin; Biophyllin†; Bronchophen; Chronophyllin; Euphyllin; Microphyllin; Nuelin; Pulmophyllin; Theo-Dur; Theoplus; Uni-Dur; Uniphyl; Vernthol†; *Singapore:* Apo-Theo; Austyn; Nuelin; Retafyllin; Theo-Dur; Theolin; *Spain:* Asmo†; Chantaline; Elixifilin; Eufilina; Histafilin; Neo Elixifilin†; Piridasmin; Pulmeno; Teodelin†; Teolixir; Theo Max; Theo-Dur; Theolair; Theoplus; Unilong; Vent Retard; *Swed.:* Euphylong; Theo-Dur; Theolair; Euphyllin; Euphylong†; Sodip-phylline; Theolair; Unifyl; Xantivent; *Thai.:* Aerobin; Almarion; Asmasolon; Franol; Med-Phylline; Nuelin; *UAE:* Theophar; *UK:* Lasma†; Nuelin; Slo-Phyllin; Theo-Dur; Uniphyllin Continus; *USA:* Accurbron; Aerolate; Aquaphyllin; Asmalix; Elixomin; Elixophyllin; Lanophyllin†; Quibron-T; Respbid; Slo-Bid; Slo-Phyllin; Sustaire; T-Phyl; Theo-24; Theo-Dur; Theo-X; Theobid Duracaps; Theochron; Theoclear; Theolair; Theospan-SR; Theostat†; Theovent; Uni-Dur; Uniphyl.

Multi-ingredient: *Aust.:* Ambredin; Asthma-Bisolvon†; Bellasthman†; Bronchisan; Eudur†; Peripherin†; Perphyllon; Theo-Lanicort†; Theo-Lanitop†; Theocaradrin†; Thilocombin; *Braz.:* Abacaterol; Alergotox; Bronquitos; CAM; Filinasma; Franol; Marax; *Canad.:* Tedral†; Theo-Bronc; *Fin.:* Theofol Comp; *Fr.:* Hypnasmine; *Ger.:* Broncho-Euphyllin; Eudur†; Neobiphyllin-Clys†; Neobiphyllin†; *Hong Kong:* Lipostabil; *Irl.:* Franol Expectorant; *Israel:* Bronchophylline; *Mex.:* Aminoefedrison NF; *Port.:* Cosmaxil†; Prelus†; *S.Afr.:* Actophlem; Alcophyllex; Diatussin; Lipostabil; Metaxol; Solphyllex; Solphyllin; Tedral†; Theophen; Theophen Comp; *Spain:* Novofilin; Teolixir Compositum; Winasma; *Switz.:* Neo-Biphyllin†; *Thai.:* Almasal; Asianbron; Bronchil; Brondil; Mila-Asma; Polyphed; Qualiton; Theosal; *UK:* Do-Do ChestEze; Franol; Franol Plus; Franolyn Expectorant; *USA:* Elixophyllin-GG; Elixophyllin-KI; Glyceryl-T; Hydrophed; Marax; Primatene Dual Action†; Quadrinal; Quibron; Slo-Phyllin GG; Tedrigen; Theodrine; Theomax DF.

Tiotropium Bromide (16866-y)

Tiotropium Bromide (*rINN*).

Ba-679BR. 6β,7β-Epoxy-3β-hydroxy-8-methyl-1αH,5αH-tropanium bromide di-2-thienylglycolate.
$C_{19}H_{22}BrNO_4S_2 = 472.4.$
CAS — 139404-48-1.

Profile

Tiotropium bromide is a quaternary ammonium antimuscarinic structurally related to ipratropium (p.766) and with a prolonged bronchodilator action. It is used in the treatment of reversible airways obstruction as capsules containing 22.5 μg of the monohydrate, equivalent to 18 μg of tiotropium, and supplying 10 μg of tiotropium from the mouthpiece of the inhaler device. The contents of one capsule are inhaled daily, at the same time of day, for the maintenance treatment of patients with chronic obstructive pulmonary disease.

◊ References.
1. Maesen FP, *et al.* Tiotropium bromide, a new long-acting antimuscarinic bronchodilator: a pharmacodynamic study in patients with chronic obstructive pulmonary disease (COPD). *Eur Respir J* 1995; **8:** 1506–13.

2. O'Connor BJ, *et al.* Prolonged effect of tiotropium bromide on methacholine-induced bronchoconstriction in asthma. *Am J Respir Crit Care Med* 1996; **154:** 876–80.

3. Casaburi R, *et al.* The spirometric efficacy of once-daily dosing with tiotropium in stable COPD: a 13-week multicenter trial. *Chest* 2000; **118:** 1294–1302.

4. van Noord JA, *et al.* A randomised controlled comparison of tiotropium and ipratropium in the treatment of chronic obstructive pulmonary disease. *Thorax* 2000; **55:** 289–94.

Tranilast (12988-j)

Tranilast (*USAN, rINN*).
MK-341; N-5'. N-(3,4-Dimethoxycinnamoyl)anthranilic acid.
$C_{18}H_{17}NO_5 = 327.3.$
CAS — 53902-12-8.

Adverse Effects and Precautions

Adverse effects reported with tranilast have included gastrointestinal disturbances, headache, drowsiness or insomnia, dizziness, malaise, and skin rashes and generalised pruritus. Rarely, liver function disturbance or jaundice, cystitis-like symptoms, anaemia, palpitations, oedema, facial flushing, and stomatitis may occur. Tranilast should be used with caution in patients with impaired hepatic function. Haematological monitoring is recommended.

The manufacturers advise against the use of tranilast in pregnancy because of teratogenicity in *animal* studies.

It should not be used for the treatment of acute asthma attacks. The general cautions described under sodium cromoglicate (p.774) also apply.

Uses and Administration

Tranilast has a stabilising action on mast cells resembling that of sodium cromoglicate (p.775). It is also stated to inhibit collagen synthesis in fibroblasts. It is used in the prophylactic management of asthma (p.757) and in allergic rhinitis (p.407) and eczema (p.1105). It is also used in the management of keloids and hypertrophic scarring, and is under investigation for the prevention of restenosis following coronary artery revascularisation procedures. Adults have been given 100 mg three times daily by mouth; 5 mg per kg body-weight daily in divided doses has been suggested for children. Eye drops containing tranilast 0.5% are administered four times daily for allergic conjunctivitis.

◊ For a mention of possible benefit from tranilast in cutaneous sarcoidosis, see p.1058.

Preparations

Proprietary Preparations (details are given in Part 3)
Jpn: Rizaben.

Tretoquinol Hydrochloride (2110-y)

Tretoquinol Hydrochloride (*pINNM*).
AQ-110 (tretoquinol); Ro-07-5965; Trimethoquinol Hydrochloride; Trimetoquinol Hydrochloride. (–)-1,2,3,4-Tetrahydro-1-(3,4,5-trimethoxybenzyl)isoquinoline-6,7-diol hydrochloride monohydrate.
$C_{19}H_{23}NO_5,HCl,H_2O = 399.9.$
CAS — 30418-38-3 (tretoquinol); 18559-59-6 (anhydrous tretoquinol hydrochloride).
Pharmacopoeias. In Jpn.

Profile

Tretoquinol is a direct-acting sympathomimetic reported to have a selective action on beta₂ receptors (a beta₂ agonist). It has properties similar to those of salbutamol (p.770). It is given as the hydrochloride for its bronchodilating properties in the management of reversible airways obstruction, as in asthma (p.757) or in some patients with chronic obstructive pulmonary disease (p.759). A usual dose by mouth is 2 to 4 mg of tretoquinol hydrochloride two to three times daily.

Preparations

Proprietary Preparations (details are given in Part 3)
Jpn: Inolin.

Tulobuterol Hydrochloride (17020-r)

Tulobuterol Hydrochloride (*BANM, rINNM*).
C-78; HN-078 (tulobuterol). 2-*tert*-Butylamino-1-*o*-chlorophenylethanol hydrochloride.
$C_{12}H_{18}ClNO,HCl = 264.2.$
CAS — 41570-61-0 (tulobuterol); 56776-01-3 (tulobuterol hydrochloride).
Pharmacopoeias. In Jpn.

Profile

Tulobuterol is a direct-acting sympathomimetic with mainly beta-adrenergic activity and a selective action on beta₂ receptors (a beta₂ agonist). It has properties similar to those of salbutamol (p.770).

Tulobuterol is used as a bronchodilator in the management of reversible airways obstruction, as in asthma (p.757) and in some patients with chronic obstructive pulmonary disease (p.759). It is given by mouth as the hydrochloride. The initial oral dose in adults is 1 or 2 mg of tulobuterol hydrochloride twice daily, increased to 2 mg three times daily if necessary. A suggested dose for children is: 6 to 10 years, 0.5 to 1 mg twice daily; over 10 years, 1 to 2 mg twice daily. Tulobuterol has also been given as the base by inhalation from a metered dose inhaler. A transdermal formulation of tulobuterol base is also available.

◊ References to the transdermal formulation of tulobuterol.
1. Uematsu T, *et al.* The pharmacokinetics of the β₂-adrenoceptor agonist, tulobuterol, given transdermally and by inhalation. *Eur J Clin Pharmacol* 1993; **44:** 361–4.

2. Iikura Y, *et al.* Pharmacokinetics and pharmacodynamics of the tulobuterol patch, HN-078, in childhood asthma. *Ann Allergy* 1995; **74:** 147–51.

Preparations

Proprietary Preparations (details are given in Part 3)
Aust.: Bremax; *Belg.:* Respacal; *Ger.:* Atenos; Brelomax; *Jpn:* Hokunalin†; *Mex.:* Bremax; *Port.:* Atenos; *UK:* Respacal†.

Zafirlukast (10561-k)

Zafirlukast (*BAN, USAN, rINN*).
ICI-204219. Cyclopentyl 3-{2-methoxy-4-[(o-tolylsulfonyl)carbamoyl]benzyl}-1-methylindole-5-carbamate.
$C_{31}H_{33}N_3O_6S = 575.7.$
CAS — 107753-78-6.
ATC — R03DC01.

Adverse Effects and Precautions

Headache, an increased incidence of respiratory-tract infection (in the elderly), and gastrointestinal disturbances have been reported with zafirlukast and other leukotriene antagonists. Other adverse effects have included generalised pain, arthralgia, myalgia, fever, and dizziness. Elevations in liver enzyme values have occurred, and rarely, symptomatic hepatitis or hyperbilirubinaemia (see also below). Hypersensitivity reactions, including urticaria and angioedema, have been reported. There have also been rare reports of agranulocytosis, bleeding, bruising and oedema. There have been a few reports of systemic eosinophilia consistent with Churg-Strauss syndrome in patients receiving zafirlukast (see below); treatment should be withdrawn in these patients.

Zafirlukast and other leukotriene antagonists should not be used for the treatment of acute asthma attacks. Zafirlukast is contra-indicated in patients with hepatic impairment or cirrhosis.

Administration in renal impairment. The UK manufacturer states that zafirlukast should be used with caution in patients with moderate or severe renal impairment because of limited experience in this group. However, the US manufacturer mentions no such caution, and states that the pharmacokinetics of zafirlukast in patients with renal impairment do not appear to differ from those in patients with normal renal function. Only about 10% of a dose is reported to be excreted in the urine.

Churg-Strauss syndrome. Pulmonary infiltrates and eosinophilia, resembling the Churg-Strauss syndrome, together with dilated cardiomyopathy, were reported following the withdrawal of corticosteroid therapy in 8 patients receiving zafirlukast.[1] Symptoms responded to withdrawal of zafirlukast and treatment with corticosteroids, with or without cyclophosphamide. It has been suggested that the patients' original asthmatic symptoms had been part of an unrecognised vasculitic syndrome that was unmasked by the corticosteroid withdrawal.[2] However, others have reported Churg-Strauss syndrome associated with zafirlukast in patients who had not been receiving corticosteroids,[3,4] although these cases were not inconsistent with the view that treatment with leukotriene antagonists was coincidental.[5] Eosinophilic syndromes have also been reported for other anti-asthma drugs including inhaled fluticasone and sodium cromoglicate, evidence supporting a non-drug-related aetiology.[5] However, the increasing number of reports with zafirlukast and the other leukotriene antagonists, montelukast[6] and pranlukast,[7] means that a particular class-effect cannot be ruled out.[8] It has been suggested that patients should be monitored carefully (e.g. by measuring erythrocyte sedimentation rate, C reactive protein, and eosinophil counts) if the introduction of an anti-asthma drug such as a leukotriene antagonist permits the reduction of oral corticosteroid dosage.[9] In addition, in patients with asthma and features of multisystem disease, the possibility of underlying Churg-Strauss syndrome (p.1049) may be worth considering.

1. Wechsler ME, *et al.* Pulmonary infiltrates, eosinophilia, and cardiomyopathy following corticosteroid withdrawal in patients with asthma receiving zafirlukast. *JAMA* 1998; **279:** 455–7.

2. Churg A, Churg J. Steroids and Churg-Strauss syndrome. *Lancet* 1998; **352:** 32–3.

3. Katz RS, Papernik M. Zafirlukast and Churg-Strauss syndrome. *JAMA* 1998; **279:** 1949.

4. Green RL, Vayonis AG. Churg-Strauss syndrome after zafirlu-kast in two patients not receiving systemic steroid treatment. *Lancet* 1999; **353:** 725–6.
5. Wechsler M, Drazen JM. Churg-Strauss syndrome. *Lancet* 1999; **353:** 1970.
6. Franco J, Artés MJ. Pulmonary eosinophilia associated with montelukast. *Thorax* 1999; **54:** 558–60.
7. Kinoshita M, *et al.* Churg-Strauss syndrome after corticosteroid withdrawal in an asthmatic patient treated with pranlukast. *J Allergy Clin Immunol* 1999; **103:** 534–5.
8. Green RL, Vayonis AG. *Lancet* 1999; **353:** 1971.
9. D'Cruz DP, *et al.* Difficult asthma or Churg-Strauss syndrome? *BMJ* 1999; **318:** 475–6.

Effects on the liver. Severe hepatitis, in one case leading to subfulminant hepatic failure requiring liver transplantation, has been reported in patients receiving zafirlukast.[1,2] In the USA, the manufacturers of zafirlukast advise stopping treatment if hepatotoxicity is suspected, and performing liver function tests; UK product information suggests that the decision to cease therapy should be based on an assessment of the individual benefits and potential risks.

1. Grieco AJ, Burstein-Stein J. Oral montelukast versus inhaled salmeterol to prevent exercise-induced bronchoconstriction. *Ann Intern Med* 2000; **133:** 392.
2. Reinus JF, *et al.* Severe liver injury after treatment with the leukotriene receptor antagonist zafirlukast. *Ann Intern Med* 2000; **133:** 964–8.

Interactions

Zafirlukast is metabolised by hepatic cytochrome P450, specifically the isoenzymes CYP2C9 and CYP3A4. Therefore concomitant use of other drugs that inhibit or are metabolised by these hepatic enzymes may result in changes in plasma concentrations of either drug and, possibly, adverse effects. Patients receiving warfarin may develop prolongation of the prothrombin time and anticoagulant dosage should be adjusted accordingly. Erythromycin, terfenadine and theophylline may reduce plasma concentrations of zafirlukast; zafirlukast has rarely been reported to increase plasma-theophylline concentrations. Increased plasma concentrations of zafirlukast have been seen when given with high doses of aspirin.

Pharmacokinetics

Peak plasma concentrations of zafirlukast occur about 3 hours after oral administration. The absolute bioavailability is uncertain, but administration with food reduces both the rate and extent of absorption, decreasing bioavailability by about 40%. Zafirlukast is about 99% bound to plasma protein. It is extensively metabolised in the liver (see Interactions, above) and excreted principally in faeces, as unchanged drug and metabolites. About 10% of a dose is excreted in urine. The terminal elimination half-life of zafirlukast is about 10 hours. Studies in *animals* suggest that small amounts cross the placenta; it is also distributed in low concentrations into breast milk.

Uses and Administration

Zafirlukast is a selective antagonist of the leukotriene D_4 receptor (p.757), stimulation of which by circulating leukotrienes is thought to play a role in the pathogenesis of asthma. It suppresses both early and late bronchoconstrictor responses to inhaled antigens or irritants, but is not suitable for the management of acute attacks of asthma.

Zafirlukast is used in the management of chronic asthma. It is given by mouth in doses of 20 mg twice daily, taken at least 1 hour before or 2 hours after meals. Children aged 7 to 11 years may be given 10 mg twice daily.

◊ General references.

1. Anonymous. Zafirlukast for asthma. *Med Lett Drugs Ther* 1996; **38:** 111–12.
2. Adkins JC, Brogden RN. Zafirlukast: a review of its pharmacology and therapeutic potential in the management of asthma. *Drugs* 1998; **55:** 121–44.
3. Anonymous. Montelukast and zafirlukast in asthma. *Drug Ther Bull* 1998; **36:** 65–8.
4. Smith LJ. A risk-benefit assessment of antileukotrienes in asthma. *Drug Safety* 1998; **19:** 205–18.
5. Lipworth BJ. Leukotriene-receptor antagonists. *Lancet* 1999; **353:** 57–62.
6. Dunn CJ, Goa KL. Zafirlukast: an update of its pharmacology and therapeutic efficacy in asthma. *Drugs* 2001; **61:** 285–315.

Asthma. Zafirlukast produces modest improvement in mild-to-moderate asthma,[1,2] which was of a similar order to that seen with inhaled sodium cromoglicate in one study,[3] but less than that of inhaled salmeterol in another.[4] Revised US guidelines for the management of asthma (p.757) permit the use of zafirlukast as an alternative to cromoglicate, nedocromil, or inhaled corticosteroids in patients with mild persistent asthma, who cannot be managed with inhaled beta$_2$ agonists on an as-needed basis alone.

1. Suissa S, *et al.* Effectiveness of the leukotriene receptor antagonist zafirlukast for mild-to-moderate asthma: a randomized, double-blind, placebo-controlled trial. *Ann Intern Med* 1997; **126:** 177–83.
2. Fish JE, *et al.* Zafirlukast for symptomatic mild-to-moderate asthma: a 13-week multicenter study. *Clin Ther* 1997; **19:** 675–90.
3. Nathan RA, *et al.* Two first-line therapies in the treatment of mild asthma: use of peak flow variability as a predictor of effectiveness. *Ann Allergy Asthma Immunol* 1999; **82:** 497–503.
4. Busse W, *et al.* Comparison of inhaled salmeterol and oral zafirlukast in patients with asthma. *J Allergy Clin Immunol* 1999; **103:** 1075–80.

Rhinitis. Zafirlukast 20 mg twice daily was not effective in seasonal allergic rhinitis (p.407) in one study.[1]

1. Pullerits T, *et al.* Randomized placebo-controlled study comparing a leukotriene receptor antagonist and a nasal glucocorticoid in seasonal allergic rhinitis. *Am J Respir Crit Care Med* 1999; **159:** 1814–18.

Preparations

Proprietary Preparations (details are given in Part 3)
Austral.: Accolate; **Belg.:** Accolate; Resma; **Canad.:** Accolate; **Fin.:** Accolate; **Hong Kong:** Accolate; **Irl.:** Accolate; **Ital.:** Accoleit; Zafirst; **Mex.:** Accolate; **Port.:** Accolate; **Singapore:** Accolate; **Spain:** Accolate; Azimax; Olmoran; **Switz.:** Accolate; **Thai.:** Accolate; **UK:** Accolate; **USA:** Accolate.

Zileuton (9332-j)

Zileuton (BAN, USAN, rINN).
A-64077; Abbott-64077. (±)-1-(1-Benzo[*b*]thien-2-ylethyl)-*N*-hydroxyurea.
$C_{11}H_{12}N_2O_2S = 236.3$.
CAS — 111406-87-2.

Adverse Effects and Precautions

Zileuton has been associated with raised liver enzyme values, gastrointestinal disturbances, urticaria, headache, and leucopenia in a few patients. It should not be used in patients with hepatic impairment or active liver disease. Hepatic transaminases should be monitored before, and periodically during, therapy. Zileuton is not suitable for the treatment of acute asthma attacks.

Interactions

Zileuton has been reported to impair the metabolism of some drugs metabolised via hepatic cytochrome P450, including propranolol, terfenadine, theophylline, and warfarin.

Pharmacokinetics

Zileuton is reported to be well absorbed from the gastrointestinal tract following oral administration, with peak plasma concentrations occurring about 2 hours after a dose. It is apparently widely distributed and is about 93% bound to plasma protein. It is extensively metabolised in the liver, and excreted in the urine, largely as glucuronide metabolites. The elimination half-life is reported to be about 2 hours.

◊ References.

1. Wong SL, *et al.* The pharmacokinetics of single oral doses of zileuton 200 to 800 mg, its enantiomers, and its metabolites, in normal healthy volunteers. *Clin Pharmacokinet* 1995; **29** (suppl 2): 9–21.
2. Awni WM, *et al.* Pharmacokinetics and pharmacodynamics of zileuton after oral administration of single and multiple dose regimens of zileuton 600 mg in healthy volunteers. *Clin Pharmacokinet* 1995; **29** (suppl 2): 22–33.
3. Braeckman RA, *et al.* The pharmacokinetics of zileuton in healthy young and elderly volunteers. *Clin Pharmacokinet* 1995; **29** (suppl 2): 42–8.
4. Awni WM, *et al.* Population pharmacokinetics of zileuton, a selective 5-lipoxygenase inhibitor, in patients with rheumatoid arthritis. *Eur J Clin Pharmacol* 1995; **48:** 155–60.

Uses and Administration

Zileuton is an orally active 5-lipoxygenase inhibitor (p.757). It is used in the management of chronic asthma but has no bronchodilator properties and is not suitable for the management of acute attacks. Zileuton is given by mouth, in doses of 600 mg 4 times daily.

It has also been tried in some other disorders including arthritis, allergic rhinitis, and inflammatory bowel disease.

Asthma. Zileuton has been found to be of some benefit in asthma, including that provoked by cold air, exercise, and NSAIDs. Revised US guidelines for the management of asthma (p.757) permit its use as an alternative to cromoglicate, nedocromil or inhaled corticosteroids in patients with mild persistent asthma who cannot be managed with inhaled beta$_2$ agonists on an as-needed basis alone.

References.

1. Israel E, *et al.* The effects of a 5-lipoxygenase inhibitor on asthma induced by cold, dry air. *N Engl J Med* 1990; **323:** 1740–4.
2. Israel E, *et al.* The effect of inhibition of 5-lipoxygenase by zileuton in mild-to-moderate asthma. *Ann Intern Med* 1993; **119:** 1059–66.
3. McGill KA, Busse WW. Zileuton. *Lancet* 1996; **348:** 519–24.
4. Israel E, *et al.* Effect of treatment with zileuton, a 5-lipoxygenase inhibitor, in patients with asthma: a randomized controlled trial. *JAMA* 1996; **275:** 931–6.

Inflammatory bowel disease. Despite initial hopes that inhibition of lipoxygenase might prove of benefit in patients with ulcerative colitis,[1] a study in patients with mild or moderately active relapsing ulcerative colitis found that the symptomatic benefits of zileuton were confined to those not already receiving sulfasalazine.[2] A subsequent study showed zileuton was not significantly better than placebo in maintaining remission.[3] For a discussion of inflammatory bowel disease and its management, see p.1205.

1. Laursen LS, *et al.* Selective 5-lipoxygenase inhibition in ulcerative colitis. *Lancet* 1990; **335:** 683–5.
2. Laursen LS, *et al.* Selective 5-lipoxygenase inhibition by zileuton in the treatment of relapsing ulcerative colitis: a randomized double-blind placebo-controlled multicentre trial. *Eur J Gastroenterol Hepatol* 1994; **6:** 209–15.
3. Hawkey CJ, *et al.* A trial of zileuton versus mesalazine or placebo in the maintenance of remission of ulcerative colitis. *Gastroenterology* 1997; **112:** 718–24.

Rhinitis. A study in 8 patients with allergic rhinitis (p.407) found that a single dose of zileuton 800 mg reduced the response to a nasal antigen challenge 3 hours later,[1] including reduced sneezing and nasal congestion.

1. Knapp HR. Reduced allergen-induced nasal congestion and leukotriene synthesis with an orally active 5-lipoxygenase inhibitor. *N Engl J Med* 1990; **323:** 1745–8.

Preparations

Proprietary Preparations (details are given in Part 3)
USA: Zyflo.

Cardiovascular Drugs

This chapter describes drugs used principally in the management of cardiovascular disorders, as well as the choice of treatment for a particular disorder. Blood products, plasma expanders, and haemostatics, which also have a role in cardiovascular disease, are described elsewhere (p.715).

Cardiovascular Drug Groups

Although very diverse, cardiovascular drugs can be broadly classified according to their pharmacological action. Basic details of the major groups follow, together with lists of the drugs described in this chapter.

ACE inhibitors

The main uses of ACE (angiotensin-converting enzyme) inhibitors are in the management of heart failure, hypertension, and myocardial infarction. Their actions and uses are discussed in more detail on p.820.

Described in this chapter are

Alacepril, p.833	Moexipril, p.935
Benazepril, p.843	Perindopril, p.953
Captopril, p.853	Quinapril, p.963
Cilazapril, p.858	Ramipril, p.966
Delapril, p.867	Spirapril, p.973
Enalapril, p.883	Temocapril, p.979
Enalaprilat, p.884	Teprotide, p.980
Fosinopril, p.892	Trandolapril, p.985
Imidapril, p.912	Zofenopril, p.999
Lisinopril, p.921	

Adrenergic neurone blockers

Adrenergic neurone blockers are used in hypertension although they have largely been superseded by other drugs less likely to cause orthostatic hypotension. They have also been used in open-angle glaucoma.

Adrenergic neurone blockers act by selectively inhibiting transmission in postganglionic adrenergic nerves. They are believed to act mainly by preventing the release of noradrenaline at nerve endings; they cause the depletion of noradrenaline stores in peripheral sympathetic nerve terminals. They do not prevent the secretion of catecholamines by the adrenal medulla.

Described in this chapter are

Betanidine, p.848	Guanadrel, p.900
Debrisoquine, p.866	Guanethidine, p.901
Guabenxan, p.900	Guanoxan, p.902

Alpha blockers

Alpha blockers are used mainly in the management of hypertension and to relieve urinary obstruction in benign prostatic hyperplasia.

Alpha blockers are also known as alpha-adrenergic antagonists or alpha-adrenergic receptor antagonists. Some have particular affinities for one of the subtypes of the alpha adrenoceptor. Drugs such as indoramin or prazosin are much more potent in blocking alpha$_1$ than alpha$_2$ adrenoceptors and are often termed selective alpha$_1$ blockers. Blockade of alpha$_1$ adrenoceptors inhibits the vasoconstriction induced by endogenous catecholamines. Both arteriolar and venous vasodilatation may occur resulting in a fall in blood pressure because of decreased peripheral resistance. Blockade of alpha$_2$ adrenoceptors with a selective drug such as yohimbine (p.1681) can conversely lead to a rise in blood pressure. With phenoxybenzamine and phentolamine, which broadly have similar affinities for both the alpha$_1$ and alpha$_2$ subtypes of receptor, any increase in blood pressure due to alpha$_2$ blockade is prevented by the inhibition of vasoconstriction caused by alpha$_1$ blockade. Alpha blockers also act at alpha adrenoceptors in nonvascular smooth muscle, for example in the bladder where alpha blockade produces decreased resistance to urinary outflow. Most alpha blockers are reversible or 'competitive' inhibitors of alpha adrenoceptors; phenoxybenzamine is an irreversible or 'non-competitive' alpha blocker and is particularly useful in phaeochromocytoma.

Described in this chapter are

Alfuzosin, p.833	Prazosin, p.958
Bunazosin, p.852	Tamsulosin, p.978
Doxazosin, p.883	Terazosin, p.980
Indoramin, p.913	Thymoxamine [Moxisylyte],
Naftopidil, p.938	p.980
Phenoxybenzamine, p.954	Tolazoline, p.984
Phentolamine, p.954	Urapidil, p.987

References.

1. Frishman WH, Kotob F. Alpha-adrenergic blocking drugs in clinical medicine. *J Clin Pharmacol* 1999; **39:** 7–16.

Angiotensin II receptor antagonists

Angiotensin II receptor antagonists are used in the management of hypertension; they may have a particular role in patients who develop cough with ACE inhibitors. Some are also under investigation in the management of heart failure. They act mainly by selective blockade of AT$_1$ receptors thus reducing the pressor effects of angiotensin II.

Described in this chapter are

Candesartan, p.853	Tasosartan, p.979
Eprosartan, p.886	Telmisartan, p.979
Irbesartan, p.914	Valsartan, p.988
Losartan, p.921	

Antiarrhythmics

Drugs used in the management of cardiac arrhythmias form a diverse group. Many of them, such as beta blockers (p.844), digoxin (p.870), lignocaine [lidocaine] (p.1313), magnesium (p.1190), and phenytoin (p.357) have important actions in addition to their antiarrhythmic properties and thus, as well as being employed in the treatment of cardiac arrhythmias, have a wide range of other clinical applications.

Various methods of classifying antiarrhythmics (formerly described as cardiac depressants) may be employed.

The most widely used classification of antiarrhythmics is that proposed by Vaughan Williams and later modified by Harrison. This classification is based largely on *in-vitro* electrophysiological effects of the drugs on myocardial cells. The action potential involved in the contraction of cardiac muscle consists of several phases (Figure 1, below) controlled by ionic movements across the myo-

cardial cell membrane. When the cell is excited it becomes depolarised due to an increase in sodium conductance and a consequent fast influx of sodium ions (phase 0) lasting a few milliseconds, followed by a transient outward current probably carried by potassium ions (phase 1). A slow influx of ions, mainly calcium ions, forms phase 2 of the cardiac action potential which is known as the 'plateau' phase. The cell finally repolarises (phase 3) due to an increase in potassium conductance and an efflux of potassium ions which returns it to its initial resting membrane potential (phase 4).

Figure 1. The action potential.

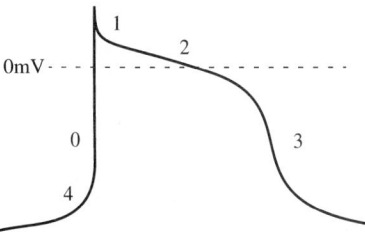

In specialised cardiac tissue such as the sino-atrial node and atrioventricular node the resting cell membrane spontaneously depolarises and initiates action potentials, due mainly to decreased potassium conductance. The tissues of the nodes are dependent predominantly on calcium transport for the depolarisation phase of the action potential, whereas the atria and ventricles are mainly sodium-dependent.

A typical normal ECG trace is shown in Figure 2, below.

Figure 2. A normal ECG trace.

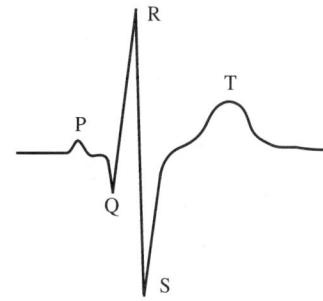

Class I includes drugs which directly interfere with depolarisation of the cell membrane (membrane-stabilising drugs) by blocking the fast inward current of sodium into cardiac cells; they also have local anaesthetic properties. They are subdivided into 3 further groups according to their effects on factors such as the duration of the cardiac action potential, the rate of change of the depolarisation phase of the cardiac action potential, the fibrillation threshold, conduction properties, and atrial and ventricular refractoriness.

Class Ia drugs slow the rate of change of the depolarisation phase of the action potential, moderately prolong the repolarisation phase, and prolong the PR, QRS, and QT intervals on ECG recording.

Described in this chapter are

Ajmaline, p.833	Pirmenol, p.956
Cibenzoline, p.857	Procainamide, p.960
Disopyramide, p.878	Quinidine, p.964
Hydroquinidine, p.912	

Class Ib drugs have a limited effect on the rate of change of the depolarisation phase of the action potential, shorten the repolarisation phase, shorten the QT interval, and elevate the fibrillation threshold.

Described in this chapter are

Aprindine, p.841	Tocainide, p.983
Mexiletine, p.932	

Class Ic drugs markedly slow the rate of change of the depolarisation phase of the action potential, have little effect on the repolarisation phase, and markedly prolong the PR and QRS intervals.

Described in this chapter are

Diprafenone, p.877	Lorcainide, p.921
Encainide, p.884	Pilsicainide, p.955
Flecainide, p.890	Propafenone, p.961

Class II drugs are characterised by beta-blocking activity, leading to a reduction in heart rate, myocardial contractility, and the rate of conduction of impulses through the conducting system.

Described in this chapter are

Beta blockers (but sotalol has predominantly class III activity), p.844	Bretylium, p.851

Class III drugs prolong the repolarisation phase of the action potential.

Described in this chapter are

Acecainide, p.825	Dofetilide, p.881
Amiodarone, p.836	Ibutilide, p.912
Azimilide, p.843	Nifekalant, p.946
Bretylium, p.851	Sotalol, p.972
Cibenzoline, p.857	

Class IV drugs block the slow inward calcium current (calcium-channel blockers) although not all drugs that fall into the broad general category of calcium-channel blockers share the same specific properties.

Described in this chapter are

Cibenzoline, p.857	Verapamil, p.989

Many antiarrhythmics have actions typical of more than one class of compound making allocation to one specific class difficult. In some cases this results in multiple classification; an example is bretylium which has class II and III actions. However, in other cases a compound has been allocated to only one class even though it does display additional properties typical of another class; thus propafenone is usually recognised as a class Ic drug although it does possess some beta-blocking activity; beta blockers such as propranolol are traditionally described as class II drugs despite possessing some class I actions; sotalol has some class II actions typical of the beta blockers generally, but has predominantly class III activity and is usually described as a class III drug. Some drugs such as adenosine and digoxin do not fit into the Vaughan Williams classification at all.

The Vaughan Williams classification has been criticised because the electrophysiological action of the antiarrhythmic drugs is not clearly related to their effectiveness in treating a particular arrhythmia in an individual patient. A more clinically useful method might be to categorise the drugs according to the cardiac tissues which each affects. Thus drugs which act on the sino-atrial node include beta blockers, class IV antiarrhythmics, and cardiac glycosides such as digoxin; class I and class III antiarrhythmics act on the ventricles; and drugs acting on atrial arrhythmias include class Ia, Ic, and III antiarrhythmics and beta blockers. Class Ia and III antiarrhythmics act on accessory pathways and drugs acting on the atrioventricular node include class Ic and IV antiarrhythmics, beta blockers, and cardiac glycosides. A simplification of this scheme is to classify drugs into those that act on both ventricular and supraventricular arrhythmias such as amiodarone, beta blockers, disopyramide, procainamide, and quinidine, those that act mainly on ventricular arrhythmias such as lignocaine [lidocaine], mexiletine, and phenytoin, and those that act mainly on supraventricular arrhythmias such as verapamil.

References.

1. Vaughan Williams EM. Classification of antidysrhythmic drugs. *Pharmacol Ther* 1975; **1**: 115–38.
2. Harrison DC. Current classification of antiarrhythmic drugs as a guide to their rational clinical use. *Drugs* 1986; **31**: 93–5.
3. Frumin H, *et al.* Classification of antiarrhythmic drugs. *J Clin Pharmacol* 1989; **29**: 387–94.
4. Nattel S. Antiarrhythmic drug classifications: a critical appraisal of their history, present status, and clinical relevance. *Drugs* 1991; **41**: 672–701.
5. Vaughan Williams EM. Classifying antiarrhythmic actions: by facts or speculation? *J Clin Pharmacol* 1992; **32**: 964–77.

Anticoagulants

Anticoagulants are used in the treatment and prophylaxis of thromboembolic disorders. They may be divided into direct anticoagulants such as the heparins, low-molecular-weight heparins, heparinoids, and direct thrombin inhibitors, and indirect anticoagulants such as the coumarin and indanedione derivatives.

Direct anticoagulants

Heparin inhibits clotting of blood *in vitro* and *in vivo* by enhancing the action of antithrombin III. Antithrombin III, which is present in plasma, inhibits the activity of activated clotting factors including thrombin (factor IIa) and activated factor X (factor Xa). With normal therapeutic doses heparin has an inhibitory effect on both thrombin and factor Xa. The low doses that are given subcutaneously for the prophylaxis of thromboembolism have a selective effect on antithrombin III's inhibition of factor Xa. Very high doses are reported to reduce the activity of antithrombin III. Heparin also has some effect on platelet function, inhibits the formation of a stable fibrin clot, and has an antilipidaemic effect.

Low-molecular-weight heparins are salts of fragments of heparin produced by chemical or enzymatic depolymerisation of the heparin molecule. Commercially available low-molecular-weight heparins differ in their method of production, molecular-weight range, and degree of sulfation. Like heparin, these compounds enhance the action of antithrombin III but they are characterised by a higher ratio of anti-factor Xa to anti-factor IIa (antithrombin activity) than heparin. Although the possibility that such selective factor-Xa inhibition would result in antithrombotic activity without anticoagulant, and hence haemorrhagic, effects has not been confirmed by clinical experience in humans, they have more predictable effects and require less monitoring than heparin. Low-molecular-weight heparins also have less effect on platelet aggregation than heparin.

Direct thrombin inhibitors such as bivalirudin, desirudin, and lepirudin are also used.

Described in this chapter are

Ardeparin, p.841	Hirudin, p.905
Argatroban, p.841	Lepirudin, p.919
Bivalirudin, p.850	Low-molecular-weight
Certoparin, p.856	Heparins, p.923
Dalteparin, p.865	Nadroparin, p.937
Desirudin, p.867	Parnaparin, p.952
Enoxaparin, p.885	Reviparin, p.968
Heparin, p.902	Tinzaparin, p.982

The term *heparinoid* includes heparin derivatives and has also been used more loosely to include naturally occurring and synthetic highly sulfated polysaccharides of similar structure, such as danaparoid and dermatan sulfate. Some compounds have been described in many ways; some of the terms used include sulfated glucosaminoglycans, glycosaminoglycan polysulfate compounds, or sulfated mucopolysaccharides.

Described in this chapter are

Danaparoid, p.866	Sodium Apolate, p.971
Dermatan Sulfate, p.867	Suleparoid, p.978
Pentosan Polysulfate Sodium, p.953	Sulodexide, p.978

Indirect anticoagulants

Indirect anticoagulants act by depressing the hepatic vitamin K-dependent synthesis of coagulation factors II (prothrombin), VII, IX, and X, and of the anticoagulant protein C and its cofactor protein S. Warfarin, a coumarin, is the main drug used, but indanediones such as phenindione are also available. Since they act indirectly, they have no effect on existing clots. Also as the coagulation factors involved have half-lives ranging from 6 to 60 hours, several hours are required before an effect is observed. A therapeutic effect is usually apparent by 24 hours, but the peak effect may not be achieved until 2 or 3 days after a dose; the overall effect may last for 5 days.

Described in this chapter are

Anisindione, p.840	Phenindione, p.954
Dicoumarol, p.869	Phenprocoumon, p.954
Ethyl Biscoumacetate, p.888	Tioclomarol, p.983
Fluindione, p.892	Warfarin, p.992
Nicoumalone [Acenocoumarol], p.940	

Antiplatelet drugs

Platelet aggregation is important in haemostasis (p.718) and is also involved in thrombus formation, particularly in the arterial circulation. Antiplatelet drugs reduce platelet aggregation and are used to prevent further thromboembolic events in patients who have suffered myocardial infarction, ischaemic stroke or transient ischaemic attacks, or unstable angina, and for primary prevention of a thromboembolic event in patients at risk. Some are also used for the prevention of reocclusion or restenosis following angioplasty and bypass procedures.

Antiplatelet drugs act through a wide range of mechanisms. Aspirin (p.14) is the most widely used and studied; it acts by irreversibly inhibiting platelet cyclo-oxygenase and thus preventing synthesis of thromboxane A_2. Reversible cyclo-oxygenase inhibitors such as indobufen are also available, and thromboxane synthase inhibitors and thromboxane receptor antagonists (sulotroban) have also been used.

Drugs that interfere with adenosine metabolism have an antiplatelet effect and those used include some prostaglandins, which act by increasing platelet cyclic adenosine monophosphate levels; clopidogrel and ticlopidine, which interfere with adenosine diphosphate mediated platelet activation; and the adenosine reuptake inhibitor dipyridamole.

Thrombin inhibitors such as heparin and the hirudins have antiplatelet and anticoagulant effects. Glycoprotein IIb/IIIa-receptor antagonists, such as abciximab, eptifibatide, and tirofiban, interfere with the final step in platelet aggregation and are used in unstable angina and as adjuncts in reperfusion and revascularisation procedures.

Described in this chapter are

Abciximab, p.819	Picotamide, p.955
Cilostazol, p.858	Sarpogrelate, p.969
Clopidogrel, p.863	Sibrafiban, p.969
Cloricromen, p.863	Sulotroban, p.978
Dipyridamole, p.877	Ticlopidine, p.981
Ditazole, p.880	Tirofiban, p.983
Eptifibatide, p.886	Trapidil, p.986
Indobufen, p.913	Triflusal, p.987
Lamifiban, p.919	Xemilofiban, p.999
Orbofiban, p.950	

References.

1. Schrör K. Antiplatelet drugs: a comparative review. *Drugs* 1995; **50**: 7–28.
2. Chong PH. Glycoprotein IIb/IIIa receptor antagonists in the management of cardiovascular diseases. *Am J Health-Syst Pharm* 1998; **55**: 2363–86.
3. Gershlick AH. Antiplatelet therapy. *Hosp Med* 2000; **61**: 15–23.
4. Sabatine MS, Jang I-K. The use of glycoprotein IIb/IIIa inhibitors in patients with coronary artery disease. *Am J Med* 2000; **109**: 224–37.

Beta blockers

Beta blockers are competitive antagonists at beta-adrenergic receptor sites and are used in the management of cardiovascular disorders such as hypertension, angina pectoris, cardiac arrhythmias, myocardial infarction, and heart failure. They are also given to control symptoms of sympathetic overactivity in alcohol withdrawal, anxiety states, hyperthyroidism, and tremor and in the prophylaxis of migraine and of bleeding associated with portal hypertension. Some beta blockers are used as eye drops to reduce raised intra-ocular pressure in glaucoma and ocular hypertension. Their actions and uses are discussed in more detail on p.844.

Described in this chapter are

Acebutolol, p.825	Labetalol, p.918
Alprenolol, p.833	Levobetaxolol, p.920
Amosulalol, p.839	Levobunolol, p.920
Arotinolol, p.841	Mepindolol, p.926
Atenolol, p.841	Metipranolol, p.930
Befunolol, p.843	Metoprolol, p.931
Betaxolol, p.848	Nadolol, p.937
Bevantolol, p.849	Nebivolol, p.938
Bisoprolol, p.850	Nipradilol, p.946
Bopindolol, p.850	Oxprenolol, p.951
Bucindolol, p.851	Penbutolol, p.952
Bunitrolol, p.852	Pindolol, p.955
Bupranolol, p.852	Practolol, p.957
Carazolol, p.855	Propranolol, p.962
Carteolol, p.855	Sotalol, p.972
Carvedilol, p.855	Talinolol, p.978
Celiprolol, p.856	Tertatolol, p.980
Epanolol, p.886	Tilisolol, p.982
Esmolol, p.887	Timolol, p.982
Indenolol, p.913	

Calcium-channel blockers

The main use of calcium-channel blockers is in the management of angina pectoris and hypertension; some are also employed in cardiac arrhythmias.

Calcium-channel blockers, also known as calcium antagonists, calcium-entry blockers, and slow-channel blockers, inhibit the cellular influx of calcium which is responsible for maintenance of the plateau phase of the action potential. Thus calcium-channel blockers primarily affect tissues in which depolarisation is dependent upon calcium rather than sodium influx, and these include vascular smooth muscle, myocardial cells, and cells within the sino-atrial (SA) and atrioventricular (AV) nodes. The main actions of the calcium-channel blockers include dilatation of coronary and peripheral arteries and arterioles with little or no effect on venous tone, a negative inotropic action, reduction of heart rate, and slowing of AV conduction. However, the effects of individual drugs, and therefore their uses, are modified by their selectivity of action at different tissue sites and by baroreceptor reflexes.

Calcium-channel blockers may be classified according to their chemical structure. There are three major groups that are highly specific blockers of calcium channels.

Dihydropyridine calcium-channel blockers (such as nifedipine) have a greater selectivity for vascular smooth muscle than for myocardium and therefore their main effect is vasodilatation. They have little or no action at the SA or AV nodes and negative inotropic activity is rarely seen at therapeutic doses. They are used for their antihypertensive and anti-anginal properties. Some dihydropyridine derivatives, for example nimodipine, cross the blood-brain barrier and are used in cerebral ischaemia.

Benzothiazepine calcium-channel blockers (such as diltiazem) and **phenylalkylamine** calcium-channel blockers (such as verapamil) have less selective vasodilator activity than dihydropyridine derivatives; they have a direct effect on myocardium causing depression of SA and AV nodal conduction. They are used for their antiarrhythmic, anti-anginal, and antihypertensive properties.

Recently, a new class of calcium-channel blockers has come under investigation. These drugs act principally on fast T-type calcium channels unlike conventional calcium-channel blockers that act on slow L-type channels. Mibefradil is an example of a T-type calcium-channel blocker but it is no longer used clinically due to serious interactions with a wide range of drugs.

For further discussion of the actions and uses of the three main groups of calcium-channel blockers, see Nifedipine, p.940, Diltiazem, p.874, and Verapamil, p.989, respectively.

Described in this chapter are

Amlodipine, p.838	Lacidipine, p.919
Anipamil, p.840	Lercanidipine, p.920
Aranidipine, p.841	Lidoflazine, p.921
Barnidipine, p.843	Manidipine, p.924
Benidipine, p.844	Mibefradil, p.933
Bepridil, p.844	Nicardipine, p.938
Cilnidipine, p.858	Nifedipine, p.940
Diltiazem, p.874	Nilvadipine, p.946
Efonidipine, p.883	Nimodipine, p.946
Felodipine, p.888	Nisoldipine, p.946
Gallopamil, p.896	Nitrendipine, p.947
Isradipine, p.916	Verapamil, p.989

References.
1. Abernethy DR, Schwartz JB. Calcium-antagonist drugs. *N Engl J Med* 1999; **341:** 1447–57.

Cardiac inotropes

Positive cardiac inotropes increase the force of contraction of the myocardium and are therefore used in the management of acute and chronic heart failure. Some inotropes also increase or decrease the heart rate (positive or negative chronotropes), provide vasodilatation (inodilators), or improve myocardial relaxation (positive lusitropes), and these additional properties influence the choice of drug in specific situations. Drugs that are used predominantly for their inotropic effects include the cardiac glycosides and phosphodiesterase inhibitors; sympathomimetics are employed as inotropes but also have other important uses.

References.
1. Feldman AM. Classification of positive inotropic agents. *J Am Coll Cardiol* 1993; **22:** 1223–7.
2. Cuthbertson BH, *et al.* Inotropic agents in the critically ill. *Br J Hosp Med* 1996; **56:** 386–91.

Cardiac glycosides, such as digoxin, possess positive inotropic activity which is mediated by inhibition of sodium-potassium adenosine triphosphatase (Na/K-ATPase). They also reduce conductivity in the heart, particularly through the atrioventricular node, and therefore have a negative chronotropic effect. The cardiac glycosides have very similar pharmacological effects but differ considerably in their speed of onset and duration of action. They are used to slow the heart rate in supraventricular arrhythmias, especially atrial fibrillation, and are also given in chronic heart failure.

Described in this chapter are

Acetyldigoxin, p.827	Digoxin, p.870
Deslanoside, p.867	Lanatoside C, p.919
Digitalis Lanata Leaf, p.869	Metildigoxin, p.930
Digitalis Leaf, p.869	Ouabain, p.950
Digitoxin, p.869	Proscillaridin, p.963
	Strophanthin-K, p.978

Phosphodiesterase inhibitors are potent inotropes; they also have vasodilator effects. They are used in the short-

term treatment of severe heart failure; long-term oral therapy with some phosphodiesterase inhibitors has been associated with increased mortality.

Described in this chapter are

Amrinone, p.839	Olprinone, p.949
Enoximone, p.885	Pimobendan, p.955
Milrinone, p.934	Vesnarinone, p.992

Centrally acting antihypertensives

Centrally acting antihypertensives include alpha$_2$-adrenoceptor agonists such as clonidine and methyldopa. Stimulation of alpha$_2$ adrenoceptors in the CNS results in a reduction in sympathetic tone and a fall in blood pressure. Heart rate is also reduced. They are used in the management of hypertension, although other drugs with fewer adverse effects are generally preferred. Some have a role in the management of glaucoma. Clonidine is also used in migraine prophylaxis and menopausal flushing, and may form part of the treatment of opioid withdrawal.

Described in this chapter are

Apraclonidine, p.840	Methyldopa, p.927
Brimonidine, p.851	Moxonidine, p.936
Clonidine, p.860	Rilmenidine, p.968
Guanabenz, p.900	Tiamenidine, p.981
Guanfacine, p.901	

Diuretics

Diuretics promote the excretion of water and electrolytes by the kidneys. They are used in the treatment of heart failure or in hepatic, renal, or pulmonary disease when salt and water retention has resulted in oedema or ascites. Diuretics are also used, either alone, or in association with other drugs, in the treatment of hypertension.

The principal groups of diuretics are as follows.

Carbonic anhydrase inhibitors are weak diuretics and are used mainly to reduce raised intra-ocular pressure.

Described in this chapter are

Acetazolamide, p.826	Dorzolamide, p.883
Brinzolamide, p.851	Methazolamide, p.927
Diclofenamide, p.869	

'Loop' or **'high-ceiling' diuretics** produce an intense, dose-dependent diuresis of relatively short duration.

Described in this chapter are

Azosemide, p.843	Frusemide [Furosemide], p.893
Bumetanide, p.852	
Etacrynic Acid, p.887	Piretanide, p.956
Etozolin, p.888	Torasemide, p.985

Osmotic diuretics raise the osmolality of plasma and renal tubular fluid. They are used to reduce or prevent cerebral oedema, to reduce raised intra-ocular pressure, and in acute renal failure.

Described in this chapter are

Isosorbide, p.915	Mannitol, p.924

Potassium-sparing diuretics have a relatively weak diuretic effect and are normally used in conjunction with thiazide or loop diuretics.

Described in this chapter are

Amiloride, p.835	Spironolactone, p.973
Canrenone, p.853	Triamterene, p.986
Potassium Canrenoate, p.957	

Thiazides (benzothiadiazines), such as bendrofluazide [bendroflumethiazide] and hydrochlorothiazide, and certain other compounds, such as metolazone, with structural similarities to the thiazides, inhibit sodium and chloride reabsorption in the kidney tubules and produce a corresponding increase in potassium excretion.

Described in this chapter are

Altizide, p.835	Hydroflumethiazide, p.911
Bemetizide, p.843	Indapamide, p.913
Bendrofluazide [Bendroflumethiazide], p.844	Mebutizide, p.925
	Mefruside, p.926
Benzthiazide, p.844	Methyclothiazide, p.927
Butizide, p.853	Meticrane, p.929
Chlorothiazide, p.856	Metolazone, p.930
Chlortalidone, p.857	Polythiazide, p.957
Clopamide, p.863	Quinethazone, p.964
Cyclopenthiazide, p.865	Teclothiazide, p.979
Cyclothiazide, p.865	Trichlormethiazide, p.987
Epitizide, p.886	Tripamide, p.987
Hydrochlorothiazide, p.907	Xipamide, p.999

Ganglion blockers

Ganglion blockers are nicotinic antagonists that inhibit the transmission of nerve impulses in both sympathetic and parasympathetic ganglia. Their antihypertensive action is due to sympathetic blockade, which produces pe-

ripheral vasodilatation; there is also a direct vasodilator effect on peripheral blood vessels.

Described in this chapter are

Mecamylamine, p.925	Trimetaphan, p.987

Lipid regulating drugs

Lipid regulating drugs are used to modify blood lipid concentrations in the management of hyperlipidaemias and for the reduction of cardiovascular risk. The principal groups of lipid regulating drugs are the statins, fibrates, bile-acid binding resins, nicotinates, and omega-3 triglycerides.

The **statins** are inhibitors of 3-hydroxy-3-methylglutaryl-coenzyme A (HMG-CoA) reductase, the rate-determining enzyme for cholesterol synthesis. They reduce cholesterol by stimulating an increase in low-density-lipoprotein (LDL)-receptors on hepatocyte membranes, thereby increasing the clearance of LDL from the circulation. Their main effect is to reduce LDL-cholesterol, but they may also reduce triglycerides to a modest extent and increase high-density-lipoprotein (HDL)-cholesterol. They are generally considered to be the most effective lipid-lowering drugs.

Described in this chapter are

Atorvastatin, p.842	Mevastatin, p.932
Cerivastatin, p.856	Pravastatin, p.957
Fluvastatin, p.892	Rosuvastatin, p.969
Lovastatin, p.922	Simvastatin, p.969

The **fibrates** include derivatives of fibric acid and related compounds. They inhibit the synthesis of cholesterol and bile acids, and enhance the secretion of cholesterol in bile. Their main effect is to reduce triglycerides by reducing the concentration of very-low-density lipoproteins (VLDL); they also increase HDL-cholesterol and have variable effects on LDL-cholesterol. They are used mainly in patients with hypertriglyceridaemia.

Described in this chapter are

Beclobrate, p.843	Fenofibrate, p.889
Bezafibrate, p.849	Gemfibrozil, p.896
Ciprofibrate, p.858	Pirifibrate, p.956
Clinofibrate, p.859	Plafibride, p.956
Clofibrate, p.859	Simfibrate, p.969
Clofibride, p.859	Tocofibrate, p.984
Etofylline Clofibrate, p.888	

Bile-acid binding resins lower cholesterol by combining with bile acids in the gastrointestinal tract and preventing their reabsorption. This leads to an increased oxidation of cholesterol to replace the lost bile acids, and an increase in LDL-receptor synthesis on hepatocytes, resulting primarily in a reduction of LDL-cholesterol.

Described in this chapter are

Colesevelam, p.863	Colestyramine, p.864
Colestipol, p.863	Divistyramine, p.880

Nicotinates include nicotinic acid (p.1372) and its derivatives. Nicotinic acid is a member of the vitamin B group and, in high doses, has beneficial effects on blood lipids; it reduces triglycerides and increases HDL-cholesterol, and may also modestly reduce LDL-cholesterol. Nicotinates are mainly used in hypertriglyceridaemia. Compounds derived from both nicotinic acid and clofibrate (nicotinate-fibrate derivatives) are also used.

Described in this chapter are

Acipimox, p.827	Pirozadil, p.956
Binifibrate, p.850	Ronifibrate, p.969
Etofibrate, p.888	Sorbinicate, p.972
Niceritrol, p.939	Tocoferil Nicotinate, p.984
Nicofibrate, p.939	

Omega-3 triglycerides are long-chain polyunsaturated fatty acids that primarily reduce triglycerides.

Described in this chapter are

Omega-3 Triglycerides, p.949	

Nitrates

Nitrates are peripheral and coronary vasodilators used in the management of angina pectoris, heart failure, and myocardial infarction. Some of them may also be used to control blood pressure during surgery. Nitrates are believed to exert their vasodilator effect through nitric oxide (p.947) stimulating guanylate cyclase in the vascular smooth muscle cells; this results in an increase in cyclic guanosine monophosphate. This nucleotide induces relaxation probably by lowering the free calcium concentration in the cytosol. Nitrates are thus termed nitrovasodilators. In their action on vascular muscle venous dilatation predominates over dilatation of the arterioles. Venous dilatation decreases venous return as a result of venous pooling and lowers left ventricular diastolic volume and pressure (termed a reduction in preload). The smaller or less important dilatation of arterioles reduces both peripheral vascular resistance and left ventricular pressure at systole (termed a reduction in afterload). The consequent effect is a reduction in the primary determinants of myocardial oxygen demand. The effect on preload is not shared by beta blockers or calcium-channel blockers. Nitrates also have a coronary vasodilator effect which improves regional coronary blood flow to ischaemic areas resulting in improved oxygen supply to the myocardium.

Described in this chapter are

Potassium-channel openers

Potassium-channel openers (potassium-channel activators) are used in the management of angina pectoris and hypertension. They have a direct relaxant effect on smooth muscle. They act at potassium channels to allow cellular efflux of potassium which hyperpolarises the cell membrane and leads to a reduction in intracellular calcium. The reduction in intracellular calcium produces relaxation of smooth muscle. Activation of potassium channels in blood vessels produces vasodilatation. Potassium-channel openers may also have potential use in other conditions caused by smooth muscle contraction, for example asthma and urinary incontinence.

Described in this chapter are

Sympathomimetics

Sympathomimetics produce either direct or indirect stimulation of adrenergic receptors and have various actions depending on the specific receptors involved. Stimulation of alpha$_1$ receptors produces smooth muscle contraction. In the cardiovascular system this leads to vasoconstriction and increased blood pressure and in the eye to mydriasis. Other affected organs include the urinary sphincter and uterus. Stimulation of beta$_1$ receptors has an inotropic effect and also increases heart rate. Stimulation of beta$_2$ receptors leads to smooth muscle relaxation and produces vasodilatation.

Sympathomimetics have a wide range of uses. In cardiovascular disorders, they are mainly used for their alpha$_1$ and beta$_1$ properties to provide haemodynamic support in the management of acute heart failure and shock. Some sympathomimetics with alpha-agonist activity, such as phenylephrine (p.1097), pseudoephedrine (p.1099), and naphazoline (p.1095), are used to produce vasoconstriction of the nasal mucosa, for the symptomatic relief of nasal congestion. Apraclonidine (p.840) and brimonidine (p.851) are examples of drugs with alpha$_2$ agonist-properties that are used to lower intra-ocular pressure and treat glaucoma.

For further discussion of the actions of sympathomimetics in general, see under Adrenaline, p.829.

Described in this chapter are

Thrombolytics

Thrombolytics are used in the treatment of thromboembolic disorders such as myocardial infarction, peripheral arterial thromboembolism, and venous thromboembolism (deep-vein thrombosis and pulmonary embolism). They are also used to clear blocked cannulas and shunts.

Thrombolytics activate plasminogen to form fibrinolysin, a proteolytic enzyme that degrades fibrin and thus produces dissolution of clots. Some thrombolytics, such as alteplase, act only on fibrin-bound plasminogen and have little effect on circulating, unbound plasminogen; these thrombolytics are termed fibrin-specific agents. Thrombolytics, such as streptokinase, that affect circulating, unbound as well as fibrin-bound plasminogen are termed fibrin-nonspecific agents.

Described in this chapter are

References.

1. Ross AM. New plasminogen activators: a clinical review. *Clin Cardiol* 1999; **22:** 165–71.
2. Verstraete M. Third-generation thrombolytic drugs. *Am J Med* 2000; **109:** 52–8.

Vasodilators

Vasodilator is a broad term applied to a wide range of drugs that produce dilatation of blood vessels. The main groups of drugs producing vasodilatation are ACE inhibitors (p.820), nitrates (above), and direct-acting vasodilators.

Direct-acting vasodilators act predominantly on the arterioles reducing peripheral resistance and producing a fall in blood pressure. Their main use is in hypertension, although other drugs are generally preferred. Some of them are used in hypertensive crises.

Described in this chapter are

Other vasodilators may be divided into those used for ischaemic heart disease and those used mainly for cerebral and peripheral vascular disorders. Some drugs originally regarded as vasodilators and used for cerebral and peripheral vascular disorders are now thought to improve microcirculatory flow disturbances by altering the rheological properties of blood or tissue metabolism.

Vasodilators used in Ischaemic Heart Disease

Described in this chapter are

Vasodilators used in Cerebral and Peripheral Vascular Disorders

Described in this chapter are

Management of Cardiovascular Disorders

Management of the main cardiovascular disorders is discussed below. These overviews focus on pharmacological therapy, but other options are also mentioned where they form an important part of treatment.

Advanced cardiac life support

Cardiac arrest is the cessation of effective cardiac mechanical activity and is usually a result of ischaemic heart disease in adults and respiratory or circulatory failure in children. It may be associated with four arrhythmias, namely **ventricular fibrillation, pulseless ventricular tachycardia, asystole,** and **electromechanical dissociation (pulseless electrical activity).** Ventricular fibrillation is the commonest in adults and asystole in children. In ventricular fibrillation and pulseless ventricular tachycardia there is chaotic electrical and mechanical activity; in asystole a total absence of both activities; and in electromechanical dissociation an absence of mechanical activity, or undetectable activity, in the presence of some electrical activity.

Cardiac arrest is an emergency situation and should be treated by the institution of full life support measures.

International guidelines[1] for advanced life support and the immediate period of cardiac arrest have been published, developed by the American Heart Association in collaboration with various resuscitation councils, including the International Liaison Committee on Resuscitation. European[2] and UK[3] guidelines have also been published; these are based on the international guidelines and, apart from some differences in detail, are broadly similar. In order to maintain cardiorespiratory function, basic life support (cardiopulmonary resuscitation) consisting of chest compression and ventilation (mouth-to-mouth/mask) should be instituted immediately and continued during the resuscitation attempt. Subsequent procedures will depend to some extent on the type of arrhythmia present. For the commonest, ventricular fibrillation, rapid defibrillation is of paramount importance and should not be delayed by other necessary measures such as the administration of oxygen, intubation, and the provision of intravenous access. Defibrillation is intended to produce momentary asystole and allow the natural pacemakers to resume normal activity. Adrenaline [epinephrine] is given principally to increase the efficacy of basic life support rather than as an adjunct to defibrillation although evidence that it improves survival is limited; through its alpha agonist effects it increases myocardial and cerebral blood flow. A dose of 1 mg of adrenaline [epinephrine] is regarded as the 'standard' dose. A higher dose of 5 mg has been used in some clinical trials, but there is no evidence that this dose is associated with an improvement in overall survival rate and it is not generally recommended. Vasopressin has been tried as an alternative although it has not been shown to be superior to adrenaline [epinephrine].[4] In the case of asystole, atropine may be given to block excess vagal tone. Amiodarone may be considered for ventricular tachycardia or fibrillation; lignocaine [lidocaine] and procainamide are alternatives. Other drugs that may be given during resuscitation attempts include buffering agents such as intravenous sodium bicarbonate for acidosis, and calcium, magnesium, or potassium salts for known deficiencies. Specific guidelines for the different types of arrhythmia are as follows.

Ventricular fibrillation and **pulseless ventricular tachycardia** are treated in the same way. The guidelines for adults emphasise that the first defibrillating shock must be administered as quickly as possible. In cases of witnessed cardiac arrest a precordial thump, which sometimes aborts the arrhythmia if given within 30 seconds of the loss of cardiac output, may be given before attaching the monitor/defibrillator, but the attachment of the defibrillator must not be delayed. The initial monophasic direct current shock (200J) is followed as necessary by a second (200J) and a third (360J) shock if the preceding shock is not successful; lower energies may be used for biphasic shocks. If the initial group of three shocks is unsuccessful, chest compression and ventilation should be continued and further shocks given. Adrenaline [epinephrine] 1 mg intravenously should be administered before the next set of three shocks (each of 360J) but should not delay further defibrillation. Endotracheal administration of adrenaline [epinephrine] may be employed if intravenous access cannot be obtained. Doses 2 to 3 times greater than those given intravenously are suggested, although studies investigating this route have had mixed results.[5,6] A single dose of vasopressin (as argipressin) 40 units intravenously has been suggested[1] as an alternative to adrenaline [epinephrine], followed by further doses of adrenaline [epinephrine] if required, but this is not universally recommended.[2,3] The loop of adrenaline [epinephrine] and up to three shocks (360J or equivalent) should be repeated as necessary. Amiodarone or other antiarrhythmics may be considered after the first loop, provided that administration does not delay further shocks. Other drugs (such as those described above) may be employed as appropriate. Meanwhile, the adrenaline [epinephrine] and 3-shock loops continue for as long as defibrillation is indicated. The total number of loops is a matter of judgement but a resuscitation attempt may reasonably last for anything from 10 minutes to 1 hour.

The basic management of **ventricular fibrillation in children** is the same as in adults, but the energies used for defibrillation and the doses of drugs used are different and a precordial thump is not generally given. The initial dose of adrenaline [epinephrine] is 10 µg per kg bodyweight by intravenous or intraosseous injection; a higher dose of 100 µg per kg may be considered for the second and subsequent doses, although there is no evidence that this improves outcome. Endotracheal administration is an alternative route if an intravenous or intraosseous access cannot be obtained; the suggested endotracheal dose is 100 µg per kg for both initial and subsequent doses.

In survivors of ventricular fibrillation and pulseless ventricular tachycardia in whom it is considered there is a high risk of **recurrence**, implantable cardioverter defibrillators may be employed. Drug therapy may also be used prophylactically as outlined under Ventricular Tachycardia in Cardiac Arrhythmias, below.

Asystole and **electromechanical dissociation** have a much less favourable prognosis than ventricular fibrillation or pulseless ventricular tachycardia, although there are certain causes such as hypovolaemia, hypoxia, pneumothorax, pulmonary embolism, drug overdose, hypothermia, and electrolyte imbalances that may respond to treatment and these should be considered and the appropriate therapy given promptly once resuscitation has been instituted. As described above, a precordial thump may be appropriate if the cardiac arrest is witnessed. Once ventricular fibrillation or tachycardia is positively excluded, cardiopulmonary resuscitation should be instituted immediately and adrenaline [epinephrine] 1 mg should be given intravenously every 3 to 5 minutes. In asystole a single dose of atropine 3 mg intravenously is also administered to block vagal activity.[2,3] In the international guidelines[1] atropine is recommended in repeated doses of 1 mg to a total of 0.04 mg per kg body-weight rather than as a single dose of 3 mg. Other drugs (such as buffering agents) may be considered. Cardiac pacing may be instituted once there is evidence of electrical activity. Resuscitation should generally continue for at least 20 to 30 minutes from the time of collapse; prolonged resuscitation is not usually undertaken as recovery rarely occurs after 15 minutes of asystole if there has been no response.

As ventricular fibrillation is unusual in **children**, a precordial thump and defibrillation are not included as routine in the paediatric guidelines for asystole or electromechanical dissociation. The initial dose of adrenaline [epinephrine] recommended is 10 µg per kg body-weight given by intravenous or intraosseous injection; as for ventricular fibrillation, higher doses have been used subsequently but are not generally recommended. Adrenaline [epinephrine] may be given by the endotracheal route in doses of 100 µg per kg. Atropine is not generally used.

1. The American Heart Association in collaboration with the International Committee on Resuscitation (ILCOR). International guidelines 2000 for cardiopulmonary resuscitation and emergency cardiovascular care: a consensus on science. *Circulation* 2000; **102** (suppl I): I1–I384. [Also published in *Resuscitation* 2000; **46**: 3–447.]
2. European Resuscitation Council. European Resuscitation Council Guidelines 2000. *Resuscitation* 2001; **48**: 199–239.
3. Resuscitation Council (UK). Resuscitation Guidelines 2000. Available at: http://www.resus.org.uk/pages/guide.htm (accessed 15/08/01).
4. Stiell IG, *et al.* Vasopressin versus epinephrine for inhospital cardiac arrest: a randomised controlled trial. *Lancet* 2001; **358**: 105–9.
5. McCrirrick A, Monk CR. Comparison of i.v. and intra-tracheal administration of adrenaline. *Br J Anaesth* 1994; **72**: 529–32.
6. Raymondos K, *et al.* Absorption and hemodynamic effects of airway administration of adrenaline in patients with severe cardiac disease. *Ann Intern Med* 2000; **132**: 800–803.

Angina pectoris

Angina pectoris is a syndrome that arises from an inadequate myocardial oxygen supply (myocardial ischaemia). The prominent symptom is transient precordial discomfort ranging from a mild ache to severe pain. Some patients may also experience dyspnoea, nausea, sweating, and left arm discomfort. Myocardial oxygen supply depends upon coronary blood flow which normally increases to meet increased oxygen demands. Ischaemia occurs when blood flow cannot be increased or is reduced and may be due to a fixed obstruction in the coronary arteries, vasoconstriction, thrombus formation, or platelet aggregation.

Three main types of angina have been described: stable angina; unstable angina; and Prinzmetal's angina. Although these are discrete groups, stable angina may become unstable, and Prinzmetal's angina may co-exist with stable or unstable angina.

Stable angina (effort angina) is angina which is usually precipitated by exertion and relieved by rest. It is often called chronic stable angina and as the name implies the frequency, intensity, and duration of the attacks are stable. The predominant underlying disorder is coronary atherosclerosis causing a fixed obstruction in one or more

coronary arteries. While the restricted coronary blood flow is still adequate for oxygenation of the unstressed heart, it is not capable of being increased to meet the increase in myocardial oxygen demand that may occur during exercise, cold exposure, emotional stress, or after eating.

Unstable angina is an acute coronary syndrome representing symptom complexes intermediate between stable angina pectoris and myocardial infarction. Three subgroups are recognised: angina that presents from the beginning as severe and frequent attacks; an increase in the frequency, intensity, and/or duration of previously stable angina, often with diminishing responsiveness to sublingual nitrates (crescendo angina); and recurring or prolonged angina at rest. In unstable angina the decreased coronary artery blood flow is usually caused by disruption of an atherosclerotic plaque which leads to platelet adhesion and aggregation, thrombus formation, and vasoconstriction, thus resulting in partial occlusion of one or more coronary arteries. The coronary blood flow can be so restricted that it does not meet the oxygenation demands of the unstressed heart, but no myocardial damage results. Non-Q wave myocardial infarction is a closely related syndrome in which some myocardial injury occurs, but to a lesser extent than in acute myocardial infarction. Patients with the different acute coronary syndromes may present similarly and definitive diagnosis is only possible retrospectively once the results of cardiac enzyme measurements are available. However, patients without the characteristic ECG change of ST-segment elevation (non-ST elevation myocardial infarction) do not generally develop Q waves and management is as for unstable angina. Patients with unstable angina are at an increased risk of sudden death and myocardial infarction, and those with rest pain are at the greatest risk.

Prinzmetal's angina (variant angina) is a rare form of angina caused by coronary vasospasm and is often associated with atherosclerosis. It occurs spontaneously at rest and with greater frequency during the night or early hours of the morning. It is associated with ST-segment elevation and carries a risk of progression to myocardial infarction. Prolonged vasospasm may also lead to ventricular arrhythmias, heart block, or death.

In addition to the types of angina described above periods of **silent myocardial ischaemia** (asymptomatic transient myocardial ischaemia) in which there is no anginal pain have been identified during ECG monitoring. In some patients all such episodes are asymptomatic. However, asymptomatic ischaemic episodes also occur in patients with angina and seem to be more common than symptomatic episodes. It is not clear why some episodes of ischaemia are symptomatic while others are not.

Treatment depends on the type of angina and involves management of acute anginal pain and long-term management to prevent angina attacks. This treatment, which is described in more detail below, includes drug therapy (nitrates, beta blockers, and calcium-channel blockers), coronary artery bypass surgery, and percutaneous transluminal coronary angioplasty. While anti-anginal treatment can abolish or control attacks of angina, it does not treat the underlying cause of the ischaemia and patients should be assessed for risk factors for cardiovascular disease. Aspirin should be given unless contra-indicated, appropriate lifestyle changes should be made, and lipid-lowering therapy should also be considered (see Cardiovascular Risk Reduction, below).

Patients with ischaemic heart disease who undergo non-cardiac surgery are at risk of complications resulting from perioperative myocardial ischaemia.[1] Perioperative use of drugs such as beta blockers or mivazerol is under investigation.

Anti-anginal drugs act in a variety of ways. Glyceryl trinitrate and other organic *nitrates* have a vasodilator effect with venodilation predominating over dilatation of the arterioles. Dilatation of veins decreases venous return as a result of venous pooling and lowers left ventricular diastolic volume and pressure (together termed a reduction in preload). The smaller or less important dilatation of arterioles reduces both peripheral vascular resistance and left ventricular pressure at systole (termed a reduction in afterload). The consequence of these effects is a reduction in myocardial oxygen demand. Also the vasodilator effect improves regional coronary blood flow to ischaemic areas, and alleviates coronary spasm. *Beta blockers* cause a slowing of the heart rate and reduction in contractility and therefore reduce myocardial oxygen demand. *Calcium-channel blockers* reduce the work of the heart by dilating peripheral arteries, and diltiazem and vera-

pamil also slow the heart rate. Calcium-channel blockers also act on the coronary circulation preventing spasm.

Percutaneous transluminal coronary *angioplasty* is a means of mechanically dilating coronary arteries using a balloon that has been passed down a catheter and inflated at the appropriate sites and is often used in conjunction with stenting. Nitrates and calcium-channel blockers may be given to alleviate coronary spasm due to the procedure. Coronary artery *bypass surgery* abolishes or reduces episodes of angina in the majority of patients but if preventative measures are not successful angina reappears after several years. Restenosis and thromboembolic complications may follow angioplasty or bypass surgery and a wide variety of drugs have been investigated for prophylaxis (see Reperfusion and Revascularisation Procedures, below). Other interventions that have been tried in refractory angina include transmyocardial revascularisation and spinal cord stimulation.

Treatment of stable angina. Management of the patient with stable angina includes treatment of contributory conditions such as anaemia, control of risk factors for atherosclerosis including lipid-lowering therapy, antiplatelet therapy, and therapy to increase blood flow to the ischaemic myocardium as well as to reduce myocardial oxygen demand.[2-6]

Treatment of infrequent angina episodes (less than about 2 attacks per week) usually consists of glyceryl trinitrate given when required, generally sublingually; alternatively, a buccal tablet or spray formulation may be used. Isosorbide dinitrate, in the form of sublingual tablets or spray, may be used, although it has a slower onset of action than glyceryl trinitrate. Glyceryl trinitrate in sublingual or buccal forms may also be used by patients before an activity or circumstance that might precipitate an attack.

When episodes occur more frequently then sublingual glyceryl trinitrate, at least on its own, may no longer be appropriate, and regular symptomatic treatment has to be considered. Such treatment includes other nitrate therapy, beta blockers, or calcium-channel blockers, and these treatments may be used individually or in combination. Choice depends upon patient characteristics and any concurrent medical conditions.

Beta blockers are the mainstay of therapy and some suggest they should be used as first-line treatment if sublingual glyceryl trinitrate is not adequate.[4] The different beta blockers appear to be equally effective in stable angina, although some[7] prefer to avoid those with intrinsic sympathomimetic activity.

A calcium-channel blocker may be used as an alternative. There has been concern regarding the safety of short-acting nifedipine preparations in patients with angina (see under Adverse Effects of Nifedipine, p.940) but recent studies indicate similar outcomes in patients receiving either long-acting calcium-channel blockers or beta blockers.[8,9] Care is required in selecting an appropriate drug since the properties of dihydropyridine calcium-channel blockers and rate-limiting calcium-channel blockers (diltiazem and verapamil) are not the same. Rate-limiting calcium-channel blockers may be used in patients unable to tolerate beta blockers. Long-acting dihydropyridines may also be used, although it has been suggested that dihydropyridines should not be used without beta blockers since response is often variable and angina may even be provoked in some patients because of the effect of increasing heart rate.[2,10,11]

Nitrate therapy for these more frequent attacks includes modified-release forms of glyceryl trinitrate, for example transdermal patches, and the long-acting nitrates such as isosorbide dinitrate or isosorbide mononitrate, and is used in patients with left ventricular dysfunction. Diminished effectiveness or tolerance occurs, particularly with nitrate preparations that produce sustained plasma concentrations, and dosage regimens including a nitrate-free period are commonly used (see Nitrate Tolerance, p.898).

Alternative drugs that may be used as monotherapy in the management of stable angina include the potassium-channel openers such as nicorandil.

Where optimal therapy with a single drug fails to control symptoms, combination therapy may be used. There is additional benefit from concomitant nitrate and beta blocker therapy, since nitrates can moderate the excessive effects that beta blockers may have in increasing left ventricular diastolic volume and pressure and in inducing bradycardia. Calcium-channel blockers may also be used with nitrates; the combination of verapamil or diltiazem with a nitrate may be preferable to a combination of nifedipine (or other dihydropyridine derivative) with nitrates as both nifedipine and nitrates cause reflex tachycardia, hypotension, and headaches.

Combination therapy with beta blockers and dihydropyridine calcium-channel blockers or diltiazem improves exercise tolerance[4] but adverse effects may be a problem. Verapamil should be avoided in such combinations as its use with a beta blocker increases the risk of impaired cardiac conduction (see Verapamil, p.990). Caution with any combination of a calcium-channel blocker with a beta blocker is particularly necessary in patients with pre-existing conduction disorders or moderate to severe left ventricular dysfunction as the use of calcium-channel blockers may actually increase mortality.[12]

Triple therapy using a nitrate, a beta blocker, and a calcium-channel blocker may sometimes be used although it is likely to be associated with more adverse effects.

If medical treatment does not control the angina the patient should be investigated to determine suitability for coronary angioplasty or coronary artery bypass surgery.[13] Angioplasty is ideally suited to patients with single-vessel disease, good left ventricular function, and stable angina, although the technique is also used in patients with more complex disease, impaired left ventricular function, and unstable angina.[14] Coronary artery bypass surgery is generally the preferred technique in patients with disease of the left main coronary artery, three-vessel disease, or impaired left ventricular function.[15] Age and other clinical factors also influence the choice of technique; angioplasty may be favoured in the elderly and others with high operative risks.[14] The role of angioplasty in patients whose symptoms are controlled with medical treatment is less clear. A comparison of angioplasty and medical treatment in patients considered suitable for either strategy suggested that greater symptomatic improvement following angioplasty may not be maintained, and that the risk of death or non-fatal infarction may be greater than for patients receiving medical treatment alone.[16]

Treatment of unstable angina. Unstable angina and non-ST segment elevation myocardial infarction are managed similarly. Unstable angina and non-ST segment elevation myocardial infarction are managed similarly. Unstable angina is generally regarded as an emergency and those patients with a change in the pattern of previously stable angina or with recurring or prolonged angina at rest should be hospitalised. The aim of treatment is to control the attacks and prevent the condition progressing to myocardial infarction and death. Once the patient has been stabilised the underlying factors can be treated or controlled and long-term prophylaxis set up to guard against any further ischaemic attacks.

Initial treatment[17-24] depends on the severity of the ischaemia. All patients with unstable angina should receive aspirin, and heparin should also be considered. Nitrates and beta blockers are given to control symptoms and to relieve ischaemia. Calcium-channel blockers may also be used if there is vasospasm or if the patient fails to respond to the other drugs.

Aspirin is routinely included in the initial treatment. It inhibits platelet aggregation and substantially reduces the incidence of myocardial infarction and death, although it has not been shown to reduce the number of ischaemic episodes or to relieve pain during the acute phase. Ticlopidine or clopidogrel may be alternatives if aspirin is not tolerated. Glycoprotein IIb/IIIa inhibitors such as abciximab, eptifibatide, and tirofiban are more potent inhibitors of platelet aggregation and may have a role in addition to aspirin. The benefit of glycoprotein IIb/IIIa inhibitors is well established in patients undergoing percutaneous coronary angioplasty (see Reperfusion and Revascularisation Procedures, p.812), but results in patients treated medically have been less consistent. Beneficial results have been reported in patients receiving tirofiban and aspirin alone[25] or in combination with heparin therapy,[26] and with eptifibatide[27] in addition to standard therapy. However, a study with abciximab[28] in addition to aspirin and heparin failed to show any additional benefit.

Heparin is given by continuous intravenous infusion to reduce thrombin generation and fibrin formation, and is generally continued for at least 48 hours.[17,20,24] It reduces the number of ischaemic episodes and major cardiovascular events during the acute phase, although it has been suggested that heparin must be started early to be effective.[18] Although some reserve heparin for high risk patients a meta-analysis[29] suggests that a combination of aspirin and heparin should be used in most patients. Re-

activation of unstable angina has been reported in patients discontinuing intravenous heparin;[30] combination with aspirin or gradual discontinuation may prevent this effect.[20] Subcutaneous heparin may be an alternative.[31] Low-molecular-weight heparins in combination with aspirin also appear to be effective[32-35] and may be given for longer periods than standard heparin. Lepirudin, a direct thrombin inhibitor, has been compared with heparin in patients with unstable angina.[36,37] Following 72 hours treatment, fewer cases of cardiovascular death, new myocardial infarction, or refractory angina were reported for lepirudin at 7 days. Bleeding episodes were more common in the lepirudin group.

The initial nitrate treatment may be given intravenously to produce a fast response and to provide better dose control than can be achieved with other routes. Glyceryl trinitrate or isosorbide dinitrate are used. Generally, the intravenous nitrate is only given during the acute phase, and once the patient is stabilised the infusion is withdrawn, usually within about 48 hours. Sublingual glyceryl trinitrate may be tried initially in patients with less severe symptoms.

Treatment with a beta blocker is started during the acute phase to reduce myocardial oxygen demand. Initially, the intravenous route may be employed and then followed by oral administration. Beta blockers with intrinsic sympathomimetic activity do not reduce resting heart rate and are not recommended.[7,24]

Calcium-channel blockers may be added to therapy although they are generally reserved for patients with angina refractory to treatment with the above drugs. However, calcium-channel blockers are the drugs of choice if the angina has a vasospastic aetiology, for example in Prinzmetal's angina. The choice of calcium-channel blocker is described under the treatment of stable angina above.

Thrombolytics such as alteplase, streptokinase, and urokinase have been given intravenously in unstable angina. Although small-scale studies reported some benefit the results were variable. Two studies have investigated alteplase (the TIMI-IIIB study[38] with 1473 patients) and anistreplase (the UNASEM study[39] involving 159 patients). Thrombolysis failed to improve outcome and was associated with an excess of bleeding complications; thrombolytic therapy is therefore not recommended for routine treatment of unstable angina.[23,24]

Drug treatment is successful in stabilising angina in about 80% of patients and these patients should continue to take aspirin and a beta blocker. Some patients are given a long-acting nitrate for long-term prophylaxis, although nitrates have not been shown to protect against subsequent cardiovascular events. Long-term oral anticoagulation has been used but is not routine therapy. A combination of warfarin with aspirin has also been tried.[40,41]

Having controlled the acute phase the patient should be assessed to see if angioplasty or coronary artery bypass surgery would be helpful. Measures should also be adopted to control recognised risk factors.

Patients with unstable angina who do not respond to full medical treatment, as above, within 48 hours should undergo emergency angiography in preparation for angioplasty or coronary artery bypass surgery.

Treatment of Prinzmetal's angina. This should be treated like unstable angina with the addition of a calcium-channel blocker; the selection of an appropriate calcium-channel blocker is described above under the treatment of stable angina. Once stabilised, maintenance should include a nitrate, or calcium-channel blocker, or both to protect against further spasm. Surgery may be considered in some patients.

Treatment of silent myocardial ischaemia. Silent myocardial ischaemia has been recognised as a potential risk factor for future cardiovascular morbidity and mortality and research has been undertaken to assess whether suppressing such episodes can improve long-term outcome. Although many of the therapies used in angina reduce the incidence of silent ischaemia it is not yet clear whether complete suppression of ischaemia affects prognosis.[9,42-44] Other studies have suggested that periods of ischaemia may protect the heart during subsequent myocardial infarction[45] and further work is needed to reconcile these findings.

1. ACC/AHA Task Force on Practice Guidelines. ACC/AHA guidelines for perioperative cardiovascular evaluation for noncardiac surgery. *Circulation* 1996; **93:** 1280–1317.
2. Shub C. Stable angina pectoris 3: medical treatment. *Mayo Clin Proc* 1990; **65:** 256–73.
3. Chan P, *et al.* The role of nitrates, beta blockers, and calcium antagonists in stable angina pectoris. *Am Heart J* 1988; **116:** 838–48.
4. North of England Stable Angina Guideline Development Group. North of England evidence based guidelines development project: summary version of evidence based guideline for the primary care management of stable angina. *BMJ* 1996; **312:** 827–32. Update available at: http://www.ncl.ac.uk/chsr/publicn/guide/angina.pdf (accessed 27/11/01).
5. de Bono D. Investigation and management of stable angina: revised guidelines 1998. *Heart* 1999; **81:** 546–55.
6. Gibbons RJ, *et al.* ACC/AHA/ACP–ASIM guidelines for the management of patients with chronic stable angina: executive summary and recommendations: a report of the American College of Cardiology/American Heart Association Task Force on Practice Guidelines (Committee on Management of Patients With Chronic Stable Angina). *Circulation* 1999; **99:** 2829–48.
7. Anonymous. Which beta-blocker? *Med Lett Drugs Ther* 2001; **43:** 9–11.
8. Rehnqvist N, *et al.* Effects of metoprolol vs verapamil in patients with stable angina pectoris: the Angina Prognosis Study in Stockholm (APSIS). *Eur Heart J* 1996; **17:** 76–81.
9. Dargie HJ, *et al.* Total Ischaemic Burden European Trial (TIBET): effects of ischaemia and treatment with atenolol, nifedipine SR and their combination on outcome in patients with chronic stable angina. *Eur Heart J* 1996; **17:** 104–12.
10. Kenny J. Calcium channel blocking agents and the heart. *BMJ* 1985; **291:** 1150–2.
11. Horowitz JD, Powell AC. Calcium antagonist drugs in the management of cardiovascular disease: current status. *Med J Aust* 1989; **150:** 591–5.
12. Packer M. Combined beta-adrenergic and calcium-entry blockade in angina pectoris. *N Engl J Med* 1989; **320:** 709–18.
13. Solomon AJ, Gersh BJ. Management of chronic stable angina: medical therapy, percutaneous transluminal coronary angioplasty, and coronary artery bypass graft surgery. *Ann Intern Med* 1998; **128:** 216–23.
14. Smith SC, *et al.* ACC/AHA guidelines for percutaneous coronary intervention: executive summary and recommendations: a report of the American College of Cardiology/American Heart Association Task Force on Practice Guidelines (Committee to Revise the 1993 Guidelines for Percutaneous Transluminal Coronary Angioplasty). *Circulation* 2001; **103:** 3019–41.
15. Eagle KA, *et al.* ACC/AHA guidelines for coronary artery bypass graft surgery: executive summary and recommendations: a report of the American College of Cardiology/American Heart Association Task Force on Practice Guidelines (Committee to Revise the 1991 Guidelines for Coronary Artery Bypass Graft Surgery). *Circulation* 1999; **100:** 1464–80.
16. RITA-2 trial participants. Coronary angioplasty versus medical therapy for angina: the second Randomised Intervention Treatment of Angina (RITA-2) trial. *Lancet* 1997; **350:** 461–8.
17. Waller D. Unstable angina and non-Q-wave myocardial infarction. *Prescribers' J* 1999; **39:** 193–201.
18. Yeghiazarians Y, *et al.* Unstable angina pectoris. *N Engl J Med* 2000; **342:** 101–14.
19. Fox KAA. Acute coronary syndromes: presentation—clinical spectrum and management. *Heart* 2000; **84:** 93–100.
20. Grubb NR, Fox KAA. Management of unstable angina. *Hosp Med* 2000; **61:** 489–94.
21. Ambrose JA, Dangas G. Unstable angina: current concepts of pathogenesis and treatment. *Arch Intern Med* 2000; **160:** 25–37.
22. Manhapra A, Borzak S. Treatment possibilities for unstable angina. *BMJ* 2000; **321:** 1269–75.
23. Braunwald E, *et al.* ACC/AHA guidelines for the management of patients with unstable angina and non-ST-segment elevation myocardial infarction: executive summary and recommendations: a report of the American College of Cardiology/American Heart Association Task Force on Practice Guidelines (Committee on Management of Patients With Unstable Angina). *Circulation* 2000; **102:** 1193–1209.
24. British Cardiac Society Guidelines and Medical Practice Committee, and Royal College of Physicians Clinical Effectiveness and Evaluation Unit. Guideline for the management of patients with acute coronary syndromes without persistent ECG ST segment elevation. *Heart* 2001; **85:** 133–42.
25. The Platelet Receptor Inhibition in Ischemic Syndrome Management (PRISM) study Investigators. A comparison of aspirin plus tirofiban with aspirin plus heparin for unstable angina. *N Engl J Med* 1998; **338:** 1498–1505.
26. The Platelet Receptor Inhibition in Ischemic Syndrome Management in Patients Limited by Unstable Signs and Symptoms (PRISM-PLUS) Study Investigators. Inhibition of the platelet glycoprotein IIb/IIIa receptor with tirofiban in unstable angina and non-Q-wave myocardial infarction. *N Engl J Med* 1998; **338:** 1488–97.
27. The PURSUIT Trial Investigators. Inhibition of platelet glycoprotein IIb/IIIa with eptifibatide in patients with acute coronary syndromes. *N Engl J Med* 1998; **339:** 436–43.
28. The GUSTO IV-ACS Investigators. Effect of glycoprotein IIb/IIIa receptor blocker abciximab on outcome in patients with acute coronary syndromes without early coronary revascularisation: the GUSTO IV-ACS randomised trial. *Lancet* 2001; **357:** 1915–24.
29. Oler A, *et al.* Adding heparin to aspirin reduces the incidence of myocardial infarction and death in patients with unstable angina: a meta-analysis. *JAMA* 1996; **276:** 811–15.
30. Théroux P, *et al.* Reactivation of unstable angina after the discontinuation of heparin. *N Engl J Med* 1992; **327:** 141–5.
31. Serneri GGN, *et al.* Randomised comparison of subcutaneous heparin, intravenous heparin, and aspirin in unstable angina. *Lancet* 1995; **345:** 1201–4. Correction. *ibid.*; **346:** 130.
32. Fragmin During Instability in Coronary Artery Disease (FRISC) Study Group. Low-molecular-weight heparin during instability in coronary artery disease. *Lancet* 1996; **347:** 561–8.
33. Gurfinkel EP, *et al.* Low molecular weight heparin versus regular heparin or aspirin in the treatment of unstable angina and silent ischaemia. *J Am Coll Cardiol* 1995; **26:** 313–18.
34. Cohen M, *et al.* A comparison of low-molecular-weight heparin with unfractionated heparin for unstable coronary artery disease. *N Engl J Med* 1997; **337:** 447–52.
35. Eikelboom JW, *et al.* Unfractionated heparin and low-molecular-weight heparin in acute coronary syndrome without ST elevation: a meta-analysis. *Lancet* 2000; **355:** 1936–42.
36. Organization to Assess Strategies for Ischemic Syndromes (OASIS) Investigators. Comparison of the effects of two doses of recombinant hirudin compared with heparin in patients with acute myocardial ischemia without ST elevation: a pilot study. *Circulation* 1997; **96:** 769–77.

37. Organisation to Assess Strategies for Ischemic Syndromes (OA-SIS-2) Investigators. Effects of recombinant hirudin (lepirudin) compared with heparin on death, myocardial infarction, refractory angina, and revascularisation procedures in patients with acute myocardial ischaemia without ST elevation: a randomised trial. *Lancet* 1999; **353:** 429–38.
38. The TIMI IIIB Investigators. Effects of tissue plasminogen activator and a comparison of early invasive and conservative strategies in unstable angina and non-Q-wave myocardial infarction: results of the TIMI IIIB trial. *Circulation* 1994; **89:** 1545–56.
39. Bär FW, *et al.* Thrombolysis in patients with unstable angina improves the angiographic but not the clinical outcome: results of UNASEM, a multicenter, randomized, placebo-controlled, clinical trial with anistreplase. *Circulation* 1992; **86:** 131–7.
40. Anand SS, *et al.* Long-term oral anticoagulant therapy in patients with unstable angina or suspected non-Q-wave myocardial infarction: Organization to Assess Strategies for Ischemic Syndromes (OASIS) pilot study results. *Circulation* 1998; **98:** 1064–70.
41. The Organization to Assess Strategies for Ischemic Syndromes (OASIS) Investigators. Effects of long-term, moderate-intensity oral anticoagulation in addition to aspirin in unstable angina. *J Am Coll Cardiol* 2001; **37:** 475–84.
42. Bertolet BD, Pepine CJ. Daily life cardiac ischaemia: should it be treated? *Drugs* 1995; **49:** 176–95.
43. Pepine CJ, *et al.* Effects of treatment on outcome in mildly symptomatic patients with ischaemia during daily life: the Atenolol Silent Ischaemia Study (ASIST). *Circulation* 1994; **90:** 762–8.
44. Davies RF, *et al.* Asymptomatic Cardiac Ischemia Pilot (ACIP) study two-year follow-up: outcomes of patients randomized to initial strategies of medical therapy versus revascularization. *Circulation* 1997; **95:** 2037–43.
45. Yellon DM, *et al.* Angina reassessed: pain or protector? *Lancet* 1996; **347:** 1159–62.

Ascites

Ascites is the accumulation of fluid within the peritoneal cavity. Although it is not strictly a cardiovascular disorder, treatment depends mainly on cardiovascular drugs. Alcoholic hepatic cirrhosis is probably the commonest underlying cause in the western world; others include malignant neoplasms, heart failure, and tuberculosis. The following discussion is restricted mainly to **cirrhotic ascites**.

The mechanism of ascites formation in hepatic cirrhosis has been explained in terms of the underfill and overflow theories, and more recently, the vasodilatation hypothesis. Whatever the mechanism, ascites formation is linked to renal sodium and water retention partly as a result of increased circulating renin and aldosterone concentrations. Portal hypertension and hypoalbuminaemia may be contributory factors. More details may be found in reviews of the pathophysiology of ascites formation.[1-3]

Small amounts of ascitic fluid may go undetected but as it accumulates abdominal distension becomes apparent, and there is a feeling of discomfort. There may be respiratory distress and cardiac dysfunction in severe cases. Peripheral oedema may, or may not, be present. Renal dysfunction may progress to severe impairment (the hepatorenal syndrome). Patients are at risk of primary (spontaneous) bacterial peritonitis (p.134).

Management[1-7] depends on the severity of ascites but the mainstays are dietary sodium restriction and diuretic treatment. In mild to moderate ascites, sodium restriction alone may sometimes be effective but most patients also require diuretics. Bed rest has been advocated but not all workers consider its value proven. Response is monitored by measuring the daily reduction in body-weight. The diuretic of choice is the aldosterone antagonist spironolactone, with the addition of a loop diuretic such as frusemide [furosemide] if necessary. Amiloride or another potassium-sparing diuretic may be used as an alternative to spironolactone if adverse effects are a problem. Spironolactone together with frusemide [furosemide] from the outset has also been employed. In tense or refractory ascites, large-volume or total paracentesis (removal of ascitic fluid by drainage) is often used initially; patients may then be maintained on diuretics or repeated paracentesis may be used. Plasma volume replacement with albumin or dextrans after paracentesis is usual, particularly if large volumes are removed. Where ascites remains refractory or repeated paracentesis is not tolerated various shunting procedures have been tried, although their role is not established. In severe cases liver transplantation may be necessary.

In **malignant ascites**, that is ascites due to malignant neoplasms, paracentesis is often necessary but spironolactone may be of benefit in some patients.

1. Roberts LR, Kamath PS. Ascites and hepatorenal syndrome: pathophysiology and management. *Mayo Clin Proc* 1996; **71:** 874–81.
2. Stanley AJ, *et al.* Pathophysiology and management of portal hypertension 2: cirrhotic ascites. *Br J Hosp Med* 1997; **58:** 74–8.
3. Jalan R, Hayes PC. Hepatic encephalopathy and ascites. *Lancet* 1997; **350:** 1309–15.
4. Gerbes AL. Medical treatment of ascites in cirrhosis. *J Hepatol* 1993; **17** (suppl 2): S4–S9.

5. Runyon BA. Care of patients with ascites. *N Engl J Med* 1994; **330:** 337–42.
6. Bataller R, *et al.* Practical recommendations for the treatment of ascites and its complications. *Drugs* 1997; **54:** 571–80.
7. Krige JEJ, Beckingham IJ. ABC of diseases of liver, pancreas, and biliary system: portal hypertension–2. Ascites, encephalopathy, and other conditions. *BMJ* 2001; **322:** 416–18.

Atherosclerosis

Atherosclerosis is the narrowing and hardening of medium and large arteries that results from the development of lipid-rich lesions (atheromas) in their intimal lining. Various types of lesion are recognised.[1,2] Early lesions include fatty streaks, which develop from infancy and are composed of lipid-filled macrophages (foam cells). Fully developed fibrous plaques consist of a core of lipid and lipid-rich macrophages surrounded by a connective-tissue matrix. These plaques may undergo calcification and may become sufficiently large to obstruct the lumen of the artery. However, occlusion occurs more commonly when there is thrombosis due to endothelial denudation or disruption of the plaque (plaque rupture or fissuring) with exposure of the thrombogenic core. Reduction or total blockage of blood supply results in ischaemia and the clinical events of angina pectoris (above), myocardial infarction (below), peripheral vascular disease (intermittent claudication) (below), and stroke (ischaemic stroke) (below). The term **ischaemic heart disease** (coronary heart or coronary artery disease) encompasses angina pectoris and myocardial infarction and is the most common manifestation of atherosclerosis; in most industrialised countries ischaemic heart disease is a leading cause of death. However, atherosclerosis is essentially a generalised condition and can affect most arteries throughout the body. Thus, the patient with peripheral vascular disease is also likely to develop or to have evidence of ischaemic heart disease and those with ischaemic heart disease may also have atherosclerotic deterioration of other arteries. The term atherosclerotic disease has been used to cover all such manifestations of atherosclerosis.

Epidemiological studies have identified various **risk factors** associated with the development of atherosclerosis. The three major modifiable risk factors are blood cholesterol concentrations, blood pressure, and smoking. Other risk factors include advancing age, male sex, diabetes, obesity, lack of exercise, and family history of atherosclerotic disease; abnormal blood clotting factors, in particular raised fibrinogen concentrations, and hyperhomocysteinaemia may also contribute but are less established. The same risk factors apply to all the main forms of atherosclerotic disease although there may be differences in their relative importance. For example the predominant risk factor for stroke is high blood pressure, whereas diabetes and smoking are most strongly linked with peripheral vascular disease. Individuals with a large increase in only one risk factor, such as those with high blood pressure or high blood-cholesterol concentrations are in a minority. Most cases of atherosclerotic disease occur in individuals with mild or moderate increases in *several* risk factors; the presence of more than one risk factor enhances the overall risk for developing atherosclerotic disease, that is, they are not simply additive. The aim is to **prevent** the development of atherosclerotic disease by abolishing or reducing these risk factors. It requires both individual intervention for those at high risk and a population approach to reduce the overall levels of risk factors in the general populace. These approaches have been the subject of guidelines[3-5] and reviews.[6-10] Most studies have been in men, but the prevention of atherosclerosis in women has also been reviewed.[11-13]

Individual intervention entails identification of those who are at high risk of developing atherosclerotic disease or who have already suffered a clinical event, and instituting measures to reduce this risk. Patients who have suffered a cardiovascular event are at high risk for further events and require treatment. Intervention in those without overt disease depends on assessment of their overall cardiovascular risk (p.797), with treatment where this is considered sufficiently high. Lifestyle and dietary changes are the mainstay of treatment and include advising patients not to smoke, to avoid obesity, to increase exercise, to moderate their alcohol intake, and to adopt a low-fat diet. The benefits of reducing blood pressure, lipid-lowering therapy, and aspirin, are also established. Women have a lower risk of atherosclerotic disease than men of a comparable age, although the difference narrows with increasing age postmenopausally. The role of HRT in reducing the incidence of cardiovascular disease in postmenopausal women is controversial (see Effects on the Cardiovascular System, p.1462).

General screening methods fail to identify all individuals at risk of atherosclerotic disease and a **population approach** is also required. This involves general health education and promotion to encourage the lifestyle changes listed above that are associated with lower risk levels. As atheroma development may begin in childhood a healthy diet should be encouraged from an early age. These efforts, though, probably produce only modest changes in risk factors.[14] The incidence of ischaemic heart disease is falling in many populations, although the WHO MONICA project (Monitoring the Trends and Determinants in Cardiovascular Diseases) found only a weak association between changes in classic risk factors and changes in event rates.[15] Thus, research continues into the pathogenesis of atherosclerosis and the identification of further risk factors.

Other possible approaches to the management of atherosclerosis include the use of drugs that interfere with atherogenesis (the development of atheromas). *Oxidation* of low-density lipoprotein (LDL) is thought to be a crucial step in atherogenesis[16-18] and dietary antioxidants such as vitamins E and C and betacarotene (see Prophylaxis of Ischaemic Heart Disease, p.1352), and polyphenol compounds found in various foods including red wine, have received much attention for their possible role in the prevention of atherosclerosis.

Hyperhomocysteinaemia may be a risk factor for atherosclerosis, although at present the mechanism by which homocysteine promotes atherosclerosis is unknown,[19] and there is growing interest in assessing the effect of folic acid in the primary or secondary prevention of atherosclerosis (see Ischaemic Heart Disease, p.1362).

Results of serological and pathological studies suggest an association between *Chlamydia pneumoniae* infection and atherosclerosis. However, prospective studies[20,21] have not supported a strong association. *C. pneumoniae* is widespread in blood vessels and any pathological effect of infection is yet to be proven; the role of antibacterials is also under investigation.[22]

Inflammation is also considered to contribute to atherosclerotic plaque formation and instability.[23] Statins may modify this process, as well as lower cholesterol levels.

Therapeutic angiogenesis (the development and growth of blood vessels) is also under investigation to improve myocardial perfusion. Preliminary studies of growth factor proteins, such as vascular endothelial growth factor (VEGF) and fibroblast growth factor (FGF), and gene therapy to stimulate VEGF production, have shown promise.[24]

1. Stary HC, *et al.* A definition of initial, fatty streak, and intermediate lesions of atherosclerosis: a report from the Committee on Vascular Lesions of the Council on Arteriosclerosis, American Heart Association. *Circulation* 1994; **89:** 2462–78.
2. Stary HC, *et al.* A definition of advanced types of atherosclerotic lesions and a histological classification of atherosclerosis: a report from the Committee on Vascular Lesions of the Council on Arteriosclerosis, American Heart Association. *Circulation* 1995; **92:** 1355–74.
3. Wood D, *et al.* Joint British recommendations on prevention of coronary heart disease in clinical practice. *Heart* 1998; **80** (suppl 2): S1–S29.
4. Wood D, *et al.* Prevention of coronary heart disease in clinical practice: recommendations of the second joint task force of European and other societies on coronary prevention. *Eur Heart J* 1998; **19:** 1434–1503.
5. Grundy SM, *et al.* Primary prevention of coronary heart disease: guidance from Framingham. A statement for healthcare professionals from the AHA task force on risk reduction. *Circulation* 1998; **97:** 1876–87.
6. Rose G. Epidemiology of atherosclerosis. In: Wolfe JHN, ed. *ABC of vascular diseases.* London: BMJ Publishing Group, 1992: 1–3.
7. Truswell AS. Reducing the risk of coronary heart disease. In: Truswell AS, ed. *ABC of nutrition.* 3rd ed. London: BMJ Publishing Group, 1999: 1–8.
8. Manson JE, *et al.* The primary prevention of myocardial infarction. *N Engl J Med* 1992; **326:** 1406–16.
9. Henderson A. Coronary heart disease: overview. *Lancet* 1996; **348:** s1–s4.
10. 27th Bethesda Conference. Matching the intensity of risk factor management with the hazard for coronary disease events. *J Am Coll Cardiol* 1996; **27:** 957–1047.
11. Wenger NK, *et al.* Cardiovascular health and disease in women. *N Engl J Med* 1993; **329:** 247–56.
12. Rich-Edwards JW, *et al.* The primary prevention of coronary heart disease in women. *N Engl J Med* 1995; **332:** 1758–66.
13. Tsang TSM, *et al.* Risks of coronary heart disease in women: current understanding and evolving concepts. *Mayo Clin Proc* 2000; **75:** 1289–1303.
14. Ebrahim S, Davey Smith G. Systematic review of randomised controlled trials of multiple risk factor interventions for preventing coronary heart disease. *BMJ* 1997; **314:** 1666–74.
15. Kuulasmaa K, *et al.* Estimation of contribution of changes in classic risk factors to trends in coronary-event rates across the WHO MONICA Project populations. *Lancet* 2000; **355:** 675–87.
16. Esterbauer H, *et al.* Lipid peroxidation and its role in atherosclerosis. *Br Med Bull* 1993; **49:** 566–76.
17. Witztum JL. The oxidation hypothesis of atherosclerosis. *Lancet* 1994; **344:** 793–5.
18. Diaz MN, *et al.* Antioxidants and atherosclerotic heart disease. *N Engl J Med* 1997; **337:** 408–16.

19. Welch GN, Loscalzo J. Homocysteine and atherothrombosis. *N Engl J Med* 1998; **338**: 1042–50.
20. Wald NJ, *et al.* Chlamydia pneumoniae infection and mortality from ischaemic heart disease: large prospective study. *BMJ* 2000; **321**: 204–7.
21. Danesh J, *et al.* Chlamydia pneumoniae IgG titres and coronary heart disease: prospective study and meta-analysis. *BMJ* 2000; **321**: 208–13.
22. Wong Y-K, *et al.* Chlamydia pneumoniae and atherosclerosis. *Heart* 1999; **81**: 232–8.
23. Ross R. Atherosclerosis – an inflammatory disease. *N Engl J Med* 1999; **340**: 115–26.
24. Sellke FW, Simons M. Angiogenesis in cardiovascular disease: current status and therapeutic potential. *Drugs* 1999; **58**: 391–6.

Cardiac arrhythmias

The heart acts as a pump and maintains circulation of the blood by alternate contraction and relaxation of cardiac muscle (the myocardium). It generally contracts at a rate of 70 to 75 beats per minute in a healthy 70-kg person at rest. The normal heart rhythm, known as *sinus rhythm*, originates in specialised cardiac cells called *pacemaker cells* in the *sino-atrial (SA)* or *sinus node* and has been defined as a sinus node rate of 60 to 100 beats per minute. Each heart beat or contraction is initiated by generation of an *action potential* (see Antiarrhythmics, p.787) in the SA node; the electrical impulse spreads over both atria, causing them to contract, and on to the *atrioventricular (AV) node*. From the AV node it spreads through the bundle of His and down the Purkinje fibres to the ventricles, causing them to contract. It is the movement of ions across the cardiac cell membrane that generates the action potential. The electrical changes involved can be recorded on an electrocardiogram (ECG). Other cardiac cells which are located outside the sinus node are also capable of initiating impulses. These cells are termed *ectopic pacemakers* and can be found in the atrioventricular junction and in the His-Purkinje system. The normal rate of impulse initiation by these ectopic pacemakers is less than that of the sinus node and therefore they do not normally initiate the heart beat but may become dominant in certain circumstances such as: if the intrinsic rate of the ectopic pacemaker rises above that of the sinus node; if the sinus node rate falls below that of the ectopic pacemaker; or when a normal sinus node impulse is prevented from being conducted through the heart (heart block) leaving the ectopic pacemaker to fire at its own intrinsic rate.

A **cardiac arrhythmia** can be defined in simple terms as any abnormality of rate, regularity, or site of origin of the cardiac impulse or as a disturbance in conduction that causes an abnormal sequence of activation. **Palpitation** is a term used to describe an unacceptable awareness of a beating heart by the patient. This may occur normally in circumstances such as emotion, exercise, or stress or may occur in association with arrhythmias. Clinically, arrhythmias may be classified by presumed site of origin, namely as **supraventricular arrhythmias** (including **atrial arrhythmias** and **atrioventricular junctional arrhythmias**) or as **ventricular arrhythmias**. Classification can also be based on rate as either bradyarrhythmias (slow) or tachyarrhythmias (fast). It is the group of tachyarrhythmias that are the main focus of the following discussion.

Bradyarrhythmias are caused by sinus node dysfunction which either depresses impulse generation or disturbs the conduction of impulses from the sinus node to the atria.[1] **Atrioventricular block** indicates disturbance of conduction of the atrial impulse to the ventricles. In first-degree block the impulse is delayed. It is usually asymptomatic but may progress to second- or third-degree block. In second-degree block the impulse is blocked intermittently and in third-degree block there is a complete block. **Atrioventricular dissociation** indicates a condition in which ventricular activity is faster, and independent of, the atrial activity. Bradyarrhythmias may be treated with either atropine or with isoprenaline, although cardiac pacing is the treatment of choice.

For **tachyarrhythmias** a classification or diagnosis based on the precise mechanism of the arrhythmia would also be desirable but this is not always clear. In many of the clinically relevant arrhythmias, however, the mechanism is one of re-entry. Re-entry occurs when the initial impulse does not die out but continues to propagate and reactivate the heart.

Diagnosis and management. Cardiac arrhythmias can range from little more than asymptomatic ECG abnormalities through to severe or life-threatening events. Treatment can be with antiarrhythmics or with non-pharmacological methods.

The precise identification of an arrhythmia is not always easy, but is important for correct management. The inappropriate use of an antiarrhythmic for a specific arrhythmia can not only be ineffective but, in view of the proarrhythmic potential of most of them, may even be deleterious. Identification and diagnosis should be based on clinical symptoms and on characteristic ECG features as well as on other specialised tests and features relevant to individual arrhythmias. A typical normal ECG trace is shown in Figure 2, p.787. An arrhythmia with a narrow QRS complex is always supraventricular in origin whereas a broad QRS complex can indicate either a supraventricular or ventricular origin, hence the diagnostic difficulties.

Ectopic beats, **extrasystoles**, or **premature contractions** can arise in either the atria or the ventricles and, although their precise meaning and definition differs, for practical purposes they can be considered equivalent. Generally, they cause few or no symptoms and usually have no prognostic value although some patients suffer distressing symptoms or palpitations.

Atrial fibrillation is the commonest cardiac arrhythmia and has been the subject of several reviews.[2-17] The mechanism of the arrhythmia in atrial fibrillation is one of re-entry. Atrial fibrillation is often associated with underlying cardiovascular disease, notably ischaemic or hypertensive heart disease, or less frequently today with rheumatic heart disease; hyperthyroidism and acute alcohol intoxication can also be causes. In some patients there is no obvious cause in which case the arrhythmia is described as 'lone' atrial fibrillation. Atrial fibrillation is relatively common following cardiothoracic surgery, but is usually self-limiting. It is characterised by an irregular and very rapid atrial rate (usually more than 300 beats per minute) and as the atrioventricular node is incapable of conducting all the impulses adequately, the increased ventricular response results in a rapid and totally irregular ventricular rate. The atrial fibrillation may be paroxysmal (intermittent) but is more usually chronic (persistent). Although atrial fibrillation can cause distressing symptoms such as severe palpitations and exercise intolerance it is not usually immediately life-threatening, but does result in long-term morbidity and mortality. The condition leads to left atrial dilatation and reduced cardiac output with stasis of blood in the left atrium. This can result in thrombus formation and subsequent systemic embolisation, notably ischaemic stroke. Thromboembolic events are relatively rare in lone atrial fibrillation but the risk is very much increased in concomitant cardiovascular disease, especially so in rheumatic heart disease.

The two main options for the management of atrial fibrillation are cardioversion followed by the maintenance of sinus rhythm, or treatment to slow the increased ventricular response while allowing atrial fibrillation to continue. Anticoagulation may also be necessary to prevent thromboembolic episodes. The relative benefits of the two approaches are not yet clear; restoration of sinus rhythm alleviates symptoms and removes the thromboembolic risk, but patients may not tolerate therapy and relapses may occur.

Rate control may have a role in the acute management of symptoms and in maintenance therapy. Digoxin has traditionally been used to slow an increased ventricular rate; however beta blockers or calcium-channel blockers such as diltiazem or verapamil are preferred by some as they are usually considered more effective, especially in controlling the increased rates that may occur during exercise. If necessary, a combination of digoxin with either a beta blocker or a calcium-channel blocker may be employed. All these drugs act by slowing the conduction through the atrioventricular node. They do not, however, have an antifibrillatory action and do not restore sinus rhythm. Catheter ablation of atrioventricular conduction pathways followed by permanent pacing may be necessary for rate control in patients intolerant or unresponsive to drug therapy.

Restoration of sinus rhythm may provide better relief of symptoms than merely controlling the increased ventricular rate, although a study[18] comparing the two methods found that both produced similar clinical effects. Sinus rhythm can be restored either by synchronised direct current cardioversion or by pharmacological cardioversion, but both methods must be preceded by anticoagulation unless fibrillation is of recent onset (less than 24 hours). Drugs employed, either orally or intravenously, are usually class I antiarrhythmics (see p.787 for an explanation of the classification of antiarrhythmics), including disopyramide, flecainide, procainamide, propaf-

enone, or quinidine. These drugs terminate atrial fibrillation by prolongation of atrial refractoriness, thus reducing the number of re-entry circuits in the atria. Amiodarone, a class III drug, may also be used and has the dual properties of ventricular rate control and antifibrillatory action. Sotalol, a beta blocker with class III antiarrhythmic activity in addition to the class II activity of beta blockers in general, also has this dual action. Newer class III drugs such as azimilide, dofetilide, and ibutilide may also be used. Direct current cardioversion has the advantage of restoring sinus rhythm more rapidly and effectively than drugs but has the disadvantage that it needs to be performed under general anaesthesia.

Once sinus rhythm has been achieved, or in cases of paroxysmal atrial fibrillation, long-term maintenance drug therapy needs to be considered. The drugs used for this are broadly similar to those used for pharmacological cardioversion, namely the class I or class III antiarrhythmics. Surgery or implantable cardioversion devices are also options available for some patients.

The problem of **thromboembolic** events, principally ischaemic stroke, resulting from atrial fibrillation has been the subject of several reviews[19-23] as well as being addressed in the general reviews quoted above. If atrial fibrillation has been present for 48 hours or more it is generally recognised that there is a potential risk of causing systemic embolisation once sinus rhythm is restored. It is therefore recommended that oral anticoagulation with warfarin should be given for 2 to 4 weeks before cardioversion is attempted. If immediate cardioversion is necessary, administration of intravenous heparin followed by transoesophageal echocardiography to exclude the presence of thrombi has been suggested.[9,11,14,24] Control of the ventricular rate as outlined above should also be undertaken during this period. Anticoagulation is usually continued for up to 4 weeks following successful cardioversion.

Anticoagulation may also be undertaken for long-term **prophylaxis of stroke** in selected patients. The risk of stroke is increased about 17 times in atrial fibrillation associated with rheumatic heart disease and the benefits of long-term prophylaxis with warfarin are well-established. For non-rheumatic heart disease the risk is less, but is still increased by about fivefold and affects many more patients, but the use of warfarin is more controversial. Meta-analysis[25] of a number of studies has clearly demonstrated a beneficial effect of warfarin in the primary and secondary prevention of stroke in patients with non-rheumatic atrial fibrillation. The design of these studies has, however, been criticised and another meta-analysis[26] of some of the trials suggested that warfarin had no significant effect on fatal stroke incidence and produced only a small reduction in major stroke incidence. The benefits of anticoagulation need to be balanced against the risk of increased bleeding episodes, notably stroke due to intracranial haemorrhage, induced by warfarin. The risk of thromboembolism is influenced by different factors and variables and should be assessed in all patients; oral anticoagulation is recommended for specific groups with high risk factors such as increasing age, ischaemic or hypertensive heart disease, heart failure, hyperthyroidism, or history or evidence of thromboembolism.[24,27] Aspirin may be used in patients at lower risk or who have contra-indications to warfarin,[24] although a number of analyses have come to different conclusions regarding its efficacy;[28-30] indobufen[31] has also been suggested as a possible alternative. Low-intensity fixed-dose warfarin regimens combined with aspirin have been tried[32,33] to reduce the risk of warfarin-induced haemorrhage, but are less effective than adjusted-dose warfarin and are not recommended.

Atrial flutter is an arrhythmia somewhat similar in nature to atrial fibrillation and has been discussed in reviews.[4,6,34] Like atrial fibrillation it is characterised by a rapid (about 300 beats per minute) atrial rate, although the atrial rhythm is more regular and organised, and by a corresponding increase in the ventricular rate. It is far less common than atrial fibrillation, to which it often degenerates if left untreated; it may revert to normal sinus rhythm in some cases. Unlike atrial fibrillation, atrial flutter has not been considered to carry an increased risk of thromboembolic episodes, but several studies have suggested this may not be the case.[35-37] Anticoagulation may therefore have a role in patients with recurrent or chronic atrial flutter,[34] and has been recommended prior to cardioversion.[24] Management strategies for atrial flutter are broadly similar to those outlined above for atrial fibrillation, namely controlling the increased ventricular response rate and cardioversion. However, in general terms drug therapy for either of these interventions is less successful in flutter than in fibrillation. Cardioversion with drug therapy has a relatively low success rate and cardiac pacing is usually employed which often results in a self-terminating atrial fibrillation. Synchronised direct current cardioversion may be employed to restore sinus rhythm if pacing fails. Radiofrequency ablation may also be used,[38] and may be the treatment of choice if long-term therapy is required.[34]

Other atrial arrhythmias include **atrial premature beats** and **atrial tachycardia**. Premature beats are usually asymptomatic but if symptoms are severe (the awareness of a pause between normal beats) beta blockers may be employed.[6] Atrial tachycardia may also be treated with beta blockers but if it is due to digoxin toxicity, withdrawal of digoxin may be all that is required.[6]

Paroxysmal supraventricular tachycardia is a re-entry arrhythmia. The term paroxysmal atrial tachycardia was used, but became obsolete when it was realised that many such arrhythmias arise in the atrioventricular junction rather than in atrial muscle.[39] The re-entry circuit can be either due to an accessory atrioventricular pathway between the atria and ventricles or re-entry can occur at the site of the node itself. It is a relatively common arrhythmia occurring in otherwise healthy individuals. It may resolve spontaneously, or reflex vagal stimulation by respiratory manoeuvres, prompt squatting, or pressure over one carotid sinus may restore normal sinus rhythm. If symptoms associated with the rapid heart rate are severe, treatment will be needed. For termination of paroxysmal supraventricular tachycardia adenosine given intravenously is often the drug of choice;[39,40] intravenous verapamil is an alternative. Digoxin or beta blockers, also given intravenously, have been tried but appear to offer no advantage over adenosine or verapamil and are less effective.[39,40] Propafenone, flecainide, procainamide, and sotalol have also been used;[41] direct current cardioversion may be necessary in some cases. Long-term maintenance therapy to prevent recurrence is required in some patients. Oral drugs are employed and may include beta blockers, digoxin, disopyramide, flecainide, quinidine, or verapamil. As discussed under atrial fibrillation above, beta blockers, digoxin, and calcium-channel blockers such as verapamil act by delaying impulses along the atrioventricular conduction system whereas the class I drugs act on atrial refractoriness. However, for symptomatic patients in whom an accessory atrioventricular pathway is the cause or for atrioventricular nodal re-entry tachycardia, radiofrequency ablation of the affected tissue is often the treatment of choice.[38,39,42]

Patients with the Wolff-Parkinson-White syndrome,[43] a congenital abnormality characterised by an accessory atrioventricular conduction pathway known as a Kent bundle, may be at special risk of developing atrial fibrillation or paroxysmal supraventricular tachycardia. Great care is necessary with the choice of antiarrhythmic in such patients and radiofrequency ablation may often be preferred.[38]

Supraventricular tachycardia can occur rarely *in utero* and is associated with hydrops fetalis and perinatal mortality and morbidity. Treatment is with antiarrhythmic drugs such as digoxin or flecainide given to the mother (transplacental therapy);[44,45] in resistant cases direct intraperitoneal or intravascular administration to the fetus may be necessary and amiodarone is often used.[44]

Ventricular tachycardia is a re-entry arrhythmia[46-50] often associated with underlying cardiovascular disease such as myocardial infarction or cardiomyopathies or with digoxin toxicity. The heart rate is about 120 to 250 beats per minute and the tachycardia, which arises in the ventricles below the atrioventricular node, can be paroxysmal consisting of short self-terminating episodes or can be sustained (lasting 30 seconds or longer). Although ventricular tachycardia can be asymptomatic (if the episodes are non-sustained) it is potentially a serious condition which may lead to reduced cardiac output, shock, and progression to **ventricular fibrillation**. It is one of the most common causes of sudden unexplained cardiac death. The ECG trace of ventricular tachycardia has sometimes been confused with that of supraventricular tachycardia but since the treatments differ markedly, every effort should be made to obtain the correct diagnosis.

The initial treatment of ventricular tachycardia depends largely on the haemodynamic status of the patient. If the patient has sustained ventricular tachycardia or has pulseless non-sustained ventricular tachycardia, both of which tend to be associated with instability and a poorer

prognosis, defibrillation, as outlined under Advanced Cardiac Life Support (above), should be initiated. In the more stable patient, intravenous drug therapy may be employed for acute termination of the tachycardia. Lignocaine [lidocaine] has been the drug of choice; other class I drugs such as disopyramide, flecainide, mexiletine, procainamide, propafenone, or quinidine are alternatives, as are bretylium, which has class II and class III activity, and the class III drug amiodarone. In some patients with non-sustained ventricular tachycardia, beta blockers may be adequate and in one study[51] sotalol appeared to be superior to lignocaine [lidocaine] for the acute termination of sustained tachycardia. Non-pharmacological methods of management include ablation either by radiofrequency or surgery, and electrical techniques such as pacing or cardioversion.

Following restoration of normal sinus rhythm maintenance therapy needs to be considered to prevent recurrences. Long-term prophylaxis is generally not warranted in low risk patients such as those who have experienced asymptomatic non-sustained ventricular tachycardia. Survivors of ventricular fibrillation and pulseless ventricular tachycardia have a high risk of recurrence of arrhythmia and until recently either an implantable cardioverter defibrillator or drug therapy has been employed in these patients prophylactically. However, a recent study in 1016 patients comparing the two methods found a greater reduction in mortality with implantable cardioverter defibrillators[52] and the American College of Cardiology/American Heart Association now recommend implantable defibrillators as preferred first-line therapy.[53] Drug therapy was formerly given empirically but choice is now generally guided by electrophysiological or electrocardiographic testing using programmed electrical stimulation or ambulatory monitoring. Drugs used have included class I drugs, beta blockers, sotalol, and amiodarone. The use of drug therapy in patients who have implantable cardioverter defibrillators to reduce activation of the device is also under investigation.

Ventricular arrhythmias may be associated with **heart disease** such as myocardial infarction or heart failure. Ventricular tachycardia and ventricular fibrillation are common early after **acute myocardial infarction**. Lignocaine [lidocaine] has been given prophylactically after myocardial infarction to patients at high risk of ventricular fibrillation, but should probably be reserved for symptomatic patients.[50] Asymptomatic premature ventricular arrhythmias in subjects who have previously suffered a myocardial infarction are also common and are recognised as a risk factor for subsequent sudden cardiac death. Suppressing such arrhythmias might be expected to reduce the incidence of sudden death but results with antiarrhythmics have not been promising; treatment with implantable cardioverter defibrillators may, however, be more effective than drug therapy.[54]

A large multicentre study was set up in the USA (the Cardiac Arrhythmia Suppression Trial known as CAST) and the class I antiarrhythmics encainide, flecainide, and moracizine were selected following a preliminary study[55] (CAPS; the Cardiac Arrhythmia Pilot Study) in which they had been shown to suppress premature ventricular depolarisations in post-infarction patients. After an average of 10 months of daily treatment with one of the active agents or placebo both the class Ic antiarrhythmics encainide and flecainide were withdrawn from the CAST study because patients receiving either of them showed a higher than expected mortality rate.[56,57] Moracizine, which is a class I antiarrhythmic with activities corresponding to a, b, and c subclasses, was not implicated in increasing mortality at the CAST I assessment,[56] so the study continued as CAST II to compare this antiarrhythmic against placebo. In late 1991 an increased mortality with moracizine was also documented and the study was halted.[58]

Following publication of the CAST studies some workers looked at other class I antiarrhythmics. A meta-analysis of trials utilising quinidine was undertaken[59] as it was believed that this drug had gained in popularity after the adverse CAST results. However, this meta-analysis suggested that quinidine was associated with at least as high a proportion of adverse events, such as death and early proarrhythmia, as the class Ic drugs flecainide and propafenone. A study of *d*-sotalol, a class III antiarrhythmic, in patients with left ventricular dysfunction following myocardial infarction was stopped early because of increased mortality in the treatment group.[60]

Until recently, meta-analyses[61,62] of prophylactic antiarrhythmic therapy have concluded that the only class of drugs with proven benefit after myocardial infarction is the beta blockers. Some limited success has been seen with amiodarone in asymptomatic arrhythmias after myocardial infarction (BASIS: the Basel Antiarrhythmic Study of Infarct Survival;[63] CAMIAT: the Canadian Amiodarone Myocardial Infarction Arrhythmia Trial,[64] and EMIAT: the European Myocardial Infarct Amiodarone Trial[65]). Both CAMIAT and EMIAT reported a reduction in risk of arrhythmic death, but neither study showed a reduction in total mortality. However, meta-analysis of studies using amiodarone found a small reduction in total mortality suggesting that it might be of benefit after myocardial infarction in patients, such as those with heart failure, at high risk of arrhythmic death.[66]

Attempts have been made to reduce deaths from ventricular arrhythmias in patients with severe **heart failure** (below); beneficial results have been reported with amiodarone but adverse effects may limit its use.

Drugs used to treat arrhythmias can have a **proarrhythmic** effect, that is they can exacerbate or induce arrhythmias of all types. **Torsade de pointes** is a potentially lethal ventricular tachycardia with a characteristic ECG pattern and is associated with prolongation of the QT interval; this may be congenital but is commonly drug-induced.[67,68] Drugs responsible include antiarrhythmics and several non-cardiac drugs[69,70] including phenothiazines, tricyclic antidepressants, antihistamines such as astemizole and terfenadine, antibacterials such as erythromycin, the antimalarial halofantrine, and the lipid lowering drug probucol. The ventricular tachycardia is often non-sustained, but may persist for long enough to cause syncope or it may even progress to ventricular fibrillation. If torsade de pointes is drug-induced, withdrawal and subsequent avoidance of the offending drug is mandatory. Electrolyte disturbances appear to contribute to torsade de pointes and initial therapy is with magnesium given intravenously together with temporary pacing of the atria or ventricles as appropriate. Isoprenaline may be given cautiously to increase the heart rate and shorten the QT interval, until pacing is instituted. Congenital long QT syndromes are usually treated with beta blockers and/or pacing.[68]

1. Mangrum JM, DiMarco JP. The evaluation and management of bradycardia. N Engl J Med 2000; 342: 703–9.
2. Pritchett ELC. Management of atrial fibrillation. N Engl J Med 1992; 326: 1264–71.
3. Clark A, Cotter L. Cardioversion in atrial fibrillation. Br J Hosp Med 1993; 49: 256–61.
4. Geraets DR, Kienzle MG. Atrial fibrillation and atrial flutter. Clin Pharm 1993; 12: 721–35.
5. Murgatroyd FD, Camm AJ. Current concepts in atrial fibrillation. Br J Hosp Med 1993; 49: 546–60.
6. Murgatroyd FD, Camm AJ. Atrial arrhythmias. Lancet 1993; 341: 1317–22.
7. Nattel S, et al. The treatment of atrial fibrillation: an evaluation of drug therapy, electrical modalities and therapeutic considerations. Drugs 1994; 48: 345–71.
8. Anonymous. The antiarrhythmic treatment of atrial fibrillation. Drug Ther Bull 1996; 34: 41–5.
9. Blackshear JL, et al. Management of atrial fibrillation in adults: prevention of thromboembolism and symptomatic treatment. Mayo Clin Proc 1996; 71: 150–60.
10. Channer KS. Treatment of atrial fibrillation. Prescribers' J 1996; 36: 146–53.
11. Gilligan DM, et al. The management of atrial fibrillation. Am J Med 1996; 101: 413–21.
12. Golzari H, et al. Atrial fibrillation: restoration and maintenance of sinus rhythm and indications for anticoagulation therapy. Ann Intern Med 1996; 125: 311–23.
13. Lip GYH, ed. ABC of atrial fibrillation. London: BMJ Publishing Group, 1996.
14. Prystowsky EN, et al. Management of patients with atrial fibrillation: a statement for healthcare professionals from the Subcommittee on Electrocardiography and Electrophysiology, American Heart Association. Circulation 1996; 93: 1262–77.
15. Narayan SM, et al. Atrial fibrillation. Lancet 1997; 350: 943–50.
16. Jung F, DiMarco JP. Treatment strategies for atrial fibrillation. Am J Med 1998; 104: 272–86.
17. Falk RH. Atrial fibrillation. N Engl J Med 2001; 344: 1067–78. Correction. ibid.; 1876.
18. Hohnloser SH, et al. Rhythm or rate control in atrial fibrillation—Pharmacological Intervention in Atrial Fibrillation (PIAF): a randomised trial. Lancet 2000; 356: 1789–94.
19. Anonymous. Warfarin or aspirin for non-rheumatic atrial fibrillation? Drug Ther Bull 1994; 32: 57–60. Correction. ibid.; 80.
20. Howard PA, Duncan PW. Primary stroke prevention in nonvalvular atrial fibrillation: implementing the clinical trial findings. Ann Pharmacother 1997; 31: 1187–96.
21. Hardman SMC, Cowie MR. Anticoagulation in heart disease. BMJ 1999; 318: 238–44.
22. Hart RG, Halperin JL. Atrial fibrillation and thromboembolism: a decade of progress in stroke prevention. Ann Intern Med 1999; 131: 688–95.
23. Lip GYH. Thromboprophylaxis for atrial fibrillation. Lancet 1999; 353: 4–6. Correction. ibid.; 1978.
24. Albers GW, et al. Antithrombotic therapy in atrial fibrillation. Chest 2001; 119 (suppl): 194S–206S.
25. Hart RG, et al. Antithrombotic therapy to prevent stroke in patients with atrial fibrillation: a meta-analysis. Ann Intern Med 1999; 131: 492–501.

796 Cardiovascular Drugs

26. Green CJ, et al. Anticoagulation in chronic nonvalvular atrial fibrillation: a critical appraisal and meta-analysis. Can J Cardiol 1997; 13: 811–15.
27. Scottish Intercollegiate Guidelines Network. Antithrombotic therapy: a national clinical guideline. Edinburgh: SIGN Secretariat, 1999.
28. The Atrial Fibrillation Investigators. The efficacy of aspirin in patients with atrial fibrillation: analysis of pooled data from 3 randomised trials. Arch Intern Med 1997; 157: 1237–40.
29. Segal JB, et al. Anticoagulants or antiplatelet therapy for non-rheumatic atrial fibrillation and flutter (updated 22 May 2001). Available in The Cochrane Library; Issue 4. Oxford: Update Software; 2001.
30. Taylor FC, et al. Systematic review of long term anticoagulation or antiplatelet treatment in patients with non-rheumatic atrial fibrillation. BMJ 2001; 322: 321–6.
31. Morocutti C, et al. Indobufen versus warfarin in the secondary prevention of major vascular events in nonrheumatic atrial fibrillation. Stroke 1997; 28: 1015–21.
32. Stroke Prevention in Atrial Fibrillation Investigators. Adjusted-dose warfarin versus low-intensity, fixed-dose warfarin plus aspirin for high-risk patients with atrial fibrillation: Stroke Prevention in Atrial Fibrillation III randomised clinical trial. Lancet 1996; 348: 633–8.
33. Gulløv AL, et al. Fixed minidose warfarin and aspirin alone and in combination vs adjusted-dose warfarin for stroke prevention in atrial fibrillation: Second Copenhagen Atrial Fibrillation, Aspirin, and Anticoagulation Study. Arch Intern Med 1998; 158: 1513–21.
34. Waldo AL. Treatment of atrial flutter. Heart 2000; 84: 227–32.
35. Lanzarotti CJ, et al. Thromboembolism in chronic atrial flutter: is the risk underestimated? J Am Coll Cardiol 1997; 30: 1506–11.
36. Wood KA, et al. Risk of thromboembolism in chronic atrial flutter. Am J Cardiol 1997; 79: 1043–7.
37. Seidl K, et al. Risk of thromboembolic events in patients with atrial flutter. Am J Cardiol 1998; 82: 580–3.
38. Morady F. Radio-frequency ablation as treatment for cardiac arrhythmias. N Engl J Med 1999; 340: 534–44.
39. Ganz LI, Friedman PL. Supraventricular tachycardia. N Engl J Med 1995; 332: 162–73.
40. Kugler JD, Danford DA. Management of infants, children, and adolescents with paroxysmal supraventricular tachycardia. J Pediatr 1996; 129: 324–38.
41. Pfammatter J-P, Bauersfeld U. Safety issues in the treatment of paediatric supraventricular tachycardias. Drug Safety 1998; 18: 345–56.
42. Kuck K-H, Schlüter M. Junctional tachycardia and the role of catheter ablation. Lancet 1993; 341: 1386–91.
43. Gaita F, et al. Wolff-Parkinson-White syndrome: identification and management. Drugs 1992; 43: 185–200.
44. Owen P, Cameron A. Fetal tachyarrhythmias. Br J Hosp Med 1997; 58: 142–4.
45. Simpson JM, Sharland GK. Fetal tachycardias: management and outcome of 127 consecutive cases. Heart 1998; 79: 576–81.
46. Dancy M. Diagnosis and management of ventricular tachycardia. Postgrad Med J 1992; 68: 406–14.
47. Campbell RWF. Ventricular ectopic beats and non-sustained ventricular tachycardia. Lancet 1993; 341: 1454–8.
48. Shenasa M, et al. Ventricular tachycardia. Lancet 1993; 341: 1512–19.
49. Welch PJ, et al. Management of ventricular arrhythmias: a trial-based approach. J Am Coll Cardiol 1999; 34: 621–30.
50. Cannom DS, Prystowsky EN. Management of ventricular arrhythmias: detection, drugs, and devices. JAMA 1999; 281: 172–9.
51. Ho DSW, et al. Double-blind trial of lignocaine versus sotalol for acute termination of spontaneous sustained ventricular tachycardia. Lancet 1994; 344: 18–23.
52. The Antiarrhythmics versus Implantable Defibrillators (AVID) Investigators. A comparison of antiarrhythmic-drug therapy with implantable defibrillators in patients resuscitated from near-fatal ventricular arrhythmias. N Engl J Med 1997; 337: 1576–83.
53. Gregoratos G, et al. ACC/AHA guidelines for implantation of cardiac pacemakers and antiarrhythmia devices: a report of the American College of Cardiology/American Heart Association Task Force on Practice Guidelines (Committee on Pacemaker Implantation). J Am Coll Cardiol 1998; 31: 1175–1209.
54. Buxton AE, et al. A randomized study of the prevention of sudden death in patients with coronary artery disease. N Engl J Med 1999; 341: 1882–90. Correction. ibid. 2000; 342: 1300.
55. The CAPS Investigators. The Cardiac Arrhythmia Pilot Study. Am J Cardiol 1986; 57: 91–5.
56. The Cardiac Arrhythmia Suppression Trial (CAST) Investigators. Preliminary report: effect of encainide and flecainide on mortality in a randomized trial of arrhythmia suppression after myocardial infarction. N Engl J Med 1989; 321: 406–12.
57. Echt DS, et al. Mortality and morbidity in patients receiving encainide, flecainide, or placebo: the Cardiac Arrhythmia Suppression Trial. N Engl J Med 1991; 324: 781–8.
58. The Cardiac Arrhythmia Suppression Trial II Investigators. Effect of the antiarrhythmic agent moricizine on survival after myocardial infarction. N Engl J Med 1992; 327: 227–33.
59. Morganroth J, Goin JE. Quinidine-related mortality in the short-to-medium-term treatment of ventricular arrhythmias: a meta-analysis. Circulation 1991; 84: 1977–83.
60. Waldo AL, et al. Effect of d-sotalol on mortality in patients with left ventricular dysfunction after recent and remote myocardial infarction. Lancet 1996; 348: 7–12. Correction. ibid.; 416.
61. Teo KK, et al. Effects of prophylactic antiarrhythmic drug therapy in acute myocardial infarction: an overview of results from randomized controlled trials. JAMA 1993; 270: 1589–95.
62. McAlister FA, Teo KK. Antiarrhythmic therapies for the prevention of sudden cardiac death. Drugs 1997; 54: 235–52.
63. Pfisterer ME, et al. Long-term benefit of 1-year amiodarone treatment for persistent complex ventricular arrhythmias after myocardial infarction. Circulation 1993; 87: 309–11.
64. Cairns JA, et al. Randomised trial of outcome after myocardial infarction in patients with frequent or repetitive ventricular premature depolarisations: CAMIAT. Lancet 1997; 349: 675–82.
65. Julian DG, et al. Randomised trial of effect of amiodarone on mortality in patients with left-ventricular dysfunction after recent myocardial infarction: EMIAT. Lancet 1997; 349: 667–74. Corrections. ibid.; 1180 and 1776.
66. Amiodarone Trials Meta-Analysis Investigators. Effect of prophylactic amiodarone on mortality after acute myocardial infarction and in congestive heart failure: meta-analysis of individual data from 6500 patients in randomised trials. Lancet 1997; 350: 1417–24.
67. Ben-David J, Zipes DP. Torsades de pointes and proarrhythmia. Lancet 1993; 341: 1578–82.
68. Viskin S. Long QT syndromes and torsade de pointes. Lancet 1999; 354: 1625–33.
69. Thomas SHL. Drugs and the QT interval. Adverse Drug React Bull 1997; 182: 691–4.
70. Doig JC. Drug-induced cardiac arrhythmias: incidence, prevention and management. Drug Safety 1997; 17: 265–75.

Cardiomyopathies

Cardiomyopathy is a term used to describe heart muscle disease. It is usually applied to a condition of unknown cause (idiopathic). Known causes of disorders of heart muscle such as systemic or pulmonary hypertension, ischaemic heart disease, valvular heart disease, congenital abnormalities, metabolic disorders, inflammatory or infectious diseases, and drug-induced conditions are excluded by some authorities when defining cardiomyopathy. Three distinct types of cardiomyopathy are generally recognised, namely dilated cardiomyopathy, hypertrophic cardiomyopathy, and restrictive cardiomyopathy; the dilated and hypertrophic forms are the two major types. The management of the individual forms has been reviewed.[1-8]

In **dilated cardiomyopathy** (previously known as congestive cardiomyopathy) the main finding is systolic dysfunction with dilated and poorly contracting ventricles and a low cardiac output. The right, left, or both ventricles may be affected. Although there may be some ventricular hypertrophy, because of the dilatation there is no overall increase in the thickness of the ventricle walls. Dilated cardiomyopathy may be asymptomatic for some time but the initial manifestations are commonly those of heart failure; chest pain, systemic and pulmonary embolism, and arrhythmias may also occur. If symptomatic heart failure is present, management should generally follow the conventional strategies for heart failure as outlined on p.798. One particular problem in dilated cardiomyopathy, because of blood stasis due to the poorly contracting ventricle, is the risk of systemic and pulmonary thromboembolism. Thus, chronic oral anticoagulation has been suggested for these patients although the current view appears to recommend it only in those with atrial fibrillation, previous systemic embolism, or severe left ventricular dysfunction.[1,9] Arrhythmias should be treated as appropriate (see under Cardiac Arrhythmias, above); amiodarone may be particularly suitable as it has no negative inotropic effect. Low-dose amiodarone may also be used in patients at high risk of sudden death, but its efficacy has not yet been confirmed.[1]

Although beta blockers have negative inotropic properties and were previously thought to be contra-indicated in patients with heart failure, they now have an accepted role in patients with stable left ventricular failure, including patients with idiopathic dilated cardiomyopathy. Early studies[10-12] in patients with dilated cardiomyopathy demonstrated significant improvements in cardiac function and symptoms, together with prevention of clinical deterioration, but failed to demonstrate a significant effect on overall mortality. However, a further trial evaluating carvedilol therapy in patients with heart failure, including patients with dilated cardiomyopathy, was terminated early because mortality was significantly reduced in the carvedilol groups[13] and the CIBIS-II trial[14] using bisoprolol was also terminated early because of favourable results. A further long-term study[15] using metoprolol has also reported a significantly higher survival rate in those receiving metoprolol for up to 7 years. Symptomatic improvement has also been reported with the calcium-channel blocker diltiazem.[16]

A number of surgical treatments have been tried but cardiac transplantation remains the principal method of improving survival in these patients. Other therapies that have been tried include growth hormone, thyroxine [levothyroxine], oxpentifylline [pentoxifylline], levocarnitine, and immunosuppressants for presumed myocarditis.

In **hypertrophic cardiomyopathy** (previously known as obstructive cardiomyopathy) there is, as the name implies, ventricular hypertrophy but the ventricles are not dilated. This leads to diastolic dysfunction since diastolic filling is impaired by the stiff hypertrophied ventricular walls. It is an inherited condition occurring as an autosomal dominant trait and can occur at any age although presentation during the second decade of life is common. Patients may be asymptomatic or may experience chest pain, syncope, dyspnoea, or arrhythmias. Sudden death associated with emotional stress or exercise is not an uncommon finding and patients should avoid strenuous exercise. However, overall life expectancy is similar to

that of the general population and many patients have little or no disability and do not require treatment.[5] Patients should be investigated for the presence of any arrhythmias and treated appropriately (see Cardiac Arrhythmias, above) although this may not necessarily prevent sudden death. Atrial fibrillation is particularly important and is probably most effectively treated with amiodarone.[4,5] Anticoagulation should be considered in all patients with sustained atrial fibrillation.[3-5]

Beta blockers may be used for control of symptoms. They curtail emotion- or exercise-induced tachycardia. Anginal pain is also reduced and syncopal attacks may be prevented. Calcium-channel blockers (usually verapamil) also improve symptoms and exercise tolerance and may be considered in those who continue to have disabling symptoms or who are unable to tolerate beta blockers.[17] However, in a crossover study[18] exercise capacity was not improved by either verapamil or nadolol, although most patients preferred one or other of the drugs rather than placebo and quality of life did appear to be improved by verapamil. Other drugs that may provide symptomatic relief include disopyramide, which is used for its negative inotropic effect. Diuretics may be needed for congestive symptoms but may also reduce cardiac output. Surgery to reduce outflow obstruction may be of benefit in some patients whose symptoms are resistant to drug therapy.[3-5]

The risk of sudden death is difficult to assess, particularly in asymptomatic patients. Neither beta blockers nor verapamil, as used for possible symptomatic relief, prevent ventricular arrhythmias. However, there is some evidence[19] that high-dose therapy with beta blockers may improve survival in children with hypertrophic cardiomyopathy. Low-dose amiodarone may have a role in high risk patients, but this remains to be confirmed;[20,21] implantable cardioverter-defibrillators are also used in some patients.[22]

In **restrictive cardiomyopathy** the filling of the ventricles is impaired, often due to endomyocardial fibrosis, resulting in predominantly diastolic dysfunction. Diuretics may improve congestive symptoms but should be used cautiously as they may decrease cardiac output. Arrhythmias should be treated if they are symptomatic and anticoagulation is advised, particularly in patients with atrial fibrillation, valvular disorders, or a low cardiac output.[6]

1. Dec GW, Fuster V. Idiopathic dilated cardiomyopathy. N Engl J Med 1994; 331: 1564–75.
2. Burch M, Runciman M. Dilated cardiomyopathy. Arch Dis Child 1996; 74: 479–81.
3. Elliott PM, McKenna WJ. Management of hypertrophic cardiomyopathy. Br J Hosp Med 1996; 55: 419–23.
4. Spirito P, et al. The management of hypertrophic cardiomyopathy. N Engl J Med 1997; 336: 775–85.
5. Maron BJ. Hypertrophic cardiomyopathy. Lancet 1997; 350: 127–33.
6. Kushwaha SS, et al. Restrictive cardiomyopathy. N Engl J Med 1997; 336: 267–76.
7. Oakley C. Aetiology, diagnosis, investigation, and management of cardiomyopathies. BMJ 1997; 315: 1520–4.
8. Elliott P. Diagnosis and management of dilated cardiomyopathy. Heart 2000; 84: 106–12.
9. Cheng JWM, Spinler SA. Should all patients with dilated cardiomyopathy receive chronic anticoagulation? Ann Pharmacother 1994; 28: 604–9.
10. Waagstein F, et al. Beneficial effects of metoprolol in idiopathic dilated cardiomyopathy. Lancet 1993; 342: 1441–6.
11. CIBIS Investigators and Committees. A randomized trial of β-blockade in heart failure: the cardiac insufficiency bisoprolol study (CIBIS). Circulation 1994; 90: 1765–73.
12. The Metoprolol in Dilated Cardiomyopathy (MDC) Trial Study Group. 3-year follow-up of patients randomised in the metoprolol in dilated cardiomyopathy trial. Lancet 1998; 351: 1180–1.
13. Packer M, et al. The effect of carvedilol on morbidity and mortality in patients with chronic heart failure. N Engl J Med 1996; 334: 1349–55.
14. CIBIS-II Investigators and Committees. The Cardiac Insufficiency Bisoprolol Study II (CIBIS-II): a randomised trial. Lancet 1999; 353: 9–13.
15. Di Lenarda A, et al. Long term survival effect of metoprolol in dilated cardiomyopathy. Heart 1998; 79: 337–44.
16. Figulla HR, et al. Diltiazem improves cardiac function and exercise capacity in patients with idiopathic dilated cardiomyopathy: results of the Diltiazem in Dilated Cardiomyopathy Trial. Circulation 1996; 94: 346–52.
17. Lorell BH. Use of calcium channel blockers in hypertrophic cardiomyopathy. Am J Med 1985; 78 (suppl 2B): 43–54.
18. Gilligan DM, et al. A double-blind, placebo-controlled crossover trial of nadolol and verapamil in mild and moderately symptomatic hypertrophic cardiomyopathy. J Am Coll Cardiol 1993; 21: 1672–9.
19. Östman-Smith I, et al. A cohort study of childhood hypertrophic cardiomyopathy: improved survival following high-dose beta-adrenoceptor antagonist treatment. J Am Coll Cardiol 1999; 34: 1813–22.
20. Clark AL, Coates AJS. Screening for hypertrophic cardiomyopathy. BMJ 1993; 306: 409–10.
21. Prasad K, Frenneaux MP. Hypertrophic cardiomyopathy: is there a role for amiodarone? Heart 1998; 79: 317–18.
22. Maron BJ, et al. Efficacy of implantable cardioverter-defibrillators for the prevention of sudden death in patients with hypertrophic cardiomyopathy. N Engl J Med 2000; 342: 365–73.

Cardiovascular risk reduction

Atherosclerotic cardiovascular disease includes coronary or ischaemic heart disease (myocardial infarction and angina pectoris), ischaemic stroke, and peripheral vascular disease. Coronary heart disease, in particular, is a major cause of mortality in developed countries, and cardiovascular disease overall is associated with considerable morbidity. The benefits of a number of interventions are well established in patients at high risk of cardiovascular disease, and identification and treatment of such people is therefore an important healthcare strategy.

Overall cardiovascular risk depends on a number of factors. Those who are at the highest risk are those with manifestations of atherosclerosis, particularly those who have already had a cardiovascular event such as a myocardial infarction or ischaemic stroke, as well as those with symptoms of angina or peripheral vascular disease. The major modifiable risk factors are tobacco smoking, raised blood pressure, and raised blood-lipid concentrations; other risk factors include age, sex, left ventricular hypertrophy, and family history. Diabetics are also at considerable risk of coronary heart disease, even when treated, and aggressive therapy to reduce risk may be appropriate.

Lifestyle and dietary modifications are the mainstay of risk reduction, particularly at a population level (see Atherosclerosis, p.793). However, in many people with high cardiovascular risk drug treatment may be required to modify risk factors. Interventions for which benefit is established include management of hypertension, modification of blood lipids, and antiplatelet therapy; tight control of blood glucose is also important in diabetic patients.

Guidelines for the treatment of hypertension and hyperlipidaemia have in the past focussed on specific levels of blood pressure and blood lipids. However, while patients with extreme hypertension or hyperlipidaemia are at substantial risk of morbidity from the disease itself and will require treatment regardless of overall risk, there is no clear cut-off between raised and normal blood pressure and lipids, and patients with only mild to moderate disease may still have an increased cardiovascular risk. Most guidelines now agree that treatment decisions should be based on the person's absolute level of cardiovascular risk. Assessment of risk is a complex procedure and risk and treatment tables are available to aid decisions about when to initiate therapy in patients without established cardiovascular disease.[1-3] They cover variables such as sex and age, and presence or absence of the risk factors of hypertension, smoking, diabetes mellitus, and left ventricular hypertrophy. Guidelines differ as to the level of risk at which treatment should be initiated; this is a matter of judgement and may depend on economic factors and the balance between benefit and risk of adverse effects in otherwise healthy people.

The assessment and treatment of *hypertension* is discussed on p.802. *Smoking cessation* is discussed on p.1642.

Hypercholesterolaemia is an established risk factor for atherosclerosis and cardiovascular disease. Epidemiological data show a progressive and continuous relationship between plasma-cholesterol concentrations and mortality from ischaemic heart disease. The 30-year follow-up of 4374 men and women from the Framingham Study[4] confirmed this continuous relationship which appeared strongest in subjects under 50 years of age, with a 9% increase in death from cardiovascular disease for each 10 mg per dL (0.26 mmol per litre) rise in total plasma-cholesterol concentration. Plasma-cholesterol concentrations of 5.2 mmol per litre (200 mg per dL) or less are associated with a low risk of ischaemic heart disease. The increased total plasma-cholesterol concentration associated with ischaemic heart disease is due mainly to raised low-density lipoprotein (LDL)-cholesterol. In contrast, high-density lipoprotein (HDL)-cholesterol is inversely associated with ischaemic heart disease. Low plasma concentrations of HDL-cholesterol (below 0.9 mmol per litre or 35 mg per dL) are generally associated with increased risk of ischaemic heart disease, whereas high concentrations are protective. There also appears to be an association between plasma-triglyceride concentrations and risk of ischaemic heart disease. Some triglyceride-rich lipoproteins such as chylomicron remnant particles and intermediate-density lipoproteins (IDL) are atherogenic and the risk of heart disease increases as triglyceride concentrations increase in patients with high total cholesterol and low HDL-cholesterol concentrations. Hypertriglyceridaemia alone (greater than

2.3 mmol per litre or 200 mg per dL) may be an independent risk factor for ischaemic heart disease, but any clinical benefit from intervention to lower triglyceride levels is yet to be established.[5]

Since the association between plasma-cholesterol concentrations and ischaemic heart disease is continuous there has been much debate over what should be considered a 'desirable' lipid concentration, at what point lipid-lowering treatment with diet and/or lipid regulating drugs is required, and how people with hyperlipidaemia should be identified (screening). British[1] and European guidelines[2] have advised that, in patients with cardiovascular disease or high cardiovascular risk, drug therapy should be added to dietary therapy if total plasma cholesterol remains above 5 mmol per litre and LDL-cholesterol above 3 mmol per litre despite dietary therapy. US guidelines[6] have suggested that drug treatment should be considered if the LDL-cholesterol level is 190 mg or more per dL. For patients with 2 or more risk factors, drug therapy should be considered if the LDL-cholesterol is 160 mg or more per dL, and for those with existing cardiovascular disease, diabetes mellitus, or particularly high risk, drug therapy should be considered if LDL-cholesterol is 130 mg or more per dL. The US guidelines also give target LDL-cholesterol levels of less than 160 mg, less than 130 mg, and less than 100 mg per dL, respectively, for the three risk groups.

Studies of cholesterol-lowering therapy have shown a reduction in coronary events, and angiography has demonstrated favourable effects on coronary artery lesions. The reduction in coronary events is seen in both dietary[7] and drug studies and has been most evident in patients at high risk, particularly those with established ischaemic heart disease (secondary prevention), and with statins.[8] There is also evidence of benefit for primary prevention of coronary heart disease,[9] and secondary prevention studies with statins have also shown a reduction in the incidence of stroke.[10-12]

There has been concern that there might be an association between low cholesterol concentrations and increased morbidity and mortality from non-cardiac causes including haemorrhagic stroke, cancer, accidents and suicide, and chronic respiratory, liver, and bowel disease.[13-18] However, meta-analyses have shown that statin therapy reduces all-cause mortality,[8] while any effect of non-statins or diet is probably not significant.[19]

Some studies[20-24] (those using drugs other than the statins) suggested that the maximum beneficial response to intervention may be delayed for several years after the start of therapy. Analysis of results of observational and randomised studies[24] indicated that little reduction in risk of ischaemic heart disease occurred in the first two years of treatment and that the full reduction took up to five years, although cholesterol concentrations had not been reduced sufficiently to produce significant reductions in ischaemic heart disease mortality. However, studies with statins[25] suggest that benefit may occur within 30 days when used for secondary prevention.

The statins have a more marked cholesterol-lowering effect than the older lipid regulating drugs such as colestyramine and clofibrate and in, for example, the large Scandinavian Simvastatin Survival Study (4S),[10,26,27] simvastatin was effective for the secondary prevention of ischaemic heart disease in patients with elevated cholesterol concentrations without increasing non-cardiac mortality. Reviews[28-30] of this and other studies have concluded that there is now clear evidence of benefit from reducing cholesterol concentrations in patients with pre-existing ischaemic heart disease. Another statin, pravastatin, has been found in the Cholesterol and Recurrent Events (CARE) Trial[31,32] and the Long-term Intervention with Pravastatin in Ischaemic Disease (LIPID) study[11] to be of benefit for secondary prevention in patients who have average, rather than elevated, cholesterol concentrations and such use has been advocated.[33] Data from the WOSCOPS trials[34-36] also indicate that pravastatin is effective for primary prevention in moderate hypercholesterolaemia. Similar findings have been published for lovastatin in patients with average cholesterol levels.[37]

The primary and secondary prevention studies have been predominantly in middle-aged men. Studies of statin therapy that have included women[11,27,37,38] have reported some benefits although the number of women studied has been too few to fully assess the effects of lipid-lowering treatment. Nevertheless, women should be assessed and treated similarly to men, depending on their level of risk.[39] Recommendations for the use of lipid-lowering

treatment in the elderly have been largely extrapolated from studies of younger patients, but secondary prevention studies including elderly patients (more than 65 years old) have reported benefits[27,40] and support these recommendations.[41]

Although most recent studies have used statins, beneficial effects for secondary prevention of ischaemic heart disease have also been reported for gemfibrozil[42] in men whose primary lipid abnormality was a low HDL-cholesterol level, and for omega-3 marine triglycerides[43] in a Mediterranean population.

Screening programmes have been introduced to identify people who require lipid-lowering therapy; in the USA it has been recommended that all adults over the age of 20 should have their blood-lipid concentrations measured every 5 years.[6] However, since the value of treatment in most of those tested is questioned, some consider that routine cholesterol measurements in healthy people are not warranted.[44,45] The risk assessment charts generally require lipid measurements for full assessment, although systems are available that use average population lipid levels and only require lipids to be measured in those who may be at high risk.[46]

A full lipoprotein analysis will identify those patients whose mild hypercholesterolaemia is due to very high plasma concentrations of HDL-cholesterol and thus avoid them undergoing inappropriate dietary or drug therapy. The triglyceride and HDL-cholesterol measurement may also influence the choice of drug as lipid regulating drugs differ in their effects on LDL- and HDL-cholesterol and triglycerides. Once a significant hyperlipidaemia has been identified then further investigations may determine whether the hyperlipidaemia is secondary to another condition or is a primary abnormality. Some secondary hyperlipidaemias respond to treatment of the underlying disease, for example hypothyroidism, whereas others may require lipid regulating therapy in addition to treatment of the primary condition, for example in diabetes mellitus and renal disease.

Other pharmacological treatments may be appropriate in specific disorders and are discussed in the individual disease reviews. The role of *antiplatelet therapy* is well established in the secondary prevention of coronary heart disease and ischaemic stroke, and aspirin has been recommended in all patients with atherosclerotic vascular disease.[1,2] Aspirin has also been tried for primary prevention of cardiovascular disease in healthy patients, but risks may outweigh benefits and it is not generally recommended (see under Myocardial Infarction, p.805, and Stroke, p.813). *ACE inhibitors* may also have a role; in the HOPE study,[47] treatment with ramipril significantly reduced the rate of death, myocardial infarction, and stroke in patients at high risk for cardiovascular disease.

1. Wood D, *et al.* Joint British recommendations on prevention of coronary heart disease in clinical practice. *Heart* 1998; **80** (suppl 2): S1–S29.
2. Wood D, *et al.* Prevention of coronary heart disease in clinical practice: recommendations of the second joint task force of European and other societies on coronary prevention. *Eur Heart J* 1998; **19**: 1434–1503.
3. Wallis EJ, *et al.* Coronary and cardiovascular risk estimation for primary prevention: validation of a new Sheffield table in the 1995 Scottish health survey population. *BMJ* 2000; **320**: 671–6. Correction. *ibid.*; 1034.
4. Anderson KM, *et al.* Cholesterol and mortality: 30 years of follow-up from the Framingham Study. *JAMA* 1987; **257**: 2176–80.
5. Sattar N, *et al.* The end of triglycerides in cardiovascular risk assessment? *BMJ* 1998; **317**: 553–4.
6. Expert Panel on Detection, Evaluation, and Treatment of High Blood Cholesterol in Adults. Executive summary of the third report of the National Cholesterol Education Program (NCEP) expert panel on detection, evaluation, and treatment of high blood cholesterol in adults (Adult Treatment Panel III). *JAMA* 2001; **285**: 2486–97.
7. Hooper L, *et al.* Dietary fat intake and prevention of cardiovascular disease: systematic review. *BMJ* 2001; **322**: 757–63.
8. LaRosa JC, *et al.* Effect of statins on risk of coronary disease: a meta-analysis of randomized controlled trials. *JAMA* 1999; **282**: 2340–6.
9. Pignone M, *et al.* Use of lipid lowering drugs for primary prevention of coronary heart disease: meta-analysis of randomised trials. *BMJ* 2000; **321**: 983–6. Correction. *ibid.*; 1519.
10. Pedersen TR, *et al.* Effect of simvastatin on ischemic signs and symptoms in the Scandinavian Simvastatin Survival Study (4S). *Am J Cardiol* 1998; **81**: 333–5.
11. The Long-Term Intervention with Pravastatin in Ischaemic Disease (LIPID) Study Group. Prevention of cardiovascular events and death with pravastatin in patients with coronary heart disease and a broad range of initial cholesterol levels. *N Engl J Med* 1998; **339**: 1349–57.
12. Plehn JF, *et al.* Reduction of stroke incidence after myocardial infarction with pravastatin: the Cholesterol and Recurrent Events (CARE) study. *Circulation* 1999; **99**: 216–23.
13. Jacobs D, *et al.* Report of the conference on low blood cholesterol: mortality associations. *Circulation* 1992; **86**: 1046–60.
14. Davey Smith G, *et al.* Plasma cholesterol concentration and mortality: the Whitehall Study. *JAMA* 1992; **267**: 70–6.
15. Law MR, *et al.* Assessing possible hazards of reducing serum cholesterol. *BMJ* 1994; **308**: 373–9.
16. Newman TB, Hulley SB. Carcinogenicity of lipid-lowering drugs. *JAMA* 1996; **275**: 55–60.

17. Zureik M, *et al.* Serum cholesterol concentration and death from suicide in men: Paris prospective study I. *BMJ* 1996; **313**: 649–51.
18. Golomb BA. Cholesterol and violence: is there a connection? *Ann Intern Med* 1998; **128**: 478–87.
19. Muldoon MF, *et al.* Cholesterol reduction and non-illness mortality: meta-analysis of randomised clinical trials. *BMJ* 2001; **322**: 11–15.
20. Oliver MF, *et al.* A co-operative trial in the primary prevention of ischaemic heart disease using clofibrate: report from the Committee of Principal Investigators. *Br Heart J* 1978; **40**: 1069–1118.
21. Lipid Research Clinics Program. The Lipid Research Clinics Coronary Primary Prevention Trial results I: reduction in incidence of coronary heart disease. *JAMA* 1984; **251**: 351–64.
22. Frick MH, *et al.* Helsinki Heart Study: primary-prevention trial with gemfibrozil in middle-aged men with dyslipidemia. *N Engl J Med* 1987; **317**: 1237–45.
23. Manninen V, *et al.* Lipid alterations and decline in the incidence of coronary heart disease in the Helsinki Heart Study. *JAMA* 1988; **260**: 641–51.
24. Law MR, *et al.* By how much and how quickly does reduction in serum cholesterol concentration lower risk of ischaemic heart disease? *BMJ* 1994; **308**: 367–73.
25. Aronow HD, *et al.* Effect of lipid-lowering therapy on early mortality after acute coronary syndromes: an observational study. *Lancet* 2001; **357**: 1063–8.
26. Scandinavian Simvastatin Survival Study Group. Randomised trial of cholesterol lowering in 4444 patients with coronary heart disease: the Scandinavian Simvastatin Survival Study (4S). *Lancet* 1994; **344**: 1383–9.
27. Miettinen TA, *et al.* Cholesterol-lowering therapy in women and elderly patients with myocardial infarction or angina pectoris: findings from the Scandinavian Simvastatin Survival Study (4S). *Circulation* 1997; **96**: 4211–18.
28. Oliver M, *et al.* Lower patients' cholesterol now. *BMJ* 1995; **310**: 1280–1.
29. van Boven AJ, *et al.* The 4S study: implications for prescribing. *Drugs* 1996; **51**: 507–14.
30. Pedersen TR, Tobert JA. Benefits and risks of HMG-CoA reductase inhibitors in the prevention of coronary heart disease: a reappraisal. *Drug Safety* 1996; **14**: 11–24.
31. Sacks FM, *et al.* The effect of pravastatin on coronary events after myocardial infarction in patients with average cholesterol levels. *N Engl J Med* 1996; **335**: 1001–9.
32. Sacks FM, *et al.* Relationship between plasma LDL concentrations during treatment with pravastatin and recurrent coronary events in the Cholesterol and Recurrent Events Trial. *Circulation* 1998; **97**: 1446–52.
33. Byrne CD, Wild SH. Lipids and secondary prevention of ischaemic heart disease. *BMJ* 1996; **313**: 1273–4.
34. Shepherd J, *et al.* Prevention of coronary heart disease with pravastatin in men with hypercholesterolemia. *N Engl J Med* 1995; **333**: 1301–7.
35. West of Scotland Coronary Prevention Group. West of Scotland Coronary Prevention Study: identification of high-risk groups and comparison with other cardiovascular intervention trials. *Lancet* 1996; **348**: 1339–42.
36. West of Scotland Coronary Prevention Study Group. Influence of pravastatin and plasma lipids on clinical events in the West of Scotland Coronary Prevention Study (WOSCOPS). *Circulation* 1998; **97**: 1440–5.
37. Downs JR, *et al.* Primary prevention of acute coronary events with lovastatin in men and women with average cholesterol levels: results of AFCAPS/TexCAPS. *JAMA* 1998; **279**: 1615–22.
38. Lewis SJ, *et al.* Effect of pravastatin on cardiovascular events in women after myocardial infarction: the Cholesterol and Recurrent Events (CARE) trial. *J Am Coll Cardiol* 1998; **32**: 140–6.
39. Mosca L, *et al.* Guide to preventive cardiology for women. *Circulation* 1999; **99**: 2480–4.
40. Lewis SJ, *et al.* Effect of pravastatin on cardiovascular events in older patients with myocardial infarction and cholesterol levels in the average range: results of the Cholesterol and Recurrent Events (CARE) trial. *Ann Intern Med* 1998; **129**: 681–9.
41. Grundy SM, *et al.* Cholesterol lowering in the elderly population. *Arch Intern Med* 1999; **159**: 1670–8.
42. Rubins HB, *et al.* Gemfibrozil for the secondary prevention of coronary heart disease in men with low levels of high-density lipoprotein cholesterol. *N Engl J Med* 1999; **341**: 410–18.
43. GISSI-Prevenzione Investigators. Dietary supplementation with n-3 polyunsaturated fatty acids and vitamin E after myocardial infarction: results of the GISSI-Prevenzione trial. *Lancet* 1999; **354**: 447–55.
44. American College of Physicians. Guidelines for using serum cholesterol, high-density lipoprotein cholesterol, and triglyceride levels as screening tests for preventing coronary heart disease in adults. *Ann Intern Med* 1996; **124**: 515–17.
45. Garber AM, *et al.* Cholesterol screening in asymptomatic adults, revisited. *Ann Intern Med* 1996; **124**: 518–31.
46. Robson J, *et al.* Estimating cardiovascular risk for primary prevention: outstanding questions for primary care. *BMJ* 2000; **320**: 702–4.
47. The Heart Outcomes Prevention Evaluation Study Investigators. Effects of an angiotensin-converting-enzyme inhibitor, ramipril, on cardiovascular events in high-risk patients. *N Engl J Med* 2000; **342**: 145–53.

Cerebrovascular disease

The term 'cerebrovascular disease' may cover disorders of the cerebral circulation such as ischaemic stroke and subarachnoid haemorrhage (see Stroke, below), but is often used to cover the rather vague concept of cerebrovascular insufficiency.

At one time it was believed that the dementia associated with Alzheimer's disease (p.1412) was due to cerebrovascular insufficiency and many drugs with vasodilator activity have been tried, but overall there is little convincing evidence of benefit. Ergot derivatives such as co-dergocrine mesilate and nicergoline have been commonly used; however, any effectiveness is now attributed to their action as metabolic enhancers or nootropic drugs rather than to vasodilatation and their place in therapy has still to be established. Calcium-channel blockers such as nimodipine are under investigation. Other vasodilators used have included buflomedil, cyclandelate, isoxsuprine, naftidrofuryl, oxpentifylline [pentoxifylline], and propentofylline.

Heart failure

Heart failure is a diagnosis made in a patient with a known or suspected cardiac disorder who presents with dyspnoea, fatigue, and oedema (peripheral and/or pulmonary).[1,2] It may be graded as mild, moderate, or severe depending upon whether symptoms such as dyspnoea and fatigue appear on ordinary physical exertion, on little exertion, or at rest, respectively. Another grading system (that of the New York Heart Association) has four grades (grades I, II, III, IV), again partly classified on appearance of symptoms in relation to exertion (with grade IV representing the most severe form). The discussion that follows focuses on the chronic form of heart failure. The management of acute heart failure resulting in cardiogenic shock is covered under Shock, below.

Heart failure is a common condition and is a consequence of cardiac abnormality, injury, or cardiovascular stress such as hypertension or valve disorders. Myocardial infarction is a leading cause of heart failure. Other cardiovascular disorders that may lead to heart failure include cardiomyopathies and cor pulmonale. Infections causing myocardial damage, and cardiotoxicity arising from alcoholism or induced by drugs may also be precipitating factors. The increased demands put on the heart by chronic severe anaemia or hyperthyroidism can also be causes.

Echocardiography is the most useful investigative procedure in patients with heart failure. It enables structural changes to be observed and rapidly identifies patients with potentially correctable abnormalities such as valvular disease. Although dysfunction of either the right or left ventricle (right- or left-sided heart failure) may occur in isolation, dysfunction of both ventricles is likely to be present to some extent; however, in most patients, and especially in those with heart failure following myocardial infarction, the predominant finding is that of a dilated and poorly contracting left ventricle. This represents left ventricular systolic dysfunction, in which both the ejection fraction and the cardiac output are low. Isolated left ventricular diastolic dysfunction, in which there is impaired ventricular filling but a normal ejection fraction, can also result in heart failure although this is less common; cardiac output may be normal but does not increase in response to exercise. Diastolic dysfunction is more common in the elderly and also occurs in some cardiomyopathies (see p.796); many patients have both diastolic and systolic dysfunction. As mentioned above, the term heart failure is usually employed to represent a symptomatic condition. However, echocardiographic investigation of some patients, especially those in the early postmyocardial infarction period, does reveal that asymptomatic left ventricular dysfunction occurs and many of these patients are treated in an attempt to prevent the development of full symptomatic disease. In theory, left ventricular systolic and diastolic dysfunction should be treated in different ways[3] and many of the guidelines are specific for systolic dysfunction. Few trials have specifically looked at patients with diastolic dysfunction; although many of the earlier drug trials were based on a clinical diagnosis of heart failure and may have included patients with diastolic dysfunction, therapy for diastolic dysfunction is not established and the discussion which follows relates to patients with systolic dysfunction unless stated otherwise.

Traditionally, heart failure has been defined as a condition in which the heart is unable to provide an adequate blood flow to meet the metabolic demands of the body and has been thought of in purely haemodynamic terms.[4] It is now appreciated that compensatory neurohormonal mechanisms play just as important a role in its development.[3-5]

Myocardial injury or impairment leads to an inability of the ventricles to empty adequately during systole. The resulting ventricular dilatation increases wall tension and initially leads to an increase in contraction while the decrease in cardiac output and blood pressure results in activation of the sympathetic nervous system, leading to an increase in the force and frequency of contraction. An increase in wall stress also occurs in the atria leading to secretion of atrial natriuretic peptide; this inhibits the release of noradrenaline but also has direct vasodilator and natriuretic actions that lower the haemodynamic load on the heart. Thus, in the short term, compensation for myocardial injury can occur and cardiac output may be maintained. In the long term, these compensatory haemodynamic and neurohormonal mechanisms become ineffective. Ventricular dilatation progresses, the sympathetic nervous system and renin-angiotensin system are persistently activated, ventricular hypertrophy occurs, and ventricular function deteriorates progressively.

Management. Heart failure is a progressively disabling condition associated with considerable morbidity and mortality. Management is aimed therefore not only at providing symptomatic relief, but also at improving prognosis. Reviews[1,2,6-11] and guidelines[12-15] have been published concerning management, although it has been suggested that the variable nature of heart failure may limit their use as absolute guidelines for therapy.[16]

Any underlying cause of heart failure should be corrected and certain non-pharmacological interventions may be beneficial. Weight reduction should be attempted in the overweight; moderate salt restriction may be undertaken; and, although in acute heart failure bed rest becomes necessary, in controlled chronic heart failure exercise should be encouraged. Immunisation with influenza and pneumococcal vaccines is advised.[12,14,15] Drug therapy of heart failure is based on the use of diuretics, ACE inhibitors, cardiac glycosides, beta blockers, and vasodilators. Other drugs that may have a role include angiotensin II receptor antagonists and spironolactone.

Diuretics have been the mainstay in the treatment of heart failure. They provide very effective symptomatic control in patients with peripheral or pulmonary oedema and rapidly relieve dyspnoea. If symptoms of fluid retention are only mild, a *thiazide diuretic*, such as *bendrofluazide [bendroflumethiazide]* or *hydrochlorothiazide*, may be adequate. However, in most cases, especially in moderate or severe fluid retention, a *loop diuretic* such as *frusemide [furosemide]* will be necessary. Combination treatment with diuretics that behave synergistically by acting at different sites (the principle of sequential nephron blockade), namely a loop diuretic with a thiazide or potassium-sparing diuretic, may be needed in some patients, especially when there is diuretic resistance.[17,18] *Spironolactone* is an aldosterone antagonist and has diuretic and, possibly, additional effects, as discussed below. However, diuretics are not a sufficient treatment on their own as clinical stability tends to deteriorate over time. In addition, there have been no long-term trials assessing the effect of diuretics on prognosis, and drugs that have been shown to have a mortality benefit are also required.

ACE inhibitors given orally produce clinical benefit in all stages of chronic heart failure additional to that seen with diuretics. They relieve symptoms such as dyspnoea and improve exercise tolerance. In addition, unlike with diuretics, studies have demonstrated that ACE inhibitors improve survival and reduce the progression of mild or moderate heart failure to more severe stages.[19] ACE inhibitors may also be beneficial in asymptomatic left ventricular dysfunction.[20] The Studies of Left Ventricular Dysfunction (SOLVD)[21] trials indicated that ACE inhibitors, in this case enalapril, might protect against myocardial infarction, unstable angina, and cardiac death in patients with either symptomatic or asymptomatic heart failure. ACE inhibitors are now recommended,[12-15,22] therefore, in all patients with symptomatic heart failure due to left ventricular systolic dysfunction, including those whose symptoms are controlled with diuretic therapy. The position in asymptomatic patients is less clear but some recommend that ACE inhibitors should be given to all patients with significantly reduced left ventricular ejection fraction, whether or not they have symptoms.

ACE inhibitors have also been given to patients shortly after suffering myocardial infarction but before the development of symptomatic heart failure and appear to be beneficial. However, it is not yet clear which patients should receive such therapy or when the optimum time to start ACE inhibitors is (see under Myocardial Infarction, below).

The precise mode of action of ACE inhibitors in heart failure is not completely understood but appears to be a result of both haemodynamic and neurohormonal mechanisms. They are vasodilators and cause both arteriolar and venous dilatation, mainly through reduction of angiotensin II formation. They also attenuate the ventricular dilatation and prevent the ventricular remodelling that develops after a myocardial injury. It has also been suggested that they may protect against the development of arrhythmias.[23]

Cardiac glycosides such as *digoxin* or *digitoxin* have an extremely long history in the management of heart failure. They are positive inotropes and increase the contractility of the heart thereby increasing cardiac output. Additional effects in heart failure appear to be due to neuroendocrine suppression such as inhibition of the sympathetic nervous system and indirect arterial vasodilatation.

The benefit of cardiac glycosides in heart failure accompanied by atrial fibrillation is not disputed although their role in patients with sinus rhythm has been debated. There is evidence that withdrawal of digoxin from patients receiving diuretics (the PROVED trial)[24] or ACE inhibitors (the RADIANCE study)[25] carries a considerable risk of clinical deterioration if they are stable on such combination therapy. The large DIG study[26] found that digoxin, given in addition to diuretics and ACE inhibitors, improved symptoms but had no effect on mortality. Digoxin may therefore have a role in patients who remain symptomatic despite ACE inhibitor, diuretic, and beta-blocker therapy,[12,13,27,28] and in those unable to tolerate ACE inhibitors.[15]

Beta blockers have negative inotropic properties and have generally been contra-indicated in patients with heart failure. However, persistent activation of the sympathetic nervous system is associated with disease progression and the benefit of beta blockers in the long-term management of heart failure is now established.[29-32] It is not clear whether all beta blockers are equally effective. Studies with *carvedilol*,[33,34] *bisoprolol*,[35] and *metoprolol*[36,37] have shown positive effects on mortality and morbidity in patients with varying degrees of heart failure and are acceptable therapy, although a meta-analysis[38] in patients with mild to moderate heart failure has suggested that vasodilating beta blockers have a greater effect on overall mortality than those that do not produce vasodilatation. The role of beta blockers in severe heart failure is less clear; a study with *bucindolol*[39] was stopped early because no mortality benefit was found, although carvedilol was found to reduce mortality in a similar study.[40] Beta blockers are now recommended[12-15] in all patients with clinically stable, mild to moderate heart failure due to left ventricular systolic dysfunction and should be given in combination with ACE inhibitors and diuretics. However, they must be introduced cautiously since symptoms may initially worsen. Beta blockers also appear to be of value in heart failure due to idiopathic dilated cardiomyopathy (see under Cardiomyopathies, above) and possibly in isolated diastolic dysfunction.

The effects of various *vasodilators* in heart failure have been studied in a series of Vasodilator-Heart Failure Trials (V-HeFT).[41] Oral nitrates, such as *isosorbide dinitrate*, produce a predominantly venous dilatation whereas *hydralazine* produces arterial vasodilatation and they are thus used in combination. They alleviate peripheral vasoconstriction and produce symptomatic control including a benefit on exercise tolerance but are of somewhat limited efficacy in long-term control. A modest improvement in long-term survival has been noted but this effect is less than that observed with the ACE inhibitors. The combination of isosorbide dinitrate with hydralazine may be considered in patients with left ventricular dysfunction who are unable to tolerate ACE inhibitors; they may also be used as adjuncts in patients who remain symptomatic despite therapy with ACE inhibitors, diuretics, beta blockers, and digoxin.

Angiotensin II receptor antagonists have been investigated as alternatives to ACE inhibitors.[42] The ELITE study,[43] which compared *losartan* with captopril in elderly patients with heart failure, found that both drugs had similar effects on renal function but other adverse effects were fewer with losartan and there was also a reduction in mortality in patients receiving losartan. However, the larger ELITE II study[44] failed to confirm any survival benefit with losartan. ACE inhibitors therefore remain first-line therapy, although other angiotensin II receptor antagonists, and the combination of angiotensin II receptor antagonists with ACE inhibitors, are being studied.[45]

Although the precise neurohormonal mechanisms leading to the development of heart failure are still not clear, there is evidence that raised levels of aldosterone may contribute to the pathophysiology.[46] ACE inhibitor therapy suppresses aldosterone production but this effect is not complete and the aldosterone antagonist *spironolactone* has been studied in combination with ACE inhibitors. In patients with severe heart failure, addition of low-dose spironolactone to therapy with ACE inhibitors and loop diuretics reduced the risk of death or hospitalisation,[47] and the use of spironolactone should therefore be considered in such patients.[12-15] However, the benefit in

patients with less severe heart failure remains to be established, and all patients receiving spironolactone with ACE inhibitors must have their plasma-potassium concentrations closely monitored.

Calcium-channel blockers, like beta blockers, have generally been contra-indicated in heart failure because of their negative inotropic activity. Despite this, their use as adjuncts has been investigated. Studies have failed to show any additional benefit with calcium-channel blockers in patients receiving standard therapy for heart failure. However, in both the PRAISE study[48] (using *amlodipine*) and the V-HeFT III study[49] (using *felodipine*), no adverse effect on morbidity or mortality was demonstrated, and amlodipine or felodipine might therefore be suitable as a treatment for angina or hypertension in patients with heart failure.

Phosphodiesterase inhibitors have a dual action being both positive inotropes and vasodilators. In theory, this is an attractive combination of mechanisms for use in heart failure but in general this group of drugs has not lived up to early expectations. Although short-term haemodynamic variables are improved, long-term oral use has been associated either with an unacceptable incidence of adverse effects (*amrinone*) or with an increased mortality rate (*enoximone*[50] and *milrinone*[51]). Thus, these phosphodiesterase inhibitors have been reserved for intravenous use in the short-term treatment of severe heart failure unresponsive to other treatment.[52-54] More recently introduced phosphodiesterase inhibitors include *vesnarinone* and *pimobendan*; they also have calcium-sensitising properties. Initial studies with vesnarinone indicated a survival benefit but a larger trial[55] has shown an increased mortality in patients receiving vesnarinone. The place of these drugs in the management of heart failure remains unclear.

Although *antiarrhythmics* are not routinely recommended in the management of heart failure, those that do not have a negative inotropic effect may have a role since sudden deaths have been attributed to ventricular arrhythmias in patients with severe heart failure. A meta-analysis[56] of 5 trials involving 1452 patients with symptomatic compensated heart failure indicated that *amiodarone* reduced the rate of arrhythmic or sudden death in high-risk patients and that this resulted in an overall reduction in mortality. However, amiodarone may have a number of adverse effects and it is not currently recommended in heart failure except in patients with symptomatic ventricular arrhythmias.

Several *miscellaneous drugs*, such as *flosequinan* (an arterial and venous vasodilator), *epoprostenol* (a prostaglandin), and *xamoterol* (a partial β_1-adrenoceptor agonist) have been tried in heart failure but have proved either disappointing or have been associated with excessive toxicity or an increased mortality rate. Pulsed β-stimulant therapy with *dobutamine* has been investigated but the oral dopamine agonist *ibopamine* appears to increase mortality in patients with severe heart failure.[57] Other drugs that are being studied in heart failure include *candoxatril*, which acts by inhibiting the metabolism of atrial natriuretic peptide, and *endothelin antagonists* such as *bosentan*. The role of *antithrombotic* therapy in patients with heart failure remains unclear.[14,58]

Many patients with chronic heart failure experience exacerbations of their condition (decompensated heart failure) requiring hospitalisation. Intravenous diuretics may be required for peripheral and pulmonary oedema; intravenous nitrates and intravenous inotropes may also be needed. Other drugs that may be used include natriuretic peptides such as nesiritide, and the calcium-sensitiser levosimendan.

Some patients with refractory heart failure may be suitable for surgical management. Heart transplantation is the optimum surgical therapy but availability is limited and a number of methods for augmenting the heart muscle or reducing ventricular dilatation are being investigated.[59]

1. Dargie HJ, McMurray JJV. Diagnosis and management of heart failure. *BMJ* 1994; **308:** 321–8.
2. Cohn JN. The management of chronic heart failure. *N Engl J Med* 1996; **335:** 490–8.
3. Gaasch WH. Diagnosis and treatment of heart failure based on left ventricular systolic or diastolic dysfunction. *JAMA* 1994; **271:** 1276–80.
4. Packer M. Pathophysiology of chronic heart failure. *Lancet* 1992; **340:** 88–92.
5. Schrier RW, Abraham WT. Hormones and hemodynamics in heart failure. *N Engl J Med* 1999; **341:** 577–85.
6. Baker DW, et al. Management of heart failure: 1. pharmacologic treatment. *JAMA* 1994; **272:** 1361–6.
7. Kleber FX, Wensel R. Current guidelines for the treatment of congestive heart failure. *Drugs* 1996; **51:** 89–98.
8. Bonarjee VVS, Dickstein K. Novel drugs and current therapeutic approaches in the treatment of heart failure. *Drugs* 1996; **51:** 347–58.
9. Forker AD. A cardiologist's perspective on evolving concepts in the management of congestive heart failure. *J Clin Pharmacol* 1996; **36:** 973–84.
10. Cleland JGF, et al. Successes and failures of current treatment of heart failure. *Lancet* 1998; **352** (suppl): 19–28.
11. Lonn E, McKelvie R. Drug treatment in heart failure. *BMJ* 2000; **320:** 1188–92. Correction. *ibid.*; **321:** 161.
12. Hunt SA, et al. ACC/AHA guidelines for the evaluation and management of chronic heart failure in the adult: a report of the American College of Cardiology/American Heart Association Task Force on Practice Guidelines (Committee to Revise the 1995 Guidelines for the Evaluation and Management of Heart Failure). Executive Summary: *J Am Coll Cardiol* 2001; **38:** 2101–13. Full version: http://www.acc.org/clinical/guidelines/failure/hf_index.htm
13. Task Force for the Diagnosis and Treatment of Chronic Heart Failure, European Society of Cardiology. Guidelines for the diagnosis and treatment of chronic heart failure. *Eur Heart J* 2001; **22:** 1527–60.
14. Packer M, Cohn JN, eds. Consensus recommendations for the management of chronic heart failure. *Am J Cardiol* 1999; **83** (suppl 2A): 1A–38A.
15. Scottish Intercollegiate Guidelines Network. *Diagnosis and treatment of heart failure due to left ventricular systolic dysfunction.* Edinburgh: SIGN Secretariat, 1999.
16. Parmley WW. Clinical practice guidelines: does the cookbook have enough recipes? *JAMA* 1994; **272:** 1374–5.
17. Ellison DH. The physiologic basis of diuretic synergism: its role in treating diuretic resistance. *Ann Intern Med* 1991; **114:** 886–94.
18. Krämer BK, et al. Diuretic treatment and diuretic resistance in heart failure. *Am J Med* 1999; **106:** 90–6.
19. Garg R, Yusuf S. Overview of randomized trials of angiotensin-converting enzyme inhibitors on mortality and morbidity in patients with heart failure. *JAMA* 1995; **273:** 1450–6.
20. Nelson KM, Yeager BF. What is the role of angiotensin-converting enzyme inhibitors in congestive heart failure and after myocardial infarction? *Ann Pharmacother* 1996; **30:** 986–93.
21. The SOLVD Investigators. Effects of enalapril on mortality and the development of heart failure in asymptomatic patients with reduced left ventricular ejection fractions. *N Engl J Med* 1992; **327:** 685–91.
22. Eccles M, et al. North of England evidence based development project; guideline for angiotensin converting enzyme inhibitors in primary care management of adults with symptomatic heart failure. *BMJ* 1998; **316:** 1369–75.
23. Campbell RWF. ACE inhibitors and arrhythmias. *Heart* 1996; **76** (suppl 3): 79–82.
24. Uretsky NF, et al. Randomized study assessing the effect of digoxin withdrawal in patients with mild to moderate chronic congestive heart failure: results of the PROVED trial. *J Am Coll Cardiol* 1993; **22:** 955–62.
25. Packer M, et al. Withdrawal of digoxin from patients with chronic heart failure treated with angiotensin-converting-enzyme inhibitors. *N Engl J Med* 1993; **329:** 1–7.
26. The Digitalis Investigation Group. The effect of digoxin on mortality and morbidity in patients with heart failure. *N Engl J Med* 1997; **336:** 525–33.
27. Packer M. End of the oldest controversy in medicine: are we ready to conclude the debate on digitalis? *N Engl J Med* 1997; **336:** 575–6.
28. Riaz K, Forker AD. Digoxin use in congestive heart failure: current status. *Drugs* 1998; **55:** 747–58.
29. Krum H. β-adrenoceptor blockers in chronic heart failure—a review. *Br J Clin Pharmacol* 1997; **44:** 111–18.
30. Eichhorn EJ. Restoring function in failing hearts: the effects of beta blockers. *Am J Med* 1998; **104:** 163–9.
31. Abraham WT. β-Blockers: the new standard of therapy for mild heart failure. *Arch Intern Med* 2000; **160:** 1237–47.
32. Hart SM. Influence of β-blockers on mortality in chronic heart failure. *Ann Pharmacother* 2000; **34:** 1440–51.
33. Packer M, et al. The effect of carvedilol on morbidity and mortality in patients with chronic heart failure. *N Engl J Med* 1996; **334:** 1349–55.
34. Australia/New Zealand Heart Failure Research Collaborative Group. Randomised, placebo-controlled trial of carvedilol in patients with congestive heart failure due to ischaemic heart disease. *Lancet* 1997; **349:** 375–80.
35. CIBIS-II Investigators and Committees. The Cardiac Insufficiency Bisoprolol Study II (CIBIS-II): a randomised trial. *Lancet* 1999; **353:** 9–13.
36. MERIT-HF Study Group. Effect of metoprolol CR/XL in chronic heart failure: Metoprolol CR/XL Randomised Intervention Trial in Congestive Heart Failure (MERIT-HF). *Lancet* 1999; **353:** 2001–7.
37. Hjalmarson Å, et al. Effects of controlled-release metoprolol on total mortality, hospitalizations, and well-being in patients with heart failure: the Metoprolol CR/XL Randomized Intervention Trial in Congestive Heart Failure (MERIT-HF). *JAMA* 2000; **283:** 1295–1302.
38. Bonet S, et al. β-Adrenergic blocking agents in heart failure: benefits of vasodilating and nonvasodilating agents according to patients' characteristics: a meta-analysis of clinical trials. *Arch Intern Med* 2000; **160:** 621–7.
39. The Beta-Blocker Evaluation of Survival Trial Investigators. A trial of the beta-blocker bucindolol in patients with advanced chronic heart failure. *N Engl J Med* 2001; **344:** 1659–67.
40. Packer M, et al. Effect of carvedilol on survival in severe chronic heart failure. *N Engl J Med* 2001; **344:** 1651–8.
41. Cohn JN. Vasodilators in heart failure: conclusions from V-HeFT II and rationale for V-HeFT III. *Drugs* 1994; **47** (suppl 4): 47–58.
42. Martineau P, Goulet J. New competition in the realm of renin–angiotensin axis inhibition; the angiotensin II receptor antagonists in congestive heart failure. *Ann Pharmacother* 2001; **35:** 71–84.
43. Pitt B, et al. Randomised trial of losartan versus captopril in patients over 65 with heart failure (Evaluation of Losartan in the Elderly Study, ELITE). *Lancet* 1997; **349:** 747–52.
44. Pitt B, et al. Effect of losartan compared with captopril on mortality in patients with symptomatic heart failure: randomised trial—the Losartan Heart Failure Survival Study ELITE II. *Lancet* 2000; **355:** 1582–7.
45. Struckman DR, Rivey MP. Combined therapy with an angiotensin II receptor blocker and an angiotensin-converting enzyme inhibitor in heart failure. *Ann Pharmacother* 2001; **35:** 242–8.
46. Struthers AD. Why does spironolactone improve mortality over and above an ACE inhibitor in chronic heart failure? *Br J Clin Pharmacol* 1999; **47:** 479–82.

47. Pitt B, *et al.* The effect of spironolactone on morbidity and mortality in patients with severe heart failure. *N Engl J Med* 1999; **341:** 709–17.
48. Packer M, *et al.* Effect of amlodipine on morbidity and mortality in severe chronic heart failure. *N Engl J Med* 1996; **335:** 1107–14.
49. Cohn JN, *et al.* Effect of the calcium antagonist felodipine as supplementary vasodilator therapy in patients with chronic heart failure treated with enalapril. V-HeFT III. *Circulation* 1997; **96:** 856–63.
50. Uretsky BF, *et al.* Multicenter trial of oral enoximone in patients with moderate to moderately severe congestive heart failure: lack of benefit compared with placebo. *Circulation* 1990; **82:** 774–80.
51. Packer M, *et al.* Effect of oral milrinone on mortality in severe chronic heart failure. *N Engl J Med* 1991; **325:** 1468–75.
52. Fischer TA, *et al.* Current status of phosphodiesterase inhibitors in the treatment of congestive heart failure. *Drugs* 1992; **44:** 928–45.
53. Packer M. The search for the ideal positive inotropic agent. *N Engl J Med* 1993; **329:** 210–2.
54. Nony P, *et al.* Evaluation of the effect of phosphodiesterase inhibitors on mortality in chronic heart failure patients: a meta-analysis. *Eur J Clin Pharmacol* 1994; **46:** 191–6.
55. Cohn JN. A dose-dependent increase in mortality with vesnarinone among patients with severe heart failure. *N Engl J Med* 1998; **339:** 1810–16.
56. Amiodarone Trials Meta-Analysis Investigators. Effect of prophylactic amiodarone on mortality after acute myocardial infarction and in congestive heart failure: meta-analysis of individual data from 6500 patients in randomised trials. *Lancet* 1997; **350:** 1417–24.
57. Hampton JR, *et al.* Randomised study of effect of ibopamine on survival in patients with advanced severe heart failure. *Lancet* 1997; **349:** 971–7.
58. Ezekowitz M. Antithrombotics for left-ventricular impairment? *Lancet* 1998; **351:** 1904.
59. Taggart DP, Westaby S. Surgical management of heart failure. *BMJ* 1997; **314:** 453–4.

High-altitude disorders

Rapid ascent (ascent without time to acclimatise) to high altitudes may produce a spectrum of illness (altitude illness) ranging from the usually benign acute mountain sickness to life-threatening pulmonary oedema and cerebral oedema. Factors influencing the development of altitude illness include rate of ascent, altitude attained, and length of stay at altitude. Individual susceptibility is also an important factor. Ascent to altitudes of 2000 to 3000 metres (6500 to 9750 feet) produces no ill-effects in most people although susceptible individuals may be affected at altitudes as low as 2000 metres.[1] Symptoms of altitude illness occur in about 50% of people ascending rapidly to altitudes of over 4000 metres (13 000 feet)[1] and in about 75% of people at 4500 metres (14 625 feet);[2] they are severe (pulmonary oedema or cerebral oedema) in about 4%.[1]

Symptoms of **acute mountain sickness** include headache, which is worse in the supine position, nausea, vomiting, anorexia, lethargy, insomnia, and dizziness. These may develop during ascent, but characteristically occur 6 to 48 hours after arrival at altitude. They are usually short-lived and resolve after a few days at altitude. In a very few people symptoms persist for longer. Chronic mountain sickness, characterised by persistent severe hypoxia and polycythaemia, may develop during prolonged residence at high altitude. The discussion that follows is limited to management of the acute forms. A small proportion of people with acute mountain sickness suddenly deteriorate and develop pulmonary oedema or cerebral oedema both of which may be life-threatening. Occasionally, pulmonary or cerebral oedema develops without symptoms of acute mountain sickness. Symptoms of **pulmonary oedema** include rapid onset of breathlessness and tachypnoea at rest, and a dry cough which may develop into haemoptysis. Symptoms of **cerebral oedema** include increasing headache, ataxia, mental disturbances, drowsiness and eventually coma. Pulmonary and cerebral oedema frequently occur together.

The **pathogenesis** of altitude illness is not fully understood, and it is not known whether the mechanisms of acute mountain sickness and pulmonary and cerebral oedema differ in nature or merely degree.[3] Hypoxia, a result of the reduced partial pressure of oxygen at high altitudes, is considered the primary stimulus in the development of altitude illness.[1-3] When ascent to high altitudes occurs gradually, the bicarbonate concentration and the pH of extracellular fluid fall progressively. The falling pH increases the sensitivity of chemoreceptors to hypoxia and so permits greater ventilation, thus allowing acclimatisation. Rapid ascent to high altitudes does not allow time for these changes to occur and although the hypoxia stimulates hyperventilation, it produces a respiratory alkalosis which limits the ventilatory response to hypoxia.[3] The hypoxaemia produced leads to alterations in fluid and electrolyte balance and haemodynamic changes responsible for the symptoms of altitude illness.

Symptoms are often worse at night when ventilation is reduced leading to a worsening of the hypoxaemia.[2]

Prophylaxis. Altitude illness may be avoided by ascending to high altitudes slowly and thereby allowing time for acclimatisation. This may be achieved by staying for 2 to 5 days at 2000 to 3000 metres and avoiding strenuous physical activity,[2,4] thus allowing the body to adapt to the reduced oxygen pressure and to ascend above 3000 metres without sickness. Acclimatisation may also be achieved when going above 3000 metres by limiting the rate of ascent to 300 metres a day with an intermediate night or two resting at a particular altitude.[1] Some recommend that after a couple of days this rate of ascent should be further reduced to 150 metres a day.[5]

However, when time for acclimatisation is limited or when abrupt arrival at high altitude (for instance by air) cannot be avoided, drug prophylaxis may be considered. Prophylaxis should also be considered for those individuals who have developed symptoms on ascending to high altitudes on previous occasions. Of the drugs tried for prophylaxis, only acetazolamide and dexamethasone have been shown to be effective.[6]

Acetazolamide is the most frequently used drug. It produces a mild metabolic acidosis which has the effect of stimulating chemoreceptors to produce an increase in the rate of respiration and tidal volume, and it therefore accelerates the process of acclimatisation. Although acetazolamide has diuretic actions it does not prevent fluid retention or prevent or protect against pulmonary or cerebral oedema. A reduction in the frequency of acute mountain sickness of about 30 to 50% has been reported with acetazolamide.[2] It improves sleep hypoxaemia and quality of sleep, reduces proteinuria, improves exercise performance, and reduces loss of muscle mass, probably by improving oxygen supply to the tissues.[3] Acetazolamide should be taken on the day of ascent or 1 or 2 days before ascent to altitudes above 3000 metres, and continued for at least 5 days at the higher altitudes.[2,4] Some have cautioned that the use of acetazolamide to prevent symptoms of acute mountain sickness may encourage too rapid an ascent and perhaps increase the risk of developing pulmonary or cerebral oedema.[3]

Dexamethasone has also been effective in the prevention of acute mountain sickness. The rationale for its use is that mild cerebral oedema is thought to contribute to the symptoms of acute mountain sickness.[2] However, as the side-effects associated with dexamethasone are more severe than those associated with acetazolamide, it is not considered suitable for prophylaxis in healthy people.[1] If it is used, dexamethasone should be taken on the day of ascent to high altitude (above 3000 metres), continued for 3 days at the higher altitudes, and then tapered over 5 days.[2]

Spironolactone has also shown some benefit, but it has only been investigated in a few people.[1]

Nifedipine has been shown to lower pulmonary artery pressure and to protect against pulmonary oedema in people susceptible to the development of pulmonary symptoms at altitude[7] but is not usually recommended for prophylaxis due to the risk of adverse effects.

Aspirin was reported[8] to reduce the incidence of headache in a small study in people with a history of headache at high altitude.

Treatment. Once symptoms of altitude illness develop the course of action should be determined by the severity and nature of the symptoms.

When symptoms are *mild* and are not suggestive of pulmonary or cerebral oedema, rest and mild analgesics for headache are usually all that is required; symptoms resolve within a few days and further ascent is possible.[2] *Acetazolamide* may have some benefit in relieving symptoms although it has only been studied in small numbers of patients.[9] If mild symptoms of pulmonary oedema are present, such as dyspnoea and cough, rest with supplementary oxygen and further oxygen at night may resolve the symptoms and allow further ascent;[4] however signs and symptoms at altitude may be confusing and it is always safest to descend. The use of hypnotics at altitude is not generally advised since there is a risk that respiratory depression may further reduce oxygen saturation. However, a small study[10] using the short-acting benzodiazepine *temazepam* reported that sleep quality was improved without an alteration in mean oxygen saturation.

When symptoms are *moderate to severe*, are progressing, or are suggestive of cerebral oedema, immediate descent is necessary. Descending by as little as 300 metres is beneficial.[2] Various drugs and therapies have been given to alleviate symptoms and to facilitate descent and should

also be employed when immediate descent is not possible. For example, *dexamethasone* can reduce the symptoms of acute mountain sickness and might be used in emergencies.[11,12] Portable hyperbaric chambers are available[1,13] and provide rapid but short-term improvement. They may be useful in combination with dexamethasone, which has a more sustained effect.[14]

If pulmonary oedema is present, oxygen, which relieves hypoxia and reduces pulmonary hypertension, should be given;[1] *nifedipine*, which suppresses the exaggerated hypoxic pulmonary vasoconstrictor response seen in people with pulmonary oedema, has provided benefit.[15,16] Positive-pressure expiration by use of a mask may also be useful;[1] it has the effect of increasing oxygen saturation and partial pressure of carbon dioxide at altitude. Inhalation of nitric oxide has also been reported to improve oxygenation but administration may not be feasible at altitude.[17]

People with cerebral oedema should be given *dexamethasone* and oxygen therapy.

1. Beeley JM, *et al.* Environmental hazards and health. *Br Med Bull* 1993; **49:** 305–25.
2. Johnson TS, Rock PB. Acute mountain sickness. *N Engl J Med* 1988; **319:** 841–5.
3. Dickinson JG. Acetazolamide in acute mountain sickness. *BMJ* 1987; **295:** 1161–2.
4. Anonymous. High altitude sickness. *Med Lett Drugs Ther* 1992; **34:** 84–6.
5. Pollard AJ. Altitude induced illness. *BMJ* 1992; **304:** 1324–5.
6. Dumont L, *et al.* Efficacy and harm of pharmacological prevention of acute mountain sickness: quantitative systematic review. *BMJ* 2000; **321:** 267–72.
7. Bärtsch P, *et al.* Prevention of high-altitude pulmonary edema by nifedipine. *N Engl J Med* 1991; **325:** 1284–9.
8. Burtscher M, *et al.* Aspirin for prophylaxis against headache at high altitudes: randomised, double blind, placebo controlled trial. *BMJ* 1998; **316:** 1057–8.
9. Grissom CK, *et al.* Acetazolamide in the treatment of acute mountain sickness: clinical efficacy and effect on gas exchange. *Ann Intern Med* 1992; **116:** 461–5.
10. Dubowitz G. Effect of temazepam on oxygen saturation and sleep quality at high altitude: randomised placebo controlled crossover trial. *BMJ* 1998; **316:** 587–9.
11. Ferrazzini G, *et al.* Successful treatment of acute mountain sickness with dexamethasone. *BMJ* 1987; **294:** 1380–2.
12. Levine BD, *et al.* Dexamethasone in the treatment of acute mountain sickness. *N Engl J Med* 1989; **321:** 1707–13.
13. Bärtsch P, *et al.* Treatment of acute mountain sickness by simulated descent: a randomised controlled trial. *BMJ* 1993; **306:** 1098–1101.
14. Keller H-R, *et al.* Simulated descent v dexamethasone in treatment of acute mountain sickness: a randomised trial. *BMJ* 1995; **310:** 1232–5.
15. Oelz O, *et al.* Nifedipine for high altitude pulmonary oedema. *Lancet* 1989; **2:** 1241–4. Correction. *ibid.* 1991; **337:** 556.
16. Jamieson A, Kerr GW. Treatment of high-altitude pulmonary oedema. *Lancet* 1992; **340:** 1468.
17. Scherrer U, *et al.* Inhaled nitric oxide for high-altitude pulmonary edema. *N Engl J Med* 1996; **334:** 624–9.

Hyperlipidaemias

Hyperlipidaemia, the elevation of lipid concentrations in plasma, is the manifestation of a disorder in the synthesis and degradation of plasma lipoproteins and may reflect a high-fat diet. A major concern in patients with hyperlipidaemia is their increased risk of ischaemic heart disease.

The **lipids** that are of relevance in hyperlipidaemias are cholesterol, an essential component of cell membranes and a precursor of steroid hormone synthesis, and triglyceride, an important energy source. They are transported in the blood as lipoproteins.

Lipoproteins are complex particles comprising a hydrophilic coat of phospholipids, free cholesterol, and specific polypeptides termed apolipoproteins (apoproteins) around a core of varying proportions of triglyceride and of cholesterol which is present as cholesteryl ester. The lipoproteins are characterised by their density which in general increases as they are metabolised and the proportion of cholesteryl ester to triglyceride increases. Table 1, below, lists the principal lipoproteins and their associated lipids. The lowest density lipoproteins are the **chylomicrons** which transport triglyceride derived from dietary fat, and the **VLDL** (very low-density lipoproteins; pre-β lipoproteins) which transport endogenous triglyceride mainly synthesised in the liver, to peripheral tissues. The triglyceride is hydrolysed in the peripheral

Table 1. Principal lipoproteins and associated lipids.

Lipoprotein	Lipid
Chylomicron	Triglyceride
VLDL	Triglyceride
IDL	Cholesterol and triglyceride
LDL	Cholesterol
HDL	Cholesterol

tissues by lipoprotein lipase, which is activated by apolipoprotein CII present in the lipoproteins. Both chylomicrons and VLDL are progressively depleted of triglyceride yielding increasingly dense lipoprotein particles termed 'remnant' particles. Chylomicron remnants are cleared rapidly from plasma by the liver where they are metabolised, releasing free cholesterol. VLDL remnants which include **IDL** (intermediate-density lipoproteins; broad β-lipoproteins) may also be cleared by the liver or converted to **LDL** (low-density lipoprotein; β-lipoprotein). **HDL** (high-density lipoproteins; α-lipoproteins) are synthesised in the liver and small intestine and have a role in the transport of cholesterol from the peripheral tissues to the liver. Cholesterol not utilised in the liver is secreted in the bile as bile acids and unesterified cholesterol. The majority is reabsorbed from the intestines and a small proportion is excreted in the faeces.

Hyperlipidaemias, sometimes referred to as dyslipidaemias, have been classified in various ways.[1] They may be described in terms of which lipid is elevated in the plasma, that is, as **hypercholesterolaemia, hypertriglyceridaemia**, or **'mixed' hyperlipidaemia** (where plasma concentrations of both cholesterol and triglyceride are raised). Alternatively, they may be described according to the lipoprotein abnormality and termed **hyperlipoproteinaemias**. This latter method, devised by Fredrickson, was adapted by the WHO and is still in common use. The WHO classification defines six types of hyperlipoproteinaemia, types I, IIa, IIb, III, IV, and V (see Table 2, above). Neither of these classification systems offers any information on the aetiology of the hyperlipidaemia, for instance, whether primary or secondary.

Primary hyperlipidaemias are those where the raised plasma-lipid concentration is the result of a genetic defect. The major primary hyperlipidaemias are given in Table 3, below. They include **monogenic hyperlipidaemias**, that is those which are the result of a single genetic defect and **polygenic** or **multifactorial hyperlipidaemias**, those where the raised plasma-lipid concentrations are the result of an interaction between genetic, dietary, and other environmental factors. The majority of people with hypercholesterolaemia fall into this latter group; the disorder is termed **common, polygenic**, or **multifactorial hypercholesterolaemia** and is generally associated with only mild or moderate elevation of plasma-cholesterol concentrations. Hyperlipidaemias caused by single genetic defects generally produce higher plasma-lipid concentrations.

Secondary hyperlipidaemias are those where the raised plasma-lipid concentration is caused by another disease state or by drug therapy. Diseases producing hypertriglyceridaemia include diabetes mellitus, chronic renal failure, and bulimia. Hypercholesterolaemia can occur in hypothyroidism, nephrotic syndrome, biliary obstruction, and anorexia nervosa. Drugs that may produce hypertriglyceridaemia and/or hypercholesterolaemia include thiazide diuretics (in high doses), beta blockers, corticosteroids, and antivirals in patients with HIV infection. Excessive alcohol intake may produce elevated plasma-triglyceride concentrations. Primary and secondary causes of hyperlipidaemia can co-exist in any individual.

The degree of hyperlipidaemia seen in patients with primary or secondary hyperlipidaemia is influenced by various factors, including, importantly, diet. A diet rich in saturated fat and cholesterol and poor in fibre can produce hypercholesterolaemia. Obesity further predisposes to hyperlipidaemia. Other factors that may influence lipid concentrations include pregnancy, lack of exercise, and smoking. Following myocardial infarction cholesterol levels may be temporarily reduced for several weeks; therefore, to measure the patient's usual level of cholesterol, blood samples should be taken within a few hours of the infarction.

The majority of people with hyperlipidaemia have plasma-lipid concentrations that are only mildly or moderately elevated, and they exhibit no **clinical symptoms**. At the other end of the spectrum, severe hypercholesterolaemia can cause tendon, tuberous, or planar xanthomas, xanthelasma, and arcus corneae; it is also associated with an increased risk of ischaemic stroke. Severe hypertriglyceridaemia can cause acute severe abdominal pain due to pancreatitis; hepatic and splenic enlargement, eruptive xanthomas, and lipaemia retinalis may also occur. Of particular significance though is the relationship between some hyperlipidaemias and premature ischaemic heart disease (before the age of 65) (see Table 3, below). In patients with very severe hypercholesterolaemia, such as familial hypercholesterolaemia, ischaemic heart disease may occur at a very young age; in those with the heterozygous form onset of heart disease during their 20s or 30s is not unusual, and in the rarer homozygous form ischaemic heart disease may develop by the age of 10. Even in people with less severe hyperlipidaemias serum cholesterol is an important determinant of cardiovascular risk (p.797) and treatment may be indicated on this basis.[2]

Treatment of hyperlipidaemias. The main aim of treatment in patients with hypercholesterolaemia is therefore to reduce the risk of developing ischaemic heart disease or the occurrence of further cardiovascular or cerebrovascular events in those with clinical evidence of ischaemic heart disease or peripheral vascular disease. In patients with severe hypertriglyceridaemia treatment is indicated to prevent attacks of acute pancreatitis. Treatment may also be indicated to promote the regression or non-progression of disfiguring xanthomas. The main methods of treating hyperlipidaemias are dietary and lifestyle changes and the administration of lipid regulating drugs. Some surgical and other procedures may also be used in familial hypercholesterolaemia (see below).

The basis of **dietary therapy** is weight reduction in the obese and a reduction in total fat intake. UK dietary recommendations include a reduction in saturated fatty acids, restriction of *trans* fatty acids, and increased consumption of long-chain n-3 polyunsaturated fatty acids; earlier restrictions on dietary intake of cholesterol and n-6 polyunsaturated fatty acids still stand.[3]

Dietary changes should be combined with other lifestyle changes such as cessation of smoking, increasing physical exercise, and moderation of alcohol intake. A reduced alcohol intake is especially advised in those with hypertriglyceridaemia. A more rigorous diet than that often recommended may be necessary for diet alone to be of much value.[4] Drug therapy is frequently necessary.

The principal groups of **lipid regulating drugs** (hypolipidaemic drugs) are the statins, fibric acid derivatives and related compounds, bile-acid binding resins, nicotinic acid and its derivatives, and the omega-3 marine triglycerides.

In general, **drug therapy** in patients without cardiovascular disease should only be initiated after an adequate trial of dietary modification has failed to reduce plasma-lipid concentrations sufficiently and should always be an adjunct to dietary modification and not a substitute for it. Patients who are likely to require drug therapy include those with severe hyperlipidaemia (familial hypercholesterolaemia, familial combined hyperlipidaemia, and familial dysbetalipoproteinaemia). Drug therapy may be started at the same time as dietary changes in those with clinical manifestations of ischaemic heart disease or peripheral vascular disease or who have undergone coronary artery bypass surgery, and those with major risk factors. Following an acute episode of unstable angina or myocardial infarction patients with raised cholesterol levels may be started on drug therapy, with dietary modification, at discharge from hospital.

The major primary hyperlipidaemias may be treated as follows.

- COMMON (POLYGENIC) HYPERCHOLESTEROLAEMIA. In this condition drug therapy may be considered if a sufficient trial of dietary modification fails to produce an adequate reduction in plasma-cholesterol concentrations. The decision to begin drug therapy depends on the estimated cardiovascular risk, including the degree of hypercholesterolaemia, other risk factors, and the presence of ischaemic heart disease or peripheral vascular disease. Treatment with one lipid regulating drug is usually sufficient. First-line drugs are now the statins; bile-acid binding resins or, if not tolerated, fibric acid derivatives, were previously used. Dextrothyroxine and neomycin have been used in patients with

Table 2. Classification of hyperlipoproteinaemias.

WHO classification	Lipoproteins elevated	Plasma lipids affected	
		Cholesterol	Triglyceride
I	Chylomicrons	Normal or elevated	Elevated
IIa	LDL	Elevated	Normal
IIb	LDL and VLDL	Elevated	Elevated
III	VLDL with abnormally high cholesterol content	Elevated	Elevated
IV	VLDL	Normal or elevated	Elevated
V	Chylomicrons and VLDL	Elevated	Elevated

Table 3. Primary hyperlipidaemias.

	WHO type	Prevalence	Typical lipid concentrations (mmol/L)		Risk of IHD	Pancreatitis
			Cholesterol	Triglyceride		
Common (polygenic) hypercholesterolaemia	IIa, IIb	Very common	6.5 to 9.0	< 2.3	+	–
Familial hypercholesterolaemia	IIa, IIb	Moderately common	7.5 to 16.0	< 2.3	+++	–
Familial hypertriglyceridaemia	IV, V	Common	6.5 to 12.0	10 to 30	?	++
Familial combined hyperlipidaemia	IIa, IIb, IV, and V	Common	6.5 to 10.0	2.3 to 12.0	++	–
Familial dysbetalipoproteinaemia or remnant hyperlipoproteinaemia	III	Uncommon	9.0 to 14.0	9.0 to 14.0	++	+
Abnormal lipoprotein lipase function	I	Rare	< 6.5	10.0 to 30.0	–	+++

+ = elevated risk; – = no risk; ? = uncertain risk; IHD = ischaemic heart disease hypercholesterolaemia but have generally been abandoned in favour of more effective or safer drugs.

- FAMILIAL HYPERCHOLESTEROLAEMIA. Patients with familial hypercholesterolaemia usually have very high plasma-cholesterol concentrations which rarely respond adequately to diet alone and drug therapy is therefore often necessary in this high-risk group. Aggressive therapy may lead to regression of atherosclerotic lesions.[5] The first-line drugs are the statins. In severe cases combination therapy is usually required. A statin together with a bile-acid binding resin may be used. A low dose of the bile-acid binding resin may be sufficient. In the homozygous form of familial hypercholesterolaemia there may be a complete lack of functional LDL-receptors and drugs that act by increasing LDL-receptors, such as statins and bile-acid binding resins, may be ineffective. However, statins may be useful as adjunctive therapy in those patients who have some LDL-receptor function. In some forms of familial hypercholesterolaemia, and where plasma-cholesterol concentrations are very high, plasma-triglyceride concentrations may also be raised. In these cases a fibric acid derivative or nicotinic acid may be effective, and in more severe cases the combination of a bile-acid binding resin together with a fibric acid derivative or a statin may be used. In patients with the homozygous form liver transplantation is the most definitive treatment. Plasma exchange (weekly or fortnightly) or more selective procedures such as LDL apheresis, including the use of heparin to precipitate LDL (the HELP system—Heparin Extracorporeal LDL Precipitation) may also be used in combination with lipid regulating drugs. Gene therapy is under investigation as a treatment for familial hypercholesterolaemia.

- FAMILIAL HYPERTRIGLYCERIDAEMIA. In patients with familial hypertriglyceridaemia dietary therapy is generally adequate, but drugs may be required if there is a high risk of acute pancreatitis or if there is a family history of atherosclerosis. The risk of acute pancreatitis is high when plasma-triglyceride concentrations are above 20 mmol per litre. Nicotinic acid or the fibric acid derivatives, particularly gemfibrozil, are generally recommended and may be used in combination in severe cases. Omega-3 marine triglycerides may also be of value. In severe intractable hypertriglyceridaemia, particularly type V hyperlipoproteinaemia, norethisterone has been suggested for women or oxandrolone for men.

- FAMILIAL COMBINED HYPERLIPIDAEMIA. Drug therapy may be used in patients who do not respond to dietary therapy alone. The choice will depend on the predominant lipid abnormality. A statin is the first choice in cases where hypercholesterolaemia is predominant. A fibric acid derivative may be first choice when hypertriglyceridaemia predominates, and nicotinic acid is useful where plasma concentrations of triglyceride and cholesterol are elevated to a similar degree. Bile-acid binding resins should not be used alone since they can aggravate hypertriglyceridaemia, but they may be useful in combination with a triglyceride-lowering drug in some patients. Treatment with a combination of drugs that lowers both cholesterol and triglyceride concentrations may be required in some patients especially in those with markedly raised plasma concentrations of triglyceride or cholesterol, as treatment of these patients with drugs effective against only one lipid may produce a rise in the plasma-concentrations of the other lipid. Many different combinations of lipid regulating drugs have been used, including combinations of statins and fibric acid derivatives; this combination is not recommended for routine use because of the possibility of increased adverse effects, but may be useful in selected patients. The choice of treatment in these cases is largely empirical as responses are not always predictable in individual patients.

- FAMILIAL DYSBETALIPOPROTEINAEMIA (remnant hyperlipoproteinaemia; remnant particle disease). In this lipid disorder the degree of hyperlipidaemia is usually severe and, although it may respond remarkably to dietary therapy, drug treatment is usually necessary. Fibric acid derivatives are the first-choice drugs. Statins or nicotinic acid may also be used.

- ABNORMAL LIPOPROTEIN LIPASE FUNCTION (chylomicronaemia). No drugs currently available are useful in this disorder. The condition is treated with severe restric-

tion of dietary fat, and the diet may be supplemented by medium chain triglycerides to improve tolerability.

1. Beaumont JL, et al. Classification of hyperlipidaemias and hyperlipoproteinaemias. Bull WHO 1970; 43: 891–915.
2. Expert Panel on Detection, Evaluation, and Treatment of High Blood Cholesterol in Adults. Executive summary of the third report of the National Cholesterol Education Program (NCEP) expert panel on detection, evaluation, and treatment of high blood cholesterol in adults (Adult Treatment Panel III). JAMA 2001; 285: 2486–97.
3. DoH. Nutritional aspects of cardiovascular disease. Report on health and social subjects 46. London: HMSO, 1994.
4. Ramsay LE, et al. Dietary reduction of serum cholesterol concentration: time to think again. BMJ 1991; 303: 953–7.
5. Smilde TJ, et al. Effect of aggressive versus conventional lipid lowering on atherosclerosis progression in familial hypercholesterolaemia (ASAP): a prospective, randomised, double-blind trial. Lancet 2001; 357: 577–81.

Hypertension

Hypertension, particularly essential or primary hypertension, is widespread and although usually asymptomatic, is a major risk factor for stroke and to some extent ischaemic heart disease. Series of reviews in Br Med Bull,[1] a 1994 Lancet octet, and a 1996 issue of JAMA have addressed various aspects of hypertension including definitions, classifications, origins, risk factors, non-pharmacological and pharmacological treatment interventions, and target-organ disease. National[2,3] and international[4,5] guidelines on management have also been published.

Definitions. The term *blood pressure* generally means arterial blood pressure, that is the pressure of the blood on artery walls. It is usually measured indirectly in the brachial artery just above the elbow using a mercury sphygmomanometer and is expressed in mmHg. Two measurements are made: *systolic* or maximum blood pressure (achieved during ventricular contraction of the heart) and *diastolic* or minimum blood pressure (achieved during ventricular dilatation). *Hypertension* means a higher than 'normal' blood pressure. Many factors influence blood pressure, resulting in a bell-shaped distribution curve in the general population, and in consequence it is difficult to define an absolute norm. An arbitrary definition of *normal* adult blood pressure[3,4] is a systolic pressure below 130 mmHg together with a diastolic pressure below 85 mmHg (i.e. below 130/85), while blood pressures of 130-139/85-89 mmHg are regarded as high normal. An *optimal* blood pressure, with respect to cardiovascular risk, of less than 120/80 mmHg has also been suggested.[3,4] Although hypertension has frequently been defined in terms of diastolic pressure alone, there is some evidence that the systolic pressure is an important predictor of risk,[6] and both are now considered to be of equal importance for guiding treatment.

Hypertension has often been classified as mild, moderate, or severe. However, these terms may be misleading since absolute cardiovascular risk is more important in determining the need for treatment and also depends on other factors (see below). In the US[3] and WHO/ISH (International Society of Hypertension)[4] guidelines a staging or grading system is preferred for classification, as follows:

stage/grade 1: 140–159/90–99 mmHg;
stage/grade 2: 160–179/100–109 mmHg;
stage/grade 3: ≥180/≥110 mmHg.

When systolic and diastolic pressure fall into different categories the higher value is used for classification purposes. Classification and subsequent treatment decisions should be based on blood pressure measurements taken on several occasions over a period that varies according to the severity of hypertension. Ambulatory blood pressure monitoring may be used in some cases.[2-4,7] However, readings tend to be lower with ambulatory monitoring than with conventional measurement and normal and abnormal values are not yet clearly established, although recommendations have been made.[2,7]

In *malignant* or *accelerated hypertension* rapidly progressing severe hypertension is associated with retinopathy and often renal impairment.

Isolated systolic hypertension occurs mainly in the elderly and has been defined as systolic pressure of 160 mmHg or higher[2] (or 140 mmHg or more[3,4]) and diastolic pressure under 90 mmHg.

Origins. In the majority of cases of hypertension the cause is unknown, and it is suspected that such *primary* or *essential* hypertension is multifactorial in origin, and that genotype, as well as external factors such as diet and body-weight, may play a role. Hypertension may also be associated with surgery and pregnancy and is prevalent in diabetics. In a limited number of cases hypertension is

secondary to some other condition, such as renal disease, Cushing's syndrome, phaeochromocytoma, or the adverse effects of drugs such as oestrogens, and such causes may be suspected particularly in resistant or malignant hypertension. Although treatment of the underlying condition will generally be desirable, the resultant hypertension will not necessarily be abolished by this.

Management of hypertension. Most of what follows relates to primary or essential hypertension in adults. Hypertensive crises and hypertension associated with surgery, diabetes, renal disease, or pregnancy are also discussed below under separate headings.

Hypertension may be discovered because of adverse vascular events, especially in the eyes, brain, kidneys, or heart, but is more often asymptomatic and only discovered on routine measurement of blood pressure. As already mentioned, the dividing line between normal and raised blood pressure is fairly arbitrary, but may be defined as the level of blood pressure above which intervention has been shown to reduce the associated cardiovascular risk. It is well-established that hypertension is a risk factor for the development of stroke, heart failure, and renal damage, and to a lesser extent ischaemic heart disease, and a reduction in blood pressure is generally beneficial, although mortality remains higher than in non-hypertensives.[8] However, it is important to assess hypertension in the context of other cardiovascular risk factors such as increasing age, male gender, postmenopausal status, previous cardiovascular events, target-organ disease such as left ventricular hypertrophy or renal disease, smoking, diabetes, dyslipidaemia, obesity, and sedentary life-style. All patients with sustained hypertension of stage/grade 2 or above can be considered at high risk and should be treated irrespective of other risk factors. For patients with 'mild' hypertension, however, the decision to treat is more complex; the absolute cardiovascular risk may range from low to high depending on what other risk factors are present, and the need for treatment depends on assessment of their overall risk.

In addition to specific antihypertensive treatment other cardiovascular risk factors should be reduced and co-existing disease dealt with. Guidelines on the management of hypertension may differ in detail, but reflect judgement on when intervention, both non-pharmacological and pharmacological, is justified.

Non-pharmacological treatment. In patients with mild hypertension and no other risk factors control of blood pressure by non-pharmacological means may be attempted and patients requiring drug therapy to reduce their blood pressure will also benefit from such life-style changes. A number of non-pharmacological options have been recommended to reduce blood pressure[2-4,9,10] and these include: reduction in excess weight; reduction in excess alcohol consumption; reduction in sodium intake; adequate exercise; reduced fat intake; and increased fruit and vegetable consumption. Tobacco smoking, a major risk factor for cardiovascular disease, should also be stopped. Other interventions tried, but with less evidence of benefit include: increased intake of potassium, magnesium, and calcium; increased polyunsaturated fat intake with reduced saturated fat intake; and relaxation therapies for stress reduction.

These life-style changes may also be promoted in the population as a whole, or in individuals most likely to develop hypertension, in strategies for the *primary prevention* of high blood pressure.

Pharmacological treatment. What needs to be decided before embarking on drug therapy of hypertension is: when to intervene with antihypertensive drugs, what the treatment goal is, and what drug regimen to choose. In patients with mild to moderate (grade 1 or 2) hypertension drug treatment should not generally be initiated until after an adequate period of observation including monitoring of blood pressure; this may extend to 3 to 6 months although the higher the blood pressure the shorter the observation period.

When to intervene with antihypertensive drugs depends on a number of factors. The guidelines differ in detail, but in general all patients with a sustained blood pressure of 160/100 mmHg or higher should be treated. For patients with a sustained blood pressure of 140/90 mmHg or higher, the decision to intervene depends on assessment of the overall cardiovascular risk. In patients who have diabetes, renal disease, or heart failure, the US guidelines[3] recommend that drug treatment should be initiated if the blood pressure is in the high normal range. For *elderly patients* (over 60 years) the benefit of treating hypertension has been established in several trials.[6,11-13]

Those with diastolic blood pressure above 90 mmHg, and those with systolic blood pressure above 160 mmHg but with diastolic below 90 mmHg (isolated systolic hypertension) should be treated with antihypertensive drugs. For those with borderline isolated systolic hypertension (systolic above 140 mmHg with diastolic below 90 mmHg) the situation is less well established and patients should be assessed individually. In the very old (those over 80 years) the benefit of initiating therapy is also less clear, although those already being treated should continue. Benefit is evident up to at least 80 years of age and a strict age limit to drug therapy is probably inappropriate. This view is supported by a meta-analysis[14] of subgroup data from controlled trials, but results of a specific trial are needed for confirmation.

Treatment goals are controversial. There has been concern that over-aggressive reduction of diastolic pressure might increase the risk of ischaemic heart disease.[15] There is now evidence that effective blood-pressure control to maintain the diastolic pressure below 90 mmHg (at about 85 mmHg) reduces the rate of cardiovascular events, but lower pressures (of around 70 mmHg) may not provide any further benefit.[16] The British Hypertension Society[2] now suggests a target of below 140/85 mmHg, with a lower target of below 140/80 mmHg in diabetics; lower targets should also be considered in patients with nephropathy. Both the US and WHO/ISH guidelines cite an optimal blood pressure of below 120/80 mmHg, although the treatment goal suggested in the US guidelines is below 140/90 mmHg. The WHO/ISH guidelines, on the other hand, suggest that blood pressure should be reduced to optimal or normal (below 130/85 mmHg) in young, middle-aged, or diabetic patients; however, this recommendation has been widely criticised.[17]

The drug regimen may include drugs from a number of groups that have antihypertensive effects. These groups have differing pharmacological actions although the precise mechanism is not understood in all cases. Thiazide diuretics and beta blockers have been the mainstay of drug therapy for hypertension, but more recently the availability of other drug groups such as calcium-channel blockers, ACE inhibitors, alpha blockers, and angiotensin II receptor antagonists, as well as concern about the possible metabolic effects of thiazides and beta blockers has led to increasing use of these newer drugs.

Choice of initial therapy has been controversial.[18,19] Studies such as the TOMHS[20] (comparing chlortalidone, acebutolol, amlodipine, enalapril, and doxazosin), and a similar study[21] (comparing hydrochlorothiazide, atenolol, diltiazem, captopril, prazosin, and clonidine), have shown that the response to the 5 main types of antihypertensive drug is similar. Each type will provide control in about 50% of patients, although the response may also depend on individual factors such as age[22] and race.[23] Tolerance of the drug groups is also similar, although results from an interim analysis[24] of the ALLHAT study have suggested that the risk of developing heart failure may be greater with doxazosin than with chlortalidone.

All of the main drug groups are therefore established as effective antihypertensives, but their effects on long-term mortality and morbidity are less clear. Only diuretics (particularly thiazides) and beta blockers have been adequately tested in long-term trials in hypertensive patients, and one systematic review[25] concluded that thiazides continue to show the best evidence of benefit. There is some evidence that other drug groups may be comparable,[26] but further studies are still required to confirm this. The UK guidelines therefore continue to recommend thiazides and beta blockers as first-line drugs; the other drug groups may be used where there are contra-indications or adverse effects, or in some co-existing diseases. The WHO/ISH guidelines, while acknowledging the lack of data supporting the newer drug groups, also point out that there is no evidence that the benefits of treating hypertension relate to the drug used rather than to the degree of blood pressure reduction obtained. They therefore suggest that all the available drug classes are suitable for initial therapy, although in some patients there are compelling or relative indications for the choice of a particular group; contra-indications should also be considered. The US guidelines follow a similar approach, although they recommend diuretics or beta blockers as first-line in uncomplicated hypertension. Compelling indications suggested include the use of ACE inhibitors in diabetics with nephropathy, diuretics or calcium-channel blockers in elderly patients, and beta blockers in patients who have had a myocardial infarction. Additional considerations include the lower efficacy of beta blockers and ACE inhibitors in Afro-Caribbean blacks. Angiotensin II receptor antagonists may be considered as an alternative to ACE inhibitors when persistent cough associated with the latter is unacceptable. The role of calcium-channel blockers is controversial;[27] although they have been widely used, the safety of short-acting dihydropyridine calcium-channel blockers has been questioned and some recommend that they should be avoided (see under Adverse Effects of Nifedipine, p.940). Long-acting dihydropyridines appear to be safe and, as mentioned above, may be a suitable choice in elderly patients.

Having decided what drug to use, treatment is started at the lowest recommended dose.[28] If this is ineffective or only partially effective the dose may be increased (except in the case of thiazide diuretics where there is generally no additional benefit, but more adverse effects); alternatively another first-line drug may either be substituted (sequential therapy) or added. Two-drug combinations will control blood pressure in a higher proportion of patients and may be necessary in most patients to achieve optimal levels, although the effects of the two drugs may not be fully additive.[29] Combination therapy also allows lower doses of the individual drugs to be used with a consequent reduction in adverse effects. The most effective combinations involve drugs that act on different physiological systems; appropriate combinations include: a diuretic plus a beta blocker, an ACE inhibitor, or an alpha blocker; a calcium-channel blocker plus an ACE inhibitor, an alpha blocker, or (except with verapamil) a beta blocker; an alpha blocker plus any other class. A 3-drug combination is often required, especially in severe hypertension. In patients who maintain an elevated diastolic blood pressure despite triple therapy the possibility of secondary hypertension should be considered, although factors such as non-compliance, NSAID use, or alcohol abuse may contribute to resistance.[30,31]

Other classes of antihypertensive drugs that are sometimes used include centrally acting drugs such as clonidine, methyldopa, and the less sedating moxonidine, and direct-acting vasodilators such as hydralazine and minoxidil. Older drugs like the adrenergic neurone blocker guanethidine and the rauwolfia alkaloid reserpine are rarely recommended now. Renin inhibitors, endopeptidase inhibitors, and endothelin antagonists are under investigation. In patients with other cardiovascular risk factors therapy with, for example, aspirin and statins should also be considered.

Withdrawal of drug treatment. It has been standard teaching that drug treatment for hypertension is continued indefinitely, but there have been some reports of successful withdrawal in selected patients.[32,33] Some guidelines[3,4] suggest that, once hypertension is controlled, a reduction in dosage or even withdrawal of antihypertensive drugs may be possible in patients with mild hypertension provided that blood pressure is consistently controlled, there is no evidence of target-organ damage, and blood pressure continues to be monitored. In these patients, non-pharmacological measures should be continued indefinitely.

Hypertensive crises. Patients with severe hypertension may be divided into those in whom there is evidence of rapid or progressive CNS, cardiovascular, or renal deterioration (hypertensive *emergencies*) and those with no evidence of target-organ damage (urgent hypertensive crises or hypertensive *urgencies*).[34,35] In the former case the goal is a reduction in mean arterial blood pressure by 25%, or a fall in diastolic blood pressure to 100 to 110 mmHg, over a period of several minutes to several hours depending on the clinical situation; intravenous therapy is often required although oral therapy may be adequate. In the latter case a drastic reduction in blood pressure is inappropriate and oral therapy is preferred, with the aim of a reduction in blood pressure over several hours to days. It should be remembered in both situations that a too rapid reduction of blood pressure may be detrimental and may lead to cerebral infarction and blindness, to deterioration in renal function, and to myocardial ischaemia.

If oral treatment can be given and there is no evidence of ongoing target-organ damage, standard initiation of antihypertensive therapy is appropriate, although the patient should be closely monitored. If there is no evidence of heart failure or asthma then a beta blocker has often been the treatment of choice.[36] A calcium-channel blocker such as nifedipine tablets, given orally, may be used as an alternative. Diuretics are less suitable since patients may initially be fluid depleted but they may be added after two to three days' treatment with other antihypertensive drugs to maintain blood pressure control.[36] Other drugs that have been used for a rapid effect include the centrally acting drug clonidine, the ACE inhibitor captopril, and the alpha blocker prazosin (especially when there are increased circulating catecholamines), but caution is needed since they may all lower blood pressure abruptly and for this reason, they are not generally recommended as initial therapy. Nifedipine and captopril have also been administered sublingually for a faster onset,[37] but again care is needed since their rapid action may be detrimental. There appears to be no clearly defined clinical advantage for sublingual as opposed to oral administration and it is generally considered that nifedipine should not be used.[3,38]

In the emergency situation, when parenteral therapy is required, choice of therapy depends on concomitant clinical conditions.[39] Sodium nitroprusside has most often been the drug of choice, given by intravenous infusion.[40,41] Alternatives include intravenous labetalol, nicardipine, hydralazine (in eclampsia), glyceryl trinitrate (in patients with coronary ischaemia), phentolamine (in phaeochromocytoma and other states associated with catecholamine excess such as the MAOI-tyramine interaction), trimetaphan,[40,41] fenoldopam,[39] and urapidil.[42] Hypertensive emergencies in children have been managed successfully with intravenous infusions of labetalol and/or sodium nitroprusside.[43]

Hypertension during surgery. Despite earlier concern over the risks of administering antihypertensive drugs to patients about to undergo surgery, substantial subsequent data have confirmed that it is not only safe but probably preferable to continue such medication up to and including the morning of surgery.[44,45]

Perioperative hypertension may occur as a result of surgery and frequently needs to be controlled with parenteral antihypertensives since oral administration in such patients may not be possible. The parenteral drug of choice is often sodium nitroprusside; others include glyceryl trinitrate (especially after coronary artery bypass), hydralazine, labetalol, enalaprilat, esmolol, fenoldopam, and nicardipine; diazoxide and methyldopa have also been used.[40,45]

Hypertension in diabetic patients. Hypertension occurs with twice the frequency in the diabetic compared with the nondiabetic population, and up to 50% of patients with type 2 diabetes mellitus become hypertensive.[46-48] The reasons proposed for this increased prevalence are controversial, but some have implicated insulin resistance.[49] In addition to being a major risk factor for atherosclerosis in large blood vessels, hypertension in diabetes appears to contribute to small vessel disease and is a risk factor for diabetic nephropathy and possibly for diabetic retinopathy. The UK Prospective Diabetes Study (UKPDS) Group has reported[50] that tight control of blood pressure (with a target of <150/85 mmHg) reduces the risk of diabetes-related death and diabetic complications, including diabetic retinopathy, in type 2 diabetics.

The threshold for intervention with drug treatment may be lower in diabetic than in non-diabetic hypertensive patients and a lower treatment goal of 140/80 mmHg (or below 130/80 mmHg in type 1 diabetics with nephropathy) has been suggested.[2] All the main groups of antihypertensive drugs can be used in diabetics. ACE inhibitors have been particularly recommended in patients with nephropathy, as there is evidence of benefit in preserving renal function; they have been reported to decrease proteinuria and preserve glomerular filtration rate in diabetic patients independently of changes in systemic blood pressure.[51] Diuretics and beta blockers have often been avoided because of their potential adverse effects on glucose and lipid metabolism, but are now generally considered a suitable choice. In the UKPDS treatment with an ACE inhibitor (captopril) or a beta blocker (atenolol) was equally effective in reducing the risk of diabetic complications, although the ACE inhibitor appeared to be better tolerated.[52]

Hypertension and renal disease. Hypertension is closely linked with the kidney—the kidney may have a role in the pathogenesis of hypertension and it may also be a prime target of damage caused by hypertension. Both renal parenchymal disorders and renovascular disorders may be associated with hypertension. In the former, hypertension is often resistant to treatment and a combination of drugs, including vasodilators, may be required. Antihypertensive therapy is also important in these patients since it may slow the decline in renal function in patients with nephropathy.[53] Although some studies[54] have suggested that ACE inhibitors have a superior effect this has not been firmly established. A suggested target blood pressure[2] for patients with nephropathy and proteinuria of over 1 g daily is below 125/75 mmHg.

Renovascular hypertension has been defined as arterial hypertension resulting from obliteration or compression of one or both renal arteries, the commonest cause being stenosis due to atherosclerosis. Underperfusion of the kidney leads to increased release of renin and a consequent rise in blood pressure. However, the relationship between renovascular hypertension and renal artery stenosis is not clear cut; the two conditions may simply coexist or hypertension may cause the stenosis rather than the other way round.[55,56]

Renovascular hypertension may be difficult to distinguish clinically, but carries a worse prognosis than essential hypertension, may be less amenable to treatment, carries a higher risk of progression to accelerated or malignant hypertension, and may result in irreversible ischaemic failure of the affected kidney.

Diagnostic methods used to detect renovascular hypertension include imaging studies such as ultrasonography and angiography, and functional tests such as the captopril-renin test (see under ACE inhibitors on p.824 for further details); renal scintigraphy with and without ACE inhibition is also used.

Blood pressure in renovascular hypertension can often be lowered by antihypertensive drugs.[57] However, medical treatment may not prevent progression of stenosis and there are concerns about possible harmful effects of blood pressure reduction on the function of the affected kidney.[55] Adverse effects on renal function are a particular concern with ACE inhibitors since, in patients with bilateral renal artery stenosis or stenosis in a solitary kidney, renal perfusion may be dependent on angiotensin II. Although some consider renovascular disease to be a contra-indication to the use of ACE inhibitors, they may be needed to control blood pressure in some patients. However, they should be used cautiously and in low doses[58] and renal function needs to be monitored with great care (see Precautions for ACE inhibitors, p.822). Alternatives to medical treatment are renal angioplasty or surgery.

Hypertension in pregnancy. Hypertension in pregnancy may be life-threatening to both mother and fetus. It may be pre-existing or may develop for the first time during pregnancy when it may range from transient hypertension late in pregnancy through to pre-eclampsia and eclampsia. Definitions vary, but hypertension presenting before 20 weeks' gestation generally continues long-term and is considered chronic hypertension. Hypertension presenting after the twentieth week (gestational hypertension) may be transient hypertension (pregnancy-induced hypertension), chronic hypertension, or pre-eclampsia. Gestational hypertension is usually defined as a blood pressure of 140/90 mmHg or more on at least two occasions in a previously normotensive woman; it is considered transient hypertension if the blood pressure has returned to normal limits by the twelfth week postpartum.[59] In pre-eclampsia, increased blood pressure occurs together with proteinuria; abnormal coagulation and liver function and oedema may also be present. Pre-eclampsia may progress to eclampsia, a convulsive phase.

Recommendations about the level of blood pressure which warrants treatment during pregnancy have been controversial. Most women with chronic hypertension will have stage 1 or stage 2 hypertension and a low risk of cardiovascular complications during the short period of pregnancy, and the benefits of treatment in such patients are not established. It is usually recommended that blood pressures of 170/110 mmHg or above should be treated; there is less agreement about lower limits but some suggest treatment of blood pressures of 140/90 mmHg or above.[2,60] However, in some cases of pre-existing hypertension it may be possible to withdraw treatment during pregnancy and only restart treatment if the blood pressure exceeds threshold values.[59] However, women with mild hypertension are at an increased risk of developing pre-eclampsia, regardless of whether they receive antihypertensives, and should be closely monitored.

Women with *pre-existing* hypertension usually continue their antihypertensive treatment although ACE inhibitors and angiotensin II receptor antagonists are contra-indicated in pregnancy. Methyldopa or beta blockers are effective first-line antihypertensives in mild to moderate hypertension and comparative studies have shown little difference between them in the outcome of pregnancy.

However, methyldopa has the advantage of reassuring long-term safety results in the infant, whereas there have been concerns about fetal growth retardation with beta blockers, particularly with atenolol.[61-63] Nifedipine may also be used.[64] Diuretics are not generally recommended for controlling hypertension in pregnancy because of the theoretical risk of exacerbating the volume depletion of pre-eclampsia; however, they appear to be safe in practice and may be used if necessary.[2,59]

In patients with *pre-eclampsia* the aim of *treatment* is to prevent maternal complications while allowing fetal maturation; delivery is the definitive treatment.[65] Oral therapy may be appropriate although intravenous antihypertensives are used in acute pre-eclampsia or when delivery is imminent. For oral treatment methyldopa or a beta blocker is considered first-line. If this fails to reduce blood pressure adequately then it is usual to add a vasodilator such as hydralazine or prazosin;[66] a calcium-channel blocker such as nifedipine is also effective.[65,67] In the emergency control of hypertension in patients with severe pre-eclampsia or eclampsia intravenous hydralazine has been widely used, although it may be less effective than other drugs.[61] Intravenous labetalol and oral nifedipine are also used, and sodium nitroprusside may be required in some patients.[59,66] Other parenteral antihypertensives tried have included diazoxide, clonidine, and glyceryl trinitrate.[67]

The management of seizures associated with eclampsia is discussed on p.341.

Prevention of pre-eclampsia. It was hoped that prevention of pre-eclampsia might be possible by reducing the local platelet aggregation thought to be responsible for some of its manifestations. Several small studies suggested that low-dose aspirin reduced the risk of pregnancy-induced hypertension and intra-uterine growth retardation in high-risk patients.[68] However, larger studies in women at lower risk generally failed to confirm this benefit[69,70] and in one[70] the risk of placental abruption was higher in those taking aspirin. Findings of the CLASP (Collaborative Low-dose Aspirin Study in Pregnancy) multicentre study[71] involving over 9000 women considered to be at increased risk of pre-eclampsia or intra-uterine growth retardation did not support the routine prophylactic or therapeutic use of antiplatelet therapy in all such women. A further study[72] in high-risk women also failed to show any benefit, although administration of aspirin appeared to be safe for mother and fetus. The CLASP workers suggested that the only women in whom low-dose aspirin may be justified are those at especially high risk of early-onset pre-eclampsia severe enough to warrant very preterm delivery. The role of calcium supplementation in the prevention of pre-eclampsia is controversial. Although small studies and a meta-analysis[73] indicated that calcium supplementation during pregnancy reduced the risk of pre-eclampsia, this was not confirmed in a larger randomised study.[74] Preliminary evidence suggests that supplementation with vitamins C and E may be beneficial in women at high risk, but confirmation is needed from larger studies.[75]

1. Reid J, Swales JD, eds. Hypertension in theory and practice. *Br Med Bull* 1994; **50:** 235–515.
2. Ramsay LE, *et al.* Guidelines for management of hypertension: report of the third working party of the British Hypertension Society. *J Hum Hypertens* 1999; **13:** 569–92.
3. Joint National Committee. The sixth report of the joint national committee on prevention, detection, evaluation, and treatment of high blood pressure (JNC VI). *Arch Intern Med* 1997; **157:** 2413–46. Correction. *ibid.* 1998; **158:** 573.
4. Guidelines Subcommittee. 1999 World Health Organization–International Society of Hypertension guidelines for the management of hypertension. *J Hypertens* 1999; **17:** 151–83.
5. WHO. Hypertension control: report of a WHO expert committee. *WHO Tech Rep Ser 862* 1996.
6. Staessen JA, *et al.* Randomised double-blind comparison of placebo and active treatment for older patients with isolated systolic hypertension. *Lancet* 1997; **350:** 757–64. Correction. *ibid.*; 1636.
7. O'Brien E, *et al.* Use and interpretation of ambulatory blood pressure monitoring: recommendations of the British Hypertension Society. *BMJ* 2000; **320:** 1128–34.
8. Andersson OK, *et al.* Survival in treated hypertension: follow up study after two decades. *BMJ* 1998; **317:** 167–71.
9. Ramsay LE, *et al.* Non-pharmacological therapy of hypertension. *Br Med Bull* 1994; **50:** 494–508.
10. Alderman MH. Non-pharmacological treatment of hypertension. *Lancet* 1994; **344:** 307–11.
11. Dahlöf B, *et al.* Morbidity and mortality in the Swedish Trial in Old Patients with Hypertension (STOP-Hypertension). *Lancet* 1991; **338:** 1281–5.
12. SHEP Cooperative Research Group. Prevention of stroke by antihypertensive drug treatment in older persons with isolated systolic hypertension: final results of the Systolic Hypertension in the Elderly Program (SHEP). *JAMA* 1991; **265:** 3255–64.
13. MRC Working Party. Medical Research Council trial of treatment of hypertension in older patients: principal results. *BMJ* 1992; **304:** 405–12.
14. Gueyffier F, *et al.* Antihypertensive drugs in very old people: a subgroup meta-analysis of randomised controlled trials. *Lancet* 1999; **353:** 793–6.
15. Staessen JA. Potential adverse effects of blood pressure lowering—J-curve revisited. *Lancet* 1996; **348:** 696–7.
16. Hansson L, *et al.* Effects of intensive blood-pressure lowering and low-dose aspirin in patients with hypertension: principal results of the Hypertension Optimal Treatment (HOT) randomised trial. *Lancet* 1998; **351:** 1755–62.
17. Woodman R. Open letter disputes WHO hypertension guidelines. *BMJ* 1999; **318:** 893.
18. Chalmers J. The treatment of hypertension. *Br J Clin Pharmacol* 1996; **42:** 29–35.
19. Kaplan NM, Gifford RW. Choice of initial therapy for hypertension. *JAMA* 1996; **275:** 1577–80.
20. Neaton JD, *et al.* Treatment of mild hypertension study: final results. *JAMA* 1993; **270:** 713–24.
21. Materson BJ, *et al.* Single-drug therapy for hypertension in men: a comparison of six antihypertensive agents with placebo. *N Engl J Med* 1993; **328:** 914–21. Correction. *ibid.* 1994; **330:** 1689.
22. Bennet NE. Hypertension in the elderly. *Lancet* 1994; **344:** 447–9.
23. Kaplan NM. Ethnic aspects of hypertension. *Lancet* 1994; **344:** 450–2.
24. The ALLHAT Officers and Coordinators for the ALLHAT Collaborative Research Group. Major cardiovascular events in hypertensive patients randomized to doxazosin vs chlorthalidone: the Antihypertensive and Lipid-Lowering Treatment to Prevent Heart Attack Trial (ALLHAT). *JAMA* 2000; **283:** 1967–75.
25. Wright JM, *et al.* Systematic review of antihypertensive therapies: does the evidence assist in choosing a first-line drug? *Can Med Assoc J* 1999; **161:** 25–32.
26. Hansson L, *et al.* Randomised trial of old and new antihypertensive drugs in elderly patients: cardiovascular mortality and morbidity the Swedish Trial in Old Patients with Hypertension-2 study. *Lancet* 1999; **354:** 1751–6.
27. Cutler JA. Calcium-channel blockers for hypertension—uncertainty continues. *N Engl J Med* 1998; **338:** 679–81.
28. Johnston GD. Selecting appropriate antihypertensive drug dosages. *Drugs* 1994; **47:** 567–75.
29. Lyons D, *et al.* Drug treatment: present and future. *Br Med Bull* 1994; **50:** 472–93.
30. McInnes GT, Semple PF. Hypertension: investigation, assessment and diagnosis. *Br Med Bull* 1994; **50:** 443–59.
31. Padfield PL. Resistant hypertension. *Prescribers' J* 1997; **37:** 69–76.
32. van den Bosch WJHM, *et al.* Withdrawal of antihypertensive drugs in selected patients. *Lancet* 1994; **343:** 1157.
33. Aylett MJ, *et al.* Withdrawing antihypertensive drugs. *Lancet* 1994; **343:** 1512.
34. Calhoun DA, Oparil S. Treatment of hypertensive crisis. *N Engl J Med* 1990; **323:** 1177–83.
35. Vaughan CJ, Delanty N. Hypertensive emergencies. *Lancet* 2000; **356:** 411–17.
36. Semple PF. Emergency treatment of hypertension. *Prescribers' J* 1989; **29:** 62–9.
37. Anonymous. Hypertensive emergencies. *Lancet* 1991; **338:** 220–1.
38. Grossman E, *et al.* Should a moratorium be placed on sublingual nifedipine capsules for hypertensive emergencies and pseudoemergencies? *JAMA* 1996; **276:** 1328–31.
39. Grossman E, *et al.* Comparative tolerability profile of hypertensive crisis treatments. *Drug Safety* 1998; **19:** 99–122.
40. Gifford RW. Management of hypertensive crises. *JAMA* 1991; **266:** 829–35.
41. Kaplan NM. Management of hypertensive emergencies. *Lancet* 1994; **344:** 1335–8.
42. Hirschl MM. Guidelines for the drug treatment of hypertensive crises. *Drugs* 1995; **50:** 991–1000.
43. Deal JE, *et al.* Management of hypertensive emergencies. *Arch Dis Child* 1992; **67:** 1089–92.
44. Goldman L. Cardiac risks and complications of noncardiac surgery. *Ann Intern Med* 1983; **98:** 504–13.
45. Erstad BL, Barletta JF. Treatment of hypertension in the perioperative patient. *Ann Pharmacother* 2000; **34:** 66–79.
46. Barnett AH. Diabetes and hypertension. *Br Med Bull* 1994; **50:** 397–407.
47. MacLeod MJ, McLay J. Drug treatment of hypertension complicating diabetes mellitus. *Drugs* 1998; **56:** 189–202.
48. Deedwania PC. Hypertension and diabetes: new therapeutic options. *Arch Intern Med* 2000; **160:** 1585–94.
49. Reaven GM, *et al.* Hypertension and associated metabolic abnormalities—the role of insulin resistance and the sympathoadrenal system. *N Engl J Med* 1996; **334:** 374–81.
50. UK Prospective Diabetes Study Group. Tight blood pressure control and risk of macrovascular and microvascular complications in type 2 diabetes: UKPDS 38. *BMJ* 1998; **317:** 703–13.
51. Kaisiske BL, *et al.* Effect of antihypertensive therapy on the kidney in patients with diabetes: a meta-regression analysis. *Ann Intern Med* 1993; **118:** 129–38.
52. UK Prospective Diabetes Study Group. Efficacy of atenolol and captopril in reducing risk of macrovascular and microvascular complications in type 2 diabetes: UKPDS 39. *BMJ* 1998; **317:** 713–20.
53. Salvetti A, *et al.* Renal protection and antihypertensive drugs: current status. *Drugs* 1999; **57:** 665–93.
54. Agodoa LY, *et al.* Effect of ramipril vs amlodipine on renal outcomes in hypertensive nephrosclerosis: a randomized controlled trial. *JAMA* 2001; **285:** 2719–28.
55. Derkx FHM, Schalekamp MADH. Renal artery stenosis and hypertension. *Lancet* 1994; **344:** 237–9.
56. Safian RD, Textor SC. Renal-artery stenosis. *N Engl J Med* 2001; **344:** 431–42.
57. Rosenthal T. Drug therapy of renovascular hypertension. *Drugs* 1993; **45:** 895–909.
58. Navis G, *et al.* ACE inhibitors and the kidney: a risk-benefit assessment. *Drug Safety* 1996; **15:** 200–211.
59. National High Blood Pressure Education Program Working Group on High Blood Pressure in Pregnancy. Report of the National High Blood Pressure Education Program Working Group on High Blood Pressure in Pregnancy. *Am J Obstet Gynecol* 2000; **183** (suppl): S1–S22. Also available from the National Institutes of Health at: http://www.nhlbi.nih.gov/health/prof/heart/hbp/hbp_preg.htm
60. Rey É. Report of the Canadian Hypertension Society Consensus Conference: pharmacologic treatment of hypertensive disorders in pregnancy. *Can Med Assoc J* 1997; **157:** 1245–54.
61. Magee LA, *et al.* Management of hypertension in pregnancy. *BMJ* 1999; **318:** 1332–6.
62. Garovic VD. Hypertension in pregnancy: diagnosis and treatment. *Mayo Clin Proc* 2000; **75:** 1071–6.
63. Magee LA. Treating hypertension in women of child-bearing age and during pregnancy. *Drug Safety* 2001; **24:** 457–74.

64. Sibai BM. Treatment of hypertension in pregnant women. *N Engl J Med* 1996; **335**: 257–65.
65. Walker JJ. Pre-eclampsia. *Lancet* 2000; **356**: 1260–5.
66. Broughton Pipkin F, Rubin PC. Pre-eclampsia—the 'disease of theories'. *Br Med Bull* 1994; **50**: 381–96.
67. Mushambi MC, *et al.* Recent developments in the pathophysiology and management of pre-eclampsia. *Br J Anaesth* 1996; **76**: 133–48.
68. Imperiale TF, Petrulis AS. A meta-analysis of low-dose aspirin for the prevention of pregnancy-induced hypertensive disease. *JAMA* 1991; **266**: 260–4.
69. Italian Study of Aspirin in Pregnancy. Low-dose aspirin in prevention and treatment of intrauterine growth retardation and pregnancy-induced hypertension. *Lancet* 1993; **341**: 396–400.
70. Sibai BM, *et al.* Prevention of preeclampsia with low-dose aspirin in healthy, nulliparous pregnant women. *N Engl J Med* 1993; **329**: 1213–18.
71. CLASP (Collaborative Low-dose Aspirin Study in Pregnancy) Collaborative Group. CLASP: a randomised trial of low-dose aspirin for the prevention and treatment of pre-eclampsia among 9364 pregnant women. *Lancet* 1994; **343**: 619–29.
72. Caritis S, *et al.* Low-dose aspirin to prevent preeclampsia in women at high risk. *N Engl J Med* 1998; **338**: 701–5.
73. Bucher HC, *et al.* Effect of calcium supplementation on pregnancy-induced hypertension and preeclampsia: a meta-analysis of randomized controlled trials. *JAMA* 1996; **275**: 1113–17. Correction. *ibid.*; **276**: 1388.
74. Levine RJ, *et al.* Trial of calcium to prevent preeclampsia. *N Engl J Med* 1997; **337**: 69–76.
75. Chappell LC, *et al.* Effect of antioxidants on the occurrence of pre-eclampsia in women at increased risk: a randomised trial. *Lancet* 1999; **354**: 810–16.

Hypotension

As discussed under Hypertension (above) many factors influence blood pressure making it difficult to define an absolute norm. An arbitrary definition of *normal* adult blood pressure[1,2] is a systolic pressure below 130 mmHg together with a diastolic pressure below 85 mmHg (i.e. below 130/85 mmHg). An *optimal* blood pressure, with respect to cardiovascular risk, of less than 120/80 mmHg has also been suggested.[1,2] Unlike hypertension, for which national and international guidelines have been developed, there does not appear to be an accepted definition of either low blood pressure or hypotension.

Despite such shortcomings over definition, the existence of several forms of hypotensive disease is recognised.

Hypotension can occur after haemorrhage or in other forms of shock and the management of this acute and potentially dangerous form of low blood pressure is usually with vasopressor sympathomimetics, notably noradrenaline [norepinephrine] or dopamine, and is described under Shock (below). Another situation in which acute hypotension can develop is during anaesthesia and surgery; spinal or epidural block is associated with a greater risk than many other forms of anaesthesia. Again, sympathomimetics, and ephedrine particularly, are used as vasopressors,[3] and this topic is discussed further on p.1091.

Chronic forms of hypotension also exist and include orthostatic (postural) hypotension and neurally mediated hypotension. The management of orthostatic hypotension is discussed on p.1070 under fludrocortisone which is usually the first pharmacological treatment to be tried in this condition. Neurally mediated hypotension, which has also been known as neurocardiogenic syncope, neurally mediated syncope, vasodepressor syncope, or vasovagal syncope, is a common cause of recurrent lightheadedness (presyncope) and syncope in persons with structurally normal hearts. It is characterised by a paradoxical neurocardiogenic reflex that ultimately results in vasodilatation, bradycardia, and hypotension. Fludrocortisone, a beta blocker (such as atenolol or metoprolol), and disopyramide are reported to be standard drugs used.[4-6] Antimuscarinics, such as propantheline bromide, have also been tried. Selective serotonin reuptake inhibitors have been suggested for refractory cases.[6] Benefit has also been reported with the alpha agonist midodrine.[7] In a few patients cardiac pacing may be required.

One contentious issue is whether general and non-specific symptoms of ill health such as mental and physical fatigue, depression, and anxiety can be attributed to a low blood pressure (for example, a systolic pressure below 110 mmHg or diastolic pressure below 60 mmHg).[8] In the UK and the USA such an association has never been accepted whereas in some European countries (e.g. Germany) a wide range of pharmaceutical preparations usually containing a sympathomimetic has been available for treatment. Some evidence has been presented to support the theory,[9,10] as well as to suggest a possible link between the chronic fatigue syndrome and neurally mediated hypotension,[4,5] although implications for treatment are far from clear.

1. Joint National Committee. The sixth report of the joint national committee on prevention, detection, evaluation, and treatment of high blood pressure (JNC VI). *Arch Intern Med* 1997; **157**: 2413–46. Correction. *ibid.* 1998; **158**: 573.

2. Guidelines Subcommittee. 1999 World Health Organization–International Society of Hypertension guidelines for the management of hypertension. *J Hypertens* 1999; **17**: 151–83.
3. McCrae AF, Wildsmith JAW. Prevention and treatment of hypotension during central neural block. *Br J Anaesth* 1993; **70**: 672–80.
4. Rowe PC, *et al.* Is neurally mediated hypotension an unrecognised cause of chronic fatigue? *Lancet* 1995; **345**: 623–4.
5. Bou-Holaigah I, *et al.* The relationship between neurally mediated hypotension and the chronic fatigue syndrome. *JAMA* 1995; **274**: 961–7.
6. Lazarus JC, Mauro VF. Syncope: pathophysiology, diagnosis, and pharmacotherapy. *Ann Pharmacother* 1996; **30**: 994–1005.
7. Ward CR, *et al.* Midodrine: a role in the management of neurocardiogenic syncope. *Heart* 1998; **79**: 45–9.
8. Mann A. Psychiatric symptoms and low blood pressure. *BMJ* 1992; **304**: 64–5.
9. Rosengren A, *et al.* Low systolic blood pressure and self perceived wellbeing in middle aged men. *BMJ* 1993; **306**: 243–6.
10. Barrett-Connor E, Palinkas LA. Low blood pressure and depression in older men: a population based study. *BMJ* 1994; **308**: 446–9.

Kawasaki disease

Cardiac effects including coronary artery abnormalities are the major complications of Kawasaki disease, also known as mucocutaneous lymph node syndrome of childhood. Normal immunoglobulin and aspirin are used in its initial management, and antiplatelet therapy, usually with aspirin, may be continued long term to prevent coronary thrombosis. Further details concerning the overall management of Kawasaki disease are provided under Normal Immunoglobulins, p.1554.

Myocardial infarction

Myocardial infarction is defined as necrosis of heart muscle caused by coronary artery occlusion, usually due to thrombosis at the site of a recently ruptured atheromatous plaque; in a few patients coronary embolism or spasm, arteritis, spontaneous thrombosis, or a sudden severe rise in blood pressure, as in phaeochromocytoma, is responsible. It is part of the spectrum of acute coronary syndromes (see Angina Pectoris, above). The immediate consequence of coronary occlusion is myocardial ischaemia which leads to impaired contractility, arrhythmias, and eventually myocardial cell death. The lay term 'heart attack' describes both sudden cardiac death and myocardial infarction. Sudden death often occurs before treatment is possible and is usually due to ventricular fibrillation. The majority of patients resuscitated from ventricular fibrillation develop features of myocardial infarction or have coronary artery disease. The initial symptoms of acute myocardial infarction are usually chest pain, breathlessness, and sweating. The chest pain is typically severe and resembles that of angina pectoris, being precordial with radiation to the neck, lower jaw, and left arm. Other signs and symptoms include nausea and vomiting, bradycardia, hypotension, and apprehension. Many myocardial infarcts are said to be silent, that is asymptomatic.

The introduction of aspirin and thrombolytics like streptokinase transformed the management of acute myocardial infarction and more people now survive the initial attack and achieve a better recovery of left ventricular function.[1] Further improvement in survival and morbidity should be possible if more candidates for thrombolysis can be identified and treated early and if the risks of recurrence and haemorrhage can be reduced as a result of the continuing development of thrombolytics and of adjunctive antiplatelet and antithrombin drugs.

Numerous large-scale studies have helped to establish various aspects of treatment and more are planned.

Guidelines for the early management of myocardial infarction[2-5] emphasise the importance of the rapid provision of life support, adequate pain relief, accurate diagnosis, immediate administration of aspirin, and, where appropriate, thrombolytic treatment ideally commencing within 90 minutes of the call for help. The immediate aims are to relieve pain and anxiety and to re-open the occluded artery (reperfusion or revascularisation) as soon as possible thus limiting damage to the heart. After reperfusion long-term management aims to maintain patency and to treat or protect against complications of the post-infarction period such as arrhythmias, left ventricular failure, persistent angina, and venous thromboembolism. Cardiac rupture and aneurysms may also occur after myocardial infarction. The ideal is of course to prevent myocardial infarction from occurring in the first place.

The **management** of myocardial infarction is discussed in more detail under the headings Early Management (of the acute phase), Long-term Management (including sec-

ondary prevention), and Primary Prevention (in healthy subjects and those with risk factors).

Early management. Those patients with myocardial infarction who develop ventricular fibrillation very quickly, often within the first hour after the onset of symptoms of infarction, die before they reach hospital; this is often referred to as sudden cardiac death. Ventricular fibrillation is treated by defibrillation followed by adrenaline [epinephrine] and possibly antiarrhythmics if defibrillation alone is unsuccessful (see under Advanced Cardiac Life Support, above, for further details). Treatment must be instituted quickly and in order to achieve this there are paramedic ambulance teams experienced in defibrillation and programmes aimed at educating the public in the basic techniques of cardiopulmonary resuscitation. Patients with suspected myocardial infarction should be admitted to hospital and where possible managed in a coronary care unit.

As already stated, the immediate priority in patients with myocardial infarction is administration of aspirin, followed by relief of pain and anxiety. Pain should be relieved with an opioid analgesic, usually diamorphine or morphine given intravenously (see Myocardial Infarction Pain, p.7); an antiemetic such as metoclopramide intravenously may also be necessary. Supplemental oxygen should also be given. An inhaled mixture of nitrous oxide and oxygen (Entonox) has sometimes been used to provide pain relief before arrival in hospital; sublingual glyceryl trinitrate or an alternative fast-acting nitrate may also be given. A benzodiazepine may be useful for anxiety.

Reperfusion is usually achieved with a thrombolytic such as streptokinase given intravenously and the antiplatelet drug aspirin by mouth;[6] the additive benefit of streptokinase and aspirin was established by, for example, the ISIS-2 study.[7] Aspirin can be given immediately and the thrombolytic as soon as an ECG has been performed to confirm the diagnosis. Some also give heparin at this stage. Alternatively, reperfusion may be achieved with angioplasty.

A *diagnosis* is made mainly from clinical history, particularly typical chest pain lasting more than 30 minutes (although this is absent in many patients), and a characteristic ECG. Rapid diagnosis is important so that, if indicated, thrombolysis can be given as soon as possible. The greatest benefit from thrombolysis appears to be achieved in patients with an ECG demonstrating ST-segment elevation or new left bundle branch block.[1,2] Other diagnostic techniques include measurement of cardiac enzymes and troponins, and echocardiography.

Thrombolysis. Thrombolytics are given intravenously to break up the thrombus or clot and restore the patency of the coronary artery, thereby limiting infarct size and irreversible damage to the myocardium. Several large studies have established that thrombolytics can preserve left ventricular function and improve short-term and one-year mortality figures;[8,9] benefit has been maintained in 5-year[10] and 10-year[11,12] follow-up studies. Reduction of ECG abnormalities and modification of ventricular remodelling may contribute to the benefits seen with thrombolytics. It is generally accepted that, subject to an appropriate ECG and provided there are no contra-indications (see Precautions under Streptokinase, p.977), the sooner thrombolytic treatment is started the better. Trials such as the GISSI-1 study[13] and the ISIS-2 study[7] helped to establish that mortality is reduced if thrombolytics are administered within 6 hours of the onset of symptoms[14] and further studies provided evidence[15,16] that patients presenting within 12 hours should receive a thrombolytic. There is insufficient experience to determine whether the benefits outweigh the risks when thrombolytics are given later than 12 hours.[14] There have been some reports of early excess mortality on days 0 to 1 ('early hazard') attributed to cardiac rupture in patients with other known risk factors for early hazard (over 64 years of age, female sex, raised blood pressure on admission) given late thrombolytic treatment (after 6 hours).[14,17,18] Thus the ideal is to give a thrombolytic as soon as possible. The British Heart Foundation Working Group[2] has recommended administration within 90 minutes of alerting the general practitioner or ambulance service ('call to needle' time); an American group[19] has recommended injection within 70 minutes. Once in hospital, the time between admission and administration of a thrombolytic (the 'door to needle' time) varies widely and could be improved; a median interval of 3 to 4½ hours between onset of pain and the start of treatment has been cited for British hospitals.[20] Prehospital thrombolysis is feasible and reduces the time to thrombolytic administration and short-term mortality.[21] Five-year follow-up of one study[22] has suggested that there is also a beneficial effect on long-term mortality.

Streptokinase has been the most widely used thrombolytic. Several large studies have compared clinical benefit in terms of improved left ventricular function and mortality and have shown no difference between streptokinase and other thrombolytics, including saruplase,[23] the tissue plasminogen activator alteplase,[24] anistreplase,[25] and reteplase[26] in overall efficacy. In the GUSTO-I study,[27] accelerated or 'front loaded' alteplase (that is, rapid intravenous administration over $1\frac{1}{2}$ hours rather than the conventional 3 hours) was more effective than streptokinase, although the study was criticised for not comparing like with like. On the other hand, alteplase might be associated with a greater risk of stroke than streptokinase.[28] Studies comparing accelerated alteplase (GUSTO-III)[29] and tenecteplase with alteplase (ASSENT-2)[30] found no difference in mortality rate. Factors such as cost, method of administration, and contra-indications help to determine the choice of thrombolytic, but ensuring that a thrombolytic is administered as soon as possible is probably more important than which is given.[6,31] If streptokinase or anistreplase, so-called antigenic thrombolytics, have been administered recently, non-antigenic drugs such as alteplase or urokinase should be given.

The overall effectiveness of thrombolytics is limited by persistent coronary occlusion, re-occlusion, and infrequent but serious bleeding complications including intracranial haemorrhage. Different thrombolytic administration regimens, such as bolus injections of reteplase, and combinations of thrombolytics, for example alteplase with streptokinase and alteplase with saruplase, are being investigated in attempts to improve patency rates. However, there has been concern that adverse effects may be higher with bolus administration. A study[32] comparing double-bolus administration of alteplase with accelerated alteplase was terminated early when excess deaths were found in the group receiving bolus injections, and a subsequent meta-analysis[33] found a higher incidence of intracranial haemorrhage associated with bolus administration of various thrombolytics. If re-occlusion occurs further thrombolytic therapy may be given. Alternatively angioplasty may be performed (see below). Antiplatelet and antithrombin drugs are given as adjuncts to thrombolytics.

Antiplatelet drugs. The value of giving aspirin by mouth, as an antiplatelet drug, was shown by the ISIS-2 study[7] in which aspirin started during the first 24 hours after myocardial infarction reduced mortality and also reduced the incidence of re-infarction and stroke. Combination with streptokinase proved to be more effective than either streptokinase or aspirin alone. Aspirin should therefore be taken as soon as possible when myocardial infarction is suspected and the tablet chewed so that some buccal absorption occurs. Despite the clear benefits of aspirin therapy, it still appears to be underused.[34,35] For patients with aspirin allergy, dipyridamole, ticlopidine, or clopidogrel are alternatives.[4,5] New antiplatelets, such as abciximab, are under investigation as adjuncts to thrombolytic therapy,[36,37] or primary angioplasty.[38]

Anticoagulants. Heparin was widely used in acute myocardial infarction before thrombolytics were available, but the necessity for adjuvant therapy with heparin in addition to aspirin is not certain.[39] Many centres administer parenteral heparin with or shortly after the thrombolytic to prevent the re-occlusion of the coronary artery often associated with thrombolysis. Alteplase appears to open occluded arteries more rapidly but to cause re-occlusion more often than streptokinase, and thus heparin has been regarded by some as particularly necessary when alteplase is used; this may also apply for reteplase and tenecteplase.[25] The ISIS-3 study[25] indicated that the addition of subcutaneous heparin (from about 4 hours after randomisation) did have a slight advantage over a thrombolytic and aspirin alone, but the benefit was not large and there was no substantial difference in mortality, whereas the incidence of major bleeds and haemorrhagic stroke was increased. An overview of randomised studies[40] found that in patients receiving aspirin, addition of heparin (either intravenous or subcutaneous) produced a small reduction in mortality but was associated with an excess of major bleeds. The authors concluded that the routine addition of heparin to aspirin could not be justified. Alternatives to heparin such as the thrombin inhibitor hirudin have been investigated although results have been disap-

pointing. Studies comparing heparin with a recombinant hirudin (desirudin in GUSTO-IIa[41] and TIMI-9A,[42] and lepirudin in HIT-III[43]) had to be stopped because of higher than expected haemorrhagic stroke rates. In GUSTO-IIa and TIMI-9A a higher stroke rate was also seen in the heparin group. Use of higher doses of heparin than in GUSTO-I and inclusion of high-risk patients may explain the stroke incidence. GUSTO-IIa and TIMI-9A restarted as GUSTO-IIb[44] and TIMI-9B,[45] respectively, using lower doses of heparin and desirudin. The results of GUSTO-IIb[44] showed that desirudin was still associated with increased haemorrhage although not with major bleeding and produced only a small benefit over heparin. TIMI-9B[45] reported no difference between heparin and desirudin. The authors suggested that desirudin may have advantages over heparin as it has a more consistent anticoagulant effect that reduces the need to adjust infusion rates and it may be useful in patients who develop heparin-induced thrombocytopenia. HIT-4,[46] which compared heparin with a lower dose of lepirudin, also reported no difference in clinical outcome and similar rates of bleeding in both groups. Other thrombin inhibitors under investigation include argatroban and bivalirudin. Heparin is also given prophylactically to myocardial infarction patients at risk of developing left ventricular mural thrombosis with subsequent systemic embolisation. Patients with complications following myocardial infarction who are likely to be immobile for several days should also receive heparin prophylaxis.

Angioplasty. Percutaneous transluminal coronary angioplasty is effective at re-opening occluded coronary arteries and immediate angioplasty (termed primary angioplasty) has been performed as an alternative method of reperfusion to thrombolysis. Studies have compared the two methods. A substudy of GUSTO-IIb suggested that angioplasty may have a small advantage over thrombolysis,[47] and a review of randomised studies comparing primary angioplasty with thrombolysis concluded that primary angioplasty was associated with lower mortality and re-infarction rates at hospital discharge or 30 days post myocardial infarction.[48] Long-term follow-up in one study[49] has found that the benefit is maintained at 5 years. Observational studies[50,51] have suggested that thrombolysis and primary angioplasty offer similar efficacy. Where angioplasty is available it may be considered, particularly for patients in whom thrombolytics are contraindicated or in patients at highest risk such as those with cardiogenic shock.[4,5] Since angioplasty is only available in specialised cardiac centres, thrombolysis will remain the method of reperfusion for the majority of patients. Angioplasty may also be considered when thrombolytic therapy has failed to unblock the artery (so-called 'rescue' angioplasty). Angioplasty has been used in attempts to abolish residual stenoses that usually remain after thrombolysis and that may re-occlude, although such use within hours or days of thrombolysis has not been successful.[52] The associated therapy, such as antithrombotic therapy, that is usually necessary in conjunction with angioplasty to prevent re-occlusion and restenosis is discussed under Reperfusion and Revascularisation Procedures (below).

Thus, at present, standard early therapy for the majority of patients with myocardial infarction is streptokinase with aspirin, and possibly heparin. Other early treatments that have been tried include beta blockers, nitrates, ACE inhibitors, magnesium, and calcium-channel blockers.

Beta blockers. Before thrombolytics were widely used the intravenous administration of beta blockers, such as atenolol and metoprolol, in the early period following myocardial infarction was associated with a reduction in mortality. Contributory mechanisms were considered to be a reduction in size of infarction or number of re-infarctions and an antiarrhythmic effect, although the ISIS-1 study[53] suggested that beta blockers improved early survival by reducing the incidence of cardiac rupture. The role of beta blockers in the thrombolytic era is less certain, but an overview of randomised studies[54] indicated that early use of intravenous beta blockers definitely reduced mortality after myocardial infarction. They appear to be less widely used in the UK than in the US.[55]

Nitrates. The use of intravenous nitrates (glyceryl trinitrate or sodium nitroprusside), started within 24 hours of the onset of pain, has been associated with a reduction in mortality in patients with acute myocardial infarction,[56] although this was before the routine use of thrombolytics, and in a more recent study molsidomine and its active metabolite linsidomine (a nitric oxide donor) had no effect on mortality.[57] Nevertheless, the empirical use of in-

travenous glyceryl trinitrate in the acute phase of myocardial infarction is widespread and appears to be safe, as was demonstrated in the GISSI-3 study;[58] these workers considered that glyceryl trinitrate could be given when clinically indicated in addition to thrombolysis, aspirin, and a beta blocker.

ACE inhibitors. Early treatment with ACE inhibitors as an adjunct to standard thrombolytic therapy is less well established than post-infarction treatment. Favourable results have been reported in the GISSI-3[58] and the ISIS-4[59] studies where lisinopril and captopril, respectively, were given by mouth starting within 24 hours of the onset of chest pain and in the Chinese Cardiac Study[60] (CCS-1) where captopril was given by mouth within 36 hours of the onset of symptoms. In the GISSI-3 study the beneficial effects were maintained at 6 months.[61] However, the CONSENSUS II study was terminated early when it was found that enalapril, given intravenously as enalaprilat and begun within 24 hours of the onset of chest pain, did not improve survival during the 180 days after infarction.[62] A substudy on some of the patients did however suggest that they may have benefited from early treatment since left ventricular dilatation was attenuated.[63] An interaction between aspirin and enalapril was postulated as one of the reasons for the overall lack of benefit seen and further analysis of the CONSENSUS II results found that the beneficial effect of enalapril was reduced in those patients already taking aspirin.[64] However, a systematic overview[65] failed to support this finding. A systematic review of the CONSENSUS II, GISSI-3, ISIS-4, and CCS-1 studies found lower 30-day cumulative mortality and incidence of non-fatal heart failure among ACE inhibitor recipients.[66] However, the size of benefit in these studies of largely unselected patients is much smaller than in the studies of patients with left ventricular dysfunction. The authors of ISIS-4[59] recommended that early treatment with an ACE inhibitor should be considered in all patients, except those with cardiogenic shock or persistent severe hypotension, and that treatment should be reviewed after a few weeks and continued in those with left ventricular dysfunction. This view is supported by the guidelines of the American College of Cardiology and American Heart Association.[4,5] Others[67,68] consider that routine early treatment with an ACE inhibitor in unselected patients is not warranted and such use should be reserved for patients with signs of heart failure (see under Long-term Management, below). The European Society of Cardiology recognises that there are valid arguments for both views and advocates the early use of an ACE inhibitor if symptoms of heart failure appear.[3]

Magnesium. Magnesium has an important physiological role in maintaining the ion balance in muscle including the myocardium. Administration of magnesium might have an antiarrhythmic effect and might protect the myocardium against reperfusion injury and in an overview of studies in patients with suspected myocardial infarction administration of intravenous magnesium, generally within 12 hours of the onset of chest pain, had reduced mortality.[69] The beneficial effect on mortality appeared to be confirmed by the LIMIT-2 study[70] and at follow-up an average of 2.7 years later;[71] there was no evidence of an antiarrhythmic effect. However, in the large ISIS-4 study[59] magnesium had no effect on mortality. No benefit was seen in any of the subgroups, including those not receiving thrombolytics. The LIMIT-2 workers[71] considered that timing of magnesium administration in relation to thrombolytic therapy or spontaneous reperfusion was likely to be critical. In their study a loading injection of magnesium was given before thrombolysis and a maintenance infusion of magnesium continued over the following 24 hours. In the ISIS-4 study magnesium was given after thrombolysis was started; it was intended that magnesium be started immediately after the early lytic phase, that is, in the first hour or so. At present, the routine use of magnesium cannot be recommended.

Calcium-channel blockers. Studies have not shown a reduction in mortality when calcium-channel blockers are given in the early phase of acute myocardial infarction. However, since myocardial stunning has been linked to intracellular calcium overload[72] there has been speculation that calcium-channel blockers might benefit patients about to undergo reperfusion. This is yet to be confirmed.

Metabolic support. Infusions containing glucose, insulin, and potassium have been used in small numbers of patients with the aim of providing metabolic support in the acute phase of myocardial infarction. A meta-analysis of randomised controlled trials that were performed before the widespread use of thrombolytics found that mortality was reduced in recipients of glucose-insulin-potassium.[73] Following a small pilot study with similar findings[74] that included patients treated with thrombolytics or primary angioplasty, a larger study is now underway. Reduced mortality has also been reported in diabetic patients with myocardial infarction given insulin-glucose infusions (see Myocardial Infarction under Insulin, p.331).

Long-term management. Patients who survive the immediate post-myocardial infarction period remain at high risk for cardiovascular mortality. The main predictors of poor outcome are the extent of left ventricular dysfunction, residual myocardial ischaemia, and ventricular arrhythmias. Follow-up should include the identification and modification of risk factors for ischaemic heart disease (see Cardiovascular Risk Reduction, above). Exercise testing can be used after myocardial infarction to help identify those at high risk for recurrent ischaemic events and to select patients needing coronary angiography.[75] In patients who develop angina soon after myocardial infarction, exercise testing may be unhelpful and potentially hazardous, although many will need angiography to determine whether angioplasty or bypass surgery is required. Myocardial imaging techniques and pharmacological stress testing may also have a role (see Ischaemic Heart Disease under Dipyridamole, p.878).

Drug therapy is also important in the long-term management of patients following myocardial infarction. *Aspirin*, given during the acute phase and then continued for one to two years, has been shown to reduce mortality and re-infarction rates. A meta-analysis[76] confirmed the benefit of prolonged antiplatelet treatment in the secondary prevention of myocardial infarction and patients should receive antiplatelet therapy indefinitely. Alternative antiplatelet drugs such as clopidogrel,[77] sulfinpyrazone, or ticlopidine may be considered in the few patients intolerant of aspirin. The routine long-term use of *oral anticoagulation* after the acute phase of myocardial infarction has been difficult to justify. In the ASPECT study,[78] such treatment had only a limited effect on mortality but did reduce the risk of cerebrovascular events and of re-infarction; as expected there was an increased incidence of bleeding complications. Those at high risk of systemic embolism because of atrial fibrillation, heart failure, or mobile mural thrombus will require prophylaxis with oral anticoagulants, but for other patients aspirin will probably be preferred.[79,80] Addition of low-dose warfarin (1 or 3 mg) to low-dose aspirin (80 mg) has not conferred clinical benefit above that achieved with moderate-dose aspirin alone (160 mg).[81] Long-term prophylactic treatment with oral *beta blockers* (most studies have used propranolol, metoprolol, or timolol) has reduced mortality and the rate of re-infarction.[82] In patients with no contra-indications to beta-blocker therapy (see Precautions, p.846) they are usually started before hospital discharge and continued for a minimum of one year; indefinite use has been recommended.[4,5] Although some only use them in patients with hypertension or angina pectoris following myocardial infarction, a recent survey of 201 752 patients who had suffered a myocardial infarction found that low-risk patients and those with conditions often considered to be contra-indications also benefited from administration of a beta blocker.[83] Beta blockers seem to be underused particularly in elderly patients even though there is clear evidence of benefit in this group.[84,85] *Calcium-channel blockers* are not routinely used in the long-term management of myocardial infarction although in selected patients without heart failure verapamil or diltiazem may be of some benefit if beta blockers are contra-indicated. *ACE inhibitors* reduce left ventricular remodelling, a process which sometimes follows myocardial infarction and is a recognised precursor of symptomatic heart failure. Myocardial infarction patients with left ventricular dysfunction benefit from long-term oral administration of ACE inhibitors such as captopril (the SAVE study),[86] ramipril (the AIRE and AIRE extension (AIREX) studies),[87-89] or trandolapril (the TRACE study)[90,91] started about 3 days, or more, after infarction. As noted under Early Management (above), favourable results have been reported with ACE inhibitors started early and continued for at least four to six weeks. An expert panel[92] recommended that all patients with signs of left ventricular dysfunction at any time after an acute myocardial infarction should receive prompt treatment with an ACE inhibitor (provided there were no contra-indications) and that such treatment should be long term. The ACE inhibitor could be started within 24 hours of onset of the infarction. The panel were unable to agree on whether all infarction patients should receive early treat-

ment with an ACE inhibitor. There is some evidence that ACE inhibitors may reduce re-infarction rates and this is being investigated in large-scale studies.[93] *Statins*, such as simvastatin and pravastatin, have a more marked cholesterol-lowering effect than older lipid regulating drugs and studies have shown them to be effective in the primary and secondary prevention of myocardial infarction in patients with both high and average cholesterol concentrations. Thus, their use has been advocated in all patients who have suffered a myocardial infarction (see Cardiovascular Risk Reduction, above). Some patients, for example those with myocardial ischaemia or poor left ventricular function may require the long-term administration of *nitrates*, but recent studies have thrown doubt on the routine use of nitrates or other nitric oxide donors. In the GISSI-3 study there was no significant benefit from the use of transdermal glyceryl trinitrate for 6 weeks post-infarction when assessed at 6 weeks[58] or 6 months.[61] In the ISIS-4 study[59] oral isosorbide mononitrate had no effect on 35-day mortality, and in the ESPRIM study[57] molsidomine had no effect on 35-day or longer term mortality. Patients with acute myocardial infarction may have magnesium deficiency and long-term treatment with *oral magnesium* has been tried, but in one study was associated with an increased risk of adverse cardiac events and could not be recommended for secondary prevention.[94]

Post-infarction problems such as heart failure (left ventricular dysfunction), angina pectoris, and arrhythmias are discussed on p.798, p.791, and p.794, respectively.

Primary prevention. Myocardial infarction is one of the principal causes of death in industrialised countries. Risk factors and general preventive measures are discussed under Cardiovascular Risk Reduction, above. See also above for the protective effect of statins.

The benefit of taking *aspirin* as an antiplatelet drug following myocardial infarction is well-established, but its role in primary prevention has been less clear. Two large studies in the UK[95] and in the US[96] in healthy male physicians produced conflicting results. In the UK study there was no reduction in the incidence of fatal and nonfatal myocardial infarction in those who had taken aspirin, while the US study did show a reduction in subjects 50 years of age or older. A large observational study in healthy US nurses[97] indicated that aspirin might reduce the risk of first myocardial infarction in women. The American Heart Association[98,99] states that aspirin may be warranted for middle-aged and older men whose risks of a first myocardial infarction outweigh the possible adverse effects of long-term use. Aspirin may also reduce the risk of first myocardial infarction in patients with stable chronic angina.[100] The Antiplatelet Trialists' Collaboration[26] concluded that aspirin or some other antiplatelet regimen offers worthwhile protection against myocardial infarction in a wide range of patients at high risk of occlusive vascular disease, but that benefit was not established for primary prevention in low risk subjects. The Thrombosis Prevention Trial[101] in males at high risk of developing occlusive vascular disease and the Hypertension Optimal Treatment (HOT) trial[102] have, more recently, confirmed that aspirin reduces the incidence of myocardial infarction in these at-risk groups. The Thrombosis Prevention Trial also investigated the use of low-intensity *warfarin* and found that its use reduced the incidence of ischaemic heart disease (defined as coronary death or myocardial infarction). A greater reduction in ischaemic heart disease incidence was seen with a combination of aspirin and low-intensity warfarin but there was increased incidence of fatal stroke. Low-intensity warfarin may be a possible alternative to aspirin therapy in high-risk males intolerant of aspirin although careful selection of subjects is necessary to minimise risk of bleeding. Studies of Left Ventricular Dysfunction (SOLVD) trials have indicated that *ACE inhibitors*, in this case enalapril,[103] might protect against myocardial infarction, unstable angina, and cardiac death in patients with symptomatic or asymptomatic heart failure.

1. Anderson HV, Willerson JT. Thrombolysis in acute myocardial infarction. *N Engl J Med* 1993; **329:** 703–9.
2. Weston CFM, *et al.* Guidelines for the early management of patients with myocardial infarction. *BMJ* 1994; **308:** 767–71.
3. The Task Force on the Management of Acute Myocardial Infarction of the European Society of Cardiology. Acute myocardial infarction: pre-hospital and in-hospital management. *Eur Heart J* 1996; **17:** 43–63.
4. Ryan TJ, *et al.* ACC/AHA guidelines for the management of patients with acute myocardial infarction: a report of the American College of Cardiology/American Heart Association Task Force on Practice Guidelines (Committee on Management of Acute Myocardial Infarction). *J Am Coll Cardiol* 1996; **28:** 1328–1428.
5. Ryan TJ, *et al.* 1999 update: ACC/AHA guidelines for the management of patients with acute myocardial infarction: a report of the American College of Cardiology/American Heart Association Task Force on Practice Guidelines (Committee on Management of Acute Myocardial Infarction). *J Am Coll Cardiol* 1999; **34:** 890–911.
6. Collins R, *et al.* Aspirin, heparin, and fibrinolytic therapy in suspected acute myocardial infarction. *N Engl J Med* 1997; **336:** 847–60.
7. Second International Study of Infarct Survival Collaborative Group. Randomised trial of intravenous streptokinase, oral aspirin, both, or neither among 17 187 cases of suspected acute myocardial infarction: ISIS-2. *Lancet* 1988; **ii:** 349–60.
8. Gruppo Italiano per lo Studio della Streptochinasi nell'Infarto Miocardico (GISSI). Long-term effects of intravenous thrombolysis in acute myocardial infarction: final report of the GISSI study. *Lancet* 1987; **ii:** 871–4.
9. Wilcox RG, *et al.* Effects of alteplase in acute myocardial infarction: 6-month results from the ASSET study. *Lancet* 1990; **335:** 1175–8.
10. Simoons ML, *et al.* Long-term benefit of early thrombolytic therapy in patients with acute myocardial infarction: 5 year follow-up of a trial conducted by the Interuniversity Cardiology Institute of the Netherlands. *J Am Coll Cardiol* 1989; **14:** 1609–15.
11. Baigent C, *et al.* ISIS-2: 10 year survival among patients with suspected acute myocardial infarction in randomised comparison of intravenous streptokinase, oral aspirin, both, or neither. *BMJ* 1998; **316:** 1337–43.
12. Franzosi MG, *et al.* Ten-year follow-up of the first megatrial testing thrombolytic therapy in patients with acute myocardial infarction: results of the Gruppo Italiano per lo Studio della Sopravvivenza nell'Infarto-1 Study. *Circulation* 1998; **98:** 2659–65.
13. Gruppo Italiano per lo Studio della Streptochinasi nell'Infarto Miocardico (GISSI). Effectiveness of intravenous thrombolytic treatment in acute myocardial infarction. *Lancet* 1986; **i:** 397–402.
14. Fibrinolytic Therapy Trialists' (FTT) Collaborative Group. Indications for fibrinolytic therapy in suspected acute myocardial infarction: collaborative overview of early mortality and major morbidity results from all randomised trials of more than 1000 patients. *Lancet* 1994; **343:** 311–22.
15. LATE Study Group. Late assessment of thrombolytic efficacy (LATE) study with alteplase 6–24 hours after onset of acute myocardial infarction. *Lancet* 1993; **342:** 759–66.
16. EMERAS (Estudio Multicéntrico Estreptoquinasa Repúblicas de América del Sur) Collaborative Group. Randomised trial of late thrombolysis in patients with suspected acute myocardial infarction. *Lancet* 1993; **342:** 767–72.
17. Davis RC. Fibrinolytic therapy in suspected acute myocardial infarction. *Lancet* 1994; **343:** 912.
18. Carlsson J, *et al.* Fibrinolytic therapy in suspected acute myocardial infarction. *Lancet* 1994; **343:** 912–13.
19. Weaver WD, *et al.* Prehospital-initiated vs hospital-initiated thrombolytic therapy: the myocardial infarction triage and intervention trial. *JAMA* 1993; **270:** 1211–16.
20. Cobbe SM. Thrombolysis in myocardial infarction. *BMJ* 1994; **308:** 216–17.
21. Morrison LJ, *et al.* Mortality and prehospital thrombolysis for acute myocardial infarction: a meta-analysis. *JAMA* 2000; **283:** 2686–92.
22. Rawles JM. Quantification of the benefit of earlier thrombolytic therapy: five-year results of the Grampian Region Early Anistreplase Trial (GREAT). *J Am Coll Cardiol* 1997; **30:** 1181–6.
23. PRIMI Trial Study Group. Randomised double-blind trial of recombinant pro-urokinase against streptokinase in acute myocardial infarction. *Lancet* 1989; **i:** 863–8.
24. GISSI-2 and International Study Group. Six-month survival in 20 891 patients with acute myocardial infarction randomized between alteplase and streptokinase with or without heparin. *Eur Heart J* 1992; **13:** 1692–7.
25. Third International Study of Infarct Survival Collaborative Group. ISIS-3: a randomised comparison of streptokinase vs tissue plasminogen activator vs anistreplase and of aspirin plus heparin vs aspirin alone among 41 299 cases of suspected acute myocardial infarction. *Lancet* 1992; **339:** 753–70.
26. International Joint Efficacy Comparison of Thrombolytics. Randomised, double-blind comparison of reteplase double-bolus administration with streptokinase in acute myocardial infarction (INJECT): trial to investigate equivalence. *Lancet* 1995; **346:** 329–36.
27. The GUSTO Investigators. An international randomized trial comparing four thrombolytic strategies for acute myocardial infarction. *N Engl J Med* 1993; **329:** 673–82.
28. Vaitkus PT, *et al.* Stroke complicating acute myocardial infarction: a meta-analysis of risk modification by anticoagulation and thrombolytic therapy. *Arch Intern Med* 1992; **152:** 2020–4.
29. The Global Use of Strategies to Open Occluded Coronary Arteries (GUSTO III) Investigators. A comparison of reteplase with alteplase for acute myocardial infarction. *N Engl J Med* 1997; **337:** 1118–23.
30. Assessment of the Safety and Efficacy of a New Thrombolytic (ASSENT-2) Investigators. Single-bolus tenecteplase compared with front-loaded alteplase in acute myocardial infarction: the ASSENT-2 double-blind randomised trial. *Lancet* 1999; **354:** 716–22.
31. Ridker PM, *et al.* Large-scale trials of thrombolytic therapy for acute myocardial infarction: GISSI-2, ISIS-3, and GUSTO-1. *Ann Intern Med* 1993; **119:** 530–2.
32. The Continuous Infusion versus Double-Bolus Administration of Alteplase (COBALT) Investigators. A comparison of continuous infusion of alteplase with double-bolus administration for acute myocardial infarction. *N Engl J Med* 1997; **337:** 1124–30.
33. Mehta SR, *et al.* Risk of intracranial haemorrhage with bolus versus infusion thrombolytic therapy: a meta-analysis. *Lancet* 2000; **356:** 449–54.
34. Moher M, Johnson N. Use of aspirin by general practitioners in suspected acute myocardial infarction. *BMJ* 1994; **308:** 760.
35. Wyllie HR, Dunn FG. Pre-hospital opiate and aspirin administration in patients with suspected myocardial infarction. *BMJ* 1994; **308:** 760–1.
36. Antman EM. Abciximab facilitates the rate and extent of thrombolysis: results of the Thrombolysis in Myocardial Infarction (TIMI) 14 trial. *Circulation* 1999; **99:** 2720–32.
37. The GUSTO V Investigators. Reperfusion therapy for acute myocardial infarction with fibrinolytic therapy or combination reduced fibrinolytic therapy and platelet glycoprotein IIb/IIIa inhibition: the GUSTO V randomised trial. *Lancet* 2001; **357:** 1905–14. Correction. *ibid.*; **358:** 512.

38. Brener SJ, et al. Randomized, placebo-controlled trial of platelet glycoprotein IIb/IIIa blockade with primary angioplasty for acute myocardial infarction. Circulation 1998; **98:** 734–41.

39. Ridker PM, et al. Are both aspirin and heparin justified as adjuncts to thrombolytic therapy for acute myocardial infarction. Lancet 1993; **341:** 1574–7.

40. Collins R, et al. Clinical effects of anticoagulant therapy in suspected acute myocardial infarction: systematic overview of randomised trials. BMJ 1996; **313:** 652–9.

41. The Global Use of Strategies to Open Occluded Coronary Arteries (GUSTO) IIa Investigators. Randomized trial of intravenous heparin versus recombinant hirudin for acute coronary syndromes. Circulation 1994; **90:** 1631–7.

42. Antman EM, et al. Hirudin in acute myocardial infarction: safety report from the Thrombolysis and Thrombin Inhibition in Myocardial Infarction (TIMI) 9A trial. Circulation 1994; **90:** 1624–30.

43. Neuhaus K-L, et al. Safety observations from the pilot phase of the randomized r-Hirudin for Improvement of Thrombolysis (HIT-III) study: a study of the Arbeitsgemeinschaft Leitender Kardiologischer Krankenhausärzte (ALKK). Circulation 1994; **90:** 1638–42.

44. The Global Use of Strategies to Open Occluded Coronary Arteries (GUSTO) IIb Investigators. A comparison of recombinant hirudin with heparin for the treatment of acute coronary syndromes. N Engl J Med 1996; **335:** 775–82.

45. Antman EM. Hirudin in acute myocardial infarction: thrombolysis and thrombin inhibition in myocardial infarction (TIMI) 9B trial. Circulation 1996; **94:** 911–21.

46. Neuhaus K-L, et al. Recombinant hirudin (lepirudin) for the improvement of thrombolysis with streptokinase in patients with acute myocardial infarction: results of the HIT-4 trial. J Am Coll Cardiol 1999; **34:** 966–73.

47. The Global Use of Strategies to Open Occluded Arteries in Acute Coronary Syndromes (GUSTO IIb) Angioplasty Substudy Investigators. A clinical trial comparing primary coronary angioplasty with tissue plasminogen activator for acute myocardial infarction. N Engl J Med 1997; **336:** 1621–8. Correction. ibid.; **337:** 287.

48. Weaver WD, et al. Comparison of primary coronary angioplasty and intravenous thrombolytic therapy for acute myocardial infarction: a quantitative review. JAMA 1997; **278:** 2093–8. Correction. 1998; **279:** 1876.

49. Zijlstra F, et al. Long-term benefit of primary angioplasty as compared with thrombolytic therapy for acute myocardial infarction. N Engl J Med 1999; **341:** 1413–19.

50. Every NR, et al. A comparison of thrombolytic therapy with primary coronary angioplasty for acute myocardial infarction. N Engl J Med 1996; **335:** 1253–60.

51. Tiefenbrunn AJ, et al. Clinical experience with primary percutaneous transluminal coronary angioplasty compared with alteplase (recombinant tissue-type plasminogen activator) in patients with acute myocardial infarction: a report from the second National Registry of Myocardial Infarction (NRMI-2). J Am Coll Cardiol 1998; **31:** 1240–5.

52. Landau C, et al. Percutaneous transluminal coronary angioplasty. N Engl J Med 1994; **330:** 981–93.

53. First International Study of Infarct Survival Collaborative Group. Mechanisms for the early mortality reduction produced by beta-blockade started early in acute myocardial infarction: ISIS-1. Lancet 1988; **i:** 921–3.

54. Teo KK, et al. Effects of prophylactic antiarrhythmic drug therapy in acute myocardial infarction: an overview of results from randomized controlled trials. JAMA 1993; **270:** 1589–95.

55. Owen A. Intravenous β blockade in acute myocardial infarction. BMJ 1989; **317:** 226–7.

56. Yusuf S, et al. Effect of intravenous nitrates on mortality in acute myocardial infarction: an overview of the randomised trials. Lancet 1988; **i:** 1088–92.

57. European Study of Prevention of Infarct with Molsidomine (ESPRIM) Group. The ESPRIM trial: short-term treatment of acute myocardial infarction with molsidomine. Lancet 1994; **344:** 91–7.

58. Gruppo Italiano per lo Studio della Sopravvivenza nell'Infarto Miocardico. GISSI-3: effects of lisinopril and transdermal glyceryl trinitrate singly and together on 6-week mortality and ventricular function after acute myocardial infarction. Lancet 1994; **343:** 1115–22.

59. ISIS-4 (Fourth International Study of Infarct Survival) Collaborative Group. ISIS-4: a randomised factorial trial assessing early oral captopril, oral mononitrate, and intravenous magnesium sulphate in 58 050 patients with suspected acute myocardial infarction. Lancet 1995; **345:** 669–85.

60. Chinese Cardiac Study collaborative group. Oral captopril versus placebo among 13 634 patients with suspected acute myocardial infarction: interim report from the Chinese Cardiac Study (CCS-1). Lancet 1995; **345:** 686–7.

61. Gruppo Italiano per lo Studio della Sopravvivenza nell'Infarto Miocardico. Six-month effects of early treatment with lisinopril and transdermal glyceryl trinitrate singly and together withdrawn six weeks after acute myocardial infarction: the GISSI-3 trial. J Am Coll Cardiol 1996; **27:** 337–44.

62. Swedberg K, et al. Effects of the early administration of enalapril on mortality in patients with acute myocardial infarction: results of the Cooperative New Scandinavian Enalapril Survival Study II (CONSENSUS II). N Engl J Med 1992; **327:** 678–84.

63. Bonarjee VVS, et al. Attenuation of left ventricular dilatation after acute myocardial infarction by early initiation of enalapril therapy. Am J Cardiol 1993; **72:** 1004–9.

64. Nguyen KN, et al. Interaction between enalapril and aspirin on mortality after acute myocardial infarction: subgroup analysis of the Cooperative New Scandinavian Enalapril Survival Study II (CONSENSUS II). Am J Cardiol 2000; **79:** 115–19.

65. Latini R, et al. Clinical effects of early angiotensin-converting enzyme inhibitor treatment for acute myocardial infarction are similar in the presence and absence of aspirin: systematic overview of individual data from 96,712 randomized patients. J Am Coll Cardiol 2000; **35:** 1801–7.

66. ACE Inhibitor Myocardial Infarction Collaborative Group. Indications for ACE inhibitors in the early treatment of acute myocardial infarction: systematic overview of individual data from 100 000 patients in randomized trials. Circulation 1998; **97:** 2202–12.

67. Ertl G, Jugdutt B. ACE inhibition after myocardial infarction: can megatrials provide answers? Lancet 1994; **344:** 1068–9.

68. Hall AS, et al. Inhibition of the renin-angiotensin system after acute myocardial infarction—treat first, select later? Heart 1996; **76** (suppl 3): 73–8.

69. Teo KK, et al. Effects of intravenous magnesium in suspected acute myocardial infarction: overview of randomised trials. BMJ 1991; **303:** 1499–1503.

70. Woods KL, et al. Intravenous magnesium sulphate in suspected acute myocardial infarction: results of the second Leicester Intravenous Magnesium Intervention Trial (LIMIT-2). Lancet 1992; **339:** 1553–8.

71. Woods KL, Fletcher S. Long-term outcome after intravenous magnesium sulphate in suspected acute myocardial infarction: the second Leicester Intravenous Magnesium Intervention Trial (LIMIT-2). Lancet 1994; **343:** 816–19.

72. Anonymous. Myocardial stunning. Lancet 1991; **337:** 585–6.

73. Fath-Ordoubadi F, Beatt KJ. Glucose-insulin-potassium therapy for treatment of acute myocardial infarction: an overview of randomized placebo-controlled trials. Circulation 1997; **96:** 1152–6.

74. Díaz R, et al. Metabolic modulation of acute myocardial infarction: the ECLA glucose-insulin-potassium pilot trial. Circulation 1998; **98:** 2227–34.

75. Northridge DB, Hall RJC. Post-myocardial-infarction exercise testing in the thrombolytic era. Lancet 1994; **343:** 1175–6.

76. Antiplatelet Trialists' Collaboration. Collaborative overview of randomised trials of antiplatelet therapy—I: prevention of death, myocardial infarction, and stroke by prolonged antiplatelet therapy in various categories of patients. BMJ 1994; **308:** 81–106. Correction. ibid.: 1540.

77. CAPRIE Steering Committee. A randomised, blinded, trial of clopidogrel versus aspirin in patients at risk of ischaemic events (CAPRIE). Lancet 1996; **348:** 1329–39.

78. Anticoagulants in the Secondary Prevention of Events in Coronary Thrombosis (ASPECT) Research Group. Effects of long-term oral anticoagulant treatment on mortality and cardiovascular morbidity after myocardial infarction. Lancet 1994; **343:** 499–503.

79. Cairns JA. Oral anticoagulants or aspirin after myocardial infarction? Lancet 1994; **343:** 497–8.

80. Julian DG, et al. A comparison of aspirin and anticoagulation following thrombolysis for myocardial infarction (the AFTER Study): a multicentre unblinded randomised clinical trial. BMJ 1996; **313:** 1429–31.

81. Coumadin Aspirin Reinfarction Study (CARS) Investigators. Randomised double-blind trial of fixed low-dose warfarin with aspirin after myocardial infarction. Lancet 1997; **350:** 389–96.

82. Freemantle N, et al. β Blockade after myocardial infarction: systematic review and meta regression analysis. BMJ 1999; **318:** 1730–7. Correction. ibid. 2000; **321:** 482.

83. Gottlieb SS, et al. Effect of beta-blockade on mortality among high-risk and low-risk patients after myocardial infarction. N Engl J Med 1998; **339:** 489–97.

84. Soumerai SB, et al. Adverse outcomes of underuse of β-blockers in elderly survivors of acute myocardial infarction. JAMA 1997; **277:** 115–21.

85. Krumholz HM, et al. National use and effectiveness of β-blockers for the treatment of elderly patients after acute myocardial infarction: National Cooperative Cardiovascular Project. JAMA 1998; **280:** 623–9. Correction. ibid. 1999; **281:** 37.

86. Pfeffer MA, et al. Effect of captopril on mortality and morbidity in patients with left ventricular dysfunction after myocardial infarction: results of the Survival and Ventricular Enlargement Trial. N Engl J Med 1992; **327:** 669–77.

87. The Acute Infarction Ramipril Efficacy (AIRE) Study Investigators. Effect of ramipril on mortality and morbidity of survivors of acute myocardial infarction with clinical evidence of heart failure. Lancet 1993; **342:** 821–8.

88. Hall AS, et al. Follow-up study of patients randomly allocated ramipril or placebo for heart failure after acute myocardial infarction: AIRE extension (AIREX) study. Lancet 1997; **349:** 1493–7.

89. Cleland JGF, et al. Effect of ramipril on morbidity and mode of death among survivors of acute myocardial infarction with clinical evidence of heart failure: a report from the AIRE study investigators. Eur Heart J 1997; **18:** 41–51.

90. Køber L, et al. A clinical trial of the angiotensin-converting-enzyme inhibitor trandolapril in patients with left ventricular dysfunction after myocardial infarction. N Engl J Med 1995; **333:** 1670–6.

91. Torp-Pedersen C, Køber L. Effect of ACE inhibitor trandolapril on life expectancy of patients with reduced left-ventricular function after acute myocardial infarction. Lancet 1999; **354:** 9–12.

92. Latini R, et al. ACE inhibitor use in patients with myocardial infarction: summary of evidence from clinical trials. Circulation 1995; **92:** 3132–7.

93. Reynolds G, et al. What have the ACE-inhibitor trials in postmyocardial patients with left ventricular dysfunction taught us? Eur J Clin Pharmacol 1996; **49:** S35–S39.

94. Galløe AM, et al. Influence of oral magnesium supplementation on cardiac events among survivors of an acute myocardial infarction. BMJ 1993; **307:** 585–7.

95. Peto R, et al. Randomised trial of prophylactic daily aspirin in British male doctors. BMJ 1988; **296:** 313–16.

96. Steering Committee of the Physicians Health Study Research Group. Final report on the aspirin component of the ongoing physicians' health study. N Engl J Med 1989; **321:** 129–35.

97. Manson JE, et al. A prospective study of aspirin use and primary prevention of cardiovascular disease in women. JAMA 1991; **266:** 521–7.

98. Fuster V, et al. Aspirin as a therapeutic agent in cardiovascular disease. Circulation 1993; **87:** 659–75.

99. Hennekens CH, et al. Aspirin as a therapeutic agent in cardiovascular disease: a statement for healthcare professionals from the American Heart Association. Circulation 1997; **96:** 2751–3.

100. Juul-Möller S, et al. Double-blind trial of aspirin in primary prevention of myocardial infarction in patients with stable chronic angina pectoris. Lancet 1992; **340:** 1421–5.

101. The Medical Research Council's General Practice Research Framework. Thrombosis prevention trial: randomised trial of low-intensity oral anticoagulation with warfarin and low-dose aspirin in the primary prevention of ischaemic heart disease in men at increased risk. Lancet 1998; **351:** 233–41.

102. Hansson L, et al. Effects of intensive blood-pressure lowering and low-dose aspirin in patients with hypertension: principal results of the Hypertension Optimal Treatment (HOT) randomised trial. Lancet 1998; **351:** 1755–62.

103. Yusuf S, et al. Effect of enalapril on myocardial infarction and unstable angina in patients with low ejection fractions. Lancet 1992; **340:** 1173–8.

Patent ductus arteriosus

The ductus arteriosus is a vascular channel present in the fetal circulation that connects the pulmonary artery and the descending aorta. In some infants the ductus arteriosus fails to close, a condition known as persistent patent ductus arteriosus. Details of its management are given on p.46.

Peripheral arterial thromboembolism

Occlusion of the peripheral arteries may occur due to embolism or thrombosis (see Thromboembolic Disorders, below). Sudden or acute occlusion causes reduction of blood flow to the distal portions of the limb and may lead to critical limb ischaemia. Emergency treatment with surgery or thrombolytic drugs is often required to restore blood flow and preserve the limb.

Acute peripheral arterial thromboembolism produces pain, pallor, and coldness in the affected limb. Numbness and paraesthesia may occur and if the clot is not removed, gangrene develops. Sudden onset is usually due to occlusion by an embolus. The heart is a frequent source of emboli; atrial fibrillation, cardiomyopathy, myocardial infarction, and valvular heart disease are all associated with peripheral arterial embolism. Peripheral arterial thrombosis often has a more gradual onset due to collateral vessels maintaining some perfusion of the limb. Thrombosis is usually the result of thrombus formation at a site of atheroma in an atherosclerotic artery; thus it may occur in patients with chronic occlusive arterial disease (see Peripheral Vascular Disease, below). Thrombosis is now more common than pure embolism although the two may co-exist.

Sudden arterial occlusion requires emergency treatment to restore circulation and to avoid gangrene and possible amputation of the limb. Where there is imminent danger to the limb surgery is necessary to rapidly restore blood flow. In patients with **embolism** in otherwise healthy arteries surgical removal of the embolus by catheter (embolectomy) is used and usually results in restoration of blood flow. Sudden arterial occlusion due to **thrombosis** where gangrene is imminent requires emergency bypass surgery to restore blood flow; surgical removal of a thrombus (thrombectomy) is not usually successful as most arterial thromboses are superimposed on atheromatous plaques, particularly in elderly patients, and thrombectomy adds to the intimal damage.

Where the risk from ischaemia is less acute, angiography may be performed to confirm the type of occlusion and intra-arterial thrombolysis may be used as initial therapy, particularly if the cause is thrombotic.[1-3] This method is particularly useful for occlusion of smaller vessels, distal occlusions in surgically inaccessible small arteries, or in patients too ill to undergo surgery. However, it is a slower method of restoring blood flow and its use in limb-threatening ischaemia is controversial.[4] The TOPAS study[5] reported no significant difference in outcomes in patients with acute arterial occlusion treated initially with thrombolysis or surgery, although the rate of bleeding complications was higher with thrombolysis. It has therefore been suggested that thrombolysis may be appropriate for initial therapy in acute occlusion, providing this will not lead to an unacceptable delay in reperfusion.[6,7] However, others[8] consider that thrombolysis should not be used as first-line therapy due to the lack of significant benefit and the increased risk of bleeding.

Thrombolytics may be administered intravenously, but intra-arterial administration of low doses of thrombolytics directly into the clot is often used. Despite the use of low doses the risk of major haemorrhage is still about 10%. Continuous intra-arterial infusion, pulse infusion, and different thrombolytics are used; the optimal technique and choice of thrombolytic are unclear. Alteplase, streptokinase, and urokinase are all used. Local treatment with low-dose streptokinase or urokinase infused into the clot is successful in about 50 to 80% of patients and recanalisation is sustained for a year in 50%. Thrombolytic therapy is more likely to be successful if it is begun soon after thrombosis occurs. If no lysis has occurred within the first 12 to 24 hours the procedure is unlikely to be successful, but where thrombolysis is occurring infusion has been continued for several days. There is rather less experience with alteplase; it is claimed to produce more rapid thrombolysis than streptokinase although studies have been too small to provide evidence of reduced limb loss or mortality.[1] On completion of thrombolytic therapy angiography should be repeated to identify the underlying abnormalities that caused the original occlusion. The lesions can then be treated by balloon angioplasty or surgical repair, and this should be done as soon as possible to avoid rethrombosis, which occurs in about 10 to 30% of patients.

Intra-arterial thrombolysis may also be used in conjunction with surgical techniques, particularly when surgery fails to restore blood flow due to distal occlusions.[9-12]

Adjunctive treatment with antithrombotics, such as heparin and aspirin, is often given to patients with peripheral arterial thromboembolism to prevent propagation of the clot and also to prevent post-operative thromboembolic complications. However, there is an increased risk of serious bleeding complications if heparin is used with thrombolytic therapy.[5] Where the occlusion has been due to embolism, the patient should be investigated for a possible source of emboli and long-term oral anticoagulation should be considered to prevent recurrent embolism.

1. Wolfe JH. Critical limb ischaemia. *Prescribers' J* 1994; **34**: 50–8.
2. Beattie DK, Davies AH. Management of the acutely ischaemic limb. *Br J Hosp Med* 1996; **55**: 204–8.
3. Ludlam CA, *et al.* Guidelines for the use of thrombolytic therapy. *Blood Coag Fibrinol* 1995; **6**: 273–85.
4. Hawkins DW, Hirsh J. Antithrombotic drugs for thromboembolic disorders: a lesson in evidence-based medicine. *Am J Health-Syst Pharm* 1997; **54**: 1992–4.
5. Ouriel K, *et al.* A comparison of recombinant urokinase with vascular surgery as initial treatment for acute arterial occlusion of the legs. *N Engl J Med* 1998; **338**: 1105–15.
6. Working Party on Thrombolysis in the Management of Limb Ischemia. Thrombolysis in the management of lower limb peripheral arterial occlusion—a consensus document. *Am J Cardiol* 1998; **81**: 207–18.
7. Jackson MR, Clagett GP. Antithrombotic therapy in peripheral arterial occlusive disease. *Chest* 2001; **119** (suppl): 283S–299S.
8. Porter JM. Thrombolysis for acute arterial occlusion of the legs. *N Engl J Med* 1998; **338**: 1148–50.
9. Earnshaw JJ, Beard JD. Intraoperative use of thrombolytic agents. *BMJ* 1993; **307**: 638–9.
10. Chester JF, *et al.* Peroperative t-PA thrombolysis. *Lancet* 1991; **337**: 861–2.
11. Verstraete M. Use of thrombolytic drugs in non-coronary disorders. *Drugs* 1989; **38**: 801–21.
12. Anonymous. Non-coronary thrombolysis. *Lancet* 1990; **335**: 691–3.

Peripheral vascular disease

The term peripheral vascular disease may be used to cover venous and arterial diseases of the limbs, but is often confined to arterial disease, as is the discussion that follows.

For details of venous diseases, see under Venous Thromboembolism, below.

Peripheral arterial disease can be divided into obstructive or occlusive disease and vasospastic disease and these two types are described in turn.

The commonest form of **occlusive arterial disease** is caused by **atherosclerosis**. It may well be only one manifestation of a generalised atherosclerotic process and sufferers also usually experience, or are at increased risk of, ischaemic heart disease. **Thromboangiitis obliterans** (Buerger's disease)[1] is also an occlusive arterial disease, but, rather than being caused by atherosclerosis, it is a result of inflammatory and proliferative lesions in medium and small arteries and veins of the limbs. The lesions are predominantly thrombotic in nature. It progresses more rapidly than atherosclerotic disease; severe ulceration and gangrene, necessitating amputation, may often occur. Sufferers are typically heavy smokers. **Intermittent claudication** is a major feature of occlusive arterial disease of the lower limbs and is characterised by pain which develops during exercise and which usually disappears at rest although it may persist in severe forms of disease. The pain is due to **ischaemia** (insufficient oxygen supply) resulting from the obstruction or vasoconstriction of peripheral arteries. Ischaemia may also result in trophic changes in the skin. In severe or advanced disease, ulceration of skin and tissues can occur and may even progress to gangrene. Although the cause of arterial obstruction is usually atherosclerosis, ischaemia is commonly precipitated by thrombosis. Smoking causes vasoconstriction and is frequently a contributory factor.

Management. Patients with occlusive arterial disease are at high risk of other cardiovascular events such as myocardial infarction and stroke, and treatment is important both to reduce this risk and to improve symptoms.[2] All patients should therefore adopt a lifestyle that minimises cardiovascular risk factors, as described under Atherosclerosis, above. They should be advised not to smoke;[3] in the case of thromboangiitis obliterans, cessation of smoking is essential to halt progression of the disease. Supervised exercise programmes may help to improve walking distance in patients with intermittent claudication.[3] In common with other atherosclerotic diseases, such as angina and myocardial infarction, antiplatelet therapy has been investigated in patients with peripheral arterial disease. Early studies indicated that *aspirin*, with or without dipyridamole, may have some effect in delaying the progression of peripheral arterial diseases. An overview of trials[4] of antiplatelet therapies demonstrated that patients with peripheral vascular disease, peripheral grafts, or peripheral angioplasty benefit additionally in terms of fewer subsequent vascular events such as myocardial infarction and stroke, although a more recent analysis[5] concluded that there was insufficient evidence to support the use of prophylactic aspirin in patients with intermittent claudication but no additional vascular risk factors. Antiplatelet therapy is generally recommended as routine prophylactic treatment in all patients with claudication.[2,3,6] The dose of aspirin generally used in the trials was 75 to 325 mg daily. Ticlopidine[4] or clopidogrel[7] may be suitable alternatives in patients unable to tolerate aspirin. Lipid lowering therapy should also be considered for cardiovascular risk reduction, although again specific evidence of benefit is limited.[2,3]

Many drugs have been employed for symptom control in occlusive arterial disease, but studies have often been unsatisfactory and their efficacy and/or overall place in management remains to be firmly established.[8]

Naftidrofuryl and *oxpentifylline [pentoxifylline]* are used in intermittent claudication to increase the time and distance walked before the onset of pain, but evidence of benefit has generally been unconvincing.[3,9-11] Limited data suggest that *cilostazol* may be of benefit and it has been recommended in patients with disabling claudication.[6] Although often described as *vasodilators*, any purported benefit with this type of drug may be due to actions on blood cells or blood rheology rather than vasodilatation. In any case, drugs with vasodilator actions do not preferentially dilate affected arteries and those to ischaemic tissue may be fully dilated already. Administration of vasodilators will result in dilatation of arteries supplying non-ischaemic tissues elsewhere in the body and thus blood may actually be diverted away from the affected ischaemic area—the so-called 'steal' phenomenon; this is a known risk with all vasodilators, but especially with powerful arterial vasodilators such as hydralazine and this type of drug is not suitable for use in peripheral arterial disease. Other drugs that have been promoted for the treatment of intermittent claudication include cinnarizine, cyclandelate, and inositol nicotinate; ginkgo biloba and levocarnitine have also been tried.

Ketanserin inhibits vasoconstriction and also changes indices of blood rheology, but results in intermittent claudication have been inconsistent.

Certain *prostaglandins* cause vasodilatation and prevent platelet aggregation and some have appeared promising in the presence of advanced disease or complications.[3] A beneficial effect on rest pain has been noted and some ulcers have either regressed or healed; in selected patients this form of therapy has avoided the need for amputation. Prostaglandins employed include *alprostadil* or *epoprostenol*, both intra-arterially or intravenously, *iloprost* intravenously, and *dinoprostone* topically. Orally active *beraprost* is under investigation.

If intermittent claudication is severe **non-pharmacological** techniques such as bypass surgery, endarterectomy, percutaneous transluminal angioplasty, or intravascular stenting should be considered. Following these procedures, treatment to prevent postoperative thrombosis and restenosis may be necessary (see Reperfusion and Revascularisation Procedures, below).

Sudden or **acute arterial occlusion** due to emboli or to thrombosis may occur in 10% of patients with atherosclerotic disease, but is rare in thromboangiitis obliterans. The initial approach has been surgical removal; dissolution of the thrombus using local or systemic thrombolytic therapy may be considered. For further details, see Peripheral Arterial Thromboembolism, above.

Vasospastic arterial disease is due to an inappropriate response to temperature, usually cold, when vasoconstriction and/or vasospasm occurs. The most important of these disorders is Raynaud's syndrome. Other vasospastic conditions include acrocyanosis, chilblains, and erythromelalgia.

In **Raynaud's syndrome**, paroxysmal attacks of pallor and cyanosis, usually of the digits, occur in response to cold, or sometimes emotional stress. Erythema replaces the cyanosis as the attacks resolve. The cause of primary Raynaud's syndrome (Raynaud's disease) is unknown. Features identified include intense vasoconstriction or vasospasm, disturbance of sympathetic nerve supply, changes in circulating catecholamines, enhanced platelet aggregation, red cell deformability, and fibrinolysis. It is probable that not all cases are due to the same mechanism. It has been suggested that the underlying defect may not be an overreaction to the initial cold insult but be a defect in the normal ensuing adaptive response. Secondary Raynaud's syndrome (Raynaud's phenomenon) frequently co-exists with arterial occlusive disease such as thromboangiitis obliterans (see above) and connective tissue disorders, in particular scleroderma (systemic sclerosis). Trauma and certain drugs, notably beta blockers and ergotamine, may also be responsible for inducing secondary Raynaud's syndrome.

Management. In mild cases of Raynaud's syndrome, where attacks are infrequent and of limited severity, protective measures to keep warm are the mainstay of treatment; this involves wearing appropriate clothing and the use of appliances such as heated gloves. Patients should also stop smoking because of the vasoconstriction caused. Any underlying or co-existing disease or cause in secondary Raynaud's syndrome should be treated. Drug therapy is indicated in more severe cases. It is directed towards producing vascular smooth muscle relaxation and vasodilatation in order to improve resting blood flow, thereby reducing the extent of tissue ischaemia. Some drugs may also act by modifying platelet aggregation or blood rheology. As with occlusive arterial disease many drugs have been tried in Raynaud's syndrome. This perhaps reflects the large number of differing mechanisms of defect that have been proposed.[12-15]

Calcium-channel blockers have been of benefit and are widely used in Raynaud's syndrome, but it is not entirely clear which of their pharmacological actions is responsible. Dihydropyridines are usually preferred; the most widely used and studied is *nifedipine*.

Thymoxamine [moxisylyte], an alpha blocker with vasodilating activity is also widely employed. Other alpha blockers, for example, phenoxybenzamine and prazosin as well as reserpine have been used although in some cases side-effects have limited their usefulness.

Cinnarizine, naftidrofuryl, oxpentifylline [pentoxifylline], and *nicotinic acid derivatives* such as inositol nicotinate have had widespread use in Raynaud's syndrome but, as for occlusive arterial disease, evidence of efficacy is lacking.

In severe Raynaud's syndrome complicated by ulceration and gangrene, as in occlusive disease, *prostaglandins* have been promising. *Alprostadil, epoprostenol,* and *iloprost* have been administered by intravenous infusion. In some cases the beneficial effects have persisted for a few months after treatment and two or three infusions given at intervals over the winter months have prevented the severe complications of Raynaud's suffered in previous years. Iloprost orally has also been reported to reduce the severity of attacks. Prostaglandins applied topically in ulcerative cases include *dinoprostone*.

Small studies or anecdotal reports have noted variable effects with many *other drugs* including the ACE inhibitors captopril and enalapril, the serotonin reuptake inhibitors fluoxetine and venlafaxine, topical nitrates such as glyceryl trinitrate, ketanserin, piracetam, and sodium nitroprusside. None of these therapies appears, however, to have come into widespread use. The potent vasodilator calcitonin gene-related peptide has shown promise.

Acrocyanosis is characterised by a persistent blue discoloration of the skin. There is an abnormal constriction of arterioles, even at normal environmental conditions and this is potentiated by cold. **Chilblains** are an inflammatory condition (perniosis) affecting the extremities and symptoms include erythema, pruritus, and ulceration; they may be acute or chronic. Chilblains occur more commonly in cold damp conditions. Acrocyanosis and chilblains do not generally require specific treatment; smoking cessation, protection from the cold, or symptomatic antipruritic treatment are often sufficient. However, if severe, the drugs described above under Raynaud's syndrome may be considered. **Erythromelalgia** is a vasospastic condition usually provoked by heat although it may also be drug-induced (secondary erythermalgia).[16] It is characterised by painful, red extremities together with a burning sensation and increased skin temperature of the affected area. Thrombocythaemia is the most common underlying cause and, indeed, erythromelalgia may be the presenting feature of this disorder; in thrombocythaemia, arteriolar occlusion may occur as a result of platelet aggregation. Small doses of aspirin have produced considerable relief in some patients, presumably by preventing platelet aggregation. Beta blockers may also be of some help. Attacks should be prevented wherever possible by avoiding exposure to heat.

1. Olin JW. Thromboangiitis obliterans (Buerger's disease). *N Engl J Med* 2000; **343:** 864–9.
2. Hiatt WR. Medical treatment of peripheral arterial disease and claudication. *N Engl J Med* 2001; **344:** 1608–21.
3. Weitz JI, *et al.* Diagnosis and treatment of chronic arterial insufficiency of the lower extremities: a critical review. *Circulation* 1996; **94:** 3026–49.
4. Antiplatelet Trialists' Collaboration. Collaborative overview of randomised trials of antiplatelet therapy—I: prevention of death, myocardial infarction, and stroke by prolonged antiplatelet therapy in various categories of patients. *BMJ* 1994; **308:** 81–106.
5. Eccles M, *et al.* North of England evidence based guideline development project: guideline on the use of aspirin as secondary prophylaxis for vascular disease in primary care. *BMJ* 1998; **316:** 1303–9.
6. Jackson MR, Clagett GP. Antithrombotic therapy in peripheral arterial occlusive disease. *Chest* 2001; **119** (suppl): 283S–299S.
7. CAPRIE Steering Committee. A randomised, blinded, trial of clopidogrel versus aspirin in patients at risk of ischaemic events (CAPRIE). *Lancet* 1996; **348:** 1329–39.
8. Moher D, *et al.* Pharmacological management of intermittent claudication: a meta-analysis of randomised trials. *Drugs* 2000; **59:** 1057–70.
9. Cameron HA, *et al.* Drug treatment of intermittent claudication: a critical analysis of the methods and findings of published clinical trials, 1965–1985. *Br J Clin Pharmacol* 1988; **26:** 569–76.
10. Radack K, Wyderski RJ. Conservative management of intermittent claudication. *Ann Intern Med* 1990; **113:** 135–46.
11. Girolami B, *et al.* Treatment of intermittent claudication with physical training, smoking cessation, pentoxifylline, or nafronyl: a meta-analysis. *Arch Intern Med* 1999; **159:** 337–45.
12. Belch JJF, Ho M. Pharmacotherapy of Raynaud's phenomenon. *Drugs* 1996; **52:** 682–95.
13. Black CM. Raynaud's phenomenon. *Prescribers' J* 1994; **34:** 125–33.
14. Isenberg DA, Black C. Raynaud's phenomenon, scleroderma, and overlap syndromes. *BMJ* 1995; **310:** 795–8.
15. Block JA, Sequeira W. Raynaud's phenomenon. *Lancet* 2001; **357:** 2042–8.
16. Drenth JPH, Michiels JJ. Three types of erythromelalgia. *BMJ* 1990; **301:** 454–5.

Phaeochromocytoma

Phaeochromocytoma is a rare catecholamine-secreting tumour of the adrenal medulla. Patients with phaeochromocytoma are usually hypertensive and suffer headache, palpitations, and excessive sweating; the hypertension may be either episodic or sustained. However, if the tumour is predominantly adrenaline-secreting, tachyarrhythmias may be associated with a normal or even decreased arterial pressure and if the tumour secretes mainly noradrenaline, vasoconstriction may lead to contraction of the venous pool and hypovolaemia. If the effects of the release of catecholamines are not controlled a life-threatening crisis ultimately ensues and may range from a shock-like syndrome with multiple organ failure to hypertensive crisis, depending on the predominance of the catecholamine secreted.

For a diagnosis of phaeochromocytoma, history and clinical symptoms are important, but a firm diagnosis requires further investigative techniques. Raised plasma or urinary concentrations of catecholamine metabolites indicate the presence of a tumour; measurement of urinary or plasma concentrations of adrenaline and noradrenaline may be necessary to confirm the diagnosis in some patients. The precise location of the tumour can be established by procedures such as computed tomography, magnetic resonance imaging, or scintigraphy with ^{131}I-iobenguane (^{131}I-*m*-iodobenzylguanidine). Other tests that may be used include administration of drugs such as clonidine which suppress catecholamine release in normal patients but not in those with phaeochromocytoma. A glucagon stimulation test may also be used but other provocative tests are generally considered obsolete.

Although surgery to remove the tumour is the ultimate treatment goal, the initial step in management must be the prevention of the pressor and other effects of catecholamines. Alpha blockers, given by mouth, are the mainstay of therapy; they both reduce the blood pressure and allow the plasma volume to return to normal. Phenoxybenzamine is the alpha blocker of choice since the long-lasting, non-competitive blockade that it produces cannot be overridden by surges of catecholamine release, as may happen with competitive blockers. In patients who are unable to tolerate phenoxybenzamine, a selective alpha$_1$-adrenoceptor blocker such as prazosin may be used; it results in less tachycardia and may be preferable if the tumour is predominantly adrenaline-secreting, but hypotension may be a problem. Phentolamine may be given intravenously in patients with hypertensive crises. The initial dose of alpha blocker should be small and should be increased gradually until all signs of pressor activity are suppressed. Once, but not until, alpha blockade is successfully established, tachycardia can be controlled by the cautious use of a beta blocker. A beta$_1$-selective blocker is preferred so that peripheral beta$_2$-mediated va-

sodilatation is unaffected. α-Methyltyrosine, which suppresses catecholamine synthesis, may be tried in selected patients such as those resistant to alpha blockade or those in whom the effects of alpha or beta blockade may be undesirable.

Once the pressor effects of catecholamine secretion are controlled, surgery can be undertaken. Drugs used for premedication and anaesthesia should be chosen so as to avoid those which may cause pressor responses or tachycardia and ideally should suppress the adrenergic response to surgical stimuli. This will still not be adequate to prevent catecholamine release when the tumour is handled and potent vasodilators such as sodium nitroprusside or glyceryl trinitrate have been given intravenously to prevent dangerously high arterial pressures; the alpha blocker phentolamine has also been advocated although tachycardia is invariably a problem. Cardioselective beta blockers such as atenolol may be given, often in high dosage, to control tachycardia during surgery.

If it proves impossible to remove all the active tissue of a phaeochromocytoma during surgery, or in patients who are unsuitable for surgery or who have malignant phaeochromocytoma, maintenance therapy with alpha and beta blockade needs to be continued or α-methyltyrosine may be used. Alternatively, ^{131}I-iobenguane has been given in high doses sufficient to cause radionecrosis; antineoplastic therapy has also been used.

References.
1. Klingler HC, *et al.* Pheochromocytoma. *Urology* 2001; **57:** 1025–32.
2. Pacak K, *et al.* Recent advances in genetics, diagnosis, localization, and treatment of pheochromocytoma. *Ann Intern Med* 2001; **134:** 315–29.

Pulmonary hypertension

Pulmonary hypertension, unless otherwise specified, refers to pulmonary arterial pressure. The criteria depend on altitude, but in a resting individual at sea level a pulmonary arterial pressure greater than 20 mmHg establishes a diagnosis; at higher altitudes, correspondingly higher pressures occur and at about 15 000 feet a value greater than 25 mmHg signifies pulmonary hypertension.

Pulmonary hypertension has usually been classified as primary or secondary, although a wider classification system based on the underlying cause may now be used.[1,2] Primary pulmonary hypertension is uncommon and patients have no underlying disease known to cause an elevation of the pulmonary arterial pressure. Secondary pulmonary hypertension, in contrast, is far more prevalent and patients have some form of cardiopulmonary disorder that can lead to the development of pulmonary hypertension.

Primary pulmonary hypertension has been reviewed.[1-7] It has been recorded in patients of all ages and in both sexes but women in the fourth decade of life are those typically seen. Initial complaints include dyspnoea on exertion, fatigue, and chest discomfort or pain. In advanced disease, cor pulmonale (an enlargement of the right ventricle due to either dilatation, hypertrophy, or both) occurs and may progress to right-sided heart failure. The pulmonary arteries may be affected by thromboembolic disease. Primary pulmonary hypertension is a progressive and incurable disease and patients appear to be prone to sudden death.

The aim of treatment is to decrease the pulmonary arterial pressure, preferably in conjunction with an increase in cardiac output. Many drugs with vasodilating effects have been investigated in pulmonary hypertension,[8,9] the rationale usually being based upon their application in systemic hypertension. Unfortunately, the vast majority have been unsatisfactory. Although most vasodilators do reduce pulmonary arterial pressure they are not selective for the pulmonary circulation and therefore also reduce systemic blood pressure producing undesirable, or sometimes intolerable, side-effects. Of all the vasodilators studied the most promising appear to be calcium-channel blockers and the prostaglandin epoprostenol. Improved survival over a 5-year period has been noted in some patients treated with high-dose *calcium-channel blockers*.[10] However, not all patients respond and because of concerns about previously reported adverse effects in patients with primary pulmonary hypertension given these drugs it has been advised that an acute response test should be performed before embarking on long term treatment.[9,10] Although oral calcium-channel blockers may be used for the test, shorter-acting vasodilators such as intravenous epoprostenol, intravenous adenosine, or inhaled nitric oxide, are generally employed.[3] *Epoproste-*

nol was originally introduced into the management of primary pulmonary hypertension to sustain patients long enough for them to have heart-lung transplantation but long-term therapy may also have a role as an alternative to transplantation.[11,12] Sustained clinical improvement and improved survival have been reported in some patients given long-term intravenous therapy using portable infusion pumps.[13-17] Continuous infusion of the more stable analogue iloprost may also be effective.[18] Administration by inhalation may avoid some of the complications of long-term intravenous access and beneficial responses have been reported with inhaled epoprostenol[19,20] and with iloprost,[19,21,22] although this route is less well established. Therapy with beraprost sodium, an epoprostenol analogue that can be given orally, has also been tried[23,24] and other prostaglandin analogues are also under investigation. The endothelin receptor antagonist *bosentan* may also be used. Lung or heart-lung transplantation may be required in patients who do not respond to vasodilator therapy.[3] Patients with primary pulmonary hypertension have an increased risk of thromboembolism and *oral anticoagulants* are recommended on a long term basis for most patients as they may improve survival.[10] *Diuretics*[10,13] and *digoxin*[10,13] are given as necessary for associated right-sided heart failure.

Secondary pulmonary hypertension occurs as a consequence of an established cardiopulmonary disorder and the clinical manifestations are dominated by those of the underlying condition. Chronic obstructive pulmonary disease is the commonest respiratory cause. Other lung disorders that may lead to pulmonary hypertension include: diseases of the lung parenchyma such as the respiratory distress syndromes, sarcoidosis, and cryptogenic fibrosing alveolitis; diseases affecting the pulmonary vessels such as thromboembolic disease and systemic lupus erythematosus; and connective tissue diseases such as scleroderma. Cardiac causes include disorders leading to impaired left ventricular function such as myocardial infarction or mitral valve disease.

Management of secondary pulmonary hypertension basically constitutes appropriate treatment of the underlying condition, although continuous intravenous epoprostenol may be of benefit in some patients.[25,26] Inhaled nitric oxide has been used in acutely ill patients.[27] Patients with underlying connective tissue disorders may require similar management to those with primary pulmonary hypertension.[28]

Persistent pulmonary hypertension of the newborn, sometimes also termed persistent fetal circulation, is, as the name implies, a form of pulmonary hypertension specifically affecting neonates. It can be primary in nature (that is, idiopathic, affecting infants with an anatomically normal heart and no pulmonary disease) or secondary, being associated with a number of cardiopulmonary conditions including congenital heart disease, diaphragmatic hernia, meconium aspiration, respiratory distress syndrome, or sepsis. The pulmonary hypertension and altered vasoreactivity lead to a right-to-left shunting of blood across the patent ductus arteriosus or foramen ovale and this often results in critical hypoxaemia.

Management generally involves high-frequency oscillatory ventilation (to achieve optimal lung inflation) and, if necessary, extracorporeal membrane oxygenation. Mechanical hyperventilation induces alkalosis and has decreased pulmonary arterial pressure and improved oxygenation in some patients.[29] Intravenous vasodilators have also been employed, but, as discussed above, their use is generally restricted because of their non-selectivity for the pulmonary circulation; inhaled *nitric oxide* which is a potent, selective pulmonary vasodilator, is now more widely used.[30] Studies[31-35] have shown that it can cause marked improvement in oxygenation and a reduction in the need for extracorporeal membrane oxygenation, but no effect on mortality has been demonstrated. Although there have been concerns that use of inhaled nitric oxide might adversely affect neurodevelopmental outcome more than conventional therapy, this has not been confirmed in infants followed up for up to 2 years.[36,37] Use of inhaled nitric oxide in combination with high-frequency oscillatory ventilation may have additional benefits.[38] Of the vasodilators tried, *tolazoline*, has been the most commonly employed. One report[39] has described the use of inhaled *epoprostenol* in two neonates, a method of administration that may overcome the problems of systemic vasodilatation. *Magnesium sulfate* intravenously has also been reported[40-42] to have potential use as a vasodilator, and intravenous *adenosine* has also been tried.[43]

1. Peacock AJ. Primary pulmonary hypertension. *Thorax* 1999; **54:** 1107–18.

2. Galiè N, Torbicki A. Pulmonary arterial hypertension: new ideas and perspectives. *Heart* 2001; **85:** 475–80.
3. Rubin LJ. Primary pulmonary hypertension. *N Engl J Med* 1997; **336:** 111–17.
4. Gaine SP, Rubin LJ. Primary pulmonary hypertension. *Lancet* 1998; **352:** 719–25. Correction. *ibid.* 1999; **353:** 74.
5. Peacock A, Raeside D. Pulmonary hypertension. *Prescribers' J* 1998; **38:** 1–6.
6. Wanstall JC, Jeffery TK. Recognition and management of pulmonary hypertension. *Drugs* 1998; **56:** 989–1007.
7. Gaine S. Pulmonary hypertension. *JAMA* 2000; **284:** 3160–8.
8. Weir EK, *et al.* The acute administration of vasodilators in primary pulmonary hypertension: experience from the National Institutes of Health Registry on Primary Pulmonary Hypertension. *Am Rev Respir Dis* 1989; **140:** 1623–30.
9. Barnes PJ, Liu SF. Regulation of pulmonary vascular tone. *Pharmacol Rev* 1995; **47:** 87–131.
10. Rich S, *et al.* The effect of high doses of calcium-channel blockers on survival in primary pulmonary hypertension. *N Engl J Med* 1992; **327:** 76–81.
11. Herner SJ, Mauro LS. Epoprostenol in primary pulmonary hypertension. *Ann Pharmacother* 1999; **33:** 340–7.
12. Barst RJ. Treatment of primary pulmonary hypertension with continuous intravenous prostacyclin. *Heart* 1997; **77:** 299–301.
13. Barst RJ, *et al.* Survival in primary pulmonary hypertension with long-term continuous intravenous prostacyclin. *Ann Intern Med* 1994; **121:** 409–15. Correction. *ibid.* 1995; **122:** 238.
14. Barst RJ, *et al.* A comparison of continuous intravenous epoprostenol (prostacyclin) with conventional therapy for primary pulmonary hypertension. *N Engl J Med* 1996; **334:** 296–301.
15. Shapiro SM, *et al.* Primary pulmonary hypertension: improved long-term effects and survival with continuous intravenous epoprostenol infusion. *J Am Coll Cardiol* 1997; **30:** 343–9.
16. McLaughlin VV, *et al.* Reduction in pulmonary vascular resistance with long-term epoprostenol (prostacyclin) therapy in primary pulmonary hypertension. *N Engl J Med* 1998; **338:** 273–7.
17. Higenbottam T, *et al.* Long term intravenous prostaglandin (epoprostenol or iloprost) for the treatment of severe pulmonary hypertension. *Heart* 1998; **80:** 151–5.
18. Higenbottam TW, *et al.* Treatment of pulmonary hypertension with the continuous infusion of a prostacyclin analogue, iloprost. *Heart* 1998; **79:** 175–9.
19. Olschewski H, *et al.* Aerosolized prostacyclin and iloprost in severe pulmonary hypertension. *Ann Intern Med* 1996; **124:** 820–4.
20. Mikhail G, *et al.* An evaluation of nebulized prostacyclin in patients with primary and secondary pulmonary hypertension. *Eur Heart J* 1997; **18:** 1499–1504.
21. Olschewski H, *et al.* Inhaled iloprost to treat severe pulmonary hypertension: an uncontrolled trial. *Ann Intern Med* 2000; **132:** 435–43.
22. Hoeper MM, *et al.* Long-term treatment of primary pulmonary hypertension with aerosolized iloprost, a prostacyclin analogue. *N Engl J Med* 2000; **342:** 1866–70.
23. Okano Y, *et al.* Orally active prostacyclin analogue in primary pulmonary hypertension. *Lancet* 1997; **349:** 1365. Correction. *ibid.*; **350:** 1406.
24. Nagaya N, *et al.* Effect of orally active prostacyclin analogue on survival of outpatients with primary pulmonary hypertension. *J Am Coll Cardiol* 1999; **34:** 1188–92.
25. McLaughlin VV, *et al.* Compassionate use of continuous prostacyclin in the management of secondary pulmonary hypertension: a case series. *Ann Intern Med* 1999; **130:** 740–3.
26. Badesch DB, *et al.* Continuous intravenous epoprostenol for pulmonary hypertension due to the scleroderma spectrum of disease: a randomized, controlled trial. *Ann Intern Med* 2000; **132:** 425–34.
27. Cuthbertson BH, *et al.* Use of inhaled nitric oxide in British intensive therapy units. *Br J Anaesth* 1997; **78:** 696–700.
28. Sanchez O, *et al.* Treatment of pulmonary hypertension secondary to connective tissue diseases. *Thorax* 1999; **54:** 273–7.
29. Kinsella JP, Abman SH. Recent developments in the pathophysiology and treatment of persistent pulmonary hypertension of the newborn. *J Pediatr* 1995; **126:** 853–64.
30. Rennie JM, Bokhari SA. Recent advances in neonatology. *Arch Dis Child* 1999; **81:** F1–F4.
31. The Neonatal Inhaled Nitric Oxide Study Group. Inhaled nitric oxide in full-term and nearly full-term infants with hypoxic respiratory failure. *N Engl J Med* 1997; **336:** 597–604.
32. Roberts JD, *et al.* Inhaled nitric oxide and persistent pulmonary hypertension of the newborn. *N Engl J Med* 1997; **336:** 605–10.
33. Davidson D, *et al.* Inhaled nitric oxide for the early treatment of persistent pulmonary hypertension of the term newborn: a randomized, double-masked, placebo-controlled, dose-response, multicenter study. *Pediatrics* 1998; **101:** 325–34.
34. Wessel DL, *et al.* Improved oxygenation in a randomized trial of inhaled nitric oxide for persistent pulmonary hypertension of the newborn. Abstract: *Pediatrics* 1997; **100:** 888. Full version: http://www.pediatrics.org/cgi/content/full/100/5/e7
35. Clark RH, *et al.* Low-dose nitric oxide therapy for persistent pulmonary hypertension of the newborn. *N Engl J Med* 2000; **342:** 469–74.
36. Rosenberg AA, *et al.* Longitudinal follow-up of a cohort of newborn infants treated with inhaled nitric oxide for persistent pulmonary hypertension. *J Pediatr* 1997; **131:** 70–5.
37. The Neonatal Inhaled Nitric Oxide Study Group. Inhaled nitric oxide in term and near-term infants: neurodevelopmental follow-up of the Neonatal Inhaled Nitric Oxide Study Group (NINOS). *J Pediatr* 2000; **136:** 611–17.
38. Kinsella JP, *et al.* Randomized, multicenter trial of inhaled nitric oxide and high-frequency oscillatory ventilation in severe, persistent pulmonary hypertension of the newborn. *J Pediatr* 1997; **131:** 55–62.
39. Bindl L, *et al.* Aerosolised prostacyclin for pulmonary hypertension in neonates. *Arch Dis Child* 1994; **71:** F214–F216.
40. Abu-Osba YK, *et al.* Treatment of severe persistent pulmonary hypertension of the newborn with magnesium sulphate. *Arch Dis Child* 1992; **67:** 31–5.
41. Tolsa J-F, *et al.* Magnesium sulphate as an alternative and safe treatment for severe persistent pulmonary hypertension of the newborn. *Arch Dis Child* 1995; **72:** F184–F187.
42. Wu T-Z, *et al.* Persistent pulmonary hypertension of the newborn treated with magnesium sulfate in premature neonates. *Pediatrics* 1995; **96:** 472–4.
43. Konduri GG, *et al.* Adenosine infusion improves oxygenation in term infants with respiratory failure. *Pediatrics* 1996; **97:** 295–300.

Raised intracranial pressure

The intracranial compartment consists of brain parenchyma, vascular tissue, and cerebrospinal fluid (CSF). Since the skull is a rigid structure a change in the volume of any one of these compartments will raise intracranial pressure. This may be due to the formation of cerebral oedema following head injury or around tumours, mass-lesions such as tumours or haemorrhage, CNS infections, or metabolic disorders. Other mechanisms which can raise intracranial pressure include increased dural sinus venous pressure, increased resistance to CSF outflow, and an increased rate of formation of CSF. In conditions such as benign intracranial hypertension there may be no obvious cause. Raised intracranial pressure (intracranial hypertension) can produce irreversible damage to the CNS and is potentially fatal; herniation of brain tissue can occur and reduced cerebral blood flow can lead to cerebral ischaemia. Symptoms of raised intracranial pressure include headache, which is frequently worse in the morning and may wake the patient from sleep, vomiting, drowsiness, and visual disturbances; most patients have papilloedema on examination.

The management of raised intracranial pressure has been reviewed.[1-4] There are several ways of reducing pressure, the choice of treatment being determined mainly by the underlying cause. Whatever the cause, in acutely raised intracranial pressure the initial aim is to reduce the volume of the intracranial contents as quickly as possible to prevent brain damage. For patients with haematoma or tumours the treatment of choice is frequently surgery but other methods may be used to control intracranial pressure before surgery.

Intracranial pressure monitoring can be helpful in guiding therapy since reducing the intracranial pressure too far is also deleterious. Patients may be sedated to avoid elevations of intracranial pressure due to unnecessary movement but if this is ineffective the use of neuromuscular blocking agents such as pancuronium or atracurium with artificial ventilation should be considered. Hyperventilation reduces the intracranial pressure by constricting the cerebral blood vessels and controlled hyperventilation may be employed. Raising the patient's head to promote venous drainage and restriction of fluid intake may be helpful to reduce intracranial pressure, but care is needed to avoid compromising the circulation. Removal of CSF through a ventricular catheter may also be effective.

The mainstay of pharmacological treatment for acutely raised intracranial pressure is diuretic therapy, usually with an osmotic diuretic. Mannitol is most commonly used but urea, glycerol, sorbitol, and hypertonic glucose solutions have also been employed.[5] Osmotic diuretics act by increasing the osmolality of plasma and drawing water out of the tissues, as well as by promoting an osmotic diuresis. They should not be given to patients with intracranial bleeding after head injury since they can exacerbate the bleeding,[6] and should also be avoided in patients who are already dehydrated. *Mannitol* has been suggested for control of raised intracranial pressure of various origins including severe head injury,[4,7] and cerebral oedema in hepatic failure,[8] and is often used to control intracranial pressure prior to surgery.[4,7,9] Mannitol has also produced beneficial responses in *children* with raised intracranial pressure from birth asphyxia,[10] diabetic ketoacidosis,[11] or Reye's syndrome.[12,13] Beneficial effects with osmotic diuretics such as mannitol or glycerol in patients following stroke have not been demonstrated (see Stroke, below). The use of osmotic diuretics to reduce intracranial pressure in patients with cerebral malaria is not routinely recommended and is controversial in other CNS infections.

In addition to its ability to lower intracranial pressure *glycerol* is reported to be able to increase blood flow to areas of brain ischaemia.[1] It has been used by mouth or intravenously in an attempt to reduce cerebral oedema and raised intracranial pressure in a variety of conditions including Reye's syndrome[14] and meningitis;[15] it has been reported to be ineffective in hepatic coma.[16] Some patients have experienced severe adverse effects including haemolysis, haemoglobinuria, and renal failure. Strongly *hyperosmotic glucose* solutions (25 to 50%) have been used to reduce raised intracranial pressure and cerebral oedema caused by delirium or acute alcohol intoxication.

If control is required for more than a few hours, repeated doses or continuous administration of osmotic diuretics may be required. Fluid and electrolyte balance and plasma osmolality should be closely monitored.

Loop diuretics such as *frusemide [furosemide]* are also effective and may be used as alternatives to osmotic diuretics, particularly where a sustained effect is required. They may increase the effect of osmotic diuretics and may be used as adjuncts, usually given after the osmotic diuretic. Frusemide [furosemide] decreases cerebral water content and possibly also reduces secretion of CSF. It may be preferred to mannitol in patients undergoing neurosurgery.[17]

Corticosteroids have an accepted and important role in the management of raised intracranial pressure associated with tumour-induced cerebral oedema. They may be used intravenously in high doses to control acutely raised intracranial pressure due to a rapidly expanding tumour. Lower doses are given orally for maintenance or where the onset of cerebral oedema is more insidious. Corticosteroids have also been tried in patients with head injury or stroke but their effectiveness is not proven and their adverse effects may outweigh any benefit. Further studies are needed to clarify their role in head injury.[18]

The use of barbiturate-induced coma with intravenous *thiopental* or *pentobarbital* for raised intracranial pressure has been controversial but it may be of benefit in patients refractory to conventional therapies. In addition to their effect on intracranial pressure barbiturates may be able to protect the brain from ischaemia. Small studies[19,20] indicated that intravenous *dimethyl sulfoxide* might be of use for raised intracranial pressure refractory to other therapy but there have been problems with fluid overload and difficulties with administration.[19] *Trometamol* is reported to lower raised intracranial pressure in patients with head injury; it may do this by causing metabolic acidosis leading to vasoconstriction of cerebral vessels.[5]

Benign intracranial hypertension (pseudotumour cerebri) is a rare disorder of unknown cause in which there is a raised intracranial pressure in the absence of an intracranial mass or obstruction to CSF outflow. Patients are often obese and tend to be young and female. Although the condition is not life-threatening and is often self-limiting, it may be a chronic condition and treatment is required to prevent visual loss and to alleviate symptoms. Management of mild symptoms usually involves diuretic treatment with frusemide [furosemide], a thiazide, or acetazolamide. Corticosteroids may be used to control acute symptoms but long-term adverse effects limit their use. Repeated lumbar puncture to remove CSF may relieve symptoms and has been used every 2 to 5 days to induce remission. In patients who cannot be controlled medically surgical methods such as lumboperitoneal shunting may be required. There has been an anecdotal report of beneficial effects with *octreotide* in a small number of patients.[21]

Acetazolamide has also been tried in the treatment of patients with chronically raised intracranial pressure due to cryptococcal meningitis.[22]

1. Dearden NM. Management of raised intracranial pressure after severe head injury. *Br J Hosp Med* 1986; **36:** 94–103.
2. Heinemeyer G. Clinical pharmacokinetic considerations in the treatment of increased intracranial pressure. *Clin Pharmacokinet* 1987; **13:** 1–25.
3. Lyons MK, Meyer FB. Cerebrospinal fluid physiology and the management of increased intracranial pressure. *Mayo Clin Proc* 1990; **65:** 684–707.
4. Woster PS, LeBlanc KL. Management of elevated intracranial pressure. *Clin Pharm* 1990; **9:** 762–72.
5. Nau R. Osmotherapy for elevated intracranial pressure: a critical reappraisal. *Clin Pharmacokinet* 2000; **38:** 23–40.
6. Williams B. Management of initial ICP after severe head injury. *Br J Hosp Med* 1987; **37:** 85.
7. Bullock R, Teasdale G. Head injuries—II. *BMJ* 1990; **300:** 1576–9.
8. Canalese J, *et al.* Controlled trial of dexamethasone and mannitol for the cerebral oedema of fulminant hepatic failure. *Gut* 1982; **23:** 625–9.
9. Andrews CJH. Intracranial aneurysms: perioperative management. *Br J Hosp Med* 1989; **41:** 485–8.
10. Levene MI, Evans DH. Medical management of raised intracranial pressure after severe birth asphyxia. *Arch Dis Child* 1985; **60:** 12–16.
11. Bello FA, Sotos JF. Cerebral oedema in diabetic ketoacidosis in children. *Lancet* 1990; **336:** 64.
12. Shaywitz BA, *et al.* Prolonged continuous monitoring of intracranial pressure in severe Reye's syndrome. *Pediatrics* 1977; **59:** 595–605.
13. Newman SL, *et al.* Reye's syndrome: success of supportive care. *N Engl J Med* 1978; **299:** 1079.
14. Nahata MC, *et al.* Variations in glycerol kinetics in Reye's syndrome. *Clin Pharmacol Ther* 1981; **29:** 782–7.
15. Kilpi T, *et al.* Oral glycerol and intravenous dexamethasone in preventing neurologic and audiologic sequelae of childhood bacterial meningitis. *Pediatr Infect Dis J* 1995; **14:** 270–8.
16. Record CO, *et al.* Glycerol therapy for cerebral oedema complicating fulminant hepatic failure. *BMJ* 1975; **ii:** 540.
17. Cottrell JE, *et al.* Furosemide- and mannitol-induced changes in intracranial pressure and serum osmolality and electrolytes. *Anesthesiology* 1977; **47:** 28–30.
18. Alderson P, Roberts I. Corticosteroids in acute traumatic brain injury: systematic review of randomised controlled trials. *BMJ* 1997; **314:** 1855–9.

19. Marshall LF, *et al.* Dimethyl sulfoxide for the treatment of intracranial hypertension: a preliminary trial. *Neurosurgery* 1984; **14:** 659–63.

20. Karaca M, *et al.* Dimethyl sulphoxide lowers ICP after closed head trauma. *Eur J Clin Pharmacol* 1991; **40:** 113–14.

21. Antaraki A, *et al.* Octreotide in benign intracranial hypertension. *Lancet* 1993; **342:** 1170.

22. Johnston SRD, *et al.* Raised intracranial pressure and visual complications in AIDS patients with cryptococcal meningitis. *J Infect* 1992; **24:** 185–9.

Reperfusion and revascularisation procedures

Percutaneous transluminal angioplasty, with or without stenting, and bypass grafting are non-pharmacological procedures employed in the management of atherosclerotic arterial disease associated with angina pectoris (above), myocardial infarction (above), and peripheral vascular disease (above) to aid revascularisation and reperfusion. Other procedures that may be used include rotational atherectomy and laser angioplasty.[1] Choice of procedure depends on various factors and is discussed under the individual diseases. Patients undergoing such revascularisation are at risk of further thromboembolic events leading to myocardial infarction, ischaemic stroke, or death either shortly after the procedure or in the long term as a consequence of restenosis of the artery.[2] Thus, adjunctive drug therapy is given with the aim of preventing perioperative thrombosis and long-term restenosis and this is the focus of the following discussion.

Heparin is given in conjunction with coronary angioplasty[3] or bypass surgery[4] to decrease the risk of perioperative thrombosis. It is given by continuous infusion, and the dose is adjusted according to clotting time. Relatively high doses are used, although lower doses have been investigated during percutaneous coronary intervention and are recommended when glycoprotein IIb/IIIa inhibitors are also used.[1,5] Administration of heparin does not prevent restenosis, although some benefit has been seen with heparin-coated stents. Low-molecular-weight heparins have also been tried but their role is not yet established.[1,5] Bivalirudin appears to be as effective as unfractionated heparin in patients undergoing percutaneous coronary interventions[6] and may be used as an alternative.[5] In one study there were fewer acute ischaemic events early after angioplasty when desirudin was given instead of heparin, but no longer term benefit was seen.[7] Oral anticoagulants such as warfarin do not appear to be used routinely either perioperatively or for long-term prophylaxis in the UK[4] or the USA[8] although they are said to be popular in parts of Europe.[4] A study[9] comparing oral anticoagulants with aspirin following peripheral bypass surgery found no difference in reocclusion or mortality, but bleeding was higher in patients receiving anticoagulants. Nitrates[3] or calcium-channel blockers[3,10] may be used during coronary angioplasty if vasospasm is likely to be a problem, but again have no routine role in long-term prevention of restenosis.

Antiplatelet drugs have a role in preventing both acute occlusion and restenosis. Aspirin is most commonly used and is usually started around the time of angioplasty or bypass grafting and continued long-term as discussed further below; clopidogrel or ticlopidine may be alternatives in patients unable to tolerate aspirin.[5] Aspirin does not completely inhibit platelet function and more potent drugs have also been studied. The benefit of glycoprotein IIb/IIIa-receptor antagonists in reducing the acute complications of percutaneous coronary interventions has been established in a number of studies,[11] although not all have shown prolonged benefit. The beneficial effect of abciximab has been demonstrated in three large studies. Two of the studies (EPIC[12] and CAPTURE[13]) included only patients at high risk of abrupt vessel closure, while the third study (EPILOG[14]) included unselected patients. Follow-up at 6 months[15] and 3 years[16] has been reported after the EPIC study and at 6 months for the EPILOG study[14] and in these studies, where abciximab was infused intravenously immediately before angioplasty and continued for 12 hours, the initial beneficial effects have been maintained at follow-up. In the CAPTURE study, where abciximab was given for 18 to 24 hours pre-procedure and for 1 hour post-procedure, the initial beneficial effects were lost at 6-month follow-up.[13] Abciximab in these studies was given in addition to aspirin and heparin. Other glycoprotein IIb/IIIa-receptor antagonists, such as eptifibatide[17] and tirofiban,[18] may also be used.[5] However, 6-month results in the tirofiban study[18] have been disappointing with no reduction in the incidence of restenosis being found, and a study[19] in patients receiving intracoronary stenting suggested that abciximab reduced major ischaemic events more than tirofiban at 30 days.

Abciximab may also have a role as an adjunct to primary angioplasty for acute myocardial infarction.[5,20]

Coronary stents (metallic mesh tubes that are inflated across a stenosis and thus permanently embedded in the vessel wall) were introduced in the early 1990s and were initially used to prevent restenosis occurring after coronary angioplasty. They are now also used increasingly as a routine adjunct to angioplasty to prevent both acute vessel closure and restenosis. Thrombotic occlusion occurring 2 to 14 days following stent implantation (subacute stent thrombosis) led to the use of intensive anticoagulation/antiplatelet regimens consisting of aspirin, dipyridamole, dextran, heparin, and warfarin.[21] However, a regimen of aspirin with ticlopidine, in addition to optimal stent deployment and heparin during the procedure, appears to be effective[22-24] and is now preferred.[25] Clopidogrel may be used as an alternative to ticlopidine,[5] and may be better tolerated.[26] Glycoprotein IIb/IIIa-receptor antagonists have also been used with coronary stenting. Abciximab reduced rates of death and myocardial infarction at 30 days,[27] 6 months,[28] and 1 year,[29] and similar results have been reported[30] with eptifibatide. Local drug delivery using heparin-coated stents is also being tried.[31]

Several pathological processes are believed to be responsible for the development of restenosis[3,32] and include platelet aggregation and thrombus formation, neointimal hyperplasia, elastic recoil, and vascular remodelling. Therefore, a wide variety of drugs has been investigated in an attempt to prevent restenosis.[32] Drugs employed have included antithrombotics (heparin, low-molecular-weight heparins, hirudin, and warfarin), antiplatelets (primarily aspirin but also dipyridamole and ticlopidine and prostaglandins such as epoprostenol and ciprostene), antiproliferatives (ACE inhibitors, colchicine, lanreotide, and trapidil), antioxidants (probucol), calcium-channel blockers, and lipid regulating drugs (fish oils and statins). Intracoronary radiotherapy has reduced the rates of restenosis after angioplasty,[33] and after stenting.[34] Local gene delivery is also under investigation as a possible treatment for restenosis. In general, with the exception of antiplatelet drugs such as aspirin, and possibly lanreotide, probucol, and trapidil, results have been either disappointing or equivocal and further evaluation is needed.

The value of antiplatelet drugs, and aspirin in particular, following coronary or peripheral angioplasty or after bypass procedures has been confirmed by the Antiplatelet Trialists' Collaboration.[35] This overview showed that such treatment reduces not only the risk of occlusion or restenosis but also reduces the incidence of major vascular events such as myocardial infarction or stroke and of death. Aspirin is sometimes started shortly before the procedures and sometimes shortly after. The rationale for delaying the initiation of therapy has been the belief that perioperative bleeding could be reduced but this does not appear to be an important factor[35] and the comment has been made[36] that trials which failed to show a benefit were those in which antiplatelet therapy had been delayed until the second or third postoperative day. The optimum dose and duration of therapy also needs to be established.[35] Other antiplatelet drugs have also been tried in addition to aspirin. Long-term administration of clopidogrel[37] reduced major cardiovascular events at 8-month follow-up, but no benefit was found in a study[38] using the oral glycoprotein IIb/IIIa inhibitor xemilofiban.

Promising results in terms of reduction in restenosis and of adverse vascular events following coronary angioplasty have been reported with lanreotide[39,40] and trapidil.[41,42] Reduction in restenosis following coronary angioplasty has also been reported with probucol.[43] The drugs have been used in addition to standard therapies such as heparin and aspirin. However, experience with them is still very limited compared with the knowledge accumulated with aspirin for long-term prophylaxis. Benefit has been observed when lanreotide was given for about 5 days around the time of angioplasty whereas trapidil was given for up to 6 months postangioplasty. Probucol was given for a month before and 6 months after angioplasty. Both lanreotide and trapidil may act by reducing smooth muscle cell proliferation thus reducing neointimal hyperplasia. Probucol may act by reducing formation of active metabolites at the angioplasty site and thus preventing endothelial dysfunction; other actions have also been proposed.

Atherosclerosis in saphenous-vein coronary bypass grafts is a frequent cause of obstruction in the years following bypass surgery, especially in patients with hyper-

lipidaemia. Aggressive lowering of LDL-cholesterol using mainly statins may be beneficial in these patients.[44]

Thrombosis may occur in the bypass grafts used to treat peripheral vascular disease. Intra-arterial administration of thrombolytics, directly into the clot, has been used in conjunction with surgery or angioplasty for acute occlusion.[45]

1. Windecker S, Meier B. Intervention in coronary artery disease. *Heart* 2000; **83:** 481–90.

2. O'Meara JJ, Dehmer GJ. Care of the patient and management of complications after percutaneous coronary interventions. *Ann Intern Med* 1997; **127:** 458–71.

3. Landau C, *et al.* Percutaneous transluminal coronary angioplasty. *N Engl J Med* 1994; **330:** 981–93.

4. Wolfe JH. Critical limb ischaemia. *Prescribers' J* 1994; **34:** 50–8.

5. Popma JJ, *et al.* Antithrombotic therapy in patients undergoing percutaneous coronary intervention. *Chest* 2001; **119** (suppl): 321S–336S.

6. Kong DF, *et al.* Clinical outcomes of bivalirudin for ischemic heart disease. *Circulation* 1999; **100:** 2049–53.

7. Serruys PW, *et al.* A comparison of hirudin with heparin in the prevention of restenosis after coronary angioplasty. *N Engl J Med* 1995; **333:** 757–63.

8. Nwasokwa ON. Coronary artery bypass graft disease. *Ann Intern Med* 1995; **123:** 528–45.

9. Dutch Bypass Oral anticoagulants or Aspirin (BOA) Study Group. Efficacy of oral anticoagulants compared with aspirin after infrainguinal bypass surgery (The Dutch Bypass Oral anticoagulants or Aspirin study): a randomised trial. *Lancet* 2000; **355:** 346–51. Correction. *ibid.;* 1104.

10. Vahanian A, Iung B. Role of calcium channel blockers in reducing acute ischaemia and preventing restenosis in PTCA. *Drugs* 1996; **52** (suppl 4): 9–16.

11. Kong DF, Califf RM. Glycoprotein IIb/IIIa receptor antagonists in non-ST elevation acute coronary syndromes and percutaneous revascularisation: a review of trial reports. *Drugs* 1999; **58:** 609–20.

12. The EPIC Investigators. Use of a monoclonal antibody directed against the platelet glycoprotein IIb/IIIa receptor in high-risk coronary angioplasty. *N Engl J Med* 1994; **330:** 956–61.

13. The CAPTURE Investigators. Randomised placebo-controlled trial of abciximab before and during coronary intervention in refractory unstable angina: the CAPTURE study. *Lancet* 1997; **349:** 1429–35. Correction. *ibid.;* **350:** 744.

14. The EPILOG Investigators. Platelet glycoprotein IIb/IIIa receptor blockade and low-dose heparin during percutaneous coronary revascularization. *N Engl J Med* 1997; **336:** 1689–96.

15. Topol EJ, *et al.* Randomised trial of coronary intervention with antibody against platelet IIb/IIIa integrin for reduction of clinical restenosis: results at six months. *Lancet* 1994; **343:** 881–6.

16. Topol EJ, *et al.* Long-term protection from myocardial ischemic events in a randomized trial of brief integrin β₃ blockade with percutaneous coronary intervention. *JAMA* 1997; **278:** 479–84.

17. The IMPACT-II Investigators. Randomised placebo-controlled trial of effect of eptifibatide on complications of percutaneous coronary intervention: IMPACT-II. *Lancet* 1997; **349:** 1422–8.

18. Gibson CM, *et al.* Six-month angiographic and clinical follow-up of patients prospectively randomized to receive either tirofiban or placebo during angioplasty in the RESTORE trial. *J Am Coll Cardiol* 1998; **32:** 28–34.

19. Topol EJ, *et al.* Comparison of two platelet glycoprotein IIb/IIIa inhibitors, tirofiban and abciximab, for the prevention of ischemic events with percutaneous coronary revascularization. *N Engl J Med* 2001; **344:** 1888–94.

20. Brener SJ, *et al.* Randomized, placebo-controlled trial of platelet glycoprotein IIb/IIIa blockade with primary angioplasty for acute myocardial infarction. *Circulation* 1998; **98:** 734–41.

21. Mauro LS, *et al.* Introduction to coronary artery stents and their pharmacotherapeutic management. *Ann Pharmacother* 1997; **31:** 1490–8.

22. Schömig A, *et al.* A randomized comparison of antiplatelet and anticoagulant therapy after the placement of coronary-artery stents. *N Engl J Med* 1996; **334:** 1084–9.

23. Hall P, *et al.* A randomized comparison of combined ticlopidine and aspirin therapy versus aspirin therapy alone after successful intravascular ultrasound-guided stent implantation. *Circulation* 1996; **93:** 215–22.

24. Leon MB, *et al.* A clinical trial comparing three antithrombotic-drug regimens after coronary-artery stenting. *N Engl J Med* 1998; **339:** 1665–71.

25. Holmes DR, *et al.* ACC Expert Consensus document on coronary artery stents. *J Am Coll Cardiol* 1998; **32:** 1471–82.

26. Bertrand ME, *et al.* Double-blind study of the safety of clopidogrel with and without a loading dose in combination with aspirin compared with ticlopidine in combination with aspirin after coronary stenting: the Clopidogrel Aspirin Stent International Cooperative Study (CLASSICS). *Circulation* 2000; **102:** 624–9.

27. The EPISTENT Investigators. Randomised placebo-controlled and balloon-angioplasty-controlled trial to assess safety of coronary stenting with use of platelet glycoprotein-IIb/IIIa blockade. *Lancet* 1998; **352:** 87–92.

28. Lincoff AM, *et al.* Complementary clinical benefits of coronary-artery stenting and blockade of platelet glycoprotein IIb/IIIa receptors. *N Engl J Med* 1999; **341:** 319–27.

29. Topol EJ, *et al.* Outcomes at 1 year and economic implications of platelet glycoprotein IIb/IIIa blockade in patients undergoing coronary stenting: results from a multicentre randomised trial. *Lancet* 1999; **354:** 2019–24.

30. O'Shea JC, *et al.* Platelet glycoprotein IIb/IIIa integrin blockade with eptifibatide in coronary stent intervention: the ESPRIT Trial: a randomized controlled trial. *JAMA* 2001; **285:** 2468–73.

31. Serruys PW, *et al.* Randomised comparison of implantation of heparin-coated stents with balloon angioplasty in selected patients with coronary artery disease (Benestent II). *Lancet* 1998; **352:** 673–81. Correction. *ibid.;* 1478.

32. Herrman J-PR, *et al.* Pharmacological approaches to the prevention of restenosis following angioplasty: the search for the holy grail? *Drugs* 1993; **46:** 18–52 and 249–62.

33. Verin V, *et al.* Endoluminal beta-radiation therapy for the prevention of coronary restenosis after balloon angioplasty. *N Engl J Med* 2001; **344:** 243–9.

34. Leon MB, *et al.* Localized intracoronary gamma-radiation therapy to inhibit the recurrence of restenosis after stenting. *N Engl J Med* 2001; **344:** 250–6.

35. Antiplatelet Trialists' Collaboration. Collaborative overview of randomised trials of antiplatelet therapy—maintenance of vascular graft or arterial patency by antiplatelet therapy. *BMJ* 1994; **308:** 159–68.
36. Underwood MJ, More RS. The aspirin papers. *BMJ* 1994; **308:** 71–2.
37. Mehta SR, *et al.* Effects of pretreatment with clopidogrel and aspirin followed by long-term therapy in patients undergoing percutaneous coronary intervention: the PCI-CURE study. *Lancet* 2001; **358:** 527–33.
38. O'Neill WW, *et al.* Long-term treatment with a platelet glycoprotein-receptor antagonist after percutaneous coronary revascularization. *N Engl J Med* 2000; **342:** 1316–24.
39. Emanuelsson H, *et al.* Long-term effects of angiopeptin treatment in coronary angioplasty: reduction of clinical events but not angiographic restenosis. *Circulation* 1995; **91:** 1689–96.
40. Eriksen U, *et al.* Randomised double-blind Scandinavian trial of angiopeptin versus placebo for the prevention of clinical events and restenosis after coronary balloon angioplasty. *Am Heart J* 1995; **130:** 1–8.
41. Okamoto S, *et al.* Effects of trapidil (triazolopyrimidine), a platelet-derived growth factor antagonist, in preventing restenosis after percutaneous transluminal coronary angioplasty. *Am Heart J* 1992; **123:** 1439–44.
42. Maresta A, *et al.* Trapidil (triazolopyrimidine), a platelet-derived growth factor antagonist, reduces restenosis after percutaneous transluminal coronary angioplasty: results of the randomized, double-blind STARC study. *Circulation* 1994; **90:** 2710–15.
43. Tardif J-C, *et al.* Probucol and multivitamins in the prevention of restenosis after coronary angioplasty. *N Engl J Med* 1997; **337:** 365–72.
44. The Post Coronary Artery Bypass Graft Trial Investigators. The effect of aggressive lowering of low-density lipoprotein cholesterol levels and low-dose anticoagulation on obstructive changes in saphenous-vein coronary-artery bypass grafts. *N Engl J Med* 1997; **336:** 153–62.
45. Greenberg RK, Ouriel K. A multi-modal approach to the management of bypass graft failure. *Vasc Med* 1998; **3:** 215–20.

Shock

Shock is a complex clinical syndrome of multiple aetiologies but the common factor in all types of shock is a failure of the circulatory system to maintain cellular perfusion and function. A traditional approach has been to place the cause of shock into one of several basic groups. Commonly used groupings are hypovolaemic shock, cardiogenic shock, septic shock, and anaphylactic shock. These are the types included below.

Hypovolaemic shock results from fluid loss and can be due to a haemorrhagic or non-haemorrhagic cause. Haemorrhagic causes include severe gastrointestinal bleeding and traumatic injury, while non-haemorrhagic causes include severe vomiting and diarrhoea, polyuria, and burns. Hypovolaemia can also be present in other forms of shock; fluid loss from the vasculature may occur due to capillary leakage in septic or anaphylactic shock, while peripheral vasodilatation may lead to relative hypovolaemia.

Cardiogenic shock usually results from acute failure of the heart, leading to an inadequate stroke volume and reduced cardiac output. It has a number of causes, but is most commonly associated with acute myocardial infarction. Other cardiac causes include valvular heart disease, cardiomyopathies, and severe cardiac arrhythmias; episodes of acute heart failure may also occur in patients with chronic heart failure. Shock due to circulatory disorders such as massive pulmonary embolism is also sometimes classified as cardiogenic. Other forms of shock may also have a cardiac component.

Septic shock occurs as a complication of infectious disease and is described and defined in more detail under Septicaemia, p.138. Hypotension occurs primarily due to peripheral vasodilatation, but fluid loss and direct effects on the heart may also be involved. *Anaphylactic shock* (p.832) is the result of a hypersensitivity reaction and is similar haemodynamically to septic shock.

The haemodynamic effects of shock thus result either from an absolute or relative reduction in plasma volume, or a reduction in cardiac output. Although compensatory mechanisms are initially able to restore the blood pressure, these become inadequate and patients in decompensated shock classically present with hypotension, tachycardia, and tachypnoea. Compensatory peripheral vasoconstriction leads to cold, clammy, cyanotic skin and impaired organ perfusion results in dulled mental alertness, which may progress to stupor or coma; oliguria or anuria, due to impaired renal perfusion, are also frequent. Pulmonary oedema may occur as a result of impaired cardiac output in cardiogenic shock. Complications of shock include disseminated intravascular coagulation due to platelet sludging and microvascular insufficiency, acute respiratory distress syndrome (previously termed 'shock lung') (p.1046), and acute renal failure. The terms multiple organ failure syndrome (MOFS) and multiple organ dysfunction syndrome (MODS) are applied to the consequences of shock where several organs or body sys-tems have become hypoperfused and are unable to maintain their normal function.

Management. The management of shock can be divided into general supportive and symptomatic measures that may be applicable in all forms of shock, and primary specific therapies directed against any underlying cause.

General measures include correction of electrolyte disturbances, correction of hypovolaemia and hypotension, and improvement of cardiac output.[1] Pain and respiratory problems often accompany shock and may necessitate the administration of intravenous opioid analgesics and oxygen therapy.

Electrolyte disturbances (p.1180) should be managed conventionally; sodium bicarbonate may be required but should be reserved for severe acidosis.[1] An adequate diuresis should be maintained in order to prevent renal failure.

Correction of hypovolaemia is important in all forms of shock. Replacement fluids available include blood products and crystalloid or colloid plasma expanders,[2,3] and the choice is not always clear. In haemorrhage, although for initial therapy volume expansion is most important, where 40% or more of the total blood volume has been lost red cell replacement is necessary. This usually takes the form of packed red cells in conjunction with plasma expanders, with other plasma components as required for severe haemorrhage. In non-haemorrhagic hypovolaemia, the choice is between crystalloid and colloid plasma expanders, and there continues to be debate over their relative merits. Crystalloids (solutions containing solutes such as glucose or sodium chloride that can pass a semipermeable membrane) rapidly expand both the intravascular and extravascular compartments. Although it has been argued that this is necessary as the interstitial space becomes depleted in hypovolaemia, large volumes are required and the duration of effect is short as fluid is rapidly redistributed. Colloids (solutions containing large molecules such as albumin, dextrans, gelatins, and etherified starches, which do not pass semipermeable membranes) expand the intravascular space more effectively; they have a longer duration of effect and smaller volumes are required. This leads to less haemodilution, although the exact significance of this has been questioned. However, colloids may cause hypersensitivity reactions including anaphylaxis, and this has been raised as a potential concern.

Studies comparing the use of crystalloids and colloids in hypovolaemia have generally been of poor quality and the results are difficult to interpret. A systematic review[4] of trials in critically ill patients concluded that there was a small increase in mortality associated with the use of colloids. However, following considerable criticism,[5,6] an update of the review[7] modified these conclusions to state that there was no evidence of a mortality benefit with colloids and therefore no support for their continued use other than in clinical trials. A further review[8] looking specifically at the use of albumin solutions also suggested that there was an increased mortality in those receiving the colloid, but this review was also criticised.[9] In practice a mixture of colloids and crystalloids tends to be given. It is unclear whether there are any significant differences in outcome associated with the various colloid solutions available,[10] but use of albumin is now generally reserved for specific indications.

Successful correction of hypovolaemia may alleviate hypotension in some cases, but cardiac output may remain depressed and signs of impaired organ perfusion may persist, necessitating additional therapy. Further measures are also frequently needed if there is profound hypotension; blood pressure in shock can be extremely low (sometimes a systolic pressure of less than 70 mmHg) despite fluid replacement. In patients with profound **hypotension** or a **low cardiac output** sympathomimetics are usually employed.[11,12] Their precise effects on the vasculature vary and choice depends on individual patient characteristics and the type of shock.[13] In cardiogenic or hypovolaemic shock cardiac output is usually low but peripheral resistance is high and drugs that have predominantly inotropic effects are most suitable. Dopamine or dobutamine are often chosen. Dopamine is widely used in all forms of shock; in low doses it may maintain renal perfusion although higher doses cause vasoconstriction, and it is often used in combination with other inotropes. Dobutamine causes peripheral vasodilatation and is useful where hypotension is not significant. Noradrenaline [norepinephrine] causes peripheral vasoconstriction and should be reserved for severe hypotension. It is particularly useful in septic shock where the cardiac output is usually high but peripheral resistance is low. It is often given in combination with more potent inotropes such as dobutamine or adrenaline [epinephrine]. Adrenaline [epinephrine] has also been used alone but renal artery vasoconstriction may limit its use, and it has also been reported to cause lactic acidosis.[14] Phosphodiesterase inhibitors such as amrinone and milrinone, which have positive inotropic activity, can also be considered in low cardiac output states;[11] like dopamine they also produce peripheral vasodilatation. Vasodilators such as intravenous glyceryl trinitrate or sodium nitroprusside can be beneficial for patients in shock with a low cardiac output but a high diastolic pressure (more than 110 mmHg),[12] and also in patients with pulmonary oedema.[1] They act by reducing cardiac afterload. Caution must however be observed because of the risk of precipitating hypotension.

In cardiogenic shock associated with **myocardial infarction**,[12,15,16] specific therapy to restore myocardial perfusion is also indicated (see p.805).

In **septic shock** appropriate antibacterial therapy should be given as outlined under Septicaemia on p.138. Methods of inhibiting endogenous mediators released in response to sepsis that are thought to be responsible for the haemodynamic effects are also under investigation but clinical benefits have not yet been demonstrated.[17,18]

Adrenaline [epinephrine] is the cornerstone of management in **anaphylactic shock** (see p.832).

1. Hinds CJ, Watson D. ABC of intensive care: circulatory support. *BMJ* 1999; **318:** 1749–52.
2. Nolan JP, Parr MJA. Aspects of resuscitation in trauma. *Br J Anaesth* 1997; **79:** 226–40.
3. Nolan J. Fluid replacement. *Br Med Bull* 1999; **55:** 821–43.
4. Schierhout G, Roberts I. Fluid resuscitation with colloid or crystalloid solutions in critically ill patients: a systematic review of randomised trials. *BMJ* 1998; **316:** 961–4.
5. Watts J. Fluid resuscitation with colloid or crystalloid solutions. *BMJ* 1998; **317:** 277.
6. Wyncoll DLA, *et al.* Fluid resuscitation with colloid or crystalloid solutions. *BMJ* 1998; **317:** 278–9.
7. Alderson P, *et al.* Colloids versus crystalloids for fluid resuscitation in critically ill patients (updated 6 September 2000). Available in The Cochrane Library; Issue 4. Oxford: Update Software; 2001.
8. Cochrane Injuries Group Albumin Reviewers. Human albumin administration in critically ill patients: systematic review of randomised controlled trials. *BMJ* 1998; **317:** 235–40.
9. Beale RJ, *et al.* Human albumin administration in critically ill patients. *BMJ* 1998; **317:** 884.
10. Bunn F, *et al.* Colloid solutions for fluid resuscitation (updated 27 February 2001). Available in The Cochrane Library; Issue 4. Oxford: Update Software; 2001.
11. Barnard MJ, Linter SPK. Acute circulatory support. *BMJ* 1993; **307:** 35–41.
12. Califf RM, Bengtson JR. Cardiogenic shock. *N Engl J Med* 1994; **330:** 1724–30.
13. Cuthbertson BH, *et al.* Inotropic agents in the critically ill. *Br J Hosp Med* 1996; **56:** 386–91.
14. Day NPJ, *et al.* The effects of dopamine and adrenaline infusions on acid-base balance and systemic haemodynamics in severe infection. *Lancet* 1996; **348:** 219–23.
15. Hollenberg SM, *et al.* Cardiogenic shock. *Ann Intern Med* 1999; **131:** 47–59.
16. Hasdai D, *et al.* Cardiogenic shock complicating acute coronary syndromes. *Lancet* 2000; **356:** 749–56.
17. Glauser MP. The inflammatory cytokines: new developments in the pathophysiology and treatment of septic shock. *Drugs* 1996; **52** (suppl 2): 9–17.
18. Astiz ME, Rackow EC. Septic shock. *Lancet* 1998; **351:** 1501–5.

Stroke

Stroke, sometimes called a cerebrovascular accident, is the major consequence of cerebrovascular disease and has been defined as an acute neurological dysfunction of vascular origin with sudden (within seconds) or at least rapid (within hours) occurrence of symptoms and signs corresponding to the involvement of focal areas of the brain.[1] If signs and symptoms persist for more than 24 hours the event is termed a completed stroke whereas if they disappear within a few minutes or hours, or at most within 24 hours, the event is termed a transient ischaemic attack.

Strokes may be ischaemic (infarction-related) or haemorrhagic. **Ischaemic stroke** is by far the commonest type and may result from arterial occlusion caused by local thrombosis in the vessels of the brain at sites of atheroma or, more often, by thromboembolism arising from outside the brain and lodging in the cerebral vessels. An example of the latter is cardio-embolic infarction associated with atrial fibrillation or acute myocardial infarction. Such arterial occlusion results in inadequate cerebral perfusion, depriving the brain of glucose and oxygen, and stroke occurs. About 20% of patients with acute ischaemic stroke experience worsening of symptoms within a few days of onset. This is termed progressing stroke, stroke-in-evolution, or unstable stroke, and occurs when the thrombotic process is incomplete. **Transient ischaemic attacks** are acute episodes of focal neurological deficit or monocular visual loss (amaurosis fugax), mainly due to ischaemia associated with atherothrombosis, but unlike stroke last less than 24 hours and often only minutes. They are usually of sudden onset with complete clinical recovery but a tendency to recur. Patients suffering these attacks are at an increased risk of stroke. **Haemorrhagic stroke** is secondary to subarachnoid or to intracerebral haemorrhage. *Subarachnoid haemorrhage* is bleeding into the fluid-filled subarachnoid space between the brain and the skull, and usually occurs after rupture of an aneurysm; other causes include arteriovenous malformations and hypertensive microaneurysms. *Intracerebral haemorrhage* is bleeding into the parenchyma of the brain, and may result from rupture of arteries damaged by chronic hypertension. Haemorrhage produces a focal haematoma causing a local increase in pressure which may lead to further bleeding and enlargement of the haematoma. The increase in pressure in the area of the haematoma may also produce local ischaemia.

Clinical presentation of stroke can vary enormously in severity and combination of signs and symptoms, and depends on the site of infarction or haemorrhage. Neurological deficits may include impairments to speech, balance, vision, touch sensation, and movement. Patients have been classed as major or minor stroke (reversible ischaemic neurological deficit) victims according to their degree of recovery at a given time after the stroke.

It is important to diagnose the type of stroke correctly because management is very different and what might be of benefit in patients with cerebral infarction might be dangerous in those with haemorrhage. Haemorrhagic stroke is typically of sudden onset with severe headaches, vomiting, and rapid deterioration of consciousness – all signs of raised intracranial pressure – but mild to moderate haemorrhage may be difficult to distinguish from infarction on the basis of clinical signs alone. Computed tomography (CT) is a surer way of distinguishing between haemorrhagic and ischaemic stroke. Magnetic resonance imaging may also be useful. Recent guidelines[2-4] have emphasised that, as in myocardial infarction, early recognition of symptoms and prompt evaluation and treatment of stroke are of vital importance; the European Ad Hoc Consensus Group[2] recommend admittance to hospital within one hour of symptom onset. Where possible patients should be managed within a stroke unit.

Diagnosis of transient ischaemic attacks usually rests on the patient's history as these short attacks are seldom witnessed by a physician and there are no objective confirmatory tests.

Management of stroke can be divided into: primary prevention, that is prior to any stroke or transient ischaemic attack in patients at risk or even apparently healthy people; treatment of acute stroke, either ischaemic or haemorrhagic; and secondary prevention, that is after a stroke or transient ischaemic attack has occurred.

Primary prevention

Primary prevention[5-7] is important, especially as treatment for acute stroke remains largely unsatisfactory. Prevention strategies require the identification of risk factors and if possible their modification in individuals at high risk and in the population as a whole. A major risk factor for stroke of any type appears to be hypertension and its treatment has reduced mortality from stroke. Atrial fibrillation, acute myocardial infarction, and valvular diseases may be sources of cardiogenic embolism[8] and are major risk factors for ischaemic stroke. Patients with these disorders may require prophylaxis with anticoagulants or antiplatelet drugs. For further details, see Cardiac Arrhythmias, above and Myocardial Infarction, above, respectively. Smoking is another major risk factor. Other risk factors identified include obesity, high fibrinogen concentrations, diabetes mellitus, oral contraceptive use (but see p.1455), diet, alcohol intake, and a family history of stroke. Many of these are also risk factors for ischaemic heart disease or atherosclerosis and similar preventive measures may apply (see Atherosclerosis, above). The relationship between plasma-cholesterol concentrations and risk of stroke is not clear, but a reduced incidence of stroke has been reported in studies of patients receiving statins[9-12] (see Cardiovascular Risk Reduction, p.797).

Endarterectomy for carotid artery stenosis is an established method for the secondary prevention of stroke, but its role in primary prevention is less clear.[13] A meta-analysis[14] of trials in patients with asymptomatic carotid stenosis concluded that carotid endarterectomy reduces

the risk of stroke more than medical treatment. However, since the overall risk of stroke in this group of patients is already low, endarterectomy cannot be recommended for primary prevention of ischaemic stroke until those patients at highest risk of stroke can be identified.

Primary prevention of stroke in healthy people has also been investigated. The US[15] and British[16] physicians' studies of aspirin in the prevention of cardiovascular and cerebrovascular disease both showed a slight non-significant increase in the number of disabling strokes which, in the US study, were attributed to cerebral haemorrhage. Although it has been suggested that aspirin may be of benefit for prevention in those at particularly high risk of ischaemic stroke, this may not be so in practice; both the Thrombosis Prevention Trial[17] in men at increased risk of ischaemic heart disease and the Hypertension Optimal Treatment (HOT) trial[18] in hypertensive patients reported little or no effect on the overall incidence of stroke.

Treatment

The treatment of **acute ischaemic stroke** has been reviewed.[19-23] The aim is early reversal or limitation of the degree of brain dysfunction by treatment, given as soon as possible after the onset of symptoms, that will re-establish cerebral blood flow, limit ischaemic neuronal injury, and reduce cerebral oedema. General supportive measures include ensuring adequate oxygenation and fluid and electrolyte balances, avoiding hypercapnia and hyperglycaemia or hypoglycaemia, abolishing seizures, and treating fever. Control of hypertension is controversial since lowering the blood pressure may reduce cerebral perfusion and worsen ischaemia, and hypertension usually resolves spontaneously without treatment.[24] Antihypertensive therapy may be indicated in specific patients, such as those with severe hypertension or those being considered for thrombolytic therapy. Many specific measures have been tried, but with the exception of aspirin, which has shown a small benefit, and possibly alteplase in selected patients, there is none that can be recommended routinely.

Antithrombotic therapy with antiplatelet drugs, heparin, and thrombolytics would be expected to be of benefit in the treatment of cerebral infarction and the re-establishment of cerebral blood flow. However, the presence of haemorrhage must be excluded and the risk of potentiating spontaneous secondary brain haemorrhage (haemorrhagic transformation) must be borne in mind.

Antiplatelet drugs. The rationale for using aspirin is based on its effectiveness in patients with myocardial infarction where the underlying vascular pathology is similar to that in ischaemic stroke. Aspirin has been evaluated in two large studies—the International Stroke Trial (IST)[25] and the Chinese Acute Stroke Trial (CAST).[26] The combined results of these studies[26] found that aspirin 160 mg[26] or 300 mg[25] daily started within 48 hours of symptom onset produced about 9 fewer deaths or nonfatal strokes per 1000 patients in the first few weeks following ischaemic stroke. Aspirin has therefore been recommended for patients with ischaemic stroke who are not receiving thrombolytic or anticoagulant therapy, and should be started within 48 hours of stroke onset.[27]

Heparin. Anticoagulation should prevent further thrombus formation and limit the size of the cerebral infarct in acute ischaemic stroke; however, any benefit may be offset by an increase in intracranial haemorrhage, and a systematic review[28] has suggested there is no evidence to support routine use. The International Stroke Trial[25] which evaluated two dosages of heparin (5000 units or 12 500 units subcutaneously twice daily) found no benefit from either regimen and the higher dose particularly was associated with haemorrhagic stroke and bleeding. It has previously been considered that patients with cardioembolic stroke are likely to benefit from heparin therapy,[29] even though there is a special risk of haemorrhagic transformation in these patients which means that early anticoagulation is often hazardous. However, the International Stroke Trial[25] failed to show any benefit in this group, and a study[30] of low-molecular-weight heparin in patients with acute ischaemic stroke and atrial fibrillation also showed no benefit. No improvement in outcome was reported after 3 months in a study of danaparoid given in acute ischaemic stroke.[31] A study[32] with ancrod found an improvement in outcome when given within 3 hours of stroke onset, but a further study was terminated due to lack of benefit. Although stroke-in-evolution has been considered as an indication for heparin therapy, the evidence for any benefit is poor.[27]

Low-dose subcutaneous heparin may be indicated to reduce the risk of venous thromboembolism (deep-vein thrombosis and pulmonary embolism) associated with stroke.

Thrombolytics. Stroke is normally considered a contraindication to the use of thrombolytics, and clearly they would be inappropriate in haemorrhagic stroke. However, when stroke is associated with thrombotic occlusion there is evidence, as with myocardial infarction, that a degree of neuronal recovery is possible if the occlusion is reversed sufficiently quickly. Some small studies suggested a fall in early death, although subsequent randomised trials produced disappointing results, with the exception of one with alteplase given within 3 hours of the onset of stroke (NINDS—National Institute of Neurological Disorders and Stroke rt-PA Stroke Trial).[33] The studies using streptokinase—MAST-E (Multicentre Acute Stroke Trial-Europe),[34] ASK (Australian Streptokinase Trial),[35] and MAST-I (Multicentre Acute Stroke Trial-Italy)[36,37]—were terminated before completion because of adverse outcomes (intracranial bleeding and increased mortality) in the treatment groups, particularly in those receiving therapy more than 3 hours after stroke onset.[35] The study investigating alteplase given within 6 hours of the onset of symptoms (ECASS I—European Cooperative Acute Stroke Study)[38] reported that, although some patients might benefit, overall alteplase was associated with higher mortality rates and an increase in some intracranial bleeding (parenchymal haemorrhage). In the NINDS randomised study,[33] alteplase given within 3 hours of the onset of ischaemic stroke appeared to improve clinical outcome despite an increased incidence of symptomatic intracerebral haemorrhage. Patients treated with alteplase were more likely to have minimal or no disability 3 months following stroke,[33] and this benefit was maintained at 12 months.[39] However, there was no difference in mortality or rate of recurrence of stroke. A second ECASS study (ECASS II)[40] that hoped to confirm the early findings of the NINDS study failed to confirm a statistical benefit for alteplase over placebo and found no significant differences between patients who received alteplase within 3 hours or between 3 and 6 hours. On the basis of the NINDS study, alteplase given within 3 hours of the onset of ischaemic stroke has been recommended for selected patients in some guidelines on stroke management[2-4] and, despite their own disappointing results, the ECASS II investigators upheld this view. However, these recommendations have been criticised.[41,42] It has been pointed out[43,44] that very few patients will be eligible for treatment with alteplase, since the time of onset of symptoms is often uncertain and in many patients more than 3 hours elapses before a definite diagnosis of ischaemic stroke is made. In addition, the NINDS study[33] excluded patients with severe stroke and those taking anticoagulants. The rationale for exclusion of patients with severe stroke is that haemorrhagic transformation is more likely to occur with large areas of infarction.[43] However, size of infarct is difficult to identify by CT scanning.[43] Anticoagulants or antiplatelets are also contra-indicated in the first 24 hours after administration of alteplase. The poor results obtained in studies using streptokinase have led to recommendations that streptokinase should be avoided in ischaemic stroke,[2,3] although an overview of thrombolytic studies[44] suggested that it may not be worse than alteplase and that the apparent hazards of streptokinase may be accounted for by differences in trial design (for example concomitant use of anticoagulants) and in patient population. Thus, while alteplase can be considered for those few patients meeting the entry criteria for the NINDS study, further large studies are required to establish more clearly the role of thrombolytics in acute ischaemic stroke. Studies of the use of alteplase outside the setting of a clinical trial have had mixed results.[45,46]

The intra-arterial administration of thrombolytics is under investigation and may be used in selected patients.[27]

Other attempts to improve cerebral blood flow have included haemodilution with *dextran* or *pentastarch,* but both of these approaches have been disappointing.

Ischaemia leads to a complex series of biochemical changes, the 'ischaemic cascade', resulting eventually in cell necrosis. The process is incompletely understood, but steps include calcium influx and release of neurotransmitters. Drugs acting at different steps in this ischaemic cascade, sometimes termed neuroprotectants, have been tried in acute ischaemic stroke in the hope of limiting the damage caused by ischaemia. Although results of studies so far have been largely disappointing, this is an area of active research and many trials of neuroprotectants are underway.[47] Recent studies are focusing more on starting treatment with these drugs in the first few hours following ischaemic stroke.[48] Drugs that are or have been under investigation include:

- *calcium-channel blockers* such as nimodipine. In addition to increasing cerebral blood flow they may prevent brain cell necrosis by limiting transcellular calcium influx, but results have been conflicting;
- *clomethiazole*, which may act through an agonist effect on GABA receptors;
- *citicoline*, a derivative of choline and cytidine, thought to prevent accumulation of toxic free fatty acids and to contribute to repair of damaged neuronal tissue;
- *fibroblast growth factors* that stimulate blood vessel formation and tissue repair processes;
- *glycine antagonists*, such as gavestinel, which block neuronal influx of calcium;
- *lipid peroxidation inhibitors* such as tirilazad (also used in subarachnoid haemorrhage) and ebselen;
- *lubeluzole*, a glutamate antagonist;
- *magnesium sulfate*;
- *naftidrofuryl*, which has a direct effect on cerebral intracellular metabolism and protects cells against the results of ischaemia;
- *N-methyl-D-aspartate (NMDA)-receptor antagonists* such as aptiganel, dextrorphan, dextromethorphan, dizocilpine, and ketamine might reduce ischaemic neuronal injury by preventing fatal influx of calcium;
- *oxpentifylline [pentoxifylline]* reduces viscosity of blood and this effect may be beneficial in ischaemic tissue.

Hypoxia and hypocapnia have been demonstrated in some patients with ischaemic stroke and are likely to contribute to ischaemic injury both directly and via cerebral vasoconstriction. There are anecdotal reports and some small studies on the use of *hyperbaric oxygen therapy* but its clinical value remains unknown.

Cerebral oedema associated with ischaemic stroke may be a mixture of intracellular oedema associated with cell damage (part of the ischaemic cascade) and interstitial vasogenic oedema. Treatment with *corticosteroids* or hyperosmolar diuretics such as *glycerol* or *mannitol* in an attempt to reduce the cerebral oedema has been disappointing.[49]

Patients who survive the acute event should be investigated to see if there is a cardiac source of emboli (see under Secondary Prevention of Stroke, below) and to determine whether surgery will be beneficial. Blood screening should also be carried out for polycythaemia, thrombocytosis, and abnormal coagulation functions.

Subarachnoid haemorrhage. Subarachnoid haemorrhage is associated with high morbidity and mortality, early deaths being due to damage from initial bleeding, recurrence of bleeding, and infarction. Infarction is often a result of vasospasm which is one of the pathophysiological mechanisms that contributes to stopping the bleeding; clot formation and increasing intracranial pressure are other processes involved. Up to a quarter of patients with subarachnoid haemorrhage develop delayed cerebral ischaemia mainly between days 5 and 14 after the initial bleed, and again vasospasm may be a contributory factor. Early medical treatment aims to prevent delayed cerebral ischaemia, to prevent rebleeding, and to stabilise the patient until surgery can be carried out to clip the aneurysm or correct the arteriovenous malformation and thus prevent further haemorrhage.[50,51] Plasma volume should be maintained to prevent delayed cerebral ischaemia; a fluid intake of 3 litres per day has been recommended. Nimodipine is of benefit and should be started as soon as possible after diagnosis of subarachnoid haemorrhage. Antifibrinolytic drug therapy with tranexamic acid or aminocaproic acid has been used to prevent rebleeding, particularly if surgery is to be delayed, although this might result in an increased incidence of cerebral ischaemic complications.[52] Paradoxically, rebleeding has been noted in patients given high doses of aminocaproic acid after subarachnoid haemorrhage (see Adverse Effects, Effects on the Blood, under Aminocaproic Acid, p.725). Headache can be managed with analgesics such as paracetamol, dextropropoxyphene, or codeine; aspirin should be avoided. Localised haematomas may be amenable to surgical evacuation. Tirilazad, a lipid peroxidation inhibitor, may be given to male patients with subarachnoid haemorrhage. It is thought to have a cytoprotective effect against radicals produced in response to tissue trauma.

Intracerebral haemorrhage. Outcome of intracerebral haemorrhage depends on the location and size of the haematoma (determined by computed tomography), on the level of consciousness, and on the progression of neurological signs, and development of increased intracranial

pressure.[53,54] Any known cause of bleeding, such as warfarin anticoagulation, should be reversed. Blood pressure should be lowered when it is very high (>180 mmHg systolic[55]), but hypoperfusion should be avoided. Drugs such as labetalol, esmolol, or sodium nitroprusside have been used to reduce blood pressure. Surgical drainage of the haematoma may sometimes be possible. Instillation of a thrombolytic to improve aspiration of the haematoma has been reported. Raised intracranial pressure must be controlled[55] (see above). Antiepileptic prophylaxis, usually with phenytoin, may be necessary in some patients.[55]

Secondary prevention

Once patients have suffered a stroke, risk factors should be identified (see Primary Prevention, above) and appropriate changes made in lifestyle. Hypertension requires treatment and surgery may be necessary in patients with aneurysms, arteriovenous malformations, or carotid stenoses. Patients who have suffered ischaemic stroke or transient ischaemic attacks are at risk of further stroke, myocardial infarction, or sudden death,[56,57] and preventative treatment may be considered (see Myocardial Infarction, p.805). Nearly 20% of ischaemic strokes are secondary to cardiogenic emboli[8] and, as mentioned for primary prevention, antithrombotic therapy may be required.

Antiplatelet drugs. Long-term prophylaxis with aspirin reduces the risk of future serious vascular events including stroke in patients who have already suffered an ischaemic stroke or transient ischaemic attack,[27,56-60] regardless of age.[61] Medium doses of 75 to 325 mg of aspirin daily have been most widely studied[58] and an analysis of trials using aspirin over a dose range of 50 to 1500 mg daily found no relationship between dose and the reduction in risk of stroke.[62] In patients undergoing carotid endarterectomy the risk of stroke, myocardial infarction, and death over 3 months may be lower for those taking medium dose aspirin compared with higher doses.[63] Dipyridamole given alone has also been shown to be effective for secondary prevention of ischaemic stroke[64] and may be used in patients unable to tolerate aspirin; the combination of aspirin and dipyridamole has produced additive protective effects.[64] Earlier studies had produced conflicting results however, possibly due to differences in dose and formulation. A meta-analysis[65] concluded that the combination did reduce the risk of stroke more than aspirin alone, but that further study is needed. Ticlopidine[66-68] or clopidogrel[69] may also be used in patients unable to tolerate aspirin and appear to be at least as effective.

Anticoagulants. The value of oral anticoagulants to prevent recurrent transient ischaemic attacks or stroke in patients with transient ischaemic attacks is unclear. One study was terminated early because of a high rate of major bleeding complications in the patients receiving an oral anticoagulant.[70] They have generally been used only in those who continue to experience transient ischaemic attacks despite treatment with aspirin.[60] Oral anticoagulants may be started in these patients following anticoagulation with heparin. Long-term aspirin therapy may then be substituted.

1. WHO. Stroke—1989: recommendations on stroke prevention, diagnosis, and therapy: report of the WHO task force on stroke and other cerebrovascular disorders. *Stroke* 1989; **20:** 1407–31.
2. The European Ad Hoc Consensus Group. European strategies for early intervention in stroke: a report of an Ad Hoc Consensus Group meeting. *Cerebrovasc Dis* 1996; **6:** 315–24.
3. Adams HP, *et al.* Guidelines for thrombolytic therapy for acute stroke: a supplement to the guidelines for the management of patients with acute ischaemic stroke. *Circulation* 1996; **94:** 1167–74 [also published in *Stroke* 1996; **27:** 1711–18].
4. The American Heart Association in collaboration with the International Committee on Resuscitation (ILCOR). International guidelines 2000 for cardiopulmonary resuscitation and emergency cardiovascular care: an international consensus on science. Part 7: the era of reperfusion. Section 2: acute stroke. *Circulation* 2000; **102** (suppl I): I204–I216 [also published in *Resuscitation* 2000; **46:** 239–52].
5. Bronner LL, *et al.* Primary prevention of stroke. *N Engl J Med* 1995; **333:** 1392–1400.
6. Gorelick PB, *et al.* Prevention of a first stroke: a review of guidelines and a multidisciplinary consensus statement from the National Stroke Association. *JAMA* 1999; **281:** 1112–20.
7. Goldstein LB, *et al.* Primary prevention of ischemic stroke: a statement for healthcare professionals from the Stroke Council of the American Heart Association. *Circulation* 2001; **103:** 163–82 [also published in *Stroke* 2001; **32:** 280–99].
8. Hart RG. Cardiogenic embolism to the brain. *Lancet* 1992; **339:** 589–94.
9. Crouse JR, *et al.* Reductase inhibitor monotherapy and stroke prevention. *Arch Intern Med* 1997; **157:** 1305–10.
10. Bucher HC, *et al.* Effect of HMGcoA reductase inhibitors on stroke: a meta-analysis of randomized, controlled trials. *Ann Intern Med* 1998; **128:** 89–95.
11. Plehn JF, *et al.* Reduction of stroke incidence after myocardial infarction with pravastatin: the Cholesterol and Recurrent Events (CARE) study. *Circulation* 1999; **99:** 216–23.
12. White HD, *et al.* Pravastatin therapy and the risk of stroke. *N Engl J Med* 2000; **343:** 317–26.
13. Biller J, *et al.* Guidelines for carotid endarterectomy: a statement for healthcare professionals from a special writing group of the Stroke Council, American Heart Association. *Stroke* 1998; **29:** 554–62.
14. Benavente O, *et al.* Carotid endarterectomy for asymptomatic carotid stenosis: a meta-analysis. *BMJ* 1998; **317:** 1477–80.
15. Steering committee of the Physicians' Health Study Research Group. Final report on the aspirin component of the ongoing physicians' health study. *N Engl J Med* 1989; **321:** 129–35.
16. Peto R, *et al.* Randomised trial of prophylactic daily aspirin in British male doctors. *BMJ* 1988; **296:** 313–16.
17. The Medical Research Council's General Practice Research Framework. Thrombosis prevention trial: randomised trial of low-intensity oral anticoagulation with warfarin and low-dose aspirin in the primary prevention of ischaemic heart disease in men at increased risk. *Lancet* 1998; **351:** 233–41.
18. Hansson L, *et al.* Effects of intensive blood-pressure lowering and low-dose aspirin in patients with hypertension: principal results of the Hypertension Optimal Treatment (HOT) randomised trial. *Lancet* 1998; **351:** 1755–62.
19. Adams HP, *et al.* Guidelines for the management of patients with acute ischaemic stroke: a statement for healthcare professionals from a special writing group of the Stroke Council, American Heart Association. *Stroke* 1994; **25:** 1901–14.
20. Alberts MJ. Diagnosis and treatment of ischemic stroke. *Am J Med* 1999; **106:** 211–21.
21. Lindley RI. Drug therapy for acute ischaemic stroke: risks versus benefits. *Drug Safety* 1998; **19:** 373–82.
22. Hill MD, Hachinski V. Stroke treatment: time is brain. *Lancet* 1998; **352** (suppl 3): 10–14.
23. Brott T, Bogousslavsky J. Treatment of acute ischemic stroke. *N Engl J Med* 2000; **343:** 710–22.
24. Goldstein LB. Should antihypertensive therapies be given to patients with acute ischaemic stroke? *Drug Safety* 2000; **22:** 13–18.
25. International Stroke Trial Collaborative Group. The International Stroke Trial (IST): a randomised trial of aspirin, subcutaneous heparin, both, or neither among 19 435 patients with acute ischaemic stroke. *Lancet* 1997; **349:** 1569–81.
26. CAST (Chinese Acute Stroke Trial) Collaborative Group. CAST: randomised placebo-controlled trial of early aspirin use in 20 000 patients with acute ischaemic stroke. *Lancet* 1997; **349:** 1641–9.
27. Albers GW, *et al.* Antithrombotic and thrombolytic therapy for ischemic stroke. *Chest* 2001; **119** (suppl): 300S–320S.
28. Gubitz G, *et al.* Anticoagulants for acute ischaemic stroke (updated 6 March 2000). Available in The Cochrane Library; Issue 4. Oxford: Update Software; 2001.
29. Sandercock PAG, *et al.* Antithrombotic therapy in acute ischaemic stroke: an overview of the completed randomised trials. *J Neurol Neurosurg Psychiatry* 1993; **56:** 17–25.
30. Berge E, *et al.* Low molecular-weight heparin versus aspirin in patients with acute ischaemic stroke and atrial fibrillation: a double-blind randomised trial. *Lancet* 2000; **355:** 1205–10.
31. The Publications Committee for the Trial of ORG 10172 in Acute Stroke Treatment (TOAST) Investigators. Low molecular weight heparinoid, ORG 10172 (danaparoid), and outcome after acute ischemic stroke: a randomized controlled trial. *JAMA* 1998; **279:** 1265–72.
32. Sherman DG, *et al.* Intravenous ancrod for treatment of acute ischemic stroke: the STAT study: a randomized controlled trial. *JAMA* 2000; **283:** 2395–2403.
33. The National Institute of Neurological Disorders and Stroke rt-PA Stroke Study Group. Tissue plasminogen activator for acute ischemic stroke. *N Engl J Med* 1995; **333:** 1581–7.
34. The Multicenter Acute Stroke Trial—Europe Study Group. Thrombolytic therapy with streptokinase in acute ischemic stroke. *N Engl J Med* 1996; **335:** 145–50.
35. Donnan GA, *et al.* Streptokinase for acute ischemic stroke with relationship to time of administration. *JAMA* 1996; **276:** 961–6.
36. Multicentre Acute Stroke Trial - Italy (MAST-I) Group. Randomised controlled trial of streptokinase, aspirin, and combination of both in treatment of acute ischaemic stroke. *Lancet* 1995; **346:** 1509–14.
37. Tognoni G, Roncaglioni MC. Dissent: an alternative interpretation of MAST-I. *Lancet* 1995; **346:** 1515.
38. Hacke W, *et al.* Intravenous thrombolysis with recombinant tissue plasminogen activator for acute hemispheric stroke: the European Cooperative Acute Stroke Study (ECASS). *JAMA* 1995; **274:** 1017–25.
39. Kwiatkowski TG, *et al.* Effects of tissue plasminogen activator for acute ischemic stroke at one year. *N Engl J Med* 1999; **340:** 1781–7.
40. Hacke W, *et al.* Randomised double-blind placebo-controlled trial of thrombolytic therapy with intravenous alteplase in acute ischaemic stroke (ECASS II). *Lancet* 1998; **352:** 1245–51.
41. Caplan LR. Stroke thrombolysis—growing pains. *Mayo Clin Proc* 1997; **72:** 1090–2.
42. Caplan LR, *et al.* Should thrombolytic therapy be the first-line treatment for acute ischemic stroke? Thrombolysis—not a panacea for ischemic stroke. *N Engl J Med* 1997; **337:** 1309–10.
43. Muir KW. Thrombolysis for stroke: pushed out of the window? *Br J Clin Pharmacol* 1996; **42:** 681–2.
44. Wardlaw JM, *et al.* Systematic review of evidence on thrombolytic therapy for acute ischaemic stroke. *Lancet* 1997; **350:** 607–14.
45. Albers GW, *et al.* Intravenous tissue-type plasminogen activator for treatment of acute stroke: the Standard Treatment with Alteplase to Reverse Stroke (STARS) Study. *JAMA* 2000; **283:** 1145–50.
46. Katzan IL, *et al.* Use of tissue-type plasminogen activator for acute ischemic stroke: the Cleveland area experience. *JAMA* 2000; **283:** 1151–8.
47. Lees KR. Neuroprotection. *Br Med Bull* 2000; **56:** 401–12.
48. Fisher M, Bogousslavsky J. Further evolution toward effective therapy for acute ischemic stroke. *JAMA* 1998; **279:** 1298–1303.
49. Anonymous. Treatment for stroke? *Lancet* 1991; **337:** 1129–31.
50. van Gijn J. Subarachnoid haemorrhage. *Lancet* 1992; **339:** 653–5.
51. Bendok BR, *et al.* Treatment of aneurysmal subarachnoid hemorrhage. *Semin Neurol* 1998; **18:** 521–31.
52. Roos YB, *et al.* Systematic review of antifibrinolytic treatment in aneurysmal subarachnoid haemorrhage. *J Neurol Neurosurg Psychiatry* 1998; **65:** 942–3.
53. Caplan LR. Intracerebral haemorrhage. *Lancet* 1992; **339:** 656–8.

54. Qureshi AI, *et al.* Spontaneous intracerebral hemorrhage. *N Engl J Med* 2001; **344:** 1450–60.
55. Broderick JP, *et al.* Guidelines for the management of spontaneous intracerebral hemorrhage: a statement for healthcare professionals from a special writing group of the Stroke Council, American Heart Association. *Stroke* 1999; **30:** 905–15.
56. American College of Physicians. Guidelines for medical treatment for stroke prevention. *Ann Intern Med* 1994; **121:** 54–5.
57. Matchar DB, *et al.* Medical treatment for stroke prevention. *Ann Intern Med* 1994; **121:** 41–53.
58. Antiplatelet Trialists' Collaboration. Collaborative overview of randomised trials of antiplatelet therapy—I: prevention of death, myocardial infarction, and stroke by prolonged antiplatelet therapy in various categories of patients. *BMJ* 1994; **308:** 81–106. Correction. *ibid.*; 1540.
59. Wolf PA, *et al.* Preventing ischemic stroke in patients with prior stroke and transient ischemic attack: a statement for healthcare professionals from the Stroke Council of the American Heart Association. *Stroke* 1999; **30:** 1991–4.
60. Albers GW, *et al.* Supplement to the guidelines for the management of transient ischemic attacks: a statement from the Ad Hoc Committee on Guidelines for the Management of Transient Ischemic Attacks, Stroke Council, American Heart Association. *Stroke* 1999; **30:** 2502–11.
61. Sivenius J, *et al.* Antiplatelet treatment in elderly people with transient ischaemic attacks or ischaemic strokes. *BMJ* 1995; **310:** 25–6.
62. Johnson ES, *et al.* A metaregression analysis of the dose-response effect of aspirin on stroke. *Arch Intern Med* 1999; **159:** 1248–53.
63. Taylor DW, *et al.* Low-dose and high-dose acetylsalicylic acid for patients undergoing carotid endarterectomy: a randomised controlled trial. *Lancet* 1999; **353:** 2179–84.
64. Diener HC, *et al.* European Stroke Prevention Study 2: dipyridamole and acetylsalicylic acid in the secondary prevention of stroke. *J Neurol Sci* 1999; **143:** 1–13.
65. Wilterdink JL, Easton JD. Dipyridamole plus aspirin in cerebrovascular disease. *Arch Neurol* 1999; **56:** 1087–92.
66. Hass WK, *et al.* A randomized trial comparing ticlopidine hydrochloride with aspirin for the prevention of stroke in high-risk patients. *N Engl J Med* 1989; **321:** 501–7.
67. Harbison JW. Ticlopidine versus aspirin for the prevention of recurrent stroke: analysis of patients with minor stroke from the ticlopidine aspirin stroke study. *Stroke* 1992; **23:** 1723–7.
68. Bellavance A. Efficacy of ticlopidine and aspirin for prevention of reversible cerebrovascular ischemic events: the ticlopidine aspirin stroke study. *Stroke* 1993; **24:** 1452–7.
69. CAPRIE Steering Committee. A randomised, blinded, trial of clopidogrel versus aspirin in patients at risk of ischaemic events (CAPRIE). *Lancet* 1996; **348:** 1329–39.
70. The Stroke Prevention in Reversible Ischemia Trial (SPIRIT) Study Group. A randomized trial of anticoagulants versus aspirin after cerebral ischemia of presumed arterial origin. *Ann Neurol* 1997; **42:** 857–65.

Thromboembolic disorders

The term thromboembolic disorder has been applied loosely to cardiovascular disorders associated with thrombus and embolus formation in blood vessels. A **thrombus** is a stationary blood clot composed of fibrin and platelets and other cellular elements. **Thrombosis** is occlusion of a vein or artery by a thrombus. An **embolus** is a fragment of blood clot, atheromatous material, or other foreign matter carried along in the blood stream. Occlusion of a blood vessel by an embolus is termed **embolism** or **thromboembolism**.

Formation of blood clots in the body is the result of a coagulation cascade (see Haemostasis and Fibrinolysis, p.718). Under normal circumstances systemic coagulation is prevented by natural antithrombotic systems that limit blood clots to sites of vascular injury. Thromboembolic disorders occur when there is an imbalance between these systems. Three factors are involved, namely damage to the endothelial lining of blood vessels, reduced blood flow, or changes in the coagulation mechanisms of the blood. A further factor that increases the risk of clotting is the presence of an artificial surface in contact with the blood, for example mechanical heart valves, intravascular catheters, or during extracorporeal circulation procedures. Thromboembolism can occur in any part of the circulation, including the heart and the capillaries, but the characteristics of the thrombi, the consequences, and the management of thromboembolism depend to a large extent upon whether the arterial or venous system is involved.

The mainstay of management for thromboembolic disorders is antithrombotic drugs. These act at different sites in the coagulation cascade and include anticoagulants and antiplatelet drugs, which are used to limit the extent of thrombosis or thromboembolism and to prevent further thromboembolic events occurring, and thrombolytics, which are used to lyse the clot.

Arterial thromboembolism is almost always a consequence of damage to the endothelium due to atherosclerosis (above); the atheroma may block the blood vessel or, more commonly, occlusion is a result of thrombus formation at a site of a recently ruptured atheromatous plaque. Arterial thrombi contain more platelets than venous thrombi and tend to remain fixed, but emboli may break off and occlude distal vessels. Arterial emboli may also result from thrombosis within the heart, for example due to arrhythmias or valvular heart disorders.

Thrombosis or thromboembolism in the arterial circulation produces ischaemia in the tissues perfused by the artery, which may lead to infarction. It may therefore result in myocardial infarction (above) or unstable angina (above) if it occurs in coronary arteries, stroke (above) if it occurs in cerebral arteries, or critical limb ischaemia if it occurs in peripheral arteries (above).

Venous thromboembolism (below) is usually a consequence of stasis of the blood, but other factors such as local trauma or coagulation activation are also required. Reduced venous blood flow occurs in many conditions, including obesity, heart failure, and during prolonged immobilisation. Abnormal clotting may occur in conditions such as malignancy, pregnancy, and the nephrotic syndrome, or during oestrogen therapy; it may also be due to inherited or acquired clotting disorders or thrombophilias (see below). Surgical operations are particularly associated with venous thromboembolism; trauma activates clotting factors and reduced blood flow may occur during the procedure and recovery period.

Venous thrombi have a 'red tail' of fibrin and red cells that may occlude the vein but which often separates to form an embolus; this is most likely during the early stages when the thrombus is only loosely attached. Thrombosis or thromboembolism in the venous circulation produces oedema or inflammation in the tissue drained by the affected vein. The commonest type of venous thrombosis is deep-vein thrombosis which is associated especially with immobility and the post-operative period. Pulmonary embolism is the most serious complication of deep-vein thrombosis and occurs when part of the thrombus migrates in the circulation and becomes lodged in the pulmonary artery. Hypercoagulable states may result in deep-vein thrombosis or more generalised clotting in microvessels (microvessel thrombosis), such as thrombotic thrombocytopenic purpura or purpura fulminans (see Thrombotic Microangiopathies, p.740).

Thrombophilias are acquired or inherited disorders of the clotting system in which the antithrombotic mechanisms are impaired. Inherited deficiencies of antithrombin III, protein C and protein S all predispose to thromboembolism. Resistance to activated protein C has been identified as a major cause of inherited thrombophilia and appears to be due to a mutation in the factor V gene (factor V Leiden). A mutation in the prothrombin (factor II) gene is associated with increased concentrations of prothrombin and risk of thrombosis. Acquired thrombophilias are more common and may occur secondary to disorders such as malignancy, infection, or collagen-vascular disorders; in many cases antiphospholipid antibodies (such as lupus anticoagulant) are present. Hyperhomocysteinaemia is another risk factor and may have both inherited and acquired causes.

Inherited thrombophilias generally result in venous thromboembolism; this is often recurrent and may occur in unusual sites or at a young age. They often present when some further risk factor is present, such as pregnancy, use of combined oral contraceptives, or surgery, but the value of screening asymptomatic patients remains unclear. Acquired thrombophilias may lead to arterial or venous thromboembolism.

Patients with thrombophilias who develop thromboembolism should be treated conventionally, with anticoagulants or thrombolytics as appropriate. There continues to be debate regarding the duration of therapy, with some authorities recommending life-long anticoagulant therapy following a single episode and others recommending life-long therapy only in those with recurrent thrombosis. If anticoagulation is not continued, thromboprophylaxis should be given during high risk situations. Thromboprophylaxis is probably also necessary during pregnancy, particularly in women with antiphospholipid antibodies who are at risk for recurrent fetal loss, but the risks to the fetus from anticoagulant therapy must also be considered (see Venous Thromboembolism, below).

References.

1. Haines ST, Bussey HI. Thrombosis and the pharmacology of antithrombotic agents. *Ann Pharmacother* 1995; **29:** 892–905.
2. Anonymous. Management of patients with thrombophilia. *Drug Ther Bull* 1995; **33:** 6–8.
3. WHO. Inherited thrombophilia: memorandum from a joint WHO/International Society on Thrombosis and Haemostasis meeting. *Bull WHO* 1997; **75:** 177–89.
4. Price DT, Ridker PM. Factor V Leiden mutation and the risks for thromboembolic disease: a clinical perspective. *Ann Intern Med* 1997; **127:** 895–903.
5. Rosendaal FR. Venous thrombosis: a multicausal disease. *Lancet* 1999; **353:** 1167–73.
6. Seligsohn U, Lubetsky A. Genetic susceptibility to venous thrombosis. *N Engl J Med* 2001; **344:** 1222–31.

Valvular heart disease

Valvular heart disease affects the normal function of the heart and leads to disorders of blood circulation. The principal cause of valvular disease world-wide is rheumatic heart disease. Other causes include congenital abnormalities, cardiovascular disorders such as ischaemic heart disease and hypertension, and degenerative disorders. Any of the heart valves may be affected but disorders of the aortic and mitral valves are most significant; more than one valve may be involved in some patients.

The symptoms of valvular heart disease depend upon the valve that is affected, and whether the problem is stenosis or regurgitation. All valve disorders place a haemodynamic burden on the heart and ultimately lead to heart failure.[1] Other consequences include the development of pulmonary hypertension and arrhythmias. Infective endocarditis and thromboembolic disorders, in particular stroke or systemic embolism, are important complications.

The main aims of treatment in patients with valvular heart disease are to reduce symptoms, prevent complications, and reduce mortality. In symptomatic patients, standard treatment for heart failure (see above) may be of benefit, although improvement is not generally sustained. Choice of therapy depends upon the valve affected. Vasodilators should not be used in patients with aortic stenosis[2] but do have a role in severe aortic regurgitation; use of nifedipine has improved outcome in asymptomatic patients with severe aortic regurgitation.[3] Arrhythmias should be treated with standard antiarrhythmics (see above). Surgical treatment is necessary in most patients and generally involves valve replacement, although valve repair may be suitable in some cases, particularly for mitral regurgitation. Valve replacement alleviates symptoms but does not remove the risks of endocarditis or thromboembolism. Bioprosthetic (tissue) or mechanical valves may be used; the latter are longer lasting, but pose a greater risk for thromboembolism.

In asymptomatic patients and in those who have had valve replacement, the main aim of therapy is to prevent the complications of bacterial endocarditis and of systemic embolism from thrombus formation within the heart.[4] Antibacterial prophylaxis should be given to all patients with valvular heart disease as indicated (see Endocarditis, p.119). Long-term thromboembolism prophylaxis is only required in patients with another risk factor for embolisation, such as concurrent atrial fibrillation, a dilated left atrium, or previous systemic embolism,[5,6] and in those with mechanical replacement valves.

Long-term treatment with an oral anticoagulant such as warfarin is generally regarded as essential for patients with a mechanical prosthetic heart valve.[4,7] The risk of thromboembolism depends upon the type and position of the valve and the presence of other risk factors. In the UK, a target INR of 3.5 is recommended,[8] but there is evidence that lower intensities may be effective while reducing the risk of bleeding.[9,10] In the USA, the recommended target INR is 2.5 to 3.5, although a lower range of 2.0 to 3.0 may be adequate for most types of valves in the aortic position when there are no other risk factors.[6,11] The value of adding an antiplatelet drug to anticoagulant therapy in patients with artificial heart valves is less clear, although it has been suggested[12] that all patients with prosthetic valves should receive low-dose aspirin given its additional benefits in preventing cardiovascular disease. There is some evidence of reduced thromboembolism with aspirin, and with dipyridamole, in patients with prosthetic valves but the risk of bleeding is increased.[13] Adjunctive antiplatelet drugs may be considered for patients with additional risk factors such as embolism while on warfarin therapy, or ischaemic heart disease.[6,11] For some types of valve the use of aspirin with warfarin adjusted to maintain a lower INR may provide adequate anticoagulation without increasing the risk of bleeding.[11]

For patients with bioprosthetic heart valves anticoagulants are recommended for the first 3 months after replacement.[4,7] Thereafter, long-term oral anticoagulant therapy is generally considered necessary only for patients with risk factors such as atrial fibrillation, a dilated left atrium, left atrial thrombus, a history of systemic embolism, and possibly those with severe left ventricular dysfunction.[6,7,11] An INR of 2.0 to 3.0 appears adequate for patients with bioprosthetic heart valves. Low-dose aspirin should be considered in patients with bioprosthetic valves who do not require oral anticoagulants.[6,11]

The use of anticoagulants is controversial in patients with infective endocarditis because of the substantial increase in risk of haemorrhage in these patients. Oral anticoagulants should generally be continued in patients who have prosthetic heart valves, unless complications occur.[5,7] Anticoagulation may also be considered for patients with endocarditis who have other risk factors for systemic embolism.

Pregnancy is a known risk-factor for thromboembolism and patients with valvular heart disease who become pregnant are therefore at increased risk. However, long-term prophylaxis with an oral anticoagulant such as warfarin presents a problem since warfarin is generally contra-indicated in pregnancy (see Adverse Effects under Warfarin, p.992). Women with mechanical prosthetic valves must continue anticoagulation but choice of therapy is unclear. A systematic review[14] found that continued use of oral anticoagulants increased the risk to the fetus, but that thromboembolic complications were higher with heparin. Guidelines therefore vary in their recommendations. It is usually recommended that subcutaneous heparin should be substituted for warfarin.[4,15] A dose of 17 500 to 20 000 units subcutaneously every 12 hours has been suggested;[15] intravenous administration is an alternative for women at high risk,[6] but low-dose subcutaneous heparin is not suitable since it provides inadequate protection against prosthetic valve thrombosis.[16] Ideally heparin should be started before conception, or as soon after as possible, and should be continued at least until the twelfth week to avoid the risk of warfarin embryopathy. If necessary, warfarin may then be reintroduced, although heparin is also recommended at term (to avoid an anticoagulated neonate). However, a retrospective study[17] suggested that outcomes were satisfactory following use of warfarin during the first trimester of pregnancy and some authorities[2] recommend continued use of oral anticoagulants throughout pregnancy in most patients, depending on the dose of warfarin. Low-molecular-weight heparins may also be an alternative to heparin in pregnant patients,[15] although there is less experience with their use. Low-dose aspirin may be used as an adjunct to subcutaneous heparin or warfarin in women at high risk of thromboembolism.[7,15]

1. Carabello BA, Crawford FA. Valvular heart disease. *N Engl J Med* 1997; **337**: 32–41.
2. Prendergast BD, *et al.* Valvular heart disease: recommendations for investigation and management. *J R Coll Physicians Lond* 1996; **30**: 309–15.
3. Scognamiglio R, *et al.* Nifedipine in asymptomatic patients with severe aortic regurgitation and normal left ventricular function. *N Engl J Med* 1994; **331**: 689–94.
4. Coulshed DS, *et al.* Drug treatment associated with heart valve replacement. *Drugs* 1995; **49**: 897–911.
5. Salem DN, *et al.* Antithrombotic therapy in valvular heart disease. *Chest* 2001; **119** (suppl): 207S–219S.
6. Bonow RO, *et al.* ACC/AHA guidelines for the management of patients with valvular heart disease. *Circulation* 1998; **98**: 1949–84.
7. Vongpatanasin W, *et al.* Prosthetic heart valves. *N Engl J Med* 1996; **335**: 407–16.
8. British Society for Haematology: British Committee for Standards in Haematology—Haemostasis and Thrombosis Task Force. Guidelines on oral anticoagulation: third edition. *Br J Haematol* 1998; **101**: 374–87.
9. Saour JN, *et al.* Trial of different intensities of anticoagulation in patients with prosthetic heart valves. *N Engl J Med* 1990; **322**: 428–32.
10. Cannegieter SC, *et al.* Optimal oral anticoagulant therapy in patients with mechanical heart valves. *N Engl J Med* 1995; **333**: 11–17.
11. Stein PD, *et al.* Antithrombotic therapy in patients with mechanical and biological prosthetic heart valves. *Chest* 2001; **119** (suppl): 220S–227S.
12. Tiede DJ, *et al.* Modern management of prosthetic valve anticoagulation. *Mayo Clin Proc* 1998; **73**: 665–80.
13. Massel D, Little SH. Risks and benefits of adding anti-platelet therapy to warfarin among patients with prosthetic heart valves: a meta-analysis. *J Am Coll Cardiol* 2001; **37**: 569–78.
14. Chan WS, *et al.* Anticoagulation of pregnant women with mechanical heart valves: a systematic review of the literature. *Arch Intern Med* 2000; **160**: 191–6.
15. Ginsberg JS, *et al.* Use of antithrombotic agents during pregnancy. *Chest* 2001; **119** (suppl): 122S–131S.
16. Maternal and Neonatal Haemostasis Working Party of the Haemostasis and Thrombosis Task. Guidelines on the prevention, investigation and management of thrombosis associated with pregnancy. *J Clin Pathol* 1993; **46**: 489–96.
17. Sbarouni E, Oakley CM. Outcome of pregnancy in women with valve prostheses. *Br Heart J* 1994; **71**: 196–201.

Venous thromboembolism

The term venous thromboembolism embraces both deep-vein thrombosis and pulmonary embolism; the two often co-exist and should be considered as a single clinical entity. In deep-vein thrombosis a thrombus forms, frequently in the pockets of valves, and blocks the veins of the lower limbs or main pelvic veins. Pulmonary embolism occurs when the thrombus or part of it migrates in the circulation and blocks the pulmonary artery. About 70% of patients with confirmed pulmonary embolism have thrombosis in their deep leg veins and about 40% of patients with confirmed deep-vein thrombosis have silent pulmonary embolism. Proximal deep-vein thrombosis is

associated with a higher risk of pulmonary embolism than distal deep-vein thrombosis.

Venous thromboembolism is a common but underdiagnosed condition and the cause of considerable morbidity and mortality, especially among hospitalised patients. Various factors underlie the development of thrombosis and there are a number of conditions that predispose patients to venous thromboembolism (see Thromboembolic Disorders, above).

Symptoms of *deep-vein thrombosis* include a tender and swollen calf; increased temperature, cyanosis, and engorgement of the superficial veins of the affected limb; fever; and tachycardia. However, about half of all cases may be symptomless. In the longer term chronic venous insufficiency and venous ulceration often occur (postphlebitic or post-thrombotic syndrome). As most clinical signs of deep-vein thrombosis are non-specific, the diagnosis should always be confirmed before committing a patient to long-term anticoagulation treatment. Noninvasive diagnostic techniques are usually adequate, although venography may be required in some patients.[1] Compression ultrasound is the preferred method, often combined with measurement of D-dimer concentrations; impedance plethysmography may also be used. *Pulmonary embolism* may present in a number of ways depending on its extent and duration. Acute massive embolism causes serious haemodynamic disturbance with a sudden reduction in cardiac output and circulatory collapse. The most common form of pulmonary embolism seen, however, is acute minor embolism where the patient may present with pleuritic pain, haemoptysis, dyspnoea, tachycardia, and fever. Diagnosis may involve perfusion/ventilation scans or angiography;[2,3] computed tomography (CT) may also be used.

Prophylaxis of venous thromboembolism. Prophylaxis with anticoagulants aims to prevent deep-vein thrombosis and hence pulmonary embolism in patients at risk. It appears to be underused.[4-7] Ideally all medical and surgical hospital inpatients should be assessed for risk factors and should receive prophylaxis according to their degree of risk at least until discharge or, for those at higher risk, after discharge. A prophylactic regimen should be chosen for a particular patient after balancing the degree of risk against the potential complications of prophylaxis. Guidelines have been published by the British Society for Haematology[8] and the American College of Chest Physicians.[9]

Patients can be categorised as being at low, medium, or high risk of venous thromboembolism according to the duration and type of operation in those undergoing surgery, to age, and to the presence of other risk factors such as cancer, heart failure, and lung disease.[9,10] Low-risk patients include young patients undergoing short operative procedures. Older age, operations lasting longer than 30 minutes, and a history of thrombophilia or previous thromboembolism indicate medium risk. Orthopaedic surgery is associated with a high risk of venous thromboembolism in all patients. Other patients at high risk include those with multiple risk factors. Non-surgical patients are also at risk of thromboembolism, particularly if they are immobile, or have major trauma or spinal cord injury. Pregnancy is also a risk factor and is discussed in more detail below.

Methods of prophylaxis may be physical or pharmacological. Physical methods, which increase venous blood flow, include elevation of the legs, early ambulation, graduated compression stockings, and intermittent pneumatic compression devices. Pharmacological methods generally involve anticoagulation with heparin, low-molecular-weight heparins, or an oral anticoagulant. Other therapies that have been used include antiplatelet drugs, dihydroergotamine, dextrans, antithrombin III, and, more recently, heparinoids such as danaparoid, and the direct thrombin inhibitor desirudin. Ancrod and argatroban have been used in patients who have developed heparin-induced thrombocytopenia or thrombosis.

For low-risk surgical patients measures such as early ambulation and the use of graduated compression stockings are generally considered adequate. Moderate- and high-risk patients require pharmacological methods, although physical methods (particularly intermittent compression devices) may be used in those who are at high risk from bleeding complications. Physical methods are not suitable in patients with significant peripheral vascular disease. In practice, a combination of mechanical methods (particularly graduated compression stockings) and pharmacological methods is often used, and may give better protection than either method alone.[9]

For moderate-risk patients, such as those undergoing general surgical procedures lasting more than 30 minutes, low-dose subcutaneous heparin ('standard heparin prophylaxis') is the most widely used pharmacological method, a typical regimen being 5000 units subcutaneously 2 hours pre-operatively, then every 8 or 12 hours postoperatively for 7 days or until the patient is mobile.[8] Subcutaneous low-molecular-weight heparins may be used as an alternative. High-risk patients may require more aggressive prophylaxis with higher doses of low-molecular-weight heparin; higher doses of unfractionated heparin with laboratory monitoring (adjusted-dose heparin) or oral anticoagulants may also be used.

The use of *low-dose subcutaneous heparin* for surgical thromboembolism prophylaxis is well established. In an overview[11] of more than 70 randomised studies in 16 000 patients heparin reduced the risk of subclinical deep-vein thrombosis by 67% in general surgery, 68% in orthopaedic surgery, and 75% in urological surgery. There was also a 40% reduction in non-fatal cases of pulmonary embolism, a 64% reduction in fatal cases, and a 47% reduction of all cases. Surgical thromboembolism prophylaxis with heparin also decreased total mortality. *Adjusted-dose heparin* may be more effective in higher risk patients but the need for laboratory monitoring and the risk of bleeding complications limit its use.

Low-molecular-weight heparins have a number of potential advantages over unfractionated heparin, including less frequent administration and no need for monitoring, and they are being used increasingly. It was hoped that they might also reduce the risk of bleeding but this has not been clearly demonstrated. Generally, studies have shown low-molecular-weight heparins to be at least as effective as unfractionated or standard heparin, but a number of meta-analyses have come to differing conclusions regarding superiority. The evidence suggests that low-molecular-weight heparins are superior in orthopaedic surgery,[12-15] particularly with regard to proximal deep-vein thrombosis.[14] In general surgery both types of heparin appear to be of equivalent efficacy, although one analysis[13] reported that low-molecular-weight heparins were superior. A large study[16] showed low-molecular-weight heparins to be as effective as heparin for prophylaxis after major abdominal surgery and to be associated with fewer bleeding complications. Two meta-analyses of 45 studies[17] and 56 studies[18] respectively evaluated the efficacy of several prophylactic methods (such as aspirin, dextran, oral anticoagulants, heparin, heparin with dihydroergotamine, low-molecular-weight heparins, and intermittent pneumatic compression) against deep-vein thrombosis following major hip surgery and concluded that low-molecular-weight heparins should be the method of choice. Low-molecular-weight heparins may also be more effective than unfractionated heparin in patients with major trauma.[19]

The optimum duration of prophylaxis is unclear. Prophylaxis is usually only continued during hospitalisation but following orthopaedic surgery there is an increased risk for deep-vein thrombosis detected by venography up to a month after discharge, which may be reduced by low-molecular-weight heparin.[20] Although the clinical significance of this finding has been questioned,[21] extended prophylaxis may have a role, particularly in high-risk patients following orthopaedic surgery, or in very high-risk general surgical patients.[9]

Oral anticoagulants have not been so widely used as subcutaneous heparin although US guidelines[9] allow the use of adjusted-dose warfarin to give an international normalised ratio (INR — see Warfarin, p.998 for further details) of 2.0 to 3.0 in patients having hip or knee replacement surgery and in selected high-risk general surgical patients. When compared[22] with low-molecular-weight heparin this 'less intense' regimen was slightly less effective in preventing deep-vein thrombosis after hip or knee replacements, but there were fewer bleeding complications with warfarin; warfarin was started on the evening of the day of surgery in an initial dose of 10 mg. A fixed 'minidose' warfarin regimen (1 mg daily) starting a mean of 20 days before surgery may be effective in gynaecological surgery[23] but not in patients having hip or knee joint replacements.[24,25] In another study[26] warfarin, in a two-stage regimen beginning 10 to 14 days before total hip replacement, was much more effective than external pneumatic compression in preventing proximal vein thrombi, but was less effective in preventing calf vein thrombosis. The dose of warfarin was adjusted to give an INR of 1.5 pre-operatively and 2.5 postoperatively.

Antiplatelet drugs such as aspirin have been considered less effective antithrombotics than anticoagulants in the venous circulation and to be of limited value in preventing venous thromboembolism. An overview[27] of randomised trials of antiplatelet therapy (mainly aspirin) available up to March 1990 and a more recent placebo-controlled trial[28] of aspirin in patients having hip surgery have suggested that antiplatelets reduce the risk of venous thromboembolism and should thus be considered in high-risk patients. However, both reports have been criticised and antiplatelet therapy alone is not routinely recommended since other methods are generally more effective.[9,29]

Of the other drugs tried for surgical thromboembolism prophylaxis, *dihydroergotamine* can reduce venous stasis by vasoconstriction of capacitance vessels and has enhanced postoperative prophylaxis when used in association with low-dose heparin, but there is a risk of peripheral ischaemia[8] and it is no longer widely used. *Dextrans* (dextran 70 or dextran 40) alone, or with dihydroergotamine, have also been used for prophylaxis, but their administration involves the infusion of 500 to 1000 mL of fluid, a procedure which is cumbersome and may interfere with fluid balance. *Antithrombin III* (an endogenous inhibitor of thrombin and the cofactor through which heparin acts) used together with heparin has reduced the risk of venous thromboembolism in patients undergoing total knee arthroplasty.[30] The direct thrombin inhibitor *desirudin* has also been shown to be effective and was reported to be superior to both low-dose subcutaneous heparin[31] and to a low-molecular-weight heparin[32] in patients undergoing hip replacement surgery. Bivalirudin has also been tried. Other drugs that are under investigation include dermatan sulfate, the oral thrombin inhibitor melagatran, and the synthetic pentasaccharide fondaparinux.

The role of prophylaxis of thromboembolism in the nonsurgical setting is less established,[33] but a meta-analysis[34] suggested that low-dose subcutaneous heparin or low-molecular-weight heparin may be of benefit, and their use should be considered in patients at high risk.[9] One study[35] showed that very-low-dose warfarin (average daily dose of 2.6 mg) was safe and effective in patients receiving chemotherapy for metastatic breast cancer, a situation in which the high risk of thromboembolic disease is well recognised. Prophylaxis with low-molecular-weight heparin has been shown to be effective in patients with immobilisation of the leg,[36] and in acutely ill medical patients with risk factors for venous thromboembolism.[37] Standard unfractionated heparin prophylaxis, however, had no effect on mortality in patients admitted to hospital with infection.[38] Although some studies[39,40] have shown an increased risk of venous thromboembolism following prolonged travel, the role of prophylaxis is unclear; compression stockings and low-dose aspirin may be considered, while low-molecular-weight heparin may be required in those at high risk.[41]

Treatment of venous thromboembolism. Treatment of *deep-vein thrombosis*[42,43] aims to prevent the development of pulmonary embolism, to prevent extension of the thrombus, and to reduce the long-term complications of chronic venous insufficiency and venous ulceration. Non-pharmacological therapy may include bed rest with the foot of the bed raised, limb exercise, and graduated compression stockings.[44] These measures may be adequate in patients with small thrombi confined to the calf veins, although this is controversial. Heparin and oral anticoagulants are the mainstay of treatment; they prevent further thrombosis while allowing natural thrombolytic mechanisms to act on the existing clot. Anticoagulants may be used in combination with non-pharmacological methods; graduated compression stockings may reduce the risk of post-phlebitic symptoms in patients receiving anticoagulants.[45] Thrombolytics, or very rarely surgical thrombectomy, may be used for very extensive thrombosis.[46]

Heparin has an immediate effect whereas oral anticoagulants such as warfarin take several days to achieve their full anticoagulant effect. Heparin is therefore used for initial therapy and oral anticoagulants are used for maintenance. Doses of unfractionated heparin and oral anticoagulants must be adjusted according to laboratory monitoring. In the initial treatment of deep-vein thrombosis, current UK recommendations[8] are for an intravenous loading dose of heparin 5000 units followed by 1000 to 2000 units per hour by continuous intravenous infusion or 15 000 units by subcutaneous injection every 12 hours. A meta-analysis suggested that heparin twice

daily by subcutaneous injection is more effective and at least as safe as continuous intravenous heparin in the initial treatment of deep-vein thrombosis.[47] In the USA,[46] a similar 5000 unit loading dose has been suggested, followed by 1400 units per hour intravenously or 17 500 units every 12 hours subcutaneously. However, low-molecular-weight heparins have a number of advantages and are now generally preferred.[48] A number of meta-analyses[49-53] have shown them to be at least as effective and safe as unfractionated heparin in the treatment of deep-vein thrombosis and pulmonary embolism. Two studies[54,55] have also shown low-molecular-weight heparins to be safe and effective for the outpatient treatment of deep-vein thrombosis and it is likely that their use will increase.

Treatment with an oral anticoagulant (usually warfarin) may be started at the same time as heparin, or 3 to 4 days before it is discontinued. A standard loading dose is usually given, and dosage is then adjusted to maintain the INR within recommended limits.[46,48,56] Heparin should be continued until the INR has been in the therapeutic range for at least 2 days;[46,48,57] a period of about 5 days is usually adequate[58] if warfarin has been started on day 1. The optimum duration of oral anticoagulation has been debated and probably depends upon the presence of risk factors. Prevention of disease recurrence must be balanced against minimising the risk of haemorrhagic complications. A multicentre study in the UK[59] indicated that, for postoperative deep-vein thrombosis or pulmonary embolism, anticoagulation for 4 weeks may be adequate; patients with idiopathic venous thromboembolism, however, may require anticoagulants for 3 months. Another multicentre study in Sweden[60] found that although six months of treatment with warfarin after a first episode of venous thromboembolism led to a lower cumulative recurrence rate than 6 weeks of treatment, this difference only occurred during active treatment and the rates remained nearly parallel thereafter. Although recommendations for duration of treatment have been made in the UK[56] and US,[46,48] there is considerable variation. For a first episode of venous thromboembolism in patients with reversible risk factors for venous thromboembolism such as surgery, trauma, or temporary immobilisation suggestions range from 6 weeks to 3 to 6 months. For patients with idiopathic venous thromboembolism periods of 3 to 6 months or longer are recommended. Longer, possibly lifelong treatment may be considered in patients with repeated thromboembolic episodes or with a continuing risk factor.

Ancrod, argatroban, or the recombinant hirudin, lepirudin, may be used as an alternative to heparin in patients who have developed heparin-induced thrombocytopenia or thrombosis. A heparinoid such as danaparoid or a low-molecular-weight heparin may also be suitable, although there may be cross-reactivity. In patients who have other contra-indications to anticoagulation or in whom thrombosis recurs despite anticoagulation, insertion of a vena caval filter may be appropriate.[46] The use of filters in conjunction with anticoagulation has also been investigated.[61] Although the incidence of pulmonary embolism was reduced during the first 12 days, no effect on mortality was shown at 2 years.

Therapy with thrombolytics such as streptokinase is controversial[62] but is generally reserved for very extensive thrombosis. Patients with more recent thrombi, incomplete occlusion, and proximal rather than distal thrombus location respond best.[63] Thrombolysis has not been shown to improve mortality in patients with deep-vein thrombosis and the main indication is to reduce the incidence of post-phlebitic syndrome. Since thrombolytic activity fades when infusion stops, heparin followed by oral anticoagulation is given to prevent re-occlusion.

Minor *pulmonary embolism* is treated with heparin and oral anticoagulants as described for deep-vein thrombosis (above). For more severe pulmonary embolism the initial bolus dose of heparin may be doubled[8] and heparin may be continued for 7 to 10 days.[46] Acute massive pulmonary embolism with major haemodynamic disturbance may be treated initially with thrombolytic therapy;[2,3] surgical methods such as embolectomy or percutaneous catheter fragmentation may be preferred in some patients.[64,65] Streptokinase, urokinase, and alteplase have all been shown to accelerate the lysis of pulmonary emboli and to decrease pulmonary vascular obstruction but no effect on mortality has yet been demonstrated, although some studies suggest improved survival in patients with massive pulmonary embolism.[3] Comparisons between thrombolytics have been difficult because the

doses used in different studies have not always been comparable. Probably more important than the choice of thrombolytic is ensuring that treatment starts quickly.[66]

Venous thromboembolism in children. Venous thromboembolism is relatively rare in children and has differing epidemiology to that in adults.[67] Although guidelines[68] for its management have been published they generally rely on extrapolation from studies in adults.

Venous thromboembolism in pregnancy. Pregnancy is a known risk factor for venous thromboembolism and, although the absolute risk is low, pulmonary embolism is the commonest cause of maternal death during pregnancy in the UK. Anticoagulation during pregnancy may be necessary either to prevent or treat venous thromboembolism; continued anticoagulation may also be needed in pregnant patients at risk of systemic embolism because of valvular heart disease or prosthetic heart valves (see above).

Oral anticoagulants such as warfarin cross the placenta and may harm the fetus; they are generally contra-indicated during pregnancy. Heparin does not appear to cross the placenta and despite potential maternal complications such as osteoporosis and thrombocytopenia remains the anticoagulant of choice in pregnancy. Low-molecular-weight heparins appear to be as safe as unfractionated heparin during pregnancy[69] and may now be preferred.[70]

The management of venous thromboembolism in pregnancy has been reviewed[71,72] and guidelines have been published in the UK[73] and the US.[70] **Prophylactic anticoagulation** is not necessary in all pregnancies, but should be considered in women at special risk of venous thromboembolism either because of a history of thromboembolism and/or a thrombophilic abnormality such as inherited deficiency of antithrombin, protein C, or protein S or acquired thrombophilia due to antiphospholipid antibodies in plasma. Patients must be managed individually and current strategies differ. In those women with a history of thromboembolism but without thrombophilic abnormalities some authors recommend prophylactic anticoagulation at delivery and for 6 weeks post partum provided there has been only one episode of thromboembolism and there are no additional risk factors; others advocate prophylaxis with subcutaneous heparin throughout pregnancy. However, a prospective study[74] has suggested that it is safe to withhold anticoagulation until after delivery in such patients, and this approach has been recommended.[70] Although standard low-dose heparin has been recommended, higher doses may be necessary during pregnancy.[70-73] Low-molecular-weight heparins may also be used.[70,72] Those with inherited or acquired thrombophilic abnormalities but no evidence of thrombosis do not necessarily require anticoagulation, but must be assessed carefully.

If acute venous thromboembolism occurs during pregnancy it should be **treated** with low-molecular-weight heparin or intravenous heparin as in non-pregnant patients (see above). Antenatal patients need to continue anticoagulation for the rest of their pregnancy, usually by substituting adjusted-dose subcutaneous heparin every 12 hours after 6 to 10 days of intravenous therapy; low-molecular-weight heparins may be an alternative.[46,72] If the patient has already had her baby, treatment can be continued with oral warfarin. Special care must be taken at delivery. Patients receiving full therapeutic doses of heparin should have their dose reduced or discontinued on the day of delivery; this may not be necessary in those on lower prophylactic doses of heparin. Low-molecular-weight heparins should be stopped 24 hours before planned delivery.[70] If possible patients receiving warfarin should be changed to heparin 2 or 3 weeks before labour or delivery and not later than 36 weeks' gestation. Anticoagulants should be continued after delivery, but can usually be stopped after 6 weeks; the total duration of treatment should be at least 3 months.[46]

During pregnancy, especially the third trimester, laboratory monitoring of anticoagulation may be less reliable because high procoagulant concentrations particularly of factor VIII and fibrinogen, may result in low activated partial thromboplastin time (APTT) values despite adequate heparin concentrations in plasma.

1. Kearon C, *et al.* Noninvasive diagnosis of deep venous thrombosis. *Ann Intern Med* 1998; **128:** 663–77.
2. British Thoracic Society, Standards of Care Committee. Suspected acute pulmonary embolism: a practical approach. *Thorax* 1997; **52** (suppl 4): S1–S24.
3. European Society of Cardiology Task Force on Pulmonary Embolism. Guidelines on diagnosis and management of acute pulmonary embolism. *Eur Heart J* 2000; **21:** 1301–36.

4. Anderson FA, *et al.* Physician practices in the prevention of venous thromboembolism. *Ann Intern Med* 1991; **115**: 591–5.
5. Thromboembolic Risk Factors (THRIFT) Consensus Group. Risk of and prophylaxis for venous thromboembolism in hospital patients. *BMJ* 1992; **305**: 567–74.
6. The Venous Thromboembolism Study Group of the Spanish Society of Clinical Pharmacology. Multicentre hospital drug utilization study on the prophylaxis of venous thromboembolism. *Br J Clin Pharmacol* 1994; **37**: 255–9.
7. Bratzler DW, *et al.* Underuse of venous thromboembolism prophylaxis for general surgery patients: physician practices in the community hospital setting. *Arch Intern Med* 1998; **158**: 1902–12.
8. Colvin BT, Barrowcliffe TW. The British Society for Haematology guidelines on the use and monitoring of heparin 1992: second revision. *J Clin Pathol* 1993; **46**: 97–103.
9. Geerts WH, *et al.* Prevention of venous thromboembolism. *Chest* 2001; **119** (suppl): 132S–175S.
10. Verstraete M. Prophylaxis of venous thromboembolism. *BMJ* 1997; **314**: 123–5.
11. Collins R, *et al.* Reduction in fatal pulmonary embolism and venous thrombosis by perioperative administration of subcutaneous heparin: overview of results of randomized trials in general, orthopedic, and urologic surgery. *N Engl J Med* 1988; **318**: 1162–73.
12. Nurmohamed MT, *et al.* Low-molecular-weight heparin versus standard heparin in general and orthopaedic surgery: a meta-analysis. *Lancet* 1992; **340**: 152–6.
13. Leizorovicz A, *et al.* Low molecular weight heparin in prevention of perioperative thrombosis. *BMJ* 1992; **305**: 913–20.
14. Anderson DR, *et al.* Efficacy and cost of low-molecular-weight heparin compared with standard heparin for the prevention of deep vein thrombosis after total hip arthroplasty. *Ann Intern Med* 1993; **119**: 1105–12.
15. Koch A, *et al.* Low molecular weight heparin and unfractionated heparin in thrombosis prophylaxis after major surgical intervention: update of previous meta-analyses. *Br J Surg* 1997; **84**: 750–9.
16. Kakkar VV, *et al.* Low molecular weight versus standard heparin for prevention of venous thromboembolism after major abdominal surgery. *Lancet* 1993; **341**: 259–65.
17. Simonneau G, Leizorovicz A. Prophylactic treatment of postoperative thrombosis: a meta-analysis of the results from trials assessing various methods used in patients undergoing major orthopaedic (hip and knee) surgery. *Clin Trials Meta-Analysis* 1993; **28**: 177–91.
18. Imperiale TF, Speroff T. A meta-analysis of methods to prevent venous thromboembolism following total hip replacement. *JAMA* 1994; **271**: 1780–5. Correction. *ibid.* 1995; **273**: 288.
19. Geerts WH, *et al.* A comparison of low-dose heparin with low-molecular-weight heparin as prophylaxis against venous thromboembolism after major trauma. *N Engl J Med* 1996; **335**: 701–7.
20. Eikelboom JW, *et al.* Extended-duration prophylaxis against venous thromboembolism after total hip or knee replacement: a meta-analysis of the randomised trials. *Lancet* 2001; **358**: 9–15.
21. Anderson DR, *et al.* Enoxaparin as prophylaxis against venous thromboembolism after total hip replacement. *N Engl J Med* 1997; **336**: 585.
22. Hull R, *et al.* A comparison of subcutaneous low-molecular-weight heparin with warfarin sodium for prophylaxis against deep-vein thrombosis after hip or knee implantation. *N Engl J Med* 1993; **329**: 1370–6.
23. Poller L, *et al.* Fixed minidose warfarin: a new approach to prophylaxis against venous thrombosis after major surgery. *BMJ* 1987; **295**: 1309–12.
24. Fordyce MJF, *et al.* Efficacy of fixed minidose warfarin prophylaxis in total hip replacement. *BMJ* 1991; **303**: 219–20.
25. Dale C, *et al.* Prevention of venous thrombosis with minidose warfarin after joint replacement. *BMJ* 1991; **303**: 224.
26. Francis CW, *et al.* Comparison of warfarin and external pneumatic compression in prevention of venous thrombosis after total hip replacement. *JAMA* 1992; **267**: 2911–15.
27. Antiplatelet Trialists' Collaboration. Collaborative overview of randomised trials of antiplatelet therapy—III: reduction in venous thrombosis and pulmonary embolism by antiplatelet prophylaxis among surgical and medical patients. *BMJ* 1994; **308**: 235–46.
28. Pulmonary Embolism Prevention (PEP) Trial Collaborative Group. Prevention of pulmonary embolism and deep vein thrombosis with low dose aspirin: Pulmonary Embolism Prevention (PEP) trial. *Lancet* 2000; **355**: 1295–1302.
29. Thomas DP. Thromboprophylaxis after replacement arthroplasty. *BMJ* 2001; **322**: 686–7.
30. Francis CW, *et al.* Prevention of venous thrombosis after total knee arthroplasty: comparison of antithrombin III and low-dose heparin with dextran. *J Bone Joint Surg (Am)* 1990; **72-A**: 976–82.
31. Eriksson BI, *et al.* Prevention of deep-vein thrombosis after total hip replacement: direct thrombin inhibition with recombinant hirudin, CGP 39393. *Lancet* 1996; **347**: 635–9.
32. Eriksson BI, *et al.* A comparison of recombinant hirudin with a low-molecular-weight heparin to prevent thromboembolic complications after total hip replacement. *N Engl J Med* 1997; **337**: 1329–35.
33. Lederle FA. Heparin prophylaxis for medical patients? *Ann Intern Med* 1998; **128**: 768–70.
34. Mismetti P, *et al.* Prevention of venous thromboembolism in internal medicine with unfractionated or low-molecular-weight heparins: a meta-analysis of randomised clinical trials. *Thromb Haemost* 2000; **83**: 14–19.
35. Levine M, *et al.* Double-blind randomised trial of very-low-dose warfarin for prevention of thromboembolism in stage IV breast cancer. *Lancet* 1994; **343**: 886–9.
36. Kock H-J, *et al.* Thromboprophylaxis with low-molecular-weight heparin in outpatients with plaster-cast immobilisation of the leg. *Lancet* 1995; **346**: 459–61.
37. Samama MM, *et al.* A comparison of enoxaparin with placebo for the prevention of venous thromboembolism in acutely ill medical patients. *N Engl J Med* 1999; **341**: 793–800.
38. Gårdlund B. Randomised, controlled trial of low-dose heparin for prevention of fatal pulmonary embolism in patients with infectious diseases. *Lancet* 1996; **347**: 1357–61.
39. Ferrari E, *et al.* Travel as a risk factor for venous thromboembolic disease: a case-control study. *Chest* 1999; **115**: 440–4.
40. Scurr JH, *et al.* Frequency and prevention of symptomless deep-vein thrombosis in long-haul flights: a randomised trial. *Lancet* 2001; **357**: 1485–9.
41. House of Lords Select Committee on Science and Technology. Fifth report on air travel and health. Available at: http://www.publications.parliament.uk (accessed 22/08/01).
42. Shetty HG. Management of deep-vein thrombosis. *Prescribers' J* 1997; **37**: 166–72.
43. Lensing AWA, *et al.* Deep-vein thrombosis. *Lancet* 1999; **353**: 479–85.
44. McCollum C. Avoiding the consequences of deep vein thrombosis. *BMJ* 1998; **317**: 696.
45. Brandjes DPM, *et al.* Randomised trial of effect of compression stockings in patients with symptomatic proximal-vein thrombosis. *Lancet* 1997; **349**: 759–62.
46. Hirsh J, Hoak J. Management of deep vein thrombosis and pulmonary embolism: a statement for healthcare professionals. *Circulation* 1996; **93**: 2212–45.
47. Hommes DW, *et al.* Subcutaneous heparin compared with continuous intravenous heparin administration in the initial treatment of deep vein thrombosis. *Ann Intern Med* 1992; **116**: 279–84.
48. Hyers TM, *et al.* Antithrombotic therapy for venous thromboembolic disease. *Chest* 2001; **119** (suppl): 176S–193S.
49. Siragusa S, *et al.* Low-molecular-weight heparins and unfractionated heparin in the treatment of patients with acute venous thromboembolism: results of a meta-analysis. *Am J Med* 1996; **100**: 269–77.
50. Leizorovicz A. Comparison of the efficacy and safety of low molecular weight heparins and unfractionated heparin in the initial treatment of deep venous thrombosis: an updated meta-analysis. *Drugs* 1996; **52** (suppl 7): 30–7.
51. Gould MK, *et al.* Low-molecular-weight heparins compared with unfractionated heparin for treatment of acute deep venous thrombosis: a meta-analysis of randomized, controlled trials. *Ann Intern Med* 1999; **130**: 800–9.
52. van den Belt AGM, *et al.* Fixed dose subcutaneous low molecular weight heparins versus adjusted dose unfractionated heparin for venous thromboembolism (updated 28 February 2001). Available in The Cochrane Library; Issue 4. Oxford: Update Software; 2001.
53. Dolovich LR, *et al.* A meta-analysis comparing low-molecular-weight heparins with unfractionated heparin in the treatment of venous thromboembolism: examining some unanswered questions regarding location of treatment, product type, and dosing frequency. *Arch Intern Med* 2000; **160**: 181–8.
54. Levine M, *et al.* A comparison of low-molecular-weight heparin administered primarily at home with unfractionated heparin administered in the hospital for proximal deep-vein thrombosis. *N Engl J Med* 1996; **334**: 677–81.
55. Koopman MMW, *et al.* Treatment of venous thrombosis with intravenous unfractionated heparin administered in the hospital as compared with subcutaneous low-molecular-weight heparin administered at home. *N Engl J Med* 1996; **334**: 682–7. Correction. *ibid.* 1997; **337**: 1251.
56. British Society for Haematology: British Committee for Standards in Haematology—Haemostasis and Thrombosis Task Force. Guidelines on oral anticoagulation: third edition. *Br J Haematol* 1998; **101**: 374–87.
57. Ginsberg JS. Management of venous thromboembolism. *N Engl J Med* 1996; **335**: 1816–28.
58. Hull RD, *et al.* Heparin for 5 days as compared with 10 days in the initial treatment of proximal venous thrombosis. *N Engl J Med* 1990; **322**: 1260–4.
59. Research Committee of the British Thoracic Society. Optimum duration of anticoagulation for deep-vein thrombosis and pulmonary embolism. *Lancet* 1992; **340**: 873–6.
60. Schulman S, *et al.* A comparison of six weeks with six months of oral anticoagulant therapy after a first episode of venous thromboembolism. *N Engl J Med* 1995; **332**: 1661–5.
61. Decousus H, *et al.* A clinical trial of vena caval filters in the prevention of pulmonary embolism in patients with proximal deep-vein thrombosis. *N Engl J Med* 1998; **338**: 409–15.
62. Hawkins DW, Hirsh J. Antithrombotic drugs for thromboembolic disorders: a lesson in evidence-based medicine. *Am J Health-Syst Pharm* 1997; **54**: 1992–4.
63. Rogers LQ, Lutcher CL. Streptokinase therapy for deep vein thrombosis: a comprehensive review of the English literature. *Am J Med* 1990; **88**: 389–95.
64. Gulba DC, *et al.* Medical compared with surgical treatment for massive pulmonary embolism. *Lancet* 1994; **343**: 576–7.
65. Goldhaber SZ. Pulmonary embolism. *N Engl J Med* 1998; **339**: 93–104.
66. Anonymous. Thrombolysis for pulmonary embolism. *Lancet* 1992; **340**: 21–2.
67. David M, Andrew M. Venous thromboembolic complications in children. *J Pediatr* 1993; **123**: 337–46.
68. Monagle P, *et al.* Antithrombotic therapy in children. *Chest* 2001; **119** (suppl): 344S–370S.
69. Sanson B-J, *et al.* Safety of low-molecular-weight heparin in pregnancy: a systematic review. *Thromb Haemost* 1999; **81**: 668–72.
70. Ginsberg JS, *et al.* Use of antithrombotic agents during pregnancy. *Chest* 2001; **119** (suppl): 122S–131S.
71. Toglia MR, Weg JG. Venous thromboembolism during pregnancy. *N Engl J Med* 1996; **335**: 108–14.
72. Greer IA. Thrombosis in pregnancy: maternal and fetal issues. *Lancet* 1999; **353**: 1258–65.
73. Maternal and Neonatal Haemostasis Working Party of the Haemostasis and Thrombosis Task. Guidelines on the prevention, investigation and management of thrombosis associated with pregnancy. *J Clin Pathol* 1993; **46**: 489–96.
74. Brill-Edwards P, *et al.* Safety of withholding heparin in pregnant women with a history of venous thromboembolism. *N Engl J Med* 2000; **343**: 1439–44.

Abciximab (14557-q)

Abciximab (BAN, USAN, rINN).

c7E3. Immunoglobulin G (human-mouse monoclonal c7E3 clone p7E3V$_H$hC$_γ$4 Fab fragment anti-human platelet glycoprotein IIb/IIIa complex), disulphide with human-mouse monoclonal c7E3 clone p7E3V$_κ$hC$_κ$ light chain.
$C_{2101}H_{3229}N_{551}O_{673}S_{15}$ = 47455.4.
CAS — 143653-53-6.
ATC — B01AC13.

Adverse Effects and Precautions

Bleeding during the first 36 hours after administration is the most common adverse effect of abciximab and therefore it should not be given to patients who are actively bleeding or to patients at increased risk of haemorrhage, including those with haemorrhagic disorders, cerebrovascular disorders, uncontrolled hypertension, or who have recently undergone major surgery. Abciximab should be discontinued if serious uncontrolled bleeding occurs or emergency surgery is required. Abciximab should not be given to patients with severe renal or hepatic impairment. Thrombocytopenia may occur and platelet counts should be monitored before and following administration of abciximab. Antibodies may develop 2 to 4 weeks after administration and hypersensitivity reactions could occur on administration of other monoclonal antibodies or following re-treatment with abciximab; thus re-administration is not generally recommended (see below). Hypersensitivity reactions have not been noted after a single administration but the possibility should be considered. Other side-effects include hypotension, nausea and vomiting, back pain, chest pain, headache, haematoma, bradycardia, fever, and vascular disorders.

Effects on the blood. Thrombocytopenia is a well documented adverse effect of abciximab therapy. In a review[1] of the major clinical trials of abciximab, mild thrombocytopenia was reported in 4.2% of patients and severe thrombocytopenia in 1.0%; patients also received treatment with heparin. There have also been a number of case reports of patients developing severe thrombocytopenia.[2] It is recommended that platelet counts should be monitored before and 2 hours after initiation of abciximab, and that the drug should be withdrawn if thrombocytopenia occurs.[2] However, pseudothrombocytopenia also occurs in some patients and should be excluded before withdrawing therapy.[3] The incidence of thrombocytopenia does not appear to be increased with other glycoprotein IIb/IIIa receptor inhibitors[1] and there have been reports of the successful use of eptifibatide[4] and tirofiban[5] in patients who developed thrombocytopenia with abciximab.

1. Dasgupta H, *et al.* Thrombocytopenia complicating treatment with intravenous glycoprotein IIb/IIIa receptor inhibitors: a pooled analysis. *Am Heart J* 2000; **140**: 206–11.
2. Bishara AI, Hagmeyer KO. Acute profound thrombocytopenia following abciximab therapy. *Ann Pharmacother* 2000; **34**: 924–30.
3. Sane DC, *et al.* Occurrence and clinical significance of pseudothrombocytopenia during abciximab therapy. *J Am Coll Cardiol* 2000; **36**: 75–83.
4. Rao J, Mascarenhas DAN. Successful use of eptifibatide as an adjunct to coronary stenting in a patient with abciximab-associated acute profound thrombocytopenia. *J Invasive Cardiol* 2001; **13**: 471–3.
5. Desai AI, Lucore CL. Uneventful use of tirofiban as an adjunct to coronary stenting in a patient with a history of abciximab-associated thrombocytopenia 10 months earlier. *J Invasive Cardiol* 2000; **12**: 109–12.

Readministration. Antibodies to abciximab develop in approximately 5.8% of patients following treatment and could lead to hypersensitivity reactions or to reduced efficacy if abciximab is readministered. In a retrospective study[1] in 164 patients who had received a second course of therapy with abciximab, efficacy was not affected and no allergic or anaphylactic reactions occurred. However, severe thrombocytopenia was noted in 4% of patients, and the incidence was highest in those receiving abciximab within 2 weeks of the first administration.

1. Madan M, *et al.* Efficacy of abciximab readministration in coronary intervention. *Am J Cardiol* 2000; **85**: 435–40.

Pharmacokinetics

Following intravenous administration of abciximab free plasma concentrations fall rapidly due to binding to platelet receptors. Platelet function recovers over about 48 hours although abciximab may remain in the circulation for 15 days or more in a platelet-bound state.

Uses and Administration

Abciximab is the Fab fragment of the chimaeric monoclonal antibody 7E3. It binds to the glycoprotein IIb/IIIa receptor on the surface of platelets. This prevents binding of fibrinogen, von Willebrand factor, and other adhesive molecules to the receptor sites and inhibits platelet aggregation. It is used as an adjunct to heparin and aspirin therapy for the prevention of acute ischaemic complications in patients undergoing percutaneous transluminal coronary procedures including angioplasty, atherectomy, and stenting. It is also used in patients with unstable angina who are candidates for such procedures.

Abciximab is given intravenously as a bolus injection over one minute in a dose of 250 µg per kg body-weight followed immediately by an infusion of 0.125 µg per kg per minute (to a maximum dose of 10 µg per minute). For stabilisation in patients with unstable angina the bolus dose followed by the infusion should be started up to 24 hours before the possible intervention and continued for 12 hours after; for other patients the bolus should be given 10 to 60 minutes before the intervention followed by the infusion for 12 hours.

◊ General references.
1. Foster RH, Wiseman LR. Abciximab: an updated review of its use in ischaemic heart disease. *Drugs* 1998; **56:** 629–65.
2. Kleiman NS. A risk-benefit assessment of abciximab in angioplasty. *Drug Safety* 1999; **20:** 43–57.

Reperfusion and revascularisation procedures. Percutaneous transluminal coronary angioplasty is a non-pharmacological procedure employed in the management of atherosclerotic arterial disease to aid revascularisation and reperfusion (p.812). Heparin is usually given during the procedure to prevent perioperative thrombosis and aspirin is given as an antiplatelet drug to reduce long-term stenosis. Abciximab has a role as an adjunct to heparin and aspirin in various groups of patients undergoing angioplasty. In the EPIC study,[1] which included only patients at high risk for abrupt vessel closure, acute ischaemic events and complications of angioplasty were reduced but there was also a significant increase in bleeding complications. In those given abciximab as a bolus injection immediately before angioplasty followed by intravenous infusion for 12 hours there was also a reduction in restenosis at 6 months[2] and at 3 years.[3] Similar results were obtained in the EPILOG study,[4] which used a lower dose of heparin and included unselected patients. However, in the CAPTURE study,[5] in which abciximab was given for 18 to 24 hours before angioplasty and for 1 hour after, the initial benefit was not maintained at 6 months. Although other glycoprotein IIb/IIIa inhibitors have a role in patients with unstable angina who are not receiving angioplasty, a large study[6] with abciximab in such patients failed to show any benefit over placebo.

Abciximab has also been used as an adjunct to angioplasty procedures involving coronary stenting. In the EPISTENT study, the combination of abciximab and stenting reduced the rates of death and myocardial infarction compared with either treatment alone; this benefit was maintained at 30 days,[7] 6 months,[8] and at 1 year[9] follow-up.

Abciximab is also being investigated as an adjunct to angioplasty[10] in patients with acute myocardial infarction, and as an adjunct to thrombolysis[11] in patients with acute myocardial infarction who are not undergoing angioplasty. In patients with acute myocardial infarction treated with primary angioplasty and coronary stenting, abciximab improved outcomes both immediately following the procedure and at 6 months.[12]

1. The EPIC Investigators. Use of a monoclonal antibody directed against the platelet glycoprotein IIb/IIIa receptor in high-risk coronary angioplasty. *N Engl J Med* 1994; **330:** 956–61.
2. Topol EJ, *et al.* Randomised trial of coronary intervention with antibody against platelet IIb/IIIa integrin for reduction of clinical restenosis: results at six months. *Lancet* 1994; **343:** 881–6.
3. Topol EJ, *et al.* Long-term protection from myocardial ischemic events in a randomized trial of brief integrin β₃ blockade with percutaneous coronary intervention. *JAMA* 1997; **278:** 479–84.
4. The EPILOG Investigators. Platelet glycoprotein IIb/IIIa receptor blockade and low-dose heparin during percutaneous coronary revascularization. *N Engl J Med* 1997; **336:** 1689–96.
5. The CAPTURE Investigators. Randomised placebo-controlled trial of abciximab before and during coronary intervention in refractory unstable angina: the CAPTURE study. *Lancet* 1997; **349:** 1429–35. Correction. *ibid.*; **350:** 744.
6. The GUSTO IV-ACS Investigators. Effect of glycoprotein IIb/IIIa receptor blocker abciximab on outcome in patients with acute coronary syndromes without early coronary revascularisation: the GUSTO IV-ACS randomised trial. *Lancet* 2001; **357:** 1915–24.
7. The EPISTENT Investigators. Randomised placebo-controlled and balloon-angioplasty-controlled trial to assess safety of coronary stenting with use of platelet glycoprotein-IIb/IIIa blockade. *Lancet* 1998; **352:** 87–92.
8. Lincoff AM, *et al.* Complementary clinical benefits of coronary-artery stenting and blockade of platelet glycoprotein-IIb/IIIa receptors. *N Engl J Med* 1999; **341:** 319–27.
9. Topol EJ, *et al.* Outcomes at 1 year and economic implications of platelet glycoprotein IIb/IIIa blockade in patients undergoing coronary stenting: results from a multicentre randomised trial. *Lancet* 1999; **354:** 2019–24. Correction. *ibid.* 2000; **355:** 1104.
10. Brener SJ, *et al.* Randomized, placebo-controlled trial of platelet glycoprotein IIb/IIIa blockade with primary angioplasty for acute myocardial infarction. *Circulation* 1998; **98:** 734–41.
11. Antman EM, *et al.* Abciximab facilitates the rate and extent of thrombolysis: results of the Thrombolysis in Myocardial Infarction (TIMI) 14 trial. *Circulation* 1999; **99:** 2720–32.
12. Montalescot G, *et al.* Platelet glycoprotein IIb/IIIa inhibition with coronary stenting for acute myocardial infarction. *N Engl J Med* 2001; **344:** 1895–1903.

Preparations

Proprietary Preparations (details are given in Part 3)
Aust.: ReoPro; **Austral.:** ReoPro; **Belg.:** ReoPro; **Canad.:** ReoPro; **Denm.:** ReoPro; **Fin.:** ReoPro; **Fr.:** ReoPro; **Ger.:** ReoPro; **Hong Kong:** ReoPro; **Irl.:** ReoPro; **Israel:** ReoPro; **Ital.:** ReoPro; **Neth.:** ReoPro; **Norw.:** ReoPro; **NZ:** ReoPro; **S.Afr.:** ReoPro; **Singapore:** ReoPro; **Spain:** ReoPro; **Swed.:** ReoPro; **Switz.:** ReoPro; **Thai.:** ReoPro; **UK:** ReoPro; **USA:** ReoPro.

Acadesine (14674-l)

Acadesine *(BAN, USAN, rINN)*.
GP-1-110; GP-1-110-0. 5-Amino-1-(β-D-ribofuranosyl)imidazole-4-carboxamide.
$C_9H_{14}N_4O_5 = 258.2$.
CAS — 2627-69-2.
ATC — C01EB13.

Profile
Acadesine is a purine nucleoside analogue reported to have cardioprotective effects. It is being investigated in the management of myocardial ischaemia particularly in patients undergoing coronary artery bypass graft surgery. Acadesine may protect against further ischaemia by influencing metabolism in ischaemic cells to enhance release of adenosine in preference to inosine following breakdown of adenosine monophosphate.

◊ References.
1. Europe/Canada Perioperative Ischemia Research Group. Multinational study of the effect of acadesine on major cardiovascular outcomes associated with CABG surgery. *J Am Coll Cardiol* 1993; **21** (suppl): 150A.
2. Leung JM, *et al.* An initial multicenter, randomized controlled trial on the safety and efficacy of acadesine in patients undergoing coronary artery bypass graft surgery. *Anesth Analg* 1994; **78:** 420–34.
3. Alkhulaifi AM, Pugsley WB. Role of acadesine in clinical myocardial protection. *Br Heart J* 1995; **73:** 304–5.
4. Mangano DT. Effects of acadesine on myocardial infarction, stroke, and death following surgery: a meta-analysis of the 5 international randomized trials. *JAMA* 1997; **277:** 325–32.

ACE Inhibitors (17463-h)

Angiotensin-converting Enzyme Inhibitors.

There appear to be few significant differences between ACE inhibitors. They may be distinguished from each other by the presence or absence of a sulfhydryl group, whether they are prodrugs or not, their route of elimination, and their affinity for angiotensin-converting enzyme in vascular and other tissue, although whether these characteristics modify pharmacodynamics and therefore clinical efficacy is uncertain. Differences in these characteristics do however influence onset and duration of action of ACE inhibitors.

Adverse Effects and Treatment
ACE inhibitors all appear to have a similar spectrum of adverse effects although at one time some, such as taste disturbances and skin reactions, were attributed to the presence of a sulfhydryl group as in captopril.

The effects include hypotension, dizziness, fatigue, headache, gastrointestinal disturbances, taste disturbances, persistent dry cough and other upper respiratory tract symptoms, skin rashes (including erythema multiforme and toxic epidermal necrolysis), angioedema, hypersensitivity reactions, renal impairment, hyperkalaemia, hyponatraemia, and blood disorders.

Pronounced hypotension may occur at the start of therapy with ACE inhibitors, particularly in patients with heart failure and in sodium- or volume-depleted patients (for example, those who have received previous diuretic therapy). In patients with ischaemic heart disease or cerebrovascular disease a severe fall in blood pressure could result in myocardial infarction or stroke.

Deterioration in renal function, including increasing blood concentrations of urea and creatinine, and reversible acute renal failure have been reported. This occurs mainly in patients with existing renal or renovascular dysfunction or heart failure and may be aggravated by hypovolaemia. Proteinuria has also occurred and in some patients has progressed to nephrotic syndrome.

Blood disorders that have been reported include neutropenia and agranulocytosis (especially in patients with renal failure and in those with collagen vascular disorders such as systemic lupus erythematosus and scleroderma), thrombocytopenia, and anaemias.

Other adverse effects reported with ACE inhibitors include chest pain, palpitations, tachycardia, stomatitis, abdominal pain, pancreatitis, hepatocellular injury or cholestatic jaundice, alopecia, muscle cramps,

paraesthesias, mood and sleep disturbances, and impotence.

ACE inhibitors may be toxic to the fetus (see Pregnancy under Precautions, below).

Most of the adverse effects of ACE inhibitors are reversible on withdrawing therapy. Symptomatic hypotension, including that following overdosage, generally responds to volume expansion with an intravenous infusion of sodium chloride 0.9%. Specific therapy with angiotensinamide (p.840) may be considered if conventional therapy is ineffective.

◊ General reviews.
1. Parish RC, Miller LJ. Adverse effects of angiotensin converting enzyme (ACE) inhibitors: an update. *Drug Safety* 1992; **7:** 14–31.
2. Alderman CP. Adverse effects of the angiotensin-converting enzyme inhibitors. *Ann Pharmacother* 1996; **30:** 55–61.

Angioedema. See under Hypersensitivity, below.

Cough. Treatment with ACE inhibitors has been associated with the development of cough in up to 20% of hypertensive patients; cough may be less troublesome in those with heart failure,[1] although the incidence may be higher.[2] The cough is reported to be persistent, paroxysmal, and non-productive; it causes irritation of the throat, may be accompanied by voice changes (hoarseness or huskiness), and is often worse when lying down.[1,3,4] It is more common in women and non-smokers, and may be delayed in onset by weeks or even months.

The majority of reports of this adverse effect concern captopril and enalapril,[3,4] but it has also occurred in patients receiving many of the other ACE inhibitors,[5] suggesting that the effect is common to all drugs of this class.

The mechanism that produces the reaction is uncertain but appears to be related to the non-specific blockade of ACE since angiotensin II receptor antagonists are associated with a much lower incidence of cough.[6] The sensitivity of the cough reflex is increased.[7] Prostaglandins released in the respiratory tract have been proposed as mediators,[3] but other mediators such as bradykinin[8] or substance P,[9] both of which are substrates for ACE, have been suggested. However, attempts to demonstrate a link between the effects of ACE inhibitors on cough, and bronchial hyperreactivity of the type found in obstructive airways disease and asthma have produced conflicting evidence, with bronchial hyperreactivity being demonstrated in some studies[10] but not in others.[11]

Where the patient can tolerate the cough, it may be reasonable to continue treatment; in some cases reducing the dose may help. Spontaneous recovery or improvement in the cough has been reported.[12] Changing to an alternative ACE inhibitor is not advised since it is rarely effective.[7] Drugs that inhibit prostaglandin synthesis including the NSAIDs sulindac[13] and indometacin,[14] and the calcium-channel blocker nifedipine[14] have been reported to suppress the cough, but NSAIDs and ACE inhibitors may interact adversely (see under Interactions, below). Inhaled bupivacaine,[15] inhaled sodium cromoglicate,[16,17] oral baclofen,[18] and oral picotamide,[19] have also been reported to be of help. However, in many patients there will be no alternative but to withdraw the ACE inhibitor.[4] Angiotensin II receptor antagonists may be a suitable alternative in patients with hypertension.

1. Anonymous. Cough caused by ACE inhibitors. *Drug Ther Bull.* 1994; **32:** 28 and 55–6.
2. Ravid D, *et al.* Angiotensin-converting enzyme inhibitors and cough: a prospective evaluation in hypertension and congestive heart failure. *J Clin Pharmacol* 1994; **34:** 1116–20.
3. Coulter DM, Edwards IR. Cough associated with captopril and enalapril. *BMJ* 1987; **294:** 1521–3.
4. Berkin KE, Ball SG. Cough and angiotensin converting enzyme inhibition. *BMJ* 1988; **296:** 1279–80.
5. Israili ZH, Hall WD. Cough and angioneurotic edema associated with angiotensin-converting enzyme inhibitor therapy. *Ann Intern Med* 1992; **117:** 234–42.
6. Pylypchuk GB. ACE inhibitor- versus angiotensin II blocker-induced cough and angioedema. *Ann Pharmacother* 1998; **32:** 1060–6.
7. Overlack A. ACE inhibitor-induced cough and bronchospasm. *Drug Safety* 1996; **15:** 72–8.
8. Ferner RE, *et al.* Effects of intradermal bradykinin after inhibition of angiotensin converting enzyme. *BMJ* 1987; **294:** 1119–20.
9. Morice AH, *et al.* Angiotensin-converting enzyme and the cough reflex. *Lancet* 1987; **ii:** 1116–18.
10. Bucknall CE, *et al.* Bronchial hyperreactivity in patients who cough after receiving angiotensin converting enzyme inhibitors. *BMJ* 1988; **296:** 86–8.
11. Boulet L-P, *et al.* Pulmonary function and airway responsiveness during long-term therapy with captopril. *JAMA* 1989; **261:** 413–16.
12. Reisin L, Schneeweiss A. Spontaneous disappearance of cough induced by angiotensin-converting enzyme inhibitors (captopril or enalapril). *Am J Cardiol* 1992; **70:** 398–9.
13. Nicholls MG, Gilchrist NL. Sulindac and cough induced by converting enzyme inhibitors. *Lancet* 1987; **i:** 872.
14. Fogari R, *et al.* Effects of nifedipine and indomethacin on cough induced by angiotensin-converting enzyme inhibitors: a double-blind, randomized, cross-over study. *J Cardiovasc Pharmacol* 1992; **19:** 670–3.
15. Brown RC, Turton CWG. Cough and angiotensin converting enzyme inhibition. *BMJ* 1988; **296:** 1741.
16. Keogh A. Sodium cromoglycate prophylaxis for angiotensin-converting enzyme inhibitor cough. *Lancet* 1993; **341:** 560.

17. Hargreaves MR, Benson MK. Inhaled sodium cromoglycate in angiotensin-converting enzyme inhibitor cough. *Lancet* 1995; **345:** 13–16.
18. Dicpinigaitis PV. Use of baclofen to suppress cough induced by angiotensin-converting enzyme inhibitors. *Ann Pharmacother* 1996; **30:** 1242–5.
19. Malini PL, *et al.* Thromboxane antagonism and cough induced by angiotensin-converting-enzyme inhibitor. *Lancet* 1997; **350:** 15–18.

Effects on the blood. A number of blood disorders have occurred in patients receiving ACE inhibitors, although there have been few reports in the literature. A reduction in haemoglobin concentration and haematocrit may occur but is not usually clinically significant. Cases of neutropenia and agranulocytosis (particularly in patients with renal or collagen vascular disorders), and thrombocytopenia have been noted. Aplastic anaemia has also occurred[1,2] and may be fatal.[2]

1. Kim CR, *et al.* Captopril and aplastic anemia. *Ann Intern Med* 1989; **111:** 187–8.
2. Harrison BD, *et al.* Fatal aplastic anaemia associated with lisinopril. *Lancet* 1995; **346:** 247–8.

Effects on the kidneys. The complex, and sometimes apparently contradictory, effects of ACE inhibitors on the kidney have been reviewed in detail.[1,2] In the normal kidney the effects of ACE inhibition depend on the state of activation of the renin-angiotensin-aldosterone system, and therefore on the state of sodium balance. In normal individuals with unrestricted sodium intake the renin-angiotensin-aldosterone system is suppressed; the increase in renal blood flow observed with captopril administration probably involves mechanisms other than ACE inhibition. Sodium restriction leads to activation of the renin-angiotensin-aldosterone system with a consequent reduction in renal blood flow and glomerular filtration rate due to renal vasoconstriction; this effect is reversed by ACE inhibitors. In patients with essential hypertension ACE inhibition has generally been reported to result in an increase in effective renal blood flow despite the reduction in arterial blood pressure. However, there are only minor changes in glomerular filtration rate, and filtration fraction falls since the pressure within the glomerulus is reduced due to the pronounced renal vasodilatation. The increase in renal blood flow is more pronounced during sodium restriction and in younger patients.

These effects increase or maintain renal blood flow and are generally beneficial. However, in patients with renovascular hypertension they may provoke problems. Severe renal function loss or even anuria have been reported in patients with a single transplanted kidney with renal artery stenosis, or patients with bilateral renal artery disease. The frequency of clinically significant renal function loss during long-term treatment with captopril in patients at risk has been reported to be about 6%. The stenotic kidney maintains its filtering capacity by preferential vasoconstriction of the efferent arterioles, a mechanism mainly mediated by the renin-angiotensin system; under ACE inhibition, vasodilatation of the efferent arterioles combined with the drop in arterial pressure can result in a critical decrease in filtration pressure. Sodium depletion contributes to renal function loss in this setting, and most patients developing renal insufficiency have been using diuretics; sodium repletion can restore renal function despite continuation of ACE inhibition.

Patients with heart failure may also be at risk of a decline in renal function on long-term ACE inhibitor therapy. This is because in chronic heart failure, angiotensin-II mediated systemic and renal vasoconstriction is more important in the maintenance of renal perfusion pressure than in normal or hypertensive persons. The decline may be alleviated by reduction of the dosage of diuretics or liberalisation of dietary salt intake, despite continuation of the ACE inhibitor. An additional risk factor in elderly patients with heart failure is the high incidence of occult renovascular disease in these patients.[3]

In addition to these pathophysiological effects ACE inhibitors may induce membranous glomerulopathy or interstitial nephritis. The former has been associated with captopril use, particularly at high doses, but is rare, and seems less likely to occur at the lower doses favoured today. The proteinuria usually clears without appreciable renal function loss irrespective of whether or not the drug is continued, although persistent proteinuria and renal function loss have been described. Proven interstitial nephritis has also been reported rarely, and may possibly be due to an allergic mechanism.

1. Gans ROB, *et al.* Renal effects of angiotensin-I converting enzyme inhibitors. *Neth J Med* 1988; **32:** 247–64.
2. Navis G, *et al.* ACE inhibitors and the kidney: a risk-benefit assessment. *Drug Safety* 1996; **15:** 200–11.
3. MacDowall P, *et al.* Risk of morbidity from renovascular disease in elderly patients with congestive cardiac failure. *Lancet* 1998; **352:** 13–16.

Effects on the liver. In a report[1] of 3 cases of liver disease apparently caused or aggravated by captopril, it was noted that jaundice due to captopril is usually predominantly cholestatic in nature but acute hepatocellular injury has also been observed. Of 29 cases of liver dysfunction due to captopril and reported to the UK Committee on Safety of Medicines, 9 had hepatocellular jaundice, with 2 deaths; 8 were cholestatic jaundice, with 1 fatality; and 3 patients had hepatorenal syndrome, all of whom died. Worldwide, excluding the UK, 164 cases of hepatic adverse reactions had been notified to the WHO by January 1989. The incidence of such reactions is estimated at 0.09 per 1000 patients but this is likely to be an underestimate. Res-

olution may take a long time and captopril should be withdrawn immediately at the earliest hint of liver sensitivity. Hepatotoxicity has also been reported with enalapril and lisinopril.[2]

1. Bellary SV, *et al.* Captopril and the liver. *Lancet* 1989; **ii:** 514.
2. Hagley MT, *et al.* Hepatotoxicity associated with angiotensin-converting enzyme inhibitors. *Ann Pharmacother* 1993; **27:** 228–31.

Effects on the mouth. Aphthous and tongue ulcers may occur during treatment with ACE inhibitors. There have been a few reports of a 'scalded mouth syndrome', described as similar to being scalded by hot liquids, associated with captopril,[1] enalapril,[1] and lisinopril[2] therapy.

1. Vlasses PH, *et al.* "Scalded mouth" caused by angiotensin-converting enzyme inhibitors. *BMJ* 1982; **284:** 1672–3.
2. Savino LB, Haushalter NM. Lisinopril-induced "scalded mouth syndrome." *Ann Pharmacother* 1992; **26:** 1381–2.

Effects on the nervous system. Encephalopathy and focal neurological signs,[1] and peripheral neuropathy,[2,3] including Guillain-Barré neuropathy,[3] have been reported in patients receiving captopril. Some CNS effects of captopril may be attributable to alterations in cerebral blood flow. In a study in patients with severe heart failure cerebral blood flow in patients aged under 65 was improved by a single dose of captopril 12.5 mg, but in patients aged over 70 there was a 13% reduction.[4] Two patients in whom captopril 6.25 mg produced impaired consciousness and paraesthesias, and dizziness, blurred vision, and aphasia, were found to have stenosis of the carotid arteries.[5] Agitation, panic, extreme depression, and insomnia was reported in a patient 4 weeks after starting treatment with enalapril; depressive episodes recurred on rechallenge.[6] There have been reports of mania possibly precipitated by captopril,[7] and visual hallucinations have been reported in association with captopril and enalapril therapy.[8]

1. Rapoport S, Zyman P. Captopril and central nervous system effects. *Ann Intern Med* 1983; **98:** 1023.
2. Samanta A, Burden AC. Peripheral neuropathy due to captopril. *BMJ* 1985; **291:** 1172.
3. Chakraborty TK, Ruddell WSJ. Guillain-Barré neuropathy during treatment with captopril. *Postgrad Med J* 1987; **63:** 221–2.
4. Britton KE, *et al.* Angiotensin-converting-enzyme inhibitors and treatment of heart failure. *Lancet* 1985; **ii:** 1236.
5. Jensen H, *et al.* Carotid artery stenosis exposed by an adverse effect of captopril. *BMJ* 1986; **293:** 1073–4.
6. Ahmad S. Enalapril-induced acute psychosis. *DICP Ann Pharmacother* 1991; **25:** 558–9.
7. Peet M, Peters S. Drug-induced mania. *Drug Safety* 1995; **12:** 146–53.
8. Haffner CA, *et al.* Hallucinations as an adverse effect of angiotensin converting enzyme inhibition. *Postgrad Med J* 1993; **69:** 240.

Effects on the pancreas. The manufacturers of captopril, enalapril, and lisinopril have all been reported[1] to have data on file on drug-associated pancreatitis. In 1994 the UK Committee on Safety of Medicines[2] noted that there had been 23 reports of pancreatitis associated with ACE inhibitors (captopril 11, enalapril 10, fosinopril 1, and quinapril 1) although whether or not this was causal was not certain.

1. Dabaghi S. ACE inhibitors and pancreatitis. *Ann Intern Med* 1991; **115:** 330–1.
2. Committee on Safety of Medicines/Medicines Control Agency. Drug-induced pancreatitis. *Current Problems* 1994; **20:** 2–3.

Effects on the respiratory system. Cough is a recognised adverse effect of ACE inhibitors but evidence for a link with bronchial hyperreactivity or airways obstruction is controversial (see Cough, above). In reports of adverse respiratory reactions to ACE inhibitors submitted to the Swedish Adverse Drug Reactions Advisory Committee and to WHO, symptoms of airway obstruction such as dyspnoea, asthma, and bronchospasm occurred rarely, usually within the first few weeks of treatment.[1] However, the evidence for a causal link between ACE inhibitors and these symptoms was questioned.[2]

Severe nasal obstruction was associated with enalapril treatment in a 45-year-old woman with a history of mild rhinorrhoea and sneezing. Symptoms cleared within 2 days of stopping enalapril and recurred on rechallenge.[3]

There have been case reports of pneumonitis associated with treatment with captopril[4] and perindopril.[5]

1. Lunde H, *et al.* Dyspnoea, asthma, and bronchospasm in relation to treatment with angiotensin converting enzyme inhibitors. *BMJ* 1994; **308:** 18–21.
2. Inman WHW, *et al.* Angiotensin converting enzyme inhibitors and asthma. *BMJ* 1994; **308:** 593–4.
3. Fennerty A, *et al.* Enalapril-induced nasal blockage. *Lancet* 1986; **ii:** 1395–6.
4. Kidney JC, *et al.* Captopril and lymphocytic alveolitis. *BMJ* 1989; **299:** 981.
5. Benard A, *et al.* Perindopril-associated pneumonitis. *Eur Respir J* 1996; **28:** 1314–16.

Effects on skeletal muscle. Severe muscle pain and weakness, accompanied by morning stiffness, was reported[1] in a patient taking enalapril. Symptoms resolved within a few days of discontinuing the drug.

1. Leloët X, *et al.* Pseudopolymyalgia rheumatica during treatment with enalapril. *BMJ* 1989; **298:** 325.

Effects on the skin. Skin rashes may occur during treatment with ACE inhibitors; they have been reported in 1 to 6% of patients receiving captopril. Angioedema is also an adverse effect of ACE inhibitors (see under Hypersensitivity, below). There have been reports of bullous pemphigoid,[1] hyperhidrosis,[2] Kaposi's sarcoma,[3] lichen planus,[4] onycholysis,[5,6] pemphigus,[7,8] and cutaneous hypersensitivity vasculitis[9] associated

with administration of captopril. Onycholysis has also occurred with enalapril[10] and pemphigus with enalapril[11,12] and ramipril.[13] Lichen planus pemphigoides has been reported with ramipril.[14] A severe cutaneous reaction, resembling early mycosis fungoides, and possibly allergic in nature, has been reported following administration of captopril or enalapril.[15] Captopril has also been reported to exacerbate psoriasis.[16] Vulvovaginal pruritus with dysuria[17] has been noted in a patient receiving enalapril.

1. Mallet L, *et al.* Bullous pemphigoid associated with captopril. *DICP Ann Pharmacother* 1989; **23:** 63.
2. Morse MH. Hyperhidrosis: a possible side effect of captopril treatment. *BMJ* 1984; **289:** 1272.
3. Puppin D, *et al.* Kaposi's sarcoma associated with captopril. *Lancet* 1990; **336:** 1251–2.
4. Cox NH, *et al.* Lichen planus associated with captopril: a further disorder demonstrating the 'tin-tack' sign. *Br J Dermatol* 1989; **120:** 319–21.
5. Brueggemeyer CD, Ramirez G. Onycholysis associated with captopril. *Lancet* 1984; **i:** 1352–3.
6. Borders JV. Captopril and onycholysis. *Ann Intern Med* 1986; **105:** 305–6.
7. Parfrey PS, *et al.* Captopril-induced pemphigus. *BMJ* 1980; **281:** 194.
8. Butt A, Burge SM. Pemphigus vulgaris induced by captopril. *Br J Dermatol* 1995; **132:** 315–16.
9. Miralles R, *et al.* Captopril and vasculitis. *Ann Intern Med* 1988; **109:** 514.
10. Gupta S, *et al.* Nail changes with enalapril. *BMJ* 1986; **293:** 140.
11. Kuechle MK, *et al.* Angiotensin-converting enzyme inhibitor-induced pemphigus: three case reports and literature review. *Mayo Clin Proc* 1994; **69:** 1166–71.
12. Frangogiannis NG, *et al.* Pemphigus of the larynx and esophagus. *Ann Intern Med* 1995; **122:** 803–4.
13. Vignes S, *et al.* Ramipril-induced superficial pemphigus. *Br J Dermatol* 1996; **135:** 657–8.
14. Ogg GS, *et al.* Ramipril-associated lichen planus pemphigoides. *Br J Dermatol* 1997; **136:** 412–14.
15. Furness PN, *et al.* Severe cutaneous reactions to captopril and enalapril; histological study and comparison with early mycosis fungoides. *J Clin Pathol* 1986; **39:** 902–7.
16. Hamlet NW, *et al.* Does captopril exacerbate psoriasis? *BMJ* 1987; **295:** 1352.
17. Heckerling PS. Enalapril and vulvovaginal pruritus. *Ann Intern Med* 1990; **112:** 879–80.

Gynaecomastia. Painful unilateral gynaecomastia was reported in a patient with systemic lupus erythematosus and impaired renal function who was given captopril for hypertension.[1] In view of reports of breast enlargement in women given penicillamine it was suggested that the sulfhydryl structure might be responsible; however, gynaecomastia has also been reported in two patients receiving enalapril,[2,3] which does not contain the sulfhydryl grouping.

1. Markusse HM, Meyboom RHB. Gynaecomastia associated with captopril. *BMJ* 1988; **296:** 1262–3.
2. Nakamura Y, *et al.* Gynaecomastia induced by angiotensin converting enzyme inhibitor. *BMJ* 1990; **300:** 541.
3. Llop R, *et al.* Gynecomastia associated with enalapril and diazepam. *Ann Pharmacother* 1994; **28:** 671–2.

Hypersensitivity. Some of the adverse effects of ACE inhibitors might be mediated by the immune system, but evidence of specific hypersensitivity reactions seems to be limited. The presence of an IgG antibody to captopril was demonstrated in the serum of 2 of 45 patients receiving the drug but the clinical significance was unclear.[1] A reaction resembling serum sickness was reported in a patient given captopril, with deposition of immune complexes in the glomerular basement membrane, and symptoms of rash, arthralgia, epidermolysis, fever, and lymphadenopathy.[2] Eosinophilia has also been reported in a number of patients.[3] The formation of antinuclear antibodies and lupus-like reactions have been described.[4,5]

Treatment with ACE inhibitors (enalapril, captopril, or lisinopril) has been associated with the development of **anaphylactoid reactions** in patients undergoing high-flux haemodialysis using polyacrylonitrile membrane (AN69).[6,7] The UK Committee on Safety of Medicines has advised that the combined use of ACE inhibitors and such membranes should be avoided.[8] Similar anaphylactoid reactions have occurred in patients taking ACE inhibitors while being treated for severe hypercholesterolaemia by extracorporeal removal of low-density lipoproteins (LDL-apheresis) with dextran sulfate columns.[9] These reactions are thought to be bradykinin-mediated. Some have averted them by prolonging the interval between the last dose of ACE inhibitor and dextran sulfate apheresis[10] whereas others found this to be ineffective, but did prevent anaphylactoid reactions in a patient using the bradykinin receptor antagonist icatibant.[11] Hypotensive reactions associated with blood transfusion through bedside leucoreduction filters in patients receiving ACE inhibitors have also been attributed to bradykinin.[12] There have also been rare reports of severe anaphylactoid reactions occurring during desensitisation with Hymenoptera venom (e.g. bee or wasp venom) in patients receiving ACE inhibitors.

Angioedema, a known adverse effect of ACE inhibitors,[13–16] is reported to occur in 0.1 to 0.2% of patients.[15,16] The incidence may be higher in black American[17] or Afro-Caribbean[18] patients. There is no evidence that it results from an immunological mechanism in these patients and it has been suggested that the effect is due to impaired kinin degradation. However, angioedema has been reported with lisinopril in a patient who had previously tolerated captopril.[19] The onset of angioedema has usually been within hours or at most a week of starting treatment with the ACE inhibitor,[15] but can occur after prolonged therapy for several months or years.[20-22] Visceral angioedema presenting as abdominal pain with diarrhoea, nausea, and vomiting, has also been reported.[23,24] If angioedema occurs the ACE inhibitor should be withdrawn and if there is swelling affecting the tongue, glottis, or larynx likely to cause airway obstruction, adrenaline [epinephrine] should be given (see p.831).

1. Coleman JW, et al. Drug-specific antibodies in patients receiving captopril. Br J Clin Pharmacol 1986; 22: 161–5.
2. Hoorntje SJ, et al. Serum-sickness-like syndrome with membranous glomerulopathy in patient on captopril. Lancet 1979; ii: 1297.
3. Kayanakis JG, et al. Eosinophilia during captopril treatment. Lancet 1980; ii: 923.
4. Schwartz D, et al. Enalapril-induced antinuclear antibodies. Lancet 1990; 336: 187.
5. Pelayo N, et al. Drug-induced lupus-like reaction and captopril. Ann Pharmacother 1993; 27: 1541–2.
6. Verresen L, et al. Angiotensin-converting-enzyme inhibitors and anaphylactoid reactions to high-flux membrane dialysis. Lancet 1990; 336: 1360–2.
7. Tielmans C, et al. ACE inhibitors and anaphylactoid reactions to high-flux membrane dialysis. Lancet 1991; 337: 370–1.
8. Committee on Safety of Medicines. Anaphylactoid reactions to high-flux polyacrylonitrile membranes in combination with ACE inhibitors. Current Problems 33 1992.
9. Olbricht CJ, et al. Anaphylactoid reactions, LDL apheresis with dextran sulphate, and ACE inhibitors. Lancet 1992; 340: 908–9.
10. Keller C, et al. LDL-apheresis with dextran sulphate and anaphylactoid reactions to ACE inhibitors. Lancet 1993; 341: 60–1.
11. Davidson DC, et al. Prevention with icatibant of anaphylactoid reactions to ACE inhibitor during LDL apheresis. Lancet 1994; 343: 1575.
12. Quillen K. Hypotensive transfusion reactions in patients taking angiotensin-converting-enzyme inhibitors. N Engl J Med 2000; 343: 1422–3.
13. Wood SM, et al. Angio-oedema and urticaria associated with angiotensin converting enzyme inhibitors. BMJ 1987; 294: 91–2.
14. Hedner T, et al. Angio-oedema in relation to treatment with angiotensin converting enzyme inhibitors. BMJ 1992; 304: 941–6.
15. Israili ZH, Hall WD. Cough and angioneurotic edema associated with angiotensin-converting enzyme inhibitor therapy: a review of the literature and pathophysiology. Ann Intern Med 1992; 117: 234–42.
16. Vleeming W, et al. ACE inhibitor-induced angioedema. Drug Safety 1998; 18: 171–88.
17. Brown NJ, et al. Black Americans have an increased rate of angiotensin converting enzyme inhibitor-associated angioedema. Clin Pharmacol Ther 1996; 60: 8–13.
18. Gibbs CR, et al. Angioedema due to ACE inhibitors: increased risk in patients of African origin. Br J Clin Pharmacol 1999; 48: 861–5.
19. McElligott S, et al. Angioedema after substituting lisinopril for captopril. Ann Intern Med 1992; 116: 426–7.
20. Chin HL, Buchan DA. Severe angioedema after long-term use of an angiotensin-converting enzyme inhibitor. Ann Intern Med 1990; 112: 312–13.
21. Edwards TB. Adverse effects of ACE inhibitors. Ann Intern Med 1993; 118: 314.
22. Chu TJ, Chow N. Adverse effects of ACE inhibitors. Ann Intern Med 1993; 118: 314.
23. Mullins RJ, et al. Visceral angioedema related to treatment with an ACE inhibitor. Med J Aust 1996; 165: 319–21.
24. Byrne TJ, et al. Isolated visceral angioedema: an underdiagnosed complication of ACE inhibitors? Mayo Clin Proc 2000; 75: 1201–4.

Overdosage. There have been reports of overdosage with captopril,[1,2] enalapril,[3-6] and lisinopril.[7,8] The main adverse effect is hypotension which usually responds to supportive treatment and volume expansion. Pressor agents are rarely required. Infusion of angiotensinamide may be considered if hypotension persists.[5,6,8]

1. Augenstein WL, et al. Captopril overdose resulting in hypotension. JAMA 1988; 259: 3302–5.
2. Graham SR, et al. Captopril overdose. Med J Aust 1989; 151: 111.
3. Waeber B, et al. Self poisoning with enalapril. BMJ 1984; 288: 287–8.
4. Lau CP. Attempted suicide with enalapril. N Engl J Med 1986; 315: 197.
5. Jackson T, et al. Enalapril overdose treated with angiotensin infusion. Lancet 1993; 341: 703.
6. Newby DE, et al. Enalapril overdose and the corrective effect of intravenous angiotensin II. Br J Clin Pharmacol 1995; 40: 103–4.
7. Dawson AH, et al. Lisinopril overdose. Lancet 1990; 335: 487–8.
8. Trilli LE, Johnson KA. Lisinopril overdose and management with intravenous angiotensin II. Ann Pharmacother 1994; 28: 1165–8.

Precautions

ACE inhibitors should not be used in patients with aortic stenosis or outflow tract obstruction. They should not generally be used in patients with renovascular disease or suspected renovascular disease, but are occasionally necessary for severe resistant hypertension in such patients when they should only be given with great caution and under close specialist supervision. It should be noted that the elderly or patients with peripheral vascular diseases or generalised atherosclerosis may be at high risk because they may have clinically silent renovascular disease. Renal function should be assessed in all patients prior to administration of ACE inhibitors and should be monitored during therapy. Patients with existing renal disease or taking high doses should be monitored regularly for proteinuria. Regular white blood cell counts may be necessary in patients with collagen vascular disorders, such as systemic lupus erythematosus and scleroderma, or in patients receiving immunosuppressive therapy, especially when they also have impaired renal function. ACE inhibitors should be used with caution in patients with a history of idiopathic or hereditary angioedema.

Patients with heart failure and patients who are likely to be salt or water depleted—for example, those receiving treatment with diuretics or dialysis—may experience symptomatic hypotension during the initial stages of ACE inhibitor therapy. Treatment should therefore be started under close medical supervision, using a low dose and with the patient in a recumbent position to minimise this effect.

Anaphylactoid reactions have occurred in patients taking ACE inhibitors during haemodialysis using high-flux polyacrylonitrile membranes, during LDL-apheresis with dextran sulfate columns, and during desensitisation with Hymenoptera venom.

ACE inhibitors have been reported to produce harmful effects in *animal* fetuses following large maternal doses and should not be used during pregnancy (see below).

Diarrhoea. Several reports have indicated that life-threatening hypotension and signs of renal failure may develop in patients receiving captopril[1-3] or enalapril[3] following volume depletion due to diarrhoea.

1. McMurray J, Matthews DM. Effect of diarrhoea on a patient taking captopril. Lancet 1985; i: 581.
2. Benett PR, Cairns SA. Captopril, diarrhoea, and hypotension. Lancet 1985; i: 1105.
3. McMurray J, Matthews DM. Consequences of fluid loss in patients treated with ACE inhibitors. Postgrad Med J 1987; 63: 385–7.

Hepatic cirrhosis. It has been suggested that in patients with cirrhosis captopril could cause a marked reduction in arterial pressure and severely compromise renal function since maintenance of glomerular filtration rate might be mediated by angiotensin II in these patients.[1] This theory was supported by a report of a reduction in glomerular filtration rate in response to a fall in mean arterial pressure in 4 patients with resistant ascites secondary to hepatic cirrhosis.[2] The fall in mean arterial pressure was associated with postural hypotension and increasing encephalopathy. Severe confusion has also been reported in 2 patients with cirrhosis during treatment with captopril 6.25 to 12.5 mg three times daily.[3]

1. Ring T. Captopril and resistant ascites: a word of caution. Lancet 1983; ii: 165.
2. Wood LJ, et al. Adverse effects of captopril in treatment of resistant ascites, a state of functional bilateral renal artery stenosis. Lancet 1985; ii: 1008–9.
3. Jørgensen F, et al. Captopril and resistant ascites. Lancet 1983; ii: 405.

Huntington's disease. The condition of a woman with Huntington's disease deteriorated dramatically during treatment with captopril and improved on withdrawal of the drug.[1]

1. Goldblatt J, Bryer A. Huntington's disease: deterioration in clinical state during treatment with angiotensin converting enzyme inhibitor. BMJ 1987; 294: 1659–60.

Peripheral vascular disease. Patients with peripheral vascular disease may have a high incidence of renal artery stenosis and are therefore at high risk of renal failure with ACE inhibitor therapy (see Effects on the Kidneys, above). Mild renal artery stenosis was found in 64 of 374 patients (17%) with peripheral vascular disease and severe renal artery stenosis in 52 (14%); the stenosis was bilateral in 43 (12%).[1] Renal function should be carefully monitored in any patient with peripheral vascular disease who receives ACE inhibitors.

1. Salmon P, Brown MA. Renal artery stenosis and peripheral vascular disease: implications for ACE inhibitor therapy. Lancet 1990; 336: 321.

Pregnancy. There is evidence from *animal* studies that administration of ACE inhibitors during pregnancy is associated with fetal toxicity and an increase in still-births.[1] Several case reports have described the development of fetal renal failure, with oligohydramnios or neonatal anuria, in the offspring of mothers receiving captopril[2-4] or enalapril;[5,6] there have been fetal[4] and neonatal[3] deaths. Withdrawal of the ACE inhibitor might result in reversal of the renal dysfunction.[6] A review of the subject has concluded that when ACE inhibitors are stopped in the first trimester the baby is likely to be born at or near term and of normal birth-weight whereas continued treatment carries a risk of early delivery and low birth-weight.[7] There are also 2 case reports in which maternal captopril[8] or enalapril[9] therapy, in association with other drugs, was associated with birth defects including defective ossification of the skull. A literature search up to the end of 1989 indicated that the use of ACE inhibitors during pregnancy can cause severe disturbances of fetal and neonatal renal function, pulmonary hypoplasia, and long-lasting neonatal anuria.[10] Analysis of pregnancy outcome in more than 100 000 women in Tennessee found that 19 had been exposed to an ACE inhibitor during pregnancy.[11] Of the 19 infants, 2 were preterm and had serious life-threatening conditions. One had prolonged anuria requiring dialysis; the mother had probably taken enalapril during the second and third trimesters, but had a renal transplant and was also receiving other drugs. The other had microcephaly and a large occipital encephalocele; the mother had probably taken captopril during the first and second trimesters.

The FDA has re-emphasised that ACE inhibitors can cause injury and even death to the developing fetus in the second and third trimester.[12] A review of the available experimental and clinical data concluded that the use of ACE inhibitors should be avoided in all trimesters of pregnancy.[13]

1. Broughton Pipkin F, et al. Possible risk with captopril in pregnancy: some animal data. Lancet 1980; i: 1256.
2. Boutroy M-J, et al. Captopril administration in pregnancy impairs fetal angiotensin converting enzyme activity and neonatal adaptation. Lancet 1984; ii: 935–6.
3. Guignard JP, et al. Persistent anuria in a neonate: a side effect of captopril? Int J Pediatr Nephrol 1981; 2: 133.
4. Knott PD, et al. Congenital renal dysgenesis possibly due to captopril. Lancet 1989; i: 451.
5. Schubiger G, et al. Enalapril for pregnancy-induced hypertension: acute renal failure in a neonate. Ann Intern Med 1988; 108: 215–16. Correction. ibid.: 777.
6. Broughton Pipkin F, et al. ACE inhibitors in pregnancy. Lancet 1989; ii: 96–7.
7. Anonymous. Are ACE inhibitors safe in pregnancy? Lancet 1989; ii: 482–3.
8. Duminy PC, Burger P du T. Fetal abnormality associated with use of captopril during pregnancy. S Afr Med J 1981; 60: 805.
9. Mehta N, Modi N. ACE inhibitors in pregnancy. Lancet 1989; ii: 96.
10. Hanssens M, et al. Fetal and neonatal effects of treatment with angiotensin-converting enzyme inhibitors in pregnancy. Obstet Gynecol 1991; 78: 128–35.
11. Piper JM, et al. Pregnancy outcome following exposure to angiotensin-converting enzyme inhibitors. Obstet Gynecol 1992; 80: 429–32.
12. Nightingale SL. Warnings on use of ACE inhibitors in second and third trimester of pregnancy. JAMA 1992; 267: 2445.
13. Shotan A, et al. Risk of angiotensin-converting enzyme inhibition during pregnancy: experimental and clinical evidence, potential mechanisms, and recommendations for use. Am J Med 1994; 96: 451–6.

Interactions

Excessive hypotension may occur when ACE inhibitors are used concurrently with diuretics, other antihypertensives, or other agents, including alcohol, that lower blood pressure. An additive hyperkalaemic effect is possible in patients receiving ACE inhibitors with potassium-sparing diuretics, potassium supplements (including potassium-containing salt substitutes), or other drugs that can cause hyperkalaemia (such as ciclosporin or indometacin) and serum-potassium concentrations should be monitored. Potassium-sparing diuretics and potassium supplements should generally be stopped before initiating ACE inhibitors in patients with heart failure. However, ACE inhibitor therapy does not obviate the possible need for potassium supplementation in patients receiving potassium-wasting diuretics and potassium concentrations should also be monitored in these patients. The adverse effects of ACE inhibitors on the kidneys may be potentiated by other drugs, such as NSAIDs, that can affect renal function.

◊ General references.

1. Shionoiri H. Pharmacokinetic drug interactions with ACE inhibitors. Clin Pharmacokinet 1993; 25: 20–58.
2. Mignat C, Unger T. ACE inhibitors: drug interactions of clinical significance. Drug Safety 1995; 12: 334–7.

Allopurinol. For reports of reactions in patients taking captopril and allopurinol, see p.398.

Antacids. Administration of captopril with antacids reduced the bioavailability of captopril although this did not significantly alter the effects on blood pressure and heart rate.[1] The bioavailability of fosinopril, and possibly other ACE inhibitors, may also be reduced by concurrent antacid administration.

1. Mäntylä R, et al. Impairment of captopril bioavailability by concomitant food and antacid intake. Int J Clin Pharmacol Ther Toxicol 1984; 22: 626–9.

Antidiabetics. Hypoglycaemia was noted in 3 type 1 diabetics when captopril was added to their therapeutic regimen; it was also seen in one type 2 diabetic, in whom withdrawal of hypoglycaemic drugs became necessary.[1] Subsequent study suggested that the effect was due to enhanced insulin sensitivity.[1] Similar instances of a reduction in blood sugar in both non-diabetic[2] and diabetic[3] patients given enalapril have occurred. Two case-control studies in diabetic patients receiving insulin or oral hypoglycaemics suggested that patients treated with ACE inhibitors were at increased risk of developing severe hypoglycaemia.[4,5] However, other studies in diabetic patients given captopril or enalapril have failed to find any significant alterations in blood-glucose control,[6,7] and ACE inhibitors are widely used in the treatment of hypertension in diabetic patients (see p.802) and also have a role in the management of diabetic complications such as nephropathy (see Kidney Disorders, below).

1. Ferriere M, *et al.* Captopril and insulin sensitivity. *Ann Intern Med* 1985; **102:** 134–5.
2. Helgeland A, *et al.* Enalapril, atenolol, and hydrochlorothiazide in mild to moderate hypertension: a comparative multicentre study in general practice in Norway. *Lancet* 1986; **i:** 872–5.
3. McMurray J, Fraser DM. Captopril, enalapril, and blood glucose. *Lancet* 1986; **i:** 1035.
4. Herings RMC, *et al.* Hypoglycaemia associated with use of inhibitors of angiotensin converting enzyme. *Lancet* 1995; **345:** 1195–8.
5. Morris AD, *et al.* ACE inhibitor use is associated with hospitalization for severe hypoglycemia in patients with diabetes. *Diabetes Care* 1997; **20:** 1363–7.
6. Passa P, *et al.* Enalapril, captopril, and blood glucose. *Lancet* 1986; **i:** 1447.
7. Winocour P, *et al.* Captopril and blood glucose. *Lancet* 1986; **ii:** 461.

Azathioprine. Leucopenia has been reported in a patient given captopril with azathioprine; the effect did not occur when either drug was given alone.[1] In a similar report, neutropenia in a patient receiving a regimen including azathioprine and captopril did not recur when captopril was reintroduced following withdrawal of azathioprine.[2]

1. Kirchertz EJ, *et al.* Successful low dose captopril rechallenge following drug-induced leucopenia. *Lancet* 1981; **i:** 1363.
2. Edwards CRW, *et al.* Successful reintroduction of captopril following neutropenia. *Lancet* 1981; **i:** 723.

Ciclosporin. An additive hyperkalaemic effect with ACE inhibitors and ciclosporin is possible. Also, acute renal failure has been reported in 2 patients receiving ciclosporin after renal transplantation following administration of enalapril.[1] Renal function recovered when the ACE inhibitor was withdrawn.

1. Murray BM, *et al.* Enalapril-associated acute renal failure in renal transplants: possible role of cyclosporine. *Am J Kidney Dis* 1990; **16:** 66–9.

Digoxin. For reports of an increase in serum-digoxin concentrations during therapy with ACE inhibitors, see p.871.

Diuretics. Excessive hypotension may occur when ACE inhibitors are used concurrently with diuretics. Deterioration in renal function has also been reported (see under Metolazone, p.931).

Epoetins. An additive hyperkalaemic effect may occur when ACE inhibitors are administered with epoetins. ACE inhibitors have also been reported to antagonise the haematopoietic effects of epoetins.

General anaesthetics. Marked hypotension may occur during general anaesthesia in patients receiving ACE inhibitors. In addition corrected cerebral blood flow was significantly lower in 11 patients who received captopril before general anaesthesia induced with thiopental and maintained with nitrous oxide and enflurane, than in 9 patients pretreated with metoprolol and 9 untreated controls.[1] Although there were no complications of anaesthesia associated with captopril pretreatment, discontinuation of ACE inhibitor therapy before anaesthesia should be considered. However, others have suggested[2] that since there is no clear evidence for stopping them, ACE inhibitors may be continued with care.

1. Jensen K, *et al.* Cerebral blood flow during anaesthesia: influence of pretreatment with metoprolol or captopril. *Br J Anaesth* 1989; **62:** 321–3.
2. Anonymous. Drugs in the peri-operative period: 4 – cardiovascular drugs. *Drug Ther Bull* 1999; **37:** 89–92.

Gold salts. The nitritoid reaction (flushing, nausea, dizziness, and hypotension associated with the first weeks of gold treatment) occurred soon after commencing treatment with an ACE inhibitor (captopril, lisinopril, or enalapril) in 4 patients who had been receiving sodium aurothiomalate for at least 2 years.[1]

1. Healey LA, Backes MB. Nitritoid reactions and angiotensin-converting-enzyme inhibitors. *N Engl J Med* 1989; **321:** 763.

Interferons. Severe granulocytopenia has been reported[1] in three patients with mixed cryoglobulinaemia treated with interferon alfa-2a who also received ACE inhibitors. The effect was considered to be due to synergistic haematological toxicity. However, in a further report,[2] two patients developed only mild granulocytopenia that was reversible despite continued therapy, while a third patient retained a normal granulocyte count.

1. Casato M, *et al.* Granulocytopenia after combined therapy with interferon and angiotensin-converting enzyme inhibitors: evidence for a synergistic hematologic toxicity. *Am J Med* 1995; **99:** 386–91.
2. Jacquot C, *et al.* Granulocytopenia after combined therapy with interferon and angiotensin-converting enzyme inhibitors: evidence for a synergistic hematologic toxicity. *Am J Med* 1996; **101:** 235–6.

Interleukin-3. Marked hypotension occurred in three patients[1] receiving ACE inhibitors who were given interleukin-3 following chemotherapy; blood pressure returned to normal when the ACE inhibitors were discontinued.

1. Dercksen MW, *et al.* Hypotension induced by interleukin-3 in patients on angiotensin-converting enzyme inhibitors. *Lancet* 1995; **345:** 448.

Lithium. For reports of lithium toxicity in patients taking ACE inhibitors, see p.294.

NSAIDs. *Indometacin* and possibly other NSAIDs, including aspirin, have been reported to reduce or abolish the hypotensive action of ACE inhibitors. NSAIDs cause sodium and water retention and thus may attenuate the effects of various antihyper-

tensives. It has also been suggested that part of the hypotensive effect of ACE inhibitors is prostaglandin-dependent, which might explain this interaction with drugs such as NSAIDs that block prostaglandin synthesis. However, in a double-blind study designed to assess the role of prostaglandins,[1] indometacin did not influence the hypotensive effect of captopril or enalapril, suggesting that the effects on prostaglandins are not significant.

The possibility of an interaction between low-dose *aspirin* and ACE inhibitors may be of concern, especially in patients with heart failure. Aspirin has been reported[2] to counteract the vasodilator activity of enalapril in patients with severe heart failure although the clinical implications for patients with less severe left ventricular dysfunction are not clear. Indeed, the benefits of both ACE inhibitors and aspirin in patients with heart failure and ischaemic heart disease are well established and thus the clinical relevance of any interaction between them is not yet established.[3-6]

The combination of NSAIDs and ACE inhibitors may also have variable effects on renal function since they act at different parts of the glomerulus.[7] When given to patients whose kidneys are underperfused, for example because of heart failure, liver cirrhosis, or haemorrhage, renal function may deteriorate. However, specific patient groups without reduced renal perfusion may benefit from combining an NSAID with an ACE inhibitor.

Indometacin, and possibly other NSAIDs, may have an additive hyperkalaemic effect.

1. Gerber JG, *et al.* The hypotensive action of captopril and enalapril is not prostacyclin dependent. *Clin Pharmacol Ther* 1993; **54:** 523–32.
2. Hall D, *et al.* Counteraction of the vasodilator effects of enalapril by aspirin in severe heart failure. *J Am Coll Cardiol* 1992; **20:** 1549–55.
3. Cleland JGF, *et al.* Is aspirin safe for patients with heart failure? *Br Heart J* 1995; **74:** 215–19.
4. Song KH, *et al.* Interaction of ACE inhibitors and aspirin in patients with congestive heart failure. *Ann Pharmacother* 1999; **33:** 375–7.
5. Stys T, *et al.* Does aspirin attenuate the beneficial effects of angiotensin-converting enzyme inhibition in heart failure? *Arch Intern Med* 2000; **160:** 1409–13.
6. Mahé I, *et al.* Interaction between aspirin and ACE inhibitors in patients with heart failure. *Drug Safety* 2001; **24:** 167–82.
7. Sturrock NDC, Struthers AD. Non-steroidal anti-inflammatory drugs and angiotensin converting enzyme inhibitors: a commonly prescribed combination with variable effects on renal function. *Br J Clin Pharmacol* 1993; **35:** 343–8.

Probenecid. Administration of probenecid to 4 healthy subjects during intravenous infusion of captopril caused increases in the steady-state plasma-captopril concentration. The interaction was considered to be due to a reduction of tubular secretion of captopril by probenecid.[1]

1. Singhvi SM, *et al.* Renal handling of captopril: effect of probenecid. *Clin Pharmacol Ther* 1982; **32:** 182–9.

Pharmacokinetics

Most ACE inhibitors are given by mouth. Apart from captopril and lisinopril, they are generally prodrugs and following absorption undergo rapid metabolism by ester hydrolysis to the active diacid form; for example, enalapril is converted to enalaprilat. Metabolism occurs mainly in the liver. Excretion as active drug or active metabolite is principally in the urine; some, such as benazeprilat and fosinoprilat are also excreted via the biliary tract. Elimination of the diacid is polyphasic and there is a prolonged terminal elimination phase, which is considered to represent binding to the angiotensin-converting enzyme at a saturable binding site. This bound fraction does not contribute to accumulation of drug following multiple doses. The terminal elimination half-life does not therefore predict the kinetics observed with multiple dosing and the effective half-life for accumulation is the value usually quoted.

◊ Reviews.

1. Burnier M, Biollaz J. Pharmacokinetic optimisation of angiotensin converting enzyme (ACE) inhibitor therapy. *Clin Pharmacokinet* 1992; **22:** 375–84.
2. Hoyer J, *et al.* Clinical pharmacokinetics of angiotensin converting enzyme (ACE) inhibitors in renal failure. *Clin Pharmacokinet* 1993; **24:** 230–54.

Uses and Administration

ACE inhibitors are antihypertensive drugs that act as vasodilators and reduce peripheral resistance. They inhibit angiotensin-converting enzyme (ACE), which is involved in the conversion of angiotensin I to angiotensin II. Angiotensin II stimulates the synthesis and secretion of aldosterone and raises blood pressure via a potent direct vasoconstrictor effect. ACE is identical to bradykininase (kininase II) and ACE inhibitors may reduce the degradation of bradykinin. They may also affect enzymes involved in the generation of

prostaglandins. The pharmacological actions of ACE inhibitors are thought to be primarily due to the inhibition of the renin-angiotensin-aldosterone system, but since they also effectively reduce blood pressure in patients with low renin concentrations other mechanisms are probably also involved. ACE inhibitors produce a reduction in both preload and afterload in patients with heart failure. They also reduce left ventricular remodelling, a process that sometimes follows myocardial infarction. Normally, renal blood flow is increased without a change in glomerular filtration rate. ACE inhibitors also reduce proteinuria associated with glomerular kidney disease.

ACE inhibitors are used in the treatment of hypertension and heart failure and are given to improve survival following myocardial infarction and for the prophylaxis of cardiovascular events in patients with certain risk factors. They are also used in the treatment of diabetic nephropathy. Administration is generally by mouth.

In some hypertensive patients there may be a precipitous fall in blood pressure when starting therapy with an ACE inhibitor and the first dose should preferably be given at bedtime; if possible, any diuretic therapy should be stopped a few days beforehand and resumed later if necessary.

In patients with heart failure taking loop diuretics, severe first-dose hypotension is common on introduction of an ACE inhibitor, but temporary withdrawal of the diuretic may cause rebound pulmonary oedema. Thus treatment should be initiated with a low dose under close medical supervision.

Action. Although the main target for ACE inhibitors was initially thought to be the endocrine renin-angiotensin system in the circulation it is now recognised that this mechanism alone cannot readily explain all the actions of ACE inhibitors.[1] It is now clear that endogenous renin-angiotensin systems exist in many tissues and that ACE inhibitors may have localised effects.[2] It is thought that this may underlie some of the long-term effects of ACE inhibition, including increased arterial wall compliance, improved left ventricular function in heart failure, regression of vascular and left ventricular hypertrophy, and delayed progression of diabetic nephropathy. Although ACE inhibitors differ in their degree of binding to tissue ACE and in their tissue distribution, there is no evidence that this is clinically significant.[1] However, novel compounds with greater tissue specificity may have new therapeutic implications.

It has been suggested[3] that ACE inhibitors may exert their antihypertensive effects, at least in part, by inhibiting calcium-mobilisation in vascular tissue. Whether this represents direct calcium-channel blocking properties or is mediated via tissue renin-angiotensin systems warrants further investigation. ACE inhibitors also have effects on the kinin system and there is some evidence that the cardiovascular actions of ACE inhibitors also involve localised accumulation of kinins.[4-6]

1. Anonymous. ACE inhibitors and tissue binding. *Lancet* 1990; **336:** 718–20.
2. Zarnke KB, Feldman RD. Direct angiotensin converting enzyme inhibitor-mediated venodilation. *Clin Pharmacol Ther* 1996; **59:** 559–68.
3. Jeremy JY, *et al.* ACE inhibitors and tissue binding. *Lancet* 1990; **336:** 1189.
4. Linz W, *et al.* Contribution of kinins to the cardiovascular actions of angiotensin-converting enzyme inhibitors. *Pharmacol Rev* 1995; **47:** 25–49.
5. Bönner G. The role of kinins in the antihypertensive and cardioprotective effects of ACE inhibitors. *Drugs* 1997; **54** (suppl 5): 23–30.
6. Gainer JV, *et al.* Effect of bradykinin-receptor blockade on the response to angiotensin-converting-enzyme inhibitor in normotensive and hypertensive subjects. *N Engl J Med* 1998; **339:** 1285–92.

Bartter's syndrome. Captopril has been reported to produce beneficial responses in patients with Bartter's syndrome[1-5] (p.1183), which is characterised by hyperaldosteronism, hypokalaemia, and hyperreninaemia, but with normal or reduced blood pressure.[1-4]

1. Aurell M, Rudin A. Effects of captopril in Bartter's syndrome. *N Engl J Med* 1981; **304:** 169.
2. Hené RJ, *et al.* Long-term treatment of Bartter's syndrome with captopril. *BMJ* 1982; **285:** 695.
3. James JM, Davies D. The use of captopril in Bartter's syndrome. *BMJ* 1984; **289:** 162.
4. Savastano A, *et al.* Treatment of Bartter's disease with captopril: a case report. *Curr Ther Res* 1986; **39:** 408–13.
5. Jest P, *et al.* Angiotensin-converting enzyme inhibition as a therapeutic principle in Bartter's syndrome. *Eur J Clin Pharmacol* 1991; **41:** 303–5.

Diabetic complications. ACE inhibitors have an established role in the management of nephropathy in patients with type 1 and type 2 diabetes (see Kidney Disorders, below).

It has been reported[1] that ACE inhibitors may reduce the progression of retinopathy in normotensive patients with type 1 diabetes mellitus (p.317). However, progression of retinopathy was a secondary end-point of the study and it was suggested that further studies were needed to confirm the beneficial results.

A preliminary report[2] has also suggested that ACE inhibitors may improve peripheral neuropathy in diabetic patients, but again further studies are needed.

ACE inhibitors have also been reported[3] to reduce the risk of major cardiovascular events in a broad range of diabetics with either a history of cardiovascular disease or at least one additional cardiovascular risk factor.

1. Chaturvedi N, *et al.* Effect of lisinopril on progression of retinopathy in normotensive people with type 1 diabetes. *Lancet* 1998; **351:** 28–31.
2. Malik RA, *et al.* Effect of angiotensin-converting-enzyme (ACE) inhibitor trandolapril on human diabetic neuropathy: randomised double-blind controlled trial. *Lancet* 1998; **352:** 1978–81.
3. Heart Outcomes Prevention Evaluation (HOPE) Study Investigators. Effects of ramipril on cardiovascular and microvascular outcomes in people with diabetes mellitus: results of the HOPE study and MICRO-HOPE substudy. *Lancet* 2000; **355:** 253–9. Correction. *ibid.*; **356:** 860.

Erythrocytosis. Erythrocytosis (polycythaemia) may occur following renal transplantation and is usually treated by phlebotomy, although ACE inhibitors and theophylline (p.784) may be alternatives. Enalapril, in a dose of 10 mg daily by mouth, was reported to be more effective than theophylline in one study.[1] A second study[2] reported effective reductions in haematocrit with a dose of enalapril 2.5 mg daily. Beneficial responses have also been reported with captopril[3] and lisinopril.[4]

1. Ok E, *et al.* Comparison of the effects of enalapril and theophylline on polycythemia after renal transplantation. *Transplantation* 1995; **59:** 1623–45.
2. Beckingham IJ, *et al.* A randomized placebo-controlled study of enalapril in the treatment of erythrocytosis after renal transplantation. *Nephrol Dial Transplant* 1995; **10:** 2316–20.
3. Hernández E, *et al.* Usefulness and safety of treatment with captopril in posttransplant erythrocytosis. *Transplant Proc* 1995; **27:** 2239–41.
4. MacGregor MS, *et al.* Treatment of postrenal transplant erythrocytosis. *Nephron* 1996; **74:** 517–21.

Heart failure. ACE inhibitors given orally produce clinical benefit in all stages of chronic heart failure (p.798) additional to that seen with diuretics. They relieve symptoms and improve survival and reduce the progression of mild or moderate heart failure to more severe stages. Thus, it is now recommended that all patients with heart failure due to left ventricular systolic dysfunction should receive ACE inhibitors, even if they are asymptomatic with diuretics alone. The studies that have shown a benefit with ACE inhibitors have tended to use higher doses than those used in practice. A study[1] with lisinopril found that higher doses reduced the combined endpoint of death or hospitalisation more than low doses and were equally well tolerated, suggesting that higher doses should be used. However, studies with enalapril have failed to show a benefit of standard doses over lower doses,[2] or high doses over standard doses,[3] and the optimum dose in patients with heart failure remains to be established. ACE inhibitors may also have a role in patients with asymptomatic left ventricular dysfunction, although this is less well established; their role in diastolic dysfunction is also not yet clear. ACE inhibitors may be beneficial in patients with heart failure associated with valve disorders.

The mechanism of action in heart failure is not established. A comparison of captopril with glyceryl trinitrate indicated that captopril is both a potent venodilator and an arterial vasodilator, which reduces both preload and afterload (in contrast to glyceryl trinitrate, which predominantly reduces preload), and it was suggested that venodilatation, rather than simply vasodilatation, may be significantly associated with improved survival in patients with heart failure.[4] The haemodynamic and neurohormonal consequences of ACE inhibition play a part[5] and there may be indirect prevention of cardiac arrhythmias.[6,7] ACE inhibitors also appear to reduce left ventricular hypertrophy. It has also been proposed that captopril's free-radical scavenging property may have a role,[8] although another study[9] did not confirm this effect.

Captopril and enalapril have both been used in infants with severe heart failure (see p.854, and p.884, respectively).

1. Packer M, *et al.* Comparative effects of low and high doses of the angiotensin-converting enzyme inhibitor, lisinopril, on morbidity and mortality in chronic heart failure. *Circulation* 1999; **100:** 2312–18.
2. The NETWORK investigators. Clinical outcome with enalapril in symptomatic chronic heart failure; a dose comparison. *Eur Heart J* 1998; **19:** 481–9.
3. Nanas JN, *et al.* Outcome of patients with congestive heart failure treated with standard versus high doses of enalapril: a multi-center study. *J Am Coll Cardiol* 2000; **36:** 2090–5.
4. Capewell S, *et al.* Acute and chronic arterial and venous effects of captopril in congestive cardiac failure. *BMJ* 1989; **299:** 942–5.
5. Deedwania PC. Angiotensin-converting enzyme inhibitors in congestive heart failure. *Arch Intern Med* 1990; **150:** 1798–1805.
6. Wesseling H, *et al.* Cardiac arrhythmias—a new indication for angiotensin-converting enzyme inhibitors? *J Hum Hypertens* 1989; **3** (suppl 1): 89–95.
7. Campbell RWF. ACE inhibitors and arrhythmias. *Heart* 1996; **76** (suppl 3): 79–82.
8. Chopra M, *et al.* Captopril: a free radical scavenger. *Br J Clin Pharmacol* 1989; **27:** 396–9.
9. Lapenna D, *et al.* Captopril has no significant scavenging antioxidant activity in human plasma in vitro or in vivo. *Br J Clin Pharmacol* 1996; **42:** 451–6.

Hypertension. The role of ACE inhibitors in the management of hypertension (p.802) has been reviewed.[1] Although beta blockers and diuretics generally remain first-line therapy in uncomplicated hypertension, since only they have been adequately studied in morbidity/mortality trials, a systematic overview has suggested that ACE inhibitors have comparable effects.[2] One study included in the overview, the Captopril Prevention Project (CAPPP) trial,[3] which compared captopril-based therapy with conventional beta blocker- or diuretic-based therapy, suggested that cardiovascular mortality was lower with captopril, although the risk of stroke was increased in those receiving captopril and overall mortality did not differ between the groups. ACE inhibitors are particularly recommended in diabetic patients with nephropathy as they may have beneficial effects on the kidney, and also in patients with heart failure. Other advantages that have been suggested include their lack of adverse effects on serum lipids, a reduction in left ventricular hypertrophy,[4] and a reduction in plasma fibrinogen levels,[5] but the clinical significance of these effects is not established.

The antihypertensive actions of ACE inhibitors may be potentiated by drugs that activate the renin-angiotensin system. Hence, combination therapy with diuretics or with calcium-channel blockers may be particularly useful.

1. Burris JF. The expanding role of angiotensin converting enzyme inhibitors in the management of hypertension. *J Clin Pharmacol* 1995; **35:** 337–42.
2. Blood Pressure Lowering Treatment Trialists' Collaboration. Effects of ACE inhibitors, calcium antagonists, and other blood-pressure-lowering drugs: results of prospectively designed overviews of randomised trials. *Lancet* 2000; **356:** 1955–64.
3. Hansson L, *et al.* Effect of angiotensin-converting-enzyme inhibition compared with conventional therapy on cardiovascular morbidity and mortality in hypertension: the Captopril Prevention Project (CAPPP) randomised trial. *Lancet* 1999; **353:** 611–16.
4. Schmieder RE, *et al.* Reversal of left ventricular hypertrophy in essential hypertension: a meta-analysis of randomized double-blind studies. *JAMA* 1996; **275:** 1507–13.
5. Fogari R, *et al.* Effects of different antihypertensive drugs on plasma fibrinogen in hypertensive patients. *Br J Clin Pharmacol* 1995; **39:** 471–6.

DIAGNOSIS OF RENOVASCULAR HYPERTENSION. Captopril has been used to diagnose renovascular hypertension: the increase in plasma renin activity following blockade of the conversion of angiotensin I to angiotensin II being greater in renovascular hypertension than in primary hypertension.[1] A review of methods for detecting renovascular hypertension[2] noted that accuracy of the captopril test may be lower in younger patients, black patients, and those with impaired renal function. However, the test may be a useful diagnostic tool for use in selected patients by specialised centres.[2,3] Captopril is also used to enhance the sensitivity and specificity of renal scintigraphy.[2,4]

1. Muller FB, *et al.* The captopril test for identifying renovascular disease in hypertensive patients. *Am J Med* 1986; **80:** 633–44.
2. Mann SJ, Pickering TG. Detection of renovascular hypertension: state of the art 1992. *Ann Intern Med* 1992; **117:** 845–53.
3. McCarthy JE, Weder AB. The captopril test and renovascular hypertension: a cautionary tale. *Arch Intern Med* 1990; **150:** 493–5.
4. Dowling RJ, *et al.* Imaging and stenting for renal artery stenosis. *Hosp Med* 1999; **60:** 329–34.

Ischaemic heart disease. ACE inhibitors have an established role in the treatment of patients after acute myocardial infarction (see below) and may also have a preventative effect; in the SAVE[1] and SOLVD[2] studies, administration of ACE inhibitors to patients with heart failure was noted to lead to a reduction in the incidence of myocardial infarction. ACE inhibitors have therefore been investigated in the management of atherosclerosis (p.793) and ischaemic heart disease but with conflicting results. In the TREND study,[3] administration of quinapril for 6 months was reported to improve endothelial dysfunction in patients with ischaemic heart disease, but apparently no effects on the progression of atherosclerosis or the incidence of cardiac events were found in the QUIET study[4] which used a lower dose of quinapril given for 3 years. However, in the HOPE study[5], treatment with ramipril significantly reduced the rate of death, myocardial infarction, and stroke in patients at high risk for cardiovascular disease, and in the QUO VADIS study,[6] administration of quinapril for 1 year in patients following coronary artery bypass grafting reduced the incidence of clinical ischaemic events although there was no effect on ischaemia during exercise testing or Holter monitoring.

A lack of acute anti-ischaemic effect has been found with short-term administration of captopril and enalapril in patients with stable angina,[7] and with enalapril in Prinzmetal's angina;[8] however, a further study[9] in patients with stable angina reported an improvement in the results of maximal exercise testing following sublingual captopril administration.

1. Pfeffer MA, *et al.* Effect of captopril on mortality and morbidity in patients with left ventricular dysfunction after myocardial infarction: results of the Survival and Ventricular Enlargement Trial. *N Engl J Med* 1992; **327:** 669–77.
2. Yusuf S, *et al.* Effect of enalapril on myocardial infarction and unstable angina in patients with low ejection fractions. *Lancet* 1992; **340:** 1173–8.
3. Mancini GBJ, *et al.* Angiotensin-converting enzyme inhibition with quinapril improves endothelial vasomotor dysfunction in patients with coronary artery disease: the TREND (Trial on Reversing Endothelial Dysfunction) study. *Circulation* 1996; **94:** 258–65.
4. Cashin-Hemphill L, *et al.* Angiotensin-converting enzyme inhibition as antiatherosclerotic therapy: no answer yet. *Am J Cardiol* 1999; **83:** 43–7.

5. The Heart Outcomes Prevention Evaluation Study Investigators. Effects of an angiotensin-converting-enzyme inhibitor, ramipril, on cardiovascular events in high-risk patients. *N Engl J Med* 2000; **342:** 145–53.
6. Oosterga M, *et al.* Effects of quinapril on clinical outcome after coronary artery bypass grafting (The QUO VADIS Study): QUInapril on Vascular Ace and Determinants of Ischemia *Am J Cardiol* 2001; **87:** 542–6.
7. Longobardi G, *et al.* Failure of protective effect of captopril and enalapril on exercise and dipyridamole-induced myocardial ischemia. *Am J Cardiol* 1995; **76:** 255–8.
8. Guazzi M, *et al.* Ineffectiveness of angiotensin converting enzyme inhibition (enalapril) on overt and silent myocardial ischemia in vasospastic angina and comparison with verapamil. *Clin Pharmacol Ther* 1996; **59:** 476–81.
9. Gemici K, *et al.* The effects of sublingual administration of captopril on parameters of exercise test and neurohormonal activation in patients with stable angina pectoris. *Int J Angiol* 1998; **7:** 238–43.

Kidney disorders. Although ACE inhibitors may adversely affect renal function (see under Adverse Effects and Treatment, above), and although pre-existing renal dysfunction is considered a reason for caution in administering these drugs, ACE inhibitors can have beneficial effects in diabetic and nondiabetic renal disease. Hypertension is closely linked with the kidney—the kidney is important in the normal control of blood pressure and may have a role in the pathogenesis of hypertension; it may also be a prime target of damage caused by hypertension.[1] ACE inhibitors tend to improve renal haemodynamics in patients with hypertension and may slow the rate of loss of renal function. However, they may also have an antiproteinuric effect that is independent of their antihypertensive action.[2-5] Proteinuria is an important indicator of glomerular kidney disease (p.1051) of various causes and may range from asymptomatic to severe. Diabetic nephropathy (p.317) is often associated with hypertension and may progress from microalbuminuria to the nephrotic syndrome and end-stage renal failure.

Most experience has been gained in patients with overt diabetic nephropathy, in whom the use of ACE inhibitors now appears to be of established benefit whether they are hypertensive or normotensive or whether they have type 1 or type 2 diabetes mellitus. They may also slow progression of microalbuminuria in early diabetic nephropathy,[4-7] and have been recommended, in conjunction with tight glycaemic control, in all diabetic patients with microalbuminuria.[8] In normotensive type 2 diabetics with normal renal albumin excretion ACE inhibitor therapy has been reported[9] to reduce the progression to albuminuria, but further studies are needed to assess the clinical significance of this effect.

ACE inhibitors may also be of benefit in renal disease unrelated to diabetes, although their role is not yet established. A number of studies[10-15] have reported that ACE inhibitors reduce both proteinuria and the rate of decline of renal function in patients with various non-diabetic renal disorders, and a meta-analysis[16] concluded that ACE inhibitors are more effective than other antihypertensives in reducing the incidence of end-stage renal disease.

Patients with systemic sclerosis (see Scleroderma, p.505) are considered to be at high risk of adverse effects from ACE inhibitors; however there is evidence that these drugs are of benefit in the management of scleroderma-associated hypertension and renal crisis.[17]

1. Raine EG. Hypertension and the kidney. *Br Med Bull* 1994; **50:** 322–41.
2. Kasiske BL, *et al.* Effect of antihypertensive therapy on the kidney in patients with diabetes: a meta-regression analysis. *Ann Intern Med* 1993; **118:** 129–38.
3. Lewis EJ. The effect of angiotensin-converting-enzyme inhibition on diabetic nephropathy. *N Engl J Med* 1993; **329:** 1456–62.
4. Ravid M, *et al.* Long-term stabilizing effect of angiotensin-converting enzyme inhibition on plasma creatinine and on proteinuria in normotensive type II diabetic patients. *Ann Intern Med* 1993; **118:** 577–81.
5. Viberti G, *et al.* Effect of captopril on progression to clinical proteinuria in patients with insulin-dependent diabetes mellitus and microalbuminuria. *JAMA* 1994; **271:** 275–9.
6. Laffel LMB, *et al.* The beneficial effect of angiotensin-converting enzyme inhibition with captopril on diabetic nephropathy in normotensive IDDM patients with microalbuminuria. *Am J Med* 1995; **99:** 497–504.
7. The EUCLID Study Group. Randomised placebo-controlled trial of lisinopril in normotensive patients with insulin-dependent diabetes and normoalbuminuria or microalbuminuria. *Lancet* 1997; **349:** 1787–92.
8. Mogensen CE, *et al.* Prevention of diabetic renal disease with special reference to microalbuminuria. *Lancet* 1995; **346:** 1080–4.
9. Ravid M, *et al.* Use of enalapril to attenuate decline in renal function in normotensive, normoalbuminuric patients with type 2 diabetes mellitus. *Ann Intern Med* 1998; **128:** 982–8.
10. Gansevoort RT, *et al.* Long-term benefits of the antiproteinuric effect of angiotensin-converting enzyme inhibition in nondiabetic renal disease. *Am J Kidney Dis* 1993; **22:** 202–6.
11. Hannedouche T, *et al.* Randomised controlled trial of enalapril and β blockers in non-diabetic chronic renal failure. *BMJ* 1994; **309:** 833–7.
12. Maschio G, *et al.* Effect of the angiotensin-converting-enzyme inhibitor benazepril on the progression of chronic renal insufficiency. *N Engl J Med* 1996; **334:** 939–45.
13. The GISEN Group (Gruppo Italiano di Studi Epidemiologici in Nefrologia). Randomised placebo-controlled trial of effect of ramipril on decline in glomerular filtration rate and risk of terminal renal failure in proteinuric, non-diabetic nephropathy. *Lancet* 1997; **349:** 1857–63.
14. Ruggenenti P, *et al.* Renal function and requirement for dialysis in chronic nephropathy patients on long-term ramipril: REIN follow-up trial. *Lancet* 1998; **352:** 1252–6.

15. Ruggenenti P, *et al.* Renoprotective properties of ACE-inhibition in non-diabetic nephropathies with non-nephrotic proteinuria. *Lancet* 1999; **354:** 359–64.
16. Giatras I, *et al.* Effect of angiotensin-converting enzyme inhibitors on the progression of nondiabetic renal disease: a meta-analysis of randomized trials. *Ann Intern Med* 1997; **127:** 337–45.
17. Steen VD, *et al.* Outcome of renal crisis in systemic sclerosis: relation to availability of angiotensin converting enzyme (ACE) inhibitors. *Ann Intern Med* 1990; **113:** 352–7.

Malignant neoplasms. *Animal* and *in vitro* studies have suggested that ACE inhibitors may protect against the development of cancer, and there has been a case report[1] of regression of Kaposi's sarcoma in a patient treated with captopril. A retrospective cohort study[2] suggested that the incidence of cancer in hypertensive patients receiving ACE inhibitors was lower than expected. However, a subsequent case control study[3] in postmenopausal women found no evidence of a reduced risk of breast cancer associated with ACE inhibitor therapy.

1. Vogt B, Frey FJ. Inhibition of angiogenesis in Kaposi's sarcoma by captopril. *Lancet* 1997; **349:** 1148.
2. Lever AF, *et al.* Do inhibitors of angiotensin-I-converting enzyme protect against risk of cancer? *Lancet* 1998; **352:** 179–84.
3. Meier CR, *et al.* Angiotensin-converting enzyme inhibitors, calcium channel blockers, and breast cancer. *Arch Intern Med* 2000; **160:** 349–53.

Myocardial infarction. ACE inhibitors may be of benefit in both the prevention and treatment of myocardial infarction (p.805). They have an established role in the management of patients following acute myocardial infarction,[1,2] particularly in patients with left ventricular dysfunction. They may also have a role in the primary or secondary prevention of myocardial infarction in certain at-risk or susceptible patient groups.

1. Borghi C, Ambrosioni E. A risk-benefit assessment of ACE inhibitor therapy post-myocardial infarction. *Drug Safety* 1996; **14:** 277–87.
2. Murdoch DR, McMurray JJV. ACE inhibitors in acute myocardial infarction. *Hosp Med* 1998; **59:** 111–15.

Peripheral vascular disease. ACE inhibitors are among many drugs that have been tried in Raynaud's syndrome, a vasospastic peripheral arterial disease (p.809). Variable effects have been reported. In a patient with Raynaud's syndrome captopril improved blood circulation in the fingers both acutely and during long-term therapy with a dose of 37.5 mg daily; the effect was apparently related to its effects on kinins rather than inhibition of angiotensin II formation.[1] However, a double-blind crossover study in 15 patients with Raynaud's phenomenon given captopril 25 mg or placebo three times daily for 6 weeks found that the drug improved blood flow but not the frequency or severity of attacks,[2] and a similar study in patients given enalapril failed to find any subjective or objective benefits.[3] It should also be borne in mind that patients with peripheral vascular disease have a high incidence of renal artery stenosis, and may be at increased risk of renal failure if given ACE inhibitors,[4] although this need not preclude their use in such patients if monitoring of renal function is adequate.[5]

In one patient, peripheral ischaemia induced by ergotamine was rapidly reversed by captopril.[6]

1. Miyazaki S, *et al.* Relief from digital vasospasm by treatment with captopril and its complete inhibition by serine proteinase inhibitors in Raynaud's phenomenon. *BMJ* 1982; **284:** 310–11.
2. Rustin MHA, *et al.* The effect of captopril on cutaneous blood flow in patients with primary Raynaud's phenomenon. *Br J Dermatol* 1987; **117:** 751–8.
3. Challenor VF, *et al.* Subjective and objective assessment of enalapril in primary Raynaud's phenomenon. *Br J Clin Pharmacol* 1991; **31:** 477–80.
4. Salmon P, Brown MA. Renal artery stenosis and peripheral vascular disease: implications for ACE inhibitor therapy. *Lancet* 1990; **336:** 321.
5. Walley T, Roberts D. ACE inhibitors and peripheral vascular disease. *Lancet* 1990; **336:** 810.
6. Zimran A, *et al.* Treatment with captopril for peripheral ischaemia induced by ergotamine. *BMJ* 1984; **288:** 364.

Acebutolol Hydrochloride (6302-q)

Acebutolol Hydrochloride (BANM, rINNM).

Acebutololi Hydrochloridum; IL-17803A; M&B-17803A. (±)-3'-Acetyl-4'-(2-hydroxy-3-isopropylaminopropoxy)butyranilide hydrochloride.
$C_{18}H_{28}N_2O_4$,HCl = 372.9.
CAS — 37517-30-9 (± *acebutolol*); 34381-68-5 (± *acebutolol hydrochloride*).

NOTE. Acebutolol is *USAN*.
Pharmacopoeias. In *Eur.* (see p.vi), *Jpn*, and *US*.

Pharmacopoeial description

Ph. Eur.: A white or almost white crystalline powder. Freely soluble in water and in alcohol; very slightly soluble in acetone and in dichloromethane; practically insoluble in ether. A 1% solution in water has a pH of 5.0 to 7.0. Protect from light.

USP 25: A white or almost white crystalline powder. Soluble in water and in alcohol; very slightly soluble in acetone and in dichloromethane; practically insoluble in ether. pH of a 1% solution in water is between 4.5 and 7.0. Store in airtight containers.

The symbol † denotes a preparation no longer actively marketed

Adverse Effects, Treatment, and Precautions
As for beta blockers, p.844.

Effects on the circulation. A report of near-fatal shock occurring within 40 minutes of acebutolol 400 mg in an elderly patient with chronic bronchitis and angina pectoris.[1]

1. Tirlapur VG, *et al.* Shock syndrome after acebutolol. *Br J Clin Pract* 1986; **40:** 33–4.

Effects on the liver. Six cases of hepatotoxicity associated with acebutolol were reported[1] in the USA to the FDA between 1985 and 1989. The syndrome consisted of markedly elevated transaminase concentrations, moderately elevated alkaline phosphatase concentrations, fever, and other constitutional symptoms. The duration of therapy before onset of symptoms ranged from 10 to 31 days; five patients received a dose of 400 mg per day; the dose was unspecified in the sixth patient. The syndrome resolved when acebutolol was discontinued. Two patients were rechallenged and the syndrome reappeared.

1. Tanner LA, *et al.* Hepatic toxicity after acebutolol therapy. *Ann Intern Med* 1989; **111:** 533–4.

Effects on respiratory function. A report of pleurisy and pulmonary granulomas in a patient receiving acebutolol and a diuretic; acebutolol was considered to be responsible.[1] Hypersensitivity pneumonitis has also been reported in a patient taking acebutolol.[2]

1. Wood GM, *et al.* Pleurisy and pulmonary granulomas after treatment with acebutolol. *BMJ* 1982; **285:** 936.
2. Akoun GM, *et al.* Acebutolol-induced hypersensitivity pneumonitis. *BMJ* 1983; **286:** 266–7.

Hypersensitivity. See under Effects on Respiratory Function, above and under Lupus, below.

Lupus. An increase in antinuclear antibodies has been observed with acebutolol.[1] A report of a lupus syndrome in an elderly patient receiving acebutolol and clonidine described remission of symptoms when acebutolol was withdrawn, but the high antinuclear antibody titre persisted for more than 9 months.[2]

1. Wilson JD. Antinuclear antibodies and cardiovascular drugs. *Drugs* 1980; **19:** 292–305.
2. Hourdebaigt-Larrusse P, *et al.* Une nouvelle observation de lupus induit par acébutolol. *Ann Cardiol Angeiol (Paris)* 1985; **34:** 421–3.

Pregnancy. Both acebutolol and its active metabolite diacetolol cross the placenta. In a study[1] in 29 pregnant women who had received acebutolol for at least one month before delivery, there was evidence of bradycardia in 12 of the 31 offspring and tachypnoea in 6.

1. Boutroy MJ, *et al.* Infants born to hypertensive mothers treated by acebutolol. *Dev Pharmacol Ther* 1982; **4** (suppl 1): 109–15.

Interactions
The interactions associated with beta blockers are discussed on p.846.

Pharmacokinetics
Acebutolol is well absorbed from the gastrointestinal tract, but undergoes extensive first-pass metabolism in the liver. Although the bioavailability of acebutolol is reported to be only about 40%, the major metabolite diacetolol is active. Following oral administration, peak plasma concentrations of acebutolol and diacetolol are reached in approximately 2 and 4 hours, respectively.

Acebutolol and diacetolol are widely distributed in the body, but they have low to moderate lipid solubility and penetration into the CSF is poor. They cross the placenta and higher concentrations are achieved in breast milk than in maternal plasma. Acebutolol is not appreciably bound to plasma proteins; it is about 50% bound to erythrocytes. The plasma elimination half-life for acebutolol and diacetolol is 3 to 4 hours and 8 to 13 hours respectively. Half-life values for acebutolol and diacetolol may be increased in the elderly and the half-life for diacetolol may be prolonged up to 32 hours in patients with severe renal impairment. Acebutolol and diacetolol are excreted in the urine and in the bile and may undergo enterohepatic recycling; acebutolol is also reported to be excreted directly from the intestinal wall. Acebutolol and diacetolol are removed by dialysis.

Uses and Administration
Acebutolol is a cardioselective beta blocker (p.844). It is reported to have some intrinsic sympathomimetic activity and membrane stabilising properties.

Acebutolol is used in the management of hypertension (p.802), angina pectoris (p.791), and cardiac arrhythmias (p.794).

Acebutolol is used as the hydrochloride, but doses are usually expressed in terms of the base. It is generally given by mouth although slow intravenous injection has been employed for the emergency treatment of arrhythmias.

In **hypertension** the usual initial dose is 400 mg once daily by mouth or 200 mg twice daily, increased if necessary after 2 weeks according to the patient's response, to 400 mg twice daily. Doses up to 1.2 g daily in divided doses may be given.

The usual dose for **angina pectoris** is 400 mg once daily by mouth or 200 mg twice daily but up to 300 mg three times daily may be required and total daily doses of 1.2 g have been given.

The usual initial dose for **cardiac arrhythmias** is 200 mg twice daily by mouth but up to 1.2 g daily in divided doses has been required.

Reduced doses may be required in patients with impaired renal function; guidelines are to reduce the dose by 50% when glomerular filtration rate is between 25 and 50 mL per minute and by 75% when glomerular filtration rate is below 25 mL per minute. Elderly patients may also require lower maintenance doses; doses greater than 800 mg daily should be avoided.

Action. Acebutolol is generally considered to be a cardioselective beta blocker but there has been considerable controversy as to the degree of its selectivity and the selectivity of its primary metabolite, diacetolol.[1-3] In a review of beta blockers,[4] acebutolol was stated to be less cardioselective than other drugs such as atenolol or metoprolol. It was proposed[5] that this may be because the metabolite accumulates during chronic dosage to reach concentrations which affect both beta$_1$ and beta$_2$ receptors since cardioselectivity is only a relative phenomenon and is dose-related. This remains uncertain and there is some evidence[6] that at least after single doses, diacetolol is actually more cardioselective than acebutolol itself.

1. Whitsett TL, *et al.* Comparison of the beta$_1$ and beta$_2$ adrenoceptor blocking properties of acebutolol and propranolol. *Chest* 1982; **82:** 668–73.
2. Nair S, *et al.* The effect of acebutolol, a beta adrenergic blocking agent, and placebo on pulmonary functions in asthmatics. *Int J Clin Pharmacol Ther Toxicol* 1981; **19:** 519–26.
3. Leary WP, *et al.* Respiratory effects of acebutolol hydrochloride: a new selective beta-adrenergic blocking agent. *S Afr Med J* 1973; **47:** 1245–8.
4. Feely J, *et al.* Beta-blockers and sympathomimetics. *BMJ* 1983; **286:** 1043–7.
5. Feely J, Maclean D. New drugs: beta blockers and sympathomimetics. *BMJ* 1983; **286:** 1972.
6. Thomas MS, Tattersfield AE. Comparison of beta-adrenoceptor selectivity of acebutolol and its metabolite diacetolol with metoprolol and propranolol in normal man. *Eur J Clin Pharmacol* 1986; **29:** 679–83.

Preparations
BP 2001: Acebutolol Capsules; Acebutolol Tablets;
USP 25: Acebutolol Hydrochloride Capsules.

Proprietary Preparations (details are given in Part 3)
Aust.: Sectral; *Belg.:* Sectral; *Canad.:* Monitan; Rhotral; Sectral; *Denm.:* Abutol†; Diasectral; *Fin.:* Diasectral; Espesil; *Fr.:* Sectral; *Ger.:* Neptal†; Prent; *Hong Kong:* Sectral; *Irl.:* Sectral; *Israel:* Sectral; *Ital.:* Acecor; Prent; Sectral; *Neth.:* Prent†; Sectral; *NZ:* ACB; Sectral; *Port.:* Prent; ACB†; Sectral; *S.Afr.:* Sectral; *Singapore:* ACB; Sectral; *Spain:* Sectral; *Switz.:* Sectral; *UK:* Sectral; *USA:* Sectral.

Multi-ingredient: *Belg.:* Sectrazide; *Ger.:* Sali-Prent; Tredalat; *Hong Kong:* Secadrex; *Irl.:* Secadrex†; *Neth.:* Secadrex; *S.Afr.:* Secadrex; *Spain:* Secadrex; *UK:* Secadrex.

Acecainide Hydrochloride (7776-m)

Acecainide Hydrochloride (USAN, rINNM).

N-Acetylprocainamide Hydrochloride; ASL-601; NAPA. 4'-[(2-Diethylaminoethyl)carbamoyl]acetanilide hydrochloride.
$C_{15}H_{23}N_3O_2$,HCl = 313.8.
CAS — 32795-44-1 (*acecainide*); 34118-92-8 (*acecainide hydrochloride*).

Profile
Acecainide is the acetylated form of procainamide (p.960) but has class III antiarrhythmic activity (p.787). It has been tried for the treatment of premature ventricular contractions and ventricular arrhythmias.

◊ References.
1. Harron DWG, Brogden RN. Acecainide (N-acetylprocainamide): a review of its pharmacodynamic and pharmacokinetic properties, and therapeutic potential in cardiac arrhythmias. *Drugs* 1990; **39:** 720–40.

Acetazolamide (2301-x)

Acetazolamide (BAN, rINN).

Acetazolam; Acetazolamidum. 5-Acetamido-1,3,4-thiadiazole-2-sulphonamide; N-(5-Sulphamoyl-1,3,4-thiadiazol-2-yl)acetamide.

$C_4H_6N_4O_3S_2 = 222.2$.

CAS — 59-66-5.

ATC — S01EC01.

Pharmacopoeias. In Chin., Eur. (see p.vi), Int., Jpn, Pol., and US.

Pharmacopoeial description

Ph. Eur.: A white or almost white, crystalline powder. Very slightly soluble in water; slightly soluble in alcohol; practically insoluble in ether. It dissolves in dilute solutions of alkali hydroxides.

USP 25: A white to faintly yellowish-white, odourless, crystalline powder. Very slightly soluble in water; sparingly soluble in practically boiling water; slightly soluble in alcohol.

Acetazolamide Sodium (2302-r)

Acetazolamide Sodium (BANM, rINNM).

Sodium Acetazolamide.

$C_4H_5N_4NaO_3S_2 = 244.2$.

CAS — 1424-27-7.

Acetazolamide sodium 275 mg is approximately equivalent to 250 mg of acetazolamide. A freshly prepared 10% solution in water has a pH of 9.0 to 10.0.

Stability. Solutions of acetazolamide sodium in glucose 5% and sodium chloride 0.9% were stable for 5 days at 25° with a loss of potency of less than 7.2%.[1] At 5° the loss of potency in both solutions was less than 6% after 44 days of storage. Small reductions in pH were recorded possibly due to the formation of acetic acid during the decomposition of acetazolamide. At −10° the loss in potency after 44 days of storage was less than 3% in both solutions. Results were similar in samples thawed in tap water and in a microwave oven.

An oral suspension of acetazolamide 25 mg per mL prepared from tablets with the aid of sorbitol solution 70% was stable for at least 79 days at 5°, 22°, and 30°. It was recommended that the formulation be maintained at pH 4 to 5 and stored in amber glass bottles.[2]

1. Parasrampuria J, *et al.* Stability of acetazolamide sodium in 5% dextrose or 0.9% sodium chloride injection. *Am J Hosp Pharm* 1987; **44**: 358–60.
2. Alexander KS, *et al.* Stability of acetazolamide in suspension compounded from tablets. *Am J Hosp Pharm* 1991; **48**: 1241–4.

Adverse Effects

Acetazolamide can commonly cause malaise, fatigue, depression, excitement, headache, weight loss, and gastrointestinal disturbances. Drowsiness and paraesthesia involving numbness and tingling of the face and extremities are common particularly with high doses. Diuresis can be troublesome, but generally abates after a few days of continuous therapy. Acidosis may develop during treatment and is generally mild but severe metabolic acidosis has occasionally been reported, especially in elderly or diabetic patients or those with impaired renal function.

Blood dyscrasias occur rarely and may include aplastic anaemia, agranulocytosis, leucopenia, thrombocytopenia, and thrombocytopenic purpura. Acetazolamide therapy can give rise to crystalluria, renal calculi, and renal colic; renal lesions, possibly due to a hypersensitivity reaction, have also been reported. Other adverse reactions include allergic skin reactions, fever, thirst, dizziness, ataxia, alterations in taste, transient myopia, and tinnitus and hearing disturbances. Hypokalaemia may occur but is generally transient and rarely clinically significant.

Intramuscular injections are painful owing to the alkalinity of the solution.

◊ A retrospective review[1] of 222 patients with glaucoma indicated that those aged 40 years or less tolerated treatment with carbonic anhydrase inhibitors much better than older patients.

1. Shrader CE, *et al.* Relationship of patient age and tolerance to carbonic anhydrase inhibitors. *Am J Ophthalmol* 1983; **96**: 730–3.

Effects on the blood. Severe, often fatal, blood dyscrasias have been reported in patients taking acetazolamide,[1-4] including thrombocytopenic purpura,[1] pancytopenia,[2] and aplastic anaemia.[4] By 1989, the National Registry of Drug-Induced Ocular Side Effects in the USA[5] had received reports of haematological reactions possibly due to carbonic anhydrase inhibitors in 139 patients of which 50 (36%) were fatal. The majority of deaths were due to aplastic anaemia. Over half the reactions occurred during the first six months of therapy. There has been considerable debate over the value of periodic blood analysis in patients taking carbonic anhydrase inhibitors for prolonged

periods;[6-11] the US National Registry has recommended[12] that initial and 6-monthly blood analysis should be undertaken.

1. Corbett JT. Acetazolamide and purpura. *BMJ* 1958; **1**: 1122–3.
2. Englund GW. Fatal pancytopenia and acetazolamide therapy. *JAMA* 1969; **210**: 2282.
3. Inman WHW. Study of fatal bone marrow depression with special reference to phenylbutazone and oxyphenbutazone. *BMJ* 1977; **1**: 1500–5.
4. Niven BI, Manoharan A. Acetazolamide-induced anaemia. *Med J Aust* 1985; **142**: 120.
5. Fraunfelder FT, Bagby GC. Possible hematologic reactions associated with carbonic anhydrase inhibitors. *JAMA* 1989; **261**: 2257.
6. Alm A, *et al.* Monitoring acetazolamide treatment. *Acta Ophthalmol (Copenh)* 1982; **60**: 24–34.
7. Johnson T, Kass MA. Hematologic reactions to carbonic anhydrase inhibitors. *Am J Ophthalmol* 1986; **101**: 128–9.
8. Zimran A, Beutler E. Can the risk of acetazolamide-induced aplastic anemia be decreased by periodic monitoring of blood cell counts? *Am J Ophthalmol* 1987; **104**: 654–8.
9. Lichter PR. Carbonic anhydrase inhibitors, blood dyscrasias, and standard-of-care. *Ophthalmology* 1988; **95**: 711–12.
10. Mogk LG, Cyrlin MN. Blood dyscrasias and carbonic anhydrase inhibitors. *Ophthalmology* 1988; **95**: 768–71.
11. Miller RD. Hematologic reactions to carbonic anhydrase inhibitors. *Am J Ophthalmol* 1985; **100**: 745–6.
12. Fraunfelder FT, *et al.* Hematologic reactions to carbonic anhydrase inhibitors. *Am J Ophthalmol* 1985; **100**: 79–81.

Effects on electrolyte balance. Acetazolamide has been reported to cause symptomatic metabolic acidosis in the elderly, in diabetic patients, and in patients with renal impairment.[1-5] Raised plasma-acetazolamide concentrations have been reported in elderly patients, probably attributable to reduced renal function, and in 6 of 9 glaucoma patients this was associated with hyperchloraemic metabolic acidosis.[6] A single-dose study[7] in 4 elderly patients indicated that acetazolamide clearance was reduced and that this correlated with renal function. Urea and electrolyte concentrations should be measured before and during treatment with acetazolamide in the elderly and in other patients such as diabetics who may have renal impairment. The elderly may require reduced doses.

1. Maisey DN, Brown RD. Acetazolamide and symptomatic metabolic acidosis in mild renal failure. *BMJ* 1981; **283**: 1527–8.
2. Goodfield M, *et al.* Acetazolamide and symptomatic metabolic acidosis in mild renal failure. *BMJ* 1982; **284**: 422.
3. Reid W, Harrower ADB. Acetazolamide and symptomatic metabolic acidosis in mild renal failure. *BMJ* 1982; **284**: 1114.
4. Heller I, *et al.* Significant metabolic acidosis induced by acetazolamide: not a rare complication. *Arch Intern Med* 1985; **145**: 1815–17.
5. Parker WA, Atkinson B. Acetazolamide therapy and acid-base disturbance. *Can J Hosp Pharm* 1987; **40**: 31–4.
6. Chapron DJ, *et al.* Acetazolamide blood concentrations are excessive in the elderly: propensity for acidosis and relationship to renal function. *J Clin Pharmacol* 1989; **29**: 348–53.
7. Chapron DJ, *et al.* Influence of advanced age on the disposition of acetazolamide. *Br J Clin Pharmacol* 1985; **19**: 363–71.

Effects on endocrine function. Hirsutism occurred in a 2½-year-old girl after treatment for 16 months with acetazolamide for congenital glaucoma.[1] There was no evidence of virilisation.

1. Weiss IS. Hirsutism after chronic administration of acetazolamide. *Am J Ophthalmol* 1974; **78**: 327–8.

Effects on the kidneys. Large reductions in glomerular filtration rate were observed during treatment with carbonic anhydrase inhibitors in 3 type 1 diabetics with nephropathy and glaucoma.[1] Kidney function improved when the carbonic anhydrase inhibitor was withdrawn.

1. Skøtt P, *et al.* Effect of carbonic anhydrase inhibitors on glomerular filtration rate in diabetic nephropathy. *BMJ* 1987; **294**: 549.

Effects on the liver. For a report of liver damage associated with use of acetazolamide, see Hypersensitivity, below.

Effects on the skin. Rashes, including severe skin reactions such as erythema multiforme, Stevens-Johnson syndrome, and toxic epidermal necrolysis, have been reported during acetazolamide administration; the fact that acetazolamide is a sulfonamide-derivative has been suggested as a cause for these reactions. Photosensitivity has also been noted rarely.

A severe exacerbation of rosacea occurred in a patient following the use of acetazolamide for glaucoma; the rosacea improved on withdrawal of acetazolamide and relapsed again on its reintroduction.[1]

1. Shah P, *et al.* Severe exacerbation of rosacea by oral acetazolamide. *Br J Dermatol* 1993; **129**: 647–8.

Extravasation. A report of extravasation in a patient following the administration of acetazolamide intravenously which resulted in severe ulceration necessitating surgical procedures to repair the skin defect.[1] It was recommended that 1 to 2 mL of sodium citrate 3.8% should be injected subcutaneously near the site of extravasation in order to neutralise the alkaline effects of the acetazolamide injection.

1. Callear J, Kirkby G. Extravasation of acetazolamide. *Br J Ophthalmol* 1994; **78**: 731.

Hypersensitivity. A 54-year-old man with glaucoma who was treated with acetazolamide 500 mg daily for 26 days developed a generalised erythematous rash and became delirious, dehydrated, markedly jaundiced, with peripheral circulatory failure, and died from cholestatic jaundice with hepatic coma and anuria.[1] Drug-induced hypersensitivity and hepatitis due to acetazolamide was suspected.

Anaphylaxis has also been reported[2] following a single oral dose in a patient who had not previously received acetazola-

mide. However, the patient was hypersensitive to sulfonamides and the reaction may have been caused by cross sensitivity.

1. Kristinsson A. Fatal reaction to acetazolamide. *Br J Ophthalmol* 1967; **51**: 348–9.
2. Tzanakis N, *et al.* Anaphylactic shock after a single oral intake of acetazolamide. *Br J Ophthalmol* 1998; **82**: 588.

Precautions

Acetazolamide is contra-indicated in the presence of sodium or potassium depletion, in hyperchloraemic acidosis, in conditions such as Addison's disease and adrenocortical insufficiency, and in marked hepatic or renal impairment. Encephalopathy may be precipitated in patients with hepatic dysfunction. It should not be used in chronic angle-closure glaucoma since it may mask deterioration of the condition. It should be given with care to patients likely to develop acidosis or with diabetes mellitus; severe metabolic acidosis may occur in the elderly and in patients with impaired renal function. Acetazolamide may increase the risk of hyperglycaemia in diabetic patients. Periodic monitoring of plasma electrolytes and blood count is recommended during long-term therapy and patients should be cautioned to report any unusual skin rashes. Acetazolamide is teratogenic in *animals*.

◊ For a brief discussion of metabolic acidosis in patients with diabetes or impaired renal function, see Effects on Electrolyte Balance under Adverse Effects, above.

For a report of renal function impairment in patients with diabetic nephropathy associated with carbonic anhydrase inhibitors, see Effects on the Kidneys under Adverse Effects, above.

The elderly. A single-dose study[1] of acetazolamide in 4 elderly subjects indicated that the elderly have a reduced capacity to clear acetazolamide from plasma correlating with creatinine clearance; that they have reduced plasma protein binding which offsets the reduced unbound clearance; and that these factors predispose the elderly to enhanced accumulation of acetazolamide in erythrocytes.

Plasma-acetazolamide concentrations exceeded the therapeutic range (5.0 to 10.0 μg per mL) in 9 of 12 elderly patients receiving acetazolamide for glaucoma or metabolic alkalosis.[2] Hyperchloraemic metabolic acidosis was detected in 6 of 9 glaucoma patients. The excessive plasma concentrations were attributed to age-related reductions in renal function. It was suggested that elderly patients may require reduced doses of acetazolamide.

For reports of symptomatic metabolic acidosis associated with use of acetazolamide in the elderly, see Effects on Electrolyte Balance under Adverse Effects, above.

1. Chapron DJ, *et al.* Influence of advanced age on the disposition of acetazolamide. *Br J Clin Pharmacol* 1985; **19**: 363–71.
2. Chapron DJ, *et al.* Acetazolamide blood concentrations are excessive in the elderly: propensity for acidosis and relationship to renal function. *J Clin Pharmacol* 1989; **29**: 348–53.

Interference with laboratory estimations. Acetazolamide interfered with an HPLC method of assay for theophylline[1] resulting in an unnecessary dose reduction and worsening apnoea in an infant. Other workers[2] pointed out that the interference depended on the solvent used in the extraction, and presented evidence to suggest that acetazolamide may not interfere with other assay methods for theophylline.

1. Mecrow IK, Goldie BP. Acetazolamide interferes with theophylline assay. *Lancet* 1987; **i**: 558.
2. Kelsey HC, *et al.* Interference by acetazolamide in theophylline assay depends on the method. *Lancet* 1987; **ii**: 403.

Interactions

By rendering the urine alkaline acetazolamide reduces the urinary excretion and so may enhance the effects of drugs such as amfetamines, ephedrine, and quinidine; urinary alkalinisation also reduces the effects of methenamine and its compounds. Acetazolamide may enhance antiepileptic-induced osteomalacia. Concurrent administration of acetazolamide and aspirin may result in severe acidosis and increase CNS toxicity. Acetazolamide may affect fluid and electrolyte balance leading to interactions similar to those of the thiazide diuretics (see Hydrochlorothiazide, p.909). Unlike thiazides, acetazolamide may increase the excretion of lithium.

Antacids. *Sodium bicarbonate* therapy enhances the risk of renal calculus formation in patients taking acetazolamide.[1]

1. Rubenstein MA, Bucy JG. Acetazolamide-induced renal calculi. *J Urol (Baltimore)* 1975; **114**: 610–12.

Antiepileptics. For severe osteomalacia in patients taking acetazolamide with *phenytoin* and other antiepileptics, see p.361. Acetazolamide may increase serum concentrations of *carbamazepine*, see p.345.

Benzodiazepines. Ventilatory depression in a mountain climber with acute mountain sickness was considered to be due to the potentiation of *triazolam* by acetazolamide.[1]

1. Masuyama S, *et al.* 'Ondine's Curse': side effect of acetazolamide? *Am J Med* 1989; **86:** 637.

Local anaesthetics. For the effect of acetazolamide on *procaine*, see p.1319.

Salicylates. Salicylates have been shown to displace acetazolamide from plasma protein binding sites and reduce its renal clearance,[1] leading to elevated plasma-acetazolamide concentrations. In addition acidosis produced by acetazolamide may increase salicylate toxicity by enhancing salicylate tissue penetration.[2] Severe metabolic acidosis has been reported[3] in patients with normal renal function during treatment with acetazolamide and salicylates.

Concurrent use of salicylates and acetazolamide should be avoided if possible, particularly if renal dysfunction is present. If the combination is used, patients should be carefully monitored for symptoms of CNS toxicity such as lethargy, confusion, somnolence, tinnitus, and anorexia.

1. Sweeney KR, *et al.* Toxic interaction between acetazolamide and salicylate: case report and a pharmacokinetic explanation. *Clin Pharmacol Ther* 1986; **40:** 518–24.
2. Anderson CJ, *et al.* Toxicity of combined therapy with carbonic anhydrase inhibitors and aspirin. *Am J Ophthalmol* 1978; **86:** 516–19.
3. Cowan RA, *et al.* Metabolic acidosis induced by carbonic anhydrase inhibitors and salicylates in patients with normal renal function. *BMJ* 1984; **289:** 347–8.

Pharmacokinetics

Acetazolamide is fairly rapidly absorbed from the gastrointestinal tract with peak plasma concentrations occurring about 2 hours after administration by mouth. It has been estimated to have a plasma half-life of about 3 to 6 hours. It is tightly bound to carbonic anhydrase and high concentrations are present in tissues containing this enzyme, particularly red blood cells and the renal cortex; it is highly bound to plasma proteins. It is excreted unchanged in the urine and has been detected in breast milk.

◊ References.

1. Lehmann B, *et al.* The pharmacokinetics of acetazolamide in relation to its use in the treatment of glaucoma and to its effects as an inhibitor of carbonic anhydrases. *Adv Biosci* 1969; **5:** 197–217.
2. Söderman P, *et al.* Acetazolamide excretion into human breast milk. *Br J Clin Pharmacol* 1984; **17:** 599–600.

Uses and Administration

Acetazolamide is an inhibitor of carbonic anhydrase with weak diuretic activity and is used mainly in the management of glaucoma. Other indications include epilepsy and high-altitude disorders.

By inhibiting the reaction catalysed by carbonic anhydrase in the renal tubules, acetazolamide increases the excretion of bicarbonate and of cations, chiefly sodium and potassium, and so promotes an alkaline diuresis. When given by mouth, its effect begins within 60 to 90 minutes and lasts for 8 to 12 hours.

Continuous administration of acetazolamide is associated with metabolic acidosis and an accompanying loss of diuretic activity. Therefore, although acetazolamide has been used as a diuretic, its effectiveness diminishes with continuous use and it has largely been superseded by drugs such as the thiazides or frusemide [furosemide]. For **diuresis** the usual dose is 250 to 375 mg by mouth and is given either daily or on alternate days; intermittent therapy is required for a continued effect.

By inhibiting carbonic anhydrase in the eye acetazolamide decreases the formation of aqueous humour and so decreases intra-ocular pressure. It is used in the pre-operative management of angle-closure **glaucoma**, or as an adjunct in the treatment of open-angle glaucoma. In the treatment of glaucoma the usual dose is 250 to 1000 mg daily by mouth; divided doses should be used for amounts greater than 250 mg daily. Modified-release preparations are also available.

Acetazolamide is also used, either alone or in association with other antiepileptics, for the treatment of various forms of **epilepsy** in doses of 250 to 1000 mg daily by mouth. A dose for children with epilepsy is 8 to 30 mg per kg body-weight daily by mouth; the total daily dose should not exceed 750 mg.

The symbol † denotes a preparation no longer actively marketed

When oral administration is impracticable, similar doses of acetazolamide sodium may be given by intramuscular or preferably by intravenous injection. Acetazolamide is also used to prevent or ameliorate the symptoms of **high-altitude disorders**. Prompt descent will still be necessary if severe symptoms such as cerebral oedema or pulmonary oedema occur. The usual dose is 500 to 1000 mg daily by mouth.

Epilepsy. Acetazolamide may be used in the treatment of epilepsy (p.338) as an alternative to conventional first-line antiepileptics for refractory partial seizures with or without secondary generalisation. It is also effective in a number of other refractory forms of epilepsy including atypical absence, tonic, atonic, myoclonic, and menstruation-related seizures (catamenial epilepsy).[1-4] Beneficial responses have also been reported with acetazolamide in combination with carbamazepine in refractory partial seizures.[5] It is believed to act by inhibition of carbonic anhydrase in glial cells in the CNS.[6] The major drawback to the chronic use of acetazolamide is the rapid development of tolerance,[6,7] but this may be delayed or prevented by using it as adjunctive therapy to other antiepileptics. Acetazolamide has been shown to have greater activity in children than in adults.[1]

1. Millichap JG. Acetazolamide in treatment of epilepsy. *Lancet* 1987; **ii:** 163.
2. Resor SR, Resor LD. Chronic acetazolamide monotherapy in the treatment of juvenile myoclonic epilepsy. *Neurology* 1990; **40:** 1677–81.
3. Shorvon SD. Medical assessment and treatment of chronic epilepsy. *BMJ* 1991; **302:** 363–6.
4. Reiss WG, Oles KS. Acetazolamide in the treatment of seizures. *Ann Pharmacother* 1996; **30:** 514–19.
5. Oles KS, *et al.* Use of acetazolamide as an adjunct to carbamazepine in refractory partial seizures. *Epilepsia* 1989; **30:** 74–8.
6. Rogawski MA, Porter RJ. Antiepileptic drugs: pharmacological mechanisms and clinical efficacy with consideration of promising developmental stage compounds. *Pharmacol Rev* 1990; **42:** 223–86.
7. Hankey GJ, Stewart-Wynne EG. Management of non-convulsive status epilepticus. *Lancet* 1987; **i:** 1427.

Glaucoma. Acetazolamide may be given orally or parenterally in the acute management of angle-closure glaucoma (p.1413) and to minimise rises in intra-ocular pressure associated with ocular surgery.[1,2] It may also be given orally in the long-term management of primary and secondary open-angle glaucoma but is usually used as a second-line drug and added to topical beta-blocker therapy. However, up to 50% of patients are unable to tolerate oral therapy because of adverse effects[3] although topical carbonic anhydrase inhibitors such as dorzolamide may be better tolerated. Attempts have been made to reduce the adverse effects of acetazolamide by modifying the dosage schedule. A single-dose study[4] showed that doses of acetazolamide greater than 63 mg produced no greater reductions in intra-ocular pressure in patients with ocular hypertension. Another study[5] reported that acetazolamide 250-mg tablets twice daily controlled intra-ocular pressure adequately while producing fewer adverse effects than 250 mg four times daily and it was suggested that there was no advantage in using the modified-release capsule formulation (500 mg twice daily). A study in patients with open-angle glaucoma[6] found that most patients were adequately controlled by a single night-time dose of acetazolamide 500 mg either as tablets or modified-release capsules. The night-time dose also reduced the severity of adverse effects compared with the same dose given in the morning, and could aid compliance.

1. Ladas ID, *et al.* Prophylactic use of acetazolamide to prevent intraocular pressure elevation following Nd-YAG laser posterior capsulotomy. *Br J Ophthalmol* 1993; **77:** 136–8.
2. Edmunds B, Canning CR. The effect of prophylactic acetazolamide in patients undergoing extensive retinal detachment repair. *Eye* 1996; **10:** 328–30.
3. Hurvitz LM, *et al.* New developments in the drug treatment of glaucoma. *Drugs* 1991; **41:** 514–32.
4. Friedland BR, *et al.* Short-term dose response characteristics of acetazolamide in man. *Arch Ophthalmol* 1977; **95:** 1809–12.
5. Ledger-Scott M, Hurst J. Comparison of the bioavailability of two acetazolamide formulations. *Pharm J* 1985; **235:** 451.
6. Joyce PW, Mills KB. Comparison of the effect of acetazolamide tablets and sustets on diurnal intraocular pressure in patients with chronic simple glaucoma. *Br J Ophthalmol* 1990; **74:** 413–16.

High-altitude disorders. Acetazolamide is the most frequently used drug for the prophylaxis of high-altitude disorders (p.800). It accelerates the process of acclimatisation, thus reducing the incidence of acute mountain sickness and associated symptoms such as headache, nausea, vomiting, and lethargy. Acetazolamide may have some benefit in relieving symptoms once they have developed although experience is limited. It does not prevent or protect against pulmonary or cerebral oedema.

Macular oedema. For mention of the use of acetazolamide to treat macular oedema associated with uveitis, see Uveitis, p.1060.

Ménière's disease. In Ménière's disease (p.407) high concentrations of carbonic anhydrase are found in the labyrinth, and acetazolamide, a carbonic anhydrase inhibitor, has been tried for both diagnosis and treatment.[1] A dose of 500 mg by intravenous injection has been suggested for diagnosis of fluc-

tuating Ménière's disease.[1] Treatment with the drug by mouth, however, has not been particularly effective and has been associated with a high incidence of side-effects.[2]

1. Brookes GB. Ménière's disease: a practical approach to management. *Drugs* 1983; **25:** 77–89.
2. Brookes GB, Booth JB. Oral acetazolamide in Ménière's disease. *J Laryngol Otol* 1984; **98:** 1087–95.

Neuromuscular disorders. Acetazolamide may be of benefit in a number of neuromuscular disorders, including hypokalaemic periodic paralysis (p.1183). Doses of 375 to 500 mg daily were effective in 2 patients with severe paralysis and were well tolerated.[1] Preliminary observations in 5 other patients given the drug showed a striking improvement in 3. In treating a further 12 patients,[2] doses of 125 mg were given three times daily to children and 250 mg two to six times daily to adults. There was dramatic improvement in 10 of the 12 and this lasted for up to 43 months. Chronic weakness between attacks in 10 patients was improved in 8.

Acetazolamide may reduce the frequency of attacks in patients with hyperkalaemic periodic paralysis (p.1182). It has also been used in episodic ataxia.[3]

1. Resnick JS, *et al.* Acetazolamide prophylaxis in hypokalemic periodic paralysis. *N Engl J Med* 1968; **278:** 582–6.
2. Griggs RC, *et al.* Acetazolamide treatment of hypokalemic periodic paralysis: prevention of attacks and improvement of persistent weakness. *Ann Intern Med* 1970; **73:** 39–48.
3. Melberg A, *et al.* Loss of control after a cup of coffee. *Lancet* 1997; **350:** 1220.

Raised intracranial pressure. Acetazolamide has been used to reduce raised intracranial pressure (p.811). It has a role in the management of benign intracranial hypertension, and has also been tried in the treatment of patients with chronically raised intracranial pressure due to cryptococcal meningitis.[1]

1. Johnston SRD, *et al.* Raised intracranial pressure and visual complications in AIDS patients with cryptococcal meningitis. *J Infect* 1992; **24:** 185–9.

Preparations

BP 2001: Acetazolamide Tablets;
USP 25: Acetazolamide for Injection; Acetazolamide Tablets.

Proprietary Preparations (details are given in Part 3)
Aust.: Diamox; *Austral.:* Diamox; *Belg.:* Diamox; *Braz.:* Diamox; *Canad.:* Diamox; Novo-Zolamide†; *Denm.:* Diamox; Glaupax; *Fin.:* Diamox; Odemin; *Fr.:* Defiltran; Diamox; *Ger.:* Diamox; Diuramid; Glaupax; *Hong Kong:* Diamox; *Irl.:* Diamox; Glaupax; *Israel:* Diamox; Uramox; *Ital.:* Diamox; *Mex.:* Acetadiazol; Akezol; Diamox; *Neth.:* Diamox; Glaupax; *Norw.:* Diamox; Glaupax; *NZ:* Diamox; *Port.:* Carbinib; *S.Afr.:* Azomid; Diamox; *Spain:* Diamox; Edemox; Smed.; *Swed.:* Diamox; Glaupax†; *Switz.:* Diamox; Glaupax; *Thai.:* Diamox; Glaupax; *UK:* Diamox; *USA:* AZM-Tab†; Dazamide; Diamox.

Acetyldigoxin (5803-x)

Desglucolanatoside C. 3β-[(*O*-3-*O*-Acetyl-2,6-dideoxy-β-D-*ribo*-hexopyranosyl-(1→4)-2,6-dideoxy-β-D-*ribo*-hexopyranosyl-(1→4)-2,6-dideoxy-β-D-*ribo*-hexopyranosyl)oxy]-12β,14-dihydroxy-5β,14β-card-20(22)-enolide (α-acetyldigoxin); 3β-[(*O*-4-*O*-Acetyl-2,6-dideoxy-β-D-*ribo*-hexopyranosyl-(1→4)-*O*-2,6-dideoxy-β-D-*ribo*-hexopyranosyl-(1→4)-2,6-dideoxy-β-D-*ribo*-hexopyranosyl)oxy]-12β,14-dihydroxy-5β,14β-card-20(22)-enolide (β-acetyldigoxin).
$C_{43}H_{66}O_{15}$ = 823.0.
CAS — 5511-98-8 (α-acetyldigoxin); 5355-48-6 (β-acetyldigoxin).
ATC — C01AA02.

Pharmacopoeias. Aust. includes a monograph for α-acetyldigoxin.

Profile

Acetyldigoxin is a cardiac glycoside with positive inotropic activity. It has the general properties of digoxin (p.870) and has been used similarly in the management of some cardiac arrhythmias (p.794) and in heart failure (p.798). Both the α- and β-isomers have been used in usual maintenance doses of 200 to 400 µg daily by mouth.

Preparations

Proprietary Preparations (details are given in Part 3)
Aust.: Corotal; Lanatilin; Novodigal; Sandolanid; *Belg.:* Novodigal†; *Ger.:* Digostada; Digotab; Digox; Digoxin "Didier"; Gladixol N; Kardiamed; Novodigal; Stillacor; *Ital.:* Cardioreg.

Multi-ingredient: *Aust.:* Digi-Aldopur; Gladixol.

Acipimox (12316-x)

Acipimox (BAN, rINN).
K-9321. 5-Methylpyrazine-2-carboxylic acid 4-oxide.
$C_6H_6N_2O_3$ = 154.1.
CAS — 51037-30-0.
ATC — C10AD06.

Adverse Effects and Precautions

Acipimox may cause peripheral vasodilatation resulting in flushing, itching, and a sensation of heat. Rash and erythema may occur. Gastrointestinal disturbances including heartburn, epigastric pain, nausea, and diarrhoea have been reported, as well as headache, malaise, and dry eye. Urticaria, angioedema, and bronchospasm may occur rarely.

Acipimox is contra-indicated in patients with peptic ulcer disease. It should not be given to patients with renal impairment if the creatinine clearance is less than 30 mL per minute; extended dose intervals should be employed if the creatinine clearance is 30 to 60 mL per minute.

◊ In a study involving 3009 hyperlipidaemic patients with type 2 diabetes,[1] adverse effects to acipimox occurred in 8.8% resulting in withdrawal in 5.5% of patients. The most frequent adverse effects involved the skin (57.6%), gastrointestinal tract (25.8%), and CNS (9.7%). Labial oedema occurred in 3 cases and an urticarial eruption, collapse, and dyspnoea in another. The incidence of adverse effects was almost twice as high in females as in males, the difference being mainly due to a greater incidence of flushing, pruritus, and skin rashes. The incidence was not affected by age. There was a mean 15.3% reduction in fasting blood-glucose concentrations and an 8.5% reduction in glycosylated haemoglobin during treatment with acipimox.

1. Lavezzari M, et al. Results of a phase IV study carried out with acipimox in type II diabetic patients with concomitant hyperlipoproteinaemia. J Int Med Res 1989; 17: 373–80.

Pharmacokinetics

Acipimox is rapidly and completely absorbed from the gastrointestinal tract and peak plasma concentrations occur within 2 hours. It does not bind to plasma proteins and the plasma half-life is about 2 hours. It is not significantly metabolised and is excreted in the urine, largely unchanged.

Uses and Administration

Acipimox is a lipid regulating drug related to nicotinic acid (p.1372). It is used in the treatment of type IIa, IIb, or IV hyperlipoproteinaemias.

It is given by mouth in usual doses of 500 to 750 mg daily in divided doses, taken with meals. Doses of up to 1200 mg daily have been used.

Hyperlipidaemias. Acipimox is used in the management of hyperlipidaemias (p.800) and produces effects on plasma lipoproteins similar to those of nicotinic acid, although it may not be as potent in its lipid modifying effect. Acipimox was developed to overcome the problems of compliance resulting from nicotinic acid's adverse effects. Its primary action is thought to be the inhibition of lipolysis thus reducing the availability of free fatty acids for the hepatic production of very-low-density lipoprotein (VLDL) and this in turn leads to a decrease in low-density lipoprotein (LDL) production. Increases in high-density lipoprotein (HDL) may also occur. The overall effect is a reduction in VLDL-triglyceride and total triglyceride concentrations and an increase in HDL-cholesterol concentrations, but only a modest reduction in LDL-cholesterol or total-cholesterol concentrations.[1-6]

Acipimox has been shown to be effective in the treatment of hyperlipidaemias in diabetic patients, and has generally produced a reduction in blood-glucose concentrations.[5,6] A patient with type A insulin-resistance syndrome, who had diabetes and severe hypertriglyceridaemia with very high fasting insulin and non-esterified fatty acids, responded to treatment with acipimox 500 mg twice daily in a modified-release form.[7]

1. Sommariva D, et al. Changes in lipoprotein cholesterol and triglycerides induced by acipimox in type IV and type II hyperlipoproteinemic patients. Curr Ther Res 1985; 37: 363–8.
2. Ball MJ, et al. Acipimox in the treatment of patients with hyperlipidaemia: a double blind trial. Eur J Clin Pharmacol 1986; 31: 201–4.
3. Taskinen M-R, Nikkilä EA. Effects of acipimox on serum lipids, lipoproteins and lipolytic enzymes in hypertriglyceridemia. Atherosclerosis 1988; 69: 249–55.
4. Crepaldi G, et al. Plasma lipid lowering activity of acipimox in patients with type II and type IV hyperlipoproteinaemia. Atherosclerosis 1988; 70: 115–21.
5. Dulbecco A, et al. Effect of acipimox on plasma glucose levels in patients with non-insulin-dependent diabetes mellitus. Curr Ther Res 1989; 46: 478–83.
6. Lavezzari M, et al. Results of a phase IV study carried out with acipimox in type II diabetic patients with concomitant hyperlipoproteinaemia. J Int Med Res 1989; 17: 373–80.
7. Kumar S, et al. Suppression of non-esterified fatty acids to treat type A insulin resistance syndrome. Lancet 1994; 343: 1073–4.

Preparations

Proprietary Preparations (details are given in Part 3)

Aust.: Olbetam; **Belg.:** Olbetam; **Braz.:** Olbetam; **Denm.:** Olbetam; **Ger.:** Olbemox; **Hong Kong:** Olbetam; **Irl.:** Olbetam; **Israel:** Olbetam; **Ital.:** Olbetam; **Mex.:** Olbetam; **Neth.:** Nedios; **NZ:** Olbetam; **S.Afr.:** Olbetam; **Singapore:** Olbetam; **Switz.:** Olbetam; **Thai.:** Olbetam; **UK:** Olbetam.

Adenosine (18724-z)

Adenosine (BAN, USAN).

Adenosinum; SR-96225. 6-Amino-9-β-D-ribofuranosyl-9H-purine.

$C_{10}H_{13}N_5O_4 = 267.2$.

CAS — 58-61-7.

ATC — C01EB10.

Pharmacopoeias. In Eur. (see p.vi) and US.

Pharmacopoeial description

Ph. Eur.: A white crystalline powder. Slightly soluble in water; soluble in hot water; practically insoluble in alcohol and in dichloromethane; dissolves in dilute mineral acids.

USP 25: A white, odourless crystalline powder. Soluble in water; practically insoluble in alcohol. Protect from light.

Stability. Adenosine was found to be stable[1] when it was mixed with glucose 5%, lactated Ringer's, sodium chloride 0.9%, or a mixture of glucose 5% and lactated Ringer's and stored in polypropylene syringes or PVC bags.

1. Ketkar VA, et al. Stability of undiluted and diluted adenosine at three temperatures in syringes and bags. Am J Health-Syst Pharm 1998; 55: 466–70.

Adverse Effects and Precautions

Adverse effects of adenosine are usually transient, lasting less than a minute, due to its very short plasma half-life. They include nausea, lightheadedness, flushing, headache, angina-like chest pain, and dyspnoea. Bronchospasm has been reported. Like other antiarrhythmics, adenosine may worsen arrhythmias. Bradycardia and heart block have been reported. The larger doses given by intravenous infusion may rarely produce hypotension and tachycardia.

Adenosine is contra-indicated in patients with second- or third-degree atrioventricular block or in those with sick sinus syndrome. It is also contra-indicated in asthmatic subjects and should be used with caution in patients with obstructive pulmonary disease. Intravenous infusion of adenosine should be used with caution in patients who may develop hypotensive complications such as those with autonomic dysfunction, pericarditis, or stenotic valvular heart disease. Patients with recent heart transplantation may have increased sensitivity to the cardiac effects of adenosine.

◊ Use of Belzer solution [University of Wisconsin (UW) solution] for the hypothermic storage of kidneys prior to transplantation has been associated with bradycardia, prolonged PR intervals, and heart block.[1,2] The solution contains hetastarch, allopurinol, glutathione, and adenosine, and adenosine was considered to be the arrhythmogenic factor. Some centres had used the solution to flush kidneys before implantation,[2] a use for which it was never intended.[3] When used properly the adenosine in solution is catabolised to hypoxanthine and inosine which do not cause cardiac problems, but this takes some time in hypothermic conditions.[3]

1. Prien T, et al. Bradyarrhythmia with University of Wisconsin preservation solution. Lancet 1989; i: 1319–20.
2. Vanrenterghem Y, et al. University of Wisconsin preservation solute and bradyarrhythmia. Lancet 1989; ii: 745.
3. Belzer FO. Correct use of University of Wisconsin preservation solution. Lancet 1990; 335: 362.

Effects on the heart. Adenosine may worsen arrhythmias. A prospective study[1] in 200 patients reported an incidence of atrial fibrillation of 12% following bolus injection of adenosine 12 mg used to terminate paroxysmal supraventricular tachycardia. Haemodynamically unstable proarrhythmia occurred in 2 patients with the Wolff-Parkinson-White syndrome and palpitations[2] after standard intravenous doses of adenosine were given.

1. Strickberger SA, et al. Adenosine-induced atrial arrhythmia: a prospective analysis. Ann Intern Med 1997; 127: 417–22.
2. Exner DV, et al. Proarrhythmia in patients with the Wolff-Parkinson-White syndrome after standard doses of intravenous adenosine. Ann Intern Med 1995; 122: 351–2.

Effects on the respiratory system. Acute exacerbation of asthma is well known following inhalation of adenosine. There have been reports of bronchospasm occurring in patients with asthma[1,2] or a history of asthma[3] following the intravenous administration of adenosine. Bronchospasm following adenosine given intravenously produced respiratory failure in a patient with obstructive pulmonary disease.[4]

1. DeGroff CG, Silka MJ. Bronchospasm after intravenous administration of adenosine in a patient with asthma. J Pediatr 1994; 125: 822–3.
2. Drake I, et al. Bronchospasm induced by intravenous adenosine. Hum Exp Toxicol 1994; 13: 263–5.
3. Hintringer F, et al. Supraventricular tachycardia. N Engl J Med 1995; 333: 323.
4. Respiratory failure following adenosine administration. Am J Emerg Med 1993; 11: 249–50.

Migraine. A 35-year-old man with a history of migraine developed symptoms identical to those of his usual episodes of

migraine immediately following two intravenous bolus doses of adenosine.[1]

1. Brown SGA, Waterer GW. Migraine precipitated by adenosine. Med J Aust 1995; 162: 389–91.

Interactions

Dipyridamole inhibits adenosine uptake and therefore may potentiate the action of adenosine; if concurrent use of the two drugs is essential the dosage of adenosine should be reduced. Theophylline and other xanthines are competitive antagonists of adenosine. The risk of atrioventricular block may be increased if adenosine is used concomitantly with other drugs that slow atrioventricular conduction.

Pharmacokinetics

Following intravenous administration adenosine is rapidly taken up by an active transport system into erythrocytes and vascular endothelial cells where it is metabolised to inosine and adenosine monophosphate. The plasma half-life is less than 10 seconds.

Uses and Administration

Adenosine is an endogenous nucleoside involved in many biological processes. It acts as an antiarrhythmic by stimulating adenosine (A_1) receptors and slowing conduction through the atrioventricular node. It does not fit into the usual classification of antiarrhythmics (p.787). It also produces peripheral and coronary vasodilatation by stimulating adenosine (A_2) receptors.

Adenosine is used to restore sinus rhythm in the treatment of paroxysmal supraventricular tachycardia including that associated with the Wolff-Parkinson-White syndrome. It is also used for the differential diagnosis of broad or narrow complex supraventricular tachycardias and in myocardial imaging.

In the treatment of **paroxysmal supraventricular tachycardia**, the usual initial dose of adenosine is 3 mg by rapid intravenous injection. If this dose is ineffective within 1 to 2 minutes, 6 mg may be given and if necessary, 12 mg after a further 1 to 2 minutes. Higher initial doses have sometimes been used. This dosage regimen is also used for differential **diagnosis of supraventricular tachycardias**. An initial dose of 50 to 100 µg per kg body-weight may be given to children; if this is not effective the dose may be increased by 50 to 100 µg per kg increments at 1 to 2 minute intervals until the arrhythmia is controlled or a dose of 300 µg per kg is reached.

In **myocardial imaging** adenosine is given by intravenous infusion in a dose of 140 µg per kg per minute for 6 minutes. The radionuclide is injected after 3 minutes of the infusion.

Adenosine triphosphate (p.1573), in the form of the disodium salt, has been used as an antiarrhythmic.

Cardiac arrhythmias. Adenosine is used for the termination of paroxysmal supraventricular tachycardia[1-4] (p.794), including that associated with the Wolff-Parkinson-White syndrome, and may often be the drug of choice. Following bolus intravenous injection of adenosine, there is a rapid response and the extremely short plasma half-life (less than 10 seconds) allows dosage titration every 1 to 2 minutes so that most episodes can be controlled within 5 minutes without the danger of drug accumulation.

Adenosine has been used successfully in pregnant women with paroxysmal supraventricular tachycardia[5-8] and cardioversion of fetal supraventricular tachycardia by direct fetal therapy with adenosine has been reported.[9,10]

Adenosine can be used for the differential **diagnosis** of broad complex tachycardia where the mechanism is not known.[1] If the cause is supraventricular, adenosine will terminate the arrhythmia or produce atrioventricular block to reveal the underlying atrial rhythm. If the cause is ventricular, adenosine will have no effect on the tachycardia, whereas if an alternative treatment such as verapamil is given to these patients severe hypotension and cardiac arrest can occur.

1. Faulds D, et al. Adenosine: an evaluation of its use in cardiac diagnostic procedures, and in the treatment of paroxysmal supraventricular tachycardia. Drugs 1991; 41: 596–624.
2. Garratt CJ, et al. Adenosine and cardiac arrhythmias. BMJ 1992; 305: 3–4.
3. Rankin AC, et al. Adenosine and the treatment of supraventricular tachycardia. Am J Med 1992; 92: 655–64.
4. Anonymous. Adenosine for acute cardiac arrhythmias. Drug Ther Bull 1993; 31: 49–50.

5. Mason BA, *et al.* Adenosine in the treatment of maternal paroxysmal supraventricular tachycardia. *Obstet Gynecol* 1992; **80:** 478–80.
6. Afridi I, *et al.* Termination of supraventricular tachycardia with intravenous adenosine in a pregnant woman with Wolff-Parkinson-White syndrome. *Obstet Gynecol* 1992; **80:** 481–3.
7. Hagley MT, Cole PL. Adenosine use in pregnant women with supraventricular tachycardia. *Ann Pharmacother* 1994; **28:** 1241–2.
8. Hagley MT, *et al.* Adenosine use in a pregnant patient with supraventricular tachycardia. *Ann Pharmacother* 1995; **29:** 938.
9. Blanch G, *et al.* Cardioversion of fetal tachyarrhythmia with adenosine. *Lancet* 1994; **344:** 1646.
10. Kohl T, *et al.* Direct fetal administration of adenosine for the termination of incessant supraventricular tachycardia. *Obstet Gynecol* 1995; **85:** 873–4.

Ischaemic heart disease. Adenosine produces coronary vasodilatation and may be used to provide a pharmacological stress in patients undergoing assessment of their ischaemic heart disease when exercise stress is inappropriate. It has been given to such patients being evaluated either by thallium-201 myocardial imaging[1] or by stress echocardiography.[2]

Adenosine is also under investigation as an adjunct to prevent reperfusion injury in the management of acute myocardial infarction.[3]

1. Mohiuddin SM, *et al.* Thallium-201 myocardial imaging in patients with coronary artery disease: comparison of intravenous adenosine and oral dipyridamole. *Ann Pharmacother* 1992; **26:** 1352–7.
2. Martin TW, *et al.* Comparison of adenosine, dipyridamole, and dobutamine in stress echocardiography. *Ann Intern Med* 1992; **116:** 190–6.
3. Mahaffey KW, *et al.* Adenosine as an adjunct to thrombolytic therapy for acute myocardial infarction: results of a multicenter, randomized, placebo-controlled trial: the Acute Myocardial Infarction STudy of ADenosine (AMISTAD) trial. *J Am Coll Cardiol* 1999; **34:** 1711–20.

Pulmonary hypertension. A number of vasodilators have been tried in persistent pulmonary hypertension of the newborn (p.810), but their use is generally restricted by their non-selectivity for the pulmonary circulation. A randomised placebo-controlled study[1] in 18 term infants with persistent pulmonary hypertension indicated that intravenous infusion of adenosine improved oxygenation without causing hypotension or tachycardia; however, larger studies were needed to assess any effect on mortality and/or the need for extracorporeal membrane oxygenation.

1. Konduri GG, *et al.* Adenosine infusion improves oxygenation in term infants with respiratory failure. *Pediatrics* 1996; **97:** 295–300.

Preparations

USP 25: Adenosine Injection.

Proprietary Preparations (details are given in Part 3)
Aust.: Adrekar†; *Austral.:* Adenocor; Adenoscan; *Belg.:* Adenocor; *Braz.:* Adenocard; *Canad.:* Adenocard; *Denm.:* Adenocor; *Fin.:* Adenocor; Adenoscan; *Fr.:* Adenoscan; Krenosin; *Ger.:* Adenoscan; Krenosin; Adrekar; *Irl.:* Adenocor; Adenoscan; *Israel:* Adenocor; *Ital.:* Adenoscan; Krenosin; *Neth.:* Adenocor; Adenoscan; *Norw.:* Adenocor; *NZ:* Adenocor; *Port.:* Adenocor; *S.Afr.:* Adenocor; *Singapore:* Adenocor; *Spain:* Adenocor; *Swed.:* Adenocor†; *Switz.:* Krenosine; *Thai.:* Adenocor; *UK:* Adenocor; Adenoscan; *USA:* Adenocard; Adenoscan.

Multi-ingredient: *Aust.:* Laevadosin; Vitasic; *Braz.:* Aminotox; Anekron; Betaliver; Biofigado; Colinvintol; Epacrosil; Eparex; Epativan B6; Epocler; Eviepar; Figadobil; Hepalin; Hepofilina; Hormo Hepatico; *Fr.:* Vitacic; Vitaphakol; *Ger.:* Hepatofalk; Vitreolent plus; *Hong Kong:* Hepatofalk; *Port.:* Vitaphakol; *Spain:* Vitaphakol; *Switz.:* Vitaphakol†.

Adrenaline (2041-c)

Adrenaline *(BAN)*.
Epinephrine *(BAN, rINN)*; Epinefrina; Epinephrinum; Epirenamine; Levorenin; Suprarenin. (R)-1-(3,4-Dihydroxyphenyl)-2-methylaminoethanol.
$C_9H_{13}NO_3 = 183.2$.
CAS — 51-43-4.
ATC — A01AD01; B02BC09; C01CA24; R03AA01; S01EA01.

NOTE. ADN and EPN are codes approved by the BP 2001 for use on single unit doses of eye drops containing adrenaline [epinephrine] where the individual container may be too small to bear all the appropriate labelling information.
Pharmacopoeias. In Br., Chin., Fr., Int., It., Jpn, Neth., Pol., and US.
US also includes the racemic substances Racepinephrine (Racepinefrine *(rINN)*) and Racepinephrine Hydrochloride (Racepinefrine Hydrochloride *(rINNM)*).

Adrenaline is an active principle of the medulla of the adrenal gland. It may be obtained from the adrenal glands of certain mammals or it may be prepared synthetically. Endogenous adrenaline and the monograph substance are the laevo isomer.

Pharmacopoeial description

BP 2001: It may be prepared by synthesis or isolated from the medulla of the suprarenal glands of certain mammals and substantially freed from noradrenaline. A white or creamy-white, sphaero-crystalline powder. It darkens in colour on exposure to air and light. Sparingly soluble in water; practically insoluble in alcohol and in ether. It dissolves in solutions of mineral acids

and in solutions of sodium or potassium hydroxide, but not in solutions of ammonia or of the alkali carbonates. It is unstable in neutral or alkaline solutions, which rapidly become red on exposure to air. Store in containers which are preferably filled with nitrogen. Protect from light.

USP 25: A white to practically white, odourless, microcrystalline powder or granules, gradually darkening on exposure to light and air. With acids, it forms salts that are readily soluble in water, and the base may be recovered by the addition of ammonia water or alkali carbonates. Very slightly soluble in water and in alcohol; insoluble in chloroform, in ether, and in fixed and volatile oils. Solutions are alkaline to litmus. Store in airtight containers. Protect from light.

Adrenaline Acid Tartrate (2042-k)

Adrenaline Acid Tartrate *(BANM)*.
Epinephrine Bitartrate *(rINNM)*; Adrenaline Bitartrate; Adrenaline Tartrate; Adrenalini Bitartras; Adrenalini Tartras; Adrenalinii Tartras; Adrenalinium Hydrogentartaricum; Epinephrine Acid Tartrate *(BANM)*; Epinephrine Hydrogen Tartrate; Epirenamine Bitartrate.
$C_9H_{13}NO_3,C_4H_6O_6 = 333.3$.
CAS — 51-42-3.
Pharmacopoeias. In Eur. (see p.vi), Int., and US.

Adrenaline [epinephrine] acid tartrate 1.8 mg is approximately equivalent to 1 mg of adrenaline [epinephrine].

Pharmacopoeial description

Ph. Eur.: A white to greyish-white, crystalline powder. Freely soluble in water; slightly soluble in alcohol; practically insoluble in ether. Store in airtight containers, or preferably in a sealed tube under vacuum or under an inert gas. Protect from light.

USP 25: A white, or greyish-white or light brownish-grey, odourless, crystalline powder. It slowly darkens on exposure to air and light. Soluble 1 in 3 of water; slightly soluble in alcohol; practically insoluble in chloroform and in ether. Its solutions in water are acid to litmus, having a pH of about 3.5. Store in airtight containers. Protect from light.

◊ Studies on the stability of adrenaline [epinephrine] injections.

1. Taylor JB, *et al.* Effect of sodium metabisulphite and anaerobic processing conditions on the oxidative degradation of adrenaline injection BP [1980]. *Pharm J* 1984; **232:** 646–8.

Adrenaline Hydrochloride (9501-z)

Adrenaline Hydrochloride *(BANM)*.
Epinephrine Hydrochloride *(BANM, rINNM)*.
$C_9H_{13}NO_3,HCl = 219.7$.
CAS — 55-31-2.

Adrenaline [epinephrine] hydrochloride 1.2 mg is approximately equivalent to 1 mg of adrenaline [epinephrine].

Adverse Effects

Adrenaline [epinephrine] is a potent sympathomimetic and may exhibit the adverse effects typical of both alpha- and beta-adrenoceptor stimulation. It can thus produce a wide range of adverse effects, most of which mimic the results of excessive stimulation of the sympathetic nervous system. Side-effects such as anxiety, dyspnoea, hyperglycaemia, restlessness, palpitations, tachycardia (sometimes with anginal pain), tremors, sweating, hypersalivation, weakness, dizziness, headache, and coldness of extremities may occur even with low doses. Overdosage may cause cardiac arrhythmias and a sharp rise in blood pressure (sometimes leading to cerebral haemorrhage and pulmonary oedema); these effects may occur at normal dosage in susceptible subjects.

Since adrenaline [epinephrine] does not readily cross the blood-brain barrier, its central effects, which encompass anxiety, fear, restlessness, insomnia, confusion, irritability, and psychotic states, may be largely a somatic response to its peripheral effects. Anorexia, nausea, and vomiting, may occur similarly.

The peripheral adverse effects of adrenaline [epinephrine] are complex and mediated via its action on the various types of adrenergic receptor (see under Uses and Administration, below). Stimulation of alpha-adrenergic (mainly alpha$_1$) receptors produces vasoconstriction leading to hypertension, and this alpha-mediated hypertension may induce reflex bradycardia. On the other hand, stimulation of beta$_1$-adrenergic receptors in the heart produces tachycardia and cardiac arrhythmias. Finally, stimulation of beta$_2$ re-

ceptors produces vasodilatation with flushing and hypotension (apparent if the vasoconstricting alpha effects are blocked).

In relation to some of the other adverse effects of adrenaline [epinephrine], difficulty in micturition with urinary retention is a characteristic of alpha$_1$-receptor stimulation whereas muscle tremor and hypokalaemia are characteristics of beta$_2$-receptor stimulation.

The potent alpha-adrenergic effects of adrenaline [epinephrine] may lead to gangrene following the vasoconstriction that is induced by infiltration of adrenaline [epinephrine]-containing local anaesthetic solutions into digits. Extravasation of parenterally administered adrenaline [epinephrine] similarly causes intense vasoconstriction, resulting in tissue necrosis and sloughing.

Topical application of adrenaline [epinephrine] to mucosal surfaces also causes vasoconstriction, which may induce hypoxia leading to compensatory rebound congestion of the mucosa.

Inhalations of adrenaline [epinephrine] have been associated with epigastric pain (which was caused by swallowing a portion of the inhalation and could be minimised by rinsing the mouth and throat with water after inhaling).

Adrenaline [epinephrine] eye drops may produce severe smarting, blurred vision, and photophobia on instillation; they may also leave melanin-like deposits in the cornea and conjunctiva, and this has led to obstruction of the naso-lachrymal ducts. Repeated ocular administration of adrenaline [epinephrine] may cause oedema, hyperaemia, and inflammation of the eyes.

Other sympathomimetics have adverse effects that resemble those of adrenaline [epinephrine] to a greater or lesser extent according to their relative agonist activities on the different receptors. For example, noradrenaline [norepinephrine], whose alpha-adrenergic effects predominate, may produce severe hypertension, whereas isoprenaline, whose beta-adrenergic effects predominate, may produce severe tachycardia.

◊ Systemic side-effects may occasionally follow the local or topical administration of sympathomimetics; this may often be in relation to the use of eye drops for the treatment of glaucoma.[1] Psychiatric side-effects including hallucinations and paranoia have also occurred following both proper and improper use of sympathomimetics in decongestant preparations.[2]

1. Everitt DE, Avorn J. Systemic effects of medications used to treat glaucoma. *Ann Intern Med* 1990; **112:** 120–5.
2. Anonymous. Drugs that cause psychiatric symptoms. *Med Lett Drugs Ther* 1993; **35:** 65–70.

Effects on the eyes. In addition to the possibility of pigment deposition and local pain (see above) adrenaline [epinephrine] eye drops have been associated with maculopathy. During 4 years, 15 patients showed reactions to adrenaline [epinephrine] eye drops, usually 2% of the hydrochloride or acid tartrate, while some used 1% epinephryl borate.[1] Blurring and distortion of vision were followed by decreased visual acuity, and by the appearance of oedema and sometimes haemorrhage in the macular region. A few patients developed cysts near the fovea. These effects appeared within a few weeks of, or several months after, commencement of therapy and were usually reversible. All except 1 of the patients were aphakic (devoid of lens). In a study of 200 consecutive patients receiving adrenaline [epinephrine] therapy, 23 were aphakic in one or both eyes, and 7 experienced these reactions to adrenaline [epinephrine].

1. Kolker AE, Becker B. Epinephrine maculopathy. *Arch Ophthalmol* 1968; **79:** 552–62.

Effects on the heart. A review of the arrhythmogenic effects of vasopressor sympathomimetics[1] concluded that dopamine and adrenaline [epinephrine] were associated with the highest risk, mainly of dose-related sinus tachycardia and ventricular arrhythmias. The clinical significance of most arrhythmias occurring with dopamine was considered questionable, however; supraventricular or ventricular arrhythmias occurring with adrenaline [epinephrine] were most likely in patients receiving general anaesthesia or with underlying disorders of cardiac conduction. The risk with noradrenaline [norepinephrine] was uncertain, though there are few clinical reports, while phenylephrine and methoxamine were thought unlikely to cause problems. Overall the frequency of serious problems with this class of drugs did not seem to be high, and benefits outweighed the risks in most patients.

Myocardial infarction has been reported in an 11-year-old boy treated with nebulised racemic adrenaline [epinephrine] for symptoms of croup.[2]

1. Tisdale JE, *et al.* Proarrhythmic effects of intravenous vasopressors. *Ann Pharmacother* 1995; **29:** 269–81.
2. Butte MJ, *et al.* Pediatric myocardial infarction after racemic epinephrine administration. Abstract: *Pediatrics* 1999; **104:** 103–4. Full version: http://www.pediatrics.org/cgi/content/full/104/1/e9

Overdosage. A report of inadvertent administration to a 13-month-old infant of a solution containing racemic adrenaline [epinephrine] meant for nebulisation.[1] The infant received the equivalent of about 327 µg per kg body-weight of *l*-adrenaline [*l*-epinephrine] intravenously. Marked pallor, pulselessness, and profound bradycardia ensued, but the child responded to cardiopulmonary resuscitation and was subsequently discharged with no evidence of long-term sequelae.

1. Kurachek SC, Rockoff MA. Inadvertent intravenous administration of racemic epinephrine. *JAMA* 1985; **253:** 1441–2.

Treatment of Adverse Effects
Because of the short duration of the adverse effects of adrenaline [epinephrine], due to inactivation in the body, treatment of severe toxic reactions in hypersensitive patients or after overdose is primarily supportive. Prompt injection of a rapidly acting alpha blocker, such as phentolamine, followed by a beta blocker such as propranolol, has been tried to counteract the pressor and arrhythmogenic effects of adrenaline [epinephrine]; rapidly-acting vasodilators such as glyceryl trinitrate have also been used.

Precautions
Adrenaline [epinephrine] should be used with great caution in patients who may be particularly susceptible to its cardiovascular actions, notably those with pre-existing arrhythmias or tachycardia, Prinzmetal's angina, thromboembolic disorders, or a history of ischaemic heart disease. Extreme care is also needed in conditions which predispose a patient to adverse effects on the heart, such as hyperthyroidism; elevated thyroid hormone concentrations may also enhance receptor sensitivity. The use of adrenaline [epinephrine] is generally inappropriate where there is pre-existing hypertension and it increases the risk of ischaemia in the extremities of patients with occlusive vascular disease. Special care is also needed in the elderly who may have pre-existing coronary or cerebrovascular disease.

Special care is also needed if adrenaline [epinephrine] is given to patients with diabetes mellitus (both because of its vasoconstrictor actions and because of its metabolic effects on blood sugar). It should be avoided in phaeochromocytoma.

Adrenaline [epinephrine] eye drops are contra-indicated in angle-closure glaucoma unless an iridectomy has been carried out.

When adrenaline [epinephrine] is used for circulatory support, correction of hypovolaemia, metabolic acidosis, and hypoxia or hypercapnia should be carried out beforehand or concomitantly.

Precautions that need to be observed for *other sympathomimetics* resemble those for adrenaline [epinephrine], but vary to a greater or lesser extent according to their relative agonist activities on the different receptors. For example, noradrenaline [norepinephrine], whose alpha-adrenergic effects predominate, is a particular hazard in hypertension, whereas a beta-adrenergic agonist such as isoprenaline is a particular hazard in tachycardia. It also needs to be borne in mind that since non-catecholamine sympathomimetics have a longer duration of action than catecholamines, side-effects are more likely to be sustained and, in particular, that any rise in blood pressure is liable to be prolonged.

Abuse. A number of sympathomimetics, particularly those available without prescription, have been subject to abuse. The use of sympathomimetics by athletes is prohibited by the International Olympic Committee,[1] although there is little evidence that they increase physical ability or stamina.

1. MacAuley D. Drugs in sport. *BMJ* 1996; **313:** 211–15.

Contact lenses. Discussion of drug-induced staining of soft-contact lenses.[1] Adrenochrome staining of contact lenses of patients using adrenaline [epinephrine] eye drops has been reported. Melanin deposits may also become locked into the lens;

such deposits may be broken down by hydrogen peroxide but in practice the lens is usually discarded. Patients prescribed drugs likely to cause this problem should be given appropriate warning. The prodrug, dipivefrine hydrochloride (p.1604) has been used without staining soft lenses.

1. Ingram DV. Spoiled soft contact lenses. *BMJ* 1986; **292:** 1619.

Infection. A small open study[1] in patients critically ill with severe sepsis or malaria has suggested that the use of adrenaline [epinephrine] as an inotrope and vasopressor in patients with severe infection causes the development of lactic acidosis. However, adrenaline [epinephrine] is widely used in the treatment of septic shock, and others have pointed out that 20 of the 23 patients involved in the former study had responded to fluids, a situation in which the use of inotropic or vasopressor support was considered questionable.[2]

1. Day NPJ, *et al.* The effects of dopamine and adrenaline infusions on acid-base balance and systemic haemodynamics in severe infection. *Lancet* 1996; **348:** 219–23. Correction. *ibid.;* 902.
2. Barry B, Bodenham A. Effects of dopamine and adrenaline infusions in severe infection. *Lancet* 1996; **348:** 1099–1100.

Interactions
Interactions with adrenaline [epinephrine] are complex and often hazardous; they stem primarily from its agonist actions on alpha and beta adrenoceptors.

Hazardous arrhythmias are a risk if adrenaline [epinephrine] is used in patients anaesthetised with *cyclopropane, halothane,* or other *volatile anaesthetics* which sensitise the myocardium to its beta-adrenergic effects.

The vasoconstrictor and pressor effects of adrenaline [epinephrine], mediated by its alpha-adrenergic action, may be enhanced by the concomitant administration of drugs with similar effects, such as *ergot alkaloids* or *oxytocin.*

Because adrenaline [epinephrine] increases blood pressure, special care is advisable in patients receiving *antihypertensive therapy.* Moreover, adrenaline [epinephrine] specifically reverses the antihypertensive effects of *adrenergic neurone blockers* such as *guanethidine* with the risk of severe hypertension. Severe hypertension (followed by reflex bradycardia) may also develop if adrenaline [epinephrine] is given with a *beta blocker (especially a non-selective beta blocker)* since the beta blocker opposes the beta-adrenergic action of adrenaline [epinephrine], leaving its alpha-adrenergic effect unopposed; for details see below. Conversely, the bronchoconstrictor effect of a *beta blocker (especially a non-selective beta blocker)* antagonises the beta$_2$ (bronchodilating) effect of adrenaline [epinephrine] and constitutes a serious hazard. It should also be noted that in patients on non-cardioselective beta blockers, severe anaphylaxis may not respond to adrenaline [epinephrine] (see below). Complex interactions also occur with *alpha blockers* such as *phenoxybenzamine* and *phentolamine* which oppose the alpha-adrenergic action of adrenaline [epinephrine] leaving its beta-adrenergic effect unopposed, thus resulting in both antihypertensive and cardiac-accelerating effects; nevertheless, use is made of this blood pressure reduction to reverse hypertension in adrenaline [epinephrine] overdosage (see also Treatment of Adverse Effects, above). For a warning concerning hypotension associated with adrenaline [epinephrine]-induced reversal of alpha-blockade in phenothiazine overdosage, see Treatment of Adverse Effects of Chlorpromazine, p.663.

Although caution is still necessary, the action of adrenaline [epinephrine] or noradrenaline [norepinephrine] may be only slightly enhanced by an *MAOI,* since they are direct acting and inactivation by uptake into nerves and tissues is not inhibited. Dangerous hypertensive interactions are, however, a risk if dopamine (which has indirect-acting properties) is given concomitantly with an *MAOI (including an RIMA).* Hazardous hypertensive interactions are also a major risk if dexamfetamine, dopexamine, ephedrine, isometheptene, mephentermine, metaraminol, methylphenidate, phentermine, phenylephrine, phenylpropanolamine, pseudoephedrine, and many other sympathomimetics are given concomitantly with an *MAOI (including an RIMA).* For additional warnings see under Phenelzine (p.305) and Moclobemide (p.299).

Administration of adrenaline [epinephrine] or noradrenaline [norepinephrine] with *tricyclic antidepressants* (which inhibit their reuptake) carries a risk of inducing hypertension and arrhythmias.

In the case of local anaesthetic preparations containing adrenaline [epinephrine] there is no clinical evidence of dangerous interactions with either *tricyclic antidepressants* or *MAOIs,* but great care needs to be taken to avoid inadvertent intravenous administration of the local anaesthetic preparations. (For a warning to avoid local anaesthetics containing noradrenaline [norepinephrine], see under Adverse Effects of Noradrenaline, p.948.)

The hypokalaemic effect of adrenaline [epinephrine] may be potentiated by other drugs that cause potassium loss, including *corticosteroids, potassium-depleting diuretics,* and *aminophylline* or *theophylline;* patients receiving high doses of beta$_2$-adrenergic agonists concomitantly should have their plasma-potassium concentration monitored (see Interactions of Salbutamol, p.771). Hypokalaemia may also result in increased susceptibility to cardiac arrhythmias caused by *digoxin* and other *cardiac glycosides.*

In addition to their interactions with *MAOIs* (cited above) the interactions of *other sympathomimetics* resemble those of adrenaline [epinephrine] to a greater or lesser extent, according to their relevant agonist activities on the different receptors. For some details of specific interactions see under individual monographs.

Beta blockers. Patients given adrenaline [epinephrine] (including the low doses used with local anaesthetics) while receiving non-selective beta blockers such as *propranolol* can develop elevated blood pressure due to alpha-mediated vasoconstriction, followed by reflex bradycardia, and occasionally cardiac arrest;[1] the bronchodilator effects of adrenaline [epinephrine] are also inhibited. In contrast, cardioselective beta blockers such as *metoprolol,* which act preferentially at beta$_1$-adrenergic receptors, do not prevent adrenaline [epinephrine]-induced vasodilatation via beta$_2$ receptors, and in consequence blood pressure and heart rate change only minimally. *Carvedilol,* which also has alpha-blocking effects, has been reported to cause hypotension with dobutamine (see p.880). Low doses of cardioselective beta blockers do not appear to interfere with sympathomimetic (isoprenaline)-induced bronchodilatation,[2] although the effect of larger doses is uncertain.

Propranolol has also been shown to inhibit the favourable pressor and bronchodilator responses to adrenaline [epinephrine] when given in anaphylaxis.[3] Thus, patients receiving long-term treatment with some non-cardioselective beta blockers who develop anaphylaxis may be relatively refractory to adrenaline [epinephrine].

1. Jay GT, Chow MSS. Interaction of epinephrine and β-blockers. *JAMA* 1995; **274:** 1830–2.
2. Decalmer PBS, *et al.* Beta blockers and asthma. *Br Heart J* 1978; **40:** 184–9.
3. Newman BR, Schultz LK. Epinephrine-resistant anaphylaxis in a patient taking propranolol hydrochloride. *Ann Allergy* 1981; **47:** 35–7.

General anaesthetics. In a review[1] in 1967 the sensitisation of the myocardium to β-adrenergic stimulation caused by some anaesthetics was considered to be of clinical importance when adrenaline [epinephrine] was injected into an operation area to reduce bleeding. It had previously been considered that adrenaline [epinephrine] could not be given when the patient had been anaesthetised with *cyclopropane, halothane,* or similar volatile anaesthetics but it had become evident that adrenaline [epinephrine] could be used so long as the dose was small and other factors likely to increase the irritability of the myocardium, such as carbon-dioxide retention, hypoxia, or the simultaneous use of cocaine were avoided. It appeared[2] that provided the solution of adrenaline [epinephrine] was not stronger than 1 in 100 000 and that the rate of injection did not exceed 10 mL per 10 minutes or 30 mL an hour no serious results should ensue under *halothane* or *trichloroethylene* anaesthesia. The technique was considered inappropriate for use with cyclopropane although some disagreed with this view admitting, however, that the risk of arrhythmias was higher with cyclopropane than with halothane or trichloroethylene.[2]

There have, however, been fatalities reported in patients who underwent surgery which involved the use of halothane and adrenaline [epinephrine].[3]

1. Anonymous. Anaesthetics and the heart. *Lancet* 1967; **i:** 484–5.
2. Katz RL, Epstein RA. The interaction of anesthetic agents and adrenergic drugs to produce cardiac arrhythmias. *Anesthesiology* 1968; **29:** 763.
3. Buzik SC. Fatal interaction? Halothane, epinephrine and tooth implant surgery. *Can Pharm J* 1990; **123:** 68–9 and 81.

Local anaesthetics. It is common practice to administer adrenaline [epinephrine] with a local anaesthetic to produce vasoconstriction; the lowest effective concentration of adrenaline [epinephrine] should be used. However, with *cocaine* there is a risk of cardiac arrhythmias and the use, for example, of cocaine and adrenaline [epinephrine] paste in otolaryngology may be hazardous. See p.1311 for references to this interaction.

Pharmacokinetics

As a result of enzymatic degradation in the gut and first-pass metabolism in the liver, adrenaline [epinephrine] is almost totally inactive when given by mouth. Systemic absorption can occur following topical application for example of eye drops. Adrenaline [epinephrine] acts rapidly following intramuscular and subcutaneous injection; this latter route is, however, sometimes considered to be slower and therefore less reliable and predictable for emergency use. Although absorption is slowed by local vasoconstriction it can be hastened by massaging the injection site.

Most adrenaline [epinephrine] that is either injected into the body or released into the circulation from the adrenal medulla, is very rapidly inactivated by processes which include uptake into adrenergic neurones, diffusion, and enzymatic degradation in the liver and body tissues. The half-life of circulating adrenaline [epinephrine] is only about 1 minute. One of the enzymes responsible for the chemical inactivation of adrenaline [epinephrine] is catechol-*O*-methyltransferase (COMT), the other is monoamine oxidase (MAO). In general, adrenaline [epinephrine] is methylated to metanephrine by COMT followed by oxidative deamination by MAO and eventual conversion to 4-hydroxy-3-methoxymandelic acid (formerly termed vanillylmandelic acid; VMA), or oxidatively deaminated by MAO and converted to 3,4-dihydroxymandelic acid which, in turn, is methylated by COMT, once again to 4-hydroxy-3-methoxymandelic acid; the metabolites are excreted in the urine mainly as their glucuronide and ethereal sulfate conjugates.

The ability of COMT to effect introduction of a methyl group is an important step in the chemical inactivation of adrenaline [epinephrine] and similar catecholamines (in particular, noradrenaline [norepinephrine]). It means that the termination of the pharmacological response of catecholamines is not simply dependent upon MAO. In its role of neurotransmitter intraneuronal catecholamine (mainly noradrenaline [norepinephrine]) is, however, enzymatically regulated by MAO.

Adrenaline [epinephrine] crosses the placenta to enter fetal circulation.

Uses and Administration

Adrenaline is an active principle of the adrenal medulla which is used as a direct-acting sympathomimetic; for an outline of the actions of sympathomimetics, see below. It has a somewhat more marked effect on beta adrenoceptors than on alpha adrenoceptors, and this property explains many aspects of its pharmacology; in addition, its actions vary considerably according to the dose given, and the consequent reflex compensating responses of the body.

In practice, major effects of adrenaline [epinephrine] include increased speed and force of cardiac contraction (with lower doses this causes increased systolic pressure yet reduced diastolic pressure since overall peripheral resistance is lowered, but with higher doses both systolic and diastolic pressure are increased as stimulation of peripheral alpha receptors increases peripheral resistance); blood flow to skeletal muscle is increased (reduced with higher doses); there is relaxation of bronchial smooth muscle; metabolic effects result in hyperglycaemia as well as markedly increased oxygen consumption; blood flow in the kidneys, mucosa, and skin is reduced; there is little direct effect on cerebral blood flow.

Adrenaline [epinephrine] has an important role in the management of acute allergic reactions and can be life-saving in patients with anaphylactic shock (be-

low). It is also used in advanced cardiac life support (below). Adrenaline [epinephrine] has been given subcutaneously in the treatment of acute asthma but more selective drugs are available, and it has no role in the chronic management of asthma (p.757). It has been given by nebulisation in severe croup (p.1049). Adrenaline [epinephrine] is used for a number of other indications including the control of minor bleeding from the skin and mucous membranes, in ophthalmology chiefly for the management of open-angle (simple) glaucoma (p.1413), and also as an adjunct to local anaesthesia (p.1304). Adrenaline [epinephrine] was formerly incorporated into creams used in the treatment of rheumatic and muscular disorders, and in rectal preparations used in the treatment of haemorrhoids. Racepinefrine (racemic adrenaline [racemic epinephrine]) or racepinefrine hydrochloride has been used for bronchodilatation.

Adrenaline [epinephrine] is given by subcutaneous or intramuscular injection. In extreme emergencies, where a more rapid effect is required, adrenaline [epinephrine] may be given as a dilute solution (1 in 10 000 or 1 in 100 000) by very slow intravenous injection or by slow intravenous infusion. Intraosseous administration, usually into the marrow of the tibia, is sometimes used as an alternative to the intravenous route. Adrenaline [epinephrine] has sometimes been injected directly in the heart; current guidelines for the management of cardiac emergencies do not include that route but recommend administration via a central vein. Endotracheal administration is occasionally employed when intravenous access cannot be obtained. Adrenaline [epinephrine] may be applied topically and can be administered by inhalation. Aqueous solutions of adrenaline [epinephrine] are usually prepared using the acid tartrate or the hydrochloride but the dosage is generally stated in terms of the equivalent content of adrenaline [epinephrine].

The usual dose of adrenaline [epinephrine] in **anaphylactic shock** is 0.5 mg (0.5 mL of a 1 in 1000 solution) by intramuscular injection repeated as necessary every 5 minutes. A dose of 0.3 mg (0.3 mL of a 1 in 1000 solution) may be appropriate for emergency self-administration. Children's doses range from 120 to 250 μg depending on age; 50 μg may be used in infants under 6 months of age. If intravenous administration is required the dose is 500 μg for adults and 10 μg per kg body-weight for children, as a more dilute 1 in 10 000 solution at a rate of 1 mL (100 μg) or less per minute.

In **advanced cardiac life support** the initial dose of adrenaline [epinephrine] for adults is 1 mg intravenously (10 mL of a 1 in 10 000 solution), preferably into a central vein, and this may be repeated as often as every 2 to 3 minutes in some circumstances for up to an hour. Depending on the arrhythmia the dose may be increased after three injections of 1 mg to 5 mg or 100 μg per kg. Children may be given intravenous doses of 10 μg per kg initially then 100 μg per kg. Intraosseous doses are the same as those used intravenously. Endotracheal doses for adults are 2 to 3 times the intravenous dose; children may be given 100 μg per kg.

Adrenaline [epinephrine] relaxes the bronchial musculature and has sometimes been injected subcutaneously or intramuscularly in the management of **acute asthmatic attacks**. However, in general, the use of adrenaline [epinephrine] in asthma has been superseded by beta₂ agonists, such as salbutamol, which can alleviate bronchospasm with fewer effects on the heart. If adrenaline [epinephrine] is to be used, the adult dose is 0.3 to 0.5 mL of a 1 in 1000 aqueous solution (300 to 500 μg); children have received 0.01 mL per kg body-weight (10 μg per kg) to a maximum of 0.5 mL (500 μg). Aqueous solutions with an adrenaline [epinephrine] content equivalent to 1 in 100 have occasionally been used by inhalation as a spray to alleviate asthmatic attacks; these solutions must never be confused with the weaker strength used for injection. Pressurised aerosols delivering metered

doses equivalent to approximately 160 μg to 275 μg of adrenaline [epinephrine] have also been used; adults have received 1 or 2 metered inhalations repeated, if necessary, after 3 hours.

Adrenaline [epinephrine] is frequently added to **local anaesthetics** to retard diffusion and limit absorption, to prolong the duration of effect, and to lessen the danger of toxicity. A concentration of 1 in 200 000 (5 μg per mL) is usually used; adrenaline [epinephrine] should not be added when procedures involve digits, ears, nose, penis, or scrotum owing to the risk of ischaemic tissue necrosis. A concentration of up to 1 in 80 000 (12.5 μg per mL) may be used in dental preparations where the total dose given is small.

Adrenaline [epinephrine] constricts arterioles and capillaries and causes blanching when applied locally to mucous membranes and exposed tissues. It is used as an aqueous solution in strengths up to a 1 in 1000 dilution to check capillary **bleeding**, epistaxis, and bleeding from superficial wounds and abrasions, but it does not stop internal haemorrhage. It is usually applied as a spray or on pledgets of cotton wool or gauze.

In ophthalmology, adrenaline [epinephrine] solutions of 0.5%, 1%, or 2% are used as eye drops instilled once or twice daily to reduce intra-ocular pressure in open-angle **glaucoma** and ocular hypertension. An adrenaline [epinephrine] borate complex is also used in ophthalmology.

Actions of sympathomimetics

Sympathomimetics have actions similar to those that follow stimulation of postganglionic sympathetic (or adrenergic) nerves. The three naturally occurring sympathomimetics are adrenaline, noradrenaline, and dopamine. All three are catecholamines, i.e. their aromatic portion is catechol (which is characterised by hydroxy groups at adjacent positions of a benzene ring) and the aliphatic portion is an amine. Despite widespread use of the term 'adrenergic' for sympathetic nerves, the physiological functions of adrenaline itself are predominantly metabolic. It is noradrenaline that is the endogenous neurotransmitter at postganglionic sympathetic nerves. Dopamine acts peripherally on the renal, mesenteric, and coronary vascular beds. Both noradrenaline and dopamine also have key roles as neurotransmitters within the CNS, but (in common with adrenaline) are highly polar and cannot cross the blood-brain barrier.

These three catecholamines differ markedly in effect according to their specificity for different adrenergic receptors.

Adrenergic receptors are divided into alpha and beta adrenoceptors. These are then subdivided into alpha₁ (postsynaptic) and alpha₂ (mainly presynaptic) types, and into beta₁, beta₂, and beta₃ receptors. A third distinct group of receptors which occur primarily within the CNS are described as dopamine receptors and at least 5 subtypes are known (see p.1160); D₁ receptors also occur within renal, mesenteric, and coronary vascular beds.

Stimulation of these different receptors produces the following effects:

- stimulation of alpha₁ receptors produces vasoconstriction, particularly in the vessels of the skin and mucosa, abdominal viscera, and kidney; this results in an increase in blood pressure, sometimes with compensatory reflex bradycardia; alpha₁ stimulation also results in contraction of other smooth muscle, including the urinary sphincter and the uterus, and induces mydriasis in the eye
- stimulation of alpha₂ receptors appears to play a role in feedback inhibition of neurotransmitter release and may be involved in the inhibition of intestinal activity; it also plays a role in the inhibition of insulin secretion
- stimulation of beta₁ receptors produces an increase in the rate and force of contraction of the heart, increased conduction velocity, and greater automaticity
- stimulation of beta₂ receptors produces vasodilatation, bronchodilatation, uterine relaxation, and a decrease in gastrointestinal motility; it also results in release of insulin and enhances gluconeogenesis and glycogenolysis
- stimulation of beta₃ receptors is thought to have a role in lipolysis and thermogenesis
- stimulation of D₁ receptors produces vasodilatation of renal, mesenteric, and coronary vessels.

The pattern of activity of the three catecholamines is complex and influenced not only by receptor specificity, but also by feedback mechanisms and receptor distribution. In broad terms:

- adrenaline is a potent agonist at both alpha and beta receptors
- noradrenaline is a potent agonist at alpha and beta$_1$ receptors, but has little effect on beta$_2$ receptors
- dopamine in low doses activates D$_1$ receptors; in higher doses it activates beta$_1$ and then alpha receptors, and also provokes release of noradrenaline from nerve terminals.

Other sympathomimetic drugs are analogues of the catecholamines and according to their structure either act directly on adrenergic receptors (e.g. phenylephrine) or indirectly (e.g. ephedrine, which also has direct actions). Indirect actions are achieved by displacing noradrenaline from storage vesicles within the nerve terminals. In practice many sympathomimetics have both direct and indirect actions.

Catecholamines have a fleeting action and are inactive by mouth whereas their analogues have a prolonged action and are active by mouth; the analogues are also less polar than the catecholamines and can often cross the blood-brain barrier. This ability to cross the blood-brain barrier explains why some sympathomimetics (e.g. dexamfetamine) have marked central stimulant effects. It may also explain the seemingly paradoxical antihypertensive effect of alpha$_2$-adrenergic agonists (e.g. clonidine) since their central effects may outweigh their effects in vascular smooth muscle.

Advanced cardiac life support. Adrenaline [epinephrine] has an important role in advanced cardiac life support (p.790) since, through its alpha agonist effects, it increases myocardial and cerebral blood flow and thereby the efficacy of cardiopulmonary resuscitation or basic life support procedures. Depending on the arrhythmia that has led to cardiac arrest treatment starts with cardiopulmonary resuscitation and defibrillation. If these measures fail to restore a conventional rhythm, the next step involves the administration of adrenaline [epinephrine].

For adults, adrenaline [epinephrine] is given in a dose of 1 mg ideally intravenously into a central vein. If such venous access is not practicable adrenaline [epinephrine] may be given through a peripheral vein followed by a flush of 20 mL or more of sodium chloride injection; however, the response is slower than with central venous injection. This intravenous dose of 1 mg may be given approximately every 3 minutes[1,2] or 3 to 5 minutes[3] in further cycles of cardiopulmonary resuscitation and, if necessary, shocks. A higher dose of 5 mg or 100 μg per kg body-weight has been given but there is insufficient evidence of benefit for this to be recommended.[1-3] In ventricular fibrillation or pulseless ventricular tachycardia, a resuscitation attempt may reasonably last for anything from 10 minutes to 1 hour with adrenaline [epinephrine] 1 mg intravenously being administered every 3 minutes during this period. Where the arrest is associated with asystole it is unlikely that a response will be achieved after 15 minutes.

The initial dose of 1 mg is reported to be based on the dose that was given by intracardiac injection, so it would be expected that a higher dose would be required for intravenous administration. However, studies[4-7] have failed to show any survival benefit with the use of doses higher than the 1-mg dose as used above.

The intravenous dose for children is 10 μg per kg as the first dose; a higher dose of 100 μg per kg[1-3] or possibly 200 μg per kg,[3] may be used for the second and subsequent doses. However, as with adults the use of the higher dose is not routinely recommended and a retrospective study[8] found no improvement in outcome.

The intraosseous route is a practicable alternative to intravenous injection for adults as well as for children, although the guidelines only give doses for children, which are identical to those given intravenously. Alternatively, adrenaline [epinephrine] can be administered through the endotracheal tube that will have been inserted, but only if the intravenous or intraosseous administration is delayed. Endotracheal doses for adults should be 2 to 3 times those used intravenously; for children doses of 100 μg per kg have been suggested. The adrenaline [epinephrine] solution should be diluted and administered deeply using a catheter; several rapid ventilations or inflations should follow. It is recognised that the endotracheal route is imperfect[1-3] and some workers consider it to be ineffective.[9]

Although covering a somewhat different clinical situation some guidelines also include resuscitation of newborn infants (during the first few hours after birth).[1-3] Adrenaline [epinephrine] may be used when the heart rate remains below 60 beats per minute despite adequate ventilation and chest compression. The dose of adrenaline [epinephrine] is 10 to 30 μg per kg, repeated every 3 to 5 minutes as required; it is administered intravenously (generally into the umbilical vein) or by the endotracheal route.

1. European Resuscitation Council. European Resuscitation Council Guidelines 2000. *Resuscitation* 2001; 48: 199–239.
2. Resuscitation Council (UK). Resuscitation Guidelines 2000. Available at: http://www.resus.org.uk/pages/guide.htm (accessed 15/08/01).
3. The American Heart Association in collaboration with the International Liaison Committee on Resuscitation (ILCOR). International guidelines 2000 for cardiopulmonary resuscitation and

emergency cardiovascular care: a consensus on science. *Circulation* 2000; 102 (suppl I): I1–I384. [Also published in *Resuscitation* 2000; 46: 3–447.]
4. Stiell IG, *et al.* High-dose epinephrine in adult cardiac arrest. *N Engl J Med* 1992; 327: 1045–50.
5. Brown CG, *et al.* A comparison of standard-dose and high-dose epinephrine in cardiac arrest outside the hospital. *N Engl J Med* 1992; 327: 1051–5.
6. Callaham M, *et al.* A randomized clinical trial of high-dose epinephrine and norepinephrine vs standard-dose epinephrine in prehospital cardiac arrest. *JAMA* 1992; 268: 2667–72.
7. Gueugniaud P-Y, *et al.* A comparison of repeated high doses and repeated standard doses of epinephrine for cardiac arrest outside the hospital. *N Engl J Med* 1998; 339: 1595–1601.
8. Carpenter TC, Stenmark KR. High-dose epinephrine is not superior to standard-dose epinephrine in pediatric in-hospital cardiopulmonary arrest. *Pediatrics* 1997; 99: 403–8.
9. McCrirrick A, Monk CR. Comparison of i.v. and intra-tracheal administration of adrenaline. *Br J Anaesth* 1994; 72: 529–32.

Anaphylactic shock. Anaphylactic shock is usually a type 1 hypersensitivity reaction (p.406) to various allergens such as drugs, foods, latex, and insect venoms. A clinically identical reaction can, however, be provoked by a type II mechanism, as in blood transfusion reactions, or a type III mechanism, as in drug-induced serum sickness reactions. It is a medical emergency and prompt treatment of laryngeal oedema, bronchospasm, and hypotension is necessary. Adrenaline [epinephrine] is the cornerstone of management[1-8] although it may not always be effective.[3]

In early anaphylaxis, vasodilatation is the main pathological change and cardiac output and blood flow to skin and muscle may be increased enabling subcutaneous and intramuscular absorption of adrenaline [epinephrine] to be sufficiently rapid and effective.[1] The intramuscular route is generally preferred although the subcutaneous route may be used, especially by patients treating themselves. Prefilled syringes for intramuscular or subcutaneous administration of adrenaline [epinephrine] are available for those known to be at high risk of developing anaphylactic shock. Such syringes mean that patients can self-administer their initial emergency treatment; they should still seek medical assistance as additional treatment may be required.[3] In the early stages adrenaline [epinephrine] may be administered by inhalation and is sometimes taken with an antihistamine.[9] However, this should not be a substitute for the administration of adrenaline [epinephrine] by injection in patients with a history of acute attacks, and the number of inhalations required may limit the use of this route in children.[10] As anaphylaxis progresses the intravascular volume becomes depleted, shock occurs, and at this stage the intravenous route is probably necessary to enable absorption.[1] The general principles used in the management of hypovolaemia and hypotension in shock are outlined on p.813.

The dose of adrenaline [epinephrine] for intramuscular injection is usually 0.5 mg (0.5 mL of a 1 in 1000 solution) which may be repeated at 5-minute intervals, according to blood pressure and pulse, until improvement occurs. Some use lower doses of 0.2 to 0.5 mg (0.2 to 0.5 mL of a 1 in 1000 solution) for intramuscular or subcutaneous injection. A more dilute solution of 1 in 10 000 is used for slow intravenous administration when the dose is 500 μg (5 mL) given at a rate of 100 μg (1 mL) per minute, stopping when a response has been obtained. Various adrenaline [epinephrine] dosage regimens have been suggested for children.[2-5,7] In one widely used regimen, the intramuscular dose for children using the 1 in 1000 solution ranges from: 50 μg (0.05 mL) for those under 6 months; 120 μg (0.12 mL) for those aged 6 months to 6 years; and 250 μg (0.25 mL) for children aged 6 to 12 years. The intravenous dose for children, employing the 1 in 10 000 solution, is 10 μg (0.1 mL) per kg body-weight.

A slow intravenous injection of an antihistamine, such as chlorpheniramine [chlorphenamine] 10 to 20 mg, may be given immediately after the adrenaline [epinephrine] and repeated over the subsequent 24 to 48 hours to prevent relapse. Although antihistamines are particularly effective in the management of angioedema, pruritus, and urticaria, they remain second-line treatment. Intravenous corticosteroids have little place in the immediate management of anaphylaxis, since their beneficial effects are delayed for several hours but in severely ill patients early administration of hydrocortisone 100 to 300 mg as the sodium succinate may help prevent deterioration after the primary treatment has been given. Also some consider that asthmatics who have relatively recently undergone regular corticosteroid treatment may benefit from hydrocortisone.[3] Patients should also receive oxygen as required.

Continuing deterioration with circulatory collapse, bronchospasm, or laryngeal oedema requires further treatment including intravenous fluids, intravenous aminophylline, a nebulised beta$_2$ agonist (such as salbutamol or terbutaline), assisted respiration (if necessary), and possibly, emergency tracheostomy. Noradrenaline [norepinephrine] may be necessary if the hypotension does not respond to adrenaline [epinephrine] and intravenous fluids.[2]

It should be remembered that patients receiving some non-cardioselective beta blockers may be relatively refractory to the effects of adrenaline [epinephrine] used for anaphylactic shock (see under Interactions for Adrenaline, above); in such cases the use of a more selective beta$_2$ agonist such as salbutamol by intravenous injection should be considered. Glucagon is another alternative to adrenaline [epinephrine] in such patients.[2,8,11]

Other measures to prevent anaphylaxis include desensitisation in patients who have reacted to bee or wasp venom.[12]

1. Fisher M. Treating anaphylaxis with sympathomimetic drugs. *BMJ* 1992; 305: 1107–8.
2. Anonymous. Adrenaline for anaphylaxis. *Drug Ther Bull* 1994; 32: 19–21.
3. Patel L, *et al.* Management of anaphylactic reactions to food. *Arch Dis Child* 1994; 71: 370–5.
4. Fisher M. Treatment of acute anaphylaxis. *BMJ* 1995; 311: 731–3. Correction. *ibid.*; 937.
5. Ewan PW. Anaphylaxis. *BMJ* 1998; 316: 1442–5. Correction. *ibid.*; 1587.
6. Ewan PW. Treatment of anaphylactic reactions. *Prescribers' J* 1997; 37: 125–32.
7. Project Team of the Resuscitation Council (UK). Emergency medical treatment of anaphylactic reactions. *J Accid Emerg Med* 1999; 16: 243–7.
8. The American Heart Association in collaboration with the International Liaison Committee on Resuscitation. Guidelines 2000 for cardiopulmonary resuscitation and emergency cardiovascular care. Part 8: advanced challenges in resuscitation: section 3: special challenges in ECC. *Circulation* 2000; 102 (suppl I): I229–1252.
9. Hourihane JO'B, Warner JO. Management of anaphylactic reactions to food. *Arch Dis Child* 1995; 72: 274.
10. Simons FER, *et al.* Can epinephrine inhalations be substituted for epinephrine injection in children at risk for systemic anaphylaxis? *Pediatrics* 2000; 106: 1040–4.
11. Lang DM. Anaphylactoid and anaphylactic reactions: hazards of β-blockers. *Drug Safety* 1995; 12: 299–304.
12. Frew AJ, *et al.* Injection immunotherapy. *BMJ* 1993; 307: 919–23.

Haemorrhage. Adrenaline [epinephrine] has a long history of being applied topically to check minor bleeding. It constricts arterioles and capillaries and causes blanching. Local injection of adrenaline [epinephrine] under endoscopic control is highly effective in controlling bleeding peptic ulcers (p.1208), and has also been combined with other therapies such as a contact thermal probe.[1]

1. Chung SSC, *et al.* Randomised comparison between adrenaline injection alone and adrenaline injection plus heat probe treatment for actively bleeding ulcers. *BMJ* 1997; 314: 1307–11.

Priapism. Aspiration of blood followed by intracavernosal irrigation with a dilute adrenaline [epinephrine] solution was reported to be effective treatment for priapism in a group of young patients (age range, 3.9 to 18.3 years) with sickle-cell disease.[1]

For reference to adrenaline [epinephrine] in low dosage and dilute solution being given by intracavernosal injection to reverse priapism caused by alprostadil, see p.1440.

1. Mantadakis E, *et al.* Outpatient penile aspiration and epinephrine irrigation for young patients with sickle cell anemia and prolonged priapism. *Blood* 2000; 95: 78–82.

Preparations

BP 2001: Adrenaline Eye Drops; Adrenaline Injection; Adrenaline Solution; Bupivacaine and Adrenaline Injection; Dilute Adrenaline Injection 1 in 10,000; Lidocaine and Adrenaline Injection;
USP 25: Cocaine and Tetracaine Hydrochlorides and Epinephrine Topical Solution; Epinephrine Bitartrate for Ophthalmic Solution; Epinephrine Bitartrate Inhalation Aerosol; Epinephrine Bitartrate Ophthalmic Solution; Epinephrine Inhalation Solution; Epinephrine Injection; Epinephrine Nasal Solution; Epinephrine Ophthalmic Solution; Epinephryl Borate Ophthalmic Solution; Lidocaine Hydrochloride and Epinephrine Injection; Prilocaine and Epinephrine Injection; Procaine Hydrochloride and Epinephrine Injection; Racepinephrine Inhalation Solution.

Proprietary Preparations (details are given in Part 3)
Aust.: Epipen; Eppystabil†; Glycirenan; Suprarenin; *Austral.:* Epipen; Medihaler-Epi†; *Belg.:* Epipen; *Canad.:* Bronkaid; Epi EZ†; Epifrin; Epipen; Vaponefrin; *Denm.:* Epipen; *Fin.:* Epipen; *Fr.:* Anahelp; Anakit; Anapen; Dyspne-Inhal; Eppy†; *Ger.:* Anaphylaxie-Besteck; Fastjekt; InfectoKrupp; Suprarenin; *Irl.:* Eppy; Simplene†; *Israel:* Epipen; *Ital.:* Eppy†; Fastjekt; Mex.: Pinadrina; *Norw.:* Epipen; *NZ:* Epipen; *Port.:* Anapen; *S.Afr.:* Ana-Guard; Epifrin†; Epipen; Eppy†; Medihaler-Epi†; Simplene†; *Spain:* Adreject; *Swed.:* Epipen; Eppy; Glaufrin†; *Switz.:* Epipen; Gingi-Pak†; Medihaler-Epi†; Orostat†; Surgident†; *UK:* Anapen; Epipen; Eppy; Medihaler-Epi†; Simplene†; *USA:* AsthmaHaler Mist; AsthmaNefrin; Bronitin Mist†; Epifrin; Epinal; Epipen; Eppy/N†; Glaucon; microNefrin; Nephron; Primatene Mist; Primatene Mist Suspension; S-2; Sus-Phrine; Vaponefrin†.

Multi-ingredient: *Austral.:* Rectinol; *Belg.:* Glaucofrin†; *Braz.:* Novaboin; *Canad.:* Ana-Kit; E-Pilo†; *Denm.:* Suprexon†; *Fr.:* Glaucadrine; Sirop Boint†; *Ger.:* Mydrial-Atropin; Suprexon; *Irl.:* Ganda; *Ital.:* Pilodren; Rinantipiol; *Neth.:* Glaucofrin†; Suprexon; *NZ:* Ana-Kit; *Port.:* Adrinex; *S.Afr.:* Ganda†; *Spain:* Coliriocilina Adren Astr; Epistaxol; *Switz.:* Glaucadrine†; Haemocortin; Medi-Kord†; Suprexon†; *UK:* Ganda; *USA:* Ana-Kit; Bronkaid Mist†; E-Pilo; Emergent-Ez; PE†.

Used as an adjunct in: Aust.: Carbostesin; Neo-Xylestesin; Neo-Xylestesin forte and Neo-Xylestesin special; Scandonest; Ubistesin; Ultracain Dental; Xylanaest; Xylocain; *Austral.:* Lignospan; Marcain; Nurocain; Nurocain with Sympathin; Scandonest; Xylocaine; *Belg.:* Citanest; Marcaine; Xylocaine; *Braz.:* Marcaina; Xylestesin; Xylocaina; *Canad.:* Astracaine; Citanest; Marcaine; Sensorcaine; Ultracaine D-S; Xylocaine; *Denm.:* Carbocain; Marcain; Scandonest; Xylocain; *Fin.:* Marcain; Ultracain D-Suprarenin; Xylocain; *Fr.:* Alphacaine; Duranest; Marcaine; Predesic; Xylocaine; *Ger.:* Anaesthol†; Carbostesin; Lidocaton†; Meaverin "A" mit Adrenalin†; Scandicain; Ubistesin; Ultracain D-S; Ultracain-Suprarenin; Xylestesin-A, Xylestesin centro; Xylestesin-S; Xylocain; *Hong Kong:* Marcaine; Xylocain; Xylocitin; Xylonest; Zingel; *Irl.:* Marcain; Xylocaine; *Israel:* Marcaine; *Ital.:* Bupiforan; Bupyl; Carbocaina; Cartidont; Citocartin; Ecocain; Lident Adrenalina; Lident Andrenor; Marcaina; Mepi-Mynol; Mepicain; Mepident; Mepiforan; Mepyl; Optocain; Scandonest;

Septanest; Ubistesin; Ultracain D-S; Xilo-Mynol; Xylocaina; Xylonor; *Mex.:* Buvacaina; Pisacaina; Xlyocaina; *Neth.:* Citanest; Marcaine; Scandicaine; Ultracain D-S; Xylocaine; *Norw.:* Marcain; Xylocain; *NZ:* Marcain; Nurocain; Xylocaine; *Port.:* Lincaina; Marcaina†; Scandinibsa; Xilonibsa; Xylocaina†; *S.Afr.:* Lignospan Special; Macaine; Scandonest; Xylotox; *Singapore:* Xylocaine; *Spain:* Anestesia Loc Braun C/A; Anestesia Topi Braun C/A; Meganest; Scandinibsa; Stoma Anestesia Dental; Ultracain; Xilonibsa; Xylonor Especial; *Swed.:* Carbocain; Citanest; Marcain; Xylocain; *Switz.:* Carbostesin; Lidocain†; Lignospan; Rapidocaine; Rudocaine; Scandicain; Scandonest; Septanest; Ubistesin; Ultracaine D-S; Xylestesin-S "special"; Xylocain; Xylonest; Xylonor†; *Thai.:* Lidocation; Lidocain; Marcaine; Xylocaine; *UAE:* Ecocain; *UK:* AccuSite†; Lignostab-A; Marcain; Septanest; Xylocaine; Xylotox; *USA:* Citanest; Duranest; Marcaine; Octocaine; Sensorcaine; Septocaine; Xylocaine.

Ajmaline (7777-b)

Ajmaline; Ajmalinum; Rauwolfine. (17R,21R)-Ajmalan-17,21-diol.

$C_{20}H_{26}N_2O_2 = 326.4.$
CAS — 4360-12-7.
ATC — C01BA05.

Pharmacopoeias. In Aust., It., and Jpn.
Aust. and It. also include Ajmaline Monohydrate and Ajmaline Monoethanolate.

Ajmaline is an alkaloid obtained from the root of *Rauwolfia serpentina* (Apocynaceae).

Adverse Effects

Ajmaline depresses the conductivity of the heart, and at high doses can cause heart block. At very high doses it may produce a negative inotropic effect. High doses may cause cardiac arrhythmias, coma, and death. Arrhythmias have also been reported after usual intravenous doses (see below). Adverse neurological effects have been reported including eye twitching, convulsions, and respiratory depression. Hepatotoxicity and agranulocytosis may occasionally occur.

Effects on the heart. Electrophysiologic study[1] in 1955 patients revealed that ajmaline 1 mg per kg body-weight given intravenously could induce arrhythmias; 63 developed a supraventricular arrhythmia and 7 an atrioventricular re-entrant tachycardia.

1. Brembilla-Perrot B, Terrier de la Chaise A. Provocation of supraventricular tachycardias by an intravenous class I antiarrhythmic drug. *Int J Cardiol* 1992; **34:** 189–98.

Precautions
As for Quinidine, p.965.

Interactions

Antiarrhythmics. Oral administration of *quinidine* with ajmaline gave considerably increased plasma concentrations of ajmaline in 4 healthy subjects; the elimination half-life of ajmaline was increased about twofold.[1] The pharmacokinetics of quinidine did not seem to be affected by ajmaline.

1. Hori R, *et al.* Quinidine-induced rise in ajmaline plasma concentration. *J Pharm Pharmacol* 1984; **36:** 202–4.

Uses and Administration
Ajmaline is a class Ia antiarrhythmic (p.787). It is used in the treatment of supraventricular and ventricular arrhythmias (p.794). Ajmaline has been given by mouth in a dose of 100 to 300 mg daily. It has also been given by intravenous injection in a dose of 1 mg per kg body-weight at a maximum rate of 10 mg per minute, or by intramuscular injection in a dose of 50 to 150 mg daily.

Ajmaline has also been used as the hydrochloride, monoethanolate, and as the phenobarbital salt.

Preparations

Proprietary Preparations (details are given in Part 3)
Aust.: Gilurytmal; *Ger.:* Gilurytmal; Tachmalin†; *Ital.:* Aritminat†; *Spain:* Gilurytmal.
Multi-ingredient: *Spain:* Diu Rauwiplus.

Alacepril (18737-x)

Alacepril (rINN).

DU-1219. N-{1-[(S)-3-Mercapto-2-methylpropionyl]-L-prolyl}-3-phenyl-L-alanine acetate (ester).
$C_{20}H_{26}N_2O_5S = 406.5.$
CAS — 74258-86-9.

Profile
Alacepril is an ACE inhibitor (p.820) used in the treatment of hypertension (p.802). It is converted to captopril and desacetylalacepril (DU-1227) in the body following oral administration. It is given by mouth in a usual dose of 25 to 75 mg daily, as a single dose or in two divided doses.

Preparations

Proprietary Preparations (details are given in Part 3)
Jpn: Cetapril.

Alfuzosin Hydrochloride (12287-p)

Alfuzosin Hydrochloride (BANM, USAN, rINNM).

Alfuzosini Hydrochloridum; SL-77499-10; SL-77499 (alfuzosin). N-{3-[4-Amino-6,7-dimethoxyquinazolin-2-yl(methyl)amino]propyl}tetrahydro-2-furamide hydrochloride.

$C_{19}H_{27}N_5O_4,HCl = 425.9.$
CAS — 81403-80-7 (alfuzosin); 81403-68-1 (alfuzosin hydrochloride).

Pharmacopoeias. In Eur. (see p.vi).

Pharmacopoeial description

Ph. Eur.: A white or almost white, slightly hygroscopic, crystalline powder. Freely soluble in water; sparingly soluble in alcohol; practically insoluble in dichloromethane. A 2% solution in water has a pH of 4.0 to 6.0. Store in airtight containers. Protect from light.

Adverse Effects, Treatment, and Precautions

As for Prazosin Hydrochloride, p.958. Alfuzosin may be more selective for the urinary tract and vasodilator effects may be less frequent. It should be avoided in severe hepatic impairment.

◊ References.

1. Lukacs B, *et al.* Safety profile of 3 months' therapy with alfuzosin in 13,389 patients suffering from benign prostatic hypertrophy. *Eur Urol* 1996; **29:** 29–35.

Pharmacokinetics
Alfuzosin is readily absorbed after oral administration and peak plasma concentrations generally occur 0.5 to 3 hours after a dose; bioavailability is about 64%. It is extensively metabolised in the liver to inactive metabolites and excreted primarily in faeces via the bile. Only about 11% of a dose is excreted unchanged in the urine. Alfuzosin has a plasma elimination half-life of 3 to 5 hours. It is 90% bound to plasma proteins.

◊ References.

1. Scott MG, *et al.* Haemodynamic and pharmacokinetic evaluation of alfuzosin in man: a dose ranging study and comparison with prazosin. *Eur J Clin Pharmacol* 1989; **37:** 53–8.

Uses and Administration
Alfuzosin is an alpha$_1$-adrenoceptor blocker (p.787) with actions similar to those of prazosin (p.959). It is used in benign prostatic hyperplasia (p.1477) to relieve symptoms of urinary obstruction and has been tried in the treatment of hypertension.

Alfuzosin is given by mouth as the hydrochloride. Like other alpha$_1$-adrenoceptor blockers, it may cause collapse in some patients after the first dose, which should therefore be given just before bedtime to reduce the risk. In benign prostatic hyperplasia, the usual dose is 2.5 mg three times daily, increased to 10 mg daily if necessary. Doses may need to be reduced in patients with hepatic impairment. Dose reduction may also be necessary in the elderly and in those with renal impairment; alternatively, modified-release preparations may be preferred.

◊ References.

1. Jardin A, *et al.* Alfuzosin for treatment of benign prostatic hypertrophy. *Lancet* 1991; **337:** 1457–61.
2. Wilde MI, *et al.* Alfuzosin: a review of its pharmacodynamic and pharmacokinetic properties, and therapeutic potential in benign prostatic hyperplasia. *Drugs* 1993; **45:** 410–29.

Preparations

Proprietary Preparations (details are given in Part 3)
Aust.: Xatral; *Belg.:* Xatral; *Braz.:* Xatral; *Denm.:* Xatral; *Fin.:* Xatral; *Fr.:* Urion; Xatral; *Ger.:* Urion; UroXatral; *Hong Kong:* Xatral; *Irl.:* Xatral; *Israel:* Xatral; *Ital.:* Benestan; Mittoval; Xatral; *Neth.:* Xatral; *Norw.:* Xatral; *Port.:* Benestan; *Singapore:* Xatral; *Spain:* Alfetim; Benestan; Dalfaz; *Swed.:* Xatral; *Switz.:* Xatral; *Thai.:* Xatral; *UK:* Xatral.

Alprenolol (20398-z)

Alprenolol (BAN, rINN).

1-(2-Allylphenoxy)-3-isopropylaminopropan-2-ol.
$C_{15}H_{23}NO_2 = 249.3.$
CAS — 13655-52-2.
ATC — C07AA01.

Alprenolol Benzoate (15827-r)

Alprenolol Benzoate (BANM, rINNM).

Alprenololi Benzoas. (±)-1-(2-Allylphenoxy)-3-isopropylaminopropan-2-ol benzoate.
$C_{22}H_{29}NO_4 = 371.5.$

Alprenolol Hydrochloride (6303-p)

Alprenolol Hydrochloride (BANM, USAN, rINNM).

Alprenololi Hydrochloridum; H56/28. (±)-1-(2-Allylphenoxy)-3-isopropylaminopropan-2-ol hydrochloride.
$C_{15}H_{23}NO_2,HCl = 285.8.$
CAS — 13707-88-5.

Pharmacopoeias. In Eur. (see p.vi) and Jpn.

Pharmacopoeial description

Ph. Eur.: A white crystalline powder or colourless crystals. Very soluble in water; freely soluble in alcohol and in dichloromethane. Protect from light.

Adverse Effects, Treatment, and Precautions

As for beta blockers, p.844.

Hypersensitivity. A report of contact eczema in workers exposed to alprenolol.[1]

1. Ekenvall L, Forsbeck M. Contact eczema produced by a β-adrenergic blocking agent (alprenolol). *Contact Dermatitis* 1978; **4:** 190–4.

Interactions
The interactions associated with beta blockers are discussed on p.846.

Pharmacokinetics
Alprenolol is almost completely absorbed from the gastrointestinal tract but is subject to considerable first-pass metabolism in the liver. Peak plasma concentrations are achieved about 1 hour after a dose. It has high lipid solubility. Alprenolol is about 85% bound to plasma proteins. It is distributed into breast milk. It is metabolised in the liver, primarily to 4-hydroxyalprenolol, which is active. The plasma half-life of alprenolol is about 3 hours and the plasma half-life of 4-hydroxyalprenolol is about 20 minutes. It is excreted in the urine mainly in the form of its metabolites.

Uses and Administration
Alprenolol is a non-cardioselective beta blocker (p.844). It is reported to have intrinsic sympathomimetic activity and some membrane-stabilising properties.

Alprenolol is used in the management of hypertension (p.802), angina pectoris (p.791), and cardiac arrhythmias (p.794).

It is given by mouth, as the benzoate or hydrochloride; doses have been expressed in terms of the base or of the hydrochloride.

In **hypertension** the usual initial dose is 200 mg daily, in divided doses by mouth, increased weekly according to the response of the patient up to a total of 800 mg daily in divided doses. The usual dose for **angina pectoris**, **cardiac arrhythmias**, and other cardiac disorders is 200 to 400 mg daily in divided doses. It may be necessary to reduce the dose in patients with renal or hepatic impairment.

Preparations

Proprietary Preparations (details are given in Part 3)
Austral.: Aptin†; *Belg.:* Aptine†; *Denm.:* Aptin†; *Ger.:* Aptin; *Neth.:* Aptine†; *Norw.:* Aptin†; *Swed.:* Aptin N†.

Alteplase (16956-z)

Alteplase (BAN, USAN, rINN).

G-11035; G-11044; G-11021 (2-chain form); Recombinant Tissue-type Plasminogen Activator; rt-PA.
CAS — 105857-23-6.
ATC — B01AD02; S01XA13.

Pharmacopoeias. In US. Eur. (see p.vi) includes Alteplase for Injection.

A glycosylated protein of 527 residues having the amino acid sequence of human tissue plasminogen activator (t-PA) and produced by recombinant DNA technology.

The symbol † denotes a preparation no longer actively marketed

Pharmacopoeial description

Ph. Eur.: Alteplase for Injection is a sterile, freeze-dried preparation of alteplase, a tissue plasminogen activator produced by recombinant DNA technology. It has a potency of not less than 500 000 units per mg of protein. It is a white or slightly yellow powder or friable mass. The reconstituted preparation has a pH of 7.1 to 7.5. Store in colourless glass containers, under vacuum or an inert gas, at a temperature between 2° and 30°. Protect from light. Alteplase consists of 527 amino acids with carbohydrate moieties attached.

USP 25: A highly purified glycosylated serine protease with fibrin-binding properties and plasminogen-specific proteolytic activities. It is produced by recombinant DNA technology. It has a potency of 522 000 to 667 000 USP units per mg of protein. Store in sealed containers, in the frozen state at a temperature of −20° or below.

◊ Incompatibility has been reported[1] between alteplase and dobutamine, dopamine, glyceryl trinitrate, and heparin, although a subsequent study found no incompatibility between alteplase and glyceryl trinitrate.[2] Another study[3] found that dilution of a proprietary preparation of alteplase (Activase) to 0.09 and 0.16 mg per mL with glucose 5% resulted in precipitation of the drug. Alteplase is formulated with arginine as a solubilising agent, and dilution with glucose 5% to concentrations below 0.5 mg of alteplase per mL makes precipitation possible. Dilution with sodium chloride 0.9% is possible to concentrations down to 0.2 mg per mL before precipitation becomes a risk. Studies[4,5] have suggested that a 1 mg per mL solution of alteplase retains its activity when frozen at −20° or below for up to 6 months.

1. Lee CY, *et al.* Visual and spectrophotometric determination of compatibility of alteplase and streptokinase with other injectable drugs. *Am J Hosp Pharm* 1990; **47:** 606–8.
2. Lam XM, *et al.* Stability and activity of alteplase with injectable drugs commonly used in cardiac therapy. *Am J Health-Syst Pharm* 1995; **52:** 1904–9.
3. Frazin BS. Maximal dilution of Activase. *Am J Hosp Pharm* 1990; **47:** 1016.
4. Calis KA, *et al.* Bioactivity of cryopreserved alteplase solutions. *Am J Health-Syst Pharm* 1999; **56:** 2056–7.
5. Wiernikowski JT, *et al.* Stability and sterility of recombinant tissue plasminogen activator at −30°C. *Lancet* 2000; **355:** 2221–2.

Units

The activity of alteplase can be measured in terms of international units using the second International Standard for tissue plasminogen activator established in 1987, although doses are generally expressed by weight. The specific activity of alteplase is 580 000 international units per mg.

Adverse Effects, Treatment, and Precautions

As for Streptokinase, p.976. Allergic reactions are less likely with alteplase than with streptokinase and repeated administration is possible.

◊ Infusion of alteplase produces considerable thrombin generation which may result from direct activation of the coagulation system by fibrinolysin (human) or by positive feedback of the coagulation system by clot-bound thrombin. This excessive thrombin generation was considered a possible cause of myocardial infarction in a patient undergoing thrombolytic therapy with alteplase for venous thrombosis.[1] Infusion of streptokinase produced no evidence of excessive thrombin generation.

1. Baglin TP, *et al.* Thrombin generation and myocardial infarction during infusion of tissue-plasminogen activator. *Lancet* 1993; **341:** 504–5.

Hypersensitivity. An anaphylactoid reaction to alteplase occurred in a patient with a history of atopy.[1] For comment on this unexpected reaction, see Hypersensitivity under the Adverse Effects of Streptokinase, p.977.

1. Purvis JA, *et al.* Anaphylactoid reaction after injection of alteplase. *Lancet* 1993; **341:** 966–7.

Interactions

As for Streptokinase, p.977.

Glyceryl trinitrate. Although thrombolytics and nitrates are both frequently used in acute myocardial infarction a report suggested that this combination may result in impaired thrombolysis. Concurrent intravenous administration of alteplase and glyceryl trinitrate to 36 patients with acute myocardial infarction produced lower plasma-antigen concentrations of tissue-plasminogen activator than alteplase given alone to 11 patients.[1] Reperfusion was sustained in only 44% of patients receiving both drugs compared with 91% of patients receiving alteplase alone. The authors of a subsequent study[2] suggested that these lower plasma concentrations may be due to increased hepatic metabolism of alteplase as a result of glyceryl trinitrate's effect of increasing hepatic blood flow.

1. Nicolini FA, *et al.* Concurrent nitroglycerin therapy impairs tissue-type plasminogen activator-induced thrombolysis in patients with acute myocardial infarction. *Am J Cardiol* 1994; **74:** 662–6.
2. Romeo F, *et al.* Concurrent nitroglycerin administration reduces the efficacy of recombinant tissue-type plasminogen activator in patients with acute anterior wall myocardial infarction. *Am Heart J* 1995; **130:** 692–7.

Pharmacokinetics

Alteplase is cleared rapidly from the plasma, mainly by metabolism in the liver.

◊ References.
1. Krause J. Catabolism of tissue-type plasminogen activator (t-PA), its variants, mutants and hybrids. *Fibrinolysis* 1988; **2:** 133–42.

Uses and Administration

Alteplase is a thrombolytic drug. It is a predominantly single-chain form of the endogenous enzyme tissue plasminogen activator and is produced by recombinant DNA technology. Like endogenous tissue plasminogen activator, alteplase converts fibrin-bound plasminogen to the active form fibrinolysin, resulting in fibrinolysis and dissolution of clots. The mechanisms of fibrinolysis are discussed further under Haemostasis and Fibrinolysis on p.718. Alteplase has relatively little effect on circulating, unbound plasminogen and thus may be termed a fibrin-specific agent. Fibrin specificity was thought to be required for reducing the risk of haemorrhage associated with the use of thrombolytics, although currently available fibrin-specific agents do not produce less bleeding than non-specific thrombolytics (see Haemorrhage under Adverse Effects of Streptokinase, p.976).

Alteplase is used similarly to streptokinase (p.977) in the treatment of thromboembolic disorders, particularly myocardial infarction (p.805) and venous thromboembolism (p.817). Alteplase may also be used in patients with acute ischaemic stroke (p.813).

In the treatment of acute **myocardial infarction**, alteplase is given intravenously as soon as possible after the onset of symptoms in a total dose of 100 mg; the total dose should not exceed 1.5 mg per kg body-weight in patients weighing less than 65 kg. The total dose of 100 mg may be given either over 1½ hours (accelerated or 'front-loaded' alteplase) or over 3 hours. The accelerated schedule has been recommended where administration is within 6 hours of myocardial infarction, while the 3-hour schedule has been recommended where administration is more than 6 hours after myocardial infarction. Administration over 1½ hours is as follows: 15 mg as an intravenous bolus, then 0.75 mg per kg body-weight, up to a maximum of 50 mg, by intravenous infusion over 30 minutes, followed by the remainder infused over the subsequent 60 minutes. Administration over 3 hours is as follows: 10 mg as an intravenous bolus, then 50 mg by intravenous infusion over 1 hour, followed by a further 40 mg infused over the subsequent 2 hours.

In the treatment of **pulmonary embolism** a total dose of 100 mg is given with the first 10 mg as an intravenous bolus and the remaining 90 mg by intravenous infusion over 2 hours; the total dose should not exceed 1.5 mg per kg in patients weighing less than 65 kg.

In acute **ischaemic stroke**, alteplase is given within 3 hours of the onset of symptoms in a dose of 0.9 mg per kg up to a maximum total dose of 90 mg. The dose is administered intravenously over 60 minutes with 10% being given as a bolus during the first minute.

◊ General references.
1. Gillis JC, *et al.* Alteplase: a reappraisal of its pharmacological properties and therapeutic use in acute myocardial infarction. *Drugs* 1995; **50:** 102–36.
2. Wagstaff AJ, *et al.* Alteplase: a reappraisal of its pharmacology and therapeutic use in vascular disorders other than acute myocardial infarction. *Drugs* 1995; **50:** 289–316.

Catheters and cannulas. Alteplase has been used successfully to clear thrombi in central venous catheters.[1,2] Doses typically employed have been 2 mg injected as a bolus into the blocked catheter. In two children[3] alteplase in doses of 0.01 to 0.05 mg per kg body-weight per hour intravenously has been used for venous thrombosis associated with indwelling intravascular catheters.

1. Paulsen D, *et al.* Use of tissue plasminogen activator for reopening of clotted dialysis catheters. *Nephron* 1993; **64:** 468–9.
2. Haire WD, *et al.* Urokinase versus recombinant tissue plasminogen activator in thrombosed central venous catheters: a double-blinded, randomized trial. *Thromb Haemost* 1994; **72:** 543–7.
3. Doyle E, *et al.* Thrombolysis with low dose tissue plasminogen activator. *Arch Dis Child* 1992; **67:** 1483–4.

Intracardiac thrombosis. Alteplase has been used, in a dose of 100 mg given intravenously over two hours, for thrombosis of prosthetic heart valves.[1]

Alteplase has been used successfully in a neonate to treat intracardiac thrombosis associated with the use of a central venous line.[2] A dose of 0.5 mg per kg body-weight given over 10 minutes was followed by infusion of 0.2 mg per kg per hour for three days.

1. Astengo D, *et al.* Recombinant tissue plasminogen activator for prosthetic mitral-valve thrombosis. *N Engl J Med* 1995; **333:** 259.
2. Van Overmeire B, *et al.* Intracardiac thrombus formation with rapidly progressive heart failure in the neonate: treatment with tissue type plasminogen activator. *Arch Dis Child* 1992; **67:** 443–5.

Microvessel thrombosis. Alteplase has been used in a number of conditions where the underlying pathology is occlusion of small blood vessels by microthrombi.

Purpura and loss of circulation in the hands of a patient recovering from **fulminant meningococcaemia**[1] responded to intra-arterial infusion of alteplase 0.02 to 0.04 mg per kg body-weight per hour for 22 hours in the right hand, and 0.02 mg per kg per hour for 11 hours in the left. Perfusion was successfully restored to both hands, and full function subsequently attained in them. Improvement was also achieved when alteplase was given to 2 infants with septic shock and purpura fulminans caused by meningococcal infection.[2]

Six patients[3] with ulcers caused by **livedoid vasculitis** and refractory to conventional treatment were treated with alteplase 10 mg infused intravenously over 4 hours daily for 14 days. Most ulcers healed rapidly; one patient required re-treatment with concomitant anticoagulation.

A 4-year-old girl[4] with **haemolytic uraemic syndrome** (see under Thrombotic Microangiopathies, p.740) responded to treatment with an intravenous infusion of alteplase 0.2 mg per kg per hour for 5 hours, subsequently reduced to 0.05 mg per kg per hour for 14 days.

Alteplase has been tried with mixed results[5-7] in a few patients with **veno-occlusive disease of the liver**, a serious complication of bone-marrow transplantation that may be caused by diffuse thrombi in the hepatic venules.

1. Keeley SR, *et al.* Tissue plasminogen activator for gangrene in fulminant meningococcaemia. *Lancet* 1991; **337:** 1359.
2. Zenz W, *et al.* Recombinant tissue plasminogen activator treatment in two infants with fulminant meningococcemia. *Pediatrics* 1995; **96:** 144–8.
3. Klein KL, Pittelkow MR. Tissue plasminogen activator for treatment of livedoid vasculitis. *Mayo Clin Proc* 1992; **67:** 923–33.
4. Kruez W, *et al.* Successful treatment of haemolytic uraemic syndrome with recombinant tissue-type plasminogen activator. *Lancet* 1993; **341:** 1665–6.
5. Laporte JP, *et al.* Alteplase for hepatic veno-occlusive disease complicating bone-marrow transplantation. *Lancet* 1992; **339:** 1057.
6. Rosti G, *et al.* Alteplase for hepatic veno-occlusive disease after bone-marrow transplantation. *Lancet* 1992; **339:** 1481–2.
7. Ringdén O, *et al.* Alteplase for hepatic veno-occlusive disease after bone-marrow transplantation. *Lancet* 1992; **340:** 546–7.

Ocular fibrinolysis. Intra-ocular alteplase has been used to treat postoperative fibrinous deposits that can form after procedures such as surgery for cataracts[1] or glaucoma,[2] including cataracts in children.[3] Doses ranging from 6 to 25 μg have been used. Intra-ocular bleeding has occurred as a complication of such use.[2,4]

1. Heiligenhaus A, *et al.* Recombinant tissue plasminogen activator in cases with fibrin formation after cataract surgery: a prospective randomised multicentre study. *Br J Ophthalmol* 1998; **82:** 810–15.
2. Lundy DC, *et al.* Intracameral tissue plasminogen activator after glaucoma surgery: indications, effectiveness, and complications. *Ophthalmology* 1996; **103:** 274–82.
3. Mehta JS, Adams GGW. Recombinant tissue plasminogen activator following paediatric cataract surgery. *Br J Ophthalmol* 2000; **84:** 983–6.
4. Azuara-Blanco A, Wilson RP. Intraocular and extraocular bleeding after intracameral injection of tissue plasminogen activator. *Br J Ophthalmol* 1998; **82:** 1345–6.

Peripheral arterial thromboembolism. Thrombolytics, including alteplase, may be used in the management of peripheral arterial thromboembolism (p.808). Alteplase has been injected intravenously or intra-arterially directly into the clot as an alternative to surgical treatment of the occlusion. It has also been infused intra-arterially to remove distal clots during a surgical procedure. Alteplase is claimed to produce more rapid thrombolysis than streptokinase although studies have been too small to provide evidence of reduced limb loss or mortality.[1] The most common dose range is 0.5 to 1 mg per hour given *intra-arterially*.[1-3]

An *intravenous* dose of 0.5 mg per kg body-weight per hour for the first hour followed by 0.25 mg per kg per hour until clot lysis occurred has been used in infants.[4] Treatment of arterial thrombosis in neonates has been reported, using doses of alteplase ranging from 0.1 to 0.5 mg per kg per hour *intravenously*.[5,6]

Where a thrombolytic is used to remove distal clots during a surgical procedure alteplase has been given *intra-arterially* as three doses of 5 mg at 10-minute intervals.[7]

1. Wolfe JH. Critical limb ischaemia. *Prescribers' J* 1994; **34:** 50–8.
2. Anonymous. Non-coronary thrombolysis. *Lancet* 1990; **335:** 691–3.

3. Ward AS, *et al.* Peripheral thrombolysis with tissue plasminogen activator: results of two treatment regimens. *Arch Surg* 1994; **129:** 861–5.
4. Zenz W, *et al.* Tissue plasminogen activator (alteplase) treatment for femoral artery thrombosis after cardiac catheterisation in infants and children. *Br Heart J* 1993; **70:** 382–5.
5. Weiner GM, *et al.* Successful treatment of neonatal arterial thromboses with recombinant tissue plasminogen activator. *J Pediatr* 1998; **133:** 133–6.
6. Farnoux C, *et al.* Recombinant tissue-type plasminogen activator therapy of thrombosis in 16 neonates. *J Pediatr* 1998; **133:** 137–40.
7. Chester JF, *et al.* Peroperative t-PA thrombolysis. *Lancet* 1991; **337:** 861–2.

Preparations

USP 25: Alteplase for Injection.

Proprietary Preparations (details are given in Part 3)
Aust.: Actilyse; Besopartin; *Austral.:* Actilyse; *Belg.:* Actilyse; *Braz.:* Actilyse; *Canad.:* Activase; *Denm.:* Actilyse; *Fr.:* Actilyse; *Ger.:* Actilyse; *Hong Kong:* Actilyse; *Irl.:* Actilyse; *Israel:* Actilyse; *Ital.:* Actilyse; Actiplas; *Mex.:* Actilyse; *Neth.:* Actilyse; *Norw.:* Actilyse; *NZ:* Actilyse; *Port.:* Actilyse; *S.Afr.:* Actilyse; *Singapore:* Actilyse; *Spain:* Actilyse; *Swed.:* Actilyse; *Switz.:* Actilyse; *Thai.:* Actilyse; *UK:* Actilyse; *USA:* Activase.

Multi-ingredient: *Fin.:* Actilyse.

Altizide   (12345-h)

Altizide *(rINN)*.

Althiazide *(USAN)*; P-1779. 3-Allylthiomethyl-6-chloro-3,4-dihydro-2*H*-1,2,4-benzothiadiazine-7-sulphonamide 1,1-dioxide.
$C_{11}H_{14}ClN_3O_4S_3 = 383.9$.
CAS — 5588-16-9.

Profile

Altizide is a thiazide diuretic (see Hydrochlorothiazide, p.907) that is used in the treatment of oedema and hypertension. It is frequently used in combination with spironolactone.

Preparations

Proprietary Preparations (details are given in Part 3)
Multi-ingredient: *Belg.:* Aldactazine; *Fr.:* Aldactazine; Practazin; Prinactizide; Spiroctazine; *Port.:* Aldactazine; *Spain:* Aldactacine.

Amezinium Metilsulfate   (12353-h)

Amezinium Metilsulfate *(rINN)*.

Amezinium Methylsulphate. 4-Amino-6-methoxy-1-phenylpyridazinium methylsulphate.
$C_{12}H_{15}N_3O_5S = 313.3$.
CAS — 30578-37-1.

Profile

Amezinium metilsulfate is a sympathomimetic (see Adrenaline, p.829) used for its vasopressor effects in the treatment of hypotensive states. It is given by mouth and also by slow intravenous injection.

Preparations

Proprietary Preparations (details are given in Part 3)
Belg.: Regulton; *Ger.:* Regulton†; Supratonin; *Jpn:* Risumic†.

Amiloride Hydrochloride   (2304-d)

Amiloride Hydrochloride *(BANM, USAN, rINNM)*.

Amiloridi Hydrochloridum; Amipramizide; Cloridrato de Amilorida; MK-870. N-Amidino-3,5-diamino-6-chloropyrazine-2-carboxamide hydrochloride dihydrate.
$C_6H_8ClN_7O,HCl,2H_2O = 302.1$.

CAS — 2609-46-3 (amiloride); 2016-88-8 (anhydrous amiloride hydrochloride); 17440-83-4 (amiloride hydrochloride dihydrate).

NOTE. Compounded preparations of amiloride hydrochloride may be represented by the following names:

• Co-amilofruse *(BAN)*—amiloride hydrochloride 1 part and frusemide [furosemide] 8 parts (w/w)

• Co-amilozide *(BAN)*—amiloride hydrochloride 1 part and hydrochlorothiazide 10 parts (w/w)

• Co-amilozide *(USP 25)*—amiloride hydrochloride and hydrochlorothiazide.

Pharmacopoeias. In *Eur.* (see p.vi), *Int.,* and *US.*

Pharmacopoeial description

Ph. Eur.: A pale yellow to greenish-yellow powder. Slightly soluble in water and in dehydrated alcohol; practically insoluble in ether. Protect from light.

USP 25: A yellow to greenish-yellow, odourless or practically odourless, powder. Slightly soluble in water; insoluble in acetone, in chloroform, in ether, and in ethyl acetate; freely soluble in dimethyl sulfoxide; sparingly soluble in methyl alcohol.

Adverse Effects

Amiloride can cause hyperkalaemia, particularly in elderly patients, diabetics, and patients with impaired

renal function. Hyponatraemia has been reported in patients receiving combination therapy with amiloride and other diuretics. Amiloride may cause nausea, vomiting, abdominal pain, diarrhoea or constipation, paraesthesia, thirst, dizziness, skin rash, pruritus, weakness, muscle cramps, headache, and minor psychiatric or visual changes. Orthostatic hypotension and rises in blood-urea-nitrogen concentrations have been reported.

Effects on electrolyte balance. Reports of metabolic acidosis associated with amiloride or triamterene[1] and with co-amilozide.[2]

1. Kushner RF, Sitrin MD. Metabolic acidosis: development in two patients receiving a potassium-sparing diuretic and total parenteral nutrition. *Arch Intern Med* 1986; **146:** 343–5.
2. Wan HH, Lye MDW. Moduretic-induced metabolic acidosis and hyperkalaemia. *Postgrad Med J* 1980; **56:** 348–50.

POTASSIUM. Hyperkalaemia is the main adverse effect when amiloride is given alone but may also occur when amiloride is given with a potassium-wasting diuretic. Severe hyperkalaemia has been reported during co-amilozide therapy, particularly in patients with impaired renal function[1,2] and has been accompanied by metabolic acidosis in one such patient.[3]

1. Whiting GFM, *et al.* Severe hyperkalaemia with Moduretic. *Med J Aust* 1979; **1:** 409.
2. Jaffey L, Martin A. Malignant hyperkalaemia after amiloride/hydrochlorothiazide treatment. *Lancet* 1981; **i:** 1272.
3. Wan HH, Lye MDW. Moduretic-induced metabolic acidosis and hyperkalaemia. *Postgrad Med J* 1980; **56:** 348–50.

SODIUM. For reports of severe hyponatraemia in patients taking amiloride with potassium-wasting diuretics, see Hydrochlorothiazide, p.908.

Effects on the skin. For a report of photosensitivity reactions in patients taking co-amilozide, see Hydrochlorothiazide, p.909.

Precautions

Amiloride has the same precautions as spironolactone with regard to hyperkalaemia (see p.974). It should be discontinued at least 3 days before glucose-tolerance tests are performed in patients who may have diabetes mellitus because of the risks of provoking severe hyperkalaemia.

Interactions

There is an increased risk of hyperkalaemia if amiloride is given concomitantly with potassium supplements or with other potassium-sparing diuretics. Hyperkalaemia may also occur in patients receiving ACE inhibitors, angiotensin II receptor antagonists, NSAIDs, ciclosporin, or trilostane concomitantly. In patients receiving amiloride with NSAIDs or ciclosporin the risk of nephrotoxicity may also be increased. Diuretics may reduce the excretion of lithium and increase the risk of lithium toxicity, but this does not appear to occur with amiloride. Severe hyponatraemia may occur in patients receiving a combination of potassium-sparing diuretic with a thiazide; this risk may be increased in patients receiving chlorpropamide. Amiloride may reduce the ulcer-healing properties of carbenoxolone. As with other diuretics, amiloride may enhance the effects of other antihypertensive drugs.

Digoxin. For the effects of amiloride on digoxin clearance, see p.872.

Quinidine. For a report of amiloride producing arrhythmias in patients receiving quinidine, see p.965.

Pharmacokinetics

Amiloride is incompletely absorbed from the gastrointestinal tract; bioavailability of about 50% is reported and is reduced by food. It is not significantly bound to plasma proteins and has a plasma half-life of 6 to 9 hours; the terminal half-life may be 20 hours or more. It is excreted unchanged by the kidneys.

◊ General references.

1. Weiss P, *et al.* The metabolism of amiloride hydrochloride in man. *Clin Pharmacol Ther* 1969; **10:** 401–6.

Hepatic impairment. In patients with acute hepatitis the terminal half-life of amiloride was 33 hours compared with 21 hours in healthy subjects.[1] The proportion of the dose excreted in the urine was increased from 49 to 80%.

1. Spahn H, *et al.* Pharmacokinetics of amiloride in renal and hepatic disease. *Eur J Clin Pharmacol* 1987; **33:** 493–8.

Renal impairment. Studies of the pharmacokinetics of amiloride[1,2] have reported an increase in terminal elimination half-life from 20 hours in healthy subjects to 100 hours in pa-

tients with end-stage renal disease. The natriuretic effect of amiloride was reduced[1] in patients with creatinine clearance below 50 mL per minute. In patients with renal impairment administration of amiloride could aggravate potassium retention due to renal disease. Studies in elderly patients have demonstrated increased half-life[3] and steady-state concentrations[4] associated with reduced renal function.

1. Knauf H, *et al.* Limitation on the use of amiloride in early renal failure. *Eur J Clin Pharmacol* 1985; **28:** 61–6.
2. Spahn H, *et al.* Pharmacokinetics of amiloride in renal and hepatic disease. *Eur J Clin Pharmacol* 1987; **33:** 493–8.
3. Sabanathan K, *et al.* A comparative study of the pharmacokinetics and pharmacodynamics of atenolol, hydrochlorothiazide and amiloride in normal young and elderly subjects and elderly hypertensive patients. *Eur J Clin Pharmacol* 1987; **32:** 53–60.
4. Ismail Z, *et al.* The pharmacokinetics of amiloride-hydrochlorothiazide combination in the young and elderly. *Eur J Clin Pharmacol* 1989; **37:** 167–71.

Uses and Administration

Amiloride is a weak diuretic which appears to act mainly on the distal renal tubules. It is described as potassium-sparing since, like spironolactone, it increases the excretion of sodium and reduces the excretion of potassium. Unlike spironolactone, however, it does not act by specifically antagonising aldosterone. Amiloride does not inhibit carbonic anhydrase. It takes effect about 2 hours after administration by mouth and its diuretic action reaches a peak in 6 to 10 hours and has been reported to persist for about 24 hours.

Amiloride diminishes the kaliuretic effects of other diuretics, and may produce an additional natriuretic effect. It is mainly used as an adjunct to thiazide diuretics such as hydrochlorothiazide and loop diuretics such as frusemide [furosemide], to conserve potassium in those at risk from hypokalaemia during the long-term treatment of oedema associated with hepatic cirrhosis (including ascites, p.793) and heart failure (p.798). It is also used in combination with other diuretics in the treatment of hypertension (p.802). Diuretic-induced hypokalaemia and its management, including the role of potassium-sparing diuretics such as amiloride, is discussed under Effects on Electrolyte Balance in the Adverse Effects of Hydrochlorothiazide, p.908. Amiloride is sometimes used to manage hypokalaemia in primary hyperaldosteronism (p.975).

Amiloride by inhalation has also been investigated in the management of cystic fibrosis patients with lung disease (see below).

In the treatment of **oedema** amiloride is given by mouth as the hydrochloride and doses are expressed in terms of the anhydrous substance. The usual dose is 5 to 10 mg daily which may be increased, if necessary, to a maximum of 20 mg daily. Similar doses are used to reduce potassium loss in patients receiving thiazide or loop diuretics.

Potassium supplements should not be given.

Cystic fibrosis. Pulmonary disease is the major cause of mortality in cystic fibrosis (p.117). Experimental treatment aimed at modifying the pulmonary disease process has included the administration of amiloride by inhalation.[1,2] No evidence of pulmonary or systemic toxicity was seen in 14 patients treated for 25 weeks.[1] The mechanism of action is unclear but could be the sodium-channel blocking effect[1] or anti-inflammatory effects[3] of amiloride. Concern has been expressed[4] over possible consequences of the inhibition of endogenous urokinase by amiloride although others[5] considered this to be unlikely at the concentrations studied. However, the addition of amiloride to standard therapy has not produced significant clinical benefits.[6,7]

1. Knowles MR, *et al.* A pilot study of aerosolized amiloride for the treatment of lung disease in cystic fibrosis. *N Engl J Med* 1990; **322:** 1189–94.
2. App EM, *et al.* Acute and long-term amiloride inhalation in cystic fibrosis lung disease: a rational approach to cystic fibrosis therapy. *Am Rev Respir Dis* 1990; **141:** 605–12.
3. Gallo RL. Aerosolized amiloride for the treatment of lung disease in cystic fibrosis. *N Engl J Med* 1990; **323:** 996–7.
4. Henkin J. Aerosolized amiloride for the treatment of lung disease in cystic fibrosis. *N Engl J Med* 1990; **323:** 997.
5. Knowles MR, *et al.* Aerosolized amiloride for the treatment of lung disease in cystic fibrosis. *N Engl J Med* 1990; **323:** 997–8.
6. Graham A, *et al.* No added benefit from nebulized amiloride in patients with cystic fibrosis. *Eur Respir J* 1993; **6:** 1243–8.
7. Bowler IM, *et al.* Nebulised amiloride in respiratory exacerbations of cystic fibrosis: a randomised controlled trial. *Arch Dis Child* 1995; **73:** 427–30.

Diabetes insipidus. Thiazide diuretics are commonly used in nephrogenic diabetes insipidus (p.1273) and NSAIDs may also be employed; both result in an overall decrease in urine production. Addition of amiloride to hydrochlorothiazide has been reported to be at least as effective as hydrochlorothiazide plus indometacin in 5 patients.[1] In addition, amiloride obviated the need for potassium supplements. The combination of hydrochlorothiazide and amiloride was also effective and well tolerated in a group of 4 children with nephrogenic diabetes insipidus who were treated for up to 5 years.[2]

1. Knoers N, Monnens LAH. Amiloride-hydrochlorothiazide versus indomethacin-hydrochlorothiazide in the treatment of nephrogenic diabetes insipidus. *J Pediatr* 1990; **117:** 499–502.
2. Kirchlechner V, *et al.* Treatment of nephrogenic diabetes insipidus with hydrochlorothiazide and amiloride. *Arch Dis Child* 1999; **80:** 548–52.

Renal calculi. Patients with idiopathic hypercalciuria and a history of renal calculi are usually given a thiazide diuretic such as hydrochlorothiazide to reduce calcium excretion (p.910). In patients with calcium oxalate calculi an inherited cellular defect in oxalate transport may also be involved and this might be corrected by amiloride.[1]

1. Baggio B, *et al.* An inheritable anomaly of red-cell oxalate transport in "primary" calcium nephrolithiasis correctable with diuretics. *N Engl J Med* 1986; **314:** 599–604.

Preparations

BP 2001: Amiloride Tablets; Co-amilofruse Tablets; Co-amilozide Oral Solution; Co-amilozide Tablets;
USP 25: Amiloride Hydrochloride and Hydrochlorothiazide Tablets; Amiloride Hydrochloride Tablets.

Proprietary Preparations (details are given in Part 3)
Aust.: Midamor; **Austral.:** Amidal†; Kaluril; Midamor; Midoride; **Canad.:** Midamor; **Denm.:** Amikal; Hydronet†; Nirulid; **Fin.:** Medamor; **Fr.:** Modamide; **Hong Kong:** Midamor; **Irl.:** Berkamil†; **Neth.:** Midamor†; **Norw.:** Midamor†; **NZ:** Midamor; **Swed.:** Amikal†; Midamor; **Switz.:** Midamor; **UK:** Amilamont; Amilospare†; Berkamil; **USA:** Midamor.

Multi-ingredient: Aust.: Aldoretic; Amiloretik; Amilorid comp; Amilostad HCT; Lanuretic; Loradur; Moducrin; Moduretic; **Austral.:** Amizide; Hydrozide†; Modizide; Moduretic; **Belg.:** Belidral; Frusamil; Kalten; Moduretic; **Braz.:** Diupress; Diurisa; Moduretic; **Canad.:** Apo-Amilzide; Moduret; Novamilor; Nu-Amilzide; **Denm.:** Amilco; Amilohyd†; Buram; Frusamil; Moduretic; Sparkal; **Fin.:** Amitrid; Diuramin; Diurex; Miloride; Moduretic; Sparkal; **Fr.:** Logirene; Moducren; Moduretic; **Ger.:** Amiduret†; Amilocomp beta; Amiloretik; Amilorid comp; Amilorid/HCT; Amilothiazid†; Amilozid; Aquaretic; Diaphal; Dignoretik; Diursan; durarese; Esmalorid; Hydrocomp; Moduren; Moducrin; Moduretik; Rhefluin†; Tensoflux; **Hong Kong:** Amilco; Amithiazide; Apo-Amilzide; Frumil; Hydrozide; Moducren; Moduretic; Navispare; **Irl.:** Amilco; Buram; Clonuretic; Fru-Co; Frumil; Lasoride; Moducren; Moduret; Moduretic; Navispare; **Israel:** Kaluril; **Ital.:** Moduretic; **Mex.:** Moducren; Moduretic; **Neth.:** Elkin; Hykaten†; Moducren†; Moduretic; **Norw.:** Moduretic Mite; Normorix; **NZ:** Amizide; Frumil; Hydrozide; Moduretic; **Port.:** Aldoretic†; Amiloride Composto; Chibretico; Diurene; Moducren; Moduretic; **S.Afr.:** Acumod†; Adco-Retic; Aldoretic; Amiloretik; Amizide; Aquadrex†; Arcanaretic†; Betaretic; Cliniretic†; Diutec; Hexaretic; Moducren; Moduretic; Servatrin; Trimolex†; **Singapore:** Apo-Amilzide; **Spain:** Ameride; Diuzine; Donicer†; Kalten; **Swed.:** Amiloferm; Normorix; Sparkal; **Switz.:** Aquarex; Aldoretic; Amilo-basan; Amilorid comp†; Betadiur; Co-Amilorid; Comilorid; Ecodurex; Escoretic; Frumil; Grodurex; Hydrolid; Kalten; Moducren; Moduretic; Rhefluin; **Thai.:** Amilhydrozide; Amilide; Hyperretic; Miduret; Milorex; Miretic; Moduretic; Poli-Uretic; Renase; Sefaretic; **UK:** Amilco; Amilmaxco; Aridil; Burinex A; Delvas; Froop Co; Fru-Co; Frumil; Frusemek; Kalten; Lasoride; Moducren; Moduret; Moduretic; Navispare; Synuretic; Zida-Co†; **USA:** Moduretic.

Amiodarone Hydrochloride (7780-f)

Amiodarone Hydrochloride (BANM, rINNM).
Amiodaroni Hydrochloridum; L-3428 (amiodarone); 51087N; SKF-33134-A (amiodarone). 2-Butylbenzofuran-3-yl 4-(2-diethylaminoethoxy)-3,5-di-iodophenyl ketone hydrochloride.
$C_{25}H_{29}I_2NO_3,HCl = 681.8$.
CAS — 1951-25-3 (amiodarone); 19774-82-4 (amiodarone hydrochloride).

NOTE. Amiodarone is *USAN*.
Pharmacopoeias. In *Chin.* and *Eur.* (see p.vi).

Pharmacopoeial description
Ph. Eur.: A white or almost white, fine crystalline powder. Very slightly soluble in water; sparingly soluble in alcohol; freely soluble in dichloromethane; soluble in methyl alcohol; very slightly soluble in petroleum spirit. Store at a temperature not exceeding 30°. Protect from light.

Adsorption. There was a rapid fall in the concentration of solutions of amiodarone hydrochloride by 10% in 3 hours followed by a steady decrease to 60% of the initial concentration after 5 days' storage in flexible PVC bags at ambient temperature.[1] When amiodarone solutions were perfused through PVC giving sets the concentration had fallen to 82% after 15 minutes. Similar losses were not observed from solutions stored in glass or rigid PVC bottles, and the losses were attributed to the presence of the plasticiser, di-2-ethylhexylphthalate.

1. Weir SJ, *et al.* Sorption of amiodarone to polyvinyl chloride infusion bags and administration sets. *Am J Hosp Pharm* 1985; **42:** 2679–83.

Incompatibility. Amiodarone injection has been reported to be incompatible with aminophylline,[1] flucloxacillin,[2] heparin,[3] and sodium bicarbonate.[4] A further study[5] reported incompatibility with ampicillin/sulbactam sodium, ceftazidime sodium, digoxin, frusemide [furosemide], imipenem/cilastatin sodium, magnesium sulfate, piperacillin sodium, piperacillin/tazobactam sodium, potassium phosphate, and sodium phosphate. The manufacturer states that it is incompatible with sodium chloride solutions.

1. Hasegawa GR, Eder JF. Visual compatibility of amiodarone hydrochloride injection with other injectable drugs. *Am J Hosp Pharm* 1984; **41:** 1379–80.
2. Taylor A, Lewis R. Amiodarone and injectable drug incompatibility. *Pharm J* 1992; **248:** 533.
3. Cairns CJ. Incompatibility of amiodarone. *Pharm J* 1986; **236:** 68.
4. Korth-Bradley JM. Incompatibility of amiodarone hydrochloride and sodium bicarbonate injections. *Am J Health-Syst Pharm* 1995; **52:** 2340.
5. Chalmers JR, *et al.* Visual compatibility of amiodarone hydrochloride injection with various intravenous drugs. *Am J Health-Syst Pharm* 2001; **58:** 504–6.

Stability. An oral suspension prepared from tablets[1] and containing amiodarone hydrochloride 5 mg per mL was stable for 3 months at 4° and 6 weeks at 25°.

1. Nahata MC. Stability of amiodarone in an oral suspension stored under refrigeration and at room temperature. *Ann Pharmacother* 1997; **31:** 851–2.

Adverse Effects and Treatment

Adverse effects are common with amiodarone; many are dose-related and reversible with reduction in dose.

Adverse cardiovascular effects associated with amiodarone include severe bradycardia, sinus arrest, and conduction disturbances. Severe hypotension may follow intravenous administration particularly, though not exclusively, at rapid infusion rates. Amiodarone may also produce ventricular tachyarrhythmias; torsade de pointes appears to be less of a problem with amiodarone than other antiarrhythmics. Rarely, heart failure may be precipitated or aggravated.

Amiodarone is reported to reduce the peripheral transformation of thyroxine [levothyroxine] (T_4) to tri-iodothyronine (T_3) and to increase the formation of reverse-T_3. It can affect thyroid function and may induce hypo- or hyperthyroidism.

There have been reports of severe pulmonary toxicity including pulmonary fibrosis and interstitial pneumonitis. These effects are usually reversible on withdrawal of amiodarone but are potentially fatal.

Amiodarone can adversely affect the liver. There may be abnormal liver function tests and cirrhosis or hepatitis; fatalities have been reported.

Prolonged treatment with amiodarone causes the development of benign yellowish-brown corneal microdeposits in the majority of patients, sometimes associated with coloured haloes of light; these are reversible on stopping therapy. Photosensitivity reactions are also common and more rarely blue-grey discoloration of the skin may occur.

Other adverse effects reported include peripheral neuropathy, paraesthesias, myopathy, ataxia, tremor, nausea, vomiting, a metallic taste, nightmares, headaches, sleeplessness, fatigue, and epididymitis.

Thrombophlebitis can occur if amiodarone is injected regularly or infused for prolonged periods into a peripheral vein. Rapid intravenous administration has been associated with anaphylactic shock, hot flushes, sweating, and nausea.

It has been suggested that amiodarone-induced phospholipidosis may explain some of its adverse effects. Amiodarone's iodine content contributes to its thyrotoxicity.

◊ Reviews of the adverse effects of amiodarone.

1. Naccarelli GV, *et al.* Adverse effects of amiodarone: pathogenesis, incidence and management. *Med Toxicol Adverse Drug Exp* 1989; **4:** 246–53.
2. Kerin NZ, *et al.* Long-term efficacy and toxicity of high- and low-dose amiodarone regimens. *J Clin Pharmacol* 1989; **29:** 418–23.
3. Perkins MW, *et al.* Intraoperative complications in patients receiving amiodarone: characteristics and risk factors. *DICP Ann Pharmacother* 1989; **23:** 757–63.
4. Vrobel TR, *et al.* A general overview of amiodarone toxicity: its prevention, detection, and management. *Prog Cardiovasc Dis* 1989; **31:** 393–426.
5. Morgan DJR. Adverse reactions profile: amiodarone. *Prescribers' J* 1991; **31:** 104–11.
6. Committee on Safety of Medicines/Medicines Control Agency. Amiodarone (Cordarone X). *Current Problems* 1996; **22:** 3–4.
7. Vorperian VR, *et al.* Adverse effects of low dose amiodarone: a meta-analysis. *J Am Coll Cardiol* 1997; **30:** 791–8.

Effects on electrolytes. Hyponatraemia associated with the syndrome of inappropriate secretion of antidiuretic hormone has been reported[1] in a patient following therapy with amiodarone for 6 months. The hyponatraemia resolved when amiodarone was discontinued.

1. Odeh M, *et al.* Hyponatremia during therapy with amiodarone. *Arch Intern Med* 1999; **159:** 2599–2600.

Effects on the eyes. Slit-lamp examination showed corneal abnormalities in 103 of 105 patients treated with amiodarone for 3 months to 7 years.[1] The most advanced abnormality comprised whorled patterns with uniform granular opacities. The corneal deposits became denser if amiodarone dosage was increased and regressed if dosage was reduced. Ocular symptoms were reported in only 12 patients. Photophobia was reported in 3 patients, while 2 had visual haloes, 1 had blurring of vision, and a further 6 had lid irritation. However, lid irritation was considered a photosensitive skin reaction and blurred vision was probably not due to amiodarone. No patient had any deterioration in visual acuity attributable to amiodarone. In 16 patients amiodarone was withdrawn with complete clearing of corneal abnormalities within 7 months and routine ophthalmological monitoring was considered unnecessary in patients without ocular symptoms. However, optic neuropathy[2] and neuritis with visual impairment have been reported in association with amiodarone and the manufacturers recommend that annual ophthalmological examinations should be performed.
A sicca syndrome with diminished tear and saliva production has been reported[3] during amiodarone treatment.

1. Ingram DV, *et al.* Ocular changes resulting from therapy with amiodarone. *Br J Ophthalmol* 1982; **66:** 676–9.
2. Feiner LA, *et al.* Optic neuropathy and amiodarone therapy. *Mayo Clin Proc* 1987; **62:** 702–17.
3. Dickinson EJ, Wolman RL. Sicca syndrome associated with amiodarone therapy. *BMJ* 1986; **293:** 510.

Effects on the genitalia. Epididymal swelling and scrotal pain have been reported with amiodarone.[1,2] Symptoms occurred 7 to 20 months after the start of treatment and resolved within 10 weeks despite continuation of amiodarone in some patients. In one patient[2] the concentration of desethylamiodarone in semen was five times the concentration in serum.
Brown discoloration of semen and sweat has also been associated with amiodarone therapy.[3]

1. Gasparich JP, *et al.* Non-infectious epididymitis associated with amiodarone therapy. *Lancet* 1984; **ii:** 1211–12.
2. Ward MJ, *et al.* Association of seminal desethylamiodarone concentration and epididymitis with amiodarone treatment. *BMJ* 1988; **296:** 19–20.
3. Adams PC, *et al.* Amiodarone in testis and semen. *Lancet* 1985; **i:** 341.

Effects on the heart. Amiodarone has the potential to provoke arrhythmias, but a review of the literature[1] indicated that the frequency of proarrhythmic events, including torsade de pointes, was low.

1. Hohnloser SH, *et al.* Amiodarone-associated proarrhythmic effects: a review with special reference to torsade de pointes tachycardia. *Ann Intern Med* 1994; **121:** 529–35.

Effects on lipids. Amiodarone increases phospholipid concentrations in tissues and this may be responsible for some of its adverse effects.[1] Although hyperlipidaemia may result from hypothyroidism, amiodarone can also increase serum-cholesterol concentrations independently of any effect on the thyroid.[2,3] The effect on triglyceride concentrations is not clear.[3]

1. Kodavanti UP, Mehendale HM. Cationic amphiphilic drugs and phospholipid storage disorder. *Pharmacol Rev* 1990; **42:** 327–54.
2. Wiersinga WM, *et al.* An increase in plasma cholesterol independent of thyroid function during long-term amiodarone therapy: a dose-dependent relationship. *Ann Intern Med* 1991; **114:** 128–32.
3. Lakhdar AA, *et al.* Long-term amiodarone therapy raises serum cholesterol. *Eur J Clin Pharmacol* 1991; **40:** 477–80.

Effects on the liver. Amiodarone-induced elevation of liver enzyme concentrations without clinical symptoms of hepatic dysfunction occurs in some patients.[1] However, hepatic injury which may be severe[2] and sometimes fatal[3-7] has been reported. Hepatitis and cirrhosis have occurred and histological changes resemble those in alcoholic liver disease. Severe reversible cholestasis with hyperbilirubinaemia has also been reported.[2] Hepatotoxicity may not occur for several years after starting amiodarone but rapidly progressive fatal hepatic failure has occurred[6] only one month after starting treatment. Liver enzymes may remain elevated and hepatic injury continue to develop for several months after discontinuing amiodarone. Acute hepatitis occurring within 24 hours of intravenous administration of amiodarone has been reported.[8] In a further patient,[9] acute hepatitis developed following intravenous amiodarone but did not recur with subsequent oral therapy, and it was suggested that the reaction may have been related to the vehicle used in the intravenous formulation.

1. Simon JB, *et al.* Amiodarone hepatotoxicity simulating alcoholic liver disease. *N Engl J Med* 1984; **311:** 167–72.
2. Morse RM, *et al.* Amiodarone-induced liver toxicity. *Ann Intern Med* 1988; **109:** 838–40.
3. Lim PK, *et al.* Neuropathy and fatal hepatitis in a patient receiving amiodarone. *BMJ* 1984; **288:** 1638–9.
4. Tordjman K, *et al.* Amiodarone and the liver. *Ann Intern Med* 1985; **102:** 411–12.
5. Rinder HM, *et al.* Amiodarone hepatotoxicity. *N Engl J Med* 1986; **314:** 318–19.
6. Lwakatare JM, *et al.* Fatal fulminating liver failure possibly related to amiodarone treatment. *Br J Hosp Med* 1990; **44:** 60–1.

7. Richer M, Robert S. Fatal hepatotoxicity following oral administration of amiodarone. *Ann Pharmacother* 1995; **29:** 582–6.
8. Pye M, *et al.* Acute hepatitis after parenteral amiodarone administration. *Br Heart J* 1988; **59:** 690–1.
9. James PR, Hardman SMC. Acute hepatitis complicating parenteral amiodarone does not preclude subsequent oral therapy. *Heart* 1997; **77:** 583–4.

Effects on the lungs. Pulmonary toxicity is one of the most severe adverse effects associated with amiodarone therapy and may occur in up to 10% of patients.[1] Interstitial and alveolar infiltration,[2] fibrosis,[3] and pneumonitis[4] have been reported. Patients often present with increasing dyspnoea, cough, and pleuritic chest pain. Most patients respond to withdrawal of amiodarone and, if necessary, treatment with corticosteroids[2] but fatalities have occurred.[3,5] Two patients with amiodarone pulmonary toxicity died less than 1 hour and 24 hours, respectively after pulmonary angiography.[6] Pulmonary toxicity appears to be dose-related[2] in some patients, but an immunological reaction occurring at low doses[4] appears to be the cause in others.

1. Martin WJ, Rosenow EC. Amiodarone pulmonary toxicity: recognition and pathogenesis. *Chest* 1988; **93:** 1067–75 (part 1) and 1242–8 (part 2).
2. Marchlinski FE, *et al.* Amiodarone pulmonary toxicity. *Ann Intern Med* 1982; **97:** 839–45.
3. Morera J, *et al.* Amiodarone and pulmonary fibrosis. *Eur J Clin Pharmacol* 1983; **24:** 591–3.
4. Venet A, *et al.* Five cases of immune-mediated amiodarone pneumonitis. *Lancet* 1984; **i:** 962–3.
5. Committee on Safety of Medicines. Recurrent ventricular tachycardia: adverse drug reactions. *BMJ* 1986; **292:** 50.
6. Wood DL, *et al.* Amiodarone pulmonary toxicity: report of two cases associated with rapidly progressive fatal adult respiratory distress syndrome after pulmonary angiography. *Mayo Clin Proc* 1985; **60:** 601–3.

Effects on mental state. Delirium occurred 17 days after starting amiodarone therapy in a 66-year-old man.[1] Mental status returned to normal on withdrawal of amiodarone.

1. Trohman RG, *et al.* Amiodarone-induced delirium. *Ann Intern Med* 1988; **108:** 68–9.

Effects on the nervous system. Of 10 patients treated with amiodarone for more than 2 years, 3 patients had evidence of peripheral neuropathy.[1] Initial results suggested that neuropathy correlated with high doses and high serum concentrations of amiodarone.

1. Fraser AG, McQueen INF. Adverse reactions during treatment with amiodarone hydrochloride. *BMJ* 1983; **287:** 612.

Effects on the pancreas. Pancreatitis has been reported[1] in a patient 4 days after the initiation of amiodarone therapy. Symptoms resolved following withdrawal of the drug but returned on re-exposure.

1. Bosch X, Bernadich O. Acute pancreatitis during treatment with amiodarone. *Lancet* 1997; **350:** 1300.

Effects on the skin and hair. The most common adverse skin reaction associated with amiodarone therapy is photosensitivity. This is a phototoxic rather than a photoallergic reaction[1-3] and the wavelengths responsible extend from the long-wave ultraviolet (UVA) into the visible light range.[1] Affected patients should be advised to wear protective clothing and avoid exposure to sunlight. Topical sunblock preparations, such as those containing zinc or titanium oxides, may reduce the risk of reaction and a reduction in amiodarone dosage may also be useful.[1] Although pyridoxine has been reported[4] to protect against amiodarone-induced photosensitivity, results from a double-blind placebo-controlled study[5] indicated that it may enhance the photosensitivity. Photosensitivity may continue for several weeks after withdrawal of amiodarone due to its extensive distribution.

Blue-grey[2,3] and golden-brown[3] pigmentation of light-exposed skin have been reported during long-term amiodarone therapy. The pigmentation is usually slowly reversible on withdrawing amiodarone but may not completely disappear. The mean concentrations of amiodarone and its desethyl metabolite in light-exposed pigmented skin have been found to be 10 times the concentrations in non-exposed skin.[2] Discoloration of semen and sweat has also been noted (see Effects on the Genitalia, above).

Cutaneous vasculitis,[6,7] exfoliative dermatitis,[8] and fatal toxic epidermal necrolysis[9] have been reported during amiodarone therapy. Alopecia[10,11] has been associated with amiodarone therapy but increased hair growth,[3] possibly due to the vasodilator activity of amiodarone, has also been reported.

1. Ferguson J, *et al.* Prevention of amiodarone-induced photosensitivity. *Lancet* 1984; **ii:** 414.
2. Zachary CB, *et al.* The pathogenesis of amiodarone-induced pigmentation and photosensitivity. *Br J Dermatol* 1984; **110:** 451–6.
3. Ferguson J, *et al.* A study of cutaneous photosensitivity induced by amiodarone. *Br J Dermatol* 1985; **113:** 537–49.
4. Kaufmann G. Pyridoxine against amiodarone-induced photosensitivity. *Lancet* 1984; **i:** 51–2.
5. Mulrow JP, *et al.* Pyridoxine and amiodarone-induced photosensitivity. *Ann Intern Med* 1985; **103:** 68–9.
6. Starke ID, Barbatis C. Cutaneous vasculitis associated with amiodarone therapy. *BMJ* 1985; **291:** 940.
7. Gutierrez R, *et al.* Vasculitis associated with amiodarone treatment. *Ann Pharmacother* 1994; **28:** 537.
8. Moots RJ, Banerjee A. Exfoliative dermatitis after amiodarone treatment. *BMJ* 1988; **296:** 1332–3.
9. Bencini PL, *et al.* Toxic epidermal necrolysis and amiodarone treatment. *Arch Dermatol* 1985; **121:** 838.

10. Samanta A, *et al.* Adverse reactions during treatment with amiodarone hydrochloride. *BMJ* 1983; **287:** 503.
11. Samuel LM, *et al.* Amiodarone and hair loss. *Postgrad Med J* 1992; **68:** 771.

Effects on thyroid function. The majority of euthyroid patients receiving amiodarone therapy remain clinically euthyroid. However, serum concentrations of thyroid hormones may be altered and can complicate the interpretation of thyroid function tests. Administration of amiodarone results in a reduction of the peripheral conversion of thyroxine (T_4) to tri-iodothyronine (T_3) with a resulting increase in T_4, a modest fall in T_3, and an increase in reverse-T_3 concentrations; the basal serum-TSH (thyroid-stimulating hormone; thyrotrophin) concentration rises transiently during the first several months of treatment.[1-4]

Occasionally patients become clinically hypo- or hyperthyroid and the prevalence appears to correlate with dietary iodine intake. The incidence of hyperthyroidism in amiodarone-treated patients in West Tuscany, Italy, an area where iodine intake is low, was 9.6% compared with an incidence of 2% in similar patients in Worcester, USA, an area where iodine intake is normal. The incidence of hypothyroidism in these patients was 5% and 22% respectively.[1] Each 200-mg tablet of amiodarone contains about 75 mg of iodine.[1,5] This large iodine load probably contributes to the development of hypo- or hyperthyroidism in patients with an underlying subclinical thyroid defect. Autoimmune mechanisms may also contribute and antithyroid antibodies have developed during amiodarone therapy.

Assessment of thyroid function is recommended in patients before starting amiodarone treatment and periodically during treatment. Patients with amiodarone-induced hyperthyroidism may present with tachycardia, tremor, weight loss, nervousness, irritability, reappearance of angina, or a worsening of arrhythmia. An ultrasensitive TSH assay should be used to confirm the diagnosis of hypo- or hyperthyroidism.

Hypothyroidism is usually treated with thyroxine [levothyroxine] starting with a low dose and gradually increasing until control is achieved; amiodarone may be continued.[1-4]

Hyperthyroidism may be treated with the thiourea drugs carbimazole, methimazole [thiamazole], or propylthiouracil;[1-6] although withdrawal of amiodarone has been advocated it may be continued if necessary. Potassium perchlorate has also been used[5] with a thiourea to reduce the thyroid iodine load. Radioiodine can be used[1] but may not be effective if the uptake of radio-iodine by the thyroid is low due to the iodine load from amiodarone. Corticosteroids may also be employed.[2-4] Thyroidectomy has been successfully used[7] in the treatment of resistant amiodarone-induced hyperthyroidism.

1. Figge HL, Figge J. The effects of amiodarone on thyroid hormone function: a review of the physiology and clinical manifestations. *J Clin Pharmacol* 1990; **30:** 588–95.
2. Kumar A, Borsey DQ. Amiodarone-related thyroid dysfunction. *Br J Hosp Med* 1994; **52:** 283–9.
3. Harjai KJ, Licata AA. Effects of amiodarone on thyroid function. *Ann Intern Med* 1997; **126:** 63–73.
4. Newman CM, *et al.* Amiodarone and the thyroid: a practical guide to the management of thyroid dysfunction induced by amiodarone therapy. *Heart* 1998; **79:** 121–7.
5. Reichert LJM, de Rooy HAM. Treatment of amiodarone induced hyperthyroidism with potassium perchlorate and methimazole during amiodarone treatment. *BMJ* 1989; **298:** 1547–8.
6. Davies PH, *et al.* Treatment of amiodarone induced thyrotoxicosis with carbimazole alone and continuation of amiodarone. *BMJ* 1992; **305:** 224–5.
7. Farwell AP, *et al.* Thyroidectomy for amiodarone-induced thyrotoxicosis. *JAMA* 1990; **263:** 1526–8.

Precautions

Amiodarone should not be given to patients with bradycardia, sino-atrial block, atrioventricular block or other severe conduction disorders (unless the patient has a pacemaker), severe hypotension, or severe respiratory failure. It may be used with caution in patients with heart failure. Electrolyte disorders should be corrected before starting treatment. The use of amiodarone should be avoided in patients with iodine sensitivity, disorders of the thyroid gland, or with a history of thyroid disorders. Patients taking amiodarone should avoid exposure to sunlight. Amiodarone is contra-indicated in breast-feeding women.

Thyroid function should be monitored regularly in order to detect amiodarone-induced hyper- or hypothyroidism. Thyroxine, tri-iodothyronine, and thyrotrophin (thyroid-stimulating hormone; TSH) concentrations should be measured; clinical assessment is important but is unreliable alone. See also under Effects on Thyroid Function in Adverse Effects and Treatment, above.

Tests of liver and pulmonary function also should be carried out regularly in patients on long-term therapy. Ophthalmological examinations should be performed annually. Although urinary excretion is not a major route for the elimination of amiodarone or its metabolites, some have nevertheless advised caution in pa-

tients with moderate or severe renal impairment because of the possibility of iodine accumulation.

Intravenous injections of amiodarone should be given slowly: if prolonged or repeated infusions are envisaged, the use of a central venous catheter should be considered.

Administration. For the problems of controlling the delivery rate of amiodarone by intravenous infusion, see under Uses and Administration, below.

Breast feeding. Amiodarone may be excreted in significant amounts in breast milk[1,2] and is therefore contra-indicated in women who are breast feeding.

1. Pitcher D, *et al.* Amiodarone in pregnancy. *Lancet* 1983; **i:** 597–8.
2. Plomp TA, *et al.* Use of amiodarone during pregnancy. *Eur J Obstet Gynecol Reprod Biol* 1992; **43:** 201–7.

Porphyria. Amiodarone is considered to be unsafe in patients with porphyria because it has been shown to be porphyrinogenic in *in-vitro* systems.

Pregnancy. Each 200-mg tablet of amiodarone contains about 75 mg of iodine. The uncertainty as to the effect of this iodine load on the fetus has largely limited the use of amiodarone in pregnancy since iodine freely crosses the placenta and may cause thyroid disorders in the fetus. There are reports[1-3] of the use of amiodarone during pregnancy without any adverse effects appearing in the neonate, although transient biochemical hyperthyroidism or hypothyroidism in 2 neonates has been reported.[4] Amiodarone and desethylamiodarone both cross the placenta and at delivery their respective concentrations in cord blood are about 10% and 25% of the maternal plasma concentrations.

1. Pitcher D, *et al.* Amiodarone in pregnancy. *Lancet* 1983; **i:** 597–8.
2. Robson DJ, *et al.* Use of amiodarone during pregnancy. *Postgrad Med J* 1985; **61:** 75–7.
3. Rey E, *et al.* Effects of amiodarone during pregnancy. *Can Med Assoc J* 1987; **136:** 959–60.
4. Plomp TA, *et al.* Use of amiodarone during pregnancy. *Eur J Obstet Gynecol Reprod Biol* 1992; **43:** 201–7.

Interactions

Amiodarone should be used with caution with other drugs liable to induce bradycardia, such as beta blockers or calcium-channel blockers, and with other antiarrhythmic drugs. Concomitant administration with arrhythmogenic drugs, for example phenothiazine antipsychotics, tricyclic antidepressants, halofantrine, and terfenadine, should be avoided. The effects of warfarin and other oral anticoagulants and of clonazepam may be enhanced by concomitant administration of amiodarone, and plasma concentrations of ciclosporin, digoxin, flecainide, phenytoin, procainamide, and quinidine may be raised. Further information on these interactions is given under the individual drug monographs. Plasma-amiodarone concentrations may be decreased by phenytoin and increased by cimetidine and other inhibitors of metabolising enzymes including HIV-protease inhibitors.

◊ Reviews.

1. Marcus FI. Drug interactions with amiodarone. *Am Heart J* 1983; **106:** 924–30.
2. Lesko LJ. Pharmacokinetic drug interactions with amiodarone. *Clin Pharmacokinet* 1989; **17:** 130–40.

Antibacterials. Palpitations and activation of an implantable cardioverter defibrillator occurred[1] in a woman receiving amiodarone therapy when treatment with *rifampicin* was added. Serum concentrations of amiodarone were found to be reduced, probably due to induction of metabolising enzymes by rifampicin.

1. Zarembski DG, *et al.* Impact of rifampin on serum amiodarone concentrations in a patient with congenital heart disease. *Pharmacotherapy* 1999; **19:** 249–51.

Antiepileptics. The interaction between *phenytoin* and amiodarone resulting in increased plasma-phenytoin concentrations is widely recognised (see p.359). However, phenytoin is a hepatic enzyme inducer and has been reported[1] to decrease serum-amiodarone concentrations by 32 and 49% after 1 and 2 weeks of concomitant administration.

1. Nolan PE, *et al.* Effect of phenytoin on the clinical pharmacokinetics of amiodarone. *J Clin Pharmacol* 1990; **30:** 1112–19.

Antivirals. A potential interaction has been suggested between amiodarone and HIV-protease inhibitors due to inhibition of amiodarone metabolism. Raised serum concentrations of amiodarone have been reported[1] in a patient who received *indinavir* for postexposure prophylaxis; no clinical signs of toxicity occurred.

1. Lohman JJHM, *et al.* Antiretroviral therapy increases serum concentrations of amiodarone. *Ann Pharmacother* 1999; **33:** 645–6.

Grapefruit juice. A study[1] in healthy subjects reported that concomitant administration with grapefruit juice decreased the metabolism of amiodarone; the area under the plasma concentration-time curve (AUC) and the maximum plasma concentration of amiodarone were both increased.

1. Libersa CC, et al. Dramatic inhibition of amiodarone metabolism induced by grapefruit juice. Br J Clin Pharmacol 2000; **49:** 373–8.

Histamine H₂-antagonists. Cimetidine inhibits hepatic metabolism and an increase in the serum-amiodarone concentration has been reported[1] in 8 out of 12 patients given amiodarone and cimetidine concurrently.

1. Hogan C, et al. Cimetidine-amiodarone interaction. J Clin Pharmacol 1988; **28:** 909.

Pharmacokinetics

Amiodarone is absorbed variably and erratically from the gastrointestinal tract. It is extensively distributed to body tissues and accumulates notably in muscle and fat; it has been reported to be 96% bound to plasma proteins. The terminal elimination half-life is about 50 days with a range of about 20 to 100 days due to its extensive tissue distribution. On stopping prolonged amiodarone therapy a pharmacological effect is evident for a month or more. One metabolite, desethylamiodarone, has been identified and this also has antiarrhythmic properties. There is very little urinary excretion of amiodarone or its metabolites, the major route of excretion being in faeces via the bile; some enterohepatic recycling may occur. Amiodarone and desethylamiodarone are reported to cross the placenta and to be distributed into breast milk.

Following intravenous injection the maximum effect is achieved within 1 to 30 minutes and persists for 1 to 3 hours.

◊ Reviews.

1. Latini R, et al. Clinical pharmacokinetics of amiodarone. Clin Pharmacokinet 1984; **9:** 136–56.

Uses and Administration

Amiodarone is predominantly a class III antiarrhythmic (p.787). It is used in the control of ventricular and supraventricular **arrhythmias**, including arrhythmias associated with Wolff-Parkinson-White syndrome. It has been tried for the prevention of arrhythmias in patients with myocardial infarction or heart failure.

Amiodarone is given by mouth as the hydrochloride in initial doses of 200 mg three times daily for a week, then 200 mg twice daily for a week, and then a usual maintenance dosage of 200 mg or less daily, according to the patient's response. Loading doses of up to 1600 mg daily for 1 to 3 weeks, followed by 600 to 800 mg daily for a month, and usual maintenance doses of up to 400 mg daily, are used in the USA. Consideration should be given to potential adverse effects, and patients should be given the minimum effective dose.

Amiodarone hydrochloride may be given intravenously where facilities for close monitoring of cardiac function and resuscitation are available. It is given by intravenous infusion usually in a dose of 5 mg per kg body-weight in 250 mL of glucose 5%, infused over 20 minutes to 2 hours; further doses may be given up to a maximum in 24 hours of 1.2 g in up to 500 mL of glucose 5%. Repeated infusions are preferably made through a central venous catheter. In emergencies it may also be given in doses of 150 to 300 mg in 10 to 20 mL of glucose by slow intravenous injection over a period of not less than 3 minutes; a second injection should not be given until at least 15 minutes after the first.

◊ General references.

1. Gill J, et al. Amiodarone: an overview of its pharmacological properties, and review of its therapeutic use in cardiac arrhythmias. Drugs 1992; **43:** 69–110.
2. Podrid PJ. Amiodarone: reevaluation of an old drug. Ann Intern Med 1995; **122:** 689–70.
3. Swanton H. Amiodarone. Br J Hosp Med 1997; **58:** 329–32.
4. Goldschlager N, et al. Practical guidelines for clinicians who treat patients with amiodarone. Arch Intern Med 2000; **160:** 1741–8.

Administration. Addition of amiodarone hydrochloride to an intravenous infusion solution reduces the drop size delivered[1,2] and the reduction in size is greater as the concentration of amiodarone is increased. This resulted[1] in a reduction of about 30% in the expected delivery rate when amiodarone hydrochloride 1200 mg was administered in 500 mL of glucose 5%. The reduction in drop size has been attributed to a reduction in sur-

face tension caused by inclusion of Tween 80 (polysorbate 80) in the commercial injection.[1] Allowances should be made for the changes in drop size causing a reduction of the delivery rate of infusions of amiodarone hydrochloride.

1. Capps PA, Robertson AL. Influence of amiodarone injection on the delivery rate of intravenous fluids. Pharm J 1985; **234:** 14–15.
2. Chouhan UM, Lynch E. Amiodarone intravenous infusion. Pharm J 1985; **235:** 466.

Cardiac arrhythmias. Amiodarone is an effective drug for the management of supraventricular and ventricular arrhythmias[1-4] (p.794). It is useful for the treatment of supraventricular arrhythmias associated with the Wolff-Parkinson-White syndrome[2,3] and for both the acute conversion and long-term management of atrial fibrillation.[5] It has been used orally and intravenously in infants and children[5,6] and has been given by various routes to terminate fetal arrhythmias.[7] It is also useful for controlling both atrial and ventricular arrhythmias associated with hypertrophic **cardiomyopathy**[2,3] and may reduce the incidence of sudden death in these patients. It is effective in the management of malignant ventricular arrhythmias, although there are few comparative studies with other antiarrhythmics,[1-3] and may also be used in the management of **cardiac arrest**[8] (see Advanced Cardiac Life Support, p.790). Amiodarone has also been tried for its antiarrhythmic effect in the management of **heart failure** (see below).

Amiodarone has also been investigated in patients with asymptomatic ventricular arrhythmias following **myocardial infarction** (BASIS: the Basel Antiarrhythmic Study of Infarct Survival,[9,10] CAMIAT: the Canadian Amiodarone Myocardial Infarction Arrhythmia Trial,[11] and EMIAT: the European Myocardial Infarct Amiodarone Trial[12]). Improved mortality rates were reported in the BASIS study,[9,10] but neither CAMIAT[11] nor EMIAT[12] showed a reduction in total mortality, although both studies reported a reduction in risk of arrhythmic death. However, meta-analysis of studies using amiodarone found a small reduction in total mortality suggesting that it might be of benefit after myocardial infarction in patients, such as those with heart failure, at high risk of arrhythmic death.[13] In patients at lower risk the role of amiodarone is not as clear; early administration of amiodarone to less-selected patients following myocardial infarction appeared to have no overall effect on mortality, although mortality was increased in the group of patients receiving a high dose.[14]

While amiodarone can cause torsade de pointes it appears to do so rarely[15,16] and patients who have experienced this form of ventricular tachycardia as a result of other antiarrhythmic therapy have been given amiodarone subsequently without a recurrence.[17] However, amiodarone has generally been withheld until other appropriate antiarrhythmics have been tried because of its toxicity and the difficulty of instituting and evaluating other therapies after discontinuation of amiodarone.[1,3] The lower doses of amiodarone employed in Europe may be more acceptable than the higher doses that have been used in the USA.

1. Mason JW. Amiodarone. N Engl J Med 1987; **316:** 455–66. Correction. ibid.; 760.
2. Counihan PJ, McKenna WJ. Risk-benefit assessment of amiodarone in the treatment of cardiac arrhythmias. Drug Safety 1990; **5:** 286–304.
3. Katritsis D, Camm AJ. Amiodarone in long term prophylaxis. Drugs 1991; **41** (suppl 2): 54–66.
4. Desai AD, et al. The role of intravenous amiodarone in the management of cardiac arrhythmias. Ann Intern Med 1997; **127:** 294–303. Correction. ibid. 1998; **128:** 505.
5. Shuler CO, et al. Efficacy and safety of amiodarone in infants. Am Heart J 1993; **125:** 1430–2.
6. Figa FH, et al. Clinical efficacy and safety of intravenous amiodarone in infants and children. Am J Cardiol 1994; **74:** 573–7.
7. Flack NJ, et al. Amiodarone given by three routes to terminate fetal atrial flutter associated with severe hydrops. Obstet Gynecol 1993; **82:** 714–16.
8. Kudenchuk PJ, et al. Amiodarone for resuscitation after out-of-hospital cardiac arrest due to ventricular fibrillation. N Engl J Med 1999; **341:** 871–8.
9. Burkart F, et al. Effect of antiarrhythmic therapy on mortality in survivors of myocardial infarction with asymptomatic complex ventricular arrhythmias: Basel Antiarrhythmic Study of Infarct Survival (BASIS). J Am Coll Cardiol 1990; **16:** 1711–18.
10. Pfisterer ME, et al. Long-term benefit of 1-year amiodarone treatment for persistent complex ventricular arrhythmias after myocardial infarction. Circulation 1993; **87:** 309–11.
11. Cairns JA, et al. Randomised trial of outcome after myocardial infarction in patients with frequent or repetitive ventricular premature depolarisations: CAMIAT. Lancet 1997; **349:** 675–82.
12. Julian DG, et al. Randomised trial of effect of amiodarone on mortality in patients with left-ventricular dysfunction after recent myocardial infarction: EMIAT. Lancet 1997; **349:** 667–74. Corrections. ibid.; 1180 and 1776.
13. Amiodarone Trials Meta-Analysis Investigators. Effect of prophylactic amiodarone on mortality after acute myocardial infarction and in congestive heart failure: meta-analysis of individual data from 6500 patients in randomised trials. Lancet 1997; **350:** 1417–24.
14. Elizari MV, et al. Morbidity and mortality following early administration of amiodarone in acute myocardial infarction. Eur Heart J 2000; **21:** 198–205.
15. Naccarelli GV, et al. Adverse effects of amiodarone: pathogenesis, incidence and management. Med Toxicol Adverse Drug Exp 1989; **4:** 246–53.
16. Hohnloser SH, et al. Amiodarone-associated proarrhythmic effects: a review with special reference to torsade de pointes tachycardia. Ann Intern Med 1994; **121:** 529–35.
17. Mattioni TA, et al. Amiodarone in patients with previous drug-mediated torsade de pointes: long-term safety and efficacy. Ann Intern Med 1989; **111:** 574–80.

Heart failure. Although antiarrhythmics are not routinely recommended in the management of heart failure (p.798), those such as amiodarone that have no significant negative inotropic effect may have a role in some patients since sudden deaths in patients with severe heart failure have been attributed to ventricular arrhythmias. In the GESICA study (Grupo de Estudio de la Sobrevida en la Insuficiencia Cardiaca en Argentina)[1] amiodarone appeared to reduce mortality in patients with severe chronic heart failure who were without symptomatic ventricular arrhythmias. An improvement in functional capacity was also noted. The decrease in mortality appeared to be greater than could be expected from antiarrhythmic activity alone. However, in the CHF-STAT study (Survival Trial of Antiarrhythmic Therapy in Congestive Heart Failure)[2] involving patients with heart failure and premature ventricular contractions, overall survival did not appear to be improved by amiodarone. A meta-analysis[3] including these and 3 further trials concluded that amiodarone reduced the rate of arrhythmic or sudden death in high-risk patients and that this resulted in an overall reduction in mortality. However, amiodarone may have a number of adverse effects and it is not currently recommended in heart failure except in patients with symptomatic ventricular arrhythmias.

1. Doval HC, et al. Randomised trial of low-dose amiodarone in severe congestive heart failure. Lancet 1994; **344:** 493–8.
2. Singh SN, et al. Amiodarone in patients with congestive heart failure and asymptomatic ventricular arrhythmia. N Engl J Med 1995; **333:** 77–82.
3. Amiodarone Trials Meta-Analysis Investigators. Effect of prophylactic amiodarone on mortality after acute myocardial infarction and in congestive heart failure: meta-analysis of individual data from 6500 patients in randomised trials. Lancet 1997; **350:** 1417–24.

Preparations

BP 2001: Amiodarone Intravenous Infusion; Amiodarone Tablets.

Proprietary Preparations (details are given in Part 3)
Aust.: Sedacoron; **Austral.:** Aratac; Cardinorm; Cordarone X; **Belg.:** Cordarone; **Braz.:** Ancoron; Angiodarona; Atlansil; Cor Mio; Miodaron; **Canad.:** Cordarone; **Denm.:** Cordarone; **Fin.:** Cordarone; **Fr.:** Corbionax; Cordarone; **Ger.:** Amiobeta; Amiodarex; Amiogamma; Amiohexal; Cordarex; Tachydaron; **Hong Kong:** Cordarone; Sedacoron; **Irl.:** Cordarone X; **Israel:** Amiodacore; Procor; **Ital.:** Amiodar; Cordarone; **Mex.:** Braxan; Cardiorona; Cordarone; Sinarona; **Neth.:** Cordarone; **Norw.:** Cordarone; **NZ:** Aratac; Cordarone; **Port.:** Cordarone; Miodrone; **S.Afr.:** Cordarone X; Hexarone; **Singapore:** Aratac; Cordarone; **Spain:** Trangorex; **Swed.:** Cordarone; **Switz.:** Cordarone; **Thai.:** Aratac; Cordarone; **UAE:** Amirone; **UK:** Amidox; Cordarone X; **USA:** Cordarone; Pacerone.

Amlodipine Besilate   (10499-b)

Amlodipine Besilate (BANM, rINNM).

Amlodipine Besylate (USAN); Amlodipini Besilas; UK-48340-26; UK-48340-11 (amlodipine maleate). 3-Ethyl 5-methyl 2-(2-aminoethoxymethyl)-4-(2-chlorophenyl)-1,4-dihydro-6-methylpyridine-3,5-dicarboxylate monobenzenesulphonate.

$C_{20}H_{25}ClN_2O_5,C_6H_6O_3S = 567.1$.

CAS — 88150-42-9 (amlodipine); 111470-99-6 (amlodipine besilate); 88150-47-4 (amlodipine maleate).

Pharmacopoeias. In Eur. (see p.vi).

Amlodipine besilate 6.9 mg is approximately equivalent to 5 mg of amlodipine.

Pharmacopoeial description

Ph. Eur.: A white or almost white powder. Slightly soluble in water and in isopropyl alcohol; sparingly soluble in dehydrated alcohol; freely soluble in methyl alcohol. Store in airtight containers. Protect from light.

Adverse Effects, Treatment, and Precautions

As for dihydropyridine calcium-channel blockers (see Nifedipine, p.940).

◊ Of 1091 patients prescribed amlodipine for hypertension, 128 (11.7%) discontinued the drug because of adverse effects.[1] The commonest side-effects were ankle oedema, flushing, headache, skin rash, and fatigue.

1. Benson E, Webster J. The tolerability of amlodipine in hypertensive patients. Br J Clin Pharmacol 1995; **39:** 578P–579P.

Heart failure. Calcium-channel blockers are normally avoided in patients with heart failure but amlodipine has not been found to have any adverse effects on morbidity or mortality in patients with severe heart failure receiving the drug.[1] Therefore, it may be a suitable treatment for angina pectoris or hypertension in such patients.

1. Packer M, et al. Effect of amlodipine on morbidity and mortality in severe chronic heart failure. N Engl J Med 1996; **335:** 1107–14.

Interactions

As for dihydropyridine calcium-channel blockers (see Nifedipine, p.942).

Pharmacokinetics

Amlodipine is well absorbed following oral administration with peak blood concentrations occurring after 6 to 12 hours. The bioavailability is about 60 to 65%. Amlodipine is reported to be about 97.5% bound to plasma proteins. It has a prolonged terminal elimination half-life of 35 to 50 hours and steady-state plasma concentrations are not achieved until after 7 to 8 days of administration. Amlodipine is extensively metabolised in the liver; metabolites are mostly excreted in urine together with less than 10% of a dose as unchanged drug.

◊ General reviews.
1. Meredith PA, Elliott HL. Clinical pharmacokinetics of amlodipine. *Clin Pharmacokinet* 1992; **22:** 22–31.

Absorption. Results of studies involving 24 healthy subjects indicated that absorption of amlodipine from a capsule was equivalent to that from a solution, suggesting that the slow transfer of amlodipine into the blood is a property of the drug not of the dosage form; it was also shown that absorption was not affected by food.[1]
1. Faulkner JK, *et al.* Absorption of amlodipine unaffected by food: solid dose equivalent to solution dose. *Arzneimittelforschung* 1989; **39:** 799–801.

Metabolism. The metabolites of amlodipine have been characterised in *animals* and in human subjects.[1] Metabolism of amlodipine is complex and extensive, and in common with other dihydropyridines oxidation to the pyridine analogue represents a major step. About 5% of a dose was recovered from urine as unchanged amlodipine.
1. Beresford AP, *et al.* Biotransformation of amlodipine. *Arzneimittelforschung* 1989; **39:** 201–9.

Uses and Administration

Amlodipine is a dihydropyridine calcium-channel blocker with actions similar to those of nifedipine (p.943). It is used in the management of hypertension (p.802) and angina pectoris (p.791).

Amlodipine is given by mouth as the besilate, but doses are usually expressed in terms of the base.

In hypertension the usual initial dose is 5 mg once daily, increased, if necessary, to 10 mg once daily. Similar doses are given in the treatment of stable angina and Prinzmetal's angina.

◊ Reviews.
1. Murdoch D, Heel RC. Amlodipine: a review of its pharmacodynamic and pharmacokinetic properties, and therapeutic use in cardiovascular disease. *Drugs* 1991; **41:** 478–505.
2. Haria M, Wagstaff AJ. Amlodipine: a reappraisal of its pharmacological properties and therapeutic use in cardiovascular disease. *Drugs* 1995; **50:** 560–86.

Preparations

Proprietary Preparations (details are given in Part 3)

Aust.: Norvasc; **Austral.:** Norvasc; **Belg.:** Amlor; **Braz.:** Cordarene; Norvasc; **Canad.:** Norvasc; **Denm.:** Norvasc; **Fin.:** Norvasc; **Fr.:** Amlor; **Ger.:** Norvasc; **Hong Kong:** Norvasc; **Irl.:** Istin; **Israel:** Norvasc; **Ital.:** Antacal; Monopina; Norvasc; **Jpn:** Amlodin†; **Mex.:** Norvas; **Neth.:** Norvasc; **Norw.:** Norvasc; **NZ:** Norvasc; **Port.:** Norvasc; **S.Afr.:** Norvasc; **Singapore:** Norvasc; **Spain:** Astudal; Norvas; **Swed.:** Norvasc; **Switz.:** Norvasc; **Thai.:** Norvasc; **UK:** Istin; **USA:** Norvasc.

Multi-ingredient: USA: Lotrel.

Amosulalol Hydrochloride   (18755-f)

Amosulalol Hydrochloride *(rINNM)*.

YM-09538.   (±)-5-(1-Hydroxy-2-{[2-(o-methoxyphenoxy)ethyl]amino}ethyl)-o-toluenesulphonamide hydrochloride.

$C_{18}H_{24}N_2O_5S,HCl = 416.9$.

CAS — 85320-68-9 *(amosulalol)*; 70958-86-0 *(amosulalol hydrochloride)*; 93633-92-2 *(amosulalol hydrochloride)*.

Profile

Amosulalol is a beta blocker (p.844). In addition, it has alpha-blocking activity. It has been given by mouth as the hydrochloride in the management of hypertension.

Preparations

Proprietary Preparations (details are given in Part 3)

Jpn: Lowgan†.

Amrinone   (12373-g)

Amrinone *(BAN, rINN)*.

Inamrinone   *(USAN)*;   Win-40680.   5-Amino-3,4'-bipyridyl-6(1H)-one.

$C_{10}H_9N_3O = 187.2$.

CAS — 60719-84-8.

ATC — C01CE01.

Pharmacopoeias. In US.

Pharmacopoeial description

USP 25: A pale yellow to tan powder; odourless or with a faint odour. Practically insoluble in water and in chloroform; slightly soluble in methyl alcohol. Protect from light.

Amrinone Lactate   (18497-x)

Amrinone Lactate *(BANM, rINNM)*.

$C_{10}H_9N_3O,C_3H_6O_3 = 277.3$.

CAS — 75898-90-7.

Amrinone lactate 1.48 mg is approximately equivalent to 1 mg of amrinone.

Incompatibilities. The manufacturer has reported that amrinone lactate injection is physically incompatible with glucose-containing solutions and with frusemide [furosemide].

Precipitation occurred[1] when amrinone was mixed with sodium bicarbonate injection, probably because of the reduced solubility of amrinone in alkaline solutions.
1. Riley CM, Junkin P. Stability of amrinone and digoxin, procainamide hydrochloride, propranolol hydrochloride, sodium bicarbonate, potassium chloride, or verapamil hydrochloride in intravenous admixtures. *Am J Hosp Pharm* 1991; **48:** 1245–52.

Adverse Effects

Amrinone produces gastrointestinal disturbances that may necessitate withdrawal of treatment. It produces dose-dependent thrombocytopenia. Hepatotoxicity may occur, particularly during long-term oral treatment. Hypotension and cardiac arrhythmias have been reported. Other adverse effects include headache, fever, chest pain, hypersensitivity reactions including myositis and vasculitis, nail discoloration, and decreased tear production. Local pain and burning may occur at the site of intravenous injection.

The adverse effects associated with oral administration have made this route unacceptable and amrinone is now only employed intravenously for short-term use. Studies with other inotropic phosphodiesterase inhibitors have shown that their prolonged oral administration can increase the mortality rate.

◊ References.
1. Wynne J, *et al.* Oral amrinone in refractory congestive heart failure. *Am J Cardiol* 1980; **45:** 1245–9.
2. Wilmshurst PT, Webb-Peploe MM. Side effects of amrinone therapy. *Br Heart J* 1983; **49:** 447–51.
3. Wilmshurst PT, *et al.* The effects of amrinone on platelet count, survival and function in patients with congestive cardiac failure. *Br J Clin Pharmacol* 1984; **17:** 317–24.
4. Silverman BD, *et al.* Clinical effects and side effects of amrinone: a study of 24 patients with chronic congestive heart failure. *Arch Intern Med* 1985; **145:** 825–9.
5. Webster MWI, Sharpe DN. Adverse effects associated with the newer inotropic agents. *Med Toxicol* 1986; **1:** 335–42.
6. Mattingly PM, *et al.* Pancytopenia secondary to short-term, high-dose intravenous infusion of amrinone. *DICP Ann Pharmacother* 1990; **24:** 1172–4.
7. Ross MP, *et al.* Amrinone-associated thrombocytopenia: pharmacokinetic analysis. *Clin Pharmacol Ther* 1993; **53:** 661–7.

Precautions

Amrinone should be used with caution in severe obstructive aortic or pulmonary valvular disease or in hypertrophic cardiomyopathy. Blood pressure and heart rate should be monitored during parenteral amrinone administration. The fluid and electrolyte balance should be maintained. Platelet counts and liver function should also be monitored.

Pharmacokinetics

Amrinone is rapidly absorbed from the gastrointestinal tract although it is no longer given orally because of an unacceptable level of adverse effects when administered by this route. The half-life is variable and after intravenous administration has been reported to be about 4 hours in healthy subjects and about 6 hours in patients with heart failure. Binding to plasma proteins is generally low. Amrinone is partially metabolised in the liver and excreted in the urine as unchanged drug and metabolites; up to about 40% is excreted as unchanged drug after intravenous admin-

istration. About 18% of an orally administered dose has been detected in the faeces over 72 hours.

◊ General references.
1. Rocci ML, Wilson H. The pharmacokinetics and pharmacodynamics of newer inotropic agents. *Clin Pharmacokinet* 1987; **13:** 91–109. Correction. *ibid.* 1988; **14:** (contents page).

Infants. For reference to the pharmacokinetics of amrinone in neonates and infants, see under Uses and Administration, below.

Renal impairment. Studies in a child with multi-organ failure and anuria[1] and in 3 adults with anuria following cardiac surgery[2] have shown that amrinone is effectively removed by haemofiltration but clearance varies widely between patients. Non-renal clearance may also be altered in critically ill patients and monitoring of plasma-amrinone concentrations has been suggested.[2]
1. Lawless S, *et al.* Effect of continuous arteriovenous haemofiltration on pharmacokinetics of amrinone. *Clin Pharmacokinet* 1993; **25:** 80–2.
2. Hellinger A, *et al.* Elimination of amrinone during continuous veno-venous haemofiltration after cardiac surgery. *Eur J Clin Pharmacol* 1995; **48:** 57–9.

Uses and Administration

Amrinone is a phosphodiesterase inhibitor which has vasodilator and positive inotropic properties. It is used in the management of heart failure (p.798). Although amrinone is effective when given orally this route has been associated with an unacceptable level of adverse effects, and the drug is now only given intravenously for the short-term management of heart failure unresponsive to other forms of therapy.

The mode of action has not been fully determined, but appears to involve an increase in cyclic adenosine monophosphate concentration secondary to inhibition of phosphodiesterase, leading to an increased contractile force in cardiac muscle.

Amrinone is administered intravenously as the lactate and doses are expressed in terms of the base. The initial loading dose is 750 µg per kg body-weight by slow intravenous injection over 2 to 3 minutes. This is followed by a maintenance infusion, although the loading dose may be repeated after 30 minutes if necessary. Maintenance doses are 5 to 10 µg per kg per minute by infusion to a usual maximum total dose (including loading doses) of 10 mg per kg in 24 hours. Doses of up to 18 mg per kg per day have been used for short periods in a limited number of patients.

◊ General references.
1. Colucci WS, *et al.* New positive inotropic agents in the treatment of congestive heart failure: mechanisms of action and recent clinical developments. *N Engl J Med* 1986; **314:** 349–58.

Administration in infants. Pharmacokinetic and pharmacodynamic studies[1,2] in infants undergoing cardiac surgery indicated that the dose needed for infants to achieve a plasma-amrinone concentration of 2 to 7 µg per mL was an initial intravenous bolus of 3.0 to 4.5 mg per kg in divided doses followed by a continuous infusion of 10 µg per kg per minute. It was suggested that neonates should receive a similar bolus dose followed by a continuous infusion of 3 to 5 µg per kg per minute. In a further study[3] that also included some older children, amrinone clearance and volume of distribution varied widely between patients but did not appear to be related to age.
1. Lawless S, *et al.* Amrinone in neonates and infants after cardiac surgery. *Crit Care Med* 1989; **17:** 751–4.
2. Lawless ST, *et al.* The acute pharmacokinetics and pharmacodynamics of amrinone in pediatric patients. *J Clin Pharmacol* 1991; **31:** 800–3.
3. Allen-Webb EM, *et al.* Age-related amrinone pharmacokinetics in a pediatric population. *Crit Care Med* 1994; **22:** 1016–24.

Preparations

USP 25: Inamrinone Injection.

Proprietary Preparations (details are given in Part 3)

Belg.: Inocor†; **Braz.:** Inocor; **Canad.:** Inocor†; **Fr.:** Inocor†; **Ger.:** Wincoram; **Israel:** Inocor; **Ital.:** Inocor; **Jpn:** Amcoral†; **Port.:** Inocor; **Spain:** Wincoram; **Swed.:** Inocor; **USA:** Inocor.

Ancrod   (4804-y)

Ancrod *(BAN, USAN, rINN)*.

CAS — 9046-56-4.

Ancrod is an enzyme obtained from the venom of the Malayan pit-viper (*Calloselasma rhodostoma = Agkistrodon rhodostoma*).

Units

The first International Reference Preparation of ancrod was established in 1976 and contains 55 units in 16.90 mg of purified ancrod (1 unit in about 307 µg).

The symbol † denotes a preparation no longer actively marketed

Adverse Effects and Treatment

Haemorrhage may occur during treatment with ancrod and usually responds to its withdrawal. If haemorrhage is severe, cryoprecipitate can be used to raise plasma fibrinogen concentrations; plasma may be used if cryoprecipitate is not available. An antivenom has been used to neutralise ancrod.

Skin rash, transient chills, and fever have been reported with the use of ancrod.

Precautions

As for Heparin, p.903.

Ancrod should not be given to patients with severe infections or disseminated intravascular coagulation. It should be used cautiously in patients with cardiovascular disorders that may be complicated by defibrination. It is very important that when ancrod is given by intravenous infusion it should be administered slowly to prevent the formation of large amounts of unstable fibrin.

Ancrod is not recommended during pregnancy; high doses in *animals* have caused placental haemorrhage and fetal death.

Interactions

Ancrod should not be administered concomitantly with antifibrinolytics such as aminocaproic acid or with plasma volume expanders such as dextrans.

Uses and Administration

Ancrod is an anticoagulant. It reduces the blood concentration of fibrinogen by the cleavage of microparticles of fibrin which are rapidly removed from the circulation by fibrinolysis or phagocytosis. It reduces blood viscosity but has no effect on established thrombi. Haemostatic concentrations of fibrinogen are normally restored in about 12 hours and normal concentrations in 10 to 20 days.

Ancrod may be used in the treatment of thromboembolic disorders (p.816), particularly in deep-vein thrombosis and to prevent thrombosis after surgery in patients requiring anticoagulation but who have developed heparin-induced thrombocytopenia or thrombosis (see p.817). It is under investigation in the treatment of ischaemic stroke and has also been given for priapism.

For treatment of thromboembolic disorders ancrod is given by intravenous infusion in an initial dose of 1 to 2 units per kg body-weight in 250 to 500 mL of sodium chloride 0.9% or glucose 5% over at least 12 hours. Maintenance doses of 0.5 to 1 unit per kg in 250 to 500 mL of infusion fluid are given over 24 hours. The blood-fibrinogen concentrations may be used to monitor treatment.

For the prevention of deep-vein thrombosis after surgery for fractured neck of a femur, 4 units per kg have been given by subcutaneous injection postoperatively, followed by 1 unit per kg daily for 4 days. Resistance has developed to ancrod.

◊ References.
1. Cole CW, *et al.* Heparin-associated thrombocytopenia and thrombosis: optimal therapy with ancrod. *Can J Surg* 1990; **33:** 207–10.
2. Demers C, *et al.* Rapid anticoagulation using ancrod for heparin-induced thrombocytopenia. *Blood* 1991; **78:** 2194–7.
3. Wright JG, Geroulakos G. Ancrod: clinical indications and methods of use. *Semin Vasc Surg* 1996; **9:** 315–28.
4. Sherman DG, *et al.* Intravenous ancrod for treatment of acute ischemic stroke: the STAT study: a randomized controlled trial. *JAMA* 2000; **283:** 2395–2403.

Preparations

Proprietary Preparations (details are given in Part 3)
Aust.: Arwin†; *Canad.:* Arvin†; Viprinex; *Ger.:* Arwin†; *Spain:* Arvin†; *UK:* Arvin†.

Angiotensinamide (2044-t)

Angiotensinamide *(BAN, rINN)*.

Angiotensin Amide *(USAN)*; NSC-107678. Asn-Arg-Val-Tyr-Val-His-Pro-Phe; [1-Asparagine,5-valine]angiotensin II.

$C_{49}H_{70}N_{14}O_{11} = 1031.2$.
CAS — 11128-99-7 (angiotensin II); 53-73-6 (angiotensinamide).
ATC — C01CX06.

Adverse Effects and Precautions

Rapid infusion of angiotensinamide may readily cause very severe hypertension. It should be given with caution to patients with cardiovascular disease or heart failure.

Interactions

Angiotensinamide should not be given to patients being treated with an MAOI or within 14 days of stopping such treatment as a hypertensive crisis may be precipitated.

Pharmacokinetics

Angiotensinamide is rapidly inactivated in the tissues and circulation by peptidase enzymes. When given intravenously it has a duration of action of only a few minutes.

Uses and Administration

Angiotensinamide is a vasopressor related to the naturally occurring peptide angiotensin II. It increases the peripheral resistance mainly in cutaneous, splanchnic, and renal blood vessels. The increased blood pressure is accompanied by a reflex reduction in heart rate, and cardiac output may also be reduced.

Angiotensinamide has been used in the treatment of hypotension associated with shock. It has also been given in the man-

agement of overdosage of ACE inhibitors, when conventional therapy has been ineffective.

For the management of hypotension, it is given by continuous intravenous infusion; concentrations have ranged from 1 to 10 mg per litre in sodium chloride 0.9%, glucose 5%, or other suitable diluent. Doses are adjusted according to blood pressure response; doses of up to 10 μg per minute may be adequate. Blood pressure must be monitored continuously during the infusion. Once the patient's condition improves the dosage should be reduced gradually before withdrawal.

◊ References.
1. Jackson T, *et al.* Enalapril overdose treated with angiotensin infusion. *Lancet* 1993; **341:** 703.
2. Newby DE, *et al.* Enalapril overdose and the corrective effect of intravenous angiotensin II. *Br J Clin Pharmacol* 1995; **40:** 103–4.
3. Yunge M, Petros A. Angiotensin for septic shock unresponsive to noradrenaline. *Arch Dis Child* 2000; **82:** 388–9.

Anipamil (3328-c)

Anipamil *(rINN)*.

2-{3-[(m-Methoxyphenethyl)methylamino]propyl}-2-(m-methoxyphenyl)-tetradecanenitrile.
$C_{34}H_{52}N_2O_2 = 520.8$.
CAS — 83200-10-6.

Profile

Anipamil is a calcium-channel blocker related to verapamil (p.989) which has been investigated in the treatment of hypertension and angina pectoris.

◊ References.
1. Dies R, *et al.* Antihypertensive efficacy of anipamil in mild to moderate hypertension. *J Cardiovasc Pharmacol* 1989; **13** (suppl 4): S36–9.
2. Sørum C, *et al.* Efficacy of anipamil, a phenylalkylamine calcium antagonist, in treatment of angina pectoris. *J Cardiovasc Pharmacol* 1994; **24:** 841–5.

Anisindione (4805-j)

Anisindione *(BAN, rINN)*.

2-(4-Methoxyphenyl)indan-1,3-dione.
$C_{16}H_{12}O_3 = 252.3$.
CAS — 117-37-3.

Profile

Anisindione is an orally administered indanedione anticoagulant with actions similar to those of warfarin (p.992). It is used in the management of thromboembolic disorders (p.816) but, as the indanediones are generally more toxic than warfarin (see Phenindione, p.954), its use is limited.

The usual initial dose is 300 mg on the first day, 200 mg on the second day, and 100 mg on the third. The maintenance dose may range from 25 to 250 mg daily according to coagulation tests.

During treatment with anisindione the urine may be coloured pink or orange.

Preparations

Proprietary Preparations (details are given in Part 3)
USA: Miradon.

Anistreplase (16996-d)

Anistreplase *(BAN, USAN, rINN)*.

Anisoylated Plasminogen Streptokinase Activator Complex; APSAC; BRL-26921. p-Anisoylated (human) lys-plasminogen streptokinase activator complex (1:1).
CAS — 81669-57-0.
ATC — B01AD03.

The manufacturer recommends that anistreplase should be **stored** at 2° to 8°.

Adverse Effects, Treatment, and Precautions

As for Streptokinase, p.976. Like streptokinase, anistreplase appears to be antigenic and may be neutralised by streptokinase antibodies.

Back pain. For references to back pain associated with anistreplase infusion, see under Streptokinase, p.976.

Interactions

As for Streptokinase, p.977.

Pharmacokinetics

Anistreplase is reported to be cleared from plasma at about half the rate of streptokinase and to have a fibrinolytic half-life of about 90 minutes. It is metabolised to the plasminogen-streptokinase complex at a steady rate.

◊ References.
1. Gemmill JD, *et al.* A comparison of the pharmacokinetic properties of streptokinase and anistreplase in acute myocardial infarction. *Br J Clin Pharmacol* 1991; **31:** 143–7.

Uses and Administration

Anistreplase is a thrombolytic drug. It consists of a complex of the lys-form of plasminogen and streptokinase with the addition of a p-anisoyl group that prevents the complex activating plasminogen to fibrinolysin. Following intravenous injection the anisoyl group undergoes deacylation at a steady rate to release the active complex which converts plasminogen to fibrinolysin, a proteolytic enzyme that has fibrinolytic effects. The mechanisms of fibrinolysis are discussed further under Haemostasis and Fibrinolysis on p.718.

Anistreplase is used similarly to streptokinase (p.977) in the treatment of thromboembolic disorders, particularly acute myocardial infarction (p.805). It is given as a single intravenous injection in a dose of 30 units over 4 to 5 minutes, as soon as possible after the onset of symptoms.

Preparations

Proprietary Preparations (details are given in Part 3)
Aust.: Eminase; *Belg.:* Eminase; *Canad.:* Eminase; *Fr.:* Eminase†; *Ger.:* Eminase†; *Israel:* Eminase; *Ital.:* Eminase†; Multilase†; *Neth.:* Eminase; *Port.:* Fibrit†; *Spain:* Iminase; *Switz.:* Eminase†; *UK:* Eminase†; *USA:* Eminase.

Apraclonidine Hydrochloride (3917-j)

Apraclonidine Hydrochloride *(BANM, USAN, rINNM)*.

AL-02145 (apraclonidine); p-Aminoclonidine Hydrochloride; Aplonidine Hydrochloride; NC-14. 2-[(4-Amino-2,6-dichlorophenyl)imino]imidazolidine hydrochloride; 2,6-Dichloro-N^1-imidazolidin-2-ylidene-p-phenylenediamine hydrochloride.
$C_9H_{10}Cl_2N_4,HCl = 281.6$.
CAS — 66711-21-5 (apraclonidine); 73218-79-8 (apraclonidine hydrochloride).

NOTE. APR is a code approved by the BP 2001 for use on single unit doses of eye drops containing apraclonidine hydrochloride where the individual container may be too small to bear all the appropriate labelling information.

Pharmacopoeias. In US.

Apraclonidine hydrochloride 11.5 mg is approximately equivalent to 10 mg of apraclonidine.

Pharmacopoeial description

USP 25: A white to off-white, odourless to practically odourless powder. Soluble 1 in 34 of water, 1 in 74 of alcohol, and 1 in 13 of methyl alcohol; insoluble in chloroform, in ethyl acetate, and in hexanes. pH of a 1% solution in water is between 5.0 and 6.6. Store in airtight containers. Protect from light.

Adverse Effects and Precautions

Adverse effects following perioperative instillation of apraclonidine into the eye include hyperaemia, lid retraction, conjunctival blanching, and mydriasis. Some patients may develop an exaggerated reduction in intra-ocular pressure. Following regular instillation an ocular intolerance reaction may occur, characterised by hyperaemia, ocular pruritus, increased lachrymation, ocular discomfort, and oedema of the lids and conjunctiva. Other adverse effects reported include dry mouth and nose, conjunctivitis, blurred vision, asthenia, headache, and taste disturbances. Systemic absorption may occur after application to the eye and may result in adverse effects similar to those of clonidine (p.860). Cardiovascular effects have been reported; therefore apraclonidine should be used with caution in patients with severe cardiovascular disease, including hypertension, and in patients with a history of vasovagal attacks. Drowsiness may also occur. Depression has rarely been associated with use of apraclonidine and it should be used with caution in depressed patients.

Interactions

Systemic absorption may occur following topical administration of apraclonidine to the eye and there is a theoretical possibility of interactions similar to those reported with clonidine (p.860). Since the effects of apraclonidine on circulating catecholamines are unknown, the concomitant use of MAOIs is contra-indicated by the manufacturer; tricyclic and related antidepressants and systemic sympathomimetics should also be avoided, or should be used with caution.

Uses and Administration

Apraclonidine is an alpha$_2$-adrenoceptor agonist derived from clonidine (p.860). It reduces intra-ocular pressure when instilled into the eye and is used in patients undergoing eye surgery and as an adjunct in the management of glaucoma. The reduction in intra-ocular pressure begins within an hour of instillation and is maximal after about three to five hours.

Apraclonidine is used as the hydrochloride, but the strength of an ophthalmic solution is usually expressed in terms of the base.

To control or prevent a postoperative increase in intra-ocular pressure in patients undergoing anterior segment laser surgery, one drop of a 1% solution is instilled into the eye one hour before surgery and a second drop is instilled immediately upon completion of surgery.

For short-term adjunctive therapy in patients with raised intra-ocular pressure not controlled by conventional therapy, one or two drops of a 0.5% solution may be instilled three times daily.

Glaucoma and ocular hypertension. Apraclonidine lowers intra-ocular pressure, probably by reducing production of aqueous humour, and is used to control intra-ocular pressure in patients undergoing eye surgery and in patients with glaucoma (p.1413). Application of apraclonidine 1% eye drops pre-operatively and/or postoperatively has minimised increases in intra-ocular pressure following ocular laser surgery[1-3] and surgical removal of cataracts.[4] Use of apraclonidine 1% with pilocarpine 4% has produced additional benefit over either drug given alone.[5] Satisfactory results have also been reported using 0.5% eye drops.[3] Although long-term use of apraclonidine has been reported[6] in patients with glaucoma, such use is limited by a high incidence of ocular adverse effects and the development of tachyphylaxis.

1. Robin AL. Argon laser trabeculoplasty medical therapy to prevent the intraocular pressure rise associated with argon laser trabeculoplasty. *Ophthalmic Surg* 1991; **22:** 31–7.
2. Rao BS, Badrinath SS. Efficacy and safety of apraclonidine in patients undergoing anterior segment laser surgery. *Br J Ophthalmol* 1989; **73:** 884–7.
3. Rosenberg LF, *et al.* Apraclonidine and anterior segment laser surgery: comparison of 0.5% versus 1.0% apraclonidine for prevention of postoperative intraocular pressure rise. *Ophthalmology* 1995; **102:** 1312–18.
4. Wiles SB, *et al.* Control of intraocular pressure with apraclonidine hydrochloride after cataract extraction. *Am J Ophthalmol* 1991; **111:** 184–8.
5. Dapling RB, *et al.* Influence of apraclonidine and pilocarpine alone and in combination on post laser trabeculoplasty pressure rise. *Br J Ophthalmol* 1994; **78:** 30–2.
6. Araujo SV, *et al.* Long term effect of apraclonidine. *Br J Ophthalmol* 1995; **79:** 1098–1101.

Preparations

USP 25: Apraclonidine Ophthalmic Solution.

Proprietary Preparations (details are given in Part 3)
Aust.: Iopidine; *Austral.:* Iopidine; *Belg.:* Iopidine; *Canad.:* Iopidine; *Denm.:* Iopidine; *Fin.:* Iopidine; *Fr.:* Iopidine; *Ger.:* Iopidine; *Hong Kong:* Iopidine; *Irl.:* Iopidine; *Israel:* Iopidine; *Ital.:* Iopidine; *Jpn:* Iopidine; *Mex.:* Iopidine; *Norw.:* Iopidine; *NZ:* Iopidine; *Port.:* Iopidine; *S.Afr.:* Iopidine; *Singapore:* Iopidine; *Spain:* Iopimax; *Swed.:* Iopidine; *Switz.:* Iopidine; *UK:* Iopidine; *USA:* Iopidine.

Aprindine Hydrochloride   (7781-d)

Aprindine Hydrochloride (*BANM, USAN, rINNM*).
AC-1802; Compound 83846; Compound 99170 (aprindine). *N*-(3-Diethylaminopropyl)-*N*-indan-2-ylaniline hydrochloride; *NN*-Diethyl-*N*′-indan-2-yl-*N*′-phenyltrimethylenediamine hydrochloride.
$C_{22}H_{30}N_2$,HCl = 358.9.
CAS — 37640-71-4 (aprindine); 33237-74-0 (aprindine hydrochloride).

Adverse Effects and Precautions

Adverse effects of aprindine are usually dose-related and most commonly affect the CNS. They include tremor, vertigo, ataxia, diplopia, memory impairment, hallucinations, and convulsions. Gastrointestinal effects include nausea, vomiting, and bloating. There have been reports of agranulocytosis which can be fatal. Hepatitis and cholestatic jaundice have occasionally been reported; blood and liver function tests should be performed during treatment.

Aprindine is contra-indicated in patients with advanced heart failure or severe conduction disturbances. Some manufacturers have recommended that aprindine should not be used in patients with parkinsonism or convulsive disorders. It should be

used with caution in patients with bradycardia, hypotension, and hepatic or renal impairment.

Interactions

Antiarrhythmics. Steady-state plasma-aprindine concentrations increased in 2 patients after the initiation of *amiodarone* therapy and coincided with the appearance of adverse effects.[1]

1. Southworth W, *et al.* Possible amiodarone-aprindine interaction. *Am Heart J* 1982; **104:** 323.

Pharmacokinetics

Aprindine is readily absorbed from the gastrointestinal tract. It has a long plasma half-life, usually between 20 and 27 hours, and is about 85 to 95% bound to plasma proteins. It is excreted in the urine and the bile.

Uses and Administration

Aprindine is a class Ib antiarrhythmic (p.787) used in the management of ventricular and supraventricular arrhythmias (p.794).

Aprindine is given as the hydrochloride in usual doses of 50 to 100 mg daily by mouth; up to 200 mg daily may be given. If necessary initial doses of up to 300 mg daily may be given under strict surveillance for the first 2 to 3 days. Therapy should be monitored by ECG during initial stabilisation of the dose and intermittently thereafter. It has also been given intravenously.

◊ References.
1. Danilo P. Aprindine. *Am Heart J* 1979; **97:** 119–24.

Preparations

Proprietary Preparations (details are given in Part 3)
Belg.: Fiboran; *Fr.:* Fiboran; *Ger.:* Amidonal; *Spain:* Fiboran.

Aranidipine   (17286-n)

Aranidipine (*rINN*).
(±)-Acetonyl methyl 1,4-dihydro-2,6-dimethyl-4-(*o*-nitrophenyl)-3,5-pyridinedicarboxylate.
$C_{19}H_{20}N_2O_7$ = 388.4.
CAS — 86780-90-7.

Profile

Aranidipine is a dihydropyridine calcium-channel blocker used in the management of hypertension.

Preparations

Proprietary Preparations (details are given in Part 3)
Jpn: Bec; Flaspas; Sapresta.

Arbutamine Hydrochloride   (14332-y)

Arbutamine Hydrochloride (*BANM, USAN, rINNM*).
GP-2-121-3 (arbutamine or arbutamine hydrochloride). (*R*)-4-(1-Hydroxy-2-[4-(4-hydroxyphenyl)butylamino]ethyl)pyrocatechol hydrochloride.
$C_{18}H_{23}NO_4$,HCl = 353.8.
CAS — 128470-16-6 (arbutamine); 125251-66-3 (arbutamine hydrochloride).

Profile

Arbutamine hydrochloride is a sympathomimetic (see Adrenaline, p.829) with beta-agonist properties and like dobutamine (p.881) has been used for cardiac stress testing in patients unable to exercise. For such a purpose an initial dose of 0.1 µg per kg body-weight is given intravenously by a computer-controlled delivery system over 1 minute, and the heart rate response is measured. The device then calculates the difference between the desired and actual heart rate and adjusts the infusion rate accordingly up to a maximum rate of 0.8 µg per kg per minute and a maximum total dose of 10 µg per kg.

◊ References.
1. Anonymous. Arbutamine for stress testing. *Med Lett Drugs Ther* 1998; **40:** 19–20.

Preparations

Proprietary Preparations (details are given in Part 3)
Swed.: Genesa†; *USA:* Genesa.

Ardeparin Sodium   (17068-j)

Ardeparin Sodium (*USAN, rINN*).
Wy-90493-RD.
CAS — 9041-08-1.

Ardeparin sodium is prepared by peroxide degradation of heparin obtained from the intestinal mucosa of pigs. The end chain structure appears to be the same as the starting material with no unusual sugar residues present. The molecular weight of 98% of the components is between 2000 and 15 000 and the average molecular weight is about 5500 to 6500. The degree of sulfation is about 2.7 per disaccharide unit.

Profile

Ardeparin sodium is a low-molecular-weight heparin (p.923) with anticoagulant activity that has been used for the prevention of postoperative venous thromboembolism.

Preparations

Proprietary Preparations (details are given in Part 3)
USA: Normiflo†.

Argatroban   (19453-c)

Argatroban (*BAN, USAN, rINN*).
DK-7419; GN-1600; MCI-9038; MD-805. (2*R*,4*R*)-4-Methyl-1-[(*S*)-*N*^{2}- {[(*RS*)-1,2,3,4-tetrahydro-3-methyl-8-quinolyl]sulfonyl}arginyl]pipecolic acid.
$C_{23}H_{36}N_6O_5S$ = 508.6.
CAS — 74863-84-6 (anhydrous argatroban); 141396-28-3 (argatroban monohydrate).

Profile

Argatroban is a synthetic thrombin inhibitor with anticoagulant and antiplatelet activity. It is used for the treatment and prophylaxis of thromboembolism in patients with heparin-induced thrombocytopenia (p.902). It has also been used in other thromboembolic disorders.

In the management of heparin-induced thrombocytopenia, argatroban is given by intravenous infusion in an initial dose of 2 µg per kg body-weight per minute, adjusted according to the activated partial thromboplastin time (APTT), to a maximum dose of 10 µg per kg per minute. The initial dose should be reduced in patients with hepatic impairment.

◊ References.
1. Kondo LM, *et al.* Argatroban for prevention and treatment of thromboembolism in heparin-induced thrombocytopenia. *Ann Pharmacother* 2001; **35:** 440–51.

Preparations

Proprietary Preparations (details are given in Part 3)
Jpn: Novastan; *USA:* Argatroban®.

Arotinolol Hydrochloride   (18779-q)

Arotinolol Hydrochloride (*rINNM*).
S-596. (±)-5-[2-{[3-(*tert*-Butylamino)-2-hydroxypropyl]thio}-4-thiazolyl]-2-thiophenecarboxamide hydrochloride.
$C_{15}H_{21}N_3O_2S_3$,HCl = 408.0.
CAS — 68377-92-4 (arotinolol).
Pharmacopoeias. In Jpn.

Profile

Arotinolol is a non-cardioselective beta blocker (p.844). In addition, it has alpha$_1$-blocking activity. It is used as the hydrochloride in the management of hypertension (p.802), angina pectoris (p.791), cardiac arrhythmias (p.794), and essential tremor (p.848). The usual dose is 20 mg daily in 2 divided doses although up to 30 mg daily may be given. The initial dose for essential tremor is 10 mg daily.

Preparations

Proprietary Preparations (details are given in Part 3)
Jpn: Almarl.

Atenolol   (6304-s)

Atenolol (*BAN, USAN, rINN*).
Atenololum; ICI-66082. 2-{*p*-[2-Hydroxy-3-(isopropylamino)propoxy]phenyl}acetamide.
$C_{14}H_{22}N_2O_3$ = 266.3.
CAS — 29122-68-7; 60966-51-0.
ATC — C07AB03.

NOTE. Compounded preparations of atenolol may be represented by the following names:

- Co-tenidone (*BAN*)—atenolol 4 parts and chlortalidone 1 part (w/w)
- Co-tenidone (*USP 25*)—atenolol and chlortalidone

Pharmacopoeias. In Chin., Eur. (see p.vi), and US.

Pharmacopoeial description

Ph. Eur.: A white or almost white powder. Sparingly soluble in water; soluble in dehydrated alcohol; slightly soluble in dichloromethane; practically insoluble in ether.

Adverse Effects, Treatment, and Precautions

As for beta blockers, p.844.

Breast feeding. For a report of bradycardia in a neonate following ingestion of atenolol in breast milk, see under Pharmacokinetics, below.

Effects on the gastrointestinal tract. Reports of sclerosing peritonitis[1] and retroperitoneal fibrosis[2] in patients taking atenolol.

1. Nielsen BV, Pedersen KG. Sclerosing peritonitis associated with atenolol. *BMJ* 1985; **290:** 518.
2. Johnson JN, McFarland J. Retroperitoneal fibrosis associated with atenolol. *BMJ* 1980; **280:** 864.

Effects on the heart. Beta blockers are used in the management of cardiac arrhythmias. However, atenolol 2.5 mg by

---

intravenous injection induced atrial fibrillation in 6 of 12 predisposed patients.[1]

1. Rassmussen K, et al. Atrial fibrillation induced by atenolol. Eur Heart J 1982; 3: 276–81.

Effects on lipid metabolism. For a report of acute pancreatitis due to hypertriglyceridaemia in a patient taking atenolol and metoprolol, see p.845.

Effects on the liver. A report of reversible cholestatic hepatitis in a patient receiving atenolol[1] and hepatic dysfunction in another.[2]

1. Schwartz MS, et al. Atenolol-associated cholestasis. Am J Gastroenterol 1989; 84: 1084–6.
2. Yusuf SW, Mishra RM. Hepatic dysfunction associated with atenolol. Lancet 1995; 346: 192.

Effects on vision. Visual symptoms without headache were associated with atenolol for migraine prophylaxis in a patient who had experienced a similar reaction with nadolol.[1]

1. Kumar KL, Cooney TG. Visual symptoms after atenolol therapy for migraine. Ann Intern Med 1990; 112: 712–13. Correction. ibid.; 113: 257.

Hypotension. Precipitous falls in blood pressure in patients with malignant hypertension may cause ischaemic damage to vital organs. Initiating treatment with 1 or 2 oral drugs is considered appropriate but not without risk. Two cases of hypotension following a single oral dose of atenolol 100 mg (27-year-old woman) and following 2 oral doses of atenolol 50 mg (51-year-old woman) have been reported.[1] The women had presented with severe hypertension, hyponatraemia, hypokalaemia, and high renin activity. There was a transient elevation of serum creatinine in both patients indicating kidney ischaemia. Renal artery thrombosis believed to be due to the hypotensive effect of atenolol was reported in a 70-year-old man with a history of circulatory and cardiac disorders.[2] He had received atenolol 100 mg for treatment of moderate hypertension.

1. Kholeif M, Isles C. Profound hypotension after atenolol in severe hypertension. BMJ 1989; 298: 161–2.
2. Shaw AB, Gopalka SK. Renal artery thrombosis caused by antihypertensive treatment. BMJ 1982; 285: 1617.

Overdosage. Ventricular asystole occurred in a man who had taken a massive overdose of atenolol.[1]

1. Stinson J, et al. Ventricular asystole and overdose with atenolol. BMJ 1992; 305: 693.

Interactions

The interactions associated with beta blockers are discussed on p.846.

Pharmacokinetics

Atenolol is incompletely absorbed from the gastrointestinal tract; following oral administration about 50% is absorbed. Peak plasma concentrations are reached in 2 to 4 hours. Atenolol has low lipid solubility. It crosses the placenta and is distributed into breast milk where concentrations higher than those in maternal plasma have been achieved. Only small amounts are reported to cross the blood-brain barrier, and plasma-protein binding is minimal. The plasma half-life is about 6 to 7 hours. Atenolol undergoes little or no hepatic metabolism and is excreted mainly in the urine.

Breast feeding. Atenolol diffuses into breast milk in concentrations similar[1] to or higher[2] than those in maternal blood. Bradycardia associated with ingestion of atenolol in breast milk has been reported in a 5-day-old term infant. The baby improved when breast feeding was discontinued.[3]

1. Thorley KJ, McAinsh J. Levels of the beta-blockers atenolol and propranolol in the breast milk of women treated for hypertension in pregnancy. Biopharm Drug Dispos 1983; 4: 299–301.
2. White WB, et al. Atenolol in human plasma and breast milk. Obstet Gynecol 1984; 63: 42S–44S.
3. Schimmel MS, et al. Toxic effects of atenolol consumed during breast feeding. J Pediatr 1989; 114: 476–8.

Pregnancy. In 6 women who had taken atenolol for at least 6 days up to the time of delivery concentrations of atenolol in maternal and umbilical serum were approximately equal. In a further woman who had discontinued treatment one day before delivery atenolol was not found in maternal or umbilical serum.[1] The half-life of atenolol in neonates born to mothers who had been receiving atenolol ranged from 10.5 to 34.6 hours (mean 16.1 hours) in a study of 35 term infants.[2] Atenolol concentrations were determined in cord blood and in neonatal blood 24 hours after delivery. The range of elimination rate was 4 times slower than in adults, a difference expected based on renal excretion of atenolol.

1. Melander A, et al. Transplacental passage of atenolol in man. Eur J Clin Pharmacol 1978; 14: 93–4.
2. Rubin PC, et al. Atenolol elimination in the neonate. Br J Clin Pharmacol 1983; 16: 659–62.

Uses and Administration

Atenolol is a cardioselective beta blocker (p.844). It is reported to lack intrinsic sympathomimetic activity and membrane-stabilising properties.

Atenolol is used in the management of hypertension (p.802), angina pectoris (p.791), cardiac arrhythmias (p.794), and myocardial infarction (p.805). It may also be used in the prophylactic treatment of migraine (p.449).

In **hypertension** atenolol is given by mouth in a dose of 50 to 100 mg daily, as a single dose, although 50 mg daily is generally adequate. The full effect is usually evident within 1 to 2 weeks.

The usual dose for **angina pectoris** is 50 to 100 mg daily by mouth, given as single or divided doses. Although up to 200 mg daily has been given for angina pectoris additional benefit is not usually obtained from higher doses of atenolol.

For the emergency treatment of **cardiac arrhythmias** atenolol may be given by intravenous injection in a dose of 2.5 mg injected at a rate of 1 mg per minute, repeated if necessary every 5 minutes to a maximum total dosage of 10 mg. Alternatively atenolol may be given by intravenous infusion, a dose of 150 μg per kg body-weight being administered over 20 minutes. The injection or infusion procedure may be repeated every 12 hours if necessary. When control is achieved maintenance doses of 50 to 100 mg daily may be given by mouth.

Atenolol is also used in the early management of acute **myocardial infarction**. Treatment should be given within 12 hours of the onset of chest pain; atenolol 5 mg should be given by slow intravenous injection at a rate of 1 mg per minute and followed after 15 minutes with 50 mg by mouth, provided no adverse effects result; alternatively the intravenous dose may be repeated after 10 minutes followed by 50 mg by mouth after a further 10 minutes. A further 50 mg may be given by mouth after 12 hours, and subsequent dosage maintained, after a further 12 hours, with 100 mg daily.

In the prophylaxis of **migraine** a dose of 50 to 100 mg daily by mouth has been used.

Reduced doses may be required in patients with impaired renal function, as follows. When creatinine clearance is 15 to 35 mL per minute the dose is 50 mg daily by mouth or 10 mg once every two days intravenously. When creatinine clearance is less than 15 mL per minute the dose is 25 mg daily or 50 mg on alternate days by mouth or 10 mg once every four days intravenously.

Preparations

BP 2001: Atenolol Injection; Atenolol Oral Solution; Atenolol Tablets; Co-tenidone Tablets;
USP 25: Atenolol Injection; Atenolol Tablets.

Proprietary Preparations (details are given in Part 3)
Aust.: Arcablock; Atehexal; Atenobene; Atenolan; Betasyn; Tenormin; **Austral.:** Anselol; Atehexal; Noten; Tenlol; Tenormin; Tensig; **Belg.:** Blokium; Tenormin; **Braz.:** Angipress; Atenol; Neotenol; **Canad.:** Apo-Atenol; Novo-Atenol; Nu-Atenol; Tenolin; Tenormin; **Denm.:** Atenet; Atenodan; Atenor; Myopax; Tenormin; Uniloc; **Fin.:** Atehexal; Atenol; Tenoblock; Tenoprin; Uniloc; **Fr.:** Betatop; Tenormine; Xaten; **Ger.:** Ate; Ate Lich; Atebeta; Atehexal; Atendol; Ateno; Atenogamma; Atenomerck†; Atereal†; Blocotenol; Cuxanorm; Dignobeta†; duratenol; Evitocor; Falitonsin; Jenatenol; Juventa; Teno; Tenormin; Tonoprotect; **Hong Kong:** Antipressan; Apo-Atenol; Ateno; Corotenol; Hypernol; Lo-Ten; Nif-Ten; Tenormin; Vascoten; Velorin; **Irl.:** Amolin; Antipressan†; Atecor; Ateni; Atenogen; Atenomel; Tenormin; Trantalol; **Israel:** Aponorm; Normalol; Normiten; **Ital.:** Atenol; Atermin; Seles Beta; Tenomax; Tenormin; **Mex.:** Tenormin; **Neth.:** Tenormin; Unibloc†; **Norw.:** Alinor; Coratol†; Tenormin; Uniloc; **NZ:** Anselol; Lo-Ten; Tenormin; **Port.:** Ancoren; Blokium; Tenormin; Tessifol; **S.Afr.:** Atenoblok; Aterol; B-Vasc; Clinaten†; Hexa-Blok; Ten-Bloka; Tenormin; Venapulse†; **Singapore:** Alonet; Apo-Atenol; Normaten; Prenolol; Tenormin; Vascoten; Velorin; **Spain:** Blokium; Neatenol; Tenormin; **Swed.:** Selinol; Tenormin; Uniloc; **Switz.:** Atenil; ateno-basan; Atesifar; Cardaxen; Selobloc; Servitenol†; Tenat; Tenormin; **Thai.:** Atenol; Noten; Oraday; Prenolol; Tenolol; Tenormin; Vascoten; Velorin; **UAE:** Tensotin; **UK:** Antipressan; Atenix; Tenormin; Totamol; **USA:** Tenormin.

Multi-ingredient: **Aust.:** Arcablock comp; Atenolan comp; Atenolol comp; Beta-Adalat; Nif-Ten; Polinorm; Tenoretic; **Belg.:** Beta-Adalat; Kalten; Tenif; Tenoretic; **Braz.:** Nifelat; Tenoretic; **Canad.:** Tenoretic; **Denm.:** Tenidon; Tenoretic; **Fin.:** Beta-Adalat; Nif-Ten; **Fr.:** Beta-Adalate; Tenordate; Tenoretic; **Ger.:** Ate Lich comp; Atehexal comp; Atel; AteNif beta; Ateno comp; Atenogamma comp; Atenolol AL comp; Atenolol comp; Atenomerck comp†; Blocotenol comp; Bresben; Diu-Atenolol; duratenolol comp†; Evitocor plus†; Nif-Ten; Nifatenol; Sigabloc; Tenoretic; TRI-Normin; **Hong Kong:** Target; Tenoret; Tenoretic; **Irl.:** Ate-Nife; Atenetic; Beta-Adalat; Cotenomel; Nif-Ten; Tenchlor†; Tenoret; Tenoretic; **Ital.:** Ataclor; Atenigron; Atinorm; Carmian; Clortanol; Diube; Eupres; Igroseles; Mixer; Nif-Ten; Nor-Pa; Nor-

mopress; Target; Tenolone; Tenoretic; **Mex.:** Plenacor; Tenoretic; **Neth.:** Hykaten†; Nif-Ten; Tenoretic; **NZ:** Tenoret; Tenoretic; **Port.:** Blokium Diu; Tenoretic; **S.Afr.:** Adco-Loten; Atenoblok Co; Ateren; Tenchlor; Tenoret†; Tenoretic; Venachlor†; **Singapore:** Nif-Ten; Nifetex; Tenoret; Tenoretic; **Spain:** Betasit Plus†; Blokium Diu; Kalten; Neatenol Diu; Neatenol Diuvas; Normopresil; Tenoretic; **Switz.:** Atedurex; ateno-basan comp.; Beta-Adalat; Cardaxen plus; Cotenolol; Kalten; Nif-Atenil; Nif-Ten; Tenoretic; **Thai.:** Tenoretic; **UK:** AtenixCo; Beta-Adalat; Kalten; Tenben; Tenchlor; Tenif; Tenoret; Tenoretic; Totaretic; **USA:** Tenoretic.

Atorvastatin Calcium (14543-n)

Atorvastatin Calcium (BANM, USAN, rINNM).
CI-981. Calcium (βR,δR)-2-(p-fluorophenyl)-β,δ-dihydroxy-5-isopropyl-3-phenyl-4-(phenylcarbamoyl)pyrrole-1-heptanoic acid (1:2) trihydrate.
$C_{66}H_{68}CaF_2N_4O_{10},3H_2O = 1209.4.$
CAS — 134523-00-5 (atorvastatin); 134523-03-8 (atorvastatin calcium).

Adverse Effects and Precautions

As for Simvastatin, p.969.

◊ General references.

1. Black DM, et al. An overview of the clinical safety profile of atorvastatin (Lipitor), a new HMG-CoA reductase inhibitor. Arch Intern Med 1998; 158: 577–84.

Effects on the blood. An immune thrombocytopenia attributed to atorvastatin has been reported in a patient.[1] Adverse haematological reactions had not been noted when the patient previously received simvastatin.

1. González-Ponte ML, et al. Atorvastatin-induced severe thrombocytopenia. Lancet 1998; 352: 1284.

Effects on the liver. Acute hepatitis was diagnosed in a woman 12 weeks after starting treatment with atorvastatin. She had previously been taking simvastatin and fenofibrate without adverse effect, but with persistent hypercholesterolaemia. Following cessation of atorvastatin, liver function tests returned to normal and the patient recommenced simvastatin therapy, again without adverse effect.[1]

1. Nakad A, et al. Atorvastatin-induced acute hepatitis with absence of cross-toxicity with simvastatin. Lancet 1999; 353: 1763–4.

Effects on skeletal muscle. Muscle disorders are well-recognised adverse effects of lipid regulating drugs such as the fibrates and statins (see Simvastatin, p.970).

A woman developed rhabdomyolysis two months after starting atorvastatin.[1] She was already taking ciclosporin following renal transplantation and had a history of systemic lupus erythematosus.

1. Maltz HC, et al. Rhabdomyolysis associated with concomitant use of atorvastatin and cyclosporine. Ann Pharmacother 1999; 33: 1176–9.

Effects on the skin. Toxic epidermal necrolysis apparently caused by atorvastatin has been reported.[1] The authors were not aware of this adverse effect previously having been associated with any of the statin lipid regulating drugs.

1. Pfeiffer CM, et al. Toxic epidermal necrolysis from atorvastatin. JAMA 1998; 279: 1613–14.

Interactions

As for Simvastatin, p.970.

Pharmacokinetics

Atorvastatin is rapidly absorbed from the gastrointestinal tract. It has low absolute bioavailability of about 12% due to presystemic clearance in the gastrointestinal mucosa and/or first-pass metabolism in the liver, its primary site of action. Atorvastatin is metabolised by the cytochrome P450 isoenzyme CYP3A4 to a number of compounds which are also active inhibitors of HMG-CoA reductase. The mean plasma elimination half-life of atorvastatin is about 14 hours although the half-life of inhibitory activity for HMG-CoA reductase is approximately 20 to 30 hours due to the contribution of the active metabolites. It is 98% bound to plasma proteins. Atorvastatin is excreted as metabolites, primarily in the bile.

Uses and Administration

Atorvastatin, a 3-hydroxy-3-methylglutaryl coenzyme A (HMG-CoA) reductase inhibitor (a statin), is a lipid regulating drug with actions on plasma lipids similar to those of simvastatin (p.970). It is used to reduce LDL-cholesterol, apolipoprotein B, and triglycerides, and to increase HDL-cholesterol in the treatment of hyperlipidaemias (p.800), including hypercholesterolaemias and combined (mixed) hyperlipidaemia (type IIa or IIb hyperlipoproteinaemias), hypertriglyceridaemia (type IV), and dysbetalipoproteinaemia (type III). Atorvastatin can also be effective as adjunctive therapy in patients with homozygous familial hypercholesterolaemia who have some LDL-receptor function.

Atorvastatin is given by mouth as the calcium salt although doses are expressed in terms of the base. The initial dose is 10 mg daily which may be adjusted at intervals of 4 weeks up to a maximum of 80 mg daily.

◊ General reviews.
1. Lea AP, McTavish D. Atorvastatin: a review of its pharmacology and therapeutic potential in the management of hyperlipidaemias. *Drugs* 1997; **53:** 828–47.
2. Malinowski JM. Atorvastatin: a hydroxymethylglutaryl-coenzyme A reductase inhibitor. *Am J Health-Syst Pharm* 1998; **55:** 2253–67.

Preparations
Proprietary Preparations (details are given in Part 3)
Aust.: Sortis; *Austral.:* Lipitor; *Belg.:* Lipitor; *Canad.:* Lipitor; *Denm.:* Zarator; *Fin.:* Lipitor; *Fr.:* Tahor; *Ger.:* Sortis; *Hong Kong:* Lipitor; *Irl.:* Lipitor; *Israel:* Lipitor; *Ital.:* Torvast; Totalip; Xarator; *Mex.:* Lipitor; *Neth.:* Lipitor; *Norw.:* Lipitor; *NZ:* Lipitor; *Port.:* Zarator; *S.Afr.:* Lipitor; *Singapore:* Lipitor; *Spain:* Cardyl; Prevencor; Zarator; *Swed.:* Lipitor; *Switz.:* Sortis; *Thai.:* Lipitor; *UK:* Lipitor; *USA:* Lipitor.

Azimilide Hydrochloride (18553-l)
Azimilide Hydrochloride (BANM, rINNM).
Azimilide Dihydrochloride (USAN); NE-10064. 1-{[5-(p-Chlorophenyl)furfurylidene]amino}-3-[4-(4-methyl-1-piperazinyl)butyl]hydantoin dihydrochloride.
$C_{23}H_{28}ClN_5O_3,2HCl = 530.9$.
CAS — 149908-53-2 (azimilide); 149888-94-8 (azimilide hydrochloride).

Profile
Azimilide hydrochloride is a class III antiarrhythmic (p.787) being studied in the management of supraventricular arrhythmias.

◊ References.
1. Clemett D, Markham A. Azimilide. *Drugs* 2000; **59:** 271–7.

Azosemide (12415-d)
Azosemide (USAN, rINN).
BM-02001; Ple-1053. 2-Chloro-5-(1*H*-tetrazol-5-yl)-4-(2-thenylamino)benzenesulphonamide.
$C_{12}H_{11}ClN_6O_2S_2 = 370.8$.
CAS — 27589-33-9.

Profile
Azosemide is a diuretic with actions similar to those of frusemide [furosemide] (p.893). It is used in the management of oedema in a usual dose of 80 mg daily by mouth.

Preparations
Proprietary Preparations (details are given in Part 3)
Ger.: Luret.

Bamethan Sulfate (9207-s)
Bamethan Sulfate (USAN, rINNM).
Bamethan Sulphate (BANM). 2-Butylamino-1-(4-hydroxyphenyl)ethanol sulphate.
$(C_{12}H_{19}NO_2)_2,H_2SO_4 = 516.6$.
CAS — 3703-79-5 (bamethan); 5716-20-1 (bamethan sulfate).
Pharmacopoeias. In Jpn and Pol.

Profile
Bamethan sulfate is a vasodilator used in the management of peripheral vascular disorders.
Bamethan nicotinate and bamethan succinate have been used similarly.

Preparations
Proprietary Preparations (details are given in Part 3)
Aust.: Provascul; Vasculat†; *Braz.:* Vasculat; *Ger.:* Emasex A; *Spain:* Vasculat.

Multi-ingredient: *Fr.:* Escinogel; *Ger.:* Emasex-N; Medigel.

Barnidipine Hydrochloride (15254-d)
Barnidipine Hydrochloride (rINNM).
LY-198561; Mepirodipine Hydrochloride; YM-730; YM-09730-5. (+)-(3′S,4S)-1-Benzyl-3-pyrrolidinyl methyl 1,4-dihydro-2,6-dimethyl-4-(*m*-nitrophenyl)-3,5-pyridinedicarboxylate hydrochloride.
$C_{27}H_{29}N_3O_6,HCl = 528.0$.
CAS — 104713-75-9 (barnidipine); 104757-53-1 (barnidipine hydrochloride).

Profile
Barnidipine is a dihydropyridine calcium-channel blocker with general properties similar to those of nifedipine (p.940). It is given by mouth as the hydrochloride in the management of hypertension (p.802) in a usual dose of 10 to 15 mg once daily.

◊ Reviews.
1. Malhotra HS, Plosker GL. Barnidipine. *Drugs* 2001; **61:** 989–96.

Preparations
Proprietary Preparations (details are given in Part 3)
Jpn: Hypoca; *Neth.:* Cyress.

Beclobrate (12421-r)
Beclobrate (BAN, rINN).
Sgd-24774. Ethyl (±)-2-(4-*p*-chlorobenzylphenoxy)-2-methylbutyrate.
$C_{20}H_{23}ClO_3 = 346.8$.
CAS — 55937-99-0.

Profile
Beclobrate, a fibric acid derivative (see Bezafibrate, p.849), was used as a lipid regulating drug, but liver toxicity led to its withdrawal.

Befunolol Hydrochloride (16528-a)
Befunolol Hydrochloride (rINNM).
BFE-60. 7-[2-Hydroxy-3-(isopropylamino)propoxy]-2-benzofuranyl methyl ketone hydrochloride.
$C_{16}H_{21}NO_4,HCl = 327.8$.
CAS — 39552-01-7 (befunolol); 39543-79-8 (befunolol hydrochloride).

Profile
Befunolol is a beta blocker (p.844). It is used as the hydrochloride in the management of ocular hypertension and open-angle glaucoma (p.1413). Eye drops containing befunolol hydrochloride 0.25% or 0.5% are instilled twice daily.

Preparations
Proprietary Preparations (details are given in Part 3)
Aust.: Glauconex; *Belg.:* Glauconex†; *Fr.:* Bentos; *Ger.:* Glauconex; *Hong Kong:* Bentos; *Ital.:* Betaclar; *Jpn:* Bentos†; *Neth.:* Glauconex†.

Bemetizide (12423-d)
Bemetizide (BAN, rINN).
Diu-60. 6-Chloro-3,4-dihydro-3-(α-methylbenzyl)-2*H*-1,2,4-benzothiadiazine-7-sulphonamide 1,1-dioxide.
$C_{15}H_{16}ClN_3O_4S_2 = 401.9$.
CAS — 1824-52-8.

Profile
Bemetizide is a thiazide diuretic (see Hydrochlorothiazide, p.907) that is used, often in combination with triamterene, in the treatment of oedema and hypertension.

Preparations
Proprietary Preparations (details are given in Part 3)
Multi-ingredient: *Aust.:* Dehydrosin†; Diucomb†; *Belg.:* Diucomb; *Fr.:* Tensigradyl†; *Ger.:* dehydro sanol tri; dehydro tri mite; Diucomb; *Switz.:* Diucomb.

Benazepril Hydrochloride (18951-m)
Benazepril Hydrochloride (BANM, USAN, rINNM).
CGS-14824A (benazepril or benazepril hydrochloride). {(3*S*)-3-[(1*S*)-1-Ethoxycarbonyl-3-phenylpropylamino]-2,3,4,5-tetrahydro-2-oxo-1*H*-1-benzazepin-1-yl}acetic acid hydrochloride; 1-Carboxymethyl-3-[1-ethoxycarbonyl-3-phenyl-(1*S*)-propylamino]-2,3,4,5-tetrahydro-1*H*-1(3*S*)-benzazepin-2-one hydrochloride.
$C_{24}H_{28}N_2O_5,HCl = 461.0$.
CAS — 86541-75-5 (benazepril); 86541-74-4 (benazepril hydrochloride).

Adverse Effects, Treatment, and Precautions
As for ACE inhibitors, p.820.

Interactions
As for ACE inhibitors, p.822.

Pharmacokinetics
Benazepril acts as a prodrug of the diacid benazeprilat, its active metabolite. Following oral administration at least 37% of a dose of benazepril is absorbed. Benazepril is almost completely metabolised in the liver to benazeprilat. Peak plasma concentrations of benazeprilat following an oral dose of benazepril have been achieved after 1 to 2 hours in the fasting state or after 2 to 4 hours in the nonfasting state. Both benazepril and benazeprilat are about 95% bound to plasma proteins. Benazeprilat is excreted mainly in the urine; about 11 to 12% is excreted in the bile. The effective half-life for accumulation of benazeprilat is 10 to 11 hours following multiple doses of benazepril. The elimination of benazeprilat is slowed in renal impairment. Small amounts of benazepril and benazeprilat are distributed into breast milk.

◊ References.
1. Kaiser G, *et al.* Pharmacokinetics of the angiotensin converting enzyme inhibitor benazepril HCl (CGS 14 824A) in healthy volunteers after single and repeated administration. *Biopharm Drug Dispos* 1989; **10:** 365–76.
2. Kaiser G, *et al.* Pharmacokinetics of a new angiotensin-converting enzyme inhibitor, benazepril hydrochloride, in special populations. *Am Heart J* 1989; **117:** 746–51.
3. Kaiser G, *et al.* Pharmacokinetics and pharmacodynamics of the ace inhibitor benazepril hydrochloride in the elderly. *Eur J Clin Pharmacol* 1990; **38:** 379–85.
4. Macdonald N-J, *et al.* A comparison in young and elderly subjects of the pharmacokinetics and pharmacodynamics of single and multiple doses of benazepril. *Br J Clin Pharmacol* 1993; **36:** 201–4.

Uses and Administration
Benazepril is an ACE inhibitor (p.820). It is used in the treatment of hypertension (p.802) and heart failure (p.798).

Benazepril owes its activity to benazeprilat to which it is converted after oral administration. The haemodynamic effects are seen within 1 hour of a single oral dose and the maximum effect occurs after about 2 to 4 hours, although the full effect may not develop for 1 to 2 weeks during chronic dosing. The haemodynamic action lasts for about 24 hours, allowing once-daily dosing. Benazepril is given by mouth as the hydrochloride, but doses are usually expressed in terms of the base.

In the treatment of **hypertension**, the usual initial dose is 10 mg once daily. An initial dose of 5 mg once daily is suggested for patients with renal impairment or who are receiving a diuretic; if possible the diuretic should be withdrawn 2 or 3 days before benazepril is started and resumed later if necessary. The usual maintenance dose is 20 to 40 mg daily, which may be given in 2 divided doses if control is inadequate with a single dose.

In the treatment of **heart failure** the usual initial dose is 2.5 mg once daily, adjusted according to response to a maximum dose of 20 mg daily.

Preparations
Proprietary Preparations (details are given in Part 3)
Aust.: Cibacen; *Belg.:* Cibacen; *Braz.:* Lotensin; *Canad.:* Lotensin; *Denm.:* Cibacen; *Fr.:* Briem; Cibacene; *Ger.:* Cibacen; *Irl.:* Cibacen; *Israel:* Cibacen; *Ital.:* Cibacen; Tensanil; Zinadril; *Mex.:* Lotensin; *Neth.:* Cibacen; *NZ:* Cibacen; *S.Afr.:* Cibace; *Spain:* Cibacen; Labopal; *Switz.:* Cibacen; *USA:* Lotensin.

Multi-ingredient: *Aust.:* Cibadrex; *Denm.:* Cibadrex; *Fr.:* Briazide; Cibadrex; *Ger.:* Cibadrex; *Ital.:* Cibadrex; Tensadiur; Zinadiur; *Neth.:* Cibadrex; *S.Afr.:* Cibadrex; *Swed.:* Cibadrex†; *Switz.:* Cibadrex; *USA:* Lotensin HCT; Lotrel.

Bencyclane Fumarate (9208-w)
Bencyclane Fumarate (rINNM).
Bencyclane Hydrogen Fumarate. 3-(1-Benzylcycloheptyloxy)-NN-dimethylpropylamine hydrogen fumarate.
$C_{19}H_{31}NO,C_4H_4O_4 = 405.5$.
CAS — 2179-37-5 (bencyclane); 14286-84-1 (bencyclane fumarate).
Pharmacopoeias. In Jpn.

Profile
Bencyclane fumarate is a vasodilator used in the management of peripheral (p.809) and cerebral vascular disorders (p.798) in usual doses of 100 to 200 mg three times daily by mouth. It has also been given intravenously.
Bencyclane acephyllinate is also used.

Preparations
Proprietary Preparations (details are given in Part 3)
Aust.: Ludilat†; *Braz.:* Fludilat; *Ger.:* Fludilat; *Hong Kong:* Fludilat; *Port.:* Fludilat; Fluxema†; *Switz.:* Fludilat†; *Thai.:* Fludilat.

Multi-ingredient: *Spain:* Dilangio Compositum†; Dilapres†.

The symbol † denotes a preparation no longer actively marketed

Bendrofluazide (2306-h)

Bendrofluazide (BAN).

Bendroflumethiazide (BAN, rINN); Bendrofluaz.; Bendroflumethiazidum; Benzydroflumethiazide; FT-81. 3-Benzyl-3,4-dihydro-6-trifluoromethyl-2H-1,2,4-benzothiadiazine-7-sulphonamide 1,1-dioxide.

$C_{15}H_{14}F_3N_3O_4S_2 = 421.4.$
CAS — 73-48-3.
ATC — C03AA01.

Pharmacopoeias. In Chin., Eur. (see p.vi), and US.

Pharmacopoeial description
Ph. Eur.: A white or almost white crystalline powder. Practically insoluble in water; soluble in alcohol; freely soluble in acetone.

USP 25: A white to cream-coloured, finely divided, crystalline powder. Is odourless or has a slight odour. Practically insoluble in water; soluble 1 in 23 of alcohol and 1 in 200 of ether; freely soluble in acetone. Store in airtight containers.

Adverse Effects, Treatment, and Precautions
As for Hydrochlorothiazide, p.907.

Overdosage. Tonic-clonic convulsions occurred in a previously healthy 14-year-old girl following ingestion of bendrofluazide [bendroflumethiazide] 150 to 200 mg.[1] The convulsions were not associated with any measurable disturbance of serum electrolytes.

1. Hine KR, et al. Bendrofluazide convulsions. Lancet 1982; i: 564.

Porphyria. Bendrofluazide [bendroflumethiazide] is considered to be unsafe in patients with porphyria because it has been shown to be porphyrinogenic in animals or in-vitro systems.

Interactions
As for Hydrochlorothiazide, p.909.

Pharmacokinetics
Bendrofluazide [bendroflumethiazide] has been reported to be completely absorbed from the gastrointestinal tract and to have a plasma half-life of about 3 or 4 hours. It is highly bound to plasma proteins. There are indications that bendrofluazide [bendroflumethiazide] is fairly extensively metabolised; about 30% is excreted unchanged in the urine.

◊ References.
1. Beermann B, et al. Pharmacokinetics of bendroflumethiazide. Clin Pharmacol Ther 1977; 22: 385–8.
2. Beermann B, et al. Pharmacokinetics of bendroflumethiazide in hypertensive patients. Eur J Clin Pharmacol 1978; 13: 119–24.

Uses and Administration
Bendrofluazide [bendroflumethiazide] is a thiazide diuretic with actions and uses similar to those of hydrochlorothiazide (p.910). It is used for oedema, including that associated with heart failure (p.798), and for hypertension (p.802). Other indications have included the suppression of lactation.

Diuresis is initiated in about 2 hours and lasts for 12 to 18 hours or longer.

In the treatment of **oedema** the usual initial dose is 5 to 10 mg by mouth daily or on alternate days; in some cases initial doses of up to 20 mg may be necessary. Maintenance dosage schedules have varied from 2.5 to 10 mg once to three times weekly in the UK to 2.5 to 5 mg daily or intermittently in the USA.

In the treatment of **hypertension** bendrofluazide [bendroflumethiazide] 2.5 mg daily, either alone or in conjunction with other antihypertensive drugs, is usually adequate although doses of up to 20 mg daily have sometimes been suggested.

An initial dose for children is up to 400 µg per kg body-weight daily, reduced to 50 to 100 µg per kg for maintenance.

Doses of 5 mg twice daily for about 5 days have been used to suppress lactation.

Preparations
BP 2001: Bendroflumethiazide Tablets;
USP 25: Bendroflumethiazide Tablets; Nadolol and Bendroflumethiazide Tablets.

Proprietary Preparations (details are given in Part 3)
Austral.: Aprinox; *Canad.:* Naturetin†; *Denm.:* Centyl; *Fr.:* Naturine†; *Irl.:* Centyl; *Norw.:* Centyl; *NZ:* Neo-NaClex; *Swed.:* Salures; *Switz.:* Sinesalin†; *UK:* Aprinox; Berkozide†; Neo-NaClex; *USA:* Naturetin.

Multi-ingredient: *Aust.:* Inderetic; Pressimedin; Sali-Aldopur; Solgeretik; *Belg.:* Inderetic; *Canad.:* Corzide†; *Denm.:* Centyl

med Kaliumklorid; *Fr.:* Precyclan; Tensionorme; *Ger.:* Docidrazin; Dociretic; Pertenso N; Sali-Aldopur; Sotaziden N; Spirostada comp; Tensoflux; *Irl.:* Centyl K; Corgaretic†; Inderetic; Prestim; *Neth.:* Inderetic; Prestim†; *Norw.:* Centyl med Kaliumklorid; *S.Afr.:* Corgaretic; Inderetic; Mendrome†; *Spain:* Betadipresan Diu; Neatenol Diu; Neatenol Diuvas; Spirometon; *Swed.:* Salures-K; *Switz.:* Corgaretic; Inderetic; Pressimed†; Saluretin; *UK:* Centyl K; Corgaretic; Inderetic; Inderex; Neo-NaClex-K; Prestim; Tenben; *USA:* Corzide; Rauzide.

Benfluorex Hydrochloride (12424-n)

Benfluorex Hydrochloride (BANM, pINNM).

Benfluorexi Hydrochloridum; JP-992; SE-780. 2-[α-Methyl-3-(trifluoromethyl)phenethylamino]ethyl benzoate hydrochloride.

$C_{19}H_{20}F_3NO_2,HCl = 387.8.$
CAS — 23602-78-0 (benfluorex); 35976-51-3 (benfluorex, ±); 23642-66-2 (benfluorex hydrochloride).

Pharmacopoeias. In Eur. (see p.vi).

Pharmacopoeial description
Ph. Eur.: A white or almost white powder. It exhibits polymorphism. Slightly soluble in water; sparingly soluble in alcohol; soluble in dichloromethane; freely soluble in methyl alcohol.

Profile
Benfluorex hydrochloride is a lipid regulating drug used in the treatment of hyperlipidaemias (p.800). It has also been used as an adjunct in the management of type 2 diabetes mellitus (p.315).

It is given in usual doses of 150 mg three times daily by mouth with meals.

Preparations
Proprietary Preparations (details are given in Part 3)
Fr.: Mediator; *Hong Kong:* Mediaxal; *Ital.:* Mediaxal; *Port.:* Mediator; *Singapore:* Mediaxal; *Spain:* Modulator; *Switz.:* Mediaxal†.

Benidipine Hydrochloride (4595-x)

Benidipine Hydrochloride (rINNM).

KW-3049; Nakadipine Hydrochloride. (±)-(R*)-3-[(R*)-1-Benzyl-3-piperidyl]methyl 1,4-dihydro-2,6-dimethyl-4-(m-nitrophenyl)-3,5-pyridinedicarboxylate hydrochloride.

$C_{28}H_{31}N_3O_6,HCl = 542.0.$
CAS — 105979-17-7 (benidipine); 91599-74-5 (benidipine hydrochloride).

Profile
Benidipine is a dihydropyridine calcium-channel blocker with general properties similar to those of nifedipine (p.940). It is given by mouth as the hydrochloride in the treatment of hypertension (p.802) and angina pectoris (p.791). In hypertension, the usual dose is 2 to 4 mg once daily, increased to 8 mg once daily if necessary. In angina pectoris, the usual dose is 4 mg twice daily.

Preparations
Proprietary Preparations (details are given in Part 3)
Jpn: Coniel.

Benzthiazide (2307-m)

Benzthiazide (BAN, rINN).

P-1393. 3-Benzylthiomethyl-6-chloro-2H-1,2,4-benzothiadiazine-7-sulphonamide 1,1-dioxide.

$C_{15}H_{14}ClN_3O_4S_3 = 431.9.$
CAS — 91-33-8.

Profile
Benzthiazide is a thiazide diuretic with properties similar to those of hydrochlorothiazide (p.907). It is used for oedema, including that associated with heart failure (p.798), and for hypertension (p.802).

Diuresis is initiated in about 2 hours and lasts for 12 to 18 hours.

The initial dose in the treatment of oedema is 50 to 200 mg by mouth daily, followed by a maintenance dose of 25 to 150 mg daily or intermittently. In the treatment of hypertension, an initial dose of 12.5 to 25 mg daily, either alone or in conjunction with other antihypertensive drugs, may be adequate although higher doses have been used. The maintenance dose should be adjusted to the lowest effective dose for the patient, but some have required up to 200 mg daily. Benzthiazide may be given in single or divided doses. An initial dose in children is 1 to 4 mg per kg body-weight daily in divided doses.

Preparations
Proprietary Preparations (details are given in Part 3)
USA: Exna.

Multi-ingredient: *Switz.:* Dyrenium compositum; *UK:* Dytide.

Bepridil Hydrochloride (12435-b)

Bepridil Hydrochloride (BANM, USAN, rINNM).

CERM-1978; Org-5730. N-Benzyl-N-(3-isobutoxy-2-pyrrolidin-1-ylpropyl)aniline hydrochloride monohydrate.

$C_{24}H_{34}N_2O,HCl,H_2O = 421.0.$
CAS — 64706-54-3 (bepridil); 49571-04-2 (bepridil); 64616-81-5 (anhydrous bepridil hydrochloride); 74764-40-2 (bepridil hydrochloride monohydrate).

Profile
Bepridil is a calcium-channel blocker (p.788) with properties similar to nifedipine (p.940). It also has antiarrhythmic activity. It is not related chemically to other calcium-channel blockers such as diltiazem, nifedipine, or verapamil.

Bepridil is used as the hydrochloride in angina pectoris (p.791) in doses of 200 to 400 mg daily by mouth. Elderly patients may require reduced doses. Ventricular arrhythmias, including torsade de pointes, and agranulocytosis have been associated with bepridil and, as a result, it is usually reserved for patients who have not responded adequately to other anti-anginal drugs.

◊ References.
1. Hollingshead LM, et al. Bepridil: a review of its pharmacological properties and therapeutic use in stable angina pectoris. Drugs 1992; 44: 835–57.
2. Awni WM, et al. Pharmacokinetics of bepridil and two of its metabolites in patients with end-stage renal disease. J Clin Pharmacol 1995; 35: 379–83.

Porphyria. Bepridil is considered to be unsafe in patients with porphyria because it has been shown to be porphyrinogenic in in-vitro systems.

Preparations
Proprietary Preparations (details are given in Part 3)
Belg.: Cordium†; *Fr.:* Cordium†; Unicordium; *USA:* Vascor.

Beta Blockers (6300-v)

Beta blockers (beta-adrenoceptor blocking drugs or antagonists) are competitive antagonists of catecholamines at beta-adrenergic receptors in a wide range of tissues. Although they have broadly similar properties they differ in their affinity for beta$_1$ or beta$_2$ receptor subtypes, intrinsic sympathomimetic activity, membrane-stabilising activity, blockade of alpha-adrenergic receptors, and pharmacokinetic properties including differences in lipid solubility (see Table 4, p.845, for some of these characteristics). These differences may affect the choice of drug in specific situations.

Adverse Effects and Treatment
The most frequent and serious adverse effects of these drugs are related to their beta-adrenergic blocking activity. Among the most serious adverse effects are heart failure, heart block, and bronchospasm. Troublesome subjective side-effects include fatigue and coldness of the extremities. Reactions may be more severe following intravenous than oral administration; ocular use has also been associated with systemic adverse effects. When beta blockers are used for long-term treatment of asymptomatic diseases such as hypertension, subjective side-effects may be an important determinant of patient compliance.

Cardiovascular effects include bradycardia and hypotension; heart failure or heart block may be precipitated in patients with underlying cardiac disorders. Abrupt withdrawal of beta blockers may exacerbate angina and may lead to sudden death. For further details on withdrawal of beta blockers, see Precautions, below. Reduced peripheral circulation can produce coldness of the extremities and may exacerbate peripheral vascular disease such as Raynaud's syndrome.

Bronchospasm may be precipitated in susceptible patients due to blockade of beta$_2$ receptors in bronchial smooth muscle. Drugs with selectivity for beta$_1$ receptors or with intrinsic sympathomimetic activity at beta$_2$ receptors may be less likely to induce bronchospasm (but see Precautions, below). Pneumonitis, pulmonary fibrosis, and pleurisy have also been reported.

CNS effects include depression, dizziness, hallucinations, confusion, and sleep disturbances including nightmares. Coma and convulsions have been reported following beta-blocker overdosage. Beta blockers which are lipid soluble are more likely to enter the brain and would be expected to be associated with a higher incidence of CNS adverse effects, although this is not proven.

Fatigue is a common side-effect experienced with beta blockers. Paraesthesia, peripheral neuropathy, and myopathies, including muscle cramps, have been reported.

Adverse gastrointestinal effects include nausea and vomiting, diarrhoea, constipation, and abdominal cramping.

Beta blockers interfere with carbohydrate and lipid metabolism and can produce hypoglycaemia, hyperglycaemia, and changes in blood concentrations of triglycerides and cholesterol (see below for further details).

Skin rash, pruritus, and reversible alopecia have occurred with use of beta blockers.

Decreased tear production, blurred vision, and soreness are among the ocular symptoms that have been reported. Adverse effects specific to ocular use are also discussed below.

Haematological reactions include nonthrombocytopenic purpura, thrombocytopenia, and rarely agranulocytosis. Transient eosinophilia can occur.

Other adverse effects reported with some beta blockers include a lupus-like syndrome, male impotence, sclerosing peritonitis, and retroperitoneal fibrosis.

For reference to the treatment of adverse effects, see under Overdosage, below.

Carcinogenicity. An apparent excess of deaths from cancer was noted in elderly men, but not women, given atenolol during a trial of antihypertensive treatment.[1] However, two subsequent studies found no evidence of a link between atenolol and cancer.[2,3]

1. MRC Working Party. Medical Research Council trial of treatment of hypertension in older adults: principal results. *BMJ* 1992; **304:** 405–12.
2. Fletcher AE, et al. Cancer mortality and atenolol treatment. *BMJ* 1993; **306:** 622–3.
3. Hole DJ, et al. Incidence of and mortality from cancer in hypertensive patients. *BMJ* 1993; **306:** 609–11.

Effects on carbohydrate metabolism. The sympathetic nervous system is involved in the control of carbohydrate metabolism and blockade of adrenergic receptors by beta blockers can interfere with carbohydrate and insulin regulation; both hypoglycaemia and hyperglycaemia have been reported.

Propranolol-induced hypoglycaemia was first noted in adult type 1 diabetic patients in the late 1960s. In a review of drug-induced hypoglycaemia,[1] 49 cases of severe hypoglycaemia associated with non-selective beta blockers were considered. These events occurred in the following circumstances: nondiabetic patients taking propranolol and undergoing regular

haemodialysis; neonates of mothers who took propranolol until a few hours before delivery; infants who received propranolol; and both diabetic and nondiabetic patients on long-term propranolol who were nutritionally compromised or had liver disease. In addition, in type 1 diabetes mellitus beta blockers mask the adrenaline-mediated symptoms of hypoglycaemia such as tachycardia and tremor, and may delay the recovery from hypoglycaemia in glucose-treated patients. In a long-term study[2] in type 2 diabetics, however, there was no difference in the incidence of hypoglycaemia in patients receiving captopril or atenolol and both significantly improved outcome. Although there have been conflicting reports, most studies have suggested that cardioselective beta blockers with little or no lipophilicity are preferred in type 2 diabetics.[3]

The use of beta blockers has also been associated with the development of hyperglycaemia[4,5] and diabetes mellitus.[6-8]

1. Seltzer HS. Drug-induced hypoglycemia. *Endocrinol Metab Clin North Am* 1989; **18:** 163–83.
2. UK Prospective Diabetes Study Group. Efficacy of atenolol and captopril in reducing risk of macrovascular and microvascular complications in type 2 diabetes: UKPDS 39. *BMJ* 1998; **317:** 713–20.
3. O'Byrne S, Feely J. Effects of drugs on glucose tolerance in non-insulin-dependent diabetics (part 1). *Drugs* 1990; **40:** 6–18.
4. Veterans Administration Cooperative Study Group on Antihypertensive Agents. Propranolol or hydrochlorothiazide alone for the initial treatment of hypertension IV: effect on plasma glucose and glucose tolerance. *Hypertension* 1985; **7:** 1008–16.
5. Pollare T, et al. Sensitivity to insulin during treatment with atenolol and metoprolol: a randomised, double blind study of effects on carbohydrate and lipoprotein metabolism in hypertensive patients. *BMJ* 1989; **298:** 1152–7.
6. Skarfors ET, et al. Do antihypertensive drugs precipitate diabetes in predisposed men? *BMJ* 1989; **298:** 1147–52.
7. Samuelsson O, et al. Diabetes mellitus in treated hypertension: incidence, predictive factors and the impact of non-selective beta-blockers and thiazide diuretics during 15 years treatment of middle-aged hypertensive men in the Primary Prevention Trial in Göteborg, Sweden. *J Hum Hypertens* 1994; **8:** 257–63.
8. Gress TW, et al. Hypertension and antihypertensive therapy as risk factors for type 2 diabetes mellitus. *N Engl J Med* 2000; **342:** 905–12.

Effects on lipid metabolism. The adrenergic system is involved in the control of lipid metabolism. Thus, beta blockers may have some effect on plasma-lipid concentrations. Plasma concentrations of very-low-density lipoprotein and triglyceride may be raised in patients taking beta blockers and concentrations of high-density lipoprotein reduced. Plasma concentrations of low-density lipoprotein are usually unchanged. These effects may be less pronounced with beta₁ cardioselective drugs, beta blockers with intrinsic sympathomimetic activity,[1] and beta blockers that also block alpha-adrenergic receptors. For example, pindolol,[2,3] a beta blocker with intrinsic sympathomimetic activity and arotinolol[4] and carvedilol,[5] which possess alpha-adrenergic blocking properties, are reported to have no adverse effects on plasma-lipid concentrations. However, a patient taking atenolol and metoprolol, both beta₁ cardioselective drugs, developed acute pancreatitis as a result of severe hypertriglyceridaemia.[6]

Exercise has been suggested to have a favourable impact on lipid profiles and 2 studies[7,8] have investigated the role of exercise in attenuating the effects of beta blockers on lipids. Neither study showed that exercise improved the lipid profile in pa-

tients given beta blockers. However, the anticipated deterioration in lipid profile may have been attenuated.[7]

1. Krone W, Nägele H. Effects of antihypertensives on plasma lipids and lipoprotein metabolism. *Am Heart J* 1988; **116:** 1729–34.
2. Hunter Hypertension Research Group. Effects of pindolol, or a pindolol/clopamide combination preparation, on plasma lipid levels in essential hypertension. *Med J Aust* 1989; **150:** 646–52.
3. Terént A, et al. Long-term effect of pindolol on plasma lipids and lipoproteins in men with newly diagnosed hypertension. *Eur J Clin Pharmacol* 1989; **36:** 347–50.
4. Sasaki J, et al. Effects of arotinolol on serum lipid and apolipoprotein levels in patients with mild essential hypertension. *Clin Ther* 1989; **11:** 580–3.
5. Hauf-Zachariou U, et al. A double-blind comparison of the effects of carvedilol and captopril on serum lipid concentrations in patients with mild to moderate essential hypertension and dyslipidaemia. *Eur J Clin Pharmacol* 1993; **45:** 95–100.
6. Durrington PN, Cairns SA. Acute pancreatitis: a complication of beta-blockade. *BMJ* 1982; **284:** 1016.
7. Morton AR, et al. Alterations in plasma lipids consequent to endurance training and beta-blockade. *Med Sci Sports Exerc* 1989; **21:** 288–92.
8. Arvan S, Rueda BG. Nonselective beta-receptor blocker effect on high density lipoprotein cholesterol after chronic exercise. *J Am Coll Cardiol* 1988; **12:** 662–8.

Effects following ophthalmic use. Ophthalmic administration of beta blockers may produce the following localised effects: ocular irritation (including hypersensitivity), blepharitis, keratitis, decreased corneal sensitivity, visual disturbances, diplopia, and ptosis. Uveitis has been reported with metipranolol eye drops.[1] A case of iris depigmentation has occurred[2] following the use of topical levobunolol.

Topical beta blockers may produce corneal anaesthesia. Older patients using these eye drops may be at greater risk of decreased corneal sensitivity or corneal anaesthesia with the consequent risk of keratitis.[3]

Systemic absorption may occur following the use of beta blockers in eye drops. Excess drug can drain into the lachrymal ducts to be absorbed through the nasal mucosa. Absorption also occurs via the ophthalmic and facial veins. Following such absorption the beta blocker reaches the systemic circulation without undergoing first-pass hepatic metabolism. The main systemic effects associated with topical ocular administration of beta blockers are on the pulmonary, cardiovascular, and central nervous systems.[4]

A number of cases of alopecia associated with ocular use of beta blockers have been reported.[5]

Beta blockers given orally can adversely affect serum-lipoprotein levels; however, a study of the effect of timolol 0.5% administered topically twice daily to both eyes of 19 patients showed no effect on lipoprotein concentrations at 5 and 15 weeks.[6]

1. Akingbehin T, Villada JR. Metipranolol-associated granulomatous anterior uveitis. *Br J Ophthalmol* 1991; **75:** 519–23.
2. Doyle E, Liu C. A case of acquired iris depigmentation as a possible complication of levobunolol eye drops. *Br J Ophthalmol* 1999; **83:** 1405–6.
3. Weissman SS, Asbell PA. Effects of topical timolol (0.5%) and betaxolol (0.5%) on corneal sensitivity. *Br J Ophthalmol* 1990; **74:** 409–12.
4. Everitt DE, Avorn J. Systemic effects of medications used to treat glaucoma. *Ann Intern Med* 1990; **112:** 120–5.
5. Fraunfelder FT, et al. Alopecia possibly secondary to topical ophthalmic β-blockers. *JAMA* 1990; **263:** 1493–4.
6. West J, Longstaff S. Topical timolol and serum lipoproteins. *Br J Ophthalmol* 1990; **74:** 663–4.

Hypersensitivity. For the suggestion that beta blockers may exacerbate anaphylactic reactions, see under Precautions, below.

Overdosage. Many cases of beta-blocker overdosage are uneventful, but some patients develop severe and occasionally fatal cardiovascular depression. Effects can include bradycardia, cardiac conduction block, hypotension, heart failure, and cardiogenic shock. Convulsions, coma, respiratory depression, and bronchoconstriction can also occur, although infrequently. Most reports of serious toxic reactions following overdosage concern beta blockers with significant membrane-stabilising activity, such as propranolol or oxprenolol.[1] Overdosage of beta blockers with intrinsic sympathomimetic activity may present with tachycardia and hypertension.[2] Overdosage of sotalol, a beta blocker with class II and III antiarrhythmic properties, usually presents as ventricular tachyarrhythmia.[1,2] **Treatment** involves gastric lavage and activated charcoal for patients presenting with a history of recent acute ingestion.[1-3] When indicated, additional measures are instituted to counter hypotension.[2,3] Mild hypotension may respond to fluid administration; if hypotension continues, glucagon or sympathomimetics may be used, either alone[1-3] or in combination.[2,3] Very large doses of sympathomimetics may be required; infusion rates of up to 333 μg per minute of isoprenaline have been used.[3] Bradycardia may be treated with atropine, sympathomimetics, or a pacemaker.

A patient who failed to respond to the usual management for beta-blocker overdosage responded to treatment with enoximone.[4] A dramatic response to calcium chloride has also been reported in a patient with electromechanical dissociation following propranolol overdosage.[5]

1. Critchley JAJH, Ungar A. The management of acute poisoning due to β-adrenoceptor antagonists. *Med Toxicol* 1989; **4:** 32–45.
2. Pentel PR, Salerno DM. Cardiac drug toxicity: digitalis glycosides and calcium-channel and β-blocking agents. *Med J Aust* 1990; **152:** 88–94.

Table 4. Characteristics of beta blockers.

Beta blocker	Beta₁ selectivity	Intrinsic sympathomimetic activity	Membrane-stabilising activity
Acebutolol	+	+	+
Alprenolol	0	+	0
Atenolol	+	0	0
Betaxolol	+	0	0
Bisoprolol	+	0	0
Carteolol	0	+	−
Celiprolol	+	+	−
Esmolol	+	0	0
Labetalol	0	0	0
Levobunolol	0	0	0
Metipranolol	0	0	0
Metoprolol	+	0	0
Nadolol	0	0	0
Oxprenolol	0	+	+
Penbutolol	0	0	0
Pindolol	0	++	0
Propranolol	0	0	++
Sotalol	0	0	0
Timolol	0	0	0

0 = absent or low; + = moderate; ++ = high; − = no information

The symbol † denotes a preparation no longer actively marketed

3. Taboulet P, et al. Pathophysiology and management of self-poisoning with beta-blockers. Clin Toxicol 1993; 31: 531–51.
4. Hoeper MM, Boeker KHW. Overdose of metoprolol treated with enoximone. N Engl J Med 1996; 335: 1538.
5. Brimacombe JR, et al. Propranolol overdose—a dramatic response to calcium chloride. Med J Aust 1991; 155: 267–8.

Precautions

Beta blockers should not be given to patients with bronchospasm or asthma or to those with a history of obstructive airways disease. This contra-indication applies even to those beta blockers considered to be cardioselective. However, some authorities consider that a cardioselective beta blocker might be used with extreme caution when there is no alternative treatment. Other contra-indications include metabolic acidosis, severe peripheral arterial disease, sinus bradycardia, and second- or third-degree atrioventricular block; caution should be observed in first-degree block. Although beta blockers are used in the management of heart failure, they should not be given to patients with uncontrolled heart failure and treatment should be initiated with great care. Patients with phaeochromocytoma should not receive beta blockers without concomitant alpha-adrenoceptor blocking therapy.

Beta blockers may mask the symptoms of hyperthyroidism and of hypoglycaemia. They may unmask myasthenia gravis. Psoriasis may be aggravated. Patients with a history of anaphylaxis to an antigen may be more reactive to repeated challenge with the antigen while taking beta blockers (see Hypersensitivity, below).

Abrupt withdrawal of beta blockers has sometimes resulted in angina, myocardial infarction, ventricular arrhythmias, and death. Patients on long-term treatment with a beta blocker should have their medication discontinued gradually over a period of 1 to 2 weeks. Cardiovascular drugs including beta blockers should generally be continued perioperatively although some authorities have advocated their gradual and temporary withdrawal in order to provide better control of the circulatory system. If beta blockers are not discontinued before anaesthesia, a drug such as atropine may be given to counter increases in vagal tone. Anaesthetics causing myocardial depression, such as ether, cyclopropane, and trichloroethylene, are best avoided. Awareness by the anaesthetist that beta blockers are being taken is of the greatest importance.

Administration of beta blockers to pregnant women shortly before delivery has occasionally resulted in bradycardia and other adverse effects such as hypoglycaemia and hypotension in the neonate. Many beta blockers are distributed into breast milk.

Similar precautions should be observed when beta blockers are applied topically as eye drops since systemic absorption can occur.

Effects on the eyes. Beta blockers may reduce tear flow, leading to irritation of the eye in wearers of contact lenses and potentially to the dehydration of soft lenses.[1] Older patients using beta blocker eye drops may be at greater risk of corneal anaesthesia. See also Effects Following Ophthalmic Use under Adverse Effects, above.
1. McGuire T. Drugs interfering with contact lenses. Aust J Hosp Pharm 1987; 17: 55–6.

Hypersensitivity. There have been reports of several patients whose anaphylactic reactions to stings or other antigens were potentiated by beta-blocker therapy.[1-3] In addition, beta blockers may antagonise the effects of adrenaline [epinephrine] in the management of anaphylaxis (see Interactions under Adrenaline, p.830).
1. Hannaway PJ, Hopper GDK. Severe anaphylaxis and drug-induced beta-blockade. N Engl J Med 1983; 308: 1536.
2. Pedersen DL. Hymenoptera stings and beta-blockers. Lancet 1989; ii: 619.
3. Lang DM. Anaphylactoid and anaphylactic reactions: hazards of β-blockers. Drug Safety 1995; 12: 299–304.

Pregnancy. The use of a beta blocker from early in pregnancy has been associated with growth retardation of the fetus.[1] However, beta blockers are still considered one of the first-line drugs in mild to moderate hypertension in pregnancy. Many beta blockers cross the placenta and administration of beta blockers to pregnant women shortly before delivery has occasionally resulted in bradycardia and other adverse effects such as hypoglycaemia and hypotension in the neonate.
1. Butters L, et al. Atenolol in essential hypertension during pregnancy. BMJ 1990; 301: 587–9.

Withdrawal. The abrupt withdrawal of beta blockers may lead to rebound hypertension or overshoot hypertension where the patient's blood pressure is higher than before treatment. Angina can be exacerbated, myocardial infarction induced, and fatalities have occurred.[1,2]
1. Houston MC, Hodge R. Beta-adrenergic blocker withdrawal syndromes in hypertension and other cardiovascular diseases. Am Heart J 1988; 116: 515–23.
2. Psaty BM, et al. The relative risk of incident coronary heart disease associated with recently stopping the use of β-blockers. JAMA 1990; 263: 1653–7.

Interactions

Both pharmacodynamic and pharmacokinetic interactions have been reported with beta blockers. **Pharmacodynamic** interactions may occur with drugs whose actions enhance or antagonise the various effects of beta blockers at beta$_1$ and beta$_2$ receptors, including their antihypertensive effect, cardiodepressant effect, effect on carbohydrate metabolism, or effect on bronchial beta$_2$ receptors. The characteristics of the individual beta blocker must therefore be borne in mind when considering likely interactions. For more details on the characteristics of different beta blockers, see Uses and Administration, below. Drugs that enhance the antihypertensive effects of beta blockers, such as ACE inhibitors, calcium-channel blockers, and clonidine may be useful in controlling hypertension. Drugs that cause hypotension such as aldesleukin and general anaesthetics also enhance the antihypertensive effects of beta blockers while other drugs, for example NSAIDs, antagonise the antihypertensive effects. Use of beta blockers with other cardiac depressants such as antiarrhythmics and rate-limiting calcium-channel blockers can precipitate bradycardia and heart block. Sotalol is particularly prone to interactions with other drugs affecting cardiac conduction (see p.972). Beta blockers may potentiate bradycardia due to digoxin. In diabetic patients beta blockers can reduce the response to insulin and oral hypoglycaemics through their effects on pancreatic beta receptors. Blockade of peripheral beta receptors interferes with the effects of sympathomimetics; patients on beta blockers, especially non-selective beta blockers, may develop elevated blood pressure if they are given adrenaline [epinephrine] and the bronchodilator effects of adrenaline [epinephrine] are also inhibited. The response to adrenaline [epinephrine] given for anaphylaxis may be reduced in patients on long-term treatment with beta blockers (see Adrenaline [epinephrine], p.830).

Pharmacokinetic interactions occur with drugs that alter the absorption or metabolism of beta blockers. Although these interactions may alter the beta blocker plasma concentration, they are not usually clinically significant since there is no association between plasma concentrations and therapeutic effect or toxicity and there are wide interindividual differences in steady-state plasma concentrations of beta blockers. Drugs that reduce absorption include aluminium salts (but see also Antacids, below) and bile-acid binding resins such as colestyramine. Metabolism of some beta blockers can be increased by concomitant treatment with drugs such as barbiturates and rifampicin and decreased with drugs such as cimetidine, erythromycin, fluvoxamine, and hydralazine. Drugs that alter hepatic blood flow also affect metabolism of some beta blockers. For example, cimetidine and hydralazine decrease hepatic blood flow and this contributes to the decreased hepatic clearance seen with these drugs. Drugs that influence hepatic metabolism affect beta blockers that are extensively metabolised, such as labetalol, propranolol, and timolol, while beta blockers that are excreted largely unchanged, for example atenolol and nadolol, are unaffected.

Since systemic absorption can occur following ocular use of beta blockers the possibility of interactions with concomitant drugs should be considered.

◊ General references.
1. McDevitt DG. Interactions that matter: 12. β-adrenoceptor antagonists. Prescribers' J 1988; 28: 25–30.
2. Blaufarb I, et al. β-Blockers: drug interactions of clinical significance. Drug Safety 1995; 13: 359–70.

Anaesthetics. Anaesthetics that cause myocardial depression, such as ether, cyclopropane, and trichloroethylene should

preferably be avoided in patients on beta blockers (see Precautions, above). The hypotensive effects of beta blockers may be potentiated by general anaesthetics.

Antacids. Bioavailability of metoprolol was increased when given concurrently with an antacid containing aluminium and magnesium salts but the bioavailability of atenolol was reduced by concurrent administration of this antacid. Variable results on bioavailability of propranolol have been reported when aluminium hydroxide was given with propranolol.[1]
1. Gugler R, Allgayer H. Effects of antacids on the clinical pharmacokinetics of drugs: an update. Clin Pharmacokinet 1990; 18: 210–19.

Antiarrhythmics. Concomitant use of beta blockers with antiarrhythmic drugs and other drugs affecting cardiac conduction can precipitate bradycardia and heart block.

Bradycardia, cardiac arrest, and ventricular fibrillation have been reported shortly after initiation of beta-blocker treatment in patients receiving amiodarone.[1] Concurrent administration of flecainide and propranolol produced additive negative inotropic effects on the heart and increased serum concentrations of both drugs.[2] In a pharmacokinetic study in 12 healthy males, concomitant administration of propafenone and propranolol resulted in increases in serum-propranolol concentrations but only modest enhancement of beta-blocking activity.[3] An increase in serum-metoprolol concentration has been reported after concurrent administration of propafenone and metoprolol.[4] The metabolism of metoprolol may be decreased by quinidine.[5] Both quinidine and beta blockers have a negative inotropic action on the heart; bradycardia[6] and hypotension[7] have occurred in patients receiving quinidine and beta blockers.

For a report of reduced clearance of disopyramide by concomitant administration of atenolol, see p.879.

The interactions of sotalol are discussed on p.972.
1. Lesko LJ. Pharmacokinetic drug interactions with amiodarone. Clin Pharmacokinet 1989; 17: 130–40.
2. Holtzman JL, et al. The pharmacodynamic and pharmacokinetic interaction of flecainide acetate with propranolol: effects on cardiac function and drug clearance. Eur J Clin Pharmacol 1987; 33: 97–9.
3. Kowey PR, et al. Interaction between propranolol and propafenone in healthy volunteers. J Clin Pharmacol 1989; 29: 512–17.
4. Wagner F, et al. Drug interaction between propafenone and metoprolol. Br J Clin Pharmacol 1987; 24: 213–20.
5. Leemann T, et al. Single-dose quinidine treatment inhibits metoprolol oxidation in extensive metabolizers. Eur J Clin Pharmacol 1986; 29: 739–41.
6. Dinai Y, et al. Bradycardia induced by interaction between quinidine and ophthalmic timolol. Ann Intern Med 1985; 103: 890–1.
7. Loon NR, et al. Orthostatic hypotension due to quinidine and propranolol. Am J Med 1986; 81: 1101–4.

Antibacterials. Serum-atenolol concentrations were reduced by concurrent administration of ampicillin given in doses of 1 g by mouth in 6 healthy subjects.[1] Plasma concentrations of propranolol,[2] metoprolol,[3] and bisoprolol[4] may be reduced by concomitant rifampicin administration.
1. Schäfer-Korting M, et al. Atenolol interaction with aspirin, allopurinol, and ampicillin. Clin Pharmacol Ther 1983; 33: 283–8.
2. Shaheen O, et al. Influence of debrisoquin phenotype on the inducibility of propranolol metabolism. Clin Pharmacol Ther 1989; 45: 439–43.
3. Bennett PN, et al. Effect of rifampicin on metoprolol and antipyrine kinetics. Br J Clin Pharmacol 1982; 13: 387–91.
4. Kirch W, et al. Interaction of bisoprolol with cimetidine and rifampicin. Eur J Clin Pharmacol 1986; 31: 59–62.

Anticoagulants. For the effect of beta blockers on the pharmacokinetics of some oral anticoagulants, see p.996.

Antidepressants. Bradycardia and heart block, occurring shortly after the introduction of treatment with fluoxetine, have been reported in patients receiving metoprolol[1] and propranolol.[2] Possible mechanisms include impaired conduction through the atrioventricular node and inhibition by fluoxetine of the oxidative metabolism of beta blockers. Concomitant use of fluoxetine also increased the plasma concentration of carvedilol in patients with heart failure but no clinical effects were noted.[3]

Fluvoxamine inhibits oxidative metabolism, and increased plasma concentrations of propranolol have been noted in patients receiving fluvoxamine.
1. Walley T, et al. Interaction of metoprolol and fluoxetine. Lancet 1993; 341: 967–8.
2. Drake WM, Gordon GD. Heart block in a patient on propranolol and fluoxetine. Lancet 1994; 343: 425–6.
3. Graff DW, et al. Effect of fluoxetine on carvedilol pharmacokinetics, CYP2D6 activity, and autonomic balance in heart failure patients. J Clin Pharmacol 2001; 41: 97–106.

Antihypertensives. An enhanced antihypertensive effect is seen when other antihypertensives are given concomitantly with beta blockers. However, some combinations should be avoided (see Calcium-channel Blockers, below). Beta blockers can potentiate the severe postural hypotension that may follow the initial dose of alpha blockers such as prazosin and can exacerbate rebound hypertension following withdrawal of clonidine treatment (see p.860).

Antimalarials. Some antimalarials, for example halofantrine, mefloquine, and quinine can cause cardiac conduction defects and caution is necessary if they are used concomitantly with beta blockers. Cardiopulmonary arrest has occurred after a single dose of mefloquine in a patient taking propranolol.[1]

1. Anonymous. Mefloquine for malaria. *Med Lett Drugs Ther* 1990; **32:** 13–14.

Antimigraine drugs. For the effect of propranolol on *rizatriptan*, see p.455.

See also under Ergot Derivatives, below, for further interactions with drugs used in the treatment of migraine.

Anxiolytics and antipsychotics. Plasma concentrations of some beta blockers may be reduced by *barbiturates*.[1-3] Increased plasma-propranolol concentrations and bioavailability and reduced metabolism have been reported in healthy subjects also given *chlorpromazine*.[4]

See p.678 for the effect of beta blockers on the pharmacokinetics of some *benzodiazepines*.

1. Sotaniemi EA, *et al.* Plasma clearance of propranolol and sotalol and hepatic drug-metabolizing enzyme activity. *Clin Pharmacol Ther* 1979; **26:** 153–61.
2. Haglund K, *et al.* Influence of pentobarbital on metoprolol plasma levels. *Clin Pharmacol Ther* 1979; **26:** 326–9.
3. Seideman P, *et al.* Decreased plasma concentrations and clinical effects of alprenolol during combined treatment with pentobarbitone in hypertension. *Br J Clin Pharmacol* 1987; **23:** 267–71.
4. Vestal RE, *et al.* Inhibition of propranolol metabolism by chlorpromazine. *Clin Pharmacol Ther* 1979; **25:** 19–24.

Calcium-channel blockers. Concurrent administration of calcium-channel blockers and beta blockers has resulted in hypotension, bradycardia, conduction defects, and heart failure.[1] Beta blockers should be avoided in combination with cardiodepressant calcium-channel blockers such as *verapamil* (see p.990) and *diltiazem*.[2] Although they are reportedly safe with dihydropyridines such as *nifedipine*,[3] heart failure and severe hypotension have been reported (see under Nifedipine, p.942). Reported pharmacokinetic interactions include increased plasma concentrations of propranolol and of metoprolol with concurrent administration of diltiazem[4] or verapamil,[1] and increased plasma concentrations of propranolol with *nicardipine*.[5]

1. Lam YWF, Shepherd AMM. Drug interactions in hypertensive patients: pharmacokinetic, pharmacodynamic and genetic considerations. *Clin Pharmacokinet* 1990; **18:** 295–317.
2. Beevers DG, Wilkins MR. Drug treatment I: first choice agents. In: *ABC of Hypertension*. 2nd ed. London: British Medical Association, 1987: 25–7.
3. Reid JL. First-line and combination treatment for hypertension. *Am J Med* 1989; **86** (suppl 4A): 2–5.
4. Tateishi T, *et al.* Effect of diltiazem on the pharmacokinetics of propranolol, metoprolol and atenolol. *Eur J Clin Pharmacol* 1989; **36:** 67–70.
5. Schoors DF, *et al.* Influence of nicardipine on the pharmacokinetics and pharmacodynamics of propranolol in healthy volunteers. *Br J Clin Pharmacol* 1990; **29:** 497–501.

Ciclosporin. For the effect of carvedilol on plasma-ciclosporin concentrations, see p.521.

Ergot derivatives. *Nicergoline* enhanced the cardiac depressant action of propranolol in healthy subjects.[1]

For reports of enhanced vasoconstrictor action in patients taking *ergot alkaloids* and beta blockers, see p.453.

1. Boismare F, *et al.* Potentiation by an alpha-adrenolytic agent, nicergoline, of the cardiac effects of propranolol. *Methods Find Exp Clin Pharmacol* 1983; **5:** 83–8.

Histamine H₂-antagonists. Plasma concentrations of propranolol and metoprolol may be increased by *cimetidine*;[1] pharmacokinetic studies indicate that cimetidine exerts its effect by reducing hepatic blood flow and impairing beta blocker metabolism. Cimetidine has been reported to increase the bioavailability of labetalol,[1] and to increase the systemic effects of timolol eye drops.[2]

1. Smith SR, Kendall MJ. Ranitidine versus cimetidine: a comparison of their potential to cause clinically important drug interactions. *Clin Pharmacokinet* 1988; **15:** 44–56.
2. Ishii Y, *et al.* Drug interaction between cimetidine and timolol ophthalmic solution: effect on heart rate and intraocular pressure in healthy Japanese volunteers. *J Clin Pharmacol* 2000; **40:** 193–9.

Local anaesthetics. For details of the effect of beta blockers in reducing the clearance of *bupivacaine*, see p.1307, and of *lignocaine [lidocaine]*, see p.1314. For the effects of propranolol with *cocaine*, see p.1311.

Neuromuscular blockers. For the effects of beta blockers on neuromuscular blockers, see under Atracurium, p.1334.

NSAIDs. The antihypertensive effect of beta blockers may be impaired by some NSAIDs, possibly due to their inhibition of renal synthesis of vasodilating prostaglandins. This interaction probably occurs with all beta blockers but may not occur with all NSAIDs. For example, *sulindac* appears to affect blood pressure control less than *indometacin*.[1]

1. Lam YWF, Shepherd AMM. Drug interactions in hypertensive patients: pharmacokinetic, pharmacodynamic and genetic considerations. *Clin Pharmacokinet* 1990; **18:** 295–317.

Opioid analgesics. Bioavailability of propranolol and metoprolol was increased in subjects given *dextropropoxyphene*.[1] Intravenous administration of *morphine* may increase serum concentrations of esmolol.[2]

1. Lundborg P, *et al.* The effect of propoxyphene pretreatment on the disposition of metoprolol and propranolol. *Clin Pharmacol Ther* 1981; **29:** 263–4.
2. Lowenthal DT, *et al.* Clinical pharmacology, pharmacodynamics and interactions with esmolol. *Am J Cardiol* 1985; **56:** 14F–17F.

Oral contraceptives. Plasma-metoprolol concentrations were increased in some women taking oral contraceptives.[1]

1. Kendall MJ, *et al.* Metoprolol pharmacokinetics and the oral contraceptive pill. *Br J Clin Pharmacol* 1982; **14:** 120–2.

Parasympathomimetics. For the effect of beta blockers on the response to *anticholinesterases*, see p.1420.

Thyroid drugs. For a discussion of thyroid status and its effect on plasma-propranolol concentrations and the effects of propranolol on *thyroid hormone* metabolism, see p.1527.

Xanthines. For details of reduced *theophylline* clearance in patients receiving beta blockers, see p.781.

Pharmacokinetics
Beta blockers differ widely in their pharmacokinetic properties. Differences in lipid solubility contribute to these varying pharmacokinetic properties. Beta blockers with low lipid solubility (hydrophilic beta blockers) include atenolol and nadolol. Beta blockers with high lipid solubility (lipophilic beta blockers) include alprenolol and propranolol. Generally, those with low lipid solubility tend to be less readily absorbed from the gastrointestinal tract, to be less extensively metabolised, to have low plasma-protein binding, to have relatively long plasma half-lives, and to cross the blood-brain barrier less readily than beta blockers with high lipid solubility. Beta blockers cross the placenta and most are known to distribute into breast milk.

There is no clear correlation between plasma concentrations of beta blockers and therapeutic activity, especially when the beta blocker undergoes metabolism to active metabolites.

Uses and Administration
Beta blockers are competitive antagonists of the effects of catecholamines at beta-adrenergic receptor sites and are used in a variety of disorders, especially those affecting the cardiovascular system.

Two subtypes of beta-adrenergic receptors are recognised: beta₁ and beta₂. Beta₁ receptors are found mainly in the heart while beta₂ receptors are found in noncardiac tissue, including bronchial tissue, peripheral blood vessels, uterus, and pancreas, although it is now recognised that in some organs, including the heart, both receptor subtypes are present. Blockade of beta₁ receptors reduces heart rate, myocardial contractility, and the rate of conduction of impulses through the conducting system. These effects are termed class II antiarrhythmic actions (p.787). Other effects of blockade of beta₁ receptors include suppression of adrenergic-induced renin release and lipolysis. Effects produced by blockade of beta₂ receptors include increased bronchial resistance and inhibition of catecholamine-induced glucose metabolism. Beta₂ receptors may also have a role in regulation of heart rate.

Beta blockers have different affinities for beta₁ or beta₂ receptors. While propranolol affects both beta₁ and beta₂ receptors, other drugs such as atenolol and metoprolol have greater affinity for beta₁ receptors and are described as cardioselective. However, selectivity is relative and, as doses are increased, activity at beta₂ receptors becomes clinically important.

Some beta blockers, such as acebutolol, celiprolol, oxprenolol, and pindolol, also possess intrinsic (partial) sympathomimetic activity in that they activate beta receptors in the absence of catecholamines and are therefore partial agonists. Beta blockers with intrinsic sympathomimetic activity produce less resting bradycardia than beta blockers without.

At high blood concentrations, propranolol and some other beta blockers also possess a membrane-stabilising effect. This effect may not be evident at therapeutic doses but may be important in overdose. Some beta blockers, such as carvedilol and labetalol, also block alpha₁ receptors and thus produce vasodilation. Other beta blockers, such as bevantolol and celiprolol, also have vasodilator properties; various mechanisms, including alpha₁ blockade, beta₂ stimulation, and direct vasodilator activity may contribute

to this effect. The non-cardioselective beta blocker sotalol also has class III antiarrhythmic activity.

Beta blockers are used in the treatment of hypertension (p.802), angina pectoris (p.791), cardiac arrhythmias (p.794), and myocardial infarction (p.805) and also have a role in heart failure (below). They are also used to control symptoms of sympathetic overactivity in the management of alcohol withdrawal (p.1131), in anxiety disorders (below), in hyperthyroidism (p.1519), and in tremor (below). Beta blockers are used in the prophylaxis of migraine (below) and of variceal bleeding associated with portal hypertension (p.1637). They are also used, in conjunction with an alpha blocker, in the initial management of phaeochromocytoma (below). Some beta blockers are instilled as eye drops in the management of glaucoma and ocular hypertension (below).

◊ The selection of a specific beta blocker for an individual patient depends on the condition being treated and patient characteristics such as liver and kidney function or existing disease such as diabetes. Patient tolerability also varies for different beta blockers. The characteristics of the beta blocker, for example, beta₁ selectivity and intrinsic sympathomimetic activity may also influence selection, as may additional pharmacological properties such as vasodilator activity. However, the clinical significance of these properties is debated.

References.

1. Hampton JR. Choosing the right β-blocker: a guide to selection. *Drugs* 1994; **48:** 549–68.
2. Brown MJ. To β block or better block? *BMJ* 1995; **311:** 701–2.
3. Anonymous. Too many beta-blockers. *Drug Ther Bull* 1996; **34:** 49–52.
4. Anonymous. Which beta-blocker? *Med Lett Drugs Ther* 2001; **43:** 9–11.

Anxiety disorders. Beta blockers have been used in patients with various anxiety disorders, including generalised anxiety disorders (p.649), panic attacks (p.649), and performance anxiety[1] (see under Phobic Disorders, p.649). However, the role of beta blockers in anxiety disorders remains to be established.[2,3] Their benefits do not appear to be particularly great and they are probably most useful in reducing symptoms such as tremor or palpitations that are mediated through beta stimulation. Improvement usually occurs within 1 to 2 hours with relatively low doses of beta blockers (propranolol 40 mg, oxprenolol 40 to 80 mg, nadolol 40 mg). Some patients require higher doses and longer periods of treatment for a beneficial effect.

1. Tyrer P. Current status of β-blocking drugs in the treatment of anxiety disorders. *Drugs* 1988; **36:** 773–83.
2. Manchanda R. Propranolol—the wonder drug for psychiatric disorders? *Br J Hosp Med* 1988; **39:** 267–71.
3. Manchanda R. Propranolol in anxiety. *Br J Hosp Med* 1988; **40:** 323.

Cardiomyopathy. See under Heart Failure, below.

Extrapyramidal disorders. Beta blockers (in low doses) have been suggested for the management of antipsychotic-induced akathisia (see under Chlorpromazine, p.662).

Glaucoma and ocular hypertension. Topical beta blockers are often the drugs of first choice[1] for the initial treatment and maintenance of open-angle glaucoma and other chronic glaucomas (p.1413). They are believed to inhibit beta receptors in the ciliary epithelium and reduce the secretion of aqueous humour. Clinical studies have established that betaxolol, carteolol, levobunolol, metipranolol, and timolol are effective, generally reducing intra-ocular pressure to a similar extent.[2-6] The possibility of systemic effects following topical use needs to be borne in mind (see above), especially in the elderly.[7]

Beta blockers are frequently combined with other ocular hypotensive drugs with different modes of action for optimum pressure control. However, in one study[8] addition of adrenaline [epinephrine] eye drops to treatment with timolol (a non-cardioselective beta blocker) did not result in an additive effect, whereas addition of adrenaline [epinephrine] to treatment with betaxolol (a cardioselective beta blocker) did result in additional benefit.

Beta blockers have also been used for prophylaxis of postoperative ocular hypertension.[9,10]

1. Frishman WH, *et al.* Topical ophthalmic β-adrenergic blockade for the treatment of glaucoma and ocular hypertension. *J Clin Pharmacol* 1994; **34:** 795–803.
2. LeBlanc RP, *et al.* Timolol: long-term Canadian Multicentre Study. *Can J Ophthalmol* 1985; **20:** 128–30.
3. Stewart RH, *et al.* Betaxolol vs timolol: a six-month double-blind comparison. *Arch Ophthalmol* 1986; **104:** 46–8.
4. Geyer O, *et al.* Levobunolol compared with timolol: a four-year study. *Br J Ophthalmol* 1988; **72:** 892–6.
5. Krieglstein GK, *et al.* Levobunolol and metipranolol: comparative ocular hypotensive efficacy, safety, and comfort. *Br J Ophthalmol* 1987; **71:** 250–3.
6. Scoville B, *et al.* A double-masked comparison of carteolol and timolol in ocular hypertension. *Am J Ophthalmol* 1988; **105:** 150–4.
7. O'Donoghue E. β Blockers and the elderly with glaucoma: are we adding insult to injury? *Br J Ophthalmol* 1995; **79:** 794–6.

8. Allen RC, Epstein DL. Additive effect of betaxolol and epinephrine in primary open angle glaucoma. *Arch Ophthalmol* 1986; **104:** 1178–84.
9. West DR, *et al.* Comparative efficacy of the β-blockers for the prevention of increased intraocular pressure after cataract extraction. *Am J Ophthalmol* 1988; **106:** 168–73.
10. Odberg T. Primary argon laser trabeculoplasty after pretreatment with timolol. *Acta Ophthalmol (Copenh)* 1990; **68:** 317–19.

Heart failure. Beta blockers have negative inotropic properties and have generally been contra-indicated in patients with heart failure (p.798). However, there is increasing evidence that they may in fact be of benefit since persistent activation of the sympathetic nervous system appears to be associated with disease progression. A systematic review[1] and meta-analyses[2,3] of trials using various beta blockers (particularly the non-cardioselective carvedilol) in the long-term management of heart failure have suggested that they improve mortality. Two larger long-term studies with the cardioselective beta blockers bisoprolol[4] and metoprolol[5] have confirmed this mortality benefit, although the role of beta blockers in older patients and those with severe heart failure is less clear. Beta blockers are now recommended[6,7] in patients with clinically stable, mild to moderate heart failure due to left ventricular systolic dysfunction and should be given in combination with ACE inhibitors and diuretics. It is not clear whether all beta blockers are equally effective, although a meta-analysis[8] has suggested that vasodilating beta blockers have a greater effect on overall mortality than those that do not produce vasodilatation. The role of beta blockers in severe heart failure is less clear; a study with bucindolol[9] was stopped early because no mortality benefit was found, although carvedilol was found to reduce mortality in a similar study.[10]

Beta blockers may also be of value in some patients with heart failure due to cardiomyopathy (p.796). A number of beta blockers have provided symptomatic benefit in idiopathic dilated cardiomyopathy, and the heart failure trials that showed a mortality benefit included patients with dilated cardiomyopathy. Beta blockers may also be of value in the symptomatic management of hypertrophic cardiomyopathy, to curtail tachycardia, reduce anginal pain, and prevent syncope.

1. Doughty RN, *et al.* Effects of beta-blocker therapy on mortality in patients with heart failure; a systematic overview of randomized controlled trials. *Eur Heart J* 1997; **18:** 560–5.
2. Heidenreich PA, *et al.* Effect of beta-blockade on mortality in patients with heart failure: a meta-analysis of randomized clinical trials. *J Am Coll Cardiol* 1997; **30:** 27–34.
3. Lechat P, *et al.* Clinical effects of β-adrenergic blockade in chronic heart failure: a meta-analysis of double-blind, placebo-controlled, randomized trials. *Circulation* 1998; **98:** 1184–91.
4. CIBIS-II Investigators and Committees. The Cardiac Insufficiency Bisoprolol Study II (CIBIS-II): a randomised trial. *Lancet* 1999; **353:** 9–13.
5. MERIT-HF Study Group. Effect of metoprolol CR/XL in chronic heart failure: Metoprolol CR/XL Randomised Intervention Trial in Congestive Heart Failure (MERIT-HF). *Lancet* 1999; **353:** 2001–7.
6. Packer M, Cohn JN, eds. Consensus recommendations for the management of chronic heart failure. *Am J Cardiol* 1999; **83** (suppl 2A): 1A–38A.
7. Scottish Intercollegiate Guidelines Network. *Diagnosis and treatment of heart failure due to left ventricular systolic dysfunction.* Edinburgh: SIGN Secretariat, 1999.
8. Bonet S, *et al.* β-Adrenergic blocking agents in heart failure: benefits of vasodilating and nonvasodilating agents according to patients' characteristics: a meta-analysis of clinical trials. *Arch Intern Med* 2000; **160:** 621–7.
9. The Beta-Blocker Evaluation of Survival Trial Investigators. A trial of the beta-blocker bucindolol in patients with advanced chronic heart failure. *N Engl J Med* 2001; **344:** 1659–67.
10. Packer M, *et al.* Effect of carvedilol on survival in severe chronic heart failure. *N Engl J Med* 2001; **344:** 1651–8.

Hypotension. A beta blocker (such as atenolol or metoprolol) is reported to be one of the standard drugs used in the management of neurally mediated hypotension (p.805). Beta blockers with partial agonist activity have been used in orthostatic hypotension due to autonomic failure (p.1070) but are potentially dangerous.

Migraine. Beta blockers (usually propranolol) are considered by many to be the drugs of choice in patients requiring prophylactic treatment for migraine (p.449). Their mechanism of action in this disorder is not fully understood. Other beta blockers reported to be effective are those that, like propranolol, possess no intrinsic sympathomimetic activity and include atenolol, metoprolol, nadolol, and timolol.

Beta blockers may sometimes also be of benefit in patients with chronic tension-type headache (p.450).

Propranolol has been tried in the treatment of children with abdominal migraine (p.455).

Peripheral vascular disease. Beta blockers may cause coldness of the extremities and have been reported to induce secondary Raynaud's syndrome. However, they may be of some help in the management of erythromelalgia (see under Peripheral Vascular Disease on p.809).

Phaeochromocytoma. Beta blockers are used, in conjunction with an alpha blocker, in the initial management of phaeochromocytoma (p.810). Beta blockers reduce the responses to the beta-adrenoceptor stimulating effects of adrenaline. Treatment must be started with the alpha blocker and only when alpha blockade is successfully established can tachycardia be

controlled by the cautious use of a beta blocker. A beta₁-selective blocker is preferred so that peripheral beta₂-mediated vasodilatation is unaffected. In most cases modest doses are sufficient although higher doses may be required for a tumour that is predominantly adrenaline-secreting.

Tension-type headache. See under Migraine, above.

Tremor. Tremor is a rhythmical oscillation of part of the body caused by involuntary contraction of opposing muscles. It may occur during action, maintenance of posture, or at rest and varies in frequency and amplitude. Resting tremor is associated mainly with parkinsonism (p.1160), whereas action tremor, which includes postural tremor and kinetic tremor, occurs in a wide variety of disorders. Treatment of the underlying disorder may remove the tremor. Drugs such as bronchodilators, tricyclic antidepressants, lithium, and caffeine may induce tremor; withdrawal of the causative drug usually alleviates the tremor. However, tremor often has no known underlying cause. Such tremor is referred to as essential tremor or benign essential tremor; it is usually postural and tends to affect the hands, head, voice, and sometimes the legs and trunk. It is exacerbated by emotional stress and anxiety. Essential tremor may appear at any age and is a lifelong condition that may progress with increasing age. In many cases there is a family history of the disorder (familial essential tremor).

Mild cases of essential tremor may not require regular drug treatment. Single doses of a beta blocker or a benzodiazepine may be useful in acute circumstances to control exacerbations provoked by stress. A single dose of propranolol usually produces a maximum effect after 1 to 2 hours and the effect may persist for several hours. Small amounts of alcohol may also provide effective temporary relief of essential tremor, although its regular use is obviously discouraged.

For more severe cases of essential tremor long-term drug treatment may be required (and may also be tried in other forms of tremor).[1-4] A beta blocker (usually a non-cardioselective beta blocker such as propranolol) is often the first drug used. Up to 70% of people have been reported to respond, although the average tremor reduction is only about 50 to 60%. The beneficial effect appears to be predominantly due to blockade of peripheral beta₂ receptors on extrafusal muscle fibres and muscle spindles, although there may also be a CNS effect. Adverse effects may be troublesome on long-term use. Primidone may also be tried[5] although there may be a high incidence of acute adverse reactions following initial doses. Concern has been expressed that patients may become tolerant to these drugs given long-term. However, three small studies found a reduced response in only a few patients.[6-8] Local injection of botulinum A toxin has been tried in refractory essential tremor. Benzodiazepines, antimuscarinics, and dopaminergic antiparkinsonian drugs may be effective in some forms of tremor.[4] Other drugs that have shown some benefit include gabapentin, theophylline, clozapine, and ondansetron.[4] In very severe disabling cases, surgery (thalamotomy or deep brain stimulation) may have to be considered.

1. Findley LJ. Essential tremor. *Br J Hosp Med* 1986; **35:** 388–92.
2. Hallett M. Classification and treatment of tremor. *JAMA* 1991; **266:** 1115–17.
3. Wills AJ. Essential tremor and related disorders. *Br J Hosp Med* 1995; **54:** 21–6.
4. Habib-ur-Rehman. Diagnosis and management of tremor. *Arch Intern Med* 2000; **160:** 2438–44.
5. Koller WC, Royse VL. Efficacy of primidone in essential tremor. *Neurology* 1986; **36:** 121–4.
6. Koller WC, Vetere-Overfield B. Acute and chronic effects of propranolol and primidone in essential tremor. *Neurology* 1989; **39:** 1587–8.
7. Calzetti S, *et al.* Clinical and computer-based assessment of long-term therapeutic efficacy of propranolol in essential tremor. *Acta Neurol Scand* 1990; **81:** 392–6.
8. Sasso E, *et al.* Primidone in the long-term treatment of essential tremor: a prospective study with computerized quantitative analysis. *Clin Neuropharmacol* 1990; **13:** 67–76.

Betanidine Sulfate (854-j)

Betanidine Sulfate (pINNM).

Betanidine Sulphate (BANM); Betanidini Sulfas; Bethanidine Sulfate (USAN); Bethanidine Sulphate; BW-467-C-60; NSC-106563. 2-Benzyl-1,3-dimethylguanidine sulphate.

$(C_{10}H_{15}N_3)_2,H_2SO_4 = 452.6$.

CAS — 55-73-2 (betanidine); 114-85-2 (betanidine sulfate).

Pharmacopoeias. In Jpn.

Profile
Betanidine is an antihypertensive with actions and uses similar to those of guanethidine (p.901), but it causes less depletion of noradrenaline stores. It has been given by mouth as the sulfate in the management of hypertension, and has also been tried in ventricular fibrillation.

Preparations
Proprietary Preparations (details are given in Part 3)
UK: Bendogen†.

Betaxolol Hydrochloride (12439-p)

Betaxolol Hydrochloride (BANM, USAN, rINNM).

ALO-1401-02; Betaxololi Hydrochloridum; SL-75212-10. 1-{4-[2-(Cyclopropylmethoxy)ethyl]phenoxy}-3-isopropylamino-propan-2-ol hydrochloride.

$C_{18}H_{29}NO_3,HCl = 343.9$.

CAS — 63659-18-7 (betaxolol); 63659-19-8 (betaxolol hydrochloride).

Pharmacopoeias. In Eur. (see p.vi) and US.

Pharmacopoeial description

Ph. Eur.: A white or almost white crystalline powder. Very soluble in water; freely soluble in alcohol; soluble in dichloromethane; practically insoluble in ether. Protect from light.

USP 25: A white crystalline powder. Freely soluble in water, in alcohol, in chloroform, and in methyl alcohol. pH of a 2% solution in water is between 4.5 and 6.5. Store in airtight containers.

Adverse Effects, Treatment, and Precautions
As for beta blockers, p.844.

◊ Myocardial infarction occurred in an 81-year-old man shortly after administration of a single eye drop of betaxolol 0.5% solution.[1] He was also taking atenolol and indapamide for hypertension.

1. Chamberlain TJ. Myocardial infarction after ophthalmic betaxolol. *N Engl J Med* 1989; **321:** 1342.

Interactions
The interactions associated with beta blockers are discussed on p.846.

Pharmacokinetics
Betaxolol is completely absorbed from the gastrointestinal tract and undergoes only minimal first-pass metabolism, resulting in a high oral bioavailability of 80 to 90%. It has high lipid solubility. Betaxolol is about 50% bound to plasma proteins. Betaxolol crosses the placenta and is distributed into breast milk where higher concentrations have been achieved than in maternal blood. The plasma elimination half-life of betaxolol ranges from 16 to 20 hours. The primary route of elimination is via hepatic metabolism and urinary excretion; only about 15% is excreted in the urine as unchanged drug.

Pregnancy and breast feeding. The pharmacokinetics of betaxolol were investigated in the perinatal period in 28 pregnant hypertensive patients receiving doses of 10 to 40 mg daily.[1] Pharmacokinetic values were similar to those observed in non-pregnant patients. Umbilical-cord concentrations were similar to maternal blood concentrations and showed a negative correlation between concentration in cord blood and timing of the last dose of betaxolol. Thus the betaxolol concentration in the newborn can be considerably reduced by discontinuing drug administration to the mother 16 to 18 hours before birth. The blood-betaxolol half-life in the neonates ranged from 14.8 to 38.5 hours. The mean apparent half-life in infants with gestational age less than 36 weeks was about 32% higher than in full-term neonates. Betaxolol concentrations in milk and/or colostrum were determined in 3 mothers. In all samples the milk-to-blood ratio was greater than 2.

1. Morselli PL, *et al.* Placental transfer and perinatal pharmacokinetics of betaxolol. *Eur J Clin Pharmacol* 1990; **38:** 477–83.

Uses and Administration
Betaxolol is a cardioselective beta blocker (p.844). It is reported to lack intrinsic sympathomimetic activity. Betaxolol has some membrane-stabilising activity.

Betaxolol is used as the hydrochloride in the management of hypertension (p.802), angina pectoris (p.791), and glaucoma (p.1413).

In **hypertension** betaxolol hydrochloride is given in initial doses of 10 to 20 mg as a single daily dose by mouth; doses may be increased if necessary after 1 to 2 weeks according to the patient's response, to 40 mg daily. Similar doses are used in **angina pectoris**.

Initial doses of 5 to 10 mg daily are suggested for elderly patients. Reduced dosages should also be used in patients with severe renal impairment.

Eye drops containing the equivalent of 0.25 or 0.5% betaxolol as the hydrochloride are instilled twice daily to reduce raised intra-ocular pressure in ocular hypertension and open-angle **glaucoma**.

◊ General references.

1. Buckley MM-T, et al. Ocular betaxolol: a review of its pharmacological properties, and therapeutic efficacy in glaucoma and ocular hypertension. Drugs 1990; 40: 75–90.

Speech disorders. A 50-year-old man who had stuttered since childhood obtained striking improvement in his stuttering when he was given betaxolol 20 mg daily for essential hypertension.[1]

1. Burris JF, et al. Betaxolol and stuttering. Lancet 1990; 335: 223.

Preparations

BP 2001: Betaxolol Eye Drops, Solution; Betaxolol Eye Drops, Suspension;
USP 25: Betaxolol Ophthalmic Solution; Betaxolol Tablets.

Proprietary Preparations (details are given in Part 3)
Aust.: Betoptic; *Austral.:* Betoptic; Betoquin; *Belg.:* Betoptic; Kerlone; *Braz.:* Betoptic; *Canad.:* Betoptic; *Denm.:* Betoptic; Kerlon; *Fin.:* Betoptic; Kerlone; *Fr.:* Betoptic; Kerlone; *Ger.:* Betoptima; Kerlone; *Hong Kong:* Betoptic; Kerlone; *Irl.:* Betoptic; *Israel:* Betoptic; Kerlone; *Ital.:* Betoptic; Kerlon; *Mex.:* Beofta; Betoptic; Bex-Hepar; *Neth.:* Betoptic†; Kerlon; *Norw.:* Betoptic; *NZ:* Betoptic; *Port.:* Bertocil; Betoptic; Davixolol; *S.Afr.:* Betoptic; *Singapore:* Betoptic; Kerlone; *Spain:* Betoptic; Oxodal; *Swed.:* Betoptic; Kerlon; *Switz.:* Betoptic-S; Kerlon; *Thai.:* Betoptic; Kerlone; *UK:* Betoptic; Kerlone; *USA:* Betoptic; Kerlone.

Multi-ingredient: *USA:* Kerledex†.

Bevantolol Hydrochloride (12440-n)

Bevantolol Hydrochloride (BANM, USAN, rINNM).
CI-775; NC-1400. 1-(3,4-Dimethoxyphenethylamino)-3-m-tolyloxypropan-2-ol hydrochloride.
$C_{20}H_{27}NO_4,HCl = 381.9$.
CAS — 59170-23-9 (bevantolol); 42864-78-8 (bevantolol hydrochloride).

Profile

Bevantolol is a cardioselective beta blocker (p.844). It is reported to be lacking in significant intrinsic sympathomimetic activity. It has weak membrane-stabilising properties and also has vasodilator activity.

Bevantolol is moderately lipid-soluble. It is reported to be virtually completely absorbed from the gastrointestinal tract and to undergo moderate first-pass metabolism, resulting in a bioavailability of about 60%. It is extensively metabolised and excreted largely in urine as metabolites and small amounts of unchanged drug; the elimination half-life has been reported as 1.5 hours.

Bevantolol has been given by mouth as the hydrochloride in the management of hypertension and angina pectoris.

◊ References.

1. Frishman WH, et al. Bevantolol: a preliminary review of its pharmacodynamic and pharmacokinetic properties, and therapeutic efficacy in hypertension and angina pectoris. Drugs 1988; 35: 1–21.

Preparations

Proprietary Preparations (details are given in Part 3)
Neth.: Ranestol†.

Multi-ingredient: *Neth.:* Ranezide†.

Bezafibrate (12441-h)

Bezafibrate (BAN, USAN, rINN).
Bezafibratum; BM-15075; LO-44. 2-[4-(2-p-Chlorobenzamidoethyl)phenoxy]-2-methylpropionic acid.
$C_{19}H_{20}ClNO_4 = 361.8$.
CAS — 41859-67-0.
ATC — C10AB02.

Pharmacopoeias. In *Eur.* (see p.vi).

Pharmacopoeial description

Ph. Eur.: A white or almost white, crystalline powder. It exhibits polymorphism. Practically insoluble in water; sparingly soluble in alcohol and in acetone; freely soluble in dimethylformamide; it dissolves in dilute solutions of alkali hydroxides.

Adverse Effects and Precautions

The commonest side-effects of bezafibrate therapy are gastrointestinal upsets including anorexia, nausea, and gastric discomfort. Other adverse effects reported to occur less frequently include headache, dizziness, vertigo, fatigue, skin rashes, pruritus, alopecia, impotence, and anaemia, leucopenia, and thrombocytopenia. Raised serum-aminotransferase concentrations have occasionally been reported. Elevated creatine phosphokinase concentrations during bezafibrate therapy may be associated with a syndrome of myositis, myopathy, and rarely rhabdomyolysis; patients with hypoalbuminaemia resulting from the nephrotic syndrome or other renal impairment may be at increased risk. Bezafibrate may increase the lithogenic index, but although there have been isolated reports of

The symbol † denotes a preparation no longer actively marketed

gallstones there is no evidence that the administration of bezafibrate is associated with an increased frequency of this adverse effect.

Bezafibrate should not be given to patients with severe hepatic impairment, primary biliary cirrhosis, gallstones or gallbladder disorders, or hypoalbuminaemic states such as the nephrotic syndrome. It should be used with caution in renal impairment.

Effects on glucose metabolism. Reductions in fasting blood-glucose concentrations and improved glucose tolerance have been reported during therapy with bezafibrate in type 2 diabetic patients with hyperlipidaemia.[1-3] It was suggested that bezafibrate may be a particularly suitable choice of lipid regulating drug in such patients.[4]

1. Rüth E, Vollmar J. Verbesserung der diabeteseinstellung unter der therapie mit bezafibrat. Dtsch Med Wochenschr 1982; 107: 1470–3.
2. Bruneder H, Klein HJ. Hyperlipoproteinämie und diabetes mellitus: langzeitbehandlung mit bezafibrat bei 115 patienten. Med Welt 1984; 35: 357–60.
3. Ogawa S, et al. Bezafibrate reduces blood glucose in type 2 diabetes mellitus. Metabolism 2000; 49: 331–4.
4. Jones IR, et al. Lowering of plasma glucose concentrations with bezafibrate in patients with moderately controlled NIDDM. Diabetes Care 1990; 13: 855–63.

Effects on the kidneys. A report of renal failure associated with bezafibrate.[1] See also Effects on Skeletal Muscle, below.

1. Lipkin GW, Tomson CRV. Severe reversible renal failure with bezafibrate. Lancet 1993; 341: 371.

Effects on the nervous system. Peripheral neuropathy occurred in a patient given bezafibrate and was substantiated by nerve conduction studies.[1]

1. Ellis CJ, et al. Peripheral neuropathy with bezafibrate. BMJ 1994; 309: 929.

Effects on skeletal muscle. The UK Committee on Safety of Medicines has noted that myositis and myopathy are well known to occur with lipid regulating drugs such as fibrates and statins.[1] Rhabdomyolysis, presenting as muscle pain with elevated creatine phosphokinase and myoglobinuria leading to renal failure, has also been reported but appears to be rare. Worldwide reporting did not indicate marked differences in the risk of the reactions with individual drugs. Patients with renal impairment, and possibly with hypothyroidism, may be at increased risk of muscle toxicity. Combined treatment with a fibrate and a *statin* may also increase the risk of serious muscle toxicity. The Committee advised that patients treated with fibrates or statins should consult their doctor if they develop muscle pain, tenderness, or weakness and treatment should be stopped if muscle toxicity is suspected clinically or if creatine phosphokinase is markedly raised or progressively rising.

1. Committee on Safety of Medicines/Medicines Control Agency. Rhabdomyolysis associated with lipid-lowering drugs. Current Problems 1995; 21: 3.

Headache. Severe recurrent headaches were associated with bezafibrate administration in a patient.[1] The headaches started about 24 hours after therapy with bezafibrate began, and recurred about 1 hour after each dose.

1. Hodgetts TJ, Tunnicliffe C. Bezafibrate-induced headache. Lancet 1989; i: 163.

Renal impairment. See under Uses and Administration, below.

Interactions

Bezafibrate and other fibrates may enhance the effects of oral anticoagulants; the dose of anticoagulant should be reduced when treatment with a fibrate is started, and then adjusted gradually if necessary. Recommendations concerning the amount that the anticoagulant dose should be reduced by vary between the manufacturers of the differing fibrates and are sometimes not even specified; the manufacturers of bezafibrate suggest a reduction of up to 50% in the dosage of anticoagulant. The mechanism of the interaction has not yet been determined. Fibrates have been reported to displace warfarin from protein binding sites but other mechanisms are probably also involved.

A number of other drugs may be displaced from plasma proteins by fibrates including tolbutamide and other sulfonylurea antidiabetics, phenytoin, and, in patients with hypoalbuminaemia, frusemide [furosemide]. The interaction with antidiabetics is complex since bezafibrate has been shown to alter glucose tolerance in both diabetic and non-diabetic patients. The dosage of antidiabetics may need adjusting during concomitant bezafibrate therapy.

There is an increased risk of myopathy if fibrates are given concurrently with statins (see Effects on Skeletal Muscle under Adverse Effects and Precautions, above).

Increased ciclosporin concentrations and associated nephrotoxicity have been reported when the drug was administered concomitantly with bezafibrate.

Pharmacokinetics

Bezafibrate is readily absorbed from the gastrointestinal tract. Plasma protein binding is about 95%. The plasma elimination half-life is about 2 hours. Most of a dose is excreted in the urine, about half as unchanged drug, the remainder as metabolites including the glucuronide conjugate. A small proportion of the dose appears in the faeces.

◊ References.

1. Abshagen U, et al. Disposition pharmacokinetics of bezafibrate in man. Eur J Clin Pharmacol 1979; 16: 31–8.
2. Abshagen U, et al. Steady-state kinetics of bezafibrate and clofibrate in healthy female volunteers. Eur J Clin Pharmacol 1980; 17: 305–8.

The elderly. In a study comparing the pharmacokinetics of bezafibrate in 19 elderly patients with younger healthy subjects,[1] maximum plasma concentrations were 1.6 times higher in the elderly group (median 12.1 mg per litre against 7.7 mg per litre) and half-life was increased by 3.8 times (median 6.6 hours against 1.7 hours). The differences could not be attributed solely to diminished renal function in elderly patients. Dosage adjustments in elderly patients should not therefore be based on renal function alone.

1. Neugebauer G, et al. Steady-state kinetics of bezafibrate retard in hyperlipidemic geriatric patients. Klin Wochenschr 1988; 66: 250–6.

Renal impairment. For a report of the half-life of bezafibrate in patients with renal impairment, see under Uses and Administration, below.

Uses and Administration

Bezafibrate, a fibric acid derivative, is a lipid regulating drug. It is used in the treatment of type IIa, type IIb, type III, type IV, and type V hyperlipoproteinaemias. It reduces elevated plasma concentrations of triglycerides by reducing the concentration of very-low-density lipoproteins (VLDL). It reduces elevated plasma concentrations of cholesterol to a lesser extent, but the effect is variable.

Bezafibrate is given in a usual dose of 200 mg three times daily by mouth taken with or after food; 200 mg twice daily may occasionally be adequate for maintenance particularly in the treatment of hypertriglyceridaemia. A 400-mg modified-release tablet is also available and is given as a single daily dose of 400 mg.

◊ General reviews.

1. Goa KL, et al. Bezafibrate: an update of its pharmacology and use in the management of dyslipidaemia. Drugs 1996; 52: 725–53.

Administration in renal impairment. The manufacturer has stated that conventional formulations of bezafibrate may be given to patients with renal impairment depending on creatinine clearance. Doses are:

- creatinine clearance (CC) 40 to 60 mL per minute, 400 mg daily
- CC 15 to 40 mL per minute, 200 mg daily or on alternate days
- CC less than 15 mL per minute, contra-indicated unless receiving dialysis
- dialysis patients, 200 mg on every third day

In a study in patients with impaired renal function[1] the half-life of bezafibrate was reported to be prolonged to 4.6 hours in 3 patients with creatinine clearance greater than 40 mL per minute, 7.8 hours in 8 patients with creatinine clearance of 20 to 40 mL per minute, and 20.1 hours in a patient with creatinine clearance of 13 mL per minute. An accelerated decline in renal function was reported[2] in 2 patients with advanced chronic renal failure during bezafibrate therapy, and it was suggested that further dosage reductions would be necessary to avoid excessive plasma-bezafibrate concentrations in uraemic patients.

1. Anderson P, Norbeck H-E. Clinical pharmacokinetics of bezafibrate in patients with impaired renal function. Eur J Clin Pharmacol 1981; 21: 209–14.
2. Williams AJ, et al. The short term effects of bezafibrate on the hypertriglyceridaemia of moderate to severe uraemia. Br J Clin Pharmacol 1984; 18: 361–7.

Hyperlipidaemias. Bezafibrate is a typical member of the fibric acid derivative group of drugs (the fibrates) used in the treatment of hyperlipidaemias (p.800). One of the primary actions of the fibrates is to promote the catabolism of triglyceride-rich lipoproteins, in particular very-low-density lipoproteins (VLDL), apparently mediated by an enhanced activity of lipoprotein lipase.[1] They may also interfere with the synthesis of VLDL, possibly by inhibiting hepatic acetyl coenzyme A carboxylase. The effect of fibrates on low-density lipoprotein (LDL)-cholesterol depends on the overall lipoprotein status of the patient. In hypertriglyceridaemic patients the response depends on underlying LDL-cholesterol concentrations and the type of lipoprotein abnormality, while in normotriglyceridaemic patients with type IIa hyperlipoproteinaemia the LDL-cholesterol tends to decrease. In these patients bezafibrate and fenofibrate may reduce LDL-cholesterol concentrations more effectively than clofibrate or gemfibrozil. High-density lipoprotein (HDL)-cholesterol concentrations are increased by fibrate therapy in both hypertriglyceridaemic and normotriglyceridaemic patients, although there have been a few reports of unexpected falls in HDL-cholesterol with bezafibrate[2,3] and ciprofibrate (see p.858).

Fibrates have three actions on sterol metabolism:[1] they inhibit the synthesis of cholesterol, they inhibit the synthesis of bile acids, and they enhance the secretion of cholesterol in bile. It is these latter two effects which are responsible for the raised cholesterol saturation of bile, which may lead to the formation of gallstones in some patients. However, other factors appear to be necessary since gallstones develop in relatively few patients.

Bezafibrate has been shown to reduce cholesterol and triglyceride concentrations in patients with type IIa, IIb, and IV hyperlipoproteinaemias and in diabetic patients with lipid abnormalities.[4] Comparative studies have shown it to be at least as effective as clofibrate and fenofibrate, and to be more so than gemfibrozil in the short, but possibly not long, term.[4] It is less effective than ciprofibrate (except for effects on HDL-cholesterol).[4]

The influence of long-term bezafibrate administration on mortality from **ischaemic heart disease** has been investigated. In the Bezafibrate Coronary Atherosclerosis Intervention Trial (BECAIT)[5,6] treatment for 5 years in young men (less than 45 years of age) following myocardial infarction resulted in fewer coronary events and slowed the progression of focal coronary atherosclerosis when compared with placebo.

1. Grundy SM, Vega GL. Fibric acids: effects on lipids and lipoprotein metabolism. *Am J Med* 1987; **83** (suppl 5B): 9–20.
2. Capps NE. Lipid profiles on fibric-acid derivatives. *Lancet* 1994; **344:** 684–5.
3. McLeod AJ, et al. Abnormal lipid profiles on fibrate derivatives. *Lancet* 1996; **347:** 261.
4. Goa KL, et al. Bezafibrate: an update of its pharmacology and use in the management of dyslipidaemia. *Drugs* 1996; **52:** 725–53.
5. Ericsson C-G, et al. Angiographic assessment of effects of bezafibrate on progression of coronary artery disease in young male postinfarction patients. *Lancet* 1996; **347:** 849–53.
6. Ericsson C-G, et al. Effect of bezafibrate treatment over five years on coronary plaques causing 20% to 50% diameter narrowing (The Bezafibrate Coronary Atherosclerosis Intervention Trial (BECAIT). *Am J Cardiol* 1997; **80:** 1125–9.

Preparations

Proprietary Preparations (details are given in Part 3)
Aust.: Bezalip; **Belg.:** Cedur; Eulitop; **Braz.:** Cedur; **Canad.:** Bezalip; **Denm.:** Bezalip; **Fin.:** Bezalip; **Fr.:** Befizal; **Ger.:** Azufibrat; Befibrat; Beza; Beza-Lande; Beza-Puren; Bezabeta; Bezacur; Bezamerck; Cedur; Durabezur†; Lipox; Regadrin B; Sklerofibrat; **Hong Kong:** Azufibrat; Bezalip; Zafibral; **Israel:** Bezalip; Norlip; **Ital.:** Bezalip; Hadiel; **Jpn:** Bezalip†; **Mex.:** Bezafisal; Bionolip; Colser; Lipocin; Redalip; Solibay; Wayfrato; **Neth.:** Bezalip; **NZ:** Bezalip; **Port.:** Bezalip; **S.Afr.:** Bezalip; **Singapore:** Bezalip; Zafibral; **Spain:** Difaterol; Eulitop; Reducterol; **Swed.:** Bezalip; **Switz.:** Cedur; **Thai.:** Bezalip; Bezamil; Polyzalip; **UAE:** Lipitrol; **UK:** Bezagen; Bezalip; Bezalip Mono; Liparol; Zimbacol.

Binifibrate (18698-g)

Binifibrate (rINN).

2-(4-Chlorophenoxy)-2-methylpropionic acid ester with 1,3-dinicotinoyloxypropan-2-ol.

$C_{25}H_{23}ClN_2O_7 = 498.9$.
CAS — 69047-39-8.

Profile
Binifibrate, a derivative of clofibrate (p.859) and nicotinic acid (p.1372), is a lipid regulating drug used in the treatment of hyperlipidaemias (p.800). The usual dose is 600 mg three times daily by mouth.

Preparations
Proprietary Preparations (details are given in Part 3)
Spain: Antopal; Biniwas; Clearon.

Bisoprolol Fumarate (18615-w)

Bisoprolol Fumarate (BANM, USAN, rINNM).

CL-297939; EMD-33512 (bisoprolol or bisoprolol fumarate). 1-[4-(2-Isopropoxyethoxymethyl)phenoxy]-3-isopropylaminopropan-2-ol fumarate.

$(C_{18}H_{31}NO_4)_2,C_4H_4O_4 = 767.0$.
CAS — 66722-44-9 (bisoprolol); 66722-45-0 (bisoprolol fumarate); 104344-23-2 (bisoprolol fumarate).

Adverse Effects, Treatment, and Precautions
As for beta blockers, p.844.

Interactions
The interactions associated with beta blockers are discussed on p.846.

Pharmacokinetics
Bisoprolol is almost completely absorbed from the gastrointestinal tract and undergoes only minimal first-pass metabolism resulting in an oral bioavailability of about 90%. Peak plasma concentrations are reached 2 to 4 hours after oral administration. Bisoprolol is about 30% bound to plasma proteins. It has a plasma elimination half-life of 10 to 12 hours. Bisoprolol is moderately lipid-soluble. Approximately 50% of a dose is metabolised in the liver and it is excreted in urine as unchanged drug and metabolites.

Uses and Administration
Bisoprolol is a cardioselective beta blocker (p.844). It is reported to be devoid of intrinsic sympathomimetic and membrane-stabilising properties.

Bisoprolol is given as the fumarate in the management of hypertension (p.802) and angina pectoris (p.791). It is also used as an adjunct to standard therapy in patients with stable chronic heart failure (p.798).

In **hypertension** or **angina pectoris** the usual dose of bisoprolol fumarate is 5 to 10 mg by mouth as a single daily dose; the maximum recommended dose is 20 mg daily. In patients with severe renal impairment (creatinine clearance less than 20 mL per minute) or severe hepatic dysfunction the dose should not exceed 10 mg daily.

In **heart failure** the initial dose of bisoprolol fumarate is 1.25 mg once daily by mouth. If tolerated, the dose should be doubled after 1 week, and then increased gradually at 1 to 4 week intervals to the maximum dose tolerated by the patient; this should not exceed 10 mg once daily.

◊ References.
1. Lancaster SG, Sorkin EM. Bisoprolol: a preliminary review of its pharmacodynamic and pharmacokinetic properties, and therapeutic efficacy in hypertension and angina pectoris. *Drugs* 1988; **36:** 256–85.
2. Johns TE, Lopez LM. Bisoprolol: is this just another beta-blocker for hypertension or angina? *Ann Pharmacother* 1995; **29:** 403–14.
3. CIBIS-II Investigators and Committees. The Cardiac Insufficiency Bisoprolol Study II (CIBIS-II): a randomised trial. *Lancet* 1999; **353:** 9–13.

Preparations
Proprietary Preparations (details are given in Part 3)
Aust.: Concor; **Belg.:** Emconcor; Isoten; **Denm.:** Bisocor; Cardicor; Emconcor; Monocor†; **Fin.:** Emconcor; **Fr.:** Cardensiel; Cardiocor; Detensiel; Soprol; **Ger.:** Biso-Puren; Bisobloc; Bisomerck; Concor; Cordalin; Fondril; **Hong Kong:** Concor; **Irl.:** Bisopine; Cardicor; Emcor; Soprol; **Israel:** Concor; **Ital.:** Concor; **Neth.:** Bisobloc; Emcor; **Port.:** Concor; **S.Afr.:** Concor; **Singapore:** Concor; **Spain:** Emconcor; Euradal; Godal; **Swed.:** Emconcor; **Switz.:** Concor; **Thai.:** Concor; **UK:** Bipranix; Cardicor; Emcor; Monocor; **USA:** Zebeta.

Multi-ingredient: Aust.: Concor Plus; **Belg.:** Emcoretic; Maxsoten; **Fin.:** Emconcor Comp; **Fr.:** Lodoz; Wytens; **Ger.:** Concor Plus; Fondril-5 HCT; **Mex.:** Biconcor; **Neth.:** Emcoretic; **Spain:** Emcoretic; **Switz.:** Concor Plus; **UK:** Monozide†; **USA:** Ziac.

Bivalirudin (17816-e)

Bivalirudin (BAN, USAN, rINN).

BG-8967; Hirulog.
$C_{98}H_{138}N_{24}O_{33} = 2180.3$.
CAS — 128270-60-0.

Adverse Effects and Precautions
The most common adverse effect of bivalirudin is bleeding.

Bivalirudin is contra-indicated in patients with active major bleeding and should be used with caution in patients at increased risk of bleeding. It should not be administered by intramuscular injection.

Interactions
Concomitant use of bivalirudin with anticoagulants or thrombolytics may increase the risk of bleeding.

Pharmacokinetics
Bivalirudin is partly metabolised and partly excreted by the kidney. Following intravenous administration the plasma half-life is about 25 minutes in patients with normal renal function but is prolonged in patients with renal impairment. Bivalirudin does not bind to plasma proteins and is removed by haemodialysis.

Uses and Administration
Bivalirudin, an analogue of the peptide hirudin (p.905), is a direct thrombin inhibitor. It is used as an anticoagulant in patients with unstable angina undergoing percutaneous transluminal coronary angioplasty (see Reperfusion and Revascularisation Procedures, p.812) and has also been investigated in unstable angina and myocardial infarction.

In the management of patients undergoing angioplasty, bivalirudin is started immediately before the procedure. The initial dose is 1 mg per kg body-weight by intravenous injection followed by an intravenous infusion of 2.5 mg per kg per hour for 4 hours. The infusion may be continued at a dose of 0.2 mg per kg per hour for up to 20 hours if required. Patients should also receive treatment with aspirin.

The dose of bivalirudin should be reduced in patients with renal impairment and the activated clotting time should be monitored. For patients with a glomerular filtration rate of 30 to 59 mL per minute the infusion dose should be reduced by 20%; for a glomerular filtration rate of 10 to 29 mL per minute the infusion dose should be reduced by 60%; and for dialysis-dependent patients the infusion dose should be reduced by 90%.

◊ References.
1. Lidón R-M, et al. A pilot, early angiographic patency study using a direct thrombin inhibitor as adjunctive therapy to streptokinase in acute myocardial infarction. *Circulation* 1995; **89:** 1567–72.
2. Fuchs J, et al. Hirulog in the treatment of unstable angina: results of the Thrombin Inhibition in Myocardial Ischemia (TIMI) 7 trial. *Circulation* 1995; **92:** 727–33.
3. Bittl JA, et al. Treatment with bivalirudin (Hirulog) as compared with heparin during coronary angioplasty for unstable or postinfarction angina. *N Engl J Med* 1995; **333:** 764–9.
4. White HD, et al. Randomized, double-blind comparison of hirulog versus heparin in patients receiving streptokinase and aspirin for acute myocardial infarction (HERO). *Circulation* 1997; **96:** 2155–61.
5. Kong DF, et al. Clinical outcomes of bivalirudin for ischemic heart disease. *Circulation* 1999; **100:** 2049–53.

Preparations
Proprietary Preparations (details are given in Part 3)
USA: Angiomax.

Bopindolol Malonate (16544-a)

Bopindolol Malonate (rINNM).

Bopindolol Hydrogen Malonate; LT-31-200. (±)-1-(tert-Butylamino)-3-[(2-methylindol-4-yl)oxy]propan-2-ol benzoate malonate.

$C_{23}H_{28}N_2O_3,C_3H_4O_4 = 484.5$.
CAS — 62658-63-3 (bopindolol); 82857-38-3 (bopindolol malonate).

Profile
Bopindolol is a non-cardioselective beta blocker (p.844). It is reported to possess some intrinsic sympathomimetic activity.

It is used as the malonate in the management of hypertension (p.802) and angina pectoris (p.791) in daily doses equivalent to 0.5 to 2 mg of bopindolol by mouth.

◊ References.
1. Harron DWG, et al. Bopindolol: a review of its pharmacodynamic and pharmacokinetic properties and therapeutic efficacy. *Drugs* 1991; **41:** 130–49.

Preparations
Proprietary Preparations (details are given in Part 3)
Aust.: Sandonorm; **Ger.:** Wandonorm†; **Switz.:** Sandonorm.

Multi-ingredient: Switz.: Sandoretic.

Bosentan (17405-z)

Bosentan (BAN, USAN, rINN).

Ro-47-0203/029. p-tert-Butyl-N-[6-(2-hydroxyethoxy)-5-(o-methoxyphenoxy)-2-(2-pyrimidinyl)-4-pyrimidinyl]benzenesulfonamide.

$C_{27}H_{29}N_5O_6S = 551.6$.
CAS — 147536-97-8 (anhydrous bosentan); 157212-55-0 (bosentan monohydrate).

Profile
Bosentan is an endothelin receptor antagonist used in the management of pulmonary hypertension (p.810). It is under investigation in heart failure and has also been studied in hypertension.

In pulmonary hypertension, bosentan is given by mouth in an initial dose of 62.5 mg twice daily, increased after 4 weeks to a maintenance dose of 125 mg twice daily. Serum aminotransferase concentrations must be measured before starting treatment and then at monthly intervals; the dose should be reduced or treatment should be withdrawn if abnormalities occur.

◊ References.
1. Krum H, et al. The effect of an endothelin-receptor antagonist, bosentan, on blood pressure in patients with essential hypertension. *N Engl J Med* 1998; **338:** 784–90.
2. Sutsch G, et al. Short-term oral endothelin-receptor antagonist therapy in conventionally treated patients with symptomatic severe chronic heart failure. *Circulation* 1998; **98:** 2262–8.
3. Weber C, et al. Multiple-dose pharmacokinetics, safety, and tolerability of bosentan, an endothelin receptor antagonist, in healthy male volunteers. *J Clin Pharmacol* 1999; **39:** 703–14.

Preparations

Proprietary Preparations (details are given in Part 3)
USA: Tracleer.

Bretylium Tosilate (855-z)

Bretylium Tosilate *(BAN, rINN).*
ASL-603; Bretylium Tosylate *(USAN)*. (2-Bromobenzyl)ethyld-imethylammonium toluene-4-sulphonate.
$C_{11}H_{17}BrN,C_7H_7O_3S = 414.4$.
CAS — 59-41-6 (bretylium); 61-75-6 (bretylium tosilate).
ATC — C01BD02.
Pharmacopoeias. In Br. and US.

Pharmacopoeial description

BP 2001: A white crystalline powder. M.p. about 98°. It exhibits polymorphism. Freely soluble in water, in alcohol, and in methyl alcohol. A 5% solution in water has a pH of 5.0 to 6.5. Store in airtight containers at a temperature not exceeding 25°. Protect from light.

USP 25: A white, hygroscopic, crystalline powder. Freely soluble in water, in alcohol, and in methyl alcohol; practically insoluble in ether, in ethyl acetate, and in hexane. Store in airtight containers.

Incompatibilities. Bretylium tosilate injection has been reported to be visually incompatible with propofol emulsion[1] and with warfarin sodium injection.[2]

1. Trissel LA, *et al.* Compatibility of propofol injectable emulsion with selected drugs during simulated Y-site administration. *Am J Health-Syst Pharm* 1997; **54:** 1287–92.
2. Bahal SM, *et al.* Visual compatibility of warfarin sodium injection with selected medications and solutions. *Am J Health-Syst Pharm* 1997; **54:** 2599–2600.

Adverse Effects and Precautions

The most common adverse effect following administration of bretylium is hypotension which may be severe. Bretylium may also cause a transient initial increase in blood pressure and heart rate, and a worsening of cardiac arrhythmias due to a release of noradrenaline. Nausea and vomiting may occur particularly during rapid intravenous infusion. Intramuscular injection of bretylium can lead to local tissue necrosis and muscle atrophy, which can be avoided by limiting the volume and varying the site of the injection (see Uses and Administration, below). Bretylium should be given with care to patients with renal impairment and doses should be reduced. Caution is also required in patients with severe aortic stenosis or pulmonary hypertension who may be unable to increase cardiac output in response to the fall in peripheral resistance produced by bretylium.

Effects on body temperature. Bretylium tosilate administered by intravenous infusion was considered to be the cause of hyperthermia in a 59-year-old-man.[1] Six similar cases had been reported to the manufacturer in the USA.

1. Thibault J. Hyperthermia associated with bretylium tosylate injection. *Clin Pharm* 1989; **8:** 145–6.

Effects on the cardiovascular system. Seven patients with recent myocardial infarction, 3 with and 4 without left ventricular failure, received bretylium tosilate 5 to 10 mg per kg body-weight intravenously.[1] Initial transient tachycardia and hypertension, and late sustained bradycardia, hypotension with decreased vascular resistance, and increased calf blood flow and venous capacitance occurred in all 7 patients. Bretylium should be used cautiously in patients with hypotension as it might cause a significant reduction in arterial pressure.

1. Chatterjee K, *et al.* Cardiovascular effects of bretylium tosylate in acute myocardial infarction. *JAMA* 1973; **223:** 757–60.

Interactions

Bretylium may exacerbate arrhythmias caused by digitalis toxicity. If sympathomimetics are required to reverse bretylium-induced hypotension, great care should be exercised since their effects may be enhanced.

Pharmacokinetics

Bretylium is incompletely absorbed from the gastrointestinal tract. It is well absorbed following intramuscular injection. It is not metabolised and is largely excreted unchanged in the urine. The half-life is reported to be between 4 and 17 hours in patients with normal renal function and is prolonged in patients with renal impairment. Bretylium is dialysable.

◊ Reviews.
1. Rapeport WG. Clinical pharmacokinetics of bretylium. *Clin Pharmacokinet* 1985; **10:** 248–56.

Uses and Administration

Bretylium is a quaternary ammonium compound with class II and class III antiarrhythmic activity (p.787); it causes an initial release of noradrenaline and then blocks adrenergic transmission by preventing noradrenaline release from adrenergic nerve endings. It suppresses ventricular fibrillation and other ventricular arrhythmias, but its exact mode of action is unknown.

It is given parenterally as the tosilate for the treatment of immediately life-threatening ventricular arrhythmias and for the short-term control of ventricular arrhythmias resistant to standard treatment (see p.794). If a positive response is to be seen in patients with ventricular fibrillation it usually occurs within minutes. However, a delay of up to several hours may occur before peak antiarrhythmic activity is achieved and therefore it should only be used in other ventricular arrhythmias if the arrhythmia is resistant to more rapidly acting drugs.

In immediately life-threatening ventricular arrhythmias such as **ventricular fibrillation** 5 mg per kg body-weight as an undiluted 5% (50 mg per mL) solution may be given by rapid intravenous injection, in association with other resuscitative measures and cardioversion, increased to 10 mg per kg if the ventricular fibrillation persists, and repeated as necessary up to a total dose of 30 mg per kg.

For the control of **ventricular arrhythmias** that are not immediately life-threatening bretylium may be given under ECG monitoring by intramuscular or slow intravenous injection. The patient should be supine or closely observed for postural hypotension. A dose of 5 to 10 mg per kg by either route may be repeated initially every 1 to 2 hours until the arrhythmia is controlled and subsequently every 6 to 8 hours for maintenance therapy. The patient should be changed to an oral antiarrhythmic as soon as possible. For intramuscular administration an undiluted 5% (50 mg per mL) solution is used; the site of intramuscular injections should be varied on repeated injection and not more than 5 mL should be given into any one site. Nausea and vomiting during intravenous administration can be avoided by administering the injection over not less than 8 minutes although a period of 15 to 30 minutes is preferred: the injection is diluted to 10 mg per mL with glucose 5% or sodium chloride 0.9%. Alternatively an intravenous infusion of 1 to 2 mg per minute has been employed.

Doses should be reduced in patients with renal impairment.

Bretylium tosilate was originally used in the treatment of hypertension but because of poor gastric absorption and the development of tolerance during long-term therapy it has been superseded by other drugs.

Preparations

BP 2001: Bretylium Injection;
USP 25: Bretylium Tosylate in Dextrose Injection; Bretylium Tosylate Injection.

Proprietary Preparations (details are given in Part 3)
Belg.: Bretylate; *Canad.:* Bretylate; *Irl.:* Bretylate; *Israel:* Bretylate; *S.Afr.:* Bretylol†; *UK:* Bretylate†; *USA:* Bretylol†.

Brimonidine Tartrate (1925-r)

Brimonidine Tartrate *(BANM, USAN, rINNM).*
AGN-190342-LF; UK-14304-18. 5-Bromo-6-(2-imidazolin-2-ylamino)quinoxaline D-tartrate.
$C_{11}H_{10}BrN_5,C_4H_6O_6 = 442.2$.
CAS — 59803-98-4 (brimonidine); 79570-19-7 (brimonidine tartrate).

Adverse Effects and Precautions

As for Apraclonidine Hydrochloride, p.840.

Interactions

As for Apraclonidine Hydrochloride, p.840.

Uses and Administration

Brimonidine is an alpha2-adrenoceptor agonist with actions and uses similar to those of apraclonidine (p.841). It is used to lower intra-ocular pressure in patients with open-angle glaucoma or ocular hypertension (p.1413), as an alternative to, or as an adjunct to, topical beta blocker therapy. The reduction in intra-ocular pressure is maximal about two hours after topical application.

Brimonidine is used as the tartrate. In the management of glaucoma or ocular hypertension one drop of a 0.2% solution is instilled two or three times daily.

◊ References.
1. Anonymous. Brimonidine—an alpha2-agonist for glaucoma. *Med Lett Drugs Ther* 1997; **39:** 54–5.
2. Adkins JC, Balfour JA. Brimonidine: a review of its pharmacological properties and clinical potential in the management of open-angle glaucoma and ocular hypertension. *Drugs Aging* 1998; **12:** 225–41.

Preparations

Proprietary Preparations (details are given in Part 3)
Aust.: Alphagan; *Austral.:* Alphagan; *Belg.:* Alphagan; *Canad.:* Alphagan; *Denm.:* Alphagan; *Fin.:* Alphagan; *Fr.:* Alphagan; *Ger.:* Alphagan; *Hong Kong:* Alphagan; *Irl.:* Alphagan; *Israel:* Alphagan; *Ital.:* Alphagan; *Mex.:* Alphagan; *NZ:* Alphagan; *Port.:* Alphagan; *S.Afr.:* Alphagan; *Singapore:* Alphagan; *Spain:* Alphagan; *Swed.:* Alphagan; *Switz.:* Alphagan; *Thai.:* Alphagan; *UK:* Alphagan; *USA:* Alphagan.

Brinzolamide (9711-h)

Brinzolamide *(BAN, USAN, rINN).*
AL-4862. (R)-4-(Ethylamino)-3,4-dihydro-2-(3-methoxypropyl)-2H-thieno[3,2-e]-1,2-thiazine-6-sulfonamide 1,1-dioxide.
$C_{12}H_{21}N_3O_5S_3 = 383.5$.
CAS — 138890-62-7.
ATC — S01EC04.

Adverse Effects and Precautions

As for Dorzolamide, p.883.

Uses and Administration

Brinzolamide is a carbonic anhydrase inhibitor with actions and uses similar to those of dorzolamide (p.883). It is used topically to reduce intra-ocular pressure in the management of open-angle glaucoma and ocular hypertension (p.1413), either alone or as adjunctive therapy with a topical beta blocker. A 1% suspension is instilled two or three times daily.

Preparations

Proprietary Preparations (details are given in Part 3)
Austral.: Azopt; *Canad.:* Azopt; *Denm.:* Azopt; *Fin.:* Azopt; *Irl.:* Azopt; *Singapore:* Azopt; *Thai.:* Azopt; *UK:* Azopt; *USA:* Azopt.

Bucindolol Hydrochloride (12462-q)

Bucindolol Hydrochloride *(BANM, USAN, rINNM).*
MJ-13105-1. 2-[2-Hydroxy-3-(2-indol-3-yl-1,1-dimethylethyl-amino)propoxy]benzonitrile hydrochloride.
$C_{22}H_{25}N_3O_2,HCl = 399.9$.
CAS — 71119-11-4 (bucindolol); 70369-47-0 (bucindolol hydrochloride).

Profile

Bucindolol is a non-cardioselective beta blocker (p.844). It is reported to possess intrinsic sympathomimetic activity as well as weak alpha1-blocking activity, and also has direct vasodilating activity. Bucindolol, as the hydrochloride, has been investigated in the management of hypertension, heart failure, and other cardiac disorders.

Buflomedil Hydrochloride (12465-w)

Buflomedil Hydrochloride *(BANM, rINNM).*
Buflomedili Hydrochloridum; LL-1656. 2′,4′,6′-Trimethoxy-4-(pyrrolidin-1-yl)butyrophenone hydrochloride.
$C_{17}H_{25}NO_4,HCl = 343.8$.
CAS — 55837-25-7 (buflomedil); 35543-24-9 (buflomedil hydrochloride).
Pharmacopoeias. In Eur. (see p.vi).

Pharmacopoeial description

Ph. Eur.: A white or almost white microcrystalline powder. Freely soluble in water; soluble in alcohol; very slightly soluble in acetone. A 5% solution in water has a pH of 4.5 to 6.5.

Adverse Effects

Buflomedil has been reported to cause gastrointestinal disturbances, headache, vertigo, syncope, rash, pruritus, and paraes-

---

thesia. Overdosage may produce severe hypotension, tachycardia, and convulsions.

◊ References.
1. Bachand RT, Dubourg AY. A review of long-term safety data with buflomedil. *J Int Med Res* 1990; **18**: 245–52.

Pharmacokinetics
Buflomedil hydrochloride is absorbed from the gastrointestinal tract and peak plasma concentrations are reached 1.5 to 4 hours following oral administration. Buflomedil is subject to first-pass metabolism; bioavailability is reported to be between 50 and 80%.

Buflomedil is widely distributed. Binding to plasma proteins is dose-dependent and varies between 60 and 80% at therapeutic concentrations. Buflomedil is metabolised in the liver and is mainly excreted in the urine both as unchanged drug and metabolites. The elimination half-life is about 2 to 3 hours. Elimination may be impaired in patients with renal or hepatic impairment.

Uses and Administration
Buflomedil hydrochloride is a vasodilator used in the treatment of cerebrovascular (p.798) and peripheral vascular disease (p.809). Usual doses by mouth are 300 to 600 mg daily, by intramuscular injection up to 100 mg daily, by slow intravenous injection up to 200 mg daily, and by intravenous infusion up to 400 mg daily.

◊ References.
1. Clissold SP, *et al.* Buflomedil: a review of its pharmacodynamic and pharmacokinetic properties, and therapeutic efficacy in peripheral and cerebral vascular diseases. *Drugs* 1987; **33**: 430–60.
2. De Backer TLM, *et al.* Buflomedil for intermittent claudication (updated 29 May 2001). Available in The Cochrane Library; Issue 4. Oxford: Update Software; 2001.

Preparations
Proprietary Preparations (details are given in Part 3)
Aust.: Buflohexal; Loftyl; *Belg.*: Loftyl; *Braz.*: Bufedil; *Fr.*: Fonzylane; Loftyl; *Ger.*: Bufedil; Buflo; Buflo-POS; Buflo-Puren; Buflo-Reu†; Buflohexal; Defluina; *Hong Kong*: Fonzylane; Irrodan; *Ital.*: Bufene†; Buflan; Buflocit; Buflofar; Bufoxin†; Emoflux; Flomed; Flupress; Irrodan; Loftyl; Medil†; Perfudan; Pirxane; *Mex.*: Loftyl; *Neth.*: Loftyl; *Port.*: Loftyl; *S.Afr.*: Loftyl; *Spain*: Lofton; Sinoxis†; *Switz.*: Loftyl; *Thai.*: Irrodan.

Bumetanide (2310-r)

Bumetanide *(BAN, USAN, rINN)*.

Bumetanidum; Ro-10-6338. 3-Butylamino-4-phenoxy-5-sulphamoylbenzoic acid.

$C_{17}H_{20}N_2O_5S = 364.4$.

CAS — 28395-03-1.

ATC — C03CA02.

Pharmacopoeias. In *Chin.*, *Eur.* (see p.vi), *Jpn*, and *US*.

Pharmacopoeial description
Ph. Eur.: A white crystalline powder. It exhibits polymorphism. Practically insoluble in water; soluble in alcohol and in acetone; slightly soluble in dichloromethane and in ether. It dissolves in dilute solutions of alkali hydroxides. Protect from light.

USP 25: A practically white powder. Slightly soluble in water; soluble in alkaline solutions. Store in airtight containers. Protect from light.

Adverse Effects
As for Frusemide [furosemide], p.893. Bumetanide may cause muscle pain, particularly at high doses.

Effects on the ears. Early reports suggested that bumetanide might be less ototoxic than frusemide [furosemide].[1] However, both drugs can cause deafness, especially when given in large doses to patients with renal impairment.

1. Ward A, Heel RC. Bumetanide: a review of its pharmacodynamic and pharmacokinetic properties and therapeutic use. *Drugs* 1984; **28**: 426–64.

Effects on the muscles. Bumetanide, particularly in high doses in patients with chronic renal impairment, may cause severe musculoskeletal pain. A curious muscle stiffness distinct from cramp, with tenderness to compression and pain on movement, was noted in association with bumetanide therapy in 4 patients with end-stage renal failure.[1] The calf muscles were the first to be affected; shoulder girdle and thigh muscle tenderness also occurred in 2 patients, and one patient also had neck stiffness. The side-effect appeared to be dose-related for the individual patients.

1. Barclay JE, Lee HA. Clinical and pharmacokinetic studies on bumetanide in chronic renal failure. *Postgrad Med J* 1975; **51** (suppl 6): 43–6.

Effects on the skin. Bullous pemphigoid developed in a patient approximately 6 weeks after starting therapy with bumetanide.[1] Healing occurred after withdrawal of the drug without the need for corticosteroid treatment.

1. Boulinguez S, *et al.* Bullous pemphigoid induced by bumetanide. *Br J Dermatol* 1998; **138**: 548–9.

Precautions
Bumetanide's precautions and contra-indications are generally dependent on its effects on fluid and electrolyte balance and are similar to those of the thiazide diuretics (see Hydrochlorothiazide, p.909).

Interactions
As for Frusemide [furosemide], p.894.

Pharmacokinetics
Bumetanide is almost completely and fairly rapidly absorbed from the gastrointestinal tract; the bioavailability is reported to be about 80 to 95%. It has a plasma elimination half-life of about 1 to 2 hours. It is about 95% bound to plasma proteins. About 80% of the dose is excreted in the urine, approximately 50% as unchanged drug, and 10 to 20% in the faeces.

◊ References to the pharmacokinetics of bumetanide in healthy subjects.
1. Halladay SC, *et al.* Diuretic effect and metabolism of bumetanide in man. *Clin Pharmacol Ther* 1977; **22**: 179–87.
2. Pentikäinen PJ, *et al.* Fate of [¹⁴C]-bumetanide in man. *Br J Clin Pharmacol* 1977; **4**: 39–44.
3. Holazo AA, *et al.* Pharmacokinetics of bumetanide following intravenous, intramuscular, and oral administrations to normal subjects. *J Pharm Sci* 1984; **73**: 1108–13.
4. McCrindle JL, *et al.* Effect of food on the absorption of frusemide and bumetanide in man. *Br J Clin Pharmacol* 1996; **42**: 743–6.

Hepatic impairment. In a study of 8 patients with chronic hepatic disease,[1] the diuretic response to bumetanide 1 mg was impaired but bumetanide excretion rates were normal.

1. Marcantonio LA, *et al.* The pharmacokinetics and pharmacodynamics of the diuretic bumetanide in hepatic and renal disease. *Br J Clin Pharmacol* 1983; **15**: 245–52.

Renal impairment. Renal excretion of bumetanide has been shown to be reduced in patients with chronic renal impairment with a subsequent attenuation of diuretic effect.[1-3] The cumulative pharmacodynamic effects of oral and intravenous doses were essentially similar in patients with renal impairment and transition from intravenous to oral maintenance regimens should pose no special problems.[2]

1. Marcantonio LA, *et al.* The pharmacokinetics and pharmacodynamics of the diuretic bumetanide in hepatic and renal disease. *Br J Clin Pharmacol* 1983; **15**: 245–52.
2. Lau HSH, *et al.* Kinetics, dynamics, and bioavailability of bumetanide in healthy subjects and patients with chronic renal failure. *Clin Pharmacol Ther* 1986; **39**: 635–45.
3. Howlett MR, *et al.* Metabolism of the diuretic bumetanide in healthy subjects and patients with renal impairment. *Eur J Clin Pharmacol* 1990; **38**: 583–6.

Uses and Administration
Although chemically unrelated, bumetanide is a loop diuretic with actions and uses similar to those of frusemide [furosemide] (p.895). Bumetanide is used in the treatment of oedema associated with heart failure (p.798) and with renal and hepatic disorders. It is given in high doses in the management of oliguria due to renal failure or insufficiency. Bumetanide has also been used in hypertension (p.802).

Diuresis is initiated within about 30 minutes to an hour after a dose by mouth, reaches a maximum at 1 to 2 hours, and lasts for about 4 hours but may be prolonged to 6 hours after high doses; after intravenous injection its effects are evident within a few minutes and last for about 2 hours. As a general guide bumetanide 1 mg produces a diuretic effect similar to frusemide [furosemide] 40 mg although this should not be used for direct substitution at higher doses.

In the treatment of **oedema** the usual dose is 1 mg by mouth in the morning or early evening; a second dose may be given 6 to 8 hours later if necessary. A dose of 0.5 mg daily may be adequate in some elderly patients.

In refractory oedema higher doses may be necessary. An initial dose of 5 mg daily has been advocated, increased by 5 mg every 12 to 24 hours as required; however other sources have suggested a maximum total dose of 10 mg daily. Twice daily dosing may be preferred at higher doses. For maintenance therapy doses may be given daily or intermittently. In an emergency or when oral therapy cannot be given 0.5 to 1 mg may be administered by intramuscular or slow intravenous injection, subsequently adjusted according to the patient's response. A dose for pulmo-

nary oedema is 1 to 2 mg by intravenous injection, repeated 20 minutes later if necessary. Alternatively, 2 to 5 mg may be given over 30 to 60 minutes in 500 mL of a suitable infusion fluid.

In the treatment of **hypertension** bumetanide has been given in doses of 0.5 to 1 mg daily by mouth, although higher doses have been used.

When very high doses of bumetanide are used careful laboratory control is essential as described under the uses for frusemide [furosemide] (p.895; high-dose therapy).

◊ General references.
1. Ward A, Heel RC. Bumetanide: a review of its pharmacodynamic and pharmacokinetic properties and therapeutic use. *Drugs* 1984; **28**: 426–64.

Preparations
BP 2001: Bumetanide and Slow Potassium Tablets; Bumetanide Injection; Bumetanide Oral Solution; Bumetanide Tablets; **USP 25:** Bumetanide Injection; Bumetanide Tablets.

Proprietary Preparations (details are given in Part 3)
Aust.: Burinex; *Austral.*: Burinex; *Belg.*: Burinex; *Braz.*: Burinax; *Canad.*: Burinex; *Denm.*: Burinex; *Fin.*: Burinex; *Fr.*: Burinex; *Ger.*: Burinex; *Hong Kong*: Burinex; *Irl.*: Burinex; *Ital.*: Fontego; *Mex.*: Bumedyl; Drenural; Durin; Miccil; *Neth.*: Burinex; *Norw.*: Burinex; *NZ*: Burinex; *S.Afr.*: Burinex; *Singapore*: Burinex; *Spain*: Farmadiuril; Fordiuran; *Swed.*: Burinex; *Switz.*: Burinex; *Thai.*: Burinex; *UK*: Betinex; Burinex; *USA*: Bumex.

Multi-ingredient: *Denm.*: Buram; Burinex med kaliumklorid; *Hong Kong*: Burinex K; *Irl.*: Buram; Burinex K; *Norw.*: Burinex K; *Singapore*: Burinex K; *UK*: Burinex A; Burinex K.

Bunazosin Hydrochloride (18560-e)

Bunazosin Hydrochloride *(rINNM)*.

E-643. 1-(4-Amino-6,7-dimethoxy-2-quinazolinyl)-4-butyryl-hexahydro-1*H*-1,4-diazepine monohydrochloride.

$C_{19}H_{27}N_5O_3, HCl = 409.9$.

CAS — 80755-51-7 (bunazosin); 52712-76-2 (bunazosin hydrochloride).

Pharmacopoeias. In *Jpn*.

Profile
Bunazosin is an alpha₁-adrenoceptor blocker (p.787) with general properties similar to those of prazosin (p.958). It is given by mouth as the hydrochloride in the management of hypertension in doses of up to 12 mg daily.

Preparations
Proprietary Preparations (details are given in Part 3)
Ger.: Andante; *Jpn*: Detantol; *Thai.*: Detantol.

Bunitrolol Hydrochloride (6307-l)

Bunitrolol Hydrochloride *(rINNM)*.

Ko-1366 (bunitrolol). 2-(3-tert-Butylamino-2-hydroxypropoxy)benzonitrile hydrochloride.

$C_{14}H_{20}N_2O_2, HCl = 284.8$.

CAS — 34915-68-9 (bunitrolol); 23093-74-5 (bunitrolol hydrochloride).

Profile
Bunitrolol is a beta blocker (p.844). It has been given as the hydrochloride by mouth in the management of cardiovascular disorders.

Preparations
Proprietary Preparations (details are given in Part 3)
Aust.: Stresson†.

Bupranolol Hydrochloride (6309-j)

Bupranolol Hydrochloride *(rINNM)*.

B-1312; KL-255. 1-tert-Butylamino-3-(6-chloro-*m*-toly-loxy)propan-2-ol hydrochloride.

$C_{14}H_{22}ClNO_2, HCl = 308.2$.

CAS — 14556-46-8 (bupranolol); 15148-80-8 (bupranolol hydrochloride).

Pharmacopoeias. In *Jpn*.

Profile
Bupranolol is a beta blocker (p.844). It is given as the hydrochloride in usual doses of 100 to 400 mg daily by mouth in the management of cardiovascular disorders.

Bupranolol eye drops have been used in the management of glaucoma.

Preparations
Proprietary Preparations (details are given in Part 3)
Aust.: Adomed†; *Ger.*: Betadrenol.

Multi-ingredient: *Aust.*: Beta-Isoket; Betamed.

Butalamine Hydrochloride (9215-s)

Butalamine Hydrochloride (BANM, rINNM).
LA-1221. NN-Dibutyl-N'-(3-phenyl-1,2,4-oxadiazol-5-yl)ethylenediamine hydrochloride.
$C_{18}H_{28}N_4O$,HCl = 352.9.
CAS — 22131-35-7 (butalamine); 56974-46-0 (butalamine hydrochloride).

Profile
Butalamine hydrochloride is a vasodilator given in the management of peripheral (p.809) and cerebral vascular disorders (p.798) in a usual dose of 80 to 240 mg daily by mouth.

Preparations
Proprietary Preparations (details are given in Part 3)
Ger.: Adrevil; *Spain*: Surem†.

Butizide (2311-f)

Butizide (rINN).
Buthiazide (USAN); Isobutylhydrochlorothiazide; Thiabutazide.
6-Chloro-3,4-dihydro-3-isobutyl-2H-1,2,4-benzothiadiazine-7-sulphonamide 1,1-dioxide.
$C_{11}H_{16}ClN_3O_4S_2$ = 353.8.
CAS — 2043-38-1.

Profile
Butizide is a thiazide diuretic with properties similar to those of hydrochlorothiazide (p.907). It is used for oedema, including that associated with heart failure (p.798), and for hypertension (p.802).

Butizide has been given by mouth in doses of 5 to 15 mg daily or on 2 or 3 days weekly for the treatment of oedema. It has also been given in doses of 2.5 to 10 mg daily for hypertension, either alone or in conjunction with other antihypertensive drugs.

Preparations
Proprietary Preparations (details are given in Part 3)
Aust.: Saltucin; *Ger.*: Saltucin†.
Multi-ingredient: *Aust.*: Aldactone Saltucin; Buti-Spirobene; Modenol†; Suprenoat; Torrat; *Ger.*: Aldactone Saltucin; Modenol; Torrat; Tri-Torrat; *Hong Kong*: Iso Triraupin; Torrat; *Ital.*: Kadiur; Saludopin; *S.Afr.*: Aldazide; Saltucin Co†; *Switz.*: Aldozone; Sali-Spiroctan; *Thai.*: Iso-Triraupin.

Cadralazine (16559-h)

Cadralazine (BAN, rINN).
CGP-18684/E; ISF-2469. Ethyl 3-{6-[ethyl(2-hydroxypropyl)amino]pyridazin-3-yl}carbazate.
$C_{12}H_{21}N_5O_3$ = 283.3.
CAS — 64241-34-5.
ATC — C02DB04.

Profile
Cadralazine is a vasodilator with actions and uses similar to those of hydralazine (p.905). In the treatment of hypertension (p.802) it is given in doses of 10 to 15 mg daily, as a single dose by mouth.

◊ Reviews.
1. McTavish D, et al. Cadralazine: a review of its pharmacodynamic and pharmacokinetic properties, and therapeutic potential in the treatment of hypertension. Drugs 1990; 40: 543–60.

◊ Cadralazine is reported not to produce the lupus-like syndrome seen in some patients receiving hydralazine.[1,2]
1. Andersson OK. Cadralazine did not produce the SLE-syndrome when hydralazine did. Eur J Clin Pharmacol 1987; 31: 741.
2. Mulder H. Conversion of drug-induced SLE-syndrome by the vasodilating agent cadralazine. Eur J Clin Pharmacol 1990; 38: 303.

Preparations
Proprietary Preparations (details are given in Part 3)
Ital.: Cadraten; Cadrilan†.

Cafedrine Hydrochloride (12500-x)

Cafedrine Hydrochloride (BANM, pINNM).
H-8351; Kafedrin Hydrochloride. 7-[2-(β-Hydroxy-α-methylphenethylamino)ethyl]theophylline hydrochloride.
$C_{18}H_{23}N_5O_3$,HCl = 393.9.
CAS — 58166-83-9 (cafedrine).

Profile
Cafedrine hydrochloride is a derivative of theophylline (p.777), used mainly in preparations with theodrenaline hydrochloride in the treatment of hypotensive states. It is given in a usual dose of 100 to 400 mg daily by mouth.

Preparations
Proprietary Preparations (details are given in Part 3)
Multi-ingredient: *Aust.*: Akrinor; *Fr.*: Praxinor; *Ger.*: Akrinor; *S.Afr.*: Akrinor; *Spain*: Bifort; *Switz.*: Akrinor†.

Calcitonin Gene-related Peptide (18900-z)

CGRP.

Profile
Calcitonin gene-related peptide is an endogenous peptide derived from the calcitonin gene. It has vasodilating activity and has been investigated in the management of peripheral vascular disease (Raynaud's syndrome), heart failure, and for ischaemia following neurosurgery for subarachnoid haemorrhage.

For details of the endogenous substance and its pharmacological effects, see under Calcitonins, p.749.

◊ References.
1. Johnston FG, et al. Effect of calcitonin-gene-related peptide on postoperative neurological deficits after subarachnoid haemorrhage. Lancet 1990; 335: 869–72.
2. Shawkett S, et al. Prolonged effect of CGRP in Raynaud's patients: a double-blind randomised comparison with prostacyclin. Br J Clin Pharmacol 1991; 32: 209–13.
3. Shekhar YC, et al. Effects of prolonged infusion of human alpha calcitonin gene-related peptide on haemodynamics, renal blood flow and hormone levels in congestive heart failure. Am J Cardiol 1991; 67: 732–6.
4. European CGRP in Subarachnoid Haemorrhage Study Group. Effect of calcitonin-gene-related peptide in patients with delayed postoperative cerebral ischaemia after aneurysmal subarachnoid haemorrhage. Lancet 1992; 339: 831–4.
5. Bunker CB, et al. Calcitonin gene-related peptide in treatment of severe peripheral vascular insufficiency in Raynaud's phenomenon. Lancet 1993; 342: 80–2.
6. Gherardini G, et al. Venous ulcers: improved healing by iontophoretic administration of calcitonin gene-related peptide and vasoactive intestinal peptide. Plast Reconstr Surg 1998; 101: 90–3.

Candesartan Cilexetil (17153-e)

Candesartan Cilexetil (BANM, USAN, rINNM).
CV-11974 (candesartan); TCV-116. (±)-1-Hydroxyethyl 2-ethoxy-1-[p-(o-1H-tetrazol-5-ylphenyl)benzyl]-7-benzimidazolecarboxylate, cyclohexyl carbonate ester.
$C_{33}H_{34}N_6O_6$ = 610.7.
CAS — 139481-59-7 (candesartan); 145040-37-5 (candesartan cilexetil).

Adverse Effects and Precautions
As for Losartan Potassium, p.921.

Pharmacokinetics
Candesartan cilexetil is an ester prodrug that is hydrolysed during absorption from the gastrointestinal tract to the active form candesartan. The absolute bioavailability for candesartan is about 40% following administration of candesartan cilexetil as a solution and about 14% following administration as tablets. Peak plasma concentrations of candesartan occur about 3 to 4 hours after oral administration. Candesartan is more than 99% bound to plasma proteins. It is excreted in urine and bile mainly as unchanged drug and a small amount of inactive metabolites. The terminal elimination half-life is approximately 9 hours.

◊ References.
1. Pfister M, et al. Pharmacokinetics and haemodynamics of candesartan cilexetil in hypertensive patients on regular haemodialysis. Br J Clin Pharmacol 1999; 47: 645–51.

Uses and Administration
Candesartan is an angiotensin II receptor antagonist with actions similar to those of losartan (p.922). It is used in the management of hypertension (p.802) and has also been investigated in heart failure.

Candesartan is administered by mouth as the ester prodrug candesartan cilexetil. The onset of antihypertensive effect occurs about 2 hours after administration and the maximum effect is achieved within about 4 weeks after initiating therapy.

In the management of hypertension candesartan cilexetil is given in an initial dose of 4 mg once daily. A lower initial dose of 2 mg once daily is suggested for patients with renal or hepatic impairment. The dose should be adjusted according to response. The usual maintenance dose is 8 mg once daily with a maximum of 16 mg once daily. In the USA higher doses are used; the usual initial dose is 16 mg once daily with a maintenance dose of 8 to 32 mg daily as a single dose or in two divided doses.

◊ Reviews.
1. Sever P, Ménard J, eds. Angiotensin II antagonism refined: candesartan cilexetil. J Hum Hypertens 1997; 11 (suppl 2): S1–S95.
2. McClellan KJ, Goa KL. Candesartan cilexetil: a review of its use in essential hypertension. Drugs 1998; 56: 847–69.

3. Stoukides CA, et al. Candesartan cilexetil: an angiotensin II receptor blocker. Ann Pharmacother 1999; 33: 1287–98.
4. See S, Stirling AL. Candesartan cilexetil: an angiotensin II-receptor blocker. Am J Health-Syst Pharm 2000; 57: 739–46.

Preparations
Proprietary Preparations (details are given in Part 3)
Aust.: Atacand; Blopress; *Austral.*: Atacand; *Belg.*: Atacand; *Canad.*: Atacand; *Denm.*: Atacand; *Fin.*: Atacand; *Fr.*: Atacand; Kenzen; *Ger.*: Atacand; Blopress; *Irl.*: Atacand; *Israel*: Atacand; *Ital.*: Blopress; Ratacand; *Mex.*: Atacand; *Neth.*: Atacand; *Norw.*: Atacand; *NZ*: Atacand; *Port.*: Atacand; Blopress; *S.Afr.*: Atacand; *Singapore*: Atacand; *Spain*: Atacand; Parapres; *Swed.*: Atacand; *Switz.*: Atacand; Blopress; *Thai.*: Blopress; *UK*: Amias; *USA*: Atacand.
Multi-ingredient: *Austral.*: Atacand Plus; *Fr.*: Cokenzen; Hytacand; *Irl.*: Atacand Plus; *Swed.*: Atacand Plus; *USA*: Atacand HCT.

Candoxatril (12037-y)

Candoxatril (BAN, USAN, rINN).
UK-79300. cis-4-{1-[(S)-2-(Indan-5-yloxycarbonyl)-3-(2-methoxyethoxy)propyl]cyclopentylcarbonylamino}cyclohexanecarboxylic acid.
$C_{29}H_{41}NO_7$ = 515.6.
CAS — 118785-03-8; 123122-55-4.

Profile
Candoxatril is an ester prodrug which is hydrolysed in the body following oral administration to its active form candoxatrilat (UK-69578). Candoxatrilat is a neutral endopeptidase (neutral metalloendopeptidase) inhibitor. It is a potent inhibitor of the endopeptidase responsible for the metabolism of atrial natriuretic peptide (ANP) (p.938); inhibition of this enzyme results in raised ANP concentrations with consequent natriuresis and suppression of the renin-angiotensin-aldosterone system. Candoxatril is under investigation in the management of hypertension and heart failure.

◊ References.
1. Newby DE, et al. Candoxatril improves exercise capacity in patients with chronic heart failure receiving angiotensin converting enzyme inhibition. Eur Heart J 1998; 19: 1808–13.
2. Westheim AS, et al. Hemodynamic and neuroendocrine effects for candoxatril and frusemide in mild stable chronic heart failure. J Am Coll Cardiol 1999; 34: 1794–1801.
3. Northridge DB, et al. Comparison of the short-term effects of candoxatril, an orally active neutral endopeptidase inhibitor, and frusemide in the treatment of patients with chronic heart failure. Am Heart J 1999; 138: 1149–57.

Canrenone (2312-d)

Canrenone (USAN, pINN).
SC-9376. 17-Hydroxy-3-oxo-17α-pregna-4,6-diene-21-carboxylic acid γ-lactone.
$C_{22}H_{28}O_3$ = 340.5.
CAS — 976-71-6.
ATC — C03DA03.

Profile
Canrenone is a potassium-sparing diuretic with properties similar to those of spironolactone (p.973) and is used in the treatment of refractory oedema associated with heart failure (p.798) or hepatic disease, and in hypertension (p.802). It is a metabolite of both spironolactone and potassium canrenoate (p.957). It is given in usual doses of 50 to 200 mg daily by mouth. Doses of up to 300 mg daily may be required in some patients.

Preparations
Proprietary Preparations (details are given in Part 3)
Belg.: Contaren; *Ital.*: Luvion.

Captopril (856-c)

Captopril (BAN, USAN, rINN).
Captoprilum; SQ-14225. 1-[(2S)-3-Mercapto-2-methylpropionyl]-L-proline.
$C_9H_{15}NO_3S$ = 217.3.
CAS — 62571-86-2.
ATC — C09AA01.

NOTE. Compounded preparations of captopril may be represented by the following names:
- Co-zidocapt (BAN)—captopril 2 parts and hydrochlorothiazide 1 part (w/w).

Pharmacopoeias. In Chin., Eur. (see p.vi), and US.

Pharmacopoeial description
Ph. Eur.: A white or almost white crystalline powder. Freely soluble in water, in dichloromethane, and in methyl alcohol. It dissolves in dilute solutions of alkali hydroxides. A 2% solution in water has a pH of 2.0 to 2.6. Store in airtight containers.

USP 25: A white or off-white crystalline powder which may have a characteristic sulfide-like odour. Freely soluble in water, in alcohol, in chloroform, and in methyl alcohol. Store in airtight containers.

The symbol † denotes a preparation no longer actively marketed

Stability. Although captopril itself is relatively stable at temperatures up to 50°,[1] and extemporaneously prepared powders (made by triturating the tablets with lactose) have been reported to be stable for at least 12 weeks at room temperature,[2] aqueous solutions are subject to oxidative degradation, mainly to captopril disulfide,[1] which increases with increase in pH above 4.[3] The manufacturers report that a liquid form prepared from pulverised tablets in distilled water containing 1 mg of captopril per mL retained 96.6% of the original concentration of drug after storage at room temperature for 5 days, but they advise that since it contains no preservative it should be used within 2 days of preparation.[4] Others have reported wide variations in stability depending upon the formulation. In one study[5] the shelf-life of a solution of captopril 1 mg per mL prepared from crushed tablets and tap water was estimated to be 27 days when stored at 5°. However, in another study[6] captopril was much less stable; in sterile water for irrigation captopril was stable for at least 3 days when stored at 5°, but in tap water it disappeared at a much faster rate. Increased stability has been reported following the addition of sodium ascorbate to the solution,[7] and with captopril powder rather than crushed tablets.[8] A 1 mg per mL preparation made with crushed tablets and undiluted syrup has also been reported to be stable for 30 days at 5° and may be more palatable than aqueous formulations.[9]

1. Lund W, Cowe HJ. Stability of dry powder formulations. *Pharm J* 1986; **237:** 179–80.
2. Taketomo CK, *et al.* Stability of captopril in powder papers under three storage conditions. *Am J Hosp Pharm* 1990; **47:** 1799–1801.
3. Timmins P, *et al.* Factors affecting captopril stability in aqueous solution. *Int J Pharmaceutics* 1982; **11:** 329–36.
4. Andrews CD, Essex A. Captopril suspension. *Pharm J* 1986; **237:** 734–5.
5. Pereira CM, Tam YK. Stability of captopril in tap water. *Am J Hosp Pharm* 1992; **49:** 612–15.
6. Anaizi NH, Swenson C. Instability of aqueous captopril solutions. *Am J Hosp Pharm* 1993; **50:** 486–8.
7. Nahata MC, *et al.* Stability of captopril in three liquid dosage forms. *Am J Hosp Pharm* 1994; **51:** 95–6.
8. Chan DS, *et al.* Degradation of captopril in solutions compounded from tablets and standard powder. *Am J Hosp Pharm* 1994; **51:** 1205–7.
9. Lye MYF, *et al.* Effects of ingredients on stability of captopril in extemporaneously prepared oral liquids. *Am J Health-Syst Pharm* 1997; **54:** 2483–7.

Adverse Effects, Treatment, and Precautions

As for ACE inhibitors, p.820.

Captopril has been reported to cause false positive results in tests for acetone in urine.

◊ Results of postmarketing surveillance in 30 515 hypertensive patients receiving captopril showed that 4.9% had their therapy discontinued because of adverse effects thought to be due to the drug. The mean initial daily dose was 46 mg; at final evaluation the mean daily dose was 58 mg. The adverse effect most commonly reported was headache (in 1.8%); others included dizziness (1.6%), rashes (1.1%), nausea (1.0%), taste disturbances (0.9%), and cough (0.8%).[1] This study excluded patients with impaired renal function but an earlier survey in 6737 patients who received captopril alone or in combination found that rash and dysgeusia were more frequent in patients with impaired renal function (occurring in 6.2% and 3.2% respectively of those receiving 150 mg daily or less of captopril) than in those with normal serum creatinine (4.3% and 2.2%). The frequency of both symptoms was somewhat higher in those given higher doses. Symptoms of hypotension occurred in about 5% of patients and were not influenced by dose or renal function.[2] The cumulative frequency of withdrawal due to adverse reactions was estimated at 5.8% in this study, which is similar to that in the larger survey. In another postmarketing surveillance study involving more than 60 000 patients, captopril was withdrawn in 8.9% because of adverse effects.[3]

For further reference to some of these adverse effects, see under ACE Inhibitors, p.820.

1. Schoenberger JA, *et al.* Efficacy, safety, and quality-of-life assessment of captopril antihypertensive therapy in clinical practice. *Arch Intern Med* 1990; **150:** 301–6.
2. Jenkins AC, *et al.* Captopril in hypertension: seven years later. *J Cardiovasc Pharmacol* 1985; **7** (suppl 1): S96–S101.
3. Chalmers D, *et al.* Postmarketing surveillance of captopril for hypertension. *Br J Clin Pharmacol* 1992; **34:** 215–23.

Porphyria. Captopril is considered to be unsafe in patients with porphyria because it has been shown to be porphyrinogenic in *in-vitro* systems.

Interactions

As for ACE inhibitors, p.822.

Pharmacokinetics

About 60 to 75% of a dose of captopril is absorbed from the gastrointestinal tract and peak plasma concentrations are achieved within about an hour. Absorption has been reported to be reduced in the presence of food, but see under Absorption, below. Captopril is about 30% bound to plasma proteins. It crosses the placenta and is found in breast milk at about 1% of maternal blood concentrations. It is largely excreted in the urine, 40 to 50% as unchanged drug, the rest as disulfide and other metabolites. The elimination half-life has been reported to be 2 to 3 hours but this is increased in renal impairment. Captopril is removed by haemodialysis.

◊ Reviews.
1. Duchin KL, *et al.* Pharmacokinetics of captopril in healthy subjects and in patients with cardiovascular diseases. *Clin Pharmacokinet* 1988; **14:** 241–59.

Absorption. The bioavailability and peak plasma concentrations of captopril have been shown to be reduced by 25 to 55% on administration with food in single dose studies[1-4] and with chronic dosing.[5] However, this may not be clinically significant since several studies[3,4,6] indicated that food intake had no effect on the antihypertensive activity of captopril.

1. Williams GM, Sugerman AA. The effect of a meal, at various times relative to drug administration, on the bioavailability of captopril. *J Clin Pharmacol* 1982; **22:** 18A.
2. Singhvi SM, *et al.* Effect of food on the bioavailability of captopril in healthy subjects. *J Clin Pharmacol* 1982; **22:** 135–40.
3. Mäntylä R, *et al.* Impairment of captopril bioavailability by concomitant food and antacid intake. *Int J Clin Pharmacol Ther Toxicol* 1984; **22:** 626–9.
4. Müller HM, *et al.* The influence of food intake on pharmacodynamics and plasma concentration of captopril. *J Hypertens* 1985; **3** (suppl 2): S135–6.
5. Öhman KP, *et al.* Effect of food intake on blood pressure during acute and chronic administration and in relation to food intake. *J Cardiovasc Pharmacol* 1985; **7** (suppl 1): S20–4.
6. Izumi Y, *et al.* Influence of food on the clinical effect of angiotensin I converting enzyme inhibitor (SQ 14225). *Tohoku J Exp Med* 1983; **139:** 279–86.

Renal impairment. A study of 9 patients with chronic renal failure undergoing dialysis found that peak plasma concentrations of captopril were 2.5 times higher and peak concentrations of the disulfide metabolites were 4 times higher than in patients with normal renal function following a single dose of captopril.[1] Peak concentrations occurred later in uraemic patients and the apparent half-life of total captopril was 46 hours in uraemic patients compared with 2.95 hours in patients with normal renal function.

1. Drummer OH, *et al.* The pharmacokinetics of captopril and captopril disulfide conjugates in uraemic patients on maintenance dialysis: comparison with patients with normal renal function. *Eur J Clin Pharmacol* 1987; **32:** 267–71.

Uses and Administration

Captopril is a sulfhydryl-containing ACE inhibitor (p.820). It is used in the management of hypertension (p.802), in heart failure (p.798), following myocardial infarction (p.805), and in diabetic nephropathy (see Kidney Disorders, p.824).

Following oral administration captopril produces a maximum effect within 1 to 2 hours, although the full effect may not develop for several weeks during chronic dosing. The duration of action is dose-dependent and may persist for 6 to 12 hours.

In the treatment of **hypertension** the initial dose is 12.5 mg twice daily by mouth, increased gradually at intervals of 2 to 4 weeks according to the response. The usual maintenance dose is 25 to 50 mg twice daily and should not normally exceed 50 mg three times daily. If hypertension is not satisfactorily controlled at this dosage, addition of a second drug or substitution of an alternative drug should be considered. In the USA higher doses of up to 150 mg three times daily have been suggested for patients with hypertension uncontrolled by lower doses of captopril in conjunction with diuretic therapy. Since there may be a precipitous fall in blood pressure in some patients when starting therapy with an ACE inhibitor, the first dose should preferably be given at bedtime and if diuretics are already being taken they should be stopped, if possible, for a few days before introducing captopril. An initial dose of 6.25 mg twice daily is recommended if captopril is given in addition to a diuretic or to elderly patients.

In the treatment of **heart failure** severe first-dose hypotension on introduction of an ACE inhibitor is common in patients on loop diuretics, but their temporary withdrawal may cause rebound pulmonary oedema. Thus an initial dose of 6.25 to 12.5 mg of captopril is given by mouth under close medical supervision; the usual maintenance dose is 25 mg two or three times daily, and doses should not normally exceed 50 mg three times daily. Again, in the USA higher doses of up to 150 mg three times daily have been suggested.

Following **myocardial infarction**, captopril is used prophylactically in clinically stable patients with symptomatic or asymptomatic left ventricular dysfunction to improve survival, delay the onset of symptomatic heart failure, and reduce recurrent infarction. It may be started 3 days after myocardial infarction in an initial dose of 6.25 mg by mouth, increased over several weeks to 150 mg daily in divided doses if tolerated.

In **diabetic nephropathy** (microalbuminuria greater than 30 mg per day) in type 1 diabetics, 75 to 100 mg of captopril may be given daily, in divided doses, by mouth. Other antihypertensives may be used with captopril if a further reduction in blood pressure is required. In patients with severe renal impairment (creatinine clearance less than 30 mL per minute) the initial dose of captopril should be 12.5 mg twice daily and if a diuretic also needs to be given a loop diuretic should be chosen rather than a thiazide.

Administration. Captopril is generally given orally. Sublingual[1] and intravenous[2,3] administration has also been tried, but these routes are not established.

1. Angeli P, *et al.* Comparison of sublingual captopril and nifedipine in immediate treatment of hypertensive emergencies: a randomized, single-blind clinical trial. *Arch Intern Med* 1991; **151:** 678–82.
2. Savi L, *et al.* A new therapy for hypertensive emergencies: intravenous captopril. *Curr Ther Res* 1990; **47:** 1073–81.
3. Langes K, *et al.* Efficacy and safety of intravenous captopril in congestive heart failure. *Curr Ther Res* 1993; **53:** 167–76.

Administration in children. Experience with captopril in children is limited. The UK manufacturers have suggested an initial dose of 0.3 mg per kg body-weight increased as necessary to a maximum of 6 mg per kg daily given in two or three divided doses. They do not recommend captopril for the treatment of mild to moderate hypertension in children.

Captopril, given in an initial dose of 0.25 mg per kg body-weight daily, increased to up to 2.5 or 3.5 mg per kg daily in 3 divided doses has also been reported to produce benefit in infants with severe heart failure secondary to congenital defects (predominantly manifesting as left-to-right shunt).[1,2]

1. Scammell AM, *et al.* Captopril in treatment of infant heart failure: a preliminary report. *Int J Cardiol* 1987; **16:** 295–301.
2. Shaw NJ, *et al.* Captopril in heart failure secondary to a left to right shunt. *Arch Dis Child* 1988; **63:** 360–3.

Nitrate tolerance. For reference to the use of captopril as a sulfhydryl donor in the management of nitrate tolerance, see under Precautions of Glyceryl Trinitrate, p.898.

Preparations

BP 2001: Captopril Tablets;
USP 25: Captopril and Hydrochlorothiazide Tablets; Captopril Tablets.

Proprietary Preparations (details are given in Part 3)
Aust.: Capace; Debax; Lopirin; *Austral.:* Acenorm; Capace; Capoten; Captohexal; Enzace; *Belg.:* Capoten; *Braz.:* Capoten; Catoprol; Hipocatril; *Canad.:* Apo-Capto; Capoten; Captril; Nu-Capto; *Denm.:* Capoten; Captodan; Captil; Catonet; *Fin.:* Capoten; Captomin; Captostad; Lopril; *Fr.:* Captirex; Captolane; Lopril; Oltens; *Ger.:* ACE-Hemmer; Acenorm; Adocor; Capto; Captodura Cor†; Capto-dura M; Captobeta; Captodoc; Captoflux; Captogamma; Captohexal; Captomerck; Captopress†; Captoreal†; Cardiagen; cor tensobon; Coronorm; Epicordin; Esparil†; Lopirin; Mundil; Sansanal; Sigacap Cor; Tensiomin; Tensiomin-Cor; Tensobon; Tensostad; *Hong Kong:* Apo-Capto; Capoten; Kimafan; Tensiomin; *Irl.:* Aceomel; Actopril; Capoten; Captor; Geroten; Tensopril; *Israel:* Aceril; Apocapen; Capti; Inhibace; *Ital.:* Acepress; Capoten; *Mex.:* Atrisol; Biodezil; Capotena; Captoser; Captral; Cardipril; Cryopril; Ecapresan; Ecapril; Ecaten; Hipertex; Kenapril; Kenolan; Lenpryl; Lowpre; Novapres; Reductel; Romir; Toprilem; Tropisol; *Neth.:* Capoten; *NZ:* Capoten; *Port.:* Calpix; Capoten; Carencil; Convertal; Hipertil; Hipotensil; Mereprine; Prilovase; Tensopril; Vidapril; *S.Afr.:* Capace; Capoten; Captohexal; Captomax; Cardiace; Zapto; *Singapore:* Capoten; Capril; Ketanine; Rilcapton; Tensoprel; *Spain:* Alopresin; Capoten; Cesplon; Dardex; Dilabar; Garanil; Tensoprel; *Swed.:* Capoten; Smico-basan; Captosol; Lopirin; Tensobon; *Thai.:* Capoten; Epsitron; Gemzil; Tensiomin; *UK:* Acepril; Capoten; Ecopace; Hytenez†; Kaplon; Tensopril; *USA:* Capoten.

Multi-ingredient: *Aust.:* Capozide; Captocomp†; Captopril Compositum; Veracapt; *Braz.:* Lopril D; *Denm.:* Capozid; *Fr.:* Captea; Ecazide; *Ger.:* Acenorm HCT; Adocomp; Capto Comp; Capto Plus; Captobeta Comp; Captogamma HCT; Captohexal Comp; Captopril Comp; Captopril HCT; Captopril Plus; Cardiagen HCT; Tensobon comp; *Irl.:* Capozide; Captor-HCT; *Ital.:* Acedlur; Aceplus; *Mex.:* Capozide; Co-Captral; *Neth.:* Aceplus; Capozide; *NZ:* Capozide; *Port.:* Lopiretic; Normotil; *S.Afr.:* Capozide; Capotoretic; Zapto Co; *Spain:* Alopresin Diu; Cesplon Plus; Decresco; Dilabar Diu; Ecadiu; Ecazide; *Swed.:* Capozid†; *Switz.:* Capozide; Tensobon comp; *UK:* Acezide; Capozide; Capto-Co; *USA:* Capozide.

Carazolol (12521-h)

Carazolol (BAN, rINN).

BM-51052. 1-(Carbazol-4-yloxy)-3-isopropylaminopropan-2-ol.

$C_{18}H_{22}N_2O_2 = 298.4.$

CAS — 57775-29-8.

Profile

Carazolol is a beta blocker (p.844). It is given in doses of 5 to 30 mg daily by mouth in the management of various cardiovascular disorders.

Preparations

Proprietary Preparations (details are given in Part 3)

Aust.: Conducton; *Ger.:* Conducton.

Carbocromen Hydrochloride (9218-l)

Carbocromen Hydrochloride (rINNM).

A-27053; AG-3; Cassella-4489; Chromonar Hydrochloride (USAN); NSC-110430. Ethyl 3-(2-diethylaminoethyl)-4-methyl-coumarin-7-yloxyacetate hydrochloride.

$C_{20}H_{27}NO_5,HCl = 397.9.$

CAS — 804-10-4 (carbocromen); 655-35-6 (carbocromen hydrochloride).

Profile

Carbocromen hydrochloride is a vasodilator used in ischaemic heart disease in usual doses of 225 to 900 mg daily by mouth. Ischaemic heart disease is discussed under Atherosclerosis (p.793) and the treatment of its clinical manifestations is described under Angina Pectoris (p.791) and Myocardial Infarction (p.805).

Preparations

Proprietary Preparations (details are given in Part 3)

Ger.: Intensain†; *Ital.:* Cardiocap.

Multi-ingredient: *Aust.:* Coro-Lanitop†.

Carperitide (15262-d)

Carperitide (rINN).

CAS — 89213-87-6.

Profile

Carperitide is a recombinant atrial natriuretic peptide (see p.938) used in the management of acute heart failure.

Preparations

Proprietary Preparations (details are given in Part 3)

Jpn: Hanp.

Carteolol Hydrochloride (12533-g)

Carteolol Hydrochloride (BANM, USAN, rINNM).

Abbott-43326; OPC-1085. 5-(3-tert-Butylamino-2-hydroxy-propoxy)-3,4-dihydroquinolin-2(1H)-one hydrochloride.

$C_{16}H_{24}N_2O_3,HCl = 328.8.$

CAS — 51781-06-7 (carteolol); 51781-21-6 (carteolol hydrochloride).

Pharmacopoeias. In Br., Jpn, and US.

Pharmacopoeial description

BP 2001: White crystals or a white crystalline powder. Soluble in water; very slightly soluble in alcohol and in glacial acetic acid; practically insoluble in ether; sparingly soluble in methyl alcohol. A 1% solution in water has a pH of 5.0 to 6.0. Store in airtight containers.

USP 25: pH of a 1% solution in water is between 5.0 and 6.0.

Adverse Effects, Treatment, and Precautions

As for beta blockers, p.844.

Interactions

The interactions associated with beta blockers are discussed on p.846.

Pharmacokinetics

Carteolol, given as the hydrochloride, is well absorbed from the gastrointestinal tract with a peak plasma concentration being reached within 1 to 3 hours of oral administration. It has low lipid solubility. Approximately 20 to 30% is protein bound. The plasma half-life is reported to be 5 to 6 hours. The major route of elimination is renal with 50 to 70% of a dose being excreted unchanged in the urine. Major metabolites are 8-hydroxycarteolol and glucuronic acid conjugates of carteolol and 8-hydroxycarteolol. The 8-hydroxycarteolol metabolite is active; its half-

The symbol † denotes a preparation no longer actively marketed

---

life is reported to be 8 to 12 hours. Because the main route of elimination is renal carteolol accumulates in patients with renal disease.

Uses and Administration

Carteolol is a non-cardioselective beta blocker (see p.844). It is reported to possess intrinsic sympathomimetic activity.

Carteolol is used as the hydrochloride in the management of glaucoma (p.1413), hypertension (p.802), and some cardiac disorders such as angina pectoris (p.791) and cardiac arrhythmias (p.794).

Eye drops containing carteolol hydrochloride 1% or 2% are instilled twice daily to reduce raised intra-ocular pressure in open-angle **glaucoma** and ocular hypertension.

In **hypertension** carteolol hydrochloride is given in initial doses of 2.5 mg once daily by mouth, increased, if necessary according to the patient's response, to 10 mg once daily. In cardiac disorders such as **angina pectoris** and **arrhythmias** carteolol hydrochloride has been employed in doses of 10 to 30 mg daily.

The oral dose of carteolol hydrochloride should be reduced in patients with renal impairment. The dosage interval should be increased from 24 hours to 48 hours in patients with a creatinine clearance of 20 to 60 mL per minute and to 72 hours in patients with a creatinine clearance of less than 20 mL per minute.

Preparations

BP 2001: Carteolol Eye Drops;

USP 25: Carteolol Hydrochloride Ophthalmic Solution; Carteolol Hydrochloride Tablets.

Proprietary Preparations (details are given in Part 3)

Aust.: Endak†; *Belg.:* Carteol; *Denm.:* Arteoptic; *Fin.:* Arteoptic; *Fr.:* Carteol; Mikelan; *Ger.:* Arteoptic; Endak; *Hong Kong:* Arteoptic; Mikelan; *Irl.:* Teoptic; *Ital.:* Carteol; *Jpn:* Mikelan; *Neth.:* Teoptic; *Port.:* Arteoptic; *S.Afr.:* Mikelan; Teoptic; *Spain:* Arteolol; Elebloc; Mikelan; *Swed.:* Arteoptic; *Switz.:* Arteoptic; *Thai.:* Arteoptic; *UK:* Teoptic; *USA:* Cartrol; Ocupress.

Multi-ingredient: *Belg.:* Carteopil; *Fr.:* Carpilo.

Carvedilol (18917-n)

Carvedilol (BAN, USAN, rINN).

BM-14190; Carvedilolum. 1-Carbazol-4-yloxy-3-[2-(2-methoxyphenoxy)ethylamino]propan-2-ol.

$C_{24}H_{26}N_2O_4 = 406.5.$

CAS — 72956-09-3.

ATC — C07AG02.

Pharmacopoeias. In Eur. (see p.vi).

Pharmacopoeial description

Ph. Eur.: A white or almost white crystalline powder. It exhibits polymorphism. Practically insoluble in water; slightly soluble in alcohol; practically insoluble in dilute acids.

Adverse Effects, Treatment, and Precautions

As for beta blockers, p.844.

Liver function abnormalities, reversible on stopping treatment with carvedilol, have been reported rarely. Carvedilol is extensively metabolised in the liver and is not recommended in patients with hepatic dysfunction. Acute renal failure and renal abnormalities have been reported in patients with heart failure who also suffered from diffuse vascular disease and/or renal impairment. The risk of hypotension may be reduced by taking carvedilol with food to decrease the rate of absorption.

Effects on lipid metabolism. Beta blockers may affect plasma-lipid concentrations (p.845), although these effects may be less pronounced with beta blockers that also block alpha-adrenergic receptors. Carvedilol has been reported to have no adverse effects on plasma-lipid concentrations.[1]

1. Hauf-Zachariou U, et al. A double-blind comparison of the effects of carvedilol and captopril on serum lipid concentrations in patients with mild to moderate essential hypertension and dyslipidaemia. *Eur J Clin Pharmacol* 1993; **45:** 95–100.

Interactions

The interactions associated with beta blockers are discussed on p.846.

Pharmacokinetics

Carvedilol is well absorbed from the gastrointestinal tract but is subject to considerable first-pass metabolism in the liver; the absolute bioavailability is about 25%. Peak plasma concentrations occur 1 to 2 hours after administration. It has high lipid solubility. Carvedilol is more than 98% bound to plasma proteins. It is extensively metabolised in the liver, the metabolites being excreted mainly in the bile. The elimination half-life is about 6 to 10 hours. Carvedilol has been shown to accumulate in breast milk in *animals*.

◊ References.

1. McTavish D, et al. Carvedilol: a review of its pharmacodynamic and pharmacokinetic properties, and therapeutic efficacy. *Drugs* 1993; **45:** 232–58.
2. Morgan T. Clinical pharmacokinetics and pharmacodynamics of carvedilol. *Clin Pharmacokinet* 1994; **26:** 335–46.
3. Tenero D, et al. Steady-state pharmacokinetics of carvedilol and its enantiomers in patients with congestive heart failure. *J Clin Pharmacol* 2000; **40:** 844–53.

Uses and Administration

Carvedilol is a non-cardioselective beta blocker (p.844). It also has vasodilating properties that are attributed mainly to its blocking activity at alpha$_1$ receptors; at higher doses calcium-channel blocking activity may contribute.

Carvedilol is used in the management of hypertension (p.802) and angina pectoris (p.791), and as an adjunct to standard therapy in symptomatic heart failure (p.798).

In **hypertension** carvedilol is given in an initial dose of 12.5 mg once daily by mouth, increased after two days to 25 mg once daily. Alternatively, an initial dose of 6.25 mg is given twice daily, increased after one to two weeks to 12.5 mg twice daily. The dose may be increased further, if necessary, at intervals of at least two weeks, to 50 mg once daily or in divided doses. A dose of 12.5 mg once daily may be adequate for elderly patients.

In **angina pectoris** an initial dose of 12.5 mg is given twice daily by mouth, increased after two days to 25 mg twice daily.

In **heart failure**, the initial dose is 3.125 mg twice daily by mouth. It should be taken with food to reduce the risk of hypotension. If tolerated, the dose should be doubled after two weeks to 6.25 mg twice daily and then increased gradually, at intervals of not less than two weeks, to the maximum dose tolerated by the patient; this should not exceed 25 mg twice daily in patients weighing less than 85 kg or 50 mg twice daily in patients weighing more than 85 kg. Patients should be monitored for 2 to 3 hours after initiation and after each dose increase.

◊ References.

1. Ruffolo RR, et al. The pharmacology of carvedilol. *Eur J Clin Pharmacol* 1990; **38:** S82–8.
2. McTavish D, et al. Carvedilol: a review of its pharmacodynamic and pharmacokinetic properties, and therapeutic efficacy. *Drugs* 1993; **45:** 232–58.
3. Morgan T. Clinical pharmacokinetics and pharmacodynamics of carvedilol. *Clin Pharmacokinet* 1994; **26:** 335–46.
4. Louis WJ, et al. A risk-benefit assessment of carvedilol in the treatment of cardiovascular disorders. *Drug Safety* 1994; **11:** 86–93.
5. Krum H, et al. Double-blind, placebo-controlled study of the long-term efficacy of carvedilol in patients with severe chronic heart failure. *Circulation* 1995; **92:** 1499–1506.
6. Packer M, et al. The effect of carvedilol on morbidity and mortality in patients with chronic heart failure. *N Engl J Med* 1996; **334:** 1349–55.
7. Australia/New Zealand Heart Failure Research Collaborative Group. Randomised, placebo-controlled trial of carvedilol in patients with congestive heart failure due to ischaemic heart disease. *Lancet* 1997; **349:** 375–80.
8. Dunn CJ, et al. Carvedilol: a reappraisal of its pharmacological properties and therapeutic use in cardiovascular disorders. *Drugs* 1997; **54:** 161–85.
9. Frishman WH. Carvedilol. *N Engl J Med* 1998; **339:** 1759–65.

Administration in the elderly. The manufacturer of carvedilol recommends an initial dose of 12.5 mg once daily in hypertension. A study in 16 elderly patients (mean age 70 years) given single doses of 12.5 mg and 25 mg found a high incidence of postural hypotension[1] and the authors suggested that a starting dose lower than 12.5 mg may be necessary in elderly patients.

1. Krum H, et al. Postural hypotension in elderly patients given carvedilol. *BMJ* 1994; **309:** 775–6.

Preparations

Proprietary Preparations (details are given in Part 3)
Aust.: Dilatrend; *Austral.:* Dilatrend; *Belg.:* Dimitone; Kredex; *Canad.:* Coreg; *Denm.:* Dimitone; *Fin.:* Cardiol; *Fr.:* Kredex; *Ger.:* Dilatrend; Querto; *Hong Kong:* Dilatrend; *Irl.:* Eucardic; *Israel:* Dimitone; *Ital.:* Carvipress; Dilatrend; Kredex†; *Mex.:* Dilatrend; *Neth.:* Eucardic; *Norw.:* Dilatrend†; Kredex; *NZ:* Dilatrend; *Port.:* Dilbloc; Kredex†; *S.Afr.:* Dilatrend; *Singapore:* Dilatrend; *Spain:* Coropres; Kredex; *Swed.:* Eucardic†; Kredex; *Switz.:* Dilatrend; *Thai.:* Dilatrend; *UK:* Eucardic; *USA:* Coreg.

Multi-ingredient: *Aust.:* Co-Dilatrend.

Celiprolol Hydrochloride (16573-d)

Celiprolol Hydrochloride *(BANM, USAN, rINNM).*
3-{3-Acetyl-4-[3-(tert-butylamino)-2-hydroxypropoxy]phenyl}-1,1-diethylurea hydrochloride.
$C_{20}H_{33}N_3O_4,HCl = 416.0$.
CAS — 56980-93-9 (celiprolol); 57470-78-7 (celiprolol hydrochloride).

Adverse Effects, Treatment, and Precautions

As for beta blockers, p.844.

Tremor and palpitations associated with intrinsic sympathomimetic activity at beta$_2$ receptors have been reported.

Interactions

The interactions associated with beta blockers are discussed on p.846.

Pharmacokinetics

Celiprolol is absorbed from the gastrointestinal tract in a non-linear fashion; the percentage of the dose absorbed increases with increasing dose. The plasma elimination half-life is about 5 to 6 hours. Celiprolol crosses the placenta. It has low lipid solubility. Metabolism is minimal and celiprolol is mainly excreted unchanged in the urine and faeces.

Uses and Administration

Celiprolol is a cardioselective beta blocker (p.844). It is reported to possess intrinsic sympathomimetic activity and direct vasodilator activity. Celiprolol is used as the hydrochloride in the management of hypertension (p.802) and angina pectoris (p.791). The usual dose of celiprolol hydrochloride is 200 to 400 mg once daily by mouth. Reduced doses may be required in patients with impaired renal function; guidelines are to reduce the dose by 50% when creatinine clearance is between 15 and 40 mL per minute, but not to use at all when it is below 15 mL per minute.

◊ References.
1. Milne RJ, Buckley MM-T. Celiprolol: an updated review of its pharmacodynamic and pharmacokinetic properties, and therapeutic efficacy in cardiovascular disease. *Drugs* 1991; **41:** 941–69.
2. Anonymous. Celiprolol: theory and practice. *Lancet* 1991; **338:** 1426–7.
3. Anonymous. Celiprolol—a better beta blocker? *Drug Ther Bull* 1992; **30:** 35–6.
4. Kendall MJ, Rajman I. A risk-benefit assessment of celiprolol in the treatment of cardiovascular disease. *Drug Safety* 1994; **10:** 220–32.
5. Riddell J. Drugs in focus 18: celiprolol. *Prescribers' J* 1996; **36:** 165–8.

Preparations

Proprietary Preparations (details are given in Part 3)
Aust.: Selectol; *Belg.:* Selectol; *Fin.:* Selectol; *Fr.:* Celectol; *Ger.:* Celipro; Selectol; *Hong Kong:* Selectol; *Irl.:* Selectol; *Ital.:* Cordiax; *Jpn:* Selectol; *Neth.:* Dilanorm; *NZ:* Celol; Selectol; *Spain:* Cardem; Moderator†; *Switz.:* Selectol; *UK:* Celectol.

Multi-ingredient: *Aust.:* Selecturon.

Cerivastatin Sodium (656-p)

Cerivastatin Sodium *(BANM, USAN, rINNM).*
Bay-W-6228. Sodium {S-[R*,S*-(E)]}-7-[4-(4-fluorophenyl)-5-(methoxymethyl)-2,6-bis(1-methylethyl)-3-pyridinyl]-3,5-dihydroxy-6-heptenoate.
$C_{26}H_{33}FNNaO_5 = 481.5$.
CAS — 143201-11-0.

Profile

Cerivastatin, a 3-hydroxy-3-methylglutaryl coenzyme A (HMG-CoA) reductase inhibitor (a statin), is a lipid regulating drug with actions on plasma lipids similar to those of simvastatin (p.970). It has been used in the treatment of hyperlipidaemi-

as but was withdrawn from the market worldwide in 2001 following reports of severe muscle toxicity, particularly when given with gemfibrozil.

◊ General reviews published before the withdrawal of cerivastatin from the market.
1. McClellan KJ, *et al.* Cerivastatin. *Drugs* 1998; **55:** 415–20.
2. Plosker GL, *et al.* Cerivastatin: a review of its pharmacological properties and therapeutic efficacy in the management of hypercholesterolaemia. *Drugs* 2000; **60:** 1179–1206.

Effects on skeletal muscle. Muscle disorders are well-recognised adverse effects of lipid regulating drugs such as fibrates and statins (see Simvastatin, p.970).
There have been a number of reports[1-6] of severe muscle toxicity in patients taking cerivastatin, and it was withdrawn from the market for this reason in 2001.
1. Rodríguez ML, *et al.* Cerivastatin-induced rhabdomyolysis. *Ann Intern Med* 2000; **132:** 598.
2. Bermingham RP, *et al.* Rhabdomyolysis in a patient receiving the combination of cerivastatin and gemfibrozil. *Am J Health-Syst Pharm* 2000; **57:** 461–4.
3. Alexandridis G, *et al.* Rhabdomyolysis due to combination therapy with cerivastatin and gemfibrozil. *Am J Med* 2000; **109:** 261–2.
4. Garcia-Valdecasas-Campelo E, *et al.* Acute rhabdomyolysis associated with cerivastatin therapy. *Arch Intern Med* 2001; **161:** 893.
5. Gemici G, *et al.* Rhabdomyolysis due to cerivastatin monotherapy. *Am J Med* 2001; **110:** 742.
6. Adverse Drug Reactions Advisory Committee (ADRAC). Cerivastatin and rhabdomyolysis—avoid gemfibrozil. *Aust Adverse Drug React Bull* 2001; **20:** 3.

Preparations

Proprietary Preparations (details are given in Part 3)
Aust.: Lipobay†; *Austral.:* Kazak; Lipobay†; *Belg.:* Cholstat; Lipobay†; *Canad.:* Baycol†; *Denm.:* Lipobay†; *Fin.:* Lipobay†; *Fr.:* Cholstat†; Staltor†; *Ger.:* Lipobay†; Zenas; *Irl.:* Lipobay; *Israel:* Lipogis; *Ital.:* Cervasta; Lipobay†; Stativa; *Neth.:* Lipobay†; *Norw.:* Lipobay†; *Port.:* Colstat; Lipobay†; *S.Afr.:* Baycol†; *Singapore:* Lipobay†; *Spain:* Lipobay†; Liposterol; Vaslip; Zenas; *Swed.:* Lipobay†; *Switz.:* Lipobay†; *Thai.:* Lipobay†; *UK:* Lipobay†; *USA:* Baycol†.

Certoparin Sodium (17408-a)

Certoparin Sodium *(BAN, rINN).*
Certoparin.

Certoparin sodium is prepared by amyl nitrite degradation of heparin obtained from the intestinal mucosa of pigs. The majority of the components have a 2-O-sulfo-α-L-idopyranosuronic acid structure at the non-reducing end and a 6-O-sulfo-2,5-anhydro-D-mannose structure at the reducing end of their chain. The molecular weight of 70% of the components is less than 10 000 and the average molecular weight is about 6000. The degree of sulfation is about 2 to 2.5 per disaccharide unit.

Units

As for Low-molecular-weight Heparins, p.923.

Adverse Effects, Treatment, and Precautions

As for Low-molecular-weight Heparins, p.923.

Interactions

As for Low-molecular-weight Heparins, p.924.

Pharmacokinetics

Certoparin sodium is rapidly and completely absorbed following subcutaneous injection. Peak plasma activity is reached within 2 to 4 hours. The half-life of anti-factor Xa activity is about 4 hours.

Uses and Administration

Certoparin sodium is a low-molecular-weight heparin (p.923) with anticoagulant activity used for the prevention of postoperative venous thromboembolism (p.817). It is given by subcutaneous injection in a dose of 3000 units 1 to 2 hours before the procedure, followed by 3000 units daily for 7 to 10 days or until the patient is fully ambulant.

◊ References.
1. Kock H-J, *et al.* Thromboprophylaxis with low-molecular-weight heparin in outpatients with plaster-cast immobilisation of the leg. *Lancet* 1995; **346:** 459–61.
2. Adolf J, *et al.* Comparison of 3,000 IU aXa of the low molecular weight heparin certoparin with 5,000 IU aXa in prevention of deep vein thrombosis after total hip replacement. *Int Angiol* 1999; **18:** 122–6.
3. Harenberg J, *et al.* Fixed-dose, body weight-independent subcutaneous LMW heparin versus adjusted dose unfractionated intravenous heparin in the initial treatment of proximal venous thrombosis. *Thromb Haemost* 2000; **83:** 652–6.

Preparations

Proprietary Preparations (details are given in Part 3)
Aust.: Sandoparin; Troparin†; *Ger.:* Mono-Embolex; *Switz.:* Sandoparine; *UK:* Alphaparin.

Multi-ingredient: *Aust.:* Embolex; Troparin compositum†; *Ger.:* Embolex NM.

Cetiedil Citrate (9217-e)

Cetiedil Citrate *(USAN, rINNM).*
2-(Perhydroazepin-1-yl)ethyl α-cyclohexyl-α-(3-thienyl)acetate dihydrogen citrate monohydrate.
$C_{20}H_{31}NO_2S,C_6H_8O_7,H_2O = 559.7$.
CAS — 14176-10-4 (cetiedil); 16286-69-4 (anhydrous cetiedil citrate).

Profile

Cetiedil citrate is a vasodilator with antimuscarinic activity used in the management of peripheral vascular disease (p.809) in doses of 400 to 600 mg daily by mouth.

Preparations

Proprietary Preparations (details are given in Part 3)
Fr.: Stratene; Vasocet†.

Chlorothiazide (2316-b)

Chlorothiazide *(BAN, rINN).*
Chlorothiazidum; Clorotiazida. 6-Chloro-2H-1,2,4-benzothiadiazine-7-sulphonamide 1,1-dioxide.
$C_7H_6ClN_3O_4S_2 = 295.7$.
CAS — 58-94-6.
ATC — C03AA04.
Pharmacopoeias. In *Eur.* (see p.vi) and *US.*

Alkaline solutions undergo decomposition due to hydrolysis upon standing or heating.

Pharmacopoeial description
Ph. Eur.: A white or almost white crystalline powder. Very slightly soluble in water; slightly soluble in alcohol; sparingly soluble in acetone. It dissolves in dilute solutions of alkali hydroxides.
USP 25: A white or practically white, odourless, crystalline powder. Very slightly soluble in water; practically insoluble in chloroform, in ether, and in benzene; freely soluble in dimethylformamide and dimethyl sulfoxide; slightly soluble in methyl alcohol and in pyridine.

Chlorothiazide Sodium (2317-v)

Chlorothiazide Sodium *(BANM, USAN, rINNM).*
Sodium Chlorothiazide.
$C_7H_5ClN_3NaO_4S_2 = 317.7$.
CAS — 7085-44-1.
Pharmacopoeias. US includes Chlorothiazide Sodium for Injection.

Chlorothiazide sodium 537 mg is approximately equivalent to 500 mg of chlorothiazide. The alkaline nature of chlorothiazide in injectable form suggests that incompatibilities with acidic drugs could be expected; the US manufacturer states that the injection may be diluted with glucose or sodium chloride solutions.

Adverse Effects, Treatment, and Precautions

As for Hydrochlorothiazide, p.907. Chlorothiazide sodium injection is alkaline: when administering chlorothiazide by intravenous infusion, care should be taken to ensure that extravasation does not occur.

Interactions

As for Hydrochlorothiazide, p.909.

Pharmacokinetics

Chlorothiazide is incompletely and variably absorbed from the gastrointestinal tract. It has been estimated to have a plasma half-life of 45 to 120 minutes although the clinical effects last for up to about 12 hours. It is excreted unchanged in the urine. Chlorothiazide crosses the placental barrier and small amounts are reported to be distributed into breast milk.

Uses and Administration

Chlorothiazide is a thiazide diuretic with actions and uses similar to those of hydrochlorothiazide (p.910). It is used for oedema, including that associated with heart failure (p.798), and for hypertension (p.802).

Following oral administration of chlorothiazide diuresis usually occurs in about 2 hours, reaches a maximum at about 4 hours, and is maintained for 6 to 12 hours.

In the treatment of **oedema** the usual dose of chlorothiazide is 0.25 to 1 g by mouth once or twice daily; therapy on alternate days or on 3 to 5 days weekly may be adequate. The dose should not normally exceed 2 g daily.

In the treatment of **hypertension** the usual initial dose is 250 to 500 mg daily by mouth, given as a single or divided dose. A dose of 125 mg may be adequate in some patients. Patients may rarely require up to 1 g daily.

A dose of chlorothiazide in children is up to 25 mg per kg body-weight by mouth daily in two divided doses. Infants up to the age of 6 months may require up to 35 mg per kg daily in two divided doses.

Chlorothiazide has also been given intravenously as the sodium salt, in doses similar to those given by mouth. It is not suitable for subcutaneous or intramuscular injection and extravasation should be avoided. The diuretic effect lasts for up to 2 hours following intravenous injection.

Preparations

USP 25: Chlorothiazide Oral Suspension; Chlorothiazide Sodium for Injection; Chlorothiazide Tablets; Methyldopa and Chlorothiazide Tablets; Reserpine and Chlorothiazide Tablets.

Proprietary Preparations (details are given in Part 3)
Austral.: Chlotride; **Denm.:** Chlotride; **Irl.:** Saluric†; **Mex.:** Pahtlisan; **Neth.:** Chlotride†; **Singapore:** Chlorzide; **UK:** Saluric†; **USA:** Diachlor†; Diurigen; Diuril.
Multi-ingredient: Canad.: Supres; **Ital.:** Ipogen†; **USA:** Aldoclor; Diupres.

Chlortalidone (2318-g)

Chlortalidone (BAN, rINN).

Chlortalidonum; Chlorthalidone (USAN); Clorotalidona; G-33182; NSC-69200. 2-Chloro-5-(1-hydroxy-3-oxoisoindolin-1-yl)benzenesulphonamide.

$C_{14}H_{11}ClN_2O_4S = 338.8$.
CAS — 77-36-1.
ATC — C03BA04.

NOTE. Compounded preparations of chlortalidone may be represented by the following names:

• Co-tenidone (BAN)—chlortalidone 1 part and atenolol 4 parts (w/w).

Pharmacopoeias. In *Eur.* (see p.vi), *Int.,* and *US.*

Pharmacopoeial description

Ph. Eur.: A white or yellowish-white powder. Practically insoluble in water and in dichloromethane; slightly soluble in alcohol; soluble in acetone and in methyl alcohol. It dissolves in dilute solutions of alkali hydroxides.

USP 25: A white or yellowish-white crystalline powder. Practically insoluble in water, in chloroform, and in ether; slightly soluble in alcohol; soluble in methyl alcohol.

Adverse Effects, Treatment, and Precautions

As for Hydrochlorothiazide, p.907.

Interactions

As for Hydrochlorothiazide, p.909.

Anticoagulants. For references to the interaction between *warfarin* and chlortalidone, see p.996.

Pharmacokinetics

Chlortalidone is erratically absorbed from the gastrointestinal tract. It has a prolonged elimination half-life from plasma and blood of 40 to 60 hours and is highly bound to red blood cells; the receptor to which it is bound has been identified as carbonic anhydrase. Chlortalidone is much less strongly bound to plasma proteins. Chlortalidone is mainly excreted unchanged in the urine. It crosses the placental barrier and is distributed into breast milk.

◊ References.
1. Riess W, *et al.* Pharmacokinetic studies with chlorthalidone (Hygroton®) in man. *Eur J Clin Pharmacol* 1977; **12:** 375–82.
2. Mulley BA, *et al.* Placental transfer of chlorthalidone and its elimination in maternal milk. *Eur J Clin Pharmacol* 1978; **13:** 129–31.
3. Fleuren HLJ, *et al.* Absolute bioavailability of chlorthalidone in man: a cross-over study after intravenous and oral administration. *Eur J Clin Pharmacol* 1979; **15:** 35–50.

4. Fleuren HLJ, *et al.* Dose-dependent urinary excretion of chlorthalidone. *Clin Pharmacol Ther* 1979; **25:** 806–12.
5. Mulley BA, *et al.* Pharmacokinetics of chlorthalidone: dependence of biological half life on blood carbonic anhydrase levels. *Eur J Clin Pharmacol* 1980; **17:** 203–7.

Uses and Administration

Chlortalidone is a diuretic with actions and uses similar to those of the thiazide diuretics (see Hydrochlorothiazide, p.910) even though it does not contain a thiazide ring system. It is used for oedema, including that associated with heart failure (p.798), and for hypertension (p.802). Other indications include diabetes insipidus (p.1273).

Diuresis is initiated in about 2 hours and lasts for 48 to 72 hours.

In the treatment of **oedema** the usual initial dose is 25 to 50 mg daily by mouth. In severe cases a daily dose of 100 to 200 mg may be given. If possible lower doses should be used for maintenance; 25 to 50 mg daily or on alternate days may be adequate.

The usual dose in the treatment of **hypertension** is 25 mg daily, given either alone or with other antihypertensives, increasing to 50 mg daily if necessary.

A dose for children is up to 2 mg per kg body-weight daily on alternate days.

In **diabetes insipidus** an initial dose of 100 mg twice daily has been employed reduced to a maintenance dose of 50 mg daily.

In the US, a preparation is available with improved bioavailability; suggested doses range from 30 to 120 mg daily for oedema and 15 to 50 mg daily for hypertension.

Preparations

BP 2001: Chlortalidone Tablets; Co-tenidone Tablets;
USP 25: Chlorthalidone Tablets; Clonidine Hydrochloride and Chlorthalidone Tablets.

Proprietary Preparations (details are given in Part 3)
Aust.: Hygroton; **Austral.:** Hygroton; **Belg.:** Hygroton; **Braz.:** Clortalil; Higroton; **Canad.:** Hygroton†; Novo-Thalidone†; **Denm.:** Hygroton; **Fr.:** Hygroton†; **Ger.:** Hydro-long; Hygroton; **Hong Kong:** Hygroton; **Israel:** Aquadon; Hygroton; **Ital.:** Igroton; Zambesil†; **Mex.:** Anilid; Diuprol; Hidrona; Higroton; **Neth.:** Hygroton; **Norw.:** Hygroton†; **NZ:** Hygroton; **Port.:** Hygroton; **S.Afr.:** Hygroton; **Spain:** Higrotona; Hygroton†; **Swed.:** Hygroton†; **Switz.:** Hygroton; **UK:** Hygroton; **USA:** Hygroton; Hylidone†; Thalitone.
Multi-ingredient: Aust.: Arcablock comp; Atenolan comp; Atenolol comp; Combipresan†; Darebon; Logroton†; Polinorm; Selecturon; Tenoretic; Trasitensin; Trepress; **Belg.:** Logroton; Tenoretic; **Braz.:** Diupress; Higroton Reserpina; Tenoretic; **Canad.:** Combipres†; Tenoretic; **Denm.:** Tenidon; Tenoretic; **Fr.:** Logroton; Tenoretic; **Ger.:** Ate Lich comp; Atehexal comp; Atel; Ateno comp; Atenogamma comp; Atenolol AL comp; Atenolol comp; Atenomerck comp†; Blocotenol comp; Combipresan; Darebon; Diu-Atenolol; duratenol comp; Evitocor plus†; Impresso; Prelis comp; Sigabloc; Teneretic; Trasitensin; Trepress; TRINormin; **Hong Kong:** Target; Tenoret; Tenoretic; **Irl.:** Atenetic; Cotenomel; Tenchlor†; Tenoret; Tenoretic; **Ital.:** Ataclor; Atenigron; Biotens†; Carmian; Clortanol; Diube; Eupres; Igroseles; Igroton-Lopresor; Igroton-Reserpina; Pressalolo Diuretico†; Target; Tenolone; Tenoretic; Trandiur; Trasitensin; **Mex.:** Higroton-Res; Tenoretic; **Neth.:** Logroton†; Tenoretic; **NZ:** Tenoret; Tenoretic; **Port.:** Blokium Diu; Tenoretic; **S.Afr.:** Adco-Loten; Atenoblok Co; Ateren; Hygroton-Reserpine; Tenchlor; Tenoret†; Tenoretic; Venachlor†; **Singapore:** Tenoret; Tenoretic; **Spain:** Aldoleo; Betasit Plus†; Blokium Diu; Higrotona Reserpina; Normopresil; Resnedal; Tenoretic; Trasitensin; **Switz.:** Atedurex; ateno-basan comp.; Cardaxen plus; Cotenolol; Hygroton-Reserpine; Logroton; Sandoretic; Slow-Trasitensine; Tenoretic; Trasitensine; Trepress†; **Thai.:** Tenoretic; **UK:** AtenixCo; Kalspare; Tenchlor; Tenoret; Tenoretic; Totaretic; **USA:** Clorpres; Combipres; Demi-Regroton; Kerledex†; Regroton; Tenoretic.

Cibenzoline (15315-x)

Cibenzoline (BAN, rINN).

Cifenline (USAN); Ro-22-7796; Ro-22-7796/001 (cibenzoline succinate); UP-339-01. (±)-2-(2,2-Diphenylcyclopropyl)-2-imidazoline.

$C_{18}H_{18}N_2 = 262.3$.
CAS — 53267-01-9 (cibenzoline); 100678-32-8 (cibenzoline succinate).
ATC — C01BG07.

Adverse Effects and Precautions

Cibenzoline may cause neurological and gastrointestinal side-effects including vertigo, tremor, nausea, vomiting, and diarrhoea. Other adverse effects include fatigue, visual disturbances, and hypoglycaemia. Like other antiarrhythmics it can cause arrhythmias and may reduce blood pressure.

Cibenzoline is contra-indicated in patients with heart block and severe heart failure. It should be used with caution in renal impairment when doses should be reduced.

Effects on the neuromuscular system. A myastheniform syndrome with acute respiratory failure occurred after a cibenzoline overdose in a patient with renal impairment.[1]
1. Similowski T, *et al.* Neuromuscular blockade with acute respiratory failure in a patient receiving cibenzoline. *Thorax* 1997; **52:** 582–4.

Hypoglycaemia. Cibenzoline therapy was associated with severe hypoglycaemia in a 67-year-old patient.[1] The plasma-cibenzoline concentration on admission to hospital was 1800 nanograms per mL which would probably be considered toxic since the accepted therapeutic trough range is 200 to 600 nanograms per mL.
1. Hilleman DE, *et al.* Cibenzoline-induced hypoglycemia. *Drug Intell Clin Pharm* 1987; **21:** 38–40.

Interactions

Histamine H_2-antagonists. Increased blood concentrations and prolonged half-lives of cibenzoline occurred in healthy subjects given *cimetidine* but the clinical importance of this was unknown.[1] The interaction did not occur with *ranitidine*. The probable reason was that cimetidine, but not ranitidine, inhibited the metabolism of cibenzoline.
1. Massarella JW. The effects of cimetidine and ranitidine on the pharmacokinetics of cibenzoline. *Br J Clin Pharmacol* 1991; **31:** 481–3.

Pharmacokinetics

Cibenzoline is well absorbed from the gastrointestinal tract following oral administration, with a bioavailability of about 90%. It is about 50 to 60% bound to plasma proteins. About 60% of a dose is excreted unchanged in the urine and the elimination half-life is reported to be about 7 hours.

◊ References.
1. Brazzell RK, *et al.* Pharmacokinetics and pharmacodynamics of intravenous cibenzoline in normal volunteers. *J Clin Pharmacol* 1985; **25:** 418–23.
2. Massarella JW, *et al.* Pharmacokinetics of cibenzoline after single and repetitive dosing in healthy volunteers. *J Clin Pharmacol* 1986; **26:** 125–30.

Uses and Administration

Cibenzoline is a class Ia antiarrhythmic that also has some class III and class IV properties (p.787). It is used in the management of ventricular and supraventricular arrhythmias (p.794).

Cibenzoline succinate is given by mouth in a dose equivalent to cibenzoline base 260 to 390 mg daily. A dosage of 130 mg daily in two divided doses is recommended in elderly patients. Cibenzoline may also be given parenterally; the usual initial dose is the equivalent of 1 mg per kg body-weight cibenzoline base over 2 minutes followed by 8 mg per kg over 24 hours by infusion, or by initiation of oral therapy. Dosage should be reduced in renal impairment.

Administration in the elderly. The renal and non-renal clearance of cibenzoline was found to decrease with increasing age in healthy subjects.[1] The mean elimination half-life was 7 hours in the 20- to 30-year age group and 10.5 hours in the 70- to 80-year age group. The reduction in renal clearance was considered to be related to the decrease in creatinine clearance with increasing age. The results suggested that older patients may need lower doses than younger patients to maintain therapeutic plasma-cibenzoline concentrations.
1. Brazzell RK, *et al.* Age and cibenzoline disposition. *Clin Pharmacol Ther* 1984; **36:** 613–19.

Administration in renal impairment. A study in patients with normal or impaired renal function has suggested that in renal impairment initial loading doses of cibenzoline may be equivalent to those used in normal renal function although maintenance doses should be reduced to about two-thirds of normal.[1]
1. Aronoff G, *et al.* Bioavailability and kinetics of cibenzoline in patients with normal and impaired renal function. *J Clin Pharmacol* 1991; **31:** 38–44.

Preparations

Proprietary Preparations (details are given in Part 3)
Belg.: Cipralan; **Fr.:** Cipralan; Exacor.

Cicletanine Hydrochloride (13232-n)

Cicletanine Hydrochloride (BANM, rINNM).

(±)-BN-1270 (cicletanine); (±)-Cycletanide Hydrochloride; Win-90000 (cicletanine). (±)-3-(p-Chlorophenyl)-1,3-dihydro-6-methylfuro[3,4-c]pyridin-7-ol hydrochloride.

$C_{14}H_{12}ClNO_2,HCl = 298.2$.
CAS — 89943-82-8 (cicletanine); 82747-56-6 (cicletanine hydrochloride).

NOTE. Cicletanine is USAN.

Profile

Cicletanine hydrochloride is a diuretic with properties similar to those of the thiazide diuretics (see Hydrochlorothiazide, p.907). It is used in the treatment of hypertension (p.802) in a usual dose of 50 to 100 mg daily by mouth.

Preparations

Proprietary Preparations (details are given in Part 3)
Fr.: Tenstaten; **Ger.:** Justar.

The symbol † denotes a preparation no longer actively marketed

Cilazapril (18620-q)

Cilazapril *(BAN, USAN, rINN)*.

Cilazaprilum; Ro-31-2848 (anhydrous cilazapril); Ro-31-2848/006 (cilazapril monohydrate). (1S,9S)-9-[(S)-1-Ethoxycarbonyl-3-phenylpropylamino]-10-oxoperhydropyridazino[1,2-a][1,2]diazepine-1-carboxylic acid monohydrate.

$C_{22}H_{31}N_3O_5,H_2O = 435.5$.

CAS — 88768-40-5 (anhydrous cilazapril); 92077-78-6 (cilazapril monohydrate).

ATC — C09AA08.

Pharmacopoeias. In Eur. (see p.vi).

Cilazapril 1.04 mg as the monohydrate is approximately equivalent to 1 mg of anhydrous cilazapril.

Pharmacopoeial description

Ph. Eur.: A white or almost white crystalline powder. Slightly soluble in water; freely soluble in dichloromethane and in methyl alcohol. Protect from light.

Adverse Effects, Treatment, and Precautions

As for ACE inhibitors, p.820.

Interactions

As for ACE inhibitors, p.822.

Pharmacokinetics

Cilazapril acts as a prodrug of the diacid cilazaprilat, its active metabolite. Following oral administration and absorption of cilazapril it is rapidly metabolised in the liver to cilazaprilat, the bioavailability of which is about 60%. Peak plasma concentrations of cilazaprilat occur within 2 hours of an oral dose of cilazapril. Cilazaprilat is eliminated unchanged in the urine. The effective half-life of cilazaprilat is reported to be 9 hours following once-daily dosing. The elimination of cilazaprilat is reduced in renal impairment. Both cilazapril and cilazaprilat are removed to a limited extent by haemodialysis.

◊ Reviews.
1. Kelly JG, O'Malley K. Clinical pharmacokinetics of the newer ACE inhibitors: a review. *Clin Pharmacokinet* 1990; **19:** 177–96.
2. Kloke HJ, *et al.* Pharmacokinetics and haemodynamic effects of the angiotensin converting enzyme inhibitor cilazapril in hypertensive patients with normal and impaired renal function. *Br J Clin Pharmacol* 1996; **42:** 615–20.

Uses and Administration

Cilazapril is an ACE inhibitor (p.820). It is used in the treatment of hypertension (p.802) and heart failure (p.798).

Cilazapril owes its activity to cilazaprilat to which it is converted after oral administration. The haemodynamic effects are seen within 1 hour of a single oral dose and the maximum effect occurs after about 3 to 7 hours. The haemodynamic action persists for about 24 hours, allowing once-daily dosing. Cilazapril is given by mouth as the monohydrate, but doses are expressed in terms of the anhydrous substance.

In the treatment of **hypertension** the initial dose is 1 mg once daily. Since there may be a precipitous fall in blood pressure in some patients when starting therapy with an ACE inhibitor, the first dose should preferably be given at bedtime. In the elderly or those taking diuretics, a usual initial dose is 0.5 mg daily. If possible the diuretic should be withdrawn 2 to 3 days before cilazapril is started and resumed later if necessary. In patients with mild to moderate renal impairment a usual initial dose is 0.5 mg daily; cilazapril should be avoided in severe renal impairment. Maintenance doses range from 2.5 to 5 mg daily.

In the treatment of **heart failure** severe first-dose hypotension on introduction of an ACE inhibitor is common in patients on loop diuretics, but their temporary withdrawal may cause rebound pulmonary oedema. Thus therapy should be initiated with a low dose under close medical supervision. Cilazapril is given in an initial dose of 0.5 mg once daily, increased if tolerated to a usual maintenance dose of 1 to 2.5 mg once daily. The usual maximum dose is 5 mg daily.

◊ References.
1. Deget F, Brogden RN. Cilazapril: a review of its pharmacodynamic and pharmacokinetic properties, and therapeutic potential in cardiovascular disease. *Drugs* 1991; **41:** 799–820.

Preparations

Proprietary Preparations (details are given in Part 3)
Aust.: Inhibace; *Austral.:* Inhibace†; *Belg.:* Inhibace; *Braz.:* Vascase; *Canad.:* Inhibace; *Fr.:* Justor; *Ger.:* Dynorm; *Hong Kong:* Inhibace; *Irl.:* Vascace; *Israel:* Vascace; *Ital.:* Inibace; Initiss; *Mex.:* Inhibace; *Neth.:* Vascase; *NZ:* Inhibace; *Port.:* Inhibace; Vascase; *S.Afr.:* Inhibace; *Singapore:* Inhibace; *Spain:* Inhibace; Inocar; *Swed.:* Inhibace; *Switz.:* Inhibace; *Thai.:* Inhibace; *UK:* Vascace.
Multi-ingredient: *Aust.:* Inhibace Plus; *Belg.:* Co-Inhibace; *Canad.:* Inhibace Plus; *Ger.:* Dynorm Plus; *Israel:* Vascace Plus; *Ital.:* Inibace Plus; Initiss Plus; *Neth.:* Vascase Plus; *NZ:* Inhibace Plus; *Port.:* Inibace Plus; Vascase Plus; *S.Afr.:* Inhibace Plus; *Spain:* Inhibace Plus; Inocar Plus; *Swed.:* Inhibace comp; *Switz.:* Inhibace Plus.

Cilnidipine (15885-p)

Cilnidipine *(rINN)*.

FRC-8653. (±)-(E)-Cinnamyl 2-methoxyethyl 1,4-dihydro-2,6-dimethyl-4-(m-nitrophenyl)-3,5-pyridinedicarboxylate.

$C_{27}H_{28}N_2O_7 = 492.5$.

CAS — 132203-70-4.

Profile

Cilnidipine is a dihydropyridine calcium-channel blocker (p.788) given by mouth in the management of hypertension (p.802). The usual dose is 5 to 10 mg once daily, increased to 20 mg once daily if necessary.

Preparations

Proprietary Preparations (details are given in Part 3)
Jpn: Cinalong.

Cilostazol (1981-g)

Cilostazol *(USAN, pINN)*.

OPC-21; OPC-13013. 6-[4-(1-Cyclohexyl-1H-tetrazol-5-yl)butoxy]-3,4-dihydrocarbostyril.

$C_{20}H_{27}N_5O_2 = 369.5$.

CAS — 73963-72-1.

Adverse Effects and Precautions

Adverse effects of cilostazol include headache, dizziness, palpitations, and diarrhoea. Cardiovascular toxicity has been reported in *animal* studies of cilostazol, and prolonged oral use of other phosphodiesterase inhibitors (such as amrinone, p.839) for treatment of heart failure has been associated with increased mortality. The use of cilostazol in patients with any degree of heart failure is therefore contra-indicated.

Interactions

Cilostazol is extensively metabolised to active and inactive metabolites by cytochrome P450 isoenzymes, mainly CYP3A4 and to a lesser extent CYP2C19. Therefore concomitant administration of other drugs that inhibit or are metabolised by these hepatic enzymes may result in changes in plasma concentrations of either drug and possibly, adverse effects. Grapefruit juice may also inhibit the metabolism of cilostazol and concomitant administration should be avoided.

Pharmacokinetics

Cilostazol is absorbed following oral administration and absorption is increased if taken with a high fat meal. Cilostazol is extensively metabolised in the liver to both active and inactive metabolites which are predominantly excreted in the urine (74%) with the remainder in the faeces (20%). The active metabolites have apparent elimination half-lives of 11 to 13 hours. Cilostazol is 95 to 98% protein bound.

Uses and Administration

Cilostazol is a phosphodiesterase inhibitor with antiplatelet and vasodilating activity. It is used in the management of peripheral vascular disease (p.809).

The dose of cilostazol for the reduction of symptoms of intermittent claudication is 100 mg orally twice daily, at least 30 minutes before or 2 hours after food. Response to treatment may occur in 2 to 4 weeks, but up to 12 weeks may be required. Cilostazol is under investigation for its antiplatelet effect following coronary stent implantation.

◊ References.
1. Ochiai M, *et al.* Uses of cilostazol, a novel antiplatelet agent, in post-Palmaz-Schatz stenting regimen. *Am J Cardiol* 1997; **79:** 1471–4.
2. Money SR, *et al.* Effect of cilostazol on walking distances in patients with intermittent claudication caused by peripheral vascular disease. *J Vasc Surg* 1998; **27:** 267–75.
3. Yoshitomi Y, *et al.* Antiplatelet treatment with cilostazol after stent implantation. *Heart* 1998; **80:** 393–6.
4. Beebe HG, *et al.* A new pharmacological treatment for intermittent claudication: results of a randomized, multicenter trial. *Arch Intern Med* 1999; **159:** 2041–50.
5. Dawson DL, *et al.* A comparison of cilostazol and pentoxifylline for treating intermittent claudication. *Am J Med* 2000; **109:** 523–30.
6. Reilly MP, Mohler ER. Cilostazol: treatment of intermittent claudication. *Ann Pharmacother* 2001; **35:** 48–56.

Preparations

Proprietary Preparations (details are given in Part 3)
Jpn: Pletaal†; *Thai.:* Pletaal; *USA:* Pletal.

Cinepazet Maleate (9219-y)

Cinepazet Maleate *(BANM, USAN, pINNM)*.

Cinepazic Acid Ethyl Ester Maleate. Ethyl 4-(3,4,5-trimethoxycinnamoyl)piperazin-1-ylacetate hydrogen maleate.

$C_{20}H_{28}N_2O_6,C_4H_4O_4 = 508.5$.

CAS — 23887-41-4 (cinepazet); 50679-07-7 (cinepazet maleate).

Profile

Cinepazet maleate is a vasodilator that has been used in angina pectoris.

Cinepazide Maleate (9220-g)

Cinepazide Maleate *(BANM, rINNM)*.

MD-67350. 1-(Pyrrolidin-1-ylcarbonylmethyl)-4-(3,4,5-trimethoxycinnamoyl)piperazine hydrogen maleate.

$C_{22}H_{31}N_3O_5,C_4H_4O_4 = 533.6$.

CAS — 23887-46-9 (cinepazide); 26328-04-1 (cinepazide maleate).

Profile

Cinepazide maleate is a vasodilator which has been used in peripheral vascular disorders, but has been withdrawn from the market in some countries following reports of agranulocytosis.

Ciprofibrate (15316-r)

Ciprofibrate *(BAN, USAN, rINN)*.

Win-35833. 2-[4-(2,2-Dichlorocyclopropyl)phenoxy]-2-methylpropionic acid.

$C_{13}H_{14}Cl_2O_3 = 289.2$.

CAS — 52214-84-3.

ATC — C10AB08.

Adverse Effects and Precautions

As for Bezafibrate, p.849.

Interactions

As for Bezafibrate, p.849.

NSAIDs. Acute renal failure due to rhabdomyolysis in a patient has been attributed to an interaction between ciprofibrate and *ibuprofen*.[1] Ibuprofen was believed to have displaced ciprofibrate from protein binding sites. The use of radiological contrast media may also have been a contributory factor.
1. Ramachandran S, *et al.* Acute renal failure due to rhabdomyolysis in presence of concurrent ciprofibrate and ibuprofen treatment. *BMJ* 1997; **314:** 1593.

Pharmacokinetics

Ciprofibrate is readily absorbed from the gastrointestinal tract; peak plasma concentrations occur within 1 to 4 hours. Ciprofibrate is highly protein bound. It is excreted in the urine as unchanged drug and as glucuronide conjugates. The elimination half-life varies from about 38 to 86 hours in patients on long-term therapy.

Uses and Administration

Ciprofibrate, a fibric acid derivative, is a lipid regulating drug with actions on plasma lipids similar to those of bezafibrate (p.849).

It is used in the treatment of type IIa, type IIb, type III, and type IV hyperlipoproteinaemias (p.800). The usual dose is 100 mg daily by mouth.

Administration in renal impairment. Ciprofibrate is contra-indicated in patients with severe renal dysfunction. The manufacturer has suggested reducing the dose to 100 mg every other day for patients with moderate renal impairment.

Renal clearance of ciprofibrate was reduced and elimination half-life approximately doubled in patients with severe renal impairment.[1] Mild renal insufficiency slowed the urinary excretion of ciprofibrate but not its extent. The clearance of ciprofibrate was unaffected by haemodialysis.
1. Ferry N, *et al.* The influence of renal insufficiency and haemodialysis on the kinetics of ciprofibrate. *Br J Clin Pharmacol* 1989; **28:** 675–81.

Hyperlipidaemias. Similarly to other fibric acid derivatives (see under Bezafibrate, p.849) ciprofibrate is stated to reduce elevated low-density lipoprotein (LDL)-cholesterol and very-low-density lipoprotein (VLDL)-triglyceride concentrations and to increase high-density lipoprotein (HDL)-cholesterol concentrations. There have, however, been reports of an abnormal response to ciprofibrate, namely a fall in HDL-cholesterol rather than the expected rise. In one patient the effect was seen when the dose of ciprofibrate was increased from 100 to 200 mg daily;[1] in another it occurred with 100 mg daily.[2]

1. Chandler HA, Batchelor AJ. Ciprofibrate and lipid profile. *Lancet* 1994; **344:** 128–9.
2. McLeod AJ, *et al.* Ciprofibrate and lipid profile. *Lancet* 1994; **344:** 955.

Preparations

Proprietary Preparations (details are given in Part 3)
Belg.: Hyperlipen; *Braz.:* Oroxadin; *Fr.:* Lipanor; *Israel:* Lipanor; *Mex.:* Oroxadin; *Neth.:* Modalim; *Port.:* Lipanor; *Singapore:* Modalim; *Switz.:* Hyperlipen; *UK:* Modalim.

Clinofibrate   (16584-m)

Clinofibrate (*rINN*).
S-8527. 2,2′-[Cyclohexylidenebis(4-phenyleneoxy)]bis[2-methylbutyric acid].
$C_{28}H_{36}O_6 = 468.6$.
CAS — 30299-08-2.
Pharmacopoeias. In Jpn.

Profile

Clinofibrate, a fibric acid derivative (see Bezafibrate, p.849), is a lipid regulating drug used in the treatment of hyperlipidaemias (p.800). The usual dose is 200 mg two or three times daily by mouth.

Preparations

Proprietary Preparations (details are given in Part 3)
Aust.: Lipoclin†; *Jpn:* Lipoclin.

Clofibrate   (1341-x)

Clofibrate (*BAN, USAN, rINN*).
AY-61123; Clofibratum; Ethyl *p*-Chlorophenoxyisobutyrate; Ethyl Clofibrate; ICI-28257; NSC-79389. Ethyl 2-(4-chlorophenoxy)-2-methylpropionate.
$C_{12}H_{15}ClO_3 = 242.7$.
CAS — 637-07-0 (clofibrate); 882-09-7 (clofibric acid).
ATC — C10AB01.
Pharmacopoeias. In Chin., Eur. (see p.vi), Jpn, and US.

Pharmacopoeial description

Ph. Eur.: A clear, almost colourless liquid. Very slightly soluble in water; miscible with alcohol and with ether.
USP 25: A colourless to pale yellow liquid with a characteristic odour. Insoluble in water; soluble in alcohol, in acetone, in chloroform, and in benzene. Store in airtight containers. Protect from light.

Aluminium Clofibrate   (1342-r)

Aluminium Clofibrate (*BAN, rINN*).
Alufibrate; Aluminum Clofibrate. Bis[2-(4-chlorophenoxy)-2-methylpropionato]hydroxyaluminium.
$C_{20}H_{21}AlCl_2O_7 = 471.3$.
CAS — 24818-79-9; 14613-01-5.
ATC — C10AB03.

Calcium Clofibrate   (16291-y)

Calcium Clofibrate (*rINN*).
$C_{20}H_{20}CaCl_2O_6 = 467.4$.
CAS — 39087-48-4.

Magnesium Clofibrate   (8041-a)

Magnesium Clofibrate (*rINN*).
Clomag; UR-112.
$C_{20}H_{20}Cl_2MgO_6 = 451.6$.
CAS — 14613-30-0.

Adverse Effects and Precautions

As for Bezafibrate, p.849.

Additional side-effects occasionally reported with clofibrate include vomiting, diarrhoea, dyspepsia, flatulence, weight gain, drowsiness, and hepatomegaly.

Large-scale long-term studies have demonstrated an increased incidence of cholecystitis, gallstones, and sometimes pancreatitis in patients receiving clofibrate, and some studies, but not all, have indicated an increased incidence of certain cardiovascular disorders, including cardiac arrhythmias. The unexpected finding of an increased mortality rate in patients taking clofibrate in the WHO study (see below) produced serious concern over its long-term safety.

◊ Doubts over the safety of clofibrate for long-term prophylaxis were raised following 2 large-scale studies: the Coronary Drug Project[1] and the WHO Cooperative Trial.[2] The Coronary Drug Project showed that while clofibrate was generally well tolerated, there was an increased incidence of serious effects over the 5-year study period. These included cholelithiasis (3.0%

The symbol † denotes a preparation no longer actively marketed

against 1.3% with placebo), pulmonary embolism or thrombophlebitis (5.2% against 3.3%), arrhythmias other than atrial fibrillation, new cases of intermittent claudication, and new angina pectoris. Other findings included an increased incidence of palpable spleen, and enlarged, firm, or tender liver. Anticoagulant therapy was required in 37% more patients taking clofibrate than placebo. Further analysis of the results[3] showed that the incidence of cholelithiasis or cholecystitis over the first 6 years was 4.0% in the clofibrate group compared with 2.6% in the placebo group.

In the WHO study[2] there was a higher incidence of cholelithiasis and a slight excess of thromboembolism, but no evidence of an increased incidence of intermittent claudication. More importantly, the long-term safety of clofibrate was thrown into doubt by the finding that, although clofibrate reduced the incidence of non-fatal myocardial infarction, the overall death rate was higher in the clofibrate group than in the control groups. The excess deaths were related to a range of disorders with no single disorder predominating. Follow-up after 9.6 years[4] and 13.2 years[5] indicated that the excess of deaths from causes other than ischaemic heart disease was almost entirely confined to the period of exposure to clofibrate; the excess during the treatment period was 47% from all causes compared with 5% after treatment ended. The causes of death were spread over a range of malignant and non-malignant disorders.

1. The Coronary Drug Project Research Group. Clofibrate and niacin in coronary heart disease. *JAMA* 1975; **231:** 360–80.
2. Oliver MF, *et al.* A co-operative trial in the primary prevention of ischaemic heart disease using clofibrate. *Br Heart J* 1978; **40:** 1069–1118.
3. The Coronary Drug Project Research Group. Gall bladder disease as a side effect of drugs influencing lipid metabolism. *N Engl J Med* 1977; **296:** 1185–90.
4. Oliver MF, *et al.* WHO cooperative trial on primary prevention of ischaemic heart disease using clofibrate to lower serum cholesterol: mortality follow-up. *Lancet* 1980; **ii:** 379–85. Correction. *ibid.*; 490.
5. Oliver MF, *et al.* WHO cooperative trial on primary prevention of ischaemic heart disease using clofibrate to lower serum cholesterol: final mortality follow-up. *Lancet* 1984; **ii:** 600–604.

Effects on the kidneys. Renal failure has been reported[1,2] in patients taking clofibrate. See also Effects on Skeletal Muscle, under Adverse Effects of Bezafibrate, p.849.

1. Dosa S, *et al.* Acute-on-chronic renal failure precipitated by clofibrate. *Lancet* 1976; **i:** 250.
2. Cumming A. Acute renal failure and interstitial nephritis after clofibrate treatment. *BMJ* 1980; **281:** 1529–30.

Effects on the nervous system. Peripheral neuropathy developed in a patient given clofibrate.[1] Symptoms resolved when clofibrate was withdrawn.

1. Gabriel R, Pearce JMS. Clofibrate-induced myopathy and neuropathy. *Lancet* 1976; **ii:** 906.

Effects on the respiratory system. Eosinophilic pneumonia in a patient associated with the use of clofibrate.[1]

1. Hendrickson RM, Simpson F. Clofibrate and eosinophilic pneumonia. *JAMA* 1982; **247:** 3082.

Interactions

As for Bezafibrate, p.849.

The manufacturers of clofibrate have suggested that, in patients taking oral anticoagulants, the dose of anticoagulant should be reduced by about 50% when treatment with clofibrate is started, and then adjusted gradually if necessary.

Pharmacokinetics

Clofibrate is readily absorbed from the gastrointestinal tract and is rapidly hydrolysed to its active metabolite, chlorophenoxyisobutyric acid (clofibric acid), which is extensively bound to plasma proteins. The plasma half-life is about 17 hours. It is excreted in the urine, predominantly in the form of a glucuronide conjugate.

◊ References.
1. Gugler R. Clinical pharmacokinetics of hypolipidaemic drugs. *Clin Pharmacokinet* 1978; **3:** 425–39.

Uses and Administration

Clofibrate, a fibric acid derivative, is a lipid regulating drug with actions on plasma lipids similar to those of bezafibrate (p.849). It is used in the treatment of type III hyperlipoproteinaemia; it may also be helpful in some patients with severe hypertriglyceridaemia due to type IIb, type IV, or type V hyperlipoproteinaemias.

The usual dose, by mouth, is 20 to 30 mg per kg body-weight daily in 2 or 3 divided doses after food. In adults, doses are commonly in the range 1.5 to 2 g daily.

The aluminium, calcium, and magnesium salts of clofibrate have also been used in the treatment of hyperlipidaemias.

Clofibrate has been used for the prophylaxis of ischaemic heart disease but is no longer recommended for this purpose because of the incidence of adverse effects during long-term treatment. For further details see under Adverse Effects, above.

Administration in renal impairment. Clofibrate should generally be avoided in patients with renal impairment.

The plasma half-life of total clofibric acid has been reported[1] to be extended from about 17 hours in healthy subjects to a mean of about 130 hours in 5 patients with renal failure undergoing haemodialysis. A dose of 1 to 1.5 g of clofibrate per week effectively lowered plasma-triglyceride concentrations without causing toxicity in 11 hypertriglyceridaemic patients undergoing haemodialysis.[2]

1. Faed EM, McQueen EG. Plasma half-life of clofibric acid in renal failure. *Br J Clin Pharmacol* 1979; **7:** 407–10.
2. Goldberg AP, *et al.* Control of clofibrate toxicity in uraemic hypertriglyceridemia. *Clin Pharmacol Ther* 1977; **21:** 317–25.

Hyperlipidaemias. Like other fibric acid derivatives clofibrate is used in the treatment of hyperlipidaemias (p.800). It reduces elevated plasma-triglyceride concentrations, probably mainly by an effect on lipoprotein lipase (see Bezafibrate, p.849).

Several studies involving clofibrate investigated whether reduction of elevated serum-lipids would reduce the incidence of **ischaemic heart disease**. The two largest long-term studies were the Coronary Drug Project[1] which involved over 8000 subjects with confirmed previous myocardial infarctions, and the WHO Cooperative Trial[2] in over 15 000 healthy men. The Coronary Drug Project found no reduction in total mortality, nor in fatal or non-fatal major ischaemic heart disease. In the WHO Cooperative Trial the overall incidence of major ischaemic heart disease was reduced in the clofibrate group compared with hyperlipidaemic controls, the difference being confined to non-fatal myocardial infarctions. The increased incidence in both cardiovascular and non-cardiovascular diseases in subjects taking clofibrate, in particular the incidence of cholelithiasis and, in the WHO study, the excess mortality in the clofibrate group[3,4] (see also under Adverse Effects, above) has meant that clofibrate is no longer used for the prophylaxis of ischaemic heart disease. Other fibric acid derivatives, for example gemfibrozil (p.897), are, however, used prophylactically.

1. The Coronary Drug Project Research Group. Clofibrate and niacin in coronary heart disease. *JAMA* 1975; **231:** 360–80.
2. Oliver MF, *et al.* A co-operative trial in the primary prevention of ischaemic heart disease using clofibrate. *Br Heart J* 1978; **40:** 1069–1118.
3. Oliver MF, *et al.* WHO cooperative trial on primary prevention of ischaemic heart disease using clofibrate to lower serum cholesterol: mortality follow-up. *Lancet* 1980; **ii:** 379–85. Correction. *ibid.*; 490.
4. Oliver MF, *et al.* WHO cooperative trial on primary prevention of ischaemic heart disease using clofibrate to lower serum cholesterol: final mortality follow-up. *Lancet* 1984; **ii:** 600–604.

Neonatal jaundice. Clofibrate has been found to be effective both in the treatment of jaundice in term infants and for prophylaxis in premature infants.[1] In a study involving 93 term infants with jaundice, clofibrate 50 mg per kg body-weight as a single oral dose reduced the intensity and duration of jaundice compared with placebo. As a prophylactic measure, clofibrate was shown to reduce the degree of jaundice in premature infants when the plasma concentration of clofibric acid reached 140 μg per mL within 24 hours of clofibrate administration. The dose required to achieve this was estimated to be 100 to 150 mg per kg.

1. Gabilan JC, *et al.* Clofibrate treatment of neonatal jaundice. *Pediatrics* 1990; **86:** 647–8.

Preparations

BP 2001: Clofibrate Capsules;
USP 25: Clofibrate Capsules.

Proprietary Preparations (details are given in Part 3)
Aust.: Arterioflexin; Regelan; *Austral.:* Atromid-S†; Col†; *Belg.:* Atromidin†; *Braz.:* Claripex AL; *Canad.:* Atromid-S; Novo-Fibrate†; *Denm.:* Atromidin†; *Fr.:* Lipavlon†; *Ger.:* Regelan N†; *Hong Kong:* Atromid-S; Lipilim; *Irl.:* Atromid-S; *Mex.:* Atromid-S; *NZ:* Atromid-S; *Port.:* Atromid-S; *S.Afr.:* Atromid-S†; *Spain:* Neo Atromid; *Swed.:* Atromidin†; *Switz.:* Regelan; *UK:* Atromid-S†; *USA:* Atromid-S.

Multi-ingredient: *Braz.:* Davistar; Lipofacton; Sinteroid; *S.Afr.:* Lipaten; *Spain:* Arteriobrate†.

Clofibride   (1345-n)

Clofibride (*rINN*).
MG-46. 3-Dimethylcarbamoylpropyl 2-(4-chlorophenoxy)-2-methylpropionate.
$C_{16}H_{22}ClNO_4 = 327.8$.
CAS — 26717-47-5.
ATC — C10AB10.

Profile

Clofibride, a fibric acid derivative (see Bezafibrate, p.849), is a lipid regulating drug that has been used in the treatment of hypercholesterolaemia and hypertriglyceridaemia.

The active metabolite of clofibride is clofibric acid (chlorophenoxyisobutyric acid). Hydroxy-4-*N*-dimethylbutyramide is an additional metabolite.

Clonidine Hydrochloride (857-k)

Clonidine Hydrochloride (*BANM, USAN, rINNM*).
Clonidini Hydrochloridum; ST-155; ST-155-BS (clonidine). 2-(2,6-Dichloroanilino)-2-imidazoline hydrochloride; 2,6-Dichloro-*N*-(imidazolidin-2-ylidene)aniline hydrochloride.
$C_9H_9Cl_2N_3,HCl = 266.6$.
CAS — 4205-90-7 (clonidine); 4205-91-8 (clonidine hydrochloride).
Pharmacopoeias. In Chin., Eur. (see p.vi), *Jpn, Pol.,* and *US.*

Pharmacopoeial description

Ph. Eur.: A white or almost white crystalline powder. Soluble in water and in dehydrated alcohol. A 5% solution in water has a pH of 4.0 to 5.0.
USP 25: pH of a 5% solution in water is between 3.5 and 5.5. Store in airtight containers.

Adverse Effects and Treatment

Drowsiness, dry mouth, dizziness, and headache commonly occur during the initial stages of therapy with clonidine. Constipation is also common, and other adverse effects which have been reported include depression, anxiety, fatigue, nausea, anorexia, parotid pain, sleep disturbances, vivid dreams, impotence and loss of libido, urinary retention or incontinence, slight orthostatic hypotension, and dry, itching, or burning sensations in the eye. Fluid retention may occur and is usually transient, but may be responsible for a reduction in the hypotensive effect during continued treatment. Clonidine may cause rashes and pruritus, and these are more common with the use of transdermal delivery systems. Less frequently, bradycardia, including sinus bradycardia with atrioventricular block, other ECG disturbances, heart failure, hallucinations, cramp, Raynaud's syndrome, gynaecomastia, and transient abnormalities in liver function tests have been reported. Large doses have been associated with initial increases in blood pressure and transient hyperglycaemia, although these do not persist during continued therapy.

Symptoms of overdosage include transient hypertension or profound hypotension, bradycardia, sedation, miosis, respiratory depression, convulsions, and coma. Treatment consists of general supportive measures. An alpha blocker may be given if necessary.

Sudden withdrawal of clonidine may produce rebound hypertension—see Precautions, below.

◊ A transdermal clonidine patch dislodged during sleep was accidentally transferred to the skin of the patient's 9-month-old child who was sharing the bed.[1] The child subsequently showed signs of somnolence, irritability, and increased fluid intake, presumably due to a dry mouth.

1. Reed MT, Hamburg EL. Person-to-person transfer of transdermal drug-delivery systems: a case report. *N Engl J Med* 1986; **314:** 1120–1.

Effects on the gastrointestinal tract. Constipation is a relatively common adverse effect of clonidine, the US manufacturer reporting an incidence of about 10%. Several cases of ileus or pseudo-obstruction of the bowel in patients receiving clonidine have been reported;[1-3] withdrawal of clonidine was associated with a return of bowel function to normal. Abdominal pain mimicking acute appendicitis occurred in another patient prescribed clonidine; symptoms recurred on restarting the drug and subsided when it was withdrawn.[4]

1. Davidov M, *et al.* The antihypertensive effects of an imidazoline compound. *Clin Pharmacol Ther* 1967; **8:** 810–16.
2. Bear R, Steer K. Pseudo-obstruction due to clonidine. *BMJ* 1976; **1:** 197.
3. Bauer GE, Hellerstrand KJ. Pseudo-obstruction due to clonidine. *BMJ* 1976; **1:** 769.
4. Mjörndal T, Mellbring G. Abdominal pain associated with clonidine. *BMJ* 1986; **292:** 174.

Effects on the heart. Clonidine has been associated with impaired atrioventricular conduction in a few patients,[1,2] although some of these may have had underlying conduction defects and had previously received digitalis, which may have contributed to their condition. Other ECG abnormalities may also occur. Sudden death has been reported in 3 children receiving clonidine and methylphenidate,[3,4] although the significance of these reports has been questioned.[5]

1. Kibler LE, Gazes PC. Effect of clonidine on atrioventricular conduction. *JAMA* 1977; **238:** 1930–2.
2. Abiuso P, Abelow G. Atrioventricular dissociation in a patient receiving clonidine. *JAMA* 1978; **240:** 108–9.

3. Maloney MJ, Schwam, JS. Clonidine and sudden death. *Pediatrics* 1995; **96:** 1176–7.
4. Fenichel RR. Combining methylphenidate and clonidine: the role of post-marketing surveillance. *J Child Adolesc Psychopharmacol* 1995; **5:** 155–6.
5. Blackman JA, *et al.* Clonidine and electrocardiograms. *Pediatrics* 1996; **98:** 1223–4.

Effects on mental function. There have been occasional reports of disturbed mental state in patients given clonidine.[1-3]

1. Lavin P, Alexander CP. Dementia associated with clonidine therapy. *BMJ* 1975; **1:** 628.
2. Enoch MD, Hammad GEM. Acute hallucinosis due to clonidine. *Curr Med Res Opin* 1977; **4:** 670–1.
3. Brown MJ, *et al.* Clonidine hallucinations. *Ann Intern Med* 1980; **93:** 456–7.

Effects on the skin. Skin reactions have been reported in up to 50% of patients receiving clonidine by a transdermal delivery system.[1] Localised erythema and irritation during early treatment are usually mild, but allergic contact dermatitis may develop.[2-4] Skin reactions may become commoner during prolonged treatment; although only mild skin reactions were observed in a trial of transdermal clonidine during 8 to 14 weeks of treatment in 15 patients, severe skin reactions occurred after an average of 20 weeks in 4 of 5 patients who continued treatment.[5] Despite a claim that skin reactions were due to a component in the delivery system and not to clonidine itself,[6] positive patch tests to clonidine have been obtained.[2,4] Subsequent reaction to oral clonidine in patients who develop skin reactions to the transdermal delivery system is reported to be rare.[7,8]

1. Carmichael AJ. Skin sensitivity and transdermal drug delivery: a review of the problem. *Drug Safety* 1994; **10:** 151–9.
2. Groth H, *et al.* Allergic skin reactions to transdermal clonidine. *Lancet* 1983; **ii:** 850–1.
3. McMahon PG, Weber MA. Allergic skin reactions to transdermal clonidine. *Lancet* 1983; **ii:** 851.
4. Boekhorst JC. Allergic contact dermatitis with transdermal clonidine. *Lancet* 1983; **ii:** 1031–2.
5. Dick JBC, *et al.* Skin reactions to long-term transdermal clonidine. *Lancet* 1987; **i:** 516.
6. Anonymous. Transdermal clonidine sensitiser identified? *Pharm J* 1984; **233:** 16.
7. Bigby M. Transdermal clonidine dermatitis. *JAMA* 1987; **258:** 1819.
8. Burris JF. Transdermal clonidine dermatitis. *JAMA* 1987; **258:** 1819–20.

PEMPHIGOID. Anogenital cicatricial pemphigoid has been reported[1] with long-term clonidine therapy.

1. van Joost T, *et al.* Drug-induced anogenital cicatricial pemphigoid. *Br J Dermatol* 1980; **102:** 715–18.

Hypersensitivity. See Effects on the Skin, above.

Overdosage. Analysis by the National Poisons Information Service[1] of poisoning by clonidine in 133 children and 37 adults revealed that there were no deaths but clinical features were often severe. Supportive measures were usually adequate but atropine was often needed for severe and persistent bradycardia. Forced diuresis was not advised because hypotension could be enhanced and there was no evidence that excretion of clonidine was increased.

Although naloxone has been suggested as an antidote for clonidine overdose, no reversal of the hypotensive effects of clonidine 300 µg was noted in 6 hypertensive subjects receiving naloxone by intravenous infusion.[2] In a retrospective analysis of 47 children with clonidine poisoning, only 3 of 19 given naloxone showed definite improvement;[3] it was concluded that naloxone is at best an inconsistent antidote for clonidine poisoning.

Severe symptoms of overdosage have also been reported following the ingestion of clonidine transdermal patches,[4] and following probable subcutaneous injection during filling of an epidural pump reservoir.[5]

1. Stein B, Volans GN. Dixarit overdose: the problem of attractive tablets. *BMJ* 1978; **2:** 667–8.
2. Rogers JF, Cubeddu LX. Naloxone does not antagonise the antihypertensive effect of clonidine in essential hypertension. *Clin Pharmacol Ther* 1983; **34:** 68–73.
3. Wiley JF, *et al.* Clonidine poisoning in young children. *J Pediatr* 1990; **116:** 654–8.
4. Raber JH, *et al.* Clonidine patch ingestion in an adult. *Ann Pharmacother* 1993; **27:** 719–22. Correction. *ibid.;* 1143.
5. Frye CB, Vance MA. Hypertensive crisis and myocardial infarction following massive clonidine overdose. *Ann Pharmacother* 2000; **34:** 611–15.

Precautions

Clonidine should be used with caution in patients with cerebrovascular disease, ischaemic heart disease including myocardial infarction, renal impairment, occlusive peripheral vascular disorders such as Raynaud's disease, or those with a history of depression.

Clonidine causes drowsiness and patients should not drive or operate machinery where loss of attention could be dangerous.

Systemic effects also occur following epidural clonidine administration and patients should be closely monitored, particularly during the first few days of therapy.

Intravenous injections of clonidine should be given slowly to avoid a possible transient pressor effect es

pecially in patients already receiving other antihypertensives such as guanethidine or reserpine.

Withdrawal of clonidine therapy should be gradual as sudden discontinuation may cause rebound hypertension, sometimes severe. Symptoms of increased catecholamine release such as agitation, sweating, tachycardia, headache, and nausea may also occur. Beta blockers can exacerbate the rebound hypertension and if clonidine is being given concurrently with a beta-blocking drug, clonidine should not be discontinued until several days after the withdrawal of the beta blocker. It has been suggested that patients should be warned of the risk of missing a dose or stopping the drug without consulting their doctor and should carry a reserve supply of tablets.

Although hypotension may occur during anaesthesia in clonidine-treated patients clonidine should not be withdrawn; indeed, if necessary it should be given intravenously during the operation to avoid the risk of rebound hypertension.

Abuse. Despite its central effects and ability to cause a form of physical dependence, WHO stated that there was no evidence of recreational use of clonidine and the likelihood of abuse was rated as very low.[1] However, clonidine may potentiate the psychoactive effects of morphine and abuse has been reported.[2]

1. WHO. WHO expert committee on drug dependence: twenty-fifth report. *WHO Tech Rep Ser 775* 1989.
2. Sullivan JT, *et al.* Does clonidine alter the abuse potential of morphine? *Clin Pharmacol Ther* 1995; **57:** 163.

Diabetes mellitus. The effects of clonidine on carbohydrate metabolism appear to be variable. Some studies suggest that clonidine does not affect carbohydrate metabolism in diabetic[1] or non-diabetic hypertensive patients.[2] Conversely, there has been a report of a diabetic patient in whom clonidine was associated with elevated fasting blood-glucose values,[3] and increased insulin requirements were noted in a diabetic child treated with clonidine for tics.[4] However, a study in 10 diabetic hypertensive patients found that although clonidine impaired response to an acute glucose load, it did not significantly affect diabetic control over a 10-week period.[5] Problems may arise when clonidine is given to diabetics with autonomic neuropathy: both severe postural hypotension[6] and paradoxical hypertension[7] have been reported.

For discussion of the use of clonidine in diabetic diarrhoea see below.

1. Nilsson-Ehle P, *et al.* Lipoproteins and metabolic control in hypertensive type II diabetics treated with clonidine. *Acta Med Scand* 1988; **224:** 131–4.
2. Molitch ME, *et al.* Effects of antihypertensive medications on carbohydrate metabolism. *Curr Ther Res* 1986; **39:** 398–407.
3. Okada S, *et al.* Effect of clonidine on insulin secretion: a case report. *J Int Med Res* 1986; **14:** 299–302.
4. Mimouni-Bloch A, Mimouni M. Clonidine-induced hyperglycemia in a young diabetic girl. *Ann Pharmacother* 1993; **27:** 980.
5. Guthrie GP, *et al.* Clonidine in patients with diabetes and mild hypertension. *Clin Pharmacol Ther* 1983; **34:** 713–17.
6. Moffat B. Postural hypotension induced by clonidine in insulin dependent diabetes. *BMJ* 1985; **290:** 822.
7. Young E, *et al.* Paradoxical hypertension from clonidine. *Ann Intern Med* 1984; **101:** 282–3.

ECT. Maximal ECT stimuli were unsuccessful in producing seizures in 4 of 7 treatment attempts in a 66-year-old patient receiving concomitant clonidine therapy.[1] It was suggested that clonidine may elevate the seizure threshold.

1. Elliott RL. Case report of a potential interaction between clonidine and electroconvulsive therapy. *Am J Psychiatry* 1983; **140:** 1237–8.

Porphyria. Clonidine hydrochloride has been associated with acute attacks of porphyria and is considered unsafe in porphyric patients.

Interactions

The hypotensive effect of clonidine may be enhanced by diuretics, other antihypertensives, and drugs that cause hypotension. However, beta blockers may exacerbate rebound hypertension following clonidine withdrawal (see Precautions, above), and tricyclic antidepressants may antagonise the hypotensive effect. The sedative effect of clonidine may be enhanced by CNS depressants.

Antidepressants. Although tricyclic antidepressants commonly cause orthostatic hypotension, they may antagonise the hypotensive effects of clonidine. In a study[1] in 5 hypertensive patients receiving clonidine and a diuretic, *desipramine* 75 mg daily resulted in a loss of blood pressure control in 4. Increase in blood pressure generally occurred in the second week of treatment, but 1 patient had a dramatic rise in blood pressure within 24 hours of starting treatment. The mechanism is thought to be due to a central interaction between clonidine and the tricyclic antidepressant, although a peripheral effect cannot be completely excluded.[2] Loss of blood pressure control also occurred in a patient receiving guanfacine, another alpha$_2$-adrenoceptor agonist, when *amitriptyline* was given concomitantly.[3] The reaction recurred with *imipramine*. However, in another study clonidine was given to 11 patients receiving *amitriptyline* or *imipramine*, and 10 achieved good blood pressure control, although 4 developed an acute rise in blood pressure when methyldopa or guanethidine was added to the regimen.[4] *Maprotiline*[5] or *mianserin*[6] do not appear to interact with clonidine.

1. Briant RH, *et al.* Interaction between clonidine and desipramine in man. *BMJ* 1973; **1:** 522–3.
2. van Spanning HW, van Zwieten PA. The interference of tricyclic antidepressants with the central hypotensive effect of clonidine. *Eur J Pharmacol* 1973; **24:** 402–4.
3. Buckley M, Feely J. Antagonism of antihypertensive effect of guanfacine by tricyclic antidepressants. *Lancet* 1991; **337:** 1173–4.
4. Raftos J, *et al.* Clonidine in the treatment of severe hypertension. *Med J Aust* 1973; **1:** 786–93.
5. Gundert-Remy U, *et al.* Lack of interaction between the tetracyclic antidepressant maprotiline and the centrally acting antihypertensive drug clonidine. *Eur J Clin Pharmacol* 1983; **25:** 595–9.
6. Elliott HL, *et al.* Absence of an effect of mianserin on the actions of clonidine or methyldopa in hypertensive patients. *Eur J Clin Pharmacol* 1983; **24:** 15–19.

Antipsychotics. Acute, severe hypotension occurred in 2 agitated hypertensive patients following administration of clonidine and either *chlorpromazine* or *haloperidol*. Both patients had mitral insufficiency.[1]

1. Fruncillo RJ, *et al.* Severe hypotension associated with concurrent clonidine and antipsychotic medication. *Am J Psychiatry* 1985; **142:** 274.

Dopaminergic antiparkinsonian drugs. For a report of the inhibition of the therapeutic effect of *levodopa* by clonidine, see Antihypertensives, p.1171.

Immunosuppressants. For a report of clonidine increasing whole blood-*ciclosporin* concentrations, see p.522.

Pharmacokinetics

Following oral administration clonidine is well absorbed from the gastrointestinal tract, with peak plasma concentrations observed after about 3 to 5 hours. About 50% of a dose is metabolised in the liver. It is excreted in the urine as unchanged drug and metabolites, 40 to 60% of an oral dose being excreted in 24 hours as unchanged drug; about 20% of a dose is excreted in the faeces, probably via enterohepatic circulation. The elimination half-life has been variously reported to range between 6 and 24 hours, extended to up to 41 hours in patients with renal impairment.

Clonidine is absorbed through the skin; absorption is reported to be better when applied to the chest or arm than when applied to the thigh. Therapeutic plasma concentrations are achieved 2 or 3 days after application of a transdermal delivery system and are roughly equivalent to trough concentrations achieved after oral dosage. Therapeutic plasma concentrations are maintained for about 8 hours after removal of the delivery system and then decline slowly over several days.

◊ Reviews.
1. Lowenthal DT, *et al.* Clinical pharmacokinetics of clonidine. *Clin Pharmacokinet* 1988; **14:** 287–310.

Pregnancy. A study in 5 pregnant women treated with clonidine for pre-eclampsia[1] reported an average ratio of cord- to plasma-concentrations of 0.87, indicating placental transfer of clonidine.

1. Boutroy MJ, *et al.* Clonidine placental transfer and neonatal adaption. *Early Hum Dev* 1988; **17:** 275–86.

Uses and Administration

Clonidine is an imidazoline antihypertensive that appears to act centrally to reduce sympathetic tone, resulting in a fall in diastolic and systolic blood pressure and a reduction in heart rate. The exact mechanism is unclear; clonidine stimulates alpha$_2$-adrenoceptors and central imidazoline receptors, but it is not known which receptors mediate which effects. It also acts peripherally, and this peripheral activity may be responsible for the transient increase in blood pressure seen during rapid intravenous administration as well as contributing to the hypotensive effect during chronic administration. Peripheral resistance is reduced during continuous treatment. Cardiovascular reflexes remain intact so postural hypotension occurs infrequently.

Clonidine is used in the management of hypertension (p.802), including hypertensive crises, although other drugs with fewer adverse effects are now generally preferred. It may be given in conjunction with a thiazide diuretic, but combination with a beta blocker should be avoided where possible. Clonidine has also been used in the prophylactic treatment of migraine or recurrent vascular headaches and in the treatment of menopausal flushing. It is used in conjunction with opioids in the management of cancer pain (p.5) and has been tried for various other forms of pain (below). Other uses of clonidine have included the symptomatic treatment of opioid withdrawal (see under Substance Dependence, below), the diagnosis of phaeochromocytoma (below), and administration as eye drops in the management of glaucoma (p.1413). It has also been tried in Tourette's syndrome (below) and numerous other disorders.

Clonidine is used as the hydrochloride. When given by mouth, its haemodynamic effects appear in about 30 to 60 minutes, reaching a maximum after 2 to 4 hours and lasting up to 8 hours. Tolerance to clonidine has been reported. Withdrawal of clonidine should be gradual because of the risk of rebound hypertension.

In **hypertension**, the usual initial dose of clonidine hydrochloride is 50 to 100 µg three times daily by mouth (or in the US, 100 µg twice daily), increased every second or third day according to the response of the patient; the usual maintenance dose is 300 to 1200 µg daily but doses of 1800 µg or more daily may sometimes be required. Clonidine may also be given in a modified-release formulation which enables once or twice daily dosage, or by transdermal delivery systems applied once a week, which each deliver 100 to 300 µg of clonidine base daily at a constant rate.

Clonidine hydrochloride may be given by slow intravenous injection over 10 to 15 minutes in hypertensive crises, usually in doses of 150 to 300 µg. The effect usually appears within 10 minutes, but transient hypertension may precede hypotension if the injection is administered too rapidly. The hypotensive effect reaches a maximum about 30 to 60 minutes after administration and the duration is about 3 to 7 hours; up to 750 µg may be given intravenously over 24 hours. Although oral administration does not produce a sufficiently rapid hypotensive effect for use in an emergency situation, a dose of 100 to 200 µg initially followed by 50 to 100 µg every hour until control of blood pressure is achieved or a maximum of 500 to 800 µg is reached, has been recommended for the control of severe hypertension.

In the prophylaxis of **migraine** or recurrent vascular headaches and in the treatment of **menopausal flushing**, a dose of 50 µg twice daily by mouth has been employed, increased, if there is no remission after 2 weeks, to 75 µg twice daily.

In the management of severe **cancer pain**, clonidine hydrochloride may be given by continuous epidural infusion in combination with an opioid, in an initial dose of 30 µg per hour, adjusted according to response.

Anxiety disorders. Clonidine has been tried in various anxiety disorders but evidence of efficacy is limited. A review[1] of the use of clonidine in panic attacks (p.649) considered that it might be useful as a last-line anxiolytic in patients unresponsive to standard treatment as occasional success had been obtained in a few patients. There have also been isolated reports of small numbers of patients with post-traumatic stress disorder (p.650) who have benefited from treatment with clonidine.[2]

1. Puzantian T, Hart LL. Clonidine in panic disorder. *Ann Pharmacother* 1993; **27:** 1351–3.
2. Harmon RJ, Riggs PD. Clonidine for posttraumatic stress disorder in preschool children. *J Am Acad Child Adolesc Psychiatry* 1996; **35:** 1247–9.

Cardiac arrhythmias. Atrial fibrillation (p.794) is managed by treatment to slow the increased ventricular responses or by cardioversion. Control of ventricular rate is usually achieved with digoxin, beta blockers, or calcium-channel blockers but clonidine, which reduces sympathetic tone and thus reduces heart rate, has also been tried.[1,2]

1. Roth A, *et al.* Clonidine for patients with rapid atrial fibrillation. *Ann Intern Med* 1992; **116:** 388–90.
2. Scardi S, *et al.* Oral clonidine for heart rate control in chronic atrial fibrillation. *Lancet* 1993; **341:** 1211–12.

Diarrhoea. Some studies have shown that clonidine possesses antidiarrhoeal properties. Clonidine may stimulate alpha$_2$-adrenoceptors on enterocytes thus promoting fluid and electrolyte absorption and inhibiting anion secretion. It may also modify intestinal motility or rectal sphincter tone.

Most experience with clonidine is in diabetic diarrhoea (p.317). Clonidine 100 to 600 µg by mouth every 12 hours reduced diabetic diarrhoea in 3 patients with type 1 diabetes[1] and good results have also been reported in such patients when transdermal clonidine was used.[2,3] Benefit has also been reported in patients with symptoms of diabetic gastroparesis in addition to diarrhoea.[3,4] However, oral (but perhaps not transdermal) clonidine may worsen orthostatic hypotension in patients with diabetic diarrhoea which may limit its usefulness.[5]

1. Fedorak RN, *et al.* Treatment of diabetic diarrhea with clonidine. *Ann Intern Med* 1985; **102:** 197–9.
2. Sacerdote A. Topical clonidine for diabetic diarrhea. *Ann Intern Med* 1986; **105:** 139.
3. Sacerdote AS. Topical clonidine and diabetic gastroparesis. *Ann Intern Med* 1990; **112:** 796.
4. Migliore A, *et al.* Diabetic diarrhea and clonidine. *Ann Intern Med* 1988; **109:** 170–1.
5. Ogbonnaya KI, Arem R. Diabetic diarrhea: pathophysiology, diagnosis, and management. *Arch Intern Med* 1990; **150:** 262–7.

Extrapyramidal disorders. There is limited evidence[1] from studies of small numbers of patients that clonidine might reduce symptoms of antipsychotic-induced akathisia and tardive dyskinesia (p.662). However, adverse effects such as sedation and hypotension may limit use.

1. Ahmed I, Takeshita J. Clonidine: a critical review of its role in the treatment of psychiatric disorders. *CNS Drugs* 1996; **6:** 53–70.

Growth retardation. Clonidine has been reported to be a stimulant of growth hormone release, presumably as a result of central alpha-adrenergic stimulation, and has been tried in the diagnosis and management of growth retardation (p.1273). It may be given orally as a provocative test for growth hormone deficiency,[1,2] particularly in children,[3] although some consider measurement of circulating somatomedins to be more useful than provocative tests. It has also been tried in growth retardation, both in children with growth hormone deficiency and in short children without proven deficiency, but results have been contradictory and largely unsatisfactory.[4-9]

1. Gil-Ad I, *et al.* Oral clonidine as a growth hormone stimulation test. *Lancet* 1979; **ii:** 278–80.
2. Hoffman WH, *et al.* Relationship of plasma clonidine to growth hormone concentrations in children and adolescents. *J Clin Pharmacol* 1990; **29:** 538–42.
3. Hindmarsh PC, Swift PGF. An assessment of growth hormone provocation tests. *Arch Dis Child* 1995; **72:** 362–8.
4. Pintor C, *et al.* Clonidine treatment for short stature. *Lancet* 1987; **i:** 1226–30.
5. Pescovitz OH, Tan E. Lack of benefit of clonidine treatment for short stature in a double-blind, placebo-controlled trial. *Lancet* 1988; **ii:** 874–7.
6. Anonymous. Alternatives to growth hormone. *Lancet* 1989; **i:** 820–2.
7. Suri D, *et al.* Clonidine for short stature. *Lancet* 1989; **i:** 508.
8. Müller EE, *et al.* Clonidine for short stature. *Lancet* 1989; **i:** 1395.
9. Allen DB. Effects of nightly clonidine administration on growth velocity in short children without growth hormone deficiency: a double-blind, placebo-controlled study. *J Pediatr* 1993; **122:** 32–6.

Hyperactivity. Drug treatment of attention deficit hyperactivity disorder (p.1505) is usually initiated with a central stimulant; clonidine has been tried mainly as an adjunct to stimulant therapy. Small studies[1,2] have suggested that clonidine may have a favourable effect, although there have probably not been controlled trials in adequate numbers of children and adverse effects may also be a problem,[3,4] either when clonidine is given alone or when given in combination with other drugs. There have been reports[5] of sudden death when clonidine has been used in combination with stimulants, but the role of the drugs in these events is unclear.

1. Hunt RD, *et al.* Clonidine benefits children with attention deficit disorder and hyperactivity: report of a double-blind placebo-crossover therapeutic trial. *J Am Acad Child Psychiatry* 1985; **24:** 617–29.
2. Hunt RD. Treatment effects of oral and transdermal clonidine in relation to methylphenidate: an open pilot study in ADD-H. *Psychopharmacol Bull* 1987; **23:** 111–14.
3. Anonymous. Clonidine for treatment of attention-deficit/hyperactivity disorder. *Med Lett Drugs Ther* 1996; **38:** 109–110.
4. Cantwell DP, *et al.* Case study: adverse response to clonidine. *J Am Acad Child Adolesc Psychiatry* 1997; **36:** 539–44.
5. Fenichel RR. Combining methylphenidate and clonidine: the role of post-marketing surveillance. *J Child Adolesc Psychopharmacol* 1995; **5:** 155–6.

Menopausal disorders. Although HRT is the mainstay of treatment for menopausal disorders (p.1464) clonidine has been of some use in countering vasomotor symptoms in patients who cannot receive hormone replacement therapy;[1,2] however, some studies have failed to demonstrate a reduction in hot flushes. The adverse effects reported in normotensive women, including orthostatic hypotension, may mean that it is best reserved for women who are also hypertensive.

Clonidine has also been tried[3] for hot flushes in women receiving tamoxifen.

1. Young RL, *et al.* Management of menopause when estrogen cannot be used. *Drugs* 1990; **40:** 220–30.
2. Lucero MA, McCloskey WW. Alternatives to estrogen for the treatment of hot flashes. *Ann Pharmacother* 1997; **31:** 915–17.
3. Pandya KJ, *et al.* Oral clonidine in postmenopausal patients with breast cancer experiencing tamoxifen-induced hot flashes: a University of Rochester Cancer Center Community Clinical Oncology Program study. *Ann Intern Med* 2000; **132:** 788–93.

Migraine. Propranolol and pizotifen are probably the most well-established drugs for prophylaxis of migraine (p.449). Many other drugs have been used, including clonidine, but a review of clinical trials[1] indicated that it was a poor first choice and seemed unlikely to work even as a last resort. It has been used in patients whose attacks may be precipitated by tyramine-containing foods.

1. Anonymous. Clonidine in migraine prophylaxis—now obsolete. *Drug Ther Bull* 1990; **28:** 79–80.

Orthostatic hypotension. Clonidine has produced beneficial effects in a few patients with orthostatic hypotension (p.1070), including orthostatic hypotension due to autonomic neuropathy.[1] Its use in this condition is somewhat paradoxical as orthostatic hypotension may occur as an adverse effect of clonidine therapy.

1. Acott PD, *et al.* Effectiveness of clonidine in congenital orthostatic hypotension. *J Pediatr* 1990; **116:** 666–7.

Pain. Administration of opioids and local anaesthetics by the epidural or intrathecal routes can produce effective analgesia but adverse effects are common. Many other drugs, including clonidine, have been tried by these routes, alone or as adjuncts. Clonidine is thought to produce analgesia by a direct action on alpha$_2$ adrenoceptors in the spinal cord. Some studies[1,2] of clonidine given *epidurally* alone in a dose of 2 µg per kg body-weight or 150 µg have produced satisfactory pain relief, although duration of action was short. Higher doses have also been used.[3] Hypotension and sedation have been reported as frequent side-effects and an editorial on epidural clonidine[4] considered it unlikely that clonidine would be useful as a sole analgesic drug although it may have a role in combination with opioids and/or local anaesthetics. Clonidine has been given epidurally in combination with various opioids and has produced satisfactory analgesia in postoperative pain,[5] neuropathic pain,[6] and labour pain;[7] the combination is also used in chronic pain due to cancer. Clonidine has also been given epidurally with local anaesthetics and enhanced analgesia has been reported in postoperative pain,[8] labour pain,[9] and in chronic pain.[10] Epidural clonidine combined with both an opioid and a local anaesthetic may increase the duration of analgesia during labour, but adverse effects on the fetal heartbeat may limit this use.[11] The combination of clonidine and bupivacaine has also produced enhanced analgesia in a study in children undergoing lower limb orthopaedic surgery;[12] clonidine was given epidurally in a dose of 2 µg per kg body-weight. Clonidine and bupivacaine have been given intrathecally[13] and may produce less urinary retention when the combination of morphine with bupivacaine.[14] Long-term intrathecal administration of clonidine in combination with midazolam has also been reported[15] and may be effective in refractory neuropathic or musculoskeletal pain.

Analgesia has also been reported following administration of clonidine by other routes. A study comparing *intravenous* and epidural clonidine 150 µg in 10 patients with back pain reported that intravenous clonidine produced better analgesia, although pain relief was poor following administration by either route.[16] However, a study[3] in postoperative patients using an initial dose of clonidine 8 µg per kg body-weight followed by bolus doses of 30 µg as required found that the epidural and intravenous routes were both effective but the epidural route produced less sedation. In another study,[17] *intramuscular* injection of clonidine 2 µg per kg was as effective as the same dose given epidurally for relief of postoperative pain. Clonidine has some effect when given *orally*[18–21] but the effect is much less marked than following parenteral administration. Premedication with oral clonidine has been reported to provide effective postoperative analgesia in children.[22] *Transdermal* clonidine has been tried for postoperative analgesia.[23] The *intra-articular* route has also been used.[24]

The role of clonidine in the management of pain remains to be established. For further discussion of pain and the management of its various types, see p.2.

1. Bonnet F, *et al.* Postoperative analgesia with extradural clonidine. *Br J Anaesth* 1989; **63:** 465–9.
2. Lund C, *et al.* Comparison of the effects of extradural clonidine with those of morphine on postoperative pain, stress responses, cardiopulmonary function and motor and sensory block. *Br J Anaesth* 1989; **63:** 516–19.
3. Bernard J-M, *et al.* Comparison of intravenous and epidural clonidine for postoperative patient-controlled analgesia. *Anesth Analg* 1995; **81:** 706–12.
4. Macdonald R. Extradural clonidine—the need for well designed controlled trials. *Br J Anaesth* 1994; **72:** 255–7.
5. Carabine UA, *et al.* Extradural clonidine infusions for analgesia after total hip replacement. *Br J Anaesth* 1992; **68:** 338–43.
6. Tamsen A, Gordh T. Epidural clonidine produces analgesia. *Lancet* 1984; **ii:** 231–2.
7. Buggy DJ, MacDowell C. Extradural analgesia with clonidine and fentanyl compared with 0.25% bupivacaine in the first stage of labour. *Br J Anaesth* 1996; **76:** 319–21.
8. Carabine UA, *et al.* Extradural clonidine and bupivacaine for postoperative analgesia. *Br J Anaesth* 1992; **68:** 132–5.
9. O'Meara ME, Gin T. Comparison of 0.125% bupivacaine with 0.125% bupivacaine and clonidine as extradural analgesia in the first stage of labour. *Br J Anaesth* 1993; **71:** 651–6.
10. Glynn C, O'Sullivan K. A double-blind randomised comparison of the effects of epidural clonidine, lignocaine and the combination of clonidine and lignocaine in patients with chronic pain. *Pain* 1995; **64:** 337–43.
11. Chassard D, *et al.* Extradural clonidine combined with sufentanil and 0.0625% bupivacaine for analgesia in labour. *Br J Anaesth* 1996; **77:** 458–62.
12. Lee JJ, Rubin AP. Comparison of a bupivacaine-clonidine mixture with plain bupivacaine for caudal analgesia in children. *Br J Anaesth* 1994; **72:** 258–62.

13. Bonnet F, *et al.* Prevention of tourniquet pain by spinal isobaric bupivacaine with clonidine. *Br J Anaesth* 1989; **63:** 93–6.
14. Gentili M, Bonnet F. Spinal clonidine produces less urinary retention than spinal morphine. *Br J Anaesth* 1996; **76:** 872–3.
15. Borg PAJ, Krijnen HJ. Long-term intrathecal administration of midazolam and clonidine. *Clin J Pain* 1996; **12:** 63–8.
16. Carroll D, *et al.* Single-dose, randomized, double-blind, double-dummy cross-over comparison of extradural and I.V. clonidine in chronic pain. *Br J Anaesth* 1993; **71:** 665–9.
17. Bonnet F, *et al.* Clonidine-induced analgesia in postoperative patients: epidural versus intramuscular administration. *Anesthesiology* 1990; **72:** 423–7.
18. Glynn CF, *et al.* Role of spinal noradrenergic system in transmission of pain in the patients with spinal cord injury. *Lancet* 1986; **ii:** 1249–50.
19. Tan Y-M, Croese J. Clonidine and diabetic patients with leg pains. *Ann Intern Med* 1986; **105:** 633–4.
20. Petros AJ, Wright RMB. Epidural and oral clonidine in domiciliary control of deafferentation pain. *Lancet* 1987; **i:** 1034.
21. Benhamou D, *et al.* Addition of oral clonidine to postoperative patient-controlled analgesia with i.v. morphine. *Br J Anaesth* 1994; **72:** 537–40.
22. Mikawa K, *et al.* Oral clonidine premedication reduces postoperative pain in children. *Anesth Analg* 1996; **82:** 225–30.
23. Segal IS, *et al.* Clinical efficacy of oral transdermal clonidine combinations during the perioperative period. *Anesthesiology* 1991; **74:** 220–5.
24. Gentili M, *et al.* Intra-articular morphine and clonidine produce comparable analgesia but the combination is not more effective. *Br J Anaesth* 1997; **79:** 660–1.

Phaeochromocytoma. Clonidine acts centrally to suppress catecholamine release and may be used[1] in the diagnosis of phaeochromocytoma (p.810). Experience gained with the clonidine suppression test and a review of published studies indicated that it is of value in selected patients with moderately elevated plasma and/or urinary catecholamine concentrations.[2]

1. Bravo EL, *et al.* Clonidine-suppression test: a useful aid in the diagnosis of pheochromocytoma. *N Engl J Med* 1981; **305:** 623–6.
2. Sjoberg RJ, *et al.* The clonidine suppression test for pheochromocytoma. *Arch Intern Med* 1992; **152:** 1193–7.

Premedication. Clonidine has been given pre-operatively for its sedative, anxiolytic, and analgesic effects and to provide haemodynamic stability and reduce anaesthetic requirements; see Pain above for some further details. Pre-operative use has also been reported[1] to reduce the incidence of postoperative vomiting in children. Clonidine may attenuate the perioperative stress response and has been shown to reduce perioperative oxygen consumption, which is a marker of sympathetic activation.[2]

1. Mikawa K, *et al.* Oral clonidine premedication reduces vomiting in children after strabismus surgery. *Can J Anaesth* 1995; **42:** 977–81.
2. Taittonen MT, *et al.* Effect of clonidine and dexmedetomidine premedication on perioperative oxygen consumption and haemodynamic state. *Br J Anaesth* 1997; **78:** 400–406.

Restless legs syndrome. Numerous drugs have been tried for the treatment of restless legs syndrome (see Parasomnias, p.653). Symptomatic improvement has been reported with clonidine in a number of case studies[1,2] and small controlled trials,[3] but side-effects may limit its use.

1. Handwerker JV, Palmer RF. Clonidine in the treatment of "restless leg" syndrome. *N Engl J Med* 1985; **313:** 1228–9.
2. Zoe A, *et al.* High-dose clonidine in a case of restless legs syndrome. *Ann Pharmacother* 1994; **28:** 878–81.
3. Wagner ML, *et al.* Randomized, double-blind, placebo-controlled study of clonidine in restless legs syndrome. *Sleep* 1996; **19:** 52–8.

Shivering. Numerous drugs, including clonidine, have been tried for the treatment of postoperative shivering (p.1255). Clonidine's central and peripheral effects could both account for its antishivering activity, but some have suggested that it acts by resetting the central threshold for shivering. In preliminary studies a small intravenous dose of clonidine 75 µg or 30 µg stopped shivering after general anaesthesia[1] or epidural anaesthesia,[2] respectively. Clonidine given pre-operatively has also been reported to reduce the incidence of postoperative shivering.[3-5]

1. Joris J, *et al.* Clonidine and ketanserin both are effective treatment for postanesthetic shivering. *Anesthesiology* 1993; **79:** 532–9.
2. Capogna G, Celleno D. IV clonidine for post-extradural shivering in parturients: a preliminary study. *Br J Anaesth* 1993; **71:** 294–5.
3. Steinfath M, *et al.* Clonidine administered intraoperatively prevents postoperative shivering. *Br J Clin Pharmacol* 1995; **39:** 580P–581P.
4. Vanderstappen I, *et al.* The effect of prophylactic clonidine on postoperative shivering: a large prospective double-blind study. *Anaesthesia* 1996; **51:** 351–5.
5. Sia S. I.v. clonidine prevents post-extradural shivering. *Br J Anaesth* 1998; **81:** 145–6.

Spasticity. Clonidine, given alone or as an adjunct to baclofen, has been tried in patients with various forms of spasticity (p.1322) including those refractory to baclofen.[1-4]

1. Nance PW, *et al.* Clonidine in spinal cord injury. *Can Med Assoc J* 1985; **133:** 41–2.
2. Donovan WH, *et al.* Clonidine effect on spasticity: a clinical trial. *Arch Phys Med Rehabil* 1988; **69:** 193–4.
3. Sandford PR, *et al.* Clonidine in the treatment of brainstem spasticity: case report. *Am J Phys Med Rehabil* 1992; **71:** 301–3.
4. Middleton JW, *et al.* Intrathecal clonidine and baclofen in the management of spasticity and neuropathic pain following spinal cord injury: a case study. *Arch Phys Med Rehabil* 1996; **77:** 824–6.

Substance dependence. ALCOHOL. Although drug treatment of alcohol withdrawal (p.1131) is usually with a benzodi-

azepine, clonidine has sometimes been used to good effect,[1,2] although it does not have any effect on convulsions or delirium tremens[3] and should not be used as sole therapy.

1. Guthrie SK. The treatment of alcohol withdrawal. *Pharmacotherapy* 1989; **9:** 131–43.
2. Ip Yam PC, *et al.* Clonidine in the treatment of alcohol withdrawal in the intensive care unit. *Br J Anaesth* 1992; **68:** 106–8.
3. Anonymous. Alcohol problems in the general hospital. *Drug Ther Bull* 1991; **29:** 69–71.

OPIOID ANALGESICS. Clonidine has been reported to be useful in controlling withdrawal symptoms following abrupt discontinuation of opioids (p.66). Treatment is required for about 10 days following methadone withdrawal and less for withdrawal from diamorphine.[1] Most studies have reported favourable results, although some[2,3] suggest that subjective response may be less favourable. However, the maximum dose of clonidine used in one of these studies[2] was 300 µg twice daily. Others used initial doses of up to 1.35 mg daily[4] and a dose of 100 to 200 µg every 4 to 6 hours has been necessary.[5] Doses of up to 17 µg per kg body-weight daily have been used.[6] The major drawback of clonidine therapy is the tendency to cause hypotension, and this may limit its usefulness in some patients.

Clonidine has been used in combination with naltrexone to shorten the withdrawal syndrome and withdrawal was achieved within 6 days.[7] Subsequent modification to the regimen allowed 38 of 40 patients addicted to methadone to withdraw completely in 4 to 5 days.[8] Patients required a mean of 2.3 mg of clonidine on the first day which reduced, but did not abolish, symptoms. A further modification was reported allowing opioid withdrawal with minimal drop-out over 2 to 3 days.[9]

Clonidine has also been used in the management of neonatal abstinence syndrome (p.67) in infants born to opioid-addicted mothers maintained on methadone.[10,11] Benefit occurred in 6 of 7 such infants given an initial clonidine dose of 0.5 to 1 µg per kg body-weight by mouth, increased over 1 to 2 days to 3 to 5 µg per kg daily in divided doses. Total length of treatment ranged from 6 to 17 days. The infant who failed to respond was born to a mother also receiving haloperidol, desipramine, and theophylline.[11]

1. Cook C, *et al.* Opiate withdrawal: inpatient versus outpatient programmes. *BMJ* 1986; **293:** 506.
2. Preston KL, *et al.* Self-administration of clonidine, oxazepam, and hydromorphone by patients undergoing methadone detoxification. *Clin Pharmacol Ther* 1985; **38:** 219–27.
3. Jasinski DR, *et al.* Clonidine in morphine withdrawal: differential effects on signs and symptoms. *Arch Gen Psychiatry* 1985; **42:** 1063–6.
4. Cami J, *et al.* Efficacy of clonidine and of methadone in the rapid detoxification of patients dependent on heroin. *Clin Pharmacol Ther* 1985; **38:** 336–41.
5. Washton AM, *et al.* Clonidine for outpatient opiate detoxification. *Lancet* 1980; **i:** 1078–9.
6. Gold MS, *et al.* Clonidine and opiate withdrawal. *Lancet* 1980; **ii:** 1078–80.
7. Charney DS, *et al.* Clonidine and naltrexone: a safe, effective, and rapid treatment of abrupt withdrawal from methadone therapy. *Arch Gen Psychiatry* 1982; **39:** 1327–32.
8. Charney DS, *et al.* The combined use of clonidine and naltrexone as a rapid, safe, and effective treatment of abrupt withdrawal from methadone. *Am J Psychiatry* 1986; **143:** 831–7.
9. Brewer C, *et al.* Opioid withdrawal and naltrexone induction in 48-72 hours with minimal drop-out, using a modification of the naltrexone-clonidine technique. *Br J Psychiatry* 1988; **153:** 340–3.
10. Hoder EL, *et al.* Clonidine in neonatal narcotic-abstinence syndrome. *N Engl J Med* 1981; **305:** 1284.
11. Hoder EL, *et al.* Clonidine treatment of neonatal narcotic abstinence syndrome. *Psychiatry Res* 1984; **13:** 243–51.

SMOKING. Nicotine dependence may be managed using behavioural or psychological counselling. In addition, nicotine replacement therapy (p.1642) can help alleviate withdrawal symptoms. A number of other drugs, including clonidine, have also been tried. A meta-analysis[1] found clonidine, given orally in doses of 150 to 450 µg daily, or transdermally in doses of 100 to 300 µg daily, to be effective; however adverse effects limit its usefulness and clonidine is usually reserved for second-line treatment in those who experience severe agitation and anxiety when stopping smoking.

Some individual studies have found clonidine to be more effective in women although the authors of the meta-analysis[1] recommended that these results be interpreted cautiously since some studies also found that women were less successful in giving up smoking unaided than men; treatment with clonidine, however, resulted in similar success rates in both men and women.

1. Gourlay SG, *et al.* Clonidine for smoking cessation (updated 30 August 2000). Available in The Cochrane Library; Issue 4. Oxford: Update Software; 2000.

Tourette's syndrome. Clonidine is one of many drugs that have been tried in the management of Tourette's syndrome (see Tics under Extrapyramidal Disorders, p.650).

Disturbance of monoamine metabolism (including dopamine, noradrenaline, and serotonin) has been implicated in Tourette's syndrome. Clonidine is thought to reduce central noradrenergic activity and may also affect other neurochemical systems and these properties may account for its beneficial effects in this disorder. Studies of clonidine in Tourette's syndrome have produced mixed results,[1-5] although this may reflect the difficulty in study design for a disease that can vary considerably in severity and presence of comorbid conditions and whose symptoms wax and wane. Nevertheless, clonidine has been used as an alternative to the commonly used dopamine antagonist antipsychotics, such as haloperidol and pimozide, when side-effects limit their use. Although it appears to be less effective than these drugs,[2] clonidine has been reported to successfully control symptoms in some children with Tourette's syndrome unresponsive to haloperidol.[1]

1. Cohen DJ, et al. Clonidine in Tourette's syndrome. Lancet 1979; ii: 551–3.
2. Shapiro AK, et al. Treatment of Gilles de la Tourette's syndrome with clonidine and neuroleptics. Arch Gen Psychiatry 1983; 40: 1235–40.
3. Leckman JF, et al. Short- and long-term treatment of Tourette's syndrome with clonidine: a clinical perspective. Neurology 1985; 35: 343–51.
4. Goetz CG, et al. Clonidine and Gilles de la Tourette's syndrome: double-blind study using objective rating methods. Ann Neurol 1987; 21: 307–10.
5. Leckman JF, et al. Clonidine treatment of Gilles de la Tourette's syndrome. Arch Gen Psychiatry 1991; 48: 324–8.

Preparations

BP 2001: Clonidine Injection; Clonidine Tablets;
USP 25: Clonidine Hydrochloride and Chlorthalidone Tablets; Clonidine Hydrochloride Tablets.

Proprietary Preparations (details are given in Part 3)
Aust.: Catanidin†; Catapressan; Dixarit†; *Austral.:* Catapres; Dixarit†; *Belg.:* Catapressan; Dixarit; *Braz.:* Atensina; *Canad.:* Catapres; Dixarit; *Denm.:* Catapresan; *Fin.:* Caprysin; Catapresan; *Fr.:* Catapressan; *Ger.:* Aruclonin; Catapresan; Clonid-Ophtal; Clonistada; Dispaclonidin; Dixarit; Haemiton; Isoglaucon; Mirfat; Paracefan; *Hong Kong:* Catapres; Dixarit; *Irl.:* Catapres; Dixarit; *Israel:* Clonnirit; Normopresan; *Ital.:* Adesipress-TTS; Catapresan; Isoglaucon; *Mex.:* Catapresan; Epiclodina; *Neth.:* Catapresan; Dixarit; *Norw.:* Catapresan; *NZ:* Catapres; Dixarit; *Port.:* Catapresan; Edolglau; *S.Afr.:* Catapres; Dixarit; *Singapore:* Dixarit; *Spain:* Catapresan; Isoglaucon; *Swed.:* Catapresan; *Switz.:* Catapresan; *Thai.:* Catapres; *UK:* Catapres; Dixarit; *USA:* Catapres; Duraclon.

Multi-ingredient: *Aust.:* Combipresan†; *Canad.:* Combipres†; *Ger.:* Combipresan; Haemiton compositum; *Spain:* Dilapres†; *USA:* Clorpres; Combipres.

Clopamide (2320-d)

Clopamide *(BAN, USAN, rINN)*.
DT-327. 4-Chloro-N-(2,6-dimethylpiperidino)-3-sulphamoyl-benzamide; *cis*-3-(Aminosulphonyl)-4-chloro-N-(2,6-dimethyl-1-piperidinyl)benzamide.
$C_{14}H_{20}ClN_3O_3S = 345.8$.
CAS — 636-54-4.
ATC — C03BA03.

Profile

Clopamide is a diuretic with properties similar to those of the thiazide diuretics (see Hydrochlorothiazide, p.907) even though it does not contain a thiazide ring system. It is used for oedema, including that associated with heart failure (p.798), and for hypertension (p.802).

Diuresis is initiated in 1 to 2 hours, reaches a maximum in about 3 to 6 hours, and lasts for up to 24 hours.

In the treatment of oedema the usual dose is 10 to 40 mg daily by mouth; frequency may be reduced for maintenance. The usual dose in the treatment of hypertension is 5 to 10 mg daily, either alone, or in conjunction with other antihypertensives.

Preparations

Proprietary Preparations (details are given in Part 3)
Denm.: Adurix; *Ger.:* Brinaldix.

Multi-ingredient: *Aust.:* Brinerdin; Viskaldix; *Belg.:* Viskaldix; *Braz.:* Viskaldix; *Fr.:* Viskaldix; *Ger.:* Briserin N; *Irl.:* Viskaldix; *Ital.:* Brinerdin†; *Neth.:* Brinerdin†; Viskaldix; *NZ:* Viskaldix; *Port.:* Brinerdine; *S.Afr.:* Brinerdin; *Spain:* Brinerdina; *Switz.:* Brinerdine; Viskaldix; *Thai.:* Bedin; Brinerdin; Hyperdine; Viskaldix; *UK:* Viskaldix.

Clopidogrel Bisulfate (3672-s)

Clopidogrel Bisulfate *(USAN, rINNM)*.
Clopidogrel Bisulphate *(BANM)*; Clopidogrel Hydrogen Sulphate; SR-25990C. Methyl (S)-2-chlorophenyl(4,5,6,7-tetrahydrothieno[3,2-c]pyridin-5-yl)acetate bisulphate; Methyl (+)-(S)-α-(o-chlorophenyl)-6,7-dihydrothieno[3,2-c]pyridine-5(4H)-acetate sulphate.
$C_{16}H_{16}ClNO_2S,H_2SO_4 = 419.9$.
CAS — 113665-84-2 (clopidogrel); 94188-84-8 (clopidogrel); 120202-66-6 (clopidogrel bisulfate).

Adverse Effects and Precautions

As for Ticlopidine, p.981. The incidence of blood dyscrasias is lower with clopidogrel.

Effects on the joints. Acute arthritis was reported in 2 patients 2 to 3 weeks after starting treatment with clopidogrel.[1] In both cases symptoms resolved following discontinuation.
1. Garg A, et al. Clopidogrel associated with acute arthritis. BMJ 2000; 320: 483.

Effects on taste. Loss of taste occurred in 2 patients 6 to 8 weeks after starting treatment with clopidogrel, but recovered fully when clopidogrel was withdrawn.[1] Rechallenge in 1 of

The symbol † denotes a preparation no longer actively marketed

the patients led to recurrence of the taste loss, which persisted when treatment was discontinued.
1. Golka K, et al. Reversible ageusia as an effect of clopidogrel treatment. Lancet 2000; 355: 465–6.

Interactions

As for Ticlopidine, p.981.

Pharmacokinetics

Clopidogrel is rapidly but incompletely absorbed following oral administration; absorption appears to be about 50%. It is a prodrug and is extensively metabolised in the liver following absorption, mainly to the inactive carboxylic acid derivative. The active metabolite appears to be a thiol derivative but has not been identified in plasma. Clopidogrel and the carboxylic acid derivative are highly protein bound. Clopidogrel and its metabolites are excreted about equally in urine and in faeces.

Uses and Administration

Clopidogrel is an analogue of ticlopidine (p.981) with similar actions and uses. It is given prophylactically as an alternative to aspirin in patients at risk of thromboembolic disorders such as myocardial infarction (p.805), peripheral arterial disease (p.808), and stroke (p.813). It is given by mouth as the bisulfate, but doses are expressed in terms of the base; the usual dose is 75 mg once daily.

◊ References.
1. CAPRIE Steering Committee. A randomised, blinded, trial of clopidogrel versus aspirin in patients at risk of ischaemic events (CAPRIE). Lancet 1996; 348: 1329–39.
2. Hankey GJ. Clopidogrel: a new safe and effective antiplatelet agent. But unanswered questions remain. Med J Aust 1997; 167: 120–1.
3. Anonymous. Clopidogrel for reduction of atherosclerotic events. Med Lett Drugs Ther 1998; 40: 59–60.
4. Sharis PJ, et al. The antiplatelet effects of ticlopidine and clopidogrel. Ann Intern Med 1998; 129: 394–405.
5. Jarvis B, Simpson K. Clopidogrel: a review of its use in the prevention of atherothrombosis. Drugs 2000; 60: 347–77.
6. The Clopidogrel in Unstable Angina to Prevent Recurrent Events Trial Investigators. Effects of clopidogrel in addition to aspirin in patients with acute coronary syndromes without ST-segment elevation. N Engl J Med 2001; 345: 494–502.

Reperfusion and revascularisation procedures. Coronary stents are being used increasingly to treat and prevent restenosis following angioplasty procedures (see p.812). Thrombotic occlusion commonly complicates their use and patients have been aggressively treated with a combination of antiplatelet drugs and anticoagulants. Recent studies, however, suggest that antiplatelet treatment alone may be adequate if the stent has been positioned correctly and the risk of thrombosis is considered to be low.

A regimen of long-term aspirin with ticlopidine for 4 weeks has been widely used. However, use of ticlopidine is associated with haematological toxicity and clopidogrel has been studied as an alternative. Observational studies[1,2] indicated that clopidogrel and ticlopidine produced similar benefits. In a subsequent randomised trial, the Clopidogrel Aspirin Stent International Cooperative Study (CLASSICS),[3] in which clopidogrel was given in a dose of 75 mg daily, with or without a 300-mg loading dose, the combination of clopidogrel with aspirin appeared to be as effective as ticlopidine with aspirin and was also better tolerated.
1. Mishkel GJ, et al. Clopidogrel as adjunctive antiplatelet therapy during coronary stenting. J Am Coll Cardiol 1999; 34: 1884–90.
2. Berger PB. Clopidogrel versus ticlopidine after intracoronary stent placement. J Am Coll Cardiol 1999; 34: 1891–4.
3. Bertrand ME, et al. Double-blind study of the safety of clopidogrel with and without a loading dose in combination with aspirin compared with ticlopidine in combination with aspirin after coronary stenting: the Clopidogrel Aspirin Stent International Cooperative Study (CLASSICS). Circulation 2000; 102: 624–9.

Preparations

Proprietary Preparations (details are given in Part 3)
Aust.: Plavix; *Austral.:* Iscover; Plavix; *Belg.:* Plavix; *Canad.:* Plavix; *Denm.:* Plavix; *Fin.:* Plavix; *Fr.:* Plavix; *Ger.:* Iscover; Plavix; *Irl.:* Plavix; *Mex.:* Plavix; *Neth.:* Plavix; *Norw.:* Plavix; *NZ:* Plavix; *Port.:* Iscover; Plavix; *Singapore:* Plavix; *Spain:* Iscover; Plavix; *Swed.:* Plavix; *Switz.:* Iscover; Plavix; *Thai.:* Plavix; *UK:* Iscover; Plavix; *USA:* Plavix.

Cloricromen (14754-l)

Cloricromen *(rINN)*.
Ethyl ({8-chloro-3-[2-(diethylamino)ethyl]-4-methyl-2-oxo-2H-1-benzopyran-7-yl}oxy)acetate.
$C_{20}H_{26}ClNO_5 = 395.9$.
CAS — 68206-94-0.
ATC — B01AC02.

Profile

Cloricromen is an antiplatelet drug with vasodilating activity

and is used in thromboembolic disorders (p.816). It is given as the hydrochloride in arterial vascular disorders where there is a risk of thrombosis. It may be given by mouth in a dose of 100 mg two or three times daily or intravenously in a dose of 30 mg daily.

Preparations

Proprietary Preparations (details are given in Part 3)
Ital.: Assogen; Proendotel.

Cloridarol (9221-q)

Cloridarol *(rINN)*.
Clobenfurol. α-(Benzofuran-2-yl)-α-(4-chlorophenyl)methanol.
$C_{15}H_{11}ClO_2 = 258.7$.
CAS — 3611-72-1.
ATC — C01DX15.

Profile

Cloridarol is a vasodilator used in ischaemic heart disease in usual doses of 250 to 500 mg daily by mouth.

Ischaemic heart disease is discussed under Atherosclerosis (p.793) and the treatment of its clinical manifestations is described under Angina Pectoris (p.791) and Myocardial Infarction (p.805).

Preparations

Proprietary Preparations (details are given in Part 3)
Spain: Menoxicor.

Colesevelam Hydrochloride (20332-x)

Colesevelam Hydrochloride *(USAN, rINNM)*.
GT31-104HB. Allylamine polymer with epichlorohydrin (1-chloro-2,3-epoxypropane), [6-(allylamino)hexyl]trimethylammonium chloride and N-allyldecylamine, hydrochloride.
CAS — 182815-44-7.

Profile

Colesevelam hydrochloride is a nonabsorbable hydrogel with bile-acid binding properties. It is used for the treatment of hypercholesterolaemia (p.800), particularly type IIa hyperlipoproteinaemia, either alone or in combination with a statin. The usual dose is 3.75 g daily by mouth, as a single dose or in two divided doses, with meals. The dose may be increased to 4.375 g daily if required. When used in combination with a statin, the dose is 2.5 to 3.75 g daily.

◊ References.
1. Davidson MH, et al. Colesevelam hydrochloride (Cholestagel): a new, potent bile acid sequestrant associated with a low incidence of gastrointestinal side effects. Arch Intern Med 1999; 159: 1893–1900.

Preparations

Proprietary Preparations (details are given in Part 3)
USA: Welchol.

Colestipol Hydrochloride (1346-h)

Colestipol Hydrochloride *(BANM, USAN, rINNM)*.
U-26597A.
CAS — 26658-42-4 (colestipol); 50925-79-6 (colestipol); 37296-80-3 (colestipol hydrochloride).
Pharmacopoeias. In Br. and US.

Pharmacopoeial description

BP 2001: A copolymer of diethylenetriamine and epichlorohydrin (1-chloro-2,3-epoxypropane). Each g binds not less than 1.1 mEq and not more than 1.7 mEq of sodium cholate, calculated as the cholate binding capacity and with reference to the dried substance. Yellow to orange hygroscopic beads. Swells but does not dissolve in water and in dilute solutions of acids or alkalis. Practically insoluble in alcohol and in dichloromethane. The supernatant of a 10% w/w suspension in water has a pH of 6.0 to 7.5. Store in airtight containers.

USP 25: A basic anion-exchange resin. It is the hydrochloride of a copolymer of diethylenetriamine and epichlorohydrin (1-chloro-2,3-epoxypropane). Each g binds not less than 1.1 mEq and not more than 1.6 mEq of sodium cholate, calculated as cholate binding capacity. Yellow to orange beads. Swells but does not dissolve in water or dilute aqueous solutions of acids or alkalis. Insoluble in common organic solvents. The supernatant of a 10% w/w suspension in water has a pH of 6.0 to 7.5. Store in airtight containers.

Adverse Effects and Precautions

As for Colestyramine, p.864.

◊ Reductions in total serum-thyroxine and thyroxine-binding globulin concentrations were found during routine monitoring of thyroid function in patients receiving colestipol and nicotinic acid, but were considered to be benign.[1]
1. Cashin-Hemphill L, et al. Alterations in serum thyroid hormonal indices with colestipol-niacin therapy. Ann Intern Med 1987; 107: 324–9.

Interactions

As for Colestyramine, p.864.

Uses and Administration

Colestipol hydrochloride is a bile-acid binding resin. It is not absorbed from the gastrointestinal tract but binds bile acids in the intestines and has actions similar to those of colestyramine (p.864).

It is a lipid regulating drug and is used in the treatment of hypercholesterolaemias, particularly type IIa hyperlipoproteinaemia.

Colestipol hydrochloride is available as granules and is administered as a suspension in water or a flavoured vehicle. The initial dose is 5 g daily or twice daily, increasing gradually at intervals of 1 to 2 months to up to 30 g daily in single or two divided doses as necessary.

In the USA, colestipol hydrochloride is also available as tablets; doses range from 2 to 16 g daily.

Hyperlipidaemias. Colestipol is a bile-acid binding resin used similarly to colestyramine (p.864) in the treatment of hyperlipidaemias (p.800).

Colestipol on its own[1] or with nicotinic acid[2,3] has been reported to be effective in the prophylaxis of **ischaemic heart disease**. The Cholesterol-Lowering Atherosclerosis Study (CLAS)[2] in middle-aged men with progressive atherosclerosis who had undergone coronary bypass surgery showed that colestipol plus nicotinic acid reduced blood concentrations of total cholesterol, triglycerides, and low-density lipoprotein (LDL)-cholesterol, and increased those of high-density lipoprotein (HDL)-cholesterol. Drug treatment also reduced progression of atherosclerosis, development of new lesions in native coronary arteries, and changes in venous bypass grafts. Benefits were maintained after 4 years.[3]

The side-effects of colestipol may be reduced by using a low-dose regimen. The dose-response curve for colestipol is nonlinear and 10 g daily can often achieve a 10 to 20% reduction in LDL-cholesterol.[4] In a study of patients with moderate hypercholesterolaemia,[5] colestipol 10 g daily (as granules in suspension), either as a single dose in the morning or evening or in two divided doses was effective and well-tolerated. In another study[6] in patients with moderate primary hypercholesterolaemia lower doses of colestipol (2.5 g three times daily) taken together with psyllium (also 2.5 g three times daily) were as effective and better tolerated than higher doses of colestipol alone (5 g three times daily).

1. Dorr AE, *et al.* Colestipol hydrochloride in hypercholesterolemic patients—effect on serum cholesterol and mortality. *J Chron Dis* 1978; **31:** 5–14.
2. Blankenhorn DH, *et al.* Beneficial effects of combined colestipol-niacin therapy on coronary atherosclerosis and coronary venous bypass grafts. *JAMA* 1987; **257:** 3233–40.
3. Cashin-Hemphill L, *et al.* Beneficial effects of colestipol-niacin on coronary atherosclerosis: a 4-year follow-up. *JAMA* 1990; **264:** 3013–17.
4. Illingworth DR. Treatment of hyperlipidaemia. *Br Med Bull* 1990; **46:** 1025–58.
5. Lyons D, *et al.* Colestipol at varying dosage intervals in the treatment of moderate hypercholesterolaemia. *Br J Clin Pharmacol* 1994; **37:** 59–62.
6. Spence JD, *et al.* Combination therapy with colestipol and psyllium mucilloid in patients with hyperlipidemia. *Ann Intern Med* 1995; **123:** 493–9.

Preparations

BP 2001: Colestipol Granules;
USP 25: Colestipol Hydrochloride for Oral Suspension.

Proprietary Preparations (details are given in Part 3)
Austral.: Colestid; *Belg.:* Colestid; *Canad.:* Colestid; *Denm.:* Lestid; *Fin.:* Lestid; *Ger.:* Cholestabyl; Colestid; *Irl.:* Colestid; *Israel:* Colestid; *Mex.:* Colestid; *Neth.:* Colestid; *Norw.:* Lestid; *NZ:* Colestid; *Port.:* Colestid; *S.Afr.:* Colestid†; *Spain:* Colestid; *Swed.:* Lestid; *Switz.:* Colestid; *UK:* Colestid; *USA:* Colestid.

Colestyramine (1344-d)

Colestyramine (BAN, rINN).
Cholestyramine; Cholestyramine Resin; MK-135.
CAS — 11041-12-6.
ATC — C10AC01.
Pharmacopoeias. In Br. and US.

Pharmacopoeial description
BP 2001: A strongly basic anion-exchange resin in the chloride form, consisting of styrene-divinylbenzene copolymer with quaternary ammonium function groups. Each g exchanges not less than 1.8 g and not more than 2.2 g of sodium glycocholate, calculated with reference to the dried material. A white to buff-coloured, fine, hygroscopic powder. Insoluble in water, in alcohol, in chloroform, and in ether. A 1% suspension in water has a pH of 4.0 to 6.0 after standing for 10 minutes. Store in airtight containers.

USP 25: A strongly basic anion-exchange resin containing quaternary ammonium functional groups which are attached to

a styrene-divinylbenzene copolymer. Each g exchanges not less than 1.8 g and not more than 2.2 g of sodium glycocholate, calculated on the dried basis. It is used in the chloride form. A white to buff-coloured, hygroscopic, fine powder, odourless or has not more than a slight amine-like odour. It loses not more than 12% of its weight on drying. Insoluble in water, in alcohol, in chloroform, and in ether. A 1% slurry in water has a pH of 4.0 to 6.0. Store in airtight containers.

Adverse Effects

The most common side-effect of colestyramine is constipation; faecal impaction may develop and haemorrhoids may be aggravated. Other gastrointestinal side-effects include abdominal discomfort or pain, heartburn, flatulence, nausea, vomiting, and diarrhoea.

Colestyramine in high doses may cause steatorrhoea by interfering with the absorption of fats from the gastrointestinal tract and therefore decreased absorption of fat-soluble vitamins, such as vitamins A, D, E, and K, may occur. Chronic use of colestyramine may thus result in an increased bleeding tendency due to hypoprothrombinaemia associated with vitamin K deficiency; it also has a potential to cause osteoporosis due to impaired calcium and vitamin D absorption.

Colestyramine is the chloride form of an anion-exchange resin and prolonged use may produce hyperchloraemic acidosis, particularly in children.

Skin rashes and pruritus of the tongue, skin, and perianal region have occasionally occurred.

◊ Results of the Lipid Research Clinics Coronary Primary Prevention Trial[1] involving 3806 men given colestyramine or placebo for an average of 7.4 years showed that gastrointestinal side-effects occurred frequently in both groups but especially in the colestyramine group. In the first year 68% of the colestyramine group experienced at least 1 gastrointestinal side-effect compared with 43% of the placebo group; by the seventh year the incidence had diminished so that approximately equal percentages of patients were affected (29% and 26% respectively). Constipation and heartburn, especially, were more frequent in the colestyramine group which also reported more abdominal pain, belching or bloating, gas, and nausea. These side-effects were usually not severe and could be dealt with by standard clinical means.

The incidence of malignant neoplasms was similar in the 2 groups although there were differences in incidence at some sites. In particular, there were 21 cases of malignancy in the gastrointestinal tract (8 fatal) in the colestyramine group compared with 11 cases (1 fatal) in the placebo group. The number of colon cancers was identical in both groups. However, the comment was made that 6 rare cancers of the buccal cavity or pharynx in the colestyramine group should not pass unnoticed.[2]

1. Lipid Research Clinics Program. The Lipid Research Clinics Coronary Primary Prevention Trial results. *JAMA* 1984; **251:** 351–64.
2. Oliver MF. Hypercholesterolaemia and coronary heart disease: an answer. *BMJ* 1984; **288:** 423–4.

Precautions

Colestyramine powder should be administered as a suspension in water or a flavoured vehicle to minimise the risk of oesophageal obstruction.

Colestyramine should not be used in patients with complete biliary obstruction as it is unlikely to be effective.

Because of the risk of vitamin deficiencies, supplements of vitamins A, D, E, and K should be considered during prolonged therapy with colestyramine; if given by mouth they need to be in a water-miscible form. Parenteral administration, particularly of vitamin K for hypoprothrombinaemia, may be necessary if a deficiency becomes established. Reduced serum-folate concentrations have also been reported in children with familial hypercholesterolaemia and supplementation with folic acid should be considered in such circumstances.

Interactions

Colestyramine may delay or reduce the absorption of other drugs, particularly acidic drugs, administered concomitantly. Enterohepatic circulation may be reduced. Delayed or reduced absorption of thiazide diuretics, propranolol, digoxin and related glycosides, loperamide, phenylbutazone, barbiturates, oestrogens, progestogens, thyroid hormones, warfarin, and some antibacterials, has either been reported or may

be expected. It is therefore recommended that other drugs should be taken at least 1 hour before, or 4 to 6 hours after, the administration of colestyramine.

Uses and Administration

Colestyramine is a bile-acid binding resin and lipid regulating drug. It is used in the treatment of hypercholesterolaemias, particularly type IIa hyperlipoproteinaemia, and for the primary prevention of ischaemic heart disease in middle-aged men with primary hypercholesterolaemia. Colestyramine is also used for the relief of diarrhoea associated with ileal resection, Crohn's disease, vagotomy, diabetic vagal neuropathy, and radiation, and to relieve the pruritus associated with the deposition in dermal tissue of excess bile acids in patients with partial biliary obstruction or primary biliary cirrhosis.

Colestyramine is not absorbed from the gastrointestinal tract but it adsorbs, and combines with, the bile acids in the intestine to form an insoluble complex that is excreted in the faeces. The normal reabsorption of bile acids is thus prevented and this leads to an increased oxidation of cholesterol to bile acids to replace those partially removed from the enterohepatic circulation. The overall effect is a reduction of total plasma-cholesterol concentration, mainly by lowering low-density lipoprotein (LDL)-cholesterol; this may be accompanied by moderate increases in plasma triglyceride and high-density lipoprotein (HDL)-cholesterol concentrations. Since the uses of colestyramine are based upon the removal of intestinal bile acids it is unlikely that a response will be achieved in patients with complete biliary obstruction.

Colestyramine may be introduced gradually over 3 to 4 weeks to minimise gastrointestinal effects.

In hyperlipidaemias and diarrhoea the usual dose by mouth is 12 to 24 g daily, administered either as a single dose or in up to 4 divided doses. Dosage should be adjusted according to the patient's response and may be increased to 36 g daily if necessary. Lower doses may be adequate in some forms of hyperlipidaemia.

In pruritus doses of 4 to 8 g daily are usually sufficient.

A dose of colestyramine for children over 6 years of age is 240 mg per kg body-weight daily in divided doses.

Colestyramine should be administered as a suspension in water or a flavoured vehicle.

Administration in children. Plasma-cholesterol concentrations were lowered in children given colestyramine alone[1] or with dietary restrictions[2,3] for periods ranging from 1 to 8 years. Long-term treatment with colestyramine had no adverse effects on physical growth[2,3] and development or sexual maturation.[2] However, compliance has been a problem with only 48% of patients complying with treatment after 8 years.[1]

1. West RJ, Lloyd JK. Long-term follow-up of children with familial hypercholesterolaemia treated with cholestyramine. *Lancet* 1980; **ii:** 873–5.
2. Glueck CJ, *et al.* Safety and efficacy of long-term diet and diet plus bile acid-binding resin cholesterol-lowering therapy in 73 children heterozygous for familial hypercholesterolemia. *Pediatrics* 1986; **78:** 338–48.
3. Tonstad S, *et al.* Efficacy and safety of cholestyramine therapy in peripubertal and prepubertal children with familial hypercholesterolemia. *J Pediatr* 1996; **129:** 42–9.

Antibiotic-associated colitis. Colestyramine binds *Clostridium difficile* toxins and has been tried as an alternative, or as an adjunct, to vancomycin or metronidazole in patients with diarrhoea associated with *C. difficile* toxins following antibiotic therapy (p.122). In general its use is not recommended.

Biliary disorders. Beneficial responses were reported with colestyramine in the management of congenital nonobstructive nonhaemolytic hyperbilirubinaemia (Crigler-Najjar disease) in 2 infants.[1,2] It has also produced a beneficial effect in a patient with sclerosing cholangitis.[3]

1. Arrowsmith WA, *et al.* Comparison of treatments for congenital nonobstructive nonhaemolytic hyperbilirubinaemia. *Arch Dis Child* 1975; **50:** 197–201.
2. Odièvre M, *et al.* Case of congenital nonobstructive, nonhaemolytic jaundice: successful long-term phototherapy at home. *Arch Dis Child* 1978; **53:** 81–2.
3. Polter DE, *et al.* Beneficial effect of cholestyramine in sclerosing cholangitis. *Gastroenterology* 1980; **79:** 326–33.

Hyperlipidaemias. Colestyramine and other bile-acid binding resins, sometimes called bile-acid sequestrants,[1-3] are used in conjunction with dietary modification in the treatment of hyperlipidaemias (p.800) in patients with raised low-density lipoprotein (LDL)-cholesterol concentrations such as occur in heterozygous familial hypercholesterolaemia. Their action is mediated through an increase in the synthesis of LDL-receptors on hepatocytes. Thus they are ineffective in patients with homozygous familial hypercholesterolaemia who lack functional LDL-receptors. They may stimulate very-low-density lipoprotein (VLDL) production and thereby increase triglyceride concentrations. If they are to be used in patients with raised triglyceride concentrations, combination with nicotinic acid or a fibric acid derivative will be necessary. These combinations also produce enhanced cholesterol-lowering effects.[4,5]

Results of the Lipid Research Clinics Coronary Primary Prevention Trial[6] in 3806 middle-aged men with primary hypercholesterolaemia (type II hyperlipoproteinaemia) demonstrated that treatment with colestyramine reduced the incidence of **ischaemic heart disease** in patients at high risk when compared with placebo, chiefly by reduction of total plasma-cholesterol and LDL-cholesterol concentrations.[7] However, there was a larger number of violent and accidental deaths in the treatment group. In the National Heart, Lung and Blood Institute (NHLBI) Type II Coronary Intervention Study in 116 patients with type II hyperlipoproteinaemia and ischaemic heart disease,[8,9] the progression of ischaemic heart disease, assessed angiographically after 5 years, was moderately reduced by colestyramine.

The side-effects of colestyramine may be reduced by using a low-dosage regimen. The dose-response curve for colestyramine is non-linear and 8 g daily can often achieve a 10 to 20% reduction in LDL-cholesterol.[10]

1. LaRosa J. Review of clinical studies of bile acid sequestrants for lowering plasma lipid levels. *Cardiology* 1989; **76** (suppl 1): 55–64.
2. Shepherd J. Mechanism of action of bile acid sequestrants and other lipid-lowering drugs. *Cardiology* 1989; **76** (suppl 1): 65–74.
3. Ast M, Frishman WH. Bile acid sequestrants. *J Clin Pharmacol* 1990; **30**: 99–106.
4. Curtis LD, *et al.* Combination treatment with cholestyramine and bezafibrate for heterozygous familial hypercholesterolaemia. *BMJ* 1988; **297**: 173–5.
5. Jones AF, *et al.* Gemfibrozil plus cholestyramine in familial hypercholesterolaemia. *Lancet* 1988; **i**: 776.
6. Lipid Research Clinics Program. The Lipid Research Clinics Coronary Primary Prevention trial results 1: reduction in incidence of coronary heart disease. *JAMA* 1984; **251**: 351–64.
7. Lipid Research Clinics Program. The Lipid Research Clinics Coronary Primary Prevention trial results 2: the relationship of reduction in incidence of coronary heart disease to cholesterol lowering. *JAMA* 1984; **251**: 365–74.
8. Brensike JF, *et al.* Effects of therapy with cholestyramine on progression of coronary arteriosclerosis: results of the NHLBI Type II Coronary Intervention Study. *Circulation* 1984; **69**: 313–24.
9. Levy RI, *et al.* The influence of changes in lipid values induced by cholestyramine and diet on progression of coronary artery disease: results of the NHLBI Type II Coronary Intervention Study. *Circulation* 1984; **69**: 325–37.
10. Illingworth DR. Treatment of hyperlipidaemia. *Br Med Bull* 1990; **46**: 1025–58.

Preparations

BP 2001: Colestyramine Oral Powder;
USP 25: Cholestyramine for Oral Suspension.

Proprietary Preparations (details are given in Part 3)
Aust.: Quantalan; *Austral.:* Questran; *Belg.:* Questran; *Braz.:* Questran; *Canad.:* Novo-Cholamine; Questran; *Denm.:* Questran; *Fin.:* Questran; *Fr.:* Questran; *Ger.:* Colesthexal; Colestyr; Lipocol; Quantalan; Vasosan; *Hong Kong:* Questran; *Irl.:* Questran; *Israel:* Chol-Less; Questran; *Ital.:* Colestrol†; Questran; *Mex.:* Questran; *Neth.:* Questran; *Norw.:* Questran; *NZ:* Questran; *Port.:* Quantalan; *S.Afr.:* Questran; *Singapore:* Questran; Resincolestiramina; *Spain:* Lismol; Questran; Resincolestiramina; *Swed.:* Questran; *Switz.:* Quantalan; *Thai.:* Questran; Resincolestiramina; *UK:* Cholemin†; Questran; *USA:* Locholest; Prevalite; Questran.

Colextran Hydrochloride (12634-e)

Colextran Hydrochloride (*rINNM*).
DEAE-dextran Hydrochloride; Detaxtran Hydrochloride; Diethylaminoethyl-dextran Hydrochloride. Dextran 2-(diethylamino)ethyl ether hydrochloride.
CAS — 9015-73-0 (colextran); 9064-91-9 (colextran hydrochloride).

Profile
Colextran hydrochloride, an anion-exchange resin, is a lipid regulating drug used in the treatment of hyperlipidaemias (p.800). It is given in a usual dose of 2 to 3 g daily by mouth in divided doses.

Preparations
Proprietary Preparations (details are given in Part 3)
Ital.: Dexide; Nolipid†; Pulsar; Rationale; *Spain:* Dexide.

Cromakalim (3034-h)

Cromakalim (*BAN, rINN*).
BRL-34915. (±)-*trans*-3,4-Dihydro-3-hydroxy-2,2-dimethyl-4-(2-oxopyrrolidin-1-yl)-2*H*-chromene-6-carbonitrile.
$C_{16}H_{18}N_2O_3 = 286.3$.
CAS — 94470-67-4 (cromakalim); 94535-50-9 (levcromakalim).

The symbol † denotes a preparation no longer actively marketed

Profile
Cromakalim is a potassium-channel opening vasodilator (p.790). Cromakalim and its (−)-enantiomer, levcromakalim (lemakalim), have been investigated in the management of hypertension and have also been tried in patients with asthma.

◊ References.
1. Williams AJ, *et al.* Attenuation of nocturnal asthma by cromakalim. *Lancet* 1990; **336**: 334–6.
2. Suzuki S, *et al.* Antihypertensive effect of levcromakalim in patients with essential hypertension: study by 24-h ambulatory blood pressure monitoring. *Arzneimittelforschung* 1995; **45**: 859–64.

Cyclandelate (9222-p)

Cyclandelate (*BAN, rINN*).
BS-572. 3,3,5-Trimethylcyclohexyl mandelate.
$C_{17}H_{24}O_3 = 276.4$.
CAS — 456-59-7.
ATC — C04AX01.
Pharmacopoeias. In Jpn.

Adverse Effects
Nausea, gastrointestinal distress, or flushing may follow high doses of cyclandelate. Other adverse effects reported include tingling, tachycardia, sweating, dizziness, and headache.

Precautions
Cyclandelate is contra-indicated in the acute phase of a cerebrovascular accident. It should be used with caution in patients with severe obliterative coronary artery disease or cerebrovascular disease.

Uses and Administration
Cyclandelate is a vasodilator used in the management of cerebrovascular (p.798) and peripheral vascular disorders (p.809). It is given by mouth in a dosage of up to 1.6 g daily in divided doses although a daily dose of 400 to 800 mg may be adequate.

Preparations
Proprietary Preparations (details are given in Part 3)
Belg.: Cyclospasmol; *Canad.:* Cyclospasmol†; *Fin.:* Cyclospasmol; *Fr.:* Cyclergine; Cyclospasmol; Novodil†; Vascunormyl; *Ger.:* Natil; Spasmocyclon; *Ital.:* Ciclospasmol; *Neth.:* Cyclospasmol†; *Port.:* Cyclospasmol; *Swed.:* Cyclomandol; *USA:* Cyclan†; Cyclospasmol†.

Multi-ingredient: *Ger.:* Eucebral-N†.

Cyclopenthiazide (2323-m)

Cyclopenthiazide (*BAN, USAN, rINN*).
Cyclopenthiaz.; NSC-107679; Su-8341. 6-Chloro-3-cyclopentylmethyl-3,4-dihydro-2*H*-1,2,4-benzothiadiazine-7-sulphonamide 1,1-dioxide.
$C_{13}H_{18}ClN_3O_4S_2 = 379.9$.
CAS — 742-20-1.
ATC — C03AA07.

NOTE. Compounded preparations of cyclopenthiazide may be represented by the following names:
• Co-prenozide (*BAN*)—cyclopenthiazide 1 part and oxprenolol hydrochloride 640 parts (w/w).
Pharmacopoeias. In Br.

Pharmacopoeial description
BP 2001: A white, odourless or almost odourless powder. Practically insoluble in water; soluble in alcohol and in acetone; practically insoluble in chloroform; very slightly soluble in ether.

Profile
Cyclopenthiazide is a thiazide diuretic with properties similar to those of hydrochlorothiazide (p.907). It is used for oedema, including that associated with heart failure (p.798), and for hypertension (p.802).

Diuresis is induced in 1 to 3 hours, reaches a maximum in 4 to 8 hours, and lasts up to about 12 hours.

In the treatment of oedema the usual initial dose is 0.25 to 0.5 mg daily by mouth; up to 1 mg daily may be given in heart failure but higher doses rarely achieve any further benefit. The dose should be reduced to the lowest effective dose for maintenance. In the treatment of hypertension the usual dose is 0.25 to 0.5 mg daily either alone, or in conjunction with other antihypertensives.

Porphyria. Cyclopenthiazide is considered to be unsafe in patients with porphyria although there is conflicting experimental evidence of porphyrinogenicity.

Preparations
BP 2001: Cyclopenthiazide Tablets.

Proprietary Preparations (details are given in Part 3)
NZ: Navidrex; Prothiazide; *UK:* Navidrex.

Multi-ingredient: *Hong Kong:* Navispare; *Irl.:* Navispare; Trasidrex; *S.Afr.:* Trasidrex; *UK:* Navispare; Trasidrex.

Cyclothiazide (2324-b)

Cyclothiazide (*BAN, USAN, rINN*).
Compound 35483; MDi-193. 6-Chloro-3,4-dihydro-3-(norborn-5-en-2-yl)-2*H*-1,2,4-benzothiadiazine-7-sulphonamide 1,1-dioxide.
$C_{14}H_{16}ClN_3O_4S_2 = 389.9$.
CAS — 2259-96-3.
ATC — C03AA09.

Profile
Cyclothiazide is a thiazide diuretic (see Hydrochlorothiazide, p.907) that has been used, usually in combination preparations, in the management of oedema and hypertension.

Preparations
Proprietary Preparations (details are given in Part 3)
Multi-ingredient: *Fr.:* Cycloteriam†.

Dalteparin Sodium (14676-j)

Dalteparin Sodium (*BAN, USAN, rINN*).
Dalteparinum Natricum; Kabi-2165.
CAS — 9041-08-1.

NOTE. The name tedelparin sodium has been applied to this substance.
Pharmacopoeias. In Eur. (see p.vi).

Pharmacopoeial description
Ph. Eur.: Dalteparin sodium is the sodium salt of a low-molecular-mass heparin that is obtained by nitrous acid depolymerisation of heparin from porcine intestinal mucosa. The majority of the components have a 2-O-sulfo-α-L-idopyranosuronic acid structure at the non-reducing end and a 6-O-sulfo-2,5-anhydro-D-mannitol structure at the reducing end of their chain. The mass-average molecular mass ranges between 5600 and 6400, with a characteristic value about 6000. The mass percentage of chains lower than 3000 is not more than 13.0% and the mass percentage of chains higher than 8000 ranges between 15.0% and 25.0%. The degree of sulfation is 2.0 to 2.5 per disaccharide unit.

The potency is not less than 110 units and not more than 210 units of anti-factor Xa activity per mg with reference to the dried substance and the ratio of anti-factor Xa activity to anti-factor IIa activity is between 1.9 and 3.2.

Units
As for Low-molecular-weight Heparins, p.923.

Adverse Effects, Treatment, and Precautions
As for Low-molecular-weight Heparins, p.923.

Severe bleeding with dalteparin may be reduced by the slow intravenous injection of protamine sulfate; 1 mg of protamine sulfate is stated to inhibit the effects of 100 units of dalteparin sodium.

Interactions
As for Low-molecular-weight Heparins, p.924.

Pharmacokinetics
Dalteparin is almost completely absorbed following subcutaneous administration, with a bioavailability of about 87%. Peak plasma concentration is reached in about 4 hours. The terminal half-life is about 2 hours following intravenous injection and 3 to 5 hours following subcutaneous injection. Dalteparin is excreted via the kidneys and the half-life is prolonged in patients with renal impairment.

Uses and Administration
Dalteparin sodium is a low-molecular-weight heparin (p.923) with anticoagulant properties. It is used in the treatment and prophylaxis of venous thromboembolism (p.817) and to prevent clotting during extracorporeal circulation. It is also used in the management of unstable angina (p.791).

Dalteparin is administered by subcutaneous or intravenous injection. Doses are expressed in terms of units of anti-factor Xa activity.

For prophylaxis of **venous thromboembolism** during surgical procedures, dalteparin is usually started pre-operatively. For patients at moderate risk of thrombosis 2500 units of dalteparin sodium are given by subcutaneous injection 1 to 2 hours before the procedure, followed by 2500 units once daily for 5 to 7 days or until the patient is fully ambulant. For patients at high risk, 2500 units are given 1 to 2 hours before and 8 to 12 hours after the procedure followed by 5000 units daily. Alternatively, 5000 units may be given the evening before surgery followed by 5000 units each subsequent evening. This dosage may be continued for up to 5 weeks following hip replacement surgery. A further option in patients undergoing hip replacement surgery is to omit the pre-operative dose; treatment is initiated with a dose of 2500 units given 4 to 8 hours postoperatively followed by 5000 units daily.

In the treatment of established deep-vein thrombosis, pulmonary embolism, or both, dalteparin sodium is given subcutaneously in a dose of 200 units per kg body-weight daily. This may be given as a single dose or, in patients at higher risk of bleeding complications, in two divided doses. The maximum recommended dose is 18 000 units daily.

For prevention of clotting in the extracorporeal circulation during **haemodialysis** or **haemofiltration** in adults with chronic renal insufficiency an intravenous injection of dalteparin sodium 30 to 40 units per kg is followed by an intravenous infusion of 10 to 15 units per kg per hour. A single injection of 5000 units may be given for a haemodialysis or haemofiltration session lasting less than 4 hours. The dose of dalteparin sodium should be reduced in patients at high risk of bleeding complications or who are in acute renal failure; in such patients an intravenous injection of 5 to 10 units per kg is followed by an infusion of 4 to 5 units per kg per hour.

In the management of **unstable angina**, dalteparin sodium is given subcutaneously in a dose of 120 units per kg every 12 hours; the maximum recommended dose is 10 000 units every 12 hours. Treatment is continued for 5 to 8 days and low-dose aspirin should be given concomitantly.

◊ References.
1. Dunn CJ, Sorkin EM. Dalteparin sodium: a review of its pharmacology and clinical use in the prevention and treatment of thromboembolic disorders. *Drugs* 1996; **52:** 276–305.
2. Howard PA. Dalteparin: a low-molecular-weight heparin. *Ann Pharmacother* 1997; **31:** 192–203.
3. Dunn CJ, Jarvis B. Dalteparin: an update of its pharmacological properties and clinical efficacy in the prophylaxis and treatment of thromboembolic disease. *Drugs* 2000; **60:** 203–37.

Preparations

Proprietary Preparations (details are given in Part 3)
Aust.: Fragmin; *Austral.:* Fragmin; *Belg.:* Fragmin; *Canad.:* Fragmin; *Denm.:* Fragmin; *Fin.:* Fragmin; *Fr.:* Fragmine; *Ger.:* Fragmin; *Hong Kong:* Fragmin; *Israel:* Fragmin; *Ital.:* Fragmin; *Neth.:* Fragmin; *Norw.:* Fragmin; *NZ:* Fragmin; *Port.:* Fragmin; *S.Afr.:* Fragmin; *Singapore:* Fragmin; *Spain:* Boxol; Fragmin; *Swed.:* Fragmin; *Switz.:* Fragmin; Low Liquemine†; *UK:* Fragmin; *USA:* Fragmin.

Danaparoid Sodium (3155-e)

Danaparoid Sodium *(BAN, USAN, rINN)*.
Org-10172.
CAS — 83513-48-8.

Danaparoid sodium is a low-molecular-weight heparinoid derived from porcine intestinal mucosa. It contains a mixture of the sodium salts of suleparoid (heparan sulfate), dermatan sulfate, and chondroitin sulfate in an approximate ratio of 21:3:1. The average molecular weight is about 5500 to 6000.

Adverse Effects and Treatment

Haemorrhage may occur after administration of danaparoid sodium, although there is a possible decreased risk of bleeding complications compared with heparin. Liver enzymes may be transiently elevated. Other adverse effects include hypersensitivity reactions, thrombocytopenia, and pain at the site of injection.

Protamine sulfate only partially neutralises the anticoagulant effect of danaparoid sodium and cannot be relied on to reverse bleeding associated with overdosage.

Precautions

As for Heparin, p.903.

Danaparoid sodium should not be administered to patients who have developed thrombocytopenia with heparin if they demonstrate cross-reactivity in an *in-vitro* test.

Pharmacokinetics

Following subcutaneous administration danaparoid sodium is well absorbed and peak anti-factor Xa activity is reached in approximately 4 to 5 hours. The elimination half-lives of anti-factor Xa and anti-factor IIa (antithrombin) activities are approximately 25 and 7 hours, respectively. Danaparoid sodium is excreted in the urine.

Uses and Administration

Danaparoid sodium is a low-molecular-weight heparinoid. It is an anticoagulant and, like heparin (p.904), enhances the action of antithrombin III. Similarly to low-molecular-weight heparins (p.923) it is characterised by a higher ratio of anti-factor Xa to anti-factor IIa (antithrombin) activity than heparin, but is reported to be a much more selective inhibitor of factor Xa than the low-molecular-weight heparins. It was therefore hoped that danaparoid might be associated with a low incidence of bleeding complications, although this is yet to be established.

Danaparoid sodium is used in the prophylaxis of venous thromboembolism (p.817) in patients undergoing surgery. It may be used as an anticoagulant for prophylaxis or treatment in patients with heparin-induced thrombocytopenia providing there is no cross-reactivity. Danaparoid has been investigated in acute ischaemic stroke.

Doses of danaparoid sodium are expressed in terms of units of anti-factor Xa activity. In the prophylaxis of venous thromboembolism it is given by subcutaneous injection in a dose of 750 units twice daily for 7 to 10 days. The first dose should be given 1 to 4 hours before surgery.

For patients with heparin-induced thrombocytopenia requiring anticoagulation, danaparoid sodium is given intravenously. The initial bolus dose is 2500 units (or 1250 units for patients weighing less than 55 kg, or 3750 units for patients weighing more than 90 kg) followed by an infusion of 400 units per hour for 2 hours, then 300 units per hour for 2 hours, then 200 units per hour for 5 days. Monitoring of plasma anti-factor Xa activity is recommended for patients with renal impairment, or those weighing more than 90 kg.

◊ References.
1. Von Bonsdorff M, *et al.* A new low molecular weight heparinoid Org 10172 as anticoagulant in hemodialysis. *Int J Artif Organs* 1990; **13:** 103–8.
2. de Valk HW, *et al.* Comparing subcutaneous danaparoid with intravenous unfractionated heparin for the treatment of venous thromboembolism: a randomized controlled trial. *Ann Intern Med* 1995; **123:** 1–9.
3. Skoutakis VA. Danaparoid in the prevention of thromboembolic complications. *Ann Pharmacother* 1997; **31:** 876–87.
4. Wilde MI, Markham A. Danaparoid: a review of its pharmacology and clinical use in the management of heparin-induced thrombocytopenia. *Drugs* 1997; **54:** 903–24.
5. The Publications Committee for the Trial of ORG 10172 in Acute Stroke Treatment (TOAST) Investigators. Low molecular weight heparinoid, ORG 10172 (danaparoid), and outcome after acute ischemic stroke: a randomized controlled trial. *JAMA* 1998; **279:** 1265–72.

Preparations

Proprietary Preparations (details are given in Part 3)
Austral.: Orgaran; *Canad.:* Orgaran; *Fr.:* Orgaran; *Ger.:* Orgaran; *Neth.:* Orgaran; *NZ:* Orgaran; *Swed.:* Orgaran; *UK:* Orgaran; *USA:* Orgaran.

Debrisoquine Sulfate (860-l)

Debrisoquine Sulfate *(rINNM)*.
Debrisoquine Sulfate *(USAN)*; Debrisoquine Sulphate *(BANM)*; Isocaramidine Sulphate; Ro-5-3307/1. 1,2,3,4-Tetrahydroisoquinoline-2-carboxamidine sulphate.
$(C_{10}H_{13}N_3)_2, H_2SO_4 = 448.5.$
CAS — 1131-64-2 (debrisoquine); 581-88-4 (debrisoquine sulfate).
Pharmacopoeias. In *Br.*

Debrisoquine sulfate 12.8 mg is approximately equivalent to 10 mg of debrisoquine.

Pharmacopoeial description
BP 2001: A white, odourless or almost odourless, crystalline powder. Sparingly soluble in water; very slightly soluble in alcohol; practically insoluble in chloroform and in ether. A 3% solution in water has a pH of 5.3 to 6.8. Protect from light.

Adverse Effects, Treatment, and Precautions

As for Guanethidine Monosulfate, p.901.

Diarrhoea is rare with debrisoquine sulfate. Abrupt cessation of treatment should be avoided as this may lead to rebound hypertension.

The metabolism of debrisoquine is subject to genetic polymorphism and non-metabolisers may show a marked response to doses that have little or no effect in metabolisers.

Interactions

As for Guanethidine Monosulfate, p.901.

Pharmacokinetics

Debrisoquine is rapidly absorbed from the gastrointestinal tract. The major metabolite is 4-hydroxydebrisoquine; metabolism is subject to genetic polymorphism.

◊ A study[1] in 15 hypertensive patients and 4 healthy subjects indicated that debrisoquine undergoes pre-systemic metabolism to 4-hydroxydebrisoquine, but the mechanism appears to be saturable and increases in the dose of debrisoquine could therefore produce disproportionate decreases in blood pressure. The estimated half-life of elimination for debrisoquine and 4-hydroxydebrisoquine ranged from 11.5 to 26 hours and from 5.8 to 14.5 hours respectively.
1. Silas JH, *et al.* The disposition of debrisoquine in hypertensive patients. *Br J Clin Pharmacol* 1978; **5:** 27–34.

Genetic polymorphism. Debrisoquine, along with sparteine and a number of other drugs, is a substrate for the cytochrome P450 isoenzyme CYP2D6, a polymorphic enzyme coded by a gene mapped to chromosome 22. Patients homozygous for the mutant allele are termed poor metabolisers and express little or no active enzyme. The prevalence of the poor-metaboliser phenotype is about 5% in most Caucasian populations, while studies in other genetic groups have indicated a range of about 2 to 10% although in some groups, such as the Japanese, poor metabolisers have yet to be identified. Poor metabolisers of debrisoquine are unable to 4-hydroxylate the drug adequately to its inactive metabolite and are thus prone to excessive hypotension. A number of other drugs are metabolised by the same enzyme, including: antidepressants such as amitriptyline, imipramine, and nortriptyline; other antihypertensives such as indoramin; antiarrhythmics such as encainide, flecainide, and propafenone; analgesics such as phenacetin; beta blockers such as metoprolol, propranolol, and timolol; hypoglycaemics such as phenformin; and opioids such as codeine and dextromethorphan. However, the clinical consequences of polymorphism in patients receiving these drugs depend on the relative activity and toxicity of parent drug and metabolite, and the availability and relative importance of other routes of metabolism. Determination of phenotype is generally performed by administration of a test drug such as debrisoquine and assay of parent drug and metabolite in urine collected over a defined period of time.
References.
1. Relling MV. Polymorphic drug metabolism. *Clin Pharm* 1989; **8:** 852–63.

Uses and Administration

Debrisoquine is an antihypertensive with actions and uses similar to those of guanethidine (p.901), but it causes less depletion of noradrenaline stores. When given by mouth, debrisoquine is reported to act within about 4 to 10 hours and to have effects lasting for 9 to 24 hours. It is used in the management of hypertension (p.802), but has largely been superseded by other drugs.

Debrisoquine is given by mouth as the sulfate, but doses are usually expressed in terms of the base.

The usual initial dose is 10 to 20 mg once or twice daily. The daily dose is then increased by 10 to 20 mg, according to the severity of the condition, every 3 or 4 days. The usual maintenance dose is 20 to 120 mg daily, but 300 mg or more daily may be given.

For reference to the use of debrisoquine in identifying metabolic phenotypes, see under Genetic Polymorphism, above.

Preparations

Proprietary Preparations (details are given in Part 3)
UK: Declinax.

Defibrotide (18626-y)

Defibrotide *(BAN, rINN)*.
ATC — B01AX01.

Polydeoxyribonucleotides from bovine lung with molecular weight between 45 000 and 55 000.

Profile

Defibrotide is a deoxyribonucleic acid derivative that has antithrombotic and fibrinolytic properties. Defibrotide's mechanism of action is uncertain; it appears to increase levels of prostaglandin E_2 and prostacyclin, to alter platelet activity, and to increase tissue plasminogen activator function at the same time as decreasing activity of tissue plasminogen activator inhibitor. It is used in the management of thromboembolic disorders. Oral and parenteral formulations have been used in doses of up to 800 mg daily.

◊ References.
1. Palmer KJ, Goa KL. Defibrotide: a review of its pharmacodynamic and pharmacokinetic properties, and therapeutic use in vascular disorders. *Drugs* 1993; **45:** 259–94.

Preparations
Proprietary Preparations (details are given in Part 3)
Ital.: Noravid; Prociclide.

Delapril Hydrochloride (2850-m)
Delapril Hydrochloride (USAN, rINNM).
Alindapril Hydrochloride; CV-3317; Indalapril Hydrochloride; REV-6000A. Ethyl (S)-2-{[(S)-1-(carboxymethyl-2-indanylcarbamoyl)ethyl]amino}-4-phenylbutyrate hydrochloride.
$C_{26}H_{32}N_2O_5,HCl = 489.0$.
CAS — 83435-66-9 (delapril); 83435-67-0 (delapril hydrochloride).

Profile
Delapril is an ACE inhibitor (p.820). It is converted in the body to two metabolites to which it owes its activity. It is given by mouth as the hydrochloride in the treatment of hypertension (p.802), in usual maintenance doses of 30 to 60 mg daily in two divided doses.

Preparations
Proprietary Preparations (details are given in Part 3)
Ital.: Delaket; *Jpn:* Adecut; *Singapore:* Cupressin; *Thai.:* Cupressin.
Multi-ingredient: *Ital.:* Delapride; Dinapres.

Denopamine (19049-b)
Denopamine (rINN).
TA-064. (−)-(R)-α-{[(3,4-Dimethoxyphenethyl)amino]methyl}-p-hydroxybenzyl alcohol.
$C_{18}H_{23}NO_4 = 317.4$.
CAS — 71771-90-9.

Profile
Denopamine is an oral sympathomimetic (see Adrenaline, p.829) with predominantly beta-adrenergic activity selective to beta₁ receptors. It acts as a partial agonist (see Xamoterol, p.998) and is used for the treatment of heart failure (p.798). The usual dose is 15 to 30 mg daily in three divided doses.

Preparations
Proprietary Preparations (details are given in Part 3)
Jpn: Kalgut.

Dermatan Sulfate (10810-a)
Dermatan Sulphate; LMW-DS (depolymerised dermatan sulfate); MF-701; OP-370 (depolymerised dermatan sulfate).
CAS — 54328-33-5 (dermatan sodium sulfate).

Profile
Dermatan sulfate is a naturally occurring glycosaminoglycan used as an anticoagulant for prophylaxis of venous thromboembolism (p.817). It is given as the sodium salt in a dose of 100 to 300 mg daily by intramuscular injection. The dose may be increased to 300 mg twice daily in patients at high risk of thromboembolism, such as those undergoing major orthopaedic surgery.
Dermatan sulfate is a component of sulodexide (p.978) and its sodium salt is a component of danaparoid sodium (p.866).
Dermatan sulfate is under investigation for the treatment of venous thromboembolism, heparin-induced thrombocytopenia, and to prevent clotting during haemodialysis. Low-molecular-weight (depolymerised) dermatan sulfate is also being studied.

◊ References.
1. Dawes J, *et al.* The pharmacokinetics of dermatan sulphate MF701 in healthy human volunteers. *Br J Clin Pharmacol* 1991; **32:** 361–6.
2. Lane DA, *et al.* Dermatan sulphate in haemodialysis. *Lancet* 1992; **339:** 334–5.
3. Cofrancesco E, *et al.* Dermatan sulphate in acute leukaemia. *Lancet* 1992; **339:** 1177–8.
4. Agnelli G, *et al.* Randomised, double-blind, placebo-controlled trial of dermatan sulphate for prevention of deep vein thrombosis in hip fracture. *Thromb Haemost* 1992; **67:** 203–8.
5. Gianese F, *et al.* The pharmacokinetics and pharmacodynamics of dermatan sulphate MF701 during haemodialysis for chronic renal failure. *Br J Clin Pharmacol* 1993; **35:** 335–9.
6. Legnani C, *et al.* Acute and chronic effects of a new low molecular weight dermatan sulphate (Desmin 370) on blood coagulation and fibrinolysis in healthy subjects. *Eur J Clin Pharmacol* 1994; **47:** 247–52.
7. Miglioli M, *et al.* Bioavailability of Desmin, a low molecular weight dermatan sulfate, after subcutaneous administration to healthy volunteers. *Int J Clin Lab Res* 1997; **27:** 195–8.
8. Taliani MR *et al.* Dermatan sulphate in patients with heparin-induced thrombocytopenia. *Br J Haematol* 1999; **104:** 87–9.
9. Di Carlo V, *et al.* Dermatan sulphate for the prevention of postoperative venous thromboembolism in patients with cancer. *Thromb Haemost* 1999; **82:** 30–4.

The symbol † denotes a preparation no longer actively marketed

Preparations
Proprietary Preparations (details are given in Part 3)
Ital.: Aclotan; Mistral.

Deserpidine (861-y)
Deserpidine (BAN, rINN).
Canescine; 11-Desmethoxyreserpine; Raunormine; Recanescine. Methyl 11-demethoxy-O-(3,4,5-trimethoxybenzoyl)reserpate.
$C_{32}H_{38}N_2O_8 = 578.7$.
CAS — 131-01-1.
ATC — C02AA05.

An ester alkaloid isolated from the root of *Rauwolfia canescens.*

Profile
Deserpidine has properties similar to those described under reserpine (p.967) and has been used in the treatment of hypertension and psychoses.

Preparations
Proprietary Preparations (details are given in Part 3)
Multi-ingredient: *Hong Kong:* Enduronyl; *Ital.:* Enduronil; *USA:* Enduronyl.

Desirudin (17413-z)
Desirudin (BAN, USAN, rINN).
CGP-39393. 63-Desulfohirudin (*Hirudo medicinalis* isoform HV1).
$C_{287}H_{440}N_{80}O_{110}S_6 = 6963.4$.
CAS — 120993-53-5.
ATC — B01AX02.

Adverse Effects and Precautions
The most common adverse effect of desirudin is bleeding. Hypersensitivity reactions have been reported. Local haematoma may occur if desirudin is administered by intramuscular injection and it should therefore not be given by this route.
Desirudin is contra-indicated in patients with active bleeding or irreversible coagulation disorders, and in those with severe renal or hepatic impairment, severe hypertension, or bacterial endocarditis. Desirudin should be used with caution in patients at increased risk of bleeding including those with haemorrhagic blood disorders, recent major bleeding, cerebrovascular disorders, or patients who have recently undergone major surgery, or biopsy or puncture of a noncompressible vessel. Teratogenicity has been observed in *animals.*

Interactions
Use of desirudin with anticoagulants or drugs that affect platelet function may increase the risk of bleeding.

Pharmacokinetics
Maximum plasma concentrations of desirudin are reached 1 to 3 hours after subcutaneous injection. Desirudin is metabolised and excreted by the kidney, and 40 to 50% of a dose is excreted unchanged in the urine. Following intravenous injection the terminal elimination half-life of desirudin is 2 to 3 hours.

◊ References.
1. Lefèvre G, *et al.* Effect of renal impairment on the pharmacokinetics and pharmacodynamics of desirudin. *Clin Pharmacol Ther* 1997; **62:** 50–9.

Uses and Administration
Desirudin is a recombinant hirudin (p.905) that is a direct inhibitor of thrombin. It is used as an anticoagulant for the prevention of postoperative venous thromboembolism (p.817) in patients undergoing hip and knee replacement surgery. It has been investigated in arterial thromboembolic disorders such as myocardial infarction and unstable angina, and as an adjunct in angioplasty procedures (see under Uses and Administration of Lepirudin, p.920).
In the prevention of venous thromboembolism, desirudin is administered subcutaneously in a dose of 15 mg twice daily. The first dose is given 5 to 15 minutes before surgery, but after induction of regional block anaesthesia, if used, and then continued until

the patient is fully ambulant, usually for 9 to a maximum of 12 days.
Response to desirudin should be monitored using activated partial thromboplastin time (APTT) in patients with renal or hepatic impairment, or increased risk of bleeding.

◊ References.
1. Matheson AJ, Goa KL. Desirudin: a review of its use in the management of thrombotic disorders. *Drugs* 2000; **60:** 679–700.

Preparations
Proprietary Preparations (details are given in Part 3)
Austral.: Revasc; *Fin.:* Revasc; *Fr.:* Revasc; *Ger.:* Revasc; *Irl.:* Revasc; *NZ:* Revasc; *Spain:* Revasc; *Swed.:* Revasc; *Switz.:* Revasc; *UK:* Revasc†.

Deslanoside (5809-m)
Deslanoside (BAN, rINN).
Deacetyl-lanatoside C; Desacetyl-lanatoside C; Deslanosídeo; Deslanosidum. 3-[(O-β-D-Glucopyranosyl-(1→4)-O-2,6-dideoxy-β-D-*ribo*-hexopyranosyl-(1→4)-O-2,6-dideoxy-β-D-*ribo*-hexopyranosyl-(1→4)-O-2,6-dideoxy-β-D-*ribo*-hexopyranosyl)oxy]-12,14-dihydroxy-3β,5β,12β-card-20(22)-enolide.
$C_{47}H_{74}O_{19} = 943.1$.
CAS — 17598-65-1.
ATC — C01AA07.
Pharmacopoeias. In Chin., Eur. (see p.vi), Jpn, and US.

Pharmacopoeial description
Ph. Eur.: A white, crystalline or finely crystalline hygroscopic powder. Practically insoluble in water and in ether; very slightly soluble in alcohol. In an atmosphere of low relative humidity, it loses water. Store in airtight, glass containers at a temperature below 10°. Protect from light.
USP 25: Store in airtight containers. Protect from light.

Profile
Deslanoside, a cardiac glycoside with positive inotropic activity, is a derivative of lanatoside C. It has the general properties of digoxin (p.870) and has been used similarly in the management of some cardiac arrhythmias (p.794) and in heart failure (p.798).
Deslanoside is usually reserved for emergency treatment although digoxin is generally preferred. Its effects occur about 5 to 10 minutes after intravenous administration and the full action on the heart is exerted after about 2 hours. It has a half-life of about 33 hours and its effects persist for 2 to 5 days.
A rapid digitalising dose of deslanoside is up to 1.6 mg given by intravenous injection as a single dose or in two divided doses. Maintenance treatment with a cardiac glycoside given by mouth may be started within 12 hours of parenteral digitalisation with deslanoside.

Preparations
USP 25: Deslanoside Injection.
Proprietary Preparations (details are given in Part 3)
Aust.: Cedilanid; *Braz.:* Cedilanide; Desacil; *Fr.:* Cedilanide†.
Multi-ingredient: *Braz.:* Gratusminal.

Dextrothyroxine Sodium (9004-r)
Dextrothyroxine Sodium (BANM, USAN, rINN).
Sodium Dextrothyroxine; 3,5,3',5'-Tetraiodo-D-thyronine Sodium; D-Thyroxine Sodium. Sodium 4-O-(4-hydroxy-3,5-di-iodophenyl)-3,5-di-iodo-D-tyrosinate hydrate.
$C_{15}H_{10}I_4NNaO_4(+ xH_2O) = 798.9$ (anhydrous).
CAS — 51-49-0 (dextrothyroxine); 137-53-1 (anhydrous dextrothyroxine sodium); 7054-08-2 (dextrothyroxine sodium hydrate).

Adverse Effects
Most adverse effects of dextrothyroxine are due to the drug's metabolic activity. Cardiac changes include angina pectoris, extrasystoles, ectopic beats, supraventricular tachycardia, and ECG evidence of ischaemic heart disease.
Other adverse effects include insomnia, nervousness, tremor, diuresis, loss of weight, sweating, flushing, fever, alopecia, menstrual irregularities, nausea, vomiting, decreased appetite, diarrhoea, constipation, skin rashes, and pruritus. The development of gallstones has also occasionally been reported. The general adverse effects of thyroid hormones are described on p.1526.

Effects on the heart. In the Coronary Drug Project, treatment with dextrothyroxine sodium was stopped after 36 months when it was found that the mortality in the 1083 patients receiving it was 18.4% higher than in those receiving placebo.[1] The excess mortality was mainly due to deaths from coronary and other cardiovascular causes, and was concentrated in a subgroup of patients with pre-existing cardiovascular disease or hypertension: the incidence of recurrent non-fatal myocardial infarction was also higher.
Adverse effects included, in addition to cardiovascular disorders, decreased glucose tolerance, possible abnormalities of hepatic function, and hypermetabolism attributable to hyper-

thyroid activity. Dextrothyroxine used in the study was shown to contain less than 0.5% of levothyroxine, equivalent to less than 30 µg of levothyroxine from the daily dose of 6 mg of dextrothyroxine. However, samples of commercially available dextrothyroxine were found to contain 0.8 to 1.0% of levothyroxine.[2]

1. The Coronary Drug Project Research Group. The Coronary Drug Project: findings leading to further modifications of its protocol with respect to dextrothyroxine. *JAMA* 1972; **220:** 996–1008.
2. Scheiffele E, Schultze KW. The Coronary Drug Project. *JAMA* 1972; **221:** 918.

Hyperthyroidism. Hyperthyroidism occurred in a patient during treatment with dextrothyroxine 4 mg daily.[1] The patient became euthyroid when dextrothyroxine was discontinued and symptoms recurred when dextrothyroxine was reintroduced.

1. Hazenburg HJA, *et al.* Dextrothyroxine induced hyperthyroidism in a patient with heterozygous familial hypercholesterolaemia. *Neth J Med* 1987; **31:** 117–21.

Precautions
Dextrothyroxine is contra-indicated in patients with hypertension or heart disease including angina pectoris, myocardial infarction, cardiac arrhythmias, and heart failure. It is also contra-indicated in patients with advanced liver or kidney disease. The precautions to be taken with thyroid hormones in general are described on p.1527.

Interactions
Dextrothyroxine may enhance the effects of anticoagulants. It may increase the requirements of insulin or oral hypoglycaemics. The interactions of thyroid hormones in general are described on p.1527.

Uses and Administration
Dextrothyroxine is the D-isomer of thyroxine [levothyroxine] but has only weak thyroid hormone activity. It is a lipid regulating drug that reduces elevated plasma-cholesterol concentrations, particularly the low-density lipoprotein (LDL) fraction.

Dextrothyroxine is used as the sodium salt in the treatment of hypercholesterolaemia in type II hyperlipoproteinaemia (p.800) but this use is severely limited by cardiotoxicity. The initial dose is 1 to 2 mg daily, increased by 1 to 2 mg at monthly intervals until a satisfactory response is achieved, up to a maximum of 4 to 8 mg daily by mouth.

Dextrothyroxine was formerly used to treat hypothyroidism.

Preparations
Proprietary Preparations (details are given in Part 3)
Canad.: Choloxin†; *Ger.:* Dynothel; *USA:* Choloxin†.

Diazoxide (862-j)

Diazoxide (*BAN, USAN, rINN*).

Diazoxidum; NSC-64198; Sch-6783; SRG-95213. 7-Chloro-3-methyl-2*H*-1,2,4-benzothiadiazine 1,1-dioxide.

$C_8H_7ClN_2O_2S = 230.7$.

CAS — 364-98-7.
ATC — C02DA01; V03AH01.

Pharmacopoeias. In Eur. (see p.vi), Int., and US.

Liquid preparations should be stored protected from light.

Pharmacopoeial description
Ph. Eur.: A white or almost white, fine or crystalline powder. Practically insoluble in water; slightly soluble in alcohol; freely soluble in dimethylformamide; practically insoluble in ether. It is very soluble in dilute solutions of alkali hydroxides.

USP 25: White or cream-white crystals or crystalline powder. Practically insoluble to sparingly soluble in water and in most organic solvents; freely soluble in dimethylformamide; very soluble in strong alkaline solutions.

Adverse Effects
In addition to inappropriate hypotension and hyperglycaemia (which includes ketoacidosis and hyperosmolar nonketotic coma), side-effects during prolonged therapy frequently include oedema due to salt and water retention, which may result in precipitation of heart failure. Other adverse effects include: dysgeusia, nausea, anorexia, and other gastrointestinal disturbances; mild hyperuricaemia; extrapyramidal symptoms; eosinophilia and thrombocytopenia; dyspnoea; hypertrichosis; and headache, dizziness, tinnitus, and blurred vision. Hypersensitivity has occurred, manifesting as rashes, leucopenia, and fever.

Alopecia has been reported in infants born to mothers taking diazoxide.

During intravenous therapy, particularly after large intravenous boluses, adverse effects may be associated with a too rapid reduction in the blood pressure and include: coronary ischaemia leading to angina, cardiac arrhythmias, marked ECG changes, tachycardia, palpitations, and bradycardia; cerebral ischaemia leading to confusion, convulsions, loss of conscious-

ness, and neurological deficit; impaired renal function; and symptoms of vasodilatation.

Diazoxide may cause a burning sensation in the vein used for injection; extravasation of the alkaline solution is painful.

Effects on the blood. A 26-year-old man with hypertension developed reversible haemolytic anaemia when treated with diazoxide by mouth on 3 separate occasions.[1]

1. Best RA, Clink HM. Haemolysis associated with diazoxide, used for the control of hypertension. *Postgrad Med J* 1975; **51:** 402–4.

Effects on the hair. *Hirsutism* and *hypertrichosis* are different types of excessive hair growth, but the terms have often been used interchangeably. Hirsutism is androgen-related whereas hypertrichosis is thought to be independent from hormone stimulation. Hypertrichosis is acknowledged to be a frequent adverse effect of diazoxide in children receiving long-term treatment for idiopathic hypoglycaemia.[1] Two such children had unusually deep (low-pitched) voices as well as marked hypertrichosis.[2] A woman on continuous diazoxide therapy who developed so-called hirsutism without signs of virilisation had raised serum concentrations of androgens.[3]

Alopecia has been reported in infants born to mothers who had been on long-term treatment with diazoxide during pregnancy.

1. Burton JL, *et al.* Hypertrichosis due to diazoxide. *Br J Dermatol* 1975; **93:** 707–11.
2. West RJ. Side effects of diazoxide. *BMJ* 1978; **2:** 506.
3. Hallengren B, Hökfelt B. Increase of serum androgens during diazoxide treatment. *Lancet* 1984; **ii:** 1044–5.

Extrapyramidal effects. In a study[1] of 100 hypertensive patients receiving diazoxide, the incidence of extrapyramidal symptoms was 15%.

1. Pohl JEF. Development and management of extrapyramidal symptoms in hypertensive patients treated with diazoxide. *Am Heart J* 1975; **89:** 401–2.

Pancreatitis. Ten patients with severe hypertension and renal failure were treated with diazoxide in a last attempt to avert nephrectomy; 1 patient developed acute pancreatitis and another diabetic ketoacidosis.[1] Both patients recovered from these effects when diazoxide was withdrawn.

1. De Broe M, *et al.* Oral diazoxide for malignant hypertension. *Lancet* 1972; **i:** 1397.

Voice changes. In addition to marked hypertrichosis, 2 children who had received diazoxide for several years were noted to have unusually deep (low-pitched) voices.[1]

1. West RJ. Side effects of diazoxide. *BMJ* 1978; **2:** 506.

Treatment of Adverse Effects
Treatment is largely symptomatic. Severe hyperglycaemia may be corrected by giving insulin: less severe hyperglycaemia may respond to oral hypoglycaemics. Hypotension may be managed with intravenous fluids. Severe hypotension may require sympathomimetics. Antiparkinsonian drugs, such as procyclidine, have been given to control extrapyramidal effects while a diuretic may be required for salt and water retention. Diazoxide can be removed from the body by dialysis but recovery is relatively low owing to extensive protein binding.

Precautions
Diazoxide should be used with care in patients with impaired cardiac or cerebral circulation and in patients with aortic coarctation, arteriovenous shunt, or other cardiac disorders in which an increase in cardiac output could be detrimental. During prolonged therapy blood-glucose concentrations and blood pressure should be monitored and the blood should be examined regularly for signs of leucopenia and thrombocytopenia; in children, bone and psychological maturation and growth should be regularly assessed. Caution is necessary in patients with renal impairment.

If given during labour, diazoxide may cause cessation of uterine contractions and delay delivery unless oxytocin is given concomitantly.

Pregnancy. Transplacental transfer of diazoxide was considered to be responsible for an inappropriately low plasma-insulin concentration in an infant whose mother had received diazoxide 150 mg daily for 47 days prior to delivery.[1]

For reports of sedation, hypotonia, hypoventilation, or apnoea among infants born to mothers given both diazoxide and clomethiazole edisilate for the treatment of toxaemia of pregnancy, see Precautions, Pregnancy, in Clomethiazole Edisilate on p.668.

1. Smith MJ, *et al.* Neonatal hyperglycaemia after prolonged maternal treatment with diazoxide. *BMJ* 1982; **284:** 1234.

Interactions
The hyperglycaemic, hyperuricaemic, and hypotensive actions of diazoxide may be enhanced by diuret-

ics. Administration of diazoxide with other antihypertensives or vasodilators may lead to increased risk of hypotension.

Chlorpromazine. A report of chlorpromazine enhancing the hyperglycaemic effect of diazoxide in a 2-year-old child.[1]

1. Aynsley-Green A, Illig R. Enhancement by chlorpromazine of hyperglycaemic action of diazoxide. *Lancet* 1975; **ii:** 658–9.

Phenytoin. For the effect of diazoxide on serum-phenytoin concentrations, see p.360.

Pharmacokinetics
Diazoxide is readily absorbed from the gastrointestinal tract and more than 90% bound to plasma proteins, although protein binding is decreased in uraemic patients. Its plasma half-life has been estimated to range from about 20 to 45 hours but values of up to 60 hours have been reported. The half-life is reported to be prolonged in renal impairment and shorter for children. The plasma half-life greatly exceeds the duration of vascular activity. Diazoxide is partly metabolised in the liver and is excreted in the urine both unchanged and in the form of metabolites; only small amounts are recovered from the faeces. It crosses the placenta and the blood-brain barrier.

Children. A pharmacokinetic study of diazoxide in 4 children with hypoglycaemia revealed a plasma half-life of 9.5 to 24 hours, which is considerably shorter than that in adults.[1]

1. Pruitt AW, *et al.* Disposition of diazoxide in children. *Clin Pharmacol Ther* 1973; **14:** 73–82.

Uses and Administration
Diazoxide increases the concentration of glucose in the plasma; it inhibits the secretion of insulin by the beta cells of the pancreas, and may increase the hepatic output of glucose. When given intravenously, it produces a fall in blood pressure by a vasodilator effect on the arterioles and a reduction in peripheral resistance. Diazoxide is closely related structurally to the thiazide diuretics, but has an antidiuretic action and thus produces fluid and electrolyte retention; a diuretic may be given concomitantly to reduce fluid retention.

Diazoxide is used by mouth in the management of intractable hypoglycaemia (p.1010) and intravenously in the management of hypertensive crises (p.802), particularly when first-line drugs such as sodium nitroprusside are ineffective or unsuitable. Diazoxide is not given by mouth in the chronic treatment of hypertension because of the severity of the adverse effects produced.

In **hypoglycaemia,** diazoxide is given in an initial dose of 3 to 5 mg per kg body-weight daily in 2 or 3 divided doses by mouth, then the dosage is adjusted according to the needs of the patient. Usual maintenance doses are from 3 to 8 mg per kg daily but total doses of up to 1 g daily have been given to adults with insulinomas (p.483). In neonates and infants, the initial dose is 5 to 10 mg per kg daily in 2 or 3 divided doses; usual maintenance doses have ranged from 8 to 15 mg per kg daily, although up to 20 mg per kg daily may be given in children with leucine-sensitive hypoglycaemia. The hyperglycaemic effect normally begins within 1 hour of administration and lasts for up to 8 hours.

In **hypertensive crises,** a single bolus intravenous injection of 300 mg will produce a rapid fall in blood pressure, but such a rapid fall may be hazardous and injection of 1 to 3 mg per kg body-weight within 30 seconds, up to a maximum dose of 150 mg, and repeated after 5 to 15 minutes if required, is now preferred.

Reduced doses may be necessary in patients with impaired renal function.

Preparations
BP 2001: Diazoxide Injection; Diazoxide Tablets;
USP 25: Diazoxide Capsules; Diazoxide Injection; Diazoxide Oral Suspension.

Proprietary Preparations (details are given in Part 3)
Belg.: Hyperstat; *Braz.:* Tensuril; *Canad.:* Hyperstat; Proglycem; *Fr.:* Hyperstat†; Proglicem; *Ger.:* Hypertonalum; Proglicem; *Ital.:* Hyperstat; Proglicem; *Mex.:* Hyperstat; Sefulken; *Neth.:* Hyperstat; Proglicem; *S.Afr.:* Hyperstat; *Spain:* Hyperstat; *Swed.:*

Hyperstat; *Switz.:* Hyperstat; Proglicem; *UK:* Eudemine; *USA:* Hyperstat; Proglycem.

Diclofenamide (2325-v)

Diclofenamide (BAN, rINN).

Dichlorphenamide; Diclofenamidum. 4,5-Dichlorobenzene-1,3-disulphonamide.

$C_6H_6Cl_2N_2O_4S_2 = 305.2$.
CAS — 120-97-8.
ATC — S01EC02.

Pharmacopoeias. In Chin., Jpn, and US.

Profile

Diclofenamide is an inhibitor of carbonic anhydrase with properties similar to those of acetazolamide (p.826). When given by mouth, its effect begins within 1 hour and lasts for 6 to 12 hours.

Diclofenamide is used to reduce intra-ocular pressure in glaucoma (p.1413). The usual initial dose is 100 to 200 mg by mouth, then 100 mg every 12 hours until the desired response is obtained, followed by a maintenance dose of 25 to 50 mg one to three times daily. Diclofenamide sodium has been given by injection.

Preparations

USP 25: Dichlorphenamide Tablets.

Proprietary Preparations (details are given in Part 3)
Aust.: Glaucol; *Austral.:* Daranide†; *Belg.:* Oratrol; *Denm.:* Oralcon; *Hong Kong:* Oratrol; *Irl.:* Daranide†; *Ital.:* Antidrasi; Fenamide; Glaumid; *Spain:* Glauconide; Oratrol; *Swed.:* Oralcon; *Switz.:* Oratrol†; *USA:* Daranide.

Dicoumarol (4811-l)

Dicoumarol (rINN).

Bishydroxycoumarin; Dicoumarin; Dicumarol (USAN); Melitoxin. 3,3′-Methylenebis(4-hydroxycoumarin).

$C_{19}H_{12}O_6 = 336.3$.
CAS — 66-76-2.
ATC — B01AA01.

Pharmacopoeias. In Int.

Adverse Effects, Treatment, and Precautions

As for Warfarin Sodium, p.992, although gastrointestinal side-effects are reported to occur more frequently. The absorption of dicoumarol is affected by food.

Interactions

The interactions associated with oral anticoagulants are discussed in detail under warfarin (p.993). Specific references to interactions involving dicoumarol can be found under the headings for the following drug groups: analgesics; antiarrhythmics; antibacterials; antidepressants; antidiabetics; antiepileptics; antigout drugs; anxiolytic sedatives; gastrointestinal drugs; lipid regulating drugs; sex hormones; and vitamins.

Pharmacokinetics

Dicoumarol is slowly and erratically absorbed from the gastrointestinal tract and is extensively bound to plasma proteins. It is metabolised in the liver and is excreted in the urine, mainly as metabolites.

Uses and Administration

Dicoumarol is an orally administered coumarin anticoagulant with actions similar to those of warfarin (p.998). It is used in the management of thromboembolic disorders (p.816). The initial dose of dicoumarol is usually 200 to 300 mg with a daily maintenance dose according to coagulation tests of 25 to 200 mg.

Because of its unpredictability of response and high incidence of gastrointestinal effects, dicoumarol has been largely replaced by warfarin.

Preparations

Proprietary Preparations (details are given in Part 3)
Swed.: Apekumarol†.

Digitalis Leaf (5812-r)

Digit. Fol.; Digit. Leaf; Digitale Pourprée; Digitalis; Digitalis Folium; Digitalis Purpureae Folium; Feuille de Digitale; Fingerhutblatt; Folha de Dedaleira; Foxglove Leaf; Hoja de Digital.

ATC — C01AA03.

NOTE. The term 'digitalis' is often used to describe the entire class of cardiac glycosides.

Pharmacopoeias. In Chin., Eur. (see p.vi), Jpn, and US.

Digitalis leaf contains a number of glycosides, including digitoxin, gitoxin, and gitaloxin.

Pharmacopoeial description

Ph. Eur.: The dried leaf of *Digitalis purpurea*. It contains not less than 0.3% of cardenolic glycosides, expressed as digitoxin, and calculated with reference to the drug dried at 100° to 105°. Protect from light and moisture.

USP 25: The dried leaf of *Digitalis purpurea* (Scrophulariaceae). The potency is such that, when assayed as directed, 100 mg

is equivalent to not less than 1 USP unit. Store in containers that protect it from absorbing moisture.

Profile

Digitalis contains cardiac glycosides with positive inotropic activity and has the general properties described under digoxin (p.870). It has been used similarly in the management of heart failure. However, when treatment with a cardiac glycoside is required a single glycoside is preferred to digitalis, and digoxin or digitoxin are most commonly used.

Digitalis is used in herbal and homoeopathic medicine.

Preparations

USP 25: Digitalis Capsules; Digitalis Tablets.

Proprietary Preparations (details are given in Part 3)
Ger.: Digophton.

Multi-ingredient: *Aust.:* Augentropfen Stulln; *Ger.:* Augentropfen Stulln Mono; Unguentum lymphaticum; *Switz.:* Augentonicum; Collypan.

Digitalis Lanata Leaf (5814-d)

Austrian Digitalis; Austrian Foxglove; Digitalis Lanatae Folium; Woolly Foxglove Leaf.

CAS — 17575-20-1 (lanatoside A).

Pharmacopoeias. In Aust.

The dried leaves of the woolly foxglove, *Digitalis lanata* (Scrophulariaceae), containing about 1 to 1.4% of a mixture of cardioactive glycosides, including digoxin, digitoxin, acetyldigoxin, acetyldigitoxin, lanatoside A, and deslanoside.

Profile

Digitalis lanata leaf is used as a source for the manufacture of digoxin and other glycosides.

◊ There have been reports[1] of toxicity following ingestion of dietary supplements contaminated with digitalis lanata.

1. Slifman NR, et al. Contamination of botanical dietary supplements by digitalis lanata. N Engl J Med 1998; 339: 806–11.

Digitoxin (5815-n)

Digitoxin (BAN, rINN).

Digitaline Cristallisée; Digitoxinum; Digitoxoside. 3β-[(O-2,6-Dideoxy-β-D-ribo-hexopyranosyl-(1→4)-O-2,6-dideoxy-β-D-ribo-hexopyranosyl-(1→4)-2,6-dideoxy-β-D-ribo-hexopyranosyl)oxy]-14β-hydroxy-5β-card-20(22)-enolide.

$C_{41}H_{64}O_{13} = 764.9$.
CAS — 71-63-6.
ATC — C01AA04.

Pharmacopoeias. In Chin., Eur. (see p.vi), Int., Jpn, and US.

Pharmacopoeial description

Ph. Eur.: A white or almost white powder. Practically insoluble in water; slightly soluble in alcohol and in methyl alcohol; freely soluble in a mixture of equal volumes of chloroform and methyl alcohol. Protect from light.

USP 25: A cardiotonic glycoside obtained from *Digitalis purpurea*, *Digitalis lanata* (Scrophulariaceae), or other suitable species of *Digitalis*. A white or pale buff-coloured, odourless, microcrystalline powder. Practically insoluble in water; soluble 1 in 150 of alcohol and 1 in 40 of chloroform; very slightly soluble in ether. Store in airtight containers.

Adsorption. Binding to an inline intravenous filter containing a cellulose ester membrane accounted for a reduction in digitoxin concentration of up to 25% from solutions of digitoxin 200 μg in 50 mL of glucose 5% or sodium chloride 0.9%.[1] Pretreatment of the filter with a polymer coating reduced adsorbance by about half.[2]

Digitoxin was found to be adsorbed onto glass and plastic in substantial amounts from simple aqueous solutions but not from solutions in 30% alcohol, or in plasma, or urine.[3]

1. Butler LD, et al. Effect of inline filtration on the potency of low-dose drugs. Am J Hosp Pharm 1980; 37: 935–41.
2. Kanke M, et al. Binding of selected drugs to a "treated" inline filter. Am J Hosp Pharm 1983; 40: 1323–8.
3. Molin L, et al. Solubility, partition, and adsorption of digitalis glycosides. Acta Pharm Suec 1983; 20: 129–44.

Adverse Effects, Treatment, and Precautions

As for Digoxin, below. Toxicity may be more prolonged after withdrawal of digitoxin because of the longer half-life.

◊ References.

1. Lely AH, van Enter CHJ. Large-scale digitoxin intoxication. BMJ 1970; 3: 737–40.
2. Gilfrich H-J, et al. Treatment of massive digitoxin overdose by charcoal haemoperfusion and cholestyramine. Lancet 1978; i: 505.
3. Pond S, et al. Treatment of digitoxin overdose with oral activated charcoal. Lancet 1981; ii: 1177–8.
4. Kurowski V, et al. Treatment of a patient with severe digitoxin intoxication by Fab fragments of anti-digitalis antibodies. Intensive Care Med 1992; 18: 439–42.
5. Schmitt K, et al. Massive digitoxin intoxication treated with digoxin-specific antibodies in a child. Pediatr Cardiol 1994; 15: 48–9.

Interactions

As for Digoxin, below. Since digitoxin is significantly metabolised in the liver it may be affected by drugs that induce micro-

somal enzymes, including rifampicin (see below) and antiepileptics such as phenobarbital.

Antibacterials. Acute heart failure has been reported in a patient taking digitoxin when treatment with *rifampicin* and isoniazid was started with plasma-digitoxin concentrations falling from a pretreatment steady-state value of 27 nanograms per mL to 10 nanograms per mL. The reduction in the digitoxin concentration was attributed to induction of digitoxin metabolism by rifampicin.[1]

Digitoxin toxicity has been described in 2 patients following addition of *azithromycin* to their therapy.[2]

1. Boman G, et al. Acute cardiac failure during treatment with digitoxin—an interaction with rifampicin. Br J Clin Pharmacol 1980; 10: 89–90.
2. Thalhammer F, et al. Azithromycin-related toxic effects of digitoxin. Br J Clin Pharmacol 1998; 45: 91–2.

Antineoplastics and immunosuppressants. A mean overall increase of 109% was seen in digitoxin clearance in 5 patients during concomitant treatment with *aminoglutethimide*. The interaction was attributed to the induction of hepatic enzymes by aminoglutethimide.[1]

1. Lønning PE, et al. Effect of aminoglutethimide on antipyrine, theophylline, and digitoxin disposition in breast cancer. Clin Pharmacol Ther 1984; 36: 796–802.

Calcium-channel blockers. Steady-state concentrations of digitoxin in the plasma increased by an average of 35% over 2 to 3 weeks in 8 of 10 patients when *verapamil* 240 mg daily was added to their therapy. Total body clearance and extra-renal clearance of digitoxin were reduced by 27% and 29% respectively although renal excretion was unchanged. Plasma-digitoxin concentrations increased by a mean of 21% in 5 of 10 patients treated with *diltiazem* but were not increased by concomitant treatment with *nifedipine*.[1]

1. Kuhlman J. Effects of verapamil, diltiazem, and nifedipine on plasma levels and renal excretion of digitoxin. Clin Pharmacol Ther 1985; 38: 667–73.

Diuretics. *Spironolactone* has been reported to decrease the half-life and the urinary elimination of unchanged digitoxin when given for at least 10 days to 8 patients on oral maintenance digitoxin therapy.[1] However, increased digitoxin half-life has been reported[2] in 3 healthy subjects when spironolactone was added to digitoxin therapy. The interaction was judged to be of minor clinical importance.

1. Wirth KE. Metabolism of digitoxin in man and its modification by spironolactone. Eur J Clin Pharmacol 1976; 9: 345–54.
2. Carruthers SG, Dujovne CA. Cholestyramine and spironolactone and their combination in digitoxin elimination. Clin Pharmacol Ther 1980; 27: 184–7.

Pharmacokinetics

Digitoxin is readily and completely absorbed from the gastrointestinal tract. Therapeutic plasma concentrations may range from 10 to 35 nanograms per mL but there is considerable interindividual variation. Digitoxin is more than 90% bound to plasma proteins. It is very slowly eliminated from the body and is metabolised in the liver. Most metabolites are inactive; the major active metabolite is digoxin. Enterohepatic recycling occurs and digitoxin is excreted in the urine, mainly as metabolites. It is also excreted in the faeces and this route becomes significant in renal impairment. Digitoxin has an elimination half-life of up to 7 days or more. The half-life is generally unchanged in renal impairment.

The pharmacokinetics of digitoxin may be affected by age and by concurrent diseases (see under Uses and Administration, below).

Uses and Administration

Digitoxin is a cardiac glycoside with positive inotropic activity. It has actions similar to those of digoxin (below) and is used in the management of some cardiac arrhythmias (p.794) and in heart failure (p.798).

Digitoxin is the most potent of the digitalis glycosides and is the most cumulative in action. The onset of its action is slower than that of the other cardiac glycosides and it may therefore be less suitable than digoxin for rapid digitalisation; following oral administration its effects may be evident in about 2 hours and its full effects in about 12 hours. Its effects persist for about 3 weeks.

As described under digoxin, dosage should be carefully adjusted to the needs of the individual patient. Steady-state therapeutic plasma concentrations of digitoxin may range from 10 to 35 nanograms per mL; higher values may be associated with toxicity. In adults an initial dose of 600 μg of digitoxin by mouth may be given for rapid digitalisation, followed by 400 μg after 4 to 6 hours, then 200 μg every 4 to 6 hours as necessary; the maximum total dose is usually 1.6 mg. For slow digitalisation 200 μg may be given twice daily for 4 days. The maintenance dose varies from 50 to 300 μg once daily, the usual dose being 150 μg daily. Digitoxin may also be given in similar doses by slow intravenous injection when vomiting or other conditions prevent administration by mouth. It has also been given intramuscularly but injections may be irritant.

Administration in children. Children were found to have a greater volume of distribution of digitoxin than adults and a shorter mean half-life, although individual variation was considerable. The increase in total clearance in children compared with adults was attributed to greater metabolic clearance. Digitalisation doses of 20 μg per kg body-weight were well tolerated.[1]

1. Larsen A, Storstein L. Digitoxin kinetics and renal excretion in children. *Clin Pharmacol Ther* 1983; **33**: 717–26.

Administration in the elderly. Digitoxin half-life, apparent volume of distribution, and clearance were not found to differ in elderly subjects compared with young adults following intravenous injection in a single-dose study. The long half-life may make once weekly dosing possible in poorly compliant patients.[1]

1. Donovan MA, *et al*. The effect of age on digitoxin pharmacokinetics. *Br J Clin Pharmacol* 1981; **11**: 401–2.

Administration in renal disease. The pharmacokinetics of digitoxin were changed significantly in 5 patients with the nephrotic syndrome. The apparent volume of distribution of digitoxin was increased and protein binding decreased. Such patients should be maintained at lower serum-digitoxin concentrations than other patients but will need larger doses because of the shortened serum half-life and the increased renal excretion of digitoxin and its cardioactive metabolites.[1]

1. Storstein L. Studies on digitalis VII: influence of nephrotic syndrome on protein binding, pharmacokinetics, and renal excretion of digitoxin and cardioactive metabolites. *Clin Pharmacol Ther* 1976; **20**: 158–66.

Preparations

BP 2001: Digitoxin Tablets;
USP 25: Digitoxin Injection; Digitoxin Tablets.

Proprietary Preparations (details are given in Part 3)
Aust.: Digimerck; Ditaven; *Belg.:* Digitaline; *Braz.:* Digitaline; Variplastic; *Canad.:* Digitaline†; *Fr.:* Digitaline; *Ger.:* Coramedan; Digimed; Digimerck; Ditaven; Tardigal; *Hong Kong:* Digitaline; *Norw.:* Digitrin†; *Swed.:* Digitrin; *USA:* Crystodigin.

Multi-ingredient: *Aust.:* Ditaven comp; *Switz.:* Augentonicum; Optazine†.

Digoxin (5801-a)

Digoxin (BAN, rINN).

Digoxinum; Digoxosidum. 3β-[(O-2,6-Dideoxy-β-D-ribo-hexopyranosyl-(1→4)-O-2,6-dideoxy-β-D-ribo-hexopyranosyl-(1→4)-2,6-dideoxy-β-D-ribo-hexopyranosyl)oxy]-12β,14β-dihydroxy-5β-card-20(22)-enolide.
$C_{41}H_{64}O_{14} = 780.9$.
CAS — 20830-75-5.
ATC — C01AA05.

Pharmacopoeias. In *Chin., Eur.* (see p.vi), *Int., Jpn, Pol.,* and *US*.

Pharmacopoeial description

Ph. Eur.: A white or almost white powder or colourless crystals. Practically insoluble in water; slightly soluble in alcohol; freely soluble in a mixture of equal volumes of dichloromethane and methyl alcohol. Protect from light.

USP 25: A cardiotonic glycoside obtained from the leaves of *Digitalis lanata* (Scrophulariaceae). Clear to white, odourless, crystals, or a white, odourless, crystalline powder. Practically insoluble in water and in ether; slightly soluble in diluted alcohol and in chloroform; freely soluble in pyridine. Store in airtight containers.

Adverse Effects

Digoxin and the other cardiac glycosides commonly produce side-effects because the margin between the therapeutic and toxic doses is small; plasma concentrations of digoxin in excess of 2 nanograms per mL are considered to be an indication that the patient is at special risk although there is considerable interindividual variation. There have been many fatalities, particularly due to cardiac toxicity.

Nausea, vomiting, and anorexia may be among the earliest symptoms of digoxin toxicity or overdosage; diarrhoea and abdominal pain may occur. Certain neurological effects are also common symptoms of digoxin overdosage and include headache, facial pain, fatigue, weakness, dizziness, drowsiness, disorientation, mental confusion, bad dreams and more rarely delirium, acute psychoses, and hallucinations. Convulsions have been reported. Visual disturbances including blurred vision may occur; colour vision may be affected with objects appearing yellow or less frequently green, red, brown, blue, or white. Hypersensitivity reactions are rare; thrombocytopenia has been reported. The cardiac glycosides may have some oestrogenic activity and occasionally cause gynaecomastia at therapeutic doses.

Rapid intravenous injection of digoxin may cause vasoconstriction and transient hypertension. Intramuscular or subcutaneous injection can cause local irritation.

The most serious adverse effects are those on the heart. Toxic doses may cause or aggravate heart failure. Supraventricular or ventricular arrhythmias and defects of conduction are common and may be an early indication of excessive dosage. In general the incidence and severity of arrhythmias is related to the severity of the underlying heart disease. Almost any arrhythmia may ensue, but particular note should be made of supraventricular tachycardia, especially atrioventricular (AV) junctional tachycardia and atrial tachycardia with block. Ventricular arrhythmias including extrasystoles, sinoatrial block, sinus bradycardia, and AV block may also occur.

Hypokalaemia predisposes to digoxin toxicity; adverse reactions to digoxin may be precipitated if hypokalaemia occurs, for example following the prolonged administration of diuretics. Hyperkalaemia occurs in acute digoxin overdosage.

As digoxin has a shorter half-life than digitalis or digitoxin any toxic effects will tend to resolve more rapidly.

◊ General references to digitalis toxicity.

1. Beller GA, *et al*. Digitalis intoxication: a prospective clinical study with serum level concentrations. *N Engl J Med* 1971; **284**: 989–97.
2. Bullock RE, Hall RJC. Digitalis toxicity and poisoning. *Adverse Drug React Acute Poisoning Rev* 1982; **1**: 201–22.
3. Aronson JK. Digitalis intoxication. *Clin Sci* 1983; **64**: 253–8.
4. George CF. Digitalis intoxication: a new approach to an old problem. *BMJ* 1983; **286**: 1533–4.
5. Pentel PR, Salerno DM. Cardiac drug toxicity: digitalis glycosides and calcium-channel and β-blocking agents. *Med J Aust* 1990; **152**: 88–94.
6. Wells TG, *et al*. Age-related differences in digoxin toxicity and its treatment. *Drug Safety* 1992; **7**: 135–51.
7. Johnston GD. Adverse reaction profile: digoxin. *Prescribers' J* 1993; **33**: 29–35.
8. Kernan WN, *et al*. Incidence of hospitalization for digitalis toxicity among elderly Americans. *Am J Med* 1994; **96**: 426–31.
9. Li-Saw-Hee FL, Lip GYH. How safe is digoxin? *Adverse Drug React Bull* 1998; (Feb): 715–18.

◊ Adverse effects reported in elderly patients with toxic plasma-digoxin concentrations have included chorea,[1] profuse watery diarrhoea,[2] and dysphagia with dysphonia.[3]

1. Mulder LJMM, *et al*. Generalised chorea due to digoxin toxicity. *BMJ* 1988; **296**: 1262.
2. Andrews PA, Wilkinson PR. Diarrhoea as a side effect of digoxin. *BMJ* 1990; **301**: 1398.
3. Cordeiro MF, Arnold KG. Digoxin toxicity presenting as dysphagia and dysphonia. *BMJ* 1991; **302**: 1025.

Effects on the blood. An association between several cardiovascular drugs, including digitalis glycosides (digoxin and acetyldigoxin), and agranulocytosis was found in an international study[1] although the incidence was low.

1. Kelly JP, *et al*. Risks of agranulocytosis and aplastic anemia in relation to the use of cardiovascular drugs: the international agranulocytosis and aplastic anemia study. *Clin Pharmacol Ther* 1991; **49**: 330–41.

Hypersensitivity. Hypersensitivity reactions to cardiac glycosides are rare but skin reactions have been reported. An 86-year-old man developed a generalised, pruritic, erythematous rash following administration of digoxin intravenously.[1] The rash recurred following rechallenge with digoxin tablets.

1. Martin SJ, Shah D. Cutaneous hypersensitivity reaction to digoxin. *JAMA* 1994; **271**: 1905.

Treatment of Adverse Effects

In *acute poisoning*, gastric lavage may be considered if the patient presents within one hour of ingestion. Activated charcoal may be given to reduce the absorption and enterohepatic recycling of cardiac glycosides and repeated doses have been used; colestyramine and colestipol have also been tried. Attempts to remove cardiac glycosides by haemodialysis or peritoneal dialysis have generally been ineffective and the value of haemoperfusion is controversial. Forced diuresis with frusemide [furosemide] is generally ineffective and may be dangerous; serious electrolyte imbalance may result from the use of such potent diuretics.

Cardiac toxicity in acute or chronic poisoning should be treated under ECG control and serum electrolytes should be monitored. Antiarrhythmic treatment may be necessary and should be determined by the specific arrhythmia present (see p.794). Atropine is given intravenously to correct bradycardia and in patients with heart block. Pacing may be necessary if atropine is not effective. Potassium chloride may be given in hypokalaemic patients provided that renal function is normal and heart block is not present. Potassium has

also been given to normokalaemic patients but caution is needed since hyperkalaemia can occur rapidly. Other electrolyte imbalance should be corrected.

In *massive overdosage* progressive hyperkalaemia occurs and is fatal unless reversed. Soluble insulin with glucose has been given and, if the hyperkalaemia is refractory, dialysis may be tried. Massive life-threatening overdosage has been treated successfully with digoxin-specific antibody fragments (p.1006).

For the treatment of *chronic poisoning* temporary withdrawal of digoxin or other cardiac glycosides may be all that is necessary, with subsequent doses adjusted according to the needs of the patient. Serum electrolytes should be measured and the ECG monitored. Potassium supplements should be given to correct hypokalaemia.

◊ References.

1. Allen NM, Dunham GD. Treatment of digitalis intoxication with emphasis on the clinical use of digoxin immune Fab. *DICP Ann Pharmacother* 1990; **24**: 991–8.
2. Dick M, *et al*. Digitalis intoxication recognition and management. *J Clin Pharmacol* 1991; **31**: 444–7.
3. Critchley JAJH, Critchley LAH. Digoxin toxicity in chronic renal failure: treatment by multiple dose activated charcoal intestinal dialysis. *Hum Exp Toxicol* 1997; **16**: 733–5.

Precautions

Digoxin is generally contra-indicated in patients with hypertrophic obstructive cardiomyopathy unless there is severe cardiac failure, since the outflow obstruction may be worsened. It is also contra-indicated in patients with the Wolff-Parkinson-White syndrome or other evidence of an accessory pathway, especially if it is accompanied by atrial fibrillation, since ventricular tachycardia or fibrillation may be precipitated. Digoxin is not an appropriate form of therapy for any ventricular arrhythmia.

Digoxin toxicity is common and may result from raised plasma concentrations or an increase in sensitivity to digoxin. Almost any deterioration in the condition of the heart or circulation may increase the sensitivity to digoxin and it should be used with caution in all patients with cardiovascular disease. Early signs of digoxin toxicity should be watched for and the heart rate should generally be maintained above 60 beats per minute. Toxicity may result from administering loading doses too rapidly and from accumulation of maintenance doses as well as from acute poisoning.

Digoxin should be used with caution in partial heart block since complete heart block may be induced; it should also be used with care in sinus node disorders. Caution is also required in acute myocarditis (such as rheumatic carditis), in acute myocardial infarction, in advanced heart failure, and in severe pulmonary disease, due to the increased myocardial sensitivity. Digoxin may also enhance the occurrence of arrhythmias in patients undergoing cardioversion and should be withdrawn 1 to 2 days before such procedures if possible. If cardioversion is essential and digoxin has already been given, low energy shocks must be used.

Electrolyte imbalances may affect the sensitivity to digoxin, as may thyroid dysfunction. The effects of digoxin are enhanced by hypokalaemia, hypomagnesaemia, hypercalcaemia, hypoxia, and hypothyroidism and doses may need to be reduced until these conditions are corrected. Resistance to the effects of digoxin may occur in hyperthyroidism. Digoxin should be given with care to patients who may have already received cardiac glycosides and it has been suggested that the initial dose should be reduced if the patient has received them in the preceding 2 weeks.

Digoxin doses should generally be reduced and plasma-digoxin concentrations monitored in patients with impaired renal function, in the elderly, and in premature infants (see Uses and Administration, below).

Gastrointestinal disorders. Absorption from tablet formulations of digoxin may be decreased in patients with malabsorption syndromes or small bowel resections due to inadequate dissolution and it has been recommended that liquid dosage forms of digoxin should be used in patients with small bowel resections.[1] However, only 40 to 60% of a digoxin dose administered as elixir was absorbed in a patient with a small bowel resection[2] compared with about 80% in patients with normal gastrointestinal function, suggesting a need for slightly increased oral maintenance doses of digoxin in patients with small bowel resections. In a further patient with a similar resection[3] a therapeutic plasma-digoxin concentration was not achieved with any oral formulation.

1. Kumer KP, *et al.* Perspectives on digoxin absorption from small bowel resections. *Drug Intell Clin Pharm* 1983; **17:** 121–3.
2. Vetticaden SJ, *et al.* Digoxin absorption in a patient with short-bowel syndrome. *Clin Pharm* 1986; **5:** 62–4.
3. Ehrenpreis ED, *et al.* Malabsorption of digoxin tablets, gel caps, and elixir in a patient with an end jejunostomy. *Ann Pharmacother* 1994; **28:** 1239–40.

Heart surgery. Patients undergoing cardiac surgery appear to have increased sensitivity to digoxin toxicity and thus an increased risk of arrhythmias.[1] Digoxin has been found[2] to be no better than placebo in preventing postoperative arrhythmias in patients following coronary artery bypass surgery and actually induced supraventricular arrhythmias in 2 patients. Arrhythmias compatible with digoxin intoxication have occurred postoperatively[1] although serum-digoxin concentrations ranged from 0 to 2.8 nanograms per mL and it may be that the surgical procedures or increased sensitivity to digoxin caused them.

1. Rose MR, *et al.* Arrhythmias following cardiac surgery: relation to serum digoxin levels. *Am Heart J* 1975; **89:** 288–94.
2. Weiner B, *et al.* Digoxin prophylaxis following coronary artery bypass surgery. *Clin Pharm* 1986; **5:** 55–8.

Interference with digoxin assays. The presence of endogenous digoxin-like substances in neonates, and in patients with liver or kidney dysfunction may be responsible for elevated values or false-positive results in some plasma-digoxin assays.[1] Some patients may have antibodies that react with the assay system and produce falsely elevated values.[2] Prednisolone[1] and spironolactone[1,3] might each interfere with plasma-digoxin assays; spironolactone may also produce actual changes in digoxin concentrations (see below).

1. Yosselson-Superstine S. Drug interferences with plasma assays in therapeutic drug monitoring. *Clin Pharmacokinet* 1984; **9:** 67–89.
2. Liendo C, *et al.* A new interference in some digoxin assays: antimurine heterophilic antibodies. *Clin Pharmacol Ther* 1996; **60:** 593–8.
3. Foukaridis GN. Influence of spironolactone and its metabolite canrenone on serum digoxin assays. *Ther Drug Monit* 1990; **12:** 82–4.

Pregnancy. There is considerable evidence that digoxin crosses the placenta freely with serum-digoxin concentrations at term similar in the newborn and mother. No significant adverse effects attributed to digoxin have been noted in the fetus or neonate although adverse fetal effects, including fetal death, have been reported in mothers with digitalis toxicity. Some concern has been expressed that maternal digitalis therapy may occasionally cause low birth-weights in infants of mothers with heart disease, but the underlying disease might also be important.[1] The presence of endogenous digoxin-like immunoreactive substances in the serum of pregnant women and neonates could make the interpretation of digoxin assays difficult. In one study,[2] high concentrations of endogenous digoxin-like immunoreactivity in cord blood suggested that it might be synthesised during delivery, in which case the placental transfer of digoxin might be overestimated.

1. Rotmensch HH, *et al.* Management of cardiac arrhythmias during pregnancy: current concepts. *Drugs* 1987; **33:** 623–33.
2. Lupoglazoff JM, *et al.* Endogenous digoxin-like immunoreactivity during pregnancy and at birth. *Br J Clin Pharmacol* 1993; **35:** 251–4.

Interactions

There may be interactions between digoxin and drugs which alter its absorption, interfere with its excretion, or have additive effects on the myocardium. Drugs which cause electrolyte disturbances increase the risk of toxicity from cardiac glycosides. Thiazides and loop *diuretics* cause hypokalaemia and also hypomagnesaemia which may lead to cardiac arrhythmias. Other causes of hypokalaemia include treatment with *corticosteroids, beta$_2$ agonists* (such as salbutamol), *amphotericin B, sodium polystyrene sulfonate, carbenoxolone,* and dialysis. Hypercalcaemia may also increase toxicity and intravenous administration of *calcium salts* is best avoided in patients taking cardiac glycosides. Serum-digoxin concentrations may be significantly increased by *quinidine, amiodarone,* and *propafenone* and reduction of digoxin dosage may be required. Other antiarrhythmic drugs may have additive effects on the myocardium increasing the likelihood of adverse effects; *beta blockers* may potentiate bradycardia due to digoxin. *Calcium-channel blockers* may increase digoxin concentrations.

The symbol † denotes a preparation no longer actively marketed

◊ Reviews of drug interactions occurring with digoxin.

1. Rodin SM, Johnson BF. Pharmacokinetic interactions with digoxin. *Clin Pharmacokinet* 1988; **15:** 227–44.
2. Magnani B, Malini PL. Cardiac glycosides: drug interactions of clinical significance. *Drug Safety* 1995; **12:** 97–109.

ACE inhibitors. Although increased serum-digoxin concentrations have been reported in patients with severe chronic heart failure given *captopril*,[1] other studies have failed to confirm this effect.[2,3] Studies with various other ACE inhibitors have also failed to show any significant effect on serum-digoxin concentrations. However, ACE inhibitors may cause a deterioration in renal function and this could lead to an increase in serum-digoxin concentration due to impaired digoxin excretion.[4]

1. Cleland JGF, *et al.* Interaction of digoxin and captopril. *Br J Clin Pharmacol* 1984; **17:** 214P.
2. Magelli C, *et al.* Lack of effect of captopril on serum digoxin in congestive heart failure. *Eur J Clin Pharmacol* 1989; **36:** 99–100.
3. Rossi GP, *et al.* Effect of acute captopril administration on digoxin pharmacokinetics in normal subjects. *Curr Ther Res* 1989; **46:** 439–44.
4. Mignat C, Unger T. ACE inhibitors: drug interactions of clinical significance. *Drug Safety* 1995; **12:** 334–47.

Alpha blockers. *Prazosin*[1] has been reported to increase the mean plasma-digoxin concentration in patients receiving a maintenance dose of digoxin.

1. Çopur S, *et al.* Effects of oral prazosin on total plasma digoxin levels. *Fundam Clin Pharmacol* 1988; **2:** 13–17.

Angiotensin II receptor antagonists. In a study[1] in healthy volunteers, *telmisartan* increased peak serum-digoxin concentrations but trough concentrations were unaffected and it was suggested that the effect was unlikely to be clinically significant. No interaction was found when digoxin was administered concomitantly with *losartan*[2] or with *eprosartan*[3] in healthy volunteers.

1. Stangier J, *et al.* The effect of telmisartan on the steady-state pharmacokinetics of digoxin in healthy male volunteers. *J Clin Pharmacol* 2000; **40:** 1373–9.
2. de Smet M, *et al.* Effect of multiple doses of losartan on the pharmacokinetics of single doses of digoxin in healthy volunteers. *Br J Clin Pharmacol* 1995; **40:** 571–5.
3. Martin DE, *et al.* Lack of effect of eprosartan on the single dose pharmacokinetics of orally administered digoxin in healthy male volunteers. *Br J Clin Pharmacol* 1997; **43:** 661–4.

Antiarrhythmics. AMIODARONE. An interaction between digoxin and amiodarone resulting in increases in plasma concentrations of digoxin has been reported[1-5] on several occasions and plasma-digoxin concentration may be doubled.[5] An increase in serum-digoxin concentrations of 68 to 800% has been reported[2] during amiodarone therapy in children. The interaction does not appear to be due to a reduction in urinary excretion alone[3,4] and seems to be dose-related. It has been recommended[1,6] that the initial dose of digoxin should be halved when amiodarone is given concurrently.

1. Moysey JO, *et al.* Amiodarone increases plasma digoxin concentrations. *BMJ* 1981; **282:** 272.
2. Koren G, *et al.* Digoxin toxicity associated with amiodarone therapy in children. *J Pediatr* 1984; **104:** 467–70.
3. Douste-Blazy P, *et al.* Influence of amiodarone on plasma and urine digoxin concentrations. *Lancet* 1984; **i:** 905.
4. Mingardi G. Amiodarone and plasma digoxin levels. *Lancet* 1984; **i:** 1238.
5. Johnston A, *et al.* The digoxin-amiodarone interaction. *Br J Clin Pharmacol* 1987; **24:** 253P.
6. Naccarelli GV, *et al.* Adverse effects of amiodarone: pathogenesis, incidence and management. *Med Toxicol Adverse Drug Exp* 1989; **4:** 246–53.

DISOPYRAMIDE. Disopyramide appears to have no clinically significant effect on the pharmacokinetics of digoxin in healthy subjects[1,2] but has been reported to modify the cardiovascular effects of digoxin.[1]

1. Elliott HL, *et al.* Pharmacodynamic and pharmacokinetic evaluation of the interaction between digoxin and disopyramide. *Br J Clin Pharmacol* 1982; **14:** 141P.
2. Risler T, *et al.* On the interaction between digoxin and disopyramide. *Clin Pharmacol Ther* 1983; **34:** 176–80.

FLECAINIDE. Administration of flecainide 200 mg twice daily to 15 healthy subjects taking digoxin caused a mean increase of 24% in predose digoxin concentrations and of 13% in digoxin concentrations 6 hours after the digoxin dose.[1] It was considered that in most cases these increases in plasma-digoxin concentrations would not present a clinical problem, but that patients with higher plasma-digoxin concentrations or atrioventricular nodal dysfunction should be monitored.

1. Weeks CE, *et al.* The effect of flecainide acetate, a new antiarrhythmic, on plasma digoxin levels. *J Clin Pharmacol* 1986; **26:** 27–31.

PROPAFENONE. Increased serum-digoxin concentrations have been reported when propafenone is given concurrently.[1-4] There is considerable interindividual variation in the extent of the interaction; increases in serum-digoxin concentrations of up to 254% have been reported. If digoxin and propafenone are given concurrently, the dose of digoxin should be reduced and serum-digoxin concentration should be monitored.

1. Nolan PE, *et al.* Effects of coadministration of propafenone on the pharmacokinetics of digoxin in healthy volunteer subjects. *J Clin Pharmacol* 1989; **29:** 46–52.
2. Calvo MV, *et al.* Interaction between digoxin and propafenone. *Ther Drug Monit* 1989; **11:** 10–15.

3. Zalzstein E, *et al.* Interaction between digoxin and propafenone in children. *J Pediatr* 1990; **116:** 310–12.
4. Bigot M-C, *et al.* Serum digoxin levels related to plasma propafenone levels during concomitant treatment. *J Clin Pharmacol* 1991; **31:** 521–6.

QUINIDINE. Quinidine causes an increase in serum-digoxin concentration in almost all patients given the two drugs concurrently.[1-3] The serum-digoxin concentration may increase by up to 500% but is usually approximately doubled.[1] Signs and symptoms of digoxin toxicity may occur although some workers[4] have suggested that these may be accounted for by an additive effect of the 2 drugs rather than by the effect on serum-digoxin concentration. The exact mechanism of interaction is not clear but a substantial decrease in the renal and nonrenal clearance of digoxin has been demonstrated.[5] The distribution volume of digoxin may also be reduced[2] reflecting impaired tissue binding, and there is increased systemic availability.[1] It is generally recommended that the dose of digoxin is halved in digitalised patients who are to be given quinidine.[2] Subsequently serum-digoxin concentrations should be monitored, especially during the first 1 to 2 weeks after which the new steady-state digoxin concentration should be achieved.[2]

1. Bigger JT, Leahey EB. Quinidine and digoxin: an important interaction. *Drugs* 1982; **24:** 229–39.
2. Pedersen KE. Digoxin interactions: the influence of quinidine and verapamil on the pharmacokinetics and receptor binding of digitalis glycosides. *Acta Med Scand* 1985; **697** (suppl): 1–40.
3. Mordel A, *et al.* Quinidine enhances digitalis toxicity at therapeutic serum digoxin levels. *Clin Pharmacol Ther* 1993; **53:** 457–62.
4. Walker AM, *et al.* Drug toxicity in patients receiving digoxin and quinidine. *Am Heart J* 1983; **105:** 1025–8.
5. Hedman A, *et al.* Interactions in the renal and biliary elimination of digoxin: stereoselective difference between quinine and quinidine. *Clin Pharmacol Ther* 1990; **47:** 20–6.

VERAPAMIL. For a discussion on the interaction between digoxin and verapamil, see under Calcium-channel Blockers, below.

Antibacterials. Approximately 10% of patients receiving digoxin may metabolise 40% or more of the drug to cardio-inactive metabolites.[1] Gut flora contribute greatly to this process, and the administration of antibacterials such as *erythromycin* or *tetracycline* to these patients appears to reduce this metabolic process resulting in higher serum concentrations.[2] Digoxin toxicity has been reported in digitalised patients given erythromycin,[3,4] *clarithromycin*,[5-7] and *roxithromycin*.[8] Oral *neomycin* may reduce serum-digoxin concentrations by reducing digoxin absorption.

Rifampicin may reduce serum-digitoxin concentrations by inducing its metabolism (see p.869). Digoxin is mainly excreted unchanged in the urine but rifampicin has been reported[9] to increase digoxin dose requirements substantially in 2 patients dependent on dialysis. When rifampicin was discontinued digoxin requirements fell by about 50%.

1. Doherty JE. A digoxin-antibiotic drug interaction. *N Engl J Med* 1981; **305:** 827–8.
2. Lindenbaum J, *et al.* Inactivation of digoxin by the gut flora: reversal by antibiotic therapy. *N Engl J Med* 1981; **305:** 789–94.
3. Maxwell DL, *et al.* Digoxin toxicity due to interaction of digoxin with erythromycin. *BMJ* 1989; **298:** 572.
4. Morton MR, Cooper JW. Erythromycin-induced digoxin toxicity. *DICP Ann Pharmacother* 1989; **23:** 668–70.
5. Midoneck SR, Etingin OR. Clarithromycin-related toxic effects of digoxin. *N Engl J Med* 1995; **333:** 1505.
6. Nawarskas JJ, *et al.* Digoxin toxicity secondary to clarithromycin therapy. *Ann Pharmacother* 1997; **31:** 864–6.
7. Laberge P, Martineau P. Clarithromycin-induced digoxin intoxication. *Ann Pharmacother* 1997; **31:** 999–1002.
8. Corallo CE, Rogers IR. Roxithromycin-induced digoxin toxicity. *Med J Aust* 1996; **165:** 433–4.
9. Gault H, *et al.* Digoxin-rifampin interaction. *Clin Pharmacol Ther* 1984; **35:** 750–4.

Antidepressants. In a study[1] in healthy male subjects, administration of *nefazodone* increased steady-state plasma-digoxin concentrations by approximately 30% but no adverse or clinical effects were associated with the increase. However, due to the narrow therapeutic range of digoxin, it was suggested that plasma-digoxin concentrations should be monitored in patients given nefazodone concomitantly. Similar recommendations have been made for *trazodone*.

1. Dockens RC, *et al.* Assessment of pharmacokinetic and pharmacodynamic drug interactions between nefazodone and digoxin in healthy male volunteers. *J Clin Pharmacol* 1996; **36:** 160–7.

Antidiabetics. Subtherapeutic plasma-digoxin concentrations were noted in a diabetic woman receiving *acarbose* and digoxin concurrently.[1] The plasma concentration of digoxin increased to a therapeutic level when acarbose was discontinued. A study[2] in healthy volunteers suggested that the interaction was due to inhibition of the absorption of digoxin by acarbose.

1. Serrano JS, *et al.* A possible interaction of potential clinical interest between digoxin and acarbose. *Clin Pharmacol Ther* 1996; **60:** 589–92.
2. Miura T, *et al.* Impairment of absorption of digoxin by acarbose. *J Clin Pharmacol* 1998; **38:** 654–7.

Antiepileptics. *Phenytoin* caused a marked decrease in steady-state serum-digoxin concentrations when administered with digoxin and acetyldigoxin to 6 healthy subjects for 7 days.[1] Total digoxin clearance was increased by an average of 27% and elimination half-life was reduced by an average of 30%. This interaction may be more likely with digitoxin, since digitoxin is more dependent on the liver for elimination. A brief report of an open study[2] in 12 subjects indicated a slight but significant decrease in digoxin bioavailability when *topira-*

mate was given concomitantly, although half-life and renal clearance of digoxin did not appear to be affected.

1. Rameis H. On the interaction between phenytoin and digoxin. *Eur J Clin Pharmacol* 1985; **29:** 49–53.
2. Liao S, Palmer M. Digoxin and topiramate drug interaction study in male volunteers. *Pharm Res* 1993; **10** (suppl): S405.

Antifungals. Two men given *itraconazole* while receiving digoxin developed signs and symptoms of digoxin toxicity and elevated serum-digoxin concentrations.[1,2] A further case report[3] suggested that the interaction was due to a reduction in the renal clearance of digoxin when itraconazole was given concomitantly.

Additive adverse effects due to hypokalaemia may occur when digoxin is given with *amphotericin B*.

1. Rex J. Itraconazole–digoxin interaction. *Ann Intern Med* 1992; **116:** 525.
2. Alderman CP, Jersmann HPA. Digoxin–itraconazole interaction. *Med J Aust* 1993; **159:** 838–9.
3. Alderman CP, Allcroft PD. Digoxin-itraconazole interaction: possible mechanisms. *Ann Pharmacother* 1997; **31:** 438–40.

Antimalarials. In 6 subjects given *quinine sulfate,* total body clearance of digoxin after an intravenous dose was decreased by 26%, primarily through a reduction in nonrenal clearance.[1] Increased urinary excretion of digoxin was consistent with alterations in the nonrenal clearance of digoxin and might be due to changes in the metabolism or biliary secretion of digoxin. Quinine increased the mean elimination half-life of digoxin from 34.2 to 51.8 hours but did not consistently change the volume of distribution.

An increase in the plasma-digoxin concentration, but without symptoms of toxicity, was noted in two women given *hydroxychloroquine* (for rheumatoid arthritis) in addition to long-term digoxin therapy.[2]

1. Wandell M, et al. Effect of quinine on digoxin kinetics. *Clin Pharmacol Ther* 1980; **28:** 425–30.
2. Leden I. Digoxin–hydroxychloroquine interaction? *Acta Med Scand* 1982; **211:** 411–12.

Antineoplastics and immunosuppressants. The absorption of digoxin from tablets was reduced by an average of 45.6% in patients undergoing antineoplastic therapy.[1] Also the steady-state concentration of digoxin after administration of β-acetyldigoxin has been reduced in patients undergoing antineoplastic therapy.[2] The interaction was considered to be due to reduced absorption of digitalis glycosides when the gastrointestinal mucosa is damaged and might be minimised by administering digoxin in the form of liquid-filled capsules[1] or by giving digitoxin.[2]

Increased serum-digoxin concentrations with symptoms of toxicity have been reported in patients when *ciclosporin* was added to their digoxin therapy.[3,4]

1. Bjornsson TD, et al. Effects of high-dose cancer chemotherapy on the absorption of digoxin in two different formulations. *Clin Pharmacol Ther* 1986; **39:** 25–8.
2. Kuhlmann J. Inhibition of digoxin absorption but not of digitoxin during cytostatic drug therapy. *Arzneimittelforschung* 1982; **32:** 698–704.
3. Dorian P, et al. Digoxin-cyclosporine interaction: severe digitalis toxicity after cyclosporine treatment. *Clin Invest Med* 1988; **ii:** 108–12.
4. Robieux I, et al. The effects of cardiac transplantation and cyclosporine therapy on digoxin pharmacokinetics. *J Clin Pharmacol* 1992; **32:** 338–43.

Antithyroid drugs. Reduced peak serum-digoxin concentrations were noted in 9 of 10 healthy subjects following administration of a single oral dose of *carbimazole* although conversely in the tenth subject digoxin concentrations rose.[1] Caution is also needed since changes in thyroid function may affect sensitivity to digoxin independently of serum concentrations (see Precautions, above).

1. Rao BR, et al. Influence of carbimazole on serum levels and haemodynamic effects of digoxin. *Clin Drug Invest* 1997; **13:** 350–4.

Benzodiazepines. Raised serum-digoxin concentrations have been reported in patients also taking *diazepam*[1] or *alprazolam*.[2,3] The clearance of digoxin was reduced by these benzodiazepines.

1. Castillo-Ferrando JR, et al. Digoxin levels and diazepam. *Lancet* 1980; **ii:** 368.
2. Tollefson G, et al. Alprazolam-related digoxin toxicity. *Am J Psychiatry* 1984; **141:** 1612–14.
3. Guven H, et al. Age-related digoxin-alprazolam interaction. *Clin Pharmacol Ther* 1993; **54:** 42–4.

Beta₂ agonists. A single intravenous[1,2] or oral[3] dose of *salbutamol* has been reported to decrease steady-state serum-digoxin concentrations by up to 16% and 22% respectively in healthy subjects. Although salbutamol had no significant effect on the concentration of digoxin in skeletal muscle, it was considered that increased binding to skeletal muscle could explain the interaction. Beta₂ agonists such as salbutamol can also cause hypokalaemia which may increase susceptibility to digoxin-induced arrhythmias.

1. Edner M, Jogestrand T. Effect of salbutamol on digoxin concentration in serum and skeletal muscle. *Eur J Clin Pharmacol* 1989; **36:** 235–8.
2. Edner M, et al. Effect of salbutamol on digoxin pharmacokinetics. *Eur J Clin Pharmacol* 1992; **42:** 197–201.
3. Edner M, Jogestrand T. Oral salbutamol decreases serum digoxin concentration. *Eur J Clin Pharmacol* 1990; **38:** 195–7.

Calcium-channel blockers. Studies on interactions between digoxin and calcium-channel blockers appear to show that *ver-* *apamil* increases plasma-digoxin concentrations[1-3] by up to 70%. The effect of *nifedipine* is not as clear. Although it has been reported[1] to produce a 45% increase in plasma-digoxin concentrations, other studies[4,5] have reported little or no increase and the interaction is unlikely to be of clinical significance for most patients. Studies on the interaction between digoxin and *diltiazem* have also produced conflicting results. Increases in plasma-digoxin concentrations of 20% and up to 59% have been reported[6,7] and an increase in metildigoxin concentrations[7] of up to 51%. However, other studies[8,9] have shown no diltiazem-induced change in digoxin pharmacokinetics or plasma concentration. *Bepridil,*[10] *gallopamil,*[1] *mibefradil,*[11] *nisoldipine,*[12] and *nitrendipine*[13] have all been reported to increase plasma-digoxin concentrations. Bepridil increased the concentration by 34% and it was recommended that patients given this combination be monitored carefully. *Felodipine*[14,15] and *isradipine*[3] have both been reported to increase peak serum-digoxin concentrations, but steady-state digoxin concentrations were not affected and the interactions were unlikely to be of clinical relevance.

The mechanism of interaction between calcium-channel blockers and digoxin is not completely understood but appears to be related to decreased renal and nonrenal clearance of digoxin. The pharmacodynamic effects of digoxin and calcium-channel blockers may also be additive.

1. Belz GG, et al. Interaction between digoxin and calcium antagonists and antiarrhythmic drugs. *Clin Pharmacol Ther* 1983; **33:** 410–17.
2. Pedersen KE, et al. Influence of verapamil on the inotropism and pharmacokinetics of digoxin. *Eur J Clin Pharmacol* 1983; **25:** 199–206.
3. Rodin SM, et al. Comparative effects of verapamil and isradipine on steady-state digoxin kinetics. *Clin Pharmacol Ther* 1988; **43:** 668–72.
4. Schwartz JB, et al. Effect of nifedipine on serum digoxin concentration and renal digoxin clearance. *Clin Pharmacol Ther* 1984; **36:** 19–24.
5. Kleinbloesem CH, et al. Interactions between digoxin and nifedipine at steady state in patients with atrial fibrillation. *Ther Drug Monit* 1985; **7:** 372–6.
6. Rameis H, et al. The diltiazem-digoxin interaction. *Clin Pharmacol Ther* 1984; **36:** 183–9.
7. Oyama Y, et al. Digoxin-diltiazem interaction. *Am J Cardiol* 1984; **53:** 1480–1.
8. Beltrami TR, et al. Lack of effects of diltiazem on digoxin pharmacokinetics. *J Clin Pharmacol* 1985; **25:** 390–2.
9. Elkayam U, et al. Effect of diltiazem on renal clearance and serum concentration of digoxin in patients with cardiac disease. *Am J Cardiol* 1985; **55:** 1393–5.
10. Belz GG, et al. Digoxin and bepridil: pharmacokinetic and pharmacodynamic interactions. *Clin Pharmacol Ther* 1986; **39:** 65–71.
11. Siepmann M, et al. The interaction of the calcium antagonist RO 40-5967 with digoxin. *Br J Clin Pharmacol* 1995; **39:** 491–6.
12. Kirch W, et al. Influence of nisoldipine on haemodynamic effects and plasma levels of digoxin. *Br J Clin Pharmacol* 1986; **22:** 155–9.
13. Kirch W, et al. Nitrendipine increases digoxin plasma levels dose dependently. *J Clin Pharmacol* 1986; **26:** 553.
14. Rehnqvist N, et al. Pharmacokinetics of felodipine and effect on digoxin plasma levels in patients with heart failure. *Drugs* 1987; **34** (suppl 3): 33–42.
15. Dunselman PHJM, et al. Digoxin-felodipine interaction in patients with congestive heart failure. *Eur J Clin Pharmacol* 1988; **35:** 461–5.

Diuretics. *Amiloride* administration increased renal clearance of digoxin and reduced the extrarenal digoxin clearance in 6 healthy subjects after a single intravenous dose of digoxin.[1] Amiloride also inhibited the digoxin-induced positive inotropic effect, but the clinical implications in cardiac patients are unknown. A further study[2] failed to confirm this effect.

Spironolactone and its metabolites have been reported to interfere with serum-digoxin determinations by radio-immunoassay or fluorescence-polarisation immunoassay resulting in falsely elevated measurements.[3,4] The interference with digoxin assays is neither consistent nor predictable and falsely low readings have also been reported.[5] Serum-digoxin concentrations should be interpreted with caution when digoxin is given concomitantly with spironolactone or *canrenoate*, especially since spironolactone has also been reported to decrease digoxin clearance by a median of 26% resulting in a true increase in serum-digoxin concentration.[6]

Diuretic therapy with *triamterene* in association with a thiazide or loop diuretic increased the mean serum-digoxin concentration; this interaction was considered unlikely to be of clinical importance, except perhaps in patients with renal impairment.[7]

1. Waldorff S, et al. Amiloride-induced changes in digoxin dynamics and kinetics: abolition of digoxin-induced inotropism with amiloride. *Clin Pharmacol Ther* 1981; **30:** 172–6.
2. Richter JP, et al. The acute effects of amiloride and potassium canrenoate on digoxin-induced positive inotropium in healthy volunteers. *Eur J Clin Pharmacol* 1993; **45:** 195–6.
3. Paladino JA, et al. Influence of spironolactone on serum digoxin concentration. *JAMA* 1984; **251:** 470–1.
4. Foukaridis GN. Influence of spironolactone and its metabolite canrenone on serum digoxin assays. *Ther Drug Monit* 1990; **12:** 82–4.
5. Steimer W, et al. Intoxication due to negative canrenone interference in digoxin drug monitoring. *Lancet* 1999; **354:** 1176–7.
6. Waldorff S, et al. Spironolactone-induced changes in digoxin kinetics. *Clin Pharmacol Ther* 1978; **24:** 162–7.
7. Impivaara O, Iisalo E. Serum digoxin concentrations in a representative digoxin-consuming adult population. *Eur J Clin Pharmacol* 1985; **27:** 627–32.

Gastrointestinal drugs. A number of gastrointestinal drugs can affect the absorption of digoxin by binding to the digoxin or by changing gastrointestinal motility. The problem has often been related to the bioavailability of the digoxin formulation and appears to be less important with currently used preparations. Some *antacids*,[1,2] particularly liquid formulations, and *adsorbents*[1] such as kaolin-pectin, can reduce the absorption of digoxin from the gastrointestinal tract and administration should probably be separated by at least 2 hours. *Activated charcoal*, and *ion-exchange resins* such as colestyramine and colestipol, also reduce digoxin absorption. *Sucralfate*[3] may also reduce the absorption of digoxin.

Omeprazole and possibly other gastric acid inhibitors may reduce the gastrointestinal metabolism and enhance the absorption of unchanged digoxin,[4] although the clinical relevance of this is uncertain.[5]

Drugs that increase gastrointestinal motility can reduce the absorption of digoxin, especially if digoxin is given as a slowly dissolving formulation. Reduced absorption of digoxin has occurred when digoxin and *metoclopramide* have been given concurrently,[6] and a similar effect has been reported with *cisapride*.[7] Conversely, *anticholinergics* reduce motility, and propantheline has increased digoxin absorption.

Sulfasalazine has been found to impair the absorption of digoxin and to reduce the serum-digoxin concentration,[8] but the mechanism is unclear.

1. Rodin SM, Johnson BF. Pharmacokinetic interactions with digoxin. *Clin Pharmacokinet* 1988; **15:** 227–44.
2. Gugler R, Allgayer H. Effects of antacids on the clinical pharmacokinetics of drugs: an update. *Clin Pharmacokinet* 1990; **18:** 210–19.
3. Rey AM, Gums JG. Altered absorption of digoxin, sustained-release quinidine, and warfarin with sucralfate administration. *DICP Ann Pharmacother* 1991; **25:** 745–6.
4. Cohen AF, et al. Influence of gastric acidity on the bioavailability of digoxin. *Ann Intern Med* 1991; **115:** 540–5.
5. Oosterhuis B, et al. Minor effect of multiple dose omeprazole on the pharmacokinetics of digoxin after a single oral dose. *Br J Clin Pharmacol* 1991; **32:** 569–72.
6. Johnson BF, et al. Effect of metoclopramide on digoxin absorption from tablets and capsules. *Clin Pharmacol Ther* 1984; **36:** 724–30.
7. Kubler PA, et al. Possible interaction between cisapride and digoxin. *Ann Pharmacother* 2001; **35:** 127–8.
8. Juhl RP, et al. Effect of sulfasalazine on digoxin bioavailability. *Clin Pharmacol Ther* 1976; **28:** 387–94.

Ginseng. Raised serum-digoxin concentrations (but without signs of digoxin toxicity) were noted in an elderly man following the use of Siberian ginseng (*Eleutherococcus senticosus*).[1] However, concentrations remained high even when digoxin was discontinued and returned to within the therapeutic range only after the ginseng was stopped. Siberian ginseng contains eleutherosides, which are chemically related to cardiac glycosides such as digoxin, and the assay may have measured these compounds, or their derivatives, as well as digoxin.

1. McRae S. Elevated serum digoxin levels in a patient taking digoxin and Siberian ginseng. *Can Med Assoc J* 1996; **155:** 293–5.

Hypericum. In a study[1] in healthy volunteers, administration of digoxin concomitantly with an extract of *Hypericum* for 10 days resulted in a significant decrease in the plasma-digoxin concentration. It was suggested that the interaction might be due to induction of the P-glycoprotein transporter.

1. Johne A, et al. Pharmacokinetic interaction of digoxin with an herbal extract from St John's wort (Hypericum perforatum). *Clin Pharmacol Ther* 1999; **66:** 338–45.

Neuromuscular blockers. *Pancuronium* or *suxamethonium* may interact with digitalis glycosides resulting in an increased incidence of arrhythmias; the interaction is more likely with pancuronium.[1]

1. Bartolone RS, Rao TLK. Dysrhythmias following muscle relaxant administration in patients receiving digitalis. *Anesthesiology* 1983; **58:** 567–9.

NSAIDs. An increase in serum-digoxin concentration has been reported with *aspirin, ibuprofen, indometacin, fenbufen,* and *diclofenac*.[1] Potentially toxic serum-digoxin concentrations occurred in preterm infants[2] with patent ductus arteriosus on digoxin therapy when given indometacin by mouth in a mean total dose of 320 µg per kg body-weight; it was recommended that the dose of digoxin should be halved initially if indometacin is also given. Lack of increase in serum-digoxin concentrations has also been reported with concomitant aspirin or indometacin, as well as with *ketoprofen*, and *tiaprofenic acid*[1] but some of these studies were in healthy subjects and it is advised that digoxin therapy be monitored carefully whenever any NSAID is initiated or discontinued in digitalised patients.

1. Verbeeck RK. Pharmacokinetic drug interactions with nonsteroidal anti-inflammatory drugs. *Clin Pharmacokinet* 1990; **19:** 44–66.
2. Koren G, et al. Effects of indomethacin on digoxin pharmacokinetics in preterm infants. *Pediatr Pharmacol* 1984; **4:** 25–30.

Pharmacokinetics

The absorption of digoxin from the gastrointestinal tract is variable depending upon the formulation used. About 70% of the administered dose is absorbed from tablets which comply with BP or USP specifications, 80% is absorbed from an elixir, and over 90% is absorbed from liquid-filled soft gelatin capsules. The generally accepted therapeutic plasma concentration range is from 0.5 to 2.0 nanograms per mL but there is considerable interindividual variation. Digoxin has a large volume of distribution and is widely distributed in tissues, including the heart, brain, erythrocytes, and skeletal muscle. The concentration of digoxin in the myocardium is considerably higher than in plasma. From 20 to 30% is bound to plasma proteins. Digoxin has been detected in CSF and breast milk; it also crosses the placenta. It has an elimination half-life of 1.5 to 2 days.

Digoxin is mainly excreted unchanged in the urine by glomerular filtration and tubular secretion; reabsorption also occurs. Extensive metabolism has been reported in a minority of patients (see under Metabolism and Excretion, below). Excretion of digoxin is proportional to the glomerular filtration rate. After intravenous injection 50 to 70% of the dose is excreted unchanged. Digoxin is not removed from the body by dialysis, and only small amounts are removed by exchange transfusion and during cardiopulmonary bypass.

◊ Reviews of the clinical pharmacokinetics of digoxin.
1. Iisalo E. Clinical pharmacokinetics of digoxin. *Clin Pharmacokinet* 1977; **2:** 1–16.
2. Aronson JK. Clinical pharmacokinetics of digoxin 1980. *Clin Pharmacokinet* 1980; **5:** 137–49.
3. Mooradian AD. Digitalis: an update of clinical pharmacokinetics, therapeutic monitoring techniques and treatment recommendations. *Clin Pharmacokinet* 1988; **15:** 165–79.

Absorption. Studies in 6 healthy subjects demonstrated that ingestion of food decreased the rate but not the extent of absorption of concurrently administered digoxin.[1]
1. Johnson BF, *et al.* Effect of a standard breakfast on digoxin absorption in normal subjects. *Clin Pharmacol Ther* 1978; **23:** 315–19.

Bioavailability. Large variations in the content, disintegration, and dissolution of solid dosage forms of digoxin preparations have led to large variations in plasma concentrations from different proprietary preparations. Other factors involved in varying bioavailability include the pharmaceutical formulation and presentation (capsules, solution, or tablets), particle size, and biological factors. Serious problems occurred in the UK[1] in 1972 and in Israel[2] in 1975 following changes in the manufacturing procedure for Lanoxin leading to a twofold increase in bioavailability.
1. Anonymous. Therapeutic non-equivalence. *BMJ* 1972; **3:** 599–600.
2. Danon A, *et al.* An outbreak of digoxin intoxication. *Clin Pharmacol Ther* 1977; **21:** 643–6.

Distribution and protein binding. Digoxin has been reported to be 5 to 60% bound to plasma proteins,[1] depending partly on the method of measurement, but the figure is usually around 20%. Protein binding is reduced in patients undergoing haemodialysis; mean reductions of about 8 and 10% have been reported.[1,2] Injection of heparin has produced a similar reduction.[2]

Digoxin is widely distributed to tissues and serum-digoxin concentrations have been reported to be increased during immobilisation[3] and decreased during exercise[4,5] due to changes in binding to tissues such as skeletal muscle.
1. Storstein L. Studies on digitalis V: the influence of impaired renal function, hemodialysis, and drug interaction on serum protein binding of digitoxin and digoxin. *Clin Pharmacol Ther* 1976; **20:** 6–14.
2. Storstein L, Janssen H. Studies on digitalis VI: the effect of heparin on serum protein binding of digitoxin and digoxin. *Clin Pharmacol Ther* 1976; **20:** 15–23.
3. Pedersen KE, *et al.* Effects of physical activity and immobilization on plasma digoxin concentration and renal digoxin clearance. *Clin Pharmacol Ther* 1983; **34:** 303–8.
4. Joreteg T, Jogestrand T. Physical exercise and digoxin binding to skeletal muscle: relation to exercise intensity. *Eur J Clin Pharmacol* 1983; **25:** 585–8.
5. Joreteg T, Jogestrand T. Physical exercise and binding of digoxin to skeletal muscle—effect of muscle activation frequency. *Eur J Clin Pharmacol* 1984; **27:** 567–70.

The elderly. For references to alterations in the pharmacokinetics of digoxin in the elderly, see under Uses and Administration, below.

Infants and neonates. Digoxin has been widely used in the treatment of cardiac disorders in neonates and infants and its pharmacokinetics in this age group have been reviewed.[1,2] In full-term neonates or infants, 80 to 90% of a dose of digoxin given by mouth in liquid form is absorbed, with peak plasma concentrations occurring within 30 to 120 minutes. The rate of absorption may be slower in preterm and low birth-weight infants, with peak concentrations achieved at 90 to 180 minutes, and may be significantly reduced in severe heart failure and in malabsorption syndromes. After the intravenous administration of digoxin there is a rapid distribution phase with an apparent half-life of 20 to 40 minutes followed by a slower exponential decay of plasma concentrations. In full-term neonates, digoxin has an apparent volume of distribution of 6 to 10 litres per kg body-weight. Low birth-weight infants have a volume of distribution of 4.3 to 5.7 litres per kg while in older infants the volume may range from 10 to 22 litres per kg which

is 1.5 to 2 times reported adult values. This large volume of distribution in full-term neonates and infants is thought to be due to increased tissue binding, a larger extracellular fluid volume, and slightly lower plasma protein binding.

The apparent plasma half-life in healthy and sick neonates is generally very long and may range from 20 to 70 hours in full-term neonates or from 40 to 180 hours in preterm neonates. Digoxin is eliminated at a considerably faster rate in infants than in neonates and, in parallel with maturation of kidney function, a marked increase in clearance rate is usually observed between the second and third month of life. The large apparent volume of distribution, higher clearance values, and greater concentrations of digoxin in the myocardial tissue and red cells of infants might justify the traditional assumption that infants tolerate digoxin better than adults and that higher doses are consequently needed in infants. However, studies have shown that in infants, as in adults, toxic signs become evident at plasma-digoxin concentrations above 3 nanograms per mL and that the therapeutic range may be 1.5 to 2 nanograms per mL.
1. Morselli PL, *et al.* Clinical pharmacokinetics in newborns and infants: age-related differences and therapeutic implications. *Clin Pharmacokinet* 1980; **5:** 485–527.
2. Besunder JB, *et al.* Principles of drug biodisposition in the neonate: a critical evaluation of the pharmacokinetic-pharmacodynamic interface. *Clin Pharmacokinet* 1988; **14:** 189–216 (part I) and 261–86 (part II).

Metabolism and excretion. Although digoxin is reported to be excreted mainly unchanged in the urine there is evidence to suggest that metabolism may sometimes be extensive. Metabolites that have been detected in the urine include digoxigenin, dihydrodigoxigenin, the mono- and bisdigitoxosides of digoxigenin, and dihydrodigoxin. Digoxigenin mono- and bisdigitoxosides are known to be cardioactive whereas dihydrodigoxin is probably much less active than digoxin.[1]

In about 10% of patients there is considerable reduction to cardio-inactive metabolites, chiefly dihydrodigoxin, and 40% or more of a dose may be excreted in the urine as dihydrodigoxin.[2-4] Bacterial flora in the gastrointestinal tract appear to be responsible for this metabolism and antibacterials can reduce the process. Oral digoxin formulations with a high bioavailability are mostly absorbed in the stomach and upper small intestine and little digoxin is available in the lower intestine for bacterial degradation to dihydrodigoxin.[4]
1. Iisalo E. Clinical pharmacokinetics of digoxin. *Clin Pharmacokinet* 1977; **2:** 1–16.
2. Doherty JE. A digoxin-antibiotic drug interaction. *N Engl J Med* 1981; **305:** 827–8.
3. Rund DG, *et al.* Decreased digoxin cardioinactive-reduced metabolites after administration of an encapsulated liquid concentrate. *Clin Pharmacol Ther* 1983; **34:** 738–43.
4. Lofts F, *et al.* Digoxin metabolism to reduced products: clinical significance. *Br J Clin Pharmacol* 1986; **21:** 600P.

Renal impairment. For references to alterations in the pharmacokinetics of digoxin in patients with renal impairment, see under Uses and Administration, below.

Uses and Administration

Digoxin is a cardiac glycoside used in the management of supraventricular arrhythmias, particularly atrial fibrillation (p.794), and in heart failure (p.798).

The principal actions of digoxin are an increase in the force of myocardial contraction (positive inotropic activity) and a reduction in the conductivity of the heart, particularly in conduction through the atrioventricular (AV) node. Digoxin also has a direct action on vascular smooth muscle and indirect effects mediated primarily by the autonomic nervous system, and particularly by an increase in vagal activity. There are also reflex alterations in autonomic activity due to the effects on the circulation. Overall, these actions result in positive inotropic effects, negative chronotropic effects, and decreased AV nodal activity.

Cardiac arrhythmias. In atrial arrhythmias direct and indirect actions cause a decrease in the conduction velocity through the AV node and an increase in the effective refractory period thus reducing ventricular rate. In addition there is a decrease in the refractory period of the cardiac muscle and depression of the sinus node partly in response to the increase in vagal activity.

Digoxin is thus given to slow the increased ventricular rate that occurs in response to atrial fibrillation, although other drugs may be preferred; treatment is usually long term. In atrial flutter, the ventricular rate is normally more difficult to control with digoxin. Direct current cardioversion is the preferred method of treatment, but treatment with digoxin may restore sinus rhythm, or it may convert the flutter to fibrillation and sinus rhythm may then be induced by subsequent withdrawal of digoxin. In patients with the Wolff-Par-

kinson-White syndrome together with atrial fibrillation, digoxin can cause rapid ventricular rates, and possibly ventricular fibrillation, and should be avoided. It may be given to relieve an attack of paroxysmal supraventricular tachycardia and has also been given to prevent further attacks.

Heart failure. Digoxin and other cardiac glycosides directly inhibit the activity of the enzyme sodium-potassium adenosine triphosphatase (Na/K-ATPase) which is required for the active transport of sodium from myocardial cells. The result is a gradual increase in the intracellular sodium concentration and a decrease in the intracellular potassium concentration. The increased concentration of sodium inside the cells leads to an increase in the intracellular calcium concentration with enhancement of mechanical contractile activity and an increased inotropic effect.

When used in heart failure the increased force of myocardial contraction results in increased cardiac output, decreased end-systolic volume, decreased heart size, and decreased end-diastolic pressure and volume. Increased blood flow through the kidneys results in diuresis with a reduction in oedema and blood volume. The decrease in pulmonary venous pressure relieves dyspnoea and orthopnoea. Digoxin may thus provide symptomatic improvement in patients with heart failure and is mainly used for adjunctive therapy.

Dosage. When given by mouth, digoxin may take effect within about 2 hours and the maximum effect may be reached in about 6 hours. Initially a loading dose may be given to digitalise the patient, although this may not be necessary in, for example, mild heart failure.

Dosage should be carefully adjusted to the needs of the individual patient. Factors which may be considered include the patient's age, lean body-mass, renal status, thyroid status, electrolyte balance, degree of tissue oxygenation, and the nature of the underlying cardiac or pulmonary disease. Bearing in mind the above factors, steady-state plasma-digoxin concentrations (in a sample taken at least 6 hours after a dose) of 0.5 to 2 nanograms per mL are generally considered acceptable. For reference to therapeutic drug monitoring, see below.

If rapid digitalisation is required then a loading dose is given to allow for the large volume of distribution. A total loading dose of 750 to 1500 μg of digoxin may be given by mouth during the initial 24-hour period; a dose towards the upper end of this range should be given in divided doses. If there is less urgency digitalisation may be achieved more slowly with doses of 250 μg once or twice daily. Steady-state plasma concentrations are achieved in about 7 days in patients with normal renal function. The usual maintenance dose of digoxin is 125 to 250 μg by mouth daily, but may range from 62.5 to 500 μg daily. In elderly patients therapy should generally be initiated gradually and with smaller doses (but see under Administration in the Elderly, below).

In urgent cases, provided that the patient has not received cardiac glycosides during the previous 2 weeks, digoxin may be given intravenously initially. The intravenous dose ranges from 500 to 1000 μg and produces a definite effect on the heart rate at about 10 minutes, reaching a maximum within about 2 hours. It is administered by intravenous infusion, either as a single dose given over 2 or more hours, or in divided doses each over 10 to 20 minutes. Maintenance treatment is then usually given by mouth. Digoxin has also been given intramuscularly but this route is not generally recommended since such injections may be painful and tissue damage has been reported. Digoxin should not be given subcutaneously as intense local irritation may occur.

Children's doses are complex. They are based on body-weight and the developmental stage of the child as well as on response. Premature infants are especially sensitive to digoxin but, along with all other neonates, infants, and children up to about 10 years of age, still require doses that are higher per kg body-weight than those used for adults. Preterm infants receive lower doses than full-term infants, while children aged 2 to 10 years require lower doses than children up to 2 years of age. As an indication of the doses employed, oral loading doses recommended by manufacturers in the UK range from 25 to 45 µg per kg body-weight over 24 hours and in the USA the range is 20 to 60 µg per kg; the range for intravenous loading doses given over 24 hours is 20 to 35 µg per kg in the UK and 15 to 50 µg per kg in the USA.

Doses should be reduced in patients with renal impairment.

◊ General reviews on the actions and uses of digoxin and the other cardiac glycosides.
1. Opie LH. Digitalis and sympathomimetic stimulants. *Lancet* 1980; i: 912–18.
2. Taggart AJ, McDevitt DG. Digitalis: its place in modern therapy. *Drugs* 1980; 20: 398–404.
3. Chamberlain DA. Digitalis: where are we now? *Br Heart J* 1985; 54: 227–33.
4. Doherty JE. Clinical use of digitalis glycosides: an update. *Cardiology* 1985; 72: 225–54.
5. Smith TW. Digitalis: mechanisms of action and clinical use. *N Engl J Med* 1988; 318: 358–65.
6. Hampton JR. Digoxin. *Br J Hosp Med* 1997; 58: 321–3.
7. Riaz K, Forker AD. Digoxin use in congestive heart failure: current status. *Drugs* 1998; 55: 747–58.

Administration in the elderly. The volume of distribution of digoxin and the elimination half-life increase with age.[1] Therefore there are problems in giving digoxin to elderly patients since steady-state plasma concentrations may not be reached for up to 2 weeks. Fears of toxicity have led some practitioners to use a fixed 'geriatric' dose of 62.5 µg daily. However, such a dose can produce subtherapeutic concentrations.[2] The routine use of very low doses of digoxin in the elderly is inappropriate and dosage should be individualised.
1. McMurray J, McDevitt DG. Treatment of heart failure in the elderly. *Br Med Bull* 1990; 46: 202–29.
2. Nolan L, et al. The need for reassessment of digoxin prescribing for the elderly. *Br J Clin Pharmacol* 1989; 27: 367–70.

Administration in renal impairment. A review of the pharmacokinetics of cardiac glycosides in patients with renal impairment.[1] The rate but not the extent of digoxin absorption is reduced in renal impairment but this is unlikely to be clinically important. Plasma-protein binding may also be reduced but since digoxin is poorly bound to these proteins and has a large apparent volume of distribution this also is unlikely to be important. The apparent volume of distribution is reduced by one-third to one-half and the loading dose of digoxin should therefore be reduced; an oral loading dose of 10 µg per kg body-weight is suggested. Non-renal clearance of digoxin is unaffected or only slightly reduced but renal clearance is reduced, the extent being closely related to creatinine clearance. The elimination half-life of digoxin is prolonged and it therefore takes longer to reach steady state and longer for toxicity to resolve. Because of the reduction in renal clearance of digoxin, maintenance doses must be reduced in line with renal function. Serum-digoxin concentration should be monitored although the presence of digoxin-like immunoreactive substances may make interpretation difficult. In addition, the presence of hyperkalaemia in patients with renal impairment may reduce sensitivity to the effects of digoxin.[2]
Since digoxin has such a large distribution volume, procedures such as peritoneal dialysis and haemodialysis remove only very small amounts of drug from the body and no dosage supplement is needed.
1. Aronson JK. Clinical pharmacokinetics of cardiac glycosides in patients with renal dysfunction. *Clin Pharmacokinet* 1983; 8: 155–78.
2. Matzke GR, Frye RF. Drug administration in patients with renal insufficiency: minimising renal and extrarenal toxicity. *Drug Safety* 1997; 16: 205–31.

Therapeutic drug monitoring. Digoxin has a narrow therapeutic index. It is generally considered that plasma-digoxin concentrations required for a therapeutic effect are usually between 0.5 and 2.0 nanograms per mL.[1-3] The factor for converting nanograms per mL to nanomoles per litre is 1.28.
Digoxin dosage can be calculated in uncomplicated cases by considering the patient's weight, renal function, and clinical status. Therapeutic drug monitoring is *not* considered to be necessary in patients with a satisfactory clinical response to conventional doses in the absence of signs or symptoms of toxicity.[1,2] Measurement of plasma-digoxin concentrations is useful if poor compliance is suspected, if response is poor or there is a deterioration in response without apparent reason, if renal function is fluctuating, when it is unknown if a cardiac glycoside has been previously taken, during drug interactions, and to confirm clinical toxicity.[1,3,4] A plasma concentration should never be considered in isolation and should be used with other patient data as an important component in clinical decision making. This is particularly important in the diagnosis of digoxin toxicity since signs and symptoms of toxicity may be difficult to distinguish from the underlying disease and can occur within the usual therapeutic range.

A number of factors may influence the response to digoxin and thus the interpretation of digoxin assays. These include renal impairment, extremes of age, thyroid disease, patient compliance, drug interactions, and electrolyte disturbances.[1-4] Variations in the bioavailability of different digoxin preparations have also caused problems. Renal impairment and hypokalaemia are two of the most important factors affecting dosage of digoxin and whenever plasma-digoxin concentrations are assayed renal function and plasma potassium should also be measured. The interpretation of digoxin assays is further confounded by the presence of digoxin-like immunoreactive substances in patients with renal or hepatic impairment, in pregnant women, and in neonates. Blood samples for digoxin assay should be taken at least 6 hours after a dose to allow for distribution.[1,3,4]
The usefulness of plasma-digoxin concentrations in the diagnosis of toxicity in children is unclear. For children older than 12 months the adult guidelines can probably be followed and for younger children the trend for increased risk of toxicity at increased plasma-digoxin concentrations appears to hold but the threshold for toxicity may be higher especially in children less than 3 months old.[1] It has been suggested that determination of electrolyte concentrations in erythrocytes (a measure of sodium-potassium ATPase inhibition) may be a more accurate means of diagnosing digoxin toxicity in adults[5] and children.[6]
1. Aronson JK. Indications for the measurement of plasma digoxin concentrations. *Drugs* 1983; 26: 230–42.
2. Lee TH, Smith TW. Serum digoxin concentration and diagnosis of digitalis toxicity: current concepts. *Clin Pharmacokinet* 1983; 8: 279–85.
3. Aronson JK, Hardman M. Digoxin. *BMJ* 1992; 305: 1149–52.
4. Brodie MJ, Feely J. Practical clinical pharmacology: therapeutic drug monitoring and clinical trials. *BMJ* 1988; 296: 1110–14.
5. van Boxtel CJ, et al. Red blood cell electrolytes for monitoring digoxin therapy in adults. *Ther Drug Monit* 1985; 7: 191–6.
6. Loes MW, et al. Relation between plasma and red-cell electrolyte concentrations and digoxin levels in children. *N Engl J Med* 1978; 299: 501–4.

Preparations

BP 2001: Digoxin Injection; Digoxin Tablets; Paediatric Digoxin Injection; Paediatric Digoxin Oral Solution;
USP 25: Digoxin Elixir; Digoxin Injection; Digoxin Tablets.

Proprietary Preparations (details are given in Part 3)
Aust.: Lanicor; Novodigal; *Austral.:* Lanoxin; *Belg.:* Lanoxin; *Braz.:* Lanoxin; *Canad.:* Lanoxin; *Fr.:* Hemigoxine Nativelle; *Ger.:* Digacin; Dilanacin; Lanicor; Lenoxin; Novodigal; *Hong Kong:* Lanoxin; *Irl.:* Lanoxin; *Israel:* Lanoxin; *Ital.:* Digomal†; Eudigox; Lanoxin; *Jpn:* Digosin; *Mex.:* Dogoxine; Lanoxin; Mapluxin; *Neth.:* Lanoxin; *Norw.:* Lanoxin; *NZ:* Lanoxin; *Port.:* Lanoxin; *S.Afr.:* Lanoxin; Purgoxin; *Singapore:* Lanoxin; *Spain:* Lanacordin; *Swed.:* Lanacrist; Lanoxin; *Switz.:* Lanoxin; *Thai.:* Grexin; Lanoxin; Toloxin; *UK:* Lanoxin; *USA:* Lanoxicaps; Lanoxin.

Multi-ingredient: *Aust.:* Gradulon†; Theo-Lanicor†; *Ger.:* Crataelanat†.

Dihydralazine Sulfate (864-c)

Dihydralazine Sulfate (rINNM).

Dihydralazine Sulphate (BANM); Dihydralazini Sulfas Hydricus; Dihydralazinum Sulfuricum; Dihydrallazine Sulphate. Phthalazine-1,4-diyldihydrazine sulphate hemipentahydrate.
$C_8H_{10}N_6, H_2SO_4, 2\frac{1}{2}H_2O = 333.3$.
CAS — 484-23-1 (dihydralazine); 7327-87-9 (dihydralazine sulfate).
Pharmacopoeias. In Eur. (see p.vi) and Pol.
Swiss includes Dihydralazine Mesilate.

Dihydralazine sulfate hemipentahydrate 28.9 mg is approximately equivalent to 25 mg of anhydrous dihydralazine sulfate.

Pharmacopoeial description
Ph. Eur.: A white or slightly yellow crystalline powder. Slightly soluble in water; practically insoluble in dehydrated alcohol. It dissolves in dilute mineral acids.

Profile
Dihydralazine is a vasodilator with actions and uses similar to those of hydralazine (p.905). It is given by mouth as the sulfate. In hypertension (p.802) the usual initial dose is 12.5 mg by mouth twice daily and the maximum recommended dose is 50 mg twice daily. Higher doses have been used in the management of heart failure.

Other salts of dihydralazine that have been used in oral preparations include the hydrochloride and the tartrate. The mesilate is given by injection.

Porphyria. Dihydralazine is considered to be unsafe in patients with porphyria because it has been shown to be porphyrinogenic in *animals* or *in-vitro* systems.

Preparations

Proprietary Preparations (details are given in Part 3)
Aust.: Nepresol; *Belg.:* Nepresol; *Braz.:* Nepresol; *Denm.:* Nepresol; *Fr.:* Nepressol†; *Ger.:* Depressan; Dihyzin; Nepresol; *Hong Kong:* Nepresol; *Israel:* Nepresol; *Neth.:* Nepresol†; *Norw.:* Nepresol; *S.Afr.:* Nepresol; *Swed.:* Nepresol; *Switz.:* Nepresol; *Thai.:* Nepresol.

Multi-ingredient: *Aust.:* Adelphan-Esidrex; Elfanex; *Braz.:* Adelfan-Esidrex; *Fr.:* Trasipressol†; *Ger.:* Adelphan-Esidrix; Obsilazin N; Tri-Torrat; Triniton; *Hong Kong:* Adelphane-Esidrex;

Israel: Pressunic Compositum; *Ital.:* Ipogen†; *S.Afr.:* Adelphane-Esidrex†; *Spain:* Adelfan-Esidrex; *Switz.:* Adelphan-Esidrex.

Di-isopropylammonium Dichloroacetate
(9223-s)

Di-isopropylamine Dichloroacetate; Di-isopropylamine Dichloroethanoate; DIPA-DCA.
$C_8H_{17}Cl_2NO_2 = 230.1$.
CAS — 660-27-5.

Profile
Di-isopropylammonium dichloroacetate is a vasodilator that has been given in peripheral and cerebral vascular disorders. Preparations containing it have sometimes been described as 'pangamic acid' (p.1647).

Preparations

Proprietary Preparations (details are given in Part 3)
Ger.: Disotat; Oxypangam; *Mex.:* Ditrei.

Multi-ingredient: *Ger.:* Neuro-Wied; *Hong Kong:* Liverall; *Spain:* Menalgil B6; Vitaber A E.

Dilazep Hydrochloride (9224-w)

Dilazep Hydrochloride (rINNM).

Asta C-4898. Perhydro-1,4-diazepin-1,4-diylbis(trimethylene 3,4,5-trimethoxybenzoate) dihydrochloride.
$C_{31}H_{44}N_2O_{10}, 2HCl = 677.6$.
CAS — 35898-87-4 (dilazep); 20153-98-4 (dilazep hydrochloride).
Pharmacopoeias. In Jpn.

Profile
Dilazep hydrochloride is a vasodilator that has been used in ischaemic heart disease.

Preparations

Proprietary Preparations (details are given in Part 3)
Ital.: Cormelian†.

Diltiazem Hydrochloride (9225-e)

Diltiazem Hydrochloride (BANM, USAN, rINNM).
CRD-401; Diltiazemi Hydrochloridum; Latiazem Hydrochloride; MK-793 (diltiazem malate). (+)-cis-3-Acetoxy-5-(2-dimethylaminoethyl)-2,3-dihydro-2-(4-methoxyphenyl)-1,5-benzothiazepin-4(5H)-one hydrochloride; (2S,3S)-5-(2-Dimethylaminoethyl)-2,3,4,5-tetrahydro-2-(4-methoxyphenyl)-4-oxo-1,5-benzothiazepin-3-yl acetate hydrochloride.
$C_{22}H_{26}N_2O_4S, HCl = 451.0$.
CAS — 42399-41-7 (diltiazem); 33286-22-5 (diltiazem hydrochloride); 144604-00-2 (diltiazem malate).
Pharmacopoeias. In Chin., Eur. (see p.vi), Jpn, and US.

Pharmacopoeial description
Ph. Eur.: A white crystalline powder. Freely soluble in water, in dichloromethane, and in methyl alcohol; slightly soluble in dehydrated alcohol. The pH of a 1% solution in water is 4.3 to 5.3. Store in airtight containers. Protect from light.
USP 25: A white, odourless, crystalline powder, or small crystals. Freely soluble in water, in chloroform, in formic acid, and in methyl alcohol; sparingly soluble in dehydrated alcohol; insoluble in ether. Store in airtight containers. Protect from light.

Adverse Effects

Treatment with diltiazem is generally well tolerated. Headache, ankle oedema, hypotension, dizziness, flushing, fatigue, and nausea and other gastrointestinal disturbances (including anorexia, vomiting, constipation or diarrhoea, taste disturbances, and weight gain) may occur. Gingival hyperplasia has been reported. Rashes, possibly due to hypersensitivity, are normally mild and transient, but in a few cases erythema multiforme or exfoliative dermatitis has developed; photosensitivity reactions may also occur. Transient elevations in liver enzyme values, and occasionally hepatitis, have been reported.

Diltiazem may depress cardiac conduction and has occasionally led to atrioventricular block, bradycardia, and rarely asystole or sinus arrest.

Overdosage with diltiazem may be associated with bradycardia, with or without atrioventricular conduction defects, and hypotension.

Diltiazem has been shown to cause teratogenicity in *animal* studies.

◊ For discussion of the possibility that calcium-channel blockers might be associated with increased cardiovascular mortality, see under Adverse Effects of Nifedipine, p.940.

Angioedema. Periorbital angioedema, accompanied by pruritus or burning and erythema developed in 2 patients given diltiazem.[1]

1. Sadick NS, et al. Angioedema from calcium channel blockers. J Am Acad Dermatol 1989; 21: 132–3.

Effects on the blood. Thrombocytopenia has been reported in association with diltiazem.[1,2]

1. Lehav M, Arav R. Diltiazem and thrombocytopenia. Ann Intern Med 1989; 110: 327.
2. Michalets EL, Jackson DV. Diltiazem-associated thrombocytopenia. Pharmacotherapy 1997; 17: 1345–8.

Effects on carbohydrate metabolism. Although raised blood-glucose concentrations and insulin requirements have been reported in a patient with type 1 diabetes mellitus during diltiazem therapy, particularly at high doses,[1] a study in 11 obese black women, who were nondiabetic but had a family history of type 2 diabetes, failed to find any effect of diltiazem 240 mg daily on plasma-glucose and C-peptide concentrations, nor any clinical signs of glucose intolerance.[2]

1. Pershadsingh HA, et al. Association of diltiazem therapy with increased insulin resistance in a patient with type I diabetes mellitus. JAMA 1987; 257: 930–1.
2. Jones BJ, et al. Effects of diltiazem hydrochloride on glucose tolerance in persons at risk for diabetes mellitus. Clin Pharm 1988; 7: 235–8.

Effects on the ears. There have been isolated reports[1] of tinnitus associated with several calcium-channel blockers including nifedipine, nicardipine, nitrendipine, diltiazem, verapamil, and cinnarizine.

1. Narváez M, et al. Tinnitus with calcium-channel blockers. Lancet 1994; 343: 1229–30.

Effects on the heart. ATRIOVENTRICULAR BLOCK. Atrioventricular block appears to be uncommon in patients receiving diltiazem, but is potentially serious when it occurs. Prescription-event monitoring of a cohort of 10 119 patients for 1 year revealed 22 reports of atrioventricular block during diltiazem treatment. At least 8 patients had third-degree heart block, and 12 required a pacemaker; 3 died within 72 hours of the onset of heart block.[1] A high proportion of these patients were also receiving beta blockers,[1] which is in line with other reports.[2,3] (See also Beta Blockers under Interactions, below.) There is some evidence that the incidence of this effect may depend on the serum concentration of diltiazem. In a study in patients receiving diltiazem after myocardial infarction, patients with serum-diltiazem concentrations greater than 150 nanograms per mL were more likely to experience atrioventricular block than patients with concentrations of diltiazem below this value.[4]

1. Waller PC, Inman WHW. Diltiazem and heart block. Lancet 1989; i: 617.
2. Hossack KF. Conduction abnormalities due to diltiazem. N Engl J Med 1982; 307: 953–4.
3. Ishikawa T, et al. Atrioventricular dissociation and sinus arrest induced by oral diltiazem. N Engl J Med 1983; 309: 1124–5.
4. Nattel S, et al. Determinants and significance of diltiazem plasma concentrations after acute myocardial infarction. Am J Cardiol 1990; 66: 1422–8.

MYOCARDIAL INFARCTION. Results from at least one large multicentre study (the Multicenter Diltiazem Postinfarction Trial) suggest that diltiazem, although apparently of benefit after myocardial infarction in patients with normal left ventricular function (as indicated by absence of pulmonary congestion), was associated with an increased risk of cardiac death or non-fatal re-infarction in patients with impaired left ventricular function.[1] Long-term follow-up[2] indicated that diltiazem also increased the risk of late-onset heart failure in postinfarction patients with left ventricular dysfunction.

1. The Multicenter Diltiazem Postinfarction Trial Research Group. The effect of diltiazem on mortality and reinfarction after myocardial infarction. N Engl J Med 1988; 319: 385–92.
2. Goldstein RE, et al. Diltiazem increases late-onset congestive heart failure in postinfarction patients with early reduction in ejection fraction. Circulation 1991; 83: 52–60.

WITHDRAWAL. Life-threatening coronary vasospasm, that was fatal in one patient, occurred in 4 patients following coronary revascularisation for unstable angina.[1] Treatment with a calcium-channel blocker (diltiazem or nifedipine) had been discontinued between 8 and 18 hours before the procedure and this abrupt withdrawal was thought to be responsible for the rebound vasospasm. The coronary vasospasm was managed with glyceryl trinitrate and nifedipine.

Withdrawal of diltiazem over a 4-day period from a patient with stable angina pectoris was followed by recurrence of anginal attacks.[2] Ambulatory ECG monitoring confirmed worsening myocardial ischaemia that responded to re-introduction of diltiazem. Two further patients experienced a similar withdrawal effect.

1. Engelman RM, et al. Rebound vasospasm after coronary revascularization in association with calcium antagonist withdrawal. Ann Thorac Surg 1984; 37: 469–72.
2. Subramanian VB, et al. Calcium antagonist withdrawal syndrome: objective demonstration with frequency-modulated ambulatory ST-segment monitoring. BMJ 1983; 286: 520–1.

Effects on the kidneys. Diltiazem may be of benefit in various kidney disorders (see under Uses, below). However, there are a few reports of acute renal failure associated with diltiazem administration.[1,2] Acute interstitial nephritis has been proposed as a mechanism.[2,3]

1. ter Wee PM, et al. Acute renal failure due to diltiazem. Lancet 1984; ii: 1337–8.

2. Abadín JA, et al. Probable diltiazem-induced acute interstitial nephritis. Ann Pharmacother 1998; 32: 656–8.
3. Achenbach V, et al. Acute renal failure due to diltiazem. Lancet 1985; i: 176.

Effects on mental function. By September 1989, the WHO collaborative programme for international drug monitoring had gathered 8 cases of mental depression (severe in 2) associated with diltiazem therapy.[1] Time of onset of symptoms varied from a few hours to a few months after starting treatment with diltiazem. There was some evidence that the problem might be dose-related as 5 of the 8 cases were receiving doses of 180 mg daily or more.

Psychoses have been reported rarely in association with diltiazem. A patient[2] who developed hallucinations (both auditory and visual) and paranoid delusions after 2 days of diltiazem therapy was subsequently treated with nifedipine without abnormal effects. Another patient[3] with bipolar affective disorder that had been well-controlled by lithium carbonate for some years developed acute psychosis with extrapyramidal symptoms of cogwheel rigidity and ataxia, which was thought to represent an interaction between diltiazem and lithium.

1. Biriell C, et al. Depression associated with diltiazem. BMJ 1989; 299: 796.
2. Bushe CJ. Organic psychosis caused by diltiazem. J R Soc Med 1988; 81: 296–7.
3. Binder EF. Diltiazem-induced psychosis and a possible diltiazem-lithium interaction. Arch Intern Med 1991; 151: 373–4.

Effects on the mouth. A study involving 115 patients given nifedipine, diltiazem, or verapamil for at least 3 months indicated that gingival hyperplasia is an important side-effect that may occur with calcium-channel blockers.[1]

1. Steele RM, et al. Calcium antagonist-induced gingival hyperplasia. Ann Intern Med 1994; 120: 663–4.

Effects on the nervous system. Akathisia has been reported in a patient the day after starting treatment with diltiazem. Symptoms disappeared when diltiazem was withdrawn and recurred on rechallenge after the third dose.[1] Similar symptoms in association with mania have also been reported in another patient given diltiazem.[2]

1. Jacobs MB. Diltiazem and akathisia. Ann Intern Med 1983; 99: 794–5.
2. Brink DD. Diltiazem and hyperactivity. Ann Intern Med 1984; 100: 459–60.

PARKINSONISM. Parkinsonism developed in an elderly patient with heart disease and hypertension when diltiazem was added to existing drug therapy.[1] Symptoms worsened over 3 months but improved significantly when diltiazem was slowly discontinued. On rechallenge severe tremor, impaired gait, and cogwheel rigidity recurred, but resolved when the drug was again discontinued except for slight residual cogwheel rigidity.

An acute parkinsonian syndrome also developed[2] in a patient taking lithium and tiotixene when diltiazem was added, and was thought to represent an interaction between lithium and diltiazem. See also under Effects on Mental Function, above.

1. Dick RS, Barold SS. Diltiazem-induced parkinsonism. Am J Med 1989; 87: 95–6.
2. Valdiserri EV. A possible interaction between lithium and diltiazem: case report. J Clin Psychiatry 1985; 46: 540–1.

Effects on the skin. A variety of skin disorders have been associated with diltiazem therapy, including acute pustular dermatitis,[1-3] cutaneous vasculitis,[4,5] erythema multiforme,[6,7] pruritic macular rashes,[3,8] severe toxic erythema,[9] and subacute lupus erythematosus-like eruptions.[10] Analysis of cutaneous adverse reactions to diltiazem indicated that acne, rash, and urticaria were among the commonest.[11] There have also been a few reports of exfoliative dermatitis, erythema multiforme, Stevens Johnson syndrome, and toxic epidermal necrolysis.[3,11]

For a report of periorbital skin rash associated with diltiazem, see under Angioedema, above.

Cross-sensitivity, manifest as a pruritic maculopapular rash, has been reported between diltiazem and amlodipine.[12]

1. Lambert DG, et al. Acute generalized exanthematous pustular dermatitis induced by diltiazem. Br J Dermatol 1988; 118: 308–9.
2. Vicente-Calleja JM, et al. Acute generalized exanthematous pustulosis due to diltiazem: confirmation by patch testing. Br J Dermatol 1997; 137: 837–9.
3. Knowles S, et al. The spectrum of cutaneous reactions associated with diltiazem: three cases and a review of the literature. J Am Acad Dermatol 1998; 38: 201–6.
4. Carmichael AJ, Paul CJ. Vasculitic leg ulcers associated with diltiazem. BMJ 1988; 297: 562.
5. Sheehan-Dare RA, Goodfield MJ. Severe cutaneous vasculitis induced by diltiazem. Br J Dermatol 1988; 119: 134.
6. Berbis P, et al. Diltiazem associated erythema multiforme. Dermatologica 1989; 179: 90.
7. Sanders CJG, Neumann HAM. Erythema multiforme, Stevens-Johnson syndrome, and diltiazem. Lancet 1993; 341: 967.
8. Wirebaugh SR, Geraets DR. Reports of erythematous macular skin eruptions associated with diltiazem therapy. DICP Ann Pharmacother 1990; 24: 1046–9.
9. Wakeel RA, et al. Severe toxic erythema caused by diltiazem. BMJ 1988; 296: 1071.
10. Crowson AN, Magro CM. Diltiazem and subacute cutaneous lupus erythematosus-like lesions. N Engl J Med 1995; 333: 1429.
11. Stern R, Khalsa JH. Cutaneous adverse reactions associated with calcium channel blockers. Arch Intern Med 1989; 149: 829–32.
12. Baker BA, Cacchione JG. Dermatologic cross-sensitivity between diltiazem and amlodipine. Ann Pharmacother 1994; 28: 118–19.

Overdosage. See under Treatment of Adverse Effects, below.

Treatment of Adverse Effects

In recent overdosage (within 1 hour) with diltiazem by mouth the stomach may be emptied by lavage; activated charcoal may be administered. Hypotension may require plasma expanders, intravenous calcium gluconate or calcium chloride, glucagon, and a sympathomimetic such as dopamine or isoprenaline. Bradycardia may be treated with atropine, isoprenaline, or cardiac pacing.

Overdosage. The consequences and treatment of diltiazem overdosage are similar to those described under nifedipine (p.942), although death and life-threatening complications might be more common with diltiazem.[1] Up to 1994, 6 cases of fatal overdose with diltiazem had been reported in the literature.[2] Measurement of diltiazem concentrations to assist in diagnosis and management of overdosage has been suggested,[2] but others[3] have disputed its value.

The following are individual reports of overdosage with diltiazem.

A patient who took approximately 10.8 g of diltiazem developed hypotension and complete heart block. Dopamine, isoprenaline, and calcium chloride were required to maintain the blood pressure. The ECG reverted to sinus rhythm after 31 hours. The plasma-diltiazem concentration was 1670 nanograms per mL 43 hours after ingestion and fell to 12.1 nanograms per mL over a further 55.5 hours with an elimination half-life of 7.9 hours.[4]

In a further case a patient took 5.88 g of diltiazem with alcohol, and developed severe junctional bradycardia, hypotension, and reduced cardiac function that did not respond to intravenous calcium gluconate. The maximum plasma-diltiazem concentration of 6090 nanograms per mL occurred 7 hours after presentation. Approximately half the dose was vomited after treatment with activated charcoal. The patient was treated with cardiac pacing and a dopamine infusion; he reverted to sinus rhythm within 24 hours, and a subsequent episode of atrial fibrillation was treated successfully with digoxin.[5]

Charcoal haemoperfusion had a limited effect in improving the clearance of diltiazem in a patient who had taken 14.94 g of diltiazem.[6] The patient developed severe hypotension, complete heart block, and acute renal failure. Supportive care included cardiac pacing and numerous vasopressors including intravenous glucagon and infusions of dopamine, adrenaline [epinephrine], and noradrenaline [norepinephrine].

1. Buckley NA, et al. Overdose with calcium channel blockers. BMJ 1994; 308: 1639.
2. Roper TA. Overdose of diltiazem. BMJ 1994; 308: 1571.
3. Lip GYH, Ferner RE. Overdose of diltiazem. BMJ 1994; 309: 193.
4. Malcolm N, et al. Massive diltiazem overdosage: clinical and pharmacokinetic observations. Drug Intell Clin Pharm 1986; 20: 888.
5. Ferner RE, et al. Pharmacokinetics and toxic effects of diltiazem in massive overdose. Hum Toxicol 1989; 8: 497–9.
6. Williamson KM, Dunham GD. Plasma concentrations of diltiazem and desacetyldiltiazem in an overdose situation. Ann Pharmacother 1996; 30: 608–11.

Precautions

Diltiazem is contra-indicated in patients with the sick sinus syndrome, pre-existing second- or third-degree atrioventricular block, or marked bradycardia, and should be used with care in patients with lesser degrees of atrioventricular block or bradycardia. Diltiazem has been associated with the development of heart failure and great care is required in patients with impaired left ventricular function. Sudden withdrawal of diltiazem might be associated with an exacerbation of angina.

Treatment with diltiazem should commence with reduced doses in elderly patients and in patients with impaired liver or kidney function.

Abuse. Abuse of diltiazem by body builders and rugby players has been alleged. Such abuse is possibly because of evidence that diltiazem increases maximum oxygen consumption after training. A body builder who admitted to taking diltiazem in high doses suffered severe abdominal cramps.[1]

1. Richards H, et al. Use of diltiazem in sport. BMJ 1993; 307: 940.

Breast feeding. Diltiazem is distributed into breast milk and should generally be avoided in women who are breast feeding. Concentrations of diltiazem were almost the same in serum and breast milk from a woman receiving diltiazem 60 mg four times daily by mouth.[1]

1. Okada M, et al. Excretion of diltiazem in human milk. N Engl J Med 1985; 312: 992–3.

Porphyria. Diltiazem is considered to be unsafe in patients with porphyria because it has been shown to be porphyrinogenic in animals or in-vitro systems.

Renal impairment. A patient with end-stage renal failure requiring haemodialysis developed hypotension, bradycardia,

The symbol † denotes a preparation no longer actively marketed

metabolic acidosis, hyperkalaemia, and acute congestive heart failure about 60 hours after his last haemodialysis.[1] The patient had been taking diltiazem 60 mg three times daily. The symptoms were attributed to diltiazem toxicity due to accumulation of diltiazem and its metabolites which are poorly dialysed and normally excreted partially in the urine.

1. Patel R, *et al.* Toxic effects of diltiazem in a patient with chronic renal failure. *J Clin Pharmacol* 1994; **34:** 273–4.

Interactions

Increased depression of cardiac conduction with risk of bradycardia and atrioventricular block may occur when diltiazem is given with drugs such as amiodarone, beta blockers, digoxin, and mefloquine. Enhanced antihypertensive effect may occur with concomitant use of other antihypertensive drugs or drugs that cause hypotension such as aldesleukin and antipsychotics. Diltiazem is extensively metabolised in the liver by the cytochrome P450 enzyme system and competitive inhibition of metabolism may occur with drugs sharing the same pathway. Interactions may also be expected with enzyme inducers, such as carbamazepine, phenobarbital, phenytoin, and rifampicin, and with enzyme inhibitors, such as cimetidine.

Antidepressants. For a report of diltiazem increasing the bioavailability of *imipramine* and *nortriptyline*, see p.277.

Antiepileptics. For reports of diltiazem administration precipitating *carbamazepine* and *phenytoin* toxicity, see p.345 and p.361, respectively.

Anxiolytics. For the effect of diltiazem on plasma-*buspirone* concentrations, see p.658.

Benzodiazepines. For a potential interaction between diltiazem and *midazolam* or *triazolam*, see Calcium-channel Blockers under Interactions of Diazepam, p.678.

Beta blockers. Profound bradycardia has been reported in a number of patients when diltiazem was prescribed with a beta blocker.[1,2] Diltiazem decreases the clearance of a single dose of *propranolol* or *metoprolol*, though not *atenolol*, and elevated concentrations of beta blocker may be responsible for the bradycardic effects.[3] This is unlikely to be the full story, however, since atenolol, which was unaffected in this study, has been implicated in producing bradycardia when diltiazem was added in a patient with myocardial ischaemia.[2]

1. Hassell AB, Creamer JE. Profound bradycardia after the addition of diltiazem to a β blocker. *BMJ* 1989; **298:** 675.
2. Nagle RE, *et al.* Diltiazem and heart block. *Lancet* 1989; **i:** 907.
3. Tateishi T, *et al.* Effect of diltiazem on the pharmacokinetics of propranolol, metoprolol and atenolol. *Eur J Clin Pharmacol* 1989; **36:** 67–70.

Calcium-channel blockers. For the effect of diltiazem and *nifedipine* on each others plasma concentrations, see p.942.

Ciclosporin. For reports of a potentially beneficial interaction between diltiazem and ciclosporin, see Transplantation under Uses and Administration, below.

Digoxin. For a discussion of interactions between digoxin and calcium-channel blockers including diltiazem, see p.872.

General anaesthetics. Two patients on diltiazem therapy developed impaired myocardial conduction during anaesthesia with *enflurane*;[1] one of the patients had severe sinus bradycardia that progressed to asystole. Additive cardiodepressant effects of diltiazem and enflurane were considered responsible.

1. Hantler CB, *et al.* Impaired myocardial conduction in patients receiving diltiazem therapy during enflurane anesthesia. *Anesthesiology* 1987; **67:** 94–6.

Histamine H₂-antagonists. *Cimetidine* administration caused increases in plasma-diltiazem concentrations and in plasma-deacetyldiltiazem concentrations in 6 subjects given a single dose of diltiazem 60 mg by mouth. *Ranitidine* produced a similar, though less marked effect.[1]

1. Winship LC, *et al.* The effect of ranitidine and cimetidine on single-dose diltiazem pharmacokinetics. *Pharmacotherapy* 1985; **5:** 16–19.

Lithium. Neurotoxicity has been reported in patients receiving lithium and diltiazem, see under Effects on Mental Function and Effects on the Nervous System, above.

Theophylline. For the effect of diltiazem on plasma-theophylline concentrations, see p.781.

Pharmacokinetics

Diltiazem is rapidly and almost completely absorbed from the gastrointestinal tract following oral administration, but undergoes extensive first-pass hepatic metabolism. The bioavailability has been reported to be about 40%, although there is considerable interindividual variation in plasma concentrations. Diltiazem is about 80% bound to plasma proteins. It is distributed into breast milk. It is extensively metabolised in the liver; one of the metabolites, desacetyldiltiazem

has been reported to have 25 to 50% of the activity of the parent compound. The half-life of diltiazem is reported to be about 3 to 5 hours. Approximately 2 to 4% of a dose is excreted in urine as unchanged diltiazem with the remainder excreted as metabolites in bile and urine. Diltiazem and its metabolites are poorly dialysable.

◊ General reviews.

1. Kelly JG, O'Malley K. Clinical pharmacokinetics of calcium antagonists: an update. *Clin Pharmacokinet* 1992; **22:** 416–33.

◊ Studies of the pharmacokinetics of diltiazem in healthy subjects after single and multiple doses,[1-3] indicating that bioavailability was increased after multiple doses, probably because of decreased presystemic elimination.[3]

1. Höglund P, Nilsson L-G. Pharmacokinetics of diltiazem and its metabolites after repeated multiple-dose treatments in healthy volunteers. *Ther Drug Monit* 1989; **11:** 543–50.
2. Höglund P, Nilsson L-G. Pharmacokinetics of diltiazem and its metabolites after repeated single dosing in healthy volunteers. *Ther Drug Monit* 1989; **11:** 551–7.
3. Höglund P, Nilsson L-G. Pharmacokinetics of diltiazem and its metabolites after single and multiple dosing in healthy volunteers. *Ther Drug Monit* 1989; **11:** 558–66.

Renal impairment. The pharmacokinetics of diltiazem and its major metabolite desacetyldiltiazem in patients with severely impaired renal function were similar to those in patients with normal renal function.[1] Nevertheless, reduced doses may be necessary in patients with renal impairment. See also under Precautions, above.

1. Pozet N, *et al.* Pharmacokinetics of diltiazem in severe renal failure. *Eur J Clin Pharmacol* 1983; **24:** 635–8.

Uses and Administration

Diltiazem hydrochloride is a benzothiazepine calcium-channel blocker (p.788). It is a peripheral and coronary vasodilator with limited negative inotropic activity but its vasodilator properties are less marked than those of the dihydropyridine calcium-channel blocker nifedipine (p.940). Unlike nifedipine, diltiazem inhibits cardiac conduction, particularly at the sino-atrial and atrioventricular nodes. Diltiazem is used in the management of angina pectoris (p.791) and hypertension (p.802). In some countries it is available for intravenous administration in the treatment of various cardiac arrhythmias (atrial fibrillation or flutter and paroxysmal supraventricular tachycardia) (p.794).

Diltiazem hydrochloride is given by mouth in the treatment of angina pectoris and hypertension and is available in a number of formulations for administration once, twice, or three times daily. The variety of formulations means that dosage is dependent on the preparation used. Reduced doses may be required in the elderly or those with impaired renal or hepatic function; the dose should not be increased if the heart rate drops below 50 beats per minute.

In **angina pectoris** an initial dose is 60 mg by mouth three times daily (or 30 mg four times daily in the USA), increased if necessary to 360 mg daily; up to 480 mg daily has sometimes been given. Formulations suitable for once- or twice-daily administration may be used in doses of 120 to 480 mg daily; up to 540 mg daily has been given.

In **hypertension** diltiazem hydrochloride may be given as modified-release capsules or tablets. Depending on the formulation, an initial dose is 60 to 120 mg twice daily, increased as required to a maximum of 360 mg daily. Formulations suitable for once-daily administration may be given in similar daily doses, although up to 540 mg daily has been given.

In **cardiac arrhythmias** an initial dose of 250 µg per kg body-weight by bolus intravenous injection over 2 minutes has been suggested; a further dose of 350 µg per kg may be administered after 15 minutes if the response is inadequate. Subsequent doses should be individualised for each patient. For those with atrial fibrillation or flutter, a continued reduction in heart rate may be achieved with an intravenous infusion of diltiazem hydrochloride after the bolus injection. An initial infusion rate of 5 to 10 mg per hour, may be increased as necessary in increments of 5 mg per hour up to a rate of 15 mg per hour. The infusion may be continued for up to 24 hours.

◊ General reviews.

1. Buckley MM-T, *et al.* Diltiazem: a reappraisal of its pharmacological properties and therapeutic use. *Drugs* 1990; **39:** 757–806.
2. Fisher M, Grotta J. New uses for calcium channel blockers: therapeutic implications. *Drugs* 1993; **46:** 961–75.
3. Weir MR. Diltiazem: ten years of clinical experience in the treatment of hypertension. *J Clin Pharmacol* 1995; **35:** 220–32.

Action. The haemodynamic and electrophysiological effects of diltiazem appear to resemble those of verapamil more than those of nifedipine.[1] It inhibits sino-atrial and atrioventricular nodal function in clinically employed doses. The effects on sino-atrial function are more pronounced than those observed after verapamil. Diltiazem causes a decrease in the rate-pressure product indicating that decreased oxygen demand is a likely mechanism of action in relieving angina pectoris. Like verapamil, but unlike nifedipine, diltiazem does not appear to cause significant increases in coronary blood flow. The negative inotropic effect of diltiazem is presumably counteracted by afterload reduction.

1. Soward AL, *et al.* The haemodynamic effects of nifedipine, verapamil and diltiazem in patients with coronary artery disease: a review. *Drugs* 1986; **32:** 66–101.

Anorectal disorders. Beneficial responses to diltiazem reported[1,2] in 2 patients with *proctalgia fugax* may have been due to smooth muscle relaxation. The resting pressure of the internal anal sphincter was decreased by a mean of 20.6% in all but 1 of 13 subjects given a single 60-mg oral dose of diltiazem.[2] Similar results have been reported[3] with oral and topical administration in healthy subjects suggesting diltiazem may be of benefit in the management of *anal fissure* (p.1325).

1. Boquet J, *et al.* Diltiazem for proctalgia fugax. *Lancet* 1986; **i:** 1493.
2. Jonard P, Essamri B. Diltiazem and internal anal sphincter. *Lancet* 1987; **i:** 754.
3. Carapeti EA, *et al.* Topical diltiazem and bethanechol decrease anal sphincter pressure without side effects. *Gut* 1999; **45:** 719–22.

Cardiomyopathies. Although calcium-channel blockers should be used with caution in patients with heart failure, symptomatic improvement has been reported in patients with dilated cardiomyopathy (p.796) given diltiazem.[1]

1. Figulla HR, *et al.* Diltiazem improves cardiac function and exercise capacity in patients with idiopathic dilated cardiomyopathy: results of the Diltiazem in Dilated Cardiomyopathy Trial. *Circulation* 1996; **94:** 346–52.

Kidney disorders. Calcium-channel blockers may be of benefit in various forms of kidney disorder (see Nifedipine, p.944). Diltiazem has been reported to reduce urinary protein excretion without exacerbating pre-existing renal dysfunction in diabetic patients.[1,2] A small study[3] in 15 hypertensive patients with type 2 diabetes mellitus, albuminuria, and renal impairment found that diltiazem only reduced urinary albumin excretion when patients received a restricted dietary sodium intake of 50 mmol daily.

Diltiazem may also reduce the nephrotoxicity associated with certain drugs. Reduced nephrotoxicity has been reported when diltiazem is given to healthy subjects receiving netilmicin,[4] but diltiazem does not appear to modify the acute renal failure associated with tubular damage which may be caused by methotrexate.[5] Diltiazem may reduce ciclosporin-induced nephrotoxicity (see Transplantation, below).

1. Bakris GL. Effects of diltiazem or lisinopril on massive proteinuria associated with diabetes mellitus. *Ann Intern Med* 1990; **112:** 707–8.
2. Demarie BK, Bakris GL. Effects of different calcium antagonists on proteinuria associated with diabetes mellitus. *Ann Intern Med* 1990; **113:** 987–8.
3. Bakris GL, Smith A. Effects of sodium intake on albumin excretion in patients with diabetic nephropathy treated with long-acting calcium antagonists. *Ann Intern Med* 1996; **125:** 201–4.
4. Lortholary O, *et al.* Calcium antagonists and aminoglycoside nephrotoxicity. *Am J Med* 1990; **88:** 445.
5. Deray G, *et al.* The effects of diltiazem on methotrexate-induced nephrotoxicity. *Eur J Clin Pharmacol* 1989; **37:** 337–40.

Migraine. For reference to the use of calcium-channel blockers, including diltiazem, in the management of migraine, see under Nifedipine, p.944.

Myocardial infarction. Studies have not shown a reduction in mortality when calcium-channel blockers are given in the **early** phase of acute myocardial infarction (p.805). However, since myocardial stunning has been linked to intracellular calcium overload[1] there has been speculation that calcium-channel blockers might benefit patients about to undergo reperfusion. This is yet to be confirmed. Diltiazem started within 24 to 72 hours after the onset of infarction and continued for up to 14 days has been reported to protect against re-infarction and refractory angina in patients recovering from acute non-Q-wave infarction.[2] Calcium-channel blockers are not routinely used in the **long-term** management of myocardial infarction although in selected patients without heart failure verapamil or diltiazem may be of some benefit. In a study by the Multicenter Diltiazem Postinfarction Trial (MDPIT) research group,[3] diltiazem (target dose 240 mg daily) reduced 1-year mortality and re-infarction rates in patients without left ventricular dysfunction, but increased such adverse events in those with left ventricular dysfunction. Re-analysis of the Multicenter Diltiazem Postinfarction Trial provided further evidence that diltiazem should be avoided in postinfarction patients with left ventricular dysfunction.[4] A more recent study[5] in patients with acute myocardial infarction treated with thrombolysis found no reduction in mortality with diltiazem started 36 to 96 hours after infarction and continued for up to 6 months, although the incidence of non-fatal cardiac events was reduced. Patients with heart failure were excluded from the trial.

1. Anonymous. Myocardial stunning. *Lancet* 1991; **337:** 585–6.
2. Gibson RS, *et al.* Diltiazem and reinfarction in patients with non-Q-wave myocardial infarction: results of a double-blind, randomized, multicenter trial. *N Engl J Med* 1986; **315:** 423–9.
3. The Multicenter Diltiazem Postinfarction Trial Research Group. The effect of diltiazem on mortality and reinfarction after myocardial infarction. *N Engl J Med* 1988; **319:** 385–92.
4. Goldstein RE, *et al.* Diltiazem increases late-onset congestive heart failure in post-infarction patients with early reduction in ejection fraction. *Circulation* 1991; **83:** 52–60.
5. Boden WE, *et al.* Diltiazem in acute myocardial infarction treated with thrombolytic agents: a randomised placebo-controlled trial. *Lancet* 2000; **355:** 1751–6.

Peripheral vascular disease. Vasospastic arterial disease (p.809) is due to an inappropriate response to temperature, usually cold, when vasoconstriction and/or vasospasm occurs. The most important of these disorders is Raynaud's syndrome. Calcium-channel blockers have been of benefit, but it is not entirely clear which of their pharmacological actions is responsible. The most widely used and studied is nifedipine (see p.945).

Although some studies have reported that diltiazem 120 or 180 mg daily in divided doses produces significant subjective improvement in the majority of patients with Raynaud's syndrome not all investigators have found similar improvement in objective parameters, and there is no evidence to date on the long-term efficacy of diltiazem or its effect on sequelae of the disease such as digital gangrene.[1]

1. Buckley MM-T, *et al.* Diltiazem: a reappraisal of its pharmacological properties and therapeutic use. *Drugs* 1990; **39:** 757–806.

Transplantation. Diltiazem increases blood-ciclosporin concentrations when given by mouth in doses of 60 to 180 mg daily to transplant patients receiving ciclosporin therapy.[1-3] In consequence, ciclosporin doses can be reduced by about one-third, at a considerable saving in cost.[2,3] However, the effect may not occur in all patients,[4] and may vary with differing formulations,[5] and it has been suggested that blood-ciclosporin concentrations should be closely monitored if diltiazem is used for this purpose. In addition to this effect, which is apparently due to non-competitive inhibition of ciclosporin metabolism by diltiazem,[6] there is evidence of improved renal graft-function in patients given the combined therapy, suggesting that diltiazem may reduce ciclosporin-induced nephrotoxicity.[1,2]

1. Wagner K, Neumayer H-H. Prevention of delayed graft function in cadaver kidney transplants by diltiazem. *Lancet* 1985; **ii:** 1355–6.
2. Neumayer H-H, Wagner K. Diltiazem and economic use of cyclosporin. *Lancet* 1986; **ii:** 523.
3. Bourge RC, *et al.* Diltiazem-cyclosporine interaction in cardiac transplant recipients: impact on cyclosporine dose and medication costs. *Am J Med* 1991; **90:** 402–4.
4. Jones TE, Morris RG. Diltiazem does not always increase blood cyclosporin concentration. *Br J Clin Pharmacol* 1996; **42:** 642–4.
5. Jones TE, *et al.* Formulation of diltiazem affects cyclosporin-sparing activity. *Eur J Clin Pharmacol* 1997; **52:** 55–8.
6. Brockmöller J, *et al.* Pharmacokinetic interaction between cyclosporin and diltiazem. *Eur J Clin Pharmacol* 1990; **38:** 237–42.

Preparations

USP 25: Diltiazem Hydrochloride Extended-release Capsules; Diltiazem Hydrochloride Tablets.

Proprietary Preparations (details are given in Part 3)
Aust.: Cardiacton; Corazem; Dilatame†; Dilzem; Gewazem; **Austral.:** Auscard; Cardcal; Cardizem; Coras; Diltahexal; Diltiamax†; Dilzem; Vasocardol; **Belg.:** Progor; Tildiem; **Braz.:** Angiolong; Balcor; Cardizem; Diltizem AP; **Canad.:** Apo-Diltiaz; Cardizem; Novo-Diltiazem; Nu-Diltiaz; Tiazac; **Denm.:** Angiact; Angicontin; Cardil; Cardizem; Dilcor; Myonil; Tilker; UnoCardil; Viazem; **Fin.:** Cardizem; Dilmin; Dilpral; Dilzem; **Fr.:** Bi-Tildiem; Deltazen; Diacor; Dilrene; Mono-Tildiem; Tildiem; **Ger.:** Corazet; Dil-Sanorania; Dilsal; Dilta; Diltabeta; Diltahexal; Diltaretard; Dilti; Diltiagamma; Diltiamerck†; Diltiuc; Dilzem; Dilzereal†; Dilzicardin; **Hong Kong:** Altiazem; Apo-Diltiaz; Dilem; Diltan; Dilzem; Herbesser; Metazem; Retalzem; Tildiem; **Irl.:** Adizem; Diltam; Dilzem; Entrydil; Metazem; Tildiem; **Israel:** Adizem; Dilatam; Levodex; **Ital.:** Altiazem; Angidil†; Angipress; Angizem; Carzem; Citizem; Diladel; Dilem; Diliter; Dilzene; Etyzem; Longazem; Tiakem; Tiazen†; Tildiem; Zilden; **Jpn:** Herbesser; **Mex.:** Angiotrofin; Tilazem; **Neth.:** Diloc; Surazem; Tiadil; Tildiem; **Norw.:** Cardizem; Diltikard; Kardil†; Tilker; **NZ:** Cardizem; Dilcard; Dilzem; **Port.:** Alandiem; Balcor; Cal-Antagon; Dilfar; Diltianginä†; Diltiem; Duplide; Etizem; Herbesser; Pentilzeno†; Tiadil; **S.Afr.:** Anzem; Diatil; Dilatam; Tilazem; Zildem; **Singapore:** Altiazem; Angizem; Cardil; Cardium; Dilatam; Diltizem; Herbesser; Metazem; Mono-Tildiem; Tildiem; **Spain:** Angiodrox; Cardiser; Carreldon; Clobendian; Convectal†; Corolater; Cronodine; Dilaclan; Diltiwas; Dinisor; Doclis; Lacerol; Masdil; Mdiltiwas; Tilker; Trumsal; Uni Masdil; **Swed.:** Cardizem; Coramil; Viazem; **Switz.:** Coridil; Dilzem; Tildiem; **Thai.:** Altiazem; Angizem; Cardil; Denazox; Dilatam; Dilem; Dilizem; Diltan; Dilzem; Dilzem; Ditizem; Herbesser; Metazem; Metazem; Mono-Tildiem; Tildiem; **UK:** Adizem; Angiozem; Angitil; Britiazim†; Calazem†; Calcicard; Dilcardia; Dilzem; Metazem; Optil; Slozem; Tildiem; Viazem XL; Zemtard; **USA:** Cardizem; Cartia; Dilacor XR; Diltia; Tiamate; Tiazac.

Multi-ingredient: UK: Adizem-XL Plus†; **USA:** Teczem.

The symbol † denotes a preparation no longer actively marketed

---

Dimetofrine Hydrochloride (2051-a)

Dimetofrine Hydrochloride (rINNM).

Dimetophrine Hydrochloride. 4-Hydroxy-3,5-dimethoxy-α-[(methylamino)methyl]benzyl alcohol hydrochloride.
$C_{11}H_{17}NO_4,HCl = 263.7$.
CAS — 22950-29-4 (dimetofrine); 22775-12-8 (dimetofrine hydrochloride).

Profile
Dimetofrine hydrochloride is a sympathomimetic (see Adrenaline, p.829) used for its vasopressor effects in usual doses of 300 to 400 mg daily by mouth in the treatment of hypotensive states; it is also given by intramuscular injection or intravenous infusion.

Preparations

Proprietary Preparations (details are given in Part 3)
Ital.: Pressamina.

Multi-ingredient: Ital.: Raffreddoremed.

Diprafenone Hydrochloride (3923-l)

Diprafenone Hydrochloride (rINNM).

(±)-2′-[2-Hydroxy-3-(*tert*-pentylamino)propoxy]-3-phenylpropiophenone hydrochloride.
$C_{23}H_{31}NO_3,HCl = 406.0$.
CAS — 81447-80-5 (diprafenone); 86342-43-0 (diprafenone hydrochloride).

Profile
Diprafenone hydrochloride is a class Ic antiarrhythmic (p.787) structurally related to propafenone. It has some beta-adrenoceptor blocking activity.

◊ References.
1. Trenk D, *et al.* Pharmacokinetic characterization of the antiarrhythmic drug diprafenone in man. *Eur J Clin Pharmacol* 1989; **37:** 313–16.
2. Wagner F, *et al.* Evaluation of the beta-adrenoceptor blocking activity of the class Ic antiarrhythmic drug diprafenone in man. *Eur J Clin Pharmacol* 1989; **36:** 579–82.
3. Koytchev R, *et al.* Influence of food on the bioavailability and some pharmacokinetic parameters of diprafenone—a novel antiarrhythmic agent. *Eur J Clin Pharmacol* 1996; **50:** 315–19.

Dipyridamole (9226-l)

Dipyridamole (BAN, USAN, rINN).

Dipyridamolum; NSC-515776; RA-8. 2,2′,2″,2‴-[(4,8-Dipiperidinopyrimido[5,4-d]pyrimidine-2,6-diyl)dinitrilo]tetraethanol.
$C_{24}H_{40}N_8O_4 = 504.6$.
CAS — 58-32-2.
ATC — B01AC07.

Pharmacopoeias. In *Chin., Eur.* (see p.vi), *Jpn, Pol.,* and *US.*

Pharmacopoeial description

Ph. Eur.: A bright yellow crystalline powder. Practically insoluble in water and in ether; soluble in dehydrated alcohol; freely soluble in acetone. It dissolves in dilute solutions of mineral acids. Protect from light.

USP 25: An intensely yellow, crystalline powder or needles. Slightly soluble in water; very soluble in chloroform, in alcohol, and in methyl alcohol; very slightly soluble in acetone and in ethyl acetate. Store in airtight containers. Protect from light.

Adverse Effects, Treatment, and Precautions

Gastric disturbances, including nausea, vomiting, and diarrhoea, headache, dizziness, faintness, facial flushing, and skin rash may occur after administration of dipyridamole. Dipyridamole can also induce chest pain or lead to a worsening of the symptoms of angina. Cardiac arrhythmias have been reported in patients given dipyridamole during thallium-201 imaging. Aminophylline may reverse some of the adverse effects.

When dipyridamole is given by mouth care is required in patients with hypotension, unstable angina, aortic stenosis, recent myocardial infarction, heart failure, or coagulation disorders. Many of these conditions may become contra-indications when dipyridamole is used intravenously and details are given under Myocardial Imaging, below.

Effects on the biliary tract. Gallstones containing unconjugated dipyridamole were removed from two patients who had been taking dipyridamole for 15 and 10 years, respectively.[1] A gallstone containing unconjugated dipyridamole recurred in a patient who continued to take the drug after endoscopic removal of a similar stone 18 months before.[2]

1. Moesch C, *et al.* Biliary drug lithiasis: dipyridamole gallstones. *Lancet* 1992; **340:** 1352–3.
2. Sautereau D, *et al.* Recurrence of biliary drug lithiasis due to dipyridamole. *Endoscopy* 1997; **29:** 421–3.

Effects on the heart. Transient myocardial ischaemia occurred in 4 patients with unstable angina and multivessel coronary artery disease during oral treatment with dipyridamole.[1] See under Myocardial Imaging, below, for additional reports.

1. Keltz TN, *et al.* Dipyridamole-induced myocardial ischemia. *JAMA* 1987; **257:** 1515–16.

Effects on the muscles. Symptoms resembling acute pseudopolymyalgia rheumatica developed in a patient taking dipyridamole.[1]

1. Chassagne P, *et al.* Pseudopolymyalgia rheumatica with dipyridamole. *BMJ* 1990; **301:** 875.

Effects on taste. A report of a disagreeable taste associated with other gastrointestinal symptoms occurring in a patient taking dipyridamole.[1] Two similar cases had been reported to the UK Committee on Safety of Medicines.

1. Willoughby JMT. Drug-induced abnormalities of taste sensation. *Adverse Drug React Bull* 1983; **100:** 368–71.

Myocardial imaging. Dipyridamole may be used in association with thallium-201 in myocardial stress imaging. Safety data from over 3900 patients has been summarised.[1] Adverse effects which occurred within 24 hours after intravenous administration of dipyridamole (mean dose 0.56 mg per kg bodyweight) were recorded. Ten patients had major adverse effects and 1820 patients experienced minor adverse effects. Myocardial infarction occurred in 4 patients, 3 of whom had unstable angina before thallium-201 myocardial scanning. Six patients developed acute bronchospasm, 4 of whom had a history of asthma or had wheezing before administration of dipyridamole. Adverse effects considered to be minor included chest pain in 19.7% of patients, ST-T-segment depression in 7.5%, ventricular extrasystoles in 5.2%, headache in 12.2%, dizziness in 11.8%, nausea in 4.6%, and hypotension in 4.6%. Aminophylline was effective in relieving symptoms of adverse effects in 97% of 454 patients.

Hypersensitivity reactions including anaphylaxis and angioedema have been reported.[2,3]

A review[4] of pharmacological stress testing suggested that with appropriate patient selection and adequate monitoring, the incidence of life-threatening adverse reactions is negligible. It was also considered that dipyridamole-thallium-201 imaging could be safely performed in the early post-myocardial infarction period. Caution should be exercised in patients with acute unstable angina or a history of bronchospasm. However, the manufacturers contra-indicate the injection of dipyridamole in subvalvular aortic stenosis, aortic disease, hypotension associated with recent myocardial infarction, significant valvular disease, uncompensated heart failure, conduction defects, or arrhythmias.

1. Ranhosky A, *et al.* The safety of intravenous dipyridamole thallium myocardial perfusion imaging. *Circulation* 1990; **81:** 1205–9.
2. Weinmann P, *et al.* Anaphylaxis-like reaction induced by dipyridamole during myocardial scintigraphy. *Am J Med* 1994; **97:** 488.
3. Angelides S, *et al.* Acute reaction to dipyridamole during myocardial scintigraphy. *N Engl J Med* 1999; **340:** 394.
4. Beller GA. Pharmacologic stress imaging. *JAMA* 1991; **265:** 633–8.

Interactions

Dipyridamole may enhance the actions of oral anticoagulants due to its antiplatelet effect. It inhibits the reuptake of adenosine and may enhance its effects; the dose of adenosine must be reduced if the two drugs are given concomitantly. Dipyridamole may also inhibit the uptake of fludarabine and may reduce its efficacy.

The absorption of dipyridamole may be reduced by drugs such as antacids that increase gastric pH.

Anticoagulants. Dipyridamole may induce bleeding in patients receiving oral anticoagulants without altering prothrombin times, see Antiplatelets, under Warfarin, Interactions, p.996.

Xanthines. Xanthines may antagonise some of the effects of dipyridamole due to their action as adenosine antagonists. *Aminophylline* may be used to reverse some of the adverse effects of dipyridamole. Administration of *caffeine* intravenously has been reported[1] to attenuate the haemodynamic response to dipyridamole and it has been suggested that caffeine should be avoided for at least 24 hours before the test in patients receiving dipyridamole for myocardial imaging.

1. Smits P, *et al.* Dose-dependent inhibition of the hemodynamic response to dipyridamole by caffeine. *Clin Pharmacol Ther* 1991; **50:** 529–37.

Pharmacokinetics

Dipyridamole is incompletely absorbed from the gastrointestinal tract with peak plasma concentrations occurring about 75 minutes after oral administration. Dipyridamole is highly bound to plasma proteins. A terminal half-life of 10 to 12 hours has been reported. Dipyridamole is metabolised in the liver and is mainly excreted as glucuronides in the bile. Excretion may be delayed by enterohepatic recirculation. A small amount is excreted in the urine.

◊ References.
1. Mahony C, et al. Dipyridamole kinetics. *Clin Pharmacol Ther* 1982; **31**: 330–8.
2. Mahony C, et al. Plasma dipyridamole concentrations after two different dosage regimens in patients. *J Clin Pharmacol* 1983; **23**: 123–6.

Uses and Administration

Dipyridamole is an adenosine reuptake inhibitor and phosphodiesterase inhibitor with antiplatelet and vasodilating activity and is used in thromboembolic disorders (p.816). Oral dipyridamole is used in association with an oral anticoagulant for the prophylaxis of thromboembolism following cardiac valve replacement (p.816). The usual adult dose is 300 to 600 mg daily by mouth in divided doses before meals. Children may be given 5 mg per kg body-weight by mouth daily in divided doses.

It has been given either alone or with aspirin in the management of myocardial infarction (p.805) and stroke (p.813). For the secondary prevention of stroke or transient ischaemic attack it may be given as a modified-release preparation in a dose of 200 mg twice daily.

Dipyridamole administered intravenously results in marked coronary vasodilatation and is used in stress testing in patients with ischaemic heart disease (see below).

◊ General references.
1. FitzGerald GA. Dipyridamole. *N Engl J Med* 1987; **316**: 1247–57.
2. Gibbs CR, Lip GYH. Do we still need dipyridamole? *Br J Clin Pharmacol* 1998; **45**: 323–8.

Ischaemic heart disease. Perfusion abnormalities due to coronary artery disease are usually absent at rest but are present during stress, and stress imaging may therefore be used in the assessment of myocardial function. The stress is usually supplied by exercise, but when exercise is inappropriate pharmacological methods such as dipyridamole may be used.

Dipyridamole has been used with thallium-201 scintigraphy and is usually given intravenously in a dose of 560 μg per kg body-weight over 4 minutes. Thallium-201 is given immediately after completion of the infusion of dipyridamole. Initial images are obtained 5 minutes after drug administration and delayed images are obtained 2.5 to 4 hours later. Dipyridamole (300 to 400 mg) has also been given as an oral suspension; thallium-201 is given about 45 minutes later to coincide with peak dipyridamole-serum concentrations.

Dipyridamole has also been used in echocardiography.[1,2] The intravenous dipyridamole dose used to obtain maximum sensitivity is often higher (750 to 840 μg per kg) than the dose used in scintigraphy.[1]
1. Beller GA. Pharmacologic stress imaging. *JAMA* 1991; **265**: 633–8.
2. Buchalter MB, et al. Dipyridamole echocardiography: the bedside stress test for coronary artery disease. *Postgrad Med J* 1990; **66**: 531–5.

Preparations

BP 2001: Dipyridamole Tablets;
USP 25: Dipyridamole Tablets.

Proprietary Preparations (details are given in Part 3)
Aust.: Persantin; *Austral.:* Persantin; *Belg.:* Didamol†; Dipyridan; Persantine; *Braz.:* Fluxocor; Persantin; Procor; *Canad.:* Novo-Dipiradol; Persantine; *Denm.:* Persantin; *Fin.:* Atrombin; Dipyrin; Persantin; *Fr.:* Cleridium; Coronarine; Perkod; Persantine; Protangix; *Ger.:* Curantyl N; Persantin; *Hong Kong:* Persantin; *Irl.:* Persantin; *Israel:* Cardoxin; *Ital.:* Corosan; Novodil†; Persantin; *Mex.:* Damosal; Dipres; Dirinol; Lodimol; Persantin; Pracem; Trepol; Trompersantin; Vadinar; *Neth.:* Persantin; *Norw.:* Persantin; *NZ:* Persantin; Pytazen; *Port.:* Persantin; *S.Afr.:* Dipyrol†; Persantin; Plato; *Singapore:* Persantin; Procardin; *Spain:* Miosen; Persantin; *Swed.:* Persantin; *Switz.:* Natyl†; Persantine; *Thai.:* Agremol; Persantin; Posanin; *UK:* Cerebrovase†; Modaplate†; Persantin; *USA:* Persantine.

Multi-ingredient: *Aust.:* Asasantin; Duplinal†; Thrombosantin; *Austral.:* Asasantin; *Belg.:* Aggrenox; *Braz.:* Persantin S Procor S; *Canad.:* Asasantine; *Fin.:* Asasantin; *Fr.:* Asasantine; *Ger.:* Asasantin; *Hong Kong:* Persantin Plus; *Ital.:* Persumbrax†; *Mex.:* Asasantin; *Neth.:* Asasantin; *Norw.:* Asasantin; *S.Afr.:* Asasantine; *Spain:* Asasantin; *Swed.:* Asasantin; *Switz.:* Asasantine; *UK:* Asasantin; *USA:* Aggrenox.

Disopyramide (7783-h)

Disopyramide (BAN, USAN, rINN).
Disopyramidum; SC-7031. 4-Di-isopropylamino-2-phenyl-2-(2-pyridyl)butyramide.
$C_{21}H_{29}N_3O = 339.5$.
CAS — 3737-09-5.
ATC — C01BA03.
Pharmacopoeias. In Eur. (see p.vi) and Jpn.

Pharmacopoeial description
Ph. Eur.: A white or almost white powder. Slightly soluble in water; soluble in alcohol; freely soluble in dichloromethane. Protect from light.

Disopyramide Phosphate (7784-m)

Disopyramide Phosphate (BANM, USAN, rINNM).
Disopyramidi Phosphas; SC-13957.
$C_{21}H_{29}N_3O,H_3PO_4 = 437.5$.
CAS — 22059-60-5.
Pharmacopoeias. In Eur. (see p.vi) and US.

Disopyramide phosphate 1.3 g is approximately equivalent to 1 g of disopyramide.

Pharmacopoeial description
Ph. Eur.: A white or almost white powder. Soluble in water; sparingly soluble in alcohol; practically insoluble in dichloromethane. A 5% solution in water has a pH of 4.0 to 5.0. Protect from light.
USP 25: A white or practically white, odourless powder. Freely soluble in water; slightly soluble in alcohol; practically insoluble in chloroform and in ether. pH of a 5% solution in water is between 4.0 and 5.0. Store in airtight containers. Protect from light.

Adverse Effects and Treatment

The adverse effects most commonly associated with disopyramide therapy relate to its antimuscarinic properties and are dose-related. They include dry mouth, blurred vision, urinary hesitancy, impotence, and constipation; the most serious effect is urinary retention. Gastrointestinal effects which are less common include nausea, bloating, and abdominal pain. Other adverse effects reported include skin rashes, hypoglycaemia, dizziness, fatigue, muscle weakness, headache, and urinary frequency. Insomnia and depression have also been associated with disopyramide administration. There have been rare reports of psychosis, cholestatic jaundice, elevated liver enzymes, thrombocytopenia, and agranulocytosis. Disopyramide has cardiac depressant properties, and may induce cardiac arrhythmias particularly ventricular tachycardia and fibrillation, heart block and conduction disturbances, heart failure, and hypotension.

Over-rapid intravenous injection of disopyramide may cause profuse sweating and severe cardiovascular depression.

In overdose cardiovascular and antimuscarinic effects are pronounced, and there may be apnoea, loss of consciousness, loss of spontaneous respiration, and asystole. Treatment of overdosage is symptomatic and supportive.

◊ A review of the adverse effects associated with the class Ia antiarrhythmic drugs disopyramide, procainamide, and quinidine, and their clinical management.[1]
1. Kim SY, Benowitz NL. Poisoning due to class IA antiarrhythmic drugs quinidine, procainamide and disopyramide. *Drug Safety* 1990; **5**: 393–420.

◊ During long-term therapy with disopyramide 400 to 1600 mg daily in 40 patients, 28 (70%) had one or more adverse effects.[1] Dry mouth occurred in 15 (38%), constipation in 12 (30%), blurred vision in 11 (28%), urinary hesitancy in 9 (23%), nausea in 9 (23%), impotence in 2 (5%), and dyspareunia in one patient (3%). In addition 3 of the 9 patients with pre-existing heart failure had worsening of their condition due to disopyramide. Adverse effects were sufficiently severe for disopyramide to be discontinued in 7 patients, and for dosage reductions in another 7.
1. Bauman JL, et al. Long-term therapy with disopyramide phosphate: side effects and effectiveness. *Am Heart J* 1986; **111**: 654–60.

Effects on the blood. Granulocytopenia was associated on 2 occasions with the use of disopyramide phosphate in a 61-year-old man.[1]
1. Conrad ME, et al. Agranulocytosis associated with disopyramide therapy. *JAMA* 1978; **240**: 1857–8.

Effects on the eyes. The antimuscarinic activity of disopyramide may cause adverse effects on the eyes such as dilated pupils,[1] severe blurring of vision,[1] and acute glaucoma.[2,3] Dis-

opyramide should be avoided in patients with glaucoma and used with caution if there is a family history of glaucoma.
1. Frucht J, et al. Ocular side effects of disopyramide. *Br J Ophthalmol* 1984; **68**: 890–1.
2. Trope GE, Hind VMD. Closed-angle glaucoma in patient on disopyramide. *Lancet* 1978; **i**: 329.
3. Ahmad S. Disopyramide: pulmonary complications and glaucoma. *Mayo Clin Proc* 1990; **65**: 1030–1.

Effects on the heart. Disopyramide has a strong negative inotropic effect and reversible heart failure has been reported[1] following administration of disopyramide. As many as 50% of patients with a previous history of heart failure may have a recurrence of the disease with an incidence of less than 5% in other patients.

As disopyramide can prolong the QT interval seen on the ECG it can induce ventricular tachyarrhythmias. A case of fatal torsade de pointes has been reported.[2]
1. Podrid PJ, et al. Congestive heart failure caused by oral disopyramide. *N Engl J Med* 1980; **302**: 614–17.
2. Schattner A, et al. Fatal torsade de pointes following jaundice in a patient treated with disopyramide. *Postgrad Med J* 1989; **65**: 333–4.

Effects on the liver. Cholestatic jaundice with raised liver enzyme values has been associated with disopyramide treatment.[1-3] Laboratory and clinical abnormalities disappear on withdrawal of disopyramide although liver enzyme values may remain elevated for several months.
Severe hepatocellular damage with disseminated intravascular coagulation[4] has also been reported.
1. Craxi A, et al. Disopyramide and cholestasis. *Ann Intern Med* 1980; **93**: 150–1.
2. Edmonds ME, Hayler AM. *Eur J Clin Pharmacol* 1980; **18**: 285–6.
3. Bakris GL, et al. Disopyramide-associated liver dysfunction. *Mayo Clin Proc* 1983; **58**: 265–7.
4. Doody PT. Disopyramide hepatotoxicity and disseminated intravascular coagulation. *South Med J* 1982; **75**: 496–8.

Effects on mental state. Agitation and distress leading to paranoia and auditory and visual hallucinations have been reported[1,2] in patients shortly after starting disopyramide therapy. Complete recovery occurred on withdrawal of disopyramide.
1. Falk RH, et al. Mental distress in patient on disopyramide. *Lancet* 1977; **i**: 858–9.
2. Padfield PL, et al. Disopyramide and acute psychosis. *Lancet* 1977; **i**: 1152.

Effects on the nervous system. Peripheral neuropathy affecting the feet and severe enough to prevent walking was associated with disopyramide in a 72-year-old patient.[1] There was gradual improvement on withdrawal of disopyramide with the patient being symptom-free after 4 months.
A 75-year-old woman with atrial fibrillation suffered a tonic-clonic seizure followed by respiratory arrest after receiving disopyramide 150 mg intravenously over a period of 10 minutes.[2] On recovery she complained of a dry mouth and blurred vision and it was considered that the seizure was caused by the antimuscarinic action of disopyramide, although it may have been due to a direct stimulant action.
1. Dawkins KD, Gibson J. Peripheral neuropathy with disopyramide. *Lancet* 1978; **i**: 329.
2. Johnson NM, et al. Epileptiform convulsion with intravenous disopyramide. *Lancet* 1978; **ii**: 848.

Effects on sexual function. Impotence in a patient taking disopyramide was abolished when the plasma concentration was reduced from 14 to 3 μg per mL.[1] This effect was probably due to the antimuscarinic activity of disopyramide although the patient did not report any other antimuscarinic symptoms.
1. McHaffie DJ, et al. Impotence in patient on disopyramide. *Lancet* 1977; **i**: 859.

Effects on the urinary tract. In a report of 9 cases of urinary retention associated with disopyramide therapy and a review of the literature,[1] it was observed that urinary retention secondary to disopyramide therapy was most likely to develop in male patients over the age of 65 in whom there was some pre-existing renal dysfunction; there was an increased risk in patients with evidence of prostatic hyperplasia.
1. Danziger LH, Horn JR. Disopyramide-induced urinary retention. *Arch Intern Med* 1983; **143**: 1683–6.

Hypersensitivity. Worsening of ventricular arrhythmia and an anaphylactoid reaction occurred in a 58-year-old man after a single dose of disopyramide 300 mg by mouth.[1] Two hours after the dose he complained of a swollen tongue and difficulty in breathing. He became cyanotic and was given diphenhydramine 25 mg intravenously, which resulted in improvement of his respiratory status.
1. Porterfield JG, et al. Respiratory difficulty after use of disopyramide. *N Engl J Med* 1980; **303**: 584.

Hypoglycaemia. Following reports to the manufacturer of hypoglycaemia associated with administration of disopyramide, 2 controlled studies were conducted in healthy subjects.[1] Disopyramide produced a small decrease in blood-glucose concentration but there were no symptoms of hypoglycaemia. It was considered that the glucose-lowering effect may be clinically significant in patients with renal or hepatic impairment.
1. Strathman I, et al. Hypoglycemia in patients receiving disopyramide phosphate. *Drug Intell Clin Pharm* 1983; **17**: 635–8.

Overdosage. A 2-year-old boy suffered hypotension, cardiac arrhythmias, and convulsions and died 28 hours after ingestion of 600 mg of disopyramide.[1] In a report[2] of 5 cases of fatal overdosage with disopyramide the most common clinical finding appeared to be an early loss of consciousness following an episode of respiratory arrest. Four of the patients initially responded to resuscitation but subsequently deteriorated rapidly, with cardiac arrhythmias and loss of spontaneous respiration; in 4 of the cases post-mortem examination demonstrated pulmonary congestion secondary to left ventricular failure.

1. Hutchison A, Kilham H. Fatal overdosage of disopyramide in a child. *Med J Aust* 1978; **2**: 335–6.
2. Hayler AM, *et al.* Fatal overdosage with disopyramide. *Lancet* 1978; **i**: 968–9.

Precautions

Disopyramide is contra-indicated in patients with complete heart block or cardiogenic shock. It should be used with extreme caution in patients with other conduction disorders or uncompensated heart failure. If disopyramide is used to treat atrial tachycardia it may be necessary to pre-treat with digoxin; see Quinidine, Precautions, p.965. Hypokalaemia should be corrected before treatment with disopyramide is initiated since the effectiveness of disopyramide may be diminished. Care should be taken in patients susceptible to hypoglycaemia, including those with heart failure, renal or hepatic impairment, and patients taking drugs that affect glucose metabolism.

Intravenous injections of disopyramide should be given slowly to avoid hypotension and it is recommended that facilities for cardiac monitoring and defibrillation should be available when the injection is used.

Dosage reduction may be necessary in patients with renal or hepatic impairment and in patients with heart failure.

Owing to its antimuscarinic properties, disopyramide should be avoided in patients with glaucoma or a tendency to urinary retention, as in benign prostatic hyperplasia, and also in patients with myasthenia gravis due to the risk of precipitating a myasthenic crisis. It should be used with caution in patients with a family history of glaucoma.

◊ For dosage adjustments in the elderly and in patients with abnormal hepatic or renal function, see under Uses and Administration, below.

Breast feeding. Disopyramide is distributed into breast milk and milk to plasma ratios of 0.4, about 0.5, and 0.9 have been reported.[1-3] Disopyramide has been detected in the plasma of breast-fed infants, but was not associated with adverse effects. Disopyramide treatment should not be considered a contra-indication to breast feeding although the infant should be monitored for adverse effects, especially antimuscarinic effects.

1. MacKintosh D, Buchanan N. Excretion of disopyramide in human breast milk. *Br J Clin Pharmacol* 1985; **19**: 856–7.
2. Hoppu K, *et al.* Disopyramide and breast feeding. *Br J Clin Pharmacol* 1986; **21**: 553.
3. Barnett DB, *et al.* Disopyramide and its N-monodesalkyl metabolite in breast milk. *Br J Clin Pharmacol* 1982; **14**: 310–12.

Pregnancy. No adverse effects were noted in a patient who received disopyramide 200 mg every 8 hours from 26 weeks' gestation until delivery,[1] although doses of 100 to 300 mg were associated with initiation of uterine contractions in another patient in week 32 of pregnancy.[2] A double-blind, placebo-controlled study[3] involving 20 women hospitalised for induction of labour confirmed that disopyramide induces uterine contractions. All 10 women given disopyramide 150 mg every 6 hours for 48 hours had initiation of contractions and in 8 delivery was induced. It was considered that disopyramide should not be used as an antiarrhythmic during pregnancy.

1. Shaxted EJ, Milton PJ. Disopyramide in pregnancy: a case report. *Curr Med Res Opin* 1979; **6**: 70–2.
2. Leonard RF, *et al.* Initiation of uterine contractions by disopyramide during pregnancy. *N Engl J Med* 1978; **299**: 84–5.
3. Tadmor OP, *et al.* The effect of disopyramide on uterine contractions during pregnancy. *Am J Obstet Gynecol* 1990; **162**: 482–6.

Interactions

Disopyramide should be used with caution in association with other cardiac depressants including beta blockers and other class I antiarrhythmics, and with other arrhythmogenic drugs. Disopyramide may be metabolised by the cytochrome P450 isoenzyme CYP3A4 and interactions may occur with inhibitors or inducers of this enzyme and with other drugs metabolised by CYP3A4. Concomitant use of disopyramide and other antimuscarinic drugs produces enhanced antimuscarinic effects.

Anti-anginals. For reference to disopyramide reducing the effectiveness of sublingual *isosorbide dinitrate*, see p.915.

The symbol † denotes a preparation no longer actively marketed

Antiarrhythmics. The cardiac depressant effects of disopyramide are additive to those of other class I antiarrhythmic drugs.[1] Disopyramide may prolong the QT interval, a factor associated with torsade de pointes, particularly when given concomitantly with other drugs that have a similar effect; this effect was noted in a few patients given *amiodarone* and disopyramide together.[2] Also the serum concentration of disopyramide has been increased by concurrent administration of *quinidine*;[3] there was a reciprocal decrease in the serum-quinidine concentration but this was less important clinically.

1. Ellrodt G, Singh BN. Adverse effects of disopyramide (Norpace): toxic interactions with other antiarrhythmic agents. *Heart Lung* 1980; **9**: 469–74.
2. Tartini R, *et al.* Dangerous interaction between amiodarone and quinidine. *Lancet* 1982; **i**: 1327–9.
3. Baker BJ, *et al.* Concurrent use of quinidine and disopyramide: evaluation of serum concentrations and electrocardiographic effects. *Am Heart J* 1983; **105**: 12–15.

Antibacterials. The metabolism of disopyramide may be increased by enzyme inducers such as *rifampicin*;[1,2] the increased clearance of disopyramide may lead to subtherapeutic plasma concentrations. Elevation of serum-disopyramide concentrations with ventricular tachycardia occurred[3] in 2 patients when *erythromycin*, an enzyme inhibitor, was added to disopyramide therapy. Ventricular fibrillation developed in a 74-year-old woman 6 days after *clarithromycin* was added to disopyramide therapy.[4] The elimination half-life of disopyramide was found to be markedly prolonged.

1. Aitio M-L, *et al.* The effect of enzyme induction on the metabolism of disopyramide in man. *Br J Clin Pharmacol* 1981; **11**: 279–85.
2. Staum JM. Enzyme induction: rifampin-disopyramide interaction. *DICP Ann Pharmacother* 1990; **24**: 701–3.
3. Ragosta M, *et al.* Potentially fatal interaction between erythromycin and disopyramide. *Am J Med* 1989; **86**: 465–6.
4. Paar D, *et al.* Life-threatening interaction between clarithromycin and disopyramide. *Lancet* 1997; **349**: 326–7.

Antiepileptics. The enzyme inducers *phenytoin*[1] and *phenobarbital* may increase the clearance of disopyramide.

1. Aitio M-L, *et al.* The effect of enzyme induction on the metabolism of disopyramide in man. *Br J Clin Pharmacol* 1981; **11**: 279–85.

Beta blockers. Bradycardia,[1,2] severe hypotension,[1] and asystole,[1] with one fatality,[1] have been reported following the intravenous injection of disopyramide 20 minutes after intravenous *practolol*. Both drugs have negative inotropic effects which are additive when they are administered in close succession, but separation of the drugs by 2 hours prevented the development of these adverse effects.[2] A pharmacokinetic interaction may also occur with beta blockers since the clearance of disopyramide has been reported[3] to be reduced by approximately 16% during concomitant treatment with *atenolol*.

1. Cumming AD, Robertson C. Interaction between disopyramide and practolol. *BMJ* 1979; **2**: 1264.
2. Gelipter D, Hazell M. Interaction between disopyramide and practolol. *BMJ* 1980; **280**: 52.
3. Bonde J, *et al.* Atenolol inhibits the elimination of disopyramide. *Eur J Clin Pharmacol* 1985; **28**: 41–3.

Pharmacokinetics

Disopyramide is readily and almost completely absorbed from the gastrointestinal tract, peak plasma concentrations being attained about 0.5 to 3 hours after oral administration.

Disopyramide is partially metabolised in the liver; the major metabolite is mono-*N*-dealkylated disopyramide which retains some antiarrhythmic and antimuscarinic activity. The major route of excretion is through the kidney, approximately 50% as the unchanged drug, 20% as the *N*-dealkylated metabolite, and 10% as other metabolites. About 10% is excreted in the faeces. The clearance of disopyramide does not appear to be influenced by urinary pH.

The therapeutic plasma concentration range is generally accepted as 2 to 6 μg per mL. Within this range, protein binding is reported to be 50 to 65%, but the degree of binding varies with the plasma concentration and this limits the usefulness of plasma concentration monitoring as a guide to therapy. Estimations of the plasma half-life of disopyramide range from about 4 to 10 hours. The half-life is increased in renal and hepatic impairment, and in cardiac failure.

Disopyramide crosses the placental barrier and is distributed into breast milk.

◊ Reviews.

1. Siddoway LA, Woosley RL. Clinical pharmacokinetics of disopyramide. *Clin Pharmacokinet* 1986; **11**: 214–22.

Metabolism. Mono-*N*-dealkylated disopyramide, the major metabolite of disopyramide, produced no substantial cardiac

effects after a single dose in healthy subjects, but produced greater antimuscarinic effects than disopyramide.[1]

1. Chiang W-T, *et al.* Kinetics and dynamics of disopyramide and its dealkylated metabolite in healthy subjects. *Clin Pharmacol Ther* 1985; **38**: 37–44.

Protein binding. The binding of disopyramide to plasma proteins shows considerable interindividual variation[1,2] and is concentration-dependent[2,3] with the unbound fraction increasing with rising plasma-disopyramide concentrations. Disopyramide is bound mostly to α1-acid glycoprotein, for which it has a high affinity, but there is also a second low-affinity binding site which may be on albumin.[1,2] Increased plasma concentrations of α1-acid glycoprotein are associated with increased binding of disopyramide;[3] significantly reduced protein binding of disopyramide is observed in Chinese subjects[4] compared with Caucasians and this is consistent with a lower concentration of α1-acid glycoprotein in Chinese people. Age also affects the protein binding of disopyramide[3] with reduced binding in neonates and increased binding in elderly patients compared with healthy adults. Decreased protein binding during the third trimester of pregnancy with increased binding one month postpartum has been reported[5] and correlates with the changes in the plasma concentration of α1-acid glycoprotein during pregnancy.

1. David BM, *et al.* Plasma binding of disopyramide. *Br J Clin Pharmacol* 1980; **9**: 614–18.
2. Giacomini KM, Blaschke TF. Effect of concentration-dependent binding to plasma proteins on the pharmacokinetics and pharmacodynamics of disopyramide. *Clin Pharmacokinet* 1984; **9** (suppl 1): 42–8.
3. Holt DW, *et al.* Effect of age and plasma concentrations of albumin and α1-acid glycoprotein on protein binding of disopyramide. *Br J Clin Pharmacol* 1983; **16**: 344–5.
4. Zhou H-H, *et al.* Differences in plasma binding of drugs between caucasians and Chinese subjects. *Clin Pharmacol Ther* 1990; **48**: 10–17.
5. Echizen H, *et al.* Plasma protein binding of disopyramide in pregnant and postpartum women, and in neonates and their mothers. *Br J Clin Pharmacol* 1990; **29**: 423–30.

Uses and Administration

Disopyramide is a class Ia antiarrhythmic (p.787) with a depressant action on the heart similar to that of quinidine (p.966). It also has antimuscarinic and negative inotropic properties.

Disopyramide is used in the management of supraventricular and ventricular **arrhythmias** (p.794).

It may be given by mouth as either the base or the phosphate or intravenously as the phosphate; doses are expressed in terms of the base. The usual oral dose is 300 to 800 mg daily in divided doses adjusted according to the patient's response. A modified-release preparation can be used, enabling 12-hourly dosage intervals. A maximum daily dose of 800 mg should not usually be exceeded. An initial loading dose of 200 to 300 mg may be given.

Disopyramide may be given by slow intravenous injection in a dose of 2 mg per kg body-weight to a maximum of 150 mg, at a rate not exceeding 30 mg per minute; this is followed by 200 mg by mouth immediately on completion of the injection and every 8 hours for 24 hours with subsequent maintenance doses usually in the range of 500 to 750 mg daily. If the arrhythmia recurs on completion of the intravenous injection it may be repeated, but a total intravenous dose of 4 mg per kg (maximum, 300 mg) should not be exceeded in the first hour, nor should the total by both intravenous and oral routes exceed 800 mg in 24 hours. Alternatively, the initial intravenous injection may be followed by intravenous infusion of 0.4 mg per kg per hour (or 20 to 30 mg per hour) to a maximum of 800 mg daily. Patients receiving disopyramide intravenously or in high oral doses should be monitored by ECG.

Dosage reduction and/or increased dosage interval may be necessary in patients with hepatic or renal impairment. Doses should also be adjusted in patients with heart failure to compensate for the prolonged half-life.

An optimum dosage regimen for children has not been fully established, but the following oral doses have been used: under 1 year, 10 to 30 mg per kg body-weight per day; age 1 to 4 years, 10 to 20 mg per kg per day; age 4 to 12 years, 10 to 15 mg per kg per day; age 12 to 18 years, 6 to 15 mg per kg per day.

◊ Reviews.

1. Brogden RN, Todd PA. Disopyramide: a reappraisal of its pharmacodynamic and pharmacokinetic properties, and therapeutic use in cardiac arrhythmias. *Drugs* 1987; **34**: 151–87.

Action. A study in 6 patients with atrial flutter suggested that the antiarrhythmic activity of racemic disopyramide resides in the S(+)-enantiomer.[1]

1. Lima JJ, et al. Antiarrhythmic activity and unbound concentrations of disopyramide enantiomers in patients. *Ther Drug Monit* 1990; **12:** 23–8.

Administration in the elderly. The clearance of disopyramide was reduced in elderly non-smoking patients compared with young subjects, but the reduction was less marked in elderly patients who smoked more than 20 cigarettes daily.[1] It was recommended that the dose of disopyramide should be reduced by approximately 30% in elderly non-smokers.

See also under Protein Binding in Pharmacokinetics, above.

1. Bonde J, et al. The influence of age and smoking on the elimination of disopyramide. *Br J Clin Pharmacol* 1985; **20:** 453–8.

Administration in hepatic impairment. Dosage reduction should be considered for patients with liver impairment who demonstrate prolonged disopyramide plasma half-lives. Also the plasma concentration of α_1-acid glycoprotein is significantly reduced in patients with liver cirrhosis[1,2] and its binding capacity for disopyramide is reduced.[1] This is associated with an increase in the free fraction of disopyramide such that measurement of total disopyramide in plasma may not be a safe indicator for dosing, and a therapeutic range 50% lower than in patients with normal hepatic function should be considered.[2]

1. Bonde J, et al. Kinetics of disopyramide in decreased hepatic function. *Eur J Clin Pharmacol* 1986; **31:** 73–7.
2. Echizen H, et al. Protein binding of disopyramide in liver cirrhosis and in nephrotic syndrome. *Clin Pharmacol Ther* 1986; **40:** 274–80.

Administration in renal impairment. Disopyramide is excreted mainly in the urine and alterations in its pharmacokinetics might be expected in renal impairment. A significant reduction in disopyramide clearance with an increase in elimination half-life has been observed[1] in patients with chronic renal failure and dosage reductions are generally recommended if creatinine clearance is less than 40 to 60 mL per minute. Patients with a creatinine clearance less than 40 mL per minute should not be given modified-release preparations of disopyramide.

At therapeutic concentrations disopyramide is not significantly removed by haemodialysis;[2] the half-life is similar both on and off dialysis (16.8 versus 16.1 hours). An increased free fraction of disopyramide has been observed[3] during haemodialysis associated with an elevation in free fatty acids in plasma and in such cases free plasma-disopyramide concentrations should be monitored.

1. Francois B, et al. Pharmacokinetics of disopyramide in patients with chronic renal failure. *Eur J Drug Metab Pharmacokinet* 1983; **8:** 85–92.
2. Sevka MJ, et al. Disopyramide hemodialysis and kinetics in patients requiring long-term hemodialysis. *Clin Pharmacol Ther* 1981; **29:** 322–6.
3. Horiuchi T, et al. Inhibitory effect of free fatty acids on plasma protein binding of disopyramide in haemodialysis patients. *Eur J Clin Pharmacol* 1989; **36:** 175–80.

Hypotension. Disopyramide is reported to be one of the standard drugs used in the management of neurally mediated hypotension (p.805).

References.

1. Milstein S, et al. Usefulness of disopyramide for prevention of upright tilt-induced hypotension-bradycardia. *Am J Cardiol* 1990; **65:** 1339–44.
2. Morillo CA, et al. A placebo-controlled trial of intravenous and oral disopyramide for prevention of neurally mediated syncope induced by head-up tilt. *J Am Coll Cardiol* 1993; **22:** 1843–8.
3. Bhaumick SK, et al. Oral disopyramide in the treatment of recurrent neurocardiogenic syncope. *Int J Clin Pract* 1997; **51:** 342.

Preparations

BP 2001: Disopyramide Capsules; Disopyramide Phosphate Capsules;
USP 25: Disopyramide Phosphate Capsules; Disopyramide Phosphate Extended-release Capsules.

Proprietary Preparations (details are given in Part 3)
Aust.: Rythmodan; *Austral.:* Norpace; Rythmodan; *Belg.:* Dirytmin; Rythmodan; *Braz.:* Dicorantil; *Canad.:* Norpace†; Rythmodan; *Denm.:* Durbis; Norpace†; *Fin.:* Disomet; Durbis; *Fr.:* Isorythm; Rythmodan; *Ger.:* Diso-Duriles; Disonorm†; Norpace; Rythmodul; *Hong Kong:* Rythmodan; *Irl.:* Rythmodan; *Israel:* Rythmical; *Ital.:* Ritmodan; *Mex.:* Dimodan; Disofarin; *Neth.:* Dirytmin; Ritmoforine; Rythmodan; *Norw.:* Durbis; *NZ:* Rythmodan; *Port.:* Ritmodan; *S.Afr.:* Norpace; Rythmodan; *Spain:* Dicorynan; *Swed.:* Dirytmin; Durbis; *Switz.:* Norpace; *Thai.:* Norpace; *UK:* Dirythmin; Isomide; Rythmodan; *USA:* Norpace.

Ditazole (2639-d)

Ditazole (*rINN*).

Diethamphenazole; S-222. 2,2'-[(4,5-Diphenyloxazol-2-yl)imino]diethanol.
$C_{19}H_{20}N_2O_3 = 324.4$.
CAS — 18471-20-0.
ATC — B01AC01.

Profile

Ditazole is an inhibitor of platelet aggregation used in the management of thromboembolic disorders (p.816) in doses of 400 mg two or three times daily by mouth.

Preparations

Proprietary Preparations (details are given in Part 3)
Port.: Fendazol†; *Spain:* Ageroplas.

Divistyramine (16609-t)

Profile

Divistyramine, a bile-acid binding resin, is a lipid regulating drug that has been used similarly to colestyramine (p.864) in the treatment of hyperlipidaemias (p.800). It has also been used for the relief of pruritus in patients with partial biliary obstruction. It has been given by mouth in usual doses of 6 to 12 g daily as a suspension in a suitable vehicle.

Preparations

Proprietary Preparations (details are given in Part 3)
Switz.: Ipocol.

Dobutamine Hydrochloride (2052-t)

Dobutamine Hydrochloride (*BANM, USAN, rINNM*).
46236; Compound 81929 (dobutamine); Dobutamini Hydrochloridum; LY-174008 (dobutamine tartrate). (±)-4-{2-[3-(4-Hydroxyphenyl)-1-methylpropylamino]ethyl}pyrocatechol hydrochloride; (±)-4-{2-[3-(4-Hydroxyphenyl)-1-methylpropylamino]ethyl}benzene-1,2-diol hydrochloride.
$C_{18}H_{23}NO_3,HCl = 337.8$.
CAS — 34368-04-2 (dobutamine); 49745-95-1 (dobutamine hydrochloride); 101626-66-8 (dobutamine tartrate).
Pharmacopoeias. In *Chin., Eur.* (see p.vi), *Jpn,* and *US.*

Pharmacopoeial description

Ph. Eur.: A white or almost white crystalline powder. Sparingly soluble in water and in alcohol; soluble in methyl alcohol. Protect from light.

USP 25: A white to practically white crystalline powder. Sparingly soluble in water and in methyl alcohol; soluble in alcohol and in pyridine. Store in airtight containers at a temperature of 15° to 30°.

Incompatibility. Dobutamine is incompatible with alkaline solutions such as sodium bicarbonate 5% and alkaline drugs such as aminophylline, frusemide [furosemide], and thiopental sodium; the manufacturers also suggest that it is physically incompatible with bumetanide, calcium gluconate, insulin, diazepam, and phenytoin, and incompatibility with heparin has also been reported.
References to the stability and compatibility of dobutamine infusions.[1-3]

1. Lee CY, et al. Visual and spectrophotometric determination of compatibility of alteplase and streptokinase with other injectable drugs. *Am J Hosp Pharm* 1990; **47:** 606–8.
2. Yamashita SK, et al. Compatibility of selected critical care drugs during simulated Y-site administration. *Am J Health-Syst Pharm* 1996; **53:** 1048–51.
3. Chiu MF, Schwartz ML. Visual compatibility of injectable drugs used in the intensive care unit. *Am J Health-Syst Pharm* 1997; **54:** 64–5.

Adverse Effects

The principal adverse effects of dobutamine are dose-related increases in heart rate and blood pressure, ectopic beats, angina or chest pain, and palpitations; dosage should be reduced or temporarily stopped if they occur. Ventricular tachycardia may occur rarely. Other adverse effects that have occurred occasionally include hypotension, dyspnoea, paraesthesias, headache, nausea and vomiting, and leg cramps.

For the adverse effects of sympathomimetics in general, see Adrenaline, p.829.

◊ For reference to fatalities occurring in patients given dobutamine, see Heart Failure in Uses and Administration, below.

Effects on body temperature. A 71-year-old woman with heart failure developed a fever on 2 separate occasions 8 to 12 hours after starting an infusion of dobutamine.[1]

1. Robison-Strane SR, Bubik JS. Dobutamine-induced fever. *Ann Pharmacother* 1992; **26:** 1523–4.

Effects on the heart. For reference to severe cardiovascular complications of dobutamine stress echocardiography, see Diagnosis and Testing, below.

Effects on the skin. A report of troublesome pruritus of the scalp associated with dobutamine infusion.[1]

1. McCauley CS, Blumenthal MS. Dobutamine and pruritus of the scalp. *Ann Intern Med* 1986; **105:** 966.

Hypersensitivity. There has been a report[1] of redness, swelling, itching and a sensation of warmth around the site of infusion of dobutamine in a patient. These symptoms recurred when the infusion was given again one week later.

1. Cernek PK. Dermal cellulitis—a hypersensitivity reaction from dobutamine hydrochloride. *Ann Pharmacother* 1994; **28:** 964.

Overdosage. A patient received an accidental overdose[1] of dobutamine when given an intravenous infusion at a rate of more than 130 µg per kg body-weight per minute for 30 minutes, this being three times the recommended maximum. Characteristic side-effects of dobutamine such as emesis, palpitations, chest pain, dyspnoea, and paraesthesia developed together with urinary incontinence, an effect not previously associated with dobutamine.

1. Paulman PM, et al. Dobutamine overdose. *JAMA* 1990; **264:** 2386–7.

Precautions

Dobutamine hydrochloride should be avoided or used only with great caution in patients with marked obstruction of cardiac ejection, such as idiopathic hypertrophic subaortic stenosis. It should also be used with caution in patients with acute myocardial infarction, and in cardiogenic shock complicated by severe hypotension. Hypovolaemia should be corrected before treatment.

For precautions to be observed with sympathomimetics in general, see Adrenaline, p.830.

Interference with diagnostic tests. Contamination of blood samples with dobutamine has been reported to produce falsely decreased creatinine values in an enzymatic test.[1] Colorimetric measurements of creatinine were not affected.

1. Daly TM, et al. "Bouncing" creatinine levels. *N Engl J Med* 1996; **334:** 1749–50.

Interactions

Although it is less likely than adrenaline [epinephrine] to produce ventricular arrhythmias, dobutamine should be used with extreme caution during anaesthesia with cyclopropane, halothane, and other volatile anaesthetics. The inotropic effects of dobutamine on the heart are reversed by beta blockade, and there may then be vasoconstriction and an increase in blood pressure due to dobutamine's alpha agonist effects.

For the interactions of sympathomimetics in general, see Adrenaline, p.830.

Beta blockers. Administration of dobutamine with beta blockers may result in hypertension due to dobutamine's alpha-agonist action. However, marked hypotension occurred[1] in a patient who had been receiving *carvedilol* for heart failure when dobutamine was given for worsening heart failure. It was suggested that the reaction may have been due to blockade of beta₁ and alpha receptors by carvedilol, leaving the beta₂-mediated vasodilatation unopposed.

1. Lindenfeld J, et al. Hypotension with dobutamine: β-adrenergic antagonist selectivity at low doses of carvedilol. *Ann Pharmacother* 1999; **33:** 1266–9.

Pharmacokinetics

Like adrenaline [epinephrine] (p.831), dobutamine is inactive when given by mouth, and it is rapidly inactivated in the body by similar processes. It has a half-life of about 2 minutes. Conjugates of dobutamine and its major metabolite 3-*O*-methyldobutamine are excreted primarily in urine, with small amounts eliminated in the faeces.

◊ The primary mechanism of clearance of dobutamine appears to be distribution to other tissues, and not metabolism or elimination. It has a half-life of about 2 minutes and plasma concentrations of dobutamine reach steady state about 10 to 12 minutes after the start of an infusion. Dobutamine is used mainly for the short-term treatment of heart failure and any pharmacokinetic changes in this condition have no clinical implications in dosage titration.[1]

A review of the pharmacokinetics of dobutamine and other cardiovascular drugs in children[2] considered that further study was required to explain the different findings that had been reported.

1. Shammas FV, Dickstein K. Clinical pharmacokinetics in heart failure: an updated review. *Clin Pharmacokinet* 1988; **15:** 94–113.
2. Steinberg C, Notterman DA. Pharmacokinetics of cardiovascular drugs in children: inotropes and vasopressors. *Clin Pharmacokinet* 1994; **27:** 345–67.

Uses and Administration

Dobutamine is a sympathomimetic (see Adrenaline, p.831) with direct effects on beta₁-adrenergic receptors, which confer upon it a prominent inotropic action on the heart. It also has some alpha- and beta₂-agonist properties. Dobutamine differs from dopamine in not having the specific dopaminergic properties of dopamine which induce renal mesenteric vasodilatation. However, like dopamine, the inotropic action of dobutamine on the heart is associated with less cardiac-accelerating effect than that of isoprenaline.

Dobutamine is used to increase the contractility of the heart in acute heart failure, as occurs in cardiogenic shock (p.813) and myocardial infarction (p.805); it is also used in septic shock. Other circumstances in which its inotropic activity may be useful are during cardiac surgery and positive end-expiratory pressure ventilation.

Dobutamine is given as the hydrochloride but doses are expressed in terms of the base. It is administered by intravenous infusion as a dilute solution (0.25 to 5 mg per mL), in glucose 5% or sodium chloride 0.9%; other fluids may also be suitable and the manufacturers' guidelines should be consulted.

In the management of **acute heart failure**, dobutamine is given at a usual rate of 2.5 to 10 µg per kg body-weight per minute, according to the patient's heart rate, blood pressure, cardiac output, and urine output. A range of 0.5 up to 40 µg per kg per minute has occasionally been required. It has been recommended that treatment with dobutamine should be discontinued gradually.

Dobutamine is also employed as an alternative to exercise in **cardiac stress testing**. A solution containing 1 mg per mL is employed for this purpose, administered via an infusion pump. A dose of 5 µg per kg per minute is infused for 8 minutes; the dose is then increased by increments of 5 µg per kg per minute up to a usual maximum of 20 µg per kg per minute, with each dose being infused for 8 minutes before the next incremental increase; higher doses of up to 40 µg per kg per minute have sometimes been employed. The ECG should be monitored continuously and the infusion terminated if arrhythmias, marked ST segment depression, or other adverse effects occur.

◊ General references.
1. Majerus TC, et al. Dobutamine: ten years later. *Pharmacotherapy* 1989; **9:** 245–59.

Action. *Animal* studies show that the ability of dobutamine to stimulate alpha₁- and beta₂-adrenergic receptors appears to be as great as its beta₁-stimulant properties, and it has been proposed that the inotropic action results from a combination of alpha-stimulant activity on myocardial alpha₁ receptors, a property residing mainly in the (−)-enantiomer, with beta₁ stimulation by the (+)-enantiomer; peripherally, alpha-mediated vasoconstriction would be opposed by the beta₂-agonist properties of the (+)-enantiomer, resulting in the net inotropic action with relatively little effect on blood pressure seen with the racemic mixture used clinically.[1]
Dobutamine has a thermogenic effect,[2] but using it to increase oxygen delivery and consumption and the cardiac index in critically ill patients did not improve patient outcome and in some cases might have been harmful.[3]
1. Ruffolo RR. The mechanism of action of dobutamine. *Ann Intern Med* 1984; **100:** 313–14.
2. Bhatt SB, et al. Effect of dobutamine on oxygen supply and uptake in healthy volunteers. *Br J Anaesth* 1992; **69:** 298–303.
3. Hayes MA, et al. Elevation of systemic oxygen delivery in the treatment of critically ill patients. *N Engl J Med* 1994; **330:** 1717–22.

Cardiac surgery. Dobutamine and dopamine are each used for inotropic support in patients undergoing cardiac surgery. A comparison in children[1] suggests that dobutamine may be preferred to dopamine since the latter could cause pulmonary vasoconstriction.
1. Booker PD, et al. Comparison of the haemodynamic effects of dopamine and dobutamine in young children undergoing cardiac surgery. *Br J Anaesth* 1995; **74:** 419–23.

Diagnosis and testing. Dynamic exercise is the established mode of stress for the assessment of cardiac function. In patients who are unable to exercise, a dobutamine infusion is one of the best alternative ways of producing a pharmacological stress.[1,2] Dobutamine stress echocardiography, which can often involve the additional administration of atropine, has been reported to be more sensitive than adenosine or dipyridamole stress echocardiography.[2,3] It also has a useful prognostic role.[4-7] However there have been instances of severe cardiovascular complications attributable to dobutamine.[8]
1. Nihoyannopoulos P. Stress echocardiography. *Br J Hosp Med* 1997; **57:** 31–5.
2. Cheitlin MD, et al. ACC/AHA guidelines for the clinical application of echocardiography: a report of the American College of Cardiology/American Heart Association Task Force on Practice Guidelines (Committee on Clinical Application of Echocardiography). *Circulation* 1997; **95:** 1686–1744.
3. Martin TW, et al. Comparison of adenosine, dipyridamole, and dobutamine in stress echocardiography. *Ann Intern Med* 1992; **116:** 190–6.

The symbol † denotes a preparation no longer actively marketed

4. Poldermans D, et al. Dobutamine-atropine stress echocardiography and clinical data for predicting late cardiac events in patients with suspected coronary artery disease. *Am J Med* 1994; **97:** 119–25.
5. Cigarroa CG, et al. Dobutamine stress echocardiography identifies hibernating myocardium and predicts recovery of left ventricular function after coronary revascularization. *Circulation* 1993; **88:** 430–6.
6. Elhendy A, et al. Relation between ST segment elevation during dobutamine stress test and myocardial viability after a recent myocardial infarction. *Heart* 1997; **77:** 115–21.
7. Pingitore A, et al. Prognostic value of pharmacological stress echocardiography in patients with known or suspected coronary artery disease: a prospective, large-scale, multicenter, head-to-head comparison between dipyridamole and dobutamine test. *J Am Coll Cardiol* 1999; **34:** 1769–77.
8. Lattanzi F, et al. Dobutamine stress echocardiography: safety in diagnosing coronary artery disease. *Drug Safety* 2000; **22:** 251–62.

Heart failure. Dobutamine may be used in the management of acute heart failure, as discussed under Shock, p.813. It may also have a role as a bridge to transplantation in patients with severe chronic heart failure (p.798). In less severe cases, conflicting results have been reported. For example, one group reported[1] that pulsed therapy with dobutamine (30 minutes daily for 4 days each week for 3 weeks) could produce similar improvements to those achieved with exercise. However, sudden death occurred in patients receiving dobutamine as infusions for 48 hours per week, and another study[2] was halted for this reason.
1. Adamopoulos S, et al. Effects of pulsed β-stimulant therapy on β-adrenoceptors and chronotropic responsiveness in chronic heart failure. *Lancet* 1995; **345:** 344–9.
2. Dies F, et al. Intermittent dobutamine in ambulatory outpatients with chronic cardiac failure. *Circulation* 1986; **74:** (suppl II): 38.

Preparations

BP 2001: Dobutamine Intravenous Infusion;
USP 25: Dobutamine for Injection; Dobutamine in Dextrose Injection; Dobutamine Injection.

Proprietary Preparations (details are given in Part 3)
Aust.: Dobutrex; Inotop; *Austral.:* Dobutrex; *Belg.:* Dobutrex; *Braz.:* Dobutrex; *Canad.:* Dobutrex; *Denm.:* Dobuject†; Dobutrex; *Fin.:* Dobuject; Dobutrex; *Fr.:* Dobutrex; *Ger.:* Dobutrex; *Hong Kong:* Dobutrex; *Irl.:* Dobutrex; Posiject; *Israel:* Butamine; Dobuject; Dobutam; Dobutrex; *Ital.:* Dobutrex; *Mex.:* Cryobutol; Dobuject; Dobutrex; Kardion; Oxiken; *Neth.:* Dobutrex; *Norw.:* Dobutrex; *NZ:* Dobutrex; *Port.:* Dobuject; Dobutina; Inotrex; *S.Afr.:* Dobutrex; Posiject; *Singapore:* Dobuject; *Spain:* Dobutrex; *Swed.:* Dobuject†; Dobutrex; *Switz.:* Dobutrex; *Thai.:* Dobucard; Dobuject; Dobutrex; *UK:* Dobutrex; *USA:* Dobutrex.

Docarpamine (6470-d)

Docarpamine *(rINN)*.
TA-870. (−)-(S)-2-Acetamido-N-(3,4-dihydroxyphenethyl)-4-(methylthio)butyramide bis(ethyl carbonate) ester.
C₂₁H₃₀N₂O₈S = 470.5.
CAS — 74639-40-0.

Profile
Docarpamine is an orally active prodrug of dopamine (below) that is used in the treatment of acute heart failure. The usual dose is 2.25 g of docarpamine daily by mouth, in 3 divided doses.

Preparations

Proprietary Preparations (details are given in Part 3)
Jpn: Tanadopa.

Dofetilide (10888-k)

Dofetilide *(BAN, USAN, rINN)*.
UK-68798. β-[(p-Methanesulfonamidophenethyl)methylamino]methanesulfono-p-phenetidide.
C₁₉H₂₇N₃O₅S₂ = 441.6.
CAS — 115256-11-6.
ATC — C01BD04.

Profile
Dofetilide is a class III antiarrhythmic (p.787) used in the treatment of atrial fibrillation and flutter (p.794). It may cause severe ventricular arrhythmias, including torsade de pointes, and is thus reserved for patients with highly symptomatic atrial fibrillation or flutter. Dofetilide is given by mouth and the dosage must be individualised according to creatinine clearance and QT interval; treatment must be initiated under ECG monitoring which must be continued for at least 3 days. The initial dose in patients with a creatinine clearance greater than 60 mL per minute and corrected QT interval of 0.44 seconds or less is 500 µg twice daily; lower doses must be used in renal impairment and the maintenance dose must be reduced if the QT interval becomes prolonged after the first dose.

◊ References.
1. McClellan KJ, Markham A. Dofetilide: a review of its use in atrial fibrillation and atrial flutter. *Drugs* 1999; **58:** 1043–59.
2. Torp-Pedersen C, et al. Dofetilide in patients with congestive heart failure and left ventricular dysfunction. *N Engl J Med* 1999; **341:** 857–65.

3. Kalus JS, Mauro VF. Dofetilide: a class III-specific antiarrhythmic agent. *Ann Pharmacother* 2000; **34:** 44–56.
4. Anonymous. Dofetilide for atrial fibrillation. *Med Lett Drugs Ther* 2000; **42:** 41–2.

Preparations

Proprietary Preparations (details are given in Part 3)
USA: Tikosyn.

Dopamine Hydrochloride (2053-x)

Dopamine Hydrochloride *(BANM, USAN, pINNM)*.
ASL-279; Dopamini Hydrochloridum; 3-Hydroxytyramine Hydrochloride. 4-(2-Aminoethyl)pyrocatechol hydrochloride; 4-(2-Aminoethyl)benzene-1,2-diol hydrochloride.
C₈H₁₁NO₂,HCl = 189.6.
CAS — 51-61-6 (dopamine); 62-31-7 (dopamine hydrochloride).
Pharmacopoeias. In *Chin., Eur.* (see p.vi), *Int., Jpn,* and *US.*

Pharmacopoeial description
Ph. Eur.: A white or almost white crystalline powder. Freely soluble in water; soluble in alcohol; sparingly soluble in acetone and in dichloromethane. Store in airtight containers. Protect from light.
USP 25: A white to off-white crystalline powder that may have a slight odour of hydrochloric acid. Freely soluble in water and in aqueous solutions of alkali hydroxides; insoluble in chloroform and in ether; soluble in methyl alcohol. pH of a 4% solution in water is between 3.0 and 5.5. Store in airtight containers.

Incompatibility. Dopamine is inactivated in alkaline solutions such as sodium bicarbonate 5% and is incompatible with alkaline drugs such as frusemide [furosemide] and thiopental sodium; incompatibility with insulin has also been reported, and the manufacturers state that it is incompatible with ampicillin and with amphotericin B, and that mixtures with gentamicin sulfate, cefalotin sodium, or oxacillin sodium should be avoided.
References to the stability and incompatibility of dopamine infusions.[1-3]
1. Lee CY, et al. Visual and spectrophotometric determination of compatibility of alteplase and streptokinase with other injectable drugs. *Am J Hosp Pharm* 1990; **47:** 606–8.
2. Yamashita SK, et al. Compatibility of selected critical care drugs during simulated Y-site administration. *Am J Health-Syst Pharm* 1996; **53:** 1048–51.
3. Chiu MF, Schwartz ML. Visual compatibility of injectable drugs used in the intensive care unit. *Am J Health-Syst Pharm* 1997; **54:** 64–5.

Adverse Effects
The most common adverse effects of dopamine infusion are ectopic beats, tachycardia, anginal pain, palpitations, hypotension, vasoconstriction, nausea and vomiting, headache, and dyspnoea. More rarely, bradycardia and cardiac conduction abnormalities, piloerection, and azotaemia have been reported; hypertension has occurred, particularly in overdosage. Extravasation may lead to tissue necrosis and sloughing.

For the adverse effects of sympathomimetics in general, see Adrenaline, p.829.

Effects on the endocrine system. Dopamine infusion, even at low doses (2.5 µg per kg body-weight per minute) was found to decrease serum concentrations of prolactin in critically ill patients.[1] This was considered undesirable because of the immunomodulatory role of prolactin in the endocrine response to stress.
1. Bailey AR, Burchett KR. Effect of low-dose dopamine on serum concentrations of prolactin in critically ill patients. *Br J Anaesth* 1997; **78:** 97–9.

Effects on the heart. For mention of the arrhythmogenic effects of dopamine on the heart, see p.829.

Ischaemia and gangrene. Ischaemia and gangrene has been reported on several occasions following dopamine infusions.[1-4] Dopamine is converted to noradrenaline [norepinephrine] which is a known powerful vasoconstrictor and is also reported to be associated with vascular problems if extravasation occurs.
1. Alexander CS, et al. Pedal gangrene associated with the use of dopamine. *N Engl J Med* 1975; **293:** 591.
2. Julka NK, Nora JR. Gangrene aggravation after use of dopamine. *JAMA* 1976; **253:** 2812–13.
3. Boltax RS, et al. Gangrene resulting from infiltrated dopamine solution. *N Engl J Med* 1977; **296:** 823.
4. Maggi JC, et al. Gangrene in a neonate following dopamine therapy. *J Pediatr* 1982; **100:** 323–5.

Treatment of Adverse Effects
Since the half-life of dopamine is only about 2 minutes most adverse effects can be corrected by discontinuing or reducing the rate of infusion. If these measures fail excessive vasoconstriction and hypertension

may be treated with an alpha blocker such as phentolamine mesilate intravenously.

Relief from tissue necrosis and pain due to extravasation may be produced by immediate infiltration with phentolamine as described under Noradrenaline, p.948.

◊ Topical glyceryl trinitrate ointment has been used successfully to improve capillary blood flow in patients with dopamine-induced ischaemia of the digits.[1,2]

1. Gibbs NM, Oh TE. Nitroglycerine ointment for dopamine induced peripheral digital ischaemia. *Lancet* 1983; **ii:** 290.
2. Coakley J. Nitroglycerin ointment for dopamine-induced peripheral ischaemia. *Lancet* 1983; **ii:** 633.

Precautions

Dopamine should not be used in patients with phaeochromocytoma or hyperthyroidism, nor in the presence of uncorrected tachyarrhythmias or ventricular fibrillation. Care is required and low doses should be used in patients with shock secondary to myocardial infarction. Patients with a history of peripheral vascular disease are at increased risk of ischaemia of the extremities. Hypovolaemia should be corrected before beginning dopamine infusion.

For precautions to be observed with sympathomimetics in general, see Adrenaline, p.830.

Withdrawal. There may be difficulty in weaning patients off dopamine. For example, there has been a report[1] of a patient in an intensive care unit with intra-abdominal sepsis who developed hypotension when withdrawal of dopamine was attempted. Withdrawal was made possible by substitution with ibopamine, a dopamine agonist.

1. Milner AR, *et al.* Ibopamine substitution in a dopamine-dependent patient. *Lancet* 1993; **342:** 1555.

Interactions

Although it is less likely than adrenaline [epinephrine] to produce ventricular arrhythmias, dopamine should be used with extreme caution during anaesthesia with cyclopropane, halothane, and other volatile anaesthetics. In patients treated with MAOIs, the dose of dopamine should be reduced substantially; a suggested starting dose is one tenth of the usual dose.

For the interactions of sympathomimetics in general, see Adrenaline, p.830.

Antiepileptics. Following a report in 1976 to the FDA of hypotension in patients given *phenytoin* in addition to dopamine infusion, a study[1] of this potential interaction found that dopamine given by intravenous infusion concomitantly with phenytoin infusion to *dogs*, did not alter the CNS effects of phenytoin nor result in hypotension and cardiovascular collapse. Large doses of phenytoin alone had a reproducible hypotensive effect which was reduced by dopamine, suggesting a possible supportive role in phenytoin-induced hypotension.

1. Smith RD, Lomas TE. Modification of cardiovascular responses to intravenous phenytoin by dopamine in dogs: evidence against an adverse interaction. *Toxicol Appl Pharmacol* 1978; **45:** 665–73.

Dopaminergics. Severe hypertension occurred[1] in a patient who had been receiving *selegiline* for Parkinson's disease when a dopamine infusion was started. Although selegiline is considered to be a selective monoamine oxidase type B inhibitor, at higher doses it also affects monoamine oxidase type A and could have reduced the metabolism of dopamine in this patient. Caution may be necessary if dopamine is given to patients who have been receiving selegiline within the previous 2 weeks.

1. Rose LM, *et al.* A hypertensive reaction induced by concurrent use of selegiline and dopamine. *Ann Pharmacother* 2000; **34:** 1020–4.

Vasodilators. Fatal hypotension occurred in a man given *tolazoline* in addition to dopamine.[1]

1. Carlon GC. Fatal association of tolazoline and dopamine. *Chest* 1979; **76:** 336.

Pharmacokinetics

The vasoconstrictor properties of dopamine preclude its administration by the subcutaneous or intramuscular route. Like adrenaline [epinephrine] (p.831) it is inactive when given by mouth, and it is rapidly inactivated in the body by similar processes, with a half-life of about 2 minutes. Dopamine is a metabolic precursor of noradrenaline and a proportion is excreted as the metabolic products of noradrenaline. Nevertheless, the majority appears to be directly metabolised into dopamine-related metabolic products.

◊ References.

1. Banner W, *et al.* Nonlinear dopamine pharmacokinetics in pediatric patients. *J Pharmacol Exp Ther* 1989; **249:** 131–3.

2. Padbury JF, *et al.* Pharmacokinetics of dopamine in critically ill newborn infants. *J Pediatr* 1990; **117:** 472–6.
3. Notterman DA, *et al.* Dopamine clearance in critically ill infants and children: effect of age and organ system dysfunction. *Clin Pharmacol Ther* 1990; **48:** 138–47.
4. Bhatt-Mehta V, *et al.* Dopamine pharmacokinetics in critically ill newborn infants. *Eur J Clin Pharmacol* 1991; **40:** 593–7.
5. Steinberg C, Notterman DA. Pharmacokinetics of cardiovascular drugs in children: inotropes and vasopressors. *Clin Pharmacokinet* 1994; **27:** 345–67.

Uses and Administration

The catecholamine, dopamine, is a sympathomimetic (see Adrenaline, p.831) with both direct and indirect effects. It is formed in the body by the decarboxylation of levodopa, and is both a neurotransmitter in its own right (notably in the brain) and a precursor of noradrenaline. Dopamine differs from adrenaline [epinephrine] and noradrenaline [norepinephrine] in dilating renal and mesenteric blood vessels and increasing urine output, apparently by a specific dopaminergic mechanism. This effect is predominant at low infusion rates (about 2 μg per kg body-weight per minute); at slightly higher infusion rates (around 2 to 10 μg per kg per minute) it also stimulates beta$_1$-adrenergic receptors in the myocardium, and at 10 to 20 μg per kg per minute the effects of alpha-adrenergic stimulation predominate, such as vasoconstriction. The inotropic action of dopamine on the heart is associated with less cardiac-accelerating effect, and a lower incidence of arrhythmias, than that of isoprenaline.

Dopamine also inhibits release of prolactin from the anterior pituitary.

Dopamine is used in acute heart failure, as occurs in cardiogenic shock (p.813) and myocardial infarction (p.805); it is also employed in renal failure, in cardiac surgery, and in septic shock.

Dopamine is administered as the hydrochloride by intravenous infusion as a dilute solution (usually 1.6 or 3.2 mg per mL, although more dilute solutions may be used where fluid expansion is not a problem), in glucose 5%, sodium chloride 0.9%, or other suitable diluents; many fluids are suitable and the manufacturers' data sheets or literature should be consulted. The initial rate is 1 to 5 μg per kg body-weight per minute, gradually increased by up to 5 to 10 μg per kg per minute according to the patient's blood pressure, cardiac output, and urine output. Up to 20 to 50 μg per kg per minute may be required in seriously ill patients; higher doses have been given. A reduction in urine flow, without hypotension, may indicate a need to reduce the dose. To avoid tissue necrosis dopamine is best administered into a large vein high up in a limb, preferably the arm. It has been recommended that on gradual discontinuation of dopamine care should be taken to avoid undue hypotension associated with very low dosage levels where vasodilatation could predominate.

Surgery and intensive care. As well as being used for its inotropic effect in cardiac surgery dopamine has been given in low doses for renal protection (sometimes termed 'renal-dose' dopamine) in patients at risk, such as those undergoing major surgery or in intensive care, and for the treatment of acute renal failure. However, the value of this use of dopamine as a renal protectant has been questioned and the evidence reviewed.[1,2] Studies in healthy *animals* and human subjects have shown that low-dose dopamine increases renal blood flow, natriuresis, diuresis, and possibly glomerular filtration rate. However, clinical studies have failed to convincingly demonstrate that low-dose dopamine is effective in either preventing acute renal failure in patients at high risk, or in improving renal function or outcome in patients with established acute renal failure. These studies were small, included uncontrolled case series, and often used surrogate markers rather than clinical outcome measures but a larger, placebo-controlled, randomised study[3] in critically-ill patients with early renal dysfunction also failed to show any benefit in those receiving dopamine. It was concluded[4] that dopamine has no role as a renal protectant in such patients, although further study is needed in patients with more severe renal failure.[5]

1. Denton MD, *et al.* "Renal-dose" dopamine for the treatment of acute renal failure: scientific rationale, experimental studies, and clinical trials. *Kidney Int* 1996; **49:** 4–14.
2. Kellum JA. The use of diuretics and dopamine in acute renal failure: a systematic review of the evidence. *Crit Care* 1997; **1:** 53–9.

3. Australian and New Zealand Intensive Care Society (ANZICS) Clinical Trials Group. Low-dose dopamine in patients with early renal dysfunction: a placebo-controlled randomised trial. *Lancet* 2000; **356:** 2139–43.
4. Galley HF. Renal-dose dopamine: will the message now get through? *Lancet* 2000; **356:** 2112–3. Correction. *ibid.* 2001; **357:** 890.
5. Romano G, Ferraccioli G. Usefulness of dopamine treatment in non-oliguric renal failure. *Lancet* 2001; **357:** 960.

Preparations

BP 2001: Dopamine Intravenous Infusion;
USP 25: Dopamine Hydrochloride and Dextrose Injection; Dopamine Hydrochloride Injection.

Proprietary Preparations (details are given in Part 3)
Belg.: Dynatra; **Braz.:** Revivan; **Canad.:** Intropin; **Denm.:** Abbodop; Dopmin; Giludop; **Fin.:** Abbodop; Dopmin; **Hong Kong:** Dopaminex; Intropin; **Irl.:** Intropin†; **Israel:** Docard; **Ital.:** Revivan; **Jpn:** Inovan; Predopa†; **Mex.:** Clorpamina Dopamina; Drynalken; Drynalquin; Inotropisa; Zetarina; **Neth.:** Dynatra; **Norw.:** Abbodop; **Port.:** Cordodopa; Medopa; **S.Afr.:** Dopamed†; Dynos; Intropin; **Singapore:** Dopmin; Intropin; **Swed.:** Abbodop; Giludop; **Thai.:** Dopamex; Dopaminex; Dopmin; Inopin; **USA:** Intropin.

Dopexamine Hydrochloride (18632-e)

Dopexamine Hydrochloride (*BANM, USAN, rINNM*).
FPL-60278; FPL-60278AR. 4-{2-[6-(Phenethylamino)hexylamino]ethyl}pyrocatechol dihydrochloride.
$C_{22}H_{32}N_2O_2,2HCl = 429.4$.
CAS — 86197-47-9 *(dopexamine)*; 86484-91-5 *(dopexamine dihydrochloride)*.

Dopexamine is inactivated in alkaline solutions such as sodium bicarbonate 5%.

Adverse Effects and Precautions

The most common adverse effect of dopexamine administration is tachycardia; transient hypotension may also occur. Other adverse effects include arrhythmias and ECG changes, exacerbation of heart failure, nausea and vomiting, tremor, headache, sweating, and dyspnoea.

Dopexamine should not be used in patients with left ventricular outlet obstruction such as aortic stenosis or in phaeochromocytoma or thrombocytopenic patients. It should be used with caution in patients with ischaemic heart disease or following myocardial infarction. Care is also required in the presence of hypokalaemia or hyperglycaemia. Pre-existing hypotension and reduced vascular resistance should be corrected before beginning dopexamine administration.

For the adverse effects of sympathomimetics in general, and precautions to be observed, see Adrenaline, p.829.

Interactions

Dopexamine may potentiate the effects of noradrenaline [norepinephrine] and some other sympathomimetics by inhibiting neuronal uptake of noradrenaline.

For the interactions of sympathomimetics in general, see Adrenaline, p.830.

Pharmacokinetics

Dopexamine has a short half-life in blood of about 6 to 7 minutes. It is excreted in bile and in urine.

Uses and Administration

Dopexamine is a sympathomimetic (see Adrenaline, p.831) with direct and indirect effects. It stimulates beta$_2$ adrenoceptors and peripheral dopamine receptors and also inhibits the neuronal reuptake of noradrenaline. These actions result in an increased cardiac output, peripheral vasodilatation, and an increase in renal and mesenteric blood flow.

Dopexamine hydrochloride is used to provide short-term haemodynamic support that may be required after cardiac surgery or in exacerbations of chronic heart failure. It is given as an intravenous infusion of either 400 or 800 μg per mL in glucose 5% or sodium chloride 0.9% through a central or large peripheral vein; more concentrated solutions may be given via a central vein but concentrations should not exceed 4 mg per mL. The initial dose is generally 0.5 μg per kg body-weight per minute and is then increased to

1 µg per kg per minute; further increases, in increments of 0.5 to 1 µg per kg per minute at intervals of not less than 15 minutes, may be made up to a total of 6 µg per kg per minute if necessary. Heart rate, blood pressure, urine output, and cardiac output should be monitored. On withdrawal, the dose of dopexamine hydrochloride should be reduced gradually.

◊ The pharmacological properties and therapeutic uses of dopexamine have been reviewed.[1,2] One set of workers[2] concluded that although dopexamine hydrochloride may prove to be a useful alternative to dopamine and dobutamine in the treatment of acute heart failure (cardiogenic shock, p.813) and the postoperative management of low cardiac output conditions, controlled studies are required to establish its efficacy and tolerability with respect to that of established therapies.[2] Much the same view was expressed in a later commentary;[3] the lack of comparative studies on the outcome of such treatment meant that it was difficult to identify advantages to employing dopexamine.

Dopexamine has also been used in acutely deteriorating chronic heart failure when it appears that systemic vasodilatation is more pronounced than with dopamine or dobutamine.[3]

1. Smith GW, Filcek SAL. Dopexamine hydrochloride: a novel dopamine receptor agonist for the acute treatment of low cardiac output states. *Cardiovasc Drug Rev* 1989; **7:** 141–59.
2. Fitton A, Benfield P. Dopexamine hydrochloride. *Drugs* 1990; **39:** 308–30.
3. Anonymous. Dopexamine after cardiac surgery. *Drug Ther Bull* 1995; **33:** 30–2.

Preparations

Proprietary Preparations (details are given in Part 3)
Denm.: Dopacard; *Fin.:* Dopacard; *Fr.:* Dopacard†; *Ger.:* Dopacard; *Irl.:* Dopacard; *NZ:* Dopacard; *Swed.:* Dopacard; *Switz.:* Dopacard; *UK:* Dopacard.

Dorzolamide Hydrochloride (17057-e)

Dorzolamide Hydrochloride (BANM, USAN, rINNM).

L-671152 (dorzolamide); MK-507; MK-0507. (4S,6S)-4-(Ethylamino)-5,6-dihydro-6-methyl-4H-thieno[2,3-b]thiopyran-2-sulphonamide 7,7-dioxide hydrochloride.

$C_{10}H_{16}N_2O_4S_3,HCl = 360.9$.

CAS — 120279-96-1 (dorzolamide); 130693-82-2 (dorzolamide hydrochloride).

Adverse Effects and Precautions
Local ocular adverse effects may occur following the use of dorzolamide eye drops and include conjunctivitis, keratitis, burning or stinging, eyelid inflammation or irritation, and blurred vision. It may be absorbed systemically, resulting in adverse effects, precautions, and interactions similar to those of acetazolamide (see p.826). Other side-effects reported are headache, bitter taste, fatigue, and nausea.

Uses and Administration
Dorzolamide is a carbonic anhydrase inhibitor with actions similar to those of acetazolamide (p.827). It is used topically in the management of open-angle **glaucoma** and ocular hypertension (p.1413), either alone or as adjunctive therapy with a topical beta blocker.

Dorzolamide is administered as eye drops containing dorzolamide hydrochloride equivalent to 2% of the base. When used as monotherapy the usual dose is one drop three times daily; a twice daily regimen is recommended when used in conjunction with a beta blocker.

Preparations

Proprietary Preparations (details are given in Part 3)
Aust.: Trusopt; *Austral.:* Trusopt; *Belg.:* Trusopt; *Canad.:* Trusopt; *Denm.:* Trusopt; *Fin.:* Trusopt; *Fr.:* Trusopt; *Ger.:* Trusopt; *Hong Kong:* Trusopt; *Irl.:* Trusopt; *Israel:* Trusopt; *Ital.:* Trusopt; *Mex.:* Trusopt; *Neth.:* Trusopt; *NZ:* Trusopt; *Port.:* Trusopt; *S.Afr.:* Trusopt; *Singapore:* Trusopt; *Spain:* Trusopt; *Swed.:* Trusopt; *Switz.:* Trusopt; *Thai.:* Trusopt; *UK:* Trusopt; *USA:* Trusopt.

Multi-ingredient: *Aust.:* Cosopt; *Belg.:* Cosopt; *Canad.:* Cosopt; *Denm.:* Cosopt; *Fin.:* Cosopt; *Fr.:* Cosopt; *Ger.:* Cosopt; *Irl.:* Cosopt; *Israel:* Cosopt; *Ital.:* Cosopt; *Mex.:* Cosopt; *Neth.:* Cosopt; *Norw.:* Cosopt; *S.Afr.:* Cosopt; *Swed.:* Cosopt; *Switz.:* Cosopt; *UK:* Cosopt; *USA:* Cosopt.

The symbol † denotes a preparation no longer actively marketed

Doxazosin Mesilate (16611-y)

Doxazosin Mesilate (BANM, rINNM).

Doxazosin Mesylate (USAN); Doxazosin Methanesulphonate; UK-33274-27. 2-[4-(2,3-Dihydro-1,4-benzodioxin-2-ylcarbonyl)piperazin-1-yl]-6,7-dimethoxyquinazolin-4-ylamine methanesulphonate; 1-(4-Amino-6,7-dimethoxyquinazolin-2-yl)-4-(1,4-benzodioxan-2-ylcarbonyl)piperazine methanesulphonate.

$C_{23}H_{25}N_5O_5,CH_3SO_3H = 547.6$.

CAS — 74191-85-8 (doxazosin); 77883-43-3 (doxazosin mesilate).

Doxazosin mesilate 1.2 mg is approximately equivalent to 1 mg of doxazosin.

Adverse Effects, Treatment, and Precautions
As for Prazosin Hydrochloride, p.958.

Effects on mental function. For a report of acute psychosis associated with doxazosin administration, see under Adverse Effects of Prazosin Hydrochloride, p.958.

Hypotension. Six of 18 hypertensive patients exhibited first-dose postural hypotension after receiving doxazosin 1 mg; three others had substantial but asymptomatic reductions in supine systolic blood pressure following the first dose.[1] The effect might have been exacerbated since all these patients were receiving concomitant beta blocker or diuretic therapy, or both. A further patient, who was also taking methyldopa, withdrew from the study with persistent postural hypotension.

1. Oliver RM, *et al.* The pharmacokinetics of doxazosin in patients with hypertension and renal impairment. *Br J Clin Pharmacol* 1990; **29:** 417–22.

Urinary incontinence. For reference to urinary incontinence associated with doxazosin, see under Adverse Effects of Prazosin Hydrochloride, p.958.

Pharmacokinetics
Doxazosin is well absorbed after oral administration, peak plasma concentrations occurring 2 hours after a dose. Oral bioavailability is about 65%. It is extensively metabolised in the liver, and excreted in faeces as metabolites and a small amount of unchanged drug. Elimination from plasma is biphasic, with a mean terminal half-life of about 22 hours. The pharmacokinetics are not altered in patients with impaired renal function. Doxazosin is extensively bound to plasma proteins and is not removed by dialysis.

◊ Reviews.
1. Elliott HL, *et al.* Pharmacokinetic overview of doxazosin. *Am J Cardiol* 1987; **59:** 78G–81G.

Uses and Administration
Doxazosin is an alpha$_1$-adrenoceptor blocker (p.787) with actions and uses similar to those of prazosin (p.959), but a longer duration of action. It is used in the management of hypertension (below) and in benign prostatic hyperplasia (p.1477) to relieve symptoms of urinary obstruction.

Doxazosin is given by mouth as the mesilate, but doses are usually expressed in terms of the base. Following an oral dose maximum reduction in blood pressure is reported to occur after 2 to 6 hours and the effects are maintained for 24 hours, permitting once daily dosage.

To avoid the risk of collapse which may occur in some patients after the first dose, the initial dose is 1 mg, preferably at bedtime. Dosage may be increased after 1 or 2 weeks according to response. Usual maintenance doses for hypertension are up to 4 mg once daily; doses of 16 mg daily should not be exceeded. For benign prostatic hyperplasia the usual maintenance dose is 2 to 4 mg daily; doses of 8 mg daily should not be exceeded.

◊ Reviews.
1. Fulton B, *et al.* Doxazosin: an update of its clinical pharmacology and therapeutic applications in hypertension and benign prostatic hyperplasia. *Drugs* 1995; **49:** 295–320.

Hypertension. Alpha blockers are among the drug groups that have been recommended as first-line therapy for hypertension (p.802). However, in the Antihypertensive and Lipid-Lowering Treatment to Prevent Heart Attack Trial (ALLHAT)[1] the doxazosin arm of the study was terminated early due to an

increased incidence of heart failure in patients receiving doxazosin compared with those receiving chlortalidone.

1. The ALLHAT Officers and Coordinators for the ALLHAT Collaborative Research Group. Major cardiovascular events in hypertensive patients randomized to doxazosin vs chlorthalidone: the Antihypertensive and Lipid-Lowering Treatment to Prevent Heart Attack Trial (ALLHAT). *JAMA* 2000; **283:** 1967–75.

Preparations

Proprietary Preparations (details are given in Part 3)
Aust.: Prostadilat; Supressin; *Austral.:* Carduran†; *Braz.:* Carduran; *Canad.:* Cardura; *Denm.:* Carduran; *Ger.:* Cardular PP; Diblocin; Doxa-Puren; Doxagamma; Doxazomerck; *Hong Kong:* Cardura; *Irl.:* Cardura; *Israel:* Cadex; Cardoral; Doxaloc; *Ital.:* Benur; Cardura; Dedralen; Normothen; *Mex.:* Cardura; *Neth.:* Cardura; *Norw.:* Carduran; *NZ:* Cardoxan; *S.Afr.:* Cardura; *Singapore:* Cardura; *Spain:* Carduran; Progandol; *Swed.:* Alfadil; *Thai.:* Cardura; *UK:* Cardura; *USA:* Cardura.

Duteplase (13784-w)

Duteplase (rINN).

245-L-Methionine Plasminogen Activator; SM-9527.
$C_{2736}H_{4174}N_{914}O_{824}S_{46} = 64529.0$.
CAS — 120608-46-0.

Profile
Duteplase is a thrombolytic drug. It is a biosynthetic derivative of endogenous tissue plasminogen activator and has been used similarly to alteplase (p.833) in the treatment of thromboembolic disorders, particularly acute myocardial infarction.

◊ References.
1. Hayashi H, *et al.* Effects of intravenous SM-9527 (double-chain tissue plasminogen activator) on left ventricular function in the chronic stage of acute myocardial infarction. *Clin Cardiol* 1993; **16:** 409–14.
2. Malcolm AD, *et al.* ESPRIT: a European study of the prevention of reocclusion after initial thrombolysis with duteplase in acute myocardial infarction. *Eur Heart J* 1996; **17:** 1522–31.

Efonidipine (15889-l)

Efonidipine (rINN).

Cyclic 2,2-dimethyltrimethylene ester of 2-(N-benzylanilino)ethyl (±)-1,4-dihydro-2,6-dimethyl-4-(m-nitrophenyl)-5-phosphononicontinate .
$C_{34}H_{38}N_3O_7P = 631.7$.
CAS — 111011-63-3.

Profile
Efonidipine is a dihydropyridine calcium-channel blocker with general properties similar to those of nifedipine (p.940) and is used in the treatment of hypertension.

Enalapril (17599-a)

Enalapril (BAN, rINN).

N-{N-[(S)-1-Ethoxycarbonyl-3-phenylpropyl]-L-alanyl}-L-proline.
$C_{20}H_{28}N_2O_5 = 376.4$.
CAS — 75847-73-3.
ATC — C09AA02.

Enalapril Maleate (12969-e)

Enalapril Maleate (BANM, USAN, rINNM).

Enalapril Maleas; MK-421. N-{N-[(S)-1-Ethoxycarbonyl-3-phenylpropyl]-L-alanyl}-L-proline hydrogen maleate.
$C_{20}H_{28}N_2O_5,C_4H_4O_4 = 492.5$.
CAS — 76095-16-4.
Pharmacopoeias. In Eur. (see p.vi) and US.

Pharmacopoeial description

Ph. Eur.: A white or almost white crystalline powder. Soluble in water; sparingly soluble in dichloromethane; freely soluble in methyl alcohol. It dissolves in dilute solutions of alkali hydroxides. A 1% solution in water has a pH of 2.4 to 2.9. Protect from light.

USP 25: An off-white crystalline powder. Sparingly soluble in water; soluble in alcohol; freely soluble in dimethylformamide and in methyl alcohol; slightly soluble in semipolar organic solvents; practically insoluble in nonpolar organic solvents.

Stability. Enalapril has been reported[1,2] to be stable for at least 56 days in extemporaneously compounded oral liquids containing enalapril maleate 1 mg per mL in a number of vehicles.

1. Nahata MC, *et al.* Stability of enalapril maleate in three extemporaneously prepared oral liquids. *Am J Health-Syst Pharm* 1998; **55:** 1155–7.
2. Allen LV, Erickson MA. Stability of alprazolam, chloroquine phosphate, cisapride, enalapril maleate, and hydralazine hydrochloride in extemporaneously compounded oral liquids. *Am J Health-Syst Pharm* 1998; **55:** 1915–20.

Enalaprilat (16618-x)

Enalaprilat (BAN, USAN, rINN).

Enalaprilic acid; MK-422. N-{N-[(S)-1-Carboxy-3-phenylpropyl]-L-alanyl}-L-proline dihydrate.

$C_{18}H_{24}N_2O_5,2H_2O = 384.4$.

CAS — 76420-72-9 (anhydrous enalaprilat); 84680-54-6 (enalaprilat dihydrate).

Pharmacopoeias. In US.

Enalaprilat 1.38 mg as the dihydrate is approximately equivalent to 1.25 mg of anhydrous enalaprilat.

Pharmacopoeial description

USP 25: A white to nearly white, hygroscopic, crystalline powder. Soluble 1 in 200 of water, 1 in 40 of dimethylformamide, and 1 in 68 of methyl alcohol; very slightly soluble in alcohol, in acetone, and in hexane; practically insoluble in acetonitrile and in chloroform; slightly soluble in isopropyl alcohol.

Incompatibility. Enalaprilat was visually incompatible with phenytoin sodium in sodium chloride 0.9%, producing a crystalline precipitate; there was also some visual evidence of incompatibility when mixed with amphotericin B in glucose 5%.[1]

1. Thompson DF, et al. Visual compatibility of enalaprilat with selected intravenous medications during simulated Y-site injection. Am J Hosp Pharm 1990; 47: 2530–1.

Adverse Effects, Treatment, and Precautions

As for ACE inhibitors, p.820.

◊ Postmarketing surveillance for enalapril was carried out by prescription-event monitoring of 12 543 patients.[1] There were 374 skin events including facial oedema or angioedema in 29 (leading to withdrawal of treatment in 10), 15 cases of photosensitivity, and urticaria in 32 (leading to withdrawal in 5). Syncope and dizziness occurred in 155 and 483 patients respectively, sometimes in association with hypotension. Hypotension occurred in 218 patients, 71 in the first month. Treatment was stopped in 121 patients with hypotension, and dosage reduced in 36. Other adverse effects reported included headache in 310 patients, paraesthesias in 126, taste disturbances in 25, conjunctivitis in 67, tachycardia in 194, cough in 360, renal failure in 82, muscle cramp in 96, diarrhoea in 236, and nausea and vomiting in 326. Of 1098 deaths only 10, due to renal failure, were thought possibly related to enalapril therapy. Dysgeusia and skin reactions appeared to be less common than has been reported for captopril, but precise comparisons were difficult; the range of adverse effects was similar.[2]

Deafness was a possible side-effect of enalapril noted earlier;[2] it was reported in 19 of the 12 543 patients monitored, but only while they were taking enalapril, there being no record of deafness after treatment stopped.

For further reference to some of these adverse effects, see under ACE Inhibitors, p.820.

1. Inman WHW, et al. Postmarketing surveillance of enalapril I: results of prescription-event monitoring. BMJ 1988; 297: 826–9.
2. Inman WHW, Rawson NSB. Deafness with enalapril and prescription event monitoring. Lancet 1987; i: 872.

Breast feeding. Following administration of a single dose of enalapril 20 mg to 5 lactating women enalaprilat was detected in breast milk in concentrations of 1 to 2.3 nanograms per mL (mean peak 1.72 nanograms per mL); enalapril was also present (mean peak 1.74 nanograms per mL). This compared with peak serum values of 39 to 112 nanograms per mL for enalaprilat and 92 to 151 nanograms per mL for enalapril. Although enalapril and its metabolite are thus present in small amounts in breast milk it was calculated that the average total daily dose to the neonate would only be about 2 µg of enalaprilat.[1]

1. Redman CWG, et al. The excretion of enalapril and enalaprilat in human breast milk. Eur J Clin Pharmacol 1990; 38: 99.

Porphyria. Enalapril has been associated with acute attacks of porphyria and is considered unsafe in porphyric patients.

Interactions

As for ACE inhibitors, p.822.

Pharmacokinetics

Enalapril acts as a prodrug of the diacid enalaprilat, its active form, which is poorly absorbed by mouth. Following oral administration about 60% of a dose of enalapril is absorbed from the gastrointestinal tract and peak plasma concentrations are achieved within about 1 hour. Enalapril is extensively hydrolysed in the liver to enalaprilat; peak plasma concentrations of enalaprilat are achieved 3 to 4 hours after an oral dose of enalapril. Enalaprilat is 50 to 60% bound to plasma proteins. About 60% of an oral dose of enalapril is excreted in urine, as enalaprilat and unchanged drug, the rest in the faeces. The elimination of enalaprilat is multiphasic but the effective half-life for accumulation following multiple doses of enalapril is reported

to be about 11 hours in patients with normal renal function. Enalaprilat is removed by haemodialysis and by peritoneal dialysis.

◊ References.

1. MacFadyen RJ, et al. Enalapril clinical pharmacokinetics and pharmacokinetic-pharmacodynamic relationships: an overview. Clin Pharmacokinet 1993; 25: 274–82.

Renal impairment. Comparison of the pharmacokinetics of enalapril in 6 diabetics with persistent proteinuria and glomerular filtration rates (GFR) of 44.1 to 58.4 mL per minute with those in 8 age-matched controls showed that in the diabetic group the peak serum concentration of enalaprilat was higher, the time to peak concentration longer, renal clearance lower, and the areas under the concentration/time curve greater than in controls.[1] Renal clearance of enalaprilat in the diabetics ranged from 56 to 66 mL per minute compared with 105 to 133 mL per minute in controls; clearance correlated with GFR.

1. Baba T, et al. Enalapril pharmacokinetics in diabetic patients. Lancet 1989; i: 226–7.

Uses and Administration

Enalapril is an ACE inhibitor (p.820) used in the treatment of hypertension (p.802) and heart failure (p.798). It may also be given prophylactically to patients with asymptomatic left ventricular dysfunction to delay the onset of symptomatic heart failure and to those with left ventricular dysfunction to reduce the incidence of coronary ischaemic events, including myocardial infarction (p.805).

Enalapril owes its activity to enalaprilat to which it is converted after oral administration. The haemodynamic effects are seen within 1 hour of a single oral dose and the maximum effect occurs after about 4 to 6 hours, although the full effect may not develop for several weeks during chronic dosing. The haemodynamic action lasts for about 24 hours, allowing once-daily dosing. Enalapril is given by mouth as the maleate.

Enalaprilat is not absorbed by mouth but is given by intravenous injection; its haemodynamic effects develop within 15 minutes of injection and reach a peak in 1 to 4 hours. The action lasts for about 6 hours at recommended doses. Enalaprilat is given as the dihydrate, but doses are expressed in terms of the anhydrous substance.

In the treatment of **hypertension**, an initial dose of 5 mg of enalapril maleate daily may be given by mouth. Since there may be a precipitous fall in blood pressure in some patients when starting therapy with an ACE inhibitor, the first dose should preferably be given at bedtime. An initial dose of 2.5 mg daily should be given to patients with renal impairment or to those who are receiving a diuretic; if possible, the diuretic should be withdrawn 2 or 3 days before enalapril is started and resumed later if necessary. An initial dose of 2.5 mg is also recommended in elderly patients. The usual maintenance dose is 10 to 20 mg given once daily, although doses of up to 40 mg daily may be required in severe hypertension. It may be given in 2 divided doses if control is inadequate with a single dose.

When oral therapy of hypertension is impractical enalaprilat may be given in a dose of 1.25 mg by slow intravenous injection over 5 minutes, repeated every 6 hours if necessary; the initial dose should be halved in patients with renal impairment (creatinine clearance less than 30 mL per minute) or those who are receiving a diuretic.

In the management of **heart failure**, severe first-dose hypotension on introduction of an ACE inhibitor is common in patients on loop diuretics, but their temporary withdrawal may cause rebound pulmonary oedema. Thus treatment should be initiated with a low dose under close medical supervision. In patients with heart failure or asymptomatic left ventricular dysfunction enalapril maleate is given by mouth in an initial dose of 2.5 mg daily. The usual maintenance dose is 20 mg daily as a single dose or in 2 divided doses although up to 40 mg daily in 2 divided doses has been given.

Administration in children. Enalapril has been given to infants with severe heart failure in doses of 0.1 to 0.5 mg per kg

body-weight daily as an oral suspension produced by suspending a crushed tablet in water.[1] In this study one infant, with severe myocarditis, developed hypotension and the drug had to be withdrawn; the remaining 7 showed clinical improvement on a mean enalapril dose of 0.26 mg per kg daily and were able markedly to reduce the dose of concomitant diuretic required. Another study in 10 infants found that enalapril was less bioavailable and probably had a shorter duration of action in infants than in adults, and that doses of 0.08 mg per kg daily were inadequate in the treatment of infant heart failure.[2] A larger study in 63 infants and children (median age 5.4 months) with heart failure found enalapril 0.36 mg per kg daily to be of benefit, whereas there was no improvement with a lower dose of 0.24 mg per kg daily.[3]

1. Frenneaux M, et al. Enalapril for severe heart failure in infancy. Arch Dis Child 1989; 64: 219–23.
2. Lloyd TR, et al. Orally administered enalapril for infants with congestive heart failure: a dose-finding study. J Pediatr 1989; 114: 650–4.
3. Leversha AM, et al. Efficacy and dosage of enalapril in congenital and acquired heart disease. Arch Dis Child 1994; 70: 35–9.

Preparations

USP 25: Enalapril Maleate and Hydrochlorothiazide Tablets; Enalapril Maleate Tablets.

Proprietary Preparations (details are given in Part 3)

Aust.: Mepril; Regomed; Renitec; **Austral.:** Alphapril; Amprace; Renitec; **Belg.:** Renitec; **Braz.:** Atens; Enapril; Eupressin; Renitec; **Canad.:** Vasotec; **Denm.:** Aceren; Alacor; Alapren†; Corodil; Enadil; Renitec; **Fin.:** Enaloc; Linatil; Renitec; **Fr.:** Renitec; **Ger.:** Benalapril; enadura; Enahexal; Enalagamma; Pres; Pres iv; Xanef; **Hong Kong:** Renitec; **Irl.:** Enap; Innomel; Innovace; Renitec; **Israel:** Convertin; **Ital.:** Converten; Enapren; Naprilene; **Mex.:** Blocatril; Enaladil; Feliberal; Glioten; Kenopril; Lipraken; Norpril; Palane; Pulsol; Renitec; **Neth.:** Renitec; **Norw.:** Renitec; **NZ:** Renitec; **Port.:** Balpril; Cetampril; Denapril; Hipten†; Renipril; Renitec; Tensazol; **S.Afr.:** Hypace; Pharmapress; Renitec; **Singapore:** Enapril; Daren; Enaril; Invoril; Renaton; Renitec; **Spain:** Acetensil; Baripril; Bitensil; Clipto; Controlvas; Corprilor; Crinoren; Dabonal; Ditensor; Herten; Hipoartel; Iecatec; Insup; Nacor; Naprilene; Neotensin; Pressitan; Reca; Renitec; Ristalen; **Swed.:** Renitec; **Switz.:** Acepril; Reniten; **Thai.:** Anapril; Enam; Enaril; Invoril; Isotopril; Korandil; Lapril; Nalopril; Naritec; Renitec; **UAE:** Narapril; **UK:** Ednyt; Enacard; Innovace; Pralenal; **USA:** Vasotec.

Multi-ingredient: Aust.: Co-Mepril; Co-Renitec; Renitec Plus; **Austral.:** Renitec Plus; **Belg.:** Co-Renitec; **Braz.:** Atens H; Co-Renitec; Eupressin H; **Canad.:** Vaseretic; **Denm.:** Co-Renitec; Corodil Comp; Synerpril; **Fin.:** Enaloc Comp; Linatil Comp; Renitec Comp; Renitec Plus; **Fr.:** Co-Renitec; **Ger.:** Pres plus; Renacor; **Hong Kong:** Co-Renitec; **Irl.:** Innozide; **Ital.:** Acesistem; Condiuren; Gentipress; Neoprex; Sinertec; Vaseretic; **Mex.:** Co-Renitec; **Neth.:** Co-Renitec; Renitec Plus; **Norw.:** Renitec Comp; **NZ:** Co-Renitec; **Port.:** Enatia; Laprilen; Renidur; **S.Afr.:** Co-Renitec; **Singapore:** Co-Renitec; **Spain:** Acediur; Acetensil Plus; Baripril Diu; Bitensil Diu; Co-Renitec; Crinoretic; Dabonal Plus; Ditenside; Hipoartel Plus; Neotensin Diu; Pressitan Plus; Renitecmax; **Swed.:** Renitec Comp; Synerpril; **Switz.:** Co-Reniten; Reniten Plus; **UK:** Innozide; **USA:** Lexxel; Teczem; Vaseretic.

Enalkiren (10781-g)

Enalkiren (USAN, rINN).

Abbott-64662. (αS)-α-[(αS)-α-(3-Amino-3-methylbutyramido)-p-methoxyhydrocinnamamido]-N-[(1S,2R,3S)-1-(cyclohexylmethyl)-2,3-dihydroxy-5-methylhexyl]imidazole-4-propionamide.

$C_{35}H_{56}N_6O_6 = 656.9$.

CAS — 113082-98-7.

Profile

Enalkiren inhibits the actions of renin and thus prevents the conversion of angiotensinogen into angiotensin I. Enalkiren is given intravenously. It has been investigated in the management of hypertension and heart failure.

◊ References.

1. Griffiths AN, et al. The hypotensive effect of increasing doses of enalkiren, a dipeptide renin inhibitor, compared with enalaprilat in hypertensive patients. Br J Clin Pharmacol 1990; 29: 614P–15P.
2. Frishman WH, et al. Renin inhibition: a new approach to cardiovascular therapy. J Clin Pharmacol 1994; 34: 873–80.
3. Rongen GA, et al. Clinical pharmacokinetics and efficacy of renin inhibitors. Clin Pharmacokinet 1995; 29: 6–14.

Encainide Hydrochloride (7785-b)

Encainide Hydrochloride (BANM, USAN, rINNM).

MJ-9067-1 (encainide). (±)-2'-[2-(1-Methyl-2-piperidyl)ethyl]-p-anisanilide hydrochloride.

$C_{22}H_{28}N_2O_2,HCl = 388.9$.

CAS — 37612-13-8 (encainide); 66778-36-7 (encainide); 66794-74-9 (encainide hydrochloride).

Profile

Encainide is a class Ic antiarrhythmic (p.787) and was used for the treatment of severe or life-threatening ventricular arrhythmias. It was withdrawn from the market as a result of an increase in mortality rates in post-infarction patients in the Cardiac Arrhythmia Suppression Trial (CAST) (p.794).

Endralazine Mesilate (12688-h)

Endralazine Mesilate (BANM, rINNM).

BQ-22-708; Compound 22-708; Endralazine Mesylate (USAN). 6-Benzoyl-5,6,7,8-tetrahydropyrido[4,3-c]pyridazin-3-ylhydrazone monomethanesulfonate.

$C_{14}H_{15}N_5O,CH_4O_3S = 365.4$.

CAS — 39715-02-1 (endralazine); 65322-72-7 (endralazine mesilate).

Profile

Endralazine is a vasodilator with properties similar to those of hydralazine (p.905). It has been used as the mesilate in the treatment of hypertension.

Preparations

Proprietary Preparations (details are given in Part 3)

Braz.: Arritlan.

Enoxaparin Sodium (13424-s)

Enoxaparin Sodium (BAN, USAN, rINN).

Enoxaparinum Natricum; PK-10169; RP-54563.

CAS — 9041-08-1.

Pharmacopoeias. In Eur. (see p.vi).

Pharmacopoeial description

Ph. Eur.: Enoxaparin sodium is the sodium salt of a low-molecular-mass heparin that is obtained by alkaline depolymerisation of the benzyl ester derivative of heparin from porcine intestinal mucosa. The majority of the components have a 4-enopyranose uronate structure at the non-reducing end of their chain. The mass-average molecular mass ranges between 3500 and 5500 with a characteristic value of about 4500. The degree of sulfation is about 2 per disaccharide unit.

The potency is not less than 90 units and not more than 125 units of anti-factor Xa activity per mg, with reference to the dried substance. The ratio of anti-factor Xa activity to anti-factor IIa activity is between 3.3 and 5.3.

Units

As for Low-molecular-weight Heparins, p.923.

Adverse Effects, Treatment, and Precautions

As for Low-molecular-weight Heparins, p.923.

Severe bleeding with enoxaparin may be reduced by the slow intravenous injection of protamine sulfate; 1 mg of protamine sulfate is stated to inhibit the effects of 1 mg (100 units) of enoxaparin sodium.

Interactions

As for Low-molecular-weight Heparins, p.924.

Pharmacokinetics

Enoxaparin is rapidly absorbed following subcutaneous injection with a bioavailability of about 92%. Peak plasma activity is reached within 1 to 5 hours. The elimination half-life is about 4 to 5 hours but anti-factor Xa activity persists for up to 24 hours following a 40-mg dose. Enoxaparin is metabolised in the liver and excreted in the urine, as unchanged drug and metabolites.

Uses and Administration

Enoxaparin sodium is a low-molecular-weight heparin (p.923) with anticoagulant properties. It is used in the treatment and prophylaxis of venous thromboembolism (p.817) and to prevent clotting during extracorporeal circulation. It is also used in the management of unstable angina (p.791).

In the prophylaxis of **venous thromboembolism** during surgical procedures, enoxaparin sodium is given by subcutaneous injection; treatment is continued for 7 to 10 days or until the patient is ambulant. Patients at low to moderate risk are given 20 mg (2000 units) once daily with the first dose approximately 2 hours pre-operatively. In patients at high risk the dose should be increased to 40 mg (4000 units) once daily with the initial dose given approximately 12 hours before the procedure. Alternatively, a dose of 30 mg (3000 units) may be given subcutaneously twice daily, starting within 12 to 24 hours after operation. Following hip replacement surgery, enoxaparin may be continued in a dose of 40 mg once daily for a further 3 weeks. For the prophylaxis of thromboembolism in immobilised medical patients, the dose is 40 mg

(4000 units) once daily for at least 6 days; treatment should be continued until the patient is fully ambulant, up to a maximum of 14 days.

For the treatment of deep-vein thrombosis enoxaparin sodium is given subcutaneously in a dose of 1 mg (100 units) per kg body-weight every 12 hours, or 1.5 mg (150 units) per kg once daily, for 5 days or until oral anticoagulation is established.

For prevention of clotting in the extracorporeal circulation during **haemodialysis**, enoxaparin sodium 1 mg (100 units) per kg is introduced into the arterial line of the circuit at the beginning of the dialysis session. A further dose of 0.5 to 1 mg (50 to 100 units) per kg may be given if required. The dose should be reduced in patients at high risk of haemorrhage.

In the management of **unstable angina**, enoxaparin sodium is given subcutaneously in a dose of 1 mg (100 units) per kg every 12 hours. Treatment is usually continued for 2 to 8 days and low-dose aspirin should be given concomitantly.

◊ References.

1. Noble S, et al. Enoxaparin: a reappraisal of its pharmacology and clinical applications in the prevention and treatment of thromboembolic disease. Drugs 1995; **49:** 388–410.
2. Noble S, Spencer CM. Enoxaparin: a review of its clinical potential in the management of coronary artery disease. Drugs 1998; **56:** 259–72.
3. Harvey DM, Offord RH. Management of venous and cardiovascular thrombosis: enoxaparin. Hosp Med 2000; **61:** 628–36.

Administration in infants and children. Increasing numbers of infants and children are receiving anticoagulants for the management of thromboembolism. Few controlled studies have been carried out and recommendations for therapy have generally been adapted from adult guidelines. Low-molecular-weight heparins may have a number of advantages in children. Enoxaparin has been used for the treatment[1,2] and prophylaxis[2] of thromboembolism in children. Use in a preterm infant has also been reported.[3] Younger children may require a higher dose than older children. A regimen[4] for treatment of thromboembolism is 1.5 mg per kg body-weight every 12 hours for those under 2 months of age and 1 mg per kg every 12 hours for those over 2 months. Doses for prophylaxis are 0.75 mg per kg every 12 hours for those under 2 months and 0.5 mg per kg every 12 hours for those over 2 months.

1. Massicotte P, et al. Low-molecular-weight heparin in pediatric patients with thrombotic disease: a dose finding study. J Pediatr 1996; **128:** 313–18.
2. Dix D, et al. The use of low molecular weight heparin in pediatric patients: a prospective cohort study. J Pediatr 2000; **136:** 439–45.
3. Dunaway KK, et al. Use of enoxaparin in a preterm infant. Ann Pharmacother 2000; **34:** 1410–13.
4. Monagle P, et al. Antithrombotic therapy in children. Chest 2001; **119** (suppl): 344S–370S.

Preparations

Proprietary Preparations (details are given in Part 3)

Aust.: Lovenox; **Austral.:** Clexane; **Belg.:** Clexane; **Braz.:** Clexane; **Canad.:** Lovenox; **Denm.:** Klexane; **Fin.:** Klexane; **Fr.:** Lovenox; **Ger.:** Clexane; **Hong Kong:** Clexane; **Irl.:** Clexane; **Israel:** Clexane; **Ital.:** Clexane; Trombenox; **Mex.:** Clexane; **Neth.:** Clexane; **Norw.:** Klexane; **NZ:** Clexane; **Port.:** Lovenox; **S.Afr.:** Clexane; **Singapore:** Clexane; **Spain:** Clexane; Decipar; **Swed.:** Klexane; **Switz.:** Clexane; Lovenox; **Thai.:** Clexane; **UK:** Clexane; **USA:** Lovenox.

Enoximone (16805-d)

Enoximone (BAN, USAN, rINN).

Fenoximone; MDL-17043; MDL-19438; RMI-17043; YMDL-17043. 4-Methyl-5-[4-(methylthio)benzoyl]-4-imidazolin-2-one.

$C_{12}H_{12}N_2O_2S = 248.3$.

CAS — 77671-31-9.

ATC — C01CE03.

Crystal formation has been observed when enoximone injection was mixed in glass containers or syringes; the manufacturer recommends that only plastic containers or syringes are used for dilutions. The manufacturer also recommends that only sodium chloride 0.9% or water be used as diluents. Glucose solutions should not be used as a diluent since crystal formation may occur.

Adverse Effects

Long-term oral treatment with enoximone has been reported to increase the mortality rate and enoximone is now only employed intravenously for short-term use.

The commonest adverse effects of enoximone affect the gastrointestinal tract and include diarrhoea, nausea, and vomiting. Other adverse effects include

headache, insomnia, chills, oliguria, fever, urinary retention, and limb pain. There have been reports of thrombocytopenia and abnormal liver enzyme values.

Enoximone may cause ventricular and supraventricular tachyarrhythmias, ectopic beats, and hypotension.

Effects on the nervous system. Tonic-clonic convulsions have been reported[1] in a patient given enoximone 6 µg per kg body-weight per minute by intravenous infusion. The convulsions subsided when enoximone was discontinued.

1. Appadurai I, et al. Convulsions induced by enoximone administered as a continuous intravenous infusion. BMJ 1990; **300:** 613–14.

Hyperosmolality. Hyperosmolality occurred in an infant during intravenous infusion of enoximone 20 µg per kg body-weight per minute. The probable cause was propylene glycol in the enoximone injection providing a dose of 2.4 mg per kg per minute.[1]

1. Huggon I, et al. Hyperosmolality related to propylene glycol in an infant treated with enoximone infusion. BMJ 1990; **301:** 19–20.

Precautions

Enoximone should be used with caution in patients with hypertrophic cardiomyopathy or severe obstructive aortic or pulmonary valvular disease.

Blood pressure, heart rate, ECG, and fluid and electrolyte status should be monitored during therapy. Platelet count and liver enzyme values should also be monitored.

The injection has a high pH (approximately 12) and must be diluted before use (but see above). Extravasation should be avoided during administration.

Hepatic and renal impairment. The elimination half-life of enoximone following intravenous administration was 2.16 hours in a patient with hepatic impairment and 1.33 hours in a patient with renal impairment. The mean elimination half-life in patients with normal hepatic and renal function was 1.26 hours. It was suggested that patients with renal impairment should be monitored and have plasma concentrations measured during continuous infusions and that in hepatic disease the dosage may need to be modified.[1] Similarly, in a study[2] in paediatric patients receiving intravenous enoximone clearance was reduced in those with renal or hepatic impairment and it was suggested that the infusion rate should be decreased in such patients.

1. Desager JP, et al. Plasma enoximone concentrations in cardiac patients. Curr Ther Res 1990; **47:** 743–52.
2. Booker PD, et al. Enoximone pharmacokinetics in infants. Br J Anaesth 2000; **85:** 205–10.

Pharmacokinetics

Enoximone is absorbed from the gastrointestinal tract but it is no longer administered orally due to an increased mortality rate in some long-term studies. The plasma elimination half-life varies widely; it may be about 1 to 4 hours in healthy volunteers and about 3 to 8 hours in patients with heart failure, but longer times have been reported. Enoximone is about 85% bound to plasma proteins. It is metabolised in the liver and is excreted in the urine, mainly as metabolites. Following intravenous administration about 70% of a dose is excreted in the urine as metabolites and less than 1% as unchanged drug.

◊ General references.

1. Rocci ML, Wilson H. The pharmacokinetics and pharmacodynamics of newer inotropic agents. Clin Pharmacokinet 1987; **13:** 91–109. Correction. ibid. 1988; **14:** (contents page).
2. Booker PD, et al. Enoximone pharmacokinetics in infants. Br J Anaesth 2000; **85:** 205–10.

Uses and Administration

Enoximone is a phosphodiesterase inhibitor similar to amrinone (p.839) with positive inotropic and vasodilator activity. It is given intravenously in the short-term management of heart failure. In some long-term studies it was given by mouth, but an increased mortality rate was reported.

The usual initial dose of enoximone by intravenous injection is 0.5 to 1.0 mg per kg body-weight given at a rate not greater than 12.5 mg per minute. This may be followed by doses of 0.5 mg per kg every 30 minutes until a satisfactory response is obtained or a total dose of 3 mg per kg has been given. Alternatively, the initial dose may be given as a continuous intravenous infusion in a dose of 90 µg per kg per minute over 10 to 30 minutes until the desired response is achieved.

For maintenance therapy the initial dose (up to a total of 3 mg per kg) may be repeated as required every 3 to 6 hours or a continuous or intermittent infusion may be given in a dose of 5 to 20 µg per kg per minute.

The total dose over 24 hours should not exceed 24 mg per kg.

Dosage may need to be reduced in patients with renal impairment.

◊ General references.
1. Vernon MW, et al. Enoximone: a review of its pharmacological properties and therapeutic potential. *Drugs* 1991; **42**: 997–1017.

Beta blocker overdosage. Enoximone, given intravenously as a bolus dose of 0.5 mg per kg body-weight followed by an infusion of 15 µg per kg per minute, successfully increased the cardiac output and stroke volume in a woman who had ingested 10 g of metoprolol.[1] It was suggested that enoximone may be useful in such patients since its action does not involve the beta-adrenergic system.
1. Hoeper MM, Boeker KHW. Overdose of metoprolol treated with enoximone. *N Engl J Med* 1996; **335**: 1538.

Heart failure. Enoximone is one of several drugs that may be used in heart failure (p.798), but because of an increased mortality rate reported following long-term oral use it is only given intravenously for short-term management of heart failure unresponsive to other treatments. In a comparison of oral enoximone and placebo in patients with moderate to moderately severe heart failure,[1] enoximone was no better than placebo in improving exercise duration over the 16-week study period. Although the overall incidence of adverse effects was similar in the two groups, 5 patients receiving enoximone died compared with none in the placebo group.
1. Uretsky BF, et al. Multicenter trial of oral enoximone in patients with moderate to moderately severe congestive heart failure: lack of benefit compared with placebo. *Circulation* 1990; **82**: 774–80.

Preparations

Proprietary Preparations (details are given in Part 3)
Belg.: Perfan; *Fr.:* Perfane; *Ger.:* Perfan; *Irl.:* Perfan; *Ital.:* Perfan; *Neth.:* Perfan; *UK:* Perfan.

Epanolol (18637-c)

Epanolol *(BAN, USAN, rINN)*.
ICI-141292. *(RS)*-N-[2-(3-o-Cyanophenoxy-2-hydroxypropylamino)ethyl]-2-(4-hydroxyphenyl)acetamide.
$C_{20}H_{23}N_3O_4 = 369.4$.
CAS — 86880-51-5.
ATC — C07AB10.

Profile
Epanolol is reported to be a cardioselective beta blocker (p.844) with some intrinsic sympathomimetic activity. It is under investigation in various cardiovascular disorders.

Epitizide (2327-q)

Epitizide *(BAN, rINN)*.
Epithiazide *(USAN)*; NSC-108164; P-2105. 6-Chloro-3,4-dihydro-3-(2,2,2-trifluoroethylthiomethyl)-2H-1,2,4-benzothiadiazine-7-sulphonamide 1,1-dioxide.
$C_{10}H_{11}ClF_3N_3O_4S_3 = 425.9$.
CAS — 1764-85-8.

Profile
Epitizide is a thiazide diuretic (see Hydrochlorothiazide, p.907) used in the treatment of oedema and hypertension, often in combination with triamterene.

Preparations
Proprietary Preparations (details are given in Part 3)
Multi-ingredient: *Belg.:* Dyta-Urese†; *Neth.:* Dyta-Urese.

Eprosartan Mesilate (17799-m)

Eprosartan Mesilate *(BANM, rINNM)*.
Eprosartan Mesylate *(USAN)*; SKF-108566-J. *(E)*-2-Butyl-1-(p-carboxybenzyl)-α-2-thenylimidazole-5-acrylic acid methanesulfonate.
$C_{23}H_{24}N_2O_4S,CH_4O_3S = 520.6$.
CAS — 133040-01-4 (eprosartan); 144143-96-4 (eprosartan mesilate).

Eprosartan mesilate 1.2 mg is approximately equivalent to 1 mg of eprosartan.

Adverse Effects and Precautions
As for Losartan Potassium, p.921.

Pharmacokinetics
Eprosartan is absorbed from the gastrointestinal tract with an absolute oral bioavailability of about 13%.

Peak plasma concentrations occur about 1 to 2 hours after an oral dose in the fasted state; administration with food delays absorption but this is not clinically significant. Eprosartan is approximately 98% bound to plasma proteins. It is excreted in the bile and in the urine, primarily as the unchanged drug; following oral administration approximately 7% of the drug is excreted in the urine, with about 2% as the acyl glucuronide. The terminal elimination half-life is about 5 to 9 hours.

Uses and Administration
Eprosartan is an angiotensin II receptor antagonist with actions similar to those of losartan (p.922). It is used in the management of hypertension (p.802).

Eprosartan is given by mouth as the mesilate but doses are expressed in terms of the base. The onset of antihypertensive effect occurs about 1 to 2 hours after administration and the maximum effect is achieved within 2 to 3 weeks after initiating therapy.

In the management of hypertension, eprosartan is given in an initial dose of 600 mg once daily. A lower initial dose of 300 mg once daily may be used in elderly patients over 75 years and in patients with renal impairment (creatinine clearance less than 60 mL per minute) or mild to moderate hepatic impairment. The dose should be adjusted according to response; the usual maintenance dose is 400 to 800 mg daily in a single dose or in two divided doses.

◊ Reviews.
1. McClellan KJ, Balfour JA. Eprosartan. *Drugs* 1998; **55**: 713–18.
2. Plosker GL, Foster RH. Eprosartan: a review of its use in the management of hypertension. *Drugs* 2000; **60**: 177–201.

Preparations
Proprietary Preparations (details are given in Part 3)
Austral.: Teveten; *Denm.:* Teveten; *Fin.:* Teveten; *Ger.:* Teveten; *Irl.:* Teveten; *Neth.:* Teveten; *Port.:* Teveten; *Spain:* Tevetens; *Swed.:* Teveten; *UK:* Teveten; *USA:* Teveten.

Eptifibatide (15030-q)

Eptifibatide *(BAN, rINN)*.
Integrelin. N^6-Amidino-N^2-(3-mercaptopropionyl)-L-lysylglycyl-L-α-aspartyl-L-tryptophyl-L-prolyl-L-cysteinamide, cyclic (1→6)-disulfide; S^1,S^6-Cyclo[N^6-carbamimidoyl-N^2-(3-sulfanylpropanoyl)-L-lysylglycyl-L-α-aspartyl-L-tryptophyl-L-prolyl-L-cysteinamide].
$C_{35}H_{49}N_{11}O_9S_2 = 832.0$.
CAS — 148031-34-9; 157630-07-4.

Adverse Effects and Precautions
Bleeding is the most common adverse effect of eptifibatide and therefore it should not be given to patients who are actively bleeding or to patients at increased risk of haemorrhage, including those with haemorrhagic disorders, cerebrovascular disorders, uncontrolled hypertension, or those who have recently undergone major surgery or severe trauma. Eptifibatide should be discontinued if serious uncontrolled bleeding occurs, or if emergency surgery or thrombolytic therapy is required. It should not be given to patients with severe renal impairment and should be used with caution in patients with hepatic impairment in whom blood coagulation could be affected. Hypotension has been reported following eptifibatide administration. Antibodies to eptifibatide have not been detected.

Pharmacokinetics
Antiplatelet effects of eptifibatide persist for about 4 hours after stopping a continuous infusion. Plasma elimination half-life is approximately 2.5 hours. Eptifibatide is about 25% bound to human plasma proteins. Renal clearance, as eptifibatide and metabolites excreted in the urine, accounts for approximately 50% of total body clearance.

Uses and Administration
Eptifibatide is an antiplatelet drug that reversibly inhibits binding of fibrinogen, von Willebrand factor, and other adhesive molecules to the glycoprotein IIb/IIIa receptor of platelets. It is used, usually in combination with aspirin and heparin, in the manage-

ment of unstable angina and in patients undergoing coronary angioplasty and stenting procedures.

In the management of **unstable angina**, eptifibatide is given in an initial dose of 180 µg per kg body-weight by intravenous injection, followed by 2 µg per kg per minute by intravenous infusion, for up to 72 hours. If percutaneous coronary intervention is performed during eptifibatide therapy, the infusion should be continued for 18 to 24 hours after the procedure, to a maximum total duration of 96 hours of therapy. A dose reduction may be considered in those with moderate renal impairment; it should not be used in those with severe impairment.

In patients undergoing **angioplasty**, though not presenting with unstable angina, eptifibatide is given in an initial dose of 180 µg per kg by intravenous injection immediately before the procedure, followed by 2 µg per kg per minute by intravenous infusion, with a second 180 µg per kg intravenous injection given 10 minutes after the first. The infusion should be continued until hospital discharge or for up to 18 to 24 hours; a minimum of 12 hours is recommended. The dose should be reduced in patients with renal impairment.

The use of eptifibatide with thrombolysis for acute myocardial infarction is under investigation.

◊ General references.
1. Goa KL, Noble S. Eptifibatide: a review of its use in patients with acute coronary syndromes and/or undergoing percutaneous coronary intervention. *Drugs* 1999; **57**: 439–62.

◊ Eptifibatide has been studied in the management of unstable angina; patients have been treated either medically or with percutaneous coronary intervention such as angioplasty.

Over 10 000 patients with ischaemic chest pain were enrolled in a study[1] comparing eptifibatide with placebo. The majority of patients also received aspirin and heparin. The incidence of death and non-fatal myocardial infarction up to 30 days after treatment was reduced in those receiving eptifibatide compared with placebo.

In a study[2] of over 4000 patients undergoing elective or scheduled percutaneous coronary revascularisation, reduced numbers of death, myocardial infarction, and further unplanned coronary intervention were also reported in those receiving eptifibatide compared with placebo. Similar results were also obtained in a further study[3] in patients who were undergoing percutaneous coronary revascularisation with stent implantation, and benefit was maintained at 6-month follow-up.[4]
1. The PURSUIT Trial Investigators. Inhibition of platelet glycoprotein IIb/IIIa with eptifibatide in patients with acute coronary syndromes. *N Engl J Med* 1998; **339**: 436–43.
2. The IMPACT-II Investigators. Randomised placebo-controlled trial of effect of eptifibatide on complications of percutaneous coronary intervention: IMPACT-II. *Lancet* 1997; **349**: 1422–8.
3. The ESPRIT Investigators. Novel dosing regimen of eptifibatide in planned coronary stent implantation (ESPRIT): a randomised, placebo-controlled trial. *Lancet* 2000; **356**: 2037–44. Correction. *ibid.* 2001; **357**: 1370.
4. O'Shea JC, et al. Platelet glycoprotein IIb/IIIa integrin blockade with eptifibatide in coronary stent intervention: the ESPRIT Trial: a randomized controlled trial. *JAMA* 2001; **285**: 2468–73.

Preparations
Proprietary Preparations (details are given in Part 3)
Canad.: Integrilin; *Denm.:* Integrilin; *Fin.:* Integrilin; *Fr.:* Integrilin; *Ger.:* Integrilin; *Irl.:* Integrilin; *Israel:* Integrilin; *Ital.:* Integrilin; *Neth.:* Integrilin; *Port.:* Integrilin; *S.Afr.:* Integrilin; *Spain:* Integrilin; *Swed.:* Integrilin; *Switz.:* Integrilin; *UK:* Integrilin; *USA:* Integrilin.

Eritrityl Tetranitrate (9229-z)

Eritrityl Tetranitrate *(rINN)*.
Erythritol Tetranitrate; Erythryl Tetranitrate *(USAN)*; Erythrol Nitrate; Erythrol Tetranitrate; Nitroerythrite; Nitroerythrol; NSC-106566; Tetranitrol. Butane-1,2,3,4-tetrol tetranitrate.
$C_4H_6(NO_3)_4 = 302.1$.
CAS — 7297-25-8.
ATC — C01DA13.

Pharmacopoeias. Diluted eritrityl tetranitrate is included in *Aust.* (25% in lactose).

Diluted eritrityl tetranitrate is a mixture of eritrityl tetranitrate and lactose or other suitable inert excipients, the excipients being added to minimise the risk of explosion.

◊ CAUTION. *Undiluted eritrityl tetranitrate can be exploded by percussion or excessive heat.*

Profile
Eritrityl tetranitrate is a vasodilator with general properties similar to those of glyceryl trinitrate (p.898). It has been used in angina pectoris.

Preparations

Proprietary Preparations (details are given in Part 3)
Ital.: Cardilate†.

Esmolol Hydrochloride (16636-f)

Esmolol Hydrochloride (BANM, USAN, rINNM).
ASL-8052. Methyl 3-[4-(2-hydroxy-3-isopropylaminopropoxy)phenyl]propionate hydrochloride.
$C_{16}H_{25}NO_4,HCl = 331.8$.
CAS — 81147-92-4 (esmolol); 84057-94-3 (esmolol); 103598-03-4 (esmolol); 81161-17-3 (esmolol hydrochloride).

Incompatibility. The manufacturers advise against admixture of esmolol hydrochloride with sodium bicarbonate because of incompatibility. There has also been a report[1] of immediate haze formation following admixture of esmolol hydrochloride with warfarin sodium.

1. Bahal SM, et al. Visual compatibility of warfarin sodium injection with selected medications and solutions. *Am J Health-Syst Pharm* 1997; **54:** 2599–2600.

Adverse Effects, Treatment, and Precautions

As for beta blockers, p.844.

Hypotension is the most frequently reported adverse effect associated with the infusion of esmolol hydrochloride; it generally resolves within 30 minutes once the dosage is reduced or the infusion is discontinued. Local irritation at the site of infusion, inflammation, induration, and thrombophlebitis have occurred and necrosis is a hazard of extravasation. These local effects have occurred with concentrations of 20 mg per mL and it is recommended that concentrations should not exceed 10 mg per mL and that the infusion should not be made into a small vein.

Effects on the CNS. Generalised tonic-clonic seizures occurred in an elderly patient given esmolol hydrochloride.[1]

1. Das G, Ferris JC. Generalized convulsions in a patient receiving ultra short-acting beta-blocker infusion. *Drug Intell Clin Pharm* 1988; **22:** 484–5.

Interactions

The interactions associated with beta blockers are discussed on p.846.

Pharmacokinetics

Following intravenous administration of esmolol hydrochloride the drug is rapidly hydrolysed by esterases in the red blood cells. Steady-state blood concentrations are reached within 30 minutes with doses of 50 to 300 µg per kg body-weight per minute. The time to steady state may be reduced to 5 minutes by the administration of an appropriate loading dose. Blood concentrations are reported to decline in a biphasic manner with a distribution half-life of about 2 minutes and an elimination half-life of about 9 minutes. Esmolol has low lipid solubility. It is excreted in urine, primarily as the de-esterified metabolite.

Uses and Administration

Esmolol is a cardioselective short-acting beta blocker (p.844). It is reported to be lacking in intrinsic sympathomimetic and membrane-stabilising properties.

Esmolol is used as the hydrochloride in the management of supraventricular arrhythmias (p.794). It is also used for the control of hypertension (p.802) and tachycardia during the perioperative period.

Esmolol hydrochloride is administered intravenously at a concentration not exceeding 10 mg per mL.

For the rapid temporary control of ventricular rate in patients with **supraventricular arrhythmias,** a loading dose of 500 µg per kg body-weight over 1 minute is followed by an initial maintenance infusion of 50 µg per kg per minute for 4 minutes. If the response is satisfactory this maintenance infusion should be continued at 50 µg per kg per minute. If a suitable response is not obtained within the initial 5 minutes a further loading dose of 500 µg per kg over 1 minute may be given and the maintenance infusion may be increased to 100 µg per kg per minute for 4 minutes. This procedure may be repeated until a satisfactory response is obtained, increasing the maintenance in-

fusion each time by 50 µg per kg per minute to a maximum of 200 µg per kg per minute. Little additional benefit is obtained from further increases in maintenance dosage. Once a satisfactory response is obtained infusion may be continued, if necessary, for up to 48 hours.

When transferring a patient to another antiarrhythmic drug, the infusion rate of esmolol hydrochloride is reduced by 50% thirty minutes after administration of the alternative drug, and may be discontinued one hour after the second dose of that drug.

In the control of perioperative **hypertension** and tachycardia, esmolol hydrochloride may be given intravenously as follows: *during* anaesthesia, a loading dose of 80 mg over 15 to 30 seconds followed by an infusion of 150 µg per kg per minute, increased as necessary up to 300 µg per kg per minute; on *waking* from anaesthesia, an infusion of 500 µg per kg per minute for 4 minutes, followed by an infusion of 300 µg per kg per minute as required; *postoperatively*, a stepped dosage schedule, as described under control of supraventricular arrhythmias above, although maintenance infusions may be increased up to 300 µg per kg per minute as necessary.

◊ References.
1. Benfield P, Sorkin EM. Esmolol: a preliminary review of its pharmacodynamic and pharmacokinetic properties, and therapeutic efficacy. *Drugs* 1987; **33:** 392–412.
2. Wiest D. Esmolol: a review of its therapeutic efficacy and pharmacokinetic characteristics. *Clin Pharmacokinet* 1995; **28:** 190–202.

Tetanus. For reference to the use of esmolol in controlling autonomic hyperactivity associated with tetanus, see under Labetalol, p.919.

Preparations

Proprietary Preparations (details are given in Part 3)
Aust.: Brevibloc; *Austral.:* Brevibloc; *Belg.:* Brevibloc; *Canad.:* Brevibloc; *Denm.:* Brevibloc; *Fin.:* Brevibloc; *Fr.:* Brevibloc; *Ger.:* Brevibloc; *Hong Kong:* Brevibloc; *Irl.:* Brevibloc; *Israel:* Brevibloc; *Mex.:* Brevibloc; *NZ:* Brevibloc; *Port.:* Brevibloc; *S.Afr.:* Brevibloc; *Singapore:* Brevibloc; *Spain:* Brevibloc; *Swed.:* Brevibloc; *Switz.:* Brevibloc; *UK:* Brevibloc; *USA:* Brevibloc.

Etacrynic Acid (2363-e)

Etacrynic Acid (BAN, rINN).
Acidum Etacrynicum; Etacrynsäure; Ethacrynic Acid (USAN); MK-595; NSC-85791. [2,3-Dichloro-4-(2-ethylacryloyl)phenoxy]acetic acid; [2,3-Dichloro-4-(2-methylene-1-oxobutyl)phenoxy]acetic acid.
$C_{13}H_{12}Cl_2O_4 = 303.1$.
CAS — 58-54-8.
ATC — C03CC01.
Pharmacopoeias. In Chin., Eur. (see p.vi), Jpn, Pol., and US.

Pharmacopoeial description
Ph. Eur.: A white or almost white, crystalline powder. Very slightly soluble in water; freely soluble in alcohol and in ether. It dissolves in ammonia and in dilute solutions of alkali hydroxides and carbonates.

USP 25: A white or practically white, odourless or practically odourless, crystalline powder. Very slightly soluble in water; soluble 1 in 1.6 of alcohol, 1 in 6 of chloroform, and 1 in 3.5 of ether.

◊ CAUTION. *Etacrynic acid, especially in the form of dust, is irritating to the skin, eyes, and mucous membranes.*

Sodium Etacrynate (2328-p)

Sodium Etacrynate (BANM, rINNM).
Etacrynate Sodium; Ethacrynate Sodium (USAN); Sodium Ethacrynate.
$C_{13}H_{11}Cl_2NaO_4 = 325.1$.
CAS — 6500-81-8.
Pharmacopoeias. In Chin.
US includes Ethacrynate Sodium for Injection.

Solutions in water of sodium etacrynate containing the equivalent of etacrynic acid 0.1% have a pH of 6.3 to 7.7. Solutions are relatively stable at about pH 7 at room temperatures for short periods and less stable at higher pH values and temperatures. They are incompatible with solutions with a pH below 5. The injection should be protected from light.

Adverse Effects

As for Frusemide, p.893. Gastrointestinal disturbances may be more common and severe with etacrynic acid; profuse watery diarrhoea is an indication for stopping therapy. Gastrointestinal bleeding has been associated with etacrynic acid and tinnitus and deafness, particularly following high dose parenteral administration may be more common. Other adverse effects in-

clude confusion, fatigue, nervousness, and apprehensiveness. Haematuria has been reported rarely.

Local irritation and pain may follow intravenous injection.

Effects on carbohydrate metabolism. Although etacrynic acid is generally considered to have less pronounced effects on carbohydrate metabolism than frusemide [furosemide] or the thiazide diuretics, adverse effects have been reported. Reductions in glucose tolerance[1] have been observed following etacrynic acid 200 mg daily for 6 weeks similar to those produced by hydrochlorothiazide 200 mg daily. The effect was most pronounced in diabetic patients. Hyperosmolar hyperglycaemic coma[2] and symptomatic hypoglycaemia with convulsions[3] have been reported in patients receiving high doses of etacrynic acid.

1. Russell RP, et al. Metabolic and hypotensive effects of etacrynic acid: comparative study with hydrochlorothiazide. *JAMA* 1968; **205:** 11–16.
2. Cowley AJ, Elkeles RS. Diabetes and therapy with potent diuretics. *Lancet* 1978; **i:** 154.
3. Maher JF, Schreiner GE. Studies on ethacrynic acid in patients with refractory edema. *Ann Intern Med* 1965; **62:** 15–29.

Effects on the ears. Drug-induced deafness occurred in 2 of 184 patients given etacrynic acid intravenously.[1,2] Deafness accompanied by nystagmus was reported in a patient[3] following an intravenous infusion of etacrynic acid orally. Symptoms resolved within 1 hour. He had previously been taking frusemide [furosemide] and etacrynic acid orally.

1. Boston Collaborative Drug Surveillance Program. Drug-induced deafness: a cooperative study. *JAMA* 1973; **224:** 515–16.
2. Porter J, Jick H. Drug-induced anaphylaxis, convulsions, deafness, and extrapyramidal symptoms. *Lancet* 1977; **i:** 587–8.
3. Gomolin IH, Garshick E. Ethacrynic acid-induced deafness accompanied by nystagmus. *N Engl J Med* 1980; **303:** 702.

Precautions

Etacrynic acid's precautions and contra-indications are generally dependent on its effects on fluid and electrolyte balance and are similar to those of the thiazide diuretics (see Hydrochlorothiazide, p.909).

Interactions

As for Frusemide, p.894. The risks of gastrointestinal bleeding may be enhanced by concurrent administration of etacrynic acid with other gastric irritants or with anticoagulants.

◊ For reference to the interaction between *warfarin* and etacrynic acid, see p.996.

Pharmacokinetics

Etacrynic acid is fairly rapidly absorbed from the gastrointestinal tract. The plasma half-life is 30 to 60 minutes. It is excreted both in the bile and the urine, partly unchanged and partly in the form of metabolites. It is extensively bound to plasma proteins.

Uses and Administration

Although chemically unrelated, etacrynic acid is a loop diuretic with actions and uses similar to those of frusemide [furosemide] (p.895). Etacrynic acid is used in the treatment of oedema associated with heart failure (p.798) and with renal and hepatic disorders.

Diuresis is initiated within about 30 minutes after a dose by mouth, and lasts for about 6 to 8 hours; after intravenous injection of its sodium salt, the effects are evident within a few minutes and last for about 2 hours.

In the treatment of **oedema,** the usual initial dose is 50 mg by mouth in the morning, taken with or immediately after food. The dose may be increased, if necessary, by 25- to 50-mg increments daily to the minimum effective dose. Severe cases have required gradual titration of the etacrynic acid dosage up to a maximum of 400 mg daily, but the effective dose range is usually between 50 and 150 mg daily. Dosage of more than 50 mg daily should be given in divided doses, and it is preferable for all doses to be taken with food. Maintenance doses may be taken daily or intermittently.

In emergencies, such as acute pulmonary oedema, or when oral therapy cannot be given, etacrynic acid may be given intravenously. It is administered as its salt, sodium etacrynate, but doses are expressed in terms of the base. The usual dose is 50 mg, or 0.5 to 1 mg per kg body-weight, as a 1 mg per mL solution in glucose 5% (provided the pH is above 5) or sodium chloride 0.9%, given by slow intravenous injection either directly or into the tubing of a running infusion. Should a subsequent injection be required the site should be changed to avoid thrombophlebitis. Single doses of 100 mg have been given intravenously in critical situations. It is not suitable for subcutaneous or intramuscular injection.

For children over 2 years of age an initial dose of etacrynic acid is 25 mg daily by mouth, cautiously increased as necessary by 25 mg daily.

If very high doses of etacrynic acid are used careful laboratory control is essential as described for frusemide [furosemide] (p.895; high-dose therapy).

Preparations

BP 2001: Sodium Etacrynate Injection;
USP 25: Ethacrynate Sodium for Injection; Ethacrynic Acid Tablets.

Proprietary Preparations (details are given in Part 3)
Aust.: Edecrin; *Austral.:* Edecril; *Canad.:* Edecrin; *Ger.:* Hydromedin; Uregyt†; *Irl.:* Edecrin; *Ital.:* Edecrin†; Reomax; *Neth.:*

The symbol † denotes a preparation no longer actively marketed

Edecrin†; *NZ:* Edecril; *Swed.:* Edecrina; *UK:* Edecrin†; *USA:* Edecrin.

Etafenone Hydrochloride (9230-p)

Etafenone Hydrochloride (rINNM).

LG-11457. 2′-(2-Diethylaminoethoxy)-3-phenylpropiophenone hydrochloride.

$C_{21}H_{27}NO_2,HCl = 361.9$.

CAS — 90-54-0 (etafenone); 2192-21-4 (etafenone hydrochloride).

Profile

Etafenone hydrochloride is a vasodilator that has been used in ischaemic heart disease.

Ethyl Biscoumacetate (4813-j)

Ethyl Biscoumacetate (BAN, rINN).

Aethylis Biscoumacetas; Ethyldicoumarol; Ethylis Biscoumacetas; Neodicumarinum. Ethyl bis(4-hydroxycoumarin-3-yl)acetate.

$C_{22}H_{16}O_8 = 408.4$.

CAS — 548-00-5.

ATC — B01AA08.

Pharmacopoeias. In Fr. and It.

Adverse Effects, Treatment, and Precautions
As for Warfarin Sodium, p.992.

Interactions
The interactions associated with oral anticoagulants are discussed in detail under warfarin (p.993). Specific references to interactions involving ethyl biscoumacetate can be found under the headings for the following drug groups: analgesics; antifungals; antigout drugs; central stimulants; corticosteroids and corticotropin; and diuretics.

Pharmacokinetics
Ethyl biscoumacetate is readily absorbed from the gastrointestinal tract and is extensively bound to plasma proteins. It is metabolised in the liver; the inactive metabolites are excreted in the urine. Reported plasma half-life ranges from 2 to 3.5 hours.

Ethyl biscoumacetate crosses the placenta and has been reported to appear in only small amounts in breast milk.

Uses and Administration
Ethyl biscoumacetate is an orally administered coumarin anticoagulant with actions similar to those of warfarin (p.998). It has been used in the management of thromboembolic disorders.

Etilefrine Hydrochloride (2061-x)

Etilefrine Hydrochloride (BANM, rINNM).

Ethyladrianol Hydrochloride; Ethylnorphenylephrine Hydrochloride; Etilefrini Hydrochloridum; M-I-36. 2-Ethylamino-1-(3-hydroxyphenyl)ethanol hydrochloride.

$C_{10}H_{15}NO_2,HCl = 217.7$.

CAS — 709-55-7 (etilefrine); 943-17-9 (etilefrine hydrochloride).

Pharmacopoeias. In Eur. (see p.vi) and Jpn.

Pharmacopoeial description
Ph. Eur.: A white, crystalline powder or colourless crystals. Freely soluble in water; soluble in alcohol; practically insoluble in dichloromethane. Store in airtight containers. Protect from light.

Profile
Etilefrine is a direct-acting sympathomimetic (see Adrenaline, p.829) with beta$_1$-agonist properties, and some alpha- and beta$_2$-agonist actions. It is used for the treatment of hypotensive states. It is given as the hydrochloride by mouth in usual doses of 5 or 10 mg three times daily; modified-release dosage forms are also employed in doses of 25 mg once or twice daily. Etilefrine hydrochloride can also be given parenterally.

Etilefrine polistirex has been used in the management of rhinitis.

Preparations
Proprietary Preparations (details are given in Part 3)
Aust.: Amphodyn mono†; Circupon; Effortil; *Belg.:* Effortil; *Braz.:* Efortil; *Fin.:* Effortil; *Fr.:* Effortil; *Ger.:* Adrenam; Bioflutin-N; Cardanat; Cardialgine; Circupon RR; Circuvit E; Confidol†; Effortil; Eti-Puren; etil; Kreislauf Katovit; Logomed Kreislauf-Tabletten†; Thomasin; Tonus-forte-Tablinen†; *Ital.:* Effortil; *Mex.:* Effortil; *Norw.:* Effortil; *Port.:* Effortil; *S.Afr.:* Effortil; *Spain:* Efortil; *Swed.:* Effortil; *Switz.:* Circupon; Effortil; *Thai.:* Effortil; Efxine; Hyprosia.

Multi-ingredient: *Aust.:* Agilan; Amphodyn; Effortil comp; Hypodyn; Influbene; *Ger.:* Agit plus; Amphodyn; Dihydergot plus; Effortil plus; Ergolefrin; Ergomimet plus; *Switz.:* Dihydergot plus; Effortil plus.

Etofibrate (12719-c)

Etofibrate (rINN).

2-Nicotinoyloxyethyl   2-(4-chlorophenoxy)-2-methylpropionate.

$C_{18}H_{18}ClNO_5 = 363.8$.

CAS — 31637-97-5.

ATC — C10AB09.

Profile
Etofibrate, a derivative of clofibrate (p.859) and nicotinic acid (p.1372), is a lipid regulating drug used in the treatment of hyperlipidaemias (p.800). The usual dose is 500 mg daily by mouth.

Preparations
Proprietary Preparations (details are given in Part 3)
Aust.: Lipo-Merz; *Braz.:* Tricerol; *Ger.:* Lipo-Merz; *Hong Kong:* Lipo-Merz; *Mex.:* Tricerol; *Port.:* Lipo-Merz; *Singapore:* Lipo-Merz; *Spain:* Afloyan†; *Switz.:* Lipo-Merz.

Etofylline Clofibrate (12720-s)

Etofylline Clofibrate (rINN).

ML-1024; Theofibrate (USAN). 2-(Theophyllin-7-yl)ethyl 2-(4-chlorophenoxy)-2-methylpropionate.

$C_{19}H_{21}ClN_4O_5 = 420.8$.

CAS — 54504-70-0.

Profile
Etofylline clofibrate, a fibric acid derivative (see Bezafibrate, p.849), is a lipid regulating drug used in the treatment of hyperlipidaemias (p.800). The usual dose is 250 mg two or three times daily by mouth.

Preparations
Proprietary Preparations (details are given in Part 3)
Aust.: Duolip; *Ger.:* Duolip; *Hong Kong:* Duolip; *Switz.:* Duolip.

Etozolin (12722-e)

Etozolin (USAN, rINN).

Gö-687; W-2900A. Ethyl (3-methyl-4-oxo-5-piperidinothiazolidin-2-ylidene)acetate.

$C_{13}H_{20}N_2O_3S = 284.4$.

CAS — 73-09-6.

ATC — C03CX01.

Profile
Etozolin is a loop diuretic with properties similar to those of frusemide [furosemide] (p.893), but with a longer duration of action. It is used in the treatment of oedema and hypertension (p.802). Etozolin is reported to be rapidly metabolised to ozolinone which also has diuretic activity.

In the treatment of oedema an initial dose of 400 to 800 mg by mouth is followed by a maintenance dose of 400 mg daily or every 2 or 3 days. In the treatment of hypertension an initial dose of 400 mg daily for 2 days is followed by a maintenance dose of 200 mg daily or on alternate days.

◊ References.

1. Knauf H, *et al.* Pharmacodynamics and kinetics of etozolin/ozolinone in hypertensive patients with normal and impaired kidney function. *Eur J Clin Pharmacol* 1984; **26:** 687–93.
2. Beermann B, Grind M. Clinical pharmacokinetics of some newer diuretics. *Clin Pharmacokinet* 1987; **13:** 254–66.

Preparations
Proprietary Preparations (details are given in Part 3)
Aust.: Elkapin†; *Ger.:* Elkapin†; *Ital.:* Elkapin; *Spain:* Elkapin†.

Fasudil Hydrochloride (15275-v)

Fasudil Hydrochloride (rINNM).

AT-877; HA-1077. Hexahydro-1-(5-isoquinolylsulfonyl)-1H-1,4-diazepine hydrochloride.

$C_{14}H_{17}N_3O_2S,HCl = 327.8$.

CAS — 103745-39-7 (fasudil); 105628-07-7 (fasudil hydrochloride).

Profile
Fasudil is a vasodilator used as the hydrochloride in the management of cerebrovascular disorders including vasospasm following surgery for subarachnoid haemorrhage.

◊ References.

1. Shibuya M, *et al.* Effect of AT877 on cerebral vasospasm after aneurysmal subarachnoid hemorrhage: results of a prospective placebo-controlled double-blind trial. *J Neurosurg* 1992; **76:** 571–7.

Preparations
Proprietary Preparations (details are given in Part 3)
Jpn: Eril.

Felodipine (16801-t)

Felodipine (BAN, USAN, rINN).

Felodipinum; H-154/82. Ethyl methyl 4-(2,3-dichlorophenyl)-1,4-dihydro-2,6-dimethylpyridine-3,5-dicarboxylate.

$C_{18}H_{19}Cl_2NO_4 = 384.3$.

CAS — 72509-76-3; 86189-69-7.

ATC — C08CA02.

Pharmacopoeias. In Eur. (see p.vi) and US.

Pharmacopoeial description
Ph. Eur.: A white or light yellow, crystalline powder. Practically insoluble in water; freely soluble in dehydrated alcohol, in acetone, in dichloromethane, and in methyl alcohol. Protect from light.

USP 25: A light yellow to yellow, crystalline powder. Insoluble in water; freely soluble in acetone and in methyl alcohol; very slightly soluble in heptane. Store in airtight containers. Protect from light.

Adverse Effects, Treatment, and Precautions
As for dihydropyridine calcium-channel blockers (see Nifedipine, p.940).

Interactions
As for dihydropyridine calcium-channel blockers (see Nifedipine, p.942).

Pharmacokinetics
Felodipine is almost completely absorbed from the gastrointestinal tract after oral administration but undergoes extensive first-pass metabolism, with a bioavailability of about 15% (range 10 to 25%). It is extensively metabolised in the gut and the liver and is excreted almost entirely as metabolites, about 70% of a dose being excreted in urine and the remainder in faeces. The terminal elimination half-life is reported to be about 11 to 16 hours following oral administration of an immediate-release preparation, but longer with a modified-release formulation. Felodipine is about 99% bound to plasma proteins (mainly albumin).

◊ General reviews.

1. Dunselman PHJM, Edgar B. Felodipine clinical pharmacokinetics. *Clin Pharmacokinet* 1991; **21:** 418–30.

Hepatic impairment. In 9 patients with liver cirrhosis given felodipine 0.75 mg by intravenous infusion over 20 minutes and 10 mg by mouth as single doses on separate occasions the mean oral bioavailability was 17.1% which was not significantly different from published values in healthy subjects, but the maximum plasma concentrations were almost twice as high as normal, apparently due to reduced systemic clearance and volume of distribution.[1] The fact that bioavailability was not increased suggests that much pre-systemic metabolism takes place in the gut rather than the liver. Although increased adverse effects were not associated with the raised felodipine concentrations in this study it is recommended that therapy in cirrhotic patients be initiated at lower doses than in patients with normal liver function.

1. Regårdh CG, *et al.* Pharmacokinetics of felodipine in patients with liver disease. *Eur J Clin Pharmacol* 1989; **36:** 473–9.

Uses and Administration
Felodipine is a dihydropyridine calcium-channel blocker with actions similar to those of nifedipine (p.943). It is used in the treatment of hypertension (p.802) and angina pectoris (p.791).

Felodipine is given by mouth, generally in a modified-release formulation for administration once daily in the morning. In **hypertension** the usual initial dose is 5 mg daily by mouth, adjusted as required; the usual maintenance dose is 2.5 to 10 mg daily and doses above 20 mg daily are not usually needed. In **angina** the usual initial dose is 5 mg daily increased if necessary to 10 mg daily.

Lower doses may be required in the elderly and in patients with impaired liver function.

◊ Reviews.

1. Saltiel E, *et al.* Felodipine: a review of its pharmacodynamic and pharmacokinetic properties, and therapeutic use in hypertension. *Drugs* 1988; **36:** 387–428.
2. Todd PA, Faulds D. Felodipine: a review of the pharmacology and therapeutic use of the extended release formulation in cardiovascular disorders. *Drugs* 1992; **44:** 251–77.
3. Walton T, Symes LR. Felodipine and isradipine: new calcium-channel-blocking agents for the treatment of hypertension. *Clin Pharm* 1993; **12:** 261–75.

Preparations

Proprietary Preparations (details are given in Part 3)
Aust.: Munobal; Plendil; *Austral.:* Agon; Felodur; Plendil; *Belg.:*
Plendil; Renedil; *Braz.:* Splendil; *Canad.:* Plendil; Renedil;
Denm.: Hydac; Plendil; *Fin.:* Hydac; Plendil; *Fr.:* Flodil; *Ger.:*
Modip; Munobal; *Hong Kong:* Plendil; *Irl.:* Plendil; *Israel:* Pen-
edil; *Ital.:* Feloday; Plendil; Prevex; *Jpn:* Splendil; *Mex.:* Muno-
bal; Plendil; *Neth.:* Plendil; Renedil; *Norw.:* Plendil; *NZ:* Agon;
Plendil; *Port.:* Preslow; *S.Afr.:* Plendil; *Singapore:* Plendil;
Spain: Fensel; Perfudal; Plendil; Preslow†; *Swed.:* Hydac;
Plendil; *Switz.:* Munobal; Plendil; *Thai.:* Plendil; *UK:* Plendil;
USA: Plendil.
Multi-ingredient: *Aust.:* Logimax; *Belg.:* Logimat; *Denm.:*
Logimax; *Fin.:* Logimax; Unimax; *Fr.:* Logimax; *Ger.:* Delmuno;
Mobloc; Unimax; *Hong Kong:* Logimax; *Mex.:* Logimax; *Neth.:*
Triapin; *Norw.:* Logimax†; *S.Afr.:* Tri-Plen; *Spain:* Logimax; Un-
imest; *Swed.:* Logimax; *Switz.:* Logimax; Unimax; *UK:* Triapin;
USA: Lexxel.

Fendiline Hydrochloride (9233-e)

Fendiline Hydrochloride (pINNM).
N-(2-Benzhydrylethyl)-α-methylbenzylamine hydrochloride.
$C_{23}H_{25}N,HCl = 351.9$.
CAS — 13042-18-7 (fendiline); 13636-18-5 (fendiline hy-drochloride).

Profile

Fendiline hydrochloride is a calcium-channel blocker used as a
vasodilator in ischaemic heart disease in usual doses of 150 mg
daily, in divided doses, by mouth.

Ischaemic heart disease is discussed under Atherosclerosis
(p.793) and the treatment of its clinical manifestations is described under Angina Pectoris (p.791) and Myocardial Infarction (p.805).

Preparations

Proprietary Preparations (details are given in Part 3)
Aust.: Sensit; *Ger.:* Sensit; *Ital.:* Difmecor†; Olbiacor; Sensit-F;
Switz.: Sensit†.

Fenofibrate (1348-b)

Fenofibrate (BAN, rINN).
LF-178; Procetofene. Isopropyl 2-[4-(4-chlorobenzoyl)phe-
noxy]-2-methylpropionate.
$C_{20}H_{21}ClO_4 = 360.8$.
CAS — 49562-28-9.
ATC — C10AB05.
Pharmacopoeias. In Chin. and Eur. (see p.vi).

Pharmacopoeial description

Ph. Eur.: A white or almost white, crystalline powder. Practically insoluble in water; slightly soluble in alcohol; very soluble in dichloromethane. M.p. 79° to 82°. Protect from light.

Adverse Effects and Precautions

As for Bezafibrate, p.849.

◊ The most common adverse effects in both long- and short-
term studies of fenofibrate have been gastrointestinal disturbances, occurring in about 3 to 5% of patients.[1] Other adverse
effects include dermatological, musculoskeletal, and neurological disorders. There has been no evidence yet of an increased
incidence of gallstones, although some increases in the indices
of bile lithogenicity have been reported.[1-3]
For a report of the half-life being prolonged in patients with
renal impairment, see Administration in Renal Impairment, under Uses and Administration, below.

1. Brown WV. Treatment of hypercholesterolaemia with fenofibrate: a review. *Curr Med Res Opin* 1989; **11:** 321–30.
2. Blane GF. Comparative toxicity and safety profile of fenofibrate
   and other fibric acid derivatives. *Am J Med* 1987; **83** (suppl 5B):
   26–36.
3. Palmer RH. Effects of fibric acid derivatives on biliary lipid composition. *Am J Med* 1987; **83** (suppl 5B): 37–43.

Interactions

As for Bezafibrate, p.849.

The manufacturers of fenofibrate suggest that in patients taking oral anticoagulants, the dose of anticoagulant should be reduced by about one-third when
treatment with fenofibrate is started, and then adjusted gradually if necessary.

Pharmacokinetics

Fenofibrate is readily absorbed from the gastrointestinal tract when taken with food; absorption is substantially reduced if fenofibrate is administered after
an overnight fast. It is rapidly hydrolysed to its active
metabolite fenofibric acid which is extensively bound
to plasma albumin. The plasma elimination half-life
is about 20 hours. Fenofibric acid is excreted predominantly in the urine, mainly as the glucuronide conju-

The symbol † denotes a preparation no longer actively marketed

gate, but also as a reduced form of fenofibric acid and
its glucuronide.

◊ References.
1. Chapman MJ. Pharmacology of fenofibrate. *Am J Med* 1987; **83**
   (suppl 5B): 21–5.

Uses and Administration

Fenofibrate, a fibric acid derivative, is a lipid regulating drug with actions on plasma lipids similar to those
of bezafibrate (p.849).

It is used in the treatment of type IIa, type IIb, type III,
type IV, and type V hyperlipoproteinaemias.

The usual initial dose, by mouth, is 300 mg daily in
divided doses with food. Doses may be adjusted according to response to between 200 and 400 mg daily.
Children may be given 5 mg per kg body-weight daily.

Preparations containing micronised fenofibrate are
available. They have improved bioavailability and
thus may allow a lower total daily dose. The initial
dose is about 200 mg daily depending upon the formulation used.

◊ General references.
1. *Am J Med* 1987; **83** (suppl 5B).
2. *Cardiology* 1989; **76** (suppl 1): 1–54.
3. Adkins JC, Faulds D. Micronised fenofibrate: a review of its
   pharmacodynamic properties and clinical efficacy in the management of dyslipidaemia. *Drugs* 1997; **54:** 615–33.
4. Guay DRP. Micronized fenofibrate: a new fibric acid hypolipidemic agent. *Ann Pharmacother* 1999; **33:** 1083–1103.

Administration in renal impairment. Fenofibrate is generally contra-indicated in patients with severe renal dysfunction, but the UK manufacturers have stated that fenofibrate may
be given in mild or moderate renal impairment in reduced doses. They have suggested doses of 134 mg of micronised fenofibrate daily for creatinine clearances of 20 to 60 mL per
minute, and 67 mg daily for creatinine clearance less than
20 mL per minute.
The plasma half-life of fenofibric acid has been shown to be
prolonged to up to about 360 hours in patients with renal disease following a single dose of fenofibrate.[1] No correlation was
found between the elimination half-life and serum creatinine
concentrations or creatinine clearance. Fenofibrate metabolites
were not removed by haemodialysis. Significant accumulation
of fenofibric acid occurs on repeated daily dosing in renal
insufficiency.

1. Desager JP, *et al.* Effect of hemodialysis on plasma kinetics of
   fenofibrate in chronic renal failure. *Nephron* 1982; **31:** 51–4.

Hyperlipidaemias. Like other fibric acid derivatives, fenofibrate is used in the treatment of hyperlipidaemias (p.800). It
reduces elevated plasma-triglyceride concentrations probably
mainly by an effect on lipoprotein lipase[1] (see Bezafibrate,
p.849). Substantial reductions in plasma-cholesterol concentrations have been reported in healthy subjects[1] and in patients
with type IIa and IIb hyperlipoproteinaemias.[2-4] Low-density
lipoprotein (LDL)-cholesterol concentrations were increased
in patients with type IV or V hyperlipoproteinaemias with low
baseline LDL-cholesterol concentrations.[5] In addition, high-
density lipoprotein (HDL)-cholesterol concentrations are generally increased.[1,3,4] A uricosuric effect has also been reported.[1]
Although patient numbers have generally been small,[1] comparative studies have suggested that fenofibrate reduces cholesterol concentrations to a greater extent than clofibrate. Overall, the
effect of fenofibrate was comparable with bezafibrate and ciprofibrate although the effects on individual lipoproteins differed somewhat. Fenofibrate was less effective than
simvastatin[6] at reducing elevated cholesterol concentrations
but more effective at reducing elevated triglyceride concentrations.

1. Balfour JA, *et al.* Fenofibrate: a review of its pharmacodynamic
   and pharmacokinetic properties and therapeutic use in dyslipidaemia. *Drugs* 1990; **40:** 260–90.
2. Brown WV, *et al.* Effects of fenofibrate on plasma lipids: double-
   blind, multicenter study in patients with type IIA or IIB hyperlipidemia. *Arteriosclerosis* 1986; **6:** 670–8.
3. Brown WV. Treatment of hypercholesterolaemia with fenofibrate: a review. *Curr Med Res Opin* 1989; **11:** 321–30.
4. Superko HR. A review of combined hyperlipidaemia and its
   treatment with fenofibrate. *J Int Med Res* 1989; **17:** 99–112.
5. Seidehamel RJ. Fenofibrate in type IV and type V hyperlipopro-
   teinemia. *Cardiology* 1989; **76** (suppl 1): 23–32.
6. Stohler R, *et al.* Effects of simvastatin and fenofibrate on serum
   lipoproteins and apolipoproteins in primary hypercholesterolaemia. *Eur J Clin Pharmacol* 1989; **37:** 199–203. Correction. *ibid.*;
   623.

Preparations

Proprietary Preparations (details are given in Part 3)
Aust.: Fenolip; Lipcor; Lipsin; *Belg.:* Fenogal; Lipanthyl; *Braz.:*
Lipanon; *Canad.:* Apo-Feno; Lipidil; *Fr.:* Fegenor; Lipanthyl; Li-
pirex; Secalip; *Ger.:* CIL; durafenat; Fenobeta; Lipanthyl; Lipidil;
Normalip pro; *Irl.:* Lipantil; *Ital.:* Fulcro; Lipanthyl; Lipidax;
Lipoclar; Lipofene; Lipsin; Nolipax; Scleril; Tilene; Volutine;
Mex.: Controlip; Lipidil; *Port.:* Catalip; Lipanthyl; Lipofen†;
S.Afr.: Lipsin; *Singapore:* Lipanthyl; *Spain:* Liparison; Secalip;

Switz.: Lipanthyl; *Thai.:* Lexemin; Lipanthyl; *UK:* Lipantil; Supralip; *USA:* Tricor.

Fenoldopam Mesilate (17955-f)

Fenoldopam Mesilate (BANM, rINNM).
Fenoldopam Mesylate (USAN); SKF-82526-j. 6-Chloro-2,3,4,5-
tetrahydro-1-(p-hydroxyphenyl)-1H-3-benzazepine-7,8-diol
methanesulfonate.
$C_{16}H_{16}ClNO_3,CH_4O_3S = 401.9$.
*CAS — 67227-56-9 (fenoldopam); 67227-57-0 (fe-
noldopam mesilate).*
Pharmacopoeias. In US.

Pharmacopoeial description

USP 25: A white to off-white powder. Soluble in water. Store
in airtight containers. Protect from moisture.

Adverse Effects and Precautions

The adverse effects of fenoldopam are mainly due to
vasodilatation and include hypotension, flushing, dizziness, headache, and reflex tachycardia. Nausea and
vomiting, and ECG abnormalities have also been reported. Hypokalaemia has occurred and serum-electrolyte concentrations should be monitored during
therapy. Fenoldopam may increase intra-ocular pressure and it should be used with caution in patients
with glaucoma. Caution is also required in patients in
whom hypotension could be deleterious, such as
those with acute cerebral infarction or haemorrhage.
Blood pressure and heart rate should be monitored.

Effects on the heart. Although fenoldopam is usually associated with reflex tachycardia, precipitous bradycardia occurred in two patients receiving fenoldopam infusion in a clinical study,[1] necessitating discontinuation of the drug.

1. Taylor AA, *et al.* Sustained hemodynamic effects of the selective
   dopamine-1 agonist, fenoldopam, during 48-hour infusions in
   hypertensive patients: a dose-tolerability study. *J Clin Pharmacol* 1999; **39:** 471–9.

Interactions

The hypotensive effects of fenoldopam may be enhanced by other drugs with hypotensive actions. Beta
blockers may block the reflex tachycardia that occurs
with fenoldopam and concomitant use is not recommended.

Pharmacokinetics

Steady-state plasma concentrations of fenoldopam
are reached about 20 minutes after commencing continuous intravenous infusion. Fenoldopam is extensively metabolised with only about 4% of a dose being excreted unchanged. It is metabolised by
conjugation (mainly glucuronidation, methylation,
and sulfation). Fenoldopam and its metabolites are
excreted predominantly in the urine, the remainder
being excreted in the faeces. The elimination half-life
of fenoldopam is about five minutes.

Uses and Administration

Fenoldopam is a dopamine agonist which is reported
to have a selective action at dopamine D_1-receptors,
leading to vasodilatation. It is given intravenously as
the mesilate in the short-term management of severe
hypertension (below). It has also been tried in heart
failure.

In the management of hypertensive crises, fenoldopam mesilate is given by continuous intravenous infusion as a solution containing 40 µg of fenoldopam per mL; doses are expressed in terms of the
base. The dose should be adjusted according to response in usual increments of 0.05 to 0.1 µg per kg
body-weight per minute at 15-minute intervals. The
usual dose range is from 0.1 to 1.6 µg per kg per
minute.

◊ Reviews.
1. Brogden RN, Markham A. Fenoldopam: a review of its pharmacodynamic and pharmacokinetic properties and intravenous clinical potential in the management of hypertensive urgencies and
   emergencies. *Drugs* 1997; **54:** 634–50.
2. Post JB, Frishman WH. Fenoldopam: a new dopamine agonist
   for the treatment of hypertensive urgencies and emergencies. *J
   Clin Pharmacol* 1998; **38:** 2–13.

Hypertension. Fenoldopam has poor oral bioavailability and
is usually given intravenously. It has a rapid onset of action and
a short elimination half-life[1] and may thus be most suitable in

patients requiring rapid blood pressure reduction. Comparative studies[2,3] with sodium nitroprusside in patients with severe hypertension requiring urgent therapy have shown fenoldopam to be effective in rapidly lowering blood pressure. Additionally, in contrast to nitroprusside, urine output, creatinine clearance, and sodium excretion were increased by fenoldopam in one of the studies.[2] Fenoldopam may therefore be particularly useful in the acute treatment of severe hypertension in patients with impaired renal function.

For a discussion of the treatment of hypertension, including hypertensive crises, see p.802.

1. Weber RR, et al. Pharmacokinetic and pharmacodynamic properties of intravenous fenoldopam, a dopamine₁-receptor agonist, in hypertensive patients. Br J Clin Pharmacol 1988; 25: 17–21.
2. Shusterman NH, et al. Fenoldopam, but not nitroprusside, improves renal function in severely hypertensive patients with impaired renal function. Am J Med 1993; 95: 161–8.
3. Panacek EA, et al. Randomized, prospective trial of fenoldopam vs sodium nitroprusside in the treatment of acute severe hypertension. Acad Emerg Med 1995; 2: 959–65.

Preparations

USP 25: Fenoldopam Mesylate Injection.

Proprietary Preparations (details are given in Part 3)
Ital.: Corlopam; **USA:** Corlopam.

Fenquizone Potassium (12745-a)

Fenquizone Potassium (rINNM).

MG-13054 (fenquizone). 7-Chloro-1,2,3,4-tetrahydro-4-oxo-2-phenylquinazoline-6-sulphonamide, monopotassium salt.

$C_{14}H_{12}ClN_3O_3S,K = 376.9$.

CAS — 20287-37-0 (fenquizone); 52246-40-9 (fenquizone potassium).

NOTE. Fenquizone is USAN.

Profile

Fenquizone potassium is a diuretic that is used in the treatment of oedema and hypertension (p.802) in doses equivalent to 10 to 20 mg of fenquizone daily by mouth.

◊ References.
1. Beermann B, Grind M. Clinical pharmacokinetics of some newer diuretics. Clin Pharmacokinet 1987; 13: 254–66.
2. Costa FV, et al. Hemodynamic and humoral effects of chronic antihypertensive treatment with fenquizone: importance of aldosterone response. J Clin Pharmacol 1990; 30: 254–61.

Preparations

Proprietary Preparations (details are given in Part 3)
Ital.: Idrolone.

Fibrinolysin (Human) (3739-I)

Fibrinolysin (Human) (rINN).

Fibrinase; Plasmin (BAN); Plasmin (Human).

CAS — 9001-90-5 (fibrinolysin); 9004-09-5 (human fibrinolysin).

Profile

Fibrinolysin (Human) is a proteolytic enzyme derived from the activation of human plasminogen. Fibrinolysin derived from cattle (bovine fibrinolysin) and other animals is also available. Fibrinolysin converts fibrin into soluble products and also hydrolyses some other proteins. Its role in the control of haemostasis is described further on p.718.

Fibrinolysin is used (generally as bovine fibrinolysin) in conjunction with deoxyribonuclease for the debridement of wounds. It was formerly given parenterally for the treatment of thrombotic disorders.

Preparations

Proprietary Preparations (details are given in Part 3)
Multi-ingredient: Aust.: Fibrolan; **Austral.:** Fibrolan; **Braz.:** Cauterex com Gentamicina; Fibrase com Clorafenicol; Gino-Cauterex; Gino-Fibrase; **Canad.:** Elase-Chloromycetin†; Elase†; **Fr.:** Elase; **Ger.:** Fibrolan; **Ital.:** Elase; **Mex.:** Fibrase; Fibrase SA; **Neth.:** Elase; **Spain:** Parkelase Chloromycetin†; Parkelase†; **Switz.:** Fibrolan; **USA:** Elase-Chloromycetin†; Elase†.

Flecainide Acetate (12753-a)

Flecainide Acetate (BANM, USAN, rINNM).

R-818.   N-(2-Piperidylmethyl)-2,5-bis(2,2,2-trifluoroethoxy)benzamide acetate.

$C_{17}H_{20}F_6N_2O_3,C_2H_4O_2 = 474.4$.

CAS — 54143-55-4 (flecainide); 54143-56-5 (flecainide acetate).

Pharmacopoeias. In Eur. (see p.vi) and US.

Pharmacopoeial description

Ph. Eur.: A white or almost white, very hygroscopic crystalline powder. Soluble in water and in dehydrated alcohol; freely soluble in dilute acetic acid; practically insoluble in dilute hydrochloric acid. A 2.5% solution in water has a pH of 6.7 to 7.1. Protect from light.

USP 25: A white to slightly off-white crystalline powder; pK_a is 9.3. Soluble in water; freely soluble in alcohol.

Stability. Storage of an extemporaneously prepared flecainide syrup in a refrigerator led to crystallisation of the drug and the administration of a toxic dose.[1] It was suggested that oral liquid formulations of flecainide should be freshly reconstituted from a powder before each dose.

1. Stuart AG, et al. Is there a genetic factor in flecainide toxicity? BMJ 1989; 298: 117–18.

Adverse Effects

The most common adverse effects caused by flecainide affect the CNS and include dizziness, visual disturbances, and lightheadedness. Nausea, vomiting, headache, tremor, peripheral neuropathy, ataxia, and paraesthesia may also occur. These effects are generally transient and respond to dosage reduction. Other adverse CNS effects that have been reported rarely include hallucinations, amnesia, confusion, depression, dyskinesias, and convulsions. Skin reactions, including rare cases of urticaria, have also occurred and there have been isolated cases of photosensitivity. Disturbances of liver function have been reported rarely. Corneal deposits, pulmonary fibrosis, and pneumonitis have occurred during long-term therapy. Cardiovascular effects are less common than those on the CNS, but can be serious and sometimes fatal. Ventricular tachyarrhythmias have been reported, particularly in patients with a history of ventricular tachyarrhythmias and taking high doses of flecainide. Flecainide produced an increased mortality rate when it was assessed for the control of asymptomatic ventricular arrhythmias in patients who had previously suffered a myocardial infarction (see Cardiac Arrhythmias under Uses and Administration, below).

◊ In a report of the non-cardiac adverse effects of flecainide from 1 short-term and 3 longer term studies,[1] the most common adverse effects during both short- and long-term studies were dizziness and visual disturbances which occurred in about 30% of patients. Headache and nausea both occurred in about 10% of patients. Other adverse effects reported include dyspnoea, chest pain, asthenia, fatigue, and tremor. Therapy was discontinued due to non-cardiac adverse effects in 10% of patients in the short-term trial, and in 6% of those in the chronic studies. A review of 60 studies using flecainide[2] reported that non-cardiac side-effects (mainly gastrointestinal and CNS adverse effects) occurred in 12% of patients. The UK Committee on Safety of Medicines had received reports of neurological (4 patients with sensory neuropathy, 2 with ataxia), corneal (2 with corneal deposits), and pulmonary (3 with pulmonary fibrosis and pneumonitis) reactions associated with the long-term use of flecainide.[3]

1. Gentzkow GD, Sullivan JY. Extracardiac adverse effects of flecainide. Am J Cardiol 1984; 53: 101B–105B.
2. Hohnloser SH, Zabel M. Short- and long-term efficacy and safety of flecainide acetate for supraventricular arrhythmias. Am J Cardiol 1992; 70: 3A–10A.
3. Committee on Safety of Medicines. Multi-system adverse reactions following long-term flecainide therapy. Current Problems 31 1991.

Effects on the blood. Severe granulocytopenia believed to be related to flecainide acetate occurred in a 66-year-old man 3 months after starting therapy with the drug.[1] Haematological findings suggested an immune-mediated reaction in which flecainide binds to normal neutrophils with subsequent recognition by specific antibodies resulting in enhanced destruction of mature granulocytes in peripheral blood and bone marrow.

1. Samlowski WE, et al. Flecainide-induced immune neutropenia: documentation of a hapten-mediated mechanism of cell destruction. Arch Intern Med 1987; 147: 383–4.

Effects on the eyes. In addition to visual disturbance, corneal deposits have been reported in association with flecainide therapy.[1]

1. Ulrik H, et al. Corneal deposits associated with flecainide. BMJ 1991; 302: 506–7.

Effects on the heart. Like many antiarrhythmics, flecainide can have proarrhythmic effects.[1,2] Further information is also given in Cardiac Arrhythmias under Uses and Administration, below.

1. Falk RH. Flecainide-induced ventricular tachycardia and fibrillation in patients treated for atrial fibrillation. Ann Intern Med 1989; 111: 107–11.
2. Herre JM, et al. Inefficacy and proarrhythmic effects of flecainide and encainide for sustained ventricular tachycardia and ventricular fibrillation. Ann Intern Med 1990; 113: 671–6.

Effects on the liver. Elevated liver enzymes and jaundice, reversible on stopping treatment, have been reported rarely in association with flecainide therapy.

Conjugated hyperbilirubinaemia with jaundice developed in a newborn infant following maternal treatment with flecainide for fetal supraventricular tachycardia.[1]

1. Vanderhal AL, et al. Conjugated hyperbilirubinemia in a newborn infant after maternal (transplacental) treatment with flecainide acetate for fetal tachycardia and fetal hydrops. J Pediatr 1995; 126: 988–90.

Effects on the lungs. There have been reports[1,2] of interstitial pneumonitis associated with flecainide therapy.

1. Akoun GM, et al. Flecainide-associated pneumonitis. Lancet 1991; 337: 49.
2. Hanston P, et al. Flecainide-associated interstitial pneumonitis. Lancet 1991; 337: 371–2.

Effects on mental state. Dysarthria and visual hallucinations were associated with elevated plasma concentration of flecainide (2500 nanograms per mL) in a patient.[1] A serial rise and fall in plasma-bilirubin concentration during flecainide therapy also suggested possible direct hepatotoxicity.

1. Ramhamadany E, et al. Dysarthria and visual hallucinations due to flecainide toxicity. Postgrad Med J 1986; 62: 61–2.

Effects on the nervous system. Peripheral neuropathy in one patient taking flecainide long term has been described; symptoms regressed after drug withdrawal.[1] The UK Committee on Safety of Medicines had received 4 other reports possibly associated with flecainide and 3 reports of aggravation of pre-existing neuropathy.[1]

1. Palace J, et al. Flecainide induced peripheral neuropathy. BMJ 1992; 305: 810.

Lupus erythematosus. A brief report of a patient who developed painful eye movement during treatment with flecainide.[1] The pain resolved when treatment was withdrawn, but recurred when flecainide was restarted, and was accompanied by lateral rectus spasm, a facial rash, and positive antinuclear factor, suggestive of lupus erythematosus.

1. Skander M, Isaacs PET. Flecainide, ocular myopathy, and antinuclear factor. BMJ 1985; 291: 450.

Treatment of Adverse Effects

In overdosage by mouth the stomach should be emptied by lavage. Treatment is largely symptomatic and supportive and may need to be continued for extended periods of time because of the long half-life and the possibility of non-linear elimination at very high doses. Haemodialysis or haemoperfusion are unlikely to enhance elimination.

Overdosage. Life-threatening ventricular tachycardia occurred in a young woman following ingestion of flecainide acetate 3.8 g, diazepam 50 mg, loperamide 20 mg, and alcohol 100 g.[1] The serum-flecainide concentration on admission, 2 hours after the overdose, was 3700 nanograms per mL. Treatment included mechanical ventilation, intravenous dopamine and an intravenous sodium load for cardiogenic shock. The stomach was emptied by lavage followed by activated charcoal and diarrhoea was induced with mannitol. Forced diuresis was performed but probably had a negligible effect owing to the extensive distribution of flecainide into the tissues. The serum-flecainide concentration 9 hours after the overdose was 1680 nanograms per mL; it continued to decline thereafter at a slower rate.

Haemoperfusion failed to reduce flecainide intoxication in a patient with terminal renal failure managed by haemodialysis.[2]

1. Winkelmann BR, Leinberger H. Life-threatening flecainide toxicity: a pharmacodynamic approach. Ann Intern Med 1987; 106: 807–14.
2. Braun J, et al. Failure of haemoperfusion to reduce flecainide intoxication: a case study. Med Toxicol 1987; 2: 463–7.

Precautions

Flecainide treatment should be instituted in hospitalised patients and pacing rescue should be available when it is used in patients with conduction defects. Its use is limited to serious or life-threatening arrhythmias and it should not be given to control asymptomatic arrhythmias especially in patients with a history of myocardial infarction (see Cardiac Arrhythmias under Uses and Administration, below). Flecainide has some negative inotropic activity and may precipitate or aggravate heart failure in patients with compromised left ventricular function; it should therefore be used with extreme caution, if at all, in patients with heart failure. Flecainide has been shown to increase the endocardial pacing threshold and should be used with caution in patients with pacemakers. Electrolyte imbalances should be corrected before initiating flecainide therapy. Reduction of dosage may be necessary in patients with renal impairment; extreme caution is needed in patients with pronounced hepatic impairment.

Pregnancy and breast feeding. Flecainide crosses the placenta and is distributed into breast milk; further details are given under Pharmacokinetics, below.

For a report of hyperbilirubinaemia in an infant following maternal treatment with flecainide, see under Effects on the Liver, above.

Interactions

Use of flecainide with other antiarrhythmics or arrhythmogenic drugs may increase the incidence of cardiac arrhythmias. Use with a beta blocker produces additive negative inotropic effects. Flecainide undergoes metabolism in the liver and its activity may be influenced by other drugs affecting the enzymes responsible for its metabolism.

Antiarrhythmics. *Amiodarone* increases the plasma-flecainide concentration when the two drugs are given concomitantly.[1] It has been recommended that the dose of flecainide should be reduced by about one-half during concomitant use, but because the effect of amiodarone differs widely between patients, plasma-flecainide concentrations should be monitored. The clearance of flecainide may be decreased by *quinidine* in patients who are extensive metabolisers, since quinidine inhibits the enzyme responsible for the metabolism of flecainide.[2] Cardiogenic shock and asystole occurred in 2 patients receiving flecainide when *verapamil* was added to their therapy.[3]

1. Shea P, *et al.* Flecainide and amiodarone interaction. *J Am Coll Cardiol* 1986; **7:** 1127–30.
2. Birgersdotter UM, *et al.* Stereoselective genetically-determined interaction between flecainide and quinidine in patients with arrhythmias. *Br J Clin Pharmacol* 1992; **33:** 275–80.
3. Buss J, *et al.* Asystole and cardiogenic shock due to combined treatment with verapamil and flecainide. *Lancet* 1992; **340:** 546.

Antimalarials. *Quinine* has been reported to inhibit metabolism of flecainide in healthy subjects without altering its renal elimination, resulting in a reduction of total clearance and prolongation of the elimination half-life.[1]

1. Munafo A, *et al.* Altered flecainide disposition in healthy volunteers taking quinine. *Eur J Clin Pharmacol* 1990; **38:** 269–73.

Beta blockers. Concurrent administration of flecainide and *propranolol* in healthy subjects increases the plasma concentration of both drugs. The negative inotropic effects of the two drugs on cardiac function are at most only additive, but treatment with this combination should be initiated with caution in patients with impaired left ventricular function.[1] Addition of *sotalol* to flecainide therapy has produced profound bradycardia and atrioventricular block followed by cardiac arrest and death in a man with ventricular tachycardia.[2]

1. Holtzman JL, *et al.* The pharmacodynamic and pharmacokinetic interaction of flecainide acetate with propranolol: effects on cardiac function and drug clearance. *Eur J Clin Pharmacol* 1987; **33:** 97–9.
2. Warren R, *et al.* Serious interactions of sotalol with amiodarone and flecainide. *Med J Aust* 1990; **152:** 277.

Food. Milk feeds reduced the absorption of flecainide in an infant who required a dose of 40 mg per kg body-weight daily to control supraventricular tachycardias. When milk feeds were replaced by glucose, the serum-flecainide concentration increased from 990 to 1824 nanograms per mL. Milk-fed infants on high doses of flecainide should have the dose reduced if milk is stopped or reduced.[1]

1. Russell GAB, Martin RP. Flecainide toxicity. *Arch Dis Child* 1989; **64:** 860–3.

Histamine H$_2$-antagonists. *Cimetidine* has been reported to increase the bioavailability of flecainide in healthy subjects, probably due to a decrease in the metabolism of flecainide. Elimination half-life and renal clearance were unchanged.[1]

1. Tjandra-Maga TB, *et al.* Altered pharmacokinetics of oral flecainide by cimetidine. *Br J Clin Pharmacol* 1986; **22:** 108–10.

Pharmacokinetics

Flecainide is almost completely absorbed after oral administration and does not undergo extensive first-pass hepatic metabolism. It is metabolised to 2 major metabolites, *m-O*-dealkylated flecainide and *m-O*-dealkylated lactam of flecainide, both of which may have some activity. Its metabolism appears to involve the cytochrome P450 isoenzyme CYP2D6 and is subject to genetic polymorphism (see Metabolism, below). Flecainide is excreted mainly in the urine, about 30% as unchanged drug and the remainder as metabolites. About 5% is excreted in the faeces. Excretion of flecainide is decreased in renal impairment, heart failure, and in alkaline urine. Haemodialysis removes only about 1% of an oral dose as unchanged flecainide.

The therapeutic plasma concentration range is generally accepted as 200 to 1000 nanograms per mL. The elimination half-life of flecainide is about 20 hours and it is about 40% bound to plasma proteins.

Flecainide crosses the placenta and is distributed into breast milk.

Breast feeding. Flecainide 100 mg every 12 hours by mouth was given to 11 healthy women beginning 1 day after delivery and continuing for 5½ days.[1] The mean milk to plasma ratios on study days 2 to 5 were 3.7, 3.2, 3.5, and 2.6 respectively but it was considered that the risk to breast-fed infants of ingesting

The symbol † denotes a preparation no longer actively marketed

toxic amounts of flecainide in breast milk was very low. The mean elimination half-life of flecainide from milk was 14.7 hours, very similar to the plasma elimination half-life.

1. McQuinn RL, *et al.* Flecainide excretion in human breast milk. *Clin Pharmacol Ther* 1990; **48:** 262–7.

Metabolism. Oxidative metabolism is an important route of flecainide elimination.[1] Several other drugs, such as sparteine and debrisoquine, which also undergo oxidative metabolism display a genetic polymorphism and extensive metabolisers and poor metabolisers can be identified. A similar type of genetic polymorphism has been demonstrated for flecainide and the 5 to 10% of the population who are poor metabolisers for sparteine and debrisoquine will also have a restricted capacity to metabolise flecainide. The mean elimination half-life of flecainide in poor metabolisers was found to be 11.8 hours compared with 6.8 hours in extensive metabolisers and the amounts of a dose excreted as unchanged drug in the urine were 51% and 31% respectively. These differences in pharmacokinetics will not be of clinical importance as long as renal function is not impaired since the reduced metabolic clearance in poor metabolisers can be compensated for by increased renal elimination. However, if patients with renal impairment are to be given flecainide their metabolic phenotype should be identified and special care taken with dosage adjustments in poor metabolisers.

1. Mikus G, *et al.* The influence of the sparteine-debrisoquin phenotype on the disposition of flecainide. *Clin Pharmacol Ther* 1989; **45:** 562–7.

Pregnancy. A study of the pharmacokinetics of flecainide, given to a mother during the third trimester of pregnancy for the treatment of fetal supraventricular tachycardia,[1] indicated that close to term flecainide crosses the placenta easily without accumulating in fetal blood, but with a high concentration in the amniotic fluid.

See also under Effects on the Liver, above.

1. Bourget P, *et al.* Flecainide distribution, transplacental passage and accumulation in the amniotic fluid during the third trimester of pregnancy. *Ann Pharmacother* 1994; **28:** 1031–4.

Uses and Administration

Flecainide is a class Ic antiarrhythmic (p.787) used for the treatment of severe symptomatic ventricular arrhythmias (sustained ventricular tachycardia or premature ventricular contractions or non-sustained ventricular tachycardia resistant to other therapy) and severe symptomatic supraventricular arrhythmias (atrioventricular nodal reciprocating tachycardia, arrhythmias associated with the Wolff-Parkinson-White syndrome, and paroxysmal atrial fibrillation).

Flecainide is administered orally or intravenously as the acetate. Treatment should be started in hospital. A suggested therapeutic plasma concentration range is 200 to 1000 nanograms per mL.

In ventricular **arrhythmias** the usual initial dose of flecainide acetate by mouth is 100 mg twice daily; the usual maximum total dose is 400 mg daily. The dose should be adjusted after 3 to 5 days and reduced once control has been achieved. In supraventricular arrhythmias the usual initial dose is 50 mg twice daily by mouth with a maximum total dose of 300 mg daily.

For rapid control of arrhythmias flecainide acetate 2 mg per kg body-weight may be administered intravenously over 10 to 30 minutes, to a maximum dose of 150 mg; the ECG should be monitored. If longer term parenteral therapy is necessary therapy is initiated by intravenous injection of 2 mg per kg over 30 minutes, as above, then continued by intravenous infusion of 1.5 mg per kg over the first hour, and 0.1 to 0.25 mg per kg per hour thereafter. The maximum cumulative dose in the first 24 hours should not exceed 600 mg. Infusion should not generally continue for more than 24 hours and oral administration should be substituted as soon as possible.

The dose of flecainide should be reduced in renal impairment. Patients with a creatinine clearance of 35 mL per minute or less should receive a maximum initial oral dose of 100 mg daily and plasma concentrations should be monitored; intravenous doses should be halved.

Children may be given flecainide in initial oral doses of 50 mg per m^2 body-surface daily in divided doses for those aged under 6 months and 100 mg per m^2 daily for those aged over 6 months. A dose of 200 mg per m^2 daily should not be exceeded.

Flecainide has also been tried in the treatment of refractory neuropathic pain.

Administration. Flecainide is usually given by mouth or intravenously, but was reported to be rapidly and reliably absorbed after rectal administration as a solution in healthy subjects.[1] The mean time to achieve peak serum concentration was 0.67 hours and the mean bioavailability was 98% compared with 1 hour and 78% for an oral solution and 4 hours and 81% for a tablet. The absorption of flecainide given rectally to 2 critically ill patients was good in one but poor in the other[2] and it was recommended that rectal administration be reserved for patients unresponsive to maximal parenteral therapy and in whom oral or nasogastric administration cannot be used.

1. Lie-A-Huen L, *et al.* Absorption kinetics of oral and rectal flecainide in healthy subjects. *Eur J Clin Pharmacol* 1990; **38:** 595–8.
2. Quattrocchi FP, Karim A. Flecainide acetate administration by enema. *DICP Ann Pharmacother* 1990; **24:** 1233–4.

Cardiac arrhythmias. Asymptomatic premature ventricular arrhythmias in subjects who have previously suffered a myocardial infarction are recognised as a risk factor for subsequent sudden cardiac death.[1] Suppressing such arrhythmias in this group might be expected to reduce the incidence of sudden death and it was to test this hypothesis that a large multicentre study was set up in the USA (the Cardiac Arrhythmia Suppression Trial known as CAST).[2,3] Encainide, flecainide, and moracizine were the antiarrhythmics studied, and all three were associated with increased mortality and it is now accepted that these drugs should not be used prophylactically in post-infarction patients with asymptomatic arrhythmias.

Licensed indications for flecainide cover severe symptomatic ventricular and supraventricular arrhythmias including sustained ventricular tachycardia, premature ventricular contractions resistant to other therapy, atrioventricular nodal reciprocating tachycardias, arrhythmias associated with the Wolff-Parkinson-White syndrome, and paroxysmal atrial fibrillation. Flecainide has been found to be effective in such arrhythmias,[4-7] and groups of patients successfully treated have included children.[8-10] Maternal administration of flecainide has been successful in treating fetal arrhythmias.[11-13]

For further discussion on the management of cardiac arrhythmias, with mention of flecainide, see p.794.

1. Task Force of the Working Group on Arrhythmias of the European Society of Cardiology. CAST and beyond: implications of the cardiac arrhythmias suppression trial. *Circulation* 1990; **81:** 1123–7. [Simultaneous publication occurred in *Eur Heart J* 1990; **11:** 194–9].
2. The Cardiac Arrhythmia Suppression Trial (CAST) Investigators. Preliminary report: effect of encainide and flecainide on mortality in a randomized trial of arrhythmia suppression after myocardial infarction. *N Engl J Med* 1989; **321:** 406–12.
3. Echt DS, *et al.* Mortality and morbidity in patients receiving encainide, flecainide, or placebo: The Cardiac Arrhythmia Suppression Trial. *N Engl J Med* 1991; **324:** 781–8.
4. Hohnloser SH, Zabel M. Short- and long-term efficacy and safety of flecainide acetate for supraventricular arrhythmias. *Am J Cardiol* 1992; **70:** 3A–10A.
5. Anderson J, *et al.* Flecainide acetate for paroxysmal supraventricular tachyarrhythmias. *Am J Cardiol* 1994; **74:** 578–84.
6. Aliot E, *et al.* Comparison of the safety and efficacy of flecainide versus propafenone in hospital out-patients with symptomatic paroxysmal atrial fibrillation/flutter. *Am J Cardiol* 1996; **77:** 66A–71A.
7. Dorian P, *et al.* A randomized comparison of flecainide versus verapamil in paroxysmal supraventricular tachycardia. *Am J Cardiol* 1996; **77:** 89A–95A.
8. Till JA, *et al.* Treatment of refractory supraventricular arrhythmias with flecainide acetate. *Arch Dis Child* 1987; **62:** 247–52.
9. Till JA, *et al.* Use of flecainide in children. *Lancet* 1989; **ii:** 326.
10. O'Sullivan JJ, *et al.* Digoxin or flecainide for prophylaxis of supraventricular tachycardia in infants? *J Am Coll Cardiol* 1995; **26:** 991–4.
11. Wren C, Hunter S. Maternal administration of flecainide to terminate and suppress fetal tachycardia. *BMJ* 1988; **296:** 249.
12. Perry JC, *et al.* Fetal supraventricular tachycardia treated with flecainide acetate. *J Pediatr* 1991; **118:** 303–5.
13. Smoleniec JS, *et al.* Intermittent fetal tachycardia and fetal hydrops. *Arch Dis Child* 1991; **66:** 1160–1.

Pain. Various drugs, including flecainide, have been tried for neuropathic pain (p.7) insensitive to opioid analgesics. Beneficial results were achieved with flecainide 100 mg twice daily by mouth in the control of severe pain associated with malignant infiltration of nerves.[1,2] A controlled trial of flecainide in neuropathic pain was abandoned[3] when an association between flecainide and increased mortality was found in a separate study in post-infarction patients. Nevertheless, flecainide may be of value in refractory neuropathic pain, usually as a second- or third-line drug in patients with advanced cancer, but with neither a history of, nor suspected, ischaemic heart disease.[4]

1. Dunlop R, *et al.* Analgesic effects of oral flecainide. *Lancet* 1988; **i:** 420–1.
2. Sinnott C, *et al.* Flecainide in cancer nerve pain. *Lancet* 1991; **337:** 1347.
3. Dunlop RJ, *et al.* Flecainide in cancer nerve pain. *Lancet* 1991; **337:** 1347.
4. Davis CL, Hardy JR. Palliative care. *BMJ* 1994; **308:** 1359–62.

Preparations

BP 2001: Flecainide Injection; Flecainide Tablets;
USP 25: Flecainide Acetate Tablets.

Proprietary Preparations (details are given in Part 3)
Aust.: Aristocor; *Austral.:* Flecatab; Tambocor; *Belg.:* Tambocor; *Canad.:* Tambocor; *Denm.:* Tambocor; *Fin.:* Tambocor; *Fr.:* Flecaine; *Ger.:* Tambocor; *Hong Kong:* Tambocor; *Irl.:* Tambocor; *Israel:* Tambocor; *Ital.:* Almarytm; *Mex.:* Tambocor; *Neth.:* Tambocor; *Norw.:* Tambocor; *NZ:* Tambocor; *Port.:* Apocard†; *S.Afr.:* Tambocor; *Singapore:* Tambocor; *Spain:* Apocard; *Swed.:* Tam-

bocor; *Switz.:* Tambocor; *Thai.:* Tambocor; *UK:* Tambocor; *USA:* Tambocor.

Flosequinan (18878-w)

Flosequinan (BAN, USAN, rINN).
BTS-49465. 7-Fluoro-1-methyl-3-methylsulphinyl-4-quinolone.
$C_{11}H_{10}FNO_2S = 239.3$.
CAS — 76568-02-0.
ATC — C01DB01.

Profile
Flosequinan is a direct-acting arteriovenous vasodilator that was used as an adjunct to the conventional treatment of heart failure, but was withdrawn from the market following findings of excess mortality.

◊ References.
1. Kamali F, Edwards C. Possible role of metabolite in flosequinan-related mortality. *Clin Pharmacokinet* 1995; **29:** 396–403.

Fluindione (4815-c)

Fluindione (rINN).
Fluorindione; LM-123. 2-(4-Fluorophenyl)indan-1,3-dione.
$C_{15}H_9FO_2 = 240.2$.
CAS — 957-56-2.

Profile
Fluindione is an orally administered indanedione anticoagulant with actions similar to those of warfarin (p.992). It is used in the management of thromboembolic disorders (p.816) but, as the indanediones are generally more toxic than warfarin (see phenindione, p.954), its use is limited.
The usual initial dose is 20 mg daily; the dose is then adjusted according to coagulation tests.

Preparations
Proprietary Preparations (details are given in Part 3)
Fr.: Previscan.

Fluvastatin Sodium (5928-w)

Fluvastatin Sodium (BANM, USAN, rINNM).
XU-62-320. Sodium $(\pm)$-$(3R^*,5S^*,6E)$-7-[3-(p-Fluorophenyl)-1-isopropylindol-2-yl]-3,5-dihydroxy-6-heptenoate.
$C_{24}H_{25}FNNaO_4 = 433.4$.
CAS — 93957-54-1 (fluvastatin); 93957-55-2 (fluvastatin sodium).

Adverse Effects and Precautions
As for Simvastatin, p.969.

Interactions
The interactions of statins with other drugs are described under simvastatin (p.970). However, similar interactions appear not to have been reported with fluvastatin although caution is advised when using such combinations. An interaction not noted with other statins is that with rifampicin, in which a decrease of about 50% in the bioavailability of fluvastatin has been recorded.

◊ General reviews.
1. Garnett WR. Interactions with hydroxymethylglutaryl-coenzyme A reductase inhibitors. *Am J Health-Syst Pharm* 1995; **52:** 1639–45.

Pharmacokinetics
Fluvastatin, unlike simvastatin or lovastatin, is active without the need for hydrolysis. It is rapidly and completely absorbed from the gastrointestinal tract and undergoes extensive first-pass metabolism in the liver, its primary site of action. An absolute bioavailability of 24% has been reported. It is more than 98% bound to plasma proteins. About 90% is excreted in the faeces with only about 6% being excreted in the urine.

◊ General reviews.
1. Desager J-P, Horsmans Y. Clinical pharmacokinetics of 3-hydroxy-3-methylglutaryl-coenzyme A reductase inhibitors. *Clin Pharmacokinet* 1996; **31:** 348–71.
2. Lennernäs H, Fager G. Pharmacodynamics and pharmacokinetics of the HMG-CoA reductase inhibitors: similarities and differences. *Clin Pharmacokinet* 1997; **32:** 403–25.

Uses and Administration
Fluvastatin, a 3-hydroxy-3-methylglutaryl coenzyme A (HMG-CoA) reductase inhibitor (a statin), is a lipid regulating drug with actions on plasma lipids similar to those of simvastatin (p.970). It is used to reduce LDL-cholesterol, apolipoprotein B, and triglycerides

in the treatment of hyperlipidaemias (p.800), including hypercholesterolaemias and combined (mixed) hyperlipidaemia (type IIa or IIb hyperlipoproteinaemias). It is also given prophylactically to hypercholesterolaemic patients with ischaemic heart disease.

Fluvastatin is given by mouth as the sodium salt, but doses are expressed in terms of the base. The initial dose is 20 to 40 mg once daily in the evening, increased if necessary at intervals of 4 weeks up to 40 mg twice daily. Modified-release preparations are also available.

◊ General reviews.
1. Deslypere JP. The role of HMG-CoA reductase inhibitors in the treatment of hyperlipidemia: a review of fluvastatin. *Curr Ther Res* 1995; **56:** 111–28.
2. Plosker GL, Wagstaff AJ. Fluvastatin: a review of its pharmacology and use in the management of hypercholesterolaemia. *Drugs* 1996; **51:** 433–59.
3. Schectman G, Hiatt J. Dose–response characteristics of cholesterol-lowering drug therapies: implications for treatment. *Ann Intern Med* 1996; **125:** 990–1000.
4. Langtry HD, Markham A. Fluvastatin: a review of its use in lipid disorders. *Drugs* 1999; **57:** 583–606.

Hyperlipidaemias. Fluvastatin, like other statins, is used in the treatment of hyperlipidaemias (p.800) and a general discussion of the lipid regulating effects of statins can be found in simvastatin (p.970).

Studies[1,2] have confirmed the ability of fluvastatin to reduce low-density lipoprotein (LDL)-cholesterol in patients with primary[1,2] or combined[2] hypercholesterolaemia; it was also well-tolerated. Hypercholesterolaemia is a risk factor for **ischaemic heart disease** and fluvastatin may be given for secondary prevention of atherosclerotic heart disease. Three large randomised, double-blind, placebo-controlled studies have found that fluvastatin may reduce the incidence of clinical events and slow the progression of atherosclerotic plaques. Fluvastatin was associated with a reduction in all cardiac events during one year of treatment in patients with hypercholesterolaemia and ischaemic heart disease.[3] In an angiographic study of change in minimum lumen diameter, fluvastatin treatment for 2.5 years significantly slowed progression of coronary atherosclerosis in patients with mildly to moderately elevated LDL-cholesterol.[4] However, a study of fluvastatin treatment following successful coronary angioplasty found no effect on restenosis or change in minimum lumen diameter, although the investigators noted a reduction in death and myocardial infarction.[5]

1. Davidson MH. Fluvastatin long-term Extension Trial (FLUENT): summary of efficacy and safety. *Am J Med* 1994; **96** (suppl 6A): 41S–44S.
2. Beil S, *et al.* Fluvastatin lipid-lowering effect in routine practice conditions (FLIRT): results of a drug surveillance study. *Clin Drug Invest* 1997; **14:** 146–53.
3. Riegger G, *et al.* The effect of fluvastatin on cardiac events in patients with symptomatic coronary artery disease during one year of treatment. *Atherosclerosis* 1999; **144:** 263–70.
4. Herd JA, *et al.* Effects of fluvastatin on coronary atherosclerosis in patients with mild to moderate cholesterol elevations (Lipoprotein and Coronary Atherosclerosis Study [LCAS]). *Am J Cardiol* 1997; **80:** 278–86.
5. Serruys PW, *et al.* A randomized placebo-controlled trial of fluvastatin for prevention of restenosis after successful coronary balloon angioplasty: final results of the fluvastatin angiographic restenosis (FLARE) trial. *Eur Heart J* 1999; **20:** 58–69.

Preparations
Proprietary Preparations (details are given in Part 3)
Aust.: Lescol; *Austral.:* Lescol; Vastin; *Belg.:* Lescol; *Braz.:* Lescol; *Canad.:* Lescol; *Denm.:* Canef; Lescol; *Fin.:* Canef; Lescol; *Fr.:* Fractal; Lescol; *Ger.:* Cranoc; LOCOL; *Hong Kong:* Lescol; *Irl.:* Lescol; *Israel:* Lescol; *Ital.:* Lipaxan; Primesin; *Jpn:* Lochol; *Mex.:* Canef; Lescol; *Neth.:* Canef; Lescol; *Norw.:* Canef; Lescol; *NZ:* Lescol; *Port.:* Canef; Cardiol; Lescol; *S.Afr.:* Lescol; *Singapore:* Lescol; *Spain:* Digaril; Lescol; Lymetel; *Swed.:* Canef; Lescol; *Switz.:* Lescol; *Thai.:* Lescol; *UK:* Lescol; *USA:* Lescol.

Fondaparinux Sodium (20172-x)

Fondaparinux Sodium (rINN).
Fondaparin Sodium (BAN); SR-90107A.
CAS — 114870-03-0.

Profile
Fondaparinux is a synthetic pentasaccharide that acts as an inhibitor of activated factor X. It is under investigation as the sodium salt as an anticoagulant in the management of venous thromboembolism.

◊ References.
1. The Rembrandt Investigators. Treatment of proximal deep vein thrombosis with a novel synthetic compound (SR90107A/ORG31540) with pure anti-factor Xa activity: a phase II evaluation. *Circulation* 2000; **102:** 2726–31.
2. Turpie AGG, *et al.* A synthetic pentasaccharide for the prevention of deep-vein thrombosis after total hip replacement. *N Engl J Med* 2001; **344:** 619–25.

Fosinopril Sodium (965-r)

Fosinopril Sodium (BANM, USAN, rINNM).
SQ-28555. (4S)-4-Cyclohexyl-1-{[(RS)-2-methyl-1-(propionyloxy)propoxy](4-phenylbutyl)phosphinoylacetyl]-L-proline, sodium salt.
$C_{30}H_{45}NNaO_7P = 585.6$.
CAS — 97825-24-6 (fosinopril); 98048-97-6 (fosinopril); 88889-14-9 (fosinopril sodium).

Adverse Effects, Treatment, and Precautions
As for ACE inhibitors, p.820.

Interactions
As for ACE inhibitors, p.822.

Pharmacokinetics
Fosinopril acts as a prodrug of the diacid fosinoprilat, its active metabolite. Following oral administration about 36% of a dose of fosinopril is absorbed. Fosinopril is rapidly and completely hydrolysed to fosinoprilat in both gastrointestinal mucosa and liver. Peak plasma concentrations of fosinoprilat are achieved about 3 hours after an oral dose of fosinopril. Fosinoprilat is more than 95% bound to plasma proteins. It is excreted both in urine and in the faeces via the bile; it has been detected in breast milk. The effective half-life for accumulation of fosinoprilat following multiple doses of fosinopril is about 11.5 hours in patients with hypertension and about 14 hours in patients with heart failure.

◊ References.
1. Singhvi SM, *et al.* Disposition of fosinopril sodium in healthy subjects. *Br J Clin Pharmacol* 1988; **25:** 9–15.
2. Kostis JB, *et al.* Fosinopril: pharmacokinetics and pharmacodynamics in congestive heart failure. *Clin Pharmacol Ther* 1995; **58:** 660–5.

Renal impairment. Total body clearance of fosinoprilat, the active metabolite of fosinopril, is slower in patients with impaired renal function. However, pharmacokinetic studies in patients with varying degrees of renal dysfunction,[1-5] including those requiring dialysis, indicate that decreases in renal clearance may be compensated for, at least in part, by increases in hepatic clearance.

1. Hui KK, *et al.* Pharmacokinetics of fosinopril in patients with various degrees of renal function. *Clin Pharmacol Ther* 1991; **49:** 457–67.
2. Gehr TWB, *et al.* Fosinopril pharmacokinetics and pharmacodynamics in chronic ambulatory peritoneal dialysis patients. *Eur J Clin Pharmacol* 1991; **41:** 165–9.
3. Sica DA, *et al.* Comparison of the steady-state pharmacokinetics of fosinopril, lisinopril and enalapril in patients with chronic renal insufficiency. *Clin Pharmacokinet* 1991; **20:** 420–7.
4. Gehr TWB, *et al.* The pharmacokinetics and pharmacodynamics of fosinopril in haemodialysis patients. *Eur J Clin Pharmacol* 1993; **45:** 431–6.
5. Greenbaum R, *et al.* Comparison of the pharmacokinetics of fosinopril with enalapril and lisinopril in patients with congestive heart failure and chronic renal insufficiency. *Br J Clin Pharmacol* 2000; **49:** 23–31.

Uses and Administration
Fosinopril is an ACE inhibitor (p.820). It is used in the treatment of hypertension (p.802) and heart failure (p.798).

Fosinopril owes its activity to fosinoprilat to which it is converted after oral administration. The haemodynamic effects are seen within 1 hour of a single oral dose and the maximum effect occurs after 2 to 6 hours, although the full effect may not develop for several weeks during chronic dosing. The haemodynamic action lasts for about 24 hours, allowing once-daily dosing. Fosinopril is given by mouth as the sodium salt.

In the treatment of **hypertension** the initial dose is 10 mg once daily. Since there may be a precipitous fall in blood pressure in some patients when starting therapy with an ACE inhibitor, the first dose should preferably be given at bedtime. Usual maintenance doses range from 10 to 40 mg once daily. In patients already receiving diuretic therapy the diuretic should be withdrawn if possible several days before commencing fosinopril, and resumed later if necessary.

In the management of **heart failure**, severe first-dose hypotension on introduction of an ACE inhibitor is common in patients on loop diuretics, but their temporary withdrawal may cause rebound pulmonary oedema. Thus treatment should be initiated with a low dose under close medical supervision. Fosinopril is given in an initial dose of 10 mg once daily and, if well tolerated, increased to up to 40 mg once daily. An initial dose of 5 mg may be given in patients at high risk of hypotension.

◊ Reviews.
1. Murdoch D, McTavish D. Fosinopril: a review of its pharmacodynamic and pharmacokinetic properties, and therapeutic potential in essential hypertension. *Drugs* 1992; **43:** 123–40.
2. Wagstaff AJ, *et al.* Fosinopril: a reappraisal of its pharmacology and therapeutic efficacy in essential hypertension. *Drugs* 1996; **51:** 777–91.
3. Davis R, *et al.* Fosinopril: a review of its pharmacology and clinical efficacy in the management of heart failure. *Drugs* 1997; **54:** 103–16.

Preparations

Proprietary Preparations (details are given in Part 3)
Aust.: Fositens; *Austral.:* Monopril; *Belg.:* Fosinil; *Braz.:* Monopril; *Canad.:* Monopril; *Denm.:* Monopril; *Fr.:* Fozitec; *Ger.:* Dynacil; *Fosinorm; **Hong Kong:** Monopril; **Israel:** Vasopril; **Ital.:*** Eliten; Fosipres; Tensogard; *Mex.:* Monopril; *Neth.:* NewAce; *Norw.:* Monopril; *Port.:* Fositen; *S.Afr.:* Monopril; *Singapore:* Monopril; *Spain:* Fosinil; Fositens; Hicarlex; Hiperlex; Tenso Stop; Tensocardil; *Swed.:* Monopril; *Switz.:* Fositen; *Thai.:* Monopril; *UK:* Staril; *USA:* Monopril.

Multi-ingredient: *Aust.:* Fosicomb; *Austral.:* Monoplus; *Belg.:* Foside; *Fr.:* Fozirétic; *Ger.:* Dynacil comp; Fosinorm comp; *Ital.:* Elidiur; Fosicombi; Tensozide; *Neth.:* Diurace; *S.Afr.:* Monozide; *Spain:* Fositens Plus; Hiperlex Plus; Tenso Stop Plus; *Swed.:* Monopril comp; *Switz.:* Fosicomp; *USA:* Monopril-HCT.

Frusemide (2331-m)

Frusemide *(BAN)*.

Furosemide *(BAN, USAN, rINN)*; Furosemidum; LB-502. 4-Chloro-N-furfuryl-5-sulphamoylanthranilic acid.
$C_{12}H_{11}ClN_2O_5S = 330.7$.
CAS — 54-31-9.
ATC — C03CA01.

NOTE. Compounded preparations of frusemide [furosemide] may be represented by the following names:
• Co-amilofruse *(BAN)*—frusemide [furosemide] 8 parts and amiloride hydrochloride 1 part (w/w).
Pharmacopoeias. In Chin., Eur. (see p.vi), Int., Jpn, Pol., and US.

Pharmacopoeial description

Ph. Eur.: A white or almost white, crystalline powder. Practically insoluble in water and in dichloromethane; sparingly soluble in alcohol; soluble in acetone; slightly soluble in ether. It dissolves in dilute solutions of alkali hydroxides. Protect from light.

USP 25: A white to slightly yellow, odourless, crystalline powder. Practically insoluble in water; sparingly soluble in alcohol; freely soluble in acetone, in dimethylformamide, and in solutions of alkali hydroxides; very slightly soluble in chloroform; slightly soluble in ether; soluble in methyl alcohol. Protect from light.

Solutions for injection are prepared with the aid of sodium hydroxide, giving solutions with a pH of 8.0 to 9.3.

Incompatibilities. Solutions for injection are alkaline and should not be mixed or diluted with glucose injection or other acidic solutions.

Frusemide [furosemide] injection has been reported[1] to be visually incompatible with injections of diltiazem hydrochloride, dobutamine hydrochloride, dopamine hydrochloride, labetalol hydrochloride, midazolam hydrochloride, milrinone lactate, nicardipine hydrochloride, and vecuronium bromide. Incompatibility has also been noted with parenteral nutrient solutions,[2] with cisatracurium besilate,[3] and with levofloxacin.[4]

1. Chiu MF, Schwartz ML. Visual compatibility of injectable drugs used in the intensive care unit. *Am J Health-Syst Pharm* 1997; **54:** 64–5.
2. Trissel LA, *et al.* Compatibility of parenteral nutrient solutions with selected drugs during simulated Y-site administration. *Am J Health-Syst Pharm* 1997; **54:** 1295–1300.
3. Trissel LA, *et al.* Compatibility of cisatracurium besylate with selected drugs during simulated Y-site administration. *Am J Health-Syst Pharm* 1997; **54:** 1735–41.
4. Saltsman CL, *et al.* Compatibility of levofloxacin with 34 medications during simulated Y-site administration. *Am J Health-Syst Pharm* 1999; **56:** 1458–9.

Adverse Effects

The most common side-effect associated with frusemide [furosemide] therapy is fluid and electrolyte imbalance including hyponatraemia, hypokalaemia, and hypochloraemic alkalosis, particularly after large doses or prolonged administration. Because of the shorter duration of action, the risk of hypokalaemia may be less with loop diuretics such as frusemide [furosemide] than with thiazide diuretics. Unlike the thiazide diuretics, frusemide [furosemide] increases the urinary excretion of calcium. Nephrocalcinosis

The symbol † denotes a preparation no longer actively marketed

has been reported when frusemide [furosemide] has been used to treat preterm infants.

Frusemide [furosemide] may provoke hyperglycaemia and glycosuria, but probably to a lesser extent than the thiazide diuretics. It may cause hyperuricaemia and precipitate attacks of gout in some patients.

Signs of electrolyte imbalance include headache, hypotension, muscle cramps, dry mouth, thirst, weakness, lethargy, drowsiness, restlessness, oliguria, cardiac arrhythmias, and gastrointestinal disturbances.

Other side-effects are relatively uncommon, and include blurred vision, yellow vision, dizziness, headache, and orthostatic hypotension. Skin rashes and photosensitivity reactions, although rare, may be severe and hypersensitivity reactions including interstitial nephritis, vasculitis, and fever occur rarely. Pancreatitis is more common at high doses and cholestatic jaundice has been reported. Bone marrow depression may occur rarely: agranulocytosis, thrombocytopenia, and leucopenia have been reported. Tinnitus and deafness may rarely occur in particular during rapid high-dose parenteral frusemide [furosemide] therapy. Rarely, deafness may be permanent particularly if frusemide [furosemide] has been given to patients taking other ototoxic drugs.

◊ Although rarely clinically important, frusemide [furosemide] may cause fluid depletion and electrolyte disturbances. These effects are dose-dependent[1,2] and serious disturbances can result from over enthusiastic use of loop diuretics in oedematous patients.[3] In a survey of 553 hospital inpatients[1] receiving frusemide [furosemide] 220 patients (40%) experienced 480 adverse reactions. Electrolyte disturbances occurred in 130 (23.5%) patients and extracellular volume depletion in 50 (9%). Adverse reactions were more common in patients with liver disease, and hepatic coma occurred in 20 patients with hepatic cirrhosis. A similar survey in 585 hospital inpatients[2] revealed 177 adverse effects in 123 patients (21%). These included volume depletion in 85 patients (14.5%), hypokalaemia in 21 (3.6%), and hyponatraemia in 6 (1%). Hypokalaemia was considered to be life-threatening in 2 patients. Hyperuricaemia occurred in 54 patients (9.2%), of whom 40 also had volume depletion, and clinical gout developed in 2.

Decreases in blood pressure and increases in haematocrit values following the introduction of frusemide [furosemide] treatment were considered to have contributed to the pathogenesis of stroke in 3 elderly patients.[4] It was suggested that the use of powerful high-ceiling diuretics such as frusemide [furosemide] could cause cerebral ischaemia and should be avoided in the treatment of hypertension in the elderly. Over enthusiastic use of frusemide [furosemide] or co-amilofruse was also considered responsible for leg ischaemia or superficial gangrene in 5 elderly patients.[5]

1. Naranjo CA, *et al.* Frusemide-induced adverse reactions during hospitalization. *Am J Hosp Pharm* 1978; **35:** 794–8.
2. Lowe J, *et al.* Adverse reactions to frusemide in hospital inpatients. *BMJ* 1979; **2:** 360–2.
3. Plumb VJ, James TN. Clinical hazards of powerful diuretics: furosemide and ethacrynic acid. *Mod Concepts Cardiovasc Dis* 1978; **47:** 91–4.
4. Jansen PAF, *et al.* Contribution of inappropriate treatment for hypertension to pathogenesis of stroke in the elderly. *BMJ* 1986; **293:** 914–17.
5. O'Rourke DA, Hede JE. Reversible leg ischaemia due to diuretics. *BMJ* 1979; **1:** 1114.

Carcinogenicity. See under Hydrochlorothiazide, p.908.

Effects on the ears. Ototoxicity and deafness during frusemide [furosemide] therapy is most frequently associated with elevated blood concentrations resulting from rapid intravenous infusion[1] or delayed excretion in patients with impaired renal function.[2] In a report[3] of 29 cases of frusemide [furosemide]-induced deafness reported to the FDA in the USA, most patients had concomitant renal disease or had received frusemide [furosemide] intravenously. Eight patients had also received another ototoxic drug. However, deafness occurred in 11 patients following oral administration, and in 4 of these hearing loss occurred in the absence of renal disease or other ototoxic drugs. Hearing loss was generally transient, lasting from one-half to 24 hours, but permanent hearing loss occurred in 3 patients, one of whom had taken frusemide [furosemide] orally. Deafness was not always associated with high doses; six patients had received a total of 200 mg or less of frusemide [furosemide].

See also Precautions, below.

1. Heidland A, Wigand ME. Einfluss hoher furosemiddosen auf die gehörfunktion bei urämie. *Klin Wochenschr* 1970; **48:** 1052–6.
2. Schwartz GH, *et al.* Ototoxicity induced by furosemide. *N Engl J Med* 1970; **282:** 1413–14.
3. Gallagher KL, Jones JK. Furosemide-induced ototoxicity. *Ann Intern Med* 1979; **91:** 744–5.

Effects on electrolyte balance. CALCIUM. Frusemide [furosemide] increases renal calcium excretion. There is a danger of hypocalcaemic tetany during frusemide [furosemide] administration in hypoparathyroid patients[1] and it has also been

reported[2] in a patient with latent hypoparathyroidism following thyroidectomy.

The decrease in serum-calcium concentrations could also induce hyperparathyroidism. In a study involving 36 patients with heart failure frusemide [furosemide] administration was associated with elevations in both parathyroid hormone and alkaline phosphatase concentrations, possibly indicating accelerated bone remodelling such as that found in primary hyperparathyroidism.[3]

For reports of hypercalciuria, rickets, renal calculi, and hyperparathyroidism in neonates treated with frusemide [furosemide], see under Effects in Infants and Neonates, below.

1. Gabow PA, *et al.* Furosemide-induced reduction in ionized calcium in hypoparathyroid patients. *Ann Intern Med* 1977; **86:** 579–81.
2. Bashey A, MacNee W. Tetany induced by frusemide in latent hypoparathyroidism. *BMJ* 1987; **295:** 960–1.
3. Elmgreen J, *et al.* Elevated serum parathyroid hormone concentration during treatment with high ceiling diuretics. *Eur J Clin Pharmacol* 1980; **18:** 363–4.

MAGNESIUM, POTASSIUM, AND SODIUM. For discussions of the effects of diuretics on these electrolytes see under the Adverse Effects of Hydrochlorothiazide, p.908.

Effects in infants and neonates. Frusemide [furosemide] is commonly used in the treatment of cardiac and pulmonary disorders in premature infants and neonates. This age group appears to be particularly susceptible to adverse effects arising from the increase in urinary calcium excretion which occurs during long-term frusemide [furosemide] therapy. Increases in parathyroid hormone concentration[1,2] and evidence of bone resorption[1,3] support the suggestion that the increased calcium loss causes secondary hyperparathyroidism. There have been reports of decreased mineral content of bone,[1,3] rickets,[4] fractures,[3] and renal calcification.[1,5-7] An observation[5] that renal calcification could be reversed by the addition of a thiazide diuretic was supported by other workers.[6] There is evidence[8] that frusemide [furosemide]-related renal calcifications in very low birth-weight infants might be associated with long-term impairment of kidney function. Renal calcification has also been reported following frusemide [furosemide] administration in older infants.[9]

It has been suggested[10] that a sodium deficit in infants treated with frusemide [furosemide] for heart failure may contribute to a failure to thrive.

Concern has been expressed over the finding[11] that frusemide [furosemide] use in premature infants with respiratory distress syndrome increases the incidence of patent ductus arteriosus. The mechanism is thought to be connected with stimulation of renal prostaglandin E_2. However, the increased incidence of patent ductus arteriosus did not adversely affect the mortality in infants treated with frusemide [furosemide], and a subsequent study[12] failed to find any increase in the incidence of patent ductus arteriosus in infants treated with frusemide [furosemide] compared with a control group. Paradoxically frusemide [furosemide] has been used in the management of delayed closure of ductus (see Patent Ductus Arteriosus under Uses and Administration, below). There is a possibility that frusemide [furosemide] may not be effective in infants receiving indometacin[13] but frusemide [furosemide] can prevent the decline in urine output which occurs during indometacin administration.[14,15]

1. Venkataraman PS, *et al.* Secondary hyperparathyroidism and bone disease in infants receiving long-term furosemide therapy. *Am J Dis Child* 1983; **187:** 1157–61.
2. Vileisis RA. Furosemide effect on mineral status of parenterally nourished premature neonates with chronic lung disease. *Pediatrics* 1990; **85:** 316–22.
3. Morgan MEI, Evans SE. Osteopenia in very low birthweight infants. *Lancet* 1986; **ii:** 1399–1400.
4. Chudley AE, *et al.* Nutritional rickets in 2 very low birthweight infants with chronic lung disease. *Arch Dis Child* 1980; **55:** 687–90.
5. Hufnagle KG, *et al.* Renal calcifications: a complication of long-term furosemide therapy in preterm infants. *Pediatrics* 1982; **70:** 360–3.
6. Noe HN, *et al.* Urolithiasis in pre-term neonates associated with furosemide therapy. *J Urol (Baltimore)* 1984; **132:** 93–4.
7. Pearse DM, *et al.* Sonographic diagnosis of furosemide-induced nephrocalcinosis in newborn infants. *J Ultrasound Med* 1984; **3:** 553–6.
8. Downing GJ, *et al.* Kidney function in very low birth weight infants with furosemide-related renal calcifications at ages 1 to 2 years. *J Pediatr* 1992; **120:** 599–604.
9. Alon US, *et al.* Nephrocalcinosis and nephrolithiasis in infants with congestive heart failure treated with furosemide. *J Pediatr* 1994; **125:** 149–51.
10. Salmon AP, *et al.* Sodium balance in infants with severe congestive heart failure. *Lancet* 1989; **ii:** 875.
11. Green TP, *et al.* Furosemide promotes patent ductus arteriosus in premature infants with respiratory-distress syndrome. *N Engl J Med* 1983; **308:** 743–8.
12. Yeh TF, *et al.* Early furosemide therapy in premature infants (≤ 2000 gm) with respiratory distress syndrome: a randomized controlled trial. *J Pediatr* 1984; **105:** 603–9.
13. Friedman Z, *et al.* Urinary excretion of prostaglandin E following the administration of furosemide and indomethacin to sick low-birth-weight infants. *J Pediatr* 1978; **93:** 512–15.
14. Yeh TF, *et al.* Furosemide prevents the renal side effects of indomethacin therapy in premature infants with patent ductus arteriosus. *J Pediatr* 1982; **101:** 433–7.
15. Nahata MC, *et al.* Furosemide can prevent decline in urine output in infants receiving indomethacin for patent ductus closure: a multidose study. *Infusion* 1988; **12:** 11–12 and 15.

Effects on lipid metabolism. Most studies into the effects of diuretics on blood-lipid concentrations have used thiazides (see Hydrochlorothiazide, p.908). The few studies into the effects of frusemide [furosemide] suggest that, like thiazides, it may adversely influence blood-lipid concentrations during short-term administration.[1]

1. Ames RP. The effects of antihypertensive drugs on serum lipids and lipoproteins I: diuretics. *Drugs* 1986; **32:** 260–78.

Precautions

Precautions and contra-indications for frusemide [furosemide] which are dependent on its effects on fluid and electrolyte balance are similar to those of the thiazide diuretics (see Hydrochlorothiazide, p.909). Although frusemide [furosemide] is used in high doses for oliguria due to chronic or acute renal insufficiency it should not be given in anuria or in renal failure caused by nephrotoxic or hepatotoxic drugs nor in renal failure associated with hepatic coma. Frusemide [furosemide] should not be given in pre-comatose states associated with hepatic cirrhosis. It should be used with care in patients with prostatic hyperplasia or impairment of micturition since it can precipitate acute urinary retention.

To reduce the risk of ototoxicity, the manufacturers recommend that frusemide [furosemide] should not be injected intravenously at a rate exceeding 4 mg per minute although some authorities advise that a single dose of up to 50 mg may be given more rapidly.

Frusemide [furosemide] should be used with caution during pregnancy and breast feeding since it crosses the placenta and also appears in breast milk. Frusemide [furosemide] may compromise placental perfusion by reducing maternal blood volume; it may also inhibit lactation.

Hepatic impairment. In patients with chronic cardiac failure and moderate liver congestion, high-dose frusemide [furosemide] therapy could produce increases in liver enzymes suggestive of hepatitis.[1] Special care should be taken with the dosage and mode of administration of frusemide [furosemide] in such patients to avoid severe ischaemic liver damage caused by a drop in systemic blood pressure.

As with the thiazides, frusemide [furosemide] should be avoided in patients with severe liver impairment.

1. Lang I, *et al.* Furosemide and increases in liver enzymes. *Ann Intern Med* 1988; **109:** 845.

Hypoparathyroidism. For comments on the possibility of hypocalcaemic tetany in hypoparathyroid patients taking frusemide [furosemide], see Effects on Electrolyte Balance, above.

Infants and neonates. Caution must be exercised in administering frusemide [furosemide] to infants, particularly for extended periods. The immaturity of the renal system can result in unexpectedly high blood concentrations and extended half-lives. Fluid and electrolyte balances should therefore be monitored carefully. Neonates appear to be particularly susceptible to increases in urinary calcium concentrations following long-term frusemide [furosemide] administration. There have also been reports[1] of an increased incidence of patent ductus arteriosus in infants given frusemide [furosemide], although this did not adversely affect the mortality.

Secondly, several studies[2-4] have shown frusemide [furosemide] to be a potent displacer of bilirubin from albumin binding sites and it should be used with caution in jaundiced infants. On a molar basis chlorothiazide, frusemide [furosemide], and etacrynic acid were at least as potent as sulfafurazole in displacing bilirubin from albumin.[3] Doses of frusemide [furosemide] 1 mg per kg body-weight probably do not produce a significant increase in free bilirubin in most jaundiced infants,[3,4] although doses greater than 1.5 mg per kg or repeated dosing could potentially do so.[4] Chlorothiazide 15 to 20 mg per kg would not be an appropriate alternative to frusemide [furosemide][3] since it could produce higher plasma bilirubin concentrations in jaundiced infants.

In addition, there is some evidence from an *in vitro* study[5] that bilirubin may displace frusemide [furosemide] from binding sites to a greater extent in neonates than in adults. The clearance of frusemide [furosemide] is much slower in neonates than in adults, with an eightfold prolongation in plasma half-life, and this should be taken into account during repeat dosing.[4]

1. Green TP, *et al.* Furosemide promotes patent ductus arteriosus in premature infants with the respiratory-distress syndrome. *N Engl J Med* 1983; **308:** 743–8.
2. Shankaran S, Poland RL. The displacement of bilirubin from albumin by furosemide. *J Pediatr* 1977; **90:** 642–6.
3. Wennberg RP, *et al.* Displacement of bilirubin from human albumin by three diuretics. *J Pediatr* 1977; **90:** 647–50.
4. Aranda JV, *et al.* Pharmacokinetic disposition and protein binding of furosemide in newborn infants. *J Pediatr* 1978; **93:** 507–11.
5. Viani A, Pacifici GM. Bilirubin displaces furosemide from serum protein: the effect is greater in newborn infants than adult subjects. *Dev Pharmacol Ther* 1990; **14:** 90–5.

Porphyria. Frusemide [furosemide] has been associated with acute attacks of porphyria and is considered unsafe in porphyric patients.

Interactions

The interactions of frusemide [furosemide] that are due to its effects on fluid and electrolyte balance are similar to those of hydrochlorothiazide (see p.909).

Frusemide [furosemide] may enhance the nephrotoxicity of cephalosporin antibacterials such as cefalotin and can enhance the ototoxicity of aminoglycoside antibacterials and other ototoxic drugs.

Antiepileptics. The diuretic effect of frusemide [furosemide] has been shown to be substantially reduced by concomitant mixed antiepileptic therapy that included *phenytoin*.[1,2] The mean diuretic effect of frusemide [furosemide] 20 mg or 40 mg by mouth in patients on such therapy was 68% and 51% that of healthy controls respectively.[1]

For the effect of frusemide [furosemide] on *phenobarbital*, see p.356.

Symptomatic hyponatraemia has been associated with the concomitant use of frusemide [furosemide] or hydrochlorothiazide with *carbamazepine*.[3]

1. Ahmad S. Renal insensitivity to frusemide caused by chronic anticonvulsant therapy. *BMJ* 1974; **3:** 657–9.
2. Fine A, *et al.* Malabsorption of frusemide caused by phenytoin. *BMJ* 1977; **2:** 1061–2.
3. Yassa R, *et al.* Carbamazepine, diuretics, and hyponatremia: a possible interaction. *J Clin Psychiatry* 1987; **48:** 281–3.

Diuretics. Severe electrolyte disturbances may occur in patients given *metolazone* concurrently with frusemide [furosemide].

Hypnotics. A syndrome of flushing, tachycardia, elevated blood pressure, and severe diaphoresis was reported following intravenous administration of frusemide [furosemide] to 6 patients who had received *cloral hydrate* orally during the preceding 24 hours.[1] The reaction recurred in 1 patient on a subsequent occasion when given both drugs but not when frusemide [furosemide] was administered without cloral hydrate. A subsequent retrospective study[2] among 43 patients who had received both cloral hydrate and frusemide [furosemide] showed that 1 patient had suffered a similar reaction; of 2 further patients who had possibly been affected, 1 had subsequently taken both drugs without adverse effects. A similar interaction has been reported in an 8-year-old child.[3]

1. Malach M, Berman N. Furosemide and chloral hydrate: adverse drug interaction. *JAMA* 1975; **232:** 638–9.
2. Pevonka MP, *et al.* Interaction of chloral hydrate and furosemide: a controlled retrospective study. *Drug Intell Clin Pharm* 1977; **11:** 332–5.
3. Dean RP, *et al.* Interaction of chloral hydrate and intravenous furosemide in a child. *Clin Pharm* 1991; **10:** 385–7.

Lithium. For reports of a possible increase in plasma-lithium concentrations in patients receiving loop diuretics, see p.295.

NSAIDs. NSAIDs may antagonise the diuretic effect of frusemide [furosemide] and other diuretics.[1] Use of NSAIDs with diuretics may increase the risk of nephrotoxicity, although it has also been suggested that frusemide [furosemide] may protect against the renal effects of *indometacin* in infants (see Effects in Infants and Neonates, above).

1. Webster J. Interactions of NSAIDs with diuretics and β-blockers: mechanisms and clinical implications. *Drugs* 1985; **30:** 32–41.

Probenecid. Probenecid has been shown[1-4] to reduce the renal clearance of frusemide [furosemide], and to reduce the diuretic effect.[2,3]

1. Honari J, *et al.* Effects of probenecid on furosemide kinetics and natriuresis in man. *Clin Pharmacol Ther* 1977; **22:** 395–401.
2. Odlind B, Beermann B. Renal tubular secretion and effects of furosemide. *Clin Pharmacol Ther* 1980; **27:** 784–90.
3. Smith DE, *et al.* Preliminary evaluation of furosemide-probenecid interaction in humans. *J Pharm Sci* 1980; **69:** 571–5.
4. Vree TB, *et al.* Probenecid inhibits the renal clearance of frusemide and its acyl glucuronide. *Br J Clin Pharmacol* 1995; **39:** 692–5.

Tobacco. The effects of tobacco smoking on the pharmacokinetics of frusemide [furosemide] have been reviewed.[1,2] Nicotine inhibits diuresis and diminishes the diuretic effect of frusemide [furosemide]. However, this effect is attenuated in habitual smokers.

1. Miller LG. Recent developments in the study of the effects of cigarette smoking on clinical pharmacokinetics and clinical pharmacodynamics. *Clin Pharmacokinet* 1989; **17:** 90–108.
2. Miller LG. Cigarettes and drug therapy: pharmacokinetic and pharmacodynamic considerations. *Clin Pharm* 1990; **9:** 125–35.

Xanthines. For the effect of frusemide [furosemide] on *theophylline*, see p.781.

Pharmacokinetics

Frusemide [furosemide] is fairly rapidly absorbed from the gastrointestinal tract; bioavailability has been reported to be about 60 to 70% but absorption is variable and erratic. The half-life of frusemide [furosemide] is up to about 2 hours although it is prolonged in neonates and in patients with renal and he-

patic insufficiency. It is up to 99% bound to plasma albumin, and is mainly excreted in the urine, largely unchanged. There is also some excretion via the bile and non-renal elimination is considerably increased in renal impairment. Frusemide [furosemide] crosses the placental barrier and is distributed into breast milk. The clearance of frusemide [furosemide] is not increased by haemodialysis.

◊ The pharmacokinetics of frusemide [furosemide] have been extensively reviewed.[1-6] The development of an analytical method using HPLC with fluorescence has produced greater sensitivity and more consistent results. Absorption following oral dosing is erratic and is subject to large inter- and intra-individual variation. It is influenced by the dosage form, underlying disease processes, and by the presence of food. Frusemide [furosemide] absorption in patients with heart failure has been reported to be even more erratic than in healthy subjects. The bioavailability of frusemide [furosemide] from oral dosage forms is also highly variable with reported values ranging from 20 to 100%. It is influenced by factors affecting absorption but the poor solubility of frusemide [furosemide] does not appear to have a major influence on bioavailability and *in vitro* dissolution data may not reflect *in vivo* bioavailability. Bioavailability tends to be decreased by about 10% in patients with renal disease, and slightly increased in liver disease. Values are erratic in patients with heart disease.

Frusemide [furosemide] is highly bound to plasma proteins, almost exclusively to albumin. The proportion of free (unbound) frusemide [furosemide] is higher in patients with heart disease, renal impairment, and cirrhosis of the liver. Patients with liver disease also have an increased apparent volume of distribution which is proportionally greater than the observed decrease in protein binding. Patients with nephrotic syndrome have significant proteinuria and secondary hypoalbuminaemia. This results in reduced protein binding in the blood, particularly at higher blood concentrations, and binding to proteins present in the urine, which may account for the resistance to frusemide [furosemide] therapy reported in these patients.

A glucuronide metabolite of frusemide [furosemide] is produced in varying amounts. The site of metabolism is unknown at present. There is debate over another potential metabolite, 4-chloro-5-sulfamoyl anthranilic acid (CSA). It has been argued[3] that it is an artefact produced during the extraction procedures although there is some evidence to refute this.[4]

A half-life for frusemide [furosemide] in healthy subjects has generally been reported in the range of 30 to 120 minutes. In patients with end-stage renal disease the average half-life is 9.7 hours. The half-life may be slightly longer in patients with hepatic dysfunction and a range of 50 to 327 minutes has been reported in patients with heart failure. In severe multi-organ failure the half-life may range from 20 to 24 hours.

Frusemide [furosemide] clearance is influenced by age, underlying disease state, and drug interactions. Clearance reduces with increasing age, probably due to declining renal function. Impaired renal function in renal or cardiac disease reduces renal clearance, although this may be compensated for by increases in non-renal clearance. Hepatic impairment has little impact on clearance. Renal and non-renal clearance may be reduced by probenecid and indometacin.

The effectiveness of frusemide [furosemide] as a diuretic depends upon it reaching its site of action, the renal tubules, unchanged. Approximately one-half to two-thirds of an intravenous dose or one-quarter to one-third of an oral dose are excreted unchanged, the difference being largely due to the poor bioavailability from the oral route. The effect of frusemide [furosemide] is more closely related to its urinary excretion than to the plasma concentration. Urinary excretion may be reduced in renal impairment due to reduced renal blood flow and reduced tubular secretion.

1. Cutler RE, Blair AD. Clinical pharmacokinetics of frusemide. *Clin Pharmacokinet* 1979; **4:** 279–96.
2. Benet LZ. Pharmacokinetics/pharmacodynamics of furosemide in man: a review. *J Pharmacokinet Biopharm* 1979; **7:** 1–27.
3. Hammarlund-Udenaes M, Benet LZ. Furosemide pharmacokinetics and pharmacodynamics in health and disease—an update. *J Pharmacokinet Biopharm* 1989; **17:** 1–46.
4. Ponto LLB, Schoenwald RD. Furosemide (frusemide): a pharmacokinetic/pharmacodynamic review (part I). *Clin Pharmacokinet* 1990; **18:** 381–408.
5. Ponto LLB, Schoenwald RD. Furosemide (frusemide): a pharmacokinetic/pharmacodynamic review (part II). *Clin Pharmacokinet* 1990; **18:** 460–71.
6. Vrhovac B, *et al.* Pharmacokinetic changes in patients with oedema. *Clin Pharmacokinet* 1995; **28:** 405–18.

Infants and neonates. The half-life of frusemide [furosemide] in term and preterm neonates is markedly prolonged compared with that in adults.[1,2] Half-lives of 4.5 to 46 hours have been reported and it has been suggested that the prolongation may be greater in preterm than in term neonates. This effect is due primarily to immature renal function and if repeated doses are necessary over a short period accumulation may occur.[1]

1. Besunder JB, *et al.* Principles of drug biodisposition in the neonate: a critical evaluation of the pharmacokinetic-pharmacodynamic interface (part II). *Clin Pharmacokinet* 1988; **14:** 261–86.
2. Aranda JV, *et al.* Pharmacokinetic disposition and protein binding of furosemide in newborn infants. *J Pediatr* 1978; **93:** 507–11.

Uses and Administration

Frusemide [furosemide] is a potent diuretic with a rapid action. Like the other loop or high-ceiling diuretics it is used in the treatment of oedema associated with heart failure (below), including pulmonary oedema, and with renal and hepatic disorders (but see Precautions, above) and may be effective in patients unresponsive to thiazide diuretics. It is also used in high doses in the management of oliguria due to renal failure or insufficiency. Frusemide [furosemide] is also used in the treatment of hypertension (p.802), either alone or together with other antihypertensives.

Frusemide [furosemide] inhibits the reabsorption of electrolytes primarily in the thick ascending limb of the loop of Henle and also in the distal renal tubules. It may also have a direct effect in the proximal tubules. Excretion of sodium, potassium, calcium, and chloride ions is increased and water excretion enhanced. It has no clinically significant effect on carbonic anhydrase. See Action, below, for further reference to its mechanism of action.

Administration and dosage. Frusemide [furosemide]'s effects are evident within 30 minutes to 1 hour after a dose by mouth, peak at 1 to 2 hours, and last for about 4 to 6 hours; after intravenous injection its effects are evident in about 5 minutes and last for about 2 hours. It is given by mouth, usually in the morning. Alternatively it may be administered intramuscularly or intravenously as the sodium salt; doses are expressed in terms of frusemide [furosemide] base. The manufacturers recommend that whether by direct intravenous injection or by infusion the rate of intravenous administration should not exceed 4 mg per minute although some authorities advise that a single dose of up to 50 mg may be given more rapidly.

Unlike the thiazide diuretics where, owing to their flat dose-response curve, very little is gained by increasing the dose, frusemide [furosemide] has a steep dose-response curve, which gives it a wide therapeutic range.

In the treatment of **oedema**, the usual initial dose is 40 mg once daily by mouth, adjusted as necessary according to response. Mild cases may respond to 20 mg daily or 40 mg on alternate days. Some patients may require doses of 80 mg or more daily given as one or two doses daily, or intermittently. Severe cases may require gradual titration of the frusemide [furosemide] dosage up to 600 mg daily. In an emergency or when oral therapy cannot be given, 20 to 50 mg of frusemide [furosemide] may be administered by intramuscular or slow intravenous injection; if necessary further doses may be given, increasing by 20-mg increments and not given more often than every 2 hours. If doses greater than 50 mg are required they should be given by slow intravenous infusion. For pulmonary oedema, if an initial slow intravenous injection of 40 mg does not produce a satisfactory response within one hour, the dose may be increased to 80 mg given slowly intravenously.

For children, the usual dose by mouth is 1 to 3 mg per kg body-weight daily up to a maximum of 40 mg daily; doses by injection are 0.5 to 1.5 mg per kg daily up to a maximum of 20 mg daily.

In the treatment of **hypertension**, frusemide [furosemide] is given in doses of 40 to 80 mg daily by mouth, either alone, or in conjunction with other antihypertensives.

High-dose therapy. In the management of **oliguria** in acute or chronic renal failure where the glomerular filtration rate is less than 20 mL per minute frusemide [furosemide] 250 mg diluted to 250 mL in a suitable diluent is infused over one hour. If urine output is insufficient within the next hour, this dose may be followed by 500 mg added to an appropriate infusion fluid, the total volume of which must be governed by the patient's state of hydration, and infused over approximately 2 hours. If a satisfactory urine output has still not been achieved within one hour of the end of the second infusion then a third dose of 1 g may be infused over approximately 4 hours. The rate of infusion should never exceed 4 mg per minute. In oliguric patients with significant fluid overload, the injection may be given without dilution directly into the vein, using a constant rate infusion pump with a micrometer screw-gauge adjustment; the rate of administration should still never exceed 4 mg per minute. Patients who do not respond to a dose of 1 g probably require dialysis. If the response to either method of administration is satisfactory, the effective dose (of up to 1 g) may then be repeated every 24 hours. Dosage adjustments should subsequently be made according to the patient's response. Alternatively, treatment may be maintained by mouth; 500 mg should be given by mouth for each 250 mg required by injection.

When used in chronic renal insufficiency, an initial dose of 250 mg may be given by mouth, increased, if necessary in steps of 250 mg every 4 to 6 hours to a maximum of 1.5 g in 24 hours; in exceptional cases up to 2 g in 24 hours may be given. Dosage adjustments should subsequently be made according to the patient's response.

During treatment with these high-dose forms of frusemide [furosemide] therapy, careful laboratory control is essential. Fluid balance and electrolytes should be carefully controlled and, in particular, in patients with shock, measures should be taken to correct the blood pressure and circulating blood volume, before commencing this type of treatment. High-dose frusemide [furosemide] therapy is contra-indicated in renal failure caused by nephrotoxic or hepatotoxic drugs, and in renal failure associated with hepatic coma.

Action. The mechanism of action of frusemide [furosemide] is not fully understood.[1] It appears to act primarily by inhibiting active reabsorption of chloride ions in the ascending limb of the loop of Henle. Urinary excretion of sodium, chloride, potassium, hydrogen, calcium, magnesium, ammonium, bicarbonate, and possibly phosphate is increased; the chloride excretion exceeds that of sodium and there is an enhanced exchange of sodium for potassium leading to greater excretion of potassium. The resulting low osmolality of the medulla inhibits the reabsorption of water by the kidney. There is a possibility that frusemide [furosemide] may also act at a more proximal site.

In addition to its diuretic actions, frusemide [furosemide] has been shown to increase peripheral venous capacitance and reduce forearm blood flow. It also reduces renal vascular resistance with a resultant increase in renal blood flow the degree of which is proportional to the renal interstitial resistance.

Frusemide [furosemide] administration has been shown to increase plasma-renin activity, plasma-noradrenaline concentrations, and plasma-arginine-vasopressin concentrations. Alterations in the renin-angiotensin-aldosterone system may play a part in the development of acute tolerance. Frusemide [furosemide] increases renal-prostaglandin concentrations but it is not known whether this is due to increased synthesis or inhibition of degradation or both. Prostaglandins appear to mediate the diuretic/natriuretic action. The primary effects appear to be alterations in renal haemodynamics with subsequent increases in electrolyte and fluid excretion.

The diuretic response to frusemide [furosemide] is related to the concentration in the urine, not to that in the plasma. Frusemide [furosemide] is delivered to the renal tubules by a nonspecific organic acid pump in the proximal tubules.[1]

In some cases sodium intake may be sufficient to overcome the diuretic effect, and limiting sodium intake could restore responsiveness.[2]

1. Ponto LLB, Schaenwald RD. Furosemide (frusemide): a pharmacokinetic/pharmacodynamic review (part I). *Clin Pharmacokinet* 1990; **18**: 381–408.
2. Brater DC. Resistance to loop diuretics: why it happens and what to do about it. *Drugs* 1985; **30**: 427–43.

Administration. Continuous intravenous infusion of loop diuretics may be more effective than intermittent intravenous bolus injection and may provide a more consistent urine flow with fewer alterations in urine balance.[1] Bumetanide was more effective by continuous infusion than by bolus administration in 8 patients with severe chronic renal insufficiency.[2] In 20 patients with chronic heart failure requiring high-dose frusemide [furosemide] therapy, frusemide [furosemide] given by continuous infusion was more effective than the same dose by bolus injection.[3] The lower plasma concentrations associated with continuous infusion may also reduce the risk of toxicity.

1. Yelton SL, *et al.* The role of continuous infusion loop diuretics. *Ann Pharmacother* 1995; **29**: 1010–14.

2. Rudy DW, *et al.* Loop diuretics for chronic renal insufficiency: a continuous infusion is more efficacious than bolus therapy. *Ann Intern Med* 1991; **115**: 360–6.
3. Dormans TPJ, *et al.* Diuretic efficacy of high dose furosemide in severe heart failure: bolus injection versus continuous infusion. *J Am Coll Cardiol* 1996; **28**: 376–82.

Ascites. Dietary sodium restriction and diuretics are mainstays of the management of cirrhotic ascites (p.793). Spironolactone is usually the diuretic of first choice, but frusemide [furosemide] may be added to therapy as necessary.

Asthma. Frusemide [furosemide] administered by oral inhalation has been found to protect against bronchoconstriction induced by exercise[1] and external stimuli,[2,3] but was not effective in improving bronchial hyperresponsiveness in a 4-week study.[4] A number of mechanisms have been suggested, including inhibition of electrolyte transport across epithelium, inhibition of inflammatory mediators, or an effect on mast cell function.[5] The potential for clinical applications remains unclear[5] and frusemide [furosemide] is not a part of the accepted schedules for the treatment of asthma (p.757).

1. Munyard P, *et al.* Inhaled frusemide and exercise-induced bronchoconstriction in children with asthma. *Thorax* 1995; **50**: 677–9.
2. Bianco S, *et al.* Protective effect of inhaled furosemide on allergen-induced early and late asthmatic reactions. *N Engl J Med* 1989; **321**: 1069–73.
3. Seidenberg J, *et al.* Inhaled furosemide against cold air induced bronchoconstriction in asthmatic children. *Arch Dis Child* 1992; **67**: 214–17.
4. Yates DH, *et al.* Effect of acute and chronic inhaled furosemide on bronchial hyperresponsiveness in mild asthma. *Am J Respir Crit Care Med* 1995; **152**: 2173–5.
5. Floreani AA, Rennard SI. Experimental treatments for asthma. *Curr Opin Pulm Med* 1997; **3**: 30–41.

Bronchopulmonary dysplasia. Bronchopulmonary dysplasia is a major cause of chronic lung disease in infants. Treatment often involves the use of corticosteroids (see p.1048). Additional supportive therapy may include the use of diuretics such as frusemide [furosemide].

Alternate-day therapy with frusemide [furosemide] 4 mg per kg by mouth has produced modest benefits in pulmonary status in the absence of a diuretic effect, and few adverse effects.[1] Improved pulmonary function has occurred in infants given frusemide [furosemide] 1 mg per kg parenterally following packed red blood cell transfusions, given to improve oxygen-carrying capacity.[2] The successful use of nebulised frusemide [furosemide] in a dose of 1 mg per kg body-weight has been reported;[3,4] again pulmonary status was improved without production of diuresis or renal side-effects. However, a single inhaled dose of 1 mg per kg failed to improve pulmonary mechanics in another study involving older infants with more severe disease.[5]

1. Rush MG, *et al.* Double-blind, placebo-controlled trial of alternate-day furosemide therapy in infants with chronic bronchopulmonary dysplasia. *J Pediatr* 1990; **117**: 112–18.
2. Stefano JL, Bhutani VK. Role of furosemide therapy after booster-packed erythrocyte transfusions in infants with bronchopulmonary dysplasia. *J Pediatr* 1990; **117**: 965–8.
3. Rastogi A, *et al.* Nebulized furosemide in infants with bronchopulmonary dysplasia. *J Pediatr* 1994; **125**: 976–9.
4. Prabhu VG, *et al.* Pulmonary function changes after nebulised and intravenous frusemide in ventilated premature infants. *Arch Dis Child* 1997; **77**: F32–F35.
5. Kugelman A, *et al.* Pulmonary effect of inhaled furosemide in ventilated infants with severe bronchopulmonary dysplasia. *Pediatrics* 1997; **99**: 71–5.

Haemolytic uraemic syndrome. Renal failure is a possible consequence of the haemolytic-uraemic syndrome (see under Thrombotic Microangiopathies, p.740). Correction of any hypovolaemic state with adequate fluids and of oliguria by inducing diuresis with frusemide [furosemide] may be used to prevent it.

Of 54 children with haemolytic-uraemic syndrome given intravenous frusemide [furosemide] 2.5 to 4 mg per kg body-weight every 3 to 4 hours immediately after diagnosis 24% eventually required dialysis.[1] In contrast, a retrospective analysis of 39 patients treated conservatively showed that 82% had required dialysis. The results therefore suggested that high-dose frusemide [furosemide] could prevent the progression of oliguria to anuria in these patients by increasing urate clearance.

1. Rousseau E, *et al.* Decreased necessity for dialysis with loop diuretic therapy in hemolytic uremic syndrome. *Clin Nephrol* 1990; **34**: 22–5.

Heart failure. Diuretics have been the mainstay in the treatment of heart failure (p.798) but drugs such as ACE inhibitors that have been shown to improve mortality are now generally recommended for first-line therapy along with diuretics. Diuretics provide very effective symptomatic control in patients with peripheral or pulmonary oedema and rapidly relieve dyspnoea. If symptoms of fluid retention are only mild, a thiazide diuretic such as bendrofluazide [bendroflumethiazide] or hydrochlorothiazide, may be adequate. However, in most cases, especially in moderate or severe fluid retention, a loop diuretic such as frusemide [furosemide] will be necessary. Combination treatment with diuretics that behave synergistically by acting at different sites (the principle of sequential nephron blockade), namely a loop diuretic with a thiazide or potassium-sparing diuretic, may be needed in some patients, especially when there is diuretic resistance.

Patients have been successfully treated using continuous intravenous infusions[1] or high doses (up to 8 g daily) of frusemide [furosemide] given by intravenous infusion[2,3] or by mouth.[3] A patient who was successfully maintained on intravenous fruse-mide [furosemide] at home has been described.[4] Combination of frusemide [furosemide] with thiazide diuretics[5] or metolazone[6,7] has been reported. There is a danger of overdiuresis with both of these strategies, and careful monitoring of electrolytes and renal function is essential.[8] Delivery of fruse-mide [furosemide] to the renal tubules may be enhanced by combined therapy with hydralazine[9] or captopril.[10] The use of captopril and frusemide [furosemide] may also correct hyponatraemia without fluid restriction.[11] In elderly patients not responding adequately to low-dose frusemide [furosemide] together with optimum doses of ACE inhibitors, increasing the dose of frusemide [furosemide] (to an average of 297 mg daily by mouth) has been reported[12] to be of benefit. However, caution is necessary when administering frusemide [furosemide] with antihypertensives and especially ACE inhibitors since these combinations can result in sudden and profound hypotension and renal toxicity. Low-dose dopamine infusion has been suggested as an alternative to high-dose frusemide [furosemide] infusion and may cause less toxicity. In a study[13] in patients with severe refractory heart failure receiving optimal therapy with ACE inhibitors, oral diuretics, nitrates, and digoxin, additional therapy with low-dose intravenous dopamine (4 μg per kg body-weight per minute) and low-dose oral fruse-mide [furosemide] (80 mg daily) was as effective as intravenous high-dose frusemide [furosemide] (10 mg per kg daily) but caused less hypokalaemia and renal impairment.

1. Lawson DH, et al. Continuous infusion of frusemide in refractory oedema. BMJ 1978; 2: 476.
2. O'Rourke MF, et al. High-dose furosemide in cardiac failure. Arch Intern Med 1984; 144: 2429.
3. Gerlag PGG, van Meijel JJM. High-dose furosemide in the treatment of refractory congestive heart failure. Arch Intern Med 1988; 148: 286–91.
4. Hattersley AT, et al. Home intravenous diuretic therapy for patient with refractory heart failure. Lancet 1989; i: 446.
5. Channer KS, et al. Thiazides with loop diuretics for severe congestive heart failure. Lancet 1990; 335: 922–3.
6. Aravot DJ, et al. Oral metolazone plus frusemide for home therapy in patients with refractory heart failure. Lancet 1989; i: 727.
7. Friedland JS, Ledingham JGG. Oral metolazone plus frusemide for home therapy in patients with refractory heart failure. Lancet 1989; i: 727–8.
8. Oster JR, et al. Combined therapy with thiazide-type and loop diuretic agents for resistant-sodium retention. Ann Intern Med 1983; 99: 405–6.
9. Nomura A, et al. Effect of furosemide in congestive heart failure. Clin Pharmacol Ther 1981; 30: 177–82.
10. Dzau VJ, Hollenberg NK. Renal response to captopril in severe heart failure: role of furosemide in natriuresis and reversal of hyponatraemia. Ann Intern Med 1984; 100: 777–82.
11. Hamilton RW, Buckalew VM. Sodium, water, and congestive heart failure. Ann Intern Med 1984; 100: 902–4.
12. Waterer G, Donaldson M. High-dose frusemide for cardiac failure. Lancet 1995; 346: 254.
13. Cotter G, et al. Increased toxicity of high-dose furosemide versus low-dose dopamine in the treatment of refractory congestive heart failure. Clin Pharmacol Ther 1997; 62: 187–93.

Hypercalcaemia. Hypercalcaemia (p.1181) usually results from an underlying disease and long-term management involves treating the cause. However, if significant symptoms are present, treatment is necessary to reduce plasma-calcium concentrations. This primarily involves rehydration, but loop diuretics such as frusemide [furosemide] have been used following rehydration to promote urinary calcium excretion.

Patent ductus arteriosus. The usual initial treatment for a haemodynamically significant ductus is reduction of fluid intake, correction of anaemia, support of respiration, and the administration of a diuretic. If that fails to control symptoms then indometacin is generally given to promote closure of the ductus (see p.46).

Frusemide [furosemide] is often chosen as the diuretic. It is effective and widely used but there has been concern that it may promote delayed ductus closure (see Effects in Infants and Neonates under Adverse Effects, above). However, the concurrent use of frusemide [furosemide] does not seem to inhibit duct closure during treatment with indometacin and may reduce adverse renal effects of indometacin, although the evidence for this is limited.[1]

1. Brion LP, Campbell DE. Furosemide for symptomatic patent ductus arteriosus in indomethacin-treated infants (updated 13 February 2001). Available in The Cochrane Library; Issue 2. Oxford: Update Software, 2001.

Raised intracranial pressure. Osmotic diuretics such as mannitol are first-line drugs for the management of raised intracranial pressure (p.811) but loop diuretics such as frusemide [furosemide] may be employed as adjuncts.

Tinnitus. Frusemide [furosemide] is one of many drugs that have been tried in tinnitus (p.1316), but although reported to be effective in some patients, it is rarely used because of problems with adverse effects.

Preparations

BP 2001: Co-amilofruse Tablets; Furosemide Injection; Furosemide Tablets;
USP 25: Furosemide Injection; Furosemide Oral Solution; Furosemide Tablets.

Proprietary Preparations (details are given in Part 3)
Aust.: Furohexal; Furon; Furostad; Furotyrol; Lasix; *Austral.:* Frusehexal; Frusid; Lasix; Uremide; Urex; *Belg.:* Lasix; *Braz.:* Diurex; Furosemida; Lasix; *Canad.:* Lasix; Novo-Semide†; *Denm.:* Diural; Furese; Furix; Furonet†; Impugan†; Lasix; *Fin.:* Furesis; Furomin; Lasix; Vesix; *Fr.:* Lasilix; *Ger.:* Diurapid; du-

rafurid; Furanthril; Furo; Furo-BASF; Furo-Puren; Furobeta; Furomed; Furorese; Furosal; Fusid; Hydro-rapid; Lasix; Odemase; Sigasalur; *Hong Kong:* Dryptal; Frusid; Lasix; Urex; *Irl.:* Dryptal†; Lasix; *Israel:* Furovite; Fusid; Lasix; Miphar; *Ital.:* Lasix; *Mex.:* Diurolan; Edenol; Frudemisan; Furmidal; Furomil; Furonex; Furosan; Furoter; Golan; Henexal; Hidrasal; Lasix; Osemin; Selectofur; Yuremid; Zafimida; *Neth.:* Fusid†; Lasiletten; Lasix; *Norw.:* Diural; Furix; Lasix; *NZ:* Diurin; Frusid; Lasix; *Port.:* Aquedux; Lasix; *S.Afr.:* Aquarid; Arcanamide†; Beurises; Hydrex; Lasix; Puresis; Uremide; *Singapore:* Dirine; Frusid; Lasix; *Spain:* Seguril; *Swed.:* Furix; Furoscand†; Impugan; Lasix; *Switz.:* Diuresal; Diurix; furo-basan; Furodrix; Furosifar; Furosel; Impugan; Lasix; Oedemex; *Thai.:* Aldic; Dirine; Frusid; Fudirine; Furetic; Furide; H-Mide; Hawkmide; Impugan; Lasix; Mediuresix; Urasin; *UAE:* Salurin; *UK:* Dryptal†; Froop; Frumax†; Frusid; Frusol; Lasix; Rusyde; Tenkafruse; *USA:* Lasix.

Multi-ingredient: *Aust.:* Furo-Aldopur; Furo-Spirobene; Furolacton; Hydrotrix; Lasilacton; Lasitace; Normotenoric; Spirono comp; Terbolan†; *Belg.:* Frusamil; *Braz.:* Diurana; Diurisa; Furosemida Composta; Hidrion; Lasilactona; Terbolan; *Denm.:* Frusamil; *Fin.:* Furesis comp; *Fr.:* Aldalix; Logirene; *Ger.:* Betasemid; Diaphal; duraspiron-comp; Furesis comp; Furo-Aldopur; Furorese Comp; Hydrotrix; Osyrol Lasix; Spiro comp; Spiro-D; Spironolacton Plus; *Hong Kong:* Frumil; *Irl.:* Diumide-K Continus; Fru-Co; Frumil; Frusene†; Lasikal†; Lasoride; *Ital.:* Fluss 40; Lasitone; Spirofur; *Mex.:* Lasilacton; *Neth.:* Elkin; *NZ:* Frumil; *Spain:* Salidur; *Switz.:* Frumil; Furosemid comp†; Furospir; Hydrotrix; Lasilactone; *UK:* Aridil; Diumide-K Continus; Froop Co; Fru-Co; Frumil; Frusemek; Frusene; Lasikal; Lasilactone; Lasix + K†; Lasoride.

Gallopamil Hydrochloride (16819-g)

Gallopamil Hydrochloride (BANM, rINNM).
D-600 (gallopamil); Methoxyverapamil Hydrochloride. 5-[N-(3,4-Dimethoxyphenethyl)-N-methylamino]-2-(3,4,5-trimethoxyphenyl)-2-isopropylvaleronitrile hydrochloride.
$C_{28}H_{40}N_2O_5,HCl = 521.1$.
CAS — 16662-47-8 (gallopamil); 16662-46-7 (gallopamil hydrochloride).

Profile
Gallopamil is a calcium-channel blocker (see p.788) with antiarrhythmic activity and is chemically related to verapamil. It is used in the management of angina pectoris (below), cardiac arrhythmias (p.794), and hypertension (p.802). Gallopamil hydrochloride is given by mouth in doses of 25 to 50 mg every 6 to 12 hours up to a maximum total dose of 200 mg daily.

◊ General references.
1. Brogden RN, Benfield P. Gallopamil: a review of its pharmacodynamic and pharmacokinetic properties, and therapeutic potential in ischaemic heart disease. Drugs 1994; 47: 93–115.

Angina pectoris. Gallopamil has been reported[1] to improve subjective and objective symptoms of angina pectoris (p.791) without causing severe adverse effects. The most frequently used dosage was gallopamil 50 mg two or three times daily, and full effectiveness was usually reached 4 weeks after the start of therapy. Therapeutic success was defined as good in 73% of cases. The most frequent adverse effects were gastric discomfort, bradycardia, and atrioventricular prolongation; therapy was discontinued in 4 patients due to cardiac adverse reactions.

Gallopamil has also been reported[2] to increase the anti-ischaemic effect of isosorbide mononitrate in patients with angina.

1. Sućić M, Schiemann J. Multizentrische gallopamil-langzeitstudie bei patienten mit koronarer herzkrankheit. Arzneimittelforschung 1984; 34: 1587–94.
2. Stauch M, et al. Lack of tolerance after chronic administration of controlled-release isosorbide-5-mononitrate: interaction of nitrate and gallopamil. Eur J Clin Pharmacol 1990; 38 (suppl 1): S31–4.

Pharmacokinetics. A single-dose study of intravenous and oral gallopamil hydrochloride in healthy subjects indicated that the drug was almost completely metabolised, only a very small amount being excreted as unchanged drug.[1] Approximately equal amounts were excreted in urine and faeces, mainly as conjugated metabolites.
1. Weymann J, et al. Metabolism of the calcium antagonist gallopamil in man. Arzneimittelforschung 1989; 39: 605–7.

Preparations

Proprietary Preparations (details are given in Part 3)
Aust.: Procorum; *Ger.:* Gallobeta; Procorum; *Ital.:* Algocor; Procorum; *Mex.:* Procorum; *Thai.:* Procorum.

Gemfibrozil (1349-v)

Gemfibrozil (BAN, USAN, rINN).
CI-719. 2,2-Dimethyl-5-(2,5-xylyloxy)valeric acid.
$C_{15}H_{22}O_3 = 250.3$.
CAS — 25812-30-0.
ATC — C10AB04.

Pharmacopoeias. In Br. and US.

Pharmacopoeial description
BP 2001: A white or almost white, slightly waxy, crystalline solid. M.p. 58° to 61°. Practically insoluble in water; freely soluble in methyl alcohol. Protect from light.

USP 25: A white waxy crystalline solid. M.p. 58° to 61°. Practically insoluble in water; soluble in alcohol, in methyl alcohol, and in chloroform. Store in airtight containers.

Adverse Effects and Precautions
As for Bezafibrate, p.849.

◊ In the Helsinki Heart Study,[1] 11.3% of 2051 patients taking gemfibrozil reported various moderate to severe upper gastrointestinal tract symptoms during the first year of treatment compared with 7% of 2030 patients taking placebo. No differences were seen between gemfibrozil and placebo groups in haemoglobin concentrations, urinary-protein, or urinary-sugar concentrations.

There was no significant difference in the total number of cancers between the gemfibrozil and placebo groups nor in the number of operations for gallstones or for cataract surgery. A higher number of deaths in the gemfibrozil group was mainly due to accident or violence and intracranial haemorrhage.

A follow-up study[2] reported that gastrointestinal symptoms remained more common in patients taking gemfibrozil. Although there was no significant difference between the gemfibrozil and placebo groups cholecystectomies were consistently more common in those receiving gemfibrozil during the entire 8.5-year observation period. Cancer occurred equally in both groups, but there was increased mortality attributable to cancer in the gemfibrozil group, mainly during the last 1.5 years of follow-up.

1. Frick MH, et al. Helsinki Heart Study: primary-prevention trial with gemfibrozil in middle-aged men with dyslipidemia: safety of treatment, changes in risk factors, and incidence of coronary heart disease. N Engl J Med 1987; 317: 1237–45.
2. Huttunen JK, et al. The Helsinki Heart Study: an 8.5-year safety and mortality follow-up. J Intern Med 1994; 235: 31–9.

Effects on glucose metabolism. There have been conflicting reports of the effects of gemfibrozil on glucose metabolism in hyperlipidaemic diabetic patients. In a study of 14 diabetic patients[1] treated with gemfibrozil for 9 to 23 weeks control of diabetes was not generally impaired and appeared in some cases to be slightly improved. Another study in 20 patients[2] reported a slight increase in antidiabetic therapy requirements in 9 and a decrease in 1. A decrease in fasting and oral glucose tolerance test-stimulated glucose concentrations has been noted[3] in patients with impaired glucose tolerance but not in those with normal glucose tolerance. No reduction in insulin secretion was noted. Two other studies[4,5] found no clinically significant changes in glucose metabolism in stable diabetics taking gemfibrozil. In another,[6] gemfibrozil was associated with decreased hyperglycaemia in diabetics whose blood-glucose concentrations were not well controlled.

1. de Salcedo I, et al. Gemfibrozil in a group of diabetics. Proc R Soc Med 1976; 69 (suppl 2): 64–70.
2. Konttinen A, et al. The effect of gemfibrozil on serum lipids in diabetic patients. Ann Clin Res 1979; 11: 240–5.
3. Testori GP, et al. Effect of gemfibrozil treatment on glucose tolerance in hypertriglyceridemic patients with normal or impaired glucose tolerance. Curr Ther Res 1990; 47: 390–5.
4. Leaf DA, et al. The hypolipidemic effects of gemfibrozil in type V hyperlipidemia. JAMA 1989; 262: 3154–60.
5. Pagani A, et al. Effect of short-term gemfibrozil administration on glucose metabolism and insulin secretion in non-insulin-dependent diabetics. Curr Ther Res 1989; 45: 14–20.
6. Notarbartolo A, et al. Effects of gemfibrozil in hyperlipidemic patients with or without diabetes. Curr Ther Res 1993; 53: 381–93.

Effects on the nervous system. The Adverse Drug Reactions Advisory Committee in Australia has received reports of paraesthesia occurring in 6 patients in association with gemfibrozil treatment.[1]
1. Anonymous. Paraesthesia and neuropathy with hypolipidaemic agents. Aust Adverse Drug React Bull 1991; 12: 6.

Effects on sexual function. Impotence and loss of libido has been reported in 3 patients[1-3] during gemfibrozil treatment. In 2 of the men[1,2] bezafibrate did not produce this adverse effect. The UK Committee on Safety of Medicines was reported to be aware of a further 6 cases.[2] Of a further 3 cases of impotence associated with gemfibrozil reported from Spain, one patient had previously reacted similarly to clofibrate.[4]
1. Pizarro S, et al. Gemfibrozil-induced impotence. Lancet 1990; 336: 1135.
2. Bain SC, et al. Gemfibrozil-induced impotence. Lancet 1990; 336: 1389.
3. Bharani A. Sexual dysfunction after gemfibrozil BMJ 1992; 305: 693.
4. Figueras A, et al. Gemfibrozil-induced impotence. Ann Pharmacother 1993; 27: 982.

Effects on skeletal muscle. For reports of rhabdomyolysis in patients taking gemfibrozil with lovastatin, and with cerivastatin, see p.923 and p.856, respectively.

Effects on the skin. Psoriasis was exacerbated in a patient within 2 weeks of starting gemfibrozil therapy and recurred when gemfibrozil was subsequently reintroduced.[1]
1. Fisher DA, et al. Exacerbation of psoriasis by the hypolipidemic agent. Arch Dermatol 1988; 124: 854–5.

Gallstones. Gemfibrozil increased the concentration of cholesterol in bile and decreased the output of bile acids in 8 normolipaemic male subjects.[1] This resulted in an increase in the lithogenic index in both gallbladder and hepatic bile, although no cholesterol crystals were detected in gallbladder bile. In the Helsinki Heart Study[2] no significant increase in gallstone operations was reported among 2051 patients taking gemfibrozil compared with 2030 taking placebo. However, a follow-up study[3] reported that cholecystectomies were consistently more common in those receiving gemfibrozil during the entire 8.5-year observation period, suggesting that gemfibrozil is lithogenic like other fibric acid derivatives.

1. Leiss O, et al. Effect of gemfibrozil on biliary lipid metabolism in normolipemic subjects. Metabolism 1985; 34: 74–82.
2. Frick MH, et al. Helsinki Heart Study: primary-prevention trial with gemfibrozil in middle-aged men with dyslipidemia: safety of treatment, changes in risk factors, and incidence of coronary heart disease. N Engl J Med 1987; 317: 1237–45.
3. Huttunen JK, et al. The Helsinki Heart Study: an 8.5-year safety and mortality follow-up. J Intern Med 1994; 235: 31–9.

Headache. Headaches occurred 30 to 90 minutes after each dose of gemfibrozil in 2 patients.[1,2] In both patients, the headaches were accompanied by dry mouth, and in 1 also by blurred vision. The headaches stopped when gemfibrozil was withdrawn and recurred one week after re-exposure.

1. Arellano F, et al. Gemfibrozil-induced headache. Lancet 1988; i: 705.
2. Alvarez-Sabin J, et al. Gemfibrozil-induced headache. Lancet 1988; ii: 1246.

Interactions

As for Bezafibrate, p.849.

Antidiabetics. For mention of the effect, in some patients, of gemfibrozil on antidiabetic therapy requirement, see Effects on Glucose Metabolism, above.

Lipid regulating drugs. The bioavailability of gemfibrozil was reduced by the concomitant administration of colestipol, but was unaffected when gemfibrozil was taken either 2 hours before or 2 hours after colestipol.[1]

For reports of rhabdomyolysis in patients taking gemfibrozil with cerivastatin or lovastatin, see Effects on Skeletal Muscle, under Cerivastatin, p.856 and under Lovastatin, p.923.

1. Forland SC, et al. Apparent reduced absorption of gemfibrozil when given with colestipol. J Clin Pharmacol 1990; 30: 29–32.

Pharmacokinetics

Gemfibrozil is readily absorbed from the gastrointestinal tract; peak concentrations in plasma occur within 1 to 2 hours; the half-life is about 1.5 hours. Plasma protein binding of gemfibrozil is about 98%. About 70% of a dose is excreted in the urine mainly as glucuronide conjugates of gemfibrozil and its metabolites; little is excreted in the faeces.

Uses and Administration

Gemfibrozil, a fibric acid derivative, is a lipid regulating drug with actions on plasma lipids similar to those of bezafibrate (p.849).

It is used in the treatment of type IIa, type IIb, type III, type IV, and type V hyperlipoproteinaemias. It is also indicated for the primary prevention of ischaemic heart disease in hyperlipidaemic middle-aged men who have not responded to dietary and other measures: in the USA this use is restricted to type IIb patients who also have low HDL-cholesterol concentrations. The usual dose, by mouth, is 1.2 g daily in 2 divided doses given 30 minutes before the morning and evening meals. The dosage range may vary between 0.9 and 1.5 g daily.

◊ Reviews.
1. Todd PA, Ward A. Gemfibrozil: a review of its pharmacodynamic and pharmacokinetic properties, and therapeutic use in dyslipidaemia. Drugs 1988; 36: 314–39.
2. Spencer CM, Barradell LB. Gemfibrozil: a reappraisal of its pharmacological properties and place in the management of dyslipidaemia. Drugs 1996; 51: 982–1018.

Administration in renal impairment. Although in the USA gemfibrozil is not recommended in patients with severe renal impairment, the UK manufacturer suggests that patients with renal impairment could be given a starting dose of 900 mg daily, adjusted according to response.

In a study[1] of the pharmacokinetics of gemfibrozil in 17 patients with stable chronic renal failure the mean plasma half-life was 1.8 and 1.9 hours after multiple and single doses respectively, which was comparable with that reported in patients with normal renal function. Gemfibrozil clearance was independent of renal function, but the kinetics of gemfibrozil metabolites were not evaluated.

Beneficial responses[2] were seen in lipid and lipoprotein concentrations in 5 of 6 uraemic patients treated with gemfibrozil 1200 mg daily for six months and in 6 nephrotic patients given gemfibrozil 800 mg daily for 4 months. No significant adverse effects or signs of organ toxicity were seen.

1. Evans JR, et al. The effect of renal function on the pharmacokinetics of gemfibrozil. J Clin Pharmacol 1987; 27: 994–1000.
2. Manninen V, et al. Gemfibrozil treatment of dyslipidaemias in renal failure with uraemia or in the nephrotic syndrome. Res Clin Forums 1982; 4: 113–18.

Hyperlipidaemias. Gemfibrozil is classified as a fibric acid derivative and is used in the treatment of hyperlipidaemias (p.800). It has effects on plasma-lipid concentrations similar to those described under bezafibrate (p.849). The major effects of gemfibrozil have been a reduction in plasma-triglyceride concentrations and an increase in high-density lipoprotein (HDL)-cholesterol concentrations. A reduction in very-low-density lipoprotein (VLDL)-triglyceride appears to be largely responsible for the fall in plasma triglyceride, although reductions in HDL- and low-density lipoprotein (LDL)-triglycerides have also been reported.[1-3] The effect of gemfibrozil on total cholesterol has been more variable. In general LDL-cholesterol may be decreased in patients with pre-existing high concentrations and raised in those with low concentrations.[1,2,4] The increase in HDL-cholesterol concentrations has resulted in favourable changes to the ratios of HDL-cholesterol to LDL-cholesterol and to total cholesterol.[4,5] Gemfibrozil has successfully raised HDL-cholesterol concentrations in patients with isolated low levels of HDL-cholesterol, but otherwise normal cholesterol concentrations.[6]

The Helsinki Heart Study[7] assessed gemfibrozil for the primary prevention of **ischaemic heart disease** in middle-aged men with hyperlipidaemia. In this study 4081 middle-aged men with raised serum concentrations of non-HDL cholesterol (Fredrickson type IIa, type IIb, and type IV hyperlipoproteinaemias) but with no coronary symptoms were randomly assigned to gemfibrozil 600 mg or placebo twice daily for 5 years; 2859 subjects completed the study, but all subjects initially randomised were followed for 5 years and included in the analysis. There was an overall reduction of 34% in the incidence of fatal and non-fatal myocardial infarctions and cardiac deaths in the gemfibrozil group compared with the placebo group, with the greatest reduction seen during years 3 to 5. On conclusion of this 5-year controlled study all participants were offered gemfibrozil with follow-up for a further 3.5 years.[8] Direct comparison with a placebo group was thus not possible, but long-term treatment with gemfibrozil seemed to postpone coronary events for about 5 years. Effects on safety and mortality were reported separately (see under Adverse Effects and Precautions, above).

The Veterans Affairs High-Density Lipoprotein Cholesterol Intervention Trial (VA-HIT)[9] assessed gemfibrozil for the secondary prevention of ischaemic heart disease in older men (mean age 64 years) whose primary lipid abnormality was a low HDL-cholesterol level. In this study 2531 men with low levels of HDL-, LDL-, and total cholesterol, and moderate levels of triglycerides were randomly assigned to gemfibrozil 1200 mg or placebo daily, with a median follow-up of 5 years. Gemfibrozil significantly increased HDL-cholesterol levels, and reduced total cholesterol and triglyceride levels; LDL-cholesterol levels were not affected. There was an overall reduction of 22% in the incidence of fatal and non-fatal myocardial infarctions and cardiac deaths in the gemfibrozil group compared with the placebo group, with the beneficial effects of gemfibrozil becoming apparent about 2 years after randomisation.

1. Olsson AG, et al. Effect of gemfibrozil on lipoprotein concentrations in different types of hyperlipoproteinaemia. Proc R Soc Med 1976; 69 (suppl 2): 28–31.
2. Nikkilä EA, et al. Gemfibrozil: effect on serum lipids, lipoproteins, postheparin plasma lipase activities and glucose tolerance in primary hypertriglyceridaemia. Proc R Soc Med 1976; 69 (suppl 2): 58–63.
3. Kesäniemi YA, Grundy SM. Influence of gemfibrozil and clofibrate on metabolism of cholesterol and plasma triglycerides in man. JAMA 1984; 251: 2241–6.
4. Manninen V, et al. Lipid alterations and decline in the incidence of coronary heart disease in the Helsinki Heart Study. JAMA 1988; 260: 641–51.
5. Lewis JE, Multicenter Collaborative Study Group. Clinical use of gemfibrozil: a controlled multicenter trial. Pract Cardiol 1983; 9: 99–118.
6. Miller M, et al. Effect of gemfibrozil in men with primary isolated low high-density lipoprotein cholesterol: a randomised, double-blind, placebo-controlled, crossover study. Am J Med 1993; 94: 7–12.
7. Frick MH, et al. Helsinki Heart Study: primary-prevention trial with gemfibrozil in middle-aged men with dyslipidemia: safety of treatment, changes in risk factors, and incidence of coronary heart disease. N Engl J Med 1987; 317: 1237–45.
8. Heinonen OP, et al. The Helsinki Heart Study: coronary heart disease incidence during an extended follow-up. J Intern Med 1994; 235: 41–9.
9. Rubins HB, et al. Gemfibrozil for the secondary prevention of coronary heart disease in men with low levels of high-density lipoprotein cholesterol. N Engl J Med 1999; 341: 410–8.

Preparations

BP 2001: Gemfibrozil Capsules; Gemfibrozil Tablets;
USP 25: Gemfibrozil Capsules; Gemfibrozil Tablets.

Proprietary Preparations (details are given in Part 3)
Aust.: Gevilon; **Austral.:** Ausgem; Gemfibromax†; Gemhexal; Jezil; Lipazil; Lopid; **Belg.:** Lopid†; **Braz.:** Lopid; **Canad.:** Lopid; **Denm.:** Lopid; **Fin.:** Gevilon; Lopid; **Fr.:** Lipur; **Ger.:** Gevilon; **Hong Kong:** Elmogan; Gemnpid; Ipolipid; Lopid; Synbrozil; **Irl.:** Lopid; **Ital.:** Fibrocit; Fibros; Gemilipid; Genlip; Genozil; Lipogen; Lipozid; Lopid; **Mex.:** Lopid; **Neth.:** Lopid; **NZ:** Gemizol; Lopid; **Port.:** Lipoite; Lopid; **S.Afr.:** Singapore: Hidil; Ipolipid; Lipofor; Lopid; Recozil; **Spain:** Bolutol; Decrelip; Litarek; Lopid; Pilder; Taborcil†; Trialmin; **Swed.:** Lopid; **Switz.:** Gevilon; **Thai.:** Deopid; Dropid; Gemfibril; Gozid; Hidil; Ipolipid; Lipidys; Lipison; Lipozil; Locholes; Lopid; Mariston; Norpid; Poli-Fibrozil; Polyxit; Tiba; **UK:** Emfib†; Lopid; **USA:** Gemcor†; Lopid.

Gepefrine Tartrate (11602-a)

Gepefrine Tartrate (rINNM).

(+)-(S)-m-(2-Aminopropyl)phenol tartrate.
$C_9H_{13}NO, C_4H_6O_6 = 301.3$.
CAS — 18840-47-6 (gepefrine).

Profile

Gepefrine is a sympathomimetic (see Adrenaline, p.829) that has been used as the tartrate in the treatment of hypotensive states.

Preparations

Proprietary Preparations (details are given in Part 3)
Ger.: Wintonin†.

Glyceryl Trinitrate (9237-z)

Glonoin; GTN; Nitroglycerin; Nitroglycerol; NTG; Trinitrin; Trinitroglycerin. Propane-1,2,3-triol trinitrate.
$C_3H_5(NO_3)_3 = 227.1$.
CAS — 55-63-0.
ATC — C01DA02; D03AX07.

Pharmacopoeias. Chin., Eur. (see p.vi), and US include glyceryl trinitrate as diluted solutions.

Pharmacopoeial description

Ph. Eur.: Glyceryl Trinitrate Solution is an ethanolic solution of glyceryl trinitrate. It is a clear, colourless or slightly yellow solution. Miscible with dehydrated alcohol and with acetone.

Pure glyceryl trinitrate is a colourless liquid. Not miscible with water; freely soluble in dehydrated alcohol; miscible with acetone.

Protect from light. Diluted solutions (1%) should be stored at 2° to 15°; more concentrated solutions may be stored at 15° to 20°.

USP 25: Diluted Nitroglycerin is a mixture of glyceryl trinitrate with lactose, glucose, alcohol, propylene glycol, or other suitable inert excipient, usually containing not more than 10% glyceryl trinitrate. When diluted in either alcohol or propylene glycol it is a clear, colourless, or pale yellow liquid. When diluted with lactose, it is a white odourless powder. Store in airtight containers protected from light at temperatures below 40°.

Undiluted glyceryl trinitrate is a white to pale yellow, thick, flammable, explosive liquid. Slightly soluble in water; soluble in alcohol, in acetone, in carbon disulfide, in chloroform, in dichloromethane, in ether, in ethyl acetate, in glacial acetic acid, in methyl alcohol, in benzene, in toluene, in nitrobenzene, and in phenol.

◊ CAUTION. Undiluted glyceryl trinitrate can be exploded by percussion or excessive heat and only exceedingly small amounts should be isolated.

Incompatibility. Studies have found glyceryl trinitrate to be incompatible with phenytoin,[1] alteplase,[2] and levofloxacin.[3]

1. Klamerus KJ, et al. Stability of nitroglycerin in intravenous admixtures. Am J Hosp Pharm 1984; 41: 303–5.
2. Lee CY, et al. Visual and spectrophotometric determination of compatibility of alteplase and streptokinase with other injectable drugs. Am J Hosp Pharm 1990; 47: 606–8.
3. Saltsman CL, et al. Compatibility of levofloxacin with 34 medications during simulated Y-site administration. Am J Health-Syst Pharm 1999; 56: 1458–9.

Stability. INTRAVENOUS SOLUTIONS. The loss of glyceryl trinitrate from solution by adsorption or absorption into some plastics of intravenous administration equipment has been recognised for some years,[1,2] although adsorption does not appear to occur to any great extent with polyolefin[3] or polyethylene.[4-6] It is not only infusion containers and plastic tubing that may be involved; some inline filters can adsorb glyceryl trinitrate.[7,8]

1. Grouthamel WG, et al. Loss of nitroglycerin from plastic intravenous bags. N Engl J Med 1978; 299: 262.
2. Roberts MS, et al. The availability of nitroglycerin from parenteral solutions. J Pharm Pharmacol 1980; 32: 237–44.
3. Wagenknecht DM, et al. Stability of nitroglycerin solutions in polyolefin and glass containers. Am J Hosp Pharm 1984; 41: 1807–11.
4. Schaber DE, et al. Nitroglycerin adsorption to a combination polyvinyl chloride, polyethylene intravenous administration set. Drug Intell Clin Pharm 1985; 19: 572–5.
5. Tracy TS, et al. Nitroglycerin delivery through a polyethylene-lined intravenous administration set. Am J Hosp Pharm 1989; 46: 2031–5.
6. Martens HJ, et al. Sorption of various drugs in polyvinyl chloride, glass, and polyethylene-lined infusion containers. Am J Hosp Pharm 1990; 47: 369–73.
7. Baaske DM, et al. Nitroglycerin compatibility with intravenous fluid filters, containers, and administration sets. Am J Hosp Pharm 1980; 37: 201–5.
8. Kanke M, et al. Binding of selected drugs to a "treated" inline filter. Am J Hosp Pharm 1983; 40: 1323–8.

TABLETS. Many studies have demonstrated that glyceryl trinitrate tablets are unstable and subject to considerable loss of potency in contact with packaging components such as adhesive labels, cotton and rayon fillers, and plastic bottles and caps. Both the Council of the Royal Pharmaceutical Society of Great Britain and the FDA in the USA have issued packaging and dispensing guidelines. Glyceryl trinitrate tablets should be dispensed only in glass containers sealed with a foil lined cap and containing no cotton wool wadding. In addition, the Council of the Royal Pharmaceutical Society of Great Britain recom-

---

mends that no more than 100 tablets should be supplied and that the container should be labelled with an indication that any tablets should be discarded after 8 weeks in use.

Adverse Effects

Glyceryl trinitrate may cause flushing of the face, dizziness, tachycardia, and throbbing headache. Large doses cause vomiting, restlessness, blurred vision, hypotension (which can be severe), syncope, and rarely cyanosis, and methaemoglobinaemia; impairment of respiration and bradycardia may ensue. Contact dermatitis has been reported in patients using topical glyceryl trinitrate preparations; local irritation and erythema may also occur. Preparations applied to the oral mucosa frequently produce a localised burning sensation.

Chronic poisoning may occur in industry but tolerance develops when glyceryl trinitrate is regularly handled and nitrate dependence can lead to severe withdrawal symptoms in subjects abruptly removed from chronic exposure. Loss of such tolerance is rapid and may cause poisoning on re-exposure. Tolerance may occur during clinical use and is usually associated with preparations that produce sustained plasma concentrations.

Effects on the heart. Tachycardia, hypotension, and bradycardia are recognised adverse cardiac effects of glyceryl trinitrate. Rarely reported adverse effects include asystole[1] and complete heart block.[2]

1. Ong EA, et al. Nitroglycerin-induced asystole. *Arch Intern Med* 1985; **145**: 954.
2. Lancaster L, Fenster PE. Complete heart block after sublingual nitroglycerin. *Chest* 1983; **84**: 111–12.

Effects on taste. A 61-year-old man experienced loss of bitter and salty taste sensations 2 weeks after addition of glyceryl trinitrate patches to his post-myocardial infarction drug regimen.[1] The patient experienced complete loss of taste after 6 weeks; his taste sensation returned to normal within one week of discontinuing glyceryl trinitrate patches. Taste sensation was again altered on rechallenge.

1. Ewing RC, et al. Ageusia associated with transdermal nitroglycerin. *Clin Pharm* 1989; **8**: 146–7.

Hypersensitivity. Contact dermatitis has been reported in patients using glyceryl trinitrate ointment and patches.[1] Both glyceryl trinitrate and formulation components may be involved in these reactions.

1. Carmichael AJ. Skin sensitivity and transdermal drug delivery: a review of the problem. *Drug Safety* 1994; **10**: 151–9.

Intravenous administration. Some commercial formulations of glyceryl trinitrate for intravenous use may contain substantial quantities of alcohol in the solvent. There have been several reports of alcohol intoxication occurring in patients during high-dose intravenous glyceryl trinitrate infusion.[1-3] In one patient[3] who required glyceryl trinitrate 2 mg per minute, a blood-alcohol concentration of 2.67 mg per mL was reported. PVC tubing had been used for the infusion and the authors suggested that adsorption of glyceryl trinitrate onto the tubing may have increased the dose requirement and thus the amount of alcohol given.

Propylene glycol is also used as a solvent in some commercial formulations of glyceryl trinitrate. Infusion of solutions with propylene glycol can lead to hyperosmolarity: see under Propylene Glycol, p.1655, for details.

1. Shook TL, et al. Ethanol intoxication complicating intravenous nitroglycerin therapy. *Ann Intern Med* 1984; **101**: 498–9.
2. Daly TJ, et al. "Cocktail"-coronary care. *N Engl J Med* 1984; **310**: 1123.
3. Korn SH, Comer JB. Intravenous nitroglycerin and ethanol intoxication. *Ann Intern Med* 1985; **102**: 274.

Treatment of Adverse Effects

Syncope and hypotension should be treated by keeping the patient in a recumbent position with the head lowered. The administration of oxygen, with assisted respiration, may be necessary in severe poisoning and infusion of plasma expanders or suitable electrolyte solutions may be required to maintain the circulation. If methaemoglobinaemia occurs methylene blue [methylthioninium chloride] may be given intravenously. In the case of severe poisoning with tablets the stomach should be emptied by lavage.

Precautions

Glyceryl trinitrate should not be used in patients with severe hypotension, hypovolaemia, marked anaemia, heart failure due to obstruction (including constrictive pericarditis), or raised intracranial pressure due to head trauma or cerebral haemorrhage. Although it has been suggested that glyceryl trinitrate may increase

intra-ocular pressure in patients with angle-closure glaucoma and should be avoided in such patients there appears to be no evidence for such a contra-indication.

It should be used with caution in patients with severely impaired renal or hepatic function, hypothyroidism, malnutrition, or hypothermia. Metal-containing transdermal systems should be removed before cardioversion or diathermy.

Nitrate tolerance. Organic nitrates can lose their anti-anginal and anti-ischaemic effects in some patients.[1] Tolerance tends to develop in the majority of patients on continuous therapy and higher nitrate doses appear to induce attenuation to a greater degree than lower doses.[2]

The mechanisms of nitrate tolerance are incompletely understood. To exert its vasodilator effect organic nitrates must be converted to nitric oxide, a process which requires the presence of cysteine or another thiol. Repeated doses of a nitrate exhaust tissue stores of sulfhydryl groups and this is one mechanism that may account for the development of tolerance.[1,3] The activation of neurohormonal systems, which releases vasoconstrictor hormones that counteract the effects of organic nitrates, has also been proposed as a mechanism.[1,3] An increase in free-radical production during nitrate therapy has also been suggested,[1] as has the nitrate-induced expansion of plasma volume leading to reversal of the effects of nitrates on ventricular preload.[1]

One method used to avoid the development of tolerance is to provide a nitrate-free interval although rebound myocardial ischaemia may occur in some during the nitrate-free period.[1] With transdermal glyceryl trinitrate systems, the patch can be removed at night. For oral, buccal, and ointment preparations, the dose given at the end of the day can be omitted. Whether a nitrate-free interval is necessary for all patients has not been determined as many patients receiving continuous nitrates do not experience clinical tolerance. A transdermal patch with a higher release rate during the first than during the second part of a 24-hour period has been tried.[4] Other methods investigated have included the administration of a sulfhydryl donor such as acetylcysteine, methionine, or captopril, and hydralazine, which may act by reducing neurohormonal activation, although none have found favour in clinical practice. Antioxidant effects of drugs, including carvedilol[5] and ascorbic acid,[6] are being studied.

1. Parker JD, Parker JO. Nitrate therapy for stable angina pectoris. *N Engl J Med* 1998; **338**: 520–31.
2. Flaherty JT. Nitrate tolerance: a review of the evidence. *Drugs* 1989; **37**: 523–50.
3. Maxwell SRJ, Kendall MJ. An update on nitrate tolerance: can it be avoided? *Postgrad Med J* 1992; **68**: 857–66.
4. Wiegand A, et al. Pharmacodynamic and pharmacokinetic evaluation of a new transdermal delivery system with a time-dependent release of glyceryl trinitrate. *J Clin Pharmacol* 1992; **32**: 77–84.
5. Watanabe H, et al. Randomized, double-blind, placebo-controlled study of carvedilol on the prevention of nitrate tolerance in patients with chronic heart failure. *J Am Coll Cardiol* 1998; **32**: 1194–1200.
6. Daniel TA, Nawarskas JJ. Vitamin C in the prevention of nitrate tolerance. *Ann Pharmacother* 2000; **34**: 1193–7.

Transdermal patches. An explosion occurred during defibrillation in a patient with a glyceryl trinitrate transdermal patch on the left side of the chest.[1] There was no visible injury to the patient. Subsequent studies suggested that this was caused by an electrical arc between the defibrillator paddle and the aluminium backing of the patch rather than explosion of the glyceryl trinitrate.

Although some recommend removal of transdermal patches prior to diathermy, a maximum rise in patch temperature of only 2.2° was reported when patches were exposed to a maximum power density of 800 watts per m².[2] It was considered that exposure of transdermal patches to microwave diathermy, for example as part of physiotherapy treatment, was unlikely to cause direct thermal injury to the wearer.[2]

1. Babka JC. Does nitroglycerin explode? *N Engl J Med* 1983; **309**: 379.
2. Moseley H, et al. The influence of microwave radiation on transdermal delivery systems. *Br J Dermatol* 1990; **122**: 361–3.

Interactions

The hypotensive effects of glyceryl trinitrate may be enhanced by alcohol, and by vasodilators and other drugs with hypotensive actions. The effectiveness of sublingual and buccal tablet preparations may be reduced by drugs that cause dry mouth since dissolution may be delayed.

◊ For the effects of glyceryl trinitrate on *alteplase*, see p.834, on *dihydroergotamine*, see p.453, and on *heparin*, see p.903.

Antimuscarinics. Delayed dissolution of glyceryl trinitrate tablets due to dry mouth has been reported in a patient taking *imipramine*[1] and in a patient treated with *atropine*;[2] this effect should be considered whenever glyceryl trinitrate sublingual tablets are given to patients taking other drugs that can cause dry mouth. Use of the lingual spray[2] rather than a sublingual

tablet or addition of 1 mL of saline under the tongue[3] may be used to overcome the problem.

1. Robbins LJ. Dry mouth and delayed dissolution of sublingual nitro-glycerin. *N Engl J Med* 1983; **309**: 985.
2. Kimchi A. Dry mouth and delayed dissolution of nitroglycerin. *N Engl J Med* 1984; **310**: 1122.
3. Rasler FE. Ineffectiveness of sublingual nitroglycerin in patients with dry mucous membranes. *N Engl J Med* 1986; **314**: 181.

Sildenafil. The concurrent use of nitrates and sildenafil is contra-indicated. Significant hypotension may occur because the vasodilator actions of nitrates are potentiated by sildenafil.[1] Deaths due to a possible interaction have been reported.[2]

1. Webb DJ, et al. Sildenafil citrate potentiates the hypotensive effects of nitric oxide donor drugs in male patients with stable angina. *J Am Coll Cardiol* 2000; **36**: 25–31.
2. Cheitlin MD, et al. Use of sildenafil (Viagra) in patients with cardiovascular disease. *J Am Coll Cardiol* 1999; **33**: 273–82. Correction. *ibid.*; **34**: 1850.

Pharmacokinetics

Glyceryl trinitrate is rapidly absorbed from the oral mucosa. It is also well absorbed from the gastrointestinal tract and through the skin. Bioavailability is less than 100% following administration by any of these routes due to pre-systemic clearance; bioavailability is further reduced after oral administration owing to extensive first-pass metabolism in the liver.

Therapeutic effect is apparent within 1 to 3 minutes of administration of sublingual tablets, sublingual spray, or buccal tablets; within 30 to 60 minutes of administration of an ointment or transdermal patch; and within 1 to 2 minutes following intravenous administration.

Duration of action is about 30 to 60 minutes with sublingual tablets or spray and 3 to 5 hours with modified-release buccal tablets. Transdermal patches are designed to release a stated amount of drug over 24 hours, while therapeutic effects following application of glyceryl trinitrate ointment 2% persist for up to 8 hours. Duration of action following intravenous administration is about 3 to 5 minutes.

Glyceryl trinitrate is widely distributed with a large apparent volume of distribution. It is taken up by smooth muscle cells of blood vessels and the nitrate group is cleaved to inorganic nitrite and then to nitric oxide. This reaction requires the presence of cysteine or another thiol. Glyceryl trinitrate also undergoes hydrolysis in plasma and is rapidly metabolised in the liver by glutathione-organic nitrate reductase to dinitrates and mononitrates. The dinitrates are less potent vasodilators than glyceryl trinitrate; the mononitrates may have some vasodilator activity.

◊ References.

1. Bogaert MG. Clinical pharmacokinetics of glyceryl trinitrate following the use of systemic and topical preparations. *Clin Pharmacokinet* 1987; **12**: 1–11.
2. Thadani U, Whitsett T. Relationship of pharmacokinetic and pharmacodynamic properties of the organic nitrates. *Clin Pharmacokinet* 1988; **15**: 32–43.
3. Ridout G, et al. Pharmacokinetic considerations in the use of newer transdermal formulations. *Clin Pharmacokinet* 1988; **15**: 114–31.

Uses and Administration

Glyceryl trinitrate is a nitrovasodilator used in the management of angina pectoris (p.791), heart failure (p.798), and myocardial infarction (below). Other indications include inducing hypotension and controlling hypertension during surgery.

Glyceryl trinitrate is believed to exert its vasodilator effect through nitric oxide stimulating guanylate cyclase in the vascular smooth muscle cells; this results in an increase in cyclic guanosine monophosphate. This nucleotide induces relaxation probably by lowering the free calcium concentration in the cytosol. In its action on vascular muscle venous dilatation predominates over dilatation of the arterioles. Venous dilatation decreases venous return as a result of venous pooling and lowers left ventricular diastolic volume and pressure (termed a reduction in preload). The smaller or less important dilatation of arterioles reduces both peripheral vascular resistance and left ventricular pressure at systole (termed a reduction in afterload). The consequent effect is a reduction in the primary determinants of myocardial oxygen demand. The effect on preload is not shared by beta blockers or calcium-channel blockers. Glyceryl trinitrate also has a coronary vasodilator effect which improves regional coronary blood flow to ischaemic areas resulting in improved oxygen supply to the myocardium.

Glyceryl trinitrate may be administered by the sublingual, buccal, oral, transdermal, or intravenous route. The dose and choice of formulation depend upon the clinical situation.

In the management of **acute angina** glyceryl trinitrate is given as sublingual tablets, a sublingual aerosol spray, or buccal tablets, which all produce a rapid onset of therapeutic effect and provide rapid relief of anginal pain. These dosage forms may also be used before an activity or stress which might provoke an attack. One sublingual tablet (usual strength 300 to 600 µg) is placed under the tongue. The dose may be repeated as required but patients should be advised to seek medical care if pain persists after a total of 3 doses within 15 minutes. If an aerosol spray is used one or two sprays of 400 µg each are directed onto or under the tongue, then the mouth is closed; three sprays may be used if necessary. Buccal tablets of glyceryl trinitrate are placed between the upper lip and gum (see below for precautions to be observed during use). A dose of 1 or 2 mg is usually sufficient, although 3 mg may be needed in some cases.

In the long-term management of **stable angina** glyceryl trinitrate is given as modified-release tablets or capsules, transdermal formulations, or buccal tablets, which all provide a long duration of action. Dosage varies according to the specific formulation. In the UK, for example, modified-release oral tablets are available that allow doses of up to 12.8 mg to be given up to three times daily. The transdermal formulations available are ointments and patches. With the ointment a measured amount ($^{1}/_{2}$ to 2 inches of glyceryl trinitrate ointment 2%) is applied 3 or 4 times daily, or every 3 to 4 hours if necessary, to the chest, arm, thigh, or back. Transdermal patches applied to the chest, upper arm, or shoulder are more convenient. Patches are generally designed to release glyceryl trinitrate at a constant rate; they are available in a range of sizes, releasing an average of 2.5 to 20 mg of glyceryl trinitrate over 24 hours (0.1 to 0.8 mg per hour). A maximum daily dose of 20 mg has been suggested. Glyceryl trinitrate ointment and patches should be applied to a fresh area of skin and several days should elapse before re-application to formerly used sites. Buccal tablets are used in doses of 1 to 5 mg three times daily. The tablets are retained in the buccal cavity; the rate of dissolution of the tablet can be increased by touching the tablet with the tongue or drinking hot liquids. It is common practice to remove the tablets at bedtime because of the risk of aspiration. Also patients using buccal tablets should be advised to alternate placement sites and pay close attention to oral hygiene to reduce the risk of dental caries. The tablets are not intended to be chewed; if the buccal tablet is inadvertently swallowed, another may be placed in the buccal cavity.

Tolerance tends to develop in the majority of patients on continuous nitrate therapy and nitrate-free intervals are often employed to avoid this problem (see above under Precautions, Nitrate Tolerance for further details).

In the management of **unstable angina** glyceryl trinitrate may be given by intravenous infusion. Manufacturers' guidelines for dilution of glyceryl trinitrate injection specify glucose 5% or sodium chloride 0.9% as the diluent. During intravenous administration of glyceryl trinitrate there should be haemodynamic monitoring of the patient with the dose being adjusted gradually to produce the desired response. The plastic used in the infusion equipment may adsorb glyceryl trinitrate (see Stability, above) and allowance may have to be made for this. The usual initial dose for unstable angina is 5 to 10 µg per minute. Most patients respond to doses between 10 and 200 µg per minute, although higher doses may be required in some cases. The sublingual and buccal routes may also be used; doses of up to 5 mg as buccal

tablets may be required to relieve pain in patients with unstable angina.

In the management of acute **heart failure** glyceryl trinitrate is given intravenously in an initial dose of 5 to 25 µg per minute. Buccal tablets have been used in doses of 5 mg repeated as needed until symptoms are controlled. In chronic heart failure buccal tablets may be given in doses of 5 to 10 mg three times daily.

Glyceryl trinitrate is also used intravenously in acute **myocardial infarction**, and to induce hypotension or control hypertension during **surgery**. The initial dose is 5 to 25 µg per minute, adjusted according to response. The usual range is 10 to 200 µg per minute but some surgical patients may require up to 400 µg per minute.

Glyceryl trinitrate has also been used as transdermal patches in the prophylactic treatment of **phlebitis and extravasation** secondary to venous cannulation. One 5-mg patch is applied distal to the intravenous site; the patch should be replaced at a different skin site either daily or after 3 to 4 days, depending on the patch. This treatment should continue only as long as the intravenous infusion is maintained.

Anal fissure. Nitrates such as glyceryl trinitrate are being studied in the treatment of chronic anal fissure (p.1325) because of their ability to relax the anal sphincter. Topical application of glyceryl trinitrate ointment in concentrations of 0.2 to 0.8% has relieved pain and aided healing of anal fissures both in uncontrolled[1-3] and controlled studies,[4,5] although it may be less effective than injection with botulinum toxin.[6] One study[5] found that a concentration of 0.6% had no additional benefit over 0.2%. Follow-up[5,7] of some of the patients indicated that after 6 to 38 months most had not experienced further problems or had had occasional recurrences (relapses of about one-quarter to one-third) which in the majority of cases had responded to further topical treatment. Encouraging results have also been obtained in an uncontrolled study using a 1% ointment of isosorbide dinitrate.[8]

1. Gorfine SR. Topical nitroglycerin therapy for anal fissures and ulcers. *N Engl J Med* 1995; **333:** 1156–7.
2. Lund JN *et al.* Use of glyceryl trinitrate ointment in the treatment of anal fissure. *Br J Surg* 1996; **83:** 776–7.
3. Watson SJ, *et al.* Topical glyceryl trinitrate in the treatment of chronic anal fissure. *Br J Surg* 1996; **83:** 771–5.
4. Lund JN, Scholefield JH. A randomised, prospective, double-blind, placebo-controlled trial of glyceryl trinitrate ointment in treatment of anal fissure. *Lancet* 1997; **349:** 11–14. Correction. *ibid.;* 656.
5. Carapeti EA, *et al.* Randomised controlled trial shows that glyceryl trinitrate heals anal fissures, higher doses are not more effective, and there is a high recurrence rate. *Gut* 1999; **44:** 727–30.
6. Brisinda G, *et al.* A comparison of injections of botulinum toxin and topical nitroglycerin ointment for the treatment of chronic anal fissure. *N Engl J Med* 1999; **341:** 65–9. Correction. *ibid.;* 624.
7. Lund JN, Scholefield JH. Follow-up of patients with chronic anal fissure treated with topical glyceryl trinitrate. *Lancet* 1998; **352:** 1681.
8. Schouten WR, *et al.* Pathophysiological aspects and clinical outcome of intra-anal application of isosorbide dinitrate in patients with chronic anal fissure. *Gut* 1996; **39:** 465–9.

Erectile dysfunction. Erectile dysfunction (p.1663) has been managed by the penile injection of drugs such as papaverine or alprostadil although oral treatment with sildenafil is now available. Penile injections are not always acceptable to the patient and a number of studies have investigated topical therapies, mostly glyceryl trinitrate applied either as ointment or as a transdermal delivery system to the penis.[1-4] Such treatment can produce erections in some subjects, although response rates vary. However, patients must wear a condom to protect their partner against potential adverse effects resulting from the transfer of glyceryl trinitrate. The mechanism of action of glyceryl trinitrate is believed to be due to smooth muscle relaxation and vasodilatation which are necessary prerequisites for penile erection.

Isosorbide dinitrate as a cream also containing aminophylline and co-dergocrine mesilate has produced some benefit[5] although a further study[6] failed to confirm these results.

It should be noted that topical nitrates must not be employed in patients already using sildenafil (see under Interactions, above).

1. Heaton JPW, *et al.* Topical glyceryl trinitrate causes measurable penile arterial dilation in impotent men. *J Urol (Baltimore)* 1990; **143:** 729–31.
2. Meyhoff HH, *et al.* Non-invasive management of impotence with transcutaneous nitroglycerin. *Br J Urol* 1992; **69:** 88–90.
3. Nunez BD, Anderson DC. Nitroglycerin ointment in the treatment of impotence. *J Urol (Baltimore)* 1993; **150:** 1241–3.
4. Anderson DC, Seifert CF. Topical nitrate treatment of impotence. *Ann Pharmacother* 1993; **27:** 1203–5.
5. Gomaa A, *et al.* Topical treatment of erectile dysfunction: randomised double blind placebo controlled trial of cream containing aminophylline, isosorbide dinitrate, and co-dergocrine mesylate. *BMJ* 1996; **312:** 1512–15.
6. Naude JH, Le Roux PJ. Topical treatment of erectile dysfunction did not show results. *BMJ* 1998; **316:** 1318.

Gallstones. Endoscopic removal of gallstones (p.1678) in a small series of 15 patients was facilitated by glyceryl trinitrate 1.2 to 3.6 mg applied as a spray to the tongue. Glyceryl trinitrate 1.2 mg was shown to relax the sphincter of Oddi to approximately 30% of its normal pressure.[1] The ability of glyceryl trinitrate to relax smooth muscle has also been employed to relieve biliary colic (p.5) in 3 patients with gallstones;[2] in one of these patients standard managements for the pain such as oral opioids had been only moderately effective.

1. Staritz M, *et al.* Nitroglycerine dilatation of sphincter of Oddi for endoscopic removal of bileduct stones. *Lancet* 1984; **i:** 956.
2. Hassel B. Treatment of biliary colic with nitroglycerin. *Lancet* 1993; **342:** 1305.

Myocardial infarction. The management of myocardial infarction (p.805) can involve numerous drug therapies including nitrates.

Nitrovasodilatation with intravenous glyceryl trinitrate or sodium nitroprusside, started within 24 hours of the onset of pain, has been associated with a reduction in mortality.[1] Its role is not certain but the empirical use of intravenous glyceryl trinitrate (in addition to standard treatment with a thrombolytic, oral aspirin, and an intravenous beta blocker) in the acute phase of myocardial infarction is widespread and appears to be safe, as was demonstrated in the GISSI-3 study.[2] In this study glyceryl trinitrate was given by intravenous infusion during the first 24 hours, starting at 5 µg per minute and increasing by 5 to 20 µg per minute every 5 minutes for the first half hour until systolic blood pressure fell by at least 10% provided it remained above 90 mmHg; after 24 hours it was replaced by a transdermal patch providing 10 mg daily.

Some patients, for example those with myocardial ischaemia or poor left ventricular function, may require the long-term administration of nitrates, but recent studies have thrown doubt on their routine use. In the GISSI-3 study there was no significant benefit from the use of transdermal glyceryl trinitrate when assessed 6 weeks[2] and 6 months[3] post-infarction and in the ISIS-4 study[4] oral isosorbide mononitrate apparently had no effect on 35-day mortality.

1. Yusuf S, *et al.* Effect of intravenous nitrates on mortality in acute myocardial infarction: an overview of the randomised trials. *Lancet* 1988; **i:** 1088–92.
2. Gruppo Italiano per lo Studio della Sopravvivenza nell'Infarto Miocardico. GISSI-3: effects of lisinopril and transdermal glyceryl trinitrate singly and together on 6-week mortality and ventricular function after acute myocardial infarction. *Lancet* 1994; **343:** 1115–22.
3. Gruppo Italiano per lo Studio della Sopravvivenza nell'Infarto Miocardico. Six-month effects of early treatment with lisinopril and transdermal glyceryl trinitrate singly and together withdrawn six weeks after myocardial infarction: the GISSI-3 trial. *J Am Coll Cardiol* 1996; **27:** 337–44.
4. ISIS-4 (Fourth International Study of Infarct Survival) Collaborative Group. ISIS-4: a randomised factorial trial assessing early oral captopril, oral mononitrate, and intravenous magnesium sulphate in 58 050 patients with suspected acute myocardial infarction. *Lancet* 1995; **345:** 669–85.

Obstetrics and gynaecology. The smooth muscle relaxant properties of glyceryl trinitrate have been employed in various obstetric or gynaecological situations although most reports are anecdotal or include small numbers of patients. The intravenous injection of glyceryl trinitrate 50 to 100 µg repeated to a total dose of 200 µg if necessary has produced sufficient uterine relaxation in postpartum women for the manual extraction of retained placentas.[1,2] Administration by sublingual spray has also been used successfully to facilitate breech extraction in a set of twins.[3]

Glyceryl trinitrate has been given as a sublingual spray to relax the cervix prior to IUD insertion. In a series of over 100 patients one or two doses of 400 µg sublingually were usually adequate.[4]

Beneficial results have been reported in women with possible premature labour (p.773) following application of glyceryl trinitrate patches to the abdomen,[5,6] and in one study[7] this was as effective as ritodrine infusion.

Transdermal glyceryl trinitrate has been tried for controlling pain in severe and moderate-to-severe dysmenorrhoea[8,9] (p.6).

Glyceryl trinitrate has been given intravenously in the management of pre-eclampsia (see under Hypertension, p.802) and is reported to reduce blood pressure without compromising uterine blood flow.[10]

Isosorbide mononitrate administered vaginally has been found to produce cervical ripening[11] and may be an alternative to prostaglandins for this purpose before first trimester termination of pregnancy (p.1439).

1. DeSimone CA, *et al.* Intravenous nitro-glycerin aids manual extraction of a retained placenta. *Anesthesiology* 1990; **73:** 787.
2. Lowenwirt IP, *et al.* Safety of intravenous glyceryl trinitrate in management of retained placenta. *Aust N Z J Obstet Gynaecol* 1997; **37:** 20–4.
3. Greenspoon JS, Kovacic A. Breech extraction facilitated by glyceryl trinitrate sublingual spray. *Lancet* 1991; **338:** 124–5.
4. Yadava RP. Sublingual glyceryl trinitrate spray facilitates IUD insertion. *Br J Sex Med* 1990; **17:** 217.
5. Lees C, *et al.* Arrest of preterm labour and prolongation of gestation with glyceryl trinitrate, a nitric oxide donor. *Lancet* 1994; **343:** 1325–6.
6. Smith GN, *et al.* Randomised, double-blind, placebo controlled pilot study assessing nitroglycerin as a tocolytic. *Br J Obstet Gynaecol* 1999; **106:** 736–9.
7. Lees CC, *et al.* Glyceryl trinitrate and ritodrine in tocolysis: an international multicenter randomized study. *Obstet Gynecol* 1999; **94:** 403–8.

8. Pittrof R, et al. Crossover study of glyceryl trinitrate patches for controlling pain in women with severe dysmenorrhoea. BMJ 1996; 312: 884.
9. The Transdermal Nitroglycerine/Dysmenorrhoea Study Group. Transdermal nitroglycerine in the management of pain associated with primary dysmenorrhoea: a multinational pilot study. J Int Med Res 1997; 25: 41–4.
10. Grunewald C, et al. Effects of nitroglycerin on the uterine and umbilical circulation in severe preeclampsia. Obstet Gynecol 1995; 86: 600–4.
11. Thomson AJ, et al. Randomised trial of nitric oxide donor versus prostaglandin for cervical ripening before first-trimester termination of pregnancy. Lancet 1998; 352: 1093–6.

Oesophageal motility disorders. Achalasia is obstruction caused by failure of the lower oesophageal sphincter to relax and permit passage of food into the stomach. Nitrates such as isosorbide dinitrate have been reported to produce effective relaxation and to reduce symptoms when administered sublingually. They have a role when mechanical dilatation of the sphincter or surgery are not feasible (see Oesophageal Motility Disorders, p.1208).

Nitrates may also be employed in oesophageal disorders such as variceal haemorrhage (see below).

Peripheral vascular disease. In peripheral vascular disease (p.809) nitrates have been tried as vasodilators and smooth muscle relaxants in order to improve resting blood flow. Glyceryl trinitrate has been applied topically in patients with Raynaud's syndrome[1-3] and in distal limb ischaemia[4] resulting in some benefit but this form of therapy is not widely used in these disorders.

1. Franks AG. Topical glyceryl trinitrate as adjunctive treatment in Raynaud's disease. Lancet 1982; i: 76–7.
2. Coppock JS, et al. Objective relief of vasospasm by glyceryl trinitrate in secondary Raynaud's phenomenon. Postgrad Med J 1986; 62: 15–18.
3. Teh LS, et al. Sustained-release transdermal glyceryl trinitrate patches as a treatment for primary and secondary Raynaud's phenomenon. Br J Rheumatol 1995; 34: 636–41.
4. Fletcher S, et al. Locally applied transdermal nitrate patches for the treatment of ischaemic rest pain. Int J Clin Pract 1997; 51: 324–5.

Pulmonary hypertension. Administration of glyceryl trinitrate to patients with primary pulmonary hypertension (p.810) results in a fall in total pulmonary resistance in most patients.[1,2] However, other vasodilators such as calcium-channel blockers or epoprostenol are generally preferred for long-term treatment.

1. Pearl RG, et al. Acute hemodynamic effects of nitroglycerin in pulmonary hypertension. Ann Intern Med 1983; 99: 9–13.
2. Weir EK, et al. The acute administration of vasodilators in primary pulmonary hypertension. Am Rev Respir Dis 1989; 140: 1623–30.

Quinine oculotoxicity. Intravenous nitrate administration has been suggested for the management of quinine oculotoxicity (p.446) and its benefit may be due to an increase in retinal vascular bed flow.[1]

1. Moore D, et al. Research into quinine ocular toxicity. Br J Ophthalmol 1992; 76: 703.

Variceal haemorrhage. The usual treatment in variceal haemorrhage (p.1637) is injection sclerotherapy or banding ligation which may be performed during the emergency endoscopy procedure. Where endoscopy is unavailable drug therapy may be used and it may also have a role when sclerotherapy fails. Vasoconstrictors that are used include vasopressin and its analogue terlipressin, given together with glyceryl trinitrate which counteracts the adverse cardiac effects of vasopressin while potentiating its beneficial effects on portal pressure; somatostatin is also used.

Prophylaxis of a first bleed in patients with portal hypertension is controversial since about 70% of patients who have varices will never bleed. It is postulated that a reduction in portal pressure to below 12 mmHg is necessary to reduce the incidence of variceal bleeding and that treatment with beta blockers alone does not achieve this. More effective drugs are being sought and isosorbide mononitrate (as adjunctive therapy with a beta blocker) is under investigation, both for prophylaxis of a first bleed[1,2] and in the prevention of rebleeding.[3] Early emergency treatment (before endoscopy) with terlipressin given intravenously and glyceryl trinitrate transdermally controlled bleeding and lowered mortality rates in patients with gastrointestinal bleeding and a history or clinical signs of cirrhosis.[4] However, combination of oral isosorbide mononitrate with somatostatin infusion for acute variceal bleeding was less effective than somatostatin alone and induced more adverse effects.[5]

1. Angelico M, et al. Isosorbide-5-mononitrate versus propranolol in the prevention of first bleeding in cirrhosis. Gastroenterology 1993; 104: 1460–5.
2. Merkel C, et al. Randomised trial of nadolol alone or with isosorbide mononitrate for primary prophylaxis of variceal bleeding in cirrhosis. Lancet 1996; 348: 1677–81.
3. Villanueva C, et al. Nadolol plus isosorbide mononitrate compared with sclerotherapy for the prevention of variceal rebleeding. N Engl J Med 1996; 334: 1624–9.
4. Levacher S, et al. Early administration of terlipressin plus glyceryl trinitrate to control active upper gastrointestinal bleeding in cirrhotic patients. Lancet 1995; 346: 865–8.
5. Junquera F, et al. Somatostatin plus isosorbide 5-mononitrate versus somatostatin in the control of acute gastro-oesophageal variceal bleeding: a double blind, randomised, placebo controlled clinical trial. Gut 2000; 46: 127–32.

Venepuncture. Glyceryl trinitrate patches applied to skin adjacent to intravenous infusion sites are used in the prophylactic treatment of phlebitis and extravasation.[1]

Local application of glyceryl trinitrate 1 to 2 mg as ointment was found to be a useful aid to venepuncture in a study of 50 patients undergoing surgery,[2] but conflicting results have been reported in children and neonates.[3,4]

1. Tjon JA, Ansani NT. Transdermal nitroglycerin for the prevention of intravenous infusion failure due to phlebitis and extravasation. Ann Pharmacother 2000; 34: 1189–92.
2. Hecker JF, et al. Nitroglycerine ointment as an aid to venepuncture. Lancet 1983; i: 332–3.
3. Vaksmann G, et al. Nitroglycerin ointment as aid to venous cannulation in children. J Pediatr 1987; 111: 89–91.
4. Maynard EC, Oh W. Topical nitroglycerin ointment as an aid to insertion of peripheral venous catheters in neonates. J Pediatr 1989; 114: 474–6.

Preparations

BP 2001: Glyceryl Trinitrate Sublingual Spray; Glyceryl Trinitrate Tablets; Glyceryl Trinitrate Transdermal Patches;
USP 25: Nitroglycerin Injection; Nitroglycerin Ointment; Nitroglycerin Tablets.

Proprietary Preparations (details are given in Part 3)
Aust.: Deponit; Minitran; Nitro Mack; Nitro Pohl; Nitro-Dur; Nitroderm; Nitrolingual; Nitronal; Nitrong; Nitrozell†; Perlinganit; *Austral.:* Anginine; Minitran; Nitradisc; Nitro-Bid; Nitro-Dur; Nitrolingual; Rectogesic; Transiderm-Nitro; *Belg.:* Deponit; Diafusor; Minitran; Nitro-Dyl; Nitroderm; Nitrolingual; Nitrong†; Nysconitrine; Trinipatch; Willlong; *Braz.:* Deponit; Nitradisc; Nitroderm TTS; *Canad.:* Minitran; Nitro-Dur; Nitrol; Nitrolingual; Nitrong; Nitrostat; Transderm-Nitro; Tridil†; Trinipatch; *Denm.:* Buccard; Discotrine; Glytrin; Nitrolingual; Nitromex; Nitrong†; Transiderm-Nitro; *Fin.:* Deponit; Minitran; Nitro; Nitromex; Perlinganit; Transiderm-Nitro; *Fr.:* Cordipatch; Corditrine†; Diafusor; Discotrine; Lenitral; Natispray; Nitriderm TTS; Optizor; Trinipatch; *Ger.:* Aquo-Trinitrosan; Corangin Nitrokapseln and Nitrospray; Coro-Nitro; Deponit; Gilustenon†; MinitranS; neos nitro OPT; Nitradisc; Nitrangin; Nitrangin forte†; Nitro Mack; Nitro Solvay; Nitro-Pflaster-ratiopharm TL; Nitroderm TTS; Nitrokapseln-ratiopharm; Nitrokor; Nitrolingual; Nitronal†; Perlinganit; Trinitrosan; Turicard†; *Hong Kong:* Angised; Deponit; Glytrin; Lenitral; Minitran; Nitro Mack; Nitro Pohl; Nitro-Dur; Nitrocine; Nitroderm TTS; Nitroglyn; Nitrolingual; Nitronal; Nitropulse; Nitrostat; Tridil; *Irl.:* Angised; Deponit; Glytrin; Nitro-Dur; Nitrocine; Nitrolingual; Nitromin; Nitronal; Suscard; Sustac; Transiderm-Nitro; Tridil†; *Israel:* Angised; Deponit; Nitrocine; Nitroderm TTS; Nitrolingual; Nitronal; Nitrovis; Trinipatch; *Ital.:* Adesitrin; Deponit; Minitran; Natispray; Nitro-Dur; Nitroderm TTS; Nitrosylon; Perganit; Top-Nitro; Triniplas; Trinitrina; Venitrin; *Jpn:* Millisrol; Vasolator†; *Mex.:* Anglix; Cardinit; Minitran; Nitradisc; Nitro-Dur; Nitroder; Nitroderm TTS; *Neth.:* Deponit; Glytrin; Minitran; Nitro Pohl; Nitro-Dur; Nitrobaat†; Nitrocine; Nitroderm TTS†; Nitrolingual; Nitronal†; Tridil; *Norw.:* Minitran; Nitradisc†; Nitro-Dur; Nitrolingual; Nitromex; Nitroven; Suscard; Transiderm-Nitro; *NZ:* Anginine; Minitran; Nitroderm; Nitrolingual; Nitronal; Port.: Nitradisc; Nitro-Dur; Nitroderm TTS; Nitromint; Plastranit; *S.Afr.:* Angised; Nitradisc†; Nitrocine; Nitroderm TTS†; Nitrolingual; Nitronal†; Tridil; *Singapore:* Angised; Deponit; Glytrin; Lenitral; Nitro Mack; *Spain:* Cardiodisco; Colenitral†; Cordiplast; Diafusor; Minitran; Nitradisc; Nitro-Dur; Nitroderm TTS; Nitropacin; Nitroplast; Nitrotard†; Solinitrina; Trinipatch; Vernies; *Swed.:* Glytrin; Minitran; Nitroglyn†; Nitrolingual; Nitromex; Nitrong; Nitroretard†; Perlinganit; Suscard; Transiderm-Nitro; *Switz.:* Deponit; Minitran; Natispray†; Niong retard; Nitro Mack; Nitro-Dur; Nitroderm TTS; Nitrolingual; Nitromint†; Nitronal; Perlinganit; Trinitrine; *Thai.:* Amitacon; Angised; Deponit; Glytrin; Minitran; Nitradisc; Nitro Mack; Nitrocine; Nitroderm; Willlong; *UK:* Coro-Nitro; Deponit; Glytrin; Minitran; Nitro-Dur; Nitrocine; Nitrolingual; Nitromin; Nitronal; Percutol; Suscard; Sustac; Transiderm-Nitro; *USA:* Deponit; Minitran; Nitrek; Nitro-Bid; Nitro-Derm; Nitro-Dur; Nitro-Time; Nitrodisc; Nitrogard; Nitroglyn; Nitrol; Nitrolingual; Nitrong; Nitrostat; NitroQuick; Nitrostat; NitroTab; NTS†; Transderm-Nitro; Transdermal-NTG; Tridil.

Multi-ingredient: *Aust.:* Myocardon; Spasmocor; *Ger.:* Angiocardyl N†; Nitrangin compositum; Nitro-cum; Nitro-Praecordin N†; *Spain:* Cafinitrina; *USA:* Emergent-Ez.

Guabenxan (12800-s)

Guabenxan (rINN).

(1,4-Benzodioxan-6-ylmethyl)guanidine.

$C_{10}H_{13}N_3O_2 = 207.2.$
CAS — 19889-45-3.

Profile
Guabenxan is an antihypertensive with properties similar to guanethidine (below). It has been given by mouth as the sulfate.

Preparations

Proprietary Preparations (details are given in Part 3)
Multi-ingredient: *Fr.:* Tensigradyl†.

Guanabenz Acetate (865-k)

Guanabenz Acetate (USAN, rINNM).

NSC-68982 (guanabenz); Wy-8678 (guanabenz). (2,6-Dichlorobenzylideneamino)guanidine acetate.

$C_8H_8Cl_2N_4,C_2H_4O_2 = 291.1.$
CAS — 5051-62-7 (guanabenz); 23256-50-0 (guanabenz acetate).
Pharmacopoeias. In Jpn and US.

Guanabenz acetate 5 mg is approximately equivalent to 4 mg of guanabenz.

Pharmacopoeial description
USP 25: A white or almost white powder with not more than a slight odour. Sparingly soluble in water and in 0.1N hydrochloric acid; soluble in alcohol and in propylene glycol. A 0.7% solution in water has a pH of 5.5 to 7.0. Store in airtight containers. Protect from light.

Adverse Effects and Precautions
As for Clonidine Hydrochloride, p.860.

Overdosage. Overdosage with guanabenz has been reported.[1] The main symptoms were lethargy, drowsiness, bradycardia, and hypotension. A 45-year-old woman who had taken 200 to 240 mg of guanabenz with alcohol recovered following gastric lavage and intravenous fluids; a 3-year-old child who had taken 12 mg of guanabenz responded to atropine and dopamine. Naloxone had little effect in either patient.

1. Hall AH, et al. Guanabenz overdose. Ann Intern Med 1985; 102: 787–8.

Pharmacokinetics
Following oral administration guanabenz is well absorbed and undergoes extensive first-pass metabolism. Peak plasma concentrations occur about 2 to 5 hours after a dose. It is about 90% bound to plasma proteins. Guanabenz is mainly excreted in urine, almost entirely as metabolites; about 10 to 30% is excreted in faeces. The average elimination half-life is reported to range from 4 to 14 hours.

Uses and Administration
Guanabenz is an alpha$_2$-adrenoceptor agonist with actions and uses similar to those of clonidine (p.861). It is used in the management of hypertension (p.802), either alone or in conjunction with other antihypertensives, particularly thiazide diuretics. Guanabenz is given by mouth as the acetate, but doses are usually expressed in terms of the base.

In hypertension, it is given in a usual dose of 4 mg twice daily initially increasing by increments of 4 to 8 mg per day every 1 to 2 weeks according to the patient's response. Doses of up to 32 mg twice daily have been used.

Preparations

USP 25: Guanabenz Acetate Tablets.

Proprietary Preparations (details are given in Part 3)
Aust.: Rexitene; Wytensin; *Braz.:* Lisapres; Tenelid; *USA:* Wytensin.

Guanadrel Sulfate (867-t)

Guanadrel Sulfate (USAN, rINNM).

CL-1388R; Guanadrel Sulphate; U-28288D. 1-(Cyclohexanespiro-2'-[1',3']dioxolan-4'-ylmethyl)guanidine sulphate; 1-(1,4-Dioxaspiro[4.5]dec-2-ylmethyl)guanidine sulphate.
$(C_{10}H_{19}N_3O_2)_2,H_2SO_4 = 524.6.$
CAS — 40580-59-4 (guanadrel); 22195-34-2 (guanadrel sulfate).
Pharmacopoeias. In US.

Pharmacopoeial description
USP 25: A white to off-white crystalline powder. Soluble in water; slightly soluble in alcohol and in acetone; sparingly soluble in methyl alcohol.

Adverse Effects, Treatment, and Precautions
As for Guanethidine Monosulfate, below. Guanadrel has been reported to cause less diarrhoea, and less orthostatic hypotension on rising in the morning, than guanethidine, but orthostatic symptoms seem to occur with a similar frequency to guanethidine during the day.

Interactions
As for Guanethidine Monosulfate, below.

Pharmacokinetics
Guanadrel is rapidly and almost completely absorbed from the gastrointestinal tract, with a reported bioavailability of about 85%. It is widely distributed throughout the body and about 20% is bound to plasma proteins. It is reported not to cross the blood-brain barrier. Plasma concentrations decline in a biphasic manner: the half-life varies widely between individuals, in the initial phase from 1 to 4 hours, and in the terminal phase from 5 to 45 hours, with a mean of about 10 hours. Guanadrel is metabolised in the liver and approximately 85% is excreted in the urine over 24 hours as the unchanged drug and its metabolites. About 40 to 50% of the drug is excreted unchanged.

Uses and Administration
Guanadrel is an antihypertensive with actions and uses similar to those of guanethidine (below). Following oral administration, guanadrel acts within 2 hours with the maximum effect after 4 to 6 hours. The hypotensive effect is reported to last for 4 to 14 hours following a single dose. It is used in the management of hypertension (p.802), although it has largely been superseded by other drugs less likely to cause orthostatic hypotension.

Guanadrel is given by mouth as the sulfate. The usual initial dose is 5 mg twice daily adjusted at weekly or monthly intervals according to the patient's response. The maintenance dose is normally in the range of 20 to 75 mg daily in two or more divided doses.

Administration in renal impairment. Renal and non-renal clearance of guanadrel were decreased in 16 patients with impaired renal function compared with 6 healthy subjects, and this was reflected in a prolongation of the terminal elimination half-life from a mean of 3.69 hours to 6.8, 12.6, and 19.2 hours in patients with mild, moderate, and severe renal insufficiency, respectively.[1] Dosage adjustment would be preferable in patients with impaired renal function given guanadrel, perhaps by giving the daily dose every 2 to 3 days in mild to moderate insufficiency and every 5 days in severe insufficiency.

1. Halstenson CE, *et al.* Disposition of guanadrel in subjects with normal and impaired renal function. *J Clin Pharmacol* 1989; **29:** 128–32.

Preparations

USP 25: Guanadrel Sulfate Tablets.

Proprietary Preparations (details are given in Part 3)
USA: Hylorel.

Guanethidine Monosulfate (869-r)

Guanethidine Monosulfate (USAN, rINNM).

Guanethidine Monosulphate (BANM); Guanethidini Monosulfas; NSC-29863 (guanethidine hemisulfate); Su-5864 (guanethidine hemisulfate). 1-[2-(Perhydroazocin-1-yl)ethyl]guanidine monosulphate.

$C_{10}H_{22}N_4,H_2SO_4 = 296.4$.

CAS — 55-65-2 (guanethidine); 60-02-6 (guanethidine hemisulfate); 645-43-2 (guanethidine monosulfate).

Pharmacopoeias. In Eur. (see p.vi), Jpn, and US.

Chin. includes the hemisulfate, $(C_{10}H_{22}N_4)_2,H_2SO_4$.

Pharmacopoeial description

Ph. Eur.: A colourless crystalline powder. Freely soluble in water; practically insoluble in alcohol and in ether. A 2% solution in water has a pH of 4.7 to 5.5. Protect from light.

USP 25: A white to off-white crystalline powder. Very soluble in water; sparingly soluble in alcohol; practically insoluble in chloroform. A 2% solution in water has a pH of 4.7 to 5.7.

Adverse Effects

The commonest side-effects with guanethidine are severe postural and exertional hypotension and diarrhoea which may be particularly troublesome during the initial stages of therapy and during dose adjustment. Dizziness, syncope, muscle weakness, and lassitude are liable to occur, especially on rising from sitting or lying. Postural hypotension may be severe enough to provoke angina, renal insufficiency, and transient cerebral ischaemia. Other frequent side-effects are bradycardia, failure of ejaculation, fatigue, headache, and salt and water retention and oedema, which may be accompanied by breathlessness and may occasionally precipitate overt heart failure.

Nausea, vomiting, dry mouth, nasal congestion, parotid tenderness, blurring of vision, depression, myalgia, muscle tremor, paraesthesia, hair loss, dermatitis, disturbed micturition, priapism, aggravation or precipitation of asthma, and exacerbation of peptic ulcer have also been reported. Guanethidine may possibly cause anaemia, leucopenia, and thrombocytopenia.

When guanethidine is used as eye drops, common side-effects are conjunctival hyperaemia and miosis. Burning sensations and ptosis have also occurred. Superficial punctate keratitis has been reported particularly following prolonged administration of concentrated solutions.

Treatment of Adverse Effects

Withdrawal of guanethidine or reduction in dosage reverses many side-effects. If overdosage occurs the stomach should be emptied by lavage and activated charcoal may be given. Diarrhoea may be controlled by reducing dosage or by giving codeine phosphate or antimuscarinics. Hypotension may respond to placing the patient in the supine position with the feet raised. If hypotension is severe it may be necessary to give intravenous fluid replacement and small doses of vasopressors may be given cautiously. The patient must be observed for several days.

Precautions

Guanethidine should not be given to patients with phaeochromocytoma, as it may cause a hypertensive crisis, or to patients with heart failure not caused by hypertension.

It should be used with caution in patients with renal impairment, cerebrovascular disorders, or ischaemic heart disease, or with a history of peptic ulceration or asthma. Exercise and heat may increase the hypotensive effect of guanethidine, and dosage requirements may be reduced in patients who develop fever.

There may be an increased risk of cardiovascular collapse or cardiac arrest in patients undergoing surgery while taking guanethidine, but authorities differ as to whether the drug should be discontinued before elective surgery. Some authorities have recommended discontinuation up to 2 or 3 weeks beforehand. In patients undergoing emergency procedures or where treatment has not been interrupted large doses of atropine should be given before induction of anaesthesia.

Patients undergoing treatment with eye drops containing guanethidine should be examined regularly for signs of conjunctival damage.

Interactions

Patients taking guanethidine may show increased sensitivity to the action of adrenaline [epinephrine], amfetamine, and other sympathomimetics resulting in exaggerated pressor effects. The hypotensive effects may also be antagonised by tricyclic antidepressants, MAOIs, and phenothiazine derivatives and related antipsychotics (although phenothiazines may also exacerbate postural hypotension, which may be more relevant clinically). In the UK the manufacturers suggest that treatment with MAOIs should be stopped at least 14 days before beginning guanethidine, although in the USA a minimum of a week has been recommended as adequate. It has been reported that oral contraceptives may reduce the hypotensive action of guanethidine. Concurrent administration of digoxin or other digitalis derivatives with guanethidine may cause excessive bradycardia.

The hypotensive effects of guanethidine may be enhanced by thiazide diuretics, other antihypertensives, and levodopa. Alcohol may cause orthostatic hypotension in patients taking guanethidine.

Pharmacokinetics

Guanethidine is variably and incompletely absorbed from the gastrointestinal tract with less than 50% of the dose reaching the systemic circulation. It is actively taken up into adrenergic neurones by the mechanism responsible for noradrenaline reuptake. A plasma concentration of 8 nanograms per mL is reported to be necessary for adrenergic blockade, but the dose required to achieve this varies between individuals due to differences in absorption and metabolism. Guanethidine is partially metabolised in the liver, and is excreted in the urine as metabolites and unchanged guanethidine. It has a terminal half-life of about 5 days. Guanethidine does not penetrate the blood-brain barrier significantly.

Uses and Administration

Guanethidine is an antihypertensive which acts by selectively inhibiting transmission in postganglionic adrenergic nerves. It is believed to act mainly by preventing the release of noradrenaline at nerve endings; it causes the depletion of noradrenaline stores in peripheral sympathetic nerve terminals. It does not prevent the secretion of catecholamines by the adrenal medulla.

When given by mouth its maximal effects may take 1 to 2 weeks to appear on continued dosing and persist for 7 to 10 days after treatment has been stopped. It causes an initial reduction in cardiac output but its main hypotensive effect is to cause peripheral vasodilatation; it reduces the vasoconstriction which normally results from standing up and which is the result of reflex sympathetic nervous activity. In the majority of patients it reduces the standing blood pressure but has a less marked effect on the supine blood pressure. When applied topically to the eye guanethidine reduces the production of aqueous humour.

Guanethidine is used in the management of hypertension (p.802) and in the topical treatment of open-angle glaucoma (p.1413). Eye drops of guanethidine have also been used for lid retraction associated with hyperthyroidism. Guanethidine may also be used in the management of neuropathic pain syndromes (see below).

Guanethidine is used in the treatment of hypertension when other drugs have proved inadequate, although it has largely been superseded by other drugs less likely to cause orthostatic hypotension. It is often given in conjunction with a diuretic or sometimes with another antihypertensive. Tolerance to guanethidine has occurred in some patients; this may be countered by intensive diuretic therapy.

In **hypertension**, the usual initial dose of guanethidine monosulfate is 10 mg daily by mouth. This is increased by increments of 10 mg every 7 days according to the response of the patient although some authorities recommend intervals of 2 to 3 weeks between increments to avoid accumulation. The usual maintenance dose varies from 25 to 50 mg daily as a single dose but up to 300 mg daily may be given.

Children have been given 200 µg per kg body-weight daily with increments of 200 µg per kg every 1 to 3 weeks until a satisfactory response is achieved; a dose of about 1.5 mg per kg daily may be required.

Smaller doses of guanethidine are needed when it is given with other antihypertensives or diuretics.

Guanethidine monosulfate has been given intramuscularly in the treatment of hypertensive crises, including severe pre-eclampsia, but more suitable drugs are available. An intramuscular dose of 10 to 20 mg is reported to produce a fall in blood pressure within 30 minutes, reaching a maximum in 1 to 2 hours and lasting for 4 to 6 hours.

Eye drops containing guanethidine monosulfate 1 or 3% together with adrenaline [epinephrine] 0.2 or 0.5%, respectively, are used in the treatment of open-angle **glaucoma**. Guanethidine monosulfate 5% eye drops, without adrenaline [epinephrine], have also been used for open-angle glaucoma and for the lid retraction which may accompany hyperthyroidism.

Pain syndromes. Sympathetic nerve blocks may be used in the management of acute or chronic pain associated with a well-defined anatomical site. Guanethidine has been used for intravenous regional sympathetic block in the management of neuropathic pain including central pain syndromes, to reduce pain and to maintain blood flow. Open studies[1,2] have shown benefit from guanethidine, and the effects of serial blocks appear to be cumulative.[3] Guanethidine has been suggested as a suitable treatment for reflex sympathetic dystrophy.[4] However, a review of the literature and a double-blind trial[5] in patients with reflex sympathetic dystrophy failed to find any benefit from guanethidine. The trial had to be terminated early due to unacceptable adverse effects. Interestingly a small double-blind study in patients with rheumatoid arthritis found that regional sympathetic blockade with guanethidine 15 mg in 13 produced a significant improvement in pain intensity and pinch strength compared with placebo in 11. Grip strength, tenderness, and morning stiffness were not improved.[6]

Intravenous regional sympathetic blockade using guanethidine has also been reported in the management of frostbite.[7]

For a discussion of sympathetic pain syndromes, see p.8.

1. Hannington-Kiff JG. Relief of causalgia in limbs by regional intravenous guanethidine. *BMJ* 1979; **2:** 367–8.
2. Loh L, *et al.* Pain due to lesions of central nervous system removed by sympathetic block. *BMJ* 1981; **282:** 1026–8.
3. Parry CBW, Withrington RH. Painful disorders of peripheral nerves. *Postgrad Med J* 1984; **60:** 869–75.
4. Yasuda JM, Schroeder DJ. Guanethidine for reflex sympathetic dystrophy. *Ann Pharmacother* 1994; **28:** 338–41.
5. Jadad AR, *et al.* Intravenous regional sympathetic blockade for pain relief in reflex sympathetic dystrophy: a systematic review and a randomized, double-blind crossover study. *J Pain Symptom Manage* 1995; **10:** 13–20.
6. Levine JD, *et al.* Clinical response to regional intravenous guanethidine in patients with rheumatoid arthritis. *J Rheumatol* 1986; **13:** 1040–3.
7. Kaplan R, *et al.* Treatment of frostbite with guanethidine. *Lancet* 1981; **ii:** 940–1.

Preparations

BP 2001: Guanethidine Tablets;
USP 25: Guanethidine Monosulfate Tablets.

Proprietary Preparations (details are given in Part 3)
Aust.: Ismelin; **Austral.:** Ismelin; **Fr.:** Ismeline†; **Ital.:** Visutensil†; **Mex.:** Ismelin; **NZ:** Ismelin; **S.Afr.:** Ismelin; **Switz.:** Ismelin†; **UK:** Ismelin; **USA:** Ismelin.

Multi-ingredient: Aust.: Thilodigon; **Denm.:** Suprexon†; **Ger.:** Esimil; Suprexon; Thilodigon; **Irl.:** Ganda; **Neth.:** Suprexon; **S.Afr.:** Ganda†; **Switz.:** Suprexon†; **UK:** Ganda; **USA:** Esimil.

Guanfacine Hydrochloride (12806-z)

Guanfacine Hydrochloride (BANM, USAN, rINNM).

BS-100-141; LON-798. N-Amidino-2-(2,6-dichlorophenyl)acetamide hydrochloride.

$C_9H_9Cl_2N_3O,HCl = 282.6$.

CAS — 29110-47-2 (guanfacine); 29110-48-3 (guanfacine hydrochloride).

Pharmacopoeias. In US.

Guanfacine hydrochloride 1.15 mg is approximately equivalent to 1 mg of guanfacine.

Pharmacopoeial description

USP 25: Store in airtight containers. Protect from light.

Adverse Effects and Precautions

As for Clonidine Hydrochloride, p.860. Rebound hypertension may occur but is delayed due to the longer half-life.

◊ Reviews.

1. Jerie P. Clinical experience with guanfacine in long-term treatment of hypertension, part II: adverse reactions to guanfacine. *Br J Clin Pharmacol* 1980; **10** (suppl 1): 157S–164S.
2. Board AW, *et al.* A postmarketing evaluation of guanfacine hydrochloride in mild to moderate hypertension. *Clin Ther* 1988; **10:** 761–75.

Withdrawal. Rapid reduction of the guanfacine dosage resulted in rebound hypertension leading to generalised seizures and coma in a 47-year-old patient with renal failure who was receiving haemodialysis.[1] Concomitant use of phenobarbital may have enhanced the metabolism of guanfacine and contributed to the development of the withdrawal effect.

1. Kiechel JR, *et al.* Pharmacokinetic aspects of guanfacine withdrawal syndrome in a hypertensive patient with chronic renal failure. *Eur J Clin Pharmacol* 1983; **25:** 463–6.

Interactions

As for Clonidine Hydrochloride, p.860.

Pharmacokinetics

Following oral administration guanfacine is rapidly absorbed, peak plasma concentrations occurring 1 to 4 hours after ingestion. The oral bioavailability is reported to be about 80%. It is about 70% bound to plasma proteins. It is excreted in urine as unchanged drug and metabolites; about 50% of a dose is reported to be eliminated unchanged. The normal elimination half-life ranges from 10 to 30 hours, tending to be longer in older patients than in young ones.

Renal impairment. Results in patients with normal and impaired renal function suggested that non-renal elimination of guanfacine plays an important role in patients with renal impairment since clearance and serum concentrations were not significantly altered in such patients.[1]

1. Kirch W, *et al.* Elimination of guanfacine in patients with normal and impaired renal function. *Br J Clin Pharmacol* 1980; **10** (suppl 1): 33S–35S.

The symbol † denotes a preparation no longer actively marketed

Uses and Administration

Guanfacine is a centrally acting alpha$_2$-adrenoceptor agonist with actions and uses similar to those of clonidine (p.861). It is used in the management of hypertension (p.802), either alone or in conjunction with other antihypertensives, particularly thiazide diuretics. However, other antihypertensives are usually preferred. It has also been tried in the management of opioid withdrawal and in hyperactivity disorders.

Guanfacine is given by mouth as the hydrochloride, but doses are usually expressed in terms of the base.

In hypertension it is given in usual initial doses of 1 mg daily increasing after 3 to 4 weeks to 2 mg daily if necessary.

◊ Reviews.
1. Cornish LA. Guanfacine hydrochloride: a centrally acting antihypertensive agent. *Clin Pharm* 1988; **7:** 187–97.

Preparations

USP 25: Guanfacine Tablets.

Proprietary Preparations (details are given in Part 3)
Belg.: Estulic; *Fr.:* Estulic; *Ger.:* Estulic; *Irl.:* Akfen; *Neth.:* Estulic; *USA:* Tenex.

Guanoxan Sulfate (871-z)

Guanoxan Sulfate *(USAN, rINNM)*.

3-01003; Guanoxan Sulphate *(BANM)*. 1-(1,4-Benzodioxan-2-ylmethyl)guanidine sulphate; 1-(2,3-Dihydro-1,4-benzodioxin-2-ylmethyl)guanidine sulphate.
$(C_{10}H_{13}N_3O_2)_2,H_2SO_4 = 512.5$.
CAS — 2165-19-7 (guanoxan); 5714-04-5 (guanoxan sulfate).

Profile

Guanoxan is an antihypertensive with properties similar to those of guanethidine (p.901). It was formerly used in the management of hypertension. Liver damage has followed treatment with guanoxan.

Adverse effects. Of 96 patients treated with guanoxan, 26 had some derangement of liver function tests, severe in 10; four of these developed jaundice and 1 of the 4 patients died with chronic hepatic necrosis.[1]
1. Cotton SG, Montuschi E. Guanoxan. *BMJ* 1967; **3:** 174.

Heparin (11401-s)

Heparin *(BAN)*.
Heparinum.
CAS — 9005-49-6.
ATC — B01AB01; C05BA03; S01XA14.

NOTE. Heparin is often described in the literature as standard heparin or unfractionated heparin to distinguish it from low-molecular-weight heparins.

Heparin is an anionic polysaccharide of mammalian origin with irregular sequence. It consists principally of alternating iduronate and glucosamine residues most of which are sulfated. It may be described as a sulfated glucosaminoglycan. Heparin has the characteristic property of delaying the clotting of freshly shed blood. It may be prepared from the lungs of oxen or the intestinal mucosa of oxen, pigs, or sheep.

Heparin Calcium (4801-w)

Heparin Calcium *(BANM)*.
Calcium Heparin; Heparinum Calcicum.
CAS — 37270-89-6.
Pharmacopoeias. In Eur. (see p.vi) and US.

Incompatibility. See Heparin Sodium, below.

Pharmacopoeial description

Ph. Eur.: The potency of heparin calcium intended for parenteral administration is not less than 150 international units per mg and the potency of heparin calcium not intended for parenteral administration is not less than 120 international units per mg, both calculated with reference to the dried substance. A white or almost white, moderately hygroscopic powder. Freely soluble in water. A 1% solution in water has a pH of 5.5 to 8.0. Store in airtight containers.

USP 25: The calcium salt of heparin with a potency, calculated on the dried basis, of not less than 140 USP units in each mg. USP heparin units are not equivalent to international units. The source of the material is usually the intestinal mucosa or other suitable tissues of domestic mammals used for food by man and should be stated on the label. A 1% solution in water has a pH of 5.0 to 7.5. Store in airtight containers at temperatures below 40°, preferably between 15 and 30°.

Heparin Sodium (4802-e)

Heparin Sodium *(BANM, rINN)*.

Heparinum Natricum; Sodium Heparin; Soluble Heparin.
CAS — 9041-08-1.
Pharmacopoeias. In Chin., Eur. (see p.vi), Jpn, and US.

Pharmacopoeial description

Ph. Eur.: The potency of heparin sodium intended for parenteral administration is not less than 150 international units per mg and the potency of heparin sodium not intended for parenteral administration is not less than 120 international units per mg, both calculated with reference to the dried substance. A white or almost white, moderately hygroscopic powder. Freely soluble in water. A 1% solution in water has a pH of 5.5 to 8.0. Store in airtight containers.

USP 25: The sodium salt of heparin with a potency, calculated on the dried basis, of not less than 140 USP units in each mg. USP heparin units are not equivalent to international units. The source of the material is usually the intestinal mucosa or other suitable tissues of domestic mammals used for food by man and should be stated on the label. A white or pale-coloured amorphous, odourless or almost odourless, hygroscopic powder. Soluble 1 in 20 of water. A 1% solution in water has a pH of 5.0 to 7.5. Store in airtight containers at temperatures below 40°, preferably between 15 and 30°.

Incompatibility. Incompatibility has been reported between heparin calcium or sodium and alteplase, amikacin sulfate, amiodarone hydrochloride, ampicillin sodium, aprotinin, benzylpenicillin potassium or sodium, cefalotin sodium, ciprofloxacin lactate, cytarabine, dacarbazine, daunorubicin hydrochloride, diazepam, dobutamine hydrochloride, doxorubicin hydrochloride, droperidol, erythromycin lactobionate, gentamicin sulfate, haloperidol lactate, hyaluronidase, hydrocortisone sodium succinate, kanamycin sulfate, meticillin sodium, netilmicin sulfate, some opioid analgesics, oxytetracycline hydrochloride, some phenothiazines, polymyxin B sulfate, streptomycin sulfate, tetracycline hydrochloride, tobramycin sulfate, vancomycin hydrochloride, and vinblastine sulfate. Heparin sodium has also been reported to be incompatible with cisatracurium besilate,[1] labetalol hydrochloride,[2] levofloxacin,[3] nicardipine hydrochloride,[4] reteplase,[5] and vinorelbine tartrate.[6] Although visually compatible,[7] cefmetazole sodium is reported to inactivate heparin sodium.

Glucose can have variable effects,[8,9] but glucose-containing solutions are generally considered suitable diluents for heparin. Incompatibility has also been reported between heparin and fat emulsion.

1. Trissel LA, *et al.* Compatibility of cisatracurium besylate with selected drugs during simulated Y-site administration. *Am J Health-Syst Pharm* 1997; **54:** 1735–41.
2. Yamashita SK, *et al.* Compatibility of selected critical care drugs during simulated Y-site administration. *Am J Health-Syst Pharm* 1996; **53:** 1048–51.
3. Saltsman CL, *et al.* Compatibility of levofloxacin with 34 medications during simulated Y-site administration. *Am J Health-Syst Pharm* 1999; **56:** 1458–9.
4. Chiu MF, Schwartz ML. Visual compatibility of injectable drugs used in the intensive care unit. *Am J Health-Syst Pharm* 1997; **54:** 64–5.
5. Committee on Safety of Medicines/Medicines Control Agency. Reteplase (Rapilysin): incompatibility with heparin. *Current Problems* 2000; **26:** 5.
6. Balthasar JP. Concentration-dependent incompatibility of vinorelbine tartrate and heparin sodium. *Am J Health-Syst Pharm* 1999; **56:** 1891.
7. Hutching SR, *et al.* Compatibility of cefmetazole sodium with commonly used drugs during Y-site delivery. *Am J Health-Syst Pharm* 1996; **53:** 2185–8.
8. Anderson W, Harthill JE. The anticoagulant activity of heparins in dextrose infusions. *J Pharm Pharmacol* 1982; **34:** 90–6.
9. Wright A, Hecker J. Long term stability of heparin in dextrose-saline intravenous fluids. *Int J Pharm Pract* 1995; **3:** 253–5.

Units

The fourth International Standard for porcine heparin was established in 1983. The USP 25 states that USP and international units are not equivalent, although doses expressed in either appear to be essentially the same.

Adverse Effects

Heparin can give rise to haemorrhage as a consequence of its action. It can also cause thrombocytopenia, either through a direct effect or through an immune effect producing a platelet-aggregating antibody. Consequent platelet aggregation and thrombosis may therefore exacerbate the condition being treated. The incidence of thrombocytopenia is reported to be greater with bovine than porcine heparin.

Hypersensitivity reactions may occur, as may local irritant effects, and skin necrosis. Alopecia and osteoporosis resulting in spontaneous fractures have occurred after prolonged use of heparin.

Effects on the adrenal glands. Heparin inhibits the secretion of aldosterone which can cause hyperkalaemia.[1] Although all patients treated with heparin may develop reduced aldosterone concentrations, most are able to compensate through the renin-angiotensin system. Patients on prolonged heparin therapy or those unable to compensate, such as patients with diabetes mellitus or renal impairment or those on concurrent therapy with potassium-sparing drugs such as ACE inhibitors may

present with symptoms. The UK Committee on Safety of Medicines suggests[2] that plasma-potassium concentration should be monitored in all patients with risk factors, particularly those receiving heparin for more than 7 days. The hyperkalaemia is usually transient or resolves when heparin is discontinued and treatment is not generally required; fludrocortisone was successfully used to treat resistant hyperkalaemia in a patient in whom continued heparin therapy was necessary.[3]

Adrenal insufficiency secondary to adrenal haemorrhage has also been associated with heparin administration; heparin-induced thrombocytopenia may be implicated.[4]

1. Oster JR, *et al.* Heparin-induced aldosterone suppression and hyperkalemia. *Am J Med* 1995; **98:** 575–86.
2. Committee on Safety of Medicines/Medicines Control Agency. Suppression of aldosterone secretion by heparin. *Current Problems* 1999; **25:** 6.
3. Sherman DS, *et al.* Fludrocortisone for the treatment of heparin-induced hyperkalemia. *Ann Pharmacother* 2000; **34:** 606–10.
4. Dahlberg PJ, *et al.* Adrenal insufficiency secondary to adrenal hemorrhage: two case reports and a review of cases confirmed by computed tomography. *Arch Intern Med* 1990; **150:** 905–9.

Effects on the blood. *Haemorrhage* is a recognised risk with heparin.[1] The risk of major bleeding may be lower with continuous intravenous infusion than with intermittent intravenous injection; risk may increase with heparin dose and age.[2]

Heparin has been associated with the development of *thrombocytopenia*. The reported incidence has varied greatly; up to 6% appears to be a reasonable estimate[3,4] although up to 10% has also been quoted.[5] Thrombocytopenia induced by heparin may be of two types. The first is an acute, but usually mild, fall in platelet count occurring within 1 to 4 days of initiation of therapy and which often resolves without cessation of treatment. A direct effect of heparin on platelet aggregation appears to be responsible. The second type of thrombocytopenia, which has an immunological basis, is more serious. It usually occurs after 5 to 11 days of heparin although its onset may be more rapid in patients previously exposed to heparin.[6] It is often associated with thromboembolic complications due to platelet-rich thrombi (the 'white clot syndrome') or, more rarely, bleeding. Of 34 cases of heparin-associated thrombocytopenia reported to the UK Committee on Safety of Medicines (CSM) from 1964 to 1989, bleeding or thromboembolic complications occurred in 11 patients, 7 of whom died.[3] This type of thrombocytopenia appears to occur more frequently with bovine heparin than with heparin from other species[7] and it has been proposed that in susceptible patients antibody reacts with heparin bound to platelets and endothelial cells.[8] Patients with lupus anticoagulant may also be more susceptible.[9] The reaction is independent of dose or route of administration; there are reports of thrombocytopenia after use of heparin flushes[10] or heparin-coated catheters.[11] The CSM recommend monitoring of platelet counts in patients given heparin for more than 5 days.[3] Patients previously exposed to heparin may be sensitised to it and after re-exposure should have a platelet count before the 5 days are up.[12]

Treatment should be stopped immediately in those who develop thrombocytopenia. It should be noted, however, that thrombosis has occurred in patients whose reduction in platelet count was relatively mild and who may not be considered to be thrombocytopenic.[13-16] On withdrawal of heparin, a heparinoid such as danaparoid[17,18] may be tried, provided that an *in-vitro* platelet aggregation test is negative, i.e. there is no cross-reactivity with heparin. Alternatively, lepirudin,[18,19] a recombinant hirudin, or the thrombin inhibitor argatroban,[18,20] may be used. Low-molecular-weight heparins have been used; they are associated with a lower incidence of induced thrombocytopenia than unfractionated heparin[21] but the rate of cross-reactivity is high and they are not generally recommended.[18,20] Alternatively, oral anticoagulation may be initiated, although an increased risk of venous limb gangrene has been reported[22] with warfarin. Ancrod[18,20] and dermatan sulfate[23] have also been used. Thrombocytopenia has been managed with aspirin and dipyridamole or with normal immunoglobulin.[24] A fibrinolytic such as urokinase has been used in a few cases of occlusive thrombosis.[25,26]

There may be a relationship between heparin-induced thrombocytopenia and skin necrosis (see below).

1. Walker AM, Jick H. Predictors of bleeding during heparin therapy. *JAMA* 1980; **244:** 1209–12.
2. Levine MN, *et al.* Hemorrhagic complications of anticoagulant treatment. *Chest* 2001; **119** (suppl): 108S–121S.
3. Committee on Safety of Medicines. Heparin-induced thrombocytopenia. *Current Problems* 28 1990.
4. Derlon A, *et al.* Thrombopénies induites par l'héparine: symptomatologie, détection, fréquence. *Therapie* 1988; **43:** 199–203.
5. Aster RH. Heparin-induced thrombocytopenia and thrombosis. *N Engl J Med* 1995; **332:** 1374–6.
6. Warkentin TE, Kelton JG. Temporal aspects of heparin-induced thrombocytopenia. *N Engl J Med* 2001; **344:** 1286–92.
7. Bell WR, Royall RM. Heparin-associated thrombocytopenia: a comparison of three heparin preparations. *N Engl J Med* 1980; **303:** 902–7.
8. Cines DB, *et al.* Immune endothelial-cell injury in heparin-associated thrombocytopenia. *N Engl J Med* 1987; **316:** 581–9.
9. Auger WR, *et al.* Lupus anticoagulant, heparin use, and thrombocytopenia in patients with chronic thromboembolic pulmonary hypertension: a preliminary report. *Am J Med* 1995; **99:** 392–6.
10. Heeger PS, Backstrom JT. Heparin flushes and thrombocytopenia. *Ann Intern Med* 1986; **105:** 143.
11. Laster JL, *et al.* Thrombocytopenia associated with heparin-coated catheters in patients with heparin-associated antiplatelet antibodies. *Arch Intern Med* 1989; **149:** 2285–7.

12. Hunter JB, *et al.* Heparin induced thrombosis: an important complication of heparin prophylaxis for thromboembolic disease in surgery. *BMJ* 1993; **307:** 53–5.
13. Phelan BK. Heparin-associated thrombosis without thrombocytopenia. *BMJ* 1999; **99:** 637–8.
14. Trono DP, *et al.* Thrombocytopenia and heparin-associated thrombosis. *Ann Intern Med* 1984; **100:** 464–5.
15. Ramirez-Lassepas M, Cipolle RJ. Heparin and thrombocytopenia. *Ann Intern Med* 1984; **100:** 613.
16. Hach-Wunderle V, *et al.* Heparin-associated thrombosis despite normal platelet counts. *Lancet* 1994; **344:** 469–70.
17. Wilde MI, Markham A. Danaparoid: a review of its pharmacology and clinical use in the management of heparin-induced thrombocytopenia. *Drugs* 1997; **54:** 903–24.
18. Januzzi JL, Jang I-K. Heparin induced thrombocytopenia: diagnosis and contemporary antithrombin management. *J Thromb Thrombolysis* 1999; **7:** 259–64.
19. Greinacher A, *et al.* Recombinant hirudin (lepirudin) provides safe and effective anticoagulation in patients with heparin-induced thrombocytopenia: a prospective study. *Circulation* 1999; **99:** 73–80.
20. Warkentin TE. Heparin-induced thrombocytopenia: pathogenesis, frequency, avoidance and management. *Drug Safety* 1997; **17:** 325–41.
21. Warkentin TE, *et al.* Heparin-induced thrombocytopenia in patients treated with low-molecular- weight heparin or unfractionated heparin. *N Engl J Med* 1995; **332:** 1330–5.
22. Warkentin TE, *et al.* The pathogenesis of venous limb gangrene associated with heparin-induced thrombocytopenia. *Ann Intern Med* 1997; **127:** 804–12.
23. Taliani MR, *et al.* Dermatan sulphate in patients with heparin-induced thrombocytopenia. *Br J Haematol* 1999; **104:** 87–9.
24. Frame JN, *et al.* Correction of severe heparin-associated thrombocytopenia with intravenous immunoglobulin. *Ann Intern Med* 1989; **111:** 946–7.
25. Krueger SK, *et al.* Thrombolysis in heparin-induced thrombocytopenia with thrombosis. *Ann Intern Med* 1985; **103:** 159.
26. Clifton GD, Smith MD. Thrombolytic therapy in heparin-associated thrombocytopenia with thrombosis. *Clin Pharm* 1986; **5:** 597–601.

Effects on the bones. Osteoporosis is a rare complication of long-term heparin therapy. Treatment and prophylaxis of thromboembolism in pregnancy is one of the few indications for long term use of heparin, so most reports and studies of heparin-induced osteoporosis have been in pregnant women.[1] The incidence of symptomatic osteoporosis in patients receiving heparin long term has been estimated to be about 2%.[1,2] Subclinical reduction in bone density occurs in up to one-third of patients,[2] but it is not possible to predict which of these patients will develop osteoporotic fractures. Pregnancy normally causes reversible bone demineralisation, so the combination of pregnancy and heparin therapy may therefore result in symptomatic osteoporosis in susceptible individuals.[1,3] Bone changes may be reversible.[1] Although some evidence suggests that bone demineralisation is dose- and duration-dependent, this has not been conclusively established.[1-3] Use of low-molecular-weight heparins may be associated with a lower risk of heparin-induced osteoporosis, but experience is limited.[1-3]

1. Nelson-Piercy C. Heparin-induced osteoporosis. *Scand J Rheumatol* 1998; **27** (suppl 107): 68–71.
2. Ginsberg JS, *et al.* Use of antithrombotic agents during pregnancy. *Chest* 2001; **119** (suppl): 122S–131S.
3. Farquharson RG. Heparin, osteoporosis and pregnancy. *Br J Hosp Med* 1997; **58:** 205–7.

Effects on electrolytes. See under Effects on the Adrenal Glands, above.

Effects on the liver. Increases in transaminase values have been reported in patients given therapeutic[1-3] or prophylactic[3] doses of heparin. The abnormality usually resolved on discontinuation of heparin.

1. Sonnenblick M, *et al.* Hyper-transaminasemia with heparin therapy. *BMJ* 1975; **3:** 77.
2. Dukes GE, *et al.* Transaminase elevations in patients receiving bovine or porcine heparin. *Ann Intern Med* 1984; **100:** 646–50.
3. Monreal M, *et al.* Adverse effects of three different forms of heparin therapy: thrombocytopenia, increased transaminases, and hyperkalaemia. *Eur J Clin Pharmacol* 1989; **37:** 415–18.

Effects on serum lipids. Administration of heparin leads to the release of lipoprotein lipase into the plasma. Postprandial lipidaemia is reduced due to increased hydrolysis of triglycerides into free fatty acids and glycerol. Raised concentrations of free fatty acids have been reported following heparin administration, but the magnitude of this effect may have been overestimated.[1] Rebound hyperlipidaemia may occur when heparin is withdrawn. With long-term administration reserves of lipoprotein lipase may be depleted; severe hypertriglyceridaemia reported in a pregnant woman was attributed to long-term heparin prophylaxis that was thought to have resulted in lipoprotein lipase deficiency.[2]

1. Riemersma RA, *et al.* Heparin-induced lipolysis, an exaggerated risk. *Lancet* 1981; **ii:** 471.
2. Watts GF, *et al.* Lipoprotein lipase deficiency due to long-term heparinization presenting as severe hypertriglyceridaemia in pregnancy. *Postgrad Med J* 1991; **67:** 1062–4.

Effects on sexual function. There have been several reports of priapism associated with the administration of heparin. The prognosis is poor, impotence following more often than in priapism of other aetiologies. The mechanism of heparin-induced priapism is unclear.[1]

1. Baños JE, *et al.* Drug-induced priapism: its aetiology, incidence and treatment. *Med Toxicol* 1989; **4:** 46–58.

Effects on the skin. Skin necrosis is a rare complication of heparin administration.[1,2] It may be a localised reaction at the site of subcutaneous injection or possibly be related to heparin-induced thrombocytopenia (see Effects on the Blood, above). An immune mechanism may be responsible.

Eczematous plaque reactions have developed several days after initiation of subcutaneous heparin. A type IV hypersensitivity reaction has been implicated.[3] Low-molecular-weight heparins may be an alternative but cross-reactivity can occur.[4]
Recurrent fixed eczematous lesions have been attributed to heparin used intravenously during haemodialysis.[5]

1. Ulrick PJ, Manoharan A. Heparin-induced skin reaction. *Med J Aust* 1984; **140:** 287–9.
2. Fowlie J, *et al.* Heparin-associated skin necrosis. *Postgrad Med J* 1990; **66:** 573–5.
3. Bircher AJ, *et al.* Eczematous infiltrated plaques to subcutaneous heparin: a type IV allergic reaction. *Br J Dermatol* 1990; **123:** 507–14.
4. O'Donnell BF, Tan CY. Delayed hypersensitivity reactions to heparin. *Br J Dermatol* 1993; **129:** 634–6.
5. Mohammed KN. Symmetric fixed eruption to heparin. *Dermatology* 1995; **190:** 91.

Treatment of Adverse Effects

Slight haemorrhage due to overdosage can usually be treated by withdrawing heparin. Severe bleeding may be reduced by the slow intravenous administration of protamine sulfate (p.1021). The dose is dependent on the amount of heparin to be neutralised and ideally should be titrated against assessments of the coagulability of the patient's blood. As heparin is being continuously excreted the dose should be reduced if more than 15 minutes have elapsed since heparin administration; for example, if protamine sulfate is given 30 minutes after heparin the dose may be reduced to about one-half. Not more than 50 mg of protamine sulfate should be injected for any one dose; patients should be carefully monitored as further doses may be required. The Ph. Eur. specifies that 1 mg of protamine sulfate precipitates not less than 100 international units of heparin sodium, but adds that this potency is based on a specific reference batch of heparin sodium. The UK manufacturer has stated that each mg of protamine sulfate will usually neutralise the anticoagulant effect of at least 80 international units of heparin (lung) or at least 100 international units of heparin (mucous). The US manufacturer has stated that each mg of protamine sulfate neutralises approximately 90 USP units of heparin (lung) or about 115 USP units of heparin (mucous).

◊ For reference to the treatment of heparin-induced thrombocytopenia and associated thromboembolic complications, see Effects on the Blood under Adverse Effects, above.

Precautions

Heparin should not be given to patients who are haemorrhaging. In general it should not be given to patients at serious risk of haemorrhage, although it has been used with very careful control; patients at risk include those with haemorrhagic blood disorders, thrombocytopenia, peptic ulcer disease, cerebrovascular disorders, bacterial endocarditis, severe hypertension, oesophageal varices, or patients who have recently undergone surgery at sites where haemorrhage would be an especial risk. Severe renal and hepatic impairment are considered by some to be contra-indications. Heparin should not be given by intramuscular injection. Since heparin has caused thrombocytopenia with severe thromboembolic complications, platelet counts should be monitored in patients receiving heparin for more than a few days. Heparin should be discontinued if thrombocytopenia develops. A test dose has been recommended for patients with a history of allergy.

Dosage of heparin may need to be reduced in the elderly; elderly women appear to be especially susceptible to haemorrhage after heparin administration.

Preservative. The preservatives used in heparin preparations have been implicated in unwanted effects. Benzyl alcohol in heparinised flushing solutions has been suspected of causing toxicity in neonates (see p.1135). Chlorobutanol present in another heparin preparation caused a sharp fall in blood pressure (see Chlorobutanol, Incompatibilities, p.1141).

Catheters and cannulas. Serum concentrations of sodium and potassium could be falsely elevated in samples obtained through heparin-bonded umbilical catheters due to release of benzalkonium chloride used in the manufacturing process of some catheters.[1] It was unknown if the amount released would be toxic to small premature neonates.

1. Gaylord MS, *et al.* Release of benzalkonium chloride from a heparin-bonded umbilical catheter with resultant factitious hypernatremia and hyperkalemia. *Pediatrics* 1991; **87:** 631–5.

Hyperkalaemia. For recommendations concerning the monitoring of patients susceptible to developing hyperkalaemia, such as those with diabetes mellitus or renal insufficiency, see Effects on the Adrenal Glands under Adverse Effects, above.

Pregnancy. Heparin does not cross the placenta, and therefore adverse effects on the fetus would not be expected.[1,2] A review[1] of the literature, however, found 2 spontaneous abortions and 17 still-births in 135 pregnancies exposed to heparin; 29 infants were premature, 10 of whom died. Another literature review[2] found adverse outcomes in 21.7% of heparin-treated patients, but this dropped to 10.4% when pregnancies with co-morbid conditions were excluded. A further drop to 3.6% was observed when cases of prematurity with normal outcome were also excluded. The death rate of 2.5% and prematurity rate of 6.8% in heparin-treated patients was similar to that found in the normal population. It was concluded that heparin appears safer for the fetus than warfarin when used during pregnancy. Similar results have also been reported with low-molecular-weight heparins; a systematic review[3] found an adverse outcome in 9.3% of 486 pregnancies in which low-molecular-weight heparin was used, but this dropped to 3.1% in women without comorbid conditions.

1. Hall JG, *et al.* Maternal and fetal sequelae of anticoagulation during pregnancy. *Am J Med* 1980; **68:** 122–40.
2. Ginsberg JS, Hirsh J. Optimum use of anticoagulants in pregnancy. *Drugs* 1988; **36:** 505–12.
3. Sanson B-J, *et al.* Safety of low-molecular-weight heparin in pregnancy: a systematic review. *Thromb Haemost* 1999; **81:** 668–72.

Spinal anaesthesia. Spinal and epidural haematomas, sometimes leading to paralysis, have occurred in patients receiving heparin or low-molecular-weight heparins in association with spinal or epidural anaesthesia or analgesia. The risk of haematoma appears to be higher in patients with indwelling epidural catheters or receiving concomitant therapy with other drugs that affect haemostasis.[1] It is generally recommended that central nerve block should be avoided in patients receiving full-dose anticoagulation.[2] However, the use of prophylactic doses of anticoagulants with central nervous blockade is less clear.[2,3] The reported risk of haematoma with low-molecular-weight heparins has been higher in the USA where higher doses have been used for prophylaxis.[3] Recommendations to reduce the risk of spinal haematoma include waiting until after blockade has been completed to administer prophylactic heparin or low-molecular-weight heparin. Where anticoagulant prophylaxis has already been given, blockade should be delayed if possible until 4 to 6 hours after heparin, and the catheter should not be removed until 4 hours after heparin.[2] For low-molecular-weight heparin it is recommended that administration should not be within 8 to 10 hours before or after central nerve block or catheter removal.[2,3]

1. Wysowski DK, *et al.* Spinal and epidural hematoma and low-molecular-weight heparin. *N Engl J Med* 1998; **338:** 1774.
2. Armstrong RF, *et al.* Epidural and spinal anaesthesia and the use of anticoagulants. *Hosp Med* 1999; **60:** 491–6.
3. Dolenska S. Neuroaxial blocks and LMWH thromboprophylaxis. *Hosp Med* 1998; **59:** 940–3.

Interactions

Heparin should be used with care in conjunction with oral anticoagulants or drugs, such as aspirin and dipyridamole, which affect platelet function. NSAIDs may also increase the risk of haemorrhage. Other drugs which affect the coagulation process and which may therefore increase the risk of haemorrhage include dextrans, thrombolytic enzymes such as streptokinase, high doses of penicillins and some cephalosporins, some contrast media, asparaginase, and epoprostenol. Estimations of oral anticoagulant control may be modified by heparin's action on prothrombin.

ACE inhibitors. For reference to hyperkalaemia in patients on heparin and ACE inhibitors, see Effects on the Adrenal Glands under Adverse Effects, above.

Alcohol. Heavy drinkers were at greater risk of major heparin-associated bleeding than moderate drinkers or non-drinkers.[1]

1. Walker AM, Jick H. Predictors of bleeding during heparin therapy. *JAMA* 1980; **244:** 1209–12.

Aprotinin. For comment on the use of heparin with aprotinin, see under Effects on Coagulation Tests in Aprotinin, p.725.

Glyceryl trinitrate. Glyceryl trinitrate has been reported to reduce the activity of heparin when both drugs are given simultaneously by the intravenous route.[1] This effect has been seen even at low doses of glyceryl trinitrate.[2] Propylene glycol present in the glyceryl trinitrate formulation may contribute to the effect,[3] or it may not.[1] No interaction was reported when glyceryl trinitrate was given immediately after heparin.[4]

1. Habbab MA, Haft JI. Heparin resistance induced by intravenous nitroglycerin. *Arch Intern Med* 1987; **147:** 857–60.
2. Brack MJ, *et al.* The effect of low dose nitroglycerine on plasma heparin concentrations and activated partial thromboplastin times. *Blood Coag Fibrinol* 1993; **4:** 183–6.
3. Col J, *et al.* Propylene glycol-induced heparin resistance during nitroglycerin infusion. *Am Heart J* 1985; **110:** 171–3.
4. Bode V, *et al.* Absence of drug interaction between heparin and nitroglycerin. *Arch Intern Med* 1990; **150:** 2117–19.

The symbol † denotes a preparation no longer actively marketed

Tobacco. Reduced half-life and increased elimination of heparin have been reported in smokers compared with non-smokers.[1]

1. Cipolle RJ, et al. Heparin kinetics: variables related to disposition and dosage. Clin Pharmacol Ther 1981; 29: 387–93.

Pharmacokinetics

Heparin is not absorbed from the gastrointestinal tract. Following intravenous or subcutaneous injection heparin is extensively bound to plasma proteins. It does not cross the placenta and it is not distributed into breast milk. The half-life of heparin depends on the dose and route of administration as well as the method of calculation and is subject to wide inter- and intra-individual variation; a range of 1 to 6 hours with an average of 1.5 hours has been cited. It may be slightly prolonged in renal impairment, decreased in patients with pulmonary embolism, and either increased or decreased in patients with liver disorders. Heparin is taken up by the reticuloendothelial system. It is excreted in the urine, mainly as metabolites, although, following administration of large doses, up to 50% may be excreted unchanged.

◊ References.
1. Estes JW. Clinical pharmacokinetics of heparin. Clin Pharmacokinet 1980; 5: 204–20.
2. Kandrotas RJ. Heparin pharmacokinetics and pharmacodynamics. Clin Pharmacokinet 1992; 22: 359–74.

Uses and Administration

Heparin is an anticoagulant used principally in the treatment and prophylaxis of thromboembolic disorders (p.816). It is often described as standard heparin or unfractionated heparin to distinguish it from low-molecular-weight heparins (p.923).

It inhibits clotting of blood in vitro and in vivo through its action on antithrombin III. Antithrombin III, which is present in plasma, inhibits the activity of activated clotting factors including thrombin (factor IIa) and activated factor X (factor Xa); heparin increases the rate of this inhibition, but in a manner that is dependent on its dose. With normal therapeutic doses heparin has an inhibitory effect on both thrombin and factor Xa. Thus the conversion of fibrinogen to fibrin is blocked through the thrombin inhibition, while the conversion of prothrombin to thrombin is blocked by the inhibition of factor Xa. The low doses that are given subcutaneously for the prophylaxis of thromboembolism have a selective effect on antithrombin III's inhibition of factor Xa. Very high doses are reported to reduce the activity of antithrombin III. Heparin also has some effect on platelet function, inhibits the formation of a stable fibrin clot, and has an antilipidaemic effect. For an explanation of the coagulation cascade, see Haemostasis and Fibrinolysis, p.718.

Heparin is used in the treatment and prophylaxis of venous thromboembolism (deep-vein thrombosis and pulmonary embolism, p.817), especially prophylaxis in surgical patients and in those pregnant women at particular risk. It is also used in the management of arterial thromboembolism including that associated with unstable angina pectoris (p.791), myocardial infarction (p.805), acute peripheral arterial occlusion (p.808), and stroke (p.813). It is often used as a precursor to oral anticoagulation and is withdrawn once the oral anticoagulant is exerting its full effect.

Heparin has been tried in the treatment of disseminated intravascular coagulation. It is also used to prevent coagulation during haemodialysis and other extracorporeal circulatory procedures such as cardiopulmonary bypass. Other uses include the anticoagulation of blood for transfusion or blood samples and the flushing of catheters and cannulas to maintain patency.

Heparin and its salts are constituents of many topical preparations for the treatment of various inflammatory disorders.

Administration and dosage. Heparin is administered intravenously, preferably by continuous infusion, or by subcutaneous injection. It may be given as the calcium or sodium salt and it is generally accepted that there is little difference in their effects. Oral formulations of heparin are under investigation.

Doses of heparin for treatment (sometimes termed 'full-dose' heparin), and in some cases prophylaxis, of thromboembolism should be monitored and determined as discussed below under Control of Heparin Therapy. The subcutaneous doses of heparin commonly used for prophylaxis and often termed 'low-dose' subcutaneous heparin do not require routine monitoring. A test dose has been recommended for patients with a history of allergy. Although international and USP units are not strictly equivalent, doses expressed in either appear to be essentially the same. The following doses of heparin are broadly in line with British Society for Haematology guidelines.

For **treatment of venous thromboembolism**, an intravenous loading dose of 5000 to 10 000 units is followed by continuous intravenous infusion of 1000 to 2000 units per hour or subcutaneous injection of 15 000 units every 12 hours. Alternatively, intermittent intravenous injection of 5000 to 10 000 units every 4 to 6 hours is suggested in some product literature. Children and small adults are given a lower intravenous loading dose followed by maintenance with continuous intravenous infusion of 15 to 25 units per kg body-weight per hour or subcutaneous injection of 250 units per kg every 12 hours.

For **prophylaxis** of **postoperative venous thromboembolism**, subcutaneous doses used are 5000 units 2 hours before surgery then every 8 to 12 hours for 7 days or until the patient is ambulant. Similar doses are used to prevent thromboembolism during pregnancy in women with a history of deep-vein thrombosis or pulmonary embolism; the dosage may need to be increased to 10 000 units every 12 hours during the third trimester.

In the management of **unstable angina** or acute **peripheral arterial embolism,** heparin may be given by continuous intravenous infusion in the same doses as those recommended for the treatment of venous thromboembolism. Doses for the prevention of re-occlusion of the coronary arteries following thrombolytic therapy in **myocardial infarction** include either 2000 units of heparin intravenously followed by 12 500 units subcutaneously every 12 hours after streptokinase, or 5000 units intravenously followed by 1000 units per hour intravenously after alteplase; a dose of 12 500 units subcutaneously every 12 hours for at least 10 days may be used to prevent mural thrombosis.

Control of Heparin Therapy. Treatment with full-dose heparin must be monitored to ensure that the dose is providing the required effect on antithrombin III. The most commonly used test to monitor the action of heparin is the activated partial thromboplastin time (APTT). The APTT of patients on full-dose heparin should generally be maintained at 1.5 to 2.5 times the control value although the optimum therapeutic range varies between individual laboratories depending on the APTT reagent in use. Regular monitoring is essential preferably on a daily basis. Prophylaxis with low-dose subcutaneous heparin is not routinely monitored; the APTT is not significantly prolonged in these patients. A dose-adjusted regimen to maintain minimal prolongation of the APTT may be required in patients with malignancy or undergoing orthopaedic surgery to ensure adequate protection against thromboembolism. Other tests used include the activated clotting time (ACT). The value of measurements of heparin concentration in the blood remains to be established.

◊ General references to anticoagulation with heparin.
1. Hirsh J. Heparin. N Engl J Med 1991; 324: 1565–74.
2. Freedman MD. Pharmacodynamics, clinical indications, and adverse effects of heparin. J Clin Pharmacol 1992; 32: 584–96.
3. Hyers TM. Heparin therapy: regimens and treatment considerations. Drugs 1992; 44: 738–49.
4. Colvin BT, Barrowcliffe TW. The British Society for Haematology guidelines on the use and monitoring of heparin 1992: second revision. J Clin Pathol 1993; 46: 97–103.
5. Hirsh J, Fuster V. Guide to anticoagulant therapy part 1: heparin. Circulation 1994; 89: 1449–68.
6. Hirsh J, et al. Heparin and low-molecular-weight heparin: mechanisms of action, pharmacokinetics, dosing, monitoring, efficacy, and safety. Chest 2001; 119 (suppl): 64S–94S.

Action. Heparin is well established as an anticoagulant and antithrombotic and acts primarily by binding to, and enhancing the activity of, antithrombin III. However, the physiological role of endogenous heparin has not been clearly defined, despite its presence in mast cells, its ability to interact with numerous proteins, and its close structural similarity to heparan sulfate (suleparoid) the ubiquitous cell-surface glycosaminoglycan.[1,2] Endogenous heparin activity may have a role in protecting against atherosclerosis.[3] Non-anticoagulant properties of heparin have been reported to include anti-inflammatory activity, with a possible application in, for example, asthma[4] or inflammatory bowel disease.[5] A major obstacle to the use of heparin itself for non-anticoagulant purposes would be the risk of bleeding.

1. Lane DA, Adams L. Non-anticoagulant uses of heparin. N Engl J Med 1993; 329: 129–30.
2. Page CP. Proteoglycans: the "Teflon" of the airways? Thorax 1997; 52: 924–5.
3. Engelberg H. Actions of heparin in the atherosclerotic process. Pharmacol Rev 1996; 48: 327–52.
4. Martineau P, Vaughan LM. Heparin inhalation for asthma. Ann Pharmacother 1995; 29: 71–2.
5. Day R, Forbes A. Heparin, cell adhesion, and pathogenesis of inflammatory bowel disease. Lancet 1999; 354: 62–5.

Administration. The activated partial thromboplastin time (APTT) is the test most commonly used to monitor intravenous full-dose heparin therapy. Heparin dosing algorithms have been developed[1,2] so that the time taken to achieve a therapeutic APTT and maintain the APTT in the therapeutic range (usually 1.5 to 2.5 times the control value) is shortened and thus the risk of recurrent thrombosis and major bleeding complications is reduced. Although use of ideal body-weight for dosage calculation in obese patients has been suggested, actual body-weight may be more appropriate,[3] but maximum bolus doses and infusion rates should be set, to avoid overdosage in morbidly obese patients.

However, the therapeutic ranges used in such algorithms are not applicable to all APTT reagents because different ones vary in their sensitivity to heparin.[4] The optimum therapeutic range therefore varies between individual laboratories depending on the APTT reagent used. Dosing algorithms may be adapted by calibrating the therapeutic APTT with heparin concentrations in patients receiving heparin.[4,5]

A weight-based algorithm for treatment doses of subcutaneous heparin in deep-vein thrombosis has also been proposed.[6]

1. Cruickshank MK, et al. A standard heparin nomogram for the management of heparin therapy. Arch Intern Med 1991; 151: 333–7.
2. Raschke RA, et al. The weight-based heparin dosing nomogram compared with a "standard care" nomogram: a randomized controlled trial. Ann Intern Med 1993; 119: 874–81.
3. Yee WP, Norton LL. Optimal weight base for a weight-based heparin dosing protocol. Am J Health-Syst Pharm 1998; 55: 159–62.
4. Brill-Edwards P, et al. Establishing a therapeutic range for heparin therapy. Ann Intern Med 1993; 119: 104–9.
5. Volles DF, et al. Establishing an institution-specific therapeutic range for heparin. Am J Health-Syst Pharm 1998; 55: 2002–6.
6. Prandoni P, et al. Use of an algorithm for administering subcutaneous heparin in the treatment of deep venous thrombosis. Ann Intern Med 1998; 129: 299–302.

Catheters and cannulas. Solutions of heparin sodium 10 or 100 units per mL in sodium chloride 0.9% are used for the flushing of intravenous catheters, cannulas, and other indwelling intravenous infusion devices (heparin locks). Several studies[1-6] and a meta-analysis[7] have, however, been unable to demonstrate any major advantage of either strength of heparin sodium solution over sodium chloride 0.9% alone in terms of maintenance of peripheral cannula patency or reduction in incidence of thrombophlebitis, and sodium chloride 0.9% is therefore recommended for cannulas intended to be in place for 48 hours or less. Reduced use of heparin flush solutions could minimise the risk of adverse effects to heparin such as thrombocytopenia and reduce the risk of incompatibilities with intravenously administered drugs.

Use of heparin-bonded catheters or the addition of heparin to intravenous fluids such as total parenteral nutrition solutions has also been tried in an attempt to maintain indwelling intravenous infusion devices (but see Catheters and Cannulas, under Precautions, above). Continuous infusion of heparin-containing fluids may prolong the patency of peripheral arterial catheters.[7]

Central venous catheters are also subject to thrombus formation and their use may be complicated by vascular thrombosis and systemic infection. A meta-analysis[8] of prophylactic heparin used with central venous and pulmonary artery catheters suggested that heparin reduces catheter-related vascular thrombosis and may reduce catheter-related infection. This analysis included a range of heparin doses and methods of administration, as well as heparin-bonded catheters, and the authors suggest that further study is needed. Very low doses of warfarin (1 mg daily) may protect against thrombosis in patients with central venous catheters.[9]

1. Epperson EL. Efficacy of 0.9% sodium chloride injection with and without heparin for maintaining indwelling intermittent injection sites. Clin Pharm 1984; 3: 626–9.

2. Hamilton RA, et al. Heparin sodium versus 0.9% sodium chloride injection for maintaining patency of indwelling intermittent infusion devices. Clin Pharm 1988; 7: 439–43.

3. Lombardi TP, et al. Efficacy of 0.9% sodium chloride injection with or without heparin sodium for maintaining patency of intravenous catheters in children. Clin Pharm 1988; 7: 832–6.

4. Shaw P, Baker D. Flushing solutions for indwelling intravenous catheters. Pharm J 1988; 241: 122–3.

5. Garrelts JC, et al. Comparison of heparin and 0.9% sodium chloride injection in the maintenance of indwelling intermittent iv devices. Clin Pharm 1989; 8: 34–9.

6. Nelson TJ, Graves SM. 0.9% Sodium chloride injection with and without heparin for maintaining peripheral indwelling intermittent-infusion devices in infants. Am J Health-Syst Pharm 1998; 55: 570–3.

7. Randolph AG, et al. Benefit of heparin in peripheral venous and arterial catheters: systematic review and meta-analysis of randomised controlled trials. BMJ 1998; 316: 969–75.

8. Randolph AG, et al. Benefit of heparin in central venous and pulmonary artery catheters: a meta-analysis of randomized controlled trials. Chest 1998; 113: 165–71.

9. Bern MM, et al. Very low doses of warfarin can prevent thrombosis in central venous catheters: a randomized prospective trial. Ann Intern Med 1990; 112: 423–8.

Disseminated intravascular coagulation. Heparin has been used with some success in disseminated intravascular coagulation (p.720) associated with a variety of conditions. However, this use is considered by some to be controversial and should be reserved for specific situations where the risk of bleeding is relatively minor in comparison with the possible beneficial effect on formation of microthromboses. The maximum dose given intravenously is usually 1000 units per hour because of the risk of bleeding.[1]

1. Colvin BT, Barrowcliffe TW. The British Society for Haematology guidelines on the use and monitoring of heparin 1992: second revision. J Clin Pathol 1993; 46: 97–103.

Extracorporeal circulation. Anticoagulation with heparin is necessary during procedures such as cardiopulmonary bypass and haemodialysis and haemofiltration.[1] In the case of bypass, heparin is added to the crystalloid solution and any stored blood used for priming the bypass machine and is given intravenously before cannulation of the heart and major blood vessels. Activated clotting time (ACT) is monitored throughout. After bypass is discontinued, anticoagulation can be reversed with protamine but caution is advised because of potential toxicity on the cardiopulmonary circulation.

At the start of haemodialysis sessions patients generally receive a loading dose of heparin followed by continuous infusion into the exit line of the extracorporeal circuit until about one hour before the end of dialysis. The dose of heparin varies widely depending on body-weight, volume of the extracorporeal circulation, dialysis membrane biocompatibility, and pump speed.

1. Colvin BT, Barrowcliffe TW. The British Society for Haematology guidelines on the use and monitoring of heparin 1992; second revision. J Clin Pathol 1993; 46: 97–103.

Idiopathic thrombocytopenic purpura. Subcutaneous administration of a low dose of heparin improved platelet counts in a small number of patients with idiopathic thrombocytopenic purpura (p.1052) that was resistant to standard corticosteroid therapy.[1] However, heparin may itself cause thrombocytopenia, even at very low doses (see Effects on the Blood under Adverse Effects, above).

1. Shen ZX, et al. Thrombocytopoietic effect of heparin given in chronic immune thrombocytopenic purpura. Lancet 1995; 346: 220–1.

Pregnancy. Heparin is the anticoagulant of choice for use in pregnancy although it is not without risk for the fetus (see Pregnancy, under Precautions, above), and for the mother.

Guidelines on thrombosis associated with pregnancy have been published.[1,2] Pregnant women may require anticoagulation for the treatment or prophylaxis of venous thromboembolism (p.817), or for the prevention of systemic thromboembolism associated with prosthetic heart valves (p.816). Patients with a history of thromboembolism or a thrombophilic abnormality such as inherited deficiencies of antithrombin III, protein C, or protein S or acquired antiphospholipid antibodies may be at particular risk. Administration of heparin to women with antiphospholipid antibodies may also decrease the risk of fetal loss that has been associated with this disorder.[3,4]

1. Maternal and Neonatal Haemostasis Working Party of the Haemostasis and Thrombosis Task. Guidelines on the prevention, investigation and management of thrombosis associated with pregnancy. J Clin Pathol 1993; 46: 489–96.

2. Ginsberg JS, et al. Use of antithrombotic agents during pregnancy. Chest 2001; 119 (suppl): 122S–131S.

3. Rosove MH, et al. Heparin therapy for pregnant women with lupus anticoagulant or anticardiolipin antibodies. Obstet Gynecol 1990; 75: 630–4.

4. Rai R, et al. Randomised controlled trial of aspirin and aspirin plus heparin in pregnant women with recurrent miscarriage associated with phospholipid antibodies (or antiphospholipid antibodies). BMJ 1997; 314: 253–7.

Reperfusion and revascularisation procedures. Heparin is widely used in patients undergoing angioplasty or bypass surgery (p.812) to prevent perioperative thrombosis of the operated artery. It is frequently used in conjunction with aspirin or other antiplatelet drugs. However, it appears to have no role in the long-term prevention of restenosis, although heparin-coated stents may have potential benefits.

The symbol † denotes a preparation no longer actively marketed

Preparations

BP 2001: Heparin Injection;
USP 25: Anticoagulant Heparin Solution; Heparin Calcium Injection; Heparin Lock Flush Solution; Heparin Sodium Injection.

Proprietary Preparations (details are given in Part 3)
Aust.: Calciparin†; Liquemin; Thrombophob; Thrombophob-S; *Austral.:* Calcihep; Calciparine; Uniparin; *Belg.:* Calparine; Liquemine; *Braz.:* Liquemine; Trombofob; *Canad.:* Calcilean†; Hepalean; Hepalean-Lok; *Fin.:* Hepaflex; Trombosol; *Fr.:* Calciparine; *Ger.:* Ariven†; Calciparin; Depot-Thrombophob-N; Embin-Venen Salbe†; Essaven 60 000; Hemeran; Hepa-Gel; Hepa-Salbe; Hepaplus; Hepathromb; Hepathrombin; Juwoment Sport; Liquemin N; Logomed Sport-Gel†; Logomed Venen-Salbe†; Perivar Venensalbe; Sportino; Thrombareduct; Thrombophob; Traumalitan; Trirutin†; Venalitan; Venelbin N†; Venoruton Emulgel; Vetren; *Hong Kong:* Lioton; *Irl.:* Calciparine; Hep-Rinse; Heplok; Hepsal; Minihep; Monoparin; Multiparin; Unihep; Uniparin; *Israel:* Calciparine; *Ital.:* Ateroclar; Calciparina; Calcipor; Chemyparin; Clarisco; Croneparina; Disebrin; Ecabil; Ecafast; Ecasolv; Emoklar; Eparical; Eparinlider; Eparinovis; Epsoclar; Hemofluss; Hepacal; Isoclar; Lioton; Liquemin; Mica; Normoparin; Reoflus; Trombolisin; Zepac; *Mex.:* Helberina; Heparth; Inhepar; Proparin; *Neth.:* Calparine; Minihep; *Norw.:* Nycoheparin; *NZ:* Minihep; Monoparin; Multiparin; *Port.:* Calciparina†; *S.Afr.:* Calciparine; Thrombophob; *Spain:* Calciparina; Menaven; *Switz.:* Calciparine; Demovarin; Gelparine; HepaGel; Lioton; Liquemine; Ruscovarin†; *UK:* Calciparine; Canusal; Hep-Flush; Heplok; Hepsal; Minihep; Monoparin; Multiparin; Pump-Hep; Unihep†; Uniparin†; *USA:* Hep-Lock; Hepflush.

Multi-ingredient: *Aust.:* Ambenat; Contractubex; Derivon; Ditaven Gel†; Dolo-Menthoneurin; Dolobene; Etrat; Ichthalgan forte; Pasta Cool; Pertrombon; Thrombophob; Venobene; Venosin; Vetren; *Braz.:* Trombofob; Venalot H; Venostasin Composto; *Canad.:* Lipactin; *Fr.:* Cirkan a la Prednacinolone; Esberiven; *Ger.:* Arnica Kneipp Salbe; Arnika plus†; Contractubex; Dolo-Menthoneurin; Dolo-Rubriment; Dolobene; Enelbin-Salbe N; Essaven; Essaven Tri-Complex; Etrat Sportgel; Fibraflex; Heparin Comp; Ichthalgan; Kelofibrase; Lipactin; NeyGeront N (Revitorgan-Dilutionen N Nr 64); Ostochont; Pe-Ce Ven N; Phlogase†; Sensicutan; Sportupac N; Trauma-Puren; Venengel; Venoplant AHS; Venostasin; *Hong Kong:* Contractubex; Dolobene; *Ital.:* Essaven; Flebs; Idracemi Eparina; Luxazone Eparina; Proctosoll; Reparil; Rubidiosin Composto; Venotrauma; Via Mal Trauma Gel; Vit Eparin; Xantervit Eparina; *Port.:* DM Gel; Etrat†; *S.Afr.:* Essaven; Thrombophob†; *Spain:* Essavenon; Recto Menaderm†; Venacol; Venoplant; *Switz.:* Assan; Assan-Thermo; Bonactin†; Butaparin; Contractubex; Dolo-Arthrosenex; Dolobene; Gorgonium; Hepabuzone; Heparinol; Hepathrombine; Keli-med; Keppur; Lipactin; Lyman; Phlebostasin compositum; Ralur; Rollbene; Sportium Emgel; Sportusal; Venalot†; Venoplant comp; Venoplant N†; Venucreme; Venugel.

Heparinoids (3872-k)

Profile
The term heparinoid includes heparin derivatives and has also been used more loosely to include naturally occurring and synthetic highly-sulfated polysaccharides of similar structure. Such compounds have been described in many ways; some of the terms used include sulfated glucosaminoglycans; glycosaminoglycan polysulfate compounds; or sulfated mucopolysaccharides.

The following anticoagulants may be described as heparinoids: danaparoid sodium (p.866), dermatan sulfate (p.867), pentosan polysulfate sodium (p.953), sodium apolate (p.971), suleparoid (p.978), and sulodexide (p.978).

Heparinoid preparations are available with uses ranging from anticoagulation to the alleviation of inflammation (applied topically); some are claimed to have hypolipidaemic properties.

The proprietary names listed below refer to preparations containing undefined or less readily defined heparinoids that are used in a range of conditions including musculoskeletal and joint disorders, haemorrhoids, lipid disorders, and thromboembolic disorders.

Preparations

Proprietary Preparations (details are given in Part 3)
Aust.: Hemeran; Hirudoid; Lasonil; *Austral.:* Hirudoid; *Belg.:* Hemeran; Hirudoid; *Braz.:* Ateroide; Hirudoid; *Denm.:* Hirudoid; *Fin.:* Hirudoid; *Ger.:* Etrat Sportsalbe MPS; Hirudoid; Lasonil N; *Hong Kong:* Hirudoid; *Ital.:* Angioflux; Ateran; Ateroid; Ateroxide; Condral; Erevan; Glicamin; Gluparin†; Hirudoid; Lasonil; Lasoven; Lipostat†; Lipostop†; Matrix; Provenal; Ravenol; Suloves†; Treparin; *Neth.:* Hirudoid; Lasonil; *Norw.:* Hirudoid; *NZ:* Hirudoid; *Port.:* Hemeran; Hirudoid; Lasonil; *Singapore:* Hirudoid; *Spain:* Dinoven; Hirudoid; *Swed.:* Hirudoid; *Switz.:* Hemeran; Hirudoid; *Thai.:* Hirudoid; Varidoid; *UK:* Bruiseze; Hirudoid; Lasonil.

Multi-ingredient: *Aust.:* Bayolin; Lemuval; Mobilat; Mobilisin; Mobilisin plus; Moviflex; *Austral.:* Lasonil; Movelat; *Belg.:* Lasonil; Mobilat; Mobilisin; *Braz.:* Ateroide; Etrat; Mobilat; Mobilisin Composto; Sinteroid; *Fin.:* Mobilat; Moviflex; *Fr.:* Bayoline†; Lasonil†; *Ger.:* Dignowell†; Dolo Mobilat; Mobilat; Mobilisin; Sanaven; Thermo Mobilisin; *Hong Kong:* Mobilat; Movilisin; Prelloran; *Israel:* Lasonil; *Ital.:* Artrocur; Flebs; Flogogin†; Herbavit; Lasonil H; Lasoproct†; Lasoreuma†; Mobilat; Mobilisin; Traumal; *Mex.:* Mobilat; *Neth.:* Mobilat; *NZ:* Lasonil; Movelat; *Port.:* Anacal; Mobilat†; Mobilisin; *S.Afr.:* Mobilat†; *Singapore:* Mobilat; *Spain:* Lasonil; Movilat; Movilisin; *Switz.:* Dolo-Veniten; Mobilat N; Mobilat†; Mobilisin; Moviflex†; Prelloran; *Thai.:* Mobilat; Movelat; *UK:* Anacal; Movelat.

Hexobendine Hydrochloride (9239-k)

Hexobendine Hydrochloride (BANM, rINNM).

ST-7090. NN′-Ethylenebis(3-methylaminopropyl 3,4,5-trimethoxybenzoate) dihydrochloride.

$C_{30}H_{44}N_2O_{10},2HCl = 665.6$.

CAS — 54-03-5 (hexobendine); 50-62-4 (hexobendine hydrochloride).

NOTE. Hexobendine is USAN.

Profile
Hexobendine hydrochloride is a vasodilator used in ischaemic heart disease in usual doses of 180 to 270 mg daily, in divided doses, by mouth. It may also be given by intravenous or intramuscular injection.

Ischaemic heart disease is discussed under Atherosclerosis (p.793) and the treatment of its clinical manifestations is described under Angina Pectoris (p.791) and Myocardial Infarction (p.805).

Preparations

Proprietary Preparations (details are given in Part 3)
Aust.: Ustimon; *Spain:* Ustimon†.

Multi-ingredient: *Aust.:* Instenon; *Hong Kong:* Instenon; *Spain:* Vasperdil†; *Thai.:* Instenon.

Hirudin (5344-s)

Hirudine.

Profile
Hirudin is a 65-amino-acid protein that is a direct inhibitor of thrombin. It has been extracted from leeches (p.919) and this form is used in various topical preparations for peripheral vascular disorders. Recombinant hirudins, such as desirudin (p.867) and lepirudin (p.919) and analogues of hirudin, such as bivalirudin (p.850), are used as anticoagulants.

Preparations

Proprietary Preparations (details are given in Part 3)
Aust.: Exhirud; Irudil; *Fr.:* Hirucreme; *Ger.:* Exhirud.

Multi-ingredient: *Ger.:* Haemo-Exhirud; *Ital.:* Hirudex.

Homonicotinic Acid (12827-x)

3-Pyridylacetic acid.

$C_7H_7NO_2 = 137.1$.

CAS — 501-81-5.

Profile
Homonicotinic acid is a lipid regulating drug.

Hydralazine Hydrochloride (878-f)

Hydralazine Hydrochloride (BANM, rINNM).

Apressinum; Hydralazini Hydrochloridum; Hydrallazine Hydrochloride; Idralazina. 1-Hydrazinophthalazine hydrochloride.

$C_8H_8N_4,HCl = 196.6$.

CAS — 86-54-4 (hydralazine); 304-20-1 (hydralazine hydrochloride).

NOTE. Hydralazine Polistirex (hydralazine and sulfonated diethenylbenzene-ethenylbenzene copolymer complex) is USAN.

Pharmacopoeias. In Eur. (see p.vi), Int., Jpn, and US.

Incompatible with glucose solutions.

Pharmacopoeial description

Ph. Eur.: A white or almost white, crystalline powder. Soluble in water; slightly soluble in alcohol; very slightly soluble in dichloromethane. A 2% solution in water has a pH of 3.5 to 4.2. Protect from light.

USP 25: A white to off-white, odourless, crystalline powder. Soluble 1 in 25 of water and 1 in 500 of alcohol; very slightly soluble in ether. A 2% solution in water has a pH of 3.5 to 4.2. Store in airtight containers.

Stability. Discoloration of hydralazine injection was observed on several occasions after storage in a syringe for up to 12 hours.[1] Hydralazine reacts with metals and therefore the injection should be prepared using a non-metal filter and should be used as quickly as possible after being drawn through a needle into a syringe.

A study of the rate of degradation of hydralazine hydrochloride, 1 mg per mL in sweetened, aqueous oral liquids showed that glucose, fructose, lactose, and maltose reduced the stability of the drug.[2] In solutions containing mannitol or sorbitol, there was less than 10% degradation of hydralazine after 3 weeks.

1. Enderlin G. Discoloration of hydralazine injection. Am J Hosp Pharm 1984; 41: 634.

2. Das Gupta V, et al. Stability of hydralazine hydrochloride in aqueous vehicles. J Clin Hosp Pharm 1986; 11: 215–23.

Adverse Effects

Adverse effects occur frequently with hydralazine, particularly tachycardia, palpitations, angina pectoris, severe headache, and gastrointestinal disturbances such as anorexia, nausea, vomiting, and diarrhoea. These adverse effects, together with flushing, dizziness, and nasal congestion, which occur less often, may be seen at the start of treatment, especially if the dose is increased quickly. They generally subside with continued treatment. Other less common side-effects include postural hypotension, fluid retention with oedema and weight gain, conjunctivitis, lachrymation, tremor, and muscle cramps.

Hydralazine may deplete pyridoxine in the body, and can produce peripheral neuropathy with numbness and tingling of the extremities. Occasionally, hepatotoxicity, blood dyscrasias, haemolytic anaemia, difficulty in urinating, glomerulonephritis, constipation, paralytic ileus, depression, and anxiety occur.

Hypersensitivity reactions including fever, chills, pruritus, and rashes have been reported, and eosinophilia may occur.

Following the prolonged use of large doses, antinuclear antibodies may develop and a condition resembling systemic lupus erythematosus may occur. The incidence is greater in slow acetylators, patients with renal impairment, women, and patients taking more than 100 mg of hydralazine daily. The symptoms usually disappear when the drug is withdrawn; some patients may require treatment with corticosteroids.

Following acute overdosage, hypotension, tachycardia, myocardial ischaemia, arrhythmias, shock, and coma may occur.

Carcinogenicity. Although earlier reports suggested that hydralazine might be carcinogenic, there was no evidence from a survey of 1978 patients with lung or colorectal cancer and 6807 controls that there was an increased risk of these neoplasms.[1]

1. Kaufman DW, et al. Hydralazine use in relation to cancers of the lung, colon, and rectum. Eur J Clin Pharmacol 1989; 36: 259–64.

Effects on the blood. Three cases of thrombocytopenia were reported[1] in neonates whose mothers had been treated with hydralazine for some months before delivery. The thrombocytopenia and bleeding was transient with full recovery occurring within a few weeks. No adverse effects were noticed in the mothers.

1. Widerlöv E, et al. Hydralazine-induced neonatal thrombocytopenia. N Engl J Med 1980; 303: 1235.

Effects on the cardiovascular system. Paradoxical severe hypertension followed administration of hydralazine by mouth or intramuscularly on 3 occasions in a patient with renal artery stenosis.[1]

1. Webb DB, White JP. Hypertension after taking hydrallazine. BMJ 1980; 280: 1582.

Effects on the kidneys. Rapidly progressive glomerulonephritis with focal and segmental lesions, usually accompanied by necrosis and crescent formation, has been reported in patients receiving hydralazine.[1-3] The condition is reported to be associated with the presence of antinuclear antibodies[3] and slow acetylator status,[2] factors associated with the development of hydralazine-induced lupus erythematosus.[4] However, renal involvement is much less common in drug-induced lupus,[4] and in a report of 15 such cases men and women and fast and slow acetylators were equally affected;[3] in addition the criteria for systemic lupus erythematosus were not usually fulfilled in these patients and it was suggested that the condition should be distinguished from lupus nephritis. Immediate withdrawal of hydralazine generally results in some improvement in renal function but complete recovery is uncommon; severe cases may require immunosuppressive therapy.[3]

1. Björck S, et al. Rapidly progressive glomerulonephritis after hydralazine. Lancet 1983; ii: 42.
2. Kincaid-Smith P, Whitworth JA. Hydralazine-associated glomerulonephritis. Lancet 1983; ii: 348.
3. Björck S, et al. Hydralazine-induced glomerulonephritis. Lancet 1985; i: 392.
4. Hughes GRV. Recent developments in drug-associated systemic lupus erythematosus. Adverse Drug React Bull 1987; (Apr.): 460–3.

Effects on the skin. Pruritus and skin rashes have been reported with hydralazine use.

A 59-year-old woman who had been taking hydralazine 25 mg three times daily for 6 months developed symptoms of Sweet's syndrome (erythematous plaques and nodules and haemorrhagic blisters).[1] Symptoms began to subside on withdrawal of hydralazine but recurred when hydralazine was reintroduced.

The condition resolved on discontinuation of hydralazine and treatment with prednisolone.

1. Gilmour E, et al. Drug-induced Sweet's syndrome (acute febrile neutrophilic dermatosis) associated with hydralazine. Br J Dermatol 1995; 133: 490–1.

Lupus erythematosus. Lupus erythematosus is a well-documented adverse effect of hydralazine therapy. Onset is typically delayed from 1 month to 5 years from the start of treatment, and the most common symptoms are arthralgia or arthritis, usually non-deforming, in up to 95% of patients, fever and myalgia in about 50%, and pleuropulmonary involvement, manifesting as pleurisy, pleural effusions, or pulmonary infiltrates in up to 30%.[1-3] Renal involvement is reported to be less common than in idiopathic systemic lupus erythematosus and there is some uncertainty as to whether the glomerulonephritis sometimes seen in patients receiving hydralazine should be considered lupus nephritis—see under Effects on the Kidneys, above. Nonetheless a 20% incidence of renal involvement has been reported.[1] Other complications and symptoms that have been associated with lupus erythematosus in patients taking hydralazine include cutaneous vasculitis,[4-6] orogenital and cutaneous ulceration,[7] bilateral retinal vasculitis,[8] reactive hypoglycaemia (although the attribution is uncertain),[9] life-threatening cardiac tamponade,[10] and hoarseness and stridor secondary to vocal cord palsy, which progressed to respiratory arrest.[11] Skin rashes are reported to be less prominent than with the idiopathic form of the disease.[1] Fatalities have occurred,[12] but appear to be rare.

Estimates of the overall incidence of hydralazine-associated lupus erythematosus vary from about 1.2 to 5% or more.[13-16] The syndrome appears to occur only in patients who develop antinuclear antibodies while receiving hydralazine, but the incidence of positive antinuclear antibody tests is much higher than that of lupus, at up to 60%, so the presence of antinuclear antibodies alone is not diagnostic.[15] There is a strong relationship with drug dose,[14,16] acetylator status,[13,15,16] and patient gender,[16] the syndrome being more common in slow acetylators and women, and in patients receiving 100 mg daily or more.

Although it has been reported that hydralazine-associated lupus was more frequent in patients with the HLA-DR4 antigen[17] this was not confirmed by others[18] and subsequent work has suggested that the association is rather with the non-expressing or null forms of the adjacent complement C4 gene.[19] Hydralazine can inactivate complement C4 in vitro[20] and might exacerbate complement deficiency (which is known to be associated with idiopathic systemic lupus erythematosus) in patients with an already low level of C4 due to a null allele.[19]

1. Hughes GRV. Recent developments in drug-associated systemic lupus erythematosus. Adverse Drug React Bull 1987; (Apr.): 460–3.
2. Cohen MG, Prowse MV. Drug-induced rheumatic syndromes: diagnosis, clinical features and management. Med Toxicol Adverse Drug Exp 1989; 4: 199–218.
3. Price EJ, Venables PJW. Drug-induced lupus. Drug Safety 1995; 12: 283–90.
4. Bernstein RM, et al. Hydralazine-induced cutaneous vasculitis. BMJ 1980; 280: 156–7.
5. Peacock A, Weatherall D. Hydralazine-induced necrotising vasculitis. BMJ 1981; 282: 1121–2.
6. Finlay AY, et al. Hydrallazine-induced necrotising vasculitis. BMJ 1981; 282: 1703–4.
7. Neville E, et al. Orogenital ulcers, SLE and hydrallazine. Postgrad Med J 1981; 57: 378–9.
8. Doherty M, et al. Hydralazine induced lupus syndrome with eye disease. BMJ 1985; 290: 675.
9. Blackshear PJ, et al. Reactive hypoglycaemia and insulin autoantibodies in drug-induced lupus erythematosus. Ann Intern Med 1983; 99: 182–4.
10. Anandadas JA, Simpson P. Cardiac tamponade associated with hydralazine therapy, in a patient with rapid acetylator status. Br J Clin Pract 1986; 40: 305–6.
11. Chong WK, et al. Acute laryngeal stridor with respiratory arrest in drug induced systemic lupus erythematosus. BMJ 1988; 297: 660–1.
12. Sturman SG, et al. Fatal hydralazine-induced systemic lupus erythematosus. Lancet 1988; ii: 1304.
13. Bing RF, et al. Hydralazine in hypertension: is there a safe dose? BMJ 1980; 281: 353–4.
14. Freestone S, et al. Incidence of hydrallazine-associated autoimmune disease. Br J Clin Pharmacol 1982; 13: 291P–292P.
15. Mansilla-Tinoco R, et al. Hydralazine, antinuclear antibodies, and the lupus syndrome. BMJ 1982; 284: 936–9.
16. Cameron HA, Ramsay LE. The lupus syndrome induced by hydralazine: a common complication with low dose treatment. BMJ 1984; 289: 410–12.
17. Batchelor JR, et al. Hydralazine-induced systemic lupus erythematosus: influence of HLA-DR and sex on susceptibility. Lancet 1980; i: 1107–9.
18. Brand C, et al. Hydralazine-induced lupus: no association with HLA-DR4. Lancet 1984; i: 462.
19. Speirs C, et al. Complement system protein C4 and susceptibility to hydralazine-induced systemic lupus erythematosus. Lancet 1989; i: 922–4.
20. Sim E, et al. Drugs that induce systemic lupus erythematosus inhibit complement component C4. Lancet 1984; ii: 422–4.

Treatment of Adverse Effects

Withdrawal of hydralazine or reduction of the dosage causes the reversal of many side-effects. Peripheral neuropathy has been reported to be alleviated by pyridoxine.

If overdosage occurs gastric lavage may be performed or activated charcoal may be given if the patient presents within one hour of ingestion. Symptomatic and supportive treatment, including plasma expanders for shock and a beta blocker for tachycardia, should be given as necessary. Hypotension may respond to placing the patient in the supine position with the feet raised. If possible, pressor drugs should be avoided. If a pressor is necessary, one should be chosen that will not cause tachycardia or exacerbate arrhythmias; adrenaline [epinephrine] should not be used.

Precautions

Hydralazine is contra-indicated in patients with severe tachycardia, dissecting aortic aneurysm, heart failure with high cardiac output, cor pulmonale, or myocardial insufficiency due to mechanical obstruction, for example aortic or mitral stenosis or constrictive pericarditis. Hydralazine is also contra-indicated in patients with idiopathic systemic lupus erythematosus and related disorders.

Hydralazine-induced vasodilatation produces myocardial stimulation. It should therefore be used with caution in patients with ischaemic heart disease since it can increase angina and it should not be given to patients following myocardial infarction until their condition has stabilised. Patients with suspected or confirmed ischaemic heart disease should be given hydralazine under cover of a beta blocker, which should be started a few days before hydralazine, in order to prevent myocardial stimulation. If given to patients with heart failure they should be monitored for postural hypotension and tachycardia during the initial stages of therapy, preferably in hospital. If treatment with hydralazine is to be stopped in patients with heart failure it should generally be withdrawn gradually. Hydralazine should be used with caution in patients with cerebrovascular disorders.

The dose of hydralazine should be reduced or the dosage interval prolonged in patients with impaired renal or hepatic function. Complete blood counts and antinuclear antibody determinations should be carried out periodically during long-term therapy. Urine analysis (for microhaematuria and proteinuria) is also recommended.

Hydralazine is teratogenic in some species of animals and should therefore be avoided during the first two trimesters of pregnancy.

Patients may experience impaired reactions, especially at the start of therapy, and should not drive or operate machinery if affected.

Porphyria. Hydralazine has been associated with acute attacks of porphyria and is considered unsafe in porphyric patients.

Pregnancy and breast feeding. Hydralazine should be avoided during the first two trimesters of pregnancy.

Hydralazine concentrations were found to be similar in maternal and umbilical-cord blood in a study of 6 women being treated with hydralazine for pronounced hypertension during pregnancy.[1] Hydralazine was determined in the breast milk of 1 mother, but amounts detected were unlikely to produce clinically relevant concentrations in the infant.

For a report of thrombocytopenia occurring in neonates following maternal treatment with hydralazine during pregnancy, see Effects on the Blood under Adverse Effects, above.

1. Liedholm H, et al. Transplacental passage and breast milk concentrations of hydralazine. Eur J Clin Pharmacol 1982; 21: 417–19.

Interactions

The hypotensive effect of hydralazine may be enhanced by other agents with a hypotensive action. Severe hypotension may occur if hydralazine and diazoxide are given concurrently. However, some interactions with antihypertensives may be beneficial: thiazide diuretics also counteract the fluid retention caused by hydralazine, and beta blockers diminish the cardiac-accelerating effects.

Indometacin. Indometacin 100 mg daily did not attenuate the hypotensive effect of hydralazine in a study in 9 healthy subjects,[1] but another study[2] showed that indometacin 200 mg daily did attenuate the hypotensive effect of hydralazine but not the effects on heart rate, renal or limb blood flow, or plasma-catecholamine concentration.

1. Jackson SHD, Pickles H. Indomethacin does not attenuate the effects of hydralazine in normal subjects. *Eur J Clin Pharmacol* 1983; **25:** 303–5.
2. Cinquegrani MP, Liang C. Indomethacin attenuates the hypotensive action of hydralazine. *Clin Pharmacol Ther* 1986; **39:** 564–70.

Pharmacokinetics

Hydralazine is rapidly absorbed from the gastrointestinal tract but undergoes considerable first-pass metabolism by acetylation in the gastrointestinal mucosa and liver. The rate of metabolism is genetically determined and depends upon the acetylator status of the individual. The bioavailability of hydralazine has been reported to be about 35% in slow acetylators and less in fast acetylators; thus plasma concentrations after a given dose are higher in slow acetylators.

Peak plasma concentrations have been reported to occur after about one hour. Hydralazine is chiefly present in plasma as a hydrazone conjugate with pyruvic acid. Plasma protein binding is about 90%. The drug is widely distributed, notably into arterial walls.

Systemic metabolism in the liver is by hydroxylation of the ring system and conjugation with glucuronic acid; most sources suggest that *N*-acetylation is not of major importance in systemic clearance and that therefore acetylator status does not affect elimination. Hydralazine is excreted mainly in urine as metabolites.

The apparent average half-life for hydralazine has been reported to vary from about 45 minutes to about 8 hours, with a number of sources giving the average as about 2 to 4 hours. Some of the variation may be due to problems with the analytical procedures—see below. The half-life is prolonged in renal impairment and may be up to 16 hours in patients with a creatinine clearance of less than 20 mL per minute.

Hydralazine crosses the placenta and is distributed into breast milk.

◊ Attempts to describe the pharmacokinetics of hydralazine have been plagued by the instability of the drug itself in plasma and in alkaline solutions, and the instability of its circulating metabolites during analysis, and has meant that many techniques for the measurement of hydralazine have proved non-selective and yield overestimates of unchanged drug.[1] Studies using less selective methods have yielded an apparent bioavailability for oral hydralazine of 38 to 69% in slow acetylators and 22 to 32% in fast acetylators; in contrast, more selective assays have yielded values of 31 to 35% and 10 to 16% for slow and rapid acetylators respectively. Similarly, hydralazine plasma clearance is lower and the half-life longer when based upon the results of non-selective assay procedures; mean elimination half-life has ranged from 2.2 to 3.6 hours based upon these methods compared with 0.67 to 0.96 hours using a more selective assay. Improved pharmacokinetic data has indicated that while the first-pass effect is dependent upon acetylator phenotype, systemic clearance is only minimally dependent upon acetylation. The formation of the pyruvic acid hydrazone, which is without significant vasodilator activity, contributes to extrahepatic phenotype-independent clearance.

Although some workers have correlated the hypotensive effect of hydralazine with the serum concentrations,[2] others have been unable to do so.[3] Moreover, the duration of hypotensive effect has been shown to exceed considerably that predicted from the rate of elimination.[4,5] Possible explanations are the accumulation of hydralazine at its sites of action in the arterial walls[6] or the existence of active metabolites.[7-9]

Concurrent intake of food has been found to enhance considerably the bioavailability of hydralazine[10] but food-related reductions in plasma-hydralazine concentrations with reduced vasodilator effect have also been reported.[11] The discrepancy was thought to be due to the greater specificity of the assay used in the latter study and to differences in the timing of food and hydralazine administration in the two studies.[12,13]

1. Ludden TM, *et al.* Clinical pharmacokinetics of hydralazine. *Clin Pharmacokinet* 1982; **7:** 185–205.
2. Zacest R, Koch-Weser J. Relation of hydralazine plasma concentration to dosage and hypotensive action. *Clin Pharmacol Ther* 1972; **13:** 420–5.
3. Talseth T, *et al.* Hydralazine slow-release: observations on serum profile and clinical efficacy in man. *Curr Ther Res* 1977; **21:** 157–68.
4. O'Malley K, *et al.* Duration of hydralazine action in hypertension. *Clin Pharmacol Ther* 1975; **18:** 581–6.
5. Shepherd AMM, *et al.* Hydralazine kinetics after single and repeated oral doses. *Clin Pharmacol Ther* 1980; **28:** 804–11.
6. Moore-Jones D, Perry HM. Radioautographic localization of hydralazine-1-C₁₄ in arterial walls. *Proc Soc Exp Biol Med* 1966; **122:** 576–9.

7. Barron K, *et al.* Comparative evaluation of the in vitro effects of hydralazine and hydralazine acetonide on arterial smooth muscle. *Br J Pharmacol* 1977; **61:** 345–9.
8. Haegele KD, *et al.* Identification of hydrallazine and hydrallazine hydrazone metabolites in human body fluids and quantitative in vitro comparisons of their smooth muscle relaxant activity. *Br J Clin Pharmacol* 1978; **5:** 489–94.
9. Reece PA, *et al.* Interference in assays for hydralazine in humans by a major plasma metabolite, hydralazine pyruvic acid hydrazone. *J Pharm Sci* 1978; **67:** 1150–3.
10. Melander A, *et al.* Enhancement of hydralazine bioavailability by food. *Clin Pharmacol Ther* 1977; **22:** 104–7.
11. Shepherd AMM, *et al.* Effect of food on blood hydralazine levels and response in hypertension. *Clin Pharmacol Ther* 1984; **36:** 14–18.
12. Melander A, *et al.* Concomitant food intake does enhance the bioavailability and effect of hydralazine. *Clin Pharmacol Ther* 1985; **38:** 475.
13. Shepherd AMM, *et al.* Concomitant food intake does enhance the bioavailability and effect of hydralazine. *Clin Pharmacol Ther* 1985; **38:** 475–6.

Uses and Administration

Hydralazine is a direct-acting vasodilator which acts predominantly on the arterioles. It reduces blood pressure and peripheral resistance but produces fluid retention. Tachycardia and an increase in cardiac output occur mainly as a reflex response to the reduction in peripheral resistance. Hydralazine tends to improve renal and cerebral blood flow and its effect on diastolic pressure is more marked than on systolic pressure.

Hydralazine hydrochloride is given by mouth for the treatment of hypertension (p.802), usually in conjunction with a beta blocker and a thiazide diuretic. In addition to an additive antihypertensive effect, this combination reduces the reflex tachycardia and fluid retention caused by hydralazine. It may be given intravenously in hypertensive crises. Hydralazine is also used together with isosorbide dinitrate in the management of heart failure (but see Precautions, above). For further discussion of this use of hydralazine, see below.

The dose of hydralazine should be reduced or the dosage interval prolonged in patients with impaired renal or hepatic function.

In **hypertension**, the usual initial dose of hydralazine hydrochloride is 40 to 50 mg daily by mouth in divided doses, increased according to the patient's response. In the UK it is recommended that the dose should not be increased above 100 mg daily without checking acetylator status, although the recommended maximum dose for hypertension is 200 mg daily; doses above 100 mg daily are associated with an increased incidence of lupus erythematosus, particularly in women and in slow acetylators.

In hypertensive crises, hydralazine hydrochloride is given intravenously. A recommended dose is 5 to 10 mg by slow intravenous injection, repeated if necessary after 20 to 30 minutes; it has been suggested that the dose should be administered over 20 minutes to avoid over-rapid reduction of blood pressure. Alternatively, it may be given by continuous intravenous infusion in an initial dose of 200 to 300 µg per minute; the usual maintenance dose range is 50 to 150 µg per minute. Hydralazine hydrochloride has also been given by intramuscular injection.

Heart failure. Hydralazine in combination with isosorbide dinitrate may have a role in the management of patients with heart failure (p.798) in whom ACE inhibitors are contra-indicated or not tolerated. Although a meta-analysis of a number of studies[1] of vasodilator therapy for heart failure failed to show a benefit in terms of improved functional status or reduced mortality in patients given hydralazine alone, there is evidence from the Veterans Administration Cooperative Study[2] of reduced mortality from the use of hydralazine with nitrates. This has been confirmed in a second study (V-HeFTII),[3] although hydralazine with isosorbide dinitrate was less effective than enalapril.

If hydralazine is used in patients with heart failure it should be started under hospital supervision (see also Precautions, above). Doses used are generally higher than those given for hypertension; in the two studies,[2,3] the dose of hydralazine was increased gradually to 300 mg daily and that of isosorbide dinitrate to 160 mg daily, provided that they were tolerated by the patient. Both drugs were given by mouth in divided doses.

Hydralazine has also been tried in children with heart failure,[4,5] but experience is limited.

1. Mulrow CD, *et al.* Relative efficacy of vasodilator therapy in chronic congestive heart failure: implications of randomized trials. *JAMA* 1988; **259:** 3422–6.

2. Cohn JN, *et al.* Effect of vasodilator therapy on mortality in chronic congestive heart failure: results of a Veterans Administration cooperative study. *N Engl J Med* 1986; **314:** 1547–52.
3. Cohn JN, *et al.* A comparison of enalapril with hydralazine-isosorbide dinitrate in the treatment of chronic congestive heart failure. *N Engl J Med* 1991; **325:** 303–10.
4. Artman M, *et al.* Hemodynamic effects of hydralazine in infants with idiopathic dilated cardiomyopathy and congestive heart failure. *Am Heart J* 1987; **113:** 144–50.
5. Rao PS, Andaya WG. Chronic afterload reduction in infants and children with primary myocardial disease. *J Pediatr* 1986; **108:** 530–4.

Preparations

BP 2001: Hydralazine Injection; Hydralazine Tablets;
USP 25: Hydralazine Hydrochloride Injection; Hydralazine Hydrochloride Oral Solution; Hydralazine Hydrochloride Tablets; Reserpine, Hydralazine Hydrochloride, and Hydrochlorothiazide Tablets.

Proprietary Preparations (details are given in Part 3)
Austral.: Alphapress; Apresoline; ***Braz.:*** Apresolina; ***Canad.:*** Apresoline; Novo-Hylazin; Nu-Hydral; ***Denm.:*** Apresolin; ***Hong Kong:*** Apresoline; ***Irl.:*** Apresoline; ***Israel:*** Alphapress; ***Neth.:*** Apresoline; ***Norw.:*** Apresolin; ***NZ:*** Apresoline; ***S.Afr.:*** Apresoline; Hyperphen; Rolazine; ***Spain:*** Hydrapres; ***Swed.:*** Apresolin; ***Thai.:*** Apresoline; Cesoline; ***UK:*** Apresoline; ***USA:*** Apresoline.

Multi-ingredient: *Aust.:* Polinorm; Trepress; Triloc; ***Canad.:*** Ser-Ap-Es†; ***Ger.:*** Docidrazin; Impresso; Pertenso N; Treloc; Trepress; TRI-Normin; ***Spain:*** Betadipresan; Betadipresan Diu; Neatenol Diuvas; Tensiocomplet; ***Switz.:*** Trepress†; ***Thai.:*** Hydrares; Hypery; Reser; Ser-Ap-Es; ***USA:*** Apresazide; Hydra-zide; Hydrap-ES; Marpres; Ser-Ap-Es; Tri-Hydroserpine.

Hydrochlorothiazide   (2333-v)

Hydrochlorothiazide (BAN, rINN).

Hidroclorotiazida; Hydrochlorothiazidum. 6-Chloro-3,4-dihydro-2*H*-1,2,4-benzothiadiazine-7-sulphonamide 1,1-dioxide.
$C_7H_8ClN_3O_4S_2 = 297.7$.
CAS — 58-93-5.
ATC — C03AA03.

NOTE. Compounded preparations of hydrochlorothiazide may be represented by the following names:

- Co-amilozide (*BAN*)—hydrochlorothiazide 10 parts and amiloride hydrochloride 1 part (w/w)
- Co-amilozide (*USP 25*)—amiloride hydrochloride and hydrochlorothiazide
- Co-spironozide (*USP 25*)—spironolactone and hydrochlorothiazide
- Co-triamterzide (*BAN*)—triamterene 2 parts and hydrochlorothiazide 1 part (w/w)
- Co-triamterzide (*USP 25*)—triamterene and hydrochlorothiazide
- Co-zidocapt (*BAN*)—hydrochlorothiazide 1 part and captopril 2 parts (w/w).

Pharmacopoeias. In *Chin.*, *Eur.* (see p.vi), *Int.*, *Jpn*, *Pol.*, and *US*.

Pharmacopoeial description

Ph. Eur.: A white or almost white, crystalline powder. Very slightly soluble in water; sparingly soluble in alcohol; soluble in acetone. It dissolves in dilute solutions of alkali hydroxides.

USP 25: A white or practically white, practically odourless crystalline powder. Slightly soluble in water; insoluble in chloroform, in ether, and in dilute mineral acids; freely soluble in dimethylformamide, in *n*-butylamine, and in sodium hydroxide solution; sparingly soluble in methyl alcohol.

Adverse Effects

Hydrochlorothiazide and other thiazide diuretics may cause a number of metabolic disturbances especially at high doses. They may provoke hyperglycaemia and glycosuria in diabetic and other susceptible patients. They may cause hyperuricaemia and precipitate attacks of gout in some patients. Administration of thiazide diuretics may be associated with electrolyte imbalances including hypochloraemic alkalosis, hyponatraemia, and hypokalaemia. Hypokalaemia intensifies the effect of digitalis on cardiac muscle and administration of digitalis or its glycosides may have to be temporarily suspended. Patients with cirrhosis of the liver are particularly at risk from hypokalaemia. Hyponatraemia may occur in patients with severe heart failure who are very oedematous, particularly with large doses in conjunction with restricted salt in the diet. The urinary excretion of calcium is reduced. Hypomagnesaemia has also occurred. Adverse changes in plasma lipids have also been noted but their clinical significance is unclear.

Signs of electrolyte imbalance include dry mouth, thirst, weakness, lethargy, drowsiness, restlessness, muscle pain and cramps, seizures, oliguria, hypotension, and gastrointestinal disturbances.

Other side-effects include anorexia, gastric irritation, nausea, vomiting, constipation, diarrhoea, sialadenitis, headache, dizziness, photosensitivity reactions, postural hypotension, paraesthesia, impotence, and yellow vision. Hypersensitivity reactions include skin rashes, fever, pulmonary oedema, pneumonitis, anaphylaxis, and toxic epidermal necrolysis. Cholestatic jaundice, pancreatitis, and blood dyscrasias including thrombocytopenia and, more rarely, granulocytopenia, leucopenia, and aplastic and haemolytic anaemia have been reported.

Intestinal ulceration has occurred following the administration of tablets containing thiazides with an enteric-coated core of potassium chloride (see also under Potassium, p.1195).

Carcinogenicity. Several studies have suggested that long-term diuretic therapy may be associated with the development of cancer. A meta-analysis[1] of 9 case control studies and 3 cohort studies found an increased risk of renal cell carcinoma in patients receiving diuretics, and a further retrospective study[2] found that the risk of colon cancer was also increased. While the risk is probably not significant in most patients, the authors suggested[1,2] that it should be taken into consideration when choosing long-term therapy for younger patients.

1. Grossman E, et al. Does diuretic therapy increase the risk of renal cell carcinoma? Am J Cardiol 1999; 83: 1090–3.
2. Tenenbaum A, et al. Is diuretic therapy associated with an increased risk of colon cancer? Am J Med 2001; 110: 143–5.

Effects on the blood. Individual case reports of intravascular immune haemolysis in patients taking hydrochlorothiazide and methyldopa.[1-3] In each of these 3 cases the hydrochlorothiazide was identified as the probable cause of haemolysis on serological data, although methyldopa could have been a contributory factor. One of these patients died[3] during the haemolytic episode although post-mortem examination failed to reveal a cause of death.

1. Vila JM, et al. Thiazide-induced immune hemolytic anemia. JAMA 1976; 236: 1723–4.
2. Garratty G, et al. Acute immune intravascular hemolysis due to hydrochlorothiazide. Am J Clin Pathol 1981; 76: 73–8.
3. Beck ML, et al. Fatal intravascular immune hemolysis induced by hydrochlorothiazide. Am J Clin Pathol 1984; 81: 791–4.

Effects on electrolyte balance. MAGNESIUM AND POTASSIUM. The clinical consequences of diuretic-induced hypokalaemia have been controversial.[1-3] Of major concern has been the possibility that diuretic-induced hypokalaemia could predispose to cardiac arrhythmias and sudden cardiac death in some patients, and it has been suggested that this could explain the lower than expected reduction in deaths due to ischaemic heart disease found in some hypertension trials. Indeed, some case-control studies[4,5] have suggested an association between an increased risk of sudden cardiac death and the use of thiazides or other non-potassium-sparing diuretics; the addition of a potassium supplement had little effect on this risk, whereas addition of a potassium-sparing diuretic to the thiazide lowered the risk.[4] However, no reduction in cardiac arrhythmias following the correction of hypokalaemia has been observed[6] nor any evidence of increased arrhythmias associated with diuretic-induced hypokalaemia.[7] Several reviews[8,9] have argued that there is no proof of a causal relationship between hypokalaemia and serious dysrhythmias and this was endorsed by a more recent randomised study.[10]

It is generally agreed that routine potassium supplementation in patients taking diuretics is unnecessary; however, supplementation will be required if the serum-potassium concentration falls below 3.0 mmol per litre. Potassium replacement or conservation is also likely to be necessary in patients at risk from the cardiac effects of hypokalaemia[11] such as those with severe heart disease, those taking digitalis preparations or high doses of diuretics, and in patients with severe liver disease.

The amount of potassium in fixed combination diuretic and potassium preparations has long been considered insufficient to correct hypokalaemia and the effectiveness of oral potassium supplements in increasing body stores of potassium has been questioned.[12-14] Hypokalaemia may be overcome by adding a potassium-sparing diuretic such as amiloride or triamterene[15] to the regimen, but there is a danger of hyperkalaemia if they are used indiscriminately. The routine use of fixed-dose combination preparations of a thiazide or loop diuretic with a potassium-sparing diuretic is considered unnecessary.[16] Potassium-sparing diuretics will not correct the potassium deficit unrelated to diuretic therapy in patients with severe heart failure.[17] Administration of a thiazide in combination with a beta blocker may ameliorate diuretic-induced hypokalaemia, but will not necessarily correct it completely. Hypokalaemia has been reported[18-20] in patients taking fixed-dose combinations of thiazides and beta blockers.

Potassium supplementation alone may not be sufficient to correct hypokalaemia in patients who are also deficient in magnesium,[21] although it is unlikely to be of clinical significance.[22] Magnesium depletion has also been implicated as a risk factor for arrhythmias.[9,23]

1. Materson BJ. Diuretic-associated hypokalemia. Arch Intern Med 1985; 145: 1966–7.

2. Kaplan NM, et al. Potassium supplementation in hypertensive patients with diuretic-induced hypokalemia. N Engl J Med 1985; 312: 746–9.
3. Kassirer JP, Harrington JT. Fending off the potassium pushers. N Engl J Med 1985; 312: 785–7.
4. Siscovick DS, et al. Diuretic therapy for hypertension and the risk of primary cardiac arrest. N Engl J Med 1994; 330: 1852–7.
5. Hoes AW, et al. Diuretics, β-blockers, and the risk for sudden cardiac death in hypertensive patients. Ann Intern Med 1995; 123: 481–7.
6. Papademetriou V, et al. Diuretic-induced hypokalemia in uncomplicated systemic hypertension: effect of plasma potassium correction on cardiac arrhythmias. Am J Cardiol 1983; 52: 1017–22.
7. Papademetriou V, et al. Thiazide therapy is not a cause of arrhythmia in patients with systemic hypertension. Arch Intern Med 1988; 148: 1272–6.
8. Harrington JT, et al. Our national obsession with potassium. Am J Med 1982; 73: 155–9.
9. Freis ED. Critique of the clinical importance of diuretic-induced hypokalaemia and elevated cholesterol level. Arch Intern Med 1989; 149: 2640–8.
10. Siegel D, et al. Diuretics, serum and intracellular electrolyte levels, and ventricular arrhythmias in hypertensive men. JAMA 1992; 267: 1083–9.
11. Anonymous. Potassium-sparing diuretics—when are they really needed? Drug Ther Bull 1985; 23: 17–20.
12. Jackson PR, et al. Relative potency of spironolactone, triamterene and potassium chloride in thiazide-induced hypokalaemia. Br J Clin Pharmacol 1982; 14: 257–63.
13. Shenfield GM. Fixed combination drug therapy. Drugs 1982; 23: 462–80.
14. Papademetriou V, et al. Effectiveness of potassium chloride or triamterene in thiazide hypokalemia. Arch Intern Med 1985; 145: 1986–90.
15. Kohvakka A. Maintenance of potassium balance during long-term diuretic therapy in chronic heart failure patients with thiazide-induced hypokalaemia: comparison of potassium supplementation with potassium chloride and potassium-sparing agents, amiloride and triamterene. Int J Clin Pharmacol Ther Toxicol 1988; 26: 273–7.
16. Anonymous. Routine use of potassium-sparing diuretics. Drug Ther Bull 1991; 29: 85–7.
17. Davidson C, et al. The effects of potassium supplements, spironolactone or amiloride on the potassium status of patients with heart failure. Postgrad Med J 1978; 54: 405–9.
18. Skehan JD, et al. Hypokalaemia induced by a combination of a beta-blocker and a thiazide. BMJ 1982; 284: 83.
19. Odugbesan O, et al. Hazards of combined beta-blocker/diuretic tablets. Lancet 1985; i: 1221–2.
20. Jacobs L. Hypokalaemia with beta-blocker/thiazide combinations. J R Coll Gen Pract 1986; 36: 39.
21. Dyckner T. Relation of cardiovascular disease to potassium and magnesium deficiencies. Am J Cardiol 1990; 65: 44–6.
22. Papademetriou V. Magnesium depletion and thiazide hypokalemia. Arch Intern Med 1986; 146: 1026.
23. Ryan MP. Diuretics and potassium/magnesium depletion: directions for treatment. Am J Med 1987; 82 (suppl 3A): 38–47.

SODIUM. Diuretic therapy is a common cause of hyponatraemia.[1-3] Dilutional hyponatraemia may occur in patients with heart failure, but hyponatraemia may also result from sodium depletion[1] or inappropriate antidiuretic hormone secretion.[4] Other suggested mechanisms include decreased renal clearance of free water, hypomagnesaemia, and intracellular potassium depletion.[3,5] There have been a number of reports suggesting that hyponatraemia may be a particular problem with combinations of hydrochlorothiazide and potassium-sparing diuretics,[6-8] especially in elderly patients. The effect may be exacerbated by the relatively high doses of thiazide present in some fixed-dose preparations.[9] The symptoms of hyponatraemia may be non-specific and include nausea, lethargy, weakness, mental confusion, and anorexia,[1,2] but it may be an important cause of morbidity.[2,5] Severe sequelae of hyponatraemia include tonic-clonic seizures[10] and clinical features resembling subarachnoid haemorrhage.[11,12] Some patients, especially the elderly, may be particularly susceptible to the hyponatraemic effects of thiazide diuretics, possibly as a result of inappropriate secretion of antidiuretic hormone.[4] Plasma electrolyte concentrations should be monitored in patients receiving long-term diuretic therapy.[3,10] Measurement of serum-sodium concentration and body-weight following a single dose of thiazide could be useful in identifying patients at increased risk of developing hyponatraemia.[5]

1. Roberts CJC, et al. Hyponatraemia: adverse effect of diuretic treatment. BMJ 1977; 1: 210.
2. Kennedy PGE, et al. Severe hyponatraemia in hospital inpatients. BMJ 1978; 2: 1251–3.
3. Walters EG, et al. Hyponatraemia associated with diuretics. Br J Clin Pract 1987; 41: 841–4.
4. Sonnenblick M, et al. Thiazide-induced hyponatremia and vasopressin release. Ann Intern Med 1989; 110: 751.
5. Friedman E, et al. Thiazide-induced hyponatremia: reproducibility by single dose rechallenge and an analysis of pathogenesis. Ann Intern Med 1989; 110: 24–30.
6. Strykers PH, et al. Hyponatremia induced by a combination of amiloride and hydrochlorothiazide. JAMA 1984; 252: 389.
7. Roberts CJC, et al. Hyponatraemia induced by a combination of hydrochlorothiazide and triamterene. BMJ 1984; 288: 1962.
8. Millson D, et al. Hyponatraemia and Moduretic (amiloride plus hydrochlorothiazide). BMJ 1984; 289: 1308–9.
9. Bayer AJ, et al. Plasma electrolytes in elderly patients taking fixed combination diuretics. Postgrad Med J 1986; 62: 159–62.
10. Johnston C, et al. Hyponatraemia and Moduretic-grand mal seizures: a review. J R Soc Med 1989; 82: 479–83.
11. Benfield GFA, et al. Dilutional hyponatraemia masquerading as subarachnoid haemorrhage in patient on hydrochlorothiazide/amiloride/timolol combined drug. Lancet 1986; ii: 341.
12. Bain PG. Thiazide-induced dilutional hyponatraemia masquerading as subarachnoid haemorrhage. Lancet 1986; ii: 634.

Effects on the gallbladder. There is an increased risk of cholecystitis in patients taking thiazide diuretics, with some indication that risk increases with the duration of treatment;[1,2]

some workers concluded that this increased risk was confined to patients with pre-existing gallstones.[2] In a study in 10 healthy subjects,[3] hydrochlorothiazide was found to induce modest changes in biliary lipid concentrations although it was not associated with supersaturation of the bile. These changes could not wholly explain any increase in gallbladder disease in patients taking thiazides. However, evidence is conflicting; other studies[4,5] have found no association between thiazide use and cholecystitis, except possibly in women who are not overweight.[5]

1. Rosenberg L, et al. Thiazides and acute cholecystitis. N Engl J Med 1980; 303: 546–8.
2. van der Linden W, et al. Acute cholecystitis and thiazides. BMJ 1984; 289: 654–5.
3. Angelin B. Effect of thiazide treatment on biliary lipid composition in healthy volunteers. Eur J Clin Pharmacol 1989; 37: 95–6.
4. Porter JB, et al. Acute cholecystitis and thiazides. N Engl J Med 1981; 304: 954–5.
5. Kakar F, et al. Thiazide use and the risk of cholecystectomy in women. Am J Epidemiol 1986; 124: 428–33.

Effects on glucose metabolism. The adverse effects of thiazide diuretics on glucose metabolism, such as insulin resistance, impaired glucose tolerance, precipitation of overt diabetes, and worsening of diabetic control, are well established but appear to be dose-related and may not be significant at lower doses (for example, hydrochlorothiazide 6.25 or 12.5 mg).[1] However, higher doses, for example bendrofluazide [bendroflumethiazide] 5 mg twice daily, as used in the Medical Research Council Study on Mild to Moderate Hypertension[2] resulted in an incidence of glucose intolerance that led to withdrawal from the study of 9.38 per 1000 patient-years in men and 6.01 per 1000 patient-years in women compared with 2.51 and 0.82 per 1000 patient-years respectively in patients taking placebo. A later prospective study[3] in non-diabetic hypertensive patients found that those taking thiazides [doses not specified] were at no greater risk for developing diabetes than those not receiving antihypertensive therapy.

In a study[4] in 16 non-diabetic hypertensive patients, bendrofluazide [bendroflumethiazide], in a dose of 1.25 mg daily, had no effect on insulin sensitivity whereas a daily dose of 5 mg produced hepatic insulin resistance.

1. Neutel JM. Metabolic manifestations of low-dose diuretics. Am J Med 1996; 101 (suppl 3A): 71S–82S.
2. Greenburg G. Adverse reactions to bendrofluazide and propranolol for the treatment of mild hypertension: report of Medical Research Council Working Party on Mild to Moderate Hypertension. Lancet 1981; ii: 539–43.
3. Gress TW, et al. Hypertension and antihypertensive therapy as risk factors for type 2 diabetes mellitus. N Engl J Med 2000; 342: 905–12.
4. Harper R, et al. Effects of low dose versus conventional dose thiazide diuretic on insulin action in essential hypertension. BMJ 1994; 309: 226–30.

Effects on the kidneys. Thiazide diuretics can produce acute renal failure either from over-enthusiastic use producing sodium depletion and hypovolaemia or, occasionally, as a result of a hypersensitivity reaction.[1] Acute interstitial nephritis has been reported.[2,3] They can occasionally cause the formation of non-opaque urate calculi.[4]

1. Curtis JR. Diseases of the urinary system: drug-induced renal disorders: I. BMJ 1977; 2: 242–4.
2. Linton AL, et al. Acute interstitial nephritis due to drugs: review of the literature with a report of nine cases. Ann Intern Med 1980; 93: 735–41.
3. Anonymous. Case records of the Massachusetts General Hospital: case 42-1983. N Engl J Med 1983; 309: 970–8.
4. Curtis JR. Diseases of the urinary system: drug-induced renal disorders: II. BMJ 1977; 2: 375–7.

Effects on lipids. Thiazide diuretics have been reported to adversely affect the plasma-lipid profile in the short term by increasing concentrations of low-density and very-low-density lipoprotein cholesterol, as well as of triglycerides, but not of high-density lipoprotein cholesterol.[1] These effects are probably dose-related[2] and it has been argued that changes in plasma lipids are likely to be slight at the relatively low doses of thiazide diuretics now used in the treatment of hypertension. The available evidence has also suggested that these lipid changes may not persist long-term,[3] but this is by no means established. In the Treatment of Mild Hypertension Study (TOMHS),[4] plasma total cholesterol concentrations were increased after 12 months in patients receiving chlortalidone but this effect was no longer present after 24 months. However, overall there is still concern in some quarters that any hyperlipidaemic effect might offset the benefits of treating hypertension in patients at risk of ischaemic heart disease.

1. Ames R. Effects of diuretic drugs on the lipid profile. Drugs 1988; 36 (suppl 2): 33–40.
2. Carlsen JE, et al. Relation between dose of bendrofluazide, antihypertensive effect, and adverse biochemical effects. BMJ 1990; 300: 975–8.
3. Freis ED. Critique of the clinical importance of diuretic-induced hypokalaemia and elevated cholesterol level. Arch Intern Med 1989; 149: 2640–8.
4. Grimm RH, et al. Long-term effects on plasma lipids of diet and drugs to treat hypertension. JAMA 1996; 275: 1549–56.

Effects on respiratory function. Acute interstitial pneumonitis and acute pulmonary oedema are rare but potentially dangerous complications of thiazide therapy and may be due to a hypersensitivity reaction. A number of cases have been reported,[1-7] frequently following a single dose of hydrochlorothiazide or chlorothiazide. The presenting symptoms could be mistakenly attributed to myocardial infarction.

1. Steinberg AD. Pulmonary edema following ingestion of hydrochlorothiazide. *JAMA* 1968; **204:** 167–9.
2. Beaudry C, Laplante L. Severe allergic pneumonitis from hydrochlorothiazide. *Ann Intern Med* 1973; **78:** 251–3.
3. Parfrey NA, Herlong HF. Pulmonary oedema after hydrochlorothiazide. *BMJ* 1984; **288:** 1880.
4. Watrigant Y, *et al.* Pneumopathie à l'hydrochlorothiazide d'évolution subaiguë: etude cytologique du lavage broncho-alvéolaire. *Rev Mal Respir* 1986; **4:** 227–9.
5. Klein MD. Noncardiogenic pulmonary edema following hydrochlorothiazide ingestion. *Ann Emerg Med* 1987; **16:** 901–3.
6. Bowden FJ. Non-cardiogenic pulmonary oedema after ingestion of chlorothiazide. *BMJ* 1989; **298:** 605.
7. Bernal C, Patarca R. Hydrochlorothiazide-induced pulmonary edema and associated immunologic changes. *Ann Pharmacother* 1999; **33:** 172–4.

Effects on sexual function. Adverse effects on sexual function have been reported in hypertensive patients receiving thiazide diuretics and other antihypertensives but it is not clear how much this is due to the underlying disease and how much is due to the drugs. In the Medical Research Council Study on Mild to Moderate Hypertension[1] the incidence of impotence in men receiving bendrofluazide [bendroflumethiazide] or placebo was 19.58 and 0.89 per 1000 patient-years, respectively. In the Treatment of Mild Hypertension Study (TOMHS),[2] which randomised patients to treatment with one of five groups of antihypertensives, the incidence of erectile dysfunction in men was relatively low but was highest in the diuretic group (chlortalidone treatment). The incidence was significantly higher in chlortalidone recipients than in placebo recipients at 24 months (17.1 and 8.1% respectively), but the difference was no longer significant at 48 months (18.3 and 16.7% respectively).

1. Greenburg G. Adverse reactions to bendrofluazide and propranolol for the treatment of mild hypertension: report of Medical Research Council Working Party on Mild to Moderate Hypertension. *Lancet* 1981; **ii:** 539–43.
2. Grimm RH, *et al.* Long-term effects on sexual function of five antihypertensive drugs and nutritional hygienic treatment in hypertensive men and women: Treatment of Mild Hypertension Study (TOMHS). *Hypertension* 1997; **29:** 8–14.

Effects on the skin. A variety of rashes and skin reactions has been reported in patients taking hydrochlorothiazide and other thiazide diuretics. *Photosensitivity* reactions are among the most frequently reported skin reactions. In Australia[1] co-amilozide was the preparation most commonly implicated in photosensitivity reactions in reports to the Australian Drug Reactions Advisory Committee, although this may reflect the high usage of this preparation. The most likely mechanism is thought to be phototoxicity[1,2] involving mainly UVA radiation although UVB may be involved in some cases.[2] Chronic photosensitivity does not usually occur following withdrawal of the drug[2] although photosensitivity may persist for longer in some patients than in others.[2,3] Eruptions resembling *lichen planus*[4] and *subacute cutaneous lupus erythematosus*[5-7] may be due to photosensitivity reactions.

Other reported skin reactions include *vasculitis*,[8,9] *erythema multiforme*,[9] and *pseudoporphyria*.[10]

1. Stone K. Photosensitivity reactions to drugs. *Aust J Pharm* 1985; **66:** 415–18.
2. Addo HA, *et al.* Thiazide-induced photosensitivity: a study of 33 subjects. *Br J Dermatol* 1987; **116:** 749–60.
3. Robinson HN, *et al.* Thiazide diuretic therapy and chronic photosensitivity. *Arch Dermatol* 1985; **121:** 522–4.
4. Graham-Brown R. Lichen planus and lichen-planus-like reactions. *Br J Hosp Med* 1986; **36:** 281–4.
5. Jones SK, *et al.* Thiazide diuretic-induced subacute cutaneous lupus-like syndrome. *Br J Dermatol* 1985; **113** (suppl 29): 25.
6. Reed BR, *et al.* Subacute cutaneous lupus erythematosus associated with hydrochlorothiazide therapy. *Ann Intern Med* 1985; **103:** 49–51.
7. Darken M, McBurney EI. Subacute cutaneous lupus erythematosus-like drug eruption due to combination diuretic hydrochlorothiazide and triamterene. *J Am Acad Dermatol* 1988; **18:** 38–42.
8. Björnberg A, Gisslén H. Thiazides: a cause of necrotising vasculitis? *Lancet* 1965; **ii:** 982–3.
9. Hardwick N, Saxe N. Patterns of dermatology referrals in a general hospital. *Br J Dermatol* 1986; **115:** 167–76.
10. Motley RS. Pseudoporphyria due to Dyazide in a patient with vitiligo. *BMJ* 1990; **300:** 1468.

Gout. Thiazide diuretics have been associated with hyperuricaemia and gout in some patients. In the Medical Research Council Study on Mild to Moderate Hypertension,[1] men receiving bendrofluazide [bendroflumethiazide] had higher incidences of gout than those receiving placebo (12.23 and 1.03 per 1000 patient-years, respectively). The risk appears to be dose-related; in a retrospective study[2] in patients aged 65 or older receiving antihypertensive therapy, there was a significantly increased risk of starting anti-gout therapy in patients receiving the equivalent of 25 mg hydrochlorothiazide or more daily, but not in those receiving lower doses.

1. Greenburg G. Adverse reactions to bendrofluazide and propranolol for the treatment of mild hypertension: report of Medical Research Council Working Party on Mild to Moderate Hypertension. *Lancet* 1981; **ii:** 539–43.
2. Gurwitz JH, *et al.* Thiazide diuretics and the initiation of anti-gout therapy. *J Clin Epidemiol* 1997; **50:** 953–9.

Withdrawal. For a report of oedema following withdrawal of thiazide diuretics, see under Precautions, below.

Treatment of Adverse Effects

Hypokalaemia in patients treated with thiazide diuretics may be avoided or treated by concurrent administration of potassium or a potassium-sparing diuretic (but see the discussion on potassium supplements, under Effects on Electrolyte Balance in Adverse Effects, above). Hypokalaemia can also be reduced by moderate sodium restriction. With the exception of patients with conditions such as liver failure or kidney disease, chloride deficiency is usually mild and does not require specific treatment. Apart from the rare occasions when it is life-threatening, dilutional hyponatraemia is best treated with water restriction rather than salt therapy; in true hyponatraemia, appropriate replacement is the treatment of choice (see p.1183).

In massive overdosage, treatment should be symptomatic and directed at fluid and electrolyte replacement. Use of activated charcoal should be considered if the patient presents within 1 hour of ingestion of hydrochlorothiazide.

Precautions

All diuretics produce changes in fluid and electrolyte balance (see under Adverse Effects, above). They should be used with caution in patients with existing fluid and electrolyte disturbances or who are at risk from changes in fluid and electrolyte balance, such as the elderly. They should be avoided in patients with severe hepatic impairment, in whom encephalopathy may be precipitated. Patients with hepatic cirrhosis are also more likely to develop hypokalaemia. Hyponatraemia may occur in patients with severe heart failure who are very oedematous, particularly with large doses of thiazides in conjunction with restricted salt in the diet. All patients should be carefully observed for signs of fluid and electrolyte imbalance, especially in the presence of vomiting or during parenteral fluid therapy. Thiazide diuretics should not be given to patients with Addison's disease.

Diuretics should also be given with caution in renal impairment since they can further reduce renal function. Most thiazide diuretics are not effective in patients with a creatinine clearance of less than 30 mL per minute. They should not be used in patients with severe renal impairment or anuria.

Thiazides may precipitate attacks of gout in susceptible patients. They may cause hyperglycaemia and aggravate or unmask diabetes mellitus. Blood-glucose concentrations should be monitored in patients taking antidiabetics, since requirements may change. Thiazides can reduce urinary excretion of calcium, sometimes resulting in mild hypercalcaemia; thiazides should not be given to patients with pre-existing hypercalcaemia. There is a possibility that thiazide diuretics may exacerbate or activate systemic lupus erythematosus in susceptible patients. For a suggestion that thiazide diuretics may increase the risk of developing gallstones, see under Effects on the Gallbladder, above.

Thiazides cross the placenta and there have been reports of neonatal jaundice, thrombocytopenia, and electrolyte imbalances following maternal treatment. Reductions in maternal blood volume could also adversely affect placental perfusion. Thiazide diuretics are distributed into breast milk. Treatment with large doses of thiazide diuretics can inhibit lactation.

Hyperparathyroidism. Hypertension is a complication of primary hyperparathyroidism but thiazides have often been withheld for fear of exacerbating hypercalcaemia. However, no differences in plasma-calcium concentrations were found in 13 patients who received thiazides intermittently for up to 18 months. It was therefore concluded that thiazide diuretics are not contra-indicated in such patients.[1] They should, however, be stopped before parathyroid function is tested.

1. Farquhar CW, *et al.* Failure of thiazide diuretics to increase plasma calcium in mild primary hyperparathyroidism. *Postgrad Med J* 1990; **66:** 714–16.

Porphyria. Hydrochlorothiazide has been associated with acute attacks of porphyria and is considered unsafe in porphyric patients.

Withdrawal. In patients with mild hypertension whose blood pressure is consistently controlled, reduction in dosage or withdrawal of antihypertensive drugs may be possible. Serious oedema occurred in 8 patients with controlled hypertension within 2 weeks of abrupt withdrawal of thiazide diuretics.[1] Thiazides were resumed and gradually tapered without recurrence of oedema.

1. Brandspigel K. Diuretic-withdrawal edema. *N Engl J Med* 1986; **314:** 515.

Interactions

Many of the interactions of hydrochlorothiazide and other thiazide diuretics are due to their effects on fluid and electrolyte balance. Diuretic-induced hypokalaemia may enhance the toxicity of digitalis glycosides and may also increase the risk of arrhythmias with drugs that prolong the QT interval, such as astemizole, terfenadine, halofantrine, pimozide, and sotalol. Thiazides may enhance the neuromuscular blocking action of competitive muscle relaxants, such as atracurium, probably by their hypokalaemic effect. The potassium-depleting effect of diuretics may be enhanced by corticosteroids, corticotropin, beta$_2$ agonists such as salbutamol, carbenoxolone, amphotericin B, or reboxetine.

Diuretics may enhance the effect of other antihypertensives, particularly the first-dose hypotension that occurs with alpha blockers or ACE inhibitors. Postural hypotension associated with diuretic therapy may be enhanced by concomitant ingestion of alcohol, barbiturates, or opioids. The antihypertensive effects of diuretics may be antagonised by drugs that cause fluid retention, such as corticosteroids, NSAIDs, or carbenoxolone. Thiazides have been reported to diminish the response to pressor amines, such as noradrenaline [norepinephrine], but the clinical significance of this effect is uncertain.

Thiazide diuretics should not usually be used with lithium since the association may lead to toxic blood concentrations of lithium. Other drugs for which increased toxicity has been reported when given with thiazides include allopurinol and tetracyclines. Thiazides may alter the requirements for hypoglycaemic drugs in diabetic patients.

Antibacterials. Severe hyponatraemia has been reported in patients taking *trimethoprim* with co-amilozide[1] and hydrochlorothiazide.[2]

1. Eastell R, Edmonds CJ. Hyponatraemia associated with trimethoprim and a diuretic. *BMJ* 1984; **289:** 1658–9.
2. Hart TL. Hyponatremia secondary to thiazide-trimethoprim interaction. *Can J Hosp Pharm* 1989; **42:** 243–6.

Antiepileptics. Report of symptomatic hyponatraemia associated with concomitant use of hydrochlorothiazide or frusemide [furosemide] and *carbamazepine*.[1]

1. Yassa R, *et al.* Carbamazepine, diuretics, and hyponatremia: a possible interaction. *J Clin Psychiatry* 1987; **48:** 281–3.

Bile-acid binding resins. Gastrointestinal absorption of both chlorothiazide and hydrochlorothiazide has been reported to be reduced by *colestipol* and *colestyramine*.[1-3] In a study in healthy subjects[2] colestyramine had the greatest effect on hydrochlorothiazide, decreasing absorption by 85% compared with a decrease of 43% with colestipol. Even when colestyramine was administered 4 hours after hydrochlorothiazide[3] reductions of absorption of at least 30 to 35% could be expected.

1. Kauffman RE, Azarnoff DL. Effect of colestipol on gastrointestinal absorption of chlorothiazide in man. *Clin Pharmacol Ther* 1973; **14:** 886–90.
2. Hunninghake DB, *et al.* The effect of cholestyramine and colestipol on the absorption of hydrochlorothiazide. *Int J Clin Pharmacol Ther Toxicol* 1982; **20:** 151–4.
3. Hunninghake DB, Hibbard DM. Influence of time intervals for cholestyramine dosing on the absorption of hydrochlorothiazide. *Clin Pharmacol Ther* 1986; **39:** 329–34.

Calcium salts. The milk-alkali syndrome, characterised by hypercalcaemia, metabolic alkalosis, and renal failure, developed in a patient taking chlorothiazide and moderately large doses of calcium carbonate.[1] Patients taking thiazide diuretics may be at increased risk of developing the milk-alkali syndrome because of their reduced ability to excrete excess calcium. Hypercalcaemia may also occur in patients taking thiazides with drugs that increase calcium levels, such as vitamin D.

1. Gora ML, *et al.* Milk-alkali syndrome associated with use of chlorothiazide and calcium carbonate. *Clin Pharm* 1989; **8:** 227–9.

Dopaminergics. For a report of increased *amantadine* toxicity associated with hydrochlorothiazide and triamterene, see p.1162.

NSAIDs. Discussion of antagonism of the diuretic actions of thiazides by NSAIDs.[1]

1. Webster J. Interactions of NSAIDs with diuretics and β-blockers: mechanisms and clinical implications. *Drugs* 1985; **30:** 32–41.

Pharmacokinetics

Hydrochlorothiazide is fairly rapidly absorbed from the gastrointestinal tract. It is reported to have a bioavailability of about 65 to 70%. It has been estimated to have a plasma half-life of between about 5 and 15 hours and appears to be preferentially bound to red blood cells. It is excreted mainly unchanged in the urine. Hydrochlorothiazide crosses the placental barrier and is distributed into breast milk.

◊ References.
1. Beermann B, et al. Absorption, metabolism, and excretion of hydrochlorothiazide. Clin Pharmacol Ther 1976; 19: 531–7.
2. Beermann B, Groschinsky-Grind M. Pharmacokinetics of hydrochlorothiazide in man. Eur J Clin Pharmacol 1977; 12: 297–303.
3. Beermann B, Groschinsky-Grind M. Pharmacokinetics of hydrochlorothiazide in patients with congestive heart failure. Br J Clin Pharmacol 1979; 7: 579–83.

Uses and Administration

Hydrochlorothiazide and the other thiazide diuretics are used in the treatment of oedema associated with heart failure (p.798) and with renal and hepatic disorders. They are also used in hypertension (p.802), either alone or together with other antihypertensives such as ACE inhibitors and beta blockers. Other indications have included the treatment of oedema accompanying the premenstrual syndrome (p.1475), the prevention of water retention associated with corticosteroids and oestrogens, the treatment of diabetes insipidus (below), and the prevention of renal calculus formation in patients with hypercalciuria (below).

Thiazides are moderately potent diuretics and exert their diuretic effect by reducing the reabsorption of electrolytes from the renal tubules, thereby increasing the excretion of sodium and chloride ions, and consequently of water. They act mainly at the beginning of the distal tubules. The excretion of other electrolytes, notably potassium and magnesium, is also increased. The excretion of calcium is reduced. They also reduce carbonic-anhydrase activity so that bicarbonate excretion is increased, but this effect is generally small compared with the effect on chloride excretion and does not appreciably alter the pH of the urine. They may also reduce the glomerular filtration rate.

Their hypotensive effect is probably partly due to a reduction in peripheral resistance; they also enhance the effects of other antihypertensives. Paradoxically, thiazides have an antidiuretic effect in patients with diabetes insipidus.

Administration and dosage. Thiazides are usually given in the morning so that sleep is not interrupted by diuresis. Diuresis is initiated in about 2 hours following the oral administration of hydrochlorothiazide, reaches a maximum in about 4 hours, and lasts for 6 to 12 hours.

The dosage of thiazides should be adjusted to the minimum effective dose, and in recent years there has been a definite trend towards lower doses. In general lower doses are required for the treatment of hypertension than for oedema, although the maximum therapeutic effect may not be seen for several weeks.

They may be given to patients with mild renal impairment, but thiazides are generally not effective at a creatinine clearance of less than 30 mL per minute. Some have recommended that the dose of hydrochlorothiazide should be halved when there is moderate renal impairment (a creatinine clearance of 30 to 70 mL per minute).

Hydrochlorothiazide is given by mouth.

In the treatment of **oedema** the usual dose is 25 to 100 mg daily, reduced to a dose of 25 to 50 mg daily or intermittently; in severe cases initial doses of up to 200 mg daily have been suggested, but the more powerful loop diuretics (see Frusemide, p.893) are preferred in such patients.

In the treatment of **hypertension** the usual dose of hydrochlorothiazide is 25 to 50 mg daily, either alone, or in conjunction with other antihypertensives. In some patients an initial dose of 12.5 mg may be sufficient. Doses of up to 100 mg have been suggested but are rarely necessary.

In the treatment of nephrogenic **diabetes insipidus** an initial dose of up to 100 mg daily may be employed.

An initial dose for children has been 1 to 2 mg per kg body-weight daily in 2 divided doses. Infants under 6 months may need doses of up to 3 mg per kg daily.

For discussion of potassium supplementation in patients taking thiazide diuretics see Effects on Electrolyte Balance, under Adverse Effects, above.

Bronchopulmonary dysplasia. Bronchopulmonary dysplasia (p.1048) is a major cause of chronic lung disease in infants. Treatment often involves the use of corticosteroids. Additional supportive therapy has included the use of diuretics such as frusemide [furosemide] (p.895); results with hydrochlorothiazide or spironolactone have been more ambiguous. No beneficial effects on lung function or oxygenation were found in a study of 12 infants after 1 week of treatment with hydrochlorothiazide and spironolactone.[1] However, hydrochlorothiazide and spironolactone therapy was found to improve total respiratory system compliance with decreased lung damage and increased survival rate in 34 premature infants with bronchopulmonary dysplasia after 8 weeks of therapy.[2] In the latter study frusemide [furosemide] was also given if clinically indicated.

1. Engelhardt B, et al. Effect of spironolactone-hydrochlorothiazide on lung function in infants with chronic bronchopulmonary dysplasia. J Pediatr 1989; 114: 619–24.
2. Albersheim SG, et al. Randomized, double-blind, controlled trial of long-term diuretic therapy for bronchopulmonary dysplasia. J Pediatr 1989; 115: 615–20.

Diabetes insipidus. Thiazide diuretics are used in nephrogenic diabetes insipidus (p.1273), sometimes combined with potassium-sparing diuretics. For instance, hydrochlorothiazide with amiloride was effective in controlling nephrogenic diabetes insipidus in 5 boys and compared favourably with treatment with hydrochlorothiazide in combination with indometacin.[1] Treatment was well tolerated in 4 patients. Abdominal pain and anorexia necessitated withdrawal of amiloride in the fifth patient after six months of treatment. The use of hydrochlorothiazide with amiloride also obviated the need for potassium supplements, which were required with hydrochlorothiazide and indometacin. The combination of hydrochlorothiazide and amiloride was also effective and well tolerated in a group of 4 children with nephrogenic diabetes insipidus who were treated for up to 5 years.[2]

1. Knoers N, Monnens LAH. Amiloride-hydrochlorothiazide versus indometacin-hydrochlorothiazide in the treatment of nephrogenic diabetes insipidus. J Pediatr 1990; 117: 499–502.
2. Kirchlechner V, et al. Treatment of nephrogenic diabetes insipidus with hydrochlorothiazide and amiloride. Arch Dis Child 1999; 80: 548–52.

Hypoparathyroidism. In hypoparathyroidism (p.747), treatment is usually with oral vitamin D compounds to correct the hypocalcaemia. Thiazide diuretics may be useful in some patients. Beneficial effects on serum-calcium concentrations in patients with hypoparathyroidism have been reported following treatment with chlortalidone plus dietary salt restriction[1] and with bendrofluazide [bendroflumethiazide].[2] However, chlortalidone has not been found to be effective in all patients,[3] and the reduction in urinary calcium excretion by thiazides has been shown to be diminished in patients with hypoparathyroidism[4] suggesting that this effect may be dependent on the presence of some parathyroid hormone. Care should be taken when administering diuretics to hypoparathyroid patients with co-existing adrenal insufficiency[3] or metabolic alkalosis.[5]

1. Porter RH, et al. Treatment of hypoparathyroid patients with chlorthalidone. N Engl J Med 1978; 298: 577–81.
2. Newman GH, et al. Effect of bendrofluazide on calcium reabsorption in hypoparathyroidism. Eur J Clin Pharmacol 1984; 27: 41–6.
3. Gertner JM, Genel M. Chlorthalidone for hypoparathyroidism. N Engl J Med 1978; 298: 1478.
4. Middler S, et al. Thiazide diuretics and calcium metabolism. Metabolism 1973; 22: 139–45.
5. Barzel US. Chlorthalidone for hypoparathyroidism. N Engl J Med 1978; 289: 1478.

Ménière's disease. In Ménière's disease (p.407) there is an excess of endolymph fluid in the ear and diuretics such as hydrochlorothiazide have been used in attempts to relieve symptoms by reducing the amount of fluid.

Osteoporosis. Although some epidemiological studies have indicated beneficial effects of thiazide diuretics on bone (reduced rates of bone loss[1] and a reduced risk of hip fracture[2–4]) a comprehensive analysis involving 9704 women over the age of 65 years[5] showed only a small effect on bone mass, no effect on the risk for falls, and no overall protective effect against fractures. Randomised, controlled studies[6,7] have confirmed that hydrochlorothiazide reduces bone loss, but again the effects were small. Thus, thiazides have no established role in the prevention or treatment of osteoporosis (p.745). They might, however, be useful to reduce hypercalciuria in patients taking glucocorticoids[8] but serum-potassium concentrations should be monitored closely.

1. Wasnich R, et al. Effect of thiazide on rates of bone mineral loss: a longitudinal study. BMJ 1990; 301: 1303–5. Correction. ibid. 1991; 302: 218.

2. Ray WA, et al. Long-term use of thiazide diuretics and risk of hip fracture. Lancet 1989; i: 687–90.
3. LaCroix AZ, et al. Thiazide diuretic agents and the incidence of hip fracture. N Engl J Med 1990; 322: 286–90.
4. Felson DT, et al. Thiazide diuretics and the risk of hip fracture: results from the Framingham Study. JAMA 1991; 265: 370–3.
5. Cauley JA, et al. Effects of thiazide diuretic therapy on bone mass, fractures, and falls. Ann Intern Med 1993; 118: 666–73.
6. Reid IR, et al. Hydrochlorothiazide reduces loss of cortical bone in normal postmenopausal women: a randomized controlled trial. Am J Med 2000; 109: 362–70.
7. LaCroix AZ, et al. Low-dose hydrochlorothiazide and preservation of bone mineral density in older adults: a randomized, double-blind, placebo-controlled trial. Ann Intern Med 2000; 133: 516–26.
8. Lukert BP, Raisz LG. Glucocorticoid-induced osteoporosis: pathogenesis and management. Ann Intern Med 1990; 112: 352–64.

Renal calculi. Normal urine contains calcium, oxalate, and phosphate in amounts greater than their normal aqueous solubility; this supersaturation is maintained by a variety of inhibitors of crystallisation, both organic and inorganic. However, increases in the concentrations of crystalline substances in the urine, or decreases in the relative proportions of crystallisation inhibitors, may render some individuals susceptible to the formation of renal calculi (kidney stones).

Renal calculi consist of crystalline components arranged around an organic matrix. They are typically formed in the calices or renal pelvis, and may become lodged in the ureter. About 1 to 5% of the population are affected, and although some patients only ever develop a single stone, between 50 and 80% of patients experience subsequent recurrences. Calcium-containing stones (usually calcium oxalate and calcium phosphate in variable proportions) account for the vast majority of occurrences although stones of other compositions including cystine, uric acid, or magnesium ammonium phosphate, are occasionally seen.

Patients with renal calculi may be asymptomatic or may pass small stones with relatively little discomfort. However, passage of a larger stone down the ureter may be accompanied by excruciating pain (renal or ureteral colic), obstruction, and trauma; there may also be associated infection.

Treatment. Treatment of existing stones, if any, is essentially surgical, while medical treatment is aimed at prevention of recurrence. In the acute episode analgesics may be required for the pain (see Biliary and Renal Colic, p.5) but if there is no obstruction, infection, or other complication conservative treatment is favoured, with the patient being monitored radiographically over several weeks to see if the stone will pass of its own accord. Where intervention is considered necessary, it may be by open or endoscopic surgery, or shock wave lithotripsy, in which focussed shock waves are used to shatter the stone. Antibacterials may be needed for infection (see p.146 for urinary-tract infections).

In the prevention of recurrence it is important to identify, and where possible correct, any underlying disease process or biochemical or anatomical abnormality. Certain general measures are also appropriate. Patients should drink a minimum of 3 litres of fluid daily in order to maintain an adequate volume of urine. In hot climates or working environments a higher volume of fluid should be taken.

Dietary restrictions may be appropriate in some cases. Traditionally, dairy products and other foods rich in calcium, as well as calcium-containing antacids and vitamin D supplements, have been avoided in patients with calcium-containing stones. However, recent studies have found an inverse relationship between dietary calcium intake and the risk of stone formation in men[1] and in women,[2] and restriction of dietary calcium is probably not necessary.[3] Conversely, calcium supplements do appear to increase the risk of stone formation and should be avoided, although the reason for this difference is not clear.[2] Limitation of the intake of animal protein and oxalate-rich foods, including tea, is also probably appropriate in such patients,[4] and sodium restriction may also be beneficial.

In patients with idiopathic hypercalciuria (i.e. when excessive calcium excretion cannot be linked to hyperparathyroidism, sarcoidosis, malignancy, or some other underlying condition) and a history of renal calculi a **thiazide diuretic** is usually given. Such therapy has generally[5,6] though not universally[7] been found effective, although the benefit may decline with time. Hydrochlorothiazide or amiloride have also been reported to be of benefit in patients with a history of calcium oxalate stones due to a defect in oxalate transport,[8] while thiazide treatment or oral phosphates have been found effective in decreasing urinary calcium excretion in patients with absorptive hypercalciuria.[9] Where thiazide treatment is ineffective treatment with sodium cellulose phosphate may be considered, together with a magnesium supplement. Sodium cellulose phosphate is of value in patients with excessive intestinal calcium absorption.[10] Phosphate salts[10] or magnesium salts[11,12] which act as non-specific inhibitors of urinary crystallisation may also be used.

In patients with reduced citrate excretion treatment with potassium citrate may be useful in preventing stone recurrence;[13] by increasing urinary pH, it may be helpful in patients with uric acid stones. Allopurinol has also been suggested, both for uric acid and for calcium oxalate stone prevention, although the latter has been a matter of debate.[14,15]

In patients with struvite (magnesium ammonium phosphate) stones, which are associated with bacterial infection and result from the action of bacterial urease, control may be difficult to achieve using antibacterials alone; acetohydroxamic acid, an inhibitor of bacterial urease, has been given as an adjunct.[16,17] Penicillamine may be of benefit in preventing cystine stones in patients with cystinuria (p.1019).

1. Curhan GC, et al. A prospective study of dietary calcium and other nutrients and the risk of symptomatic kidney stones. N Engl J Med 1993; 328: 833–8.
2. Curhan GC, et al. Comparison of dietary calcium with supplemental calcium and other nutrients as factors affecting the risk for kidney stones in women. Ann Intern Med 1997; 126: 497–504.
3. Coe FL, et al. Diet and calcium: the end of an era? Ann Intern Med 1997; 126: 553–5.
4. Lemann J. Composition of the diet and calcium kidney stones. N Engl J Med 1993; 328: 880–2.
5. Yendt ER, et al. The use of thiazides in the prevention of renal calculi. Can Med Assoc J 1970; 102: 614–20.
6. Laerum E, Larsen S. Thiazide prophylaxis of urolithiasis: a double-blind study in general practice. Acta Med Scand 1984; 215: 383–9.
7. Scholz D, et al. Double-blind study with thiazide in recurrent calcium lithiasis. J Urol (Baltimore) 1982; 128: 903–7.
8. Baggio B, et al. An inheritable anomaly of red-cell oxalate transport in "primary" calcium nephrolithiasis correctable with diuretics. N Engl J Med 1986; 314: 599–604.
9. Insogna KL, et al. Trichlormethiazide and oral phosphate therapy in patients with absorptive hypercalciuria. J Urol (Baltimore) 1989; 141: 269–74.
10. Pak CYC. Formation of renal stones may be prevented by restoring normal urinary composition. Proc Eur Dial Transplant Assoc 1983; 20: 371–85.
11. Melnick I, et al. Magnesium therapy for recurring calcium oxalate urinary calculi. J Urol (Baltimore) 1971; 105: 119–22.
12. Johansson G, et al. Biochemical and clinical effects of the prophylactic treatment of renal calcium stones with magnesium hydroxide. J Urol (Baltimore) 1980; 124: 770–4.
13. Pak CYC, Fuller C. Idiopathic hypocalciuric calcium-oxalate nephrolithiasis successfully treated with potassium citrate. Ann Intern Med 1986; 104: 33–7.
14. Ettinger B, et al. Randomized trial of allopurinol in the prevention of calcium oxalate calculi. N Engl J Med 1986; 315: 1386–9.
15. Tiselius H-G, et al. Clinical results of allopurinol treatment in prevention of calcium oxalate stone formation. J Urol (Baltimore) 1986; 136: 50–3.
16. Martelli A, et al. Acetohydroxamic acid therapy in infected renal stones. Urology 1981; 17: 320–2.
17. Williams JJ, et al. A randomized double-blind study of acetohydroxamic acid in struvite nephrolithiasis. N Engl J Med 1984; 311: 760–4.

Preparations

BP 2001: Co-amilozide Oral Solution; Co-amilozide Tablets; Co-triamterzide Tablets; Hydrochlorothiazide Tablets;
USP 25: Amiloride Hydrochloride and Hydrochlorothiazide Tablets; Captopril and Hydrochlorothiazide Tablets; Enalapril Maleate and Hydrochlorothiazide Tablets; Hydrochlorothiazide Tablets; Methyldopa and Hydrochlorothiazide Tablets; Metoprolol Tartrate and Hydrochlorothiazide Tablets; Propranolol Hydrochloride and Hydrochlorothiazide Tablets; Propranolol Hydrochloride and Hydrochlorothiazide Extended-release Capsules; Reserpine and Hydrochlorothiazide Tablets; Reserpine, Hydralazine Hydrochloride, and Hydrochlorothiazide Tablets; Spironolactone and Hydrochlorothiazide Tablets; Timolol Maleate and Hydrochlorothiazide Tablets; Triamterene and Hydrochlorothiazide Capsules; Triamterene and Hydrochlorothiazide Tablets.

Proprietary Preparations (details are given in Part 3)
Aust.: Dithiazid; Esidrex; *Austral.:* Dichlotride; *Belg.:* Dichlotride; Esidrex†; *Braz.:* Clorana; Diurezin; Drenol; Tenadren; *Canad.:* Apo-Hydro; HydroDiuril; Novo-Hydrazide†; *Denm.:* Dichlotride; Hydronet†; *Fin.:* Hydrex; *Fr.:* Esidrex; *Ger.:* Disalunil; diu-melusin; Esidrix; HCT; HCT-ISIS; *Hong Kong:* Hydrozide; *Irl.:* HydroSaluric; *Israel:* Esidrex; *Ital.:* Esidrex; *Mex.:* Diclotride; *Neth.:* Dichlotride†; Esidrex; *Norw.:* Dichlotride; Esidrex†; *Port.:* Dichlotride; *S.Afr.:* Dichlotride; *Singapore:* Apo-Hydro; Di-Ertride; Didralin; Hydrozide; *Spain:* Acuretic; Esidrex; Hidrosaluretil; *Swed.:* Dichlotride; Esidrex; *Switz.:* Esidrex; *Thai.:* Dichlotride; Didralin; Diuret-P; Hydrozide; Servithiazid; *UK:* HydroSaluric†; *USA:* Diaqua†; Esidrix; Hydro-Chlor†; Hydro-Z†; HydroDiuril; Hydromal†; Hydrozide†; Microzide; Mictrin; Oretic; Thiuretic†.

Multi-ingredient: *Aust.:* Accuzide; Acecomb; Adelphan-Esidrex; Adoretic; Amiloretik; Amilorid comp; Amilostad HCT; Beloc comp; Capozide; Captopril Compositum; Cibadrex; Co-Acetan; Co-Dilatrend; Co-Diovan; Co-Mepril; Co-Renitec; Concor Plus; Confit; Corindocomb†; Cosaar Plus; Deverol mit Thiazid; Diurid; Dytide H; Elfanex; Fosicomb; Hypren plus; Inderal comp; Inhibace Plus; Lanuretic; Loradur; Metolol compositum; Moducrin; Moduretic; Prinzide†; Renitec Plus; Resaltex; Salodiur; Seloken retard Plus; Supergan; Supracid; Tardurol†; Triamteren comp; Triastad HCT; Trilok; Tritazide; Zestoretic; *Austral.:* Amizide; Atacand Plus; Avapro HCT; Dyazide; Hydrene; Hydrozide†; Karvezide; Modizide; Moduretic; Monoplus; Renitec Plus; *Belg.:* Accuretic; Belidral; Co-Diovane; Co-Inhibace; Co-Renitec; Cosaar Plus; Dytenzide; Emcoretic; Foside; Kalten; Loortan Plus; Maxsoten; Maxzide; Moduretic; Novazyd; Sectrazide; Selozide; Tritazide; Uractazide; Zestoretic; Zok-Zid; *Braz.:* Adelfan-Esidrex; Aldazida; Atens H; Co-Renitec; Eupressin H; Hydromet; Iguassina; Lopril D; Moduretic; Prinzide; Selopress; Zestoretic; *Canad.:* Accuretic; Aldactazide; Aldoril†; Apo-Amilzide; Apo-Methazide; Apo-Triazide; Diovan HCT; Dyazide; Hydropres†; Hyzaar; Inderide; Inhibace Plus; Moduret; Novamilor; Novo-Doparil†; Novo-Spirozine; Novo-Triamzide; Nu-Amilzide; Nu-Triazide; Prinzide; Ser-Ap-Es†; Timolide; Vaseretic; Viskazide; Zestoretic; *Denm.:* Amilco; Amilohyd†; Capozid;

Cibadrex; Co-Renitec; CoAprovel; Corodil Comp; Cozaar Comp; Diovan Comp; Fortzaar; Moduretic; Sparkal; Synerpril; Triatec Comp; Vivazid; Zestoretic; Zok-Zid; *Fin.:* Accupro Comp; Acercomp; Amitrid; Cardace Comp; Cozaar Comp; Diovan Comp; Diuramin; Diurex; Emconcor Comp; Enaloc Comp; Linatil Comp; Lisipril Comp; Miloride; Moduretic; Renitec Comp; Renitec Plus; Selocomp ZOC; Sparkal; Vivatec Comp; *Fr.:* Acuilix; Briazide; Captea; Cibadrex; Co-Renitec; CoAprovel; Cokenzen; Cotareg; Ecazide; Fortzaar; Foziretic; Hytacand; Hyzaar; Koretic; Lodoz; Moducren; Moduretic; Nisisco; Prestole; Prinzide; Wytens; Zestoretic; *Ger.:* Accuzide; Acenorm HCT; Acercomp; Adelphan-Esidrix; Adocomp; Amiduret†; Amilocomp beta; Amiloretik; Amilorid comp; Amilorid/HCT; Amilothiazid†; Amilozid; Aquaretic; Azumetop HCT; Barotonal; Beloc comp†; Beloc-Zok comp; Beta-Nephral†; Beta-Turfa; Betathiazid; Betathiazid A; Capozide; Capto Comp; Capto Plus; Captobeta Comp; Captogamma HCT; Captohexal Comp; Captopril Comp; Captopril HCT; Captopril Plus; Cardiagen HCT; Cibadrex; Co-Diovan; Coprovel; Concor Plus; Coric Plus; Corindocomb; Delix plus; Dignoretik; Disalpin; Diu Venostasin; Diuretikum Verla; Diursan; Diutensat; Diutensat comp; Dociteren; duradiuret; durarese; Dynacil comp; Dynorm Plus; Dytide H; Esimil; Esiteren; Fempress Plus; Fondril-5 HCT; Fosinorm comp; Haemiton compositum; Hydrocomp; Hypertorr; Isoptin plus; Jenateren comp; Karvezide; Lorzaar plus; Manimon; Meto comp; Meto-comp†; meto-thiazid; Metobeta comp; Metodura comp; Metohexal comp; Metostad Comp; Modu-Puren; Moducrin; Moduretik; Nephral; Pres plus; Propra comp; Provas comp; Renacor; Resaltex†; Rhefluin†; Risicordin; Sali-Puren; Spironothiazid; Tensobon comp; Thiazid-comp; Treloc; Tri-Thiazid; Tri-Thiazid Reserpin; Triampur; Triamteren comp; Triamteren-H; Triamteren/HCT; Triarese; triazid; Triniton; Turfa; Veratide; Vesdil plus; *Hong Kong:* Adelphane-Esidrex; Amilco; Amithiazide; Apo-Amilzide; Apo-Triazide; Betaloc Comp; Co-Renitec; Dyazide; Hydrozide; Hyzaar; Moducren; Moduretic; Secadrex; Triam-Co; Trizid; Zestoretic; *Irl.:* Accuretic; Amilco; Atacand Plus; Capozide; Captor-HCT; Carace Plus; Clonuretic; Co-Betaloc; Co-Diovan; CoAprovel; Cozaar Comp; Dyazide; Hydromet†; Innozide; Moducren; Moduret; Moduretic; Secadrex†; Zestoretic; *Israel:* Kaluril; Ocsaar Plus; Vascace Plus; *Ital.:* Accuretic; Acediur; Aceplus; Acequide; Acesistem; Aldactazide; Cibadrex; CoAprovel; Combisartan; Condiuren; Cotareg; Elidiur; Femipres Plus; Fosicombi; Gentipress; Hizaar; Idroquark; Inibace Plus; Initiss Plus; Karvezide; Losazid; Medozide; Moduretic; Nalapres; Neo-Lotan Plus; Neoprex; Prinzide; Quinazide; Selozide; Sinertec; Spiridazide; Tensadiur; Tensozide; Triatec HCT; Vasoretic; Zestoretic; Zinadiur; *Mex.:* Biconcor; Capozide; Co-Captral; Co-Renitec; Diovan HCT; Dyazide; Hyzaar; Moducren; Moduretic; Prinzide; Selopres; Tritazide; Zestoretic; *Neth.:* Aceplus; Acuzide; Capozide; Cibadrex; Co-Diovan; Co-Renitec; CoAprovel; Diurace; Dytenzide; Emcoretic; Hydromet†; Hykaten†; Hyzaar; Moducren†; Moduretic; Novazyd; Ranezide†; Renitec Plus; Secadrex; Selokomb; Tritazide; Vascase Plus; Zestoretic; *Norw.:* CoAprovel; Cozaar Comp; Diovan Comp; Moduretic Mite; Normorix; Renitec Comp; Vivatec Comp; Zestoretic; *NZ:* Amizide; Capozide; Co-Renitec; Dyazide; Hydrozide; Inhibace Plus; Moduretic; Prinzide; Triamizide; Trizid; Zestoretic; *Port.:* Acuretic; Aldoretic†; Amiloride Composto; Chibretico; Co-Diovan; CoAprovel; Cozaar Plus; Diurene; Dyazide; Enatia; Inibace Plus; Laprilen; Lopiretic; Lortaan Plus; Moducren; Moduretic; Normotil; Ondolen; Prinzide; Renidur; Triam-Tiazida R; Triatec Composto; Vascase Plus; Zestoretic; *S.Afr.:* Accuretic; Acumod†; Adco-Retic; Adelphane-Esidrex†; Aldoretic; Amiloretic; Amizide; Aquadrex†; Arcanaretic†; Betaretic; Capozide; Captoretic; Cibadrex; Cliniretic†; Co-Diovan; Co-Renitec; Cozaar Comp; Diutec; Dyazide; Hexaretic; Inhibace Plus; Loretic†; Moducren; Moduretic; Monozide; Renezide; Secadrex; Servatrin; Sotazide†; Trimolex†; Urirex-K; Urizide; Zapto Co; Zestoretic; Ziak; *Singapore:* Apo-Amilzide; Apo-Triazide; Co-Diovan; Co-Renitec; Dyazide; Hyzaar; *Spain:* Acediur; Acetensil Plus; Adelfan-Esidrex; Alopresin Diu; Ameride; Baripril Diu; Bicetil; Bitensil Diu; Cesplon Plus; Co-Diovan; Co-Renitec; Co-Vals; Co-Aprovel; Cozaar Plus; Crinoretic; Dabonal Plus; Decresco; Dilabar Diu; Dilapres†; Ditenside; Diu Rauwiplus; Diuzine; Doneka Plus; Donicer†; Ecadiu; Ecazide; Emcoretic; Flebo Stop; Fositens Plus; Hiperlex Plus; Hipoartel Plus; Inhibace Plus; Inocar Plus; Kalpress Plus; Kalten; Karvezide; Lidaltrin Diu; Miscidon; Neotensin Diu; Pressitan Diu; Prinivil Plus; Renitecmax; Rulun; Secadrex; Secubar Diu; Selopresin; Tensiocomplet; Tenso Stop Plus; Urocaudal Tiazida; Zestoretic; *Swed.:* Accupro Comp; Amiloferm; Atacand Plus; Capozid†; Cibadrex†; CoAprovel; Cozaar Comp; Diovan Comp; Hydromet†; Inhibace comp; Moduretic; Monopril comp; Normorix; Renitec Comp; Sparkal; Synerpril; Triatec Comp; Zestoretic; *Switz.:* Accuretic; Adelphan-Esidrex; Agorex; Aldoretic; Amilo-basan; Amilorid comp†; Betadiur; Capozide; Cibadrex; Co-Amiloretic; Co-Diovan; Co-Renitec; Co-Aprovel; Comilorid; Concor Plus; Cosaar Plus; Dyazide; Ecodurex; Escoretic; Fosicomp; Grodurex; Hydrolid; Inhibace Plus; Kalten; Moducren; Moduretic; Prinzide; Reniten Plus; Rhefluin; Spironothiazid; Synureticum†; t/h-basan; Tensobon comp; Triatec Comp; Zestoretic; *Thai.:* Amilhydrozide; Amilide; Co-Diovan; Dinazide; Dyazide; Dyterene; Hydrares; Hyperretic; Hypery; Hyzaar; Medeserpine Co; Miduret; Milorex; Miretic; Moduretic; Poli-Uretic; Renase; Reser; Sefaretic; Ser-Ap-Es; Skezide; *UK:* Accuretic; Acezide; Adizem-XL Plus†; Amilco; Amilmaxco; Capozide; Capto-Co; Carace Plus; Co-Betaloc; CoAprovel; Cozaar Comp; Delvas; Dyazide; Innozide; Kalten; Moducren; Moduret; Moduretic; Monozide†; Secadrex; Synuretic; Triamaxco; Triamco; Zestoretic; Zida-Co†; *USA:* Accuretic; Aldactazide; Aldoril; Apresazide; Atacand HCT; Avalide; Capozide; Diovan HCT; Dyazide; Esimil; Hydra-zide; Hydrap-ES; Hydro-Serp; Hydropres; Hydroserpine; Hyzaar; Inderide; Lopressor HCT; Lotensin HCT; Marpres; Maxzide; Micardis HCT; Moduretic; Monopril-HCT; Prinzide; Ser-Ap-Es; Timolide; Tri-Hydroserpine; Uniretic; Vaseretic; Zestoretic; Ziac.

Hydroflumethiazide (2334-g)

Hydroflumethiazide (BAN, rINN).

Hydroflumethiazidum; Trifluoromethylhydrothiazide. 3,4-Dihydro-6-trifluoromethyl-2H-1,2,4-benzothiadiazine-7-sulphonamide 1,1-dioxide.

$C_8H_8F_3N_3O_4S_2 = 331.3$.

CAS — 135-09-1.

ATC — C03AA02.

NOTE. Compounded preparations of hydroflumethiazide may be represented by the following names:

• Co-flumactone (BAN)—hydroflumethiazide and spironolactone in equal parts (w/w).

Pharmacopoeias. In Br. and US.

Pharmacopoeial description

BP 2001: White or almost white, odourless or almost odourless, glistening crystals or crystalline powder. Practically insoluble in water; soluble in alcohol; practically insoluble in chloroform and in ether.

USP 25: A white to cream-coloured, odourless, finely divided crystalline powder. Very slightly soluble in water and in chloroform; soluble 1 in 39 of alcohol and 1 in 2500 of ether; freely soluble in acetone. A 1% dispersion in water has a pH of 4.5 to 7.5. Store in airtight containers.

Adverse Effects, Treatment, and Precautions

As for Hydrochlorothiazide, p.907.

Interactions

As for Hydrochlorothiazide, p.909.

Pharmacokinetics

Hydroflumethiazide is incompletely but fairly rapidly absorbed from the gastrointestinal tract. It is reported to have a beta-phase biological half-life of about 17 hours and a metabolite with a longer half-life which is extensively bound to red blood cells. Hydroflumethiazide is excreted in the urine; its metabolite has also been detected in the urine.

◊ References.
1. Yakatan GJ, et al. Pharmacokinetics of orally administered hydroflumethiazide in man. J Clin Pharmacol 1977; 17: 37–47.
2. McNamara PJ, et al. Absorption kinetics of hydroflumethiazide. J Clin Pharmacol 1978; 18: 190–3.
3. Brørs O, et al. Pharmacokinetics of a single dose of hydroflumethiazide in health and in cardiac failure. Eur J Clin Pharmacol 1978; 14: 29–37.
4. Brørs O, et al. Excretion of hydroflumethiazide in bile and urine of man. Eur J Clin Pharmacol 1979; 15: 287–9.
5. Brørs O, Jacobsen S. Distribution and elimination of hydroflumethiazide in man. Eur J Clin Pharmacol 1979; 16: 125–31.

Uses and Administration

Hydroflumethiazide is a thiazide diuretic with actions and uses similar to those of hydrochlorothiazide (p.910). It is used for oedema, including that associated with heart failure (p.798), and for hypertension (p.802).

Diuresis is initiated in about 2 hours and has been reported to last for up to 24 hours.

In the treatment of **oedema** the usual initial dose by mouth is 50 to 100 mg daily, in one or two divided doses, reduced to a dose of 25 to 50 mg on alternate days or intermittently. Doses of up to 200 mg daily may be required by some patients. In the treatment of **hypertension** the usual dose is 25 to 50 mg daily either alone, or in conjunction with other antihypertensives. An initial dose of 12.5 mg may be employed.

An initial dose for children is 1 mg per kg bodyweight daily, reduced for maintenance.

Preparations

BP 2001: Hydroflumethiazide Tablets;
USP 25: Hydroflumethiazide Tablets.

Proprietary Preparations (details are given in Part 3)
UK: Hydrenox†; *USA:* Diucardin; Saluron.

Multi-ingredient: *Irl.:* Aldactide; *S.Afr.:* Protensin-M; *UK:* Aldactide; Spiro-Co; *USA:* Salutensin.

The symbol † denotes a preparation no longer actively marketed

Hydroquinidine Hydrochloride (7786-v)

Dihydrochinidin Hydrochloride; Dihydroquinidine Hydrochloride; Hydroconchinine Hydrochloride. (8R,9S)-10,11-Dihydro-6'-methoxycinchonan-9-ol hydrochloride.

$C_{20}H_{26}N_2O_2,HCl = 362.9$.

CAS — 1435-55-8 (hydroquinidine); 1476-98-8 (hydroquinidine hydrochloride).

Pharmacopoeias. In *Fr.*

Profile

Hydroquinidine is an antiarrhythmic with actions and uses similar to those of quinidine (p.964). It is given as the hydrochloride in a usual maintenance dose of 600 mg daily by mouth in divided doses.

Hydroquinidine alginate and quinalbital (the hydroquinidine salt of amobarbital) have also been used in the treatment of cardiac arrhythmias.

Preparations

Proprietary Preparations (details are given in Part 3)

Fr.: Serecor; *Spain:* Lentoquine.

Ibopamine Hydrochloride (12838-d)

Ibopamine Hydrochloride (BANM, rINNM).

SB-7505 (ibopamine); SKF-100168 (ibopamine). 4-(2-Methylaminoethyl)-o-phenylene di-isobutyrate hydrochloride.

$C_{17}H_{25}NO_4,HCl = 343.8$.

CAS — 66195-31-1 (ibopamine); 75011-65-3 (ibopamine hydrochloride).

NOTE. Ibopamine is *USAN*.

Adverse Effects and Precautions

Ibopamine should not be used in patients with severe heart failure in whom, similarly to xamoterol (p.998), it has been reported to increase the risk of death.

For the adverse effects of sympathomimetics in general, and precautions to be observed, see Adrenaline, p.829.

◊ A multicentre study (PRIME II) of the use of ibopamine in patients with severe (NYHA class III or IV) heart failure found that the drug was associated with an increased risk of death:[1] the study was stopped early. Subgroup analysis found that use of an antiarrhythmic drug was independently predictive of an adverse effect in ibopamine-treated patients. Excess mortality in heart failure has also been reported with dobutamine and xamoterol, and with flosequinan and the phosphodiesterase inhibitors amrinone, enoximone, milrinone, and vesnarinone, all of which produce positive inotropic effects through catecholamine-receptor stimulation or post-receptor pathway stimulation.[2] The association with antiarrhythmic therapy in the ibopamine study might reflect an interaction with amiodarone, the most commonly used antiarrhythmic in this study, or might simply be a marker for patients at risk of ibopamine-induced tachyarrhythmias.

1. Hampton JR, *et al.* Randomised study of effect of ibopamine on survival in patients with advanced severe heart failure. *Lancet* 1997; **349:** 971–7.
2. Niebauer J, Coats AJS. Treating chronic heart failure: time to take stock. *Lancet* 1997; **349:** 966–7.

Interactions

It has been recommended that ibopamine should not be given to patients receiving amiodarone in the light of the increased mortality seen in the PRIME II study in patients receiving both drugs (see above), although it is not clear that this represents a genuine interaction.

For the interactions of sympathomimetics in general, see Adrenaline, p.830.

Uses and Administration

Ibopamine is rapidly converted after oral administration to its active metabolite, epinine, which is a peripheral dopamine agonist with vasodilating properties and a weak positive inotropic effect; at high concentrations it has a stimulant action on alpha and beta adrenoceptors.

Ibopamine has been used in the management of heart failure (p.798). It is given as the hydrochloride but doses are often expressed in terms of the base. Doses of 100 to 200 mg by mouth two or three times daily have been used, in combination with a diuretic.

Ibopamine is also used topically as a mydriatic (p.460) in the form of eye drops containing ibopamine hydrochloride 2%.

◊ References.

1. Henwood JM, Todd PA. Ibopamine: a preliminary review of its pharmacodynamic and pharmacokinetic properties and therapeutic efficacy. *Drugs* 1988; **36:** 11–31.
2. Spencer C, *et al.* Ibopamine: a review of its pharmacodynamic and pharmacokinetic properties, and therapeutic use in congestive heart failure. *Drugs Aging* 1993; **3:** 556–84.
3. Rousseau MF, *et al.* Progression of left ventricular dysfunction secondary to coronary artery disease, sustained neurohormonal activation and effects of ibopamine therapy during long-term therapy with angiotensin-converting enzyme inhibitor. *Am J Cardiol* 1994; **73:** 488–93.
4. Dohmen HJM, *et al.* Comparison of captopril and ibopamine in mild to moderate heart failure. *Heart* 1997; **78:** 285–90.

Preparations

Proprietary Preparations (details are given in Part 3)

Aust.: Escandine; *Belg.:* Idopamil; Scandine; *Braz.:* Escandine; *Ital.:* Inopamil; Scandine; Trazyl; *Neth.:* Inopamil; *Port.:* Scandine; *Spain:* Erfolgan; Escandine.

Ibutilide Fumarate (13799-k)

Ibutilide Fumarate (BANM, USAN, rINNM).

U-70226E. (±)-4'-[4-(Ethylheptylamino)-1-hydroxybutyl]methanesulfonanilide fumarate (2:1).

$(C_{20}H_{36}N_2O_3S)_2,C_4H_4O_4 = 885.2$.

CAS — 122647-31-8 (ibutilide); 122647-32-9 (ibutilide fumarate).

Adverse Effects

Adverse cardiovascular effects associated with ibutilide include heart block, hypotension, hypertension, and bradycardia. Like other antiarrhythmics it can cause arrhythmias, including torsade de pointes. Other adverse effects include nausea and vomiting.

Effects on the kidneys. Acute renal failure with biopsy evidence of acute tubular necrosis developed in a 52-year-old man shortly after he received 2 doses of ibutilide for an episode of atrial flutter.[1] Renal function returned to normal following 4 sessions of haemodialysis.

1. Franz M, *et al.* Acute renal failure after ibutilide. *Lancet* 1999; **353:** 467.

Precautions

ECG monitoring should be carried out during, and for at least 4 hours after, administration of ibutilide. Electrolyte abnormalities should be corrected before treatment is started.

Interactions

Use of ibutilide with other antiarrhythmics or drugs that prolong the QT interval, for example tricyclic antidepressants and phenothiazines, should be avoided.

Pharmacokinetics

Ibutilide is widely distributed in the body after intravenous administration. It has low plasma protein binding (about 40%) and undergoes extensive metabolism in the liver to form several metabolites. Ibutilide is excreted mainly in the urine as metabolites with about 19% being excreted in the faeces. The elimination half-life is reported to range from 2 to 12 hours.

Uses and Administration

Ibutilide is a class III antiarrhythmic (p.787) used in the management of **atrial fibrillation** or **flutter** (p.794).

Ibutilide is given intravenously as the fumarate. The dose for patients weighing 60 kg or more is 1 mg of ibutilide fumarate given intravenously over 10 minutes. This dose may be repeated, if necessary, 10 minutes after completion of the first dose. The infusion should be stopped as soon as the arrhythmia is terminated. A dose of 10 μg per kg body-weight should be used in patients weighing less than 60 kg.

◊ References.

1. Foster RH, *et al.* Ibutilide: a review of its pharmacological properties and clinical potential in the acute management of atrial flutter and fibrillation. *Drugs* 1997; **54:** 312–30.
2. Granberry MC. Ibutilide: a new class III antiarrhythmic agent. *Am J Health-Syst Pharm* 1998; **55:** 255–60.
3. Howard PA. Ibutilide: an antiarrhythmic agent for the treatment of atrial fibrillation or flutter. *Ann Pharmacother* 1999; **33:** 38–47.

Preparations

Proprietary Preparations (details are given in Part 3)

Aust.: Corvert; *Fin.:* Corvert; *Fr.:* Corvert; *Ital.:* Corvert; *Neth.:* Corvert; *Norw.:* Corvert; *Swed.:* Corvert; *Switz.:* Corvert; *USA:* Corvert.

Ifenprodil Tartrate (9241-e)

Ifenprodil Tartrate (rINNM).

RC-61-91. (±)-2-(4-Benzylpiperidino)-1-(4-hydroxyphenyl)propan-1-ol tartrate.

$(C_{21}H_{27}NO_2)_2,C_4H_6O_6 = 801.0$.

CAS — 23210-56-2 (ifenprodil); 23210-58-4 (ifenprodil tartrate).

Pharmacopoeias. In *Jpn.*

Profile

Ifenprodil tartrate is a vasodilator, with alpha-adrenoceptor blocking properties, used in peripheral vascular disease (p.809). It is given in usual doses of 40 to 60 mg daily by mouth or up to 15 mg daily by deep intramuscular injection, slow intravenous injection, or intravenous infusion.

Preparations

Proprietary Preparations (details are given in Part 3)

Fr.: Vadilex; *Hong Kong:* Vadilex; *Singapore:* Vadilex.

Imidapril Hydrochloride (17996-p)

Imidapril Hydrochloride (BANM, rINNM).

TA-6366. (S)-3-{N-[(S)-1-Ethoxycarbonyl-3-phenylpropyl]-L-alanyl}-1-methyl-2-oxoimidazoline-4-carboxylic acid hydrochloride.

$C_{20}H_{27}N_3O_6,HCl = 441.9$.

CAS — 89371-37-9 (imidapril); 89396-94-1 (imidapril hydrochloride).

Adverse Effects, Treatment, and Precautions

As for ACE inhibitors, p.820.

Interactions

As for ACE inhibitors, p.822.

Pharmacokinetics

Imidapril acts as a prodrug of the diacid imidaprilat, its active metabolite. Following oral administration, imidapril is rapidly but incompletely absorbed; absorption is about 70% and is reduced in the presence of food. Imidapril is metabolised in the liver to imidaprilat. The bioavailability of imidaprilat is about 42% following oral imidapril administration, and peak plasma concentrations of imidaprilat are reached in about 7 hours. Both imidapril and imidaprilat are moderately bound to plasma proteins. About 40% of an oral dose is excreted in the urine, the rest in the faeces. The terminal half-life of imidaprilat is more than 24 hours. Imidapril and imidaprilat are removed by haemodialysis.

◊ References.

1. Hoogkamer JFW, *et al.* Pharmacokinetics of imidapril and its active metabolite imidaprilat following single dose and during steady state in patients with impaired liver function. *Eur J Clin Pharmacol* 1997; **51:** 489–91.
2. Hoogkamer JFW, *et al.* Pharmacokinetics of imidapril and its active metabolite imidaprilat following single dose and during steady state in patients with chronic renal failure. *Eur J Clin Pharmacol* 1998; **54:** 59–61.
3. Harder S, *et al.* Single dose and steady state pharmacokinetics and pharmacodynamics of the ACE-inhibitor imidapril in hypertensive patients. *Br J Clin Pharmacol* 1998; **45:** 377–80.

Uses and Administration

Imidapril is an ACE inhibitor (p.820). It is used in the treatment of hypertension (p.802). Imidapril owes its activity to imidaprilat, to which it is converted after oral administration. The maximum haemodynamic effect occurs 6 to 8 hours after administration, although the full effect may not develop for several weeks during chronic dosing. Imidapril is given by mouth as the hydrochloride.

In the treatment of hypertension, the usual initial dose of imidapril hydrochloride is 5 mg once daily, before food. Since there may be a precipitous fall in blood pressure in some patients when starting therapy with an ACE inhibitor, the first dose should preferably be given at bedtime. An initial dose of 2.5 mg daily should be used in the elderly, in patients with renal or hepatic impairment, or in those receiving a diuretic; if possible, the diuretic should be withdrawn 2 or 3 days before imidapril is started and resumed later if necessary. The usual maintenance dose is 10 mg daily, although up to 20 mg daily may be given if required. The maximum dose for elderly patients is 10 mg daily.

Preparations

Proprietary Preparations (details are given in Part 3)
Aust.: Tanatril; *Fin.:* Tanatril; *Fr.:* Tanatril; *Ger.:* Tanatril; *Ital.:* Tanatril; *Jpn:* Novarok†; Tanatril; *Singapore:* Tanatril; *Thai.:* Tanatril; *UK:* Tanatril.

Indapamide (2335-q)

Indapamide (BAN, USAN, rINN).
Indapamidum; SE-1520. 4-Chloro-N-(2-methylindolin-1-yl)-3-sulphamoylbenzamide.
$C_{16}H_{16}ClN_3O_3S = 365.8$.
CAS — 26807-65-8 (anhydrous indapamide).
ATC — C03BA11.
Pharmacopoeias. In Eur. (see p.vi) and US.

Pharmacopoeial description

Ph. Eur.: A white or almost white powder. Practically insoluble in water; soluble in alcohol; slightly soluble in ether. Protect from light.

USP 25: A white to off-white crystalline powder. Practically insoluble in water, soluble in alcohol, in glacial acetic acid, in acetonitrile, in ethyl acetate, and in methyl alcohol; very slightly soluble in chloroform and in ether.

Adverse Effects, Treatment, and Precautions

As for Hydrochlorothiazide, p.907.

◊ It has been claimed that indapamide produces few adverse biochemical effects at the usual dose of 2.5 mg daily. However, adverse biochemical effects have been reported in individual patients, including severe hypokalaemia[1] and hyponatraemia,[2,3] and with the trend towards using lower doses of thiazide diuretics in hypertension, it may be that indapamide has no clinical advantage over low-dose thiazide diuretics.

Several studies have reported no changes in blood-glucose concentrations during indapamide treatment,[4-6] although elevated blood-glucose concentrations have been reported in individual patients.[7,8] There have been reports of increases in total cholesterol[5] and of no change.[6]

1. Rodat O, Hamelin J-P. Hypokaliémie au cours d'un traitement par l'indapamide. *Nouv Presse Med* 1978; **7:** 3054.
2. Read SJ, *et al.* Hyponatraemia and raised creatine kinase level associated with indapamide. *Med J Aust* 1994; **161:** 607–8.
3. Chan TYK. Indapamide-induced severe hyponatraemia and hypokalemia. *Ann Pharmacother* 1995; **29:** 1124–8.
4. Velussi M, *et al.* Treatment of mild-to-moderate hypertension with indapamide in type II diabetics: midterm (six months) evaluation. *Curr Ther Res* 1988; **44:** 1076–86.
5. Prisant LM, *et al.* Biochemical, endocrine, and mineral effects of indapamide in black women. *J Clin Pharmacol* 1990; **30:** 121–6.
6. Leonetti G, *et al.* Long-term effects of indapamide: final results of a two-year Italian multicenter study in systemic hypertension. *Am J Cardiol* 1990; **65:** 674–714.
7. Slotkoff L. Clinical efficacy and safety of indapamide in the treatment of edema. *Am Heart J* 1983; **106:** 233–7.
8. Beling S, *et al.* Long term experience with indapamide. *Am Heart J* 1983; **106:** 258–62.

Effects on the kidneys. Acute interstitial nephritis was associated with indapamide treatment in a 74-year-old patient.[1]

1. Newstead CG, *et al.* Interstitial nephritis associated with indapamide. *BMJ* 1990; **300:** 1344.

Effects on the skin. Sixteen cases of skin rash attributed to indapamide had been reported to the Netherlands Centre for Monitoring of Adverse Reactions to Drugs.[1] All patients had taken indapamide 2.5 mg daily for hypertension. The skin rash was accompanied by fever in 5 cases. In all cases the rash subsided within 14 days of indapamide being stopped, and 11 patients subsequently took thiazides, frusemide [furosemide], or clopamide without recurrence. Among 188 cases of skin rash attributed to indapamide reported to the WHO Collaborating Centre for International Drug Monitoring were 4 cases of erythema multiforme and 2 of epidermal necrolysis. A further case of toxic epidermal necrolysis was reported by independent authors.[2]

1. Stricker BHC, Biriell C. Skin reactions and fever with indapamide. *BMJ* 1987; **295:** 1313–14.
2. Black RJ, *et al.* Toxic epidermal necrolysis associated with indapamide. *BMJ* 1990; **301:** 1280–1.

Interactions

As for Hydrochlorothiazide, p.909.

Pharmacokinetics

Indapamide is rapidly and completely absorbed from the gastrointestinal tract. Elimination is biphasic with a half-life in whole blood of about 14 hours. Indapamide is strongly bound to red blood cells. It is extensively metabolised. About 60 to 70% of the dose has been reported to be excreted in the urine; only about 5 to 7% is excreted unchanged. About 16 to 23% of

the administered dose is excreted in the faeces. Indapamide is not removed by haemodialysis but does not accumulate in patients with impaired renal function.

◊ References.
1. Beermann B, Grind M. Clinical pharmacokinetics of some newer diuretics. *Clin Pharmacokinet* 1987; **13:** 254–66.

Uses and Administration

Indapamide is a diuretic with actions and uses similar to those of the thiazide diuretics (see Hydrochlorothiazide, p.910) even though it does not contain a thiazide ring system. It is used for hypertension (p.802), and also for oedema, including that associated with heart failure (p.798).

In some countries indapamide is described as the hemihydrate. In the treatment of **hypertension** the usual dose by mouth is 1.25 to 2.5 mg once daily, either alone, or in conjunction with other antihypertensives; at higher doses the diuretic effect may become apparent without appreciable additional antihypertensive effect although the US manufacturers have suggested that the dose may be increased to 5 mg after 4 weeks. In the treatment of **oedema** the usual dose is 2.5 mg once daily increasing to 5 mg daily after 1 week if necessary.

◊ Reviews.
1. Chaffman M, *et al.* Indapamide: a review of its pharmacodynamic properties and therapeutic efficacy in hypertension. *Drugs* 1984; **28:** 189–235.

Preparations

USP 25: Indapamide Tablets.

Proprietary Preparations (details are given in Part 3)
Aust.: Fludex; *Austral.:* Dapa-Tabs; Indahexal; Insig; Napamide; Naride; Natrilix; *Belg.:* Fludex; *Braz.:* Natrilix; *Canad.:* Lozide; *Denm.:* Fludex; Natrilix; *Fin.:* Natrilix; *Fr.:* Fludex; *Ger.:* Natrilix; Sicco; *Hong Kong:* Agelan; Dapa-Tabs; Frumeron; Millibar; Napamide; Natrilix; *Irl.:* Agelan; Clonilix; Inamide; Natrilix; *Israel:* Pamid; *Ital.:* Damide; Indaflex; Indamol; Indolin; Ipamix; Millibar; Natrilix; Pressural; Veroxil; *Neth.:* Fludex; *NZ:* Napamide; Naplin; Natrilix; *Port.:* Fludex; Fluidema; Tandix; *S.Afr.:* Dapamax; Daptril; Hydro-Less; Indalix; Natrilix; *Singapore:* Dapa-Tabs; Millibar; Napamide; Natrilix; *Spain:* Extur; Tertensif; *Switz.:* Fludapamide; Fludex; *Thai.:* Frumeron; Lorvas; Napamide; Natrilix; *UAE:* Indanorm; *UK:* Natramid; Natrilix; Nindaxa; Opumide†; *USA:* Lozol.

Multi-ingredient: *Fr.:* Bipreterax; Preterax; *Ital.:* Atinorm; Delapride; Dinapres; Nor-Pa; Normopress.

Indenolol Hydrochloride (12849-m)

Indenolol Hydrochloride (BANM, rINNM).
Sch-28316Z (indenolol); YB-2.
$C_{15}H_{21}NO_2,HCl = 283.8$.
CAS — 60607-68-3 (indenolol); 68906-88-7 (indenolol hydrochloride).
Pharmacopoeias. In Jpn.

A 2:1 tautomeric mixture of 1-(inden-7-yloxy)-3-isopropylaminopropan-2-ol hydrochloride and 1-(inden-4-yloxy)-3-isopropylaminopropan-2-ol hydrochloride.

Profile

Indenolol is a non-cardioselective beta blocker (p.844). It is reported to possess potent membrane-stabilising properties and intrinsic sympathomimetic activity.

Indenolol is used as the hydrochloride in the management of various cardiovascular disorders in doses of 30 to 180 mg daily by mouth.

Preparations

Proprietary Preparations (details are given in Part 3)
Ital.: Securpres; *Jpn:* Pulsan†.

Indobufen (12850-t)

Indobufen (rINN).
K-3920. (±)-2-[4-(1-Oxo-isoindolin-2-yl)phenyl]butyric acid.
$C_{18}H_{17}NO_3 = 295.3$.
CAS — 63610-08-2.
ATC — B01AC10.

Profile

Indobufen is an inhibitor of platelet aggregation used in various thromboembolic disorders (p.816) in doses of 200 to 400 mg daily by mouth given in 2 divided doses. It is also given parenterally as the sodium salt in similar doses. For patients with renal impairment or those over the age of 65, the dose should be reduced to 100 to 200 mg daily.

◊ References.
1. Wiseman LR, *et al.* Indobufen: a review of its pharmacodynamic and pharmacokinetic properties, and therapeutic efficacy in cerebral, peripheral and coronary vascular disease. *Drugs* 1992; **44:** 445–64.

Preparations

Proprietary Preparations (details are given in Part 3)
Aust.: Ibustrin; *Ital.:* Ibustrin; *Mex.:* Ibustrin; *Port.:* Ibustrin; *Thai.:* Ibustrin.

Indoramin Hydrochloride (879-d)

Indoramin Hydrochloride (BANM, USAN, rINNM).
Wy-21901 (indoramin). N-[1-(2-Indol-3-ylethyl)-4-piperidyl]benzamide hydrochloride.
$C_{22}H_{25}N_3O,HCl = 383.9$.
CAS — 26844-12-2 (indoramin); 33124-53-7 (indoramin hydrochloride); 38821-52-2 (indoramin hydrochloride).
Pharmacopoeias. In Br.

Indoramin hydrochloride 11.0 mg is approximately equivalent to 10 mg of indoramin.

Pharmacopoeial description

BP 2001: A white or almost white powder. It exhibits polymorphism. Slightly soluble in water; sparingly soluble in alcohol; very slightly soluble in ether; soluble in methyl alcohol. A 2% suspension in water has a pH of 4.0 to 5.5. Protect from light.

Adverse Effects, Treatment, and Precautions

The most common adverse effects in patients receiving indoramin are sedation and dizziness; dry mouth, nasal congestion, headache, fatigue, depression, weight gain (almost certainly due to fluid retention), and failure of ejaculation may also occur. Tachycardia does not seem to be a problem with therapeutic doses. Extrapyramidal disturbances have been reported.

Following overdosage, coma, convulsions, and hypotension may occur; hypothermia has been reported in *animals*. In acute poisoning the stomach should be emptied by lavage and appropriate symptomatic and supportive care given.

Indoramin should be avoided in patients with heart failure; it has been recommended that incipient heart failure should be controlled before giving indoramin. Caution should be observed in patients with hepatic or renal insufficiency, a history of depression, epilepsy, or Parkinson's disease. Elderly patients may respond to lower doses.

Because indoramin can cause drowsiness care should be taken in patients who drive or operate machinery.

Effects on mental function. Sleep disturbances and vivid dreams were reported during a study in hypertensive patients when indoramin was added to therapy with a thiazide diuretic and a beta blocker.[1]

1. Marshall AJ, *et al.* Evaluation of indoramin added to oxprenolol and bendrofluazide as a third agent in severe hypertension. *Br J Clin Pharmacol* 1980; **10:** 217–21.

Overdosage. A 43-year-old woman with a long history of heavy alcohol intake died after taking 100 tablets of indoramin 25 mg.[1] The main clinical features were deep sedation, respiratory depression, hypotension, and convulsions. Although the hypotension was satisfactorily controlled the effects on the CNS were resistant to treatment and proved fatal. Other clinical features included areflexia, metabolic acidosis, tachycardia, and later bradyarrhythmias.

1. Hunter R. Death due to overdose of indoramin. *BMJ* 1982; **285:** 1011.

Interactions

The hypotensive effects of indoramin may be enhanced by the concomitant administration of diuretics and other antihypertensives. It has been reported that the concomitant ingestion of alcohol can increase the rate and extent of absorption and the sedative effects of indoramin (see below) and that indoramin should not be given to patients already receiving MAOIs.

Alcohol. In a study in 9 healthy subjects alcohol 0.5 g per kg body-weight significantly enhanced plasma concentrations of indoramin following ingestion of indoramin 50 mg compared with placebo.[1] The effect was most marked in the early period, corresponding to the absorptive phase. The mean maximum plasma concentration of indoramin was increased from 15.0 to 23.7 nanograms per mL by concomitant alcohol administration; the area under the concentration/time curve was increased by 25%. Alcohol did not affect the pharmacokinetics of intravenous indoramin. The results suggest that alcohol increases indoramin bioavailability either by enhancing absorption or reducing first-pass metabolism. Since the combination was more sedative than either drug alone patients taking indoramin

The symbol † denotes a preparation no longer actively marketed

should be advised not to drink alcohol if they intend to drive or operate machinery.

1. Abrams SML, *et al.* Pharmacokinetic interaction between indoramin and ethanol. *Hum Toxicol* 1989; **8:** 237–41.

Pharmacokinetics

Indoramin is readily absorbed from the gastrointestinal tract and undergoes extensive first-pass metabolism. It is reported to be about 90% bound to plasma proteins. It has a half-life of about 5 hours which is reported to be prolonged in elderly patients. It is extensively metabolised and is excreted mainly as metabolites in the urine and faeces. There is evidence to suggest that some metabolites may retain some alpha-adrenoceptor blocking activity.

The elderly. The plasma half-life of indoramin in 5 healthy elderly subjects following a single oral dose ranged from 6.6 to 32.8 hours with a mean of 14.7 hours.[1] The increased half-life may have been caused by reduced clearance in elderly patients.

1. Norbury HM, *et al.* Pharmacokinetics of oral indoramin in elderly and middle-aged female volunteers. *Eur J Clin Pharmacol* 1984; **27:** 247–9.

Uses and Administration

Indoramin is a selective and competitive $alpha_1$-adrenoceptor blocker (p.787) with actions similar to those of prazosin (p.959); it is also reported to have membrane-stabilising properties and to be a competitive antagonist at histamine H_1 and 5-hydroxytryptamine receptors. Indoramin is used in the management of hypertension (p.802) and in benign prostatic hyperplasia (p.1477) to relieve symptoms of urinary obstruction. It has also been used in the prophylactic treatment of migraine.

Indoramin is given by mouth as the hydrochloride, but doses are usually expressed in terms of the base.

In **hypertension**, the initial dose is 25 mg twice daily, increased in steps of 25 or 50 mg at intervals of 2 weeks to a maximum of 200 mg daily in 2 or 3 divided doses.

In **benign prostatic hyperplasia**, the initial dose is 20 mg twice daily, increased if necessary by 20 mg at 2-week intervals, to a maximum of 100 mg daily in divided doses.

Lower doses may be required in the elderly.

◊ Reviews.
1. Holmes B, Sorkin EM. Indoramin: a review of its pharmacodynamic and pharmacokinetic properties, and therapeutic efficacy in hypertension and related vascular, cardiovascular and airway diseases. *Drugs* 1986; **31:** 467–99.

Migraine. Propranolol and pizotifen are probably the most well-established drugs for prophylaxis of migraine (p.449). Many other drugs have been used including indoramin. In a double-blind study,[1] indoramin in a dose of 25 mg twice daily was reported to be as effective as dihydroergotamine mesilate in reducing the frequency of migraine attacks.

1. Pradalier A, *et al.* Etude comparative indoramine versus dihydroergotamine dans le traitement préventif de la migraine. *Therapie* 1988; **43:** 293–7.

Preparations

BP 2001: Indoramin Tablets.

Proprietary Preparations (details are given in Part 3)
Aust.: Wypresin; *Fr.:* Vidora; *Ger.:* Wydora; *Irl.:* Baratol; Doralese; *S.Afr.:* Baratol; *Spain:* Orfidora†; *UK:* Baratol; Doralese.

Inositol Nicotinate (9243-y)

Inositol Nicotinate (BAN, rINN).

Inositol Niacinate (USAN); NSC-49506; Win-9154. *meso*-Inositol hexanicotinate; *myo*-Inositol hexanicotinate.
$C_{42}H_{30}N_6O_{12} = 810.7$.
CAS — 6556-11-2.
ATC — C04AC03.
Pharmacopoeias. In Br.

Pharmacopoeial description

BP 2001: A white or almost white odourless or almost odourless powder. Practically insoluble in water, in alcohol, in acetone, and in ether; sparingly soluble in chloroform. It dissolves in dilute mineral acids.

Profile

Inositol nicotinate is a vasodilator and is believed to be slowly hydrolysed to nicotinic acid. It is given by mouth in the management of peripheral vascular disease (p.809). The usual dose is 3 g daily given in divided doses. The dose may be increased to 4 g daily if necessary.

Inositol nicotinate has been used in hyperlipidaemias.

Preparations

BP 2001: Inositol Nicotinate Tablets.

Proprietary Preparations (details are given in Part 3)
Ger.: Hamovannad; Hexanicit; Nicolip; *Irl.:* Hexogen; Hexopal; *Swed.:* Hexanicit; *UK:* Hexopal.

Multi-ingredient: *Aust.:* Prospervital†; *Canad.:* Formula CI†; *Ger.:* Veno-Hexanicit†; Zellaforte N Plus; *S.Afr.:* Geratar; *Spain:* Venosan; Vertigum†; *Switz.:* Hexafene†; Venosan†.

Irbesartan (17634-v)

Irbesartan (BAN, USAN, rINN).
BMS-186295; SR-47436. 2-Butyl-3-[p-(o-1H-tetrazol-5-ylphenyl)benzyl]-1,3-diazaspiro[4.4]non-1-en-4-one.
$C_{25}H_{28}N_6O = 428.5$.
CAS — 138402-11-6.
ATC — C09CA04.

Adverse Effects and Precautions

As for Losartan Potassium, p.921.

Pharmacokinetics

Irbesartan is rapidly absorbed from the gastrointestinal tract with an oral bioavailability of 60 to 80%. It undergoes some metabolism in the liver, primarily by the cytochrome P450 isoenzyme CYP2C9, to inactive metabolites. Peak plasma concentrations of irbesartan occur 1.5 to 2 hours after an oral dose. Irbesartan is about 96% bound to plasma proteins. It is excreted as unchanged drug and metabolites in the bile and in urine; after oral or intravenous administration approximately 20% of the dose is excreted in the urine, with less than 2% as unchanged drug. The terminal elimination half-life is about 11 to 15 hours.

◊ References.
1. Sica DA, *et al.* The pharmacokinetics of irbesartan in renal failure and maintenance hemodialysis. *Clin Pharmacol Ther* 1997; **62:** 610–18.
2. Marino MR, *et al.* Pharmacokinetics and pharmacodynamics of irbesartan in healthy subjects. *J Clin Pharmacol* 1998; **38:** 246–55.
3. Marino MR, *et al.* Pharmacokinetics and pharmacodynamics of irbesartan in patients with hepatic cirrhosis. *J Clin Pharmacol* 1998; **38:** 347–56.
4. Vachharajani NN, *et al.* Oral bioavailability and disposition characteristics of irbesartan, an angiotensin antagonist, in healthy volunteers. *J Clin Pharmacol* 1998; **38:** 702–7.
5. Vachharajani NN, *et al.* The effects of age and gender on the pharmacokinetics of irbesartan. *Br J Clin Pharmacol* 1998; **46:** 611–13.

Uses and Administration

Irbesartan is an angiotensin II receptor antagonist with actions similar to those of losartan (p.922). It is used in the management of hypertension (p.802) and is under investigation in diabetic nephropathy.

Irbesartan is administered by mouth. Following an oral dose the hypotensive effect peaks within 3 to 6 hours and persists for at least 24 hours. The maximum hypotensive effect is achieved within 4 to 6 weeks after initiating therapy.

In hypertension, irbesartan is given in a dose of 150 mg once daily increased, if necessary, to 300 mg once daily. A lower initial dose of 75 mg once daily may be considered in elderly patients over 75 years, for patients with intravascular volume depletion, and for those receiving haemodialysis.

◊ Reviews.
1. Gillis JC, Markham A. Irbesartan: a review of its pharmacodynamic and pharmacokinetic properties and therapeutic use in the management of hypertension. *Drugs* 1997; **54:** 885–902.
2. Brown MJ. Irbesartan treatment in hypertension. *Hosp Med* 1998; **59:** 808–11.
3. Markham A, *et al.* Irbesartan: an updated review of its use in cardiovascular disorders. *Drugs* 2000; **59:** 1187–1206.

Preparations

Proprietary Preparations (details are given in Part 3)
Austral.: Avapro; Karvea; *Belg.:* Aprovel; *Canad.:* Avapro; *Denm.:* Aprovel; *Fin.:* Aprovel; *Fr.:* Aprovel; *Ger.:* Aprovel; Karvea; *Hong Kong:* Aprovel; *Irl.:* Aprovel; *Israel:* Irban; *Ital.:* Aprovel; Karvea; *Mex.:* Aprovel; *Neth.:* Aprovel; *Norw.:* Aprovel; *Port.:* Aprovel; *S.Afr.:* Aprovel; *Singapore:* Aprovel; *Spain:* Aprovel; Karvea; *Swed.:* Aprovel; *Switz.:* Aprovel; *Thai.:* Aprovel; *UK:* Aprovel; *USA:* Avapro.

Multi-ingredient: *Austral.:* Avapro HCT; Karvezide; *Denm.:* CoAprovel; *Fr.:* CoAprovel; *Ger.:* CoAprovel; Karvezide; *Irl.:* CoAprovel; *Ital.:* CoAprovel; *Neth.:* CoAprovel; *Norw.:* CoAprovel; *Port.:* CoAprovel; *Spain:* CoAprovel; Karvezide; *Swed.:* CoAprovel; *Switz.:* CoAprovel; *UK:* CoAprovel; *USA:* Avalide.

Isoprenaline (14807-s)

Isoprenaline (BAN, rINN).
Isopropylarterenol; Isopropylnoradrenaline; Isoproterenol. 1-(3,4-Dihydroxyphenyl)-2-isopropylaminoethanol.
$C_{11}H_{17}NO_3 = 211.3$.
CAS — 7683-59-2.
ATC — C01CA02; R03AB02; R03CB01.

Isoprenaline Hydrochloride (2074-h)

Isoprenaline Hydrochloride (BANM, rINNM).
Isopropylarterenol Hydrochloride; Isopropylnoradrenaline Hydrochloride; Isoproterenol Hydrochloride.
$C_{11}H_{17}NO_3,HCl = 247.7$.
CAS — 51-30-9.
Pharmacopoeias. In Chin., Eur. (see p.vi), Int., Jpn, and US.

Pharmacopoeial description

Ph. Eur.: A white or almost white crystalline powder. Freely soluble in water; sparingly soluble in alcohol; practically insoluble in dichloromethane. A 5% solution in water has a pH of 4.3 to 5.5. Store in airtight containers. Protect from light.

USP 25: A white to practically white, odourless, crystalline powder. It gradually darkens on exposure to air and light. Soluble 1 in 3 of water and 1 in 50 of alcohol; less soluble in dehydrated alcohol; insoluble in chloroform and in ether. A 1% solution in water has a pH of about 5. Solutions become pink to brownish-pink on standing exposed to air and almost immediately so when made alkaline. Store in airtight containers. Protect from light.

Isoprenaline Sulfate (2075-m)

Isoprenaline Sulfate (rINNM).
Isoprenaline Sulphate (BANM); Isoprenalini Sulfas; Isopropylarterenol Sulphate; Isopropylnoradrenaline Sulphate; Isoproterenol Sulfate.
$(C_{11}H_{17}NO_3)_2,H_2SO_4,2H_2O = 556.6$.
CAS — 299-95-6 (anhydrous isoprenaline sulfate); 6700-39-6 (isoprenaline sulfate dihydrate).
Pharmacopoeias. In Eur. (see p.vi), Int., Pol., and US.

Isoprenaline sulfate 1.32 mg is approximately equivalent to 1 mg of isoprenaline or to 1.17 mg of the hydrochloride.

Pharmacopoeial description

Ph. Eur.: A white or almost white crystalline powder. Freely soluble in water; very slightly soluble in alcohol. A 5% solution in water has a pH of 4.3 to 5.5. Store in airtight containers. Protect from light.

USP 25: A white to practically white, odourless, crystalline powder. It gradually darkens on exposure to light and air. Soluble 1 in 4 of water; very slightly soluble in alcohol, in chloroform, in ether, and in benzene. A 1% solution in water has a pH of about 5. Solutions become pink to brownish-pink on standing exposed to air, and almost immediately so when made alkaline. Store in airtight containers. Protect from light.

Adverse Effects and Precautions

The adverse effects of isoprenaline may include tachycardia and cardiac arrhythmias, palpitations, hypotension, tremor, headache, sweating, and facial flushing. Prolonged use of isoprenaline has been associated with swelling of the parotid glands. Special caution is needed in the presence of ischaemic heart disease, diabetes mellitus, and hyperthyroidism.

Prolonged use of isoprenaline tablets sublingually has been reported to cause severe damage to the teeth due to the acidic nature of the drug. Sublingual use or inhalation may colour the saliva or sputum red.

For the adverse effects of sympathomimetics in general, and precautions for their use, see Adrenaline, p.829.

Increased mortality. For a discussion of the increased mortality and morbidity that has sometimes been observed in asthmatic patients and reference to an early epidemic associated with isoprenaline inhalers, see Fenoterol, p.765.

Interactions

Isoprenaline should not be used with other potent $beta_1$ agonists such as adrenaline [epinephrine].

For the interactions of sympathomimetics in general, see Adrenaline, p.830.

Theophylline. For reports of increased theophylline clearance following concomitant use of isoprenaline, see p.782.

Pharmacokinetics

As a result of sulfate conjugation in the gut, isoprenaline is considerably less active following administration by mouth than following parenteral administration. It is absorbed through the oral mucosa and has accordingly been given sublingually, but absorption by this route remains very erratic. Isoprenaline in the body is resistant to metabolism by monoamine oxidase, but is metabolised by catechol-*O*-methyltransferase in the liver, lungs, and other tissues, this metabolite being subsequently conjugated before excretion in the urine. Whereas the sulfate conjugate of isoprenaline is inactive the methylated metabolite exhibits weak activity.

Following intravenous injection isoprenaline has a plasma half-life of about one to several minutes according to whether the rate of injection is rapid or slow; it is almost entirely excreted in the urine as unchanged drug and metabolites within 24 hours. A much slower onset of action and a more extended initial half-life has been demonstrated following oral administration. Isoprenaline is reported to have a duration of action of up to about 2 hours after inhalation; it has been demonstrated that a large proportion of an inhaled dose is swallowed.

◊ References.
1. Blackwell EW, *et al*. The fate of isoprenaline administered by pressurized aerosols. *Br J Pharmacol* 1970; **39:** 194P–195P.
2. Conolly ME, *et al*. Metabolism of isoprenaline in dog and man. *Br J Pharmacol* 1972; **46:** 458–72.
3. Blackwell EW, *et al*. Metabolism of isoprenaline after aerosol and direct intrabronchial administration in man and dog. *Br J Pharmacol* 1974; **50:** 587–91.
4. Reyes G, *et al*. The pharmacokinetics of isoproterenol in critically ill pediatric patients. *J Clin Pharmacol* 1993; **33:** 29–34.

Uses and Administration

Isoprenaline is a sympathomimetic (see Adrenaline, p.831) that acts almost exclusively on beta-adrenergic receptors. It stimulates the CNS. It has a powerful stimulating action on the heart and increases cardiac output, excitability, and rate; it also causes peripheral vasodilatation and produces a fall in diastolic blood pressure and usually maintains or slightly increases systolic blood pressure. In addition, isoprenaline has bronchodilating properties.

Isoprenaline has been used in a variety of cardiac disorders. It may be used for the temporary prevention or control of Stokes-Adams attacks although for long-term management the use of a pacemaker is preferable. Isoprenaline may be useful in severe bradycardia unresponsive to atropine, although again cardiac pacing is preferred. It has also been advocated as an adjunct for other cardiac disorders including shock (p.813) and torsade de pointes (see Cardiac Arrhythmias, p.794). It has been used in the diagnosis of congenital heart defects.

In the management of **cardiac disorders**, isoprenaline is usually given as the hydrochloride by slow intravenous infusion under ECG control. Infusion rates may range from 0.5 to 10 µg per minute depending on the clinical condition of the patient; 1 to 4 µg per minute may be adequate to correct bradycardia but higher rates of 4 to 8 µg per minute may be required for acute Stokes-Adams attacks. Isoprenaline hydrochloride can be given by intracardiac injection in extreme cases. It has also been given subcutaneously or intramuscularly in initial doses of 200 µg (as 1 mL of a 0.02% solution) and by slow intravenous injection in initial doses of 20 to 60 µg (as 1 to 3 mL of a 0.002% solution); doses are subsequently adjusted according to ventricular rate. Tablets of isoprenaline hydrochloride have been administered by mouth or sublingually.

Isoprenaline has been used as a bronchodilator in the management of **reversible airways obstruction** but sympathomimetics with a selective action on beta$_2$ receptors, such as salbutamol, are now preferred (see Asthma, p.757). It has been given as the sulfate or hydrochloride usually by inhalation; sublingual tablets and intravenous injections have also been used. The adult dosage has generally been 1 to 3 inhalations of isoprenaline sulfate 80 µg by metered dose inhaler, repeated if necessary after not less than 30 minutes up to a maximum of 8 treatments in 24 hours. An aerosol inhaler which delivers metered doses of 400 µg has also been employed. Solutions containing about 0.1%

isoprenaline hydrochloride have been administered by nebulisation; solutions up to 1% have been used in a hand-bulb nebuliser. Isoprenaline hydrochloride has also been given by sublingual administration in the management of bronchospasm.

Preparations

BP 2001: Isoprenaline Injection;
USP 25: Acetylcysteine and Isoproterenol Hydrochloride Inhalation Solution; Isoproterenol Hydrochloride and Phenylephrine Bitartrate Inhalation Aerosol; Isoproterenol Hydrochloride Inhalation Aerosol; Isoproterenol Hydrochloride Injection; Isoproterenol Hydrochloride Tablets; Isoproterenol Inhalation Solution; Isoproterenol Sulfate Inhalation Aerosol; Isoproterenol Sulfate Inhalation Solution.

Proprietary Preparations (details are given in Part 3)
Aust.: Ingelan; Medihaler-Iso†; *Austral.:* Isuprel; *Belg.:* Isuprel; Medihaler-Iso†; *Canad.:* Isuprel; *Fr.:* Isuprel; *Ger.:* Ingelan; Kattwilon N; *Hong Kong:* Saventrine; *Irl.:* Saventrine; *Israel:* Isuprel; *Neth.:* Medihaler-Iso†; *NZ:* Isuprel; *Port.:* Medihaler-Iso†; *S.Afr.:* Imuprel; Lenoprel†; Medihaler-Iso†; Saventrine†; *Singapore:* Isuprel; Saventrine; *Spain:* Aleudrina; *Thai.:* Isuprel; *UK:* Medihaler-Iso†; Saventrine; *USA:* Isuprel; Medihaler-Iso.

Multi-ingredient: *Aust.:* Ingelan; *Ger.:* Ingelan; *Port.:* Prelus†; *Spain:* Aldo Asma; Frenal Compositum; *Switz.:* Mucobronchyl†; *USA:* Duo-Medihaler†; Norisodrine with Calcium Iodide.

Isosorbide (2336-p)

Isosorbide *(BAN, USAN, rINN)*.
AT-101; NSC-40725. 1,4:3,6-Dianhydro-D-glucitol.
$C_6H_{10}O_4 = 146.1$.
CAS — 652-67-5.
Pharmacopoeias. In Jpn.
US includes Isosorbide Concentrate.

Pharmacopoeial description

USP 25: Isosorbide Concentrate is an aqueous solution containing 70.0 to 80.0% w/w of isosorbide. A colourless to slightly yellow liquid. Soluble in water and in alcohol. Store in airtight containers. Protect from light.

Profile

Isosorbide is an osmotic diuretic with properties similar to those of mannitol (p.924). It is reported to cause less nausea and vomiting than other oral osmotic diuretics.

Isosorbide is used for short-term reduction of intra-ocular pressure in acute glaucoma or prior to surgery (p.1413). The usual dose is 1 to 3 g per kg body-weight by mouth 2 to 4 times daily. The onset of action is usually within 30 minutes and lasts for up to 5 or 6 hours.

Preparations

USP 25: Isosorbide Concentrate; Isosorbide Oral Solution.

Proprietary Preparations (details are given in Part 3)
USA: Ismotic.

Isosorbide Dinitrate (9245-z)

Isosorbide Dinitrate *(BAN, USAN, rINN)*.
ISDN; Isosorbidi Dinitras; Sorbide Nitrate. 1,4:3,6-Dianhydro-D-glucitol 2,5-dinitrate.
$C_6H_8N_2O_8 = 236.1$.
CAS — 87-33-2.
ATC — C01DA08; D03AX08.
Pharmacopoeias. In Chin., Jpn, and Pol.
Eur. (see p.vi) and US include diluted isosorbide dinitrate.

Pharmacopoeial description

Ph. Eur.: Diluted Isosorbide Dinitrate is a dry mixture of isosorbide dinitrate and lactose monohydrate or mannitol. The solubility of the diluted product depends on the diluent and its concentration. Protect from light.

Undiluted isosorbide dinitrate is a fine, white, crystalline powder. Very slightly soluble in water; sparingly soluble in alcohol; very soluble in acetone.

USP 25: Diluted Isosorbide Dinitrate is a dry mixture of isosorbide dinitrate (usually about 25%) with lactose, mannitol, or other suitable inert excipients, the latter being added to minimise the risk of explosion. It may contain up to 1% of a suitable stabiliser such as ammonium phosphate. It is an ivory-white, odourless powder. Store in airtight containers.

Undiluted isosorbide dinitrate occurs as white crystalline rosettes. Very slightly soluble in water; sparingly soluble in alcohol; very soluble in acetone; freely soluble in chloroform.

◊ CAUTION. *Undiluted isosorbide dinitrate may explode if subjected to percussion or excessive heat.*

Stability. The loss of isosorbide dinitrate from solution during infusion was found to be 30% with PVC plastic intravenous infusion sets but negligible when polyolefin or glass delivery systems were used.[1] Another study reported a 23% decrease in isosorbide dinitrate concentration after 24 hours of storage at 21° in PVC containers; most of the loss occurred in the first 6 hours. Loss of potency was not noted when isosorbide dinitrate

was stored under similar conditions in glass bottles or polyethylene, nylon, and polypropylene laminated bags.[2]
1. Kowaluk EA, *et al*. Drug loss in polyolefin infusion systems. *Am J Hosp Pharm* 1983; **40:** 118–19.
2. Martens HJ, *et al*. Sorption of various drugs in polyvinyl chloride, glass, and polyethylene-lined infusion containers. *Am J Hosp Pharm* 1990; **47:** 369–73.

Adverse Effects, Treatment, and Precautions

As for Glyceryl Trinitrate, p.898.

Effects on the blood. Haemolysis occurred in 2 patients with glucose-6-phosphate dehydrogenase deficiency during treatment with isosorbide dinitrate.[1]
1. Aderka D, *et al*. Isosorbide dinitrate-induced hemolysis in G6PD-deficient subjects. *Acta Haematol (Basel)* 1983; **69:** 63–4.

Headache. The most common adverse effect of nitrate therapy is headache which usually decreases after a few days. There has been a report[1] of a severe continuous unilateral headache with an oculosympathetic paresis on the same side associated with isosorbide dinitrate therapy.
1. Mueller RA, Meienberg O. Hemicrania with oculosympathetic paresis from isosorbide dinitrate. *N Engl J Med* 1983; **308:** 458–9.

Hypersensitivity. Laryngeal oedema developed on two occasions in a woman following the administration of isosorbide dinitrate spray;[1] nifedipine was also given sublingually which on the second occasion caused a noticeable increase in the laryngeal swelling induced by the nitrate.
1. Silfvast T, *et al*. Laryngeal oedema after isosorbide dinitrate spray and sublingual nifedipine. *BMJ* 1995; **311:** 232.

Oedema. Reports of ankle oedema associated with isosorbide dinitrate therapy in 3 patients with cardiac failure.[1]
1. Rodger JC. Peripheral oedema in patients treated with isosorbide dinitrate. *BMJ* 1981; **283:** 1365–6.

Tolerance. Continuous administration of organic nitrates is associated with tolerance to their haemodynamic effects; for an overview of nitrate tolerance, see under Precautions for Glyceryl Trinitrate, p.898.

A study in 12 patients with chronic stable angina[1] showed that following treatment for one week with isosorbide dinitrate 30 mg two or three times daily, treadmill-walking time was longer throughout a 5-hour testing period compared with placebo. In contrast, after treatment for one week with isosorbide dinitrate 30 mg four times daily, treadmill-walking time was prolonged at one hour but not at 3 or 5 hours. These results support the concept that clinical efficacy of isosorbide dinitrate is maintained if administered in a dose schedule which provides a nitrate-free or a low-nitrate period.

The effect of sublingual isosorbide dinitrate in patients receiving chronic therapy with isosorbide dinitrate was evaluated in 24 patients with angina.[2] Sublingual administration produced less reduction of aortic systolic pressure and left ventricular end-diastolic pressure and less dilatation of coronary artery diameter in patients who received chronic isosorbide dinitrate therapy compared with patients not receiving chronic therapy.
1. Parker JO, *et al*. Effect of intervals between doses on the development of tolerance to isosorbide dinitrate. *N Engl J Med* 1987; **316:** 1440–4.
2. Naito H, *et al*. Effects of sublingual nitrate in patients receiving sustained therapy of isosorbide dinitrate for coronary artery disease. *Am J Cardiol* 1989; **64:** 565–68.

Interactions

As for Glyceryl Trinitrate, p.898.

Disopyramide. The effectiveness of sublingual isosorbide dinitrate was reduced in a patient taking disopyramide.[1] The interaction was considered to be due to diminished salivary secretions caused by the antimuscarinic action of disopyramide which inhibited the dissolution of the sublingual isosorbide dinitrate tablet.
1. Barletta MA, Eisen H. Isosorbide dinitrate-disopyramide phosphate interaction. *Drug Intell Clin Pharm* 1985; **19:** 764.

Pharmacokinetics

Like glyceryl trinitrate, isosorbide dinitrate is readily absorbed from the oral mucosa. Isosorbide dinitrate is also readily absorbed when given by mouth but owing to extensive first-pass metabolism in the liver and presystemic clearance its bioavailability is reduced. Isosorbide dinitrate is also absorbed through the skin from an ointment basis.

Following sublingual administration, anti-anginal effect is apparent within 2 to 5 minutes and persists for about 2 hours. Following oral administration of conventional tablets, anti-anginal activity is present in less than one hour and lasts for 4 to 6 hours.

Isosorbide dinitrate is widely distributed with a large apparent volume of distribution. It is taken up by smooth muscle cells of blood vessels and the nitrate group is cleaved to inorganic nitrite and then to nitric oxide. It is also rapidly metabolised in the liver to the major active metabolites isosorbide 2-mononitrate and isosorbide 5-mononitrate (see Isosorbide Mononitrate, below).

After sublingual administration, isosorbide dinitrate has a plasma half-life of 45 to 60 minutes. Plasma half-lives of 20 minutes and 4 hours have been reported following intravenous and oral administration, respectively. During prolonged administration, the half-life is increased due to accumulation of the isosorbide 5-mononitrate metabolite which reduces hepatic isosorbide dinitrate extraction. Both primary metabolites have longer half-lives than the parent compound.

◊ References.
1. Abshagen U, et al. Pharmacokinetics and metabolism of isosorbide-dinitrate after intravenous and oral administration. Eur J Clin Pharmacol 1985; 27: 637–44.
2. Straehl P, Galeazzi RL. Isosorbide dinitrate bioavailability, kinetics, and metabolism. Clin Pharmacol Ther 1985; 38: 140–9.
3. Thadani U, Whitsett T. Relationship of pharmacokinetic and pharmacodynamic properties of the organic nitrates. Clin Pharmacokinet 1988; 15: 32–43.
4. Schneider W, et al. Concentrations of isosorbide dinitrate, isosorbide-2-mononitrate and isosorbide-5-mononitrate in human vascular and muscle tissue under steady-state conditions. Eur J Clin Pharmacol 1990; 38: 145–7.
5. Vogt D, et al. Pharmacokinetics and haemodynamic effects of ISDN following different dosage forms and routes of administration. Eur J Clin Pharmacol 1994; 46: 319–24.
6. Bergami A, et al. Pharmacokinetics of isosorbide dinitrate in healthy volunteers after 24-hour intravenous infusion. J Clin Pharmacol 1997; 37: 828–33.

Uses and Administration
Isosorbide dinitrate is a vasodilator with general properties similar to those of glyceryl trinitrate (p.898). It is used in the management of angina pectoris (p.791) and of heart failure (p.798). It has also been investigated in myocardial infarction (p.805).

Isosorbide dinitrate may be administered by the sublingual, oral, transdermal, or intravenous route.

In **angina** isosorbide dinitrate may be given as sublingual tablets or spray for the relief of an acute attack, although glyceryl trinitrate may be preferred because it has a faster onset of action. Isosorbide dinitrate may also be used before an activity or stress which might provoke an attack. The usual dose in acute angina is 2.5 to 10 mg sublingually. As an alternative, one to three sprays (1.25 mg per spray) may be directed under the tongue.

Isosorbide dinitrate is also used in the long-term management of angina in oral doses of 30 to 120 mg daily in divided doses according to the patient's needs. Increases in dosage should be gradual to avoid side-effects. Up to 240 mg daily in divided doses may be necessary. Modified-release formulations may be used in equivalent doses. Transdermal preparations such as topical sprays or ointments may also be used.

Isosorbide dinitrate is given by intravenous infusion for unstable angina. The dose is titrated according to patient response; doses in the range of 2 to 12 mg per hour are usually suitable but up to 20 mg per hour may be necessary in some patients. The plastic used in the infusion equipment may adsorb isosorbide dinitrate (see Stability, above) and allowance may have to be made for this.

During percutaneous transluminal coronary angioplasty isosorbide dinitrate may be given by the intracoronary route to allow prolonged balloon inflation and to prevent or relieve coronary spasm. Only injections of isosorbide dinitrate which are approved for intracoronary administration should be given by this route as preparations intended for normal intravenous administration may contain additives that are harmful if injected into diseased coronary vessels. The usual dose is 1 mg as a bolus before balloon inflation. The maximum recommended dose is 5 mg within a 30-minute time period.

Isosorbide dinitrate is also used in the management of **heart failure**. It is given in doses of 5 to 15 mg sublingually every 2 to 3 hours, or in oral doses of 30 to 160 mg daily in divided doses. Oral doses of up to 240 mg daily may be required. The intravenous route may also be employed using the intravenous doses given above for angina.

◊ As well as being used in cardiovascular disorders, nitrates such as isosorbide dinitrate have been tried in a number of other conditions including anal fissure, erectile dysfunction, and oesophageal motility disorders such as achalasia and spasm. Further details of these uses are given under Glyceryl Trinitrate (p.899).

Preparations
BP 2001: Isosorbide Dinitrate Sublingual Tablets; Isosorbide Dinitrate Tablets;
USP 25: Isosorbide Dinitrate Chewable Tablets; Isosorbide Dinitrate Extended-release Capsules; Isosorbide Dinitrate Extended-release Tablets; Isosorbide Dinitrate Sublingual Tablets; Isosorbide Dinitrate Tablets.

Proprietary Preparations (details are given in Part 3)
Aust.: Cedocard; Hexanitrat; Iso Mack; Isoket; Isostad; Maydil†; Sorbidilat; Vasorbate; **Austral.:** Isogen†; Isordil; Sorbidin; **Belg.:** Cedocard; Isocard†; Isordil; Sorbitrate†; **Braz.:** Elantan; Isocord; Isordil; **Canad.:** Apo-ISDN; Cedocard; Coradur†; Isordil; Novo-Sorbide†; **Denm.:** Cardopax; Iso Mack; **Fin.:** Dinit; Nitrosid; **Fr.:** Disorlon†; Isocard; Langoran; Risordan; **Ger.:** Corovliss†; Dignonitrat†; duranitrat; Iso Mack; Iso-Puren; Isodinit; Isoket; Isostenase; Jenacard; Maycor; Nitro-Tablinen†; Nitrosorbon; TD Spray Iso Mack; **Hong Kong:** Iso Mack; Isoket; Isordil; Isorem; Nitorol; **Irl.:** Cedocard; Imtack†; Isoket; Isordil; Soni-Slo; **Israel:** Cordil; Isocardide; Isoket; Isotard; **Ital.:** Carvasin; Diniket; Nitrosorbide; **Jpn:** Nitorol; **Mex.:** Isoket; Isorbid; **Neth.:** Cedocard; Isordil; Prodicard; **Norw.:** Sorbangil; **NZ:** Carvasin; Coronex; **Port.:** Flindix; Isoket; Isopront; **S.Afr.:** Angi-Spray; Dilanid; Isoket; Isordil; **Singapore:** Apo-ISDN; Iso Mack; Isobib; Isoket; Isordil; Nitrosorbide; **Spain:** Iso; Maycor†; Redil; **Swed.:** Sorbangil; **Switz.:** Acordin; Iso Mack; Isoday†; Isoket; Sorbidilat; **Thai.:** Angitrit; Cedocard; Hartsorb; Iso Mack; Isobinate; Isoket; Isordil; Isorem; Isotrate; Izo; Sorbidin; Sorbitrate; Sornil; **UK:** Angitak; Cedocard; Imtack†; Isocard; Isoket; Isordil; Jeridin†; Soni-Slo†; Sorbichew†; Sorbid†; Sorbitrate†; **USA:** Dilatrate; Isordil; Isotrate†; Sorbitrate.

Multi-ingredient: Aust.: Acordin†; Beta-Isoket; Viskenit; **Ger.:** Stenoptin†.

Isosorbide Mononitrate (15336-h)

Isosorbide Mononitrate (BAN, USAN, rINN).
AHR-4698; BM-22145; IS-5-MN; Isosorbide-5-mononitrate; Isosorbidi Mononitras. 1,4:3,6-Dianhydro-D-glucitol 5-nitrate.
$C_6H_9NO_6 = 191.1$.
CAS — 16051-77-7.
ATC — C01DA14.

Pharmacopoeias. Eur. (see p.vi) includes diluted isosorbide mononitrate.

Pharmacopoeial description
Ph. Eur.: Diluted Isosorbide Mononitrate is a dry mixture of isosorbide mononitrate and lactose monohydrate or mannitol. The solubility of the diluted product depends on the diluent and its concentration. Protect from light.
Undiluted isosorbide mononitrate is a white crystalline powder. Freely soluble in water, in alcohol, in acetone, and in dichloromethane.

Adverse Effects, Treatment, and Precautions
As for Glyceryl Trinitrate, p.898.

Interactions
As for Glyceryl Trinitrate, p.898.

Pharmacokinetics
Isosorbide mononitrate is readily absorbed from the gastrointestinal tract. Following oral administration of conventional tablets, peak plasma levels are reached in about 1 hour; onset of action occurs within 20 minutes and lasts for about 8 to 10 hours. Unlike isosorbide dinitrate, isosorbide mononitrate does not undergo first-pass hepatic metabolism and bioavailability is nearly 100%. Isosorbide mononitrate is widely distributed with a large apparent volume of distribution. It is taken up by smooth muscle cells of blood vessels and the nitrate group is cleaved to inorganic nitrite and then to nitric oxide. Isosorbide mononitrate is metabolised to inactive metabolites, including isosorbide and isosorbide glucuronide. Only about 2% of isosorbide mononitrate is excreted unchanged in the urine. An elimination half-life of about 4 to 5 hours has been reported.

◊ References.
1. Taylor T, et al. Isosorbide 5-mononitrate pharmacokinetics in humans. Biopharm Drug Dispos 1981; 2: 255–63.
2. Thadani U, Whitsett T. Relationship of pharmacokinetic and pharmacodynamic properties of the organic nitrates. Clin Pharmacokinet 1988; 15: 32–43.
3. McClennen W, et al. The plasma concentrations of isosorbide 5-mononitrate (5-ISMN) administered in an extended-release form to patients with acute myocardial infarction. Br J Clin Pharmacol 1995; 39: 704–8.

4. Hutt V, et al. Evaluation of the pharmacokinetics and absolute bioavailability of three isosorbide-5-mononitrate preparations in healthy volunteers. Arzneimittelforschung 1995; 45: 142–5.
5. Baxter T, Eadie CJ. Twenty-four hour plasma profile of sustained-release isosorbide mononitrate in healthy volunteers and in patients with chronic stable angina: two open label trials. Br J Clin Pharmacol 1997; 43: 333–5.

Uses and Administration
Isosorbide mononitrate is an active metabolite of the vasodilator isosorbide dinitrate and is used in the long-term management of angina pectoris (p.791) and heart failure (p.798). It has also been investigated in myocardial infarction (below).

The usual oral dose is 20 mg two or three times daily, although doses ranging from 20 to 120 mg daily have been given. Modified-release oral preparations have been developed for use in angina.

Myocardial infarction. Long-term management of myocardial infarction (p.805) can involve numerous drug therapies and some patients, for example those with myocardial ischaemia or poor left ventricular function, may require the long-term administration of nitrates, although recent studies have thrown doubt on their routine use. In the GISSI-3 study[1] there was no significant benefit from the use of transdermal glyceryl trinitrate when assessed 6 weeks post-infarction and in the ISIS-4 study[2] oral isosorbide mononitrate apparently had no effect on 35-day mortality.
1. Gruppo Italiano per lo Studio della Sopravvivenza nell'Infarto Miocardico. GISSI-3: effects of lisinopril and transdermal glyceryl trinitrate singly and together on 6-week mortality and ventricular function after acute myocardial infarction. Lancet 1994; 343: 1115–22.
2. ISIS-4 (Fourth International Study of Infarct Survival) Collaborative Group. ISIS-4: a randomised factorial trial assessing early oral captopril, oral mononitrate, and intravenous magnesium sulphate in 58 050 patients with suspected acute myocardial infarction. Lancet 1995; 345: 669–85.

Termination of pregnancy. For mention of the use of isosorbide mononitrate to ripen the cervix before termination of pregnancy, see Obstetrics and Gynaecology, under Glyceryl Trinitrate, p.899.

Variceal haemorrhage. For reference to the use of isosorbide mononitrate in the management of variceal haemorrhage, see under Glyceryl Trinitrate, p.900.

Preparations
BP 2001: Isosorbide Mononitrate Tablets.

Proprietary Preparations (details are given in Part 3)
Aust.: Corangin; Elantan; Epicordin; Imdur; Isomonat; Mono Mack; Monoket; Myocardon mono; Olicardin; Sorbimon; **Austral.:** Duride; Imdur; Imtrate; Isomonit; Monodur; **Belg.:** Pentacard†; Promocard; **Braz.:** Monocordil; **Canad.:** Ismo; Imdur; **Denm.:** Fem-Mono; Imdur; Ismo†; Isodur; Isomonit; **Fin.:** Imdur; Isangina; Ismexin; Ismox; Ormox; **Fr.:** Monicor; **Ger.:** Coleb; Conpin; Corangin; duramonitat; Elantan; IS 5 Mono; Ismo; Isomonit; Isomonoreal†; Moni; Monit-Puren; mono corax; Mono Mack; Mono Maycor; Mono Wolff; Monobeta; Monoclair; Monolong; Mononitrat; Monopur; Monostenase; Olicard; Orasorbil; Sigacora; Turimonit; **Hong Kong:** Corangin; Elantan; Imdur; Ismo; Isotrate; Mono Mack; Monocinque; **Irl.:** Elantan; Imdur; Isomel; Isomonit; Isotrate; Sormon; **Israel:** Ismo; Monocord; Monolong; Mononit; **Ital.:** Duronitrin; Elan; Ismo; Kiton; Leicester Retard; Monocinque; Monoket; Nitrex; Orasorbil; Vasdilat; **Mex.:** Elantan; Imdur; Mono Mack; **Neth.:** Ismo†; Mono Mack†; Mono-Cedocard; Promocard; **Norw.:** Imdur; Ismo; Monoket; **NZ:** Corangin; Duride; Imdur; Imtrate; Ismo; **Port.:** Amplexol; Imdur; Ismo; Monoket; Mononitril; Monopront; Orasorbil; **S.Afr.:** Angitrate; Elantan; Imdur; Ismo; **Singapore:** Elantan; Imdex; Imdur; Ismo; Isotrate; Mono Mack; Monotrate; **Spain:** Cardionil; Cardiovas; Coronur; Dolak; Isonitril; Olicard; Pancardiol†; Percorina; Pertil; Titrane†; Uniket; **Swed.:** Fem-Mono; Imdur; Ismo; Isodur; Monoket; **Switz.:** Corangine; Elantan; Etimonis†; Imdur; Ismo; **Thai.:** Elantan; Imdur; Ismo; Isopen; Mono Mack; Monolin; Monotrate; Pentacard; **UK:** Angeze; Chemydur; Dynamin; Elantan; Imdur; Isib; Ismo; Isodur; Isotard; Isotrate; MCR-50; Modisal; Monit; Mono-Cedocard†; Monomax; Monosorb; Xismox; **USA:** Imdur; Ismo; Monoket.

Multi-ingredient: UK: Imazin.

Isradipine (19367-a)

Isradipine (BAN, USAN, rINN).
PN-200-110. Isopropyl methyl 4-(2,1,3-benzoxadiazol-4-yl)-1,4-dihydro-2,6-dimethylpyridine-3,5-dicarboxylate.
$C_{19}H_{21}N_3O_5 = 371.4$.
CAS — 75695-93-1.
ATC — C08CA03.

Pharmacopoeias. In Br. and US.

Pharmacopoeial description
BP 2001: A yellow crystalline powder. Practically insoluble in water and in n-hexane; freely soluble in acetone; soluble in acetonitrile and in methyl alcohol. Protect from light.

USP 25: A yellow fine crystalline powder. Protect from light.

Stability. An oral preparation of isradipine 1 mg per mL, prepared using the powder from capsules of isradipine suspended in syrup[1] and stored at 4°, was stable when tested at 7, 16, 22, 28, and 35 days after preparation.

1. MacDonald JL, et al. Stability of isradipine in an extemporaneously compounded oral liquid. Am J Hosp Pharm 1994; **51:** 2409–11.

Adverse Effects, Treatment, and Precautions

As for dihydropyridine calcium-channel blockers (see Nifedipine, p.940).

◊ In a multicentre study involving 74 patients allocated to antihypertensive therapy with isradipine 2.5 to 10 mg twice daily, and 72 allocated to treatment with hydrochlorothiazide, adverse effects were reported in 44 of the isradipine group but only 29 of the thiazide group.[1] Flushing, palpitation, and oedema were more common in patients receiving isradipine, while headache, dizziness, and dyspnoea were reported in both groups with similar frequency. In another study,[2] spontaneously reported adverse effects occurred less frequently in patients taking isradipine (18.4% of 103 patients) than in those taking amlodipine (33.3% of 102 patients). In particular, ankle oedema was more frequent, severe, and prolonged than the oedema reported in patients taking isradipine. A multicentre study comparing isradipine and enalapril antihypertensive therapy[3] reported adverse effects in 51% of 71 patients taking isradipine and 45% of 64 patients taking enalapril. The commonest side-effects with isradipine were dizziness (14%), oedema (10%), fatigue (9%), headache (9%), and pruritus (7%).

1. Carlsen JE, Køber L. Blood pressure lowering effect and adverse events during treatment of arterial hypertension with isradipine and hydrochlorothiazide. Drug Invest 1990; **2:** 10–16.
2. Hermans L, et al. At equipotent doses, isradipine is better tolerated than amlodipine in patients with mild-to-moderate hypertension: a double-blind, randomized, parallel-group study. Br J Clin Pharmacol 1994; **38:** 335–40.
3. Johnson BF, et al. A multicenter comparison of adverse reaction profiles of isradipine and enalapril at equipotent doses in patients with essential hypertension. J Clin Pharmacol 1995; **35:** 484–92.

Interactions

As for dihydropyridine calcium-channel blockers (see Nifedipine, p.942).

Pharmacokinetics

Isradipine is almost completely absorbed from the gastrointestinal tract following a dose by mouth but undergoes extensive first-pass metabolism; the bioavailability is reported to be 15 to 24%. Peak plasma concentrations occur about 2 hours after oral administration. It is about 95% bound to plasma proteins. Isradipine is extensively metabolised in the liver. About 70% of an oral dose is reported to be excreted in urine, the remainder in faeces as metabolites. The terminal elimination half-life is often stated to be about 8 hours although a value of less than 4 hours has also been reported.

◊ In single-dose and steady-state studies of the pharmacokinetics of isradipine in 9 hypertensive subjects using a specific high performance liquid chromatographic assay, isradipine was found to be rapidly absorbed with peak concentrations occurring 1.2 (steady state) to 1.5 (single dose) hours after administration.[1] The mean terminal elimination half-life at steady state was 3.8 hours, suggesting that duration of action is likely to be short and that isradipine would need to be administered at least twice daily. There was considerable interindividual variation in the pharmacokinetics. In an earlier study[2] in healthy subjects the effective half-life of isradipine was calculated to be 8.8 hours, but radiolabelled isradipine was used and the assay method might have been less specific for unchanged drug.

1. Shenfield GM, et al. The pharmacokinetics of isradipine in hypertensive subjects. Eur J Clin Pharmacol 1990; **38:** 209–11.
2. Tse FLS, Jaffe JM. Pharmacokinetics of PN 200-110 (isradipine), a new calcium antagonist, after oral administration in man. Eur J Clin Pharmacol 1987; **32:** 361–5.

Hepatic impairment. Systemic availability following a radiolabelled dose of isradipine 5 mg by mouth was no different at 15.6% in 7 patients with non-cirrhotic chronic liver disease from the value of 16.5% in 8 healthy subjects.[1] However, in 8 patients with cirrhosis of the liver availability was markedly increased to a mean of 36.9%; this was associated with decreased clearance (1.6 litres per minute, compared with 9.9 in controls). Terminal half-life, as measured after intravenous administration, was greater at 11.9 hours in cirrhotic patients than the 5.1 hours seen in controls.

1. Cotting J, et al. Pharmacokinetics of isradipine in patients with chronic liver disease. Eur J Clin Pharmacol 1990; **38:** 599–603.

Uses and Administration

Isradipine is a dihydropyridine calcium-channel blocker with actions similar to those of nifedipine (p.943). It is used in the treatment of hypertension (p.802).

The usual initial dose of isradipine is 2.5 mg by mouth twice daily increased if necessary after 3 to 4 weeks to 5 mg twice daily. Some patients may require 10 mg twice daily. In elderly patients and those with impaired hepatic or renal function an initial dose of 1.25 mg twice daily may be preferable; a maintenance dose of 2.5 or 5 mg once daily may sometimes be sufficient.

A modified-release preparation allowing once-daily dosing is available in some countries.

◊ Reviews.

1. Fitton A, Benfield P. Isradipine: a review of its pharmacodynamic and pharmacokinetic properties, and therapeutic use in cardiovascular disease. Drugs 1990; **40:** 31–74.
2. Walton T, Symes LR. Felodipine and isradipine: new calcium-channel blocking agents for the treatment of hypertension. Clin Pharm 1993; **12:** 261–75.
3. Brogden RN, Sorkin EM. Isradipine: an update of its pharmacodynamic and pharmacokinetic properties and therapeutic efficacy in the treatment of mild to moderate hypertension. Drugs 1995; **49:** 618–49.

Preparations

BP 2001: Isradipine Tablets.

Proprietary Preparations (details are given in Part 3)
Aust.: Lomir; **Belg.:** Lomir; **Braz.:** Lomir; **Denm.:** Lomir; **Fin.:** Lomir; **Fr.:** Icaz; **Ger.:** Vascal; **Hong Kong:** Dynacirc; **Irl.:** Prescal†; **Ital.:** Cliveten; Esradin; Lomir; **Mex.:** Dynacirc; **Neth.:** Lomir; **Norw.:** Lomir; **NZ:** Dynacirc; **Port.:** Dilatol; Lomir; **S.Afr.:** Dynacirc; **Singapore:** Dynacirc; **Spain:** Lomir; Vaslan†; **Swed.:** Lomir; **Switz.:** Lomir; **Thai.:** Dynacirc; **UK:** Prescal; **USA:** Dynacirc.

Ketanserin Tartrate   (12881-m)

Ketanserin Tartrate (BANM, rINNM).
R-49945; R-41468 (ketanserin). 3-{2-[4-(4-Fluorobenzoyl)piperidino]ethyl}quinazoline-2,4(1H,3H)-dione tartrate.
$C_{22}H_{22}FN_3O_3,C_4H_6O_6 = 545.5$.
CAS — 74050-98-9 (ketanserin); 83846-83-7 (ketanserin tartrate).

NOTE. Ketanserin is USAN.

Ketanserin tartrate 27.6 mg is approximately equivalent to 20 mg of ketanserin.

Adverse Effects and Precautions

Ketanserin has been reported to cause sedation, fatigue, light-headedness, dizziness, headache, dry mouth, and gastrointestinal disturbances. Oedema has been reported rarely. In patients with predisposing factors chronic administration of ketanserin has been associated with the development of ventricular arrhythmias; ketanserin should be used with caution in patients taking antiarrhythmics or those with second- or third-degree atrioventricular block. Care should be taken to avoid the development of hypokalaemia in patients taking ketanserin, for example if diuretics are given concomitantly.

Because ketanserin may cause drowsiness care should be taken in patients who drive or operate machinery.

Ketanserin is reported to be better tolerated in elderly than in younger patients.

Hypotension. Profound hypotension occurred in 2 patients one hour after taking ketanserin 40 mg by mouth.[1] Both patients were also taking a beta blocker which may have exacerbated the reaction.

1. Waller PC, et al. Profound hypotension after the first dose of ketanserin. Postgrad Med J 1987; **63:** 305–7.

Interactions

The hypotensive effects of ketanserin may be enhanced by diuretics and other antihypertensives. Ketanserin should be used with caution in patients taking antiarrhythmics or drugs that cause hypokalaemia since the risk of arrhythmias is increased.

Pharmacokinetics

Ketanserin is rapidly absorbed from the gastrointestinal tract but has a bioavailability of about 50% due to first-pass hepatic metabolism. Peak plasma concentrations occur between 30 and 120 minutes after a dose by mouth. Ketanserin is about 95% bound to plasma proteins. The terminal half-life is stated to be between 13 and 18 hours but some studies report that following multiple doses the half-life is 19 to 29 hours. The metabolite ketanserinol has a terminal half-life of 31 to 35 hours following multiple doses, and it has been suggested that reconversion of ketanserinol to ketanserin may be responsible for the prolonged half-life of the parent compound during chronic administration.

Following oral administration about 68% of a dose is excreted in urine, and 24% in faeces, mainly as metabolites. Studies in animals suggest that ketanserin may cross the placenta and that some is present, together with metabolites, in breast milk.

◊ References.

1. Kurowski M. Bioavailability and pharmacokinetics of ketanserin in elderly subjects. Eur J Clin Pharmacol 1985; **28:** 411–17.
2. Persson B, et al. Pharmacokinetics of ketanserin in patients with essential hypertension. Eur J Clin Pharmacol 1987; **32:** 259–65.
3. Persson B, et al. Clinical pharmacokinetics of ketanserin. Clin Pharmacokinet 1991; **20:** 263–79.

Uses and Administration

Ketanserin is a serotonin antagonist with a high affinity for peripheral serotonin-2 (5-HT$_2$) receptors and thus inhibits serotonin-induced vasoconstriction, bronchoconstriction, and platelet aggregation. It also has some alpha$_1$-antagonist and histamine H$_1$-antagonist properties, but the clinical significance of these is controversial.

Ketanserin is used in the management of hypertension (p.802) and has also been tried in a variety of other conditions (see below).

Ketanserin is given as the tartrate, but doses are usually expressed in terms of the base.

Ketanserin produces a gradual hypotensive effect when administered by mouth, and 2 or 3 months of therapy may be required to produce the maximum reduction in blood pressure. Following intravenous injection a fall in blood pressure is generally produced in one or two minutes and lasts for 30 to 60 minutes.

In **hypertension** the usual initial dose is 20 mg twice daily by mouth, increasing, if necessary, after 1 month, to 40 mg twice daily. It has also been given by intravenous or intramuscular injection.

Action. Ketanserin has antagonist activity at both 5-HT$_2$ and alpha$_1$-adrenergic receptors, and the relative contribution of these and other mechanisms, including depression of the renin-angiotensin-aldosterone system, sympathetic inhibition, depletion of monoamine stores, and CNS effects to the antihypertensive effect is still being investigated.[1] Experiments with ritanserin suggest that 5-HT$_2$ antagonism alone, either at central or peripheral sites, does not lower arterial pressure. Evidence for a role of alpha$_1$-adrenoceptor antagonism is conflicting, but there is some evidence that these two mechanisms of action act to potentiate antihypertensive effects. There is no clear unconflicting evidence for any central effect or for action on the renin-angiotensin system; an apparent partial depletion of catecholamine and indoleamine stores has been noted, as well as evidence for a direct effect on transmembrane sodium transport systems, but the contribution, if any, of these actions to the drug's antihypertensive effects remains to be determined.

1. Brogden RN, Sorkin EM. Ketanserin: a review of its pharmacodynamic and pharmacokinetic properties, and therapeutic potential in hypertension and peripheral vascular disease. Drugs 1990; **40:** 903–49.

Administration in hepatic impairment. The half-life and volume of distribution of ketanserin were decreased in patients with cirrhosis but the area under the concentration-time curve was markedly increased. The rate of metabolism was reduced. The results suggested that the dosage should be reduced or the dosage interval increased when ketanserin is given to patients with cirrhosis.[1]

1. Lebrec D, et al. Pharmacokinetics of ketanserin in patients with cirrhosis. Clin Pharmacokinet 1990; **19:** 160–6.

Administration in renal impairment. Results from a study in 12 patients with chronic renal impairment, of whom 6 required haemodialysis, suggested that no adjustment of the standard dose of ketanserin 20 mg twice daily was required in patients with renal impairment.[1]

1. Barendregt JNM, et al. Ketanserin pharmacokinetics in patients with renal failure. Br J Clin Pharmacol 1990; **29:** 715–23.

Glaucoma and ocular hypertension. Although ketanserin, as 0.5% eye drops, can reduce intra-ocular pressure in normal and glaucomatous eyes,[1] its value, if any, in the treatment of glaucoma and ocular hypertension remains to be determined.

1. Costagliola C, et al. Effect of topical ketanserin administration on intraocular pressure. Br J Ophthalmol 1993; **77:** 344–8.

Peripheral vascular disease. Ketanserin is one of many drugs that have been tried in the management of peripheral vascular disease (p.809) but results have been contradictory. Evidence of benefit from ketanserin in patients with intermittent claudication is equivocal. One study[1] reported improvement in claudication distance and blood flow, but other studies[2,3] have failed to show a beneficial effect. The multicentre Prevention of Atherosclerotic Complications with Ketanserin Trial (PACK),[4] involving 3899 patients with intermittent claudication, suggested that ketanserin might be of benefit in preventing limb amputation in some patients, although this was the result of subgroup analysis. Conflicting results have also been reported in patients with *Raynaud's syndrome*; some studies[5-7] have demonstrated evidence of clinical improvement, but in others[8,9] no benefit has been found. Doses used in both indications have been fairly high (up to 40 mg three times daily) and some studies have found adverse effects to be common. A systematic review[10] found that ketanserin led to a small improvement in Raynaud's syndrome in patients with systemic sclerosis but that adverse effects increased; the authors concluded that ketanserin was not clinically beneficial in such patients.

Ketanserin has also been tried in other conditions associated with impaired peripheral blood flow: see Wounds and Ulcers, below.

1. De Cree J, et al. Placebo-controlled double-blind trial of ketanserin in treatment of intermittent claudication. Lancet 1984; **ii:** 775–9.
2. Bounameaux H, et al. Placebo-controlled, double-blind, two-centre trial of ketanserin in intermittent claudication. Lancet 1985; **ii:** 1268–71.
3. Beckers RCY, et al. Effect of ketanserin on macrocirculatory and microcirculatory blood flow in patients with intermittent claudication: a prospective randomized study. Eur J Clin Pharmacol 1989; **37:** 295–6.

The symbol † denotes a preparation no longer actively marketed

4. Prevention of Atherosclerotic Complications with Ketanserin Trial Group. Prevention of atherosclerotic complications: controlled trial of ketanserin. *BMJ* 1989; **298:** 424–30. Correction. *ibid.:* 644.
5. Roald OK, Seem E. Treatment of Raynaud's phenomenon with ketanserin in patients with connective tissue disorders. *BMJ* 1984; **289:** 577–9.
6. Codella O, *et al.* Controlled comparison of ketanserin and nifedipine in Raynaud's phenomenon. *Angiology* 1989; **40:** 114–21.
7. Coffman JD, *et al.* International study of ketanserin in Raynaud's phenomenon. *Am J Med* 1989; **87:** 264–8.
8. Kirch W, *et al.* Ketanserin versus nifedipine in secondary Raynaud's phenomenon. *Vasa* 1987; **16:** 77–80.
9. Engelhart M. Ketanserin in the treatment of Raynaud's phenomenon associated with generalized scleroderma. *Br J Dermatol* 1988; **119:** 751–4.
10. Pope J, *et al.* Ketanserin for Raynaud's phenomenon in progressive systemic sclerosis (updated 29 August 2001). Available in The Cochrane Library; Issue 4. Oxford: Update Software; 2001.

Shivering. Numerous drugs, including ketanserin, have been tried for the treatment of postoperative shivering (p.1255). In a preliminary study ketanserin 10 mg intravenously stopped shivering after general anaesthesia.[1]

1. Joris J, *et al.* Clonidine and ketanserin both are effective treatment for postanesthetic shivering. *Anesthesiology* 1993; **79:** 532–9.

Wounds and ulcers. Systemic administration of ketanserin has been reported to improve healing in various ulcers (p.1108) associated with impaired blood flow,[1,2] although others have found little benefit.[3] Several placebo-controlled studies[4-6] have reported improved healing of decubitus, venous, and ischaemic ulcers following the application of ketanserin as a 2% ointment. However, when ketanserin was applied topically as a 2% gel to surgical wounds no improvement in healing rate was found and it was suggested that ketanserin is only of benefit where the blood supply is compromised.[7]

1. Roald OK, Seem E. Treatment of Raynaud's phenomenon with ketanserin in patients with connective tissue disorders. *BMJ* 1984; **289:** 577–9.
2. Rustin MHA, *et al.* Chronic leg ulceration with livedoid vasculitis, and response to oral ketanserin. *Br J Dermatol* 1989; **120:** 101–5.
3. Cox NH, Dufton PA. Treatment of Raynaud's phenomenon with ketanserin. *BMJ* 1984; **289:** 1078–9.
4. Tytgat H, van Asch H. Topical ketanserin in the treatment of decubitus ulcers: a double-blind study with 2% ketanserin ointment against placebo. *Adv Therapy* 1988; **5:** 143–52.
5. Roelens P. Double-blind placebo-controlled study with topical 2% ketanserin ointment in the treatment of venous ulcers. *Dermatologica* 1989; **178:** 98–102.
6. Janssen PAJ, *et al.* Use of topical ketanserin in the treatment of skin ulcers: a double-blind study. *J Am Acad Dermatol* 1989; **21:** 85–90.
7. Lawrence CM, *et al.* The effect of ketanserin on healing of fresh surgical wounds. *Br J Dermatol* 1995; **132:** 580–6.

Preparations

Proprietary Preparations (details are given in Part 3)
Belg.: Sufrexal; *Ital.:* Perketan; Serepress; Sufrexal; *Mex.:* Sufrexal; *Neth.:* Ketensin; *Port.:* Sufrexal; *Thai.:* Sufrexal.

Labetalol Hydrochloride (6311-p)

Labetalol Hydrochloride (BANM, USAN, rINNM).

AH-5158A; Ibidomide Hydrochloride; Labetaloli Hydrochloridum; Sch-15719W. 5-[1-Hydroxy-2-(1-methyl-3-phenylpropylamino)ethyl]salicylamide hydrochloride; 2-Hydroxy-5-[1-hydroxy-2-(1-methyl-3-phenylpropylamino)ethyl]benzamide hydrochloride.

$C_{19}H_{24}N_2O_3,HCl = 364.9$.

CAS — 36894-69-6 (labetalol); 32780-64-6 (labetalol hydrochloride).

Pharmacopoeias. In Eur. (see p.vi) *and US.*

Pharmacopoeial description

Ph. Eur.: A white or almost white powder. Sparingly soluble in water and in alcohol; practically insoluble in dichloromethane and in ether. A 1% solution in water has a pH of 4.0 to 5.0.

USP 25: A white to off-white powder. Soluble in water and in alcohol; insoluble in chloroform and in ether. A 1% solution in water has a pH of 4.0 to 5.0. Store in airtight containers. Protect from light.

Incompatibility. Labetalol hydrochloride is compatible with standard intravenous solutions such as glucose 5% and sodium chloride 0.9%. However, precipitation has been reported when labetalol hydrochloride is added to sodium bicarbonate injection 5%.[1] The precipitate is probably labetalol base.[2] Incompatibilities have been reported with frusemide [furosemide],[3] heparin,[4] insulin,[4] and thiopental.[3] In all cases a white precipitate formed immediately on mixing with labetalol hydrochloride 5 mg per mL (in glucose 5%). There has also been a report of immediate haze following admixture of labetalol hydrochloride (0.8 mg per mL) with warfarin sodium.[5]

1. Yuen P-HC, *et al.* Compatibility and stability of labetalol hydrochloride in commonly used intravenous solutions. *Am J Hosp Pharm* 1983; **40:** 1007–9.
2. Alam AS. Identification of labetalol precipitate. *Am J Hosp Pharm* 1984; **41:** 74.
3. Chiu MF, Schwartz ML. Visual compatibility of injectable drugs used in the intensive care unit. *Am J Health-Syst Pharm* 1997; **54:** 64–5.

4. Yamashita SK, *et al.* Compatibility of selected critical care drugs during simulated Y-site administration. *Am J Health-Syst Pharm* 1996; **53:** 1048–51.
5. Bahal SM, *et al.* Visual compatibility of warfarin sodium injection with selected medications and solutions. *Am J Health-Syst Pharm* 1997; **54:** 2599–2600.

Adverse Effects

The adverse effects associated with beta blockers are described on p.844. Labetalol also has alpha-blocking activity which contributes to its adverse effects and these effects may predominate. Postural hypotension may be a problem with high doses or at the start of treatment. Other effects include scalp tingling, nasal congestion, muscle weakness, dyspnoea, tremor, urinary retention, hepatitis, and jaundice. Male sexual function may be impaired to a greater extent than with beta blockade alone.

Effects on the liver. By 1990, the FDA had received 11 reports of hepatocellular damage associated with labetalol therapy.[1] Three patients died. Liver function should be monitored and labetalol discontinued in patients who develop liver function abnormalities. The *R,R*-isomer of labetalol, dilevalol, was withdrawn from the market because of hepatotoxicity.[2]

1. Clark JA, *et al.* Labetalol hepatotoxicity. *Ann Intern Med* 1990; **113:** 210–13.
2. Harvengt C. Labetalol hepatotoxicity. *Ann Intern Med* 1991; **114:** 341.

Hypersensitivity. Hypersensitivity reactions associated with labetalol may manifest as fever.[1] Anaphylactoid reaction to labetalol has also been reported.[2]

1. D'Arcy PF. Drug reactions and interactions: drug fever with labetalol. *Int Pharm J* 1987; **1:** 43–4.
2. Ferree CE. Apparent anaphylaxis from labetalol. *Ann Intern Med* 1986; **104:** 729–30.

Overdosage. Acute oliguric renal failure developed after a short period of moderate hypotension in a patient who ingested labetalol 16 g. Renal function subsequently recovered.[1] Renal failure has also been reported[2] following ingestion of labetalol 6 g. The patient recovered following treatment with glucagon, isoprenaline, and dialysis.

1. Smit AJ, *et al.* Acute renal failure after overdose of labetalol. *BMJ* 1986; **293:** 1142–3.
2. Korzets A, *et al.* Acute renal failure associated with a labetalol overdose. *Postgrad Med J* 1990; **66:** 66–7.

Precautions

As for beta blockers, p.846.

Because labetalol causes postural hypotension it is recommended that injections are administered to patients when they are lying down and that patients should remain lying down for the following 3 hours.

Labetalol should be withdrawn from patients who develop signs of liver impairment.

Interactions

The interactions associated with beta blockers are discussed on p.846.

Pharmacokinetics

Labetalol is readily absorbed from the gastrointestinal tract, but is subject to considerable first-pass metabolism. Bioavailability varies widely between patients and may be increased in the presence of food. Peak plasma concentrations occur about 1 to 2 hours after an oral dose. Labetalol has low lipid solubility and only very small amounts appear to cross the blood-brain barrier in *animals*. It is about 50% protein bound. Labetalol crosses the placenta and is distributed into breast milk. Labetalol is metabolised predominantly in the liver, the metabolites being excreted in the urine together with only small amounts of unchanged labetalol; its major metabolite has not been found to have significant alpha- or beta-adrenoceptor blocking effects. Excretion also occurs in the faeces via the bile. The elimination half-life at steady state is reported to be about 8 hours. Following intravenous infusion, the elimination half-life is about 5.5 hours. Labetalol is not removed by dialysis.

The elderly. Data from 4 single-dose studies and 3 multidose studies were analysed to determine the effect of age on the pharmacokinetics of labetalol hydrochloride given by mouth.[1] Age did not appear to be a significant factor in oral clearance in elderly patients receiving labetalol for long-term management of hypertension.

1. Rocci ML, *et al.* Effects of age on the elimination of labetalol. *Clin Pharmacokinet* 1989; **17:** 452–7.

Pregnancy and breast feeding. The concentration of labetalol hydrochloride has been found to be lower in amniotic fluid and fetal plasma than in maternal plasma. A ratio of infant to maternal drug concentration of 0.2 to 0.8 has been reported[1] based on concentration in infant cord blood at delivery [time since last maternal dose not stated]. In another study,[2] however, higher concentrations were found in cord plasma than in maternal plasma at delivery when infants were delivered 12 to 24 hours after the last maternal dose.

The half-life of labetalol was reported as 24 hours in a neonate of 37 weeks' gestation whose mother had received labetalol 600 mg daily for 11 weeks prior to delivery.[3]

In 2 of 3 studies, the concentration of labetalol in breast milk was substantially less than in maternal plasma. In the third study, the concentration of drug in milk exceeded maternal plasma concentration in 2 of 3 mothers. In one infant, the plasma-labetalol concentration was similar to that of the mother.[1]

1. Goa KL, *et al.* Labetalol: a reappraisal of its pharmacology, pharmacokinetics and therapeutic use in hypertension and ischaemic heart disease. *Drugs* 1989; **37:** 583–627.
2. Boulton DW, *et al.* Transplacental distribution of labetalol stereoisomers at delivery. *Br J Clin Pharmacol* 1999; **47:** 573–4.
3. Haraldsson A, Geven W. Half-life of maternal labetalol in a premature infant. *Pharm Weekbl (Sci)* 1989; **11:** 229–31.

Uses and Administration

Labetalol is a non-cardioselective beta blocker (p.844). It is reported to possess some intrinsic sympathomimetic and membrane-stabilising activity. In addition, it has selective alpha₁-blocking properties which decrease peripheral vascular resistance. The ratio of alpha- to beta-blocking activity has been estimated to be about 1:3 following oral administration and 1:7 following intravenous administration.

Labetalol is used as the hydrochloride in the management of hypertension (p.802). It is also used to induce hypotension during surgery. Labetalol decreases blood pressure more rapidly than other beta blockers; the full antihypertensive effect may be seen within 1 to 3 hours of an oral dose.

In **hypertension** labetalol hydrochloride is usually given in an initial dose of 100 mg twice daily by mouth with food, gradually increased if necessary according to the response of the patient and standing blood pressure, to 200 to 400 mg twice daily; total daily doses of 2.4 g have occasionally been required. An initial dose of 50 mg twice daily has been recommended for elderly patients.

For the emergency treatment of hypertension labetalol hydrochloride may be given by slow intravenous injection. In the UK a dose of 50 mg, over a period of at least 1 minute, is recommended; if necessary this dose may be repeated at intervals of 5 minutes until a total of 200 mg has been given. In the USA an initial dose of 20 mg is recommended, given over 2 minutes; subsequent doses of 40 to 80 mg may be given every 10 minutes if necessary up to a maximum of 300 mg. Blood pressure should be monitored, and the patient should remain supine during intravenous administration and for 3 hours afterwards, to avoid excessive postural hypotension. Following bolus intravenous injection a maximum effect is usually obtained within 5 minutes and usually lasts up to 6 hours, although it may extend as long as 18 hours.

Labetalol hydrochloride has also been given by intravenous infusion in usual doses of 2 mg per minute. Suggested concentrations for intravenous infusions are 1 mg per mL or 2 mg per 3 mL of suitable diluent. In hypertension in pregnancy, labetalol infusion may be started at the rate of 20 mg per hour, then doubled every 30 minutes until a satisfactory response is obtained or a dose of 160 mg per hour is reached. In hypertension following myocardial infarction, labetalol infusion may be started at the rate of 15 mg per hour and gradually increased until a satisfactory response is obtained or a dose of 120 mg per hour is reached.

The initial dose in **hypotensive anaesthesia** is 10 to 20 mg intravenously, with increments of 5 to 10 mg if satisfactory hypotension is not achieved after 5 minutes. A higher initial dose may be required if halothane anaesthesia is not used (see under Interactions of Beta Blockers, p.846).

◊ General references.

1. Goa KL, *et al.* Labetalol: a reappraisal of its pharmacology, pharmacokinetics and therapeutic use in hypertension and ischaemic heart disease. *Drugs* 1989; **37:** 583–627.

Action. Labetalol hydrochloride has 2 optical centres; it is used as the racemic mixture of the 4 stereoisomers. The R,R-isomer is responsible for the beta-blocking activity and has limited alpha-blocking activity; it also has beta-adrenergic mediated peripheral vasodilating activity. The S,R-isomer has the most potent alpha-blocking activity. The S,S-isomer has some alpha-blocking activity and the R,S-isomer does not appear to have either alpha- or beta-adrenergic blocking effect.[1] The R,R-isomer, dilevalol, was withdrawn from the market because of hepatotoxicity.

1. Gold EH, *et al.* Synthesis and comparison of some cardiovascular properties of the stereoisomers of labetalol. *J Med Chem* 1982; **25:** 1363–70.

Tetanus. Autonomic overactivity, usually due to excessive catecholamine release, may occur as a complication of tetanus. Intravenous labetalol has been used successfully to control the cardiovascular effects.[1] Labetalol has both alpha- and beta-blocking properties. Unopposed beta blockade may produce severe hypertension and is thus not usually recommended, although esmolol, a short-acting beta blocker has been used.[2]

Management of the neuromuscular manifestations of tetanus is discussed on p.1332.

1. Domenighetti GM, *et al.* Hyperadrenergic syndrome in severe tetanus: extreme rise in catecholamines responsive to labetalol. *BMJ* 1984; **288:** 1483–4.
2. King WW, Cave DR. Use of esmolol to control autonomic instability of tetanus. *Am J Med* 1991; **91:** 425–8.

Preparations

BP 2001: Labetalol Injection; Labetalol Tablets;
USP 25: Labetalol Hydrochloride Injection; Labetalol Hydrochloride Tablets.

Proprietary Preparations (details are given in Part 3)
Aust.: Trandate; **Austral.:** Presolol; Trandate; **Belg.:** Trandate; **Canad.:** Trandate; **Denm.:** Trandate; **Fin.:** Albetol; **Fr.:** Trandate; **Hong Kong:** Trandate; **Irl.:** Trandate; **Israel:** Trandate; **Ital.:** Abetol†; Alfabetal†; Amipress; Ipolab; Pressalolo†; Trandate; **Neth.:** Trandate; **Norw.:** Trandate; **NZ:** Hybloc; Trandate; **Port.:** Trandate; **S.Afr.:** Trandate; **Singapore:** Trandate; **Spain:** Trandate; **Swed.:** Trandate; **Switz.:** Trandate; **UK:** Labrocol; Trandate; **USA:** Normodyne; Trandate.

Multi-ingredient: *Ital.:* Biotens†; Pressalolo Diuretico†; Trandiur.

Lacidipine (2495-d)

Lacidipine (BAN, USAN, rINN).
GR-43659X; GX-1048. Diethyl 4-{2-[(*tert*-butoxycarbonyl)vinyl]phenyl}-1,4-dihydro-2,6-dimethylpyridine-3,5-dicarboxylate.
$C_{26}H_{33}NO_6 = 455.5$.
CAS — 103890-78-4.
ATC — C08CA09.

Adverse Effects, Treatment, and Precautions
As for dihydropyridine calcium-channel blockers (see Nifedipine, p.940).

Interactions
As for dihydropyridine calcium-channel blockers (see Nifedipine, p.942).

Pharmacokinetics
Lacidipine is rapidly but poorly absorbed from the gastrointestinal tract following oral administration and undergoes extensive first-pass metabolism; the bioavailability has been reported to be 2 to 9%, or 18.5% (range 4 to 52%) using a more sensitive assay method. It is more than 95% bound to plasma proteins. Lacidipine is eliminated by metabolism in the liver and metabolites are excreted mainly by the biliary route. About 70% of an oral dose is eliminated in the faeces, the remainder in the urine. The average steady-state terminal elimination half-life of lacidipine is 13 to 19 hours.

Uses and Administration
Lacidipine is a dihydropyridine calcium-channel blocker with actions similar to those of nifedipine (p.943). It is used in the treatment of hypertension (p.802).

The usual initial dose of lacidipine is 2 mg once daily by mouth increased if necessary after 3 to 4 weeks or more to 4 mg daily; a further increase in dose to 6 mg daily may be necessary in some patients.

The symbol † denotes a preparation no longer actively marketed

◊ Reviews.
1. Lee CR, Bryson HM. Lacidipine: a review of its pharmacodynamic and pharmacokinetic properties and therapeutic potential in the treatment of hypertension. *Drugs* 1994; **48:** 274–96.
2. Zanchetti A, ed. Cardiovascular advantages of a third generation calcium antagonist: symposium on lacidipine. *Drugs* 1999; **57** (suppl 1): 1–29.

Preparations

Proprietary Preparations (details are given in Part 3)
Belg.: Motens; **Braz.:** Lacipil; **Denm.:** Midotens; **Fr.:** Caldine; **Ger.:** Motens; **Hong Kong:** Lacipil; **Ital.:** Aponil; Lacipil; Lacirex; Ladip; Viapres; **Mex.:** Lacipil; Midotens; **Neth.:** Motens; **Port.:** Lacipil; Tens; **S.Afr.:** Zascal†; **Singapore:** Lacipil; **Spain:** Lacimen; Lacipil; Motens; **Swed.:** Midotens; **Switz.:** Motens; **Thai.:** Motens; **UK:** Motens.

Lamifiban (17727-w)

Lamifiban (USAN, rINN).
Ro-44-9883; Ro-44-9883/000. ({1-[*N*-(*p*-Amidinobenzoyl)-L-tyrosyl]-4-piperidyl}oxy)acetic acid.
$C_{24}H_{28}N_4O_6 = 468.5$.
CAS — 144412-49-7 (lamifiban); 243835-65-6 (lamifiban hydrochloride).

Profile
Lamifiban is a glycoprotein IIb/IIIa-receptor antagonist. It is under investigation as an antiplatelet drug given intravenously for the management of thromboembolic disorders, such as unstable angina and myocardial infarction.

◊ References.
1. Théroux P, *et al.* Platelet membrane receptor glycoprotein IIb/IIIa antagonism in unstable angina: the Canadian Lamifiban Study. *Circulation* 1996; **94:** 899–905.
2. The PARAGON Investigators. International, randomized, controlled trial of lamifiban (a platelet glycoprotein IIb/IIIa inhibitor), heparin, or both in unstable angina. *Circulation* 1998; **97:** 2386–95.
3. The PARADIGM Investigators. Combining thrombolysis with the platelet glycoprotein IIb/IIIa inhibitor lamifiban: results of the Platelet Aggregation Receptor Antagonist Dose Investigation and Reperfusion Gain in Myocardial Infarction (PARADIGM) trial. *J Am Coll Cardiol* 1998; **32:** 2003–10.

Lanatoside C (5819-v)

Lanatoside C (BAN, rINN).
Celanide; Celanidum; Lanatosidum C. 3-[(*O*-β-D-Glucopyranosyl-(1→4)-*O*-3-acetyl-2,6-dideoxy-β-D-*ribo*-hexopyranosyl-(1→4)-*O*-2,6-dideoxy-β-D-*ribo*-hexopyranosyl-(1→4)-*O*-2,6-dideoxy-β-D-*ribo*-hexopyranosyl)oxy]-12,14-dihydroxy-3β,5β,12β-card-20(22)-enolide.
$C_{49}H_{76}O_{20} = 985.1$.
CAS — 17575-22-3.
ATC — C01AA06.
Pharmacopoeias. In Jpn and Pol.

A glycoside obtained from digitalis lanata leaf.

Profile
Lanatoside C is a cardiac glycoside with positive inotropic activity. It has general properties similar to those of digoxin (p.870) and has been used in the treatment of some cardiac arrhythmias and in heart failure.

Mixtures of lanatosides A, B, and C have also been used.

Preparations

Proprietary Preparations (details are given in Part 3)
Aust.: Cedilanid.

Lanoteplase (9235-y)

Lanoteplase (USAN, rINN).
BMS-200980; Sun-9216. *N*-[*N*²-(*N*-Glycyl-L-alanyl)-L-arginyl]-117-L-glutamine-245-L-methionine-(1-5)-(87-527)-plasminogen activator (human tissue-type protein moiety).
$C_{2184}H_{3323}N_{633}O_{666}S_{29} = 50032.5$.
CAS — 171870-23-8.

Profile
Lanoteplase is a thrombolytic under investigation in acute myocardial infarction.

◊ References.
1. Anonymous. Intravenous NPA for the treatment of infarcting myocardium early: InTIME-II, a double-blind comparison of single-bolus lanoteplase vs accelerated alteplase for the treatment of patients with acute myocardial infarction. *Eur Heart J* 2000; **21:** 2005–13.

Leech (4816-k)

Blutegel; Hirudo; Sangsue; Sanguessugas; Sanguisuga.
Pharmacopoeias. In Chin.

Hirudo medicinalis is the leech commonly used in medicine and is a fresh-water annelid.

Profile
Leeches are used for withdrawing blood from congested areas and have been found to be of value in plastic surgery. The buc-

cal secretion of the leech contains the anticoagulant hirudin (p.905). The part to be bitten may be moistened with sugar solution before applying the leech. Once used a leech should not be applied to another patient.

There have been reports of wound infection from *Aeromonas hydrophila* transmitted by leeches. Prolonged bleeding may occur from the site of attachment after removal of the leech.

◊ References.
1. Braidwood PS. The medicinal leech. *Pharm J* 1987; **239:** 766–7.
2. Abrutyn E. Hospital-associated infection from leeches. *Ann Intern Med* 1988; **109:** 356–8.
3. Adams SL. The medicinal leech; a page from the annelids of internal medicine. *Ann Intern Med* 1988; **109:** 399–405.
4. Menage MJ, Wright G. Use of leeches in a case of severe periorbital haematoma. *Br J Ophthalmol* 1991; **75:** 755–6.
5. Utley DS, *et al.* The failing flap in facial plastic and reconstructive surgery: role of the medicinal leech. *Laryngoscope* 1998; **108:** 1129–35.

Precautions. Wound infection by *Aeromonas hydrophila*, an organism normally found in the gut of the leech, is a recognised complication of the use of leeches for decongestion following plastic surgery.[1] Infections have caused minor wound drainage, cellulitis, abscess, tissue loss, and sepsis. Cephalosporins such as cefotaxime have been used for prophylaxis and treatment.

Other organisms have also caused cellulitis during treatment with leeches. *Aeromonas sobria* infection in a patient was treated with ceftazidime and ciprofloxacin.[2] *Serratia marcescens* infection in another patient was treated with ciprofloxacin.[3]

1. Lineaweaver WC, *et al.* Aeromonas hydrophila infections following use of medicinal leeches in replantation and flap surgery. *Ann Plast Surg* 1992; **29:** 238–44.
2. Fenollar F, *et al.* Unusual case of Aeromonas sobria cellulitis associated with the use of leeches. *Eur J Clin Microbiol Infect Dis* 1999; **18:** 72–3.
3. Pereira JA, *et al.* Leech-borne Serratia marcescens infection following complex hand injury. *Br J Plast Surg* 1998; **51:** 640–1.

Lepirudin (19770-g)

Lepirudin (BAN, rINN).
HBW-023. 1-L-Leucine-2-L-threonine-63-desulfohirudin (*Hirudo medicinalis* isoform HV1).
$C_{287}H_{440}N_{80}O_{111}S_6 = 6979.4$.
CAS — 138068-37-8.
ATC — B01AX03.

Adverse Effects and Precautions
The most frequent adverse effect of lepirudin is bleeding. Hypersensitivity reactions and fever have been reported.

Lepirudin should be used with caution in patients who are bleeding or at serious risk of bleeding including those with haemorrhagic blood disorders, recent major bleeding, cerebrovascular disorders, bacterial endocarditis, severe hypertension, or patients who have recently undergone major surgery or puncture of large vessels or organ biopsy. In patients with renal impairment the dose of lepirudin must be reduced and infusions should be avoided in those on haemodialysis.

Interactions
Concomitant use of lepirudin with thrombolytics, oral anticoagulants, or drugs that affect platelet function may increase the risk of bleeding.

Pharmacokinetics
Lepirudin is metabolised and excreted by the kidney. Following intravenous administration about 45% of a dose is detected in the urine and about 35% is excreted unchanged. The terminal elimination half-life of lepirudin is about 1.3 hours. In patients with severe renal impairment the half-life may be prolonged to about 2 days.

Breast feeding. The concentration of hirudin was measured in the breast milk of a woman who was treated with lepirudin 50 mg subcutaneously twice daily for deep-vein thrombosis and heparin-induced thrombocytopenia.[1] Three hours after injection plasma concentrations of hirudin in the woman were 0.5 to 1 mg per litre but no hirudin was detected in the breast milk.
1. Lindhoff-Last E, *et al.* Hirudin treatment in a breastfeeding woman. *Lancet* 2000; **355:** 467–8.

Uses and Administration
Lepirudin is a recombinant hirudin (p.905) that is a direct inhibitor of thrombin. It is used as an anticoagulant in the management of venous thromboembolism (p.817) in patients with heparin-induced thrombocytopenia. It is being investigated in arterial

thromboembolic disorders such as myocardial infarction and unstable angina.

In the management of thromboembolism in patients with heparin-induced thrombocytopenia lepirudin is given in an initial dose of 400 μg per kg body-weight (to a maximum dose of 44 mg) by slow intravenous injection. This is followed by a maintenance dose of 150 μg per kg per hour (to a maximum dose per hour of 16.5 mg) by continuous intravenous infusion, adjusted according to response, usually for 2 to 10 days.

Doses of lepirudin should be reduced in patients with renal impairment. The initial dose is reduced to 200 μg per kg, and the maintenance infusion rate is reduced according to creatinine clearance: for creatinine clearance of 45 to 60 mL per minute, infusion rate 50% of normal rate; 30 to 44 mL per minute, 30% of normal rate; 15 to 29 mL per minute, 15% of normal rate. In patients with creatinine clearance below 15 mL per minute infusion of lepirudin should be avoided, although further intravenous bolus doses of 100 μg per kg may be used on alternate days, according to response.

◊ Studies[1] have shown lepirudin to be effective for the management of venous thromboembolism in patients with heparin-induced thrombocytopenia. Recombinant hirudins are also under investigation as alternatives to heparin in the early management of myocardial infarction (p.805). Initial studies comparing heparin with the recombinant hirudins desirudin[2,3] (p.867) or lepirudin[4] had to be stopped because of higher than expected haemorrhagic stroke rates,[5,6] and subsequent studies using lower doses of desirudin[7,8] or lepirudin[9] failed to show a clear benefit over heparin. The role of hirudins therefore remains to be confirmed.

Desirudin has been investigated in unstable angina[10] (p.791) and studies in patients with acute ischaemic syndromes suggest that lepirudin is superior to heparin in preventing cardiovascular death, myocardial infarction, and refractory angina.[11,12] Desirudin has also been studied in patients undergoing percutaneous transluminal angioplasty[13] (p.812).

1. Greinacher A, et al. Recombinant hirudin (lepirudin) provides safe and effective anticoagulation in patients with heparin-induced thrombocytopenia: a prospective study. Circulation 1999; 99: 73–80.
2. The Global Use of Strategies to Open Occluded Coronary Arteries (GUSTO) IIa Investigators. Randomized trial of intravenous heparin versus recombinant hirudin for acute coronary syndromes. Circulation 1994; 90: 1631–7.
3. Antman EM, et al. Hirudin in acute myocardial infarction: safety report from the Thrombolysis and Thrombin Inhibition in Myocardial Infarction (TIMI) 9A trial. Circulation 1994; 90: 1624–30.
4. Neuhaus K-L, et al. Safety observations from the pilot phase of the randomized r-Hirudin for Improvement of Thrombolysis (HIT-III) study: a study of the Arbeitsgemeinschaft Leitender Kardiologischer Krankenhausärzte (ALKK). Circulation 1994; 90: 1638–42.
5. Zeymer U, Neuhaus K-L. Hirudin and excess bleeding: implications for future use. Drug Safety 1995; 12: 234–9.
6. Conrad KA. Clinical pharmacology and drug safety: lessons from hirudin. Clin Pharmacol Ther 1995; 58: 123–6.
7. The Global Use of Strategies to Open Occluded Coronary Arteries (GUSTO) IIb Investigators. A comparison of recombinant hirudin with heparin for the treatment of acute coronary syndromes. N Engl J Med 1996; 335: 775–82.
8. Antman EM. Hirudin in acute myocardial infarction: thrombolysis and thrombin inhibition in myocardial infarction (TIMI) 9B trial. Circulation 1996; 94: 911–21.
9. Neuhaus K-L, et al. Recombinant hirudin (lepirudin) for the improvement of thrombolysis with streptokinase in patients with acute myocardial infarction: results of the HIT-4 trial. J Am Coll Cardiol 1999; 34: 966–73.
10. Topol EJ, et al. Recombinant hirudin for unstable angina pectoris: a multicenter, randomized angiographic trial. Circulation 1994; 89: 1557–66.
11. Organization to Assess Strategies for Ischemic Syndromes (OASIS) Investigators. Comparison of the effects of two doses of recombinant hirudin compared with heparin in patients with acute myocardial ischemia without ST elevation: a pilot study. Circulation 1997; 96: 769–77.
12. Organisation to Assess Strategies for Ischemic Syndromes (OASIS-2) Investigators. Effects of recombinant hirudin (lepirudin) compared with heparin on death, myocardial infarction, refractory angina, and revascularisation procedures in patients with acute myocardial ischaemia without ST elevation: a randomised trial. Lancet 1999; 353: 429–38.
13. Serruys PW, et al. A comparison of hirudin with heparin in the prevention of restenosis after coronary angioplasty. N Engl J Med 1995; 333: 757–63.

Preparations

Proprietary Preparations (details are given in Part 3)
Aust.: Refludan; *Austral.:* Refludan; *Belg.:* Refludan; *Denm.:* Refludan; *Fin.:* Refludan; *Fr.:* Refludan; *Irl.:* Refludan; *Ital.:* Refludan; *Neth.:* Refludan; *Norw.:* Refludan; *Port.:* Refludan; *S.Afr.:* Refludin; *Spain:* Refludan; *Swed.:* Refludan; *Switz.:* Refludan; *UK:* Refludan; *USA:* Refludan.

Lercanidipine Hydrochloride (17047-s)

Lercanidipine Hydrochloride (BANM, rINNM).

Masnidipine Hydrochloride; R-75; Rec-15-2375. (±)-2-[(3,3-Diphenylpropyl)methylamino]-1,1-dimethylethyl methyl 1,4-dihydro-2,6-dimethyl-4-(m-nitrophenyl)-3,5-pyridinedicarboxylate hydrochloride.

$C_{36}H_{41}N_3O_6$,HCl = 648.2.

CAS — 100427-26-7 (lercanidipine); 132866-11-6 (lercanidipine hydrochloride).

Adverse Effects, Treatment, and Precautions

As for dihydropyridine calcium-channel blockers (see Nifedipine, p.940).

Interactions

As for dihydropyridine calcium-channel blockers (see Nifedipine, p.942).

Pharmacokinetics

Lercanidipine is completely absorbed from the gastrointestinal tract following oral administration but undergoes extensive saturable first-pass metabolism. Peak plasma concentrations occur about 1.5 to 3 hours after oral administration. Lercanidipine is rapidly and widely distributed. It is more than 98% bound to plasma proteins. Lercanidipine is extensively metabolised mainly to inactive metabolites and about 50% of an oral dose is excreted in the urine. The terminal elimination half-life is about 2 to 5 hours.

Uses and Administration

Lercanidipine is a dihydropyridine calcium-channel blocker with actions similar to those of nifedipine (p.943). It is used in the treatment of hypertension (p.802).

Lercanidipine is given by mouth as the hydrochloride in a usual initial dose of 10 mg once daily before food increased if necessary after at least 2 weeks to 20 mg daily.

◊ Reviews.
1. McClellan KJ, Jarvis B. Lercanidipine: a review of its use in hypertension. Drugs 2000; 60: 1123–40.

Preparations

Proprietary Preparations (details are given in Part 3)
Aust.: Zanidip; *Belg.:* Zanidip; *Denm.:* Zanidip; *Fin.:* Zanidip; *Fr.:* Lercan; Zanidip; *Israel:* Vasodip; *Ital.:* Cardiovasc; Lercadip; Zanedip; *Neth.:* Lerdip; *Spain:* Lercadip; Lerzam; Zanidip; *Swed.:* Zanidip; *UK:* Zanidip.

Levobetaxolol Hydrochloride

(11011-a)

Levobetaxolol Hydrochloride (USAN, rINNM).

AL-1577A (levobetaxolol or levobetaxolol hydrochloride). (-)-(S)-1-{p-[2-(Cyclopropylmethoxy)ethyl]phenoxy}-3-isopropylaminopropan-2-ol hydrochloride.

$C_{18}H_{29}NO_3$,HCl = 343.9.

CAS — 93221-48-8 (levobetaxolol); 116209-55-3 (levobetaxolol hydrochloride).

Adverse Effects, Treatment, and Precautions

As for beta blockers, p.844.

Interactions

The interactions associated with beta blockers are discussed on p.846.

Uses and Administration

Levobetaxolol, the S-isomer of betaxolol (p.848) is a cardioselective beta blocker (p.844). It is reported to lack intrinsic sympathomimetic activity and to have no significant membrane-stabilising properties.

Levobetaxolol is used as the hydrochloride to reduce raised intra-ocular pressure in open-angle glaucoma and ocular hypertension (p.1413). It is used topically as a suspension containing the equivalent of 0.5% levobetaxolol instilled twice daily.

Preparations

Proprietary Preparations (details are given in Part 3)
USA: Betaxon.

Levobunolol Hydrochloride (6312-s)

Levobunolol Hydrochloride (BANM, USAN, rINNM).

(-)-Bunolol Hydrochloride; l-Bunolol Hydrochloride; W-7000A. (-)-5-(3-tert-Butylamino-2-hydroxypropoxy)-1,2,3,4-tetrahydronaphthalen-1-one hydrochloride.

$C_{17}H_{25}NO_3$,HCl = 327.8.

CAS — 47141-42-4 (levobunolol); 27912-14-7 (levobunolol hydrochloride).

Pharmacopoeias. In Br. and US.

Pharmacopoeial description

BP 2001: A white or pinkish-white crystalline powder. Freely soluble in water; sparingly soluble in alcohol. A 5% solution in water has a pH of between 4.5 and 6.5. Protect from light.

USP 25: A white odourless crystalline powder. Soluble in water and in methyl alcohol; slightly soluble in alcohol and in chloroform. A 5% solution in water has a pH between 4.5 and 6.5.

Adverse Effects, Treatment, and Precautions

As for beta blockers, p.844.

Effects on respiratory function. A 42-year-old female developed a wheeze, which lasted about 20 minutes, approximately 8 hours after starting treatment with one drop in each eye of levobunolol 0.25%.[1] A second dose was instilled 12 hours after the first dose and after about 2½ hours the patient developed severe respiratory distress requiring hospitalisation.
1. Stubbs GM. Betagan drops. Med J Aust 1994; 161: 576.

Interactions

The interactions associated with beta blockers are discussed on p.846.

Pharmacokinetics

Some systemic absorption is reported to occur following topical application to the eye. Following oral administration levobunolol is rapidly and almost completely absorbed from the gastrointestinal tract. It is extensively metabolised in the liver; the principal metabolite, dihydrolevobunolol, is reported to possess beta-blocking activity. The metabolites and some unchanged drug are excreted in the urine.

Uses and Administration

Levobunolol is a non-cardioselective beta blocker (p.844). It is reported to lack intrinsic sympathomimetic activity and membrane-stabilising properties.

Levobunolol is used as the hydrochloride to reduce raised intra-ocular pressure in open-angle glaucoma and ocular hypertension (p.1413). It is usually used as a 0.5% ophthalmic solution instilled once or twice daily; alternatively a 0.25% solution may be instilled twice daily.

Preparations

BP 2001: Levobunolol Eye Drops;
USP 25: Levobunolol Hydrochloride Ophthalmic Solution.
Proprietary Preparations (details are given in Part 3)
Aust.: Vistagan; *Austral.:* Betagan; *Belg.:* Betagan; *Braz.:* Betagan; *Canad.:* Betagan; Ophtho-Bunolol; *Denm.:* Betagan; *Fr.:* Betagan; *Ger.:* Vistagan; *Hong Kong:* Betagan; *Irl.:* Betagan; *Israel:* Betagan; *Ital.:* Vistagan; *Mex.:* Betagan; *Neth.:* Betagan†; *NZ:* Betagan; *Port.:* Betagan; *S.Afr.:* Betagan; *Singapore:* Betagan; *Spain:* Betagan; *Swed.:* Betagan†; *Switz.:* Vistagan; *Thai.:* Betagan; *UK:* Betagan; *USA:* Ak-Beta; Betagan.
Multi-ingredient: *Canad.:* Probeta.

Levosimendan (17095-k)

Levosimendan (USAN, rINN).

(-)-OR-1259. Mesoxalonitrile (-)-{p-[(R)-1,4,5,6-tetrahydro-4-methyl-6-oxo-3-pyridazinyl]phenyl}hydrazone.

$C_{14}H_{12}N_6O$ = 280.3.

CAS — 141505-33-1.

Profile

Levosimendan is a cardiac inotrope and vasodilator used in the management of acute heart failure (p.798). It is given intravenously in a loading dose of 12 μg per kg body-weight over 10 minutes followed by a continuous infusion of 0.05 to 0.2 μg per kg per minute, adjusted according to response.

◊ References.
1. Figgitt DP, et al. Levosimendan. Drugs 2001; 61: 613–27.

Preparations

Proprietary Preparations (details are given in Part 3)
Swed.: Simdax.

Lidoflazine (9250-I)

Lidoflazine *(BAN, USAN, rINN)*.
McN-JR-7904; Ordiflazine; R-7904. 4-[3-(4,4′-Difluorobenzhydryl)propyl]piperazin-1-ylaceto-2′,6′-xylidide.
$C_{30}H_{35}F_2N_3O = 491.6$.
CAS — 3416-26-0.
ATC — C08EX01.
Pharmacopoeias. In Belg.

Profile
Lidoflazine is a calcium-channel blocker (p.788) that reduces atrioventricular conduction. It has been used in angina pectoris.

Lifibrol (13818-b)

Lifibrol *(USAN, rINN)*.
K-12148. (±)-*p*-[4-(*p-tert*-Butylphenyl)-2-hydroxybutoxy]benzoic acid.
$C_{21}H_{26}O_4 = 342.4$.
CAS — 96609-16-4.

Profile
Lifibrol is under investigation as a lipid regulating drug for the treatment of hypercholesterolaemia.

◊ References.
1. Schwandt P, *et al.* Safety and efficacy of lifibrol upon four-week administration to patients with primary hypercholesterolaemia. *Eur J Clin Pharmacol* 1994; **47:** 133–8.
2. Locker PK, *et al.* Lifibrol: a novel lipid-lowering drug for the therapy of hypercholesterolemia. *Clin Pharmacol Ther* 1995; **57:** 73–88.

Linsidomine Hydrochloride (5469-f)

Linsidomine Hydrochloride *(rINNM)*.
3-Morpholinosydnonimine hydrochloride.
$C_6H_{10}N_4O_2,HCl = 206.6$.
CAS — 33876-97-0 (linsidomine); 16142-27-1 (linsidomine hydrochloride).

Profile
Linsidomine is a nitrovasodilator and a metabolite of molsidomine (p.936). It is given as the hydrochloride via the intracoronary route in doses of 0.6 to 1 mg in the management of coronary artery spasm and to facilitate vasodilatation during coronary angiography. Additional doses may be required; the maximum total dose is 2 mg. It is also given by intravenous infusion in the management of unstable angina (p.791), in an initial dose of 1 mg per hour, adjusted according to response.

◊ References.
1. Delonca J, *et al.* Comparative efficacy of the intravenous administration of linsidomine, a direct nitric oxide donor, and isosorbide dinitrate in severe unstable angina: a French multicentre study. *Eur Heart J* 1997; **18:** 1300–6.

Preparations
Proprietary Preparations (details are given in Part 3)
Fr.: Corvasal.

Lisinopril (16878-k)

Lisinopril *(BAN, USAN, rINN)*.
Lisinoprilum; MK-521. N-{N-[(S)-1-Carboxy-3-phenylpropyl]-L-lysyl}-L-proline dihydrate.
$C_{21}H_{31}N_3O_5,2H_2O = 441.5$.
CAS — 76547-98-3 (anhydrous lisinopril); 83915-83-7 (lisinopril dihydrate).
ATC — C09AA03.

Pharmacopoeias. In Eur. (see p.vi) and US.

Lisinopril 2.72 mg as the dihydrate is approximately equivalent to 2.5 mg of anhydrous lisinopril.

Pharmacopoeial description
Ph. Eur.: A white crystalline powder. Soluble in water; practically insoluble in dehydrated alcohol and in acetone; sparingly soluble in methyl alcohol.

USP 25: A white crystalline powder. Soluble 1 in 10 of water and 1 in 70 of methyl alcohol; practically insoluble in alcohol, in acetone, in acetonitrile, in chloroform, and in ether.

Adverse Effects, Treatment, and Precautions
As for ACE inhibitors, p.820.

Porphyria. Lisinopril has been associated with acute attacks of porphyria and is considered unsafe in porphyric patients.

Interactions
As for ACE inhibitors, p.822.

The symbol † denotes a preparation no longer actively marketed

---

Pharmacokinetics
Lisinopril is slowly and incompletely absorbed following oral administration. About 25% of a given dose is absorbed on average, but the absorption varies considerably between individuals, ranging from about 6 to 60%. It is already an active diacid and does not need to be metabolised *in vivo*. Peak concentrations in plasma are reported to occur after about 7 hours. Lisinopril is reported not to be significantly bound to plasma proteins. It is excreted unchanged in the urine. The effective half-life for accumulation following multiple doses is 12 hours in patients with normal renal function. Lisinopril is removed by haemodialysis.

◊ References.
1. Till AE, *et al.* The pharmacokinetics of lisinopril in hospitalized patients with congestive heart failure. *Br J Clin Pharmacol* 1989; **27:** 199–204.
2. Neubeck M, *et al.* Pharmacokinetics and pharmacodynamics of lisinopril in advanced renal failure: consequence of dose adjustment. *Eur J Clin Pharmacol* 1994; **46:** 537–43.

Uses and Administration
Lisinopril is an ACE inhibitor (p.820). It is used in the treatment of hypertension (p.802) and heart failure (p.798), prophylactically after myocardial infarction (p.805), and in diabetic nephropathy (see Kidney Disorders, p.824).

The haemodynamic effects of lisinopril are seen within 1 to 2 hours of a single oral dose and the maximum effect occurs after about 6 hours, although the full effect may not develop for several weeks during chronic dosing. The haemodynamic action lasts for about 24 hours following once-daily dosing. Lisinopril is given by mouth as the dihydrate, but doses are expressed in terms of the anhydrous substance.

In the treatment of **hypertension** the initial dose is 2.5 mg daily; if possible, diuretic therapy should be withdrawn 2 or 3 days before lisinopril is started and resumed later if required. Since there may be a precipitous fall in blood pressure in some patients when starting therapy with an ACE inhibitor, the first dose should preferably be given at bedtime. Higher initial doses have been used and in the USA 10 mg of lisinopril daily is suggested for patients with uncomplicated hypertension, not on diuretic therapy, and without substantial renal impairment. The usual maintenance dose is 10 to 20 mg given once daily, though up to 40 mg daily may be given if necessary.

In the management of **heart failure**, severe first-dose hypotension on introduction of an ACE inhibitor is common in patients on loop diuretics, but their temporary withdrawal may cause rebound pulmonary oedema. Thus treatment should be initiated with a low dose under close medical supervision. Lisinopril is given by mouth in an initial dose of 2.5 mg daily. In the USA an initial dose of 5 mg daily is suggested. Usual maintenance doses range from 5 to 40 mg daily.

Following **myocardial infarction**, treatment with lisinopril may be started within 24 hours of the onset of symptoms in an initial dose of 5 mg once daily for two days, then increased to 10 mg once daily. An initial dose of 2.5 mg once daily is recommended for patients with a low systolic blood pressure.

In **diabetic nephropathy**, the initial dose is 2.5 mg once daily. In normotensive insulin-dependent diabetics the maintenance dose is 10 mg daily, increased to 20 mg daily if necessary to achieve a sitting diastolic blood pressure below 75 mmHg. In hypertensive non-insulin-dependent diabetics, the dose should be adjusted to achieve a sitting diastolic blood pressure below 90 mmHg.

◊ Reviews.
1. Noble TA, Murray KM. Lisinopril: a nonsulfhydryl angiotensin-converting enzyme inhibitor. *Clin Pharm* 1988; **7:** 659–69.
2. Armayor GM, Lopez LM. Lisinopril: a new angiotensin-converting enzyme inhibitor. *Drug Intell Clin Pharm* 1988; **22:** 365–72.
3. Lancaster SG, Todd PA. Lisinopril: a preliminary review of its pharmacodynamic and pharmacokinetic properties, and therapeutic use in hypertension and congestive heart failure. *Drugs* 1988; **35:** 646–69.
4. Goa KL, *et al.* Lisinopril: a review of its pharmacology and clinical efficacy in the early management of acute myocardial infarction. *Drugs* 1996; **52:** 564–88.

---

5. Goa KL, *et al.* Lisinopril: a review of its pharmacology and use in the management of the complications of diabetes mellitus. *Drugs* 1997; **53:** 1081–1105.
6. Simpson K, Jarvis B. Lisinopril: a review of its use in congestive heart failure. *Drugs* 2000; **59:** 1149–67.

Preparations
BP 2001: Lisinopril Tablets;
USP 25: Lisinopril Tablets.

Proprietary Preparations (details are given in Part 3)
Aust.: Acemin; Acetan; Prinivil†; *Austral.:* Fibsol; Lisodur; Prinivil; Zestril; *Belg.:* Novatec; Zestril; *Braz.:* Novral; Prinivil; Zestril; *Canad.:* Apo-Lisinopril; Acepril; Lanatin; Vivatec; Zestril; *Fin.:* Lisipril; Vivatec; Zestril; *Fr.:* Prinivil; Zestril; *Ger.:* Acerbon; Coric; Lisigamma; Lisihexal; Lisodura; *Hong Kong:* Prinivil; Zestril; *Irl.:* Carace; Zestril; *Israel:* Tensopril; *Ital.:* Alapril; Prinivil; Zestril; *Mex.:* Prinivil; Zestril; *Neth.:* Novatec; Zestril; *Norw.:* Vivatec; Zestril; *NZ:* Prinivil; Zestril; *Port.:* Farpresse; Lipril; Prinivil; Zestril; *S.Afr.:* Prinivil; Zestomax; Zestril; *Singapore:* Prinivil; Zestril; *Spain:* Doneka; Iricil; Likenil; Prinivil; Secubar; Tensikey; Zestril; *Swed.:* Vivatec; Zestril; *Switz.:* Prinil; Zestril; *Thai.:* Lispril; *UK:* Carace; Zestril; *USA:* Prinivil; Zestril.

Multi-ingredient: *Aust.:* Acecomb; Co-Acetan; Prinzide†; Zestoretic; *Belg.:* Novazyd; Zestoretic; *Braz.:* Prinzide; Zestoretic; *Canad.:* Prinzide; Zestoretic; *Denm.:* Vivazid; Zestoretic; *Fin.:* Acercomp; Lisipril Comp; Vivatec Comp; *Fr.:* Prinzide; Zestoretic; *Ger.:* Acercomp; Coric Plus; *Hong Kong:* Zestoretic; *Irl.:* Carace Plus; Zestoretic; *Ital.:* Nalapres; Prinzide; Zestoretic; *Mex.:* Prinzide; Zestoretic; *Neth.:* Novazyd; Zestoretic; *Norw.:* Vivatec Comp; Zestoretic; *NZ:* Prinzide; Zestoretic; *Port.:* Prinzide; Zestoretic; *S.Afr.:* Zestoretic; *Spain:* Doneka Plus; Prinivil Plus; Secubar Diu; Zestoretic; *Swed.:* Zestoretic; *Switz.:* Prinzide; Zestoretic; *UK:* Carace Plus; Zestoretic; *USA:* Prinzide; Zestoretic.

Lorcainide Hydrochloride (7788-q)

Lorcainide Hydrochloride *(BANM, USAN, rINNM)*.
Isocainide Hydrochloride; R-15889; Socainide Hydrochloride. 4′-Chloro-N-(1-isopropyl-4-piperidyl)-2-phenylacetanilide hydrochloride.
$C_{22}H_{27}ClN_2O,HCl = 407.4$.
CAS — 59729-31-6 (lorcainide); 58934-46-6 (lorcainide hydrochloride).

Profile
Lorcainide is a class Ic antiarrhythmic (p.787) that has been used for the management of ventricular and supraventricular arrhythmias. It has been given by mouth and by intravenous infusion as the hydrochloride.

Losartan Potassium (11145-s)

Losartan Potassium *(BANM, USAN, rINNM)*.
DuP-753; E-3340; MK-0954. 2-Butyl-4-chloro-1-[*p*-(o-1H-tetrazol-5-ylphenyl)benzyl]imidazole-5-methanol potassium.
$C_{22}H_{22}ClKN_6O = 461.0$.
CAS — 114798-26-4 (losartan); 124750-99-8 (losartan potassium).

Adverse Effects
Adverse effects of losartan have been reported to be usually mild and transient, and include dizziness and dose-related orthostatic hypotension. Hypotension may occur particularly in patients with volume depletion (for example those who have received high-dose diuretics). Impaired renal function and, rarely, rash, angioedema, and raised liver enzyme values may occur. Hyperkalaemia and myalgia have been reported. Losartan appears less likely than ACE inhibitors to cause cough. Other adverse effects that have been reported with angiotensin II receptor antagonists include respiratory-tract disorders, back pain, gastrointestinal disturbances, fatigue, and neutropenia.

◊ Reviews.
1. Mazzolai L, Burnier M. Comparative safety and tolerability of angiotensin II receptor antagonists. *Drug Safety* 1999; **21:** 23–33.

Angioedema. Angioedema is a recognised adverse effect of ACE inhibitors and is thought to be due to accumulation of bradykinins. However losartan, which does not affect bradykinin levels, has been associated with reports[1-3] of angioedema. In some cases patients had previously experienced angioedema with ACE inhibitors and caution is advised when using angiotensin II receptor antagonists in such patients.[4]

1. Acker CG, Greenberg A. Angioedema induced by the angiotensin II blocker losartan. *N Engl J Med* 1995; **333:** 1572.
2. van Rijnsoever EW, *et al.* Angioneurotic edema attributed to the use of losartan. *Arch Intern Med* 1998; **158:** 2063–5.
3. Adverse Drug Reactions Advisory Committee. Angiotensin II receptor antagonists. *Aust Adverse Drug React Bull* 1999; **18:** 2.
4. Warner KK, *et al.* Angiotensin II receptor blockers in patients with ACE inhibitor-induced angioedema. *Ann Pharmacother* 2000; **34:** 526–8.

Effects on the blood. Symptomatic anaemia occurred[1] in a patient with a renal transplant 6 weeks after commencing therapy with losartan. Decreased haemoglobin concentrations have also been reported[2] in patients with severe renal impairment undergoing haemodialysis.

1. Horn S, et al. Losartan and renal transplantation. *Lancet* 1998; **351:** 111.
2. Schwarzbeck A, et al. Anaemia in dialysis patients as a side-effect of sartanes. *Lancet* 1998; **352:** 286.

Effects on the liver. Raised liver enzyme values have occurred rarely in patients receiving losartan. Severe, acute hepatotoxicity developed in a patient one month after losartan was substituted for enalapril because of ACE inhibitor-induced cough.[1] The patient recovered when losartan was withdrawn but symptoms and raised liver enzyme concentrations recurred following rechallenge. Acute, reversible hepatotoxicity also occurred in a patient who had been taking losartan in a dose of 150 mg daily for 6 weeks.[2] A case of cholestatic jaundice associated with irbesartan therapy has also been reported;[3] the jaundice resolved slowly once irbesartan was withdrawn.

1. Bosch X. Losartan-induced hepatotoxicity. *JAMA* 1997; **278:** 1572.
2. Andrade RJ, et al. Hepatic injury associated with losartan. *Ann Pharmacother* 1998; **32:** 1371.
3. Hariraj R, et al. Prolonged cholestasis associated with irbesartan. *BMJ* 2000; **321:** 547.

Effects on the skin. Atypical cutaneous lymphoid infiltrates developed in two patients while they were receiving losartan for hypertension.[1] In both cases the lesions disappeared within a few weeks of stopping the drug.

1. Viraben R, et al. Losartan-associated atypical cutaneous lymphoid hyperplasia. *Lancet* 1997; **350:** 1366.

Effects on taste. Taste disturbances, in some cases progressing to complete taste loss, have occurred[1,2] in patients receiving losartan for hypertension. In each case taste returned to normal after discontinuing losartan therapy.

1. Schlienger RG, et al. Reversible ageusia associated with losartan. *Lancet* 1996; **347:** 471–2.
2. Heeringa M, van Puijenbroek EP. Reversible dysgeusia attributed to losartan. *Ann Intern Med* 1998; **129:** 72.

Migraine. Severe migraine has been reported[1] in a patient following administration of losartan. The patient had no history of migraine and symptoms recurred on rechallenge.

1. Ahmad S. Losartan and severe migraine. *JAMA* 1995; **274:** 1266–7.

Pancreatitis. Acute pancreatitis has been reported[1,2] in two patients receiving losartan. However, one of the patients subsequently developed pancreatitis unrelated to losartan.[3] The other patient[2] had also developed acute pancreatitis during enalapril therapy.

1. Bosch X. Losartan-induced acute pancreatitis. *Ann Intern Med* 1997; **127:** 1043–4.
2. Birck R, et al. Pancreatitis after losartan. *Lancet* 1998; **351:** 1178.
3. Bosch X. Correction: losartan, pancreatitis, and microlithiasis. *Ann Intern Med* 1998; **129:** 755.

Precautions

Losartan is contra-indicated in pregnancy and should be used with care, if at all, during breast feeding. It should be used with caution in patients with renal artery stenosis. Reduced doses may be required in patients with renal impairment and should be considered in patients with hepatic impairment. Patients with volume depletion (for example those who have received high-dose diuretic therapy) may experience hypotension, which may be minimised by initiating treatment with a low dose of losartan. Since hyperkalaemia may occur, serum-potassium concentrations should be monitored, especially in the elderly and patients with renal impairment, and the concomitant use of potassium-sparing diuretics should generally be avoided.

Pregnancy. Losartan is contra-indicated in pregnancy since it has been associated with fetal toxicity in *animal* studies and other drugs such as ACE inhibitors that act on the renin-angiotensin system have been associated with fetal toxicity in humans (see p.822). Oligohydramnios with subsequent fetal death occurred in a patient who received losartan during weeks 20 to 31 of pregnancy;[1] the effects on the fetus were similar to those reported with ACE inhibitors. A number of similar cases have subsequently been reported with losartan,[2,3] candesartan,[4] and valsartan.[3,5]

1. Saji H, et al. Losartan and fetal toxic effects. *Lancet* 2001; **357:** 363.
2. Lambot M-A, et al. Angiotensin-II-receptor inhibitors in pregnancy. *Lancet* 2001; **357:** 1619–20.
3. Martinovic J, et al. Fetal toxic effects and angiotensin-II-receptor antagonists. *Lancet* 2001; **358:** 241–2.
4. Hinsberger A, et al. Angiotensin-II-receptor inhibitors in pregnancy. *Lancet* 2001; **357:** 1620.
5. Briggs GG, Nageotte MP. Fatal fetal outcome with the combined use of valsartan and atenolol. *Ann Pharmacother* 2001; **35:** 859–61.

Pharmacokinetics

Losartan is readily absorbed from the gastrointestinal tract following oral administration, with an oral bioavailability of about 33%. It undergoes first-pass metabolism to form an active carboxylic acid metabolite E-3174 (EXP-3174), which has greater pharmacological activity than losartan, and some inactive metabolites. Metabolism is primarily by cytochrome P450 isoenzymes CYP2C9 and CYP3A4. Peak plasma concentrations of losartan and E-3174 occur about 1 hour and 3 to 4 hours, respectively, after an oral dose. Both losartan and E-3174 are more than 98% bound to plasma proteins. Losartan is excreted in the urine, and in the faeces via bile, as unchanged drug and metabolites. Following oral dosing about 35% of the dose is excreted in the urine and about 60% in the faeces. The terminal elimination half-lives of losartan and E-3174 are about 1.5 to 2.5 hours and 3 to 9 hours, respectively.

◊ References.

1. Ohtawa M, et al. Pharmacokinetics and biochemical efficacy after single and multiple oral administration of losartan, an orally active nonpeptide angiotensin II receptor antagonist, in humans. *Br J Clin Pharmacol* 1993; **35:** 290–7.
2. Lo M-W, et al. Pharmacokinetics of losartan, an angiotensin II receptor antagonist, and its active metabolite EXP3174 in humans. *Clin Pharmacol Ther* 1995; **58:** 641–9.
3. Csajka C, et al. Pharmacokinetic-pharmacodynamic profile of angiotensin II receptor antagonists. *Clin Pharmacokinet* 1997; **32:** 1–29.
4. Sica DA, et al. Pharmacokinetics and blood pressure response of losartan in end-stage renal disease. *Clin Pharmacokinet* 2000; **38:** 519–26.
5. Pedro AA, et al. The pharmacokinetics and pharmacodynamics of losartan in continuous ambulatory peritoneal dialysis. *J Clin Pharmacol* 2000; **40:** 389–95.

Uses and Administration

Losartan is an angiotensin II receptor antagonist with antihypertensive activity due mainly to selective blockade of AT_1 receptors and the consequent reduced pressor effect of angiotensin II. It is used in the management of hypertension (p.802) and may have a role in patients who develop cough with ACE inhibitors. It has also been tried in heart failure (below) and in myocardial infarction (p.805), and is under investigation in diabetic nephropathy.

Losartan is given by mouth as the potassium salt. The maximum hypotensive effect is achieved in about 3 to 6 weeks after initiating treatment.

In hypertension the usual dose is 50 mg once daily. The dose may be increased, if necessary, to 100 mg daily as a single dose or in two divided doses. An initial dose of 25 mg once daily may be used in the elderly over 75 years, and for patients with moderate to severe renal impairment (creatinine clearance less than 20 mL per minute), or intravascular fluid depletion. A reduced dose should also be considered for patients with hepatic impairment.

◊ References.

1. Anonymous. Losartan—a new antihypertensive. *Drug Ther Bull* 1995; **33:** 73–4.
2. Johnston CI. Angiotensin receptor antagonists: focus on losartan. *Lancet* 1995; **346:** 1403–7.
3. Carr AA, Prisant LM. Losartan: first of a new class of angiotensin antagonists for the management of hypertension. *J Clin Pharmacol* 1996; **36:** 3–12.
4. Goa KL, Wagstaff AJ. Losartan potassium: a review of its pharmacology, clinical efficacy and tolerability in the management of hypertension. *Drugs* 1996; **51:** 820–45.
5. Schaefer KL, Porter JA. Angiotensin II receptor antagonists: the prototype losartan. *Ann Pharmacother* 1996; **30:** 625–36.
6. Burrell LM. A risk-benefit assessment of losartan potassium in the treatment of hypertension. *Drug Safety* 1997; **16:** 56–65.
7. McConnaughey MM, et al. Practical considerations of the pharmacology of angiotensin receptor blockers. *J Clin Pharmacol* 1999; **39:** 547–59.
8. Burnier M, Brunner HR. Angiotensin II receptor antagonists. *Lancet* 2000; **355:** 637–45.

Heart failure. Diuretics, ACE inhibitors, and beta blockers are the standard drugs used in the management of heart failure (p.798). Angiotensin II receptor antagonists have been studied as an alternative to ACE inhibitors since they may be better tolerated. In the ELITE study,[1] which compared losartan with captopril, both drugs had similar effects on renal function but other adverse effects were fewer with losartan and there was also a reduction in mortality in patients receiving losartan. However, the larger ELITE II study[2] failed to confirm any survival benefit with losartan and ACE inhibitors remain first-line therapy. Other angiotensin II receptor antagonists are also be-

ing investigated in heart failure, and the combination of angiotensin II receptor antagonists with ACE inhibitors is also being studied.

1. Pitt B, et al. Randomised trial of losartan versus captopril in patients over 65 with heart failure (Evaluation of Losartan in the Elderly Study, ELITE). *Lancet* 1997; **349:** 747–52.
2. Pitt B, et al. Effect of losartan compared with captopril on mortality in patients with symptomatic heart failure: randomised trial—the Losartan Heart Failure Survival Study ELITE II. *Lancet* 2000; **355:** 1582–7.

Uricosuric action. In a study[1] in healthy subjects losartan was found to reduce serum uric acid concentration and increase urinary uric acid excretion in a dose-dependent manner. However, in a further study[2] in hypertensive subjects, losartan produced only a small increase in uric acid excretion, and there was no significant change in serum uric acid concentration.

1. Nakashima M, et al. Pilot study of the uricosuric effect of DuP-753, a new angiotensin II receptor antagonist, in healthy subjects. *Eur J Clin Pharmacol* 1992; **42:** 333–5.
2. Puig JG, et al. Effect of eprosartan and losartan on uric acid metabolism in patients with essential hypertension. *J Hypertens* 1999; **17:** 1033–9.

Preparations

Proprietary Preparations (details are given in Part 3)

Aust.: Cosaar; *Austral.:* Cozaar; *Belg.:* Cozaar; Loortan; *Braz.:* Cozaar; *Canad.:* Cozaar; *Denm.:* Cozaar; *Fin.:* Cozaar; *Fr.:* Cozaar; *Ger.:* Lorzaar; *Hong Kong:* Cozaar; *Irl.:* Cozaar; *Israel:* Ocsaar; *Ital.:* Lortaan; Losaprex; Neo-Lotan; *Jpn:* Nu-Lotan; *Mex.:* Cozaar; *Neth.:* Cozaar; *Norw.:* Cozaar; *NZ:* Cozaar; *Port.:* Cozaar; Lortaan; *S.Afr.:* Cozaar; *Singapore:* Cozaar; *Spain:* Cozaar; *Swed.:* Cozaar; *Switz.:* Cosaar; *Thai.:* Cozaar; *UK:* Cozaar; *USA:* Cozaar.

Multi-ingredient: *Aust.:* Cosaar Plus; *Belg.:* Cozaar Plus; Loortan Plus; *Canad.:* Hyzaar; *Denm.:* Cozaar Comp; Fortzaar; *Fin.:* Cozaar Comp; *Fr.:* Fortzaar; Hyzaar; *Ger.:* Lorzaar plus; *Hong Kong:* Hyzaar; *Irl.:* Cozaar Comp; *Israel:* Ocsaar Plus; *Ital.:* Hizaar; Losazid; Neo-Lotan Plus; *Mex.:* Hyzaar; *Neth.:* Hyzaar; *Norw.:* Cozaar Comp; *Port.:* Cozaar Plus; Lortaan Plus; *S.Afr.:* Cozaar Comp; *Singapore:* Hyzaar; *Spain:* Cozaar Plus; *Swed.:* Cozaar Comp; *Switz.:* Cozaar Plus; *Thai.:* Hyzaar; *UK:* Cozaar Comp; *USA:* Hyzaar.

Lovastatin (16894-k)

Lovastatin (BAN, USAN, rINN)

L-154803; Lovastatinum; MB-530B; 6α-Methylcompactin; Mevinolin; MK-803; Monacolin K; MSD-803. (3R,5R)-7-{(1S,2S,6R,8S,8aR)-1,2,6,7,8,8a-Hexahydro-2,6-dimethyl-8-[(S)-2-methylbutyryloxy]-1-naphthyl}-3-hydroxyheptan-5-olide.

$C_{24}H_{36}O_5 = 404.5$.

CAS — 75330-75-5.

ATC — C10AA02.

Pharmacopoeias. In *Eur.* (see p.vi) and US.

Pharmacopoeial description

Ph. Eur.: A white or almost white crystalline powder. Practically insoluble in water; sparingly soluble in dehydrated alcohol; soluble in acetone. Store under nitrogen at a temperature of 2° to 8°.

USP 25: A white to off-white crystalline powder. Insoluble in water; sparingly soluble in alcohol; practically insoluble in petroleum spirit; freely soluble in chloroform; soluble in acetone, in acetonitrile, and in methyl alcohol. Store under nitrogen in airtight containers at a temperature not exceeding 8°.

Adverse Effects and Precautions

As for Simvastatin, p.969.

◊ Adverse effects led to withdrawal of lovastatin in 21 of 745 patients receiving the drug for about 5 years.[1] They included asymptomatic elevation of hepatic aminotransferases in 10 patients, gastrointestinal symptoms in 3, rash in 2, myopathy in 2, myalgia in 1, arthralgia in 1, insomnia in 1, and weight gain in 1.

1. Lovastatin Study Groups. Lovastatin 5-year safety and efficacy study: Lovastatin Study Groups I through IV. *Arch Intern Med* 1993; **153:** 1079–87.

Children. Bile-acid binding resins such as colestyramine have traditionally been used to treat heterozygous familial hyperlipidaemia in children and adolescents. Limited information suggests that statins are effective at lowering total cholesterol and low-density lipoprotein (LDL)-cholesterol in children older than 10 years.[1] However, there are concerns about the potential adverse effects of statins on growth and sexual development, because these patients require life-long therapy.[2] A placebo-controlled study[3] of lovastatin in 132 adolescent males reported significant reduction in LDL-cholesterol compared with placebo, but no significant differences between the groups in measures of growth and sexual maturation. However, patients were studied for one year only, and the authors acknowledge that further study is needed.

1. Duplaga BA. Treatment of childhood hypercholesterolemia with HMG-CoA reductase inhibitors. *Ann Pharmacother* 1999; **33:** 1224–7.

2. Rifkind BM, *et al.* When should patients with heterozygous familial hypercholesterolemia be treated? *JAMA* 1999; **281:** 180–1.
3. Stein EA, *et al.* Efficacy and safety of lovastatin in adolescent males with heterozygous familial hypercholesterolemia: a randomized controlled trial. *JAMA* 1999; **281:** 137–44.

Effects on the blood. Haemolytic anaemia in a patient has been attributed to lovastatin;[1] no adverse effect was seen when the patient was given simvastatin.

1. Robbins MJ, *et al.* Lovastatin-induced hemolytic anemia; not a class-specific reaction. *Am J Med* 1995; **99:** 328–9.

Effects on the eyes. Lens opacities were found in 13 of 101 patients taking lovastatin following an 18-week study.[1] However, no further deterioration was seen in 11 of these patients who continued to take lovastatin at follow-up after an average of 26 months from the start of treatment.

No differences were found in the development of lens opacities or in changes in visual acuity between patients treated with lovastatin for 48 weeks and patients taking placebo in a study of 8245 patients.[2]

1. Hunninghake DB, *et al.* Lovastatin: follow-up ophthalmologic data. *JAMA* 1988; **259:** 354–5.
2. Laties AM, *et al.* The human lens after 48 weeks of treatment with lovastatin. *N Engl J Med* 1990; **323:** 683–4.

Effects on the nervous system. Paraesthesias developed in a 47-year-old woman about two years after starting treatment with lovastatin.[1] Symptoms disappeared a few weeks after treatment was discontinued, but reappeared two weeks after starting treatment with pravastatin. Symptoms again abated a few weeks after pravastatin was discontinued.

1. Jacobs MB. HMG-CoA reductase inhibitor therapy and peripheral neuropathy. *Ann Intern Med* 1994; **120:** 970.

Effects on sexual function. Low sperm count associated with lovastatin therapy was reported in a patient.[1]

1. Hildebrand RD, Hepperlen TW. Lovastatin and hypospermia. *Ann Intern Med* 1990; **112:** 549–50.

Effects on skeletal muscle. Muscle disorders are well-recognised adverse effects of lipid regulating drugs such as the fibrates and statins (see Simvastatin, p.970).

There have been reports of myopathy and rhabdomyolysis in patients receiving lovastatin in combination with azithromycin,[1] clarithromycin,[1] danazol,[2] erythromycin,[3] gemfibrozil,[4-6] itraconazole,[7] and nicotinic acid,[8] and in patients receiving immunosuppressive therapy (often including ciclosporin) following transplant surgery.[9-11] There has also been a report of rhabdomyolysis in a patient taking lovastatin on its own.[12] Muscle weakness and soreness associated with lovastatin was relieved in a patient by the administration of ubidecarenone.[13]

1. Grunden JW, Fisher KA. Lovastatin-induced rhabdomyolysis possibly associated with clarithromycin and azithromycin. *Ann Pharmacother* 1997; **31:** 859–63.
2. Dallaire M, Chamberland M. Rhabdomyolyse sévère chez un patient recevant lovastatine, danazol et doxycycline. *Can Med Assoc J* 1994; **150:** 1991–4.
3. Ayanian JZ, *et al.* Lovastatin and rhabdomyolysis. *Ann Intern Med* 1988; **109:** 682–3.
4. Kogan AD, Orenstein S. Lovastatin-induced acute rhabdomyolysis. *Postgrad Med J* 1990; **66:** 294–6.
5. Marais GE, Larson KK. Rhabdomyolysis and acute renal failure induced by combination lovastatin and gemfibrozil therapy. *Ann Intern Med* 1990; **112:** 228–30.
6. Pierce LR, *et al.* Myopathy and rhabdomyolysis associated with lovastatin-gemfibrozil combination therapy. *JAMA* 1990; **264:** 71–5.
7. Lees RS, Lees AM. Rhabdomyolysis from the coadministration of lovastatin and the antifungal agent itraconazole. *N Engl J Med* 1995; **333:** 664–5.
8. Reaven P, Witztum JL. Lovastatin, nicotinic acid, and rhabdomyolysis. *Ann Intern Med* 1988; **109:** 597–8.
9. Norman DJ, *et al.* Myolysis and acute renal failure in a heart-transplant recipient receiving lovastatin. *N Engl J Med* 1988; **318:** 46–7.
10. East C, *et al.* Rhabdomyolysis in patients receiving lovastatin after cardiac transplantation. *N Engl J Med* 1988; **318:** 47–8.
11. Corpier CL, *et al.* Rhabdomyolysis and renal injury with lovastatin use: report of two cases in cardiac transplant recipients. *JAMA* 1988; **260:** 239–41.
12. Wallace CS, Mueller BA. Lovastatin-induced rhabdomyolysis in the absence of concomitant drugs. *Ann Pharmacother* 1992; **26:** 190–2.
13. Walravens PA, *et al.* Lovastatin, isoprenes, and myopathy. *Lancet* 1989; **ii:** 1097–8.

Effects on sleep patterns. For reports of the effects of statins, including lovastatin, on sleep patterns, see Simvastatin, p.970.

Pregnancy. For a report suggesting that exposure to lovastatin during pregnancy has no adverse outcome, see Simvastatin, p.970.

Interactions
As for Simvastatin, p.970.

◊ General reviews.
1. Garnett WR. Interactions with hydroxymethylglutaryl-coenzyme A reductase inhibitors. *Am J Health-Syst Pharm* 1995; **52:** 1639–45.

◊ Raised concentrations of lovastatin have occurred in patients also given *mibefradil.* Lovastatin has been associated with both hyperthyroidism[1] and hypothyroidism[2] in patients taking *thyroxine [levothyroxine].* Bleeding and increases in prothrombin time have been reported in patients taking lovastatin with coumarin *anticoagulants* (see under Warfarin, p.997).

The symbol † denotes a preparation no longer actively marketed

For reports of interactions of lovastatin with *azithromycin, clarithromycin, danazol, erythromycin, gemfibrozil, immunosuppressants, itraconazole,* and *nicotinic acid,* see Effects on Skeletal Muscle, above.

1. Lustgarten BP. Catabolic response to lovastatin therapy. *Ann Intern Med* 1988; **109:** 171–2.
2. Demke DM. Drug interaction between thyroxine and lovastatin. *N Engl J Med* 1989; **321:** 1341–2.

Pharmacokinetics
Lovastatin is absorbed from the gastrointestinal tract and is hydrolysed in the liver to its active β-hydroxy-acid form. Three other metabolites have also been isolated. Lovastatin undergoes extensive first-pass metabolism in the liver, its primary site of action, and less than 5% of the oral dose has been reported to reach the circulation. Lovastatin is metabolised by the cytochrome P450 isoenzyme CYP3A4. Peak plasma concentrations occur within 2 to 4 hours, and steady-state concentrations are achieved after 2 to 3 days with daily administration. Both lovastatin and its β-hydroxyacid metabolite are more than 95% bound to plasma proteins. It is mainly excreted in the bile; about 85% of the administered dose has been recovered from the faeces and about 10% from the urine. The half-life of the active metabolite is 1 to 2 hours.

◊ General reviews.
1. Desager J-P, Horsmans Y. Clinical pharmacokinetics of 3-hydroxy-3-methylglutaryl-coenzyme A reductase inhibitors. *Clin Pharmacokinet* 1996; **31:** 348–71.
2. Lennernäs H, Fager G. Pharmacodynamics and pharmacokinetics of the HMG-CoA reductase inhibitors: similarities and differences. *Clin Pharmacokinet* 1997; **32:** 403–25.

Uses and Administration
Lovastatin, a 3-hydroxy-3-methylglutaryl coenzyme A (HMG-CoA) reductase inhibitor (a statin), is a lipid regulating drug with actions on plasma lipids similar to those of simvastatin (p.970).

Lovastatin is used to reduce cholesterol in the treatment of hyperlipidaemias (below), particularly in type IIa and IIb hyperlipoproteinaemias. It is also given prophylactically for both primary and secondary prevention of ischaemic heart disease.

Lovastatin is given in an initial dose of 10 to 20 mg daily in the evening with food, increased, if necessary, at intervals of 4 weeks or more to 80 mg daily in single or divided doses. In patients taking ciclosporin an initial dose of 10 mg daily should be used. The daily dose should not exceed 20 mg in patients taking ciclosporin, fibric acid derivatives, or nicotinic acid, and the risk of myopathy must be considered. Doses above 20 mg daily should be used cautiously in patients with severe renal impairment.

◊ General reviews.
1. McKenney JM. Lovastatin: a new cholesterol-lowering agent. *Clin Pharm* 1988; **7:** 21–36.
2. Henwood JM, Heel RC. Lovastatin: a preliminary review of its pharmacodynamic properties and therapeutic use in hyperlipidaemia. *Drugs* 1988; **36:** 429–54.
3. Frishman WH, *et al.* Lovastatin and other HMG-CoA reductase inhibitors. *J Clin Pharmacol* 1989; **29:** 975–82.
4. Schectman G, Hiatt J. Dose–response characteristics of cholesterol-lowering drug therapies: implications for treatment. *Ann Intern Med* 1996; **125:** 990–1000.

Adrenoleucodystrophy. A preliminary study[1] has shown that lovastatin may be useful in the treatment of adrenoleucodystrophy (p.1629). Lovastatin reduced the plasma levels of very-long-chain fatty acids which are known to be elevated in patients with this rare metabolic disorder.

1. Pai GS, *et al.* Lovastatin therapy for X-linked adrenoleukodystrophy: clinical and biochemical observations on 12 patients. *Mol Genet Metab* 2000; **69:** 312–22.

Hyperlipidaemias. Lovastatin, like other statins, is used in the treatment of hyperlipidaemias (p.800) and a general discussion of the lipid regulating effects of statins can be found in simvastatin (p.970).

Lovastatin is effective in the treatment of primary hypercholesterolaemia. In the Expanded Clinical Evaluation of Lovastatin (EXCEL) study[1,2] involving more than 8000 patients with moderate hypercholesterolaemia, lovastatin lowered low-density lipoprotein (LDL)-cholesterol, total cholesterol, and triglyceride concentrations and increased high-density lipoprotein (HDL)-cholesterol concentrations in both men and women; benefit was maintained in those followed up for 2 years.[3] Lovastatin appeared to be more effective than nicotinic acid at reducing LDL-cholesterol in patients with primary hypercholesterolaemia, but less effective at increasing HDL-cholesterol; lovastatin was better tolerated.[4] Hypercholesterolaemia is a risk factor for **ischaemic heart disease** and lovastatin may be given for the secondary prevention of atherosclerotic heart dis-

ease. In the Asymptomatic Carotid Artery Progression Study (ACAPS)[5] lovastatin appeared to be of benefit in patients with early carotid artery atherosclerosis, although in another study it failed to prevent restenosis after coronary angioplasty.[6] Benefit has also been demonstrated[7] with lovastatin in primary prevention of coronary disease in men and women and even in those with only average cholesterol levels.

1. Bradford RH, *et al.* Expanded clinical evaluation of lovastatin (EXCEL) study results: I. efficacy in modifying plasma lipoproteins and adverse event profile in 8245 patients with moderate hypercholesterolemia. *Arch Intern Med* 1991; **151:** 43–9.
2. Bradford RH, *et al.* Efficacy and tolerability of lovastatin in 3390 women with moderate hypercholesterolemia. *Ann Intern Med* 1993; **118:** 850–5.
3. Bradford RH, *et al.* Expanded clinical evaluation of lovastatin (EXCEL) study results: two-year efficacy and safety follow-up. *Am J Cardiol* 1994; **74:** 667–73.
4. Illingworth DR, *et al.* Comparative effects of lovastatin and niacin in primary hypercholesterolemia. *Arch Intern Med* 1994; **154:** 1586–95.
5. Furberg CD, *et al.* Effect of lovastatin on early carotid atherosclerosis and cardiovascular events. *Circulation* 1994; **90:** 1679–87.
6. Weintraub WS, *et al.* Lack of effect of lovastatin on restenosis after coronary angioplasty. *N Engl J Med* 1994; **331:** 1331–7.
7. Downs JR, *et al.* Primary prevention of acute coronary events with lovastatin in men and women with average cholesterol levels: results of AFCAPS/TexCAPS. *JAMA* 1998; **279:** 1615–22.

Preparations
USP 25: Lovastatin Tablets.

Proprietary Preparations (details are given in Part 3)
Aust.: Mevacor; *Braz.:* Mevacor; Reducol; *Canad.:* Mevacor; *Denm.:* Lipivas†; Mevacor; *Fin.:* Lovacol; Mevacor; *Ger.:* Mevinacor; Mevinacor; Mevacor; *Hong Kong:* Medostatin; Mevacor; *Israel:* Lovalip; *Mex.:* Mevacor; *Norw.:* Mevacor; *Port.:* Lipus; Mevinacor; Mevlor; Tecnolip; *Singapore:* Lostatin; Rovacor; *Spain:* Lipofren; Liposcler; Mevacor; Nergadan; Taucor; *USA:* Mevacor.

Low-molecular-weight Heparins

(18636-z)

Depolymerised Heparins; Heparina Massae Molecularis Minoris; LMW Heparins; Low-molecular-mass Heparins.

Pharmacopoeias. In Eur. (see p.vi).

Pharmacopoeial description
Ph. Eur.: Low-molecular-weight heparins are salts of sulfated glucosaminoglycans and have a mass-average molecular mass less than 8000. They are obtained by fractionation or depolymerisation of heparin of natural origin and display different chemical structures at the reducing or the non-reducing end of the polysaccharide chains.
The potency is not less than 70 units of anti-factor Xa activity per mg with reference to the dried substance and the ratio of anti-factor Xa activity to anti-factor IIa (antithrombin) activity is not less than 1.5.
A white or almost white hygroscopic powder. Freely soluble in water. A 1% solution in water has a pH of 5.5 to 8.0. Store in airtight containers.

Units
The first International Standard for low-molecular-weight heparin was established in 1986 and is used to calibrate products for both anti-factor Xa and anti-factor IIa activities. Potency is expressed in terms of units of anti-factor Xa activity per mg and the ratio of anti-factor Xa to anti-factor IIa activity. This ratio differs for individual low-molecular-weight heparins and neither they nor unfractionated heparin can be used interchangeably unit for unit.

Adverse Effects
As for Heparin, p.902.

Effects on the adrenal glands. Hyperkalaemia related to hypoaldosteronism has been reported in patients treated with low-molecular-weight heparins.[1-3] The UK Committee on Safety of Medicines suggests that plasma-potassium concentrations should be monitored in all patients with risk factors for hyperkalaemia, particularly those receiving low-molecular-weight heparins for more than 7 days[4] (see Heparin, p.902).

1. Levesque H, *et al.* Low molecular weight heparins and hypoaldosteronism. *BMJ* 1990; **300:** 1437–8.
2. Canova CR, *et al.* Effect of low-molecular-weight heparin on serum potassium. *Lancet* 1997; **349:** 1447–8.
3. Wiggam MI, Beringer TRO. Effect of low-molecular-weight heparin on serum concentrations of potassium. *Lancet* 1997; **350:** 292–3.
4. Committee on Safety of Medicines/Medicines Control Agency. Suppression of aldosterone secretion by heparin. *Current Problems* 1999; **25:** 6.

Effects on the blood. It was hoped that, because of their higher ratio of anti-factor Xa to anti-thrombin activity compared with heparin, low-molecular-weight heparins might cause less bleeding while maintaining their antithrombotic activity. Some large studies[1,2] have suggested less bleeding with low-molecular-weight heparins than with unfractionated heparin. However, meta-analyses and reviews[3,4] have been unable to confirm a significant reduction in major haemorrhage in patients treated with low-molecular-weight heparins, compared with heparin, for venous thromboembolism, although they confirmed that low-molecular-weight heparins are not associated with an increase in risk.

Thrombocytopenia has also been reported with low-molecular-weight heparins[5-7] although in one study the incidence was less than with unfractionated heparin.[8]

There has also been a report of thrombocytosis in a patient receiving enoxaparin.[9]

1. Levine MN, et al. Prevention of deep vein thrombosis after elective hip surgery: a randomized trial comparing low molecular weight heparin with standard unfractionated heparin. Ann Intern Med 1991; 114: 545–51.
2. Hull RD, et al. Subcutaneous low-molecular-weight heparin compared with continuous intravenous heparin in the treatment of proximal-vein thrombosis. N Engl J Med 1992; 326: 975–82. Correction. ibid. 327: 140.
3. Gould MK, et al. Low-molecular-weight heparins compared with unfractionated heparin for treatment of acute deep venous thrombosis: a meta-analysis of randomized, controlled trials. Ann Intern Med 1999; 130: 800–809.
4. Levine MN, et al. Hemorrhagic complications of anticoagulant treatment. Chest 2001; 119 (suppl): 108S–121S.
5. Eichinger S, et al. Thrombocytopenia associated with low-molecular-weight heparin. Lancet 1991; 337: 1425–6.
6. Lecompte T, et al. Thrombocytopenia associated with low-molecular-weight heparin. Lancet 1991; 338: 1217.
7. Tardy B, et al. Thrombocytopenia associated with low-molecular-weight heparin. Lancet 1991; 338: 1217.
8. Warkentin TE, et al. Heparin-induced thrombocytopenia in patients treated with low-molecular-weight heparin or unfractionated heparin. N Engl J Med 1995; 332: 1330–5.
9. Rizzieri DA, et al. Thrombocytosis associated with low-molecular-weight heparin. Ann Intern Med 1996; 125: 157.

Effects on the skin. Adverse effects of low-molecular-weight heparins on the skin have been reviewed[1] and are estimated to be rare. Most low-molecular-weight heparins have been implicated. Urticarial rash or immediate hypersensitivity has been reported (see below). Delayed hypersensitivity skin reactions have occurred mainly in women. These women were generally postmenopausal, pregnant, or in the postpartum period, suggesting a hormonal influence on pathogenesis. About half of these patients also had a history of allergy to unfractionated heparin.

Skin necrosis reactions are usually localised to the subcutaneous injection site of the low-molecular-weight heparin, although distant lesions have also been reported.

1. Wütschert R, et al. Adverse skin reactions to low molecular weight heparins: frequency, management and prevention. Drug Safety 1999; 20: 515–25.

Hypersensitivity. Reports of hypersensitivity reactions associated with low-molecular-weight heparins are rare. However, a patient being treated with enoxaparin 20 mg subcutaneously daily developed a widespread pruritic urticaria and swelling of lips and tongue after three days of treatment.[1] Antihistamines and prednisone given with enoxaparin failed to control the reaction and enoxaparin treatment was stopped after a further three days. Urticaria and angioedema rapidly resolved on withdrawal of enoxaparin.

Delayed hypersensitivity skin reactions have also been reported (see above).

1. Odeh M, Oliven A. Urticaria and angioedema induced by low-molecular-weight heparin. Lancet 1992; 340: 972–3.

Treatment of Adverse Effects

Severe bleeding with low-molecular-weight heparins, usually caused by accidental overdosage, may be reduced by the slow intravenous administration of protamine sulfate (p.1021). The recommended doses of protamine sulfate are given in the individual monographs and should completely neutralise the antithrombin effect of the low-molecular-weight heparin but will only partially neutralise the anti-factor-Xa effect. Not more than 50 mg of protamine sulfate should be injected for any one dose.

Precautions

As for Heparin, p.903.

Low-molecular-weight heparins should not be given to patients who have developed thrombocytopenia with heparin and who have a positive in-vitro platelet aggregation test (that is, cross-reactivity) with the particular low-molecular-weight heparin to be used.

Spinal anaesthesia. Spinal and epidural haematomas, sometimes leading to paralysis, have occurred in patients receiving low-molecular-weight heparin in association with spinal or epidural anaesthesia or analgesia (see p.903).

Interactions

As for Heparin, p.903.

Pharmacokinetics

Although the precise pharmacokinetic parameters of different low-molecular-weight heparins vary (see individual monographs), they generally have a greater bioavailability after subcutaneous injection and a longer half-life than heparin.

◊ References.
1. Kandrotas RJ. Heparin pharmacokinetics and pharmacodynamics. Clin Pharmacokinet 1992; 22: 359–74.

Uses and Administration

Low-molecular-weight heparins are salts of fragments of heparin produced by chemical or enzymatic depolymerisation of the heparin molecule. Commercially available low-molecular-weight heparins differ in their method of production, molecular-weight range, and degree of sulfation. Like heparin (p.904), these compounds enhance the action of antithrombin III but they are characterised by a higher ratio of anti-factor Xa to anti-factor IIa (antithrombin) activity than heparin. Low-molecular-weight heparins have less effect on platelet aggregation than heparin. They have no significant effect on blood coagulation tests such as activated partial thromboplastin time (APTT). Therapy may be monitored by measurement of plasma-anti-factor-Xa activity but monitoring is less frequently required than with heparin since low-molecular-weight heparins have a more predictable effect.

Low-molecular-weight heparins are used in the managment of venous thromboembolism (deep-vein thrombosis and pulmonary embolism, p.817). They are used for prophylaxis, particularly during surgery, and for treatment of established thromboembolism. They are administered by subcutaneous injection once or twice daily. They are also given intravenously to prevent coagulation during haemodialysis and other extracorporeal circulatory procedures, and subcutaneously in the management of unstable angina (p.791).

Doses are expressed either in terms of the weight of low-molecular-weight heparin or in terms of units of anti-factor Xa activity. Since low-molecular-weight heparins differ in their relative inhibition of factor Xa and thrombin, doses, even when expressed in terms of anti-factor-Xa activity, cannot be equated. Different preparations of the same low-molecular-weight heparin may also have different doses depending on the reference preparation used.

◊ References.
1. Colvin BT, Barrowcliffe TW. The British Society for Haematology guidelines on the use and monitoring of heparin 1992: second revision. J Clin Pathol 1993; 46: 97–103.
2. Green D, et al. Low molecular weight heparin: a critical analysis of clinical trials. Pharmacol Rev 1994; 46: 89–109.
3. Nurmohamed MT, et al. Low molecular weight heparin(oid)s: clinical investigations and practical recommendations. Drugs 1997; 53: 736–51.
4. Weitz JI. Low-molecular-weight heparins. N Engl J Med 1997; 337: 688–98. Correction. ibid.: 1567.
5. Hirsh J, et al. Heparin and low-molecular-weight heparin: mechanisms of action, pharmacokinetics, dosing, monitoring, efficacy, and safety. Chest 2001; 119 (suppl): 64S–94S.

Lubeluzole (17435-r)

Lubeluzole (BAN, USAN, rINN).

R-87926. (S)-1-{4-[1,3-Benzothiazol-2-yl(methyl)amino]piperidino}-3-(3,4-difluorophenoxy)propan-2-ol.
$C_{22}H_{25}F_2N_3O_2S = 433.5$.
CAS — 144665-07-6.

Profile
Lubeluzole is a neuroprotectant under investigation for ischaemic stroke but results have been disappointing.

◊ References.
1. Grotta J. Lubeluzole treatment of acute ischemic stroke. Stroke 1997; 28: 2338–46.
2. Diener HC. Multinational randomised controlled trial of lubeluzole in acute ischaemic stroke. Cerebrovasc Dis 1998; 8: 172–81.
3. Diener HC, et al. Lubeluzole in acute ischemic stroke treatment: a double-blind study with an 8-hour inclusion window comparing a 10-mg daily dose of lubeluzole with placebo. Stroke 2000; 31: 2543–51.

Manidipine Hydrochloride (6487-s)

Manidipine Hydrochloride (rINNM).
CV-4093; Franidipine Hydrochloride. 2-[4-(Diphenylmethyl)-1-piperazinyl]ethyl methyl (±)-1,4-dihydro-2,6-dimethyl-4-(m-nitrophenyl)-3,5-pyridinedicarboxylate dihydrochloride.
$C_{35}H_{38}N_4O_6,2HCl = 683.6$.
CAS — 120092-68-4 (manidipine); 89226-75-5 (manidipine hydrochloride); 126229-12-7 (manidipine hydrochloride).

Profile
Manidipine is a dihydropyridine calcium-channel blocker (see Nifedipine, p.940). It is given by mouth as the hydrochloride in the management of hypertension (p.802) in a usual dose of 10 to 20 mg once daily.

◊ References.
1. Takabatake T, et al. Renal effects of manidipine hydrochloride: a new calcium antagonist in hypertensive patients. Eur J Clin Pharmacol 1993; 45: 321–5.

Preparations
Proprietary Preparations (details are given in Part 3)
Ital.: Iperten; Vascoman; **Jpn:** Calslot; **Thai.:** Madiplot.

Mannitol (2338-w)

Cordycepic Acid; E421; Manita; Manitol; Manna Sugar; Mannite; Mannitolum. D-Mannitol.
$C_6H_{14}O_6 = 182.2$.
CAS — 69-65-8.
ATC — A06AD16; B05BC01; B05CX04.
Pharmacopoeias. In Chin., Eur. (see p.vi), Int., Jpn, Pol., and US.

A hexahydric alcohol related to mannose ($C_6H_{12}O_6 = 180.2$). It is isomeric with sorbitol.

Supersaturated aqueous solutions are prepared with the aid of heat. Any crystals which form during storage of the injection should be dissolved by warming before use; this may be a particular problem with the 20 and 25% injections which are supersaturated. A 5.07% solution in water is iso-osmotic with serum.

Pharmacopoeial description

Ph. Eur.: A white or almost white crystalline powder or free-flowing granules. It exhibits polymorphism. Freely soluble in water; very slightly soluble in alcohol.

USP 25: A white odourless crystalline powder or free-flowing granules with a sweet taste. Soluble 1 in 5.5 of water; very slightly soluble in alcohol; practically insoluble in ether; slightly soluble in pyridine; soluble in alkaline solutions.

Incompatibility. Mannitol should never be added to whole blood for transfusion or given through the same set by which blood is being infused. For details of the adverse effects of mannitol on red blood cells, see Effects on the Blood under Adverse Effects, below.

Adverse Effects

The most common side-effect associated with mannitol therapy is fluid and electrolyte imbalance including circulatory overload and acidosis at high doses. The expansion of extracellular volume can precipitate pulmonary oedema and patients with diminished cardiac reserve are at special risk. The shift of fluid from the intracellular to extracellular compartment can cause tissue dehydration; dehydration of the brain, particularly in patients with renal failure, may give rise to CNS symptoms.

When given by mouth, mannitol causes diarrhoea. Intravenous infusion of mannitol has been associated with nausea, vomiting, thirst, headache, dizziness, chills, fever, tachycardia, chest pain, hyponatraemia, dehydration, blurred vision, urticaria, and hypotension or hypertension. Large doses have been associated rarely with acute renal failure. Hypersensitivity reactions have occurred.

Extravasation of the solution may cause oedema and skin necrosis; thrombophlebitis may occur.

Effects on the blood. Agglutination and irreversible crenation of erythrocytes occurred when blood was mixed with varying proportions of a 10% mannitol solution.[1] It was suggested that intravenous infusions should be carefully controlled and administered at a slow rate. This observation could have particular relevance to patients with sickle-cell disease.[2,3] Although agglutination and crenation had been observed in vitro, dilutional effects would make in-vivo interaction with blood cells less likely.[4]

1. Roberts BE, Smith PH. Hazards of mannitol infusions. Lancet 1966; ii: 421–2.
2. Konotey-Ahulu FID. Hazards of mannitol infusions. Lancet 1966; ii: 591.

3. Roberts BE, Smith PH. Hazards of mannitol infusions. *Lancet* 1966; **ii:** 591.
4. Samson JH. Hazards of mannitol infusions. *Lancet* 1966; **ii:** 1191.

Effects on the gastrointestinal tract. Potentially explosive intracolonic concentrations of hydrogen gas have been measured in patients given mannitol prior to colonoscopy,[1,2] and cases of colonic explosion, including fatalities, have been reported in patients undergoing colonoscopic electrocautery, who had received mannitol bowel preparation. However, the risk of explosion was considered to be small when air or carbon dioxide insufflation and suction were used during the colonoscopy procedure.[2,3]
Colonic perforation and subsequent death has been attributed to the use of mannitol for the treatment of constipation.[4]

1. La Brooy SJ, *et al.* Potentially explosive colonic concentrations of hydrogen after bowel preparation with mannitol. *Lancet* 1981; **i:** 634–6.
2. Avgerinos A, *et al.* Bowel preparation and the risk of explosion during colonoscopic polypectomy. *Gut* 1984; **25:** 361–4.
3. Trotman I, Walt R. Mannitol and explosions. *Lancet* 1981; **i:** 848.
4. Moses FM. Colonic perforation due to oral mannitol. *JAMA* 1988; **260:** 640.

Effects on the kidneys. Focal osmotic nephrosis occurred in a patient who received mannitol 20% intravenously.[1]
Acute oliguric renal failure has been associated with the administration of large doses of mannitol to patients with previously normal renal function.[2-4]

1. Goodwin WE, Latta H. Focal osmotic nephrosis due to the therapeutic use of mannitol: a case of perirenal hematoma after renal biopsy. *J Urol (Baltimore)* 1970; **103:** 11–14.
2. Whelan TV, *et al.* Acute renal failure associated with mannitol intoxication. *Arch Intern Med* 1984; **144:** 2053–5.
3. Goldwasser P, Fotino S. Acute renal failure following massive mannitol infusion: appropriate response of tubuloglomerular feedback? *Arch Intern Med* 1984; **144:** 2214–16.
4. Rabetoy GM, *et al.* Where the kidney is concerned, how much mannitol is too much? *Ann Pharmacother* 1993; **27:** 25–8.

Overdosage. Severe mannitol intoxication was reported in 8 patients with renal failure who had received large, and sometimes enormous, amounts of mannitol intravenously over 1 to 3 days.[1] These patients had CNS involvement out of proportion to uraemia, severe hyponatraemia, a large osmolality gap, and fluid overload. Six patients were treated with haemodialysis and this was considered to be more effective than peritoneal dialysis, which was used in 1 patient.

1. Borges HF, *et al.* Mannitol intoxication in patients with renal failure. *Arch Intern Med* 1982; **142:** 63–6.

Precautions

Mannitol is contra-indicated in patients with pulmonary congestion or pulmonary oedema, intracranial bleeding (except during craniotomy), heart failure (in patients with diminished cardiac reserve, expansion of the extracellular fluid may lead to fulminating heart failure), and in patients with renal failure unless a test dose has produced a diuretic response (if urine flow is inadequate, expansion of the extracellular fluid may lead to acute water intoxication).

Mannitol should not be given with whole blood.

All patients given mannitol should be carefully observed for signs of fluid and electrolyte imbalance and renal function should be monitored.

Pharmacokinetics

Only small amounts of mannitol are absorbed from the gastrointestinal tract. Following intravenous injection mannitol is excreted rapidly by the kidneys before any very significant metabolism can take place in the liver. Mannitol does not cross the blood-brain barrier or penetrate the eye. An elimination half-life of about 100 minutes has been reported.

Uses and Administration

Mannitol is an osmotic agent. Although an isomer of sorbitol, it has little energy value, since it is largely eliminated from the body before any metabolism can take place.

Mannitol is mainly used, with adequate rehydration, to increase urine flow in patients with acute renal failure and to reduce raised intracranial pressure (p.811) and treat cerebral oedema. It is also used in the short-term management of glaucoma (p.1413), especially to reduce intra-ocular pressure prior to ophthalmic surgery, and to promote the excretion of toxic substances by forced diuresis.

Other indications include bladder irrigation during transurethral resection of the prostate in order to reduce haemolysis and oral administration as an osmotic laxative for bowel preparation. Mannitol is used as

a diluent and excipient in pharmaceutical preparations and as a bulk sweetener.

When given parenterally, mannitol raises the osmotic pressure of the plasma thus drawing water out of body tissues and produces an osmotic diuresis. Reduction of cerebrospinal and intra-ocular fluid pressure occurs within 15 minutes of the start of a mannitol infusion and lasts for 3 to 8 hours after the infusion is discontinued; diuresis occurs after 1 to 3 hours.

When used as an osmotic diuretic, mannitol is administered by intravenous infusion. Careful monitoring of fluid balance, electrolytes, renal function, and vital signs is necessary during infusion to prevent fluid and electrolyte imbalance, including circulatory overload and tissue dehydration. Solutions containing more than 15% of mannitol may crystallise during storage, particularly at low temperatures; crystals may be redissolved by warming before use; the administration set should include a filter.

Mannitol may be used to treat patients with **renal failure** (oliguria) or those suspected of inadequate renal function after correction of plasma volume, provided a test dose of about 200 mg per kg body-weight given by rapid intravenous infusion of a 15 to 25% solution over 3 to 5 minutes produces a diuresis of at least 30 to 50 mL per hour during the next 2 to 3 hours; a second test dose is permitted if the response to the first is inadequate. The usual adult dose of mannitol ranges from 50 to 100 g by intravenous infusion of a 5 to 25% solution. The rate of administration is usually adjusted to maintain a urine flow of at least 30 to 50 mL per hour.

For children, a dose of 0.25 to 2 g per kg body-weight has been used.

The total dosage, the concentration, and the rate of administration depend on the fluid requirement, the urinary output, and the nature and severity of the condition being treated. Mannitol infusion has also been used to prevent acute renal failure during cardiovascular and other types of surgery, or following trauma.

To reduce **raised intracranial** or **intra-ocular pressure** mannitol may be given by intravenous infusion as a 15 to 25% solution in a dose of 0.25 to 2 g per kg body-weight over 30 to 60 minutes. Rebound increases in intracranial or intra-ocular pressure may occur but are less frequent than with urea.

During **transurethral prostatic resection** a 2.5 to 5% solution of mannitol has been used for irrigating the bladder.

Ciguatera poisoning. Ciguatera poisoning occurs as a result of the consumption of certain fish contaminated with ciguatoxin found throughout the Caribbean and Indopacific. Symptoms can be severe, including a bizarre reversal of hot and cold sensation. Some neurological symptoms, pruritus, arthralgia, and fatigue, may persist for years.[1] Treatment is usually symptomatic since there is no specific antidote. Dramatic reversal of neuromuscular symptoms with slower resolution of gastrointestinal upset has been reported following administration of mannitol 1 g per kg body-weight by intravenous infusion over 30 to 45 minutes in the acute phase of the illness.[2-4] Treatment with mannitol may also be beneficial up to a week after poisoning.[5] Amitriptyline has been found on several occasions[6-8] to relieve neurological symptoms (dysaesthesia and paraesthesias) and pruritus. Gabapentin has also been reported to be of benefit.[9]

1. Lehane L. Ciguatera update. *Med J Aust* 2000; **172:** 176–9.
2. Palafox NA, *et al.* Successful treatment of ciguatera fish poisoning with intravenous mannitol. *JAMA* 1988; **259:** 2740–2.
3. Pearn JH, *et al.* Ciguatera and mannitol: experience with a new treatment regimen. *Med J Aust* 1989; **151:** 77–80.
4. Williamson J. Ciguatera and mannitol: a successful treatment. *Med J Aust* 1990; **153:** 306–7.
5. Fenner PJ, *et al.* A Queensland family with ciguatera after eating coral trout. *Med J Aust* 1997; **166:** 473–5.
6. Bowman PB. Amitriptyline and ciguatera. *Med J Aust* 1984; **140:** 802.
7. Davis RT, Villar LA. Symptomatic improvement with amitriptyline in ciguatera fish poisoning. *N Engl J Med* 1986; **315:** 65.
8. Calvert GM, *et al.* Treatment of ciguatera fish poisoning with amitriptyline and nifedipine. *J Toxicol Clin Toxicol* 1987; **25:** 423–8.
9. Perez CM, *et al.* Treatment of ciguatera poisoning with gabapentin. *N Engl J Med* 2001; **344:** 692–3.

Gastrointestinal disorders. BOWEL PREPARATION. Mannitol, 1000 mL of a 10% solution or 500 mL of 10 or 20% solution by mouth, has been used to prepare the bowel for surgical and diagnostic procedures.[1,2] The potential for formation of explo-

sive gas in the bowel should be borne in mind (see under Adverse Effects, above).

1. Palmer KR, Khan AN. Oral mannitol: a simple and effective bowel preparation for barium enema. *BMJ* 1979; **2:** 1038.
2. Newstead GL, Morgan BP. Bowel preparation with mannitol. *Med J Aust* 1979; **2:** 582–3.

DIAGNOSIS AND TESTING. Mannitol has been used in combination with lactulose[1,2] and with cellobiose[3,4] in the detection of abnormal small bowel permeability, particularly that occurring in coeliac disease. For further information on the use of differential sugar absorption tests, see Lactulose, p.1230.

1. Pearson ADJ, *et al.* The gluten challenge—biopsy v permeability. *Arch Dis Child* 1983; **58:** 653.
2. Cooper BT. Intestinal permeability in coeliac disease. *Lancet* 1983; **1:** 658–9.
3. Juby LD, *et al.* Cellobiose/mannitol sugar test—a sensitive tubeless test for coeliac disease: results on 1010 unselected patients. *Gut* 1989; **30:** 476–80.
4. Hodges S, *et al.* Cellobiose: mannitol differential permeability in small bowel disease. *Arch Dis Child* 1989; **64:** 853–5.

Preparations

BP 2001: Mannitol Intravenous Infusion;
USP 25: Mannitol in Sodium Chloride Injection; Mannitol Injection.

Proprietary Preparations (details are given in Part 3)
Aust.: Osmofundin 20%; **Austral.:** Mede-Prep; Osmitrol; **Canad.:** Osmitrol; **Fr.:** Manicol†; **Ger.:** Mannit-Losung; Osmofundin 15% N; Osmosteril 20%; Thomaemannit; **Ital.:** Isotol; Mannistol; **Mex.:** Osmorol; **NZ:** Mede-Prep; Resectisol; **Port.:** Osmofundina; **Spain:** Osmofundina Concentrada; **Switz.:** Mannite; **Thai.:** Maniton; **USA:** Osmitrol; Resectisol.

Multi-ingredient: Aust.: Osmofundin 10%; Resectal; **Fin.:** Somanol + Ethanol; **Fr.:** Lyptocodine†; **Ger.:** Freka-Drainjet Purisole; Osmofundin 10%; Osmosteril 10%; **Hong Kong:** Lederscon; **Ital.:** Levoplus; Naturalass; **Port.:** Purisole; Xarope de Macas Rainetas; **Spain:** Jorkil†; Osmofundina; Salcedogen; Salcemetic; Salmagne; **Swed.:** Somanol†; **Switz.:** Bigasan†; Cital†; Purisole†.

Mebutamate (7063-c)

Mebutamate (BAN, USAN, rINN).
W-583. 2-sec-Butyl-2-methyltrimethylene dicarbamate.
$C_{10}H_{20}N_2O_4 = 232.3$.
CAS — 64-55-1.
ATC — N05BC04.

Profile
Mebutamate is a carbamate with general properties similar to those of meprobamate (p.691). It has been given by mouth as an adjunct in the treatment of hypertension in doses of 300 mg up to four times daily.

Preparations
Proprietary Preparations (details are given in Part 3)
Ital.: Sigmafon.

Mebutizide (2339-e)

Mebutizide (rINN).
6-Chloro-3-(1,2-dimethylbutyl)-3,4-dihydro-2H-1,2,4-benzothiadiazine-7-sulphonamide 1,1-dioxide.
$C_{13}H_{20}ClN_3O_4S_2 = 381.9$.
CAS — 3568-00-1.
ATC — C03AA13.

Profile
Mebutizide is a thiazide diuretic (see Hydrochlorothiazide, p.907) which is used in the treatment of oedema and hypertension.

Preparations
Proprietary Preparations (details are given in Part 3)
Belg.: Neoniagar†.

Multi-ingredient: Spain: Triniagar.

Mecamylamine Hydrochloride (880-c)

Mecamylamine Hydrochloride (BANM, rINNM).
Mecamine Hydrochloride. N-Methyl-2,3,3-trimethylbicyclo[2.2.1]hept-2-ylamine hydrochloride.
$C_{11}H_{21}N,HCl = 203.8$.
CAS — 60-40-2 (mecamylamine); 826-39-1 (mecamylamine hydrochloride).
Pharmacopoeias. In US.

Pharmacopoeial description
USP 25: Store in airtight containers.

Adverse Effects, Treatment, and Precautions
As for Trimetaphan Camsilate, p.987. The administration of mecamylamine may also cause tremor, convulsions, choreiform movements, insomnia, sedation, dysarthria, and mental aberrations.

Pharmacokinetics
Mecamylamine hydrochloride is almost completely absorbed from the gastrointestinal tract. It diffuses across the placenta and crosses the blood-brain barrier. About 50% of the dose is

excreted unchanged in the urine over 24 hours, but the rate is diminished in alkaline urine.

Uses and Administration
Mecamylamine hydrochloride is a ganglion blocker with actions similar to those of trimetaphan (p.987). It is used in the management of hypertension (p.802), although other antihypertensives with fewer adverse effects are preferred.

The usual initial dosage is 2.5 mg twice daily by mouth, gradually increased or decreased, usually in steps of 2.5 mg at intervals of not less than 2 days, until a satisfactory response is obtained. The average maintenance dose is 25 mg daily in three divided doses. Tolerance may develop.

Smoking cessation. Mecamylamine acts centrally as a nicotinic antagonist and might be of some benefit in assisting withdrawal from smoking. Two studies[1,2] have shown that addition of oral mecamylamine therapy appeared to enhance the effectiveness of nicotine skin patches. Smoking cessation is discussed under Nicotine, p.1642.

1. Rose JE, et al. Mecamylamine combined with nicotine skin patch facilitates smoking cessation beyond nicotine patch treatment alone. *Clin Pharmacol Ther* 1994; **56:** 86–99.
2. Rose JE, et al. Nicotine-mecamylamine treatment for smoking cessation: the role of pre-cessation therapy. *Exp Clin Psychopharmacol* 1998; **6:** 331–43.

Preparations
USP 25: Mecamylamine Hydrochloride Tablets.

Proprietary Preparations (details are given in Part 3)
USA: Inversine.

Mefruside (2340-b)
Mefruside (BAN, USAN, rINN).

Bay-1500; FBA-1500. 4-Chloro-N^1-methyl-N^1-(tetrahydro-2-methylfurfuryl)benzene-1,3-disulphonamide.
$C_{13}H_{19}ClN_2O_5S_2 = 382.9$.
CAS — 7195-27-9.
ATC — C03BA05.

Pharmacopoeias. In Jpn.

Profile
Mefruside is a diuretic with properties similar to those of the thiazide diuretics (see Hydrochlorothiazide, p.907) even though it does not contain a thiazide ring system. It is used for oedema, including that associated with heart failure (p.798), and for hypertension (p.802).

Diuresis is initiated in about 2 to 4 hours and reaches a maximum between 6 and 12 hours.

In the treatment of oedema the usual dose is 25 to 50 mg daily by mouth, increasing if necessary to 75 to 100 mg. For long-term therapy a dose of 25 to 50 mg every second or third day is preferable.

In the treatment of hypertension the usual dose is 25 mg daily, either alone, or in conjunction with other antihypertensives; initial doses of 25 to 50 mg daily have been recommended; alternate-day maintenance dosage may be used.

Preparations
Proprietary Preparations (details are given in Part 3)
Denm.: Baycaron; *Ger.:* Baycaron†; *Irl.:* Baycaron; *Neth.:* Baycaron; *Norw.:* Baycaron†; *UK:* Baycaron†.

Multi-ingredient: *Ger.:* Bendigon N; duranifin Sali; Nifehexal Sali†; Sali-Adalat; Sali-Prent; Sali-Presinol†.

Meglutol (18802-y)
Meglutol (USAN, rINN).

CB-337. 3-Hydroxy-3-methylglutaric acid.
$C_6H_{10}O_5 = 162.1$.
CAS — 503-49-1.
ATC — C10AX05.

Profile
Meglutol is a lipid regulating drug used in the treatment of hyperlipidaemias (p.800). The usual dose is 1.5 to 3 g daily in divided doses by mouth.

Preparations
Proprietary Preparations (details are given in Part 3)
Ital.: Mevalon.

Melinamide (16885-c)
Melinamide (rINN).

AC-223. N-(α-Methylbenzyl)linoleamide.
$C_{26}H_{41}NO = 383.6$.
CAS — 14417-88-0.

Profile
Melinamide is a lipid regulating drug that has been used in the treatment of hyperlipidaemias.

Mephentermine Sulfate (2078-g)
Mephentermine Sulfate (rINNM).

Mephentermine Sulphate (BANM); Mephentermini Sulfas; Mephedrine Sulphate; Sulfato de Mefentermina. N,α,α-Trimethylphenethylamine sulphate dihydrate.
$(C_{11}H_{17}N)_2,H_2SO_4,2H_2O = 460.6$.
CAS — 100-92-5 (mephentermine); 1212-72-2 (anhydrous mephentermine sulfate); 6190-60-9 (mephentermine sulfate dihydrate).

Pharmacopoeias. In Chin.

Mephentermine base 15 mg is approximately equivalent to 21 mg of mephentermine sulfate.

Adverse Effects, Treatment, and Precautions
Mephentermine may produce CNS stimulation, especially in overdosage; anxiety, drowsiness, incoherence, hallucinations, and convulsions have been reported.

Although the central stimulant effects of mephentermine are much less than those of amfetamine its use may lead to dependence of the amfetamine type.

The hypertensive effects of mephentermine may be treated with an alpha blocker such as phentolamine mesilate.

For the adverse effects of sympathomimetics in general, and precautions to be observed, see Adrenaline, p.829.

Interactions
For the interactions of sympathomimetics in general, see Adrenaline, p.830.

Pharmacokinetics
Mephentermine acts in about 5 to 15 minutes following intramuscular injection and has a duration of action of up to about 4 hours; it acts almost immediately following intravenous injection with a duration of action of up to about 30 minutes. It is rapidly metabolised in the body by demethylation; hydroxylation may follow. It is excreted as unchanged drug and metabolites in the urine; excretion is more rapid in acidic urine.

Uses and Administration
Mephentermine is a sympathomimetic (see Adrenaline, p.831) with mainly indirect effects on adrenergic receptors. It has alpha- and beta-adrenergic activity, and a slight stimulating effect on the CNS. It has an inotropic effect on the heart.

Mephentermine sulfate has been used to maintain blood pressure in hypotensive states, for example following spinal anaesthesia. Typical doses are the equivalent of up to 45 mg of mephentermine base by slow intravenous injection, or 15 to 30 mg intramuscularly.

Preparations
Proprietary Preparations (details are given in Part 3)
USA: Wyamine.

Multi-ingredient: *USA:* Emergent-Ez.

Mepindolol Sulfate (12928-h)
Mepindolol Sulfate (rINNM).

LF-17895 (mepindolol); Mepindolol Sulphate (BANM); SHE-222. 1-Isopropylamino-3-(2-methylindol-4-yloxy)propan-2-ol sulphate.
$(C_{15}H_{22}N_2O_2)_2,H_2SO_4 = 622.8$.
CAS — 23694-81-7 (mepindolol); 56396-94-2 (mepindolol sulfate).

Profile
Mepindolol, the methyl analogue of pindolol, is a non-cardioselective beta blocker (p.844). It is reported to possess intrinsic sympathomimetic activity.

Mepindolol is used by mouth as the sulfate in the management of various cardiovascular disorders, including hypertension, in usual doses of 2.5 to 10 mg daily.

Preparations
Proprietary Preparations (details are given in Part 3)
Aust.: Corindolan; *Ger.:* Corindolan; *Ital.:* Betagon.

Multi-ingredient: *Aust.:* Corindocomb†; *Ger.:* Corindocomb.

Mersalyl Acid (2345-s)
Acidum Mersalylicum; Mersal. Acid; Mersalylum Acidum. A mixture of {3-[2-(carboxymethoxy)benzamido]-2-methoxypropyl}hydroxymercury and its anhydrides.
$C_{13}H_{17}HgNO_6 = 483.9$.
CAS — 486-67-9.

Mersalyl Sodium (2346-w)
Mersalyl (pINN). The sodium salt of mersalyl acid.
$C_{13}H_{16}HgNNaO_6 = 505.8$.
CAS — 492-18-2.
ATC — C03BC01.

Profile
Mersalyl acid, in the form of its salts, is a powerful diuretic that acts on the renal tubules, increasing the excretion of sodium and chloride, in approximately equal amounts, and of water. Organic mercurial diuretics were widely used prior to the introduction of thiazide and other diuretics but have now been almost completely superseded by these orally active drugs which

are both potent and less toxic. The most frequently occurring adverse effects of mersalyl are stomatitis, gastric disturbance, vertigo, febrile reactions, and skin eruptions and irritation. Thrombocytopenia, neutropenia, and agranulocytosis have followed the use of mercurial diuretics. Intravenous injection may cause severe hypotension and cardiac arrhythmias and has been followed by sudden death.

Mersalyl acid was usually given by injection as the sodium salt in conjunction with theophylline as this lessened the local irritant reaction and increased absorption. It was given by deep intramuscular injection after a test dose for hypersensitivity. Other organic mercurial diuretics include chlormerodrin, meralluride, mercaptomerin sodium, mercurophylline sodium, and merethoxylline procaine. They were mainly administered by intramuscular injection or, for those which were less irritant, subcutaneous injection.

Metaraminol Tartrate (2079-q)
Metaraminol Tartrate (BANM, rINNM).

Hydroxynorephedrine Bitartrate; Metadrine Bitartrate; Metaraminol Acid Tartrate; Metaraminol Bitartrate. (−)-2-Amino-1-(3-hydroxyphenyl)propan-1-ol hydrogen tartrate.
$C_9H_{13}NO_2,C_4H_6O_6 = 317.3$.
CAS — 54-49-9 (metaraminol); 33402-03-8 (metaraminol tartrate).

Pharmacopoeias. In Br., Chin., and US.

Metaraminol tartrate 9.5 mg is approximately equivalent to 5 mg of metaraminol.

Pharmacopoeial description

BP 2001: An odourless or almost odourless, white, crystalline powder. Freely soluble in water; sparingly soluble in alcohol; practically insoluble in chloroform and in ether. A 5% solution in water has a pH of 3.2 to 3.5.

USP 25: A 5% solution in water has a pH of between 3.2 and 3.5.

Adverse Effects, Treatment, and Precautions
Metaraminol has a longer duration of action than adrenaline [epinephrine] or noradrenaline [norepinephrine] and therefore an excessive vasopressor response may cause a prolonged rise in blood pressure. Tachycardia or other arrhythmias may also occur. Metaraminol may reduce placental perfusion and should be avoided during pregnancy.

The hypertensive effects of metaraminol may be treated with an alpha blocker such as phentolamine.

Tissue necrosis can occur as a result of accidental extravasation during intravenous injection. Infiltration with phentolamine may be beneficial if extravasation occurs.

For the adverse effects of sympathomimetics in general, and precautions to be observed, see Adrenaline, p.829.

Interactions
For the interactions of sympathomimetics in general, see Adrenaline, p.830.

Pharmacokinetics
Metaraminol acts about 10 minutes after intramuscular injection with a duration of action of up to about 1 hour. Effects are seen 1 to 2 minutes after intravenous injection with a duration of action of about 20 minutes.

Uses and Administration
Metaraminol is a sympathomimetic (see Adrenaline, p.831) with direct and indirect effects on adrenergic receptors. It has alpha- and beta-adrenergic activity, the former being predominant. Metaraminol has an inotropic effect and acts as a peripheral vasoconstrictor, thus increasing cardiac output, peripheral resistance, and blood pressure. Coronary blood flow is increased and the heart rate slowed.

Metaraminol tartrate is used for its pressor action in **hypotensive states** such as those that may occur following spinal anaesthesia. Doses are expressed in terms of the base. An intravenous infusion of 15 to 100 mg per 500 mL of glucose 5% or sodium chloride 0.9% may be used for maintaining the blood pressure, the rate of administration being adjusted according to blood pressure response. Higher concentrations have been given. As the maximum effects are not immediately apparent, at least 10 minutes should elapse before increasing the dose and the possibility of a cumulative effect should be borne in mind. In an emergency an initial dose of 0.5 to 5 mg may be given by direct intravenous injection followed by an intravenous infusion as above.

Metaraminol tartrate has also been given by intramuscular or subcutaneous injection for the prevention of hypotension in doses equivalent to 2 to 10 mg of metaraminol. Subcutaneous injection increases the risk of local tissue necrosis and sloughing.

Diagnosis and testing. The use of metaraminol as a provocative test in the diagnosis of familial Mediterranean fever has been described.[1] Intravenous infusion of metaraminol 10 mg in 500 mL of sodium chloride 0.9% provoked typical symptoms of the disease in 21 patients but this did not occur in 21 control subjects. However, the use of metaraminol for such a purpose has been questioned in terms of safety and possible adverse effects that may be produced.[2,3] Additionally, the specificity, and therefore the reliability, of the test has been doubted.[4]

1. Barakat MH, *et al.* Metaraminol provocative test: a specific diagnostic test for familial Mediterranean fever. *Lancet* 1984; **i:** 656–7.
2. Cattan D, *et al.* Metaraminol provocation test for familial Mediterranean fever. *Lancet* 1984; **i:** 1130–1.
3. Buades J, *et al.* The metaraminol test and adverse cardiac effects. *Ann Intern Med* 1989; **111:** 259–60.
4. Ben-Chetrit E, *et al.* Dopamine-β-hydroxylase activity in familial Mediterranean fever. *Lancet* 1990; **335:** 176.

Priapism. Metaraminol in low dosage and dilute solution, by intracavernosal injection, has been used successfully to treat priapism associated with a variety of conditions; these have included drug-induced priapism,[1] as a complication of chronic myeloid leukaemia,[2] associated with haemodialysis,[3] and during spinal block[4] or fentanyl-induced general anaesthesia.[4] It may be used to reverse the effects of alprostadil or papaverine given for the management of some types of erectile dysfunction. However, this use of metaraminol by intracavernosal injection has been associated with fatal hypertensive crisis (see also Alprostadil, p.1440).

Alternatives include the use of corporal aspiration followed by intracavernosal phenylephrine in low dosage and dilute solution in patients with low-flow priapism (due to decreased penile venous outflow);[5] in high-flow priapism (due to increased arterial inflow), which is less of an emergency, embolisation of the source of abnormal inflow is used. Surgery is usually favoured in low-flow priapism unresponsive to drug therapy. Phenylpropanolamine[5] and pseudoephedrine[6] have both been given by mouth as an alternative to phenylephrine or metaraminol injection. Intracavernosal irrigation with a dilute adrenaline [epinephrine] solution has been used for priapism caused by sickle-cell disease (see p.832).

1. Brindley GS. New treatment for priapism. *Lancet* 1984; **ii:** 220–1.
2. Stanners A, Colin-Jones D. Metaraminol for priapism. *Lancet* 1984; **ii:** 978.
3. Branger B, *et al.* Metaraminol for haemodialysis-associated priapism. *Lancet* 1985; **i:** 641.
4. Tsai SK, Hong CY. Intracavernosal metaraminol for treatment of intraoperative penile erection. *Postgrad Med J* 1990; **66:** 831–3.
5. Harmon WJ, Nehra A. Priapism: diagnosis and management. *Mayo Clin Proc* 1997; **72:** 350–5.
6. Millard RJ, *et al.* Risks of self-injection therapy for impotence. *Med J Aust* 1996; **165:** 117–18.

Preparations

BP 2001: Metaraminol Injection;
USP 25: Metaraminol Bitartrate Injection.

Proprietary Preparations (details are given in Part 3)
Austral.: Aramine; *Belg.:* Aramine; *Braz.:* Aramin; *Hong Kong:* Aramine; *Ital.:* Levicor†; *Norw.:* Aramine; *NZ:* Aramine; *Thai.:* Aramine; *UK:* Aramine; *USA:* Aramine.

Methazolamide (2347-e)

Methazolamide (BAN, rINN).
N-(4-Methyl-2-sulphamoyl-Δ²-1,3,4-thiadiazolin-5-ylidene)acetamide.
$C_5H_8N_4O_3S_2 = 236.3.$
CAS — 554-57-4.
Pharmacopoeias. In US.

Pharmacopoeial description

USP 25: A white or faintly yellow crystalline powder with a slight odour. Very slightly soluble in water and in alcohol; slightly soluble in acetone; soluble in dimethylformamide. Protect from light.

Adverse Effects and Precautions

As for Acetazolamide, p.826.

◊ Cholestatic hepatitis with jaundice, rash, and subsequent pure red cell aplasia was associated with methazolamide in a patient.[1] Drug-induced hypersensitivity was suspected as the cause of the reaction.

1. Krivoy N, *et al.* Methazolamide-induced hepatitis and pure RBC aplasia. *Arch Intern Med* 1981; **141:** 1229–30.

Pharmacokinetics

Methazolamide is absorbed from the gastrointestinal tract more slowly than acetazolamide. It has been reported not to be extensively bound to plasma protein, and to have a half-life of about 14 hours. About 15 to 30% of the dose is excreted in the urine; the fate of the remainder is unknown.

Uses and Administration

Methazolamide is an inhibitor of carbonic anhydrase with actions similar to those of acetazolamide (p.827). It is used in the management of glaucoma (p.1413) in doses of 50 to 100 mg two or three times daily by mouth. Its action is less prompt but of longer duration than that of acetazolamide, lasting for 10 to 18 hours.

The diuretic activity of methazolamide is less pronounced than that of acetazolamide.

Preparations

USP 25: Methazolamide Tablets.

Proprietary Preparations (details are given in Part 3)
Austral.: Neptazane; *Canad.:* Neptazane; *Israel:* Neptazane; *Thai.:* Neptazane; *USA:* GlaucTabs; MZM; Neptazane.

Methoxamine Hydrochloride (2080-d)

Methoxamine Hydrochloride (BANM, rINNM).
Methoxamedrine Hydrochloride. 2-Amino-1-(2,5-dimethoxyphenyl)propan-1-ol hydrochloride.
$C_{11}H_{17}NO_3,HCl = 247.7.$
CAS — 390-28-3 (methoxamine); 61-16-5 (methoxamine hydrochloride).
Pharmacopoeias. In Br. and Chin.

Pharmacopoeial description

BP 2001: Colourless crystals or white plate-like crystals or white crystalline powder; odourless or almost odourless. Freely soluble in water; soluble in alcohol; very slightly soluble in chloroform and in ether. A 2% solution in water has a pH of 4.0 to 6.0.

Adverse Effects, Treatment, and Precautions

Methoxamine may induce a desire to micturate and a pilomotor reaction (goose flesh). The hypertensive effects of methoxamine may be treated with an alpha blocker such as phentolamine. Atropine may be given if reflex bradycardia is significant.

For the adverse effects of sympathomimetics in general, and precautions to be observed, see Adrenaline, p.829.

Interactions

For the interactions of sympathomimetics in general, see Adrenaline, p.830.

Pharmacokinetics

Methoxamine acts within about 2 minutes of intravenous injection and within about 15 to 20 minutes of intramuscular injection; the duration of action of these two routes is about 10 to 15 minutes and about 1.5 hours respectively.

Uses and Administration

Methoxamine is a sympathomimetic (see Adrenaline, p.831) with mainly direct effects on adrenergic receptors. It has alpha-adrenergic activity entirely; beta-adrenergic activity is not demonstrable and beta-adrenoceptor blockade has been postulated. Methoxamine causes prolonged peripheral vasoconstriction and consequently a rise in arterial blood pressure. It has little effect on the heart, though reflex bradycardia may occasionally occur. It has a marked pilomotor effect but does not stimulate the CNS or cause bronchodilatation. It markedly reduces blood flow to the kidney.

Methoxamine hydrochloride is used for its pressor action in **hypotensive states** (p.805), notably in general or spinal anaesthesia; it may be used in patients who have received cyclopropane or halothane anaesthesia. It is given intramuscularly in usual doses of 10 to 15 mg (range 5 to 20 mg). As the maximum effects are not immediately apparent, about 15 minutes should elapse before repeating a dose. In an emergency 3 to 5 mg may be given by slow intravenous injection (at a rate of 1 mg per minute); doses of up to 10 mg have been employed. In children, doses of 70 to 280 μg per kg body-weight intramuscularly or 40

---

to 70 μg per kg by slow intravenous injection have been employed.

Methoxamine hydrochloride may be given for **paroxysmal supraventricular tachycardia** unresponsive to other therapies (p.794) in doses of 10 mg by slow intravenous injection over 3 to 5 minutes.

Methoxamine hydrochloride has also been used for its vasoconstrictor effect in the management of **nasal congestion** (p.1082). It has been administered by nasal drops or a spray.

Preparations

BP 2001: Methoxamine Injection.

Proprietary Preparations (details are given in Part 3)
Aust.: Vasoxine†; *Austral.:* Vasylox Junior†; *Canad.:* Vasoxyl; *Irl.:* Vasoxine; *UK:* Vasoxine; *USA:* Vasoxyl.

Methyclothiazide (2348-I)

Methyclothiazide (BAN, USAN, rINN).
NSC-110431. 6-Chloro-3-chloromethyl-3,4-dihydro-2-methyl-2H-1,2,4-benzothiadiazine-7-sulphonamide 1,1-dioxide.
$C_9H_{11}Cl_2N_3O_4S_2 = 360.2.$
CAS — 135-07-9.
ATC — C03AA08.
Pharmacopoeias. In US.

Pharmacopoeial description

USP 25: A white or practically white crystalline powder, odourless or with a slight odour. Very slightly soluble to practically insoluble in water and in chloroform; soluble 1 in 92.5 of alcohol and 1 in 2700 of ether; freely soluble in acetone and in pyridine; sparingly soluble in methyl alcohol; very slightly soluble in benzene.

Profile

Methyclothiazide is a thiazide diuretic with properties similar to those of hydrochlorothiazide (see p.907). It is used for oedema, including that associated with heart failure (p.798), and for hypertension (p.802).

Diuresis is initiated in about 2 hours, reaches a peak at about 6 hours, and lasts for 24 hours or more.

In the treatment of oedema the usual initial dose is 2.5 to 5 mg by mouth daily, increasing to a maximum dose of 10 mg daily if necessary. In the treatment of hypertension the usual dose is 2.5 to 5 mg daily, either alone, or in conjunction with other antihypertensives. Doses of up to 10 mg daily have been suggested, but this may not result in an increased hypotensive effect. Children have been given a dose of 50 to 200 μg per kg body-weight daily.

Preparations

USP 25: Methyclothiazide Tablets.

Proprietary Preparations (details are given in Part 3)
Austral.: Enduron†; *Hong Kong:* Enduron; *USA:* Aquatensen; Enduron.

Multi-ingredient: *Fr.:* Isobar; *Hong Kong:* Enduronyl; *Ital.:* Enduronil; *USA:* Diutensen-R; Enduronyl.

Methyldopa (882-a)

Methyldopa (BAN, USAN, rINN).
Alpha-methyldopa; Methyldopum; Methyldopum Hydratum; Metildop; MK-351. (−)-3-(3,4-Dihydroxyphenyl)-2-methyl-L-alanine sesquihydrate; (−)-2-Amino-2-(3,4-dihydroxybenzyl)propionic acid sesquihydrate.
$C_{10}H_{13}NO_4,1\frac{1}{2}H_2O = 238.2.$
CAS — 555-30-6 (anhydrous methyldopa); 41372-08-1 (methyldopa sesquihydrate).
Pharmacopoeias. In Eur. (see p.vi), Int., Jpn, and US.

Methyldopa sesquihydrate 1.13 g is approximately equivalent to 1 g of anhydrous methyldopa.

Pharmacopoeial description

Ph. Eur.: Colourless or almost colourless crystals or a white to yellowish-white crystalline powder. Slightly soluble in water; very slightly soluble in alcohol; practically insoluble in ether; freely soluble in dilute mineral acids. Protect from light.

USP 25: A white to yellowish-white odourless fine powder which may contain friable lumps. Sparingly soluble in water; slightly soluble in alcohol; practically insoluble in ether; very soluble in 3N hydrochloric acid. Protect from light.

Methyldopate Hydrochloride (883-t)

Methyldopate Hydrochloride (BANM, USAN).
Cloridrato de Metildopato. The hydrochloride of the ethyl ester of anhydrous methyldopa; Ethyl (−)-2-amino-2-(3,4-dihydroxybenzyl)propionate hydrochloride.
$C_{12}H_{17}NO_4,HCl = 275.7.$
CAS — 2544-09-4 (methyldopate); 2508-79-4 (methyldopate hydrochloride).
Pharmacopoeias. In Br. and US.

The symbol † denotes a preparation no longer actively marketed

Pharmacopoeial description

BP 2001: A white or almost white, odourless or almost odourless, crystalline powder. Freely soluble in water, in alcohol, and in methyl alcohol; slightly soluble in chloroform; practically insoluble in ether. A 1% solution in water has a pH of 3.0 to 5.0. Protect from light.

USP 25: A white or almost white, odourless or almost odourless, crystalline powder. Freely soluble in water, in alcohol, and in methyl alcohol; slightly soluble in chloroform; practically insoluble in ether. A 1% solution in water has a pH of between 3.0 and 5.0.

Incompatibility. A haze developed over 3 hours when methyldopate hydrochloride 1 g per litre was mixed with amphotericin B 200 mg per litre in glucose injection; crystals were produced with methohexital sodium 200 mg per litre in sodium chloride injection, but a haze developed when they were mixed in glucose injection. A crystalline precipitate occurred with tetracycline hydrochloride 1 g per litre in glucose injection, and with sulfadiazine sodium 4 g per litre in glucose injection or sodium chloride injection.[1]

1. Riley BB. Incompatibilities in intravenous solutions. *J Hosp Pharm* 1970; **28:** 228–40.

Adverse Effects

The adverse effects of methyldopa are mostly consequences of its pharmacological action. The incidence of adverse effects overall may be as high as 60% but most are transient or reversible. Drowsiness is common, especially initially and following an increase in dosage. Dizziness and lightheadedness may be associated with postural hypotension; nausea, headache, weakness and fatigue, and decreased libido and impotence have also been reported quite frequently.

The mental and neurological effects of methyldopa have included impaired concentration and memory, mild psychoses, depression, disturbed sleep and nightmares, paraesthesias, Bell's palsy, involuntary choreoathetotic movements, and parkinsonism.

In addition to postural hypotension, methyldopa is frequently associated with fluid retention and oedema, which responds to diuretics but may rarely progress to heart failure. Angina pectoris may be aggravated. Bradycardia, syncope, and prolonged carotid sinus hypersensitivity have been reported. Intravenous administration of methyldopate has been associated with a paradoxical rise in blood pressure.

Methyldopa may produce gastrointestinal disturbances including nausea and vomiting, diarrhoea, constipation, and rarely pancreatitis and colitis. A black or sore tongue, and inflammation of the salivary glands, have occurred, and dry mouth is quite common.

A positive Coombs' test may occur in 10 to 20% of all patients on prolonged therapy but only a small proportion develop haemolytic anaemia. Thrombocytopenia and leucopenia, notably granulocytopenia, have occurred and warrant prompt discontinuation. Other hypersensitivity effects have included myocarditis, fever, eosinophilia, and disturbances of liver function. Hepatitis may develop, particularly in the first 2 or 3 months of therapy, and is generally reversible on discontinuation, but fatal hepatic necrosis has occurred. Antinuclear antibodies may develop and cases of a lupus-like syndrome have been reported.

Other adverse effects that have been reported in patients receiving methyldopa include rashes, lichenoid and granulomatous eruptions, toxic epidermal necrolysis, a flu-like syndrome (of fever, myalgia, and mild arthralgia), nocturia, uraemia, nasal congestion, and retroperitoneal fibrosis. Hyperprolactinaemia may occur, with breast enlargement or gynaecomastia, galactorrhoea, and amenorrhoea.

Methyldopa may occasionally cause urine to darken on exposure to the air because of the breakdown of the drug or its metabolites.

◊ Reviews.
1. Furhoff A-K. Adverse reactions with methyldopa—a decade's reports. *Acta Med Scand* 1978; **203:** 425–8.
2. Lawson DH, *et al.* Adverse reactions to methyldopa with particular reference to hypotension. *Am Heart J* 1978; **96:** 572–9.

Effects on the blood. An analysis of drug-induced blood dyscrasias reported to the Swedish Adverse Drug Reaction Committee for the 10-year period 1966-75 showed that haemolytic anaemia attributable to methyldopa had been reported on 69 occasions and had caused 3 deaths. This represented the vast majority of all the reports of drug-induced haemolytic anae-

mia.[1] However, the actual incidence of haemolytic anaemia in patients receiving methyldopa is quite low; data from the Boston Collaborative Drug Surveillance Program indicated that only 2 of 1067 patients receiving methyldopa developed haemolytic anaemia,[2] an incidence of about 0.2%. The proportion of patients with a positive Coombs' test is much higher, being variously reported[3-5] at 10 to 20%. It has been suggested that the high incidence of autoantibody formation may be due to inhibition of suppressor T-cells by methyldopa[4] while the relatively low incidence of resultant haemolysis may be due to drug-associated impairment of the reticuloendothelial system which would normally clear the antibody-sensitised cells from the circulation.[5]

1. Böttiger LE, *et al.* Drug-induced blood dyscrasias. *Acta Med Scand* 1979; **205:** 457–61.
2. Lawson DH, *et al.* Adverse reactions to methyldopa with particular reference to hypotension. *Am Heart J* 1978; **96:** 572–9.
3. Carstairs K, *et al.* Methyldopa and haemolytic anaemia. *Lancet* 1966; **i:** 201.
4. Kirtland HH, *et al.* Methyldopa inhibition of suppressor-lymphocyte function: a proposed cause of autoimmune hemolytic anemia. *N Engl J Med* 1980; **302:** 825–32.
5. Kelton JG. Impaired reticuloendothelial function in patients treated with methyldopa. *N Engl J Med* 1985; **313:** 596–600.

Effects on the gastrointestinal tract. COLITIS. There has been a report of 6 cases of colitis associated with methyldopa.[1] An auto-immune mechanism was proposed.

1. Graham CF, *et al.* Acute colitis with methyldopa. *N Engl J Med* 1981; **304:** 1044–5.

DIARRHOEA. Severe chronic diarrhoea over a 2-year period in a 62-year-old woman was associated with methyldopa therapy. Diarrhoea stopped immediately after discontinuation of methyldopa.[1] In another case[2] progressively severe diarrhoea in an elderly senile patient, which had persisted for 7 years, stopped when methyldopa was withdrawn and recurred, after a delay, when the drug was resumed in a lower dose. Discontinuation of methyldopa resulted in complete freedom from diarrhoea and faecal incontinence within 7 days.

1. Quart BD, Guglielmo BJ. Prolonged diarrhea secondary to methyldopa therapy. *Drug Intell Clin Pharm* 1983; **17:** 462.
2. Gloth FM, Busby MJ. Methyldopa-induced diarrhea: a case of iatrogenic diarrhea leading to request for nursing home placement. *Am J Med* 1989; **87:** 480–1.

PANCREATITIS. Increases in serum- and urinary-amylase activity accompanied by fever and suggestive of pancreatitis were associated with methyldopa in 2 patients,[1] one of whom had symptoms of severe pancreatitis. Symptoms reappeared on rechallenge in both patients. A further report of acute pancreatitis in a patient who had recently begun methyldopa therapy (with a diuretic) also confirmed a recurrence of symptoms on rechallenge.[2] In contrast to the acute form, chronic pancreatitis is not generally attributable to drug treatment.[3] However, a case of florid chronic pancreatitis, with exocrine and endocrine insufficiency and heavy calcification over 30 months, associated with 2 periods of methyldopa treatment, has been reported.[4] Symptoms in this patient, who was also receiving a thiazide, included severe diabetic ketoacidosis.

1. van der Heide H, *et al.* Pancreatitis caused by methyldopa. *BMJ* 1981; **282:** 1930–1.
2. Anderson JR, *et al.* Drug-associated recurrent pancreatitis. *Dig Surg* 1985; **2:** 24–6.
3. Banergee AK, *et al.* Drug-induced acute pancreatitis. *Med Toxicol Adverse Drug Exp* 1989; **4:** 186–98.
4. Ramsay LE, *et al.* Methyldopa-induced chronic pancreatitis. *Practitioner* 1982; **226:** 1166–9.

Effects on the heart. Sudden death in a number of patients receiving methyldopa has been associated with myocarditis, often in association with hepatitis and pneumonitis.[1,2] The effect is thought to be due to hypersensitivity. Hypersensitivity myocarditis is generally marked by ECG changes, a slight rise in cardiac enzymes, cardiomegaly, and persistent sinus tachycardia, along with peripheral blood eosinophilia, and most patients will recover within days if the drug is withdrawn in time.[3]

1. Mullick FG, McAllister HA. Myocarditis associated with methyldopa therapy. *JAMA* 1977; **237:** 1699–1701. Correction. *ibid.*; **238:** 399.
2. Seeverens H, *et al.* Myocarditis and methyldopa. *Acta Med Scand* 1982; **211:** 233–5.
3. Anonymous. Myocarditis related to drug hypersensitivity. *Lancet* 1985; **ii:** 1165–6.

Effects on the liver. In a report of 6 cases of hepatitis in patients taking methyldopa, including a review of 77 cases from the literature,[1] most patients presented with symptoms including malaise, fatigue, anorexia, weight loss, nausea, and vomiting, and histopathological changes resembling those of viral hepatitis. Fever occurred in 28 of the 83 patients; rashes and eosinophilia occurred rarely. Symptoms usually began 1 to 4 weeks after the first dose of methyldopa. Clinically apparent jaundice occurred as early as 1 week and as late as 3 years after the initiation of therapy, although only 6 or 7 patients presented with jaundice later than 3 months. Liver damage was not dose-related and had features suggestive of an immunologically-mediated hypersensitivity reaction. The histological changes included chronic active hepatitis, massive fatal necrosis, and cirrhosis.

In a further analysis of 36 patients with liver damage due to methyldopa, hepatic injury tended to occur in 2 phases—acute and chronic.[2] Acute liver damage developed within a few months of starting treatment with methyldopa, and was considered to be an allergic reaction to methyldopa metabolites. The

chronic form usually occurred at least a year after starting methyldopa, and was characterised by an accumulation of fat in the liver. Recovery after withdrawal of methyldopa was directly related to duration of exposure and degree of liver damage. There was also a suggestion of genetic predisposition, as acute methyldopa-induced liver damage occurred in 4 members of a family. Idiosyncratic metabolism of methyldopa in susceptible patients may be responsible for expression of an antigen on the surface of liver cells with which circulating antibodies react.[3]

See also under Fever, below.

1. Rodman JS, *et al.* Methyldopa hepatitis: a report of six cases and review of the literature. *Am J Med* 1976; **60:** 941–8.
2. Sotaniemi EA, *et al.* Hepatic injury and drug metabolism in patients with alpha-methyldopa-induced liver damage. *Eur J Clin Pharmacol* 1977; **12:** 429–35.
3. Neuberger J, *et al.* Antibody mediated hepatocyte injury in methyldopa induced hepatotoxicity. *Gut* 1985; **26:** 1233–9.

Effects on mental function. Anecdotal reports have implicated methyldopa in the production of disturbances of mental acuity including inability to concentrate, an impaired calculating ability, and forgetfulness.[1-3] These have been confirmed to some extent by psychometric studies. Impaired verbal memory but not visual memory has been reported in 10 patients receiving methyldopa with a diuretic.[4] A crossover study in 16 patients also indicated impairment of cognitive function by methyldopa.[5]

1. Adler S. Methyldopa-induced decrease in mental activity. *JAMA* 1974; **230:** 1428–9.
2. Ghosh SK. Methyldopa and forgetfulness. *Lancet* 1976; **i:** 202–3.
3. Fernandez PG. Alpha methyldopa and forgetfulness. *Ann Intern Med* 1976; **85:** 128.
4. Solomon S, *et al.* Impairment of memory function by antihypertensive medication. *Arch Gen Psychiatry* 1983; **40:** 1109–12.
5. Johnson B, *et al.* Effects of methyldopa on psychometric performance. *J Clin Pharmacol* 1990; **30:** 1102–5.

DEPRESSION. Depression has been associated with methyldopa therapy, although the exact relationship is unclear.[1] One review[2] reported the incidence to be 3.6% and suggested that depression was more common in patients with a previous history.

1. Patten SB, Love EJ. Drug-induced depression. *Drug Safety* 1994; **10:** 203–19.
2. Paykel ES, *et al.* Psychiatric side effects of antihypertensive drugs other than reserpine. *J Clin Psychopharmacol* 1982; **2:** 14–39.

Effects on the nervous system. Involuntary choreoathetotic movements resembling those of Huntington's chorea began in a 59-year-old man with cerebrovascular disease following increase of his methyldopa dose from 1 to 1.5 g daily. He recovered when methyldopa therapy was withdrawn.[1] In another report methyldopa was associated with the development of bilateral choreiform movements in a patient without cerebrovascular disease but with chronic renal failure.[2]

1. Yamadori A, Albert ML. Involuntary movement disorder caused by methyldopa. *N Engl J Med* 1972; **286:** 610.
2. Neil EM, Waters AK. Generalized choreiform movements as a complication of methyldopa therapy in chronic renal failure. *Postgrad Med J* 1981; **57:** 732–3.

Effects on sexual function. Methyldopa has been associated with numerous cases of sexual dysfunction. In males failure to maintain erection, decreased libido, impaired ejaculation, and gynaecomastia have occurred, while in females decreased libido, painful breast enlargement, and delayed or absent orgasm have been reported.[1] The reported incidence varies and there is some evidence[2] that sexual dysfunction may be underreported: while only 2 of 30 men receiving methyldopa spontaneously reported erection failure the actual incidence on questioning was 16 of 30.

1. Stevenson JG, Umstead GS. Sexual dysfunction due to antihypertensive agents. *Drug Intell Clin Pharm* 1984; **18:** 113–21.
2. Alexander WD, Evans JI. Side effects of methyldopa. *BMJ* 1975; **2:** 501.

Fever. In a report of 78 cases of methyldopa-induced fever,[1] fever occurred 5 to 35 days after the first exposure to methyldopa in 77 patients and one day after recommencing methyldopa in the remaining patient. Rigors, headache, and myalgia were common accompanying symptoms, but eosinophilia and skin rashes were not seen. The majority of patients did not appear seriously ill, but 4 patients presented the picture of septic shock. Biochemical evidence of liver damage was found in 61% of patients but jaundice was uncommon. In the majority of patients, symptoms were relieved within 48 hours of the withdrawal of the drug.

1. Stanley P, Mijch A. Methyldopa: an often overlooked cause of fever and transient hepatocellular dysfunction. *Med J Aust* 1986; **144:** 603–5.

Lupus erythematosus. The incidence of antinuclear antibodies was 13% in 269 hypertensive patients taking methyldopa (irrespective of other medication), compared with 3.8% in 448 hypertensive patients not taking methyldopa.[1] Apart from the occasional case of methyldopa-induced lupus, however, patients do not appear to be at risk.

1. Wilson JD, *et al.* Antinuclear antibodies in patients receiving non-practolol beta-blockers. *BMJ* 1978; **1:** 14–16.

Overdosage. Ingestion of methyldopa 2.5 g produced coma, hypothermia, hypotension, bradycardia, and dry mouth in a 19-year-old man.[1] The serum-methyldopa concentration 10 hours after ingestion was 19.2 µg per mL compared with serum concentrations of approximately 2 µg per mL in patients receiving therapeutic doses of methyldopa. The patient recovered following treatment with intravenous fluids.

1. Shnaps Y, et al. Methyldopa poisoning. *J Toxicol Clin Toxicol* 1982; **19:** 501–3.

Retroperitoneal fibrosis. A 60-year-old patient developed retroperitoneal fibrosis and a positive direct Coombs' test associated with methyldopa given in a daily dose of 750 mg with bendrofluazide [bendroflumethiazide] 2.5 mg for about 5 years.[1]

1. Iversen BM, et al. Retroperitoneal fibrosis during treatment with methyldopa. *Lancet* 1975; **ii:** 302–4.

Treatment of Adverse Effects

Withdrawal of methyldopa or reduction in dosage causes the reversal of many side-effects. If overdosage occurs activated charcoal may be given or the stomach may be emptied by lavage. Treatment is largely symptomatic, but if necessary, intravenous fluid infusions may be given to promote urinary excretion, and vasopressors given cautiously. Severe hypotension may respond to placing the patient in the supine position with the feet raised.

Methyldopa is dialysable.

Precautions

Methyldopa should be used with caution in patients with impaired renal or hepatic function or with a history of haemolytic anaemia, liver disease, or depression. Care is also advisable in patients with parkinsonism. It should not be given to patients with active liver disease or depression and it is not recommended for phaeochromocytoma.

It is advisable to make periodic blood counts and to perform liver function tests at intervals during the first 6 to 12 weeks of treatment or if the patient develops an unexplained fever. Patients taking methyldopa may produce a positive response to a direct Coombs' test; if blood transfusion is required, prior knowledge of a positive direct Coombs' test reaction will aid cross-matching.

Methyldopa may cause sedation; if affected patients should not drive or operate machinery.

Porphyria. Methyldopa has been associated with acute attacks of porphyria and is considered unsafe in porphyric patients.

Pregnancy and breast feeding. Methyldopa is commonly used in the management of hypertension occurring during pregnancy (p.802). There is little evidence of adverse effects on fetal development. However, methyldopa crosses the placenta[1] and reduced blood pressure has been reported in infants born to mothers receiving methyldopa.[2] There has also been a report of tremor in 7 infants associated with maternal methyldopa therapy during pregnancy.[3] Depressed noradrenaline concentrations in the CSF were noted in the 3 infants examined leading to successful treatment of the other 4 infants with atropine: tremor was abolished in 2 and substantially reduced in the other 2 infants.

A small amount of methyldopa may be distributed into breast milk.[1]

1. Jones HMR, Cummings AJ. A study of the transfer of α-methyldopa to the human foetus and newborn infants. *Br J Clin Pharmacol* 1978; **6:** 432–4.
2. Whitelaw A. Maternal methyldopa treatment and neonatal blood pressure. *BMJ* 1981; **283:** 471.
3. Bódis J, et al. Methyldopa in pregnancy hypertension and the newborn. *Lancet* 1982; **ii:** 498–9.

Interactions

The hypotensive effects of methyldopa are potentiated by diuretics, other antihypertensives, and drugs with hypotensive effects. However, there have been reports of paradoxical antagonism of the hypotensive effects by tricyclic antidepressants, antipsychotics, and beta blockers. Sympathomimetics may also antagonise the hypotensive effects.

There may be an interaction between methyldopa and MAOIs and care is required if they are given concomitantly. Caution is also needed with entacapone since it might inhibit the metabolism of methyldopa.

Patients receiving methyldopa may require lower doses of general anaesthetics.

Alpha blockers. Urinary incontinence occurred on concomitant administration of methyldopa and *phenoxybenzamine* in a patient who had undergone bilateral lumbar sympathectomy.[1]

1. Fernandez PG, et al. Urinary incontinence due to interaction of phenoxybenzamine and α-methyldopa. *Can Med Assoc J* 1981; **124:** 174–5.

The symbol † denotes a preparation no longer actively marketed

Antipsychotics. Antipsychotics may enhance the hypotensive effects of methyldopa but a paradoxical increase in blood pressure has also been reported. A woman with systemic lupus erythematosus taking *trifluoperazine* up to 15 mg daily and prednisone up to 120 mg daily was given methyldopa up to 2 g and triamterene for high blood pressure.[1] Her blood pressure rose further to 200/140 mmHg. After discontinuation of trifluoperazine blood pressure returned to 160/100 mmHg.

In another report, 2 patients with essential hypertension who had been receiving methyldopa for 3 years and 18 months respectively developed symptoms of dementia within days of concurrent administration of *haloperidol* for anxiety.[2] In both patients the symptoms resolved rapidly on discontinuation of haloperidol.

1. Westervelt FB, Atuk NO. Methyldopa-induced hypertension. *JAMA* 1974; 557.
2. Thornton WE. Dementia induced by methyldopa with haloperidol. *N Engl J Med* 1976; **294:** 1222.

Cephalosporins. A pustular pruritic eruption occurred following administration of *cefazolin sodium* to a patient receiving methyldopa.[1] A previous similar case has been reported in a patient receiving *cefradine* and methyldopa.

1. Stough D, et al. Pustular eruptions following administration of cefazolin: a possible interaction with methyldopa. *J Am Acad Dermatol* 1987; **16:** 1051–2.

Digoxin. Syncope associated with carotid sinus hypersensitivity has been reported to be possibly enhanced by methyldopa in a patient taking digoxin and chlortalidone.[1] In another report,[2] sinus bradycardia developed in 2 patients taking methyldopa and digoxin concomitantly.

1. Bauernfeind R, et al. Carotid sinus hypersensitivity with alpha methyldopa. *Ann Intern Med* 1978; **88:** 214–15.
2. Davis JC, et al. Sinus node dysfunction caused by methyldopa and digoxin. *JAMA* 1981; **245:** 1241–3.

Iron. Following results in healthy subjects which indicated that the absorption of methyldopa was reduced by 73% and 61% respectively when taken with a dose of *ferrous sulfate* or *ferrous gluconate*, 5 hypertensive patients receiving methyldopa were also given ferrous sulfate 325 mg three times daily for 2 weeks.[1] All patients experienced a rise in systolic pressure, and 4 had a rise in diastolic pressure, associated with ferrous sulfate administration, amounting to more than 15/10 mmHg in some patients after 2 weeks. Blood pressure fell again when the iron therapy was discontinued.

1. Campbell N, et al. Alteration of methyldopa absorption, metabolism, and blood pressure control caused by ferrous sulfate and ferrous gluconate. *Clin Pharmacol Ther* 1988; **43:** 381–6.

Levodopa. For reference to a mutual interaction between methyldopa and levodopa, see Antihypertensives, under Levodopa, Interactions, p.1171.

Lithium. For reference to the development of lithium toxicity on concurrent administration of methyldopa, see p.295.

Sympathomimetics. A 31-year-old man whose hypertension was well controlled with methyldopa and oxprenolol suffered a severe hypertensive episode when he took a preparation for a cold containing *phenylpropanolamine*.[1]

1. McLaren EH. Severe hypertension produced by interaction of phenylpropanolamine with methyldopa and oxprenolol. *BMJ* 1976; **2:** 283–4.

Pharmacokinetics

Following oral administration methyldopa is variably and incompletely absorbed, apparently by an amino-acid active transport system. The mean bioavailability has been reported to be about 50%. It is extensively metabolised and is excreted in urine mainly as unchanged drug and the *O*-sulfate conjugate. It crosses the blood-brain barrier and is decarboxylated in the CNS to active alpha-methylnoradrenaline.

The elimination is biphasic with a half-life of about 1.7 hours in the initial phase; the second phase is more prolonged. Clearance is decreased and half-life prolonged in renal impairment. Plasma protein binding is reported to be minimal. Methyldopa crosses the placenta; small amounts are distributed into breast milk.

Uses and Administration

Methyldopa is an antihypertensive that is thought to have a predominantly central action. It is decarboxylated in the CNS to alpha-methylnoradrenaline which is thought to stimulate alpha$_2$ adrenoceptors resulting in a reduction in sympathetic tone and a fall in blood pressure. It may also act as a false neurotransmitter, and have some inhibitory actions on plasma renin activity. Methyldopa reduces the tissue concentrations of dopamine, noradrenaline, adrenaline, and serotonin.

Methyldopa is used in the management of hypertension (p.802), although other drugs with fewer adverse

effects are generally preferred. Methyldopa may, however, be the treatment of choice for hypertension in pregnancy. Oedema and tolerance sometimes associated with methyldopa therapy may be reduced when it is given with a thiazide diuretic.

Methyldopa is given by mouth as the sesquihydrate, but doses are usually expressed in terms of anhydrous methyldopa. For hypertensive crises, methyldopa has been given intravenously as methyldopate hydrochloride.

When methyldopa is given by mouth its effects reach a maximum in 4 to 6 hours following a single dose, although the maximum hypotensive effect may not occur until the second or third day of continuous treatment; some effect is usually apparent for 48 hours after withdrawal of methyldopa. When given intravenously the hypotensive effect may be obtained within 4 to 6 hours and last for 10 to 16 hours. It lowers the standing, and to a lesser extent the supine, blood pressure.

In **hypertension**, the usual initial adult dose by mouth is 250 mg of methyldopa two or three times daily for 2 days; this is then adjusted by small increments or decrements, not more frequently than every 2 days, according to the response of the patient. Although higher doses have been given, it is generally considered that no advantage can be gained by giving doses larger than 3 g daily. The usual maintenance dosage is 0.5 to 2 g of methyldopa daily. In the elderly an initial dose of 125 mg twice daily has been used; this dose may be increased gradually if necessary, but should not exceed 2 g daily.

An initial dose for children is 10 mg per kg body-weight daily in 2 to 4 divided doses, increased as necessary to a maximum of 65 mg per kg or 3 g daily, whichever is less.

The usual adult dose by intravenous injection is 250 to 500 mg of methyldopate hydrochloride in 100 mL of glucose 5% administered over 30 to 60 minutes every 6 hours; the dose should not exceed 1 g every 6 hours. Children may be given 5 to 10 mg per kg every 6 hours. The maximum daily dose for children is 65 mg per kg or 3 g, whichever is less.

Preparations

BP 2001: Methyldopa Tablets; Methyldopate Injection;
USP 25: Methyldopa and Chlorothiazide Tablets; Methyldopa and Hydrochlorothiazide Tablets; Methyldopa Oral Suspension; Methyldopa Tablets; Methyldopate Hydrochloride Injection.

Proprietary Preparations (details are given in Part 3)
Aust.: Aldometil; Presinol; *Austral.:* Aldomet; Aldopren; Hydopa; Nudopa†; *Belg.:* Aldomet; *Braz.:* Aldomet; Cardin; *Canad.:* Aldomet; Novo-Medopa; Nu-Medopa; *Denm.:* Aldomet; Dopamet†; *Fr.:* Aldomet; *Ger.:* Dopegyt; Presinol; Sembrina†; *Hong Kong:* Aldomet; Dopamet; Dopegyt; *Irl.:* Aldomet; Dopamet†; Meldopa; *Israel:* Aldomin; *Ital.:* Aldomet; Medopren; *Mex.:* Aldomet; Amender; Ehlindopa; Hipten; Medopal; Prodop; Pulsoton; Selm; Tenzona; Toparal; Yuremetil D; *Neth.:* Aldomet; Sembrina†; *Norw.:* Aldomet; Dopamet†; *NZ:* Aldomet; Prodopa; *Port.:* Aldomet; *S.Afr.:* Aldomet; Alphamex†; Arcanadopa†; Hy-Po-Tone; Normopress; Pharmet†; Sinepress; *Singapore:* Dopegyt; *Spain:* Aldomet; *Swed.:* Aldomet; *Switz.:* Aldomet; Dopamet†; *Thai.:* Aldomet; Dopamed; Dopasian; Dopegyt; Isomet; Medopa; Medopate; Mefpa; Servidopa; Siamdopa; *UK:* Aldomet; Dopamet†; *USA:* Medomet; Metalpha†; *USA:* Aldoclor.

Multi-ingredient: *Aust.:* Aldoretic; *Braz.:* Hydromet; *Canad.:* Aldoril†; Apo-Methazide; Novo-Doparil†; Supres; *Ger.:* Sali-Presinol†; *Irl.:* Hydromet†; *Ital.:* Medozide; Saludopin; *Neth.:* Hydromet†; *Port.:* Aldoretic†; *S.Afr.:* Aldoretic; *Swed.:* Hydromet†; *Switz.:* Aldoretic; *USA:* Aldoclor; Aldoril.

Meticrane (12953-m)

Meticrane *(rINN)*.

SD-17102. 6-Methylthiochroman-7-sulphonamide 1,1-dioxide.
$C_{10}H_{13}NO_4S_2 = 275.3$.
CAS — 1084-65-7.
ATC — C03BA09.

Pharmacopoeias. In Jpn.

Profile

Meticrane is a thiazide diuretic (see Hydrochlorothiazide, p.907) that has been used in the treatment of hypertension.

Metildigoxin (5820-r)

Metildigoxin (rINN).

Medigoxin (BAN); β-Methyl Digoxin; β-Methyldigoxin. 3β-[(O-2,6-Dideoxy-4-O-methyl-D-ribo-hexopyranosyl-(1→4)-O-2,6-dideoxy-D-ribo-hexopyranosyl-(1→4)-2,6-dideoxy-D-ribo-hexopyranosyl)oxy]-12β,14-dihydroxy-5β,14β-card-20(22)-enolide.

$C_{42}H_{66}O_{14}$ = 795.0.
CAS — 30685-43-9.
ATC — C01AA08.

Pharmacopoeias. In Jpn. as $C_{42}H_{66}O_{14}, \frac{1}{2}C_3H_6O$.

Adverse Effects, Treatment, and Precautions
As for Digoxin, p.870.

Interactions
As for Digoxin, p.871.

Calcium-channel blockers. For a report of an interaction between metildigoxin and *diltiazem*, see Calcium-channel Blockers, under Interactions of Digoxin, p.872.

Pharmacokinetics
Metildigoxin is rapidly and almost completely absorbed from the gastrointestinal tract and at steady state a half-life of 54 to 60 hours has been reported. Demethylation to digoxin occurs. About 60% of an oral or intravenous dose is excreted in the urine as unchanged drug and metabolites over 7 days.

Hepatic impairment. Hepatic demethylation of metildigoxin was reduced in 12 patients with cirrhosis of the liver compared with 12 healthy subjects. This resulted in a reduction in metildigoxin clearance, a smaller volume of distribution, and a significantly higher serum concentration.[1]

1. Rameis H, et al. Changes in metildigoxin pharmacokinetics in cirrhosis of the liver: a comparison with β-acetyldigoxin. *Int J Clin Pharmacol Ther Toxicol* 1984; **22:** 145–51.

Renal impairment. For reference to the pharmacokinetics of metildigoxin in patients with renal impairment, see under Uses and Administration, below.

Uses and Administration
Metildigoxin is a cardiac glycoside with positive inotropic activity. It has actions similar to those of digoxin (p.873) and may be used in the treatment of some cardiac arrhythmias (p.794) and in heart failure (p.798).

The onset of action of metildigoxin is more rapid than that of digoxin. When metildigoxin is given by mouth an effect may appear within 5 to 20 minutes and a maximum effect on the myocardium may be seen in 15 to 30 minutes. The duration of action is similar to or a little longer than that of digoxin; therapeutic plasma concentrations are also similar. In stabilised patients a dose of 300 µg of metildigoxin is as effective as 500 µg of digoxin.

Metildigoxin may be given by mouth or intravenously. Initial doses of 150 to 600 µg daily by mouth may be given depending upon whether rapid or slow digitalisation is desired; digitalisation is usually performed over 2 to 4 days and the larger doses are given in divided daily doses. A daily dose of 400 µg intravenously for 3 days may also be employed. Maintenance therapy is continued with 50 to 300 µg daily by mouth in divided doses.

Dosage should be reduced in patients with renal impairment.

Administration in renal impairment. Fairly good non-linear correlation was found between creatinine clearance and metildigoxin half-life in a study of 15 patients with chronic renal impairment, including 8 undergoing haemodialysis, and 4 patients with heart failure and unimpaired renal function. The mean elimination half-life was 5.62 days in patients undergoing dialysis (clearance essentially 0 mL per minute) and 3.41 days in the other patients with chronic renal impairment (clearance 15 to 50 mL per minute) compared with 1.49 days in patients with normal renal function (clearance 62 to 96 mL per minute). It was recommended that patients undergoing dialysis should be given 30 to 50% of the usual dose initially.[1] Other studies have suggested[2] that dose reduction may be necessary in renal impairment when creatinine clearance is below 50 mL per minute per 1.48 m^2 body-surface.

1. Trovato GM, et al. Relationship between β-methyl-digoxin pharmacokinetic and degree of renal impairment. *Curr Ther Res* 1983; **33:** 158–64.
2. Tsutsumi K, et al. Pharmacokinetics of beta-methyldigoxin in subjects with normal and impaired renal function. *J Clin Pharmacol* 1993; **33:** 154–60.

Preparations

Proprietary Preparations (details are given in Part 3)
Aust.: Lanitop; *Belg.:* Lanitop; *Braz.:* Lanitop; *Ger.:* Lanitop; *Hong Kong:* Lanitop; *Ital.:* Cardiolan†; Lanitop; Miopat; *Jpn:* Lanirapid†; *Port.:* Lanitop; *Spain:* Lanirapid; *Switz.:* Lanitop.

Multi-ingredient: *Aust.:* Coro-Lanitop†; Theo-Lanitop†.

Metipranolol (6313-w)

Metipranolol (BAN, USAN, rINN).
BMOI-004; Methypranolol; VUAB-6453 (SPOFA); VUFB-6453. 1-(4-Acetoxy-2,3,5-trimethylphenoxy)-3-isopropylaminopropan-2-ol; 4-(2-Hydroxy-3-isopropylaminopropoxy)-2,3,6-trimethylphenyl acetate.
$C_{17}H_{27}NO_4$ = 309.4.
CAS — 22664-55-7.
ATC — S01ED04.

NOTE. MPR is a code approved by the BP 2001 for use on single unit doses of eye drops containing metipranolol where the individual container may be too small to bear all the appropriate labelling information.
Pharmacopoeias. In Br.

Pharmacopoeial description
BP 2001: A white crystalline powder. Practically insoluble in water; soluble in alcohol, in acetone, and in methyl alcohol; dissolves in dilute mineral acids. The filtrate of a 2.5% suspension in water has a pH of 9.0 to 10.0. Protect from light.

Adverse Effects, Treatment, and Precautions
As for beta blockers, p.844.

Conjunctivitis, conjunctival leukoplakia, transient stinging, as well as other ocular adverse effects have been reported with metipranolol eye drops. Granulomatous anterior uveitis has been reported mainly in the UK and it has been suggested that this effect may be associated with changes induced by radiation sterilisation of metipranolol eye drops in their final container.

Effects on the lungs. Acute pulmonary oedema, secondary to the negative inotropic and chronotropic effects of beta blockade, developed in a 72-year-old woman who had been instilling one drop daily of metipranolol 0.3% eye drops into each eye for about six weeks.[1] Symptoms cleared over about 10 hours, but reappeared following accidental rechallenge. It was suggested that drug had accumulated over the six-week period, possibly due to deficient metabolism.

1. Johns MD, Ponte CD. Acute pulmonary edema associated with ocular metipranolol use. *Ann Pharmacother* 1995; **29:** 370–3.

Interactions
The interactions associated with beta blockers are discussed on p.846.

Uses and Administration
Metipranolol is a non-cardioselective beta blocker (p.844). It is reported to be largely lacking in intrinsic sympathomimetic activity and membrane-stabilising properties.

Metipranolol is used in the management of open-angle glaucoma (p.1413). It has also been used in the management of cardiovascular disorders.

To reduce raised intra-ocular pressure in open-angle glaucoma and ocular hypertension, eye drops containing metipranolol 0.1 or 0.3% are used twice daily.

Preparations

BP 2001: Metipranolol Eye Drops.

Proprietary Preparations (details are given in Part 3)
Aust.: Beta-Ophtiole; *Belg.:* Beta-Ophtiole; *Ger.:* Betamann; *Ital.:* Turoptin; *Mon.:* Betanol; *Neth.:* Beta-Ophtiole; *Port.:* Beta-Ophtiole; *S.Afr.:* Beta-Ophtiole; *Singapore:* Beta-Ophtiole; *Switz.:* Turoptin; *Thai.:* Beta-Ophtiole; *USA:* OptiPranolol.

Multi-ingredient: *Aust.:* Betacarpin; Torrat; *Belg.:* Normoglaucon; *Ger.:* Normoglaucon; Torrat; Tri-Torrat; *Hong Kong:* Torrat; *Ital.:* Ripix; *Neth.:* Normoglaucon; *Port.:* Normoglaucon; *Singapore:* Normoglaucon; *Switz.:* Ripix; *Thai.:* Normoglaucon.

Metirosine (15325-f)

Metirosine (BAN, rINN).
L-588357-0; Metyrosine (USAN); MK-781. (−)-α-Methyl-L-tyrosine; 4-Hydroxy-α-methylphenylalanine.
$C_{10}H_{13}NO_3$ = 195.2.
CAS — 672-87-7 (metirosine); 620-30-4 (racemetirosine).
ATC — C02KB01.

NOTE. The term α-methyltyrosine (α-MPT; α-MT; α-methyl-*p*-tyrosine) is used below since although metirosine, the (−)-isomer, is the active form the manufacturers state that some racemate (racemetirosine; (±)-α-methyl-DL-tyrosine) is produced during synthesis but that the material supplied contains mainly (−)-isomer with a small amount of (+)-isomer.
The code name MK-781, applied to earlier investigational material, may have described a racemate or a preparation containing a smaller proportion of (−)-isomer than the product now available commercially.

Potency of the proprietary preparation (Demser) is expressed in terms of metirosine.
Pharmacopoeias. In US.

Adverse Effects
Sedation occurs in almost all patients receiving α-methyltyrosine. Other adverse effects include extrapyramidal symptoms, such as trismus and frank parkinsonism; anxiety, depression, and psychic disturbances including hallucinations, disorientation, and confusion; and diarrhoea, which may be severe. Crystalluria, transient dysuria, and haematuria have been seen in a few patients. There have also been occasional reports of slight swelling of the breast, galactorrhoea, nasal congestion, decreased salivation, gastrointestinal disturbances, headache, impotence or failure of ejaculation, and hypersensitivity reactions. Eosinophilia, raised serum aspartate aminotransferase, and peripheral oedema have been reported rarely.

◊ Neuroleptic malignant syndrome occurred after the use of the dopamine-depleting drugs tetrabenazine and α-methyltyrosine in a patient with Huntington's chorea.[1]

1. Burke RE, et al. Neuroleptic malignant syndrome caused by dopamine-depleting drugs in a patient with Huntington disease. *Neurology* 1981; **31:** 1022–6.

Precautions
To minimise the risk of crystalluria, patients receiving α-methyltyrosine should have a fluid intake sufficient to maintain a urine volume of at least 2 litres daily and their urine should be examined regularly for the presence of crystals.

α-Methyltyrosine has sedative effects and patients should be warned of the hazards of driving a motor vehicle or operating machinery while receiving the drug. Symptoms of psychic stimulation and insomnia may occur when α-methyltyrosine is withdrawn.

When α-methyltyrosine is used pre-operatively in patients with phaeochromocytoma, blood pressure and the ECG should be monitored continuously during surgery as the danger of hypertensive crises and arrhythmias is not obviated. Concomitant alpha blockade (e.g. with phentolamine) may be required; a beta blocker or lignocaine [lidocaine] may be needed for the management of arrhythmias. Blood volume must be maintained during and after surgery, particularly if an alpha blocker is used concurrently, in order to avoid hypotension.

Interactions
The sedative effects of α-methyltyrosine may be potentiated by alcohol and other CNS depressants. Concomitant administration with phenothiazines or haloperidol may exacerbate extrapyramidal effects.

Pharmacokinetics
α-Methyltyrosine is well absorbed from the gastrointestinal tract and is excreted mainly unchanged by the kidneys. A plasma half-life of 3.4 to 7.2 hours has been reported. Less than 1% of a dose may be excreted as the metabolites α-methyldopa, α-methyldopamine, α-methylnoradrenaline, and α-methyltyramine.

Uses and Administration
α-Methyltyrosine is an inhibitor of the enzyme tyrosine hydroxylase, and consequently of the synthesis of catecholamines. It is used to control the symptoms of excessive sympathetic stimulation in patients with phaeochromocytoma (p.810) and decreases the frequency and severity of hypertensive attacks and related symptoms in most patients. It may be given for pre-operative preparation, or for long-term management in those for whom surgery is contra-indicated or who have malignant phaeochromocytoma.

In the management of phaeochromocytoma, α-methyltyrosine is given by mouth in a dose of 250 mg four times daily, increased daily by 250 mg or 500 mg to a maximum of 4 g daily in divided doses. The optimum dose, achieved by monitoring clinical symptoms and catecholamine excretion, is usually in the range of 2 to 3 g daily and when used pre-operatively it should be given for at least 5 to 7 days before surgery. The concomitant use of alpha blockers may be necessary.

α-Methyltyrosine is not effective in controlling essential hypertension.

α-Methyltyrosine has also been tried in patients with schizophrenia.

Preparations

USP 25: Metyrosine Capsules.

Proprietary Preparations (details are given in Part 3)
Neth.: Demser†; *UK:* Demser†; *USA:* Demser.

Metolazone (2349-y)

Metolazone (BAN, USAN, rINN).
SR-720-22. 7-Chloro-1,2,3,4-tetrahydro-2-methyl-4-oxo-3-o-tolylquinazoline-6-sulphonamide.
$C_{16}H_{16}ClN_3O_3S$ = 365.8.
CAS — 17560-51-9.
ATC — C03BA08.
Pharmacopoeias. In US.

Pharmacopoeial description
USP 25: Store in airtight containers. Protect from light.

Adverse Effects and Treatment

As for Hydrochlorothiazide, p.907. Metolazone has also been reported to cause palpitations, chest pain, and chills.

Effects on the blood. Profound neutropenia was observed in a 58-year-old woman within 10 days of starting treatment with metolazone.[1] Neutropenia persisted for a further 10 days after metolazone was withdrawn. No other haematological abnormalities were observed.

1. Donovan KL. Neutropenia and metolazone. *BMJ* 1989; **299:** 981.

Effects on the nervous system. Two patients experienced acute muscle cramps with impairment of consciousness and epileptiform movements after taking metolazone 5 mg (single dose) or 2.5 mg daily for 3 days.[1]

1. Fitzgerald MX, Brennan NJ. Muscle cramps, collapse, and seizures in two patients taking metolazone. *BMJ* 1976; **1:** 1381–2.

Precautions

As for Hydrochlorothiazide, p.909.

Interactions

As for Hydrochlorothiazide, p.909. Severe electrolyte disturbances may occur when metolazone and frusemide [furosemide] are used concurrently.

ACE inhibitors. Deterioration in renal function occurred in a 65-year-old woman when metolazone 5 mg [daily] was added to treatment with *captopril*, frusemide [furosemide], spironolactone, and digoxin for heart failure.[1] An interaction between captopril and metolazone was suspected and both drugs were discontinued with a subsequent return to normal renal function. It was suggested that natriuresis and a fall in blood pressure caused by the diuretic may have compromised an already low renal perfusion pressure when autoregulatory mechanisms were blocked by captopril.

1. Hogg KJ, Hillis WS. Captopril/metolazone induced renal failure. *Lancet* 1986; **i:** 501–2.

Antidiabetics. Hypoglycaemia occurred in a patient with type 2 diabetes mellitus controlled with *glibenclamide* 40 hours after initiation of therapy with metolazone 5 mg daily.[1] Studies of protein binding *in vitro* did not reveal any evidence of displacement of glibenclamide from binding sites.

1. George S, *et al.* Possible protein binding displacement interaction between glibenclamide and metolazone. *Eur J Clin Pharmacol* 1990; **38:** 93–5.

Ciclosporin. An increase in serum-creatinine concentration in a renal transplant patient was attributed to a toxic drug interaction between metolazone and ciclosporin.[1] Serum-creatinine concentrations returned to pretreatment values when metolazone was discontinued.

1. Christensen P, Leski M. Nephrotoxic drug interaction between metolazone and cyclosporin. *BMJ* 1987; **294:** 578.

Pharmacokinetics

Metolazone is slowly and incompletely absorbed from the gastrointestinal tract. An average of about 65% of a dose has been reported to be absorbed after oral administration in healthy subjects, and an average of about 40% in patients with cardiac disease. In some countries a formulation with enhanced bioavailability is available. About 95% of the drug is bound in the circulation; about 50 to 70% to the red blood cells and between 15 and 33% to plasma proteins. The half-life has been reported to be 8 to 10 hours in whole blood, and 4 to 5 hours in plasma, but the diuretic effect persists for up to 24 hours or more. About 70 to 80% of the amount of metolazone absorbed is excreted in the urine, of which 80 to 95% is excreted unchanged. The remainder is excreted in the bile and some enterohepatic circulation has been reported. Metolazone crosses the placental barrier and is distributed into breast milk.

◊ References.

1. Tilstone WJ, *et al.* Pharmacokinetics of metolazone in normal subjects and in patients with cardiac or renal failure. *Clin Pharmacol Ther* 1974; **16:** 322–9.

Uses and Administration

Metolazone is a diuretic with actions and uses similar to those of the thiazide diuretics (see Hydrochlorothiazide, p.910) even though it does not contain a thiazide ring system. It is used for oedema, including that associated with heart failure (p.798), and for hypertension (p.802).

Unlike thiazides in general, metolazone is reported to be effective in patients with a glomerular filtration rate of less than 20 mL per minute. Diuresis is initiat-

ed in about 1 hour, reaches a peak in about 2 hours, and lasts for 12 to 24 hours depending on the dose.

In some countries a preparation is available with enhanced bioavailability which is effective in lower doses than conventional formulations. Doses given in *Martindale* refer to the conventional tablet formulation unless otherwise stated.

In the treatment of **oedema** the usual dose is 5 to 10 mg by mouth daily; in some cases doses of 20 mg or more may be required. No more than 80 mg should be given in any 24-hour period. In refractory cases, metolazone has been used in combination with frusemide [furosemide] or other loop diuretics, but the electrolyte balance should be monitored closely.

In the treatment of **hypertension** the usual dose is 2.5 to 5 mg daily either alone, or in conjunction with other antihypertensives. An initial dose of 1.25 mg has also been employed. The dosage may be adjusted after 3 to 4 weeks according to response. A maintenance dose of 5 mg on alternate days has been used. Formulations with enhanced bioavailability are given in doses of 0.5 to 1 mg daily in the treatment of hypertension. They are not bioequivalent to the conventional tablet formulation and should not be used interchangeably.

Preparations

USP 25: Metolazone Tablets.

Proprietary Preparations (details are given in Part 3)
Aust.: Birobin; *Austral.:* Diulo†; *Canad.:* Zaroxolyn; *Ger.:* Zaroxolyn; *Irl.:* Zaroxolyn†; *Ital.:* Zaroxolyn; *Mex.:* Zaroxolyn; *Port.:* Diulo; *S.Afr.:* Zaroxolyn; *Spain:* Diondel†; *Swed.:* Zaroxolyn; *Switz.:* Zaroxolyne; *UK:* Metenix 5; *USA:* Diulo†; Mykrox; Zaroxolyn.

Metoprolol Tartrate (6314-e)

Metoprolol Tartrate (BANM, USAN, rINNM).

CGP-2175E; H-93/26; Metoprololi Tartras. (±)-1-Isopropylamino-3-[4-(2-methoxyethyl)phenoxy]propan-2-ol tartrate. $(C_{15}H_{25}NO_3)_2,C_4H_6O_6 = 684.8$.

CAS — 54163-88-1 (metoprolol); 37350-58-6 (metoprolol); 98418-47-4 (metoprolol succinate); 56392-17-7 (metoprolol tartrate).

Pharmacopoeias. In *Chin., Eur.* (see p.vi) and *US.*
US also includes Metoprolol Fumarate. *Eur.* and *US* also include Metoprolol Succinate.

Pharmacopoeial description

Ph. Eur.: A white crystalline powder or colourless crystals. It exhibits polymorphism. Very soluble in water; freely soluble in alcohol. A 2% solution in water has a pH of between 6.0 and 7.0. Protect from light.

USP 25: A white crystalline powder. Very soluble in water; freely soluble in alcohol, in chloroform, and in dichloromethane; slightly soluble in acetone; insoluble in ether. A 10% solution in water has a pH of between 6.0 and 7.0. Store in airtight containers. Protect from light.

Stability. Metoprolol tartrate 0.4 mg per mL in glucose 5% or sodium chloride 0.9% was stable for 36 hours when stored at 24° in PVC bags.[1]

1. Belliveau PP, *et al.* Stability of metoprolol tartrate in 5% dextrose injection or 0.9% sodium chloride injection. *Am J Hosp Pharm* 1993; **50:** 950–2.

Adverse Effects, Treatment, and Precautions

As for beta blockers, p.844.

Effects on bones and joints. Five cases of arthralgia associated with the use of metoprolol had been reported to the FDA; 6 reports of similar symptoms associated with propranolol, and one with atenolol, had been reported.[1] A case of polymyalgia rheumatic-like syndrome has also been reported.[2]

1. Sills JM, Bosco L. Arthralgia associated with β-adrenergic blockade. *JAMA* 1986; **255:** 198–9.
2. Snyder S. Metoprolol-induced polymyalgia-like syndrome. *Ann Intern Med* 1991; **114:** 96–7.

Effects on the gastrointestinal tract. Reports of retroperitoneal fibrosis in a patient who had been taking metoprolol and nifedipine[1] and of sclerosing peritonitis in a patient receiving metoprolol.[2]

1. Thompson J, Julian DG. Retroperitoneal fibrosis associated with metoprolol. *BMJ* 1982; **284:** 83–4.
2. Clark CV, Terris R. Sclerosing peritonitis associated with metoprolol. *Lancet* 1983; **i:** 937.

Effects on hearing. Loss of hearing in a patient receiving metoprolol appeared to be dose-related;[1] hearing gradually improved over several months once the drug was withdrawn.

1. Fäldt R, *et al.* β Blockers and loss of hearing. *BMJ* 1984; **289:** 1490–2.

Effects on lipid metabolism. Beta blockers may increase serum-triglyceride concentrations. For a report of acute pancreatitis provoked by severe hypertriglyceridaemia in a patient taking atenolol and metoprolol, see p.845.

Effects on the liver. Acute hepatitis associated with metoprolol has been reported in a 56-year-old woman.[1] The hepatotoxicity could not be explained by deficient oxidation of metoprolol; drug oxidation phenotyping showed she was an extensive metaboliser of debrisoquine and hence metoprolol.

For debate as to whether the polymorphic oxidation of metoprolol contributes to the incidence of adverse effects, see Metabolism, under Pharmacokinetics, below.

1. Larrey D, *et al.* Metoprolol-induced hepatitis: rechallenge and drug oxidation phenotyping. *Ann Intern Med* 1988; **108:** 67–8.

Interactions

The interactions associated with beta blockers are discussed on p.846.

Pharmacokinetics

Metoprolol is readily and completely absorbed from the gastrointestinal tract but is subject to considerable first-pass metabolism. Peak plasma concentrations vary widely and occur about 1.5 to 2 hours after a single oral dose. It is moderately lipid-soluble.

Metoprolol is widely distributed; it crosses the blood-brain barrier, the placenta, and is distributed into breast milk. It is slightly bound to plasma protein. It is extensively metabolised in the liver by oxidative deamination, O-dealkylation followed by oxidation, and aliphatic hydroxylation. The metabolites are excreted in the urine together with only small amounts of unchanged metoprolol. The rate of hydroxylation to α-hydroxymetoprolol is determined by genetic polymorphism; the half-life of metoprolol in fast hydroxylators is stated to be 3 to 4 hours, whereas in poor hydroxylators it is about 7 hours.

The elderly. Several studies[1-3] indicate that age-related physiological changes have negligible effects on the pharmacokinetics of metoprolol.

1. Quarterman CP, *et al.* The effect of age on the pharmacokinetics of metoprolol and its metabolites. *Br J Clin Pharmacol* 1981; **11:** 287–94.
2. Regårdh CG, *et al.* Pharmacokinetics of metoprolol and its metabolite α-OH-metoprolol in healthy, non-smoking, elderly individuals. *Eur J Clin Pharmacol* 1983; **24:** 221–6.
3. Larsson M, *et al.* Pharmacokinetics of metoprolol in healthy, elderly, non-smoking individuals after a single dose and two weeks of treatment. *Eur J Clin Pharmacol* 1984; **27:** 217–22.

Metabolism. Metoprolol exhibits a debrisoquine-type genetic polymorphism with poor metabolisers of metoprolol also being poor metabolisers of debrisoquine.[1-3] However, the clinical relevance of the polymorphism has been questioned, since there has been no correlation shown between poor metaboliser status and increased incidence of adverse effects.[4,5]

The subject may be further confused by variations in the phenotype between ethnic groups. Although the incidence of the poor metaboliser phenotype in whites of European origin is reported to be about 9%, a study in 138 Nigerians[6] failed to identify evidence of polymorphic metabolism, and the authors caution against extrapolation of data between different racial groups.

1. Lennard MS, *et al.* Defective metabolism of metoprolol in poor hydroxylators of debrisoquine. *Br J Clin Pharmacol* 1982; **14:** 301–3.
2. Lennard MS, *et al.* Oxidation phenotype—a major determinant of metoprolol metabolism and response. *N Engl J Med* 1982; **307:** 1558–60.
3. McGourty JC, *et al.* Metoprolol metabolism and debrisoquine oxidation polymorphism—population and family studies. *Br J Clin Pharmacol* 1985; **20:** 555–66.
4. Regårdh CG, Johnsson G. Interindividual variations in metoprolol metabolism—some clinical and other observations. *Br J Clin Pharmacol* 1984; **17:** 495–6.
5. Clark DWJ, *et al.* Adverse effects from metoprolol are not generally associated with oxidation status. *Br J Clin Pharmacol* 1984; **18:** 965–6.
6. Iyun AO, *et al.* Metoprolol and debrisoquin metabolism in Nigerians: lack of evidence for polymorphic oxidation. *Clin Pharmacol Ther* 1986; **40:** 387–94.

Pregnancy and breast feeding. The clearance of metoprolol was increased fourfold in 5 pregnant women during the last trimester, compared with that some months after delivery; this was probably due to enhanced hepatic metabolism in the pregnant state.[1]

The disposition of metoprolol was investigated in newborn infants of mothers treated with metoprolol 50 to 100 mg twice daily.[2] In 15 of the 17 neonates plasma-metoprolol concentrations increased in the first 2 to 5 hours of the postnatal period, then declined over the next 15 hours; 5 of these infants had no detectable metoprolol concentrations in the umbilical plasma. No infant demonstrated signs of beta blockade.

The symbol † denotes a preparation no longer actively marketed

Only a small amount of metoprolol appears to be distributed into breast milk.

1. Högstedt S, *et al.* Increased oral clearance of metoprolol in pregnancy. *Eur J Clin Pharmacol* 1983; **24**: 217–20.
2. Lundborg P, *et al.* Disposition of metoprolol in the newborn. *Br J Clin Pharmacol* 1981; **12**: 598–600.

Renal impairment. A study[1] of the pharmacokinetics of metoprolol and its renally excreted metabolite α-hydroxymetoprolol in normal subjects and subjects with renal impairment showed that a single dose of a modified-release tablet of metoprolol produced similar plasma-metoprolol concentrations and values for the area under the concentration/time curve in both groups. Mean plasma concentrations of α-hydroxymetoprolol were increased two to threefold in subjects with renal impairment compared with normal subjects but such a rise was not considered likely to contribute to beta blockade.

1. Lloyd P, *et al.* The effect of impaired renal function on the pharmacokinetics of metoprolol after single administration of a 14/190 metoprolol OROS system. *Am Heart J* 1990; **120**: 478–82.

Uses and Administration

Metoprolol is a cardioselective beta blocker (p.844). It is reported to lack intrinsic sympathomimetic activity and to have little or no membrane-stabilising activity.

It is used in the management of hypertension (p.802), angina pectoris (p.791), cardiac arrhythmias (p.794), myocardial infarction (p.805), and heart failure (p.798). It is also used in the management of hyperthyroidism (p.1519) and in the prophylactic treatment of migraine (p.449). Metoprolol is under investigation in dilated cardiomyopathy (p.796).

Metoprolol is given as the tartrate. The fumarate and succinate salts are used in some modified-release tablets.

Reduced doses should be given to patients with hepatic dysfunction.

In **hypertension** metoprolol tartrate is usually given in an initial dose of 100 mg daily by mouth, increased weekly according to the response of the patient to 400 mg daily; it may be taken as a single daily dose or twice daily. A usual maintenance dose is 100 to 200 mg daily. Some manufacturers recommend that the dose should be taken with or immediately following a meal.

The usual dose for **angina pectoris** is 50 to 100 mg two or three times daily by mouth.

In the treatment of **cardiac arrhythmias** the usual dose is 50 mg two or three times daily by mouth, increased if necessary up to 300 mg daily in divided doses.

For the emergency treatment of cardiac arrhythmias metoprolol tartrate may be given intravenously in an initial dose of up to 5 mg administered at a rate of 1 to 2 mg per minute; this may be repeated, if necessary, at intervals of 5 minutes to a total dose of 10 to 15 mg. When acute arrhythmias have been controlled, maintenance therapy may be started with doses not exceeding 50 mg three times daily by mouth 4 to 6 hours after intravenous therapy.

Arrhythmias may be prevented on induction of anaesthesia or controlled during anaesthesia, by the slow intravenous injection of 2 to 4 mg; further injections of 2 mg may be repeated as necessary to a maximum total dose of 10 mg.

Metoprolol is also used as an adjunct in the early management of acute **myocardial infarction.** Treatment should be given within 12 hours of the onset of chest pain; metoprolol tartrate 5 mg should be given intravenously at 2-minute intervals to a total of 15 mg, where tolerated. This should be followed, after 15 minutes, by the commencement of oral treatment, in patients who have received the full intravenous dose, with 50 mg every 6 hours for 2 days. In patients who have failed to tolerate the full intravenous dose a reduced oral dose should be given as and when their condition permits. Subsequent maintenance dosage is 100 mg given twice daily by mouth. In patients who did not receive metoprolol by intravenous injection as part of the early management of myocardial infarction, metoprolol 100 mg twice daily by

mouth may be started once the clinical condition of the patient stabilises.

As an adjunct in the treatment of **hyperthyroidism** metoprolol tartrate may be given in doses of 50 mg four times daily by mouth. Doses of 100 to 200 mg are given daily in divided doses for **migraine** prophylaxis.

◊ General references.

1. Plosker GL, Clissold SP. Controlled release metoprolol formulations: a review of their pharmacodynamic and pharmacokinetic properties, and therapeutic use in hypertension and ischaemic heart disease. *Drugs* 1992; **43**: 382–414.
2. Prakash A, Markham A. Metoprolol: a review of its use in chronic heart failure. *Drugs* 2000; **60**: 647–78.

Preparations

BP 2001: Metoprolol Injection; Metoprolol Tartrate Tablets;
USP 25: Metoprolol Succinate Extended-Release Tablets; Metoprolol Tartrate and Hydrochlorothiazide Tablets; Metoprolol Tartrate Injection; Metoprolol Tartrate Tablets.

Proprietary Preparations (details are given in Part 3)
Aust.: Beloc; Lanoc; Lopresor; Metohexal; Metolol; Metoros; Metotyrol; Seloken; *Austral.:* Betaloc; Lopresor; Metohexal; Metolol; Minax; *Belg.:* Lopresor; Selo-Zok; Seloken; Slow-Lopresor; *Braz.:* Lopressor; Seloken; *Canad.:* Betaloc; Lopresor; Novo-Metoprol; Nu-Metop; *Denm.:* Dura-Zok; Mepronet; Metozoc; Selo-Zok; Seloken; *Fin.:* Metblock; Metoprolin; Metozoc; Seloken; Seloken ZOC; Selopral; Spesicor; *Fr.:* Lopressor; Seloken; *Ger.:* Azumetop; Beloc; Beloc-Zok; Dignometoprol†; Jeprolol; Lopresor; Meprolol; Meto; Meto-Tablinen; Metobeta; Metodura; Metohexal; Metomerck; Metoprogamma; Prelis; Sigaprolol; *Hong Kong:* Betaloc; Minax; *Irl.:* Betaloc; Betazok; Lopresor; Metocor; Metop; Topromel; *Israel:* Lopressor; Metopress; Neobloc; *Ital.:* Lopresor; Seloken; *Jpn.:* Seloken; *Mex.:* Eurolol; Kenaprol; Leptoprol; Letoprol; Metozzard; Proken M; Prolaken; Ritmolol; Selectadril; Seloken; Sermetrol; *Neth.:* Lopresor; Selokeen; *Norw.:* Metozoc; Selo-Zok; Seloken; *NZ:* Betaloc; Lopressor; Slow-Lopresor; *Port.:* Lopresor; *S.Afr.:* Lopresor; *Singapore:* Betaloc; Denex; *Spain:* Lopresor; Seloken; *Swed.:* Metoproferm†; Seloken; Seloken ZOC; *Switz.:* Beloc COR; Beloc-Zok; Lopresor; Metopress; *Thai.:* Betaloc; Cardeloc; Cardoxone; Denex; Melol; Metoblock; Metolol; *UK:* Arbralene; Betaloc; Lopresor; Mepranix†; *USA:* Lopressor; Toprol XL.

Multi-ingredient: *Aust.:* Beloc comp; Logimax; Logroton†; Metolol compositum; Seloken retard Plus; Triloc; *Belg.:* Logimat; Logroton; Selozide; Zok-Zid; *Braz.:* Selopress; *Denm.:* Logimax; Zok-Zid; *Fin.:* Logimax; Selocomp ZOC; Seloken ZOC/ASA; *Fr.:* Logimax; Logroton; *Ger.:* Azumetop HCT; Belnif; Beloc comp†; Beloc-Zok comp; Meto comp; Meto-comp†; meto-thiazid; Metobeta comp; Metodura comp; Metohexal comp; Metostad Comp; Mobloc; Prelis comp; Treloc; *Hong Kong:* Betaloc Comp; Logimax; *Irl.:* Co-Betaloc; *Ital.:* Igroton-Lopresor; Selozide; *Mex.:* Logimax; Selopres; *Neth.:* Logroton†; Selokomb; *Norw.:* Logimax†; *Spain:* Logimax; Selopresin; *Swed.:* Logimax; Seloken ZOC/ASA; *Switz.:* Logimax; Logroton; *UK:* Co-Betaloc; *USA:* Lopressor HCT.

Mevastatin (16591-h)

Mevastatin *(rINN)*.

Compactin; CS-500; ML-236B. (1S,7S,8S,8aR)-1,2,3,7,8,8a-Hexahydro-7-methyl-8-{2-[(2R,4R)-tetrahydro-4-hydroxy-6-oxo-2H-pyran-2-yl]ethyl}-1-naphthyl (S)-2-methylbutyrate.
$C_{23}H_{34}O_5$ = 390.5.
CAS — 73573-88-3.

Profile
Mevastatin, which has been isolated from *Penicillium citrinum,* is a lipid regulating drug. It is a 3-hydroxy-3-methylglutaryl coenzyme A (HMG-CoA) reductase inhibitor (a statin) (see Simvastatin, p.969) but is no longer used in clinical practice because of reports of toxicity in *animals.*

Mexiletine Hydrochloride (7789-p)

Mexiletine Hydrochloride *(BANM, USAN, rINNM)*.
Kö-1173; Mexiletini Hydrochloridum. 1-Methyl-2-(2,6-xylyloxy)ethylamine hydrochloride.
$C_{11}H_{17}NO,HCl$ = 215.7.
CAS — 31828-71-4 *(mexiletine)*; 5370-01-4 *(mexiletine hydrochloride)*.
Pharmacopoeias. In *Chin., Eur.* (see p.vi), *Jpn,* and *US.*

Pharmacopoeial description
Ph. Eur.: A white or almost white, crystalline powder. It exhibits polymorphism. Freely soluble in water and in methyl alcohol; sparingly soluble in dichloromethane; practically insoluble in ether. A 10% solution in water has a pH of 4.0 to 5.5.

USP 25: A white powder. Freely soluble in water and in dehydrated alcohol; practically insoluble in ether; slightly soluble in acetonitrile. A 10% solution in water has a pH of between 3.5 and 5.5. Store in airtight containers.

Adverse Effects and Treatment
Mexiletine has a narrow therapeutic ratio; many adverse effects of mexiletine are dose-related and will respond to dosage reduction but may be severe

enough to necessitate discontinuation of mexiletine and the institution of symptomatic and supportive therapy. Toxicity is commonly seen with oral or parenteral loading doses when plasma concentrations are high.

The most common adverse effects involve the gastrointestinal tract and CNS. Effects on the gastrointestinal tract include nausea, vomiting, constipation, and diarrhoea. Effects on the nervous system include tremor, confusion, lightheadedness, dizziness, blurred vision and other visual disturbances, sleep disturbances, and speech difficulties. The most frequent cardiovascular effects are hypotension, sinus bradycardia, atrioventricular dissociation, and atrial fibrillation. As with other antiarrhythmics mexiletine may exacerbate arrhythmias. Other adverse effects which have been reported include skin rashes, abnormal liver function tests, thrombocytopenia, positive antinuclear factor titres, and convulsions. The Stevens-Johnson syndrome has been reported rarely.

◊ In a study involving 100 patients with ventricular arrhythmias given mexiletine, the drug had to be discontinued in 49 patients due to intolerable adverse effects.[1] The most common intolerable effects affected the gastrointestinal system (27%) and included nausea (10%), vomiting (6%), heartburn (6%), and oesophageal spasm (3%). Intolerable adverse effects affecting the CNS occurred in 10% of patients and these were most commonly tremor (4%), ataxia (2%), dyskinesia (1%), and tinnitus (1%). When mexiletine was used with another antiarrhythmic, the incidence of intolerable adverse effects was 56%.

Tolerable adverse effects with mexiletine alone were transient and dose-dependent and occurred in 18% of patients. They most commonly affected the gastrointestinal tract. No irreversible adverse effects were reported and no proarrhythmic effects were seen.

1. Kerin NZ, *et al.* Mexiletine: long-term efficacy and side effects in patients with chronic drug-resistant potentially lethal ventricular arrhythmias. *Arch Intern Med* 1990; **150**: 381–4.

Effects on the lungs. Pulmonary fibrosis has been reported in an elderly patient receiving mexiletine; the manufacturer was aware of three other cases.[1]

1. Bero CJ, Rihn TL. Possible association of pulmonary fibrosis with mexiletine. *DICP Ann Pharmacother* 1991; **25**: 1329–31.

Precautions
Mexiletine should be used with special caution in patients with sinus node dysfunction, conduction disorders, bradycardia, hypotension, cardiogenic shock, heart failure, or hepatic impairment. ECG and blood pressure monitoring should be carried out during treatment.

Absorption of mexiletine may be delayed after myocardial infarction.

Pregnancy. A normal infant was born to a woman given mexiletine with propranolol for the control of ventricular tachycardia during the third trimester of pregnancy.[1] During the first 6 hours after delivery the infant had a heart rate of only 90 beats per minute, probably due to the propranolol; it was normal thereafter. At delivery the concentration of mexiletine in the serum of the mother and the infant was the same.

1. Timmis AD, *et al.* Mexiletine for control of ventricular dysrhythmias in pregnancy. *Lancet* 1980; **ii**: 647–8.

Interactions
Mexiletine undergoes extensive metabolism in the liver and interactions may occur with other drugs metabolised by the same enzymes. Plasma concentrations of mexiletine may be reduced by drugs which induce hepatic enzymes such as phenytoin and rifampicin; increased plasma concentrations may occur with enzyme inhibitors.

Absorption of mexilitine may be delayed by drugs that slow gastric emptying such as opioid analgesics and atropine. The rate of absorption may be increased by metoclopramide; the extent of absorption is unaffected.

Drugs that acidify or alkalinise the urine enhance or reduce the rate of elimination of mexiletine, respectively.

There may be an increased risk of arrhythmias if mexiletine is given concurrently with other antiarrhythmics or with arrhythmogenic drugs.

Mexiletine has been reported to increase theophylline concentrations (p.780) and to precipitate lignocaine [lidocaine] toxicity (p.1314).

◊ References.
1. Wing LMH, *et al.* The effect of metoclopramide and atropine on the absorption of orally administered mexiletine. *Br J Clin Pharmacol* 1980; **9**: 505–9.
2. Begg EJ, *et al.* Enhanced metabolism of mexiletine after phenytoin administration. *Br J Clin Pharmacol* 1982; **14**: 219–23.
3. Pentikäinen PJ, *et al.* Effect of rifampicin treatment on the kinetics of mexiletine. *Eur J Clin Pharmacol* 1982; **23**: 261–6.

Pharmacokinetics

Mexiletine is readily and almost completely absorbed from the gastrointestinal tract although absorption may be delayed after myocardial infarction.

Mexiletine is metabolised in the liver to a number of metabolites; metabolism may involve cytochrome P450 isoenzymes CYP1A2, CYP2D6, and CYP3A4. It is excreted in the urine, mainly in the form of its metabolites with about 10% excreted as unchanged mexiletine; the clearance of mexiletine is increased in acid urine.

Mexiletine is widely distributed throughout the body and is about 50 to 70% bound to plasma proteins. Mexiletine crosses the placenta and is distributed into breast milk. It has an elimination half-life of about 10 hours in healthy subjects but this may be prolonged in patients with heart disease, hepatic impairment, or severe renal impairment. Its therapeutic effect has been correlated with plasma concentrations of 0.5 to 2 µg per mL, but the margin between therapeutic and toxic concentrations is narrow, and severe toxicity may occur within this range.

◊ References.
1. Labbé L, Turgeon J. Clinical pharmacokinetics of mexiletine. *Clin Pharmacokinet* 1999; **37**: 361–84.

Uses and Administration

Mexiletine is a class Ib antiarrhythmic (p.787) with actions similar to those of lignocaine [lidocaine] (p.1315), to which it is structurally related. Unlike lignocaine [lidocaine] it undergoes little hepatic first-pass metabolism and is suitable for oral administration.

Mexiletine is used for the treatment of ventricular **arrhythmias**.

It is given by mouth as the hydrochloride in an initial loading dose of 400 mg followed by 200 to 250 mg three or four times daily, starting 2 hours after the loading dose. Higher loading doses (for example, of 600 mg) may be necessary in patients after myocardial infarction to overcome delayed absorption, especially if they have received an opioid analgesic. The usual maintenance dosage of mexiletine is 600 to 900 mg daily in divided doses; doses up to 1200 mg daily may be given. Use of a modified-release preparation allows administration every 12 hours.

Mexiletine may be given by slow intravenous injection of the hydrochloride in doses of 100 to 250 mg at a rate of 25 mg per minute, followed by an infusion at a rate of 250 mg over 1 hour, 250 mg over the next 2 hours, and then at about 0.5 mg per minute for maintenance, according to the patient's response; when appropriate the patient may be transferred to oral therapy with doses of 200 to 250 mg of the hydrochloride three or four times daily. Alternatively, an initial intravenous dose of 200 mg at a rate of 25 mg per minute, may be followed by an oral dose of 400 mg on completion of the injection, with subsequent oral therapy as before.

Mexiletine has also been tried in the treatment of refractory neuropathic **pain**.

◊ Reviews.
1. Campbell RWF. Mexiletine. *N Engl J Med* 1987; **316**: 29–34.
2. Monk JP, Brogden RN. Mexiletine: a review of its pharmacodynamic and pharmacokinetic properties, and therapeutic use in the treatment of arrhythmias. *Drugs* 1990; **40**: 374–411. Correction. *ibid.* 1991; **41**: 377.

Administration in children. The dose of mexiletine in children should be titrated according to the concentration in plasma.[1] In a 2-week-old girl and a 20-month-old boy high oral doses of 25 and 15 mg per kg body-weight daily, respectively, were needed to produce therapeutic concentrations in plasma and control of tachycardia.
1. Holt DW, *et al.* Paediatric use of mexiletine and disopyramide. *BMJ* 1979; **2**: 1476–7.

The symbol † denotes a preparation no longer actively marketed

Administration in the elderly. The rate of absorption of mexiletine was slower in a group of 7 elderly subjects compared with 8 young subjects given mexiletine 100 mg by mouth, but the extent of absorption was probably not affected.[1] Elimination of mexiletine was not significantly different between the 2 groups and there was no pharmacokinetic basis for dosage modification of mexiletine in the elderly.
1. Grech-Bélanger O, *et al.* Pharmacokinetics of mexiletine in the elderly. *J Clin Pharmacol* 1989; **29**: 311–15.

Administration in renal impairment. The pharmacokinetics of mexiletine were not significantly modified in patients with chronic renal impairment when the creatinine clearance was above 10 mL per minute and these patients could be given usual doses of mexiletine.[1] However, in patients with a creatinine clearance below 10 mL per minute the steady-state plasma concentration and half-life were increased and in these patients mexiletine dosage should be adjusted according to plasma-mexiletine concentrations.

Continuous ambulatory peritoneal dialysis did not influence the clearance of mexiletine in a patient with chronic renal failure.[2]
1. El Allaf D, *et al.* Pharmacokinetics of mexiletine in renal insufficiency. *Br J Clin Pharmacol* 1982; **14**: 431–5.
2. Guay DRP, *et al.* Mexiletine clearance during peritoneal dialysis. *Br J Clin Pharmacol* 1985; **19**: 857–8.

Cardiac arrhythmias. Several studies[1-4] showed that mexiletine could reduce the incidence of ventricular arrhythmias (p.794) after acute myocardial infarction but no significant reduction in mortality was demonstrated.

The long-term efficacy of mexiletine in the treatment of ventricular arrhythmias refractory to other drug therapy has also been the subject of several studies,[5-8] but, although it may be effective in the treatment of some such patients, adverse effects may limit its usefulness.
1. Chamberlain DA, *et al.* Oral mexiletine in high-risk patients after myocardial infarction. *Lancet* 1980; **ii** 1324–7.
2. Bell JA, *et al.* A trial of prophylactic mexiletine in home coronary care. *Br Heart J* 1982; **48**: 285–90.
3. Halinen MO, *et al.* Antiarrhythmic efficacy of combined intravenous and oral mexiletine in acute myocardial infarction: a double blind placebo-controlled study. *Eur Heart J* 1984; **5**: 675–83.
4. IMPACT Research Group. International mexiletine and placebo antiarrhythmic coronary trial: I: report on arrhythmia and other findings. *J Am Coll Cardiol* 1984; **4**: 1148–63.
5. Stein J, *et al.* Long-term mexiletine for ventricular arrhythmia. *Am Heart J* 1984; **107**: 1091–8.
6. Rutledge JC, *et al.* Clinical evaluation of oral mexiletine therapy in the treatment of ventricular arrhythmias. *J Am Coll Cardiol* 1985; **6**: 780–4.
7. Nademanee K, *et al.* Mexiletine: double-blind comparison with procainamide in PVC suppression and open-label sequential comparison with amiodarone in life-threatening ventricular arrhythmias. *Am Heart J* 1985; **110**: 923–31.
8. Poole JE, *et al.* Intolerance and ineffectiveness of mexiletine in patients with serious ventricular arrhythmias. *Am Heart J* 1986; **112**: 322–6.

Pain. Neuropathic pain is often insensitive to opioid analgesics and various drugs, including mexiletine, have been tried. Mexiletine has been tried in painful diabetic neuropathy (p.5) although results have been conflicting.[1-5] Two of the studies that reported no difference between treatment and placebo found that a subset of patients (those with stabbing or burning pain, heat sensations, and formication) appeared to benefit.[2,3]

Other painful states in which mexiletine has been reported to be of benefit include: Dercum's disease (a condition involving painful fatty deposits),[6] central post-stroke pain (thalamic pain syndrome)[7] (p.5), and severe scrotal and inguinal pain after radiation for prostate cancer.[8]
1. Dejgård A, *et al.* Mexiletine for treatment of chronic painful diabetic neuropathy. *Lancet* 1988; **i**: 9–11.
2. Stracke H, *et al.* Mexiletine in the treatment of diabetic neuropathy. *Diabetes Care* 1992; **15**: 1550–5.
3. Wright JM, *et al.* Mexiletine in the symptomatic treatment of diabetic peripheral neuropathy. *Ann Pharmacother* 1997; **31**: 29–34.
4. Oskarsson P, *et al.* Efficacy and safety of mexiletine in the treatment of painful diabetic neuropathy. *Diabetes Care* 1997; **20**: 1594–7.
5. Jarvis B, Coukell AJ. Mexiletine: a review of its therapeutic use in painful diabetic neuropathy. *Drugs* 1998; **56**: 691–707.
6. Petersen P, *et al.* Treating the pain of Dercum's disease. *BMJ* 1984; **288**: 1880.
7. Awerbuch GI, Sandyk R. Mexiletine for thalamic pain syndrome. *Int J Neurosci* 1990; **55**: 129–33.
8. Colclough G, *et al.* Mexiletine for chronic pain. *Lancet* 1993; **342**: 1484–5.

Preparations

BP 2001: Mexiletine Capsules; Mexiletine Injection;
USP 25: Mexiletine Hydrochloride Capsules.

Proprietary Preparations (details are given in Part 3)
Aust.: Mexitil; *Austral.:* Mexitil; *Belg.:* Mexitil; *Braz.:* Mexitil; *Canad.:* Mexitil; *Denm.:* Mexitil; *Fin.:* Mexetil; *Fr.:* Mexitil; *Ger.:* Mexitil; *Hong Kong:* Mexitil; *Irl.:* Mexitil; *Israel:* Mexilen; *Ital.:* Mexitil; *Mex.:* Mexitil; *Neth.:* Mexitil†; *Norw.:* Mexitil; *NZ:* Mexitil; *S.Afr.:* Mexitil; *Spain:* Mexitil; *Swed.:* Mexitil; *Switz.:* Mexitil†; *Thai.:* Mexitil; *UK:* Mexitil; *USA:* Mexitil.

Mibefradil Hydrochloride (19405-p)

Mibefradil Hydrochloride (*BANM, rINNM*).

Mibefradil Dihydrochloride (*USAN*); Ro-40-5967 (mibefradil); Ro-40-5967/001 (mibefradil hydrochloride). (1S,2S)-(2-{[3-(2-Benzimidazolyl)propyl]methylamino}ethyl)-6-fluoro-1,2,3,4-tetrahydro-1-isopropyl-2-naphthyl methoxyacetate dihydrochloride.
$C_{29}H_{38}FN_3O_3,2HCl = 568.6$.
CAS — 116644-53-2 (mibefradil); 116666-63-8 (mibefradil hydrochloride).

Profile

Mibefradil is a calcium-channel blocker that acts principally on fast T-type calcium channels unlike conventional calcium-channel blockers that act on slow L-type channels (see p.788). Mibefradil was introduced for the management of hypertension and angina pectoris but was withdrawn worldwide several months later due to increasing reports of serious interactions with a wide range of drugs.

Preparations

Proprietary Preparations (details are given in Part 3)
Austral.: Posicor†; *Irl.:* Posicor†; *Neth.:* Posicor†; *UK:* Posicor†; *USA:* Posicor†.

Midodrine Hydrochloride (12959-s)

Midodrine Hydrochloride (*BANM, USAN, rINNM*).

A-4020 Linz; ST-1085 (midodrine or midodrine hydrochloride); St. Peter-224. 2-Amino-N-(β-hydroxy-2,5-dimethoxyphenethyl)acetamide hydrochloride; (RS)-N¹-(β-Hydroxy-2,5-dimethoxyphenethyl)glycinamide hydrochloride.
$C_{12}H_{18}N_2O_4,HCl = 290.7$.
CAS — 42794-76-3 (midodrine); 3092-17-9 (midodrine hydrochloride).

Adverse Effects, Treatment, and Precautions

The most serious adverse effect of midodrine is supine hypertension. Paraesthesias, dysuria, pilomotor reaction (goose flesh), pruritus and rashes have been reported. The hypertensive effects of midodrine may be treated with an alpha blocker such as phentolamine.

For the adverse effects of sympathomimetics in general, and precautions to be observed, see Adrenaline, p.829.

Interactions

For the interactions of sympathomimetics in general, see Adrenaline, p.830.

Pharmacokinetics

Midodrine is well absorbed from the gastrointestinal tract and undergoes enzymatic hydrolysis in the systemic circulation to its active metabolite, deglymidodrine (desglymidodrine; ST-1059). Midodrine itself reaches its peak plasma concentrations about half an hour after a dose by mouth, and has a plasma half-life of about 25 minutes. The active metabolite reaches its peak plasma concentration about an hour after oral administration and has a terminal elimination half-life of about 3 hours. Deglymidodrine undergoes some further metabolism in the liver. Midodrine is primarily excreted in the urine as metabolites and a small amount of unchanged drug.

Uses and Administration

Midodrine is a direct-acting sympathomimetic (see Adrenaline, p.831) with selective alpha-agonist activity; the main active moiety has been stated to be its major metabolite, deglymidodrine. It acts as a peripheral vasoconstrictor but has no direct cardiac stimulatory effects.

Midodrine hydrochloride is used in the treatment of hypotensive states (p.805) and in particular of orthostatic hypotension (p.1070). Alpha-agonist drugs such as midodrine have also been used as an adjunct in the management of urinary incontinence (p.459).

In **hypotensive states**, a usual initial dose of midodrine hydrochloride is 2.5 mg twice daily by mouth adjusted gradually according to the patient's response; up to 10 mg three times daily may be required. The potential for supine hypertension is reduced by taking the last dose of the day at least 4 hours before bedtime.

A dose for **urinary incontinence** is 2.5 to 5 mg by mouth two or three times daily.

Midodrine hydrochloride can also be given in similar doses by slow intravenous injection. It has also been used in the treatment of retrograde ejaculation in a dose of 10 to 40 mg intravenously.

◊ References.
1. McTavish D, Goa KL. Midodrine: a review of its pharmacological properties and therapeutic use in orthostatic hypotension and secondary hypotensive disorders. *Drugs* 1989; **38**: 757–77.
2. Jankovic J, *et al.* Neurogenic orthostatic hypotension: a double-blind, placebo-controlled study with midodrine. *Am J Med* 1993; **95**: 38–48.
3. Fouad-Tarazi FM, *et al.* Alpha sympathomimetic treatment of autonomic insufficiency with orthostatic hypotension. *Am J Med* 1995; **99**: 604–10.
4. Low PA, *et al.* Efficacy of midodrine vs placebo in neurogenic orthostatic hypotension: a randomized, double-blind multicenter study. *JAMA* 1997; **277**: 1046–51. Correction. *ibid.*; **278**: 388.

5. Ward CR, *et al.* Midodrine: a role in the management of neuro-cardiogenic syncope. *Heart* 1998; **79:** 45–9.
6. McClellan KJ, *et al.* Midodrine: a review of its therapeutic use in the management of orthostatic hypotension. *Drugs Aging* 1998; **12:** 76–86.

Preparations

Proprietary Preparations (details are given in Part 3)
Aust.: Gutron; **Canad.:** Amatine; **Fr.:** Gutron; **Ger.:** Gutron; **Hong Kong:** Gutron; **Irl.:** Midon; **Israel:** Gutron; **Ital.:** Gutron; **Mex.:** Gutron; **NZ:** Gutron; **Port.:** Gutron; **Switz.:** Gutron; **Thai.:** Gutron; **USA:** ProAmatine.

Milrinone (16896-t)

Milrinone (BAN, USAN, rINN).

Win-47203-2. 1,6-Dihydro-2-methyl-6-oxo[3,4′-bipyridine]-5-carbonitrile.

$C_{12}H_9N_3O = 211.2$.

CAS — 78415-72-2.

ATC — C01CE02.

Milrinone Lactate (13500-v)

Milrinone Lactate (BANM, rINNM).

$C_{12}H_9N_3O,C_3H_6O_3 = 301.3$.

Milrinone lactate injection is reported to be **incompatible** with frusemide [furosemide] and bumetanide, and it should not be diluted with sodium bicarbonate injection. Milrinone lactate 1.43 mg is approximately equivalent to 1 mg of milrinone.

Adverse Effects and Precautions

Prolonged oral treatment with milrinone has increased the mortality rate and milrinone is now only employed intravenously for short-term use.

Supraventricular and ventricular arrhythmias, hypotension, angina-like chest pain, and headache have been reported. Hypokalaemia, tremor, and thrombocytopenia may occur.

Milrinone should be used with caution in patients with severe obstructive aortic or pulmonary valvular disease or with hypertrophic cardiomyopathy. Since milrinone may facilitate conduction through the atrioventricular node it can increase the ventricular response rate in patients with atrial flutter or fibrillation. Digitalisation should be considered in these patients before milrinone therapy is started.

Blood pressure, heart rate, ECG, and fluid and electrolyte balance should be monitored during milrinone therapy.

Pharmacokinetics

Milrinone is rapidly and almost completely absorbed from the gastrointestinal tract, but is only given intravenously because of an increased mortality rate associated with prolonged administration via the oral route. It is about 70% bound to plasma proteins. Elimination occurs mainly via the urine; about 83% of a dose is excreted as unchanged drug. The elimination half-life is about 2.3 hours.

◊ General references.
1. Rocci ML, Wilson H. The pharmacokinetics and pharmacodynamics of newer inotropic agents. *Clin Pharmacokinet* 1987; **13:** 91–109. Correction. *ibid.* 1988; **14:** (contents page).

Uses and Administration

Milrinone is a phosphodiesterase inhibitor similar to amrinone (p.839) with positive inotropic and vasodilator activity. It is, however, reported to have greater positive inotropic activity than amrinone. It is given intravenously, as the lactate, in the short-term management of severe heart failure unresponsive to other forms of therapy and in acute heart failure following cardiac surgery. In some longer-term studies milrinone was given by mouth, but an increased mortality rate was reported.

Doses of milrinone lactate are expressed in terms of the base. The initial loading dose is 50 μg per kg body-weight given over 10 minutes followed by a continuous maintenance infusion. The maintenance infusion may be titrated between 0.375 and 0.75 μg per kg per minute but a total daily dose of 1.13 mg per kg should not be exceeded.

Dosage should be reduced in patients with renal impairment.

Administration in children. Pharmacokinetic studies[1,2] have suggested that steady-state plasma concentrations of milrinone are lower in children than in adults given similar doses, and that milrinone clearance is faster in children. It has been suggested[1] that in children an initial loading dose of 75 μg per kg body-weight should be administered, followed by maintenance infusions of 0.75 μg per kg per minute, increased to 1.0 μg per kg per minute if required. An additional bolus dose of 25 μg per kg was recommended before each increase of 0.25 μg per kg per minute in infusion rate.

1. Lindsay CA, *et al.* Pharmacokinetics and pharmacodynamics of milrinone lactate in pediatric patients with septic shock. *J Pediatr* 1998; **132:** 329–34.
2. Ramamoorthy C, *et al.* Pharmacokinetics and side effects of milrinone in infants and children after open heart surgery. *Anesth Analg* 1998; **86:** 283–9.

Heart failure. Milrinone is one of several drugs that may be used in heart failure (p.798), but because of an increased mortality rate reported following long-term oral use it is usually only given intravenously for short-term management of heart failure unresponsive to other treatments. The PROMISE (Prospective Randomized Milrinone Survival Evaluation) study[1] showed that oral milrinone increased morbidity and mortality in patients with severe chronic heart failure. However, more recently longer-term continuous intravenous administration for up to 8 weeks has been studied in patients awaiting heart transplantation and appeared to be well tolerated.[2] Intermittent use on several days a week has also been tried.[3]

1. Packer M, *et al.* Effect of oral milrinone on mortality in severe chronic heart failure. *N Engl J Med* 1991; **325:** 1468–75.
2. Mehra MR, *et al.* Safety and clinical utility of long-term intravenous milrinone in advanced heart failure. *Am J Cardiol* 1997; **80:** 61–4.
3. Cesario D, *et al.* Beneficial effects of intermittent home administration of the inotrope/vasodilator milrinone in patients with end-stage congestive heart failure: a preliminary study. *Am Heart J* 1998; **135:** 121–9.

Preparations

Proprietary Preparations (details are given in Part 3)
Aust.: Corotrop; **Austral.:** Primacor; **Belg.:** Corotrope; **Braz.:** Primacor; **Canad.:** Primacor; **Fr.:** Corotrope; **Ger.:** Corotrop; **Hong Kong:** Primacor; **Israel:** Primacor; **Jpn:** Milrila; **Neth.:** Corotrope; **NZ:** Primacor; **Singapore:** Primacor; **Spain:** Corotrope; **Swed.:** Corotrop; **Switz.:** Corotrop; **Thai.:** Primacor; **UK:** Primacor; **USA:** Primacor.

Minoxidil (884-x)

Minoxidil (BAN, USAN, rINN).

Minoxidilum; U-10858. 2,6-Diamino-4-piperidinopyrimidine 1-oxide.

$C_9H_{15}N_5O = 209.2$.

CAS — 38304-91-5.

ATC — C02DC01; D11AX01.

Pharmacopoeias. In Eur. (see p.vi) and US.

Pharmacopoeial description

Ph. Eur.: A white or almost white crystalline powder. Slightly soluble in water; very slightly soluble in ether; soluble in methyl alcohol and in propylene glycol. Protect from light.

USP 25: A white or off-white crystalline powder. Slightly soluble in water; soluble in alcohol and in propylene glycol; practically insoluble in acetone, in chloroform, in ethyl acetate, and in petroleum spirit; sparingly soluble in methyl alcohol.

Adverse Effects and Treatment

Adverse effects commonly caused by minoxidil include reflex tachycardia, fluid retention accompanied by weight gain, oedema, and sometimes deterioration of existing heart failure and changes in the ECG. Hypertrichosis develops in up to 80% of patients within 3 to 6 weeks of the start of minoxidil therapy but is slowly reversible on discontinuation. Pericardial effusion, sometimes with associated tamponade, has been reported in about 3% of patients. Pericarditis may also occur. Minoxidil may aggravate or uncover angina pectoris. Other less frequent adverse effects include headache, nausea, gynaecomastia and breast tenderness, polymenorrhoea, allergic skin rashes, Stevens-Johnson syndrome, and thrombocytopenia.

Reflex tachycardia can be overcome by the concomitant administration of a beta blocker, or alternatively methyldopa, and a diuretic (usually a loop diuretic) is used to reduce fluid retention. If excessive hypotension occurs, an intravenous infusion of normal saline can be given to maintain the blood pressure. If a pressor agent is necessary, drugs such as adrenaline [epinephrine] which can aggravate tachycardia should be avoided; phenylephrine, angiotensinamide, vasopressin, or dopamine may be given if there is evidence of inadequate perfusion of a vital organ.

Topical application of minoxidil may be associated with contact dermatitis, pruritus, local burning, and flushing; sufficient may be absorbed to produce systemic adverse effects.

◊ Two haemorrhagic lesions with Kaposi's features appeared on the forehead, an unusual location for HIV-associated Kaposi's sarcoma, in an HIV-positive patient who had applied topical minoxidil there for 3 months.[1] In another, healthy, patient an angioma of the scalp developed after 2 months of topical minoxidil therapy. The patient had had a similar lesion as a baby. Minoxidil may induce angiogenesis or may stimulate endothelial cells, fibroblasts, and muscle cells to proliferate. Care should be taken when minoxidil is applied to the skin of people who are predisposed to neo-angiogenesis, or who are HIV-positive.

For other effects of minoxidil on the skin following topical application, see below.
1. Pavlovitch JH, *et al.* Angiogenesis and minoxidil. *Lancet* 1990; **336:** 889.

Effects on the eyes. Bilateral optic neuritis and retinitis occurred in a patient during treatment with minoxidil for hypertension following a renal transplant.[1] The patient was also taking prednisolone and azathioprine.
1. Gombos GM. Bilateral optic neuritis following minoxidil administration. *Ann Ophthalmol* 1983; **15:** 259–61.

Effects on the hair. The hypertrichosis associated with minoxidil taken orally makes it unsuitable generally for use in women. As well as frequent hypertrichosis, there have been reports of changes in hair colour in patients receiving minoxidil.[1] In addition a case has been reported of increased hair loss, followed by subsequent regrowth of differently-coloured hair.[2] Substantial hair loss occurred in a female patient following withdrawal of minoxidil and she had to wear a wig.[3] Severe hypertrichosis has also been reported in 35 of 56 women applying minoxidil 5% solution topically for androgenetic alopecia.[4] Facial, arm, and leg hypertrichosis were reported 2 to 3 months after starting treatment. Hypertrichosis had disappeared 5 months after discontinuation of minoxidil.

1. Traub YM, *et al.* Treatment of severe hypertension with minoxidil. *Isr J Med Sci* 1975; **11:** 991–8.
2. Ingles RM, Kahn T. Unusual hair changes with minoxidil therapy. *Int J Dermatol* 1983; **22:** 120–2.
3. Kidwai BJ, George M. Hair loss with minoxidil withdrawal. *Lancet* 1992; **340:** 609–10.
4. Peluso AM, *et al.* Diffuse hypertrichosis during treatment with 5% topical minoxidil. *Br J Dermatol* 1997; **136:** 118–20.

Effects on skeletal muscle. A polymyalgia syndrome, manifesting as fatigue, anorexia, weight loss, and severe pain in the shoulders and pelvic girdle was seen in 4 men using topical minoxidil.[1] All symptoms improved within 2 to 4 weeks of withdrawing the drug. In 2 of the patients rechallenge produced a relapse of the symptoms.
1. Colamarino R, *et al.* Polymyalgia and minoxidil. *Ann Intern Med* 1990; **113:** 256–7.

Effects on the skin. Although skin reactions to systemic minoxidil do not appear to be common, a case of classic Stevens-Johnson syndrome has been reported in a patient receiving minoxidil.[1] The syndrome responded to withdrawal and corticosteroid therapy; subsequent rechallenge provoked a recurrence. In another patient extensive erythematous weeping rash, with lesions consistent with actinic keratosis also appeared to be due to minoxidil; bullous lesions recurred on re-exposure.[2] Following topical application itching, scaling, flushing, and dermatitis have been the most common adverse effects; allergic contact dermatitis has been reported in rare instances.[3]

For other lesions associated with Kaposi's sarcoma and angioma and for effects on the hair, see above.
1. DiSantis DJ, Flanagan J. Minoxidil-induced Stevens-Johnson syndrome. *Arch Intern Med* 1981; **141:** 1515.
2. Ackerman BH, *et al.* Pruritic rash with actinic keratosis and impending exfoliation in a patient with hypertension managed with minoxidil. *Drug Intell Clin Pharm* 1988; **22:** 702–3.
3. Clissold SP, Heel RC. Topical minoxidil: a preliminary review of its pharmacodynamic properties and therapeutic efficacy in alopecia areata and alopecia androgenetica. *Drugs* 1987; **33:** 107–22.

Precautions

Minoxidil is contra-indicated in phaeochromocytoma. It should be used with caution after a recent myocardial infarction, and in patients with pulmonary hypertension, angina pectoris, chronic heart failure, and significant renal impairment.

Topical application of minoxidil should be restricted to the scalp; it should not be applied to inflamed scalp skin or areas affected by psoriasis, severe sunburn, or severe excoriations, due to the risk of increased absorption. Patients being treated for hypertension should be monitored if topical minoxidil is used concurrently.

AIDS. For recommendations that topical minoxidil should be used with caution in HIV-positive patients, see under Adverse Effects, above.

Porphyria. Minoxidil is considered to be unsafe in patients with porphyria because it has been shown to be porphyrinogenic in *animals* or *in-vitro* systems.

Pregnancy and breast feeding. A patient who took minoxidil, propranolol, and frusemide [furosemide] throughout pregnancy delivered a normal infant at 37 weeks. Pregnancy was uneventful.[1] Subsequent studies showed that minoxidil was rapidly distributed into breast milk achieving similar concentrations to those in the plasma. No adverse effects were seen in the infant after 2 months but it was considered that prolonged exposure during breast feeding could be deleterious to the infant.

1. Valdivieso A, *et al.* Minoxidil in breast milk. *Ann Intern Med* 1985; **102:** 135.

Interactions

The antihypertensive effect of minoxidil may be enhanced by concomitant use of other hypotensive drugs. Severe orthostatic hypotension may occur if minoxidil and sympathetic blocking drugs such as guanethidine or betanidine are given concurrently.

Topical minoxidil should not be used with other topical agents known to enhance absorption, such as corticosteroids, retinoids, or occlusive ointment bases.

Pharmacokinetics

About 90% of an oral dose of minoxidil has been reported to be absorbed from the gastrointestinal tract. The plasma half-life is about 4.2 hours although the haemodynamic effect may persist for up to 75 hours, presumably due to accumulation at its site of action. Minoxidil is not bound to plasma proteins. It is distributed into breast milk. Minoxidil is extensively metabolised by the liver. It requires sulfation to become active, but the major metabolite is a glucuronide conjugate. Minoxidil is excreted predominantly in the urine mainly in the form of metabolites. Minoxidil and its metabolites are dialysable.

Following topical application between 0.3 and 4.5% of the total applied dose of minoxidil is absorbed from intact scalp.

◊ References.

1. Pacifici GM, *et al.* Minoxidil sulphation in human liver and platelets: a study of interindividual variability. *Eur J Clin Pharmacol* 1993; **45:** 337–41.

Uses and Administration

Minoxidil is an antihypertensive that acts predominantly by causing direct peripheral vasodilatation of the arterioles. It produces effects on the cardiovascular system similar to those of hydralazine (p.907). Minoxidil is administered by mouth for the treatment of severe hypertension unresponsive to standard therapy (p.802). When applied topically to the scalp minoxidil may stimulate hair growth to a limited extent and is used in the treatment of alopecia.

In the treatment of **hypertension** minoxidil is given with a beta blocker, or with methyldopa, to diminish the cardiac-accelerating effects, and with a diuretic, usually a loop diuretic, to control oedema. Following a single dose by mouth, the maximum hypotensive effect usually occurs after 2 to 3 hours, although the full effects may not occur until after 3 to 7 days of continuous treatment. The action may persist for up to 75 hours. An initial dose of 5 mg of minoxidil daily (or 2.5 mg daily in the elderly) is gradually increased at intervals of not less than 3 days to 40 or 50 mg daily according to the patient's response; in exceptional circumstances up to 100 mg daily has been given. If more rapid control of blood pressure is required, dosage adjustments may be made every 6 hours with careful monitoring. The daily dose may be given as a single dose or in 2 divided doses. For children, the initial dose is 200 µg per kg body-weight daily, increased in steps of 100 to 200 µg per kg at intervals of not less than 3 days, until control of blood pressure has been achieved or a maximum of 1 mg per kg or 50 mg daily has been reached.

Reduced doses may be required in patients with impaired renal function.

In the treatment of **male-pattern baldness** (alopecia androgenetica) 1 mL of a 2% or 5% solution of minoxidil is applied twice daily to the scalp.

Administration in renal impairment. A study of the pharmacokinetics of minoxidil in patients with varying degrees of renal impairment found that the non-renal clearance was also impaired as renal function worsened.[1] Substantial accumulation of minoxidil might occur in these patients during multiple-dose therapy. It was advised that minoxidil therapy be initiated with smaller doses or a longer dose interval in patients with renal insufficiency.

1. Halstenson CE, *et al.* Disposition of minoxidil in patients with various degrees of renal function. *J Clin Pharmacol* 1989; **29:** 798–802.

Alopecia. Although topical minoxidil clearly has some effect on hair growth in alopecia (p.1104), increases in pigmented non-vellus hair may be due to thickening and pigmentation of existing vellus hair rather than new growth.[1] As a result cosmetically acceptable hair growth may occur in less than 10% of patients with male-pattern baldness (alopecia androgenetica),[2-4] and fewer still among those with alopecia areata,[4] despite the fact that higher-strength 5% solutions have been tried in the latter condition.[4] One study indicated that combination of topical minoxidil with 0.5% dithranol cream was more effective than either treatment alone in patients with alopecia areata.[5] The hair is lost again when treatment is stopped,[2-4] and even with continued use there is a waning of effect.[2,4] Minoxidil may be more effective in retarding the progression of male-pattern baldness than in reversing it,[1] and users are advised to abandon treatment if there is insufficient benefit after a year.[3]

A review of controlled trials, that were conducted mostly in men,[6] concluded that topical minoxidil 2% had only a minimal to modest effect on promoting hair regrowth in alopecia androgenetica and needed to be used indefinitely; some workers believed it to be more effective in females than in males, although another review of controlled studies in women[7] concluded that the effectiveness of minoxidil in female alopecia androgenetica was yet to be demonstrated and that larger trials were required. Minoxidil appeared to have no beneficial effect on alopecia areata.[6]

1. Katz HI. Topical minoxidil: review of efficacy and safety. *Cutis* 1989; **43:** 94–8.
2. de Groot AC, *et al.* Minoxidil: hope for the bald? *Lancet* 1987; **i:** 1019–22.
3. Shrank AB. Treating young men with hair loss. *BMJ* 1989; **298:** 847–8.
4. Anonymous. Topical minoxidil does little for baldness. *Drug Ther Bull* 1989; **27:** 74–5.
5. Fiedler VC, *et al.* Treatment-resistant alopecia areata. *Arch Dermatol* 1990; **126:** 756–9.
6. Anonymous. Topical minoxidil for baldness: a reappraisal. *Med Lett Drugs Ther* 1994; **36:** 9–10.
7. Wong WM, Seifert L. Minoxidil used in female alopecia. *Ann Pharmacother* 1994; **28:** 890–1.

CHEMOTHERAPY-INDUCED ALOPECIA. Minoxidil 2% solution was applied daily to the scalp of a boy with acute lymphoblastic leukaemia whose hair had failed to regrow satisfactorily following intensive chemotherapy.[1] Almost normal hair growth, achieved over a period of 9 months, was attributed to the application of minoxidil.

A small study[2] in women undergoing combination chemotherapy including doxorubicin found that topical minoxidil applied throughout the duration of antineoplastic therapy and for up to 4 months afterwards reduced the duration of alopecia by an average of 50 days.

Other methods for reducing chemotherapy-induced alopecia are described under the Treatment of Adverse Effects of Antineoplastics, p.480.

1. Vickers MA, Barton CJ. Minoxidil induced hair growth after leukaemia treatment? *Arch Dis Child* 1995; **73:** 184.
2. Duvic M, *et al.* A randomized trial of minoxidil in chemotherapy-induced alopecia. *J Am Acad Dermatol* 1996; **35:** 74–8.

Preparations

BP 2001: Minoxidil Scalp Application;
USP 25: Minoxidil Tablets; Minoxidil Topical Solution.

Proprietary Preparations (details are given in Part 3)
Aust.: Loniten; Moxiral; Regaine; Rogaine; *Austral.:* Loniten; Ralogaine†; Regaine; *Belg.:* Lonnoten; Neoxidil; Regaine; *Braz.:* Loniten; Minoxidine; Neoxidil; Regaine; *Canad.:* Apo-Gain; Loniten; Minox; Minoxigaine†; Rogaine; *Denm.:* Regaine; *Fin.:* Minona; Regaine; *Fr.:* Alopexy; Alostil; Lonoten; Neoxidil; Regaine; Unipexil; *Ger.:* Lonolox; *Hong Kong:* Apo-Gain; Headway; Loniten; Neoxidil; Regaine; *Irl.:* Loniten; Regaine; *Israel:* Apohair; Hairgaine; Minoxi; Regaine; *Ital.:* Aloxidil; Loniten; Minovital; Minoximen; Normoxidil; Regaine; Tricoxidil; *Mex.:* Folcress; Neoxil; Regaine; *Neth.:* Lonnoten; Regaine; *Norw.:* Regaine; *NZ:* Apo-Gain; Headway; Loniten; Regaine; *Port.:* Crinalsofex†; Loniten; Mantai; Minocalve; Minox; Regaine; Tricovivax; *S.Afr.:* Loniten; Regaine; *Singapore:* Loniten; Minoxitrim; Neoxidil; Regaine; Regro; *Spain:* Kapodin†; Kresse†; Lacovin; Loniten; Pilovital†; Regaine; Riteban; *Swed.:* Regaine; *Switz.:* Alopexy; Loniten; Neocapil; Piloxil; Regaine; *Thai.:* Loniten; Minoxitrim; Modil; Neoxidil; Noxidil; Nuhair; Regaine; *UK:* Loniten; Regaine; *USA:* Loniten; Rogaine.

Mivazerol (14644-g)

Mivazerol (rINN).
UCB-22073.
CAS — 125472-02-8.

Profile

Mivazerol is an alpha$_2$-adrenoceptor agonist that has been in-

vestigated for the prevention of perioperative complications resulting from myocardial ischaemia in patients with ischaemic heart disease undergoing non-cardiac surgery.

◊ References.

1. Oliver MF, *et al.* Effect of mivazerol on perioperative cardiac complications during non-cardiac surgery in patients with coronary heart disease: the European Mivazerol Trial (EMIT). *Anesthesiology* 1999; **91:** 951–61.

Moexipril Hydrochloride (17803-g)

Moexipril Hydrochloride *(BANM, USAN, rINNM)*.
CI-925; RS-10085-197; SPM-925. (3S-{2[R*(R*)],3R*})-2-(2-{[1-(Ethoxycarbonyl)-3-phenylpropyl]amino}-1-oxopropyl)-1,2,3,4-tetrahydro-6,7-dimethoxy-3-isoquinoline-carboxylic acid hydrochloride.
$C_{27}H_{34}N_2O_7,HCl$ = 535.0.
CAS — 103775-10-6 *(moexipril)*; 82586-52-5 *(moexipril hydrochloride)*.

Adverse Effects, Treatment, and Precautions

As for ACE inhibitors, p.820.

Interactions

As for ACE inhibitors, p.822.

Pharmacokinetics

Moexipril acts as a prodrug of the diacid moexiprilat, its active metabolite. Following oral administration moexipril is rapidly but incompletely absorbed and is metabolised to moexiprilat in the gastrointestinal mucosa and liver. Absorption is reduced in the presence of food. The bioavailability of moexiprilat is about 13% following oral moexipril administration, and peak plasma concentrations of moexiprilat are reached in about 1.5 hours. Both moexipril and moexiprilat are moderately bound to plasma proteins. Moexipril is excreted predominantly in the urine as moexiprilat, unchanged drug, and other metabolites; some moexiprilat may also be excreted in the faeces. The functional elimination half-life of moexiprilat is about 12 hours.

Uses and Administration

Moexipril is an ACE inhibitor (p.820). It is used in the treatment of hypertension (p.802).

Moexipril owes its activity to moexiprilat, to which it is converted after oral administration. The haemodynamic effects are seen about 1 hour after an oral dose and the maximum effect occurs after about 3 to 6 hours, although the full effect may not develop for 2 to 4 weeks during chronic dosing. Moexipril is given by mouth as the hydrochloride.

In the treatment of **hypertension**, the usual initial dose of moexipril hydrochloride is 7.5 mg once daily. Since there may be a precipitous fall in blood pressure in some patients when starting therapy with an ACE inhibitor, the first dose should preferably be given at bedtime. An initial dose of 3.75 mg once daily, given under close medical supervision, is suggested for patients who are receiving a diuretic; if possible the diuretic should be withdrawn 2 or 3 days before moexipril is started and resumed later if necessary. An initial dose of 3.75 mg once daily is also recommended for patients with renal or liver impairment and for the elderly. The usual maintenance dose is 7.5 to 30 mg daily, which may be given in 2 divided doses if control is inadequate with a single dose.

◊ Reviews.

1. Brogden RN, Wiseman LR. Moexipril: a review of its use in the management of essential hypertension. *Drugs* 1998; **55:** 845–60.

Preparations

Proprietary Preparations (details are given in Part 3)
Denm.: Moex†; Perdix; *Fin.:* Perdix; *Fr.:* Moex; *Ger.:* Fempress; *Ital.:* Femipres; Primoxil; *Swed.:* Perdix; *Switz.:* Fempress; *UK:* Perdix; *USA:* Univasc.

Multi-ingredient: *Ger.:* Fempress Plus; *Ital.:* Femipres Plus; *USA:* Uniretic.

The symbol † denotes a preparation no longer actively marketed

Molsidomine (12971-v)

Molsidomine (BAN, USAN, rINN).
CAS-276; Morsydomine; SIN-10. N-Ethoxycarbonyl-3-morpholinosydnonimine.
$C_9H_{14}N_4O_4 = 242.2$.
CAS — 25717-80-0.
ATC — C01DX12.

Profile
Molsidomine is a nitrovasodilator used in angina pectoris (p.791). It may also be used in heart failure (p.798) and following myocardial infarction (p.805).

It is given by mouth in usual doses of 1 to 4 mg two to four times daily. Modified-release preparations are also available. It is also given by injection in single doses of 2 to 4 mg and doses of 2 mg may be repeated at intervals of at least 2 hours if necessary; total doses of up to 40 mg daily have been given. Infusions may be employed at a rate of up to 3 mg per hour.

Molsidomine is metabolised to linsidomine (p.921), an active metabolite.

◊ The pharmacokinetics of molsidomine have been reviewed.[1] Molsidomine is metabolised in the liver to linsidomine and other morpholine derivatives. Prolonged elimination half-lives of molsidomine and linsidomine due to reduced plasma clearance have been reported in patients with liver cirrhosis.[2]

Molsidomine tends to degrade into morpholine (even when protected from the light), a compound considered potentially carcinogenic. This finding led to the suspension of marketing of one molsidomine formulation;[3] an earlier temporary suspension was related to evidence of carcinogenicity in some animals, although this has not been confirmed in humans.

1. Rosenkranz B, et al. Clinical pharmacokinetics of molsidomine. Clin Pharmacokinet 1996; **30:** 372–84.
2. Spreux-Varoquaux O, et al. Pharmacokinetics of molsidomine and its active metabolite, linsidomine, in patients with liver cirrhosis. Br J Clin Pharmacol 1991; **32:** 399–401.
3. Anonymous. Corvaton Tropfen. Dtsch Apotheker Ztg 1989; **129** (49): VI.

Myocardial infarction. Although intravenous nitrates (glyceryl trinitrate or sodium nitroprusside) may be used in the management of acute myocardial infarction (p.805), molsidomine and its active metabolite linsidomine (a nitric oxide donor) had no effect on mortality.[1]

1. European Study of Prevention of Infarct with Molsidomine (ESPRIM) Group. The ESPRIM trial: short-term treatment of acute myocardial infarction with molsidomine. Lancet 1994; **344:** 91–7.

Preparations
Proprietary Preparations (details are given in Part 3)
Aust.: Molsidolat; Molsihexal; **Belg.:** Corvasal; Molsidirex; **Ger.:** Corvaton; duracoron; Molsi-Azu; Molsi-Puren; Molsicor; Molsihexal; molsiket; **Spain:** Corpea; Molsidain; **Switz.:** Corvaton.

Monteplase (17638-s)

Monteplase (rINN).
E-6010.
$C_{2569}H_{3896}N_{746}O_{783}S_{39} = 59009.5$.
CAS — 156616-23-8.

Profile
Monteplase is a thrombolytic related to alteplase (p.833) used in acute myocardial infarction (p.805). The usual dose is 27 500 units per kg body-weight, given by intravenous injection as soon as possible after the onset of symptoms.

◊ References.
1. Kawai C, et al. A prospective, randomized, double-blind multicenter trial of a single bolus injection of the novel modified t-PA E6010 in the treatment of acute myocardial infarction: comparison with native t-PA. J Am Coll Cardiol 1997; **29:** 1447–53.

Preparations
Proprietary Preparations (details are given in Part 3)
Jpn.: Cleactor.

Moracizine Hydrochloride (12978-l)

Moracizine Hydrochloride (BANM, rINNM).
EN-313 (moracizine). Ethyl [10-(3-morpholinopropionyl)phenothiazin-2-yl]carbamate hydrochloride.
$C_{22}H_{25}N_3O_4S,HCl = 464.0$.
CAS — 31883-05-3 (moracizine); 29560-58-5 (moracizine hydrochloride).
NOTE. Moricizine is USAN.
Pharmacopoeias. In US.

Pharmacopoeial description
USP 25: A white to off-white crystalline powder. Soluble in water and in alcohol. Store in airtight containers.

Adverse Effects
The most common adverse effects associated with moracizine therapy affect the CNS and the gastrointestinal tract and include dizziness, headache, fatigue, nausea, and abdominal pain. Other adverse effects include dyspnoea, dry mouth, blurred vision, impotence, and urinary-tract disorders. There

have been occasional reports of fever, thrombocytopenia, hepatic dysfunction, hypothermia, and skin rash.

Like other antiarrhythmics moracizine can provoke or worsen arrhythmias. This may range from an increase in the frequency of premature ventricular contractions to induction or worsening of ventricular tachycardia.

An increased mortality rate occurred when moracizine was tested in the control of asymptomatic ventricular arrhythmias in post-infarction patients (see Cardiac Arrhythmias under Uses and Administration, below).

◊ Fever with elevated creatine phosphokinase and hepatic transaminase concentrations was associated with moracizine administration in 2 patients.[1] The fever abated within 48 hours of withdrawing moracizine and recurred within 24 hours of re-challenge in both patients. Results suggested a similarity to the neuroleptic malignant syndrome which has been attributed to other phenothiazine derivatives.

1. Miura DS, et al. Ethmozine toxicity: fever of unknown origin. J Clin Pharmacol 1986; **26:** 153–5.

Precautions
As for Flecainide Acetate, p.890.

Interactions
Concomitant administration of moracizine with other antiarrhythmics or arrhythmogenic drugs may increase the incidence of cardiac arrhythmias. Moracizine undergoes metabolism in the liver and its activity may be influenced by other drugs affecting the enzymes responsible for its metabolism; it is an enzyme inducer and may also affect the activity of other hepatically-metabolised drugs.

Pharmacokinetics
Moracizine is readily and almost completely absorbed from the gastrointestinal tract. It undergoes significant first-pass hepatic metabolism so that the bioavailability following oral administration is about 38%. Moracizine is extensively metabolised and some of the numerous metabolites may be active. It induces its own metabolism; the plasma elimination half-life is about 2 hours following multiple doses. Although plasma concentrations are reduced with multiple dosing, clinical response is not affected. It is about 95% bound to plasma proteins. Moracizine is distributed into breast milk. Approximately 56% of a dose is excreted in the faeces and approximately 39% in the urine.

◊ References.
1. Benedek IH, et al. Enzyme induction by moricizine: time course and extent in healthy subjects. J Clin Pharmacol 1994; **34:** 167–75.

Uses and Administration
Moracizine is a phenothiazine compound with class I antiarrhythmic activity (p.787) but which does not readily fall into the subclasses a, b, or c. It is used as the hydrochloride in the treatment of serious symptomatic ventricular **arrhythmias**. Moracizine hydrochloride is given in a usual dose of 600 to 900 mg daily by mouth in 2 or 3 divided doses. Doses, which should be given initially in hospital, should be adjusted at intervals of not less than 3 days. If rapid control of life-threatening arrhythmias is essential an initial dose of 400 to 500 mg followed by 200 mg every 8 hours may be given.

Patients with hepatic or renal impairment should be started on a dosage of 600 mg or less daily and monitored closely.

◊ General reviews of moracizine published before[1-3] and after[4] the results of the Cardiac Arrhythmia Suppression Trial (CAST II), in which moracizine was associated with increased mortality (see Cardiac Arrhythmias, below).
1. Fitton A, Buckley MM-T. Moricizine: a review of its pharmacological properties, and therapeutic efficacy in cardiac arrhythmias. Drugs 1990; **40:** 138–67.
2. Carnes CA, Coyle JD. Moricizine: a novel antiarrhythmic agent. DICP Ann Pharmacother 1990; **24:** 745–53.
3. Mann HJ. Moricizine: a new class I antiarrhythmic. Clin Pharm 1990; **9:** 842–52.
4. Clyne CA, et al. Moricizine. N Engl J Med 1992; **327:** 255–60.

Cardiac arrhythmias. Asymptomatic premature ventricular arrhythmias in subjects who have previously suffered a myocardial infarction are recognised as a risk factor for subsequent sudden cardiac death.[1] Suppressing such arrhythmias in this group might be expected to reduce the incidence of sudden death and it was to test this hypothesis that a large multicentre study was set up in the USA (the Cardiac Arrhythmia Suppression Trial known as CAST).[2,3] Encainide, flecainide, and moracizine were the antiarrhythmics studied, but encainide and flecainide, and later moracizine,[4] were all associated with increased mortality. It is now accepted that these drugs should not be used prophylactically in post-infarction patients with asymptomatic arrhythmias.

Licensed indications for moracizine cover severe symptomatic ventricular arrhythmias (p.794).

1. Task Force of the Working Group on Arrhythmias of the European Society of Cardiology. CAST and beyond: implications of the cardiac arrhythmias suppression trial. Circulation 1990; **81:** 1123–7. [Simultaneous publication occurred in Eur Heart J 1990; **11:** 194–9.]
2. The Cardiac Arrhythmia Suppression Trial (CAST) Investigators. Preliminary report: effect of encainide and flecainide on mortality in a randomized trial of arrhythmia suppression after myocardial infarction. N Engl J Med 1989; **321:** 406–12.

3. Echt DS, et al. Mortality and morbidity in patients receiving encainide, flecainide, or placebo: the Cardiac Arrhythmia Suppression Trial. N Engl J Med 1991; **324:** 781–8.
4. The Cardiac Arrhythmia Suppression Trial II Investigators. Effect of the antiarrhythmic agent moricizine on survival after myocardial infarction. N Engl J Med 1992; **327:** 227–33.

Preparations
USP 25: Moricizine Hydrochloride Tablets.
Proprietary Preparations (details are given in Part 3)
Irl.: Ethmozine; **UK:** Ethmozine†; **USA:** Ethmozine.

Moxonidine (19534-k)

Moxonidine (BAN, USAN, rINN).
BDF-5895; BDF-5896; BE-5895; LY-326869. 4-Chloro-5-(2-imidazolin-2-ylamino)-6-methoxy-2-methylpyrimidine.
$C_9H_{12}ClN_5O = 241.7$.
CAS — 75438-57-2.
ATC — C02AC05.

Adverse Effects and Treatment
Moxonidine has similar adverse effects to clonidine (p.860) but causes less sedation. The incidence of dry mouth may also be lower.

Precautions
Moxonidine should not be used in patients with conduction disorders, bradycardia, severe arrhythmias, severe heart failure, severe ischaemic heart disease, severe hepatic or renal impairment, or a history of angioedema. The manufacturer suggests that it should also be avoided in patients with intermittent claudication or Raynaud's disease, Parkinson's disease, epilepsy, glaucoma, and depression. Moxonidine is distributed into breast milk and should not be used during breast feeding.

Although rebound hypertension has not been reported following moxonidine withdrawal it should not be stopped abruptly but should be withdrawn gradually over 2 weeks. In patients who are receiving a beta blocker concomitantly, the beta blocker should be stopped several days before moxonidine is withdrawn.

Interactions
The hypotensive effect of moxonidine may be enhanced by other antihypertensives and drugs that cause hypotension. The effect of sedatives and hypnotics, including benzodiazepines, may be enhanced by moxonidine.

Pharmacokinetics
Moxonidine is well absorbed following oral administration and has a bioavailability of about 88%. Peak plasma concentrations occur 0.5 to 3 hours after an oral dose. It is excreted almost entirely in the urine as unchanged drug and metabolites; about 50 to 75% of an oral dose is excreted as unchanged drug. The mean plasma elimination half-life is 2 to 3 hours and is prolonged in renal impairment. Moxonidine is about 7% bound to plasma proteins. It is distributed into breast milk.

Uses and Administration
Moxonidine is a centrally acting antihypertensive structurally related to clonidine (p.860). It appears to act through stimulation of central imidazoline receptors to reduce sympathetic tone, and also has alpha$_2$-adrenoceptor agonist activity. It is used in the treatment of hypertension (p.802) and has also been investigated for heart failure.

In the treatment of hypertension, moxonidine is given by mouth in a usual initial dose of 200 μg once daily. The dose may be increased if necessary, after 3 weeks, to 400 μg daily as a single dose or in two divided doses, and after a further 3 weeks, to a maximum dose of 600 μg daily in two divided doses. The dose should be reduced in patients with renal impairment.

◊ References.
1. Chrisp P, Faulds D. Moxonidine: a review of its pharmacology, and therapeutic use in essential hypertension. Drugs 1992; **44:** 993–1012.

2. Schachter M, *et al.* Safety and tolerability of moxonidine in the treatment of hypertension. *Drug Safety* 1998; **19:** 191–203.
3. Bousquet P, Feldman J. Drugs acting on imidazoline receptors: a review of their pharmacology, their use in blood pressure control and their potential interest in cardioprotection. *Drugs* 1999; **58:** 799–812.
4. Schachter M. Moxonidine. *Prescribers' J* 1999; **39:** 113–17.

Preparations

Proprietary Preparations (details are given in Part 3)
Aust.: Normoxin; **Belg.:** Moxon; **Braz.:** Cynt; **Denm.:** Physiotens; **Fin.:** Physiotens; **Fr.:** Physiotens; **Ger.:** Physiotens; **Neth.:** Normatens; **Norw.:** Physiotens; **S.Afr.:** Physiotens; **Spain:** Cynt; Moxon; **Swed.:** Physiotens; **Switz.:** Physiotens; **UK:** Physiotens.

Nadolol (6315-I)

Nadolol *(BAN, USAN, rINN)*.
SQ-11725. (2R,3S)-5-(3-*tert*-Butylamino-2-hydroxypropoxy)-1,2,3,4-tetrahydronaphthalene-2,3-diol.
$C_{17}H_{27}NO_4 = 309.4$.
CAS — 42200-33-9.
ATC — C07AA12.
Pharmacopoeias. In Jpn and US.

Pharmacopoeial description

USP 25: White or off-white, practically odourless, crystalline powder. Soluble in water at pH 2; slightly soluble in water at pH 7 to 10; freely soluble in alcohol and in methyl alcohol; insoluble in acetone, in ether, in petroleum spirit, in trichloroethane, and in benzene; slightly soluble in chloroform, in dichloromethane, and in isopropyl alcohol.

Adverse Effects, Treatment, and Precautions

As for beta blockers, p.844.

Hypersensitivity. Hypersensitivity pneumonitis was associated with nadolol in a patient prescribed the drug for migraine.[1] Symptoms improved when nadolol was withdrawn.

1. Levy MB, *et al.* Nadolol and hypersensitivity pneumonitis. *Ann Intern Med* 1986; **105:** 806–7.

Interactions

The interactions associated with beta blockers are discussed on p.846.

Pharmacokinetics

Nadolol is incompletely absorbed from the gastrointestinal tract to give peak plasma concentrations about 3 or 4 hours after a dose. It has low lipid solubility. Nadolol is widely distributed and concentrations found in breast milk have been higher than those in serum. It is only about 30% bound to plasma proteins. It does not appear to be metabolised and is excreted mainly in the urine. The plasma half-life has been reported as ranging from about 12 to 24 hours. Nadolol is reported to be dialysable.

◊ In 4 patients with mild hypertension given nadolol 2 mg by mouth or intravenously, the elimination half-life from plasma was an average of 10 to 12 hours (a range of 5.9 to 12.2 hours following intravenous administration, and a range of 9.6 to 14.2 hours following oral administration). Calculations based on urinary excretion and plasma concentration data suggested that about 33% was absorbed after oral administration. There was evidence of biliary as well as urinary excretion since after intravenous administration about 73% was excreted in urine and 23% in faeces. Nadolol did not appear to be metabolised.[1] In a similar study of therapeutic oral doses, terminal half-lives ranging from 14 to 17 hours were reported for nadolol 80 mg given as a single dose and the same dose daily in a multiple dosage regimen.[2]

1. Dreyfuss J, *et al.* Metabolic studies in patients with nadolol: oral and intravenous administration. *J Clin Pharmacol* 1977; **17:** 300–7.
2. Dreyfuss J, *et al.* Pharmacokinetics of nadolol, a beta-receptor antagonist: administration of therapeutic single- and multiple-dosage regimens to hypertensive patients. *J Clin Pharmacol* 1979; **19:** 712–20.

Breast feeding. Concentrations of nadolol in breast milk were determined in 12 lactating normotensive women who took nadolol 80 mg daily by mouth for 5 days.[1] The mean nadolol concentration in milk for the 24 hours after the last dose was 357 nanograms per mL; the equivalent mean serum-nadolol concentration was only 77 nanograms per mL.

1. Devlin RG, Fleiss PM. Nadolol excretion in human milk. *Clin Pharmacol Ther* 1981; **29:** 240.

Children. The pharmacokinetics of nadolol given intravenously and orally were studied in six children aged 3 months to 14 years.[1] The elimination half-lives for the two oldest children aged 10 and 14 years were 7.3 and 15.7 hours, respectively. These values are similar to those reported for adults whereas in the children 22 months of age or younger, shorter half-lives of 3.2 to 4.3 hours were found. The authors considered that the shorter half-lives were probably a result of a reduction in the

total apparent volume of distribution of nadolol in the youngest children. Elimination rates were similar after either intravenous or oral administration.

1. Mehta AV, *et al.* Pharmacokinetics of nadolol in children with supraventricular tachycardia. *J Clin Pharmacol* 1992; **32:** 1023–7.

Uses and Administration

Nadolol is a non-cardioselective beta blocker (p.844). It is reported to lack intrinsic sympathomimetic and membrane-stabilising activity. Nadolol is used in the management of hypertension (p.802), angina pectoris (p.791), and cardiac arrhythmias (p.794). It is also used in the management of hyperthyroidism (p.1519) and in the prophylactic treatment of migraine (p.449).

In the treatment of **hypertension**, nadolol is usually given in an initial dose of 40 to 80 mg daily by mouth, increased weekly according to the response of the patient to 240 mg or more daily.

In **angina pectoris**, the usual initial dose is 40 mg daily, increased weekly according to the response of the patient to usual doses of up to 160 mg daily; some patients may require up to 240 mg daily. Doses of 40 to 160 mg daily have also been given for **cardiac arrhythmias**.

Similar doses of 40 to 160 mg daily are used in **migraine** prophylaxis.

In the management of **hyperthyroidism**, doses of 80 to 160 mg daily have been given; most patients are reported to require the higher dose.

Patients with renal impairment may require a lower dose or less frequent administration. One method of dose adjustment is to increase the dosage interval according to the patient's creatinine clearance. For patients with a creatinine clearance between 31 and 50 mL per minute, nadolol is given every 24 to 36 hours; for patients with a clearance between 10 and 30 mL per minute, administration is every 24 to 48 hours; for those with a clearance of less than 10 mL per minute, the dosage interval is 40 to 60 hours.

Preparations

USP 25: Nadolol and Bendroflumethiazide Tablets; Nadolol Tablets.

Proprietary Preparations (details are given in Part 3)
Aust.: Solgol; **Belg.:** Corgard; **Braz.:** Corgard; **Canad.:** Apo-Nadol; **Corgard; Fr.:** Corgard; **Ger.:** Solgol; **Hong Kong:** Apo-Nadol; Corgard; **Irl.:** Corgard†; **Ital.:** Corgard; **NZ:** Corgard; **S.Afr.:** Corgard; **Spain:** Corgard; Solgol; **Switz.:** Corgard; **UK:** Corgard; **USA:** Corgard.

Multi-ingredient: Aust.: Solgeretik; **Canad.:** Corzide†; **Ger.:** Sotaziden N; **Irl.:** Corgaretic†; **S.Afr.:** Corgaretic; **Switz.:** Corgaretic; **UK:** Corgaretic; **USA:** Corzide.

Nadoxolol Hydrochloride (12992-w)

Nadoxolol Hydrochloride *(rINNM)*.
LL-1530. 3-Hydroxy-4-(1-naphthyloxy)butyramide oxime hydrochloride.
$C_{14}H_{16}N_2O_3,HCl = 296.7$.
CAS — 54063-51-3 (nadoxolol); 35991-93-6 (nadoxolol hydrochloride).

Profile

Nadoxolol hydrochloride is an antiarrhythmic used in doses of 0.75 to 1.5 g daily by mouth.

Preparations

Proprietary Preparations (details are given in Part 3)
Fr.: Bradyl.

Nadroparin Calcium (4871-n)

Nadroparin Calcium *(BAN, rINN)*.
CY-216; Nadroparinum Calcicum.
Pharmacopoeias. In Eur. (see p.vi).

Pharmacopoeial description

Ph. Eur.: Nadroparin calcium is prepared by nitrous acid depolymerisation of heparin obtained from the intestinal mucosa of pigs. The majority of the components have a 2-*O*-sulfo-α-L-idopyranosuronic acid structure at the non-reducing end and a 6-*O*-sulfo-2,5-anhydro-D-mannitol structure at the reducing end of their chain. The mass-average molecular mass ranges between 3600 and 5000, with a characteristic value of 4300. The mass percentage of chains lower than 2000 is not more than 15%. The degree of sulfation is about 2 per disaccharide unit.

The potency is not less than 95 units and not more than 130 units of anti-factor Xa activity per mg with reference to the

dried substance, and the ratio of anti-factor Xa activity to anti-factor IIa (antithrombin) activity is between 2.5 and 4.0.

Profile

Nadroparin calcium is a low-molecular-weight heparin (p.923) with anticoagulant properties. It is used in the treatment and prophylaxis of venous thromboembolism (p.817) and to prevent clotting during extracorporeal circulation.

Doses are expressed in terms of anti-factor Xa activity (anti-Xa units) although different values may be encountered in the literature depending upon the reference preparation used. For prophylaxis of venous thromboembolism during surgery, patients at moderate risk of thrombosis are given 2850 units of nadroparin calcium by subcutaneous injection daily for at least 7 days or until the patient is ambulant; the first dose is given 2 to 4 hours before the procedure. For patients at high risk of thrombosis the dose is adjusted according to body-weight. Usual doses are 38 units per kg 12 hours before surgery, 12 hours postoperatively and then daily until 3 days after the procedure; the dose is then increased by 50% to 57 units per kg daily. The total duration of treatment should be at least 10 days.

For the treatment of thromboembolism, nadroparin calcium is given in a dose of 85 units per kg by subcutaneous injection every 12 hours for 10 days. Alternatively, a dose of 171 units per kg is given once daily.

For prevention of clotting in the extracorporeal circulation during haemodialysis sessions lasting less than 4 hours, nadroparin calcium is administered into the arterial line of the circuit at the beginning of the dialysis session. The usual dose is 2850 units for patients weighing less than 50 kg, 3800 units for patients weighing 50 to 69 kg, and 5700 units for patients weighing 70 kg or more. Doses should be reduced in patients at high risk of haemorrhage.

◊ References.

1. Barradell LB, Buckley MM. Nadroparin calcium: a review of its pharmacology and clinical applications in the prevention and treatment of thromboembolic disorders. *Drugs* 1992; **44:** 858–88.

Preparations

Proprietary Preparations (details are given in Part 3)
Aust.: Fraxiparin; **Austral.:** Fraxiparine; **Belg.:** Fraxiparine; **Braz.:** Fraxiparina; **Canad.:** Fraxiparine; **Denm.:** Fraxiparine†; **Fin.:** Fraxiparine; **Fr.:** Fraxiparine; Fraxodi; **Ger.:** Fraxiparin; **Hong Kong:** Fraxiparine; **Ital.:** Fraxiparina; Seleparina; **Mex.:** Fraxiparine; **Neth.:** Fraxiparine; Fraxodi; **Norw.:** Fraxiparin; **NZ:** Fraxiparine; **Port.:** Fraxiparina; **Singapore:** Fraxiparine; **Spain:** Fraxiparina; **Swed.:** Fraxiparine; **Switz.:** Fraxiforte; Fraxiparine; **Thai.:** Fraxiparine.

Naftidrofuryl Oxalate (9256-a)

Naftidrofuryl Oxalate *(BANM, rINNM)*.
EU-1806; LS-121; Nafronyl Oxalate *(USAN)*; Naftidrofuryl Hydrogen Oxalate; Naftidrofuryli Hydrogenooxalas. 2-Diethylaminoethyl 3-(1-naphthyl)-2-tetrahydrofurfurylpropionate hydrogen oxalate.
$C_{24}H_{33}NO_3,C_2H_2O_4 = 473.6$.
CAS — 31329-57-4 (naftidrofuryl); 3200-06-4 (naftidrofuryl oxalate).
Pharmacopoeias. In Eur. (see p.vi).

Pharmacopoeial description

Ph. Eur.: A white or almost white powder. Freely soluble in water and in alcohol; slightly or sparingly soluble in acetone.

Adverse Effects

Naftidrofuryl oxalate given orally may cause nausea and epigastric pain. Rash has been reported occasionally. Hepatitis or hepatic failure has occurred rarely. Convulsions may occur at high doses. Depression of cardiac conduction may occur following overdose. Following intravenous administration cardiac arrhythmias, hypotension, and convulsions have been reported and intravenous preparations have been withdrawn from the market (see below).

◊ In early 1995 the UK Committee on Safety of Medicines (CSM) published details of adverse reactions to naftidrofuryl.[1] Following parenteral administration of naftidrofuryl 47 reports of 79 reactions had been received, the most serious consequences being 9 cases of cardiac arrhythmias, 3 of convulsions, and 2 of hypotension. It was also noted that 2 fatal cases of cardiac arrest had occurred in Germany following bolus intravenous doses and it was stressed that the drug must not be given as a bolus but as a slow intravenous infusion. Additionally, 16 reports, including one fatality, of hepatitis or hepatic failure associated with oral naftidrofuryl had been received although this appeared to be a rare reaction.

Later in 1995, following a review conducted in the UK and Europe, it was announced by the CSM that intravenous naftidrofuryl was to be withdrawn.[2] It was considered that the risks of cardiac and neurological toxicity outweighed the benefits of intravenous administration in peripheral vascular disease. The oral form of naftidrofuryl would remain available.

1. Committee on Safety of Medicines/Medicines Control Agency. Adverse reactions with naftidrofuryl (Praxilene). *Current Problems* 1995; **21:** 2.
2. Committee on Safety of Medicines/Medicines Control Agency. Withdrawal of naftidrofuryl infusion (Praxilene Forte). *Current Problems* 1995; **21:** 7.

Effects on the kidneys. Calcium oxalate crystals in the renal tubules of 2 patients with acute renal failure[1] were associated with the high amounts of oxalate they had received when naftidrofuryl oxalate was administered intravenously.

1. Moesch C, *et al.* Renal intratubular crystallisation of calcium oxalate and naftidrofuryl oxalate. *Lancet* 1991; **338:** 1219–20.

Uses and Administration

Naftidrofuryl oxalate is used as a vasodilator in the treatment of peripheral (p.809) and cerebral vascular disorders (p.798). It is also claimed to enhance cellular oxidative capacity thereby protecting cells against the results of ischaemia.

Naftidrofuryl oxalate is given by mouth in usual doses of 100 to 200 mg three times daily for peripheral vascular disorders and 100 mg three times daily for cerebrovascular disorders.

Naftidrofuryl oxalate has also been administered parenterally. However, intravenous administration has been associated with serious adverse effects (see above) and intravenous preparations have been withdrawn.

Stroke. Naftidrofuryl is one of many drugs (sometimes referred to as neuroprotectants) that have been tried in acute ischaemic stroke (p.813). It has been suggested that any beneficial effect might be due to cerebral intracellular metabolism protecting the cells against the results of ischaemia. Results of a double-blind placebo-controlled study of naftidrofuryl in 91 patients with acute stroke indicated that the extent of recovery was greater following 12 weeks of treatment with oral naftidrofuryl and patients were able to leave hospital on average 25 days sooner than patients taking placebo.[1] However, a later, similar study[2] in 100 patients found no significant difference in mortality or recovery. A placebo-controlled study[3] in 100 patients with acute stroke given naftidrofuryl initially by intravenous infusion [preparation no longer available] for 10 days followed by 9 months of oral treatment, showed no effect on death rate but an improvement was seen in neurological recovery.

1. Admani AK. New approach to treatment of recent stroke. *BMJ* 1978; **2:** 1678–9.
2. Gray CS, *et al.* A randomized double-blind controlled trial of naftidrofuryl in acute stroke. *Age Ageing* 1990; **19:** 356–63.
3. Steiner TJ, Rose FC. Towards a model stroke trial: the single-centre naftidrofuryl study. *Neuroepidemiology* 1986; **5:** 121–47.

Preparations

BP 2001: Naftidrofuryl Capsules.

Proprietary Preparations (details are given in Part 3)
Aust.: Dusodril; Naftodril; *Belg.:* Praxilene; *Fr.:* Di-Actane; Gevatran; Naftilux; Praxilene; *Ger.:* Artocoron; Azunaftil; Dusodril; Luctor; Nafti; Naftilong; *Hong Kong:* Praxilene; *Irl.:* Praxilene; *Ital.:* Esedril†; Praxilene; *Port.:* Praxilene; *Singapore:* Praxilene; *Spain:* Praxilene; *Switz.:* Praxilene; Sodipryl retard; *Thai.:* Praxilene; *UK:* Praxilene; Stimlor.

Naftopidil (2756-v)

Naftopidil (*rINN*).

BM-15275; KT-611. (±)-4-(*o*-Methoxyphenyl)-α-[(1-naphthyloxy)methyl]-1-piperazineethanol.
$C_{24}H_{28}N_2O_3 = 392.5$.
$CAS — 57149-07-2$.

Profile
Naftopidil is a peripheral alpha$_1$-adrenoceptor blocker which is structurally related to urapidil (p.987) and has similar general properties. It is under investigation in the management of hypertension and in benign prostatic hyperplasia to relieve symptoms of urinary obstruction.

Preparations

Proprietary Preparations (details are given in Part 3)
Jpn: Avishot; Flivas.

Nasaruplase (17099-r)

Nasaruplase (*rINN*).

Prourokinase (enzyme-activating) (human clone pA3/pD2/pF1 protein moiety), glycosylated.
$CAS — 99821-44-0$.

Profile
Nasaruplase is a thrombolytic under investigation in acute ischaemic stroke.

◊ References.
1. Furlan A, *et al.* Intra-arterial prourokinase for acute ischemic stroke. The PROACT II study: a randomized controlled trial. *JAMA* 1999; **282:** 2003–11.

Natriuretic Peptides (3930-e)

Profile
Natriuretic peptides are endogenous substances that possess diuretic, natriuretic, and vasodilator properties. Three types are known: atrial natriuretic peptide (ANP), which is also known as atrial natriuretic factor (ANF), atriopeptin, auriculin, or cardionatrin, and is produced mainly in the cardiac atria; brain natriuretic peptide (BNP; B-type natriuretic peptide), which was originally isolated from brain tissue but is now known to be mainly produced by the cardiac ventricles; and C-type natriuretic peptide (CNP), which is produced by the endothelium

and appears to act locally as a vasodilator but has little natriuretic effect. Ularitide (urodilatin) is an endogenous form of atrial natriuretic peptide that is produced in the kidney.

Natriuretic peptides have an important physiological role in fluid and electrolyte homoeostasis and in the regulation of blood pressure, and they interact closely with other complex systems such as the renin-angiotensin-aldosterone cascade. Plasma concentrations of atrial natriuretic peptide and brain natriuretic peptide are altered in some pathological states and have been used as indicators of cardiac function. Natriuretic peptides that are being investigated for therapeutic use include anaritide, a synthetic form of atrial natriuretic peptide, and ularitide, both of which have been studied in acute renal failure. Recombinant forms of atrial natriuretic peptide (carperitide, p.855) and brain natriuretic peptide (nesiritide, p.938) are used in the management of acute heart failure.

The currently available natriuretic peptides have short half-lives and have to be given parenterally. Other approaches to manipulating their effects are under investigation and include the use of atriopeptidase inhibitors (neutral endopeptidase inhibitors; neutral metalloendopeptidase inhibitors), such as candoxatrilat (p.853) and ecadotril (sinorphan) to prolong the half-life of endogenous atrial natriuretic peptide. Compounds such as omapatrilat (p.949) that inhibit both neutral endopeptidase and angiotensin-converting enzyme are also being studied.

◊ References.
1. Tan ACITL, *et al.* Atrial natriuretic peptide: an overview of clinical pharmacology and pharmacokinetics. *Clin Pharmacokinet* 1993; **24:** 28–45.
2. Deutsch A, *et al.* Atrial natriuretic peptide and its potential role in pharmacotherapy. *J Clin Pharmacol* 1994; **34:** 1133–47.
3. Struthers AD. Ten years of natriuretic peptide research: a new dawn for their diagnostic and therapeutic use? *BMJ* 1994; **308:** 1615–19.
4. Richards AM. The renin-angiotensin-aldosterone system and the cardiac natriuretic peptides. *Heart* 1996; **76** (suppl 3): 36–44.
5. Wilkins MR, *et al.* The natriuretic-peptide family. *Lancet* 1997; **349:** 1307–10.
6. Allgren RL, *et al.* Anaritide in acute tubular necrosis. *N Engl J Med* 1997; **336:** 828–34.
7. Levin ER, *et al.* Natriuretic peptides. *N Engl J Med* 1998; **339:** 321–8.

Nebivolol Hydrochloride (2966-z)

Nebivolol Hydrochloride (*BANM, rINNM*).

R-67555; R-65824 (nebivolol). (1*RS*,1′*RS*)-1,1′-[(2*RS*,2′*SR*)-Bis(6-fluorochroman-2-yl)]-2,2′-iminodiethanol hydrochloride.
$C_{22}H_{25}F_2NO_4,HCl = 441.9$.
$CAS — 99200-09-6 (nebivolol)$.

NOTE. Nebivolol is *USAN*.

Adverse Effects, Treatment, and Precautions
As for beta blockers, p.844. Nebivolol should not be used in patients with hepatic impairment.

Interactions
The interactions associated with beta blockers are discussed on p.846.

Pharmacokinetics
Nebivolol is rapidly absorbed following oral administration. It is extensively metabolised in the liver by alicyclic and aromatic hydroxylation, *N*-dealkylation, and glucuronidation; the hydroxy metabolites are reported to be active. The rate of aromatic hydroxylation by cytochrome P450 isoenzyme CYP2D6 is subject to genetic polymorphism and bioavailability and half-life vary widely. In fast metabolisers the elimination half-life of nebivolol is about 10 hours and of the hydroxy metabolites is about 24 hours. Peak plasma concentrations of unchanged drug plus active metabolites are 1.3 to 1.4 times higher in slow metabolisers and the half-lives of nebivolol and its hydroxy metabolites are prolonged.

Nebivolol is about 98% bound to plasma proteins. It is excreted in the urine and faeces, almost entirely as metabolites. Nebivolol is distributed into breast milk in *animal* studies.

Uses and Administration
Nebivolol is a cardioselective beta blocker (p.844). It is also reported to have vasodilating activity but to lack intrinsic sympathomimetic and membrane-stabilising activity.

Nebivolol is used in the management of hypertension (p.802). It is given by mouth as the hydrochloride although doses are expressed in terms of the base. The

usual dose is 5 mg daily. An initial dose of 2.5 mg daily is employed in the elderly and in patients with renal impairment.

◊ References.
1. McNeely W, Goa KL. Nebivolol in the management of essential hypertension: a review. *Drugs* 1999; **57:** 633–51. Correction. *ibid.:* 870.

Preparations

Proprietary Preparations (details are given in Part 3)
Aust.: Nebilet†; *Ger.:* Nebilet; *Irl.:* Nebilet; *Ital.:* Lobivon; Nebilox; *Neth.:* Nebilet; *Port.:* Nebilet; *Spain:* Lobivon; *Switz.:* Nebilet; *UK:* Nebilet.

Nesiritide (20221-y)

Nesiritide (*USAN, rINN*).
$C_{143}H_{244}N_{50}O_{42}S_4 = 3464.0$.
$CAS — 124584-08-3 (nesiritide); 189032-40-4 (nesiritide citrate)$.

NOTE. Nesiritide Citrate is *USAN*.

Profile
Nesiritide is a recombinant brain natriuretic peptide (see p.938) used in the management of acutely decompensated heart failure (p.798). It is given intravenously as the citrate, but dosage is expressed in terms of the base. The initial dose of nesiritide is 2 μg per kg body-weight by intravenous injection over 1 minute, followed by a maintenance infusion of 0.01 μg per kg per minute.

◊ References.
1. Colucci WS, *et al.* Intravenous nesiritide, a natriuretic peptide, in the treatment of decompensated congestive heart failure. *N Engl J Med* 2000; **343:** 246–53. Correction. *ibid.;* 1504.

Preparations

Proprietary Preparations (details are given in Part 3)
USA: Natrecor.

Nicardipine Hydrochloride (13008-c)

Nicardipine Hydrochloride (*BANM, USAN, rINNM*).

RS-69216; RS-69216-XX-07-0; YC-93. 2-[Benzyl(methyl)amino]ethyl methyl 1,4-dihydro-2,6-dimethyl-4-(3-nitrophenyl)pyridine-3,5-dicarboxylate hydrochloride.
$C_{26}H_{29}N_3O_6,HCl = 516.0$.
$CAS — 55985-32-5 (nicardipine); 54527-84-3 (nicardipine hydrochloride)$.

Pharmacopoeias. In *Jpn*.

Incompatibilities. The manufacturers recommend that a solution containing nicardipine hydrochloride 0.1 mg per mL is used for intravenous infusion. Suitable diluents are solutions of glucose or sodium chloride; sodium bicarbonate and lactated Ringer's are incompatible with nicardipine infusion.

Nicardipine hydrochloride (1 mg per mL in glucose 5%) has been reported[1] to be visually incompatible with frusemide [furosemide], heparin, and thiopental.

1. Chiu MF, Schwartz ML. Visual compatibility of injectable drugs used in the intensive care unit. *Am J Health-Syst Pharm* 1997; **54:** 64–5.

Adverse Effects, Treatment, and Precautions
As for dihydropyridine calcium-channel blockers (see Nifedipine, p.940).

Interactions
As for dihydropyridine calcium-channel blockers (see Nifedipine, p.942).

Pharmacokinetics
Nicardipine is rapidly absorbed from the gastrointestinal tract but is subject to saturable first-pass hepatic metabolism. Bioavailability of about 35% has been reported following a 30-mg dose at steady state. The pharmacokinetics of nicardipine are non-linear due to the saturable first-pass hepatic metabolism and an increase in dose may produce a disproportionate increase in plasma concentration. There is also considerable interindividual variation in plasma-nicardipine concentrations. Nicardipine is more than 95% bound to plasma proteins. Nicardipine is extensively metabolised in the liver and is excreted in the urine and faeces, mainly as inactive metabolites. The terminal plasma half-life is about 8.6 hours, thus steady-state plasma concentrations are achieved after 2 to 3 days of dosing three times daily.

◊ References.
1. Graham DJM, *et al.* Pharmacokinetics of nicardipine following oral and intravenous administration in man. *Postgrad Med J* 1984; **60** (suppl 4): 7–10.
2. Graham DJM, *et al.* The metabolism and pharmacokinetics of nicardipine hydrochloride in man. *Br J Clin Pharmacol* 1985; **20**: 23S–28S.
3. Razak TA, *et al.* The effect of hepatic cirrhosis on the pharmacokinetics and blood pressure response to nicardipine. *Clin Pharmacol Ther* 1990; **47**: 463–9.
4. Porchet HC, Dayer P. Serum concentrations and effects of (±)-nicardipine compared with nifedipine in a population of healthy subjects. *Clin Pharmacol Ther* 1990; **48**: 155–60.

Uses and Administration

Nicardipine is a dihydropyridine calcium-channel blocker with actions and uses similar to nifedipine (p.943). It is used in the management of hypertension (p.802) and angina pectoris (p.791).

Nicardipine hydrochloride is generally given by mouth although the intravenous route has been employed for the short-term treatment of hypertension.

Oral doses of nicardipine hydrochloride are similar for both **hypertension** and **angina**. The initial dose is 20 mg by mouth three times daily and may be increased at intervals of at least 3 days until the required effect is achieved. The usual maintenance dose is 30 mg three times daily, but daily doses of between 60 and 120 mg in divided doses may be given. Modified-release preparations of nicardipine hydrochloride for administration twice daily are also available.

Nicardipine hydrochloride may be administered by slow intravenous infusion as a 0.1 mg per mL solution in the short-term treatment of hypertension. An initial infusion rate of 5 mg per hour is recommended, increased, as necessary, up to a maximum of 15 mg per hour and subsequently reduced to 3 mg per hour.

Reduced doses of nicardipine hydrochloride and longer dosing intervals may be necessary in patients with impaired liver function.

◊ General reviews.
1. Sorkin EM, Clissold SP. Nicardipine: a review of its pharmacodynamic and pharmacokinetic properties, and therapeutic efficacy, in the treatment of angina pectoris, hypertension and related cardiovascular disorders. *Drugs* 1987; **33**: 296–345.
2. Frishman WH. New therapeutic modalities in hypertension: focus on a new calcium antagonist—nicardipine. *J Clin Pharmacol* 1989; **29**: 481–7.

Administration in neonates. Intravenous infusion of nicardipine was used successfully in 8 preterm infants (gestational age 28 to 36 weeks) for the management of hypertension.[1] Infusions were continued for periods of 3 to 36 days. No hypotension, oedema, or tachycardia were observed.
1. Gouyon JB, *et al.* Intravenous nicardipine in hypertensive preterm infants. *Arch Dis Child* 1997; **76**: F126–F127.

Cerebrovascular disorders. Nicardipine has been reported to increase cerebral blood flow[1] and has been investigated for possible benefit in haemorrhagic[2] and ischaemic stroke[3,4] (p.813), although nimodipine (p.946) is the dihydropyridine calcium-channel blocker usually used. Nicardipine has also been tried[5] in patients with cerebrovascular insufficiency. However, studies have produced inconclusive results.
1. Savage I, James I. The effect of nicardipine hydrochloride on cerebral blood flow in normotensive volunteers. *Br J Clin Pharmacol* 1986; **21**: 591P–592P.
2. Feigin VL, *et al.* Calcium antagonists in patients with aneurysmal subarachnoid hemorrhage: a systematic review. *Neurology* 1998; **50**: 876–83.
3. Yao L, Ding D. Effect of nicardipine on somatosensory evoked potentials in patients with acute cerebral infarction. *J Neurol Neurosurg Psychiatry* 1990; **53**: 844–6.
4. Rosenbaum D, *et al.* Early treatment of ischemic stroke with a calcium antagonist. *Stroke* 1991; **22**: 437–41.
5. Silva APE, Diament CK. Nicardipine versus cinnarizine in cerebrovascular insufficiency. *Curr Ther Res* 1988; **43**: 888–99.

Transplantation. Like other calcium-channel blockers nicardipine increases blood-ciclosporin concentrations when the 2 drugs are given concurrently.[1,2] However, in contrast to reports of benefit from the concurrent use of nifedipine and ciclosporin (p.945), no improvement in renal function was noted when nicardipine and ciclosporin were given together in renal transplant patients.[2]
1. Todd P, *et al.* Nicardipine interacts with cyclosporin. *Br J Dermatol* 1991; **121**: 820.
2. Kessler M, *et al.* Influence of nicardipine on renal function and plasma cyclosporin in renal transplant patients. *Eur J Clin Pharmacol* 1989; **36**: 637–8.

Preparations

Proprietary Preparations (details are given in Part 3)
Aust.: Karden; *Belg.:* Rydene; *Canad.:* Cardene; *Fr.:* Loxen; *Ger.:* Antagonil; *Irl.:* Cardene; *Ital.:* Bionicard; Cardioten; Cardip; Cordipina; Lisanirc; Neucor; Nicant; Nicapress; Nicardal; Nicardium; Nicarpin; Nimicor; Niven; Perdipina; Ranvil; Vasod-

in; Vasonorm; *Jpn:* Perdipine; *Mex.:* Ridene; *Neth.:* Cardene; *Port.:* Nerdipina; *Singapore:* Cardibloc; *Spain:* Dagan; Flusemide; Lecibral; Lincil; Lucenfal; Nerdipina; Vasonase; Vatrasin; *Thai.:* Cardepine; Cenpine; *UK:* Cardene; *USA:* Cardene.

Niceritrol (9258-x)

Niceritrol (*BAN, rINN*).

PETN. Pentaerythritol tetranicotinate; 2,2-Bis(hydroxymethyl)propane-1,3-diol tetranicotinate.
$C_{29}H_{24}N_4O_8 = 556.5.$
CAS — 5868-05-3.
ATC — C10AD01.

NOTE. The synonym PETN has been applied to both niceritrol and pentaerithrityl tetranitrate.
Pharmacopoeias. In Jpn.

Profile

Niceritrol, an ester of pentaerythritol and nicotinic acid, has general properties similar to those of nicotinic acid (p.1372), to which it is slowly hydrolysed. Niceritrol is used as a lipid regulating drug in hyperlipidaemias (p.800) in initial doses of 250 mg three times daily by mouth, gradually increased to 1 g three times daily.

It has also been used as a vasodilator in the treatment of peripheral vascular disease (p.809).

◊ References.
1. Curtis LD, *et al.* Clinical and laboratory responses to niceritrol in the treatment of hypercholesterolaemia. *Postgrad Med J* 1988; **64**: 672–5.
2. Suefuji H, *et al.* Effect of niceritrol on fibrinolysis and lipoprotein (a) levels in patients with coronary artery disease. *Coron Artery Dis* 1996; **7**: 167–72.

Preparations

Proprietary Preparations (details are given in Part 3)
Swed.: Perycit.

Nicofibrate Hydrochloride (1353-n)

Nicofibrate Hydrochloride (*rINNM*).

Clofenpyride Hydrochloride. 3-Pyridylmethyl 2-(4-chlorophenoxy)-2-methylpropionate hydrochloride.
$C_{16}H_{16}ClNO_3,HCl = 342.2.$
CAS — 31980-29-7 (nicofibrate); 17413-51-3 (nicofibrate hydrochloride).

Profile

Nicofibrate hydrochloride, a derivative of clofibrate (p.859) and nicotinic acid (p.1372), is a lipid regulating drug that has been used in the treatment of hyperlipidaemias.

Preparations

Proprietary Preparations (details are given in Part 3)
Spain: Arterium†.

Nicorandil (16912-m)

Nicorandil (*BAN, USAN, rINN*).

SG-75. N-[2-(Nitroxy)ethyl]-3-pyridinecarboxamide.
$C_8H_9N_3O_4 = 211.2.$
CAS — 65141-46-0.
ATC — C01DX16.

Adverse Effects and Precautions

Adverse effects reported with nicorandil are headache which is usually transitory and occurring at the start of therapy, cutaneous vasodilatation and flushing, nausea, vomiting, dizziness, and weakness. A reduction in blood pressure and/or an increase in heart rate may occur with high doses.

Nicorandil is contra-indicated in patients with cardiogenic shock, left ventricular failure with low filling pressures, and hypotension. It should be avoided, or used only with caution, in patients with hypovolaemia, low systolic blood pressure, or acute pulmonary oedema.

Oral ulceration. Painful, large aphthous ulcers on the tongue and oral mucosa have been reported[1-3] in patients receiving nicorandil for angina. The ulcers were usually resistant to treatment but all healed when nicorandil was withdrawn. Colchicine or thalidomide treatment has improved ulcers associated with nicorandil in a few patients, but relapse occurred when the colchicine or thalidomide was stopped.[3]
1. Cribier B, *et al.* Chronic buccal ulceration induced by nicorandil. *Br J Dermatol* 1998; **138**: 372–3.
2. Desruelles F, *et al.* Giant oral aphthous ulcers induced by nicorandil. *Br J Dermatol* 1998; **138**: 712–13.
3. Agbo-Godeau S, *et al.* Association of major aphthous ulcers and nicorandil. *Lancet* 1998; **352**: 1598–9.

Interactions

Nicorandil should not be used with sildenafil as the hypotensive effect of nicorandil may be significantly enhanced.

Pharmacokinetics

Nicorandil is well absorbed from the gastrointestinal tract and maximum plasma concentrations are achieved 30 to 60 minutes after administration by mouth. Metabolism is mainly by deni-

tration and approximately 20% of an administered dose is excreted in the urine mainly as metabolites. The elimination half-life is about one hour. Nicorandil is only slightly bound to plasma proteins.

Uses and Administration

Nicorandil is a nitrate derivative of nicotinamide (p.1372) and acts as a vasodilator. It is a potassium-channel opener (p.790) providing vasodilatation of arterioles and large coronary arteries and its nitrate component produces venous vasodilatation through stimulation of guanylate cyclase. It is used in angina pectoris (p.791). The usual initial dose by mouth is 10 mg twice daily (or 5 mg twice daily in patients susceptible to headache), increased as necessary to a maximum of 30 mg twice daily; the usual therapeutic dose is in the range of 10 to 20 mg twice daily.

◊ References.
1. Frampton J, *et al.* Nicorandil: a review of its pharmacology and therapeutic efficacy in angina pectoris. *Drugs* 1992; **44**: 625–55.
2. Anonymous. Nicorandil for angina. *Drug Ther Bull* 1995; **33**: 89–92.
3. Goldschmidt M, *et al.* Nicorandil: a potassium channel opening drug for treatment of ischemic heart disease. *J Clin Pharmacol* 1996; **36**: 559–72.
4. Purcell H, Fox K. Drugs in focus: nicorandil. *Prescribers' J* 1999; **39**: 39–43.
5. Markham A, *et al.* Nicorandil: an updated review of its use in ischaemic heart disease with emphasis on its cardioprotective effects. *Drugs* 2000; **60**: 955–74.

Preparations

Proprietary Preparations (details are given in Part 3)
Aust.: Dancor; *Austral.:* Ikorel; *Denm.:* Angicor; *Fr.:* Adancor; Ikorel; *Irl.:* Ikorel; *Jpn:* Sigmart; *Neth.:* Dancor†; Ikorel; *NZ:* Ikorel; *Port.:* Dancor; Nikoril; *Spain:* Dancor; *Switz.:* Dancor; *UK:* Ikorel.

Nicotinyl Alcohol (9261-z)

Nicotinyl Alcohol (*BAN, USAN*).

3-Hydroxymethylpyridine; Nicotinic Alcohol; NSC-526046; NU-2121; 3-Pyridinemethanol; β-Pyridylcarbinol; Ro-1-5155. 3-Pyridylmethanol.
$C_6H_7NO = 109.1.$
CAS — 100-55-0.
ATC — C04AC02; C10AD05.

Nicotinyl Alcohol Tartrate (9262-c)

Nicotinyl Alcohol Tartrate (*BANM*).

Nicotinyl Tartrate. 3-Pyridylmethanol hydrogen tartrate; 3-Pyridylmethanol hydrogen (2R,3R)-tartrate.
$C_6H_7NO,C_4H_6O_6 = 259.2.$
CAS — 6164-87-0.
Pharmacopoeias. In Br.

Nicotinyl alcohol tartrate 2.4 g is approximately equivalent to 1 g of nicotinyl alcohol.

Pharmacopoeial description

BP 2001: A white or almost white odourless or almost odourless crystalline powder. Freely soluble in water; slightly soluble in alcohol; practically insoluble in chloroform and in ether. A 5% solution in water has a pH of 2.8 to 3.7.

Adverse Effects and Precautions

Nicotinyl alcohol may cause flushing of the skin of the face and neck, pruritus, faintness, nausea and vomiting, and hypotension. Skin rashes and urticaria have been reported. Abnormal liver function tests indicating hepatotoxicity have been reported when high doses are used for long periods.

Glucose tolerance may be impaired particularly at higher doses, and therefore nicotinyl alcohol should be used with care in diabetic or pre-diabetic patients.

Effects on the liver. A report of hepatic lesions in 2 patients following long-term administration of nicotinyl alcohol (1.35 to 1.5 g daily).[1]
1. Keller C, *et al.* Unusual but reversible hepatic lesions following long-term treatment with pyridylcarbinol for familial hypercholesterolemia. *Klin Wochenschr* 1988; **66**: 647–50.

Uses and Administration

Nicotinyl alcohol is a vasodilator and lipid regulating drug with general properties similar to those of nicotinic acid (p.1373), to which it is partly hydrolysed.

Nicotinyl alcohol tartrate is given by mouth in the management of peripheral vascular disease (p.809) in usual doses equivalent to 25 to 50 mg of nicotinyl alcohol 4 times daily. It has been given as a modified-release preparation in doses equivalent to 150 to 300 mg of nicotinyl alcohol twice daily.

Nicotinyl alcohol tartrate is also used in Ménière's disease and in hyperlipidaemias.

Preparations

BP 2001: Nicotinyl Alcohol Tablets.

Proprietary Preparations (details are given in Part 3)
Ger.: Radecol; *UK:* Ronicol†.

Multi-ingredient: *Aust.:* Thilocombin; *Braz.:* Lipofacton; *S.Afr.:* Lipaten.

Nicoumalone (4817-a)

Nicoumalone *(BAN)*.

Acenocoumarol *(BAN, rINN)*; Acenocumarin; G-23350. 4-Hy-droxy-3-[1-(4-nitrophenyl)-3-oxobutyl]coumarin.

$C_{19}H_{15}NO_6 = 353.3$.

CAS — 152-72-7.

ATC — B01AA07.

Pharmacopoeias. In Br.

Pharmacopoeial description

BP 2001: An almost white to buff-coloured odourless or almost odourless powder. It exhibits polymorphism. Practically insoluble in water and in ether; slightly soluble in alcohol and in chloroform; dissolves in aqueous solutions of alkali hydroxides.

Adverse Effects, Treatment, and Precautions

As for Warfarin Sodium, p.992.

Effects on the fetus. Fetal outcome has been reported for a group of women who received nicoumalone [acenocoumarol] for anticoagulant prophylaxis of mechanical heart valves during pregnancy.[1] Fetal loss occurred in 13 of 61 pregnancies where oral anticoagulation was continued during the first trimester. No malformations were reported in the remaining neonates, although there was one case of hydrocephalus.

1. Meschengieser SS, *et al.* Anticoagulation in pregnant women with mechanical heart valve prostheses. *Heart* 1999; **82:** 23–6.

Interactions

The interactions associated with oral anticoagulants are discussed in detail under warfarin (p.993). Specific references to interactions involving nicoumalone [acenocoumarol] can be found there under the headings for the following drug groups: analgesics; antiarrhythmics; antibacterials; antifungals; antigout drugs; antihistamines; antineoplastics; antiplatelets; antivirals; diuretics; gastrointestinal drugs; lipid regulating drugs; prostaglandins; sex hormones; and vaccines.

Pharmacokinetics

Nicoumalone [acenocoumarol] is readily absorbed from the gastrointestinal tract and is excreted chiefly in the urine mainly as metabolites. It is extensively bound to plasma proteins. Figures reported for elimination half-life vary; 8 to 11 hours appears a reasonable range. Nicoumalone [acenocoumarol] crosses the placenta; only small quantities have been detected in breast milk. It is administered as a racemic mixture; the *R*-isomer is reported to be more potent. The stereo-isomers have different pharmacokinetics.

Uses and Administration

Nicoumalone [acenocoumarol] is an orally administered coumarin anticoagulant with actions similar to those of warfarin (p.998). It is used in the management of thromboembolic disorders (p.816). The usual dose is 8 to 12 mg on the first day and 4 to 8 mg on the second day; subsequent maintenance doses range from 1 to 8 mg depending on the response. Nicoumalone [acenocoumarol] is given in a single dose at the same time every day.

Preparations

BP 2001: Acenocoumarol Tablets.

Proprietary Preparations (details are given in Part 3)
Aust.: Sintrom; *Belg.:* Sintrom; *Canad.:* Sintrom; *Fr.:* Mini-sintrom; Sintrom; *Israel:* Sintrom; *Ital.:* Sintrom; *Mex.:* Sintrom; *Neth.:* Sintrom Mitis; *Port.:* Sintrom; *Spain:* Sintrom; *Switz.:* Sintrom; *UK:* Sinthrome.

Nifedipine (9263-k)

Nifedipine *(BAN, USAN, rINN)*.

Bay-a-1040; Nifedipina; Nifedipinum. Dimethyl 1,4-dihydro-2,6-dimethyl-4-(2-nitrophenyl)pyridine-3,5-dicarboxylate.

$C_{17}H_{18}N_2O_6 = 346.3$.

CAS — 21829-25-4.

ATC — C08CA05.

Pharmacopoeias. In Chin., Eur. (see p.vi), Jpn, and US.

Pharmacopoeial description

Ph. Eur.: A yellow crystalline powder. Practically insoluble in water; sparingly soluble in dehydrated alcohol; freely soluble in acetone. When exposed to daylight or to certain wavelengths of artificial light it is converted to a nitrosophenylpyridine derivative, while exposure to ultraviolet light leads to formation of a nitrophenylpyridine derivative. Solutions should be prepared in the dark or under light of wavelength greater than 420 nm, immediately before use. Protect from light.

USP 25: A yellow powder. Practically insoluble in water; soluble 1 in 10 of acetone. When exposed to daylight or to certain wavelengths of artificial light it is converted to a nitrosophenylpyridine derivative, while exposure to ultraviolet light leads to formation of a nitrophenylpyridine derivative. Store in airtight containers. Protect from light.

Stability. Mention of the use of yellow food colourings such as curcumin to slow photodegradation of nifedipine solutions.[1]

1. Thoma K, Klimek R. Photostabilization of drugs in dosage forms without protection from packaging materials. *Int J Pharmaceutics* 1991; **67:** 169–75.

Adverse Effects

The most common adverse effects of nifedipine are associated with its vasodilator action and often diminish on continued therapy. They include dizziness, flushing, headache, hypotension, peripheral oedema, tachycardia, and palpitations. Nausea and other gastrointestinal disturbances, increased micturition frequency, lethargy, eye pain, and mental depression have also occurred. A paradoxical increase in ischaemic chest pain may occur at the start of treatment and in a few patients excessive fall in blood pressure has led to cerebral or myocardial ischaemia or transient blindness.

There have been reports of rashes (including erythema multiforme), fever, and abnormalities in liver function, including cholestasis, due to hypersensitivity reactions. Gingival hyperplasia, myalgia, tremor, and impotence have been reported.

Overdosage may be associated with bradycardia and hypotension.

Nifedipine has been reported to be teratogenic in *animals*.

◊ Since 1995 there have been reports and reviews that have implicated calcium-channel blockers (particularly short-acting nifedipine and high doses) in increasing cardiovascular[1] and overall mortality[2] and risks of cancer and haemorrhage. Other safety concerns include links with depression and suicide. In response, the US National Heart, Lung, and Blood Institute issued a statement warning that short-acting nifedipine should be used with great caution (if at all), especially at higher doses, in the treatment of hypertension, angina, and myocardial infarction,[3] and in some countries short-acting nifedipine preparations have been withdrawn. However, there has been much debate and controversy over the reports that questioned the safety of calcium-channel blockers.[4-6]

A review by the WHO/ISH pointed out that much of the evidence for adverse effects comes from observational studies or small randomised studies and concluded that, as there was insufficient evidence to confirm either benefit or harm, current recommendations on the management of angina, hypertension, and myocardial infarction should remain unchanged.[7] In addition, many of the studies that have led to the negative reports employed the older short-acting calcium-channel blockers. The calcium-channel blockers used now are largely modified-release formulations of short half-life blockers or are calcium-channel blockers with long half-lives.

Since the WHO/ISH review was published, further studies have been completed. A placebo-controlled study investigating the effects of calcium-channel blockers on cardiovascular events (SYST-EUR) reported[8] a reduction in incidence of stroke and cardiovascular events in 4695 elderly patients treated with nitrendipine (and enalapril and hydrochlorothiazide in addition if necessary) for isolated systolic hypertension. A retrospective cohort study[9] in post-myocardial infarction patients failed to show any increase in mortality after one year in those receiving calcium-channel blockers. However, a meta-analysis[10] of randomised trials comparing calcium-channel blockers with other antihypertensives in patients with hypertension suggested that calcium-channel blockers were associated with an increased risk of major cardiovascular events (except stroke) although all-cause mortality was not increased. Two further large long-term randomised studies in hypertension are underway—the Antihypertensive and Lipid Lowering treatment to prevent Heart Attack Trial (ALLHAT) and the Anglo-Scandinavian Coronary Outcomes Trial (ASCOT)—that should clarify the effects of calcium-channel blockers on morbidity and mortality.

1. Psaty BM, *et al.* The risk of myocardial infarction associated with antihypertensive drug therapies. *JAMA* 1995; **274:** 620–5.
2. Furberg CD, *et al.* Nifedipine: dose-related increase in mortality in patients with coronary heart disease. *Circulation* 1995; **92:** 1326–31.
3. McCarthy M. US NIH issues warning on nifedipine. *Lancet* 1995; **346:** 689–90.
4. Opie LH, Messerli FH. Nifedipine and mortality: grave defects in the dossier. *Circulation* 1995; **92:** 1068–72.
5. Grossman E, Messerli FH. Calcium antagonists in cardiovascular disease: a necessary controversy but an unnecessary panic. *Am J Med* 1997; **102:** 147–9.
6. Stanton AV. Calcium channel blockers. *BMJ* 1998; **316:** 1471–3.
7. Ad Hoc Subcommittee of the Liaison Committee of the World Health Organisation and the International Society of Hypertension. Effects of calcium antagonists on the risks of coronary heart disease, cancer, and bleeding. *J Hypertens* 1997; **15:** 105–15.
8. Staessen JA, *et al.* Randomised double-blind comparison of placebo and active treatment for older patients with isolated systolic hypertension. *Lancet* 1997; **350:** 757–64. Correction. *ibid.;* 1636.
9. Jollis JG, *et al.* Calcium channel blockers and mortality in elderly patients with myocardial infarction. *Arch Intern Med* 1999; **159:** 2341–8.
10. Pahor M, *et al.* Health outcomes associated with calcium antagonists compared with other first-line antihypertensive therapies: a meta-analysis of randomised controlled trials. *Lancet* 2000; **356:** 1949–54.

Cancer occurrence. An observational study carried out between 1988 and 1992 suggested that calcium-channel blockers are associated with an increased risk of cancer.[1] Subsequent studies have failed to support this finding.[2-7] A review by the WHO/ISH concluded that there is no good evidence that calcium-channel blockers increase cancer risk,[8] and the biological basis for an effect of calcium-channel blockers on cancer risk has also been questioned.[9] Long-term morbidity and mortality studies are currently underway that should yield further information.[10]

1. Pahor M, *et al.* Calcium-channel blockade and incidence of cancer in aged populations. *Lancet* 1996; **348:** 493–7.
2. Jick H, *et al.* Calcium-channel blockers and risk of cancer. *Lancet* 1997; **349:** 525–8.
3. Rosenberg L, *et al.* Calcium channel blockers and the risk of cancer. *JAMA* 1998; **279:** 1000–4.
4. Braun S, *et al.* Calcium channel blocking agents and risk of cancer in patients with coronary heart disease. *J Am Coll Cardiol* 1998; **31:** 804–8.
5. Sajadieh A, *et al.* Verapamil and risk of cancer in patients with coronary artery disease. *Am J Cardiol* 1999; **83:** 1419–22.
6. Meier CR, *et al.* Angiotensin-converting enzyme inhibitors, calcium channel blockers, and breast cancer. *Arch Intern Med* 2000; **160:** 349–53.
7. Cohen HJ, *et al.* Calcium channel blockers and cancer. *Am J Med* 2000; **108:** 210–15.
8. Ad Hoc Subcommittee of the Liaison Committee of the World Health Organisation and the International Society of Hypertension. Effects of calcium antagonists on the risks of coronary heart disease, cancer and bleeding. *J Hypertens* 1997; **15:** 105–15.
9. Mason RP. Calcium channel blockers, apoptosis and cancer: is there a biologic relationship? *J Am Coll Cardiol* 1999; **34:** 1857–66.
10. Howes LG, Edwards CT. Calcium antagonists and cancer: is there really a link? *Drug Safety* 1998; **18:** 1–7.

Effects on the blood. Treatment with nifedipine significantly reduces the ability of platelets to aggregate *in vitro*[1] and results indicating inhibition of platelet function in healthy subjects receiving oral (but not intravenous) nifedipine have been reported.[2,3] Thus, concern has been expressed[4] that calcium-channel blockers may have the potential to produce haemorrhagic complications in surgical patients (specifically, those undergoing coronary bypass surgery). Major surgical bleeding was associated with nimodipine in patients undergoing cardiac valve replacement,[5] although it has been used in other situations apparently without an increased risk of bleeding.[6]

Conflicting results have been reported with regard to the risk of gastrointestinal bleeding. A prospective cohort study in 1636 elderly hypertensive patients,[7] and a subsequent case-control study,[8] reported that calcium-channel blockers were associated with an increased risk of gastrointestinal haemorrhage compared with beta blockers. However, it was suggested[9] that this may have been due to a protective effect of beta blockers rather than an adverse effect of calcium-channel blockers, and another study[10] also suggested that the risk of gastrointestinal bleeding was not materially increased by calcium-channel blockers.

Calcium-channel blockers have also been associated with a number of blood dyscrasias; there have been case reports of aplastic anaemia with nifedipine,[11] and of thrombocytopenia with amlodipine[12] and with diltiazem.[13,14]

1. Ośmiałwska Z, *et al.* Effect of nifedipine monotherapy on platelet aggregation in patients with untreated essential hypertension. *Eur J Clin Pharmacol* 1990; **39:** 403–4.
2. Winther K, *et al.* Dose-dependent effects of verapamil and nifedipine on in vivo platelet function in normal volunteers. *Eur J Clin Pharmacol* 1990; **39:** 291–3.
3. Walley TJ, *et al.* The effects of intravenous and oral nifedipine on ex vivo platelet function. *Eur J Clin Pharmacol* 1989; **37:** 449–52.
4. Becker RC, Alpert JS. The impact of medical therapy on hemorrhagic complications following coronary artery bypass grafting. *Arch Intern Med* 1990; **150:** 2016–21.
5. Wagenknecht LE, *et al.* Surgical bleeding: unexpected effect of a calcium antagonist. *BMJ* 1995; **310:** 776–7.
6. Öhman J and others. Surgical bleeding and calcium antagonists. *BMJ* 1995; **311:** 388–9. (Several letters.)
7. Pahor M, *et al.* Risk of gastrointestinal haemorrhage with calcium antagonists in hypertensive persons over 67 years old. *Lancet* 1996; **347:** 1061–5.
8. Kaplan RC, *et al.* Use of calcium channel blockers and risk of hospitalized gastrointestinal tract bleeding. *Arch Intern Med* 2000; **160:** 1849–55.
9. Suissa S, *et al.* Antihypertensive drugs and the risk of gastrointestinal bleeding. *Am J Med* 1998; **105:** 230–5.
10. Kelly JP, *et al.* Major upper gastrointestinal bleeding and the use of calcium channel blockers. *Lancet* 1999; **353:** 559.
11. Laporte J-R, *et al.* Fatal aplastic anaemia associated with nifedipine. *Lancet* 1998; **352:** 619–20.
12. Usalan C, *et al.* Severe thrombocytopenia associated with amlodipine treatment. *Ann Pharmacother* 1999; **33:** 1126–7.
13. Lehav M, Arav R. Diltiazem and thrombocytopenia. *Ann Intern Med* 1989; **110:** 327.
14. Michalets EL, Jackson DV. Diltiazem-associated thrombocytopenia. *Pharmacotherapy* 1997; **17:** 1345–8.

Effects on the brain. Cerebral ischaemia[1,2] has been reported in small numbers of patients given nifedipine.

1. Nobile-Orazio E, Sterzi R. Cerebral ischaemia after nifedipine treatment. *BMJ* 1981; **283:** 948.
2. Schwartz M, *et al.* Oral nifedipine in the treatment of hypertensive urgency: cerebrovascular accident following a single dose. *Arch Intern Med* 1990; **150:** 686–7.

Effects on carbohydrate metabolism. There are reports of deterioration of diabetes,[1] reduction in glucose tolerance,[2] and development of diabetes[1,3] in patients receiving treatment with nifedipine. Nifedipine has also been reported to increase plasma-glucose concentrations.[3,4] However, other reports and studies have found no change in glucose tolerance in either diabetic or non-diabetic patients taking nifedipine.[5-10]

See also Diabetes Mellitus under Precautions, below.

1. Bhatnagar SK, et al. Diabetogenic effects of nifedipine. BMJ 1984; 289: 19.
2. Giugliano D, et al. Impairment of insulin secretion in man by nifedipine. Eur J Clin Pharmacol 1980; 18: 395–8.
3. Zezulka AV, et al. Diabetogenic effects of nifedipine. BMJ 1984; 289: 437–8.
4. Charles S, et al. Hyperglycaemic effect of nifedipine. BMJ 1981; 283: 19–20.
5. Harrower ADB, Donnelly T. Hyperglycaemic effect of nifedipine. BMJ 1981; 283: 796.
6. Greenwood RH. Hyperglycaemic effect of nifedipine. BMJ 1982; 284: 50.
7. Abadie E, Passa P. Diabetogenic effects of nifedipine. BMJ 1984; 289: 438.
8. Antonelli D. Nifedipine and fasting glycemia. Ann Intern Med 1985; 104: 125–6.
9. Whitcroft I, et al. Calcium antagonists do not impair long-term glucose control in hypertensive non-insulin dependent diabetics (NIDDS). Br J Clin Pharmacol 1986; 22: 208P.
10. Tentorio A, et al. Insulin secretion and glucose tolerance in non-insulin dependent diabetic patients after chronic nifedipine treatment. Eur J Clin Pharmacol 1989; 36: 311–13.

Effects on the ears. There have been isolated reports[1] of tinnitus associated with several calcium-channel blockers including nifedipine, nicardipine, nitrendipine, diltiazem, verapamil, and cinnarizine.

1. Narváez M, et al. Tinnitus with calcium-channel blockers. Lancet 1994; 343: 1229–30.

Effects on the eyes. Individual reports have implicated nifedipine in the development of transient retinal ischaemia and blindness,[1] and of periorbital oedema.[2] In a postmarketing survey painful or stinging eyes were more common in patients receiving nifedipine (178 of 757 evaluable) than in those given captopril (45 of 289), although the cause was uncertain.[3] Nifedipine has also been suggested as a risk factor in the development of cataract,[4,5] but the numbers involved in this analysis are small[6] and it is possible that the risk, if it exists,[7] relates to hypertension rather than nifedipine treatment.[6]

1. Pitlik S, et al. Transient retinal ischaemia induced by nifedipine. BMJ 1983; 287: 1845–6.
2. Silverstone PH. Periorbital oedema caused by nifedipine. BMJ 1984; 288: 1654.
3. Coulter DM. Eye pain with nifedipine and disturbance of taste with captopril: a mutually controlled study showing a method of postmarketing surveillance. BMJ 1988; 296: 1086–8.
4. van Heyningen R, Harding JJ. Do aspirin-like analgesics protect against cataract? Lancet 1986; i: 1111–13.
5. Harding JJ, van Heyningen R. Drugs, including alcohol, that act as risk factors for cataract, and possible protection against cataract by aspirin-like analgesics and cyclopenthiazide. Br J Ophthalmol 1988; 72: 809–14.
6. van Heyningen R, Harding JJ. Aspirin-like analgesics and cataract. Lancet 1986; ii: 283.
7. Kewitz H, et al. Aspirin and cataract. Lancet 1986; ii: 689.

Effects on the heart. The use of nifedipine has been associated with the development of various heart disorders in some patients. Complete heart block has been reported in an elderly patient who had previously developed heart block with verapamil,[1] and sudden circulatory collapse has been reported in 4 patients receiving nifedipine who underwent routine coronary bypass surgery.[2] One patient died despite all attempts at resuscitation.[2] However, probably the majority of reports have concerned the development or aggravation of cardiac ischaemia, up to and including frank myocardial infarction following administration of short-acting nifedipine.[3-6] Such cases appear to be chiefly associated with a too-rapid fall in blood pressure following the use of sublingual nifedipine for hypertensive urgencies or emergencies,[5,6] or occur in patients with a history of ischaemic heart disease.[3,4]

For discussion of the effects of calcium-channel blockers on cardiovascular mortality, see under Adverse Effects, above.

1. Chopra DA, Maxwell RT. Complete heart block with low dose nifedipine. BMJ 1984; 288: 760.
2. Goiti JJ. Calcium channel blocking agents and the heart. BMJ 1985; 291: 1505.
3. Sia STB, et al. Aggravation of myocardial ischaemia by nifedipine. Med J Aust 1985; 142: 48–50.
4. Boden WE, et al. Nifedipine-induced hypotension and myocardial ischemia in refractory angina pectoris. JAMA 1985; 253: 1131–5.
5. O'Mailia JJ, et al. Nifedipine-associated myocardial ischemia or infarction in the treatment of hypertensive urgencies. Ann Intern Med 1987; 107: 185–6.
6. Leavitt AD, Zweifler AJ. Nifedipine, hypotension, and myocardial injury. Ann Intern Med 1988; 108: 305–6.

WITHDRAWAL. Exacerbation of coronary ischaemia and thrombosis of arteriovenous graft could have resulted from withdrawal of nifedipine in a patient.[1] Abrupt withdrawal of nisoldipine from 15 patients with stable angina pectoris after 6 weeks of therapy resulted in severe unstable angina in 2 patients and acute myocardial infarction in another.[2] It was postulated that the withdrawal effect could be due to an increase in sensitivity of vascular α_2 adrenoceptors to circulating adrenaline.[2]

1. Mysliwiec M, et al. Calcium antagonist withdrawal syndrome. BMJ 1983; 286: 1898.
2. Mehta J, Lopez LM. Calcium-blocker withdrawal phenomenon: increase in affinity of alpha₂ adrenoceptors for agonist as a potential mechanism. Am J Cardiol 1986; 58: 242–6.

Effects on the kidneys. Calcium-channel blockers may be of benefit in various forms of kidney disorder (see under Uses and Administration, below). However, reversible deterioration in renal function without any appreciable accompanying decline in systemic arterial blood pressure has been reported in 4 patients with underlying renal insufficiency receiving nifedipine[1] and nifedipine increased urinary protein excretion and exacerbated renal impairment in 14 type 2 diabetic patients.[2] Excessive diuresis occurred in a patient given nifedipine for angina pectoris[3] and nocturia in 9 patients referred for prostatic surgery was also attributed to nifedipine.[4]

1. Diamond JR, et al. Nifedipine-induced renal dysfunction: alterations in renal hemodynamics. Am J Med 1984; 77: 905–9.
2. Demarie BK, Bakris GL. Effects of different calcium antagonists on proteinuria associated with diabetes mellitus. Ann Intern Med 1990; 113: 987–8.
3. Antonelli D, et al. Excessive nifedipine diuretic effect. BMJ 1984; 288: 760.
4. Williams G, Donaldson RM. Nifedipine and nocturia. Lancet 1986; i: 738.

Effects on the liver. A number of cases of hepatitis, apparently due to a hypersensitivity reaction, and frequently accompanied by fever, sweating, chills, rigor, and arthritic symptoms, have been reported in patients receiving nifedipine.[1-4]

1. Rotmensch HH, et al. Lymphocyte sensitisation in nifedipine-induced hepatitis. BMJ 1980; 281: 976–7.
2. Davidson AR. Lymphocyte sensitisation in nifedipine-induced hepatitis. BMJ 1980; 281: 1354.
3. Abramson M, Littlejohn GO. Hepatic reactions to nifedipine. Med J Aust 1985; 142: 47–8.
4. Shaw DR, et al. Nifedipine hepatitis. Aust N Z J Med 1987; 17: 447–8.

Effects on the menstrual cycle. Menorrhagia in 2 women[1] and menstrual irregularity with heavy bleeding in another[2] have been reported in association with nifedipine treatment.

1. Rodger JC, Torrance TC. Can nifedipine provoke menorrhagia? Lancet 1983; ii: 460.
2. Singh G, et al. Can nifedipine provoke menorrhagia? Lancet 1983; ii: 1022.

Effects on mental function. Insomnia, hyperexcitability, pacing, agitation, and depression were reported[1] in a patient in association with nifedipine therapy. The symptoms disappeared within 2 days of withdrawal of nifedipine. Four further cases of major depression, which developed within a week of commencing the drug, and resolved within a week of discontinuing the drug, have been reported.[2]

Recently, 2 epidemiological studies suggested that calcium-channel blockers may promote suicide.[3] However a subsequent study[4] found no evidence of an association between depression and the use of calcium-channel blockers, and the number of suicides was low. A further study[5] also failed to find an increased risk of suicide with calcium-channel blockers compared with other antihypertensive drugs.

1. Ahmad S. Nifedipine-induced acute psychosis. J Am Geriatr Soc 1984; 32: 408.
2. Hullett FJ, et al. Depression associated with nifedipine-induced calcium channel blockade. Am J Psychiatry 1988; 145: 1277–9.
3. Lindberg G, et al. Use of calcium channel blockers and risk of suicide: ecological findings confirmed in population based cohort study. BMJ 1998; 316: 741–5.
4. Dunn NR, et al. Cohort study on calcium channel blockers, other cardiovascular agents, and the prevalence of depression. Br J Clin Pharmacol 1999; 48: 230–3.
5. Gasse C, et al. Risk of suicide among users of calcium channel blockers: population based, nested case-control study. BMJ 2000; 320: 1251.

Effects on the mouth. GINGIVAL HYPERPLASIA. A number of reports have implicated nifedipine in the development of gingival hyperplasia.[1-4] In most cases it has occurred about 1 to 6 months after starting nifedipine and has resolved following withdrawal of nifedipine. A patient who had taken nifedipine for 12 years developed gingival hyperplasia shortly after the dosage of nifedipine was increased.[5] Amlodipine has also induced gingival overgrowth.[6] A study involving 115 patients who had received nifedipine, diltiazem, or verapamil for at least 3 months indicated that gingival hyperplasia is an important side-effect that may occur with calcium-channel blockers in general.[7] Dihydropyridine calcium-channel blockers were among the most common drugs associated with reports of gingival hyperplasia in the Australian Adverse Drug Reactions Advisory Committee database.[8]

1. Ramon Y, et al. Gingival hyperplasia caused by nifedipine—a preliminary report. Int J Cardiol 1984; 5: 195–204.
2. van der Wall EE, et al. Gingival hyperplasia induced by nifedipine, an arterial vasodilating drug. Oral Surg 1985; 60: 38–40.
3. Shaftic AA, et al. Nifedipine-induced gingival hyperplasia. Drug Intell Clin Pharm 1986; 20: 602–5.
4. Jones CM. Gingival hyperplasia associated with nifedipine. Br Dent J 1986; 160: 416–17.
5. Johnson RB. Nifedipine-induced gingival overgrowth. Ann Pharmacother 1997; 31: 935.
6. Ellis JS, et al. Gingival sequestration of amlodipine and amlodipine-induced gingival overgrowth. Lancet 1993; 341: 1102–3.
7. Steele RM, et al. Calcium antagonist-induced gingival hyperplasia. Ann Intern Med 1994; 120: 663–4.
8. Adverse Drug Reactions Advisory Committee. Drug-induced gingival overgrowth. Aust Adverse Drug React Bull 1999; 18: 6–7.

PAROTITIS. Acute swelling of the parotid glands occurred in a patient after sublingual administration of nifedipine.[1]

1. Bosch X, et al. Nifedipine-induced parotitis. Lancet 1986; ii: 467.

Effects on the neuromuscular system. Severe muscle cramps have been reported in a few patients taking nifedipine;[1,2] in one patient[2] the cramps were associated with widespread paraesthesia. Reversible myoclonic dystonia associated with nifedipine has been reported in a patient.[3] Severe rhabdomyolysis developed in a patient with a transplanted kidney who was receiving an intravenous infusion of nifedipine.[4] The patient recovered rapidly once the infusion was stopped. There has also been a report[5] of myopathy, myalgia, and arthralgia associated with amlodipine, and of arthralgia in a patient[6] receiving diltiazem.

1. Keidar S, et al. Muscle cramps during treatment with nifedipine. BMJ 1982; 285: 1241–2.
2. Macdonald JB. Muscle cramps during treatment with nifedipine. BMJ 1982; 285: 1744.
3. de Medina A, et al. Nifedipine and myoclonic dystonia. Ann Intern Med 1985; 104: 125.
4. Horn S, et al. Severe rhabdomyolysis in a kidney-transplant recipient receiving intravenous nifedipine. Lancet 1995; 346: 848–9.
5. Phillips BB, Muller BA. Severe neuromuscular complications possibly associated with amlodipine. Ann Pharmacother 1998; 32: 1165–7.
6. Smith KM. Arthralgia associated with calcium-channel blockers. Am J Health-Syst Pharm 2000; 57: 55–7.

Effects on the peripheral circulation. An erythromelalgia-like eruption occurred in a patient 8 weeks after starting therapy with nifedipine. Symptoms included severe burning pain and swelling in the feet and lower legs, which were fiery red, tender, and warm to the touch. Symptoms resolved in 2 days when nifedipine was discontinued.[1] Similar effects have been reported in other patients on nifedipine.[2-4] Erythromelalgia has also been reported with nicardipine.[5] This type of erythromelalgia may be termed secondary erythermalgia.[6]

1. Fisher JR, et al. Nifedipine and erythromelalgia. Ann Intern Med 1983; 98: 671–2.
2. Grunwald Z. Painful edema, erythematous rash, and burning sensation due to nifedipine. Drug Intell Clin Pharm 1982; 16: 492.
3. Brodmerkel GJ. Nifedipine and erythromelalgia. Ann Intern Med 1983; 99: 415.
4. Sunahara JF, et al. Possible erythromelalgia-like syndrome associated with nifedipine in a patient with Raynaud's phenomenon. Ann Pharmacother 1996; 30: 484–6.
5. Levesque H, et al. Erythromelalgia induced by nicardipine (inverse Raynaud's phenomenon?) BMJ 1989; 298: 1252–3.
6. Drenth JPH, Michiels JJ. Three types of erythromelalgia. BMJ 1990; 301: 454–5.

Effects on the respiratory system. There have been some reports of pulmonary oedema being precipitated by nifedipine therapy in patients with aortic stenosis.[1,2] Nifedipine has also been reported to exacerbate impaired tissue oxygenation in patients with cor pulmonale secondary to obstructive airways disease.[3]

For a report of exacerbation of laryngeal oedema, see under Hypersensitivity, below.

1. Gillmar DJ, Kark P. Pulmonary oedema precipitated by nifedipine. BMJ 1980; 280: 1420–1.
2. Aderka D, Pinkhas J. Pulmonary oedema precipitated by nifedipine. BMJ 1984; 289: 1272.
3. Kalra L, Bone MF. Nifedipine and impaired oxygenation in patients with chronic bronchitis and cor pulmonale. Lancet 1989; i: 1135–6.

Effects on the skin. The commonest skin reactions to nifedipine have been rash, pruritus, urticaria, alopecia, and exfoliative dermatitis;[1] there have been a few reports of erythema multiforme and the Stevens-Johnson syndrome.[1] Erythema multiforme occurred in a patient following substitution of amlodipine for nifedipine[2] and cross-sensitivity, manifest as a pruritic maculopapular rash, has been reported between amlodipine and diltiazem.[3] Generalised pruritus has been reported with amlodipine.[4] Severe photosensitivity reactions,[5] nonthrombocytopenic purpuric rashes,[6] and telangiectasias,[7] including photodistributed telangiectasias with amlodipine[8,9] and with nifedipine[10] (that recurred 3 years later with amlodipine[8]), have also been reported.

For reference to erythromelalgia, see under Effects on the Peripheral Circulation, above.

1. Stern R, Khalsa JH. Cutaneous adverse reactions associated with calcium channel blockers. Arch Intern Med 1989; 149: 829–32.
2. Bewley AP, et al. Erythema multiforme following substitution of amlodipine for nifedipine. BMJ 1993; 307: 241.
3. Baker BA, Cacchione JG. Dermatologic cross-sensitivity between diltiazem and amlodipine. Ann Pharmacother 1994; 28: 118–19.
4. Orme S, et al. Generalised pruritus associated with amlodipine. BMJ 1997; 315: 463.
5. Thomas SE, Wood ML. Photosensitivity reactions associated with nifedipine. BMJ 1986; 292: 992.
6. Oren R, et al. Nifedipine-induced nonthrombocytopenic purpura. DICP Ann Pharmacother 1989; 23: 88.
7. Tsele E, Chu AC. Nifedipine and telangiectasias. Lancet 1992; 339: 365–6.
8. Basarab T, et al. Calcium antagonist-induced photo-exposed telangiectasia. Br J Dermatol 1997; 136: 974–5.
9. Grabczynska SA, Cowley N. Amlodipine induced-photosensitivity presenting as telangiectasia. Br J Dermatol 2000; 142: 1255–6.
10. Collins P, Ferguson J. Photodistributed nifedipine-induced facial telangiectasia. Br J Dermatol 1993; 129: 630–3.

Effects on taste. Although distortion of taste and smell has been reported in 2 patients taking nifedipine,[1] a large survey involving 922 patients receiving nifedipine and 343 taking captopril did not show any association of taste disturbances with nifedipine.[2]

1. Levenson JL, Kennedy K. Dysomia, dysgeusia, and nifedipine. *Ann Intern Med* 1985; **102**: 135–6.
2. Coulter DM. Eye pain with nifedipine and disturbance of taste with captopril: a mutually controlled study showing a method of postmarketing surveillance. *BMJ* 1988; **296**: 1086–8.

Gynaecomastia. Unilateral gynaecomastia developed in 3 men 4, 6, and 26 weeks after starting nifedipine therapy.[1]

1. Clyne CAC. Unilateral gynaecomastia and nifedipine. *BMJ* 1986; **292**: 380.

Haemorrhage. See under Effects on the Blood, above.

Hypersensitivity. Nifedipine is associated with various hypersensitivity reactions including skin rashes and effects on the liver (see above).

Nifedipine, given sublingually, exacerbated laryngeal swelling that developed in a woman following the use of isosorbide dinitrate spray.[1]

1. Silfvast T, *et al.* Laryngeal oedema after isosorbide dinitrate spray and sublingual nifedipine. *BMJ* 1995; **311**: 232.

Oedema. Peripheral oedema of the feet and ankles is a common side-effect of nifedipine and other dihydropyridine calcium-channel blockers. It occurs typically 2 or more weeks after starting treatment and is caused by pre-capillary arteriolar dilatation rather than fluid retention.[1] Evidence from a study in 10 diabetic subjects beginning nifedipine therapy, 5 of whom developed ankle oedema, suggested that nifedipine abolished the reflex vasoconstriction produced when the feet are below the level of the heart which is believed to prevent excessive fluid filtration into the tissues.[2]

The oedema may respond to simple measures such as elevation of the feet or to a reduction in dosage but if it persists the calcium-channel blocker should be withdrawn.[1]

1. Maclean D, MacConnachie AM. Selective side-effects: peripheral oedema with dihydropyridine calcium antagonists. *Prescribers' J* 1991; **31**: 4–6.
2. Williams SA, *et al.* Dependent oedema and attenuation of postural vasoconstriction associated with nifedipine therapy for hypertension in diabetic patients. *Eur J Clin Pharmacol* 1989; **37**: 333–5.

Treatment of Adverse Effects

In recent overdosage (within 1 hour) with nifedipine by mouth the stomach may be emptied by lavage; activated charcoal may be administered. Supportive and symptomatic care should be given. Hypotension may respond to placing the patient in the supine position with the feet raised and the administration of plasma expanders, although cardiac overload should be avoided. If hypotension is not corrected, calcium gluconate or calcium chloride should be given intravenously. Glucagon may also be used. If hypotension persists, intravenous administration of a sympathomimetic such as isoprenaline, dopamine, or noradrenaline [norepinephrine] may also be necessary. Bradycardia may be treated with atropine, isoprenaline, or cardiac pacing. Dialysis is not useful as nifedipine is highly protein bound. Plasmapheresis may be beneficial.

Overdosage. Although the consequences and management of overdosage with all calcium-channel blockers are similar,[1] non-dihydropyridines have been suggested to cause more severe effects and to require more aggressive treatment.[2]

Most reports of overdosage have been with verapamil,[3] although there have been a few published reports of nifedipine overdosage. In one, hypotension, tachycardia, and flushing, followed by hypokalaemia, were seen in a patient who took nifedipine 600 mg as modified-release tablets together with an overdose of paracetamol, but there was no evidence of heart block.[4] The patient was given calcium gluconate intravenously and subsequently activated charcoal and lactulose. Absorption of nifedipine was essentially complete 10 hours after ingestion. Potassium chloride was given by mouth to treat hypokalaemia and acetylcysteine was used to manage the paracetamol poisoning.

Third-degree atrioventricular block, progressing to asystole, developed in a 14-month-old child who ingested approximately 800 mg of nifedipine.[5] During cardiopulmonary resuscitation a total of 700 mg of calcium chloride was given, together with atropine, adrenaline [epinephrine], and sodium bicarbonate. The stomach was subsequently emptied by gastric lavage and activated charcoal given. The patient remained tachycardic and hypotensive, with evidence of pulmonary oedema and hyperglycaemia, and was given intravenous electrolytes and dopamine infusions and assisted ventilation, together with treatment to control subsequent tonic-clonic seizures. She eventually made an apparently complete recovery apart from a moderate speech delay.

Case reports[6,7] have suggested that administration of insulin infusion, with glucose if required to maintain normal blood-glu-

cose concentrations, may be beneficial in patients in whom myocardial function fails to improve with conventional therapy.

1. Kenny J. Treating overdose with calcium channel blockers. *BMJ* 1994; **308**: 992–3.
2. Buckley NA, *et al.* Overdose with calcium channel blockers. *BMJ* 1994; **308**: 1639.
3. Howarth DM, *et al.* Calcium channel blocking drug overdose: an Australian series. *Hum Exp Toxicol* 1994; **13**: 161–6.
4. Ferner RE, *et al.* Pharmacokinetics and toxic effects of nifedipine in massive overdose. *Hum Exp Toxicol* 1990; **9**: 309–11.
5. Wells TG, *et al.* Nifedipine poisoning in a child. *Pediatrics* 1990; **86**: 91–4.
6. Yuan TH, *et al.* Insulin-glucose as adjunctive therapy for severe calcium channel antagonist poisoning. *J Toxicol Clin Toxicol* 1999; **37**: 463–74.
7. Boyer EW, Shannon M. Treatment of calcium-channel-blocker intoxication with insulin infusion. *N Engl J Med* 2001; **344**: 1721–2.

Precautions

Nifedipine should be used with caution in patients with hypotension, in patients whose cardiac reserve is poor, and in those with heart failure since deterioration of heart failure has been noted. Nifedipine should not be used in cardiogenic shock, in patients who have recently suffered a myocardial infarction, or in acute unstable angina. Nifedipine should not be used to treat an anginal attack in chronic stable angina. In patients with severe aortic stenosis nifedipine may increase the risk of developing heart failure. Sudden withdrawal of nifedipine might be associated with an exacerbation of angina. The dose may need to be reduced in patients with hepatic impairment.

Nifedipine should be discontinued in patients who experience ischaemic pain following its administration.

Nifedipine is reported to be teratogenic in *animals* and may inhibit labour, but it has been used in hypertension in pregnancy (see Hypertension, under Uses and Administration, below).

Diabetes mellitus. Nifedipine may modify insulin and glucose responses (see Effects on Carbohydrate Metabolism under Adverse Effects, above) calling for adjustments in antidiabetic therapy. Also some studies have suggested that nifedipine may worsen proteinuria and renal dysfunction in diabetic patients with some degree of renal insufficiency,[1,2] but other studies, (see Kidney Disorders under Uses and Administration, below), have suggested that nifedipine treatment may prevent or retard the progression of albuminuria.

Some studies have suggested that patients with diabetes mellitus[3,4] or impaired glucose metabolism[5] may be more susceptible to adverse cardiovascular effects of calcium-channel blockers (see above). The calcium-channel blockers used in these studies were nisoldipine, amlodipine, and isradipine (long-acting or intermediate-acting calcium-channel blockers). However, two of the studies[3,4] compared the calcium-channel blocker with an ACE inhibitor and it has been suggested that ACE inhibitors may have a protective effect in patients with diabetes that is additional to their antihypertensive action. Thus, ACE inhibitors may be particularly beneficial in these patients rather than calcium-channel blockers being particularly harmful.[6] Large randomised studies are underway that should provide further information.

1. Mimran A, *et al.* Contrasting effects of captopril and nifedipine in normotensive patients with incipient diabetic nephropathy. *J Hypertens* 1988; **6**: 919–23.
2. Demarie BK, Bakris GL. Effects of different calcium antagonists on proteinuria associated with diabetes mellitus. *Ann Intern Med* 1990; **113**: 987–8.
3. Estacio RO, *et al.* The effect of nisoldipine as compared with enalapril on cardiovascular outcomes in patients with non-insulin-dependent diabetes and hypertension. *N Engl J Med* 1998; **338**: 645–52. Correction. *ibid.*; **339**: 1339.
4. Tatti P, *et al.* Outcome results of the fosinopril versus amlodipine cardiovascular events randomized trial (FACET) in patients with hypertension and NIDDM. *Diabetes Care* 1998; **21**: 597–603.
5. Byington RP, *et al.* Isradipine, raised glycosylated haemoglobin, and risk of cardiovascular events. *Lancet* 1997; **350**: 1075–6.
6. Poulter NR. Calcium channel blockers and cardiovascular risk in diabetes. *Lancet* 1998; **351**: 1809–10.

Interference with laboratory estimations. Nifedipine may give falsely elevated spectrophotometric values of urinary vanillylmandelic acid; HPLC estimations are unaffected.

Porphyria. Nifedipine has been associated with acute attacks of porphyria and is considered unsafe in porphyric patients.

Withdrawal. Sudden withdrawal of nifedipine might be associated with an exacerbation of angina.

For a report of life-threatening coronary vasospasm occurring following withdrawal of nifedipine before a revascularisation procedure, see under Effects on the Heart, in Diltiazem, p.875.

Interactions

Nifedipine may enhance the antihypertensive effects of other antihypertensive drugs such as beta blockers although the combination is generally well tolerated. Enhanced antihypertensive effects may also be seen

with concomitant use of drugs such as aldesleukin and antipsychotics that cause hypotension. Nifedipine may modify insulin and glucose responses (see Effects on Carbohydrate Metabolism, above) and therefore diabetic patients may need to adjust their antidiabetic treatment when receiving nifedipine. Nifedipine is extensively metabolised in the liver by the cytochrome P450 enzyme system, and interactions may occur with other drugs, such as quinidine, sharing the same metabolic pathway, and with enzyme inducers, such as carbamazepine, phenytoin, and rifampicin, and enzyme inhibitors, such as cimetidine and erythromycin.

Alcohol. A study involving 10 healthy subjects showed that the area under the concentration-time profile for nifedipine 20 mg by mouth was increased by 54% when taken with alcohol, and maximum pulse rate was achieved more rapidly, which was in line with *animal* and *in-vitro* studies suggesting that the metabolism of nifedipine is inhibited by alcohol.[1]

1. Qureshi S, *et al.* Nifedipine-alcohol interaction. *JAMA* 1990; **264**: 1660–1.

Antiarrhythmics. Nifedipine and *quinidine* probably have a common metabolic pathway in the liver and might be expected to interact if given concurrently. In one study,[1] quinidine appeared to inhibit nifedipine metabolism resulting in increased serum concentrations of nifedipine; quinidine concentrations were unchanged. However, conflicting effects on serum-quinidine concentrations have been reported, see p.965.

1. Bowles SK, *et al.* Evaluation of the pharmacokinetic and pharmacodynamic interaction between quinidine and nifedipine. *J Clin Pharmacol* 1993; **33**: 727–31.

Antidiabetics. See Diabetes Mellitus under Precautions and Effects on Carbohydrate Metabolism under Adverse Effects, above.

Antiepileptics. The effects of dihydropyridine calcium-channel blockers may be reduced by enzyme-inducing antiepileptics such as *carbamazepine, phenobarbital,* and *phenytoin.*[1-3] In contrast, *sodium valproate* has been reported to increase plasma-nimodipine concentrations.[3]

For reports of an interaction between nifedipine and *phenytoin* resulting in raised serum-phenytoin concentration, see p.361.

1. Capewell S, *et al.* Reduced felodipine bioavailability in patients taking anticonvulsants. *Lancet* 1988; **ii**: 480–2.
2. Schellens JHM, *et al.* Influence of enzyme induction and inhibition on the oxidation of nifedipine, sparteine, mephenytoin and antipyrine in humans as assessed by a "cocktail" study design. *J Pharmacol Exp Ther* 1989; **249**: 638–45.
3. Tartara A, *et al.* Differential effects of valproic acid and enzyme-inducing anticonvulsants on nimodipine pharmacokinetics in epileptic patients. *Br J Clin Pharmacol* 1991; **32**: 335–40.

Antifungals. Azole antifungals inhibit the cytochrome P450 enzyme system and may therefore interfere with metabolism of calcium-channel blockers. Two women who had been taking felodipine for about a year developed peripheral oedema a few days after starting treatment with *itraconazole.*[1] Plasma-felodipine concentrations were measured in one of the women before and during a subsequent course of itraconazole and increased considerably when the two drugs were used together. A similar interaction occurred when itraconazole therapy was started in a patient already taking nifedipine.[2] Potentiation of the effects of nifedipine by *fluconazole* has also been reported.[3]

1. Neuvonen PJ, Suhonen R. Itraconazole interacts with felodipine. *J Am Acad Dermatol* 1995; **33**: 134–5.
2. Tailor SAN, *et al.* Peripheral edema due to nifedipine-itraconazole interaction: a case report. *Arch Dermatol* 1996; **132**: 350–2.
3. Kremens B, *et al.* Loss of blood pressure control on withdrawal of fluconazole during nifedipine therapy. *Br J Clin Pharmacol* 1999; **47**: 707–8.

Antihistamines. Severe angina developed in a patient stabilised on nifedipine who took *terfenadine* 60 mg for seasonal allergy. The pain resolved within an hour or two.[1]

1. Falkenberg HM. Possible interaction report. *Can Pharm J* 1988; **121**: 294.

Antineoplastics. For a report of increased *vincristine* toxicity in children also receiving itraconazole and nifedipine concomitantly, see p.579.

Beta blockers. Although nifedipine is often used with beta blockers without untoward effects, heart failure has been reported in a few patients with angina who were given nifedipine and a beta blocker.[1,2] Severe hypotension has been reported in 1 of 15 angina patients given nifedipine and *atenolol;*[3] withdrawal of the beta blocker precipitated severe unstable angina in this patient. Severe hypotension in a patient was attributed to the use of nifedipine with *propranolol*, and was thought to have contributed to fatal myocardial infarction.[4]

1. Anastassiades CJ. Nifedipine and beta-blocker drugs. *BMJ* 1980; **281**: 1251–2.
2. Robson RH, Vishwanath MC. Nifedipine and beta-blockade as a cause of cardiac failure. *BMJ* 1982; **284**: 104.
3. Opie LH, White DA. Adverse interaction between nifedipine and β-blockade. *BMJ* 1980; **281**: 1462.
4. Staffurth JS, Emery P. Adverse interaction between nifedipine and beta-blockade. *BMJ* 1981; **282**: 225.

Calcium-channel blockers. Plasma concentrations of nifedipine were increased in a study in 6 healthy subjects when pretreated with *diltiazem*; the elimination half-life of nifedipine was prolonged from 2.54 hours to 3.40 hours after pretreatment with diltiazem 30 mg daily and to 3.47 hours after 90 mg daily. The effect was probably due to reduced hepatic metabolism of nifedipine.[1] Nifedipine and diltiazem are reported to be metabolised by the same hepatic enzyme and, conversely, pretreatment with nifedipine has resulted in increased concentrations of diltiazem.[2]

1. Tateishi T, *et al.* Dose dependent effect of diltiazem on the pharmacokinetics of nifedipine. *J Clin Pharmacol* 1989; **29:** 994–7.
2. Tateishi T, *et al.* The effect of nifedipine on the pharmacokinetics and dynamics of diltiazem: the preliminary study in normal volunteers. *J Clin Pharmacol* 1993; **33:** 738–40.

Digoxin. For the effect of nifedipine and other dihydropyridine calcium-channel blockers on digoxin, see p.872.

Grapefruit juice. Grapefruit juice inhibits the cytochrome P450 enzyme system, particularly in the intestinal wall, and oral administration with calcium-channel blockers has been shown to increase markedly bioavailability of the calcium-channel blocker;[1-3] calcium-channel blockers given intravenously appear to be unaffected.[4] Most calcium-channel blockers should not therefore be taken orally at the same time as grapefruit juice.[5]

See also Absorption under Pharmacokinetics, below.

1. Bailey DG, *et al.* Interaction of citrus juices with felodipine and nifedipine. *Lancet* 1991; **337:** 268–9.
2. Bailey DG, *et al.* Effect of grapefruit juice and naringin on nisoldipine pharmacokinetics. *Clin Pharmacol Ther* 1993; **54:** 589–94.
3. Lundahl J, *et al.* Relationship between time of intake of grapefruit juice and its effect on pharmacokinetics and pharmacodynamics of felodipine in healthy subjects. *Eur J Clin Pharmacol* 1995; **49:** 61–7.
4. Rashid TJ, *et al.* Factors affecting the absolute bioavailability of nifedipine. *Br J Clin Pharmacol* 1995; **40:** 51–8.
5. Committee on Safety of Medicines/Medicines Control Agency. Drug interactions with grapefruit juice. *Current Problems* 1997; **23:** 2.

Histamine H₂-antagonists. Pharmacokinetic studies have indicated that concurrent administration of nifedipine and *cimetidine* can increase the bioavailability of nifedipine.[1-4] An increase in the area under the plasma concentration-time curve of between 77 and 92% has been reported.[2,3] Potentiation of the hypotensive effect of nifedipine by cimetidine was also shown in 7 hypertensive patients.[1] The mechanism of the interaction was thought to be due to inhibition of the cytochrome P450 system by cimetidine and thus inhibition of the metabolism of nifedipine.

Ranitidine was found to have little effect on the pharmacokinetics of nifedipine, although there was an increase in the bioavailability of nifedipine during ranitidine administration.[5] *Famotidine* has been reported not to interact with nifedipine.[6]

1. Kirch W, *et al.* Einflußvon cimetidin und ranitidin auf pharmakokinetik und antihypertensiven effekt von nifedipin. *Dtsch Med Wochenschr* 1983; **108:** 1757–61.
2. Renwick AG, *et al.* Factors affecting the pharmacokinetics of nifedipine. *Eur J Clin Pharmacol* 1987; **32:** 351–5.
3. Smith SR, *et al.* Ranitidine and cimetidine: drug interactions with single dose and steady-state nifedipine administration. *Br J Clin Pharmacol* 1987; **23:** 311–15.
4. Schwartz JB, *et al.* Effect of cimetidine or ranitidine administration on nifedipine pharmacokinetics and pharmacodynamics. *Clin Pharmacol Ther* 1988; **43:** 673–80.
5. Kirch W, *et al.* Ranitidine increases bioavailability of nifedipine. *Clin Pharmacol Ther* 1985; **37:** 204.
6. Kirch W, *et al.* Negative effects of famotidine on cardiac performance assessed by noninvasive hemodynamic measurements. *Gastroenterology* 1989; **96:** 1388–92.

Immunosuppressants. Flushing, paraesthesias, and rashes were reported in 2 patients given nifedipine 40 mg daily while taking *ciclosporin* for psoriasis.[1] A study in 8 psoriatic patients indicated that administration of nifedipine with ciclosporin resulted in reduced recovery of the principal metabolite of nifedipine, presumably because ciclosporin reduced nifedipine metabolism through competition for the cytochrome P450 metabolising enzymes.

For reference to the effects of calcium-channel blockers on ciclosporin concentrations in blood, see p.521. For the possible protective effect of nifedipine against ciclosporin-induced nephrotoxicity, see Transplantation under Uses and Administration, below.

For the effect of nifedipine on *tacrolimus*, see p.570.

1. McFadden JP, *et al.* Cyclosporin decreases nifedipine metabolism. *BMJ* 1989; **299:** 1224.

Magnesium salts. Profound hypotension has been reported in 2 women in whom a single dose of nifedipine 10 mg by mouth was added to treatment with magnesium sulfate infusion for pre-eclampsia; both women were also receiving methyldopa.[1] Neuromuscular blockade has been reported in 2 women following concomitant use of nifedipine and intravenous magnesium sulfate. In one woman receiving nifedipine as a tocolytic, symptoms of neuromuscular blockade occurred immediately on injection of magnesium sulfate and resolved within 25 minutes of stopping the injection.[2] In another woman who was receiving a magnesium sulfate infusion for pre-eclampsia, symptoms developed 30 minutes after the second of 2 doses of nifedipine had been administered and improved following administration of calcium gluconate injection.[3]

1. Waisman GD, *et al.* Magnesium plus nifedipine: potentiation of hypotensive effect in pre-eclampsia? *Am J Obstet Gynecol* 1988; **159:** 308–9.

2. Snyder SW, Cardwell MS. Neuromuscular blockade with magnesium sulfate and nifedipine. *Am J Obstet Gynecol* 1989; **161:** 35–6.
3. Ben-Ami M, *et al.* The combination of magnesium sulphate and nifedipine: a cause of neuromuscular blockade. *Br J Obstet Gynaecol* 1994; **101:** 262–3.

Tobacco. In a study of the effects of cigarette smoking and the treatment of angina with nifedipine, propranolol, or atenolol, smoking was shown to have direct and adverse effects on the heart and to interfere with the efficacy of all 3 anti-anginal drugs, with nifedipine being the most affected.[1]

1. Deanfield J, *et al.* Cigarette smoking and the treatment of angina with propranolol, atenolol, and nifedipine. *N Engl J Med* 1984; **310:** 951–4.

Xanthines. For the effect of nifedipine on *theophylline*, see p.781.

Pharmacokinetics

Nifedipine is rapidly and almost completely absorbed from the gastrointestinal tract, but undergoes extensive hepatic first-pass metabolism. Bioavailability after oral administration of liquid-filled capsules is between 45 and 75%, but is lower for longer-acting formulations. Following administration by mouth peak blood concentrations are reported to occur after 30 minutes with liquid-filled capsules.

Nifedipine is about 92 to 98% bound to plasma proteins. It is distributed into breast milk. It is extensively metabolised in the liver and 70 to 80% of a dose is excreted in the urine almost entirely as inactive metabolites. The half-life is about 2 hours following intravenous administration or administration of liquid-filled capsules.

◊ General reviews.
1. Kelly JG, O'Malley K. Clinical pharmacokinetics of calcium antagonists: an update. *Clin Pharmacokinet* 1992; **22:** 416–33.

◊ A review of the pharmacokinetics of nifedipine.[1] Studies of the pharmacokinetics of nifedipine have been complicated by the difficulty in preparing a stable intravenous formulation and the problems in developing a sufficiently sensitive and specific method of analysis. Nearly 100% of an oral dose of nifedipine is absorbed in the small intestine although the bioavailability from capsules is 45 to 68%. The rate of absorption from both oral and sublingual capsules varies widely among individuals: there has been a report that high plasma-nifedipine concentrations are achieved more rapidly if the capsule is bitten and swallowed than from standard oral and sublingual administration. The absorption of nifedipine from tablets is slower than from capsules, with maximum plasma concentrations occurring at 1.6 to 4.2 hours compared with 0.5 to 2.17 hours, and absorption may still be occurring at 24 to 32 hours after administration.

Nifedipine undergoes almost complete hepatic oxidation to 3 pharmacologically inactive metabolites which are excreted in the urine. It has been reported that following oral administration 30 to 40% of the amount absorbed is metabolised during the first pass through the liver. The elimination half-life of nifedipine is apparently dependent upon the dosage form in which it is administered, with half-lives of 6 to 11 hours, 2 to 3.4 hours, and 1.3 to 1.8 hours measured after oral tablet, oral capsule, and intravenous administration respectively. The total systemic clearance of nifedipine from plasma ranges from 27 to about 66 litres per hour. Renal impairment does not substantially alter nifedipine pharmacokinetics.

1. Sorkin EM, *et al.* Nifedipine: a review of its pharmacodynamic and pharmacokinetic properties, and therapeutic efficacy, in ischaemic heart disease, hypertension and related cardiovascular disorders. *Drugs* 1985; **30:** 182–274.

Absorption. Although studies have indicated that the absorption of nifedipine may be affected by administration with food the results appear to vary depending upon the preparation used. A reduction in peak plasma-nifedipine concentrations, and a delay in achieving them, was reported[1] when nifedipine *capsules* were given after a meal compared with 30 minutes before. In contrast, the bioavailability and maximum serum concentrations of nifedipine were markedly increased when a *modified-release tablet* (Adalat L) was given after a meal rather than fasting.[2] A *modified-release capsule* containing uncoated and enteric-coated granules (Sepamit R) was reported to have essentially the same bioavailability when taken before or after a meal.[3]

See also under Interactions, Grapefruit Juice, above.

1. Hirasawa K, *et al.* Effect of food ingestion on nifedipine absorption and haemodynamic response. *Eur J Clin Pharmacol* 1985; **28:** 105–7.
2. Ueno K, *et al.* Effect of food on nifedipine sustained-release preparation. *DICP Ann Pharmacother* 1989; **23:** 662–5.
3. Ueno K, *et al.* Effect of a light breakfast on the bioavailability of sustained-release nifedipine. *DICP Ann Pharmacother* 1991; **25:** 317–19.

Hepatic impairment. The pharmacokinetics of nifedipine were found to be considerably altered in 7 patients with liver cirrhosis.[1] Systemic plasma clearance was substantially reduced and the elimination half-life was considerably longer than in healthy subjects. In addition, systemic availability of

oral nifedipine was much higher in patients with cirrhosis and was complete in 3 patients with surgical portacaval shunt. Patients with liver cirrhosis seemed to be more sensitive to the effects of nifedipine on diastolic blood pressure and heart rate, and this could be explained by the higher free drug concentrations observed. It was concluded that lower doses of nifedipine may be required in patients with liver cirrhosis, and the patient's response should be closely monitored.

1. Kleinbloesem CH, *et al.* Nifedipine: kinetics and hemodynamic effects in patients with liver cirrhosis after intravenous and oral administration. *Clin Pharmacol Ther* 1986; **40:** 21–8.

Interindividual variation. A study in 53 Dutch subjects found a bimodal distribution of plasma concentrations of nifedipine following a single oral dose; it was proposed that the higher plasma concentrations in 17% of subjects represented a slow metaboliser phenotype, with the majority of the population being fast metabolisers.[1] Although further studies[2,3] in European populations have not confirmed these results, a study in 12 Mexican subjects supported the concept of polymorphic metabolism, with 5 fast and 7 slow metabolisers, a much higher proportion of slow metabolisers than in the European studies.[4] Studies have also reported a markedly increased area under the concentration-time curve in South Asian,[5,6] Mexican,[7] and Nigerian[8] subjects compared with Caucasians. The difference did not appear to be due to diet.[5,6] The initial dose of nifedipine might need to be lower in these ethnic groups.

1. Kleinbloesem CH, *et al.* Variability in nifedipine pharmacokinetics and dynamics: a new oxidation polymorphism in man. *Biochem Pharmacol* 1984; **33:** 3721–4.
2. Renwick AG, *et al.* The pharmacokinetics of oral nifedipine—a population study. *Br J Clin Pharmacol* 1988; **25:** 701–8.
3. Lobo J, *et al.* The intra- and inter-subject variability of nifedipine pharmacokinetics in young volunteers. *Eur J Clin Pharmacol* 1986; **30:** 57–60.
4. Hoyo-Vadillo C, *et al.* Pharmacokinetics of nifedipine slow release tablet in Mexican subjects: further evidence for an oxidation polymorphism. *J Clin Pharmacol* 1989; **29:** 816–20.
5. Ahsan CH, *et al.* Ethnic differences in the pharmacokinetics of oral nifedipine. *Br J Clin Pharmacol* 1991; **31:** 399–403.
6. Ahsan CH, *et al.* The influences of dose and ethnic origins on the pharmacokinetics of nifedipine. *Clin Pharmacol Ther* 1993; **54:** 329–38.
7. Castañeda-Hernández G, *et al.* Interethnic variability in nifedipine disposition: reduced systemic plasma clearance in Mexican subjects. *Br J Clin Pharmacol* 1996; **41:** 433–4.
8. Sowunmi A, *et al.* Ethnic differences in nifedipine kinetics: comparisons between Nigerians, Caucasians and South Asians. *Br J Clin Pharmacol* 1995; **40:** 489–93.

Uses and Administration

Nifedipine is a dihydropyridine calcium-channel blocker (p.788). It is a peripheral and coronary vasodilator, but, unlike the calcium-channel blockers verapamil or diltiazem, has little or no effect on cardiac conduction and negative inotropic activity is rarely seen at therapeutic doses. Administration of nifedipine results primarily in vasodilatation, with reduced peripheral resistance, blood pressure, and afterload, increased coronary blood flow, and a reflex increase in heart rate. This in turn results in an increase in myocardial oxygen supply and cardiac output. Nifedipine has no antiarrhythmic activity. Nicardipine and newer dihydropyridines such as amlodipine, felodipine, isradipine, and lacidipine may be even more selective than nifedipine for vascular smooth muscle. Nimodipine acts particularly on cerebral blood vessels. Most of the dihydropyridine calcium-channel blockers (nifedipine and lacidipine are exceptions) are chiral compounds used as racemic mixtures.

Nifedipine is used in the management of hypertension; in the prophylaxis of angina pectoris (p.791), particularly when a vasospastic element is present, as in Prinzmetal's angina; and in the treatment of Raynaud's syndrome. Nifedipine has also been tried in numerous non-vascular disorders.

Nifedipine is usually given by mouth. It is available in a number of formulations. Liquid-filled capsules with a relatively rapid onset but short duration of action are administered three times daily. This short-acting preparation is not recommended for the management of hypertension (see below). There are also tablets and capsules with a slower onset and longer duration of action, enabling twice-daily administration; although these are often referred to by nomenclature implying extended or sustained release they should be distinguished from the true extended-release preparations available in some countries that allow administration once daily. Nifedipine is normally given with or after food.

Doses of nifedipine are dependent upon the formulation used; they may need to be reduced in the elderly or those with impaired liver function.

In the management of **hypertension** a long-acting preparation of nifedipine may be given in doses of 10 to 40 mg twice daily, or 20 to 90 mg once daily, depending on the preparation used.

In the management of **angina pectoris**, nifedipine may be given as a long-acting preparation in a dose of 10 to 40 mg twice daily or 30 to 90 mg once daily, depending on the preparation. Alternatively, the liquid-filled capsules have been given in a dose of 5 to 20 mg three times daily, but longer-acting preparations are preferred.

Nifedipine has been administered by injection via a coronary catheter for the treatment of coronary spasm during coronary angiography and balloon angioplasty. Blood pressure and heart rate should be monitored carefully.

In the management of **Raynaud's syndrome**, nifedipine may be given as liquid-filled capsules in a dose of 5 to 20 mg three times daily.

◊ General reviews.
1. Sorkin EM, et al. Nifedipine. Drugs 1985; 30: 182–274.
2. Anonymous. Nifedipine in myocardial ischaemia, systemic hypertension, and other cardiovascular disorders. Ann Intern Med 1986; 105: 714–29.
3. Anonymous. Calcium antagonists for cardiovascular disease. Drug Ther Bull 1993; 31: 81–4.
4. Fisher M, Grotta J. New uses for calcium channel blockers: therapeutic implications. Drugs 1993; 46: 961–75.

Administration in children. Nifedipine has been administered sublingually[1] to children aged 6 to 15 years with acute severe hypertension in a mean dose of 240 μg per kg bodyweight (range 180 to 320 μg per kg). Sublingual administration is difficult in younger children, but nifedipine has successfully been administered rectally,[2] as a pierced capsule with sufficient of the contents withdrawn to give a dose in the range 200 to 500 μg per kg body-weight; it has also been given intranasally[3] in a dose of 400 μg per kg.
1. Evans JHC, et al. Sublingual nifedipine in acute severe hypertension. Arch Dis Child 1988; 63: 975–7.
2. Uchiyama M, Ogawa I. Rectal nifedipine in acute severe hypertension in young children. Arch Dis Child 1989; 64: 632–3.
3. Lopez-Herce J, et al. Treatment of hypertensive crisis with intranasal nifedipine. Crit Care Med 1988; 9: 914.

Amaurosis fugax. Relief of vasospasm might explain the efficacy of the calcium-channel blockers nifedipine and verapamil in a few patients with amaurosis fugax (see under Stroke, p.813) unresponsive to anticoagulants or antiplatelet agents.[1]
1. Winterkorn JMS, et al. Brief report: treatment of vasospastic amaurosis fugax with calcium-channel blockers. N Engl J Med 1993; 329: 396–8.

Anal fissure. Calcium antagonists such as nifedipine have been tried in the treatment of chronic anal fissure (p.1325).

Atherosclerosis. The use of drugs that interfere with atherogenesis (the development of atheromas) has been suggested as a means of reducing diseases associated with atherosclerosis (p.793). Calcium is thought to be necessary for several steps in atherogenesis and studies in *animals* have shown that calcium-channel blockers slow the development and progression of atherosclerotic lesions. However, studies in humans have been less convincing.[1] In one study,[2] amlodipine had no demonstrable effect on angiographic progression of coronary atherosclerosis or the risk of major cardiovascular events although it was associated with fewer admissions to hospital for unstable angina and revascularisation.
1. Borcherding SM, et al. Calcium-channel antagonists for prevention of atherosclerosis. Ann Pharmacother 1993; 27: 61–7.
2. Pitt B, et al. Effect of amlodipine on the progression of atherosclerosis and the occurrence of clinical events. Circulation 2000; 102: 1503–10.

Cardiomyopathies. Calcium-channel blockers may have a role in some forms of cardiomyopathy (p.796). In *hypertrophic cardiomyopathy* verapamil is probably the calcium-channel blocker of choice (see p.991). Nifedipine does not appear to reduce left ventricular outflow tract obstruction, and conflicting results have been demonstrated with respect to improvement in the diastolic function abnormality with this drug.[1] The use of calcium-channel blockers is not standard therapy in *dilated cardiomyopathy* although symptomatic improvement has been reported[2] with diltiazem.
1. Richardson PJ. Calcium antagonists in cardiomyopathy. Br J Clin Pract 1988; 42 (suppl 60): 33–7.
2. Figulla HR, et al. Diltiazem improves cardiac function and exercise capacity in patients with idiopathic dilated cardiomyopathy: results of the Diltiazem in Dilated Cardiomyopathy Trial. Circulation 1996; 94: 346–52.

Cough. Nifedipine has been reported to reduce the severity of cough induced by captopril,[1] possibly by inhibiting prostaglandin synthesis. For further details on cough associated with ACE inhibitors, see p.820.
1. Fogari R, et al. Effects of nifedipine and indomethacin on cough induced by angiotensin-converting enzyme inhibitors: a double-blind, randomized, cross-over study. J Cardiovasc Pharmacol 1992; 19: 670–3.

Epilepsy. Calcium-channel blockers have been tried in various forms of epilepsy but are not the usual therapy (see p.338). There were preliminary reports of beneficial results with nifedipine in patients with refractory epilepsy.[1,2] However, neither nifedipine[3] nor nimodipine,[4] which has greater CNS penetration, were of benefit when given as adjunctive therapy in controlled studies of patients with refractory epilepsy.
1. Larkin JG, et al. Nifedipine for epilepsy: a pilot study. BMJ 1988; 296: 530–1.
2. Sander JWAS, Shorvon SD. Nifedipine for epilepsy? BMJ 1988; 296: 1070.
3. Brodie MJ, et al. A double-blind, crossover, placebo-controlled trial of adjuvant nifedipine in refractory epilepsy. Br J Clin Pharmacol 1990; 29: 592P-593P.
4. Meyer FB, et al. Nimodipine as an add-on therapy for intractable epilepsy. Mayo Clin Proc 1995; 70: 623–7.

Gastrointestinal spasm. Nifedipine 20 mg by mouth produced complete pain relief within 2 hours in 11 of 14 patients with acute intestinal colic (p.1204) due to bacillary or amoebic dysentery.[1] This compared with pain relief in only 2 of 14 control patients given placebo. The results suggest a spasmolytic activity of nifedipine on intestinal muscles. A similar mechanism has been proposed for calcium-channel blockers in the management of irritable bowel syndrome (p.1206), but the results of small trials have not been encouraging.
1. Al-Waili NSD. Nifedipine in intestinal colic. JAMA 1990; 263: 3258.

Hiccup. Hiccups (p.667) result from involuntary spasmodic contraction of the diaphragm. Intractable hiccups resolved completely with nifedipine 20 mg every 8 hours in a patient.[1] In a further 7 such patients,[2] nifedipine in doses of 20 to 80 mg daily stopped hiccups in 4 and improved them in another. Resolution of intractable hiccups has also been reported[3] in 2 patients given nimodipine; the drug was administered orally in one patient and intravenously in the other.
1. Mukhopadhyay P, et al. Nifedipine for intractable hiccups. N Engl J Med 1986; 314: 1256.
2. Lipps DC, et al. Nifedipine for intractable hiccups. Neurology 1990; 40: 531–2.
3. Hernández JL, et al. Nimodipine treatment for intractable hiccups. Am J Med 1999; 106: 600.

High-altitude disorders. Nifedipine lowers pulmonary artery pressure and is one of several drugs that are used in high-altitude disorders (p.800), success being reported for both the treatment[1,2] and prevention[2,3] of symptoms of pulmonary oedema. In a study conducted at 4559 m above sea-level[1] nifedipine 10 mg sublingually, then 20 mg as a modified-release dosage form was given to 6 subjects with symptoms of high-altitude pulmonary oedema. The sublingual dose was repeated if tolerated after 15 minutes and the subjects subsequently received modified-release nifedipine 20 mg every 6 hours while they remained at high altitude. Symptoms of high-altitude pulmonary oedema were relieved within 1 hour of beginning nifedipine and radiographic signs of oedema regressed during treatment despite remaining at high altitude for 36 hours and participating in mountaineering activities. Raised pulmonary arterial pressure was also reduced to control values by nifedipine. Successful treatment of pulmonary oedema in a climber at 6550 m has been described with doses of 20 mg every 8 hours for 36 hours and such doses also prevented the development of symptoms in 2 climbers who had taken nifedipine from the start of the climb.[2] Doses of 20 mg every 8 hours have been reported to allow rapid ascent to 4559 m without development of pulmonary oedema in 9 of 10 subjects who received nifedipine compared with 4 of 11 who received only placebo.[3] However, the point has been made that although it is reasonable that many climbers carry nifedipine in case of an attack, prophylactic nifedipine should not be considered an alternative to slow ascent and acclimatisation.[4]
1. Oelz O, et al. Nifedipine for high altitude pulmonary oedema. Lancet 1989; ii: 1241–4. Correction. ibid. 1991; 337: 556.
2. Jamieson A, Kerr GW. Treatment of high-altitude pulmonary oedema. Lancet 1992; 340: 1468.
3. Bärtsch P, et al. Prevention of high-altitude pulmonary oedema by nifedipine. N Engl J Med 1991; 325: 1284–9.
4. A'Court CHD, et al. Doctor on a mountaineering expedition. BMJ 1995; 310: 1248–52.

Hypertension. Although diuretics and beta blockers are generally considered to be first-line therapy in uncomplicated hypertension (p.802) calcium-channel blockers may be used as an alternative in selected patients. The use of short-acting calcium-channel blockers is not recommended (see under Adverse Effects, above). Combination therapy may be necessary in many patients and suitable combinations include a dihydropyridine calcium-channel blocker plus a beta blocker or an ACE inhibitor.

In **hypertensive crises**, where oral treatment is suitable, a calcium-channel blocker such as nifedipine has been widely used. Nifedipine has also been administered sublingually, or by biting the capsule and swallowing the contents,[1] but such use may cause dangerous hypotension and is no longer recommended. Some calcium-channel blockers, for example nicardipine, are available for intravenous administration and may be given when a parenteral antihypertensive drug is considered necessary. One study concluded that intravenous nicardipine was as effective as sodium nitroprusside in the treatment of postoperative hypertension.[2]

For **hypertension in pregnancy**, first-line treatment is usually methyldopa or a beta blocker but calcium-channel blockers may also be used. Nifedipine is reported to be teratogenic in *animals* and may inhibit labour; but it has been tried in a limited number of patients with pre-eclampsia. Although a high rate of caesarean deliveries, premature births, and small-for-date infants was reported[3] in patients given nifedipine as a second-line drug, assessment of the role of nifedipine is difficult because outcome is often poor in such severely compromised pregnancies.[4] Fetal nifedipine concentrations have been reported to be 75% of maternal values 2 to 3 hours after sublingual administration.[5] However, nifedipine in a single 20-mg oral dose lowered blood pressure without compromising blood flow in the fetus in 9 women in the third trimester with normal haemodynamics.[4] This is in line with other reports,[6] although there has also been a report[7] of severe hypotension and fetal distress following sublingual nifedipine administration. In a randomised controlled study,[8] nifedipine 10 to 30 mg sublingually followed by 10 mg as capsules by mouth every 6 hours increasing to 20 mg every 4 hours if necessary, was compared with hydralazine 12.5 mg intravenously as required followed by 20 to 30 mg by mouth every 6 hours, with added methyldopa if necessary. Both groups also received intravenous magnesium sulfate. Effective control of blood pressure was achieved in 23 of 24 patients given nifedipine compared with only 17 of 25 given hydralazine and 9 nifedipine patients achieved term delivery compared with only 2 of those receiving hydralazine. The average gestational age was greater in infants in the nifedipine group; hence these neonates weighed more and had fewer neonatal complications when compared with neonates from the hydralazine treated group.
1. Gifford RW. Management of hypertensive crises. JAMA 1991; 266: 829–35.
2. Halpern NA, et al. Postoperative hypertension: a multicenter, prospective, randomized comparison between intravenous nicardipine and sodium nitroprusside. Crit Care Med 1992; 20: 1637–43.
3. Constantine G, et al. Nifedipine as a second line antihypertensive drug in pregnancy. Br J Obstet Gynaecol 1987; 94: 1136–42.
4. Hanretty KP, et al. Effect of nifedipine on Doppler flow velocity waveforms in severe pre-eclampsia. BMJ 1989; 299: 1205–6.
5. Pirhonen JP, et al. Single dose of nifedipine in normotensive pregnancy: nifedipine concentrations, hemodynamic responses, and uterine and fetal flow velocity waveforms. Obstet Gynecol 1990; 76: 807–11.
6. Pirhonen JP, et al. Uterine and fetal flow velocity wave forms in hypertensive pregnancy: the effect of a single dose of nifedipine. Obstet Gynecol 1990; 76: 37–41.
7. Impey L. Severe hypotension and fetal distress following sublingual administration of nifedipine to a patient with severe pregnancy induced hypertension at 33 weeks. Br J Obstet Gynaecol 1993; 100: 959–61.
8. Fenakel K, et al. Nifedipine in the treatment of severe preeclampsia. Obstet Gynecol 1991; 77: 331–7.

Kidney disorders. Although nifedipine may adversely affect renal function (see under Adverse Effects, above) there is evidence that calcium-channel blockers may be of benefit in various forms of kidney disorder. Proteinuria is an important indicator of glomerular kidney disease (p.1051) of various causes and the effects of calcium-channel blockers on proteinuria and renal dysfunction have been studied in a variety of patients. Results have been mixed,[1-5] and it is not clear whether any protective effect of calcium-channel blockers on renal function is only due to their antihypertensive action or whether they also have additional effects. The benefits of ACE inhibitors in kidney disorders are much better established (see p.824) and a study[6] in African American hypertensives was stopped early when treatment with ramipril was found to be superior to treatment with amlodipine.

Nifedipine has also been reported to protect against ciclosporin-induced nephrotoxicity in renal transplant patients (see Transplantation, below).
1. Demarie BK, Bakris GL. Effects of different calcium antagonists on proteinuria associated with diabetes mellitus. Ann Intern Med 1990; 113: 987–8.
2. Melbourne Diabetic Nephropathy Study Group. Comparison between perindopril and nifedipine in hypertensive and normotensive diabetic patients with microalbuminuria. BMJ 1991; 302: 210–16.
3. Reams G, et al. The effect of nifedipine GITS on renal function in hypertensive patients with renal insufficiency. J Clin Pharmacol 1991; 31: 468–72.
4. Abbott K, et al. Effects of dihydropyridine calcium antagonists on albuminuria in patients with diabetes. J Clin Pharmacol 1996; 36: 274–9.
5. Bouhanick B, et al. Equivalent effects of nicardipine and captopril on urinary albumin excretion of type 2, non-insulin-dependent diabetic subjects with mild to moderate hypertension. Therapie 1996; 51: 41–7.
6. Agodoa LY, et al. Effect of ramipril vs amlodipine on renal outcomes in hypertensive nephrosclerosis: a randomized controlled trial. JAMA 2001; 285: 2719–28.

Migraine and cluster headache. Drugs with calcium-channel blocking activity have been given in the management of headaches considered to have a vascular component such as migraine (p.449) and cluster headache (p.449).

In migraine prophylaxis, of those drugs with calcium-channel blocking activity studied, flunarizine (p.418) has the best documented efficacy, and verapamil may be useful. Other calcium-channel blockers such as diltiazem, nifedipine, and nimodipine have been tried, but results have been conflicting. Verapamil has also been given intravenously to treat a patient with hemiplegic migraine.[1]

Beneficial effects have been reported[2-4] with calcium-channel blockers in the prevention of cluster headache during cluster periods. Verapamil appears to have been the most widely used. In one double-blind study it was found to be of similar efficacy to lithium[5] and appeared to produce fewer adverse effects.

1. Ng TMH, *et al.* The effect of intravenous verapamil on cerebral hemodynamics in a migraine patient with hemiplegia. *Ann Pharmacother* 2000; **34:** 39–43.
2. Jónsdóttir M, *et al.* Efficacy, side effects and tolerance compared during headache treatment with three different calcium blockers. *Headache* 1987; **27:** 364–9.
3. Gabai IJ, Spierings ELH. Prophylactic treatment of cluster headache with verapamil. *Headache* 1989; **29:** 167–8.
4. Leone M, *et al.*. Verapamil in the prophylaxis of episodic cluster headache: a double-blind study versus placebo. *Neurology* 2000; **54:** 1382–5.
5. Bussone G, *et al.* Double blind comparison of lithium and verapamil in cluster headache prophylaxis. *Headache* 1990; **30:** 411–17.

Oesophageal motility disorders. Results from a number of studies have indicated that nifedipine, usually in doses of 10 to 20 mg sublingually may be of benefit in patients with achalasia, reducing lower oesophageal sphincter pressure and producing some symptomatic improvement.[1-5] Nifedipine has a role when mechanical dilatation of the sphincter or surgery are not feasible (see Oesophageal Motility Disorders, p.1208).

1. Bortolotti M, Labò G. Clinical and manometric effects of nifedipine in patients with esophageal achalasia. *Gastroenterology* 1981; **80:** 39–44.
2. Gelfond M, *et al.* Isosorbide dinitrate and nifedipine treatment of achalasia: a clinical, manometric and radionuclide evaluation. *Gastroenterology* 1982; **83:** 963–9.
3. Traube M, *et al.* Effects of nifedipine in achalasia and in patients with high-amplitude peristaltic esophageal contractions. *JAMA* 1984; **252:** 1733–6.
4. Román FJ, *et al.* Effects of nifedipine in achalasia and patients with high-amplitude peristaltic esophageal contractions. *JAMA* 1985; **253:** 2046.
5. Coccia G, *et al.* Prospective clinical and manometric study comparing pneumatic dilatation and sublingual nifedipine in the treatment of oesophageal achalasia. *Gut* 1991; **32:** 604–6.

Peripheral vascular disease. Vasospastic arterial disease (p.809) is due to an inappropriate response to temperature, usually cold, when vasoconstriction and/or vasospasm occurs. The most important of these disorders is Raynaud's syndrome. Calcium-channel blockers have been of benefit in Raynaud's syndrome, but it is not entirely clear which of their pharmacological actions is responsible. The most widely used and studied is nifedipine. Evidence of subjective benefit has been seen both in primary idiopathic disease[1-4] and in Raynaud's phenomenon secondary to systemic sclerosis,[2,3,5,6] systemic lupus erythematosus,[2,3] rheumatoid arthritis,[3] and cancer chemotherapy.[7] Objective improvement as demonstrated by evidence of improved digital blood flow has been demonstrated in some[4,5,8,9] but not all[6] studies. Doses have varied; 10 mg of nifedipine twice daily initially, increased after a week to a maximum of 20 mg twice daily has been suggested,[10] but in many studies doses of up to 60 mg daily have been used, although side-effects have proved intolerable in some patients given such doses.[6] A modified-release preparation has also been used[11] and may reduce the incidence of adverse effects.

Nifedipine in doses of 20 to 60 mg daily has also been reported to be of benefit in the treatment of another vasospastic condition, chilblains, both for established chilblains and in the prevention of relapse.[12]

1. Roath S. Management of Raynaud's phenomenon: focus on newer treatments. *Drugs* 1989; **37:** 700–12.
2. Smith CD, McKendry RJR. Controlled trial of nifedipine in the treatment of Raynaud's phenomenon. *Lancet* 1982; **ii:** 1299–1301.
3. Kahan A, *et al.* Nifedipine for Raynaud's phenomenon. *Lancet* 1983; **i:** 131.
4. Gasser P. Reaction of capillary blood cell velocity in nailfold capillaries to nifedipine and ketanserin in patients with vasospastic disease. *J Int Med Res* 1991; **19:** 24–31.
5. Thomas RHM, *et al.* Nifedipine in the treatment of Raynaud's phenomenon in patients with systemic sclerosis. *Br J Dermatol* 1987; **117:** 237–41.
6. Rademaker M, *et al.* Comparison of intravenous infusions of iloprost and oral nifedipine in treatment of Raynaud's phenomenon in patients with systemic sclerosis: a double blind randomised study. *BMJ* 1989; **298:** 561–4.
7. Hantel A, *et al.* Nifedipine and oncologic Raynaud phenomenon. *Ann Intern Med* 1988; **108:** 767.
8. Nilsson H, *et al.* Treatment of digital vasospastic disease with the calcium-entry blocker nifedipine. *Acta Med Scand* 1984; **215:** 135–9.
9. Finch MB, *et al.* The peripheral vascular effects of nifedipine in Raynaud's disease. *Br J Clin Pharmacol* 1986; **21:** 100P–101P.
10. Grigg MH, Wolfe JHN. Raynaud's syndrome and similar conditions. *BMJ* 1991; **303:** 913–16.
11. Raynaud's Treatment Study Investigators. Comparison of sustained-release nifedipine and temperature biofeedback for treatment of primary Raynaud phenomenon: results from a randomized clinical trial with 1-year follow-up. *Arch Intern Med* 2000; **160:** 1101–8.
12. Rustin MHA, *et al.* The treatment of chilblains with nifedipine: the results of a pilot study, a double-blind placebo-controlled randomized study and a long-term open trial. *Br J Dermatol* 1989; **120:** 267–75.

Phaeochromocytoma. Pharmacological management of phaeochromocytoma (p.810) is principally achieved by alpha-

adrenergic blockade and tachycardia may subsequently be controlled by cautious addition of a beta blocker. There is also some limited experience with nifedipine. A patient with a noradrenaline-secreting phaeochromocytoma experienced great improvement in cardiovascular symptoms during treatment with nifedipine.[1] Symptomatic relief was associated with a pronounced decline in elevated urinary noradrenaline concentrations and it was suggested that nifedipine could interfere with the release of noradrenaline from phaeochromocytoma tissue. However, high plasma concentrations of noradrenaline have been reported in some patients with phaeochromocytoma despite abolition of the associated increase in blood pressure by nifedipine.[2,3] It was suggested that nifedipine was interfering with the action of noradrenaline by acting directly on the vascular smooth muscle.[2] In a review of 10 cases of childhood phaeochromocytoma 4 were reported to have been treated with nifedipine but adequate pre-operative control of blood pressure was achieved with nifedipine alone only in 2. Nonetheless, although phenoxybenzamine and propranolol remained the drug of first choice for catecholamine blockade, results with nifedipine were considered encouraging.[4]

1. Serfas D, *et al.* Phaeochromocytoma and hypertrophic cardiomyopathy: apparent suppression of symptoms and noradrenaline secretion by calcium-channel blockade. *Lancet* 1983; **ii:** 711–13.
2. Lenders JWM, *et al.* Treatment of a phaeochromocytoma of the urinary bladder with nifedipine. *BMJ* 1985; **290:** 1624–5.
3. Favre L, Vallotton MB. Nifedipine in pheochromocytoma. *Ann Intern Med* 1986; **104:** 125.
4. Deal JE, *et al.* Phaeochromocytoma—investigation and management of 10 cases. *Arch Dis Child* 1990; **65:** 269–74.

Premature labour. Although beta$_2$-adrenoceptor agonists are the drugs most commonly used as tocolytics to postpone premature labour (p.773), some success has been achieved with calcium-channel blockers such as nifedipine, either given alone or added to beta$_2$ agonists. Case reports and small studies have reported beneficial effects. Labour was successfully postponed in a patient treated with nifedipine 20 mg three times daily and terbutaline 5 mg 4-hourly by mouth.[1] Terbutaline 0.25 mg up to 4 times daily by subcutaneous injection was also occasionally necessary. Nifedipine was administered from the twenty-sixth week of pregnancy for 55 days. A normal, healthy infant was delivered in the thirty-sixth week of pregnancy. In a study[2] in 20 patients, nifedipine 30 mg initially, then 20 mg every 8 hours by mouth, was more effective in suppressing premature labour than ritodrine given intravenously or no treatment. However, a similar study[3] in 33 patients found nifedipine to be no more effective than ritodrine infusion, although associated with a lower incidence of adverse effects. A meta-analysis[4] concluded that nifedipine was at least as effective as beta$_2$ agonists and was associated with fewer maternal adverse effects, and this was supported by the results of a further study[5] in 185 women using nifedipine in an initial dose of up to 40 mg followed by 60 to 160 mg daily. Similar results have been reported with nicardipine.[6]

1. Kaul AF, *et al.* The management of preterm labor with the calcium channel-blocking agent nifedipine combined with the β-mimetic terbutaline. *Drug Intell Clin Pharm* 1985; **19:** 369–71.
2. Read MD, Wellby DE. The use of a calcium antagonist (nifedipine) to suppress preterm labour. *Br J Obstet Gynaecol* 1986; **93:** 933–7.
3. Ferguson JE, *et al.* A comparison of tocolysis with nifedipine or ritodrine: analysis of efficacy and maternal, fetal, and neonatal outcome. *Am J Obstet Gynecol* 1990; **163:** 105–11.
4. Ray JG. Meta-analysis of nifedipine versus beta-sympathomimetic agents for tocolysis during preterm labour. *J Soc Obstet Gynaecol Can* 1998; **20:** 259–69.
5. Papatsonis DNM, *et al.* Nifedipine and ritodrine in the management of preterm labor: a randomized multicenter trial. *Obstet Gynecol* 1997; **90:** 230–4.
6. Jannet D, *et al.* Nicardipine versus salbutamol in the treatment of premature labor: a prospective randomized study. *Eur J Obstet Gynecol Reprod Biol* 1997; **73:** 11–16.

Pulmonary hypertension. Vasodilators have been tried in primary pulmonary hypertension (p.810) on the premise that pulmonary vasoconstriction is an important component of the condition. Calcium-channel blockers are the most widely-used. Improved survival over a 5-year period has been noted in a study in patients treated with high doses of calcium-channel blockers (nifedipine or diltiazem).[1] However, treatment failures have occurred with nifedipine, and at least one death has been reported shortly after starting therapy.[2] Other reports have also stressed the potentially deleterious effects of nifedipine (or other vasodilator) therapy in pulmonary hypertension. Increased dyspnoea and a fall in arterial PO$_2$ have been reported in a patient with primary pulmonary hypertension given nifedipine, probably due to preferential vasodilatation of underventilated hypoxic tissues resulting in an increased physiological shunt.[3] Invasive investigations, notably blood-gas monitoring, is therefore recommended when giving nifedipine to these patients[2,3] and it has been advised that an acute response test should be performed before embarking on long-term treatment.[1]

1. Rich S, *et al.* The effect of high doses of calcium-channel blockers on survival in primary pulmonary hypertension. *N Engl J Med* 1992; **327:** 76–81.
2. McLeod AA, Jewitt DE. Drug treatment of primary pulmonary hypertension. *Drugs* 1986; **31:** 177–84.
3. Krol RC, *et al.* Primary pulmonary hypotension, nifedipine, and hypoxemia. *Ann Intern Med* 1984; **100:** 163.

Tardive dyskinesia. Calcium-channel blockers have been tried in the treatment of tardive dyskinesia[1] (see under Extrapy-

ramidal Disorders, p.662). However, results have been mixed and there is concern that, if their action is mediated through an antidopaminergic effect, they may only temporarily mask symptoms or exacerbate them in the long term.[1]

1. Cates M, *et al.* Are calcium-channel blockers effective in the treatment of tardive dyskinesia? *Ann Pharmacother* 1993; **27:** 191–6.

Transplantation. The main adverse effect of ciclosporin is reversible, dose-related nephrotoxicity. There is some evidence that nifedipine may be of value in protecting against this effect. Retrospective analysis[1] of 106 ciclosporin-treated renal transplant patients found that patients receiving nifedipine for hypertension had better graft function, despite having shorter graft duration and therefore requiring higher dosage of ciclosporin, than hypertensive patients receiving other drug treatment. Subsequent studies have similarly reported improved graft function[2] in patients receiving nifedipine and suggest that graft survival is also improved.[3,4] A nephroprotective effect has also been reported with nitrendipine,[5] felodipine,[6] and with the non-dihydropyridine diltiazem (see p.877), although a study[7] with nicardipine failed to demonstrate any improvement in graft function.

See also Kidney Disorders, above.

For a report of adverse effects attributed to reduced metabolism of nifedipine in patients taking ciclosporin, see Immunosuppressants, under Interactions, above.

1. Feehally J, *et al.* Does nifedipine ameliorate cyclosporin A nephrotoxicity? *BMJ* 1987; **295:** 310.
2. Shin GT, *et al.* Effect of nifedipine on renal allograft function and survival beyond one year. *Clin Nephrol* 1997; **47:** 33–6.
3. Weinrauch LA, *et al.* Role of calcium channel blockers in diabetic renal transplant patients: preliminary observations on protection from sepsis. *Clin Nephrol* 1995; **44:** 185–92.
4. Mehrens T, *et al.* The beneficial effects of calcium channel blockers on long-term kidney transplant survival are independent of blood-pressure reduction. *Clin Transplant* 2000; **14:** 257–61.
5. Rahn K-H, *et al.* Effect of nitrendipine on renal function in renal-transplant patients treated with cyclosporin: a randomised trial. *Lancet* 1999; **354:** 1415–20.
6. Madsen JK, *et al.* The effect of felodipine on renal function and blood pressure in cyclosporin-treated renal transplant recipients during the first three months after transplantation. *Nephrol Dial Transplant* 1998; **13:** 2327–34.
7. Kessler M, *et al.* Influence of nicardipine on renal function and plasma cyclosporin in renal transplant patients. *Eur J Clin Pharmacol* 1989; **36:** 637–8.

Urticaria. Oral antihistamines are the main drugs used in the management of urticaria (p.1107). Addition of a calcium-channel blocker, such as nifedipine, has been suggested for patients unresponsive to treatment with oral antihistamines alone, but results have been mixed.[1,2]

1. Lawlor F, *et al.* Calcium antagonist in the treatment of symptomatic dermographism: low-dose and high-dose studies with nifedipine. *Dermatologica* 1988; **177:** 287–91.
2. Bressler RB, *et al.* Therapy of chronic idiopathic urticaria with nifedipine: demonstration of beneficial effect in a double-blinded, placebo-controlled, crossover trial. *J Allergy Clin Immunol* 1989; **83:** 756–63.

Preparations

BP 2001: Nifedipine Capsules;
USP 25: Nifedipine Capsules; Nifedipine Extended-release Tablets.

Proprietary Preparations (details are given in Part 3)

Aust.: Adalat; Buconif; Einalat†; Fedip; Gewadilat†; Majolat; Nifebene; Nifecard; Nifehexal; Ospocard; Unidipin†; *Austral.:* Adalat; Adapine; Nifecard; Nifehexal; Nyefax; *Belg.:* Adalat; *Braz.:* Adalat; Biocord; Cardalin; Dilaflux; Oxcord; *Canad.:* Adalat; Apo-Nifed; Novo-Nifedin; Nu-Nifed; *Denm.:* Adalat; Hexadilat; Nifecodan; Nycopin; *Fin.:* Adalat; Nifangin; Nifdemin; Nifecor; *Fr.:* Adalate; Chronadalate; *Ger.:* Adalat; Aprical; Cisday; Cordicant; Corinfar; Corotrend; Dignokonstant; duranifin; Jedipin; Nife; nife uno; Nifeclair; Nifecor; Nifedipat; Nifedipat uno; Nifehexal; Nifelat; Nifical; Nifirat†; Pidilat; *Hong Kong:* Adalat; Coracten; Nadipinia; Nif-Ten; Nifecard; *Irl.:* Adalat; Nifedalat; Nifelease; Nifensar†; Pinifed; Systepin; Vasofed; *Israel:* Aprical; Megalat; Osmo-Adalat; Pressolat; *Ital.:* Adalat; Anifed†; Bionif; Citilat; Coral; Fenidina; Nifedicor; Nifedicron; Nifedin; Nifexal; Nipin; *Mex.:* Adalat; Aldar; Cordilat; Corogal; Corotrend; Elocor; Feniken; Nifedigel; Nifedipres; Nifezzard; *Neth.:* Adalat; *Norw.:* Adalat; Nycopin; *NZ:* Adalat; Nyefax; *Port.:* Adalat; Medipina†; Nifedate; Zenusin; *S.Afr.:* Adalat; Anginor†; Cardifen; Cardilat; Clinolat†; Nifedalat; Nifidine; Vascard; Vasofed; *Singapore:* Adalat; Apo-Nifed; Fenamon; Nifedi-Denk; Nifelat; Vasdalat; *Spain:* Adalat; Cordilan; Dari; Dilcor; Pertensal; *Swed.:* Adalat; *Switz.:* Adalat; Aldipin; Cardipin; Corotrend; Ecodipine; Fedip†; nife-basan; Nifedicor; *Thai.:* Adalat; Calcigard; Coracten; Fenamon; Jedipin; Nelapine; Nifecard; Nifelat; Nificard; Nyefax; Servidipine; Zenusin; *UK:* Adalat; Adipine; Angiopine; Calanif; Cardilate; Cardilate MR; Coracten; Coraday; Fortipine; Hypolar Retard; Nifedipress; Nifedotard†; Nifelease†; Nifopress; Nimodipin; Nivaten; Slofedipine; Tensipine; Unipine XL†; *USA:* Adalat; Nifedical; Procardia.

Multi-ingredient: *Aust.:* Beta-Adalat; Nif-Ten; Pontuc; *Belg.:* Beta-Adalat; Tenif; *Braz.:* Nifelat; *Fin.:* Adalat; Nif-Ten; *Fr.:* Beta-Adalate; Tenordate; *Ger.:* AteNif beta; Belnif; Bresben; duranifin Sali; Nifatenol; Nifehexal Sali†; Pontuc; Sali-Adalat; Tredalat; *Irl.:* Ate-Nife; Beta-Adalat; Nif-Ten; *Ital.:* Mixer; Nif-Ten; *Mex.:* Plenacor; *Neth.:* Nif-Ten; *Singapore:* Nif-Ten; Nifetex; *Switz.:* Beta-Adalat; Nif-Atenil; Nif-Ten; *UK:* Beta-Adalat; Tenif.

The symbol † denotes a preparation no longer actively marketed

Nifekalant Hydrochloride (15778-v)

Nifekalant Hydrochloride (rINNM).

MS-551. 6-[(2-{(2-Hydroxyethyl)[3-(p-nitrophenyl)propyl]amino}ethyl)amino]-1,3-dimethyluracil hydrochloride.

$C_{19}H_{27}N_5O_5$,HCl = 441.9.

CAS — 130636-43-0 (nifekalant); 130656-51-8 (nifekalant hydrochloride).

Profile

Nifekalant is a class III antiarrhythmic (p.787) used intravenously as the hydrochloride in the management of life-threatening ventricular arrhythmias (p.794). The usual dose is 300 µg per kg body-weight by intravenous injection over 5 minutes under continuous ECG monitoring; this may be followed by a maintenance dose of 400 µg per kg per hour by intravenous infusion if required, under ECG monitoring.

Preparations

Proprietary Preparations (details are given in Part 3)
Jpn: Shinbit.

Nilvadipine (2192-p)

Nilvadipine (USAN, rINN).

CL-287389; FK-235; Nivadipine; SKF-102362. 5-Isopropyl 3-methyl 2-cyano-1,4-dihydro-6-methyl-4-(m-nitrophenyl)-3,5-pyridinedicarboxylate.

$C_{19}H_{19}N_3O_6$ = 385.4.

CAS — 75530-68-6.

ATC — C08CA10.

Profile

Nilvadipine is a dihydropyridine calcium-channel blocker with general properties similar to those of nifedipine (p.940). It is used in the management of hypertension (p.802). Nilvadipine is given by mouth as a modified-release preparation in a usual dose of up to 16 mg daily.

◊ References.

1. Takata Y, *et al.* Elevated plasma nilvadipine concentration after single and chronic oral administration to patients with chronic liver disease. *Eur J Clin Pharmacol* 1992; **42:** 475–9.

Preparations

Proprietary Preparations (details are given in Part 3)
Aust.: Arcadipin†; Tensan; *Denm.:* Escort†; *Fin.:* Escor; *Ger.:* Escor; Nivadil; *Hong Kong:* Escor; *Irl.:* Nivadil; *Jpn:* Nivadil; *Port.:* Nivadil; *Switz.:* Nivadil.

Nimodipine (16914-v)

Nimodipine (BAN, USAN, rINN).

Bay-e-9736; Nimodipinum. Isopropyl 2-methoxyethyl 1,4-dihydro-2,6-dimethyl-4-(3-nitrophenyl)pyridine-3,5-dicarboxylate.

$C_{21}H_{26}N_2O_7$ = 418.4.

CAS — 66085-59-4.

ATC — C08CA06.

Pharmacopoeias. In *Eur.* (see p.vi).

The manufacturer states that solutions of nimodipine are incompatible with some plastics, including PVC.

Pharmacopoeial description

Ph. Eur.: A light yellow or yellow crystalline powder. It exhibits polymorphism. Practically insoluble in water; sparingly soluble in dehydrated alcohol; freely soluble in ethyl acetate. Exposure to ultraviolet light leads to formation of a nitrophenylpyridine derivative. Solutions should be prepared in the dark or under light of wavelength greater than 420 nm, immediately before use. Protect from light.

Adverse Effects, Treatment, and Precautions

As for dihydropyridine calcium-channel blockers (see Nifedipine, p.940).

Nimodipine should be administered with caution to patients with cerebral oedema or severely raised intracranial pressure.

◊ Marked bradycardia developed in a patient with acute ischaemic stroke during treatment with nimodipine and was suspected to be related to the drug therapy.[1]

1. Fagan SC, Nacci N. Nimodipine and bradycardia in acute stroke—drug or disease? *DICP Ann Pharmacother* 1991; **25:** 247—9.

Interactions

As for dihydropyridine calcium-channel blockers (see Nifedipine, p.942).

Pharmacokinetics

Nimodipine is rapidly absorbed from the gastrointestinal tract following oral administration but undergoes extensive first-pass metabolism in the liver. The oral bioavailability is reported to be about 13%. Nimodipine is about 95% bound to plasma proteins. It

readily crosses the blood-brain barrier. Nimodipine is extensively metabolised in the liver. It is excreted in faeces via the bile, and in urine, almost entirely as metabolites. The terminal elimination half-life is reported to be about 9 hours but the initial decline in plasma concentrations is very much more rapid, equivalent to a half-life of 1 to 2 hours.

Uses and Administration

Nimodipine is a dihydropyridine calcium-channel blocker that has the general properties of nifedipine (p.943), but acts particularly on cerebral blood vessels. It is used in cerebrovascular disorders (see below), particularly in the prevention and treatment of ischaemic neurological deficits following aneurysmal or traumatic subarachnoid haemorrhage.

For the prophylaxis of neurological deficit following aneurysmal haemorrhage nimodipine is given by mouth in a dose of 60 mg every 4 hours. Treatment should begin within 4 days of onset of haemorrhage and should continue for 21 days. In patients with impaired hepatic function the initial dose may be halved to 30 mg every 4 hours and blood pressure should be closely monitored. If cerebral ischaemia occurs during prophylactic administration, oral therapy may be continued to complete a 21-day course or intravenous administration may be substituted as outlined below although the total duration of nimodipine use should not exceed 21 days.

If cerebral ischaemia has already occurred following either aneurysmal or traumatic haemorrhage, neurological deficit may be treated by intravenous infusion of nimodipine. It should be given via a bypass into a running intravenous infusion into a central vein. The initial dose should be nimodipine 1 mg per hour for 2 hours, increased (provided that no severe decrease in blood pressure is observed) to 2 mg per hour. The starting dose should be reduced to 0.5 mg or less per hour in patients weighing less than 70 kg, in those with unstable blood pressure, or in those with impaired hepatic function. In aneurysmal haemorrhage infusion should be started as soon as possible and continued for at least 5 and no more than 14 days. In traumatic haemorrhage infusion should be started within 12 hours of the trauma and continued for 7 to 10 days; this should then be followed by oral therapy for 11 to 14 days to complete a total of 21 days of treatment.

◊ General reviews.

1. Langley MS, Sorkin EM. Nimodipine: a review of its pharmacodynamic and pharmacokinetic properties, and therapeutic potential in cerebrovascular disease. *Drugs* 1989; **37:** 669–99.

Cerebrovascular disorders. Nimodipine is used orally and intravenously in the prevention and treatment of ischaemic neurological deficits caused by arterial vasospasm following aneurysmal[1] and traumatic[2] subarachnoid haemorrhage (see Stroke, p.813). In addition to dilating cerebral blood vessels and improving cerebral blood flow, nimodipine may also prevent or reverse ischaemic damage to the brain by limiting transcellular calcium influx.

These effects have led to the investigation of nimodipine in other conditions associated with cerebral ischaemia. Studies of nimodipine given orally following ischaemic stroke have produced conflicting results.[3,4] A meta-analysis[5] of controlled studies suggested that nimodipine is beneficial if given within 12 hours of stroke onset but a further study[6] failed to confirm these findings. In a controlled study of 155 patients suffering a cardiac arrest, nimodipine was given by intravenous infusion for 24 hours.[7] Nimodipine had no effect on overall survival, although it did improve survival of patients in whom advanced life support was delayed for more than 10 minutes after arrest. Nimodipine has also been tried in dementia (p.1412). Two multicentre studies involving a total of 755 patients with dementia of vascular or degenerative origin given nimodipine for up to 6 months reported improvements in cognitive function and disability.[8]

1. Feigin VL, *et al.* Calcium antagonists in patients with aneurysmal subarachnoid hemorrhage: a systematic review. *Neurology* 1998; **50:** 876–83.
2. Harders A, *et al.* Traumatic subarachnoid hemorrhage and its treatment with nimodipine. *J Neurosurg* 1996; **85:** 82–9.
3. Gelmers HJ, *et al.* A controlled trial of nimodipine in acute ischemic stroke. *N Engl J Med* 1988; **318:** 203–7.
4. Trust Study Group. Randomised, double-blind, placebo-controlled trial of nimodipine in acute stroke. *Lancet* 1990; **336:** 1205–9.
5. Mohr JP, *et al.* Meta-analysis of oral nimodipine trials in acute ischemic stroke. *Cerebrovasc Dis* 1994; **4:** 197–203.

6. Horn J, *et al.* Very Early Nimodipine Use in Stroke (VENUS): a randomized, double-blind, placebo-controlled trial. *Stroke* 2001; **32:** 461–5.
7. Roine RO, *et al.* Nimodipine after resuscitation from out-of-hospital ventricular fibrillation: a placebo-controlled, double-blind, randomized trial. *JAMA* 1990; **264:** 3171–7.
8. Parnetti L, *et al.* Mental deterioration in old age: results of two multicenter, clinical trials with nimodipine. *Clin Ther* 1993; **15:** 394–406.

Migraine. For reference to the use of calcium-channel blockers, including nimodipine, in the management of migraine, see under Nifedipine, p.944.

Preparations

BP 2001: Nimodipine Intravenous Infusion; Nimodipine Tablets.

Proprietary Preparations (details are given in Part 3)
Aust.: Nimotop; *Austral.:* Nimotop; *Belg.:* Nimotop; *Braz.:* Nimotop; Noodipina; Norton; Oxigen; *Canad.:* Nimotop; *Denm.:* Nimotop; *Fin.:* Nimotop; *Fr.:* Nimotop; *Ger.:* Nimotop; *Hong Kong:* Nimotop; *Irl.:* Nimotop; *Israel:* Nimotop; *Ital.:* Nimotop; Periplum; *Mex.:* Nimotop; *Neth.:* Nimotop; *Norw.:* Nimotop; *NZ:* Nimotop; *Port.:* Brainox; Modina; Nimotop; Sobrepina; Trinalion; *S.Afr.:* Nimotop; *Singapore:* Nimotop; *Spain:* Admon; Brainal; Calnit; Kenesil; Modus; Nimotop; Remontal; *Swed.:* Nimotop; *Switz.:* Nimotop; *Thai.:* Nimotop; *UK:* Nimotop; *USA:* Nimotop.

Nipradilol (19579-q)

Nipradilol (rINN).

K-351; Nipradolol. 8-[2-Hydroxy-3-(isopropylamino)propoxy]-3-chromanol 3-nitrate.

$C_{15}H_{22}N_2O_6$ = 326.3.

CAS — 81486-22-8.

Profile

Nipradilol is a beta blocker (p.844). It is also reported to have direct vasodilating activity. It is used in the management of ocular hypertension and glaucoma (p.1413); eye drops containing nipradilol 0.05% are instilled twice daily. It has been used in the management of hypertension and angina pectoris.

Preparations

Proprietary Preparations (details are given in Part 3)
Jpn: Hypadil.

Nisoldipine (13022-j)

Nisoldipine (BAN, USAN, rINN).

Bay-k-5552. Isobutyl methyl 1,4-dihydro-2,6-dimethyl-4-(2-nitrophenyl)pyridine-3,5-dicarboxylate.

$C_{20}H_{24}N_2O_6$ = 388.4.

CAS — 63675-72-9.

ATC — C08CA07.

Adverse Effects, Treatment, and Precautions

As for dihydropyridine calcium-channel blockers (see Nifedipine, p.940).

Interactions

As for dihydropyridine calcium-channel blockers (see Nifedipine, p.942).

Pharmacokinetics

Nisoldipine is well absorbed from the gastrointestinal tract after oral administration, but undergoes rapid and extensive first-pass metabolism in the gut wall and liver and bioavailability has been reported to be only about 4 to 8%. About 60 to 80% of an oral dose is excreted in the urine and the remainder in the faeces, mainly as metabolites. The terminal elimination half-life is about 7 to 12 hours. Nisoldipine is about 99% bound to plasma proteins.

◊ The results of a study[1] in 11 patients receiving nisoldipine 10 mg once or twice daily by mouth indicated that the pharmacokinetics of nisoldipine could best be described by an open 2-compartment model. Peak plasma concentrations occurred 1 hour after a single oral dose, and varied greatly between the patients. The mean plasma elimination half-life was 11.4 hours after a single dose and 14.0 hours after repeated dosing, which was longer than had been previously reported, perhaps reflecting the greater sensitivity of the assay.

In another study oral, but not intravenous, administration of nisoldipine increased liver blood flow in 10 healthy subjects and thus affected its own systemic availability.[2] Variations in liver blood flow may account for the interindividual variation in the pharmacokinetics of nisoldipine.

1. Ottosson A-M, *et al.* Analysis and pharmacokinetics of nisoldipine in hypertensive patients. *Curr Ther Res* 1989; **45:** 347–58.
2. van Harten J, *et al.* Variability in the pharmacokinetics of nisoldipine as caused by differences in liver blood flow response. *J Clin Pharmacol* 1989; **29:** 714–21.

Uses and Administration

Nisoldipine is a dihydropyridine calcium-channel blocker with actions and uses similar to those of nifedipine (p.943). It is used in the management of hypertension (p.802) and angina pectoris (p.791).

Nisoldipine is given by mouth usually as a modified-release preparation. Doses are similar for both hypertension and angina. The initial dose is 10 mg once daily and the usual maintenance dose is 20 to 40 mg once daily before food.

◊ Reviews.
1. Mitchell J, et al. Nisoldipine: a new dihydropyridine calcium-channel blocker. *J Clin Pharmacol* 1993; **33:** 46–52.
2. Plosker GL, Faulds D. Nisoldipine coat-core: a review of its pharmacology and therapeutic efficacy in hypertension. *Drugs* 1996; **52:** 232–53.
3. Langtry HD, Spencer CM. Nisoldipine coat-core; a review of its pharmacodynamic and pharmacokinetic properties and clinical efficacy in the management of ischaemic heart disease. *Drugs* 1997; **53:** 867–84.

Preparations

Proprietary Preparations (details are given in Part 3)
Aust.: Syscor; **Belg.:** Sular; Syscor; **Fin.:** Syscor; **Ger.:** Baymycard; **Ital.:** Syscor; Zadipina; **Mex.:** Sular; Syscor; **Neth.:** Sular; Syscor; **S.Afr.:** Syscor; **Spain:** Cornel; Sular; Syscor; **Swed.:** Syscor†; **Switz.:** Syscor; **UK:** Syscor; **USA:** Sular.

Nitrendipine (16915-g)

Nitrendipine (BAN, USAN, rINN).
Bay-e-5009; Nitrendipinum. Ethyl methyl 1,4-dihydro-2,6-dimethyl-4-(3-nitrophenyl)pyridine-3,5-dicarboxylate.
$C_{18}H_{20}N_2O_6 = 360.4$.
CAS — 39562-70-4.
ATC — C08CA08.
Pharmacopoeias. In *Eur.* (see p.vi).

Pharmacopoeial description

Ph. Eur.: A yellow crystalline powder. It exhibits polymorphism. Practically insoluble in water; sparingly soluble in dehydrated alcohol and in methyl alcohol; freely soluble in ethyl acetate. Exposure to ultraviolet light leads to formation of a nitrophenylpyridine derivative. Solutions should be prepared in the dark or under light of wavelength greater than 420 nm, immediately before use. Protect from light.

Adverse Effects, Treatment, and Precautions

As for dihydropyridine calcium-channel blockers (see Nifedipine, p.940).

Interactions

As for dihydropyridine calcium-channel blockers (see Nifedipine, p.942).

Pharmacokinetics

Nitrendipine is reported to be well absorbed following oral administration but undergoes extensive first-pass metabolism; the absolute oral bioavailability is reported to range from about 10 to 20%, depending in part on the dosage form. Nitrendipine is about 98% bound to plasma proteins. It is extensively metabolised in the liver and is excreted as metabolites, mainly in urine, with small amounts in the faeces. Although early studies reported a terminal elimination half-life of about 2 to 4 hours, later studies, using more sensitive assay procedures, have recorded values between about 10 and 22 hours.

◊ References.
1. Soons PA, Breimer DD. Stereoselective pharmacokinetics of oral and intravenous nitrendipine in healthy male subjects. *Br J Clin Pharmacol* 1991; **32:** 11–16.

Uses and Administration

Nitrendipine is a dihydropyridine calcium-channel blocker with actions similar to those of nifedipine (p.943). It is used in the treatment of hypertension (p.802).

The usual dose is 20 mg daily as a single dose by mouth or as 2 divided doses. The dose may be increased to 20 mg twice daily if necessary for the control of resistant hypertension. In the elderly, and in patients with liver disease, an initial dose of 10 mg daily should be used.

◊ Reviews.
1. Goa KL, Sorkin EM. Nitrendipine: a review of its pharmacodynamic and pharmacokinetic properties, and therapeutic efficacy in the treatment of hypertension. *Drugs* 1987; **33:** 123–55.
2. Santiago TM, Lopez LM. Nitrendipine: a new dihydropyridine calcium-channel antagonist for the treatment of hypertension. *DICP Ann Pharmacother* 1990; **24:** 167–75.

Preparations

Proprietary Preparations (details are given in Part 3)
Aust.: Baypress; **Belg.:** Baypress; **Braz.:** Caltren; Nitrencord; Nitrenpress; **Denm.:** Baypress; **Fr.:** Baypress; Nidrel; **Ger.:** Bayotensin; Nitre-Puren; Nitregamma; Nitren Lich; Nitrendepat; Nitrendimerck; Nitrensal; Nitrepress; **Hong Kong:** Baypress; **Ital.:** Baypress; Deiten; **Mex.:** Baypress; **Neth.:** Baypress; **Port.:** Farnitran; Hiperdipina; Hipertenol; **Spain:** Balminil; Baypresol; Gericin; Monopress†; Niprina; Sub Tensin; Tensogradal; Trendinol; Vastensium; **Switz.:** Baypress; **Thai.:** Baypress; Ditrenil; Miniten.

Nitric Oxide (15530-b)

Nitric Oxide (USAN).
Mononitrogen Monoxide; Nitrogen Monoxide; Nitrogenii Oxidum; OHM-11771.
NO = 30.01.
CAS — 10102-43-9.
Pharmacopoeias. In *Eur.* (see p.vi).

Pharmacopoeial description

Ph. Eur.: A colourless gas which turns brown when exposed to air. At 20° and at a pressure of 101 kPa, 1 volume dissolves in about 21 volumes of water. Store compressed at a pressure not exceeding 2.5 MPa measured at 15° in suitable containers.

Adverse Effects

Inhaled nitric oxide may lead to the development of methaemoglobinaemia, particularly at higher doses. Although it is a selective pulmonary vasodilator, systemic hypotension may occur. Abrupt withdrawal of therapy may lead to a deterioration in oxygenation and the development of rebound pulmonary hypertension.

Nitrogen dioxide produced when nitric oxide combines with oxygen can cause acute lung injury; high concentrations of inhaled nitric oxide are directly irritant to the lungs.

◊ A potential complication of inhaled nitric oxide is methaemoglobinaemia but this is probably related to the dose and the risk does not appear to be increased during low-dose (20 ppm) therapy.[1] Another possible adverse event is an increased risk of bleeding due to inhibition of platelet aggregation by nitric oxide.[2-5] Rebound pulmonary hypertension[6] and deterioration in oxygenation[7,8] have been reported in some children following withdrawal of nitric oxide therapy. Severe systemic hypotension has also been reported[9] following initiation of inhaled nitric oxide therapy in a neonate with severe left ventricular dysfunction. Motor neurone disease in a patient with alcoholism has been partly attributed[10] to the use of nitric oxide for pulmonary hypertension.

1. Kinsella JP, Abman SH. Methaemoglobin during nitric oxide therapy with high-frequency ventilation. *Lancet* 1993; **342:** 615.
2. Högman M, et al. Bleeding time prolongation and NO inhalation. *Lancet* 1993; **341:** 1664–5.
3. Joannidis M, et al. Inhaled nitric oxide. *Lancet* 1996; **348:** 1448–9.
4. Cheung P-Y, et al. Inhaled nitric oxide and inhibition of platelet aggregation in critically ill neonates. *Lancet* 1998; **351:** 1181–2.
5. George TN, et al. The effect of inhaled nitric oxide therapy on bleeding time and platelet aggregation in neonates. *J Pediatr* 1998; **132:** 731–4.
6. Miller OI, et al. Rebound pulmonary hypertension on withdrawal from inhaled nitric oxide. *Lancet* 1995; **346:** 51–2.
7. Aly H, et al. Weaning strategy with inhaled nitric oxide therapy in persistent pulmonary hypertension of the newborn. *Arch Dis Child* 1997; **76:** F118–F122.
8. Davidson D, et al. Safety of withdrawing inhaled nitric oxide therapy in persistent pulmonary hypertension of the newborn. *Pediatrics* 1999; **104:** 231–6.
9. Henrichsen T, et al. Inhaled nitric oxide can cause severe systemic hypotension. *J Pediatr* 1996; **129:** 183.
10. Tsai GE, Gastfriend DR. Nitric oxide-induced motor neuron disease in a patient with alcoholism. *N Engl J Med* 1995; **332:** 1036.

Precautions

Patients receiving inhaled nitric should be monitored for methaemoglobinaemia and oxygenation. Inspired nitric oxide and nitrogen dioxide levels should also be monitored. Treatment should not be discontinued abruptly since rebound pulmonary hypertension and deterioration in oxygenation may occur. Consideration should be given to limiting the exposure of healthcare workers to nitric oxide and nitrogen dioxide.

◊ References.
1. Committee on Safety of Medicines/Medicines Control Agency. Inhaled nitric oxide. *Current Problems* 1996; **22:** 8.
2. Cuthbertson BH, et al. Use of inhaled nitric oxide in British intensive therapy units. *Br J Anaesth* 1997; **78:** 696–700.
3. Phillips ML, et al. Assessment of medical personnel exposure to nitrogen oxides during inhaled nitric oxide treatment of neonatal and pediatric patients. *Pediatrics* 1999; **104:** 1095–1100.

Pharmacokinetics

Nitric oxide is absorbed systemically after inhalation but is rapidly inactivated by reaction with haemoglobin to form methaemoglobin and nitrate; it has a half-life of only a few seconds. It is excreted predominantly in the urine as nitrate.

Uses and Administration

Nitric oxide is an endogenous chemical messenger that acts predominantly by stimulating guanylate cyclase in smooth muscle to cause vasodilatation. It is also involved in platelet aggregation, neurotransmission, and the immune system, and possesses antimicrobial, antitumour, and antiviral activity.

Endogenous nitric oxide is synthesised from L-arginine and is now recognised to be the same substance as endothelium-derived relaxing factor (EDRF). Synthesis from L-arginine is by the enzyme, nitric oxide synthase. Three isoforms of this enzyme have been identified. Constitutive isoforms occur in endothelial cells (such as in vascular endothelium, platelets, and the heart) and neuronal cells (in some central and peripheral neurones). Small amounts of nitric oxide are regularly produced by these systems. In contrast, an inducible nitric oxide synthase isoform is expressed only after activation by external stimuli such as in infection or inflammation and larger amounts of nitric oxide are produced. This inducible nitric oxide synthase may be expressed in a wide range of cells, including macrophages and cells in vascular smooth muscle, the heart, gastrointestinal tract, and liver.

Inhaled nitric oxide is a highly selective pulmonary vasodilator. It is used in the management of term and near-term neonates with hypoxic respiratory failure associated with pulmonary hypertension. It is also being studied in a variety of other bronchopulmonary disorders and in different age groups.

In the management of hypoxic respiratory failure in neonates, nitric oxide is given by inhalation in a usual concentration of 20 ppm. Doses have been titrated above and below this concentration but due to the risk of methaemoglobinaemia, doses above 20 ppm are not generally recommended. The concentration should be reduced gradually before discontinuing nitric oxide treatment.

◊ General reviews.
1. Änggård E. Nitric oxide: mediator, murderer, and medicine. *Lancet* 1994; **343:** 1199–1206.
2. Holden K. Nitric oxide—from exhaust fumes to medical revolution. *Pharm J* 1994; **252:** 402–7.
3. Lowenstein CJ, et al. Nitric oxide: a physiologic messenger. *Ann Intern Med* 1994; **120:** 227–37.
4. Vallance P, Collier J. Biology and clinical relevance of nitric oxide. *BMJ* 1994; **309:** 453–7.
5. Edwards AD. The pharmacology of inhaled nitric oxide. *Arch Dis Child* 1995; **72:** F127–F130.
6. Lunn RJ. Inhaled nitric oxide therapy. *Mayo Clin Proc* 1995; **70:** 247–55.
7. Quinn AC, et al. Nitric oxide: an endogenous gas. *Br J Anaesth* 1995; **74:** 443–51.
8. Zoritch B. Nitric oxide and asthma. *Arch Dis Child* 1995; **72:** 259–62.
9. Loscalzo J. Nitric oxide and vascular disease. *N Engl J Med* 1995; **333:** 251–3.
10. Brett SJ, Evans TW. Nitric oxide: physiological roles and therapeutic implications in the lung. *Br J Hosp Med* 1996; **55:** 487–90.
11. Finer N. Inhaled nitric oxide in neonates. *Arch Dis Child* 1997; **77:** F81–F84.
12. American Academy of Pediatrics Committee on Fetus and Newborn. Use of inhaled nitric oxide. *Pediatrics* 2000; **106:** 344–5.
13. Vallance P, Chan N. Endothelial function and nitric oxide: clinical relevance. *Heart* 2001; **85:** 342–50.

◊ Inhaled nitric oxide is a potent and highly selective pulmonary vasodilator used in the management of persistent pulmonary hypertension of the newborn (below) and other conditions leading to hypoxic respiratory failure in neonates.

Nitric oxide is also under investigation in children and adults with acute respiratory distress syndrome (below), respiratory failure,[1] acute severe asthma,[2] primary pulmonary hypertension,[3,4] and in pulmonary hypertension associated with a wide range of conditions including heart failure,[5] post-cardiac surgery,[6,7] and high-altitude disorders.[8]

1. Dobyns EL, et al. Multicenter randomized controlled trial of the effects of inhaled nitric oxide therapy on gas exchange in children with acute hypoxemic respiratory failure. *J Pediatr* 1999; **134:** 406–12.
2. Nakagawa TA, et al. Life-threatening status asthmaticus treated with inhaled nitric oxide. *J Pediatr* 1999; **137:** 119–22.
3. Kinsella JP, et al. Selective and sustained pulmonary vasodilation with inhalational nitric oxide therapy in a child with idiopathic pulmonary hypertension. *J Pediatr* 1993; **122:** 803–6.
4. Goldman AP, et al. Is it time to consider domiciliary nitric oxide? *Lancet* 1995; **345:** 199–200.
5. Matsumoto A, et al. Inhaled nitric oxide and exercise capacity in congestive heart failure. *Lancet* 1997; **349:** 999–1000. Correction. *ibid.*; **350:** 818.
6. Haydar A, et al. Inhaled nitric oxide for postoperative pulmonary hypertension in patients with congenital heart defects. *Lancet* 1992; **340:** 1545.
7. Miller OI, et al. Inhaled nitric oxide and prevention of pulmonary hypertension after congenital heart surgery: a randomised double-blind study. *Lancet* 2000; **356:** 1464–9.
8. Scherrer U, et al. Inhaled nitric oxide for high-altitude pulmonary edema. *N Engl J Med* 1996; **334:** 624–9.

Acute respiratory distress syndrome. Although inhalation of nitric oxide has been reported[1,2] to improve oxygenation in patients with acute respiratory distress syndrome (p.1046), a small randomised trial[3] and a multicentre study[2] have reported no effect on mortality; other studies have shown that response to nitric oxide therapy is very variable. Further studies are underway to confirm the benefits of nitric oxide in patients with the acute respiratory distress syndrome.[4] Various dosage regimens have been studied[5,6] in children but results have been inconsistent. Simultaneous intravenous administration of almitrine, a pulmonary vasoconstrictor, has been reported to increase arterial oxygenation more than nitric oxide alone.[7]

1. Rossaint R, et al. Inhaled nitric oxide for the adult respiratory distress syndrome. N Engl J Med 1993; **328:** 399–405.
2. Dellinger RP, et al. Effects of inhaled nitric oxide in patients with acute respiratory distress syndrome: results of a randomized phase II trial. Crit Care Med 1998; **26:** 15–23.
3. Troncy E, et al. Should we treat acute respiratory distress syndrome with inhaled nitric oxide? Lancet 1997; **350:** 111–12.
4. Young JD. The use of inhaled nitric oxide in the acute respiratory distress syndrome. Br J Hosp Med 1997; **57:** 126–7.
5. Nakagawa TA, et al. Dose response to inhaled nitric oxide in pediatric patients with pulmonary hypertension and acute respiratory distress syndrome. J Pediatr 1997; **131:** 63–9.
6. Tang SF, et al. Randomised trial of three doses of inhaled nitric oxide in acute respiratory distress syndrome. Arch Dis Child 1998; **79:** 415–18.
7. Wysocki M, et al. Additive effect on gas exchange of inhaled nitric oxide and intravenous almitrine bismesylate in the adult respiratory distress syndrome. Intensive Care Med 1994; **20:** 254–9.

Respiratory disorders in neonates. Inhaled nitric oxide may have a role[1-3] in the management of persistent pulmonary hypertension of the newborn (p.810) and other disorders associated with hypoxic respiratory failure in neonates. Studies have shown marked improvement in oxygenation[4,5] although one study suggested this may not be sustained.[6] Multicentre controlled studies[7-9] have found that inhaled nitric oxide reduces the use of extracorporeal membrane oxygenation but have not shown any effect on mortality. Some neonates may not respond to nitric oxide therapy; one study found that neonates with pulmonary hypoplasia and dysplasia may have decreased sensitivity to nitric oxide.[6] Another study reported that some neonates who failed to respond to nitric oxide were successfully treated with a combination of nitric oxide and high-frequency oscillatory ventilation.[10] No benefit was found with inhaled nitric oxide in neonates with hypoxic respiratory failure associated with congenital diaphragmatic hernia.[9,11] There have been concerns that use of inhaled nitric oxide might adversely affect neurodevelopmental outcome more than conventional therapy, but this has not been confirmed in infants followed up for up to 2 years.[12,13]

Inhaled nitric oxide has also been reported to improve oxygenation in premature neonates with hypoxic respiratory failure[14,15] or respiratory distress syndrome.[16,17] However, no improvement in mortality has been shown and one study[18] has reported poor neurodevelopmental outcome in premature neonates who received nitric oxide treatment.

1. Kinsella JP, Abman SH. Recent developments in the pathophysiology and treatment of persistent pulmonary hypertension of the newborn. J Pediatr 1995; **126:** 853–64.
2. Mupanemunda RH, Edwards AD. Treatment of newborn infants with inhaled nitric oxide. Arch Dis Child 1995; **72:** F131–F134.
3. Kinsella JP, Abman SH. Clinical approach to inhaled nitric oxide therapy in the newborn with hypoxemia. J Pediatr 2000; **136:** 717–26.
4. Davidson D, et al. Inhaled nitric oxide for the early treatment of persistent pulmonary hypertension of the term newborn: a randomized, double-masked, placebo-controlled, dose-response, multicenter study. Pediatrics 1998; **101:** 325–34.
5. Wessel DL, et al. Improved oxygenation in a randomized trial of inhaled nitric oxide for persistent pulmonary hypertension of the newborn. Abstract: Pediatrics 1997; **100:** 888. Full version: http://www.pediatrics.org/cgi/content/full/100/5/e7
6. Goldman AP, et al. Four patterns of response to inhaled nitric oxide for persistent pulmonary hypertension of the newborn. Pediatrics 1996; **98:** 706–13.
7. The Neonatal Inhaled Nitric Oxide Study Group. Inhaled nitric oxide in full-term and nearly full-term infants with hypoxic respiratory failure. N Engl J Med 1997; **336:** 597–604. Correction. ibid.; **337:** 434.
8. Roberts JD, et al. Inhaled nitric oxide and persistent pulmonary hypertension of the newborn. N Engl J Med 1997; **336:** 605–10.
9. Clark RH, et al. Low-dose nitric oxide therapy for persistent pulmonary hypertension of the newborn. N Engl J Med 2000; **342:** 469–74.
10. Kinsella JP, et al. Randomized, multicenter trial of inhaled nitric oxide and high-frequency oscillatory ventilation in severe, persistent pulmonary hypertension of the newborn. J Pediatr 1997; **131:** 55–62.
11. The Neonatal Inhaled Nitric Oxide Study Group. Inhaled nitric oxide and hypoxic respiratory failure in infants with congenital diaphragmatic hernia. Pediatrics 1997; **99:** 838–45.
12. Rosenberg AA, et al. Longitudinal follow-up of a cohort of newborn infants treated with inhaled nitric oxide for persistent pulmonary hypertension. J Pediatr 1997; **131:** 70–5.
13. The Neonatal Inhaled Nitric Oxide Study Group. Inhaled nitric oxide in term and near-term infants: neurodevelopmental follow-up of the Neonatal Inhaled Nitric Oxide Study Group (NINOS). J Pediatr 2000; **136:** 611–17.
14. Kinsella JP, et al. Inhaled nitric oxide in premature neonates with severe hypoxaemic respiratory failure: a randomised controlled trial. Lancet 1999; **354:** 1061–5.
15. The Franco-Belgium Collaborative NO Trial Group. Early compared with delayed inhaled nitric oxide in moderately hypoxaemic neonates with respiratory failure: a randomised controlled trial. Lancet 1999; **354:** 1066–71.
16. Peliowski A, et al. Inhaled nitric oxide for premature infants after prolonged rupture of the membranes. J Pediatr 1995; **126:** 450–3.
17. Skimming JW, et al. Nitric oxide inhalation in infants with respiratory distress syndrome. J Pediatr 1997; **130:** 225–30.
18. Cheung P-Y, et al. The outcome of very low birth weight neonates (≤1500g) rescued by inhaled nitric oxide: neurodevelopment in early childhood. J Pediatr 1998; **133:** 735–9.

Preparations

Proprietary Preparations (details are given in Part 3)
USA: INOmax.

Noradrenaline (9506-x)

Noradrenaline (BAN).
Norepinephrine (BAN, rINN); Norepirenamine. (R)-2-Amino-1-(3,4-dihydroxyphenyl)ethanol.
$C_8H_{11}NO_3 = 169.2$.
CAS — 51-41-2.
ATC — C01CA03.
Pharmacopoeias. Jpn includes the racemic form.

Noradrenaline Acid Tartrate (2087-q)

Noradrenaline Acid Tartrate (BANM).
Norepinephrine Bitartrate (USAN, rINNM); Arterenol Acid Tartrate; l-Arterenol Bitartrate; Levarterenol Acid Tartrate; Levarterenol Bitartrate; Levarterenoli Bitartras; Noradrenaline Bitartrate; Noradrenaline Tartrate; Noradrenalini Tartras; Norepinephrine Acid Tartrate (BANM); l-Norepinephrine Bitartrate.
$C_8H_{11}NO_3, C_4H_6O_6, H_2O = 337.3$.
CAS — 51-40-1 (anhydrous noradrenaline [norepinephrine] acid tartrate); 69815-49-2 (noradrenaline [norepinephrine] acid tartrate monohydrate).
Pharmacopoeias. In Chin., Eur. (see p.vi), Pol., and US.

Noradrenaline [norepinephrine] acid tartrate 2 μg is approximately equivalent to 1 μg of noradrenaline [norepinephrine].

Pharmacopoeial description

Ph. Eur.: A white or almost white, odourless, crystalline powder. Freely soluble in water; slightly soluble in alcohol; practically insoluble in ether. Store in airtight containers, or preferably, in a sealed tube under vacuum or an inert gas. Protect from light.

USP 25: A white or faintly grey, odourless, crystalline powder. It slowly darkens on exposure to air and light. Soluble 1 in 2.5 of water and 1 in 300 of alcohol; practically insoluble in chloroform and in ether. Its solutions in water have a pH of about 3.5. Store in airtight containers. Protect from light.

Incompatibility. Noradrenaline [norepinephrine] acid tartrate is strongly acidic in solution, and would be expected to be incompatible with drugs having an alkaline pH. The manufacturers in the UK state that solutions are reportedly incompatible with alkalis and oxidising agents, barbiturates, chlorpheniramine [chlorphenamine], chlorothiazide, nitrofurantoin, novobiocin, phenytoin, sodium bicarbonate, sodium iodide, and streptomycin. Incompatibility with insulin has also been reported.[1]

1. Yamashita SK, et al. Compatibility of selected critical care drugs during simulated Y-site administration. Am J Health-Syst Pharm 1996; **53:** 1048–51.

Noradrenaline Hydrochloride (9505-t)

Noradrenaline Hydrochloride (BANM).
Norepinephrine Hydrochloride (BANM, rINNM); Noradrenalini Hydrochloridum.
$C_8H_{11}NO_3, HCl = 205.6$.
CAS — 329-56-6.
Pharmacopoeias. In Eur. (see p.vi).

Noradrenaline [norepinephrine] hydrochloride 1.2 μg is approximately equivalent to 1 μg of noradrenaline [norepinephrine].

Pharmacopoeial description

Ph. Eur.: A white or brownish-white, crystalline powder. It becomes coloured on exposure to air and light. Very soluble in water; slightly soluble in alcohol. A 2% solution in water has a pH of 3.5 to 4.5. Store in airtight containers, or preferably, in a sealed tube under vacuum or an inert gas. Protect from light.

Adverse Effects

Noradrenaline [norepinephrine] is an extremely potent peripheral vasoconstrictor and hypertension (possibly associated with reflex bradycardia), headache, and peripheral ischaemia, which may be severe enough to result in gangrene of the extremities, are among the potential adverse effects.

Noradrenaline [norepinephrine] is a severe tissue irritant and only very dilute solutions should be injected. The needle must be inserted well into the vein to avoid extravasation, otherwise severe phlebitis and sloughing may occur.

For the adverse effects of sympathomimetics in general, see Adrenaline, p.829.

◊ Severe headache, once with fatal cerebral haemorrhage, had been reported in dental patients who had received injections of lignocaine [lidocaine] 2% with noradrenaline [norepinephrine] 1 in 25 000. It was suggested that a concentration of noradrenaline [norepinephrine] 1 in 25 000 was too high and could not be justified and that a concentration of 1 in 80 000 was to be preferred.[1] However, authorities in the UK now consider that noradrenaline [norepinephrine] should not be used as a vasoconstrictor in local anaesthetic solutions since it presents no advantages over adrenaline [epinephrine] and carries additional hazard.

1. Boakes AJ, et al. Adverse reactions to local anaesthetic/vasoconstrictor preparations: a study of the cardiovascular responses to Xylestesin and Hostacain-with-Noradrenaline. Br Dent J 1972; **133:** 137–40.

Treatment of Adverse Effects

The hypertensive effects of noradrenaline [norepinephrine] may be treated with an alpha blocker such as phentolamine. If extravasation occurs, infiltration with phentolamine (see p.955) as soon as possible, and certainly within 12 hours, may relieve pain and prevent tissue necrosis.

Precautions

Noradrenaline [norepinephrine] must be avoided in the presence of hypertension and blood pressure and infusion rate must be monitored frequently. Noradrenaline [norepinephrine]-induced cardiac arrhythmias are more likely in patients with hypoxia or hypercapnia. Hypovolaemia should be corrected before starting noradrenaline [norepinephrine] infusion.

Noradrenaline [norepinephrine] may reduce placental perfusion throughout pregnancy and some consider that it and similar vasoconstrictor sympathomimetics are best avoided; also in late pregnancy noradrenaline [norepinephrine] provokes uterine contractions which can result in fetal asphyxia.

For the precautions to be observed with sympathomimetics in general, see Adrenaline, p.830.

Interactions

For the interactions of the sympathomimetics in general, see Adrenaline, p.830.

Pharmacokinetics

Like adrenaline [epinephrine] (p.831), noradrenaline [norepinephrine] is inactive when given by mouth, and it is rapidly inactivated in the body by similar processes. When given intravenously it is extensively metabolised and only small amounts are excreted unchanged in the urine of healthy subjects.

Uses and Administration

The catecholamine, noradrenaline, is a direct-acting sympathomimetic (see Adrenaline, p.831) with pronounced effects on alpha-adrenergic receptors and less marked effects on beta-adrenergic receptors. It is a neurotransmitter, stored in granules in nerve axons, which is released at the terminations of post ganglionic adrenergic nerve fibres when they are stimulated; some is also present in the adrenal medulla from which it is liberated together with adrenaline. A major effect of noradrenaline is to raise systolic and diastolic blood pressure (which is accompanied by reflex slowing of the heart rate). This is a result of its alpha-stimulant effects which cause vasoconstriction, with reduced blood flow in the kidneys, liver, skin, and usually skeletal muscle. The pregnant uterus also contracts; high doses liberate glucose from the liver and have other hormonal effects similar to those of adrenaline. There is little stimulation of the CNS. Beta-stimulant effects of noradrenaline have a positive inotropic action on the heart, but there is little bronchodilator effect.

Noradrenaline [norepinephrine] is used for the emergency restoration of blood pressure in acute hypotensive states such as shock (p.813). It has been used in local anaesthesia to diminish the absorption and localise the effect of the local anaesthetic (p.1304) but adrenaline [epinephrine] is now preferred (see also under Adverse Effects, above). Locally applied solutions have been used to control bleeding in upper gastrointestinal haemorrhage and similar disorders.

In **acute hypotensive states**, noradrenaline [norepinephrine] is administered as the acid tartrate by intravenous infusion of a solution containing the equivalent of 4 µg of the base per mL in glucose 5%, or sodium chloride 0.9% and glucose 5%. To avoid tissue necrosis the infusion should be given through a central venous catheter or into a large vein high up in a limb, preferably the arm. Some sources have suggested that addition of phentolamine 5 to 10 mg per litre to the infusion may prevent sloughing, should extravasation occur, without affecting the vasopressor action. The infusion is usually given initially at a rate of 2 to 3 mL per minute (8 to 12 µg per minute) and adjusted according to the blood pressure response. Blood pressure is initially recorded every 2 minutes and the rate of infusion continuously monitored. The infusion must not be stopped suddenly but should be gradually withdrawn to avoid disastrous falls in blood pressure. The average maintenance dose is 0.5 to 1 mL per minute (2 to 4 µg per minute), but there is a wide variation and higher doses may be required. The concentration of the infusion may be altered according to clinical needs. Alternatively a solution containing the equivalent of 40 µg of the base per mL may be given at an initial rate of 0.16 to 0.33 mL per minute via a central venous catheter, using a syringe pump or drip counter. Noradrenaline [norepinephrine] may also be given parenterally as the hydrochloride in the management of hypotensive states.

Similar doses may be given to restore blood pressure following **cardiac arrest**. In patients with cardiac standstill, a more concentrated solution of the acid tartrate equivalent to 100 µg of the base per mL can be given by rapid intravenous or intracardiac injection; a dose of 0.5 to 0.75 mL (50 to 75 µg of noradrenaline [norepinephrine]) has been suggested which may be repeated if necessary.

Preparations

BP 2001: Noradrenaline Injection;
USP 25: Norepinephrine Bitartrate Injection; Propoxycaine and Procaine Hydrochlorides and Norepinephrine Bitartrate Injection.

Proprietary Preparations (details are given in Part 3)
Austral.: Levophed; *Belg.:* Levophed; *Canad.:* Levophed; *Ger.:* Arterenol; *Hong Kong:* Levophed; *Irl.:* Levophed; *Israel:* Levophed; *Mex.:* Naprina; Pridam; *NZ:* Levophed; *Singapore:* Levophed; *Spain:* Adrenor†; *UK:* Levophed; *USA:* Levophed.

Used as an adjunct in: *Aust.:* Neo-Xylestesin forte and Neo-Xylestesin special; Scandonest; *Austral.:* Nurocain with Sympathin; *Braz.:* Xylocaina; *Ger.:* Anaesthol†; Meaverin "N" mit Noradrenaline†; Neo-Lidocaton†; Nor-Anaesthol†; Xylestesin-S; Xylestesin, Xylestesin-F; *Ital.:* Lident Andrenor; Xylonor; *Port.:* Xiloniba; *S.Afr.:* Scandonest; Xylotox; *Spain:* Llorentecaina Noradrenal; Stoma Anestesia Dental; Xylonor Especial; *Switz.:* Scandonest; Xylestesin-F; Xylestesin-S "special"; Xylonor†; *Thai.:* Neo-Lidocaton; *USA:* Ravocaine and Novocain†.

Norfenefrine Hydrochloride (2089-s)

Norfenefrine Hydrochloride *(rINNM)*.

Norphenylephrine Hydrochloride; *m*-Norsynephrine Hydrochloride; WV-569. 2-Amino-1-(3-hydroxyphenyl)ethanol hydrochloride.
$C_8H_{11}NO_2,HCl = 189.6$.
CAS — 536-21-0 (norfenefrine); 15308-34-6 (norfenefrine hydrochloride).

NOTE. *m*-Octopamine has been used as a synonym for norfenefrine. Care should be taken to avoid confusion between the 2 compounds.

Profile
Norfenefrine is a sympathomimetic (see Adrenaline, p.829) with predominantly alpha-adrenergic activity. It is used as the hydrochloride for its vasopressor effect in the treatment of hypotensive states (p.805). The usual dose is 15 mg three times daily by mouth, as a controlled-release preparation, but doses of up to 45 mg three times daily have been given. Norfenefrine hydrochloride has also been given by injection.

Preparations

Proprietary Preparations (details are given in Part 3)
Aust.: Novadral; *Ger.:* Energona; Novadral; *Mex.:* AS Cor; *Switz.:* Novadral.

Multi-ingredient: *Ger.:* Adyston; Normotin-R; Ordinal Forte; *Switz.:* Ortho-Maren retard.

Octodrine (6344-k)

Octodrine *(USAN, rINN)*.
SKF-51. 1,5-Dimethylhexylamine.
$C_8H_{19}N = 129.2$.
CAS — 543-82-8.

Profile
Octodrine is a sympathomimetic (see Adrenaline, p.829) with predominantly alpha-adrenergic activity. It is given by mouth as the camsilate, in combination with norfenefrine (p.949), in the treatment of hypotensive states. Octodrine phosphate has been used as an ingredient of preparations for obstructive airways disease.

Preparations

Proprietary Preparations (details are given in Part 3)
Multi-ingredient: *Aust.:* Ambredin; *Ger.:* Ordinal Forte.

Octopamine (2090-h)

Octopamine *(rINN)*.

β,4-Dihydroxyphenethylamine; *p*-Hydroxymandelamine; ND-50; Noroxedrine; *p*-Norsynephrine. 2-Amino-1-(4-hydroxyphenyl)ethanol.
$C_8H_{11}NO_2 = 153.2$.
CAS — 104-14-3.
ATC — C01CA18.

NOTE. *m*-Octopamine has been used as a synonym for norfenefrine. Care should be taken to avoid confusion between the 2 compounds.

Profile
Octopamine is a sympathomimetic (see Adrenaline, p.829) with predominantly alpha-adrenergic activity. It has been given by mouth as the hydrochloride or the tartrate in the treatment of hypotensive states.

Olprinone Hydrochloride (20337-h)

Olprinone Hydrochloride *(rINNM)*.

1,2-Dihydro-5-imidazo[1,2-*a*]pyridin-6-yl-6-methyl-2-oxonicotinonitrile hydrochloride.
$C_{14}H_{10}N_4O,HCl = 286.7$.
CAS — 106730-54-5 (olprinone); 119615-63-3 (olprinone hydrochloride).

Profile
Olprinone is a phosphodiesterase inhibitor used as a cardiac inotrope in acute heart failure (p.798). It is administered intravenously as the hydrochloride in an initial dose of 10 µg per kg body-weight given over 5 minutes, followed by a continuous infusion at a rate of 0.1 to 0.4 µg per kg per minute, according to response.

Preparations

Proprietary Preparations (details are given in Part 3)
Jpn: Coretec.

Omapatrilat (19905-v)

Omapatrilat *(BAN, USAN, rINN)*.

BMS-186716; BMS-186716-01. (4S,7S,10aS)-Octahydro-4-[(S)-α-mercaptohydrocinnamamido]-5-oxo-7H-pyrido[2,1-b][1,3]thiazepine-7-carboxylic acid.
$C_{19}H_{24}N_2O_4S_2 = 408.5$.
CAS — 167305-00-2.

Profile
Omapatrilat is a vasopeptidase inhibitor. It inhibits both angiotensin-converting enzyme and neutral endopeptidase and is under investigation in the management of hypertension and heart failure. However, it has been associated with severe angioedema which may limit its use.

◊ References.
1. Messerli FH, Nussberger J. Vasopeptidase inhibition and angioedema. *Lancet* 2000; **356:** 608–9.
2. Rouleau JL, *et al.* Comparison of vasopeptidase inhibitor, omapatrilat, and lisinopril on exercise tolerance and morbidity in patients with heart failure: IMPRESS randomised trial. *Lancet* 2000; **356:** 615–20. Correction. *ibid.*; 1774.

Omega-3 Triglycerides (3897-m)

ATC — C10AX06.

Docosahexaenoic Acid (16610-l)

DHA. Docosahexa-4,7,10,13,16,19-enoic acid.
$C_{22}H_{32}O_2 = 328.5$.

NOTE. DHA is also used as a synonym for dihydroxyacetone.

Eicosapentaenoic Acid (12685-f)

EPA. Eicosapenta-5,8,11,14,17-enoic acid.
$C_{20}H_{30}O_2 = 302.5$.
CAS — 25378-27-2.

NOTE. EPA is also used as a synonym for pheneturide.

Omega-3 Marine Triglycerides (3899-v)

Omega-3 Marine Triglycerides *(BAN)*.
Pharmacopoeias. In Eur. (see p.vi).

Pharmacopoeial description
Ph. Eur.: A mixture of mono-, di-, and triesters of omega-3 acids with glycerol containing mainly triesters. They are obtained by esterification of concentrated and purified omega-3 acids with glycerol or by transesterification of the omega-3 acid ethyl esters with glycerol. The omega-3 acids are from the body oil of fatty fish species coming from families such as Engraulidae, Carangidae, Clupeidae, Osmeridae, Salmonidae, and Scrombroidae. The acids consist of alpha-linolenic acid, moroctic acid, eicosatetraenoic acid, eicosapentaenoic acid (timnodonic acid), heneicosapentaenoic acid, clupanodonic acid, and docosahexaenoic acid (cervonic acid). The total amount of omega-3 acids expressed as triglycerides is not less than 60% and that of both eicosapentaenoic acid and docosahexaenoic acid together, expressed as triglycerides, is not less than 45%. Tocopherol may be added as an antioxidant.
A pale yellow liquid. Practically insoluble in water; slightly soluble in dehydrated alcohol; very soluble in acetone and in heptane. Store in well-filled, airtight containers under inert gas. Protect from light.

Adverse Effects and Precautions
Omega-3 marine triglycerides and similar preparations may cause nausea and eructation, particularly at higher doses. Some preparations may also contain significant amounts of vitamins A and D and long-term use can cause toxicity. There is also a theoretical possibility of vitamin E deficiency with long-term use. Some concern has been expressed over the high calorific value and cholesterol content of some preparations.

Omega-3 triglycerides have antithrombotic activity and should be given with caution to patients with haemorrhagic disorders or to those receiving anticoagulants or other drugs affecting coagulation. They should also be used with caution in asthmatic patients sensitive to aspirin.

◊ Fever, myalgia, sore throat, and tender lymphadenopathy lasting for 3 weeks were associated with omega-3 triglycerides in a 68-year-old woman.[1] Symptoms recurred within 48 hours of restarting administration.
1. Ogden P, *et al.* Reactive lymphoid hyperplasia after omega-3 fatty acid supplementation. *Ann Intern Med* 1988; **109:** 843–4.

Effects on the blood. Epistaxis was associated with omega-3 marine triglyceride treatment in 8 of 11 patients.[1] Prolonged bleeding time was noted in 3 patients.
1. Clarke JTR, *et al.* Increased incidence of epistaxis in adolescents with familial hypercholesterolemia treated with fish oil. *J Pediatr* 1990; **116:** 139–41.

Effects on the gastrointestinal tract. High-dose purified eicosapentaenoic acid ethyl ester produced loose motions with passage of unabsorbed oil in the stool.[1]
1. Hawthorne AB, *et al.* Fish oil revisited. *Lancet* 1989; **ii:** 811.

Effects on glucose metabolism. A deterioration in glycaemic control has been reported in both type 1 and type 2 diabetic patients taking omega-3 marine triglycerides and fish oil preparations.[1-6] However, improved insulin sensitivity has also been reported.[7]
1. Glauber H, *et al.* Adverse metabolic effect of omega-3 fatty acids in non-insulin-dependent diabetes mellitus. *Ann Intern Med* 1988; **108:** 663–8.
2. Kasim SE, *et al.* Effects of omega-3 fish oils on lipid metabolism, glycemic control, and blood pressure in type II diabetic patients. *J Clin Endocrinol Metab* 1988; **67:** 1–5.
3. Schectman G, *et al.* Effect of fish oil concentrate on lipoprotein composition in NIDDM. *Diabetes* 1988; **37:** 1567–73.
4. Hendra TJ, *et al.* Effects of fish oil supplements in NIDDM subjects: controlled study. *Diabetes Care* 1990; **13:** 821–9.
5. Vessby B, Boberg M. Dietary supplementation with n-3 fatty acids may impair glucose homeostasis in patients with non-insulin-dependent diabetes mellitus. *J Intern Med* 1990; **228:** 165–71.
6. Stacpoole PW, *et al.* Dose-response effects of dietary marine oil on carbohydrate and lipid metabolism in normal subjects and patients with hypertriglyceridemia. *Metabolism* 1989; **38:** 946–56.
7. Popp-Snijders C, *et al.* Dietary supplementation of omega-3 polyunsaturated fatty acids improves insulin sensitivity in non-insulin-dependent diabetics. *Diabetes Res* 1987; **4:** 141–7.

Uses and Administration
The omega-3 marine triglycerides contain triglycerides of the omega-3 fatty acids, particularly eicosapentaenoic acid and docosahexaenoic acid. These long-chain n-3 polyunsaturated fatty acids are precursors of eicosanoids in *fish* and when taken by man

---

The symbol † denotes a preparation no longer actively marketed

they compete with the precursor arachidonic acid. Their actions in man include a hypolipidaemic action, especially a reduction in plasma triglycerides; an anti-inflammatory action; and an antiplatelet effect.

Fish oils are a source of omega-3 triglycerides and preparations such as omega-3 marine triglycerides are thus used in patients with severe hypertriglyceridaemia. They are also marketed as dietary supplements.

A wide range of doses have been employed. The usual dose by mouth is 5 g twice daily with food.

◊ Fish oils and other omega-3 fatty acid preparations have been widely promoted as dietary supplements and a wide range of preparations of varying composition and potency is available. The interest in marine fish oils arose following observations that populations with a diet rich in marine fish oils generally have a low incidence of cardiovascular disease. In addition the incidence of asthma, psoriasis, and auto-immune diseases has been reported to be lower among Eskimos than in populations consuming a typical western diet, although the incidence of haemorrhagic stroke and epilepsy may be higher.

The omega-3 fatty acids eicosapentaenoic acid and docosahexaenoic acid are long-chain n-3 polyunsaturated fatty acids. They compete with arachidonic acid for inclusion in cyclo-oxygenase and lipoxygenase pathways: their antithrombotic activity is attributed to effects on prostanoid synthesis, promoting vasodilatation, a reduction in platelet aggregation, increased bleeding time and decreased platelet counts. Their anti-inflammatory activity is attributed to effects on leukotriene synthesis. Omega-3 fatty acids also have hypolipidaemic activity (below). Other effects reported include an increase in erythrocyte deformability, a decrease in blood viscosity, and a reduction in blood pressure.[1-4] Beneficial effects have been reported with omega-3 fatty acids in some inflammatory and auto-immune disorders including rheumatoid arthritis (p.9)[5-7] and psoriasis (p.1106),[8,9] but in later studies neither administration by the oral[10] nor the topical[11] route was effective in psoriasis. Other conditions in which some response has been noted include Behçet's syndrome,[12] Raynaud's syndrome (p.809),[13] Crohn's disease[14] and ulcerative colitis (p.1205),[15] renal transplantation (p.503),[16] and glomerular kidney disease.[17]

Overall, it would appear that an increase in seafood in the diet could have a beneficial effect in many people, but it is not clear if healthy people gain any benefit from going a stage further by taking supplements of fish oil or omega-3 triglycerides.

1. Knapp HR, FitzGerald GA. The antihypertensive effects of fish oils: a controlled study of polyunsaturated fatty acid supplements in essential hypertension. N Engl J Med 1989; 320: 1037–43.
2. Bønaa KH, et al. Effect of eicosapentaenoic and docosahexaenoic acids on blood pressure in hypertension: a population-based intervention trial from the Tromsø study. N Engl J Med 1990; 322: 795–801.
3. Appel LJ, et al. Does supplementation of diet with 'fish oil' reduce blood pressure? A meta-analysis of controlled clinical trials. Arch Intern Med 1993; 153: 1429–38.
4. Morris MC, et al. Does fish oil lower blood pressure? A meta-analysis of controlled trials. Circulation 1993; 88: 523–33.
5. Kremer JM, et al. Fish-oil fatty acid supplementation in active rheumatoid arthritis: a double-blinded, controlled, crossover study. Ann Intern Med 1987; 106: 497–503.
6. Lau CS, et al. Effects of fish oil supplementation on non-steroidal anti-inflammatory drug requirement in patients with mild rheumatoid arthritis—a double-blind placebo controlled study. Br J Rheumatol 1993; 32: 982–9.
7. Geusens P, et al. Long-term effect of omega-3 fatty acid supplementation in active rheumatoid arthritis: a 12-month, double-blind, controlled study. Arthritis Rheum 1994; 37: 824–9.
8. Gupta AK, et al. Double-blind, placebo-controlled study to evaluate the efficacy of fish oil and low-dose UVB in the treatment of psoriasis. Br J Dermatol 1989; 120: 801–7.
9. Lassus A, et al. Effects of dietary supplementation with polyunsaturated ethyl ester lipids (Angiosen) in patients with psoriasis and psoriatic arthritis. J Int Med Res 1990; 18: 68–73.
10. Søyland E, et al. Effect of dietary supplementation with very-long-chain n-3 fatty acids in patients with psoriasis. N Engl J Med 1993; 328: 1812–16.
11. Henneicke-von Zepelin H-H, et al. Highly purified omega-3 polyunsaturated fatty acids for topical treatment of psoriasis: results of a double-blind, placebo-controlled multicentre study. Br J Dermatol 1993; 129: 713–17.
12. Kürkçüoğlu N, Tandoğdu R. The effect of "MaxEPA" in the treatment of patients with Behcet's disease. Br J Dermatol 1989; 121: 667–8.
13. DiGiacomo RA, et al. Fish-oil dietary supplementation in patients with Raynaud's phenomenon: a double-blind, controlled, prospective study. Am J Med 1989; 86: 158–64.
14. Belluzzi A, et al. Effect of an enteric-coated fish-oil preparation on relapses in Crohn's disease. N Engl J Med 1996; 334: 1557–60.
15. Salomon P, et al. Treatment of ulcerative colitis with fish oil n-3-ω-fatty acid: an open trial. J Clin Gastroenterol 1990; 12: 157–61.
16. Homan van der Heide JJ, et al. Effect of dietary fish oil on renal function and rejection in cyclosporine-treated recipients of renal transplants. N Engl J Med 1993; 329: 769–73.
17. Donadio JV, et al. A controlled trial of fish oil in IgA nephropathy. N Engl J Med 1994; 331: 1194–9.

Hyperlipidaemias. The omega-3 fatty acids eicosapentaenoic acid and docosahexaenoic acid have hypolipidaemic activity. The most consistent effect is a dose-dependent reduction in triglyceride concentrations due to a reduction in very-low-density lipoproteins (VLDL). Variable responses have been seen in

cholesterol, low-density lipoprotein (LDL)-cholesterol, and high-density lipoprotein (HDL)-cholesterol concentrations. However, the results of early studies may have been confounded by the cholesterol content of fish oils used. The hypolipidaemic effects from studies using omega-3 fatty acid preparations have been more consistent. There is some doubt as to whether the hypotriglyceridaemic effect is sustained during long-term therapy.

Omega-3 fatty acids are used in the treatment of hypertriglyceridaemia (p.800) and there is some evidence of benefit in secondary prevention of **ischaemic heart disease**. Following myocardial infarction, long-term use of omega-3 fatty acid supplements reduced the risk of fatal cardiovascular events in a large group of Italian patients studied for 3.5 years.[1] Supplements taken for 2 years in another smaller study[2] had a modest beneficial effect on progression of coronary atherosclerosis, assessed by angiography, compared with placebo. Some,[3,4] but not other[5] studies have shown a decrease in coronary vessel restenosis after angioplasty. However, in a large long-term cohort study increased dietary intake of omega-3 fatty acids, as fish consumption, did not substantially reduce the risk of ischaemic heart disease in men who had initially been free of known cardiovascular disease.[6]

1. GISSI-Prevenzione Investigators. Dietary supplementation with n-3 polyunsaturated fatty acids and vitamin E after myocardial infarction: results of the GISSI-Prevenzione trial. Lancet 1999; 354: 447–55. Correction. ibid. 2001; 357: 642.
2. von Schacky C, et al. The effect of dietary ω-3 fatty acids on coronary atherosclerosis: a randomized, double-blind, placebo-controlled trial. Ann Intern Med 1999; 130: 554–62.
3. Dehmer GJ, et al. Reduction in the rate of early restenosis after coronary angioplasty by a diet supplemented with n-3 fatty acids. N Engl J Med 1988; 319: 733–40.
4. Gapinski JP, et al. Preventing restenosis with fish oils following coronary angioplasty: a meta-analysis. Arch Intern Med 1993; 153: 1595–1601.
5. Reis GJ, et al. Randomised trial of fish oil for prevention of restenosis after coronary angioplasty. Lancet 1989; ii: 177–81.
6. Ascherio A, et al. Dietary intake of marine n-3 fatty acids, fish intake, and the risk of coronary disease among men. N Engl J Med 1995; 332: 977–82.

Preparations

Proprietary Preparations (details are given in Part 3)
Aust.: Eicosapen; Omegaven; *Austral.:* Ethical Nutrients Maxepa; Fishaphos; Maxepa; Natures Own Maxepa; Natures Way Omega 3; *Fr.:* Maxepa; Mega 65; Omega 3+; Omegaven; *Ger.:* Bilatin Fischol; Eicosapen; Lipiscor; Omegaven; *Hong Kong:* Lipomega; Maxepa; *Ital.:* Esapent; Eskim†; Fish Factor; Maxepa; Omegaven; Seacor; Triglicen; Triolip; Triomar; *Norw.:* Omacor; *Port.:* Omegaven; *Swed.:* Omegaven; *Switz.:* Ameu; Eicosapen; Epacaps; Omega-3; Omegaven; Omesan; *UK:* Best EPA; Flowmega; Gamma EPA; Marinepa; Maxepa; Pure Omega; Triomar; *USA:* Cardi-Omega 3; Maxepa; Promega; Tricol Softgels†.

Multi-ingredient: *Austral.:* APR Cream; Arthriforte; Bioglan Arthri Plus; Bioglan E-Plus†; Bioglan Maxepa; Bioglan Zellulean with Escin; Efacal; Efamol Marine†; Epo + Maxepa + Vitamin E Herbal Plus Formula 8†; Ethical Nutrients Antioxidant Fish Oil Garlic Plus; Himega; Lifechange Circulation Aid; Lifesystem Herbal Plus Formula 9 Fatty Acids And Vitamin E†; Macro Maxepa; Maxepa & EPO; Maxepa Plus; Naudicelle Marine; Naudicelle Plus†; Pre Natal; Vita-Preg; *Braz.:* Lipcor; *Fr.:* Bionagrol Plus; Elteans; Omegacoeur; Synerbiol; *Hong Kong:* Himega; *Ital.:* Agedin Plus; Derman-Oil; Dermana; Fotrec DHA; Gammaplus; Ictom 3; Trofinerv; Trofinerv Antiox; Venactive; *NZ:* Efacal; Efamol Marine; *UK:* Efacal; Efamarine; Efatime; EPOC Marine†; Epopa; Galmarin; Gamma Marine; Naudicelle Forte; Naudicelle Plus; Naudicelle SL; Super GammaOil Marine; *USA:* Marine Lipid Concentrate; Sea-Omega; SuperEPA.

Orbofiban Acetate (5599-s)

Orbofiban Acetate (USAN, rINNM).

SC-57099-B. N-{[(3S)-1-(p-Amidinophenyl)-2-oxo-3-pyrrolidinyl]carbamoyl}-β-alanine ethyl ester monoacetate quadrantihydrate.

$C_{17}H_{23}N_5O_4,C_2H_4O_2,\frac{1}{4}H_2O = 426.0$.
CAS — 163250-90-6 (orbofiban); 165800-05-5 (orbofiban acetate).

Profile
Orbofiban is a glycoprotein IIb/IIIa-receptor antagonist. It has been investigated as an oral antiplatelet drug in unstable angina and myocardial infarction but has been associated with an increase in mortality.

◊ References.

1. Cannon CP, et al. Oral glycoprotein IIb/IIIa inhibition with orbofiban in patients with unstable coronary syndromes (OPUS-TIMI 16) trial. Circulation 2000; 102: 149–56.

Ouabain (5823-n)

Acocantherin; G-Strophanthin; Ouabainum; Strophanthin-G; Strophanthinum; Strophanthoside-G; Uabaina; Ubaína. 3β-(α-L-Rhamnopyranosyloxy)-1β,5,11α,14,19-pentahydroxy-5β,14β-card-20(22)-enolide octahydrate.

$C_{29}H_{44}O_{12},8H_2O = 728.8$.
CAS — 630-60-4 (anhydrous ouabain); 11018-89-6 (ouabain octahydrate).
ATC — C01AC01.
Pharmacopoeias. In Eur. (see p.vi), Jpn, and Pol.

A glycoside obtained from the seeds of *Strophanthus gratus* or from the wood of *Acokanthera schimperi* or *A. ouabaio* (Apocynaceae).

Pharmacopoeial description
Ph. Eur.: Colourless crystals or white, crystalline powder. Sparingly soluble in water and in dehydrated alcohol; practically insoluble in ether and in ethyl acetate. Protect from light.

Profile
Ouabain is a cardiac glycoside with positive inotropic activity. It has general properties similar to those of digoxin (p.870) and may be used in the treatment of heart failure (p.798). Ouabain is given by mouth in a dose of up to 24 mg daily; it has also been given intravenously.

Preparations
Proprietary Preparations (details are given in Part 3)
Ger.: Strodival; Strophocor N†.

Oxedrine (9510-c)

Oxedrine (BAN).

Sympaethaminum; Synephrine. (RS)-1-(4-Hydroxyphenyl)-2-(methylamino)ethanol.
$C_9H_{13}NO_2 = 167.2$.
CAS — 94-07-5.
ATC — C01CA08; S01GA06.

NOTE. *m*-Synephrine has been used as a synonym for phenylephrine. Care should be taken to avoid confusion between the two compounds.

Oxedrine Hydrochloride (11485-g)

Oxedrine Hydrochloride (BANM).
$C_9H_{13}NO_2,HCl = 203.7$.

Oxedrine Tartrate (2092-b)

Oxedrine Tartrate (BANM).

Aetaphen. Tartrat.; Aethaphenum Tartaricum; Oxedrini Tartras; Oxyphenylmethylaminoethanol Tartrate; Sinefrina Tartrato; Synephrine Tartrate.
$(C_9H_{13}NO_2)_2,C_4H_6O_6 = 484.5$.
CAS — 16589-24-5 (oxedrine tartrate); 67-04-9 (oxedrine tartrate, ±).
Pharmacopoeias. In It.

Profile
Oxedrine is a sympathomimetic (see Adrenaline, p.829) given as the tartrate in the treatment of hypotensive states in doses of about 100 to 150 mg three times daily by mouth; it has also been given by subcutaneous, intramuscular, or intravenous injection.

The tartrate is used in eye drops as an ocular decongestant, usually in a concentration of 0.5% in combination preparations. The hydrochloride has also been used in eye drops.

Preparations
Proprietary Preparations (details are given in Part 3)
Aust.: Sympatol; *Ger.:* Sympatol†; *Hong Kong:* Ocuton; *Ital.:* Sympatol; *Switz.:* Sympalept.

Multi-ingredient: *Aust.:* Dacrin; Pasuma-Dragees†; *Fr.:* Antalyre; Dacryne; Dacryoboraline; Dacryoseptil; Polyfra; Posine; Sedacollyre; Uvicol; *Ger.:* Dacrin; Ophtalmin; Pasgensin; Solupen-D; *Port.:* Dacrine; *Switz.:* Chibro-Boraline; Dacrine.

Oxilofrine Hydrochloride (11409-k)

Oxilofrine Hydrochloride (rINNM).

p-Hydroxyephedrine Hydrochloride; Methylsynephrine Hydrochloride; Oxyephedrine Hydrochloride. erythro-p-Hydroxy-α-[1-(methylamino)ethyl]benzyl alcohol hydrochloride.
$C_{10}H_{15}NO_2,HCl = 217.7$.
CAS — 942-51-8.

Profile
Oxilofrine is a sympathomimetic related to ephedrine (p.1090). It is used as the hydrochloride in the treatment of hypotensive states in usual doses of 16 mg three times daily by mouth, although higher doses have been given. Its salts have been used in antitussive preparations.

Preparations
Proprietary Preparations (details are given in Part 3)
Aust.: Carnigen; *Ger.:* Carnigen.

Multi-ingredient: *Canad.:* Cophylac.

Oxpentifylline (9267-r)

Oxpentifylline (BAN).

Pentoxifylline (BAN, USAN, rINN); BL-191; Pentoxifyllinum. 3,7-Dimethyl-1-(5-oxohexyl)xanthine.
$C_{13}H_{18}N_4O_3 = 278.3$.
CAS — 6493-05-6.
ATC — C04AD03.
Pharmacopoeias. In Eur. (see p.vi) and Jpn.

Pharmacopoeial description

Ph. Eur.: A white or almost white crystalline powder. Soluble in water; sparingly soluble in alcohol; freely soluble in dichloromethane; very slightly soluble in ether. Protect from light.

Adverse Effects

Oxpentifylline [pentoxifylline] can cause nausea, gastrointestinal disturbances, dizziness, and headache. Flushing, angina, palpitations, cardiac arrhythmias, and hypersensitivity reactions may also occur. Bleeding events have been reported rarely, usually in association with bleeding risk factors.

Overdosage with oxpentifylline [pentoxifylline] may be associated with fever, faintness, flushing, hypotension, drowsiness, agitation, and seizures.

Haemorrhage. Three major bleeding episodes including 2 fatal cerebral haemorrhages were reported in a group of patients receiving oxpentifylline [pentoxifylline] 400 mg three times daily together with nicoumalone [acenocoumarol] for intermittent claudication.[1] Gastrointestinal bleeding occurred in a 67-year-old patient with a history of duodenal ulcer following a single dose of oxpentifylline [pentoxifylline] for optic neuropathy.[2]

1. APIC Study Group. Acenocoumarol and pentoxifylline in intermittent claudication: a controlled clinical study. *Angiology* 1989; **40:** 237–48.
2. Oren R, *et al.* Pentoxifylline-induced gastrointestinal bleeding. *DICP Ann Pharmacother* 1991; **25:** 315–16.

Overdosage. A 22-year-old woman who took oxpentifylline [pentoxifylline] 4 to 6 g with suicidal intent experienced severe bradycardia and first- and second-degree atrioventricular block; other side-effects included nausea, vomiting, abdominal cramps, hypokalaemia, excitation, and insomnia.[1] She recovered after intensive supportive and symptomatic treatment.

1. Sznajder IJ, *et al.* First and second degree atrioventricular block in oxpentifylline overdose. *BMJ* 1984; **288:** 26.

Precautions

Oxpentifylline [pentoxifylline] should be avoided in cerebral haemorrhage, extensive retinal haemorrhage, and acute myocardial infarction. It should be used with caution in patients with ischaemic heart disease or hypotension. The dose of oxpentifylline [pentoxifylline] may need to be adjusted in patients with impaired renal function or severe liver impairment.

Hepatic impairment. The elimination half-life of oxpentifylline [pentoxifylline] and the 5-hydroxyhexyl metabolite is prolonged in patients with cirrhosis.[1]

1. Rames A, *et al.* Pharmacokinetics of intravenous and oral pentoxifylline in healthy volunteers and in cirrhotic patients. *Clin Pharmacol Ther* 1990; **47:** 354–9.

Porphyria. Oxpentifylline [pentoxifylline] is considered to be unsafe in patients with porphyria because it has been shown to be porphyrinogenic in *in-vitro* systems.

Interactions

Oxpentifylline [pentoxifylline] may potentiate the effect of antihypertensives. High parenteral doses of oxpentifylline [pentoxifylline] may enhance the hypoglycaemic action of insulin in diabetic patients. Oxpentifylline [pentoxifylline] should not be given concomitantly with ketorolac as there is reported to be an increased risk of bleeding and/or prolongation of the prothrombin time. There may also be an increased risk of bleeding during concomitant use with meloxicam. Serum levels of theophylline may be raised by oxpentifylline [pentoxifylline].

Pharmacokinetics

Oxpentifylline [pentoxifylline] is readily absorbed from the gastrointestinal tract but undergoes first-pass hepatic metabolism. Some metabolites are active. The apparent plasma half-life of oxpentifylline [pentoxifylline] is reported to be 0.4 to 0.8 hours; that of the metabolites varies from 1.0 to 1.6 hours. In 24 hours most of a dose is excreted in the urine mainly as metabolites and less than 4% is recovered in the faeces. Elimination of oxpentifylline [pentoxifylline] is decreased in elderly patients and patients with hepatic disease. Oxpentifylline [pentoxifylline] and its metabolites are distributed into breast milk.

◊ References.

1. Beermann B, *et al.* Kinetics of intravenous and oral pentoxifylline in healthy subjects. *Clin Pharmacol Ther* 1985; **37:** 25–8.
2. Smith RV, *et al.* Pharmacokinetics of orally administered pentoxifylline in humans. *J Pharm Sci* 1986; **75:** 47–52.
3. Witter FR, Smith RV. The excretion of pentoxifylline and its metabolites into human breast milk. *Am J Obstet Gynecol* 1985; **151:** 1094–7.
4. Paap CM, *et al.* Multiple-dose pharmacokinetics of pentoxifylline and its metabolites during renal insufficiency. *Ann Pharmacother* 1996; **30:** 724–9.

Uses and Administration

Oxpentifylline [pentoxifylline] is a xanthine derivative used as a vasodilator in the treatment of peripheral (p.809) and cerebral vascular disorders (p.798). It also reduces blood viscosity probably by effects on erythrocyte deformability, platelet adhesion, and platelet aggregation. Oxpentifylline [pentoxifylline] is reported to increase blood flow to ischaemic tissues and improve tissue oxygenation in patients with peripheral vascular disease and to increase oxygen tension in the cerebral cortex and in the cerebrospinal fluid. Oxpentifylline [pentoxifylline] inhibits production of the cytokine, tumour necrosis factor alpha (TNF-α) and this property is under investigation in a number of diseases (see below).

The symbol † denotes a preparation no longer actively marketed

---

In the treatment of peripheral vascular disease the usual dose of oxpentifylline [pentoxifylline] is 400 mg three times daily by mouth in a modified-release formulation, reducing to 400 mg twice daily if adverse effects are troublesome. Doses should be taken with meals to reduce gastrointestinal disturbances. Beneficial effects may not be evident until after 2 to 6 weeks of treatment. Oxpentifylline [pentoxifylline] may also be administered parenterally.

◊ General references.

1. Ward A, Clissold SP. Pentoxifylline: a review of its pharmacodynamic and pharmacokinetic properties, and its therapeutic efficacy. *Drugs* 1987; **34:** 50–97.
2. Samlaska CP, Winfield EA. Pentoxifylline. *J Am Acad Dermatol* 1994; **30:** 603–21.

◊ Oxpentifylline [pentoxifylline] inhibits production of tumour necrosis factor alpha (TNFα), a cytokine that is implicated in the pathogenesis of many diseases and investigative work with oxpentifylline [pentoxifylline] is being, or has been, carried out in many such disorders. Studies have been performed in patients with AIDS,[1,2] acute respiratory distress syndrome,[3] alcoholic hepatitis,[4] cerebral malaria,[5,6] diabetes mellitus,[7-12] inflammatory bowel disease,[13] infertility (males),[14,15] severe sepsis or septic shock,[16] recurrent aphthous stomatitis,[17] toxic epidermal necrolysis,[18] and various vasculitic syndromes.[19,20] Oxpentifylline [pentoxifylline] has also been tried for reducing the toxicity of procedures and treatments associated with bone-marrow transplantation[21,22] including graft-versus-host disease. Although promising results have been reported in some of these studies, the place of oxpentifylline [pentoxifylline] in the overall management of these disorders remains to be established.

1. Luke DR, *et al.* Phase I/II study of pentoxifylline with zidovudine on HIV-1 growth in AIDS patients. *Int J Clin Pharmacol Ther Toxicol* 1993; **31:** 343–50.
2. Reeves GEM, *et al.* Pentoxifylline to treat Mycobacterium avium complex exacerbation in late-stage HIV infection. *Med J Aust* 1997; **166:** 446.
3. Ardizzoia A, *et al.* Respiratory distress syndrome in patients with advanced cancer treated with pentoxifylline: a randomized study. *Support Care Cancer* 1993; **1:** 331–3.
4. Akriviadis E, *et al.* Pentoxifylline improves short-term survival in severe acute alcoholic hepatitis: a double-blind, placebo-controlled trial. *Gastroenterology* 2000; **119:** 1637–48.
5. Di Perri G, *et al.* Pentoxifylline as a supportive agent in the treatment of cerebral malaria in children. *J Infect Dis* 1995; **171:** 1317–22.
6. Looareesuwan S, *et al.* Pentoxifylline as an ancillary treatment for severe falciparum malaria in Thailand. *Am J Trop Med Hyg* 1998; **58:** 348–53.
7. Sulerte SB, Ferrari E. Diabetic retinal vascular complications and erythrocyte filtrability: results of a 2-year follow-up study with pentoxifylline. *Pharmatherapeutica* 1985; **4:** 341–50.
8. White JR, *et al.* Effects of pentoxifylline on proteinuria in normotensive patients with diabetes mellitus. *DICP Ann Pharmacother* 1990; **24:** 1043–5.
9. Campbell RK. Clinical update on pentoxifylline therapy for diabetes-induced peripheral vascular disease. *Ann Pharmacother* 1993; **27:** 1099–1105.
10. MacDonald MJ, *et al.* Pentoxifylline in the treatment of children with new-onset type I diabetes mellitus. *JAMA* 1994; **271:** 27–8.
11. Sebag J, *et al.* Effects of pentoxifylline on choroidal blood flow in nonproliferative diabetic retinopathy. *Angiology* 1994; **45:** 429–33.
12. Guerrero-Romero F, *et al.* Pentoxifylline reduces proteinuria in insulin-dependent and non-insulin dependent diabetic patients. *Clin Nephrol* 1995; **43:** 116–21.
13. Bauditz J, *et al.* Treatment with tumour necrosis factor inhibitor oxpentifylline does not improve corticosteroid dependent chronic active Crohn's disease. *Gut* 1997; **40:** 470–4.
14. Craft I, Shrivastav P. Treatment of male infertility. *Lancet* 1994; **344:** 191–2.
15. Rizk B, *et al.* Successful use of pentoxifylline in male-factor infertility and previous failure of in vitro fertilization: a prospective randomized study. *J Assist Reprod Genet* 1995; **12:** 710–4.
16. Staubach K-H, *et al.* Effect of pentoxifylline in severe sepsis: results of a randomized, double-blind, placebo-controlled study. *Arch Surg* 1998; **133:** 94–100.
17. Pizarro A, *et al.* Treatment of recurrent aphthous stomatitis with pentoxifylline. *Br J Dermatol* 1995; **133:** 659–60.
18. Redondo P, *et al.* Toxic epidermal necrolysis: treatment with pentoxifylline. *Br J Dermatol* 1994; **130:** 688–9.
19. Calderón MJ, *et al.* Successful treatment of cutaneous PAN with pentoxifylline. *Br J Dermatol* 1993; **128:** 706–7.
20. Nürnberg W, *et al.* Synergistic effects of pentoxifylline and dapsone in leucocytoclastic vasculitis. *Lancet* 1994; **343:** 491.
21. Clift RA, *et al.* A randomized controlled trial of pentoxifylline for the prevention of regimen-related toxicities in patients undergoing allogeneic marrow transplantation. *Blood* 1993; **82:** 2025–30.
22. Ferrà C, *et al.* Pentoxifylline, ciprofloxacin and prednisone failed to prevent transplant-related toxicities in bone marrow transplant recipients and were associated with an increased incidence of infectious complications. *Bone Marrow Transplant* 1997; **20:** 1075–80.

Preparations

Proprietary Preparations (details are given in Part 3)

Aust.: Haemodyn; Pentohexal; Pentomer; Pentoxi; Trental; Vasonit; *Austral.:* Trental; *Belg.:* Torental; *Braz.:* Pentox; Trental; *Canad.:* Trental; *Denm.:* Trental; *Fin.:* Artal; Pentoxin; Trental; *Fr.:* Pentoflux; Torental; *Ger.:* Agapurin; Azupentat; Claudicat; durapental; Pento; Pento-Puren; Pentohexal; Pentox; Pentoxy; Ralofekt; Rentylin; Trental; *Hong Kong:* Trental; *Irl.:* Trental; *Israel:* Oxopurin; Trental; *Ital.:* Trental; *Mex.:* Fixoten; Kentadin; Peridane; Sufisal; Trental; Vasofyl; *Neth.:* Trental; *Norw.:* Trental; *NZ:* Trental; *Port.:* Claudicat; Trental; *S.Afr.:* Trental; *Singapore:* Flexital; Trenlin; Trental; *Spain:* Elorgan; Hemovas; Retimax; *Switz.:* Dinostral; Pentoxi; Trental; *Thai.:* Elastab; Flexital; Herden; Penlol; Sipental; Trental; *UK:* Trental; *USA:* Trental.

Oxprenolol Hydrochloride (6317-j)

Oxprenolol Hydrochloride (BANM, USAN, rINNM).

Ba-39089; Oxprenololi Hydrochloridum; Oxprenolol Hydrochloride. 1-(o-Allyloxyphenoxy)-3-isopropylaminopropan-2-ol hydrochloride.

$C_{15}H_{23}NO_3$,HCl = 301.8.

CAS — 6452-71-7 (oxprenolol); 6452-73-9 (oxprenolol hydrochloride).

NOTE. Compounded preparations of oxprenolol hydrochloride may be represented by the following names:

• Co-prenozide (*BAN*)—oxprenolol hydrochloride 640 parts and cyclopenthiazide 1 part (w/w).

Pharmacopoeias. In *Eur.* (see p.vi), *Jpn, Pol.,* and *US.*

Pharmacopoeial description

Ph. Eur.: A white or almost white, crystalline powder. Very soluble in water; freely soluble in alcohol; practically insoluble in ether. A 10% solution in water has a pH of 4.5 to 6.0. Protect from light.

USP 25: A white crystalline powder. Freely soluble in water, in alcohol, and in chloroform; sparingly soluble in acetone; practically insoluble in ether. A 10% solution in water has a pH of 4.0 to 6.0.

Adverse Effects, Treatment, and Precautions

As for beta blockers, p.844.

Effects on the gastrointestinal tract. Retroperitoneal fibrosis has been reported[1] in a patient who was taking oxprenolol.

1. McCluskey DR, *et al.* Oxprenolol and retroperitoneal fibrosis. *BMJ* 1980; **281:** 1459–60.

Hypersensitivity. A report of oxprenolol-induced drug fever in a patient which was confirmed by a challenge test.[1]

1. Hasegawa K, *et al.* Drug fever due to oxprenolol. *BMJ* 1980; **281:** 27–8.

Overdosage. A report of rhabdomyolysis and myoglobinuria complicating severe overdosage with oxprenolol.[1]

1. Schofield PM, *et al.* Recovery after severe oxprenolol overdose complicated by rhabdomyolysis. *Hum Toxicol* 1985; **4:** 57–60.

Interactions

The interactions associated with beta blockers are discussed on p.846.

Pharmacokinetics

Oxprenolol is well absorbed from the gastrointestinal tract, but is subject to first-pass metabolism resulting in variable bioavailability (20 to 70%). Peak plasma concentrations have been reported to occur about 1 or 2 hours after a dose. Oxprenolol is 80% bound to plasma proteins. Oxprenolol is metabolised in the liver and almost entirely excreted in the urine. Oxprenolol diffuses across the placenta and is present in breast milk. It is moderately lipid-soluble and crosses the blood-brain barrier. An elimination half-life of 1 to 2 hours has been reported.

Pregnancy and breast feeding. A study of the placental transfer of oxprenolol and its passage into breast milk in 32 pregnant women receiving a preparation containing oxprenolol and dihydralazine (Trasipressol).[1] At delivery the mean maternal plasma concentration was 0.386 nanomoles per mL compared with 0.071 and 0.081 nanomoles per mL in plasma from the umbilical artery and vein respectively. Oxprenolol plasma concentrations in the newborn ranged from 0 to 0.186 nanomoles per mL during the first 24 hours of life. The concentrations of oxprenolol in breast milk 3 to 6 days after delivery ranged from 0 to 1.342 nanomoles per mL, and the milk to plasma concentration ratio was 0.45:1. Based on the highest milk concentration observed it was calculated that a breast-fed infant could receive, at a maximum, a daily dose at least sixty times less than an average daily dose (240 mg daily) taken by a hypertensive adult.

1. Sioufi A, *et al.* Oxprenolol placental transfer, plasma concentrations in newborns and passage into breast milk. *Br J Clin Pharmacol* 1984; **18:** 453–6.

Uses and Administration

Oxprenolol is a non-cardioselective beta blocker (p.844). It is reported to possess intrinsic sympathomimetic and membrane-stabilising activity.

Oxprenolol is used as the hydrochloride in the management of hypertension (p.802), angina pectoris (p.791), and cardiac arrhythmias (p.794). It is also used in anxiety disorders (p.649).

In **hypertension** oxprenolol hydrochloride is given by mouth in a usual dose of 80 to 160 mg daily in two or three divided doses. The dose may be increased at weekly or fortnightly intervals until a satisfactory response is achieved. The usual maximum dose is 320 mg daily although up to 480 mg daily has been allowed. Modified-release tablets may be given once daily in a dose of up to 320 mg.

The usual dose for **angina pectoris** is 80 to 160 mg daily in two or three divided doses with a usual maximum of 320 mg daily. For **cardiac arrhythmias** a dose of 40 mg daily to not more than 240 mg daily in two or three divided doses may be used.

For the emergency treatment of cardiac arrhythmias oxprenolol hydrochloride has been given by slow intravenous injection or by the intramuscular route.

Oxprenolol hydrochloride is given by mouth in usual doses of 40 to 80 mg daily, either as a single dose or in two divided doses, to relieve **anxiety** in stressful situations.

Preparations

BP 2001: Oxprenolol Tablets;
USP 25: Oxprenolol Hydrochloride Extended-release Tablets; Oxprenolol Hydrochloride Tablets.

Proprietary Preparations (details are given in Part 3)
Aust.: Trasicor; *Austral.:* Corbeton; *Belg.:* Trasicor; *Canad.:* Slow-Trasicor; Trasicor; *Denm.:* Trasicor; *Fr.:* Trasicor; *Ger.:* Trasicor; *Irl.:* Slow-Trasicor; Trasicor; *Israel:* Tevacor; Trasicor; *Neth.:* Trasicor; *Norw.:* Trasicor†; *NZ:* Captol; Slow-Trasicor; Trasicor; *S.Afr.:* Trasicor; *Spain:* Trasicor; *Switz.:* Slow-Trasicor; Trasicor; *UK:* Apsolox†; Oxyprenix†; Slow-Trasicor; Trasicor.

Multi-ingredient: *Aust.:* Trasitensin; Trepress; *Fr.:* Trasipressol†; Trasitensine; *Ger.:* Impresso; Trasitensin; Trepress; *Irl.:* Trasidrex; *Ital.:* Trasitensin; *S.Afr.:* Trasidrex; *Spain:* Trasitensin; *Switz.:* Slow-Trasitensine; Trasitensine; Trepress†; *UK:* Trasidrex.

Oxyfedrine Hydrochloride (9268-f)

Oxyfedrine Hydrochloride (BANM, rINNM).
D-563; Oxifedrini Chloridum. L-3-(β-Hydroxy-α-methylphenethylamino)-3′-methoxypropiophenone hydrochloride.
$C_{19}H_{23}NO_3,HCl = 349.9$.
CAS — 15687-41-9 (oxyfedrine); 16777-42-7 (oxyfedrine hydrochloride).

Profile

Oxyfedrine hydrochloride has vasodilator properties and is used in angina pectoris (p.791), and myocardial infarction (p.805).

It is given in doses of 8 to 24 mg three times daily by mouth. It may also be given by slow intravenous injection or intravenous infusion. Oxyfedrine is metabolised to phenylpropanolamine (p.1098).

Preparations

Proprietary Preparations (details are given in Part 3)
Aust.: Ildamen; *Ger.:* Ildamen; Myofedrin; *Hong Kong:* Ildamen; *Port.:* Ildamen.

Pamabrom (13073-h)

Pamabrom (USAN).
2-Amino-2-methylpropan-1-ol 8-bromotheophyllinate.
$C_4H_{11}NO,C_7H_7BrN_4O_2 = 348.2$.
CAS — 606-04-2.
Pharmacopoeias. In US.

Profile

Pamabrom is a weak diuretic that has been used, in combination with analgesics and antihistamines, for symptomatic relief of the premenstrual syndrome.

Preparations

Proprietary Preparations (details are given in Part 3)
USA: Fluidex with Pamabrom†; Maximum Strength Aqua-Ban.

Multi-ingredient: *Canad.:* Midol PMS Extra Strength; Pamprin; Trendar PMS; Tylenol Menstrual; *USA:* Bayer Select Maximum Strength Menstrual†; Fem-1; Fem-Etts†; Lurline PMS; Midol PMS; Pamprin; Premsyn PMS; Teen Midol†; Womens Tylenol Multi-Symptom Menstrual Relief.

Pantethine (13075-b)

(R)-NN′-[Dithiobis(ethyleneiminocarbonylethylene)]bis(2,4-dihydroxy-3,3-dimethylbutyramide).
$C_{22}H_{42}N_4O_8S_2 = 554.7$.
CAS — 16816-67-4.
ATC — A11HA32.
Pharmacopoeias. In Jpn.

Profile

Pantethine is a component of coenzyme A. It is a lipid regulating drug used in the treatment of hyperlipidaemias (p.800). The usual dose is 600 to 1200 mg daily by mouth in divided doses.

Preparations

Proprietary Preparations (details are given in Part 3)
Hong Kong: Pantomin; *Ital.:* Analip†; Lipodel†; Pantetina; *Jpn:* Pantomin; *Spain:* Atarone†; Liponet; Obliterol.

Multi-ingredient: *Ital.:* Carpantin.

Pargyline Hydrochloride (886-f)

Pargyline Hydrochloride (BANM, USAN, rINNM).
A-19120; MO-911; NSC-43798. N-Methyl-N-2-propynylbenzylamine hydrochloride; Benzylmethylprop-2-ynylamine hydrochloride.
$C_{11}H_{13}N,HCl = 195.7$.
CAS — 555-57-7 (pargyline); 306-07-0 (pargyline hydrochloride).

Profile

Pargyline hydrochloride is an MAOI (see Phenelzine Sulfate, p.303) that was formerly used in the treatment of moderate to severe hypertension.

Parnaparin Sodium (10349-y)

Parnaparin Sodium (BAN, rINN).
OP-21-23; Parnaparinum Natricum.
CAS — 9041-08-1.
Pharmacopoeias. In Eur. (see p.vi).

Pharmacopoeial description

Ph. Eur.: Parnaparin sodium is prepared by hydrogen peroxide and cupric salt depolymerisation of heparin obtained from the intestinal mucosa of pigs and cattle. The majority of the components have a 2-O-sulfo-α-L-idopyranosuronic acid structure at the non-reducing end and a 2-N,6-O-disulfo-D-glucosamine structure at the reducing end of their chain. The mass-average molecular mass ranges between 4000 and 6000, with a characteristic value of about 5000. The mass percentage of chains lower than 3000 is not more than 30%. The degree of sulfation is 2.0 to 2.6 per disaccharide unit. Potency is not less than 75 units and not more than 110 units of anti-factor Xa activity per mg with reference to the dried substance, and the ratio of anti-factor Xa activity to anti-factor IIa (antithrombin) activity is between 1.5 and 3.0.

Profile

Parnaparin sodium is a low-molecular-weight heparin (p.923) with anticoagulant activity used in the prevention of postoperative venous thromboembolism (p.817). For general surgical procedures it is given by subcutaneous injection in a dose of 3200 units 2 hours before the procedure, followed by 3200 units once daily for 7 days or until the patient is fully ambulant. For higher risk or orthopaedic patients a dose of 4250 units is given 12 hours before the procedure, followed by 4250 units 12 hours postoperatively and then once daily for 10 days.

◊ References.
1. Frampton JE, Faulds D. Parnaparin: a review of its pharmacology, and clinical application in the prevention and treatment of thromboembolic and other vascular disorders. *Drugs* 1994; **47:** 652–76.

Preparations

Proprietary Preparations (details are given in Part 3)
Ital.: Fluxum; Minidalton†.

Penbutolol Sulfate (6318-z)

Penbutolol Sulfate (USAN, rINNM).
Hoe-39-893d; Hoe-893d; Levopenbutolol Sulphate; Penbutolol Hemisulphate; Penbutolol Sulphate (BANM); Penbutololi Sulfas. (S)-1-tert-Butylamino-3-(2-cyclopentylphenoxy)propan-2-ol hemisulphate.
$(C_{18}H_{29}NO_2)_2,H_2SO_4 = 680.9$.
CAS — 38363-40-5 (penbutolol); 38363-32-5 (penbutolol sulfate).
Pharmacopoeias. In Eur. (see p.vi), Jpn, and US.

Pharmacopoeial description

Ph. Eur.: A white or almost white, crystalline powder. Slightly soluble in water; practically insoluble in cyclohexane; soluble in methyl alcohol. Protect from light.

USP 25: A white to off-white, crystalline powder. Soluble in water and in methyl alcohol. Store in airtight containers. Protect from light.

Adverse Effects, Treatment, and Precautions

As for beta blockers, p.844.

Interactions

The interactions associated with beta blockers are discussed on p.846.

Pharmacokinetics

Penbutolol is readily absorbed from the gastrointestinal tract and peak plasma concentrations occur about 1 to 3 hours after a dose. Penbutolol is 80 to 98% bound to plasma proteins. It has a high lipid solubility. It is extensively metabolised in the liver by hydroxylation and glucuronidation, the metabolites being excreted in the urine together with only small amounts of unchanged penbutolol. A plasma elimination half-life of about 20 hours has been reported.

Renal impairment. Glucuronidation was considered more prominent than hydroxylation in the metabolism of penbutolol and its activity was not altered in patients with renal insufficiency.[1]
1. Bernard N, *et al.* Pharmacokinetics of penbutolol and its metabolites in renal insufficiency. *Eur J Clin Pharmacol* 1985; **29:** 215–19.

Uses and Administration

Penbutolol is a non-cardioselective beta blocker (p.844). It is reported to possess some intrinsic sympathomimetic activity but lacks membrane-stabilising properties.

Penbutolol is used as the sulfate in the management of hypertension (p.802). It may also be used in cardiac disorders such as angina pectoris (p.791).

In **hypertension** penbutolol sulfate is given in initial doses of 20 mg daily by mouth; the dose may be increased if necessary to 40 to 80 mg daily. Maximum antihypertensive efficacy is reported to occur within 2 weeks in patients given a dose of 20 mg daily but about 4 weeks may be required for maximum effect in patients given 10 mg daily.

Penbutolol sulfate has also been used in similar doses in cardiac disorders such as **angina**.

◊ References.
1. Frishman WH, Covey S. Penbutolol and carteolol: two new beta-adrenergic blockers with partial agonism. *J Clin Pharmacol* 1990; **30:** 412–21.
2. Schlanz KD, Thomas RL. Penbutolol: a new β-adrenergic blocking agent. *DICP Ann Pharmacother* 1990; **24:** 403–8.

Preparations

USP 25: Penbutolol Sulfate Tablets.

Proprietary Preparations (details are given in Part 3)
Aust.: Betapressin†; *Fr.:* Betapressine†; *Ger.:* Betapressin; *Mex.:* Betapresin; *USA:* Levatol.

Multi-ingredient: *Aust.:* Normotensin; *Ger.:* Betarelix; Betasemid.

Pentaerithrityl Tetranitrate (9270-c)

Pentaerithrityl Tetranitrate (BAN, rINN).
Erynite; Nitropentaerythrol; Nitropenthrite; Pentaerythritol Tetranitrate; Pentaerythritolum Tetranitricum; Pentanitrol; PETN. 2,2-Bis(hydroxymethyl)propane-1,3-diol tetranitrate.
$C_5H_8N_4O_{12} = 316.1$.
CAS — 78-11-5.
ATC — C01DA05.
NOTE. The synonym PETN has been applied to both niceritrol and pentaerithrityl tetranitrate.
Pharmacopoeias. In Pol.
Eur. (see p.vi) includes as diluted pentaerithrityl tetranitrate.

Pharmacopoeial description

Ph. Eur.: Undiluted pentaerithrityl tetranitrate is a white or slightly yellowish powder. Practically insoluble in water; slightly soluble in alcohol; soluble in acetone.

Diluted pentaerithrityl tetranitrate is a mixture of pentaerithrityl tetranitrate with lactose monohydrate or mannitol. Protect from light and heat.

◊ CAUTION. *Undiluted pentaerithrityl tetranitrate can be exploded by percussion or excessive heat.*

Profile

Pentaerithrityl tetranitrate is a vasodilator with general properties similar to those of glyceryl trinitrate (p.898) but its duration of action is more prolonged.

It is used in angina pectoris (p.791) in oral doses of 40 to 240 mg daily, in divided doses, before a meal. It is also given as modified-release preparations.

Pentaerithrityl trinitrate, an active metabolite of pentaerithrityl tetranitrate, has also been used clinically under the name pentrinitrol.

Preparations

Proprietary Preparations (details are given in Part 3)
Aust.: Dilcoran†; *Canad.:* Peritrate†; *Fr.:* Nitrodex; *Ger.:* Dilcoran; Nirason N; Pentalong; *Irl.:* Mycardol†; *Ital.:* Peritrate;

S.Afr.: Peritrate†; *Switz.:* Nitrodex; *Thai.:* Peritrate; *UK:* Mycardol†; *USA:* Pentylan†.

Multi-ingredient: *Aust.:* Spasmocor; *Ger.:* Nitro-Crataegutt; Nitro-Obsidan; VisanoCor N.

Pentifylline (639-q)

Pentifylline *(BAN, rINN)*.

I-Hexyltheobromine; SK7. I-Hexyl-3,7-dimethylxanthine.
$C_{13}H_{20}N_4O_2 = 264.3$.
CAS — 1028-33-7.
ATC — C04AD01.

Profile
Pentifylline is a xanthine derivative used as a vasodilator in the management of peripheral or cerebral vascular disorders.

Preparations
Proprietary Preparations (details are given in Part 3)
Ger.: Cosaldon.

Multi-ingredient: *Aust.:* Cosaldon; *Ger.:* Cosaldon A; *S.Afr.:* Cosaldon.

Pentosan Polysulfate Sodium (4821-j)

Pentosan Polysulfate Sodium *(BAN, USAN, rINN)*.

Pentosan Polysulphate Sodium; PZ-68; Sodium Pentosan Polysulphate; Sodium Xylanpolysulphate; SP-54.
CAS — 37319-17-8; 116001-96-8.
ATC — C05BA04.

A mixture of linear polymers of β-1→4-linked xylose, usually sulfated at the 2- and 3-positions and occasionally (approximately 1 in every 4 residues) substituted at the 2-position with 4-*O*-methyl-α-D-glucuronic acid 2,3-*O*-sulfate. The average molecular weight lies between 4000 and 6000 with a total molecular weight range of 1000 to 40 000.

Adverse Effects and Precautions
As for Heparin, p.902. Gastrointestinal disturbances may also occur.

Uses and Administration
Pentosan polysulfate sodium is a heparinoid with anticoagulant and fibrinolytic properties; it may also have hypolipidaemic and anti-inflammatory effects. It is used in thromboembolic disorders, although its anticoagulant effect is less than that of heparin. It is also used in the management of interstitial cystitis (see below) and has been tried in a number of other conditions. Pentosan polysulfate sodium has been administered orally, parenterally, and by topical application.

In the management of interstitial cystitis, pentosan polysulfate sodium is given orally in a dose of 100 mg three times daily.

Cystitis. Pentosan polysulfate sodium has been used in inflammatory conditions of the bladder, including interstitial cystitis (see under Uses and Administration of Dimethyl Sulfoxide, p.1402), and is postulated to act by enhancing the protective effect of mucins at the bladder surface. Studies have differed concerning its efficacy in the treatment of interstitial cystitis and an analysis[1] of placebo-controlled trials concluded that pentosan polysulfate sodium was more effective in treating pain, urgency, and frequency, but that the difference was small. Any benefit is usually apparent within 3 to 6 months of commencing treatment and only occurs in a minority of patients.[2] Pentosan polysulfate sodium was reported[3] to have minimal long-term efficacy in a group of patients with severe or refractory interstitial cystitis.

Administration of pentosan polysulfate sodium by mouth controlled haemorrhage in 5 patients with radiation cystitis.[4] An improvement in symptoms has also been reported[5] in an uncontrolled study of oral pentosan polysulfate sodium in men with chronic nonbacterial prostatitis.

1. Hwang P, *et al.* Efficacy of pentosan polysulfate in the treatment of interstitial cystitis: a meta-analysis. *Urology* 1997; **50:** 39–43.
2. Anonymous. Pentosan for interstitial cystitis. *Med Lett Drugs Ther* 1997; **39:** 56.
3. Jepsen JV, *et al.* Long-term experience with pentosanpolysulfate in interstitial cystitis. *Urology* 1998; **51:** 381–7.
4. Parsons CL. Successful management of radiation cystitis with sodium pentosanpolysulfate. *J Urol (Baltimore)* 1986; **136:** 813–14.
5. Nickel JC, *et al.* Pentosan polysulfate therapy for chronic nonbacterial prostatitis (chronic pelvic pain syndrome category IIIA): a prospective multicenter clinical trial. *Urology* 2000; **56:** 413–17.

Preparations
Proprietary Preparations (details are given in Part 3)
Aust.: Polyanion; *Austral.:* Elmiron; *Canad.:* Elmiron; *Fr.:* Hemoclar; *Ger.:* Fibrezym; *Hong Kong:* Elmiron; SP54; *Ital.:* Fibrase; *Port.:* Fibrocide†; *S.Afr.:* Tavan-SP 54; *Spain:* Fibrocid; *USA:* Elmiron.

Multi-ingredient: *Aust.:* Flexurat; Thrombocid; *Fr.:* Collyrex; Keratosane; *Ger.:* Flexurat†; Thrombocid; *Hong Kong:* Anso; Thrombocid; *Port.:* Thrombocid; *Spain:* Anso; Plasmaclar†; Rulun; Thrombocid; *Switz.:* Thrombocid.

Perhexiline Maleate (9272-a)

Perhexiline Maleate *(BANM, USAN, rINNM)*.

WSM-3978G. 2-(2,2-Dicyclohexylethyl)piperidine hydrogen maleate.
$C_{19}H_{35}N,C_4H_4O_4 = 393.6$.
CAS — 6621-47-2 (perhexiline); 6724-53-4 (perhexiline maleate).

Profile
Perhexiline maleate may be used in the long-term management of severe angina pectoris (p.791) in patients who have not responded to other anti-anginal drugs. Its mode of action is complex.

The usual dose is 100 to 200 mg daily by mouth in 2 divided doses; it is generally recommended not to administer more than 300 mg daily although doses of 400 mg daily have been necessary in some patients. The maintenance of plasma-perhexiline concentrations between 0.15 and 0.60 μg per mL has been recommended.

Perhexiline occasionally produces severe adverse effects including peripheral neuropathy affecting all four limbs with associated papilloedema, severe and occasionally fatal hepatic toxicity, and metabolic abnormalities with marked weight loss, hypertriglyceridaemia, and profound hypoglycaemia. It is contra-indicated in patients with impaired hepatic or renal function. Perhexiline should be administered with caution to diabetic patients. Hepatic metabolism of perhexiline is mediated by the cytochrome P450 isoenzyme CYP2D6. Therefore caution is advised if perhexiline is used with other drugs that inhibit or are metabolised by this enzyme; perhexiline toxicity has been reported in patients also receiving the SSRIs fluoxetine or paroxetine.

Porphyria. Perhexiline is considered to be unsafe in patients with porphyria because it has been shown to be porphyrinogenic in *animals* or *in-vitro* systems.

Preparations
Proprietary Preparations (details are given in Part 3)
Austral.: Pexid; Pexsig; *Belg.:* Pexid†; *NZ:* Pexid.

Perindopril (729-s)

Perindopril *(BAN, USAN, rINN)*.

McN-A-2833; S-9490. (2S,3aS,7aS)-1-{*N*-[(*S*)-1-Ethoxycarbonylbutyl]-L-alanyl}perhydroindole-2-carboxylic acid.
$C_{19}H_{32}N_2O_5 = 368.5$.
CAS — 82834-16-0.
ATC — C09AA04.

Perindopril Erbumine (13519-c)

Perindopril Erbumine *(BANM, USAN, rINNM)*.

McN-A-2833-109; Perindopril *tert*-Butylamine; S-9490-3.
$C_{19}H_{32}N_2O_5,C_4H_{11}N = 441.6$.
CAS — 107133-36-8.

Adverse Effects, Treatment, and Precautions
As for ACE inhibitors, p.820.

◊ In a postmarketing surveillance study[1] of 47 351 patients receiving perindopril for hypertension, no unexpected adverse effects were reported and serious reactions were rare; 1587 (6.3%) women and 782 (3.5%) men withdrew from therapy due to adverse effects.

Although a study[2] of perindopril administration to patients with stable chronic heart failure reported no significant first-dose hypotension, there has been a case report[3] of ischaemic stroke possibly associated with hypotension in a patient with post-infarction heart failure following a single dose of perindopril. Standard precautions as for other ACE inhibitors (p.822) should be followed when initiating perindopril therapy.

1. Speirs C, *et al.* Perindopril postmarketing surveillance: a 12 month study in 47 351 hypertensive patients. *Br J Clin Pharmacol* 1998; **46:** 63–70.
2. MacFadyen RJ, *et al.* Differences in first dose response to angiotensin converting enzyme inhibition in congestive heart failure: a placebo controlled study. *Br Heart J* 1991; **66:** 206–11.
3. Bagger JP. Adverse event with first-dose perindopril in congestive heart failure. *Lancet* 1997; **349:** 1671–2.

Interactions
As for ACE inhibitors, p.822.

Pharmacokinetics
Perindopril acts as a prodrug of the diacid perindoprilat, its active form. Following oral administration perindopril is rapidly absorbed and extensively metabolised, mainly in the liver, to perindoprilat and inactive metabolites including glucuronides. The presence of food is reported to reduce the conversion of perindopril to perindoprilat. Peak plasma concentrations of perindoprilat are achieved 3 to 4 hours after an oral dose of perindopril. Perindoprilat is about 10 to 20% bound to plasma proteins. About 75% of an oral dose of perindopril is excreted in the urine as unchanged drug, as perindoprilat, and as other metabolites; the remainder is excreted in the faeces. The elimination of perindoprilat is biphasic with a distribution half-life of about 5 hours and an elimination half-life of 25 to 30 hours, the latter half-life probably representing strong binding to angiotensin-converting enzyme. The excretion of perindoprilat is decreased in renal impairment. Both perindopril and perindoprilat are removed by dialysis.

◊ References.
1. Lecocq B, *et al.* Influence of food on the pharmacokinetics of perindopril and the time course of angiotensin-converting enzyme inhibition in serum. *Clin Pharmacol Ther* 1990; **47:** 397–402.
2. Verpooten GA, *et al.* Single dose pharmacokinetics of perindopril and its metabolites in hypertensive patients with various degrees of renal insufficiency. *Br J Clin Pharmacol* 1991; **32:** 187–92.
3. Sennesael J, *et al.* The pharmacokinetics of perindopril and its effects on serum angiotensin converting enzyme activity in hypertensive patients with chronic renal failure. *Br J Clin Pharmacol* 1992; **33:** 93–9.
4. Thiollet M, *et al.* The pharmacokinetics of perindopril in patients with liver cirrhosis. *Br J Clin Pharmacol* 1992; **33:** 326–8.
5. Guérin A, *et al.* The effect of haemodialysis on the pharmacokinetics of perindoprilat after long-term perindopril. *Eur J Clin Pharmacol* 1993; **44:** 183–7.

Uses and Administration
Perindopril is an ACE inhibitor (p.820). It is used in the treatment of hypertension (p.802) and heart failure (p.798)

Perindopril is converted in the body into its active metabolite perindoprilat. ACE inhibition is reported to occur within 1 hour of a dose, to be at a maximum at about 4 to 8 hours, and to be maintained for 24 hours. Perindopril is given by mouth as the erbumine salt and should be taken before food.

In the treatment of **hypertension** perindopril erbumine is given in an initial dose of 2 mg once daily. Since there may be a precipitous fall in blood pressure in some patients when starting therapy with an ACE inhibitor, the first dose should preferably be given at bedtime. The dose may be increased according to response to a maximum of 8 mg daily. The usual maintenance dose is 4 mg daily. Higher doses are suggested in the USA, with an initial dose of 4 mg once daily and a maximum dose of 16 mg daily in uncomplicated hypertensive patients. Patients receiving diuretics should have the diuretic discontinued 2 or 3 days before starting perindopril if possible, and resumed later if necessary.

In the management of **heart failure**, severe first-dose hypotension on introduction of an ACE inhibitor is common in patients on loop diuretics, but their temporary withdrawal may cause rebound pulmonary oedema. Thus treatment should be initiated with a low dose under close medical supervision. Perindopril is given in an initial dose of 2 mg in the morning. The usual maintenance dose is 4 mg daily.

A reduction in dosage may be necessary in patients with impaired renal function; in the UK the recommended maintenance dose is 2 mg daily or on alternate days, depending on the degree of impairment.

◊ References.
1. Todd PA, Fitton A. Perindopril: a review of its pharmacological properties and therapeutic use in cardiovascular disorders. *Drugs* 1991; **42:** 90–114.
2. Doyle AE, ed. Angiotensin-converting enzyme (ACE) inhibition: benefits beyond blood pressure control. *Am J Med* 1992; **92** (suppl 4B): 1S–107S.
3. Hurst M, Jarvis B. Perindopril: an updated review of its use in hypertension. *Drugs* 2001; **61** 867–96.

Preparations
Proprietary Preparations (details are given in Part 3)
Aust.: Coversum; *Austral.:* Coversyl; *Belg.:* Coversyl; *Canad.:* Coversyl; *Denm.:* Coversyl; *Fin.:* Coversyl; *Fr.:* Coversyl; *Ger.:* Coversum; *Hong Kong:* Acertil; *Irl.:* Coversyl; *Ital.:* Coversyl; Procaptan; *Jpn:* Coversyl; *Mex.:* Coversyl; *Neth.:* Coversyl; *NZ:* Coversyl; *Port.:* Coversyl; *S.Afr.:* Coversyl; *Singapore:* Coversyl; *Spain:* Coversyl; *Switz.:* Coversum; *Thai.:* Coversyl; *UK:* Coversyl; *USA:* Aceon.

Multi-ingredient: *Fr.:* Bipreterax; Preterax.

The symbol † denotes a preparation no longer actively marketed

Phenindione (4818-t)

Phenindione (BAN, rINN).

Fenindione; Phenylindanedione; Phenylinium. 2-Phenylindan-1,3-dione.

$C_{15}H_{10}O_2 = 222.2$.

CAS — 83-12-5.

ATC — B01AA02.

Pharmacopoeias. In Br. and Fr.

Pharmacopoeial description

BP 2001: Soft, odourless or almost odourless, white or creamy-white crystals. Very slightly soluble in water; slightly soluble in alcohol and in ether; freely soluble in chloroform. Solutions are yellow to red.

Adverse Effects and Treatment

As for Warfarin Sodium, p.992. However, phenindione and the other indanediones are generally more toxic than warfarin with hypersensitivity reactions involving many organs and sometimes resulting in death. Some of the reactions include skin rashes and exfoliative dermatitis, pyrexia, diarrhoea, vomiting, sore throat, liver and kidney damage, myocarditis, agranulocytosis, leucopenia, eosinophilia, and a leukaemoid syndrome. Phenindione may discolour the urine pink or orange and this is independent of any haematuria. Taste disturbances have been reported.

Effects on the gastrointestinal tract. There have been cases of paralytic ileus, one fatal, associated with phenindione.[1,2]

1. Menon IS. Phenindione and paralytic ileus. Lancet 1966; i: 1421–2.
2. Nash AG. Phenindione and paralytic ileus. Lancet 1966; ii: 51–2.

Precautions

As for Warfarin Sodium, p.993.

Phenindione is not recommended in pregnancy. Unlike warfarin significant quantities have been detected in breast milk so it should not be given to breast-feeding women.

Interactions

The interactions associated with oral anticoagulants are described in detail under warfarin (p.993). Specific references to interactions involving phenindione can be found there under the headings for the following drug groups: analgesics; antibacterials; antifungals; antiplatelets; anxiolytic sedatives; gastrointestinal drugs; lipid regulating drugs; and sex hormones.

Pharmacokinetics

Phenindione is absorbed from the gastrointestinal tract. It diffuses across the placenta and is distributed into breast milk. Metabolites of phenindione excreted in the urine are responsible for any discoloration that may occur.

Uses and Administration

Phenindione is an orally administered indanedione anticoagulant with actions similar to those of warfarin (p.998). It is used in the management of thromboembolic disorders (p.816), but because of its higher incidence of severe adverse effects it is now rarely employed.

The usual initial dose of phenindione is 200 mg on the first day, 100 mg on the second day, and then maintenance doses of 50 to 150 mg daily according to coagulation tests.

Preparations

BP 2001: Phenindione Tablets.

Proprietary Preparations (details are given in Part 3)
Austral.: Dindevan; *Fr.:* Pindione; *UK:* Dindevan†.

Phenoxybenzamine Hydrochloride

(892-x)

Phenoxybenzamine Hydrochloride (BANM, rINNM).

SKF-688A. Benzyl(2-chloroethyl)(1-methyl-2-phenoxyethyl)amine hydrochloride.

$C_{18}H_{22}ClNO,HCl = 340.3$.

CAS — 59-96-1 (phenoxybenzamine); 63-92-3 (phenoxybenzamine hydrochloride).

Pharmacopoeias. In Br., Chin., and US.

Pharmacopoeial description

BP 2001: A white or almost white, odourless or almost odourless, crystalline powder. Sparingly soluble in water; freely soluble in alcohol and in chloroform.

Adverse Effects and Treatment

The adverse effects of phenoxybenzamine are primarily due to its alpha-adrenoceptor blocking activity. They include postural hypotension and dizziness, reflex tachycardia, nasal congestion, and miosis. Inhibition of ejaculation may occur. These effects may be minimised by using a low initial dose of phenoxybenzamine, and may diminish with continued administration, but the hypotensive effect can be exaggerated by exercise, heat, a large meal, or alcohol ingestion. Other side-effects include dryness of the mouth, decreased sweating, drowsiness, fatigue, and confusion.

Gastrointestinal effects are usually slight. When phenoxybenzamine is administered intravenously, idiosyncratic profound hypotension can occur within a few minutes of starting the infusion. Convulsions have been reported after rapid intravenous infusion of phenoxybenzamine.

Severe hypotension may occur in overdose and treatment includes support of the circulation by postural measures and parenteral fluid volume replacement. Sympathomimetics are considered to be of little value, and adrenaline [epinephrine] is contra-indicated since it also stimulates beta receptors causing increased hypotension and tachycardia. Sources differ as to the value of noradrenaline [norepinephrine] in overcoming alpha-receptor blockade.

Phenoxybenzamine has been shown to be mutagenic in *in vitro* tests and carcinogenic in *rodents*.

Precautions

Phenoxybenzamine should be given with care to patients with heart failure, ischaemic heart disease, cerebrovascular disease, or renal impairment, and should be avoided if a fall in blood pressure would be dangerous. Phenoxybenzamine may aggravate the symptoms of respiratory infections.

When given intravenously, phenoxybenzamine hydrochloride should always be diluted and given by infusion. Intravenous fluids must always be given beforehand to ensure an adequate circulating blood volume and to prevent a precipitous fall in blood pressure. Care should be taken to avoid extravasation. Contamination of the skin should also be avoided since contact sensitisation may occur.

Porphyria. Phenoxybenzamine is considered to be unsafe in patients with porphyria because it has been shown to be porphyrinogenic in *in-vitro* systems.

Interactions

Since phenoxybenzamine only blocks alpha receptors, leaving the beta receptors unopposed, concomitant administration of drugs such as adrenaline [epinephrine] that also stimulate beta receptors may enhance the cardiac-accelerating and hypotensive action of phenoxybenzamine.

Pharmacokinetics

Phenoxybenzamine is incompletely and variably absorbed from the gastrointestinal tract. The maximum effect is attained in about 1 hour after an intravenous dose. Following oral administration the onset of action is gradual over several hours and persists for 3 or 4 days following a single dose. The plasma half-life is about 24 hours. Phenoxybenzamine is metabolised in the liver and excreted in the urine and bile, but small amounts remain in the body for several days. The duration of action is thought to depend on the rate of synthesis of new alpha receptors following irreversible covalent bonding to existing alpha receptors by a reactive intermediate of phenoxybenzamine.

Uses and Administration

Phenoxybenzamine is a powerful alpha-adrenoceptor blocker (p.787) with a prolonged duration of action; it binds covalently to alpha receptors in smooth muscle to produce an irreversible ('non-competitive') blockade. A single large dose of phenoxybenzamine can cause alpha-adrenoceptor blockade for 3 days or longer.

Phenoxybenzamine is used in the management of phaeochromocytoma (p.810). It has also been employed in severe shock (p.813) and in the treatment of urinary retention (p.459).

Phenoxybenzamine is used as the hydrochloride. It is given by mouth or by intravenous infusion as a dilute solution.

In **phaeochromocytoma** it is used to control the hypertension associated with excessive catecholamine release during the pre-operative period and in patients whose tumours are inoperable. A beta blocker may also be given to control tachycardia, but not before

alpha blockade has completely suppressed the pressor effects of the phaeochromocytoma. The usual initial dose of phenoxybenzamine hydrochloride is 10 mg once or twice daily by mouth, increased gradually, according to the patient's response, to a usual dose of 1 to 2 mg per kg body-weight daily in 2 divided doses. It may be given intravenously for operative cover in patients with phaeochromocytoma in a daily dose of 1 mg per kg in 200 mL of sodium chloride 0.9% infused over at least 2 hours. A similar intravenous dose in 200 to 500 mL of sodium chloride 0.9% has been given in the management of severe **shock**.

For **urinary retention** due to neurogenic bladder a dose of 10 mg twice daily by mouth has been given.

Preparations

BP 2001: Phenoxybenzamine Capsules;
USP 25: Phenoxybenzamine Hydrochloride Capsules.

Proprietary Preparations (details are given in Part 3)
Aust.: Dibenzyran; *Austral.:* Dibenyline; *Belg.:* Dibenyline; *Ger.:* Dibenzyran; *Hong Kong:* Dibenyline; *Israel:* Dibenyline; *Neth.:* Dibenyline; *NZ:* Dibenyline; *UK:* Dibenyline; *USA:* Dibenzyline†.

Phenprocoumon (4819-x)

Phenprocoumon (BAN, USAN, rINN).

Phenylpropylhydroxycoumarin. 4-Hydroxy-3-(1-phenylpropyl)coumarin.

$C_{18}H_{16}O_3 = 280.3$.

CAS — 435-97-2.

ATC — B01AA04.

Adverse Effects, Treatment, and Precautions

As for Warfarin Sodium, p.992.

Effects on the liver. A woman who had twice previously developed jaundice while taking phenprocoumon developed jaundice and parenchymal liver damage when, after some years, phenprocoumon was again given.[1] Two other cases of phenprocoumon-associated hepatitis have been reported.[2]

1. den Boer W, Loeliger EA. Phenprocoumon-induced jaundice. Lancet 1976; i: 912.
2. Slagboom G, Loeliger EA. Coumarin-associated hepatitis: report of two cases. Arch Intern Med 1980; 140: 1028–9.

Interactions

The interactions associated with oral anticoagulants are discussed in detail under warfarin (p.993). Specific references to interactions involving phenprocoumon can be found there under the headings for the following drug groups: analgesics; antiarrhythmics; antidepressants; antidiabetics; antigout drugs; antineoplastics; gastrointestinal drugs; lipid regulating drugs; prostaglandins; and sex hormones.

Pharmacokinetics

Phenprocoumon is readily absorbed from the gastrointestinal tract and is extensively bound to plasma proteins. A half-life of 5 to 6 days has been reported. It is excreted in the urine and faeces as conjugated hydroxy metabolites and parent compound. Phenprocoumon is administered as a racemic mixture; the S-isomer is reported to be more potent. The stereo-isomers have different pharmacokinetics.

◊ References.
1. Husted S, Andreasen F. Individual variation in the response to phenprocoumon. Eur J Clin Pharmacol 1977; 11: 351–8.
2. Toon S, et al. Metabolic fate of phenprocoumon in humans. J Pharm Sci 1985; 74: 1037–40.

Uses and Administration

Phenprocoumon is an orally administered coumarin anticoagulant with actions similar to those of warfarin (p.998). It is used in the management of thromboembolic disorders (p.816). Initial doses of up to 15 mg on the first day followed by up to 9 mg on the second day are used. Maintenance doses are usually from 1.5 to 6 mg daily, depending on the response.

Preparations

Proprietary Preparations (details are given in Part 3)
Aust.: Marcoumar; *Belg.:* Marcoumar; *Braz.:* Marcoumar; *Denm.:* Marcoumar; *Ger.:* Falithrom; Marcumar; marcuphen; Phenpro; *Neth.:* Marcoumar; *Switz.:* Marcoumar.

Phentolamine Mesilate (894-f)

Phentolamine Mesilate (BANM, rINNM).

Phentolamine Mesylate; Phentolamine Methanesulphonate; Phentolamini Mesilas. 3-[N-(2-Imidazolin-2-ylmethyl)-p-toluidino]phenol methanesulphonate.

$C_{17}H_{19}N_3O,CH_4SO_3 = 377.5$.

CAS — 50-60-2 (phentolamine); 73-05-2 (phentolamine hydrochloride); 65-28-1 (phentolamine mesilate).

Pharmacopoeias. In Chin., Eur. (see p.vi), and US.

Pharmacopoeial description

Ph. Eur.: A white, slightly hygroscopic, crystalline powder. Freely soluble in water and in alcohol; practically insoluble in dichloromethane. Store in airtight containers. Protect from light.

USP 25: A white or off-white, odourless crystalline powder. Soluble 1 in 1 of water, 1 in 4 of alcohol, and 1 in 700 of chloroform. Its solutions in water have a pH of about 5 and slowly deteriorate. Store in airtight containers. Protect from light.

Adverse Effects and Treatment

The adverse effects of phentolamine are primarily due to its alpha-adrenoceptor blocking activity and include orthostatic hypotension and tachycardia. Myocardial infarction and cerebrovascular spasm or occlusion have been reported occasionally, usually in association with marked hypotension; flushing, sweating, and feelings of apprehension may accompany hypotensive episodes. Anginal pain and arrhythmias have been reported rarely. Nausea, vomiting, and diarrhoea may also occur. Other side-effects include weakness, dizziness, flushing, and nasal congestion. Hypoglycaemia has been reported following overdosage.

Severe hypotension may occur in overdosage although phentolamine has a short duration of action. Treatment may include keeping the patient's legs raised and the administration of a plasma expander. Noradrenaline [norepinephrine] may be administered cautiously to overcome alpha-adrenoceptor blockade. Adrenaline [epinephrine] is contra-indicated since it also stimulates beta receptors causing increased hypotension and tachycardia.

When injected into the corpus cavernosum of the penis phentolamine has been associated with local pain; induration and fibrosis may occur with repeated use. Priapism has occurred.

Precautions

Phentolamine should not generally be given to patients with angina pectoris or other evidence of ischaemic heart disease. Care should be taken in patients with peptic ulcer disease, which may be exacerbated.

Interactions

Since phentolamine only blocks alpha receptors, concomitant use of drugs such as adrenaline [epinephrine] may lead to severe hypotension and tachycardia due to unopposed beta-adrenoceptor stimulation.

Pharmacokinetics

Following intravenous administration, the half-life of phentolamine has been reported to be 19 minutes. It is extensively metabolised and about 13% of an intravenous dose is excreted unchanged in the urine.

Uses and Administration

Phentolamine is an alpha-adrenoceptor blocker (p.787) which also has a direct action on vascular smooth muscle. It produces vasodilatation, an increase in cardiac output, and has a positive inotropic effect, but is reported to have little effect on the blood pressure of patients with essential hypertension. The alpha-receptor blocking action is reversible ('competitive') and non-selective, and the duration of effect is relatively short.

Phentolamine is given in the management of hypertensive crises due to excessive catecholamine release associated with surgery for phaeochromocytoma (p.810). It has been employed for the differential diagnosis of phaeochromocytoma, but has largely been superseded by estimations of catecholamines in blood and urine.

Phentolamine is also used to prevent or treat dermal necrosis and sloughing associated with the intravenous infusion or extravasation of noradrenaline [norepinephrine]. It has been used in the treatment of erectile dysfunction (p.1663).

Phentolamine is given by injection as the mesilate.

In patients with hypertensive crises during surgery for **phaeochromocytoma**, a dose of 2 to 5 mg of phentolamine mesilate is given intravenously and repeated if necessary; blood pressure should be monitored. A dose of 1 mg intravenously is used for children. The intramuscular route may be used pre-operatively and for diagnostic procedures.

For prevention of **dermal necrosis** during intravenous infusion of noradrenaline [norepinephrine], 10 mg of phentolamine mesilate is added to each litre of solution containing noradrenaline [norepinephrine]. For treatment following extravasation of noradrenaline [norepinephrine], 5 to 10 mg of phentolamine mesilate in 10 mL of sodium chloride 0.9% is injected into the affected area.

Injections of phentolamine mesilate, usually in association with papaverine, into the corpora cavernosa of the penis, have been used in the treatment of **erectile dysfunction**. Other approaches that are under investigation include administration by the oral route and intracavernosal use in combination with vasoactive intestinal polypeptide.

Pancreatic pain. Pain due to pancreatitis (p.7) is usually treated with opioid analgesics. Long-term relief of pain has been reported in a patient with chronic pancreatitis following an intravenous infusion of phentolamine.[1]

1. McCleane GJ. Phentolamine abolishes the pain of chronic pancreatitis. *Br J Hosp Med* 1996; **55:** 521.

Preparations

BP 2001: Phentolamine Injection;
USP 25: Phentolamine Mesylate for Injection.

Proprietary Preparations (details are given in Part 3)
Austral.: Regitine; *Belg.:* Regitine; *Canad.:* Regitine; *Denm.:* Regitin; *Hong Kong:* Q-Tech; *Israel:* Regitine; *Mex.:* Z-Max; *Neth.:* Regitine; *NZ:* Regitine; *S.Afr.:* Regitine; *Switz.:* Regitine; *UK:* Rogitine; *USA:* Regitine.

Multi-ingredient: *Aust.:* Androskat; *Neth.:* Androskat.

Pholedrine Sulfate   (2096-p)

Pholedrine Sulfate (rINNM).

Isodrine Sulphate; Pholedrine Sulphate (BANM); Sympropaminum (pholedrine). 4-(2-Methylaminopropyl)phenol sulphate.
$(C_{10}H_{15}NO)_2,H_2SO_4 = 428.5.$
CAS — 370-14-9 (pholedrine); 6114-26-7 (pholedrine sulfate).

Profile

Pholedrine is a sympathomimetic (see Adrenaline, p.829) given by mouth as the sulfate in combination with other drugs in the treatment of hypotensive states. It is also an ingredient of preparations promoted for vascular disorders.

Preparations

Proprietary Preparations (details are given in Part 3)
Multi-ingredient: *Ger.:* Adyston; Zellaforte N Plus; *Spain:* Venosan; *Switz.:* Ortho-Maren retard; Venosan†.

Picotamide   (3939-x)

Picotamide (BAN).

G-137; Picotamidum Monohydricum. 4-Methoxy-N,N'-bis(3-pyridinylmethyl)-1,3-benzenedicarboxamide monohydrate.
$C_{21}H_{20}N_4O_3,H_2O = 394.4.$
CAS — 32828-81-2 (anhydrous picotamide); 80530-63-8 (picotamide monohydrate); 86247-87-2 (picotamide tartrate).
ATC — B01AC03.

Pharmacopoeias. In *Eur.* (see p.vi).

Pharmacopoeial description

Ph. Eur.: A white or almost white, polymorphic, crystalline powder. Slightly soluble in water; soluble in dehydrated alcohol and in dichloromethane; dissolves in dilute mineral acids.

Profile

Picotamide is a thromboxane synthase inhibitor and thromboxane receptor antagonist with antiplatelet activity. It is given by mouth in thromboembolic disorders (p.816) in initial doses of 900 to 1200 mg daily in divided doses, reducing to a maintenance dose of 300 to 600 mg daily.

ACE inhibitor-induced cough. Cough is a recognised adverse effect of ACE inhibitor administration and has been treated with a number of drugs (see p.820). Administration of picotamide led to the disappearance of cough in 8 of 9 patients receiving enalapril for hypertension,[1] suggesting that thromboxanes may be involved in the aetiology of ACE inhibitor-induced cough.

1. Malini PL, *et al.* Thromboxane antagonism and cough induced by angiotensin-converting-enzyme inhibitor. *Lancet* 1997; **350:** 15–18.

Preparations

Proprietary Preparations (details are given in Part 3)
Ital.: Plactidil.

Pilsicainide Hydrochloride   (991-d)

Pilsicainide Hydrochloride (rINNM).

SUN-1165. Tetrahydro-1H-pyrrolizine-7a(5H)-aceto-2',6'-xylidide hydrochloride.
$C_{17}H_{24}N_2O,HCl = 308.8.$
CAS — 88069-67-4 (pilsicainide); 88069-49-2 (pilsicainide hydrochloride).

Profile

Pilsicainide hydrochloride is an antiarrhythmic with class Ic activity (p.787).

◊ References.
1. Takabatake T, *et al.* Pharmacokinetics of SUN 1165, a new antiarrhythmic agent, in renal dysfunction. *Eur J Clin Pharmacol* 1991; **40:** 411–14.
2. Okishige K, *et al.* Pilsicainide for conversion and maintenance of sinus rhythm in chronic atrial fibrillation: a placebo-controlled, multicenter study. *Am Heart J* 2000; **140:** 437–44.
3. Kumagai K, *et al.* Single oral administration of pilsicainide versus infusion of disopyramide for termination of paroxysmal atrial fibrillation: a multicenter trial. *Pacing Clin Electrophysiol* 2000; **23:** 1880–2.

Preparations

Proprietary Preparations (details are given in Part 3)
Jpn: Sunrythm.

Pimobendan   (19663-m)

Pimobendan (USAN, rINN).

UDCG-115. 4,5-Dihydro-6-[2-(p-methyoxyphenyl)-5-benzimidazolyl]-5-methyl-3(2H)-pyridazinone.
$C_{19}H_{18}N_4O_2 = 334.4.$
CAS — 74150-27-9; 118428-36-7.

Profile

Pimobendan is a phosphodiesterase inhibitor with calcium-sensitising properties. It has positive inotropic and vasodilator activity and is used as an adjunct to standard therapy in the management of heart failure (p.798). It is given orally in a dose of 1.25 to 2.5 mg twice daily.

Studies with other inotropic phosphodiesterase inhibitors have shown that their prolonged oral use can increase the mortality rate.

◊ References.
1. Przechera M, *et al.* Pharmacokinetic profile and tolerability of pimobendan in patients with terminal renal insufficiency. *Eur J Clin Pharmacol* 1991; **40:** 107–11.
2. The Pimobendan in Congestive Heart Failure (PICO) Investigators. Effect of pimobendan on exercise capacity in patients with heart failure: main results from the Pimobendan in Congestive Heart Failure (PICO) trial. *Heart* 1996; **76:** 223–31.

Preparations

Proprietary Preparations (details are given in Part 3)
Jpn: Acardi.

Pinacidil   (16954-y)

Pinacidil (USAN, rINN).

P-1134.   (±)-2-Cyano-1-(4-pyridyl)-3-(1,2,2-trimethylpropyl)guanidine.
$C_{13}H_{19}N_5 = 245.3.$
CAS — 60560-33-0 (anhydrous pinacidil); 85371-64-8 (pinacidil monohydrate).
ATC — C02DG01.

Profile

Pinacidil is a potassium-channel opener (p.790) that produces direct peripheral vasodilatation of the arterioles. It has been used in the management of hypertension. It reduces blood pressure and peripheral resistance and produces fluid retention. Tachycardia and an increase in cardiac output occur mainly as a reflex response to the reduction in peripheral resistance.

◊ Reviews.
1. Friedel HA, Brogden RN. Pinacidil: a review of its pharmacodynamic and pharmacokinetic properties, and therapeutic potential in the treatment of hypertension. *Drugs* 1990; **39:** 929–67.

Preparations

Proprietary Preparations (details are given in Part 3)
Denm.: Pindac†; *Irl.:* Pindac†.

Pindolol   (6319-c)

Pindolol (BAN, USAN, rINN).

LB-46; Pindololum; Prindolol; Prinodolol. 1-(Indol-4-yloxy)-3-isopropylaminopropan-2-ol.
$C_{14}H_{20}N_2O_2 = 248.3.$
CAS — 13523-86-9.
ATC — C07AA03.

Pharmacopoeias. In *Eur.* (see p.vi), *Jpn*, and *US*.

Pharmacopoeial description

Ph. Eur.: A white or almost white, crystalline powder. Practically insoluble in water; slightly soluble in methyl alcohol; dissolves in dilute mineral acids. Protect from light.

USP 25: A white to off-white, crystalline powder with a faint odour. Practically insoluble in water; very slightly soluble in chloroform; slightly soluble in methyl alcohol. Protect from light.

Adverse Effects, Treatment, and Precautions

As for beta blockers, p.844.

Effects on lipid metabolism. Beta blockers can affect plasma-lipid concentrations, although these effects may be less pronounced with beta blockers having intrinsic sympathomimetic activity (p.845). Use of pindolol in patients with hypertension is not associated with any increases in total plasma-cholesterol concentrations or falls in high-density lipoprotein fraction.[1,2]

1. Hunter Hypertension Research Group. Effects of pindolol, or a pindolol/clopamide combination preparation, on plasma lipid levels in essential hypertension. *Med J Aust* 1989; **150:** 646–52.
2. Terént A, *et al.* Long-term effect of pindolol on lipids and lipoproteins in men with newly diagnosed hypertension. *Eur J Clin Pharmacol* 1989; **36:** 347–50.

Tremor. Fine tremor in the extremities of 5 patients during pindolol therapy was considered to have been due to its partial agonist activity.[1]

1. Hod H, *et al.* Pindolol-induced tremor. *Postgrad Med J* 1980; **56:** 346–7.

Interactions

The interactions associated with beta blockers are discussed on p.846.

Pharmacokinetics

Pindolol is almost completely absorbed from the gastrointestinal tract and peak plasma concentrations are obtained about 1 to 2 hours after an oral dose. About 40 to 60% is reported to be bound to plasma proteins. It is moderately lipid-soluble. Pindolol is distributed into breast milk. It is only partially metabolised in the liver and is excreted in the urine both unchanged and in the form of metabolites. A plasma elimination half-life of 3 to 4 hours has been reported in healthy adults. The half-life may be prolonged in elderly hypertensive patients and in patients with renal or hepatic impairment.

Uses and Administration

Pindolol is a non-cardioselective beta blocker (p.844). It is reported to have intrinsic sympathomimetic activity but little membrane-stabilising activity.

Pindolol is used in the management of hypertension (p.802), angina pectoris (p.791), and other cardiovascular disorders. It is also used in glaucoma (p.1413).

In **hypertension** pindolol is usually given initially in a dosage of 5 mg two or three times daily by mouth, subsequently increased according to the patient's response; additional benefit is rarely obtained from doses higher than 45 mg daily, although doses up to 60 mg daily have been given. A once-daily dosage regimen has been reported to be adequate for some patients.

The usual dose for **angina pectoris** is 2.5 to 5 mg up to three times daily; however, doses of up to 10 mg three times daily have been used.

Pindolol eye drops in concentrations of 0.5 to 1% are used in the management of **glaucoma**.

Depression. Pindolol has been studied as an augmentation agent with serotonergic antidepressants in the treatment of refractory depression (p.271).

References.

1. Artigas F, *et al.* Pindolol induces a rapid improvement of depressed patients treated with serotonin reuptake inhibitors. *Arch Gen Psychiatry* 1994; **51:** 248–51.
2. Blier P, Bergeron R. Effectiveness of pindolol with selected antidepressant drugs in the treatment of major depression. *J Clin Psychopharmacol* 1995; **15:** 217–22.
3. Pérez V, *et al.* Randomised, double-blind, placebo-controlled trial of pindolol in combination with fluoxetine antidepressant treatment. *Lancet* 1997; **349:** 1594–7.
4. Maes M, *et al.* Pindolol and mianserin augment the antidepressant activity of fluoxetine in hospitalized major depressed patients, including those with treatment resistance. *J Clin Psychopharmacol* 1999; **19:** 177–82.

Orthostatic hypotension. Many drugs have been tried in the management of orthostatic hypotension (p.1070) although none is entirely satisfactory. The successful treatment of 4 patients, with severe orthostatic hypotension because of chronic autonomic failure, with pindolol has been reported.[1] However, pindolol was of no benefit in 5 patients with postural hypotension due to autonomic failure associated with multiple system atrophy.[2] Others[3] have also reported lack of effect.

1. Man in't Veld AJ, *et al.* Effects of β-adrenoceptor agonists and antagonists in patients with peripheral autonomic neuropathy. *Br J Clin Pharmacol* 1982; **13:** 367S–74S.
2. Davies B, *et al.* Pindolol in postural hypotension: the case for caution. *Lancet* 1981; **ii:** 982–3.
3. Goldstraw P, Waller DG. Pindolol in orthostatic hypotension. *BMJ* 1981; **283:** 310.

Preparations

BP 2001: Pindolol Tablets;
USP 25: Pindolol Tablets.

Proprietary Preparations (details are given in Part 3)
Aust.: Visken; *Austral.:* Barbloc; Visken; *Belg.:* Visken; *Braz.:* Visken; *Canad.:* Apo-Pindol; Novo-Pindol; Nu-Pindol; Visken; *Denm.:* Hexapindol; Visken; *Fin.:* Pindocor; Pinloc; Visken; *Fr.:* Visken; *Ger.:* durapindol; Glauco-Stulln; Pindoptan; Pindorealt; Visken; *Hong Kong:* Visken; *Irl.:* Visken; *Israel:* Pinden; Visken; *Ital.:* Visken; *Neth.:* Viskeen; *Norw.:* Hexapindolt; Viskent; *NZ:* Pindol; Visken; *S.Afr.:* Visken; *Swed.:* Hexapindolt; Visken; *Switz.:* Betapindol; Viskene; *Thai.:* Pinsken; *UK:* Visken; *USA:* Visken.

Multi-ingredient: *Aust.:* Viskaldix; Viskenit; *Belg.:* Viskaldix; *Braz.:* Viskaldix; *Canad.:* Viskazide; *Fr.:* Viskaldix; *Ger.:* Viskaldix; *Irl.:* Viskaldix; *Neth.:* Viskaldix; *NZ:* Viskaldix; *Switz.:* Viskaldix; *Thai.:* Viskaldix; *UK:* Viskaldix.

Pipratecol (9274-x)

Pipratecol (rINN).

711-SE. 1-(3,4-Dihydroxyphenyl)-2-[4-(2-methoxyphenyl)piperazin-1-yl]ethanol.
$C_{19}H_{24}N_2O_4 = 344.4$.
CAS — 15534-05-1.

Profile

Pipratecol is a vasodilator that has been given in conjunction with raubasine (p.967) in the treatment of cerebrovascular disorders.

Piretanide (13130-a)

Piretanide (BAN, USAN, rINN).

Hoe-118; Piretanidum; S73-4118. 4-Phenoxy-3-(pyrrolidin-1-yl)-5-sulphamoylbenzoic acid.
$C_{17}H_{18}N_2O_5S = 362.4$.
CAS — 55837-27-9.
ATC — C03CA03.
Pharmacopoeias. In *Eur.* (see p.vi).

Pharmacopoeial description

Ph. Eur.: A yellowish-white to yellowish powder. It exhibits polymorphism. Very slightly soluble in water; sparingly soluble in dehydrated alcohol. Protect from light.

Adverse Effects

As for Frusemide, p.893. Muscle cramps have been reported following high doses of piretanide.

Precautions

Piretanide's precautions and contra-indications, which are dependent on its effects on fluid and electrolyte balance, are similar to those of the thiazide diuretics (see Hydrochlorothiazide, p.909). Patients with impaired micturition or prostatic hyperplasia may develop retention of urine with piretanide.

Interactions

As for Frusemide, p.894.

Pharmacokinetics

Piretanide has been reported to be almost completely absorbed following oral administration. It is extensively bound to plasma proteins, and is reported to have a half-life of about 1 hour.

◊ References.

1. Beermann B, Grind M. Clinical pharmacokinetics of some newer diuretics. *Clin Pharmacokinet* 1987; **13:** 254–66.

Uses and Administration

Piretanide is a loop diuretic with actions and uses similar to those of frusemide [furosemide] (p.895). In the treatment of hypertension (p.802) it is given in a usual dose of 6 to 12 mg daily by mouth. The sodium salt is given by injection.

◊ References.

1. Clissold SP, Brogden RN. Piretanide: a preliminary review of its pharmacodynamic and pharmacokinetic properties, and therapeutic efficacy. *Drugs* 1985; **29:** 489–530.

Preparations

Proprietary Preparations (details are given in Part 3)
Aust.: Arelix; *Braz.:* Arelix; *Fr.:* Eurelix; *Ger.:* Arelix; *Irl.:* Arelix; *Ital.:* Tauliz; *Mex.:* Diural; *S.Afr.:* Arelix; *Spain:* Midatent; Perbilen; *Switz.:* Arelix; Pirenext; *UK:* Arelixt.

Multi-ingredient: *Aust.:* Trialix; *Ger.:* Arelix ACE; Betarelix; *Irl.:* Trialix; *Ital.:* Prilace; *Switz.:* Trialix.

Pirifibrate (13134-f)

Pirifibrate (rINN).

EL-466. 6-Hydroxymethyl-2-pyridylmethyl 2-(4-chlorophenoxy)-2-methylpropionate.
$C_{17}H_{18}ClNO_4 = 335.8$.
CAS — 55285-45-5.

Profile

Pirifibrate, a fibric acid derivative (see Bezafibrate, p.849), is a lipid regulating drug used in the treatment of hyperlipidaemias (p.800). The usual dose is 750 mg twice daily by mouth.

Preparations

Proprietary Preparations (details are given in Part 3)
Spain: Bratenol.

Pirmenol Hydrochloride (16955-j)

Pirmenol Hydrochloride (USAN, rINNM).

CI-845. (±)-cis-2,6-Dimethyl-α-phenyl-α-2-pyridyl-1-piperidinebutanol hydrochloride.
$C_{22}H_{30}N_2O,HCl = 374.9$.
CAS — 68252-19-7 (pirmenol); 61477-94-9 (pirmenol hydrochloride).

Profile

Pirmenol hydrochloride is an antiarrhythmic with class Ia activity (p.787).

◊ References.

1. Hampton EM, *et al.* Initial and long-term outpatient experience with pirmenol for control of ventricular arrhythmias. *Eur J Clin Pharmacol* 1986; **31:** 15–22.
2. Stringer KA, *et al.* Enhanced pirmenol elimination by rifampin. *J Clin Pharmacol* 1988; **28:** 1094–7.
3. Janiczek N, *et al.* Pharmacokinetics of pirmenol enantiomers and pharmacodynamics of pirmenol racemate in patients with premature ventricular contractions. *J Clin Pharmacol* 1997; **37:** 502–13.

Pirozadil (3912-s)

Pirozadil (rINN).

722-D. 2,6-Pyridinediyldimethylene bis(3,4,5-trimethoxybenzoate).
$C_{27}H_{29}NO_{10} = 527.5$.
CAS — 54110-25-7.

Profile

Pirozadil, a nicotinic acid derivative, is a lipid regulating drug that has been used in the treatment of hyperlipidaemias.

◊ Pirozadil has been shown to reduce total and low-density lipoprotein-cholesterol concentrations in patients with hypercholesterolaemias.[1,2] Adverse effects in 2 of 15 patients[1] included oedema, palpitations, and numbness of the extremities. This latter effect was sufficiently severe to necessitate withdrawal of treatment in 1 patient.

1. Shinomiya M, *et al.* Effect of pirozadil on lipids, lipoproteins and apolipoproteins in Japanese with type IIa hyperlipoproteinaemia. *Arzneimittelforschung* 1987; **37:** 1069–71.
2. Masana L, *et al.* Treatment of diet-resistant polygenic hypercholesterolaemic patients with a new nicotinate derivative: in vivo and in vitro low density lipoprotein metabolic studies. *J Clin Pharmacol* 1989; **29:** 201–6.

Preparations

Proprietary Preparations (details are given in Part 3)
Spain: Pemix†.

Plafibride (13139-b)

Plafibride (rINN).

ITA-104. 1-[2-(4-Chlorophenoxy)-2-methylpropionyl]-3-morpholinomethylurea.
$C_{16}H_{22}ClN_3O_4 = 355.8$.
CAS — 63394-05-8.

Profile

Plafibride, a fibric acid derivative (see Bezafibrate, p.849), is a lipid regulating drug that has been used in the treatment of hyperlipidaemias.

Plasminogen (13140-x)

Plasminogen (BAN).

CAS — 9001-91-6.

Profile

Plasminogen is the specific substance derived from plasma which, when activated to fibrinolysin, has the property of lysing fibrinogen, fibrin, and some other proteins. Its role in the control of haemostasis is described further on p.718. Plasminogen has been investigated as a thrombolytic and has been used in combination with other blood products in wound-sealant preparations.

Preparations

Proprietary Preparations (details are given in Part 3)
Multi-ingredient: _Aust.:_ Tissucol; Tissucol Duo Quick; **_Canad.:_** Tisseel; Tisseel Duo Quick; **_Denm.:_** Tisseel Duo Quick; **_Fin.:_** Tisseel Duo Quick; **_Ger.:_** Tissucol Duo S; Tissucol Fibrinkleber tiefgefroren†; Tissucol-Kit; **_Hong Kong:_** Tisseel; **_Israel:_** Tisseel; **_Spain:_** Tissucol; **_Swed.:_** Tisseel Duo Quick; **_Switz.:_** Tissucol; Tissucol Duo S; **_UK:_** Tisseel.

Polythiazide   (2352-p)

Polythiazide (BAN, USAN, rINN).
NSC-108161; P-2525. 6-Chloro-3,4-dihydro-2-methyl-3-(2,2,2-trifluoroethylthiomethyl)-2H-1,2,4-benzothiadiazine-7-sulphonamide 1,1-dioxide.
$C_{11}H_{13}ClF_3N_3O_4S_3 = 439.9.$
CAS — 346-18-9.
ATC — C03AA05.
Pharmacopoeias. In Br.

Pharmacopoeial description

BP 2001: A white or almost white, crystalline powder with an alliaceous odour. Practically insoluble in water and in chloroform; sparingly soluble in alcohol.

Adverse Effects, Treatment, and Precautions

As for Hydrochlorothiazide, p.907.

Interactions

As for Hydrochlorothiazide, p.909.

Pharmacokinetics

Polythiazide is fairly readily absorbed from the gastrointestinal tract. It has been estimated to have a plasma elimination half-life of about 26 hours. More than 80% may be bound to plasma proteins. It is excreted mainly in the urine as unchanged polythiazide and metabolites.

◊ References.
1. Hobbs DC, Twomey TM. Kinetics of polythiazide. *Clin Pharmacol Ther* 1978; **23:** 241–6.

Uses and Administration

Polythiazide is a thiazide diuretic with actions and uses similar to those of hydrochlorothiazide (p.910). It is used for oedema, including that associated with heart failure (p.798), and for hypertension (p.802).

Diuresis is initiated within about 2 hours after administration, and lasts for 24 to 48 hours.

In the treatment of **oedema** the usual dose is 1 to 4 mg by mouth daily. In the treatment of **hypertension** the usual dose is stated to be 2 to 4 mg daily, either alone or in conjunction with other antihypertensives although doses of only 0.5 to 1 mg may be adequate.

Preparations

BP 2001: Polythiazide Tablets.
Proprietary Preparations (details are given in Part 3)
Belg.: Renese; **_Irl.:_** Nephril; **_UK:_** Nephril; **_USA:_** Renese.
Multi-ingredient: _Ger.:_ Polypress; **_USA:_** Minizide; Renese R.

Potassium Canrenoate   (2313-n)

Potassium Canrenoate (BANM, rINN).
Aldadiene Potassium; Canrenoate Potassium (USAN); MF-465a; SC-14266. Potassium 17-hydroxy-3-oxo-17α-pregna-4,6-diene-21-carboxylate.
$C_{22}H_{29}KO_4 = 396.6.$
CAS — 4138-96-9 (canrenoic acid); 2181-04-6 (potassium canrenoate).
ATC — C03DA02.
Pharmacopoeias. In Jpn.

Adverse Effects and Precautions

As for Spironolactone, p.973. Irritation or pain may occur at the site of injection.

Effects on endocrine function. A lower incidence of gynaecomastia has been reported in patients with hepatic cirrhosis and ascites during treatment with potassium canrenoate compared with equivalent doses of spironolactone[1] and spironolactone-induced gynaecomastia disappeared when spironolactone was replaced by potassium canrenoate in a patient with hyperaldosteronism.[2] This suggests that metabolites other than canrenone (a common metabolite of both canrenoate and spironolactone thought to be responsible for their activity)

or possibly spironolactone itself may be responsible for the anti-androgenic effects of spironolactone.[3,4]

1. Bellati G, Idéo G. Gynaecomastia after spironolactone and potassium canrenoate. *Lancet* 1986; **i:** 626.
2. Dupont A. Disappearance of spironolactone-induced gynaecomastia during treatment with potassium canrenoate. *Lancet* 1985; **ii:** 731.
3. Gardiner P. Spironolactone and potassium canrenoate metabolism. *Lancet* 1985; **ii:** 1432.
4. Overdiek JWPM, Merkus FWHM. Spironolactone metabolism and gynaecomastia. *Lancet* 1986; **i:** 1103.

Interactions

As for Spironolactone, p.974.

Uses and Administration

Potassium canrenoate is a potassium-sparing diuretic with actions and uses similar to those of spironolactone (p.974). Canrenone (p.853) is a metabolite common to both drugs, but its contribution to the pharmacological action is unclear. Potassium canrenoate is used in the treatment of refractory oedema associated with heart failure (p.798) or hepatic disease when an injectable aldosterone antagonist is required. It may be given in doses of 200 to 400 mg daily, increasing to 800 mg daily in exceptional cases, by slow intravenous injection over a period of 2 to 3 minutes per 200 mg or by intravenous infusion in glucose 5% or sodium chloride 0.9%.

Preparations

Proprietary Preparations (details are given in Part 3)
Aust.: Aldactone; Osiren; **_Belg.:_** Canrenol; Soldactone; **_Denm.:_** Soldactone; **_Fin.:_** Soldactone; **_Fr.:_** Soldactone; **_Ger.:_** Aldactone; Kalium-Can; Osyrol; **_Ital.:_** Kanrenol; Luvion; Venactone; **_Neth.:_** Soldactone; **_Norw.:_** Soldactone; **_Swed.:_** Soldactone; **_Switz.:_** Soldactone; Spiroctan; **_UK:_** Spiroctan-M†.
Multi-ingredient: _Ital.:_ Kadiur.

Practolol   (6320-s)

Practolol (BAN, USAN, pINN).
AY-21011; ICI-50172. 4′-(2-Hydroxy-3-isopropylaminopropoxy)acetanilide.
$C_{14}H_{22}N_2O_3 = 266.3.$
CAS — 6673-35-4.
ATC — C07AB01.

Profile

Practolol is a cardioselective beta blocker (p.844). It is reported to possess intrinsic sympathomimetic activity. Its use was restricted by its serious adverse effects, in particular the potentially fatal 'oculomucocutaneous syndrome' comprising serious adverse effects on the skin, eyes, and mucous membranes, deafness, systemic lupus erythematosus, and sclerosing peritonitis.

Prajmalium Bitartrate   (7790-n)

Prajmalium Bitartrate (BAN, rINN).
GT-1012; NPAB. N-Propylajmalinium hydrogen tartrate.
$C_{23}H_{33}N_2O_2,C_4H_5O_6 = 518.6.$
CAS — 35080-11-6 (prajmalium); 2589-47-1 (prajmalium bitartrate).

Adverse Effects and Precautions

As for Ajmaline, p.833.

Effects on the liver. Cholestatic jaundice associated with pruritus, chills, and eosinophilia[1] was attributed to an allergic reaction to prajmalium bitartrate in a patient 20 days after the start of treatment.

1. Rotmensch HH, et al. Cholestatic jaundice: an immune response to prajmalium bitartrate. *Postgrad Med J* 1980; **56:** 738–41.

Effects on mental state. Confusion and disorientation in time and place[1] occurred on 2 occasions in a 67-year-old man given prajmalium bitartrate 100 mg daily for the control of tachycardia; the confusion rapidly disappeared when prajmalium was withdrawn.

1. Lessing JB, Copperman IJ. Severe cerebral confusion produced by prajmalium bitartrate. *BMJ* 1977; **2:** 675.

Uses and Administration

Prajmalium is a class I antiarrhythmic (p.787) and is the N-propyl derivative of ajmaline (p.833). It is given by mouth as the bitartrate in the management of supraventricular and ventricular arrhythmias (p.794) in initial doses of 60 to 80 mg daily. Maintenance doses of 20 to 40 mg daily in divided doses are used.

Preparations

Proprietary Preparations (details are given in Part 3)
Aust.: Neo-Gilurytmal; **_Ger.:_** Neo-Gilurytmal; **_Israel:_** Neo-Gilurythmal; Neorythmin; **_Ital.:_** Neo Aritmina†; **_Spain:_** Neo-Gilurytmal.

Multi-ingredient: _Spain:_ Cresophene.

Pravastatin Sodium   (3758-z)

Pravastatin Sodium (BANM, USAN, rINNM).
CS-514; Eptastatin Sodium; 3β-Hydroxycompactin Sodium; SQ-31000. Sodium (3R,5R)-7-{(1S,2S,6S,8S,8aR)-1,2,6,7,8,8a-hexahydro-6-hydroxy-2-methyl-8-[(S)-2-methylbutyryloxy]-1-naphthyl}-3,5-dihydroxyheptanoate.
$C_{23}H_{35}O_7Na = 446.5.$
CAS — 81093-37-0 (pravastatin); 81131-70-6 (pravastatin sodium).

Adverse Effects and Precautions

As for Simvastatin, p.969.

Effects on mental function. For comments on the depressive symptoms reported in patients receiving statins, including pravastatin, see under Simvastatin, p.969.

Effects on the nervous system. For a report of paraesthesias associated with pravastatin therapy, see under Lovastatin, p.923.

Effects on skeletal muscle. Muscle disorders are well-recognised adverse effects of lipid regulating drugs such as the fibrates and statins (see under Simvastatin, p.970).

An inflammatory myopathy resembling dermatomyositis developed in a woman treated for 5 months with pravastatin.[1]

1. Schalke BB, et al. Pravastatin-associated inflammatory myopathy. *N Engl J Med* 1992; **327:** 649–50.

Interactions

The interactions of statins with other drugs are described under simvastatin (p.970). However, similar interactions appear not to have been reported with pravastatin although caution is advised when using such combinations.

◊ General reviews.
1. Garnett WR. Interactions with hydroxymethylglutaryl-coenzyme A reductase inhibitors. *Am J Health-Syst Pharm* 1995; **52:** 1639–45.

Pharmacokinetics

Pravastatin, unlike simvastatin or lovastatin, is active without the need for hydrolysis. Following absorption from the gastrointestinal tract it undergoes extensive first-pass metabolism in the liver, its primary site of action. The absolute bioavailability of pravastatin is 17%. Approximately 50% of the circulating drug is bound to plasma proteins. The plasma elimination half-life of pravastatin is 1.5 to 2 hours. About 70% of pravastatin is excreted in the faeces via the bile and about 20% is excreted in the urine.

◊ General reviews.
1. Quion JAV, Jones PH. Clinical pharmacokinetics of pravastatin. *Clin Pharmacokinet* 1994; **27:** 94–103.
2. Desager J-P, Horsmans Y. Clinical pharmacokinetics of 3-hydroxy-3-methylglutaryl-coenzyme A reductase inhibitors. *Clin Pharmacokinet* 1996; **31:** 348–71.
3. Lennernäs H, Fager G. Pharmacodynamics and pharmacokinetics of the HMG-CoA reductase inhibitors: similarities and differences. *Clin Pharmacokinet* 1997; **32:** 403–25.

Uses and Administration

Pravastatin, a 3-hydroxy-3-methylglutaryl coenzyme A (HMG-CoA) reductase inhibitor (a statin), is a lipid regulating drug with actions on plasma lipids similar to those of simvastatin (p.970).

Pravastatin is used to reduce LDL-cholesterol, apolipoprotein B, and triglycerides in the treatment of hyperlipidaemias (below), including hypercholesterolaemias and combined (mixed) hyperlipidaemia (type IIa or IIb hyperlipoproteinaemias), hypertriglyceridaemia (type IV), and dysbetalipoproteinaemia (type III). It is also given prophylactically to hypercholesterolaemic patients for both primary and secondary prevention of ischaemic heart disease. It is also used in patients with a previous myocardial infarction or unstable angina to reduce the risk of stroke.

Pravastatin is given by mouth as the sodium salt in usual doses of 10 to 40 mg once daily at bedtime. The dose may be adjusted at intervals of not less than 4 weeks.

◊ General reviews.
1. Raasch RH. Pravastatin sodium, a new HMG-CoA reductase inhibitor. *DICP Ann Pharmacother* 1991; **25:** 388–94.
2. McTavish D, Sorkin EM. Pravastatin: a review of its pharmacological properties and therapeutic potential in hypercholesterolaemia. *Drugs* 1991; **42:** 65–89.
3. Jungnickel PW, et al. Pravastatin: a new drug for the treatment of hypercholesterolemia. *Clin Pharm* 1992; **11:** 677–89.

The symbol † denotes a preparation no longer actively marketed

4. Schectman G, Hiatt J. Dose–response characteristics of choles-
terol-lowering drug therapies: implications for treatment. *Ann Intern Med* 1996; **125**: 990–1000.
5. Haria M, McTavish D. Pravastatin: a reappraisal of its pharma-
cological properties and clinical effectiveness in the management of coronary heart disease. *Drugs* 1997; **53**: 299–336.

Hyperlipidaemias. Pravastatin, like other statins, is used in the treatment of hyperlipidaemias (p.800) and a general discussion of the effects of statins can be found in simvastatin (p.970).

Pravastatin is effective for the treatment of primary hypercholesterolaemia; it lowers low-density lipoprotein (LDL)-choles-
terol concentrations and also increases high-density lipoprotein (HDL)-cholesterol.[1] Hypercholesterolaemia is a risk factor for **ischaemic heart disease** and pravastatin has been shown to have a protective effect in men with moderate hypercholesterolaemia and no history of myocardial infarction.[2-4] Benefit has also been demonstrated for secondary prevention in patients with average cholesterol concentrations.[5-7] Lowering lipid con-
centrations in patients with previous myocardial infarction[7,8] or unstable angina[7] has also reduced the frequency of **stroke**.

1. Rubenfire M, *et al.* The effect of pravastatin on plasma lipopro-
tein and apolipoprotein levels in primary hypercholesterolemia. *Arch Intern Med* 1991; **151**: 2234–40.
2. Shepherd J, *et al.* Prevention of coronary heart disease with prav-
astatin in men with hypercholesterolemia. *N Engl J Med* 1995; **333**: 1301–7.
3. West of Scotland Coronary Prevention Group. West of Scotland Coronary Prevention Study: identification of high-risk groups and comparison with other cardiovascular intervention trials. *Lancet* 1996; **348**: 1339–42.
4. West of Scotland Coronary Prevention Study Group. Influence of pravastatin and plasma lipids on clinical events in the West of Scotland Coronary Prevention Study (WOSCOPS). *Circulation* 1998; **97**: 1440–5.
5. Sacks FM, *et al.* The effect of pravastatin on coronary events after myocardial infarction in patients with average cholesterol levels. *N Engl J Med* 1996; **335**: 1001–9.
6. Sacks FM, *et al.* Relationship between plasma LDL concentra-
tions during treatment with pravastatin and recurrent coronary events in the Cholesterol and Recurrent Events Trial. *Circulation* 1998; **97**: 1446–52.
7. The Long-Term Intervention with Pravastatin in Ischaemic Dis-
ease (LIPID) Study Group. Prevention of cardiovascular events and death with pravastatin in patients with coronary heart disease and a broad range of initial cholesterol levels. *N Engl J Med* 1998; **339**: 1349–57.
8. Plehn JF, *et al.* Reduction of stroke incidence after myocardial infarction with pravastatin: the Cholesterol and Recurrent Events (CARE) study. *Circulation* 1999; **99**: 216–23.

Preparations

Proprietary Preparations (details are given in Part 3)
Aust.: Pravachol; Sanaprav; Selipran; **Austral.:** Pravachol; **Belg.:** Pravasine; **Braz.:** Pravacol; **Canad.:** Pravachol; **Denm.:** Prava-
chol; **Fin.:** Pravachol; **Fr.:** Elisor; Vasten; **Ger.:** Liprevil; Mevalo-
tin; Pravasin; **Hong Kong:** Pravachol; **Irl.:** Lipostat; **Israel:** Lipi-
dal; Lipostat; **Ital.:** Aplactin; Prasterol; Pravaselect; Sanaprav; Selectin; **Jpn:** Mevalotin; **Mex.:** Pravacol; **Neth.:** Selektine; **Norw.:** Pravachol; **NZ:** Lipostat; **Port.:** Pravacol; Sanaprav; **S.Afr.:** Prava; **Singapore:** Pravachol; **Spain:** Bristacol; Lipemol; Liplat; Praeduct; **Swed.:** Pravachol; **Switz.:** Mevalotin; Selipran; **Thai.:** Mevalotin; **UK:** Lipostat; **USA:** Pravachol.

Prazosin Hydrochloride (896-n)

Prazosin Hydrochloride *(BANM, USAN, rINNM)*.
CP-12299-1; Furazosin Hydrochloride; Prazosini Hydrochlori-
dum. 2-[4-(2-Furoyl)piperazin-1-yl]-6,7-dimethoxyquinazolin-
4-ylamine hydrochloride.
$C_{19}H_{21}N_5O_4$,HCl = 419.9.
CAS — 19216-56-9 (prazosin); 19237-84-4 (prazosin hy-
drochloride).
Pharmacopoeias. In *Chin.*, *Eur.* (see p.vi), and *US*.

Prazosin hydrochloride 1.1 mg is approximately equivalent to 1 mg of prazosin.

Pharmacopoeial description

Ph. Eur.: A white or almost white powder. Very slightly solu-
ble in water; slightly soluble in alcohol and in methyl alcohol; practically insoluble in acetone. Protect from light.

USP 25: A white to tan powder. Slightly soluble in water, in dimethylacetamide, in dimethylformamide, and in methyl alcohol; very slightly soluble in alcohol; practically insoluble in ac-
etone and in chloroform. Store in airtight containers. Protect from light.

Adverse Effects

Prazosin hydrochloride can cause postural hypotension and it may be severe and produce syncope following the initial dose; it may be preceded by tachy-
cardia. This reaction can be avoided by starting treatment with a low dose, preferably at night (see Uses and Administration, below).

The more common side-effects include dizziness, drowsiness, headache, lack of energy, nausea, and palpitations, and may diminish with continued prazosin therapy or with a reduction in dosage. Other ad-
verse effects include oedema, chest pain, dyspnoea,

---

constipation, diarrhoea, vomiting, depression and nervousness, sleep disturbances, vertigo, hallucinations, paraesthesia, nasal congestion, epistaxis, dry-
ness of mouth, urinary frequency and incontinence, reddened sclera, blurred vision, tinnitus, abnormal liver enzyme values, pancreatitis, arthralgia, skin rashes, pruritus, and diaphoresis. Impotence and priapism have also been reported.

◊ General reviews.
1. Carruthers SG. Adverse effects of α₁-adrenergic blocking drugs. *Drug Safety* 1994; **11**: 12–20.

Effects on the cardiovascular system. Postural hypotension, preceded by tachycardia and sometimes producing synco-
pe, is an established side-effect of prazosin following the initial dose. Sinus bradycardia was associated with prazosin in a patient who experienced light headedness following each daily dose.[1]
1. Ball J. Symptomatic sinus bradycardia due to prazosin. *Lancet* 1994; **343**: 121.

Effects on the gastrointestinal tract. Faecal incontinence in a 52-year-old man receiving prazosin was exacerbated by haemorrhoidectomy and appeared to be due to diminished resting anal tone, presumably because of smooth muscle relaxation secondary to alpha-adrenoceptor blockade.[1] Symptoms ceased almost immediately on discontinuing the drug.
1. Holmes SAV, *et al.* Faecal incontinence resulting from α₁-adren-
oceptor blockade. *Lancet* 1990; **336**: 685–6.

Effects on mental function. Psychiatric symptoms including confusion, paranoia, and hallucinations developed in 3 pa-
tients associated with prazosin treatment.[1] Two of the patients had chronic renal failure and the renal function of the third was mildly impaired. Acute psychosis has also been reported with doxazosin.[2]
1. Chin DKF, *et al.* Neuropsychiatric complications related to use of prazosin in patients with renal failure. *BMJ* 1986; **293**: 1347.
2. Evans M, *et al.* Drug induced psychosis with doxazosin. *BMJ* 1997; **314**: 1869.

Hypersensitivity. Urticaria and angioedema were attributed to prazosin in a 70-year-old woman.[1]
1. Ruzicka T, Ring J. Hypersensitivity to prazosin. *Lancet* 1983; **i**: 473–4.

Lupus erythematosus. One study has reported the forma-
tion of antinuclear antibodies in patients receiving prazosin,[1] but this is not in agreement with other reports,[2,3] and commentators consider the association unproven.[4] There is no evidence of the development of lupus erythematosus.[4]
1. Marshall AJ, *et al.* Positive antinuclear factor tests with prazosin. *BMJ* 1979; **1**: 165–6.
2. Wilson JD, *et al.* Antinuclear factor in patients on prazosin. *BMJ* 1979; **1**: 553–4.
3. Melkild A, Gaarder PI. Does prazosin induce formation of anti-
nuclear factor? *BMJ* 1979; **1**: 620–1.
4. Kristensen BØ. Does prazosin induce formation of antinuclear factor? *BMJ* 1979; **1**: 621.

Urinary incontinence. There have been reports of urinary incontinence developing in patients receiving prazosin. Analysis[1] of 56 cases reported to the Australian Adverse Drug Reactions Advisory Committee indicated that typically symp-
toms appeared within a day or two of the commencement of prazosin and persisted until the drug was withdrawn or the dose reduced. Both stress and urge incontinence were experienced, sometimes in the same patient. Of the 56 patients, 51 were women and most were elderly. In a study[2] in women attending a hypertension clinic urinary incontinence was reported in 40.8% of 49 women receiving alpha blockers (prazosin, terazosin, or doxazosin) and in 16.3% of controls. Incontinence might be due to a reduction in urethral pressure induced by alpha-adrenoceptor blockade.
Interestingly, faecal incontinence has also been reported with prazosin—see Effects on the Gastrointestinal Tract, above.
1. Mathew TH, *et al.* Urinary incontinence secondary to prazosin. *Med J Aust* 1988; **148**: 305–6.
2. Marshall HJ, Beevers DG. α-Adrenoceptor blocking drugs and female urinary incontinence: prevalence and reversibility. *Br J Clin Pharmacol* 1996; **42**: 507–9.

Treatment of Adverse Effects

If overdosage occurs activated charcoal should be given if the patient presents within 1 hour of inges-
tion. Severe hypotension may respond to placing the patient in the supine position with the feet raised. The effects of gross overdosage may be treated by infusions of volume expanders, and if necessary cautious intravenous infusion of a vasopressor. Prazosin is not removed by dialysis.

Precautions

Treatment with prazosin should be introduced cautiously because of the risk of sudden collapse follow-
ing the initial dose. Especial caution is necessary in patients with renal or hepatic impairment and in the elderly.

Prazosin is not recommended for the treatment of heart failure caused by mechanical obstruction, for example aortic or mitral valve stenosis, pulmonary embolism, and restrictive pericardial disease. It should be used with caution in patients with angina pectoris. Prazosin may cause drowsiness or dizziness; patients so affected should not drive or operate machinery.

Cerebral haemorrhage. Hypotension with disturbance of consciousness[1] occurred in 3 patients with recent cerebral haemorrhage following an initial dose of prazosin 0.5 mg.
1. Lin M-S, Hsieh W-J. Prazosin-induced first-dose phenomenon possibly associated with hemorrhagic stroke: a report of three cases. *Drug Intell Clin Pharm* 1987; **21**: 723–6.

Tolerance. Although favourable reponses to prazosin may oc-
cur initially in patients with chronic heart failure, a number of studies[1,2] have reported the development of tolerance to its haemodynamic effects on prolonged therapy. The mechanism by which this occurs remains to be determined.
1. Packer M, *et al.* Role of the renin-angiotensin system in the de-
velopment of hemodynamic and clinical tolerance to long-term prazosin therapy in patients with severe chronic heart failure. *J Am Coll Cardiol* 1986; **7**: 671–80.
2. Bayliss J, *et al.* Clinical importance of the renin-angiotensin sys-
tem in chronic heart failure: double blind comparison of captopril and prazosin. *BMJ* 1985; **290**: 1861–5.

Interactions

The hypotensive effects of prazosin may be enhanced by the concomitant administration of diuretics and other antihypertensives, and by alcohol and other drugs that cause hypotension. The risk of first-dose hypotension may be particularly increased in patients receiving beta blockers or calcium-channel blockers.

Analgesics. *Indometacin* reduced prazosin-induced hypotension in 4 of 9 subjects.[1]
1. Rubin P, *et al.* Studies on the clinical pharmacology of prazosin II: the influence of indomethacin and of propranolol on the action and disposition of prazosin. *Br J Clin Pharmacol* 1980; **10**: 33–9.

Antidepressants and antipsychotics. A patient who was taking *amitriptyline* and *chlorpromazine* developed acute agitation on receiving prazosin.[1] The symptoms settled rapidly when prazosin was discontinued. Antidepressants and antipsychotics may enhance the hypotensive effect of prazosin and other alpha blockers.
1. Bolli P, Simpson FO. New vasodilator drugs for hypertension. *BMJ* 1974; **1**: 637.

Calcium-channel blockers. An enhanced hypotensive ef-
fect has been reported in normotensive subjects given prazosin and *verapamil* concurrently; the effect may be due in part to enhanced bioavailability of prazosin.[1] Markedly increased hypotensive responses have also been reported with combined use of prazosin and *nifedipine*,[2,3] although the validity of such reports has been questioned.[4]
1. Pasanisi F, *et al.* Combined alpha adrenoceptor antagonism and calcium channel blockade in normal subjects. *Clin Pharmacol Ther* 1984; **36**: 716–23.
2. Jee LD, Opie LH. Acute hypotensive response to nifedipine add-
ed to prazosin in treatment of hypertension. *BMJ* 1983; **287**: 1514.
3. Jee LD, Opie LH. Acute hypotensive response to nifedipine added to prazosin. *BMJ* 1984; **288**: 238–9.
4. Elliott HL, *et al.* Acute hypotensive response to nifedipine added to prazosin. *BMJ* 1984; **288**: 238.

Digoxin. For reference to the effect of prazosin on serum-digoxin concentrations, see under Digoxin, p.871.

Pharmacokinetics

Prazosin is readily absorbed from the gastrointestinal tract with peak plasma concentrations occurring 1 to 3 hours after an oral dose. The bioavailability is variable and a range of 43 to 85% has been reported. Pra-
zosin is highly bound to plasma proteins. It is exten-
sively metabolised in the liver and some of the metabolites are reported to have hypotensive activity. It is excreted as the metabolites and 5 to 11% as un-
changed prazosin mainly in the faeces via the bile. Less than 10% is excreted in the urine. Small amounts are distributed into breast milk. Its duration of action is longer than would be predicted from its relatively short plasma half-life of about 2 to 4 hours. Half-life is reported to be increased to about 7 hours in patients with heart failure.

The elderly. The bioavailability of prazosin was significantly reduced in the elderly, about 40% less unchanged drug reaching the systemic circulation compared with the young.[1] This was attributed to a reduction in the absorption from the gastrointestinal tract. The half-life was also prolonged in the elderly and this was associated with an increase in the volume of dis-

tribution at steady state. However, it was considered unlikely that these effects would have major clinical significance.

1. Rubin PC, *et al.* Prazosin disposition in young and elderly subjects. *Br J Clin Pharmacol* 1981; **12:** 401–4.

Protein binding. Although it was reported that prazosin was about 80 to 85% bound to serum albumin and only about 10 to 30% bound to α_1-acid glycoprotein *in vitro*,[1] the study did not take account of potential interactions between the binding proteins *in vivo*, and binding to α_1-acid glycoprotein might be more significant in clinical practice. A subsequent study indicated that variations in prazosin protein binding pre- and postoperatively were related to variations in concentration of the glycoprotein.[2]

1. Brunner F, Müller WE. Prazosin binding to human α_1-acid glycoprotein (orosomucoid), human serum albumin, and human serum: further characterisation of the 'single drug binding site' of orosomucoid. *J Pharm Pharmacol* 1985; **37:** 305–9.
2. Sager G, *et al.* Binding of prazosin and propranolol at variable α_1-acid glycoprotein and albumin concentrations. *Br J Clin Pharmacol* 1989; **27:** 229–34.

Uses and Administration

Prazosin is an alpha blocker (p.787) that acts by selective blockade of alpha$_1$-adrenoceptors. It is used in the management of hypertension (p.802), in Raynaud's syndrome (below), and to relieve symptoms of urinary obstruction in benign prostatic hyperplasia (p.1477). It has also been used in heart failure (p.798).

Prazosin produces peripheral dilatation of both arterioles and veins and reduction of peripheral resistance, usually without reflex tachycardia. It reduces both standing and supine blood pressure with a greater effect on the diastolic pressure. It is reported to have no effect on renal blood flow or glomerular filtration rate, and has little effect on cardiac output in hypertensive patients. In patients with heart failure, prazosin reduces both preload and afterload and produces an improvement in cardiac output, although tolerance may develop. In benign prostatic hyperplasia, prazosin may relieve the symptoms of urinary obstruction by reducing smooth muscle tone in the prostate and bladder neck.

Prazosin is given by mouth as the hydrochloride, but doses are usually expressed in terms of the base. Following oral administration the hypotensive effect is seen within 2 to 4 hours and persists for several hours.

A low starting dose is given in the evening to lessen the risk of collapse which may occur in some patients after the first dose (see Adverse Effects, above). Doses may need to be reduced in the elderly and in patients with renal or hepatic impairment.

In **hypertension**, the usual initial dose in the UK is 500 µg two or three times daily for 3 to 7 days; if tolerated the dose may then be increased to 1 mg two or three times daily for a further 3 to 7 days, and thereafter gradually increased, according to the patient's response, to a usual maximum of 20 mg daily in divided doses. In the US the recommended starting dose is 1 mg two or three times daily and up to 40 mg daily in divided doses has been given; however, the usual maintenance dose is between 6 and 15 mg daily. Smaller doses may be required in patients concurrently taking other antihypertensive drugs. Modified-release preparations may allow once daily dosing.

In **Raynaud's syndrome** and in **benign prostatic hyperplasia** an initial dose of 500 µg twice daily may be given increasing to a maintenance dose not exceeding 2 mg twice daily.

In **heart failure**, treatment has been started with 500 µg two to four times daily and increased gradually according to response; the usual maintenance dose has been 4 to 20 mg daily.

Erectile dysfunction. Prazosin has been administered transurethrally in combination[1] with alprostadil in the management of erectile dysfunction (p.1663).

1. Peterson CA, *et al.* Erectile response to transurethral alprostadil, prazosin and alprostadil-prazosin combinations. *J Urol (Baltimore)* 1998; **159:** 1523–8.

Muscle cramp. Skeletal muscle cramp may occur during haemodialysis, possibly due to activation of the sympathetic nervous system. Prazosin was reported[1] to reduce the incidence of cramp in 4 of 5 patients with frequent haemodialysis-associated muscle cramp. However, the incidence of hypotension was

also increased and might limit the use of prazosin for this indication.

1. Sidhom OA, *et al.* Low-dose prazosin in patients with muscle cramps during hemodialysis. *Clin Pharmacol Ther* 1994; **56:** 445–51.

Peripheral vascular disease. Alpha blockers, including prazosin, may be used in the management of Raynaud's syndrome (p.809). Studies of the benefits of prazosin have produced varying results. A short-term reduction in number and duration of attacks was reported in 5 of 7 patients given prazosin 2 mg daily but only 1 patient had complete relief from attacks and few could tolerate doses higher than 6 mg daily.[1] Improvements were not maintained during continued treatment for 2 months. Others[2,3] have reported benefit from prazosin 1 mg two or three times daily in the majority of patients, with one study suggesting greater benefit in Raynaud's disease (the primary, idiopathic form) than in secondary Raynaud's syndrome.[2] In a subsequent study, higher doses of prazosin (2 mg or 4 mg three times daily) were no more effective than 1 mg three times daily, and were associated with a significantly greater incidence of adverse effects.[4]

1. Nielsen SL, *et al.* Prazosin treatment of primary Raynaud's phenomenon. *Eur J Clin Pharmacol* 1983; **24:** 421–3.
2. Allegra C, *et al.* Pharmacological treatment of Raynaud's phenomenon: a new therapeutic approach. *Curr Ther Res* 1986; **40:** 303–11.
3. Wollersheim H, *et al.* Double-blind, placebo-controlled study of prazosin in Raynaud's phenomenon. *Clin Pharmacol Ther* 1986; **40:** 219–25.
4. Wollersheim H, Thien T. Dose-response study of prazosin in Raynaud's phenomenon: clinical effectiveness versus side effects. *J Clin Pharmacol* 1988; **28:** 1089–93.

Scorpion stings. Stings from the Indian red scorpion (*Mesobuthus tamulus*) are potentially fatal. The scorpion venom is a potent sympathetic stimulator resulting in high circulating catecholamines, hypertension, arrhythmias, pulmonary oedema, and circulatory failure. Antivenom is generally ineffective and treatment for cardiotoxicity is supportive (see p.1563). Prazosin, given orally, appears to be beneficial and has been suggested[1] as first-line treatment, except in cases of severe pulmonary oedema.

1. Bawaskar HS, Bawaskar PH. Scorpion envenoming and the cardiovascular system. *Trop Doct* 1997; **27:** 6–9.

Preparations

BP 2001: Prazosin Tablets;
USP 25: Prazosin Hydrochloride Capsules.

Proprietary Preparations (details are given in Part 3)
Aust.: Minipress; *Austral.:* Minipress; Mipraz; Prasig; Pratsiol; Prazohexal; Pressin; *Belg.:* Minipress; *Braz.:* Minipress; *Canad.:* Apo-Prazo; Minipress; Novo-Prazin; Nu-Prazo; *Denm.:* Hexapress; Peripress; Prazac; *Fin.:* Patsolin; Minipress; Pratsiol; Prazocor; *Fr.:* Alpress; Minipress; *Ger.:* Adversuten; duramipress; Eurex; Minipress; *Hong Kong:* Apo-Prazo; Minipress; Pratsiol; *Irl.:* Hypovase; *Israel:* Hypotens; *Mex.:* Minipres; Sinozzard; *Neth.:* Minipress; *NZ:* Hyprosin; Pratsiol; *S.Afr.:* Minipress; Pratsiol; *Singapore:* Minipress; *Spain:* Minipres; *Swed.:* Peripress†; *Switz.:* Minipress; *Thai.:* Atodel; Lopress; Minima; Minipress; Mysial; Parabowl; Polypress; Pratsiol; Pressin; *UK:* Alphavase; Hypovase; *USA:* Minipress.

Multi-ingredient: *Ger.:* Polypress; *USA:* Minizide.

Prenalterol Hydrochloride   (13164-v)

Prenalterol Hydrochloride (*BANM, USAN, rINNM*).

C-50005/A-Ba (racemate); CGP-7760B; H133/22; H-80/62 (racemate). (*S*)-1-(4-Hydroxyphenoxy)-3-isopropylaminopropan-2-ol hydrochloride.
$C_{12}H_{19}NO_3,HCl = 261.7$.
CAS — 57526-81-5 (prenalterol); 61260-05-7 (prenalterol hydrochloride).

Profile

Prenalterol is a sympathomimetic (see Adrenaline, p.829) with stimulant effects on beta$_1$ adrenoceptors. It has an inotropic action on the heart with relatively little chronotropic effect. Prenalterol hydrochloride has been administered parenterally in the treatment of heart failure and shock. It has also been promoted for the reversal of beta blockade.

Preparations

Proprietary Preparations (details are given in Part 3)
Denm.: Hyprenan†; *Norw.:* Hyprenan†; *Swed.:* Hyprenan†.

Probucol   (1356-b)

Probucol (*BAN, USAN, rINN*).

DH-581. 4,4'-(Isopropylidenedithio)bis(2,6-di-*tert*-butylphenol).
$C_{31}H_{48}O_2S_2 = 516.8$.
CAS — 23288-49-5.
ATC — C10AX02.

Pharmacopoeias. In US.

Pharmacopoeial description

USP 25: A white to off-white, crystalline powder. Insoluble in water; soluble in alcohol and in petroleum spirit; freely soluble in chloroform and in propyl alcohol. Protect from light.

Adverse Effects and Precautions

The commonest side-effects of probucol therapy are gastrointestinal upsets with diarrhoea occurring in about 10% of patients; flatulence, abdominal pain, nausea, and vomiting may also occur. Hypersensitivity reactions including angioedema have been reported.

Fatal cardiac arrhythmias have been reported in *animals* and prolonged QT intervals in man. Probucol should be given with caution to patients with recent myocardial damage, severe ventricular arrhythmias, cardiovascular-associated syncope, or prolonged QT interval. The risk of arrhythmias may be increased in patients taking tricyclic antidepressants, class I or III antiarrhythmics, or phenothiazines.

◊ Side-effects reported during a 1-year study involving 88 patients given probucol decreased after the first 3 months of therapy.[1] The most common was loose stools or diarrhoea; constipation was reported much less frequently. Other side-effects which occurred were flatulence, vertigo, dizziness, a different odour of the skin, and pruritus. No patient withdrew from the study because of side-effects.

1. McCaughan D. Nine years of treatment with probucol. *Artery* 1982; **10:** 56–70.

Effects on the heart. Evaluation of 198 patients[1] who had received probucol for 5 years or more, revealed that changes in the QT interval had occurred with increases predominating. In 42 patients studied[2] for up to 2 years, no correlation was found between blood concentrations of probucol and lengthening of the QT interval; although nearly half the patients showed a lengthening of the QT interval on probucol the overall change was not statistically significant. There was no clinical or electrocardiographic evidence of arrhythmias in any patient. In an analysis of 48 men[3] who had taken probucol as part of a multifactorial primary prevention study, probucol was found to increase QT interval compared with controls. However, prolongations were modest. Correlation was seen between QT changes and serum triglyceride concentrations. Although serious cardiac arrhythmias were not noted in these studies, there have been individual reports[4,5] of potentially fatal polymorphic ventricular tachycardia (torsade de pointes) in patients with probucol-associated prolongation of the QT interval.

1. Troendle G, *et al.* Probucol and the QT interval. *Lancet* 1982; **i:** 1179.
2. Dujovne CA, *et al.* Electrocardiographic effects of probucol: a controlled prospective clinical trial. *Eur J Clin Pharmacol* 1984; **26:** 735–9.
3. Naukkarinen V, *et al.* Probucol-induced electrocardiographic changes in a five-year primary prevention of vascular diseases. *Curr Ther Res* 1989; **45:** 232–7.
4. Gohn DC, Simmons TW. Polymorphic ventricular tachycardia (torsade de pointes) associated with the use of probucol. *N Engl J Med* 1992; **326:** 1435–6.
5. Kajinami K, *et al.* Propranolol for probucol-induced QT prolongation with polymorphic ventricular tachycardia. *Lancet* 1993; **341:** 124–5.

Interactions

The risk of arrhythmias in patients receiving probucol may be increased in those taking arrhythmogenic drugs concurrently (see Adverse Effects and Precautions, above).

Ciclosporin. For reference to the effect of probucol on ciclosporin concentrations, see p.522.

Pharmacokinetics

The absorption of probucol from the gastrointestinal tract is limited and variable, and is stated to be at a maximum if taken with food. Concentrations in blood rise slowly and reach steady state after 3 to 4 months of continuous treatment. Probucol accumulates in adipose tissue and concentrations fall only slowly, over several months, when treatment is withdrawn. Excretion is considered to be chiefly by the biliary system into the faeces.

Uses and Administration

Probucol is a lipid regulating drug that has been used in the treatment of hypercholesterolaemia, particularly type IIa hyperlipoproteinaemia. It lowers total plasma-cholesterol concentrations, mainly by reducing low-density lipoprotein (LDL)-cholesterol and high-density lipoprotein (HDL)-cholesterol concentrations. It has little effect on triglyceride or very-low-density lipoprotein (VLDL)-cholesterol concentrations. It may cause regression of xanthomas.

The usual dose by mouth is 500 mg twice daily, given with the morning and evening meals.

Administration in the elderly. Probucol reduced total cholesterol and LDL-cholesterol concentrations more markedly in patients over 65 years of age than in younger patients.[1]

1. Morisaki N, *et al.* Effects of long-term treatment with probucol on serum lipoproteins in cases of familial hypercholesterolemia in the elderly. *J Am Geriatr Soc* 1990; **38:** 15–18.

Hyperlipidaemias. Probucol has been used in the treatment of hyperlipidaemias (p.800). It lowers plasma concentrations of low-density lipoprotein (LDL)-cholesterol by about 10 to 20% and high-density lipoprotein (HDL)-cholesterol by about 30% in hyperlipidaemic subjects.[1] The reduction in LDL-cholesterol appears to be mainly due to an increase in the fractional catabolic rate of LDL. An independent antioxidant effect may also contribute to the clinical action of probucol.[1,2] Hypercholesterolaemia is a known risk factor for atherosclerosis and reduction of raised LDL-cholesterol concentrations is of benefit in the secondary prevention of **ischaemic heart disease**. The antioxidant effect of probucol could be of additional benefit. The significance of the reduction in HDL-cholesterol is not yet known: such a reduction could be expected to increase the risk, although this has not been observed in clinical studies.[1,2] Probucol has been reported to reduce the rate of restenosis after coronary angioplasty.[3]

1. Buckley MM-T, et al. Probucol: a reappraisal of its pharmacological properties and therapeutic use in hypercholesterolaemia. Drugs 1989; 37: 761–800.
2. Zimetbaum P, et al. Probucol: pharmacology and clinical application. J Clin Pharmacol 1990; 30: 3–9.
3. Tardif J-C, et al. Probucol and multivitamins in the prevention of restenosis after coronary angioplasty. N Engl J Med 1997; 337: 365–72.

Preparations

USP 25: Probucol Tablets.

Proprietary Preparations (details are given in Part 3)
Austral.: Lurselle; *Braz.:* Lesterol; *Ger.:* Lurselle†; *Hong Kong:* Lurselle; *Mex.:* Colbuzer; Lesterol; Serterol; *S.Afr.:* Lurselle; *Spain:* Bifenabid†; Superlipid; *Thai.:* Lurselle.

Procainamide Hydrochloride (7791-h)

Procainamide Hydrochloride (BANM, rINNM).
Novocainamidum; Procainamidi Chloridum; Procainamidi Hydrochloridum. 4-Amino-N-(2-diethylaminoethyl)benzamide hydrochloride.
$C_{13}H_{21}N_3O,HCl = 271.8$.
CAS — 51-06-9 (procainamide); 614-39-1 (procainamide hydrochloride).
Pharmacopoeias. In Chin., Eur. (see p.vi), Int., Jpn, Pol., and US.

Pharmacopoeial description
Ph. Eur.: A white or very slightly yellow, hygroscopic, crystalline powder. Very soluble in water; freely soluble in alcohol; slightly soluble in acetone; practically insoluble in ether. A 10% solution in water has a pH of 5.6 to 6.3. Store in airtight containers. Protect from light.

USP 25: A white to tan, odourless, crystalline powder. Very soluble in water; soluble in alcohol; slightly soluble in chloroform; very slightly soluble in ether and in benzene. A 10% solution in water has a pH of 5.0 to 6.5. Store in airtight containers.

Stability. Procainamide is more stable in neutral solutions, such as sodium chloride, than in acidic solutions, such as glucose, but patients requiring intravenous procainamide often have heart failure and cannot tolerate the sodium load associated with sodium chloride injections. The stability of procainamide in glucose 5% is improved by neutralising the glucose using sodium bicarbonate, or storing the admixture at 5°. The concentration of procainamide remained above 90% of the initial concentration for 24 hours if the glucose was first neutralised and this was considered more practical than refrigeration if extended stability was required.[1]
The compound formed by mixing procainamide hydrochloride with glucose 5% was shown to be a mixture of α- and β-glucosylamines[2] and about 10 to 15% of the procainamide was lost in this way after 10 hours at room temperature.
An oral liquid,[3] prepared from procainamide capsules, containing 5, 50, or 100 mg per mL of the hydrochloride was stable for at least 6 months when stored at 4 to 6°.

1. Raymond GG, et al. Stability of procainamide hydrochloride in neutralized 5% dextrose injection. Am J Hosp Pharm 1988; 45: 2513–17.
2. Sianipar A, et al. Chemical incompatibility between procainamide hydrochloride and glucose following intravenous admixture. J Pharm Pharmacol 1994; 46: 951–5.
3. Metras JI, et al. Stability of procainamide hydrochloride in an extemporaneously compounded oral liquid. Am J Hosp Pharm 1992; 49: 1720–4.

Adverse Effects

Cardiac effects occur particularly during intravenous administration of procainamide and in overdose. Rapid intravenous administration may result in severe hypotension, ventricular fibrillation, and asystole. High plasma concentrations are also associated with impaired cardiac conduction.

Hypersensitivity reactions to procainamide are common. Procainamide is a frequent cause of drug-induced systemic lupus erythematosus (SLE) and the incidence has been reported to be as high as 30% in patients taking procainamide over prolonged periods. Antinuclear antibodies may be detected in a high proportion of patients, but they do not necessarily develop the symptoms of SLE, which include arthralgia, arthritis, myalgia, pleural effusion, pericarditis, and fever. Agranulocytosis, eosinophilia, neutropenia, thrombocytopenia, and haemolytic anaemia have been reported. Other symptoms of hypersensitivity not necessarily related to SLE may also occur including hepatomegaly, angioedema, skin rashes, pruritus, urticaria, flushing, and hypergammaglobulinaemia.

Anorexia, nausea, vomiting, a bitter taste, and diarrhoea are more common with higher oral doses. Effects on the CNS such as mental depression, dizziness, and psychosis with hallucinations, have been reported.

◊ Out of 488 hospitalised patients in the Boston Collaborative Drug Surveillance Program who had received procainamide, 45 experienced acute adverse effects attributed to the drug.[1] Life-threatening reactions included heart block in 3, tachyarrhythmias in 2, and bradycardia and/or hypotension in 2. Other reactions included gastrointestinal upsets in 19, pyrexia in 8, bradycardia and hypotension in 5, tachyarrhythmias in 3, heart block in 1, eosinophilia in 1, and urticaria in 1 patient.

1. Lawson DH, Jick H. Adverse reactions to procainamide. Br J Clin Pharmacol 1977; 4: 507–11.

Effects on the blood. Adverse haematological effects reported during procainamide therapy include neutropenia,[1-3] agranulocytosis,[2-6] thrombocytopenia,[5] haemolytic anaemia,[7] and pancytopenia.[8] These disorders are usually reversible on withdrawing procainamide although some fatalities have been reported.[3,4] It has been suggested[2,6] that agranulocytosis or severe neutropenia is more likely in patients taking modified-release preparations, but others have found no difference in the incidence between modified-release and conventional-release preparations.[3] An increased risk of agranulocytosis with procainamide has been documented in one large study.[9] Although the precise estimate of excess risk could not be calculated, the order of magnitude was about 3 per million exposed for up to one week. This excess risk was low and of little relevance in the initial choice of therapy.

1. Riker J, et al. Bone marrow granulomas and neutropenia associated with procainamide. Arch Intern Med 1978; 138: 1731–2.
2. Ellrodt AG, et al. Severe neutropenia associated with sustained-release procainamide. Ann Intern Med 1984; 100: 197–201.
3. Meyers DG, et al. Severe neutropenia associated with procainamide: comparison of sustained release and conventional preparations. Am Heart J 1985; 109: 1393–5.
4. Fleet S. Agranulocytosis, procainamide, and phenytoin. Ann Intern Med 1984; 100: 616–17.
5. Christensen DJ, et al. Agranulocytosis, thrombocytopenia, and procainamide. Ann Intern Med 1984; 100: 918.
6. Thompson JF, et al. Procainamide agranulocytosis: a case report and review of the literature. Curr Ther Res 1988; 44: 872–81.
7. Kleinman S, et al. Positive direct antiglobulin tests and immune hemolytic anemia in patients receiving procainamide. N Engl J Med 1984; 311: 809–12.
8. Bluming AZ, et al. Severe transient pancytopenia associated with procainamide ingestion. JAMA 1976; 236: 2520–1.
9. Kelly JP, et al. Risks of agranulocytosis and aplastic anemia in relation to the use of cardiovascular drugs: The International Agranulocytosis and Aplastic Anemia Study. Clin Pharmacol Ther 1991; 49: 330–41.

Effects on the gastrointestinal tract. Pseudo-obstruction of the bowel occurred in a diabetic patient when given procainamide both orally and intravenously. It was believed that the anticholinergic properties of procainamide, together with the diabetic state, contributed to the severe hypomotility of the gastrointestinal tract.[1]

1. Peterson AM, et al. Procainamide-induced pseudo-obstruction in a diabetic patient. DICP Ann Pharmacother 1991; 25: 1334–5.

Effects on the heart. Procainamide has been associated with the development of torsade de pointes.[1,2] Elevated plasma concentrations of the major metabolite N-acetylprocainamide were present in 1 patient[1] and haemodialysis was used to reduce the plasma concentration and control the arrhythmia.

1. Nguyen KPV, et al. N-Acetylprocainamide, torsades de pointes, and hemodialysis. Ann Intern Med 1986; 104: 283–4.
2. Habbab MA, El-Sherif N. Drug-induced torsades de pointes: role of early afterdepolarizations and dispersion of repolarization. Am J Med 1990; 89: 241–6.

Effects on the liver. There have been reports of granulomatous hepatitis[1] and intrahepatic cholestasis[2,3] due to hypersensitivity reactions in patients taking procainamide. Fever and elevation of liver enzyme values also occurred. The reactions were reversible on withdrawing procainamide.

1. Rotmensch HH, et al. Granulomatous hepatitis: a hypersensitivity response to procainamide. Ann Intern Med 1978; 89: 646–7.
2. Ahn C-S, Tow DE. Intrahepatic cholestasis due to hypersensitivity reaction to procainamide. Arch Intern Med 1990; 150: 2589–90.
3. Chuang LC, et al. Possible case of procainamide-induced intrahepatic cholestatic jaundice. Ann Pharmacother 1993; 27: 434–7.

Effects on mental function. Acute psychosis has been reported[1] in patients receiving therapy with procainamide.

1. Bizjak ED, et al. Procainamide-induced psychosis: a case report and review of the literature. Ann Pharmacother 1999; 33: 948–51.

Effects on the muscles. Procainamide may affect neuromuscular transmission and there have been reports of severe generalised skeletal muscle weakness[1-3] in patients receiving procainamide. In 2 patients this was associated with respiratory failure[1,2] and developed shortly after starting therapy. Concentrations of procainamide and its N-acetyl metabolite exceeded the normal therapeutic ranges and rapid cycling peritoneal dialysis was used to remove the drug in 1 patient.[2] Adverse muscle symptoms are a feature of procainamide-induced lupus ery-

thematosus (see below), but in such instances symptoms usually develop on long-term treatment.

1. Lewis CA, et al. Myopathy after short term administration of procainamide. BMJ 1986; 292: 593–4.
2. Javaheri S, et al. Diaphragmatic paralysis. Am J Med 1989; 86: 623–4.
3. Sayler DJ, DeJong DJ. Possible procainamide-induced myopathy. DICP Ann Pharmacother 1991; 25: 436.

Lupus erythematosus. Procainamide is one of the most common causes of drug-induced lupus erythematosus.[1-3] Antinuclear antibodies are present in the majority of patients on long-term therapy but the clinical syndrome develops in only up to 30%. The development of antinuclear antibodies is more likely in slow acetylators than in rapid acetylators; also the antibodies appear earlier in treatment in slow acetylators.[4] The clinical syndrome may include fever, polyarthritis, arthralgia, myalgia, and pleuropulmonary and pericardial features, and is usually spontaneously reversible on withdrawal of procainamide.

1. Hughes GRV. Recent developments in drug-associated systemic lupus erythematosus. Adverse Drug React Bull 1987; (Apr.): 460–3.
2. Mitchell JA, et al. Immunotoxic side-effects of drug therapy. Drug Safety 1990; 5: 168–78.
3. Price EJ, Venables PJW. Drug-induced lupus. Drug Safety 1995; 12: 283–90.
4. Woosley RL, et al. Effect of acetylator phenotype on the rate at which procainamide induces antinuclear antibodies and the lupus syndrome. N Engl J Med 1978; 298: 1157–9.

Treatment of Adverse Effects

In overdosage treatment is largely symptomatic and supportive. The ECG, blood pressure, and renal function should be monitored. Supportive measures include correction of hypotension, assisted ventilation, and electrical pacing. Haemodialysis or haemoperfusion increase the elimination of procainamide and N-acetylprocainamide.

Systemic lupus erythematosus will normally respond to withdrawal of procainamide but corticosteroids may be required.

Dialysis. There are reports of haemodialysis and haemoperfusion being effective in reducing concentrations of procainamide and N-acetylprocainamide.[1-3]

1. Atkinson AJ, et al. Hemodialysis for severe procainamide toxicity: clinical and pharmacokinetic observations. Clin Pharmacol Ther 1976; 20: 585–92.
2. Braden GL, et al. Hemoperfusion for treatment of N-acetylprocainamide intoxication. Ann Intern Med 1986; 105: 64–5.
3. Domoto DT, et al. Removal of toxic levels of N-acetylprocainamide with continuous arteriovenous hemofiltration or continuous arteriovenous hemodiafiltration. Ann Intern Med 1987; 106: 550–2.

Precautions

Procainamide is contra-indicated in patients with heart block or systemic lupus erythematosus, and should be used with caution in those with myocardial damage or severe organic heart disease. Some authorities consider that it should not be used in heart failure or hypotension. Patients with torsade de pointes may deteriorate if given procainamide. If procainamide is used to treat atrial tachycardia it may be necessary to pre-treat with digoxin. Procainamide should preferably not be used in patients with myasthenia gravis or digoxin toxicity. There may be cross-sensitivity between procaine and procainamide.

Accumulation of procainamide may occur in patients with heart failure, renal insufficiency, or hepatic impairment and dosage reduction may be necessary.

Regular blood tests should be carried out in patients receiving procainamide, and screening for lupus erythematosus and serum antinuclear factor should be carried out before and regularly during therapy.

Grave hypotension may follow intravenous administration of procainamide; it should be injected slowly under ECG control.

Breast feeding. There was evidence of accumulation of procainamide and N-acetylprocainamide in the breast milk of a woman taking procainamide 500 mg four times daily.[1] However, it was considered that the amount ingested by an infant would not be expected to yield clinically significant plasma concentrations.

1. Pittard WB, Glazier H. Procainamide excretion in human milk. J Pediatr 1983; 102: 631–3.

Interactions

Procainamide may enhance the effects of antihypertensives, other antiarrhythmics and arrhythmogenic drugs, antimuscarinics, and neuromuscular blocking drugs, and diminish those of parasympathomimetics, such as neostigmine. Procainamide is actively secreted by kidney tubules and interactions are possible with other drugs secreted by the same pathway, such as cimetidine and trimethoprim.

Alcohol. The total body clearance of procainamide is increased by alcohol[1] and the elimination half-life reduced. The acetylation rate of procainamide is also increased resulting in a greater proportion of drug present as the active metabolite N-acetylprocainamide.

1. Olsen H, Mørland J. Ethanol-induced increase in procainamide acetylation in man. *Br J Clin Pharmacol* 1982; **13**: 203–8.

Antacids. Adsorption of procainamide by *antacids*[1] can reduce the bioavailability of procainamide and it is recommended that they are not administered concomitantly.

1. Al-Shora HI, *et al.* Interactions of procainamide, verapamil, guanethidine and hydralazine with adsorbent antacids and antidiarrhoeal mixtures. *Int J Pharmaceutics* 1988; **47**: 209–13.

Antiarrhythmics. *Amiodarone* given orally alters the pharmacokinetic properties of an intravenous dose of procainamide,[1] decreasing clearance and prolonging the plasma elimination half-life. The dosage of intravenous procainamide should be reduced by 20 to 30% during concurrent use.

1. Windle J, *et al.* Pharmacokinetic and electrophysiologic interactions of amiodarone and procainamide. *Clin Pharmacol Ther* 1987; **41**: 603–10.

Antibacterials. The renal clearance of procainamide and N-acetylprocainamide is reduced by *trimethoprim*[1] through competition for renal tubular secretion. Serum concentrations may be increased with a resulting increase in pharmacodynamic response.

1. Vlasses PH, *et al.* Trimethoprim decreases the renal clearance of procainamide and N-acetylprocainamide. *Clin Pharmacol Ther* 1986; **39**: 233.

Histamine H₂-antagonists. Histamine H₂-antagonists compete with other basic drugs for renal tubular secretion. *Cimetidine* reduces the renal clearance of procainamide and N-acetylprocainamide[1,2] and a dosage reduction may be necessary. Increases[3,4] and decreases[4] in renal and metabolic clearances of procainamide have been reported when *ranitidine* is used concomitantly.

1. Christian CD, *et al.* Cimetidine inhibits renal procainamide clearance. *Clin Pharmacol Ther* 1984; **36**: 221–7.
2. Somogyi A, *et al.* Cimetidine-procainamide pharmacokinetic interaction in man: evidence of competition for tubular secretion of basic drugs. *Eur J Clin Pharmacol* 1983; **25**: 339–45.
3. Somogyi A, Bochner F. Dose and concentration dependent effect of ranitidine on procainamide disposition and renal clearance in man. *Br J Clin Pharmacol* 1984; **18**: 175–81.
4. Rocci ML, *et al.* Ranitidine-induced changes in the renal and hepatic clearances of procainamide are correlated. *J Pharmacol Exp Ther* 1989; **248**: 923–8.

Pharmacokinetics

Procainamide is readily and almost completely absorbed from the gastrointestinal tract. It is widely distributed throughout the body and is only about 15 to 20% bound to plasma proteins. The therapeutic effect of procainamide has been correlated with plasma concentrations of about 3 to 10 μg per mL in most patients, progressively severe toxicity being noted at concentrations above 12 μg per mL.

Some procainamide undergoes acetylation in the liver to N-acetylprocainamide (acecainide, p.825). This metabolite also has antiarrhythmic properties. The rate of acetylation of procainamide is genetically determined, there being slow and fast acetylators. Procainamide also undergoes hydrolysis in plasma to para-aminobenzoic acid.

Procainamide is excreted in the urine following active renal secretion, 30 to 70% as unchanged procainamide, with the remainder as N-acetylprocainamide and other metabolites. The elimination half-life of procainamide is 2.5 to 5 hours and that of its acetyl metabolite 6 to 7 hours. N-Acetylprocainamide may represent a significant fraction of the total drug in the circulation.

Procainamide crosses the placental barrier and is distributed into breast milk.

◊ References.
1. Grasela TH, Sheiner LB. Population pharmacokinetics of procainamide from routine clinical data. *Clin Pharmacokinet* 1984; **9**: 545–54.

Bioavailability. Modified-release procainamide preparations have been shown[1] to produce similar steady-state serum concentrations of procainamide and N-acetylprocainamide when compared with equivalent total doses of immediate-release capsules. However, tablet matrices of a modified-release preparation have been recovered from the stools of a patient with

diarrhoea[2] and 3.5 g of procainamide was recovered in these matrices over an 18-hour collection period; the patient had correspondingly low plasma-procainamide concentrations.

1. Vlasses PH, *et al.* Immediate-release and sustained-release procainamide: bioavailability at steady state in cardiac patients. *Ann Intern Med* 1983; **98**: 613–14.
2. Woosley RL, *et al.* Antiarrhythmic therapy: clinical pharmacology update. *J Clin Pharmacol* 1984; **24**: 295–305.

Uses and Administration

Procainamide hydrochloride is a class Ia antiarrhythmic (p.787); it has properties similar to those of quinidine (p.966).

Procainamide hydrochloride tends to be used for the short-term management of severe or symptomatic **arrhythmias** (p.794). It is used for the treatment of ventricular arrhythmias particularly those resistant to lignocaine [lidocaine] and those following myocardial infarction. It may also be used to maintain sinus rhythm after cardioversion of atrial fibrillation.

Therapeutic effect is generally associated with plasma concentrations of 3 to 10 μg per mL. The dose of procainamide hydrochloride required will depend on the age, renal and hepatic function, and underlying cardiac condition of the patient: an adult with normal renal function generally requires up to 50 mg per kg body-weight daily by mouth in divided doses every 3 to 6 hours. Higher doses may be necessary for atrial arrhythmias. Modified-release preparations are available. A dose of 40 to 60 mg per kg body-weight daily by mouth in 4 to 6 divided doses has been used in children.

In an emergency and under continuous ECG and blood pressure monitoring, procainamide hydrochloride may be given intravenously. The injection should be diluted in a 5% solution of glucose to permit better control of the speed of injection, and should be given in doses of 100 mg every 5 minutes at a rate not exceeding 50 mg per minute until the arrhythmia has been suppressed or a maximum dose of 1 g has been reached. A response may be obtained after 100 to 200 mg has been given and more than 500 or 600 mg is not generally required. Alternatively, procainamide hydrochloride may be administered by continuous infusion of 500 to 600 mg over 25 to 30 minutes. Therapeutic plasma concentrations may then be maintained by giving an infusion in a 5% solution of glucose, at a rate of 2 to 6 mg per minute. When transferring to oral therapy, a period of about 3 to 4 hours should elapse between the last intravenous dose and the first oral dose.

Procainamide hydrochloride has also been given intramuscularly.

Administration in children. In a study in 5 children treated with procainamide for various cardiac arrhythmias the mean elimination half-life was found to be 1.7 hours, and the plasma clearance was higher than that reported in adults.[1] In contrast the total serum clearance of procainamide in 3 neonates with supraventricular tachycardia was found to be similar to that in adults and the mean elimination half-life was 5.3 hours.[2] A loading dose of 10 to 12 mg per kg body-weight intravenously was given followed by a continuous infusion of 20 to 75 μg per kg per minute.

1. Singh S, *et al.* Procainamide elimination kinetics in pediatric patients. *Clin Pharmacol Ther* 1982; **32**: 607–11.
2. Bryson SM, *et al.* Therapeutic monitoring and pharmacokinetic evaluation of procainamide in neonates. *DICP Ann Pharmacother* 1991; **25**: 68–71.

Administration in the elderly. Reduced renal clearance of procainamide has been reported in the elderly.[1]

1. Reidenberg MM, *et al.* Aging and renal clearance of procainamide and acetylprocainamide. *Clin Pharmacol Ther* 1980; **28**: 732–5.

Administration in hepatic impairment. In 20 healthy subjects and 20 patients with chronic liver disease given a single dose of procainamide hydrochloride 500 mg by mouth about 64 and 33% respectively of the administered dose was excreted in the urine within 6 hours.[1] Decreased procainamide acetylation in the patients compared with the control group was not correlated with the severity of liver disease whereas decreased procainamide hydrolysis and increased procainamide-derived aminobenzoic acid acetylation appeared to be related to the degree of hepatic impairment. It was suggested that the decrease in excretion of procainamide and its metabolites in the urine of the patients with liver disease could be due to an im-

pairment in oral absorption since renal function was within the normal range but the variations in acetylation and hydrolysis were related to hepatic function.

1. du Souich P, Erill S. Metabolism of procainamide and p-aminobenzoic acid in patients with chronic liver disease. *Clin Pharmacol Ther* 1977; **22**: 588–95.

Administration in renal impairment. Procainamide is excreted in the urine, largely as unchanged drug, and accumulation, especially of the active acetyl metabolite,[1] may occur in renal insufficiency. Haemodialysis and haemoperfusion increase the clearance of procainamide and N-acetylprocainamide (see Treatment of Adverse Effects, above).

1. Vlasses PH, *et al.* Lethal accumulation of procainamide metabolite in renal insufficiency. *Drug Intell Clin Pharm* 1984; **18**: 493–4.

Preparations

BP 2001: Procainamide Injection; Procainamide Tablets;
USP 25: Procainamide Hydrochloride Capsules; Procainamide Hydrochloride Extended-release Tablets; Procainamide Hydrochloride Injection; Procainamide Hydrochloride Tablets.

Proprietary Preparations (details are given in Part 3)
Austral.: Pronestyl; **Braz.:** Procamide; **Canad.:** Procan; Pronestyl; **Hong Kong:** Pronestyl; **Irl.:** Pronestyl; **Israel:** Pronestyl; **Ital.:** Procamide†; **Neth.:** Pronestyl; **NZ:** Pronestyl; **S.Afr.:** Pronestyl†; **Spain:** Biocoryl; **Switz.:** Pronestyl; **Thai.:** Pronestyl; **UK:** Pronestyl; **USA:** Procanbid; Pronestyl.

Propafenone Hydrochloride (13177-w)

Propafenone Hydrochloride (BANM, USAN, rINNM).
Fenopraine Hydrochloride; SA-79; WZ-884642; WZ-884643. 2′-(2-Hydroxy-3-propylaminopropoxy)-3-phenylpropiophenone hydrochloride.
$C_{21}H_{27}NO_3,HCl = 377.9$.
CAS — 54063-53-5 (propafenone); 34183-22-7 (propafenone hydrochloride).
Pharmacopoeias. In Chin. and US.

Pharmacopoeial description

USP 25: A white powder. Soluble in hot water and in methyl alcohol; slightly soluble in alcohol and in chloroform; very slightly soluble in acetone; insoluble in ether and in toluene. A 0.5% solution in water has a pH of 5.0 to 6.2. Store in airtight containers. Protect from light.

Adverse Effects

Propafenone can cause disturbances in cardiac conduction which can result in bradycardia, heart block, and sinus arrest. It may aggravate heart failure and may cause hypotension. In common with other antiarrhythmics, propafenone may induce or worsen arrhythmias in some patients.

Among the most common adverse effects are gastrointestinal intolerance, dry mouth, a bitter or metallic taste, dizziness, blurred vision, headache, and fatigue. Convulsions, blood dyscrasias, liver disorders, lupus erythematosus, skin rashes, impotence, and increased breathlessness and worsening of asthma have also been reported.

Effects on the heart. Fatal exacerbation of ventricular tachycardia was associated with propafenone therapy in a 63-year-old man.[1]

1. Nathan AW, *et al.* Fatal ventricular tachycardia in association with propafenone, a new class IC antiarrhythmic agent. *Postgrad Med J* 1984; **60**: 155–6.

Effects on the liver. A review of liver injury secondary to propafenone therapy has concluded it is a rare occurrence and appears to be due to hepatocellular injury, cholestasis, or a combination.[1]

1. Spinler SA, *et al.* Propafenone-induced liver injury. *Ann Pharmacother* 1992; **26**: 926–8.

Effects on mental function. Delusions, hallucinations, and paranoia have been reported in an elderly patient following two doses of propafenone. The manufacturer had received reports of mania and psychosis.[1] Amnesia developed in a 61-year-old man six days after starting treatment with propafenone.[2] Symptoms resolved 6 to 7 hours after discontinuing the drug.

1. Robinson AJ. Paranoia after propafenone. *Pharm J* 1991; **247**: 556.
2. Jones RJ, *et al.* Probable propafenone-induced transient global amnesia. *Ann Pharmacother* 1995; **29**: 586–90.

Effects on the nervous system. Myoclonus has been reported in a patient receiving propafenone.[1] In another patient peripheral neuropathy developed 10 months after starting treatment but symptoms had resolved 6 months after stopping the drug.[2]

1. Chua TP, *et al.* Myoclonus associated with propafenone. *BMJ* 1994; **308**: 113.
2. Galasso PJ, *et al.* Propafenone-induced peripheral neuropathy. *Mayo Clin Proc* 1995; **70**: 469–72.

Lupus erythematosus. Symptoms of lupus erythematosus and raised antinuclear antibody titres were associated with propafenone therapy on 2 occasions in a 63-year-old woman.[1]

1. Guindo J, et al. Propafenone and a syndrome of the lupus erythematosus type. Ann Intern Med 1986; 104: 589.

Precautions

Propafenone is contra-indicated in patients with uncontrolled heart failure, conduction disturbances including heart block unless controlled by artificial pacing, cardiogenic shock (unless arrhythmia-induced), severe bradycardia, or pronounced hypotension. It may alter the endocardial pacing threshold and adjustment may be necessary in patients with pacemakers.

Propafenone's beta-blocking activity can exacerbate obstructive airways disease; it should be used with great caution in patients with this disease and if the disease is severe then propafenone is contra-indicated. Propafenone may aggravate myasthenia gravis and should be avoided in patients with this condition. Electrolyte disturbances should be corrected before initiating propafenone treatment. Propafenone should be used with caution in patients with hepatic or renal impairment.

Pregnancy and breast feeding. Experience in a patient given propafenone throughout the last trimester of pregnancy indicated that despite transplacental diffusion propafenone could safely be used at this time without harm to the fetus. Propafenone and its metabolite were excreted in breast milk although it was considered that the amount would have represented a markedly subtherapeutic dose to the infant who in any case was not breast fed.[1]

1. Libardoni M, et al. Transfer of propafenone and 5-OH-propafenone to foetal plasma and maternal milk. Br J Clin Pharmacol 1991; 32: 527–8.

Interactions

Propafenone is extensively metabolised by the hepatic mixed function oxidase system and plasma-propafenone concentrations may be reduced by inducers of this system such as rifampicin; enzyme inhibitors, such as cimetidine, quinidine, and HIV-protease inhibitors, may increase plasma-propafenone concentrations. Propafenone itself may alter the plasma concentrations of other drugs given concomitantly, possibly by interfering with their metabolism. Drugs affected include beta blockers, ciclosporin, desipramine, digoxin, theophylline, and warfarin. Details are given under the individual drug monographs. There may be an increased risk of arrhythmias if propafenone is given concomitantly with other antiarrhythmics or arrhythmogenic drugs.

Antiarrhythmics. *Quinidine* inhibits the hepatic metabolism of propafenone and has raised plasma-propafenone concentrations in extensive metabolisers;[1] the plasma concentration of the active 5-hydroxy metabolite was reduced and that of the N-depropyl metabolite increased but there was no change in the clinical response.

1. Funck-Brentano C, et al. Genetically-determined interaction between propafenone and low dose quinidine: role of active metabolites in modulating net drug effect. Br J Clin Pharmacol 1989; 27: 435–44.

Antibacterials. *Rifampicin* has lowered steady-state plasma concentrations of propafenone with the reappearance of arrhythmia.[1]

1. Castel JM, et al. Rifampicin lowers plasma concentrations of propafenone and its antiarrhythmic effect. Br J Clin Pharmacol 1990; 30: 155–6.

Histamine H₂-antagonists. *Cimetidine* has been reported[1] to raise plasma-propafenone concentrations. The mean steady-state concentration increased by 22% but the wide interindividual variability meant this change was not significant.

1. Pritchett ELC, et al. Pharmacokinetic and pharmacodynamic interactions of propafenone and cimetidine. J Clin Pharmacol 1988; 28: 619–24.

Pharmacokinetics

Propafenone is readily and almost completely absorbed from the gastrointestinal tract. It is metabolised in the liver and the extent of metabolism is genetically determined. In subjects with the extensive metaboliser phenotype there is extensive first-pass metabolism to two active metabolites, 5-hydroxypropafenone and N-depropylpropafenone, and to other minor inactive metabolites. In the small proportion of subjects with the slow metaboliser phenotype little or no 5-hydroxypropafenone is formed. The bioavail-

ability of propafenone is dependent upon metaboliser phenotype but more importantly on dosage as the first-pass metabolism is saturable. In practice doses are high enough to compensate for differences in phenotype. Propafenone and its metabolites also undergo glucuronidation.

Propafenone is more than 95% protein bound.

Propafenone is excreted in the urine and faeces mainly in the form of conjugated metabolites. The elimination half-life is reported to be 2 to 10 hours in extensive metabolisers and 10 to 32 hours in slow metabolisers.

Propafenone crosses the placenta and is distributed into breast milk.

◊ General references.

1. Hii JTY, et al. Clinical pharmacokinetics of propafenone. Clin Pharmacokinet 1991; 21: 1–10.

Uses and Administration

Propafenone hydrochloride is a class Ic antiarrhythmic (p.787) with some negative inotropic and beta-adrenoceptor blocking activity. It is used in the management of supraventricular and ventricular **arrhythmias**.

The usual initial dose by mouth is 150 mg three times daily and this may be increased, if necessary, at intervals of 3 to 4 days up to a maximum of 300 mg three times daily. Patients of less than 70 kg body-weight should be given reduced doses; the elderly may also respond to reduced doses. Doses may need to be reduced if hepatic function is impaired.

Propafenone hydrochloride has also been given by slow intravenous injection or by infusion.

◊ General references.

1. Bryson HM, et al. Propafenone: a reappraisal of its pharmacology, pharmacokinetics and therapeutic use in cardiac arrhythmias. Drugs 1993; 45: 85–130.

Administration in renal impairment. Propafenone is extensively metabolised and its metabolites are excreted in the urine and faeces. A study of the effect of renal function on disposition of propafenone found that renal impairment did not alter the pharmacokinetics of propafenone or 5-hydroxypropafenone.[1] Nevertheless, the manufacturers advise that caution is necessary if propafenone is given to patients with renal impairment.

1. Fromm MF, et al. Influence of renal function on the steady-state pharmacokinetics of the antiarrhythmic propafenone and its phase I and phase II metabolites. Eur J Clin Pharmacol 1995; 48: 279–83.

Cardiac arrhythmias. Early reviews[1-4] showed propafenone, a class Ic antiarrhythmic, to be effective in a large variety of cardiac arrhythmias (p.794) including ventricular arrhythmias and supraventricular arrhythmias such as atrial flutter and atrial fibrillation. It has been used successfully to treat arrhythmias in children.[5,6] However, the results of the Cardiac Arrhythmia Suppression Trial (known as CAST), demonstrating that other class I antiarrhythmics (encainide, flecainide, and moracizine) were associated with an increased mortality rate when used for asymptomatic ventricular arrhythmias in post-infarction patients, led to many drugs of this class being restricted to severe or life-threatening ventricular arrhythmias; this restriction has also applied to propafenone in many countries although, in some, use in supraventricular arrhythmias is permitted. As well as having antiarrhythmic actions propafenone also has some beta-adrenoceptor blocking activity and this theoretically may be beneficial in post-infarction patients, but in the absence of data showing safety and efficacy of propafenone in this situation such use is not considered warranted.[4] A more recent review[7] acknowledges a general trend against the use of class Ic antiarrhythmics, including propafenone, in patients with nonsustained ventricular arrhythmias. Others[8,9] support its use in supraventricular arrhythmias.

1. Siddoway LA, Woosley RL. Propafenone: a promising new antiarrhythmic agent. Cardiovasc Rev Rep 1986; 7: 153–5 and 158–9.
2. Harron DWG, Brogden RN. Propafenone: a review of its pharmacodynamic and pharmacokinetic properties, and therapeutic use in the treatment of arrhythmias. Drugs 1987; 34: 617–47.
3. Chow MSS, et al. Propafenone: a new antiarrhythmic agent. Clin Pharm 1988; 7: 869–77.
4. Funck-Brentano C, et al. Propafenone. N Engl J Med 1990; 322: 518–25.
5. Heusch A, et al. Clinical experience with propafenone for cardiac arrhythmias in the young. Eur Heart J 1994; 15: 1050–6.
6. Janoušek J, Paul T. Safety of oral propafenone in the treatment of arrhythmias in infants and children (European Retrospective Multicenter Study). Am J Cardiol 1998; 81: 1121–4.
7. Capucci A, Boriani G. Propafenone in the treatment of cardiac arrhythmias: a risk-benefit appraisal. Drug Safety 1995; 12: 55–72.

8. Kishore AGR, Camm AJ. Guidelines for the use of propafenone in treating supraventricular arrhythmias. Drugs 1995; 50: 250–62.
9. Reimold SC, et al. Propafenone for the treatment of supraventricular tachycardia and atrial fibrillation: a meta-analysis. Am J Cardiol 1998; 82: 66N–71N.

Preparations

Proprietary Preparations (details are given in Part 3)
Aust.: Asonacor†; Metronom†; Rhythmocor; Rytmonorma; **Belg.**: Rytmonorm; **Braz.**: Ritmonorm; **Canad.**: Rythmol; **Denm.**: Rytmonorm; **Fin.**: Rytmonorm; **Fr.**: Rythmol; **Ger.**: Cuxafenon; Propafen; Propamerck; Propastad†; Prorynorm; Rytmo-Puren; Rytmogenat; Rytmonorm; Tachyfenon†; **Hong Kong:** Rytmonorm; **Irl.**: Arythmol; **Israel:** Rythmex; **Ital.**: Rytmonorm; **Mex.**: Kenona; Nistaken; Norfenon; **Neth.**: Rytmonorm; **NZ**: Rytmonorm; **Port.**: Rytmonorm; **S.Afr.**: Rythmol; **Singapore:** Rytmonorm; **Spain**: Rytmonorm; **Swed.**: Rytmonorm; **Switz.**: Rytmonorm; **Thai.**: Rytmonorm; **UK**: Arythmol; **USA**: Rythmol.

Propatylnitrate (9276-f)

Propatylnitrate (BAN, rINN).

ETTN; Etriol Trinitrate; Propatyl Nitrate (USAN); Trinetriol; Win-9317. 2-Ethyl-2-hydroxymethylpropane-1,3-diol trinitrate.
$C_6H_{11}N_3O_9 = 269.2.$
CAS — 2921-92-8.
ATC — C01DA07.

Profile

Propatylnitrate is a vasodilator with general properties similar to those of glyceryl trinitrate (p.898) that has been used in angina pectoris.

Preparations

Proprietary Preparations (details are given in Part 3)
Braz.: Sustrate.

Propentofylline (239-j)

Propentofylline (BAN, rINN).

HWA-285. 3-Methyl-1-(5-oxohexyl)-7-propylxanthine.
$C_{15}H_{22}N_4O_3 = 306.4.$
CAS — 55242-55-2.
ATC — N06BC02.

Profile

Propentofylline is a xanthine derivative that has been investigated in cerebrovascular disorders including dementia. It is also used in veterinary medicine.

Propranolol Hydrochloride (6301-g)

Propranolol Hydrochloride (BANM, USAN, rINNM).

AY-64043; ICI-45520; NSC-91523; Propranololi Hydrochloridum. (±)-1-Isopropylamino-3-(1-naphthyloxy)propan-2-ol hydrochloride.
$C_{16}H_{21}NO_2,HCl = 295.8.$
CAS — 525-66-6 (propranolol); 13013-17-7 (propranolol); 318-98-9 (propranolol hydrochloride); 3506-09-0 (propranolol hydrochloride).

Pharmacopoeias. In Chin., Eur. (see p.vi), Int., Jpn, Pol., and US.

In aqueous solutions propranolol decomposes with oxidation of the isopropylamine side-chain, accompanied by a reduction in pH and discoloration of the solution. Solutions are most stable at pH 3 and decompose rapidly when alkaline.

Pharmacopoeial description

Ph. Eur.: A white or almost white powder. Soluble in water and in alcohol.

USP 25: A white to off-white, odourless, crystalline powder. Soluble in water and in alcohol; slightly soluble in chloroform; practically insoluble in ether.

Adverse Effects, Treatment, and Precautions

As for beta blockers, p.844.

Effects on the gastrointestinal tract. A report of retroperitoneal fibrosis associated with propranolol in a patient.[1]

1. Pierce JR, et al. Propranolol and retroperitoneal fibrosis. Ann Intern Med 1981; 95: 244.

Interactions

The interactions associated with beta blockers are discussed on p.846.

Pharmacokinetics

Propranolol is almost completely absorbed from the gastrointestinal tract, but is subject to considerable hepatic tissue binding and first-pass metabolism. Peak plasma concentrations occur about 1 to 2 hours after an oral dose. Plasma concentrations vary greatly between individuals. It has high lipid solubility. Propranolol crosses the blood-brain barrier and the placenta. The drug is distributed into breast milk. Propranolol is more than 90% bound to plasma proteins. It is metabolised in the liver and at least one of its metabolites (4-hydroxypropranolol) is considered to be biologically active, but the contribution of metabolites to its overall activity is uncertain. The metabolites and small amounts of unchanged drug are excreted in the urine. The plasma half-life of propranolol is about 3 to 6 hours. Propranolol is reported not to be significantly dialysable.

Breast feeding. Propranolol is distributed into breast milk. A milk/plasma ratio range of 0.33 to 1.65 was reported in a study of 3 lactating women.[1] It was calculated that the maximum dose likely to be ingested by a breast-fed infant would be less than 0.1% of the maternal dose.

1. Smith MT, et al. Propranolol, propranolol glucuronide, and naphthoxylactic acid in breast milk and plasma. Ther Drug Monit 1983; 5: 87–93.

Pregnancy. A study in 6 pregnant patients (32 to 36 weeks' gestation) showed that the disposition of propranolol 120 mg by mouth and 10 mg intravenously was not altered in pregnancy compared with the postnatal period.[1] Another study[2] in 13 pregnant patients given propranolol to control hypertension demonstrated that the pharmacokinetics of propranolol and most of its major metabolites were not altered during pregnancy. Samples at term[3] in 10 of the women showed that propranolol and all of its known metabolites were present in maternal plasma, cord plasma, and neonatal plasma. At delivery plasma protein binding of propranolol was reported as 87.5% in maternal plasma and 67.2% in cord plasma. Similar results for maternal and cord plasma protein binding have been reported by others.[4]

1. O'Hare MFO, et al. Pharmacokinetics of propranolol during pregnancy. Eur J Clin Pharmacol 1984; 27: 583–7.
2. Smith MT, et al. Chronic propranolol administration during pregnancy: maternal pharmacokinetics. Eur J Clin Pharmacol 1983; 25: 481–90.
3. Smith MT, et al. Metabolism of propranolol in the human maternal-placental-foetal unit. Eur J Clin Pharmacol 1983; 24: 727–32.
4. Wood M, Wood AJJ. Changes in plasma drug binding and α_1-acid glycoprotein in mother and newborn infant. Clin Pharmacol Ther 1981; 29: 522–6.

Uses and Administration

Propranolol is a non-cardioselective beta blocker (p.844). It is reported to have membrane-stabilising properties, but does not possess intrinsic sympathomimetic activity.

Propranolol is used as the hydrochloride in the management of hypertension (p.802), phaeochromocytoma (p.810), angina pectoris (p.791), myocardial infarction (p.805), and cardiac arrhythmias (p.794). It is also used in hypertrophic subaortic stenosis. It is used to control symptoms of sympathetic overactivity in the management of hyperthyroidism (p.1519), anxiety disorders (p.649), and tremor (p.848). Other indications include the prophylaxis of migraine (p.449) and of upper gastrointestinal bleeding in patients with portal hypertension (see Variceal Haemorrhage under Monoethanolamine Oleate, p.1637).

Propranolol hydrochloride is usually given by mouth. In **hypertension** propranolol hydrochloride is given in initial doses of 40 to 80 mg twice daily increased as required to a usual range of 160 to 320 mg daily; some patients may require up to 640 mg daily. Propranolol is *not* suitable for the emergency treatment of hypertension; it should not be given intravenously in hypertension.

In **phaeochromocytoma**, 60 mg daily may be given on 3 pre-operative days always in association with alpha blockade. If the tumour is inoperable prolonged treatment may be given with a daily dose of 30 mg.

In **angina**, initial doses of propranolol hydrochloride 40 mg given 2 or 3 times daily are increased as required to a usual range of 120 to 240 mg daily. Some patients may require up to 320 mg daily.

Propranolol hydrochloride is administered within 5 to 21 days of **myocardial infarction** in doses of 40 mg given four times daily for 2 or 3 days followed by 80 mg twice daily. Another regimen is to give 180 to 240 mg daily in divided doses.

Propranolol may be given in doses of 30 to 160 mg daily in divided doses in the long-term management of **cardiac arrhythmias**. For the emergency treatment of cardiac arrhythmias, propranolol hydrochlo-

ride may be given by slow intravenous injection in a dose of 1 mg injected over a period of 1 minute, repeated if necessary every 2 minutes until a maximum total of 10 mg has been given in conscious patients and 5 mg in patients under anaesthesia. Patients receiving propranolol intravenously should be carefully monitored.

In **hypertrophic subaortic stenosis,** the usual dose of propranolol hydrochloride is 10 to 40 mg given three or four times daily.

In **hyperthyroidism** propranolol hydrochloride is given in doses of 10 to 40 mg three or four times daily. Intravenous administration may be necessary; the dose is 1 mg injected over 1 minute, repeated at 2-minute intervals until a response is observed or to a maximum dose of 10 mg in conscious patients or 5 mg in patients under anaesthesia.

The dose for **anxiety** is 40 mg daily; this may be increased to 40 mg two or three times daily.

Essential tremor may be treated with 40 mg given two or three times daily; the dose can be increased at weekly intervals to 160 mg daily although doses up to 320 mg daily may be necessary.

An initial dose of 40 mg two or three times daily is used in **migraine** prophylaxis; the dose can be increased at weekly intervals up to 160 mg daily. Some patients have been given 240 mg daily.

In **portal hypertension,** propranolol hydrochloride should be given in initial doses of 40 mg twice daily; the dose may be increased as required up to 160 mg twice daily.

Children. Propranolol hydrochloride has been used in the treatment of hypertension in children in initial doses of 1 mg per kg body-weight daily in divided doses by mouth, increased as required to a usual range of 2 to 4 mg per kg daily in divided doses. For arrhythmias, phaeochromocytoma, and hyperthyroidism, the dose is 250 to 500 µg per kg three or four times daily by mouth. Children requiring intravenous administration may be given 25 to 50 µg per kg injected slowly with appropriate monitoring; this dose may be repeated three or four times daily. Children under 12 years of age may be given 20 mg two or three times daily for the prophylactic management of migraine.

Administration in hepatic impairment. A study of the effects of cirrhosis on the disposition of propranolol during steady-state oral administration in 9 normal subjects and 7 with cirrhosis demonstrated a mean threefold increase in unbound propranolol concentrations in the blood in patients with cirrhosis when compared with the controls. Mean half-lives for the 2 groups were 11.2 and 4 hours respectively.[1] Another study of the pharmacokinetics of propranolol given as a single dose of a 20-mg tablet and a 160-mg modified-release preparation daily for 7 days in 10 patients with cirrhosis and portal hypertension demonstrated higher plasma concentrations in patients with severe liver disease compared with those reported in normal controls.[2] Similar pharmacokinetic findings have been reported by others.[3]

In patients with severe liver disease, it has been suggested that propranolol therapy be started at a low dose such as 20 mg three times daily, or 80 mg of a modified-release preparation given once daily,[2] or 160 mg of a modified-release preparation given every other day.[3] Monitoring of beta blockade is essential; checking the heart rate[2] or exercise testing[3] have been suggested as suitable methods to assess the extent of beta blockade in patients with cirrhosis.

1. Wood AJJ, et al. The influence of cirrhosis on steady-state blood concentrations of unbound propranolol after oral administration. Clin Pharmacokinet 1978; 3: 478–87.
2. Arthur MJP, et al. Pharmacology of propranolol in patients with cirrhosis and portal hypertension. Gut 1985; 26: 14–19.
3. Calès P, et al. Pharmacodynamic and pharmacokinetic study of propranolol in patients with cirrhosis and portal hypertension. Br J Clin Pharmacol 1989; 27: 763–70.

Administration in renal impairment. A study of the pharmacokinetics of propranolol in 11 patients with chronic renal insufficiency showed no impairment in the elimination kinetics of propranolol compared with 8 subjects with normal renal function.[1] Peak concentrations of propranolol reported in patients with chronic renal failure have been 2 to 3 times higher than those reported in patients receiving dialysis or normal subjects.[1,2] Additional studies indicate that there is no pharmacokinetic reason to amend the dosage of propranolol in patients with renal impairment.[3]

Findings from a study in 8 patients on haemodialysis include a slight elevation of propranolol-plasma concentrations, no ele-

vation of plasma concentration of 4-hydroxypropranolol, but extremely high plasma concentrations of other propranolol metabolites.[4]

1. Lowenthal DT, et al. Pharmacokinetics of oral propranolol in chronic renal disease. Clin Pharmacol Ther 1974; 16: 761–9.
2. Bianchetti G, et al. Pharmacokinetics and effects of propranolol in terminal uraemic patients and in patients undergoing regular dialysis treatment. Clin Pharmacokinet 1976; 1: 373–84.
3. Wood AJJ, et al. Propranolol disposition in renal failure. Br J Clin Pharmacol 1980; 10: 561–6.
4. Stone WJ, Walle T. Massive propranolol metabolite retention during maintenance hemodialysis. Clin Pharmacol Ther 1980; 28: 449–55.

Preparations

BP 2001: Prolonged-release Propranolol Capsules; Propranolol Injection; Propranolol Tablets;

USP 25: Propranolol Hydrochloride and Hydrochlorothiazide Extended-release Capsules; Propranolol Hydrochloride and Hydrochlorothiazide Tablets; Propranolol Hydrochloride Extended-release Capsules; Propranolol Hydrochloride Injection; Propranolol Hydrochloride Tablets.

Proprietary Preparations (details are given in Part 3)

Aust.: Inderal; Proprahexal; *Austral.:* Deralin; Inderal; *Belg.:* Inderal; *Braz.:* Inderal; Tenadren; *Canad.:* Inderal; Novo-Pranol†; *Denm.:* Inderal; Propal; Propranet†; *Fin.:* Inderal; Propral; Ranoprin; *Fr.:* Adrexan; Avlocardyl; Hemipralon; *Ger.:* Beta-Tablinen; Dociton; Efektolol; Elbrol; Indobloc; Obsidan; Propabloc; Prophylux; propra; Propra-ratiopharm; Propranur; *Hong Kong:* Angilol; Antarol; Berkolol; Inderal; Inpanol; Propa; *Irl.:* Berkolol†; Half Inderal; Inderal; Tiperal; *Israel:* Deralin; Inderal; Prolol; Slow Deralin; *Ital.:* Inderal; *Mex.:* Europranolol; Inderalici; Prochor; Propalem; Propalen; Propalgin; Propol; *Neth.:* Inderal; Norw.: Inderal; Pranolol; Pronovan†; *NZ:* Angilol; Cardinol; *Port.:* Corpendol; Inderal; *S.Afr.:* Cardiblok; Cardimax†; Cardispare; Dynablok†; Hipranol†; Inderal; Indoblok†; Nolol; Norpro†; Pressanol†; Prodorol; Pur-Bloka; Rexigen†; *Singapore:* Inderal; Inpanol; Spain: Sumial; Swed.: Inderal; Switz.: Betaprol; Inderal; Thai.: Atensin; Betalol; Betapress; Cardenol; Emforal; Inderal; Normpress; Palon; Perlol; Pralol; Prolol; Pronosil; Servanolol; Syntonol; UK: Angilol; Apsolol†; Bedranol; Berkolol†; Beta-Prograne; Betadur CR; Cardinol†; Half Beta-Prograne; Half Betadur CR; Half Inderal; Inderal; Lopranol LA; Probeta LA; Propanix†; Syprol; *USA:* Betachron†; Inderal.

Multi-ingredient: *Aust.:* Inderal comp; Inderetic; Tardurol†; *Belg.:* Inderetic; *Canad.:* Inderide; *Ger.:* Beta-Nephral†; Beta-Turfa; Betathiazid; Betathiazid A; Diutensan comp; Docidrazin; Dociretic; Dociteren; Manimon; Nitro-Obsidan; Obsilazin N; Pertenso N; Propra comp; *Irl.:* Inderetic; *Neth.:* Inderetic; *S.Afr.:* Inderetic; *Spain:* Betadipresan; Betadipresan Diu; *Switz.:* Inderetic; *UK:* Inderetic; Inderex; *USA:* Inderide.

Proscillaridin (5826-b)

Proscillaridin (BAN, USAN, rINN).

2936; A-32686; Proscillaridin A; PSC-801. 14-Hydroxy-3β-(α-L-rhamnopyranosyloxy)-14β-bufa-4,20,22-trienolide.

$C_{30}H_{42}O_8 = 530.6$.
CAS — 466-06-8.
ATC — C01AB01.

A glycoside obtained from *Drimia maritima* (Liliaceae).

Profile
Proscillaridin is a cardiac glycoside and positive inotrope with general properties similar to those of digoxin (p.870). It is reported to have a rapid onset and a short duration of action.

Proscillaridin is used in the treatment of heart failure (p.798). It is given by mouth in usual initial and usual maintenance doses of 1 to 1.5 mg daily; maintenance doses may range from 0.5 to 2.5 mg daily as required.

Preparations

Proprietary Preparations (details are given in Part 3)
Aust.: Caradrin; *Austral.:* Talusin; *Fin.:* Talusin; *Ger.:* Talusin; *S.Afr.:* Talusin†; *Switz.:* Talusin.

Multi-ingredient: *Aust.:* Theocaradrin†; *Switz.:* Theo-Talusin.

Quinapril Hydrochloride (491-m)

Quinapril Hydrochloride (BANM, USAN, rINNM).

CI-906 (quinapril). (3S)-2-{N-[(S)-1-Ethoxycarbonyl-3-phenylpropyl]-L-alanyl}-1,2,3,4-tetrahydro-isoquinoline-3-carboxylic acid hydrochloride.

$C_{25}H_{30}N_2O_5,HCl = 475.0$.
CAS — 85441-61-8 (quinapril); 82586-55-8 (quinapril hydrochloride).

Quinapril hydrochloride 10.8 mg is approximately equivalent to 10.0 mg of quinapril.

Adverse Effects, Treatment, and Precautions
As for ACE inhibitors, p.820.

Interactions
As for ACE inhibitors, p.822.

Antibacterials. Quinapril has been reported to reduce the absorption of *tetracyclines* due to the presence of magnesium carbonate in the tablet formulation.

Pharmacokinetics

Quinapril acts as a prodrug of the diacid quinaprilat, its active metabolite. Following oral administration about 60% of a dose is absorbed. Quinapril is metabolised mainly in the liver to quinaprilat and inactive metabolites. Peak plasma concentrations of quinaprilat are achieved within 2 hours of an oral dose of quinapril. Quinaprilat is about 97% bound to plasma proteins. Up to 60% of an oral dose of quinapril is excreted in the urine as quinaprilat, other metabolites, and unchanged drug, with the rest being excreted in the faeces. The effective half-life for accumulation of quinaprilat is approximately 3 hours following multiple doses of quinapril; a long terminal phase half-life of 25 hours may represent strong binding of quinaprilat to angiotensin-converting enzyme.

The pharmacokinetics of both quinapril and quinaprilat are affected by renal and hepatic impairment.

◊ References.
1. Begg EJ, *et al.* The pharmacokinetics and pharmacodynamics of quinapril and quinaprilat in renal impairment. *Br J Clin Pharmacol* 1990; **30**: 213–20.
2. Halstenson CE, *et al.* The pharmacokinetics of quinapril and its active metabolite, quinaprilat, in patients with various degrees of renal function. *J Clin Pharmacol* 1992; **32**: 344–50.
3. Wolter K, Fritschka E. Pharmacokinetics and pharmacodynamics of quinaprilat after low dose quinapril in patients with terminal renal failure. *Eur J Clin Pharmacol* 1993; **44** (suppl 1): S53–6.
4. Begg EJ, *et al.* The pharmacokinetics of quinapril and quinaprilat in patients with congestive heart failure. *Br J Clin Pharmacol* 1994; **37**: 302–4.
5. Squire IB, *et al.* Haemodynamic response and pharmacokinetics after the first dose of quinapril in patients with congestive heart failure. *Br J Clin Pharmacol* 1994; **38**: 117–23.
6. Breslin E, *et al.* A pharmacodynamic and pharmacokinetic comparison of intravenous quinaprilat and oral quinapril. *J Clin Pharmacol* 1996; **36**: 414–21.

Uses and Administration

Quinapril is an ACE inhibitor (p.820). It is used in the treatment of hypertension (p.802) and heart failure (p.798).

Quinapril is converted in the body to its active metabolite quinaprilat. The haemodynamic effects are seen within 1 hour of a single dose by mouth and the maximum effect occurs after about 2 to 4 hours, although the full effect may not develop for 1 to 2 weeks during chronic administration. The haemodynamic action persists for about 24 hours, allowing once-daily dosing. Quinapril is given by mouth as the hydrochloride, but doses are expressed in terms of quinapril.

In the treatment of **hypertension** the initial dose is 10 mg once daily. Since there may be a precipitous fall in blood pressure in some patients when starting therapy with an ACE inhibitor, the first dose should preferably be given at bedtime. An initial dose of 2.5 mg daily is recommended in the elderly, in patients with renal impairment, or in those receiving a diuretic; if possible, the diuretic should be withdrawn 2 or 3 days before quinapril is started and resumed later if necessary. The usual maintenance dose is 20 to 40 mg daily, as a single dose or divided into 2 doses, although up to 80 mg daily has been given.

In the management of **heart failure**, severe first-dose hypotension on introduction of an ACE inhibitor is common in patients on loop diuretics, but their temporary withdrawal may cause rebound pulmonary oedema. Thus treatment should be initiated with a low dose under close medical supervision. Quinapril is given in an initial dose of 2.5 mg daily. Usual maintenance doses range from 10 to 20 mg daily, as a single dose or divided into 2 doses; up to 40 mg daily has been given.

Quinaprilat is given intravenously.

◊ Reviews.
1. Wadworth AN, Brogden RN. Quinapril: a review of its pharmacological properties, and therapeutic efficacy in cardiovascular disorders. *Drugs* 1991; **41**: 378–99.
2. Plosker GL, Sorkin EM. Quinapril: a reappraisal of its pharmacology and therapeutic efficacy in cardiovascular disorders. *Drugs* 1994; **48**: 227–52.

Preparations

Proprietary Preparations (details are given in Part 3)
Aust.: Accupro; Continucor; ***Austral.:*** Accupril; Asig; ***Belg.:*** Accupril; ***Canad.:*** Accupril; ***Denm.:*** Accupro; ***Fin.:*** Accupro; ***Fr.:*** Acuitel; Korec; ***Ger.:*** Accupro; ***Hong Kong:*** Accupril; ***Irl.:*** Accupro; ***Ital.:*** Accuprin; Acequin; Quinazil; ***Mex.:*** Acupril; ***Neth.:*** Acupril; ***NZ:*** Accupril; ***Port.:*** Acupril; ***S.Afr.:*** Accupril; ***Singapore:*** Accupril; ***Swed.:*** Accupro; ***Switz.:*** Accupro; ***Thai.:*** Accupril; ***UK:*** Accupro; ***USA:*** Accupril.

Multi-ingredient: ***Aust.:*** Accuzide; ***Belg.:*** Accuretic; ***Canad.:*** Accuretic; ***Fin.:*** Accupro Comp; ***Fr.:*** Acuilix; Koretic; Quinimax; ***Ger.:*** Accuzide; ***Irl.:*** Accuretic; ***Ital.:*** Accuretic; Acuzide; Quinazide; ***Neth.:*** Acuzide; ***Port.:*** Acuretic; ***S.Afr.:*** Accuretic; ***Spain:*** Bicetil; Lidaltrin Diu; ***Swed.:*** Accupro Comp; ***Switz.:*** Accuretic; ***UK:*** Accuretic; ***USA:*** Accuretic.

Quinethazone (2354-w)

Quinethazone (BAN, rINN).

Chinethazonum. 7-Chloro-2-ethyl-1,2,3,4-tetrahydro-4-oxo-quinazoline-6-sulphonamide.

$C_{10}H_{12}ClN_3O_3S = 289.7$.

CAS — 73-49-4.

ATC — C03BA02.

Profile

Quinethazone is a diuretic which is related chemically to metolazone and has properties similar to those of the thiazide diuretics (see Hydrochlorothiazide, p.907). It is used for oedema, including that associated with heart failure (p.798), and for hypertension (p.802).

Diuresis is initiated within about 2 hours after administration, reaches a peak after 6 hours, and lasts for 18 to 24 hours.

In the treatment of oedema the usual dose is 50 to 100 mg by mouth daily; in some cases doses of 200 mg daily may be necessary.

In the treatment of hypertension the usual dose is 50 to 100 mg daily, either alone, or in conjunction with other antihypertensives. An initial dose of 25 mg daily has also been used.

Preparations

Proprietary Preparations (details are given in Part 3)
USA: Hydromox.

Quinidine (7771-r)

Quinidine (BAN).

Chinidinum; Quinidina. (8R,9S)-6′-Methoxycinchonan-9-ol; (+)-(αS)-α-(6-Methoxy-4-quinolyl)-α-[(2R,4S,5R)-(5-vinylquinuclidin-2-yl)]methanol.

$C_{20}H_{24}N_2O_2 = 324.4$.

CAS — 56-54-2 (anhydrous quinidine); 63717-04-4 (quinidine dihydrate); 72402-50-7 (± quinidine).

ATC — C01BA01.

An isomer of quinine, obtained from the bark of species of *Cinchona* and their hybrids; it may also be obtained from *Remijia pedunculata*, or prepared from quinine. It may contain some hydroquinidine, a closely allied base with similar chemical, physical, and physiological properties.

Quinidine Bisulfate (7772-f)

Quinidine Bisulphate (BANM).

$C_{20}H_{24}N_2O_2,H_2SO_4 = 422.5$.

CAS — 747-45-5 (anhydrous quinidine bisulfate); 6151-39-9 (quinidine bisulfate tetrahydrate).

Pharmacopoeias. In Br.

Quinidine bisulfate (anhydrous) 260 mg is approximately equivalent to 200 mg of quinidine (anhydrous).

Pharmacopoeial description

BP 2001: Colourless, odourless or almost odourless, crystals. It contains not more than 15% of hydroquinidine bisulfate. Freely soluble in water and in alcohol; practically insoluble in ether. A 1% solution in water has a pH of 2.6 to 3.6. Protect from light.

Quinidine Gluconate (7773-d)

Quinidine Gluconate (BANM).

Quinidinium Gluconate.

$C_{20}H_{24}N_2O_2,C_6H_{12}O_7 = 520.6$.

CAS — 7054-25-3.

Pharmacopoeias. In US.

Quinidine gluconate (anhydrous) 321 mg is approximately equivalent to 200 mg of quinidine (anhydrous).

Pharmacopoeial description

USP 25: A white, odourless powder. It contains not more than 20% of hydroquinidine gluconate. Freely soluble in water; slightly soluble in alcohol. Protect from light.

◊ More than 40% of a dose of quinidine gluconate was lost when the drug was administered by intravenous infusion using a PVC infusion bag and tubing.[1]

1. Darbar D, *et al.* Loss of quinidine gluconate injection in a polyvinyl chloride infusion system. *Am J Health-Syst Pharm* 1996; **53**: 655–8.

Quinidine Polygalacturonate (7774-n)

Quinidine poly(D-galacturonate) hydrate.

$C_{20}H_{24}N_2O_2,(C_6H_{10}O_7)_x,xH_2O$.

CAS — 27555-34-6 (anhydrous quinidine polygalacturonate); 65484-56-2 (quinidine polygalacturonate hydrate).

Quinidine Sulfate (7775-h)

Chinidini Sulfas; Chinidinsulfate; Chinidinum Sulfuricum; Quinidine Sulphate (BANM); Quinidini Sulfas.

$(C_{20}H_{24}N_2O_2)_2,H_2SO_4,2H_2O = 782.9$.

CAS — 50-54-4 (anhydrous quinidine sulfate); 6591-63-5 (quinidine sulfate dihydrate).

Pharmacopoeias. In Eur. (see p.vi), Int., Jpn, Pol., and US.

Quinidine sulfate (dihydrate) 241 mg and quinidine sulfate (anhydrous) 230 mg are each approximately equivalent to 200 mg of quinidine (anhydrous).

Pharmacopoeial description

Ph. Eur.: White or almost white, crystalline powder, or silky, colourless needles. It contains not more than 15% of hydroquinidine sulfate. Slightly soluble in water; soluble in boiling water and in alcohol; practically insoluble in acetone. A 1% solution in water has a pH of 6.0 to 6.8. Protect from light.

USP 25: Fine, needle-like, white crystals, frequently cohering in masses, or a fine, white powder. It is odourless and darkens on exposure to light. It contains not more than 20% of hydroquinidine sulfate. Its solutions are neutral or alkaline to litmus. Soluble 1 in 100 of water, 1 in 10 of alcohol, and 1 in 15 of chloroform; insoluble in ether. Protect from light.

Stability. Quinidine sulfate was reported[1] to be stable for up to 60 days in a number of extemporaneously prepared oral liquid formulations.

1. Allen LV, Erickson MA. Stability of bethanechol chloride, pyrazinamide, quinidine sulfate, rifampin, and tetracycline hydrochloride in extemporaneously compounded oral liquids. *Am J Health-Syst Pharm* 1998; **55**: 1804–9.

Adverse Effects and Treatment

Quinidine and its salts cause both cardiac and non-cardiac adverse effects. They commonly cause gastrointestinal irritation with nausea, vomiting, and diarrhoea.

Hypersensitivity similar to that occurring with quinine may also occur and a test dose should be given to each patient (see Uses and Administration, below). Reactions include respiratory difficulties, urticaria, pruritus, skin rashes, purpura, thrombocytopenia and other blood dyscrasias, and, rarely, fever and anaphylaxis. Granulomatous hepatitis and a lupus-like syndrome have been reported.

Quinidine may give rise to cinchonism (see Quinine, p.445) with tinnitus, impaired hearing, visual disturbances, headache, confusion, vertigo, vomiting, and abdominal pain; it is usually associated with large doses, but may occur in idiosyncratic subjects given small doses.

Quinidine may induce hypotension; this is a special risk with intravenous administration. It may precipitate ventricular arrhythmias, including torsade de pointes.

In quinidine overdosage, the cardiac symptoms of intoxication predominate. Quinidine is cumulative in action and inappropriately high plasma concentrations may induce ECG changes, heart block, asystole, ventricular tachycardia, ventricular fibrillation, syncope, seizures, coma, and sometimes death. Treatment of adverse effects and overdosage is symptomatic and supportive.

◊ A review of adverse effects associated with the class Ia antiarrhythmic drugs quinidine, disopyramide, and procainamide, and their clinical management.[1]

1. Kim SY, Benowitz NL. Poisoning due to class IA antiarrhythmic drugs quinidine, procainamide and disopyramide. *Drug Safety* 1990; **5**: 393–420.

Effects on the blood. Quinidine-induced thrombocytopenia is not uncommon and it is one of the best documented drugs known to cause drug-dependent thrombocytopenia. The reaction is considered to be a hypersensitivity reaction probably due to the binding of quinidine to the platelet surface causing production of autoantibodies and subsequent platelet lysis.[1] The antigenic constituent of the platelet membrane may be glycoprotein Ib although other surface glycoproteins have also been implicated.[2] Highly specific quinidine-dependent platelet antibodies have been found in the serum of patients with quinidine-induced thrombocytopenia;[3] the antibodies reacted with quinidine and the isomerically similar desmethoxy derivative cinchonine, but not with quinine. Once formed such antibodies may remain detectable for over 2 years.

A second mechanism has been proposed in which quinidine-autoantibody complexes are formed and then deposited on the platelet causing lysis.[2]

1. Mitchell JA, *et al.* Immunotoxic side-effects of drug therapy. *Drug Safety* 1990; **5:** 168–78.
2. Stricker RB, Shuman MA. Quinidine purpura: evidence that glycoprotein V is a target platelet antigen. *Blood* 1986; **67:** 1377–81.
3. Reid DM, Shulman NR. Drug purpura due to surreptitious quinidine intake. *Ann Intern Med* 1988; **108:** 206–8.

Effects on the eyes. Corneal deposits resembling those found in keratopathy developed in a patient who had been taking quinidine for 2 years.[1] Symptoms had improved and both corneas had cleared completely within 2 months of stopping the drug.

A small number of patients have also been identified[2] who developed uveitis during quinidine treatment.

1. Zaidman GW. Quinidine keratopathy. *Am J Ophthalmol* 1984; **97:** 247–9.
2. Fraunfelder FW, Rosenbaum JT. Drug-induced uveitis: incidence, prevention and treatment. *Drug Safety* 1997; **17:** 197–207.

Effects on the joints. Quinidine has been associated with the development of reversible, symmetrical polyarthritis in several patients.[1-3] No biochemical or immunological abnormalities were found and the reaction was considered to be distinct from quinidine-induced lupus erythematosus (see below). Symptoms resolved within 1 week of withdrawing quinidine.

1. Kertes P, Hunt D. Polyarthritis complicating quinidine treatment. *BMJ* 1982; **284:** 1373–4.
2. Cohen MG, *et al.* Two distinct quinidine-induced rheumatic syndromes. *Ann Intern Med* 1988; **108:** 369–71.
3. Naschitz JE, Yeshurun D. Quinidine and rheumatic syndromes. *Ann Intern Med* 1988; **109:** 248–9.

Effects on the liver. Hypersensitivity reactions involving the liver have been reported in about 2% of patients receiving quinidine.[1,2] The main clinical symptom is fever[1-3] but skin rash,[1,3] purpura,[2] and hepatomegaly[1] may also occur. Liver enzyme values are raised[1-4] and the platelet count may be reduced.[3] The reaction is reversible on withdrawing quinidine with fever resolving in about 48 hours and liver enzymes values returning to normal within about 2 weeks. Liver biopsy often shows granulomatous hepatitis,[1-3] but other inflammatory changes[2] and cholestatic jaundice[4] have been found.

1. Geltner D, *et al.* Quinidine hypersensitivity and liver involvement: a survey of 32 patients. *Gastroenterology* 1976; **70:** 650–2.
2. Knobler H, *et al.* Quinidine-induced hepatitis. *Arch Intern Med* 1986; **146:** 526–8.
3. Bramlet DA, *et al.* Granulomatous hepatitis as a manifestation of quinidine hypersensitivity. *Arch Intern Med* 1980; **140:** 395–7.
4. Hogan DB, *et al.* Unusual hepatotoxic reaction to quinidine. *Can Med Assoc J* 1984; **130:** 973.

Effects on mental state. Gradually progressive cerebral dysfunction characterised by intermittent confusion, agitation, restlessness, personality change, and paranoid features occurred in a 62-year-old man who had taken quinidine for about 15 years.[1] Within 24 hours of discontinuing quinidine there was a marked improvement and after 5 days he had returned to normal with no cognitive deficits. It was considered that quinidine precipitated or exacerbated the functional psychosis in this patient.

1. Johnson AG, *et al.* A functional psychosis precipitated by quinidine. *Med J Aust* 1990; **153:** 47–9.

Effects on the skin. Skin reactions reported with quinidine include exacerbation of psoriasis,[1] blue-grey pigmentation,[2] and photosensitivity.[3] Purpuric bruising has occurred in a person who was subjected to inhalation of quinidine dust in the workplace.[4]

1. Harwell WB. Quinidine-induced psoriasis. *J Am Acad Dermatol* 1983; **9:** 278.
2. Mahler R, *et al.* Pigmentation induced by quinidine therapy. *Arch Dermatol* 1986; **122:** 1062–4.
3. Marx JL, *et al.* Quinidine photosensitivity. *Arch Dermatol* 1983; **119:** 39–43.
4. Salom IL. Purpura due to inhaled quinidine. *JAMA* 1991; **266:** 1220.

Hypoglycaemia. Mean plasma-insulin concentrations increased and mean plasma-glucose concentrations decreased in 8 healthy subjects and 10 patients with malaria given quinidine intravenously.[1] Profound hypoglycaemia occurred in one patient with cerebral malaria and acute renal failure. These effects were considered to be associated with stimulation of β-cell secretion of insulin by quinidine and it was concluded that hypoglycaemia may occur in any severely ill fasting patient given parenteral quinidine.

1. Phillips RE, *et al.* Hypoglycaemia and antimalarial drugs: quinidine and release of insulin. *BMJ* 1986; **292:** 1319–21.

Lupus erythematosus. There are several well-documented reports of quinidine-induced lupus erythematosus.[1-4] The syndrome involves polyarthritis with a positive antinuclear antibody test. Symptoms do not usually occur until several months after starting quinidine and resolve slowly on withdrawing the drug. A recurrence of lupus-like symptoms has occurred in patients with a previous reaction to procainamide.[2]

1. West SG, *et al.* Quinidine-induced lupus erythematosus. *Ann Intern Med* 1984; **100:** 840–2.
2. Amadio P, *et al.* Procainamide, quinidine, and lupus erythematosus. *Ann Intern Med* 1985; **102:** 419.

3. Lavie CJ, *et al.* Systemic lupus erythematosus (SLE) induced by quinidine. *Arch Intern Med* 1985; **145:** 446–8.
4. Cohen MG, *et al.* Two distinct quinidine-induced rheumatic syndromes. *Ann Intern Med* 1988; **108:** 369–71.

Oesophageal stricture. Oesophageal ulceration and stricture formation have been reported[1] in patients taking quinidine and reviews[1,2] suggest that quinidine is one of the most common causes of drug-induced oesophageal damage.

1. McCord GS, Clouse RE. Pill-induced esophageal strictures: clinical features and risk factors for development. *Am J Med* 1990; **88:** 512–18.
2. Jaspersen D. Drug-induced oesophageal disorders: pathogenesis, incidence, prevention and management. *Drug Safety* 2000; **22:** 237–49.

Precautions

Quinidine sulfate is contra-indicated in patients with complete heart block. An initial test dose of quinidine should always be given to detect hypersensitivity; positive responders should not be given quinidine nor should patients who have previously experienced quinidine hypersensitivity. It should be used with extreme caution in patients with incomplete heart block or uncompensated heart failure. Care is also required in patients with myasthenia gravis as it can exacerbate the symptoms and may reduce the effectiveness of parasympathomimetic drugs. Antiarrhythmic therapy with quinidine should be initiated with extreme caution, if at all, during acute infections or fever as hypersensitivity reactions may be masked.

When quinidine is used to treat atrial flutter or fibrillation, the reduction in atrioventricular block may result in a very rapid ventricular rate. This can be avoided by prior digitalisation or concomitant administration of a rate-limiting calcium-channel blocker or beta blocker. However, quinidine is contraindicated in digitalis overdosage as concomitant administration of quinidine with digoxin results in markedly increased plasma concentrations of digoxin.

Reduced dosage should be considered for the elderly, for patients with hepatic or renal impairment, and on the occasions when it is used in heart failure.

Pregnancy and breast feeding. In a report[1] on the administration of quinidine sulfate to a woman throughout pregnancy, concentrations in the infant's serum at delivery were similar to the mother's although amniotic fluid concentrations were raised. Quinidine diffused freely into the mother's milk and, although the infant would have received a dose far below the therapeutic dose, she was advised not to breast feed because of potential quinidine accumulation in the immature newborn liver.

1. Hill LM, Malkasian GD. The use of quinidine sulfate throughout pregnancy. *Obstet Gynecol* 1979; **54:** 366–8.

Interactions

Quinidine is used in combination with other antiarrhythmic drugs but caution is required with such combinations (see below). Concomitant use with other arrhythmogenic drugs should be avoided.

Quinidine is metabolised in the liver, mainly by the cytochrome P450 isoenzyme CYP3A4, and interactions may occur through inhibition or enhancement of hepatic metabolism. Rifampicin, phenobarbital, and phenytoin increase hepatic metabolism of quinidine and increased doses of quinidine may be needed if one of these drugs is added to quinidine therapy. The HIV-protease inhibitors nelfinavir and ritonavir may produce toxic concentrations of quinidine when given concomitantly.

Urinary excretion of quinidine is dependent on urinary pH; drugs which increase urinary pH such as sodium bicarbonate, some antacids, and carbonic anhydrase inhibitors tend to increase the plasma concentration of quinidine since the proportion of nonionised drug in the urine is increased allowing greater renal tubular reabsorption.

As well as being affected by a range of drugs quinidine can in its turn affect other compounds which include oral anticoagulants, antihypertensives, antimuscarinics, beta blockers, digoxin, muscle relaxants, and parasympathomimetics. These interactions are discussed under the monographs for those drugs. Quinidine also inhibits the cytochrome P450

isoenzyme CYP2D6 and may affect drugs metabolised by this route.

Antiarrhythmics. *Amiodarone* may increase the plasma concentration of quinidine, increasing the risk of toxicity; prolongation of the QT interval with torsade de pointes has been reported.[1] This interaction is probably due to amiodarone inhibiting hepatic or renal clearance of quinidine or displacing quinidine from binding sites. If the two drugs are used together the dose of quinidine may need to be reduced and the patient should be closely monitored. *Verapamil* given intravenously has been reported[2] to cause severe hypotension in patients also receiving quinidine by mouth. Studies *in vitro* suggest this is due to the additive blockade of α-adrenergic receptors by both drugs and the simultaneous blockade of calcium channels by verapamil; verapamil may also increase the plasma concentration of quinidine. Quinidine may increase the plasma concentration of other antiarrhythmics when administered concomitantly (see Ajmaline, p.833, Digoxin, p.871, Disopyramide, p.879, Flecainide Acetate, p.891, and Propafenone Hydrochloride, p.962).

1. Lesko LJ. Pharmacokinetic drug interactions with amiodarone. *Clin Pharmacokinet* 1989; **17:** 130–40.
2. Maisel AS, *et al.* Hypotension after quinidine plus verapamil. *N Engl J Med* 1985; **312:** 167–70.

Antibacterials. *Erythromycin* might inhibit the hepatic metabolism of quinidine.[1]

1. Spinler SA, *et al.* Possible inhibition of hepatic metabolism of quinidine by erythromycin. *Clin Pharmacol Ther* 1995; **57:** 89–94.

Antifungals. *Ketoconazole* temporarily increased the plasma-quinidine concentration in a patient through reduced hepatic elimination.[1] Another antifungal that inhibits hepatic metabolism, *itraconazole*, has also been reported[2] to increase plasma-quinidine concentrations.

1. McNulty RM, *et al.* Transient increase in plasma quinidine concentrations during ketoconazole-quinidine therapy. *Clin Pharm* 1989; **8:** 222–5.
2. Kaukonen K-M, *et al.* Itraconazole increases plasma concentrations of quinidine. *Clin Pharmacol Ther* 1997; **62:** 510–17.

Beta blockers. Sinus bradycardia in a patient prescribed quinidine by mouth and *timolol* eye drops,[1] and orthostatic hypotension with quinidine and *atenolol*[2] have occurred. Administration of quinidine or the beta blocker alone was well tolerated in each case with no adverse effects.

1. Dinai Y, *et al.* Bradycardia induced by interaction between quinidine and ophthalmic timolol. *Ann Intern Med* 1985; **103:** 890–1.
2. Manolis AS, Estes NAM. Orthostatic hypotension due to quinidine and atenolol. *Am J Med* 1987; **82:** 1083–4.

Calcium-channel blockers. *Nifedipine* has been reported[1] to reduce plasma-quinidine concentrations and up to 20 mg of quinidine per kg body-weight failed to increase the plasma concentration. Withdrawal of nifedipine resulted in a doubling of the quinidine concentration. A pharmacokinetic and pharmacodynamic study in healthy subjects, however, failed to show that modified-release *felodipine* or nifedipine had any effect on quinidine disposition.[2] Another study in healthy subjects suggested that quinidine may inhibit nifedipine metabolism.[3] *Diltiazem* has also been reported[4] to decrease the clearance and increase the half-life of quinidine in healthy subjects, although it was noted that another study had failed to show any interaction.

For the effects of *verapamil* on quinidine, see under Antiarrhythmics, above.

1. Green JA, *et al.* Nifedipine-quinidine interaction. *Clin Pharm* 1983; **2:** 461–5.
2. Bailey DG, *et al.* Quinidine interaction with nifedipine and felodipine: pharmacokinetic and pharmacodynamic evaluation. *Clin Pharmacol Ther* 1993; **53:** 354–9.
3. Bowles SK, *et al.* Evaluation of the pharmacokinetic and pharmacodynamic interaction between quinidine and nifedipine. *J Clin Pharmacol* 1993; **33:** 727–31.
4. Laganière S, *et al.* Pharmacokinetic and pharmacodynamic interactions between diltiazem and quinidine. *Clin Pharmacol Ther* 1996; **60:** 255–64.

Diuretics. *Carbonic anhydrase inhibitors* tend to increase plasma-quinidine concentrations due to increased renal tubular reabsorption of quinidine.

Administration of *amiloride* to 10 patients receiving quinidine therapy produced arrhythmias in 4 of them.[1] It was suggested that additive sodium-channel blockade may be responsible.

1. Wang L, *et al.* Amiloride-quinidine interaction: adverse outcomes. *Clin Pharmacol Ther* 1994; **56:** 659–67.

Histamine H₂-antagonists. *Cimetidine* inhibits the hepatic metabolism of quinidine and increases in plasma concentration and half-life with a reduction in clearance have been reported.[1-3]

1. Hardy BG, *et al.* Effect of cimetidine on the pharmacokinetics and pharmacodynamics of quinidine. *Am J Cardiol* 1983; **52:** 172–5.
2. Kolb KW, *et al.* Effect of cimetidine on quinidine clearance. *Ther Drug Monit* 1984; **6:** 306–12.
3. MacKichan JJ, *et al.* Effect of cimetidine on quinidine bioavailability. *Biopharm Drug Dispos* 1989; **10:** 121–5.

Pharmacokinetics

Quinidine is rapidly absorbed from the gastrointestinal tract, peak plasma concentrations being achieved about 1.5 hours after oral administration of quinidine sulfate and about 4 hours after quinidine gluconate; its bioavailability is variable, owing to first-pass metabolism in the liver.

Quinidine is metabolised in the liver, mainly by the cytochrome P450 isoenzyme CYP3A4, to a number of metabolites, at least some of which are pharmacologically active. It is excreted in the urine, mainly in the form of its metabolites. The proportion excreted unchanged is dependent on urinary pH; in acidic urine about 20% is excreted as unchanged quinidine but in alkaline urine this is reduced to about 5% due to increased renal tubular reabsorption.

Quinidine is widely distributed throughout the body and is 80 to 90% bound to plasma proteins including α_1-acid glycoprotein. It has a plasma half-life of about 6 to 8 hours but this may show wide variation. Its therapeutic effect has been correlated with plasma concentrations of about 2 to 7 µg per mL. However, plasma concentrations can be misleading as, depending on the assay method, quinidine may not be differentiated from its metabolites. It has been suggested that with specific assays quinidine concentrations of 1 µg or less per mL may be all that are required.

Quinidine crosses the placenta and is distributed into breast milk. Small amounts are removed by haemodialysis.

◊ Considerable intersubject and intrasubject variability in the pharmacokinetics of quinidine have been noted;[1] in one study the half-life ranged from about 1 to 16 hours regardless of whether the drug was administered as a tablet, capsule, oral solution, or intramuscular injection. There may also be considerable variations in absorption pharmacokinetic parameters depending upon the formulation and the salt used.[2,3] The effect of food on absorption is not clear.[4,5] The heart condition being treated or associated with the arrhythmia may alter quinidine's pharmacokinetics[6,7] as may the age of the patient.[8-10] Hepatic impairment may affect protein binding and prolong quinidine's half-life.[11] Protein binding increases in patients with renal impairment, although it returns to normal during dialysis procedures.[12] Accumulation of quinidine metabolites may occur in patients with renal dysfunction.[13-15]

1. Mason WD, et al. Comparative plasma concentrations of quinidine following administration of one intramuscular and three oral formulations to 13 human subjects. J Pharm Sci 1976; 65: 1325–9.
2. Frigo GM, et al. Comparison of quinidine plasma concentration curves following oral administration of some short- and long-acting formulations. Br J Clin Pharmacol 1977; 4: 449–54.
3. Mahon WA, et al. Comparative bioavailability study of three sustained release quinidine formulations. Clin Pharmacokinet 1987; 13: 118–24.
4. Woo E, Greenblatt DJ. Effect of food on enteral absorption of quinidine. Clin Pharmacol Ther 1980; 27: 188–93.
5. Martinez MN, et al. Effect of dietary fat content on the bioavailability of a sustained release quinidine gluconate tablet. Biopharm Drug Dispos 1990; 11: 17–29.
6. Ueda CT, Dzindzio BS. Quinidine kinetics in congestive heart failure. Clin Pharmacol Ther 1978; 23: 158–64.
7. Ueda CT, Dzindzio BS. Bioavailability of quinidine in congestive heart failure. Br J Clin Pharmacol 1981; 11: 571–7.
8. Drayer DE, et al. Prevalence of high (3S)-3-hydroxyquinidine/quinidine ratios in serum, and clearance of quinidine in cardiac patients with age. Clin Pharmacol Ther 1980; 27: 72–5.
9. Szefler SJ, et al. Rapid elimination of quinidine in pediatric patients. Pediatrics 1982; 70: 370–5.
10. Pickoff AS, et al. Age-related differences in the protein binding of quinidine. Dev Pharmacol Ther 1981; 3: 108–15.
11. Kessler KM, et al. Quinidine pharmacokinetics in patients with cirrhosis or receiving propranolol. Am Heart J 1978; 96: 627–35.
12. Kessler KM, Perez GO. Decreased quinidine plasma protein binding during haemodialysis. Clin Pharmacol Ther 1981; 30: 121–6.
13. Kessler KM, et al. Quinidine elimination in patients with congestive heart failure or poor renal function. N Engl J Med 1974; 290: 706–9.
14. Drayer DE, et al. Steady-state serum levels of quinidine and active metabolites in cardiac patients with varying degrees of renal function. Clin Pharmacol Ther 1978; 24: 31–9.
15. Hall K, et al. Clearance of quinidine during peritoneal dialysis. Am Heart J 1982; 104: 646–7.

Uses and Administration

Quinidine is a class Ia antiarrhythmic (p.787). It also has antimuscarinic and alpha-adrenoceptor blocking properties. Quinidine is used to maintain sinus rhythm after cardioversion of atrial fibrillation, and for the suppression of supraventricular and ventricular **arrhythmias**.

Quinidine is an isomer of quinine and may be used as an alternative to quinine in the treatment of **malaria** when quinine is not immediately available.

Strengths of preparations and doses of quinidine salts used have been expressed in a variety of ways; as well

as expressing in terms of the salt actually being employed, equivalences in terms of anhydrous quinidine base or quinidine sulfate dihydrate have commonly been used.

For the management of cardiac arrhythmias, quinidine sulfate is given by mouth. An initial test dose of 200 mg should always be given to detect hypersensitivity. The usual dose is then 200 to 400 mg three or four times daily. Doses of up to 600 mg every 2 to 4 hours have been given for the treatment of supraventricular tachycardias to a maximum of 4 g daily; these higher doses should only be given with frequent monitoring of the ECG and plasma concentration.

Quinidine is also given by mouth as a range of salts including the bisulfate, the gluconate, and the polygalacturonate.

Modified-release formulations are generally preferred as the plasma concentration profile is smoother and doses can be given at 8- to 12-hourly intervals.

Quinidine has been given intramuscularly or by slow intravenous injection, but absorption from the intramuscular route can be erratic and incomplete, and the intravenous route is associated with a risk of severe hypotension. Parenteral doses of quinidine gluconate are: intramuscularly, 600 mg initially then up to 400 mg repeated every 2 hours if necessary; by intravenous infusion 800 mg diluted to a volume of 50 mL with glucose 5% and given at a rate of 1 mL per minute with ECG and blood-pressure monitoring.

◊ General references.
1. Grace AA, Camm AJ. Quinidine. N Engl J Med 1998; 338: 35–45.

Cardiac arrhythmias. Quinidine is a class Ia antiarrhythmic and has been used in the management of supraventricular and ventricular arrhythmias (p.794), although occasionally it may precipitate arrhythmias. The CAST (Cardiac Arrhythmia Suppression Trial) studies demonstrated that other class I antiarrhythmics (encainide, flecainide, and moracizine) were associated with an increased mortality rate when used for asymptomatic ventricular arrhythmias in post-infarction patients and led to many drugs of this class being restricted to severe or life-threatening arrhythmias. A meta-analysis of trials utilising quinidine was undertaken as it was believed this drug had gained in popularity after the adverse CAST results. This meta-analysis[1] suggested that quinidine was associated with at least as high a proportion of adverse events, such as death and early proarrhythmia, as the class Ic drugs flecainide and propafenone. It was, however, emphasised that these results do not necessarily apply to the use of quinidine for the treatment of life-threatening or sustained ventricular arrhythmias.

1. Morganroth J, Goin JE. Quinidine-related mortality in the short-to-medium-term treatment of ventricular arrhythmias: a meta-analysis. Circulation 1991; 84: 1977–83.

Congenital myasthenia. Although quinidine may exacerbate the symptoms of myasthenia gravis and should be used with great caution in such patients, beneficial responses have been reported in patients with the slow-channel congenital myasthenic syndrome (see p.1416).

Cramps. Although quinidine would be expected to have similar efficacy to quinine in preventing nocturnal cramps, quinine is preferred due to its lower potential for cardiotoxicity.[1] For a discussion of the usual treatment of nocturnal cramp, see under Muscle Spasm, p.1322.

1. Beeley L. BMJ 1991; 302: 33.

Hiccup. Quinidine is one of several drugs that have been tried in intractable hiccups. For details of a protocol for the control of hiccups see under Chlorpromazine, p.667.

Malaria. Although quinidine might theoretically be superior to quinine as an antimalarial it is more likely to cause cardiac toxicity and hypersensitivity and WHO[1] has recommended that parenteral formulations of quinidine should only be used when parenteral quinine or artemisinin derivatives are not immediately available. In these situations intravenous infusions of quinidine could be used to initiate treatment for severe chloroquine-resistant malaria. Patients should be transferred to oral therapy with quinine as soon as possible to complete a 7-day course; alternatively a single oral treatment of pyrimethamine-sulfadoxine may be given.

In the USA, the Centers for Disease Control[2,3] have recommended parenteral quinidine gluconate as the drug of choice for the treatment of complicated falciparum malaria, but only because of the lack of availability of parenteral quinine.

Quinidine is given intravenously as the gluconate and doses have been expressed in terms of the base or salt; it should be given under close control, preferably with continuous ECG monitoring and frequent measurements of blood pressure. Regimens used include one[1,4] where the equivalent of 15 mg of the base per kg body-weight is infused over 4 hours as a loading dose followed by the equivalent of 7.5 mg of the base per kg

every 8 hours as infusions over 4 hours; the patient should be transferred to an oral form of antimalarial as soon as possible. An alternative regimen[5] consists of a loading dose of 10 mg of quinidine gluconate per kg given by intravenous infusion over a period of 1 to 2 hours followed by a constant intravenous infusion of 0.02 mg per kg per minute for a maximum of 72 hours or until oral therapy with quinine can be instituted to complete a total 3-day course of treatment. It is generally recommended that loading doses should not be used if the patient has received quinine or quinidine within the previous 24 hours or mefloquine within the preceding 7 days.

The overall management of malaria is discussed in the chapter on Antimalarials, p.428.

1. WHO. Management of severe malaria: a practical handbook. Geneva: WHO, 2000.
2. Centers for Disease Control. Treatment with quinidine gluconate of persons with severe Plasmodium falciparum infection: discontinuation of parenteral quinine from CDC drug service. MMWR 1991; 40 (RR-4): 21–3.
3. Centers for Disease Control. Availability and use of parenteral quinidine gluconate for severe or complicated malaria. MMWR 2000; 49: 1138–40.
4. Phillips RE, et al. Intravenous quinidine for the treatment of severe falciparum malaria: clinical pharmacokinetic studies. N Engl J Med 1985; 312: 1273–8.
5. Miller KD, et al. Treatment of severe malaria in the United States with a continuous infusion of quinidine gluconate and exchange transfusion. N Engl J Med 1989; 321: 65–70.

Preparations

BP 2001: Quinidine Sulphate Tablets;
USP 25: Quinidine Gluconate Extended-release Tablets; Quinidine Gluconate Injection; Quinidine Sulfate Capsules; Quinidine Sulfate Extended-release Tablets; Quinidine Sulfate Tablets.

Proprietary Preparations (details are given in Part 3)
Aust.: Galactoquin†; **Austral.:** Kinidin; **Belg.:** Kinidine Durettes; **Braz.:** Natisedine; Quinicardine; **Canad.:** Biquin; Cardioquin; Natisedine†; Quinate†; Quinidex; Quinobarb†; **Denm.:** Kinidin; **Fin.:** Kinidin; Kiniduron; **Fr.:** Cardioquine†; Longacor†; Quinidurule; **Ger.:** Optochinidin retard†; **Hong Kong:** Kinidin; **Irl.:** Kinidin; **Israel:** Quiniduran; **Ital.:** Chinteina; Longachin; Naticardina; Natisedina; Ritmocor; **Mex.:** Quineuron; Quini; **Neth.:** Cardioquin; Kiditard†; Kinidine; **Norw.:** Kinidin†; Systodin†; **NZ:** Kinidin; **S.Afr.:** Quinaglute; **Spain:** Cardioquine; Longacor; Quinicardina†; **Swed.:** Kinidin; **Switz.:** Kinidin; Longacor; **Thai.:** Kinidin; **UK:** Kinidin; Quinora; **USA:** Cardioquin†; Quinaglute; Quinalant†; Quinidex; Quinora.

Multi-ingredient: Fr.: Quinimax; Ger.: Cordichin.

Ramipril (16975-a)

Ramipril (BAN, USAN, rINN).

Hoe-498; Ramiprilum. (2S,3aS,6aS)-1-{N-[(S)-1-Ethoxycarbonyl-3-phenylpropyl]L-alanyl}perhydrocyclopenta[b]pyrrole-2-carboxylic acid.
$C_{23}H_{32}N_2O_5 = 416.5$.
CAS — 87333-19-5.
ATC — C09AA05.

Pharmacopoeias. in Eur. (see p.vi).

Pharmacopoeial description

Ph. Eur.: A white or almost white, crystalline powder. Sparingly soluble in water; freely soluble in methyl alcohol. Protect from light.

Adverse Effects, Treatment, and Precautions

As for ACE inhibitors, p.820.

Interactions

As for ACE inhibitors, p.822.

Pharmacokinetics

Ramipril acts as a prodrug of the diacid ramiprilat, its active metabolite. Following oral administration at least 50 to 60% is absorbed. Ramipril is metabolised in the liver to ramiprilat; other metabolites are inactive. Peak plasma concentrations of ramiprilat are achieved 2 to 4 hours after an oral dose of ramipril. Ramiprilat is about 56% bound to plasma proteins. About 60% of an oral dose of ramipril is excreted in the urine, the rest in the faeces. The effective half-life for accumulation of ramiprilat is 13 to 17 hours following multiple doses of ramipril 5 to 10 mg, but is much longer for doses of 1.25 to 2.5 mg daily. The clearance of ramiprilat is reduced in renal impairment.

◊ Reviews.
1. Meisel S, et al. Clinical pharmacokinetics of ramipril. Clin Pharmacokinet 1994; 26: 7–15.
2. van Griensven JMT, et al. Pharmacokinetics, pharmacodynamics and bioavailability of the ACE inhibitor ramipril. Eur J Clin Pharmacol 1995; 47: 513–8.
3. Fillastre JP, et al. Kinetics, safety, and efficacy of ramipril after long-term administration in hemodialyzed patients. J Cardiovasc Pharmacol 1996; 27: 269–74.

Uses and Administration

Ramipril is an ACE inhibitor (p.820). It is used in the treatment of hypertension (p.802), heart failure (p.798), and following myocardial infarction (p.805) to improve survival in patients with clinical evidence of heart failure. It is also used to reduce the risk of cardiovascular events in patients with certain risk factors.

Ramipril owes its activity to ramiprilat to which it is converted after oral administration. The haemodynamic effects are seen within 1 to 2 hours of a single oral dose and the maximum effect occurs after about 3 to 6 hours, although the full effect may not develop for several weeks during chronic dosing. The haemodynamic effect is maintained for at least 24 hours, allowing once-daily dosing.

In the treatment of **hypertension** an initial dose of 1.25 mg once daily is given by mouth. Since there may be a precipitous fall in blood pressure when starting therapy with an ACE inhibitor, the first dose should preferably be given at bedtime. Patients receiving diuretics should, if possible, have the diuretic discontinued 2 to 3 days before starting ramipril, and resumed later if necessary. The usual maintenance dose is 2.5 to 5 mg daily as a single dose, although up to 10 mg daily may be required. In the USA an initial dose of 2.5 mg once daily in hypertensive patients not receiving a diuretic and a maintenance dose of 2.5 to 20 mg daily have been suggested.

In the management of **heart failure**, severe first-dose hypotension on introduction of an ACE inhibitor is common in patients on loop diuretics, but their temporary withdrawal may cause rebound pulmonary oedema. Thus treatment should be initiated with a low dose under close medical supervision; high doses of diuretics should be reduced before starting ramipril. Ramipril is given in an initial dose of 1.25 mg once daily. The usual maximum dose is 10 mg daily; doses of 2.5 mg or more daily may be taken in 1 or 2 divided doses.

Following **myocardial infarction**, treatment with ramipril may be started in hospital 3 to 10 days after the infarction at a usual initial dose of 2.5 mg twice daily, increased after two days to 5 mg twice daily. The usual maintenance dose is 2.5 to 5 mg twice daily.

For the **prophylaxis of cardiovascular events** in patients considered to be at high risk, ramipril is given in an initial dose of 2.5 mg once daily. The dose should be increased, if tolerated, to 5 mg once daily after 1 week, then to the usual maintenance dose of 10 mg once daily after a further 3 weeks. In patients with hypertension or recent myocardial infarction it may also be given in divided doses.

A reduction in dosage of ramipril may be necessary in patients with impaired renal function.

◊ References.
1. Todd PA, Benfield P. Ramipril: a review of its pharmacological properties and therapeutic efficacy in cardiovascular disorders. *Drugs* 1990; **39:** 110–35.
2. The Acute Infarction Ramipril Efficacy (AIRE) Study Investigators. Effect of ramipril on mortality and morbidity of survivors of acute myocardial infarction with clinical evidence of heart failure. *Lancet* 1993; **342:** 821–8.
3. Frampton JE, Peters DH. Ramipril: an updated review of its therapeutic use in essential hypertension and heart failure. *Drugs* 1995; **49:** 440–66.
4. The Heart Outcomes Prevention Evaluation Study Investigators. Effects of an angiotensin-converting-enzyme inhibitor, ramipril, on cardiovascular events in high-risk patients. *N Engl J Med* 2000; **342:** 145–53.

Preparations

Proprietary Preparations (details are given in Part 3)
Aust.: Hypren; Tritace; *Austral.:* Ramace; Tritace; *Belg.:* Ramace; Tritace; *Braz.:* Triatec; *Canad.:* Altace; *Denm.:* Ramace; Triatec; *Fin.:* Cardace; Ramace; *Fr.:* Triatec; *Ger.:* Delix; Vesdil; *Hong Kong:* Tritace; *Irl.:* Tritace; *Israel:* Tritace; *Ital.:* Quark; Tritace; Unipril; *Mex.:* Ramace; Tritace; *Neth.:* Tritace; *Norw.:* Triatec; *Port.:* Triatec; *S.Afr.:* Ramace; Tritace; *Singapore:* Tritace; *Spain:* Acovil; Carasel; *Swed.:* Pramace; Triatec; *Switz.:* Vesdil; *Thai.:* Tritace; *UK:* Tritace; *USA:* Altace.

Multi-ingredient: *Aust.:* Hypren plus; Lasitace; Trialix; Tritazide; *Belg.:* Tritazide; *Denm.:* Triatec Comp; *Fin.:* Cardace Comp; Unimax; *Ger.:* Arelix ACE; Delix plus; Delmuno; Unimax; Vesdil plus; *Irl.:* Trialix; *Ital.:* Idroquark; Prilace; Triatec HCT; *Mex.:* Tritazide; *Neth.:* Triapin; Tritazide; *Port.:* Triatec

The symbol † denotes a preparation no longer actively marketed

---

Composto; *S.Afr.:* Tri-Plen; *Spain:* Unimest; *Swed.:* Triatec Comp; *Switz.:* Trialix; Triatec Comp; Unimax; *UK:* Triapin.

Ranolazine Hydrochloride (3760-s)

Ranolazine Hydrochloride *(USAN, rINNM)*.
RS-43285. (±)-4-[2-Hydroxy-3-(o-methoxyphenoxy)propyl]-1-piperazineaceto-2',6'-xylidide dihydrochloride.
$C_{24}H_{33}N_3O_4,2HCl = 500.5$.
CAS — 95635-55-5 (ranolazine); 95635-56-6 (ranolazine hydrochloride).

Profile
Ranolazine hydrochloride is under investigation for use in angina pectoris.

◊ References.
1. McCormack JG, *et al.* Ranolazine: a novel metabolic modulator for the treatment of angina. *Gen Pharmacol* 1998; **30:** 639–45.
2. Pepine CJ, Wolff AA. A controlled trial with a novel anti-ischemic agent, ranolazine, in chronic stable angina pectoris that is responsive to conventional antianginal agents. *Am J Cardiol* 1999; **84:** 46–50.

Raubasine (9277-d)

Ajmalicine; Alkaloid F; δ-Yohimbine. Methyl 16,17-didehydro-19α-methyl-18-oxayohimban-16-carboxylate.
$C_{21}H_{24}N_2O_3 = 352.4$.
CAS — 483-04-5.

Raubasine is an alkaloid obtained from *Rauwolfia serpentina* (Apocynaceae).

Profile
Raubasine is a vasodilator related chemically to reserpine (p.967). It has been given by mouth and by injection in peripheral and cerebral vascular disorders.

Preparations

Proprietary Preparations (details are given in Part 3)
Aust.: Lamuran; *Ital.:* Lamuran; *S.Afr.:* Melanex†.

Multi-ingredient: *Aust.:* Defluina; Modenol†; *Braz.:* Vasofluina; *Fr.:* Duxil; Iskedyl; *Hong Kong:* Duxaril; Iso Triraupin; *Port.:* Duxil; Transoxyl; *S.Afr.:* Saltucin Co†; *Singapore:* Duxaril; *Spain:* Duxor; Iskedyl; Isquebral; Salvalion; *Thai.:* Duxaril; Iso-Triraupin.

Rauwolfia Serpentina (898-m)

Chotachand; Rauvolfia; Rauwolfia; Rauwolfiae Radix; Rauwolfiawurzel.
CAS — 8063-17-0 (rauwolfia).
Pharmacopoeias. In Ger. (not less than 1% of total alkaloids) and US. US also includes Powdered Rauwolfia Serpentina.

Rauwolfia serpentina contains numerous alkaloids, the most active as hypotensive agents being the ester alkaloids, reserpine and rescinnamine. Other alkaloids present have structures related to reserpic acid, but are not esterified, and include ajmaline (rauwolfine), ajmalinine, ajmalicine, isoajmaline (isorauwolfine), serpentine, rauwolfinine, and sarpagine.

Pharmacopoeial description

USP 25: The dried roots of *Rauwolfia serpentina* (Apocynaceae). It contains not less than 0.15% of reserpine-rescinnamine group alkaloids calculated as reserpine. Store at 15° to 30° in a dry place.

Powdered Rauwolfia Serpentina contains 0.15 to 0.20% of reserpine-rescinnamine group alkaloids, calculated as reserpine. A fine or very fine powder adjusted with lactose or starch or with powdered rauwolfia serpentina containing a higher or lower content of alkaloids. Store at 15° to 30° in a dry place.

Profile
The actions of rauwolfia serpentina are those of its alkaloids and it has been used for the same purposes as reserpine, p.967. It has been administered by mouth as the powdered whole root. Rauwolfia vomitoria has also been used.

A crude form of rauwolfia serpentina has been used in India for centuries as preparations such as Sarpagandha, in the treatment of insomnia and certain forms of mental illness.

Preparations

USP 25: Rauwolfia Serpentina Tablets.

Proprietary Preparations (details are given in Part 3)
Ger.: Arte Rautin forte S.

Multi-ingredient: *Ger.:* Hyperforat-forte; Raufuncton N; Rauwoplant; *Spain:* Diu Rauwiplus; Rulun; *USA:* Rauzide.

Remikiren (15920-a)

Remikiren *(rINN)*.
Ro-42-5892. (αS)-α-[(αS)-α-[(tert-Butylsulfonyl)methyl]hydrocinnamamido]-N-[(1S,2R,3S)-1-(cyclohexylmethyl)-3-cyclopropyl-2,3-dihydroxypropyl]imidazole-4-propionamide.
$C_{33}H_{50}N_4O_6S = 630.8$.
CAS — 126222-34-2.
ATC — C09XA01.

Profile
Remikiren inhibits the actions of renin and thus prevents the conversion of angiotensinogen into angiotensin I. It is active by mouth and is under investigation in the management of hypertension and heart failure.

◊ A number of renin antagonists are under investigation as specific inhibitors of the renin-angiotensin system.[1,2] Remikiren is a nonpeptide that is active intravenously and orally, but it is reported to have a very low oral bioavailability.
1. Frishman WH, *et al.* Renin inhibition: a new approach to cardiovascular therapy. *J Clin Pharmacol* 1994; **34:** 873–80.
2. Rongen GA, *et al.* Clinical pharmacokinetics and efficacy of renin inhibitors. *Clin Pharmacokinet* 1995; **29:** 6–14.

Rescinnamine (900-b)

Rescinnamine *(BAN, rINN)*.
Methyl-O-(3,4,5-trimethoxycinnamoyl)reserpate.
$C_{35}H_{42}N_2O_9 = 634.7$.
CAS — 24815-24-5.
ATC — C02AA01.

An ester alkaloid isolated from the root of *Rauwolfia serpentina* or *R. vomitoria*.

Profile
Rescinnamine has properties similar to those described under reserpine (below) and has been used in the treatment of hypertension.

Preparations

Proprietary Preparations (details are given in Part 3)
Multi-ingredient: *Aust.:* Modenol†; *Hong Kong:* Iso Triraupin; *S.Afr.:* Saltucin Co†; *Spain:* Diu Rauwiplus; *Thai.:* Iso-Triraupin.

Reserpine (901-v)

Reserpine *(BAN, rINN)*.
Reserpinum. Methyl 11,17α-dimethoxy-18β-(3,4,5-trimethoxybenzoyloxy)-3β,20α-yohimbane-16β-carboxylate; Methyl O-(3,4,5-trimethoxybenzoyl)reserpate.
$C_{33}H_{40}N_2O_9 = 608.7$.
CAS — 50-55-5.
ATC — C02AA02.
Pharmacopoeias. In Chin., Eur. (see p.vi), Int., Jpn, Pol., and US.

An alkaloid obtained from the roots of certain species of *Rauwolfia* (Apocynaceae), mainly *Rauwolfia serpentina* and *R. vomitoria,* or by synthesis. The material obtained from natural sources may contain closely related alkaloids. Reserpine is unstable in the presence of alkalis, particularly when the drug is in solution.

Pharmacopoeial description

Ph. Eur.: It occurs as small, white to slightly yellow crystals or a crystalline powder. It darkens slowly on exposure to light. Practically insoluble in water and in ether; very slightly soluble in alcohol. Protect from light.

USP 25: A white or pale buff to slightly yellowish, odourless, crystalline powder. It darkens slowly on exposure to light, but more rapidly when in solution. Insoluble in water; soluble 1 in 1800 of alcohol and 1 in 6 of chloroform; freely soluble in acetic acid; very slightly soluble in ether; slightly soluble in benzene. Store in airtight containers. Protect from light.

Adverse Effects
Side-effects commonly include nasal congestion, headache, and CNS symptoms including depression, drowsiness, dizziness, lethargy, nightmares, and symptoms of increased gastrointestinal tract motility including diarrhoea, abdominal cramps, and, at higher doses, increased gastric acid secretion. Respiratory distress, cyanosis, anorexia, and lethargy may occur in infants whose mothers have received reserpine prior to delivery.

Higher doses may cause flushing, bradycardia, severe depression which may lead to suicide, and extrapyramidal effects. Hypotension, coma, convulsions, respiratory depression and hypothermia also occur in overdosage. Hypotension is also more common in patients following a cerebrovascular accident.

Breast engorgement and galactorrhoea, gynaecomastia, increased prolactin concentrations, decreased libido, impotence, sodium retention, oedema, decreased or increased appetite, weight gain, miosis, dry mouth, sialorrhoea, dysuria, rashes, pruritus, and thrombocytopenic purpura have also been reported.

Reserpine has been shown to be tumorigenic in *rodents* following administration of large doses. Several reports have suggested an association between the ingestion of reserpine and the development of neoplasms of the breast (see below) but other surveys have failed to confirm the association.

Neoplasms of the breast. Epidemiological studies[1-4] suggested that the incidence of breast cancer was up to 3 to 4 times greater in hypertensive women treated with rauwolfia preparations than in control groups. Other studies, however, have failed to find an association between reserpine and breast cancer[5-11] and no firm conclusion has been made.
1. Boston Collaborative Drug Surveillance Program. Reserpine and breast cancer. *Lancet* 1974; **ii:** 669–71.

2. Armstrong B, *et al.* Retrospective study of the association between use of rauwolfia derivatives and breast cancer in English women. *Lancet* 1974; **ii**: 672–5.
3. Heinonen OP, *et al.* Reserpine use in relation to breast cancer. *Lancet* 1974; **ii**: 675–7.
4. Armstrong B, *et al.* Rauwolfia derivatives and breast cancer in hypertensive women. *Lancet* 1976; **ii**: 8–12.
5. Mack TM, *et al.* Reserpine and breast cancer in a retirement community. *N Engl J Med* 1975; **292**: 1366–71.
6. O'Fallon WM, *et al.* Rauwolfia derivatives and breast cancer. *Lancet* 1975; **ii**: 292–6.
7. Laska EM, *et al.* Matched-pairs study of reserpine use and breast cancer. *Lancet* 1975; **ii**: 296–300.
8. Christopher LJ, *et al.* A multicentre study of rauwolfia derivates and breast cancer. *Eur J Clin Pharmacol* 1977; **11**: 409–17.
9. Labarthe DR, O'Fallon WM. Reserpine and breast cancer: a community-based longitudinal study of 2000 hypertensive women. *JAMA* 1980; **243**: 2304–10.
10. Curb JD, *et al.* Reserpine and breast cancer in the Hypertensive Detection and Follow-up Program. *Hypertension* 1982; **4**: 307–11.
11. Friedman GD. Rauwolfia and breast cancer: no relation found in long term users age fifty and over. *J Chron Dis* 1983; **36**: 367–70.

Treatment of Adverse Effects

Withdrawal of reserpine or reduction of the dosage causes the reversal of many side-effects although mental disorders may persist for months and hypotensive effects may persist for weeks after the cessation of treatment. If overdosage occurs the stomach should be emptied by lavage even if several hours have elapsed after ingestion. Treatment is generally supportive and symptomatic. Severe hypotension may respond to placing the patient in the supine position with the feet raised. Direct-acting sympathomimetics may be effective for treatment of severe hypotension, but should be given with caution. The patient must be observed for at least 72 hours.

Precautions

Reserpine should not be used in patients with depression or a history of depression, with active peptic ulcer or ulcerative colitis, or in patients with Parkinson's disease. It should also be avoided in phaeochromocytoma.

It should be used with caution in debilitated or elderly patients, and in the presence of cardiac arrhythmias, myocardial infarction, renal insufficiency, gallstones, epilepsy, or allergic conditions such as bronchial asthma.

Reserpine is contra-indicated in patients receiving electroconvulsive therapy; if electroconvulsive therapy is required in patients who have been taking reserpine an interval of at least 7 to 14 days should be allowed to elapse between the last dose of reserpine and the commencement of the shock treatment.

It is probably not necessary to discontinue treatment with reserpine during anaesthesia, although the effects of CNS depressants may be enhanced by reserpine.

Interactions

Patients taking reserpine may be hypersensitive to adrenaline [epinephrine] and other direct-acting sympathomimetics which should not be given except to antagonise reserpine. The effects of indirect-acting sympathomimetics such as ephedrine may be decreased by reserpine. The hypotensive effects of reserpine are enhanced by thiazide diuretics and other antihypertensives. Reserpine may cause excitation and hypertension in patients receiving MAOIs. Concurrent administration of digitalis or quinidine may cause cardiac arrhythmias. Reserpine may enhance the effects of CNS depressants.

Pharmacokinetics

Reserpine is absorbed from the gastrointestinal tract with a reported bioavailability of 50%. It is extensively metabolised and is excreted slowly in the urine and faeces. About 8% has been reported to be excreted in the urine in the first 4 days, mainly as metabolites; about 60% has been reported to be excreted in the faeces in the first 4 days, mainly unchanged. Reserpine crosses the placenta and the blood-brain barrier and also appears in breast milk.

Uses and Administration

Reserpine is an antihypertensive drug that causes depletion of noradrenaline stores in peripheral sympathetic nerve terminals and depletion of catecholamine and serotonin stores in the brain, heart, and many other organs resulting in a reduction in blood pressure, bradycardia, and CNS depression. The hypotensive effect is mainly due to a reduction in cardiac output and a reduction in peripheral resistance. Cardiovascular reflexes are partially inhibited, but postural hypotension is rarely a problem at the doses used in hypertension. When given by mouth the full effect is only reached after several weeks of continued treatment and persists for up to 6 weeks after treatment is discontinued.

Reserpine has been used in the management of hypertension (p.802) and in chronic psychoses (p.650) such as schizophrenia. It has also been tried in the treatment of Raynaud's syndrome (p.809).

In **hypertension**, reserpine is given by mouth in an initial dose of up to 500 μg daily for about 2 weeks, subsequently reduced to the lowest dose necessary to maintain the response; some sources have recommended an initial dose of 100 μg. A maintenance dose of about 250 μg daily is usually adequate and 500 μg should not normally be exceeded. To reduce side-effects and tolerance smaller doses of reserpine may be given in conjunction with a thiazide diuretic.

Reserpine has been used in chronic **psychoses** in daily doses of up to 1 mg.

Preparations

USP 25: Reserpine and Chlorothiazide Tablets; Reserpine and Hydrochlorothiazide Tablets; Reserpine Elixir; Reserpine Injection; Reserpine Tablets; Reserpine, Hydralazine Hydrochloride, and Hydrochlorothiazide Tablets.

Proprietary Preparations (details are given in Part 3)

Braz.: Ortoserpina; Rauserpin; **Canad.:** Serpasil†; **Port.:** Serfinato†; **Thai.:** Reserpina; **USA:** Serpalan†.

Multi-ingredient: **Aust.:** Adelphan-Esidrex; Brinerdin; Darebon; Elfanex; Modenol†; Pressimedin; Resaltex; Supergan; Suprenoat; Terbolan†; **Braz.:** Adelfan-Esidrex; Higroton Reserpina; Id Sedin; Terbolan; Vagoplex; **Canad.:** Hydropres†; Ser-Ap-Es†; **Fr.:** Tensionorme; **Ger.:** Adelphan-Esidrix; Barotonal; Bendigon N; Briserin N; Darebon; Disalpin; Durotan; Modenol; Resaltex†; Tri-Thiazid Reserpin; Triniton; **Hong Kong:** Adelphane-Esidrex; Iso Triraupin; **Israel:** Pressunic Compositum; **Ital.:** Brinerdina; Igroton-Reserpina; **Mex.:** Higroton-Res; **Neth.:** Brinerdin†; **Port.:** Brinerdine; **S.Afr.:** Adelphane-Esidrex†; Brinerdin; Hygroton-Reserpine; Protensin-M; Saltucin Co†; **Spain:** Adelfan-Esidrex; Brinerdina; Diu Rauwiplus; Higrotona Reserpina; Resnedal; Tensiocomplet; **Switz.:** Adelphan-Esidrex; Brinerdine; Hygroton-Reserpine; Pressimed†; **Thai.:** Bedin; Brinerdin; Hydrares; Hyperdine; Hypery; Iso-Triraupin; Medeserpine Co; Reser; Ser-Ap-Es; **USA:** Demi-Regroton; Diupres; Diutensen-R; Hydrap-ES; Hydro-Serp; Hydropres; Hydroserpine; Marpres; Metatensin; Regroton; Renese R; Salutensin; Ser-Ap-Es; Tri-Hydroserpine.

Reteplase (17311-s)

Reteplase (BAN, USAN, rINN).
BM-06.022; rPA. 173-L-Serine-174-L-tyrosine-175-L-glutamine-173–527-plasminogen activator (human tissue-type).
$C_{1736}H_{2653}N_{499}O_{522}S_{22} = 39571.1$.
CAS — 133652-38-7.
ATC — B01AD07.

A nonglycosylated protein produced by recombinant DNA technology that consists of selected domains of human tissue plasminogen activator.

Incompatibility. Reteplase may precipitate out of solution if it is given with heparin in the same intravenous line.[1] Reteplase and heparin must therefore be given separately; if a single intravenous line is used it must be flushed thoroughly with sodium chloride 0.9% or with glucose 5% prior to, and following, reteplase injection.

1. Committee on Safety of Medicines/Medicines Control Agency. Reteplase (Rapilysin): incompatibility with heparin. *Current Problems* 2000; **26**: 5.

Adverse Effects, Treatment, and Precautions

As for Streptokinase, p.976. Allergic reactions may be less likely to occur with reteplase than with streptokinase.

Interactions

As for Streptokinase, p.977.

Pharmacokinetics

Reteplase is reported to have a fibrinolytic half-life of about 1.6 hours in patients with myocardial infarction.

Uses and Administration

Reteplase is a thrombolytic drug. It converts plasminogen to fibrinolysin, a proteolytic enzyme which has fibrinolytic effects. The mechanisms of fibrinolysis are discussed further under Haemostasis and Fibrinolysis on p.718.

Reteplase is used similarly to streptokinase (p.977) in acute myocardial infarction (p.805). It is given intravenously as soon as possible after the onset of symptoms. The dose is 10 units given by slow intravenous injection (but over not more than 2 minutes) and this dose of 10 units is repeated once, 30 minutes after the start of the first injection.

◊ General references.

1. Noble S, McTavish D. Reteplase: a review of its pharmacological properties and clinical efficacy in the management of acute myocardial infarction. *Drugs* 1996; **52**: 589–605.
2. Wooster MB, Luzier AB. Reteplase: a new thrombolytic for the treatment of acute myocardial infarction. *Ann Pharmacother* 1999; **33**: 318–24.

Preparations

Proprietary Preparations (details are given in Part 3)

Aust.: Rapilysin; **Austral.:** Rapilysin; **Belg.:** Rapilysin; **Canad.:** Retavase; **Denm.:** Rapilysin; **Fin.:** Rapilysin; **Fr.:** Rapilysin; **Ger.:** Rapilysin; **Irl.:** Rapilysin; **Ital.:** Rapilysin; **Neth.:** Rapilysin; **Norw.:** Rapilysin; **NZ:** Rapilysin; **Port.:** Rapilysin; **Spain:** Rapilysin; **Swed.:** Rapilysin; **Switz.:** Rapilysin; **UK:** Rapilysin; **USA:** Retavase.

Reviparin Sodium (15402-t)

Reviparin Sodium (BAN, rINN).
CAS — 9041-08-1.

Reviparin sodium is prepared by nitrous acid depolymerisation of heparin obtained from the intestinal mucosa of pigs. The majority of the components have a 2-O-sulfo-α-L-idopyranosuronic acid structure at the non-reducing end and a 6-O-sulfo-2,5-anhydro-D-mannitol structure at the reducing end of their chain. The mass-average molecular mass ranges between 3150 and 5150 with a characteristic value of about 4150. The degree of sulfation is about 2.1 per disaccharide unit.

Units

As for Low-molecular-weight Heparins, p.923.

Adverse Effects, Treatment, and Precautions

As for Low-molecular-weight Heparins, p.923.

Severe bleeding with reviparin sodium may be reduced by the slow intravenous injection of protamine sulfate; about 17.5 mg of protamine sulfate is stated to inhibit the effect of 1432 units of reviparin sodium.

Interactions

As for Low-molecular-weight Heparins, p.924.

Pharmacokinetics

Reviparin sodium is absorbed following subcutaneous administration with a bioavailability of about 95%. Peak plasma concentrations are reached after about 3 hours. Reviparin sodium is excreted predominantly in the urine; the elimination half-life is about 3 hours.

Uses and Administration

Reviparin sodium is a low-molecular-weight heparin (p.923) with anticoagulant activity. It is used in the prevention and treatment of venous thromboembolism (p.817) and to prevent coagulation during haemodialysis.

In the prophylaxis of **venous thromboembolism** during surgery, reviparin sodium is given subcutaneously in a dose of 1432 units once daily, with the first dose given 2 hours before surgery. Patients at high risk of thromboembolism may be given a dose of 3436 units once daily, beginning 12 hours before surgery. For treatment of thromboembolism, a dose of 71 units per kg body-weight is given subcutaneously twice daily.

For prevention of clotting in the extracorporeal circulation during **haemodialysis**, reviparin sodium is administered into the arterial side of the dialyser in an initial dose of 70 units per kg; doses for subsequent sessions should be adjusted according to response. The maximum recommended dose is 82 units per kg.

◊ References.

1. The Columbus Investigators. Low-molecular-weight heparin in the treatment of patients with venous thromboembolism. *N Engl J Med* 1997; **337**: 657–62.
2. Breddin HK, *et al.* Effects of a low-molecular-weight heparin on thrombus regression and recurrent thromboembolism in patients with deep-vein thrombosis. *N Engl J Med* 2001; **344**: 626–31.

Preparations

Proprietary Preparations (details are given in Part 3)

Denm.: Clivarin; **Fin.:** Clivarin; **Fr.:** Clivarine; **Ger.:** Clivarin; **Norw.:** Clivarin; **Port.:** Clivarin; **Swed.:** Clivarin; **UK:** Clivarine.

Rilmenidine Phosphate (14744-w)

Rilmenidine Phosphate (rINNM).
Oxaminozoline Phosphate; Rilmenidine Acid Phosphate; Rilmenidine Hydrogen Phosphate; S-3341-3. 2-[(Dicyclopropylmethyl)amino]-2-oxazoline phosphate.
$C_{10}H_{16}N_2O,H_3PO_4 = 278.2$.
CAS — 54187-04-1 (rilmenidine); 85409-38-5 (rilmenidine phosphate).

Profile

Rilmenidine is a centrally acting antihypertensive that appears to act through stimulation of central imidazoline receptors and also has alpha$_2$-adrenoceptor agonist activity. It has general properties similar to those of clonidine (p.860), but is reported to cause less sedation and central adverse effects. In the management of hypertension (p.802) it has been given as the phosphate, in doses equivalent to 1 mg of base daily, as a single dose by mouth; this may be increased if necessary, after 1 month, to 2 mg daily in divided doses.

◊ References.
1. Fillastre JP, Vanhoutte PM, eds. Second international symposium on rilmenidine. *Am J Med* 1989; **87** (suppl 3C): 1S–74S.
2. Bousquet P, Feldman J. Drugs acting on imidazoline receptors: a review of their pharmacology, their use in blood pressure control and their potential interest in cardioprotection. *Drugs* 1999; **58**: 799–812.

Preparations

Proprietary Preparations (details are given in Part 3)
Fr.: Hyperium; *Port.:* Hyperium.

Ronifibrate (2922-m)

Ronifibrate (*rINN*).
I-612. 3-Hydroxypropyl nicotinate 2-(4-chlorophenoxy)-2-methylpropionate.
$C_{19}H_{20}ClNO_5 = 377.8.$
CAS — 42597-57-9.
ATC — C10AB07.

Profile

Ronifibrate, a derivative of clofibrate (p.859) and nicotinic acid (p.1372), is a lipid regulating drug that has been used in the treatment of hyperlipidaemias.

Preparations

Proprietary Preparations (details are given in Part 3)
Ital.: Cloprane†.

Rosuvastatin (19945-y)

Rosuvastatin (*BAN, rINN*).
S-4522 (rosuvastatin calcium); ZD-4522. (*E*)-(3*R*,5*S*)-7-{4-(4-Fluorophenyl)-6-isopropyl-2-[methyl(methylsulfonyl)amino]pyrimidin-5-yl}-3,5-dihydroxyhept-6-enoic acid.
$C_{22}H_{28}FN_3O_6S = 481.5.$
CAS — 147098-20-2 (rosuvastatin calcium).

NOTE. Rosuvastatin Calcium is *USAN*.

Profile

Rosuvastatin, a hydroxymethylglutaryl coenzyme A (HMG-CoA) reductase inhibitor (a statin), is a lipid regulating drug with similar properties to simvastatin (p.969). It is under investigation for the treatment of hyperlipidaemias.

Saralasin Acetate (902-g)

Saralasin Acetate (*BANM, USAN, rINNM*).
P-113; The acetate of I-Sar-8-Ala-angiotensin II. The hydrated acetate of Sar-Arg-Val-Tyr-Val-His-Pro-Ala; [1-(*N*-Methylglycine)-5-L-valine-8-L-alanine]-angiotensin II acetate hydrate.
$C_{42}H_{65}N_{13}O_{10}, xCH_3COOH, xH_2O = 912.0$ (saralasin).
CAS — 34273-10-4 (saralasin); 54194-01-3 (anhydrous saralasin); 39698-78-7 (saralasin acetate hydrate).

Profile

Saralasin acetate is a competitive antagonist of angiotensin II and thus blocks its pressor action. It is also a partial agonist and causes a transient initial rise in blood pressure. Saralasin has a short half-life and has been used in the differential diagnosis of renovascular hypertension but its use has largely been superseded by the ACE inhibitors.

Sarpogrelate Hydrochloride (14655-s)

Sarpogrelate Hydrochloride (*rINNM*).
(±)-2-(Dimethylamino)-1-{[*o*-(*m*-methoxyphenethyl)phenoxy]methyl}ethyl hydrogen succinate hydrochloride.
$C_{24}H_{31}NO_6,HCl = 466.0.$
CAS — 125926-17-2 (sarpogrelate).

Profile

Sarpogrelate is an inhibitor of platelet aggregation used in thromboembolic disorders. It is used for occlusive arterial disease (p.809) in doses of 100 mg of the hydrochloride, by mouth, three times daily.

Preparations

Proprietary Preparations (details are given in Part 3)
Jpn: Anplag.

Saruplase (248-z)

Saruplase (*BAN, rINN*).
Prourokinase (enzyme-activating) (human clone pUK4/pUK18), non-glycosylated; Recombinant Human Single-Chain Urokinase-type Plasminogen Activator; scuPA.
$C_{2031}H_{3121}N_{585}O_{601}S_{31} = 46343.1.$
CAS — 99149-95-8.
ATC — B01AD08.

Profile

Saruplase is a thrombolytic drug. It is a urokinase-type plasminogen activator with a single chain structure prepared via recombinant DNA technology and is converted to urokinase

The symbol † denotes a preparation no longer actively marketed

(p.988) in the body by fibrinolysin. It also has some intrinsic plasminogen-activating properties and is reported to have greater selectivity for fibrin-bound plasminogen than for plasma plasminogen. Saruplase is under investigation in acute myocardial infarction.

◊ References.
1. Koster RW, *et al.* Pharmacokinetics and pharmacodynamics of saruplase, an unglycosylated single-chain urokinase-type plasminogen activator, in patients with acute myocardial infarction. *Thromb Haemost* 1994; **72**: 740–4.
2. Tebbe U, *et al.* Randomized, double-blind study comparing saruplase with streptokinase therapy in acute myocardial infarction: the COMPASS equivalence trial. *J Am Coll Cardiol* 1998; **31**: 487–93.

Sibrafiban (10240-d)

Sibrafiban (*BAN, USAN, rINN*).
Ro-48-3657/001. Ethyl (*Z*)-[(1-{*N*-[(*p*-hydroxyamidino)benzoyl]-L-alanyl}-4-piperidyl)oxy] acetate.
$C_{20}H_{28}N_4O_6 = 420.5.$
CAS — 172927-65-0.

Profile

Sibrafiban is a glycoprotein IIb/IIIa-receptor antagonist. It has been investigated as an oral antiplatelet drug in unstable angina and myocardial infarction but results have been disappointing.

◊ References.
1. Cannon CP, *et al.* Randomized trial of an oral platelet glycoprotein IIb/IIIa antagonist, sibrafiban, in patients after an acute coronary syndrome: results of the TIMI 12 trial. *Circulation* 1998; **97**: 340–9.
2. Newby LK. Long-term oral platelet glycoprotein IIb/IIIa receptor antagonism with sibrafiban after acute coronary syndromes: study design of the sibrafiban versus aspirin to yield maximum protection from ischemic heart events post-acute coronary syndromes (SYMPHONY) trial. *Am Heart J* 1999; **138**: 210–8.
3. The SYMPHONY Investigators. Comparison of sibrafiban with aspirin for prevention of cardiovascular events after acute coronary syndromes: a randomised trial. *Lancet* 2000; **355**: 337–45.
4. Second SYMPHONY Investigators. Randomized trial of aspirin, sibrafiban, or both for secondary prevention after acute coronary syndromes. *Circulation* 2001; **103**: 1727–33.

Simfibrate (1358-g)

Simfibrate (*rINN*).
CLY-503; Diclofibrate. Trimethylene bis[2-(4-chlorophenoxy)-2-methylpropionate].
$C_{23}H_{26}Cl_2O_6 = 469.4.$
CAS — 14929-11-4.
ATC — C10AB06.
Pharmacopoeias. In Jpn.

Profile

Simfibrate, a fibric acid derivative (see Bezafibrate, p.849), is a lipid regulating drug that has been used in the treatment of hyperlipidaemias.

Preparations

Proprietary Preparations (details are given in Part 3)
Ital.: Cholesolvin†; *Jpn:* Cholesolvin†.

Simvastatin (2452-l)

Simvastatin (*BAN, USAN, rINN*).
L-644128-000U; MK-733; Simvastatinum; Synvinolin; Velastatin. (1*S*,3*R*,7*S*,8*S*,8a*R*)-1,2,3,7,8,8a-Hexahydro-3,7-dimethyl-8-{2-[(2*R*,4*R*)-tetrahydro-4-hydroxy-6-oxo-2*H*-pyran-2-yl]ethyl}-1-naphthyl 2,2-dimethylbutyrate.
$C_{25}H_{38}O_5 = 418.6.$
CAS — 79902-63-9.
ATC — C10AA01.

Pharmacopoeias. In Eur. (see p.vi) and US.

Pharmacopoeial description

Ph. Eur.: A white or almost white crystalline powder. Practically insoluble in water; freely soluble in alcohol; very soluble in dichloromethane. Store under nitrogen in airtight containers. Protect from light.

USP 25: A white to off-white powder. Practically insoluble in water; freely soluble in alcohol, in chloroform, and in methyl alcohol; sparingly soluble in propylene glycol; very slightly soluble in petroleum spirit. Store under nitrogen.

Adverse Effects and Precautions

The commonest adverse effects of therapy with simvastatin and other statins are gastrointestinal disturbances. Other adverse effects reported include headache, skin rashes, dizziness, blurred vision, insomnia, and dysgeusia. Reversible increases in serum-aminotransferase concentrations may occur and liver function should be assessed before treatment is initiated and then monitored periodically until one year

after the last elevation in dose. Hepatitis and pancreatitis have been reported. A hypersensitivity syndrome whose features have included angioedema has been reported. Myopathy, characterised by myalgia and muscle weakness and associated with increased creatine phosphokinase concentrations, has been reported, especially in patients taking simvastatin concurrently with ciclosporin, fibric acid derivatives, or nicotinic acid. Rarely, rhabdomyolysis with acute renal failure may develop.

Simvastatin should not be given to patients with acute liver disease or unexplained persistently raised serum-aminotransferase concentrations. It should be avoided during pregnancy since there is a possibility that it could interfere with fetal sterol synthesis; there have been a few reports of congenital abnormalities associated with statins (but see Pregnancy, below). It should be discontinued if marked or persistent increases in serum-aminotransferase or creatine phosphokinase concentrations occur. It should be used with caution in patients with severe renal impairment.

◊ In February 1992 the UK Committee on Safety of Medicines (CSM) briefly reviewed[1] the adverse effects that had been reported to it since simvastatin was made available in the UK in May 1989. There had been 257 000 prescriptions and 738 reports to the CSM. Abnormal hepatic function and myalgia were 2 of the most frequently reported reactions, with 36 and 48 reports respectively, including 5 reports of hepatitis and 2 of jaundice. Other muscle effects included 3 reports of myositis, 10 of myopathy, and 7 reports of asymptomatic increases in serum creatine kinase concentrations. Gastrointestinal side-effects accounted for 20% of the reports; skin, neurological and musculoskeletal effects for 15% each; psychiatric effects for 10%; liver effects for 7%; and visual effects for 4%.
1. Committee on Safety of Medicines. Simvastatin. *Current Problems* 33 1992.

Effects on the blood. Thrombotic thrombocytopenic purpura has been described in a patient within 24 hours of taking the second dose of newly-initiated simvastatin therapy.[1] No other precipitating factor was apparent.
1. McCarthy LJ, *et al.* Thrombotic thrombocytopenic purpura and simvastatin. *Lancet* 1998; **352**: 1284–5.

Effects on the hair. Since its introduction in Australia 16 cases of alopecia in association with the use of simvastatin had been reported to the Adverse Drug Reactions Advisory Committee.[1] Most cases involved either excessive hair loss or hair thinning, although two cases of hair loss in patches and one resembling alopecia areata were reported. Onset occurred between 3 days and 15 months of starting therapy.
1. Anonymous. Simvastatin and alopecia. *Aust Adverse Drug React Bull* 1993; **12**: 7.

Effects on the kidneys. Proteinuria was reported in 10 patients taking simvastatin 40 mg daily.[1] The protein loss was of a pattern typical for increased glomerular permeability. In 2 patients proteinuria disappeared when simvastatin was withdrawn and recurred on its subsequent reintroduction.
Renal failure due to rhabdomyolysis has been reported rarely (see under Effects on Skeletal Muscle, below).
1. Deslypere JP, *et al.* Proteinuria as complication of simvastatin treatment. *Lancet* 1990; **336**: 1453.

Effects on mental function. A few cases have been reported of depressive symptoms developing in patients treated with pravastatin[1] or simvastatin.[2] The symptoms appeared during the first few weeks or months of treatment. However, a randomised placebo-controlled study[3] involving over 600 patients did not find that simvastatin treatment was associated with mood disturbances.
1. Lechleitner M, *et al.* Depressive symptoms in hypercholesterolaemic patients treated with pravastatin. *Lancet* 1992; **340**: 910.
2. Duits N, Bos FM. Depressive symptoms and cholesterol-lowering drugs. *Lancet* 1993; **341**: 114.
3. Wardle J, *et al.* Randomised placebo controlled trial of effect on mood of lowering cholesterol concentration. *BMJ* 1996; **313**: 75–8.

Effects on the nervous system. Since its introduction in Australia 22 cases of paraesthesia associated with simvastatin had been reported to the Adverse Drug Reactions Advisory Committee.[1] Symptoms most frequently involved the face, scalp, tongue, and limbs and ranged from hypoaesthetic to hyperaesthetic sensations. In a few cases symptoms occurred immediately on starting treatment while in others they appeared up to one year after initiating therapy. Symptoms disappeared shortly after treatment was withdrawn; in 5 cases symptoms recurred on rechallenge. Four cases of more serious neurological damage had also been reported.
1. Anonymous. Paraesthesia and neuropathy with hypolipidaemic agents. *Aust Adverse Drug React Bull* 1993; **12**: 6.

Effects on sexual function. Impotence has been reported[1] in 5 men receiving simvastatin. No sexual difficulties were noted when fluvastatin was substituted in 4 of them. Others[2] suggest that simvastatin is unlikely to cause impotence, based on the number of men reporting impotence or sexual dysfunction during the Scandinavian Simvastatin Survival Study.

1. Jackson G. Simvastatin and impotence. *BMJ* 1997; **315:** 31.
2. Pedersen TR, Færgeman O. Simvastatin seems unlikely to cause impotence. *BMJ* 1999; **318:** 192.

Effects on skeletal muscle. The UK Committee on Safety of Medicines has noted that myositis and myopathy are well known to occur with lipid regulating drugs such as fibrates and statins.[1] Rhabdomyolysis, presenting as muscle pain with elevated creatine phosphokinase and myoglobinuria leading to renal failure, has also been reported but appears to be rare. Worldwide reporting did not indicate marked differences in the risk of the reactions with individual drugs. [However, the incidence may be higher with cerivastatin, which was withdrawn worldwide in 2001 following reports of severe muscle toxicity, see p.856.] Patients with renal impairment and possibly with hypothyroidism may be at increased risk of muscle toxicity, as may those given *ciclosporin* and a statin concomitantly. Combined treatment with a *fibrate* and a statin may also increase the risk of serious muscle toxicity. The Committee advised that patients treated with fibrates or statins should consult their doctor if they develop muscle pain, tenderness, or weakness and treatment should be stopped if muscle toxicity is suspected clinically or if creatine phosphokinase is markedly raised or progressively rising. Cases of rhabdomyolysis have been reported in patients receiving simvastatin concomitantly with enzyme inhibitors including *itraconazole*,[2,3] *ketoconazole*,[4] and *nefazodone*.[5]

The problem of muscle disorders, as a class effect, associated with statins (namely fluvastatin, pravastatin, and simvastatin) has also been noted by the Adverse Drug Reactions Advisory Committee in Australia.[6]

1. Committee on Safety of Medicines/Medicines Control Agency. Rhabdomyolysis associated with lipid-lowering drugs. *Current Problems* 1995; **21:** 3.
2. Segaert MF, *et al.* Drug-interaction-induced rhabdomyolysis. *Nephrol Dial Transplant* 1996; **11:** 1846–7.
3. Horn M. Coadministration of itraconazole with hypolipidemic agents may induce rhabdomyolysis in healthy individuals. *Arch Dermatol* 1996; **132:** 1254.
4. Gilad R, Lampl Y. Rhabdomyolysis induced by simvastatin and ketoconazole treatment. *Clin Neuropharmacol* 1999; **22:** 295–7.
5. Jacobson RH, *et al.* Myositis and rhabdomyolysis associated with concurrent use of simvastatin and nefazodone. *JAMA* 1997; **277:** 296.
6. Adverse Drug Reactions Advisory Committee (ADRAC). Fluvastatin and muscle disorders—a class effect. *Aust Adverse Drug React Bull* 1997; **16:** 3.

Effects on sleep patterns. Patients taking lovastatin have been reported to experience a reduction in the length of continuous sleep while no such effect was observed with pravastatin.[1] A similar sleep disturbance has been reported with simvastatin.[2] It was suggested that pravastatin might be less likely to affect sleep since it is hydrophilic and does not penetrate the brain easily. However, there have been conflicting reports: in other studies neither lovastatin,[3] pravastatin,[4] nor simvastatin,[3-5] had any adverse effect on sleep, but there have been further individual reports of sleep disturbances with lovastatin.[6,7]

1. Schaefer EJ. HMG-CoA reductase inhibitors for hypercholesterolemia. *N Engl J Med* 1988; **319:** 1222.
2. Barth JD, *et al.* Inhibitors of hydroxymethylglutaryl coenzyme A reductase for treating hypercholesterolaemia. *BMJ* 1990; **301:** 669.
3. Black DM, *et al.* Sleep disturbances and HMG CoA reductase inhibitors. *JAMA* 1990; **264:** 1105.
4. Eckernäs S-Å, *et al.* The effects of simvastatin and pravastatin on objective and subjective measures of nocturnal sleep: a comparison of two structurally different HMG CoA reductase inhibitors in patients with primary moderate hypercholesterolaemia. *Br J Clin Pharmacol* 1993; **35:** 284–9.
5. Keech AC, *et al.* Absence of effects of prolonged simvastatin therapy on nocturnal sleep in a large randomized placebo-controlled study. *Br J Clin Pharmacol* 1996; **42:** 483–90.
6. Rosenson RS, Goranson NL. Lovastatin-associated sleep and mood disturbances. *Am J Med* 1993; **95:** 548–9.
7. Sinzinger H, *et al.* Sleep disturbance and appetite loss after lovastatin. *Lancet* 1994; **343:** 973.

Porphyria. Simvastatin is considered to be unsafe in patients with porphyria because it has been shown to be porphyrinogenic in *animals*.

Pregnancy. Postmarketing surveillance identified 134 cases of unintentional exposure to lovastatin or simvastatin during pregnancy in which the outcome was known.[1] Although there were 9 reports of congenital anomalies these consisted of a spectrum of unrelated malformations and the frequency did not exceed that expected in the general population. It was therefore considered that these drugs did not adversely affect outcome of pregnancy.

1. Manson JM, *et al.* Postmarketing surveillance of lovastatin and simvastatin exposure during pregnancy. *Reprod Toxicol* 1996; **10:** 439–46.

Interactions

There is an increased risk of myopathy if certain drugs are given concurrently with statins. Concomitant administration of drugs that inhibit the cytochrome P450 isoenzyme CYP3A4, such as ciclosporin, itraconazole, ketoconazole, erythromycin, clarithromycin, HIV-protease inhibitors, and nefazodone, might produce high plasma levels of simvastatin, thus increasing the risk of myopathy. Drugs that alone can cause myopathy, such as fibric acid derivatives or nicotinic acid, can increase the risk of this reaction when given with simvastatin. For further details see Effects on Skeletal Muscle, under Adverse Effects, above. Bleeding and increases in prothrombin time have been reported in patients taking simvastatin with coumarin anticoagulants. Raised concentrations of simvastatin have occurred in patients also given mibefradil.

◊ General reviews.

1. Garnett WR. Interactions with hydroxymethylglutaryl-coenzyme A reductase inhibitors. *Am J Health-Syst Pharm* 1995; **52:** 1639–45.

Pharmacokinetics

Simvastatin is absorbed from the gastrointestinal tract and is hydrolysed to its active β-hydroxyacid form. Other active metabolites have been detected and a number of inactive metabolites are also formed. Simvastatin undergoes extensive first-pass metabolism in the liver, its primary site of action. Less than 5% of the oral dose has been reported to reach the circulation as active metabolites. Both simvastatin and its β-hydroxyacid metabolite are about 95% bound to plasma proteins. It is mainly excreted in the faeces via the bile as metabolites. About 10 to 15% is recovered in the urine, mainly in inactive forms. The half-life of the active metabolite is 1.9 hours.

◊ General reviews.

1. Mauro VF. Clinical pharmacokinetics and practical applications of simvastatin. *Clin Pharmacokinet* 1993; **24:** 195–202.
2. Desager J-P, Horsmans Y. Clinical pharmacokinetics of 3-hydroxy-3-methylglutaryl-coenzyme A reductase inhibitors. *Clin Pharmacokinet* 1996; **31:** 348–71.
3. Lennernäs H, Fager G. Pharmacodynamics and pharmacokinetics of the HMG-CoA reductase inhibitors: similarities and differences. *Clin Pharmacokinet* 1997; **32:** 403–25.

Uses and Administration

Simvastatin is a lipid regulating drug; it is a competitive inhibitor of 3-hydroxy-3-methylglutaryl coenzyme A reductase (HMG-CoA reductase), the rate-determining enzyme for cholesterol synthesis. HMG-CoA reductase inhibitors (also called statins) reduce total cholesterol, low-density lipoprotein (LDL)-cholesterol, and very-low-density lipoprotein (VLDL)-cholesterol concentrations in plasma. They also tend to reduce triglycerides and to increase high-density lipoprotein (HDL)-cholesterol concentrations. They are considered to exert their hypocholesterolaemic action by stimulating an increase in LDL-receptors on hepatocyte membranes thereby increasing the clearance of LDL from the circulation.

Simvastatin is used to reduce LDL-cholesterol, apolipoprotein B, and triglycerides, and to increase HDL-cholesterol in the treatment of hyperlipidaemias (below), including hypercholesterolaemias and combined (mixed) hyperlipidaemia (type IIa or IIb hyperlipoproteinaemias). Statins can be effective as adjunct therapy in patients with homozygous familial hypercholesterolaemia who have some LDL-receptor function. Simvastatin is also given prophylactically to hypercholesterolaemic patients with ischaemic heart disease.

Simvastatin is given by mouth in an initial dose of 5 to 10 mg in the evening; an initial dose of 20 mg may be used in patients with ischaemic heart disease. The dose may be adjusted at intervals of not less than 4 weeks up to a maximum of 80 mg once daily in the evening. Patients with homozygous familial hypercholesterolaemia may be treated with 40 mg once daily in the evening, or 80 mg daily in three divided doses of 20 mg, 20 mg, and an evening dose of 40 mg. A maximum of 10 mg daily is recommended in those taking ciclosporin, fibric acid derivatives, or nicotinic acid, and the risk of myopathy must be considered.

◊ General reviews.

1. Mauro VF, MacDonald JL. Simvastatin: a review of its pharmacology and clinical use. *DICP Ann Pharmacother* 1991; **25:** 257–64.
2. Plosker GL, McTavish D. Simvastatin: a reappraisal of its pharmacology and therapeutic efficacy in hypercholesterolaemia. *Drugs* 1995; **50:** 334–63.

3. Schectman G, Hiatt J. Dose–response characteristics of cholesterol-lowering drug therapies: implications for treatment. *Ann Intern Med* 1996; **125:** 990–1000.
4. White CM. Pharmacological effects of HMG CoA reductase inhibitors other than lipoprotein modulation. *J Clin Pharmacol* 1999; **39:** 111–18.

Hyperlipidaemias. Statins, including simvastatin, are used in the treatment of hyperlipidaemias (p.800) and are effective in reducing total cholesterol and low-density lipoprotein (LDL)-cholesterol concentrations in patients with hypercholesterolaemia.[1-4] They are also of value in the prevention of ischaemic heart disease.

Statins have been shown to be more effective in reducing LDL-cholesterol concentrations than bile-acid binding resins or fibric acid derivatives, typically achieving reductions of 20 to 40%. Concentrations of high-density lipoprotein (HDL)-cholesterol are increased, or unchanged, resulting in an improvement of the LDL:HDL-cholesterol ratio. Combination of statins with bile-acid binding resins has been shown to produce additional reductions in LDL-cholesterol concentrations of up to about 60%. However, there is concern over enhanced adverse effects with combinations of statins and nicotinic acid or fibric acid derivatives.

STUDIES WITH SIMVASTATIN. An interim report of the 5-year Oxford Cholesterol Study in over 600 patients at increased risk of ischaemic heart disease confirmed the efficacy and safety of simvastatin as a lipid regulating drug at follow-up after 3 years.[5] Total cholesterol, LDL-cholesterol, and triglyceride concentrations were all substantially reduced and there were small increases in HDL-cholesterol. Since hypercholesterolaemia is a known risk factor for atherosclerosis, there is much interest in the value of this lipid regulating effect in the prophylaxis of **ischaemic heart disease**. Large placebo-controlled studies with simvastatin for the secondary prevention of ischaemic heart disease, the Multicentre Anti-Atheroma Study (MAAS)[6] and the Scandinavian Simvastatin Survival Study (4S)[7-9] have indicated a beneficial effect when cholesterol levels are reduced in patients with ischaemic heart disease. In MAAS, reduction of atherogenic lipoproteins was claimed to slow the coronary atherosclerotic process in patients with moderate hypercholesterolaemia and known ischaemic heart disease. Overall, in 4S, simvastatin was associated with improved survival and no apparent increase in non-cardiac mortality in patients with angina pectoris or previous myocardial infarction. The risk for major coronary events in this trial was reduced for women as well as for men although there were too few women studied to assess effects on mortality. Additionally, there was some evidence[9] that simvastatin retarded progression of **non-cardiac atherosclerosis** as the risk of peripheral vascular disease (such as intermittent claudication) and cerebrovascular disease (stroke and transient ischaemic attacks) was reduced.

1. Hoeg JM, Brewer HB. 3-Hydroxy-3-methylglutaryl-coenzyme A reductase inhibitors in the treatment of hypercholesterolemia. *JAMA* 1987; **258:** 3532–6.
2. Illingworth DR, Bacon S. Hypolipidemic effects of HMG-CoA reductase inhibitors in patients with hypercholesterolemia. *Am J Cardiol* 1987; **60:** 33G–42G.
3. Grundy SM. HMG-CoA reductase inhibitors for treatment of hypercholesterolemia. *N Engl J Med* 1988; **319:** 24–33.
4. Slater EE, MacDonald JS. Mechanism of action and biological profile of HMG CoA reductase inhibitors. *Drugs* 1988; **36** (suppl 3): 72–82.
5. Keech A, *et al.* Three-year follow-up of the Oxford Cholesterol Study: assessment of the efficacy and safety of simvastatin in preparation for a large mortality study. *Eur Heart J* 1994; **15:** 255–69.
6. MAAS Investigators. Effect of simvastatin on coronary atheroma: the Multicentre Anti-Atheroma Study (MAAS). *Lancet* 1994; **344:** 633–8. Correction. *ibid.*: 762.
7. Scandinavian Simvastatin Survival Study Group. Randomised trial of cholesterol lowering in 4444 patients with coronary heart disease: the Scandinavian Simvastatin Survival Study (4S). *Lancet* 1994; **344:** 1383–9.
8. Miettinen TA, *et al.* Cholesterol-lowering therapy in women and elderly patients with myocardial infarction or angina pectoris: findings from the Scandinavian Simvastatin Survival Study (4S). *Circulation* 1997; **96:** 4211–18.
9. Pedersen TR, *et al.* Effect of simvastatin on ischemic signs and symptoms in the Scandinavian Simvastatin Survival Study (4S). *Am J Cardiol* 1998; **81:** 333–5.

Preparations

USP 25: Simvastatin Tablets.

Proprietary Preparations (details are given in Part 3)
Aust.: Zocord; *Austral.:* Lipex; Zocor; *Belg.:* Zocor; *Braz.:* Zocor; *Canad.:* Zocor; *Denm.:* Zocor; *Fin.:* Corolin; Zocor; *Fr.:* Lodales; Zocor; *Ger.:* Denan; Zocor; *Hong Kong:* Zocor; *Irl.:* Zocor; *Israel:* Simovil; *Ital.:* Liponorm; Medipo; Sinvacor; Sivastin; Zocor; *Mex.:* Zocor; *Neth.:* Zocor; *Norw.:* Zocor; *NZ:* Zocor; *Port.:* Zocor; *S.Afr.:* Zocor; *Singapore:* Zocor; *Spain:* Colemin; Pantok; Zocor; *Swed.:* Zocord; *Switz.:* Zocor; *Thai.:* Zocor; *UAE:* Simvast; *UK:* Zocor; *USA:* Zocor.

Sitosterol (1359-q)

β-Sitosterin; β-Sitosterol. Stigmast-5-en-3β-ol.
$C_{29}H_{50}O = 414.7$.
CAS — 83-46-5.

Profile

Sitosterol is a naturally occurring phytosterol that is used as a lipid regulating drug in the treatment of hyperlipidaemias (p.800). The usual dose is 3 to 6 g daily in divided doses by mouth. Sitosterol has been incorporated into margarine for use in the dietary management of hypercholesterolaemia (see also Stanol Esters, p.1379).

It is also used in benign prostatic hyperplasia (p.1477) in usual initial doses of 20 mg three times daily by mouth reducing to 10 mg three times daily for long-term therapy.

◊ References.
1. Berges RR, *et al.* Randomised, placebo-controlled, double-blind clinical trial of β-sitosterol in patients with benign prostatic hyperplasia. *Lancet* 1995; **345:** 1529–32.
2. Klippel KF, *et al.* A multicentric, placebo-controlled, double-blind clinical trial of β-sitosterol (phytosterol) for the treatment of benign prostatic hyperplasia. *Br J Urol* 1997; **80:** 427–32.
3. Wilt TJ, *et al.* β-Sitosterol for the treatment of benign prostatic hyperplasia: a systematic review. *BJU Int* 1999; **83:** 976–83.

Preparations

Proprietary Preparations (details are given in Part 3)
Aust.: Harzol; **Ger.:** Azuprostat M; Flemun; Harzol; Liposit†; LP-Truw mono†; Prostasal; Sito-Lande; Triastonal; **Thai.:** Mebo; **UAE:** Mebo.

Multi-ingredient: UK: Cholasitrol; Kolestop; **USA:** Beta Prostate; Cholesterol Support; Prostate Support.

Sodium Apolate (13240-n)

Sodium Apolate (BAN, rINN).

Lyapolate Sodium (USAN); Sodium Lyapolate. Poly(sodium ethylenesulphonate).

$(C_2H_3NaO_3S)_n$.

CAS — 25053-27-4.
ATC — C05BA02.

Profile

Sodium apolate is a synthetic heparinoid anticoagulant. It has been used in the topical treatment of haematomas and superficial thromboses and for the relief of sprains and contusions.

Preparations

Proprietary Preparations (details are given in Part 3)
Multi-ingredient: Braz.: Pergalen.

Sodium Nitroprusside (903-q)

Disodium (OC-6-22)-Pentakis(cyano-C)nitrosylferrate Dihydrate; Natrii Nitroprussias; Sodium Nitroferricyanide Dihydrate; Sodium Nitroprussiate. Sodium nitrosylpentacyanoferrate(III) dihydrate.

$Na_2Fe(CN)_5NO,2H_2O = 297.9$.

CAS — 14402-89-2 (anhydrous sodium nitroprusside); 13755-38-9 (sodium nitroprusside dihydrate).
Pharmacopoeias. In Chin., Eur. (see p.vi), Int., and US.

Pharmacopoeial description
Ph. Eur.: Reddish-brown crystals or powder. Freely soluble in water; slightly soluble in alcohol. Protect from light.

USP 25: Reddish-brown, practically odourless crystals or powder. Freely soluble in water; slightly soluble in alcohol; very slightly soluble in chloroform; insoluble in benzene. Store in airtight containers. Protect from light.

◊ CAUTION. *Solutions of sodium nitroprusside decompose when exposed to light and must be protected during infusion by wrapping the container with aluminium foil or some other light-proof material. Nitroprusside will react with minute quantities of organic and inorganic substances forming highly coloured products. If this occurs the solution should be discarded. Solutions should not be used more than 24 hours after preparation.*

Incompatibility. Sodium nitroprusside has been reported to be visually incompatible with cisatracurium besilate[1] and with levofloxacin[2] during simulated Y-site administration.
1. Trissel LA, *et al.* Compatibility of cisatracurium besylate with selected drugs during simulated Y-site administration. *Am J Health-Syst Pharm* 1997; **54:** 1735–41.
2. Saltsman CL, *et al.* Compatibility of levofloxacin with 34 medications during simulated Y-site administration. *Am J Health-Syst Pharm* 1999; **56:** 1458–9.

Stability in solution. The instability of sodium nitroprusside solutions has been the subject of considerable investigation. Although stated to be more stable in acid than in alkaline solution,[1] a later study[2] found that whereas the initial light-induced darkening of a 1% solution was independent of pH, further degradation leading to the development of a blue precipitate required an acid pH. If protected from light by wrapping in aluminium foil sodium nitroprusside 50 or 100 µg per mL was found to be stable in 5% glucose, lactated Ringer's, and normal saline solutions for 48 hours.[3] In clinical practice the infusion container should be opaque or protected with foil, but an amber giving set may be used in conjunction, which allows visual monitoring of the infusion.[4,5]

Various substances have been reported to increase the stability of nitroprusside solutions, including dimethyl sulfoxide,[6] glycerol,[1] sodium citrate,[1] and other salts with anionic chelating potential such as sodium acetate or phosphate.[1] In contrast

sodium bisulfite and the hydroxybenzoates are reported to reduce stability.[1]
1. Schumacher GE. Sodium nitroprusside injection. *Am J Hosp Pharm* 1966; **23:** 532.
2. Hargrave RE. Degradation of solutions of sodium nitroprusside. *J Hosp Pharm* 1974; **32:** 188–91.
3. Mahony C, *et al.* In vitro stability of sodium nitroprusside solutions for intravenous administration. *J Pharm Sci* 1984; **73:** 838–9.
4. Davidson SW, Lyall D. Sodium nitroprusside stability in light-protective solutions. *Pharm J* 1987; **239:** 599–601.
5. Lyall D. Sodium nitroprusside stability. *Pharm J* 1988; **240:** 5.
6. Asker AF, Gragg R. Dimethyl sulfoxide as a photoprotective agent for sodium nitroprusside solutions. *Drug Dev Ind Pharm* 1983; **9:** 837–48.

Adverse Effects

Sodium nitroprusside rapidly reduces blood pressure and is converted in the body to cyanide and then thiocyanate. Its adverse effects can be attributed mainly to excessive hypotension and excessive cyanide accumulation; thiocyanate toxicity may also occur, especially in patients with renal impairment. Intravenous infusion of sodium nitroprusside may produce nausea and vomiting, apprehension, headache, dizziness, restlessness, perspiration, palpitations, retrosternal discomfort, abdominal pain, and muscle twitching, but these effects may be reduced by slowing the rate of infusion.

An excessive amount of cyanide in plasma (more than 0.08 µg per mL), because of overdosage or depletion of endogenous thiosulfate (which converts cyanide to thiocyanate *in vivo*), may result in tachycardia, sweating, hyperventilation, arrhythmias, and profound metabolic acidosis. Metabolic acidosis may be the first sign of cyanide toxicity. Methaemoglobinaemia may also occur.

Adverse effects attributed to thiocyanate include tinnitus, miosis, and hyperreflexia; confusion, hallucinations, and convulsions have also been reported.

Other adverse effects include thrombocytopenia and phlebitis.

Effects on the blood. THROMBOCYTOPENIA. Platelet counts decreased in 7 of 8 patients with heart failure 1 to 6 hours after intravenous infusion of nitroprusside was started.[1] The counts began to return to normal 24 hours after the infusion was stopped.
1. Mehta P, *et al.* Nitroprusside lowers platelet count. *N Engl J Med* 1978; **299:** 1134.

Effects on the gastrointestinal tract. Five out of 38 patients who were given sodium nitroprusside intravenously for controlled hypotension during surgery developed symptoms of adynamic ileus postoperatively.[1] The symptoms could have been secondary to intestinal ischaemia due to diminished mesenteric arterial blood flow. However, other explanations have been proposed including sympathetic stimulation[2,3] or the concomitant use of opioid analgesics.[4]
1. Chen JW, *et al.* Adynamic ileus following induced hypotension. *JAMA* 1985; **253:** 633.
2. Gelman S. Adynamic ileus following induced hypotension. *JAMA* 1985; **254:** 1721.
3. Lampert BA. Adynamic ileus following induced hypotension. *JAMA* 1985; **254:** 1721.
4. Lemmo J, Karnes J. Adynamic ileus following induced hypotension. *JAMA* 1985; **254:** 1721.

Effects on intracranial pressure. A significant increase in intracranial pressure while the mean blood pressure was 90 or 80% of initial values was reported[1] in 14 normocapnic patients given an infusion of sodium nitroprusside to produce controlled hypotension prior to neurosurgery; values reverted towards normal at mean blood pressures of 70% of controls. A similar but insignificant trend occurred in 5 hypocapnic patients. In another report[2] a rise in intracranial pressure was noted following the use of nitroprusside in a patient with Reye's syndrome.
1. Turner JM, *et al.* Intracranial pressure changes in neurosurgical patients during hypotension induced with sodium nitroprusside or trimetaphan. *Br J Anaesth* 1977; **49:** 419–24.
2. Griswold WR, *et al.* Nitroprusside-induced intracranial hypertension. *JAMA* 1981; **246:** 2679–80.

Phlebitis. Acute transient phlebitis has occurred following sodium nitroprusside administration.[1]
1. Miller R, Stark DCC. Acute phlebitis from nitroprusside. *Anesthesiology* 1978; **49:** 372.

Treatment of Adverse Effects

Side-effects due to excessive hypotension may be treated by slowing or discontinuing the infusion.

For details of the treatment of cyanide poisoning see Hydrocyanic Acid, p.1433. Thiocyanate can be removed by dialysis.

Precautions

Sodium nitroprusside should not be used in the presence of compensatory hypertension (for example, in arteriovenous shunts or coarctation of the aorta). It should be used with caution, if at all, in patients with hepatic impairment, and in patients with low plasma-cobalamin concentrations or Leber's optic atrophy. It should also be used with caution in patients with impaired renal or pulmonary function and with particular caution in patients with impaired cerebrovascular circulation. Thiocyanate, a metabolite of sodium nitroprusside, inhibits iodine binding and uptake and sodium nitroprusside should be used with caution in patients with hypothyroidism. The plasma-thiocyanate concentration should be monitored if treatment continues for more than 3 days and should not exceed 100 µg per mL although toxicity may be apparent at lower thiocyanate concentrations. Thiocyanate concentrations do not reflect cyanide toxicity and cyanide concentrations should also be monitored; the blood concentration of cyanide should not exceed 1 µg per mL and the plasma concentration should not exceed 0.08 µg per mL. The acid-base balance should also be monitored. Care should be taken to ensure that extravasation does not occur. Sodium nitroprusside should not be withdrawn abruptly due to the risk of rebound effects.

Tachyphylaxis. Tachyphylaxis to sodium nitroprusside was associated with high plasma concentrations of cyanide without metabolic acidosis in 3 patients undergoing hypotensive anaesthesia.[1]
1. Cottrell JE, *et al.* Nitroprusside tachyphylaxis without acidosis. *Anesthesiology* 1978; **49:** 141–2.

Withdrawal. Rebound haemodynamic changes, including hypertension and increased heart rate, occurred 10 to 30 minutes after discontinuation of intravenous sodium nitroprusside infusion in a study in 20 patients with heart failure.[1] The changes generally resolved spontaneously within 1 to 3 hours after drug withdrawal and produced only minimal exacerbation of symptoms in most patients, although 3 patients developed pulmonary oedema 20 to 30 minutes after stopping the nitroprusside infusion that required reinstitution of nitroprusside in 2 of them. A study investigating a possible mechanism for this effect[2] found that plasma-renin concentrations were increased during infusion of nitroprusside and remained elevated for 30 minutes after the infusion was stopped. It was suggested that this persistence of elevated plasma-renin concentrations after clearance of short-lived nitroprusside may be responsible for the rebound effects.
1. Packer M, *et al.* Rebound hemodynamic events after the abrupt withdrawal of nitroprusside in patients with severe chronic heart failure. *N Engl J Med* 1979; **301:** 1193–7.
2. Cottrell JE, *et al.* Rebound hypertension after sodium nitroprusside-induced hypotension. *Clin Pharmacol Ther* 1980; **27:** 32–6.

Interactions

Enhanced hypotension should be expected if sodium nitroprusside is used concomitantly with other antihypertensives or drugs that produce hypotension.

Alteplase. Sodium nitroprusside infusion prolonged the fibrinolytic activity of alteplase when given concomitantly to *animals*; use of nitrovasodilators with alteplase may be responsible for the enhanced bleeding tendency seen in some patients on thrombolytic therapy.[1]
1. Korbut R, *et al.* Prolongation of fibrinolytic activity of tissue plasminogen activator by nitrovasodilators. *Lancet* 1990; **335:** 669.

Pharmacokinetics

Sodium nitroprusside is converted in the erythrocytes to cyanide. Nitric oxide is also released *in vivo*. Cyanide is metabolised in the liver to thiocyanate by the enzyme rhodanase in the presence of thiosulfate and slowly excreted in the urine. The plasma half-life of thiocyanate is reported to be about 3 days, but may be much longer in patients with renal impairment.

◊ Reviews.
1. Schulz V. Clinical pharmacokinetics of nitroprusside, cyanide, thiosulphate and thiocyanate. *Clin Pharmacokinet* 1984; **9:** 239–51.

Metabolism. Although the liberation of cyanide from nitroprusside *in vivo* has been questioned, and reported values have been attributed to photodecomposition prior to infusion of nitroprusside, flaws in the assay technique, or both,[1,2] others have shown that incubation of nitroprusside with blood (but not with assay reagents) produced significant amounts of cyanide

---

The symbol † denotes a preparation no longer actively marketed

in vitro,[3] and have provided further evidence for breakdown of nitroprusside to cyanide *in vivo*.[4]

1. Bisset WIK, *et al.* Sodium nitroprusside and cyanide release: reasons for re-appraisal. *Br J Anaesth* 1981; **53**: 1015–18.
2. Butler AR, *et al.* Sodium nitroprusside and cyanide release. *Br J Anaesth* 1982; **54**: 792–3.
3. Vesey CJ, *et al.* Decay of nitroprusside I: in vitro. *Br J Anaesth* 1990; **64**: 696–703.
4. Vesey CJ, *et al.* Decay of nitroprusside II: in vivo. *Br J Anaesth* 1990; **64**: 704–9.

Uses and Administration

Sodium nitroprusside is a short-acting hypotensive drug with a duration of action of 1 to 10 minutes. It produces peripheral vasodilatation and reduces peripheral resistance by a direct action on both veins and arterioles. It has been termed a nitrovasodilator because it releases nitric oxide *in vivo*. Its effects appear within a few seconds of intravenous infusion. Sodium nitroprusside is used in the treatment of hypertensive crises (p.802) and to produce controlled hypotension during general anaesthesia. It has also been used to reduce preload and afterload in severe heart failure (p.798) including that associated with myocardial infarction (p.805).

It is given by continuous intravenous infusion of a solution containing 50 to 200 μg per mL. A controlled infusion device must be used. The solution should be prepared immediately before use by dissolving sodium nitroprusside in glucose 5% and then diluting with glucose 5%; the solution must be protected from light during administration. Blood pressure should be monitored closely during administration and care should be taken to prevent extravasation. In general, treatment should not continue for more than 72 hours. If required for several days blood and plasma concentrations of cyanide should be monitored and should not exceed 1 μg per mL and 0.08 μg per mL respectively; thiocyanate concentrations in serum should also be measured if infusion continues for more than 72 hours and should not exceed 100 μg per mL. Since rebound hypertension has been reported when sodium nitroprusside is withdrawn, the infusion should be tailed off gradually over 10 to 30 minutes.

For **hypertensive crises** in patients not receiving antihypertensive drugs, an initial dose of 0.3 to 1.5 μg per kg body-weight per minute may be given, increasing gradually under close supervision until the desired reduction in blood pressure is achieved. The average dose required to maintain the blood pressure 30 to 40% below the pretreatment diastolic blood pressure is 3 μg per kg per minute and the usual dose range is 0.5 to 6 μg per kg per minute. Lower doses should be used in patients already receiving other antihypertensives. The maximum recommended rate is about 8 μg per kg per minute in the UK, and 10 μg per kg per minute in the USA; infusions at these rates should be used for no longer than 10 minutes and should be stopped after 10 minutes if there is no response. If there is a response, sodium nitroprusside should ideally be given for only a few hours to avoid the risk of cyanide toxicity. An alternative antihypertensive that can be given by mouth should be introduced as soon as possible.

For the **induction of hypotension** during anaesthesia a maximum dose of 1.5 μg per kg body-weight per minute is recommended.

In **heart failure** an initial dose of 10 to 15 μg per minute has been used increasing by increments of 10 to 15 μg per minute every 5 to 10 minutes until the initial response is seen. The usual dosage range is 10 to 200 μg per minute and the dose should not exceed 280 μg per minute (or 4 μg per kg body-weight per minute).

Sodium nitroprusside is also used as a reagent for detecting ketones in urine.

Administration in children. Although experience is more limited than with adults, sodium nitroprusside has been successfully used in infants and children. Continuous infusion of nitroprusside at a rate of 2 to 4 μg per kg body-weight per minute for 28 days was reported[1] in an 11-year-old child with refractory hypertension, without any signs of thiocyanate toxicity. In a series of 58 neonates with cardiovascular disorders or respiratory distress syndrome,[2] sodium nitroprusside was given

in a usual initial dose of 0.25 to 0.5 μg per kg per minute, and the rate was then repeatedly doubled at intervals of 15 to 20 minutes until the desired effect was achieved, adverse effects supervened, or it was judged ineffective. The maximum rate did not exceed 6 μg per kg per minute. Infusion of sodium nitroprusside in doses of 0.5 to 8 μg per kg per minute to produce controlled reduction of blood pressure has also been reported[3] in 28 children with hypertensive crises; 16 had also received labetalol.[3]

1. Luderer JR, *et al.* Long-term administration of sodium nitroprusside in childhood. *J Pediatr* 1977; **91**: 490–1.
2. Benitz WE, *et al.* Use of sodium nitroprusside in neonates: efficacy and safety. *J Pediatr* 1985; **106**: 102–10.
3. Deal JE, *et al.* Management of hypertensive emergencies. *Arch Dis Child* 1992; **67**: 1089–92.

Ergotamine poisoning. For the use of sodium nitroprusside in the treatment of cyanosis of the extremities due to ergotamine overdosage, see p.452.

Preparations

BP 2001: Sodium Nitroprusside Intravenous Infusion;
USP 25: Sodium Nitroprusside for Injection.

Proprietary Preparations (details are given in Part 3)
Braz.: Nipride; *Canad.:* Nipride; *Fr.:* Nitriate; *Ger.:* Nipruss; *Irl.:* Nipride; *Israel:* Nipride; Niprus; *Jpn:* Nitopro; *Neth.:* Nipride†; *S.Afr.:* Hypoten; *Spain:* Nitroprussiat; *Swed.:* Nipride†; *USA:* Nitropress.

Sorbinicate (13262-q)

Sorbinicate (rINN).
D-Glucitol hexanicotinate.
$C_{42}H_{32}N_6O_{12} = 812.7$.
CAS — 6184-06-1.

Profile

Sorbinicate, a derivative of nicotinic acid, is a lipid regulating drug that has been used in the treatment of hyperlipidaemias.

Sotalol Hydrochloride (6322-e)

Sotalol Hydrochloride (BANM, USAN, rINNM).
MJ-1999; d,l-Sotalol Hydrochloride; Sotaloli Hydrochloridum.
4′-(1-Hydroxy-2-isopropylaminoethyl)methanesulphonanilide hydrochloride.
$C_{12}H_{20}N_2O_3S,HCl = 308.8$.
CAS — 3930-20-9 (sotalol); 959-24-0 (sotalol hydrochloride).
Pharmacopoeias. In *Eur.* (see p.vi).

Pharmacopoeial description

Ph. Eur.: A white or almost white powder. Freely soluble in water; soluble in alcohol; practically insoluble in dichloromethane. A 5% solution in water has a pH of 4.0 to 5.0. Protect from light.

Adverse Effects, Treatment, and Precautions

As for beta blockers, p.844.

Torsade de pointes has been reported in patients given sotalol, usually due to prolongation of the QT interval. The QT interval should be monitored; extreme caution is required if the QT interval exceeds 0.50 seconds and sotalol should be discontinued or the dose reduced if the QT interval exceeds 0.55 seconds. As hypokalaemia or hypomagnesaemia may predispose patients to arrhythmias, serum-electrolyte concentrations should be monitored before and during treatment with sotalol.

Sotalol is contra-indicated in patients with renal impairment whose creatinine clearance is less than 10 mL per minute.

Effects on the gastrointestinal tract. A report of retroperitoneal fibrosis associated with the use of sotalol.[1]

1. Laakso M, *et al.* Retroperitoneal fibrosis associated with sotalol. *BMJ* 1982; **285**: 1085–6.

Effects on the heart. Atypical ventricular tachycardia ('torsade de pointes') has been reported in patients receiving sotalol and may be associated with prolongation of the QT interval.[1,2] Hypokalaemia may contribute to sotalol's proarrhythmic effect and was considered relevant in 8 of 12 patients who developed ventricular tachycardia when given sotalol in association with hydrochlorothiazide; 4 patients were also receiving other drugs known to prolong the QT interval.[3] A meta-analysis[4] of 22 clinical trials involving 3135 patients who had taken sotalol orally found women to be at increased risk of developing torsade de pointes. Torsade de pointes developed in 44 (1.9%) of 2336 men and in 33 (4.1%) of 799 women.

In one patient torsade de pointes was treated successfully with magnesium sulfate by intravenous infusion and withdrawal of sotalol.[5]

1. Kontopoulos A, *et al.* Sotalol-induced torsade de pointes. *Postgrad Med J* 1981; **57**: 321–3.
2. Krapf R, Gertsch M. Torsade de pointes induced by sotalol despite therapeutic plasma sotalol concentrations. *BMJ* 1985; **290**: 1784–5.
3. McKibbin JK, *et al.* Sotalol, hypokalaemia, syncope, and torsade de pointes. *Br Heart J* 1984; **541**: 157–62.
4. Lehmann MH, *et al.* Sex difference in risk of torsade de pointes with d,l-sotalol. *Circulation* 1996; **94**: 2534–41.
5. Arstall MA, *et al.* Sotalol-induced torsade de pointes: management with magnesium infusion. *Postgrad Med J* 1992; **68**: 289–90.

Interactions

Sotalol should not be given concurrently with other drugs that prolong the QT interval due to the increased risk of precipitating ventricular arrhythmias. Thus sotalol should not be given with antiarrhythmics that prolong the QT interval (such as amiodarone, disopyramide, procainamide, or quinidine), phenothiazine antipsychotics, tricyclic antidepressants, certain antihistamines (astemizole, mizolastine, and terfenadine), cisapride, erythromycin, halofantrine, pentamidine, sultopride, or vincamine. Also, sotalol should be given with great caution with drugs that cause electrolyte disturbances such as diuretics.

Other interactions associated with beta blockers are discussed on p.846.

Pharmacokinetics

Sotalol is virtually completely absorbed from the gastrointestinal tract and peak plasma concentrations are obtained about 2 to 4 hours after a dose. The plasma elimination half-life is about 10 to 20 hours. Sotalol has low lipid solubility. Very little is metabolised and it is excreted unchanged in the urine. Binding to plasma proteins is reported to be low. It crosses the placenta and is distributed into breast milk where higher concentrations have been achieved than in maternal serum. Only small amounts are reported to cross the blood-brain barrier and enter the CSF. Sotalol is removed by dialysis.

◊ General references.

1. Singh BN, *et al.* Sotalol: a review of its pharmacodynamic and pharmacokinetic properties, and therapeutic use. *Drugs* 1987; **34**: 311–49.
2. Fitton A, Sorkin EM. Sotalol: an updated review of its pharmacological properties and therapeutic use in cardiac arrhythmias. *Drugs* 1993; **46**: 678–719.

Breast feeding. Sotalol is distributed into breast milk. Milk to serum ratios have been reported[1] to range from 2.43 to 5.64. It was calculated that a breast-fed infant may receive 20 to 23% of a maternal dose.

1. Hackett LP, *et al.* Excretion of sotalol in breast milk. *Br J Clin Pharmacol* 1990; **29**: 277–8.

Pregnancy. The pharmacokinetics of sotalol in 6 healthy pregnant subjects have been reported.[1] The systemic clearance of sotalol following an intravenous dose was significantly higher during pregnancy than in the postnatal period, and the mean elimination half-life shorter (6.6 versus 9.3 hours) although the latter difference was not significant. Clearance following an oral dose was also higher during pregnancy than afterwards, but half-lives (10.9 versus 10.3 hours) and mean bioavailability were similar. The changes were probably due to alterations in renal function in the antenatal period.

1. O'Hare MF, *et al.* Pharmacokinetics of sotalol during pregnancy. *Eur J Clin Pharmacol* 1983; **24**: 521–4.

Stereo-isomers. In a pharmacokinetic study, 6 subjects were given *d*-sotalol (dexsotalol) in doses of 0.25 to 2 mg per kg body-weight by intravenous infusion and a single dose of 100 mg by mouth.[1] Results suggest that it has a linear pharmacokinetic profile over the doses studied. The oral absorption of *d*-sotalol was almost complete; peak concentrations were reached between 3 and 4 hours after oral administration. Unchanged *d*-sotalol was mainly excreted in the urine; an average of 75% of an intravenous dose was excreted in the urine within 48 hours. The elimination half-life averaged 7.2 and 7.5 hours following intravenous and oral administration respectively.

See under Action in Uses and Administration, below for further information on the stereo-isomers of sotalol.

1. Poirier JM, *et al.* The pharmacokinetics of d-sotalol and d,l-sotalol in healthy volunteers. *Eur J Clin Pharmacol* 1990; **38**: 579–82.

Uses and Administration

Sotalol is a non-cardioselective beta blocker (p.844). It is reported to lack both intrinsic sympathomimetic and membrane-stabilising properties. In addition to the class II antiarrhythmic activity of beta blockers, sotalol lengthens the duration of the action potential resulting in class III antiarrhythmic activity. For a classification and explanation of antiarrhythmic activity, see p.787.

Sotalol is used in the management of ventricular and supraventricular **arrhythmias** (p.794). It was also formerly used in the management of angina pectoris, hypertension, and myocardial infarction but, because of its proarrhythmic effect, it is no longer recommended for these indications. Its use in arrhythmias is restricted to severe disturbances. It should not be used in patients with asymptomatic ventricular arrhythmias.

Sotalol is usually given orally as the hydrochloride. Initiation of treatment should be in hospital with suitable monitoring facilities. The QT interval is monitored before the start of treatment and whenever the dosage is adjusted (see Precautions above). Plasma-electrolyte concentrations and renal function should also be monitored. The dosage is individualised according to the response of the patient. Doses are increased gradually allowing two or three days between dosing increments. The initial dose of sotalol hydrochloride is 80 mg daily by mouth given as a single dose or in two divided doses. Most patients respond to doses of 160 to 320 mg daily (usually given in two divided doses). Some patients may require doses as high as 640 mg daily.

Sotalol may be given intravenously as the hydrochloride to control acute arrhythmias, to substitute for oral therapy, and for programmed electrical stimulation. To control acute arrhythmias, a dose of 20 to 120 mg (0.5 to 1.5 mg per kg body-weight) is given intravenously over 10 minutes. This dose may be repeated every six hours if necessary. To substitute for oral therapy an intravenous infusion of 0.2 to 0.5 mg per kg per hour may be used. The total daily dose should not exceed 640 mg. For programmed electrical stimulation (to test antiarrhythmic efficacy) an initial dose of 1.5 mg per kg of sotalol hydrochloride is given over 10 to 20 minutes, followed by an intravenous infusion of 0.2 to 0.5 mg per kg per hour.

The dose should be reduced in patients with renal impairment. The following dosage reductions may be used for both the oral and intravenous routes: half the dose in patients whose creatinine clearance is between 30 and 60 mL per minute, and quarter the dose in patients whose creatinine clearance is between 10 and 30 mL per minute. Alternatively, when sotalol is given orally the dosage interval may be increased. At least five or six doses should be given before incremental dosage adjustments are made.

The use of sotalol as described above is as the racemic mixture; *d*-sotalol (dexsotalol; (+)-sotalol) has been investigated as an antiarrhythmic (see under Action, below).

◊ General references.
1. Fitton A, Sorkin EM. Sotalol: an updated review of its pharmacological properties and therapeutic use in cardiac arrhythmias. *Drugs* 1993; **46:** 678–719.
2. Nappi JM, McCollam PL. Sotalol: a breakthrough antiarrhythmic? *Ann Pharmacother* 1993; **27:** 1359–68.
3. Zanetti LAF. Sotalol: a new class III antiarrhythmic agent. *Clin Pharm* 1993; **12:** 883–91.
4. Hohnloser SH, Woosley RL. Sotalol. *N Engl J Med* 1994; **331:** 31–8.

Action. Sotalol is used as the racemic mixture of the two stereoisomers, *d*-sotalol (dexsotalol; (+)-sotalol) and *l*-sotalol ((−)-sotalol). A comparison of the effects of *d*-sotalol and racemic sotalol in 6 healthy subjects[1] showed that the beta-blocking activity resided almost entirely in the *l*-isomer, while the effects on the QT interval, which are consistent with type III antiarrhythmic activity, appear to be due to both isomers. A study in 8 healthy subjects also showed a lack of beta blockade by *d*-sotalol.[2] This would suggest that the electrophysiological effects of sotalol are unrelated to its beta-blocking properties. *d*-Sotalol has been investigated as an antiarrhythmic.[3] However, a preliminary placebo-controlled study in patients with myocardial infarction at high risk of arrhythmia due to impaired left ventricular function was terminated early when increased mortality was seen in the treatment group.[4,5]

1. Johnston GD, *et al.* A comparison of the cardiovascular effects of (+)-sotalol and (±)-sotalol following intravenous administration in normal volunteers. *Br J Clin Pharmacol* 1985; **20:** 507–10.

---

2. Yasuda SU, *et al.* d-Sotalol reduces heart rate in vivo through a β-adrenergic receptor-independent mechanism. *Clin Pharmacol Ther* 1993; **53:** 436–42.
3. Advani SV, Singh BN. Pharmacodynamic, pharmacokinetic and antiarrhythmic properties of d-sotalol, the dextro-isomer of sotalol. *Drugs* 1995; **49:** 664–79.
4. Choo V. SWORD slashed. *Lancet* 1994; **344:** 1358.
5. Waldo AL, *et al.* Effect of d-sotalol on mortality in patients with left ventricular dysfunction after recent and remote myocardial infarction. *Lancet* 1996; **348:** 7–12. Correction. *ibid.;* 416.

Administration in renal impairment. Sotalol is excreted mainly by the renal route and elimination is therefore slower in patients with reduced renal function. Reduced doses or increased dosage intervals should be used (see above). In a study of 10 hypertensive patients with varying degrees of renal impairment,[1] the apparent first-order elimination rate constant and plasma clearance of sotalol correlated with glomerular filtration rate. Another study[2] compared kinetics in patients with normal renal function, renal insufficiency, and renal failure. Elimination half-lives of 8.1 and 24.2 hours were reported in patients with creatinine clearance values above 39 mL per minute and clearance values between 8 and 38 mL per minute, respectively. It was suggested that an increase in the dosage interval to 48 or 72 hours may be necessary to compensate for longer half-lives. Caution is required when sotalol is administered to patients on dialysis; a half-life of 33.9 hours was reported in patients with renal failure but this fell to 5.8 hours during dialysis which removed approximately 43% of sotalol.

1. Berglund G, *et al.* Pharmacokinetics of sotalol after chronic administration to patients with renal insufficiency. *Eur J Clin Pharmacol* 1980; **18:** 321–6.
2. Blair AD, *et al.* Sotalol kinetics in renal insufficiency. *Clin Pharmacol Ther* 1981; **29:** 457–63.

Preparations

BP 2001: Sotalol Injection; Sotalol Tablets.

Proprietary Preparations (details are given in Part 3)
Aust.: Darob; Sotacor; Sotamed; Sotastad; **Austral.:** Cardol; Sotab; Sotacor; Sotahexal; **Belg.:** Sotalex; **Braz.:** Sotacor; **Canad.:** Rylosol; Sotacor; Sotamol; **Denm.:** Dutacor; Sotabet; Sotacor; **Fin.:** Sotacor; Sotalin; **Fr.:** Sotalex; **Ger.:** CorSotalol; Darob; Favorex; Gilucor; Rentibloc; Sota; Sota Lich; Sota-Gry; Sota-Puren; Sota-saar; Sotabeta; Sotagamma; Sotahexal; Sotalex; Sotaryt; Sotastad; Tachytalol; **Hong Kong:** Sotacor; **Irl.:** Sotacor; **Israel:** Sotacor; **Ital.:** Betades; Rytmobeta; Sotalex; **Jpn:** Sotacor; **Mex.:** Sotaper; **Neth.:** Sotacor; **Norw.:** Sotacor; **NZ:** Sotacor; **Port.:** Darob; **S.Afr.:** Sotacor; Sotahexal; **Singapore:** Sotacor; **Spain:** Sotapor; **Swed.:** Darob†; Sotacor; **Switz.:** Sotalex; **Thai.:** Sotacor; **UK:** Beta-Cardone; Sotacor; **USA:** Betapace.

Multi-ingredient: **S.Afr.:** Sotazide†; **Swed.:** Sotacor/ASA†.

Spirapril Hydrochloride (2542-j)

Spirapril Hydrochloride (BANM, USAN, rINNM).

Sch-33844. (S)-7-{N-[(S)-1-Ethoxycarbonyl-3-phenylpropyl]-L-alanyl}-1,4-dithia-7-azaspiro[4.4]nonane-8-carboxylic acid hydrochloride.

$C_{22}H_{30}N_2O_5S_2,HCl = 503.1$.
CAS — 83647-97-6 (spirapril); 94841-17-5 (spirapril hydrochloride).

Profile
Spirapril is an ACE inhibitor (p.820) that is used in the management of hypertension (p.802). It owes its activity to the diacid spiraprilat, to which it is converted after oral administration. It is given by mouth as the hydrochloride in a usual maintenance dose of 6 mg once daily.

◊ References.
1. Noble S, Sorkin EM. Spirapril: a preliminary review of its pharmacology and therapeutic efficacy in the treatment of hypertension. *Drugs* 1995; **49:** 750–66.
2. Widimský J, *et al.* Czech and Slovak spirapril intervention study (CASSIS): a randomized, placebo and active-controlled, double-blind multicentre trial in patients with congestive heart failure. *Eur J Clin Pharmacol* 1995; **49:** 95–102.

Preparations

Proprietary Preparations (details are given in Part 3)
Aust.: Quadropril; Sandopril†; **Ger.:** Quadropril; **Ital.:** Renormax; Setrilan; **Spain:** Renormax; Renpress; **Switz.:** Cardiopril.

Spironolactone (2355-e)

Spironolactone (BAN, rINN).

Espironolactona; SC-9420; Spiralactone; Spironolactonum. 7α-Acetylthio-3-oxo-17α-pregn-4-ene-21,17β-carbolactone; (7α,17α)-7-(Acetylthio)-17-hydroxy-3-oxo-pregn-4-ene-21-carboxylic acid γ-lactone.
$C_{24}H_{32}O_4S = 416.6$.
CAS — 52-01-7.
ATC — C03DA01.

NOTE. Compounded preparations of spironolactone may be represented by the following names:

• Co-flumactone (*BAN*)—spironolactone and hydroflumethiazide in equal parts (w/w)

• Co-spironozide (*USP 25*)—spironolactone and hydrochlorothiazide.

Pharmacopoeias. In *Chin.*, *Eur.* (see p.vi), *Int.*, *Jpn*, *Pol.*, and *US*.

Pharmacopoeial description

Ph. Eur.: A white or yellowish-white powder. Practically insoluble in water; soluble in alcohol; slightly soluble in ether. It exhibits polymorphism. Protect from light.

USP 25: A light cream-coloured to light tan, crystalline powder with a faint to mild mercaptan-like odour. Practically insoluble in water; soluble in alcohol and in ethyl acetate; freely soluble in chloroform and in benzene; slightly soluble in methyl alcohol and in fixed oils.

Stability. There was no appreciable loss of spironolactone from extemporaneously prepared suspensions of spironolactone, 2.5, 5 and 10 mg per mL, in a cherry syrup after storage for 2 weeks at 5° or 30° or at ambient room temperature under intense fluorescent light.[1] Degradation was less than 5% for samples stored for 4 weeks, but was more noticeable in suspensions with a higher initial concentration. There were no changes in colour or odour. Bacterial and fungal counts were well within acceptable limits after 4 weeks at 30°.

1. Mathur LK, Wickman A. Stability of extemporaneously compounded spironolactone suspensions. *Am J Hosp Pharm* 1989; **46:** 2040–2.

Adverse Effects

Spironolactone may give rise to headache and drowsiness, and gastrointestinal disturbances, including cramp and diarrhoea. Ataxia, mental confusion, and skin rashes have been reported as side-effects. Gynaecomastia is not uncommon and in rare cases breast enlargement may persist. Other endocrine disorders include hirsutism, deepening of the voice, menstrual irregularities, and impotence. Transient increases in blood-urea-nitrogen concentrations may occur and mild acidosis has been reported. Spironolactone has been demonstrated to cause tumours in *rats*.

Spironolactone may cause hyponatraemia and hyperkalaemia.

◊ A survey indicated that of 788 patients who received spironolactone 164 developed side-effects.[1] These included hyperkalaemia in 8.6%, dehydration in 3.4%, hyponatraemia in 2.4%, gastrointestinal disorders in 2.3%, neurological disorders in 2%, rash, and gynaecomastia. Hyperkalaemia was associated with renal insufficiency and the administration of potassium supplements: only 2.8% of nonazotaemic patients not receiving potassium chloride developed hyperkalaemia, while 42.1% of those with marked azotaemia and treated with potassium chloride became hyperkalaemic.

In a study of 54 patients (53 female, 1 male) taking spironolactone 200 mg daily for hirsutism or acne adverse effects were reported in 91%.[2] Menstrual disturbances occurred in 72% of patients, breast tenderness in 39%, dry skin in 39%, and breast enlargement in 24%. Other adverse effects included nausea and vomiting, dizziness, headache, drowsiness, and skin rashes. Two patients developed a chloasma-like pigmentation of the face. The gynaecological effects were reduced in patients taking oral contraceptives.

1. Greenblatt DG, Koch-Weser J. Adverse reactions to spironolactone: a report from the Boston Collaborative Drug Surveillance Program. *JAMA* 1973; **225:** 40–3.
2. Hughes BR, Cunliffe WJ. Tolerance of spironolactone. *Br J Dermatol* 1988; **118:** 687–91.

Carcinogenicity. Breast cancer was reported in 5 patients taking spironolactone and hydrochlorothiazide for prolonged periods[1] although it has been suggested[2] that the association with spironolactone therapy was unlikely to be causal.

Although the *rat* may not be an appropriate model for determining long-term safety in man,[3,4] evidence of carcinogenicity in this species prompted the UK Committee on Safety of Medicines to limit the product licences of spironolactone-containing products to exclude use in essential hypertension or idiopathic oedema.[5]

1. Loube SD, Quirk RA. Breast cancer associated with administration of spironolactone. *Lancet* 1975; **i:** 1428–9.
2. Jick H, Armstrong B. Breast cancer and spironolactone. *Lancet* 1975; **ii:** 368–9.
3. Lumb G, *et al.* Effects in animals of chronic administration of spironolactone—a review. *J Environ Pathol Toxicol* 1978; **i:** 641–60.
4. Wagner BM. Long-term toxicology studies of spironolactone in animals and comparison with potassium canrenoate. *J Drug Dev* 1987; **1** (suppl 2): 7–11.
5. Committee on Safety of Medicines. Spironolactone. *Current Problems* 1988; 21.

Effects on the blood. Agranulocytosis has been reported[1,2] in association with the administration of spironolactone.

1. Stricker BHC, Oei TT. Agranulocytosis caused by spironolactone. *BMJ* 1984; **289:** 731.
2. Whitling AM, *et al.* Spironolactone-induced agranulocytosis. *Ann Pharmacother* 1997; **31:** 582–5.

Effects on electrolyte balance. CALCIUM. A report[1] suggested that spironolactone may have a calcium-sparing effect, in addition to its well known potassium-sparing properties.

1. Puig JG, *et al.* Hydrochlorothiazide versus spironolactone: long-term metabolic modifications in patients with essential hypertension. *J Clin Pharmacol* 1991; **31:** 455–61.

The symbol † denotes a preparation no longer actively marketed

POTASSIUM. There have been a number of reports[1-3] of severe hyperkalaemia in patients taking spironolactone, including those with impaired renal function and those with a high potassium intake from either dietary sources or as potassium supplements. In the Boston Collaborative Drug Surveillance Program[4] hyperkalaemia was reported in 42.1% of patients with uraemia taking spironolactone and receiving potassium supplements compared with 2.8% of those without uraemia and not receiving potassium supplements. Two deaths were attributed to hyperkalaemia in patients taking spironolactone and potassium chloride. Potassium supplements should be avoided in patients receiving spironolactone, and plasma-potassium concentrations should be carefully monitored in those with impaired renal function.

1. Pongpaew C, *et al.* Hyperkalemic cardiac arrhythmia secondary to spironolactone. *Chest* 1973; **63**: 1023–5.
2. Udezue EO, Harrold BP. Hyperkalaemic paralysis due to spironolactone. *Postgrad Med J* 1980; **56**: 254–5.
3. O'Reilly PH, *et al.* Life-threatening hyperkalaemia after bladder decompression for high pressure chronic retention. *Lancet* 1987; **ii**: 859.
4. Greenblatt DJ, Koch-Weser J. Adverse reactions to spironolactone: a report from the Boston Collaborative Drug Surveillance Program. *JAMA* 1973; **225**: 40–3.

Effects on endocrine function. Spironolactone has been associated with a number of disturbances of endocrine function. The most prominent in men is gynaecomastia which appears to be related to both dose and duration of treatment. Incidences of 62%[1] and 100%[2] have been reported. Gynaecomastia has also been accompanied by impotence.[3,4] The effects are generally reversible on discontinuing treatment. Reversal of male-pattern baldness has also been reported.[5]

In women symptoms include breast enlargement and tenderness.[6] The incidence of menstrual abnormalities may be high: unspecified disturbances have been reported in 33 of 53 women,[6] secondary amenorrhoea in 6 of 9,[7] and secondary and primary amenorrhoea in 1 and 2 patients, respectively.[8] The incidence of gynaecological disturbances has been found to be lower in women taking oral contraceptives than in those using other methods of contraception.[6]

The mechanism of the effects of spironolactone on the endocrine system is unclear. Some workers[9] suggested that although spironolactone affects testosterone synthesis, the more likely explanation was its anti-androgenic action, and reduction in 17-hydroxylase activity. Others[10] demonstrated an alteration in the testosterone/oestrogen ratio due to an increase in testosterone clearance and increased peripheral conversion to estradiol. In addition, spironolactone is reported to inhibit binding of dihydrotestosterone to receptors.

1. Huffman DH, *et al.* Gynecomastia induced in normal males by spironolactone. *Clin Pharmacol Ther* 1978; **24**: 465–73.
2. Bellati G, Idéo G. Gynaecomastia after spironolactone and potassium canrenoate. *Lancet* 1986; **i**: 626.
3. Greenblatt DJ, Koch-Weser J. Gynecomastia and impotence complications of spironolactone therapy. *JAMA* 1973; **223**: 82.
4. Greenlaw C. Spironolactone induced gynecomastia: a case report. *Drug Intell Clin Pharm* 1977; **11**: 70–3.
5. Thomas PS. Hair: wanted and unwanted. *BMJ* 1986; **293**: 698.
6. Hughes BR, Cunliffe WJ. Tolerance of spironolactone. *Br J Dermatol* 1988; **118**: 687–91.
7. Levitt JI. Spironolactone therapy and amenorrhea. *JAMA* 1970; **211**: 2014–15.
8. Potter C, *et al.* Primary and secondary amenorrhea associated with spironolactone therapy in chronic liver disease. *J Pediatr* 1992; **121**: 141–3.
9. Loriaux DL, *et al.* Spironolactone and endocrine dysfunction. *Ann Intern Med* 1976; **85**: 630–6.
10. Rose LI, *et al.* Pathophysiology of spironolactone-induced gynecomastia. *Ann Intern Med* 1977; **87**: 398–403.

Effects on lipid metabolism. Unlike thiazide diuretics, spironolactone appeared not to increase serum-cholesterol concentrations in a study of 23 patients.[1]

1. Ames RP, Peacock PB. Serum cholesterol during treatment of hypertension with diuretic drugs. *Arch Intern Med* 1984; **144**: 710–14.

Effects on the liver. Hepatotoxicity characterised by cholestatic lesions has been reported in a patient receiving spironolactone.[1] Only one other published case of spironolactone-associated hepatic toxicity was known to the authors.

1. Renkes P, *et al.* Spironolactone and hepatic toxicity. *JAMA* 1995; **273**: 376–7.

Effects on the skin. A report of lichen-planus-like skin eruptions which developed in a 62-year-old woman who was taking digoxin, propranolol, diazepam, spironolactone, and iron tablets.[1] Flares of the lichen-planus-like eruption seemed to be associated with administration of spironolactone and there was evidence of resolution when spironolactone was withdrawn. Cutaneous vasculitis was associated with spironolactone treatment on 3 occasions in an 80-year-old man.[2] A chloasma-like pigmentation of the face was reported in 2 patients receiving spironolactone for hirsutism or acne.[3]

1. Downham TF. Spironolactone-induced lichen planus. *JAMA* 1978; **240**: 1138.
2. Phillips GWL, Williams AJ. Spironolactone induced vasculitis. *BMJ* 1984; **288**: 368.
3. Hughes BR, Cunliffe WJ. Tolerance of spironolactone. *Br J Dermatol* 1988; **118**: 687–91.

Hypersensitivity. Eosinophilia and a rash developed in 2 patients with alcoholic cirrhosis while taking spironolactone.[1]

1. Wathen CG, *et al.* Eosinophilia associated with spironolactone. *Lancet* 1986; **i**: 919–20.

Precautions

Spironolactone should not be used in patients with hyperkalaemia or severe renal impairment. It should be used with care in patients who are at increased risk of developing hyperkalaemia; such patients include the elderly, those with diabetes mellitus, and those with some degree of renal or hepatic impairment. It should also be given with care to patients likely to develop acidosis. Serum electrolytes and blood-urea-nitrogen should be measured periodically. Spironolactone is not suitable for breast-feeding mothers.

Diabetes mellitus. Severe hyperkalaemia in a type 1 diabetic woman with hyporeninaemic hypoaldosteronism given spironolactone.[1]

1. Large DM, *et al.* Hyperkalaemia in diabetes mellitus—potential hazards of coexisting hyporeninaemic hypoaldosteronism. *Postgrad Med J* 1984; **60**: 370–3.

Interference with laboratory estimations. Spironolactone and canrenone can interfere with some assays for plasma-digoxin concentrations.[1-3] However, spironolactone may also produce actual changes in digoxin concentrations (see p.872) and results of assays should be interpreted with caution.

1. Yosselson-Superstine S. Drug interferences with plasma assays in therapeutic drug monitoring. *Clin Pharmacokinet* 1984; **9**: 67–87.
2. Foukaridis GN. Influence of spironolactone and its metabolite canrenone on serum digoxin assays. *Ther Drug Monit* 1990; **12**: 82–4.
3. Steimer W, *et al.* Intoxication due to negative canrenone interference in digoxin drug monitoring. *Lancet* 1999; **354**: 1176–7.

Porphyria. Spironolactone has been associated with acute attacks of porphyria and is considered unsafe in porphyric patients.

Interactions

There is an increased risk of hyperkalaemia if spironolactone is given concomitantly with potassium supplements or with other potassium-sparing diuretics. Hyperkalaemia may also occur in patients receiving ACE inhibitors, angiotensin II receptor antagonists, NSAIDs, ciclosporin, or trilostane concomitantly. In patients receiving spironolactone with NSAIDs or ciclosporin the risk of nephrotoxicity may also be increased. Diuretics may reduce the excretion of lithium and increase the risk of lithium toxicity. Hyponatraemia may occur in patients receiving a combination of potassium-sparing diuretic with a thiazide; this risk may be increased in patients receiving chlorpropamide. Spironolactone may reduce the ulcer-healing properties of carbenoxolone. As with other diuretics, spironolactone may enhance the effects of other antihypertensive drugs and may diminish vascular reponses to noradrenaline [norepinephrine].

ACE inhibitors. Hyperkalaemia causing complete heart block was associated with concomitant administration of spironolactone and *captopril*[1] in a 72-year-old woman. A similar fatal reaction has been reported in a patient taking spironolactone and *enalapril*.[2] Hyperkalaemia in a 55-year-old patient taking spironolactone and enalapril[3] persisted for over 48 hours despite discontinuation of the drugs and treatment with ion-exchange resin and intravenous glucose and insulin.

1. Lo TCN, Cryer RJ. Complete heart block induced by hyperkalaemia associated with treatment with a combination of captopril and spironolactone. *BMJ* 1986; **292**: 1672.
2. Lakhani M. Complete heart block induced by hyperkalaemia associated with treatment with a combination of captopril and spironolactone. *BMJ* 1986; **293**: 271.
3. Morton AR, Crook SA. Hyperkalaemia and spironolactone. *Lancet* 1987; **ii**: 1525.

Aspirin. Administration of aspirin to healthy subjects taking spironolactone has been shown to produce substantial reductions in sodium excretion[1] and to reduce the excretion of spironolactone's active metabolite, canrenone.[2] However, administration of aspirin in therapeutic amounts to hypertensive patients[3] did not alter the effect of spironolactone on blood pressure, serum electrolytes, blood urea nitrogen, or plasma-renin activity.

1. Tweeddale MG, Ogilvie RI. Antagonism of spironolactone-induced natriuresis by aspirin in man. *N Engl J Med* 1973; **289**: 198–200.
2. Ramsay LE, *et al.* Influence of acetylsalicylic acid on the renal handling of a spironolactone metabolite in healthy subjects. *Eur J Clin Pharmacol* 1976; **10**: 43–8.
3. Hollifield JW. Failure of aspirin to antagonize the antihypertensive effect of spironolactone in low-renin hypertension. *South Med J* 1976; **69**: 1034–6.

Cardiac glycosides. For discussions of the effects of spironolactone on *digoxin* and *digitoxin*, see p.872 and p.869, respectively. See also Interference with Laboratory Estimations, under Precautions, above.

Mitotane. For a report of the inhibition of the action of mitotane by concomitant administration of spironolactone, see p.559.

Warfarin. For reference to the interaction between warfarin and spironolactone, see p.996.

Pharmacokinetics

Spironolactone is fairly rapidly absorbed from the gastrointestinal tract, the extent of absorption depending on particle size and formulation. Modern formulations are reported to provide a bioavailability of about 90%. It is about 90% bound to plasma proteins.

Spironolactone is metabolised extensively to a number of metabolites including canrenone and the sulfur-containing 7α-thiomethylspirolactone, both of which are pharmacologically active. The major metabolite may be 7α-thiomethylspirolactone, although it is uncertain to what extent the actions of spironolactone are dependent on the parent compound or its metabolites.

Spironolactone is excreted mainly in the urine and also in the faeces, in the form of metabolites. Spironolactone or its metabolites may cross the placental barrier, and canrenone is distributed into breast milk.

◊ References.
1. Overdiek HWPM, Merkus FWHM. The metabolism and biopharmaceutics of spironolactone in man. *Rev Drug Metab Drug Interact* 1987; **5**: 273–302.
2. Gardiner P, *et al.* Spironolactone metabolism: steady-state serum levels of the sulfur-containing metabolites. *J Clin Pharmacol* 1989; **29**: 342–7.
3. Sungaila I, *et al.* Spironolactone pharmacokinetics and pharmacodynamics in patients with cirrhotic ascites. *Gastroenterology* 1992; **102**: 1680–5.

Uses and Administration

Spironolactone, a steroid with a structure resembling that of the natural adrenocortical hormone, aldosterone, acts on the distal portion of the renal tubule as a competitive antagonist of aldosterone. It acts as a potassium-sparing diuretic, increasing sodium and water excretion and reducing potassium excretion.

Spironolactone is reported to have a relatively slow onset of action, requiring 2 or 3 days for maximum effect, and a similarly slow diminishment of action over 2 or 3 days on discontinuation.

Spironolactone is used in the treatment of refractory oedema associated with heart failure (below), cirrhosis of the liver (with or without ascites, p.793), or the nephrotic syndrome, and in ascites associated with malignancy. It is frequently given with the thiazides, frusemide [furosemide], or similar diuretics, where it adds to their natriuretic but diminishes their kaliuretic effects, hence conserving potassium in those at risk from hypokalaemia. Diuretic-induced hypokalaemia and its management, including the role of potassium-sparing diuretics, is discussed under Effects on the Electrolyte Balance in the Adverse Effects of Hydrochlorothiazide, p.908. It has been used in the treatment of essential hypertension (in lower doses than for oedema), but in the UK is no longer recommended for use in either essential hypertension or idiopathic oedema; doubts have been expressed over its safety during long-term administration.

Spironolactone is also used in the diagnosis and treatment of primary hyperaldosteronism (below).

Other conditions in which spironolactone has been tried on the basis of its anti-androgenic properties include hirsutism, particularly in the polycystic ovary syndrome.

In the treatment of **oedema**, spironolactone is usually given in an initial dose of 100 mg daily by mouth, subsequently adjusted as necessary; some patients may require doses of up to 400 mg daily. In hepatic cirrhosis with ascites and oedema, patients with a urinary sodium/potassium ratio greater than 1 may be given an initial dose of spironolactone 100 mg daily while patients with a ratio of less than 1 may be given initial doses of 200 to 400 mg daily.

Spironolactone is given in doses of 400 mg daily in the presumptive diagnosis of primary **hyperaldosteronism**; in doses of 100 to 400 mg daily for the pre-operative management of hyperaldosteronism; and in the lowest effective dosage for long-term maintenance therapy in the absence of surgery.

An initial dose of spironolactone for children is 1.5 to 3 mg per kg body-weight daily, in divided doses.

Potassium supplements should not be given with spironolactone.

◊ Reviews.
1. Ochs HR, *et al.* Spironolactone. *Am Heart J* 1978; **96:** 389–400.
2. Skluth HA, Gums JG. Spironolactone: a re-examination. *DICP Ann Pharmacother* 1990; **24:** 52–9.

Acne. Spironolactone has been used for its anti-androgenic properties in some cases of acne (p.1103) where standard therapy is unsuccessful. Beneficial responses to oral therapy have been reported in patients with acne from both open[1] and placebo-controlled[2,3] studies. Topical application has been tried[4,5] but response has been variable. It is possible that the vehicle may affect the response. In women, spironolactone may be useful when treatment with an oestrogen is contra-indicated.
1. Burke BM, Cunliffe WJ. Oral spironolactone therapy for female patients with acne, hirsutism or androgenic alopecia. *Br J Dermatol* 1985; **112:** 124–5.
2. Goodfellow A, *et al.* Oral spironolactone improves acne vulgaris and reduces sebum excretion. *Br J Dermatol* 1984; **111:** 209–14.
3. Muhlemann MF, *et al.* Oral spironolactone: an effective treatment for acne vulgaris in women. *Br J Dermatol* 1986; **115:** 227–32.
4. Messina M, *et al.* A new therapeutic approach to acne: an antiandrogen percutaneous treatment with spironolactone. *Curr Ther Res* 1983; **34:** 319–24.
5. Walton S, *et al.* Lack of effect of topical spironolactone on sebum excretion. *Br J Dermatol* 1986; **114:** 261–4.

Bartter's syndrome. Spironolactone may be used to reduce potassium wasting in patients with Bartter's syndrome (p.1183).

Bronchopulmonary dysplasia. Bronchopulmonary dysplasia (p.1048) is a major cause of chronic lung disease in infants. Treatment often involves the use of corticosteroids. Additional supportive therapy has included the use of diuretics such as frusemide [furosemide] (p.895); results with hydrochlorothiazide or spironolactone have been more ambiguous (p.910).

Heart failure. Drug therapy of heart failure (p.798) is based on the use of diuretics, ACE inhibitors, cardiac glycosides, beta blockers, and vasodilators. Spironolactone has been used as a diuretic for refractory oedema, but it may also have an additional role as an aldosterone antagonist. Although the precise neurohormonal mechanisms leading to the development of heart failure are still not clear, there is evidence that raised levels of aldosterone may contribute to the pathophysiology.[1] ACE inhibitor therapy suppresses aldosterone production but this effect is not complete and spironolactone has therefore been studied in combination with ACE inhibitors. In patients with severe heart failure, addition of spironolactone in a dose of 25 to 50 mg daily to therapy with ACE inhibitors and loop diuretics reduced the risk of death or hospitalisation,[2] and the use of spironolactone should therefore be considered in such patients.[3,4] However, concomitant use of spironolactone with ACE inhibitors may lead to hyperkalaemia and careful monitoring of potassium concentrations is required.[5]
1. Struthers AD. Why does spironolactone improve mortality over and above an ACE inhibitor in chronic heart failure? *Br J Clin Pharmacol* 1999; **47:** 479–82.
2. Pitt B, *et al.* The effect of spironolactone on morbidity and mortality in patients with severe heart failure. *N Engl J Med* 1999; **341:** 709–17.
3. Packer M, Cohn JN, eds. Consensus recommendations for the management of chronic heart failure. *Am J Cardiol* 1999; **83** (suppl 2A): 1A–38A.
4. Scottish Intercollegiate Guidelines Network. *Diagnosis and treatment of heart failure due to left ventricular systolic dysfunction.* Edinburgh: SIGN Secretariat, 1999.
5. Georges B, *et al.* Spironolactone and congestive heart-failure. *Lancet* 2000; **355:** 1369–70.

High-altitude disorders. Acetazolamide is generally the drug of choice for prophylaxis of high-altitude disorders (p.800). Anecdotal reports[1-4] and a small-scale double-blind study[5] suggested that spironolactone could be useful in preventing acute mountain sickness, although a deterioration in pulmonary function despite spironolactone prophylaxis has been noted in 1 patient.[6]
1. Currie TT, *et al.* Spironolactone and acute mountain sickness. *Med J Aust* 1976; **2:** 168–70.
2. Snell JA, Cordner EP. Spironolactone and acute mountain sickness. *Med J Aust* 1977; **1:** 828.
3. Turnbull G. Spironolactone prophylaxis in mountain sickness. *BMJ* 1980; **280:** 1453.
4. Rutter LD. Spironolactone prophylaxis in mountain sickness. *BMJ* 1980; **281:** 618.
5. Brown GV, *et al.* Spironolactone in acute mountain sickness. *Lancet* 1977; **i:** 855.
6. Meyers DH. Spironolactone prophylaxis of mountain sickness. *BMJ* 1980; **281:** 1569.

Hirsutism. Hirsutism (p.1468) is frequently treated with antiandrogenic drug therapy, usually cyproterone or spironolactone. Spironolactone in doses of 50 to 200 mg daily has produced both subjective and objective improvement in hirsutism in patients with idiopathic hirsutism or polycystic ovary syn-

The symbol † denotes a preparation no longer actively marketed

drome.[1-4] It is preferably used in combination with oral contraceptives,[5,6] to improve efficacy and menstrual irregularity and to avoid the risk of feminisation to a male fetus. A double-blind placebo-controlled study[7] failed to demonstrate any benefit with spironolactone 100 mg daily in idiopathic hirsutism, whereas another randomised study (not placebo-controlled) found spironolactone 100 mg daily and cyproterone 100 mg daily to be equally effective.[8] Most studies have involved premenopausal women and it has been suggested[4,9] that spironolactone would be useful in women in whom cyproterone is contra-indicated or not tolerated. A meta-analysis of the use of spironolactone in hirsutism was unable to determine its effectiveness.[10]
1. Cumming DC, *et al.* Treatment of hirsutism with spironolactone. *JAMA* 1982; **247:** 1295–8.
2. Burke BM, Cunliffe WJ. Oral spironolactone therapy for female patients with acne, hirsutism or androgenic alopecia. *Br J Dermatol* 1985; **112:** 124–5.
3. Evans DJ, Burke CW. Spironolactone in the treatment of idiopathic hirsutism and the polycystic ovary syndrome. *J R Soc Med* 1986; **79:** 451–3.
4. Barth JH, *et al.* Spironolactone therapy for hirsute women. *Br J Dermatol* 1988; **119** (suppl 33): 17.
5. Chapman MG, *et al.* Spironolactone in combination with an oral contraceptive: an alternative treatment for hirsutism. *Br J Obstet Gynaecol* 1985; **92:** 983–5.
6. Rittmaster RS. Hirsutism. *Lancet* 1997; **349:** 191–5.
7. McLellan AR, *et al.* Lack of effect of spironolactone on hair shaft diameter in hirsute females. *Postgrad Med J* 1989; **65:** 459–62.
8. O'Brien RC, *et al.* Comparison of sequential cyproterone acetate/estrogen versus spironolactone/oral contraceptive in the treatment of hirsutism. *J Clin Endocrinol Metab* 1991; **72:** 1008–13.
9. West TET. Does spironolactone have a place in treating facial hirsutism in women? *BMJ* 1988; **296:** 1456.
10. Lee O, *et al.* Spironolactone versus placebo or in combination with steroids for hirsutism and/or acne (updated 28 May 2001). Available in The Cochrane Library; Issue 2. Oxford: Update Software; 2001.

Hyperaldosteronism. Hyperaldosteronism (aldosteronism) is a disorder characterised by mineralocorticoid excess due to high circulating levels of aldosterone. Mineralocorticoid excess due to other mineralocorticoids is rare. Primary hyperaldosteronism is usually caused by an aldosterone-producing adenoma (Conn's syndrome) or primary adrenal hyperplasia. Other causes include aldosterone-producing adrenal carcinoma and glucocorticoid-suppressible hyperaldosteronism.

Secondary hyperaldosteronism is more common and results from conditions in which there is activation of the renin-angiotensin-aldosterone system, including diuretic therapy, and oedematous conditions such as heart failure, hepatic cirrhosis, and nephrotic syndrome. Bartter's syndrome (p.1183) also results in hyperaldosteronism.

Most patients with primary hyperaldosteronism are asymptomatic, although they may present with signs or symptoms of mineralocorticoid excess (p.1039). Diagnosis often follows the incidental discovery of hypokalaemia. Symptomatic hypokalaemia (p.1182) may develop in some patients, particularly those receiving diuretic therapy.

Diagnosis is confirmed by the presence of raised plasma and urinary aldosterone concentrations. However, the concentrations may be affected by serum-potassium concentration, posture, and time of day, and interpretation may be difficult. The plasma aldosterone:renin ratio may also be measured. In primary hyperaldosteronism the aldosterone concentration is raised but renin is suppressed whereas in secondary hyperaldosteronism both are raised. Radiological and nuclear imaging are useful for further differentiating between adenoma and hyperplasia.

Hyperaldosteronism due to an aldosterone-producing adenoma is usually treated surgically. The aldosterone antagonist spironolactone may be given pre-operatively to lower the blood pressure and normalise the serum potassium. In patients who are not suitable for surgery, long-term medical management involves spironolactone, initially in high doses but reduced to the lowest dose for maintenance. If spironolactone is not tolerated, amiloride may be used as an alternative, but high doses are required. Trilostane, an adrenal suppressant, has also been used to inhibit aldosterone synthesis.

In primary adrenal hyperplasia surgery is not usually effective and medical management with spironolactone or amiloride is required. Additional antihypertensive therapy may also be needed. Glucocorticoid-suppressible hyperaldosteronism is a rare autosomal dominant form and may be treated with dexamethasone. However, this may not control the blood pressure and spironolactone or amiloride may be required in addition.

In secondary hyperaldosteronism the underlying condition should be treated, but spironolactone may be of benefit as part of the therapy.

References.
1. Ganguly A. Primary aldosteronism. *N Engl J Med* 1998; **339:** 1828–34.
2. Stewart PM. Mineralocorticoid hypertension. *Lancet* 1999; **353:** 1341–7.

Precocious puberty. Spironolactone (as an anti-androgen) and testolactone were given to boys with familial precocious puberty (p.1277) for periods of up to 18 months. Rates of growth and bone maturation were restored to normal during combination therapy but not with either drug given alone.[1]

However, after further treatment for 2.0 to 4.2 years there was a diminishing response manifested by the recurrence of clinical features of puberty and an increase in the bone maturation rate.[2] Addition of deslorelin appeared to restore the control.
1. Laue L, *et al.* Treatment of familial male precocious puberty with spironolactone and testolactone. *N Engl J Med* 1989; **320:** 496–502.
2. Laue L, *et al.* Treatment of familial male precocious puberty with spironolactone, testolactone, and deslorelin. *J Clin Endocrinol Metab* 1993; **76:** 151–5.

Premenstrual syndrome. Spironolactone has been used for its diuretic and anti-androgenic properties in premenstrual syndrome (p.1475).

Preparations

BP 2001: Spironolactone Tablets;
USP 25: Spironolactone and Hydrochlorothiazide Tablets; Spironolactone Tablets.

Proprietary Preparations (details are given in Part 3)
Aust.: Aldactone; Aldopur; Deverol; Osiren; Spirobene; Spirohexal; Spirox; **Austral.:** Aldactone; Spiractin; **Belg.:** Aldactone; Uractone; **Braz.:** Aldactone; **Canad.:** Aldactone; Novo-Spiroton; **Denm.:** Hexalacton; Spilacnet†; Spirix; Spiron; **Fin.:** Aldactone; Spiresis; Spirix; **Fr.:** Aldactone; Flumach; Practon; Spiroctan; Spironone; **Ger.:** Aldactone; Aldopur†; Aquareduct; duraspiron; Jenaspiron; Osyrol; spiro; Spiro-Tablinen†; Spirono; verospiron; **Hong Kong:** Aldactone; **Irl.:** Aldactone; Melactone†; **Israel:** Aldactone; Aldospirone; Spironol; **Ital.:** Aldactone; Idrolattone†; Spiroderm; Spirolang; Uractone; **Mex.:** Aldactone; Quimolactona; **Neth.:** Aldactone; Norw.: Aldactone; Spirix; Spiropal; **NZ:** Aldactone; Spirotone; **Port.:** Aldactone; Aldonar; Nefrolactona; **S.Afr.:** Aldactone; Spiractin; Tensin; **Singapore:** Aldactone; Spiridon; Uractonum; **Spain:** Aldactone; Swed.: Aldactone; Spirix; Spiroscand; **Switz.:** Aldactone; Spiroctan; Xenalon; **Thai.:** Aldactone; Altone; Berlactone; Spironex; **UK:** Aldactone; Laractone; Spiretic; Spiroctan†; Spirolone†; Spirospare; **USA:** Alatone†; Aldactone.

Multi-ingredient: Aust.: Aldactone Saltucin; Buti-Spirobene; Deverol mit Thiazid; Digi-Aldopur; Furo-Aldopur; Furo-Spirobene; Furolacton; Lasilacton; Sali-Aldopur; Spirono comp; Supracid; Suprenoat; **Belg.:** Aldactazine; Uractazide; **Braz.:** Aldazida; Lasilactona; **Canad.:** Aldactazide; Novo-Spirozine; **Fr.:** Aldactazine; Aldalix; Practazin; Prinactizide; Spiroctazine; **Ger.:** Aldactone Saltucin; duraspiron-comp; Furo-Aldopur; Furorese Comp; Osyrol Lasix; Risicordin; Sali-Aldopur; Spiro comp; Spiro-D; Spironolacton Plus; Spironothiazid; Spirostada comp; **Irl.:** Aldactide; **Ital.:** Aldactazide; Lasitone; Spiridazide; Spirofur; **Mex.:** Lasilacton; **Port.:** Aldactazine; Ondolen; **S.Afr.:** Aldazide; **Spain:** Aldactacine; Aldoleo; Miscidon; Resnedal; Spirometon; **Switz.:** Aldozone; Furosemid comp†; Furospir; Lasilactone; Sali-Spiroctan; Saluretin; Spironothiazid; Synureticum†; **UK:** Aldactide; Lasilactone; Spiro-Co; **USA:** Aldactazide.

Staphylokinase (17142-p)

Profile
Staphylokinase is a thrombolytic under investigation for the treatment of thromboembolic disorders, including acute myocardial infarction.

◊ References.
1. Vanderschueren S, *et al.* Thrombolytic therapy of peripheral arterial occlusion with recombinant staphylokinase. *Circulation* 1995; **92:** 2050–57.
2. Vanderschueren S, *et al.* Randomized coronary patency trial of double-bolus recombinant staphylokinase versus front-loaded alteplase in acute myocardial infarction. *Am Heart J* 1997; **134:** 213–19.

Streptokinase (3746-e)

Streptokinase (BAN, rINN).

Estreptoquinasa; Plasminokinase; Streptokinasum.
CAS — 9002-01-1.
ATC — B01AD01.

Pharmacopoeias. In Eur. (see p.vi).

Pharmacopoeial description

Ph. Eur.: A protein obtained from culture filtrates of certain strains of *Streptococcus haemolyticus* group C. It has the property of combining with human plasminogen to form plasminogen activator and has been purified to contain not less than 600 international units of streptokinase activity per µg of nitrogen. After purification it is usually mixed with a buffer and may be stabilised by the addition of suitable substances such as albumin.

A hygroscopic, white powder or friable solid. Freely soluble in water. A solution in water containing 5000 units per mL has a pH of 6.8 to 7.5. Store in sealed containers and protect from light.

Stability. The incorporation of albumin in commercial preparations of streptokinase has reduced the incidence of flocculation with streptokinase solutions. However, flocculation has occurred with small volumes prepared with sodium chloride 0.9% in sterilised glass containers apparently because of residual acid buffers that remain in empty evacuated containers following sterilisation.[1]
1. Thibault L. Streptokinase flocculation in evacuated glass bottles. *Am J Hosp Pharm* 1985; **42:** 278.

Units

The potency of streptokinase is expressed in international units and preparations are assayed using the second International Standard (1989).

The Christensen unit is the quantity of streptokinase that will lyse a standard blood clot completely in 10 minutes and is equivalent to the international unit.

Adverse Effects

In common with other thrombolytics streptokinase may cause haemorrhage, particularly from puncture sites; severe internal bleeding has occurred and may be difficult to control. Streptokinase is antigenic, and allergic reactions ranging from rashes to rarer, but more serious, anaphylactoid and serum-sickness-like symptoms have occurred. Fever, sometimes high, and associated symptoms such as chills and back or abdominal pain are quite frequent. Nausea and vomiting may occur. There have been a few reports of Guillain-Barré syndrome.

Streptokinase infusion may be associated with hypotension, both direct or as a result of reperfusion; bradycardia and arrhythmias may also occur due to reperfusion. The break-up of existing clots may occasionally produce emboli elsewhere; pulmonary embolism and acute renal failure due to cholesterol embolisation have been reported.

Back pain. Streptokinase infusion has been associated with the development of very severe low back pain, which resolves within a few minutes of stopping the infusion, and may be severe enough to warrant opioid analgesia.[1-3] The back pain may represent a hypersensitivity reaction. Providing that the pain is controlled and that dissecting aortic aneurysm is not suspected, it may still be possible to complete the streptokinase infusion.[4] Alternatively, immediate substitution with a different thrombolytic has been suggested.[5]

There have also been a few reports of low back pain associated with anistreplase infusion.[6,7]

1. Shah M, Taylor RT. Low back pain associated with streptokinase. *BMJ* 1990; **301**: 1219.
2. Dickinson RJ, Rosser A. Low back pain associated with streptokinase. *BMJ* 1991; **302**: 111–12.
3. Porter NJ, Nikoletatos K. Low back pain associated with streptokinase. *BMJ* 1991; **302**: 112.
4. Lear J, *et al.* Low back pain associated with streptokinase. *Lancet* 1992; **340**: 851.
5. Fishwick D, *et al.* Thrombolysis and low back pain. *BMJ* 1995; **310**: 504.
6. Hannaford P, Kay CR. Back pain and thrombolysis. *BMJ* 1992; **304**: 915.
7. Lear J, Rajapakse R. Low back pain associated with anistreplase. *BMJ* 1993; **306**: 896.

Effects on the blood. Although falls in the haemoglobin value of patients receiving thrombolytics are most likely to be due to blood loss from haemorrhage, there has been a report of a patient who had signs of haemolytic anaemia following intravenous infusion of streptokinase.[1] In a subsequent test *in vitro* the patient's serum caused strong agglutination of streptokinase-treated red blood cells, supporting the view that streptokinase was responsible for the haemolysis.

1. Mathiesen O, Grunnet N. Haemolysis after intravenous streptokinase. *Lancet* 1989; **i**: 1016–17.

Effects on the eyes. Acute uveitis[1,2] and iritis,[3,4] associated with transient renal impairment in one patient,[3] have followed treatment of myocardial infarction with intravenous streptokinase. In one case uveitis was associated with serum sickness[2] and in all of them hypersensitivity to streptokinase was suspected.

1. Kinshuck D. Bilateral hypopyon in streptokinase. *BMJ* 1992; **305**: 1332.
2. Proctor BD, Joondeph BC. Bilateral anterior uveitis: a feature of streptokinase-induced serum sickness. *N Engl J Med* 1994; **330**: 576–7.
3. Birnbaum Y, *et al.* Acute iritis and transient renal impairment following thrombolytic therapy for acute myocardial infarction. *Ann Pharmacother* 1993; **27**: 1539–40.
4. Gray MY, Lazarus JH. Iritis after treatment with streptokinase. *BMJ* 1993; **309**: 97.

Effects on the kidneys. Transient proteinuria has been reported following the administration of streptokinase. In some patients proteinuria and impaired renal function have developed about 7 days after thrombolytic therapy and have been associated with a syndrome resembling serum sickness,[1,2] suggesting a delayed hypersensitivity reaction; a similar case in a patient receiving anistreplase was associated with Henoch-Schönlein-like vasculitis.[3] These delayed reactions should be distinguished from the transient and apparently self-limiting proteinuria that has been reported in some patients in the first 24 to 72 hours after beginning streptokinase.[4,5] Proteinuria within the first 24 hours has been attributed to deposition of an immune complex in the glomeruli,[6] although haemodynamic and neurohormonal changes associated with acute myocardial infarction may be responsible since proteinuria has occurred in patients not receiving thrombolytic therapy.[7,8]

Streptokinase infusion has also been associated with acute oliguric renal failure due to acute tubular necrosis, apparently as a result of hypotension during the infusion, in a patient with existing renovascular narrowing.[9] Interestingly, it has been pointed out that a variant streptokinase may be the pathogenic agent in glomerulonephritis occurring after *Streptococcus pyogenes* infection.[10]

Renal failure has developed as a consequence of a streptokinase-induced cholesterol embolism, see under Embolism, below.

1. Payne ST, *et al.* Transient impairment of renal function after streptokinase therapy. *Lancet* 1989; **ii**: 1398.
2. Callan MFC, *et al.* Proteinuria and thrombolytic agents. *Lancet* 1990; **335**: 106.
3. Ali A, *et al.* Proteinuria and thrombolytic agents. *Lancet* 1990; **335**: 106–7.
4. Argent N, Adams PC. Proteinuria and thrombolytic agents. *Lancet* 1990; **335**: 106.
5. More RS, Peacock F. Haematuria and proteinuria after thrombolytic therapy. *Lancet* 1990; **336**: 1454.
6. Lynch M, *et al.* Proteinuria with streptokinase. *Lancet* 1993; **341**: 1024.
7. Pickett TM, Hilton PJ. Proteinuria and streptokinase. *Lancet* 1993; **341**: 1538.
8. von Eyben FE, *et al.* Albuminuria with or without streptokinase. *Lancet* 1993; **342**: 365–6.
9. Kalra PA, *et al.* Acute tubular necrosis induced by coronary thrombolytic therapy. *Postgrad Med J* 1991; **67**: 212.
10. Barnham M. Hypersensitivity and streptokinase. *Lancet* 1990; **335**: 535.

Effects on the liver. Raised serum-alanine aminotransferase values, and in some cases raised aspartate aminotransferase activity, were seen more frequently in 95 patients who received streptokinase than in 94 given placebo as part of a study in patients with myocardial infarction.[1] The mechanism for the raised aminotransferase activity was not clear; a concomitant rise in γ-glutamyltransferase activity and bilirubin concentration suggested an hepatic source.

For references to rupture of the liver occurring during treatment with streptokinase, see under Haemorrhage, below.

1. Maclennan AC, *et al.* Activities of aminotransferases after treatment with streptokinase for acute myocardial infarction. *BMJ* 1990; **301**: 321–2.

Effects on the nervous system. There have been a few reports of Guillain-Barré syndrome following treatment with streptokinase.[1-4] Whether streptokinase was the cause is not certain although its antigenic properties do suggest that induction of an immunological reaction might be responsible.[3]

For discussion of cerebrovascular effects of streptokinase, see under Haemorrhage, below.

1. Eden KV. Possible association of Guillain-Barré syndrome with thrombolytic therapy. *JAMA* 1983; **249**: 2020–1.
2. Leaf DA, *et al.* Streptokinase and the Guillain-Barré syndrome. *Ann Intern Med* 1984; **100**: 617.
3. Barnes D, Hughes RAC. Guillain-Barré syndrome after treatment with streptokinase. *BMJ* 1992; **304**: 1225.
4. Taylor BV, *et al.* Guillain-Barré syndrome complicating treatment with streptokinase. *Med J Aust* 1995; **162**: 214–15.

Effects on the respiratory system. Fatal acute respiratory distress syndrome occurred in a patient given streptokinase for pulmonary embolism.[1] It was suggested that streptokinase may have caused the pulmonary injury by altering vascular permeability due to generation of fibrinolytic products or via reperfusion oedema.

1. Martin TR, *et al.* Adult respiratory distress syndrome following thrombolytic therapy for pulmonary embolism. *Chest* 1983; **83**: 151–3.

Effects on the skin. Rashes may occur as an allergic reaction to streptokinase. For a report of skin necrosis possibly associated with cholesterol embolisation, see Embolism, below.

Embolism. Thrombolytic therapy has occasionally and paradoxically been associated with further embolism in the patients receiving it. Such embolism may be due to clots that break away from the thrombus being treated, or to cholesterol crystals released following removal of fibrin from atheromatous plaques by thrombolysis.

Fatal pulmonary embolism has been reported,[1] apparently due to breakaway from a deep-vein thrombus under treatment. However, comparative studies have suggested that there is no evidence of a higher rate of such complications with streptokinase than with heparin.[2] When they do occur a good clinical response is usually seen to continued streptokinase.[2] Complications due to multiple microemboli were reported[3] in 7 of 475 consecutive patients treated with streptokinase or anistreplase for acute myocardial infarction. The sites of embolism were the legs (in 4) and brain (in 3); one patient apparently had systemic effects with skin infarction and impaired renal function. Five of the 7 patients died.

Cholesterol embolisation can have many clinical manifestations depending on the location of the emboli. A classic presentation is livedo reticularis, gangrenous lower extremities, and acute renal failure.[4,5] Symptoms may appear within a few hours of starting thrombolytic treatment,[6] although in some cases they may not become evident for several days.[7-10]

1. Hill LN. Streptokinase therapy and breakaway pulmonary emboli. *Am J Med* 1991; **90**: 411–12.
2. Rogers LQ, Lutcher CL. Streptokinase therapy and breakaway pulmonary emboli. *Am J Med* 1991; **90**: 412–13.
3. Stafford PJ, *et al.* Multiple microemboli after disintegration of clot during thrombolysis for acute myocardial infarction. *BMJ* 1989; **299**: 1310–12.

4. Blankenship JC. Cholesterol embolisation after thrombolytic therapy. *Drug Safety* 1996; **14**: 78–84.
5. Wong FKM, *et al.* Acute renal failure after streptokinase therapy in a patient with acute myocardial infarction. *Am J Kidney Dis* 1995; **26**: 508–10.
6. Pochmalicki G, *et al.* Cholesterol embolisation syndrome after thrombolytic therapy for myocardial infarction. *Lancet* 1992; **339**: 58–9.
7. Ridker PM, Michel T. Streptokinase therapy and cholesterol embolization. *Am J Med* 1989; **87**: 357–8.
8. Pirson Y, *et al.* Cholesterol embolism in a renal graft after treatment with streptokinase. *BMJ* 1988; **296**: 394–5.
9. Dass H, Fescharek R. Skin necrosis induced by streptokinase. *BMJ* 1994; **309**: 1513–14.
10. Penswick J, Wright AL. Skin necrosis induced by streptokinase. *BMJ* 1994; **309**: 378.

Haemorrhage. Haemorrhage is a common adverse effect of thrombolytic therapy, particularly where there is existing or concomitant trauma: bleeding or severe bruising has been associated with various therapeutic manipulations including vascular puncture (e.g. injection, phlebotomy, or catheterisation),[1] intramuscular injection of analgesics,[2] the use of an automatic blood-pressure measuring machine,[3] a pre-existing prosthetic abdominal aortic graft,[4] and recent dental extraction.[5] In addition, other disease states may contribute: haemospermia has been reported following thrombolysis in a patient with mild prostatic symptoms,[6] haemorrhagic bullae have been reported in a patient with lichen sclerosus et atrophicus,[7] and diabetic patients are at risk of retinal haemorrhage if they have diabetic retinopathy,[8] although any increase in risk seems to be small.[9]

The problem and its management have been reviewed.[1] Thrombolytics can produce a 'lytic state' due to depletion of the natural fibrinolysin inhibitor α_2-antiplasmin by excess fibrinolysin production, although this correlates only weakly, if at all, with bleeding. Currently available 'fibrin-specific' agents such as alteplase do not produce less bleeding than non-specific thrombolytics such as streptokinase. More than 70% of bleeding episodes occur at vascular puncture sites, so invasive procedures should be avoided if possible; if catheterisation is considered essential meticulous care of the vascular puncture site is necessary. A review of the GUSTO-I Study[10] (40 903 patients) confirmed that invasive procedures are a risk factor for bleeding. Older age, low body-weight, female sex, and African ancestry were other factors that increased the risk of haemorrhage.

Of particular concern is the possibility of intracranial haemorrhage leading to cerebrovascular events. There has been contradictory evidence of the relative risk with streptokinase and other thrombolytics. Assessment of individual patient data collected from national registries and various large-scale studies confirm that thrombolytic therapy does cause intracranial haemorrhage in a small number of patients. Risk factors include older age, hypertension on admission, a history of stroke, low body-weight, female sex, black ethnicity, and thrombolysis with current alteplase regimens.[11-14] The benefits and risks must be assessed for each patient and thrombolytic therapy should still be given to the elderly and to those with hypertension if the expected benefits are great.

In the NINDS study of alteplase for stroke clinical outcome appeared to be improved despite an increased incidence of symptomatic intracerebral haemorrhage. Subgroup analysis[15] suggested that severe neurological deficit, brain oedema, and mass effect, before treatment, were risks associated with the increased incidence of haemorrhage.

Rupture of the spleen[16,17] and liver[18] has been reported in patients receiving thrombolytic therapy, and rupture of a follicle has been reported in a menstruating woman.[19] Rupture of the heart with fatal consequences has been reported. A review of randomised studies[20] did not suggest that thrombolytic therapy following myocardial infarction increases the overall risk of cardiac rupture, although women may be at increased risk for early rupture.[21]

1. Sane DC, *et al.* Bleeding during thrombolytic therapy for acute myocardial infarction: mechanisms and management. *Ann Intern Med* 1989; **111**: 1010–22.
2. Morris GC, Sterry MJG. [case report]. *BMJ* 1991; **302**: 246.
3. Gibson P. [case report]. *BMJ* 1991; **302**: 1412.
4. London NJM, *et al.* Systemic thrombolysis causing haemorrhage around a prosthetic abdominal aortic graft. *BMJ* 1993; **306**: 1530–1.
5. Lustig JP, *et al.* Thrombolytic therapy for acute myocardial infarction after oral surgery. *Oral Surg Oral Med Oral Pathol* 1993; **75**: 547–8.
6. Keeling PJ, Lawson CS. Haemospermia: a complication of thrombolytic therapy. *Br J Hosp Med* 1990; **44**: 244.
7. Dunn HM, Fulton RA. Haemorrhagic bullae in a patient with lichen sclerosus et atrophicus treated with streptokinase. *Heart* 1996; **76**: 448.
8. Caramelli B, *et al.* Retinal haemorrhage after thrombolytic therapy. *Lancet* 1991; **337**: 1356–7.
9. Ward H, Yudkin JS. Thrombolysis in patients with diabetes. *BMJ* 1995; **310**: 3–4.
10. Berkowitz SD, *et al.* Incidence and predictors of bleeding after contemporary thrombolytic therapy for myocardial infarction. *Circulation* 1997; **95**: 2508–16.
11. Simoons ML, *et al.* Individual risk assessment for intracranial haemorrhage during thrombolytic therapy. *Lancet* 1993; **342**: 1523–8.
12. Aylward PE, *et al.* Relation of increased arterial blood pressure to mortality and stroke in the context of contemporary thrombolytic therapy for acute myocardial infarction: a randomized trial. *Ann Intern Med* 1996; **125**: 891–900.
13. Bovill EG, *et al.* Hemorrhagic events during therapy with recombinant tissue-type plasminogen activator, heparin, and aspirin for unstable angina (Thrombolysis in Myocardial Ischemia, Phase IIIB trial). *Am J Cardiol* 1997; **79**: 391–6.

14. Gurwitz JH, *et al.* Risk for intracranial hemorrhage after tissue plasminogen activator treatment for acute myocardial infarction. *Ann Intern Med* 1998; **129:** 597–604.
15. The NINDS t-PA Stroke Study Group. Intracerebral hemorrhage after intravenous t-PA therapy for ischemic stroke. *Stroke* 1997; **28:** 2109–18.
16. Wiener RS, Ong LS. Streptokinase and splenic rupture. *Am J Med* 1989; **86:** 249.
17. Blankenship JC, Indeck M. Spontaneous splenic rupture complicating anticoagulant or thrombolytic therapy. *Am J Med* 1993; **94:** 433–7.
18. Eklöf B, *et al.* Spontaneous rupture of liver and spleen with severe intra-abdominal bleeding during streptokinase treatment of deep venous thrombosis. *Vasa* 1977; **6:** 369–71.
19. Müller C-H, *et al.* Near-fatal intra-abdominal bleeding from a ruptured follicle during thrombolytic therapy. *Lancet* 1996; **347:** 1697.
20. Massel DR. How sound is the evidence that thrombolysis increases the risk of cardiac rupture? *Br Heart J* 1993; **69:** 284–7.
21. Becker RC, *et al.* Fatal cardiac rupture among patients treated with thrombolytic agents and adjunctive thrombin antagonists: observations from the Thrombolysis and Thrombin Inhibition in Myocardial Infarction 9 Study. *J Am Coll Cardiol* 1999; **33:** 479–87.

Hypersensitivity. Streptokinase is a bacterial protein and has antigenic activity. The formation of streptokinase-neutralising antibodies may reduce the efficacy of subsequent doses and increase the risk of hypersensitivity reactions.

In a series of 25 patients given intravenous streptokinase for myocardial infarction, titres of streptokinase-neutralising antibodies rose from a mean neutralisation capacity of 0.16 million units before treatment to a mean of 25.54 million units 2 weeks after treatment, the highest individual titre being 93 million units. After 12 weeks the neutralisation capacity was still sufficient in 24 patients to have neutralised a standard 1.5-million-unit dose of streptokinase. After 17 to 34 weeks titres were still high enough in 18 of 20 patients examined to neutralise at least half a standard dose.[1] As these results indicate, administration of standard doses of streptokinase within up to a year of a previous course may lead to reduced effect. Thus, the period in which it should not be repeated is usually between 5 days and 12 months post infarction (see Precautions, below). However, high titres of neutralising antibodies persisting for up to 7.5 years after administration of streptokinase have been reported.[2-4] Since readministration also increases the risk of hypersensitivity reactions, it has been suggested[2,5] that repeat courses should not be given within 4 or more years, and that if a repeat course is needed a non-antigenic thrombolytic such as alteplase or urokinase should be used until it is known whether or not high *in-vitro* titres affect efficacy. Increased titres of streptokinase-neutralising antibodies have also been measured in patients receiving topical streptokinase for wounds.[6]

Anistreplase also appears susceptible to neutralisation by streptokinase antibodies.[7]

Plasmacytosis,[8,9] serum-sickness,[8,10,11] rhabdomyolysis,[12] impaired renal function (see under Effects on the Kidneys, above), uveitis (see under Effects on the Eyes, above), arthritis,[13] and anaphylaxis[14-17] have been reported in patients receiving streptokinase and are thought to represent hypersensitivity reactions, in some cases perhaps due to previous exposure to streptococcal antigens during infection. Back pain (see above) may also represent a hypersensitivity reaction. In some patients there may be a delay of between 1 and 10 days before appearance of the reaction.[18] The incidence of severe hypersensitivity reactions is probably fairly low, however; in the GISSI study anaphylaxis was reported in only 7 of 5860 patients although other hypersensitivity reactions leading to withdrawal of streptokinase were reported in 99 patients, with a further 42 such reactions after completion of the infusion.[15] Some episodes of apparent anaphylaxis seen with streptokinase administration may be fibrinolysin-mediated rather than antibody-antigen reactions. Administration of alteplase, which is considered nonantigenic, produced an anaphylactoid reaction in a patient who had a history of atopy.[19] Fibrinolysin, which activates complement cascade and the kinin system, is formed in quantity after the administration of a thrombolytic. In most patients these effects are clinically insignificant, but in those who are strongly atopic there is the possibility of precipitating an anaphylactoid reaction.

1. Jalihal S, Morris GK. Antistreptokinase titres after intravenous streptokinase. *Lancet* 1990; **335:** 184–5.
2. Elliott JM, *et al.* Neutralizing antibodies to streptokinase four years after intravenous thrombolytic therapy. *Am J Cardiol* 1993; **71:** 640–5.
3. Lee HS, *et al.* Raised levels of antistreptokinase antibody and neutralization titres from 4 days to 54 months after administration of streptokinase or anistreplase. *Eur Heart J* 1993; **14:** 84–9.
4. Squire IB, *et al.* Humoral and cellular immune responses up to 7.5 years after administration of streptokinase for acute myocardial infarction. *Eur Heart J* 1999; **20:** 1245–52.
5. Jennings K. Antibodies to streptokinase. *BMJ* 1996; **312:** 393–4.
6. Green C. Antistreptokinase titres after topical streptokinase. *Lancet* 1993; **341:** 1602–3.
7. Binette MJ, Agnone FA. Failure of APSAC thrombolysis. *Ann Intern Med* 1993; **119:** 637.
8. Straub PW, *et al.* Plasmozytose nach thrombolytischer Therapie mit Streptokinase. *Schweiz Med Wochenschr* 1974; **104:** 1891–2.
9. Chan NS, *et al.* Plasmacytosis and renal failure after readministration of streptokinase for threatened myocardial reinfarction. *BMJ* 1988; **297:** 717–18.
10. Payne ST, *et al.* Transient impairment of renal function after streptokinase therapy. *Lancet* 1989; **ii:** 1398.
11. Callan MFC, *et al.* Proteinuria and thrombolytic agents. *Lancet* 1990; **335:** 106.
12. Montgomery HE, *et al.* Rhabdomyolysis and multiple system organ failure with streptokinase. *BMJ* 1995; **311:** 1472.
13. Kelly MP, Bielawska C. Recurrence of a reactive arthritis following streptokinase therapy. *Postgrad Med J* 1991; **67:** 402.
14. McGrath KG, Patterson R. Anaphylactic reactivity to streptokinase. *JAMA* 1984; **252:** 1314–17.
15. Gruppo Italiano per lo Studio della Streptochinasi nell'Infarto Miocardico. Effectiveness of intravenous thrombolytic treatment in acute myocardial infarction. *Lancet* 1986; **i:** 397–401.
16. Bednarczyk EM, *et al.* Anaphylactic reaction to streptokinase with first exposure: case report and review of the literature. *DICP Ann Pharmacother* 1989; **23:** 869–72.
17. Tisdale JE, *et al.* Streptokinase-induced anaphylaxis. *DICP Ann Pharmacother* 1989; **23:** 984–7.
18. Seibert WJ, *et al.* Streptokinase morbidity—more common than previously recognised. *Aust N Z J Med* 1992; **22:** 129–33.
19. Purvis JA, *et al.* Anaphylactoid reaction after injection of alteplase. *Lancet* 1993; **341:** 966–7.

Treatment of Adverse Effects
Allergic reactions may require treatment with antihistamines and corticosteroids, which have sometimes been given prophylactically to reduce the risk of such reactions. Anaphylaxis requires the administration of adrenaline [epinephrine] (for further details, see Anaphylactic Shock, p.832).

Severe haemorrhage not controlled by local pressure requires discontinuation of the streptokinase infusion. Tranexamic acid, aminocaproic acid, or aprotinin may be of benefit. Packed red blood cells may be preferable to whole blood for replacement therapy; factor VIII preparations may also be given. Volume expansion may be necessary, but the use of dextrans should be avoided because of their platelet-inhibiting properties.

Precautions
Streptokinase should be used with great care, if at all, in patients at increased risk of bleeding, or those in whom haemorrhage is likely to prove particularly dangerous. It should thus be avoided in patients with active internal bleeding or a recent history of peptic ulcer disease, oesophageal varices, ulcerative colitis or other bleeding gastrointestinal lesions, in patients with pancreatitis, in patients with subacute bacterial endocarditis, in patients with coagulation defects including those due to liver or kidney disease, or after recent surgery, childbirth, or trauma. It should not be given to patients at increased risk of cerebral bleeding including those with severe hypertension, haemorrhage or recent stroke, or to patients with cerebral neoplasm. It should not be given in pregnancy, particularly in the first 18 weeks because of the risk of placental separation and it has been suggested that it should not be used during heavy vaginal bleeding.

Invasive procedures, including intramuscular injections, should be avoided during, and immediately before and after, streptokinase therapy as they may increase the risk of bleeding. It should be used with care in elderly patients and in patients with diabetic retinopathy. Patients with mitral stenosis associated with atrial fibrillation are more likely to have left heart thrombus which may lead to cerebral embolism following thrombolytic therapy.

Anti-streptokinase antibodies are formed following streptokinase use, with antibody titres rising abruptly after about 5 days. These antibodies may cause resistance or hypersensitivity to subsequent doses of streptokinase. Therefore, further doses of streptokinase should not be given in the period between 5 days and 12 months after the initial dose (even longer periods have been suggested, see Hypersensitivity, under Adverse Effects, above); if thrombolytic therapy is required in this period an alternative non-antigenic drug should be used. Some streptococcal infections such as acute rheumatic fever or acute glomerulonephritis may also result in high titres of anti-streptokinase antibodies, such that similar precautions may be necessary.

Administration. Overinfusion of streptokinase may occur if a drop-counting infusion pump is employed.[1] This arises as a result of flocculation of the streptokinase solution producing translucent fibres that affect the drop-forming mechanism so increasing the drop size.

For a comment on the incidence of flocculation in streptokinase solutions, see under Stability, above.

1. Schad RF, Jennings RH. Overinfusions of streptokinase. *Am J Hosp Pharm* 1982; **39:** 1850.

Aortic dissection. A report of 4 cases of the inappropriate use of streptokinase in patients with aortic dissection misdiagnosed as myocardial infarction.[1] Thrombolytics are likely to extend aortic dissection and adversely affect the outcome. Of the 2 patients who died, one, who would have been suitable for early operation, died through the delay caused by impaired clotting. Although early intervention with thrombolytics may be of major benefit in acute myocardial infarction it is important that accurate differential diagnosis takes place to exclude conditions such as aortic dissection and prevent avoidable deaths.

1. Butler J, *et al.* Streptokinase in acute aortic dissection. *BMJ* 1990; **300:** 517–19.

Cardiopulmonary resuscitation. Thrombolytics are not recommended after prolonged or traumatic cardiopulmonary resuscitation because of the risk of haemorrhage. However, no clinically significant bleeding complications were found in a study in 39 patients with acute myocardial infarction who had a cardiac arrest before or shortly after receiving thrombolysis.[1]

1. Cross SJ, *et al.* Safety of thrombolysis in association with cardiopulmonary resuscitation. *BMJ* 1991; **303:** 1242.

Pregnancy. Thrombolytics are contra-indicated in pregnancy, although there are a few reports of their use which have been briefly reviewed.[1] In most cases, thrombolytics were given at 28 weeks of pregnancy or later to patients with deep-vein thrombosis, pulmonary embolism, or prosthetic valve thrombosis. There were some reports of favourable maternal and fetal outcomes although therapy was associated with maternal haemorrhage, including spontaneous abortion and minor vaginal bleeding, especially when given near the time of delivery. There was one report of abruptio placentae with fetal death.

1. Roth A, Elkayam U. Acute myocardial infarction associated with pregnancy. *Ann Intern Med* 1996; **125:** 751–62.

Interactions
Oral anticoagulants, heparin, and antiplatelet drugs such as aspirin are often used in conjunction with streptokinase, but may increase the risk of haemorrhage. Other drugs which affect platelet function may do likewise, including allopurinol, dextrans, quinidine, sex hormones, sulfonamides, tetracyclines, valproic acid, and some essential oils.

◊ References.
1. Harder S, Klinkhardt U. Thrombolytics: drug interactions of clinical significance. *Drug Safety* 2000; **23:** 391–9.

Pharmacokinetics
Streptokinase is rapidly cleared from the circulation following intravenous administration. Clearance is biphasic with the initial and more rapid phase being due to specific antibodies. A half-life of 23 minutes has been reported for the streptokinase-activator complex.

◊ References.
1. Grierson DS, Bjornsson TD. Pharmacokinetics of streptokinase in patients based on amidolytic activator complex activity. *Clin Pharmacol Ther* 1987; **41:** 304–13.
2. Gemmill JD, *et al.* A comparison of the pharmacokinetic properties of streptokinase and anistreplase in acute myocardial infarction. *Br J Clin Pharmacol* 1991; **31:** 143–7.

Uses and Administration
Streptokinase is a thrombolytic drug derived from various streptococci. It rapidly activates endogenous plasminogen, indirectly by means of a streptokinase-plasminogen complex, to fibrinolysin (p.890), which has fibrinolytic effects and can dissolve intravascular blood clots. The mechanisms of fibrinolysis are discussed further under Haemostasis and Fibrinolysis on p.718. Streptokinase affects circulating, unbound plasminogen as well as fibrin-bound plasminogen and thus may be termed a fibrin-nonspecific thrombolytic agent. This action was thought to contribute to the risk of haemorrhage, although currently available fibrin-specific agents, such as alteplase, do not produce less bleeding than nonspecific thrombolytics (see Haemorrhage under Adverse Effects, above).

Streptokinase is given by intravenous or sometimes intra-arterial infusion in the treatment of thromboembolic disorders such as myocardial infarction (p.805), peripheral arterial thromboembolism (below), and venous thromboembolism (deep-vein thrombosis and pulmonary embolism) (p.817). It has also been tried in unstable angina (p.791) and in ischaemic stroke (p.813), but these uses are less well-established.

Streptokinase may be used to clear cannulas and shunts and is used topically in conjunction with streptodornase to clear clots and purulent matter.

In acute **myocardial infarction** streptokinase is usually given intravenously as a single dose of 1.5 million units infused over 1 hour as soon as possible after the onset of symptoms. Streptokinase may also be given by intracoronary infusion but coronary catheterisation with the aid of angiography is required, thus restricting administration to suitably equipped centres. An initial intracoronary dose of 10 000 to 25 000 units has been given as a bolus injection followed by an infusion of 2000 to 4000 units per minute. Infusion has been continued until reperfusion has been achieved (usually within about 30 minutes) and for 30 to 60 minutes thereafter, or for 60 to 75 minutes if reperfusion has not been achieved.

In the treatment of **pulmonary embolism** and other **arteriovenous occlusions** an initial loading dose of streptokinase, normally 250 000 units infused intravenously over 30 minutes, is given to overcome any resistance due to circulating antibodies. This is followed by infusion of a maintenance dose of 100 000 units per hour for 12 to 72 hours, depending on the condition to be treated. Treatment should be controlled by monitoring the thrombin clotting time, which should be maintained at 2 to 4 times normal values. Since thrombolytic activity rapidly fades when the infusion stops, streptokinase treatment is generally followed by intravenous heparin infusion, and then oral anticoagulation, to prevent re-occlusion. In children, the initial dose should be estimated according to the streptokinase resistance; maintenance doses of 1300 to 1400 units per kg body-weight per hour or 20 units per mL of blood volume per hour have been employed.

Streptokinase, as a solution containing 1000 units per mL, is used to clear shunts of occluding thrombi; 250 000 units in 2 mL is used to clear occluded cannulas.

◊ General references.
1. Fears R. Biochemical pharmacology and therapeutic aspects of thrombolytic agents. *Pharmacol Rev* 1990; **42:** 201–21.
2. Stringer KA. Beyond thrombolysis: other effects of thrombolytic drugs. *Ann Pharmacother* 1994; **28:** 752–6.
3. Ludlam CA, et al. Guidelines for the use of thrombolytic therapy. *Blood Coag Fibrinol* 1995; **6:** 273–85.

Empyema and pleural effusion. Thoracic empyema is treated with antibacterials and pleural drainage. Efficient removal of fluid may be impaired by fibrinous clots within the pleural cavity. Intrapleural instillation of streptokinase (100 000 to 750 000 units in up to 100 mL of sodium chloride 0.9%)[1] or urokinase (100 000 to 250 000 units in 100 mL of sodium chloride 0.9%)[1] has been reported to be effective in small series of patients.[1-4] Intrapleural streptokinase has also been employed successfully in a few patients with malignant multiloculated pleural effusion resistant to standard pleural drainage.[5]
Intrapericardial instillation of thrombolytics has been tried in a few patients with pericardial empyema to prevent the development of constrictive pericarditis.[6,7]
1. Temes RT, et al. Intrapleural fibrinolytics in management of empyema thoracis. *Chest* 1996; **110:** 102–6.
2. Bouros D, et al. Role of streptokinase in the treatment of acute loculated parapneumonic pleural effusions and empyema. *Thorax* 1994; **49:** 852–5.
3. Davies RJO, et al. Randomised controlled trial of intrapleural streptokinase in community acquired pleural infection. *Thorax* 1997; **52:** 416–21.
4. Bouros D, et al. Intrapleural streptokinase versus urokinase in the treatment of complicated parapneumonic effusions: a prospective, double-blind study. *Am J Respir Crit Care Med* 1997; **155:** 291–5.
5. Davies CWH, et al. Intrapleural streptokinase in the management of malignant multiloculated pleural effusions. *Chest* 1999; **115:** 729–33.
6. Winkler W-B, et al. Treatment of exudative fibrinous pericarditis with intrapericardial urokinase. *Lancet* 1994; **344:** 1541–2.
7. Juneja R, et al. Intrapericardial streptokinase in purulent pericarditis. *Arch Dis Child* 1999; **80:** 275–7.

Intracardiac thrombosis. Thrombosis of prosthetic heart valves is usually managed surgically. In left-sided prosthetic valve thrombosis, thrombolytic therapy may be used in critically ill patients who are at high risk of complications from surgery. Thrombolysis for low risk patients remains controversial. Streptokinase or urokinase are the thrombolytics usually employed, although alteplase has also been used.[1]
1. Lengyel M, et al. Guidelines for management of left-sided prosthetic valve thrombosis: a role for thrombolytic therapy. *J Am Coll Cardiol* 1997; **30:** 1521–6.

Peripheral arterial thromboembolism. Thrombolytics including streptokinase may be used in the management of peripheral arterial thromboembolism (p.808). Streptokinase has been injected intravenously or intra-arterially directly into the clot as an alternative to surgical treatment of the occlusion. It has also been infused intra-arterially to remove distal clots during a surgical procedure. The *intravenous* dose generally used is 250 000 units over 30 minutes followed by 100 000 units per hour. A lower dose of 5000 units per hour has been used *intra-arterially* directly into the clot[1] and for removal of distal clots during a surgical procedure streptokinase has been given intra-arterially in a dose of 100 000 units over 30 minutes or as five bolus doses of 20 000 units at 5-minute intervals.[2]
1. Anonymous. Non-coronary thrombolysis. *Lancet* 1990; **335:** 691–3.
2. Earnshaw JJ, Beard JD. Intraoperative use of thrombolytic agents. *BMJ* 1993; **307:** 638–9.

Preparations

BP 2001: Streptokinase Injection.

Proprietary Preparations (details are given in Part 3)
Aust.: Kabikinase; Streptase; *Austral.:* Kabikinase; Streptase; *Belg.:* Kabikinase; Streptase; *Braz.:* Kabikinase; Streptase; *Canad.:* Kabikinase; Streptase; *Denm.:* Kabikinase; Streptase; *Fin.:* Kabikinase; Streptase; *Fr.:* Kabikinase; Streptase; *Ger.:* Kabikinase; Streptase; *Hong Kong:* Kabikinase; Streptase; *Irl.:* Kabikinase; Streptase; *Israel:* Kabikinase; Streptase; *Ital.:* Streptase; *Mex.:* Kabikinase; Streptase; *Neth.:* Kabikinase; Streptase; *Norw.:* Kabikinase; Streptase; *NZ:* Kabikinase; Streptase; *Port.:* Kabikinase†; Streptase; *S.Afr.:* Kabikinase; Streptase; *Singapore:* Kabikinase; Streptase; *Spain:* Kabikinase; Streptase; *Swed.:* Kabikinase†; Streptase; *Switz.:* Kabikinase; Streptase; *Thai.:* Kabikinase†; Streptase; *UK:* Kabikinase†; Streptase; *USA:* Kabikinase†; Streptase.

Multi-ingredient: *Aust.:* Varidase; *Austral.:* Varidase; *Belg.:* Varidase; *Denm.:* Varidase; *Fin.:* Varidase; *Ger.:* Varidase; *Irl.:* Varidase; *Israel:* Varidase; *Ital.:* Varidase; *Mex.:* Varidasa; *Neth.:* Varidase; *Norw.:* Varidase; *NZ:* Varidase; *Port.:* Varidasa; *S.Afr.:* Varidase; *Spain:* Ernodasa; Varibiotic; Varidasa; *Swed.:* Varidase; *UK:* Varidase.

Strophanthin-K (5827-v)

Estrofantina; Kombé Strophanthin; Strophanthin; Strophanthoside-K.
CAS — 11005-63-3.

NOTE. Do not confuse with K-strophanthin-α which is Cymarin.
Pharmacopoeias. In Aust. and It.

A mixture of cardiac glycosides from strophanthus, the seeds of *Strophanthus kombé* (Apocynaceae) or other spp., adjusted by admixture with a suitable diluent such as lactose so as generally to possess 40% of the activity of anhydrous ouabain.

Profile
Strophanthin-K is a positive inotrope with general properties similar to those of digoxin (p.870). It is poorly absorbed from the gastrointestinal tract but may be given intravenously in doses of 125 to 500 µg daily in the management of heart failure (p.798).

Preparations
Proprietary Preparations (details are given in Part 3)
Aust.: Laevostrophan; *Ger.:* Kombetin†; *Ital.:* Kombetin.

Multi-ingredient: *Aust.:* Laevostrophan compositum.

Suleparoid (19289-x)

Suleparoid (rINNM).
Heparan Sulfate; Heparan Sulphate; Heparitin Sulfate.
CAS — 9050-30-0 (suleparoid); 57459-72-0 (suleparoid sodium).

NOTE. Suleparoid Sodium is rINN.

Profile
Suleparoid is a naturally occurring glycosaminoglycan given orally in the management of thromboembolic disorders. Suleparoid sodium is a component of danaparoid sodium (p.866).

Preparations
Proprietary Preparations (details are given in Part 3)
Ital.: Aremin; Arteven; Clarema; Hemovasal; Iparen; Leparan; Tavidan; Tromir; Tronan; Vas; Vasorema; Vepar†.

Suloctidil (9278-n)

Suloctidil (BAN, USAN, rINN).
CP-556S; MJF-12637. 1-(4-Isopropylthiophenyl)-2-octylaminopropan-1-ol.
$C_{20}H_{35}NOS = 337.6$.
CAS — 54063-56-8.

Profile
Suloctidil is a vasodilator that was formerly used in the management of peripheral and cerebral vascular disorders. It is hepatotoxic and fatalities have occurred.

Sulodexide (13285-j)

Sulodexide (rINN).
Glucurono-2-amino-2-deoxyglucoglucan sulphate.
CAS — 57821-29-1.
ATC — B01AB11.

Profile
Sulodexide is a heparinoid consisting of a mixture of low-molecular-weight heparin and dermatan sulfate. It is used as a hypolipidaemic and antithrombotic and has been administered by mouth and parenterally for peripheral vascular disease and cerebrovascular disease. It is also included in preparations used topically for local vascular inflammation and soft-tissue disorders. Sulodexide is also under investigation for the treatment of diabetic nephropathy.

◊ References.
1. Ofosu FA. Pharmacological actions of sulodexide. *Semin Thromb Hemost* 1998; **24:** 127–38.

Preparations
Proprietary Preparations (details are given in Part 3)
Ital.: Clarens; Vessel Due F; *Spain:* Aterina; Luzone.

Multi-ingredient: *Ital.:* Dermoangiopan; Vessiflex.

Sulotroban (18855-m)

Sulotroban (BAN, USAN, rINN).
BM-13177; SKF-95587. [p-(2-Benzenesulfonamidoethyl)phenoxy]acetic acid.
$C_{16}H_{17}NO_5S = 335.4$.
CAS — 72131-33-0.

Profile
Sulotroban is a thromboxane A_2 antagonist under investigation as an antiplatelet drug.

◊ References.
1. Piper C, et al. Pharmacokinetics of the thromboxane A_2 receptor antagonist sulotroban (BM 13177) in renal failure. *Br J Clin Pharmacol* 1989; **28:** 281–8.
2. Pierucci A, et al. Improvement of renal function with selective thromboxane antagonism in lupus nephritis. *N Engl J Med* 1989; **320:** 421–5.
3. Savage MP, et al. Multi-hospital Eastern Atlantic Restenosis trial II: a placebo-controlled trial of thromboxane blockage in the prevention of restenosis following coronary angioplasty. *Am Heart J* 1991; **122:** 1239–44.
4. Savage MP, et al. Effect of thromboxane A_2 blockade on clinical outcome and restenosis after successful coronary angioplasty: Multi-Hospital Eastern Atlantic Restenosis Trial (M-HEART II). *Circulation* 1995; **92:** 3194–3200.

Syrosingopine (905-s)

Syrosingopine (BAN, rINN).
Methyl Carbethoxysyringoyl Reserpate; Su-3118. Methyl O-(4-ethoxycarbonyloxy-3,5-dimethoxybenzoyl)reserpate.
$C_{35}H_{42}N_2O_{11} = 666.7$.
CAS — 84-36-6.

Profile
Syrosingopine is a derivative of reserpine (p.967) that has been used in the treatment of hypertension.

Talinolol (1015-g)

Talinolol (rINN).
(±)-1-{p-[3-(tert-Butylamino)-2-hydroxypropoxy]phenyl}-3-cyclohexylurea.
$C_{20}H_{33}N_3O_3 = 363.5$.
CAS — 57460-41-0.

Profile
Talinolol is a cardioselective beta blocker (p.844). It is given by mouth in the management of hypertension and other cardiovascular disorders. It may also be given intravenously.

Preparations
Proprietary Preparations (details are given in Part 3)
Ger.: Cordanum.

Tamsulosin Hydrochloride (1543-q)

Tamsulosin Hydrochloride (BANM, USAN, rINNM).
LY-253351; YM-617; R-(−)-YM-12617; YM-12617-1. (−)-(R)-5-(2-{[2-(o-Ethoxyphenoxy)ethyl]amino}-propyl)-2-methoxybenzenesulfonamide hydrochloride.
$C_{20}H_{28}N_2O_5S,HCl = 445.0$.
CAS — 106133-20-4 (tamsulosin); 106463-17-6 (tamsulosin hydrochloride).

Adverse Effects, Treatment, and Precautions
As for Prazosin Hydrochloride, p.958. Tamsulosin should be avoided in severe liver impairment.

Pharmacokinetics

Tamsulosin is absorbed from the gastrointestinal tract and is almost completely bioavailable. The extent and rate of absorption are reduced in the presence of food. Following oral administration of an immediate-release preparation, peak plasma concentrations occur about 1 hour after a dose. Tamsulosin is metabolised slowly in the liver and is excreted mainly in the urine as metabolites and some unchanged drug. The plasma elimination half-life has been reported to be between 4 and 5.5 hours. Tamsulosin is about 99% bound to plasma proteins.

Some of the pharmacokinetic values cited above may be altered when tamsulosin is administered as a modified-release preparation, the form in which it is usually employed; for instance, peak plasma concentrations occur about 6 hours after a dose and the apparent elimination half-life may be 10 to 13 hours.

Renal impairment. Plasma-tamsulosin concentrations were reported to be increased in patients with renal impairment when compared with subjects with normal renal function.[1,2] However, plasma concentrations of unbound, pharmacologically active drug were similar in both groups and it was suggested that the raised total plasma concentrations were due to an increase in plasma protein binding.

1. Koiso K, *et al.* Pharmacokinetics of tamsulosin hydrochloride in patients with renal impairment: effects of α_1-acid glycoprotein. *J Clin Pharmacol* 1996; **36:** 1029–38.
2. Wolzt M, *et al.* Pharmacokinetics of tamsulosin in subjects with normal and varying degrees of impaired renal function: an open-label single-dose and multiple-dose study. *Eur J Clin Pharmacol* 1998; **54:** 367–73.

Uses and Administration

Tamsulosin is an alpha$_1$-adrenoceptor blocker (p.787) with actions similar to those of prazosin (p.959); it is reported to be more selective for the alpha$_{1A}$-adrenoceptor subtype. It is used in benign prostatic hyperplasia (p.1477) to relieve symptoms of urinary obstruction.

Tamsulosin is given by mouth as the hydrochloride. In benign prostatic hyperplasia it is administered in a modified-release formulation, in a dose of 400 µg once daily, after the same meal each day. The dose may be increased after 2 to 4 weeks, if necessary, to 800 µg once daily.

◊ Reviews.
1. Wilde MI, McTavish D. Tamsulosin: a review of its pharmacological properties and therapeutic potential in the management of symptomatic benign prostatic hyperplasia. *Drugs* 1996; **52:** 883–98.
2. Lee M. Tamsulosin for the treatment of benign prostatic hypertrophy. *Ann Pharmacother* 2000; **34:** 188–99.

Preparations

Proprietary Preparations (details are given in Part 3)
Aust.: Alna; *Austral.:* Flomax; *Canad.:* Flomax; *Denm.:* Omnic; *Fin.:* Expros; Omnic; *Fr.:* Josir; Omix; *Ger.:* Alna; Omnic; *Irl.:* Omnic; *Israel:* Omnic; *Ital.:* Omnic; Pradif; *Jpn:* Harnal; *Mex.:* Secotex; *Neth.:* Omnic; *Norw.:* Omnic; *NZ:* Omnic; *Port.:* Omnic; Pradif; *S.Afr.:* Flomax; *Spain:* Omnic; Urolosin; *Switz.:* Pradif; *Thai.:* Harnal; *UK:* Flomax; *USA:* Flomax.

Tasosartan   (17859-f)

Tasosartan *(BAN, USAN, rINN)*.

WAY-ANA-756. 5,8-Dihydro-2,4-dimethyl-8-[*p*-(*o*-1*H*-tetrazol-5-ylphenyl)benzyl]pyrido[2,3-*d*]pyrimidin-7(6*H*)-one.

$C_{23}H_{21}N_7O = 411.5$.
CAS — 145733-36-4.
ATC — C09CA05.

Profile

Tasosartan is an angiotensin II receptor antagonist that has been investigated for the management of hypertension.

◊ References.
1. Oparil S, *et al.* Tolerability profile of tasosartan, a long-acting angiotensin II AT$_1$ receptor blocker, in the treatment of patients with essential hypertension. *Curr Ther Res* 1997; **58:** 930–43.
2. Lacourciere Y, *et al.* A randomized, double-blind, placebo-controlled, parallel-group, multicenter trial of four doses of tasosartan in patients with essential hypertension. Tasosartan Investigators Group. *Am J Hypertens* 1998; **11:** 454–61.
3. Neutel JM, *et al.* Efficacy and tolerability of tasosartan, a novel angiotensin II receptor blocker: results from a 10-week, double-blind, placebo-controlled, dose-titration study. Tasosartan Investigators Group. *Am Heart J* 1999; **137:** 118–25.

The symbol † denotes a preparation no longer actively marketed

---

Teclothiazide Potassium   (2356-I)

Teclothiazide Potassium *(BANM, rINNM)*.

Tetrachlormethiazide. 6-Chloro-3,4-dihydro-3-trichloromethyl-2*H*-1,2,4-benzothiadiazine-7-sulphonamide 1,1-dioxide, potassium salt.

$C_8H_7Cl_4N_3O_4S_2,K = 454.2$.
CAS — 4267-05-4 (teclothiazide); 5306-80-9 (teclothiazide potassium).

Profile

Teclothiazide potassium is a thiazide diuretic (see Hydrochlorothiazide, p.907) used in the treatment of oedema.

Preparations

Proprietary Preparations (details are given in Part 3)
Multi-ingredient: *Spain:* Quimodril.

Telmisartan   (17450-x)

Telmisartan *(BAN, USAN, rINN)*.

BIBR-277-SE. 4′-{[4-Methyl-6-(1-methyl-2-benzimidazolyl)-2-propyl-1-benzimidazolyl]methyl}-2-biphenylcarboxylic acid.

$C_{33}H_{30}N_4O_2 = 514.6$.
CAS — 144701-48-4.
ATC — C09CA07.

Adverse Effects and Precautions

As for Losartan Potassium, p.921. Telmisartan should be used with caution in patients with hepatic impairment or biliary obstruction.

Pharmacokinetics

Telmisartan is rapidly absorbed from the gastrointestinal tract; the absolute oral bioavailability is dose-dependent and is about 42% following a 40-mg dose and 58% following a 160-mg dose. Peak plasma concentrations of telmisartan are reached about 0.5 to 1 hour after an oral dose. Telmisartan is over 99% bound to plasma proteins. It is excreted almost entirely in the faeces via bile, mainly as unchanged drug. The terminal elimination half-life of telmisartan is about 24 hours.

◊ References.
1. Stangier J, *et al.* Absorption, metabolism, and excretion of intravenously and orally administered [^{14}C]telmisartan in healthy volunteers. *J Clin Pharmacol* 2000; **40:** 1312–22.

Uses and Administration

Telmisartan is an angiotensin II receptor antagonist with actions similar to those of losartan (p.922). It is used in the management of hypertension (p.802).

Telmisartan is administered by mouth. Following an oral dose the hypotensive effect peaks within 3 hours and persists for at least 24 hours. The maximum hypotensive effect is achieved within about 4 to 8 weeks after initiating therapy.

In hypertension, telmisartan is given in an initial dose of 40 mg once daily. This may be increased, if necessary, to a maximum dose of 80 mg once daily.

◊ Reviews.
1. McClellan KJ, Markham A. Telmisartan. *Drugs* 1998; **56:** 1039–44.
2. Sharpe M, *et al.* Telmisartan: a review of its use in hypertension. *Drugs* 2001; **61:** 1501–29.

Administration in hepatic impairment. Administration of telmisartan to patients with hepatic impairment resulted in an increase in bioavailability and a reduction in clearance compared with healthy volunteers.[1] Although telmisartan was well tolerated, it was suggested that lower doses should be considered in patients with hepatic impairment.

1. Stangier J, *et al.* Pharmacokinetics and safety of intravenous and oral telmisartan 20 mg and 120 mg in subjects with hepatic impairment compared with healthy volunteers. *J Clin Pharmacol* 2000; **40:** 1355–64.

Preparations

Proprietary Preparations (details are given in Part 3)
Austral.: Micardis; Pritor; *Belg.:* Micardis; *Denm.:* Micardis; *Fr.:* Micardis; Pritor; *Ger.:* Micardis; *Irl.:* Micardis; *Ital.:* Micardis; Pritor; *Neth.:* Micardis; *Port.:* Micardis; *S.Afr.:* Micardis; *Spain:* Micardis; Pritor; *Switz.:* Micardis; *UK:* Micardis; *USA:* Micardis.

Multi-ingredient: *USA:* Micardis HCT.

Temocapril Hydrochloride   (10960-s)

Temocapril Hydrochloride *(BANM, USAN, rINNM)*.

CS-622. (+)-(2*S*,6*R*)-6-{[(1*S*)-1-Carboxy-3-phenyl-propyl]amino}tetrahydro-5-oxo-2-(2-thienyl)-1,4-thiazepine-4(5*H*)-acetic acid, 6-ethyl ester, hydrochloride.

$C_{23}H_{28}N_2O_5S_2,HCl = 513.1$.
CAS — 111902-57-9 (temocapril); 110221-44-8 (temocapril hydrochloride).

Profile

Temocapril is an ACE inhibitor (p.820) that is used in the treatment of hypertension (p.802). It owes its activity to the diacid temocaprilat to which it is converted after oral administration. It is given by mouth as the hydrochloride in a usual initial dose of 1 mg daily, increased to a maintenance dose of 2 to 4 mg daily as necessary.

◊ References.
1. Nakashima M, *et al.* Pharmacokinetics of temocapril hydrochloride, a novel angiotensin converting enzyme inhibitor, in renal insufficiency. *Eur J Clin Pharmacol* 1992; **43:** 657–9.
2. Oguchi H, *et al.* Pharmacokinetics of temocapril and enalapril in patients with various degrees of renal insufficiency. *Clin Pharmacokinet* 1993; **24:** 421–7.
3. Furuta S, *et al.* Pharmacokinetics of temocapril, an ACE inhibitor with preferential biliary excretion, in patients with impaired liver function. *Eur J Clin Pharmacol* 1993; **44:** 383–5.

Preparations

Proprietary Preparations (details are given in Part 3)
Jpn: Acecol.

Tenecteplase   (20185-h)

Tenecteplase *(BAN, USAN, rINN)*.

TNK-tPA. [103-L-Asparagine-117-L-glutamine-296-L-alanine-297-L-alanine-298-L-alanine-299-L-alanine]plasminogen activator (human tissue-type).
CAS — 191588-94-0.

A 527 amino acid glycoprotein produced by recombinant DNA technology. It is a modified form of human tissue plasminogen activator.

Adverse Effects, Treatment, and Precautions

As for Streptokinase, p.976

Interactions

As for Streptokinase, p.977

Pharmacokinetics

Following intravenous injection, tenecteplase has a biphasic clearance from plasma with an initial half-life of 20 to 24 minutes and a terminal phase half-life of 90 to 130 minutes. It is cleared predominantly by hepatic metabolism.

◊ References.
1. Modi NB, *et al.* Pharmacokinetics and pharmacodynamics of tenecteplase: results from a phase II study in patients with acute myocardial infarction. *J Clin Pharmacol* 2000; **40:** 508–15.

Uses and Administration

Tenecteplase is a thrombolytic drug. It converts plasminogen to fibrinolysin, a proteolytic enzyme which has fibrinolytic effects. The mechanisms of fibrinolysis are discussed further under Haemostasis and Fibrinolysis on p.718. Tenecteplase is a fibrin-specific thrombolytic. Fibrin specificity was thought to be required for reducing the risk of haemorrhage associated with the use of thrombolytics, although currently available fibrin-specific agents do not produce less bleeding than non-specific thrombolytics (see Haemorrhage under Adverse Effects of Streptokinase, p.976).

Tenecteplase is used similarly to streptokinase (p.977) in acute myocardial infarction (p.805). It is given intravenously as a single bolus dose over 5 to 10 seconds as soon as possible after the onset of symptoms. The dose is based on body-weight and ranges from 30 to 50 mg; a total dose of 50 mg should not be exceeded.

◊ References.
1. Cannon CP, *et al.* TNK-tissue plasminogen activator compared with front-loaded alteplase in acute myocardial infarction: results of the TIMI 10B trial. *Circulation* 1998; **98:** 2805–14.
2. Assessment of the Safety and Efficacy of a New Thrombolytic (ASSENT-2) Investigators. Single-bolus tenecteplase compared with front-loaded alteplase in acute myocardial infarction: the ASSENT-2 double-blind randomised trial. *Lancet* 1999; **354:** 716–22.

Preparations

Proprietary Preparations (details are given in Part 3)
Austral.: Metalyse; *UK:* Metalyse; *USA:* TNKase.

Tenitramine   (13304-n)

NNN'N'-Tetrakis(2-hydroxyethyl)ethylenediamine tetranitrate.
$C_{10}H_{20}N_6O_{12} = 416.3$.
CAS — 21946-79-2.
ATC — C01DA38.

Profile

Tenitramine is a vasodilator with general properties similar to those of glyceryl trinitrate (p.898) and is used in angina pectoris (p.791). It is given in a usual dose of 10 mg by mouth for acute attacks and 10 mg every six hours for long-term management.

Preparations

Proprietary Preparations (details are given in Part 3)
Braz.: Ditran; *Ital.:* Tenitran.

Teprotide   (906-w)

Teprotide *(BAN, USAN, rINN)*.

BPF$_{9a}$; L-Pyroglutamyl-L-tryptophyl-L-prolyl-L-arginyl-L-prolyl-L-glutaminyl-L-isoleucyl-L-prolyl-L-proline; SQ-20881; 2-L-Tryptophan-3-de-L-leucine-4-de-L-proline-8-L-glutaminebradykinin potentiator B. 5-oxo-Pro-Trp-Pro-Arg-Pro-Gln-Ile-Pro-Pro.
$C_{53}H_{76}N_{14}O_{12} = 1101.3$.
CAS — 35115-60-7.

Profile

Teprotide is a nonapeptide originally found in the venom of *Bothrops jararaca*, a South American pit-viper. It is an ACE inhibitor that was given parenterally. It has a short duration of action and has been used as an investigational tool.

Terazosin Hydrochloride   (13306-m)

Terazosin Hydrochloride *(BANM, USAN, rINN)*.

Abbott-45975.   1-(4-Amino-6,7-dimethoxyquinazolin-2-yl)-4-(tetrahydro-2-furoyl)piperazine hydrochloride dihydrate; 6,7-Dimethoxy-2-[4-(tetrahydrofuran-2-carbonyl)piperazin-1-yl]quinazolin-4-ylamine hydrochloride dihydrate.
$C_{19}H_{25}N_5O_4,HCl,2H_2O = 459.9$.

CAS — 63590-64-7 (terazosin); 63074-08-8 (anhydrous terazosin hydrochloride); 70024-40-7 (terazosin hydrochloride dihydrate).

Terazosin hydrochloride 1.2 mg is approximately equivalent to 1 mg of terazosin.

Adverse Effects, Treatment, and Precautions

As for Prazosin Hydrochloride, p.958.

Urinary incontinence. For reference to urinary incontinence associated with terazosin, see under Adverse Effects of Prazosin Hydrochloride, p.958.

Interactions

As for Prazosin Hydrochloride, p.958.

Pharmacokinetics

Terazosin is rapidly and almost completely absorbed from the gastrointestinal tract after oral administration; the bioavailability is reported to be about 90%. Peak plasma concentrations are achieved in about one hour. It is metabolised in the liver; one of the metabolites is reported to possess antihypertensive activity. The half-life in plasma is approximately 12 hours. It is excreted in faeces via the bile, and in the urine, as unchanged drug and metabolites. Terazosin is 90 to 94% protein bound.

Uses and Administration

Terazosin is an alpha$_1$-adrenoceptor blocker (p.787) with actions similar to those of prazosin (p.959), but a longer duration of action.

It is used in the management of hypertension (p.802) and in benign prostatic hyperplasia (p.1477) to relieve symptoms of urinary obstruction.

Terazosin is given by mouth as the hydrochloride, but doses are usually expressed in terms of the base. Following oral administration its hypotensive effects are seen within 15 minutes and may last for up to 24 hours, permitting once daily dosage.

To avoid the risk of collapse which may occur in some patients after the first dose the initial dose for both hypertension and benign prostatic hyperplasia is 1 mg of terazosin at bedtime, increasing gradually at intervals of 7 days according to the patient's response. For **hypertension** the usual maintenance dose is 2 to 10 mg once daily and the usual maximum dose is 20 mg daily in a single dose or two divided doses. For **benign prostatic hyperplasia** the usual maintenance dose is 5 to 10 mg once daily.

◊ Reviews.
1. Titmarsh S, Monk JP. Terazosin: a review of its pharmacodynamic and pharmacokinetic properties, and therapeutic efficacy in essential hypertension. *Drugs* 1987; **33:** 461–77.
2. Achari R, Laddu A. Terazosin: a new alpha adrenoceptor blocking drug. *J Clin Pharmacol* 1992; **32:** 520–3.

Preparations

Proprietary Preparations (details are given in Part 3)
Aust.: Uroflo; Vicard; *Austral.:* Hytrin; *Belg.:* Hytrin; *Braz.:* Hytrin; *Canad.:* Hytrin; *Denm.:* Sinalfa; *Fr.:* Dysalfa; Hytrine; *Ger.:* Flotrin; Heitrin; *Hong Kong:* Hytrin; *Irl.:* Hytrin; *Israel:* Hytrin; *Ital.:* Ezosina; Itrin; Teraprost; Unoprost; Urodie; *Mex.:* Adecur; Hytrin; *Neth.:* Hytrin; *Norw.:* Sinalfa; *NZ:* Hytrin; *Port.:* Hytrin; *S.Afr.:* Hytrin; *Singapore:* Hytrin; *Spain:* Deflox; Magnurol; *Swed.:* Hytrinex; Sinalfa; *Switz.:* Hytrin BPH; *Thai.:* Hytrin; *UK:* Hytrin; *USA:* Hytrin.

Tertatolol Hydrochloride   (1143-j)

Tertatolol Hydrochloride *(BANM, rINN)*.

S-2395 (tertatolol or tertatolol hydrochloride); SE-2395 (tertatolol or tertatolol hydrochloride). (±)-1-(tert-Butylamino)-3-(thiochroman-8-yloxy)propan-2-ol hydrochloride.
$C_{16}H_{25}NO_2S,HCl = 331.9$.
CAS — 34784-64-0 (tertatolol); 33580-30-2 (tertatolol hydrochloride).

Profile

Tertatolol is a non-cardioselective beta blocker (p.844). It is reported to lack intrinsic sympathomimetic activity.

Tertatolol is given by mouth as the hydrochloride in the management of hypertension (p.802) in single doses of 5 mg daily.

Preparations

Proprietary Preparations (details are given in Part 3)
Belg.: Artex†; *Denm.:* Artexal; *Fr.:* Artex; *Ger.:* Prenalex; *Irl.:* Artexal; *Neth.:* Artex; *Port.:* Artex.

Tezosentan   (20394-e)

Tezosentan *(rINN)*.

N-{6-(2-Hydroxyethoxy)-5-(o-methoxyphenoxy)-2-[2-(1H-tetrazol-5-yl)-4-pyridyl]-4-pyrimidinyl}-5-isopropyl-2-pyridinesulfonamide.
$C_{27}H_{27}N_9O_6S = 605.6$.
CAS — 180384-57-0.

Profile

Tezosentan is an endothelin receptor antagonist under investigation for acute heart failure.

◊ References.
1. Torre-Amione G, *et al.* Hemodynamic effects of tezosentan, an intravenous dual endothelin receptor antagonist, in patients with class III to IV congestive heart failure. *Circulation* 2001; **103:** 973–80.

Thymoxamine Hydrochloride   (9280-a)

Thymoxamine Hydrochloride *(BANM)*.

Moxisylyte Hydrochloride *(BANM, rINNM)*; Moxisilita Clorhidrato. 4-(2-Dimethylaminoethoxy)-5-isopropyl-2-methylphenyl acetate hydrochloride.
$C_{16}H_{25}NO_3,HCl = 315.8$.
CAS — 54-32-0 (thymoxamine [moxisylyte]); 964-52-3 (thymoxamine [moxisylyte] hydrochloride).

NOTE. THY is a code approved by the BP 2001 for use on single unit doses of eye drops containing thymoxamine [moxisylyte] hydrochloride where the individual container may be too small to bear all the appropriate labelling information.
Pharmacopoeias. In Br. and Jpn.

Thymoxamine [moxisylyte] hydrochloride 45.2 mg is approximately equivalent to 40 mg of thymoxamine [moxisylyte].

Pharmacopoeial description

BP 2001: A white, odourless or almost odourless, crystalline powder. Freely soluble in water and in chloroform; soluble in alcohol; practically insoluble in ether and in petroleum spirit. A 5% solution in water has a pH of 4.5 to 5.5. Protect from light.

Adverse Effects

Thymoxamine [moxisylyte] hydrochloride may cause nausea, diarrhoea, headache, vertigo, flushing of the skin, dry mouth, and nasal congestion. Hepatotoxicity has been reported. Overdosage may cause hypotension.

Transient ptosis has occurred occasionally following ophthalmic application. Prolonged erections or priapism have occurred rarely following intracavernosal injection and systemic effects may also occur.

Effects on the liver. Hepatic adverse reactions have been noted with thymoxamine [moxisylyte]. These first appeared in France following its use in benign prostatic hyperplasia, a condition in which relatively high doses were employed (up to 480 mg daily compared with up to 320 mg daily for peripheral vascular disease). Since then the UK Committee on Safety of Medicines has received reports associated with lower doses.[1] Thirteen hepatic reactions, accounting for 17% of all reports of suspected adverse reactions to thymoxamine [moxisylyte], had been received. These comprised 3 cases of hepatic function abnormalities, 3 of jaundice, 4 of cholestatic jaundice, 2 of hepatitis, and 1 of hepatitis with jaundice. In most cases the reaction occurred within 5 weeks of the start of treatment and resolved on drug withdrawal. In 9 cases the dosage of thymoxamine [moxisylyte] was known and varied from 80 to 320 mg daily with 7 patients receiving 160 mg or less daily.
1. Committee on Safety of Medicines/Medicines Control Agency. Hepatic reactions with thymoxamine (Opilon). *Current Problems* 1993; **19:** 11–12.

Precautions

Thymoxamine [moxisylyte] hydrochloride should not be given to patients with active liver disease and should be given with care to patients with diabetes mellitus. Monitoring of liver function is recommended, especially if therapy is prolonged or if high doses are being employed. Intracavernosal injection of thymoxamine [moxisylyte] is contra-indicated in patients with conditions that predispose to priapism.

Interactions

Thymoxamine [moxisylyte] may enhance the effects of antihypertensives and the hypotensive effect of thymoxamine [moxisylyte] may be enhanced by tricyclic antidepressants.

Uses and Administration

Thymoxamine [moxisylyte] is an alpha-adrenoceptor blocker with vasodilating activity that is used by mouth in the treatment of peripheral vascular disease (p.809) and by intracavernosal injection in erectile dysfunction (p.1663).

Thymoxamine [moxisylyte] is used as the hydrochloride but the dose may be expressed in terms of the base.

In the management of **peripheral vascular disease**, the usual dose is the equivalent of 40 mg of thymoxamine [moxisylyte] four times daily by mouth increased if necessary to 80 mg four times daily. It should be withdrawn if there is no response in 2 weeks.

In the management of **erectile dysfunction**, thymoxamine [moxisylyte] is self-administered by intracavernosal injection The initial dose is 10 mg of thymoxamine [moxisylyte] hydrochloride; if this is unsuccessful a dose of 20 mg may be used. Thymoxamine [moxisylyte] should not be injected intracavernosally more than three times each week and there should be at least 24 hours between injections.

Thymoxamine [moxisylyte] has been used locally in the eye to reverse the mydriasis caused by phenylephrine and other sympathomimetics. It has also been used orally in benign prostatic hyperplasia, although such use has been associated with reports of hepatotoxicity; the doses used in prostatic hyperplasia were generally higher than those in peripheral vascular disease.

◊ Reviews.
1. Marquer C, Bressolle F. Moxisylyte: a review of its pharmacodynamic and pharmacokinetic properties, and its therapeutic use in impotence. *Fundam Clin Pharmacol* 1998; **12:** 377–87.

Preparations

BP 2001: Moxisylyte Tablets.

Proprietary Preparations (details are given in Part 3)
Fr.: Carlytene; Icavex; *Irl.:* Opilon; *Ital.:* Arlitene†; *UK:* Erecnos†; Opilon.

Tiadenol   (1360-d)

Tiadenol *(rINN)*.

LL-1558. 2,2'-(Decamethylenedithio)diethanol.
$C_{14}H_{30}O_2S_2 = 294.5$.
CAS — 6964-20-1.
ATC — C10AX03.

Profile

Tiadenol is a lipid regulating drug used in the treatment of hyperlipidaemias (p.800). The usual dose is 1.2 to 2.4 g daily by mouth in divided doses.

Preparations

Proprietary Preparations (details are given in Part 3)
Fr.: Fonlipol; *Ital.:* Eulip†; Tiabrenolo; Tiaden; *Spain:* Endol†.

Tiamenidine Hydrochloride (13336-s)

Tiamenidine Hydrochloride (BANM, USAN, rINNM).

Hoe-42-440; Hoe-440 (tiamenidine). (2-Chloro-4-methyl-3-thienyl)-2-imidazolin-2-ylamine hydrochloride.

$C_8H_{10}ClN_3S,HCl = 252.2$.

CAS — 31428-61-2 (tiamenidine); 51274-83-0 (tiamenidine hydrochloride); 31428-62-3 (tiamenidine hydrochloride).

Profile

Tiamenidine hydrochloride is an alpha₂-adrenoceptor agonist with general properties similar to those of clonidine (p.860). It has been used in the treatment of hypertension.

Ticlopidine Hydrochloride (13343-p)

Ticlopidine Hydrochloride (BANM, USAN, rINNM).

4-C-32; 53-32C; Ticlopidini Hydrochloridum. 5-(2-Chlorobenzyl)-4,5,6,7-tetrahydrothieno[3,2-c]pyridine hydrochloride.

$C_{14}H_{14}ClNS,HCl = 300.2$.

CAS — 55142-85-3 (ticlopidine); 53885-35-1 (ticlopidine hydrochloride).

Pharmacopoeias. In Eur. (see p.vi) and Jpn.

Pharmacopoeial description

Ph. Eur.: A white or almost white, crystalline powder. Sparingly soluble in water and in dehydrated alcohol; practically insoluble in ether; very slightly soluble in ethyl acetate. A 2.5% solution in water has a pH of 3.5 to 4.0.

Adverse Effects and Precautions

Gastrointestinal disturbances and skin rashes are the most commonly reported side-effects associated with ticlopidine therapy. Blood dyscrasias, including neutropenia and thrombotic thrombocytopenic purpura, and haemorrhagic disorders have also occurred. There have been reports of hepatitis and cholestatic jaundice. Blood-lipid concentrations may increase during long-term therapy.

Ticlopidine should not be administered to patients with haematopoietic disorders such as neutropenia or thrombocytopenia, haemorrhagic diathesis or other haemorrhagic disorders associated with a prolonged bleeding time, or conditions with an increased risk of bleeding such as gastrointestinal ulcers, acute cerebral haemorrhage, or severe liver dysfunction. Full blood counts should be performed before starting treatment and every 2 weeks during the first 3 months of therapy. If ticlopidine is discontinued during this period, a full blood count should be performed within 2 weeks of stopping treatment. Consideration should be given to stopping ticlopidine therapy 10 to 14 days before elective surgery.

Effects on the blood. Severe *neutropenia* or *agranulocytosis* may occur in about 1% of patients given ticlopidine[1] and fatal infection has been reported.[2] Neutropenia usually develops within the first three months of therapy and is reversible on discontinuation of ticlopidine, but there has been a report[3] of a delayed reaction that occurred 18 days after ticlopidine was discontinued. Isolated *thrombocytopenia* occurs in about 0.4% of patients and *thrombotic thrombocytopenic purpura*, sometimes fatal, has occurred.[1,4-7] Cases of thrombotic thrombocytopenic purpura and haemolytic uraemic syndrome have also been reported[8,9] with clopidogrel, although the association is less well established.[10] Conversely, good results have been achieved with ticlopidine as a treatment for thrombotic thrombocytopenic purpura,[11,12] but it should only be used with extreme caution.[13] Aplastic anaemia has occurred rarely with ticlopidine[1,14] and with clopidogrel.[15]

1. Love BB, et al. Adverse haematological effects of ticlopidine: prevention, recognition and management. Drug Safety 1998; 19: 89–98.
2. Carlson JA, Maesner JE. Fatal neutropenia and thrombocytopenia associated with ticlopidine. Ann Pharmacother 1994; 28: 1236–8.
3. Farver DK, Hansen LA. Delayed neutropenia with ticlopidine. Ann Pharmacother 1994; 28: 1344–6.
4. Bennett CL, et al. Thrombotic thrombocytopenic purpura associated with ticlopidine: a review of 60 cases. Ann Intern Med 1998; 128: 541–4.
5. Bennett CL, et al. Thrombotic thrombocytopenic purpura after stenting and ticlopidine. Lancet 1998; 352: 1036–7.
6. Steinhubl SR, et al. Incidence and clinical course of thrombotic thrombocytopenic purpura due to ticlopidine following coronary stenting. JAMA 1999; 281: 806–10.
7. Bennett CL, et al. Thrombotic thrombocytopenic purpura associated with ticlopidine in the setting of coronary artery stents and stroke prevention. Arch Intern Med 1999; 159: 2524–8.
8. Bennett CL, et al. Thrombotic thrombocytopenic purpura associated with clopidogrel. N Engl J Med 2000; 342: 1773–7.
9. Oomen PHN, et al. Hemolytic uremic syndrome in a patient treated with clopidogrel. Ann Intern Med 2000; 132: 1006.
10. Hankey GJ. Clopidogrel and thrombotic thrombocytopenic purpura. Lancet 2000; 356: 269–70.

---

11. Vianelli N, et al. Thrombotic thrombocytopenic purpura and ticlopidine. Lancet 1991; 337: 1219.
12. Bobbio-Pallavicini E, et al. Antiplatelet agents in thrombotic thrombocytopenic purpura (TTP): results of a randomized multicenter trial by the Italian Cooperative Group for TTP. Haematologica 1997; 82: 429–35.
13. Rock G, et al. Thrombotic thrombocytopenic purpura treatment in year 2000. Haematologica 2000; 85: 410–19.
14. Yeh S-P, et al. Ticlopidine-associated aplastic anemia: a case report and review of literature. Ann Hematol 1998; 76: 87–90.
15. Trivier J-M, et al. Fatal aplastic anaemia associated with clopidogrel. Lancet 2001; 357: 446.

Effects on the gastrointestinal tract. Diarrhoea is a common side-effect of ticlopidine therapy; it usually occurs during the first few months of therapy and resolves within 1 to 2 weeks without stopping therapy. However, there has been a report[1] of diarrhoea and weight loss of 2 months duration that first presented 2 years after ticlopidine was started; diarrhoea resolved when ticlopidine was withdrawn.

1. Mansoor GA, Aziz K. Delayed chronic diarrhea and weight loss possibly due to ticlopidine therapy. Ann Pharmacother 1997; 31: 870–2.

Effects on the kidneys. A reversible deterioration in renal function has been reported in patients receiving ticlopidine following coronary stent implantation.[1,2] There has also been a report[3] of membranous nephropathy with nephrotic syndrome in a patient receiving clopidogrel.

1. Elsman P, Zijlstra F. Ticlopidine and renal function. Lancet 1996; 348: 273–4.
2. Virdee M, et al. Ticlopidine and renal function. Lancet 1996; 348: 1031–2.
3. Tholl U, et al. Clopidogrel and membranous nephropathy. Lancet 1999; 354: 1443–4.

Effects on the liver. Cholestatic hepatitis has been reported in patients receiving ticlopidine and is usually reversible when ticlopidine is stopped.[1,2] However, there has been a report of persistent cholestasis following ticlopidine withdrawal.[3] A case of granulomatous hepatitis has also been reported.[4] Clopidogrel was substituted for ticlopidine in a patient who had developed raised liver enzymes during ticlopidine treatment;[5] liver enzyme values returned to normal during continued clopidogrel therapy.

1. Cassidy LJ, et al. Probable ticlopidine-induced cholestatic hepatitis. Ann Pharmacother 1995; 29: 30–2.
2. Pérez-Balsa AM, et al. Hepatotoxicity due to ticlopidine. Ann Pharmacother 1998; 32: 1250–1.
3. Colivicchi F, et al. Ticlopidine-induced chronic cholestatic hepatitis: a case report. Curr Ther Res 1994; 55: 929–31.
4. Ruiz-Valverde P, et al. Ticlopidine-induced granulomatous hepatitis. Ann Pharmacother 1995; 29: 633–4.
5. Zeolla MM, Carson JJ. Successful use of clopidogrel for cerebrovascular accident in a patient with suspected ticlopidine-induced hepatotoxicity. Ann Pharmacother 1999; 33: 939–41.

Effects on the lungs. Bronchiolitis obliterans-organising pneumonia developed in a 76-year-old woman receiving ticlopidine and prednisone for temporal arteritis.[1] The condition resolved over several months when ticlopidine was withdrawn.

1. Alonso-Martinez JL, et al. Bronchiolitis obliterans-organizing pneumonia caused by ticlopidine. Ann Intern Med 1998; 129: 71–2.

Interactions

Ticlopidine should be used with caution in patients receiving other drugs, such as anticoagulants and antiplatelets, that increase the risk of bleeding. Ticlopidine may inhibit the metabolism of other drugs that are metabolised in the liver. The clearance of ticlopidine may be reduced by concomitant cimetidine therapy. Corticosteroids may antagonise the effect of ticlopidine on bleeding time.

Anticoagulants. Concomitant use of ticlopidine with anticoagulants may increase the risk of bleeding. However, ticlopidine has been reported to antagonise the effect of *nicoumalone [acenocoumarol]* (see Interactions under Warfarin, p.996).

Antiepileptics. For a report of acute *phenytoin* toxicity in a well-stabilised patient following addition of ticlopidine, see p.361.

Xanthines. For reference to the effect of ticlopidine on *theophylline* half-life, see p.782.

Pharmacokinetics

Ticlopidine is rapidly and almost completely absorbed from the gastrointestinal tract. It is extensively bound to plasma proteins. The terminal half-life during chronic dosing is reported to be about 30 to 50 hours. Ticlopidine is extensively metabolised in the liver. About 60% of a dose is excreted in the urine as metabolites and 25% in the faeces.

◊ References.

1. Desager J-P. Clinical pharmacokinetics of ticlopidine. Clin Pharmacokinet 1994; 26: 347–55.
2. Buur T, et al. Pharmacokinetics and effect of ticlopidine on platelet aggregation in subjects with normal and impaired renal function. J Clin Pharmacol 1997; 37: 108–15.

Uses and Administration

Ticlopidine hydrochloride is an antiplatelet drug used in thromboembolic disorders (p.816). It appears to act by inhibiting adenosine diphosphate-mediated platelet aggregation. It is given prophylactically as an alternative to aspirin in patients at risk of thrombotic stroke (p.813) and in the management of intermittent claudication and ischaemic heart disease. It is also used as an adjunct to aspirin for the prevention of subacute stent occlusion after intracoronary stenting (see Reperfusion and Revascularisation Procedures, p.812). Ticlopidine may also be used to prevent platelet loss during extracorporeal circulatory procedures.

In the prevention of thrombotic stroke, ticlopidine hydrochloride is given in a dose of 250 mg twice daily by mouth, with meals. For the prevention of subacute stent occlusion after intracoronary stenting ticlopidine hydrochloride is given in a dose of 250 mg twice daily for 4 weeks, starting at the time of stent placement.

Regular haematological monitoring is required during ticlopidine therapy (see Adverse Effects and Precautions, above).

◊ References.

1. McTavish D, et al. Ticlopidine: an updated review of its pharmacology and therapeutic use in platelet-dependent disorders. Drugs 1990; 40: 238–59.
2. Flores-Runk P, Raasch RH. Ticlopidine and antiplatelet therapy. Ann Pharmacother 1993; 27: 1090–8.
3. Sharis PJ, et al. The antiplatelet effects of ticlopidine and clopidogrel. Ann Intern Med 1998; 129: 394–405.

Reperfusion and revascularisation procedures. Coronary stents are being used increasingly to treat and prevent restenosis following angioplasty procedures. Thrombotic occlusion commonly complicates their use and patients have been aggressively treated with a combination of antiplatelet drugs and anticoagulants. Recent studies, however, suggest that antiplatelet treatment alone may be adequate if the stent has been positioned correctly and the risk of thrombosis is considered to be low.

In a study[1] comparing a combination of long-term aspirin with 4 weeks treatment with either ticlopidine or phenprocoumon, fewer cardiac events and fewer haemorrhagic complications occurred in the antiplatelet group. At 6-months follow-up,[2] however, there was no significant difference in rates of restenosis or repeat revascularisation between the groups. Similar short-term benefits have also been reported[3] in a study comparing antiplatelet with anticoagulant therapy for 6 weeks following coronary stenting. A larger study[4] also found antiplatelet therapy in the 30 days following coronary stent placement to be beneficial. The rate of stent thrombosis was reduced in the group treated with aspirin and ticlopidine compared with those treated with aspirin and warfarin or aspirin alone. However, the incidence of haemorrhagic complications was not significantly different for the ticlopidine and warfarin groups, but was significantly lower in the group treated with aspirin alone. An earlier small study[5] had suggested that aspirin alone may be as effective as ticlopidine with aspirin.

Shorter courses of ticlopidine for 2 weeks following intracoronary stent placement may reduce the risk of neutropenia caused by the drug without increasing the risk of stent thrombosis.[6]

Ticlopidine has also been reported[7] to improve the long-term patency of saphenous vein bypass grafts used to treat peripheral vascular disease in the legs.

1. Schömig A, et al. A randomized comparison of antiplatelet and anticoagulant therapy after the placement of coronary-artery stents. N Engl J Med 1996; 334: 1084–9.
2. Kastrati A, et al. Restenosis after coronary stent placement and randomization to a 4-week combined antiplatelet or anticoagulant therapy: six-month angiographic follow-up of the Intracoronary Stenting and Antithrombotic Regimen (ISAR) trial. Circulation 1997; 96: 462–7.
3. Bertrand ME, et al. Randomized multicenter comparison of conventional anticoagulation versus antiplatelet therapy in unplanned and elective coronary stenting: the Full Anticoagulation versus Aspirin and Ticlopidine (FANTASTIC) study. Circulation 1998; 98: 1597–1603.
4. Leon MB, et al. A clinical trial comparing three antithrombotic-drug regimens after coronary-artery stenting. N Engl J Med 1998; 339: 1665–71.
5. Hall P, et al. A randomized comparison of combined ticlopidine and aspirin therapy versus aspirin therapy alone after successful intravascular ultrasound-guided stent implantation. Circulation 1996; 93: 215–22.
6. Berger PB, et al. Safety and efficacy of ticlopidine for only 2 weeks after successful intracoronary stent placement. Circulation 1999; 99: 248–53.
7. Becquemin J-P. Effect of ticlopidine on the long-term patency of saphenous-vein bypass grafts in the legs. N Engl J Med 1997; 337: 1726–31.

Preparations

Proprietary Preparations (details are given in Part 3)

Aust.: Thrombodine; Ticlodone†; Tiklid; **Austral.:** Ticlid; Tilodene; **Belg.:** Ticlid; **Braz.:** Ticlobal; **Canad.:** Ticlid; **Fr.:** Ticlid; **Ger.:** Desiticlopidin; Tiklyd; **Hong Kong:** Ticlid; **Israel:** Ticlidil; **Ital.:** Anagregal; Antigreg; Aplaket; Clox; Fluilast; Klodin; Opter-

---

on; Parsilid; Ticlodone; Ticlogi; Ticloproge; Tiklid; *Mex.*: Ticlid; *Norw.*: Ticlid; *NZ:* Ticlid; *Port.*: Isaxion; Movin; Plaquetal; Ticlodix; Tiklyd; Trombopat; *S.Afr.*: Ticlid; *Singapore:* Antigreg; Aplaket; Tacron; Ticlid; Tipidin; *Spain:* Ticlodone; Tiklid; *Swed.*: Ticlid; *Switz.*: Ticlid†; *Thai.*: Aplaket; Ticlid; *UK:* Ticlid; *USA:* Ticlid.

Tienilic Acid (2357-y)

Tienilic Acid (BAN, rINN).
SKF-62698; Ticrynafen (USAN). [2,3-Dichloro-4-(2-thenoyl)phenoxy]acetic acid.
$C_{13}H_8Cl_2O_4S = 331.2$.
CAS — 40180-04-9.
ATC — C03CC02.

Profile
Tienilic acid is a diuretic and was formerly used in the treatment of oedema and hypertension. It has been withdrawn from the market because of reports of severe, sometimes fatal, liver damage.

Tilisolol (3768-k)

Tilisolol (rINN).
N-696 (tilisolol hydrochloride). (±)-4-[3-(tert-Butylamino)-2-hydroxypropoxy]-2-methylisocarbostyril.
$C_{17}H_{24}N_2O_3 = 304.4$.
CAS — 85136-71-6.

Profile
Tilisolol is a non-cardioselective beta blocker (p.844). It is reported to lack intrinsic sympathomimetic activity. It also has direct vasodilator activity.

Tilisolol has been used as the hydrochloride in the management of hypertension.

Timolol Maleate (6323-l)

Timolol Maleate (BANM, USAN, rINNM).
MK-950; Timololi Maleas. (S)-1-tert-Butylamino-3-(4-morpholino-1,2,5-thiadiazol-3-yloxy)propan-2-ol maleate.
$C_{13}H_{24}N_4O_3S, C_4H_4O_4 = 432.5$.
CAS — 26839-75-8 (timolol); 91524-16-2 (timolol hemihydrate); 26921-17-5 (timolol maleate).

NOTE. TIM is a code approved by the BP 2001 for use on single unit doses of eye drops containing timolol maleate where the individual container may be too small to bear all the appropriate labelling information.
Pharmacopoeias. In Chin., Eur. (see p.vi), Int., and US.

Pharmacopoeial description
Ph. Eur.: A white or almost white, crystalline powder or colourless crystals. Soluble in water and in alcohol; practically insoluble in ether. A 2% solution in water has a pH of 3.8 to 4.3. Protect from light.
USP 25: A white to practically white, odourless or practically odourless powder. Soluble in water, in alcohol, and in methyl alcohol; sparingly soluble in chloroform and in propylene glycol; insoluble in cyclohexane and in ether. A 2% solution in water has a pH of 3.8 to 4.3.

Adverse Effects, Treatment, and Precautions
As for beta blockers, p.844.

Effects on the gastrointestinal tract. Sclerosing peritonitis[1] and retroperitoneal fibrosis[2] have been reported in patients receiving timolol.
1. Baxter-Smith DC, *et al.* Sclerosing peritonitis in patient on timolol. *Lancet* 1978; **ii:** 149.
2. Rimmer E, *et al.* Retroperitoneal fibrosis associated with timolol. *Lancet* 1983; **i:** 300.

Effects following ophthalmic use. Treatment with timolol eye drops for glaucoma was associated with depression and bradycardia in a 74-year-old woman.[1] Rapid withdrawal of the eye drops was followed by a rise in blood pressure and neurological signs of stroke. Severe nausea and vomiting which occurred in a woman being treated with timolol eye drops resolved within a few days of withdrawing treatment.[2] Symptoms recurred on rechallenge.
1. Rao MR, *et al.* Systemic hazards of ocular timolol. *Br J Hosp Med* 1993; **50:** 553.
2. Wolfhagen FHJ, *et al.* Severe nausea and vomiting with timolol eye drops. *Lancet* 1998; **352:** 373.

Interactions
The interactions associated with beta blockers are discussed on p.846.

Pharmacokinetics
Timolol is almost completely absorbed from the gastrointestinal tract but is subject to moderate first-pass metabolism. Peak plasma concentrations occur about

1 to 2 hours after a dose. Timolol has low to moderate lipid solubility. Protein binding is reported to be low. A plasma half-life of 4 hours has been reported. Timolol is extensively metabolised in the liver, the metabolites being excreted in the urine together with some unchanged timolol. It crosses the placenta and is distributed into breast milk.

◊ References to the metabolism of timolol being influenced by genetic polymorphism.[1-3]
1. McGourty JC, *et al.* Pharmacokinetics and beta-blocking effects of timolol in poor and extensive metabolizers of debrisoquin. *Clin Pharmacol Ther* 1985; **38:** 409–13.
2. Lewis RV, *et al.* Timolol and atenolol: relationships between oxidation phenotype, pharmacokinetics and pharmacodynamics. *Br J Clin Pharmacol* 1985; **19:** 329–33.
3. Lennard MS, *et al.* Timolol metabolism and debrisoquine oxidation polymorphism: a population study. *Br J Clin Pharmacol* 1989; **27:** 429–34.

Breast feeding. Following instillation of timolol 0.5% eye drops twice daily, concentrations of timolol in breast milk of a lactating woman were approximately six times greater than those in serum, the values being 5.6 and 0.93 nanograms per mL respectively.[1]
1. Lustgarten JS, Podos SM. Topical timolol and the nursing mother. *Arch Ophthalmol* 1983; **101:** 1381–2.

Uses and Administration
Timolol is a non-cardioselective beta blocker (p.844). It is reported to lack intrinsic sympathomimetic and membrane-stabilising activity.

Timolol is used as the maleate in the management of glaucoma (p.1413), hypertension (p.802), angina pectoris (p.791), and myocardial infarction (p.805). It is also used in the prophylactic treatment of migraine (p.449). The hemihydrate is also used.

Eye drops containing timolol maleate or hemihydrate equivalent to 0.25 and 0.5% of timolol are instilled twice daily to reduce **raised intra-ocular pressure** in open-angle **glaucoma** and ocular hypertension. Once-daily instillation may suffice when the intra-ocular pressure has been controlled. Gel-forming eye drops are also available that are instilled once daily.

In **hypertension** timolol maleate is usually given in initial doses of 10 mg daily by mouth, increased according to response at intervals of 7 or more days; usual maintenance doses are 10 to 40 mg daily in single or divided doses, but doses up to 60 mg daily may be required in some patients.

In **angina pectoris** an initial dose of 5 mg two or three times daily has been recommended, increased at intervals of 3 or more days by no more than 10 mg daily initially and 15 mg daily subsequently, in divided doses. Most patients respond to 35 to 45 mg daily in divided doses, but some patients may require up to 60 mg daily.

In patients who have had a **myocardial infarction** timolol maleate is given in initial doses of 5 mg twice daily for 2 days, starting 7 to 28 days after infarction, and increased subsequently in the absence of any contra-indicating adverse effects, to 10 mg twice daily.

Doses of 10 to 20 mg daily of timolol maleate are used in the prophylaxis of **migraine**.

Reduced doses may be required in renal or hepatic impairment.

Preparations
BP 2001: Timolol Eye Drops; Timolol Tablets;
USP 25: Timolol Maleate and Hydrochlorothiazide Tablets; Timolol Maleate Ophthalmic Solution; Timolol Maleate Tablets.

Proprietary Preparations (details are given in Part 3)
Aust.: Blocadren; Dispatim; Tim-Ophtal; Timabak; Timoftal; Timohexal; Timoptic; *Austral.*: Blocadren†; Optimol; Tenopt; Timoptol; Timoptol-XE; *Belg.*: Blocadren; Timoptol; *Braz.*: Glautimol; Timoptol; *Canad.*: Apo-Timol; Apo-Timop; Beta-Tim†; Blocadren; Novo-Timol; Tim-Ak; Timoptic; *Denm.*: Aquanil; Oftamolol; Optimol; Timacar; *Fin.*: Aquanil; Blocanol; Timosan; *Fr.*: Digaol; Nyolol; Ophtim; Timabak; Timacor; Timoptol; *Ger.*: Arutimol; Chibro-Timoptol; Dispatim; duratimol†; Tim-Ophtal; Timo-COMOD; Timo-Stulln; TimoEDO; Timohexal; Timomann; Timosine; *Hong Kong:* Blocadren; Cusimolol; Nyolol; Timabak; Timoptol; *Irl.*: Blocadren†; Cusimolol; Nyolol; Timoptol; *Israel:* Apotil; Nyolol; Octil; Oftan; Tiloptic; V-Optic; *Ital.*: Blocadren; Cusimolol; Droptimol; Oftimolo; Timoptol; *Mex.*: Blocadren; Cusimolol; Shemol; Timoptol; Timozzard; Tiof; *Mon.*: Gaoptol; *Neth.*: Blocadren†; Loptomit†; Timo-COMOD; Timoptol; *Norw.*: Aquanil; Betim†; Blocadren; Oftan; *NZ:* Timoptol; Hypermol; Timoptol; *Port.*: Blocadren; Cusimolol; Nyolol; Timoglau; Timolen; Timoptol; *S.Afr.*: Blocadren; Glaucosan; Timoptol; *Singapore:* Nyolol; Timabak; Timoptol; *Spain:* Cusimolol; Nyolol†; Timoftol; Unitimoftol; *Swed.*: Aquanil; Blo-

cadren; Optimol; *Switz.*: Blocadren; Oftan; Timisol; Timoptic; *Thai.*: Glauco-Oph; Nyolol; Oftan; Timodrop; Timoptol; Timosil; *UK:* Betim; Blocadren†; Glau-opt; Glaucol; Timoptol; *USA:* Betimol; Blocadren; Timoptic.

Multi-ingredient: *Aust.:* Cosopt; Moducrin; Timpilo; *Austral.*: Timpilo; *Belg.*: Cosopt; *Canad.:* Cosopt; Timolide; Timpilo; *Denm.:* Cosopt; Fotil; Timpilo; *Fin.:* Cosopt; Fotil; Timpilo; *Fr.*: Cosopt; Moducren; Timpilo; *Ger.:* Cosopt; Fotil; Moducrin; Timpilo; TP-Ophtal; *Hong Kong:* Moducren; Timpilo; *Irl.:* Cosopt; Moducren; Prestim; *Israel:* Timpilo; *Ital.:* Cosopt; Equiton; Pilobl8oc; Timicon; *Mex.:* Cosopt; Moducren; Timpilo; *Neth.:* Cosopt; Moducren†; Prestim†; Timpilo; *Norw.:* Cosopt; Fotil; Timpilo; *NZ:* Timpilo; *Port.:* Moducren; Timoglau Plus; *S.Afr.:* Cosopt; Fotil; Timpilo; Moducren; Servatrin; *Singapore:* Timpilo; *Swed.:* Cosopt; Fotil; Timpilo; *Switz.:* Cosopt; Fotil; Moducren; Timpilo; *Thai.:* Fotil; *UK:* Cosopt; Moducren; Prestim; Xalacom; *USA:* Cosopt; Timolide.

Tinzaparin Sodium (14909-z)

Tinzaparin Sodium (BAN, USAN, rINN).
Tinzaparinum Natricum.
CAS — 9041-08-1.
Pharmacopoeias. In Eur. (see p.vi).

Pharmacopoeial description
Ph. Eur.: Tinzaparin sodium is prepared by enzymatic depolymerisation, using heparinase from *Flavobacterium heparinum*, of heparin obtained from the intestinal mucosa of pigs. The majority of the components have a 2-O-sulfo-4-enepyranosuronic acid structure at the non-reducing end and a 2-N,6-O-disulfo-D-glucosamine structure at the reducing end of their chain. The mass-average molecular mass ranges between 5500 and 7500, with a characteristic value of about 6500. The mass percentage of chains lower than 2000 is not more than 10%. The degree of sulfation is 1.8 to 2.5 per disaccharide unit.
The potency is not less than 70 units and not more than 120 units of anti-factor Xa activity per mg with reference to the dried substance and the ratio of anti-factor Xa activity to anti-factor IIa (antithrombin) activity is between 1.5 and 2.5.

Units
As for Low-molecular-weight Heparins, p.923.

Adverse Effects, Treatment, and Precautions
As for Low-molecular-weight Heparins, p.923.

Severe bleeding with tinzaparin sodium may be reduced by the slow intravenous injection of protamine sulfate; 1 mg of protamine sulfate is stated to inhibit the effects of 100 units of tinzaparin sodium.

Interactions
As for Low-molecular-weight Heparins, p.924.

Pharmacokinetics
Tinzaparin sodium is absorbed following subcutaneous injection with a bioavailability of about 90%. Peak plasma activity is reached within 4 to 6 hours. The elimination half-life is about 90 minutes but detectable anti-factor Xa activity persists for up to 24 hours.

Uses and Administration
Tinzaparin sodium is a low-molecular-weight heparin (p.923) with anticoagulant properties. It is used in the treatment and prophylaxis of venous thromboembolism (p.817) and to prevent clotting during extracorporeal circulation.

For prophylaxis of **venous thromboembolism** during general surgical procedures 3500 units of tinzaparin sodium are given by subcutaneous injection 2 hours before the procedure, followed by 3500 units once daily for 7 to 10 days. In patients undergoing orthopaedic surgery a dose of 50 units per kg body-weight has been recommended; alternatively, a dose of 4500 units may be given 12 hours before surgery, followed by 4500 units once daily. For the treatment of venous thromboembolism tinzaparin sodium is given in a dose of 175 units per kg by subcutaneous injection once daily for at least 6 days and until adequate oral anticoagulation is established.

For prevention of clotting in the extracorporeal circulation during **haemodialysis**, tinzaparin sodium may be administered into the arterial side of the dialyser or intravenously. The dialyser may be primed with 500 to 1000 mL sodium chloride 0.9% containing 5000 units tinzaparin sodium per litre. For dialysis sessions lasting less than 4 hours a single dose of 2000 to 2500 units tinzaparin sodium is given; for longer sessions an initial dose of 2500 units is followed by an infusion of 750 units per hour.

◊ References.
1. Friedel HA, Balfour JA. Tinzaparin: a review of its pharmacology and clinical potential in the prevention and treatment of thrombo-embolic disorders. *Drugs* 1994; **48:** 638–60.
2. Fegan CD. Tinzaparin as an antithrombotic: an overview. *Hosp Med* 1998; **59:** 145–8.

Preparations
Proprietary Preparations (details are given in Part 3)
Aust.: Logiparin; *Belg.:* Innohep; *Canad.:* Innohep; *Denm.:* Innohep; *Fin.:* Innohep; *Fr.:* Innohep; *Ger.:* Innohep; *Irl.:* Innohep; *Ital.:* Innohep†; *Neth.:* Innohep; *Norw.:* Innohep; *NZ:* Innohep; *Port.:* Innohep; *S.Afr.:* Logiparin†; *Singapore:* Innohep; *Spain:* Innohep; *Swed.:* Innohep; *UK:* Innohep; *USA:* Innohep.

Tioclomarol (13347-l)
Tioclomarol *(rINN)*.
LM-550. 3-[5-Chloro-α-(4-chloro-β-hydroxyphenethyl)-2-thenyl]-4-hydroxycoumarin.
$C_{22}H_{16}Cl_2O_4S = 447.3$.
CAS — 22619-35-8.
ATC — B01AA11.

Profile
Tioclomarol is an orally administered coumarin anticoagulant with actions similar to those of warfarin (p.992) and is used in the management of thromboembolic disorders (p.816). The usual initial dose is 4 mg daily, and maintenance doses usually range from 1 to 8 mg daily depending on response.

Preparations
Proprietary Preparations (details are given in Part 3)
Fr.: Apegmone.

Tirilazad Mesilate (5845-q)
Tirilazad Mesilate *(BANM, rINNM)*.
Tirilazad Mesylate *(USAN)*; U-74006F (tirilazad or tirilazad mesilate). 21-[4-(2,6-Di-1-pyrrolidinyl-4-pyrimidinyl)-1-piperazinyl]-16α-methylpregna-1,4,9(11)-triene-3,20-dione monomethanesulfonate hydrate.
$C_{38}H_{52}N_6O_2,CH_4O_3S,xH_2O = 721.0$ (anhydrous).
CAS — 110101-66-1 (tirilazad); 111793-42-1 (tirilazad mesilate); 149042-61-5 (tirilazad mesilate).

Profile
Tirilazad, a lazaroid, is an inhibitor of lipid peroxidation thought to have a cytoprotective effect against radicals produced in response to tissue trauma. It may be used in the prevention of secondary tissue damage in subarachnoid haemorrhage (see Stroke, p.813). It is under investigation in spinal cord injuries (p.1058). It has also been investigated in head injuries and ischaemic stroke.

In subarachnoid haemorrhage the dose is 1.5 mg per kg body-weight of tirilazad mesilate by intravenous infusion every 6 hours for 8 to 10 days, starting within 48 hours of the onset of haemorrhage. Each dose should be infused over 10 to 30 minutes. This dosage regimen is only recommended for males; tirilazad clearance is higher in females than males and this dosage is ineffective in females.

◊ References.
1. Fleishaker JC, *et al.* Evaluation of the pharmacokinetics and tolerability of tirilazad mesylate, a 21-aminosteroid free radical scavenger: multiple-dose administration. *J Clin Pharmacol* 1993; **33:** 182–90.
2. Hulst LK, *et al.* Effect of age and gender on tirilazad pharmacokinetics in humans. *Clin Pharmacol Ther* 1994; **55:** 378–84.
3. The STIPAS Investigators. Safety study of tirilazad mesylate in patients with acute ischemic stroke (STIPAS). *Stroke* 1994; **25:** 418–23.
4. Haley EC, *et al.* Phase II trial of tirilazad in aneurysmal subarachnoid haemorrhage: a report of the Cooperative Aneurysm Study. *J Neurosurg* 1995; **82:** 786–90.
5. Clark WM, *et al.* Lazaroid: CNS pharmacology and current research. *Drugs* 1995; **50:** 971–83.
6. Marshall LF, *et al.* A multicenter trial on the efficacy of using tirilazad mesylate in cases of head injury. *J Neurosurg* 1998; **89:** 519–25.
7. Fleishaker JC, *et al.* Hormonal effects on tirilazad clearance in women: assessment of the role of CYP3A. *J Clin Pharmacol* 1999; **39:** 260–7.

Preparations
Proprietary Preparations (details are given in Part 3)
Aust.: Freedox; *Austral.:* Freedox; *Belg.:* Freedox; *Denm.:* Freedox†; *Fin.:* Freedox; *Norw.:* Freedox; *S.Afr.:* Freedox; *Swed.:* Freedox; *Switz.:* Freedox.

Tirofiban Hydrochloride (19429-c)
Tirofiban Hydrochloride *(BANM, USAN, rINNM)*.
L-700462; MK-383; MK-0383. N-(Butylsulfonyl)-4-[4-(4-piperidyl)butoxy]-L-phenylalanine hydrochloride monohydrate.
$C_{22}H_{36}N_2O_5S,HCl,H_2O = 495.1$.
CAS — 144494-65-5 (tirofiban); 142373-60-2 (anhydrous tirofiban hydrochloride); 150915-40-5 (tirofiban hydrochloride monohydrate);.

Adverse Effects and Precautions
Bleeding is the most common adverse effect of tirofiban and therefore it should not be given to patients who are actively bleeding or to patients at increased risk of haemorrhage, including those with haemorrhagic disorders, cerebrovascular disorders, acute pericarditis, vasculitis, haemorrhagic retinopathy, uncontrolled hypertension, or to those who have recently undergone major surgery or severe trauma. Tirofiban should be discontinued if serious uncontrolled bleeding occurs, or if emergency surgery or thrombolytic therapy is required. Tirofiban should not be given to patients with severe hepatic impairment; dose reduction is recommended for patients with severe renal impairment. Thrombocytopenia may occur and platelet counts should be monitored before and following administration of tirofiban. Other side-effects include nausea, headache, fever, and rashes.

Pharmacokinetics
After stopping an infusion of tirofiban, the antiplatelet effect persists for about 4 to 8 hours. Tirofiban is eliminated largely unchanged in the urine, with some biliary excretion in the faeces. The plasma half-life is about 2 hours. Tirofiban is removed by haemodialysis.

Uses and Administration
Tirofiban hydrochloride is an antiplatelet drug that reversibly inhibits binding of fibrinogen to the glycoprotein IIb/IIIa receptors of platelets. It is given in combination with heparin and aspirin for the management of unstable angina. It is also under investigation in patients undergoing coronary angioplasty. Tirofiban is used as the hydrochloride, but the dose is expressed in terms of the base.

Tirofiban is administered intravenously, at an initial rate of 0.4 µg per kg body-weight per minute for 30 minutes, and then continued at 0.1 µg per kg per minute. The recommended duration of treatment is at least 48 hours. Tirofiban infusion may be continued during coronary angiography, and should be maintained for 12 to 24 hours after angioplasty or atherectomy. The entire duration of treatment should not exceed 108 hours.

Patients with severe renal impairment (creatinine clearance less than 30 mL per minute) should receive half the usual dose.

◊ General references.
1. McClellan KJ, Goa KL. Tirofiban: a review of its use in acute coronary syndromes. *Drugs* 1998; **56:** 1067–80.

◊ Beneficial results have been reported in patients receiving tirofiban in combination with heparin and aspirin. A study[1] comparing tirofiban with heparin in the medical management of unstable angina or non-Q-wave myocardial infarction reported an initial benefit, at 2 days, of reduced risk of refractory ischaemia, myocardial infarction, or death with tirofiban. However, this benefit was not maintained at 7 or 30 days following treatment. In another study,[2] the combination of heparin and tirofiban also reduced the risk of this composite end-point, compared with heparin alone, which was maintained at 6 months. About half of these patients also underwent revascularisation procedures or surgery if required.

Tirofiban has also been studied in patients who undergo angioplasty or atherectomy within 72 hours of presentation with unstable angina or myocardial infarction.[3] Compared with heparin alone, tirofiban with heparin reduced the risk of death, non-fatal myocardial infarction, or repeat revascularisation at 2 and 7 days, but this benefit was not maintained at 30 days following treatment. Follow-up at 6 months showed no reduction in the incidence of restenosis.

1. The Platelet Receptor Inhibition in Ischemic Syndrome Management (PRISM) Study Investigators. A comparison of aspirin plus tirofiban with aspirin plus heparin for unstable angina. *N Engl J Med* 1998; **338:** 1498–1505.
2. The Platelet Receptor Inhibition in Ischemic Syndrome Management in Patients Limited by Unstable Signs and Symptoms (PRISM-PLUS) Study Investigators. Inhibition of the platelet glycoprotein IIb/IIIa receptor with tirofiban in unstable angina and non-Q-wave myocardial infarction. *N Engl J Med* 1998; **338:** 1488–97.
3. Gibson CM, *et al.* Six-month angiographic and clinical follow-up of patients prospectively randomized to receive either tirofiban or placebo during angioplasty in the RESTORE trial. *J Am Coll Cardiol* 1998; **32:** 28–34.

Preparations
Proprietary Preparations (details are given in Part 3)
Austral.: Aggrastat; *Belg.:* Aggrastat; *Denm.:* Aggrastat; *Fin.:* Aggrastat; *Fr.:* Agrastat; *Ger.:* Aggrastat; *Irl.:* Aggrastat; *Ital.:* Aggrastat; *Mex.:* Agrastat; *Neth.:* Aggrastat; *NZ:* Aggrastat; *S.Afr.:* Aggrastat; *Singapore:* Aggrastat; *Spain:* Agrastat; *Swed.:* Aggrastat; *Switz.:* Aggrastat; *UK:* Aggrastat; *USA:* Aggrastat.

Tocainide Hydrochloride (7793-b)
Tocainide Hydrochloride *(BANM, rINNM)*.
W-36095 (tocainide). 2-Aminopropiono-2′,6′-xylidide hydrochloride.
$C_{11}H_{16}N_2O,HCl = 228.7$.
CAS — 41708-72-9 (tocainide); 35891-93-1 (tocainide hydrochloride).
NOTE. Tocainide is *USAN.*
Pharmacopoeias. In *Chin.* and *US.*

Pharmacopoeial description
USP 25: A fine, white, odourless powder. Freely soluble in water and in alcohol; practically insoluble in chloroform and in ether.

Adverse Effects
Tocainide causes severe haematological toxicity leading to neutropenia, agranulocytosis, thrombocytopenia, and aplastic anaemia; fatalities have occurred. Pulmonary toxicity has also proved fatal; patients have developed interstitial pneumonitis, pulmonary fibrosis, and other respiratory disorders.

The most common side-effects are dose-related CNS and gastrointestinal effects including tremor, dizziness, paraesthesia, lightheadedness, blurred vision, and nausea. These may occur particularly in the initial stages of therapy and may be transient. Other less frequent gastrointestinal side-effects include vomiting, anorexia, constipation, and diarrhoea. Various mental changes and ataxia have been reported.

Other adverse effects reported include skin rash, lupus erythematosus, sweating, tinnitus, taste disturbances, and liver disorders.

As with other antiarrhythmics, tocainide can cause various cardiac arrhythmias and disturbances of conduction. Bradycardia and hypotension may occur particularly after intravenous administration.

◊ A review of the adverse effects associated with the class Ib antiarrhythmics tocainide, lignocaine [lidocaine], and mexiletine, with guidelines for the clinical management of toxicity.[1]

1. Denaro CP, Benowitz NL. Poisoning due to class IB antiarrhythmic drugs: lignocaine, mexiletine and tocainide. *Med Toxicol Adverse Drug Exp* 1989; **4:** 412–28.

Effects on the blood. Adverse haematological effects associated with tocainide are serious and have caused fatalities.[1-3] They include agranulocytosis, aplastic anaemia, thrombocytopenia, and neutropenia. The US manufacturer has declared that haematological reactions occur in up to 0.18% of patients and that the mortality rate of patients who develop agranulocytosis is 25%.

These haematological reactions usually occur in the first 12 weeks of treatment and it is therefore recommended that full blood counts are performed weekly during this time and monthly thereafter. Patients should be advised to report promptly any unusual bleeding or bruising, or signs of infection such as fever, sore throat, or chills. The seriousness of these adverse effects limits the use of tocainide.

1. Holmes GI, *et al.* Drug therapy: flecainide and tocainide. *N Engl J Med* 1987; **316:** 344.
2. Volosin K, *et al.* Tocainide associated agranulocytosis. *Am Heart J* 1985; **109:** 1392–3.
3. Morrill GB. Tocainide-induced aplastic anemia. *DICP Ann Pharmacother* 1989; **23:** 90–1.

Effects on the liver. Acute hepatocellular damage in one patient[1] and granulomatous hepatitis in another[2] have been associated with tocainide therapy.

1. Farquhar DL, Davidson NM. Possible hepatotoxicity of tocainide. *Scott Med J* 1984; **29:** 238.
2. Tucker LE. Tocainide-induced granulomatous hepatitis. *JAMA* 1986; **255:** 3362.

The symbol † denotes a preparation no longer actively marketed

Effects on the lungs. Interstitial pneumonitis[1-3] and pulmonary fibrosis[4,5] have been reported in small numbers of patients receiving tocainide.

1. Perlow GM, et al. Tocainide-associated interstitial pneumonitis. Ann Intern Med 1981; 94: 489.
2. Van Natta B, et al. Irreversible interstitial pneumonitis associated with tocainide therapy. West J Med 1988; 149: 91–2.
3. Ahmad S. Tocainide: interstitial pneumonitis. J Am Coll Cardiol 1990; 15: 1458.
4. Subauste CS, et al. Tocainide-induced pulmonary toxicity. Illinois Med J 1988; 174: 287–9.
5. Feinberg L, et al. Pulmonary fibrosis associated with tocainide: report of a case with literature review. Am Rev Respir Dis 1990; 141: 505–8.

Effects on mental state. Confusion, paranoia, and hallucinations have been reported[1-3] in a few patients receiving tocainide at recommended doses; all symptoms resolved on discontinuing tocainide. In one patient the reaction was confirmed by rechallenge with tocainide.

1. Currie P, Ramsdale DR. Paranoid psychosis induced by tocainide. BMJ 1984; 288: 606–7.
2. Harrison DJ, Wathen CG. Paranoid psychosis induced by tocainide. BMJ 1984; 288: 1010–11.
3. Clarke CWF, El-Mahdi EO. Confusion and paranoia associated with oral tocainide. Postgrad Med J 1985; 61: 79–81.

Effects on the skin. The US FDA received 21 reports of severe dermatologic reactions associated with tocainide therapy during 1985 and 1986.[1] These included erythema multiforme, Stevens-Johnson syndrome, and exfoliative dermatitis. The reaction occurred within 3 weeks of starting tocainide in 67% of patients for whom the duration of treatment was given. Seventeen patients recovered on withdrawal of tocainide, 2 patients died, and the outcome was not available for 2 patients.

1. Arrowsmith JB, et al. Severe dermatologic reactions reported after treatment with tocainide. Ann Intern Med 1987; 107: 693–6.

Overdosage. In overdosage with tocainide there may be convulsions, complete heart block, and asystole. Treatment is symptomatic and supportive. Haemodialysis and possibly charcoal haemoperfusion may be helpful. Treatment may need to be continued for a prolonged period due to tocainide's long half-life.

Fatal overdose occurred in a 70-year-old man after taking tocainide 16 g by mouth.[1] Postmortem tocainide concentrations were 384.8 µmol per mL in the blood and 2860 µmol per mL in the urine. Toxic effects included convulsions, complete heart block, multiple ventricular ectopic beats, profound hypotension, evidence of ischaemic cardiac changes, and multiple episodes of asystole which was eventually unresponsive to cardiac pacing.

1. Clarke CWF, El-Mahdi EO. Fatal oral tocainide overdosage. BMJ 1984; 288: 760.

Precautions

Tocainide should not be used in patients with second- or third-degree atrioventricular block in the absence of a pacemaker, or in patients with hypersensitivity to amide-type drugs. It should be used with caution in patients with uncompensated heart failure and in patients receiving other antiarrhythmics. Blood counts should be monitored weekly during the first 12 weeks of therapy and monthly thereafter. Tocainide should be given with caution to patients with impaired renal or hepatic function. Hypokalaemia should be corrected before initiating tocainide therapy.

Interactions

Tocainide is structurally related to lignocaine [lidocaine] and concomitant use may produce additive CNS side-effects. Tocainide is metabolised in the liver and enzyme-inducing drugs may reduce the elimination half-life of tocainide.

Tocainide may have a modest inhibitory effect on theophylline metabolism (p.780).

Antibacterials. *Rifampicin* increased the total clearance and reduced the elimination half-life of tocainide in 8 healthy subjects,[1] probably due to an increase in hepatic metabolism of tocainide.

1. Rice TL, et al. Influence of rifampin on tocainide pharmacokinetics in humans. Clin Pharm 1989; 8: 200–5.

Histamine H$_2$-antagonists. *Cimetidine* has been reported[1] to decrease the bioavailability of tocainide without affecting the renal clearance or half-life. The exact mechanism of the interaction could not be determined but may have been due to reduced absorption of tocainide secondary to a cimetidine-induced increase in gastrointestinal pH; however, no interaction was observed with *ranitidine*.

1. North DS, et al. The effect of histamine-2 receptor antagonists on tocainide pharmacokinetics. J Clin Pharmacol 1988; 28: 640–3.

Pharmacokinetics

Tocainide is readily and almost completely absorbed from the gastrointestinal tract. It is widely distributed throughout the body and is reported to be about 10% bound to plasma proteins.

Tocainide is metabolised to a number of apparently inactive metabolites and is excreted mainly in the urine, 30 to 50% as unchanged drug. It has an elimination half-life of about 10 to 20 hours; renal clearance is reduced in alkaline urine but acidification has no effect on excretion. Its therapeutic effect has been correlated with plasma concentrations of about 3 to 10 µg per mL.

◊ Tocainide exists as 2 optically active enantiomers although a 1:1 racemic mixture is used clinically. The pharmacokinetics of the enantiomers are different;[1-3] the *R*(−)-enantiomer has a faster clearance and shorter elimination half-life than the *S*(+)-enantiomer. Stereoselective metabolism by liver enzymes has been suggested to explain this difference. The slower clearance of the *S*(+)-enantiomer means that the *S:R* plasma concentration ratio will increase with continued administration of tocainide[2] but the clinical significance, if any, has not been established.

In anephric patients[3] both enantiomers are cleared more slowly than in healthy subjects, but the clearance of the *S*(+)-enantiomer shows a greater relative reduction. Haemodialysis effectively removes both enantiomers.[3]

1. Edgar B, et al. The pharmacokinetics of R- and S-tocainide in healthy subjects. Br J Clin Pharmacol 1984; 17: 216P.
2. Thomson AH, et al. Pharmacokinetics of R- and S-tocainide in patients with acute ventricular arrhythmias. Br J Clin Pharmacol 1986; 21: 149–54.
3. McErlane KM, et al. Stereoselective pharmacokinetics of tocainide in human uraemic patients and in healthy subjects. Eur J Clin Pharmacol 1990; 39: 373–6.

Uses and Administration

Tocainide is a class Ib antiarrhythmic (p.787) with actions similar to those of lignocaine [lidocaine] (p.1315) to which it is structurally related. Unlike lignocaine [lidocaine], it undergoes negligible first-pass metabolism and can be given by mouth. Because of its toxicity (see Adverse Effects, above) tocainide is generally restricted to the treatment of life-threatening ventricular **arrhythmias** (p.794) that cannot be treated by other means.

For treatment of chronic arrhythmias tocainide hydrochloride 1.2 g is given by mouth daily, divided in 2 or 3 doses, the dose being adjusted according to the patient's tolerance and response. Doses above 2.4 g daily are not normally required. Treatment should be initiated in hospital under ECG monitoring. Doses may need to be reduced in patients with renal or hepatic insufficiency. Tocainide hydrochloride was also formerly given intravenously for rapid control of acute arrhythmias.

◊ General references.

1. Holmes B, et al. Tocainide: a review of its pharmacological properties and therapeutic efficacy. Drugs 1983; 26: 93–123.
2. Kutalek SP, et al. Tocainide: a new oral antiarrhythmic agent. Ann Intern Med 1985; 103: 387–91.
3. Roden DM, Woosley RL. Tocainide. N Engl J Med 1986; 315: 41–5.

Administration in renal impairment. Tocainide is mainly excreted in the urine, and in patients with renal insufficiency the elimination of tocainide is impaired and the half-life prolonged.[1,2] Alterations of urine pH can cause clinically significant alterations in tocainide excretion in patients with mild to moderate renal insufficiency.[2] It has been recommended[1] that the dose of tocainide should be reduced by 50% in patients with severe renal impairment; smaller reductions may be necessary in patients with less severe renal impairment.

Haemodialysis has been reported[1] to remove 25% of tocainide present in the body and a half-life of 8.5 hours was reported; patients may need a supplemental dose of tocainide following haemodialysis.

1. Wiegers U, et al. Pharmacokinetics of tocainide in patients with renal dysfunction and during haemodialysis. Eur J Clin Pharmacol 1983; 24: 503–7.
2. Braun J, et al. Pharmacokinetics of tocainide in patients with severe renal failure. Eur J Clin Pharmacol 1985; 28: 665–70.

Preparations

USP 25: Tocainide Hydrochloride Tablets.

Proprietary Preparations (details are given in Part 3)
Canad.: Tonocard; *Ger.:* Xylotocan; *Hong Kong:* Tonocard; *Irl.:* Tonocard†; *Neth.:* Tonocard; *Swed.:* Tonocard; *Thai.:* Tonocard; *UK:* Tonocard†; *USA:* Tonocard.

Tocoferil Nicotinate (7899-j)

Tocopheryl Nicotinate; Vitamin E Nicotinate. (±)-α-Tocopherol nicotinate.

$C_{35}H_{53}NO_3 = 535.8.$
CAS — 51898-34-1; 16676-75-8.
Pharmacopoeias. In Jpn.

Profile

Tocoferil nicotinate is a lipid regulating drug and a vasodilator. It is used in the treatment of hyperlipidaemias (p.800). The usual dose is 100 to 200 mg three times daily by mouth.

Preparations

Proprietary Preparations (details are given in Part 3)
Hong Kong: Hijuven; *Jpn:* Juvela; *Port.:* Nicojuvel; Reoferol; *Spain:* Disclar†; Vitaber PP + E†; *Thai.:* Hijuven.
Multi-ingredient: *Fr.:* Anaphase; *Ital.:* Evitex; *Spain:* Evitex A E Fuerte.

Tocofibrate (3916-y)

Tocofibrate (rINN).
2,5,7,8-Tetramethyl-2-(4,8,12-trimethyltridecyl)-6-chromanyl 2-(4-chlorophenoxy)-2-methylpropionate.
$C_{39}H_{59}ClO_4 = 627.3.$
CAS — 50465-39-9.

Profile

Tocofibrate, a fibric acid derivative (see Bezafibrate, p.849), is a lipid regulating drug that has been used in the treatment of hyperlipidaemias.

Preparations

Proprietary Preparations (details are given in Part 3)
Spain: Transferal†.

Todralazine Hydrochloride (13358-z)

Todralazine Hydrochloride (BANM, pINNM).
BT-621; CEPH; Ecarazine Hydrochloride. Ethyl 3-(phthalazin-1-yl)carbazate hydrochloride monohydrate.
$C_{11}H_{12}N_4O_2,HCl,H_2O = 286.7.$
CAS — 14679-73-3 (todralazine); 3778-76-5 (anhydrous todralazine hydrochloride).
Pharmacopoeias. In Jpn and Pol.

Profile

Todralazine hydrochloride is an antihypertensive structurally related to hydralazine (p.905) and with similar properties.

Tolazoline Hydrochloride (9281-t)

Tolazoline Hydrochloride (BANM, rINNM).
Benzazoline Hydrochloride; Tolazol. Hydrochlor.; Tolazolinium Chloratum. 2-Benzyl-2-imidazoline hydrochloride.
$C_{10}H_{12}N_2,HCl = 196.7.$
CAS — 59-98-3 (tolazoline); 59-97-2 (tolazoline hydrochloride).
Pharmacopoeias. In Aust., It., Pol., and US.

Pharmacopoeial description

USP 25: A white to off-white, crystalline powder. Its solutions are slightly acid to litmus. Soluble 1 in less than 1 of water, 1 in 2 of alcohol, 1 in 3 of chloroform, and 1 in 10 000 of ether.

Adverse Effects

Side-effects of tolazoline include piloerection, headache, flushing, tachycardia, cardiac arrhythmias, tingling, chilliness, shivering, sweating, nausea, vomiting, diarrhoea, and epigastric pain. Orthostatic hypotension or marked hypertension may occur, especially with large doses. Tolazoline stimulates gastric acid and may exacerbate ulcers. Oliguria, haematuria, myocardial infarction, gastrointestinal haemorrhage, thrombocytopenia and other blood dyscrasias have been reported.

Intra-arterial injection has been followed by a burning sensation in the limb.

Effects in the neonate. Hypochloraemic metabolic alkalosis,[1] acute renal failure,[2] and duodenal perforation[3] have been reported in neonates given tolazoline.

1. Adams JM, et al. Hypochloremic metabolic alkalosis following tolazoline-induced gastric hypersecretion. Pediatrics 1980; 65: 298–300.
2. Trompeter RS, et al. Tolazoline and acute renal failure in the newborn. Lancet 1981; i: 1219.
3. Wilson RG, et al. Duodenal perforation associated with tolazoline. Arch Dis Child 1985; 60: 878–9.

Treatment of Adverse Effects

In the event of overdosage hypotension is best treated by keeping the patient recumbent with the head lowered. If necessary the circulation may be maintained by infusion of suitable electrolyte solutions. Hypotension may be treated with ephedrine. Adrenaline [epinephrine] is not suitable for the reversal of hypotension induced by alpha blockers since it may exacerbate the hypotension by stimulating beta receptors.

Precautions

Tolazoline should not be given to patients with ischaemic heart disease, hypotension, or after a cerebrovascular accident. Since tolazoline stimulates gastric secretion of hydrochloric acid, it should not be used in the presence of peptic ulcer disease. Pre-treatment of infants with antacids may prevent gastrointestinal bleeding. Tolazoline should be used with caution in patients with mitral stenosis.

Interactions

Tolazoline should not be administered concomitantly with drugs such as adrenaline [epinephrine] since the hypotensive effect may be potentiated due to unopposed beta-adrenoceptor stimulation. Tolazoline may cause a disulfiram-like reaction if given with alcohol.

Dopamine. For the effect of tolazoline on dopamine, see p.882.

Ranitidine. Intravenous administration of ranitidine reversed the falls in pulmonary and systemic vascular resistances in 12 children who had been given tolazoline as a pulmonary vasodilator.[1]

1. Bush A, et al. Cardiovascular effects of tolazoline and ranitidine. Arch Dis Child 1987; 62: 241–6.

Pharmacokinetics

Tolazoline is absorbed from the gastrointestinal tract. It is more rapidly absorbed after intramuscular injection. A plasma half-life in neonates of 3 to 10 hours has been reported, although it may be as high as about 40 hours and is inversely related to urine output. Tolazoline is rapidly excreted in the urine, largely unchanged.

Uses and Administration

Tolazoline hydrochloride is a vasodilator that has a direct dilator action on the peripheral blood vessels. It has some alpha-adrenoceptor blocking activity and also stimulates smooth muscle in the gastrointestinal tract, increases gastrointestinal secretion, can cause mydriasis, and has a stimulant effect on the heart.

Tolazoline hydrochloride is used to reduce pulmonary artery pressure in persistent pulmonary hypertension in newborn infants with persistent fetal circulation. It has also been used in the treatment of peripheral vascular disease (p.809) and in some ophthalmic conditions.

In pulmonary hypertension in neonates, the usual dose is 1 to 2 mg per kg body-weight over 10 minutes by intravenous infusion followed by 1 to 2 mg per kg per hour thereafter. Infants with reduced urine output may require lower maintenance doses. For additional details on administration in infants, see below.

In peripheral vascular disease doses of 25 to 50 mg have been given four times daily by mouth. Doses of up to 50 mg have been given by subcutaneous, intramuscular, intravenous, or slow intra-arterial injection.

Pulmonary hypertension. Tolazoline and other vasodilators have been tried in persistent pulmonary hypertension in the newborn (p.810) in an attempt to induce selective pulmonary vasodilatation and improve gas exchange. The response is variable and often unsuccessful due to concomitant systemic hypotension, a failure to achieve or sustain pulmonary vasodilatation, and adverse effects, and other therapies such as high-frequency oscillatory ventilation, extracorporeal membrane oxygenation, and inhaled nitric oxide are now more widely used. The high incidence of adverse effects seen in neonates given tolazoline has led to several studies investigating the administration of lower doses. One group suggested that a loading dose of 0.5 mg per kg body-weight given intravenously followed by a continuous infusion of 0.5 mg per kg per hour was more appropriate and safer than standard doses.[1] Another study indicated that constant plasma concentrations of tolazoline can be maintained by a dose of 0.16 mg per kg per hour for each 1-mg per kg loading dose.[2]

1. Monin P, et al. Treatment of persistent fetal circulation syndrome of the newborn: comparison of different doses of tolazoline. Eur J Clin Pharmacol 1987; 31: 569–73.
2. Ward RM, et al. Oliguria and tolazoline pharmacokinetics in the newborn. Pediatrics 1986; 77: 307–15.

Preparations

USP 25: Tolazoline Hydrochloride Injection.

Proprietary Preparations (details are given in Part 3)
Aust.: Vaso-Dilatan; *Austral.:* Priscoline†; *Ger.:* Priscol; *NZ:* Priscoline; *USA:* Priscoline.

Multi-ingredient: *Switz.:* Lunadon.

Torasemide (1272-d)

Torasemide (BAN, rINN).

AC-4464; BM-02015; Torsemide (USAN). 1-Isopropyl-3-(4-m-toluidinopyridine-3-sulphonyl)urea.

$C_{16}H_{20}N_4O_3S = 348.4$.

CAS — 56211-40-6 (torasemide); 72810-59-4 (torasemide sodium).

ATC — C03CA04.

Pharmacopoeias. In US.

Pharmacopoeial description

USP 25: A white to off-white, crystalline powder. Practically insoluble in water and in ether; slightly soluble in alcohol, in methyl alcohol, in 0.1N sodium hydroxide, and in 0.1N hydrochloric acid; very slightly soluble in acetone and in chloroform.

Adverse Effects and Precautions

As for Frusemide, p.893.

Interactions

As for Frusemide, p.894.

Pharmacokinetics

Torasemide is well absorbed from the gastrointestinal tract. Peak serum concentrations are achieved within one hour of administration by mouth. Torasemide is metabolised in the liver and inactive metabolites are excreted in the urine. The elimination half-life of torasemide is approximately 3.5 hours. Torasemide is extensively bound to plasma proteins. In patients with heart failure both hepatic and renal clearance are reduced. In patients with renal impairment, the renal clearance is reduced but total plasma clearance is not significantly altered.

◊ References.
1. Knauf H, Mutschler E. Clinical pharmacokinetics and pharmacodynamics of torasemide. Clin Pharmacokinet 1998; 34: 1–24.

Uses and Administration

Torasemide is a loop diuretic with actions similar to those of frusemide [furosemide] (p.895).

Torasemide is used for oedema associated with heart failure (p.798), including pulmonary oedema, and with renal and hepatic disorders. It is also used in the treatment of hypertension (p.802), either alone or together with other antihypertensives.

Diuresis following oral administration is initiated within 1 hour, reaches a maximum in about 1 to 2 hours, and lasts for up to 8 hours; after intravenous injection its effects are evident within 10 minutes but like oral administration can last up to 8 hours.

In the treatment of **oedema** the usual dose is 5 mg once daily by mouth increased according to response to 20 mg once daily; doses of up to 40 mg daily have been required in some patients. Torasemide may also be given intravenously in usual doses of 10 to 20 mg daily. Higher intravenous doses may sometimes be necessary, especially in oedema of renal origin when an initial dose of 20 mg daily may be increased stepwise as necessary to a maximum of 200 mg daily, although doses should not exceed 40 mg daily in patients with hepatic cirrhosis.

In the treatment of **hypertension** torasemide is given in doses of 2.5 to 5 mg daily by mouth; sources in the USA have suggested that doses of up to 10 mg daily may be employed although in the UK doses above 5 mg are considered unlikely to produce additional benefit.

◊ Reviews.
1. Blose JS, et al. Torsemide: a pyridine-sulfonylurea loop diuretic. Ann Pharmacother 1995; 29: 396–402.
2. Dunn CJ, et al. Torasemide: an update of its pharmacological properties and therapeutic efficacy. Drugs 1995; 49: 121–42.
3. Brater DC. Benefits and risks of torsemide in congestive heart failure and essential hypertension. Drug Safety 1996; 14: 104–120.

Preparations

Proprietary Preparations (details are given in Part 3)
Belg.: Torrem; *Canad.:* Demadex†; *Ger.:* Torem; Unat; *Hong Kong:* Unat; *Ital.:* Diuremid; Diuresix; Toradiur; *Mex.:* Unat; *Neth.:* Torem†; *S.Afr.:* Unat; *Spain:* Dilutol; Isodiur; Sutril; *Swed.:* Torem; *Switz.:* Torem; *UK:* Torem; *USA:* Demadex.

Trandolapril (2831-d)

Trandolapril (BAN, rINN).

RU-44570. Ethyl (2S,3aR,7aS)-1-{(S)-N-[(S)-1-carboxy-3-phenylpropyl]alanyl}hexahydro-2-indolinecarboxylate; (2S,3aR,7aS)-1-{N-[(S)-1-Ethoxycarbonyl-3-phenylpropyl]-L-alanyl}perhydroindole-2-carboxylic acid.

$C_{24}H_{34}N_2O_5 = 430.5$.

CAS — 87679-37-6.

ATC — C09AA10.

Adverse Effects, Treatment, and Precautions

As for ACE inhibitors, p.820.

Interactions

As for ACE inhibitors, p.822.

Pharmacokinetics

Trandolapril acts as a prodrug of the diacid trandolaprilat, its active metabolite. Following oral administration of trandolapril the bioavailability of trandolaprilat is 40 to 60%. Trandolapril is metabolised in the liver to trandolaprilat and to some inactive metabolites. Peak plasma concentrations of trandolaprilat are achieved 4 to 6 hours after an oral dose of trandolapril. Trandolaprilat is more than 80% bound to plasma proteins. About 33% of an oral dose of trandolapril is excreted in the urine, mainly as trandolaprilat, the rest is excreted in the faeces. The effective half-life for accumulation of trandolaprilat is 16 to 24 hours following multiple doses of trandolapril. Impaired renal function decreases the excretion of trandolaprilat.

◊ References.
1. Bevan EG, et al. Effect of renal function on the pharmacokinetics and pharmacodynamics of trandolapril. Br J Clin Pharmacol 1993; 35: 128–35.

Uses and Administration

Trandolapril is an ACE inhibitor (p.820). It is used in the treatment of hypertension (p.802) and in left ventricular dysfunction following myocardial infarction (p.805).

Trandolapril owes its activity to trandolaprilat to which it is converted after oral administration. The haemodynamic effects are seen about 1 hour after an oral dose and the maximum effect occurs after 8 to 12 hours. The haemodynamic action lasts for at least 24 hours, allowing once-daily dosing.

In the treatment of **hypertension** the initial dose is 0.5 mg once daily by mouth. Since there may be a precipitous fall in blood pressure in some patients when starting therapy with an ACE inhibitor, the first dose should preferably be given at bedtime. In patients already receiving diuretic therapy, the diuretic should be discontinued, if possible, 2 to 3 days before starting trandolapril and resumed later if necessary. In patients with co-existing heart failure treatment with trandolapril should begin under close medical supervision. The usual maintenance dose for hypertension is 1 to 2 mg once daily, although up to 4 mg daily may be given, as a single dose or in 2 divided doses.

Following **myocardial infarction**, treatment with trandolapril may be started 3 days after the infarction in an initial dose of 0.5 mg once daily, gradually increased to a maximum of 4 mg once daily.

A reduction in dosage may be necessary in patients with renal impairment.

◊ References.
1. Zannad F. Trandolapril: How does it differ from other angiotensin converting enzyme inhibitors? Drugs 1993; 46 (suppl 2): 172–82.
2. Wiseman LR, McTavish D. Trandolapril: a review of its pharmacodynamic and pharmacokinetic properties, and therapeutic use in essential hypertension. Drugs 1994; 48: 71–90.
3. Køber L, et al. A clinical trial of the angiotensin-converting-enzyme inhibitor trandolapril in patients with left ventricular dysfunction after myocardial infarction. N Engl J Med 1995; 333: 1670–6.
4. Peters DC, et al. Trandolapril: an update of its pharmacology and therapeutic use in cardiovascular disorders. Drugs 1998; 56: 871–93.

Preparations

Proprietary Preparations (details are given in Part 3)
Austral.: Gopten; Odrik; *Braz.:* Gopten; *Canad.:* Mavik; *Denm.:* Gopten; Odrik; *Fin.:* Gopten; *Fr.:* Gopten; Odrik; *Ger.:* Gopten; Udrik; *Irl.:* Gopten; Odrik; *Ital.:* Gopten; Zeddan†; *Jpn:* Odric; Preran; *Mex.:* Gopten; *Neth.:* Gopten; *Norw.:* Gopten; *NZ:* Gopten; Odrik; *Port.:* Gopten; Odrik; *S.Afr.:* Gopten; *Spain:* Gopten; Odrik; *Swed.:* Gopten; *Switz.:* Gopten; *UK:* Gopten; Odrik; *USA:* Mavik.

Multi-ingredient: *Denm.:* Tarka; *Fin.:* Tarka; *Fr.:* Ocadrix; Tarka; *Ger.:* Tarka; Udramil; *Ital.:* Tarka; *Mex.:* Tarka; *Neth.:* Tarka; *S.Afr.:* Tarka; *Spain:* Tarka; Tricen; *Swed.:* Tarka; *Switz.:* Tarka; *UK:* Tarka; *USA:* Tarka.

The symbol † denotes a preparation no longer actively marketed

Trapidil (13366-z)

Trapidil (BAN, rINN).

AR-12008; Trapidilum. 7-Diethylamino-5-methyl-1,2,4-triazo-lo[1,5-a]pyrimidine.
$C_{10}H_{15}N_5 = 205.3$.
CAS — 15421-84-8.
ATC — C01DX11.

Pharmacopoeias. In Eur. (see p.vi) and Jpn.

Pharmacopoeial description

Ph. Eur.: A white or almost white crystalline powder. Freely soluble in water; soluble in dehydrated alcohol and in dichloromethane. Protect from light.

Profile

Trapidil is a vasodilator and an inhibitor of platelet aggregation. It is also an antagonist of platelet-derived growth factor. It is used in the management of ischaemic heart disease in doses of 300 to 600 mg daily, in divided doses, by mouth. It may also be given by intravenous injection. Ischaemic heart disease is discussed under Atherosclerosis (p.793) and the treatment of its clinical manifestations is described under Angina Pectoris (p.791) and Myocardial Infarction (p.805). Trapidil may also be used to prevent restenosis following angioplasty (p.812).

◊ References.
1. Okamoto S, *et al.* Effects of trapidil (triazolopyrimidine), a platelet-derived growth factor antagonist, in preventing restenosis after percutaneous transluminal coronary angioplasty. *Am Heart J* 1992; **123:** 1439–44.
2. Maresta A, *et al.* Trapidil (triazolopyrimidine), a platelet-derived growth factor antagonist, reduces restenosis after percutaneous transluminal coronary angioplasty: results of the randomized, double-blind STARC study. *Circulation* 1994; **90:** 2710–15.
3. Harder S, *et al.* Pharmacokinetics of trapidil, an antagonist of platelet derived growth factor, in healthy subjects and in patients with liver cirrhosis. *Br J Clin Pharmacol* 1996; **42:** 443–9.
4. Yasue H, *et al.* Effects of aspirin and trapidil on cardiovascular events after acute myocardial infarction: Japanese Antiplatelets Myocardial Infarction Study (JAMIS) Investigators. *Am J Cardiol* 1999; **83:** 1308–13.

Preparations

Proprietary Preparations (details are given in Part 3)
Ger.: Rocornal; *Ital.:* Avantrin; Travisco.

Triamterene (2358-j)

Triamterene (BAN, USAN, rINN).

NSC-77625; SKF-8542; Triamterenum; Triantereno. 6-Phenylpteridine-2,4,7-triamine; 2,4,7-Triamino-6-phenylpteridine.
$C_{12}H_{11}N_7 = 253.3$.
CAS — 396-01-0.
ATC — C03DB02.

NOTE. Compounded preparations of triamterene may be represented by the following names:

• Co-triamterzide (BAN)—triamterene 2 parts and hydrochlorothiazide 1 part (w/w)

• Co-triamterzide (USP 25)—triamterene and hydrochlorothiazide.

Pharmacopoeias. In Chin., Eur. (see p.vi), Jpn, and US.

Pharmacopoeial description

Ph. Eur.: A yellow, crystalline powder. Very slightly soluble in water and in alcohol; practically insoluble in ether. Acidified solutions give a blue fluorescence. Protect from light.

USP 25: A yellow, odourless, crystalline powder. Practically insoluble in water, in chloroform, in ether, in benzene, and in dilute alkali hydroxides; very slightly soluble in alcohol, in acetic acid, and in dilute mineral acids; soluble 1 in 30 of formic acid and 1 in 85 of 2-methoxyethanol. Store in airtight containers. Protect from light.

Adverse Effects

As for Amiloride Hydrochloride, p.835. Triamterene has also been reported to cause photosensitivity reactions, increases in uric acid concentrations, and blood dyscrasias. Renal calculi may occur in susceptible patients, and megaloblastic anaemia has been reported in patients with depleted folic acid stores such as those with hepatic cirrhosis. Reversible renal failure, due either to acute interstitial nephritis or to an interaction with NSAIDs (see under Interactions, below) has occurred.

◊ In a postmarketing surveillance study of 70 898 patients[1] taking a combination of triamterene and hydrochlorothiazide the most common adverse effects were fatigue, dizziness, and nausea. Adverse effects necessitated withdrawal in 8.1% of patients. A subgroup analysis of 21 731 patients[2] indicated that

---

hyperkalaemia was more common in elderly patients and in those with diabetes mellitus.
1. Hollenberg NK, Mickiewicz CW. Postmarketing surveillance in 70,898 patients treated with a triamterene/hydrochlorothiazide combination (Maxzide). *Am J Cardiol* 1989; **63:** 37B–41B.
2. Hollenberg NK, Mickiewicz CW. Hyperkalemia in diabetes mellitus: effect of a triamterene-hydrochlorothiazide combination. *Arch Intern Med* 1989; **149:** 1327–30.

Effects on the blood. Case reports of pancytopenia associated with triamterene therapy.[1,2] Some patients had hepatic cirrhosis and the antifolate activity of triamterene was considered responsible.[2]
1. Castellano G, *et al.* Pancitopenia aguda y megaloblastosis medular durante el tratemiento con triamterene de la ascitis causada por cirrosis hepática: aportación de dos casos. *Gastroenterol Hepatol* 1983; **6:** 540–4.
2. Remacha A, *et al.* Triamterene-induced megaloblastosis: report of two new cases, and review of the literature. *Biol Clin Hematol* 1983; **5:** 127–34.

Effects on the kidneys. There have been a number of reports[1-4] of renal calculi containing triamterene or its metabolites, generally in patients taking the drug with hydrochlorothiazide. An abnormal urinary sediment was described which was thought to represent precipitated triamterene.[5] These observations were expanded in a crossover study:[6] abnormal urinary sediment was seen in 14 of 26 patients while taking triamterene but in none while taking amiloride. Triamterene and its metabolites had been identified by others in 181 of 50 000 renal calculi.[7] Triamterene either formed the nucleus of the stone or was deposited with calcium oxalate or uric acid. One-third of the 181 stones were entirely or predominantly composed of triamterene and its metabolites. In a case report, crystal deposition causing intrarenal obstruction and a direct nephrotoxic effect were considered responsible for acute oliguric renal failure following overdosage with triamterene and hydrochlorothiazide.[8] Deposition of triamterene in the urine may also play a part in the development of interstitial nephritis.[6,9]
No evidence of abnormal excretion or metabolism of triamterene has been detected in patients with renal stones,[10,11] but the concentration of the sulfate metabolite has exceeded the apparent maximum solubility.[10-12] It has been suggested that supersaturation of the urine with triamterene and its metabolites could provide suitable nuclei for the crystallisation of calcium oxalate.[12] However, other workers were unable to demonstrate this and suggested that triamterene and its metabolites could become incorporated into the protein matrix of existing stones.[13] In addition, an epidemiological study[14] found no evidence that triamterene use was associated with an increased incidence of renal stones. Some authors[15] have therefore considered that contra-indicating the drug in patients with a history of recurrent renal calculi was not yet warranted.
Triamterene has also been associated with transient decline in renal function and the development of renal failure.[16,17] Several mechanisms may be responsible including interstitial nephritis, intrarenal obstruction by crystalline deposits, and an interaction with NSAIDs (see under Interactions, below).[17] Elderly patients may be particularly at risk.[16]
1. Ettinger B, *et al.* Triamterene-induced nephrolithiasis. *Ann Intern Med* 1979; **91:** 745–6.
2. Socolow EL. Triamterene-induced nephrolithiasis. *Ann Intern Med* 1980; **92:** 437.
3. Gault MH, *et al.* Triamterene urolithiasis. *Can Med Assoc J* 1981; **124:** 1556–7.
4. Grunberg RW, Silberg SJ. Triamterene-induced nephrolithiasis. *JAMA* 1981; **245:** 2494–5.
5. Fairley KF, *et al.* Abnormal urinary sediment in patients on triamterene. *Lancet* 1983; **i:** 421–2.
6. Spence JD, *et al.* Effects of triamterene and amiloride on urinary sediment in hypertensive patients taking hydrochlorothiazide. *Lancet* 1985; **ii:** 73–5.
7. Ettinger B, *et al.* Triamterene nephrolithiasis. *JAMA* 1980; **244:** 2443–5.
8. Farge D, *et al.* Dyazide-induced reversible acute renal failure associated with intracellular crystal deposition. *Am J Kidney Dis* 1986; **8:** 445–9.
9. Anonymous. Triamterene and the kidney. *Lancet* 1986; **i:** 424.
10. Ettinger B. Excretion of triamterene and its metabolite in triamterene stone patients. *J Clin Pharmacol* 1985; **25:** 365–8.
11. Sörgel F, *et al.* Metabolic fate and solubility of triamterene—not an explanation for triamterene nephrolithiasis. *J Pharm Sci* 1986; **75:** 129–32.
12. White DJ, Nancollas GH. Triamterene and renal stone formation. *J Urol (Baltimore)* 1982; **127:** 593–7.
13. Werness PG, *et al.* Triamterene urolithiasis: solubility, pK, effect on crystal formation, and matrix binding of triamterene and its metabolites. *J Lab Clin Med* 1982; **99:** 254–62.
14. Jick H, *et al.* Triamterene and renal stones. *J Urol (Baltimore)* 1982; **127:** 224–5.
15. Woolfson RG, Mansell MA. Does triamterene cause renal calculi? *BMJ* 1991; **303:** 1217–18.
16. Lynn KL, *et al.* Renal failure with potassium-sparing diuretics. *N Z Med J* 1985; **98:** 629–33.
17. Sica DA, Gehr TWB. Triamterene and the kidney. *Nephron* 1989; **51:** 454–61.

Effects on the skin. Photodermatitis has been reported in a patient receiving triamterene.[1] Pseudoporphyria, possibly associated with exposure to sunlight, occurred in a patient with vitiligo during treatment with triamterene and hydrochlorothiazide.[2]
1. Fernández de Corres L, *et al.* Photodermatitis from triamterene. *Contact Dermatitis* 1987; **17:** 114–15.
2. Motley RJ. Pseudoporphyria due to Dyazide in a patient with vitiligo. *BMJ* 1990; **300:** 1468.

Precautions

As for Amiloride Hydrochloride, p.835. Triamterene should also be given with caution to patients with hyperuricaemia or gout, or a history of renal calculi. Patients with depleted folic acid stores such as those with hepatic cirrhosis may be at increased risk of megaloblastic anaemia.

Triamterene may interfere with the fluorescent measurement of quinidine. It may slightly colour the urine blue.

Interactions

As for Amiloride Hydrochloride, p.835.

Digoxin. For a report of the effect of triamterene on digoxin, see p.872.

Dopaminergics. For a report of increased *amantadine* toxicity associated with hydrochlorothiazide and triamterene, see p.1162.

NSAIDs. There have been several reports of renal failure in patients taking triamterene and NSAIDs.[1,2] Both types of drug are nephrotoxic and in combination the effect appears to be additive.[3-5] It has been suggested that the suppression of urinary prostaglandins by NSAIDs could potentiate the nephrotoxic effects of triamterene.[1]
NSAIDs may also antagonise the diuretic action of triamterene.[6]
1. Favre L, *et al.* Reversible acute renal failure from combined triamterene and indomethacin: a study in healthy subjects. *Ann Intern Med* 1982; **96:** 317–20.
2. Härkönen M, Ekblom-Kullberg S. Reversible deterioration of renal function after diclofenac in patient receiving triamterene. *BMJ* 1986; **293:** 698–9.
3. Bailey RR. Adverse renal reactions to non-steroidal anti-inflammatory drugs and potassium-sparing diuretics. *Adverse Drug React Bull* 1988; (Aug.): 492–5.
4. Lynn KL, *et al.* Renal failure with potassium-sparing diuretics. *N Z Med J* 1985; **98:** 629–33.
5. Sica DA, Gehr TWB. Triamterene and the kidney. *Nephron* 1989; **51:** 454–61.
6. Webster J. Interactions of NSAIDs with diuretics and β-blockers: mechanisms and clinical implications. *Drugs* 1985; **30:** 32–41.

Pharmacokinetics

Triamterene is variably but fairly rapidly absorbed from the gastrointestinal tract. The bioavailability has been reported to be about 50%. The plasma half-life has been reported to be about 2 hours. It is estimated to be about 60% bound to plasma proteins. It is extensively metabolised and is mainly excreted in the urine in the form of metabolites with some unchanged triamterene. Triamterene crosses the placental barrier and may be distributed into breast milk.

◊ References.
1. Pruitt AW, *et al.* Variations in the fate of triamterene. *Clin Pharmacol Ther* 1977; **21:** 610–19.
2. Gundert-Remy U, *et al.* Plasma and urinary levels of triamterene and certain metabolites after oral administration to man. *Eur J Clin Pharmacol* 1979; **16:** 39–44.
3. Gilfrich HJ, *et al.* Pharmacokinetics of triamterene after iv administration to man: determination of bioavailability. *Eur J Clin Pharmacol* 1983; **25:** 237–41.
4. Sörgel F, *et al.* Oral triamterene disposition. *Clin Pharmacol Ther* 1985; **38:** 306–12.

Hepatic impairment. Triamterene clearance was markedly decreased in 7 patients with alcoholic cirrhosis and ascites.[1] The diuretic effect lasted for up to 48 hours in cirrhotic patients compared with 8 hours in healthy controls.
1. Villeneuve JP, *et al.* Triamterene kinetics and dynamics in cirrhosis. *Clin Pharmacol Ther* 1984; **35:** 831–7.

Renal impairment. Urinary excretion of triamterene and its metabolite, hydroxytriamterene sulfate, was significantly reduced in patients with renal impairment[1] and in the elderly whose renal function was reduced.[2] Accumulation of the active metabolite was possible in patients with renal impairment.[1]
1. Knauf H, *et al.* Delayed elimination of triamterene and its active metabolite in chronic renal failure. *Eur J Clin Pharmacol* 1983; **24:** 453–6.
2. Williams RL, *et al.* Absorption and disposition of two combination formulations of hydrochlorothiazide and triamterene: influence of age and renal function. *Clin Pharmacol Ther* 1986; **40:** 226–32.

Uses and Administration

Triamterene is a weak diuretic with potassium-sparing properties which has actions and uses similar to those of amiloride (p.835). It produces a diuresis in about 2 to 4 hours, with a duration of 7 to 9 hours. The full therapeutic effect may be delayed until after several days of treatment.

Triamterene adds to the natriuretic but diminishes the kaliuretic effects of other diuretics. It is mainly used, as an adjunct to thiazide diuretics such as hydrochlorothiazide and loop diuretics such as frusemide [furosemide], to conserve potassium in those at risk from hypokalaemia during the treatment of refractory oedema associated with hepatic cirrhosis, heart failure (p.798), and the nephrotic syndrome. It is also used in combination with other diuretics in the treatment of hypertension (p.802).

When triamterene is given alone in the treatment of **oedema**, the dosage range is 150 to 250 mg daily by mouth; 100 mg twice daily, after breakfast and lunch, is considered to be the optimum dose, preferably on alternate days for maintenance therapy. More than 300 mg daily should not be given.

Smaller doses are used initially when other diuretics are also being given. When used with hydrochlorothiazide, for example, in the treatment of **hypertension**, an initial dose of 50 mg of triamterene daily may be employed.

Potassium supplements should not be given.

Preparations

BP 2001: Co-triamterzide Tablets; Triamterene Capsules;
USP 25: Triamterene and Hydrochlorothiazide Capsules; Triamterene and Hydrochlorothiazide Tablets; Triamterene Capsules.

Proprietary Preparations (details are given in Part 3)
Canad.: Dyrenium; **Ger.:** Jatropur†; **Neth.:** Dytac; **Spain:** Urocaudal; **Switz.:** Dyrenium†; **UK:** Dytac; **USA:** Dyrenium.

Multi-ingredient: Aust.: Confit; Dehydrosin†; Diucomb†; Diurid; Dytide H; Hydrotrix; Inderal comp; Resaltex; Salodiur; Tardurol†; Triamteren comp; Triastad HCT; **Austral.:** Dyazide; Hydrene; **Belg.:** Diucomb; Dyta-Urese†; Dytenzide; Maxzide; **Braz.:** Diurana; Iguassina; **Canad.:** Apo-Triazide; Dyazide; Novo-Triamzide; Nu-Triazide; **Fin.:** Furesis comp; Uretren Comp; **Fr.:** Cycloteriam†; Isobar; Prestole; **Ger.:** Beta-Nephral†; Beta-Turfa; Betathiazid; dehydro sanol tri; dehydro tri mite; Diu Venostasin; Diucomb; Diuretikum Verla; Diutensat; Diutensat comp; Dociteren; duradiuret; Dytide H; Esiteren; Furesis comp; Haemiton compositum; Hydrotrix; Hypertorr; Jenateren comp; Manimon; Neotri; Nephral; Propra comp; Resaltex†; Sali-Puren; Thiazid-comp; Tri-Thiazid; Tri-Thiazid Reserpin; Triampur; Triamteren comp; Triamteren-H; Triamteren/HCT; Triarese; triazid; Turfa; Veratide; **Hong Kong:** Apo-Triazide; Dyazide; Triam-Co; Trizid; **Irl.:** Dyazide; Frusene†; **Ital.:** Fluss 40; **Mex.:** Dyazide; **Neth.:** Dyta-Urese; Dytenzide; **NZ:** Dyazide; Triamizide; Trizid; **Port.:** Dyazide; Triam-Tiazida R; **S.Afr.:** Dyazide; Loretic†; Renezide; Urizide; **Singapore:** Apo-Triazide; Dyazide; **Spain:** Salidur; Triniagar; Urocaudal Tiazida; **Switz.:** Diucomb; Dyazide; Dyrenium compositum; Hydrotrix; t/h-basan; **Thai.:** Dinazide; Dyazide; Dyterene; Skezide; **UK:** Dyazide; Dytide; Frusene; Kalspare; Triamaxco; Triamco; **USA:** Dyazide; Maxzide.

Trichlormethiazide   (2359-z)

Trichlormethiazide (rINN).

Trichlormethiazidum. 6-Chloro-3-dichloromethyl-3,4-dihydro-2H-1,2,4-benzothiadiazine-7-sulphonamide 1,1-dioxide.
$C_8H_8Cl_3N_3O_4S_2 = 380.7$.
CAS — 133-67-5.
ATC — C03AA06.

Pharmacopoeias. In Jpn and US.

Pharmacopoeial description

USP 25: A white or practically white, crystalline powder, odourless or with a slight characteristic odour. Soluble 1 in 1100 of water, 1 in 48 of alcohol, 1 in 5000 of chloroform, 1 in about 4 of dimethylformamide, 1 in about 9 of dioxan, and 1 in 1400 of ether; freely soluble in acetone; soluble in methyl alcohol.

Profile

Trichlormethiazide is a thiazide diuretic with properties similar to those of hydrochlorothiazide (p.907). It is used for oedema, including that associated with heart failure (p.798), and for hypertension (p.802).

Diuresis is initiated in about 2 hours, and lasts about 24 hours.

In the treatment of oedema the usual dose by mouth is 1 to 4 mg daily or intermittently. In the treatment of hypertension the usual dose is 2 to 4 mg daily, either alone, or in conjunction with other antihypertensives. In some patients 1 mg daily may be adequate. In children over 6 months of age a dose of 70 µg per kg body-weight daily in one or two doses has been used.

Preparations

USP 25: Trichlormethiazide Tablets.

Proprietary Preparations (details are given in Part 3)
USA: Diurese; Metahydrin; Naqua.

Multi-ingredient: Fin.: Uretren Comp; **Ger.:** Esmalorid; **Spain:** Rulun; **USA:** Metatensin.

The symbol † denotes a preparation no longer actively marketed

Triflusal   (13379-x)

Triflusal (BAN, rINN).

Triflusalum; UR-1501. 2-Acetoxy-4-trifluoromethylbenzoic acid; O-Acetyl-4-(trifluoromethyl)salicylic acid.
$C_{10}H_7F_3O_4 = 248.2$.
CAS — 322-79-2.
ATC — B01AC18.

Pharmacopoeias. In Eur. (see p.vi).

Pharmacopoeial description

Ph. Eur.: A white or almost white powder. Practically insoluble in water; very soluble in dehydrated alcohol; freely soluble in dichloromethane. Store in airtight containers at a temperature not exceeding 25°.

Profile

Triflusal is an inhibitor of platelet aggregation used for the prophylaxis of thromboembolic disorders (p.816) in doses of 300 mg daily by mouth and in maintenance therapy in usual doses of 300 to 900 mg daily.

◊ References.
1. McNeely W, Goa KL. Triflusal. *Drugs* 1998; **55:** 823–33.
2. Cruz-Fernández JM, *et al.* Randomized comparative trial of triflusal and aspirin following acute myocardial infarction. *Eur Heart J* 2000; **21:** 457–65.

Preparations

Proprietary Preparations (details are given in Part 3)
Braz.: Disgren; **Ital.:** Disgren†; Triflux; **Mex.:** Disgren; **Port.:** Tecnosal; **Spain:** Disgren.

Trimetaphan Camsilate   (911-q)

Trimetaphan Camsilate (BAN, rINN).

Méthioplégium; Trimetaphan Camphorsulphonate; Trimetaphan Camsylate; Trimetaphani Camsylas; Trimethaphan Camsylate.   (+)-1,3-Dibenzylperhydro-2-oxothieno[1',2':1,2]thieno[3,4-d]-imidazol-5-ium 2-oxobornane-10-sulphonate;   4,6-Dibenzyl-4,6-diaza-1-thioniatricyclo[6.3.0.0^{3.7}]undecan-5-one 2-oxobornane-10-sulphonate.
$C_{22}H_{25}N_2OS,C_{10}H_{15}O_4S = 596.8$.
CAS — 7187-66-8 (trimetaphan); 68-91-7 (trimetaphan camsilate).

Pharmacopoeias. In It. and Jpn.

Incompatible with thiopental sodium, gallamine triethiodide, iodides, bromides, and strongly alkaline solutions.

Adverse Effects and Treatment
The adverse effects of trimetaphan are mainly due to ganglionic blockade. A reduction in gastrointestinal motility may result in constipation and, on prolonged administration, paralytic ileus. Urinary retention, cycloplegia, mydriasis, tachycardia, precipitation of angina, and gastrointestinal disturbances may occur. Orthostatic hypotension may be severe. Rapid intravenous infusion at rates greater than 5 mg per minute can result in respiratory arrest. Other adverse effects include raised intraocular pressure, dry mouth, hypoglycaemia, hypokalaemia, fluid retention, weakness, urticaria, and itching. Trimetaphan crosses the placenta and can cause paralytic or meconium ileus in the neonate.

If severe hypotension occurs, administration of trimetaphan should be stopped and the patient positioned with the head lower than the feet. A vasopressor may be given cautiously if necessary.

Effects on the eyes. Although trimetaphan may increase intra-ocular pressure, a sudden and dramatic reduction of intra-ocular pressure to very low levels was noted in 5 patients undergoing surgery when the systolic blood pressure was reduced to 60 mmHg with trimetaphan infusion.[1]
1. Dias PLR, *et al.* Effect on the intraocular pressure of hypotensive anaesthesia with intravenous trimetaphan. *Br J Ophthalmol* 1982; **66:** 721–4.

Precautions
Trimetaphan should be avoided in patients with asphyxia or respiratory insufficiency, uncorrected anaemia, shock or hypovolaemia, severe arteriosclerosis, severe ischaemic heart disease, or pyloric stenosis and should only be used with extreme caution in those with impaired hepatic or renal function, degenerative disease of the CNS, Addison's disease, prostatic hyperplasia, glaucoma, cerebral or coronary vascular insufficiency, and diabetes. It should be used with care in elderly or debilitated patients and should be avoided in pregnancy. Owing to a histamine-liberating effect it should be used with caution in allergic subjects.

Interactions
Trimetaphan should be used with caution in patients being treated with other antihypertensives, drugs which depress cardiac function, muscle relaxants, and in those taking corticosteroids. The hypotensive effect is enhanced by general and spinal anaesthetics. Adrenaline [epinephrine] should not be infiltrated locally at the site of incision when trimetaphan is being given since this may antagonise the effect of trimetaphan.

Neuromuscular blockers. For a reference to possible potentiation of neuromuscular blockade by trimetaphan, see Ganglion Blockers, under Interactions of Atracurium, p.1335.

Uses and Administration
Trimetaphan is a ganglion blocker which inhibits the transmission of nerve impulses in both sympathetic and parasympathetic ganglia. The sympathetic blockade produces peripheral vasodilatation. Trimetaphan also has a direct vasodilator effect on peripheral blood vessels. It is used for inducing controlled hypotension during surgical procedures although sodium nitroprusside is usually preferred. It acts rapidly to produce a hypotensive response which persists for about 10 to 15 minutes.

Trimetaphan camsilate is administered by slow intravenous infusion of a solution usually containing 1 mg per mL. The infusion is started at the rate of 3 to 4 mg per minute and then adjusted according to the response of the patient. Blood pressure should be closely monitored and should be allowed to rise before wound closure.

Trimetaphan has also been used for the emergency treatment of hypertensive crises (p.802), especially in the presence of pulmonary oedema or acute dissecting aortic aneurysms, but sodium nitroprusside is often preferred.

Preparations

Proprietary Preparations (details are given in Part 3)
UK: Arfonad.

Trimetazidine Hydrochloride   (9282-x)

Trimetazidine Hydrochloride (BANM, rINNM).

Trimetazidine Dihydrochloride; Trimetazidini Dihydrochloridum; Trimetazine Hydrochloride. 1-(2,3,4-Trimethoxybenzyl)piperazine dihydrochloride.
$C_{14}H_{22}N_2O_3,2HCl = 339.3$.
CAS — 5011-34-7 (trimetazidine); 13171-25-0 (trimetazidine hydrochloride).

Pharmacopoeias. In Eur. (see p.vi) and Jpn.

Pharmacopoeial description

Ph. Eur.: A slightly hygroscopic, white or almost white crystalline powder. Freely soluble in water; sparingly soluble in alcohol. Store in airtight containers.

Profile

Trimetazidine hydrochloride is used in angina pectoris (p.791) and in ischaemia of neurosensorial tissues as in Ménière's disease (p.407); 40 to 60 mg is given daily by mouth in divided doses.

◊ References.
1. McClellan KJ, Plosker GL. Trimetazidine: a review of its use in stable angina pectoris and other coronary conditions. *Drugs* 1999; **58:** 143–57.

Preparations

Proprietary Preparations (details are given in Part 3)
Denm.: Vastarel; **Fr.:** Cardiazidine; Centrophene; Oxygirex; Vastarel; **Hong Kong:** Vastarel; **Irl.:** Vastarel; **Ital.:** Vastarel; **Port.:** Vastarel; **Singapore:** Vastarel; **Spain:** Idaptan; **Thai.:** Vastarel; Vastinol.

Tripamide   (1293-v)

Tripamide (USAN, rINN).

ADR-033; E-614. 4-Chloro-N-(endo-hexahydro-4,7-methanoisoindolin-2-yl)-3-sulphamoylbenzamide.
$C_{16}H_{20}ClN_3O_3S = 369.9$.
CAS — 73803-48-2.

Profile

Tripamide is a diuretic structurally related to indapamide. It is used in the treatment of hypertension.

Preparations

Proprietary Preparations (details are given in Part 3)
Jpn: Normalol†; **Thai.:** Normonal.

Urapidil   (11586-e)

Urapidil (BAN, rINN).

B-66256M. 6-[3-(4-o-Methoxyphenylpiperazin-1-yl)propylamino]-1,3-dimethyluracil.
$C_{20}H_{29}N_5O_3 = 387.5$.
CAS — 34661-75-1.
ATC — C02CA06.

Urapidil Hydrochloride   (14001-k)

Urapidil Hydrochloride (BANM, rINNM).
$C_{20}H_{29}N_5O_3,HCl = 423.9$.
CAS — 64887-14-5.

Adverse Effects and Precautions
Urapidil is reported to be well-tolerated, with adverse effects generally transient and most frequent at the beginning of therapy. Dizziness, nausea, headache, fatigue, orthostatic hypotension, palpitations, nervousness, pruritus, and allergic skin reactions have been reported.

It should be used with care in elderly patients and those with severe hepatic insufficiency. Intravenous urapidil should not be used in patients with aortic stenosis.

Urinary incontinence. A report of enuresis associated with the use of urapidil in 2 elderly patients.[1]

1. Jonville A-P, *et al.* Urapidil and enuresis. *Lancet* 1992; **339:** 688.

Pharmacokinetics

Following oral administration urapidil is rapidly absorbed with a reported bioavailability of 70 to 80%. It is extensively metabolised in the liver, principally by hydroxylation, and excreted mostly in urine, as metabolites and 10 to 20% of unchanged drug. Urapidil is reported to be about 80% bound to plasma proteins. The elimination half-life is reported to be about 4.7 hours following oral administration as capsules and about 2.7 hours following intravenous administration.

◊ Reviews.

1. Kirsten R, *et al.* Clinical pharmacokinetics of urapidil. *Clin Pharmacokinet* 1988; **14:** 129–40.

Uses and Administration

Urapidil is an antihypertensive drug that is reported to block peripheral alpha$_1$-adrenoceptors (p.787) and to have central actions. It produces a reduction in peripheral resistance and a fall in systolic and diastolic blood pressure, usually without reflex tachycardia.

Urapidil is used in the management of hypertension (p.802), including hypertensive crises.

Urapidil is given by mouth as the base and intravenously as the hydrochloride, but doses are usually expressed in terms of the base. Urapidil fumarate has also been given by mouth.

In hypertension doses of 30 to 90 mg are given twice daily by mouth. In hypertensive crises a suggested regimen is to give an initial dose of 25 mg by slow intravenous injection over 20 seconds, repeated if necessary, followed by a maintenance infusion of 9 to 30 mg per hour.

◊ Reviews.

1. Langtry HD, *et al.* Urapidil: a review of its therapeutic potential in the treatment of hypertension. *Drugs* 1989; **38:** 900–40.
2. Dooley M, Goa KL. Urapidil: a reappraisal of its use in the management of hypertension. *Drugs* 1998; **56:** 929–55.

Preparations

Proprietary Preparations (details are given in Part 3)
Aust.: Ebrantil; *Belg.:* Ebrantil; *Braz.:* Ebrantil; *Fr.:* Eupressyl; Mediatensyl; *Ger.:* Alpha-Depressan†; Ebrantil; *Ital.:* Ebrantil; *Neth.:* Ebrantil; *Port.:* Ebrantil; *Spain:* Elgadil; *Switz.:* Ebrantil.

Urokinase (3752-s)

Urokinase *(BAN, USAN, rINN).*

Urokinasum.

CAS — 9039-53-6.

ATC — B01AD04.

Pharmacopoeias. In *Eur.* (see p.vi) and *Jpn.*

Pharmacopoeial description

Ph. Eur.: An enzyme isolated from human urine that activates plasminogen. It consists of a mixture of low (33 000) and high (54 000) molecular mass forms, the high molecular mass form being predominant. The potency is not less than 70 000 international units per mg of protein. A white or almost white, amorphous powder. Soluble in water. Store in airtight containers at a temperature not exceeding 8°. Protect from light.

Stability. Despite a slight fall in thrombolytic activity after 7 days a mixture of heparin with urokinase suitable for maintaining vascular access devices free of thrombi was stable on incubation at 37° for 21 days.[1]

Urokinase is diluted before administration with glucose 5% or sodium chloride 0.9%. A study[2] of the effects of diluent, container, giving set, and drug concentration on adsorption of urokinase found a loss of 15 to 20% of urokinase activity in solutions of glucose 5% containing 1500 units of urokinase per mL stored in polyvinyl chloride (PVC) containers. No loss of activity was measured in solutions of urokinase in sodium chloride 0.9% or in solutions of glucose 5% containing 5000 units of urokinase per mL.

1. Morgan GJ, *et al.* Stability of a heparin urokinase mixture. *Intensive Therapy Clin Monit* 1987; **8:** 189.
2. Patel JP, *et al.* Activity of urokinase diluted in 0.9% sodium chloride injection or 5% dextrose injection and stored in glass or plastic syringes. *Am J Hosp Pharm* 1991; **48:** 1511–14.

Units

The potency of urokinase is expressed in international units. Preparations are assayed using the first International Reference Preparation (1968), a mixture of low-molecular-weight and high-molecular-weight urokinases. The first International Standard for high-molecular-weight urokinase was established in 1989 for use with preparations of this type of urokinase.

Potency used to be expressed in Ploug or Plough units or in CTA units, but these now appear to be obsolete.

Adverse Effects, Treatment, and Precautions

As for Streptokinase, p.976. Serious allergic reactions may be less likely to occur with urokinase than with streptokinase.

Hypersensitivity. Allergic reactions are considered to be less frequent with urokinase than with streptokinase. However, in a series of six patients who had previously been treated with streptokinase,[1] thrombolytic therapy with urokinase for recurrent myocardial infarction was associated with rigors in four patients, two of whom also developed bronchospasm. None of the patients had any history of atopy.

1. Matsis P, Mann S. Rigors and bronchospasm with urokinase after streptokinase. *Lancet* 1992; **340:** 1552.

Transmission of infection. Some preparations of urokinase are produced in cultures of human cells and there is a risk of transmission of infection associated with their use.

Interactions

As for Streptokinase, p.977.

Pharmacokinetics

Following intravenous infusion urokinase is cleared rapidly from the circulation by the liver. A plasma half-life of up to 20 minutes has been reported.

Uses and Administration

Urokinase is a thrombolytic drug. It directly converts plasminogen to fibrinolysin, a proteolytic enzyme which has fibrinolytic effects. The mechanisms of fibrinolysis are discussed further under Haemostasis and Fibrinolysis on p.718. Urokinase affects circulating, unbound plasminogen as well as fibrin-bound plasminogen and thus may be termed a fibrin-nonspecific thrombolytic agent. This action was thought to contribute to the risk of haemorrhage, although currently available fibrin-specific agents, such as alteplase, do not produce less bleeding than nonspecific thrombolytics (see Haemorrhage under Adverse Effects of Streptokinase, p.976).

Urokinase is used similarly to streptokinase (p.977) in the management of thromboembolic disorders including venous thromboembolism (deep-vein thrombosis and pulmonary embolism) (p.817) and acute myocardial infarction (p.805). It is also used in peripheral arterial thromboembolism (p.808) and has a specific use in clearing clots following haemorrhage within the eye. Like streptokinase it is used to clear cannulas and shunts of occluding thrombi.

In the treatment of **pulmonary embolism** urokinase is given by intravenous infusion in initial doses of 4400 units per kg body-weight over 10 minutes, followed by 4400 units per kg per hour for 12 hours. Similar doses are used in **deep-vein thrombosis.** Alternatively, 15 000 units per kg may be given as a bolus injection into the pulmonary artery, repeated if necessary at 24-hour intervals for up to three doses; subsequent doses may be adjusted if necessary.

In acute **myocardial infarction** infusion into the coronary arteries of urokinase in a dose of 6000 units per minute, for up to 2 hours, has been performed; coronary infusion should be preceded by intravenous heparin. Alternatively, urokinase has been given intravenously in usual doses of 2 to 3 million units over 45 to 90 minutes.

In the treatment of **peripheral arterial thromboembolism** urokinase is infused into the clot via a catheter at a rate of 4000 units per minute as a solution containing 2500 units per mL; the catheter is advanced into the remaining occlusion every 2 hours until flow resumes, and is then partially withdrawn and an infusion of 1000 units per minute given until the remaining clot has lysed.

To break down clots within the anterior chamber of the eye following internal haemorrhage (hyphaema), solutions of urokinase have been instilled through an incision and the clot fragments removed by aspiration. A dose of 5000 units dissolved in 2 mL of sodium chloride 0.9% has been employed for irrigation of clots in the anterior chamber.

For the clearance of occluded cannulas and shunts up to 25 000 units in 2 to 3 mL of sodium chloride 0.9%

may be instilled into the affected device and clamped off for 2 to 4 hours; the lysate is then aspirated.

Catheters and cannulas. In a study[1] in 227 paediatric patients with a total of 254 right atrial catheters, occlusion occurred in 58 catheters over 1 year. Clot lysis was achieved in 44 by bolus instillation of 5000 units (1 mL) of urokinase, followed if necessary after 4 hours by a second bolus of 10 000 units in 2 mL. The remaining catheters that remained blocked were infused directly with a solution of urokinase supplying 200 units per kg body-weight per lumen per hour for 24 to 48 hours (or in one patient considered at high risk of intracranial haemorrhage, 100 units per kg per hour) and of the 12 catheters actually studied, 11 were cleared by this low-dose infusion, with a mean infusion time of 28.7 hours. Blood coagulation profiles were not significantly affected by the urokinase infusion.

Of 434 neonates[2] with central venous catheters, thrombosis developed in 26. Urokinase, given as a bolus of 4400 units per kg over 10 minutes followed by continuous infusion of 4400 units per kg per hour, achieved thrombolysis in 16 of the neonates.

1. Bagnall HA, *et al.* Continuous infusion of low-dose urokinase in the treatment of central venous catheter thrombosis in infants and children. *Pediatrics* 1989; **83:** 963–6.
2. Wever MLG, *et al.* Urokinase therapy in neonates with catheter related central venous thrombosis. *Thromb Haemost* 1995; **73:** 180–5.

Empyema. For the use of urokinase in the management of pericardial and thoracic empyema, see under Streptokinase, p.978.

Intracardiac thrombosis. For the use of urokinase in the management of thrombosis associated with prosthetic heart valves, see under Streptokinase, p.978.

Peritonitis. Antibacterial therapy, given intraperitoneally, is the usual treatment for peritonitis in patients on continuous ambulatory peritoneal dialysis (CAPD), but some patients relapse. Thrombolytics have been tried in recurrent or persistent peritonitis in patients on CAPD.[1] In case reports and small studies, urokinase has been given intraperitoneally in typical doses of 5000 to 7500 units, followed by a course of antibacterial treatment. The mode of action of urokinase in these cases is uncertain, although the rationale for using it has been that lysis of fibrin within the peritoneum and/or catheter might expose bacteria protected by it thus allowing antibacterials to act.

An advisory committee on peritonitis management recommended that thrombolytic therapy has only a limited role in treatment of CAPD peritonitis.[2]

1. Worland MA, *et al.* Intraperitoneal thrombolytic therapy for peritoneal dialysis-associated peritonitis. *Ann Pharmacother* 1998; **32:** 1216–20.
2. Keane WF, *et al.* Peritoneal dialysis-related peritonitis treatment recommendations: 1996 update. *Perit Dial Int* 1996; **16:** 557–73.

Preparations

Proprietary Preparations (details are given in Part 3)
Aust.: Abbokinase; Actosolv; Ukidan; *Austral.:* Ukidan; *Belg.:* Actosolv; *Canad.:* Abbokinase; *Denm.:* Trombolysin; *Fr.:* Actosolv; *Ger.:* Actosolv; Alphakinase†; Corase; rheotromb; *Hong Kong:* Ukidan; *Israel:* Abbokinase; Actosolv; Ukidan; *Ital.:* Actosolv; Alfakinasi; Kisolv; Persolv Richter; Purochin; Ukidan; *NZ:* Ukidan; *Port.:* Ukidan†; *S.Afr.:* Ukidan†; *Spain:* Abbokinase†; Uroquidan; *Swed.:* Abbokinase; Ukidan; *Switz.:* Ukidan; *UK:* Ukidan†; *USA:* Abbokinase.

Valsartan (17122-b)

Valsartan *(BAN, USAN, rINN).*

CGP-48933. *N*-[p-(o-1*H*-Tetrazol-5-ylphenyl)benzyl]-*N*-valeryl-L-valine; *N*-Pentanoyl-*N*-[2′-(1*H*-tetrazol-5-yl)biphenyl-4-yl-methyl]-L-valine.

$C_{24}H_{29}N_5O_3 = 435.5.$

CAS — 137862-53-4.

ATC — C09CA03.

Adverse Effects and Precautions

As for Losartan Potassium, p.921. Valsartan is contraindicated in patients with severe hepatic impairment, cirrhosis, or biliary obstruction.

Pharmacokinetics

Valsartan is rapidly absorbed following oral administration, with a bioavailability of about 23%. Peak plasma concentrations of valsartan occur 2 to 4 hours after an oral dose. It is between 94 and 97% bound to plasma proteins. Valsartan is not significantly metabolised and is excreted mainly via the bile as unchanged drug. The terminal elimination half-life is about 5 to 9 hours. Following an oral dose about 83% is excreted in the faeces and 13% in urine.

◊ References.

1. Brookman LJ, *et al.* Pharmacokinetics of valsartan in patients with liver disease. *Clin Pharmacol Ther* 1997; **62:** 272–8.

Uses and Administration

Valsartan is an angiotensin II receptor antagonist with actions similar to those of losartan (p.922). It is used in the management of hypertension (p.802) and is under investigation in heart failure.

Valsartan is administered by mouth. Following an oral dose the hypotensive effect occurs within 2 hours, is maximal within 4 to 6 hours, and persists for over 24 hours. The maximum hypotensive effect is achieved within 2 to 4 weeks.

In hypertension, valsartan is given in an initial dose of 80 mg once daily. This may be increased, if necessary, to 160 mg once daily, although doses of up to 320 mg once daily have been used. A lower initial dose of 40 mg once daily may be used in elderly patients over 75 years, and in those with moderate to severe renal impairment (creatinine clearance less than 20 mL per minute), intravascular volume depletion, or hepatic impairment.

◊ References.
1. Markham A, Goa KL. Valsartan: a review of its pharmacology and therapeutic use in essential hypertension. *Drugs* 1997; **54:** 299–311.

Preparations

Proprietary Preparations (details are given in Part 3)
Aust.: Diovan; *Belg.:* Diovane; *Canad.:* Diovan; *Denm.:* Diovan; *Fin.:* Diovan; *Fr.:* Nisis; Tareg; *Ger.:* Provas; *Hong Kong:* Diovan; *Irl.:* Diovan; *Israel:* Diovan; *Ital.:* Tareg; Valpression; *Mex.:* Diovan; *Neth.:* Diovan; *Norw.:* Diovan; *NZ:* Diovan; *Port.:* Diovan; *S.Afr.:* Diovan; *Singapore:* Diovan; *Spain:* Diovan; Kalpress; Vals; *Swed.:* Diovan; *Switz.:* Diovan; *Thai.:* Diovan; *UK:* Diovan; *USA:* Diovan.

Multi-ingredient: *Aust.:* Co-Diovan; *Belg.:* Co-Diovane; *Canad.:* Diovan HCT; *Denm.:* Diovan Comp; *Fin.:* Diovan Comp; *Fr.:* Cotareg; Nisisco; *Ger.:* Co-Diovan; Provas comp; *Irl.:* Co-Diovan; *Ital.:* Combisartan; Cotareg; *Mex.:* Diovan HCT; *Neth.:* Co-Diovan; *Norw.:* Diovan Comp; *Port.:* Co-Diovan; *S.Afr.:* Co-Diovan; *Singapore:* Co-Diovan; *Spain:* Co-Diovan; Co-Vals; Kalpress Plus; *Swed.:* Diovon Comp; *Switz.:* Co-Diovan; *Thai.:* Co-Diovan; *USA:* Diovan HCT.

Verapamil Hydrochloride (7794-v)

Verapamil Hydrochloride *(BANM, USAN, rINNM)*.

CP-16533-1 (verapamil); D-365 (verapamil); Iproveratril Hydrochloride; Verapamili Hydrochloridum. 5-[*N*-(3,4-Dimethoxyphenethyl)-*N*-methylamino]-2-(3,4-dimethoxyphenyl)-2-isopropylvaleronitrile hydrochloride.

$C_{27}H_{38}N_2O_4,HCl = 491.1.$

CAS — 52-53-9 (verapamil); 152-11-4 (verapamil hydrochloride).

Pharmacopoeias. In Chin., Eur. (see p.vi), Int., Jpn, and US.

Pharmacopoeial description
Ph. Eur.: A white, crystalline powder. Soluble in water; sparingly soluble in alcohol; freely soluble in methyl alcohol. A 5% solution in water has a pH of 4.5 to 6.0. Protect from light.

USP 25: A white or practically white, practically odourless, crystalline powder. Soluble in water; sparingly soluble in alcohol; freely soluble in chloroform; practically insoluble in ether. A 5% solution in water has a pH of 4.5 to 6.5. Store in airtight containers. Protect from light.

Incompatibility. Verapamil hydrochloride will precipitate in alkaline solutions. There have been reports of incompatibility with solutions of aminophylline,[1] nafcillin sodium,[2] and sodium bicarbonate.[3]
1. Johnson CE, *et al.* Compatibility of aminophylline and verapamil in intravenous admixtures. *Am J Hosp Pharm* 1989; **46:** 97–100.
2. Tucker R, Gentile JF. Precipitation of verapamil in an intravenous line. *Ann Intern Med* 1984; **101:** 880.
3. Cutie MR. Verapamil precipitation. *Ann Intern Med* 1983; **98:** 672.

Adverse Effects

Treatment with verapamil is generally well tolerated, but adverse effects connected with verapamil's pharmacological effects on cardiac conduction can arise and may be particularly severe in patients with hypertrophic cardiomyopathies. Adverse effects on the heart include bradycardia, atrioventricular block, worsening heart failure, and transient asystole. These effects are more common with parenteral than with oral therapy.

The most troublesome non-cardiac adverse effect is constipation. Nausea may occur but is less frequently reported. Other adverse effects include hypotension, dizziness, flushing, headaches, fatigue, dyspnoea, and peripheral oedema. There have been reports of skin reactions and some cases of abnormal liver function

The symbol † denotes a preparation no longer actively marketed

and hepatotoxicity. Gingival hyperplasia has occurred. Gynaecomastia has been reported rarely.

In overdosage there may be severe cardiotoxicity and profound hypotension.

◊ For discussion of the possibility that calcium-channel blockers might be associated with increased cardiovascular mortality, see under Adverse Effects of Nifedipine, p.940.

Cancer occurrence. See under Adverse Effects of Nifedipine, p.940.

Effects on the cardiovascular system. Verapamil has vasodilating properties and negative inotropic activity and may cause adverse cardiovascular effects with worsening of arrhythmias. As discussed below under Precautions certain cardiac disorders put the patient at risk of severe toxicity.
Some references.
1. Radford D. Side effects of verapamil in infants. *Arch Dis Child* 1983; **58:** 465–6.
2. Perrot B, *et al.* Verapamil: a cause of sudden death in a patient with hypertrophic cardiomyopathy. *Br Heart J* 1984; **51:** 352–4.
3. Kirk CR, *et al.* Cardiovascular collapse after verapamil in supraventricular tachycardia. *Arch Dis Child* 1987; **62:** 1265–6.
4. Mohindra SK, Udeani GO. Long-acting verapamil and heart failure. *JAMA* 1989; **261:** 994.
5. Garratt C, *et al.* Degeneration of junctional tachycardia to pre-excited atrial fibrillation after intravenous verapamil. *Lancet* 1989; **ii:** 219.

Effects on the ears. There have been isolated reports[1] of tinnitus associated with several calcium-channel blockers including nifedipine, nicardipine, nitrendipine, diltiazem, verapamil, and cinnarizine.
1. Narváez M, *et al.* Tinnitus with calcium-channel blockers. *Lancet* 1994; **343:** 1229–30.

Effects on the endocrine system. There have been reports of a few patients developing elevated serum-prolactin concentrations during verapamil therapy;[1,2] one of these patients experienced galactorrhoea.[2]

Hyperglycaemia, metabolic acidosis, hyperkalaemia, and bradycardia have occurred[3] following a single dose of modified-release verapamil in a non-diabetic patient who had previously tolerated regular verapamil.

Verapamil has been reported not to affect the release of calcitonin,[4] thyroxine, tri-iodothyronine, thyrotrophin (TSH), follicle-stimulating hormone (FSH), luteinising hormone (LH), or testosterone when given by mouth;[1] however, intravenous administration has been reported to have an inhibitory effect on the release of FSH, LH, and TSH.[5]
1. Semple CG, *et al.* Calcium antagonists and endocrine status: lack of effect of oral verapamil on pituitary-testicular and pituitary-thyroid function. *Br J Clin Pharmacol* 1984; **17:** 179–82.
2. Gluskin LE, *et al.* Verapamil-induced hyperprolactinemia and galactorrhea. *Ann Intern Med* 1981; **95:** 66–7.
3. Roth A, *et al.* Slow-release verapamil and hyperglycemic metabolic acidosis. *Ann Intern Med* 1989; **110:** 171–2.
4. Amado JA, *et al.* No effect of verapamil on calcium stimulated calcitonin release. *Postgrad Med J* 1987; **63:** 23–4.
5. Barbarino A, De Marinis L. Calcium antagonists and hormone release II: effects of verapamil on basal, gonadotrophin-releasing hormone- and thyrotrophin-releasing hormone-induced pituitary hormone release in normal subjects. *J Clin Endocrinol Metab* 1980; **51:** 749–53.

Effects on the liver. Elevated serum concentrations of liver enzymes and bilirubin have been reported during verapamil therapy.[1-4] Clinical symptoms of hepatotoxicity such as abdominal pain, fever, darkened urine, and malaise may occur.[2-4] These reactions might have been due to a hypersensitivity reaction and were reversible on discontinuing verapamil.
1. Brodsky SJ, *et al.* Hepatotoxicity due to treatment with verapamil. *Ann Intern Med* 1981; **94:** 490–1.
2. Stern EH, *et al.* Possible hepatitis from verapamil. *N Engl J Med* 1982; **306:** 612–13.
3. Nash DT, Feer TD. Hepatic injury possibly induced by verapamil. *JAMA* 1983; **249:** 395–6.
4. Guarascio P, *et al.* Liver damage from verapamil. *BMJ* 1984; **288:** 362–3.

Effects on the mouth. Gingival hyperplasia[1] and oral mucosal injury[2] have been associated with verapamil therapy. A study involving 115 patients who had received nifedipine, diltiazem, or verapamil for at least 3 months indicated that gingival hyperplasia is an important side-effect that may occur with calcium-channel blockers in general.[3]
1. Pernu HE, *et al.* Verapamil-induced gingival overgrowth: a clinical, histologic, and biochemic approach. *J Oral Pathol Med* 1989; **18:** 422–5.
2. Guttenberg SA. Chemical injury of the oral mucosa from verapamil. *N Engl J Med* 1990; **323:** 615.
3. Steele RM, *et al.* Calcium antagonist-induced gingival hyperplasia. *Ann Intern Med* 1994; **120:** 663–4.

Effects on the nervous system. A report of 3 patients who complained of unusual perceptual symptoms, described as painful coldness and numbness or bursting feelings, especially in the legs, in association with oral verapamil therapy.[1]
1. Kumana CR, Mahon WA. Bizarre perceptual disorder of extremities in patients taking verapamil. *Lancet* 1981; **i:** 1324–5.

Effects on the neuromuscular system. A myoclonic, dystonic movement disorder was apparently induced by verapamil in a 70-year-old man.[1]
1. Hicks CB, Abraham K. Verapamil and myoclonic dystonia. *Ann Intern Med* 1985; **103:** 154.

Effects on the peripheral circulation. Persistent disabling burning pain and severe erythema and swelling of the feet occurred in a patient receiving verapamil;[1] it resolved when the drug was discontinued. The condition was diagnosed as secondary erythermalgia, a type of erythromelalgia secondary to a variety of diseases and to vasoactive drugs,[2] including the calcium-channel blocker nifedipine.[1]
1. Drenth JPH, *et al.* Verapamil-induced secondary erythermalgia. *Br J Dermatol* 1992; **127:** 292–4.
2. Drenth JPH, Michiels JJ. Three types of erythromelalgia. *BMJ* 1990; **301:** 454–5.

Effects on the respiratory tract. A patient with a history of bronchial asthma developed symptoms of acute asthma following administration of a modified-release verapamil preparation;[1] it was possible that excipients, notably alginate, may have been responsible for the reaction.
1. Ben-Noun L. Acute asthma associated with sustained-release verapamil. *Ann Pharmacother* 1997; **31:** 593–5.

Effects on sexual function. Impotence was associated with verapamil therapy in 3 out of 14 men. In one patient normal sexual function returned when verapamil was discontinued and a recurrence of impotence was reported when verapamil therapy was re-instituted.[1]
1. King BD, *et al.* Impotence during therapy with verapamil. *Arch Intern Med* 1983; **143:** 1248–9.

Effects on the skin and hair. The commonest skin reactions to verapamil have been rash, pruritus, alopecia, and urticaria;[1] there have been a few reports of erythema multiforme, the Stevens-Johnson syndrome, and exfoliative dermatitis.[1] Hypertrichosis, over many parts of the body, has been reported in a male patient within about one month of starting verapamil therapy.[2] In a female patient who had been prematurely grey for about 40 years administration of verapamil caused portions of the hair to regrow in its original natural black colour.[3]
1. Stern R, Khalsa JH. Cutaneous adverse reactions associated with calcium channel blockers. *Arch Intern Med* 1989; **149:** 829–32.
2. Sever PS. Hypertrichosis and verapamil. *Lancet* 1991; **338:** 1215–16.
3. Read GM. Verapamil and hair colour change. *Lancet* 1991; **338:** 1520.

Extrapyramidal disorders. Tremor (postural and at rest) diagnosed as parkinsonism developed in a 70-year-old patient 4 months after starting treatment with verapamil. A 79-year-old patient developed symptoms including parkinsonism, rigidity, and bradykinesia 2 years after beginning verapamil therapy. Symptoms disappeared or improved considerably when verapamil was discontinued.[1] Calcium-channel blockers have been tried in the treatment of tardive dyskinesia (see under Uses of Nifedipine, p.945).
1. Padrell MD, *et al.* Verapamil-induced parkinsonism. *Am J Med* 1995; **99:** 436.

Haemorrhage. See Effects on the Blood under Adverse Effects of Nifedipine, p.940.

Overdosage. Acute overdosage with verapamil generally produces cardiovascular symptoms[1-3] such as severe bradycardia, heart block, profound hypotension, and diminished peripheral perfusion with loss of peripheral pulses, cyanosis, and cold hands and feet. Overdosage may be fatal.[3] Haematemesis and gastric ulcers have been reported[4] following ingestion of verapamil 3.2 g.

Long-term treatment with verapamil 240 mg daily[5] in a patient with cirrhosis of the liver led to loss of consciousness, cardiogenic shock, cyanosis, hypotension, severe acidosis, hyperkalaemia, hypothermia, and renal failure. The patient recovered following treatment with high doses of dopamine, noradrenaline [norepinephrine], sodium bicarbonate, and sodium chloride.

See also Treatment of Adverse Effects, below.
1. Perkins CM. Serious verapamil poisoning: treatment with intravenous calcium gluconate. *BMJ* 1978; **2:** 1127.
2. Crump BJ, *et al.* Lack of response to intravenous calcium in severe verapamil poisoning. *Lancet* 1982; **ii:** 939–40.
3. Orr GM, *et al.* Fatal verapamil overdose. *Lancet* 1982; **ii:** 1218–19.
4. Miller ARO, Ingamells CJ. Gastrointestinal haemorrhage associated with an overdose of verapamil. *BMJ* 1984; **288:** 1346.
5. Stehle G, *et al.* Cardiogenic shock associated with verapamil in a patient with liver cirrhosis. *Lancet* 1990; **336:** 1079.

Treatment of Adverse Effects

In overdosage with verapamil by mouth the stomach should be emptied by lavage; activated charcoal may be administered. Verapamil is not removed by dialysis. Treatment of cardiovascular effects is supportive and symptomatic. Intravenous infusion of calcium salts is recommended as a specific antagonist to verapamil and may reverse the haemodynamic and electrophysiological effects. A slow intravenous injection or an infusion of calcium gluconate in a dose of 10 to 20 mL of a 10% solution has been suggested; alternatively calcium chloride in a dose of 1 g may be used. If hypotension persists, intravenous administration of a sympathomimetic such as isoprenaline, dopamine, or noradrenaline [norepinephrine] may also be necessary. Bradycardia may be treated with atropine, iso-prenaline, or cardiac pacing.

◊ Although the consequences and management of overdosage with all calcium-channel blockers are similar,[1] non-dihydropy-ridines such as verapamil have been suggested to cause more severe effects and to require more aggressive treatment,[2] including thorough gastrointestinal decontamination and high doses of calcium intravenously.[3] The importance of these measures was also noted in a review of intoxication specifically with verapamil.[4] Other treatment of possible benefit in verapamil overdosage includes glucagon,[5] and the specific antidote fampridine.[6]

Overdosage with modified-release preparations of verapamil may result in prolonged toxicity of delayed onset.[7] Conventional-release preparations may also produce prolonged toxicity; elimination half-life was reported to be prolonged to 15 hours and peak plasma concentrations delayed to 6 to 7 hours in a 59-year-old man following ingestion of 2.4 g of verapamil.[8] Rate-limiting absorption at high doses was considered to be the cause.

Pretreatment with calcium salts has been suggested[9] before intravenous administration of verapamil in patients for whom hypotension might result in serious adverse effects.

1. Kenny J. Treating overdose with calcium channel blockers. *BMJ* 1994; **308**: 992–3.
2. Buckley NA, *et al.* Overdose with calcium channel blockers. *BMJ* 1994; **308**: 1639.
3. Howarth DM, *et al.* Calcium channel blocking drug overdose: an Australian series. *Hum Exp Toxicol* 1994; **13**: 161–6.
4. Hofer CA, *et al.* Verapamil intoxication: a literature review of overdoses and discussions of therapeutic options. *Am J Med* 1993; **95**: 431–8.
5. White CM. A review of potential cardiovascular uses of intravenous glucagon administration. *J Clin Pharmacol* 1999; **39**: 442–7.
6. Stevens JJWM, Ghosh S. Overdose of calcium channel blockers. *BMJ* 1994; **309**: 193.
7. Barrow PM, *et al.* Overdose of sustained-release verapamil. *Br J Anaesth* 1994; **72**: 361–5.
8. Buckley JG, Aronson JK. Prolonged half-life of verapamil in a case of overdose: implications for therapy. *Br J Clin Pharmacol* 1995; **39**: 680–3.
9. Moser LR, *et al.* The use of calcium salts in the prevention and management of verapamil-induced hypotension. *Ann Pharmacother* 2000; **34**: 622–9.

Precautions

Verapamil is contra-indicated in hypotension, in cardiogenic shock, in marked bradycardia, in second- or third-degree atrioventricular block, and in uncompensated heart failure. It is also contra-indicated in the sick-sinus syndrome unless a pacemaker is fitted. There is an increased incidence of adverse cardiac effects in patients with hypertrophic cardiomyopathy. In patients with atrial flutter or fibrillation and an accessory pathway with anterograde conduction, for example Wolff-Parkinson-White syndrome, verapamil may induce severe ventricular tachycardia and some authorities contra-indicate its use in such patients.

Special care is required in using verapamil as an antiarrhythmic in infants as they may be more susceptible to verapamil-induced arrhythmias.

Doses of verapamil should be reduced in patients with impaired liver function.

Sudden withdrawal of verapamil might be associated with an exacerbation of angina.

Muscular disorders. Sudden respiratory failure was believed to have been precipitated by intravenous verapamil therapy in a patient with Duchenne's muscular dystrophy.[1]

1. Zalman F, *et al.* Acute respiratory failure following intravenous verapamil in Duchenne's muscular dystrophy. *Am Heart J* 1983; **105**: 510–11.

Porphyria. Verapamil has been associated with acute attacks of porphyria and is considered unsafe in porphyric patients.

Interactions

Verapamil should be used with caution in combination with other drugs that have antiarrhythmic or beta-blocking effects. The combination of intravenous verapamil with a beta blocker is especially hazardous (see below). Verapamil is extensively metabolised in the liver and interactions may occur with drugs that inhibit or enhance liver metabolism. Verapamil can itself affect the pharmacokinetics of other drugs, particularly by inhibition of the cytochrome P450 isoenzyme CYP3A4 and by inhibition of P-glycoprotein. Increased plasma concentrations of many drugs, including carbamazepine, ciclosporin, digoxin, midazolam, and theophylline may occur, and the plasma concentration of alcohol may also be increased. For

details of these interactions, see under the individual drug monographs.

Analgesics. For a possible interaction of verapamil with *aspirin*, see under Antiplatelets, below.

Antiarrhythmics. Cardiogenic shock and asystole has been described in two patients receiving *flecainide* when verapamil was added to their therapy.[1] Verapamil given intravenously has been reported to cause severe hypotension in patients also receiving *quinidine* by mouth.[2]

1. Buss J, *et al.* Asystole and cardiogenic shock due to combined treatment with verapamil and flecainide. *Lancet* 1992; **340**: 546.
2. Maisel AS, *et al.* Hypotension after quinidine plus verapamil. *N Engl J Med* 1985; **312**: 167–70.

Antibacterials. Acute verapamil toxicity manifested by complete heart block has been reported in a patient following the administration of *ceftriaxone* and *clindamycin*.[1] Displacement of verapamil from binding sites was postulated as the probable mechanism of action. *Rifampicin* is an enzyme-inducing drug and has been reported[2,3] to reduce plasma-verapamil concentrations. A verapamil dose of 1920 mg was required to control supraventricular tachycardia in a patient also taking rifampicin[3] and when rifampicin was withdrawn the plasma-verapamil concentration 9 days later was almost four times higher. A patient taking propranolol and verapamil developed symptomatic bradycardia a few days after starting treatment with *clarithromycin* and on another occasion after starting treatment with *erythromycin*.[4] Inhibition of verapamil metabolism by the antibacterials was proposed as the mechanism for the interaction. A further case of severe hypotension and bradycardia has also been reported[5] in a patient shortly after beginning therapy with clarithromycin and verapamil.

1. Kishore K, *et al.* Acute verapamil toxicity in a patient with chronic toxicity: possible interaction with ceftriaxone and clindamycin. *Ann Pharmacother* 1993; **27**: 877–80.
2. Rahn KH, *et al.* Reduction of bioavailability of verapamil by rifampin. *N Engl J Med* 1985; **312**: 920–1.
3. Barbarash RA. Verapamil-rifampin interaction. *Drug Intell Clin Pharm* 1985; **19**: 559–60.
4. Steenbergen JA, Stauffer VL. Potential macrolide interaction with verapamil. *Ann Pharmacother* 1998; **32**: 387–8.
5. Kaeser YA, *et al.* Severe hypotension and bradycardia associated with verapamil and clarithromycin. *Am J Health-Syst Pharm* 1998; **55**: 2417–18.

Antiepileptics. *Phenobarbital* is a hepatic enzyme-inducing drug and has been reported[1] to increase the clearance of oral and intravenous verapamil and to reduce oral bioavailability in healthy subjects. Plasma protein binding of verapamil was also reduced. Dosage adjustment of verapamil may be needed in patients also taking phenobarbital. Marked reduction in verapamil concentrations has occurred with *phenytoin*.[2]

1. Rutledge DR, *et al.* Effects of chronic phenobarbital on verapamil disposition in humans. *J Pharmacol Exp Ther* 1988; **246**: 7–13.
2. Woodcock BG, *et al.* A reduction in verapamil concentrations with phenytoin. *N Engl J Med* 1991; **325**: 1179.

Antiplatelets. Calcium-channel blockers can inhibit platelet function (see Effects on the Blood under Adverse Effects of Nifedipine, p.940). Concurrent use of verapamil and *aspirin* in an 85-year-old man was considered to be the cause of ecchymoses and retroperitoneal bleeding that developed about 3 weeks after starting treatment with the combination.[1]

1. Verzino E, *et al.* Verapamil-aspirin interaction. *Ann Pharmacother* 1994; **28**: 536–7.

Anxiolytics. For the effect of verapamil on plasma-*buspirone* concentrations, see p.658.

Beta blockers. Oral verapamil and beta blockers have been used together in the treatment of angina and hypertension but both drugs have cardiodepressant activity and the combination, if used at all, must be used with extreme caution; bradycardia, heart block, and left ventricular failure have been reported.[1-4] Bradycardia has also been reported[5] in a patient treated with *timolol* eye drops and oral verapamil. Patients with severe ischaemic heart disease or heart failure are particularly at risk.[6] The risks are increased when verapamil is given intravenously and the interaction is especially hazardous when both verapamil and the beta blocker are given by this route. Treatment with beta blockers should be discontinued for at least 24 hours before administration of intravenous verapamil.[6]

1. Eisenberg JNH, Oakley GDG. Probable adverse interaction between oral metoprolol and verapamil. *Postgrad Med J* 1984; **60**: 705–6.
2. Hutchison SJ, *et al.* β blockers and verapamil: a cautionary tale. *BMJ* 1984; **289**: 659–60.
3. Findlay IN, *et al.* β blockers and verapamil: a cautionary tale. *BMJ* 1984; **289**: 1074.
4. McGourty JC, Silas JH. β blockers and verapamil: a cautionary tale. *BMJ* 1984; **289**: 1624.
5. Pringle SD, MacEwen CJ. Severe bradycardia due to interaction of timolol eye drops and verapamil. *BMJ* 1987; **294**: 155–6.
6. McInnes GT. Interactions that matter: calcium blockers. *Prescribers' J* 1988; **28**: 60–4.

Calcium salts. Calcium salts antagonise the pharmacological response to verapamil and are given intravenously to treat adverse effects of verapamil (see Treatment of Adverse Effects, above). Recurrence of atrial fibrillation has occurred[1] during maintenance verapamil treatment when calcium adipinate and calciferol were given by mouth.

1. Bar-Or D, Yoel G. Calcium and calciferol antagonise effect of verapamil in atrial fibrillation. *BMJ* 1981; **282**: 1585–6.

Histamine H₂-antagonists. Studies in healthy subjects using single doses of verapamil following pretreatment with *cimetidine* for up to 8 days have produced conflicting results. The pharmacokinetics of intravenous verapamil were unaltered by cimetidine in some studies,[1,2] but a 21% reduction in clearance and a 50% increase in the elimination half-life were also reported.[3] The pharmacokinetics of oral verapamil were unchanged in one study[2] but two others[1,4] reported a significant increase in bioavailability. Although one of these studies[1] found the interaction had no clinical effects, the other[4] reported an increased clinical effect in 5 of 6 subjects. The interaction with cimetidine appears to be stereoselective since the oral bioavailability of the *S*-enantiomer increased by 35% and that of the *R*-enantiomer by 15%.[4] The clinical significance of this interaction in patients and during long-term verapamil treatment is unknown, but cimetidine should be used with caution in patients receiving verapamil.

1. Smith MS, *et al.* Influence of cimetidine on verapamil kinetics and dynamics. *Clin Pharmacol Ther* 1984; **36**: 551–4.
2. Abernethy DR, *et al.* Lack of interaction between verapamil and cimetidine. *Clin Pharmacol Ther* 1985; **38**: 342–9.
3. Loi C-M, *et al.* Effect of cimetidine on verapamil disposition. *Clin Pharmacol Ther* 1985; **37**: 654–7.
4. Mikus G, *et al.* Interaction of verapamil and cimetidine: stereo-chemical aspects of drug metabolism, drug disposition and drug action. *J Pharmacol Exp Ther* 1990; **253**: 1042–8.

Lithium. Neurotoxicity has been reported in a patient receiving lithium following the addition of verapamil.[1] Serum-lithium concentrations were still inside the accepted therapeutic range and it was considered that the similar actions of lithium and verapamil on neurosecretory processes may have been responsible. Verapamil has also been reported to decrease serum-lithium concentrations.[2]

1. Price WA, Giannini AJ. Neurotoxicity caused by lithium-verapamil synergism. *J Clin Pharmacol* 1986; **26**: 717–19.
2. Weinrauch LA, *et al.* Decreased serum lithium during verapamil therapy. *Am Heart J* 1984; **108**: 1378–80.

Pharmacokinetics

Verapamil is approximately 90% absorbed from the gastrointestinal tract, but is subject to very considerable first-pass metabolism in the liver and the bioavailability is only about 20%.

Verapamil exhibits bi- or tri-phasic elimination kinetics and is reported to have a terminal plasma half-life of 2 to 8 hours following a single oral dose or after intravenous administration. After repeated oral doses this increases to 4.5 to 12 hours. Verapamil acts within 5 minutes of intravenous administration and in 1 to 2 hours after oral administration; peak plasma concentrations occur 1 to 2 hours after an oral dose. There is considerable interindividual variation in plasma concentrations.

Verapamil is about 90% bound to plasma proteins. It is extensively metabolised in the liver to at least 12 metabolites of which norverapamil has been shown to have some activity. About 70% of a dose is excreted by the kidneys in the form of its metabolites but about 16% is excreted in the bile into the faeces. Less than 4% is excreted unchanged. Verapamil crosses the placenta and is distributed into breast milk.

◊ Reviews.

1. Hamann SR, *et al.* Clinical pharmacokinetics of verapamil. *Clin Pharmacokinet* 1984; **9**: 26–41.
2. Kelly JG, O'Malley K. Clinical pharmacokinetics of calcium antagonists: an update. *Clin Pharmacokinet* 1992; **22**: 416–33.

Breast feeding. Verapamil concentrations in breast milk similar to those found in plasma have been reported[1] in a woman taking verapamil 80 mg four times daily. The maximum concentration measured in breast milk was 300 nanograms per mL. However, the average concentration in milk in another woman[2] taking 80 mg three times daily was 23% of that in serum. The serum concentration of verapamil in the breast-fed child was 2.1 nanograms per mL during treatment and undetectable 38 hours after the last maternal dose. In another patient[3] taking the same dose, the average steady-state concentrations of verapamil and norverapamil in milk were, respectively, 60% and 16% of the concentration in plasma. The ratio between milk and plasma varied during a dosage interval and it is therefore important to know when a sample was obtained if valid conclusions about distribution into breast milk are to be made. No verapamil or norverapamil could be detected in the plasma of the infant.

1. Inoue H, *et al.* Level of verapamil in human milk. *Eur J Clin Pharmacol* 1984; **26**: 657–8.
2. Andersen HJ. Excretion of verapamil in human milk. *Eur J Clin Pharmacol* 1983; **25**: 279–80.
3. Anderson P, *et al.* Verapamil and norverapamil in plasma and breast milk during breast feeding. *Eur J Clin Pharmacol* 1987; **31**: 625–7.

The elderly. Total verapamil clearance was found to be decreased in elderly (61 years of age or older) hypertensive patients compared with that in young patients, and the elimination half-life was prolonged.[1]

1. Abernethy DR, *et al.* Verapamil pharmacodynamics and disposition in young and elderly hypertensive patients: altered electrocardiographic and hypotensive responses. *Ann Intern Med* 1986; **105:** 329–36.

Stereospecificity. Verapamil is used as a racemic mixture. A series of studies have been carried out to determine whether differences in the pharmacokinetics of the *R*- and *S*-isomers of verapamil could account for observed differences in the plasma concentration-response curve following oral and intravenous administration. After intravenous administration, there were pronounced differences in the pharmacokinetics and protein binding of the 2 isomers;[1] the volume of distribution and total systemic clearance of *S*-verapamil were much higher than those of the *R*-isomer although the terminal half-life was similar. After oral administration of a mixture of *R*- and *S*-verapamil, plasma concentrations of the *R*-isomer were found to be substantially higher than those of the *S*-isomer[2] suggesting stereospecific first-pass hepatic metabolism. Following oral dosing total verapamil concentrations thus consist of a smaller proportion of the more potent *S*-isomer accounting for the apparent lower potency of verapamil when given orally. The proportion of *S*-isomer also depends on the oral formulation; modified-release formulations produce lower proportions of *S*-isomer in plasma than conventional formulations.[3] It has been shown[4] that *S*-verapamil is 3.3 times more potent than the racemic mixture and 11 times more potent than *R*-verapamil. Thus it was concluded that the cardiac effects of verapamil are related not to the total plasma-verapamil concentration but to the concentration of the *S*-isomer, and conventional plasma concentration monitoring will be of little value in establishing therapeutic plasma concentrations during multiple oral dosing.

1. Eichelbaum M, *et al.* Pharmacokinetics of (+)-, (−)- and (±)-verapamil after intravenous administration. *Br J Clin Pharmacol* 1984; **17:** 453–8.
2. Vogelgesang B, *et al.* Stereoselective first-pass metabolism of highly cleared drugs: studies of the bioavailability of L- and D-verapamil examined with a stable isotope technique. *Br J Clin Pharmacol* 1984; **18:** 733–40.
3. Karim A, Piergies A. Verapamil stereoisomerism: enantiomeric ratios in plasma dependent on peak concentrations, oral input rate, or both. *Clin Pharmacol Ther* 1995; **58:** 174–84.
4. Echizen H, *et al.* Effects of d,l-verapamil on atrioventricular conduction in relation to its stereoselective first-pass metabolism. *Clin Pharmacol Ther* 1985; **38:** 71–6.

Uses and Administration

Verapamil is a calcium-channel blocker (p.788) and a class IV antiarrhythmic (p.787). Verapamil slows conduction through the atrioventricular node, and thus slows the increased ventricular response rate that occurs in atrial fibrillation and flutter. A decrease in both coronary and peripheral vascular resistance together with a sparing effect on myocardial intracellular oxygen consumption appear to be the modes of action in angina. The decrease in peripheral vascular resistance may explain the antihypertensive effect of verapamil. It is used in the control of supraventricular arrhythmias and in the management of angina pectoris and hypertension. It may also be used in the management of myocardial infarction.

Verapamil may be given intravenously or by mouth as the hydrochloride for the control of supraventricular **arrhythmias**. Intravenous injections should be given under continuous ECG monitoring. When given intravenously a dose of 5 to 10 mg is injected over a period of 2 to 3 minutes; if necessary, a further 5 mg may be injected 5 to 10 minutes after the first. In the USA a second dose of 10 mg given after 30 minutes if required is suggested. Children should be treated with great care; intravenous doses given over at least 2 minutes are: up to 1 year of age, 100 to 200 µg per kg body-weight; children aged 1 to 15 years, 100 to 300 µg per kg (to a maximum dose of 5 mg). The dose may be repeated after 30 minutes if necessary. Smaller doses may be adequate and the injection should be stopped when a response has been obtained.

Oral doses for the treatment of supraventricular arrhythmias are 120 to 480 mg daily in 3 or 4 divided doses, according to the severity of the condition and the patient's response. Oral doses for children are: up to 2 years of age, 20 mg two or three times daily; 2 years and over, 40 to 120 mg two or three times daily according to age and response; great care is still required.

In the management of **angina pectoris**, verapamil hydrochloride is given by mouth in doses of 120 mg three times daily; some patients with angina of effort may respond to 80 mg three times daily, but this lower

dose is not likely to be effective in angina at rest or Prinzmetal's variant angina. Modified-release preparations may be given in doses of up to 480 mg daily.

In **hypertension** the dose of verapamil hydrochloride is generally 160 mg twice daily by mouth with a range of 240 mg to 480 mg daily. Modified-release preparations may be given in similar daily doses. A dose of up to 10 mg per kg body-weight daily in divided doses may be employed for children.

In the management of **myocardial infarction**, verapamil hydrochloride, as a modified-release oral preparation, may be started at least one week after acute infarction (in patients without heart failure) in a dose of 360 mg daily in divided doses.

Doses of verapamil should be reduced to about one-third of the usual dose in patients with impaired liver function.

◊ General reviews.

1. McTavish D, Sorkin EM. Verapamil: an updated review of its pharmacodynamic and pharmacokinetic properties, and therapeutic use in hypertension. *Drugs* 1989; **38:** 19–76.
2. Anonymous. Calcium antagonists for cardiovascular disease. *Drug Ther Bull* 1993; **31:** 81–4.
3. Fisher M, Grotta J. New uses for calcium channel blockers: therapeutic implications. *Drugs* 1993; **46:** 961–75.
4. Brogden RN, Benfield P. Verapamil: a review of its pharmacological properties and therapeutic use in coronary artery disease. *Drugs* 1996; **51:** 792–819.

Administration in the elderly. For a report that the pharmacokinetics of verapamil are altered in the elderly, see Pharmacokinetics, above.

Administration in hepatic impairment. In patients with liver cirrhosis steady-state plasma concentrations of verapamil were double those seen in patients with normal liver function following intravenous administration and 5 times the normal concentration when given by mouth and verapamil dosage must be drastically reduced in these patients, especially when given orally.[1] The elimination half-life was prolonged about fourfold following oral or intravenous administration and thus steady-state plasma concentration will not be reached in patients with liver cirrhosis until about 56 hours after therapy has started.

1. Somogyi A, *et al.* Pharmacokinetics, bioavailability and ECG response of verapamil in patients with liver cirrhosis. *Br J Clin Pharmacol* 1981; **12:** 51–60.

Administration in renal impairment. The pharmacokinetics and pharmacodynamic effects of verapamil are not significantly altered by renal impairment[1] and dosage adjustment is not considered to be necessary. The elimination of verapamil is not altered by haemodialysis,[1,2] haemofiltration,[2] or peritoneal dialysis[2] and no dosage supplement is required in patients undergoing these procedures.

1. Mooy J, *et al.* Pharmacokinetics of verapamil in patients with renal failure. *Eur J Clin Pharmacol* 1985; **28:** 405–10.
2. Beyerlein C, *et al.* Verapamil in antihypertensive treatment of patients on renal replacement therapy—clinical implications and pharmacokinetics. *Eur J Clin Pharmacol* 1990; **39** (suppl 1): S35–S37.

Amaurosis fugax. Relief of vasospasm might explain the efficacy of the calcium-channel blockers nifedipine and verapamil in a few patients with amaurosis fugax unresponsive to anticoagulants or antiplatelets.[1]

1. Winterkorn JMS, *et al.* Brief report: treatment of vasospastic amaurosis fugax with calcium-channel blockers. *N Engl J Med* 1993; **329:** 396–8.

Angina pectoris. Treatment of angina pectoris (p.791) depends on the type of angina and may include the use of nitrates, beta blockers, and calcium-channel blockers such as verapamil either alone or in combination. However, combination of verapamil with a beta blocker has produced adverse effects and this is discussed under Interactions, above.

Bipolar disorder. Although lithium is the mainstay of therapy in bipolar disorder (p.271) it cannot be used in some patients because of undue toxicity, and is ineffective in others. Verapamil is one of several drugs that have been studied as an alternative.[1] Beneficial responses to verapamil 80 to 120 mg two to four times daily have been reported.[2-5]

1. Höschl C. Do calcium antagonists have a place in the treatment of mood disorders? *Drugs* 1991; **42:** 721–29.
2. Dubovsky SL, *et al.* Effectiveness of verapamil in the treatment of a manic patient. *Am J Psychiatry* 1982; **139:** 502–4.
3. Giannini AJ, *et al.* Antimanic effects of verapamil. *Am J Psychiatry* 1984; **141:** 1602–3.
4. Dubovsky SL, *et al.* Calcium antagonists in mania: a double-blind study of verapamil. *Psychiatry Res* 1986; **18:** 309–20.
5. Giannini AJ, *et al.* Verapamil and lithium in maintenance therapy of manic patients. *J Clin Pharmacol* 1987; **27:** 980–2.

Box jellyfish sting. Stings by the box jellyfish (*Chironex fleckeri*) (p.1546) can be fatal due to the effects of the venom on the cardiovascular and respiratory systems and on the kidneys. Studies in *rodents* have reported a beneficial effect of intravenous verapamil in the treatment of box jellyfish envenomation. It has been suggested that intravenous verapamil be used in the acute management of patients with serious box jellyfish stings since it may reverse the cardiotoxic effects of the venom

and allow more time for additional supportive care and for the antivenom to exert its action.[1]

1. Burnett JW. The use of verapamil to treat box-jellyfish stings. *Med J Aust* 1990; **153:** 363.

Cardiac arrhythmias. Verapamil may be used to control supraventricular arrhythmias such as atrial fibrillation and flutter and paroxysmal supraventricular tachycardia (p.794).

It reduces ventricular rate during atrial fibrillation, but should not be used when fibrillation or flutter is associated with an accessory pathway as in the Wolff-Parkinson-White syndrome. Intravenous verapamil has a more rapid onset than digitalis and has a direct depressant effect on the atrioventricular node which persists to a greater extent than that of digitalis during stress and exercise. A bolus dose of 10 mg of verapamil has commonly been recommended for the treatment of acute atrial fibrillation, but some workers[1] have preferred to give 1 mg by slow injection, repeated at 1-minute intervals. Ventricular fibrillation and severe hypotension have been reported[2] following the administration of intravenous verapamil 5 to 10 mg to patients with the Wolff-Parkinson-White syndrome.

Verapamil may also be given to terminate paroxysmal supraventricular tachycardia, although adenosine may be preferred.

Verapamil has been given to the mother in combination with digoxin in the management of fetal atrial flutter or supraventricular tachycardia.[3] Caution is necessary when verapamil is given to infants to treat their arrhythmias, see Precautions, above.

1. Klein HO, Kaplinsky E. Digitalis and verapamil in atrial fibrillation and flutter: is verapamil now the preferred agent? *Drugs* 1986; **31:** 185–97.
2. McGovern B, *et al.* Precipitation of cardiac arrest by verapamil in patients with Wolff-Parkinson-White syndrome. *Ann Intern Med* 1986; **104:** 791–4.
3. Maxwell DJ, *et al.* Obstetric importance, diagnosis, and management of fetal tachycardias. *BMJ* 1988; **297:** 107–10.

Cardiomyopathies. Clinical trials have suggested that long-term administration of verapamil improves symptoms and exercise tolerance in many patients with *hypertrophic cardiomyopathy* and it may be considered for the treatment of those patients who continue to have disabling symptoms or who are unable to tolerate beta blockers.[1] However, in a crossover study exercise capacity was not improved by either verapamil or nadolol, although most patients preferred one or other of the drugs rather than placebo and quality of life did appear to be improved by verapamil.[2] The incidence of serious ventricular or supraventricular arrhythmias does not appear to be reduced by verapamil and caution is also required since patients with hypertrophic cardiomyopathy are especially susceptible to conduction disturbances associated with verapamil. This is because loss of the synchronised contribution of atrial contraction may cause diminished filling of the stiff left ventricle and result in hypotension.[1]

The use of calcium-channel blockers is not standard therapy in *dilated cardiomyopathy* and has resulted in clinical and haemodynamic deterioration.[3] However, symptomatic improvement has been reported with diltiazem over a 24-month period.

For a discussion of the management of cardiomyopathies in general, see p.796.

1. Lorell BH. Use of calcium channel blockers in hypertrophic cardiomyopathy. *Am J Med* 1985; **78** (suppl 2B): 43–54.
2. Gilligan DM, *et al.* A double-blind, placebo-controlled crossover trial of nadolol and verapamil in mild and moderately symptomatic hypertrophic cardiomyopathy. *J Am Coll Cardiol* 1993; **21:** 1672–9.
3. Richardson PJ. Calcium antagonists in cardiomyopathy. *Br J Clin Pract* 1988; **42** (suppl 60): 33–7.

Hypertension. Verapamil may be used for the initial treatment of mild to moderate hypertension (p.802), but is not usually the drug of first choice.[1,2] It may be used as a modified-release or conventional-release formulation. Verapamil may be more effective in elderly patients than in younger patients. Verapamil has been used in pregnant women with severe gestational proteinuric hypertension.[3]

It may also be used in multiple drug regimens to control severe or refractory hypertension[1,2] and will usually have at least an additive effect with other antihypertensives. Extreme caution is needed if verapamil is used in combination with a beta blocker (see under Interactions, above).

1. McTavish D, Sorkin EM. Verapamil: an updated review of its pharmacodynamic and pharmacokinetic properties, and therapeutic use in hypertension. *Drugs* 1989; **38:** 19–76.
2. Kaplan NM. Calcium entry blockers in the treatment of hypertension: current status and future prospects. *JAMA* 1989; **262:** 817–23.
3. Belfort MA, *et al.* Hemodynamic changes associated with intravenous infusion of the calcium antagonists verapamil in the treatment of severe gestational proteinuric hypertension. *Obstet Gynecol* 1990; **75:** 970–4.

Kidney disorders. Calcium-channel blockers may be of benefit in various forms of kidney disorder (see Nifedipine, p.944). Verapamil may also reduce the nephrotoxicity associated with certain drugs. For example, verapamil can prevent ciclosporin-induced deterioration in renal function (see under Transplantation, below) and may possibly reduce nephrotoxicity associated with the aminoglycoside gentamicin.[1]

1. Kazierad DJ, *et al.* The effect of verapamil on the nephrotoxic potential of gentamicin as measured by urinary enzyme excretion in healthy volunteers. *J Clin Pharmacol* 1995; **35:** 196–201.

Malignant neoplasms. Verapamil has been shown to reverse multidrug resistance to antineoplastics in cultured cells and in *animal* studies,[1] but studies in which verapamil was added to therapy for small cell lung cancer[2] or multiple myeloma[3] failed to demonstrate any benefit.

1. Ford JM, Hait WN. Pharmacology of drugs that alter multidrug resistance in cancer. *Pharmacol Rev* 1990; **42**: 155–99.
2. Milroy R, *et al.* A randomised clinical study of verapamil in addition to combination chemotherapy in small cell lung cancer. *Br J Cancer* 1993; **68**: 813–18.
3. Dalton WS, *et al.* A phase III randomized study of oral verapamil as a chemosensitizer to reverse drug resistance in patients with refractory myeloma: a Southwest Oncology Group Study. *Cancer* 1995; **75**: 815–20.

Migraine. For reference to the use of calcium-channel blockers, including verapamil, in the management of migraine and cluster headache, see under Nifedipine, p.944.

Myocardial infarction. Studies have not shown a reduction in mortality when calcium-channel blockers are given in the early phase of acute myocardial infarction (p.805). Results of the Danish Verapamil Infarction Trial (DAVIT I) suggested that early intervention (on admission to hospital) with verapamil might be harmful.[1] However, since myocardial stunning has been linked to intracellular calcium overload[2] there has been speculation that calcium-channel blockers might benefit patients about to undergo reperfusion. This is yet to be confirmed. Calcium-channel blockers are not routinely used in the long-term management of myocardial infarction although in selected patients without heart failure verapamil or diltiazem may be of some benefit. In the DAVIT II study[3] late intervention with verapamil (started in the second week after admission) reduced overall mortality, cardiac events, and re-infarction in such patients although another study[4] found only a benefit in re-infarction rate and not in overall mortality.

1. The Danish Study Group on Verapamil in Myocardial Infarction. The Danish studies on verapamil in acute myocardial infarction. *Br J Clin Pharmacol* 1986; **21**: 197S–204S.
2. Anonymous. Myocardial stunning. *Lancet* 1991; **337**: 585–6.
3. The Danish Study Group on Verapamil in Myocardial Infarction. Effect of verapamil on mortality and major events after acute myocardial infarction (the Danish Verapamil Infarction Trial II–DAVIT II). *Am J Cardiol* 1990; **66**: 779–85.
4. Rengo F, *et al.* A controlled trial of verapamil in patients after acute myocardial infarction: results of the calcium antagonist reinfarction Italian study (CRIS). *Am J Cardiol* 1996; **77**: 365–9.

Transplantation. Ciclosporin is widely used in transplantation to prevent rejection but its use is limited by its nephrotoxicity. A series of studies in renal[1] and heart or lung[2] transplant recipients suggested that verapamil can prevent ciclosporin-induced deterioration in renal function. Although the concentration of ciclosporin in blood was increased by verapamil, kidney function was improved. The incidence of transplant rejection was also reduced by verapamil. The beneficial effect of verapamil therapy on transplant outcome may be related to its ability to protect cells from ischaemia, selective vasodilatation of the afferent renal arterioles, elevation of plasma-ciclosporin concentrations, and inherent immunosuppressive properties. Concomitant use of verapamil also allows lower doses of ciclosporin to be employed.[2]

1. Dawidson I, Rooth P. Improvement of cadaver renal transplantation outcomes with verapamil: a review. *Am J Med* 1991; **90** (suppl 5A): 37S–41S.
2. Chan C, *et al.* A randomized controlled trial of verapamil on cyclosporine nephrotoxicity in heart and lung transplant recipients. *Transplantation* 1997; **63**: 1435–40.

Preparations

BP 2001: Prolonged-release Verapamil Tablets; Verapamil Injection; Verapamil Tablets;
USP 25: Verapamil Hydrochloride Extended-release Tablets; Verapamil Hydrochloride Injection; Verapamil Hydrochloride Tablets.

Proprietary Preparations (details are given in Part 3)
Aust.: Isoptin; Verapabene; Verexamil; *Austral.:* Anpec; Cordilox; Isoptin; Veracaps; Verahexal; *Belg.:* Isoptin; Lodixal; *Braz.:* Dilacoron; Veracoron; *Canad.:* Apo-Verap; Chronovera; Isoptin; Novo-Veramil; Nu-Verap; Verelan; *Denm.:* Geangin; Hexasoptin; Isoptin; Veraloc; *Fin.:* Isoptin; Vermin; Veraptor; Verpamil; *Fr.:* Arpamyl LP; Isoptine; Novapamyl†; *Ger.:* Azupamil; Cardioprotect; Dignover†; durasoptin; Falicard; Isoptin; Jenapamil; Praecicor†; Vera; Vera-Lich; Verabeta; Veragamma; Verahexal; Veramex; Veranorm; Verasal; Veroptinstada; *Hong Kong:* Akilen; Isoptin; *Irl.:* Berkatens†; Isoptin; Veramil; Verelan; Verisop; *Israel:* Apoacor; Ikacor; Ikapress; Veracor; Verapress; *Ital.:* Isoptin; Quasar; *Jpn:* Vasolan†; *Mex.:* Cronovera; Dilacoran; Euritmin; Galenpamil; Veraken; Veralan; *Neth.:* Isoptin; Norw.: Geangin†; Isoptin; Verakard; *NZ:* Civicor; Isoptin; Verpamil; *Port.:* Isoptin; *S.Afr.:* Bonceur; Calcicard; Iso-Card†; Isoptin; Ravamil; Vasomil; Verahexal†; Verpamil; *Singapore:* Civicor; Isoptin; Verpamil; *Spain:* Manidon; Redupres; Veratensin; *Swed.:* Isoptin; Veraloc; *Switz.:* Corpamil; Flamon; Isoptin; Veracim†; Verasifar; *Thai.:* Caveril; Civicor; Isopamil; Isoptin; Vasopten; Verapin; Vermine; *UK:* Isoptin; Berkatens†; Cordilox; Ethimil; Half Securon; Securon; Univer; Verapress; Vertab; Zolvera; *USA:* Calan; Covera; Isoptin; Verelan.

Multi-ingredient: *Aust.:* Captocomp†; Confit; Gradulon†; Veracapt; *Denm.:* Tarka; *Fin.:* Tarka; *Fr.:* Ocadrik; Tarka; *Ger.:* Cordichin; Isoptin plus; Stenoptin†; Tarka; Udramil; Veratide; *Ital.:* Tarka; *Mex.:* Tarka; *Neth.:* Tarka; *S.Afr.:* Tarka; *Spain:* Tarka; Tricen; *Swed.:* Tarka; *Switz.:* Tarka; *UK:* Tarka; *USA:* Tarka.

Vesnarinone (3772-y)

Vesnarinone (USAN, rINN).
OPC-8212. 1-(1,2,3,4-Tetrahydro-2-oxo-6-quinolyl)-4-veratroylpiperazine.
$C_{22}H_{25}N_3O_4 = 395.5$.
CAS — 81840-15-5.

Profile

Vesnarinone is a phosphodiesterase inhibitor with calcium-sensitising properties. It has positive inotropic activity and has been tried by mouth in the management of heart failure.

◊ Studies with other inotropic phosphodiesterase inhibitors have shown that their prolonged oral use can increase the mortality rate. In a multicentre study of vesnarinone,[1] treatment of 120 mg daily resulted in increased mortality whereas 60 mg daily for 6 months was associated with lower morbidity and mortality. Reversible neutropenia occurred in 2.5% of the patients given 60 mg daily. However, in a subsequent larger study,[2] increased mortality was also reported with doses of 30 and 60 mg daily.

1. Feldman AM, *et al.* Effects of vesnarinone on morbidity and mortality in patients with heart failure. *N Engl J Med* 1993; **329**: 149–55.
2. Cohn JN, *et al.* A dose-dependent increase in mortality with vesnarinone among patients with severe heart failure. *N Engl J Med* 1998; **339**: 1810–16.

Preparations

Proprietary Preparations (details are given in Part 3)
Jpn: Arkin-Z†.

Warfarin Sodium (14736-w)

Warfarin Sodium (BANM, rINNM).
Sodium Warfarin; Warfarinum Natricum. The sodium salt of 4-hydroxy-3-(3-oxo-1-phenylbutyl)coumarin .
$C_{19}H_{15}NaO_4 = 330.3$.
CAS — 81-81-2 (warfarin); 2610-86-8 (warfarin potassium); 129-06-6 (warfarin sodium).

Pharmacopoeias. In Chin., Eur. (see p.vi), Int., and US.
Chin., Int., and US permit either warfarin sodium or warfarin sodium clathrate. Eur. has a separate monograph for warfarin sodium clathrate (see below).
Jpn includes Warfarin Potassium.

NOTE. Commercial warfarin sodium is racemic.

Pharmacopoeial description
Ph. Eur.: A white, hygroscopic powder. Very soluble in water and in alcohol; soluble in acetone; very slightly soluble in dichloromethane and in ether. A 1% solution in water has a pH of 7.6 to 8.6. Store in airtight containers. Protect from light.
USP 25: A white, odourless, amorphous solid or a crystalline clathrate which is discoloured by light. Very soluble in water; freely soluble in alcohol; very slightly soluble in chloroform and in ether. A 1% solution in water has a pH of 7.2 to 8.3. Protect from light.

Adsorption. Studies carried out for periods of 24 hours to 3 months have demonstrated some adsorption of warfarin sodium by PVC when dissolved in 0.9% sodium chloride solution[1,2] or in 5% glucose solution.[3] In one of these studies,[1] adsorption was decreased by buffering the solution from its initial pH of 6.7 to a pH of 7.4. The second study[2] could demonstrate no adsorption onto polyethylene-lined or glass infusion containers.

1. Kowaluk EA, *et al.* Interactions between drugs and polyvinyl chloride infusion bags. *Am J Hosp Pharm* 1981; **38**: 1308–14.
2. Martens HJ, *et al.* Sorption of various drugs in polyvinyl chloride, glass, and polyethylene-lined infusion containers. *Am J Hosp Pharm* 1990; **47**: 369–73.
3. Moorhatch P, Chiou WL. Interactions between drugs and plastic intravenous fluid bags: part i: sorption studies on 17 drugs. *Am J Hosp Pharm* 1974; **31**: 72–8.

Incompatibilities. Solutions of warfarin sodium have been reported to be incompatible with adrenaline [epinephrine] hydrochloride, amikacin sulfate, metaraminol tartrate, oxytocin, promazine hydrochloride, and tetracycline hydrochloride. Visual incompatibility has been reported[1] with solutions of warfarin sodium mixed with solutions of aminophylline, bretylium tosilate, ceftazidime, cimetidine hydrochloride, ciprofloxacin lactate, dobutamine hydrochloride, esmolol hydrochloride, gentamicin sulfate, labetalol hydrochloride, metronidazole hydrochloride, or vancomycin hydrochloride. Haze was also reported after 24 hours with sodium chloride 0.9%.

1. Bahal SM, *et al.* Visual compatibility of warfarin sodium injection with selected medications and solutions. *Am J Health-Syst Pharm* 1997; **54**: 2599–2600.

Warfarin Sodium Clathrate (4823-c)

Warfarin Sodium Clathrate (BANM).
Warfarinum Natricum Clathratum. The clathrate of warfarin sodium with isopropyl alcohol in the molecular proportions 2 to 1 respectively.

Pharmacopoeias. In Eur. (see p.vi).
Chin., Int., and US permit either warfarin sodium or warfarin sodium clathrate.

NOTE. Until 1991 the BP, like the USP, allowed the use of either warfarin sodium or warfarin sodium clathrate in the definition of warfarin sodium. The use of the term warfarin sodium in *Martindale* should generally be taken to include the sodium clathrate.

Pharmacopoeial description
Ph. Eur.: A white powder. Very soluble in water; freely soluble in alcohol; soluble in acetone; very slightly soluble in dichloromethane and in ether. A 1% solution in water has a pH of 7.6 to 8.6. Store in airtight containers. Protect from light.
Warfarin sodium clathrate contains approximately 92% of warfarin sodium.

Adverse Effects

The major risk from warfarin therapy is of haemorrhage from almost any organ of the body with the consequent effects of haematomas as well as anaemia. Although good control of warfarin anticoagulation is essential in preventing haemorrhage, bleeding has occurred at therapeutic international normalised ratio (INR) values. In such cases the possibility of an underlying cause such as renal or alimentary tract disease should be investigated. Skin necrosis, and purple discoloration of the toes (due to cholesterol embolisation) have occasionally occurred. Hypersensitivity reactions are extremely rare. Other effects not necessarily associated with haemorrhage include alopecia, fever, nausea, vomiting, diarrhoea, skin reactions, jaundice, hepatic dysfunction, and pancreatitis.

Warfarin is a recognised teratogen. Given in the first trimester of pregnancy it can cause a fetal warfarin syndrome or warfarin embryopathy characterised by bone stippling (chondrodysplasia punctata) and nasal hypoplasia. CNS abnormalities may develop following use in any trimester but appear most likely after use in the second or third trimester. Use of warfarin during pregnancy has been associated with an increased rate of abortion and still-birth, although this may, in part, be the consequence of an underlying maternal condition. Use in the late stages of pregnancy is associated with fetal haemorrhage. Reported incidences of the above complications have varied; one estimate is that if a coumarin anticoagulant is taken during pregnancy, one-sixth of pregnancies will result in an abnormal liveborn infant, and one-sixth will result in abortion or still-birth.

Effects on the blood. The incidence and risk of haemorrhage during long-term oral anticoagulation has been studied in patients in clinical trials[1] and in population-based studies.[2-5] The risk of bleeding was generally higher with more intense anticoagulation and in the presence of other risk factors but the relationship with age was less clear. Some studies have shown higher rates of bleeding in elderly patients, but others have not; the risk of intracranial bleeding, however, does seem to be higher in the elderly.[1,5] Although cumulative risk of bleeding was related to duration of anticoagulation therapy, risk may be highest early in the course.[1]
Withdrawal of warfarin therapy may lead to rebound hypercoagulability and it has been suggested[6] that warfarin should be withdrawn gradually, although there is no clinical evidence to support this.
For the risk of corpus luteum haemorrhage or haematoma associated with ovulation in patients on oral anticoagulants, see under Precautions, below.

1. Levine MN, *et al.* Hemorrhagic complications of anticoagulant treatment. *Chest* 2001; **119** (suppl): 108S–121S.
2. Gitter MJ, *et al.* Bleeding and thromboembolism during anticoagulant therapy: a population-based study in Rochester, Minnesota. *Mayo Clin Proc* 1995; **70**: 725–33.
3. Fihn SD, *et al.* The risk for and severity of bleeding complications in elderly patients treated with warfarin. *Ann Intern Med* 1996; **124**: 970–9.
4. Palareti G, *et al.* Bleeding complications of oral anticoagulant treatment: an inception-cohort, prospective collaborative study (ISCOAT). *Lancet* 1996; **348**: 423–8.
5. Palareti G, *et al.* Oral anticoagulation treatment in the elderly: a nested, prospective, case-control study. *Arch Intern Med* 2000; **160**: 470–8.
6. Palareti G, Legnani C. Warfarin withdrawal: pharmacokinetic-pharmacodynamic considerations. *Clin Pharmacokinet* 1996; **30**: 300–13.

Effects on the bones. Vitamin K is involved in bone metabolism and vitamin K deficiency is associated with an increased risk of osteoporotic fractures. It has been suggested, therefore, that patients on long-term treatment with oral anticoagulants, which are vitamin K antagonists, may be at increased risk of osteoporosis and fractures. However, two large observational studies in older women have produced conflicting results. A prospective study[1] of both users and nonusers of warfarin found that warfarin was not associated with decrease in bone density or increase in fracture rates. A retrospective study[2] reported an association between long-term anticoagulant use and increased risk of vertebral and rib fractures, compared with the general population. Overall, however, the risk of any fracture was not significantly increased.

1. Jamal SA, *et al.* Warfarin use and risk for osteoporosis in elderly women. *Ann Intern Med* 1998; **128:** 829–32.
2. Caraballo PJ, *et al.* Long-term use of oral anticoagulants and the risk of fracture. *Arch Intern Med* 1999; **159:** 1750–6.

Effects on the fetus. Reviews of reported fetal complications following exposure to coumarin anticoagulants during pregnancy.

1. Hall JG, *et al.* Maternal and fetal sequelae of anticoagulation during pregnancy. *Am J Med* 1980; **68:** 122–40.
2. Chan WS, *et al.* Anticoagulation of pregnant women with mechanical heart valves: a systematic review of the literature. *Arch Intern Med* 2000; **160:** 191–6.
3. Ginsberg JS, *et al.* Use of antithrombotic agents during pregnancy. *Chest* 2001; **119** (suppl): 122S–131S.

Effects on the liver. There have been a few isolated reports of cholestatic liver damage in patients taking warfarin sodium.[1-3] In these cases hepatic injury resolved on withdrawal of the drug.

1. Rehnqvist N. Intrahepatic jaundice due to warfarin therapy. *Acta Med Scand* 1978; **204:** 335–6.
2. Jones DB, *et al.* Jaundice following warfarin therapy. *Postgrad Med J* 1980; **56:** 671.
3. Adler E, *et al.* Cholestatic hepatic injury related to warfarin exposure. *Arch Intern Med* 1986; **146:** 1837–9.

Effects on sexual function. There have been reports[1-3] of priapism in patients taking oral anticoagulants such as warfarin.

1. Baños JE, *et al.* Drug-induced priapism: its aetiology, incidence and treatment. *Med Toxicol* 1989; **4:** 46–58.
2. Daryanani S, Wilde JT. Priapism in a patient with protein C deficiency. *Clin Lab Haematol* 1997; **19:** 213–14.
3. Zimbelman J, *et al.* Unusual complications of warfarin therapy: skin necrosis and priapism. *J Pediatr* 2000; **137:** 266–8.

Effects on the skin and hair. Necrosis of skin and soft tissue associated with coumarin anticoagulant therapy has been reviewed.[1,2] Coumarin-induced necrosis occurs rarely and is characterised by a localised, painful skin lesion, initially erythematous or haemorrhagic in appearance, that becomes bullous and eventually culminates in gangrenous necrosis. Fatalities have occurred. Areas of increased subcutaneous fat such as breast, thigh, and buttocks have most often been involved. The aetiology appears to be thrombotic but the exact pathophysiology is not known. Patients with protein C deficiency appear to be at highest risk. Treatment with coumarin anticoagulants should be discontinued on appearance of skin lesions and vitamin K should be given to reverse their effect. Heparin should be administered to provide anticoagulation. Fresh frozen plasma or protein C concentrates may also have a role in reversing the condition. Surgical intervention is usually required if necrosis does develop.

Other skin reactions have also been reported with coumarins. Vasculitis affecting both legs developed in a 74-year-old woman a few weeks after starting treatment with nicoumalone [acenocoumarol] for deep-vein thrombosis and pulmonary embolism.[3] Nicoumalone [acenocoumarol] treatment was stopped and the skin lesions steadily improved over 15 days. However, the skin lesions reappeared a few hours after re-exposure to a single dose of nicoumalone [acenocoumarol]. The patient had also been taking amiodarone which may have contributed to the reaction.

Increased shedding of telogen hair has been stated to occur in patients given coumarin anticoagulants.[4]

1. Cole MS, *et al.* Coumarin necrosis—a review of the literature. *Surgery* 1988; **103:** 271–7.
2. Comp PC. Coumarin-induced skin necrosis: incidence, mechanisms, management and avoidance. *Drug Safety* 1993; **8:** 128–35.
3. Susano R, *et al.* Hypersensitivity vasculitis related to nicoumalone. *BMJ* 1993; **306:** 973.
4. Smith AG. Drug-induced disorders of hair and nails. *Adverse Drug React Bull* 1995 (173); 655–8.

Treatment of Adverse Effects

The methods used to manage bleeding and/or excessive anticoagulation during warfarin therapy, or following warfarin overdosage, depend upon the degree of bleeding, the value of the international normalised ratio (INR), and the degree of thromboembolic risk.

If the INR is greater than 5.0 but there is no bleeding or only minor bleeding, warfarin should be temporarily withheld until the INR falls to below 5.0. In some cases where the INR is between 5.0 and 6.0 a reduction in warfarin dose, rather than withdrawal, may be sufficient. For an INR greater than 8.0 administration of phytomenadione (vitamin K$_1$) should also be considered if there are other risk factors for bleeding; typical doses of phytomenadione are 0.5 mg intravenously or up to 5 mg orally.

If there is any major bleeding warfarin should be stopped and phytomenadione 5 mg by slow intravenous injection given together with a concentrate of factors II, VII, IX, and X. The dose of concentrate

should be calculated based on 50 units of factor IX per kg body-weight. If no concentrate is available fresh frozen plasma should be infused (about one litre for an adult), but may not be as effective. Higher doses of phytomenadione have been used (see Over-anticoagulation, p.1397) but it should be remembered that phytomenadione takes several hours to act and large doses may reduce the response to resumed therapy with anticoagulants for a week or more.

If bleeding occurs unexpectedly at therapeutic INR values, the possibility of an underlying cause such as renal or alimentary tract disease should be investigated.

See under Effects on the Skin and Hair, above, for the management of skin and soft tissue necrosis.

Precautions

Warfarin should not be given to patients who are haemorrhaging. In general it should not be given to patients at serious risk of haemorrhage, although it has been used with very careful control; patients at risk include those with haemorrhagic blood disorders, peptic ulcer disease, severe wounds (including surgical wounds), cerebrovascular disorders, and bacterial endocarditis. Severe renal and hepatic impairment as well as severe hypertension are considered by some to be contra-indications. Pregnancy is also generally considered to be a contra-indication, especially in the first trimester and during the last few weeks of pregnancy (see Adverse Effects, above).

Many factors may affect anticoagulant control with warfarin. These include vitamin K status, thyroid status, renal function, bioavailability differences between warfarin preparations, factors affecting absorption of warfarin, and drug interactions. Such factors may be responsible for apparent resistance to warfarin and a few patients have displayed hereditary resistance. Dosage alterations should be guided by regular monitoring of oral anticoagulant therapy and clinical status. Patients should carry anticoagulant treatment booklets.

◊ A discussion of factors affecting the anticoagulant effect of warfarin sodium.[1]

1. Shetty HGM, *et al.* Clinical pharmacokinetic considerations in the control of oral anticoagulant therapy. *Clin Pharmacokinet* 1989; **16:** 238–53.

◊ Corpus luteum haematoma or haemorrhage was associated with ovulation in 3 women being treated with coumarin anticoagulants.[1] It was suggested that suppression of ovulation be considered for women on anticoagulants during their fertile years, even if sterilisation had been performed.

See Sex Hormones under Interactions, below, for the effect of oral contraceptives on the activity of oral anticoagulants.

1. Bogers J-W, *et al.* Complications of anticoagulant therapy in ovulatory women. *Lancet* 1991; **337:** 618–19.

Interactions

Many compounds interact with warfarin and other oral anticoagulants. Details of these interactions are given below for all oral anticoagulants with different groups of drugs; if the anticoagulant is other than warfarin, then its identity is specified. The major interactions are summarised in the tables, above. Readers should be aware that while interactions of a pharmacodynamic nature occurring with one anticoagulant may well apply to another, this is not necessarily the case with interactions of a pharmacokinetic nature.

An interaction may be due to increased or decreased anticoagulant metabolism; with warfarin some interacting drugs such as cimetidine, co-trimoxazole, or phenylbutazone have a selective effect on its stereoisomers. Altered absorption may sometimes play a part, as with colestyramine. Displacement of oral anticoagulants from plasma protein binding sites has been reported with many drugs, including some analgesics. Not all reports that have recorded an alteration in the pharmacokinetics of the anticoagulant have, however, shown a corresponding change in clinical response.

Interference with the coagulation process may be responsible for the increased risk of haemorrhage when

Drugs generally recognised as diminishing the effects of oral anticoagulants are included in the following list. Further information on the interactions with these drugs and others where the interaction is not so well recognised is provided in the referenced section below.

acetomenaphthone	ethchlorvynol
alcohol (chronic ingestion without liver impairment)	glutethimide
	griseofulvin
aminoglutethimide	nafcillin
barbiturates	phytomenadione
carbamazepine	rifampicin
dichloralphenazone	

Drugs recognised or generally reported as enhancing oral anticoagulants are included in the following list. Further information on the interactions with these drugs and others where the interaction is not so well recognised is provided in the referenced section below.

alcohol (acute ingestion or chronic ingestion with liver impairment)	etacrynic acid
	ethylestrenol
	fluconazole
allopurinol	glucagon
amiodarone	itraconazole
aspirin	ketoconazole
cefamandole	metronidazole
chloramphenicol	miconazole
cimetidine	norethandrolone
clofibrate	NSAIDs
cloral hydrate	oxymetholone
co-trimoxazole	quinidine
danazol	stanozolol
dextropropoxyphene	sulfinpyrazone
dextrothyroxine	tamoxifen
dipyridamole	thyroid agents
disulfiram	tienilic acid
erythromycin	triclofos sodium

aspirin, clofibrate, or thyroid hormones are used with anticoagulants. Many other compounds, such as asparaginase, some contrast media, epoprostenol, streptokinase, and urokinase also carry this risk; while interactions between these compounds and anticoagulants are not discussed further below, the possibility of an increased risk of haemorrhage should be considered when they are used together.

Where there is a risk of serious haemorrhage from an interaction, then use of the 2 drugs is best avoided. In other instances the anticoagulant activity should be carefully monitored so as to increase or decrease the anticoagulant dose as required. Critical periods are when patients stabilised on an anticoagulant commence treatment with an interacting drug, or when patients stabilised on a regimen of an interacting drug and anticoagulant have the interacting drug withdrawn. Depending on the mechanism of the interaction, the clinical response to the interaction may be rapid or may take some days. Interactions involving displacement from plasma protein binding sites are often transient. Readers should also be aware that some interacting drugs do not produce predictable effects; there have for instance been reports of increased as well as decreased anticoagulant activity with disopyramide, phenytoin, quinidine, and oral contraceptives. Another problem occurs with dipyridamole; it can cause bleeding when given to patients taking anticoagulants but without any changes in the measures used for anticoagulant control.

◊ Reviews.

1. Harder S, Thürmann P. Clinically important drug interactions with anticoagulants: an update. *Clin Pharmacokinet* 1996; **30:** 416–44.

Alcohol. Alcohol has a variable effect on warfarin. Heavy regular drinkers may experience a diminished effect, perhaps through enzyme induction, although the effect of warfarin may be increased in the presence of liver impairment; acute inges-

The symbol † denotes a preparation no longer actively marketed

tion has enhanced the effect of warfarin. A moderate alcohol intake is generally not considered to cause problems.

Analgesics and NSAIDs. All NSAIDs should be used with caution or not at all in patients on warfarin. Many NSAIDs inhibit platelet function to some extent and have an irritant effect on the gastrointestinal tract, so increasing the risk of haemorrhage. Furthermore, some NSAIDs increase the hypoprothrombinaemic effect of warfarin, possibly by an intrinsic effect on coagulation or by displacement of warfarin from plasma protein-binding sites. Many studies have compared the relative displacing action of a range of NSAIDs *in vitro*, but such studies cannot easily be extrapolated to the clinical situation. Changes in plasma concentration of unbound warfarin resulting from displacement from plasma protein-binding sites are usually transient and are most likely to occur in the first few weeks after an NSAID is added to or withdrawn from warfarin therapy; monitoring of anticoagulant therapy is, therefore, most critical during this period.

High doses of *aspirin* and some other *salicylates* enhance the hypoprothrombinaemic effect of warfarin and should generally be avoided in patients on oral anticoagulant therapy. Low-dose aspirin with warfarin may have a role in some patients but the risk of gastrointestinal bleeding is increased. The possibility of an interaction with topical salicylates should also be considered.[1,2]

Concurrent administration of *phenylbutazone* and warfarin has led to serious haemorrhage and should be avoided. Phenylbutazone affects the metabolism of the *R*- and *S*- isomers of warfarin in complex and different ways with the net effect of enhancing its anticoagulant activity.[3] Related drugs such as *oxyphenbutazone*, *azapropazone*,[4-6] and *feprazone*[7] behave similarly and should also be avoided.

For the following NSAIDs there are a few studies or isolated reports suggesting that they may enhance the hypoprothrombinaemic effect of warfarin or other specified oral anticoagulant: *diflunisal* (with nicoumalone [acenocoumarol][8] or warfarin[9]), *flurbiprofen* (with nicoumalone [acenocoumarol]),[10] *indometacin*,[11,12] *ketoprofen*,[13] *meclofenamate sodium*,[14] *mefenamic acid*,[15] *piroxicam*, (with warfarin[16] or nicoumalone [acenocoumarol][17]), *sulindac*,[18,19] *tiaprofenic acid* (with nicoumalone [acenocoumarol]),[20] and *tolmetin sodium*.[21] In many cases the result of concomitant therapy was an increased prothrombin time which may or may not be clinically significant; in other cases haemorrhage occurred. It should also be noted that for many of the above NSAIDs, perhaps particularly indometacin, there are studies (not cited) in which no enhancement of warfarin activity could be demonstrated. NSAIDs with an apparently minimal effect on warfarin activity include *etodolac*, *ibuprofen*, and *naproxen*.

Although a study in healthy volunteers indicated that there was no interaction between warfarin and *celecoxib*, a selective inhibitor of cyclo-oxygenase-2, there have been several reports[22-24] of an increase in the INR with concomitant therapy; bleeding has also been reported in some patients.[24] A small increase in INR has also been reported in a study[25] of warfarin with *rofecoxib*.

In view of the above considerations, *paracetamol* is recommended as the general analgesic and antipyretic of choice in patients on oral anticoagulant therapy. Caution should, however, be observed since, although it has no effect on the gastric mucosa or on platelet function, some studies (with warfarin, anisindione, dicoumarol, or phenprocoumon)[26,27] and isolated reports[28] have demonstrated an increased risk of bleeding in patients taking regular doses of paracetamol while on an oral anticoagulant.

Opioid analgesics do not generally cause problems, although there have been reports of enhanced anticoagulant activity in patients receiving *tramadol* with warfarin[29] or phenprocoumon.[30] *Co-proxamol*, a combination of *dextropropoxyphene* and paracetamol, has increased the effect of warfarin.[31-33] *Co-codamol*, a combination of *codeine* and paracetamol, has also enhanced warfarin activity.[34]

Amongst other analgesics, *cinchophen* (with dicoumarol, ethyl biscoumacetate, or phenindione)[35] and *fenyramidol* (with warfarin, dicoumarol, or phenindione)[36] have been reported to enhance the activity of oral anticoagulants and there is the possibility of such an effect with *glafenine* (with phenprocoumon).[37] *Phenazone*, an inducer of enzyme metabolism, reduces plasma concentrations of warfarin and, in contrast with most other analgesics, may necessitate an increase in warfarin dosage.[38]

1. Chow WH, *et al.* Potentiation of warfarin anticoagulation by topical methylsalicylate ointment. *J R Soc Med* 1989; **82:** 501–2.
2. Littleton F. Warfarin and topical salicylates. *JAMA* 1990; **263:** 2888.
3. Banfield C, *et al.* Phenylbutazone-warfarin interaction in man: further stereochemical and metabolic considerations. *Br J Clin Pharmacol* 1983; **16:** 669–75.
4. Powell-Jackson PR. Interaction between azapropazone and warfarin. *BMJ* 1977; **1:** 1193–4.
5. Green AE, *et al.* Potentiation of warfarin by azapropazone. *BMJ* 1977; **1:** 1532.
6. Win N, Mitchell DC. Azapropazone and warfarin. *BMJ* 1991; **302:** 969–70.
7. Chierichetti S, *et al.* Comparison of feprazone and phenylbutazone interaction with warfarin in man. *Curr Ther Res* 1975; **18:** 568–72.

8. Tempero KF, *et al.* Diflunisal: a review of pharmacokinetic and pharmacodynamic properties, drug interactions, and special tolerability studies in humans. *Br J Clin Pharmacol* 1977; **4:** 31S–36S.
9. Serlin MJ, *et al.* The effect of diflunisal on the steady state pharmacodynamics and pharmacokinetics of warfarin. *Br J Clin Pharmacol* 1980; **9:** 287P–8P.
10. Stricker BHC, Delhez JL. Interaction between flurbiprofen and coumarins. *BMJ* 1982; **285:** 812–13.
11. Koch-Weser J. Hemorrhagic reactions and drug interactions in 500 warfarin-treated patients. *Clin Pharmacol Ther* 1973; **14:** 139.
12. Self TH, *et al.* Drug enhancement of warfarin activity. *Lancet* 1975; **ii:** 557–8.
13. Flessner MF. Prolongation of prothrombin time and severe gastrointestinal bleeding associated with combined use of warfarin and ketoprofen. *JAMA* 1988; **259:** 353.
14. Baragar FD, Smith TC. Drug interaction studies with sodium meclofenamate (Meclomen®). *Curr Ther Res* 1978; **23** (suppl 4): S51–S59.
15. Holmes EL. Pharmacology of the fenamates: IV toleration by normal human subjects. *Ann Phys Med* 1966; **9** (suppl): 36–49.
16. Rhodes RS, *et al.* A warfarin-piroxicam drug interaction. *Drug Intell Clin Pharm* 1985; **19:** 556–8.
17. Bonnabry P, *et al.* Stereoselective interaction between piroxicam and acenocoumarol. *Br J Clin Pharmacol* 1996; **41:** 525–30.
18. Carter SA. Potential effect of sulindac on response of prothrombin-time to oral anticoagulants. *Lancet* 1979; **ii:** 698–9.
19. Ross JRY, Beeley L. Sulindac, prothrombin time, and anticoagulants. *Lancet* 1979; **ii:** 1075.
20. Whittaker SJ, *et al.* A severe, potentially fatal, interaction between tiaprofenic acid and nicoumalone. *Br J Clin Pract* 1986; **40:** 440.
21. Koren JF, *et al.* Tolmetin-warfarin interaction. *Am J Med* 1987; **82:** 1278–9.
22. Mersfelder TL, Stewart LR. Warfarin and celecoxib interaction. *Ann Pharmacother* 2000; **34:** 325–7.
23. Haase KK, *et al.* Potential interaction between celecoxib and warfarin. *Ann Pharmacother* 2000; **34:** 666–7.
24. Adverse Drug Reactions Advisory Committee. Interaction of celecoxib and warfarin. *Aust Adverse Drug React Bull* 2001; **20:** 2.
25. Schwartz JI, *et al.* The effect of rofecoxib on the pharmacodynamics and pharmacokinetics of warfarin. *Clin Pharmacol Ther* 2000; **68:** 626–36.
26. Antlitz AM, *et al.* Potentiation of oral anticoagulant therapy by acetaminophen. *Curr Ther Res* 1968; **10:** 501–7.
27. Hylek EM, *et al.* Acetaminophen and other risk factors for excessive warfarin anticoagulation. *JAMA* 1998; **279:** 657–62.
28. Boeijinga JJ, *et al.* Interaction between paracetamol and coumarin anticoagulants. *Lancet* 1982; **i:** 506.
29. Scher ML, *et al.* Potential interaction between tramadol and warfarin. *Ann Pharmacother* 1997; **31:** 646–7.
30. Madsen H, *et al.* Interaction between tramadol and phenprocoumon. *Lancet* 1997; **350:** 637.
31. Orme M, *et al.* Warfarin and Distalgesic interaction. *BMJ* 1976; **1:** 200.
32. Jones RV. Warfarin and Distalgesic interaction. *BMJ* 1976; **1:** 460.
33. Smith R, *et al.* Propoxyphene and warfarin interaction. *Drug Intell Clin Pharm* 1984; **18:** 822.
34. Bartle WR, Blakely JA. Potentiation of warfarin anticoagulation by acetaminophen. *JAMA* 1991; **265:** 1260.
35. Jarnum S. Cinchophen and acetylsalicylic acid in anticoagulant treatment. *Scand J Clin Lab Invest* 1954; **6:** 91–3.
36. Carter SA. Potentiation of the effect of orally administered anticoagulants by phenyramidol hydrochloride. *N Engl J Med* 1965; **273:** 423–6.
37. Boeijinga JK, van der Vijgh WJF. Double blind study of the effect of glafenine (Glifanan®) on oral anticoagulant therapy with phenprocoumon (Marcumar®). *J Clin Pharmacol* 1977; **12:** 291–6.
38. Whitfield JB, *et al.* Changes in plasma γ-glutamyl transpeptidase activity associated with alterations in drug metabolism in man. *BMJ* 1973; **1:** 316–18.

Antiarrhythmics. *Amiodarone* has been shown in several studies to increase the activity of warfarin[1-5] and nicoumalone [acenocoumarol],[6,7] probably through inhibition of metabolism. The potentiating effect of amiodarone has been reported to persist for up to 4 months after its withdrawal.[1] There is a report of phenprocoumon being affected by amiodarone.[8] Isolated reports with *disopyramide*[9] and *quinidine*[10] have suggested that these drugs can enhance the anticoagulant effect of warfarin. In 7 patients on warfarin or dicoumarol treated with disopyramide or quinidine, however, all but one needed a small increase in the weekly anticoagulant dose suggesting that the antiarrhythmic had reduced the anticoagulant effect.[11] Since the effect was observed after conversion of atrial fibrillation to sinus rhythm an involvement of haemodynamic factors was postulated. Several studies (not cited) have failed to show an effect of quinidine on warfarin. There are also reports indicating that *propafenone*[12] and *moracizine*[13] can enhance warfarin.

1. Martinowitz U, *et al.* Interaction between warfarin sodium and amiodarone. *N Engl J Med* 1981; **304:** 671–2.
2. Almog S, *et al.* Mechanism of warfarin potentiation by amiodarone: dose—and concentration—dependent inhibition of warfarin elimination. *Eur J Clin Pharmacol* 1985; **28:** 257–61.
3. Watt AH, *et al.* Amiodarone reduces plasma warfarin clearance in man. *Br J Clin Pharmacol* 1985; **20:** 707–9.
4. O'Reilly RA, *et al.* Interaction of amiodarone with racemic warfarin and its separated enantiomorphs in humans. *Clin Pharmacol Ther* 1987; **42:** 290–4.
5. Kerin NZ, *et al.* The incidence, magnitude, and time course of the amiodarone-warfarin interaction. *Arch Intern Med* 1988; **148:** 1779–81.
6. Arboix M, *et al.* The potentiation of acenocoumarol anticoagulant effect by amiodarone. *Br J Clin Pharmacol* 1984; **18:** 355–60.
7. Richard C, *et al.* Prospective study of the potentiation of acenocoumarol by amiodarone. *Eur J Clin Pharmacol* 1985; **28:** 625–9.
8. Verstraete M, *et al.* Dissimilar effect of two anti-anginal drugs belonging to the benzofuran group on the action of coumarin derivatives. *Arch Int Pharmacodyn Ther* 1968; **176:** 33–41.
9. Haworth E, Burroughs AK. Disopyramide and warfarin interaction. *BMJ* 1977; **2:** 866–7.
10. Gazzaniga AB, Stewart DR. Possible quinidine-induced hemorrhage in a patient on warfarin sodium. *N Engl J Med* 1969; **280:** 711–12.
11. Sylvén C, Anderson P. Evidence that disopyramide does not interact with warfarin. *BMJ* 1983; **286:** 1181.
12. Kates RE, *et al.* Interaction between warfarin and propafenone in healthy volunteer subjects. *Clin Pharmacol Ther* 1987; **42:** 305–11.
13. Serpa MD, *et al.* Moricizine: a possible drug interaction. *Ann Pharmacother* 1992; **26:** 127.

Antibacterials. Several antibacterials have been involved in interactions with warfarin. Only a few reports are of serious effects and it is unlikely that any of the drugs need to be contraindicated with warfarin; careful control should suffice.

Most of the drugs enhance the effects of warfarin. Apart from possible effects on the metabolism or plasma-protein binding of warfarin, some antibacterials may interfere with platelet function or with the bacterial synthesis of vitamin K in the gastrointestinal tract and thus have an anticoagulant effect of their own. This is generally considered unlikely to be of clinical significance except, perhaps, in patients with an inadequate vitamin K intake. Fever itself may increase the catabolism of clotting factors and exaggerate a potential antibacterial-warfarin interaction.

There are several reports of an enhanced warfarin response with *co-trimoxazole*; stereospecific inhibition of warfarin metabolism is probably responsible.[1] The interaction is generally attributed to the *sulfamethoxazole* moiety and there are isolated reports suggesting that the activity of warfarin (or other specified oral anticoagulant) may be enhanced by other sulfonamides including *sulfafurazole*,[2] *sulfamethizole*,[3] and *sulfaphenazole* (with phenindione).[4]

There are several reports of potentiation of the effects of warfarin by *erythromycin* or its salts; inhibition of warfarin metabolism probably occurs. Although no clinically-significant increase in prothrombin time could be demonstrated in 8 non-infected patients, the potential for an interaction was recognised.[5] An enhanced response to warfarin has also been reported with *azithromycin*[6,7] and with *roxithromycin*,[8] including reports of spontaneous bleeding with the latter. *Clarithromycin* may potentiate the effect of nicoumalone [acenocoumarol][9] and of warfarin,[10] although other factors may also have been involved in this case.

Cefamandole has been reported to enhance the hypoprothrombinaemic response to warfarin.[11,12] Interference with vitamin K synthesis in the gastrointestinal tract and/or liver has been implicated. Related cephalosporins with an *N*-methylthiotetrazole side-chain such as *cefmetazole*, *cefmenoxime*, *cefoperazone*, and *latamoxef* may be expected to behave similarly although there appear to be no reports of an interaction. *Cefazolin*, which has a similar side-chain, may also enhance the effect of warfarin to some extent.[12]

There have been a few reports of increased activity of warfarin (or other specified oral anticoagulant) by quinolone antibacterials including *nalidixic acid* (with warfarin[13,14] or nicoumalone [acenocoumarol][15]), *ciprofloxacin*,[16,17] *norfloxacin*,[18] and *ofloxacin*,[19,20] although for some of these there are also studies indicating no effect (not cited). *Enoxacin* has been reported to decrease the clearance of *R*-warfarin but not *S*-warfarin; no prolongation of prothrombin time occurred.[21]

There are isolated reports suggesting an enhanced effect of warfarin (or other specified oral anticoagulant) with *aminosalicylic acid*,[22] *benzylpenicillin*,[23] *chloramphenicol* (with dicoumarol),[24] *doxycycline*,[25] *isoniazid*,[26] and *neomycin*.[27] Prothrombin times might be prolonged by broad-spectrum antibacterials such as *ampicillin*, but published reports are lacking. Manufacturers' warnings of potentiation of warfarin by *aztreonam*, *trimethoprim*, and *tetracyclines* other than doxycycline appear to have only a theoretical basis. *Metronidazole* is discussed under Antiprotozoals, below.

Rifampicin diminishes the effect of warfarin by induction of metabolising enzymes in the liver. There are several reports of a similar effect with *nafcillin*[28-30] and with *dicloxacillin sodium*.[31,32]

1. O'Reilly RA. Stereo selective interaction of trimethoprim-sulfamethoxazole with the separated enantiomorphs of racemic warfarin in man. *N Engl J Med* 1980; **302** 33–5.
2. Sioris LJ, *et al.* Potentiation of warfarin anticoagulation by sulfisoxazole. *Arch Intern Med* 1980; **140:** 546–7.
3. Lumholtz B, *et al.* Sulfamethizole-induced inhibition of diphenylhydantoin, tolbutamide, and warfarin metabolism. *Clin Pharmacol Ther* 1975; **17:** 731–4.
4. Varma DR, *et al.* Prothrombin response to phenindione during hypoalbuminaemia. *Br J Clin Pharmacol* 1975; **2:** 467–8.
5. Weibert RT, *et al.* Effect of erythromycin in patients receiving long-term warfarin therapy. *Clin Pharm* 1989; **8:** 210–14.
6. Lane G. Increased hypoprothrombinemic effect of warfarin possibly induced by azithromycin. *Ann Pharmacother* 1996; **30:** 884–5.
7. Woldtvedt BR, *et al.* Possible increased anticoagulation effect of warfarin induced by azithromycin. *Ann Pharmacother* 1998; **32:** 269–70.
8. Anonymous. Interaction of warfarin with macrolide antibiotics. *Aust Adverse Drug React Bull* 1995; **14:** 11.
9. Grau E, *et al.* Interaction between clarithromycin and oral anticoagulants. *Ann Pharmacother* 1996; **30:** 1495–6.
10. Recker MW, Kier KL. Potential interaction between clarithromycin and warfarin. *Ann Pharmacother* 1997; **31:** 996–8.
11. Angaran DM, *et al.* The influence of prophylactic antibiotics on the warfarin anticoagulation response in the postoperative prosthetic cardiac valve patient. *Ann Surg* 1984; **199:** 107–11.

12. Angaran DM, *et al.* The comparative influence of prophylactic antibiotics on the prothrombin response to warfarin in the postoperative prosthetic cardiac valve patient: cefamandole, cefazoline, vancomycin. *Ann Surg* 1987; **206:** 155–61.
13. Hoffbrand BI. Interaction of nalidixic acid and warfarin. *BMJ* 1974; **2:** 666.
14. Leor J, *et al.* Interaction between nalidixic acid and warfarin. *Ann Intern Med* 1987; **107:** 601.
15. Potasman I, Bassan H. Nicoumalone and nalidixic acid interaction. *Ann Intern Med* 1980; **92:** 571.
16. Mott FE, *et al.* Ciprofloxacin and warfarin. *Ann Intern Med* 1989; **111:** 542–3.
17. Kamada AK. Possible interaction between ciprofloxacin and warfarin. *DICP Ann Pharmacother* 1990; **24:** 27–8.
18. Linville T, Matanin D. Norfloxacin and warfarin. *Ann Intern Med* 1989; **110:** 751–2.
19. Leor J, Matetzki S. Ofloxacin and warfarin. *Ann Intern Med* 1988; **109:** 761.
20. Baciewicz AM, *et al.* Interaction of ofloxacin and warfarin. *Ann Intern Med* 1993; **119:** 1223.
21. Toon S, *et al.* Enoxacin-warfarin interaction: pharmacokinetic and stereochemical aspects. *Clin Pharmacol Ther* 1987; **42:** 33–41.
22. Self TH. Interaction of warfarin and aminosalicylic acid. *JAMA* 1973; **223:** 1285.
23. Brown MA, *et al.* Interaction of penicillin-G and warfarin? *Can J Hosp Pharm* 1979; **32:** 18–19.
24. Christensen LK, Skovsted L. Inhibition of drug metabolism by chloramphenicol. *Lancet* 1969; **ii:** 1397–9.
25. Westfall LK, *et al.* Potentiation of warfarin by tetracycline. *Am J Hosp Pharm* 1980; **37:** 1620 and 1625.
26. Rosenthal AR, *et al.* Interaction of isoniazid and warfarin. *JAMA* 1977; **238:** 2177.
27. Udall JA. Drug interference with warfarin therapy. *Clin Med* 1970; **77** (Aug.): 20–5.
28. Qureshi GD, *et al.* Warfarin resistance with nafcillin therapy. *Ann Intern Med* 1984; **100:** 527–9.
29. Fraser GL, *et al.* Warfarin resistance associated with nafcillin therapy. *Am J Med* 1989; **87:** 237–8.
30. Davis RL, *et al.* Warfarin-nafcillin interaction. *J Pediatr* 1991; **118:** 300–3.
31. Krstenansky PM, *et al.* Effect of dicloxacillin sodium on the hypoprothrombinemic response to warfarin sodium. *Clin Pharm* 1987; **6:** 804–6.
32. Mailloux A, *et al.* Potential interaction between warfarin and dicloxacillin. *Ann Pharmacother* 1996; **30:** 1402–7.

Antidepressants. *Amitriptyline* and *nortriptyline* have been reported to prolong the half-life of dicoumarol in healthy subjects.[1,2] The few reports investigating the effect of tricyclic antidepressants on warfarin have not been able to conclude that a significant interaction exists. *Mianserin* and phenprocoumon have been reported not to interact.[3]

Some authorities consider that there is a theoretical risk of increased warfarin activity with *MAOIs* and with *fluvoxamine* and other SSRIs. Increased warfarin activity has been reported in a few patients taking *fluoxetine*.[4]

An increase in the dose of warfarin has been required by patients also taking *trazodone*.[5,6]

1. Vesell ES, *et al.* Impairment of drug metabolism in man by allopurinol and nortriptyline. *N Engl J Med* 1970; **283:** 1484–8.
2. Pond SM, *et al.* Effects of tricyclic antidepressants on drug metabolism. *Clin Pharmacol Ther* 1975; **18:** 191–9.
3. Kopera H, *et al.* Phenprocoumon requirement, whole blood coagulation time, bleeding time and plasma γ-GT in patients receiving mianserin. *Eur J Clin Pharmacol* 1978; **13:** 351–6.
4. Woolfrey S, *et al.* Fluoxetine-warfarin interaction. *BMJ* 1993; **307:** 241.
5. Hardy J-L, Sirois A. Reduction of prothrombin and partial thromboplastin times with trazodone. *Can Med Assoc J* 1986; **135:** 1372.
6. Small NL, Giamonna KA. Interaction between warfarin and trazodone. *Ann Pharmacother* 2000; **34:** 734–6.

Antidiabetics. There have been a few early instances of *tolbutamide* enhancing the activity of dicoumarol.[1] However, this effect has not been observed in later studies involving dicoumarol,[1–3] warfarin,[2] and phenprocoumon,[4] although one study did demonstrate altered dicoumarol pharmacokinetics.[3] An absence of effect has been documented for phenprocoumon and *insulin*, *glibenclamide*, or *glibornuride*,[4] but there is a report of glibenclamide enhancing the effect of warfarin.[5]

There has been an isolated report of bleeding in a patient taking *phenformin* and warfarin.[6] *Metformin* has been reported to diminish phenprocoumon activity.[7]

An enhanced response to warfarin has been reported in a patient receiving *troglitazone*.[8]

Coumarin anticoagulants may increase the hypoglycaemic effect of *sulfonylureas* (see p.336).

1. Chaplin H, Cassell M. Studies on the possible relationship of tolbutamide to dicumarol in anticoagulant therapy. *Am J Med Sci* 1958; **235:** 706–16.
2. Poucher RL, Vecchio TJ. Absence of tolbutamide effect on anticoagulant therapy. *JAMA* 1966; **197:** 1069–70.
3. Jähnchen E, *et al.* Pharmacokinetic analysis of the interaction between dicoumarol and tolbutamide in man. *Eur J Clin Pharmacol* 1976; **10:** 349–56.
4. Heine P, *et al.* The influence of hypoglycaemic sulphonylureas on elimination and efficacy of phenprocoumon following a single oral dose in diabetic patients. *Eur J Clin Pharmacol* 1976; **10:** 31–6.
5. Jassal SV. *BMJ* 1991; **303:** 789.
6. Hamblin TJ. Interaction between warfarin and phenformin. *Lancet* 1971; **ii:** 1323.
7. Ohnhaus EE, *et al.* The influence of dimethylbiguanide on phenprocoumon elimination and its mode of action: a drug interaction study. *Klin Wochenschr* 1983; **61:** 851–8.
8. Plowman BK, Morreale AP. Possible troglitazone—warfarin interaction. *Am J Health-Syst Pharm* 1998; **55:** 1071.

Antiepileptics. Barbiturates such as *phenobarbital* and *primidone* diminish the activity of warfarin and other coumarins through increased metabolism. *Carbamazepine* is reported to have a similar effect.[1,2] Reports of the effect of *phenytoin* on anticoagulants do not provide a clear picture. There are reports of phenytoin enhancing the effects of warfarin[3,4] and a report of initial enhancement followed by decreased anticoagulant action.[5] Phenytoin has been reported to diminish the effect of dicoumarol.[6] Addition of *felbamate* to the therapy of a patient has been reported[7] to necessitate a reduction in warfarin dosage in order to maintain a target INR. In another patient there was a transient increase in warfarin activity when *valproic acid* was commenced.[8] Valproate also inhibits platelet function and caution is required when it is given concomitantly with warfarin.

For the effect of oral anticoagulants on phenytoin, see p.360.

1. Hansen JM, *et al.* Carbamazepine-induced acceleration of diphenylhydantoin and warfarin metabolism in man. *Clin Pharmacol Ther* 1971; **12:** 539–43.
2. Ross JRY, Beeley L. Interaction between carbamazepine and warfarin. *BMJ* 1980; **280:** 1415–16.
3. Nappi JM. Warfarin and phenytoin interaction. *Ann Intern Med* 1979; **90:** 852.
4. Panegyres PK, Rischbieth RH. Fatal phenytoin warfarin interaction. *Postgrad Med J* 1991; **67:** 98.
5. Levine M, Sheppard I. Biphasic interaction of phenytoin with warfarin. *Clin Pharm* 1984; **3:** 200–3.
6. Hansen JM, *et al.* Effect of diphenylhydantoin on the metabolism of dicoumarol in man. *Acta Med Scand* 1971; **189:** 15–19.
7. Tisdel KA, *et al.* Warfarin—felbamate interaction: first report. *Ann Pharmacother* 1994; **28:** 805.
8. Guthrie SK, *et al.* Hypothesized interaction between valproic acid and warfarin. *J Clin Psychopharmacol* 1995; **15:** 138–9.

Antifungals. *Griseofulvin* has been reported to diminish the activity of warfarin.[1-3] There are several reports indicating that *miconazole*, given either systemically or topically as the oral gel, may enhance the activity of oral anticoagulants (warfarin, ethyl biscoumacetate, nicoumalone [acenocoumarol], phenindione, and tioclomarol).[4-11] Absorption of miconazole after intravaginal administration may have enhanced the activity of nicoumalone [acenocoumarol] in 2 elderly women.[12] Studies in healthy subjects given a single warfarin dose[13,14] support case reports[15-17] suggesting that *fluconazole* may increase the anticoagulant activity of warfarin. There are isolated reports of the potentiation of warfarin by *itraconazole*[18] and *ketoconazole*.[19] There has been a case report of a reduction in the effect of warfarin by *terbinafine*,[20] although a study[21] in healthy subjects found no clinically significant interaction, and others[22] considered that no interaction usually occurs. A case of potentiation of warfarin by terbinafine has also been reported;[23] the authors speculate that concomitant cimetidine may have contributed to the interaction by increasing plasma-terbinafine concentrations.

1. Cullen SI, Catalano PM. Griseofulvin-warfarin antagonism. *JAMA* 1967; **199:** 582–3.
2. Udall JA. Drug interference with warfarin therapy. *Clin Med* 1970; **77** (Aug.): 20–5.
3. Okino K, Weibert RT. Warfarin-griseofulvin interaction. *Drug Intell Clin Pharm* 1986; **20:** 291–3.
4. Loupi E, *et al.* Interactions médicamenteuses et miconazole: a propos de 10 observations. *Therapie* 1982; **37:** 437–41.
5. Watson PG, *et al.* Drug interaction with coumarin derivative anticoagulants. *BMJ* 1982; **285:** 1045–6.
6. Colquhoun MC, *et al.* Interaction between warfarin and miconazole oral gel. *Lancet* 1987; **i:** 695–6.
7. Bailey GM, *et al.* Miconazole and warfarin interaction. *Pharm J* 1989; **242:** 183.
8. Ariyaratnam S, *et al.* Potentiation of warfarin anticoagulant activity by miconazole oral gel. *BMJ* 1997; **314:** 349.
9. Evans J, *et al.* Treating oral candidiasis: potentially fatal. *Br Dent J* 1997; **182:** 452.
10. Pemberton MN, *et al.* Derangement of warfarin anticoagulation by miconazole oral gel. *Br Dent J* 1998; **184:** 68–9.
11. Ortín M, *et al.* Miconazole oral gel enhances acenocoumarol anticoagulant activity: a report of three cases. *Ann Pharmacother* 1999; **33:** 175–7.
12. Lansdorp D, *et al.* Potentiation of acenocoumarol during vaginal administration of miconazole. *Br J Clin Pharmacol* 1999; **47:** 225–6.
13. Lazar JD, Wilner KD. Drug interactions with fluconazole. *Rev Infect Dis* 1990; **12** (suppl 3): S327–S333.
14. Black DJ, *et al.* Warfarin–fluconazole II: a metabolically based drug interaction: in vivo studies. *Drug Metab Dispos* 1996; **24:** 422–8.
15. Seaton TL, *et al.* Possible potentiation of warfarin by fluconazole. *DICP Ann Pharmacother* 1990; **24:** 1177–8.
16. Gericke KR. Possible interaction between warfarin and fluconazole. *Pharmacotherapy* 1993; **13:** 508–9.
17. Baciewicz AM, *et al.* Fluconazole—warfarin interaction. *Ann Pharmacother* 1994; **28:** 1111.
18. Yeh J, *et al.* Potentiation of action of warfarin by itraconazole. *BMJ* 1990; **301:** 669.
19. Smith AG. Potentiation of oral anticoagulants by ketoconazole. *BMJ* 1984; **288:** 188–9. Correction. *ibid.*; 608.
20. Warwick JA, Corrall RJ. Serious interaction between warfarin and oral terbinafine. *BMJ* 1998; **316:** 440.
21. Guerret M, *et al.* Evaluation of effects of terbinafine on single oral dose pharmacokinetics and anticoagulant actions of warfarin in healthy volunteers. *Pharmacotherapy* 1997; **17:** 767–73.
22. Stockley IH. Terbinafine and warfarin mystery. *Pharm J* 1998; **260:** 408.
23. Gupta AK, Ross GS. Interaction between terbinafine and warfarin. *Dermatology* 1998; **196:** 266–7.

Antigout drugs. The two drugs in this group that have mostly been implicated in interactions with anticoagulants are allopurinol and sulfinpyrazone.

With *allopurinol* there are conflicting reports of patients experiencing no interaction or an enhanced anticoagulant effect with dicoumarol,[1] phenprocoumon,[2] or warfarin.[3,4]

Interactions with *sulfinpyrazone* have usually involved warfarin and, apart from a case of a mixed response,[5] have involved increased anticoagulant activity, sometimes with haemorrhage, so calling for careful control. It is still not clear how sulfinpyrazone exerts its effect, but studies point to a stereoselective effect on warfarin metabolism where the *S*-isomer's metabolic clearance is inhibited.[6] It should also be remembered that sulfinpyrazone affects platelets. Sulfinpyrazone has also enhanced the anticoagulant activity of nicoumalone [acenocoumarol].[7] A significant interaction with phenprocoumon appears unlikely.[8]

Administration of *probenecid* has accelerated the elimination of a single dose of phenprocoumon without effect on the prothrombin time.[9]

Benziodarone has been reported to enhance the effects of warfarin, diphenadione, ethyl biscoumacetate, and nicoumalone [acenocoumarol], but not of dicoumarol, phenindione, or phenprocoumon.[10] A further study[11] confirmed that benziodarone could increase the half-life of ethyl biscoumacetate, but also found that the effect of phenprocoumon was enhanced.

1. Vesell ES, *et al.* Impairment of drug metabolism in man by allopurinol and nortriptyline. *N Engl J Med* 1970; **283:** 1484–8.
2. Jähnchen E, *et al.* Interaction of allopurinol with phenprocoumon in man. *Klin Wochenschr* 1977; **55:** 759–61.
3. Rawlins MD, Smith SE. Influence of allopurinol on drug metabolism in man. *Br J Pharmacol* 1973; **48:** 693–8.
4. Pond SM, *et al.* The effects of allopurinol and clofibrate on the elimination of coumarin anticoagulants in man. *Aust N Z J Med* 1975; **5:** 324–8.
5. Nenci GG, *et al.* Biphasic sulphinpyrazone-warfarin interaction. *BMJ* 1981; **282:** 1361–2.
6. Toon S, *et al.* The warfarin-sulfinpyrazone interaction: stereochemical considerations. *Clin Pharmacol Ther* 1986; **39:** 15–24.
7. Michot F, *et al.* Über die Beeinflussung der gerinnungshemmenden Wirkung von Acenocoumarol durch Sulfinpyrazon. *Schweiz Med Wochenschr* 1981; **111:** 255–60.
8. Heimark LD, *et al.* The effect of sulfinpyrazone on the disposition of pseudoracemic phenprocoumon in humans. *Clin Pharmacol Ther* 1987; **42:** 312–19.
9. Mönig H, *et al.* The effects of frusemide and probenecid on the pharmacokinetics of phenprocoumon. *Eur J Clin Pharmacol* 1990; **39:** 261–5.
10. Pyörälä K, *et al.* Benziodarone (Amplivix®) and anticoagulant therapy. *Acta Med Scand* 1963; **173:** 385–9.
11. Verstraete M, *et al.* Dissimilar effect of two anti-anginal drugs belonging to the benzofuran group on the action of coumarin derivatives. *Arch Int Pharmacodyn Ther* 1968; **176:** 33–41.

Antihistamines. There has been a report[1] of a raised INR and severe epistaxis in a patient receiving long-term nicoumalone [acenocoumarol] following the addition of *cetirizine* to his therapy.

1. Berod T, Mathiot I. Probable interaction between cetirizine and acenocoumarol. *Ann Pharmacother* 1997; **31:** 122.

Antimalarials. The ingestion of large amounts of tonic water by 2 patients necessitated a reduction in their warfarin dosage. The enhanced effect was attributed to the *quinine* content of the tonic water.[1] A woman stabilised on warfarin developed haematuria and a high prothrombin ratio after taking *proguanil* for malaria prophylaxis.[2]

1. Clark DJ. Clinical curio: warfarin and tonic water. *BMJ* 1983; **286:** 1258.
2. Armstrong G, *et al.* Warfarin potentiated by proguanil. *BMJ* 1991; **303:** 789.

Antineoplastics and immunosuppressants. There have been several reports of interactions between warfarin and antineoplastics. No clear picture emerges from these reports which is not surprising considering that antineoplastics are often given in combination and that they can exert their own haematological effects. *Cyclophosphamide* for instance has been associated with an increase in warfarin's activity when given with *methotrexate* and *fluorouracil*,[1] but with a decrease when given with nonantineoplastic drugs.[2] An increase in the activity of warfarin and mucous membrane bleeding occurred in a patient who received 4 courses of fluorouracil and folic acid at weekly intervals.[3] The patient was also taking indometacin. Warfarin dosage had to be reduced in 5 patients who received fluorouracil-based antineoplastic regimens.[4] Fluorouracil has also been reported to increase the effect of warfarin when given with levamisole (see below). The manufacturers of *capecitabine* state that altered coagulation parameters and bleeding have been reported in patients taking capecitabine and warfarin or phenprocoumon. In one patient, concurrent therapy with warfarin and *ciclosporin* was associated with reduced effect of both drugs;[5] the patient was, however, also receiving phenobarbital. Increased effects of both drugs were observed in another patient receiving ciclosporin and nicoumalone [acenocoumarol].[6] *Etoposide* with *vindesine*[7] or with *carboplatin*,[8] *ifosfamide* with *mesna*,[9] and *tamoxifen*[10-12] have all produced an increased anticoagulant effect. *Aminoglutethimide* has led to decreased activity of warfarin or nicoumalone [acenocoumarol],[13,14] probably due to increased warfarin metabolism. The manufacturers of the anti-androgen *flutamide* state that increases in prothrombin time have been reported after initiation of flutamide therapy in patients on long-term warfarin. *Mercaptopurine*[15] and *mitotane*[16] have also decreased warfarin activity. Severe bleeding occurred in a patient on long-term warfarin treatment after discontinuing *azathioprine*,[17] while another patient[18] required an increased dose of warfarin when azathioprine was given concomitantly.

1. Seifter EJ, *et al.* Possible interactions between warfarin and antineoplastic drugs. *Cancer Treat Rep* 1985; **69:** 244–5.
2. Tashima CK. Cyclophosphamide effect on coumarin anticoagulation. *South Med J* 1979; **72:** 633–4.
3. Brown MC. Multisite mucous membrane bleeding due to a possible interaction between warfarin and 5-fluorouracil. *Pharmacotherapy* 1997; **17:** 631–3.

4. Kolesar JM, *et al*. Warfarin–5-FU interaction—a consecutive case series. *Pharmacotherapy* 1999; **19**: 1445–9.
5. Snyder DS. Interaction between cyclosporine and warfarin. *Ann Intern Med* 1988; **108**: 311.
6. Campistol JM, *et al*. Interaction between ciclosporin A and Sintrom. *Nephron* 1989; **53**: 291–2.
7. Ward K, Bitran JD. Warfarin, etoposide, and vindesine interactions. *Cancer Treat Rep* 1984; **68**: 817–18.
8. Le AT, *et al*. Enhancement of warfarin response in a patient receiving etoposide and carboplatin chemotherapy. *Ann Pharmacother* 1997; **31**: 1006–8.
9. Hall G, *et al*. Intravenous infusions of ifosfamide/mesna and perturbation of warfarin anticoagulant control. *Postgrad Med J* 1990; **66**: 860–1.
10. Lodwick R, *et al*. Life threatening interaction between tamoxifen and warfarin. *BMJ* 1987; **295**: 1141.
11. Tenni P, *et al*. Life threatening interaction between tamoxifen and warfarin. *BMJ* 1989; **298**: 93.
12. Ritchie LD, Grant SMT. Tamoxifen-warfarin interaction: the Aberdeen hospitals drug file. *BMJ* 1989; **298**: 1253.
13. Lønning PE, *et al*. The influence of a graded dose schedule of aminoglutethimide on the disposition of the optical enantiomers of warfarin in patients with breast cancer. *Cancer Chemother Pharmacol* 1986; **17**: 177–81.
14. Bruning PF, Bonfrèr JGM. Aminoglutethimide and oral anticoagulant therapy. *Lancet* 1983; **ii**: 582.
15. Spiers ASD, Mibashan RS. Increased warfarin requirement during mercaptopurine therapy: a new drug interaction. *Lancet* 1974; **ii**: 221–2.
16. Cuddy PG, *et al*. Influence of mitotane on the hypoprothrombinemic effect of warfarin. *South Med J* 1986; **79**: 387–8.
17. Singleton JD, Conyers L. Warfarin and azathioprine: an important drug interaction. *Am J Med* 1992; **92**: 217.
18. Rotenberg M, *et al*. Effect of azathioprine on the anticoagulant activity of warfarin. *Ann Pharmacother* 2000; **34**: 120–2.

Antiplatelets. The interaction between anticoagulants and *dipyridamole* is an oddity in that bleeding can occur without any alteration in prothrombin times; special care is therefore required as the usual method of monitoring the anticoagulant effect is of no value. This interaction has involved a small number of patients taking dipyridamole and warfarin or phenindione;[1] inhibition of platelet function by dipyridamole has been implicated. However, in general it does not appear to increase the risk of bleeding.[2]

Interestingly, in a group of patients receiving nicoumalone [acenocoumarol] for thromboprophylaxis, addition of *ticlopidine* was found to significantly increase nicoumalone [acenocoumarol] requirements.[3]

See also under Analgesics and NSAIDs (above).

1. Kalowski S, Kincaid-Smith P. Interaction of dipyridamole with anticoagulants in the treatment of glomerulonephritis. *Med J Aust* 1973; **2**: 164–6.
2. Levine MN, *et al*. Hemorrhagic complications of long-term anticoagulant therapy. *Chest* 1989; **95** (suppl): 26S–36S.
3. Salar A, *et al*. Ticlopidine antagonizes acenocoumarol treatment. *Thromb Haemost* 1997; **77**: 223–4.

Antiprotozoals. *Metronidazole* enhances the activity of warfarin[1,2] through selective inhibition of the metabolism of its *S*-isomer.[3]

1. Kazmier FJ. A significant interaction between metronidazole and warfarin. *Mayo Clin Proc* 1976; **51**: 782–4.
2. Dean RP, Talbert RL. Bleeding associated with concurrent warfarin and metronidazole therapy. *Drug Intell Clin Pharm* 1980; **14**: 864–6.
3. O'Reilly RA. The stereoselective interaction of warfarin and metronidazole in man. *N Engl J Med* 1976; **295**: 354–7.

Antithyroid drugs. See under Thyroid and Antithyroid Drugs, below.

Antivirals. Reductions in dosage of either warfarin[1] or nicoumalone [acenocoumarol][2] were necessary in 2 patients receiving *interferon alfa* for hepatitis C. The interactions may have been due to decreased metabolism of the anticoagulant. A similar need for a reduced warfarin dose had also been noted in other patients taking *interferon alfa-2b* or *interferon beta*.[1]

An enhanced response to warfarin has been reported[3] in a patient taking *saquinavir* concomitantly. The mechanism may involve competitive inhibition of warfarin metabolism and might also occur with other HIV-protease inhibitors. However, a decreased response to warfarin seemed to be caused by *ritonavir* when it was added to the multidrug therapy of a patient.[4]

1. Adachi Y, *et al*. Potentiation of warfarin by interferon. *BMJ* 1995; **311**: 292.
2. Serratrice J, *et al*. Interferon-alpha 2b interaction with acenocoumarol. *Am J Hematol* 1998; **57**: 89.
3. Darlington MR. Hypoprothrombinemia during concomitant therapy with warfarin and saquinavir. *Ann Pharmacother* 1997; **31**: 647.
4. Knoell KR, *et al*. Potential interaction involving warfarin and ritonavir. *Ann Pharmacother* 1998; **32**: 1299–1302.

Anxiolytic sedatives, hypnotics, and antipsychotics. *Barbiturates*, by inducing liver metabolism, can reduce the activity of anticoagulants; *glutethimide* has a similar action. The *benzodiazepines* on the other hand do not generally have any effect although there is the rare report of increased or decreased activity.

Although there is a report suggesting that *cloral hydrate* may decrease the effect of dicoumarol by enzyme induction,[1] other studies and experience indicate an increase in the anticoagulant activity of warfarin.[2-4] However, the increase is only transient and is probably the result of displacement of warfarin from plasma protein binding sites by the metabolite trichloroacetic

acid.[2] *Triclofos sodium* appears to increase the activity of warfarin in a similar way.[5]

Reduced anticoagulant activity has been reported with *dichloralphenazone*,[6,7] *ethchlorvynol* (with dicoumarol),[8] and *haloperidol* (with phenindione).[9] Compounds such as *meprobamate* and *methaqualone* appear to have no effect on anticoagulants.

1. Cucinell SA, *et al*. The effect of chloral hydrate on bishydroxycoumarin metabolism: a fatal outcome. *JAMA* 1966; **197**: 366–8.
2. Sellers EM, Koch-Weser J. Kinetics and clinical importance of displacement of warfarin from albumin by acidic drugs. *Ann N Y Acad Sci* 1971; **179**: 213–25.
3. Boston Collaborative Drug Surveillance Program. Interaction between chloral hydrate and warfarin. *N Engl J Med* 1972; **286**: 53–5.
4. Udall JA. Warfarin-chloral hydrate interaction: pharmacological activity and clinical significance. *Ann Intern Med* 1974; **81**: 341–4.
5. Sellers EM, *et al*. Enhancement of warfarin-induced hypoprothrombinemia by triclofos. *Clin Pharmacol Ther* 1972; **13**: 911–15.
6. Breckenridge A, Orme M. Clinical implications of enzyme induction. *Ann N Y Acad Sci* 1971; **179**: 421–3.
7. Whitfield JB, *et al*. Changes in plasma α-glutamyl transpeptidase activity associated with alterations in drug metabolism in man. *BMJ* 1973; **1**: 316–18.
8. Johansson S-A. Apparent resistance to oral anticoagulant therapy and influence of hypnotics on some coagulation factors. *Acta Med Scand* 1968; **184**: 297–300.
9. Oakley DP, Lautch H. Haloperidol and anticoagulant treatment. *Lancet* 1963; **ii**: 1231.

Beta blockers. Possible potentiation of the effect of warfarin by *propranolol*[1] has been reported. Beta blockers, particularly those with a high lipid solubility such as propranolol, may inhibit the metabolism of warfarin.[2] However, although a number of studies have shown pharmacokinetic interactions between some beta blockers and oral anticoagulants, no effect on anticoagulant activity has been found.

1. Bax NDS, *et al*. Inhibition of drug metabolism by β-adrenoceptor antagonists. *Drugs* 1983; **25** (suppl 2): 121–6.
2. Mantero F, *et al*. Effect of atenolol and metoprolol on the anticoagulant activity of acenocoumarin. *Br J Clin Pharmacol* 1984; **17**: 94S–96S.

Central stimulants. While *methylphenidate* has been reported to increase the half-life of ethyl biscoumacetate,[1] it has also been reported to have no effect on the half-life or on the anticoagulant activity of ethyl biscoumacetate.[2] *Prolintane* also had no effect on ethyl biscoumacetate.[2]

1. Garrettson LK, *et al*. Methylphenidate interaction with both anticonvulsants and ethyl biscoumacetate: a new action of methylphenidate. *JAMA* 1969; **207**: 2053.
2. Hague DE, *et al*. The effect of methylphenidate and prolintane on the metabolism of ethyl biscoumacetate. *Clin Pharmacol Ther* 1971; **12**: 259–62.

Corticosteroids and corticotropin. There are several reports of corticosteroids or corticotropin either enhancing[1,2] or diminishing[3] the effects of anticoagulants. Matters are further confused by corticosteroids being associated with an increase in the coagulability of the blood. However, the extensive use of corticosteroids and anticoagulants, and very few reports of interaction, suggests that any problems are rare.

1. Van Cauwenberge H, Jaques LB. Haemorrhagic effect of ACTH with anticoagulants. *Can Med Assoc J* 1958; **79**: 536–40.
2. Costedoat-Chalumeau N, *et al*. Potentiation of vitamin K antagonists by high-dose intravenous methylprednisolone. *Ann Intern Med* 2000; **132**: 631–5.
3. Chatterjea JB, Salomon L. Antagonistic effect of ACTH and cortisone on the anticoagulant activity of ethyl biscoumacetate. *BMJ* 1954; **2**: 790–2.

Dermatological drugs. A patient's warfarin dose had to be increased when he started treatment with *etretinate*.[1]

1. Ostlere LS, *et al*. Reduced therapeutic effect of warfarin caused by etretinate. *Br J Dermatol* 1991; **124**: 505–10.

Disulfiram. Two reports suggesting that disulfiram enhances the activity of warfarin[1,2] were confirmed by a study in 8 healthy subjects.[3] Although inhibition of liver enzymes by disulfiram was considered responsible,[3] a later study[4] suggested that disulfiram acts directly on the liver to increase hypoprothrombinaemia. This interaction is complicated by the variable effects of alcohol on warfarin (see above). Special care is therefore called for when these drugs are used together.

1. Rothstein E. Warfarin effect enhanced by disulfiram. *JAMA* 1968; **206**: 1574–5.
2. Rothstein E. Warfarin effect enhanced by disulfiram (Antabuse). *JAMA* 1972; **221**: 1052–3.
3. O'Reilly RA. Interaction of sodium warfarin and disulfiram (Antabuse®) in man. *Ann Intern Med* 1973; **78**: 73–6.
4. O'Reilly RA. Dynamic interaction between disulfiram and separated enantiomorphs of racemic warfarin. *Clin Pharmacol Ther* 1981; **29**: 332–6.

Diuretics. There have been a number of studies on the effects of diuretics on anticoagulants. *Tienilic acid* produces the most serious interaction enhancing the activity of ethyl biscoumacetate,[1] nicoumalone [acenocoumarol],[2] and warfarin[3] and has led to haemorrhage. *Etacrynic acid* has also been reported to enhance the activity of warfarin,[4] but reports do not show as severe an effect as with tienilic acid.

Chlortalidone[5] and *spironolactone*[6] have both been associated with a reduction in warfarin's activity in healthy subjects and it has been suggested that this might be a consequence of the diuresis concentrating the circulating clotting factors. However,

bumetanide, frusemide [furosemide], and the *thiazides* appear to have no effect on warfarin.

1. Detilleux M, *et al*. Potentialisation de l'effet des anticoagulants coumariniques par un nouveau diurétique, l'acide tiénilique. *Nouv Presse Med* 1976; **5**: 2395.
2. Grand A, *et al*. Potentialisation de l'action anticoagulante des anti-vitamines K par l'acide tiénilique. *Nouv Presse Med* 1977; **6**: 2691.
3. McLain DA, *et al*. Adverse reactions associated with ticrynafen use. *JAMA* 1980; **243**: 763–4.
4. Petrick RJ, *et al*. Interaction between warfarin and ethacrynic acid. *JAMA* 1975; **231**: 843–4.
5. O'Reilly RA, *et al*. Impact of aspirin and chlorthalidone on the pharmacodynamics of oral anticoagulant drugs in man. *Ann N Y Acad Sci* 1971; **179**: 173–86.
6. O'Reilly RA. Spironolactone and warfarin interaction. *Clin Pharmacol Ther* 1980; **27**: 198–201.

Gastrointestinal drugs. Antacids may or may not interact with warfarin. *Bismuth carbonate* and *magnesium trisilicate* for example have been reported to reduce warfarin's absorption,[1] but *aluminium hydroxide* has been observed to have no effect on warfarin or dicoumarol.[2] *Psyllium*[3] and *magnesium hydroxide*[2] have also been reported to have no effect on warfarin, but the latter has increased the plasma concentrations of dicoumarol.[2]

There have been occasional reports of *sucralfate* diminishing the effect of warfarin.[4-6]

Histamine H_2-antagonists have been widely studied. There are several reports indicating that *cimetidine* can enhance the anticoagulant effect of warfarin and haemorrhage has occurred. A number of studies show that cimetidine can increase the plasma concentration and half-life of warfarin and that there is a selective inhibitory effect on the metabolism of its *R*-isomer.[7-10] Not all these studies have, however, demonstrated an increase in prothrombin time. The effect of cimetidine on warfarin appears to be dose-dependent[7] and to be subject to interindividual variation;[9,10] the need for careful monitoring of patients receiving both drugs is, therefore, evident. Limited evidence suggests that cimetidine has a similar effect on the metabolism of nicoumalone [acenocoumarol][11,12] and phenindione[11] but not of phenprocoumon.[13] Studies with *ranitidine* have generally been unable to demonstrate an effect on the metabolism of warfarin,[10,14] although in one study warfarin clearance was reduced.[7] There is a case report suggesting that potentiation of warfarin by ranitidine may occasionally occur.[15]

One study has suggested that *omeprazole* could inhibit the metabolism of *R*-warfarin although a clinically significant effect on the activity of warfarin was unlikely.[16] No evidence of an interaction was found in a retrospective study[17] of patients on nicoumalone [acenocoumarol] who received omeprazole therapy. Similarly, *pantoprazole* appears to have no effect on the pharmacokinetics or pharmacodynamics of warfarin[18] or phenprocoumon.[19]

A marked increase in the effect of warfarin has been reported in a patient when *cisapride* was added to his therapy.[20]

A reduction in the response to warfarin with development of venous thrombosis has been reported in a patient receiving *mesalazine*,[21] and in another patient receiving *sulfasalazine*.[22]

1. McElnay JC, *et al*. Interaction of warfarin with antacid constituents. *BMJ* 1978; **2**: 1166.
2. Ambre JJ, Fischer LJ. Effect of coadministration of aluminum and magnesium hydroxides on absorption of anticoagulants in man. *Clin Pharmacol Ther* 1973; **14**: 231–7.
3. Robinson DS. Interaction of warfarin and nonsystemic gastrointestinal drugs. *Clin Pharmacol Ther* 1971; **12**: 491–5.
4. Mungall D, *et al*. Sucralfate and warfarin. *Ann Intern Med* 1983; **98**: 557.
5. Rey AM, Gums JG. Altered absorption of digoxin, sustained-release quinidine, and warfarin with sucralfate administration. *DICP Ann Pharmacother* 1991; **25**: 745–6.
6. Parrish RH, *et al*. Sucralfate-warfarin interaction. *Ann Pharmacother* 1992; **26**: 1015–16.
7. Desmond PV, *et al*. Decreased oral warfarin clearance after ranitidine and cimetidine. *Clin Pharmacol Ther* 1984; **35**: 338–41.
8. Choonara IA, *et al*. Stereoselective interaction between the R enantiomer of warfarin and cimetidine. *Br J Clin Pharmacol* 1986; **21**: 271–7.
9. Sax MJ, *et al*. Effect of two cimetidine regimens on prothrombin time and warfarin pharmacokinetics during long-term warfarin therapy. *Clin Pharm* 1987; **6**: 492–5.
10. Toon S, *et al*. Comparative effects of ranitidine and cimetidine on the pharmacokinetics and pharmacodynamics of warfarin in man. *Eur J Clin Pharmacol* 1987; **32**: 165–72.
11. Serlin MJ, *et al*. Cimetidine: interaction with oral anticoagulants in man. *Lancet* 1979; **ii**: 317–19.
12. Gill TS, *et al*. Cimetidine-nicoumalone interaction in man: stereochemical considerations. *Br J Clin Pharmacol* 1989; **27**: 469–74.
13. Harenberg J, *et al*. Cimetidine does not increase the anticoagulant effect of phenprocoumon. *Br J Clin Pharmacol* 1982; **14**: 292–3.
14. Serlin MJ, *et al*. Lack of effect of ranitidine on warfarin action. *Br J Clin Pharmacol* 1981; **12**: 791–4.
15. Baciewicz AM, Morgan PJ. Ranitidine-warfarin interaction. *Ann Intern Med* 1990; **112**: 76–7.
16. Sutfin T, *et al*. Stereoselective interaction of omeprazole with warfarin in healthy men. *Ther Drug Monit* 1989; **11**: 176–84.
17. Vreeburg EM, *et al*. Lack of effect of omeprazole on oral acenocoumarol anticoagulant therapy. *Scand J Gastroenterol* 1997; **32**: 991–4.
18. Duursema L, *et al*. Lack of effect of pantoprazole on the pharmacodynamics and pharmacokinetics of warfarin. *Br J Clin Pharmacol* 1995; **39**: 700–3.
19. Ehrlich A, *et al*. Lack of pharmacodynamic and pharmacokinetic interaction between pantoprazole and phenprocoumon in man. *Eur J Clin Pharmacol* 1996; **51**: 277–81.
20. Darlington MR. Hypoprothrombinemia induced by warfarin sodium and cisapride. *Am J Health-Syst Pharm* 1997; **54**: 320–1.

21. Marinella MA. Mesalamine and warfarin therapy resulting in decreased warfarin effect. *Ann Pharmacother* 1998; **32:** 841–2.
22. Teefy AM, *et al.* Warfarin resistance due to sulfasalazine. *Ann Pharmacother* 2000; **34:** 1265–8.

Ginseng. Reduction in the response to warfarin was reported in a patient after he started taking a ginseng preparation.[1]

1. Janetzky K, Morreale AP. Probable interaction between warfarin and ginseng. *Am J Health-Syst Pharm* 1997; **54:** 692–3.

Glucagon. A dose-dependent enhancement of warfarin's anticoagulant activity has been reported with glucagon.[1]

1. Koch-Weser J. Potentiation by glucagon of the hypoprothrombinemic action of warfarin. *Ann Intern Med* 1970; **72:** 331–5.

Hypericum. Hypericum has been reported to reduce the anticoagulant effect of warfarin.[1]

1. Yue Q-Y, *et al.* Safety of St John's wort (Hypericum perforatum). *Lancet* 2000; **355:** 576–7.

Leukotriene antagonists. *Zafirlukast* is reported to decrease the clearance of *S*-warfarin.[1] The manufacturers of zafirlukast state that it probably inhibits the cytochrome P450 isoenzyme CYP2C9 which is involved in the metabolism of warfarin. Patients receiving warfarin may develop prolongation of the prothrombin time when zafirlukast is added and warfarin dosage should be adjusted accordingly.

A study[2] of *montelukast* and warfarin found no significant interaction between the two drugs.

1. Suttle AB, *et al.* Effect of zafirlukast on the pharmacokinetics of R- and S-warfarin in healthy men. *Clin Pharmacol Ther* 1997; **61:** 186.
2. Van Hecken, *et al.* Effect of montelukast on the pharmacokinetics and pharmacodynamics of warfarin in healthy volunteers. *J Clin Pharmacol* 1999; **39:** 495–500.

Levamisole. An increased INR has been reported[1] in a patient receiving chronic warfarin therapy after addition of *levamisole* and fluorouracil. Inhibition of warfarin metabolism was postulated as the mechanism responsible for the interaction. In a second patient, a similar reaction was reported[2] following administration of levamisole and fluorouracil and an episode of bleeding subsequently occurred after administration of levamisole alone.

1. Scarfe MA, Israel MK. Possible drug interaction between warfarin and combination of levamisole and fluorouracil. *Ann Pharmacother* 1994; **28:** 464–7.
2. Wehbe TW, Warth JA. A case of bleeding requiring hospitalization that was likely caused by an interaction between warfarin and levamisole. *Clin Pharmacol Ther* 1996; **59:** 360–2.

Lipid regulating drugs. *Clofibrate* can enhance the activity of warfarin, sometimes to the point of haemorrhage. The mechanism of this interaction is not clear, but it does not appear to be connected with any pharmacokinetic effect. Similar enhancement of activity has been reported when clofibrate is given to patients taking dicoumarol or phenindione. *Bezafibrate* has been reported to enhance the effect of phenprocoumon[1] and warfarin,[2] and *fenofibrate*[3] and *gemfibrozil*[4] have been reported to enhance the effect of warfarin.

Hypoprothrombinaemia and bleeding has been reported in 2 patients on warfarin given *lovastatin*.[5] An increased response to warfarin has also been reported[6,7] in a number of patients receiving *fluvastatin* concomitantly. The manufacturers of *simvastatin* state that it has slightly enhanced the effect of coumarin anticoagulants. Simvastatin has been reported[8] to potentiate the effect of nicoumalone [acenocoumarol] in a patient. However, the INR in a patient on long-term warfarin remained stable on the addition of treatment with simvastatin.[9] The manufacturers of *pravastatin* have not observed any change in warfarin activity in patients given both drugs. However, there has been a report[10] of bleeding in a patient receiving fluindione when pravastatin was added. In a study[11] of 46 patients on warfarin who had been converted from pravastatin to *simvastatin*, the mean INR increased, but the median weekly warfarin dose did not differ significantly and no episodes of bleeding were reported.

Dextrothyroxine increases the anticoagulant effect of warfarin sodium[12,13] and dicoumarol.[14]

An opposite effect may occur with *colestyramine* which has reduced warfarin's serum concentration[15] and half-life[16] as well as its activity.[15,16] The mechanisms of this interaction include binding of warfarin to colestyramine and reduced absorption;[15] the enterohepatic recycling of warfarin may also be interrupted.[16] Phenprocoumon's activity has also been reduced by colestyramine.[17] It should be remembered, however, that colestyramine can also reduce vitamin K absorption, which may result in hypoprothrombinaemia and bleeding.

Benfluorex[18] and *colestipol*[19] have been reported not to interact with phenprocoumon.

1. Zimmermann R, *et al.* The effect of bezafibrate on the fibrinolytic enzyme system and the drug interaction with racemic phenprocoumon. *Atherosclerosis* 1978; **29:** 477–85.
2. Beringer TRO. Warfarin potentiation with bezafibrate. *Postgrad Med J* 1997; **73:** 657–8.
3. Ascah KJ, *et al.* Interaction between fenofibrate and warfarin. *Ann Pharmacother* 1998; **32:** 765–8.
4. Ahmad S. Gemfibrozil interaction with warfarin sodium (Coumadin). *Chest* 1990; **98:** 1041–2.
5. Ahmad S. Lovastatin: warfarin interaction. *Arch Intern Med* 1990; **150:** 2407.
6. Trilli LE, *et al.* Potential interaction between warfarin and fluvastatin. *Ann Pharmacother* 1996; **30:** 1399–1402.
7. Kline SS, Harrell CC. Potential warfarin-fluvastatin interaction. *Ann Pharmacother* 1997; **31:** 790–1.
8. Grau E, *et al.* Simvastatin-oral anticoagulant interaction. *Lancet* 1996; **347:** 405–6.
9. Gaw A, Wosornu D. Simvastatin during warfarin therapy in hyperlipoproteinaemia. *Lancet* 1992; **340:** 979–80.
10. Trenque T, *et al.* Pravastatin: interaction with oral anticoagulant? *BMJ* 1996; **312:** 886.
11. Lin JC, *et al.* The effect of converting from pravastatin to simvastatin on the pharmacodynamics of warfarin. *J Clin Pharmacol* 1999; **39:** 86–90.
12. Owens JC, *et al.* Effect of sodium dextrothyroxine in patients receiving anticoagulants. *N Engl J Med* 1962; **266:** 76–9.
13. Solomon HM, Schrogie JJ. Change in receptor site affinity: a proposed explanation for the potentiating effect of D-thyroxine on the anticoagulant response to warfarin. *Clin Pharmacol Ther* 1967; **8:** 797–9.
14. Schrogie JJ, Solomon HM. The anticoagulant response to bishydroxycoumarin: II. The effect of D-thyroxine, clofibrate, and norethandrolone. *Clin Pharmacol Ther* 1967; **8:** 70–7.
15. Robinson DS, *et al.* Interaction of warfarin and nonsystemic gastrointestinal drugs. *Clin Pharmacol Ther* 1971; **12:** 491–5.
16. Jähnchen E, *et al.* Enhanced elimination of warfarin during treatment with cholestyramine. *Br J Clin Pharmacol* 1978; **5:** 437–40.
17. Meinertz T, *et al.* Interruption of the enterohepatic circulation of phenprocoumon by cholestyramine. *Clin Pharmacol Ther* 1977; **21:** 731–5.
18. De Witte P, Brems HM. Co-administration of benfluorex with oral anticoagulant therapy. *Curr Med Res Opin* 1980; **6:** 478–80.
19. Harvengt C, Desager JP. Effect of colestipol, a new bile acid sequestrant, on the absorption of phenprocoumon in man. *Eur J Clin Pharmacol* 1973; **6:** 19–21.

Pesticides. Chlorinated insecticides diminished the activity of warfarin in a patient.[1]

1. Jeffery WH, *et al.* Loss of warfarin effect after occupational insecticide exposure. *JAMA* 1976; **236:** 2881–2.

Piracetam. Piracetam caused an increase in prothrombin time in a patient who had been stabilised on warfarin.[1]

1. Pan HYM, Ng RP. The effect of Nootropil in a patient on warfarin. *Eur J Clin Pharmacol* 1983; **24:** 711.

Sex hormones. There have been a number of reports of steroids with anabolic or androgenic properties enhancing the activity of anticoagulants to the point of haemorrhage. Reports have covered *oxymetholone* enhancing warfarin[1-3] and nicoumalone [acenocoumarol];[4] *stanozolol* enhancing warfarin[5,6] and dicoumarol;[7] *ethylestrenol* enhancing phenindione;[8] *norethandrolone* enhancing dicoumarol;[9] *methyltestosterone* enhancing phenprocoumon;[10] and *danazol* enhancing warfarin.[11-13] The mechanism of this interaction is not clear although it is considered that it is not due to altered pharmacokinetics. Steroids with a 17-α-alkyl substituent appear to be most involved, but there has been a report of topically applied testosterone, which does not have such a substituent, enhancing warfarin.[14]

Oral contraceptives have also been implicated in interactions. However, while the effects of dicoumarol were diminished by a combined oral contraceptive,[15] those of nicoumalone [acenocoumarol] were enhanced by other preparations.[16] Combined oral contraceptives have increased the clearance of phenprocoumon without altering the anticoagulant effect.[17] There has also been a report[18] of a single course of *levonorgestrel* for emergency contraception increasing the effect of warfarin.

1. Robinson BHB, *et al.* Decreased anticoagulant tolerance with oxymetholone. *Lancet* 1971; **i:** 1356.
2. Longridge RGM, *et al.* Decreased anticoagulant tolerance with oxymetholone. *Lancet* 1971; **ii:** 90.
3. Edwards MS, Curtis JR. Decreased anticoagulant tolerance with oxymetholone. *Lancet* 1971; **ii:** 221.
4. de Oya JC, *et al.* Decreased anticoagulant tolerance with oxymetholone in paroxysmal nocturnal haemoglobinuria. *Lancet* 1971; **ii:** 259.
5. Acomb C, Shaw PW. A significant interaction between warfarin and stanozolol. *Pharm J* 1985; **234:** 73–4.
6. Shaw PW, Smith AM. Possible interaction of warfarin and stanozolol. *Clin Pharm* 1987; **6:** 500–2.
7. Howard W, *et al.* Anabolic steroids and anticoagulants. *BMJ* 1977; **1:** 1659–60.
8. Vere DW, Fearnley GR. Suspected interaction between phenindione and ethyloestrenol. *Lancet* 1968; **i:** 281.
9. Schrogie JJ, Solomon HM. The anticoagulant response to bishydroxycoumarin: II. The effect of D-thyroxine, clofibrate, and norethandrolone. *Clin Pharmacol Ther* 1967; **8:** 70–7.
10. Husted S, *et al.* Increased sensitivity to phenprocoumon during methyltestosterone therapy. *Eur J Clin Pharmacol* 1976; **10:** 209–16.
11. Goulbourne IA, Macleod DAD. Interaction between danazol and warfarin: case report. *Br J Obstet Gynaecol* 1981; **88:** 950–1.
12. Meeks ML, *et al.* Danazol increases the anticoagulant effect of warfarin. *Ann Pharmacother* 1992; **26:** 641–2.
13. Booth CD. A drug interaction between danazol and warfarin. *Pharm J* 1993; **250:** 439–40.
14. Lorentz SMcQ, Weibert RT. Potentiation of warfarin anticoagulation by topical testosterone ointment. *Clin Pharm* 1985; **4:** 332–4.
15. Schrogie JJ, *et al.* Effect of oral contraceptives on vitamin K-dependent clotting activity. *Clin Pharmacol Ther* 1967; **8:** 670–5.
16. de Teresa E, *et al.* Interaction between anticoagulants and contraceptives: an unsuspected finding. *BMJ* 1979; **2:** 1260–1.
17. Mönig H, *et al.* Effect of oral contraceptive steroids on the pharmacokinetics of phenprocoumon. *Br J Clin Pharmacol* 1990; **30:** 115–18.
18. Ellison J, *et al.* Apparent interaction between warfarin and levonorgestrel used for emergency contraception. *BMJ* 2000; **321:** 1382.

Thyroid and antithyroid drugs. Since response to oral anticoagulants is dependent on thyroid status an interaction between oral anticoagulants and thyroid or antithyroid drugs might be expected. Thyroid compounds do enhance the activity of oral anticoagulants possibly by increased metabolism of clotting factors. Dextrothyroxine is discussed under Lipid Regulating Drugs, above. Antithyroid compounds have not, however, been reported to diminish the effect of anticoagulants and paradoxically *propylthiouracil* has been reported to have caused hypoprothrombinaemia (see Effects on the Blood, under Carbimazole, p.1521).

Tobacco. Although tobacco smoking may increase warfarin clearance,[1] an appreciable effect on anticoagulant activity appears unlikely.[1,2] However, there has been a report[3] of an increase in INR in a patient receiving warfarin when he stopped smoking.

1. Bachmann K, *et al.* Smoking and warfarin disposition. *Clin Pharmacol Ther* 1979; **25:** 309–15.
2. Weiner B, *et al.* Warfarin dosage following prosthetic valve replacement: effect of smoking history. *Drug Intell Clin Pharm* 1984; **18:** 904–6.
3. Colucci VJ, Knapp JF. Increase in international normalized ratio associated with smoking cessation. *Ann Pharmacother* 2001; **35:** 385–6.

Ubidecarenone. Decreased INR values and reduced effect of warfarin has been reported[1] in 3 patients after the addition of ubidecarenone to their therapy.

1. Spigset O. Reduced effect of warfarin caused by ubidecarenone. *Lancet* 1994; **344:** 1372–3.

Vaccines. There have been a few reports of increased prothrombin time and bleeding in warfarin-stabilised patients following *influenza vaccination*. Studies investigating this possible interaction have found only a small or inconsistent increase in warfarin activity[1,2] or no effect.[3-5] One study suggested that influenza vaccine decreases rather than increases the prothrombin time.[6] In a group of patients on long-term nicoumalone [acenocoumarol] therapy, influenza vaccination had no effect on nicoumalone [acenocoumarol] activity.[7]

1. Kramer P, *et al.* Effect of influenza vaccine on warfarin anticoagulation. *Clin Pharmacol Ther* 1984; **35:** 416–18.
2. Weibert RT, *et al.* Effect on influenza vaccine in patients receiving long-term warfarin therapy. *Clin Pharm* 1986; **5:** 499–503.
3. Lipsky BA, *et al.* Influenza vaccination and warfarin anticoagulation. *Ann Intern Med* 1984; **100:** 835–7.
4. Scott AK, *et al.* Lack of effect of influenza vaccination on warfarin in healthy volunteers. *Br J Clin Pharmacol* 1985; **19:** 144P–145P.
5. Gomolin IH. Lack of effect of influenza vaccination on warfarin anticoagulation in the elderly. *Can Med Assoc J* 1986; **135:** 39–41.
6. Bussey HI, Saklad JJ. Effect of influenza vaccine on chronic warfarin therapy. *Drug Intell Clin Pharm* 1988; **22:** 198–201.
7. Souto JC, *et al.* Lack of effect of influenza vaccine on anticoagulation by acenocoumarol. *Ann Pharmacother* 1993; **27:** 365–8.

Vitamins. Since vitamin K reverses the effects of oral anticoagulants, it is not surprising that there have been reports of *acetomenaphthone* and *phytomenadione* reducing anticoagulant activity, or of foods or nutritional preparations containing vitamin K compounds doing the same.

Occasional reports of *ascorbic acid* reducing the activity of warfarin[1,2] have not been confirmed in subsequent studies.[3,4] There have also been isolated reports suggesting that *vitamin E* may enhance the activity of warfarin[5] or dicoumarol,[6] although no effect was found in a study[7] of patients receiving warfarin and vitamin E.

1. Rosenthal G. Interaction of ascorbic acid and warfarin. *JAMA* 1971; **215:** 1671.
2. Smith EC, *et al.* Interaction of ascorbic acid and warfarin. *JAMA* 1972; **221:** 1166.
3. Hume R, *et al.* Interaction of ascorbic acid and warfarin. *JAMA* 1972; **219:** 1479.
4. Feetam CL, *et al.* Lack of clinically important interaction between warfarin and ascorbic acid. *Toxicol Appl Pharmacol* 1975; **31:** 544–7.
5. Corrigan JJ, Marcus FI. Coagulopathy associated with vitamin E ingestion. *JAMA* 1974; **230:** 1300–1.
6. Schrogie JJ. Coagulopathy and fat-soluble vitamins. *JAMA* 1975; **232:** 19.
7. Kim JM, White RH. Effect of vitamin E on the anticoagulant response to warfarin. *Am J Cardiol* 1996; **77:** 545–6.

Pharmacokinetics

Warfarin sodium is readily absorbed from the gastrointestinal tract; it can also be absorbed through the skin. It is extensively bound to plasma proteins and its plasma half-life is about 37 hours. It crosses the placenta but does not occur in significant quantities in breast milk. Warfarin is used as a racemic mixture; the *S*-isomer is reported to be more potent. The *R*- and *S*-isomers are both metabolised in the liver, the *S*-isomer more rapidly than the *R*-isomer; the stereo-isomers may also be affected differently by other drugs (see Interactions, above). Metabolites, with negligible or no anticoagulant activity, are excreted in the urine following reabsorption from the bile.

◊ References.

1. Mungall DR, *et al.* Population pharmacokinetics of racemic warfarin in adult patients. *J Pharmacokinet Biopharm* 1985; **13:** 213–27.
2. Holford NHG. Clinical pharmacokinetics and pharmacodynamics of warfarin: understanding the dose-effect relationship. *Clin Pharmacokinet* 1986; **11:** 483–504.

Uses and Administration

Warfarin is a coumarin anticoagulant used in the treatment and prophylaxis of thromboembolic disorders (p.816). It acts by depressing the hepatic vitamin K-dependent synthesis of coagulation factors II (prothrombin), VII, IX, and X, and of the anticoagulant protein C and its cofactor protein S. For an explanation of the coagulation cascade, see Haemostasis and Fibrinolysis, p.718. Since warfarin acts indirectly, it has no effect on existing clots. Also as the coagulation factors involved have half-lives ranging from 6 to 60 hours, several hours are required before an effect is observed. A therapeutic effect is usually apparent by 24 hours, but the peak effect may not be achieved until 2 or 3 days after a dose; the overall effect may last for 5 days.

Warfarin is used in the prevention and treatment of venous thromboembolism (deep-vein thrombosis and pulmonary embolism, p.817). If an immediate effect on blood coagulation is required, heparin should be given intravenously or subcutaneously to cover the first 2 to 3 days. Warfarin therapy may be initiated concomitantly with or shortly after the initial heparin treatment. Warfarin is also used for the prevention of systemic thromboembolism and ischaemic stroke in some patients with atrial fibrillation (p.794), prosthetic heart valves (see Valvular Heart Disease, p.816), or who have suffered a myocardial infarction (p.805). It may also have a role in the prevention of myocardial infarction and in the management of stroke or transient ischaemic attacks (p.813). Antiplatelet drugs may be given concomitantly.

Some patients may show a hereditary resistance to warfarin. Warfarin is a potent rodenticide although resistance has been reported in *rats*.

Administration and dosage. Warfarin is equally effective either orally or intravenously, but is usually given by mouth. Dosage must be determined individually as discussed below under Control of Anticoagulant Therapy. When rapid anticoagulation is required, an initial dose of warfarin sodium 10 mg daily for 2 days may be used. However, in many cases an initial dose of 5 mg daily is adequate. Initial doses of less than 5 mg daily may be used in elderly patients and in those at increased risk of bleeding (see Precautions, above). Subsequent maintenance doses usually range from 3 to 9 mg daily. If necessary the same dose may be given by slow intravenous injection. Doses of warfarin sodium should be given at the same time each day. Theoretically, sudden discontinuation of warfarin may result in rebound hypercoagulability with risk of thrombosis. Therefore some clinicians tail off long-term treatment over several weeks but the need for this is unclear. Anticoagulant treatment booklets should be carried by patients.

Warfarin has also been given as the potassium salt; warfarin-deanol has been tried.

Control of Oral Anticoagulant Therapy. Treatment with oral anticoagulants must be monitored to ensure that the dose is providing the required effect on the vitamin-K-dependent clotting factors; too small a dose provides inadequate anticoagulation, too large a dose puts the patient at risk of haemorrhage. This monitoring is commonly carried out by checking the clotting property of the patient's plasma using a suitable preparation of thromboplastin and a source of calcium. The time taken for the clot to form due to the effect of the thromboplastin preparation on prothrombin is known as the prothrombin time (PT). The prothrombin time ratio (PTR) is the prothrombin time of the patient's plasma divided by that for a standard plasma sample.

So that there is some consistency in prothrombin time ratios measured at different times or at different laboratories, it is now common practice for the manufacturer or control laboratory to calibrate their batches of thromboplastin against the international reference preparation. This calibration produces an international sensitivity index (ISI) appropriate to that thromboplastin. The laboratory measuring the clotting capacity of a sample of plasma is thus able to convert the prothrombin time ratio to an international normalised ratio (INR) using the sensitivity index through the formula

$$INR = PTR^{(ISI)}$$

Thus a prothrombin time ratio of 2.0 obtained with a thromboplastin with a declared international sensitivity index of 1.5 would be converted to an international normalised ratio of 2.8. An international normalised ratio is therefore equivalent to a prothrombin time ratio carried out using the primary international reference preparation of thromboplastin.

This method of standardisation has taken over from methods involving use of a standard reagent such as the British or Manchester comparative thromboplastin. Also preparations of thromboplastin derived from *rabbit* brain have superseded or are superseding those from human brain because of the dangers of viral transmission.

Recommended target values or ranges of international normalised ratio for patients receiving anticoagulant treatment or cover for various conditions or procedures are given by the British Society for Haematology in the UK and the American College of Chest Physicians and the National Heart, Lung and Blood Institute in the USA. These are given in Table 5, below. An INR within 0.5 units of the target value in the UK is generally considered satisfactory. In the USA it is recommended that the INR be maintained at the mid-level of the range. An INR less than 2.0 represents inadequate anticoagulation and an INR greater than 4.5 represents risk of haemorrhage.

Measurements should be carried out before treatment and then daily or on alternate days in the early stages of treatment. Once the dose has been established and

the patient well stabilised the measurement can be made at greater but regular intervals, for example every 8 weeks; allowances should be made for any events that might influence the activity of the anticoagulant.

◊ General references.
1. Harrington R, Ansell J. Risk-benefit assessment of anticoagulant therapy. *Drug Safety* 1991; **6:** 54–69.
2. Le DT, *et al.* The international normalized ratio (INR) for monitoring warfarin therapy: reliability and relation to other monitoring methods. *Ann Intern Med* 1994; **120:** 552–8.
3. Hirsh J, Fuster V. Guide to anticoagulants therapy part 2: oral anticoagulants. *Circulation* 1994; **89:** 1469–80.
4. Routledge PA. Practical prescribing: warfarin. *Prescribers' J* 1997; **37:** 173–9.
5. British Society for Haematology: British Committee for Standards in Haematology—Haemostasis and Thrombosis Task Force. Guidelines on oral anticoagulation: third edition. *Br J Haematol* 1998; **101:** 374–87.
6. Hardman SMC, Cowie MR. Anticoagulation in heart disease. *BMJ* 1999; **318:** 238–44.
7. Gage BF, *et al.* Management and dosing of warfarin therapy. *Am J Med* 2000; **109:** 481–8.
8. Hirsh J, *et al.* Oral anticoagulants: mechanism of action, clinical effectiveness, and optimal therapeutic range. *Chest* 2001; **119** (suppl): 8S–21S.
9. Ansell J, *et al.* Managing oral anticoagulant therapy. *Chest* 2001; **119** (suppl): 22S–38S.

Administration and dosage. Algorithms and guidelines have been developed for the initiation of anticoagulant therapy, based on the method of Fennerty *et al.*[1] Although a loading dose of 10 mg daily for 2 days (depending on the INR) has been widely used, lower doses may be more appropriate. Studies[2-4] have compared warfarin loading doses of 5 and 10 mg and found that for both groups a therapeutic INR in the range of 2.0 to 3.0 was reached in most patients by day 5 of treatment.

In outpatient and community settings, when rapid anticoagulation is not necessary, loading doses may not be required. A low-dose regimen for elderly patients requiring anticoagulation prophylaxis has been described.[5] Warfarin was started at a dose of 2 mg daily for 2 weeks followed by weekly adjustment using an algorithm until the target INR was reached.

1. Fennerty A, *et al.* Flexible induction dose regimen for warfarin and prediction of maintenance dose. *BMJ* 1984; **288:** 1268–70.
2. Harrison L, *et al.* Comparison of 5-mg and 10-mg doses used in initiation of warfarin therapy. *Ann Intern Med* 1997; **126:** 133–6.
3. Crowther MA, *et al.* Warfarin: less may be better. *Ann Intern Med* 1997; **127:** 333.
4. Crowther MA, *et al.* A randomized trial comparing 5-mg and 10-mg warfarin loading doses. *Arch Intern Med* 1999; **159:** 46–8.
5. Oates A, *et al.* A new regimen for starting warfarin therapy in out-patients. *Br J Clin Pharmacol* 1998; **46:** 157–61.

Administration in infants and children. Increasing numbers of infants and children are receiving anticoagulants for prophylaxis and treatment of thromboembolism. Doses of warfarin and therapeutic INR ranges have been adapted from adult therapy but cohort studies[1,2] of paediatric patients have found that warfarin requirements may be affected by a number of factors including age, and the use of infant formulas supplemented with vitamin K. Recommendations[3] for the use of oral anticoagulants in children have been published.

1. Tait RC, *et al.* Oral anticoagulation in paediatric patients: dose requirements and complications. *Arch Dis Child* 1996; **74:** 228–31.
2. Streif W, *et al.* Analysis of warfarin therapy in pediatric patients: a prospective cohort study of 319 patients. *Blood* 1999; **94:** 3007–14.
3. Monagle P, *et al.* Antithrombotic therapy in children. *Chest* 2001; **119** (suppl): 344S–370S.

Catheters and cannulas. For mention of the use of oral anticoagulants to prevent thrombosis in patients with indwelling infusion devices, see Heparin Sodium, p.904.

Connective tissue and muscular disorders. Warfarin has been proposed to treat subcutaneous calcium deposition (calcinosis cutis) in patients with dermatomyositis, but its value is disputed, see Polymyositis and Dermatomyositis, p.1057.

Preparations

BP 2001: Warfarin Tablets.
USP 25: Warfarin Sodium for Injection; Warfarin Sodium Tablets.

Proprietary Preparations (details are given in Part 3)
Austral.: Coumadin; Marevan; *Belg.:* Marevan; *Braz.:* Marevan; *Canad.:* Coumadin; Warfilone; *Denm.:* Marevan; *Fin.:* Marevan; *Fr.:* Coumadine; *Ger.:* Coumadin; *Irl.:* Warfant; *Israel:* Coumadin; *Ital.:* Coumadin; *Mex.:* Romesa; *Norw.:* Marevan; *NZ:* Coumadin; Marevan; *Port.:* Varfine; *S.Afr.:* Coumadin†; *Singapore:* Coumadin; *Spain:* Aldocumar; *Swed.:* Waran; *Thai.:* Orfarin; *UK:* Marevan; *USA:* Coumadin.

Xamoterol Fumarate (17133-q)

Xamoterol Fumarate (BANM, USAN, rINNM)
ICI-118587. N-{2-[2-Hydroxy-3-(4-hydroxyphenoxy)propylamino]ethyl}morpholine-4-carboxamide fumarate.
$(C_{16}H_{25}N_3O_5)_2,C_4H_4O_4 = 794.8$.
CAS — 81801-12-9 (xamoterol); 90730-93-1 (xamoterol fumarate).

Profile
Xamoterol is a beta-adrenoceptor partial agonist with a selec-

---

Table 5. Recommended International Normalised Ratios (INR).

	INR	Condition or procedure
UK	2.5	Pulmonary embolism; deep-vein thrombosis; recurrence of venous thromboembolism when no longer on warfarin; symptomatic inherited thrombophilia; atrial fibrillation; cardioversion; mural thrombus; cardiomyopathy.
	3.5	Recurrence of venous thromboembolism when on warfarin; antiphospholipid syndrome; mechanical prosthetic heart valves.
US	2.0 to 3.0	Prophylaxis of venous thromboembolism in high-risk surgical patients; treatment of venous thrombosis and pulmonary embolism; prophylaxis of systemic embolism in patients with atrial fibrillation, valvular heart disease, bioprosthetic heart valves, or acute myocardial infarction.
	2.5 to 3.5	Prophylaxis in patients with mechanical prosthetic heart valves; prevention of recurrent myocardial infarction.

tive action on beta₁ receptors. As a partial agonist it exerts predominantly agonist activity at rest and under conditions of low sympathetic drive which results in improved ventricular function and increased cardiac output; during exercise and during conditions of increased sympathetic drive, such as that occurring in severe heart failure, xamoterol exerts beta-blocking activity. It therefore has the properties of both sympathomimetics (see Adrenaline, p.829) and beta blockers (see p.844).

Xamoterol has been used in the management of chronic mild heart failure but was associated with deterioration and an excess of deaths in those with more severe disease. It has also been used in orthostatic hypotension secondary to autonomic failure.

◊ References.
1. Anonymous. Xamoterol—more trouble than it's worth? *Drug Ther Bull* 1990; **28**: 53–4.
2. Anonymous. New evidence on xamoterol. *Lancet* 1990; **336**: 24.
3. The Xamoterol in Severe Heart Failure Study Group. Xamoterol in severe heart failure. *Lancet* 1990; **336**: 1–6.

Preparations
Proprietary Preparations (details are given in Part 3)
Aust.: Corwil†; *Belg.:* Corwin†; *UK:* Corwin†.

Xantinol Nicotinate (9285-d)
Xantinol Nicotinate (BAN, rINN).
SK-331A; Xantinol Niacinate (USAN); Xantinol Nicotinate. 7-{2-Hydroxy-3-[(2-hydroxyethyl)methylamino]propyl}theophylline nicotinate.
$C_{13}H_{21}N_5O_4,C_6H_5NO_2 = 434.4$.
CAS — 437-74-1.
ATC — C04AD02.
Pharmacopoeias. In Pol.

Profile
Xantinol nicotinate is a vasodilator with general properties similar to those of nicotinic acid (p.1372), to which it is slowly hydrolysed. It is used in the management of peripheral (p.809) and cerebral vascular disorders (p.798) and in hyperlipidaemias (p.800). Doses of up to 3 g daily may be given by mouth. It has also been given by intramuscular or slow intravenous injection.

Preparations
Proprietary Preparations (details are given in Part 3)
Aust.: Complamin†; Frigol; *Belg.:* Complamin; *Canad.:* Complamin†; *Ger.:* Complamin; Complamin spezial; *Ital.:* Complamin; Vedrin; *Neth.:* Complamin; *Swed.:* Complamin; *Switz.:* Complamin.

Multi-ingredient: *Spain:* Plasmaclar†; Rulun.

Xemilofiban Hydrochloride (18566-k)
Xemilofiban Hydrochloride (USAN, rINNM).
SC-54684A. Ethyl (3S)-3-{3-[(p-amidinophenyl)carbamoyl]propionamido}-4-pentynoate monohydrochloride.
$C_{18}H_{22}N_4O_4,HCl = 394.9$.
CAS — 149620-74-6 (xemilofiban); 156586-91-3 (xemilofiban hydrochloride).

Profile
Xemilofiban is a glycoprotein IIb/IIIa-receptor antagonist. It has been investigated as an oral antiplatelet drug for the management of thromboembolic disorders such as unstable angina, and following angioplasty, but results have been disappointing.

◊ References.
1. O'Neill WW, *et al.* Long-term treatment with a platelet glycoprotein-receptor antagonist after percutaneous coronary revascularization. *N Engl J Med* 2000; **342**: 1316–24.

Xipamide (2362-w)
Xipamide (BAN, USAN, rINN).
Be-1293; MJF-10938. 4-Chloro-5-sulphamoylsalicylo-2′,6′-xylidide; 5-(Aminosulphonyl)-4-chloro-N-(2,6-dimethylphenyl)-2-hydroxy-benzamide.
$C_{15}H_{15}ClN_2O_4S = 354.8$.
CAS — 14293-44-8.
ATC — C03BA10.

Adverse Effects, Treatment, and Precautions
As for Hydrochlorothiazide, p.907.

Effects on electrolyte balance. Although reductions in plasma-potassium concentrations with xipamide have been shown to be on average comparable with those produced by thiazide and loop diuretics at equipotent doses,[1] there have been several reports of marked hypokalaemia in individual patients. Asymptomatic hypokalaemia was reported in 4 of 5 patients[2] (serum-potassium concentrations of less than 3.4 mmol per litre) and in 3 of 13 patients[3] (serum-potassium concentrations of less than 3.0 mmol per litre). Severe hypokalaemia resulting in ventricular arrhythmias has been reported following xipamide alone[4] or in combination with indapamide.[5] Profound electrolyte disturbances with altered consciousness and ventricular extrasystoles occurred in a patient taking digoxin following the addition of xipamide for 10 days.[6] A case of hypokalaemic periodic paralysis associated with xipamide administration has also been reported.[7]
1. Prichard BNC, Brogden RN. Xipamide: a review of its pharmacodynamic and pharmacokinetic properties and therapeutic efficacy. *Drugs* 1985; **30**: 313–32.
2. Weissberg P, Kendall MJ. Hypokalaemia and xipamide. *BMJ* 1982; **284**: 975.
3. Raftery EB, *et al.* A study of the antihypertensive action of xipamide using ambulatory intra-arterial monitoring. *Br J Clin Pharmacol* 1981; **12**: 381–5.
4. Altmann P, Hamblin JJ. Ventricular fibrillation induced by xipamide. *BMJ* 1982; **284**: 494.
5. Boulton AJM, Hardisty CA. Ventricular arrhythmias precipitated by treatment with non-thiazide diuretics. *Practitioner* 1982; **226**: 125–8.
6. Bentley J. Hypokalaemia and xipamide. *BMJ* 1982; **284**: 975.
7. Boulton AJM, Hardisty CA. Hypokalaemic periodic paralysis precipitated by diuretic therapy and minor surgery. *Postgrad Med J* 1982; **58**: 106–7.

Hepatic impairment. For a recommendation that xipamide should be given with caution to patients with liver disease, see under Pharmacokinetics, below.

Interactions
As for Hydrochlorothiazide, p.909.

Pharmacokinetics
Xipamide has been reported to be well absorbed from the gastrointestinal tract. Absorption is fairly rapid with peak plasma concentrations occurring within 1 or 2 hours of oral administration. It is 99% bound to plasma proteins, and is excreted in the urine, partly unchanged and partly in the form of the glucuronide metabolite. It is reported to have a plasma half-life of about 5 to 8 hours. In patients with renal impairment excretion in the bile becomes more prominent.

◊ References.
1. Beermann B, Grind M. Clinical pharmacokinetics of some newer diuretics. *Clin Pharmacokinet* 1987; **13**: 254–66.

Hepatic impairment. Xipamide was present in the plasma and in ascitic fluid in patients with liver cirrhosis in proportion to the protein content of the respective compartments.[1] The amount of drug excreted into the urine was much greater in patients with liver disease than in healthy control subjects. This was attributed to a diminution in hepatic elimination, which could result in significant effects on the clinical response to xipamide. Thus patients with cholestasis could have an enhanced response to xipamide. On the other hand cirrhotic patients with the hepatorenal syndrome may be resistant to diuretics. Xipamide should be used with caution in patients with liver disease.
1. Knauf H, *et al.* Xipamide disposition in liver cirrhosis. *Clin Pharmacol Ther* 1990; **48**: 628–32.

Renal impairment. Following single oral and intravenous doses of xipamide 20 mg the drug appeared to be completely absorbed from the gastrointestinal tract.[1] The mean elimination half-life in healthy subjects was 7 hours and two-thirds of the clearance was by extrarenal routes. There was some accumulation in patients with chronic renal failure, with a calculated elimination half-life of 9 hours in end-stage renal disease.
1. Knauf H, Mutschler E. Pharmacodynamics and pharmacokinetics of xipamide in patients with normal and impaired kidney function. *Eur J Clin Pharmacol* 1984; **26**: 513–20.

Uses and Administration
Xipamide is a diuretic, structurally related to indapamide, with actions and uses similar to those of the thiazide diuretics (see Hydrochlorothiazide, p.910). It is used for oedema, including that associated with heart failure (p.798), and for hypertension (p.802).

Diuresis is initiated in about 1 or 2 hours, reaches a peak at 4 to 6 hours, and lasts for about 12 hours.

In the treatment of **oedema** the usual initial dose is 40 mg by mouth daily, subsequently reduced to 20 mg daily, according to the patient's response; in resistant cases doses of 80 mg daily may be required. In the treatment of **hypertension** the usual dose is 20 mg daily, as a single morning dose, either alone, or in conjunction with other antihypertensives. In some patients a dose of 10 mg daily may be adequate.

◊ References.
1. Prichard BNC, Brogden RN. Xipamide: a review of its pharmacodynamic and pharmacokinetic properties and therapeutic efficacy. *Drugs* 1985; **30**: 313–32.

Preparations
Proprietary Preparations (details are given in Part 3)
Aust.: Aquaphoril; *Belg.:* Diurexan; *Fr.:* Chronexan†; Lumitens; *Ger.:* Aquaphor; *Hong Kong:* Diurexan; *Irl.:* Diurexan; *Ital.:* Aquafor; *Port.:* Diurexan; *S.Afr.:* Diurexan; *Spain:* Demiax; Diurex; *UK:* Diurexan.

Multi-ingredient: *Ger.:* Durotan; Neotri.

Zofenopril Calcium (3660-v)
Zofenopril Calcium (BANM, USAN, rINNM).
SQ-26991. Calcium salt of (4S)-1-[(2S)-3-(Benzylthio)-2-methylpropionyl]-4-(phenylthio)-L-proline.
$C_{44}H_{44}CaN_2O_8S_4 = 897.2$.
CAS — 81872-10-8 (zofenopril); 81938-43-4 (zofenopril calcium).

Profile
Zofenopril is an ACE inhibitor (p.820) that is used as the calcium salt in the management of hypertension and myocardial infarction. It owes its activity to the active metabolite SQ-26333 to which it is converted after oral administration.

◊ References.
1. Ambrosioni E, *et al.* The effect of the angiotensin-converting-enzyme inhibitor zofenopril on mortality and morbidity after anterior myocardial infarction. *N Engl J Med* 1995; **332**: 80–5.
2. Borghi C, *et al.* Effects of the administration of an angiotensin-converting enzyme inhibitor during the acute phase of myocardial infarction in patients with arterial hypertension: the SMILE study investigators: Survival of Myocardial Infarction Long-term Evaluation. *Am J Hypertens* 1999; **12**: 665–72.

Chelators Antidotes and Antagonists

The drugs included in this chapter act in a variety of ways to counter the toxic effects of exogenous and endogenous substances in the body. They are therefore used in the management of poisoning and overdosage, to protect against the toxicity of drugs such as antineoplastics, and in the management of metabolic disorders such as Wilson's disease where toxic substances accumulate. Some are antagonists, such as the opioid antagonist naloxone, that compete with the poison for receptor sites. Others inhibit the toxin by reacting with it to form less active or inactive complexes or by interfering with its metabolism; chelators are typical examples of the first group and methionine is an example of the second. Other compounds with a role in the treatment of specific types of poisoning include those such as atropine (p.460) that block essential receptors mediating the toxic effects, or those that reduce the rate of conversion of the poison to a more toxic compound, such as alcohol (p.1130) in methyl alcohol poisoning, or those that bypass the effect of the drug as happens with calcium folinate (p.1363) in methotrexate overdosage. Acetylcysteine (p.1082) is an antagonist used in paracetamol poisoning.

Acute poisoning

In the management of suspected acute poisoning it is often impossible to determine the identity of the poison or the size of the dose received with any certainty. Moreover, specific antidotes and methods of elimination are available for relatively few poisons and the mainstay of treatment for patients with suspected acute poisoning is therefore supportive and symptomatic therapy; in many cases nothing further is required. Symptoms of acute poisoning are frequently non-specific, particularly in the early stages. Maintenance of the airway and ventilation is the most important initial measure; other treatment, for example for cardiovascular or neurological symptoms, may be added as appropriate. Patients who are unconsciousness may be given naloxone if opioid overdosage is suspected. Some centres also recommend the routine administration of glucose to all unconscious patients since hypoglycaemia may be a cause of unconsciousness; thiamine is given in addition since glucose may precipitate Wernicke's encephalopathy.

Specific antidotes are available for a number of poisons and are the primary treatment where there is severe poisoning with a known toxin. They may be life-saving in such cases but their use is not without hazard and in many situations they are not necessary; their use does not preclude relevant supportive treatment.

Measures to reduce or prevent the absorption of the poison are widely advocated. For inhalational poisoning the victim is removed from the source of poisoning. Some toxins, in particular pesticides, may be absorbed through the skin and clothing is removed and the skin thoroughly washed to avoid continued absorption. Caustic substances are removed from the skin or eyes with copious irrigation. Orally ingested poisons may be actively removed from the stomach by emesis or by gastric lavage, although these measures are of limited value (see p.1093). Activated charcoal may be administered to adsorb the toxin.

Induction of emesis has been used in the home situation although its value is questioned; the preferred emetic agent is syrup of ipecacuanha. It should only be used in fully conscious patients and should not be used if the poison is corrosive or petroleum based, or if the poison is removed by treatment with activated charcoal. Gastric lavage may be indicated for ingestion of non-caustic poisons if less than one hour has elapsed since ingestion and is followed by activated charcoal. Lavage should not be attempted if the airway is not adequately protected. Whole-bowel irrigation using a non-absorbable osmotic agent such as a macrogol has been used following ingestion of substances that pass beyond the stomach before being absorbed, such as iron preparations or enteric-coated or modified-release formulations. A single oral dose of activated charcoal is effective for a wide range of toxins, particularly if it is given within one hour of ingestion, although delayed use may still be beneficial particularly for modified-release preparations or for drugs which slow gastrointestinal transit time such as those with

antimuscarinic properties; it is generally well tolerated although vomiting is common and there is a risk of aspiration if the airway is not adequately protected.

Techniques intended to promote the elimination of poisons from the body such as haemodialysis or haemoperfusion are only of value for a limited number of poisons in a few severely poisoned patients; forced diuresis is generally no longer recommended. Repeated oral doses of activated charcoal may often be as effective as these more invasive methods.

Poisons Information Centres exist in many countries and should be consulted for more detailed information in specific situations.

Acetylcholinesterase (11228-i)

Profile
Acetylcholinesterase is an endogenous enzyme which hydrolyses acetylcholine (p.1415) and thus plays an essential role in cholinergic transmission. It is chiefly found at cholinergic synapses and in the neurones. Unlike the more widely distributed plasma cholinesterase (pseudocholinesterase; butyrylcholinesterase), which can hydrolyse other esters, its actions are relatively selective for choline esters. Acetylcholinesterase has been given by intravenous injection to counteract the effect of overdosage or poisoning with suxamethonium or organophosphorus pesticides.

Preparations

Proprietary Preparations (details are given in Part 3)
Ger.: Serum-Cholinesterase†.

Activated Charcoal (686-j)

Carbo Activatus; Decolorising Charcoal.
CAS — 16291-96-6 (charcoal).
Pharmacopoeias. In Chin., Eur. (see p.vi), Int., Jpn, and US.

Pharmacopoeial description

Ph. Eur.: It is obtained from vegetable matter by suitable carbonisation processes intended to confer a high adsorption power. A black, light powder free from grittiness. Practically insoluble in all usual solvents. It adsorbs not less than 40% of its own weight of phenazone, calculated with reference to the dried substance. Store in airtight containers.

USP 25: The residue from the destructive distillation of various organic materials, treated to increase its adsorptive power. A fine, black, odourless, tasteless powder, free from gritty matter. The USP 25 has tests for adsorptive power in respect of alkaloids and dyes.

Adverse Effects and Precautions

Activated charcoal is relatively non-toxic when given by mouth but gastrointestinal disturbances such as vomiting, constipation, or diarrhoea have been reported. It may colour the faeces black.

Haemoperfusion with activated charcoal has produced various adverse effects including platelet aggregation, charcoal embolism, thrombocytopenia, haemorrhage, hypoglycaemia, hypocalcaemia, hypothermia, and hypotension.

Activated charcoal is contra-indicated when specific oral antidotes such as methionine are used (see Interactions, below).

Effects on the gastrointestinal tract. Intestinal obstruction[1-4] or faecal impaction, in one case resulting in rectal ulceration,[5] has been reported following multiple oral doses of activated charcoal. Special care should be taken when treating overdoses of drugs with antimuscarinic activity, such as tricyclic antidepressants and phenothiazines.[2] Two cases of pseudo-obstruction, one of which was fatal, have also been reported[6] following the use of activated charcoal and sorbitol with opioid sedation for theophylline poisoning. Care should also be taken to prevent pulmonary aspiration (see below).

1. Watson WA, *et al.* Gastrointestinal obstruction associated with multiple-dose activated charcoal. *J Emerg Med* 1986; **4:** 401–7.
2. Anderson IM, Ware C. Syrup of ipecacuanha. *BMJ* 1987; **294:** 578.
3. Ray MJ, *et al.* Charcoal bezoar: small-bowel obstruction secondary to amitriptyline overdose therapy. *Dig Dis Sci* 1988; **33:** 106–7.
4. Atkinson SW, *et al.* Treatment with activated charcoal complicated by gastrointestinal obstruction requiring surgery. *BMJ* 1992; **305:** 563.

5. Mizutani T, *et al.* Rectal ulcer with massive haemorrhage due to activated charcoal treatment in oral organophosphate poisoning. *Hum Exp Toxicol* 1991; **10:** 385–6.
6. Longdon P, Henderson A. Intestinal pseudo-obstruction following the use of enteral charcoal and sorbitol and mechanical ventilation with papaveretum sedation for theophylline poisoning. *Drug Safety* 1992; **7:** 74–7.

Effects on the lungs. Pulmonary aspiration of activated charcoal, sometimes with fatal results, has been reported following oral administration for the treatment of acute poisoning.[1-4] Vomiting has been reported to be fairly common by some,[1,5] but not all,[6] correspondents following use of activated charcoal; the water load resulting from repeated administration of charcoal slurry could contribute to any nausea and vomiting[5] and the use of sorbitol-containing preparations has also been said to contribute to the vomiting.[7] The use of a cuffed endotracheal tube has been recommended for any patient with impaired laryngeal reflexes to prevent aspiration.[4,8]

1. Hoffman JR. Charcoal for gastrointestinal clearance of drugs. *N Engl J Med* 1983; **308:** 157.
2. Harsch HH. Aspiration of activated charcoal. *N Engl J Med* 1986; **314:** 318.
3. Menzies DG, *et al.* Fatal pulmonary aspiration of oral activated charcoal. *BMJ* 1988; **297:** 459–60.
4. Rau NR, *et al.* Fatal pulmonary aspiration of oral activated charcoal. *BMJ* 1988; **297:** 918–19.
5. Danel V. Fatal pulmonary aspiration of oral activated charcoal. *BMJ* 1988; **297:** 684.
6. Levy G. Charcoal for gastrointestinal clearance of drugs. *N Engl J Med* 1983; **308:** 157.
7. McFarland AK, Chyka PA. Selection of activated charcoal products for the treatment of poisonings. *Ann Pharmacother* 1993; **27:** 358–61.
8. Power KJ. Fatal pulmonary aspiration of oral activated charcoal. *BMJ* 1988; **297:** 919.

Interactions

Activated charcoal has the potential to reduce the absorption of many drugs from the gastrointestinal tract and simultaneous oral therapy should therefore be avoided. In the management of acute poisoning, concurrent medication should be given parenterally. Activated charcoal should not be used when a specific oral antidote such as methionine is given since adsorption of the antidote may decrease effectiveness.

Uses and Administration

Activated charcoal can adsorb a wide range of plant and inorganic poisons and many drugs including salicylates, paracetamol, barbiturates, and tricyclic antidepressants; thus when given by mouth it reduces their systemic absorption from the gastrointestinal tract and is used in the treatment of acute oral poisoning. It is of no value in the treatment of poisoning by strong acids, alkalis, or other corrosive substances and its adsorptive capacity is too low to be of use in poisoning with iron salts, cyanides, lithium, malathion, clofenotane, and some organic solvents such as methyl alcohol or ethylene glycol. Adsorption characteristics can be influenced by charcoal's particle size, thus different responses may be obtained with different preparations.

Activated charcoal is given by mouth usually as a slurry in water. The usual dose is 50 g, but higher doses have been used. For maximum efficacy, activated charcoal should be administered as soon as possible (within 1 hour) after ingestion of the toxic compound. However, it may be effective several hours after poisoning with certain drugs that slow gastric emptying. In the case of drugs that undergo enterohepatic or enteroenteric recycling (e.g. phenobarbital and theophylline) *repeated doses* of activated charcoal are of value in enhancing faecal elimination. Doses for repeated administration have varied but typically 50 g may be given every 4 hours or 25 g every 2 hours. Administration may also be via a nasogastric tube.

Mixtures such as 'universal antidote' that contained activated charcoal, magnesium oxide, and tannic acid should not be used; activated charcoal alone is more effective and tannic acid may cause hepatotoxicity.

In treatment of poisoning using charcoal haemoperfusion, activated charcoal is used to remove drugs from the blood stream. It may be of value in acute severe poisoning by drugs such as the barbiturates, glutethimide, or theophylline when other intensive measures fail to improve the condition of the patient.

Activated charcoal is used in dressings for ulcers and suppurating wounds (p.1108) to reduce malodour and may improve the rate of healing.

Activated charcoal has been used as a marker of intestinal transit and has also been tried in the treatment of flatulence. Both activated charcoal and vegetable charcoal (wood charcoal; carbo ligni) are included in preparations for various gastrointestinal disorders.

Technical grades of activated charcoal have been used as purifying and decolorising agents, for the removal of residual gases in low-pressure apparatus, and in respirators as a protection against toxic gases.

Administration. Activated charcoal is most commonly given as a slurry in water but this is often found to be unpalatable because of the colour, gritty taste, lack of flavour, and difficulty in swallowing.[1] Efforts have therefore been made to improve its palatability but studies *in vitro* or in healthy subjects indicated that some foods such as ice cream, milk, and cocoa might inhibit the adsorptive capacity of activated charcoal whereas starches and jams appeared to have no effect.[2,3] Carmellose has improved palatability although it might also reduce the adsorptive power of activated charcoal.[4-6] Activated charcoal formulations containing sorbitol, carmellose sodium, or starch were more palatable and essentially equivalent to the aqueous slurry formulation in efficacy.[1] When chocolate syrup was used as a sweet flavouring agent it had to be added just before administration as the sweetness and flavour disappeared after a few minutes of contact with the activated charcoal.[1] Saccharin sodium, sucrose, or sorbitol might be suitable flavours for activated charcoal formulations.[7] A survey[8] of commercially available ready-to-use charcoal preparations in the USA indicated that although differences did exist between the formulations, the clinical significance of such variations was unknown. The problems associated with sorbitol-containing products (see also under Poisoning, below) were highlighted and caution made against their use, especially for repeated-dose therapy.

1. Scholtz EC, *et al.* Evaluation of five activated charcoal formulations for inhibition of aspirin absorption and palatability in man. *Am J Hosp Pharm* 1978; **35:** 1355–9.
2. Levy G, *et al.* Inhibition by ice cream of the antidotal efficacy of activated charcoal. *Am J Hosp Pharm* 1975; **32:** 289–91.
3. De Neve R. Antidotal efficacy of activated charcoal in presence of jam, starch and milk. *Am J Hosp Pharm* 1976; **33:** 965–6.
4. Mathur LK, *et al.* Activated charcoal–carboxymethylcellulose gel formulation as an antidotal agent for orally ingested aspirin. *Am J Hosp Pharm* 1976; **33:** 717–19.
5. Manes M. Effect of carboxymethylcellulose on the adsorptive capacity of charcoal. *Am J Hosp Pharm* 1976; **33:** 1120, 1122.
6. Mathur LK, *et al.* Effect of carboxymethylcellulose on the adsorptive capacity of charcoal. *Am J Hosp Pharm* 1976; **33:** 1122.
7. Cooney DO. Palatability of sucrose-, sorbitol-, and saccharin-sweetened activated charcoal formulations. *Am J Hosp Pharm* 1980; **37:** 237–9.
8. McFarland AK, Chyka PA. Selection of activated charcoal products for the treatment of poisonings. *Ann Pharmacother* 1993; **27:** 358–61.

Poisoning. The management of acute poisoning is discussed on p.1000. The administration of a *single oral dose* of activated charcoal has become a widespread method of preventing the absorption of ingested compounds[1] and may be superior to gastric emptying.[2,3] In addition, *multiple oral doses* of activated charcoal have been found to enhance the elimination of some drugs and toxic substances even after systemic absorption.[4-13] Mechanisms by which activated charcoal may increase drug elimination from the body include interruption of the enterohepatic circulation of drugs excreted into the bile, reduction of the reabsorption of drugs which diffuse or are actively secreted into the intestines, and increased elimination of the drug via the gastrointestinal tract when co-administered with a laxative to decrease gastrointestinal transit time,[6] although the practice of giving charcoal with a laxative has been questioned.[9,14] Repeated oral doses of activated charcoal may therefore be considered for compounds that undergo enterohepatic or enteroenteric circulation, have a small volume of distribution, are not extensively bound to plasma proteins, and have a low endogenous clearance. Anecdotal reports and studies in acutely poisoned patients indicate that a technique of giving multiple doses of charcoal may offer an alternative to charcoal haemoperfusion or haemodialysis. However, while activated charcoal is generally well tolerated, major complications do occasionally occur, including pulmonary aspiration and bowel obstruction.[15] Also, use of multiple doses of charcoal preparations containing sorbitol or sodium bicarbonate can result in increased vomiting[16] or in electrolyte disturbances.[9-11]

1. American Academy of Clinical Toxicology, European Association of Poisons Centres and Clinical Toxicologists. Position statement: single-dose activated charcoal. *Clin Toxicol* 1997; **35:** 721–41.
2. Pond SM, *et al.* Gastric emptying in acute overdose: a prospective randomised controlled trial. *Med J Aust* 1995; **163:** 345–9.
3. Albertson TE, *et al.* Superiority of activated charcoal alone compared with ipecac and activated charcoal in the treatment of acute toxic ingestions. *Ann Emerg Med* 1989; **18:** 56–9.
4. Levy G. Gastrointestinal clearance of drugs with activated charcoal. *N Engl J Med* 1982; **307:** 676–8.
5. Park GD, *et al.* Expanded role of charcoal therapy in the poisoned and overdosed patient. *Arch Intern Med* 1986; **146:** 969–73.
6. Pond SM. Role of repeated oral doses of activated charcoal in clinical toxicology. *Med Toxicol* 1986; **1:** 3–11.

7. Anonymous. Repeated oral activated charcoal in acute poisoning. *Lancet* 1987; **i:** 1013–15.
8. Katona BG, *et al.* The new black magic: activated charcoal and new therapeutic uses. *J Emerg Med* 1987; **5:** 9–18.
9. Neuvonen PJ, Olkkola KT. Oral activated charcoal in the treatment of intoxications: role of single and repeated doses. *Med Toxicol* 1988; **3:** 33–58.
10. McLuckie A, *et al.* Role of repeated doses of oral activated charcoal in the treatment of acute intoxications. *Anaesth Intensive Care* 1990; **18:** 375–84.
11. Tenenbein M. Multiple doses of activated charcoal: time for reappraisal? *Ann Emerg Med* 1991; **20:** 529–31.
12. Vale JA, Proudfoot AT. How useful is activated charcoal? *BMJ* 1993; **306:** 78–9.
13. Bayly GR, Ferner RE. Activated charcoal for drug overdose. *Prescribers' J* 1995; **35:** 12–17.
14. Neuvonen PJ, Olkkola KT. Effect of purgatives on antidotal efficacy of oral activated charcoal. *Hum Toxicol* 1986; **5:** 255–63.
15. Palatnick W, Tenenbein M. Activated charcoal in the treatment of drug overdose: an update. *Drug Safety* 1992; **7:** 3–7.
16. McFarland AK, Chyka PA. Selection of activated charcoal products for the treatment of poisonings. *Ann Pharmacother* 1993; **27:** 358–61.

HAEMOPERFUSION. Haemoperfusion involves the passage of blood through an adsorbent material such as activated charcoal or synthetic hydrophobic polystyrene resins which can retain certain drugs and toxic agents. Early problems with charcoal haemoperfusion such as charcoal embolism, marked thrombocytopenia, fibrinogen loss, and pyrogen reactions have been largely overcome by purification procedures and by coating the carbon with biocompatible polymers. However, transient falls in platelet count, leucocyte count, and circulatory concentrations of clotting factors, calcium, glucose, urea, creatinine, and urate have been reported during haemoperfusion. While there is no substitute for supportive measures, haemoperfusion can significantly reduce the body burden of certain compounds with a low volume of distribution within 4 to 6 hours in some severely poisoned patients; haemoperfusion is not effective for drugs or poisons with very large volumes of distribution.

References.

1. Widdop B, Vale JA. The clinical application and risk-benefit of haemoperfusion. *Hum Toxicol* 1985; **4:** 345.
2. Webb D. Charcoal haemoperfusion in drug intoxication. *Br J Hosp Med* 1993; **49:** 493–6.

Porphyria. Activated charcoal may be used as part of the management of erythropoietic protoporphyria, one of the non-acute porphyrias (p.1011). It acts as a sorbent in the gut lumen, interrupting the enterohepatic recycling of protoporphyrin. It has also been tried in a patient with photomutilation diagnosed as having congenital erythropoietic porphyria, a very rare porphyria.[1] Activated charcoal 30 g given by mouth every 3 hours for 36 hours reduced the plasma-porphyrin concentration to normal values by 20 hours and was more effective than colestyramine or transfusional therapy. After discontinuation of activated charcoal, plasma-porphyrin concentrations rose rapidly to near pretreatment levels within 10 days. Long-term treatment with oral charcoal over a 9-month period effected a clinical remission with low concentrations of plasma and skin porphyrin and an absence of photocutaneous activity. The optimal dose was determined to be 60 g three times daily. However, exacerbation following an initial period of remission has been reported in another patient[2] and total lack of efficacy in a third.[3]

1. Pimstone NR, *et al.* Therapeutic efficacy of oral charcoal in congenital erythropoietic porphyria. *N Engl J Med* 1987; **316:** 390–3.
2. Hift RJ, *et al.* The effect of oral activated charcoal on the course of congenital erythropoietic porphyria. *Br J Dermatol* 1993; **129:** 14–17.
3. Minder EI, *et al.* Lack of effect of oral charcoal in congenital erythropoietic porphyria. *N Engl J Med* 1994; **330:** 1092–4.

Pruritus. Pruritus (p.1106) is usually treated symptomatically. Activated charcoal has been tried in pruritus associated with renal failure. In a double-blind crossover study, administration of activated charcoal 6 g daily by mouth for 8 weeks was more effective than placebo in relieving generalised pruritus in 11 patients undergoing maintenance haemodialysis.[1]

1. Pederson JA, *et al.* Relief of idiopathic generalized pruritus in dialysis patients treated with activated oral charcoal. *Ann Intern Med* 1980; **93:** 446–8.

Preparations

Proprietary Preparations (details are given in Part 3)
Aust.: Kolemed; Norit; Norit-Carbomix; ***Austral.:*** Ad-Sorb; Carbosorb; Charcocaps; Charcotabs; Karbons; Prodiarrhoea†; ***Belg.:*** Norit; Norit-Carbomix; ***Canad.:*** Charcodote Aqueous; ***Fin.:*** Carbomix; ***Fr.:*** Actisorb†; Carbactive; Carbomix; Carbonet; Charbon de Belloc; Formocarbine; Mandocarbine†; Splenocarbine; ***Ger.:*** Kohle-Compretten; Kohle-Hevert; Kohle-Pulvis; Kohle-Tabletten; Ultracarbon; ***Irl.:*** Carbomix; Carbonet; Norit; ***Ital.:*** Carbomix; Neo Carbone Belloc†; ***Neth.:*** Norit; ***NZ:*** Carbosorb; ***Singapore:*** Aqueous Charcodote; Ultracarbon; ***Spain:*** Arkocapsulas Carbon Veg; Ultracarbon; ***Swed.:*** Carbomix; Kolsuspension; Medikol; ***Thai.:*** Ca-R-Bob; Ultracarbon; ***UK:*** Actidose-Aqua; Bragg's; Carbomix; Carbonet; Charcodote; Clinisorb; Liqui-Char; Lyofoam C; Medicoal; Modern Herbals Trapped Wind & Indigestion; ***USA:*** Actidose-Aqua; Charcoaid; Charcoal Plus; Charcocaps; Liqui-Char.

Multi-ingredient: ***Aust.:*** Eucarbon; Intestinol; ***Austral.:*** Carbosorb S; Kaltocarb†; No Gas; ***Belg.:*** Carbobel; Eucarbon; ***Braz.:*** Passicarbone; ***Canad.:*** Charcodote; ***Fr.:*** Acticarbine; Actisorb Plus; Carbolevure; Carbophagix; Carbophos; Carbosylane; Carbosymag; Quinocarbine; ***Ger.:*** Carboyoghurt; Hevert-Carmin symbio; ***Hong Kong:*** Biscasil; ***Irl.:*** Actisorb Plus; ***Israel:*** Carbosylane; Eucarbon; Kaltocarb; Novicarbon; ***Ital.:*** Actisorb Plus; Carbondifer; Carbonesia; Carbotiol†; Carboyoghurt; Cura†; No-Gas; ***NZ:*** Carbosorb S; ***Port.:*** Carboflex; ***S.Afr.:*** Rubilax; ***Switz.:***

Carbolevure; Carboticon; Eucarbon†; ***Thai.:*** Belacid; Bicobon; Biodan; Carbonpectate; Papytazyme; Pepsitase; Polyenzyme-I; ***UK:*** Acidosis; Actisorb Plus; Carbellon; Kaltocarb†; Papaya Plus; ***USA:*** Actidose with Sorbitol; Flatulex; Poison Antidote Kit.

Amifostine   (17040-h)

Amifostine (BAN, USAN, rINN).

Ethiofos; Gammaphos; NSC-296961; WR-2721. S-[2-(3-Aminopropylamino)ethyl] dihydrogen phosphorothioate.
$C_5H_{15}N_2O_3PS = 214.2$.

CAS — 20537-88-6 (amifostine); 63717-27-1 (amifostine monohydrate).
ATC — V03AF05.

Pharmacopoeias. In US.

Pharmacopoeial description

USP 25: A white crystalline powder. Freely soluble in water. pH of a 5% solution in water is between 6.5 and 7.5. Store in airtight containers at a temperature of 2° to 8°. Protect from light.

Incompatibilities. Amifostine has been reported[1] to be physically incompatible with aciclovir sodium, amphotericin B, cefoperazone sodium, chlorpromazine hydrochloride, cisplatin, ganciclovir sodium, hydroxyzine hydrochloride, minocycline hydrochloride, and prochlorperazine edisilate during simulated Y-site administration.

1. Trissel LA, Martinez JF. Compatibility of amifostine with selected drugs during simulated Y-site administration. *Am J Health-Syst Pharm* 1995; **52:** 2208–12.

Adverse Effects, Treatment, and Precautions

Amifostine may cause a transient reduction, usually in systolic, or, less frequently, in diastolic blood pressure. However, more pronounced reductions in blood pressure may occur and transient loss of consciousness has been reported very rarely. To minimise hypotension, patients should be adequately hydrated before treatment with amifostine begins and should be in a supine position. Amifostine is contra-indicated in patients who are hypotensive or dehydrated. Patients taking antihypertensive drugs should discontinue treatment 24 hours before administration of amifostine. Arterial blood pressure must be monitored during the amifostine infusion and if systolic blood pressure decreases significantly, infusion must stop. It may be continued if blood pressure returns to normal within 5 minutes.

Nausea and vomiting are frequently reported and concurrent antiemetic therapy is recommended.

Amifostine reduces serum-calcium concentrations, although clinical hypocalcaemia has occurred only very rarely in patients who received multiple doses of amifostine within 24 hours. Serum-calcium concentrations should be monitored in patients at risk of hypocalcaemia.

Other side-effects include flushing, chills, somnolence, hiccups, sneezing, and mild skin rashes.

Administration of amifostine over a longer period than the recommended 15 minutes is associated with a higher incidence of side-effects.

Pharmacokinetics

Amifostine is rapidly cleared from the plasma following intravenous administration and is dephosphorylated by alkaline phosphatase to the active metabolite WR-1065, a free thiol compound. The elimination half-life of amifostine after a 15-minute infusion is less than 10 minutes. About 6% or less of a dose is excreted in the urine.

Uses and Administration

Amifostine, an aminothiol compound, is a cytoprotective agent. It is converted in the body to its active metabolite WR-1065 which protects noncancerous cells against the toxic effects of antineoplastics and ionising radiation. It is used in patients with advanced ovarian cancer to reduce neutropenia-related infection associated with cyclophosphamide and cisplatin therapy and, in patients with advanced solid tumours of non-germ cell origin, to reduce the cumulative renal toxicity associated with repeated cisplatin administration. It is also used to reduce the incidence of xerostomia (dry mouth) in patients undergoing radiation therapy for head and neck cancer. Amifostine is under investigation in ameliorating the adverse effects of other antineoplastics.

In chemotherapy, amifostine is given by intravenous infusion over 15 minutes starting no more than 30 minutes before administration of antineoplastic therapy. The recommended dose in adults is 910 mg per m^2 body-surface once daily. The dose should be reduced to 740 mg per m^2 in patients unable to tolerate the full dose. This lower dose of 740 mg per m^2 is also recommended for the reduction of renal toxicity of cisplatin if doses of cisplatin of less than 100 mg per m^2 are used.

In the prevention of xerostomia, amifostine is given in a dose of 200 mg per m^2 daily as a 3-minute intravenous infusion started 15 to 30 minutes before radiotherapy.

Adjunct in antineoplastic therapy. WR-1065, the active metabolite of amifostine, readily enters non-malignant cells where it deactivates cytotoxics such as alkylating and platinum-containing antineoplastics and protects against the effects of ionising radiation. The cytoprotective effects of amifostine are reported to be selective for normal cells and not to interfere with the cytotoxic effects of antineoplastics and radiation on malignant cells. Several factors contribute to this selectivity; malignant tumours contain less alkaline phosphatase than normal tissue and WR-1065 is less readily transported into malignant cells.

References.
1. Foster-Nora JA, Siden R. Amifostine for protection from antineoplastic drug toxicity. *Am J Health-Syst Pharm* 1997; **54:** 787–800.
2. Mabro M, *et al.* A risk-benefit assessment of amifostine in cytoprotection. *Drug Safety* 1999; **21:** 367–87.
3. Culy CR, Spencer CM. Amifostine: an update on its clinical status as a cytoprotectant in patients with cancer receiving chemotherapy or radiotherapy and its potential therapeutic application in myelodysplastic syndrome. *Drugs* 2001; **61:** 641–84.

Preparations

Proprietary Preparations (details are given in Part 3)
Austral.: Ethyol; *Belg.:* Ethyol; *Canad.:* Ethyol; *Denm.:* Ethyol; *Fin.:* Ethyol; *Fr.:* Ethyol; *Ger.:* Ethyol; *Hong Kong:* Ethyol; *Israel:* Ethyol; *Ital.:* Ethyol; *Mex.:* Ethyol; *Neth.:* Ethyol; *NZ:* Ethyol; *Port.:* Ethyol; *S.Afr.:* Ethyol; *Singapore:* Ethyol; *Spain:* Ethyol; *Swed.:* Ethyol; *Switz.:* Ethyol; *Thai.:* Ethyol; *UK:* Ethyol; *USA:* Ethyol.

Ammonium Tetrathiomolybdate (10500-b)

$(NH_4)_2MoS_4 = 260.3$.
CAS — 15060-55-6.

Profile
Ammonium tetrathiomolybdate is a chelator that aids the elimination of copper from the body. It is under investigation in the treatment of Wilson's disease.

Wilson's disease. Ammonium tetrathiomolybdate forms a complex with protein and copper. When it is taken with food it blocks the intestinal absorption of copper, and when given between meals it combines with albumin- and caeruloplasmin-bound copper. Ammonium tetrathiomolybdate is under investigation for the initial reduction of copper levels in patients with Wilson's disease (p.1019); it may be particularly suitable for patients with neurological symptoms.[1,2] Reversible bone marrow depression has been reported in two patients treated with ammonium tetrathiomolybdate.[3]

1. Brewer GJ, *et al.* Treatment of Wilson's disease with ammonium tetrathiomolybdate I: initial therapy in 17 neurologically affected patients. *Arch Neurol* 1994; **51:** 545–54.
2. Brewer GJ, *et al.* Treatment of Wilson disease with ammonium tetrathiomolybdate II: initial therapy in 33 neurologically affected patients and follow-up with zinc therapy. *Arch Neurol* 1996; **53:** 1017–25.
3. Harper PL, Walshe JM. Reversible pancytopenia secondary to treatment with tetrathiomolybdate. *Br J Haematol* 1986; **64:** 851–3.

Amyl Nitrite (9205-q)

Amylis Nitris; Amylium Nitrosum; Azotito de Amilo; Isoamyl Nitrite; Isopentyl Nitrite; Nitrito de Amilo; Pentanolis Nitris.
$C_5H_{11}NO_2 = 117.1$.
ATC — V03AB22.
Pharmacopoeias. In Aust., It., Jpn, and US.

It is liable to decompose with evolution of nitrogen, particularly if it has become acid in reaction.

Pharmacopoeial description
USP 25: A mixture of the nitrite esters of 3-methyl-1-butanol and 2-methyl-1-butanol. A clear, yellowish liquid having a peculiar, ethereal, fruity odour. It is very flammable. It is volatile even at low temperatures. B.p. about 96°. Practically insoluble

in water; miscible with alcohol and with ether. Store in a cool place in airtight containers. Protect from light.

◊ CAUTION. *Amyl nitrite is very flammable and must not be used where it may be ignited.*

Adverse Effects, Treatment, and Precautions
Amyl nitrite inhalation commonly causes flushing, headache, and dizziness; nausea and vomiting, hypotension, restlessness, and tachycardia may also occur. Overdosage may result in cyanosis, syncope, dyspnoea, and muscular weakness, due to vasodilatation and methaemoglobinaemia. Methylene blue [methylthioninium chloride] administration may be required for severe methaemoglobinaemia but should not be used if cyanide poisoning is suspected since cyanide may be displaced.

Amyl nitrite may increase intra-ocular and intracranial pressure and should be used with caution in patients with glaucoma, recent head trauma, or cerebral haemorrhage.

Abuse. Volatile nitrites (commonly known as 'poppers') have been abused, in the belief that they expand creativity, stimulate music appreciation, promote a sense of abandon in dancing, and intensify sexual experience.[1,2]

Inhalation of amyl, butyl, or isobutyl nitrite has caused headache, tachycardia, syncope, acute psychosis, increased intraocular pressure, transient hemiparesis, methaemoglobinaemia, coma, and, rarely, sudden death.[3]

Haemolytic anaemia has been reported in subjects after abuse of volatile nitrites;[4,5] in some subjects, Heinz body formation has been detected.[4] Methaemoglobinaemia has been reported following ingestion of volatile nitrites.[6-9] Symptoms are similar to those of hypoxia[8] and may be reversed by administration of methylene blue [methylthioninium chloride].[6-9]

Exposure to amyl nitrite inhalation has led to severe and extensive contact dermatitis around the face with secondary spread elsewhere on the body.[10]

1. Sigell LT, *et al.* Popping and snorting volatile nitrites: a current fad for getting high. *Am J Psychiatry* 1978; **135:** 1216–18.
2. Lockwood B. Poppers: volatile nitrite inhalants. *Pharm J* 1996; **257:** 154–5.
3. Anonymous. Treatment of acute drug abuse reactions. *Med Lett Drugs Ther* 1987; **29:** 83–6.
4. Romeril KR, Concannon AJ. Heinz body haemolytic anaemia after sniffing volatile nitrites. *Med J Aust* 1981; **1:** 302–3.
5. Brandes JC, *et al.* Amyl nitrite-induced hemolytic anemia. *Am J Med* 1989; **86:** 252–4.
6. Laaban JP, *et al.* Amyl nitrite poppers and methemoglobinemia. *Ann Intern Med* 1985; **103:** 804–5.
7. Osterloh J, Olson K. Toxicities of alkyl nitrites. *Ann Intern Med* 1986; **104:** 727.
8. Pierce JMT, Nielsen MS. Acute acquired methaemoglobinaemia after amyl nitrite poisoning. *BMJ* 1989; **298:** 1566.
9. Forsyth RJ, Moulden A. Methaemoglobinaemia after ingestion of amyl nitrite. *Arch Dis Child* 1991; **66:** 152.
10. Bos JD, *et al.* Allergic contact dermatitis to amyl nitrite ('poppers'). *Contact Dermatitis* 1985; **12:** 109.

Uses and Administration
Amyl nitrite is rapidly absorbed on inhalation and has been employed in the immediate treatment of patients with definite cyanide poisoning (p.1433) to induce the formation of methaemoglobin, which combines with the cyanide to form non-toxic cyanmethaemoglobin. The value of such treatment has been questioned since only low levels of methaemoglobin are formed, but other mechanisms may also be important. A suggested procedure has been to administer amyl nitrite by inhalation for up to 30 seconds every minute until other measures can be instituted. It has also been suggested for use in the management of hydrogen sulfide poisoning (p.1199).

Amyl nitrite has an action similar to that of glyceryl trinitrate (p.898) and used to be given by inhalation for the relief of acute attacks of angina pectoris but is seldom used now.

Amyl nitrite is used in homoeopathic medicine.

Preparations

USP 25: Amyl Nitrite Inhalant.

Proprietary Preparations (details are given in Part 3)
Multi-ingredient: *S.Afr.:* Tripac-Cyano; *USA:* Cyanide Antidote Package; Emergent-Ez.

Asoxime Chloride (19298-r)

HI-6. 1-({[4-(Aminocarbonyl)pyridinio]methoxy}methyl)-2-[(hydroxyimino)methyl]pyridinium dichloride.
$C_{14}H_{16}Cl_2N_4O_3 = 359.2$.
CAS — 34433-31-3.

Profile
Asoxime chloride is a cholinesterase reactivator which has been tried in the treatment of poisoning by organophosphorus pesticides and related compounds.

◊ References.
1. Jovanović D, *et al.* A case of unusual suicidal poisoning by the organophosphorus insecticide dimethoate. *Hum Exp Toxicol* 1990; **9:** 49–51.
2. Kušić R, *et al.* HI-6 in man: efficacy of the oxime in poisoning by organophosphorus insecticides. *Hum Exp Toxicol* 1991; **10:** 113–18.

Atipamezole Hydrochloride (5005-y)

Atipamezole Hydrochloride (BANM, rINNM).
MPV-1248 (atipamezole). 4-(2-Ethyl-2-indanyl)imidazole hydrochloride.
$C_{14}H_{16}N_2,HCl = 248.8$.
CAS — 104054-27-5 (atipamezole); 104075-48-1 (atipamezole hydrochloride).
NOTE. Atipamezole is USAN.

Profile
Atipamezole hydrochloride is a selective alpha$_2$-adrenergic receptor antagonist that is used in veterinary medicine to reverse the sedative effects of medetomidine.

Calcium Polystyrene Sulfonate

(5004-l)

Calcium Polystyrene Sulphonate.
CAS — 37286-92-3.
Pharmacopoeias. In Br. and Jpn.

The calcium salt of sulfonated styrene polymer.

Pharmacopoeial description
BP 2001: A cream to light brown, fine powder. The calcium content is not less than 6.5% and not more than 9.5%, calculated with reference to the dried substance. Each g exchanges not less than 1.3 mmol and not more than 2.0 mmol of potassium, calculated with reference to the dried substance. Practically insoluble in water and in alcohol. Store in airtight containers.

Adverse Effects and Precautions
As for Sodium Polystyrene Sulfonate, p.1023. Sorbitol should not be used with calcium polystyrene sulfonate due to the risk of colonic necrosis. Sodium overloading is not a problem with calcium polystyrene sulfonate, but calcium overloading and hypercalcaemia may occur. It should therefore be avoided in patients with conditions such as hyperparathyroidism, multiple myeloma, sarcoidosis, or metastatic carcinoma who may present with renal failure together with hypercalcaemia. Patients should be monitored for electrolyte disturbances, especially hypokalaemia and hypercalcaemia.

Effects on the lungs. An elderly man who died from cardiac arrest was found at necropsy to have bronchopneumonia associated with inhalation of calcium polystyrene sulfonate;[1] the resin had been given by mouth to treat hyperkalaemia.
1. Chaplin AJ, Millard PR. Calcium polystyrene sulphonate: an unusual cause of inhalation pneumonia. *BMJ* 1975; **3:** 77–8.

Interactions
As for Sodium Polystyrene Sulfonate, p.1024. Calcium ions are released from the resin in the gastrointestinal tract and this may reduce the absorption of tetracycline given by mouth.

Uses and Administration
Calcium polystyrene sulfonate is a cation-exchange resin which exchanges calcium ions for potassium ions and other cations in the gastrointestinal tract. It is used similarly to sodium polystyrene sulfonate (p.1024) to enhance potassium excretion in the treatment of hyperkalaemia (p.1182) and may be preferred to the sodium resin in patients who cannot tolerate an increase in their sodium load. It is estimated that 1 g of calcium polystyrene sulfonate could bind 1.3 to 2 mmol of potassium but it is unlikely that such figures could be achieved in practice.

It is given by mouth, in a dose of 15 g up to four times daily, as a suspension in water or syrup or as a sweetened paste. It should not be given in fruit juices that have a high potassium content. A dose for children is up to 1 g per kg body-weight daily in divided doses for acute hyperkalaemia, reduced to a maintenance dose of 500 mg per kg daily in divided doses; the oral route is not recommended for neonates.

When oral administration is difficult, calcium polystyrene sulfonate may be administered rectally as an enema. The usual daily dose is 30 g given as a suspension in 100 mL of 2% methylcellulose '450' and 100 mL of water and retained, if possible, for at least 9 hours. Initial therapy may constitute administration by both oral and rectal routes. Following retention of the enema the colon should be irrigated to remove the resin. Children and neonates may be given rectal doses similar to those suggested for children by mouth.

Preparations

Proprietary Preparations (details are given in Part 3)
Aust.: CPS Pulver; Sorbisterit; *Austral.:* Calcium Resonium; *Belg.:* Kayexalate Calcium; *Braz.:* Sorcal; *Canad.:* Resonium Calcium; *Denm.:* Resonium Calcium; *Fr.:* Calcium-Sorbisterit†; *Ger.:* Anti-Kalium; Calcium Resonium; CPS Pulver; Elutit-Calcium; Sorbisterit; *Hong Kong:* Calcium Resonium; *Irl.:* Calcium Resonium; *Jpn:* Kalimate; *Neth.:* Calcium Resonium†; *Norw.:* Resonium Calcium; *NZ:* Calcium Resonium; *Spain:* Resincalcio; *Swed.:* Resonium Calcium; *Switz.:* Sorbisterit; *UK:* Calcium Resonium.

Multi-ingredient: *Port.:* Resical.

Calcium Trisodium Pentetate   (1032-q)

Calcium Trisodium Pentetate *(BAN, rINN)*.

Calcium Trisodium DTPA; NSC-34249; Pentetate Calcium Trisodium *(USAN)*; Trisodium Calcium Diethylenetriaminepentaacetate. Calcium trisodium nitrilodiethylenedinitrilopenta-acetate.

$C_{14}H_{18}CaN_3Na_3O_{10} = 497.4$.

CAS — 12111-24-9 (calcium trisodium pentetate); 67-43-6 (pentetic acid).

NOTE. Pentetic acid is *BAN, USAN,* and *rINN.*

Pharmacopoeias. US includes Pentetic Acid.

Profile

Pentetic acid and its salts are chelators with the general properties of the edetates (see Sodium Calcium Edetate, p.1022). Calcium trisodium pentetate is used in the treatment of poisoning by heavy metals and radioactive metals such as plutonium. Doses of 1 g daily have been administered by slow intravenous infusion for 3 to 5 days. Further treatment may be given after an interval of 3 days.

Calcium pentetate has also been used.

Pentetates, labelled with metallic radionuclides, are used in nuclear medicine (see Indium-111, p.1449, and Technetium-99m, p.1451).

Thalassaemia. Calcium pentetate, 0.5 to 1 g by subcutaneous infusion on alternate days or for 5 days each week, was given to 5 patients with thalassaemia (p.718) in whom desferrioxamine had to be withdrawn because of high-tone deafness.[1] Calcium pentetate was as effective as desferrioxamine at increasing iron excretion. Hearing improved during treatment. Oral zinc supplements were necessary during treatment with calcium pentetate to maintain adequate plasma-zinc concentrations.

1. Wonke B, *et al.* Reversal of desferrioxamine induced auditory neurotoxicity during treatment with Ca-DTPA. *Arch Dis Child* 1989; **64:** 77–82.

Preparations

Proprietary Preparations (details are given in Part 3)
Ger.: Ditripentat-Heyl.

Deferiprone   (3851-l)

Deferiprone *(BAN, rINN)*.

Dimethylhydroxypyridone; L1. 1,2-Dimethyl-3-hydroxypyrid-4-one; 3-Hydroxy-1,2-dimethyl-4-pyridone.

$C_7H_9NO_2 = 139.2$.
CAS — 30652-11-0.
ATC — V03AC02.

Profile

Deferiprone is an orally active iron chelator used in the treatment of iron overload in patients with thalassaemia for whom desferrioxamine is unsuitable. It is given by mouth in doses of 25 mg per kg body-weight three times daily; dosage should be calculated to the nearest half tablet. Doses above 100 mg per kg daily are not recommended.

Iron overload. Although desferrioxamine is effective in the treatment of iron overload such as that associated with thalassaemia (p.718), compliance is limited by the need for regular injections. Deferiprone is an orally effective iron chelator that was developed with the aim of overcoming this problem. Beneficial responses have been reported,[1-6] although a small study[7] indicated that deferiprone did not adequately control body iron burden long term in patients with thalassaemia and might worsen hepatic fibrosis. The manufacturer concedes that the efficacy of deferiprone may be less than that of desferrioxamine and consequently its use is limited to those unsuitable for therapy with desferrioxamine.

Concern has also been expressed over the potential toxicity of deferiprone. Preclinical testing in *animals* revealed embryotoxicity, teratogenicity, organ atrophy, and haematological toxicity,[8] and reversible neutropenia or agranulocytosis has been reported in patients.[5,6,9,10] In addition, a case of fatal systemic lupus erythematosus has been reported[11] although this could have been related to the patient's thalassaemia rather than to the drug.[12,13] Other reported adverse effects include musculoske-

The symbol † denotes a preparation no longer actively marketed

letal and joint pain,[5,6,9,10,14] gastrointestinal intolerance,[5,6,9,10] transient liver enzyme abnormalities,[6] and zinc deficiency.[6]

1. Kontoghiorghes GJ, *et al.* 1,2-dimethyl-3-hydroxypyrid-4-one, an orally active chelator for treatment of iron overload. *Lancet* 1987; **i:** 1294–5.
2. Kontoghiorghes GJ, Hoffbrand AV. Clinical trials with oral iron chelator L1. *Lancet* 1989; **ii:** 1516–17.
3. Agarwal MB, *et al.* Oral iron chelation with L1. *Lancet* 1990; **335:** 601.
4. Olivieri NF, *et al.* Comparison of oral iron chelator L1 and desferrioxamine in iron-loaded patients. *Lancet* 1990; **336:** 1275–9.
5. Olivieri NF, *et al.* Iron-chelator therapy with oral deferiprone in patients with thalassaemia major. *N Engl J Med* 1995; **332:** 918–22.
6. Al-Refaie FN, *et al.* Results of long-term deferiprone (L1) therapy: a report by the International Study Group on Oral Iron Chelators. *Br J Haematol* 1995; **91:** 224–9.
7. Olivieri NF, *et al.* Long-term safety and effectiveness of iron-chelation therapy with deferiprone for thalassemia major. *N Engl J Med* 1998; **339:** 417–23.
8. Berdoukas V, *et al.* Toxicity of oral iron chelator L1. *Lancet* 1993; **341:** 1088.
9. Hershko C. Development of oral iron chelator L1. *Lancet* 1993; **341:** 1088–9.
10. Kontoghiorghes GJ, *et al.* Future of oral iron chelator deferiprone (L1). *Lancet* 1993; **341:** 1479–80.
11. Mehta J, *et al.* Fatal systemic lupus erythematosus in patient taking oral iron chelator L1. *Lancet* 1991; **337:** 298.
12. Berdoukas V. Antinuclear antibodies in patients taking L1. *Lancet* 1991; **337:** 672.
13. Olivieri NF, *et al.* Rarity of systemic lupus erythematosus after oral iron chelator L1. *Lancet* 1991; **337:** 924.
14. Berkovitch M, *et al.* Arthropathy in thalassaemia patients receiving deferiprone. *Lancet* 1994; **343:** 1471–2.

Preparations

Proprietary Preparations (details are given in Part 3)
Fr.: Ferriprox; *Ital.:* Ferriprox; *UK:* Ferriprox.

Desferrioxamine Mesilate   (1034-s)

Desferrioxamine Mesilate *(BANM)*.

Deferoxamine Mesilate *(pINNM)*; Ba-33112; Ba-29837 (desferrioxamine hydrochloride); Deferoxamine Mesylate *(USAN)*; Deferoxamini Mesilas; Desferrioxamine Mesylate; Desferrioxamine Methanesulphonate; NSC-527604 (desferrioxamine). 30-Amino-3,14,25-trihydroxy-3,9,14,20,25-penta-azatriacontane-2,10,13,21,24-pentaone methanesulphonate; *N′*-{5-[(4-{[5-(Acetylhydroxyamino)pentyl]amino}-1,4-dioxobutyl)hydroxyamino]pentyl}-*N*-(5-aminopentyl)-*N*-hydroxy-butanediamide monomethanesulphonate.

$C_{25}H_{48}N_6O_8,CH_3SO_3H = 656.8$.

CAS — 70-51-9 (desferrioxamine); 138-14-7 (desferrioxamine mesilate); 1950-39-6 (desferrioxamine hydrochloride).

Pharmacopoeias. In *Eur.* (see p.vi), *Int., Jpn,* and *US.*

Pharmacopoeial description

Ph. Eur.: A white or almost white powder. Freely soluble in water; very slightly soluble in alcohol; practically insoluble in ether; slightly soluble in methyl alcohol. A freshly prepared 10% solution in water has a pH of 3.7 to 5.5. Store at 2° to 8°. Protect from light.

USP 25: A white to off-white powder. Freely soluble in water; slightly soluble in methyl alcohol. pH of a 1% solution in water is between 4.0 and 6.0. Store in airtight containers.

Incompatibility. The manufacturers report that desferrioxamine solutions are incompatible with heparin.

Adverse Effects and Treatment

Rapid intravenous injection of desferrioxamine may cause flushing, urticaria, hypotension, and shock. Local pain may occur with subcutaneous or intramuscular injections and pruritus, erythema, and swelling have occurred after prolonged subcutaneous administration. Gastrointestinal disorders, dysuria, fever, allergic skin rashes, tachycardia, cardiac arrhythmias, convulsions, and leg cramps have been reported. Visual disturbances, including retinal changes, and hearing loss may occur and may be reversible if desferrioxamine is withdrawn. Cataract formation has also been reported. Desferrioxamine therapy may retard growth in very young children.

◊ Reviews of the adverse effects of desferrioxamine.

1. Bentur Y, *et al.* Deferoxamine (desferrioxamine): new toxicities for an old drug. *Drug Safety* 1991; **6:** 37–46.

Effects on the blood. A patient with end-stage renal disease developed reversible thrombocytopenia on 3 separate occasions after intravenous infusions of desferrioxamine for dialysis osteomalacia.[1] Acute fatal aplastic anaemia occurred in a 16-year-old girl with thalassaemia following intravenous administration of high doses of desferrioxamine (80 mg per kg body-weight daily) for 20 days.[2]

1. Walker JA, *et al.* Thrombocytopenia associated with intravenous desferrioxamine. *Am J Kidney Dis* 1985; **6:** 254–6.
2. Sofroniadou K, *et al.* Acute bone marrow aplasia associated with intravenous administration of deferoxamine (desferrioxamine). *Drug Safety* 1990; **5:** 152–4.

Effects on the ear and eye. Lens opacities, retinal pigmentary changes and other retinal abnormalities, and ocular disturbances including loss of colour vision, night blindness, decreased visual acuity, and field defects have been reported in patients receiving long-term or high-dose treatment with desferrioxamine.[1-4] In assessments of patients on long-term therapy with desferrioxamine the incidence of symptomatic and asymptomatic ocular changes has varied from 4% of 52 patients[5] to 66% of 15 patients.[6]

Sensorineural hearing impairment has also been reported.[5,7-12] Tinnitus has been reported in a few patients.[11,13]

Both ophthalmic and auditory abnormalities can improve when desferrioxamine is withdrawn,[1,3,5-10] although sometimes the effects may be irreversible[14] or recovery may only be partial.[8,9]

Several mechanisms for desferrioxamine neurotoxicity have been suggested.[6,8,11,15-18]

1. Davies SC, *et al.* Ocular toxicity of high-dose intravenous desferrioxamine. *Lancet* 1983; **ii:** 181–4.
2. Simon P, *et al.* Desferrioxamine, ocular toxicity, and trace metals. *Lancet* 1983; **ii:** 512–13.
3. Borgna-Pignatti C, *et al.* Visual loss in patient on high-dose subcutaneous desferrioxamine. *Lancet* 1984; **i:** 681.
4. Rubinstein M, *et al.* Ocular toxicity of desferrioxamine. *Lancet* 1985; **i:** 817–18.
5. Cohen A, *et al.* Vision and hearing during deferoxamine therapy. *J Pediatr* 1990; **117:** 326–30.
6. De Virgiliis S, *et al.* Depletion of trace elements and acute ocular toxicity induced by desferrioxamine in patients with thalassaemia. *Arch Dis Child* 1988; **63:** 250–5.
7. Guerin A, *et al.* Acute deafness and desferrioxamine. *Lancet* 1985; **ii:** 39.
8. Olivieri NF, *et al.* Visual and auditory neurotoxicity in patients receiving subcutaneous deferoxamine infusions. *N Engl J Med* 1986; **314:** 869–73.
9. Barratt PS, Toogood IRG. Hearing loss attributed to desferrioxamine in patients with beta-thalassaemia major. *Med J Aust* 1987; **147:** 177–9.
10. Wonke B, *et al.* Reversal of desferrioxamine induced auditory neurotoxicity during treatment with Ca-DTPA. *Arch Dis Child* 1989; **64:** 77–82.
11. Porter JB, *et al.* Desferrioxamine ototoxicity: evaluation of risk factors in thalassaemic patients and guidelines for safe dosage. *Br J Haematol* 1989; **73:** 403–9.
12. Argiolu F, *et al.* Hearing impairment during deferoxamine therapy for thalassemia major. *J Pediatr* 1991; **118:** 826.
13. Marsh MN, *et al.* Tinnitus in a patient with beta-thalassaemia intermedia on long-term treatment with desferrioxamine. *Postgrad Med J* 1981; **57:** 582–4.
14. Bene C, *et al.* Irreversible ocular toxicity from single "challenge" dose of deferoxamine. *Clin Nephrol* 1989; **31:** 45–8.
15. Arden GB, *et al.* Ocular changes in patients undergoing long-term desferrioxamine treatment. *Br J Ophthalmol* 1984; **68:** 873–7.
16. Rahi AHS, *et al.* Ocular toxicity of desferrioxamine: light microscopic histochemical and ultrastructural findings. *Br J Ophthalmol* 1986; **70:** 373–81.
17. Pall H, *et al.* Ocular toxicity of desferrioxamine – an example of copper promoted auto-oxidative damage? *Br J Ophthalmol* 1989; **73:** 42–7.
18. Bentur Y, *et al.* Comparison of deferoxamine pharmacokinetics between asymptomatic thalassemic children and those exhibiting severe neurotoxicity. *Clin Pharmacol Ther* 1990; **47:** 478–82.

Effects on growth rate. Growth retardation has been noted in thalassaemic children undergoing desferrioxamine therapy.[1,2] Growth retardation was related to dose[1,2] and inversely related to iron stores.[1] Also retardation was greater in those who started receiving desferrioxamine at the start of transfusion therapy at approximately 9 months old than in those who started desferrioxamine once iron accumulation was established, after about 3 years. A sharp increase in growth velocity was reported in 15 patients with low ferritin levels following a 50% reduction in desferrioxamine dose.[1]

1. Piga A, *et al.* High-dose desferrioxamine as a cause of growth failure in thalassaemic patients. *Eur J Haematol* 1988; **40:** 380–1.
2. De Virgiliis S, *et al.* Deferoxamine-induced growth retardation in patients with thalassaemia major. *J Pediatr* 1988; **113:** 661–9.

Effects on the kidneys. A 14-year-old boy with thalassaemia major and haemosiderosis developed acute renal insufficiency during intravenous infusion of desferrioxamine.[1] Acute decreases in renal function were reported in 3 patients following infusions of desferrioxamine.[2] Two of these patients had received 180 mg per kg body-weight daily and it was suggested[3] that the nephrotoxicity could be related to these high doses, although others reported also having seen reductions in glomerular filtration rates following regular doses.[4]

1. Batey R, *et al.* Acute renal insufficiency occurring during intravenous desferrioxamine therapy. *Scand J Haematol* 1979; **22:** 277–9.
2. Koren G, *et al.* Acute changes in renal function associated with deferoxamine therapy. *Am J Dis Child* 1989; **143:** 1077–80.
3. Li Volti S, *et al.* Acute changes in renal function associated with deferoxamine therapy. *Am J Dis Child* 1990; **144:** 1069–70.
4. Koren G, Bentur Y. Acute changes in renal function associated with deferoxamine. *Am J Dis Child* 1990; **144:** 1070.

Effects on the lungs. A pulmonary syndrome with tachypnoea, hypoxaemia, reduced pulmonary function, and radiographic evidence of diffuse interstitial pneumonia has been reported in patients receiving high-dose intravenous therapy with desferrioxamine.[1,2] It has been suggested that a hypersensitivity reaction was involved.[1,2]

Fatal acute respiratory distress syndrome has occurred in 4 patients; in these cases desferrioxamine infusions had been given for 65 to 92 hours. Pulmonary complications had not been noted in patients given desferrioxamine for less than 24 hours.[3] This report did, however, generate subsequent correspondence disagreeing with the view that prolonged use of desferrioxamine was the cause of the toxicity. Alternative explanations for the pulmonary injury included the administration of above maximum daily doses of desferrioxamine[4] as well as inadequate desferrioxamine therapy.[5]

1. Freedman MH, *et al.* Pulmonary syndrome in patients with thalassemia major receiving intravenous deferoxamine infusions. *Am J Dis Child* 1990; **144:** 565–9.
2. Scanderbeg AC, *et al.* Pulmonary syndrome and intravenous high-dose desferrioxamine. *Lancet* 1990; **336:** 1511.
3. Tenenbein M, *et al.* Pulmonary toxic effects of continuous desferrioxamine administration in acute iron poisoning. *Lancet* 1992; **339:** 699–701.
4. Macarol V, Yawalkar SJ. Desferrioxamine in acute iron poisoning. *Lancet* 1992; **339:** 1601.
5. Shannon M. Desferrioxamine in acute iron poisoning. *Lancet* 1992; **339:** 1601.

Effects on the skin. Desferrioxamine may be used in the management of porphyria cutanea tarda (see p.1011). However, lesions resembling porphyria cutanea tarda developed in 3 patients during long-term therapy with desferrioxamine for aluminium toxicity.[1] The lesions worsened on exposure to sun and resolved when desferrioxamine treatment was completed. It was also possible that the lesions were associated with aluminium accumulation. Alopecia was noted in one patient but an association with desferrioxamine therapy could not be established.

1. McCarthy JT, *et al.* Clinical experience with desferrioxamine in dialysis patients with aluminium toxicity. *Q J Med* 1990; **74:** 257–76.

Hypersensitivity. Individual cases of anaphylactoid reactions to desferrioxamine have been reported.[1,2] Rapid intravenous desensitisation was successful in two patients.[1,2] Effects on the lungs have also been attributed to hypersensitivity (see above).

1. Miller KB, *et al.* Rapid desensitisation for desferrioxamine anaphylactic reaction. *Lancet* 1981; **i:** 1059.
2. Bousquet J, *et al.* Rapid desensitisation for desferrioxamine anaphylactoid reactions. *Lancet* 1983; **ii:** 859–60.

Treatment of adverse effects. The adverse effects of desferrioxamine generally respond to dosage reduction. In acute overdosage desferrioxamine may be removed by haemodialysis.

Isoniazid, 50 or 100 mg with pyridoxine, suppressed intolerable adverse effects of desferrioxamine in a patient with Alzheimer's disease.[1] The adverse effects, anorexia and weight loss, were attributed to a toxic metabolite of desferrioxamine generated by the plasma monoamine oxidase enzyme system and isoniazid reduced the formation of this suspect metabolite.

1. Kruck TPA, *et al.* Suppression of deferoxamine mesylate treatment-induced side effects by coadministration of isoniazid in a patient with Alzheimer's disease subject to aluminum removal by ionspecific chelation. *Clin Pharmacol Ther* 1990; **48:** 439–46.

Precautions

Desferrioxamine should be used with caution in patients with impaired renal function since the metal complexes are excreted by the kidneys (in those with severe renal impairment dialysis increases elimination). The desferrioxamine-iron complex excreted by the kidneys may colour the urine reddish-brown. Desferrioxamine may exacerbate aluminium-related encephalopathy and precipitate seizures. Prophylactic treatment with antiepileptics such as clonazepam has been suggested for patients judged to be at risk. An increased susceptibility to infection, particularly with *Yersinia* species, has been reported in patients with iron overload treated with desferrioxamine. Severe fungal infections have also been reported, predominantly in patients undergoing dialysis. If infection is suspected, treatment with desferrioxamine should be stopped and appropriate antimicrobial treatment given. Skeletal fetal anomalies have occurred in *animals.*

The urinary excretion of iron should be regularly monitored during treatment and periodic ophthalmological and audiological examinations are recommended for patients on long-term therapy. Monitoring of cardiac function is also recommended for patients receiving combined treatment with ascorbic acid (see also under Interactions, below).

Inappropriately high dosage in children with low ferritin levels may retard growth and therefore regular checks on height and weight are recommended for children.

Aluminium encephalopathy. The precipitation of dialysis dementia with some fatal outcomes[1-3] has been associated with desferrioxamine treatment for aluminium overload in dialysis patients. Some workers[2] suggested that the effect could be dose related, but others[3] reported exacerbation of aluminium encephalopathy following the low dose of 0.5 g twice weekly. Yet other authors[1] suggested that the onset of symptoms could be associated with high concentrations of aluminium observed af-

ter desferrioxamine administration and recommended the use of low doses (for example 10 mg per kg body-weight) given immediately before dialysis in affected patients in conjunction with charcoal haemoperfusion to avoid high serum-aluminium concentrations.

1. Sherrard DJ, *et al.* Precipitation of dialysis dementia by deferoxamine treatment of aluminum related bone disease. *Am J Kidney Dis* 1988; **12:** 126–30.
2. McCauley J, Sorkin I. Exacerbation of aluminium encephalopathy after treatment with desferrioxamine. *Nephrol Dial Transplant* 1989; **4:** 110–14.
3. Lillevang ST, Pedersen FB. Exacerbation of aluminium encephalopathy after treatment with desferrioxamine. *Nephrol Dial Transplant* 1989; **4:** 676.

Diagnostic tests. Desferrioxamine could interfere with estimations of total iron-binding capacity.[1] It may also interfere with colorimetric iron assays.

Desferrioxamine may distort the results of gallium-67 imaging studies.

1. Bentur Y, *et al.* Misinterpretation of iron-binding capacity in the presence of deferoxamine. *J Pediatr* 1991; **118:** 139–42.

Infection susceptibility. *Yersinia enterocolitica* is one of the most iron-dependent of all microbes, but unlike most other aerobic bacteria, it produces no detectable iron-binding compounds, or siderophores.[1] Exogenous siderophores, such as desferrioxamine, may enable *Y. enterocolitica* to overcome this handicap[2] and the apparent increased susceptibility to yersiniosis in patients with severe iron overload may therefore be attributable at least in part to desferrioxamine therapy rather than just the increased availability of iron. Infections due to *Y. enterocolitica* have been reported in patients receiving desferrioxamine for acute iron overdosage[3] or for chronic iron overload.[2,4-7] Severe infection with *Y. pseudotuberculosis* has also been reported in a thalassaemic patient on long-term desferrioxamine therapy.[8]

Treatment with desferrioxamine may also increase susceptibility to mucormycosis. Infections have occurred both in patients with iron overload disorders[9,10] and in those who do not have excessive iron stores.[11-13] A review[10] of 26 cases of mucormycosis in patients undergoing treatment revealed that 23 patients died; in 19 cases the diagnosis was only made at necropsy and only 9 patients received potentially effective treatment (surgery and/or amphotericin B). The organisms responsible were *Rhizopus* species in 13 cases and *Cunninghamella bertholletiae* in 3. In another review of 24 cases of mucormycosis in patients on dialysis,[14] at least 21 were receiving desferrioxamine; infection was fatal in 21 of the 24 patients.

In view of the serious nature of these infections it is important that they should be recognised and treated promptly. It has been suggested that a short course of a suitable antibacterial could be given as prophylaxis to young children from areas with a high incidence of yersiniosis (see Yersinia Enteritis, p.124) who require treatment with desferrioxamine.[15]

1. Anonymous. Yersiniosis today. *Lancet* 1984; **i:** 84–5.
2. Robins-Browne RM, Prpic JK. Desferrioxamine and systemic yersiniosis. *Lancet* 1983; **ii:** 1372.
3. Melby K, *et al.* Septicaemia due to Yersinia enterocolitica after oral overdoses of iron. *BMJ* 1982; **285:** 467–8.
4. Scharnetzky M, *et al.* Prophylaxis of systemic yersinosis in thalassaemia major. *Lancet* 1984; **i:** 791.
5. Chiu HY, *et al.* Infection with Yersinia enterocolitica in patients with iron overload. *BMJ* 1986; **292:** 97.
6. Kelly D, *et al.* Yersinia and iron overload. *BMJ* 1986; **292:** 413.
7. Gallant T, *et al.* Yersinia sepsis in patients with iron overload treated with deferoxamine. *N Engl J Med* 1986; **314:** 1643.
8. Gordts B, *et al.* Yersinia pseudotuberculosis septicaemia in thalassaemia major. *Lancet* 1984; **i:** 41–2.
9. Sane A, *et al.* Deferoxamine as a risk factor for zygomycete infection. *J Infect Dis* 1989; **159:** 151–2.
10. Daly AL, *et al.* Mucormycosis: association with deferoxamine therapy. *Am J Med* 1989; **87:** 468–71.
11. Goodill JJ, Abuelo JG. Mucormycosis–a new risk of deferoxamine therapy in dialysis patients with aluminum overload? *N Engl J Med* 1987; **316:** 54.
12. Windus DW, *et al.* Fatal rhizopus infections in hemodialysis patients receiving deferoxamine. *Ann Intern Med* 1987; **107:** 678–80.
13. Boelaert JR, *et al.* Mucormycosis infections in dialysis patients. *Ann Intern Med* 1987; **107:** 782–3.
14. Boelaert JR, *et al.* Mucormycosis among patients on dialysis. *N Engl J Med* 1989; **321:** 190–1.
15. Hadjiminas JM. Yersiniosis in acutely iron-loaded children treated with desferrioxamine. *J Antimicrob Chemother* 1988; **21:** 680–1.

Pregnancy. Abnormalities in *animals* have been noted following the administration of desferrioxamine in pregnancy. Thus the outcome following iron overdose during pregnancy was studied in 66 patients reported to the UK Teratology Information Service of whom 35 received desferrioxamine.[1] Seven infants of the 66 pregnancies had malformations (severe in only one) and all were associated with maternal overdoses after the first trimester and therefore could not be directly related to either iron or desferrioxamine. It was concluded that treatment of iron overdose with desferrioxamine should not be withheld solely on the grounds of pregnancy.

1. McElhatton PR, *et al.* Outcome of pregnancy following deliberate iron overdose by the mother. *Hum Exp Toxicol* 1993; **12:** 579.

Interactions

Desferrioxamine is usually administered parenterally and thus drug interactions due to chelation with oral metal ions are not a problem.

Ascorbic acid. Ascorbic acid is often given in addition to desferrioxamine to patients with iron overload to achieve better iron excretion. However, early on in treatment when there is excess tissue iron there is some evidence that ascorbic acid may worsen the iron toxicity, particularly to the heart. Thus, ascorbic acid should not be given for the first month after starting desferrioxamine treatment.

Phenothiazines. Neurological symptoms including loss of consciousness, occurred in 2 patients who received *prochlorperazine* during desferrioxamine administration.[1] Concomitant use should be avoided.

1. Blake DR, *et al.* Cerebral and ocular toxicity induced by desferrioxamine. *Q J Med* 1985; **56:** 345–55.

Pharmacokinetics

Desferrioxamine mesilate is poorly absorbed from the gastrointestinal tract. Following parenteral administration, desferrioxamine forms chelates with metal ions and is also metabolised, primarily in the plasma. The iron-desferrioxamine chelate is excreted in the urine and bile. Desferrioxamine is absorbed during peritoneal dialysis if added to the dialysis fluid.

◊ References.

1. Summers MR, *et al.* Studies in desferrioxamine and ferrioxamine metabolism in normal and iron-loaded subjects. *Br J Haematol* 1979; **42:** 547–55.
2. Allain P, *et al.* Pharmacokinetics and renal elimination of desferrioxamine and ferrioxamine in healthy subjects and patients with haemochromatosis. *Br J Clin Pharmacol* 1987; **24:** 207–12.

Uses and Administration

Desferrioxamine is a chelator which has a high affinity for ferric iron. When given by injection it forms a stable water-soluble iron-complex (ferrioxamine) which is readily excreted in the urine and bile. Desferrioxamine appears to remove both free iron and bound iron from haemosiderin and ferritin but not from haemoglobin, transferrin, or cytochromes. It is estimated that 100 mg of desferrioxamine mesilate could bind about 8.5 mg of iron but it is unlikely that such a figure could be achieved in practice. Desferrioxamine also has an affinity for other trivalent metal ions including aluminium and theoretically 100 mg of the mesilate could bind 4.1 mg of aluminium.

Desferrioxamine increases the excretion of iron from the body and is used in conditions associated with chronic iron overload (such as the iron storage disorders haemochromatosis and haemosiderosis and following repeated transfusions as in thalassaemia) and in acute iron poisoning. It has been used as eye drops in the management of ocular siderosis and corneal rust stains. It is also used to reduce aluminium overload in patients with end-stage renal failure on maintenance dialysis.

Desferrioxamine is administered as the mesilate and may be given by subcutaneous or intravenous infusion, by intramuscular injection, or intraperitoneally. It may also be given orally in acute iron poisoning.

In the treatment of **chronic iron overload** the dosage and route of administration should be determined for each patient by monitoring urinary iron excretion, with the aim of normalising serum-ferritin concentrations. Continuous subcutaneous infusions, preferably with the aid of a small portable infusion pump, are particularly convenient for ambulant patients and are more effective than intramuscular injections. Continuous intravenous infusion has been recommended for patients incapable of continuing subcutaneous infusions or for those with cardiac problems secondary to iron overload. An initial daily dose of desferrioxamine mesilate 0.5 g may be given by subcutaneous infusion or intravenous infusion, increasing until a plateau of iron excretion is reached. The usual effective dose range is 20 to 60 mg per kg body-weight daily. Subcutaneous infusions are administered 4 to 7 times a week depending on the degree of iron overload and are given over 8 to 12 hours, or over 24 hours in some patients. When given by intramuscular injection the initial dose has been 0.5 to 1 g daily as 1 or 2 injections, but again the maintenance dose is determined by response. It has been suggested that in addition to intramuscular treatment, up to 2 g of desferrioxamine mesilate should be given by intravenous infusion for each unit of blood transfused, at a rate not more than 15 mg per kg body-weight per hour at the time of each blood transfusion. Desferrioxamine should be administered separately from the blood. The co-administration of ascorbic acid supplements can enhance the excretion of iron, but, to reduce the risk of toxicity, should not be started until 1 month after starting desferrioxamine treatment (see under Interactions, above). Ascorbic acid is given in doses of 200 mg daily for adults or 100 mg daily for infants; it should be administered separately from food since it also enhances iron absorption.

Desferrioxamine has been used as a *diagnostic test* for iron storage disease in patients with normal renal function by injecting 0.5 g of the mesilate intramuscularly and estimating the excretion of iron in the urine collected over the next 6 hours; an excretion of more than 1 mg of iron by the patient under test is suggestive of iron storage disease and more than 1.5 mg can be regarded as pathological.

In the treatment of **acute iron poisoning** the following doses and routes are suggested. In the UK, desferrioxamine mesilate 5 to 10 g in 50 to 100 mL of water may be given by mouth, or by stomach tube, to chelate any iron left in the stomach and prevent further absorption following gastric lavage. To eliminate iron already absorbed, desferrioxamine mesilate should be given intramuscularly or, if the patient is hypotensive or in shock, intravenously by slow infusion. The dose and route of parenteral administration should be adjusted according to the severity of the poisoning, preferably as indicated by the serum-iron concentration and total iron binding capacity, if available, although chelation therapy should be started in patients with significant symptoms without waiting for the results of blood concentrations. In the UK, the usual dose of desferrioxamine mesilate is 2 g in adults or 1 g in children by intramuscular injection. Alternatively, it may be given by slow intravenous infusion of up to 15 mg per kg body-weight per hour, reducing after 4 to 6 hours to provide a total dose not exceeding 80 mg per kg in 24 hours, although larger doses may be tolerated. In the USA, a recommended procedure is to give desferrioxamine mesilate 1 g initially by intramuscular injection followed by 0.5 g every 4 hours for 2 doses. Subsequent doses of 0.5 g may be administered every 4 to 12 hours to a maximum of 6 g in 24 hours. Alternatively, the same doses may be given by slow intravenous infusion at a rate of not more than 15 mg per kg per hour, but this route of administration is only recommended for patients in a state of cardiovascular collapse.

In the treatment of **aluminium overload** in patients with end-stage renal failure, those undergoing maintenance haemodialysis or haemofiltration may be given desferrioxamine mesilate 5 mg per kg once a week by slow intravenous infusion during the last hour of a dialysis. In patients on peritoneal dialysis (CAPD or CCPD) desferrioxamine mesilate 5 mg per kg may be given once a week, by slow intravenous infusion, subcutaneously, intramuscularly, or intraperitoneally (the recommended route) before the final exchange of the day. For the *diagnosis* of aluminium overload desferrioxamine mesilate 5 mg per kg is administered by slow intravenous infusion during the last hour of haemodialysis. An increase in serum-aluminium concentration above baseline of more than 150 nanograms per mL (measured at the start of the next dialysis session) suggests aluminium overload.

Eye drops containing desferrioxamine mesilate 10% have been administered for the treatment of ocular siderosis and corneal rust stains.

Administration. Attempts have been made to overcome compliance problems encountered with standard parenteral administration of desferrioxamine by developing oral,[1-3] rectal,[4] or intranasal[5] regimens. Although most regimens produced an increase in urinary iron excretion above baseline, the amount excreted was generally considered to be insufficient to be clinically useful, particularly in young children with low iron stores.[3] However, these alternate routes of administration could be useful as an adjunct in selected patients.[1,5]

Greater success has been reported with daily intravenous infusion of desferrioxamine 6 to 12 g over 12 hours[6] or intermittent intravenous infusions in addition to subcutaneous administration[7] in patients poorly compliant with conventional subcutaneous therapy. No major disturbances in vision or hearing were encountered in 8 patients undergoing intensive intravenous treatment for up to 24 months,[6] and established iron-induced heart disease in 2 of these patients improved during therapy. Administration by twice-daily subcutaneous bolus injection has also been reported.[8]

Intraperitoneal administration of desferrioxamine may be used to reduce aluminium levels in patients receiving peritoneal dialysis for chronic renal failure. Good results have also been reported[9] in a patient with haemochromatosis complicated by cirrhosis and cardiomyopathy, in whom a chronic peritoneal dialysis catheter was used to control ascites and to administer desferrioxamine.

1. Callender ST, Weatherall DJ. Iron chelation with oral desferrioxamine. *Lancet* 1980; **ii:** 689.
2. Jacobs A, Chang Ting W. Iron chelation with oral desferrioxamine. *Lancet* 1980; **ii:** 794.
3. Kattamis C, *et al.* Oral desferrioxamine in young patients with thalassaemia. *Lancet* 1981; **i:** 51.
4. Kontoghiorghes G, *et al.* Desferrioxamine suppositories. *Lancet* 1983; **ii:** 454.
5. Gordon GS, *et al.* Intranasal administration of deferoxamine to iron overloaded patients. *Am J Med Sci* 1989; **297:** 280–4.
6. Cohen AR, *et al.* Rapid removal of excessive iron with daily, high-dose intravenous chelation therapy. *J Pediatr* 1989; **115:** 151–5.
7. Sabatino D. Rapid removal of excessive iron in thalassemia by high-dose intravenous chelation therapy. *J Pediatr* 1990; **116:** 157–8.
8. Borgna-Pignatti C, Cohen A. Evaluation of a new method of administration of the iron chelating agent deferoxamine. *J Pediatr* 1997; **130:** 86–8.
9. Swartz RD, Legault DJ. Long-term intraperitoneal deferoxamine for hemochromatosis. *Am J Med* 1996; **100:** 308–12.

Aluminium overload. Aluminium has been implicated in a number of disorders[1] including renal osteodystrophy, dialysis dementia, and Alzheimer's disease (p.1412). Patients with chronic renal failure may be exposed to aluminium from the use of aluminium-containing phosphate binders and from the high concentrations of aluminium sometimes found in tap water used to prepare dialysis fluids. Sources of aluminium in other patients include aluminium-containing antacids, preparations for total parenteral nutrition, contaminated albumin solutions, and environmental and industrial sources.[1] Further references to aluminium toxicity are included under Aluminium (see p.1577).

In patients with chronic renal failure the major sources of aluminium can be substantially reduced by the use of alternative phosphate binders (see Renal Osteodystrophy, p.746) and by reduction in the aluminium concentration of dialysis fluids by reverse osmosis and deionisation.[1] Desferrioxamine may also be used (but see under Precautions, above, for a discussion of aluminium toxicity being exacerbated by desferrioxamine).

Desferrioxamine can greatly increase the removal of aluminium by adsorbent haemoperfusion or haemodialysis.[2] In the treatment of dialysis encephalopathy, desferrioxamine has been reported to have beneficial effects by mobilising and removing aluminium when administered in doses of up to 6 g once a week via the arterial line during the first 2 hours of haemodialysis.[3,4] In a study of 11 patients with dialysis encephalopathy 5 treated with deionised or reverse-osmosis water alone and all died. The other 6 were treated similarly but were also given desferrioxamine 6 to 10 g intravenously each week at dialysis; 4 of these patients improved but 2 died of progressive dementia.[5]

Although the total amount of aluminium removed with desferrioxamine treatment during peritoneal dialysis may be small compared with the amounts removed during haemodialysis, substantial improvement in early aluminium encephalopathy has been achieved in a patient on continuous ambulatory peritoneal dialysis by using intraperitoneal desferrioxamine.[6] In a study of 27 patients undergoing haemodialysis but without clinical encephalopathy impaired cerebral function associated with only mildly elevated plasma-aluminium concentrations was noted.[7] Administration of desferrioxamine to 15 of these patients for 3 months improved psychomotor performance.

Desferrioxamine has produced rapid clinical improvement in patients with dialysis-related bone disease.[8-10] Reduction in the aluminium content of bone was reported in two studies involving 7 patients,[10] and 9 patients,[9] respectively. However, such findings were not replicated in a further 2 patients.[8] Measurement of plasma-aluminium concentrations 24 and 44 hours after administration of desferrioxamine 40 mg per kg body-weight has been used to diagnose aluminium-related osteodystrophy[9,11] but a study,[10] using a lower dose of desferrioxamine (28.5 mg per kg) and measuring plasma aluminium 5 hours later, found similar increases in patients both with and without bone-aluminium accumulation.

Desferrioxamine therapy has also produced beneficial results in dialysis patients with anaemia[12-14] and has also been found to reverse aluminium-induced resistance to erythropoietin.[15,16]

Prurigo nodularis in chronic aluminium overload has responded to desferrioxamine with resolution of itch and skin lesions.[17]

Sustained low doses of desferrioxamine were found to slow the progression of the dementia of Alzheimer's disease in a study

of 48 patients[18] although these results have been questioned.[19,20]

1. Monteagudo FSE, *et al.* Recent developments in aluminium toxicology. *Med Toxicol* 1989; **4:** 1–16.
2. Chang TMS, Barre P. Effect of desferrioxamine on removal of aluminium and iron by coated charcoal haemoperfusion and haemodialysis. *Lancet* 1983; **ii:** 1051–3.
3. Ackrill P, *et al.* Successful removal of aluminium from patient with dialysis encephalopathy. *Lancet* 1980; **ii:** 692–3.
4. Arze RS, *et al.* Reversal of aluminium dialysis encephalopathy after desferrioxamine treatment. *Lancet* 1981; **ii:** 1116.
5. Milne FJ, *et al.* Low aluminium water, desferrioxamine, and dialysis encephalopathy. *Lancet* 1982; **ii:** 502.
6. Payton CD, *et al.* Successful treatment of aluminium encephalopathy by intraperitoneal desferrioxamine. *Lancet* 1984; **i:** 1132–3.
7. Altmann P, *et al.* Disturbance of cerebral function by aluminium in haemodialysis patients without overt aluminium toxicity. *Lancet* 1989; **ii:** 7–12.
8. Brown DJ, *et al.* Treatment of dialysis osteomalacia with desferrioxamine. *Lancet* 1982; **ii:** 343–5.
9. McCarthy JT, *et al.* Clinical experience with desferrioxamine in dialysis patients with aluminium toxicity. *Q J Med* 1990; **74:** 257–76.
10. Malluche HH, *et al.* The use of deferoxamine in the management of aluminium accumulation in bone in patients with renal failure. *N Engl J Med* 1984; **311:** 140–4.
11. Milliner DS, *et al.* Use of desferrioxamine infusion test in the diagnosis of aluminium-related osteodystrophy. *Ann Intern Med* 1984; **101:** 775–80.
12. de la Serna F-J, *et al.* Improvement in the erythropoiesis of chronic haemodialysis patients with desferrioxamine. *Lancet* 1988; **i:** 1009–11.
13. Altmann P, *et al.* Aluminium chelation therapy in dialysis patients: evidence for inhibition of haemoglobin synthesis by low levels of aluminium. *Lancet* 1988; **i:** 1012–15.
14. Padovese P, *et al.* Desferrioxamine versus erythropoietin for treatment of dialysis anaemia. *Lancet* 1990; **335:** 1465.
15. Rosenlöf K, *et al.* Erythropoietin, aluminium, and anaemia in patients on haemodialysis. *Lancet* 1990; **335:** 247–9.
16. Zachée P, *et al.* Erythropoietin, aluminium, and anaemia in patients on haemodialysis. *Lancet* 1990; **335:** 1038–9.
17. Brown MA, *et al.* Prurigo nodularis and aluminium overload in maintenance haemodialysis. *Lancet* 1992; **340:** 48.
18. McLachlan DRC, *et al.* Intramuscular desferrioxamine in patients with Alzheimer's disease. *Lancet* 1991; **337:** 1304–8. Correction. *ibid.*: 1618.
19. Davies P. Desferrioxamine for Alzheimer's disease. *Lancet* 1991; **338:** 325.
20. Holleman DR, Goldstone JR. Desferrioxamine for Alzheimer's disease. *Lancet* 1991; **338:** 325.

Iron overload. Chronic iron overload can be caused by inappropriately increased gastrointestinal absorption, by grossly excessive oral intake over long periods, or by parenteral administration of iron, for example from transfused blood.[1] Excess iron is stored in the form of ferritin and haemosiderin. The term *haemosiderosis* is applied to the accumulation of haemosiderin in body tissues without associated tissue damage; *haemochromatosis* refers to a chronic disease state in which iron overload leads to tissue damage, predominantly in the heart, liver, and pancreas.[1-3] Primary or hereditary haemochromatosis is caused by a genetic defect in iron metabolism which results in excessive gastrointestinal absorption of iron. The treatment of choice for primary haemochromatosis is phlebotomy,[1-4] but chelation therapy may be needed in patients with anaemia, hypoproteinaemia, or severe cardiac disease.[1,3] Secondary or acquired haemochromatosis is commonly associated with chronic anaemias, in particular thalassaemia, in which excessive iron uptake due to disordered erythropoiesis and excess iron from repeated blood transfusions contribute to iron overload. In these patients the usual therapy is iron chelation with desferrioxamine (see below).

1. Halliday JW, Basset ML. Treatment of iron storage disorders. *Drugs* 1980; **20:** 2077–15.
2. Crawford DHG, Halliday JW. Current concepts in rational therapy for haemochromatosis. *Drugs* 1991; **41:** 875–82.
3. Kirking MH. Treatment of chronic iron overload. *Clin Pharm* 1991; **10:** 775–83.
4. Barton JC, *et al.* Management of hemochromatosis. *Ann Intern Med* 1998; **129:** 932–9.

THALASSAEMIA. Patients homozygous for β-thalassaemia (p.718) have severe anaemia requiring regular blood transfusions. As a consequence of this treatment iron overload develops and the excessive deposition of iron in the myocardium usually results in these patients dying in their second or third decade from arrhythmias or cardiac failure. Desferrioxamine is used to retard the accumulation of iron, the greatest increase in iron excretion being seen in patients given the drug by continuous subcutaneous infusion than intramuscular bolus. Better iron excretion may be achieved if patients are given ascorbic acid 100 to 200 mg daily in addition to desferrioxamine (but see Interactions, above).

Desferrioxamine has been shown to improve survival in thalassaemic children given regular systemic therapy,[1-3] and there has also been some evidence that impaired organ function might improve with intensive desferrioxamine therapy. A reduction in liver-iron concentrations and an improvement in liver function was reported in some patients with transfusional iron overload treated with desferrioxamine 2 to 4 g by slow subcutaneous infusion over 12 hours on 6 nights a week,[4] although in another study[5] improvement in the degree of hepatic fibrosis was observed in only 2 of 7 patients given desferrioxamine up to 85 mg per kg body-weight daily by subcutaneous injection after 3 to 5 years, despite reductions in iron concentrations. Beginning chelation therapy before puberty could help to ensure normal sexual development in patients with thalassaemia major.[6] Studies indicating that desferrioxamine treatment might preserve or possibly improve cardiac function impaired by iron overload in thalassaemic patients[7-9] have been supported by a decrease in mortality from cardiac disease since the introduction of desferrioxamine in Italy,[1] although this continues to be the main cause of death in patients with thalassaemia.[1,2] A further study[3] in patients with β-thalassaemia demonstrated a markedly improved prognosis for survival without cardiac disease in patients who began chelation therapy with desferrioxamine before iron loading was severe and in whom reduced serum-ferritin concentrations were maintained over a long period. Failure to prevent the accumulation of excess iron or to remove large stores of iron was associated with a poor prognosis at any age. Thus, it is considered advisable to begin chelation therapy as early as possible (in practice usually at 2 to 3 years of age when iron overload becomes significant) to try to prevent organ damage developing.

1. Zurlo MG, et al. Survival and causes of death in thalassaemia major. Lancet 1989; ii: 27–30.
2. Ehlers KH, et al. Prolonged survival in patients with beta-thalassemia major treated with deferoxamine. J Pediatr 1991; 118: 540–5.
3. Olivieri NF, et al. Survival in medically treated patients with homozygous β-thalassemia. N Engl J Med 1994; 331: 574–8.
4. Hoffbrand AV, et al. Improvement in status and liver function in patients with transfusional iron overload with long-term subcutaneous desferrioxamine. Lancet 1979; i: 947–9.
5. Maurer HS, et al. A prospective evaluation of iron chelation therapy in children with severe β-thalassemia: a six-year study. Am J Dis Child 1988; 142: 287–92.
6. Bronspiegel-Weintrob N, et al. Effect of age at the start of iron chelation therapy on gonadal function in β-thalassemia major. N Engl J Med 1990; 323: 713–19.
7. Freeman AP, et al. Early left ventricular dysfunction and chelation therapy in thalassemia major. Ann Intern Med 1983; 99: 450–4.
8. Marcus RE, et al. Desferrioxamine to improve cardiac function in iron-overloaded patients with thalassaemia major. Lancet 1984; i: 392–3.
9. Wolfe L, et al. Prevention of cardiac disease by subcutaneous deferoxamine in patients with thalassemia major. N Engl J Med 1985; 312: 1600–3.

Iron poisoning. Despite the frequency of acute poisoning with iron preparations, no universally accepted treatment protocol exists. It is often difficult to determine the amount of iron ingested, and assessment of clinical symptoms can be misleading since patients may exhibit mild symptoms despite having ingested potentially toxic quantities of iron. Measurement of the serum-iron concentration and the total iron-binding capacity (TIBC) is useful in assessing the severity of poisoning but may not be immediately available and may be misleading. The desferrioxamine challenge test entails giving desferrioxamine 50 mg per kg body-weight (to a maximum dose of 1 g) intramuscularly; if free iron is present, ferrioxamine will be excreted in the urine imparting a classic 'vin rosé' colour. However, the results can be difficult to interpret and a negative result does not rule out iron toxicity.

The initial stage of treatment entails removal of unabsorbed iron from the gastrointestinal tract by gastric lavage, with whole-bowel irrigation as a treatment option in patients suspected of ingesting modified-release preparations or those with radiographic evidence of unabsorbed tablets remaining after gastric lavage. The addition of desferrioxamine to the lavage fluid is controversial since there is little evidence of its efficacy and concern over possible toxic effects of ferrioxamine. Supportive care should be given as appropriate and may be all that is required in mild poisoning. Activated charcoal is not effective in iron poisoning.

Chelation therapy with desferrioxamine given intramuscularly or intravenously is indicated in patients with impaired consciousness, shock or hypotension; in those with other symptoms of severe poisoning, for example leucocytosis; in those in whom the serum-iron concentration exceeds the TIBC; in those with a positive desferrioxamine challenge test; and those with a serum-iron concentration above 350 μg per 100 mL if TIBC estimations are unavailable. In severe toxicity intravenous desferrioxamine is given immediately without waiting for the results of serum-iron measurements. There is no general agreement on the duration of chelation therapy; among the suggested end-points are the disappearance of the vin rosé coloration of the urine, 24 hours after the disappearance of coloration, and reduction of serum-iron concentrations to less than 100 μg per 100 mL.

General references.
1. Proudfoot AT, et al. Management of acute iron poisoning. Med Toxicol 1986; 1: 83–100.
2. Engle JP, et al. Acute iron intoxication: treatment controversies. Drug Intell Clin Pharm 1987; 21: 153–9.
3. Mann KV, et al. Management of acute iron overdose. Clin Pharm 1989; 8: 428–40.

Malaria. Following the suggestion that iron-deficiency anaemia may offer some protection against infections (see Infections in the Precautions for Iron, p.1367), desferrioxamine was tried in a few patients with malaria.[1,2] Any antimalarial effect of desferrioxamine was thought to be as a result of chelation of parasite-associated iron rather than reduction in body-iron concentrations in the patient. Desferrioxamine given intravenously was reported[3] to shorten the time to regain consciousness in children with cerebral malaria receiving standard therapy with intravenous quinine and oral pyrimethamine-sulfadoxine. However, in a more recent study[4] there was no evidence of a beneficial effect on mortality when desferrioxamine was added to an antimalarial treatment regimen that included a loading dose of quinine.

1. Gordeuk VR, et al. Iron chelation as a chemotherapeutic strategy for falciparum malaria. Am J Trop Med Hyg 1993; 48: 193–7.
2. Thompson DF. Deferoxamine treatment of malaria. Ann Pharmacother 1994; 28: 602–3.
3. Gordeuk V, et al. Effect of iron chelation therapy on recovery from deep coma, in children with cerebral malaria. N Engl J Med 1992; 327: 1473–7.
4. Thuma PE, et al. Effect of iron chelation therapy on mortality in Zambian children with cerebral malaria. Trans R Soc Trop Med Hyg 1998; 92: 214–18.

Porphyria. The management of various forms of porphyria is discussed on p.1011. Desferrioxamine may be used to reduce serum-iron concentrations in porphyria cutanea tarda if phlebotomy is contra-indicated. In a study of 25 patients with porphyria cutanea tarda,[1] subcutaneous infusion of desferrioxamine was found to be as effective as repeated phlebotomies in normalising porphyrin excretion and iron storage. Desferrioxamine was also used successfully to treat haemodialysis-related porphyria cutanea tarda in a 22-year-old man in whom venesection therapy was contra-indicated because of severe anaemia requiring multiple blood transfusion.[2] Each course of intravenous desferrioxamine therapy after the end of 3 haemodialysis sessions was accompanied by a marked decrease in plasma porphyrins, a sharp increase in haematocrit values, and a simultaneous improvement in skin lesions.

1. Rocchi E, et al. Iron removal therapy in porphyria cutanea tarda: phlebotomy versus slow subcutaneous desferrioxamine infusion. Br J Dermatol 1986; 114: 621–9.
2. Praga M, et al. Treatment of hemodialysis-related porphyria cutanea tarda with deferoxamine. N Engl J Med 1987; 316: 547–8.

Preparations

BP 2001: Desferrioxamine Injection;
USP 25: Deferoxamine Mesylate for Injection.

Proprietary Preparations (details are given in Part 3)
Aust.: Desferal; **Austral.:** Desferal; **Belg.:** Desferal; **Braz.:** Desferal; **Canad.:** Desferal; **Denm.:** Desferal; **Fin.:** Desferal; **Fr.:** Desferal; **Ger.:** Desferal; **Hong Kong:** Desferal; **Irl.:** Desferal; **Israel:** Desferal; **Ital.:** Desferal; **Neth.:** Desferal; **Norw.:** Desferal; **NZ:** Desferal; **Port.:** Desferal; **S.Afr.:** Desferal; **Singapore:** Desferal; **Spain:** Desferin; **Swed.:** Desferal; **Switz.:** Desferal; **Thai.:** Desferal; **UK:** Desferal; **USA:** Desferal.

Dexrazoxane (19333-p)

Dexrazoxane (BAN, USAN, rINN).
ADR-529; ICRF-187; NSC-169780. (+)-(S)-4,4′-Propylenebis(piperazine-2,6-dione).
$C_{11}H_{16}N_4O_4 = 268.3$.
CAS — 24584-09-6.
ATC — V03AF02.

Adverse Effects and Precautions

Dexrazoxane may add to the bone-marrow depression caused by antineoplastics given concurrently and frequent complete blood counts are recommended during therapy. Although dexrazoxane protects against the cardiotoxic effects of anthracyclines cardiac function should continue to be monitored when dexrazoxane is used. Pain on injection has been reported.

It has been recommended that dexrazoxane should only be given to patients who have received a cumulative dose of doxorubicin of 300 mg per m² body-surface and who require continued administration, since there is some evidence that dexrazoxane may reduce the efficacy of the antineoplastic regimen.

◊ Severe cutaneous and subcutaneous necrosis has been reported[1] in a patient who received dexrazoxane by infusion into a peripheral forearm vein, followed by intravenous injection of doxorubicin at a different site in the same arm. Local pain occurred during the dexrazoxane infusion but there was no evidence of extravasation.

1. Lossos IS, Ben-Yehuda D. Cutaneous and subcutaneous necrosis following dexrazoxane-CHOP therapy. Ann Pharmacother 1999; 33: 253–4.

Pharmacokinetics

Dexrazoxane is mainly excreted in the urine as unchanged drug and metabolites. The elimination half-life is reported to be about 2 hours.

Uses and Administration

Dexrazoxane is the (+)-enantiomorph of the antineoplastic drug razoxane (p.567) and is a cytoprotective agent that is used to reduce the cardiotoxicity of doxorubicin and other anthracyclines (see Effects on the Heart, p.535). It is hydrolysed to an active metabolite that is similar to edetic acid. This chelates iron within the cells and appears to prevent the formation of the anthracycline-iron complex that is thought to be responsible for cardiotoxicity.

Dexrazoxane is used to reduce the incidence and severity of cardiomyopathy associated with doxorubicin in women with metastatic breast cancer who have received cumulative doses of doxorubicin of 300 mg per m² body-surface and who require continued administration. It is administered as the hydrochloride, by slow intravenous injection or rapid intravenous infusion, starting within 30 minutes before doxorubicin administration. The dose is expressed as the base, calculated on a 10:1 ratio with doxorubicin; typically, 500 mg per m² of dexrazoxane is given for every 50 mg per m² of doxorubicin.

Dexrazoxane is also being investigated for use with doxorubicin in various other malignancies.

◊ References.
1. Wiseman LR, Spencer CM. Dexrazoxane: a review of its use as a cardioprotective agent in patients receiving anthracycline-based chemotherapy. Drugs 1998; 56: 385–403.
2. Links M, Lewis C. Chemoprotectants: a review of their clinical pharmacology and therapeutic efficacy. Drugs 1999; 57: 293–308.

Preparations

Proprietary Preparations (details are given in Part 3)
Canad.: Zinecard; **Denm.:** Cardioxane; **Fr.:** Cardioxane; **Israel:** Cardioxane; **Ital.:** Cardioxane; Eucardion†; **USA:** Zinecard.

Dicobalt Edetate (1033-p)

Dicobalt Edetate (BAN, rINN).

Cobalt Edetate; Cobalt EDTA; Cobalt Tetracemate. Cobalt [ethylenediaminetetra-acetato(4—)-N,N′,O,O′]cobalt(II).
$C_{10}H_{12}Co_2N_2O_8 = 406.1$.
CAS — 36499-65-7.

Adverse Effects and Precautions

Dicobalt edetate may cause hypotension, tachycardia, and vomiting. Anaphylactic reactions have occurred; oedema of the face and neck, sweating, chest pain, cardiac irregularities, and skin rashes have been reported.

The adverse effects of dicobalt edetate are more severe in the absence of cyanide. Therefore, dicobalt edetate should not be given unless cyanide poisoning is definitely confirmed and poisoning is moderate or severe, that is, when consciousness is impaired.

Oedema. A patient with cyanide toxicity developed severe facial and pulmonary oedema after treatment with dicobalt edetate.[1] It has been suggested that when dicobalt edetate is used, facilities for intubation and resuscitation should be immediately available.

1. Dodds C, McKnight C. Cyanide toxicity after immersion and the hazards of dicobalt edetate. BMJ 1985; 291: 785–6.

Uses and Administration

Dicobalt edetate is a chelator used in the treatment of severe cyanide poisoning (p.1433). Its use arises from the property of cobalt salts to form a relatively non-toxic stable ion-complex with cyanide. Owing to its toxicity, dicobalt edetate should be used only in confirmed cyanide poisoning and never as a precautionary measure. Cyanide poisoning must be treated as quickly as possible. A suggested dose is 300 mg given by intravenous injection, over about 1 minute, repeated if the response is inadequate; a further dose of 300 mg of dicobalt edetate may be given 5 minutes later if required. For less severe poisoning the injection should be given over 5 minutes. Each injection of dicobalt edetate may be followed immediately by 50 mL of glucose 50% intravenously to reduce toxicity, though the value of giving glucose has been questioned.

Preparations

Proprietary Preparations (details are given in Part 3)
Austral.: Kelocyanor†; **Fr.:** Kelocyanor; **Irl.:** Kelocyanor; **S.Afr.:** Kelocyanor†; **UK:** Kelocyanor.

Digoxin-specific Antibody Fragments (19076-q)

Digoxin Immune Fab (Ovine); F(ab).

Adverse Effects and Precautions

Allergic reactions to digoxin-specific antibody fragments have been reported rarely. Patients known to be allergic to sheep protein and patients who have previously received digoxin-specific antibody fragments are likely to be at greater risk of developing an allergic reaction. Blood pressure, ECG, and potassium concentrations should be monitored closely during and after administration.

Uses and Administration

Digoxin-specific antibody fragments are derived from antibodies produced in sheep immunised to digoxin. Digoxin has greater affinity for the antibodies than for tissue-binding sites, and the digoxin-antibody complex is then rapidly excreted in the urine. Digoxin-specific antibody fragments are generally restricted to the treatment of life-threatening digoxin or digitoxin intoxication in which conventional treatment is ineffective. Successful treatment of lanatoside C poisoning has also been reported.

It is estimated that 38 mg of antibody fragments could bind about 0.5 mg of digoxin or digitoxin and the dose calculation is based on this estimate and the body-load of digoxin (based on the amount ingested or ideally from the steady-state plasma concentration). Administration is by intravenous infusion over a 30-minute period. If cardiac arrest is imminent the dose may be given as a bolus. In the case of incomplete reversal or recurrence of toxicity a further dose can be given. In patients considered to be at high risk of an allergic response an intradermal or skin scratch test may be performed.

◊ Clinical studies and reviews of the use of digoxin-specific antibody fragments have confirmed their effectiveness in the treatment of severe digitalis toxicity in the majority of patients.[1-4] An initial response is usually seen within 30 minutes of the end of the infusion with a maximum response after 3 to 4 hours.[3] The main causes of treatment failure or partial response are incorrect diagnosis of digitalis intoxication, inadequate dosage of antibody fragments, and administration to patients already moribund.[3,4] Few adverse reactions have been attributed to the administration of digoxin-specific antibody fragments; a few cases of minor allergic reactions have been reported including erythema, facial swelling, urticaria, and rashes,[2,3] but no anaphylactic reactions have been reported.[1-4] Haemodynamic status normally improves, but withdrawal of the inotropic support provided by digoxin may produce a decline in cardiac function in some patients. There may be dramatic reductions in plasma potassium concentrations.

Treatment has been successful in patients with varying degrees of renal impairment.[2,3,5] Elimination of the antibody-digoxin complex may be markedly delayed in severe renal impairment and prolonged monitoring may be required in such patients.[6] Measurement of free serum-digoxin concentrations may be useful.[7] Experience with digoxin-specific antibody fragments in a patient with chronic renal failure receiving haemodialysis has been reported.[8] The patient had a good clinical response but haemodialysis did not remove the antibody fragment-digoxin complex.

In patients with adequate renal function the half-life of the antibody fragment-digoxin complex has been reported to be about 16 to 20 hours[2] although longer half-lives have been reported.[9] It has been suggested[10] that the administration of digoxin-specific antibody fragments by infusion over 7 hours following an initial loading dose could be useful in ensuring adequate antibody concentrations are maintained to bind digoxin as it is released from tissue stores over a prolonged period.

Use of the antibody fragments has also been effective in children with severe digitalis intoxication.[11]

For reference to the use of digoxin-specific antibody fragments to treat poisoning due to common or yellow oleander, see Oleander, p.1643.

1. Smith TW, et al. Treatment of life-threatening digitalis intoxication with digoxin-specific Fab antibody fragments: experience in 26 cases. N Engl J Med 1982; 307: 1357–62.
2. Wenger TL, et al. Treatment of 63 severely digitalis-toxic patients with digoxin-specific antibody fragments. J Am Coll Cardiol 1985; 5: 118A–123A.
3. Stolshek BS, et al. The role of digoxin-specific antibodies in the treatment of digitalis poisoning. Med Toxicol 1988; 3: 167–71.
4. Antman EM, et al. Treatment of 150 cases of life-threatening digitalis intoxication with digoxin-specific Fab antibody fragments: final report of a multicenter study. Circulation 1990; 81: 1744–52.
5. Allen NM, et al. Clinical and pharmacokinetic profiles of digoxin immune Fab in four patients with renal impairment. DICP Ann Pharmacother 1991; 25: 1315–20.
6. Ujhelyi MR, et al. Disposition of digoxin immune Fab in patients with kidney failure. Clin Pharmacol Ther 1993; 54: 388–94.
7. Ujhelyi MR, Robert S. Pharmacokinetic aspects of digoxin-specific Fab therapy in the management of digitalis toxicity. Clin Pharmacokinet 1995; 28: 483–93.
8. Clifton GD, et al. Free and total serum digoxin concentrations in a renal failure patient after treatment with digoxin immune Fab. Clin Pharm 1989; 8: 441–5.
9. Gibb I, Parnham A. A star treatment for digoxin overdose? BMJ 1986; 293: 1171–2.
10. Schaumann W, et al. Kinetics of the Fab fragments of digoxin antibodies and of bound digoxin in patients with severe digoxin intoxication. Eur J Clin Pharmacol 1986; 30: 527–33.
11. Woolf AD, et al. The use of digoxin-specific Fab fragments for severe digitalis intoxication in children. N Engl J Med 1992; 326: 1739–44.

The symbol † denotes a preparation no longer actively marketed

Preparations

Proprietary Preparations (details are given in Part 3)
Aust.: Digitalis Antidot; *Austral.:* Digibind; *Belg.:* Digitalis Antidot; *Canad.:* Digibind; *Ger.:* Digitalis Antidote; *Singapore:* Digitalis Antidote; *Swed.:* Digitalis Antidot; *Switz.:* Antidote Anti-Digitale BM; *UK:* Digibind; *USA:* Digibind.

Dimercaprol (1036-e)

Dimercaprol (BAN, rINN).
BAL; British Anti-Lewisite; Dimercaprolum. 2,3-Dimercaptopropan-1-ol.
$C_3H_8OS_2 = 124.2$.
CAS — 59-52-9.
ATC — V03AB09.
Pharmacopoeias. In Chin., Eur. (see p.vi), Int., Jpn, and US.

Pharmacopoeial description
Ph. Eur.: A clear colourless or slightly yellow liquid. Soluble in water and in arachis oil; miscible with alcohol and with benzyl benzoate. Store at 2° to 8° in well-filled airtight containers. Protect from light.
USP 25: A colourless or practically colourless liquid, having a disagreeable, mercaptan-like odour. Soluble 1 in 20 of water; soluble in alcohol, in benzyl benzoate, and in methyl alcohol. Store at a temperature not exceeding 8° in airtight containers. Protect from light.

Adverse Effects and Treatment

The most consistent side-effects produced by dimercaprol are hypertension and tachycardia. Other side-effects include nausea, vomiting, headache, burning sensation of the lips, mouth, throat, and eyes, lachrymation and salivation, tingling of the extremities, a sensation of constriction in the throat and chest, muscle pains and muscle spasm, rhinorrhoea, conjunctivitis, sweating, restlessness, and abdominal pain. Transient reductions in the leucocyte count have also been reported. Pain may occur at the injection site and sterile abscesses occasionally develop. In children, fever commonly occurs and persists during therapy.

Side-effects are dose-related, relatively frequent, and usually reversible. It has been suggested that oral administration of ephedrine sulfate 30 to 60 mg thirty minutes before each injection of dimercaprol may reduce side-effects; antihistamines may alleviate some of the symptoms.

Precautions

Dimercaprol should be used with care in patients with hypertension or renal impairment. It should be discontinued, or continued with extreme caution, if acute renal insufficiency develops during therapy. Alkalinisation of the urine may protect the kidney during therapy by stabilising the dimercaprol-metal complex. Dimercaprol should not be used in patients with hepatic impairment unless due to arsenic poisoning. It should not be used in the treatment of poisoning due to cadmium, iron, or selenium as the dimercaprol-metal complexes formed are more toxic than the metals themselves.

Glucose-6-phosphate dehydrogenase deficiency. A report[1] of haemolysis during chelation therapy with dimercaprol and sodium calcium edetate for high blood-lead concentrations in 2 children with a deficiency of glucose-6-phosphate dehydrogenase.

1. Janakiraman N, et al. Hemolysis during BAL chelation therapy for high blood lead levels in two G6PD deficient children. Clin Pediatr (Phila) 1978; 17: 485–7.

Interactions

Iron supplements should not be given during dimercaprol therapy as toxic dimercaprol-metal complexes are formed.

Pharmacokinetics

After intramuscular injection, maximum blood concentrations of dimercaprol may be attained within 30 to 60 minutes. Dimercaprol is rapidly metabolised and the metabolites and dimercaprol-metal chelates are excreted in the urine and bile. Elimination is essentially complete within 4 hours of a single dose.

Uses and Administration

Dimercaprol is a chelator used in the treatment of acute poisoning by arsenic (p.1582), gold (p.83), and

mercury (p.1634); its role in the treatment of poisoning by antimony, bismuth, and thallium is less well established. It is also used, in conjunction with sodium calcium edetate, in acute lead poisoning (p.1627).

The sulfhydryl groups on dimercaprol compete with endogenous sulfhydryl groups on proteins such as enzymes to combine with these metals; chelation by dimercaprol therefore prevents or reverses any inhibition of the sulfhydryl enzymes by the metal and the dimercaprol-metal complex formed is readily excreted by the kidney. Since the complex may dissociate, particularly at acid pH, or be oxidised, the aim of treatment is to provide an excess of dimercaprol in body fluids until the excretion of the metal is complete.

Dimercaprol should be administered by deep intramuscular injection and the injections should be given at different sites. Various dosage schedules are in use.

In the UK a recommended schedule for adults is to give doses of 400 to 800 mg on the first day of treatment, 200 to 400 mg on the second and third days, and 100 to 200 mg on the fourth and subsequent days, all administered in divided doses. Within these dose ranges, the individual dose is determined by body-weight, severity of symptoms, and the causative agent. Single doses should not generally exceed 3 mg per kg body-weight but single doses of up to 5 mg per kg may be required initially in patients with severe acute poisoning. The dose for children is based on body-weight using a similar dose per kg as for adults. A minimum interval of 4 hours between doses appears to reduce side-effects.

In the USA a recommended schedule for severe arsenical or gold poisoning is 3 mg per kg body-weight given at 4-hourly intervals throughout the first 2 days, 4 doses are given on the third day, and 2 doses on each of the next 10 days. In milder cases 2.5 mg per kg is given 4 times daily on each of the first 2 days, twice daily on the third day, and once daily on subsequent days for 10 days. For acute mercurial poisoning an initial injection of 5 mg per kg is followed by 2.5 mg per kg once or twice daily for 10 days.

Some authorities have suggested that doses of up to 5 mg per kg every 4 hours may be required during the first 1 or 2 days of treatment in severe poisoning with gold, mercury, or arsenic.

Dimercaprol is also used in conjunction with sodium calcium edetate (p.1022) in the treatment of lead poisoning. It can be of particular value in the treatment of acute lead encephalopathy and a suggested procedure is to administer an initial dose of dimercaprol 4 mg per kg alone followed at 4-hourly intervals by dimercaprol 3 to 4 mg per kg with concomitant doses of sodium calcium edetate administered at a separate site; treatment may be maintained for 2 to 7 days depending on the clinical response.

Preparations

BP 2001: Dimercaprol Injection;
USP 25: Dimercaprol Injection.

4-Dimethylaminophenol Hydrochloride

(12658-t)

Dimetamfenol Hydrochloride; 4-DMAP.
$C_8H_{11}NO,HCl = 173.6$.
CAS — 619-60-3 (4-dimethylaminophenol); 5882-48-4 (4-dimethylaminophenol hydrochloride).

Profile

4-Dimethylaminophenol hydrochloride is reported to oxidise haemoglobin to methaemoglobin and has been used in conjunction with sodium thiosulfate as an alternative to sodium nitrite (p.1023) in the treatment of cyanide poisoning. Doses of 3 to 4 mg per kg body-weight have been given intravenously.

◊ References.
1. Weger NP. Treatment of cyanide poisoning with 4-dimethylaminophenol (DMAP)–experimental and clinical overview. Fundam Appl Toxicol 1983; 3: 387–96.

Preparations

Proprietary Preparations (details are given in Part 3)
Ger.: 4-DMAP; *Neth.:* 4-DMAP.

Diprenorphine Hydrochloride (7302-z)

Diprenorphine Hydrochloride (BANM, rINNM).

M5050. (6R,7R,14S)-17-Cyclopropylmethyl-7,8-dihydro-7-(1-hydroxy-1-methylethyl)-6-O-methyl-6,14-ethano-17-normorphine hydrochloride; 2-[(−)-(5R,6R,7R,14S)-9a-Cyclopropylmethyl-4,5-epoxy-3-hydroxy-6-methoxy-6,14-ethanomorphinan-7-yl]propan-2-ol hydrochloride.

$C_{26}H_{35}NO_4,HCl = 462.0$.

CAS — 14357-78-9 (diprenorphine); 16808-86-9 (diprenorphine hydrochloride).

Pharmacopoeias. In BP(Vet).

Pharmacopoeial description

BP(Vet) 2001: A white or almost white crystalline powder. Sparingly soluble in water; slightly soluble in alcohol; very slightly soluble in chloroform; practically insoluble in ether. A 2% solution in water has a pH of 4.5 to 6.0. Protect from light.

Profile

Diprenorphine hydrochloride is an opioid antagonist used in veterinary medicine to reverse the effects of etorphine hydrochloride.

Disodium Edetate (1038-y)

Disodium Edetate (BAN).

Disodium Edathamil; Disodium EDTA; Disodium Tetracemate; Edetate Disodium; Natrii Edetas; Sodium Versenate. Disodium dihydrogen ethylenediaminetetra-acetate dihydrate .

$C_{10}H_{14}N_2Na_2O_8,2H_2O = 372.2$.

CAS — 139-33-3 (anhydrous disodium edetate); 6381-92-6 (disodium edetate dihydrate).

NOTE. The term sodium edetate has been used in the literature for various sodium salts of edetic acid.

Pharmacopoeias. In Eur. (see p.vi), Int., Jpn, Pol., and US.

Pharmacopoeial description

Ph. Eur.: A white, crystalline powder. Soluble in water; sparingly soluble in alcohol; practically insoluble in ether. A 5% solution in water has a pH of 4.0 to 5.5.

USP 25: A white crystalline powder. Soluble in water. pH of a 5% solution in water is between 4.0 and 6.0.

Trisodium Edetate (16285-z)

Edetate Trisodium (USAN). Trisodium hydrogen ethylenediaminetetra-acetate.

$C_{10}H_{13}N_2Na_3O_8 = 358.2$.
CAS — 150-38-9.

Adverse Effects and Precautions

Disodium and trisodium edetate have similar adverse effects and precautions to sodium calcium edetate (p.1022) and, when used as pharmaceutical excipients, to edetic acid (p.1008).

Hypocalcaemia can occur if disodium or trisodium edetate is administered by intravenous infusion too rapidly or in too concentrated a solution and tetany, convulsions, respiratory arrest, and cardiac arrhythmias may result. Plasma-electrolyte concentrations, particularly of ionised calcium, should be monitored.

In addition, edetates should be used with caution in patients with tuberculosis, impaired cardiac function, or a history of seizures, and are contra-indicated in renal insufficiency.

The rate of infusion should be decreased if signs of muscle reactivity occur. The infusion should be discontinued if tetany occurs and should only be restarted cautiously after plasma ionised and total calcium concentrations indicate a need for further treatment and tetany has stopped.

Interactions

Edetates chelate bivalent and trivalent metal ions and may affect the activity of agents such as zinc insulin that contain such ions.

◊ For reference to the inactivation of phenylmercuric salts by disodium edetate, see Phenylmercuric Nitrate, p.1154. For reports of edetates reducing the antimicrobial efficacy of thiomersal, see p.1158.

Uses and Administration

Disodium and trisodium edetate are chelators with a high affinity for calcium, with which they form a stable, soluble complex that is readily excreted by the kidneys. They have been administered intravenously

in the emergency treatment of hypercalcaemia (p.1181) and have been used to control digitalis-induced cardiac arrhythmias although less toxic agents are generally preferred (p.870). They are also used to treat calcium deposits in the eye.

Disodium and trisodium edetate also chelate other polyvalent metals but, unlike sodium calcium edetate, which is saturated with calcium, they are not used for the treatment of heavy metal poisoning since hypocalcaemia rapidly develops.

In the treatment of hypercalcaemia, injections containing varying amounts of disodium and trisodium edetate are used. In the UK, the trisodium salt is generally used. A dose of up to 70 mg per kg bodyweight daily has been suggested for adults; children may be given up to 60 mg per kg daily. It should be given by slow intravenous infusion over 2 to 3 hours and each gram of trisodium edetate should be diluted with 100 mL of glucose 5% or sodium chloride 0.9%. In the USA, disodium edetate is administered as a mixture of the disodium and trisodium salts. A dose of 50 mg per kg body-weight of disodium edetate in 24 hours by slow intravenous infusion has been suggested for adults with a maximum daily dose of 3 g. Children may be given 40 to 70 mg per kg in 24 hours. The injection should be diluted with 500 mL of sodium chloride 0.9% or glucose 5% for adults or a concentration not greater than 3% for children, and infused over 3 hours or more, preferably 4 to 6 hours. The dosage may be repeated for a further 4 days followed by a two-day interval before subsequent courses of treatment. If necessary, up to fifteen doses may be given in total.

Disodium and trisodium edetate are used in the treatment of calcium deposits from calcium oxide or calcium hydroxide burns of the eye and in the treatment of calcified corneal opacities, either by topical application after removing the appropriate area of corneal epithelium or by iontophoresis. Irrigation has also been suggested for zinc chloride injury to the eye, but treatment may be ineffective unless started within 2 minutes. In the UK a 0.4% solution of the trisodium salt is used for topical application to the eye; in the USA a 0.35 to 1.85% solution of a mixture of the disodium and trisodium salts has been suggested.

Disodium and trisodium edetate are also used in cleaners for contact lenses and as antioxidant synergists in cosmetic and pharmaceutical preparations.

Atherosclerosis. Calcium is thought to be necessary for several steps in atherogenesis and removal of calcium from atherosclerotic plaques using a chelator such as disodium edetate has been proposed.[1,2] However, there is little objective evidence of efficacy and reports of beneficial clinical responses are largely anecdotal or from small, short-term, or uncontrolled clinical studies,[2-4] and in view of the potential toxicity of such treatment it cannot be recommended;[1-3,5-7] there is a report of fatal renal failure in a patient who has undergone such therapy.[5]

1. Scott J. Chelation therapy—evolution or devolution of a nostrum? N Z Med J 1988; 101: 109–10.
2. Grier MT, Meyers DG. So much writing, so little science: a review of 37 years of literature on edetate sodium chelation therapy. Ann Pharmacother 1993; 27: 1504–9.
3. Rathmann KL, Golightly LK. Chelation therapy of atherosclerosis. Drug Intell Clin Pharm 1984; 18: 1000–3.
4. Elihu N, et al. Chelation therapy in cardiovascular disease: ethylenediaminetetraacetic acid, deferoxamine, and dexrazoxane. J Clin Pharmacol 1998; 38: 101–5.
5. Magee R. Chelation treatment of atherosclerosis. Med J Aust 1985; 142: 514–15.
6. Wirebaugh SR, Geraets DR. Apparent failure of edetic acid chelation therapy for the treatment of coronary atherosclerosis. DICP Ann Pharmacother 1990; 24: 22–5.
7. Anonymous. EDTA chelation therapy for atherosclerotic cardiovascular disease. Med Lett Drugs Ther 1994; 36: 48.

Preparations

BP 2001: Trisodium Edetate Intravenous Infusion;
USP 25: Edetate Disodium Injection.

Proprietary Preparations (details are given in Part 3)
Fr.: Chelatran; Tracemate†; Irl.: Limclair; UK: Limclair; USA: Disotate†; Endrate.

Multi-ingredient: Braz.: Flex-Care; Ger.: Complete†; Duracare†; Oxysept†; Israel: Cleaner No 4; Mex.: Adapettes; UK: Uriflex G; Uriflex R.

Edetic Acid (1039-j)

Edetic Acid (BAN, rINN).

Acidum Edeticum; Edathamil; EDTA; Tetracemic Acid. Ethylenediaminetetra-acetic acid.

$C_{10}H_{16}N_2O_8 = 292.2$.
CAS — 60-00-4.

Pharmacopoeias. In Eur. (see p.vi). Also in USNF.

Pharmacopoeial description

Ph. Eur.: A white, crystalline powder or colourless crystals. Practically insoluble in water and in alcohol. It dissolves in dilute solutions of alkali hydroxides.

USNF 20: A white crystalline powder. Very slightly soluble in water; soluble in solutions of alkali hydroxides.

Adverse Effects and Precautions

Edetic acid, used as a pharmaceutical excipient, is generally well tolerated. Adverse effects have been reported following inhalation of solutions containing edetic acid.

Asthma. Inhalation of an ipratropium nebuliser solution, that contained edetic acid as one of the preservatives, caused bronchoconstriction in 6 of 22 patients with asthma.[1] Inhalation of edetic acid alone produced dose-related bronchoconstriction which persisted for longer than 60 minutes.

1. Beasley CRW, et al. Bronchoconstrictor properties of preservatives in ipratropium bromide (Atrovent) nebuliser solution. BMJ 1987; 294: 1197–8.

Blood testing. Edetic acid may induce platelet clumping in some specimens collected for blood-cell counting leading to diagnostic errors. The recognition of pseudothrombocytopenia resulting from the use of edetic acid as the anticoagulant in blood samples and the use of alternative anticoagulants have been discussed.[1,2]

1. Lombarts AJPF, de Kieviet W. Recognition and prevention of pseudothrombocytopenia and concomitant pseudoleukocytosis. Am J Clin Pathol 1988; 89: 634–9.
2. Lippi U, et al. EDTA-induced platelet aggregation can be avoided by a new anticoagulant also suitable for automated complete blood count. Haematologica 1990; 75: 38–41.

Interactions

Edetic acid and its salts chelate polyvalent metal ions and may affect the activity of agents that contain such ions.

Disinfectants. Edetic acid has been reported to enhance the antimicrobial efficacy of some disinfectants such as chloroxylenol (p.1142). However, for a report of edetates reducing the antimicrobial efficacy of thiomersal, see p.1158.

Uses

Edetic acid and its salts are chelators used in pharmaceutical manufacturing and as anticoagulants for blood taken for haematological investigations. Edetates have many industrial applications as chelators; for their use in medicine see Disodium Edetate, p.1008, and Sodium Calcium Edetate, p.1022.

Gallstones. Edetic acid has been suggested as a possible solvent for non-cholesterol gallstones (p.1678).

Preparations

Proprietary Preparations (details are given in Part 3)
Multi-ingredient: Ital.: Conta-Lens Wetting; USA: Summers Eve Post-Menstrual; Triv; Zonite.

Flumazenil (13215-d)

Flumazenil (BAN, USAN, rINN).

Flumazenilum; Flumazepil; Ro-15-1788; Ro-15-1788/000. Ethyl 8-fluoro-5,6-dihydro-5-methyl-6-oxo-4H-imidazo[1,5-a][1,4]benzodiazepine-3-carboxylate.

$C_{15}H_{14}FN_3O_3 = 303.3$.
CAS — 78755-81-4.
ATC — V03AB25.

Pharmacopoeias. In Eur. (see p.vi).

Pharmacopoeial description

Ph. Eur.: A white or almost white crystalline powder. Very slightly soluble in water; freely soluble in dichloromethane; sparingly soluble in methyl alcohol.

Adverse Effects and Precautions

The adverse effects of flumazenil are generally due to the reversal of benzodiazepine effects and resemble benzodiazepine withdrawal symptoms (see p.675). Nausea, vomiting, dizziness, blurred vision, headache, and flushing may occur. Anxiety, fear, and agitation have been reported following too rapid reversal of sedation. There have been reports of seizures, especially in epileptics. Transient increases in blood pressure and heart rate have been observed. Patients who have received benzodiazepines for prolonged periods are particularly at risk of experiencing withdrawal symptoms and rapid injection of flumazenil should be avoided in such patients.

Because of its short duration of action, patients given flumazenil to reverse benzodiazepine-induced sedation should be kept under close observation; further doses of flumazenil may be necessary. Flumazenil is contra-indicated in patients who are receiving benzodiazepines to control potentially life-threatening conditions and should not be given to epileptic patients who have been receiving benzodiazepines for a prolonged period to control seizures.

In cases of mixed overdose, administration of flumazenil may unmask adverse effects of other psychotropic drugs. In particular, flumazenil should not be used in the presence of severe intoxication with tricyclic and related antidepressants.

Flumazenil should not be given to patients who have received neuromuscular blockers until the effects of neuromuscular blockade have fully cleared. Dosage should be adjusted individually. In high-risk or anxious patients, and after major surgery, it may be preferable to maintain some sedation during the early postoperative period. The risk of raising intracranial pressure in patients with head injuries needs to be borne in mind.

Careful titration of dosage is recommended in hepatic impairment.

◊ Cardiac arrhythmias,[1] sometimes preceded by tonic-clonic (grand mal) seizures[2,3] and occasionally fatal,[2] have been reported in several patients following the administration of flumazenil for mixed overdoses with benzodiazepines and other psychotropics. Heart block has also been reported[4] following flumazenil administration in a patient who had taken benzodiazepines, paracetamol, nifedipine, and atenolol. Death from refractory tonic-clonic seizures has been reported in a patient[5] following the use of flumazenil for a mixed overdose with a benzodiazepine and a tricyclic antidepressant.

Death from respiratory failure occurred in an 83-year-old woman following sedation with midazolam[6] despite flumazenil administration, although some[7] considered that this did not represent a failure by flumazenil to reverse the depressive effects on respiration of midazolam. Ventricular fibrillation followed by asystole and death has been reported in a patient given flumazenil during weaning from assisted ventilation (a period during which diazepam had been administered).[8]

1. Short TG, et al. Ventricular arrhythmia precipitated by flumazenil. BMJ 1988; 296: 1070–1.
2. Burr W, et al. Death after flumazenil. BMJ 1989; 298: 1713.
3. Marchant B, et al. Flumazenil causing convulsions and ventricular tachycardia. BMJ 1989; 299: 860.
4. Herd B, Clarke F. Complete heart block after flumazenil. Hum Exp Toxicol 1991; 10: 289.
5. Haverkos GP, et al. Fatal seizures after flumazenil administration in a patient with mixed overdose. Ann Pharmacother 1994; 28: 1347–9.
6. Lim AG. Death after flumazenil. BMJ 1989; 299: 858–9. Correction. ibid.: 1531.
7. Birch BRP, Miller RA. Death after flumazenil? BMJ 1990; 300: 467–8.
8. Katz Y, et al. Cardiac arrest associated with flumazenil. BMJ 1992; 304: 1415.

Effects on mental function. A severe acute psychotic disorder, which developed during treatment with flumazenil in a patient with hepatic encephalopathy, resolved when flumazenil was discontinued.[1]

1. Seebach J, Jost R. Flumazenil-induced psychotic disorder in hepatic encephalopathy. Lancet 1992; 339: 488–9.

Pharmacokinetics

Flumazenil is well absorbed from the gastrointestinal tract but undergoes extensive first-pass hepatic metabolism and has a systemic bioavailability of about 20%. It is about 50% bound to plasma proteins. Following intravenous administration it is extensively metabolised in the liver to the inactive carboxylic acid form, which is excreted predominantly in the urine. The elimination half-life is reported to be about 40 to 80 minutes. In patients with impaired hepatic function the clearance of flumazenil is decreased with a resultant prolongation of half-life.

◊ References.
1. Klotz U, et al. Pharmacokinetics of the selective benzodiazepine antagonist Ro 15-1788 in man. Eur J Clin Pharmacol 1984; 27: 115–17.
2. Roncari G, et al. Pharmacokinetics of the new benzodiazepine antagonist Ro 15-1788 in man following intravenous and oral administration. Br J Clin Pharmacol 1986; 22: 421–8.
3. Breimer LTM, et al. Pharmacokinetics and EEG effects of flumazenil in volunteers. Clin Pharmacokinet 1991; 20: 491–6.
4. Jones RDM, et al. Pharmacokinetics of flumazenil and midazolam. Br J Anaesth 1993; 70: 286–92.
5. Roncari G, et al. Flumazenil kinetics in the elderly. Eur J Clin Pharmacol 1993; 45: 585–7.

The symbol † denotes a preparation no longer actively marketed

Uses and Administration

Flumazenil is a benzodiazepine antagonist which acts competitively at CNS benzodiazepine receptors. It is used in anaesthesia and intensive care to reverse benzodiazepine-induced sedation; it may also be used to treat benzodiazepine overdosage (but see warnings in Precautions, above, and under Benzodiazepine Antagonism: Overdosage, below).

Flumazenil should be administered by slow intravenous injection or infusion.

The usual initial dose for the reversal of benzodiazepine-induced sedation is 200 μg given over 15 seconds, followed at intervals of 60 seconds by further doses of 100 to 200 μg if required, to a maximum total dose of 1 mg or occasionally 2 mg (usual range, 0.3 to 1 mg). If drowsiness recurs an intravenous infusion may be used, at a rate of 100 to 400 μg per hour, adjusted according to response. Alternatively, further doses of up to 1 mg, administered in boluses of 200 μg as above, may be given at 20-minute intervals to a maximum of 3 mg in one hour. Patients at risk from the effects of benzodiazepine reversal, such as those dependent on benzodiazepines, should receive smaller bolus injections of 100 μg.

The usual initial dose for the management of benzodiazepine overdose is 200 μg given intravenously over 30 seconds. A further dose of 300 μg can be given after another 30 seconds and can be followed by doses of 500 μg at one-minute intervals if required, to a total dose of 3 mg or occasionally 5 mg. The manufacturers consider that if a dose of up to 5 mg produces no response then further doses are unlikely to be effective. If symptoms of intoxication recur one or two doses of 500 μg may be given as above, with a one-minute interval between doses. This procedure may be repeated at 20-minute intervals to a maximum of 3 mg in one hour. As before a slower rate of administration may be used for 'at risk' patients.

If signs of overstimulation occur during the use of flumazenil, diazepam or midazolam may be given by slow intravenous injection.

◊ General references.
1. Brogden RN, Goa KL. Flumazenil: a reappraisal of its pharmacological properties and therapeutic efficacy as a benzodiazepine antagonist. Drugs 1991; 42: 1061–89.
2. Hoffman EJ, Warren EW. Flumazenil: a benzodiazepine antagonist. Clin Pharm 1993; 12: 641–56.
3. Krenzelok EP. Judicious use of flumazenil. Clin Pharm 1993; 12: 691–2.

Benzodiazepine antagonism. Flumazenil is a specific benzodiazepine antagonist which binds competitively with benzodiazepine receptors. Flumazenil reverses the centrally mediated effects of benzodiazepines. Its effects are evident within a few minutes of intravenous administration, even after substantial doses of benzodiazepines, and last for up to 3 hours depending on the dose and on the characteristics of the benzodiazepine intoxication. In patients who have received benzodiazepines for prolonged periods, flumazenil may precipitate withdrawal syndromes.

SEDATION. Flumazenil reduces postoperative sedation and amnesia following induction or maintenance of general anaesthesia with benzodiazepines; however, use in some patients has increased analgesic requirements, and some patients have experienced anxiety. Reversal of benzodiazepine sedation and amnesia may also be useful in some patients following minor surgery or diagnostic procedures. However, although flumazenil may antagonise the obvious effects of sedation, higher cognitive functions may still be impaired and the patient may be unfit to be discharged safely unaccompanied.[1] There is also a risk that sedation may recur if long-acting benzodiazepines have been used.[2-4] Patients who might benefit from sedation reversal include those at increased risk of postoperative complications, those in whom postoperative neurological evaluation would be beneficial, and those who are particularly sensitive to the effects of benzodiazepines.[2,3] Although experience with flumazenil in children is limited, it appears to be well tolerated and effective.[5] In an intensive care unit, flumazenil may assist in weaning sedated patients from mechanical ventilation and in extubation,[3,4,6,7] but multiple doses or an infusion may be required due to the short duration of action.[6]

OVERDOSAGE. Flumazenil may be used as an adjunct in the management of benzodiazepine overdose including overdose involving multiple agents. However, its use may unmask the effects of other intoxicants,[2-4,6-8] and since benzodiazepine overdose is rarely lethal and may even protect against the toxicity of other drugs, flumazenil should be used with great caution in mixed overdose, particularly when involving tricyclic antidepressants.[9] Repeated doses of flumazenil may be re-

quired to maintain consciousness depending on the benzodiazepine responsible and the magnitude of the overdose.

1. Sanders LD, et al. Reversal of benzodiazepine sedation with the antagonist flumazenil. Br J Anaesth 1991; 66: 445–53.
2. Anonymous. Flumazenil. Lancet 1988; ii: 828–30.
3. Klotz U, Kanto J. Pharmacokinetics and clinical use of flumazenil (Ro 15-1788). Clin Pharmacokinet 1988; 14: 1–12.
4. Karavokiros KAT, Tsipis GB. Flumazenil: a benzodiazepine antagonist. DICP Ann Pharmacother 1990; 24: 976–81.
5. Shannon M, et al. Safety and efficacy of flumazenil in the reversal of benzodiazepine-induced conscious sedation. J Pediatr 1997; 131: 582–6.
6. Amrein R, et al. Flumazenil in benzodiazepine antagonism: actions and clinical use in intoxications and anaesthesiology. Med Toxicol 1987; 2: 411–29.
7. Anonymous. Flumazenil—the first benzodiazepine antagonist. Drug Ther Bull 1989; 27: 39–40.
8. Weinbroum AA, et al. A risk-benefit assessment of flumazenil in the management of benzodiazepine overdose. Drug Safety 1997; 17: 181–96.
9. Hoffman RS, Goldfrank LR. The poisoned patient with altered consciousness: controversies in the use of a 'coma cocktail'. JAMA 1995; 274: 562–9.

Hepatic encephalopathy. Flumazenil has been tried in hepatic encephalopathy (p.1205) because of the suspected role of benzodiazepine-like agonists in the pathogenesis of the disorder. However, benefits have generally been modest, and its role remains to be determined.

References.
1. Grimm G, et al. Improvement of hepatic encephalopathy treated with flumazenil. Lancet 1988; ii: 1392–4.
2. Basile AS, et al. The pathogenesis and treatment of hepatic encephalopathy: evidence for the involvement of benzodiazepine receptor ligands. Pharmacol Rev 1991; 43: 27–71.
3. Pomier-Layrargues G, et al. Flumazenil in cirrhotic patients in hepatic coma: a randomized double-blind placebo-controlled crossover trial. Hepatology 1994; 19: 32–7.
4. Gyr K, et al. Evaluation of the efficacy and safety of flumazenil in the treatment of portal systemic encephalopathy: a double-blind, randomised, placebo controlled multicentre study. Gut 1996; 39: 319–24.
5. Barbaro G, et al. Flumazenil for hepatic encephalopathy grade III and IVa in patients with cirrhosis: an Italian multicenter double-blind, placebo-controlled, cross-over study. Hepatology 1998; 28: 374–8.

Non-benzodiazepine antagonism. Flumazenil blocks the effects of non-benzodiazepines, such as zopiclone and zolpidem, that act via the benzodiazepine receptor. In a double-blind study[1] in healthy volunteers, flumazenil rapidly antagonised clinical sedation induced by zolpidem.

1. Patat A, et al. Flumazenil antagonizes the central effects of zolpidem, an imidazopyridine hypnotic. Clin Pharmacol Ther 1994; 56: 430–6.

Preparations

Proprietary Preparations (details are given in Part 3)
Aust.: Anexate; *Austral.:* Anexate; *Belg.:* Anexate; *Braz.:* Lanexat; *Canad.:* Anexate; *Denm.:* Lanexat; *Fin.:* Lanexat; *Fr.:* Anexate; *Ger.:* Anexate; *Hong Kong:* Anexate; *Irl.:* Anexate; *Israel:* Anexate; *Ital.:* Anexate; *Mex.:* Lanexat; *Neth.:* Anexate; *Norw.:* Anexate; *NZ:* Anexate; *Port.:* Anexate; *S.Afr.:* Anexate; *Singapore:* Anexate; *Spain:* Anexate; *Swed.:* Lanexat; *Switz.:* Anexate; *Thai.:* Anexate; *UK:* Anexate; *USA:* Romazicon.

Fomepizole   (2184-p)

Fomepizole (BAN, USAN, rINN).

4-Methylpyrazole; 4-MP. 4-Methyl-1H-pyrazole.

$C_4H_6N_2 = 82.10$.

CAS — 7554-65-6.

Profile

Fomepizole is an inhibitor of alcohol dehydrogenase. It is used for the treatment of poisoning by ethylene glycol (p.1609), which is converted to toxic metabolites by alcohol dehydrogenase. Fomepizole is given in a loading dose of 15 mg per kg body-weight followed by 10 mg per kg every 12 hours for 4 doses, then 15 mg per kg every 12 hours until serum concentrations of ethylene glycol are less than 20 mg per 100 mL. All doses should be given by intravenous infusion over 30 minutes. Fomepizole has also been given in the treatment of methyl alcohol poisoning.

◊ References.
1. Jacobsen D, et al. Non-linear kinetics of 4-methylpyrazole in healthy human subjects. Eur J Clin Pharmacol 1989; 37: 599–604.
2. Harry P, et al. Efficacy of 4-methylpyrazole in ethylene glycol poisoning: clinical and toxicokinetic aspects. Hum Exp Toxicol 1994; 13: 61–4.
3. Burns MJ, et al. Treatment of methanol poisoning with intravenous 4-methylpyrazole. Ann Emerg Med 1997; 30: 829–32.
4. Harry P, et al. Ethylene glycol poisoning in a child treated with 4-methylpyrazole. Pediatrics 1998; 102: 627. Full version: http://www.pediatrics.org/cgi/content/full/102/3/e31
5. Brent J, et al. Fomepizole for the treatment of ethylene glycol poisoning. N Engl J Med 1999; 340: 832–8.
6. Borron SW, et al. Fomepizole in treatment of uncomplicated ethylene glycol poisoning. Lancet 1999; 354: 831.
7. Brent J, et al. Fomepizole for the treatment of methanol poisoning. N Engl J Med 2001; 344: 424–9.

Preparations

Proprietary Preparations (details are given in Part 3)
Israel: Antizol; *UK:* Antizol; *USA:* Antizol.

Fuller's Earth (1610-h)

Terra Fullonica.

CAS — 8031-18-3.

Consists largely of montmorillonite, a native hydrated aluminium silicate, with which very finely divided calcite (calcium carbonate) may be associated.

Profile

Fuller's earth is an adsorbent which is used in dusting powders, toilet powders, and lotions. Fuller's earth of high adsorptive capacity is used in industry as a clarifying and filtering medium. It has been used in the treatment of paraquat poisoning (p.1435). A dose of 200 to 500 mL of a 30% suspension was administered orally every 2 hours for 3 doses, in association with magnesium sulfate or mannitol to promote diarrhoea and empty the gut.

Preparations

Proprietary Preparations (details are given in Part 3)
Multi-ingredient: *Braz.:* Camomila.

Glucagon (7711-s)

Glucagon (BAN, rINN).

Glucagonum; HGF. His-Ser-Gln-Gly-Thr-Phe-Thr-Ser-Asp-Tyr-Ser-Lys-Tyr-Leu-Asp-Ser-Arg-Arg-Ala-Gln-Asp-Phe-Val-Gln-Trp-Leu-Met-Asn-Thr.

$C_{153}H_{225}N_{43}O_{49}S = 3482.7.$

CAS — 16941-32-5.

ATC — H04AA01.

Pharmacopoeias. In *Eur.* (see p.vi) and *US.*

A recombinant glucagon is available in some countries.

Pharmacopoeial description

Ph. Eur.: A polypeptide hormone obtained from beef or pork pancreas. A white or almost white powder. Practically insoluble in water and in most organic solvents; it dissolves in dilute mineral acids and in dilute solutions of alkali hydroxides. Store in airtight containers at a temperature below 8° and preferably at −20°.

USP 25: A polypeptide hormone obtained from porcine and bovine pancreas glands. A fine, white or faintly coloured, practically odourless, crystalline powder. Soluble in dilute alkali and acid solutions; insoluble in most organic solvents. Store under nitrogen in airtight glass containers at a temperature of 2° to 8°.

Adverse Effects

Nausea and vomiting may occur following administration of glucagon. Hypersensitivity reactions and hypokalaemia have also been reported.

Precautions

Glucagon should generally not be given to patients with phaeochromocytoma since it can cause a release of catecholamines producing marked hypertension. Glucagon should be administered with caution to patients with insulinoma as it may induce hypoglycaemia due to its insulin-releasing effect. Glucagon was formerly used to diagnose phaeochromocytoma and insulinoma but this use has been largely abandoned. Caution is also required when it is being employed as a diagnostic aid in diabetic patients or in elderly patients with heart disease.

Glucagon is not effective in patients with marked depletion of liver glycogen stores, as in starvation, adrenal insufficiency, alcohol-induced hypoglycaemia, or chronic hypoglycaemia.

Interactions

Warfarin. For a report of glucagon enhancing the anticoagulant effect of warfarin, see p.997.

Pharmacokinetics

Glucagon has a plasma half-life of about 3 to 6 minutes. It is inactivated in the liver, kidneys, and plasma.

Bioavailability. In a study in healthy subjects and diabetic patients the bioavailability following intranasal administration of glucagon was about 30% of that following intramuscular administration.[1] However the apparent half-life following intramuscular injection was 28.6 and 31.4 minutes respectively in the two groups, three to four times longer than that after either intravenous or intranasal administration, possibly due to slow release of glucagon from the injection site. It was also recognised that the quicker onset of activity with the intranasal route might be of value in an emergency.

1. Pontiroli AE, *et al.* Pharmacokinetics of intranasal, intramuscular and intravenous glucagon in healthy subjects and diabetic patients. *Eur J Clin Pharmacol* 1993; **45:** 555–8.

Uses and Administration

Glucagon is a polypeptide hormone which is produced by the alpha cells of the pancreatic islets of Langerhans. It is a hyperglycaemic which mobilises glucose by activating hepatic glycogenolysis. It can to a lesser extent stimulate the secretion of pancreatic insulin. Glucagon is given as the hydrochloride; doses are usually expressed as glucagon (note that 1 unit is equivalent to 1 mg of glucagon). Glucagon is used in the treatment of severe hypoglycaemic reactions when the patient cannot take glucose by mouth and intravenous glucose is not feasible. It is given by subcutaneous, intramuscular, or intravenous injection in a dose of 1 mg (or 0.5 mg in patients under about 20 kg body-weight). If there is no response within 10 to 15 minutes, intravenous glucose should be given, although there is no contra-indication to repeating the dose of glucagon. Once the patient has responded sufficiently to take carbohydrate by mouth this should be given to restore liver glycogen stores and prevent secondary hypoglycaemia.

As glucagon reduces the motility of the gastrointestinal tract it is used as a diagnostic aid in gastrointestinal examinations. The route of administration and dose is dependent upon the diagnostic procedure. A dose of 1 to 2 mg administered intramuscularly has an onset of action of 4 to 15 minutes and a duration of effect of 10 to 40 minutes; 0.2 to 2 mg given intravenously produces an effect within one minute that lasts for 5 to 25 minutes.

Glucagon possesses positive cardiac inotropic activity but is not generally considered suitable for heart failure. However, as it can bypass blocked beta receptors, it is used in the treatment of beta-blocker overdosage, see Cardiovascular Effects, below.

Intranasal preparations have been studied.

Administration. References to intranasal administration of glucagon in healthy subjects and diabetics.

1. Freychet L, *et al.* Effect of intranasal glucagon on blood glucose levels in healthy subjects and hypoglycaemic patients with insulin-dependent diabetes. *Lancet* 1988; **i:** 1364–6.
2. Pontiroli AE, *et al.* Intranasal glucagon is a remedy for hypoglycemia: studies in healthy subjects and type I diabetic patients. *Diabetes Care* 1989; **12:** 604–8.
3. Pontiroli AE, *et al.* Nasal administration of glucagon and human calcitonin to healthy subjects: a comparison of powders and spray solutions and of different enhancing agents. *Eur J Clin Pharmacol* 1989; **37:** 427–30.
4. Hvidberg A, *et al.* Glucose recovery after intranasal glucagon during hypoglycaemia in man. *Eur J Clin Pharmacol* 1994; **46:** 15–17.

Cardiovascular effects. Glucagon has chronotropic and inotropic effects due to its ability to raise cyclic AMP concentrations independently of a response to catecholamines. It is used in the management of beta-blocker overdosage (see p.845); doses of 50 to 150 µg per kg body-weight (or 5 to 10 mg) by intravenous injection, followed by an infusion of 1 to 5 mg per hour if required, have been suggested.

Glucagon may be effective in the management of anaphylactic reactions to contrast media in patients receiving beta blockers.[1,2] A dramatic improvement in refractory hypotension during an anaphylactic reaction to contrast media was described in a 75-year-old man receiving beta blockers following intravenous administration of glucagon.[3]

While it is not regarded as standard treatment for overdosage with calcium-channel blockers, intravenous administration of glucagon 10 mg has been reported to be beneficial.[4]

1. Lieber JJ. Risk for anaphylactoid reaction from contrast media. *Ann Intern Med* 1991; **115:** 985.
2. Lang DM, *et al.* Risk for anaphylactoid reaction from contrast media. *Ann Intern Med* 1991; **115:** 985.
3. Zaloga GP, *et al.* Glucagon reversal of hypotension in a case of anaphylactic shock. *Ann Intern Med* 1986; **105:** 65–6.
4. Walter FG, *et al.* Amelioration of nifedipine poisoning associated with glucagon therapy. *Ann Emerg Med* 1993; **22:** 1234–7.

Diagnosis and testing. PITUITARY FUNCTION. Glucagon stimulates secretion of growth hormone and cortisol (hydrocortisone) and has been used both alone[1,2] and in combination with a beta blocker[3,4] as a test of pituitary function. The test is contra-indicated in patients with heart block, asthma, heart failure, and diabetes mellitus,[4] and severe secondary hypoglycaemia and death has been reported in a 2-year-old child following a glucagon test for growth hormone secretion.[5] In a review of growth hormone provocation tests,[6] the glucagon test and the insulin-tolerance test were regarded as being less useful than the clonidine test.

1. Milner RDG, Burns EC. Investigation of suspected growth hormone deficiency. *Arch Dis Child* 1982; **57:** 944–7.
2. Anonymous. Testing anterior pituitary function. *Lancet* 1986; **i:** 839–41.

3. Colle M, *et al.* Betaxolol and propranolol in glucagon stimulation of growth hormone. *Arch Dis Child* 1984; **59:** 670–2.
4. Abboud CF. Laboratory diagnosis of hypopituitarism. *Mayo Clin Proc* 1986; **61:** 35–48.
5. Shah A, *et al.* Hazards of pharmacologic tests of growth hormone secretion in childhood. *BMJ* 1992; **304:** 173–4.
6. Hindmarsh PC, Swift PGF. An assessment of growth hormone provocation tests. *Arch Dis Child* 1995; **72:** 362–8.

Gastrointestinal disorders. The relaxant effect of glucagon on smooth muscle has been used to stop hiccups resulting from distension of the gallbladder[1] and to facilitate passage of swallowed foreign bodies and impacted food boluses which have become lodged in the lower oesophagus.[2,3] Glucagon has also been tried in the management of biliary colic.[4]

1. Gardner AMN. Glucagon stops hiccups. *BMJ* 1985; **290:** 822.
2. Cooke MW, Glucksman EE. Swallowed coins. *BMJ* 1991; **302:** 1607.
3. Farrugia M, *et al.* Radiological treatment of acute oesophageal food impaction. *Br J Hosp Med* 1995; **54:** 410–11.
4. Grossi E, *et al.* Different pharmacological approaches to the treatment of acute biliary colic. *Curr Ther Res* 1986; **40:** 876–82.

Hypoglycaemia. Hypoglycaemia most commonly occurs in diabetic patients, particularly those receiving insulin therapy. Other rare causes include alcohol ingestion and tumours such as insulinomas. Neonatal hypoglycaemia occurs in small-for-gestational-age infants or infants of diabetic mothers. Persistent or recurrent hypoglycaemia in neonates is usually due to an endocrine or metabolic disorder, such as nesidioblastosis.

Glucose is the treatment of choice for acute hypoglycaemia since it corrects the problem at source. Glucagon is generally used as an alternative to parenteral glucose in hypoglycaemic patients whose consciousness is impaired and who cannot therefore take glucose by mouth, or in other situations where glucose administration is not possible. Some have advocated the use of glucagon as a first-line treatment in patients requiring parenteral therapy since it is more convenient and easier to give than parenteral glucose.[1] However, this does not seem to be the general view. The action of glucagon relies upon the patient having adequate hepatic glycogen stores which may not always be the case; for example, glycogen stores are depleted in patients with alcohol-induced hypoglycaemia or with insulinoma and glucagon is not effective.

Hypoglycaemia in neonates is usually managed by adjusting the enteral feeds or by administration of parenteral glucose in symptomatic infants. Glucagon may be used if parenteral glucose is not effective or cannot be given.[2,3]

Continuous infusion of glucagon was reported to be effective in the management of hypoglycaemia in a patient with an extrapancreatic tumour.[4]

1. Gibbins RL. Treating hypoglycaemia in general practice. *BMJ* 1993; **306:** 600–1.
2. Carter PE, *et al.* Glucagon for hypoglycaemia in infants small for gestational age. *Arch Dis Child* 1988; **63:** 1264.
3. Williams AF. Hypoglycaemia of the newborn: a review. *Bull WHO* 1997; **75:** 261–90.
4. Samaan NA, *et al.* Successful treatment of hypoglycemia using glucagon in a patient with an extrapancreatic tumor. *Ann Intern Med* 1990; **113:** 404–6.

Liver disorders. For references to the use of glucagon with insulin in the treatment of liver disorders, see under Insulin, p.331.

Preparations

BP 2001: Glucagon Injection;
USP 25: Glucagon for Injection.

Proprietary Preparations (details are given in Part 3)
Aust.: GlucaGen; *Austral.:* GlucaGen; *Belg.:* GlucaGen; *Denm.:* GlucaGen; *Fin.:* GlucaGen; *Fr.:* GlucaGen; *Ger.:* GlucaGen; *Hong Kong:* GlucaGen; *Irl.:* GlucaGen; *Israel:* GlucaGen; *Ital.:* GlucaGen; *Mex.:* Glucagon; *NZ:* GlucaGen; *Port.:* GlucaGen; *S.Afr.:* GlucaGen; *Switz.:* GlucaGen; *Thai.:* GlucaGen; *UK:* GlucaGen; Glucagon.

Glutathione (588-l)

GSH. *N*-(*N*-L-γ-Glutamyl-L-cysteinyl)glycine.

$C_{10}H_{17}N_3O_6S = 307.3.$

CAS — 70-18-8.

ATC — V03AB32.

Profile

Glutathione is an endogenous peptide with antioxidant and other metabolic functions. It has been used in the treatment of poisoning with a number of compounds including heavy metals. Glutathione sodium has been used similarly. Glutathione has also been tried in idiopathic pulmonary fibrosis and has been used in other conditions such as liver disorders, corneal disorders, eczema, and for mitigation of the adverse effects of antineoplastic therapy including the neurotoxicity of cisplatin.

◊ Reviews.

1. Lomaestro BM, Malone M. Glutathione in health and disease: pharmacotherapeutic issues. *Ann Pharmacother* 1995; **29:** 1263–73.

Antineoplastic toxicity. Glutathione has been reported to reduce the incidence of neurotoxicity induced by cisplatin therapy. In a double-blind, randomised trial[1] in 50 patients receiving cisplatin for advanced gastric cancer, administration of glutathione significantly reduced the incidence of neuropathy assessed within one week of completing cisplatin therapy. There did not appear to be any reduction in cytotoxic activity.

1. Cascinu S, et al. Neuroprotective effect of reduced glutathione on cisplatin-based chemotherapy in advanced gastric cancer: a randomized double-blind placebo-controlled trial. *J Clin Oncol* 1995; **13:** 26–32.

Lung disorders. Glutathione is an important extracellular antioxidant in the lung and high concentrations are found in lung epithelial lining fluid. A deficiency of glutathione may contribute to the epithelial damage that occurs in cryptogenic fibrosing alveolitis (idiopathic pulmonary fibrosis) and to the increased susceptibility to lung infections that occurs in patients with HIV infection. Preliminary studies have demonstrated beneficial biochemical results with glutathione delivered by aerosol in 10 patients with cryptogenic fibrosing alveolitis,[1] and in 14 HIV-seropositive patients,[2] but no clinical effects have been reported.

1. Borok Z, et al. Effect of glutathione aerosol on oxidant-antioxidant imbalance in idiopathic pulmonary fibrosis. *Lancet* 1991; **338:** 215–16.
2. Holroyd KJ, et al. Correction of glutathione deficiency in the lower respiratory tract of HIV seropositive individuals by glutathione aerosol treatment. *Thorax* 1993; **48:** 985–9.

Preparations

Proprietary Preparations (details are given in Part 3)
Hong Kong: TAD; *Ital.:* Gluko†; Glutamed†; Glutanil; Glutasan; Gluthion; Glutoxil; Ipatox; Maglut; Novatox†; Ridutox; Rition; Scavenger; TAD; Tationil; Thioxene; *Jpn.:* Atomolan†; Tathion†; *Spain:* Tition; *USA:* Cachexon.

Multi-ingredient: *Belg.:* Vitathion†; *Canad.:* Vitathion-ATP; *Fr.:* Vita-Iodurol ATP†; Vita-Iodurol†; *Hong Kong:* BSS Plus; *Spain:* Higado Potenciado Medic†.

Haem Derivatives (2164-b)

Heme Derivatives.

Profile

Haem is the iron protoporphyrin constituent of haemoglobin and is responsible for its colour and oxygen-carrying capacity. It is used in the management of porphyrias (below). Haem is administered intravenously as its derivatives, although there is some confusion over their terminology. The names haematin (hematin) and haemin (hemin) have been used interchangeably although chemically haematin is the hydroxy derivative, formed by the reaction of haemin and sodium carbonate in solution. The arginine salt (haem arginate; haemin arginate; heme arginate) is reported to be more stable.

Haem arginate is used alone or with tin-protoporphyrin (p.1673) in the treatment of acute intermittent porphyria. It is administered by slow intravenous infusion in a dose of 3 mg per kg body-weight daily, infused over at least 30 minutes.

Haematin is used intravenously for the amelioration of acute intermittent porphyria associated with the menstrual cycle in patients unresponsive to other therapy. It is given in a dose of 1 to 4 mg per kg daily for 3 to 14 days as an intravenous infusion over 10 to 15 minutes.

Phlebitis may occur after injection of haematin into small arm veins.

Porphyrias. The porphyrias are a group of inherited and acquired disorders of haem biosynthesis. Deficiencies occur in specific enzymes leading to the accumulation of different porphyrins and porphyrin precursors. They are generally classified as acute or non-acute, reflecting their clinical presentation, or as hepatic or erythropoietic, depending on the site of the enzyme defect. The three most common forms are acute intermittent porphyria, porphyria cutanea tarda, and erythropoietic protoporphyria.

ACUTE PORPHYRIAS. These are inherited disorders characterised by the accumulation of porphyrin precursors, leading to acute attacks of neurovisceral symptoms. The most common form is *acute intermittent porphyria* (acute hepatic porphyria); *variegate porphyria* and *hereditary coproporphyria* are generally less common forms in which there is accumulation of both porphyrin precursors and porphyrins, leading to acute attacks in conjunction with cutaneous symptoms similar to those seen in non-acute porphyrias (see below).

In acute porphyrias the enzyme defect is not complete and only becomes apparent when demand for hepatic haem is increased by drugs, hormones, or nutritional factors. Attacks are rare before puberty and the disorder may remain latent in many patients. The presenting symptom is most commonly severe abdominal pain; other gastrointestinal symptoms such as nausea and vomiting also occur, along with autonomic effects including hypertension, tachycardia, sweating, pallor, and pyrexia. Convulsions may occur at the peak of an attack and may persist

The symbol † denotes a preparation no longer actively marketed

---

between attacks. Neuropathy leads to weakness and paralysis and may progress rapidly to respiratory distress. Psychiatric symptoms are also common, particularly agitation, anxiety, and behavioural disturbances. Attacks are usually precipitated by drugs, alcohol, steroid hormones, reduced caloric intake, or infection. They typically last for several days and are followed by complete recovery, although in some patients chronic abdominal pain may persist without other symptoms.

The primary management of an attack is to remove precipitants and to provide intensive support. *Symptomatic treatment* is complicated by the wide range of drugs that may precipitate porphyria. High doses of parenteral opioids may be required for pain and there is a danger of addiction occurring, particularly if attacks are frequent or if pain persists between attacks. Phenothiazines such as chlorpromazine are useful to control nausea and agitation and their sedative effect may also be beneficial. High doses of propranolol may be required for cardiovascular symptoms. Assisted ventilation may be necessary. Convulsions usually disappear as the attack resolves; management of patients who experience convulsions between attacks is a therapeutic problem since many antiepileptics are porphyrinogenic (see Porphyria, p.342). *Specific therapy* is aimed at suppressing the haem biosynthetic pathway. A high carbohydrate intake should be ensured in all patients to suppress precursor production; this is given orally to prevent fluid overload but intravenous glucose may be required in patients who are vomiting. Haem administration is also effective; it is given as haematin or as haem arginate and tin-protoporphyrin may be used in conjunction. Prevention of attacks involves avoiding drugs which precipitate porphyria and maintaining an adequate carbohydrate intake. Gonadorelin analogues, such as buserelin, may have a role in preventing attacks related to the menstrual cycle.

NON-ACUTE PORPHYRIAS. These are characterised by the accumulation of porphyrins and usually present with cutaneous symptoms although porphyrins also accumulate in the liver and liver damage commonly occurs. *Porphyria cutanea tarda* (cutaneous hepatic porphyria) is the most common form of porphyria. It is usually an acquired disorder and in most cases there is a history of moderate or heavy alcohol intake. There is usually a raised serum-iron concentration and oestrogen administration has also been implicated. The main clinical symptom is cutaneous photosensitivity leading to bullous dermatosis, pruritus, and skin fragility, in areas exposed to sunlight. *Management* involves protecting the skin from sunlight and trauma and avoiding causative agents such as alcohol and iron. Sunscreen preparations must be based on zinc oxide or titanium dioxide to be effective. Reduction of serum-iron concentrations by phlebotomy is effective in most patients and should be carried out at weekly intervals until remission occurs; desferrioxamine is an alternative method to aid iron excretion but is less effective. Chloroquine and hydroxychloroquine have also been used and may be effective where phlebotomy is contra-indicated; they appear to act by complexing with porphyrins and increasing their excretion but low doses are necessary to avoid exacerbating the condition.

Erythropoietic protoporphyria is a less common non-acute porphyria and is an inherited disorder leading to accumulation of protoporphyrin. Symptoms are cutaneous and there is an acute reaction to sunlight leading to urticaria, pruritus, swelling, redness, and a severe burning sensation; liver damage may also occur. *Management* involves protection of the skin, as for porphyria cutanea tarda. Betacarotene produces benefit in most patients with photosensitivity and canthaxanthin may also be used. Haem administration, as haematin or haem arginate, may be beneficial in suppressing protoporphyrin production. Colestyramine and activated charcoal reduce protoporphyrin levels by interrupting enterohepatic recycling; they also bind other porphyrins and may have a role in rare forms of porphyria such as *congenital erythropoietic porphyria*.

References.
1. Todd DJ. Erythropoietic protoporphyria. *Br J Dermatol* 1994; **131:** 751–66.
2. Elder GH, et al. The acute porphyrias. *Lancet* 1997; **349:** 1613–17.
3. Gorchein A. Drug treatment in acute porphyria. *Br J Clin Pharmacol* 1997; **44:** 427–34.
4. Murphy GM. The cutaneous porphyrias: a review. *Br J Dermatol* 1999; **140:** 573–81.
5. Thadani H, et al. Diagnosis and management of porphyria. *BMJ* 2000; **320:** 1647–51.

◊ References to haem derivatives in the management of porphyrias.
1. Anonymous. Hemin infusions in acute intermittent porphyria. *Med Lett Drugs Ther* 1984; **26:** 42.
2. Mustajoki P, et al. Haem arginate in the treatment of acute hepatic porphyrias. *BMJ* 1986; **293:** 538–9.
3. Kordač V, Martásek P. Haem arginate in acute hepatic porphyrias. *BMJ* 1986; **293:** 1098.
4. Tokola O, et al. Haem arginate improves hepatic oxidative metabolism in variegate porphyria. *Br J Clin Pharmacol* 1988; **26:** 753–7.
5. Volin L, et al. Heme arginate: effects on hemostasis. *Blood* 1988; **71:** 625–8.
6. Herrick AL, et al. Controlled trial of haem arginate in acute hepatic porphyria. *Lancet* 1989; **i:** 1295–7.
7. Dover SB, et al. Haem-arginate plus tin-protoporphyrin for acute hepatic porphyria. *Lancet* 1991; **338:** 263.
8. Mustajoki P, Nordmann Y. Early administration of heme arginate for acute porphyric attacks. *Arch Intern Med* 1993; **153:** 2004–8.

Preparations

Proprietary Preparations (details are given in Part 3)
Austral.: Panhematin; *Fin.:* Normosang; *Fr.:* Normosang; *Ger.:* Normosang; *Switz.:* Normosang; *UK:* Normosang; *USA:* Panhematin.

Lofexidine Hydrochloride (12901-j)

Lofexidine Hydrochloride (BANM, USAN, rINNM).
Ba-168; MDL-14042; MDL-14042A; RMI-14042A. 2-[1-(2,6-Dichlorophenoxy)ethyl]-2-imidazoline hydrochloride.
$C_{11}H_{12}Cl_2N_2O,HCl = 295.6$.
CAS — 31036-80-3 (lofexidine); 21498-08-8 (lofexidine hydrochloride).

Adverse Effects

Lofexidine has central alpha-adrenergic effects and may cause drowsiness, dryness of the mouth, throat, and nose, hypotension, and bradycardia. Symptoms of overdosage with lofexidine include sedation and coma.

Sudden withdrawal of lofexidine may produce rebound hypertension.

Precautions

Lofexidine should be used with caution in patients with cerebrovascular disease, ischaemic heart disease including recent myocardial infarction, bradycardia, renal impairment, or a history of depression.

It may cause drowsiness and if affected, patients should not drive or operate machinery.

Withdrawal of lofexidine therapy should be gradual over 2 to 4 days or more to reduce the risk of rebound hypertension.

Interactions

Lofexidine may enhance the central depressant effects of sedative agents including alcohol. Tricyclic antidepressants administered concomitantly may reduce the efficacy of lofexidine.

Uses and Administration

Lofexidine is an alpha$_2$-adrenoceptor agonist structurally related to clonidine (p.860). It has antihypertensive activity, but is used mainly in the control of opioid withdrawal symptoms.

In opioid withdrawal lofexidine is given as the hydrochloride in an initial dose of 200 μg twice daily by mouth. The dose may be increased gradually by 200 to 400 μg daily to a maximum of 2.4 mg daily. After 7 to 10 days, or longer in some cases, treatment is withdrawn gradually over at least 2 to 4 days.

Opioid dependence. The use of lofexidine in the treatment of opioid dependence (p.66) has been reviewed.[1] It appears to be a useful addition to the range of treatments available, and may be more acceptable to patients than clonidine, though perhaps less acceptable than methadone.

1. Strang J, et al. Lofexidine for opiate detoxification: review of recent randomised and open controlled trials. *Am J Addict* 1999; **8:** 337–48.

Preparations

Proprietary Preparations (details are given in Part 3)
UK: Britlofex.

Mesna (3726-q)

Mesna (BAN, USAN, rINN).
D-7093; Mesnum; UCB-3983. Sodium 2-mercaptoethanesulphonate.
$C_2H_5NaO_3S_2 = 164.2$.
CAS — 19767-45-4.
ATC — R05CB05; V03AF01.

Stability. There was no evidence of degradation of mesna when stored in solution with ifosfamide in polyethylene infusion bags at room temperature for 7 hours[1] or in polypropylene syringes at room temperature or at 4° for 4 weeks.[2] However, in the latter study ifosfamide concentrations fell by about 3% after 7 days and 12% after 4 weeks at both temperatures.

1. Shaw IC, Rose JWP. Infusion of ifosfamide plus mesna. *Lancet* 1984; **i:** 1353–4.
2. Rowland CG, et al. Infusion of ifosfamide plus mesna. *Lancet* 1984; **ii:** 468.

Adverse Effects and Precautions

Adverse effects which may occur after use of mesna include gastrointestinal effects, headache, fatigue, limb pains, depression, irritability, hypotension and tachycardia (but see below), and skin rash. Bronchospasm has been reported after administration by nebuliser.

Mesna may produce a false positive result in diagnostic tests for urinary ketones and may produce a false positive or false negative result in diagnostic tests for urinary erythrocytes.

Effects on the blood pressure. Severe hypertension occurred following administration of mesna both in combination with ifosfamide and alone.[1]

1. Gilleece MH, Davies JM. Mesna therapy and hypertension. *DICP Ann Pharmacother* 1991; **25:** 867.

Effects on the nervous system. For reports of severe encephalopathy in patients receiving mesna and ifosfamide, see p.546.

Hypersensitivity. Hypersensitivity reactions including rash, fever, nausea, facial and periorbital oedema, ulceration of mucous membranes, and tachycardia have been attributed to mesna.[1-4]

1. Lang E, Goos M. Hypersensitivity to mesna. *Lancet* 1985; **ii:** 329.
2. Seidel A, *et al.* Allergic reactions to mesna. *Lancet* 1991; **338:** 381.
3. Gross WL, *et al.* Allergic reactions to mesna. *Lancet* 1991; **338:** 381–2.
4. D'Cruz D, *et al.* Allergic reactions to mesna. *Lancet* 1991; **338:** 705–6.

Pharmacokinetics

Mesna is rapidly excreted in the urine after oral or intravenous administration as the unchanged drug and as the metabolite mesna disulfide (dimesna). The half-lives of mesna and dimesna are reported to be about 20 minutes and 70 minutes respectively.

◊ References.
1. Burkert H, *et al.* Bioavailability of orally administered mesna. *Arzneimittelforschung* 1984; **34:** 1597–1600.
2. James CA, *et al.* Pharmacokinetics of intravenous and oral sodium 2-mercaptoethane sulphonate (mesna) in normal subjects. *Br J Clin Pharmacol* 1987; **23:** 561–8.
3. El-Yazigi A, *et al.* Pharmacokinetics of mesna and dimesna after simultaneous intravenous bolus and infusion administration in patients undergoing bone marrow transplantation. *J Clin Pharmacol* 1997; **37:** 618–24.

Uses and Administration

Mesna is used for the prophylaxis of urothelial toxicity in patients being treated with the antineoplastics ifosfamide or cyclophosphamide. In the kidney, mesna disulfide, the inactive metabolite of mesna, is reduced to free mesna which has thiol groups that react with the metabolites of ifosfamide and cyclophosphamide, including acrolein, considered to be responsible for the toxic effects on the bladder.

The aim of mesna therapy is to ensure adequate levels of mesna in the urine throughout the period during which these toxic metabolites are present and the duration of mesna treatment should therefore be equal that of the antineoplastic treatment plus the time taken for the concentration of antineoplastic metabolites in the urine to fall to non-toxic levels. Urinary output should be maintained and the urine monitored for haematuria and proteinuria throughout the treatment period. However, frequent emptying of the bladder should be avoided.

Mesna may be given intravenously or orally for the prophylaxis of urothelial toxicity, the dosage and frequency depending on the antineoplastic regimen used. Following oral administration, availability of mesna in urine is approximately 50% of that following intravenous administration and excretion in urine is delayed up to 2 hours and is more prolonged. The intravenous preparation may be given orally when it should be added to a flavoured drink; this mixture may be stored in a sealed container in a refrigerator for up to 24 hours. Alternatively, tablets are available.

Intravenous bolus antineoplastic regimens. If ifosfamide or cyclophosphamide is given as an intravenous bolus, the *intravenous dose of mesna* is 20% of the dose of the antineoplastic on a weight for weight basis given on 3 occasions over 15 to 30 minutes at intervals of 4 hours beginning at the same time as the antineoplastic injection; thus a total dose of mesna equivalent to 60% of the antineoplastic is given. This regimen is repeated each time the antineoplastic is used. The individual dose of mesna may be increased to 40% of the dose of the antineoplastic and given 4 times at intervals of 3 hours for children and patients at high risk of urotoxicity; in such cases the total dose of mesna is equivalent to 160% of the antineoplastic given. The *oral dose of mesna* is 40% of the dose of the antineoplastic given on 3 occasions at intervals of 4 hours beginning two hours before the antineoplastic injection; thus a total dose of mesna equivalent to

120% of the antineoplastic is given. Alternatively, the initial dose of mesna (20% of the dose of the antineoplastic) may be given *intravenously* followed by two *oral doses* (each 40% of the dose of the antineoplastic) given 2 and 6 hours after the intravenous dose. Any of these regimens may be used if **cyclophosphamide** is given **orally**.

Intravenous infusion antineoplastic regimens. If the antineoplastic is given as an intravenous infusion over 24 hours, an initial *intravenous injection* of mesna as 20% of the total antineoplastic dose is followed by 100% of the total dose by intravenous infusion over 24 hours, followed by 60% by intravenous infusion over a further 12 hours. The final 12-hour infusion may be replaced either by 3 intravenous injections each of 20% of the antineoplastic dose at intervals of 4 hours, the first injection being given 4 hours after the infusion has been stopped, or by *oral mesna* given in 3 doses each of 40% of the antineoplastic dose, the first dose being given when the 24-hour infusion is stopped, and the second and third doses being given 2 and 6 hours later.

Mesna is also administered by inhalation as a mucolytic in the management of some respiratory-tract disorders. The usual daily dose is 0.6 to 1.2 g administered by a nebuliser; it may also be given by direct endotracheal instillation.

◊ General references.
1. Schoenike SE, Dana WJ. Ifosfamide and mesna. *Clin Pharm* 1990; **9:** 179–91.

Preparations

Proprietary Preparations (details are given in Part 3)
Aust.: Mistabron; Uromitexan; *Austral.:* Uromitexan; *Belg.:* Mistabron; Uromitexan; *Braz.:* Mitexan; *Canad.:* Uromitexan; *Denm.:* Uromitexan; *Fin.:* Uromitexan; *Fr.:* Mucofluid; Uromitexan; *Ger.:* Mistabronco; Uromitexan; *Hong Kong:* Mistabron; Uromitexan; *Irl.:* Uromitexan; *Israel:* Mexan; *Ital.:* Ausobronc†; Mucofluid; Mucolene; Uromitexan; *Mex.:* Filesna; Mesnil; Uromitexan; Ziken; *Neth.:* Mistabron; Uromitexan; *Norw.:* Uromitexan; *NZ:* Uromitexan; *Port.:* Uromitexan; *S.Afr.:* Mistabron; Uromitexan; *Singapore:* Mistabron; Uromitexan; *Spain:* Mucofluid; Uromitexan; *Swed.:* Uromitexan; *Switz.:* Mistabron; Uromitexan; *Thai.:* Mistabron; Uromitexan; *UK:* Uromitexan; *USA:* Mesnex.

Methionine (605-x)

Methionine (*USAN, rINN*).
M; S-Methionine; L-Methionine; Methioninum. L-2-Amino-4-(methylthio)butyric acid.
$C_5H_{11}NO_2S = 149.2$.
CAS — 63-68-3.
ATC — V03AB26.
Pharmacopoeias. In *Eur.* (see p.vi), *Jpn, Pol.,* and *US.*

Pharmacopoeial description
Ph. Eur.: A white or almost white, crystalline powder or colourless crystals. Soluble in water; very slightly soluble in alcohol; practically insoluble in ether. A 2.5% solution in water has a pH of 5.5 to 6.5. Protect from light.
USP 25: White crystals having a characteristic odour. Soluble in water, in warm dilute alcohol, and in dilute mineral acids; insoluble in dehydrated alcohol, in acetone, in ether, and in benzene. pH of a 1% solution in water is between 5.6 and 6.1.

DL-Methionine (606-r)

DL-Methioninum; Racemethionine (*USAN*). DL-2-Amino-4-(methylthio)butyric acid.
$C_5H_{11}NO_2S = 149.2$.
CAS — 59-51-8.

NOTE. The name methionine is often applied to DL-methionine. Compounded preparations of DL-methionine may be represented by the following names:

• Co-methiamol *x/y* (*BAN*)—where *x* and *y* are the strengths in milligrams of DL-methionine and paracetamol respectively.
Pharmacopoeias. In *Eur.* (see p.vi).

Pharmacopoeial description
Ph. Eur.: An almost white crystalline powder or small flakes. Sparingly soluble in water; very slightly soluble in alcohol; practically insoluble in ether; dissolves in dilute acids and in dilute solutions of alkali hydroxides. A 2% solution in water has a pH of 5.4 to 6.1. Protect from light.

Adverse Effects and Precautions

Methionine may cause nausea, vomiting, drowsiness, and irritability. It should not be used in patients with acidosis. Methionine may aggravate hepatic encepha-

lopathy in patients with established liver damage; it should be used with caution in patients with severe liver disease.

Interactions

Orally administered methionine may be adsorbed by activated charcoal leading to a diminished effect of methionine if they are given concurrently.

Dopaminergics. For the antagonism of the antiparkinsonian effect of *levodopa* by methionine, see Nutritional Agents, under Interactions of Levodopa, p.1172.

Uses and Administration

L-Methionine is an amino acid which is an essential constituent of the diet and is incorporated into amino-acid solutions for parenteral nutrition (p.1351).

Methionine also enhances the synthesis of glutathione and is used as an alternative to acetylcysteine in the treatment of paracetamol poisoning to prevent hepatic damage (see p.71). The literature relating to the use of methionine in paracetamol poisoning is, in general, imprecise as to the form of methionine used. In the UK the usual dose of DL-methionine is 2.5 g by mouth every 4 hours for 4 doses starting less than 10 to 12 hours after ingestion of the paracetamol. Children under 6 years old may be given 1 g every 4 hours for 4 doses. Methionine has also been given intravenously. Preparations containing both methionine and paracetamol have been formulated for use in situations where overdosage may occur. However, the issue of whether methionine should be routinely added to paracetamol preparations is contentious for medical and ethical reasons.

Methionine has also been given by mouth to lower urinary pH and as an adjunct in the treatment of liver disorders.

Preparations

Proprietary Preparations (details are given in Part 3)
Aust.: Acimethin; *Austral.:* Methnine; *Ger.:* Acimethin; *Switz.:* Acimethin; *USA:* M-Caps; Pedameth; Uracid.

Multi-ingredient: *Austral.:* Berberis Complex; Liv-Detox; *Belg.:* Verrulyse-Methionine†; *Braz.:* Aminotox; Anekron; Betaliver; Biofigado; Colinvitol; Epacrosil; Eparex; Epativan B6; Epocler; Eviepar; Extrato Hepatico Composto; Figadobil; Hepalin; Hepasedan; Hepatocler; Hepatotris; Hormo Hepatico; Mesitol; Metiocolin B12; Metionina Composta; Necrohepat; Neofarmotox; Panvitrop; Silimalon; Xantina B12; Xantinon B12; *Canad.:* Amino-Cerv; Selenium Plus; *Fr.:* Cysti-Z; Forcapil; Lobamine-Cysteine; Verrulyse-Methionine†; *Ger.:* Hepalipon N†; Hepar-Pasc duo; Hepar-Pasc N†; Lipovitan; *Hong Kong:* Bilsan; Lipochol; *Ital.:* Agedin Plus; Lozione Same AS†; Meziv; *Mex.:* Lipovitasi-Or; *Port.:* Drenomade; Metionina; *S.Afr.:* Hepavite; *Spain:* Dertrase; *Switz.:* Lobamine-Cysteine†; Mechovit; *Thai.:* Bio-Vitas; Lipochol; Liporon; *UK:* Fat-Solv; Lipotropic Factors; Pameton†; Paradote; *USA:* Amino-Cerv.

Methylene Blue (1042-s)

Methylene Blue (*BAN*).
Methylthioninium Chloride (*BAN, rINN*); Azul de Metileno; Blu di Metilene; CI Basic Blue 9; Colour Index No. 52015; Methylenii Caeruleum; Methylthioninii Chloridum; Schultz No. 1038; Tetramethylthionine Chloride Trihydrate. 3,7-Bis(dimethylamino)phenazathionium chloride trihydrate.
$C_{16}H_{18}ClN_3S,3H_2O = 373.9$.
CAS — 61-73-4 (*anhydrous methylene blue [methylthioninium chloride]*); 7220-79-3 (*methylene blue [methylthioninium chloride] trihydrate*).
ATC — V03AB17; V04CG05.
Pharmacopoeias. In *Chin.* and *US;* in *Eur.* (see p.vi) (as xH_2O); in *Int.* (as anhydrous or 3H_2O).

Pharmacopoeial description
Ph. Eur.: A dark blue, crystalline powder with a copper-coloured sheen, or green crystals with a bronze-coloured sheen. Soluble in water; slightly soluble in alcohol. Store in airtight containers. Protect from light.
USP 25: Dark green crystals or crystalline powder with a bronze-like lustre. Is odourless or practically so. Solutions in water or alcohol are deep blue in colour. Soluble 1 in 25 of water and 1 in 65 of alcohol; soluble in chloroform.

◊ NOTE. *Commercial methylene blue [methylthioninium chloride] may consist of the double chloride of tetramethylthionine and zinc, and is not suitable for medicinal use.*

Adverse Effects and Precautions

After intravenous administration of high doses, methylene blue [methylthioninium chloride] may cause nausea, vomiting, abdominal and chest pain, head-ache, dizziness, mental confusion, profuse sweating, dyspnoea, and hypertension; methaemoglobinaemia and haemolysis may occur. Haemolytic anaemia and hyperbilirubinaemia have been reported in newborn infants following intra-amniotic injection. Oral administration may cause gastrointestinal disturbances and dysuria.

Methylene blue [methylthioninium chloride] should not be injected subcutaneously as it has been associated with isolated cases of necrotic abscesses. It should not be given by intrathecal injection as neural damage has occurred. Methylene blue [methylthioninium chloride] should be used with caution in patients with severe renal impairment and is contra-indicated in patients with glucose-6-phosphate dehydrogenase deficiency (see Uses, below). Methylene blue [methylthioninium chloride] is used to treat methaemoglobinaemia but in large doses it can itself produce methaemoglobinaemia and methaemoglobin concentration should therefore be closely monitored during treatment. Methylene blue [methylthioninium chloride] should not be used to treat methaemoglobinaemia induced by sodium nitrite during the treatment of cyanide poisoning, since cyanide binding will be reduced with resultant increased toxicity. It has also been contra-indicated in methaemoglobinaemia due to chlorate poisoning because of the risk that the more toxic hypochlorite may be formed, although several authorities consider its use to treat methaemoglobinaemia in severe chlorate poisoning appropriate.

Methylene blue [methylthioninium chloride] imparts a blue colour to saliva, urine, faeces, and skin, which may hinder a diagnosis of cyanosis.

◊ Methylene blue [methylthioninium chloride] should be used with caution in the treatment of aniline-induced methaemoglobinaemia since it may precipitate Heinz body formation and haemolytic anaemia.[1] Methylene blue [methylthioninium chloride] may reduce methaemoglobin concentrations, but repeated doses could aggravate haemolysis without further reducing methaemoglobinaemia.

1. Harvey JW, Keitt AS. Studies of the efficacy and potential hazards of methylene blue therapy in aniline-induced methaemoglobinaemia. *Br J Haematol* 1983; **54:** 29–41.

Pregnancy. Although intra-amniotic injection of methylene blue [methylthioninium chloride] has been used to diagnose premature rupture of fetal membranes or to identify separate amniotic sacs in twin pregnancies, there have been several reports of haemolytic anaemia (Heinz-body anaemia) and hyperbilirubinaemia in neonates who had been exposed to methylene blue [methylthioninium chloride] in the amniotic cavity.[1-5] In most cases, exchange transfusions and/or phototherapy were required to control the jaundice; in one case phototherapy led to a phototoxic reaction.[5] Some[3] have considered that the use of methylene blue [methylthioninium chloride] for detecting premature rupture of the membranes should be avoided.

Multiple ileal occlusions have been reported in babies born to mothers who had twin pregnancies and who had received methylene blue [methylthioninium chloride] by amniocentesis;[4,6,7] in some cases it was possible to determine that methylene blue [methylthioninium chloride] had been injected into the amniotic sac of the affected twin. Analysis of data from the EURO-CAT registries[8] for 1980 to 1988 which surveyed pregnancy outcomes in 11 countries found a slightly higher risk of ileal and jejunal atresia or stenosis in twins regardless of whether they had received methylene blue [methylthioninium chloride], but the use of methylene blue [methylthioninium chloride] was rare and no increased risk could be shown in babies exposed to it. A further difficulty in using methylene blue [methylthioninium chloride] by amniocentesis for the diagnosis of premature rupture of the membranes is that the resultant staining of the skin and mucous membranes of the neonate hinders assessment of hypoxia including the use of pulse oximetry.[9]

1. Cowett RM, *et al.* Untoward neonatal effect of intraamniotic administration of methylene blue. *Obstet Gynecol* 1976; **48** (suppl): 74s–75s.
2. Serota FT, *et al.* The methylene-blue baby. *Lancet* 1979; **ii:** 1142–3.
3. Crooks J. Haemolytic jaundice in a neonate after intra-amniotic injection of methylene blue. *Arch Dis Child* 1982; **57:** 872–3.
4. Nicolini V, Monni G. Intestinal obstruction in babies exposed in utero to methylene blue. *Lancet* 1990; **336:** 1258–9.
5. Porat R, *et al.* Methylene blue-induced phototoxicity: an unrecognized complication. *Pediatrics* 1996; **97:** 717–21.
6. van der Pol JG, *et al.* Jejunal atresia related to the use of methylene blue in genetic amniocentesis in twins. *Br J Obstet Gynaecol* 1992; **99:** 141–3.
7. Lancaster PAL, *et al.* Intra-amniotic methylene blue and intestinal atresia in twins. *J Perinat Med* 1992; **20** (suppl 1): 262.
8. Dolk H. Methylene blue and atresia or stenosis of ileum and jejunum. *Lancet* 1991; **338:** 1021–2.
9. Troche BT. The methylene blue baby. *N Engl J Med* 1989; **320:** 1756–7.

Pharmacokinetics
Methylene blue [methylthioninium chloride] is absorbed from the gastrointestinal tract. It is believed to be reduced in the tissues to the leuco form which is slowly excreted, mainly in the urine, together with some unchanged drug.

Uses and Administration
Methylene blue [methylthioninium chloride] is a thiazine dye that is used in the treatment of methaemoglobinaemia; it is also used as an antiseptic and in diagnostic procedures.

In patients with methaemoglobinaemia, therapeutic doses of methylene blue [methylthioninium chloride] can lower the levels of methaemoglobin in the red blood cells. It activates a normally dormant reductase enzyme system which reduces the methylene blue [methylthioninium chloride] to leucomethylene blue, which in turn is able to reduce methaemoglobin to haemoglobin. However, in large doses methylene blue [methylthioninium chloride] can itself produce methaemoglobinaemia and methaemoglobin concentration should therefore be closely monitored during treatment. Methylene blue [methylthioninium chloride] is not effective for the treatment of methaemoglobinaemia in patients with glucose-6-phosphate dehydrogenase deficiency as these patients have a diminished capacity to reduce methylene blue [methylthioninium chloride] to leucomethylene blue; it is also potentially harmful as patients with glucose-6-phosphate dehydrogenase deficiency are particularly susceptible to the haemolytic anaemias induced by methylene blue [methylthioninium chloride].

In the treatment of drug-induced methaemoglobinaemia, as in nitrite poisoning, methylene blue [methylthioninium chloride] is given intravenously as a 1% solution in doses of 1 to 2 mg per kg body-weight injected over a period of several minutes. A repeat dose may be given after one hour if required. It may be of some value in inherited methaemoglobinaemia; doses of up to 300 mg daily by mouth have been used.

Methylene blue [methylthioninium chloride] has a mildly antiseptic action and has been given by mouth in doses of 65 to 130 mg three times daily in minor urinary-tract infections and to prevent the formation of urinary oxalate stones. It is also included in some mixed preparations intended for application to the eye, mouth and pharynx, and skin.

Methylene blue [methylthioninium chloride] is also used as a bacteriological stain, as a dye in diagnostic procedures such as fistula detection and the diagnosis of ruptured amniotic membranes (but see Pregnancy under Adverse Effects and Precautions, above) and for the delineation of certain body tissues during surgery. The blue colour can be removed from the skin with hypochlorite solution. It was formerly used in a renal-function test.

Glutaricaciduria. Methylene blue [methylthioninium chloride] may be of benefit in glutaricaciduria. A response has been observed in one infant[1] with neonatal glutaricaciduria type II. Following the observation in one patient that ifosfamide neurotoxicity (encephalopathy) was associated with glutaricaciduria, methylene blue [methylthioninium chloride] was used successfully in 3 patients to reverse or prevent ifosfamide neurotoxicity.[2,3] In glutaricaciduria, where there is, or is likely to be, an absence of electron-transferring flavoproteins, methylene blue [methylthioninium chloride] may act as an electron acceptor.

1. Harpey J-P, *et al.* Methylene-blue for riboflavine-unresponsive glutaricaciduria type II. *Lancet* 1986; **i:** 391.
2. Küpfer A, *et al.* Prophylaxis and reversal of ifosfamide encephalopathy with methylene-blue. *Lancet* 1994; **343:** 763–4.
3. Zulian GB, *et al.* Methylene blue for ifosfamide-associated encephalopathy. *N Engl J Med* 1995; **332:** 1239–40.

Ifosfamide encephalopathy. See under Glutaricaciduria, above.

Methaemoglobinaemia. Methaemoglobinaemia is a rare disorder of the blood in which there is an increase in the proportion of haemoglobin present in the oxidised form. It may be inherited, due either to a deficiency of methaemoglobin reductase or to a structural abnormality of haemoglobin, or may be acquired, usually secondary to exposure to drugs or chemicals that oxidise haemoglobin. Agents that may cause methaemoglobinaemia include nitrates and nitrites, sodium nitroprusside, dapsone, sulfonamides, phenacetin, and some local anaesthetics such as prilocaine. Administration of low doses over pro-

longed periods may lead to chronic methaemoglobinaemia whereas large doses may lead to an acute effect.

Methaemoglobinaemia has a profound effect on oxygen transport by the blood; there is an increase in oxygen affinity leading to reduced tissue delivery and varying degrees of cyanosis. The presence of symptoms depends upon the degree and rapidity of methaemoglobin formation. Chronic mild methaemoglobinaemia is generally well tolerated although patients may appear cyanotic. Acute methaemoglobinaemia, particularly where methaemoglobin levels exceed 20%, is associated with dyspnoea, headache, malaise, giddiness, and altered mental state; methaemoglobin levels above 50% may lead to vascular collapse, coma, and death.

Patients with inherited methaemoglobinaemia are usually asymptomatic but treatment may be given for cosmetic purposes to reduce the cyanotic skin colour. Patients with reductase deficiency generally respond to oral therapy with drugs that promote the reduction of methaemoglobin to haemoglobin, such as ascorbic acid, riboflavin, or methylene blue [methylthioninium chloride]; methylene blue [methylthioninium chloride] may also be given intravenously. Patients with structural abnormalities of haemoglobin do not respond. In acquired methaemoglobinaemia the causative agent should be identified and removed. Chronic or mild cases may not require treatment but acute symptomatic methaemoglobinaemia may be life-threatening and patients should be given intravenous methylene blue [methylthioninium chloride]. Toxicity is uncommon with methylene blue [methylthioninium chloride] but it should not be used for methaemoglobinaemia due to the use of nitrites for cyanide poisoning since increased toxicity may result (for debate about its use after chlorate poisoning, see Adverse Effects and Precautions, above). Severe methaemoglobinaemia may require exchange transfusion; exchange transfusion with haemodialysis is the treatment of choice in patients with acute methaemoglobinaemia and haemolysis. Ascorbic acid is not useful in the acute situation since it acts too slowly but it may be of benefit where maintenance therapy is required.

References.
1. Coleman MD, Coleman NA. Drug-induced methaemoglobinaemia: treatment issues. *Drug Safety* 1996; **14:** 394–405.

ADMINISTRATION. In acute methaemoglobinaemia, methylene blue [methylthioninium chloride] is usually administered by intravenous bolus injection, but repeated doses may be needed. Methylene blue [methylthioninium chloride] was administered by continuous intravenous infusion at a dose of 7.5 to 10 mg per hour for 43 hours to control methaemoglobinaemia following dapsone poisoning.[1] The patient had responded to two bolus doses of 100 mg but methaemoglobinaemia had subsequently increased again owing to the long half-life of dapsone. Additional therapy included repeated doses of activated charcoal. A dosing schedule for methylene blue [methylthioninium chloride] of 1 to 2 mg per kg body-weight as a bolus followed by a continuous infusion at an initial rate of 0.1 to 0.15 mg per kg per hour was suggested.

1. Dawson AH, Whyte IM. Management of dapsone poisoning complicated by methaemoglobinaemia. *Med Toxicol Adverse Drug Exp* 1989; **4:** 387–92.

Septic shock. Nitric oxide may play a role in the hypotension that occurs in septicaemia (p.138). Methylene blue [methylthioninium chloride] is a guanylate cyclase inhibitor and may block the vasodilator effects of nitric oxide. In an uncontrolled study[1] in 14 patients with septic shock, administration of methylene blue [methylthioninium chloride] increased arterial blood pressure, but cardiac output and tissue oxygenation did not improve; the study was not designed to show an effect on mortality. Improvement in blood pressure has also been reported[2] following use of methylene blue [methylthioninium chloride] in 5 neonates with refractory hypotension assumed to be due to septic shock. However, nitric oxide is only one of many mediators that may be involved in septic shock and further randomised studies are required to determine whether methylene blue [methylthioninium chloride] has any effect on outcome.

1. Preiser J-C, *et al.* Methylene blue administration in septic shock: a clinical trial. *Crit Care Med* 1995; **23:** 259–64.
2. Driscoll W, *et al.* Effect of methylene blue on refractory neonatal hypotension. *J Pediatr* 1996; **129:** 904–8.

Surgery. References to the use of methylene blue [methylthioninium chloride] to stain and identify the parathyroid glands prior to surgery.

1. Dudley NE. Methylene blue for rapid identification of the parathyroid. *BMJ* 1971; **3:** 680–1.
2. Rowntree T. Parathyroids—a personal series. *J R Soc Med* 1980; **73:** 14–18.
3. Bainbridge ET, Barnes AD. Some changing aspects of primary hyperparathyroidism. *Ann R Coll Surg Engl* 1983; **65:** 67–70.
4. Young AE. Intraoperative methods. *Br J Hosp Med* 1984; **31:** 198, 200–3.

Preparations
USP 25: Methylene Blue Injection.

Proprietary Preparations (details are given in Part 3)
Fr.: Collubleu; Vitableu†; *Mex.:* Zumetil; *Spain:* Azul Metile†; *USA:* Urolene Blue.

Multi-ingredient: *Aust.:* Methyment; *Austral.:* Mackenzies Menthoids†; *Braz.:* Acridin; Cezane; Colyrazul; Cystex; Mirabel; Oftazul; Paludil; Pilulas De Witt's; Sepurin; Urosalin; Uroseptin; Vislin; Visodin; Visolux; *Canad.:* Blue Collyrium†; Collyre Bleu; *Fr.:* Antiseptique-Calmante; Collyre Bleu; Mictasol Bleu; Pastilles Monleon; Stilla; *Israel:* Pronaestin; *Ital.:* Mictasol Bleu; Visustrin; *NZ:* De Witts Pills; *Spain:* Argentofenol; Azulina; Bleukawine†; Centilux; Ojosbel Azul; Tivitis; *Switz.:* Collyre Bleu Laiter; *USA:* Atrosept; Dolsed; Prosed/DS; Trac Tabs 2X; UAA; Uridon Modified; Urimar-T; Urimax; Urised; Urogesic Blue.

Nalmefene Hydrochloride (19740-d)

Nalmefene Hydrochloride *(BANM, pINNM)*.

6-Desoxy-6-methylene-naltrexone hydrochloride; JF-I (nalmefene); Nalmetrene Hydrochloride; ORF-11676 (nalmefene). (5R)-9a-Cyclopropylmethyl-4,5-epoxy-6-methylenemorphinan-3,14-diol hydrochloride.

$C_{21}H_{25}NO_3, HCl = 375.9$.

CAS — 58895-64-0.

NOTE. Nalmefene is *USAN*.

Adverse Effects

Nausea, vomiting, tachycardia, hypertension, fever, and dizziness have been reported with therapeutic doses of nalmefene. At higher doses or in patients later found to be physically dependent on opioids, symptoms suggestive of opioid withdrawal have been noted; these have included abdominal cramps, chills, dysphoria, myalgia, and joint pain.

Precautions

Nalmefene should be used with caution in patients who are physically dependent on opioids or who have received large doses of opioids, as an acute withdrawal syndrome may be precipitated (see Dependence under Opioid Analgesics, p.66). Nalmefene should also be used with caution in patients with cardiovascular disease or receiving cardiotoxic drugs since opioid antagonists have been associated with adverse cardiovascular effects in some patients (see Adverse Effects under Naloxone, p.1014). Incremental doses of nalmefene should be administered slowly in patients with renal impairment.

Pharmacokinetics

Nalmefene is absorbed following oral administration, but bioavailability is not complete owing to significant first-pass metabolism. It is metabolised in the liver, mainly to the inactive glucuronide, and is excreted in the urine. Some of the dose is excreted in the faeces and it may undergo enterohepatic recycling. The plasma elimination half-life is reported to be about 10 hours.

◊ References.
1. Dixon R, *et al.* Nalmefene: intravenous safety and kinetics of a new opioid antagonist. *Clin Pharmacol Ther* 1986; **39:** 49–53.
2. Dixon R, *et al.* Nalmefene: safety and kinetics after single and multiple oral doses of a new opioid antagonist. *J Clin Pharmacol* 1987; **27:** 233–9.
3. Frye RF, *et al.* The effect of age on the pharmacokinetics of the opioid antagonist nalmefene. *Br J Clin Pharmacol* 1996; **42:** 301–6.
4. Frye RF, *et al.* Effects of liver disease on the disposition of the opioid antagonist nalmefene. *Clin Pharmacol Ther* 1997; **61:** 15–23.

Uses and Administration

Nalmefene is a derivative of naltrexone and is a specific opioid antagonist with actions and uses similar to those of naloxone (p.1015), but with a longer duration of action. It is administered as the hydrochloride but doses are expressed in terms of the base. It is usually administered intravenously for a rapid onset of action; subcutaneous or intramuscular administration is also effective but has a slower onset. Nalmefene has also been given orally.

For the reversal of postoperative central depression due to the use of opioids, nalmefene is administered intravenously, at a concentration of 100 μg per mL, in an initial dose of 0.25 μg per kg body-weight. Further doses of 0.25 μg per kg may be given at intervals of 2 to 5 minutes until the desired level of opioid reversal is reached; cumulative doses above 1 μg per kg do not provide additional benefit. In patients with an increased cardiovascular risk a concentration of 50 μg per mL and doses of 0.1 μg per kg are recommended.

In the management of known or suspected opioid overdosage, nalmefene is administered intravenously

at a concentration of 1 mg per mL. An initial dose of 0.5 mg per 70 kg is recommended, followed by a second dose of 1 mg per 70 kg after 2 to 5 minutes if necessary. If a total dose of 1.5 mg per 70 kg is not effective then additional doses are unlikely to have an effect. If the patient is suspected of being physically dependent on opioids an initial dose of 0.1 mg per 70 kg is recommended; if there is no evidence of withdrawal symptoms within 2 minutes the usual dosage may be used.

Although nalmefene has a longer duration of action than naloxone, all patients should be closely observed and if respiratory depression does recur, the dose of nalmefene should be titrated as above to avoid over-reversal of opioid effects.

Alcohol withdrawal and abstinence. Nalmefene is being studied[1] as an alternative to naltrexone in the adjunctive management of patients with alcohol dependence (p.1131).
1. Mason BJ, *et al.* A double-blind, placebo-controlled pilot study to evaluate the efficacy and safety of oral nalmefene HCl for alcohol dependence. *Alcohol Clin Exp Res* 1994; **18:** 1162–7.

Pruritus. It has been hypothesised that because central opioid receptors modulate itch, an opioid antagonist might block pruritus, and a number of opioid antagonists have been reported to be of benefit, although they are not part of the usual management of pruritus (p.1106).

Rapid improvement of severe pruritus was reported following a single oral dose of *nalmefene* 10 or 20 mg in a double-blind study of 80 patients with either chronic urticaria or atopic dermatitis.[1] Pruritus was almost completely eliminated in up to 60% of patients receiving nalmefene. Adverse effects occurred in 67% of patients and included dizziness or lightheadedness, fatigue, and nausea. In another study,[2] 14 patients with resistant pruritus secondary to cholestatic liver disease were treated with oral nalmefene for 2 to 26 months. The initial dose was 2 mg twice daily and the dose was increased gradually as necessary. Although 13 of the patients reported some amelioration of pruritus, 5 found that increasing doses were required to produce any benefit, and in 3 tolerance appeared to develop.

Continuous infusion of *naloxone* 0.2 μg per kg body-weight per minute was reported to reduce perception of pruritus and scratching activity in a double-blind study of 29 patients with pruritus due to cholestasis.[3] Although naloxone infusion is unlikely to have a role in the long-term management of this condition, longer acting oral opioid antagonists may be useful. In a double-blind study in 15 haemodialysis patients with severe resistant pruritus, administration of *naltrexone* 50 mg daily by mouth significantly reduced pruritus scores. However, the long term safety and benefit in this situation was not known.[4]
1. Monroe EW. Efficacy and safety of nalmefene in patients with severe pruritus caused by chronic urticaria and atopic dermatitis. *J Am Acad Dermatol* 1989; **21:** 135–6.
2. Bergasa NV, *et al.* Open-label trial of oral nalmefene therapy for the pruritus of cholestasis. *Hepatology* 1998; **27:** 679–84.
3. Bergasa NV, *et al.* Effects of naloxone infusions in patients with the pruritus of cholestasis. *Ann Intern Med* 1995; **123:** 161–7.
4. Peer G, *et al.* Randomised crossover trial of naltrexone in uraemic pruritus. *Lancet* 1996; **348:** 1552–4.

Preparations

Proprietary Preparations (details are given in Part 3)
USA: Revex.

Nalorphine (17967-m)

Nalorphine *(BAN, rINN)*.

(–)-(5R,6S)-9a-Allyl-4,5-epoxymorphin-7-en-3,6-diol; 17-Allyl-17-normorphine.

$C_{19}H_{21}NO_3 = 311.4$.

CAS — 62-67-9.
ATC — V03AB02.

Nalorphine Hydrobromide (7304-k)

Nalorphine Hydrobromide *(BANM, rINNM)*.

$C_{19}H_{21}NO_3, HBr = 392.3$.

Pharmacopoeias. In Chin. and It.

Nalorphine Hydrochloride (7305-a)

Nalorphine Hydrochloride *(BANM, rINNM)*.

Nalorphini Hydrochloridum; Nalorphinium Chloride.

$C_{19}H_{21}NO_3, HCl = 347.8$.

CAS — 57-29-4.
Pharmacopoeias. In US.

Pharmacopoeial description

USP 25: Store in airtight containers. Protect from light.

Adverse Effects and Precautions

Nalorphine may give rise to drowsiness, respiratory depression, miosis, dysphoria, and lethargy.

Nalorphine can induce an acute withdrawal syndrome in opioid-dependent patients.

Uses and Administration

Nalorphine is an opioid antagonist with properties similar to those of naloxone (below); in addition it also possesses some agonist properties. It reverses severe opioid-induced respiratory depression but may exacerbate respiratory depression such as that induced by alcohol or other non-opioid central depressants.

Nalorphine has been used as the hydrobromide or hydrochloride in the treatment of opioid-induced respiratory depression. A dose of 5 to 10 mg has been given by intravenous injection, repeated every 10 to 15 minutes as necessary until respiration is restored, with a maximum total dosage of 40 mg. It has also been given intramuscularly.

Preparations

USP 25: Nalorphine Hydrochloride Injection.

Naloxone Hydrochloride (7306-t)

Naloxone Hydrochloride *(BANM, USAN, rINNM)*.

N-Allylnoroxymorphone Hydrochloride; Cloridrato de Naloxona; EN-15304; Naloxoni Hydrochloridum. 17-Allyl-6-deoxy-7,8-dihydro-14-hydroxy-6-oxo-17-normorphine hydrochloride dihydrate; (–)-(5R,14S)-9a-Allyl-4,5-epoxy-3,14-dihydroxymorphinan-6-one hydrochloride dihydrate.

$C_{19}H_{21}NO_4, HCl, 2H_2O = 399.9$.

CAS — 465-65-6 (naloxone); 357-08-4 (anhydrous naloxone hydrochloride); 51481-60-8 (naloxone hydrochloride dihydrate).

Pharmacopoeias. In Eur. (see p.vi), Int., and US. Forms specified may be anhydrous, dihydrate, or both.

Pharmacopoeial description

Ph. Eur.: It contains two molecules of water of hydration. A white or almost white, hygroscopic, crystalline powder. Freely soluble in water; soluble in alcohol; practically insoluble in toluene. Store in airtight containers. Protect from light.

USP 25: It is anhydrous or contains two molecules of water of hydration. A white to slightly off-white powder. Soluble in water, in dilute acids, and in strong alkali; slightly soluble in alcohol; practically insoluble in chloroform and in ether. Its aqueous solution is acidic. Store in airtight containers. Protect from light.

Incompatibility. It is recommended that infusions of naloxone hydrochloride should not be mixed with preparations containing bisulfite, metabisulfite, long-chain or high-molecular-weight anions, or solutions with an alkaline pH.

Adverse Effects

Nausea and vomiting have occurred with naloxone. Some adverse effects may be associated with opioid withdrawal. There have been individual reports of hypotension, hypertension, cardiac arrhythmias, and pulmonary oedema, generally in patients given naloxone postoperatively. Seizures have also been reported infrequently.

◊ Hypertension,[1,2] pulmonary oedema,[3] and cardiac arrhythmias including ventricular tachycardia and fibrillation[4] have been reported following the use of naloxone postoperatively, generally in patients with pre-existing heart disease undergoing cardiac surgery. However, pulmonary oedema has also been reported in 2 healthy young men[5,6] following naloxone administration, in one case fatal,[6] although the role of naloxone in these cases has been questioned.[7]

Hypotension, bradycardia, and precipitation of focal seizures have been reported in patients receiving naloxone 4 mg per kg body-weight initially then a 24-hour infusion of 2 mg per kg per hour following acute stroke.[8]

Ventricular fibrillation has been observed in an opioid addict after administration of naloxone to reverse the effects of diamorphine.[9] However, this patient was later shown to have hepatic cirrhosis and alcoholic cardiomyopathy and the National Poisons Information Service in London noted that it had never been informed of such a suspected adverse reaction despite being contacted in about 800 cases of opioid poisoning each year.[10] More recently, severe adverse effects were reported to have occurred in 6 of 453 subjects given naloxone to reverse diamorphine intoxication.[11] The effects were: asystole (1 case), generalised convulsions (3 cases), pulmonary oedema (1 case), and violent behaviour (1 case).
1. Tanaka GY. Hypertensive reaction to naloxone. *JAMA* 1974; **228:** 25–6.
2. Azar I, Turndorf H. Severe hypertension and multiple atrial premature contractions following naloxone administration. *Anesth Analg* 1979; **58:** 524–5.
3. Flacke JW, *et al.* Acute pulmonary edema following naloxone reversal of high-dose morphine anesthesia. *Anesthesiology* 1977; **47:** 376–8.
4. Michaelis LL, *et al.* Ventricular irritability associated with the use of naloxone hydrochloride: two case reports and laboratory assessment of the effects of the drug on cardiac excitability. *Ann Thorac Surg* 1974; **18:** 608–14.
5. Taff RH. Pulmonary edema following naloxone administration in a patient without heart disease. *Anesthesiology* 1983; **59:** 576–7.

6. Wride SRN, *et al.* A fatal case of pulmonary oedema in a healthy young male following naloxone administration. *Anaesth Intensive Care* 1989; **17:** 374–7.
7. Allen T. No adverse reaction. *Ann Emerg Med* 1989; **18:** 116.
8. Barsan WG, *et al.* Use of high dose naloxone in acute stroke: possible side effects. *Crit Care Med* 1989; **17:** 762–7.
9. Cuss FM, *et al.* Cardiac arrest after reversal of effects of opiates with naloxone. *BMJ* 1984; **288:** 363–4.
10. Barret L, *et al.* Cardiac arrest following naloxone. *BMJ* 1984; **288:** 936.
11. Osterwalder JJ. Naloxone—for intoxications with intravenous heroin and heroin mixtures—harmless or hazardous? A prospective clinical study. *Clin Toxicol* 1996; **34:** 409–16.

Precautions

Naloxone should be used with caution in patients physically dependent on opioids, or who have received large doses of opioids, as an acute withdrawal syndrome may be precipitated (see Dependence under Opioid Analgesics, p.66). A withdrawal syndrome may also be precipitated in newborn infants of opioid-dependent mothers.

Naloxone should be used with caution in patients with cardiac problems or those receiving cardiotoxic drugs.

The duration of action of some opioids exceeds that of naloxone; patients should therefore be carefully observed after administration in case of relapse.

Pharmacokinetics

Naloxone is absorbed from the gastrointestinal tract but it is subject to considerable first-pass metabolism. It is metabolised in the liver, mainly by glucuronide conjugation, and excreted in the urine. It has a short plasma half-life of approximately one hour after parenteral administration.

Pregnancy and the neonate. A study in 30 mothers given a single intravenous dose of naloxone during the second stage of labour, indicated that naloxone rapidly crossed the placental barrier so that some therapeutic effect might be anticipated in most babies.[1] Placental transfer in 7 further mothers given naloxone intramuscularly was considered to be too variable for therapeutic purposes.

In 12 newborn infants given naloxone hydrochloride 35 or 70 μg intravenously via the umbilical vein, the mean plasma half-life of naloxone was 3.53 and 2.65 hours respectively.[2] These half-lives were 2 to 3 times longer than those reported for adults, possibly due to a diminished ability of the newborn to metabolise drugs by conjugation with glucuronic acid. Mean peak plasma concentrations of 8.2 nanograms per mL in those given 35 μg, and 13.7 nanograms per mL in those given 70 μg, were reached within 40 minutes of administration but this time was very variable, and in 5 infants peak plasma concentrations were reached within 5 minutes. When naloxone hydrochloride 200 μg was administered intramuscularly to 17 further newborn infants, peak concentrations of 7.4 to 34.6 nanograms per mL occurred at 0.5 to 2 hours.

1. Hibbard BM, *et al.* Placental transfer of naloxone. *Br J Anaesth* 1986; **58:** 45–8.
2. Moreland TA, *et al.* Naloxone pharmacokinetics in the newborn. *Br J Clin Pharmacol* 1980; **9:** 609–12.

Uses and Administration

Naloxone is a specific opioid antagonist that acts competitively at opioid receptors. It is an effective antagonist of opioids with agonist or mixed agonist-antagonist activity though larger doses may be needed for compounds with the latter activity and for codeine, dextropropoxyphene, and methadone. It is used to reverse opioid central depression, including respiratory depression, induced by natural or synthetic opioids in the following situations: in the treatment of known or suspected opioid overdosage; postoperatively following the use of opioids during surgery; in neonates following the administration of opioid analgesics to the mother during labour.

Naloxone hydrochloride is usually given intravenously for a rapid onset of action which occurs within 2 minutes. The onset of action is only slightly less rapid when it is given intramuscularly or subcutaneously; sublingual and endotracheal administration have also been suggested. The duration of action of naloxone is dependent on the dose and route of administration; it may be 1 to 4 hours or much shorter.

In the treatment of known or suspected **opioid overdosage**, the initial dose of naloxone hydrochloride is 0.4 to 2 mg given intravenously and repeated if necessary at intervals of 2 to 3 minutes. If no response has been observed after a total dose of 10 mg then the

diagnosis of overdosage with drugs other than opioids should be considered. If the patient is suspected of being physically dependent on opioids the dose may be reduced to 0.1 to 0.2 mg to avoid precipitating withdrawal symptoms. In children, the usual initial dose is 10 μg per kg body-weight intravenously followed, if necessary, by a larger dose of 100 μg per kg (for an alternative children's dose suggested in the USA to treat opioid intoxication, see under Administration, below). In both adults and children, if the intravenous route is not feasible the intramuscular or subcutaneous route can be used.

Naloxone hydrochloride may also be used **postoperatively** to reverse central depression resulting from the use of opioids during surgery. A dose of 100 to 200 μg (1.5 to 3 μg per kg) may be given intravenously at intervals of at least 2 minutes, titrated for each patient in order to obtain an optimum respiratory response while maintaining adequate analgesia.

All patients receiving naloxone should be closely observed as the duration of action of some opioids exceeds that of naloxone and repeated doses by intravenous, intramuscular, or subcutaneous injection may be required. Alternatively, to sustain opioid antagonism, an intravenous infusion of naloxone hydrochloride has been suggested. Naloxone hydrochloride 4 μg per mL in sodium chloride 0.9% or glucose 5% may be infused at a rate titrated in accordance with the patient's response, both to the infusion and previous bolus injections; a rate of 0.4 to 0.8 mg per hour has been suggested.

Opioid-induced depression in **neonates** resulting from the administration of opioid analgesics to the mother during labour may be reversed by administering naloxone hydrochloride 10 μg per kg body-weight to the infant by intravenous, intramuscular, or subcutaneous injection, repeated at intervals of 2 to 3 minutes if necessary. Alternatively, a single intramuscular dose of about 60 μg per kg may be given at birth for a more prolonged action. Naloxone should be given with caution to the infants of opioid dependent mothers since withdrawal symptoms can result.

Some opioid analgesics have been formulated in combination with naloxone hydrochloride to reduce their potential for parenteral abuse. Naloxone hydrochloride has also been used cautiously in small doses to diagnose opioid dependence by precipitating the withdrawal syndrome (see below and under Naltrexone Hydrochloride, p.1016).

Administration. INFANTS AND CHILDREN. The Committee on Drugs of the American Academy of Pediatrics[1,2] has recommended a dose of 100 μg of naloxone per kg body-weight by intravenous or intratracheal administration for neonates, including premature infants, to the age of 5 years or 20 kg bodyweight for treatment of *opioid intoxication*. Children over 5 years or 20 kg body-weight should be given a minimum of 2 mg. These doses may be repeated as necessary to maintain opioid reversal. The use of injections containing 0.02 mg per mL of naloxone hydrochloride are no longer recommended because of the fluid load involved at these doses, especially in small neonates.

1. American Academy of Pediatrics. Emergency drug doses for infants and children and naloxone use in newborns: classification. *Pediatrics* 1989; **83:** 803.
2. American Academy of Pediatrics. Naloxone dosage and route of administration for infants and children: addendum to emergency drug doses for infants and children. *Pediatrics* 1990; **86:** 484–5.

Eating disorders. Endogenous opioids may have a role in the pathophysiology of eating disorders,[1] thus opioid antagonists such as naloxone and naltrexone have been tried in their management. However, their role appears to be limited and opioid antagonists do not form part of the usual management of these conditions.

1. de Zwaan M, Mitchell JE. Opiate antagonists and eating behavior in humans: a review. *J Clin Pharmacol* 1992; **32:** 1060–72.

Non-opioid overdosage. In addition to reversing the effects of exogenous opioids, naloxone also antagonises the action of endogenous opioids. This may explain the varying responses reported to naloxone used in the treatment of overdosage with non-opioids, some of which may modulate endogenous opioids.

Naloxone was successfully used to reverse intoxication with *camylofin* in 2 infants.[1]

The response of patients with *clonidine* intoxication to naloxone has been inconsistent. There have been reports of benefit in some patients,[2-7] while other studies have been una-

ble to demonstrate any beneficial effects;[8,9] hypertension has been reported in some patients.[4,6,7]

Results suggesting that naloxone may reverse sedation and respiratory depression produced by *benzodiazepines*[10] have not been supported.[11,12]

1. Schvartsman S, *et al.* Camylofin intoxication reversed by naloxone. *Lancet* 1988; **ii:** 1246.
2. Kulig K, *et al.* Naloxone for treatment of clonidine overdose. *JAMA* 1982; **247:** 1697.
3. Niemann JT, *et al.* Reversal of clonidine toxicity by naloxone. *Ann Emerg Med* 1986; **15:** 1229–31.
4. Gremse DA, *et al.* Hypertension associated with naloxone treatment for clonidine poisoning. *J Pediatr* 1986; **108:** 776–8.
5. Wedin GP, Edwards JL. Clonidine poisoning treated with naloxone. *Am J Emerg Med* 1989; **7:** 343–4.
6. Fiser DH, *et al.* Critical care for clonidine poisoning in toddlers. *Crit Care Med* 1990; **18:** 1124–8.
7. Wiley JF, *et al.* Clonidine poisoning in young children. *J Pediatr* 1990; **116:** 654–8.
8. Rogers JF, Cubeddu LX. Naloxone does not antagonize the antihypertensive effect of clonidine in essential hypertension. *Clin Pharmacol Ther* 1983; **34:** 68–73.
9. Banner W, *et al.* Failure of naloxone to reverse clonidine toxic effect. *Am J Dis Child* 1983; **137:** 1170–1.
10. Jordan C, *et al.* Effect of naloxone on respiratory changes after diazepam. *Br J Anaesth* 1979; **51:** 570P.
11. Christensen KN, Hüttel M. Naloxone does not antagonize diazepam-induced sedation. *Anesthesiology* 1979; **51:** 187.
12. Forster A, *et al.* Respiratory depressant effects of different doses of midazolam and lack of reversal with naloxone—a double-blind randomized study. *Anesth Analg* 1983; **62:** 920–4.

Postoperative use. Naloxone is used postoperatively to reverse central depression resulting from the use of opioids during surgery. However, it may antagonise the analgesic effects of the opioids in the control of postoperative pain, and the increasing use of short-acting intravenous opioid analgesics should reduce the need for its use.

Pruritus. For reference to the use of opioid antagonists, including naloxone, in the management of pruritus, see under Nalmefene Hydrochloride, p.1014

Reversal of opioid effects. Naloxone has been reported to alleviate some of the adverse effects of opioids without loss of therapeutic efficacy. Naloxone reversed respiratory depression in a patient given intrathecal morphine,[1] and urinary retention in 3 patients after epidural morphine,[2] without reversing analgesia. Naloxone given intravenously has been shown to reverse the delay in gastric emptying induced by opioid analgesics in healthy subjects[3] and in women during labour.[4] Continuous intravenous infusion of naloxone reduced the incidence of adverse effects in patients receiving morphine by patient-controlled analgesia for postoperative pain.[5] Pain control was not compromised and the lower dose of naloxone used (0.25 μg per kg body-weight hourly as opposed to 1 μg per kg hourly) appeared to have an opioid-sparing effect. In patients receiving long-term opioids, oral naloxone in a daily dose equivalent to 20 to 40% of the daily opioid dose relieved opioid-induced constipation without compromising analgesic control.[6,7] Doses equivalent to 10% or less of the opioid dose were ineffective.[8] Other opioid antagonists that are under investigation for similar indications include methylnaltrexone.[9]

See also Postoperative Use, above.

1. Jones RDM, Jones JG. Intrathecal morphine: naloxone reverses respiratory depression but not analgesia. *BMJ* 1980; **281:** 645–6.
2. Rawal N, *et al.* Naloxone reversal of urinary retention after epidural morphine. *Lancet* 1981; **ii:** 1411.
3. Nimmo WS, *et al.* Reversal of narcotic-induced delay in gastric emptying and paracetamol absorption by naloxone. *BMJ* 1979; **2:** 1189.
4. Frame WT, *et al.* Effect of naloxone on gastric emptying during labour. *Br J Anaesth* 1984; **56:** 263–5.
5. Gan TJ, *et al.* Opioid-sparing effects of a low-dose infusion of naloxone in patient-administered morphine sulfate. *Anesthesiology* 1997; **87:** 1075–81.
6. Sykes NP. Oral naloxone in opioid-associated constipation. *Lancet* 1991; **337:** 1475.
7. Sykes NP. Oral naloxone in opioid-associated constipation. *Lancet* 1991; **338:** 582.
8. Robinson BA, *et al.* Oral naloxone in opioid-associated constipation. *Lancet* 1991; **338:** 581–2.
9. Yuan C-S, *et al.* The safety and efficacy of oral methylnaltrexone in preventing morphine-induced delay in oral-cecal transit time. *Clin Pharmacol Ther* 1997; **61:** 467–75.

DIAGNOSTIC USE. Naloxone is used to reverse opioid effects in the diagnosis of opioid overdose, although some workers have recommended that administration should be restricted to those patients with clinical signs of opioid overdose.[1]

Naloxone has been given intravenously, to precipitate withdrawal symptoms in the diagnosis of opioid dependence and methods that do not induce acute withdrawal have also been investigated. One study[2] reported that pupillary dilatation in response to naloxone hydrochloride solution 1 mg per mL applied conjunctivally could distinguish patients with a physical dependence from non-dependent patients who had received opioids on a single occasion as pre-operative medication, but this response was not confirmed in another study[3] using naloxone 0.4 mg per mL solution. Furthermore there has been a report[4] of withdrawal syndrome and pupillary dilatation occurring in 4 opioid dependent subjects following instillation of naloxone solution 40 mg per mL.

1. Hoffman JR, *et al.* The empiric use of naloxone in patients with altered mental status: a reappraisal. *Ann Emerg Med* 1991; **20:** 246–52.
2. Creighton FJ, Ghodse AH. Naloxone applied to conjunctiva as a test for physical opiate dependence. *Lancet* 1989; **i:** 748–50.

3. Loimer N, *et al.* Conjunctival naloxone is no decision aid in opioid addiction. *Lancet* 1990; **335:** 1107–8.
4. Sanchez-Ramos JR, Senay EC. Ophthalmic naloxone elicits abstinence in opioid-dependent subjects. *Br J Addict* 1987; **82:** 313–15.

Preparations

BP 2001: Naloxone Injection; Neonatal Naloxone Injection;
USP 25: Naloxone Hydrochloride Injection; Pentazocine and Naloxone Hydrochlorides Tablets.

Proprietary Preparations (details are given in Part 3)

Aust.: Narcanti; *Austral.:* Narcan; *Belg.:* Narcan; *Braz.:* Narcan; *Canad.:* Narcan; *Denm.:* Narcanti; *Fin.:* Narcanti; *Fr.:* Nalone; Narcan; *Ger.:* Narcanti; *Hong Kong:* Narcan; *Irl.:* Narcan; *Israel:* Narcan; *Ital.:* Narcan; *Mex.:* Narcanti; *Norw.:* Narcanti; *NZ:* Narcan; *Port.:* Narcan; Naxolan; *S.Afr.:* Narcan; Zynox; *Singapore:* Narcan; *Swed.:* Narcanti; *Switz.:* Narcan; *Thai.:* Narcan; *UK:* Narcan; *USA:* Narcan.

Multi-ingredient: *Ger.:* Andolor; Nalidin; *Israel:* Rafazocine X.

Used as an adjunct in: Belg.: Valtran; *Ger.:* Findol N; Gruntin Tropfen; Tili; Tili-Puren; Tilicomp; Tilidalor; Tilidin comp; Tilidin N; Tilidin plus; Tilidin-saar; Tiligetic; Tilimerck; tilnalox; Valoron N; *Israel:* Talwin NX; *NZ:* Temgesic-nx; *USA:* Talwin NX.

Naltrexone Hydrochloride (7307-x)

Naltrexone Hydrochloride (BANM, rINNM).

EN-1639A. (5R)-9a-Cyclopropylmethyl-3,14-dihydroxy-4,5-epoxymorphinan-6-one hydrochloride; 17-(Cyclopropylmethyl)-4,5α-epoxy-3,14-dihydroxymorphinan-6-one hydrochloride.

$C_{20}H_{23}NO_4,HCl = 377.9$.

CAS — 16590-41-3 (naltrexone); 16676-29-2 (naltrexone hydrochloride).

NOTE. Naltrexone is *USAN.*

Pharmacopoeias. In *US.*

Pharmacopoeial description

USP 25: Store in airtight containers.

Adverse Effects

Difficulty in sleeping, loss of energy, anxiety, dysphoria, abdominal pain, nausea, vomiting, reduction in appetite, joint and muscle pain, and headache may occur with naltrexone. Other side-effects including dizziness, constipation, diarrhoea, skin rashes, and reduced potency and ejaculatory difficulties have also been reported. Some adverse effects may be associated with opioid withdrawal. Thrombocytopenic purpura has occurred rarely. High doses may cause hepatocellular injury.

Effects on the liver. Increased liver enzyme values were reported in 6 of 40 obese patients receiving naltrexone 50 or 100 mg daily for eight weeks.[1] Five of the six patients had minimally abnormal liver function before naltrexone was administered and liver function tests returned to baseline values or better on discontinuing naltrexone.

Raised transaminase levels were noted in 5 of 26 obese patients after 3 weeks' treatment with naltrexone 300 mg daily; transaminase activity returned to normal when treatment was stopped.[2]

1. Atkinson RL, *et al.* Effects of long-term therapy with naltrexone on body weight in obesity. *Clin Pharmacol Ther* 1985; **38:** 419–22.
2. Mitchell JE. Naltrexone and hepatotoxicity. *Lancet* 1986; **i:** 1215.

Precautions

Naltrexone should be avoided in patients taking opioids for medication or abuse as an acute withdrawal syndrome may be precipitated (see Dependence under Opioid Analgesics, p.66). Withdrawal symptoms may develop within 5 minutes and last up to 48 hours. Naltrexone should be discontinued at least 48 hours before elective surgery involving opioid analgesia. For further precautions when administering naltrexone as an adjunct in the treatment of opioid dependence, see under Uses and Administration, below.

When analgesia is required, larger doses than usual of opioids will be needed and there is an increased risk of respiratory depression and other adverse effects.

Naltrexone should be used with caution in patients with hepatic dysfunction and is contra-indicated in patients with acute hepatitis or liver failure. Regular monitoring of hepatic function has been recommended. Naltrexone should be given with caution to patients with impaired renal function.

Pharmacokinetics

Naltrexone is well absorbed from the gastrointestinal tract but is subject to considerable first-pass metabolism and may undergo enterohepatic recycling. It is extensively metabolised in the liver and the major metabolite, 6-β-naltrexol may also possess weak opioid antagonist activity. Maximum plasma concentrations of naltrexone and 6-β-naltrexol are achieved in about 1 hour and naltrexone is about 20% bound to plasma proteins at therapeutic doses. The elimination half-life of naltrexone is approximately 4 hours and that of 6-β-naltrexol about 13 hours. Naltrexone and its metabolites are excreted mainly in the urine. Less than 1% of an oral dose of naltrexone is excreted unchanged.

◊ References.

1. Verebey K, *et al.* Naltrexone: disposition, metabolism, and effects after acute and chronic dosing. *Clin Pharmacol Ther* 1976; **20:** 315–28.
2. Wall ME, *et al.* Metabolism and disposition of naltrexone in man after oral and intravenous administration. *Drug Metab Dispos* 1981; **9:** 369–75.
3. Wall ME, *et al.* Naltrexone disposition in man after subcutaneous administration. *Drug Metab Dispos* 1984; **12:** 677–82.
4. Meyer MC, *et al.* Bioequivalence, dose-proportionality, and pharmacokinetics of naltrexone after oral administration. *J Clin Psychiatry* 1984; **45:** 15–19.
5. Chiang CN, *et al.* Kinetics of a naltrexone sustained-release preparation. *Clin Pharmacol Ther* 1984; **36:** 704–8.

Uses and Administration

Naltrexone is a specific opioid antagonist with actions similar to those of naloxone (p.1015); however, it is more potent than naloxone and has a longer duration of action.

It is used in the treatment of **opioid dependence** as an aid to maintaining abstinence following opioid withdrawal. Naltrexone treatment should not be started until the patient has been detoxified and abstinent from opioids for at least 7 to 10 days because of the risk of acute withdrawal; abstinence should be verified by analysis of the patient's urine. A *naloxone challenge test* should then be administered to confirm the absence of opioid dependence, as follows: naloxone hydrochloride 200 µg is administered intravenously and the patient observed for 30 seconds for evidence of withdrawal symptoms; if none occur a further dose of 600 µg is given and the patient observed for 30 minutes. A confirmatory rechallenge with naloxone hydrochloride 1.6 mg intravenously may be considered if results are ambiguous. Sources in the USA suggest a naloxone challenge test with a single dose of 800 µg given subcutaneously as an alternative to the intravenous route.

Once a negative naloxone challenge test has been obtained, naltrexone hydrochloride is given by mouth to *treat* opioid dependence. Treatment may be initiated with a dose of 25 mg. If no signs of opioid withdrawal occur subsequent doses may be increased to 50 mg daily. The usual maintenance dose of naltrexone hydrochloride is 350 mg weekly administered as 50 mg daily, but the dosing interval may be lengthened to improve compliance; for example, doses of 100 mg on Monday and Wednesday and 150 mg on Friday may be effective and various other intermittent dosage regimens have been used. Patients should be carefully counselled and warned that attempts to overcome the opioid blockade with large doses of opioids could result in fatal opioid intoxication.

Naltrexone hydrochloride is also used as an adjunct in the management of **alcohol dependence** and the recommended dose is 50 mg daily.

Alcohol withdrawal and abstinence. Naltrexone may be of use as an adjunct to psychotherapy in maintaining abstinence after alcohol withdrawal in patients with alcohol dependence (p.1131). Short-term studies[1,2] of 12 weeks' duration indicate that it is of benefit for reducing alcohol craving and the severity and number of relapses. Data on long-term efficacy are limited but some benefit may persist after withdrawal of treatment.[3] Reports[4] from patients who continued to drink during therapy suggest that naltrexone may reduce the pleasure associated with drinking, possibly by blocking the effect of endorphins released as a result of alcohol consumption.[5] It has been suggested[6] that naltrexone should be given for a minimum of 6 months because of the high relapse rates usually seen during the first 3 to 6 months following alcohol withdrawal. Although

naltrexone does not appear to be hepatotoxic at the dosage of 50 mg daily used for alcohol dependence caution is recommended in patients with liver disease.[6] Concurrent use with disulfiram, which is potentially hepatotoxic, is not usually recommended.[5]

1. Volpicelli JR, *et al.* Naltrexone in the treatment of alcohol dependence. *Arch Gen Psychiatry* 1992; **49:** 876–80.
2. O'Malley SS, *et al.* Naltrexone and coping skills therapy for alcohol dependence: a controlled study. *Arch Gen Psychiatry* 1992; **49:** 881–7.
3. O'Malley SS, *et al.* Six-month follow-up of naltrexone and psychotherapy for alcohol dependence. *Arch Gen Psychiatry* 1996; **53:** 217–24.
4. Volpicelli JR, *et al.* Effect of naltrexone on alcohol "high" in alcoholics. *Am J Psychiatry* 1995; **152:** 613–15.
5. Anonymous. Naltrexone for alcohol dependence. *Med Lett Drugs Ther* 1995; **37:** 64–6.
6. Berg BJ, *et al.* A risk-benefit assessment of naltrexone in the treatment of alcohol dependence. *Drug Safety* 1996; **15:** 274–82.

Opioid dependence. MAINTENANCE. Naltrexone is a long-acting, non-addictive oral opioid antagonist. Although it can be effective in maintaining abstinence in opioid addicts following detoxification, compliance with therapy is difficult to maintain because although it blocks the euphoriant effects of opioids it does not block the craving for narcotics. It is thus most effective in highly motivated addicts with good sociological and psychological support to discourage impulsive use of opioids.

For a discussion of the management of opioid dependence, see p.66.

References.

1. Crabtree BL. Review of naltrexone, a long-acting opiate antagonist. *Clin Pharm* 1984; **3:** 273–80.
2. Anonymous. Naltrexone for opioid addiction. *Med Lett Drugs Ther* 1985; **27:** 11–12.
3. Ginzburg HM, MacDonald MG. The role of naltrexone in the management of drug abuse. *Med Toxicol* 1987; **2:** 83–92.
4. Gonzalez JP, Brogden RN. Naltrexone: a review of its pharmacodynamic and pharmacokinetic properties and therapeutic efficacy in the management of opioid dependence. *Drugs* 1988; **35:** 192–213.
5. Kirchmayer U, *et al.* Naltrexone maintenance treatment for opioid dependence (updated 29 August 2001). Available in The Cochrane Library; Issue 4. Oxford: Update Software; 2001.

RAPID DETOXIFICATION. Use of clonidine with naltrexone enabled 38 of 40 opioid addicts to withdraw completely from long-term methadone therapy within 4 or 5 days.[1] Modification of the regimen allowed opioid withdrawal over 2 to 3 days.[2] The experimental technique of rapid detoxification with naltrexone while the patient is anaesthetised is controversial.

1. Charney DS, *et al.* The combined use of clonidine and naltrexone as a rapid, safe and effective treatment of abrupt withdrawal from methadone. *Am J Psychiatry* 1986; **143:** 831–7.
2. Brewer C, *et al.* Opioid withdrawal and naltrexone induction in 48–72 hours with minimal drop-out, using a modification of the naltrexone-clonidine technique. *Br J Psychiatry* 1988; **153:** 340–3.

Pruritus. For reference to the use of opioid antagonists, including naltrexone, in pruritus, see under Nalmefene Hydrochloride, p.1014.

Preparations

USP 25: Naltrexone Hydrochloride Tablets.

Proprietary Preparations (details are given in Part 3)

Aust.: Nemexin; Revia; *Austral.:* Revia; *Canad.:* Revia; *Denm.:* Revia; *Fin.:* Revia; *Fr.:* Nalorex; *Ger.:* Nemexin; *Hong Kong:* Trexan; *Irl.:* Nalorex; Revia; *Israel:* Antaxone; Nalorex; Narcoral; *Port.:* Antaxone; Basinal; Nalorex; *Singapore:* Trexan; *Spain:* Antaxone; Celupan; Revia; *Switz.:* Nemexin; *Thai.:* Revia; *UK:* Nalorex; *USA:* Depade; Revia; Trexan.

Obidoxime Chloride (1043-w)

Obidoxime Chloride (USAN, rINN).

LüH6. 1,1'-[Oxybis(methylene)]bis[4-(hydroxyimino)methyl]pyridinium dichloride.

$C_{14}H_{16}Cl_2N_4O_3 = 359.2$.

CAS — 7683-36-5 (obidoxime); 114-90-9 (obidoxime chloride).

Profile

Obidoxime chloride is a cholinesterase reactivator with similar actions and uses to pralidoxime (p.1020). It is given in conjunction with atropine in the treatment of organophosphorus poisoning in usual adult doses of 250 mg by slow intravenous injection; it has also been given by intramuscular injection.

◊ References.

1. Thiermann H, *et al.* Cholinesterase status, pharmacokinetics and laboratory findings during obidoxime therapy in organophosphate poisoned patients. *Hum Exp Toxicol* 1997; **16:** 473–80.

Preparations

Proprietary Preparations (details are given in Part 3)

Aust.: Toxogonin; *Denm.:* Toxogonin; *Ger.:* Toxogonin; *Neth.:* Toxogonin; *S.Afr.:* Toxogonin; *Swed.:* Toxogonin; *Switz.:* Toxogonin†.

Penicillamine (1045-I)

Penicillamine (BAN, USAN, rINN).

D-Penicillamine; Penicillaminum. D-3,3-Dimethylcysteine; D-3-Mercaptovaline.

$C_5H_{11}NO_2S = 149.2$.

CAS — 52-67-5 (penicillamine); 2219-30-9 (penicillamine hydrochloride).

ATC — M01CC01.

Pharmacopoeias. In Eur. (see p.vi), Int., Pol., and US.

Pharmacopoeial description

Ph. Eur.: A white or almost white, crystalline powder. Freely soluble in water; slightly soluble in alcohol; practically insoluble in ether. A 1% solution in water has a pH of 4.5 to 5.5.

USP 25: A white or practically white, crystalline powder having a slight characteristic odour. Freely soluble in water; slightly soluble in alcohol; insoluble in chloroform and in ether. pH of a 1% solution in water is between 4.5 and 5.5. Store in airtight containers.

Adverse Effects and Treatment

Side-effects of penicillamine are frequent. Gastrointestinal disturbances including anorexia, nausea, and vomiting may occur; oral ulceration and stomatitis have been reported and impaired taste sensitivity is common.

Skin rashes occurring early in treatment are commonly allergic and may be associated with pruritus, urticaria, and fever; they are usually transient but temporary drug withdrawal and treatment with corticosteroids or antihistamines may be required. Lupus erythematosus and pemphigus have been reported. A Stevens-Johnson-like syndrome has been observed during penicillamine treatment. Prolonged use of high doses may affect skin collagen and elastin, resulting in increased skin friability, eruptions resembling elastosis perforans serpiginosa, and a late rash or acquired epidermolysis bullosa (penicillamine dermatopathy) that may necessitate dosage reduction or discontinuation.

Haematological side-effects have included thrombocytopenia and less frequently leucopenia; these are usually reversible but agranulocytosis and aplastic anaemia have occurred and fatalities have been reported. Haemolytic anaemia has also occurred.

Proteinuria occurs frequently and in some patients may progress to glomerulonephritis or nephrotic syndrome. Penicillamine-induced haematuria is rare but normally requires immediate discontinuation.

Other side-effects associated with penicillamine include Goodpasture's syndrome, bronchiolitis and pneumonitis, myasthenia gravis, polymyositis (rarely with cardiac involvement), intrahepatic cholestasis, and pancreatitis.

◊ References describing the range and incidence of adverse effects associated with of D-penicillamine.[1,2] The L or DL forms are much more toxic.[3]

1. Kean WF, et al. Efficacy and toxicity of D-penicillamine for rheumatoid disease in the elderly. J Am Geriatr Soc 1982; 30: 94–100.
2. Steen VD, et al. The toxicity of D-penicillamine in systemic sclerosis. Ann Intern Med 1986; 104: 699–705.
3. Kean WF, et al. Chirality in antirheumatic drugs. Lancet 1991; 338: 1565–8.

Effects on the blood. Of the 18 deaths ascribed to penicillamine reported to the UK Committee on Safety of Medicines between January 1964 and December 1977, 14 were apparently due to blood disorders, at least 7 of them being marrow aplasias. The myelotoxicity of penicillamine was reviewed in 10 patients with confirmed or suspected marrow depression during penicillamine treatment for rheumatoid arthritis or scleroderma; 6 of these 10 patients died.[1]

An incidence of 12 to 27% of penicillamine-induced thrombocytopenia has been reported in patients with rheumatoid arthritis.[2] Thrombocytopenia appeared to be due to bone-marrow suppression and a reduced platelet-production rate. There have been isolated reports[3-5] of thrombotic thrombocytopenic purpura attributed to the use of penicillamine with some fatalities.

For a brief discussion of the genetic factors influencing myelotoxicity, see under Genetic Factors, below.

1. Kay AGL. Myelotoxicity of D-penicillamine. Ann Rheum Dis 1979; 38: 232–6.
2. Thomas D, et al. Thrombokinetics in patients with rheumatoid arthritis treated with D-penicillamine. Ann Rheum Dis 1984; 43: 402–6.
3. Ahmed F, et al. Thrombohemolytic thrombocytopenic purpura during penicillamine therapy. Arch Intern Med 1978; 138: 1292–3.

4. Speth PAJ, et al. Thrombotic thrombocytopenic purpura associated with D-penicillamine treatment in rheumatoid arthritis. J Rheumatol 1982; 9: 812–13.
5. Trice JM, et al. Thrombotic thrombocytopenic purpura during penicillamine therapy in rheumatoid arthritis. Arch Intern Med 1983; 143: 1487–8.

Effects on the breast. Breast enlargement has been reported both in women[1-4] and in men[5] taking penicillamine and may be a rare complication of penicillamine therapy. In some patients breast enlargement was prolonged with poor resolution and others required surgery. Danazol has been used successfully to treat penicillamine-induced breast gigantism.[2-4]

1. Thew DCN, Stewart IM. D penicillamine and breast enlargement. Ann Rheum Dis 1980; 39: 200.
2. Taylor PJ, et al. Successful treatment of D-penicillamine-induced breast gigantism with danazol. BMJ 1981; 282: 362–3.
3. Rooney PJ, Cleland J. Successful treatment of D-penicillamine-induced breast gigantism with danazol. BMJ 1981; 282: 1627–8.
4. Craig HR. Penicillamine induced mammary hyperplasia: report of a case and review of the literature. J Rheumatol 1988; 15: 1294–7.
5. Reid DM, et al. Reversible gynaecomastia associated with D-penicillamine in a man with rheumatoid arthritis. BMJ 1982; 285: 1083–4.

Effects on the gastrointestinal tract. There have been isolated reports of acute colitis in patients taking penicillamine.[1,2] Ileal ulceration and stenosis in a patient with Wilson's disease was considered to be related to elastosis probably resulting from long-term penicillamine therapy.[3]

1. Hickling P, Fuller J. Penicillamine causing acute colitis. BMJ 1979; 2: 367.
2. Grant GB. Penicillamine causing acute colitis. BMJ 1979; 2: 555.
3. Wassef M, et al. Unusual digestive lesions in a patient with Wilson's disease treated with long-term penicillamine. N Engl J Med 1985; 313: 49.

Effects on the heart. For reports of heart block, Stokes-Adams syndrome, and fatal myocarditis in patients taking penicillamine, see Polymyositis under Effects on the Muscles and the Neuromuscular System, below.

Effects on the kidneys. Proteinuria associated with penicillamine has usually occurred within 4 to 18 months of starting therapy though onset can be later. A greater incidence has been found in patients with rheumatoid arthritis and cystinuria than in those with Wilson's disease. The severity of proteinuria varies; proteinuria of nephrotic proportions usually develops rapidly but resolves on drug cessation. Minimal change, mesangioproliferative, and membranous nephropathy have all been associated with penicillamine treatment and progressive glomerulonephritis has been observed in a few patients who had developed features of Goodpasture's syndrome.[1]

Although there is some evidence of a relationship between nephropathy and penicillamine dose and its rate of increase,[1] a study of 33 rheumatoid arthritis patients with penicillamine-induced nephropathy found no correlation with the dose or duration of treatment.[2] Appreciable proteinuria could still be detected 12 months after stopping penicillamine in 40% of their patients, but subsequently resolved in those whose proteinuria was solely related to penicillamine.

Penicillamine was successfully reintroduced and administered for at least 13 months in 5 patients with rheumatoid arthritis who had developed proteinuria during the first course of therapy. Proteinuria did not recur.[3]

Corticosteroids have been used in patients developing rapidly progressive glomerulonephritis[4] but may be unnecessary and potentially hazardous in patients who develop the nephrotic syndrome.[2]

For reports of Goodpasture's syndrome in patients taking penicillamine, see also under Effects on the Respiratory System, below.

For a brief discussion of the genetic factors influencing renal toxicity, see under Genetic Factors, below.

1. Anonymous. Penicillamine nephropathy. BMJ 1981; 282: 761–2.
2. Hall CL, et al. Natural course of penicillamine nephropathy: a long term study of 33 patients. BMJ 1988; 296: 1083–6.
3. Hill H, et al. Resumption of treatment with penicillamine after proteinuria. Ann Rheum Dis 1979; 38: 229–31.
4. Ntoso KA, et al. Penicillamine-induced rapidly progressive glomerulonephritis in patients with progressive systemic sclerosis: successful treatment of two patients and a review of the literature. Am J Kidney Dis 1986; 8: 159–63.

Effects on the liver. In a report of a patient with penicillamine-associated hepatotoxicity and a review of other reports,[1] the 9 patients considered all had liver function profiles consistent with intrahepatic cholestasis; one patient died of acute renal failure but the others improved rapidly after drug withdrawal.[1] In a later report,[2] a 72-year-old man with rheumatoid arthritis developed jaundice approximately 4 weeks after starting penicillamine therapy. Liver biopsy indicated a slight degree of cholangitis with eosinophils in the portal tracts and severe predominantly intrahepatocellular cholestasis. Jaundice cleared within 3 weeks of stopping penicillamine and liver enzyme values approached normal after 6 weeks. Monitoring of liver function and eosinophil counts in the early weeks of penicillamine therapy was recommended.[1]

1. Seibold JR, et al. Cholestasis associated with D-penicillamine therapy: case report and review of the literature. Arthritis Rheum 1981; 24: 554–6.
2. Devogelaer JP, et al. A case of cholestatic hepatitis associated with D-penicillamine therapy for rheumatoid arthritis. Int J Clin Pharmacol Res 1985; 5: 35–8.

Effects on the muscles and the neuromuscular system. Neuromyotonia[1] and profound sensory and motor neuropathy have been reported in patients taking penicillamine. Symptoms improved rapidly after the initiation of pyridoxine supplementation.[2] Low back pain in conjunction with fever and rash developed in a patient during penicillamine treatment.[3] Fever and back pain recurred on rechallenge with penicillamine. It was suggested that an allergic mechanism was involved.

1. Reeback J, et al. Penicillamine-induced neuromyotonia. BMJ 1979; 1: 1464–5.
2. Pool KD, et al. Penicillamine-induced neuropathy in rheumatoid arthritis. Ann Intern Med 1981; 95: 457–8.
3. Bannwarth B, et al. Low back pain associated with penicillamine. BMJ 1991; 303: 525.

MYASTHENIA. Myasthenia gravis is a well recognised, though uncommon, complication of long-term penicillamine therapy.[1] Symptoms are similar to those seen with spontaneous myasthenia gravis and include ptosis and diplopia, and generalised weakness, occasionally affecting the respiratory muscles.[1-3] The onset of symptoms usually occurs within 6 to 7 months but may be delayed for a number of years.[3] Myasthenic symptoms usually resolve spontaneously once penicillamine is withdrawn, but some patients require anticholinesterase therapy.[1-3] Acetylcholine receptor antibodies are found in about 75% of affected patients.[2,3] Patients with HLA antigens DRI and Bw35 may have a genetic predisposition to developing myasthenia.[4] Patients with auto-immune diseases may well display an increased susceptibility to drug-induced myasthenia.[5]

1. Delamere JP, et al. Penicillamine-induced myasthenia in rheumatoid arthritis: its clinical and genetic features. Ann Rheum Dis 1983; 42: 500–4.
2. Carter H, et al. La myasthénie au cours du traitement de la polyarthrite rhumatoïde par la D-pénicillamine. Therapie 1984; 39: 689–95.
3. Katz LJ, et al. Ocular myasthenia gravis after D-penicillamine administration. Br J Ophthalmol 1989; 73: 1015–18.
4. Garlepp MJ, et al. HLA antigens and acetylcholine receptor antibodies in penicillamine induced myasthenia gravis. BMJ 1983; 286: 338–40.

POLYMYOSITIS. Penicillamine therapy has been associated rarely with polymyositis and dermatomyositis,[1-6] usually reversible but in some cases fatal.[2] At least two deaths have resulted from myocarditis,[2] and complete heart block and severe Stokes-Adams attacks have been reported[4] in patients with polymyositis. It is possible that some patients may have a genetically determined susceptibility to this complication.[5]

1. Wojnarowska F. Dermatomyositis induced by penicillamine. J R Soc Med 1980; 73: 885–6.
2. Doyle DR, et al. Fatal polymyositis in D-penicillamine-treated rheumatoid arthritis. Ann Intern Med 1983; 98: 327–30.
3. Renier JC, et al. Polymyosite induite par la D-pénicillamine. Therapie 1984; 39: 697–703.
4. Christensen PD, Sørensen KE. Penicillamine-induced polymyositis with complete heart block. Eur Heart J 1989; 10: 1041–4.
5. Carroll GJ, et al. Penicillamine induced polymyositis and dermatomyositis. J Rheumatol 1987; 14: 995–1001.
6. Aydintug AO, et al. Polymyositis complicating D-penicillamine treatment. Postgrad Med J 1991; 67: 1018–20.

Effects on the respiratory system. Reports of pulmonary haemorrhage associated with progressive renal failure in individual patients treated with penicillamine have commonly been classified as Goodpasture's syndrome,[1,2] although an immune complex syndrome has been suggested.[3] There have been rare reports of obliterative bronchiolitis in patients with rheumatoid arthritis treated with penicillamine.[4-6]

1. Sternlieb I, et al. D-Penicillamine induced Goodpasture's syndrome in Wilson's disease. Ann Intern Med 1975; 82: 673–6.
2. Gibson T, et al. Goodpasture syndrome and D-penicillamine. Ann Intern Med 1976; 84: 100.
3. Turner-Warwick M. Adverse reactions affecting the lung: possible association with D-penicillamine. J Rheumatol 1981; 8 (suppl 7): 166–8.
4. Lyle WH. D-Penicillamine and fatal obliterative bronchiolitis. BMJ 1977; 1: 105.
5. Epler GR, et al. Bronchiolitis and bronchitis in connective tissue disease: a possible relationship to the use of penicillamine. JAMA 1979; 242: 528–32.
6. Murphy KC, et al. Obliterative bronchiolitis in two rheumatoid arthritis patients treated with penicillamine. Arthritis Rheum 1981; 24: 557–60.

RHINITIS. Nasal blockage due to grossly oedematous nasal linings and severe disabling watery nasal discharge associated with penicillamine administration was reported in a 76-year-old patient.[1] The patient also had pemphigus foliaceus. The rhinitis resolved promptly when penicillamine was discontinued, as did concurrent bilateral blepharitis.

1. Presley AP. Penicillamine induced rhinitis. BMJ 1988; 296: 1332.

Effects on the skin. Penicillamine-induced skin lesions have been reviewed.[1] Reactions observed during penicillamine therapy include those resulting from interference with collagen and elastin such as penicillamine dermatopathy, elastosis perforans serpiginosa, and cutis laxa; those associated with auto-immune mechanisms such as pemphigus, pemphigoid, lupus erythematosus, and dermatomyositis; and those classified as acute sensitivity reactions including macular or papular eruptions and urticaria. The effects on collagen and elastin (see below) tend to occur only after prolonged treatment with high doses, as in patients with Wilson's disease or cystinuria, whereas patients with diseases characterised by altered immune systems, such as rheumatoid arthritis, are more prone to develop the antibody-related adverse skin reactions. Acute hypersensitivity reactions tend to occur early in penicillamine treatment, usually within the first 7 to 10 days, and appear not to be dose-related. Lichenoid reactions, stomatitis, nail changes, and adverse effects on hair have also occurred.

1. Levy RS, et al. Penicillamine: review and cutaneous manifestations. J Am Acad Dermatol 1983; **8:** 548–58.

INTERFERENCE WITH COLLAGEN AND ELASTIN. Long-term, high-dose treatment with penicillamine can interfere with elastin and collagen production giving rise to increased skin friability, haemorrhagic lesions, miliary papules, and excessive wrinkling and laxity of the skin.[1] Penicillamine dermatopathy, characterised by wrinkling and purpura over bony prominences, has been described.[2] In addition, lesions resembling pseudoxanthoma elasticum have been reported.[3,4] Abnormal elastic tissue has also been reported in patients taking low doses of penicillamine (less than 1 g daily), not only in the skin but also in joint capsules,[5] and elastosis perforans serpiginosa has been reported[6] in a child receiving a low cumulative dose over a short period. In all these cases, histological findings generally show damage to elastic fibres giving them a typical appearance described as 'lumpy-bumpy' or 'bramble-bush'.

For reports of cutis laxa in neonates, see under Pregnancy in Precautions, below.

1. Levy RS, et al. Penicillamine: review and cutaneous manifestations. J Am Acad Dermatol 1983; **8:** 548–58.
2. Sternlieb I, Scheinberg IH. Penicillamine therapy for hepatolenticular degeneration. JAMA 1964; **189:** 748–54.
3. Thomas RHM, et al. Pseudoxanthoma elasticum-like skin changes induced by penicillamine. J R Soc Med 1984; **77:** 794–8.
4. Bentley-Phillips B. Pseudoxanthoma elasticum-like skin changes induced by penicillamine. J R Soc Med 1985; **78:** 787.
5. Dalziel KL, et al. Elastic fibre damage induced by low-dose D-penicillamine. Br J Dermatol 1990; **123:** 305–12.
6. Sahn EE, et al. D-Penicillamine-induced elastosis perforans serpiginosa in a child with juvenile rheumatoid arthritis. J Am Acad Dermatol 1989; **20:** 979–88.

LICHEN PLANUS. Observations in some patients reported in the 1980s led to the suggestion that penicillamine might exacerbate or unmask lichen planus.[1,2] However, there do not appear to have been subsequent reports.

1. Powell FC, Rogers RS. Primary biliary cirrhosis, penicillamine, and lichen planus. Lancet 1981; **ii:** 525.
2. Powell FC, et al. Lichen planus, primary biliary cirrhosis and penicillamine. Br J Dermatol 1982; **107:** 616.

PEMPHIGUS. Pemphigus vulgaris[1] and a number of variants including pemphigus foliaceus,[1] herpetiform pemphigus,[2] pemphigus erythematosus,[3] benign mucous membrane pemphigoid,[4] cicatricial pemphigoid,[5] and combined pemphigus and pemphigoid features[6] have been reported with penicillamine therapy.

1. Zone J, et al. Penicillamine-induced pemphigus. JAMA 1982; **247:** 2705–7.
2. Marsden RA, et al. Herpetiform pemphigus induced by penicillamine. Br J Dermatol 1977; **97:** 451–2.
3. de Jong MCJM, et al. Immunohistochemical findings in a patient with penicillamine pemphigus. Br J Dermatol 1980; **102:** 333–7.
4. Lever LR, Wojnarowska F. Benign mucous membrane pemphigoid and penicillamine. Br J Dermatol 1985; **113** (suppl 29): 88–9.
5. Shuttleworth D, Graham-Brown RAC. Cicatricial pemphigoid in a D-penicillamine treated patient with rheumatoid arthritis. Br J Dermatol 1985; **113** (suppl 29): 89–90.
6. Velthuis PJ, et al. Combined features of pemphigus and pemphigoid induced by penicillamine. Br J Dermatol 1985; **112:** 615–19.

PSORIASIFORM ERUPTIONS. Two patients with rheumatoid arthritis developed psoriasiform eruptions during penicillamine treatment.[1] In one patient the eruption resolved when penicillamine was stopped but worsened when treatment was restarted.

1. Forgie JC, Highet AS. Psoriasiform eruptions associated with penicillamine. BMJ 1987; **294:** 1101.

SYSTEMIC SCLEROSIS. Penicillamine has been used in the treatment of scleroderma and systemic sclerosis (see under Uses, below). However, systemic sclerosis-like lesions developed in a 14-year-old boy with Wilson's disease who had been treated with penicillamine for 11 years[1] and the suitability of penicillamine for this indication has therefore been questioned.

1. Miyagawa S, et al. Systemic sclerosis-like lesions during long-term penicillamine therapy for Wilson's disease. Br J Dermatol 1987; **116:** 95–100.

TOXIC EPIDERMAL NECROLYSIS. A 56-year-old woman developed agranulocytosis and toxic epidermal necrolysis 7 weeks after starting therapy with penicillamine 250 mg daily for primary biliary cirrhosis.[1]

1. Ward K, Weir DG. Life threatening agranulocytosis and toxic epidermal necrolysis during low dose penicillamine therapy. Ir J Med Sci 1981; **150:** 252–3.

Genetic factors.
There is evidence that some patients may have a genetically determined increased susceptibility to the adverse effects of penicillamine. Several studies have suggested that rheumatoid arthritis patients with a poor capacity for producing sulfoxides may be more susceptible to the toxic effects of penicillamine.[1,2] The poor sulfoxidation capacity found in patients with primary biliary cirrhosis could partly explain their high incidence of adverse reactions to penicillamine,[3] although no association between penicillamine toxicity and sulfoxidation status was found in a study of 20 such patients.[4]

In addition to poor sulfoxidation, increased toxicity was noted in patients possessing the histocompatibility antigen HLA-DR3.[5] Other studies have shown associations between pro-

teinuria and HLA antigens B8 and DR3,[6,7] myasthenia gravis and Bw35 and DR1,[8] thrombocytopenia and HLA antigens DR4,[6,7] A1,[6] and C4BQO,[6] and polymyositis or dermatomyositis and HLA antigens B18, B35, and DR4.[9] However, such associations are insufficiently strong and testing procedures too expensive to make testing sulfoxidation status or HLA-typing useful for identifying high-risk patients.[7,10]

1. Panayi GS, et al. Deficient sulphoxidation status and d-penicillamine toxicity. Lancet 1983; **i:** 414.
2. Emery P, et al. Sulphoxidation status of rheumatoid patients manifesting untoward reactions to chronic D-penicillamine therapy. Br J Clin Pharmacol 1984; **18:** 286P.
3. Olomu A, et al. Poor sulphoxidation in primary biliary cirrhosis. Lancet 1985; **i:** 1504.
4. Mitchison HC, et al. D-penicillamine-induced toxicity in primary biliary cirrhosis (PBC): the role of sulphoxidation status. Gut 1986; **27:** A622.
5. Emery P, et al. D-Penicillamine induced toxicity in rheumatoid arthritis: the role of sulphoxidation status and HLA-DR3. J Rheumatol 1984; **11:** 626–32.
6. Stockman A, et al. Genetic markers in rheumatoid arthritis: relationship to toxicity from D-penicillamine. J Rheumatol 1986; **13:** 269–73.
7. Moens HJB, et al. Longterm followup of treatment with D-penicillamine for rheumatoid arthritis: effectivity and toxicity in relation to HLA antigens. J Rheumatol 1987; **14:** 1115–19.
8. Garlepp MJ, et al. HLA antigens and acetylcholine receptor antibodies in penicillamine induced myasthenia gravis. BMJ 1983; **286:** 338–40.
9. Carroll GJ, et al. Penicillamine induced polymyositis and dermatomyositis. J Rheumatol 1987; **14:** 995–1001.
10. Hall CL. Penicillamine nephropathy. BMJ 1988; **297:** 137.

Systemic lupus erythematosus.
A syndrome resembling lupus erythematosus developed in 6 women with long-standing severe rheumatoid arthritis while being treated with penicillamine;[1] these patients represented an approximate frequency of penicillamine-induced lupus erythematosus of 2%. All 6 had developed previous cutaneous reactions to gold therapy. A case of bullous systemic lupus erythematosus associated with penicillamine administration has also been reported.[2]

1. Chalmers A, et al. Systemic lupus erythematosus during penicillamine therapy for rheumatoid arthritis. Ann Intern Med 1982; **97:** 659–63.
2. Condon C, et al. Penicillamine-induced type II bullous systemic lupus erythematosus. Br J Dermatol 1997; **136:** 474–5.

Precautions

Penicillamine is contra-indicated in patients with lupus erythematosus or a history of penicillamine-induced agranulocytosis, aplastic anaemia, or severe thrombocytopenia. It should be used with care, if at all, in patients with renal impairment.

Penicillamine should not be given with other drugs capable of causing similar serious haematological or renal adverse effects, for example gold salts, chloroquine or hydroxychloroquine, or immunosuppressive drugs. Patients who are allergic to penicillin may react similarly to penicillamine but cross-sensitivity appears to be rare (see below).

Patients need to be carefully supervised and observed for side-effects. In particular full blood counts and urinalysis should be carried out; one recommendation is to perform such checks weekly for the first 2 months of treatment and after any change in dosage, and monthly thereafter. Treatment should be withdrawn if there is a fall in white cell or platelet count, or if progressive or serious proteinuria or haematuria occur. Liver function tests have also been recommended at 6-monthly intervals and renal function should be monitored.

Pyridoxine 25 mg daily may be given to patients on long-term therapy, especially if they are on a restricted diet, since penicillamine increases the requirement for this vitamin.

Because of the effect of penicillamine on collagen and elastin and a possible delay in wound healing, it has been suggested that the dose should be reduced to 250 mg daily for 6 weeks prior to surgery and during the postoperative period until healing has taken place.

Anaesthesia.
Penicillamine-induced myasthenia in a 57-year-old woman led to prolonged postoperative apnoea necessitating artificial ventilation.[1] The significance of this report in planning anaesthesia for patients with rheumatoid arthritis treated with penicillamine was discussed.

1. Fried MJ, Protheroe DT. D-Penicillamine induced myasthenia gravis: its relevance for the anaesthetist. Br J Anaesth 1986; **58:** 1191–3.

Penicillin allergy.
Penicillamine is a degradation product of penicillin and patients with penicillin allergy may theoretically have a cross-sensitivity to penicillamine. Reactions due to contamination of penicillamine with trace amounts of penicillin have been eliminated by the use of synthetic penicillamine. Results of a study in 40 patients with penicillin allergy[1] suggested that while cutaneous cross-reactivity with penicillamine had

been documented, the risk of a severe allergic reaction to penicillamine in penicillin-allergic patients was probably quite low.

1. Bell CL, Graziano FM. The safety of administration of penicillamine to penicillin-sensitive individuals. Arthritis Rheum 1983; **26:** 801–3.

Pregnancy.
Penicillamine teratogenicity has been reviewed.[1] Evidence of the embryotoxicity of maternal penicillamine exposure in animal studies has been confirmed in humans by 5 reports of cutis laxa in neonates of mothers who had taken penicillamine during pregnancy; 3 further reports of intra-uterine brain injury were less characteristic. Nevertheless most pregnancy outcomes were normal. No birth defects have been reported when penicillamine was discontinued in early pregnancy. Unless a safer therapy could be confirmed, penicillamine management of women with Wilson's disease should be continued throughout pregnancy since the benefits outweighed the risks. However, for conditions for which there were safer alternatives it would be prudent to discontinue penicillamine during pregnancy.

1. Rosa FW. Teratogen update: penicillamine. Teratology 1986; **33:** 127–31.

Interactions

Penicillamine forms chelates with metal ions and oral absorption of penicillamine may be reduced by concomitant administration of iron and other metals, antacids, and food. Penicillamine should be taken on an empty stomach and it has been recommended that there should be an interval of at least 2 hours between taking penicillamine and iron supplements.

Antacids.
In a single-dose study in 6 healthy subjects, penicillamine given by mouth immediately after food, an oral dose of ferrous sulfate, or a dose of an antacid mixture (aluminium hydroxide, magnesium hydroxide, and simeticone), resulted in plasma concentrations of penicillamine that were 52%, 35%, and 66%, respectively, of those obtained after administration in a fasting state. Results suggested that the reduction in plasma-penicillamine concentrations was associated with decreased penicillamine absorption.[1] Another study[2] showed that the reduction of penicillamine plasma concentrations produced by aluminium- and magnesium-containing antacids did not occur with sodium bicarbonate, and thus the interaction was probably a result of chelation rather than a pH effect.

1. Osman MA, et al. Reduction in oral penicillamine absorption by food, antacid, and ferrous sulphate. Clin Pharmacol Ther 1983; **33:** 465–70.
2. Ifan A, Welling PG. Pharmacokinetics of oral 500 mg penicillamine: effect of antacids on absorption. Biopharm Drug Dispos 1986; **7:** 401–5.

Diazepam.
For a report of exacerbation of intravenous diazepam-induced phlebitis by oral penicillamine, see under Diazepam, p.679.

Gold.
There have been conflicting reports on the effect of previous gold therapy on the subsequent development of penicillamine toxicity in patients with rheumatoid arthritis.

A multicentre trial group[1] found no evidence of any interaction between gold and penicillamine but others[2] found that although the overall incidence of side-effects with penicillamine appeared unaffected by prior gold therapy, bone-marrow depression and rashes were more common in those patients previously treated with gold. Patients who had to stop gold therapy because of adverse effects were reported[3] to be more prone to develop major adverse effects to penicillamine and a study[4] indicated that patients who reacted adversely to gold were more likely to develop side-effects to penicillamine. The mean interval between finishing gold and beginning penicillamine in patients who developed identical adverse reactions to both drugs was found to be significantly shorter than in those who developed different side-effects or no side-effects;[4] this supported the theory that some adverse reactions to penicillamine might result from the mobilisation of gold previously stored in the tissues during gold therapy. An interval of at least 6 months between gold and penicillamine therapy in patients who had adverse reactions to gold was recommended. In contrast, others[5] found no evidence that the interval between gold and penicillamine therapy had any influence on the subsequent development of penicillamine toxicity. A genetic susceptibility in certain patients to react adversely to either drug was suggested. However, in a prospective study,[6] prior gold, penicillamine, or levamisole treatment had no influence on the subsequent efficacy or toxicity of any one of these alternative drugs.

There has been a report of gold therapy causing a recurrence of myasthenia that had previously occurred with penicillamine.[7]

1. Multi-centre Trial Group. Absence of toxic or therapeutic interaction between penicillamine and previously administered gold in a trial of penicillamine in rheumatoid disease. Postgrad Med J 1974; **50** (suppl 2): 77–8.
2. Webley M, Coomes EN. Is penicillamine therapy in rheumatoid arthritis influenced by previous treatment with gold? BMJ 1978; **2:** 91.
3. Hill H. Penicillamine and previous treatment with gold. BMJ 1978; **2:** 961.
4. Dodd MJ, et al. Adverse reactions to D-penicillamine after gold toxicity. BMJ 1980; **280:** 1498–1500.
5. Smith PJ, et al. Influence of previous gold toxicity on subsequent development of penicillamine toxicity. BMJ 1982; **285:** 595–6.

6. Steven MM, *et al.* Does the order of second-line treatment in rheumatoid arthritis matter? *BMJ* 1982; **284:** 79–81.
7. Moore AP, *et al.* Penicillamine induced myasthenia reactivated by gold. *BMJ* 1984; **288:** 192–3.

Insulin. Unexplained hypoglycaemia in 2 patients with type 1 diabetes occurred 6 to 8 weeks after penicillamine treatment for rheumatoid arthritis was started.[1] Both patients required a reduction in their insulin dose. A possible mechanism has been proposed.[2]

1. Elling P, Elling H. Penicillamine, captopril, and hypoglycemia. *Ann Intern Med* 1985; **103:** 644–5.
2. Becker RC, Martin RG. Penicillamine-induced insulin antibodies. *Ann Intern Med* 1986; **104:** 127–8.

Iron. Penicillamine plasma concentrations were reduced by 52% when penicillamine was administered after a dose of ferrous sulfate in healthy subjects.[1] Patients stabilised on penicillamine while on oral iron therapy were considered unlikely to respond fully to penicillamine and would be exposed to a large increase in penicillamine absorption with possible adverse reactions if the iron was stopped.[2]

1. Osman MA, *et al.* Reduction in oral penicillamine absorption by food, antacid, and ferrous sulfate. *Clin Pharmacol Ther* 1983; **33:** 465–70.
2. Harkness JAL, Blake DR. Penicillamine nephropathy and iron. *Lancet* 1982; **ii:** 1368–9.

Probenecid. Probenecid reduced the beneficial effects of penicillamine in cystinuria; co-administration in hyperuricaemic cystinuric patients was contra-indicated.[1]

1. Yu T-F, *et al.* Studies on the metabolism of D-penicillamine and its interaction with probenecid in cystinuria and rheumatoid arthritis. *J Rheumatol* 1984; **11:** 467–70.

Pharmacokinetics

Penicillamine is readily absorbed from the gastrointestinal tract and reaches peak concentrations in the blood within 1 to 3 hours. It is reported to be more than 80% bound to plasma proteins. It is metabolised in the liver and excreted in the urine and faeces mainly as metabolites. Elimination is biphasic with an initial elimination half-life of about 1 to 3 hours followed by a slower phase, suggesting gradual release from tissues.

◊ Reviews.

1. Netter P, *et al.* Clinical pharmacokinetics of D-penicillamine. *Clin Pharmacokinet* 1987; **13:** 317–33.

Uses and Administration

Penicillamine is a chelator which aids the elimination from the body of certain heavy-metal ions, including copper, lead, and mercury, by forming stable soluble complexes with them that are readily excreted by the kidney. It is used in the treatment of Wilson's disease (to promote the excretion of copper), in heavy-metal poisoning such as lead poisoning, in cystinuria (to reduce urinary concentrations of cystine), in severe active rheumatoid arthritis, and in chronic active hepatitis.

Penicillamine is administered by mouth and should be taken on an empty stomach. A low initial dose increased gradually to the minimum optimal maintenance dosage may reduce the incidence of side-effects as well as provide closer control of the condition being treated.

In the treatment of **Wilson's disease**, a dose of 1.5 to 2 g daily in divided doses may be given initially. The optimal dosage to achieve a negative copper balance should be determined initially by regular analysis of 24-hour urinary copper excretion and subsequently by monitoring free copper in the serum. A maintenance dose of 0.75 to 1 g daily may be adequate once remission is achieved and should be continued indefinitely; the UK manufacturers recommend that a maintenance dose of 2 g daily should not be continued for more than a year. In children, a suggested dose is up to 20 mg per kg body-weight daily (minimum 500 mg daily) in divided doses. A dose of up to 20 mg per kg daily is also suggested for the elderly.

In the management of **lead poisoning**, penicillamine may be given in doses of 1 to 2 g daily in divided doses until the urinary lead concentration is stabilised at less than 0.5 mg per day. Children may be given 20 to 25 mg per kg daily in divided doses and the elderly 20 mg per kg daily.

In **cystinuria**, doses of penicillamine are adjusted according to cystine concentrations in the urine. For the *treatment* of cystinuria and cystine calculi, the dose is usually in the range of 1 to 4 g daily in divided doses; a suggested dose for children is up to 30 mg per kg daily in divided doses. For the *prevention* of cystine calculi, lower doses of 0.5 to 1 g at bedtime may be given. An adequate fluid intake is essential to maintain urine flow during penicillamine administration for cystinuria.

In the treatment of **severe active rheumatoid arthritis**, an initial dose of penicillamine 125 to 250 mg daily is increased gradually by the same amount at intervals of 4 to 12 weeks. Remission is usually achieved with maintenance doses of 500 to 750 mg daily in divided doses, but up to 1.5 g daily may be required. Improvement may not occur for several months; the USA manufacturers suggest that penicillamine should be discontinued if there is no response after treatment for 3 to 4 months with 1 to 1.5 g daily; in the UK a trial for 12 months is suggested. After remission has been sustained for 6 months an attempt may be made gradually to reduce the dose by 125 to 250 mg daily every 2 to 3 months but relapse may occur. Lower doses may be required in the elderly who may be more susceptible to developing adverse effects. Initial doses of 50 to 125 mg daily have been recommended, gradually increased to a maximum of 1 g daily if necessary. In children the maintenance dose is 15 to 20 mg per kg daily; a suggested initial dose is 2.5 to 5 mg per kg or 50 mg daily for one month increased gradually at 4-weekly intervals.

In the management of **chronic active hepatitis**, an initial dose of penicillamine 500 mg daily in divided doses may be given after liver function tests have indicated that the disease has been controlled by corticosteroids; the dose is gradually increased over 3 months to 1.25 g daily with a concurrent reduction in the corticosteroid dose.

Acetylpenicillamine has been used in mercury poisoning.

Chronic active hepatitis. Penicillamine has been tried in chronic active hepatitis (p.1048) as an alternative to prolonged corticosteroid maintenance therapy once control of the disease is achieved. The dose of penicillamine is increased over several months to a suitable maintenance dose with a concurrent reduction in the corticosteroid dose.

Cystinuria. Cystinuria is an inherited disorder of renal amino-acid excretion in which there is excessive excretion of cystine (cysteine disulfide), along with ornithine, lysine, and arginine. The low solubility of cystine leads to the formation of cystine stones in the kidney, resulting in pain, haematuria, renal obstruction, and infection. Treatment is primarily aimed at reducing the urinary concentration of cystine to below its solubility limit of 300 to 400 mg per litre at neutral pH. Patients with cystinuria excrete 400 to 1200 mg cystine daily and should be advised to drink at least 3 litres of water daily, including at night, to maintain a dilute urine. Cystine is more soluble in alkaline urine and urinary alkalinisers such as sodium bicarbonate, sodium citrate, or potassium citrate may be used; however, high doses are required and calcium stone formation may be promoted. In patients where these measures are ineffective or not tolerated, penicillamine may be used; it complexes with cysteine to form a more soluble mixed disulfide, therefore reducing cystine excretion, preventing cystine stone formation, and promoting the gradual dissolution of existing stones. Adverse effects are common and tiopronin, which has a similar action, may be used as an alternative. Surgical removal may be necessary for established stones but lithotripsy is not very effective.

Lead poisoning. Penicillamine may be used to treat asymptomatic lead intoxication and to achieve desirable lead-tissue levels in patients with symptomatic lead poisoning once they have received treatment with sodium calcium edetate and dimercaprol (see p.1627).

Primary biliary cirrhosis. Copper accumulation in the liver has been noted in patients with primary biliary cirrhosis (p.501) and therapy with penicillamine to reduce liver-copper concentrations has been studied. Despite good preliminary results, most trials have found it to be ineffective and any benefit appears to be offset by the high incidence of side-effects.[1]

1. James OFW. D-Penicillamine for primary biliary cirrhosis. *Gut* 1985; **26:** 109–13.

Retinopathy of prematurity. Penicillamine has been investigated for the prophylaxis of retinopathy of prematurity (p.1395) in infants considered to be at risk, and a systematic review of 2 such studies considered that there was evidence for a reduced incidence of acute retinopathy.[1] Further studies were considered justified, with careful attention to possible adverse effects.

1. Phelps DL, *et al.* D-Penicillamine for preventing retinopathy of prematurity in preterm infants (updated 5 December 2000). Available in The Cochrane Library; Issue 4. Oxford: Update Software; 2001.

Rheumatoid arthritis. *Rheumatoid arthritis* (p.9) and *juvenile idiopathic arthritis* (p.9) are generally treated using the same methods. Penicillamine is one of a diverse group of disease-modifying antirheumatic drugs used in an attempt to suppress the rate of cartilage erosion or alter the course of the disease. However, early enthusiasm for penicillamine has been tempered by a high incidence of adverse effects.[1] During long-term therapy as many as 50% of patients taking penicillamine have been reported to withdraw from treatment as a consequence of adverse effects.[2] Low doses of penicillamine to reduce the incidence of side-effects have been tried and while doses as low as 125 mg daily have been claimed to be effective in some patients with *rheumatoid arthritis*, a 36-week multi-centre double-blind study[3] involving 225 patients concluded that a dose of penicillamine 500 mg daily was only slightly more effective than placebo. A dose of 125 mg daily was not significantly different from either the 500 mg dose or placebo. However, a 5-year open study[4] comparing penicillamine in doses up to 500 mg daily with hydroxychloroquine, sodium aurothiomalate, or auranofin in rheumatoid arthritis found penicillamine to be as effective as the other drugs and well tolerated, with 53% of the patients randomised to penicillamine still receiving it at 5 years, as opposed to about 30 to 35% of those randomised to other drugs.

In patients with *juvenile idiopathic arthritis* it has been suggested that gold therapy may be preferred to penicillamine.[5]

1. Suarez-Almazor ME, *et al.* Penicillamine for rheumatoid arthritis (updated 29 August 2001). Available in The Cochrane Library; Issue 4. Oxford: Update Software; 2001.
2. Moens HJB, *et al.* Longterm followup of treatment with D-penicillamine for rheumatoid arthritis: effectivity and toxicity in relation to HLA antigens. *J Rheumatol* 1987; **14:** 1115–19.
3. Williams HJ, *et al.* Low-dose D-penicillamine therapy in rheumatoid arthritis: a controlled, double-blind clinical trial. *Arthritis Rheum* 1983; **26:** 581–92.
4. Jessop JD, *et al.* A long-term five-year randomized controlled trial of hydroxychloroquine, sodium aurothiomalate, auranofin and penicillamine in the treatment of patients with rheumatoid arthritis. *Br J Rheumatol* 1998; **37:** 992–1002.
5. Rosenberg AM. Advanced drug therapy for juvenile rheumatoid arthritis. *J Pediatr* 1989; **114:** 171–8.

Scleroderma. Despite the lack of conclusive evidence in its favour penicillamine, which affects the cross-linking of collagen,[1] has been widely thought to be of benefit in scleroderma (p.505), and perhaps in some visceral manifestations of systemic sclerosis.[2,3] If used, treatment should probably be begun early and continued for several years; therapy for 6 to 12 months is required before any benefit can be observed. A dose of 250 to 500 mg of penicillamine daily has been used.[2]

For a report of sclerodermatous lesions in a patient taking penicillamine for Wilson's disease, see Systemic Sclerosis, under Effects on the Skin, above.

1. Herbert CM, *et al.* Biosynthesis and maturation of skin collagen in scleroderma, and effect of D-penicillamine. *Lancet* 1974; **i:** 187–92.
2. Oliver GF, Winkelmann RK. The current treatment of scleroderma. *Drugs* 1989; **37:** 87–96.
3. Steen VD, *et al.* D-Penicillamine therapy in progressive systemic sclerosis (scleroderma): a retrospective analysis. *Ann Intern Med* 1982; **97:** 652–9.

Wilson's disease. Wilson's disease, or hepatolenticular degeneration, is a rare autosomal disorder of copper accumulation. Excretion of excess copper, which normally occurs via the bile, is impaired and total body copper progressively increases. The excess copper accumulates in the liver, brain, and other organs including the kidneys and corneas, and eventually causes tissue damage.

Effective treatment of Wilson's disease involves the use of copper-reducing drugs to establish a negative copper balance. This prevents deposition of more copper and also mobilises excess copper that has already been deposited making it available for excretion. Once negative copper balance has been achieved, maintenance treatment must be continued lifelong. Dietary restriction of copper is not generally considered to be an important part of the treatment of Wilson's disease although patients may be advised to avoid copper-rich foods, such as liver and shellfish, during the first year of treatment and to restrict their consumption thereafter. Symptomatic recovery from copper overload occurs slowly, but is usually complete if treatment is started early enough, and a normal life expectancy can be achieved. However, once irreversible organ damage such as liver cirrhosis has occurred, treatment can only prevent further deterioration; those presenting with end-stage liver disease do not benefit from copper-reducing therapy, and liver transplantation is necessary (although successful medical treatment has been reported in children). The drugs used to reduce copper concentrations in the treatment of Wilson's disease are penicillamine, trientine, and zinc. Ammonium tetrathiomolybdate is under investigation.

Penicillamine reduces copper concentrations in several ways. Its main action is to chelate circulating copper which is then excreted in the urine. In addition penicillamine reduces the affinity of copper for proteins and polypeptides, allowing removal of copper from tissues. It also induces hepatic synthesis of metallothionein, a protein that combines with copper to form a non-toxic product. *Trientine* is a less potent copper chelator than penicillamine; it competes for copper bound to serum albumin and increases copper excretion. *Zinc* induces synthesis of metallothionein in the intestine so that absorption of copper from the gastrointestinal tract is blocked. It is usually given as the acetate as this form is less irritating to the stomach than the sulfate. *Ammonium tetrathiomolybdate* forms a complex with protein and copper. When it is given with food it blocks the intestinal absorption of copper, and when taken between meals it combines with albumin- and caeruloplasmin-bound copper.

CHOICE OF DRUG. Penicillamine is generally regarded as the drug of choice for the initial management of Wilson's disease as it produces a rapid reduction in copper levels. However, it may initially exacerbate neurological symptoms (possibly due to transiently increased brain and blood copper concentrations) and some practitioners therefore suggest starting with zinc; zinc is not suitable in those requiring rapid reduction of copper levels as it has a slow onset of action. Trientine, which may also exacerbate neurological symptoms, is used in patients intolerant of penicillamine. Ammonium tetrathiomolybdate is under investigation for the initial reduction of copper levels; it may be particularly suitable for patients with neurological symptoms.

Once a negative copper balance is achieved, maintenance therapy must be continued for life. Penicillamine, trientine, and zinc are all used for maintenance treatment. Patients taking penicillamine are also given pyridoxine to prevent deficiency (see under Precautions, above). The adverse effects of penicillamine may be a problem during long-term use and zinc, which has low toxicity, is often preferred. Zinc is also used in patients in the asymptomatic stage of the disease.

References.
1. Tankanow RM. Pathophysiology and treatment of Wilson's disease. *Clin Pharm* 1991; **10:** 839–49.
2. Stremmel W, *et al.* Wilson disease: clinical presentation, treatment, and survival. *Ann Intern Med* 1991; **115:** 720–6.
3. Brewer GJ. Practical recommendations and new therapies for Wilson's disease. *Drugs* 1995; **50:** 240–9.
4. Santos Silva EE, *et al.* Successful medical treatment of severely decompensated Wilson disease. *J Pediatr* 1996; **128:** 285–7.

Preparations

BP 2001: Penicillamine Tablets;
USP 25: Penicillamine Capsules; Penicillamine Tablets.

Proprietary Preparations (details are given in Part 3)
Aust.: Artamin†; Distamine†; *Austral.:* D-Penamine; *Belg.:* Kelatin; *Braz.:* Cuprimine; *Canad.:* Cuprimine; Depen; *Denm.:* Atamir; Rhumantin†; *Fr.:* Trolovol; *Ger.:* Metalcaptase; Trisorcin; Trolovol; *Irl.:* Distamine; *Israel:* Pemine; *Ital.:* Pemine; *Mex.:* Adalken; Sufortan; *Neth.:* Cuprimine†; Distamine†; Kelatin; *Norw.:* Cuprimine; *NZ:* D-Penamine; *Port.:* Kelatine; *S.Afr.:* Metalcaptase; *Singapore:* Artamin; *Spain:* Cupripen; Sufortanon; *Swed.:* Cuprimine; *Switz.:* Mercaptyl; *Thai.:* Cuprimine; *UK:* Distamine; Pendramine†; *USA:* Cuprimine; Depen.

Potassium Polystyrene Sulfonate (13157-g)

Potassium Polystyrene Sulphonate.
CAS — 9011-99-8.

The potassium salt of sulfonated styrene polymer.

Profile
Potassium polystyrene sulfonate is a cation-exchange resin that exchanges potassium ions for calcium ions and other cations and is used in the management of hypercalciuria and renal calculi.

Preparations

Proprietary Preparations (details are given in Part 3)
Ger.: Campanyl.

Multi-ingredient: *Ger.:* Ujostabil.

Pralidoxime (13533-j)

Pralidoxime *(BAN).*
2-Hydroxyiminomethyl-1-methylpyridinium.
$C_7H_9N_2O = 137.2.$
CAS — 6735-59-7; 495-94-3.
ATC — V03AB04.

Pralidoxime Chloride (1050-s)

Pralidoxime Chloride *(BANM, USAN).*
2-Formyl-1-methylpyridinium Chloride Oxime; 2-PAM; 2-PAM Chloride; 2-PAMCl; 2-Pyridine Aldoxime Methochloride.
$C_7H_9ClN_2O = 172.6.$
CAS — 51-15-0.
Pharmacopoeias. In US.

Pharmacopoeial description
USP 25: A white to pale yellow, odourless, crystalline powder. Freely soluble in water.

Pralidoxime Iodide (1048-z)

Pralidoxime Iodide *(BANM, USAN, rINN).*
NSC-7760; 2-PAM Iodide; 2-PAMI.
$C_7H_9IN_2O = 264.1.$
CAS — 94-63-3.
Pharmacopoeias. In Chin.

Pralidoxime Mesilate (1049-c)

2-PAMM; Pralidoxime Mesylate *(BANM, USAN);* Pralidoxime Methanesulphonate; P2S.
$C_7H_9N_2O,CH_3O_3S = 232.3.$
CAS — 154-97-2.

Pralidoxime Metilsulfate (1047-j)

Pralidoxime Methylsulphate *(BANM).*
$C_7H_9N_2O,CH_3SO_4 = 248.3.$
CAS — 1200-55-1.
Pharmacopoeias. In It.

Adverse Effects
Use of pralidoxime may be associated with drowsiness, dizziness, disturbances of vision, nausea, tachycardia, headache, hyperventilation, and muscular weakness. Tachycardia, laryngospasm, and muscle rigidity have been attributed to giving pralidoxime intravenously at too rapid a rate. Large doses of pralidoxime may cause transient neuromuscular blockade.

Precautions
Pralidoxime should be used cautiously in patients with renal impairment; a reduction in dosage may be necessary. Caution is also required in giving pralidoxime to patients with myasthenia gravis as it may precipitate a myasthenic crisis. Pralidoxime should not be used to treat poisoning by carbamate pesticides.

When atropine and pralidoxime are given together, the signs of atropinisation may occur earlier than might be expected when atropine is used alone.

Pharmacokinetics
Pralidoxime is not bound to plasma proteins, does not readily pass into the CNS, and is rapidly excreted in the urine partly unchanged and partly as a metabolite. The elimination half-life is about 1 to 3 hours.

◊ References.
1. Sidell FR, Groff WA. Intramuscular and intravenous administration of small doses of 2-pyridinium aldoxime methochloride to man. *J Pharm Sci* 1971; **60:** 1224–8.
2. Siddell FR, *et al.* Pralidoxime methansulfonate: plasma levels and pharmacokinetics after oral administration to man. *J Pharm Sci* 1972; **61:** 1136–40.
3. Swartz RD, *et al.* Effects of heat and exercise on the elimination of pralidoxime in man. *Clin Pharmacol Ther* 1973; **14:** 83–9.

Uses and Administration
Pralidoxime is a cholinesterase reactivator. It is used as an adjunct to, but *not* as a substitute for, atropine in the treatment of poisoning by certain cholinesterase inhibitors. Its main indication is in poisoning due to organophosphorus insecticides or related compounds (see p.1435). These compounds phosphorylate and consequently inactivate cholinesterase, causing acetylcholine accumulation and muscle paralysis. Pralidoxime acts principally to reactivate cholinesterase, restoring the enzymatic destruction of acetylcholine at the neuromuscular junction and relieving muscle paralysis. However, concomitant administration of atropine is required to counteract directly the adverse effects of acetylcholine accumulation, particularly at the respiratory centre. Pralidoxime is not equally antagonistic to all organophosphorus anticholinesterases as reactivation is dependent on the nature of the phosphoryl group and the rate at which inhibition becomes irreversible. It is not effective in the treatment of poisoning due to phosphorus, inorganic phosphates, or organophosphates without anticholinesterase activity. It has usually been contra-indicated in the treatment of poisoning by carbamate insecticides (including carbaryl poisoning) as it may increase toxicity (see p.1429). The use of pralidoxime has been suggested for the treatment of overdosage by anticholinesterase drugs, including those used to treat

myasthenia gravis such as neostigmine; however, it is only slightly effective and its use is not generally recommended.

Pralidoxime is usually given as the chloride or mesilate but the iodide and metilsulfate salts have also been used. Doses are expressed in terms of the salts.

Pralidoxime may be administered by slow intravenous injection over 5 to 10 minutes, by intravenous infusion over 15 to 30 minutes, or by subcutaneous or intramuscular injection; it has also been given orally.

In the treatment of **organophosphorus poisoning** pralidoxime should be given within 24 hours of poisoning to be fully effective as cholinesterase inactivation usually becomes irreversible after this time; however patients with severe poisoning may occasionally respond up to 36 hours or longer after exposure. Injections of *atropine* should be given intravenously or intramuscularly and repeated as necessary until the patient shows signs of atropine toxicity; atropinisation should then be maintained for 48 hours or more. Large amounts of atropine may be required. See under Atropine Sulfate, p.462, for details of dosages. Concomitantly, 1 to 2 g of *pralidoxime*, as the chloride, iodide, or mesilate, should be given intramuscularly or intravenously and repeated if necessary according to the patient's condition (alternatively, a dose of pralidoxime mesilate of 30 mg per kg body-weight by slow intravenous injection is recommended by the *British National Formulary*). Additional doses may be required every 3 to 8 hours in cases of ingestion (alternatively, in severe poisoning, a continuous infusion of 200 to 500 mg per hour may be administered, titrated against response). A maximum dose of 12 g in 24 hours has been suggested. In children pralidoxime mesilate 20 to 60 mg per kg body-weight may be given depending on the severity of poisoning and response to treatment. The dose of pralidoxime may need to be reduced in patients with renal impairment.

Treatment should preferably be monitored by the determination of blood-cholinesterase concentrations and clinical symptoms. Patients should be closely observed for at least 24 hours following resolution of symptoms.

Other oximes with cholinesterase reactivating properties that have been used similarly include obidoxime chloride (p.1016), diacetyl monoxime, and trimedoxime bromide (TMB-4).

Administration. Pralidoxime was administered by continuous intravenous infusion in a dose of 9 to 19 mg per kg body-weight per hour immediately after a loading dose of 15 to 50 mg per kg to 7 children with symptomatic organophosphorus intoxication.[1] Continuous infusion for 18 to 60 hours was effective and well tolerated. In adults, rates of up to 500 mg per hour have been used for prolonged nicotinic symptoms.[2]
1. Farrar HC, *et al.* Use of continuous infusion of pralidoxime for treatment of organophosphate poisoning in children. *J Pediatr* 1990; **116:** 658–61.
2. Tush GM, Anstead MI. Pralidoxime continuous infusion in the treatment of organophosphate poisoning. *Ann Pharmacother* 1997; **31:** 441–4.

Preparations

USP 25: Pralidoxime Chloride for Injection.

Proprietary Preparations (details are given in Part 3)
Braz.: Contrathion; *Canad.:* Protopam; *Fr.:* Contrathion; *Ital.:* Contrathion; *USA:* Protopam.

Protamine (4999-k)

CAS — 9012-00-4.
ATC — V03AB14.

Protamine Hydrochloride (11518-f)

Protamine Hydrochloride *(BANM).*
Cloridrato de Protamina; Protamini Hydrochloridum.
Pharmacopoeias. In Eur. (see p.vi).

Pharmacopoeial description
Ph. Eur.: A mixture of the hydrochlorides of basic peptides prepared from the sperm or roe of suitable species of fish, usually from the families Clupeidae or Salmonidae. A white or almost white hygroscopic powder. Soluble in water; practically insoluble in alcohol and in ether. Store in airtight containers.

Protamine Sulfate (1051-w)

Protamine Sulfate (rINN).

Protamine Sulphate (BAN); Protamini Sulfas; Sulfato de Protamina.
CAS — 9009-65-8.
Pharmacopoeias. In Chin., Eur. (see p.vi), Jpn, and US.

Pharmacopoeial description
Ph. Eur.: A mixture of the sulfates of basic peptides prepared from the sperm or roe of suitable species of fish, usually from the families Clupeidae or Salmonidae. A white or almost white hygroscopic powder. Sparingly soluble in water; practically insoluble in alcohol and in ether. Store in airtight containers.
USP 25: A purified mixture of simple protein principles obtained from the sperm or testes of suitable species of fish. Store at 2° to 8° in airtight containers.

Adverse Effects and Precautions
Intravenous injections of protamine sulfate, particularly if given rapidly, may cause hypotension, bradycardia, and dyspnoea. A sensation of warmth, transitory flushing, nausea and vomiting, and lassitude may also occur.

Hypersensitivity reactions can occur; patients at risk include diabetics who have received protamine-insulin preparations, those who have previously undergone procedures such as coronary angioplasty or cardiopulmonary bypass surgery, those allergic to fish, and men who are infertile or who have had a vasectomy. Anaphylactoid reactions have been reported.

Protamine has an anticoagulant effect when administered in the absence of heparin.

When repeated doses of protamine are used to neutralise large doses of heparin, rebound bleeding which responds to further doses of protamine, may occur. Clotting parameters should be closely monitored in patients receiving such prolonged therapy.

◊ In a report on 4 patients who received protamine sulfate after cardiac surgery to neutralise the effect of heparin severe adverse reactions including marked hypotension, vascular collapse, and pulmonary oedema were described.[1] Previous reports of similar reactions to protamine were reviewed. A total of 17 patients had immediate anaphylactic reactions; in 1 patient a complement-dependent IgG antibody-mediated reaction had been demonstrated and 3 patients tested for allergy to protamine had positive skin tests. In 15 of these 17 patients there was evidence of previous exposure to protamine; those with a high risk of sensitisation included leucopheresis donors who had received the drug, diabetics using insulin containing protamine, and patients with fish allergy. Suspected reactions to protamine occurred in a further 10 patients after cardiac surgery. However, these reactions were characterised by severe vascular damage manifested as noncardiogenic pulmonary oedema or persistent hypotension and onset was delayed for 30 minutes to several hours. Evidence suggested that these reactions were not antibody mediated; only 2 of 7 evaluable patients had previous exposure. All patients required aggressive therapy.

In a review of the toxicity of protamine[2] adverse cardiovascular responses were considered to be of 3 types: transient hypotension related to rapid drug administration, occasional anaphylactoid responses, and rarely, catastrophic pulmonary vasoconstriction.

1. Holland CL, et al. Adverse reactions to protamine sulfate following cardiac surgery. Clin Cardiol 1984; 7: 157–62.
2. Horrow JC. Protamine: a review of its toxicity. Anesth Analg 1985; 64: 348–61.

Uses and Administration
Protamine is a basic protein which combines with heparin to form a stable inactive complex. Protamine is used to neutralise the anticoagulant action of heparin in the treatment of haemorrhage resulting from severe heparin or low-molecular-weight heparin overdosage. It is also used to neutralise the effect of heparin given before surgery and during extracorporeal circulation as in dialysis or cardiac surgery. Protamine is used in some insulin preparations to prolong the effects of insulin. Protamine is usually given as the sulfate, although the hydrochloride may also be used.

Protamine sulfate is given by slow intravenous injection over a period of about 10 minutes. The dose is dependent on the amount of heparin to be neutralised and ideally should be titrated against the coagulability of the patient's blood. Protamine sulfate has weak anticoagulating properties and if given in gross excess its anticoagulant action could be significant. As

The symbol † denotes a preparation no longer actively marketed

heparin is being continuously excreted the dose should be reduced if more than 15 minutes have elapsed since heparin administration; for example, if protamine sulfate is given 30 minutes after heparin the dose may be reduced to about one-half. Not more than 50 mg of protamine sulfate should be injected for any one dose; patients should be carefully monitored as further doses may be required. The Ph. Eur. specifies that 1 mg of protamine sulfate precipitates not less than 100 units of heparin sodium, but adds that this potency is based on a specific reference batch of heparin sodium. One UK manufacturer has stated that each mg of protamine sulfate will usually neutralise the anticoagulant effect of at least 80 international units of heparin (lung) or at least 100 international units of heparin (mucous). The US manufacturer has stated that each mg of protamine sulfate neutralises about 90 USP units of heparin (lung) or about 115 USP units of heparin (mucous). One UK manufacturer has stated that each mg of protamine sulfate will usually neutralise the anticoagulant effect of at least 80 international units of heparin (lung) or at least 100 international units of heparin (mucous). The US manufacturer has stated that each mg of protamine sulfate neutralises about 90 USP units of heparin (lung) or about 115 USP units of heparin (mucous).

Protamine neutralises the anti-thrombin activity of low-molecular-weight heparins but only partially neutralises the anti-factor-Xa effect; 1 mg of protamine sulfate is stated to inhibit the effects of 100 units of dalteparin sodium or 1 mg (100 units) of enoxaparin sodium.

Protamine hydrochloride may be used similarly.

Haemorrhagic disorders. Endogenous production of heparin-like substances may, rarely, be responsible for some bleeding disorders. Protamine could be useful as a diagnostic aid in vitro and could be administered intravenously to transiently control bleeding in such patients.[1,2]

1. Tefferi A, et al. Circulating heparin-like anticoagulants: report of five consecutive cases and a review. Am J Med 1990; 88: 184–8.
2. Bayly PJM, Thick M. Reversal of post-reperfusion coagulopathy by protamine sulphate in orthotopic liver transplantation. Br J Anaesth 1994; 73: 840–2.

Preparations
BP 2001: Protamine Sulphate Injection;
USP 25: Protamine Sulfate for Injection; Protamine Sulfate Injection.

Proprietary Preparations (details are given in Part 3)
Hong Kong: Prosulf; **Israel:** Prosulf; **UK:** Prosulf.

Prussian Blue (13186-e)

Berlin Blue; CI Pigment Blue 27; Colour Index No. 77510; Ferric Ferrocyanide; Ferric Hexacyanoferrate (II).
$Fe_4[Fe(CN)_6]_3 = 859.2$.
CAS — 14038-43-8; 12240-15-2.
ATC — V03AB31.

NOTE. The name Prussian Blue (CI Pigment Blue 27) is applied to both ferric hexacyanoferrate (II) and to potassium ferric hexacyanoferrate (II), $KFe[Fe(CN)_6] = 306.9$ (Colour Index No. 77520).

Profile
Prussian blue is used in the treatment of thallium poisoning (see p.1671). When administered by mouth it forms a non-absorbable complex with thallium in the gastrointestinal tract which is excreted in the faeces. A suggested dose of Prussian blue is 10 g, or 125 mg per kg body-weight, twice daily by mouth or duodenal tube until the urinary excretion of thallium falls to 0.5 mg or less per 24 hours. It has been used similarly for the removal of radiocaesium from the body.

Preparations
Proprietary Preparations (details are given in Part 3)
Ger.: Antidotum Thallii-Heyl; Radiogardase-Cs.

Sevelamer Hydrochloride (9348-f)

Sevelamer Hydrochloride (BANM, USAN, rINNM).
GT16-026A. Allylamine polymer with 1-chloro-2,3-epoxypropane hydrochloride.
CAS — 52757-95-6 (sevelamer); 182683-00-7 (sevelamer hydrochloride).

Profile
Sevelamer hydrochloride is a phosphate binder used for hyperphosphataemia in patients with chronic renal failure on haemodialysis. The usual initial dose is 800 to 1600 mg of sevelamer hydrochloride three times daily with each meal, depending on the severity of hyperphosphataemia. Doses thereafter should be adjusted according to phosphate concentrations in the plasma.

◊ References.
1. Burke SK. Renagel®: reducing serum phosphorus in haemodialysis patients. Hosp Med 2000; 61: 622–7.

Preparations
Proprietary Preparations (details are given in Part 3)
Fr.: Renagel; **Irl.:** Renagel; **UK:** Renagel; **USA:** Renagel.

Silymarin (13236-v)

A mixture of the isomers silibinin, silicristin, and silidianin.
CAS — 65666-07-1.
ATC — A05BA03.
Pharmacopoeias. Ger. includes Milk Thistle Fruit, the ripe liberated fruit of Silybum marianum containing not less than 1.5% of silymarin calculated as silibinin. USNF includes Milk Thistle and Powdered Milk Thistle.

The active principle from the fruit of Silybum marianum (=Carduus marianus) (Compositae). The principal components are the flavonolignans silibinin, silicristin, and silidianin of which silibinin is the major component.

Silibinin (929-k)

Silibinin (rINN).
Silybin; Silybum Substance E₆. 3,5,7-Trihydroxy-2-[3-(4-hydroxy-3-methoxyphenyl)-2-(hydroxymethyl)-1,4-benzodioxan-6-yl]-4-chromanone.
$C_{25}H_{22}O_{10} = 482.4$.
CAS — 22888-70-6.

NOTE. The name silymarin has also been used to denote silibinin.

Silicristin (15705-e)

Silicristin (rINN).
Silychristin. 2-[2,3-Dihydro-7-hydroxy-2-(4-hydroxy-3-methoxyphenyl)-3-(hydroxymethyl)-5-benzofuranyl]-3,5,7-trihydroxy-4-chromanone.
$C_{25}H_{22}O_{10} = 482.4$.
CAS — 33889-69-9.

Silidianin (15706-l)

Silidianin (rINN).
Silydianin. (+)-2,3α,3aα,7a-Tetrahydro-7aα-hydroxy-8(R*)-(4-hydroxy-3-methoxyphenyl)-4-(3α,5,7-trihydroxy-4-oxo-2β-chromanyl)-3,6-methanobenzofuran-7(6αH)-one.
$C_{25}H_{22}O_{10} = 482.4$.
CAS — 29782-68-1.

Profile
Silymarin is claimed to be a free radical scavenger and has been used for the treatment of hepatic disorders. Silibinin, one of the active constituents of silymarin, has been used as the disodium dihemisuccinate salt in Amanita phalloides poisoning (p.1639). Silymarin is poorly water-soluble and has been given by mouth; disodium silibinin dihemisuccinate is water-soluble and has been given by intravenous injection. Silymarin in doses of up to 140 mg (equivalent to silibinin 60 mg) two or three times daily by mouth has been suggested for hepatic disorders. A dose of silibinin 20 mg per kg body-weight daily by intravenous infusion in 4 divided doses as the disodium dihemisuccinate has been suggested in Amanita phalloides poisoning.

Amanita poisoning. Silymarin and silibinin have been found to be effective in preventing hepatic damage following amanita poisoning.[1-3]

1. Vogel G. The anti-amanita effect of silymarin. In: Faulstich H, et al., eds. Amanita toxins and poisoning. Baden-Baden: Verlag Gerhad Witzstrock, 1980: 180–7.
2. Lorenz D. Über die anwending von silibinin bei der knollenblätterpilzvergiftung. Dtsch Arzt 1982; 79: 43–5.
3. Hruby K, et al. Chemotherapy of Amanita phalloides poisoning with intravenous silibinin. Hum Toxicol 1983; 2: 183–90.

Hepatic disorders. References to the use of silymarin in patients with liver disorders.
1. Cavalieri S. Valutazione clinica controllata del legalon. Gazz Med Ital 1974; 133: 628–35.
2. Salmi HA, Sarna S. Effect of silymarin on chemical, functional, and morphological alterations of the liver: a double-blind controlled study. Scand J Gastroenterol 1982; 17: 517–21.
3. Ferenci P, et al. Randomized controlled trial of silymarin treatment in patients with cirrhosis of the liver. J Hepatol 1989; 9: 105–13.

Preparations
Proprietary Preparations (details are given in Part 3)
Aust.: Apihepar; Biogelat Leberschutz; Hepar Pasc Mono; Legalon; Silyhexal; **Austral.:** Bioglan Liver-Vite; Herbal Liver Formula; Liver Tonic Capsules; Prol; Silymarin Phytosome; **Belg.:** Legalon; Legalon SIL; **Braz.:** Eleparon; Siliver; **Fr.:** Legalon; **Ger.:** Alepa; Ardeyhepan N; Carduus-monoplant†; Cefasliymarin; Divinal-Hepa†; durasilymarin; Hegrimarin†; Heliplant†; Hepa-loges N; Hepa-Merz Sil; Hepaduran V; Hepar-Pasc; Heparano N; Heparsyx N; Hepatorell; Hepatos; Heplant; Legalon; Legalon SIL; Logomed Leber-Kapseln†; Mariendistel Curarina; Phytohepar; Poikicholan; Probiophyt V; Silibene; Silicur; Silimarit; Silmar†; Silvaysan; SX Cardus; Vit-o-Mar†; **Hong Kong:** Legalon; **Ital.:** Eparsil†; Legalon; Locasil†; Marsil†; Silepar; Silimarin; Silirex; Silliver; Trissil†; **Mex.:** Legalon; **Neth.:** Venoplant†; **Port.:** Cholagutt; Legalon; **S.Afr.:** Legalon; Legalon; Silarine; Silimazu; **Switz.:** Legalon; Legalon SIL; **Thai.:** Legalon.

Multi-ingredient: **Aust.:** Aristochol; Bakanasan Leber-Galle; Hepabene; Pascopankreat; Sanhelios Leber-Galle; Sidroga Leber-Galle-Tee; **Austral.:** Antioxidant Forte Tablets; Extralife Liva-

Care; Herbal Cleanse; Lifesystem Herbal Formula 7 Liver Tonic; Liver Tonic Herbal Formula 6; Silybum Complex; St Mary's Thistle Plus; Super B Plus Liver Tonic; T & T Antioxidant; *Braz.:* Silimalon; *Ger.:* Bilisan C3†; Bilisan Duo; Cefachol; Cheiranthol; Cholhepan N; Cholosom-Tee; Doppelherz Magenstarkung†; Esberigal N†; Gallexier; Galloselect M; Hepar-Pasc duo; Hepar-Pasc N†; Hepaticum-Medice H; Hepatimed N†; Hepatofalk Planta N; Heumann Leber- und Gallentee Solu-Hepar NT; Heusin; Hevert-Gall S; Iberogast; JuCholan S†; Legapas comp†; Marianon; Pankreaplex Neu; Pascohepan novo; Pascopankreat novo; Presselin Hepaticum P; Schwohepan S; Vasesana-Vasoregulans; Venacton; *Hong Kong:* Hepatofalk Planta; Simepar; *Ital.:* Castindia; Venoplant†; Venoplus; *Port.:* Synchrorose; *Singapore:* Hepatofalk Planta; Noricaven; Simepar; *Spain:* Venoplant; *Switz.:* Boldocynara N; Demonatur Gouttes pour le foie et la bile; Iberogast; Lapidar 14†; Phytomed Hepato; Simepar; Tisane hepatique et biliaire.

Sodium Calcium Edetate   (1052-e)

Sodium Calcium Edetate *(BAN, rINN)*.

Calcium Disodium Edathamil; Calcium Disodium Edetate; Calcium Disodium Ethylenediaminetetra-acetate; Calcium Disodium Versenate; Calcium EDTA; Disodium Calcium Tetracemate; E385; Edetate Calcium Disodium *(USAN)*; Natrii Calcii Edetas; Sodium Calciumedetate. The calcium chelate of disodium ethylenediaminetetra-acetate; Disodium[(ethylenedinitrilo)tetraacetato]calciate(2−) hydrate.

$C_{10}H_{12}CaN_2Na_2O_8,xH_2O = 374.3$ (anhydrous).

CAS — 23411-34-9 *(sodium calcium edetate, hydrate)*; 62-33-9 *(anhydrous sodium calcium edetate)*.

Pharmacopoeias. In *Eur.* (see p.vi), *Pol.*, and *US*.
US specifies a mixture of the dihydrate and trihydrate but predominantly the dihydrate. *Int.* specifies the dihydrate.

Pharmacopoeial description

Ph. Eur.: A white or almost white, hygroscopic, powder. Freely soluble in water; practically insoluble in alcohol and in ether. A 20% solution in water has a pH of 6.5 to 8.0.

USP 25: A mixture of the dihydrate and trihydrate, predominantly the dihydrate. White, slightly hygroscopic, odourless, crystalline powder or granules. Freely soluble in water. pH of a 20% solution in water is between 6.5 and 8.0. Store in airtight containers.

Adverse Effects

Sodium calcium edetate is nephrotoxic and may cause renal tubular necrosis. Nausea and cramp may also occur. Thrombophlebitis has followed intravenous infusion and may be related to the concentration of the injection. Pain at the intramuscular injection site has been reported. Other side-effects that have been reported include fever, malaise, headache, myalgia, histamine-like responses such as sneezing, nasal congestion, and lachrymation, skin eruptions, transient hypotension, and ECG abnormalities.

Sodium calcium edetate chelates zinc within the body and zinc deficiency has been reported. Displacement of calcium from sodium calcium edetate may lead to hypercalcaemia.

Effects on the kidneys. Of 130 children with lead poisoning who received combined chelation therapy of sodium calcium edetate (25 mg per kg body-weight intramuscularly every 12 hours) and dimercaprol (3 mg per kg intramuscularly every 4 hours) for a total of 5 days, 21 developed clinical evidence of nephrotoxicity and in 4 severe oliguric acute renal failure began 1 or 2 days after chelation therapy was discontinued.[1] Nephrotoxicity was probably attributable to the use of sodium calcium edetate.

1. Moel DI, Kumar K. Reversible nephrotic reactions to a combined 2,3-dimercapto-l-propanol and calcium disodium ethylenediaminetetraacetic acid regimen in asymptomatic children with elevated blood lead levels. *Pediatrics* 1982; **70:** 259–62.

Precautions

Sodium calcium edetate should be used with caution, if at all, in patients with renal impairment. Daily urinalysis to monitor proteinuria and haematuria and regular monitoring of renal function has been recommended.

Sodium calcium edetate can chelate with several endogenous metals, including zinc, and may increase their excretion; therapy should be intermittent to prevent severe deficiency developing and monitoring of zinc levels may be required (see below).

Sodium calcium edetate should not be given by mouth in the treatment of lead poisoning as it has been suggested that absorption of lead may be increased as a result.

◊ Sodium calcium edetate 500 mg per m² body-surface was administered by deep intramuscular injection every 12 hours for 5 days to 10 children with asymptomatic lead poisoning.[1] Lead concentrations in blood decreased to about 58% of the pretreatment values after 5 days of treatment and were essentially unchanged for up to 60 hours after the last dose. Sodium calcium edetate also produced a marked fall in the mean plasma concentration of zinc but this rebounded rapidly after cessation of treatment. Mean urinary-lead excretion increased about 21-fold during the first 24 hours of therapy and urinary-zinc excretion increased about 17-fold. Sodium calcium edetate had little effect on the plasma concentrations or urinary excretion of copper. The results suggested that careful monitoring of zinc was required during treatment with sodium calcium edetate.

1. Thomas DJ, Chisolm JJ. Lead, zinc and copper decorporation during calcium disodium ethylenediamine tetraacetate treatment of lead-poisoned children. *J Pharmacol Exp Ther* 1986; **239:** 829–35.

Pharmacokinetics

Sodium calcium edetate is poorly absorbed from the gastrointestinal tract. It distributes primarily to the extracellular fluid and does not penetrate cells. It is not significantly metabolised; after intravenous injection about 50% of a dose is excreted in the urine in 1 hour and over 95% in 24 hours.

Uses and Administration

Sodium calcium edetate is the calcium chelate of disodium edetate and is a chelator used in the treatment of lead poisoning (see Lead, Treatment of Adverse Effects, p.1627). It mobilises lead from bone and tissues and aids elimination from the body by forming a stable, water-soluble, lead complex which is readily excreted by the kidneys. It may be used as a diagnostic test for lead poisoning but measurement of blood-lead concentrations is generally preferred.

Sodium calcium edetate is also a chelator of other heavy-metal polyvalent ions, including chromium. A cream containing sodium calcium edetate 10% has been used in the treatment of chrome ulcers and skin sensitivity reactions due to contact with heavy metals.

Edetates have been labelled with metallic radionuclides and used in nuclear medicine. Sodium calcium edetate is also used as a pharmaceutical excipient and as a food additive.

In the treatment of *lead poisoning*, sodium calcium edetate may be administered by intramuscular injection or by intravenous infusion. The intramuscular route may be preferred in patients with lead encephalopathy and increased intracranial pressure in whom excess fluids must be avoided, and also in children, who have an increased risk of incipient encephalopathy. Sodium calcium edetate may initially aggravate the symptoms of lead toxicity due to mobilisation of stored lead and it is commonly given with dimercaprol (p.1007) in patients who are symptomatic; the first dose of dimercaprol should preferably be given at least 4 hours before the sodium calcium edetate.

For administration by intravenous infusion, 1 g of sodium calcium edetate should be diluted with 250 to 500 mL of glucose 5% or sodium chloride 0.9%; a concentration of 3% should not be exceeded. The infusion should be administered over a period of at least one hour and infusion times of 8 to 12 hours or longer have been recommended. In the UK, the usual dose is 60 to 80 mg per kg body-weight daily given in two divided doses. In the USA, a dose of 1000 mg per m² body-surface daily is suggested for asymptomatic adults and children; a daily dose of 1500 mg per m² may be used in patients with symptomatic poisoning. Treatment is given for up to 5 days, repeated if necessary after an interval of at least 2 days. Any further treatment with sodium calcium edetate should then not be recommended for at least 7 days.

Alternatively, the same daily dose of sodium calcium edetate may be given intramuscularly in 2 to 4 divided doses as a 20% solution. Intramuscular injection of sodium calcium edetate is painful and it is recommended that preservative-free procaine hydrochloride should be added to a concentration of 0.5 to 1.5% to minimise pain; alternatively, lignocaine [lidocaine] may be added to a concentration of 0.5%.

As excretion is predominantly renal, an adequate urinary flow must be established and maintained during treatment. In patients with renal impairment, smaller and less frequent doses have been recommended.

Preparations

BP 2001: Sodium Calcium Edetate Intravenous Infusion;
USP 25: Edetate Calcium Disodium Injection.

Proprietary Preparations (details are given in Part 3)
Ger.: Calcium Vitis; *Irl.:* Ledclair; *Switz.:* Chelintox; *UK:* Ledclair.

Sodium Cellulose Phosphate   (1053-l)

Cellulose Sodium Phosphate *(USAN)*.
CAS — 9038-41-9; 68444-58-6.
ATC — V03AG01.
Pharmacopoeias. In *US*.

The sodium salt of the phosphate ester of cellulose.

Pharmacopoeial description

USP 25: It is prepared by the phosphorylation of alpha cellulose. A free-flowing, cream-coloured, odourless, powder. Insoluble in water, in dilute acids, and in most organic solvents. The pH of a filtrate of a 5% mixture in water is between 6.0 and 9.0. The inorganic bound phosphate content is not less than 31.0% and not more than 36.0%; the free phosphate content is not more than 3.5%; and the sodium content is not less than 9.5% and not more than 13.0%, all calculated on the dried basis. The calcium binding capacity, calculated on the dried basis, is not less than 1.8 mmol per g.

Adverse Effects and Precautions

Diarrhoea and other gastrointestinal disturbances have been reported.

Sodium cellulose phosphate should not be administered to patients with primary or secondary hyperparathyroidism, hypomagnesaemia, hypocalcaemia, bone disease, or enteric hyperoxaluria. It should be administered cautiously to pregnant women and children, since they have high calcium requirements.

Patients should be monitored for electrolyte disturbances. Uptake of sodium and phosphate may increase and sodium cellulose phosphate should not be given to patients with renal failure or conditions requiring a restricted sodium intake such as heart failure. Theoretically, long-term treatment could result in calcium deficiency; regular monitoring of calcium and parathyroid hormone has therefore been recommended. Sodium cellulose phosphate is not a totally selective exchange resin and the intestinal absorption of other dietary cations may be reduced; magnesium deficiency has been reported but may be corrected by dosage reduction or oral magnesium supplements. Urinary excretion of oxalate may increase and dietary restriction of oxalate intake may be necessary.

◊ Potential complications of long-term sodium cellulose phosphate therapy include secondary hyperparathyroidism and bone disease; deficiency of magnesium, copper, zinc, and iron; and hyperoxaluria. A study in 18 patients[1] with absorptive hypercalciuria and recurrent renal stones indicated that these complications could largely be avoided if therapy was confined to those with absorptive hypercalciuria (hypercalciuria, intestinal hyperabsorption of calcium, and normal or suppressed parathyroid function); if the dose was adjusted so as not to reduce intestinal calcium absorption or urinary calcium subnormally (the optimal maintenance dose in most patients was 10 g daily); if oral magnesium supplements were provided; and if a moderate dietary restriction of calcium and oxalate was imposed. There was no evidence of zinc, copper, or iron deficiency.
1. Pak CYC. Clinical pharmacology of sodium cellulose phosphate. *J Clin Pharmacol* 1979; **19:** 451–7.

Interactions

Sodium cellulose phosphate binds with calcium and other cations. Administration with calcium or magnesium salts, including cation-donating antacids or laxatives, may reduce the effectiveness of sodium cellulose phosphate. Magnesium supplements are often required in patients receiving sodium cellulose phosphate but should be administered at least one hour before or after any dose of the resin since the absorption of the magnesium may otherwise be impaired.

Uses and Administration

Sodium cellulose phosphate is a cation-exchange resin that exchanges sodium ions for calcium and other divalent cations. When administered by mouth, it binds calcium ions within the stomach and intestine to form a non-absorbable complex which is excreted in the faeces. Theoretically a 5 g dose will bind approximately 350 mg calcium. It is used in the treatment of absorptive hypercalciuria and recurrent formation of calcium-containing renal calculi (p.910), usually in conjunction with a low calcium diet. Sodium cellulose phosphate is also used in the treatment of hypercalcaemia associated with osteopetrosis, sarcoidosis, and vitamin D intoxication, and in idiopathic hypercalcaemia of infancy, although other more effective agents are usually used (see p.1181).

The usual initial dose is 15 g daily by mouth in 3 divided doses with meals reducing to 10 g daily for maintenance. A suggested dose for children is 10 g daily (but see under Adverse Effects and Precautions, above). The powder may be taken dispersed in water or sprinkled onto food. Oral magnesium supplements equivalent to about 60 or 90 mg (about 2.4 or 3.6 mmol) of elemental magnesium twice daily have been recommended for patients taking daily doses of sodium cellulose phosphate 10 or 15 g respectively. The magnesium supplement should not be given simultaneously with sodium cellulose phosphate.

Sodium cellulose phosphate may also be used for the investigation of calcium absorption.

Preparations

USP 25: Cellulose Sodium Phosphate for Oral Suspension.

Proprietary Preparations (details are given in Part 3)
Austral.: Calcisorb; *Belg.:* Calcisorb†; *Israel:* Calcisorb; *Neth.:* Calcisorb; *NZ:* Calcisorb; *S.Afr.:* Calcisorb†; *Spain:* Anacalcit; *UK:* Calcisorb†; *USA:* Calcibind.

Sodium Fytate (1056-z)

Sodium Fytate *(rINNM)*.

Phytate Sodium *(USAN)*; Sodium Phytate; SQ-9343. The nonasodium salt of *myo*-inositol hexakis(dihydrogen phosphate); Sodium cyclohexanehexyl(hexaphosphate).
$C_6H_9Na_9O_{24}P_6 = 857.9$.
CAS — 83-86-3 (phytic acid); 7205-52-9 (sodium fytate).

Profile

Sodium fytate reacts with calcium in the gastrointestinal tract to form non-absorbable calcium phytate which is excreted in the faeces. Sodium fytate is used in a similar manner to sodium cellulose phosphate (p.1022) to reduce the absorption of calcium from the gut in the treatment of hypercalciuria.

Preparations

Proprietary Preparations (details are given in Part 3)
Fr.: Phytat†.

Multi-ingredient: *Ital.:* Lightening; Phytic Acid.

Sodium Nitrite (1055-j)

E250; Natrii Nitris; Natrium Nitrosum.
$NaNO_2 = 69.00$.
CAS — 7632-00-0.
ATC — V03AB08.
Pharmacopoeias. In Chin., Eur. (see p.vi), Int., and US.

Pharmacopoeial description

Ph. Eur.: Hygroscopic, colourless crystals or mass or yellowish rods. Freely soluble in water; soluble in alcohol. Store in airtight containers.

USP 25: A white to slightly yellow, granular powder, or white or practically white, opaque, fused masses or sticks. It is deliquescent in air. Soluble 1 in 1.5 of water; sparingly soluble in alcohol. Its solutions are alkaline to litmus. Store in airtight containers.

Adverse Effects

Sodium nitrite may cause nausea and vomiting, abdominal pain, dizziness, headache, flushing, cyanosis, tachypnoea, and dyspnoea; vasodilatation resulting in syncope, hypotension, and tachycardia may occur. Overdosage may result in cardiovascular collapse, coma, convulsions, and death. Ionised nitrites readily oxidise haemoglobin to methaemoglobin, causing methaemoglobinaemia.

Sodium nitrite is a precursor for the formation of nitrosamines many of which are carcinogenic in *animals*, but a relationship with human cancer has not been established.

◊ Methaemoglobinaemia has been reported following the consumption of nitrite-contaminated meat.[1,2]
1. Walley T, Flanagan M. Nitrite-induced methaemoglobinaemia. *Postgrad Med J* 1987; **63:** 643–44.
2. Kennedy N, *et al.* Faulty sausage production causing methaemoglobinaemia. *Arch Dis Child* 1997; **76:** 367–8.

Treatment of Adverse Effects

When toxicity results from the ingestion of nitrites, treatment is supportive and symptomatic; oxygen and methylene blue [methylthioninium chloride] may be required for methaemoglobinaemia although methylene blue [methylthioninium chloride] should not be administered if cyanide poisoning is suspected since cyanide may be displaced. Exchange transfusion may be considered when methaemoglobinaemia is severe.

Uses and Administration

Sodium nitrite is used in conjunction with sodium thiosulfate in the treatment of cyanide poisoning (p.1433). The sodium nitrite produces methaemoglobinaemia; it is postulated that the cyanide ions combine with the methaemoglobin to produce cyanmethaemoglobin, thus protecting cytochrome oxidase from the cyanide ions, although other mechanisms may have a significant role. As the cyanmethaemoglobin slowly dissociates, the cyanide is converted to relatively non-toxic thiocyanate and is excreted in the urine. Sodium thiosulfate provides an additional source of sulfur for this reaction and this accelerates the process.

The usual dosage regimen in adults is 300 mg of *sodium nitrite* (10 mL of a 3% solution) given by intravenous injection over 3 to 5 minutes followed by 12.5 g of *sodium thiosulfate* (50 mL of a 25% solution or 25 mL of a 50% solution) given intravenously over a period of about 10 minutes. A suggested dosage regimen in children is 0.15 to 0.33 mL per kg body-weight, or 6 to 8 mL per m^2 body-surface, of a 3% solution of *sodium nitrite* (approximately 4.5 to 10 mg per kg) to a maximum of 10 mL, followed by 1.65 mL per kg, or 28 mL per m^2, of a 25% solution of *sodium thiosulfate* (412.5 mg per kg) to a maximum of 50 mL. The methaemoglobin concentration should not be allowed to exceed 30 to 40%. If symptoms of cyanide toxicity recur, it has been suggested that the injections of nitrite and thiosulfate may be repeated after 30 minutes at half the initial doses.

Sodium nitrite has also been suggested in the treatment of hydrogen sulfide poisoning (see p.1199).

Sodium nitrite has been used as a rust inhibitor. It is also used as a preservative in foods such as cured meats but should not be used in food for infants under the age of 3 months due to the risk of methaemoglobinaemia. Potassium nitrite is also used as a food preservative.

Preparations

USP 25: Sodium Nitrite Injection.

Proprietary Preparations (details are given in Part 3)
Austral.: O A R.

Multi-ingredient: *Canad.:* Sporex; *Ital.:* Benzogen Ferri; Citrosil Alcolico Azzuro; Esoform Ferri Alcolico†; Esoform Ferri†; *S.Afr.:* Tripac-Cyano; *USA:* Cyanide Antidote Package.

Sodium Polystyrene Sulfonate

(5009-k)

Sodium Polystyrene Sulphonate.
CAS — 9003-59-2; 9080-79-9; 25704-18-1.
Pharmacopoeias. In Br., Jpn, and US.

The sodium salt of sulfonated styrene copolymer with divinylbenzene.

Pharmacopoeial description

BP 2001: A cream to light brown, fine powder. It contains not less than 9.4% and not more than 11.0% of sodium, calculated with reference to the dried substance. Each g exchanges not less than 2.8 mmol and not more than 3.4 mmol of potassium, calculated with reference to the dried substance. Practically insoluble in water and in alcohol. Store in airtight containers.

USP 25: A golden brown, fine, odourless powder containing not more than 10% of water. The sodium content is not less than 9.4% and not more than 11.5%, calculated on the anhydrous basis. Each g exchanges not less than 110 mg and not more than 135 mg of potassium, calculated on the anhydrous basis. Insoluble in water.

Adverse Effects

Anorexia, nausea, vomiting, constipation, and occasionally diarrhoea may develop during treatment with sodium polystyrene sulfonate. Constipation may be severe; large doses in elderly patients and in children may result in faecal impaction and gastrointestinal concretions have occurred following oral administration to neonates. If necessary a mild laxative may be used to prevent or treat constipation; magnesium-containing laxatives should not be used (see Interactions, below).

Serious potassium deficiency can occur with sodium polystyrene sulfonate and signs of severe hypokalaemia may include irritability, confusion, ECG abnormalities, cardiac arrhythmias, and severe muscle weakness. Like other cation-exchange resins, sodium polystyrene sulfonate is not totally selective and its use may result in other electrolyte disturbances such as hypocalcaemia. Significant sodium retention may also occur, especially in patients with impaired renal function, and may lead to heart failure.

Effects on the gastrointestinal tract. Colonic necrosis has been reported[1,2] in 6 patients following administration of sodium polystyrene sulfonate in sorbitol as enemas. The inclusion of sorbitol was considered to contribute to this effect,[1,2] although it was subsequently pointed out that colonic irrigation, as recommended by the manufacturer, had not been carried out to remove the residual resin.[3,4]
1. Lillemoe KD, *et al.* Intestinal necrosis due to sodium polystyrene (Kayexalate) in sorbitol enemas: clinical and experimental support for the hypothesis. *Surgery* 1987; **101:** 267–72.
2. Wootton FT, *et al.* Colonic necrosis with Kayexalate-sorbitol enemas after renal transplantation. *Ann Intern Med* 1989; **111:** 947–9.
3. Burnett RJ. Sodium polystyrene-sorbitol enemas. *Ann Intern Med* 1990; **112:** 311–12.
4. Shepard KV. Cleansing enemas after sodium polystyrene sulfonate enemas. *Ann Intern Med* 1990; **112:** 711.

Effects on the lungs. Particles of sodium polystyrene sulfonate were found at autopsy in the lungs of 3 patients who had taken the resin by mouth and were associated with acute bronchitis and bronchopneumonia in 2 and with early bronchitis in the third.[1] It was suggested that rectal administration of sodium polystyrene sulfonate may be preferable, but if administration by mouth is necessary the patient should be positioned carefully to facilitate ingestion of the resin and avoid aspiration.
1. Haupt HM, Hutchins GM. Sodium polystyrene sulfonate pneumonitis. *Arch Intern Med* 1982; **142:** 379–81.

Precautions

Sodium polystyrene sulfonate should not be administered orally to neonates, and is contra-indicated by any route in neonates with reduced gut motility or in any patient with obstructive bowel disease. Care is also needed with rectal administration to neonates and children in order to avoid impaction of the resin. Treatment should be discontinued if clinically significant constipation develops. Sorbitol has been recommended for the prophylaxis and treatment of constipation (but see Effects on the Gastrointestinal Tract, above); magnesium-containing laxatives should not be used (see Interactions, below).

Patients receiving sodium polystyrene sulfonate should be monitored for electrolyte disturbances, especially hypokalaemia. Since serum concentrations may not always reflect intracellular potassium deficiency, symptoms of hypokalaemia should also be watched for and the decision to stop treatment assessed individually.

Use of sodium polystyrene sulfonate can result in sodium overloading and it should be used cautiously in patients with renal failure or conditions requiring a restricted sodium intake, such as heart failure and severe hypertension; calcium polystyrene sulfonate (p.1002) may be preferred in these patients.

The possible effects of sodium polystyrene sulfonate on serum electrolytes should be considered when diagnostic measurements are contemplated in patients receiving such treatment.

Following the administration of sodium polystyrene sulfonate retention enemas, the colon should be irrigated to ensure removal of the resin.

Interactions

Sodium polystyrene sulfonate is not totally selective for potassium and may also bind other cations. Metabolic alkalosis has been reported in patients, particularly those with renal impairment, after the concomitant oral administration of sodium polystyrene sulfonate and cation-donating antacids and laxatives such as magnesium hydroxide, aluminium hydroxide, or calcium carbonate; binding of the cation by the resin prevents neutralisation of bicarbonate ions in the small intestine. The potassium-lowering effect of the resin will also be diminished.

Ion-exchange resins may also bind other drugs given concomitantly, reducing their absorption. For reference to such an effect with thyroxine [levothyroxine], see p.1528.

Hypokalaemia may exacerbate the adverse effects of digoxin and sodium polystyrene sulfonate should be used with caution in patients receiving cardiac glycosides.

Uses and Administration

Sodium polystyrene sulfonate is a cation-exchange resin which exchanges sodium ions for potassium ions and other cations in the gastrointestinal tract following oral or rectal administration. The exchanged resin is then excreted in the faeces. Each gram of resin exchanges about 3 mmol of potassium *in vitro*, and about 1 mmol *in vivo*.

Sodium polystyrene sulfonate is used to enhance potassium excretion in the treatment of hyperkalaemia, including that associated with anuria or severe oliguria (caution is demanded due to the sodium content). An effect may not be evident for several hours or longer, and in severe hyperkalaemia, where a rapid effect is required, other measures must also be considered (see p.1182).

Serum-electrolyte concentrations should be monitored throughout treatment and doses given according to the patient's response.

The usual oral dose is 15 g up to four times daily as a suspension in water or syrup or as a sweetened paste. It should not be given in fruit juices that have a high potassium content. A suggested dose for children is up to 1 g per kg body-weight daily by mouth in divided doses for acute hyperkalaemia, reduced to a maintenance dose of 500 mg per kg daily; the oral route is not recommended for neonates.

When oral administration is difficult, sodium polystyrene sulfonate may be administered rectally as an enema. The usual daily dose is 30 g given as a suspension in 100 mL of 2% methylcellulose '450' and 100 mL of water and retained, if possible, for at least 9 hours; higher doses, shorter retention times, and alternative vehicles have also been used. Following retention of the enema the colon should be irrigated to remove the resin. Initial therapy may constitute administration by both oral and rectal routes. Children and neonates may be given rectal doses similar to those suggested for children by mouth; particular care is needed with rectal administration in children as excessive dosage or inadequate dilution could result in impaction of resin.

Other polystyrene sulfonate resins include calcium polystyrene sulfonate (p.1002), which is used similarly to the sodium form; potassium polystyrene sulfonate (p.1020), which is used in the treatment of hypercalciuria; aluminium polystyrene sulfonate, which was formerly used in the treatment of hyperkalaemia; and ammonium polystyrene sulfonate, which was formerly used to reduce the absorption of sodium ions.

Preparations

USP 25: Sodium Polystyrene Sulfonate Suspension.

Proprietary Preparations (details are given in Part 3)
Aust.: Resonium A; *Austral.:* Resonium A; *Belg.:* Kayexalate Sodium; *Canad.:* Kayexalate; *Denm.:* Resonium; *Fin.:* Resonium; *Fr.:* Kayexalate; *Ger.:* Elutit-Natrium; *Hong Kong:* Resonium A; *Irl.:* Resonium A; *Israel:* Kayexalate; *Ital.:* Kayexalate; *Neth.:* Resonium A; *NZ:* Resonium A; *Port.:* Resonium; *S.Afr.:* Kexelate; *Singapore:* Resinsodio; *Spain:* Resinsodio;
Swed.: Resonium; *Switz.:* Resonium A; *Thai.:* Kayexalate; Resinsodio; Resonium A; *UK:* Resonium A; *USA:* Kayexalate; Kionex; SPS.

Multi-ingredient: *Ger.:* Ujostabil.

Sodium Thiosulfate (1057-c)

Natrii Thiosulfas; Natrium Thiosulfuricum; Sodium Hyposulphite; Sodium Thiosulphate.
$Na_2S_2O_3,5H_2O = 248.2$.
CAS — 7772-98-7 (anhydrous sodium thiosulfate); 10102-17-7 (sodium thiosulfate pentahydrate).
Pharmacopoeias. In *Chin.*, *Eur.* (see p.vi), *Int.*, *Jpn*, *Pol.*, and *US*.

Pharmacopoeial description
Ph. Eur.: Colourless transparent crystals; efflorescent in dry air. It dissolves in its own water of crystallisation at about 49°. Very soluble in water; practically insoluble in alcohol. A 10% solution in water has a pH of 6.0 to 8.4. Store in airtight containers.
USP 25: Large, colourless crystals, or a coarse, crystalline powder. Is deliquescent in moist air and effloresces in dry air at temperatures exceeding 33°. Soluble 1 in 0.5 of water; insoluble in alcohol. Its solutions are neutral or faintly alkaline to litmus. Store in airtight containers.

Stability. Solutions of sodium thiosulfate 50% stored in air developed cloudiness or a deposit after autoclaving.[1] Addition of sodium phosphate 0.5% or 1.2% improved stability but solutions became cloudy or developed a deposit after 12 and 6 weeks respectively at 25°. Solutions containing sodium bicarbonate 0.5% became cloudy or developed a deposit after 12 weeks at 25°. No significant improvement in stability was obtained when the concentration of sodium thiosulfate was reduced to 30% or 15%, or when the injection was sealed under nitrogen.
1. Anonymous. Sodium thiosulphate injection–effect of additives on stability. *PSGB Lab Rep* P/75/3 1975.

Adverse Effects

Apart from osmotic disturbances sodium thiosulfate is relatively non-toxic. Large doses by mouth have a cathartic action.

Interactions

◊ For reference to the inactivation of phenylmercuric salts by sodium thiosulfate, see Phenylmercuric Nitrate, p.1154.

Pharmacokinetics

Sodium thiosulfate is poorly absorbed from the gastrointestinal tract. After intravenous injection it is distributed throughout the extracellular fluid and rapidly excreted in the urine.

◊ An intravenous infusion of sodium thiosulfate 12 g per m² body-surface was administered over 6 hours to 8 patients receiving intraperitoneal antineoplastic therapy;[1] in 6 of the patients it was given in conjunction with cisplatin to protect against the adverse effects of cisplatin. The thiosulfate was rapidly eliminated, 95% being excreted within 4 hours of stopping the infusion; on average only 28.5% of the dose was recovered unchanged in the urine. The mean plasma elimination half-life was 80 minutes.
1. Shea M, *et al.* Kinetics of sodium thiosulfate, a cisplatin neutralizer. *Clin Pharmacol Ther* 1984; **35:** 419–25.

Uses and Administration

Sodium thiosulfate is used in the treatment of cyanide poisoning (p.1433). Sodium thiosulfate may be effective alone in less severe cases of cyanide poisoning, but it is often used after administration of sodium nitrite (p.1023).

Sodium thiosulfate acts as a sulfur-donating substrate for the enzyme rhodanese, which catalyses the conversion of cyanide to relatively non-toxic thiocyanate, and thus accelerates the detoxification of cyanide.

The usual dosage regimen in adults is 300 mg of *sodium nitrite* (10 mL of a 3% solution) given by intravenous injection over 3 to 5 minutes followed by 12.5 g of *sodium thiosulfate* (50 mL of a 25% solution or 25 mL of a 50% solution) given intravenously over a period of about 10 minutes. A suggested dosage regimen in children is 0.15 to 0.33 mL per kg body-weight, or 6 to 8 mL per m² body-surface, of a 3% solution of *sodium nitrite* (about 4.5 to 10 mg per kg) to a maximum of 10 mL, followed by 1.65 mL per kg, or 28 mL per m², of a 25% solution of *sodium thiosulfate* (412.5 mg per kg) to a maximum of 50 mL. The methaemoglobin concentration should
not be allowed to exceed 30 to 40%. If symptoms of cyanide toxicity recur, it has been suggested that the injections of nitrite and thiosulfate may be repeated after 30 minutes at half the initial doses.

Sodium thiosulfate is used as an isotonic 4% solution in the management of extravasation of mustine [chlormethine] and has been tried in the management of extravasation of some other antineoplastics (although this is a contentious area, see p.480).

Sodium thiosulfate has been used for its antifungal properties. Sodium thiosulfate and magnesium thiosulfate are included in mixed preparations for a variety of disorders.

Antineoplastic toxicity. Sodium thiosulfate may be used in the management of extravasation of mustine [chlormethine] and some other antineoplastics (see p.480).
Sodium thiosulfate given by intravenous infusion has been reported to reduce the incidence of nephrotoxicity associated with intraperitoneal cisplatin (see under Adverse Effects in Cisplatin, p.525) and to reduce hearing loss associated with carboplatin (see Effects on the Ears, p.515).

Bromate poisoning. Sodium thiosulfate has been used in the treatment of bromate poisoning[1,2] although its clinical efficacy is unclear.[3] Sodium thiosulfate is thought to act by reducing bromate to the less toxic bromide ion, but evidence is lacking.[3] However, the high morbidity and mortality associated with bromate poisoning may justify the use of this relatively innocuous drug in some clinical circumstances.[4]
1. Lue JN, *et al.* Bromate poisoning from ingestion of professional hair-care neutralizer. *Clin Pharm* 1988; **7:** 66–70.
2. Lichtenberg R, *et al.* Bromate poisoning. *J Pediatr* 1989; **114:** 891–4.
3. McElwee NE, Kearney TE. Sodium thiosulfate unproven as bromate antidote. *Clin Pharm* 1988; **7:** 570, 572.
4. Johnson CE. Sodium thiosulfate unproven as bromate antidote. *Clin Pharm* 1988; **7:** 572.

Preparations

BP 2001: Sodium Thiosulphate Injection;
USP 25: Sodium Thiosulfate Injection.

Proprietary Preparations (details are given in Part 3)
Canad.: Consept Step 2; *Mex.:* Hiposul.

Multi-ingredient: *Aust.:* Schwefelbad Dr Klopfer; *Belg.:* ITC†; *Braz.:* Alersan; Desensibilizante Chauvin; Osmogenol; *Canad.:* Adasept; *Fr.:* Desintex; Desintex Infantile; Desintex-Choline; Rhino-Sulfuryl; Vagostabyl; *Ger.:* Corti Jaikal; Jaikal; Schwefelbad Dr Klopfer; *Hong Kong:* Colircusi Iodine-Thio-Calcic; *S.Afr.:* Tripac-Cyano; *Spain:* Yodo Tio Calci; *Switz.:* Thiorubrol; *USA:* Cyanide Antidote Package; Tinver; Versiclear.

Succimer (1058-k)

Succimer (*BAN, USAN, rINN*).
DIM-SA; DMSA. meso-2,3-Dimercaptosuccinic acid; (R^*,S^*)-2,3-Dimercapto-butanedioic acid.
$C_4H_6O_4S_2 = 182.2$.
CAS — 304-55-2.

Adverse Effects and Precautions

Succimer may cause gastrointestinal disorders, skin rashes, increases in serum transaminase, flu-like symptoms, drowsiness, and dizziness. Mild to moderate neutropenia has been reported in some patients and regular full blood counts are recommended during therapy. Succimer should be used with caution in patients with renal impairment or a history of hepatic disease.

Pharmacokinetics

Succimer is rapidly but incompletely absorbed after oral administration. It undergoes rapid and extensive metabolism and is excreted mainly in the urine with small amounts excreted in the bile and via the lungs.

◊ References.
1. Dart RC, *et al.* Pharmacokinetics of meso-2,3-dimercaptosuccinic acid in patients with lead poisoning and in healthy adults. *J Pediatr* 1994; **125:** 309–16.

Uses and Administration

Succimer is a chelator structurally related to dimercaprol (p.1007). It forms water-soluble chelates with heavy metals and is used in the treatment of lead poisoning. It has also been used in the treatment of poisoning with arsenic and mercury.

Succimer, labelled with a radionuclide, is used in nuclear medicine.

In the treatment of lead poisoning, succimer is given by mouth in a suggested dose of 10 mg per kg body-weight or 350 mg per m² body-surface every 8 hours for 5 days then every 12 hours for an additional 14 days. The course of treatment may be repeated if necessary, usually after an interval of not less than 2 weeks.

Lead poisoning. The use of succimer in lead poisoning has been reviewed.[1,2] Although, in children, succimer is generally only indicated if blood-lead concentrations are greater than 45 µg per 100 mL,[3] promising results have also been reported in those with lower concentrations.[4] A number of dosage regimens have been studied.[5] For the management of lead poisoning, see Lead, Treatment of Adverse Effects, p.1627.

1. Anonymous. Succimer—an oral drug for lead poisoning. *Med Lett Drugs Ther* 1991; **33:** 78.
2. Mann KV, Travers JD. Succimer, an oral lead chelator. *Clin Pharm* 1991; **10:** 914–22.
3. Rogan WJ, *et al.* The effect of chelation therapy with succimer on neuropsychological development in children exposed to lead. *N Engl J Med* 2001; **344:** 1421–6.
4. Besunder JB, *et al.* Short-term efficacy of oral dimercaptosuccinic acid in children with low to moderate lead intoxication. *Pediatrics* 1995; **96:** 683–7.
5. Farrar HC, *et al.* A comparison of two dosing regimens of succimer in children with chronic lead poisoning. *J Clin Pharmacol* 1999; **39:** 180–3.

Mercury poisoning. Extracorporeal infusion of succimer into the arterial blood line during haemodialysis, a procedure known as extracorporeal regional complexing haemodialysis, produced a substantial clearance of mercury in an anuric patient following intoxication with inorganic mercury.[1] Clearance was approximately ten times greater than that achieved with haemodialysis following intramuscular administration of dimercaprol. For the management of mercury poisoning, see Mercury, Treatment of Adverse Effects, p.1634.

1. Kostyniak PJ, *et al.* Extracorporeal regional complexing haemodialysis treatment of acute inorganic mercury intoxication. *Hum Toxicol* 1990; **9:** 137–41.

Preparations

Proprietary Preparations (details are given in Part 3)
Aust.: Chemet; *Fr.:* Succicaptal; *USA:* Chemet.

Tiopronin (13349-j)

Tiopronin (*rINN*).
Thiopronine. *N*-(2-Mercaptopropionyl)glycine.
$C_5H_9NO_3S = 163.2$.
CAS — 1953-02-2.
ATC — R05CB12.

Adverse Effects and Precautions

Tiopronin has similar adverse effects and precautions to those of penicillamine (p.1017).

◊ In a study of 140 patients[1] with rheumatoid arthritis receiving long-term treatment with tiopronin, adverse effects necessitated withdrawal of treatment in 56 patients (40%). The majority of adverse effects occurred within the first 6 months of treatment. The most common were those affecting the skin and mucous membranes (46 patients) including stomatitis, pruritus, erythema, and 1 case of pemphigus. Proteinuria developed in 5 patients and nephrotic syndrome in 3. Haematological disorders developed in 13 patients. Gastrointestinal disorders and ageusia were also reported.

In another study of 74 patients[2] with rheumatoid arthritis adverse effects were reported in 32 patients (43%) and necessitated withdrawal in 24%. The most common adverse effects were ageusia (21%), mucocutaneous lesions (16%), and gastrointestinal disturbances (14%). Haematological disorders occurred in 5 patients and proteinuria in 3 patients.

In a comparative study in 200 patients,[3] treatment was withdrawn due to toxicity in 27% of patients taking tiopronin and 21% of patients treated with gold.

1. Sany J, *et al.* Etude de la tolérance à long terme de la thiopronine (Acadione) dans le traitement de la polyarthrite rhumatoïde: a propos de 140 cas personnels. *Rev Rhum* 1990; **57:** 105–11.
2. Ehrhart A, *et al.* Effets secondaires dus au traitement par la tiopronine de 74 polyarthrites rhumatoïdes. *Rev Rhum* 1991; **58:** 193–7.
3. Ferraccioli GF, *et al.* Long-term outcome with gold thiosulphate and tiopronin in 200 rheumatoid patients. *Clin Exp Rheumatol* 1989; **7:** 577–81.

Effects on the blood. Leucopenia or thrombocytopenia has been reported in 13 of 140 patients[1] and 5 of 74 patients[2] during long-term studies of tiopronin.

Isolated cases of agranulocytosis[3] and bone marrow aplasia[4] have been reported.

1. Sany J, *et al.* Etude de la tolérance à long terme de la thiopronine (Acadione) dans le traitement de la polyarthrite rhumatoïde: a propos de 140 cas personnels. *Rev Rhum* 1990; **57:** 105–11.
2. Ehrhart A, *et al.* Effets secondaires dus au traitement par la tiopronine de 74 polyarthrites rhumatoïdes. *Rev Rhum* 1991; **58:** 193–7.
3. Corda C, *et al.* Thiopronin-induced agranulocytosis. *Therapie* 1985; **40:** 161.
4. Taillan B, *et al.* Aplasie médullaire au cours d'une polyarthrite rhumatoïde traitée par tiopronine. *Rev Rhum* 1990; **57:** 443–4.

The symbol † denotes a preparation no longer actively marketed

---

Effects on the kidneys. Proteinuria developed in 3 patients 4 to 14 months after starting treatment with tiopronin for cystinuria.[1] None of the patients had clinical symptoms of nephrotic syndrome. Renal biopsies in 2 patients demonstrated membranous glomerulonephritis. Proteinuria disappeared in all 3 patients 4 to 5 months after tiopronin was discontinued. However, there was histological evidence of irreversible changes and signs of progressive glomerular lesions in one patient.

Proteinuria was reported in 5 patients and nephrotic syndrome in 3 of 140 patients receiving tiopronin long term.[2]

1. Lindell A, *et al.* Membranous glomerulonephritis induced by 2-mercaptopropionylglycine (2-MPG). *Clin Nephrol* 1990; **34:** 108–15.
2. Sany J, *et al.* Etude de la tolérance à long terme de la thiopronine (Acadione) dans le traitement de la polyarthrite rhumatoïde: a propos de 140 cas personnels. *Rev Rhum* 1990; **57:** 105–11.

Effects on the liver. Acute liver damage often leading to jaundice has developed in patients given tiopronin; this has led to the Japanese authorities contra-indicating it in patients with a history of hypersensitivity and recommending that serial liver function tests be carried out during treatment.[1]

1. Anonymous. Tiopronin and liver damage. *WHO Drug Inf* 1989; **3:** 139.

Effects on the skin. Mucocutaneous lesions are among the most common adverse effects of tiopronin (see above). Lichenoid eruptions in a patient developed after 2 years of treatment with tiopronin and resolved when tiopronin was withdrawn.[1] Skin patch testing gave a positive response not only to tiopronin but also to penicillamine and captopril, neither of which the patient had taken. It was suggested that the lichenoid reaction was immunologically mediated and that the sulfhydryl group, which is common to all three compounds, could have been responsible.

Skin lesions resembling pemphigus have been reported in a few patients receiving tiopronin.[2,3] The lesions may improve when tiopronin is discontinued;[2] the remaining patients require treatment with a corticosteroid or other immunosuppressant drug, or both.[3]

1. Kurumaji Y, Miyazaki K. Tiopronin-induced lichenoid eruption in a patient with liver disease and positive patch test reaction to drugs with sulfhydryl group. *J Dermatol* 1990; **17:** 176–81.
2. Trotta F, *et al.* Thiopronine-induced pemphigus vulgaris in rheumatoid arthritis. *Scand J Rheumatol* 1984; **13:** 93–5.
3. Verdier-Sevrain S, *et al.* Thiopronine-induced herpetiform pemphigus: report of a case studied by immunoelectron microscopy and immunoblot analysis. *Br J Dermatol* 1994; **130:** 238–40.

Pharmacokinetics

Tiopronin is absorbed from the gastrointestinal tract. Up to 48% of the dose is reported to be excreted in the urine during the first 4 hours and up to 78% by 72 hours.

◊ References.

1. Carlsson SM, *et al.* Pharmacokinetics of intravenous 2-mercaptopropionylglycine in man. *Eur J Clin Pharmacol* 1990; **38:** 499–503.
2. Carlsson MS, *et al.* Pharmacokinetics of oral tiopronin. *Eur J Clin Pharmacol* 1993; **45:** 79–84.

Uses and Administration

Tiopronin is a sulfhydryl compound and chelator with properties similar to those of penicillamine (p.1019). It is given by mouth in the management of cystinuria, in conjunction with adequate hydration and alkalinisation of the urine, in usual doses of 0.8 to 1 g daily in divided doses, rising to 2 g if necessary. Tiopronin should be given on an empty stomach. Tiopronin is used in similar doses in rheumatoid arthritis. It has been tried in hepatic disorders, heavy-metal poisoning, and as a mucolytic in respiratory disorders, when it may be given by inhalation. It may also be given rectally or by intravenous or intramuscular injection.

The sodium salt has also been used.

Cystinuria. Tiopronin may be used as an alternative to penicillamine in the management of cystinuria (p.1019). In a multicentre study,[1] 66 patients with cystine nephrolithiasis were treated with tiopronin in doses of up to 2 g daily (mean 1.193 g); ongoing alkali therapy was continued and the same dietary and fluid regimens were maintained. Tiopronin significantly reduced urinary-cystine concentrations and the new stone formation rate. The adverse effects of tiopronin and penicillamine were compared in 49 patients who had been treated with penicillamine before starting the study. Both drugs had similar side-effects; 41 patients had side-effects to penicillamine of which 34 required cessation of drug therapy and 37 patients had side-effects to tiopronin of which 15 required drug withdrawal. However of the 34 patients who had to stop penicillamine therapy because of adverse effects, 22 were able to continue treatment with tiopronin. Of the 17 patients without a history of penicillamine therapy, 11 had adverse effects to tiopronin and 1 discontinued treatment because of proteinuria.

1. Pak CYC, *et al.* Management of cystine nephrolithiasis with alpha-mercaptopropionylglycine. *J Urol (Baltimore)* 1986; **136:** 1003–8.

Lead poisoning. Parenteral administration of tiopronin (30 g over a period of 10 days) to 27 men with symptoms of chronic lead poisoning had a beneficial effect on the biochemical indices of lead poisoning.[1] The mechanism of action was not clear since urinary lead excretion did not change. The usual treatment of lead poisoning is discussed on p.1627.

1. Candura F, *et al.* Sulphydryl compounds in lead poisoning. *Lancet* 1979; **i:** 330.

Mucolytic activity. Studies on the mucolytic activity of tiopronin.

1. Costantini D, *et al.* Evaluation of the therapeutic effectiveness of thiopronine in children with cystic fibrosis. *Curr Ther Res* 1982; **31:** 714–17.
2. Carratù L, *et al.* Clinico-functional and rheological research on mucolytic activity of thiopronine in chronic broncho-pneumopathies. *Curr Ther Res* 1982; **32:** 529–43.

Rheumatoid arthritis. Tiopronin has been reported to have activity comparable to that of gold salts[1] and penicillamine[2] in patients with rheumatoid disease, and could be tried cautiously to treat rheumatoid arthritis (p.9) in patients intolerant of penicillamine.

1. Ferraccioli GF, *et al.* Long-term outcome with gold thiosulphate and tiopronin in 200 rheumatoid patients. *Clin Exp Rheumatol* 1989; **7:** 577–81.
2. Sany J, *et al.* Etude de la tolérance à long terme de la thiopronine (Acadione) dans le traitement de la polyarthrite rhumatoïde: a propos de 140 cas personnels. *Rev Rhum* 1990; **57:** 105–11.

Preparations

Proprietary Preparations (details are given in Part 3)
Fr.: Acadione; *Ger.:* Captimer; *Hong Kong:* Thiola; *Ital.:* Mucolysin; Mucosyt; Thiola; Thiosol; *Switz.:* Mucolysin; *USA:* Thiola.
Multi-ingredient: *Spain:* Hepadigest†.

Trientine Dihydrochloride (13377-a)

Trientine Dihydrochloride (*BAN, rINNM*).
MK-0681; Trien Hydrochloride; Trientine Hydrochloride (*USAN*); Triethylenetetramine Dihydrochloride. 2,2′-Ethylenediiminobis(ethylamine) dihydrochloride; *N,N′*-bis(2-Aminoethyl)-1,2-ethanediamine dihydrochloride.
$C_6H_{18}N_4,2HCl = 219.2$.
CAS — 112-24-3 (trientine); 38260-01-4 (trientine dihydrochloride).
Pharmacopoeias. In *US*.

Pharmacopoeial description

USP 25: A white to pale yellow crystalline powder. Freely soluble in water; slightly soluble in alcohol; insoluble in chloroform and in ether; soluble in methyl alcohol. pH of a 1% solution in water is between 7.0 and 8.5. Store under an inert gas in airtight containers at 2° to 8°. Protect from light.

Adverse Effects and Precautions

Trientine dihydrochloride may cause nausea. Iron deficiency may occur; if iron supplements are given an interval of at least 2 hours between the administration of a dose of trientine and iron has been recommended. Recurrence of symptoms of systemic lupus erythematosus has been reported in a patient who had previously reacted to penicillamine.

Interactions

Chelation of trientine with metal ions in the diet or in mineral supplements may impair the absorption of both. Trientine should not be taken with mineral supplements and should be taken at least one hour apart from food, other drugs, or milk, to reduce the likelihood of absorption being affected. Iron supplements should be taken at least 2 hours before or after trientine.

Uses and Administration

Trientine dihydrochloride is a copper chelator used in a similar way to penicillamine in the treatment of Wilson's disease (p.1019). It tends to be used in patients intolerant of penicillamine.

Trientine dihydrochloride is administered by mouth, preferably on an empty stomach. In the USA the usual initial dose in adults is 0.75 to 1.25 g daily in 2 to 4 divided doses increasing to a maximum of 2 g daily if required; daily doses of 1.2 to 2.4 g have been recommended in the UK. In children, the usual initial dose is 0.5 to 0.75 g daily increasing to a maximum of 1.5 g daily if required.

Preparations

USP 25: Trientine Hydrochloride Capsules.

Proprietary Preparations (details are given in Part 3)
USA: Syprine.

Unithiol (1059-a)

DMPS; Unitiol. Sodium 2,3-dimercaptopropanesulfonate .
$C_3H_7NaO_3S_3 = 210.3$.
CAS — 4076-02-2.

Profile

Unithiol is a chelator structurally related to dimercaprol (p.1007). It is water soluble and reported to be less toxic than dimercaprol. Unithiol is used in the treatment of poisoning by heavy metals including arsenic, lead, inorganic and organic mercury compounds, and chromium. It may be less effective in cadmium poisoning.

Unithiol is given by mouth in doses of 100 mg three or four times daily in chronic poisoning. A dose of 1.2 to 2.4 g has been suggested in acute poisoning. It has also been administered parenterally.

◊ Reviews.
1. Aposhian HV. DMSA and DMPS—water soluble antidotes for heavy metal poisoning. *Ann Rev Pharmacol Toxicol* 1983; **23:** 193–215.
2. Hruby K, Donner A. 2,3-Dimercapto-1-propanesulphonate in heavy metal poisoning. *Med Toxicol* 1987; **2:** 317–23.

Lead poisoning. Unithiol has been tried in chronic lead poisoning. In a study of twelve children[1] it reduced lead concentrations in blood but did not affect the concentrations of copper or zinc in plasma, although the urinary excretion of lead, copper, and zinc was increased during treatment.

The usual chelators used in the management of lead poisoning are discussed under Lead, Treatment of Adverse Effects, on p.1627.
1. Chisolm JJ, Thomas DJ. Use of 2,3-dimercaptopropane-1-sulfonate in treatment of lead poisoning in children. *J Pharmacol Exp Ther* 1985; **235:** 665–9.

Mercury poisoning. Unithiol 100 mg given twice daily by mouth for a maximum of 15 days enhanced urinary elimination of mercury in 7 patients with mercury poisoning.[1] The urinary elimination of copper and zinc was also increased in most patients and two developed skin rashes. Unithiol, 50 mg per 10 kg body-weight by intramuscular injection three times daily reducing to 50 mg per 10 kg once daily by the third day of treatment, effectively reduced the half-life of mercury in the blood following poisoning with methylmercury.[2]

There has been a more recent report of 4 weeks of intravenous treatment followed by 3 weeks of oral treatment with unithiol in the successful management of a patient with severe poisoning with mercuric chloride.[3]

For the management of mercury poisoning, see Mercury, Treatment of Adverse Effects, p.1634.

1. Mant TGK. Clinical studies with dimercaptopropane sulphonate in mercury poisoning. *Hum Toxicol* 1985; **4:** 346.

2. Clarkson TW, *et al*. Tests of efficacy of antidotes for removal of methylmercury in human poisoning during the Iraq outbreak. *J Pharmacol Exp Ther* 1981; **218:** 74–83.
3. Toet AE, *et al*. Mercury kinetics in a case of severe mercuric chloride poisoning treated with dimercapto-1-propane sulphonate (DMPS). *Hum Exp Toxicol* 1994; **13:** 11–16.

Wilson's disease. Unithiol 200 mg twice daily[1] was used successfully to maintain cupriuresis in a 13-year-old boy with Wilson's disease (see p.1019) after he developed systemic lupus during treatment with penicillamine and with trientine dihydrochloride. Unithiol was started in two similar patients[1] but both withdrew from treatment, one because of fever and a fall in leucocyte count following a test dose and the other because of intense nausea and taste impairment.

1. Walshe JM. Unithiol in Wilson's disease. *BMJ* 1985; **290:** 673–4.

Preparations

Proprietary Preparations (details are given in Part 3)
Ger.: Dimaval; Mercuval.

Colouring Agents

Colouring agents have long been used in foods and cosmetics in an attempt to improve the appearance of the product or subject. They are also used in medicinal preparations with the aim of improving their acceptability to patients and this chapter describes the colouring agents used in medicines as well as those used in foods and cosmetics. Such uses are now widely controlled and this has resulted in restrictions on the extent to which colouring agents may be used. Matters of concern that have received considerable publicity include sensitivity reactions (see Tartrazine, p.1029) and hyperactive behaviour (see below).

Colouring agents can be broadly categorised into synthetic dyes and into natural agents (such as canthaxanthin, caramel, carmine, chlorophyll, cochineal, saffron, and turmeric, all of which are described in this chapter). Other compounds which may be used as cosmetic colours or food colours (and which are themselves the natural pigments of the foodstuffs) are anthocyanins (E163) and carotenoids. In this latter group are included bixin (E160b) and norbixin (E160b) which are obtained from annatto (E160b), capsanthin (E160c) which is an extract of paprika, carotenes (E160a) (see Betacarotene, p.1355), lycopene (E160d), beta-apo-8′-carotenal (E160e), and the ethyl ester of beta-apo-8′-carotenoic acid (E160f); lutein (E161b), like canthaxanthin, can be classified either as a carotenoid or as a xanthophyll.

Other agents described in *Martindale* that may be used as food colours include aluminium (p.1577), gold (p.1617), indigo carmine (p.1623), patent blue V (p.1649), riboflavin (p.1386), silver (p.1664), and titanium dioxide (p.1126).

Hyperactivity. The role of foods and food additives in hyperactive behaviour (p.1505) is not clear. In one double-blind placebo-controlled study,[1] children whose poor behaviour was attributed, by their parents, to the intake of food additives, were given oral challenges with food colours (amaranth, carmoisine, sunset yellow, and tartrazine) in doses far in excess of estimated normal daily intakes. Although the study investigators could measure a worsening of behavioural scores after the food colours, the parents did not note the difference between challenge and placebo periods. Another study[2] of similar design detected a dose-dependent association between tartrazine intake and behavioural changes (irritability, restlessness, and sleep disturbances).

1. Pollock I, Warner JO. Effect of artificial food colours on childhood behaviour. *Arch Dis Child* 1990; **65:** 74–7.
2. Rowe KS, Rowe KJ. Synthetic food coloring and behavior: a dose response effect in a double-blind, placebo-controlled, repeated-measures study. *J Pediatr* 1994; **125:** 691–8.

Allura Red AC (2372-l)

CI Food Red 17; Colour Index No. 16035; E129; FD & C Red No. 40. Disodium 6-hydroxy-5-(6-methoxy-4-sulphonato-*m*-tolylazo)naphthalene-2-sulphonate.
$C_{18}H_{14}N_2Na_2O_8S_2 = 496.4.$
CAS — 25956-17-6.

Profile
Allura red AC is used as a colouring agent in cosmetics and foodstuffs.

Amaranth (2373-y)

Bordeaux S; CI Acid Red 27; CI Food Red 9; Colour Index No. 16185; E123. It consists mainly of trisodium 3-hydroxy-4-(4-sulphonato-1-naphthylazo)naphthalene-2,7-disulphonate.
$C_{20}H_{11}N_2Na_3O_{10}S_3 = 604.5.$
CAS — 915-67-3.
Pharmacopoeias. In Fr.

Profile
Amaranth is used as a colouring agent in medicines, foodstuffs, and cosmetics.

◊ Although some evidence of carcinogenicity was found in early *animal* studies, subsequent work failed to confirm these findings and in the UK amaranth is considered suitable for use as a food colour.[1]

1. MAFF. Food advisory committee: final report on the review of the colouring matter in food regulations 1973. *FdAC/REP/4.* London: HMSO, 1987.

Beetroot Red (10150-r)

Beet Red; E162.

Beetroot red is obtained from the roots of red beets, *Beta vulgaris* var. *rubra* (Chenopodiaceae). The main colouring principle consists of betacyanins of which betanine is the main constituent.

Profile
Beetroot red is used as a colouring agent for foodstuffs and cosmetics.

Black PN (2375-z)

Brilliant Black BN; Brilliant Black PN; CI Food Black 1; Colour Index No. 28440; E151; Noir Brillant BN. It consists mainly of tetrasodium 4-acetamido-5-hydroxy-6-[7-sulphonato-4-(4-sulphonatophenylazo)-1-naphthylazo]naphthalene-1,7-disulphonate.
$C_{28}H_{17}N_5Na_4O_{14}S_4 = 867.7.$
CAS — 2519-30-4.
Pharmacopoeias. In Fr.

Profile
Black PN is used as a colouring agent in medicines, cosmetics, and foods.

Bordeaux B (2376-c)

Azorubrum; CI Acid Red 17; Colour Index No. 16180. It consists mainly of disodium 3-hydroxy-4-(1-naphthylazo)naphthalene-2,7-disulphonate.
$C_{20}H_{12}N_2Na_2O_7S_2 = 502.4.$
CAS — 5858-33-3.

Profile
Bordeaux B was formerly used as a colouring agent for medicines and foods but has been replaced by other colours.

Brilliant Blue FCF (2377-k)

Blue EGS; CI Acid Blue 9; CI Food Blue 2; Colour Index No. 42090; E133; FD & C Blue No. 1; Patent Blue AC. Disodium 4′,4″-bis(*N*-ethyl-3-sulphonatobenzylamino)triphenylmethylium-2-sulphonate.
$C_{37}H_{34}N_2Na_2O_9S_3 = 792.8.$
CAS — 3844-45-9.

Profile
Brilliant blue FCF is used as a colouring agent in medicines, cosmetics, and foodstuffs.

◊ Blue discoloration of the skin, initially attributed to cyanosis, has been reported[1] in a child who received a large quantity of brilliant blue FCF as a colouring in an enteral feed.

1. Zillich AJ, *et al.* Skin discoloration with blue food colouring. *Ann Pharmacother* 2000; **34:** 868–70.

Brown FK (2378-a)

Chocolate Brown FK; CI Food Brown 1; E154. A mixture of 6 azo dyes: sodium 2′,4′-diaminoazobenzene-4-sulphonate; sodium 2′,4′-diamino-5′-methylazobenzene-4-sulphonate; disodium 4,4′-(4,6-diamino-1,3-phenylenebisazo) dibenzenesulphonate; disodium 4,4′-(2,4-diamino-1,3-phenylenebisazo) dibenzenesulphonate; disodium 4,4′-(2,4-diamino-5-methyl-1,3-phenylenebisazo) dibenzenesulphonate; trisodium 4,4′,4″-(2,4-diaminobenzene-1,3,5-triazo)tribenzenesulphonate.
CAS — 8062-14-4.

Profile
Brown FK is used as a colouring agent for foodstuffs.

Brown HT (2386-a)

Chocolate Brown HT; CI Food Brown 3; Colour Index No. 20285; E155. Disodium 4,4′-(2,4-dihydroxy-5-hydroxymethyl-1,3-phenylenebisazo)di(naphthalene-1-sulphonate).
$C_{27}H_{18}N_4Na_2O_9S_2 = 652.6.$
CAS — 4553-89-3.

Profile
Brown HT is used as a colouring agent for foodstuffs.

Canthaxanthin (2380-l)

CI Food Orange 8; Colour Index No. 40850; E161(g). β,β-Carotene-4,4′-dione.
$C_{40}H_{52}O_2 = 564.8.$
CAS — 514-78-3.

Profile
Canthaxanthin is a carotenoid but unlike betacarotene or β-apo-8′-carotenal it possesses no vitamin A activity. It is given to salmon or trout to colour their flesh. It is also used in cosmetics.

Canthaxanthin has also been given by mouth to produce an artificial suntan, and as an adjunct to betacarotene in the management of erythropoietic protoporphyria (p.1011). Such use has led to retinal deposits and in some cases to impairment of vision.

◊ In the UK canthaxanthin has been considered to be suitable for use as a food colour; it was, however, believed that it should be restricted to use as a feed additive for farmed salmon and trout in order to produce a coloration of the fish flesh.[1] This restriction was based partly on reports of retinal changes in humans who had taken canthaxanthin orally, either for the production of an artificial tan by means of pigment deposition in the skin or for the medical treatment of erythropoietic protoporphyria. The retinal changes were an accumulation of bright yellow particles around the macula ('gold speck' maculopathy) and have been associated with altered function of the eye and visual deterioration.[1,2] Although a temporary acceptable daily intake for canthaxanthin was established by the FAO/WHO in 1987 this was not extended in 1990.[2] Long-term toxicity studies in *animals* had indicated a potential for hepatotoxicity although it was acknowledged that the primary problem associated with canthaxanthin was the possible retinal damage.[2] However, subsequent studies failed to confirm hepatotoxicity in humans and an acceptable daily intake was established by the FAO/WHO in 1995.[3]

There has also been a report of fatal aplastic anaemia in a patient who took canthaxanthin in order to produce an artificial tan.[4]

1. MAFF. Food advisory committee: final report on the review of the colouring matter in food regulations 1973. *FdAC/REP/4.* London: HMSO, 1987.
2. FAO/WHO. Evaluation of certain food additives and contaminants: thirty-fifth report of the joint FAO/WHO expert committee on food additives. *WHO Tech Rep Ser 789* 1990.
3. FAO/WHO. Evaluation of certain food additives and contaminants: forty-fourth report of the joint FAO/WHO expert committee on food additives. *WHO Tech Rep Ser 859* 1995.
4. Bluhm R, *et al.* Aplastic anemia associated with canthaxanthin ingested for 'tanning' purposes. *JAMA* 1990; **264:** 1141–2.

Preparations

Proprietary Preparations (details are given in Part 3)
Multi-ingredient: *Fr.:* Phenoro; *Switz.:* Apotrin.

Caramel (2381-y)

Burnt Sugar; E150; Sacch. Ust.; Saccharum Ustum.
CAS — 8028-89-5.
Pharmacopoeias. In USNF.

Caramels used as food colours are complex mixtures of compounds prepared by heating carbohydrates (food-grade sweeteners consisting of glucose, fructose, or polymers of these) either alone or in the presence of acids or alkalis (food-grade citric or sulfuric acids or calcium, potassium, or sodium hydroxides, or mixtures of these). The caramels can be classified according to the reactants used in the manufacturing process:
Class I (E150a, plain caramel, spirit caramel, or caustic caramel); no ammonium or sulfite compounds are employed.
Class II (E150b or caustic sulfite caramel); sulfate compounds employed but not ammonium compounds.
Class III (E150c, ammonia caramel, or beer caramel); ammonium compounds employed but not sulfite compounds
Class IV (E150d, sulfite ammonia caramel, or soft-drink caramel); both ammonium and sulfite compounds employed.

Pharmacopoeial description

USNF 20: A concentrated solution of the product obtained by heating sugar or glucose until the sweet taste is destroyed and a uniform dark brown mass results, a small amount of alkali or of alkaline carbonate or a trace of mineral acid being added while heating. It is a thick, dark brown liquid, having the characteristic odour of burnt sugar, and a pleasant bitter taste. One part dissolved in 1000 parts of water yields a clear solution having a distinct yellowish-orange colour. The colour of this solution is not changed and no precipitate is formed after exposure to sunlight for 6 hours. When spread as a thin layer on a glass plate, it appears homogeneous, reddish-brown, and transparent. Miscible with water; immiscible with ether, with chloroform, with acetone, with petroleum spirit, and with benzene; soluble in dilute alcohol up to 55%. Store in airtight containers.

Profile
Caramel is used as a colouring agent to produce pale yellow to dark brown colours; it is used as a food colour. It has no calorific value.

Some caramels also have flavouring properties.

Carmine (2382-j)

CI Natural Red 4; Colour Index No. 75470; E120.
CAS — 1390-65-4.
Pharmacopoeias. In Swiss which specifies the aluminium-calcium lake.

An aluminium lake of the colouring matter of cochineal. It contains carminic acid, an anthraquinone glycoside. Unless precautions are taken during manufacture and transport to prevent contamination, carmine may be infected with salmonella micro-organisms.

Profile
Carmine and some of its salts are used as colouring agents in medicines, foodstuffs, and cosmetics.

Carmine passes through the gastrointestinal tract unchanged and has been used as a faecal 'marker' in a dose of 200 to 500 mg.

◊ Extrinsic allergic alveolitis has been described (1 patient) due to occupational exposure to carmine used as a food additive.[1] Additionally, severe anaphylactic reactions have occurred following the ingestion of food[2,3] (2 patients) and drink[4] (1 patient) containing carmine as a colour.

1. Dietemann-Molard A, *et al.* Extrinsic allergic alveolitis secondary to carmine. *Lancet* 1991; **338:** 460.
2. Beaudouin E, *et al.* Food anaphylaxis following ingestion of carmine. *Ann Allergy Asthma Immunol* 1995; **74:** 427–30.
3. Baldwin JL, *et al.* Popsicle-induced anaphylaxis due to carmine dye allergy. *Ann Allergy Asthma Immunol* 1997; **79:** 415–19.
4. Kägi MK, *et al.* Campari-orange anaphylaxis due to carmine allergy. *Lancet* 1994; **344:** 60–1.

Carmoisine (2384-c)

Azorubine; CI Food Red 3; Colour Index No. 14720; E122. It consists mainly of disodium 4-hydroxy-3-(4-sulphonato-1-naphthylazo)naphthalene-1-sulphonate.
$C_{20}H_{12}N_2Na_2O_7S_2 = 502.4.$
CAS — 3567-69-9.
Pharmacopoeias. In Fr.

Profile
Carmoisine is used as a colouring agent in foods, medicines, and cosmetics.

Chlorophyll (2385-k)

CI Natural Green 3; Colour Index No. 75810; E140.
CAS — 479-61-8 (chlorophyll a); 519-62-0 (chlorophyll b).
Pharmacopoeias. US includes Chlorophyllin Copper Complex Sodium.

Chlorophyll is a green colouring matter of plants that contains two closely related substances, chlorophyll a ($C_{55}H_{72}MgN_4O_5 = 893.5$) and chlorophyll b ($C_{55}H_{70}MgN_4O_6 = 907.5$). The only difference between the 2 chlorophylls is that a methyl side-chain in chlorophyll a is replaced by a formyl group in chlorophyll b.

Oil-soluble chlorophyll derivatives. Replacement of the magnesium atom in the chlorophylls by 2 hydrogen atoms using dilute mineral acids produces olive-green water-insoluble phaeophytins. Copper phaeophytins (sometimes called copper chlorophyll complex; E141) can be formed; these are more stable to acids and to light than the chlorophylls.

Water-soluble chlorophyll derivatives. When the chlorophylls are hydrolysed with alkali, phytyl alcohol and methyl alcohol are split off and green water-soluble chlorophyllins are formed as the potassium or sodium salts. Similar water-soluble compounds can be prepared in which the magnesium is replaced by copper to give copper chlorophyllin complex (E141).

Profile
Chlorophylls and chlorophyllins, as well as the copper complexes of these compounds, are employed principally as colouring agents, in foods, medicines, and cosmetics.

Chlorophyll is used as an external application in the treatment of wounds and ulcers. There is no clear evidence that it accelerates healing but it is considered to have a deodorant action. Chlorophyllin and copper chlorophyllin complex are used similarly.

Preparations
Proprietary Preparations (details are given in Part 3)
Ger.: Anti-Geruchs; **USA:** Chloresium; Derifil; Innerfresh Pro†; Pals.

Multi-ingredient: Belg.: Ex'ail†; **Braz.:** Anapyon; Broncopinol; Gargosedans; Gargotrat; Higienex; Massageol; Mentolatun; Napiro; Sanador; Sanoclorofila; **Fr.:** Ex'ail; **Ger.:** Bagnisan med Heilbad; Chlorophyl liquid "Schuh"; Chlorophyllin Salbe "Schuh"; Ginseng-Complex "Schuh"; Stomasal Med; **Hong Kong:** Crema-U; **Ital.:** Dentovax†; **Spain:** Balneogel; Odontocromil c Sulfamida; Vitavox Pastillas; **Thai.:** Sanaco; **UK:** Chlorophyll; **USA:** Panafil; Prophyllin.

Cochineal (2387-t)

CI Natural Red 4; Coccionella; Coccus; Coccus Cacti; Colour Index No. 75470; E120.
CAS — 1343-78-8.
Pharmacopoeias. In Br.

Pharmacopoeial description
BP 2001: The dried female insect, *Dactylopius coccus* containing eggs and larvae. It has a characteristic odour. It complies with a test for contamination with *Escherichia coli* and salmonellae.

Profile
Cochineal, which is a source of carmine, is used as a red colouring agent in food, medicines, and cosmetics.
Cochineal is also used in homoeopathic medicine.

Curcumin (10200-z)

Colour Index No. 75300; E100. 1,7-Bis(4-hydroxy-3-methoxy-phenyl)hepta-1,6-diene-3,5-dione.
$C_{21}H_{20}O_6 = 368.4.$

Curcumin is the main colouring component of turmeric (p.1029).

Profile
Curcumin is used as a colouring agent for foodstuffs and cosmetics.

Eosin (2391-z)

CI Acid Red 87; Colour Index No. 45380; D & C Red No. 22; Eosin Y; Éosine Disodique. The disodium salt of 2′,4′,5′,7′-tetra-bromofluorescein.
$C_{20}H_6Br_4Na_2O_5 = 691.9.$
CAS — 548-26-5; 17372-87-1.
ATC — D08AX02.
Pharmacopoeias. In Fr.

Profile
Eosin has been incorporated in solution-tablets to give a distinctive colour to solutions prepared from them. It is also used in cosmetics.

Erythrosine (2392-c)

CI Food Red 14; Colour Index No. 45430; E127; Erythrosine BS; Erythrosine Sodium; FD & C Red No. 3. The monohydrate of the disodium salt of 2′,4′,5′,7′-tetraiodofluorescein.
$C_{20}H_6I_4Na_2O_5,H_2O = 897.9.$
CAS — 568-63-8 (anhydrous erythrosine sodium); 16423-68-0 (anhydrous erythrosine sodium); 49746-10-3 (erythrosine sodium monohydrate).
Pharmacopoeias. Fr. permits disodium or dipotassium salts.

Red or brownish-red odourless hygroscopic powder. Soluble in water forming a bluish-red solution that shows no fluorescence in ordinary light.

Profile
Erythrosine is used as a colouring agent for medicines and foods. It is also used in cosmetics and as a disclosing agent for plaque on teeth.

◊ Although early *animal* studies had indicated that erythrosine might have an adverse effect on the thyroid gland some authorities,[1] on re-assessing the evidence together with later studies, consider that erythrosine is not genotoxic or mutagenic and that it is suitable for use as a food colour.

1. MAFF. Food advisory committee: final report on the review of the colouring matter in food regulations 1973. *FdAC/REP/4.* London: HMSO, 1987.

Preparations
Proprietary Preparations (details are given in Part 3)
Austral.: Disclo-Gel; Disclo-Tabs; **UK:** Ceplac.

Ferric Oxide (5038-f)

E172 (iron oxides or hydroxides).
CAS — 51274-00-1; 1309-37-1.
Pharmacopoeias. Fr. includes monographs for black, brown, red, and yellow forms of ferric oxide. It. includes both red and yellow ferric oxide. USNF allows the basic colours of red or yellow ferric oxide or mixtures of these.

Pharmacopoeial description
USNF 20: A powder exhibiting two basic colours (red and yellow), or other shades produced on blending the basic colours. Insoluble in water and in organic solvents; dissolves in hydrochloric acid upon warming, a small amount of insoluble residue usually remaining.

Profile
Ferric oxide is used for tinting pharmaceutical preparations and foodstuffs.

Preparations
Proprietary Preparations (details are given in Part 3)
Multi-ingredient: Port.: Filter Oil Free.

Green S (2394-a)

Acid Brilliant Green BS; Acid Green S; CI Food Green 4; Colour Index No. 44090; E142; Lissamine Green; Wool Green B. Sodium 1-[4-dimethylamino-α-(4-dimethyliminiocyclohexa-2,5-dienylidene)benzyl]-2-hydroxynaphthalene-3,6-disulphonate.
$C_{27}H_{25}N_2NaO_7S_2 = 576.6.$
CAS — 3087-16-9.

Profile
Green S is used as a colouring agent in medicines, cosmetics, and foodstuffs.

◊ Studies in *animals* indicated that there is some absorption of green S and caecal enlargement but it was considered that there is a very large margin of safety between the highest estimated intake of green S of 130 μg per person daily and the level at which changes were seen in *animal* studies (500 mg per kg body-weight daily). It was recommended that the use of green S in food is acceptable.[1]

1. MAFF. Food advisory committee: final report on the review of the colouring matter in food regulations 1973. *FdAC/REP/4.* London: HMSO, 1987.

Pigment Rubine (10167-q)

E180; Lithol Rubine BK.

Profile
Pigment rubine is used as a colouring agent for foodstuffs.

Ponceau 4R (2397-r)

Brilliant Ponceau 4RC; Brilliant Scarlet; CI Food Red 7; Coccine Nouvelle; Cochineal Red A; Colour Index No. 16255; E124; Rouge Cochenille A. Trisodium 7-hydroxy-8-(4-sulphonato-1-naphthylazo)naphthalene-1,3-disulphonate.
$C_{20}H_{11}N_2Na_3O_{10}S_3 = 604.5.$
CAS — 2611-82-7.
Pharmacopoeias. In Fr.

Profile
Ponceau 4R is used as a colouring agent in medicines, cosmetics, and foods. Sensitivity reactions have been reported.

Quinoline Yellow (2398-f)

Canary Yellow; CI Acid Yellow 3; CI Food Yellow 13; Colour Index No. 47005; E104; Jaune De Quinoléine. The sodium salts of a mixture of the mono- and disulfonic acids of quinophthalone or 2-(2-quinolyl)indanedione.
CAS — 8004-92-0.

NOTE. D & C yellow No. 10 is used as a synonym for quinoline yellow, but describes a mixture consisting mainly of the mono-sulfonic acid of quinophthalone.
Pharmacopoeias. In Fr.

Profile
Quinoline yellow is used as a colouring agent in medicines, cosmetics, and foodstuffs.

◊ A severe urticarial reaction[1] in a patient has been attributed to quinoline yellow (E104).

1. Bell T. Colourants and drug reactions. *Lancet* 1991; **338:** 55–6.

Raspberry (2399-d)

Framboise; Fructus Rubi Idaei; Himbeer; Rubus Idaeus.
CAS — 8027-46-1.

The fresh ripe fruit of *Rubus idaeus* (Rosaceae).

Profile
Raspberry is used as a colouring and flavouring agent in medicines and foodstuffs.

Preparations
Proprietary Preparations (details are given in Part 3)
Multi-ingredient: Fr.: IgeE.

Red 2G (2400-d)

Acid Red 1; CI Food Red 10; Colour Index No. 18050; E128; Ext. D & C Red No. 11; Geranine 2G. Disodium 5-acetamido-4-hydroxy-3-phenylazonaphthalene-2,7-disulphonate.
$C_{18}H_{13}N_3Na_2O_8S_2 = 509.4.$
CAS — 3734-67-6.

Profile
Red 2G is used as a colouring agent in medicines, cosmetics, and foods.

◊ There has been concern that red 2G might produce haemolysis in subjects deficient in glucose-6-phosphate dehydrogenase, but investigations have not confirmed such a risk. However, red 2G might hydrolyse in acid solution to red 10B about which there is inadequate data. Therefore, in the UK it is considered undesirable to use red 2G in foods of high acidity that are subjected to a high temperature during processing and is recommended that the use of red 2G is confined to certain meat products.[1]

1. MAFF. Food advisory committee: final report on the review of the colouring matter in food regulations 1973. *FdAC/REP/4.* London: HMSO, 1987.

Red Cherry (2401-n)

Acerola; Cerasus; Cerise Rouge; Ginja; Griottier.

Pharmacopoeias. In Fr.

The fresh ripe fruit of varieties of the red or sour cherry, *Prunus cerasus* (Rosaceae).

Profile
Red cherry is used as a colouring and flavouring agent. It has also been used in herbal preparations.

Preparations
Proprietary Preparations (details are given in Part 3)
Multi-ingredient: *Austral.:* Bio C; Bio-C Complex; *Switz.:* A Vogel Capsules polyvitaminees; *UK:* Vitamin C; *USA:* Bio-Acerola C Complex†; Citrus-flav C; Ester-C Plus; Ester-C Plus Multi-Mineral; Super Complex C†.

Red-Poppy Petal (2402-h)

Coquelicot; Klatschrose; Petalos de Amapola; Rhoead. Pet.; Rhoeados Petalum.

The dried petals of *Papaver rhoeas* (Papaveraceae).

Profile
Red-poppy petal has been used as a colouring agent. It is also included in several herbal preparations.

Preparations
Proprietary Preparations (details are given in Part 3)
Multi-ingredient: *Fr.:* Actisane Nervosite†; Astressane†; Nocvalene; *Ital.:* Normalax†; Relaten†; *Switz.:* Baume; Melissa Tonic†; Tisane pectorale et antitussive.

Red-Rose Petal (2403-m)

Fleur de Rose; Flos Rosae; Red Rose Petals; Ros. Pet.; Rosae Gallicae Petala; Rosae Petalum; Rosenblüte.

The petals of the red or Provins rose, *Rosa gallica* (Rosaceae).

Profile
Red-rose petal has been employed as a colouring agent and for its mild astringent properties.

Preparations
Proprietary Preparations (details are given in Part 3)
Multi-ingredient: *Braz.:* Broncmel; *Fr.:* Ophtalmine; *Ger.:* Melrosum Hustensirup N.

Saffron (2407-q)

Açafrão; Azafrán; CI Natural Yellow 6; Colour Index No. 75100; Croci Stigma; Crocus; Estigmas de Azafrán; Safran.

Pharmacopoeias. In Aust., Chin., and Jpn.

The dried stigmas and tops of the styles of *Crocus sativus* (Iridaceae), containing crocines, crocetins, and picrocrocine.

Profile
Saffron is used as a food and cosmetic dye and flavouring agent. In some circles it is considered to be a food. It was once widely used for colouring medicines. Saffron has been included in preparations for teething pain. There have been reports of poisoning with saffron.

Saffron is also used in homoeopathic medicine.

Preparations
Proprietary Preparations (details are given in Part 3)
Multi-ingredient: *Belg.:* Calmant Martou†; *Fr.:* Delabarre.; *Ger.:* Infi-tract N; Schwedentrunk mit Ginseng†; Schwedentrunk†; *Ital.:* Fluxoten†; *Spain:* Dentol Topico; Dentomicin; Nani Pre Dental.

Sunset Yellow FCF (2410-h)

CI Food Yellow 3; Colour Index No. 15985; E110; FD & C Yellow No. 6; Jaune Orangé S; Jaune Soleil; Orange Yellow S. Disodium 6-hydroxy-5-(4-sulphonatophenylazo)naphthalene-2-sulphonate.
$C_{16}H_{10}N_2Na_2O_7S_2 = 452.4.$
CAS — 2783-94-0.
Pharmacopoeias. In Fr.

Profile
Sunset yellow FCF is used as a colouring agent in foods, medicines, and cosmetics. Sensitivity reactions have been reported.

◊ Although some evidence of carcinogenicity was found in early *animal* studies subsequent work failed to confirm these findings and in the UK sunset yellow FCF is considered suitable for use as a food colour.[1]

1. MAFF. Food advisory committee: final report on the review of the colouring matter in food regulations 1973. *FdAC/REP/4.* London: HMSO, 1987.

◊ Hypersensitivity reactions including severe abdominal cramps[1] and Quincke's oedema[2] have been recorded in individual patients receiving medication that was coloured with sunset yellow FCF.

1. Gross PA, *et al.* Additive allergy: allergic gastroenteritis due to yellow dye #6. *Ann Intern Med* 1989; **111:** 87–8.
2. Lévesque H, *et al.* Reporting adverse drug reactions by proprietary name. *Lancet* 1991; **338:** 393.

Preparations
BP 1980: Compound Tartrazine Solution.

Tartrazine (2411-m)

CI Food Yellow 4; Colour Index No. 19140; E102; FD & C Yellow No. 5; Jaune Tartrique; Tartrazin.; Tartrazol Yellow. It consists mainly of trisodium 5-hydroxy-1-(4-sulphonatophenyl)-4-(4-sulphonatophenylazo)pyrazole-3-carboxylate.
$C_{16}H_9N_4Na_3O_9S_2 = 534.4.$
CAS — 1934-21-0.
Pharmacopoeias. In Fr.

Profile
Tartrazine is used as a colouring agent in foods, cosmetics, and medicines. Some patients may experience sensitivity reactions.

◊ There have been numerous reports of reactions to tartrazine and these cover angioedema, asthma, urticaria, and anaphylactic shock. Some of the reports have dealt with cross-sensitivity, especially with aspirin, although the connection with aspirin has been questioned.[1] A suggested incidence[2] of tartrazine sensitivity is 1 in 10 000. The mechanism of the reactions may not necessarily be immunological.[3]
In considering the reports of tartrazine sensitivity or intolerance the Food Advisory Committee in the UK[1] reported that similar evidence of intolerance might well be obtained for a variety of natural food ingredients if as many studies were conducted on them as on tartrazine. The Committee considered that tartrazine posed no more problems than other colours or food ingredients and recommended that the continued use of tartrazine in food is acceptable. However, use of tartrazine in medicines appears to be diminishing.

1. MAFF. Food advisory committee: final report on the review of the colouring matter in food regulations 1973. *FdAC/REP/4.* London: HMSO, 1987.
2. Anonymous. Tartrazine: a yellow hazard. *Drug Ther Bull* 1980; **18:** 53–5.
3. Murdoch RD, *et al.* Tartrazine induced histamine release in vivo in normal subjects. *J R Coll Physicians Lond* 1987; **21:** 257–61.

Preparations
BP 1980: Compound Tartrazine Solution.

Turmeric (2415-q)

CI Natural Yellow 3; Curcuma; Indian Saffron.

CAS — 458-37-7.

Pharmacopoeias. In Chin.
Eur. (see p.vi) includes Javanese Turmeric (Curcumae Xanthorrhizae Rhizoma).

The dried rhizome of *Curcuma longa* (Zingiberaceae).

Pharmacopoeial description
Ph. Eur.: Javanese Turmeric consists of the dried rhizome, cut in slices, of *Curcuma xanthorrhiza*. It contains not less than 5% v/w of essential oil and not less than 1% of dicinnamoyl methane derivatives expressed as curcumin, both calculated with reference to the anhydrous drug. It has an aromatic odour. Protect from light.

Profile
Turmeric is used principally as a constituent of curry powders and other condiments. Turmeric and its main ingredient curcumin (p.1028) are used as yellow colouring agents in foods. Turmeric has also been used as an ingredient of preparations indicated for biliary and gastrointestinal disorders.

◊ There has been some concern about the safety of turmeric oleoresin, an extract of turmeric, following reports of adverse thyroid changes in *pigs.*[1,2]

1. MAFF. Food advisory committee: final report on the review of the colouring matter in food regulations 1973. *FdAC/REP/4.* London: HMSO, 1987.
2. FAO/WHO. Evaluation of certain food additives and contaminants: thirty-fifth report of the joint FAO/WHO expert committee on food additives. *WHO Tech Rep Ser 789* 1990.

Preparations
Proprietary Preparations (details are given in Part 3)
Ger.: Aristochol CC; Choldestal; Meteophyt N; Sergast.

Multi-ingredient: *Aust.:* Aktiv Leber- und Gallentee; Bakanasan Leber-Galle; Claim; Gallo Merz; Kneipp Galle- und Leber-Tee; Krautertee Nr 17; Sanhelios Leber-Galle; Sanvita Leber-Galle; Spasmo Claim; *Austral.:* Arthriforte; Bioglan Joint Mobility; Extralife Arthri-Care; Extralife Liva-Care; Herbal Digestive Formula; *Fr.:* Hepatoum; *Ger.:* Chol-Arbuz N; Cholagogum F; Cholagogum N; Cholosolm Phyto; Digest-Merz; Gallo Merz N; Gastrol S; Hepaticum-Medice H; Hevert-Gall S; Horvilan N†; Kneipp Galle- und Leber-Tee N; Opobyl-phyto; Pankreaticum; Paverysat forte; spasmo gallo sanol; Steigal; Ventracid N; *Hong Kong:* Hepatofalk Planta; Lipochol; *Singapore:* Artrex; *Switz.:* Stago.

Vegetable Carbon (10105-c)

Carbon Black; E153; Vegetable Black.

NOTE. The name Carbon Black has also been used as a synonym for Channel Black, a colouring agent not used in food; care should be taken to avoid confusion between the two compounds.

Profile
Vegetable carbon, which consists essentially of finely divided carbon, is produced by the carbonisation of vegetable material such as peat. It is used as a colouring agent for foodstuffs and cosmetics.

Yellow 2G (2419-e)

107; Acid Light Yellow 2G; Acid Yellow 17; CI Food Yellow 5; Colour Index No. 18965. Disodium 2,5-dichloro-4-[5-hydroxy-3-methyl-4-(4-sulphonatophenylazo)pyrazol-1-yl]benzenesulphonate.
$C_{16}H_{10}Cl_2N_4Na_2O_7S_2 = 551.3.$
CAS — 6359-98-4.

Profile
Yellow 2G is used as a colouring agent in cosmetics.

Contrast Media

Contrast media are agents that enhance the images obtained from visualisation techniques such as radiography (X-ray imaging, including computed tomography), magnetic resonance imaging, or ultrasound imaging.

In **radiography**, contrast media may be used to increase the absorption of X-rays as they pass through the body, and this is described as *positive contrast*. A gas (air, oxygen, or carbon dioxide) may also be used for visualisation and this is referred to as *negative contrast*. When both gas and contrast medium are used concomitantly the procedure is called *double contrast*. Radiographic contrast media are described further below. Radiographic contrast media may also be used to enhance **computed tomography** images. Tomography is the procedure whereby a selected plane of the subject is visualised using X-rays.

Magnetic resonance imaging also provides sectional images. Contrast agents in magnetic resonance imaging (see below) enhance the images obtained from the absorption of radio waves by atomic nuclei.

In **ultrasound**, contrast agents enhance the images obtained from the reflection of sound waves by different tissues by providing air-liquid interfaces (see below).

Radiographic Contrast Media

Radiographic contrast media contain elements with high atomic numbers that absorb X-rays. The agents most commonly used are *iodinated organic compounds*, whose degree of opacity or radiodensity is directly proportional to their iodine content. *Barium sulfate* is a metal salt with a long established use as a contrast medium. Other heavy atoms have been investigated, but many, such as thorium dioxide and tantalum, were unsuitable due to acute or chronic toxicity.

The iodinated contrast media may be classified as either ionic or nonionic, and additionally as monomeric or dimeric.

The *ionic monomeric* media, such as the amidotrizoates, iodamide, and iopanoic acid, generally have very high osmolality when given in concentrations suitable for radiographic visualisation and the resulting hypertonic solutions are associated with a relatively high incidence of adverse effects. Since radiodensity depends solely upon the iodine concentration, and osmolality solely upon the number of particles present in a given weight of solvent, the osmolality of contrast medium solutions can be reduced for a given radiodensity by using an *ionic dimeric* medium, such as adipiodone or ioxaglic acid, that contains twice the number of iodine atoms in each molecule, or by using a *nonionic* medium that does not dissociate into cation and anion. Nonionic media may be *monomeric*, such as iohexol, iopamidol, iopromide, and ioversol, or *dimeric*, for example iotrolan. Thus the best ratio of radiodensity to osmolality is achieved with the nonionic dimeric media.

Choice of radiographic contrast medium. Radiographic techniques to visualise particular structures within the body depend upon the physical and chemical properties of the contrast medium used and upon the way in which it is administered. Some radiographic procedures and the specific contrast media used in them are described below. The likelihood of adverse effects is greater with the older iodinated ionic contrast media, especially in high risk patients (see below), and this also influences the choice of contrast medium.

For **urography** (visualisation of the kidneys and urinary tract) the molecule must be small and highly water-soluble, with low protein-binding, so that glomerular filtration is encouraged with subsequent passage through the urinary tract. For good visualisation high concentrations must be achieved in the urinary tract from the start, and this in turn means high plasma concentrations: contrast media for urography are thus invariably given by the intravenous route. Examples of ionic urographic media include the amidotrizoates, iotalamates, and metrizoates. These ionic monomeric media have a relatively high incidence of adverse effects, due in part to their high osmolality, and better tolerance may be achieved with compounds of lower osmolality, such as ionic dimeric media (ioxaglic acid) and nonionic media (iohexol, iopamidol, and iopromide).

The requirements for **angiography** (visualisation of the circulatory system) are similar to those for urography in that a water-soluble molecule is required that can be readily distributed through the blood vessels. In addition, the solution should be of low viscosity to facilitate rapid injection and of high radiodensity to counteract the diluting effects of the blood. There are no particular differences between requirements for visualisation of veins (**phlebography** or **venography**) and those for arteries (**arteriography**); however, for **angiocardiography** (visualisation of the heart and heart vessels), or **digital subtraction angiography** where movement of a bolus of contrast medium through the circulation is studied over a period of time, the heart may be exposed to higher-than-usual concentrations of contrast medium and low cardiotoxicity is particularly important. There has been a general trend towards the use of low osmolality media for all types of angiography, since greatly improved tolerance, and in particular less pain on injection, means that procedures can be carried out without general anaesthesia and with less risk of serious adverse effects. Examples of angiographic media include iodixanol, iohexol, iopamidol, iopromide, and ioversol.

For **gastrointestinal radiography** the principal requirements are that the contrast medium should not be absorbed but should form an even, homogeneous coat on the gastrointestinal mucosa, without interacting with gut secretions or producing misleading radiographic artifacts. The chief contrast medium for this purpose is barium sulfate, and much effort has been devoted to the production of suitable formulations to improve its coating properties and reduce the formation of bubbles, cracks, and other radiographic artifacts.

The requirements for **cholecystography** and **cholangiography** (visualisation of the gallbladder and biliary tract) depend to some degree on the intended route of administration. In order that the molecule should be preferentially excreted in the bile it should be sufficiently large for biliary excretion and must possess a free carboxy or other acidic group, since the biliary active transport mechanism is an anion transfer process. In addition, the molecule should be protected by virtue of its size or by protein binding from the more rapid renal excretion processes. However, the oral cholecystographic agents need to be absorbed from the gastrointestinal tract before they become effective, and this imposes a second, and to some extent conflicting, set of requirements. For optimal enteral absorption, molecules should be of relatively small size, sufficiently soluble in gastrointestinal fluids, and sufficiently lipophilic to pass the cell membranes of the mucosa. Examples of *oral* cholecystographic media include the iopodates, iocetamic acid, iopanoic acid, and sodium tyropanoate. These are relatively small, monomeric molecules and therefore they require conjugation with glucuronic acid within the body to achieve sufficient molecular weight for biliary excretion. They are often given after a fatty meal to enhance absorption and reduce the incidence of inadequate visualisation. The *intravenous* cholecystographic agents do not have to meet the above requirements for enteral absorption and are mostly larger, dimeric molecules that do not require conjugation. They are generally more effective than the oral media. Examples of intravenous cholecystographic media include salts of adipiodone and iotroxic acid.

For **myelography** (visualisation of the structures of the spinal cord) no special requirements other than good tolerance are necessary. Although visualisation was at one time achieved with oily media such as iofendylate these have now mostly been replaced with nonionic water-soluble media. These offer improved tolerance, better visualisation since they are miscible with cerebrospinal fluid, and, unlike the oil-based media, are removed from the subarachnoid space by normal pharmacokinetic mechanisms. Examples include iohexol and iopamidol.

Arthrography (visualisation of the joint capsule) may be performed with many different contrast media provided they are well-diluted before use.

Bronchography (examination of the bronchial tree) has been performed with oily or aqueous media, such as iopydol or iopydone, instilled through a catheter or bronchoscope to coat the airways.

For **hysterosalpingography** (visualisation of the uterus and fallopian tubes) a water-soluble contrast medium is required. Examples include iotrolan, ioxaglic acid, and metrizoic acid.

Very high radiodensity is required to obtain good visualisation of the lymphatic structures in radiography of the lymphatic system (**lymphography** or **lymphangiography**). In addition, water-soluble media rapidly leave the system and only particulate or water-insoluble media or very large molecules persist within the lymphatic vessels for any length of time. The medium that has been most frequently used is iodised oil. It gives good visualisation of that part of the lymphatic system between the point at which it is infused and the point at which it enters the general circulation, but it is not distributed throughout the whole lymphatic space and has the potential for a number of severe side-effects.

Adverse effects. The adverse effects of iodinated contrast media are described under Amidotrizoic Acid, p.1031. Many of the adverse effects[1,2] of iodinated ionic contrast media are associated with their high osmolality. The newer nonionic, low-

osmolal contrast media have a lower incidence of adverse effects than the older ionic, high-osmolal agents.[1,3,4] There is evidence from studies in Australia[3] and Japan[4] which suggests that 'low-risk' patients given conventional ionic media are at greater risk of adverse effects than patients considered 'at-risk' who are given nonionic media.

Cost considerations mean that low-osmolal media tend to be reserved for patients considered to be at high risk of adverse effects (see Precautions under Amidotrizoic Acid, p.1031).

1. Thomsen HS, Bush WH. Adverse effects of contrast media: incidence, prevention and management. *Drug Safety* 1998; **19:** 313–24.
2. Ansell G. Adverse reactions profile: intravascular iodinated radiocontrast media. *Prescribers' J* 1993; **33:** 82–8.
3. Palmer FJ. The RACR Survey of intravenous contrast media reactions: final report. *Australas Radiol* 1988; **32:** 426–8.
4. Katayama H, *et al.* Adverse reactions to ionic and nonionic contrast media: a report from the Japanese Committee on the Safety of Contrast Media. *Radiology* 1990; **175:** 621–8.

HYPERSENSITIVITY. Anaphylactoid reactions to iodinated contrast media are more common with the ionic agents than the nonionic media of lower osmolality. Patients at increased risk are those with a history of asthma or allergy, drug hypersensitivity, adrenal suppression, heart disease, previous reaction to a contrast medium, and those receiving beta blockers or interleukin-2 therapy. In such patients, nonionic media are preferred. Discontinuation of beta blockers should be considered in patients with other risk factors.

Pretreatment with corticosteroids may be considered for preventing anaphylactoid reactions in high-risk patients and an antihistamine may be given. However, the value is uncertain.

References.
1. Greenberger PA, *et al.* Effects of beta-adrenergic and calcium antagonists on the development of anaphylactoid reactions from radiographic contrast media during cardiac angiography. *J Allergy Clin Immunol* 1987; **80:** 698–702.
2. Lang DM, *et al.* Increased risk for anaphylactoid reaction from contrast media in patients on β-adrenergic blockers or with asthma. *Ann Intern Med* 1991; **115:** 270–6.
3. Ansell G. Adverse reactions profile: intravascular iodinated radiocontrast media. *Prescribers' J* 1993; **33:** 82–8.
4. Wittbrodt ET, Spinler SA. Prevention of anaphylactoid reactions in high-risk patients receiving radiographic contrast media. *Ann Pharmacother* 1994; **28:** 236–41.
5. Sidhu PS, Dawson P. Corticosteroid prophylaxis in contrast examinations. *Br J Hosp Med* 1997; **58:** 304–6.

THROMBOEMBOLISM. Angiography is associated with a risk of thromboembolism. It has been suggested[1-3] that nonionic contrast media, which are the preferred agents in angiography (see above), may contribute to this risk since they have less anticoagulant activity than the ionic contrast media. It is recommended that great care should be taken to prevent mixing of blood and contrast media before injection in angiography.

1. Robertson HJ. Thrombogenic potential of nonionic contrast media. *Mayo Clin Proc* 1990; **65:** 603–4.
2. King BF. Thrombogenic potential of nonionic contrast media. *Mayo Clin Proc* 1990; **65:** 604.
3. Anonymous. Thromboembolism during angiography. *Lancet* 1992; **339:** 1576–8.

Magnetic Resonance Contrast Media

Magnetic resonance contrast media are paramagnetic or superparamagnetic agents that enhance the magnetic resonance image by interfering with the relaxation times of adjacent nuclei. Paramagnetic contrast media include the gadolinium complexes, gadodiamide, gadopentetic acid, and gadoteridol, and the manganese complex mangafodipir trisodium. Superparamagnetic contrast media include the iron compounds ferristene, ferumoxides, and ferumoxsil.

◊ References.
1. Armstrong P, Keevil SF. Magnetic resonance imaging—1: basic principles of image production. *BMJ* 1991; **303:** 35–40.
2. Armstrong P, Keevil SF. Magnetic resonance imaging—2: clinical uses. *BMJ* 1991; **303:** 105–9.
3. Edelman RR, Warach S. Magnetic resonance imaging (first of two parts). *N Engl J Med* 1993; **328:** 708–15.
4. Edelman RR, Warach S. Magnetic resonance imaging (second of two parts). *N Engl J Med* 1993; **328:** 785–91.

Ultrasound Contrast Media

Contrast agents for use in ultrasound imaging, termed echocontrast agents or echo-enhancers, have recently been introduced. Microbubbles of gas encapsulated in albumin (p.724), galactose, or fluorocarbons such as perflenapent and perflisopent are examples.

◊ References.
1. Blomley H, Cosgrove D. Contrast agents in ultrasound. *Br J Hosp Med* 1996; **55:** 6–7.
2. Blomley MJK, *et al.* Microbubble contrast agents: a new era in ultrasound. *BMJ* 2001; **322:** 1222–5.

Adipiodone (1525-v)

Adipiodone (BAN, rINN).

Iodipamide. 3,3'-Adipoyldiaminobis(2,4,6-tri-iodobenzoic acid).
$C_{20}H_{14}I_6N_2O_6 = 1139.8$.
CAS — 606-17-7.
ATC — V08AC04.

Pharmacopoeias. In Chin., Pol., and US.

Adipiodone contains approximately 66.8% of I.

Pharmacopoeial description

USP 25: A white, practically odourless, crystalline powder.
Very slightly soluble in water, in chloroform, and in ether;
slightly soluble in alcohol.

Meglumine Adipiodone (1563-e)

Meglumine Adipiodone (rINNM).

Adipiodone Meglumine (BANM); Dimeglumine Iodipamide;
Iodipamide Meglumine; Meglumine Iodipamide. The di(N-meth-
ylglucamine) salt of adipiodone.
$C_{20}H_{14}I_6N_2O_6,(C_7H_{17}NO_5)_2 = 1530.2$.
CAS — 3521-84-4.

Pharmacopoeias. US includes only as an injection.

Meglumine adipiodone contains approximately 49.8% of I.
Incompatibilities have been reported with some antihistamines.

Adverse Effects, Treatment, and Precautions
See under the amidotrizoates, p.1031. The incidence of adverse
effects may be increased following rapid administration.

Adipiodone may show some uricosuric activity.

Effects on the liver. Of 149 patients who received the dose
of adipiodone recommended by the manufacturer 13 developed
elevated serum aspartate aminotransferase (SGOT) values; of
126 who received twice the dose, 23 developed elevated values.[1] Hepatotoxicity has also been reported[2-4] on isolated occasions in patients given meglumine adipiodone.

1. Scholz FJ, et al. Hepatotoxicity in cholangiography. JAMA 1974;
   229: 1724.
2. Stillman AE. Hepatotoxic reaction to iodipamide meglumine injection. JAMA 1974; **228:** 1420–1.
3. Sutherland LR, et al. Meglumine iodipamide (Cholografin)
   hepatotoxicity. Ann Intern Med 1977; **86:** 437–9.
4. Imoto S. Meglumine hepatotoxicity. Ann Intern Med 1978; **88:**
   129.

Pharmacokinetics
Meglumine adipiodone is rapidly distributed in extracellular
fluid following slow intravenous injection and is reported to be
extensively bound to plasma proteins. It appears in the bile
ducts within about 10 to 15 minutes after injection, with peak
opacity at about 40 to 80 minutes, and reaches the gallbladder
by about 1 hour, peak opacification occurring after about 2
hours. About 80 to 95% is excreted unchanged in the faeces;
small amounts are excreted unchanged in urine. A terminal
half-life of about 2 hours has been reported.

Uses and Administration
Adipiodone is an iodinated ionic dimeric contrast medium that
is used as its meglumine salt for cholecystography and cholangiography (p.1030).

It is administered by slow intravenous injection as a solution
containing 52% of the meglumine salt over an average of 10
minutes; the usual dose of meglumine adipiodone used is about
10 g.

Preparations

BP 2001: Meglumine Iodipamide Injection;
USP 25: Iodipamide Meglumine Injection.

Proprietary Preparations (details are given in Part 3)
Belg.: Transbilix†; *Canad.:* Cholografin†; *Fr.:* Transbilix†; *USA:*
Cholografin.

Multi-ingredient: *Canad.:* Sinografin†; *USA:* Sinografin.

Amidotrizoic Acid (1554-w)

Amidotrizoic Acid (BAN).

Acidum Amidotrizoicum; Diatrizoic Acid (USAN); NSC-
262168. 3,5-Diacetamido-2,4,6-tri-iodobenzoic acid.
$C_{11}H_9I_3N_2O_4,2H_2O = 649.9$.
CAS — 117-96-4 (anhydrous amidotrizoic acid); 50978-
11-5 (amidotrizoic acid dihydrate).
ATC — V08AA01.

Pharmacopoeias. In Eur. (see p.vi), Int., Jpn, and US.

It contains approximately 62% of I calculated on the anhydrous
substance.

Pharmacopoeial description

Ph. Eur.: A white or almost white, crystalline powder. Very
slightly soluble in water and in alcohol; practically insoluble in
ether; dissolves in dilute solutions of alkali hydroxides. Protect
from light.

USP 25: It is anhydrous or contains two molecules of water of
hydration. A white, odourless, powder. Very slightly soluble in
water and in alcohol; soluble in dimethylformamide and in alkali hydroxide solutions.

The symbol † denotes a preparation no longer actively marketed

Meglumine Amidotrizoate (1555-e)

Meglumine Amidotrizoate (BANM).

Diatrizoate Meglumine; Meglumine Diatrizoate; Methylglucamine Diatrizoate. N-Methylglucamine 3,5-diacetamido-2,4,6-
tri-iodobenzoate.
$C_{11}H_9I_3N_2O_4,C_7H_{17}NO_5 = 809.1$.
CAS — 131-49-7.

Pharmacopoeias. In US.

It contains approximately 47.1% of I.

Pharmacopoeial description

USP 25: A white, odourless, powder. Freely soluble in water.

Sodium Amidotrizoate (1556-l)

Sodium Amidotrizoate (BANM, rINN).

Diatrizoate Sodium; Natrii Amidotrizoas; NSC-61815; Sodium
Diatrizoate. Sodium 3,5-diacetamido-2,4,6-tri-iodobenzoate.
$C_{11}H_8I_3N_2NaO_4 = 635.9$.
CAS — 737-31-5.

Pharmacopoeias. In Eur. (see p.vi), Int., Pol., and US.

It contains approximately 59.9% of I calculated on the anhydrous substance.

Incompatibilities with some antihistamines have been reported.

Pharmacopoeial description

Ph. Eur.: A white or almost white powder. Freely soluble in
water; slightly soluble in alcohol; practically insoluble in acetone. A 50% solution in water has a pH of 7.5 to 9.5. Protect
from light.

USP 25: A white, odourless, powder. Soluble in water; slightly
soluble in alcohol; practically insoluble in acetone and in ether.

Adverse Effects and Treatment
Many of the effects of iodinated ionic monomeric contrast media can be attributed to the high osmolality which is a feature
of these agents; reducing the osmolality through altering the
ionic or molecular profile produces a reduced incidence of adverse effects (see p.1030). The route and speed of administration, and the volume, concentration, and viscosity of the
solution also affect the incidence of adverse effects. Most reactions occur within 5 to 10 minutes of injection, but they may be
delayed.

Hyperthyroidism has been reported following administration
of iodinated contrast media, presumably due to small amounts
of iodine present as a contaminant or released by any breakdown of the medium in the body. For the effects of iodine on
the thyroid gland, see p.1522.

When given by injection the amidotrizoates may cause nausea,
a metallic taste, vomiting, flushing and sensations of heat,
weakness, dizziness, headache, coughing, rhinitis, sweating,
sneezing, lachrymation, visual disturbances, pruritus, salivary
gland enlargement, pallor, tachycardia, bradycardia, transient
ECG abnormalities, haemodynamic disturbances, and hypotension. Rarely, more severe adverse effects, including convulsions, paralysis, coma, rigors, ventricular fibrillation,
pulmonary oedema, circulatory failure, and cardiac arrest have
occurred. Occasionally anaphylactoid or hypersensitivity reactions occur; dyspnoea, bronchospasm, angioedema, and severe
urticaria have been reported, and reactions have sometimes
been fatal. Injection of amidotrizoates into the CNS produces
severe neurotoxicity.

Deaths have also been recorded due to acute renal failure,
which may follow intravenous administration, particularly in
dehydrated patients and patients with other predisposing factors (see also under Effects on the Kidneys, and Precautions,
below).

Pain may occur at the injection site; extravasation may be followed by tissue damage, thrombophlebitis, thrombosis, venospasm, and embolism (see p.1030).

Fibrinolysis and a possible depressant effect on blood coagulation factors has been reported. Disseminated intravascular coagulation has occurred. Meglumine salts are reportedly better
tolerated and produce less pain on injection than sodium salts,
but the sodium salts may be associated with a lower incidence
of arrhythmias. As a result, the sodium and meglumine salts are
often given in combination to minimise adverse effects.

Mild diarrhoea may follow the oral or rectal administration of
sodium and meglumine amidotrizoates for gastrointestinal examinations. The accidental aspiration of solutions of these salts
has caused fatal pulmonary oedema.

Adverse effects are treated symptomatically and adequate resuscitative facilities should be available when radiographic
procedures are to be employed.

Effects on the blood. Reports of amidotrizoates adversely
affecting the blood.

1. Catterall JR, et al. Intravascular haemolysis with acute renal failure after angiocardiography. BMJ 1981; **282:** 779–80.
2. Shojania AM. Immune-mediated thrombocytopenia due to an iodinated contrast medium (diatrizoate). Can Med Assoc J 1985;
   133: 123.
3. Fairley S, Ihle BU. Thrombotic microangiopathy and acute renal
   failure associated with arteriography. BMJ 1986; **293:** 922–3.

Effects on the kidneys. Administration of contrast media
may be associated with renal toxicity.[1-3] Estimates of the inci-

dence of nephrotoxicity vary widely, but the figure is probably
less than 1% of all patients receiving contrast media and does
not appear to differ significantly with ionic or nonionic media.
In the majority of patients who develop contrast-medium-in-
duced renal impairment the condition develops within about 24
hours of the procedure, is asymptomatic, and resolves completely within about 10 days. However, the condition may occasionally be severe, producing oliguria and renal failure that
requires dialysis; fatalities have occurred.

The mechanism of nephrotoxicity is not well understood and it
seems probable that more than one type of lesion may contribute to the overall incidence of toxicity. Possible mechanisms
are tubular necrosis (including that due to anaphylaxis or cardiovascular collapse), traumatic occlusion of the renal arteries,
cholesterol embolism, and obstruction of the tubules by protein
casts (as in patients with multiple myeloma).

Risk factors include pre-existing renal impairment, especially
in patients with diabetes mellitus, and conditions where there is
reduced renal blood flow, such as heart failure and dehydration.
Old age, repeated administration (over a short period of time),
multiple myeloma, and pre-existing hepatic impairment have
also been proposed as risk factors.

1. Brezis M, Epstein FH. A closer look at radiocontrast-induced nephropathy. N Engl J Med 1989; **320:** 179–81.
2. Parfrey PS, et al. Contrast material-induced renal failure in patients with diabetes mellitus, renal insufficiency, or both. N Engl
   J Med 1989; **320:** 143–9.
3. Schwab SJ, et al. Contrast nephrotoxicity: a randomized controlled trial of a nonionic and an ionic radiographic contrast agent.
   N Engl J Med 1989; **320:** 149–53.

Precautions
The amidotrizoates and similar contrast media should be administered with great caution to patients with asthma or a history of allergy and should be avoided in patients with known
hypersensitivity to contrast media or to iodine. An intravenous
injection of 0.5 to 1 mL of contrast medium has been given as
a test for sensitivity before administration of the main dose but
it does not predict hypersensitivity with certainty and severe
reactions and fatalities have followed the test dose. Pretreatment with corticosteroids may be considered in patients considered 'at risk' but its value is uncertain (see Hypersensitivity
under Adverse Effects of Radiographic Contrast Media,
p.1030). An antihistamine may be given with the corticosteroid.

Caution is needed in patients with severe hepatic or renal impairment or others who may be at increased risk of renal failure; dehydrated patients should have their fluid and electrolyte
balance corrected before contrast medium administration. Patients with multiple myeloma may be at particular risk if dehydrated, since precipitation of protein in the renal tubules may
lead to anuria and fatal renal failure.

An increased risk of adverse effects has also been reported in
patients with severe hypertension, advanced cardiac disease,
phaeochromocytoma, sickle-cell disease, or hyperthyroidism.
Debilitated, severely ill, very old, or very young patients are
also at risk.

Certain problems may be associated with particular radiographic techniques. Administration of amidotrizoates or similar hypertonic media into the CNS, e.g. for myelography,
should be avoided, and use for cerebral angiography or
computed tomography of the brain is contra-indicated in
patients with subarachnoid haemorrhage. All intravascular
administration requires caution in patients with occlusive vascular disorders. These media should not be given for hysterosalpingography in the presence of infection or inflammation of
the pelvic cavity, nor during menstruation or in pregnancy (but
all abdominal radiography should be avoided in any case during pregnancy because of the risks of radiation to the fetus).

The administration of iodine-containing contrast media may
interfere with thyroid function tests. There may also be interference with blood coagulation tests and certain urine tests.

Neonates. The use of meglumine amidotrizoate might have
contributed to the death, with bowel necrosis, perforation, and
peritonitis, of 2 infants with meconium ileus.[1]

1. Leonidas JC, et al. Possible adverse effects of methylglucamine
   diatrizoate compounds on the bowel of newborn infants with
   meconium ileus. Radiology 1976; **121:** 693–6.

Pharmacokinetics
Amidotrizoates are very poorly absorbed from the gastrointestinal tract. Amidotrizoates in the circulation are not significantly bound to plasma proteins. If renal function is not impaired,
unchanged amidotrizoate is rapidly excreted by glomerular filtration; over 95% of an intravascular dose is reported to be excreted in urine within 24 hours, and about 1 to 2% of a dose
may be excreted in faeces. Trace amounts may be detected in
other body fluids including tears and saliva. Faecal excretion
may increase to 10 to 50% in severe renal impairment. The
half-life of amidotrizoates has been reported to be 30 to 60 minutes, which can increase to 20 to 140 hours in severe renal impairment. They are removed by haemodialysis and peritoneal
dialysis.

The amidotrizoates cross the placenta and have been reported
to be present in breast milk.

Uses and Administration

The amidotrizoates are iodinated ionic monomeric contrast media (p.1030). Both the sodium and the meglumine salt have been widely used in diagnostic radiography including computed tomography (p.1030), but a mixture of both is often preferred to minimise side-effects.

The amidotrizoates are used in an extensive range of procedures. The route of administration and the dose employed depend on the type of procedure and the degree and extent of contrast required. They may be given by many routes including the oral, intravenous, intramuscular, subcutaneous, intra-arterial, intra-articular, and intra-osseous. For some procedures, they may be injected into the gallbladder, biliary ducts, or spleen.

Solutions of amidotrizoates have also been given as an enema in the treatment of uncomplicated meconium ileus.

Calcium amidotrizoate and lysine amidotrizoate have also been used as contrast media.

Intussusception. Contrast medium enemas, usually amidotrizoate or barium sulfate (p.1032) have been administered as an initial treatment for ileocolic intussusception in children.[1] Surgery is performed if the hydrostatic pressure produced by the enema fails to reduce the intussusception.

1. Collins DL, et al. Hydrostatic reduction of ileocolic intussusception: a second attempt in the operating room with general anesthesia. J Pediatr 1989; **115:** 204–7.

Preparations

BP 2001: Meglumine Amidotrizoate Injection; Sodium Amidotrizoate Injection;
USP 25: Diatrizoate Meglumine and Diatrizoate Sodium Injection; Diatrizoate Meglumine and Diatrizoate Sodium Solution; Diatrizoate Meglumine Injection; Diatrizoate Sodium Injection; Diatrizoate Sodium Solution.

Proprietary Preparations (details are given in Part 3)
Aust.: Angiografin†; Gastrografin; Peritrast; Urografin; Urovison; *Austral.:* MD-60; MD-76; MD-Gastroview; *Belg.:* Urografine; *Braz.:* Hypaque; Pielograf; Plenigraf; Reliev; Trazograf; Urografina; *Canad.:* Gastrografin†; Hypaque; Hypaque-M; MD-76; Reno-M†; Renografin†; *Denm.:* Urografin; Urografin Meglumin; *Fr.:* Gastrografin; *Fr.:* Angiografine†; Gastrografine; Radioselectan; *Ger.:* Angiografin; Ethibloc Okklusions-Emulsion; Gastrografin; Gastrolux; Peritrast; Peritrast comp; Peritrast-Infusio 160/32%; Peritrast-Infusio 180/31%; Peritrast-Oral CT; Peritrast-Oral-GI; Peritrast-RE; Urografin; Urolux Retro; Urovison; *Irl.:* Hypaque†; *Israel:* Urografin; *Ital.:* Gastrografin; Selectografin†; *Neth.:* Angiografin; Gastrografin; Urografin; Urovison; *Norw.:* Gastrografin; *NZ:* Gastrografin; Urografin; *Port.:* Gastrografina; Urografina; *S.Afr.:* Angiografin; Gastrografin; Urografin; *Spain:* Gastrografin; Pielograf; Plenigraf; Radialar 280; Trazograf; Uro Angiografin; Urografin; *Swed.:* Gastrografin; Urografin; *Switz.:* Ethibloc†; Gastrografin; Urografin; *UK:* Gastrografin; Hypaque; Urografin 150, 325, and 370; *USA:* Angiovist 282†; Angiovist 292, Angiovist 370†; Cystografin; Gastrografin; Hypaque; Hypaque-M, Hypaque-76; MD-76; MD-Gastroview; Reno-M; Renografin; Renovist†; Urovist†.

Multi-ingredient: *Braz.:* Hypaque-M; *Canad.:* Sinografin†; *USA:* Sinografin.

Barium Sulfate   (1552-p)

Barii Sulfas; Barii Sulphas; Barium Sulfuricum; Barium Sulphate; Baryum (Sulfate de).
$BaSO_4 = 233.4$.
CAS — 7727-43-7.
Pharmacopoeias. In *Chin., Eur.* (see p.vi), *Int., Jpn, Pol.,* and *US.*

Pharmacopoeial description

Ph. Eur.: A fine, heavy, white powder, free from gritty particles. Practically insoluble in water and in organic solvents; very slightly soluble in acids and in solutions of alkali hydroxides.

USP 25: A fine, white, odourless, bulky powder, free from grittiness. Practically insoluble in water, in organic solvents, and in solutions of acids and of alkalis. pH in a 10% w/w aqueous suspension is between 3.5 and 10.0.

Adverse Effects

Because barium sulfate is almost insoluble it lacks the severe toxicity characteristic of the barium ion; deaths have occurred following the administration of the more soluble barium sulfide in error for the sulfate.

Constipation may occur after oral or rectal barium sulfate administration; impaction, obstruction, and appendicitis have occurred. Surgical removal of faecaliths has sometimes been necessary. Cramping or diarrhoea have also been reported. Venous intravasation has led to the formation of emboli; deaths have occurred. Perforation of the bowel has led to peritonitis, adhesions, granulomas, and a high mortality rate.

ECG abnormalities have occurred during the use of barium sulfate enemas.

Accidental aspiration into the lungs has led to pneumonitis or granuloma formation.

Hypersensitivity. A survey of hypersensitivity reactions to barium preparations found that although barium is inert many of the additives used in formulation have the potential to cause reactions.[1] Of 106 reactions reported or found in the literature, 61% involved the skin and only 8% the respiratory tract; unconsciousness was reported in 8% of cases. In view of the frequency of use of barium preparations, such adverse reactions must be very rare, but radiologists should be aware that they may be somewhat more common than is usually appreciated. A

number of severe reactions associated with the use of barium enemas supplied with an inflatable latex cuff may have been due to leaching of components from the latex.[2]

1. Janower ML. Hypersensitivity reactions after barium studies of the upper and lower gastrointestinal tract. *Radiology* 1986; **161:** 139–40.
2. Nightingale SL. Severe adverse reactions to barium enema procedures. *JAMA* 1990; **264:** 2863.

Precautions

Barium sulfate should not be given to patients with intestinal obstruction and care is needed in those with conditions such as pyloric stenosis or lesions which may predispose to obstruction. Adequate hydration should be ensured after the procedure to prevent severe constipation.

It is contra-indicated in patients with gastrointestinal perforation, and should be avoided, particularly when given rectally, in those at risk of perforation as in acute ulcerative colitis or diverticulitis and following rectal or colonic biopsy, sigmoidoscopy, or radiotherapy.

Uses and Administration

Barium sulfate is used as a contrast medium for X-ray examination of the gastrointestinal tract involving single- or double-contrast techniques or computed tomography (p.1030).

The dose of barium sulfate is dependent upon the type of examination and technique employed. For examination of the oesophagus, up to 150 mL of a 50 to 200% w/v suspension may be given by mouth. For examination of the stomach and duodenum, up to 300 mL of a 30 to 200% w/v suspension may be given by mouth. For examination of the small intestine, up to 300 mL of a 30 to 200% w/v suspension may be given by mouth. For examination of the colon, up to 2 litres of a 20 to 130% w/v suspension may be administered as an enema.

For double-contrast examination, gas can be introduced into the gastrointestinal tract by using suspensions of barium sulfate containing carbon dioxide; separate gas-producing preparations based on sodium bicarbonate are also available. Air administered via a tube may be used as an alternative to carbon dioxide.

◊ Reviews.

1. Bentley A, Piper K. Barium sulphate preparations. *Pharm J* 1987; **238:** 138–9.
2. Nolan DJ. Barium examination of the small intestine. *Br J Hosp Med* 1994; **52:** 136–41.

Intussusception. Barium enemas have been recommended in the investigation of children with suspected acute intussusception, a condition where part of the intestine prolapses into the lumen of an adjacent part causing an obstruction. In some cases, the hydrostatic pressure exerted by the enema may reduce the intussusception thus avoiding the need for surgery.[1,2]

1. Anonymous. Acute intussusception in childhood. *Lancet* 1985; **ii:** 250–1.
2. Collins DL, et al. Hydrostatic reduction of ileocolic intussusception: a second attempt in the operating room with general anesthesia. *J Pediatr* 1989; **115:** 204–7.

Preparations

BP 2001: Barium Sulphate Oral Suspension;
USP 25: Barium Sulfate Paste; Barium Sulfate for Suspension; Barium Sulfate Suspension; Barium Sulfate Tablets.

Proprietary Preparations (details are given in Part 3)
Aust.: Micropaque†; Microtrast†; Prontobario; Scannotrast; Unibaryt†; *Austral.:* Medebar; Medescan; Tixobar; *Belg.:* E-Z-Paque; Micropaque; Polibar; *Braz.:* Bariogel; Baritest; Baropac; Celobar; Duplobar; Neobar; Telebar; *Canad.:* E-Z-Cat†; Ultra-R†; Unibar†; *Denm.:* Micropaque; Mixobar; *Fin.:* Mixobar; *Fr.:* Micropaque; Microtrast; *Ger.:* Barilux; Micropaque; Microtrast; *Israel:* E-Z-HD; Polibar ACB; *Ital.:* Mixobar; Prontobario; TAC Esofago; *Neth.:* Micropaque†; *Norw.:* Mixobar; *NZ:* Medebar; *Port.:* Duogast†; E-Z-Cat; E-Z-HD; Gastrobario; Micropaque; Microtrast; Polibar; Prontobario; *Spain:* Barigraf; Barigraf Tac; Bario Dif; Bario Faes Ultra†; Bario Faes†; Bario Llorente; Bariopacin; Disperbarium; Justebarin; Micropaque; *Swed.:* Barytgen†; Mixobar; *Switz.:* CAT-Barium (E-Z-CAT); Microbar-Colon; Microbar-HD (E-Z-HD); Micropaque; Polibar ACB; *UK:* Baritop; E-Z-Cat; E-Z-HD; E-Z-Paque; Micropaque†; Polibar; Polibar Rapid; Polibar Viscous; *USA:* Anatrast; Baricon; Baro-cat; Baroflave†; Barosperse; Enecat†; Entrobar; Epi-C; Flo-Coat; HD 200 Plus; HD 85; Liquipaket; Prepcat; Tomocat; Tonopaque.

Multi-ingredient: *Aust.:* Barilux; *Switz.:* Calcipulpe†; Endomethasone†.

Ferristene   (17904-e)

Ferristene *(BAN, USAN)*.
$C_8H_{11}NO_3S, (Fe_2O_3)_{0.725}$.
CAS — 155773-56-1.
ATC — V08CB02.

Iron ferrite crystals carried on monosized spheres of cross-linked poly(ammonium styrenesulfonate).

Ferristene 100 mg contains approximately 23.4 mg Fe.

Adverse Effects and Precautions

Nausea, vomiting, and constipation or loose stools may occur. Ferristene should not be used in patients with gastrointestinal obstruction or perforation and should be used with care in patients prone to developing these conditions.

Uses and Administration

Ferristene is a superparamagnetic agent used orally for contrast enhancement in magnetic resonance imaging (p.1030) of the abdomen. It is usually given in a dose of 400 to 800 mL of a suspension containing 0.117 mg of iron per mL.

Preparations

Proprietary Preparations (details are given in Part 3)
Aust.: Abdoscan; *Denm.:* Abdoscan; *Fin.:* Abdoscan; *Ger.:* Abdoscan; *Norw.:* Abdoscan; *Spain:* Abdoscan; *Swed.:* Abdoscan; *Switz.:* Abdoscan; *UK:* Abdoscan.

Ferumoxides   (17059-y)

Ferumoxides *(BAN, USAN)*.
AMI-25.
$(Fe_2O_3)_m(FeO)_n$.
CAS — 119683-68-0.

Profile

Ferumoxides is a superparamagnetic agent used intravenously for contrast enhancement in magnetic resonance imaging (p.1030) of the liver. The usual dose contains the equivalent of up to 0.84 mg of iron per kg body-weight, and is administered in 100 mL of glucose 5% over at least 30 minutes.

Preparations

Proprietary Preparations (details are given in Part 3)
Aust.: Endorem; *Belg.:* Endorem; *Denm.:* Endorem; *Fin.:* Endorem; *Fr.:* Endorem; *Ger.:* Endorem; *Israel:* Feridex; *Ital.:* Endorem; *Jpn:* Feridex; *Neth.:* Endorem†; *Norw.:* Endorem; *Port.:* Endorem; *Spain:* Endorem; *Swed.:* Endorem; *Switz.:* Endorem; *USA:* Feridex.

Ferumoxsil   (17060-g)

Ferumoxsil *(BAN, USAN)*.
AMI-121.
ATC — V08CB01.

Profile

Ferumoxsil is a superparamagnetic agent used for contrast enhancement in magnetic resonance imaging (p.1030) of the gastrointestinal tract. It is usually given orally in a dose of 600 to 900 mL of a suspension containing 0.175 mg of iron per mL. A dose of 300 to 600 mL is used rectally.

Preparations

Proprietary Preparations (details are given in Part 3)
Aust.: Lumirem†; *Denm.:* Lumirem; *Fin.:* Lumirem; *Fr.:* Lumirem; *Ger.:* Lumirem; *Ital.:* Lumirem; *Neth.:* Lumirem†; *Swed.:* Lumirem; *Switz.:* Lumirem†.

Gadobenic Acid   (15276-g)

Gadobenic Acid *(BAN, rINN)*.
B-19036;   Gd-BOPTA.   [2-(Benzyloxymethyl)-6-(carboxylatomethyl-κO)-3,9-bis(carboxymethyl-κO)-3,6,9-triazaundecanedioato-κ$^3N^{3,6,9}$,κ$^2O^{1,11}$] gadolinium (III).
$C_{22}H_{28}GdN_3O_{11} = 667.7$.
CAS — 113662-23-0.
ATC — V08CA08.

Meglumine Gadobenate   (17562-v)

B-19036/7; Gadobenate Dimeglumine *(USAN)*. Dihydrogen [(±)-4-carboxy-5,8,11-tris(carboxymethyl)-1-phenyl-2-oxa-5,8,11-triaza-tridecan-13-oato(5-)]gadolinate(2-) compound with 1-deoxy-1-(methylamino)-D-glucitol (1:2).
$C_{22}H_{28}GdN_3O_{11}, 2C_7H_{17}NO_5 = 1058.1$.
CAS — 127000-20-8.

Profile

Gadobenic acid is an ionic paramagnetic agent used, as meglumine gadobenate, for contrast enhancement in magnetic resonance imaging (p.1030) of the liver and CNS.

Meglumine gadobenate is available as a solution containing 529 mg (0.5 mmol) per mL. The usual dose is 0.1 mL (0.05 mmol) per kg body-weight intravenously for imaging of the liver, and 0.2 mL (0.1 mmol) per kg intravenously for imaging of the brain or spine.

Preparations

Proprietary Preparations (details are given in Part 3)
Aust.: MultiHance; *Belg.:* MultiHance; *Ger.:* MultiHance; *Ital.:* MultiHance; *Neth.:* MultiHance; *Swed.:* MultiHance; *UK:* MultiHance.

Gadodiamide   (14637-q)

Gadodiamide (BAN, rINN).

GdDTPA-BMA; S-041. Aqua[6-carboxylatomethyl-3,9-bis(methylcarbamoylmethyl-κ-O)-3,6,9-triazaundecanedioato-κ³-N³,N⁶,N⁹-κ³-O¹,O⁶,O¹¹(3-)gadolinium(III)]; a complex of gadolinium with diethylenetriamine penta-acetic acid bismethylamide.

$C_{16}H_{28}GdN_5O_9,xH_2O = 591.7$ (anhydrous).
CAS — 131410-48-5 (anhydrous gadodiamide); 122795-43-1 (gadodiamide hydrate).
ATC — V08CA03.

NOTE. Anhydrous Gadodiamide is USAN.

Pharmacopoeias. In US.

Pharmacopoeial description

USP 25: A white, odourless, powder. Freely soluble in water and in methyl alcohol; soluble in alcohol; slightly soluble in acetone and in chloroform.

Adverse Effects and Precautions

As for Gadopentetic Acid, below.

Effects on the pancreas. There has been a report[1] of acute pancreatitis developing in a patient shortly after injection of gadodiamide for imaging of his liver.

1. Terzi C, Sökmen S. Acute pancreatitis induced by magnetic-resonance-imaging contrast agent. Lancet 1999; 354: 1789–90. Correction. ibid. 2000; 355: 660.

Pharmacokinetics

Gadodiamide is rapidly distributed into extracellular fluid. About 96% of a dose is excreted unchanged in the urine within 24 hours. An elimination half-life of approximately 70 minutes has been reported. Gadodiamide is not bound to plasma proteins.

Uses and Administration

Gadodiamide is a nonionic paramagnetic agent used for contrast enhancement in magnetic resonance imaging (p.1030) of cranial and spinal structures.

Gadodiamide is available as a solution containing 287 mg (0.5 mmol) per mL. The usual dose in adults is 0.2 mL (0.1 mmol) per kg body-weight intravenously.

Preparations

USP 25: Gadodiamide Injection.

Proprietary Preparations (details are given in Part 3)
Aust.: Omniscan; Austral.: Omniscan; Belg.: Omniscan; Canad.: Omniscan; Denm.: Omniscan; Fin.: Omniscan; Fr.: Omniscan; Ger.: Omniscan; Ital.: Omniscan; Jpn: Omniscan; Neth.: Omniscan†; Norw.: Omniscan; NZ: Omniscan; Spain: Omniscan; Swed.: Omniscan; Switz.: Omniscan; UK: Omniscan; USA: Omniscan.

Gadopentetic Acid   (3798-d)

Gadopentetic Acid (BAN, rINN).

Gadolinium-DTPA. {N′,N″-Bis(carboxymethyl)-N′,N″-[(aceta to)iminodiethylene]diglycinato-O,-O′,O″,N,-N′,N″}gadolinium(3+); a complex of gadolinium with diethylenetriamine penta-acetic acid.

$C_{14}H_{20}GdN_3O_{10} = 547.6$.
CAS — 80529-93-7.
ATC — V08CA01.

Meglumine Gadopentetate   (10657-h)

Dimeglumine Gadopentetate; Gadopentetate Dimeglumine (USAN); Gadopentetate Meglumine; SH-L-451-A. The di(N-methylglucamine) salt of gadopentetic acid.

$C_{14}H_{20}GdN_3O_{10},(C_7H_{17}NO_5)_2 = 938.0$.
CAS — 86050-77-3.

Pharmacopoeias. US includes only as an injection.

Adverse Effects

There may be headache, nausea, vomiting, and transient sensations of heat or cold or taste disturbances following injection of gadopentetate. Rarely, convulsions, hypotension, allergic or anaphylactoid reactions, and shock may occur. Paraesthesias, dizziness, and localised pain have also been reported. Transient elevations of serum iron and bilirubin values have been observed.

◊ General references.
1. Nelson KL, et al. Clinical safety of gadopentetate dimeglumine. Radiology 1995; 196: 439–43.

Hypersensitivity. A report of anaphylactic shock in a patient following the intravenous administration of meglumine gadopentetate.[1] The patient had a history of pollen allergy and had experienced anaphylactic shock when given an iodine-based contrast agent intravenously 2 months earlier.

1. Tardy B, et al. Anaphylactic shock induced by intravenous gadopentetate dimeglumine. Lancet 1992; 339: 494.

Precautions

Gadopentetate should be given with care to patients with severe renal impairment, epilepsy, hypotension, or a history of hypersensitivity, asthma, or other allergic respiratory disorders. Care should be taken to avoid extravasation. Gadopentetate may interfere with tests of serum iron or bilirubin concentrations.

The symbol † denotes a preparation no longer actively marketed

Myasthenia gravis. A report of acute deterioration of myasthenia gravis in a patient after magnetic resonance imaging of the brain using gadopentetate as the contrast medium.[1]
1. Nordenbo AM, Somnier FE. Acute deterioration of myasthenia gravis after intravenous administration of gadolinium-DTPA. Lancet 1992; 340: 1168.

Pharmacokinetics

Gadopentetate is rapidly distributed into extracellular space following intravenous injection. An elimination half-life of 1.6 hours has been reported. It is not metabolised and about 90% of a dose is excreted in the urine within 24 hours. A small amount is distributed into breast milk. Gadopentetate is removed by haemodialysis.

Uses and Administration

Gadopentetic acid is an ionic paramagnetic agent used, as meglumine gadopentetate, for contrast enhancement in magnetic resonance imaging (p.1030) of cranial and spinal structures, of the whole body, and of the gastrointestinal tract; it may also be employed for the evaluation of renal function.

Meglumine gadopentetate is used intravenously for cranial, spinal, and whole body imaging as a solution containing 469.01 mg (0.5 mmol) per mL. The usual dose in adults, children, and neonates is 0.2 mL (0.1 mmol) per kg body-weight intravenously. For cranial and spinal imaging, a further dose of 0.2 mL (0.1 mmol) per kg may be given within 30 minutes if necessary; in adults this second dose may be 0.4 mL (0.2 mmol) per kg. For whole body imaging in adults and children over 2 years, a dose of 0.4 mL (0.2 mmol) per kg may be needed in some cases to produce adequate contrast and in special circumstances a dose of 0.6 mL (0.3 mmol) per kg may be used in adults.

Meglumine gadopentetate is administered orally and rectally for gastrointestinal imaging. A solution containing 9.38 mg per mL is diluted before use (100 mL with 900 mL of water) and doses in the range of 100 to 1000 mL of this diluted solution are used in adults depending upon the organ or tissue being investigated.

Preparations

USP 25: Gadopentetate Dimeglumine Injection.

Proprietary Preparations (details are given in Part 3)
Aust.: Magnevist; Belg.: Magnevist; Braz.: Magnevistan; Canad.: Magnevist; Denm.: Magnevist; Fin.: Magnevist; Fr.: Magnevist; Ger.: Magnevist; Ital.: Magnevist; Neth.: Magnevist; Norw.: Magnevist; NZ: Magnevist; Port.: Magnevist; Spain: Magnevist; Magnograf; Swed.: Magnevist; Switz.: Magnevist; UK: Magnevist; USA: Magnevist.

Gadoteric Acid   (6479-s)

Gadoteric Acid (BAN, rINN).

ZK-112004. Hydrogen [1,4,7,10-tetraazacyclododecane-1,4,7,10-tetraaceto(4–)]gadolinate(1–); Hydrogen [1,4,7,10-tetrakis(carboxylatomethyl)-1,4,7,10-tetra-azacyclododecane-κ⁴N]gadolinate(1–).

$C_{16}H_{25}GdN_4O_8 = 558.6$.
CAS — 72573-82-1.
ATC — V08CA02.

Meglumine Gadoterate   (17390-n)

Gadoterate Meglumine.

Profile

Gadoteric acid is an ionic paramagnetic contrast medium with actions similar to those of gadopentetic acid (above). It is used, as meglumine gadoterate, for contrast enhancement in cranial, spinal, and hepatic magnetic resonance imaging (p.1030).

Meglumine gadoterate is available as a solution containing 377 mg (0.5 mmol) per mL. The usual dose in adults and children is 0.2 mL (0.1 mmol) per kg body-weight by intravenous injection.

Preparations

Proprietary Preparations (details are given in Part 3)
Aust.: Dotarem; Belg.: Dotarem; Braz.: Dotarem; Denm.: Dotarem; Fin.: Dotarem; Fr.: Dotarem; Israel: Dotarem; Ital.: Dotarem; Neth.: Dotarem†; Norw.: Dotarem; Port.: Dotarem; Spain: Dotarem; Swed.: Dotarem; Switz.: Dotarem.

Gadoteridol   (15277-q)

Gadoteridol (BAN, USAN, rINN).

SQ-32692. (±)-[10-(2-Hydroxypropyl)-1,4,7,10-tetraazacyclododecane-1,4,7-triacetato(3–)]gadolinium.

$C_{17}H_{29}GdN_4O_7 = 558.7$.
CAS — 120066-54-8.
ATC — V08CA04.

Pharmacopoeias. In US.

Pharmacopoeial description

USP 25: A white to off-white, odourless, crystalline powder. Freely soluble in water and in methyl alcohol; soluble in isopropyl alcohol. Store in airtight containers. Protect from light.

Adverse Effects and Precautions

As for Gadopentetic Acid, above.

Hypersensitivity. Vasovagal response and anaphylactoid reaction has been reported during intravenous use of gadoteridol.[1]
1. Shellock FG, et al. Adverse reaction to intravenous gadoteridol. Radiology 1993; 189: 151–2.

Pharmacokinetics

About 94% of a dose of gadoteridol is excreted unchanged in the urine within 24 hours. An elimination half-life of about 1.57 hours has been reported.

Uses and Administration

Gadoteridol is a nonionic paramagnetic agent used for contrast enhancement in magnetic resonance imaging (p.1030) of cranial and spinal structures.

Gadoteridol is available as a solution containing 279.3 mg (0.5 mmol) per mL. The usual adult dose is 0.2 mL (0.1 mmol) per kg body-weight intravenously; an additional dose of up to 0.4 mL (0.2 mmol) per kg may be given approximately 30 minutes after the first if necessary. A single dose of 0.2 mL per kg is used in children from 6 months of age.

Preparations

USP 25: Gadoteridol Injection.

Proprietary Preparations (details are given in Part 3)
Aust.: Prohance; Belg.: Prohance; Canad.: Prohance†; Denm.: Prohance; Fr.: Prohance; Ger.: Prohance; Ital.: Prohance; Neth.: Prohance; Norw.: Prohance; Spain: Prohance; Swed.: Prohance; Switz.: Prohance; UK: Prohance; USA: Prohance.

Galactose   (12778-b)

Galactose (USAN).

D-Galactopyranose; D-Galactose; Galactosum.
$C_6H_{12}O_6 = 180.2$.
CAS — 59-23-4 (D-galactose); 3646-73-9 (α-D-galactose).
ATC — V04CE01.

Pharmacopoeias. In Eur. (see p.vi).

Pharmacopoeial description

Ph. Eur.: A white, crystalline or finely granulated powder. Freely soluble or soluble in water; very slightly soluble in alcohol.

Profile

Galactose is a naturally occurring monosaccharide used as an ultrasound contrast medium (p.1030). It is administered intravenously or transcervically as a microbubble-microparticle suspension to enhance ultrasound images of the heart or female genital tract, respectively. Palmitic acid may be included to stabilise the microbubbles.

The clearance of galactose following intravenous administration has been used as a measure of liver function.

Preparations

Proprietary Preparations (details are given in Part 3)
Aust.: Echovist; Levovist; Canad.: Echovist; Levovist; Denm.: Echovist†; Levovist; Fin.: Echovist; Levovist; Fr.: Echovist; Levovist; Ger.: Echovist; Levovist; Israel: Echovist; Levovist; Ital.: Levovist; Neth.: Echovist; Levovist; Norw.: Echovist; Levovist; NZ: Echovist; Levovist; Port.: Levovist; S.Afr.: Echovist; Spain: Levograf; Levovist; Swed.: Echovist; Levovist; Switz.: Echovist; Levovist; UK: Echovist; Levovist.

Iobitridol   (17092-j)

Iobitridol (BAN, rINN).

N,N′-Bis(2,3-dihydroxypropyl)-5-[2-(hydroxymethyl)hydracrylamido]-2,4,6-triiodo-N,N′-dimethylisophthalamide; N,N′-Bis(2,3-dihydroxypropyl)-5-(3-hydroxy-2-hydroxymethylpropionamido)-2,4,6-tri-iodo-N,N′-dimethylisophthalamide.
$C_{20}H_{28}I_3N_3O_9 = 835.2$.
CAS — 136949-58-1.
ATC — V08AB11.

Profile

Iobitridol is an iodinated nonionic monomeric contrast medium used parenterally for a wide range of radiographic diagnostic procedures (p.1030).

Preparations

Proprietary Preparations (details are given in Part 3)
Aust.: Xenetix; Belg.: Xenetix; Denm.: Xenetix; Fin.: Xenetix; Fr.: Xenetix; Ger.: Xenetix; Israel: Xenetix; Ital.: Xenetix; Neth.: Xenetix†; Norw.: Xenetix; Port.: Xenetix; Spain: Xenetix; Swed.: Xenetix; Switz.: Xenetix.

Iocetamic Acid   (1561-s)

Iocetamic Acid (BAN, USAN, pINN).

DRC-1201; MP-620. N-Acetyl-N-(3-amino-2,4,6-tri-iodophenyl)-2-methyl-β-alanine; 2-[N-(3-Amino-2,4,6-tri-iodophenyl)acetamidomethyl]-propionic acid.
$C_{12}H_{13}I_3N_2O_3 = 614.0$.
CAS — 16034-77-8.
ATC — V08AC07.

Iocetamic acid contains approximately 62% of I.

Adverse Effects and Precautions

As for Iopanoic Acid, p.1035.

Pharmacokinetics
Iocetamic acid is variably absorbed from the gastrointestinal tract. It is conjugated in the liver with glucuronic acid, and is excreted in the bile and concentrated in the gallbladder; about 62% of a dose is excreted in the urine within 48 hours.

Uses and Administration
Iocetamic acid is an iodinated ionic monomeric contrast medium and is used mainly for cholecystography (p.1030). A dose of 3.0 or 4.5 g is given by mouth 10 to 15 hours before examination. If visualisation is unsuccessful a further dose may be given on the evening of the first examination, and the examination repeated on the following day.

Preparations
Proprietary Preparations (details are given in Part 3)
Braz.: Colebrina; *Neth.*: Cholebrine; *Swed.*: Cholebrin†; *USA*: Cholebrine†.

Iodamide (1523-m)
Iodamide (BAN, USAN, rINN).
Ametriodinic Acid; B-4130; SH-926. α,5-Diacetamido-2,4,6-triiodo-*m*-toluic acid; 3-Acetamido-5-acetamidomethyl-2,4,6-triiodobenzoic acid.
$C_{12}H_{11}I_3N_2O_4 = 627.9$.
CAS — 440-58-4.
ATC — V08AA03.
Pharmacopoeias. In Jpn.

Iodamide contains approximately 60.6% of I.

Meglumine Iodamide (1524-b)
Iodamide Meglumine (USAN). The *N*-methylglucamine salt of iodamide.
$C_{12}H_{11}I_3N_2O_4,C_7H_{17}NO_5 = 823.2$.
CAS — 18656-21-8.

Meglumine iodamide contains approximately 46.3% of I.

Sodium Iodamide (1562-w)
Iodamide Sodium.
$C_{12}H_{10}I_3N_2NaO_4 = 649.9$.
CAS — 10098-82-5.

Sodium iodamide contains approximately 58.6% of I.

Profile
Iodamide is an iodinated ionic monomeric contrast medium given by intravenous or local administration in a variety of radiographic diagnostic procedures (p.1030).

It is given as a 65% solution of the meglumine salt, as an approximately 53% concentration of the sodium salt, or as a mixture of the sodium and meglumine salts. The dose varies according to the procedure and route of administration. A 24% solution of the meglumine salt has been used for contrast enhancement in computed tomography of the brain.

Preparations
Proprietary Preparations (details are given in Part 3)
Aust.: Uromiro; *Braz.*: Uromiron; *Ital.*: Isteropac ER; Opacist ER; Uromiro 24%, 36%, and 300; Uromiro 300 Sodico; Uromiro 340 and 420; *Neth.*: Urombrine 420†; Urombrine†; *Port.*: Uromiro; *Switz.*: Isteropac; Opacist ER; Uromiro; *USA*: Renovue†.

Iodised Oil (1564-l)
Ethiodized Oil.
CAS — 8001-40-9 (iodised oil); 8008-53-5 (ethiodized oil injection).

An iodine addition product of the ethyl esters of the fatty acids obtained from poppy-seed oil. It contains about 35 to 39% of combined iodine.

Because of its solvent action on polystyrene, iodised oil injection should not be administered in plastic syringes made with polystyrene.

Adverse Effects and Precautions
The risk of hypersensitivity reactions or iodism is greater after the use of iodised oil than after water-soluble iodinated contrast media such as the amidotrizoates. Pulmonary oil embolism is reported to be relatively frequent following lymphography but is not usually severe; however, hypotension, tachycardia, and pulmonary oedema and infarction may occur rarely and deaths have been reported in patients with pulmonary disease. Chemical pneumonitis, oedema, granuloma formation, and goitre have occurred.

Great care should be taken to avoid vascular structures, because of the danger of oil embolism; it should not therefore be used in areas affected by haemorrhage or local trauma. Iodised oil should be used with care in patients with thyroid dysfunction or a history of allergic reactions. The administration of iodised oil may interfere with thyroid-function tests for several months.

◊ The use of oily contrast media for hysterosalpingography was considered dangerous and unnecessary.[1] Oil embolism and pelvic adhesions had occurred. In the presence of unsuspected pel-

vic tuberculosis there have been violent reactions with pelvic abscess formation. Several patients had been seen with bilateral tubal occlusion following an original investigation, using iodised oil, which had shown tubal patency.

1. Wright FW, Stallworthy J. Female sterility produced by investigation. *BMJ* 1973; **3**: 632.

Pharmacokinetics
Iodised oil may persist in the body for several weeks or months after administration. It is only slowly absorbed from most body sites, although absorption from the peritoneal cavity is stated to be relatively rapid. It is reported to be slowly metabolised to fatty acids and iodine.

Uses and Administration
Iodised oil is an iodinated contrast medium that is used mainly for lymphography although it has also been used in various other radiographic diagnostic procedures (p.1030). It has been used for hysterosalpingography but water-soluble agents are preferred. The dose is dependent upon the procedure. The fluid injection of iodised oil is unsuitable for use in bronchography. Because it is slowly metabolised to release iodine, iodised oil is used in the management of iodine deficiency (p.1523).

Malignant neoplasms. Injection of iodised oil into the hepatic artery is followed by selective and long-lasting retention within hepatic carcinomas and used with computed tomography is considered to be more sensitive than other imaging techniques.[1] The sensitivity of this method also enables the imaging of very small satellite nodules, which if undetected are responsible for high early rates of recurrence after resection. Iodised oil has also been used to provide targeted delivery of lipophilic antineoplastics or radioactive iodine to hepatic[1-4] or breast tumours.[5]

1. Anonymous. Lipiodol computed tomography for small hepatocellular carcinomas. *Lancet* 1991; **337**: 333–4.
2. Novell R, *et al.* Ablation of recurrent primary liver cancer using ^{131}I-lipiodol. *Postgrad Med J* 1991; **67**: 393–5.
3. Group d'Etude et de Traitement du Carcinome Hépatocellulaire. A comparison of Lipiodol chemoembolization and conservative treatment for unresectable hepatocellular carcinoma. *N Engl J Med* 1995; **332**: 1256–61.
4. Lau WY, *et al.* Adjuvant intra-arterial iodine-131-labelled lipiodol for resectable hepatocellular carcinoma: a prospective randomised trial. *Lancet* 1999; **353**: 797–801.
5. Novell JR, *et al.* Targeted therapy for recurrent breast carcinoma with regional 'Lipiodol'/epirubicin infusion. *Lancet* 1990; **336**: 1383.

Preparations
BP 2001: Iodised Oil Fluid Injection;
USP 25: Ethiodized Oil Injection.

Proprietary Preparations (details are given in Part 3)
Aust.: Lipiodol†; *Austral.*: Lipiodol; *Belg.*: Lipiodol; *Braz.*: Lipiodol; *Denm.*: Lipiodol; *Fr.*: Lipiodol; *Ger.*: Lipiodol; *Israel*: Lipiodol; *Ital.*: Lipiodol; *Neth.*: Lipiodol†; *Norw.*: Lipiodol; *NZ*: Lipiodol; *Port.*: Lipiodol; *UK*: Lipiodol; *USA*: Ethiodol.

Iodixanol (2807-d)
Iodixanol (BAN, USAN, rINN).
2-5410-3A. 5,5'-[(2-Hydroxytrimethylene)bis(acetylimino)]bis[*N,N'*-bis(2,3-dihydroxypropyl)-2,4,6-triiodoisophthalamide].
$C_{35}H_{44}I_6N_6O_{15} = 1550.2$.
CAS — 92339-11-2.
ATC — V08AB09.

Iodixanol contains approximately 49.1% of I.

Adverse Effects, Treatment, and Precautions
See under the amidotrizoates, p.1031.

Pharmacokinetics
Iodixanol is rapidly distributed into extracellular fluid following intravenous injection. It is not bound to plasma proteins. It is not metabolised and about 97% of a dose is excreted in the urine within 24 hours. A terminal elimination half-life of about 2 hours has been reported. Iodixanol is removed by dialysis.

Uses and Administration
Iodixanol is an iodinated nonionic dimeric contrast medium that is used for angiography and urography and for contrast enhancement during computed tomography (p.1030).

Iodixanol is given by injection as a solution usually containing between 30.5 and 65.2% of iodixanol (equivalent to between 150 and 320 mg of iodine per mL). The dose and strength used vary according to the procedure and route of injection.

◊ References.
1. Spencer CM, Goa KL. Iodixanol: a review of its pharmacodynamic and pharmacokinetic properties and diagnostic use as an x-ray contrast medium. *Drugs* 1996; **52**: 899–927.

Preparations
Proprietary Preparations (details are given in Part 3)
Aust.: Visipaque; *Austral.*: Visipaque; *Belg.*: Visipaque; *Canad.*: Visipaque; *Denm.*: Visipaque; *Fin.*: Visipaque; *Fr.*: Visipaque; *Ger.*: Visipaque; *Ital.*: Visipaque; *Neth.*: Visipaque†; *Norw.*: Visipaque; *NZ*: Visipaque; *Spain*: Visipaque; *Swed.*: Visipaque; *Switz.*: Visipaque; *UK*: Visipaque; *USA*: Visipaque.

Iodoxamic Acid (1527-q)
Iodoxamic Acid (BAN, USAN, rINN).
B-10610; SQ-21982. 3,3'-(4,7,10,13-Tetraoxahexadecanedioyldiamino)bis(2,4,6-tri-iodobenzoic acid).
$C_{26}H_{26}I_6N_2O_{10} = 1287.9$.
CAS — 31127-82-9.
ATC — V08AC01.

Iodoxamic acid contains approximately 59.1% of I.

Meglumine Iodoxamate (1567-z)
Meglumine Iodoxamate (BANM).
Dimeglumine Iodoxamate; Iodoxamate Meglumine (USAN). The di(*N*-methylglucamine) salt of iodoxamic acid.
$C_{26}H_{26}I_6N_2O_{10}.(C_7H_{17}NO_5)_2 = 1678.3$.
CAS — 51764-33-1.

Meglumine iodoxamate contains approximately 45.4% of I.

Profile
Iodoxamic acid is an iodinated ionic dimeric contrast medium that has been used as the meglumine salt for cholecystography and cholangiography (p.1030).

Preparations
Proprietary Preparations (details are given in Part 3)
Aust.: Endobil†; *Irl.*: Endobil.

Iofendylate (1571-e)
Iofendylate (BAN, rINN).
Ethyl Iodophenylundecylate; Iodophendylate; Iophendylate. A mixture of stereoisomers of ethyl 10-(4-iodophenyl)undecanoate.
$C_{19}H_{29}IO_2 = 416.3$.
CAS — 99-79-6; 1320-11-2.
ATC — V08AD04.
Pharmacopoeias. In Chin. and US.

It contains about 30.5% of I.

Pharmacopoeial description
USP 25: A colourless to pale yellow, viscous liquid, darkening on long exposure to air. Is odourless or has a faintly ethereal odour. Very slightly soluble in water; freely soluble in alcohol, in chloroform, in ether, and in benzene. Store in airtight containers. Protect from light.

Incompatibility. Polystyrene was soluble in iofendylate and syringes made from polystyrene were rapidly attacked.[1] Syringes made from polypropylene appeared to be unaffected.
1. Irving JD, Reynolds PV. Disposable syringe danger. *Lancet* 1966; **i**: 362.

Profile
Iofendylate is an iodinated ionic monomeric contrast medium that was formerly used mainly for myelography (p.1030); it was also formerly used for examination of the third and fourth ventricles, and to visualise the fetus in the amniotic sac prior to intra-uterine blood transfusion. However, serious side-effects including allergy, arachnoiditis, and aseptic meningitis have occurred with its use and it has been superseded by nonionic media such as iohexol (p.1035). Residues of iofendylate remaining years after myelography have been associated with adverse effects.

Preparations
BP 2001: Iofendylate Injection;
USP 25: Iophendylate Injection.

Ioglicic Acid (10491-t)
Ioglicic Acid (BAN, USAN, rINN).
SH-H-200-AB. 5-Acetamido-2,4,6-tri-iodo-*N*-(methylcarbamoylmethyl)isophthalamic acid.
$C_{13}H_{12}I_3N_3O_5 = 671.0$.
CAS — 49755-67-1.
ATC — V08AA06.

Ioglicic acid contains approximately 56.7% of I.

Meglumine Ioglicate (11450-a)
Ioglicate Meglumine. The *N*-methylglucamine salt of ioglicic acid.
$C_{13}H_{12}I_3N_3O_5,C_7H_{17}NO_5 = 866.2$.

Meglumine ioglicate contains approximately 44.0% of I.

Sodium Ioglicate (12855-n)
Ioglicate Sodium.
$C_{13}H_{11}I_3N_3NaO_5 = 692.9$.

Sodium ioglicate contains approximately 54.9% of I.

Profile
Ioglicic acid is an iodinated ionic monomeric contrast medium that has been given by injection, as the meglumine and sodium salts, for urography, angiography, and related procedures (p.1030).

Preparations

Proprietary Preparations (details are given in Part 3)
Aust.: Rayvist 180; *Braz.:* Biligrama; *Switz.:* Rayvist†.

Iohexol (12856-h)

Iohexol *(BAN, USAN, rINN)*.

Iohexolum; Win-39424. *N,N′*-Bis(2,3-dihydroxypropyl)-5-[N-(2,3-dihydroxypropyl)acetamido]-2,4,6-tri-iodoisophthalamide.
$C_{19}H_{26}I_3N_3O_9 = 821.1$.
CAS — 66108-95-0.
ATC — V08AB02.

Pharmacopoeias. In *Eur.* (see p.vi), *Int.*, and *US.*

Iohexol contains approximately 46.4% of I.

Pharmacopoeial description

Ph. Eur.: A white or greyish-white, hygroscopic powder. Very soluble in water; practically insoluble in dichloromethane and in ether; freely soluble in methyl alcohol. Store in airtight containers. Protect from light.

USP 25: A white to off-white, hygroscopic, odourless powder. Very soluble in water and in methyl alcohol; practically insoluble or insoluble in chloroform and in ether. Protect from light.

Adverse Effects and Precautions

See under the amidotrizoates, p.1031.

Additional neurological adverse effects may occur when iodinated nonionic contrast media such as iohexol are used for myelography. These include severe headache, backache, neck stiffness, dizziness, and leg or sciatic-type pain. Convulsions, aseptic meningitis, and mild and transitory perceptual aberrations, such as visual and speech disturbances, and confusion, may occur occasionally; rarely, more severe mental disturbances have occurred. Urinary retention has also been reported.

Effects on the nervous system. Encephalopathy which developed in a 48-year-old man with sciatica within 9 hours of iohexol administration for lumbar myelography had largely resolved 48 hours after the myelogram; complete resolution took 4 days.[1] However, recovery was slow in a patient who developed paraplegia and areflexia in the legs after a similar procedure. Five months later the patient still complained of paraesthesia in her legs and could not stand without support.[2]
1. Donaghy M, *et al.* Encephalopathy after iohexol myelography. *Lancet* 1985; ii: 887.
2. Noda K, *et al.* Prolonged paraplegia after iohexol myelography. *Lancet* 1991; 337: 681.

Pharmacokinetics

Following intravascular administration, 90% or more of iohexol is eliminated unchanged in the urine within 24 hours. An elimination half-life of approximately 2 hours in patients with normal renal function has been reported. Protein binding in blood is reported to be very low.

Pregnancy. Contrast material was detected[1] in the intestines of twin neonates who were born 17 hours after administration of iohexol to their mother for angiography, suggesting that transplacental transfer had taken place.
1. Moon AJ, *et al.* Transplacental passage of iohexol. *J Pediatr* 2000; 136: 548–9.

Uses and Administration

Iohexol is an iodinated nonionic monomeric contrast medium that is used by injection and locally for a wide range of diagnostic procedures including myelography, angiography, urography, arthrography, and visualisation of the gastrointestinal tract and body cavities (p.1030). Iohexol is also used to produce contrast enhancement during computed tomography.

Iohexol is usually available as solutions containing 30.2 to 75.5% of iohexol (equivalent to 140 to 350 mg of iodine per mL) and the dose and strength used vary according to the procedure and the route of administration.

Preparations

USP 25: Iohexol Injection.

Proprietary Preparations (details are given in Part 3)
Aust.: Omnipaque; *Austral.:* Omnipaque; *Belg.:* Omnipaque; *Braz.:* Omnipaque; *Canad.:* Omnipaque; *Denm.:* Omnipaque; *Fin.:* Omnipaque; *Fr.:* Accupaque; Omnipaque; *Ger.:* Accupaque; Omnipaque; *Ital.:* Omnipaque; *Neth.:* Omnipaque†; *Norw.:* Omnipaque; *NZ:* Omnipaque; *Spain:* Omnigraf; Omnipaque; Omnitrast; *Swed.:* Omnipaque; *Switz.:* Omnipaque; *UK:* Omnipaque; *USA:* Omnipaque.

Iomeprol (2865-w)

Iomeprol *(BAN, USAN, rINN)*.

N,N′-Bis(2,3-dihydroxypropyl)-2,4,6-triiodo-5-(N-methylglycolamido)-isophthalamide.
$C_{17}H_{22}I_3N_3O_8 = 777.1$.
CAS — 78649-41-9.
ATC — V08AB10.

Iomeprol contains approximately 49% of I.

Profile

Iomeprol is an iodinated nonionic monomeric contrast medium that is used for a wide range of radiographic procedures

The symbol † denotes a preparation no longer actively marketed

(p.1030) including myelography, angiography, urography, and arthrography. It is also used to produce contrast enhancement during computed tomography.

Iomeprol is usually available as solutions containing 30.62 to 81.65% of iomeprol (equivalent to 150 to 400 mg of iodine per mL) and the dose and strength used vary according to the procedure and the route of administration.

◊ Reviews.
1. Dooley M, Jarvis B. Iomeprol: a review of its use as a contrast medium. *Drugs* 2000; 59: 1169–86.

Preparations

Proprietary Preparations (details are given in Part 3)
Aust.: Iomeron; *Austral.:* Iomeron; *Belg.:* Iomeron; *Denm.:* Iomeron; *Fin.:* Iomeron; *Fr.:* Iomeron; *Ger.:* Imeron; *Israel:* Iomeron; *Ital.:* Iomeron; *Jpn:* Iomeron; *Neth.:* Iomeron; *Norw.:* Iomeron; *NZ:* Iomeron; *Port.:* Iomeron; *Spain:* Iomeron; *Swed.:* Iomeron; *Switz.:* Iomeron; *UK:* Iomeron.

Iopamidol (14037-g)

Iopamidol *(BAN, USAN, rINN)*.

B-15000; Iopamidolum; SQ-13396. (S)-N,N′-Bis[2-hydroxy-1-(hydroxymethyl)ethyl]-2,4,6-tri-iodo-5-lactamidoisophthalamide.
$C_{17}H_{22}I_3N_3O_8 = 777.1$.
CAS — 60166-93-0; 62883-00-5.
ATC — V08AB04.

Pharmacopoeias. In *Eur.* (see p.vi) and *US.*

Iopamidol contains approximately 49% of I.

Pharmacopoeial description

Ph. Eur.: A white or almost white powder. Freely soluble in water; practically insoluble in alcohol and in dichloromethane; very slightly soluble in methyl alcohol. Protect from light.

USP 25: A white to off-white, practically odourless, powder. Very soluble in water; practically insoluble in alcohol and in chloroform; sparingly soluble in methyl alcohol. Protect from light.

Adverse Effects and Precautions

As for the amidotrizoates, p.1031. For the adverse effects relating to the use of iopamidol for myelography, see under Iohexol, p.1035.

Effects on the nervous system. Reports of serious neurological sequelae to lumbar myelography with iopamidol.
1. Wallers K, *et al.* Severe meningeal irritation after intrathecal injection of iopamidol. *BMJ* 1985; 291: 1688.
2. Robinson C, Fon G. Adverse reaction to iopamidol. *Med J Aust* 1986; 144: 553.
3. Bell JA, McIlwaine GG. Postmyelographic lateral rectus palsy associated with iopamidol. *BMJ* 1990; 300: 1343–4.
4. Mallat Z, *et al.* Aseptic meningoencephalitis after iopamidol myelography. *Lancet* 1991; 338: 252.
5. Bain PG, *et al.* Paraplegia after iopamidol myelography. *Lancet* 1991; 338: 252–3.

Uses and Administration

Iopamidol is an iodinated nonionic monomeric contrast medium used by injection for a variety of radiographic procedures including angiography, arthrography, myelography, and urography (p.1030). Iopamidol is also used for contrast enhancement during computed tomography.

Iopamidol is usually available as solutions containing 26.1 to 75.5% of iopamidol (equivalent to 128 to 370 mg of iodine per mL) and the dose and strength used vary according to the procedure and route of administration.

Iopamidol has also been administered orally or by enema for visualisation of the gastrointestinal tract.

Preparations

USP 25: Iopamidol Injection.

Proprietary Preparations (details are given in Part 3)
Aust.: Gastromiro; Jopamiro; *Austral.:* Isovue; *Braz.:* Iopamiron; *Canad.:* Isovue†; *Denm.:* Iopamiro; *Fin.:* Iopamiro; *Fr.:* Iopamiron; *Ger.:* Solutrast; Unilux; *Irl.:* Gastromiro; Niopam; *Israel:* Gastromiro; Iopamiro; *Ital.:* Gastromiro; Iopamiro; *Neth.:* Iopamiro†; *Norw.:* Iopamiro; *Port.:* Gastromiro; Iopamiro; *Spain:* Iopamiro; Iopamiro; *Swed.:* Iopamiro; *Switz.:* Iopamiro; *UK:* Gastromiro; Niopam; *USA:* Isovue.

Iopanoic Acid (1570-w)

Iopanoic Acid *(BAN, rINN)*.

Acidum Iopanoicum; Iodopanoic Acid. 2-(3-Amino-2,4,6-tri-iodobenzyl)butyric acid.
$C_{11}H_{12}I_3NO_2 = 570.9$.
CAS — 96-83-3.
ATC — V08AC06.

Pharmacopoeias. In *Chin.*, *Eur.* (see p.vi), *Int.*, *Jpn*, and *US.*

It contains approximately 66.7% of I.

Pharmacopoeial description

Ph. Eur.: A white or yellowish-white powder. Practically insoluble in water; soluble in dehydrated alcohol, in ether, and in methyl alcohol; dissolves in dilute solutions of alkali hydroxides. Protect from light.

USP 25: A cream-coloured powder, with a faint characteristic odour. Insoluble in water; soluble in alcohol, in chloroform, in ether, and in solutions of alkali hydroxides and carbonates. Store in airtight containers. Protect from light.

Adverse Effects

Gastrointestinal disturbances such as nausea, vomiting, abdominal cramp, and diarrhoea are reported to occur in up to 40% of patients but are usually mild and transient. Mild stinging or burning on micturition, and skin rashes and flushing have occurred occasionally. Acute renal failure, thrombocytopenia, and hypersensitivity reactions have been reported.

Iopanoic acid has potent uricosuric and anticholinesterase effects.

Precautions

Iopanoic acid is contra-indicated in severe hepatic or renal disease; doses higher than 3 g should not be given to patients with renal impairment. It should not be used in the presence of acute gastrointestinal disorders that may impair absorption. It should be used with caution in patients with a history of hypersensitivity to iodine or to other contrast media, severe hyperthyroidism, hyperuricaemia, or cholangitis. In the light of its cholinergic action premedication with atropine has been suggested in some countries for patients with coronary heart disease. The administration of iodine-containing contrast media may interfere with thyroid-function tests and with some blood and urine tests.

Pharmacokinetics

Iopanoic acid is variably absorbed from the gastrointestinal tract and is strongly and extensively bound to plasma proteins. It is conjugated in the liver to the glucuronide and excreted largely in the bile and the remainder (about one-third of the dose) in the urine. It appears in the gallbladder about 4 hours after a dose is taken and maximum concentrations occur after about 17 hours. About 50% of a dose is excreted in 24 hours, but elevated protein-bound iodine concentrations may persist for several months.

Uses and Administration

Iopanoic acid is an iodinated ionic monomeric contrast medium used for cholecystography and cholangiography (p.1030). Usual doses of 3 g are given by mouth with plenty of water about 10 to 14 hours before X-ray examination. For repeat examinations an additional 3 g may be administered on the same day. Alternatively, repeat examination may be carried out after an interval of 5 to 7 days with a single 6 g dose. No more than 6 g of iopanoic acid should be taken during any 24-hour period, and doses over 3 g should be avoided in renal impairment. Adequate visualisation is achieved in the majority of patients with a single dose.

Preparations

BP 2001: Iopanoic Acid Tablets;
USP 25: Iopanoic Acid Tablets.

Proprietary Preparations (details are given in Part 3)
Austral.: Telepaque; *Braz.:* Telepaque; *Canad.:* Telepaque†; *Ital.:* Cistobil; *Spain:* Colegraf; Neocontrast†; *Switz.:* Cistobil†; *UK:* Telepaque†; *USA:* Telepaque.

Iopentol (2172-b)

Iopentol *(BAN, USAN, rINN)*.

Compound 5411. *N,N′*-Bis(2,3-dihydroxypropyl)-5-[N-(2-hydroxy-3-methoxypropyl)acetamido]-2,4,6-tri-iodoisophthalamide.
$C_{20}H_{28}I_3N_3O_9 = 835.2$.
CAS — 89797-00-2.
ATC — V08AB08.

Iopentol contains approximately 45.6% of I.

Profile

Iopentol is an iodinated nonionic monomeric contrast medium that is used for a variety of radiographic procedures including enhancement of computed tomography (p.1030).

Preparations

Proprietary Preparations (details are given in Part 3)
Aust.: Imagopaque; *Fin.:* Imagopaque; *Fr.:* Ivepaque; *Ger.:* Imagopaque; *Ital.:* Imagopaque; *Norw.:* Imagopaque†; *Spain:* Imagopaque; *Switz.:* Imagopaque.

Iopodic Acid (10912-n)

Ipodic Acid. 3-(3-Dimethylaminomethyleneamino-2,4,6-tri-iodophenyl)propionic acid.
$C_{12}H_{13}I_3N_2O_2 = 598.0$.
CAS — 5587-89-3.

Calcium Iopodate (1553-s)

Calcium Ipodate; Ipodate Calcium. Calcium 3-(3-dimethylaminomethyleneamino-2,4,6-tri-iodophenyl)propionate.
$(C_{12}H_{12}I_3N_2O_2)_2Ca = 1234.0$.
CAS — 1151-11-7.
ATC — V08AC10.

It contains approximately 61.7% of I.

Sodium Iopodate (1585-k)

Sodium Iopodate (BAN, rINN).

Ipodate Sodium (USAN); NSC-106962; Sodium Ipodate. Sodium 3-(3-dimethylaminomethyleneamino-2,4,6-tri-iodophenyl)propionate.
$C_{12}H_{12}I_3N_2NaO_2 = 619.9$.
CAS — 1221-56-3.
ATC — V08AC08.

Pharmacopoeias. In Jpn and US.

It contains about 61.4% of I.

Pharmacopoeial description

USP 25: A fine, white or off-white, odourless, crystalline powder. Soluble 1 in less than 1 of water, 1 in 2 of alcohol, 1 in 2 of dimethylacetamide, and 1 in 3.5 of dimethylformamide and of dimethyl sulfoxide; very slightly soluble in chloroform; freely soluble in methyl alcohol. Store in airtight containers.

Adverse Effects and Precautions

As for Iopanoic Acid, above. Effects on the gastrointestinal tract may be less with iopodate salts than with iopanoic acid.

Pharmacokinetics

The iopodate salts are absorbed from the gastrointestinal tract following oral or rectal administration, and almost completely metabolised. Protein binding to plasma proteins is reported to be high. Elimination is by the renal and hepatic routes; about half of an oral dose is stated to be excreted in the urine within 24 hours.

Uses and Administration

Iopodic acid is an iodinated ionic monomeric contrast medium given by mouth as the calcium and sodium salts for cholecystography and cholangiography (p.1030). Calcium iopodate is administered as a freshly-prepared suspension; the sodium salt is normally given as capsules. Following administration, optimal visualisation of the bile ducts usually occurs after 1 to 3 hours and that of the gallbladder after 10 to 12 hours.

For routine cholecystography they are given by mouth in a dose of 3 g of either salt in the evening, 10 to 12 hours before the examination; in fractionated oral cholecystography this may be followed by a second similar dose the following day, 3 hours before examination. In rapid cholecystography a single dose of 3 or 6 g may be given.

For cholangiography, a single dose of 6 g may be given.

Preparations

USP 25: Ipodate Sodium Capsules.

Proprietary Preparations (details are given in Part 3)
Aust.: Biloptin; Ger.: Biloptin; Port.: Biloptin; S.Afr.: Biloptin; Switz.: Biloptin†; UK: Biloptin; Solu-Biloptin; USA: Bilivist†; Oragrafin†.

Iopromide (18651-j)

Iopromide (BAN, USAN, rINN).

ZK-35760. N,N′-Bis(2,3-dihydroxypropyl)-2,4,6-tri-iodo-5-(2-methoxyacetamido)-N-methylisophthalamide.
$C_{18}H_{24}I_3N_3O_8 = 791.1$.
CAS — 73334-07-3.
ATC — V08AB05.

Pharmacopoeias. In US.

It contains about 48.1% of I.

Pharmacopoeial description

USP 25: A white to slightly yellow powder. Freely soluble in water and in dimethyl sulfoxide; practically insoluble in alcohol, in acetone, and in ether. Protect from light.

Adverse Effects and Precautions

See under the amidotrizoates, p.1031.

Uses and Administration

Iopromide is an iodinated nonionic monomeric contrast medium that is used for angiography, urography, arthrography, and the visualisation of body cavities (p.1030). It is also used for contrast enhancement during computed tomography, and to check functioning of a dialysis shunt.

Iopromide is administered locally and by injection. It is usually available as solutions containing 31.2 to 76.9% of iopromide (equivalent to 150 to 370 mg of iodine per mL) and the dose and strength used vary according to the procedure and route of administration.

Preparations

USP 25: Iopromide Injection.

Proprietary Preparations (details are given in Part 3)
Aust.: Ultravist; Austral.: Ultravist; Belg.: Ultravist; Canad.: Ultravist; Denm.: Ultravist; Fin.: Ultravist; Fr.: Ultravist; Ger.: Ultravist; Israel: Ultravist; Ital.: Ultravist; Jpn: Proscope; Neth.: Ultravist; Norw.: Ultravist; NZ: Ultravist; Port.: Ultravist; S.Afr.: Ultravist; Spain: Clarograf; Ultravist; Swed.: Ultravist; Switz.: Ultravist; UK: Ultravist; USA: Ultravist.

Iopydol (1573-y)

Iopydol (BAN, USAN).

1-(2,3-Dihydroxypropyl)-3,5-di-iodo-4-pyridone.
$C_8H_9I_2NO_3 = 421.0$.
CAS — 5579-92-0.
ATC — V08AD02.

Iopydol contains approximately 60.3% of I.

Profile

Iopydol is an iodinated contrast medium that has been used in conjunction with iopydone for bronchography (p.1030).

Preparations

Proprietary Preparations (details are given in Part 3)
Multi-ingredient: Braz.: Hytrast; Fr.: Hytrast†; Ger.: Hytrast†.

Iopydone (1574-j)

Iopydone (BAN, USAN).

3,5-Di-iodo-4-pyridone.
$C_5H_3I_2NO = 346.9$.
CAS — 5579-93-1.

Iopydone contains approximately 73.2% of I.

Profile

Iopydone is an iodinated contrast medium that has been used in conjunction with iopydol for bronchography (p.1030).

Preparations

Proprietary Preparations (details are given in Part 3)
Multi-ingredient: Braz.: Hytrast; Fr.: Hytrast†; Ger.: Hytrast†.

Iotalamic Acid (1530-h)

Iotalamic Acid (BAN, rINN).

Acidum Iotalamicum; Iothalamic Acid (USAN); Methalamic Acid; MI-216. 5-Acetamido-2,4,6-tri-iodo-N-methylisophthalamic acid.
$C_{11}H_9I_3N_2O_4 = 613.9$.
CAS — 2276-90-6.
ATC — V08AA04.

Pharmacopoeias. In Chin., Eur. (see p.vi), Jpn, and US.

It contains approximately 62% of I.

Pharmacopoeial description

Ph. Eur.: A white or almost white powder. Slightly soluble in water and in alcohol; practically insoluble in ether; dissolves in dilute solutions of alkali hydroxides. Protect from light.

USP 25: A white, odourless, powder. Slightly soluble in water and in alcohol; soluble in solutions of alkali hydroxides.

Meglumine Iotalamate (1531-m)

Meglumine Iotalamate (BANM, rINNM).

Iothalamate Meglumine; Meglumine Iothalamate. The N-methylglucamine salt of iotalamic acid.
$C_{11}H_9I_3N_2O_4,C_7H_{17}NO_5 = 809.1$.
CAS — 13087-53-1.

Pharmacopoeias. US includes only as various injections.

Meglumine iotalamate contains approximately 47.1% of I.

Sodium Iotalamate (1575-z)

Sodium Iotalamate (BANM, rINNM).

Iothalamate Sodium; Sodium Iothalamate.
$C_{11}H_8I_3N_2NaO_4 = 635.9$.
CAS — 17692-74-9; 1225-20-3.

Pharmacopoeias. US includes only as various injections.

Sodium iotalamate contains approximately 59.9% of I.

Adverse Effects, Treatment, and Precautions

As for the amidotrizoates, p.1031.

◊ In 40 patients who underwent phlebography with 60% meglumine iotalamate minor adverse reactions were common despite the use of saline flushing and muscle contraction to clear the veins after examination.[1] The commonest effect was pain at the site of injection, or in the calf or foot; 15 patients of those who had pain in the calf or foot were found to have venous thrombosis. Serious complications to phlebography appear to be rare but can cause serious morbidity; examination of 200 case notes and a retrospective study involving 3060 patients revealed 4 cases of necrosis in the skin of the foot and gangrene of the foot in 2.

1. Thomas ML, MacDonald LM. Complications of ascending phlebography of the leg. BMJ 1978; ii: 317–18.

Pharmacokinetics

Following intravascular administration the iotalamates are rapidly distributed; suitable concentrations for urography reach the urinary tract within 3 to 8 minutes of a bolus intravenous injection. Protein binding of both the sodium and meglumine salts is reported to be low. The iotalamates are eliminated by the kidneys. In patients with normal renal function more than 90% of the dose injected is excreted in urine within 24 hours.

Small amounts are reported to be excreted via the bile in the faeces. The iotalamates are removed by peritoneal dialysis and haemodialysis.

Uses and Administration

Iotalamic acid is an iodinated ionic monomeric contrast medium with actions similar to the amidotrizoates (p.1032). It is given locally and by injection for a wide range of radiographic procedures, including angiography, arthrography, cholangiography, urography, and for contrast enhancement during computed tomography (p.1030); oral or rectal administration has been used to visualise the gastrointestinal tract.

Iotalamic acid is usually available as solutions containing up to 80% of sodium iotalamate or up to 60% of meglumine iotalamate. The dose and strength used vary according to the procedure and route of administration. A mixture of the two salts is often preferred to minimise side-effects.

Iotalamates are not suitable for injection into the subarachnoid space.

Preparations

BP 2001: Meglumine Iotalamate Injection; Sodium Iotalamate Injection;
USP 25: Iothalamate Meglumine and Iothalamate Sodium Injection; Iothalamate Meglumine Injection; Iothalamate Sodium Injection.

Proprietary Preparations (details are given in Part 3)
Austral.: Conray 280; Conray 420†; Belg.: Contrix†; Canad.: Conray; Cysto-Conray; Ger.: Conray 30; Conray 60; Conray 70; Conray FL; Ital.: Angio-Conray†; Norw.: Conray; UK: Conray; Conray 325; Conray 420; USA: Angio-Conray†; Conray; Cysto-Conray; Vascoray†.

Iotrolan (3807-p)

Iotrolan (BAN, USAN, rINN).

Iotrol; Iotrolum; ZK-39482. N,N′,N″,N‴-Tetrakis(2,3-dihydroxy-1-hydroxymethylpropyl)-2,2′,4,4′,6,6′-hexaiodo-5,5′-(N,N′-dimethylmalonyldi-imino)di-isophthalamide.
$C_{37}H_{48}I_6N_6O_{18} = 1626.2$.
CAS — 79770-24-4.
ATC — V08AB06.

Iotrolan contains approximately 46.8% of I.

Adverse Effects and Precautions

As for the amidotrizoates, p.1031. For the adverse effects relating to the use of iotrolan for myelography, see under Iohexol, p.1035.

Uses and Administration

Iotrolan is an iodinated nonionic dimeric contrast medium that is given locally or by injection for a wide range of diagnostic procedures, including myelography, lymphography, arthrography, hysterosalpingography, cholangiopancreatography, and for visualisation of the mammary ducts and the gastrointestinal tract (p.1030). It is also used for contrast enhancement during computed tomography.

Iotrolan is usually available as solutions containing 51.3% or 64.1% of iotrolan (equivalent to 240 mg or 300 mg of iodine per mL, respectively) and the dose and strength used vary according to the procedure and route of administration.

Preparations

Proprietary Preparations (details are given in Part 3)
Aust.: Isovist; Canad.: Osmovist; Denm.: Isovist; Fin.: Isovist; Ger.: Isovist; Ital.: Isovist†; Neth.: Isovist; Norw.: Isovist†; NZ: Isovist; Port.: Iotrovist†; S.Afr.: Isovist; Swed.: Isovist†; Switz.: Isovist; UK: Isovist.

Iotroxic Acid (12859-v)

Iotroxic Acid (BAN, USAN, rINN).

SH-213AB. 3,3′-(3,6,9-Trioxaundecanedioyldi-imino)bis(2,4,6-tri-iodobenzoic acid).
$C_{22}H_{18}I_6N_2O_9 = 1215.8$.
CAS — 51022-74-3.
ATC — V08AC02.

Pharmacopoeias. In Int. and Jpn.

Iotroxic acid contains approximately 62.6% of I.

Meglumine Iotroxate (12860-r)

Meglumine Iotroxate (BANM).

Dimeglumine Iotroxate; Iotroxate Meglumine; Meglumine Iotroxinate. The di(N-methylglucamine)salt of iotroxic acid.
$C_{22}H_{18}I_6N_2O_9,2C_7H_{17}NO_5 = 1606.2$.
CAS — 68890-05-1.

Meglumine iotroxate contains approximately 47.4% of I.

Adverse Effects, Treatment, and Precautions

See under the amidotrizoates, p.1031.

Uses and Administration

Iotroxic acid is an iodinated ionic dimeric contrast medium that is used intravenously as the meglumine salt for cholecystography and cholangiography (p.1030).

Meglumine iotroxate is given by intravenous infusion in a dose equivalent to about 5 g of iodine usually as a 10.5% solution. The infusion should be administered over not less than 15 minutes.

Preparations

Proprietary Preparations (details are given in Part 3)
Aust.: Biliscopin; **Braz.:** Biliscopin; **Ger.:** Biliscopin; **Neth.:** Biliscopin†; **NZ:** Biliscopin; **Spain:** Bilisegrol; **Swed.:** Biliscopin; **Switz.:** Biliscopin; **UK:** Biliscopin.

Ioversol (2494-f)

Ioversol (BAN, USAN, rINN).
MP-328.   N,N′-Bis(2,3-dihydroxypropyl)-5-[N-(2-hydroxyethyl)glycolamido]-2,4,6-tri-iodoisophthalamide.
$C_{18}H_{24}I_3N_3O_9 = 807.1$.
CAS — 87771-40-2.
ATC — V08AB07.
Pharmacopoeias. In US.

Ioversol contains approximately 47.2% of I.

Adverse Effects, Treatment, and Precautions
See under the amidotrizoates, p.1031.

Uses and Administration
Ioversol is an iodinated nonionic monomeric contrast medium that is used by injection in angiography and urography (p.1030). It is also used for contrast enhancement during computed tomography. It is usually available as a solution containing 34 to 74% (equivalent to 160 to 350 mg of iodine per mL). The dose and strength used vary according to the procedure and route of administration.

Preparations
USP 25: Ioversol Injection.

Proprietary Preparations (details are given in Part 3)
Aust.: Optiray; **Austral.:** Optiray; **Belg.:** Optiject; Optiray; **Canad.:** Optiray; **Denm.:** Optiray; **Fin.:** Optiray; **Fr.:** Optiject; Optiray; **Ger.:** Optiray; **Israel:** Optiray; **Ital.:** Optiray; **Port.:** Optiray; **Spain:** Optiray; **Swed.:** Optiray; **Switz.:** Optiray; **USA:** Optiray.

Ioxaglic Acid (12861-f)

Ioxaglic Acid (BAN, USAN, rINN).
Acidum Ioxaglicum; P-286. N-(2-Hydroxyethyl)-2,4,6-tri-iodo-5-[2′,4′,6′-tri-iodo-3′-(N-methylacetamido)-5′-methylcarbamoylhippuramido]isophthalamic acid.
$C_{24}H_{21}I_6N_5O_8 = 1268.9$.
CAS — 59017-64-0.
ATC — V08AB03.
Pharmacopoeias. In Eur. (see p.vi) and US.

Ioxaglic acid contains approximately 60% of I.

Pharmacopoeial description
Ph. Eur.: A white or almost white hygroscopic powder. Very slightly soluble in water and in dichloromethane; slightly soluble in alcohol. It dissolves in dilute solutions of alkali hydroxides. Store in airtight containers. Protect from light.

Meglumine Ioxaglate (15337-m)

Meglumine Ioxaglate (BANM).
Ioxaglate Meglumine (USAN); MP-302 (with sodium ioxaglate). The N-methylglucamine salt of ioxaglic acid.
$C_{24}H_{21}I_6N_5O_8,C_7H_{17}NO_5 = 1464.1$.
CAS — 59018-13-2.

Meglumine ioxaglate contains approximately 52% of I.

Sodium Ioxaglate (15338-b)

Sodium Ioxaglate (BANM).
Ioxaglate Sodium (USAN); MP-302 (with meglumine ioxaglate).
$C_{24}H_{20}I_6N_5NaO_8 = 1290.9$.
CAS — 67992-58-9.

Sodium ioxaglate contains approximately 59% of I.

Adverse Effects, Treatment, and Precautions
See under the amidotrizoates, p.1031.

Pharmacokinetics
Following intravascular administration, ioxaglates are rapidly distributed throughout the extracellular fluid. Protein binding is reported to be very low. About 90% of a dose is excreted unchanged in the urine within 24 hours. An elimination half-life of about 90 minutes has been reported, which may be prolonged in renal impairment. Ioxaglates cross the placenta and are distributed into breast milk. They are removed by haemodialysis and peritoneal dialysis.

Uses and Administration
Ioxaglic acid is an iodinated ionic dimeric contrast medium that is given locally and by injection as a combined solution of its meglumine and sodium salts for a wide range of diagnostic procedures, including angiography, arthrography, hysterosalpingography, and urography (p.1030). It is also used for contrast enhancement during computed tomography.
The dose and strength used depend upon the procedure and route of administration. Commonly used solutions contain

39.3% of meglumine ioxaglate and 19.6% of sodium ioxaglate (equivalent to 320 mg of iodine per mL) or 24.6% of meglumine ioxaglate and 12.3% of sodium ioxaglate (equivalent to 200 mg of iodine per mL).

Ioxaglate is unsuitable for myelography and should not be given by the subarachnoid or epidural routes.

Preparations
USP 25: Ioxaglate Meglumine and Ioxaglate Sodium Injection.

Proprietary Preparations (details are given in Part 3)
Aust.: Hexabrix†; **Austral.:** Hexabrix; **Belg.:** Hexabrix; **Braz.:** Hexabrix; **Canad.:** Hexabrix; **Denm.:** Hexabrix; **Fin.:** Hexabrix; **Fr.:** Hexabrix; **Ger.:** Hexabrix; **Israel:** Hexabrix; **Ital.:** Hexabrix; **Neth.:** Hexabrix†; **Norw.:** Hexabrix; **NZ:** Hexabrix; **Port.:** Hexabrix; **Spain:** Hexabrix; **Swed.:** Hexabrix; **Switz.:** Hexabrix; **UK:** Hexabrix; **USA:** Hexabrix.

Ioxilan (6484-g)

Ioxilan (USAN, rINN).
N-(2,3-Dihydroxypropyl)-5-[N-(2,3-dihydroxypropyl)acetamido]-N′-(2-hydroxyethyl)-2,4,6-triiodoisophthalamide.
$C_{18}H_{24}I_3N_3O_8 = 791.1$.
CAS — 107793-72-6.
Pharmacopoeias. In US.

Ioxilan contains approximately 48.1% of I.

Pharmacopoeial description
USP 25: A white to off-white, practically odourless, powder. Soluble in water and in methyl alcohol. pH of a 10% solution in water is between 5.0 and 7.5. Protect from light.

Profile
Ioxilan is an iodinated nonionic monomeric contrast medium used for various radiographic procedures including enhancement of computed tomography (p.1030). It is given by injection.

Preparations
USP 25: Ioxilan Injection.

Ioxitalamic Acid (1532-b)

Ioxitalamic Acid (rINN).
AG-58107; Ioxithalamic Acid. 5-Acetamido-N-(2-hydroxyethyl)-2,4,6-tri-iodoisophthalamic acid.
$C_{12}H_{11}I_3N_2O_5 = 643.9$.
CAS — 28179-44-4.
ATC — V08AA05.
Pharmacopoeias. In Fr.

Ioxitalamic acid contains approximately 59.1% of I.

Meglumine Ioxitalamate (1533-v)

Ioxitalamate Meglumine. The N-methylglucamine salt of ioxitalamic acid.
$C_{12}H_{11}I_3N_2O_5,C_7H_{17}NO_5 = 839.2$.
CAS — 29288-99-1.

Meglumine ioxitalamate contains approximately 45.4% of I.

Sodium Ioxitalamate (1576-c)

Ioxitalamate Sodium.
$C_{12}H_{10}I_3N_2NaO_5 = 665.9$.
CAS — 33954-26-6.

Sodium ioxitalamate contains approximately 57.2% of I.

Profile
Ioxitalamic acid is an iodinated ionic monomeric contrast medium with actions similar to those of the amidotrizoates (p.1031). It is used as its meglumine and sodium salts locally and by injection for a wide range of diagnostic procedures, including angiography, cholangiography, hysterosalpingography, and urography (p.1030). It may be given by mouth or rectally for visualisation of the gastrointestinal tract. It is also used for contrast enhancement during computed tomography.
Monoethanolamine ioxitalamate has also been used.

Preparations

Proprietary Preparations (details are given in Part 3)
Aust.: Telebrix†; **Belg.:** Telebrix; Telebrix Gastro; Telebrix Hystero; **Braz.:** Telebrix 30; Telebrix 38; Telebrix Coronar; Telebrix TC; Vasobrix; Vasurix Polividona; **Canad.:** Telebrix; **Denm.:** Telebrix†; **Fr.:** Telebrix 12; Telebrix 30; Telebrix 35; Telebrix Gastro; Telebrix Hystero; **Ger.:** Telebrix Gastro; Telebrix N 180 and 300; **Israel:** Telebrix Gastro; **Ital.:** Telebrix 30†; Telebrix 38†; **Neth.:** Telebrix 12†; Telebrix 30†; Telebrix 350†; Telebrix Gastro†; Telebrix Polyvidone†; **Port.:** Telebrix 12; Telebrix 350; Telebrix Gastro; Telebrix Hystero; **Switz.:** Telebrix 12; Telebrix 30; Telebrix 35; Telebrix Gastro.

Mangafodipir Trisodium (5032-c)

Mangafodipir Trisodium (BANM, USAN, rINNM).
MnDPDP (mangafodipir); S-095 (mangafodipir); WIN-59010; Win-59010-2 (mangafodipir). Trisodium trihydrogen (OC-6-13)-{[N,N-′-ethylenebis(N-{[3-hydroxy-5-(hydroxymethyl)-2-methyl-4-pyridyl]methyl}glycine)   5,5′-bis(phosphato)](8-)}manganate(6-); Trisodium trihydrogen (OC-6-13)-N,N′-ethane-1,2-diylbis{N-[2-methyl-3-oxido-κO-5-(phosphonatooxymethyl)-4-pyridylmethyl]glycinato(O,N)}manganate(II).
$C_{22}H_{27}MnN_4Na_3O_{14}P_2 = 757.3$.
CAS — 155319-91-8 (mangafodipir); 140678-14-4 (mangafodipir trisodium).

Profile
Mangafodipir trisodium is a paramagnetic agent used intravenously for contrast enhancement in magnetic resonance imaging (p.1030) of the liver and pancreas.
Mangafodipir trisodium is available as a solution containing 7.57 mg (10 μmol) per mL. The usual dose in adults is 0.5 mL (5 μmol) per kg body-weight given by intravenous infusion at a rate of 2 to 3 mL per minute for imaging of the liver and 4 to 6 mL per minute for imaging of the pancreas.

Preparations
Proprietary Preparations (details are given in Part 3)
Aust.: Teslascan; **Belg.:** Teslascan; **Denm.:** Teslascan; **Fin.:** Teslascan; **Fr.:** Teslascan; **Ger.:** Teslascan; **Norw.:** Teslascan; **NZ:** Teslascan; **Spain:** Teslascan; **Swed.:** Teslascan; **UK:** Teslascan; **USA:** Teslascan.

Metrizamide (1578-a)

Metrizamide (BAN, USAN, rINN).
Win-39103. 2-[3-Acetamido-2,4,6-tri-iodo-5-(N-methylacetamido)benzamido]-2-deoxy-D-glucose.
$C_{18}H_{22}I_3N_3O_8 = 789.1$.
CAS — 31112-62-6 (metrizamide); 55134-11-7 (metrizamide, glucopyranose form).
ATC — V08AB01.

Metrizamide contains approximately 48.2% of I.

Adverse Effects and Precautions
As for the amidotrizoates, p.1031. For the adverse effects relating to the use of metrizamide for myelography, see under Iohexol, p.1035.

Pharmacokinetics
Following intrathecal administration metrizamide diffuses upwards through the CSF and enters the extracellular fluid of the brain. Most of a dose is eliminated from the CSF within several hours. It enters the blood and is eliminated primarily in urine; in patients with normal renal function 60% or more of an intrathecal dose is excreted in urine within 48 hours. Small amounts are excreted in bile. Metrizamide is not significantly bound to plasma proteins. It has been reported to be distributed into breast milk.

Uses and Administration
Metrizamide is an iodinated nonionic monomeric contrast medium that has been used in myelography, angiography, intravenous urography, and arthrography (p.1030), and also for contrast enhancement during computed tomography. The dose and strength used depend upon the procedure and route of administration.

Preparations
Proprietary Preparations (details are given in Part 3)
USA: Amipaque†.

Metrizoic Acid (1534-g)

3-Acetamido-2,4,6-tri-iodo-5-(N-methylacetamido)benzoic acid.
$C_{12}H_{11}I_3N_2O_4 = 627.9$.
CAS — 1949-45-7.
ATC — V08AA02.

Metrizoic acid contains approximately 60.6% of I.

Meglumine Metrizoate (1535-q)

Metrizoate Meglumine. The N-methylglucamine salt of metrizoic acid.
$C_{12}H_{11}I_3N_2O_4,C_7H_{17}NO_5 = 823.2$.
CAS — 7241-11-4.

Meglumine metrizoate contains approximately 46.3% of I.

Sodium Metrizoate (1579-t)

Sodium Metrizoate (BAN, rINN).
Metrizoate Sodium (USAN); NSC-107431.
$C_{12}H_{10}I_3N_2NaO_4 = 649.9$.
CAS — 7225-61-8.

Sodium metrizoate contains approximately 58.6% of I.

Profile
Metrizoic acid is an iodinated ionic monomeric contrast medium with actions similar to those of the amidotrizoates (p.1031). It is used as the meglumine and sodium salts, often together

---

The symbol † denotes a preparation no longer actively marketed

with calcium metrizoate and magnesium metrizoate, for a variety of diagnostic procedures including angiography, cholangiography, and hysterosalpingography (p.1030).

Preparations

Proprietary Preparations (details are given in Part 3)
Belg.: Isopaque†; **Denm.:** Isopaque†; **Norw.:** Isopaque Cysto†; **Swed.:** Isopaque Amin†; Isopaque Cysto†; **UK:** Isopaque Cysto.

Perflenapent (7208-k)

Perflenapent (USAN, rINN).
Dodecafluoropentane.
$C_5F_{12} = 288.0$.
CAS — 678-26-2.
ATC — V08DA03.

Profile

Perflenapent is a fluorocarbon ultrasound contrast medium (p.1030) used with perflisopent (below) for echocardiography.

◊ References.
1. Robbin ML, Eisenfeld AJ. Perflenapent emulsion: a US contrast agent for diagnostic radiology—multicenter, double-blind comparison with a placebo. *Radiology* 1998; **207:** 717–22.

Perflisopent (20110-g)

Perflisopent (USAN, rINN).
Nonafluoro-2-(trifluoromethyl)butane.
$C_5F_{12} = 288.0$.
CAS — 594-91-2.

Profile

Perflisopent is a fluorocarbon ultrasound contrast medium (p.1030) used with perflenapent (above) for echocardiography.

Propyliodone (1582-j)

Propyliodone (rINN).
Propyliodonum. Propyl 1,4-dihydro-3,5-di-iodo-4-oxo-1-pyridylacetate.
$C_{10}H_{11}I_2NO_3 = 447.0$.
CAS — 587-61-1.
ATC — V08AD03.
Pharmacopoeias. In *Int.* and *US.*

It contains about 56.8% of I.

Pharmacopoeial description

USP 25: A white or almost white, crystalline powder. Is odourless or has a faint odour. Practically insoluble in water; soluble in alcohol, in acetone, and in ether. Store in airtight containers. Protect from light.

Adverse Effects

Propyliodone may cause transient pyrexia, sometimes associated with malaise and aching of the joints, especially with the aqueous suspension, lasting 48 hours and sometimes accompanied by coughing. In a few cases, dyspnoea, atelectasis, or pneumonia have occurred. Hypersensitivity reactions may occur rarely.

Precautions

Propyliodone should be used with great care where there is hypersensitivity to iodine and is contra-indicated in patients with severe heart disease. It should also be used with caution in patients with asthma, bronchiectasis, or pulmonary emphysema, or in whom pulmonary function is otherwise reduced. If bilateral examination of the bronchial tract is necessary in such patients an interval of several days should elapse between the examinations. Use of an excessive volume or too-rapid administration may result in lobar collapse.

The administration of iodine-containing contrast media may interfere with thyroid-function tests.

Pharmacokinetics

After instillation into the lungs some propyliodone may be expectorated and swallowed but the remainder is absorbed into the blood. It is rapidly hydrolysed and is excreted in the urine as di-iodopyridone acetate. Approximately 50% of the administered dose is reported to be eliminated in the urine within 3 days.

Uses and Administration

Propyliodone is an iodinated contrast medium that has been used for bronchography (p.1030) as either a 50% aqueous suspension or as a 60% oily suspension.

Preparations

USP 25: Propyliodone Injectable Oil Suspension.
Proprietary Preparations (details are given in Part 3)
Israel: Dionosil; **USA:** Dionosil Oily†.

Sodium Tyropanoate (1586-a)

Sodium Tyropanoate (BAN, rINN).
NSC-107434; Tyropanoate Sodium (USAN); Win-8851-2. Sodium 2-(3-butyramido-2,4,6-tri-iodobenzyl)butyrate.
$C_{15}H_{17}I_3NNaO_3 = 663.0$.
CAS — 27293-82-9 (tyropanoic acid); 7246-21-1 (sodium tyropanoate).

It contains approximately 57.4% of I.

Profile

Sodium tyropanoate is an iodinated ionic monomeric contrast medium with actions similar to those of iopanoic acid (p.1035) and has been used for cholecystography and cholangiography (p.1030).

Preparations

Proprietary Preparations (details are given in Part 3)
USA: Bilopaque†.

Corticosteroids

The adrenal cortex synthesises a number of steroids, which may be divided into corticosteroids, based on a 21-carbon nucleus, and sex corticoids, primarily androgens, based on a 19-carbon nucleus. The corticosteroids are traditionally divided into those with predominantly glucocorticoid actions, of which cortisol (hydrocortisone) is the most important endogenous example, and those which are primarily mineralocorticoid, of which aldosterone is much the most important.

The endogenous glucocorticoids are under regulatory control from the hypothalamus and pituitary, via the releasing hormones corticorelin (p.1280) and corticotropin or ACTH (see p.1280). In return the glucocorticoids act to inhibit production and release of these releasing hormones by a negative feedback mechanism. The system is known collectively as the hypothalamic-pituitary-adrenal (HPA) axis. Aldosterone secretion, by contrast, is under the control of the renin-angiotensin system.

The main **mineralocorticoid** actions are on fluid and electrolyte balance. They enhance sodium reabsorption in the kidney and hence expand the extracellular fluid volume, and they enhance renal excretion of potassium and H^+.

The **glucocorticoid** actions are wide-ranging. They have potent anti-inflammatory and immunosuppressive effects, at least partly through inhibition of the release of various cytokines, and it is primarily these that are made use of clinically (see p.1044). They also have profound metabolic effects: blood glucose concentrations are maintained or increased by a decrease in peripheral glucose utilization and an increase in gluconeogenesis; glycogen deposition, protein breakdown, and lipolysis are increased, and effects on calcium uptake and excretion lead to a decrease in body calcium stores. Glucocorticoids play a facilitative or permissive role in the function of many other active endogenous substances, and have effects on the function of cardiovascular system, kidneys, skeletal muscle and CNS.

Many synthetic congeners and derivatives of the corticosteroids are available. The main corticosteroids used systemically are hydroxy compounds (alcohols). They are relatively insoluble in water and the sodium salt of the phosphate or succinate ester is generally used to provide water-soluble forms for injections or solutions. Such esters are readily hydrolysed in the body.

Various structure-activity relationships are understood for the corticosteroids and have been made use of in the development of new compounds. The presence of a hydroxyl group at position 11 seems to be essential for glucocorticoid activity, while a hydroxyl at position 21 is required for mineralocorticoid activity. Fluorination at position 9 enhances both mineralocorticoid and glucocorticoid activity. Substitution at carbon 16 (as in betamethasone, dexamethasone, or triamcinolone) virtually eliminates mineralocorticoid activity. Esterification of corticosteroids at the 17 or 21 positions with fatty acids generally increases the topical activity. The formation of cyclic acetonides at the 16 and 17 positions further increases topical anti-inflammatory activity, usually without increasing systemic glucocorticoid activity.

In the medical and pharmacological literature the names of unesterified corticosteroids have frequently been used indiscriminately for both the unesterified and esterified forms and it is not always apparent to which form reference is being made. The unesterified form is sometimes qualified by the phrase 'free alcohol'.

Adverse Effects of Corticosteroids and their Treatment

The adverse effects of corticosteroids may result from unwanted mineralocorticoid or glucocorticoid actions, or from inhibition of the hypothalamic-pituitary-adrenal axis.

Mineralocorticoid adverse effects are manifest in the retention of sodium and water, with oedema and hypertension, and in the increased excretion of potassium with the possibility of hypokalaemic alkalosis. In susceptible patients, cardiac failure may be induced. Disturbances of electrolyte balance are common with the naturally occurring corticosteroids, such as cortisone and hydrocortisone, but are less frequent with many synthetic glucocorticoids, which have little or no mineralocorticoid activity.

Adverse **glucocorticoid** effects lead to mobilisation of calcium and phosphorus, with osteoporosis and spontaneous fractures; muscle wasting and nitrogen depletion; and hyperglycaemia with accentuation or precipitation of the diabetic state. The insulin requirements of diabetic patients are increased. Increased appetite is often reported.

Impaired tissue repair and immune function can lead to delayed wound healing, and increased susceptibility to infection. Increased susceptibility to all kinds of infection, including septicaemia, tuberculosis, fungal infections, and viral infections, has been reported in patients on corticosteroid therapy. Infections may also be masked by the anti-inflammatory, analgesic, and antipyretic effects of glucocorticoids. Recent attention has focussed on the increased severity of varicella, with a possible fatal outcome in non-immune patients receiving systemic corticosteroid therapy.

Other adverse effects include menstrual irregularities, amenorrhoea, hyperhidrosis, skin thinning, ocular changes including development of glaucoma and cataract, mental and neurological disturbances, benign intracranial hypertension, acute pancreatitis, and avascular necrosis of bone. An increase in the coagulability of the blood may lead to thromboembolic complications. Peptic ulceration has been reported but reviews of the literature do not always agree that corticosteroids are responsible for an increased incidence.

The negative feedback effects of glucocorticoids on the hypothalamic-pituitary-adrenal (HPA) axis may lead to adrenal atrophy, in some cases after therapy for as little as 7 days. This produces secondary adrenocortical insufficiency, which may become manifest following overly rapid withdrawal of treatment or be precipitated by some stress such as infection or trauma. Patients vary considerably in the degree and duration of adrenal suppression following a given course of corticosteroid, but adrenal atrophy may persist for months or years, and withdrawal should be gradual in those who have been treated for any length of time (see also Withdrawal, below). High doses of corticosteroids administered during pregnancy may cause fetal or neonatal adrenal suppression. Although the precise mechanism is uncertain, growth retardation may follow the administration of even relatively small doses of corticosteroids to children.

Large doses of corticosteroids, or of corticotropin, may produce Cushingoid symptoms typical of hyperactivity of the adrenal cortex, with moon-face, sometimes with hirsutism, buffalo hump, flushing, increased bruising, ecchymoses, striae, and acne (see also Cushing's Syndrome, p.1272). Rapid intravenous administration of large doses of corticosteroids may cause cardiovascular collapse.

Hypersensitivity reactions have occurred with corticosteroids, mainly when administered topically.

Adverse effects occur, in general, fairly equally with all systemic corticosteroid preparations and their incidence rises steeply if dosage increases much above physiological values, traditionally considered to be about 7.5 mg daily of prednisolone or its equivalent (see under Uses and Administration, below, for equivalent doses of other corticosteroids). Short courses at high dosage for emergencies appear to cause fewer side-effects than prolonged courses with lower doses.

Most topically applied (including inhaled) corticosteroids may, under certain circumstances, be absorbed in sufficient amounts to produce systemic effects. The topical application of corticosteroid preparations to the eyes has produced corneal ulcers, raised intra-ocular pressure, and reduced visual function. Application of corticosteroids to the skin has led to loss of skin collagen and subcutaneous atrophy; local hypopigmentation of deeply pigmented skins has been reported following both the intradermal injection and topical application of potent corticosteroids. Dryness, irritation, epistaxis, and rarely ulceration or perforation of the nasal septum have followed intranasal use; smell and taste disturbances may also occur. Hoarseness and candidiasis of the mouth or throat may occur in patients receiving inhaled corticosteroids.

Intrathecal administration (including inadvertent intrathecal administration after attempted epidural injection) has been associated with arachnoiditis.

Adverse effects should be treated symptomatically, with the corticosteroid dosage reduced or slowly withdrawn where possible.

Adrenal suppression. The inhibition of hypothalamic-pituitary-adrenocortical function associated with corticosteroid use may persist for a year or more after treatment is withdrawn and may cause acute adrenocortical insufficiency with circulatory collapse during stress. The degree of suppression depends on a number of factors, including length of treatment, time of day of administration, type of corticosteroid preparation used, route of administration, dose administered, and dosing interval. In general, suppression of secretion of adrenocorticotrophic hormone and atrophy of the adrenal gland become progressively more definite as doses of corticosteroid exceed physiological amounts (see under Uses and Administration, below), and as the duration of therapy increases (significant suppression is likely in patients receiving more than 3 weeks of therapy). It is less when the corticosteroid is given as a single dose in the morning, and even less if this morning dose is given on alternate days or less frequently. In patients taking high enough doses of corticosteroids to suppress the adrenals the dose should be increased during any form of stress (for example, illness or surgery); similarly those treated with such doses within the last 2 or 3 months should be restarted on therapy. Where the interval since treatment is greater than 3 months, resumption of treatment depends on clinical assessment of signs of adrenocortical insufficiency.

To avoid precipitating acute adrenocortical insufficiency, withdrawal of corticosteroid treatment should be carried out gradually, differing regimens being used according to the disease being treated and the duration of therapy. Examples of withdrawal

regimens that have been used are described under Withdrawal, below.

Adrenal suppression may occur after very short courses of high-dose therapy and since many patients undergoing such therapy will be under continuing stress when the drugs are stopped, gradual withdrawal of corticosteroids over 5 to 7 days is preferable.

It should also be remembered that corticosteroid-induced adrenal suppression has been associated not only with systemic therapy, but has followed topical application of corticosteroid preparations, particularly those containing potent corticosteroids. Some degree of adrenal suppression is also associated with the use of high dose inhalants and nasal preparations, and has followed the topical application of eye drops and eye ointments.

Effects on bones and joints. Corticosteroid-induced **avascular necrosis** of bone is an uncommon but disabling complication of therapy.[1-3] The incidence may vary in patients with different disease states; alcoholics, and patients with connective tissue disease (especially systemic lupus erythematosus) may have increased susceptibility.[3,4] There may be a relationship with corticosteroid dose: even short courses of high-dose corticosteroids may be associated with its development.[1-3] There is also a report of avascular necrosis associated with topical application of corticosteroids.[5]

Corticosteroids may also produce **osteoporosis**. A review[6] of data obtained from studies published between 1970 and 1990 established that osteoporosis is a common consequence of long-term treatment with corticosteroids, occurring in approximately 50% of patients. Bone loss is more rapid during the early stages of therapy and is most rapid in areas of the skeleton containing the greatest proportion of trabecular bone such as the spine, hip, distal radius, pelvis, and ribs.

Reviews and guidelines[7-11] on the prevention and management of corticosteroid-induced osteoporosis suggest that the dose should be minimised, as oral doses above 7.5 mg of prednisolone or prednisone (or the equivalent) daily are associated with more significant bone loss and increased fracture risk.[12] Alternate-day therapy, although desirable for its reduced effect on the hypothalamic-pituitary-adrenal axis, does not reduce the risk of bone loss. Patients should maintain an adequate intake of calcium and vitamin D, should take regular exercise, and avoid smoking and excessive alcohol intake. Hormone replacement therapy is advocated in postmenopausal women. In high risk patients in whom hormone replacement therapy is inappropriate or contra-indicated the prophylactic use of bisphosphonates, calcitriol, or calcitonin should be considered. Recent evidence increasingly favours use of bisphosphonates for prevention and treatment of corticosteroid-induced bone loss,[13] although there is less evidence for a consequent reduction in fracture rates. A thiazide diuretic may be helpful in controlling hypercalciuria in patients not receiving calcitriol. Whether some corticosteroids have reduced effects on the bone is unclear.[10]

1. Nixon JE. Early diagnosis and treatment of steroid induced avascular necrosis of bone. *BMJ* 1984; **288**: 741–4.
2. Anonymous. Transplant osteonecrosis. *Lancet* 1985; **i**: 965–6.
3. Capell H. Selected side-effects: 5. steroid therapy and osteonecrosis. *Prescribers' J* 1992; **32**: 32–4.
4. Knight A. Images in clinical medicine: corticosteroid osteonecrosis. *N Engl J Med* 1995; **333**: 130.
5. McLean CJ, *et al*. Cataracts, glaucoma, and femoral avascular necrosis caused by topical corticosteroid ointment. *Lancet* 1995; **345**: 330.
6. Lukert BP, Raisz LG. Glucocorticoid-induced osteoporosis: pathogenesis and management. *Ann Intern Med* 1990; **112**: 352–64.
7. Picado C, Luengo M. Corticosteroid-induced bone loss: prevention and management. *Drug Safety* 1996; **15**: 347–59.
8. Anonymous. Corticosteroid-induced osteoporosis. *Drug Ther Bull* 1996; **34**: 84–6.
9. American College of Rheumatology Ad Hoc Committee on Glucocorticoid-Induced Osteoporosis. Recommendations for the prevention and treatment of glucocorticoid-induced osteoporosis. *Arthritis Rheum* 2001; **44**: 1496–1503.
10. Eastell R. Management of corticosteroid-induced osteoporosis. *J Intern Med* 1995; **237**: 439–47.
11. Eastell R, *et al*. A UK Consensus Group on management of corticosteroid-induced osteoporosis: an update. *J Intern Med* 1998; **244**: 271–92.
12. van Staa, *et al*. Oral corticosteroids and fracture risk: relationship to daily and cumulative doses. *Rheumatology* 2000; **39**: 1383–9.
13. Homik J, *et al*. Bisphosphonates for steroid induced osteoporosis (updated 9 May 2001). Available in The Cochrane Library; Issue 3. Oxford: Update Software; 2001.

Effects on carbohydrate and protein metabolism. Corticosteroids produce glucose intolerance[1-4] and protein catabolism.[5,6] Although mainly associated with systemic use, there is a report of deterioration in diabetic control associated with high-dose inhaled corticosteroid treatment.[7]

1. Hurel SJ, Taylor R. Drugs and glucose tolerance. *Adverse Drug React Bull* 1995; (Oct.): 659–62.
2. Landy HJ, *et al*. The effect of chronic steroid therapy on glucose tolerance in pregnancy. *Am J Obstet Gynecol* 1988; **159**: 612–15.
3. O'Byrne S, Feely J. Effects of drugs on glucose tolerance in non-insulin-dependent diabetics (part I). *Drugs* 1990; **40**: 6–18.
4. Bruno A, *et al*. Serum glucose, insulin and C-peptide response to oral glucose after intravenous administration of hydrocortisone and methylprednisolone in man. *Eur J Clin Pharmacol* 1994; **46**: 411–5.
5. Brownlee KG, *et al*. Catabolic effect of dexamethasone in the preterm baby. *Arch Dis Child* 1992; **67**: 1–4.

6. Van Goudoever JB, *et al*. Effect of dexamethasone on protein metabolism in infants with bronchopulmonary dysplasia. *J Pediatr* 1994; **124**: 112–18.
7. Faul JL, *et al*. High dose inhaled corticosteroids and dose dependent loss of diabetic control *BMJ* 1998; **317**: 1491.

Effects on the cerebrovascular system. Despite being used in high doses to treat benign intracranial hypertension, corticosteroids may also occasionally cause this disorder. Children receiving long-term therapy are mainly affected, an increase in dosage often being responsible. Symptoms usually subside when dosage is reduced.[1]

1. Gibberd B. Drug-induced benign intracranial hypertension. *Prescribers' J* 1991; **31**: 118–21.

Effects on the eyes. Ocular adverse effects of corticosteroids include raised intra-ocular pressure. Most reports implicate prolonged topical administration to the eye or face.[1-3] Young children (less than 8 years of age) may be at increased risk.[4] Increases in intra-ocular pressure appear to be less marked in patients receiving systemic corticosteroids.[5] However, there is evidence of an increased risk in patients receiving inhaled corticosteroids.[6] Again, prolonged or high-dose administration seems to be generally implicated. A recent study in elderly patients has also demonstrated a dose-related increase in the risk of raised intra-ocular pressure or open-angle glaucoma.[7]

Topical administration of corticosteroids to patients with ocular herpes simplex infection can alleviate the symptoms but allow the infection to develop with the risk of irreversible corneal scarring[1] that may lead to loss of vision, or even loss of the eye. Warnings have been sounded about the ocular risks of applying corticosteroid ointments to skin near the eyes.[8]

Cataract formation[2,3,9-12] is another risk from corticosteroid use; this hazard is associated with systemic corticosteroid absorption. Again, there is evidence that cataract formation may also be associated with use of inhaled corticosteroids.[13,14] Individual susceptibility to this effect appears to vary, but it may be more important than dosage and duration of treatment. Again, children may be more likely to develop cataract than adults.[5]

Systemic corticosteroid use has also been associated with damage to the retinal pigment epithelial barrier, predisposing the patient to serous retinal detachment.[15]

1. Anonymous. Avoiding eye damage from topical corticosteroids. *Drug Ther Bull* 1987; **25**: 29–30.
2. Butcher JM, *et al*. Bilateral cataracts and glaucoma induced by long term use of steroid eye drops. *BMJ* 1994; **309**: 43.
3. McLean CJ, *et al*. Cataracts, glaucoma, and femoral avascular necrosis caused by topical corticosteroid ointment. *Lancet* 1995; **345**: 330.
4. Lam DSC, *et al*. Accelerated ocular hypertensive response to topical steroids in children. *Br J Ophthalmol* 1997; **81**: 422–3.
5. Rennie IG. Clinically important ocular reactions to systemic drug therapy. *Drug Safety* 1993; **9**: 196–211.
6. Garbe E, *et al*. Inhaled and nasal glucocorticoids and the risks of ocular hypertension or open-angle glaucoma. *JAMA* 1997; **277**: 722–7.
7. Garbe E, *et al*. Risk of ocular hypertension or open-angle glaucoma in elderly patients on oral glucocorticoids. *Lancet* 1997; **350**: 979–82.
8. Chong NHV. Glaucoma induced by steroids. *BMJ* 1994; **309**: 343.
9. Allen M, *et al*. Steroid aerosols and cataract formation. *BMJ* 1989; **299**: 432–3.
10. Karim AKA, *et al*. Steroid aerosols and cataract formation. *BMJ* 1989; **299**: 918.
11. Ghanchi F. Young patients on inhaled steroids and cataract. *Lancet* 1993; **342**: 1306–7.
12. Costagliola C, *et al*. Cataracts associated with long-term topical steroids. *Br J Dermatol* 1989; **120**: 472–3.
13. Cumming RG, *et al*. Use of inhaled corticosteroids and the risk of cataracts. *N Engl J Med* 1997; **337**: 8–14.
14. Garbe E, *et al*. Association of inhaled corticosteroid use with cataract extraction in elderly patients. *JAMA* 1998; **280**: 539–43. Correction. *ibid*.; 1830.
15. Polak BCP, *et al*. Diffuse retinal pigment epitheliopathy complicating systemic corticosteroid treatment. *Br J Ophthalmol* 1995; **79**: 922–5.

Effects on the gastrointestinal tract. It has long been considered that treatment with corticosteroids might lead to peptic ulcers. Some years ago a review of the data then available suggested that since an ulcer developed in 1% of control patients not receiving corticosteroids, the 2% incidence for patients receiving corticosteroids did not warrant the prophylactic use of anti-ulcer drugs in all patients.[1] Others have found little evidence of an increased risk of peptic ulcer produced by corticosteroids alone although there is some increase in risk associated with the concomitant use of corticosteroids and NSAIDs.[2] It has been suggested that it might be prudent to avoid such combination therapy whenever possible.[3]

Doubt has therefore been cast on the prophylactic value of anti-ulcer therapy given concomitantly with corticosteroids.[1,4] If an ulcer does develop and there is good reason to continue treatment then corticosteroids may be continued along with some form of ulcer therapy.[1]

There have been several reports of corticosteroids being associated with gastrointestinal perforation.[5-8] There is a risk that the anti-inflammatory properties of corticosteroids may mask the signs of perforation and delay diagnosis with potentially fatal results.

1. Spiro HM. Is the steroid ulcer a myth? *N Engl J Med* 1983; **309**: 45–7.
2. Piper JM. Corticosteroid use and peptic ulcer disease: role of nonsteroidal anti-inflammatory drugs. *Ann Intern Med* 1991; **114**: 735–40.
3. Guslandi M, Tittobello A. Steroid ulcers: a myth revisited. *BMJ* 1992; **304**: 655–6.

4. Marcus P, McCauley DL. Steroid therapy and H$_2$-receptor antagonists: pharmacoeconomic implications. *Clin Pharmacol Ther* 1997; **61**: 503–8.
5. Arsura EL. Corticosteroid-associated perforation of colonic diverticula. *Arch Intern Med* 1990; **150**: 1337–8.
6. Ng PC, *et al.* Gastroduodenal perforation in preterm babies treated with dexamethasone for bronchopulmonary dysplasia. *Arch Dis Child* 1991; **66**: 1164–6.
7. O'Neil EA, *et al.* Dexamethasone treatment during ventilator dependency: possible life threatening gastrointestinal complications. *Arch Dis Child* 1992; **67**: 10–11.
8. Epstein A, *et al.* Perforation of colon diverticula during corticosteroid therapy for pemphigus vulgaris. *Ann Pharmacother* 1993; **27**: 979–80.

Effects on growth. Corticosteroids impair normal growth in children when given systemically,[1,2] and although alternate day therapy may reduce the effect on growth it does not abolish it. Recent concerns have centred on the possible effects of inhaled corticosteroids on growth.[1,3] Some studies have not found an effect of inhaled corticosteroids on growth if doses are modest, even when treatment is prolonged.[1,4,5] Others have found that inhaled corticosteroids, particularly in high doses, do have some effect on growth parameters,[4,6-9] but it is unclear whether this has long-term effects on the child's ultimate height, and the alternative in children requiring such high-dose therapy is likely to be an oral corticosteroid, with its consequent effects. Nonetheless, in the light of the increasing number of studies suggesting some effects of inhaled or intranasal corticosteroids on growth the FDA has required the inclusion of a warning in US labelling that such products may slow growth rates. For a suggestion that inhalation of a single dose of budesonide in the morning had less effect on growth than twice daily dosage, see Administration, p.1064.

1. Allen DB, *et al.* A meta-analysis of the effect of oral and inhaled corticosteroids on growth. *J Allergy Clin Immunol* 1994; **93**: 967–76.
2. Lai H-C, *et al.* Risk of persistent growth impairment after alternate-day prednisone treatment in children with cystic fibrosis. *N Engl J Med* 2000; **342**: 851–9.
3. Hanania NA, *et al.* Adverse effects of inhaled corticosteroids. *Am J Med* 1995; **98**: 196–208.
4. Wolthers OD, Pedersen S. Controlled study of linear growth in asthmatic children during treatment with inhaled glucocorticosteroids. *Pediatrics* 1992; **89**: 839–42.
5. Volovitz B, *et al.* Growth and pituitary-adrenal function in children with severe asthma treated with inhaled budesonide. *N Engl J Med* 1993; **329**: 1703–8.
6. Wolthers OD, Pedersen S. Short term growth during treatment with inhaled fluticasone propionate and beclomethasone dipropionate. *Arch Dis Child* 1993; **68**: 673–6.
7. Todd G, *et al.* Growth and adrenal suppression in asthmatic children treated with high-dose fluticasone propionate. *Lancet* 1996; **348**: 27–9.
8. McCowan C, *et al.* Effect of asthma and its treatment on growth: four year follow up of cohort of children from general practices in Tayside, Scotland. *BMJ* 1998; **316**: 668–72.
9. Sharek PJ, Bergman DA. The effect of inhaled steroids on the linear growth of children with asthma: a meta-analysis. Abstract: *Pediatrics* 2000; **106**: 129. Full version: http://www.pediatrics.org/cgi/content/full/106/1/e8

Effects on immune response. Owing to their immunosuppressant effect administration of corticosteroids in doses greater than those required for physiological replacement therapy is associated with increased susceptibility to infection, aggravation of existing infection, and activation of latent infection. An additional problem is that the anti-inflammatory effect of corticosteroids may mask symptoms until the infection has progressed to an advanced stage; the altered response of the body may also permit the bizarre spread of infections, frequently in aberrant forms, such as disseminated parasitic infections. The risk is greater in patients receiving high doses, or associated therapy with other immunosuppressants such as cytotoxic drugs, and in those who are already debilitated. Children receiving high doses of corticosteroids are at special risk from childhood diseases, such as chickenpox, but vaccination with living organisms is contra-indicated since infection may be induced (killed vaccines or toxoids may be given but the response may be reduced). This increased susceptibility to infection coupled with masking of symptoms may also be caused by topical or local corticosteroid therapy. Thus, topical application to the skin has led to unusual changes such as atypical ringworm infection. Fungal infections (particularly candidiasis), generally restricted to the mouth and throat, are associated with corticosteroid inhalations. Severe damage to the eye has followed the ocular use of corticosteroids in herpetic infections, and a similar generalised spread of herpes infection may follow application to the mouth in the presence of herpes infection.

Conversely, the effect of corticosteroids on the symptoms and course of some infections may be life-saving (see Uses and Administration, below). Before embarking on a long-term course of corticosteroid therapy general measures for the reduction of risk of infection include a diligent search for active or quiescent infection and, where appropriate, prevention or eradication of the infection before starting, or concurrent administration of chemoprophylaxis during corticosteroid treatment.

Effects on lipid metabolism. Glucocorticoids have potent effects on lipid metabolism, facilitating the effects of growth hormone and endogenous stimulants of lipolysis. As a result they increase both high- and low-density lipoprotein cholesterol concentrations in the blood.

On prolonged administration glucocorticoids also have a dramatic effect on body fat distribution, resulting in the character-

istic Cushingoid appearance of moon face, and increased fat at the back of the neck and supraclavicular area.

Effects on mental state. Reviews and reports of the effects of corticosteroids on mental state[1-7] suggest a causative link between corticosteroid therapy, particularly in high doses, and certain cases of mental disturbance. These disturbances have included psychosis, euphoria, and depression. Impairment of memory has been associated with pulsed intravenous methylprednisolone.[8]

1. Mitchell DM, Collins JV. Do corticosteroids really alter mood? *Postgrad Med J* 1984; **60**: 467–70.
2. Sultzer DL, Cummings JL. Drug-induced mania—causative agents, clinical characteristics and management: a retrospective analysis of the literature. *Med Toxicol Adverse Drug Exp* 1989; **4**: 127–43.
3. d'Orbán PT. Steroid-induced psychosis. *Lancet* 1989; **ii**: 694.
4. Wolkowitz OM, Rapaport M. Long-lasting behavioral changes following prednisone withdrawal. *JAMA* 1989; **261**: 1731–2.
5. Anonymous. Drugs that cause psychiatric symptoms. *Med Lett Drugs Ther* 1993; **35**: 65–70.
6. Patten SB, Love EJ. Drug-induced depression: incidence, avoidance and management. *Drug Safety* 1994; **10**: 203–19.
7. Patten SB, Neutel CI. Corticosteroid-induced adverse psychiatric effects: incidence, diagnosis and management. *Drug Safety* 2000; **22**: 111–22.
8. Oliveri RL, *et al.* Pulsed methylprednisolone induces a reversible impairment of memory in patients with relapsing-remitting multiple sclerosis. *Acta Neurol Scand* 1998; **97**: 366–9.

Effects on the neonate. Various adverse effects have been reported in premature neonates given corticosteroids, see under Dexamethasone, p.1067.

Effects on the nervous system. Paraesthesia and irritation, most commonly occurring in the anogenital region, have been associated with the intravenous administration of dexamethasone sodium phosphate[1] and hydrocortisone sodium phosphate,[2] but not with hydrocortisone sodium succinate.[2] Further comments and discussions on this topic are listed below.[3-5] Also listed below are references to epidural lipomatosis with severe neurological complications following systemic corticosteroid therapy.[6,7]

1. Czerwinski AW, *et al.* Effects of a single, large, intravenous injection of dexamethasone. *Clin Pharmacol Ther* 1972; **13**: 638–42.
2. Novak E, *et al.* Anorectal pruritus after intravenous hydrocortisone sodium succinate and sodium phosphate. *Clin Pharmacol Ther* 1976; **20**: 109–12.
3. Anonymous. Which form of intravenous hydrocortisone. *Drug Ther Bull* 1979; **17**: 71–2.
4. Thomas VL. More on dexamethasone-induced perineal irritation. *N Engl J Med* 1986; **314**: 1643.
5. Allan SG, Leonard RCF. Dexamethasone antiemesis and side-effects. *Lancet* 1986; **i**: 1035.
6. Butcher DL, Sahn SA. Epidural lipomatosis: a complication of corticosteroid therapy. *Ann Intern Med* 1979; **90**: 60.
7. George WE, *et al.* Medical management of steroid-induced epidural lipomatosis. *N Engl J Med* 1983; **308**: 316–19.

Effects on the pancreas. Acute pancreatitis has been associated with corticosteroid use,[1-3] although evidence supporting the association has been challenged on a number of grounds, both clinical and experimental.[2]

1. Nakashima Y, Howard JM. Drug-induced acute pancreatitis. *Surg Gynecol Obstet* 1977; **145**: 105–9.
2. Banerjee AK, *et al.* Drug-induced acute pancreatitis: a critical review. *Med Toxicol Adverse Drug Exp* 1989; **4**: 186–98.
3. Felig DM, Topazian M. Corticosteroid-induced pancreatitis. *Ann Intern Med* 1996; **124**: 1016.

Effects on the skin. Topical corticosteroids are associated with a number of local adverse effects on the skin, principally due to their antiproliferative effects on keratinocytes and fibroblasts (leading to skin thinning and atrophy), and to possible interference with the skin flora (leading to increased risk of superinfection or opportunistic infection).[1] Skin thinning is more likely if corticosteroids are applied under occlusion (this is especially true of halogenated corticosteroids which are more resistant to inactivation by enzymes in the epidermis). Striae, which occur usually in intertriginous areas such as axillae and groin where skin is thin, moist, and occluded, are the most readily appreciable manifestation of skin atrophy, and are irreversible, unlike more minor degrees of atrophy. Other local adverse effects include telangiectasias and purpura. The balance between benefit and the likelihood of local or systemic adverse effects following topical application of corticosteroids will depend on the chemical structure of the drug (i.e. its lipophilicity and resistance to enzymic degradation), the formulation of the vehicle, the way in which it is applied, and the nature of the skin to be treated.[1]

Skin thinning and purpura have also been reported in patients receiving inhaled corticosteroids.[2,3]

The adverse skin effects arising from systemic corticosteroids also include striae and skin thinning as well as acneiform eruptions. Somewhat counter-intuitively a case-control study has suggested an increased risk of Stevens-Johnson syndrome or toxic epidermal necrolysis in patients receiving corticosteroids, particularly in the period shortly after beginning therapy.[4]

Skin reactions are occasionally observed with inhaled corticosteroids.[5]

1. Mori M, *et al.* Topical corticosteroids and unwanted local effects: improving the benefit/risk ratio. *Drug Safety* 1994; **10**: 406–12.
2. Shuttleworth D, *et al.* Inhaled corticosteroids and skin thinning. *Br J Dermatol* 1990; **122**: 268.

3. Capewell S, *et al.* Purpura and dermal thinning associated with high dose inhaled corticosteroids. *BMJ* 1990; **300**: 1548–51.
4. Roujeau J-C, *et al.* Medication use and the risk of Stevens-Johnson syndrome or toxic epidermal necrolysis. *N Engl J Med* 1995; **333**: 1600–7.
5. Isaksson M. Skin reactions to inhaled corticosteroids: incidence, avoidance and management. *Drug Safety* 2001; **24**: 369–73.

Effects on the voice. Dysphonia may be associated with inhaled corticosteroids.[1-5] Although oropharyngeal candidiasis may be one possible cause of such hoarseness, most patients with dysphonia are reported not to have candidiasis.[5]

1. Anonymous. Inhaled steroids and dysphonia. *Lancet* 1984; **i**: 375–6.
2. Dash CH, Pover GM. Inhaled steroids and dysphonia. *Lancet* 1984; **i**: 458.
3. Campbell IA. Inhaled steroids and dysphonia. *Lancet* 1984; **i**: 744.
4. Streeton JA. Inhaled steroids and dysphonia. *Lancet* 1984; **i**: 963.
5. Crompton GK. Local adverse effects of inhaled corticosteroids. *Prescribers' J* 1995; **35**: 225.

Hypersensitivity and anaphylaxis. There have been occasional reports of hypersensitivity reactions, and sometimes anaphylaxis, caused by corticosteroids.[1] Reactions have occurred with any route, although the topical route is mainly involved. It has been observed that the incidence of hypersensitivity is increasing[2] and it has been suggested that a lack of response in chronic eczema might be due to a reaction to the corticosteroid treatment.[2] Fluorinated corticosteroids may be less likely to induce a contact hypersensitivity reaction than non-fluorinated compounds.[3]

1. Kamm GL, Hagmeyer KO. Allergic-type reactions to corticosteroids. *Ann Pharmacother* 1999; **33**: 451–60.
2. Dooms-Goossens A. Sensitivity to corticosteroids: consequences for anti-inflammatory therapy. *Drug Safety* 1995; **13**: 123–9.
3. Thomson KF, *et al.* The prevalence of corticosteroid allergy in two U.K. centres: prescribing implications. *Br J Dermatol* 1999; **141**: 863–6.

Tumour lysis syndrome. Reports of corticosteroid-induced tumour lysis syndrome.[1-3]

1. Sparano J, *et al.* Increasing recognition of corticosteroid-induced tumour lysis syndrome in non-Hodgkin's lymphoma. *Cancer* 1990; **65**: 1072–3.
2. Smith RE, Stoiber TR. Acute tumor lysis syndrome in prolymphocytic leukemia. *Am J Med* 1990; **88**: 547–8.
3. Haller C, Dhadly M. The tumor lysis syndrome. *Ann Intern Med* 1991; **114**: 808–9.

Withdrawal of Corticosteroids

The use of pharmacological doses of corticosteroids suppresses the endogenous secretion of corticotropin by the anterior pituitary, with the result that the adrenal cortex becomes atrophied. Sudden withdrawal or reduction in dosage, or an increase in corticosteroid requirements associated with the stress of infection or accidental or surgical trauma, may then precipitate acute adrenocortical insufficiency; deaths have followed the abrupt withdrawal of corticosteroids. (Adrenocortical insufficiency has also occurred following the effective reduction in systemic corticosteroid concentrations produced by overly rapid transfer from oral to inhaled corticosteroid therapy.) For the emergency treatment of acute adrenocortical insufficiency caused by abrupt withdrawal of corticosteroids, see under Adrenocortical Insufficiency, p.1046.

In some instances, withdrawal symptoms may involve or resemble a clinical relapse of the disease for which the patient has been undergoing treatment. Other effects that may occur during withdrawal or change of corticosteroid therapy include fever, myalgia, arthralgia, weight loss, benign intracranial hypertension with headache and vomiting, and papilloedema caused by cerebral oedema. Latent rhinitis or eczema may be unmasked.

Duration of treatment and dosage are important factors in determining suppression of the pituitary-adrenal response to stress on cessation of corticosteroid treatment, and individual liability to suppression is also important.

Following short courses at moderate doses it may be appropriate to withdraw corticosteroids without tapering the dose (see below). However, after high-dose or prolonged therapy, withdrawal should be gradual, the rate depending upon the individual patient's response, the dose, the disease being treated, and the duration of therapy. Recommendations for initial reduction, stated in terms of prednisolone, have varied from as little as steps of 1 mg monthly to 2.5 to 5 mg every 2 to 7 days. Provided the disease is unlikely to relapse the dose of systemic corticosteroid may be reduced rapidly to physiological values; dose reduction should then be slower to allow recovery of pituitary-adrenal function. Symptoms attributable to over-rapid withdrawal should be countered by resuming a higher dose and continuing the reduction at a slower rate. The administration of corticotropin does not help to re-establish adrenal responsiveness.

This gradual withdrawal of corticosteroid therapy permits a return of adrenal function adequate for daily needs, but years may sometimes be required for the return of function necessary to meet the stress of infection, surgical operations, or trauma. On such occasions patients with a history of recent corticosteroid withdrawal should be protected by means of supplementary corticosteroid therapy as described under Precautions, below.

◊ The UK Committee on Safety of Medicines recommends that moderate dosage with corticosteroids (up to 40 mg daily of prednisolone, or equivalent), for up to 3 weeks, may be stopped without tapering provided that the original disease is unlikely to relapse, although prophylactic cover may be required for any stress within a week of finishing the course.[1] However, it should be borne in mind that individuals vary widely in their response to corticosteroids and their ability to tolerate withdrawal. Gradual withdrawal should be considered, even after shorter courses, if higher doses are given, or in patients with other risk factors for adrenocortical insufficiency, including those who have had repeated courses of systemic corticosteroids, those who receive a course within one year of finishing long-term corticosteroid therapy, or those who regularly take doses in the evening, when their suppressive effect is greater. Withdrawal should not be abrupt in any patient who receives systemic corticosteroids for more than 3 weeks.[1]

How dose reduction is carried out depends largely on the likelihood of relapse of the original disease. If this is unlikely, the dose of systemic corticosteroid may be reduced rapidly to physiological values (traditionally considered to be 7.5 mg of prednisolone daily or equivalent). It should then be reduced more slowly to allow the hypothalamic-pituitary-adrenal axis to recover.[1] Where disease relapse is a possibility even the initial reduction may need to be more cautious. Long-term treatment may require withdrawal over many months (such as a reduction of 1 mg in the daily dose of prednisolone every 3 to 4 weeks).

In reviews of the inhibition of hypothalamic-pituitary-adrenocortical function associated with corticosteroid administration, further regimens for corticosteroid withdrawal are described.[2-4] For example, patients who have been treated for weeks or months may have their daily dose of prednisolone reduced by 2.5 to 5 mg every 2 or 3 days, or, for those on longer-term treatment, the reduction may be more gradual at a rate of 2.5 mg every 1 to 3 weeks and possibly less. When the dose has reached 10 mg daily decrements may be made with 1-mg tablets. Another approach may be to convert daily therapy gradually into alternate-day therapy by progressively reducing the amount of corticosteroid received on every second day, and once alternate-day therapy is established the dose may be further reduced until, for example, a dose of 1 mg on alternate days for one week is attained.

1. Committee on Safety of Medicines/Medicines Control Agency. Withdrawal of systemic corticosteroids. *Current Problems* 1998; **24:** 5–7.
2. Anonymous. Corticosteroids and hypothalamic-pituitary-adrenocortical function. *BMJ* 1980; **280:** 813–14.
3. Helfer EL, Rose LI. Corticosteroids and adrenal suppression: characterising and avoiding the problem. *Drugs* 1989; **38:** 838–45.
4. Page RC. How to wean a patient off corticosteroids. *Prescribers' J* 1997; **37:** 11–16.

Precautions for Corticosteroids

Corticosteroids should only be used systemically with great caution in the presence of heart failure, recent myocardial infarction, or hypertension, in patients with diabetes mellitus, epilepsy (but see below for use in infantile seizures), glaucoma, hypothyroidism, hepatic failure, osteoporosis, peptic ulceration, psychoses or severe affective disorders, and renal impairment. Children may be at increased risk of some adverse effects; in addition, corticosteroids may cause growth retardation, and prolonged administration is rarely justified. The elderly too may be at greater risk from adverse effects.

Corticosteroids are usually contra-indicated in the presence of acute infections uncontrolled by appropriate antimicrobial chemotherapy. Similarly, patients already receiving corticosteroid therapy are more susceptible to infection, the symptoms of which, moreover, may be masked until an advanced stage has been reached. Patients with active or doubtfully quiescent tuberculosis should not be given corticosteroids except, very rarely, as adjuncts to treat-

ment with antitubercular drugs. Patients with quiescent tuberculosis should be observed closely and should receive chemoprophylaxis if corticosteroid therapy is prolonged.

The risks of chickenpox and probably of severe herpes zoster are increased in non-immune patients receiving therapeutic doses of systemic corticosteroids, and patients should avoid close personal contact with either infection. Passive immunisation is recommended for non-immune patients who do come into contact with chickenpox. Similar precautions apply to measles. Live vaccines should not be given to patients receiving high-dose systemic corticosteroid therapy nor for at least 3 months afterwards; killed vaccines or toxoids may be given although the response may be attenuated.

During prolonged courses of corticosteroid therapy, patients should be examined regularly. Sodium intake may need to be reduced and calcium and potassium supplements may be necessary. Monitoring of the fluid intake and output, and daily weight records may give early warning of fluid retention. Back pain may signify osteoporosis. Children are at special risk from raised intracranial pressure. Patients should carry cards (and preferably also wear bracelets) giving full details of their corticosteroid therapy; they and their relatives should be fully conversant with the implications of their therapy and the precautions to be taken.

Measures to compensate for the adrenals' inability to respond to stress (see Withdrawal, above) include increasing the dose to cover minor intercurrent illnesses or trauma such as surgery (with intramuscular administration to cover vomiting). For details of dosages used, see Uses and Administration, below.

Rapid intravenous injection of massive doses of corticosteroids may sometimes cause cardiovascular collapse and injections should therefore be given slowly or by infusion.

Many drugs have been reported to interfere with certain assay procedures for corticosteroids in body fluids and corticosteroids themselves may interfere with or alter the results of assays for some endogenous substances or drugs.

The risk of systemic absorption should always be considered when applying corticosteroids topically. They should not be applied with an occlusive dressing to large areas of the body. Long-term topical use is best avoided, especially in children. Also they should not be used for the treatment of ulcerative conditions, nor of rosacea, and should not be used indiscriminately for pruritus. Occasionally they may be used with the addition of a suitable antimicrobial substance in the treatment of infected skin but there is a risk of sensitivity reactions occurring.

Height should be monitored in children receiving prolonged therapy with inhaled or nasal corticosteroids. High doses of inhaled corticosteroids should preferably be inhaled using large-volume spacer devices to reduce oropharyngeal deposition and hence the incidence of candidiasis; rinsing the mouth with water after inhalation may also be helpful. In addition the use of spacer devices may reduce systemic absorption (see also Inhalation Therapy, under Uses and Administration, below). Paradoxical bronchospasm has occurred with inhaled corticosteroids and may require discontinuation of therapy, although if mild it may be prevented by inhalation of a beta$_2$ adrenoceptor agonist, or by transfer from an aerosol to a dry powder formulation.

Caution is required when corticosteroids are used locally to treat eye disorders (see below).

◊ A report of two cases of Cushing's syndrome associated with inappropriately prolonged use of corticosteroid nasal drops in children.[1] Such drops should not be prescribed on a repeat prescription basis. See also Adrenal Suppression, under Adverse Effects, above.

1. Findlay CA, *et al.* Childhood Cushing's syndrome induced by betamethasone nose drops, and repeat prescriptions. *BMJ* 1998; **317:** 739–40.

Contraception. There are some isolated case reports of contraceptive failure in women using intra-uterine devices and receiving corticosteroid therapy.[1-3]

1. Zerner J, *et al.* Failure of an intrauterine device concurrent with administration of corticosteroids. *Fertil Steril* 1976; **27:** 1467–8.
2. Inkeles DM, Hansen RI. Unexpected pregnancy in a woman using an intrauterine device and receiving steroid therapy. *Ann Ophthalmol* 1982; **14:** 975.
3. Buhler M, Papiernik E. Successive pregnancies in women fitted with intrauterine devices who take anti-inflammatory drugs. *Lancet* 1983; **i:** 483.

Eye disorders. Topical corticosteroids have transformed the management of inflammatory disease of the anterior segment of the eye and it should be noted that their proper use may be sight-saving but that their inappropriate use is potentially blinding.[1] The dangers include the conversion of a simple dendritic herpes simplex epithelial lesion into an extensive amoeboid ulcer with the likelihood of permanent corneal scarring and loss of vision and also the risk of potentiation of bacterial and fungal infections. Other dangers include the development of open-angle glaucoma and cataracts. Topical corticosteroids are used by ophthalmologists in herpes simplex keratitis but always under appropriate antiviral cover and their use requires considerable experience. Topical corticosteroids should never be given for an undiagnosed red eye and many consultant ophthalmic surgeons believe that general practitioners should never initiate therapy without an ophthalmic opinion.

Further studies and discussions on the inappropriate use of corticosteroids to treat eye disorders are listed below.[2-10]

1. St Clair Roberts D. Steroids, the eye, and general practitioners. *BMJ* 1986; **292:** 1414–15.
2. Lavin MJ, Rose GE. Use of steroid eye drops in general practice. *BMJ* 1986; **292:** 1448–50.
3. Claoué CMP, Stevenson KE. Incidence of inappropriate treatment of herpes simplex keratitis with topical steroids. *BMJ* 1986; **292:** 1450–1.
4. Livingstone A. Steroids, the eye, and general practitioners. *BMJ* 1986; **292:** 1737.
5. Lawrence M. Steroids, the eye, and general practitioners. *BMJ* 1986; **292:** 1737–8.
6. Trevor-Roper P. Steroids, the eye, and general practitioners. *BMJ* 1986; **292:** 1738.
7. Jay B. Steroids, the eye, and general practitioners. *BMJ* 1986; **293:** 205.
8. Rose GE, Lavin MJ. Steroids, the eye, and general practitioners. *BMJ* 1986; **293:** 205.
9. O'Day DM. Corticosteroids: an unresolved debate. *Ophthalmology* 1991; **98:** 845–6.
10. Stern GA, Buttross M. Use of corticosteroids in combination with antimicrobial drugs in the treatment of infectious corneal disease. *Ophthalmology* 1991; **98:** 847–53.

Porphyria. Corticosteroids are generally considered to be safe in patients with porphyria although there is conflicting evidence of porphyrinogenicity. In a review[1] of drug-induced porphyrias it was noted that a report suggesting that corticosteroids may have a role in treating the acute attack together with many reports attesting to their safety, contrasted with their repeated incrimination as the offending agent in producing such episodes. It was considered that as corticosteroids may be life-saving, they should be used if really indicated.

1. Moore MR, Disler PB. Drug-induction of the acute porphyrias. *Adverse Drug React Acute Poisoning Rev* 1983; **2:** 149–89.

Pregnancy and breast feeding. Studies have shown that corticosteroids administered to pregnant women did not have adverse effects on the fetus in terms of psychological development[1] or growth and general health factors.[2] However, there has been an isolated report[3] wherein the topical administration of triamcinolone to a pregnant woman for treatment of eczema was considered to have caused fetal growth retardation. In another study[4] of 11 women with placenta praevia given intramuscular betamethasone 12 mg repeated 24 hours later, there were two cases of constriction of the ductus arteriosus; neither case was severe.

Early studies in *animals* have demonstrated an increase in fetal cleft palate following maternal ingestion of high corticosteroid doses, and cortisone has been used widely as a tool for the investigation of mechanisms responsible for cleft lip and palate. With doses used in clinical practice, however, the risk appears to be low. In an analysis of several hundred cases reported in the literature[5] it was concluded that the incidence of cleft palate in exposed children was slightly higher than in a random sample, but that in the small selected group studied, this higher incidence might be fallacious. Although an increased incidence of malformations in the children of asthmatic mothers given prednisolone 2.5 to 30 mg daily during pregnancy was noted,[6] others[7] have suggested that the outcome might have been worse in untreated asthmatic mothers. Moreover, no significant increase in the risk of fetal or maternal complications was found in a study of asthmatic mothers given prednisone 2.5 to 20 mg daily.[8] More recently, no evidence of a teratogenic effect for corticosteroids was noted in a comparison of the maternal drug histories of the mothers of 764 infants born with anomalies of the CNS and 764 controls,[9] and in another study[10] there were no striking differences in birth-weight and frequency of 'small for dates' infants born to mothers who received systemic corticosteroids during pregnancy for pemphigoid gestationis and those who did not.

Fears concerning the use of corticosteroids during late pregnancy relate to their direct adverse effects on the fetus. These involve the known side-effects of corticosteroids, such as increased risk of infection and adrenal insufficiency. No such adverse effects were noted in the infants of 70 exposed pregnancies,[8] although there have been individual reports.[11,12] The potential dangers of maternal diabetogenic effects have been demonstrated in a study of metabolic changes induced in diabetic women by salbutamol (used in the prevention of premature labour) which could be exacerbated by concomitant use of dexamethasone (to promote maturation of the fetal lung) with consequent danger to the fetus.[13]

A review[14] by the UK Committee on Safety of Medicines concluded that there was no convincing evidence that corticosteroids caused an increased incidence of congenital abnormality. Prolonged or repeated use during pregnancy did increase the risk of intra-uterine growth retardation but this did not seem to be a problem following short-term treatment. It was noted that the ability of different corticosteroids to cross the placenta varied very markedly. It was also remarked that sufficient prednisolone was distributed into breast milk (see p.1078) that infants of mothers receiving 40 mg or more daily should be monitored for signs of adrenal suppression; it was not known if this applied to other corticosteroids.

1. Schmand B, et al. Psychological development of children who were treated antenatally with corticosteroids to prevent respiratory distress syndrome. Pediatrics 1990; 86: 58–64.
2. Doyle LW, et al. Antenatal steroid therapy and 5-year outcome of extremely low birth weight infants. Obstet Gynecol 1989; 73: 743–6.
3. Katz VL, et al. Severe symmetric intrauterine growth retardation associated with the topical use of triamcinolone. Am J Obstet Gynecol 1990; 162: 396–7.
4. Wasserstrum N, et al. Betamethasone and the human fetal ductus arteriosus. Obstet Gynecol 1989; 74: 897–900.
5. Popert AJ. Pregnancy and adrenocortical hormones: some aspects of their interaction in rheumatic diseases. BMJ 1962; 1: 967–72.
6. Warrell DW, Taylor R. Outcome for the foetus of mothers receiving prednisolone during pregnancy. Lancet 1968; i: 117–18.
7. Scott JK. Foetal risk with maternal prednisolone. Lancet 1968; i: 201.
8. Schatz M, et al. Corticosteroid therapy for the pregnant asthmatic patient. JAMA 1975; 233: 804–7.
9. Winship KA, et al. Maternal drug histories and central nervous system anomalies. Arch Dis Child 1984; 59: 1052–60.
10. Holmes RC, Black MM. The fetal prognosis in pemphigoid gestationis (herpes gestationis). Br J Dermatol 1984; 110: 67–72.
11. Grajwer LA, et al. Neonatal subclinical adrenal insufficiency: result of maternal steroid therapy. JAMA 1977; 238: 1279–80.
12. Evans TJ, et al. Congenital cytomegalovirus infection after maternal renal transplantation. Lancet 1975; i: 1359–60.
13. Gündoğdu AS, et al. Comparison of hormonal and metabolic effects of salbutamol infusion in normal subjects and insulin-requiring diabetics. Lancet 1979; ii: 1317–21.
14. Committee on Safety of Medicines/Medicines Control Agency. Systemic corticosteroids in pregnancy and lactation. Current Problems 1998; 24: 9.

Septic shock. Some manufacturers recommend that corticosteroids should not be given to patients with septic shock and references to the controversial use of high-dose corticosteroids are given under Septic Shock, in Uses and Administration, below.

Sickle-cell disease. Sickle-cell crisis was reported to have been precipitated by corticosteroids in 2 patients with sickle C disease.[1] The crises in these patients were considered to have started with ischaemic necrosis of the bone marrow leading to fat embolism, cerebral hypoxia, and coma.

For mention of the use of corticosteroids in sickle-cell crisis, see under Sickle-cell Disease, in Uses and Administration, below.

1. Huang JC, et al. Sickling crisis, fat embolism, and coma after steroids. Lancet 1994; 344: 951–2.

Tooth erosion. The increased incidence of tooth erosion seen in patients with asthma might be related to the pH of inhaled powder (but not aerosol) formulations.[1] Beclometasone dipropionate and fluticasone had pHs of 4.76 as powder formulations, whereas the aerosols were well above the pH of 5.5 at which tooth substance begins to dissolve. Budesonide was less acidic in its powder formulation (pH 6.47).

1. O'Sullivan EA, Curzon MEJ. Drug treatments for asthma may cause erosive tooth damage. BMJ 1998; 317: 820.

Varicella. A number of cases of fatal or near fatal chickenpox have been reported in patients receiving corticosteroids.[1-3] Although mostly associated with systemic use, severe disseminated varicella and staphylococcal pericarditis have been reported in an infant following a single application of a potent topical corticosteroid cream.[4] Guidelines issued by the UK Committee on Safety of Medicines state that all patients taking systemic corticosteroids for purposes other than replacement, and who have not had chickenpox, should be regarded as being at risk of severe chickenpox, irrespective of the dose or duration of treatment.[2,5] Passive immunisation with varicella-zoster immunoglobulin should be given to non-immune patients who are receiving corticosteroids, or who have received them within the last 3 months, if they are exposed to chickenpox. Passive immunisation should preferably be given within 3 days and not later than 10 days from exposure.[2] They consider there is currently no good evidence that topical, inhaled, or rectal corticosteroids are associated with an increased risk of severe chickenpox.

1. Rice P, et al. Near fatal chickenpox during prednisolone treatment. BMJ 1994; 309: 1069–70.
2. Committee on Safety of Medicines/Medicines Control Agency. Severe chickenpox associated with systemic corticosteroids. Current Problems 1994; 20: 1–2.

3. Dowell SF, Breese JS. Severe varicella associated with steroid use. Pediatrics 1993; 92: 223–8.
4. Brumund MR, et al. Disseminated varicella and staphylococcal pericarditis after topical steroids. J Pediatr 1997; 131: 162–3.
5. Ellender D, et al. Severe chickenpox during treatment with corticosteroids. BMJ 1995; 310: 327.

Interactions of Corticosteroids

Concurrent use of barbiturates, carbamazepine, phenytoin, primidone, or rifampicin may enhance the metabolism and reduce the effects of systemic corticosteroids. Conversely oral contraceptives or ritonavir may increase plasma concentrations of corticosteroids. Use of corticosteroids with potassium-depleting diuretics, such as thiazides or frusemide [furosemide], may cause excessive potassium loss. There is also an increased risk of hypokalaemia with concurrent amphotericin B or bronchodilator therapy with xanthines or beta$_2$ agonists. There may be an increased incidence of gastrointestinal bleeding and ulceration when corticosteroids are given with NSAIDs. Response to anticoagulants may be altered by corticosteroids and requirements of antidiabetic drugs and antihypertensives may be increased. Corticosteroids may decrease serum concentrations of salicylates and may decrease the effect of antimuscarinics in myasthenia gravis.

Analgesics. For the effect of corticosteroids on salicylates, see Aspirin, Interactions, p.16.

Antibacterials. Rifampicin reduces the activity of corticosteroids[1-8] by accelerating their metabolism, and a similar effect would be expected with other rifamycins. There is limited evidence that the macrolide antibacterials troleandomycin,[9-11] and perhaps erythromycin,[12] may inhibit the metabolism of methylprednisolone, but not of prednisolone.[10] Dosage reduction should be made as necessary if troleandomycin and methylprednisolone are used concurrently. There is no evidence of a clinically significant interaction between these macrolides and other corticosteroids.

For reference to corticosteroids lowering plasma concentrations of isoniazid and enhancing its renal clearance, see p.217.

1. Edwards OM, et al. Changes in cortisol metabolism following rifampicin therapy. Lancet 1974; ii: 549–51.
2. Maisey DN, et al. Rifampicin and cortisone replacement therapy. Lancet 1974; ii: 896–7.
3. Steenbergen GJ, Pfaltzgraff RE. Treatment of neuritis in borderline leprosy with rifampicin and corticosteroids—a pilot trial. Lepr Rev 1975; 46: 115–18.
4. Buffington GA, et al. Interaction of rifampin and glucocorticoids: adverse effect on renal allograft function. JAMA 1976; 236: 1958–60.
5. Hendrickse W, et al. Rifampicin-induced non-responsiveness to corticosteroid treatment in nephrotic syndrome. BMJ 1979; 1: 306.
6. van Marle W, et al. Concurrent steroid and rifampicin therapy. BMJ 1979; 1: 1020.
7. Jopline WH, Pettit JHS. Interaction between rifampicin, steroids and oral contraceptives. Lepr Rev 1979; 50: 331–2.
8. McAllister WAC, et al. Rifampicin reduces effectiveness and bioavailability of prednisolone. BMJ 1983; 286: 923–5.
9. Szefler SJ, et al. The effect of troleandomycin on methylprednisolone elimination. J Allergy Clin Immunol 1980; 66: 447–51.
10. Szefler SJ, et al. Steroid-specific and anticonvulsant interaction aspects of troleandomycin-steroid therapy. J Allergy Clin Immunol 1982; 69: 455–60.
11. Kamada AK, et al. Glucocorticoid reduction with troleandomycin in chronic severe asthmatic children: implication for future trials and clinical application. J Allergy Clin Immunol 1992; 89: 285.
12. LaForce CF, et al. Inhibition of methylprednisolone elimination in the presence of erythromycin therapy. J Allergy Clin Immunol 1983; 72: 34–9.

Anticoagulants. For the various effects of corticosteroids on anticoagulants, see under Warfarin Sodium, p.996.

Antiepileptics. Reduced efficacy of corticosteroids has been noted in asthmatic, arthritic, renal transplant, and other patients who also received phenytoin or phenobarbital,[1-3] and the clearance of corticosteroids has also been reported to be markedly increased by concurrent use of carbamazepine.[3] Induction of microsomal liver enzymes by the antiepileptic drug, resulting in enhanced metabolism of the corticosteroid is believed to be the underlying mechanism. Different corticosteroids appear to be affected to different degrees, but the disease state, doses, and other determinants such as diet, sex, and other drugs used may also be contributory factors. An increase in the dosage of the corticosteroids may be necessary in order to maintain the desired therapeutic response.[1]

1. Brooks SM, et al. Adverse effects of phenobarbital on corticosteroid metabolism in patients with bronchial asthma. N Engl J Med 1972; 286: 1125–8.
2. Nation RL, et al. Pharmacokinetic drug interactions with phenytoin (part II). Clin Pharmacokinet 1990; 18: 131–50.
3. Bartoszek M, et al. Prednisolone and methylprednisolone kinetics in children receiving anticonvulsant therapy. Clin Pharmacol Ther 1987; 42: 424–32.

Antifungals. Ketoconazole[1,2] and itraconazole[3,4] increase serum-methylprednisolone concentrations and enhance methylprednisolone's adrenal suppressive effects. A 50% reduction in intravenous methylprednisolone dose was suggested during

concomitant ketoconazole therapy.[2] A similar effect was not evident when prednisone was given by mouth[4,5] although some workers[6] found that ketoconazole reduced the total clearance of prednisolone given intravenously and of prednisone given by mouth.

1. Glynn AM, et al. Effects of ketoconazole on methylprednisolone pharmacokinetics and cortisol secretion. Clin Pharmacol Ther 1986; 39: 654–9.
2. Kandrotas RJ, et al. Ketoconazole effects on methylprednisolone disposition and their joint suppression of endogenous cortisol. Clin Pharmacol Ther 1987; 42: 465–70.
3. Varis T, et al. Plasma concentrations and effects of oral methylprednisolone are considerably increased by itraconazole. Clin Pharmacol Ther 1998; 64: 363–8.
4. Lebrun-Vignes B, et al. Effect of itraconazole on the pharmacokinetics of prednisolone and methylprednisolone and cortisol secretion in healthy subjects. Br J Clin Pharmacol 2001; 51: 443–50.
5. Ludwig EA, et al. Steroid-specific effects of ketoconazole on corticosteroid disposition: unaltered prednisolone elimination. DICP Ann Pharmacother 1989; 23: 858–61.
6. Zürcher RM, et al. Impact of ketoconazole on the metabolism of prednisolone. Clin Pharmacol Ther 1989; 45: 366–72.

Antineoplastics and immunosuppressants. It has been suggested that mutual inhibition of metabolism occurs between ciclosporin and corticosteroids, and may increase the plasma concentrations of either drug.[1,2] A review[3] cited studies supporting this conclusion but also mentioned studies which showed that ciclosporin did not significantly decrease clearance of prednisolone[4] and that corticosteroids either did not change, or decreased, ciclosporin concentrations.[5,6] Some of these conflicting results may be due to differences in the methods used to measure ciclosporin concentrations.

For reference to single doses of prednisone inhibiting the activation of cyclophosphamide (but longer-term treatment increasing its activation), see Cyclophosphamide, p.528.

1. Ost L. Effects of cyclosporin on prednisolone metabolism. Lancet 1984; i: 451.
2. Klintmalm G, Säwe J. High dose methylprednisolone increases plasma cyclosporin levels in renal transplant recipients. Lancet 1984; i: 731.
3. Yee GC, McGuire TR. Pharmacokinetic drug interactions with cyclosporin (part II). Clin Pharmacokinet 1990; 19: 400–15.
4. Frey FJ, et al. Evidence that cyclosporine does not affect the metabolism of prednisolone after renal transplantation. Transplantation 1987; 43: 494–8.
5. Ptachcinski RJ, et al. Cyclosporine - high-dose steroid interaction in renal transplant recipients: assessment by HPLC. Transplant Proc 1987; 19: 1728–9.
6. Hricik DE, et al. Association of the absence of steroid therapy with increased cyclosporine blood levels in renal transplant recipients. Transplantation 1990; 49: 221–3.

Antivirals. For a possible effect of corticosteroids on the metabolism of HIV-protease inhibitors, see p.627.

Lipid regulating drugs. Addition of colestipol to the therapy of a patient with hypopituitarism receiving maintenance therapy with hydrocortisone resulted in headaches, ataxia, and lethargy.[1] Mental status returned to normal within hours of an intravenous dose of hydrocortisone 100 mg, and colestipol was subsequently withdrawn uneventfully.

1. Neki KE, Aron DC. Hydrocortisone-colestipol interaction. Ann Pharmacother 1993; 27: 980–1.

Neuromuscular blockers. For reference to corticosteroids antagonising the effects of competitive neuromuscular blockers, see under Atracurium, p.1335.

Sex hormones. Reviews[1,2] discussing several reports of an enhanced effect of corticosteroids in women also receiving oestrogens or oral contraceptives and commenting that the dose of corticosteroids in some cases may need to be reduced. There is some evidence that budesonide may be less affected by concurrent use of oral contraceptives than prednisolone.[3]

1. Shenfield GM. Drug interactions with oral contraceptive preparations. Med J Aust 1986; 144: 205–10.
2. Back DJ, Orme ML'E. Pharmacokinetic drug interactions with oral contraceptives. Clin Pharmacokinet 1990; 18: 472–84.
3. Seidegård J, et al. Effect of an oral contraceptive on the plasma levels of budesonide and prednisolone and the influence on plasma cortisol. Clin Pharmacol Ther 2000; 67: 373–81.

Smoking. There was a report of an appreciable and consistent increase in plasma corticosteroids after cigarette smoking in man.[1] However, a review concerning the clinical importance of smoking and drug interactions[2] concluded that in the majority of examples, including corticosteroids, there was little evidence of a recognisable hazard from the interaction.

1. Kershbaum A, et al. Effect of smoking and nicotine on adrenocortical secretion. JAMA 1968; 203: 275–8.
2. D'Arcy PF. Tobacco smoking and drugs: a clinically important interaction? Drug Intell Clin Pharm 1984; 18: 302–7.

Sympathomimetics. Studies in 21 asthmatic patients suggested that the plasma half-life of dexamethasone was decreased when it was given with ephedrine.[1] More significantly, concomitant use of corticosteroids with beta$_2$ agonists may potentiate any hypokalaemic effects.[2]

1. Brooks SM, et al. The effects of ephedrine and theophylline on dexamethasone metabolism in bronchial asthma. J Clin Pharmacol 1977; 17: 308–18.
2. Committee on Safety of Medicines. β$_2$ agonists, xanthines and hypokalaemia. Current Problems 28 1990.

Thalidomide. In a double-blind crossover study of thalidomide in the treatment of severe chronic erythema nodosum leprosum,[1] the dose of prednisolone necessary to suppress symptoms was considerably reduced in 9 of 10 patients while they were receiving thalidomide; there has been a comment[2] that prednisolone should not be given with thalidomide.

For reference to a possible interaction between thalidomide and dexamethasone, see under Effects on the Skin in Adverse Effects of Thalidomide, p.1670.

1. Waters MFR. An internally-controlled double blind trial of thalidomide in severe erythema nodosum leprosum. *Lepr Rev* 1971; **42:** 26–42.
2. WHO, Regional Office for the Western Pacific. Final report on the first regional working group on leprosy, Manila, Philippines, 7–12 December, 1978. *Lepr Rev* 1979; **50:** 326–9.

Xanthines. For the effect of corticosteroids on *theophylline*, see p.781.

Pharmacokinetics of Corticosteroids

Corticosteroids are, in general, readily absorbed from the gastrointestinal tract. They are also absorbed from sites of local administration. When used topically, particularly under an occlusive dressing or when the skin is broken, or as a rectal enema, sufficient corticosteroid may be absorbed to give systemic effects; this is also a possibility with other local routes of administration such as inhalation. Water-soluble forms of corticosteroids are given by intravenous injection for a rapid response; more prolonged effects are achieved using lipid-soluble forms of corticosteroids by intramuscular injection.

Corticosteroids are rapidly distributed to all body tissues. They cross the placenta to varying degrees and may be excreted in small amounts in breast milk.

Most corticosteroids in the circulation are extensively bound to plasma proteins, mainly to globulin and less so to albumin. The corticosteroid-binding globulin (transcortin) has high affinity but low binding capacity, while albumin has low affinity but large binding capacity. The synthetic corticosteroids are less extensively protein bound than hydrocortisone (cortisol). They also tend to have longer half-lives.

Corticosteroids are metabolised mainly in the liver but also in other tissues, and are excreted in the urine. The slower metabolism of the synthetic corticosteroids with their lower protein-binding affinity may account for their increased potency compared with the natural corticosteroids.

◊ Reviews.
1. Begg EJ, *et al.* The pharmacokinetics of corticosteroid agents. *Med J Aust* 1987; **146:** 37–41.
2. McGhee CNJ. Pharmacokinetics of ophthalmic corticosteroids. *Br J Ophthalmol* 1992; **76:** 681–4.
3. Jusko WJ. Pharmacokinetics and receptor-mediated pharmacodynamics of corticosteroids. *Toxicology* 1995; **102:** 189–96.
4. Derendorf H, *et al.* Pharmacokinetics and pharmacodynamics of inhaled corticosteroids. *J Allergy Clin Immunol* 1998; **101** (suppl 2): S440–6.

Uses and Administration of Corticosteroids

The corticosteroids are used in physiological doses for replacement therapy in adrenal insufficiency. Pharmacological doses are used when palliative anti-inflammatory or immunosuppressant effects are required. Before instituting therapy the benefits and risks of corticosteroids should be considered; where appropriate, local rather than systemic therapy should be used. The lowest dose of corticosteroids that is effective should be used for the shortest possible duration of time; high doses may be needed for life-threatening situations.

The effects of different corticosteroids vary qualitatively as well as quantitatively, and it may not be possible to substitute one for another in equal therapeutic amounts without provoking side-effects. Thus, whereas cortisone and hydrocortisone have very appreciable mineralocorticoid (or sodium-retaining) properties relative to their glucocorticoid (or anti-inflammatory) properties, prednisolone and prednisone have considerably less, and others, such as betamethasone and dexamethasone, have none or virtually none. In contrast, the mineralocorticoid properties of fludrocortisone are so pronounced that its glucocorticoid effects are considered to have no clinical significance.

As a rough guide, the approximate **equivalent doses** of the main corticosteroids in terms of their glucocorticoid (or anti-inflammatory) properties alone, are:

• betamethasone 0.75 mg
• cortisone acetate 25 mg
• dexamethasone 0.75 mg
• hydrocortisone 20 mg
• methylprednisolone 4 mg
• prednisolone 5 mg
• prednisone 5 mg
• triamcinolone 4 mg.

The mineralocorticoid properties of corticosteroids (see p.1039) are rarely used. Exceptions include the treatment of primary adrenocortical insufficiency, in which both mineralocorticoid and glucocorticoid replacement is necessary, usually in the form of fludrocortisone with hydrocortisone (for details, see p.1046). The mineralocorticoid properties of fludrocortisone are also used to maintain blood pressure in patients with orthostatic hypotension (see p.1070).

The anti-inflammatory and immunosuppressant glucocorticoid properties of corticosteroids (see p.1039) are used to suppress the clinical manifestations of disease in a wide range of disorders considered to have inflammatory or immunological components. For these purposes, the synthetic analogues with their considerably reduced mineralocorticoid properties linked with enhanced glucocorticoid properties, are preferred. Despite the existence of very powerful synthetic glucocorticoids with virtually no mineralocorticoid activity, the hazards of inappropriately high glucocorticoid therapy are such that the less powerful prednisolone and prednisone are the glucocorticoids of choice for most conditions, since they allow for a greater margin of safety. There is little to choose between prednisolone and prednisone; prednisolone is usually recommended in the UK since it exists in a metabolically active form, whereas prednisone is inactive and must be converted into its active form by the liver; hence, particularly in some liver disorders, bioavailability of prednisone is less reliable (but see under Precautions of Prednisolone, p.1078).

Because the therapeutic effects of corticosteroids seem to be of longer duration than the metabolic effects, intermittent treatment with corticosteroids has been used to allow the metabolic rhythm of the body to become re-established while maintaining the therapeutic effects. Regimens of intermittent therapy have usually consisted of short courses of treatment or of the administration of single doses on alternate days. Such alternate-day therapy, however, is only appropriate for corticosteroids with a relatively short duration of action and small mineralocorticoid effect, such as prednisolone, and only in certain disease states. Corticosteroids are also given in single daily doses at times coinciding with maximum or minimum function of the adrenal cortex in order to obtain the desired effect on the adrenals (see under Administration, below).

Doses of corticosteroids higher than those required for physiological replacement will eventually lead to some degree of adrenal suppression, the extent depending on the dose given, and the route, frequency, time, and duration of administration. The adrenal glands are traditionally considered to have a daily output equivalent to approximately 20 mg of hydrocortisone (cortisol), but individual blood-cortisol concentrations may vary widely, and can increase up to tenfold or more during stress. Therefore, during periods of stress or trauma, such as during and after surgery and when suffering from intercurrent infections, the corticosteroid dosage of patients must be increased. In patients on long-term corticosteroid therapy undergoing surgery this is usually provided by parenteral hydrocortisone; graduated regimens tailored to the severity of surgery (see p.1074) are now preferred to the former high-dose standard regimens tapered over 5 days, whose use has been questioned (see Surgery, under Administration, below).

Although the empirical use of a corticosteroid is appropriate in a life-threatening situation, generally it is advisable not to begin corticosteroid therapy until a definite diagnosis has been made, for otherwise symptoms may be masked to such an extent that a true diagnosis becomes extremely difficult to make and the disease may reach an advanced stage before detection.

Systemic therapy is indicated in a wide variety of conditions. Where possible the oral route is preferred but parenteral administration may be used if the disease is severe or an emergency arises. Intravenous therapy is generally employed for intensive emergency treatment as the onset of action is relatively fast although intramuscular injections, often formulated as longer-acting depot preparations, may also be used to provide subsequent cover. Examples of conditions treated with systemic corticosteroids include:

• as an adjunct to adrenaline [epinephrine] in life-threatening allergic reactions such as angioedema or anaphylaxis (see p.832)
• some blood disorders, including auto-immune haemolytic anaemia (p.716) and idiopathic thrombocytopenic purpura (p.1052)
• selected connective tissue and muscle disorders, such as Behçet's syndrome (p.1047), polymyalgia rheumatica (p.1056), polymyositis (p.1057), systemic lupus erythematosus (p.1059), and the vasculitic syndromes (p.1060)
• some inflammatory eye disorders, particularly those affecting the posterior chamber
• inflammatory gastrointestinal disorders, such as Crohn's disease and ulcerative colitis, although administration by the rectal route may be preferred in some circumstances (see p.1205)
• infections accompanied by a severe inflammatory component provided that appropriate anti-infective chemotherapy is also given and that the benefits of corticosteroid therapy outweigh the possible risk of disseminated infection; examples of conditions where corticosteroid may be considered include helminthic infections, the Jarisch-Herxheimer reaction, and tuberculous meningitis
• selected kidney disorders including lupus nephritis (p.1059) and various glomerular disorders (p.1051)
• selected liver disorders, including auto-immune chronic active hepatitis (p.1048)
• some neurological disorders such as infantile seizures and subacute demyelinating polyneuropathy; also in cerebral oedema (p.1048), including that associated with malignancy
• some respiratory disorders, such as asthma (see p.757, although inhaled corticosteroids are preferred to oral therapy for prophylaxis), diffuse parenchymal lung disease (p.1050), pulmonary sarcoid (p.1058), and neonatal respiratory distress syndrome (p.1055)
• some cases of rheumatoid arthritis, where recent evidence suggests there may be value in early treatment of active disease (see p.1057)
• severe skin disorders such as pemphigus and pemphigoid (p.1106).

Glucocorticoids are also used in conjunction with antineoplastics in regimens for the management of malignant disease. They are also given to reduce immune responses after organ transplantations, often in conjunction with other immunosuppressants (see p.502).

Corticosteroids are not now considered useful in patients with aspiration syndromes, stroke, or septic shock, although they have been used in these conditions.

Intra-articular injection, in the absence of infection and with full aseptic precautions, may be used, for example, in the treatment of rheumatoid arthritis (p.9), osteoarthritis (p.9), and ankylosing spondylitis (p.10). Either hydrocortisone acetate or one of the esters of the synthetic corticosteroids is used. It should be noted that there have been several reports of joint damage after the intra-articular injection of corticosteroids into load-bearing joints.

Topical application often produces dramatic suppression of skin diseases, such as eczema, seborrhoeic dermatitis, and some forms of psoriasis, in which inflammation is a prominent feature. However, the disease may return or be exacerbated when corticosteroids are withdrawn and this appears to be a particular problem in some of the forms of psoriasis. Occasionally, corticosteroids may be used with the addition of a suitable antimicrobial substance, such as neomycin, in the treatment of infected skin. For comments on the topical application of preparations containing a corticosteroid and neomycin, see Neomycin Sulfate, p.228.

Intralesional injection sometimes hastens the resolution of chronic skin lesions such as lichen planus, lichen simplex, and keloids.

Topical application to the eye in inflammatory and traumatic disorders has led to dramatic results, but the occurrence of herpetic and fungal infections of the cornea and other serious complications are considerable obstacles, and eye drops containing corticosteroids should be used under strict ophthalmic supervision with regular checks of intra-ocular pressure. Care is also required when corticosteroids are given by **subconjunctival injection** in inflammatory eye disorders.

Ear drops containing corticosteroids are used in the treatment of otitis externa (see p.132).

Inhalational therapy is widely used in the prophylaxis of asthma (see p.757).

Nasal application is used in the prophylaxis and treatment of allergic and non-allergic rhinitis (see p.407).

Rectal administration, by either suppository or enema, may be used for some corticosteroids, notably in the treatment of inflammatory bowel disease (p.1205).

Administration
It has long been known that the diurnal rhythm of the adrenal cortex leads to about 70% of the daily secretion being made between midnight and 9 am.[1] In the treatment of adrenal cortical hyperplasia a dose of hydrocortisone given at night will be nearly twice as suppressive as the same dose given during the day. However, in treating allergic or collagen disease when suppression of adrenal cortical activity is best avoided a dose of hydrocortisone at about 8 am is indicated. When reducing corticosteroid dosage after treatment, a single dose given at 8 am will be most beneficial and will not inhibit corticotropin secretion. Also, for similar reasons,[2] when used for replacement therapy corticosteroids are given in unequal doses during the day (two-thirds of the daily dose in the morning, and one-third at night).

1. Demos CH, *et al.* A modified (once a day) corticosteroid dosage regimen. *Clin Pharmacol Ther* 1964; **5:** 721–7.
2. Aronson JK. Chronopharmacology: reflections on time and a new text. *Lancet* 1990; **335:** 1515–16.

Epidural route. Reviews[1,2] of the epidural use of corticosteroids in sciatica concluded that reported clinical complications were uncommon but that their role is unclear. Another study[3] suggested that although epidural injection of methylprednisolone acetate produced short-term improvement in pain and sensory deficit, treatment resulted in no functional benefit and did not reduce the need for surgery.

It should be noted that inadvertent intrathecal administration of corticosteroids has resulted in severe neurological complications.

1. Bogduk N, Cherry D. Epidural corticosteroid agents for sciatica. *Med J Aust* 1985; **143:** 402–6.
2. Tonkovich-Quaranta LA, Winkler SR. Use of epidural corticosteroids in low back pain. *Ann Pharmacother* 2000; **34:** 1165–72. Correction. *ibid.*; 1489.
3. Carette S, *et al.* Epidural corticosteroid injections for sciatica due to herniated nucleus pulposus. *N Engl J Med* 1997; **336:** 1634–40.

Inhalational therapy. The majority of patients taking inhaled corticosteroids for asthma only require standard doses. A discussion on high-dose inhaled corticosteroids in asthma therapy,[1] published in 1987, concluded that improvement in asthma control could be achieved in patients with severe or chronic asthma when the dose was increased. In some patients dependent upon oral corticosteroids significant reductions in the oral dose could be made by increasing the inhaled dose.[1] Some doubt was cast on this view by a later multicentre study which found that high doses of inhaled beclometasone dipropionate, given via a spacer device, were no better at permitting a reduction in oral corticosteroid dosage than were low doses.[2] Another study found that although increasing the

inhaled doses of beclometasone or fluticasone did improve pulmonary function, the changes were insufficiently great to be of much clinical significance.[3] However, accepted guidelines for the treatment of asthma include instructions to increase the dose of inhaled corticosteroid should the standard dose not produce improvement (see p.757), and in clinical practice improved asthma control can often be achieved by increasing the dose.

Different inhaled corticosteroids differ in their potency, though there is little evidence of a difference in efficacy at recommended doses.[4] Of those widely available by inhalation, flunisolide is less potent than beclometasone while budesonide is considered more potent, and fluticasone more potent still. (However, a general practice study in New Zealand has suggested that budesonide is less potent than beclometasone.[5]) The ability to use fewer inhalations with more potent drugs might enhance compliance.[4] For inhaled corticosteroids to be effective in the prophylaxis of asthma they must be taken regularly and patient compliance is important.

Efficient delivery to the bronchial tree is crucial and a number of different devices are available for administration. The pressurised aerosol inhaler remains the most convenient and acceptable if the patient's technique is satisfactory. However, many patients, especially children, find that administration by inhalation is made much easier by fitting a spacer device to the inhaler.[6] Such a device is recommended when high doses are to be inhaled, to prevent oropharyngeal deposition and subsequent systemic absorption. However, the type of spacer used and the method of use may dramatically alter the amount of drug available for inhalation. The drug should be introduced into the spacer by single actuations, each followed by inhalation, with the delay between actuation of the inhaler and inhalation from the spacer kept to a minimum. In some spacers static electricity accumulates, and the build up of charge reduces drug delivery: this can be controlled by washing and drying the spacer in air before beginning use.[7] Considerable differences in the dose delivered to the airways may also be seen between different types of nebuliser, and between nebulisers and spacer devices.[8]

Changes in formulation of the propellant, to remove chlorofluorocarbons, may also affect drug availability; it is reported to be increased, requiring dose reduction with new formulations.[9]

It should be borne in mind that apparent differences in the dose supplied from inhaler devices in different countries may in some cases be artefacts, due to variations in the way the dose is measured or expressed. In the UK, for example, the dose supplied from a metered-dose inhaler is generally quoted as the amount released into the mouthpiece from the valve. In the USA, however, doses may be stated in terms of the amount of drug emitted from the mouthpiece, which due to drug deposition will be slightly less than the amount released from the valve.

1. Smith MJ. The place of high-dose inhaled corticosteroids in asthma therapy. *Drugs* 1987; **33:** 423–9.
2. Hummel S, *et al.* Comparison of oral-steroid sparing by high-dose and low-dose inhaled steroid in maintenance treatment of severe asthma. *Lancet* 1992; **340:** 1483–7.
3. Boe J, *et al.* High-dose inhaled steroids in asthmatics: moderate efficacy gain and suppression of the hypothalamic-pituitary-adrenal axis. *Eur Respir J* 1994; **7:** 2179–84.
4. Kelly HW. Comparison of inhaled corticosteroids. *Ann Pharmacother* 1998; **32:** 220–32.
5. Pethica BD, *et al.* Comparison of potency of inhaled beclomethasone and budesonide in New Zealand: retrospective study of computerised general practice records. *BMJ* 1998; **317:** 986–90.
6. Keeley D. Large volume plastic spacers in asthma. *BMJ* 1992; **305:** 598–9.
7. O'Callaghan C, Barry P. Spacer devices in the treatment of asthma. *BMJ* 1997; **314:** 1061–2.
8. O'Callaghan C, Barry P. Delivering inhaled corticosteroids to patients. *BMJ* 1999; **318:** 410–11.
9. Legge A. Shift to CFC-free inhalers may require change in doses. *BMJ* 1997; **315:** 1179.

Intra-articular route. Intra-articular and periarticular injection of corticosteroids is an established treatment for a variety of joint and soft-tissue lesions.[1-3] Pain and inflammation associated with rheumatoid and juvenile idiopathic arthritis, crystal arthropathies such as gout, and osteoarthritis can be alleviated by injection of a suitable corticosteroid, and in some cases the benefits may be quite prolonged. The longer-acting esters methylprednisolone acetate, triamcinolone acetonide, and triamcinolone hexacetonide are generally preferred. In some cases these may be combined with a local anaesthetic and a short-acting soluble corticosteroid for more rapid relief and to reduce the risk of a post-injection flare.

The risks associated with this technique have been reviewed.[4] Accurate injection technique is essential, and vigorous skin cleansing and an aseptic technique are required to avoid the introduction of infection into the joint; pre-existing joint infection is a contra-indication to corticosteroid injection. Intra-articular injections may be repeated if necessary but it has been suggested that a single joint should not be injected more than 3 or 4 times a year.

Periarticular injection is also employed in various soft tissue disorders such as bursitis, capsulitis (painful shoulder syndromes), epicondylitis, tenosynovitis, and carpal tunnel syndrome. Particular care is required when injecting to avoid injection directly into a tendon, which may cause the tendon to rupture. A shorter-acting corticosteroid such as hydrocortisone acetate may be more suitable for extra-articular lesions.

1. Anonymous. Articular and periarticular corticosteroid injections. *Drug Ther Bull* 1995; **33:** 67–70.
2. Caldwell JR. Intra-articular corticosteroids: guide to selection and indications for use. *Drugs* 1996; **52:** 507–14.
3. Pullar T. Routes of drug administration: intra-articular route. *Prescribers' J* 1998; **38:** 123–6.
4. Hunter JA, Blyth TH. A risk-benefit assessment of intra-articular corticosteroids in rheumatic disorders. *Drug Safety* 1999; **21:** 353–65.

Surgery. In the light of what was known about the adrenal stress response to surgery a discussion on the appropriate glucocorticoid supplementation for patients receiving corticosteroids who undergo surgery concluded that some recommendations were excessive.[1] (At this time in the UK recommended regimens consisted of the equivalent of 100 mg of hydrocortisone, usually as the sodium succinate, intravenously or intramuscularly before surgery, repeated every 8 hours, with the dose being tapered over 5 days to 20 or 30 mg daily.) It was suggested that for minor surgery 25 mg of hydrocortisone or its equivalent pre-operatively was adequate; where surgical stress was likely to be moderate, 50 to 75 mg of hydrocortisone or its equivalent daily in divided doses for 1 to 2 days was suggested. For major surgical stress, a target of 100 to 150 mg of hydrocortisone or its equivalent should be given daily in divided doses for 2 to 3 days, although less might be given if the patient's pre-operative glucocorticoid dose was low. It was also considered that the practice of gradually reducing postoperative coverage over several days was not supported by evidence except in cases of high-dose glucocorticoid administration for prolonged periods.

For currently recommended regimens see p.1074.

1. Salem M, *et al.* Perioperative glucocorticoid coverage: a reassessment 42 years after emergence of a problem. *Ann Surg* 1994; **219:** 416–25.

Topical application. Guidelines[1,2] for the correct use of topical corticosteroids recommend that an appropriately potent preparation to bring the skin disorder under control should be used. Some recommend use of the lowest potency which will control the disorder, while others have advocated starting treatment with a more potent preparation, treatment may then be continued with a less potent preparation and with less frequent application, once control is obtained. The most potent topical corticosteroids are generally reserved for recalcitrant dermatoses. Once the skin has healed, treatment should be tailed off. Particular care is necessary in the use of topical corticosteroids in children, and the more potent preparations are contra-indicated in infants under 1 year of age, although potent preparations may be needed briefly in older children. It has been suggested that a 'steroid holiday' of at least 2 weeks be considered in children after each 2 or 3 weeks of daily topical therapy to allow thinned epidermis to restore itself and maintain its barrier function.[3]

Care is also necessary in applying corticosteroids to certain anatomical sites such as the face and flexures; some advocate using only hydrocortisone 0.5 or 1% on the face. Patients should be advised that topical corticosteroids should be applied sparingly in thin layers, by smoothing gently into the skin preferably after a bath, and that no benefit is gained from more frequent than twice daily application or by vigorous rubbing.

In a study to determine the requirement of topical corticosteroids,[4] 16 adult patients with eczema were treated with a variety of topical preparations until substantial clearing had occurred (up to 10 days). Results indicated that the mean requirement of preparation, regardless of potency or vehicle, was 6.86 g per m² body-surface. Using this value the calculated quantities of topical corticosteroid to the nearest 5 g required for twice daily application for one week for the whole body, arms and legs only, and trunk only respectively were as follows:

- 6 months of age, 35 g, 20 g, and 15 g
- 1 year, 45 g, 25 g, and 15 g
- 4 years, 60 g, 35 g, and 20 g
- 8 years, 90 g, 50 g, and 35 g
- 12 years, 120 g, 65 g, and 45 g
- 16 years, 155 g, 85 g, and 55 g
- adult (70-kg male), 170 g, 90 g, and 60 g.

Calculated quantities for the same application schedule for an adult (70-kg male) for individual portions of the body were: face and neck, 10 g; one arm, 15 g; one leg, 30 g; hands and feet, 10 g.

Table 1, below, is a guide to the potency of topical corticosteroids. There may be some degree of overlap between these groups and, not surprisingly, there are minor variations to this classification. For example, some authorities consider fluocinolone acetonide 0.2% to be potent rather than very potent and halcinonide 0.1% to be potent rather than very potent.

It has been suggested, however, that the advent of non-fluorinated double esters such as hydrocortisone and methylprednisolone aceponates, or prednicarbate, has resulted in corticosteroids whose topical anti-inflammatory potency is not as closely related to their potential atrophic effects on skin, and that a classification taking both into account would be desirable.[5,6]

1. Miller JA, Munro DD. Topical corticosteroids: clinical pharmacology and therapeutic use. *Drugs* 1980; 19: 119–34.
2. Savin JA. Some guidelines to the use of topical corticosteroids. *BMJ* 1985; 290: 1607–8.
3. Hepburn D, *et al.* Topical steroid holiday. *Pediatrics* 1995; 95: 455.
4. Maurice PDL, Saihan EM. Topical steroid requirement in inflammatory skin conditions. *Br J Clin Pract* 1985; 39: 441–2.
5. Mori M, *et al.* Topical corticosteroids and unwanted local effects: improving the benefit/risk ratio. *Drug Safety* 1994; 10: 406–12.
6. Schäfer-Korting M, *et al.* Topical glucocorticoids with improved risk-benefit ratio: rationale of a new concept. *Drug Safety* 1996; 14: 375–85.

Acute respiratory distress syndrome

Acute respiratory distress syndrome (ARDS) is characterised by areas of lung damage leading to decreased compliance, pulmonary oedema associated with increased capillary and alveolar permeability, and refractory hypoxaemia. Diffuse pulmonary infiltrates are seen on radiography, and patients exhibit dyspnoea, tachypnoea, or both. Diagnosis is primarily clinical, and there has been some disagreement as to what should be included in the syndrome;[1] it is now seen as forming the most severe end of a spectrum of symptoms due to lung inflammation and increased permeability known as acute lung injury.[2-4] ARDS is sometimes considered to refer to 'adult respiratory distress syndrome' but it is not confined to adult patients.

ARDS may be caused by a variety of pulmonary or systemic insults but is particularly frequent in patients with sepsis; because of an association with failure of other organs it has been suggested that it represents the pulmonary component of multiple organ failure syndrome.[5] A wide variety of inflammatory mediators have been implicated in its pathogenesis but evidence suggests that re-

cruitment of neutrophils by interleukin-8 plays an important role.[6,7]

Management. Therapy for ARDS is essentially supportive and despite improving understanding of the pathogenesis, mortality rates have remained high. Mechanical ventilation is necessary in most cases, and circulatory support may require fluids, cardiac inotropes, and vasodilators. Optimum management may include diuretics and fluid restriction provided that cardiac output and oxygen delivery are maintained.[3,8] Because of the association with sepsis antibacterial therapy may be important, but studies of anti-endotoxin antibodies have produced disappointing results.[4]

Numerous drugs have been proposed for the management of ARDS, but, although case reports are often encouraging, none has been conclusively shown to improve mortality in controlled trials. Among the drugs which have proved disappointing in this regard are acetylcysteine,[9,10] alprostadil,[11,12] pulmonary surfactants,[13-15] and nitric oxide[16] (which may, however, improve oxygenation to some degree). Corticosteroids do not appear to reduce acute mortality,[3-5] although they may be tried in the later phases of the syndrome (5 or more days from onset) to try to prevent fibroproliferative lung changes.[3,17] Good results have been reported with inhaled epoprostenol,[18,19] but these results await confirmation from larger controlled studies.

There is evidence that ketoconazole may prevent development of ARDS in patients considered at risk,[20,21] but it does not appear to be effective as a treatment for ARDS or acute lung injury.[22]

1. Rocker GM, *et al.* Diagnostic criteria for adult respiratory distress syndrome: time for reappraisal. *Lancet* 1989; i: 120–3.
2. Bernard GR, *et al.* The American-European Consensus Conference on ARDS: definitions, mechanisms, relevant outcomes, and clinical trial coordination. *Am J Respir Crit Care Med* 1994; 149: 818–24.
3. Kollef MH, Schuster DP. The acute respiratory distress syndrome. *N Engl J Med* 1995; 332: 27–37.
4. Bigatello LM, Zapol WM. New approaches to acute lung injury. *Br J Anaesth* 1996; 77: 99–109.
5. Weinberger SE. Recent advances in pulmonary medicine (part 2). *N Engl J Med* 1993; 328: 1462–70.
6. Repine JE. Scientific perspectives on adult respiratory distress syndrome. *Lancet* 1992; 339: 466–9.
7. Donnelly SC, *et al.* Interleukin-8 and development of adult respiratory distress syndrome in at-risk patient groups. *Lancet* 1993; 341: 643–7.
8. Elsasser S, *et al.* Adjunctive drug treatment in severe hypoxic respiratory failure. *Drugs* 1999; 58: 429–46.
9. Jepsen S, *et al.* Antioxidant treatment with N-acetylcysteine during adult respiratory distress syndrome: a prospective, randomized, placebo-controlled study. *Crit Care Med* 1992; 20: 918–23.
10. Domenighetti G, *et al.* Treatment with N-acetylcysteine during acute respiratory distress syndrome: a randomized, double-blind, placebo-controlled clinical study. *J Crit Care* 1997; 12: 177–82.
11. Bone RC, *et al.* Randomized double-blind, multicenter study of prostaglandin E₁ in patients with the adult respiratory distress syndrome. *Chest* 1989; 96: 114–19.
12. Abraham E, *et al.* Liposomal prostaglandin E₁, in acute respiratory distress syndrome: a placebo-controlled, randomized, double-blind, multicenter clinical trial. *Crit Care Med* 1996; 24: 10–15.
13. Haslam PL, *et al.* Surfactant replacement therapy in late-stage adult respiratory distress syndrome. *Lancet* 1994; 343: 1009–11.
14. Weg JG, *et al.* Safety and potential efficacy of an aerosolized surfactant in human sepsis-induced adult respiratory distress syndrome. *JAMA* 1994; 272: 1433–8.
15. Anzueto A, *et al.* Aerosolized surfactant in adults with sepsis-induced acute respiratory distress syndrome. *N Engl J Med* 1996; 334: 1417–21.
16. Sokol J, *et al.* Inhaled nitric oxide for acute hypoxemic respiratory failure in children and adults (updated 30 May 2001). Available in The Cochrane Library; Issue 3. Oxford: Update Software; 2001.
17. Meduri GU, *et al.* Effect of prolonged methylprednisolone therapy in unresolving acute respiratory distress syndrome: a randomized controlled trial. *JAMA* 1998; 280: 159–65.
18. Walmrath D, *et al.* Aerosolised prostacyclin in adult respiratory distress syndrome. *Lancet* 1993; 342: 961–2.
19. Walmrath D, *et al.* Direct comparison of inhaled nitric oxide and aerosolized prostacyclin in acute respiratory distress syndrome. *Am J Respir Crit Care Med* 1996; 153: 991–6.
20. Yu M, Tomasa G. A double-blind, prospective, randomized trial of ketoconazole, a thromboxane synthetase inhibitor, in the prophylaxis of the adult respiratory distress syndrome. *Crit Care Med* 1993; 21: 1635–42.
21. Sinuff T, *et al.* Development, implementation, and evaluation of a ketoconazole practice guideline for ARDS prophylaxis. *J Crit Care* 1999; 14: 1–6.
22. The ARDS Network Authors. Ketoconazole for early treatment of acute lung injury and acute respiratory distress syndrome: a randomized controlled trial. *JAMA* 2000; 283: 1995–2002.

Adrenal hyperplasia, congenital
See Congenital Adrenal Hyperplasia, below.

Adrenocortical insufficiency
The major function of the adrenal cortex is the production of glucocorticoid and mineralocorticoid hormones, of which cortisol (hydrocortisone) and aldosterone respectively are the most important. Glucocorticoid production is regulated by the hypothalamic-pituitary-adrenal axis, being stimulated by the release of ACTH (adrenocorticotrophic hormone; corticotropin) from the pituitary, while mineralocorticoid production is primarily controlled by the renin-angiotensin system.

Adrenocortical insufficiency is defined as inadequate production of endogenous corticosteroids. It may be primary (Addison's disease), due to destruction of the adrenal cortex by some cause; or secondary, due to hypothalamic or pituitary disease, or corticosteroid therapy which suppresses ACTH release. Diagnosis can be difficult, even with the aid of hormone tests such as the tetracosactide stimulation test.

Clinical manifestations of adrenocortical insufficiency are usually seen once about 90% of the adrenal cortex is destroyed. Weight loss, anorexia, weakness, and fatigue may be accompanied by gastrointestinal symptoms such as abdominal pain, nausea, vomiting, and diarrhoea, as well as electrolyte abnormalities (hyponatraemia, hyperkalaemia), salt craving, and postural hypotension. In acute cases, abdominal pain and rigidity, fever, volume depletion, hypotension, and shock may occur. Hyperpigmentation, especially of skin creases, exposed areas, and scars is a distinguishing feature of primary, but not secondary, insufficiency. Hypoglycaemia is more likely in secondary deficiency due to lack of growth hormone, and failure of other pituitary hormones usually accompanies secondary adrenocortical insufficiency.

Treatment for acute insufficiency should be with intravenous hydrocortisone as the sodium succinate, sodium phosphate or other readily soluble ester: the usual dose is the equivalent of 100 mg every 6 to 8 hours for 24 hours. Volume depletion, dehydration, hypotension and hy-

Table 1. Guide to potencies of topical corticosteroids.

Very potent	Potent	Moderately potent	Mild
Clobetasol propionate 0.05%	Amcinonide 0.1%	Alclometasone dipropionate 0.05%	Fluocinolone acetonide 0.0025%
Diflucortolone valerate 0.3%	Beclometasone dipropionate 0.025%	Betamethasone valerate 0.025%	Hydrocortisone 0.5% and 1%
Fluocinolone acetonide 0.2%	Betamethasone benzoate 0.025%	Clobetasone butyrate 0.05%	Hydrocortisone acetate 1%
Halcinonide 0.1%	Betamethasone dipropionate 0.05%	Desoximetasone 0.05%	Methylprednisolone acetate 0.25%
Ulobetasol propionate 0.05%	Betamethasone valerate 0.1%	Flumetasone pivalate 0.02%	
	Budesonide 0.025%	Fluocinolone acetonide 0.00625% and 0.01%	
	Desonide 0.05%	Fluocortin butyl 0.75%	
	Desoximetasone 0.25%	Fluocortolone preparations (caproate with pivalate, each 0.1%	
	Diflorasone diacetate 0.05%	and caproate with either free alcohol or pivalate, each 0.25%)	
	Diflucortolone valerate 0.1%	Flurandrenolone 0.0125%	
	Fluclorolone acetonide 0.025%	Hydrocortisone aceponate 0.1%	
	Fluocinolone acetonide 0.025%	Prednicarbate 0.25%	
	Fluocinonide 0.05%		
	Fluprednidene acetate 0.1%		
	Fluticasone propionate 0.005% and 0.05%		
	Hydrocortisone butyrate 0.1%		
	Methylprednisolone aceponate 0.1%		
	Mometasone furoate 0.1%		
	Triamcinolone acetonide 0.1%		

poglycaemia should be corrected with intravenous saline and glucose, and precipitating factors, such as infection, should be dealt with appropriately. Provided no complications occur, the dosage of hydrocortisone can be tapered over 4 or 5 days to maintenance therapy by mouth. For chronic insufficiency the usual dosage of **maintenance** or **replacement therapy** is hydrocortisone 20 to 30 mg by mouth, preferably divided unequally, e.g. 30 mg as 20 mg in the morning and 10 mg in the evening, in an attempt to mimic the natural pattern of secretion. Other corticosteroids have been used, including cortisone acetate, prednisolone, prednisone, and dexamethasone, but offer no advantage over hydrocortisone. Patients with primary insufficiency also require additional mineralocorticoid replacement with fludrocortisone, usually in a dose of 0.1 mg daily. Mineralocorticoid replacement is not usually necessary in secondary insufficiency. There has been some evidence of benefit from studies of adjunctive oral administration of prasterone, another steroidal compound secreted by the adrenal glands, in patients with primary or secondary adrenal insufficiency.

Corticosteroid cover. An increase in replacement therapy is required during periods of stress. In mild infection, a doubling of the maintenance dose of hydrocortisone may be appropriate but for major infection, or severe stress such as surgery, parenteral therapy is required. It is generally considered safer to overestimate rather than underestimate the appropriate cover. For regimens used to provide cover in patients with secondary insufficiency due to corticosteroid therapy see Uses and Administration of Hydrocortisone, p.1074.

AIDS
For the use of corticosteroids in AIDS patients with *Pneumocystis carinii* pneumonia, see p.1056.

Alopecia
The management of alopecia (p.1104) is often difficult. In alopecia areata intralesional corticosteroids, most commonly triamcinolone, will induce hair growth although they are not suitable when more than 50% of the scalp is involved.[1] Regrowth is confined to the site of injection and therefore patchy, although soon concealed by spontaneous growth from uninjected regions. Some atrophy of the scalp is inevitable. Topical corticosteroids are mostly reported to be ineffective although some consider them beneficial; the use of systemic corticosteroids is controversial, given their adverse effects and a lack of evidence that they alter the long-term prognosis.

1. Shapiro J. Alopecia areata: update on therapy. *Dermatol Clin* 1993; **11:** 35–46.

Anaemias
For reference to the use of immunosuppressants, including corticosteroid-containing regimens, as an alternative to bone-marrow transplantation in the management of aplastic anaemia, see p.715; for the use of corticosteroids in haemolytic anaemias, including cold haemagglutinin disease, see p.716.

Anaphylactic shock
For the use of corticosteroids in the management of anaphylactic shock, see p.832. Intravenous corticosteroids are given following initial treatment with adrenaline [epinephrine] as part of the management of anaphylaxis; their effects are delayed, and they are not suited for immediate relief, but early use may help prevent deterioration after primary treatment has been given.

Aspiration syndromes
For a review of the management of aspiration syndromes, including reference to the probable lack of value of corticosteroids, see p.1202.

Asthma
The cornerstones of current asthma therapy, as discussed in more detail on p.757, are the beta$_2$-adrenoceptor agonists and the corticosteroids. Drug therapy for **chronic asthma** is managed by a stepwise approach. Patients requiring only occasional relief from symptoms may be managed with an inhaled short-acting beta$_2$ agonist as required. An inhaled corticosteroid such as beclometasone dipropionate, budesonide, or fluticasone may be added to therapy if symptomatic relief is needed more than once daily but regular use is important since corticosteroids

take several hours to exert an effect in asthma. If control is still inadequate, the dose of inhaled corticosteroid may be increased and given by means of a large volume spacer device, or a long-acting beta$_2$ agonist or theophylline, and possibly cromoglicate or nedocromil, may be added to therapy. Severe asthma may require regular bronchodilator therapy as well as high-dose inhaled corticosteroids, while in the most severe cases, regular oral corticosteroids may also be required. A short 'rescue' course of oral corticosteroid may be needed at any stage for an acute exacerbation. Corticosteroids should be used cautiously in children because of possible adverse effects on growth. While increasing the dose of inhaled corticosteroid is part of this schedule of treatment, it has proved difficult to demonstrate the benefits in controlled studies (see Inhalational Therapy, under Administration, above).

Acute severe asthma (status asthmaticus) is potentially life-threatening and is treated with inhaled oxygen and beta$_2$ agonists, as well as systemic corticosteroids; ipratropium bromide, and intravenous xanthine or beta$_2$ agonist may need to be added. Once lung function is stabilised the patient can be discharged on a regimen of oral and inhaled corticosteroids, inhaled or nebulised beta$_2$ agonists as required, and oral theophylline, long-acting beta$_2$ agonists, or inhaled ipratropium bromide as necessary.

Behçet's syndrome
Behçet's syndrome (or Behçet's disease) is a recurrent multifocal disorder most prevalent in Japan and countries of the Mediterranean and Middle East, although it is also found elsewhere.

The clinical features include oral and genital ulceration, skin lesions, arthritis, vasculitis leading to thromboembolic disorders and aneurysms, ocular lesions (including uveitis, hypopyon, and iridocyclitis leading eventually to blindness), and CNS involvement (meningomyelitis, dementia, extrapyramidal symptoms, and paralysis, sometimes fatal). Gastrointestinal disturbances and involvement of other body systems have been reported. However, the complete gamut of symptoms is unlikely in a single patient, and the disease has been classified into mucocutaneous, arthritic, neurological, and ocular forms depending on the predominant symptoms. Diagnosis can be difficult, but oral ulceration, together with recurrent genital ulceration, ocular involvement, and skin lesions or a positive pathergy test are considered the major diagnostic criteria.[1]

Treatment of Behçet's syndrome is essentially symptomatic and empirical. Controlled studies are mostly lacking, which has hindered meta-analysis.[2] Where possible topical treatment of local lesions should be attempted before embarking on systemic therapy. Topical application of potent corticosteroids or a tetracycline solution may be tried for oral ulceration.[1] Ocular involvement may be treated with a mydriatic and corticosteroid eye drops or local injections.[1,3]

Corticosteroids are widely used for systemic treatment of Behçet's syndrome although their use has been less favoured in some countries, notably Japan,[4] and good evidence of benefit, particularly for ocular symptoms, is lacking.[2,5] Prednisone or prednisolone is given by mouth, usually in doses of up to 60 mg initially, which is reduced to a minimum effective maintenance dose as the patient responds.

Long-term maintenance with corticosteroids poses problems of toxicity and various cytotoxic immunosuppressants have been tried for disease control, either alone or as corticosteroid-sparing agents to permit a reduction in the dosage of concomitant corticosteroid therapy. Drugs that may be of benefit include azathioprine,[2,6] chlorambucil,[3,5] cyclophosphamide,[4] and ciclosporin.[2,7] Pulsed cyclophosphamide may be of benefit for vasculitic symptoms,[1,3] alone or combined with corticosteroids. Such therapy carries its own risks of toxicity, including the possibility of the development of malignancy with long-term use, which must be weighed against its value in delaying the most crippling symptoms of Behçet's syndrome, eye disease and blindness.

An alternative is the use of colchicine. This is reportedly beneficial in the treatment of mucocutaneous lesions,[1,3,8] although ciclosporin is more effective for ocular disease,[7] and a small meta-analysis failed to find any evidence of benefit from colchicine treatment.[2] Colchicine has been used in combination with systemic and topical corticosteroids in acute exacerbations, followed by colchicine maintenance;[9] colchicine with aspirin has also been recommended to prevent acute exacerbations,[10] and

colchicine with benzathine benzylpenicillin has reportedly been found effective.[11]

Other drugs that have been tried include dapsone, interferon alfa-2b (for ocular disease and arthritis), levamisole, omega-3 fatty acids, oxpentifylline [pentoxifylline], stanozolol (for vascular symptoms), and thalidomide, which is effective for mucocutaneous symptoms,[12] although relapses occur on cessation of therapy. Sulfasalazine has been given for colitis associated with Behçet's syndrome, and mesalazine has been applied topically to cutaneous lesions in one patient with some success.

1. Kaklamani VG, et al. Behçet's disease. *Semin Arthritis Rheum* 1998; **27:** 197–217.
2. Saenz A, et al. Pharmacotherapy for Behçet's syndrome (updated 30 August 2000). Available in The Cochrane Library; Issue 3. Oxford: Update Software; 2001.
3. Sakane T, et al. Behçet's disease. *N Engl J Med* 1999; **341:** 1284–91.
4. Oniki S, et al. Immunosuppressive treatment of Behçet's disease with cyclophosphamide. *Jpn J Ophthalmol* 1976; **20:** 32–40.
5. Kaklamani VG, Kaklamanis PG. Treatment of Behçet's disease—an update. *Semin Arthritis Rheum* 2001; **30:** 299–312.
6. Yazici H, et al. A controlled trial of azathioprine in Behçet's syndrome. *N Engl J Med* 1990; **322:** 281–5.
7. Masuda K, et al. Double-masked trial of cyclosporin versus colchicine and long-term open study of cyclosporin in Behçet's disease. *Lancet* 1989; **i:** 1093–6.
8. Miyachi Y, et al. Colchicine in the treatment of the cutaneous manifestations of Behçet's disease. *Br J Dermatol* 1981; **104:** 67–9.
9. Rakover Y, et al. Behcet disease: long-term follow-up of three children and review of the literature. *Pediatrics* 1989; **83:** 986–92.
10. Wechsler B, Piette JC. Behçet's disease. *BMJ* 1992; **304:** 1199–1200.
11. Çalgüneri M, et al. Effect of prophylactic benzathine penicillin on mucocutaneous symptoms of Behçet's disease. *Dermatology* 1996; **192:** 125–8.
12. Hamuryudan V, et al. Thalidomide in the treatment of the mucocutaneous lesions of the Behçet syndrome; a randomized, double-blind, placebo-controlled trial. *Ann Intern Med* 1998; **128:** 443–50.

Bell's palsy
Bell's palsy is a condition which may be caused[1] by herpes simplex virus 1. It affects the facial nerves and results in facial muscle weakness and paralysis. It is often accompanied by pain and lachrymation. Untreated, over 80% of all patients recover completely or almost so, while in a smaller number facial weakness persists; complete failure of motor recovery is very rare.

Corticosteroids dramatically relieve the pain of Bell's palsy,[2] and their use in treatment is widely accepted.[3] The suggested dose of prednisone for adults is 1 mg per kg body-weight daily by mouth in divided doses morning and evening; if the paralysis remains incomplete after 5 or 6 days the prednisone is gradually withdrawn over the next 5 days but if the paralysis is complete the initial dosage should be continued for another 10 days and then gradually withdrawn.[2] However, the benefits of corticosteroids in this condition have never been established by a large controlled trial,[4,5] although a systematic review of 4 small studies suggested an increased rate of complete recovery with corticosteroid treatment.[6] There is some suggestion that addition of aciclovir to corticosteroid treatment may improve outcome,[3] although again substantive evidence is lacking.

1. Murakami S, et al. Bell palsy and herpes simplex virus: identification of viral DNA in endoneurial fluid and muscle. *Ann Intern Med* 1996; **124:** 27–30.
2. Adour KK. Current concepts in neurology: diagnosis and management of facial paralysis. *N Engl J Med* 1982; **307:** 348–51.
3. Knox GW. Treatment controversies in Bell palsy. *Arch Otolaryngol Head Neck Surg* 1998; **124:** 821–3.
4. Karis R. Facial paralysis. *N Engl J Med* 1982; **307:** 1647.
5. Staal A, et al. Facial paralysis. *N Engl J Med* 1982; **307:** 1647.
6. Williamson IG, Whelan TR. The clinical problem of Bell's palsy: is treatment with steroids effective? *Br J Gen Pract* 1996; **46:** 743–7.

Bites and stings
Corticosteroids (prednisone 100 mg daily) have been recommended for the stabilisation of erythrocyte membranes in the management of systemic envenomation by the brown recluse spider (*Loxosceles reclusa*).[1] They have also been given following stings by some species of scorpion, although their value is not certain.[1] Corticosteroids are considered to have no place in snake venom poisoning.[2] Topical corticosteroids may be useful for mild itching of healing skin after some types of jelly fish sting, while systemic corticosteroids have been used for delayed hypersensitivity reactions.[3]

1. Binder LS. Acute arthropod envenomation: incidence, clinical features and management. *Med Toxicol Adverse Drug Exp* 1989; **4:** 163–73.
2. Nelson BK. Snake envenomation: incidence, clinical presentation and management. *Med Toxicol* 1989; **4:** 17–31.
3. Fenner PJ, Williamson JA. Worldwide deaths and severe envenomation from jelly fish stings. *Med J Aust* 1996; **165:** 658–61.

Bone cysts

Methylprednisolone acetate 40 to 200 mg injected into unicameral bone cysts under brief general anaesthesia stimulates bone formation to obliterate the cyst or promote sufficient healing to prevent further fractures.[1] A single injection is sufficient for healing in 10 to 25% of cysts; only rarely will greater than 4 injections be needed. (Systemic corticosteroids are, of course, generally associated with bone loss rather than bone formation—see Effects on Bones and Joints, p.1040).

1. Weinert CR. Administering steroids in unicameral bone cysts. *West J Med* 1989; **150:** 684–5.

Brain injury

See under Spinal Cord Injury, p.1058.

Bronchiolitis

Acute bronchiolitis is usually caused by respiratory syncytial virus (RSV) infection (p.612) in children, and may contribute to the subsequent development of asthma. Supportive therapy, where necessary, may involve the use of oxygen and bronchodilators (see also p.772). Numerous studies have failed to show a benefit from corticosteroid therapy, and it has generally been considered that corticosteroids have no role in the management of the condition. Although one study did find that oral prednisolone might be of benefit,[1] it was suggested that the results might be due to inclusion of children with asthma among the study population.[2] However, a subsequent meta-analysis also showed that systemic corticosteroids could be of benefit.[3] Inhaled corticosteroids seem to be of little value.[4]

1. van Woensel JBM, *et al.* Randomised double blind placebo controlled trial of prednisolone in children admitted to hospital with respiratory syncytial virus bronchiolitis. *Thorax* 1997; **52:** 634–7.
2. Milner AD. The role of corticosteroids in bronchiolitis and croup. *Thorax* 1997; **52:** 595–7.
3. Garrison MM, *et al.* Systemic corticosteroids in infant bronchiolitis: a meta-analysis. Abstract: *Pediatrics* 2000; **105:** 849. Full version: http://www.pediatrics.org/cgi/content/full/105/4/e44
4. Richter H, Seddon P. Early nebulized budesonide in the treatment of bronchiolitis and the prevention of postbronchiolitic wheezing. *J Pediatr* 1998; **132:** 849–53.

Bronchopulmonary dysplasia

Bronchopulmonary dysplasia is the major cause of chronic lung disease (defined as the need for supplementary oxygen more than 28 days after birth) in neonates. It is considered to comprise 4 radiographically distinct stages: stage 1 is effectively indistinguishable from neonatal respiratory distress syndrome (see p.1055), with which it is usually associated. A 'bubbly' appearance of the lung is seen in radiographs of advanced disease. Bronchopulmonary dysplasia is invariably associated with prolonged mechanical ventilation, but it is uncertain whether it plays a causative role, or whether the disease develops anyway in infants with respiratory failure severe enough to need prolonged ventilation.[1]

Treatment. Corticosteroids,[2-9] usually in the form of intravenous dexamethasone, have been widely used in premature infants with bronchopulmonary dysplasia, or who are considered to be at high risk of it (the borderline between treatment and prophylaxis in studies in these mechanically ventilated infants is not always clear[6]). Dexamethasone has been reported to improve pulmonary outcome, allowing more rapid weaning from mechanical ventilation, and in some studies was reported to improve neurological outcome as well.[3] However, some investigators consider its benefits in the long term inadequately established,[6,8,10] and there remains some concern about possible adverse effects, especially on long-term development.[11] One meta-analysis suggests that use is associated with a high incidence of cerebral palsy and neurodevelopmental impairment, and should be abandoned.[12] Many studies have favoured an initial dose of 0.5 mg per kg body-weight daily intravenously, tapered over a period of days to weeks, but it is not always clear if this is expressed in terms of the base or one of its esters,[13] and in any case regimens have varied between studies and the optimum has yet to be determined.[14] Despite suggestions that beginning therapy shortly after birth might minimise lung injury, evidence suggests that early therapy offers no advantage,[10,15] and may be more hazardous.[10,16,17] Meta-analysis has suggested that while beginning dexamethasone at any time between birth and 14 days of age reduced the risk of chronic lung disease, mortality was only reduced in the group who began treatment between 7 and 14 days of age.[18] However, a subsequent systematic review concluded that the benefits of therapy started between 7 to 14 days may not outweigh the adverse effects.[17] Inhaled corticosteroids have also been investigated. A systematic review of inhaled corticosteroid did not demonstrate any reduction in the incidence of chronic lung disease; however, inhaled therapy was associated with less need for systemic corticosteroids.[19] A systematic review of controlled studies found that inhaled corticosteroids may improve the rate of extubation in infants.[20]

Additional therapy is essentially supportive, including fluid restriction, nutritional supplementation, bronchodilators, and diuretics. In general, diuretics are indicated for episodes of associated cardiac failure but their long-term value is uncertain; if used, consideration should be given to a calcium-sparing regimen.[14] Improved pulmonary status has been reported with frusemide [furosemide] in established dysplasia,[21,22] although routine or sustained use cannot be recommended at present. Results with hydrochlorothiazide and spironolactone are more ambiguous.[23,24] Anaemia in infants with bronchopulmonary dysplasia has benefited from erythropoietin.[25] Although vitamin A deficiency has been implicated in the pathogenesis of bronchopulmonary dysplasia, vitamin A supplementation has not been found to produce overall benefit.[26,27] However, there is some preliminary evidence that treatment with alpha$_1$-proteinase inhibitor may be of value.[28]

1. Bancalari E, *et al.* Bronchopulmonary dysplasia: clinical presentation. *J Pediatr* 1979; **95:** 819–23.
2. Mammel MC, *et al.* Controlled trial of dexamethasone therapy in infants with bronchopulmonary dysplasia. *Lancet* 1983; **i:** 1356–8.
3. Cummings JJ, *et al.* A controlled trial of dexamethasone therapy in preterm infants with bronchopulmonary dysplasia. *N Engl J Med* 1989; **320:** 1505–10.
4. Kazzi NJ, *et al.* Dexamethasone effects on the hospital course of infants with bronchopulmonary dysplasia who are dependent on artificial ventilation. *Pediatrics* 1990; **86:** 722–7.
5. Collaborative Dexamethasone Trial Group. Dexamethasone therapy in neonatal chronic lung disease: an international placebo-controlled trial. *Pediatrics* 1991; **88:** 421–7.
6. Kari MA, *et al.* Dexamethasone treatment in preterm infants at risk for bronchopulmonary dysplasia. *Arch Dis Child* 1993; **68:** 566–9.
7. Durand M, *et al.* Effects of early dexamethasone therapy on pulmonary mechanics and chronic lung disease in very low birth weight infants: a randomized, controlled trial. *Pediatrics* 1995; **95:** 584–90.
8. Jones R, *et al.* Controlled trial of dexamethasone in neonatal chronic lung disease: a 3-year follow-up. *Pediatrics* 1995; **96:** 897–906.
9. Rastogi A, *et al.* A controlled trial of dexamethasone to prevent bronchopulmonary dysplasia in surfactant-treated infants. *Pediatrics* 1996; **98:** 204–10.
10. Papile L-A, *et al.* A multicenter trial of two dexamethasone regimens in ventilator-dependent premature infants. *N Engl J Med* 1998; **338:** 1112–18.
11. Greenough A. Gains and losses from dexamethasone for neonatal chronic lung disease. *Lancet* 1998; **352:** 835–6.
12. Barrington KJ. The adverse neuro-developmental effects of postnatal steroids in the preterm infant: a systematic review of RCTs. Available at: http://www.biomedcentral.com/1471–2431/1/1
13. Jones RAK, Grant AM. The "dose" question. *Pediatrics* 1992; **90:** 781.
14. Report of a Joint Working Group of the British Association of Perinatal Medicine and the Research Unit of the Royal College of Physicians. Development of audit measures and guidelines for good practice in the management of neonatal respiratory distress syndrome. *Arch Dis Child* 1992; **67:** 1221–7.
15. Tapia JL, *et al.* The effect of early dexamethasone administration on bronchopulmonary dysplasia in preterm infants with respiratory distress syndrome. *J Pediatr* 1998; **132:** 48–52.
16. Halliday HL, Ehrenkranz RA. Early postnatal (<96 hours) corticosteroids for preventing chronic lung disease in preterm infants (updated 13 February 2001). Available in The Cochrane Library; Issue 3. Oxford: Update Software; 2001.
17. Halliday HL, Ehrenkranz RA. Moderately early (7-14 days) postnatal corticosteroids for preventing chronic lung disease in preterm infants (updated 13 February 2001). Available in The Cochrane Library; Issue 3. Oxford: Update Software; 2001.
18. Bhuta T, Ohlsson A. Systematic review and meta-analysis of early postnatal dexamethasone for prevention of chronic lung disease. *Arch Dis Child Fetal Neonatal Ed* 1998; **79:** F26–F33.
19. Shah V, *et al.* Early administration of inhaled corticosteroids for preventing chronic lung disease in ventilated very low birth weight preterm neonates (updated 27 February 2001). Available in The Cochrane Library; Issue 3. Oxford: Update Software; 2001.
20. Lister P, *et al.* Inhaled steroids for neonatal chronic lung disease (updated 30 May 2001). Available in The Cochrane Library; Issue 3. Oxford: Update Software; 2001.
21. Brion LP, *et al.* Aerosolized diuretics for preterm infants with (or developing) chronic lung disease (updated 28 February 2001). Available in The Cochrane Library; Issue 3. Oxford: Update Software; 2001.
22. Brion LP, Primhak RA. Intravenous or enteral loop diuretics for preterm infants with (or developing) chronic lung disease (updated 27 February 2001). Available in The Cochrane Library; Issue 3. Oxford: Update Software; 2001.
23. Engelhardt B, *et al.* Effect of spironolactone-hydrochlorothiazide on lung function in infants with chronic bronchopulmonary dysplasia. *J Pediatr* 1989; **114:** 619–24.
24. Albersheim SG, *et al.* Randomized, double-blind, controlled trial of long-term diuretic therapy for bronchopulmonary dysplasia. *J Pediatr* 1989; **115:** 615–20.
25. Ohls RK, *et al.* A randomized double-blind, placebo-controlled trial of recombinant erythropoietin in treatment of the anemia of bronchopulmonary dysplasia. *J Pediatr* 1993; **123:** 996–1000.
26. Pearson E, *et al.* Trial of vitamin A supplementation in very low birth weight infants at risk for bronchopulmonary dysplasia. *J Pediatr* 1992; **121:** 420–7.
27. Tyson JE, *et al.* Vitamin A supplementation for extremely-low-birth-weight infants. *N Engl J Med* 1999; **340:** 1962–8.
28. Stiskal JA, *et al.* α$_1$-Proteinase inhibitor therapy for the prevention of chronic lung disease of prematurity: a randomized, controlled trial. *Pediatrics* 1998; **101:** 89–94.

Cachexia

For mention of the use of corticosteroids in cancer-related cachexia see p.1481.

Cerebral oedema

Corticosteroids (usually dexamethasone) play an important role in the treatment of cerebral oedema caused by malignancy and dexamethasone is advocated for the cerebral oedema associated with high-altitude disorders (see p.800). Corticosteroids have also been used for the management of raised intracranial pressure in patients with head injuries or stroke, but despite earlier small studies showing them to be beneficial in some patients, more recent evidence shows that survival and neurological outcome is not improved in these conditions. Current opinion is that corticosteroids are not useful in head injuries (see also under Spinal Cord Injury, p.1058) or stroke, and that their adverse effects may outweigh any possible benefit. The management of raised intracranial pressure and the usual drugs used to treat it are discussed on p.811.

References.
1. Sila CA, Furlan AJ. Drug treatment of stroke: current status and future prospects. *Drugs* 1988; **35:** 468–76.
2. Anonymous. A fresh look at some old stroke treatments. *Pharm J* 1990; **244:** 202.
3. Lyons MK, Meyer FB. Cerebrospinal fluid physiology and the management of increased intracranial pressure. *Mayo Clin Proc* 1990; **65:** 684–707.
4. Woster PS, LeBlanc KL. Management of elevated intracranial pressure. *Clin Pharm* 1990; **9:** 762–72.
5. Jeevaratnam DR, Menon DK. Survey of intensive care of severely head injured patients in the United Kingdom. *BMJ* 1996; **312:** 944–7.

Chronic active hepatitis

Chronic hepatitis is characterised by liver cell necrosis and inflammation which persists for more than 6 to 12 months. Probably the most serious form is chronic active hepatitis in which inflammatory infiltrates (mononuclear and plasma cells) are found within and around the portal areas, with piecemeal necrosis of adjacent liver cells, and in severe cases bands of necrotic tissue between portal tracts or to the central vein (bridging necrosis). Symptoms are essentially non-specific and include fatigue, malaise, fever, anorexia, jaundice, and raised serum aminotransferase values; biopsy is required for accurate diagnosis. The causes of chronic active hepatitis vary and may include: infection with hepatitis viruses; adverse effects of drugs such as isoniazid, methyldopa, or nitrofurantoin; or, particularly in women, an apparently idiopathic form, auto-immune hepatitis.

Treatment with corticosteroids is widely used in patients with auto-immune hepatitis.[1,2] A moderate initial dose of 20 to 30 mg of prednisolone or prednisone daily by mouth or a higher dose of 60 mg daily may be used,[3,4] and is then slowly tapered over several months to the minimum required for maintenance. Daily maintenance therapy appears more effective than alternate day regimens. Patients who respond (as shown by a return of serum aminotransferase values to the normal or near normal range and a reduction in the inflammatory processes on biopsy) usually require prolonged treatment; although some patients remain in remission for months to years after withdrawal, relapse generally occurs, and therapy should be reinstated when the disease becomes active again.[1]

Combined treatment including azathioprine is frequently given and may be the preferred initial treatment in some patients;[4] such treatment is at least as effective as a corticosteroid alone,[2] can produce[5,6] and maintain[7,8] remission, and permits a reduction in corticosteroid dosage in a group of patients who will require long-term drug treatment.[1] There has been some dispute about the value of azathioprine alone, but combined therapy has generally been found to be superior.[5] However azathioprine has been used alone in high doses to maintain remission.[8]

In contrast to the fairly extensive experience with azathioprine, ciclosporin is little used in this condition; once started it appears to be required indefinitely.[4] It may be an alternative in severe disease where corticosteroids alone or with azathioprine cannot suffice. Some investigators have also used cyclophosphamide successfully,[3] and tacrolimus is under investigation.[9]

As an alternative to prolonged use of corticosteroid maintenance therapy, penicillamine has been tried, the dose of penicillamine being gradually increased over several months to a suitable maintenance dose as the dosage of corticosteroid is tapered off.

It is generally agreed that immunosuppression is not suitable in patients with viral chronic active hepatitis.[1,10] However, combination therapy has been reported to produce benefit in patients positive for HBsAg,[5] and it has been reported[11] that patients with chronic active hepatitis of unknown cause, at least some of whom may have hepatitis C,[10] respond as well to corticosteroids or combined therapy as patients with proven auto-immune disease.

1. Krawitt EL. Autoimmune hepatitis. *N Engl J Med* 1996; **334:** 897–903.
2. Stavinoha MW, Soloway RD. Current therapy of chronic liver disease. *Drugs* 1990; **39:** 814–40.
3. Meyer zum Büschenfelde KH, Lohse AW. Autoimmune hepatitis. *N Engl J Med* 1995; **333:** 1004–5.
4. Czaja AJ. Drug therapy in the management of type 1 autoimmune hepatitis. *Drugs* 1999; **57:** 49–68.
5. Giusti G, *et al.* Immunosuppressive therapy in chronic active hepatitis (CAH): a multicentric retrospective study on 867 patients. *Hepatogastroenterology* 1984; **31:** 24–9.
6. Vegnente A, *et al.* Duration of chronic active hepatitis and the development of cirrhosis. *Arch Dis Child* 1984; **59:** 330–5.
7. Stellon AJ, *et al.* Randomised controlled trial of azathioprine withdrawal in autoimmune chronic active hepatitis. *Lancet* 1985; **i:** 668–70.
8. Johnson PJ, *et al.* Azathioprine for long-term maintenance of remission in autoimmune hepatitis. *N Engl J Med* 1995; **333:** 958–63.
9. Van Thiel DH, *et al.* Tacrolimus: a potential new treatment for autoimmune chronic active hepatitis: results of an open-label preliminary trial. *Am J Gastroenterol* 1995; **90:** 771–6.
10. Gitnick G. Cryptogenic versus autoimmune chronic hepatitis: to split or to lump? *Mayo Clin Proc* 1990; **65:** 119–21.
11. Czaja AJ. Clinical features and prognostic implications of severe corticosteroid-treated cryptogenic chronic active hepatitis. *Mayo Clin Proc* 1990; **65:** 23–30.

Chronic obstructive pulmonary disease

Corticosteroids play some part in the symptomatic and palliative management of chronic obstructive pulmonary disease (COPD—p.759), although there is controversy as to their value. Most patients do not respond to corticosteroids but in about 10% of those receiving maximal bronchodilator therapy a short course of oral corticosteroid therapy can improve airflow further. In these patients maintenance therapy may be given, preferably by inhalation. However, whether corticosteroids slow the deterioration rate and improve long-term outcome in COPD, regardless of corticosteroid responsiveness, remains to be confirmed. One 6-month study[1] has reported a trend towards a reduction in acute exacerbations of COPD with inhaled fluticasone therapy. A large randomised trial of high-dose fluticasone in patients with moderate to severe COPD also reported fewer acute exacerbations of the disease and a slower decline in health status.[2] An analysis[3] of data from 3 small studies suggested that inhaled budesonide or beclometasone may also reduce the decline in lung function. However, recent evidence from larger studies in patients without significant bronchodilator[4] or corticosteroid[5,6] responsiveness suggests that standard- or high-dose inhaled budesonide had limited benefits in terms of decline in lung function. Therefore, some commentators have suggested corticosteroids are unlikely to have a role in the long-term management of COPD.[7]

Short courses of systemic corticosteroids are commonly used for acute exacerbations of COPD, despite limited evidence of clinical benefit. A recent study[8] found that a 2-week course of corticosteroids in patients hospitalised for acute exacerbations did result in moderate reductions in treatment failures and length of hospital stay; a longer course of 8 weeks was no more effective than 2 weeks. Another smaller study also produced evidence of benefit for a 2-week course.[9]

1. Paggiaro PL, *et al.* Multicentre randomised placebo-controlled trial of inhaled fluticasone propionate in patients with chronic obstructive pulmonary disease. *Lancet* 1998; **351:** 773–80.
2. Burge PS, *et al.* Randomised, double blind, placebo controlled study of fluticasone propionate in patients with moderate to severe chronic obstructive pulmonary disease: the ISOLDE trial. *BMJ* 2000; **320:** 1297–1303.
3. van Grunsven PM, *et al.* Long term effects of inhaled corticosteroids in chronic obstructive pulmonary disease: a meta-analysis. *Thorax* 1999; **54:** 7–14.
4. Pauwels RA, *et al.* Long-term treatment with inhaled budesonide in persons with mild chronic obstructive pulmonary disease who continue smoking. *N Engl J Med* 1999; **340:** 1948–53.
5. Bourbeau J, *et al.* Randomised controlled trial of inhaled corticosteroids in patients with chronic obstructive pulmonary disease. *Thorax* 1998; **53:** 477–82.
6. Vestbo J, *et al.* Long-term effect of inhaled budesonide in mild and moderate chronic obstructive pulmonary disease: a randomised controlled trial. *Lancet* 1999; **353:** 1819–23.
7. Burge PS. EUROSCOP, ISOLDE and the Copenhagen City Lung Study. *Thorax* 1999; **54:** 287–8.

8. Niewoehner DE, *et al.*. Effect of systemic glucocorticoids on exacerbations of chronic obstructive pulmonary disease. *N Engl J Med* 1999; **340:** 1941–7.
9. Davies L, *et al.* Oral corticosteroids in patients admitted to hospital with exacerbations of chronic obstructive pulmonary disease: a prospective randomised controlled trial. *Lancet* 1999; **354:** 456–60.

Churg-Strauss syndrome

The Churg-Strauss syndrome is sometimes classified with polyarteritis nodosa (see p.1056), although, unlike the latter, pulmonary manifestations are relatively common in Churg-Strauss syndrome. Patients commonly have a history of allergic disease (rhinitis, sinusitis, and asthma), and intractable asthma and eosinophilia together with granulomatous vasculitis characterise the syndrome.

Treatment is similar to that of polyarteritis nodosa, being based on systemic corticosteroids and, where necessary, cyclophosphamide.[1-3] When cyclophosphamide is used, administration as intravenous pulse therapy is coming to be preferred to continuous oral administration,[3] as it has been shown to reduce adverse effects.[4] Azathioprine has been used but has been largely superseded by cyclophosphamide.[1] Interferon alfa may also be of benefit.[5]

1. Taylor HG, Samanta A. Treatment of vasculitis. *Br J Clin Pharmacol* 1993; **35:** 93–104.
2. Guillevin L, *et al.* Treatment of polyarteritis nodosa and Churg-Strauss syndrome: a meta-analysis of 3 prospective controlled trials including 182 patients over 12 years. *Ann Med Interne (Paris)* 1992; **143:** 405–16.
3. Guillevin L, Lhote F. Classification and management of necrotising vasculitides. *Drugs* 1997; **53:** 805–16.
4. Chow C-C, *et al.* Allergic granulomatosis and angiitis (Churg-Strauss syndrome): response to 'pulse' intravenous cyclophosphamide. *Ann Rheum Dis* 1989; **48:** 605–8.
5. Tatsis E, *et al.* Interferon-α treatment of four patients with the Churg-Strauss syndrome. *Ann Intern Med* 1998; **129:** 370–4.

Cogan's syndrome

Corticosteroids are useful in the treatment of Cogan's syndrome, a condition characterised by non-syphilitic interstitial keratitis and audiovestibular symptoms including deafness.[1-3] The deafness, although often irreversible, may respond to systemic corticosteroids initiated within 2 weeks of onset of symptoms (prednisolone or prednisone, at least 1.5 mg per kg body-weight daily for 2 weeks is advised) and ocular involvement benefits from topical corticosteroid therapy (e.g. prednisolone 1% at a rate of 1 drop every hour for 1 to 2 weeks).[3] Improvement in ocular symptoms has also been seen with sodium cromoglicate eye drops.[4] For patients with severe Cogan's syndrome including large-vessel vasculitis, corticosteroids have been used in conjunction with other immunosuppressants such as azathioprine, ciclosporin and cyclophosphamide.[5] Methotrexate has also been tried.[6]

1. Anonymous. Cogan's syndrome. *Lancet* 1991; **337:** 1011–12.
2. Vollertsen RS, *et al.* Cogan's syndrome: 18 cases and a review of the literature. *Mayo Clin Proc* 1986; **61:** 344–61.
3. St Clair EW, McCallum RM. Cogan's syndrome. *Curr Opin Rheumatol* 1999; **11:** 47–52.
4. Carter F, Nabarro J. Cromoglycate for Cogan's syndrome. *Lancet* 1987; **i:** 888.
5. Allen NB, *et al.* Use of immunosuppressive agents in the treatment of severe ocular and vascular manifestations of Cogan's syndrome. *Am J Med* 1990; **88:** 296–301.
6. Riente L, *et al.* Efficacy of methotrexate in Cogan's syndrome. *J Rheumatol* 1996; **23:** 1830–1.

Congenital adrenal hyperplasia

Congenital adrenal hyperplasia comprises a heterogeneous group of disorders due to inherited defects of steroid synthesis in the adrenal gland, the most frequent of which are defects involving 21-hydroxylase or 11-β-hydroxylase. Defective enzyme production blocks the formation of cortisol and aldosterone; the pituitary produces increased amounts of ACTH in an attempt to compensate, but this results in excessive adrenal androgen production. Presentation varies from virilisation and abnormal genital formation at birth to mild cryptic forms that may be detected only later in life. Salt-losing forms (due to lack of aldosterone or the accumulation of precursors with antagonist activity) may lead to hyperkalaemia, acidosis, and dehydration. Patients with 11-β-hydroxylase defect are also prone to hypertension.

Neonates with **salt-losing forms** of congenital adrenal hyperplasia require urgent treatment. Treatment usually consists of a mineralocorticoid, fludrocortisone, and a glucocorticoid (usually hydrocortisone) in regimens similar to those for adrenocortical insufficiency (see p.1046).[1-4] Saline infusion or addition of salt to the feed is required initially.

Even where salt-losing symptoms are not overt or marked, control is reportedly better with a mineralocor-

ticoid added to therapy, rather than with hydrocortisone alone,[1] and it has been recommended that children with salt-losing congenital adrenal hyperplasia should continue to receive combined therapy at least until adult life.[2] Careful titration of dosage is important to avoid growth retardation and toxicity, and potent synthetic glucocorticoids such as betamethasone and dexamethasone are probably inappropriate in infants and children with the condition, even in the non-salt-losing form. An alternative approach is the use of flutamide and testolactone to block androgenic effects, together with a reduced dose of hydrocortisone.[5]

Patients with **non-salt-losing congenital adrenal hyperplasia** may be adequately managed with glucocorticoids alone, and in mild late-onset forms a single dose daily in the late evening (when its suppressive effect on ACTH production is greatest) may be sufficient. In adults who do not require mineralocorticoid treatment betamethasone or dexamethasone may be useful because of their lack of mineralocorticoid actions.

Surgical correction may be necessary in females with masculinised external genitalia. Administration of a glucocorticoid to pregnant women whose offspring are considered at risk has been tried in an attempt to prevent virilisation:[4,6-8] dexamethasone is preferred to hydrocortisone because of a lack of placental degradation.[7]

1. Hughes IA, *et al.* Continuing the need for mineralocorticoid therapy in salt-losing congenital adrenal hyperplasia. *Arch Dis Child* 1979; **54:** 350–5.
2. Griffiths KD, *et al.* Plasma renin activity in the management of congenital adrenal hyperplasia. *Arch Dis Child* 1984; **59:** 360–5.
3. Young MC, Hughes IA. Response to treatment of congenital adrenal hyperplasia in infancy. *Arch Dis Child* 1990; **65:** 441–4.
4. American Academy of Pediatrics. Technical report: congenital adrenal hyperplasia. *Pediatrics* 2000; **106:** 1511–18. Correction. *ibid.* 2001; **107:** 1450.
5. Merke DP, Cutler GB. New approaches to the treatment of congenital adrenal hyperplasia. *JAMA* 1997; **277:** 1073–6.
6. David M, Forest MG. Prenatal treatment of congenital adrenal hyperplasia resulting from 21-hydroxylase deficiency. *J Pediatr* 1984; **105:** 799–803.
7. Evans MI, *et al.* Pharmacologic suppression of the fetal adrenal gland in utero: attempted prevention of abnormal external genital masculinization in suspected congenital adrenal hyperplasia. *JAMA* 1985; **253:** 1015–20.
8. Anonymous. Prenatal treatment of congenital adrenal hyperplasia. *Lancet* 1990; **335:** 510–11.

Corneal graft rejection

Corticosteroids are the mainstay of postoperative prophylaxis and treatment of corneal graft rejection.[1] Topical and subconjunctival corticosteroids are widely employed, but in acute rejection episodes involving the endothelium systemic therapy is usually necessary. A single 500-mg intravenous pulse of methylprednisolone appears to be as effective as up to 2 weeks' treatment with oral prednisolone 60 to 80 mg daily for the management of severe endothelial rejection.[2]

In high-risk patients corticosteroids alone provide insufficient immunosuppression and systemic ciclosporin is occasionally used.[1] Topical ciclosporin has also been investigated.[3]

For discussions of the role of corticosteroids in other forms of organ and tissue grafting, see Organ and Tissue Transplantation, p.502.

1. Hill JC. Immunosuppression in corneal transplantation. *Eye* 1995; **9:** 247–53.
2. Hill JC, *et al.* Corticosteroids in corneal graft rejection: oral versus single pulse therapy. *Ophthalmology* 1991; **98:** 329–33.
3. Zhao JC, Jim XY. Local therapy of corneal allograft rejection with cyclosporine. *Am J Ophthalmol* 1995; **19:** 189–94.

Croup

Croup is an acute syndrome of upper respiratory tract inflammation (laryngotracheobronchitis) associated with viral infection, usually by parainfluenza virus although other viruses may also produce the syndrome. It is characterised by harsh, barking cough, stridor, and hoarseness, most usually occurring at night in children aged 6 months to 4 years.[1,2]

Traditional home management has revolved around the inhalation of steam, despite a lack of evidence for effectiveness, but symptoms may be sufficiently alarming to result in presentation to a hospital.

In severe croup there is some evidence that treatment with a systemic corticosteroid reduces symptoms and decreases the need for intubation.[3-5] Nebulised budesonide has also been reported to be effective,[6-8] and of similar efficacy to inhalation of nebulised adrenaline [epinephrine];[9] however despite the theoretical attraction of this route, studies have failed to find any significant difference in effectiveness between nebulised budesonide

2 mg and oral dexamethasone 0.6 mg per kg body-weight,[10] or combination therapy with both,[11] and another study found 0.6 mg per kg of dexamethasone given intramuscularly to be more effective than 4 mg of nebulised budesonide.[12] In contrast, others have found that addition of nebulised budesonide to oral dexamethasone produced more rapid improvement than the latter alone.[13] Studies have also shown a significant benefit from corticosteroids in children with mild to moderate croup,[10,14,15] and although the use of such potent drugs in children with a mild, largely self-limiting condition has been questioned,[16] a review of the risks and benefits concluded that oral dexamethasone 0.15 mg per kg, or nebulised budesonide 2 mg were the treatment of choice in mild to moderate croup while oral prednisolone 1 mg per kg should be given for croup requiring intubation.[2] However, nebulised adrenaline [epinephrine] is probably the drug of choice where rapid relief of obstructive symptoms is required.[17]

1. Doull I. Corticosteroids in the management of croup. *BMJ* 1995; **311:** 1244.
2. Yates RW, Doull IJM. A risk-benefit assessment of corticosteroids in the management of croup. *Drug Safety* 1997; **16:** 48–55.
3. Kairys SW, et al. Steroid treatment of laryngotracheitis: a meta-analysis of the evidence from randomized trials. *Pediatrics* 1989; **83:** 683–93.
4. Freezer NJ, et al. Steroids in croup: do they increase the incidence of successful extubation? *Anaesth Intensive Care* 1990; **18:** 224–8.
5. Geelhoed GC. Sixteen years of croup in a Western Australian teaching hospital: effects of routine steroid treatment. *Ann Emerg Med* 1996; **28:** 621–6.
6. Klassen TP, et al. Nebulized budesonide for children with mild-to-moderate croup. *N Engl J Med* 1994; **331:** 285–9.
7. Husby S, et al. Treatment of croup with nebulised steroid (budesonide): a double blind, placebo controlled study. *Arch Dis Child* 1993; **68:** 352–5.
8. Godden CW, et al. Double blind placebo controlled trial of nebulised budesonide for croup. *Arch Dis Child* 1997; **76:** 155–8.
9. Fitzgerald D, et al. Nebulized budesonide is as effective as nebulized adrenaline in moderately severe croup. *Pediatrics* 1996; **97:** 722–5.
10. Geelhoed GC, MacDonald WBG. Oral and inhaled steroids in croup: a randomized placebo-controlled trial. *Pediatr Pulmonol* 1995; **20:** 355–61.
11. Klassen TP, et al. Nebulized budesonide and oral dexamethasone for treatment of croup: a randomized controlled trial. *JAMA* 1998; **279:** 1629–32.
12. Johnson DW, et al. A comparison of nebulised budesonide, intramuscular dexamethasone, and placebo for moderately severe croup. *N Engl J Med* 1998; **339:** 498–503.
13. Klassen TP, et al. The efficacy of nebulized budesonide in dexamethasone-treated outpatients with croup. *Pediatrics* 1996; **97:** 463–6.
14. Geelhoed GC, et al. Efficacy of a small single dose of oral dexamethasone for outpatient croup: a double blind placebo controlled clinical trial. *BMJ* 1996; **313:** 140–2.
15. Ausejo M, et al. Glucocorticoids for croup (updated 29 May 2000). Available in The Cochrane Library; Issue 3. Oxford: Update Software; 2001.
16. Macfarlane PI, Suri S. Steroids in the management of croup. *BMJ* 1996; **312:** 510.
17. Anonymous. Inhaled budesonide and adrenaline for croup. *Drug Ther Bull* 1996; **34:** 23–4.

Cystic fibrosis

Corticosteroids have been used by mouth or by inhalation in the management of the inflammatory response of the lungs in cystic fibrosis (see p.117).

Deafness

For references to the use of corticosteroids in the treatment of deafness associated with Cogan's syndrome, see above.

Dermatomyositis

For references to the treatment of dermatomyositis with corticosteroids, see Polymyositis and Dermatomyositis, p.1057.

Diffuse parenchymal lung disease

Diffuse parenchymal lung disease (DPLD; interstitial lung disease) represents a large and heterogeneous group of inflammatory disorders which have in common thickening of the interstitial walls between alveoli. In some cases, particularly in the early stages, this is due to accumulation of inflammatory cells in the interstitium, and control of inflammation can reverse the changes; however, when fibrotic changes to the alveolar walls take place these are usually irreversible. The causes of chronic DPLD are numerous and include pneumoconioses due to inhalation of inorganic dusts (as in asbestosis and silicosis); extrinsic allergic alveolitis due to inhalation of, usually, organic antigens (as in farmers' lung, bird fanciers' lung, and many similar occupational disorders); cryptogenic fibrosing alveolitis (idiopathic pulmonary fibrosis); adverse effects of drugs such as bleomycin; sarcoidosis; lung disease associated with collagen vascular disorders such as rheumatoid arthritis and systemic lupus

erythematosus, or with the vasculitides; histiocytic syndromes; and pulmonary eosinophilic syndromes. Cryptogenic fibrosing alveolitis (below) and sarcoidosis (p.1058) are probably the most common chronic DPLDs.[1]

The symptoms of DPLD are usually insidious and non-specific, and may include dyspnoea of varying severity, usually first noticed on exertion, cough, and fatigue; fine crackling sounds (rales) on breathing and finger clubbing occur in some forms. If disease progresses respiratory failure becomes more severe, and eventually may prove fatal.

Where a causative agent can be identified, initial treatment is to prevent exposure but where inflammation persists, or where the causation is uncertain, corticosteroids are the mainstay of treatment (despite a lack of controlled trials for efficacy),[2–4] in an attempt to control inflammation and preserve as much normal tissue as possible. The management of cryptogenic fibrosing alveolitis is discussed in more detail below.

Cryptogenic fibrosing alveolitis (idiopathic pulmonary fibrosis) is a form of DPLD of uncertain origin, associated with alveolitis and thickening of the interstitial walls by oedema, cellular exudate, and fibrosis. The clinical course is variable but the mean survival is only 3 to 5 years.[3,5,6] Cryptogenic fibrosing alveolitis itself appears to represent a spectrum of disorders; some have advocated that usual interstitial pneumonia (the most common form) should be distinguished from forms such as nonspecific or desquamative interstitial pneumonia, or bronchiolitis obliterans organising pneumonia (BOOP), which may respond better to corticosteroid therapy.[7]

The British Thoracic Society has recommended[1] that where therapy is considered appropriate (rapid disease progression, increasing symptomatology, or results from computed tomography scans suggestive of a responsive pathology) initial treatment should be with oral prednisolone 0.5 mg per kg body-weight plus azathioprine. Azathioprine may be used alone where corticosteroid therapy is problematic, or cyclophosphamide may be combined with the corticosteroid if azathioprine is not tolerated. About 50% of patients with cryptogenic fibrosing alveolitis show a symptomatic response to corticosteroids and about 25% show an improvement in lung function; however, in the absence of placebo-controlled trials there is no clear evidence that treatment improves survival. Survival does seem to be improved following treatment with corticosteroids plus azathioprine, compared with corticosteroids alone. It should also be borne in mind that patients defined as having cryptogenic fibrosing alveolitis are a heterogeneous group, with some forms appearing to respond better to treatment than others, which makes comparison of studies difficult. If the condition stabilises, the dose of corticosteroid may be reduced gradually for maintenance. Corticosteroid therapy is usually continued lifelong; attempts at withdrawal should be gradual and cautious and if clinical deterioration ensues aggressive therapy with corticosteroids and cytotoxic immunosuppressants should be reinstituted immediately.[5]

A variety of other drugs have been tried in patients with cryptogenic fibrosing alveolitis;[1] responses have been reported in a few patients given ciclosporin or penicillamine, and there is some evidence suggesting that colchicine may be as effective as a corticosteroid.

In patients in whom other options fail, lung transplantation should be considered.[1,8]

1. British Thoracic Society. The diagnosis, assessment and treatment of diffuse parenchymal lung disease in adults. *Thorax* 1999; **54:** (suppl 1): S1–S30.
2. Crystal RG, et al. Interstitial lung diseases of unknown cause: disorders characterized by chronic inflammation of the lower respiratory tract. *N Engl J Med* 1984; **310:** 154–66 and 235–44.
3. Trembath PW. Corticosteroid therapy in respiratory disorders. *Med J Aust* 1985; **143:** 607–9.
4. Johnston IDA, et al. British Thoracic Society study of cryptogenic fibrosing alveolitis: current presentation and initial management. *Thorax* 1997; **52:** 38–44.
5. Panos RJ, et al. Clinical deterioration in patients with idiopathic pulmonary fibrosis: causes and assessment. *Am J Med* 1990; **88:** 396–404.
6. Chan-Yeung M, Müller NL. Cryptogenic fibrosing alveolitis. *Lancet* 1997; **350:** 651–6.
7. Ryu JH, et al. Idiopathic pulmonary fibrosis: current concepts. *Mayo Clin Proc* 1998; **73:** 1085–1101.
8. Nicod LP. Recognition and treatment of idiopathic pulmonary fibrosis. *Drugs* 1998; **55:** 555–62.

Eczema

Several treatments may be used in the management of atopic eczema (p.1105) but topical corticosteroids are the mainstay. The least potent preparation that is effective

should be used, combined with regular use of an emollient; in mild to moderate disease the topical corticosteroid is only given for 1 to 2 weeks at a time. Most patients with mild to moderate eczema respond to treatment with a mildly potent preparation such as 1% hydrocortisone ointment. For older children and adults with refractory disease, a more potent topical corticosteroid should be considered for long enough to bring the disease under control, followed by a weaker preparation as the condition improves.

The use of systemic corticosteroids is a treatment of last resort in resistant severe eczema, usually for short periods to control the disease, and very rarely for maintenance.

Epidermolysis bullosa

High-dose oral corticosteroids may be tried to control blistering in severe forms of epidermolysis bullosa (p.1105).

Epilepsy

Corticosteroids and corticotropin have been commonly used to treat **infantile spasms**,[1] which are generally unresponsive to conventional antiepileptics. One study[2] indicated that high-dose corticotropin was preferable to prednisone. However, as discussed on p.338, corticotropin and corticosteroids are associated with frequent and severe adverse effects, and some now prefer newer antiepileptics such as vigabatrin.

It has been suggested that high doses of corticosteroids may produce a response in epilepsia partialis continua (a form of **status epilepticus**) refractory to standard antiepileptics (see p.341).

1. Robinson RO. Seizures and steroids. *Arch Dis Child* 1985; **60:** 94–5.
2. Baram TZ, et al. High-dose corticotropin (ACTH) versus prednisone for infantile spasms: a prospective, randomized, blinded study. *Pediatrics* 1996; **97:** 375–9.

Erythema multiforme

In the management of erythema multiforme (p.1105) systemic corticosteroids may be considered in severe reactions but there has been controversy about their value.

Giant cell arteritis

Giant cell arteritis (temporal arteritis; cranial arteritis) is a vasculitic disorder which is frequently associated with polymyalgia rheumatica (p.1056). It occurs mainly in persons over 50 years of age of European, particularly Scandinavian, extraction and is more common in women than men. It is characterised by inflammatory, granulomatous lesions with giant mononuclear cell infiltrates affecting large and medium sized arteries, particularly those supplying the neck and extracranial structures of head and arms. Symptoms vary but may include headache, scalp tenderness, claudication of the jaw, swelling and absence of pulse in the temporal artery, fever, weight loss, malaise, anaemia, visual disturbances, and irreversible blindness. About a third of all patients also exhibit polymyalgia rheumatica.

Treatment is with corticosteroids,[1–5] and early diagnosis and treatment is desirable to reduce the risk of sudden blindness. Most regimens have involved high initial doses of corticosteroid to control the disease followed by reduction to a maintenance dose, but both initial and maintenance doses have varied considerably. The current view seems to be that prednisolone 40 mg daily by mouth initially is adequate in uncomplicated cases without visual symptoms;[2,5,6] this can be reduced after one month to 30 mg daily, after a further month to 20 mg daily, and then more gradually to 10 mg daily or less depending on the patient's response.[2]

Patients presenting with visual symptoms should receive at least 60 mg of prednisolone daily, and one suggested regimen in this group is hydrocortisone 250 mg intravenously at first followed by prednisolone 80 mg by mouth daily for 3 days; the daily prednisolone dose is then reduced to 60 mg for 3 days, then 40 mg for 4 days, and subsequently decreased by 5 mg per week until a maintenance dose of 10 mg daily is reached.[1,2] Some ophthalmologists recommend 80 mg (or 1 mg per kg body-weight) of prednisolone daily as an initial dose in all patients with giant cell arteritis;[5,7] in patients with overt anterior ischaemic optic neuropathy an initial 1-g intravenous infusion of methylprednisolone has also been suggested, followed by high-dose oral corticosteroids.[7]

Maintenance treatment is usually required for at least 2 years. While a small number require indefinite treatment, most patients should be able to discontinue treatment within 4 to 5 years;[8] however relapses are not uncommon.

Because of the need for prolonged corticosteroid therapy side-effects are common, and their management may be the most difficult aspect of treatment.[2,8] Azathioprine has been added to corticosteroid therapy for its modest 'steroid-sparing' effect,[9] and there is evidence of similar benefit from the use of low-dose methotrexate.[10] Other cytotoxic immunosuppressants do not appear to be used. The prognosis is excellent in adequately-treated patients, as the life expectancy of patients with giant cell arteritis is the same as the general population.[11]

1. Clearkin LG, Watts MT. Ocular involvement in giant cell arteritis. *Br J Hosp Med* 1990; **43:** 373–6.
2. Taylor HG, Samanta A. Treatment of vasculitis. *Br J Clin Pharmacol* 1993; **35:** 93–104.
3. Pountain G, Hazleman B. Polymyalgia rheumatica and giant cell arteritis. *BMJ* 1995; **310:** 1057–9.
4. Zilko PJ. Polymyalgia rheumatica and giant cell arteritis. *Med J Aust* 1996; **165:** 438–42.
5. Swannell AJ. Polymyalgia rheumatica and temporal arteritis: diagnosis and management. *BMJ* 1997; **314:** 1329–32.
6. Kyle V, Hazleman BL. Treatment of polymyalgia rheumatica and giant cell arteritis I: steroid regimens in the first two months. *Ann Rheum Dis* 1989; **48:** 658–61.
7. Ferris J, Lamb R. Polymyalgia rheumatica and giant cell arteritis. *BMJ* 1995; **311:** 455.
8. Kyle V, Hazleman BL. Stopping steroids in polymyalgia rheumatica and giant cell arteritis. *BMJ* 1990; **300:** 344–5.
9. De Silva M, Hazleman BL. Azathioprine in giant cell arteritis/polymyalgia rheumatica: a double blind study. *Ann Rheum Dis* 1986; **45:** 136–8.
10. Hernández-García C, *et al.* Methotrexate treatment in the management of giant cell arteritis. *Scand J Rheumatol* 1994; **23:** 295–8.
11. Matteson EL, *et al.* Long-term survival of patients with giant cell arteritis in the American College of Rheumatology giant cell arteritis classification criteria cohort. *Am J Med* 1996; **100:** 193–6.

Glomerular kidney disease

Glomerular disease accounts for a considerable proportion of all kidney disease. Various forms of primary glomerular disease (glomerulopathy) are known, and are discussed below; in addition, numerous systemic diseases (connective-tissue disorders such as systemic lupus erythematosus as well as malignancy and conditions such as diabetes), may result in secondary glomerular disorders. Despite the various potential causes it is thought that many of these diseases act by common immunological mechanisms to damage the glomerulus, either by accumulation of antigen-antibody complexes (immune-complex nephritis) or more rarely by the formation of antibodies to the glomerular basement membrane (anti-GBM nephritis).

Since the kidney can respond in only a limited number of ways to glomerular damage certain common presentations are seen, regardless of aetiology, including **acute glomerulonephritis** (acute nephritis syndrome), which is marked by haematuria and proteinuria of abrupt onset, usually with impaired renal function (a decrease in glomerular filtration rate), salt and water retention, and hypertension; and the **nephrotic syndrome**, which is marked by severe proteinuria, hypoalbuminaemia, and oedema. Other, less dramatic presentations of glomerular disease are asymptomatic proteinuria or microscopic haematuria; alternatively, glomerular disease may be one of the many potential causes of chronic renal failure. Appropriate management of these conditions depends to a considerable extent on the underlying disease.

• MANAGEMENT OF PRIMARY GLOMERULAR DISEASE.

Minimal change nephropathy (MCN; minimal change disease). This condition occurs mainly in children, the highest incidence being at 2 to 4 years, and is the main cause of childhood nephrotic syndrome. It also accounts for about 20% of adult cases of nephrotic syndrome.[1] It is treated with a corticosteroid. Regimens vary somewhat but a suggested regimen for adults has been 60 mg prednisolone daily by mouth for 4 days, reduced to 40 mg daily until remission occurs (which in 90% of patients will be within 3 weeks) and then tapered off.[1] In children, initial doses of 60 mg of prednisolone or prednisone per m[2] body-surface daily have been used,[2] which may be given for anything up to 4 weeks before switching to 40 mg per m[2] given on alternate days for a further 4 weeks, and then tapered off.[3] A modification to the children's dose is to give 60 mg of prednisolone per m[2] daily until there is a response when the dose is reduced to 40 mg per m[2] on alternate days for the next 4 weeks. If there is no response within 4 weeks' treatment with the 60 mg per m[2] dose then the drug should be withdrawn and the child considered to be corticosteroid resistant.[4] A

meta-analysis of treatment regimens found that children with their first episode of nephropathy should be treated with prednisone for at least 3, and possibly up to 7 months to reduce the risk of relapse.[5]

Relapse is common and occurs in about 60% of cases; relapses usually respond to a further course of corticosteroids, but if a third relapse occurs cyclophosphamide 2 to 3 mg per kg body-weight daily for 8 weeks may be added to a course of corticosteroid therapy.[1,2,6] Deflazacort may also be effective in corticosteroid-sensitive patients who do not respond to prednisone.[5]

Prognosis is relatively good: even in those patients who relapse repeatedly there is no evidence of deterioration in renal function,[6] and the potential adverse effects of therapy must be considered. Pulsed intravenous methylprednisolone, followed by low-dose oral prednisone, has been suggested as an alternative to conventional oral doses of corticosteroids in an attempt to reduce adverse effects.[7] Cytotoxic immunosuppressants are reserved for relapsing or corticosteroid-dependent cases because of their potential for severe toxicity, including carcinogenesis; cyclophosphamide appears to be preferred to chlorambucil because it is perceived as entailing a somewhat lower risk, although both are effective. Levamisole has also been tried.[3]

A minority of patients have minimal change disease resistant to corticosteroids: ciclosporin has been added successfully in both adults[8] and children[9] with this rare form of the disease but must be used with caution because of its own potential for nephrotoxicity.

Focal glomerulosclerosis. Focal glomerulosclerosis is a sclerosing lesion affecting parts of the glomeruli which occurs in some patients who otherwise have symptoms characteristic of minimal change nephropathy, and some authorities do not regard it as a distinct disease. It is common in abusers of diamorphine and has also been linked with the nephropathy that can occur in patients with AIDS. Treatment is similar to that for minimal change nephropathy but only about 20% of cases respond to corticosteroids; addition of a cytotoxic immunosuppressant such as cyclophosphamide improves the prospect of remission. In patients who fail to respond, progression to renal failure may occur over several years, but renal transplantation may not be helpful as disease can recur in the transplanted kidney. Responses to ciclosporin have been seen.[8,9]

Membranous nephropathy (membranous glomerulonephritis). This is a disease predominantly of adults, in whom it is the single most important cause of the nephrotic syndrome, accounting for about 50% of cases. It is characterised by diffuse thickening of the glomerular basement membrane following subepithelial deposition of immune complexes. Unlike minimal change nephropathy, whose treatment is fairly well established, treatment of membranous nephropathy is a contentious area. The course of disease is variable and often slow, with some spontaneous remissions, which makes the benefits of treatment difficult to demonstrate and the use of potentially toxic drugs difficult to justify. Cyclophosphamide or chlorambucil combined with a corticosteroid appears to produce some clinical improvement, and stabilisation of progressive disease;[10-12] it is not clear if corticosteroids alone are effective.[13-15] Ciclosporin alone has been tried in a few patients and was associated with complete or partial remission in about half;[16] a small controlled study has also reported benefits.[17] Treatment of any kind tends to be reserved for patients with progressive renal dysfunction.[18]

Mesangiocapillary glomerulonephritis (MCGN; membranoproliferative glomerulonephritis; MPGN). Mesangiocapillary glomerulonephritis comprises 2 separate diseases, known as type I and type II, which both occur in children and young adults and usually result in nephrotic syndrome, although about 20% of cases present with acute glomerulonephritis. Both forms show proliferation of mesangial cells and thickening of glomerular walls with formation of deposits (in type I disease due to immune complexes) in capillary walls and basement membranes. There is no established treatment regimen: some improvement or stabilisation of renal function may occur with corticosteroids and cytotoxic immunosuppressants, but about half of all patients develop end-stage renal failure within 15 to 20 years (type I disease) or 6 to 10 years (type II disease). Antiplatelet drugs and anticoagulants have also been tried but as with other therapies there is little evidence of benefit, and some centres do not recommend any specific therapy, al-

though prednisolone and cyclophosphamide may be offered to those with a rapidly progressive course.[19]

IGA nephropathy (Berger's disease) is the commonest cause of primary glomerular disease in developed countries, and is most common in young men. It results in focal, segmental proliferative glomerulonephritis associated with mesangial formation of immune deposits largely composed of IgA. The usual presentation is acute glomerulonephritis with gross haematuria, often during or just after viral upper-respiratory-tract infection. Some patients develop rapidly progressive disease similar to idiopathic rapidly progressive glomerulonephritis, with renal failure within 6 months, but in many others the syndrome is benign, and requires only observation. No form of therapy has been unequivocally shown to be of value, but control of associated hypertension is considered important. Corticosteroids and cytotoxic immunosuppressants may be tried in severe rapidly progressive disease;[20-22] mycophenolate mofetil has been reported to be effective in 2 patients.[23] Some promising results have been seen with the use of n-3 fatty acids from fish oil,[24] and there is also a report of benefit with normal immunoglobulin.[25]

Idiopathic rapidly progressive glomerulonephritis (RPGN). Although rapidly progressive glomerulonephritis (crescentic glomerulonephritis) may be a feature of other forms of glomerular disease such as IgA nephropathy (see above) or Goodpasture's syndrome (see below) it also occurs in an idiopathic form. The disease is characterised by the formation of glomerular crescents associated with leakage of fibrin from damaged capillaries, and loss of renal function is very rapid, sometimes with renal failure within weeks. Oral corticosteroids are of little value alone, but pulsed intravenous methylprednisolone followed by oral prednisone or prednisone and cyclophosphamide over several months has produced some impressive responses;[26,27] an alternative is the use of intensive plasma exchange together with a corticosteroid and cytotoxic immunosuppressants.[28] Controlled trials of these therapies are mostly lacking, although a small prospective study[29] found lymphocytapheresis to be more effective than pulsed methylprednisolone as an addition to prednisolone and cyclophosphamide therapy for reduction of glomerular injury.

Goodpasture's syndrome. Goodpasture's syndrome is a form of anti-GBM nephritis in which rapidly progressive glomerulonephritis is accompanied by pulmonary haemorrhage due to reaction of the same antibody responsible for the renal symptoms with the membranes of the alveoli. It is a disease predominantly of young adults. Pulmonary haemorrhage responds to high dose oral prednisolone or prednisone, or pulsed intravenous methylprednisolone, but corticosteroids are of little value in controlling renal lesions, which requires vigorous plasma exchange therapy with corticosteroids and cyclophosphamide on a daily or alternate day basis for several weeks, until antibody is no longer detectable and disease progression has halted; it is important to begin therapy before renal damage becomes irreversible.

• MANAGEMENT OF SECONDARY GLOMERULAR DISEASE.

Post-infectious glomerulonephritis. The classical form of post-infectious glomerulonephritis is post-streptococcal glomerulonephritis, which produces an immune-complex-mediated acute glomerulonephritis, but glomerular disease may follow other bacterial infections, as well as protozoal infections such as malaria (malaria-associated nephrotic syndrome is familiar in endemic regions) and viral infections such as AIDS (see Focal Glomerulosclerosis, above). In most cases no additional treatment beyond appropriate management of infection and general supportive care is warranted, and corticosteroids and cytotoxic immunosuppressants are not generally used and may in some cases be harmful.[30] Nonetheless, delayed progressive renal disease may occur in a minority of patients, and has prompted efforts to treat.

Other secondary glomerulopathies. Where glomerular disease is secondary to other diseases (connective tissue disorders such as systemic lupus erythematosus, the vasculitides, Henoch-Schönlein purpura, thrombotic thrombocytopenic purpura, or others such as rheumatoid arthritis, amyloidosis, neoplasia, sickle-cell disease, gout, or diabetes mellitus) most treatment is directed at the underlying disease. In addition, symptomatic management such as the use of sodium restriction for the oedema of nephrotic syndrome may be appropriate; diuretics should be used cautiously because of the risk of hypovolaemia.[2] Proteinuria of various causes may respond to the use of ACE inhibitors or NSAIDs,[1,31] although care is required in patients with renal artery stenosis or renal failure respectively. Associated hypertension and hypercholesterolaemia should be treated, and anticoagulants may be required for associated coagulation disorders (it has been suggested that warfarin may be more appropriate than heparin, although both have been used[31]). Renal toxicity can arise from various drug treatments and this should also be treated symptomatically.

1. Boulton-Jones M. Management of nephrotic syndrome. *Prescribers' J* 1993; **33**: 96–102. Correction. *ibid.*; 176.
2. Melvin T, Bennett W. Management of nephrotic syndrome in childhood. *Drugs* 1991; **42**: 30–51.
3. Hogg RJ, *et al.* Evaluation and management of proteinuria and nephrotic syndrome in children: recommendations from a pediatric nephrology panel established at the National Kidney Foundation conference on proteinuria, albuminuria, risk, assessment, detection, and elimination (PARADE). *Pediatrics* 2000; **105**: 1242–9.
4. Report of a Workshop by the British Association for Paediatric Nephrology and Research Unit, Royal College of Physicians. Consensus statement on management and audit potential for steroid responsive nephrotic syndrome. *Arch Dis Child* 1994; **70**: 151–7.
5. Hodson EM, *et al.* Corticosteroid therapy for nephrotic syndrome in children (updated 23 May 2001). Available in The Cochrane Library; Issue 3. Oxford: Update Software; 2001.
6. Trompeter RS, *et al.* Long-term outcome for children with minimal-change nephrotic syndrome. *Lancet* 1985; **i**: 368–70.
7. Imbasciati E, *et al.* Controlled trial of methylprednisolone pulses and low dose oral prednisone for the minimal change nephrotic syndrome. *BMJ* 1985; **291**: 1305–8.
8. Nyrop M, Olgaard K. Cyclosporin A treatment of severe steroid resistant nephrotic syndrome in adults. *J Intern Med* 1990; **227**: 65–8.
9. Niaudet P, *et al.* Steroid-resistant idiopathic nephrotic syndrome and ciclosporin. *Nephron* 1991; **57**: 481.
10. Mathieson PW, *et al.* Prednisolone and chlorambucil treatment in idiopathic membranous nephropathy with deteriorating renal function. *Lancet* 1985; **ii**: 869–72.
11. Ponticelli C, *et al.* A 10-year follow-up of a randomized study with methylprednisolone and chlorambucil in membranous nephropathy. *Kidney Int* 1995; **48**: 1600–4.
12. Bruns FJ, *et al.* Sustained remission of membranous glomerulonephritis after cyclophosphamide and prednisone. *Ann Intern Med* 1991; **114**: 725–30.
13. Cattran DC, *et al.* A randomized controlled trial of prednisone in patients with idiopathic membranous nephropathy. *N Engl J Med* 1989; **320**: 210–15.
14. Ponticelli C, *et al.* Methylprednisolone plus chlorambucil as compared with methylprednisolone alone for the treatment of idiopathic membranous nephropathy. *N Engl J Med* 1992; **327**: 599–603.
15. Falk RJ, *et al.* Treatment of progressive membranous glomerulopathy: a randomized trial comparing cyclophosphamide and corticosteroids with corticosteroids alone. *Ann Intern Med* 1992; **116**: 438–45.
16. Rostoker G, *et al.* Cyclosporin in idiopathic steroid-resistant membranous glomerulonephritis. *Lancet* 1989; **ii**: 975–6.
17. Cattran DC, *et al.* A controlled trial of cyclosporine in patients with progressive membranous nephropathy. *Kidney Int* 1995; **47**: 1130–5.
18. Lewis EJ. Idiopathic membranous nephropathy—to treat or not to treat? *N Engl J Med* 1993; **329**: 127–9.
19. Mason PD, Pusey CD. Glomerulonephritis: diagnosis and treatment. *BMJ* 1994; **309**: 1557–63. Correction. *ibid* 1995; **310**: 116.
20. Goumenos D, *et al.* Can immunosuppressive drugs slow the progression of IgA nephropathy? *Nephrol Dial Transplant* 1995; **10**: 1173–81.
21. Faedda R, *et al.* Immunosuppressive treatment of Berger's disease. *Clin Pharmacol Ther* 1996; **60**: 561–7.
22. Kobayashi Y, *et al.* Steroid therapy during the early stage of progressive IgA nephropathy: a 10-year follow-up study. *Nephron* 1996; **72**: 237–42.
23. Nowack R, *et al.* Mycophenolate mofetil for systemic vasculitis and IgA nephropathy. *Lancet* 1997; **349**: 774.
24. Donadio JV, *et al.* A controlled trial of fish oil in IgA nephropathy. *N Engl J Med* 1994; **331**: 1194–9.
25. Rostoker G, *et al.* High-dose immunoglobulin therapy for severe IgA nephropathy and Henoch-Schönlein purpura. *Ann Intern Med* 1994; **120**: 476–84.
26. Bolton WK, Sturgill BC. Methylprednisolone therapy for acute crescentic rapidly progressive glomerulonephritis. *Am J Nephrol* 1989; **9**: 368–75.
27. Bruns FJ, *et al.* Long-term follow-up of aggressively treated idiopathic rapidly progressive glomerulonephritis. *Am J Med* 1989; **86**: 400–6.
28. Gianviti A, *et al.* Retrospective study of plasma exchange in patients with idiopathic rapidly progressive glomerulonephritis and vasculitis. *Arch Dis Child* 1996; **75**: 186–90.
29. Furuta T, *et al.* Lymphocytapheresis to treat rapidly progressive glomerulonephritis: a randomised comparison with steroid-pulse treatment. *Lancet* 1998; **352**: 203–4.
30. Adeniyi A, *et al.* A controlled trial of cyclophosphamide and azathioprine in Nigerian children with the nephrotic syndrome and poorly selective proteinuria. *Arch Dis Child* 1979; **54**: 204–7.
31. Alaniz C, *et al.* Pharmacologic management of adult idiopathic nephrotic syndrome. *Clin Pharm* 1993; **12**: 429–39.

Graves' ophthalmopathy

As discussed under Hyperthyroidism, p.1519, patients with moderate to severe ophthalmopathy may be treated with high-dose systemic corticosteroids or with orbital radiotherapy, which appear to be equally effective. It has also been reported that concomitant therapy with a corticosteroid can prevent the transient exacerbation of Graves' ophthalmopathy that may be caused by radioiodine treatment in hyperthyroid patients.[1]

1. Bartalena L, *et al.* Relation between therapy for hyperthyroidism and the course of Graves' ophthalmopathy. *N Engl J Med* 1998; **338**: 73–8.

Haemangioma

Haemangiomas are benign vascular neoplasms of the skin which may enlarge dramatically before regressing spontaneously. Although no treatment is normally required, occasional complications due to ocular or visceral involvement, or associated thrombocytopenia due to platelet trapping (the Kasabach-Merritt syndrome), may merit treatment, generally with corticosteroids. Response is variable.[1-7] A common technique is intralesional injection of a mixture of triamcinolone with betamethasone.[8] There has been a report of 2 infants responding to vincristine after corticosteroids had failed.[9] Interferon alfa has also been tried,[10] as has phototherapy with a pulsed dye laser.[11]

1. Evans J, *et al.* Haemangioma with coagulopathy: sustained response to prednisone. *Arch Dis Child* 1975; **50**: 809–12.
2. Sloan GM, *et al.* Intralesional corticosteroid therapy for infantile hemangiomas. *Plast Reconstr Surg* 1989; **83**: 459–66.
3. Morrell AJ, Willshaw HE. Normalisation of refractive error after steroid injection for adnexal haemangiomas. *Br J Ophthalmol* 1991; **75**: 301–5.
4. David TJ, *et al.* Haemangioma with thrombocytopenia (Kasabach-Merritt syndrome). *Arch Dis Child* 1983; **58**: 1022–3.
5. Enjoiras O, *et al.* Management of alarming hemangiomas in infancy: a review of 25 cases. *Pediatrics* 1990; **85**: 491–8.
6. Sadan N, Wolach B. Treatment of hemangiomas of infants with high doses of prednisone. *J Pediatr* 1996; **128**: 141–6.
7. Drolet BA, *et al.* Hemangiomas in children. *N Engl J Med* 1999; **341**: 173–81.
8. Yap E-Y, *et al.* Periocular capillary hemangioma: a review for pediatricians and family physicians. *Mayo Clin Proc* 1998; **73**: 753–9.
9. Payarols JP, *et al.* Treatment of life-threatening infantile hemangiomas with vincristine. *N Engl J Med* 1995; **333**: 69.
10. Ezekowitz RAB, *et al.* Interferon alfa-2a therapy for life-threatening hemangiomas of infancy. *N Engl J Med* 1992; **326**: 1456–63. Correction. *ibid.* 1995; **333**: 595–6.
11. Barlow RJ, *et al.* Treatment of proliferative haemangiomas with the 585 nm pulsed dye laser. *Br J Dermatol* 1996; **34**: 700–4.

Headache

Corticosteroids have a limited role in the management of some types of headache. Although their long-term use is not considered desirable, short courses of prednisolone or prednisone in doses of 20 to 40 mg daily can be an effective alternative to standard drugs such as ergotamine in the prevention of cluster headache attacks during cluster periods (p.449). Corticosteroids have also been used for the emergency treatment of prolonged severe attacks of migraine (status migrainosus) (p.449) refractory to other drugs.

Herpes infections

Although corticosteroids alone are contra-indicated for most forms of ocular herpes simplex infection (p.607), which should be treated with a topical antiviral such as aciclovir, a combination of corticosteroid and antiviral may be useful in some cases.

Hypercalcaemia

For a description of the treatment of hypercalcaemia, including the specific role of corticosteroids, see p.1181.

Hypersensitivity vasculitis

Hypersensitivity vasculitis is usually associated with an antigenic stimulus, either exogenous such as a drug or microbe, or endogenous such as an immune complex associated with connective tissue disease. The term covers a heterogeneous group of disorders, many of which are associated with some underlying disease process (including infections, malignant neoplasms and disorders such as rheumatoid arthritis or systemic lupus erythematosus), as well as vasculitis of less clear aetiology such as Henoch-Schönlein purpura, a disease typically seen in prepubertal males. There is a suggestion that such a broad grouping is inappropriate, and that the term 'hypersensitivity vasculitis' should not be used;[1] however, at present it continues to be employed in the literature.

Hypersensitivity vasculitis is characterised by small vessel involvement (arterioles and venules), particularly of the skin, and skin manifestations such as purpura, rashes, and urticaria predominate. Neutrophil debris is typically present around the vessel (**leucocytoclastic vasculitis**). However other organ systems may also be involved: in **Henoch-Schönlein purpura**, the skin lesions are associated with arthralgia, abdominal pain and other gastrointestinal symptoms, and glomerulonephritis (usually without impairment of renal function).[2]

The prognosis is typically much better in hypersensitivity vasculitis than in the other major vasculitic syndromes, and most cases resolve spontaneously. Where a recognised antigenic stimulus is present it should be removed if possible, e.g. by withdrawal of a drug or by appropriate therapy of infection. Hypersensitivity vasculitis generally responds less well to conventional drug therapy than other vasculitic syndromes. Nonetheless, where disease persists or results in organ dysfunction, a corticosteroid should be given, typically prednisone or prednisolone 60 mg, or 1 mg per kg body-weight, by mouth daily, tapered rapidly until therapy can be discontinued. Plasmapheresis has also been used, but the use of cytotoxic immunosuppressants is less well established. Anecdotal reports of excellent responses to dapsone in Henoch-Schönlein purpura exist.[3] Other drugs that have been tried include danazol,[4] oxpentifylline [pentoxifylline],[5] the latter sometimes in conjunction with dapsone,[5] and normal immunoglobulin.[6]

1. Jennette JC, *et al.* Nomenclature of systemic vasculitides: proposal of an international consensus conference. *Arthritis Rheum* 1994; **37**: 187–92.
2. Tizard EJ. Henoch-Schönlein purpura. *Arch Dis Child* 1999; **80**: 380–3.
3. Hoffbrand BI. Dapsone in Henoch-Schönlein purpura—worth a trial. *Postgrad Med J* 1991; **67**: 961–2.
4. Lee YJ, *et al.* Danazol for Henoch-Schönlein purpura. *Ann Intern Med* 1993; **118**: 827.
5. Nürnberg W, *et al.* Synergistic effects of pentoxifylline and dapsone in leucocytoclastic vasculitis. *Lancet* 1994; **343**: 491.
6. Rostoker G, *et al.* High-dose immunoglobulin therapy for severe IgA nephropathy and Henoch-Schönlein purpura. *Ann Intern Med* 1994; **120**: 476–84.

Idiopathic thrombocytopenic purpura

Idiopathic thrombocytopenic purpura (ITP; sometimes referred to as auto-immune thrombocytopenic purpura[1]) is an auto-immune bleeding disorder characterised by the development of antibodies to the body's own platelets, with consequent sequestration and destruction of platelets. Both acute and chronic forms are seen; the acute form, which is usually self-limiting and follows viral or other infection, is the usual form in children, whereas chronic and sometimes more serious disease is more likely in adults, particularly young or middle-aged women. Patients develop petechiae, ecchymoses, and epistaxis, and women may develop menorrhagia; death due to haemorrhage is not unknown.

Treatment. For both adults and children with mild thrombocytopenia (counts of 20 to 30 000 per mm^3 or more) and no severe bruising or haemorrhage, no treatment is required.[2-6] In many cases the platelet count will return to normal or remain in a safe range despite the lack of therapy, and spontaneous remission can occur, even after a period of years.[7]

Where treatment is required in chronic disease, corticosteroids are the mainstay of therapy in adults.[2-4,8] Prednisolone (or prednisone) 1 mg per kg body-weight daily is often used, continued until response occurs (sometimes not for a week or more[1]) and then tapered down. If there is no response within 3 weeks the drug should be gradually discontinued as it is unlikely to be effective. About 70 to 80% of adult patients with chronic disease exhibit some response, although not always a sufficient one, but most will relapse when the drug is withdrawn and may require long-term low-dose maintenance, perhaps using alternate day administration.[2] Good responses have also been reported with the use of high-dose oral or intravenous methylprednisolone for 3 to 7 days,[9-13] (this has also been tried in children with the acute form[14] although a controlled study[15] found intravenous normal immunoglobulin to be more effective) and pulsed treatment with high-dose dexamethasone looks promising,[6,16] although it is not clear how great the benefits will be in children.[17-19]

Use of corticosteroids for acute or chronic ITP in children is in any case controversial. Some consider low daily doses of prednisolone (0.25 mg per kg) to be as effective as higher ones,[3] while others consider high doses (prednisone 4 mg per kg) to be necessary.[20,21] Some centres consider that corticosteroids are of at best temporary benefit in children.[22]

In patients with chronic disease and symptoms of bleeding who fail to respond to first-line therapy, splenectomy should be considered.[2-6,8,22] About 70% of patients will respond but the operative and postoperative risks (notably of sepsis) must be considered, particularly in children.

Responses can also be achieved with intravenous normal immunoglobulin, which in practice is often preferred to corticosteroids for initial drug therapy of acute ITP in children.[23] An increase in platelet count is usually achievable with doses of 400 mg per kg daily for 5 days although the effect may be transient; some patients refractory to these doses respond to high-dose therapy (800 mg to 1 g per kg daily).[2] Response is often achievable even in patients refractory to other therapies, but treatment must be repeated periodically. It is perhaps most useful when acute symptoms supervene, because of its rapid activity, and it is recommended that it be reserved for patients with acute severe bleeding, as pre-operative prophylaxis in patients with severe thrombocytopenia, or for patients with bleeding symptoms refractory to corticosteroids.[3-6] A response to normal immunoglobulin has been reported to be a good predictor of benefit from splenectomy.[24] An alternative to normal immunoglobulin in rhesus-positive patients may be the use of anti-D immunoglobulin,[25] although there are conflicting views as to its effectiveness,[8,21,25-28] and it has been associated with haemoglobinuria and haemoglobinaemia.[29]

Various other second-line drugs have been tried in the minority of patients with refractory chronic disease, but few have been well evaluated. Generally,[30-33] but not universally,[34] good results have been reported with danazol, particularly in older patients. It may have advantages for long-term maintenance, and is a potential alternative to splenectomy, at least in selected patients.[32,33] It can be used as a 'steroid-sparing' drug, permitting reduction in corticosteroid maintenance doses.[32]

Antineoplastic and immunosuppressive drugs have been tried in refractory disease, but their potential toxicity has meant that they have often been reserved for older patients, as a treatment of last resort. Cyclophosphamide or azathioprine have been given by mouth in doses of 50 to 150 mg daily; responses to cyclophosphamide generally occur within 8 weeks but for azathioprine several months' treatment is generally necessary before response can be assessed.[2,6] High-dose cyclophosphamide has also been tried in refractory, life-threatening disease.[6] Although some patients have responded to intravenous injection of vincristine, responses have tended to be partial and inadequate, and somewhat better results have been achieved with infusions of platelets incubated with vinblastine or vincristine to encourage binding and permit selective drug delivery to the macrophages responsible for platelet destruction.[35-37] Although the developers of this technique have reported long-lasting remission in 38% of patients,[37] enthusiasm elsewhere appears to be muted.[2,38] Combination chemotherapy (cyclophosphamide and prednisone plus vincristine, vincristine and procarbazine, or etoposide) has produced prolonged remission in a few patients,[6,39,40] but such aggressive treatment would be difficult to justify in most cases.

Other reports of benefit exist for colchicine,[41-43] heparin,[44] and ascorbic acid,[45] the latter having at least the advantage that it is relatively non-toxic, but such therapies remain experimental.

Thrombopoietin can now be produced and this may offer a future new approach to treatment.[46]

Tranexamic acid may be helpful in the symptomatic management of menorrhagia, although hysterectomy is occasionally necessary.

In pregnancy. Particular problems arise in the management of ITP in pregnancy, since antiplatelet antibodies can cross the placenta and produce thrombocytopenia in the fetus. The risk is greater when disease exists before pregnancy than when it develops in the course of pregnancy.

If therapy is considered necessary the mother may be given prednisolone or normal immunoglobulin, with platelet infusions for more serious, unresponsive symptoms.[2] A course of intravenous immunoglobulin before delivery is useful in protecting against postpartum complications. Treatment may be required for the neonate[2] if there are complications or the platelet count falls below 50 000 per mm³. Delivery by caesarean section may be considered.[4]

1. Karpatkin S. Autoimmune (idiopathic) thrombocytopenic purpura. *Lancet* 1997; **349:** 1531–6.
2. Provan AB. Management of adult idiopathic thrombocytopenic purpura. *Prescribers' J* 1992; **32:** 193–200.
3. Eden OB, Lilleyman JS. Guidelines for management of idiopathic thrombocytopenic purpura. *Arch Dis Child* 1992; **67:** 1056–8.
4. The American Society of Hematology ITP Practice Guideline Panel. Diagnosis and treatment of idiopathic thrombocytopenic purpura: recommendations of the American Society of Hematology. *Ann Intern Med* 1997; **126:** 319–26.
5. Gillis S. The thrombocytopenic purpuras: recognition and management. *Drugs* 1996; **51:** 942–53.
6. McMillan R. Therapy for adults with refractory chronic immune thrombocytopenic purpura. *Ann Intern Med* 1997; **126:** 307–14.
7. Tait RC, Evans DIK. Late spontaneous recovery of chronic thrombocytopenia. *Arch Dis Child* 1993; **68:** 680–1.
8. Stasi R, et al. Long-term observation of 208 adults with chronic idiopathic thrombocytopenic purpura. *Am J Med* 1995; **98:** 436–42.
9. von dem Borne AEGK, et al. High dose intravenous methylprednisolone or high dose intravenous gammaglobulin for autoimmune thrombocytopenia. *BMJ* 1988; **296:** 249–50.
10. Özsoylu Ş, et al. Megadose methylprednisolone for chronic idiopathic thrombocytopenic purpura. *Lancet* 1990; **336:** 1078–9.
11. Akoğlu T, et al. Megadose methylprednisolone pulse therapy in adult idiopathic thrombocytopenic purpura. *Lancet* 1991; **337:** 56.
12. Özsoylu S. Mega-dose methylprednisolone for chronic idiopathic thrombocytopenic purpura. *Lancet* 1991; **337:** 1611–12.
13. Alpdoğan Ö, et al. Efficacy of high-dose methylprednisolone as a first-line therapy in adult patients with idiopathic thrombocytopenic purpura. *Br J Haematol* 1998; **103:** 1061–3.
14. Albayrak D, et al. Acute immune thrombocytopenic purpura: a comparative study of very high oral doses of methylprednisolone and intravenously administered immune globulin. *J Pediatr* 1994; **125:** 1004–7.
15. Rosthøj S, et al. Randomized trial comparing intravenous immunoglobulin with methylprednisolone pulse therapy in acute idiopathic thrombocytopenic purpura. *Acta Paediatr* 1996; **85:** 910–15.
16. Andersen JC. Response of resistant idiopathic thrombocytopenic purpura to pulsed high-dose dexamethasone therapy. *N Engl J Med* 1994; **330:** 1560–4.
17. Adams DM, et al. High-dose oral dexamethasone therapy for chronic childhood idiopathic thrombocytopenic purpura. *J Pediatr* 1996; **128:** 281–3.
18. Borgna-Pignatti C, et al. A trial of high-dose dexamethasone therapy for chronic idiopathic thrombocytopenic purpura in childhood. *J Pediatr* 1997; **130:** 13–16.
19. Kühne T, et al. Platelet and immune responses to oral cyclic dexamethasone therapy in childhood chronic immune thrombocytopenic purpura. *J Pediatr* 1997; **130:** 17–24.
20. Blanchette VS, et al. A prospective, randomized trial of high-dose intravenous immune globulin G therapy, oral prednisone therapy, and no therapy in childhood acute immune thrombocytopenic purpura. *J Pediatr* 1993; **123:** 989–95.
21. Blanchette V, et al. Randomised trial of intravenous immunoglobulin G, intravenous anti-D, and oral prednisone in childhood acute immune thrombocytopenic purpura. *Lancet* 1994; **344:** 703–7.
22. Reid MM. Chronic idiopathic thrombocytopenic purpura: incidence, treatment, and outcome. *Arch Dis Child* 1995; **72:** 125–8.
23. Bolton-Maggs PHB, Moon I. Assessment of UK practice for management of acute childhood idiopathic thrombocytopenic purpura against published guidelines. *Lancet* 1997; **350:** 620–3.
24. Law C, et al. High-dose intravenous immune globulin and the response to splenectomy in patients with idiopathic thrombocytopenic purpura. *N Engl J Med* 1997; **336:** 1494–8.
25. Anonymous. Rho(D) immune globulin iv for prevention of Rh isoimmunization and for treatment of ITP. *Med Lett Drugs Ther* 1996; **38:** 6–8.
26. Andrew M, et al. A multicenter study of the treatment of childhood chronic idiopathic thrombocytopenic purpura with anti-D. *J Pediatr* 1992; **120:** 522–7.
27. Zunich KM, et al. Intravenous anti-D immunoglobulin for childhood acute immune thrombocytopenic purpura. *Lancet* 1995; **346:** 1363–4.
28. Blanchette V, Wang E. Intravenous anti-D immunoglobulin for childhood acute immune thrombocytopenic purpura. *Lancet* 1995; **346:** 1364–5.
29. Gaines AR. Acute onset hemoglobinemia and/or hemoglobinuria and sequelae following Rh₀(D) immune globulin intravenous administration in immune thrombocytopenic purpura patients. *Blood* 2000; **95:** 2523–9.
30. Buelli M, et al. Danazol for the treatment of idiopathic thrombocytopenic purpura. *Acta Haematol (Basel)* 1985; **74:** 97–8.
31. Mylvaganam R, et al. Very low dose danazol in idiopathic thrombocytopenic purpura and its role as an immune modulator. *Am J Med Sci* 1989; **298:** 215–20.
32. Ahn YS, et al. Long-term danazol therapy in autoimmune thrombocytopenia: unmaintained remission and age-dependent response in women. *Ann Intern Med* 1989; **111:** 723–9.
33. Edelmann DZ, et al. Danazol in non-splenectomized patients with refractory idiopathic thrombocytopenic purpura. *Postgrad Med J* 1990; **66:** 827–30.
34. McVerry BA, et al. The use of danazol in the management of chronic immune thrombocytopenic purpura. *Br J Haematol* 1985; **61:** 145–8.
35. Ahn YS, et al. The treatment of idiopathic thrombocytopenia with vinblastine-loaded platelets. *N Engl J Med* 1978; **298:** 1101–7.
36. Agnelli G, et al. Vinca-loaded platelets. *N Engl J Med* 1984; **311:** 599.
37. Ahn YS, et al. Vinca-loaded platelets. *N Engl J Med* 1984; **311:** 599–600.
38. Rosse WF. Whatever happened to vinca-loaded platelets? *N Engl J Med* 1984; **310:** 1051–2.
39. Figueroa M, et al. Combination chemotherapy in refractory immune thrombocytopenic purpura. *N Engl J Med* 1993; **328:** 1226–9.
40. McMillan R. Long-term outcomes after treatment for refractory immune thrombocytopenic purpura. *N Engl J Med* 2001; **344:** 1402–3.
41. Strother SV, et al. Colchicine therapy for refractory idiopathic thrombocytopenic purpura. *Arch Intern Med* 1984; **144:** 2198–2200.
42. Jim RTS. Therapeutic use of colchicine in thrombocytopenia. *Hawaii Med J* 1986; **45:** 221–6.
43. Baker RI, Manoharan A. Colchicine therapy for idiopathic thrombocytopenic purpura—an inexpensive alternative. *Aust N Z J Med* 1989; **19:** 412–13.
44. Shen ZX, et al. Thrombocytopoietic effect of heparin given in chronic immune thrombocytopenic purpura. *Lancet* 1995; **346:** 220–1.
45. Cohen HA, et al. Treatment of chronic idiopathic thrombocytopenic purpura with ascorbate. *Clin Pediatr (Phila)* 1993; **32:** 300–2.
46. Schick BP. Hope for treatment of thrombocytopenia. *N Engl J Med* 1994; **331:** 875–6.

Infections

Although long-term corticosteroid therapy has an adverse effect on the body's response to infection (see Effects on Immune Response, under Adverse Effects, p.1041), the judicious use of corticosteroids, usually on a short-term basis, and in conjunction with appropriate chemotherapeutic agents, may have a beneficial effect on the symptoms of selected acute infections, and may on occasions be life-saving. Guidelines have been published concerning a number of infections and whether corticosteroids should be employed or not.[1]

For further comment on the use of corticosteroids in ocular herpes infections, infectious mononucleosis, leishmaniasis, leprosy, meningitis, *Pneumocystis carinii* pneumonia in AIDS patients, septic shock, and tuberculosis, see under the relevant headings in this section.

1. McGowan JE, et al. Report by the Working Group on Steroid Use, Antimicrobial Agents Committee, Infectious Diseases Society of America: Guidelines for the use of systemic glucocorticoids in the management of selected infections. *J Infect Dis* 1992; **165:** 1–13.

Infectious mononucleosis

In a short discussion on the use of corticosteroids in infectious mononucleosis (glandular fever—see Epstein-Barr Virus Infections, p.607) it was considered that although all cases would respond promptly to therapy, only patients with an unduly prolonged infection and those with an exceptionally severe sore throat that interferes with either respiratory function or eating should be treated with a corticosteroid.[1] Most experts would use corticosteroids in patients with severe thrombocytopenia, haemolytic anaemia, encephalitis, pericarditis, or myocarditis associated with infection by the Epstein-Barr virus. Doses of prednisone may be 80 mg daily initially, decreasing gradually and withdrawn after 14 days. Prednisone is very safe in infectious mononucleosis but the theoretical risk of impairing immunity is a concern as there might be an increased risk of Epstein-Barr virus-related tumours in later life.[1] Others have also expressed a relatively negative view of the value of corticosteroids.[2]

1. Sheagren JN. Corticosteroids for treatment of mononucleosis and aphthous stomatitis. *JAMA* 1986; **256:** 1051.
2. McGowan JE, et al. Report by the Working Group on Steroid Use, Antimicrobial Agents Committee, Infectious Diseases Society of America: Guidelines for the use of systemic glucocorticoids in the management of selected infections. *J Infect Dis* 1992; **165:** 1–13.

Inflammatory bowel disease

Together with aminosalicylates, the corticosteroids form the mainstay of treatment for active ulcerative colitis and Crohn's disease (see Inflammatory Bowel Disease, p.1205). In moderate to severe acute disease systemic corticosteroids are indicated for initial management, either orally or in the most severe cases intravenously. Doses are high initially and are gradually reduced as symptoms resolve. In patients with disease confined to the distal colon or rectum, local topical therapy with suppositories or enemas of corticosteroids are appropriate. Oral or rectal formulations of poorly absorbed or rapidly metabolised corticosteroids such as beclometasone, budesonide, or tixocortol have been developed in the hope of producing local improvement without systemic effects.

Juvenile osteopetrosis

Osteopetrosis is a rare set of heterogeneous disorders characterised by an increase in bone density, generally due to a failure of the osteoclasts to resorb mineralised bone. In the severe forms there is reduction in the bone marrow space, leading to anaemia, hepatosplenomegaly, and nerve compression which may produce blindness and deafness; early death often results.

Bone marrow transplantation may be curative if a suitable donor can be found.[1] Corticosteroids are used palliatively. Benefit has been reported in 3 of 4 children treated with prednisone 1 mg per kg body-weight daily by mouth, together with phosphate supplements and a low-calcium diet.[2] Some patients have also benefited from the use of high-dose calcitriol, again with a low-calcium diet.[3]

Another study, in 14 patients, found that treatment with interferon gamma-1b increased bone resorption.[4] In 11 who received this treatment for 18 months there were stabilisation or improvement in clinical condition and a reduction in the frequency of serious infection.

1. Gerritsen EJ, et al. Bone marrow transplantation for autosomal recessive osteopetrosis: a report from the Working Party on Inborn Errors of the European Bone Marrow Transplantation Group. *J Pediatr* 1994; **125:** 896–902.
2. Dorantes LM, et al. Juvenile osteopetrosis: effects on blood and bone of prednisone and a low calcium, high phosphate diet. *Arch Dis Child* 1986; **61:** 666–70.
3. Key LL, Ries WL. Osteopetrosis: the pharmaco-physiologic basis of therapy. *Clin Orthop* 1993; **294:** 85–9.
4. Key LL, et al. Long-term treatment of osteopetrosis with recombinant human interferon gamma. *N Engl J Med* 1995; **332:** 1594–9.

Leishmaniasis

Corticosteroids may be required to control severe inflammation in patients with mucocutaneous leishmaniasis (p.584), although pentavalent antimony is the drug used for initial treatment.

Leprosy

Type I lepra (reversal) reactions in patients with leprosy (p.126) frequently respond to high-dose corticosteroids (for example 40 to 60 mg of prednisolone daily) started immediately and given for several days.[1] Doses may be reduced over several weeks or months. Corticosteroids may also be used for type II reactions.

Corticosteroid treatment of nerve function impairment should be started within 6 months of onset, as the earlier that treatment is started, the more likely it is that function will be restored. A standardised regimen in which the usual adult dose was 40 mg daily of prednisolone for 4 weeks, tapered over the following 12 weeks, has been successfully used in the field management of acute nerve function impairment,[2] as has a regimen consisting of 30 mg of prednisone for 2 weeks tapered down with a minimum duration of 10 weeks.[3]

1. WHO. WHO expert committee on leprosy. *WHO Tech Rep Ser* 874 1998.
2. Croft RP, *et al.* Field treatment of acute nerve function impairment in leprosy using a standardized corticosteroid regimen—first year's experience with 100 patients. *Lepr Rev* 1997; **68:** 316–25.
3. Bernink EHM, Voskens JEJ. Study on the detection of leprosy reactions and the effect of prednisone on various nerves, Indonesia. *Lepr Rev* 1997; **68:** 225–32.

Lichen

Lichen planus (p.1106) is generally controlled with corticosteroids applied topically, or occasionally, injected intralesionally; systemic corticosteroids (usually prednisone or prednisolone) are used for severe erosive lichen planus.[1,2] Prednisone has generally been used in oral doses of 30 to 60 mg daily, for courses of 4 to 6 weeks.[1] Shorter courses may be of value: prednisolone (30 mg daily for 10 days) was reported to be effective and safe for mild or moderately severe lichen planus.[3]

The use of topically applied corticosteroids in the treatment of lichen sclerosus (a degenerative disease of upper dermal connective tissue, particularly around the genitals) has been discussed.[4] Relief from vulvar pruritus is obtained in most cases with a potent corticosteroid preparation, such as clobetasol propionate, applied twice daily for up to 3 months before tapering the dose.[4]

1. Cribier B, *et al.* Treatment of lichen planus: an evidence-based medicine analysis of efficacy. *Arch Dermatol* 1998; **134:** 1521–30.
2. Edwards L. Vulvar lichen planus. *Arch Dermatol* 1989; **125:** 1677–80.
3. Kellett JK, Ead RD. Treatment of lichen planus with a short course of oral prednisolone. *Br J Dermatol* 1990; **123:** 550–1.
4. Powell JJ, Wojnarowska F. Lichen sclerosus. *Lancet* 1999; **353:** 1777–83.

Liver disorders

Corticosteroids are considered to be useful in chronic active hepatitis (p.1048). There is some disagreement over the benefit from corticosteroid therapy in alcoholic liver disease with hepatic encephalopathy,[1-6] and they do not appear to be of benefit in acute hepatic failure.[7] Corticosteroid therapy may however be of benefit in sclerosing cholangitis.[8]

No treatment has proven unequivocally successful in the management of primary biliary cirrhosis (p.501). Corticosteroids are one of a number of drugs for which reports of benefit exist, but their use has been restricted as they may exacerbate bone disease.

1. Black M, Tavill AS. Corticosteroids in severe alcoholic hepatitis. *Ann Intern Med* 1989; **110:** 677–80.
2. Imperiale TF, McCullough AJ. Do corticosteroids reduce mortality from alcoholic hepatitis? A meta-analysis of the randomized trials. *Ann Intern Med* 1990; **113:** 299–307.
3. Thomson AD, *et al.* Alcoholic liver disease. *Gut* 1991; (suppl): S97–103.
4. Ramond M-J, *et al.* A randomized trial of prednisolone in patients with severe alcoholic hepatitis. *N Engl J Med* 1992; **326:** 507–12.
5. Wrona SA, Tankanow RM. Corticosteroids in the management of alcoholic hepatitis. *Am J Hosp Pharm* 1994; **51:** 347–53.
6. Christensen E, Gluud C. Glucocorticoids are ineffective in alcoholic hepatitis: a meta-analysis adjusting for confounding variables. *Gut* 1995; **37:** 113–18.
7. Caraceni P, Van Thiel DH. Acute liver failure. *Lancet* 1995; **345:** 163–9.
8. Lindor KD, *et al.* Advances in primary sclerosing cholangitis. *Am J Med* 1990; **89:** 73–80.

Male infertility

Immunosuppressive treatment with corticosteroids is given for male infertility (p.1275) due to low-grade autoimmune orchitis.[1] Examples of regimens after which pregnancy has been successfully achieved in female partners include oral methylprednisolone 96 mg daily for 7 days beginning on day 21 of the partner's menstrual cycle[2] and oral prednisolone 20 mg twice daily on days 1 to 10 of the partner's menstrual cycle plus 5 mg on days 11 and 12.[3] However, there is a lack of evidence from substantial controlled trials of benefit from corticosteroid therapy in men with auto-immune causes of infertility.

1. Haidl G, Schill W-B. Guidelines for drug treatment of male infertility. *Drugs* 1991; **41:** 60–8.
2. Shulman JF, Shulman S. Methylprednisolone treatment of immunologic infertility in the male. *Fertil Steril* 1982; **38:** 591–9.
3. Hendry WF, *et al.* Comparison of prednisolone and placebo in subfertile men with antibodies to spermatozoa. *Lancet* 1990; **335:** 85–8.

Malignant neoplasms

Corticosteroids are extensively prescribed in malignant disease for the relief of pain, nerve compression, or raised intracranial pressure; to alleviate dyspnoea, effusion, or hypercalcaemia; to counteract adverse effects of other therapies such as antineoplastic-induced nausea and vomiting or radiation-induced inflammation; and in the management of cachexia and to improve mood and sense of well-being.[1] In addition they form an important part of multidrug anticancer regimens used for various haematological malignancies such as acute lymphoblastic leukaemia (p.484) and Hodgkin's disease (p.487).

1. Twycross R. The risks and benefits of corticosteroids in advanced cancer. *Drug Safety* 1994; **11:** 163–78.

Meningitis

Corticosteroids may be given as adjuncts to antibacterial therapy in bacterial meningitis (p.128), in the hope of moderating any neurological sequelae; there is some evidence that dexamethasone, especially if given early, may reduce the risk of deafness in children with Haemophilus meningitis, although evidence of benefit in pneumococcal and meningococcal meningitis is scanty.

Mouth ulceration

Local treatment of mouth ulcers (p.1206) often involves a topical corticosteroid for symptomatic relief. Systemic corticosteroids have occasionally been given where there is severe underlying disease.

Multiple sclerosis

Corticosteroids are often employed in the management of multiple sclerosis (p.633). Corticosteroid therapy reduces the duration of the relapse and accelerates recovery from acute relapses, but it is not known whether it alters the course of the disease in the long term.[1,2] Methylprednisolone has superseded corticotropin and prednisolone as the drug of choice. Methylprednisolone is usually given intravenously in high doses (typically 1 g daily) for 3 to 5 days, sometimes followed by a tapering dose of oral prednisolone. Doses of up to 2 g of methylprednisolone daily have been tried.[3] In patients with acute optic neuritis (frequently the first manifestation of multiple sclerosis), methylprednisolone delayed the onset of other symptoms of multiple sclerosis[4] although the effect was not sustained beyond 2 years.[5] Beneficial responses have also been reported with oral methylprednisolone at doses including 500 mg once daily for 5 days followed by a tapering dose over 10 days[6] and 48 mg once daily for 7 days followed by a tapering dose over 14 days.[7]

In patients with primary progressive disease, the benefits of short-course methylprednisolone lasted no longer than 3 months[8] although in patients with secondary progressive disease, a preliminary study has suggested that progression may be delayed by intermittent high-dose methylprednisolone therapy.[9]

1. Rudick RA, *et al.* Management of multiple sclerosis. *N Engl Med J* 1997; **337:** 1604–11.
2. Filippini G, *et al.* Corticosteroids or ACTH for acute exacerbations in multiple sclerosis (updated 29 May 2001). Available in The Cochrane Library; Issue 3. Oxford: Update Software; 2001.
3. Oliveri RL, *et al.* Randomized trial comparing two different high doses of methylprednisolone in MS: a clinical and MRI study. *Neurology* 1998; **50:** 1833–6.
4. Beck RW, *et al.* The effect of corticosteroids for acute optic neuritis on the subsequent development of multiple sclerosis. *N Engl J Med* 1993; **329:** 1764–9.
5. Beck RW, *et al.* The optic neuritis treatment trial: three-year follow-up results. *Arch Ophthalmol* 1995; **113:** 136–7.
6. Sellebjerg F, *et al.* Double-blind, randomized, placebo-controlled study of oral, high-dose methylprednisolone in attacks of MS. *Neurology* 1998; **51:** 529–34.

7. Barnes D, *et al.* Randomised trial of oral and intravenous methylprednisolone in acute relapses of multiple sclerosis. *Lancet* 1997; **349:** 902–6.
8. Cazzato G, *et al.* Double-blind, placebo-controlled, randomized, crossover trial of high-dose methylprednisolone in patients with chronic progressive form of multiple sclerosis. *Eur Neurol* 1995; **35:** 193–8.
9. Goodkin DE, *et al.* A phase II study of IV methylprednisolone in secondary-progressive multiple sclerosis. *Neurology* 1998; **51:** 239–45.

Muscular dystrophies

Muscular dystrophies are a range of inherited myopathies in which there is progressive degeneration of muscle fibres and associated muscle weakness. They may be classified according to the mode of inheritance. The most common type is the fatal recessive X-linked **Duchenne muscular dystrophy** (DMD) in which there is a deficiency in the structural muscle protein dystrophin. There is no effective therapy that affects the ultimate outcome of the various muscular dystrophies. Management is mainly through the use of physiotherapy, supports, and surgery. Drug treatment has been tried for symptomatic management, but generally the number of patients studied has been small. However, prednisone given in doses of up to 2 mg per kg body-weight daily has been effective in increasing muscle strength in children and slowing the progression of Duchenne muscular dystrophy;[1-5] improvement does not appear to be sustained to the same degree with alternate day therapy.[4] Benefit has also been seen with deflazacort.[6] It has been suggested that the failure of azathioprine to produce any beneficial effect when used alone or added to prednisone treatment might indicate that prednisone's effectiveness is not due to immunosuppression.[5] There have also been reports of benefit in small numbers of patients given ciclosporin; evidence to support the use of most other drugs (e.g. allopurinol) is either conflicting or unconvincing. The possible use of gene therapy is being studied.

1. DeSilva S, *et al.* Prednisone treatment in Duchenne muscular dystrophy: long-term benefit. *Arch Neurol* 1987; **44:** 818–22.
2. Mendell JR, *et al.* Randomized double-blind six-month trial of prednisone in Duchenne's muscular dystrophy. *N Engl J Med* 1989; **320:** 1592–7.
3. Griggs RC, *et al.* Prednisone in Duchenne dystrophy: a randomized, controlled trial defining the time course and dose response. *Arch Neurol* 1991; **48:** 383–8.
4. Fenichel GM, *et al.* A comparison of daily and alternate-day prednisone therapy in the treatment of Duchenne muscular dystrophy. *Arch Neurol* 1991; **48:** 575–9.
5. Griggs RC, *et al.* Duchenne dystrophy: randomized, controlled trial of prednisone (18 months) and azathioprine (12 months). *Neurology* 1993; **43:** 520–7.
6. Bigger WD, *et al.* Deflazacort treatment of Duchenne muscular dystrophy. *J Pediatr* 2001; **138:** 45–50.

Myasthenia gravis

Corticosteroids are the main immunosuppressants used in the management of myasthenia gravis (p.1414), and are employed in patients who are seriously ill prior to thymectomy or insufficiently improved after thymectomy, as well as in those who are unsuitable for surgical treatment.

Nasal polyps

Nasal polyps are outgrowths of the nasal mucosa, typically pale, smooth, translucent, and round or pear-shaped.[1,2] They are often associated with a history of rhinitis or asthma; the triad of nasal polyps, asthma, and hypersensitivity to aspirin may occur. Patients typically present with obstruction, loss of smell, and often rhinorrhoea and postnasal drip.

Corticosteroids are extremely effective in reducing polyp size, either by intranasal[3] or systemic administration. In the former case beginning with betamethasone sodium phosphate nasal drops, and subsequently maintaining the reduction with an intranasal spray such as beclometasone, budesonide, or fluticasone, has been suggested.[1] Alternatively prednisone, prednisolone, or dexamethasone can be given by mouth: suggested regimens have included prednisone 60 mg daily, tapered over 10 or 14 days and followed by intranasal corticosteroids,[2] or dexamethasone 12, 8, and 4 mg daily, each for 3 days.[1] Surgery may be necessary where there is marked obstruction, and most patients require it at some point,[1] although polyps usually recur. Pre-operative administration of systemic corticosteroids may help reduce recurrence.[2] Continued use of topical corticosteroids may reduce the frequency of relapses.[3]

1. Lund VJ. Diagnosis and treatment of nasal polyps. *BMJ* 1995; **311:** 1411–14.
2. Slavin RG. Nasal polyps and sinusitis. *JAMA* 1997; **278:** 1849–54.
3. Badia L, Lund V. Topical corticosteroids in nasal polyposis. *Drugs* 2001; **61:** 573–8.

Nausea and vomiting

Corticosteroids, usually in the form of dexamethasone, play an important role in antiemetic regimens (see p.1206) used to combat the effects of moderately to severely emetogenic cancer chemotherapy: they have been shown to enhance the effects of both metoclopramide- and 5-HT$_3$ antagonist-based regimens. Dexamethasone is probably the most effective single agent available against delayed emesis at present.

Neonatal intraventricular haemorrhage

For the suggestion that antenatal corticosteroids may reduce the incidence of intraventricular haemorrhage in neonates, see p.723.

Neonatal respiratory distress syndrome

Neonatal respiratory distress syndrome is a condition of increasing respiratory distress occurring at, or shortly after, birth and marked by cyanosis, tachypnoea, expiratory grunting and sternal retraction. Symptoms increase in severity with progressive collapse of the lung (atelectasis), leakage of plasma into alveolar spaces, and the formation of hyaline membranes, until death occurs or slow recovery takes place from about the 2nd to 4th day. The syndrome affects primarily premature infants and its incidence increases with the degree of prematurity; severe problems are most likely in those delivered before 30 weeks' gestation. Symptoms are thought to be at least partly due to inadequate amounts of surfactant in the premature lung resulting in high internal surface tension and increased risk of alveolar collapse, but in very immature infants other factors, possibly including impaired sodium and fluid absorption from the lung, may play a role.[1]

Treatment. The optimum treatment is prevention, and UK guidelines[2] recommend the administration of betamethasone or dexamethasone twice daily by intramuscular injection for 2 days to women in whom delivery before 32 weeks of gestation is likely. Results are best if treatment is given more than 24 hours but less than 7 days before delivery. Similar recommendations apply elsewhere. In the USA, for example, antenatal corticosteroid treatment is recommended for women between 24 and 34 weeks of pregnancy who show signs of premature delivery.[3] An overview of studies of antenatal corticosteroid therapy suggests that it may reduce the risk of respiratory distress syndrome by about 50% overall;[4] the risk of death, and of periventricular haemorrhage and necrotising enterocolitis is also reduced. Whether repeat courses should be considered as uncertain, although the practice has become widespread; it has been recommended that it be restricted to patients in clinical trials.[5] Delaying delivery with beta$_2$ agonists (see Premature Labour, p.773) may be considered to increase the time available for management with antenatal corticosteroids.[2] Reported benefit from adding protirelin to antenatal corticosteroids has not been borne out by 2 large multicentre studies.[6-8] The earlier of these studies actually found neonatal outcome and maternal morbidity to be worse in those who also received protirelin,[6,7] but this conclusion has been questioned.[9,10]

In infants born with the syndrome rapid supportive care is required, which may include correction of metabolic acidosis, circulatory support, oxygen supplementation, and assisted ventilation, although there is a lack of consensus about the most appropriate method for these.[2] It has been suggested that ventilation using a helium-oxygen mixture gives better results than a nitrogen-oxygen mix.[11] Another alternative may be the use of partial liquid ventilation with the fluorocarbon compound perflubron.[12] Meta-analysis suggests that inhaled nitric oxide improves outcomes in infants born at or near term who are hypoxaemic,[13] but evidence of benefit in preterm infants has not been shown.[14] The majority of infants survive the acute episode with careful management, although associated complications may subsequently develop, including bronchopulmonary dysplasia (see p.1048), retinopathy of prematurity (p.1395), and cerebral palsy. There is some evidence that supplementation with inositol can reduce the incidence of adverse outcomes in preterm infants.[15]

Since deficiency of surfactant is considered to play an important role in the neonatal respiratory distress syndrome, the use of surfactant replacement therapy has been intensively investigated, and is now accepted as reducing the risk of death from the disease and the development of pneumothorax and other lung complications.[2,16,17] Both natural and synthetic surfactants have

been used: although both are effective there is some evidence that results are better with the preparations of natural origin.[18-20] Natural surfactants of differing origins may also vary in their properties: poractant,[21] or calfactant,[22] have both been reported to give better responses than beractant. Surfactant is given as a suspension by endotracheal tube directly into the infant's lung, although other means of administration, such as nebulisers, have been investigated. Most surfactants are given in recommended doses of 100 to 200 mg phospholipids per kg birth-weight. Repeat doses may be given if necessary, and a meta-analysis[23] of data from two randomised controlled trials utilising preparations of natural surfactant extract in neonates with established disease found a more favourable clinical outcome, including a decreased risk of pneumothorax, with multiple rather than single doses. However, in clinical practice the number of doses and the dosage interval varies. One large study found that a dose of 100 mg per kg, repeated twice, was as effective as 200 mg per kg followed by up to four further doses of 100 mg per kg.[24] Another found that 3 doses, given at 12-hour intervals with the first dose shortly after birth were more effective than the first dose alone in improving physiological findings and mortality rates in low birth-weight infants.[25] One large multicentre randomised controlled trial[26] investigated the difference between administering repeat doses of a surfactant (calfactant) at a low threshold of respiratory support, as recommended by the manufacturer, versus a higher threshold. The conclusion was that efficacy was not compromised by delaying surfactant re-treatment in infants with uncomplicated respiratory distress syndrome until they had reached a higher level of respiratory support than is currently recommended, but infants with complications should continue to be treated by the currently recommended low-threshold strategy.

There has been debate whether 'prophylactic' early therapy, given immediately after birth to all infants deemed at risk of the syndrome, or delayed therapy given 2 or more hours after birth to intubated infants who have developed symptoms, is the more appropriate,[2,27] but the large OSIRIS study,[28] and later systematic reviews,[29,30] found in favour of early intervention.

1. Barker PM, et al. Decreased sodium ion absorption across nasal epithelium of very premature infants with respiratory distress syndrome. J Pediatr 1997; 130: 373–7.
2. Report of a Joint Working Group of the British Association of Perinatal Medicine and the Research Unit of the Royal College of Physicians. Development of audit measures and guidelines for good practice in the management of neonatal respiratory distress syndrome. Arch Dis Child 1992; 67: 1221–7.
3. NIH Consensus Development Panel on the Effect of Corticosteroids for Fetal Maturation on Perinatal Outcomes. Effect of corticosteroids for fetal maturation on perinatal outcomes. JAMA 1995; 273: 413–18.
4. Crowley PA. Antenatal corticosteroid therapy: a meta-analysis of the randomized trials, 1972 to 1994. Am J Obstet Gynecol 1995; 173: 322–35.
5. National Institutes of Health. Consensus development conference statement—antenatal corticosteroids revisited: repeat courses. Available at: http://odp.od.nih.gov/consensus/cons/112/112_statement.htm (accessed 14/06/01).
6. ACTOBAT Study Group. Australian collaborative trial of antenatal thyrotropin-releasing hormone (ACTOBAT) for prevention of neonatal respiratory disease. Lancet 1995; 345: 877–82.
7. Crowther CA, et al. Australian Collaborative Trial of antenatal thyrotropin-releasing hormone: adverse effects at 12-month follow-up. Pediatrics 1997; 99: 311–17.
8. Ballard RA, et al. Antenatal thyrotropin-releasing hormone to prevent lung disease in preterm infants. N Engl J Med 1998; 338: 493–8.
9. Moya FR, Maturana A. Thyrotropin-releasing hormone for prevention of neonatal respiration disease. Lancet 1995; 345: 1572–3.
10. McCormick MC. The credibility of the ACTOBAT follow-up study. Pediatrics 1997; 99: 476–8.
11. Elleau C, et al. Helium-oxygen mixture in respiratory distress syndrome: a double-blind study. J Pediatr 1993; 122: 132–6.
12. Leach CL, et al. Partial liquid ventilation with perflubron in premature infants with severe respiratory distress syndrome. N Engl J Med 1996; 335: 761–7.
13. Finer NN, et al. Nitric oxide for respiratory failure in infants born at or near term (updated 13 February 2001). Available in The Cochrane Library; Issue 3. Oxford: Update Software; 2001.
14. Barrington KJ, Finer NN. Inhaled nitric oxide for respiratory failure in preterm infants (updated 14 May 2001). Available in The Cochrane Library; Issue 3. Oxford: Update Software; 2001.
15. Howlett A, Ohlsson A. Inositol for respiratory distress syndrome in preterm infants (updated 27 February 2001). Available in The Cochrane Library; Issue 3. Oxford: Update Software; 2001.
16. Schwartz RM, et al. Effect of surfactant on morbidity, mortality, and resource use in newborn infants weighing 500 to 1500 g. N Engl J Med 1994; 330: 1476–80.
17. Walti H, Monset-Couchard M. A risk-benefit assessment of natural and synthetic exogenous surfactants in the management of neonatal respiratory distress syndrome. Drug Safety 1998; 18: 321–37.
18. Halliday HL. Natural vs synthetic surfactants in neonatal respiratory distress syndrome. Drugs 1996; 51: 226–37.
19. Hudak ML, et al. A multicenter randomized, masked comparison trial of natural versus synthetic surfactant for the treatment of respiratory distress syndrome. J Pediatr 1996; 128: 396–406.
20. Soll RF, Blanco F. Natural surfactant extract versus synthetic surfactant for neonatal respiratory distress syndrome (updated 26 February 2001). Available in The Cochrane Library; Issue 3. Oxford: Update Software; 2001.
21. Speer CP, et al. Randomised clinical trial of two treatment regimens of natural surfactant preparations in neonatal respiratory distress syndrome. Arch Dis Child 1995; 72: F8–F13.
22. Bloom BT, et al. Randomized double-blind multicenter trial of Survanta (SURV) and Infasurf (IS). Pediatr Res 1994; 35: 326.
23. Soll RF. Multiple versus single dose natural surfactant extract for severe neonatal respiratory distress syndrome (updated 27 February 2001). Available in The Cochrane Library; Issue 3. Oxford: Update Software; 2001.
24. Halliday HL, et al. Multicentre randomised trial comparing high and low dose surfactant regimens for the treatment of respiratory distress syndrome (the Curosurf 4 trial). Arch Dis Child 1993; 69: 276–80.
25. Corbet A, et al. Double-blind, randomized trial of one versus three prophylactic doses of synthetic surfactant in 826 neonates weighing 700 to 1100 grams: effects on mortality rate. J Pediatr 1995; 126: 969–74.
26. Kattwinkel J, et al. High- versus low-threshold surfactant re-treatment for neonatal respiratory distress syndrome. Pediatrics 2000; 106: 282–8.
27. Dunn MS. Surfactant replacement therapy: prophylaxis or treatment? Pediatrics 1993; 92: 148–50.
28. The OSIRIS Collaborative Group (Open Study of Infants at high risk of or with Respiratory Insufficiency—the role of surfactant). Early versus delayed neonatal administration of a synthetic surfactant—the judgement of OSIRIS. Lancet 1992; 340: 1363–9.
29. Morley CJ. Systematic review of prophylactic vs rescue surfactant. Arch Dis Child 1997; 77: F70–4.
30. Yost CC, Soll RF. Early versus delayed selective surfactant treatment for neonatal respiratory distress syndrome (updated 16 November 2001). Available in The Cochrane Library; Issue 3. Oxford: Update Software; 2001.

Optic neuropathies

Improvement in vision was reported in patients with auto-immune optic neuropathy following 5 to 7 days of treatment with high doses of intravenous methylprednisolone (1 to 2 g daily) or oral prednisolone (80 to 400 mg daily).[1] In some patients, recurrent visual loss required repeated high-dose intravenous methylprednisolone, an increase in oral prednisolone dosage, or additional immunosuppressants, but in many patients visual benefits were maintained even when treatment was withdrawn. Visual recovery has also been reported in patients with optic neuritis of unknown aetiology receiving intravenous methylprednisolone 250 or 500 mg every 6 hours for 3 to 7 days.[2] One study has found oral prednisone alone (1 mg per kg body-weight daily for 14 days) to be ineffective whereas intravenous methylprednisolone (1 g daily for 3 days) followed by oral prednisone (1 mg per kg daily for 11 days) was beneficial in the treatment of acute optic neuritis.[3] A review of corticosteroid use in optic neuritis concluded that high-dose oral or parenteral methylprednisolone, or corticotropin, were of value in the treatment of acute disease. However, their long-term benefit could not be determined.[4]

1. Kupersmith MJ, et al. Autoimmune optic neuropathy: evaluation and treatment. J Neurol Neurosurg Psychiatry 1988; 51: 1381–6.
2. Spoor TC, Rockwell DL. Treatment of optic neuritis with intravenous megadose corticosteroids: a consecutive series. Ophthalmology 1988; 95: 131–4.
3. Beck RW, et al. A randomized, controlled trial of corticosteroids in the treatment of acute optic neuritis. N Engl J Med 1992; 326: 581–8.
4. Kaufman DI, et al. Practice parameter: the role of corticosteroids in the management of acute monosymptomatic optic neuritis: report of the quality standards subcommittee of the American Academy of Neurology. Neurology 2000; 54: 2039–44.

Organ and tissue transplantation

For a discussion of organ and tissue transplantation, including the role of corticosteroids, see under Choice of Immunosuppressant, p.502.

Osteoarthritis

In contrast to rheumatoid arthritis, systemic corticosteroids are not considered to have a place in the management of osteoarthritis (p.9); intra-articular or peri-articular injection, although controversial, may be of some help in patients with localised inflammation. Such injections should be given only infrequently and as adjunctive therapy.

Pain

Corticosteroids have produced improvement, often substantial, in neuropathic pain, including pain due to nerve damage and sympathetically maintained pain, and are widely used in conditions such as chronic low back pain and cancer pain. Dexamethasone, methylprednisolone, and prednisolone have been used for pain management, sometimes in the form of long-acting depot injections administered locally. The exact mechanism of action of corticosteroids in analgesia is not clear but may involve relief of pressure on nervous tissue by reduction of inflammation and oedema.

For discussions of pain and its management, see p.2.

Pancreatitis

Corticosteroids are generally contra-indicated for pancreatitis (p.1646), but a response has been reported[1,2] in patients with acute episodes caused by sarcoidosis (p.1058).

1. McCormick PA, et al. Pancreatitis in sarcoidosis. BMJ 1985; 290: 1472–3.
2. Limaye AP, et al. Sarcoidosis associated with recurrent pancreatitis. South Med J 1997; 90: 431–3.

Pemphigus and pemphigoid

Systemic corticosteroids are the mainstay of management of pemphigus and pemphigoid (p.1106). Initially high doses are used to control blistering and doses up to 400 mg of prednisolone daily have been suggested, although most dermatologists attempt to keep the dose below 120 mg daily. Adjuvant therapy with an immunosuppressant such as azathioprine, cyclophosphamide, or gold may be used.[1] Maintenance treatment must be individualised, but in general the dose of prednisolone should be reduced by 50% every 2 to 3 weeks. When the daily dose has been lowered to 80 mg daily it is desirable to convert gradually to alternate-day therapy. During this period topical therapy with potent corticosteroids is useful and is also a valuable first-line treatment for early relapses. A combined corticosteroid-antibacterial preparation also reduces the chance of infection. Therapy for mucous membranes is also based on the use of corticosteroids, applied topically, sucked as lozenges, or possibly inhaled. High dose oral prednisolone and oral cyclophosphamide have also been found to be effective in relieving inflammation in patients with ocular cicatricial pemphigoid, although they may not completely prevent cicatrisation.[2]

With the aim of reducing adverse effects, corticosteroids have been given in lower initial doses by mouth (prednisolone 45 to 60 mg daily)[3] or by intravenous pulse therapy (dexamethasone 136 mg given over 1 to 2 hours daily for 3 days, repeated at least monthly, with intravenous cyclophosphamide 500 mg infused on day 1);[4] pemphigus responded to both of these regimens.

Bullous pemphigoid has responded to high potency corticosteroids applied topically.[5]

1. Carson PJ, et al. Influence of treatment on the clinical course of pemphigus vulgaris. J Am Acad Dermatol 1996; 34: 645–52.
2. Elder MJ, et al. Role of cyclophosphamide and high dose steroid in ocular cicatricial pemphigoid. Br J Ophthalmol 1995; 79: 264–6.
3. Ratnam KV, et al. Pemphigus therapy with oral prednisolone regimens. Int J Dermatol 1990; 29: 363–7.
4. Kaur S, Kanwar AJ. Dexamethasone–cyclophosphamide pulse therapy in pemphigus. Int J Dermatol 1990; 29: 371–4.
5. Westerhof W. Treatment of bullous pemphigoid with topical clobetasol propionate. J Am Acad Dermatol 1989; 20: 458–61.

Pneumocystis carinii pneumonia

The management of Pneumocystis carinii pneumonia (p.375) is primarily with either co-trimoxazole or pentamidine. In patients with moderate or severe attacks, adjuvant therapy with high-dose oral or intravenous corticosteroids reduces both the risk of respiratory failure and the risk of death.[1,2] Concerns about the potential for further immunosuppression with such adjuvant therapy in patients with HIV infection[3] do not seem to have been borne out: a comparative study noted no increase in mortality or the risk of developing other opportunistic infections.[4]

1. Miller RF, et al. Pneumocystis carinii infection: current treatment and prevention. J Antimicrob Chemother 1996; 37 (suppl B): 33–53.
2. Bye MR, et al. Markedly reduced mortality associated with corticosteroid therapy of Pneumocystis carinii pneumonia in children with acquired immunodeficiency syndrome. Arch Pediatr Adolesc Med 1994; 148: 638–41.
3. Nelson MR, et al. Treatment with corticosteroids—a risk factor for the development of clinical cytomegalovirus disease in AIDS. AIDS 1993; 7: 375–8.
4. Gallant JE, et al. The effect of adjunctive corticosteroids for the treatment of Pneumocystis carinii pneumonia on mortality and subsequent complications. Chest 1998; 114: 1258–63.

Polyarteritis nodosa and microscopic polyangiitis

Polyarteritis nodosa is considered the prototype of systemic necrotising vasculitis. It may occur at any age but is more common in white patients and in men. It is characterised by inflammation throughout the arterial wall with fibrinoid necrosis of the arterial media, particularly in medium-sized vessels, partial occlusion of the vessel due to proliferation of the intima (possibly leading to thrombosis and infarction), fibrosis, and the formation of aneurysms. Microscopic polyangiitis, in which small vessels are primarily involved, with frequent renal and pulmonary involvement, has been seen as part of the spectrum of polyarteritis nodosa but is now considered an entity in its own right, although patients may have features of both. Antineutrophil cytoplasmic antibodies (ANCA) are common in patients with microscopic polyangiitis but not in classic polyarteritis nodosa.

Symptoms vary depending on the vessels affected but most patients have fever, weight loss, myalgia, and arthralgia. Gastrointestinal involvement may be marked by mouth ulceration, diarrhoea, visceral pain, haemorrhage, or sometimes infarction of the bowel, while involvement of liver can lead to hepatomegaly or hepatic necrosis and pancreatic involvement may simulate pancreatitis. Renal involvement may present as acute glomerulonephritis and renal failure or as nephrotic syndrome; like pulmonary involvement it is a feature particularly of microscopic polyarteritis, and associated with a poor prognosis. Skin lesions, peripheral neuropathies, alterations in mental function, convulsions, episcleritis or scleritis and retinal vasculitis, ischaemic heart disease, heart failure, Raynaud's phenomenon, and hypertension are among other potential symptoms. If untreated, death, usually due to renal or cardiac involvement, occurs in about 90% of patients within 5 years.

Classic polyarteritis nodosa may respond to treatment with a corticosteroid given alone, typically prednisone or prednisolone in a dose of 40 to 60 mg daily; however, although the benefits of adding a cytotoxic to the regimen have been queried,[1,2] a combined regimen with cyclophosphamide is often preferred.[1,3,4] In patients with microscopic polyangiitis a combined regimen is recommended. One suggested regimen is prednisone or prednisolone 1 mg per kg body-weight together with cyclophosphamide 2 mg per kg, both daily by mouth, for initial induction of remission.[5] The corticosteroid dose is gradually tapered to about 10 mg daily or less over 6 months; once disease remission is established azathioprine is substituted for cyclophosphamide. There is a trend towards the use of shorter courses of cyclophosphamide, and to the use of intravenous pulsed cyclophosphamide rather than oral administration, in an attempt to reduce adverse effects.[5] Mycophenolate mofetil has been tried in a few patients as an alternative to cyclophosphamide in combination therapy after initial induction.[6]

A monoclonal anti-CD4 antibody, alemtuzumab, has produced benefit in a patient with a systemic vasculitis (not identified as polyarteritis nodosa) refractory to standard therapy[7] and it may be that monoclonal antibodies will prove useful in this disease; results in microscopic polyarteritis are encouraging (see below). Polyarteritis nodosa may be associated with hepatitis B infection; the vasculitis responds in most cases to treatment with antiviral agents and plasma exchange.[3]

Alemtuzumab and other anti-CD4 monoclonal antibodies have been used successfully in patients with microscopic polyarteritis unresponsive to conventional treatment.[8] Another therapy that has been tried in this group and produced clinical improvement is high dose intravenous normal immunoglobulin,[5] but with ambiguous results.

Vasodilators such as calcium-channel blockers, inhibitors of platelet activation, or drugs that improve blood flow may be useful to improve local ischaemia.[9] Skin lesions in a patient with cutaneous polyarteritis nodosa have reportedly responded to oral oxpentifylline [pentoxifylline].[10]

1. Taylor HG, Samanta A. Treatment of vasculitis. Br J Clin Pharmacol 1993; 35: 93–104.
2. Conn DL. Role of cyclophosphamide in treatment of polyarteritis nodosa? J Rheumatol 1991; 18: 489–90.
3. Guillevin L, et al. Treatment of polyarteritis nodosa and Churg-Strauss syndrome: a meta-analysis of 3 prospective controlled trials including 182 patients over 12 years. Ann Med Interne (Paris) 1992; 143: 405–16.
4. Guillevin L, et al. Longterm follow up after treatment of polyarteritis nodosa and Churg-Strauss syndrome with comparison of steroids, plasma exchange and cyclophosphamide to steroids and plasma exchange: a prospective randomized trial of 71 patients. J Rheumatol 1991; 18: 567–74.
5. Savage COS, et al. Primary systemic vasculitis. Lancet 1997; 349: 553–8.
6. Nowack R, et al. Mycophenolate mofetil for systemic vasculitis and IgA nephropathy. Lancet 1997; 349: 774.
7. Mathieson PW, et al. Monoclonal-antibody therapy in systemic vasculitis. N Engl J Med 1990; 323: 250–4.
8. Lockwood CM, et al. Long-term remission of intractable systemic vasculitis with monoclonal antibody therapy. Lancet 1993; 341: 1620–2.

9. Conn DL. Update on systemic necrotizing vasculitis Mayo Clin Proc 1989; 64: 535–43.
10. Calderón MJ, et al. Successful treatment of cutaneous PAN with pentoxifylline. Br J Dermatol 1993; 128: 706–7.

Polychondritis

Relapsing polychondritis is a rare systemic disease which results in inflammation and destruction of cartilage in various parts of the body, most seriously in the respiratory system (e.g. nose, larynx, and trachea). Airway narrowing and obstruction due to loss of cartilaginous support results, and may be complicated by pneumonia: fatalities have resulted. Relatively high doses of corticosteroid may improve symptoms in active disease, but do not appear to retard progression. Methotrexate may be of value in reducing corticosteroid requirements.[1] Dapsone,[2] and CD4 antibodies[3,4] have also been tried.

1. Trentham DE, Le CH. Relapsing polychondritis. Ann Intern Med 1998; 129: 114–22.
2. Espinoza LR, et al. Immune complex-mediated renal involvement in relapsing polychondritis. Am J Med 1981; 71: 181–3.
3. van der Lubbe PA, et al. Anti-CD4 monoclonal antibody for relapsing polychondritis. Lancet 1991; 337: 1349.
4. Choy EHS, et al. Chimaeric anti-CD4 monoclonal antibody for relapsing polychondritis. Lancet 1991; 338: 450.

Polymyalgia rheumatica

Polymyalgia rheumatica is a rheumatic disorder of uncertain aetiology. It occurs mainly in persons over 50 years of age of European, especially Scandinavian, extraction and is more common in women than in men. The disease is characterised by myalgia and severe morning stiffness in the neck and shoulder girdle and in the hips and pelvic girdle, which may spread in more advanced cases to the muscles of the thighs, chest, and arms. Stiffness and pain are worse after periods of inactivity. There may be some joint involvement; other symptoms include fatigue, weight loss, and fever, and anaemia and raised erythrocyte sedimentation rate are seen. In some patients polymyalgia rheumatica is associated with giant cell arteritis (p.1050).

Treatment. Although NSAIDs may improve the symptoms of polymyalgia rheumatica they do not control the disease process, and corticosteroids are preferred;[1-7] in particular, corticosteroid therapy is essential where giant cell arteritis is present.

The usual initial dose is prednisolone or prednisone 10 to 20 mg daily by mouth, depending on the severity of symptoms; higher doses are needed where giant cell arteritis is also present, particularly if there are ophthalmic symptoms. After 2 to 3 months a reduction in dosage is usually possible provided symptoms are well controlled. Dosage reduction should be gradual: one suggestion is a reduction of 0.5 to 1 mg every 3 or 4 weeks if dosage levels are low (10 mg daily) or 2.5 to 5 mg weekly at higher doses (40 to 50 mg daily).[1] Most patients in large studies are taking 6 to 7.5 mg daily at one year.[3]

Maintenance therapy may need to be prolonged. Although about a third to a half of all patients may be able to have corticosteroids withdrawn within about 2 years,[5] maintenance can be required for considerably longer periods ranging from 4 to 8 years or more.[1,8] Intramuscular methylprednisolone has also been found to be effective in polymyalgia rheumatica; because the cumulative dose with prolonged therapy is lower it has been suggested that this has advantages over the use of oral corticosteroids.[9] Relapse is not uncommon and is most likely within one year of corticosteroid withdrawal.[5,6] It may be associated with arteritic symptoms,[1] but arteritic relapses are unusual in patients whose original presentation was pure polymyalgia.[5,8] Methotrexate or azathioprine may be used for their corticosteroid-sparing effect in patients in whom withdrawal is difficult.[5,6]

1. Hart FD. Polymyalgia rheumatica: its correct diagnosis and treatment. Drugs 1987; 33: 280–87.
2. Anonymous. The management of polymyalgia rheumatica and giant cell arteritis. Drug Ther Bull 1993; 31: 65–8.
3. Kyle V. Polymyalgia rheumatica. Prescribers' J 1997; 37: 138–44.
4. Pountain G, Hazleman B. Polymyalgia rheumatica and giant cell arteritis. BMJ 1995; 310: 1057–9.
5. Swannell AJ. Polymyalgia rheumatica and temporal arteritis: diagnosis and management. BMJ 1997; 314: 1329–32.
6. Zilko PJ. Polymyalgia rheumatica and giant cell arteritis. Med J Aust 1996; 165: 438–42.
7. Salvarani C, et al. Polymyalgia rheumatica. Lancet 1997; 350: 43–7.
8. Kyle V, Hazelman BL. Stopping steroids in polymyalgia rheumatica and giant cell arteritis. BMJ 1990; 300: 344–5.
9. Dasgupta B, et al. An initially double-blind controlled 96 week trial of depot methylprednisolone against oral prednisolone in the treatment of polymyalgia rheumatica. Br J Rheumatol 1998; 37: 189–95.

Polymyositis and dermatomyositis

The term polymyositis has been used to describe several types of rare idiopathic inflammatory muscle disorders (myopathies).

The cardinal symptom of polymyositis is symmetrical progressive muscle weakness, usually starting in the shoulder girdle and neck, and pelvic girdle. Onset is usually gradual over a period of months, and accompanied by mild pain and tenderness, although more rapidly evolving disease with intense muscle pain is known. With progression, weakness may prevent the patient from moving their limbs, and muscle atrophy and contracture can develop. Dysphagia, pulmonary aspiration, and hypoventilation may occur, and some patients develop fibrosing alveolitis; pulmonary involvement, especially aspiration pneumonia, can be fatal. ECG abnormalities, usually asymptomatic, are common, and some patients develop Raynaud's syndrome. Primary disease may be associated with skin rashes, in which case it is known as dermatomyositis. Purplish scaly rashes on knees, elbows, and knuckles, and a characteristic purplish ('heliotrope') coloration and oedema of the eyelids may occur. A childhood form known as juvenile dermatomyositis exists, in which additional signs include vasculitis and subcutaneous calcium deposition (calcinosis cutis), and gastrointestinal haemorrhage and perforation may occur.

Treatment. Patients with active disease require bed rest, with the head elevated in patients at risk of aspiration. Physiotherapy to maintain muscle tone and avoid the development of contractures may be required.

Initial drug therapy is based on corticosteroids.[1-4] The usual choice is oral prednisone or prednisolone 40 to 60 mg or more, or 1 to 2 mg per kg body-weight, daily. This usually produces improvement within one to two months. The dose may then be gradually tapered off to the minimum required for disease control; some patients with well controlled disease may be satisfactorily maintained on an alternate-day regimen. Maintenance therapy may need to be prolonged (it is considered unwise to attempt discontinuation until disease has been controlled for at least a year[1]) and a reduction in corticosteroid dosage to the minimum is therefore desirable, but too early or too rapid a reduction may lead to relapse.

Up to 25% of patients do not respond to corticosteroids, or develop unacceptable adverse effects,[1] and in these cases the second-line drugs are cytotoxic immunosuppressants.[1-4] There is considerable experience with the use of methotrexate, by mouth or intravenously, usually at weekly intervals; it may be combined with corticosteroids, permitting a reduction in corticosteroid dose. Azathioprine may also be given with corticosteroids, again permitting a reduction in corticosteroid dosage, and the combination has also been shown to be superior to a corticosteroid alone for long-term maintenance (although this was only apparent after more than a year of therapy).[5]

Some authorities consider that corticosteroid therapy should be combined with a cytotoxic immunosuppressant such as azathioprine or methotrexate from the outset of treatment. There is some evidence that methotrexate may be superior to azathioprine in patients unresponsive to prednisone alone.[6]

The role of other drugs is less well defined. Opinions differ as to the value of cyclophosphamide,[1-4,7] although it may have a role in disease associated with lung fibrosis,[2,3] while chlorambucil and mercaptopurine have produced benefit in individual cases but have not been formally assessed. There have been reports of ciclosporin producing a response in refractory disease.[8,9] Normal immunoglobulin has also produced responses,[10,11] but remains an experimental therapy at present.

Cutaneous symptoms in patients with dermatomyositis do not always respond satisfactorily to corticosteroids, but hydroxychloroquine is reputed to be of benefit in patients with rash,[12] probably due to a photoprotective effect.[13] Calcinosis, which can cause considerable morbidity, is particularly difficult to treat: some cases have responded to treatment with aluminium hydroxide.[14-16] Warfarin therapy has been used,[17,18] but its value for calcinosis is disputed.[19]

1. Oddis CV, Medsger TA. Current management of polymyositis and dermatomyositis. *Drugs* 1989; **37:** 382–90.
2. Kaye SA, Isenberg DA. Treatment of polymyositis and dermatomyositis. *Br J Hosp Med* 1994; **52:** 463–8.
3. Plotz PH, *et al.* Myositis: immunologic contributions to understanding cause, pathogenesis, and therapy. *Ann Intern Med* 1995; **122:** 715–24.
4. Bunch TW. Polymyositis: a case history approach to the differential diagnosis and treatment. *Mayo Clin Proc* 1990; **65:** 1480–97.
5. Bunch TW. Prednisone and azathioprine for polymyositis: long-term followup. *Arthritis Rheum* 1981; **24:** 45–8.
6. Joffe MM, *et al.* Drug therapy of the idiopathic inflammatory myopathies: predictors of response to prednisone, azathioprine, and methotrexate and a comparison of their efficacy. *Am J Med* 1993; **94:** 379–87.
7. Bombardieri S, *et al.* Cyclophosphamide in severe polymyositis. *Lancet* 1989; **i:** 1138–9.
8. Heckmatt J, *et al.* Cyclosporin in juvenile dermatomyositis. *Lancet* 1989; **i:** 1063–6.
9. Lueck CJ, *et al.* Cyclosporin in the management of polymyositis and dermatomyositis. *J Neurol Neurosurg Psychiatry* 1991; **54:** 1007–8.
10. Cherin P, *et al.* Efficacy of intravenous gammaglobulin therapy in chronic refractory polymyositis and dermatomyositis: an open study with 20 adult patients. *Am J Med* 1991; **91:** 162–8.
11. Dalakas MC, *et al.* A controlled trial of high-dose intravenous immune globulin infusions as treatment for dermatomyositis. *N Engl J Med* 1993; **329:** 1993–2000.
12. Woo TY, *et al.* Cutaneous lesions of dermatomyositis are improved by hydroxychloroquine. *J Am Acad Dermatol* 1984; **10:** 592–600.
13. Cox NH. Amyopathic dermatomyositis, photosensitivity and hydroxychloroquine. *Br J Dermatol* 1995; **132:** 1016–17.
14. Wang W-J, *et al.* Calcinosis cutis in juvenile dermatomyositis: remarkable response to aluminium therapy. *Arch Dermatol* 1988; **124:** 1721–2.
15. Nakagawa T, Takaiwa T. Calcinosis cutis in juvenile dermatomyositis responsive to aluminium hydroxide treatment. *J Dermatol* 1993; **20:** 558–60.
16. Wananukul S, *et al.* Calcinosis cutis presenting years before other clinical manifestations for juvenile dermatomyositis: report of two cases. *Australas J Dermatol* 1997; **38:** 202–5.
17. Berger RG, Hadler NM. Treatment of calcinosis universalis secondary to dermatomyositis or scleroderma with low dose warfarin. *Arthritis Rheum* 1983; **26** (suppl): S11.
18. Martinez-Cordero E, *et al.* Calcinosis in childhood dermatomyositis. *Clin Exp Rheumatol* 1990; **8:** 198–200.
19. Ansell B. Is there a treatment for the calcinosis of juvenile dermatomyositis? *Br J Rheumatol* 1990; **29:** 263.

Polyneuropathies

A report of 10 patients with subacute demyelinating polyneuropathy who obtained a beneficial response to corticosteroid therapy.[1] In one patient the response was initially slight, but became dramatic when azathioprine was added. Prednisone was given in initial single daily doses of 40 to 150 mg, until definite clinical improvement was obtained, and followed by a single-dose alternate-day regimen. In reviewing different forms of polyneuropathy, including the Guillain-Barré syndrome (p.1554), and their response to corticosteroid therapy, it was concluded that subacute demyelinating neuropathy appeared to be a distinct and clinically identifiable entity in which corticosteroid therapy is indicated. High-dose intravenous methylprednisolone has proved ineffective in patients with Guillain-Barré syndrome.[2]

1. Oh SJ. Subacute demyelinating polyneuropathy responding to corticosteroid treatment. *Arch Neurol* 1978; **35:** 509–16.
2. Hughes RAC, van der Meché FGA. Corticosteroids for treating Guillain-Barré syndrome (updated 27 February 2001). Available in The Cochrane Library; Issue 3. Oxford: Update Software; 2001.

Postoperative ocular inflammation

Corticosteroid eye drops are used to control the inflammatory response commonly observed following cataract surgery; prednisolone is usually used but dexamethasone may be necessary if the inflammation is severe.

Corticosteroids should only be used with care and for short periods for topical control of postoperative ocular inflammation, as discussed on p.66.

Pregnancy

Although some adverse effects have been recorded and certain precautions need to be observed regarding the use of corticosteroids during pregnancy (see under Precautions, p.1042) they may appropriately be given during pregnancy to promote foetal maturation where there is a risk of premature delivery (see Neonatal Respiratory Distress Syndrome, above). In addition, in those maternal conditions serious enough to require administration of systemic corticosteroids the risk to both mother and offspring of discontinuing therapy is often greater than that of corticosteroid administration during pregnancy.

Psoriasis

Reviews of psoriasis (p.1106) and its management[1-4] include topical corticosteroids among first-line treatments. However, the adverse effects of corticosteroids, including in some cases exacerbation of psoriasis, or a rebound after treatment is stopped, mean that topical corticosteroid therapy is a problematic first-line choice for the treatment of psoriasis and most UK dermatologists now reserve it for special circumstances. In the USA it has been reported to be the most widely used treatment for psoria- sis. Combination therapy using corticosteroids with other topical treatments, such as calcipotriol or tazarotene, may be used to reduce adverse effects and improve efficacy of both drugs.[5]

Intralesional injection of corticosteroids has been used for small, localised, recalcitrant plaques of psoriasis but caution is required to avoid skin atrophy or depigmentation.[1] Systemic corticosteroids are not generally recommended, but have been used for short periods in extreme or rare cases; there is a risk of systemic adverse effects and of rebound psoriasis occurring on stopping therapy.[2]

1. Menter A, Barker JNWN. Psoriasis in practice. *Lancet* 1991; **338:** 231–4.
2. Williams REA, *et al.* Workshop of the Research Unit of the Royal College of Physicians of London. Guidelines for management of patients with psoriasis. *BMJ* 1991; **303:** 829–35.
3. Linden KG, Weinstein GD. Psoriasis: current perspectives with an emphasis on treatment. *Am J Med* 1999; **107:** 595–605.
4. Peters BP, *et al.* Pathophysiology and treatment of psoriasis. *Am J Health-Syst Pharm* 2000; **57:** 645–62.
5. Trozak DJ. Topical corticosteroid therapy in psoriasis vulgaris: update and new strategies. *Cutis* 1999; **64:** 315–18.

Pyoderma gangrenosum

A systemic corticosteroid is one of the treatments that has been tried in pyoderma gangrenosum (p.1107). Six of eight patients with severe refractory pyoderma gangrenosum responded favourably to treatment with high-dose systemic corticosteroid pulse therapy;[1] none had serious complications. However, pulse therapy needs very careful use and monitoring, as it is not without adverse effects.[2] Healing of superficial granulomatous pyoderma has occurred following intralesional injection of triamcinolone,[3,4] oral administration of prednisolone,[3,4] and following long-term topical corticosteroids.[4]

1. Prystowsky JH, *et al.* Present status of pyoderma gangrenosum: review of 21 cases. *Arch Dermatol* 1989; **125:** 57–64.
2. Callen JP. Pyoderma gangrenosum. *Lancet* 1998; **351:** 581–5.
3. Quimby SR, *et al.* Superficial granulomatous pyoderma: clinico-pathologic spectrum. *Mayo Clin Proc* 1989; **64:** 37–43.
4. Hardwick N, Cerio R. Superficial granulomatous pyoderma: a report of two cases. *Br J Dermatol* 1993; **129:** 718–22.

Respiratory disorders

Although corticosteroids have been employed in the management of many forms of respiratory disorder, their use has frequently been on an empirical and uncontrolled basis, and evidence of benefit is often somewhat mixed. Thus, while an established role exists for corticosteroids in the management of asthma (p.757), the antenatal prevention of neonatal respiratory distress syndrome (p.1055), and probably in croup (p.1049) they are no longer used in aspiration syndromes (p.1202) and their role in diffuse parenchymal lung disorders (see p.1050 and under Sarcoidosis, below) and in acute respiratory distress syndrome (p.1046) is uncertain. Other disorders in which they have been tried with varying success include chronic obstructive pulmonary disease (see p.1049), fat embolism syndrome,[1] bronchiolitis (p.1048), acute eosinophilic pneumonia[2] and pulmonary eosinophilia,[3] diffuse alveolar haemorrhage,[4] and 'ice hockey lung' (due to nitrogen dioxide).[5]

1. Van Besouw J-P, Hinds CJ. Fat embolism syndrome. *Br J Hosp Med* 1989; **42:** 304–11.
2. Anonymous. Acute eosinophilic pneumonia. *Lancet* 1990; **335:** 947.
3. Anonymous. Pulmonary eosinophilia. *Lancet* 1990; **335:** 512.
4. Metcalf JP, *et al.* Corticosteroids as adjunctive therapy for diffuse alveolar hemorrhage associated with bone marrow transplantation. *Am J Med* 1994; **96:** 327–34.
5. Anonymous. Ice hockey lung: NO_2 poisoning. *Lancet* 1990; **335:** 1191.

Retinal vasculitis

In the treatment of retinal vasculitis, corticosteroids are the most useful drugs for the management of inflammation and its sequelae when vision is compromised.[1] For uniocular disease treatment with orbital floor injection of corticosteroids such as methylprednisolone acetate may be possible. For bilateral disease systemic therapy is required, with additional immunosuppressant cover if relapse occurs despite high-dose corticosteroid therapy.

1. Anonymous. Retinal vasculitis. *Lancet* 1989; **i:** 823–4.

Rheumatoid arthritis

The use of corticosteroids in rheumatoid arthritis (p.9) is controversial. Systemic corticosteroids can suppress symptoms of the disease, but their value is limited by their adverse effects and they have usually been reserved for severe rapidly progressing disease unresponsive to therapy with NSAIDs and disease-modifying antirheumatic drugs (DMARDs). They may also be used temporarily to control disease activity during initiation of therapy with DMARDs, or in disease accompanied by severe extra-articular effects. However, recent results indicate that there may be advantages to the early use of low doses of corticosteroids in active disease. Intra-articular injection of corticosteroids may be used when an acute flare affects one or two individual joints but should be given infrequently.

References.
1. Gotzsche PC, Johansen HK. Short-term low-dose corticosteroids vs placebo and nonsteroidal antiinflammatory drugs in rheumatoid arthritis (updated 1 March 2001). Available in The Cochrane Library; Issue 3. Oxford: Update Software; 2001.
2. Criswell LA, et al. Moderate-term, low-dose corticosteroids for rheumatoid arthritis (updated 30 August 2000). Available in The Cochrane Library; Issue 3. Oxford: Update Software; 2001.

Rhinitis

For a brief description of rhinitis and a discussion of its management including the use of corticosteroids, see p.407. A recent systematic review of 16 randomised controlled trials found that intranasal corticosteroids produced greater relief of the nasal symptoms of allergic rhinitis than oral antihistamines, and there was no difference between the two treatments in relief of eye symptoms.[1]

1. Weiner JM, et al. Intranasal corticosteroids versus oral H_1 receptor antagonists in allergic rhinitis: systematic review of randomised controlled trials. BMJ 1998; 317: 1624–9.

Sarcoidosis

Sarcoidosis is a disorder involving the development of multiple granulomas in a variety of organs, which may subsequently resolve or progress to chronic fibrosis.[1] Almost any organ can be affected, but manifestations in lymph nodes, lungs, skin, joints, and eyes are common. The disease is frequently asymptomatic, and since it usually regresses spontaneously estimating the incidence is difficult, but it appears to vary considerably in different countries. It is most often seen in young adults and is slightly more common in female than male and in black than white patients.

Symptoms vary enormously, depending on the organ affected, and as already mentioned it is often asymptomatic. Lymphadenopathy, some decrease in pulmonary function, dyspnoea, and cough may mark lung and lymph node involvement. Skin manifestations include erythema nodosum, macular or papular lesions due to granuloma formation in the skin, and violaceous plaques on fingers, nose, ears, and cheeks known as lupus pernio. Arthropathy, with painful joint swellings, may be associated with erythema nodosum and fever in acute presentations; bone lesions are most common in fingers and toes. Involvement of the nervous system may be particularly difficult to diagnose because of its protean manifestations. Involvement of the eyes is usually marked by uveitis although other symptoms include keratoconjunctivitis sicca. Symptomatic disease involving the gastrointestinal tract, liver, pancreas, heart, or kidneys is rare, although asymptomatic involvement may occur.

In addition to symptoms directly due to the disease, sarcoidosis is often associated with hypercalcaemia and hypersensitivity to the effects of vitamin D (for discussion of the symptoms of hypercalcaemia, see p.1181). Other biochemical abnormalities include raised serum concentrations of angiotensin-converting enzyme (ACE), and there are abnormalities of some aspects of immune function.

Diagnosis of sarcoidosis is problematic because of its multiple manifestations and the fact that it is so often clinically silent. It is often detected by accident, when radiography is performed for other reasons, but biopsy is often needed to help confirm the disease. The Kveim test, in which an antigen derived from patients with sarcoidosis (see p.1626) is given intradermally and produces a delayed reaction in patients with the disease, is now rarely used because of its perceived lack of precision, although some workers still consider it useful.[2]

Treatment. Asymptomatic disease requires no therapy, and since spontaneous remission can occur, corticosteroids, which are the usual therapy,[1] are generally reserved for patients in whom the disease is interfering with the function of a vital organ or for patients with hypercalcaemia. NSAIDs alone may be adequate to control the fever and arthropathy of acute disease. Where corticosteroids are called for a typical regimen is prednisolone or prednisone 30 to 40 mg daily by mouth, the dose being reduced after several weeks as the patient improves. Therapy should be continued (at the minimum effective maintenance dose) for 12 to 18 months before any at-

tempt is made to withdraw it.[3] Some workers favour alternate-day administration, usually beginning at 40 mg every other day.[4] There is some evidence[5] that relapse may be more likely following withdrawal of corticosteroids than in patients who do not receive corticosteroid therapy, but this may simply reflect the natural course of disease in this group. There also remains some dispute about the value of oral corticosteroids in pulmonary disease: although they are useful in the short term their long-term benefits are more uncertain.[6] Inhaled corticosteroids have also been investigated in pulmonary sarcoidosis; they appear less reliable than oral therapy for primary treatment, but may have a role as maintenance therapy.[7] In patients with ocular disease corticosteroid drops and ointment are used for anterior uveitis; resistant cases, or patients with posterior uveitis, require systemic corticosteroids. Skin lesions usually respond to corticosteroids but the high doses that may be required for suppression of lupus pernio may produce changes in appearance as disfiguring as the disease.[3]

Other drugs have occasionally been used in sarcoidosis but are very much second-line. In patients in whom corticosteroids are not effective or not tolerated cytotoxic immunosuppressants such as methotrexate, chlorambucil, azathioprine, or ciclosporin have been given, with variable results.[1,3] Methotrexate has perhaps been most useful, having been found to be effective in low doses (up to 22.5 mg weekly) by mouth in refractory cutaneous sarcoidosis,[8,9] and with reports of benefit from intramuscular administration in nervous system involvement.[10] The antimalarials have also been tried as adjuncts or alternatives to corticosteroid therapy,[11-13] and there is evidence that they reduce the effects of the disease on calcium metabolism[11,12,14] as well as reports of benefit in cutaneous disease.[13,15,16] Other reports of benefit in cutaneous sarcoidosis have involved allopurinol,[17] thalidomide,[18] and tranilast,[19] while there is report of response to melatonin in 2 patients with refractory sarcoidosis.[20]

1. Newman LS, et al. Sarcoidosis. N Engl J Med 1997; 336: 1224–34. Correction. ibid.; 337: 139.
2. du Bois RM, et al. Moratorium on Kveim test. Lancet 1993; 342: 173.
3. Muthiah MM, Macfarlane JT. Current concepts in the management of sarcoidosis. Drugs 1990; 40: 231–7.
4. DeRemee RA. Sarcoidosis. Mayo Clin Proc 1995; 70: 177–81.
5. Gottlieb JE, et al. Outcome in sarcoidosis: the relationship of relapse to corticosteroid therapy. Chest 1997; 111: 623–31.
6. Paramothayan NS, Jones PW. Corticosteroids for pulmonary sarcoidosis (updated 30 May 2001). Available in The Cochrane Library; Issue 3. Oxford: Update Software; 2001.
7. British Thoracic Society. The diagnosis, assessment and treatment of diffuse parenchymal lung disease in adults. Thorax 1999; 54 (suppl 1): S1–30a.
8. Webster GF, et al. Methotrexate therapy in cutaneous sarcoidosis. Ann Intern Med 1989; 111: 538–9.
9. Baughman RP, Lower EE. A clinical approach to the use of methotrexate for sarcoidosis. Thorax 1999; 54: 742–6.
10. Soriano FG, et al. Neurosarcoidosis: therapeutic success with methotrexate. Postgrad Med J 1990; 66: 142–3.
11. DeSimone DP, et al. Granulomatous infiltration of the talus and abnormal vitamin D and calcium metabolism in a patient with sarcoidosis: successful treatment with hydroxychloroquine. Am J Med 1989; 87: 694–6.
12. O'Leary TJ, et al. The effects of chloroquine on serum 1,25-dihydroxyvitamin D and calcium metabolism in sarcoidosis. N Engl J Med 1986; 315: 727–30.
13. Zic JA, et al. Treatment of cutaneous sarcoidosis with chloroquine: review of the literature. Arch Dermatol 1991; 127: 1034–40.
14. Adams JS, et al. Effective reduction in the serum 1,25-dihydroxy-vitamin D and calcium concentration in sarcoidosis-associated hypercalcemia with short-course chloroquine therapy. Ann Intern Med 1989; 111: 437–3.
15. Spiteri MA, et al. Lupus pernio: a clinico-radiological study of thirty-five cases. Br J Dermatol 1985; 112: 315–22.
16. Jones E, Callen JP. Hydroxychloroquine is effective therapy for control of cutaneous sarcoidal granulomas. J Am Acad Dermatol 1990; 23: 487–9.
17. Brechtel B, et al. Allopurinol: a therapeutic alternative for disseminated cutaneous sarcoidosis. Br J Dermatol 1996; 135: 307–9.
18. Carlesimo M, et al. Treatment of cutaneous and pulmonary sarcoidosis with thalidomide. J Am Acad Dermatol 1995; 32: 866–9.
19. Yamada H, et al. Treatment of cutaneous sarcoidosis with tranilast. J Dermatol 1995; 22: 149–52.
20. Cagnoni ML, et al. Melatonin for treatment of chronic refractory sarcoidosis. Lancet 1995; 346: 1229–30.

Sciatica

For mention of the use of epidural corticosteroid injections to treat sciatica, and doubts about the extent of benefit, see Administration, Epidural Route, p.1045.

Scleritis

Scleritis and episcleritis are inflammatory diseases of the sclera often associated with various systemic diseases. Episcleritis tends to be a benign superficial condition but treatment can be difficult and it tends to recur. The use of topical corticosteroids and topical NSAIDs are sometimes of temporary benefit. Scleritis is a rarer more deep-

seated inflammation. Initial treatment of non-necrotising scleritis is with NSAIDs; high dose systemic corticosteroids (usually prednisolone 60 to 80 mg by mouth daily) have been used successfully in many patients unresponsive to NSAIDs.[1,2] If necessary, to reduce any attendant adverse effects, corticosteroids have been given by orbital floor injection (methylprednisolone acetate 40 mg)[1] or at a reduced systemic dosage with an additional immunosuppressant such as ciclosporin,[2] methotrexate, cyclophosphamide, or azathioprine.[3] Immunosuppressants may also be of value alone in severe or unresponsive disease.[3,4] It has been suggested that immunosuppressant therapy should be the initial choice in necrotising scleritis, as therapeutic failure is very common with less aggressive regimens.[3]

1. Hakin KN, et al. Use of orbital floor steroids in the management of patients with uniocular non-necrotising scleritis. Br J Ophthalmol 1991; 75: 337–9.
2. Hakin KN, et al. Use of cyclosporin in the management of steroid-dependent non-necrotising scleritis. Br J Ophthalmol 1991; 75: 340–1.
3. Sainz de la Maza M, et al. An analysis of therapeutic decision for scleritis. Ophthalmology 1993; 100: 1372–6.
4. Wakefield D, McCluskey P. Cyclosporin therapy for severe scleritis. Br J Ophthalmol 1989; 73: 743–6.

Seborrhoeic dermatitis

Topical corticosteroids are used, together with an antifungal imidazole, in the management of seborrhoeic dermatitis (p.1107).

Septic shock

Although early studies reported both beneficial[1] and detrimental[2] effects, current opinion appears to be that corticosteroids are ineffective in septic shock[2,3] and may worsen secondary infection.[4-7]

1. Sprung CL, et al. The effects of high-dose corticosteroids in patients with septic shock: a prospective, controlled study. N Engl J Med 1984; 311: 1137–43.
2. Bone RC, et al. A controlled clinical trial of high-dose methylprednisolone in the treatment of severe sepsis and septic shock. N Engl J Med 1987; 317: 653–8.
3. The Veterans Administration Systemic Sepsis Cooperative Study Group. Effect of high-dose glucocorticoid therapy on mortality in patients with clinical signs of systemic sepsis. N Engl J Med 1987; 317: 659–65.
4. Anonymous. No evidence that corticosteroids help in septic shock. Drug Ther Bull 1990; 28: 74–5.
5. Rackow EC, Astiz ME. Pathophysiology and treatment of septic shock. JAMA 1991; 266: 548–54.
6. Cohen J, Glauser MP. Septic shock: treatment. Lancet 1991; 338: 736–9.
7. McGowan JE, et al. Report by the Working Group on Steroid Use, Antimicrobial Agents Committee, Infectious Diseases Society of America: Guidelines for the use of systemic glucocorticoids in the management of selected infections. J Infect Dis 1992; 165: 1–13.

Sickle-cell disease

A study[1] has suggested that a short course of high-dose methylprednisolone might be a useful adjunct in controlling pain in sickle-cell crisis (p.7). However, the use of corticosteroids in sickle-cell disease is problematic; apart from the usual adverse effects, including the risk of exacerbating underlying infection, corticosteroid therapy has been reported to provoke sickle-cell crisis in patients with sickle C disease—see under Precautions, p.1043.

1. Griffin TC, et al. High-dose intravenous methylprednisolone therapy for pain in children and adolescents with sickle cell disease. N Engl J Med 1994; 330: 733–7.

Skin disorders

For some guidelines to the use of topical application of corticosteroids in skin disorders, see under Administration, p.1045. For discussion of the use of corticosteroids in individual skin disorders see under the relevant headings in this section.

Spinal cord injury

Results of a multicentre placebo-controlled study in the USA[1] indicated that high-dose intravenous corticosteroids resulted in improvements in neurological function if given within 8 hours of spinal cord injury. Methylprednisolone was given in an initial dose of 30 mg per kg body-weight followed by 5.4 mg per kg per hour for 23 hours. A subsequent study found that although this regimen was adequate if begun within 3 hours of injury, better results were obtained by continuing methylprednisolone for 48 hours in patients in whom therapy commenced 3 to 8 hours after injury.[2,3] The lazaroid tirilazad, given for 48 hours, had some benefit in this study, although it was less effective than 48 hours treatment with methylprednisolone in the doses used. In contrast, a systematic review found that high-dose methylprednisolone did not improve neurological function in patients, and might potentially have a deleterious effect.[4] There is little evidence that corticosteroids or tirilazad are of any value in acute traumatic brain injury.[5,6]

1. Bracken MB, *et al.* A randomized, controlled trial of methylprednisolone or naloxone in the treatment of acute spinal-cord injury: results of the Second National Acute Spinal Cord Injury Study. *N Engl J Med* 1990; **322:** 1405–11.
2. Bracken MB, *et al.* Administration of methylprednisolone for 24 or 48 hours or tirilazad mesylate for 48 hours in the treatment of acute spinal cord injury: results of the third National Acute Spinal Cord Injury Randomized Controlled Trial. *JAMA* 1997; **277:** 1597–1604.
3. Bracken MB, *et al.* Methylprednisolone or tirilazad mesylate administration after acute spinal cord injury: 1-year follow up. Results of the third National Acute Spinal Cord Injury randomized controlled trial. *J Neurosurg* 1998; **89:** 699–706.
4. Short DJ, *et al.* High dose methylprednisolone in the management of acute spinal cord injury—a systematic review from a clinical perspective. *Spinal Cord* 2000; **38:** 273–86.
5. Newell DW, *et al.* Corticosteroids in acute traumatic brain injury. *BMJ* 1998; **316:** 396.
6. Alderson P, Roberts I. Corticosteroids for acute traumatic brain injury (updated 6 February 2001). Available in The Cochrane Library; Issue 3. Oxford: Update Software; 2001.

Spondyloarthropathies

Intra-articular injections of corticosteroids have been given in ankylosing spondylitis (see Spondyloarthropathies, p.10).

Systemic lupus erythematosus

Systemic lupus erythematosus (SLE) is an auto-immune disease of unknown aetiology characterised by autoantibodies which participate in the mediation of tissue damage affecting joints, skin, kidney, CNS, and other organs. It is far more common in women than in men, the evidence suggesting that male hormones have a protective effect, and peak onset is usually in women in their 20s and 30s.

The commonest symptom in patients with SLE is arthralgia or arthritis; fatigue, fever, weight loss, rashes (characteristically a so-called 'butterfly rash' on the cheeks and bridge of the nose), CNS involvement including personality changes, anaemia, nephritis, and pulmonary symptoms (notable pleurisy) are also frequent, while other symptoms include myalgia, alopecia, Raynaud's syndrome, convulsions, coma, stroke, pneumonitis, pericarditis, myocarditis with tachycardia, leucopenia, thrombocytopenia, coagulation disorders (both thrombosis and haemorrhage), hepatomegaly, splenomegaly, and lymphadenopathy. Thrombotic symptoms and recurrent abortion may represent an 'antiphospholipid antibody syndrome' due to antibodies against phospholipids, which occurs in about a third of all patients with SLE but may also occur independently.[1]

Management. The management of patients with SLE must be adjusted individually depending on the manifestations of disease and their severity. Since the disease is characterised by exacerbation and remission careful monitoring of the patient and appropriate treatment of symptoms as and when they occur are required. Treatment is largely empirical and symptomatic, and there have been few controlled studies.

In addition to any specific treatment, patients require emotional support, extensive rest, and avoidance where possible of stimuli that may provoke disease exacerbation, including ultraviolet light, certain drugs or foods rich in psoralens, infections, and psychological stress.

Mild disease may require no treatment, or may be managed simply with NSAIDs for muscular and joint symptoms.[2] In more severe, but not-life-threatening disease chloroquine or, more often, hydroxychloroquine is effective, particularly for cutaneous and joint manifestations,[3,4] although disease flare may occur on withdrawal.[5] Retinoids such as acitretin have also been shown to be of use in some patients.[6]

Many patients require treatment with corticosteroids at some point, although in such patients they can be a major cause of morbidity.[4,7] It is usual to employ a corticosteroid when treatment with NSAIDs or antimalarials has failed, or when life or vital organs are threatened.[2] They are usually employed in high doses (1 mg or more of prednisone or prednisolone per kg body-weight daily, sometimes preceded by a course of intravenous methylprednisolone) for life-threatening manifestations such as high fever, severe thrombocytopenia, coma, seizures, or involvement of a major organ such as the kidney[3] (see also Lupus Nephritis, below). Non-life-threatening symptoms that fail to respond to other measures will usually respond to lower corticosteroid doses (not more than 0.5 mg of prednisolone or prednisone per kg daily). Once

a response is achieved the dose should be tapered to the lowest required to control symptoms, ideally in the form of alternate-day dosage.[3] Raising the maintenance corticosteroid dose temporarily to counteract any increases in the concentration of antibodies to double-stranded DNA may reduce the number of relapses,[8] but the design and conclusions of this study are open to criticism.

Prolonged corticosteroid therapy, particularly at the higher doses, is associated with adverse effects such as aseptic bone necrosis and an increased susceptibility to infection, and other drugs have been added to corticosteroid therapy in an attempt to lower the corticosteroid dose but maintain disease control. In particular the immunosuppressant azathioprine has been used for its corticosteroid-sparing effect;[2,9] immunosuppressants such as cyclophosphamide are considered to pose more of a risk of long-term toxicity but cyclophosphamide has been used with some success to treat severe acute organ involvement in patients with disease refractory to corticosteroids alone.[10-14] Recent results have suggested that methotrexate, too, may be helpful in some patients, such as those with joint disease.[15] The antimalarials may also be combined with corticosteroid therapy, and in addition to a corticosteroid-sparing effect there is a suggestion that hydroxychloroquine may counter the adverse effects of corticosteroids on serum-lipid profiles.[2,16] Prasterone is under investigation for the treatment of severe disease.[17]

Thrombotic symptoms due to antiphospholipid antibodies require adequate long-term anticoagulation with warfarin or low-dose aspirin, and it should be borne in mind that stroke and related CNS symptoms will not respond to corticosteroids. In patients with other severe CNS symptoms that fail to respond to corticosteroids intravenous cyclophosphamide may be helpful,[11,14] but response is unpredictable. Intravenous immunoglobulin has been used as an adjunct in CNS lupus, although its role is unclear; it may also be used in the management of thrombocytopenic symptoms.[18]

In patients with severe and potentially fatal symptoms plasma exchange may provide temporary benefit by removing circulating antibodies.

Lupus nephritis. Renal disease is probably the best studied symptom of SLE. Almost all patients develop some renal involvement, with clinical nephritis in up to 75%. Usual manifestations of renal disease include hypertension, oedema, proteinuria or frank nephrotic syndrome, and oliguria; more severe disease is usually associated with focal or diffuse proliferative glomerulonephritis on biopsy.[19,20]

Patients with active disease (worsening renal function, proteinuria, and urinary sediment) require aggressive treatment to prevent irreversible renal damage. It is generally accepted that the combination of a cytotoxic immunosuppressant drug with a corticosteroid is more effective than the use of corticosteroids alone in controlling nephritis and the risk of end-stage renal failure, although corticosteroids alone may be used for less severe disease.[18,21]

One suggested outline for treatment in severe active disease is to begin with pulsed intravenous methylprednisolone as 3 doses of 1g, followed by prednisone by mouth (initially 0.8 to 1 mg per kg daily, gradually reduced to 0.4 mg per kg daily) accompanied if necessary by cyclophosphamide or azathioprine. Provided disease activity is controlled subsequent maintenance can be reduced to alternate-day prednisone.[19] An alternative approach is to begin therapy with intermittent intravenous cyclophosphamide,[22-24] which appears to be more effective than pulsed methylprednisolone[25,26] and maintain patients with low-dose oral prednisone plus intravenous cyclophosphamide every 3 months. Ciclosporin has also been investigated, with preliminary results suggestive of benefit,[27,28] but has been viewed with caution because of its nephrotoxicity.[19]

Pregnancy. Although symptoms of SLE do not appear to be exacerbated in most patients during pregnancy,[29,30] it is considered advisable that pregnancy be deferred until the disease is in remission or controlled by therapy since complications are more likely in active disease.[29] Cyclophosphamide or methotrexate are contra-indicated in pregnancy because of the risk of teratogenesis but corticosteroids, azathioprine, and hydroxychloroquine may be used if necessary;[2,31] the risks of miscarriage, stillbirth, growth retardation, or preterm delivery due to the disease are considered greater than the risks to the fetus of continued therapy. The use of low-dose aspirin (75 mg daily) has been recommended in women with renal in-

volvement or a history of pre-eclampsia or fetal growth retardation;[31] in women with antiphospholipid antibodies, low-dose aspirin together with subcutaneous heparin markedly improves the live birth rate.[32] The use of high-dose prednisone, with or without aspirin, to suppress antiphospholipid antibodies, while reportedly effective in some women with bad obstetric histories,[33,34] has been found by others to be of no benefit,[35] and is associated with unacceptable maternal morbidity.[36] Warfarin prophylaxis, which appears effective in other patients with the antiphospholipid antibody syndrome,[37] is unsuited to pregnant women because of the teratogenic effects of warfarin.[38]

Postpartum exacerbation is well recognised,[29,31] and some workers favour prophylactic corticosteroid cover during the puerperium. A small proportion of neonates born to mothers with lupus exhibit a neonatal lupus syndrome,[39] manifesting most seriously as heart block which may require a permanent pacemaker.

1. Hughes GRV. The antiphospholipid syndrome: ten years on. *Lancet* 1993; **342:** 341–4.
2. Anonymous. Systemic lupus erythematosus. *Drug Ther Bull* 1996; **34:** 20–3.
3. Lockshin MD. Therapy for systemic lupus erythematosus. *N Engl J Med* 1991; **324:** 189–91.
4. Hay EM, Snaith ML. Systemic lupus erythematosus and lupus-like syndromes. *BMJ* 1995; **310:** 1257–61.
5. The Canadian Hydroxychloroquine Study Group. A randomized study of the effect of withdrawing hydroxychloroquine sulfate in systemic lupus erythematosus. *N Engl J Med* 1991; **324:** 150–4.
6. Ruzicka T, *et al.* Treatment of cutaneous lupus erythematosus with acitretin and hydroxychloroquine. *Br J Dermatol* 1992; **127:** 513–18.
7. Mills JA. Systemic lupus erythematosus. *N Engl J Med* 1994; **330:** 1871–9.
8. Bootsma H, *et al.* Prevention of relapses in systemic lupus erythematosus. *Lancet* 1995; **345:** 1595–9. Correction. *ibid.*; **346:** 516.
9. Callen JP, *et al.* Azathioprine: an effective corticosteroid-sparing therapy for patients with recalcitrant cutaneous lupus erythematosus or with recalcitrant cutaneous leukocytoclastic vasculitis. *Arch Dermatol* 1991; **127:** 515–22.
10. Sigal LH. Chronic inflammatory polyneuropathy complicating SLE: successful treatment with monthly oral pulse cyclophosphamide. *J Rheumatol* 1989; **16:** 1518–19.
11. Fricchione GL, *et al.* Electroconvulsive therapy and cyclophosphamide in combination for severe neuropsychiatric lupus with catatonia. *Am J Med* 1990; **88:** 442–3.
12. Boumpas DT, *et al.* Intermittent cyclophosphamide for the treatment of autoimmune thrombocytopenia in systemic lupus erythematosus. *Ann Intern Med* 1990; **112:** 674–7.
13. Barr WG, *et al.* Plasmapheresis and pulse cyclophosphamide in systemic lupus erythematosus. *Ann Intern Med* 1988; **108:** 152–3.
14. Neuwelt CM, *et al.* Role of intravenous cyclophosphamide in the treatment of severe neuropsychiatric systemic lupus erythematosus. *Am J Med* 1995; **98:** 32–41.
15. Wilson K, Abeles M. A 2 year, open ended trial of methotrexate in systemic lupus erythematosus. *J Rheumatol* 1994; **21:** 1674–7.
16. Hodis HN, *et al.* The lipid, lipoprotein, and apolipoprotein effects of hydroxychloroquine in systemic lupus erythematosus. *J Rheumatol* 1993; **20:** 661–5.
17. van Vollenhoven RF. Dehydroepiandrosterone in systemic lupus erythematosus. *Rheum Dis Clin North Am* 2000; **26:** 349–62.
18. Boumpas DT, *et al.* Systemic lupus erythematosus: emerging concepts. *Ann Intern Med* 1995; **122:** 940–50 and **123:** 42–53.
19. Ponticelli C. Current treatment recommendations for lupus nephritis. *Drugs* 1990; **40:** 19–30.
20. Dhillon VB, *et al.* Lupus nephritis: a review. *Postgrad Med J* 1989; **65:** 336–43.
21. Venables PJW. Diagnosis and treatment of systemic lupus erythematosus. *BMJ* 1993; **307:** 663–6.
22. Austin HA, *et al.* Therapy of lupus nephritis: controlled trial of prednisone and cytotoxic drugs. *N Engl J Med* 1986; **314:** 614–19.
23. McCune WJ, *et al.* Clinical and immunologic effects of monthly administration of intravenous cyclophosphamide in severe systemic lupus erythematosus. *N Engl J Med* 1988; **318:** 1423–31.
24. Lehman TJA, *et al.* Intermittent intravenous cyclophosphamide therapy for lupus nephritis. *J Pediatr* 1989; **114:** 1055–60.
25. Boumpas DT, *et al.* Controlled trial of pulse methylprednisolone versus two regimens of pulse cyclophosphamide in severe lupus nephritis. *Lancet* 1992; **340:** 741–5.
26. Gourley MF, *et al.* Methylprednisolone and cyclophosphamide, alone or in combination, in patients with lupus nephritis: a randomized, controlled trial. *Ann Intern Med* 1996; **125:** 549–57.
27. Fu LW, *et al.* Clinical efficacy of cyclosporin A Neoral in the treatment of paediatric lupus nephritis with heavy proteinuria. *Br J Rheumatol* 1998; **37:** 217–21.
28. Tam LS, *et al.* Long-term treatment of lupus nephritis with cyclosporin A. *Q J Med* 1998; **91:** 573–80.
29. Anonymous. Systemic lupus erythematosus in pregnancy. *Lancet* 1991; **338:** 87–8.
30. Yell JA, Burge SM. The effect of hormonal changes on cutaneous disease in lupus erythematosus. *Br J Dermatol* 1993; **129:** 18–22.
31. Hunt BJ, Lakasing L. Management of pre-existing disorders in pregnancy: connective-tissue disorders. *Prescribers' J* 1997; **37:** 54–60.
32. Rai R, *et al.* Randomised controlled trial of aspirin and aspirin plus heparin in pregnant women with recurrent miscarriage associated with phospholipid antibodies (or antiphospholipid antibodies). *BMJ* 1997; **314:** 253–7.
33. Lubbe WF, *et al.* Fetal survival after prednisone suppression of maternal lupus-anticoagulant. *Lancet* 1983; **i:** 1361–3.
34. Branch DW, *et al.* Obstetric complications associated with the lupus anticoagulant. *N Engl J Med* 1985; **313:** 1322–6.
35. Laskin CA, *et al.* Prednisone and aspirin in women with autoantibodies and unexplained recurrent fetal loss. *N Engl J Med* 1997; **148:** 148–53.
36. Greaves M. Antiphospholipid antibodies and thrombosis. *Lancet* 1999; **353:** 1348–53.

37. Khamashta MA, *et al.* The management of thrombosis in the antiphospholipid-antibody syndrome. *N Engl J Med* 1995; **332:** 993–7.
38. Lockshin MD. Answers to the antiphospholipid-antibody syndrome? *N Engl J Med* 1995; **332:** 1025–7.
39. Anonymous. Neonatal lupus syndrome. *Lancet* 1987; **ii:** 489–90.

Takayasu's arteritis

Takayasu's arteritis is a vasculitis of the aorta and its branches seen particularly in young women and in Oriental patients. It is characterised by vasculitis followed by fibrosis, leading to stenosis or occlusion of the vessel. Symptoms vary depending on the anatomical site, but include constitutional symptoms such as fever, malaise, and arthralgia, syncope, dyspnoea, palpitations, loss of pulses, intermittent claudication, and visual disturbances.

Active inflammatory disease may respond to corticosteroids: doses of 1 mg per kg body-weight daily of prednisone, tapered after one month in patients who respond, have been suggested.[1] In patients who do not respond, low-dose oral cyclophosphamide has been added, although opinions vary as to the necessity of cytotoxic agents in these patients.[1,2] Widely varying estimates of mortality and aggressiveness exist for Takayasu's arteritis, and in the absence of large controlled studies it is difficult to assess the benefits of drug therapy. The course may be very prolonged, and minimising the maintenance dosage (e.g. by alternate-day corticosteroid therapy) is important to avoid adverse effects.[3]

Surgical reconstruction of affected vessels has been carried out in patients at risk of ischaemic compromise.[4] Angioplasty has been tried.

1. Shelhamer JH, *et al.* Takayasu's arteritis and its therapy. *Ann Intern Med* 1985; **103:** 121–6.
2. Hall S, Hunder GG. Treatment of Takayasu's arteritis. *Ann Intern Med* 1986; **104:** 288.
3. Taylor HG, Samanta A. Treatment of vasculitis. *Br J Clin Pharmacol* 1993; **35:** 93–104.
4. Kerr GS, *et al.* Takayasu arteritis. *Ann Intern Med* 1994; **120:** 919–29.

Tuberculosis

The use of corticosteroids in tuberculosis (p.143) is controversial.[1-3] They should never be given to patients with active disease without protective chemotherapy cover, and must be used with caution in patients with dormant disease as it may be reactivated. Administration of corticosteroids in pulmonary tuberculosis is to be avoided except in life-threatening disease. WHO suggests that corticosteroids may be useful adjuvants to antituberculous therapy in selected conditions including tuberculous meningitis, pericarditis, pleural effusion, or laryngitis, or tuberculosis of the renal tract, adrenocortical insufficiency due to adrenal gland tuberculosis, massive lymph node enlargement, or to control drug hypersensitivity. They are also likely to be of benefit in patients with HIV infection and the above conditions.[4] Similar recommendations are made by the British Thoracic Society.[5] However, systematic reviews of tuberculous pleurisy,[6] pericarditis,[7] and meningitis[8] have concluded that there is insufficient evidence to support the use of corticosteroids in these conditions.

1. Horne NW, ed. *Modern drug treatment of tuberculosis.* 7th ed. London: The Chest, Heart and Stroke Association, 1990.
2. McGowan JE, *et al.* Report by the Working Group on Steroid Use, Antimicrobial Agents Committee, Infectious Diseases Society of America: Guidelines for the use of systemic glucocorticoids in the management of selected infections. *J Infect Dis* 1992; **165:** 1–13.
3. Alzeer AH, FitzGerald JM. Corticosteroids and tuberculosis: risks and use as adjunct therapy. *Tubercle Lung Dis* 1993; **74:** 6–11.
4. WHO. *TB/HIV: a clinical manual.* Geneva: WHO, 1996.
5. Joint Tuberculosis Committee of the British Thoracic Society. Chemotherapy and management of tuberculosis in the United Kingdom: recommendations 1998. *Thorax* 1998; **53:** 536–48.
6. Matchaba PT, Volmink J. Steroids for treating tuberculous pleurisy (updated 24 February 2001). Available in The Cochrane Library; Issue 3. Oxford: Update Software; 2001.
7. Mayosi BM, *et al.* Interventions for treating tuberculous pericarditis (updated 30 May 2001). Available in The Cochrane Library; Issue 3. Oxford: Update Software; 2001.
8. Prasad K, *et al.* Steroids for treating tuberculous meningitis (updated 7 December 2000). Available in The Cochrane Library; Issue 3. Oxford: Update Software; 2001.

Urticaria and angioedema

Oral antihistamines are the mainstay of treatment for urticaria (p.1107). Severe attacks refractory to standard therapy may require a short course of oral corticosteroid therapy.

When angioedema affecting the larynx (laryngeal oedema) is present, the patients should be treated with adren-

aline [epinephrine] as an allergic emergency (see under Anaphylactic Shock, p.832).

Uveitis

Uveitis is inflammation of the uveal tract of the eye which comprises the choroid, ciliary body, and the iris. It is usually idiopathic but may be secondary to infection, allergy, or inflammatory disorders with an auto-immune component.

In anterior uveitis, also referred to as iridocyclitis, there is inflammation of the iris (iritis) and the ciliary body (cyclitis). It tends to be acute and self-limiting and is likely to be associated with infection. The iris becomes spongy and hyperaemic and exudates may result in adhesions between the iris and the lens (posterior synechiae). Chronic anterior uveitis is associated with formation of cataracts and glaucoma. Posterior uveitis can be acute or chronic and may just affect the choroid (choroiditis) or may also involve the retina (chorioretinitis). It is more likely to be an auto-immune condition.

The treatment of uveitis has been reviewed.[1-5]

Corticosteroids given topically and, when necessary, systemically are the mainstay of treatment for acute anterior uveitis. Cycloplegics and mydriatics such as atropine, cyclopentolate, and homatropine are used adjunctively to rest the ciliary body and iris, diminish hyperaemia, and to prevent the formation of posterior synechiae. Antibacterials should be used to treat any infection. In children with chronic anterior uveitis associated with juvenile idiopathic arthritis, corticosteroids are supplemented with chronic use of an oral NSAID if inflammation persists after 90 days of treatment and attempted corticosteroid withdrawal.[6] In the 30% or so of cases which do not respond to corticosteroids and NSAIDs, low-dose weekly methotrexate (with folic acid supplements daily) is advocated, with other immunosuppressants being substituted or used adjunctively when methotrexate fails or is not tolerated.

Treatment of posterior uveitis is less satisfactory than that of acute anterior uveitis since gross damage to the retina often occurs before the condition can be controlled. Corticosteroids are usually required given either as periocular injections or as high-dose systemic therapy. A suggested protocol[4] involves the use of high-dose systemic corticosteroids to control active disease; long-term control is then maintained primarily with low-dose ciclosporin, corticosteroids being tapered to a low dose or eventually withdrawn. Certain patients may require an additional immunosuppressant, usually azathioprine although methotrexate or cyclophosphamide may be considered. Other immunosuppressants being studied include tacrolimus. There is also a report that mycophenolate mofetil produces improvement in refractory uveitis.[7]

Visual impairment in chronic uveitis is often the result of macular oedema and is not necessarily prevented by immunosuppressants. Short-term treatment with acetazolamide is considered to have produced some encouraging results in reducing chronic uveitic macular oedema but its long-term efficacy or efficacy with low-dose corticosteroids remains to be determined.[8] Although systemic and topical NSAIDs have been shown to reduce cystoid macular oedema in post cataract extraction (see Postoperative Inflammatory Ocular Disorders, p.66) their role in the treatment of macular oedema associated with uveitis is less clear.

1. Herman DC. Endogenous uveitis: current concepts of treatment. *Mayo Clin Proc* 1990; **65:** 671–83.
2. Lightman S. Uveitis: management. *Lancet* 1991; **338:** 1501–4.
3. Anglade E, Whitcup SM. The diagnosis and management of uveitis. *Drugs* 1995; **49:** 213–23.
4. Dick AD, *et al.* Immunosuppressive therapy for chronic uveitis: optimising therapy with steroids and cyclosporin A. *Br J Ophthalmol* 1997; **81:** 1107–12.
5. McCluskey PJ, *et al.* Management of chronic uveitis. *BMJ* 2000; **320:** 555–8.
6. Nguyen QD, Foster S. Saving the vision of children with juvenile rheumatoid arthritis-associated uveitis. *JAMA* 1998; **280:** 1133–4.
7. Kilmartin DJ, *et al.* Rescue therapy with mycophenolate mofetil in refractory uveitis. *Lancet* 1998; **352:** 35–6.
8. Dick AD. The treatment of chronic uveitic macular oedema. *Br J Ophthalmol* 1994; **78:** 1–2.

Vasculitic syndromes

Vasculitis may be defined as inflammation of the blood vessel wall, and the term has been applied in describing a wide range of diseases involving blood vessels of various sizes and types. Vasculitis may occur as part of a systemic disease such as rheumatoid arthritis or systemic lupus erythematosus, or may itself be the primary disorder,

and symptoms may vary from superficial cutaneous disease, with purpura and urticaria, to progressive and fatal systemic vasculitides such as Wegener's granulomatosis. In some forms of vasculitis, such as giant cell arteritis, mononuclear giant cells may be seen, while in granulomatous vasculitis the mononuclear cells form granulomata adjacent to the damaged vessel wall. Necrotising vasculitis is used to describe inflammation associated with necrosis of the media, the middle part of the vessel wall, while polyarteritis implies inflammation of the full thickness of an arterial wall.

Because of the heterogeneous nature of this group of diseases and the degree of overlap which exists between some of them, and between them and other diseases, classification has been difficult. Classification has often been based on the size of the affected vessel, as well as the presence or absence of granulomata and antineutrophil cytoplasmic antibodies (ANCA), and whether the vasculitis is primary or secondary. Of the major primary vasculitic syndromes, giant cell arteritis (p.1050) and Takayasu's arteritis (p.1060) are examples of large vessel disease; classic polyarteritis nodosa (p.1056) affects medium-sized vessels; Churg-Strauss syndrome (p.1049), microscopic polyangiitis (p.1056), and Wegener's granulomatosis (below) are diseases of small or medium-sized vessels; the so-called 'hypersensitivity vasculitides', including Henoch-Schönlein purpura, are small vessel diseases (p.1052), though usually limited in extent.

Treatment depends on the type of vasculitis, its severity, and prognosis. Treatment of the systemic vasculitides has revolved around corticosteroids and cyclophosphamide; other cytotoxic immunosuppressants, normal immunoglobulins, NSAIDs, anticoagulants, dapsone, and colchicine have been tried in various forms of disease.

Vitiligo

Topical corticosteroids are sometimes effective in inducing repigmentation in patients with vitiligo (p.1106 under Pigmentation Disorders).

Wegener's granulomatosis

Wegener's granulomatosis is a form of granulomatous vasculitis which occurs more frequently in men and in white patients. It is characterised by necrotising vasculitis of small arteries and veins, accompanied by granuloma formation, and affecting particularly the respiratory tract and kidneys. It is usually associated with antineutrophil cytoplasmic antibodies (ANCA). Symptoms include rhinorrhoea, sinusitis, cough and dyspnoea (signs of pulmonary infiltration which is seen in the majority of patients at presentation); renal manifestations include haematuria, proteinuria, uraemia, and oedema of the lower limbs due to a focal glomerulonephritis which can progress to crescentic glomerulonephritis and rapidly progressive renal failure. Other organ systems may be involved, with effects similar to those of polyarteritis nodosa (see p.1056). If untreated, the disease is fatal.

Treatment is with a combination regimen based on cyclophosphamide with a corticosteroid. A standard regimen has been low-dose (1 to 2 mg per kg body-weight daily) oral cyclophosphamide, together with prednisolone or prednisone 1 mg per kg daily by mouth initially, subsequently tapered to an alternate-day regimen and eventually discontinued.[1-3] Cyclophosphamide is usually continued for at least a year before considering gradual discontinuation but there is a trend in Europe towards the use of shorter courses of cyclophosphamide.[4] Regimens similar to the standard regimen, but substituting azathioprine for cyclophosphamide once remission is achieved (usually after 4 to 6 months) and continuing with low-dose corticosteroids concomitantly have been employed. Standard treatment regimens produce improvement or remissions in about 90% of patients.[1-5] Relapses may subsequently occur in about half, and require re-treatment; prompt intensification of treatment when serum ANCA concentrations begin to rise may avert relapse.[6] There is evidence from one controlled study that addition of co-trimoxazole to maintenance regimens reduces the incidence of relapse,[7] although another suggested that it might actually increase the risk of relapse.[8]

Despite the success of regimens based on low-dose oral cyclophosphamide there is considerable concern about their toxicity, particularly since prolonged administration may be necessary. Intermittent high-dose intravenous ('pulse') cyclophosphamide has been suggested as an alternative to the oral regimen with fewer adverse effects,[9] but results in practice seem to have been variable.[10,11]

Other drugs, such as methotrexate, have been tried and addition of low-dose weekly methotrexate to a corticosteroid may be a possible treatment option.[8,12,13] Ciclosporin has been reported to reverse acute renal failure in 2 patients with Wegener's granulomatosis, as well as controlling fulminant symptoms unresponsive to cyclophosphamide and corticosteroids in one of them,[14] but others have found ciclosporin plus a corticosteroid to be ineffective in suppressing disease activity.[15] Etoposide has also been successfully used to induce remission in cyclophosphamide-resistant disease.[16] Other drugs which have been investigated include high-dose intravenous immunoglobulin,[17] and mycophenolate mofetil,[18] while anti-CD4 monoclonal antibodies have proved useful in patients with microscopic polyarteritis, which has some similarities to Wegener's granulomatosis, but the role of such investigational regimens remains to be determined.

1. Fauci AS, et al. Wegener's granulomatosis: prospective clinical and therapeutic experience with 85 patients for 21 years. Ann Intern Med 1983; 98: 76–85.
2. Hoffman GS, et al. Wegener granulomatosis: an analysis of 158 patients. Ann Intern Med 1992; 116: 488–98.
3. Langford CA, Hoffman GS. Wegener's granulomatosis. Thorax 1999; 54: 629–37.
4. Savage COS, et al. Primary systemic vasculitis. Lancet 1997; 349: 553–8.
5. Rottem M, et al. Wegener granulomatosis in children and adolescents: clinical presentation and outcome. J Pediatr 1993 122: 26–31.
6. Tervaert JWC, et al. Prevention of relapses in Wegener's granulomatosis by treatment based on antineutrophil cytoplasmic antibody titre. Lancet 1990; 336: 709–11.
7. Stegeman CA, et al. Trimethoprim-sulfamethoxazole (co-trimoxazole) for the prevention of relapses of Wegener's granulomatosis. N Engl J Med 1996; 335: 16–20.
8. de Groot K, et al. Therapy for the maintenance of remission in sixty-five patients with generalized Wegener's granulomatosis: methotrexate versus trimethoprim/sulfamethoxazole. Arthritis Rheum 1996; 39: 2052–61.
9. Cupps TR. Cyclophosphamide: to pulse or not to pulse? Am J Med 1990; 89: 399–402.
10. Hoffman GS, et al. Treatment of Wegener's granulomatosis with intermittent high-dose intravenous cyclophosphamide. Am J Med 1990; 89: 403–10.
11. Reinhold-Keller E, et al. Influence of disease manifestation and antineutrophil cytoplasmic antibody titre on the response to pulse cyclophosphamide therapy in patients with Wegener's granulomatosis. Arthritis Rheum 1994; 37: 919–24.
12. Sneller MC. Wegener's granulomatosis. JAMA 1995; 273: 1288–91.
13. Gottlieb BS, et al. Methotrexate treatment of Wegener granulomatosis in children. J Pediatr 1996; 129: 604–7.
14. Gremmel F, et al. Cyclosporin in Wegener granulomatosis. Ann Intern Med 1988; 108: 491.
15. Inoue K-I, et al. Successful treatment with combination therapy of cyclophosphamide and cyclosporin for late recurrence of Wegener granulomatosis. Arch Intern Med 2000; 160: 393–4.
16. D'Cruz D, et al. Response of cyclophosphamide-resistant Wegener's granulomatosis to etoposide. Lancet 1997; 340: 425–6.
17. Jayne DRW, et al. Treatment of systemic vasculitis with pooled intravenous immunoglobulin. Lancet 1991; 337: 1137–9.
18. Nowack R, et al. Mycophenolate mofetil for systemic vasculitis and IgA nephropathy. Lancet 1997; 349: 774.

Alclometasone Dipropionate (12338-m)

Alclometasone Dipropionate (BANM, USAN, rINNM).
Sch-22219. 7α-Chloro-11β,17α,21-trihydroxy-16α-methylpregna-1,4-diene-3,20-dione 17,21-dipropionate.
$C_{28}H_{37}ClO_7 = 521.0$.
CAS — 67452-97-5 (alclometasone); 66734-13-2 (alclometasone dipropionate).
Pharmacopoeias. In US.

Pharmacopoeial description
USP 25: Store in airtight containers.

Profile
Alclometasone dipropionate is a corticosteroid used topically for its glucocorticoid activity (p.1039) in the treatment of various skin disorders. It is usually employed as a cream or ointment containing 0.05%.

When applied topically, particularly to large areas, when the skin is broken, or under occlusive dressings, corticosteroids may be absorbed in sufficient amounts to cause systemic effects (p.1039). The effects of topical corticosteroids on the skin are described on p.1041. For recommendations concerning the correct use of corticosteroids on the skin, and a rough guide to the clinical potencies of topical corticosteroids, see p.1045.

Preparations
USP 25: Alclometasone Dipropionate Cream; Alclometasone Dipropionate Ointment.

Proprietary Preparations (details are given in Part 3)
Austral.: Logoderm; Denm.: Legederm; Fin.: Legederm; Fr.: Aclosone; Ger.: Delonal; Hong Kong: Perderm; Irl.: Modrasone; Ital.: Legederm; Mex.: Logoderm; Neth.: Aclosone; NZ: Logoderm; Port.: Miloderme; S.Afr.: Aclosone; Singapore: Perderm; Swed.: Legederm; Switz.: Delonal; UK: Modrasone; USA: Aclovate.

Aldosterone (1061-l)

Aldosterone (BAN, rINN).
Electrocortin. 11β,18-Epoxy-18,21-dihydroxypregn-4-ene-3,20-dione.
$C_{21}H_{28}O_5 = 360.4$.
CAS — 52-39-1.
ATC — H02AA01.

Adverse Effects
Aldosterone has very pronounced mineralocorticoid actions and little effect on carbohydrate metabolism. It may therefore exhibit the mineralocorticoid adverse effects described for the corticosteroids in general (p.1039).

Uses and Administration
Aldosterone is the main mineralocorticoid (p.1039) secreted by the adrenal cortex. It has no significant glucocorticoid (anti-inflammatory) properties.

Aldosterone has been given by intramuscular or intravenous injection, in association with a glucocorticoid, in the treatment of primary adrenocortical insufficiency (p.1046) but synthetic mineralocorticoids such as fludrocortisone (p.1070), which can be given by mouth, are usually preferred. It has also been used as the sodium succinate.

Preparations
Proprietary Preparations (details are given in Part 3)
Multi-ingredient: Ital.: Sinsurrene†.

Amcinonide (12351-d)

Amcinonide (BAN, USAN, rINN).
Amcinopol; CL-34699. 16α,17α-Cyclopentylidenedioxy-9α-fluoro-11β,21-dihydroxypregna-1,4-diene-3,20-dione 21-acetate.
$C_{28}H_{35}FO_7 = 502.6$.
CAS — 51022-69-6.
ATC — D07AC11.
Pharmacopoeias. In US.

Profile
Amcinonide is a corticosteroid used topically for its glucocorticoid activity (p.1039) in the treatment of various skin disorders. It is usually used as a cream, lotion, or ointment containing 0.1%.

When applied topically, particularly to large areas, when the skin is broken, or under occlusive dressings, corticosteroids may be absorbed in sufficient amounts to cause systemic effects (p.1039). The effects of topical corticosteroids on the skin are described on p.1041. For recommendations concerning the correct use of corticosteroids on the skin, and a rough guide to the clinical potencies of topical corticosteroids, see p.1045.

Preparations
USP 25: Amcinonide Cream; Amcinonide Ointment.

Proprietary Preparations (details are given in Part 3)
Belg.: Amicla; Canad.: Cyclocort; Fr.: Penticort; Ger.: Amciderm; Ital.: Amcinil; Mex.: Visderm; Neth.: Amicla†; Thai.: Amciderm; Visderm; USA: Cyclocort.

Multi-ingredient: Fr.: Penticort Neomycine†.

Beclometasone Dipropionate

(1062-y)

Beclometasone Dipropionate (BANM, rINNM).
Beclometasoni Dipropionas; Beclomethasone Dipropionate (USAN); 9α-Chloro-16β-methylprednisolone Dipropionate; Sch-18020W. 9α-Chloro-11β,17α,21-trihydroxy-16β-methylpregna-1,4-diene-3,20-dione 17,21-dipropionate.
$C_{28}H_{37}ClO_7 = 521.0$.
CAS — 4419-39-0 (beclometasone); 5534-09-8 (beclometasone dipropionate).
Pharmacopoeias. In Chin., Eur. (see p.vi), Int., and Jpn.
US allows either the anhydrous or monohydrate form. Br. includes a separate monograph for the monohydrate.

Pharmacopoeial description
Ph. Eur.: A white or almost white, crystalline powder. Practically insoluble in water; sparingly soluble in alcohol; freely soluble in acetone. Protect from light.

BP 2001: Beclometasone dipropionate monohydrate is a white or almost white, crystalline powder. It exhibits polymorphism. Practically insoluble in water; sparingly soluble in alcohol; freely soluble in acetone and in chloroform. Protect from light.

USP 25: It is anhydrous or contains one molecule of water of hydration. A white to cream white, odourless powder. Very slightly soluble in water; freely soluble in alcohol and in acetone; very soluble in chloroform.

Adverse Effects, Treatment, Withdrawal, and Precautions
As for corticosteroids in general (p.1039).

Adrenal suppression may occur in some patients treated with high-dose long-term inhalation therapy for asthma. It has been stated that in the majority of patients no significant suppression is likely to occur when total daily doses of less than 1.5 mg are employed (but see under Adrenal Suppression, below).

When applied topically, particularly to large areas, when the skin is broken, or under occlusive dressings, corticosteroids may be absorbed in sufficient amounts to cause systemic effects. Systemic absorption may also follow nasal administration, particularly if high doses are used or treatment is prolonged.

Adrenal suppression. The problem of adrenal suppression with corticosteroids is discussed on p.1040. Listed below are some references and correspondence concerning adrenal suppression due to beclometasone inhalation therapy,[1-9] in some cases occurring with doses below 1.5 mg daily.[7] However, one study found that function of the hypothalamic-pituitary-adrenal axis remained normal in most patients at beclometasone doses below 3 mg daily.[10]

1. Grant IWB, Crompton GK. Becloforte inhaler. BMJ 1983; 286: 644–5.
2. Slessor IM. Becloforte inhaler. BMJ 1983; 286: 645.
3. Ebden P, Davies BH. High-dose corticosteroid inhalers for asthma. Lancet 1984; ii: 576.
4. Law CM, et al. Nocturnal adrenal suppression in asthmatic children taking inhaled beclomethasone dipropionate. Lancet 1986; i: 942–4.
5. Brown HM. Nocturnal adrenal suppression in children inhaling beclomethasone dipropionate. Lancet 1986; i: 1269.
6. Littlewood JM, et al. Growth retardation in asthmatic children treated with inhaled beclomethasone dipropionate. Lancet 1988; i: 115–16.
7. Maxwell DL, Webb J. Adverse effects of inhaled corticosteroids. BMJ 1989; 298: 827–8.
8. Priftis K, et al. Adrenal function in asthma. Arch Dis Child 1990; 65: 838–40.
9. Tabachnik E, Zadik Z. Diurnal cortisol secretion during therapy with inhaled beclomethasone dipropionate in children with asthma. J Pediatr 1991; 118: 294–7.
10. Brown PH, et al. Large volume spacer devices and the influence of high dose beclomethasone dipropionate on hypothalamo-pituitary-adrenal axis function. Thorax 1993; 48: 233–8.

Candidiasis. Results of a study involving 229 asthmatic children indicated that the presence of a sore throat or a hoarse voice was not related to the presence of Candida or to treatment with inhaled beclometasone.[1] The occurrence of only one clinical case of oral candidiasis in 129 of the children receiving beclometasone confirmed previous observations that it is an uncommon finding in children compared with the reported incidence of between 4.5 and 13% in adults. The incidence of colonisation with Candida was greater in those children who received corticosteroids than in those who did not but was not affected by either the dose used or type of inhaler employed.

1. Shaw NJ, Edmunds AT. Inhaled beclomethasone and oral candidiasis. Arch Dis Child 1986; 61: 788–90.

Effects on the bones. The adverse effects of corticosteroids in general on bones are discussed on p.1040.

Studies in healthy subjects have shown that beclometasone dipropionate can suppress bone metabolism.[1-3] High-dose inhalation therapy (2000 μg daily) for 2 weeks resulted in a decrease in serum-osteocalcin concentrations.[1] Continuation of treatment for 4 weeks produced a more marked decrease in bone metabolism (using serum alkaline phosphatase activity and urinary hydroxyproline-creatinine ratio as markers).[2] Doses ranging from 400 to 2000 μg daily also decreased serum osteocalcin, with a dose-dependent effect up to 1400 μg daily.[3] Another study found that markers of collagen turnover, but not osteocalcin, were reduced by beclometasone or budesonide 800 μg daily in mildly asthmatic children.[4] Results are difficult to interpret since osteocalcin concentrations are reduced in patients with asthma regardless of treatment,[5] and it is uncertain whether significant bone loss does occur in practice.

1. Pouw EM, et al. Beclomethasone inhalation decreases serum osteocalcin concentrations. BMJ 1991; 302: 627–8.
2. Ali N, et al. Beclomethasone and osteocalcin. BMJ 1991; 302: 1080.
3. Teelucksingh S, et al. Inhaled corticosteroids, bone formation and osteocalcin. Lancet 1991; 338: 60–1.
4. Birkebæk NH, et al. Bone and collagen turnover during treatment with inhaled dry powder budesonide and beclomethasone dipropionate. Arch Dis Child 1995; 73: 524–7.
5. König P, et al. Bone metabolism in children with asthma treated with inhaled beclomethasone dipropionate. J Pediatr 1993; 122: 219–26.

Effects on growth. Meta-analysis of 3 eligible studies (out of 92 examined) concluded that inhaled beclometasone therapy at a dose of 400 μg daily may cause a 1.54 cm per year decrease in growth in children with mild to moderate asthma.[1] The long-term effects of treatment are unknown, and therefore it is not clear whether catch-up growth will occur upon cessation of therapy. The lowest possible dose of corticosteroid therapy should be used in asthma, and growth should be monitored.[1] For further details of the effects of corticosteroids on growth, see p.1041.

1. Sharek PJ, et al. Beclomethasone for asthma in children: effects on linear growth (updated 30 May 2001). Available in The Cochrane Library; Issue 3. Oxford: Update Software; 2001.

Effects on the lungs. References to the development of pulmonary eosinophilia in patients treated with inhaled beclometasone.

1. Paterson IC, *et al.* Pulmonary eosinophilia after substitution of aerosol for oral corticosteroid therapy. *Br J Dis Chest* 1975; **69:** 217–22.
2. Hudgel DW, Spector SL. Pulmonary infiltration with eosinophilia: recurrence in an asthmatic patient treated with beclomethasone dipropionate. *Chest* 1977; **72:** 359–60.
3. Klotz LR, *et al.* The use of beclomethasone dipropionate inhaler complicated by the development of an eosinophilic pneumonia reaction. *Ann Allergy* 1977; **39:** 133–6.
4. Mollura JL, *et al.* Pulmonary eosinophilia in a patient receiving beclomethasone dipropionate aerosol. *Ann Allergy* 1979; **42:** 326–9.

Hypersensitivity. Reports of asthmatic responses to beclometasone dipropionate inhalations, possibly associated with materials used in their formulation, or with the containers.

1. Maddern PJ, *et al.* Adverse reaction after aerosol inhalation. *Med J Aust* 1978; **1:** 274.
2. Godin J, Malo JL. Acute bronchoconstriction caused by Beclovent and not Vanceril. *Clin Allergy* 1979; **9:** 585–9.
3. Clark RJ. Exacerbation of asthma after nebulised beclomethasone dipropionate. *Lancet* 1986; **ii:** 574–5.
4. Beasley R, *et al.* Benzalkonium chloride and bronchoconstriction. *Lancet* 1986; **ii:** 1227.

Reformulation. Reformulation of some metered-dose inhalers to use a chlorofluorocarbon (CFC)-free propellant has resulted in a change of efficacy. One CFC-free product (Qvar, UK) is reported to be effective at approximately half the dose[1] required with the standard product (see Uses and Administration, below) and the UK Committee on Safety of Medicines has issued a reminder of the need for dosage reduction when converting from the conventional formulation to this product.[2] This dose reduction does not apply to all CFC-free formulations of beclometasone. However, an open-label, crossover study in healthy volunteers also found higher beclometasone plasma concentrations following the use of another brand (Beclozone, Eire) of CFC-free product.[3]

1. Davies RJ, Donnell D. HFA-beclomethasone (BDP) extrafine aerosol improves therapeutic index. *Thorax* 1997; **52** (suppl 6): A58.
2. Committee on Safety of Medicines/Medicines Control Agency. Dose of CFC-free inhaled beclomethasone (Qvar). *Current Problems* 1999; **25:** 5–6.
3. Lipworth BJ, Jackson CM. Pharmacokinetics of chlorofluorocarbon and hydrofluoroalkane metered-dose inhaler formulations of beclomethasone dipropionate. *Br J Clin Pharmacol* 1999; **48:** 866–8.

Interactions

The interactions of corticosteroids in general are described on p.1043.

Pharmacokinetics

For a brief outline of the pharmacokinetics of corticosteroids, see p.1044. Beclometasone is stated to be readily absorbed from sites of local application, and rapidly distributed to all body tissues. It is metabolised principally in the liver, but also in other tissues including gastrointestinal tract and lung; enzymatic hydrolysis rapidly produces the monopropionate (which has some glucocorticoid activity) and, more slowly, the free alcohol, which is virtually devoid of activity. Only a small proportion of an absorbed dose is excreted in urine, the remainder being excreted in the faeces mainly as metabolites.

Uses and Administration

Beclometasone dipropionate is a corticosteroid with mainly glucocorticoid activity (p.1039) that is stated to exert a topical effect on the lungs without significant systemic activity at recommended doses (but see Adrenal Suppression under Adverse Effects, above). It is used by inhalation, generally from a metered-dose aerosol, for the prophylaxis of asthma (see below).

A wide variety of formulations is now available, with differing dosage regimens, and the appropriate product literature should be consulted before initiating therapy or changing to another formulation. Furthermore in the UK the doses of beclometasone dipropionate for asthma and rhinitis are expressed in units of 50 µg or multiples thereof (dose supplied into the mouthpiece per actuation) whereas in the USA the dose-unit is 42 µg or multiples thereof (dose emitted from the mouthpiece); recommended doses therefore appear somewhat lower in the USA than the UK doses given below, although in practical terms there is probably no difference.

In the UK the adult dosage of the **conventional aerosol** and some dry powder inhalers is usually 400 µg

daily, inhaled in 2 to 4 divided doses for maintenance treatment; if necessary, 600 to 800 µg may be inhaled daily initially, subsequently adjusted according to the patient's response. In patients with severe asthma or in those showing only a partial response to standard inhalation doses, high-dose inhalation therapy may be considered; doses of 1 mg daily (250 µg four times daily or 500 µg twice daily) may be used and may be increased to 1.5 to 2 mg daily (500 µg three or four times daily) if necessary; a maximum of 2 mg daily should not be exceeded. In children, 50 or 100 µg may be inhaled 2 to 4 times daily according to the response or alternatively, 100 or 200 µg may be inhaled twice daily.

Although beclometasone dipropionate is generally inhaled in aerosol form, **inhalation capsules** or **discs** containing powder for inhalation are available for patients who experience difficulty in using the aerosol. Owing to differences in the relative bioavailability to the lungs of the preparations a 100-µg dose from an inhalation capsule or disc is approximately equivalent in activity to a 50-µg dose from a conventional aerosol. Recommended maintenance doses of beclometasone dipropionate from inhalation capsules or discs are therefore 200 µg inhaled 3 or 4 times daily or 400 µg inhaled twice daily for adults, and 100 µg inhaled 2 to 4 times daily or 200 µg inhaled twice daily for children. Up to 800 µg twice daily may be inhaled if necessary in adults requiring high-dose therapy.

In some countries beclometasone dipropionate is now available as a **CFC-free aerosol.** Because of changes in particle size the dose required from some such inhalers may be *lower* than that from a conventional aerosol: typical UK doses for one product (Qvar) range from 100 to 200 µg daily in mild asthma to 400 to 800 µg daily in severe asthma, given as 2 divided doses.

Inhalation of **nebulised** beclometasone dipropionate has also been used in the management of asthma in children.

Beclometasone dipropionate is also used as a **nasal spray** in the prophylaxis and treatment of allergic and non-allergic rhinitis (p.407). Usual doses are 100 µg in each nostril twice daily or 50 µg in each nostril 3 or 4 times daily; a total of 400 µg daily should not generally be exceeded. The nasal spray is also used in the prevention of recurrence of nasal polyps following surgical removal (p.1054).

Beclometasone dipropionate is also used **topically** in the treatment of various skin disorders. It is generally applied as a cream or ointment containing 0.025%. Beclometasone salicylate has also been used topically. For recommendations concerning the correct use of corticosteroids on the skin, and a rough guide to the clinical potencies of topical corticosteroids, see p.1045.

Adenoidal hypertrophy. Although normally managed by surgery (or if less severe simply by symptomatic relief) adenoidal hypertrophy in children was reported to respond to aqueous nasal beclometasone 336 µg daily in an 8-week crossover study.[1] Improvements in adenoidal obstruction and symptom scores were enhanced in a subsequent 16-week follow-on study using 168 µg daily.

1. Demain JG, Goetz DW. Pediatric adenoidal hypertrophy and nasal airway obstruction: reduction with aqueous nasal beclomethasone. *Pediatrics* 1995; **95:** 355–64.

Asthma. Corticosteroids and beta₂-adrenoceptor agonists form the cornerstone of the management of asthma (p.757). Patients requiring only occasional relief from symptoms may be managed with an inhaled short-acting beta₂ agonist, and an inhaled corticosteroid such as beclometasone is added if symptomatic relief is needed more than once daily. The dose of inhaled corticosteroid is increased in more severe asthma, often together with the addition of other drugs.

High-dose regimens may pose problems of compliance if beclometasone must be inhaled several times daily. However, one study[1] found once-daily inhalation to be as effective as the same dose divided into 2 daily inhalations in short-term control of moderate asthma. Also there have been doubts that increasing the dose of inhaled beclometasone brings about increased benefits,[2] but guidelines and clinical practice suggest that improved control can often be achieved by increasing the dose. A systematic review[3] noted that while there was little evidence of an effect of dose titration, evidence was lacking in patients with

more severe disease (who are more likely to be given high-dose therapy), and studies were needed to resolve the question.

Inhalation of beclometasone dipropionate as a nebulised solution has been found to be useful in the management of severe asthma in children aged 2 years or under previously unresponsive to other drugs.[4] Nebulised beclometasone dipropionate was also effective in the management of recurrent episodes of bronchopulmonary obstruction following bronchiolitis in children under 2 years of age.[5] However, in other reports nebulised beclometasone dipropionate, although more effective than saline in pre-school children, produced a response less than that usually observed with inhalation of beclometasone from an aerosol or capsules,[6] or no benefit at all.[7] This may have been due to beclometasone somehow failing to reach the lungs.[8] In pre-school children able to use a spacer device with a metered aerosol, intermittent therapy with high-dose beclometasone dipropionate, given at the first sign of symptoms, reduced the severity of acute episodic asthma.[9]

1. Gagnon M, *et al.* Comparative safety and efficacy of single or twice daily administration of inhaled beclomethasone in moderate asthma. *Chest* 1994; **105:** 1732–7.
2. Boe J, *et al.* High-dose inhaled steroids in asthmatics: moderate efficacy gain and suppression of the hypothalamic-pituitary-adrenal axis. *Eur Respir J* 1994; **7:** 2179–84.
3. Adams NP, *et al.* Inhaled beclomethasone versus placebo for chronic asthma (updated 30 May 2001). Available in The Cochrane Library; Issue 3. Oxford: Update Software; 2001.
4. Pedersen W, Prahl P. Jet-nebulized beclomethasone dipropionate in the management of bronchial asthma: topical steroids for asthmatic children younger than 4 years. *Allergy* 1987; **42:** 272–5.
5. Carlsen KH, *et al.* Nebulised beclomethasone dipropionate in recurrent obstructive episodes after acute bronchiolitis. *Arch Dis Child* 1988; **63:** 1428–33.
6. Storr J, *et al.* Nebulised beclomethasone dipropionate in preschool asthma. *Arch Dis Child* 1986; **61:** 270–3.
7. Webb MSC, *et al.* Nebulised beclomethasone dipropionate suspension. *Arch Dis Child* 1986; **61:** 1108–10.
8. Clarke SW. Nebulised beclomethasone dipropionate suspension: commentary. *Arch Dis Child* 1986; **61:** 1110.
9. Wilson NM, Silverman M. Treatment of acute, episodic asthma in preschool children using intermittent high dose inhaled steroids at home. *Arch Dis Child* 1990; **65:** 407–10.

Bronchopulmonary dysplasia. For mention of the use of beclometasone in infants at risk of bronchopulmonary dysplasia, see p.1048.

Chronic obstructive pulmonary disease. For discussion of the value of inhaled corticosteroids in chronic obstructive pulmonary disease, including reference to the use of beclometasone, see p.1049.

Cough. In children with recurrent cough (p.1082) inhalation of beclometasone 200 µg twice daily from a conventional aerosol or salbutamol 200 µg twice daily had no effect on cough frequency or severity.[1]

1. Chang AB, *et al.* A randomised, placebo controlled trial of inhaled salbutamol and beclomethasone for recurrent cough. *Arch Dis Child* 1998; **79:** 6–11.

Graft-versus-host disease. Beclometasone is under investigation for its topical effect in the treatment of intestinal graft-versus-host disease (GVHD). A study[1] in patients with acute intestinal GVHD after bone marrow transplantation (p.502) found that addition of oral beclometasone to prednisolone therapy was associated with a greater proportion of durable responses after 30 days.

1. McDonald GB, *et al.* Oral beclomethasone dipropionate for treatment of intestinal graft-versus-host disease: a randomized, controlled trial. *Gastroenterology* 1998; **115:** 28–35.

Inflammatory bowel disease. Beclometasone 0.5 mg administered nightly as an enema was as effective as betamethasone 5 mg enemas in the treatment of acute attacks of distal ulcerative colitis.[1] Although betamethasone produced slightly superior histological improvement and faster disappearance of blood from the stools, systemic adverse effects observed with betamethasone therapy were absent in patients treated with beclometasone.

A comparison of beclometasone dipropionate enemas (3 mg) with prednisolone sodium phosphate enemas (30 mg) found them to be equally effective.[2] The incidence of adverse effects in both groups was low.

For a review of the management of inflammatory bowel disease, including the role of corticosteroids, see p.1205.

1. Halpern Z, *et al.* A controlled trial of beclomethasone versus betamethasone enemas in distal ulcerative colitis. *J Clin Gastroenterol* 1991; **13:** 38–41.
2. Campieri M, *et al.* Beclomethasone dipropionate enemas versus prednisolone sodium phosphate enemas in the treatment of distal ulcerative colitis. *Aliment Pharmacol Ther* 1998; **121:** 361–6.

Preparations

BP 2001: Beclomethasone Cream; Beclomethasone Nasal Spray; Beclomethasone Ointment; Beclomethasone Pressurised Inhalation.

Proprietary Preparations (details are given in Part 3)
Aust.: Beclomet; Beconase; Becotide; *Austral.:* Aldecin; Becloforte; Beconase; Becotide; *Belg.:* Aldecin†; Beconase; Becotide; *Braz.:* Aldecina; Beclosol; *Canad.:* Beclodisk; Becloforte; Beclovent; Beconase; Gen-Beclo; Propaderm; Rivanase; Vancenase; Vanceril†; *Denm.:* AeroBec; Aldecin; Andion†; Becloforte†; Beclomet; Becocent†; Beconase; Becotide†; *Fin.:* AeroBec; Beclomet; Beclonasal; Beconase; Becotide; *Fr.:* Asmabec; Beclo-Rhino; Beclojet; Beclone; Beconase; Becotide; Bemedrex; Prolair; Qvar; Rhinirex; Spir; *Ger.:* AeroBec; Beclomet; Beclorhinol; Becloturmant; Beconase Aquosum; Bronchocort; Cyclocaps; Junik; ratioAllerg; Rhinivict; Sanasth-

max; Sanasthmyl; Ventolair; Viarox; **Hong Kong:** Aldecin; Atomase; Beclo Asma; Becloforte; Becodisks; Beconase; Becotide; Clenil; Nasobec; Rino Clenil; *Irl.*: AeroBec; Asmabec; Beclazone; Beclo-Rhino; Becodisks; Beconase; Becotide; Nasobec; Qvar; **Israel:** Becloforte; Becotide; Rhinocort; Viarex; *Ital.*: Becotide; Becotide A; Bronco-Turbinal; Cleniderm†; Clenil; Clipper; Menaderm Simplex; Rino Clenil; Topster; Turbinal; *Mex.*: AeroBec; Beconase; Becotide; **Neth.:** AeroBec; Aldecin†; Becloforte; Beconase; Becotide; Qvar; **Norw.:** Beclomet; Beconase; Becotide; Qvar; **NZ:** Alanase; Aldecin; Atomase; Atomide; Becloforte; Becodisk; Beconase; Becotide; Qvar; Respocort; Sinase; *Port.*: Aldecina; Beclotaide; Beconase; Becotide; *S.Afr.*: AeroBec; Anceron; Beceze; Beclate; Becloforte; Becodisks; Beconase; Becotide; Clenil; Nobec; Propaderm†; Qvar; Rinaze; Ventnaze; Ventzone; Viarox; *Singapore:* Aldecin; Beclazone; Becloforte; Beclomet; Beconase; Becotide; Clenil; Rino Clenil; **Spain:** Beclo Asma; Beclo Rino; Becloforte; Beclosona; Beconase; Betsuril; Broncivent; Decasona; Dereme; Dermisone Beclo†; Menaderm Simple; Novahaler; Recto Menaderm NF; **Swed.:** Beclomet; Becotide; *Switz.*: Aldecin†; Becloforte; Beclomet; Becodisk; Beconase; Beconasol; Becotide; **Thai.:** Atomase; Becloforte; Beclomet; Becodisk; Beconase; Becotide; Clenil; **UK:** AeroBec; Asmabec; Beceze†; Beclazone; Beclo Aqua; Becloforte; Beclogen; Becodisks; Beconase; Becotide; Filair; Hayfever Relief; Nasal Spray for Hayfever; Nasal-Bec; Nasobec; Pollenase Hayfever; Propaderm; Qvar; Zonivent†; *USA:* Beclovent; Beconase; Qvar; Vancenase; Vanceril.

Multi-ingredient: Aust.: Duospirel†; Ventide; **Braz.:** Aerotide; **Hong Kong:** Ventide; **Ital.:** Clenil Compositum; Menaderm; Ventolin Flogo; **Mex.:** Propaderm-C†; **Singapore:** Clenil Compositum; Ventide; **Spain:** Butosol; Menaderm Clio; Menaderm Neomicina; Menaderm Otologico; Recto Menaderm†; **Switz.:** Beclonarin; **Thai.:** Clenil Compositum; Ventide; **UK:** Ventide.

Bendacort   (6589-z)

AF-2071; Cortazac; Hydrocortisone Bendazac.
$C_{37}H_{42}N_2O_7 = 626.7$.
CAS — 53716-43-1.

Profile
Bendacort is the 21-ester of hydrocortisone with bendazac (p.19). It has been applied topically for its glucocorticoid activity (p.1039) in the management of various skin disorders.

Betamethasone   (1063-j)

Betamethasone *(BAN, USAN, rINN).*
Betadexamethasone; Betamethasonum; Flubenisolone; Flubenisolonum; 9α-Fluoro-16β-methylprednisolone; β-Methasone; NSC-39470; Sch-4831. 9α-Fluoro-11β,17α,21-trihydroxy-16β-methylpregna-1,4-diene-3,20-dione.
$C_{22}H_{29}FO_5 = 392.5$.
CAS — 378-44-9.
ATC — A07EA04; C05AA05; D07AC01; D07XC01; H02AB01; R01AD06; R03BA04; S01BA06; S01CB04; S02BA07.

Pharmacopoeias. In Chin., Eur. (see p.vi), Int., Jpn, and US.

Pharmacopoeial description
Ph. Eur.: A white or almost white, crystalline powder. Practically insoluble in water; sparingly soluble in dehydrated alcohol; very slightly soluble in dichloromethane. Protect from light.
USP 25: A white to practically white, odourless, crystalline powder. Soluble 1 in 5300 of water, 1 in 65 of alcohol, 1 in 15 of warm alcohol, 1 in 325 of chloroform, and 1 in 3 of methyl alcohol; sparingly soluble in acetone and in dioxan; very slightly soluble in ether.

Betamethasone Acetate   (1064-z)

Betamethasone Acetate *(BANM, rINNM).*
Betamethasoni Acetas. Betamethasone 21-acetate.
$C_{24}H_{31}FO_6 = 434.5$.
CAS — 987-24-6.
Pharmacopoeias. In Eur. (see p.vi) and US.

Betamethasone acetate 1.1 mg is approximately equivalent to 1 mg of betamethasone.

Pharmacopoeial description
Ph. Eur.: A white or almost white, crystalline powder. Practically insoluble in water; soluble in alcohol and in dichloromethane; freely soluble in acetone. It shows polymorphism. Protect from light.
USP 25: A white to creamy-white, odourless powder. Soluble 1 in 2000 of water, 1 in 9 of alcohol, and 1 in 16 of chloroform; freely soluble in acetone. Store in airtight containers.

Betamethasone Benzoate   (1065-c)

Betamethasone Benzoate *(BANM, USAN, rINNM).*
W-5975. Betamethasone 17α-benzoate.
$C_{29}H_{33}FO_6 = 496.6$.
CAS — 22298-29-9.
Pharmacopoeias. In US.

Betamethasone benzoate 1.3 mg is approximately equivalent to 1 mg of betamethasone.

Pharmacopoeial description
USP 25: A white to practically white, practically odourless, powder. Insoluble in water; soluble in alcohol, in chloroform, and in methyl alcohol. Store in airtight containers.

Betamethasone Dipropionate   (1066-k)

Betamethasone Dipropionate *(BANM, USAN, rINNM).*
Betamethasoni Dipropionas; Sch-11460. Betamethasone 17α,21-dipropionate.
$C_{28}H_{37}FO_7 = 504.6$.
CAS — 5593-20-4.

NOTE. Compounded preparations of betamethasone dipropionate may be represented by the following names:

• Co-climasone (*USP 25*)—clotrimazole and betamethasone dipropionate.

Pharmacopoeias. In Eur. (see p.vi), Jpn, and US.

Betamethasone dipropionate 1.3 mg is approximately equivalent to 1 mg of betamethasone.

Pharmacopoeial description
Ph. Eur.: A white or almost white, crystalline powder. Practically insoluble in water; sparingly soluble in alcohol; freely soluble in acetone and in dichloromethane. Protect from light.
USP 25: A white to cream-white, odourless powder. Insoluble in water; sparingly soluble in alcohol; freely soluble in acetone and in chloroform.

Betamethasone Sodium Phosphate   (1067-a)

Betamethasone Sodium Phosphate *(BANM, rINNM).*
Betamethasone Disodium Phosphate; Betamethasoni Natrii Phosphas. Betamethasone 21-(disodium phosphate).
$C_{22}H_{28}FNa_2O_8P = 516.4$.
CAS — 360-63-4 (betamethasone phosphate); 151-73-5 (betamethasone sodium phosphate).

NOTE. BET is a code approved by the BP 2001 for use on single unit doses of eye drops containing betamethasone sodium phosphate where the individual container may be too small to bear all the appropriate labelling information.
Pharmacopoeias. In Eur. (see p.vi), Jpn, and US.

Betamethasone sodium phosphate 1.3 mg is approximately equivalent to 1 mg of betamethasone.

Pharmacopoeial description
Ph. Eur.: A white or almost white, very hygroscopic, powder. Freely soluble in water; slightly soluble in alcohol; practically insoluble in dichloromethane and in ether. A 1% solution in water has a pH of 7.5 to 9.0. Store in airtight containers. Protect from light.
USP 25: A white to practically white, odourless, hygroscopic, powder. Soluble 1 in 2 of water and 1 in 470 of alcohol; freely soluble in methyl alcohol; practically insoluble in acetone and in chloroform. Store in airtight containers.

Betamethasone Valerate   (1068-t)

Betamethasone Valerate *(BANM, USAN, rINNM).*
Betamethasoni Valeras. Betamethasone 17α-valerate.
$C_{27}H_{37}FO_6 = 476.6$.
CAS — 2152-44-5.
Pharmacopoeias. In Eur. (see p.vi), Int., Jpn, and US.

Betamethasone valerate 1.2 mg is approximately equivalent to 1 mg of betamethasone.

Pharmacopoeial description
Ph. Eur.: A white or almost white, crystalline powder. Practically insoluble in water; soluble in alcohol; freely soluble in acetone and in dichloromethane. Protect from light.
USP 25: A white to practically white, odourless, powder. Practically insoluble in water; soluble 1 in 16 of alcohol, 1 in less than 10 of chloroform, and 1 in 400 of ether; freely soluble in acetone; slightly soluble in benzene. Store in airtight containers.

Adverse Effects, Treatment, Withdrawal, and Precautions

As for corticosteroids in general (see p.1039).

Betamethasone has little or no effects on sodium and water retention.

When applied topically, particularly to large areas, when the skin is broken, or under occlusive dressings, or when given intranasally, corticosteroids may be absorbed in sufficient amounts to cause systemic effects. Prolonged application to the eye of preparations containing corticosteroids has caused raised intra-ocular pressure and reduced visual function.

Anosmia. A report of anosmia occurring in two patients following the use of nasal drops containing betamethasone and neomycin sulfate.[1] The anosmia was complete and, in one patient, showed no sign of resolving one year later. The reaction was thought to be due to thiomersal present in the drops as a preservative, although it was noted that neomycin could exert a toxic effect on the olfactory mucosa and that there have been several reports of anosmia associated with the use of betamethasone alone.

1. Whittet HB, *et al.* Anosmia due to nasal administration of corticosteroid. *BMJ* 1991; **303:** 651.

Interactions
The interactions of corticosteroids in general are described on p.1043.

Pharmacokinetics
For a brief outline of the pharmacokinetics of corticosteroids, see p.1044. Betamethasone crosses the placenta.

Uses and Administration
Betamethasone is a corticosteroid with mainly glucocorticoid activity, as described under Corticosteroids, p.1039; the anti-inflammatory activity of 750 µg of betamethasone is equivalent to about 5 mg of prednisolone. It has been used, either in the form of the free alcohol or in one of the esterified forms, in the treatment of conditions for which corticosteroid therapy is indicated (p.1044), except adrenal-deficiency states for which hydrocortisone with supplementary fludrocortisone is preferred. Its virtual lack of mineralocorticoid properties makes betamethasone particularly suitable for treating conditions in which water retention would be a disadvantage.

For administration by mouth betamethasone or betamethasone sodium phosphate is used; the usual dose, expressed in terms of betamethasone, ranges from 0.5 to 5 mg daily.

For parenteral administration the sodium phosphate ester may be given intravenously by injection or infusion or intramuscularly by injection in doses equivalent to 4 to 20 mg of betamethasone. It may also be given by local injection into soft tissues in doses equivalent to 4 to 8 mg of betamethasone. Doses in children, as a slow intravenous injection, are, in infants aged up to 1 year the equivalent of 1 mg of betamethasone; children aged 1 to 5 years, 2 mg; 6 to 12 years, 4 mg. Doses may be repeated 3 or 4 times in 24 hours if necessary, depending on the condition being treated and the clinical response. The sodium phosphate ester is also sometimes used in conjunction with the acetate or dipropionate esters, which have a slower and more prolonged action.

Betamethasone sodium phosphate is also used in the topical treatment of allergic and inflammatory conditions of the eyes, ears, or nose, usually as drops or ointment containing 0.1%.

For topical application in the treatment of various skin disorders the dipropionate and valerate esters of betamethasone are extensively used; the usual concentrations available are the equivalent of 0.05% of betamethasone as the dipropionate, and 0.025 or 0.1% as the valerate. For recommendations concerning the correct use of corticosteroids on the skin, and a rough guide to the clinical potencies of topical corticosteroids, see p.1045.

Betamethasone valerate has also been used by inhalation for the prophylaxis of asthma.

Other esters of betamethasone which have occasionally been used include the benzoate, butyrate propionate, phosphate, salicylate (cortobenzolone), and valero-acetate.

Betamethasone adamantoate has been used in veterinary practice.

Haemangioma. For reference to the use of a mixture of betamethasone and triamcinolone for the intralesional injection of haemangiomas, see p.1052.

Inflammatory bowel disease. For a comparison of betamethasone and beclometasone enemas in the treatment of ulcerative colitis, see under Beclometasone, p.1062. Corticosteroids are one of the mainstays of treatment of inflammatory bowel disease, the general management of which is discussed on p.1205.

Preparations
BP 2001: Betamethasone and Clioquinol Cream; Betamethasone and Clioquinol Ointment; Betamethasone Eye Drops; Betamethasone Injection; Betamethasone Sodium Phosphate Tablets; Betamethasone Tablets; Betamethasone Valerate Cream; Betamethasone

The symbol † denotes a preparation no longer actively marketed

Valerate Lotion; Betamethasone Valerate Ointment; Betamethasone Valerate Scalp Application;
USP 25: Betamethasone Benzoate Gel; Betamethasone Cream; Betamethasone Dipropionate Cream; Betamethasone Dipropionate Lotion; Betamethasone Dipropionate Ointment; Betamethasone Dipropionate Topical Aerosol; Betamethasone Sodium Phosphate and Betamethasone Acetate Injectable Suspension; Betamethasone Sodium Phosphate Injection; Betamethasone Syrup; Betamethasone Tablets; Betamethasone Valerate Cream; Betamethasone Valerate Lotion; Betamethasone Valerate Ointment; Clotrimazole and Betamethasone Dipropionate Cream.

Proprietary Preparations (details are given in Part 3)
Aust.: Betnesol; Betnovate; Celestan; Diproderm; Diproforte; Diprophos; Solu-Celestan; *Austral.:* Antroquoril; Betnovate; Celestone Chronodose; Celestone M; Celestone V; Diprosone; Eleuphrat; *Belg.:* Betnelan-V; Betnesol; Celestone; Celestone Chronodose; Diprolene; Diprosone; *Braz.:* Bebyderm; Betaderm; Betnelan; Betnovate; Celestone; Celestone Soluspan; Clenil; Dermoval; Dermovate; Diprosone; Epidermil; Sensitex; *Canad.:* Beben†; Betacort†; Betaderm; Betaject; Betnesol; Celestoderm; Celestone Soluspan; Celestone†; Diprolene Glycol; Diprosone; Ectosone; Occlucort†; Prevex B; Rivasone†; Rolene†; Rosone†; Taro-Sone; Topilene; Topisone; Valisone; *Denm.:* Betnovat; Betoid; Bettamousse; Celeston; Diproderm; Diprolen; Diprospan; *Fin.:* Bemetson; Betapred; Betnovat; Bettamousse; Celestoderm; Celeston Chronodose; Diproderm; Diprolen; Diprosalic; *Fr.:* Betnesol; Betneval; Celestene; Celestene Chronodose; Celestoderm; Diprolene; Diprosone; *Ger.:* Bemon; Beta-Stulln; BetaCreme; Betagalen; Betam-Ophtal; BetaSalbe; Betnesol; Betnesol-V; Celestamine N; Celestan solubile; Celestan-V; Cordes Beta; Diprosis; Diprosone; Euvaderm†; Lygal E Creme; Pentacort; Soderm; *Hong Kong:* Betasone; Betnovate; Celestoderm-V; Celestone; Diprocel; Diprosone; Diprospan; Topilene; *Irl.:* Betacap; Betnelan; Betnesol; Betnovate; Bettamousse; Diprosone; *Israel:* Betacorten; Betnesol; Betnovate; Celestoderm-V; Celestone Chronodose; Dicorten; Diprolene; Diprosone; Diprospan; *Ital.:* Beben; Bentelan; Beta 21; Betamesol; Bettamousse; Celestoderm-V; Celestene Cronodose; Celestone; Diprosone; Ecoval; *Mex.:* Betnovate; Celestoderm-V; Celestone; Celestone Soluspan; Dermoval; Diprosone; Diprospan; *Neth.:* Betnelan; Betnesol; Celestoderm; Celestone; Celestone Chronodose; Diprolene; Diprosone; *Norw.:* Betnovat; Betoid; Celeston; Diproderm; *NZ:* Beta Scalp; Betnesol; Betnovate; Bivate; Celestone Chronodose; Diprolene; Diprosone; *Port.:* Betnasol†; Betnovate; Celesdepot; Celestone; Cilestoderme; Dibetop; Diprofos; Diprosone; Soluderme; Vabeta; *S.Afr.:* Betanoid; Betnelan†; Betnesol; Betnovate; Celestoderm-V; Celestone; Celestone Soluspan; Diprolene; Diprosone; Lenasone; Lenovate; Persivate; Steromien; Topivate; *Singapore:* Beprogel; Beprosone; Besone; Betacorten; Celestoderm-V; Celestone; Dibetasol; Diprocel; Diprosone; Diprospan; Medobeta; Uniflex; *Spain:* Betamatil; Betnovate; Bettamousse; Celestoderm; Celestoderm-V; Celestone; Celestone Cronodose; Diproderm; *Swed.:* Betapred; Betnovat; Betoid; Bettamousse; Celeston; Celeston valerat; Diproderm; *Switz.:* Betnesol; Betnovate; Celestoderm-V; Celestone; Celestone Chronodose; Diprolene; Diprosone; *Thai.:* Bennasone; Beprosone; Besone; Bessasone; Beta; Betameth; Bethasone; Betnovate; Betosone; Bipro; Celestamine; Celestone; Derzid; Diprosone; Diprospan; Diprotop; Sebo; Valbet; *UAE:* Betasone; *UK:* Betacap; Betnelan; Betnesol; Betnovate; Betnovate RD (Ready Diluted); Bettamousse; Diprosone; Vista-Methasone; *USA:* Alphatrex; Beta-Val; Betatrex; Cel-U-Jec; Celestone; Celestone Soluspan; Diprolene; Diprosone; Luxiq; Maxivate; Psorion†; Teladar; Valisone.

Multi-ingredient: *Aust.:* Betnesol-N; Betnovate-N; Celestamine; *Austral.:* Celestone VG; *Belg.:* Betnelan-VC; Betnelan-VN†; Diprophos; Diprosalic; Fucicort; Garasone; Lotriderm; *Braz.:* Betazon; Betnovate-N; Betnovate-Q; Candicort; Celestamine; Clenil Compositum; Diprogenta; Diprosalic; Diprospan; Garasone; Gentacort; Novacort; Oto Betnovate; Quadriderm; Quadrilo; Reumix-G; *Canad.:* Diprogen; Diprosalic; Garasone; Lotriderm; Valisone-G; *Denm.:* Betnovat med Chinoform; Betnovat Rektal; Celeston med Chinoform; Clotrason; Diproform; Diprosalic; Fucicort; *Fin.:* Betnovat Comp; Betnovat-C; Celestoderm cum Chinoform; Celestoderm cum Garamycin; Fucicort; *Fr.:* Betnesalic; Betneval-Neomycine; Celestamine; Diprosalic; Diprosept; Diprosone Neomycine; Diprostene; Gentasone; *Ger.:* Betadermic; Betagentam; Betamethason Plus; Betnesalic; Celestamine; Celestan Depot; Diprogenta; Diprosalic; Diprosone Depot; Euvaderm N†; Euvaderm†; Fucicort; Lotricomb; Lygal E Tinktur; Sulmycin mit Celestan-V; *Hong Kong:* Bechlomin; Beclomin; Betnesalic; Betnovate-C; Betnovate-N; Celestamine; Celestoderm-V with Garamycin; Celestoderm-V with Neomycin; Diprogenta; Diprosalic; Fucicort; Garasone; Quadriderm; Synbetamine; Triderm; *Irl.:* Betnesol-N; Betnovate-C; Betnovate-N; Diprosalic; Fucibet; Lotriderm; Vista-Methasone N; *Israel:* Betacorten-G; Betnesol-N; Betnovate-N; Celestoderm-V with Garamycin; Diprogenta; Diprosalic; Fucicort; Triderm; *Ital.:* Alfaflor; Apsor†; Beben Clorossina; Betabioptal; Biorinil; Brumeton Colloidale S; Deltavagin; Dermatar; Diproform; Diprogenta†; Diprosalic; Ecoval con Neomicina; Eubetal; Eubetal Antibiotico; Fluororinil; Gentalyn Beta; Micutrin Beta; Psorinase; Rinojet; Stranoval; Viobeta; Visublefarite; Visumetazone Antibiotico; Visumidriatic Antiflogistico†; *Mex.:* Celestamine; Celestamine-F; Clio-Betnovate; Diprosalic; Diprosone G; Diprosone-Y; Fucicort; Garamicina V; Garasone; Genrex-B; Quadriderm NF; *Neth.:* Betnelan Clioquinol†; Betnelan Neomycine†; Celestoderm met Neomycine; Celestoform; Diprosalic; Betnovat med Chinoform; Diprosalic; *NZ:* Betnesol Aqueous; Betnesol-N; Betnovate-C; Diprosalic; Fucicort; Lotricomb; Ultrazon N; *Port.:* Celestoderm-V; Betnovate-N; Dibetop Q; Diprogenta; Diprosalic; Epione; Flotiran; Fucicort; Psodermil; Quadriderme; *S.Afr.:* Betnesol-N; Betnovate-C; Betnovate-N; Celestamine; Celestoderm-V with Garamycin; Diprogenta; Diprosalic; Garasone; Lotriderm; Quadriderm; *Singapore:* B-Tasone-G; Beprogent; Beprosalic; Besone-N; Betnovate-C; Betnovate-GM; Betnovate-M; Celestoderm-V with Garamycin; Celestoderm-V with Neomycin; Combiderm; Conazole; Diprogenta; Diprosalic; Fucicort; Garasone; Gentrisone; Neoderm; Quadriderm; Tri-Micon; Triderm; Uniflex-N; *Spain:* Alergical; Beta Micoter; Betamatil con Neomicina; Betamida;

Betartrinovo†; Bronsal; Celesemine; Celestoderm Gentamicina; Celestone S; Clotrasone; Cuatroderm; Diprogenta; Diprosalic; Fucibet; Nasotic Oto; Resorborina; Sclane; Visublefarite†; *Swed.:* Betnovat med Chinoform; Betnovat med Neomycin; Celeston bifas; Celeston valerat comp; Celeston valerat med chinoform; Celeston valerat med gentamicin; Diprosalic; *Switz.:* Betnesalic; Betnovate-C; Betnovate-N; Celestamine; Diprogenta; Diprosalic; Diprosalic; Fucicort; Ophtasone; Quadriderm; Triderm; *Thai.:* Benn; Beprogenta; Besone-N; Beta-C; Beta-S; Beta-S; Betamina-EN; Bethasone-N; Betnesalic; Betnovate-C; Betnovate-N; Betosalic; Betosone-CE; Canasone; Canazol-BE; Celestoderm-V with Neomycin; Clotrasone; Diprogenta; Diprosalic; Fucicort; Fungiderm-B; Quadriderm; Valbet-N; *UAE:* Futasone; Supraproct-S; *UK:* Betnesol-N; Betnovate Rectal Ointment; Betnovate-C; Betnovate-N; Diprosalic; Fucibet; Lotriderm†; Vipsogal; Vista-Methasone N; *USA:* Lotrisone.

Budesonide (12463-p)

Budesonide *(BAN, USAN, rINN)*.

S-1320. An epimeric mixture of the α- and β-propyl forms of 16α,17α-butylidenedioxy-11β,21-dihydroxypregna-1,4-diene-3,20-dione.

$C_{25}H_{34}O_6 = 430.5.$

CAS — 51333-22-3 (11β,16α); 51372-29-3 (11β,16α(R)); 51372-28-2 (11β,16α(S)).
ATC — A07EA06; D07AC09; H02AB16; R01AD05; R03BA02.

Pharmacopoeias. In Eur. (see p.vi).

Pharmacopoeial description

Ph. Eur.: A white or almost white, crystalline powder. Practically insoluble in water; sparingly soluble in alcohol; freely soluble in dichloromethane.

Adverse Effects, Treatment, Withdrawal, and Precautions

As for corticosteroids in general (see p.1039).

Inhalation of high doses of budesonide is associated with some adrenal suppression. Systemic absorption may follow nasal administration, particularly if high doses are used or treatment is prolonged.

When applied topically, particularly to large areas, when the skin is broken, or under occlusive dressings, or when given intranasally, corticosteroids may be absorbed in sufficient amounts to cause systemic effects.

Effects on the bones. For mention of a reduction in markers of collagen turnover in mildly asthmatic children receiving budesonide by inhalation, see under Adverse Effects of Beclometasone, p.1061. For the suggestion that inhalation once-a-day in the morning may have less marked effects on growth and collagen turnover than twice-daily inhalation, see Administration, below.

Effects on the nervous system. Psychotic behaviour has been reported following use of inhaled budesonide.[1-3]

1. Lewis LD, Cochrane GM. Psychosis in a child inhaling budesonide. *Lancet* 1983; **ii:** 634.
2. Meyboom RHB, de Graff-Breederveld N. Budesonide and psychic side effects. *Ann Intern Med* 1988; **109:** 683.
3. Connett G, Lenney W. Inhaled budesonide and behavioural disturbances. *Lancet* 1991; **338:** 634–5.

Hypersensitivity. Contact dermatitis has been reported to topical or intranasal budesonide.[1]

1. Quintiliani R. Hypersensitivity and adverse reactions associated with the use of newer intranasal corticosteroids for allergic rhinitis. *Curr Ther Res* 1996; **57:** 478–88.

Interactions

The interactions of corticosteroids in general are described on p.1043.

Pharmacokinetics

For a brief outline of the pharmacokinetics of corticosteroids, see p.1044. Budesonide is rapidly and almost completely absorbed following administration by mouth, but has poor systemic availability (about 10%) due to extensive first-pass metabolism in the liver. The major metabolites, 6-β-hydroxybudesonide and 16-α-hydroxyprednisolone have less than 1% of the glucocorticoid activity of unchanged budesonide. Budesonide is reported to have a terminal half-life of about 4 hours.

Uses and Administration

Budesonide is a corticosteroid with mainly glucocorticoid activity (p.1039). It is used by inhalation in the management of asthma, in usual doses of 400 µg daily in 2 divided doses from a metered-dose aerosol; in severe asthma the dosage may be increased up to a

total of 1.6 mg daily, and guidelines for the management of asthma permit up to 2 mg daily (see p.757). Maintenance doses may be less than 400 µg daily but should not be below 200 µg daily. A dose for children is 50 to 400 µg inhaled twice daily. Budesonide is also available for the management of asthma in the form of a dry powder inhaler; doses are 200 to 800 µg daily, as 2 divided doses or a single daily dose; up to 800 µg twice daily may be given to adults if necessary. Patients for whom administration of budesonide from a pressurised inhaler or dry powder formulation is unsatisfactory may use a nebulised solution. The usual adult dosage by this method is 1 to 2 mg inhaled twice daily. This may be increased if asthma is severe. Maintenance doses are 0.5 to 1 mg inhaled twice daily. For children between 3 months and 12 years of age, an initial dose is 0.5 to 1 mg twice daily with a maintenance dose of 0.25 to 0.5 mg twice daily.

Budesonide is also given by inhalation as a nebulised solution in the management of childhood croup (p.1049). The usual dose is 2 mg, as a single inhaled dose or 2 doses of 1 mg, given 30 minutes apart.

Budesonide is used topically in the treatment of various skin disorders, as a cream or ointment containing 0.025%. For recommendations concerning the correct use of corticosteroids on the skin, and a rough guide to the clinical potencies of topical corticosteroids, see p.1045.

Budesonide is also used as a nasal spray for the prophylaxis and treatment of rhinitis (p.407), and in the management of nasal polyps (p.1054). In the UK it is used for rhinitis in a usual initial dose of 200 µg into each nostril once daily, subsequently reduced to the lowest dose adequate to control symptoms which may be 100 µg into each nostril daily. Alternatively, the initial dose may be 100 µg into each nostril twice daily. The latter dose is given for up to three months in the treatment of nasal polyps. In the USA and some other countries the intranasal dose may be expressed in multiples of 32 µg, which is the quantity of budesonide delivered from the nasal adaptor. When given from a nasal inhaler an initial dose of 128 µg daily in each nostril, reduced once control is established, is recommended in adults and children over 6 years of age. An alternative regimen, beginning with 32 µg daily in each nostril and increasing as necessary up to a maximum of 128 µg daily in each nostril for adults or half this amount in children, is recommended when the dose is given as an aqueous nasal spray.

Local formulations of budesonide are used in the management of inflammatory bowel disease (see below). In mild to moderate Crohn's disease affecting the ileum or ascending colon it is given by mouth as modified-release capsules intended for a topical effect on the gastrointestinal tract. The recommended dose is 9 mg daily for up to 8 weeks. The dosage should be reduced 2 to 4 weeks before discontinuing budesonide therapy. An enema solution containing 0.002% is also available; it is administered at bedtime for 4 weeks in the treatment of ulcerative colitis at a dose of 2 mg.

◊ General references.

1. Brogden RN, McTavish D. Budesonide: an updated review of its pharmacological properties, and therapeutic efficacy in asthma and rhinitis. *Drugs* 1992; **44:** 375–407 and 1012.
2. Hvizdos KM, Jarvis B. Budesonide inhalation suspension: a review of its use in infants, children and adults with inflammatory respiratory disorders. *Drugs* 2000; **60:** 1141–78.

Administration. INHALATIONAL ROUTE. One study in 6 children aged up to 30 months found that about 75% of the nominal dose of nebulised budesonide was deposited in the nebuliser system,[1] while a study in 126 older children indicated that maintenance doses of budesonide could be halved when the dose was given by dry powder inhaler rather than nebuliser,[2] without any loss of asthma control. Although oropharyngeal deposition is thought to play a role in the systemic effects of inhaled corticosteroids, another study[3] indicated that only about 20% of the systemically available drug appeared to be derived from oropharyngeal deposition following inhalation from a dry powder inhaler.

There is evidence that the timing of inhaled therapy might influence some systemic effects. A study[4] in children with mild asthma found that 800 µg of budesonide inhaled in the morning had less effect on measurements of short-term growth and collagen turnover than inhalation of 400 µg twice daily.

1. Carlsen KCL, *et al.* How much nebulised budesonide reaches infants and toddlers? *Arch Dis Child* 1992; **67:** 1077–9.
2. Agertoft L, Pedersen S. Importance of the inhalation device on the effect of budesonide. *Arch Dis Child* 1993; **69:** 130–3.
3. Pedersen S, *et al.* The influence of orally deposited budesonide on the systemic availability of budesonide after inhalation from a Turbuhaler. *Br J Clin Pharmacol* 1993; **36:** 211–14.
4. Heuck C, *et al.* Adverse effects of inhaled budesonide (800 µg) on growth and collagen turnover in children with asthma: a double-blind comparison of once-daily versus twice-daily administration. *J Pediatr* 1998; **133:** 608–12.

Asthma. References to the use of budesonide in asthma.[1,2]

1. Baker JW, *et al.* A multiple-dosing, placebo-controlled study of budesonide inhalation suspension given once or twice daily for treatment of persistent asthma in young children and infants. *Pediatrics* 1999; **103:** 414–21.
2. The Childhood Asthma Management Program Research Group. Long-term effects of budesonide or nedocromil in children with asthma. *N Engl J Med* 2000; **343:** 1054–63.

Chronic obstructive pulmonary disease. For discussion of the value of inhaled corticosteroids in chronic obstructive pulmonary disease, including reference to the use of budesonide, see p.1049.

Cystic fibrosis. Cystic fibrosis (p.117) is associated with bronchial hyper-responsiveness; a small study[1] has suggested that inhalation of budesonide 1.6 mg daily for 6 weeks improves hyper-responsiveness slightly and leads to improvement in cough and dyspnoea.

1. Van Haren EHJ, *et al.* The effects of the inhaled corticosteroid budesonide on lung function and bronchial hyperresponsiveness in adult patients with cystic fibrosis. *Respir Med* 1995; **89:** 209–14.

Inflammatory bowel disease. Budesonide has been given as an enema for the treatment of distal ulcerative colitis, in which context its potency, high aqueous solubility, and low systemic availability are advantageous.[1,2] It is also available as a modified-release oral dosage form for the management of active Crohn's disease,[3-6] and has been investigated for its potential in delaying relapse in quiescent disease,[7-9] although any benefit appears short-term. Similarly, oral budesonide was ineffective in preventing postoperative recurrence after resection for Crohn's disease.[10] Oral budesonide has also been tried as an alternative to conventional systemic corticosteroids in ulcerative colitis.[11]

For a discussion of inflammatory bowel disease, see p.1205.

1. Sachar DB. Budesonide for inflammatory bowel disease: is it a magic bullet? *N Engl J Med* 1994; **331:** 873–4.
2. Spencer CM, McTavish D. Budesonide: a review of its pharmacological properties and therapeutic efficacy in inflammatory bowel disease. *Drugs* 1995; **50:** 854–72.
3. Greenberg GR, *et al.* Oral budesonide for active Crohn's disease. *N Engl J Med* 1994; **331:** 836–41.
4. Rutgeerts P, *et al.* A comparison of budesonide with prednisolone for active Crohn's disease. *N Engl J Med* 1994; **331:** 842–5.
5. Campieri M, *et al.* Oral budesonide is as effective as oral prednisolone in active Crohn's disease. *Gut* 1997; **41:** 209–14.
6. Thomsen OØ, *et al.* A comparison of budesonide and mesalamine for active Crohn's disease. *N Engl J Med* 1998; **339:** 370–4.
7. Greenberg GR, *et al.* Oral budesonide as maintenance treatment for Crohn's disease: a placebo-controlled dose-ranging study. *Gastroenterology* 1996; **110:** 45–51.
8. Löfberg R, *et al.* Budesonide prolongs time to relapse in ileal and ileocaecal Crohn's disease: a placebo controlled one year study. *Gut* 1996; **39:** 82–6.
9. Gross V, *et al.* Low dose oral pH modified release budesonide for maintenance of steroid induced remission in Crohn's disease. *Gut* 1998; **42:** 493–6.
10. Hellers G, *et al.* Oral budesonide for prevention of postsurgical recurrence in Crohn's disease. *Gastroenterology* 1999; **116:** 294–300.
11. Keller R, *et al.* Oral budesonide therapy for steroid-dependent ulcerative colitis: a pilot trial. *Aliment Pharmacol Ther* 1997; **11:** 1047–52.

Preparations

Proprietary Preparations (details are given in Part 3)
Aust.: Budo-san; Entocort; Pulmicort; Rhinocortol; *Austral.:* Budamax; Entocort; Pulmicort; Rhinocort; *Belg.:* Preferid†; Pulmicort; Entocort; *Canad.:* Entocort; Pulmicort; Rhinocort; *Denm.:* Entocort; Miflonide; Rhinocort; Rhinosol; Spirocort; *Fin.:* Cortivent; Entocort; Pulmicort; Rhinocort; *Fr.:* Entocort; Pulmicort; *Ger.:* Benosid; Bronchocux; Budapp; Budecort; Budefat; Budenofalk; Budepur E; Budes; Budon; Entocort; Pulmicort; Respicort; *Hong Kong:* Eltair; Entocort; Pulmicort; Rhinocort; *Irl.:* Entocort; Preferid; Pulmicort; Rhinocort; *Israel:* Budeson; Budicort; Entocort; Nasocort; Pulmotide; *Ital.:* Aircort; Bidien; Miflonide; Preferid; Pulmaxan; Rhinocort; *Mex.:* Pulmicort; Rhinocort; *Neth.:* Entocort; Preferid†; Pulmicort; Rhinocort; *Norw.:* Entocort; Preferid†; Pulmicort; Rhinocort; *NZ:* Butacort; Eltair; Entocort; Hayclear; Pulmicort; Rhinocort; *Port.:* Miflonide; Pulmicort; *S.Afr.:* Budeflam; Entocord; Inflammide; Pulmicort; Rhinocort; *Singapore:* Eltair; Entocort; Inflammide; Pulmicort; Rhinocort; *Spain:* Demotest; Entocord; Neo Rinactive; Olfex; Pulmicort; Pulmictan; Rhinocort; Ribujet; Ribusol†; Rinactive†; *Swed.:* Entocort; Preferid†; Pulmicort; Rhinocort; *Switz.:* Budenofalk; Entocort; Preferid†; Pulmicort; Rhinocort; *Thai.:* Eltair; Inflammide; Pulmicort; Rhinocort; *UK:* Budenofalk; Entocort; Pulmicort; Rhinocort; *USA:* Pulmicort; Rhinocort.

Multi-ingredient: *UK:* Symbicort.

Ciprocinonide   (3439-d)

Ciprocinonide *(USAN, rINN).*
RS-2386. (6α,11β,16α)-21-[(cyclopropylcarbonyl)oxy]-6,9-difluoro-11-hydroxy-16,17-[(1-methylethylidene)-bis(oxy)]-pregna-1,4-diene-3,20-dione.
$C_{28}H_{34}F_2O_7 = 520.6.$
CAS — 58524-83-7.

Profile
Ciprocinonide is a derivative of fluocinolone acetonide (p.1071) which has been applied topically in combination with fluocinonide and procinonide in the management of various skin disorders.

Preparations
Proprietary Preparations (details are given in Part 3)
Multi-ingredient: *Canad.:* Trisyn†.

Clobetasol Propionate   (1069-x)

Clobetasol Propionate *(BANM, USAN, rINN).*
CCI-4725; GR-2/925. 21-Chloro-9α-fluoro-11β,17α-dihydroxy-16β-methylpregna-1,4-diene-3,20-dione 17-propionate.
$C_{25}H_{32}ClFO_5 = 467.0.$
CAS — 25122-41-2 (clobetasol); 25122-46-7 (clobetasol propionate).
Pharmacopoeias. In Br. and US.

Pharmacopoeial description
BP 2001: A white or almost white, crystalline powder. Practically insoluble in water; sparingly soluble in alcohol; freely soluble in acetone and in dichloromethane. Protect from light.

USP 25: A white to cream crystalline powder. Practically insoluble in water; sparingly soluble in dehydrated alcohol; soluble in acetone, in chloroform, in dimethyl sulfoxide, in dioxan, and in methyl alcohol; slightly soluble in benzene and in ether. Store in airtight containers. Protect from light.

Profile
Clobetasol propionate is a corticosteroid used topically for its glucocorticoid activity (p.1039) in the treatment of various skin disorders. It is usually employed as a cream, ointment, or scalp application containing 0.05%.

When applied topically, particularly to large areas, when the skin is broken, or under occlusive dressings, corticosteroids may be absorbed in sufficient amounts to cause systemic effects (p.1039). The effects of topical corticosteroids on the skin are described on p.1041. For recommendations concerning the correct use of corticosteroids on the skin, and a rough guide to the clinical potencies of topical corticosteroids, see p.1045.

Preparations
BP 2001: Clobetasol Cream; Clobetasol Ointment;
USP 25: Clobetasol Propionate Cream; Clobetasol Propionate Ointment; Clobetasol Propionate Topical Solution.

Proprietary Preparations (details are given in Part 3)
Aust.: Dermovate; *Belg.:* Dermovate; *Braz.:* Psorex; *Canad.:* Dermasone; Dermovate; *Denm.:* Dermovat; *Fin.:* Dermovat; *Fr.:* Dermoval; *Ger.:* Clobegalen; Dermoxin; Dermoxinale; Karison; *Hong Kong:* Dermasone; Dermovate; Medodermone; *Irl.:* Dermovate; *Israel:* Dermovate; *Ital.:* Clobesol; *Mex.:* Dermatovate; *Neth.:* Dermovate; *Norw.:* Dermovat; *NZ:* Dermol; Dermovate; *Port.:* Dermovate; *S.Afr.:* Dermovate; Dovate; Xenovate; *Singapore:* Clobeson; Cloderm; Dermovate; Dhabesol; Medodermone; Uniderm; Univate; *Spain:* Clovate; Decloban; *Swed.:* Dermovate; *Switz.:* Dermovate; *Thai.:* Betasol; Clobasone; Clobet; Clobetate; Clonovate; Dermasil; Dermovate; Medodermone; Stivate; *UAE:* Gamavate; *UK:* Dermovate; *USA:* Cormax; Embeline E; Entocort; Olux; Temovate.

Multi-ingredient: *Port.:* Dermovate-NN; *Switz.:* Dermovate-NN; *UK:* Dermovate-NN.

Clobetasone Butyrate   (1070-y)

Clobetasone Butyrate *(BANM, USAN, rINN).*
CCI-5537; Clobetasoni Butyras; GR-2/1214. 21-Chloro-9α-fluoro-17α-hydroxy-16β-methylpregna-1,4-diene-3,11,20-trione 17-butyrate.
$C_{26}H_{32}ClFO_5 = 479.0.$
CAS — 54063-32-0 (clobetasone); 25122-57-0 (clobetasone butyrate).
Pharmacopoeias. In Eur. (see p.vi).

Pharmacopoeial description
Ph. Eur.: A white or almost white powder. Practically insoluble in water; slightly soluble in alcohol; freely soluble in acetone and in dichloromethane. Protect from light.

Profile
Clobetasone butyrate is a corticosteroid used topically for its glucocorticoid activity (p.1039) in the treatment of various skin disorders. It is usually employed as a cream or ointment containing 0.05%. When applied topically, particularly to large areas, when the skin is broken, or under occlusive dressings, corticosteroids may be absorbed in sufficient amounts to cause systemic effects (p.1039). The effects of topical corticosteroids on the skin are described on p.1041. For recommendations con-

cerning the correct use of corticosteroids on the skin, and a rough guide to the clinical potencies of topical corticosteroids, see p.1045.

Clobetasone butyrate is also used for inflammatory eye disorders, as eye drops containing 0.1%. Prolonged application to the eye of preparations containing corticosteroids has caused raised intra-ocular pressure and reduced visual function.

Preparations
BP 2001: Clobetasone Cream; Clobetasone Ointment.

Proprietary Preparations (details are given in Part 3)
Aust.: Emovate; *Belg.:* Eumovate; *Braz.:* Eumovate; *Canad.:* Eumovate; *Denm.:* Emovat; *Fin.:* Emovat; *Ger.:* Emovate; *Hong Kong:* Eumovate; *Irl.:* Eumovate; *Israel:* Eucorten; Eumovate; *Ital.:* Clobet; Eumovate; Visucloben; *Neth.:* Emovate; *Norw.:* Cloptison; *NZ:* Eumovate; *Port.:* Emovate; *S.Afr.:* Eumovate; *Singapore:* Amisol; Eumovate; *Spain:* Cortoftal; Emovate; *Swed.:* Emovat; *Switz.:* Cloptison; Emovate; *Thai.:* Eumovate; *UK:* Cloburate; Eumovate.

Multi-ingredient: *Israel:* Cicloderm-C; *Ital.:* Visucloben Antibiotico; Visucloben Decongestionante; *Switz.:* Cloptison-N†; *UK:* Cloburate-N†; Trimovate.

Clocortolone Pivalate   (12584-k)

Clocortolone Pivalate *(USAN, rINN).*
CL-68; SH-863. 9α-Chloro-6α-fluoro-11β,21-dihydroxy-16α-methylpregna-1,4-diene-3,20-dione 21-pivalate.
$C_{27}H_{36}ClFO_5 = 495.0.$
CAS — 4828-27-7 (clocortolone); 34097-16-0 (clocortolone pivalate).
Pharmacopoeias. In US.

Pharmacopoeial description
USP 25: A white to yellowish-white, odourless powder. Sparingly soluble in alcohol; soluble in acetone; freely soluble in chloroform and in dioxan; slightly soluble in ether and in benzene. Store in airtight containers. Protect from light.

Profile
Clocortolone pivalate is a corticosteroid used topically for its glucocorticoid activity (p.1039), as a 0.1% cream or ointment, in the treatment of various skin disorders. Clocortolone caproate has been used in combination with the pivalate.

When applied topically, particularly to large areas, where the skin is broken, or under occlusive dressings, corticosteroids may be absorbed in sufficient amounts to cause systemic effects (p.1039). The effects of topical corticosteroids on the skin are described on p.1041. For recommendations concerning the correct use of corticosteroids on the skin, see p.1045.

Preparations
USP 25: Clocortolone Pivalate Cream.

Proprietary Preparations (details are given in Part 3)
Aust.: Glimbal; *USA:* Cloderm.

Multi-ingredient: *Ger.:* Corto-Tavegil; Crino-Kaban N; Kaban; Kabanimat; Procto-Kaban.

Cloprednol   (1071-j)

Cloprednol *(BAN, USAN, rINN).*
RS-4691. 6-Chloro-11β,17α,21-trihydroxypregna-1,4,6-triene-3,20-dione.
$C_{21}H_{25}ClO_5 = 392.9.$
CAS — 5251-34-3.
ATC — H02AB14.

Profile
Cloprednol is a corticosteroid with mainly glucocorticoid activity (p.1039); the anti-inflammatory activity of 2.5 mg of cloprednol is equivalent to about 5 mg of prednisolone. Cloprednol is given by mouth in various disorders for which corticosteroid therapy is helpful (p.1044), in usual doses ranging from 1.25 to 12.5 mg daily.

Preparations
Proprietary Preparations (details are given in Part 3)
Ger.: Syntestan; *Ital.:* Cloradryn†; *Mex.:* Novacort.

Cortisone Acetate   (1072-z)

Cortisone Acetate *(BANM, rINN).*
Compound E Acetate; Cortisoni Acetas; 11-Dehydro-17-hydroxycorticosterone Acetate. 17α,21-Dihydroxypregn-4-ene-3,11,20-trione 21-acetate.
$C_{23}H_{30}O_6 = 402.5.$
CAS — 53-06-5 (cortisone); 50-04-4 (cortisone acetate).
Pharmacopoeias. In Chin., Eur. (see p.vi), Jpn, Pol., and US.

Pharmacopoeial description
Ph. Eur.: A white or almost white, crystalline powder. It shows polymorphism. Practically insoluble in water; slightly soluble in alcohol and in methyl alcohol; sparingly soluble in acetone; freely soluble in dichloromethane; soluble in dioxan. Protect from light.

USP 25: A white or practically white, odourless, crystalline powder. Insoluble in water; soluble 1 in 350 of alcohol, 1 in 75 of acetone, 1 in 4 of chloroform, and 1 in 30 of dioxan.

The symbol † denotes a preparation no longer actively marketed

Adverse Effects, Treatment, Withdrawal, and Precautions
As for corticosteroids in general (see p.1039).

Interactions
The interactions of corticosteroids in general are described on p.1043.

Pharmacokinetics
For a brief outline of the pharmacokinetics of corticosteroids, see p.1044.

Cortisone acetate is readily absorbed from the gastrointestinal tract and the cortisone is rapidly converted in the liver to its active metabolite, hydrocortisone (cortisol). The biological half-life of cortisone itself is only about 30 minutes. Absorption of cortisone acetate from intramuscular sites is considerably slower than following oral administration.

Uses and Administration
Cortisone is a corticosteroid secreted by the adrenal cortex. It has glucocorticoid activity (p.1039), as well as appreciable mineralocorticoid activity; 25 mg of cortisone acetate is equivalent in anti-inflammatory activity to about 5 mg of prednisolone.

Cortisone acetate is rapidly effective when given by mouth, and more slowly by intramuscular injection.

Cortisone acetate has been used mainly for replacement therapy in adrenocortical insufficiency (p.1046), but hydrocortisone (p.1073) is generally preferred since cortisone itself is inactive and must be converted by the liver to hydrocortisone, its active metabolite; hence, in some liver disorders the activity of cortisone may be less reliable. Doses of cortisone acetate by mouth for replacement therapy are 12.5 to 37.5 mg daily in divided doses, together with fludrocortisone if additional mineralocorticoid activity is required.

Cortisone acetate has been used in the treatment of many of the allergic and inflammatory disorders for which corticosteroid therapy is helpful (p.1044) but prednisolone or other synthetic glucocorticoids are generally preferred. Doses of cortisone acetate employed have generally ranged from about 25 to 300 mg daily by mouth or by intramuscular injection.

Preparations
BP 2001: Cortisone Tablets;
USP 25: Cortisone Acetate Injectable Suspension; Cortisone Acetate Tablets.

Proprietary Preparations (details are given in Part 3)
Aust.: Cortone; **Austral.:** Cortate; **Belg.:** Adreson; **Canad.:** Cortone; **Ital.:** Cortone; **Norw.:** Cortone; **S.Afr.:** Cortogen; **Spain:** Altesona; **Swed.:** Cortal; **Cortone; UK:** Cortisyl; **USA:** Cortone.

Multi-ingredient: Braz.: Corciclen; **Ital.:** Dutimelan†; **Spain:** Antiblefarica; Blefarida; Gingilone; **Switz.:** Septicortin†.

Cortivazol (1073-c)
Cortivazol (USAN, pINN).
H-3625; MK-650; NSC-80998. 11β,17α,21-Trihydroxy-6,16α-dimethyl-2′-phenyl-2′H-pregna-2,4,6-trieno[3,2-c]pyrazol-20-one 21-acetate.
$C_{32}H_{38}N_2O_5 = 530.7$.
CAS — 1110-40-3.
ATC — H02AB17.

Profile
Cortivazol is a corticosteroid with mainly glucocorticoid activity (p.1039); 300 µg of cortivazol is equivalent in anti-inflammatory activity to about 5 mg of prednisolone. It is given in the treatment of musculoskeletal and joint disorders by intra-articular, periarticular, or epidural injection in doses of about 1.25 to 3.75 mg, according to the size of the joint, usually at intervals of 1 to 3 weeks. It has also been given by mouth.

Preparations
Proprietary Preparations (details are given in Part 3)
Fr.: Altim.

Deflazacort (12627-l)
Deflazacort (BAN, USAN, rINN).
Azacort; DL-458-IT; L-5458; MDL-458; Oxazacort. 11β,21-Dihydroxy-2′-methyl-5′βH-pregna-1,4-dieno[17,16-d]oxazole-3,20-dione 21-acetate.
$C_{25}H_{31}NO_6 = 441.5$.
CAS — 14484-47-0.
ATC — H02AB13.

Profile
Deflazacort is a corticosteroid with mainly glucocorticoid activity (p.1039); 6 mg of deflazacort is reportedly equivalent in anti-inflammatory activity to about 5 mg of prednisolone (but see Action, below).

Deflazacort is used for its anti-inflammatory properties in conditions responsive to corticosteroid therapy (p.1044). It is given by mouth in initial doses of up to 120 mg daily; usual mainte-

nance doses are 3 to 18 mg daily. Doses of 0.25 to 1.5 mg per kg body-weight daily have been used in children.

◊ References.
1. Markham A, Bryson HM. Deflazacort: a review of its pharmacological properties and therapeutic efficacy. *Drugs* 1995; **50:** 317–33.

Action. Although it has been suggested that deflazacort produces fewer adverse effects than some conventional corticosteroids such as prednisolone, a study in healthy subjects found that the ratio of efficacy for deflazacort compared with prednisolone was higher than the 1.2 : 1 previously assumed,[1] implying that lower effective doses of deflazacort had been used in such comparisons. All systemic corticosteroids may produce clinically significant adverse reactions (see also p.1039) which are primarily dependent on dose and duration of use.
1. Babadjanova G, *et al.* Comparison of the pharmacodynamic effects of deflazacort and prednisolone in healthy subjects. *Eur J Clin Pharmacol* 1996; **51:** 53–7.

Preparations
Proprietary Preparations (details are given in Part 3)
Braz.: Calcort; **Ger.:** Calcort; **Irl.:** Calcort; **Ital.:** Deflan; Flantadin; **Mex.:** Calcort; **Port.:** Rosilan; **Spain:** Dezacor; Zamene; **Switz.:** Calcort; **UK:** Calcort.

Deprodone (6900-g)
Deprodone (BAN, rINN).
11β,17α-Dihydroxypregna-1,4-diene-3,20-dione.
$C_{21}H_{28}O_4 = 344.4$.
CAS — 20423-99-8 (deprodone); 20424-00-4 (deprodone propionate).

Profile
Deprodone is a corticosteroid that has been used topically as the propionate.

Desonide (1076-t)
Desonide (BAN, USAN, rINN).
D-2083; Desfluorotriamcinolone Acetonide; 16-Hydroxyprednisolone 16,17-Acetonide; Prednacinolone Acetonide. 11β,21-Dihydroxy-16α,17α-isopropylidenedioxypregna-1,4-diene-3,20-dione.
$C_{24}H_{32}O_6 = 416.5$.
CAS — 638-94-8.
ATC — D07AB08; S01BA11.

Profile
Desonide is a corticosteroid used topically for its glucocorticoid activity (p.1039) in the treatment of various skin disorders. It is usually used as a cream or ointment containing 0.05%. The pivalate and the sodium phosphate esters have also been used.

When applied topically, particularly to large areas, when the skin is broken, or under occlusive dressings, corticosteroids may be absorbed in sufficient amounts to cause systemic effects (p.1039). The effects of topical corticosteroids on the skin are described on p.1041. For recommendations concerning the correct use of corticosteroids on the skin, and a rough guide to the clinical potencies of topical corticosteroids, see p.1045.

Preparations
Proprietary Preparations (details are given in Part 3)
Austral.: DesOwen; **Belg.:** Sterax; **Braz.:** Desonol; Epidex; Steronide; **Canad.:** Desocort; Tridesilon; **Fin.:** Apolar; **Fr.:** Locapred; Locatop; Tridesonit; **Ger.:** Sterax; Prenacid; **Hong Kong:** DesOwen; Ital.: PR 100; Prenacid; Reticus; **Mex.:** DesOwen; **Norw.:** Apolar; **NZ:** DesOwen; **Port.:** Locapred; Zotinar; **Singapore:** DesOwen; **Swed.:** Apolar; **Switz.:** Locapred; Locatop; Sterax; **USA:** DesOwen; Tridesilon.

Multi-ingredient: Fr.: Cirkan a la Prednacinolone; **Ital.:** PR 100-Cloressidina; **Norw.:** Apolar med dekvalon; **USA:** Tridesilon.

Desoximetasone (1077-x)
Desoximetasone (BAN, USAN, rINN).
A-41-304; Desoxymethasone; Hoe-304; R-2113. 9α-Fluoro-11β,21-dihydroxy-16α-methylpregna-1,4-diene-3,20-dione.
$C_{22}H_{29}FO_4 = 376.5$.
CAS — 382-67-2.
ATC — D07AC03; D07XC02.
Pharmacopoeias. In US.

Pharmacopoeial description
USP 25: A white to practically white, odourless, crystalline powder. Insoluble in water; freely soluble in alcohol, in acetone, and in chloroform.

Profile
Desoximetasone is a corticosteroid used topically for its glucocorticoid activity (p.1039) in the treatment of various skin disorders. It is usually employed as a cream, gel, lotion, or ointment; concentrations used range from 0.05 to 0.25%.

When applied topically, particularly to large areas, when the skin is broken, or under occlusive dressings, corticosteroids may be absorbed in sufficient amounts to cause systemic effects (p.1039). The effects of topical corticosteroids on the skin are described on p.1041. For recommendations concerning the correct use of corticosteroids on the skin, and a rough guide to the clinical potencies of topical corticosteroids, see p.1045.

Adverse effects. A photosensitivity reaction occurred in a patient treated for psoriasis with topical desoximetasone; rechallenge led to a recurrence.[1] The patient was also receiving propranolol hydrochloride.
1. Stierstorfer MB, Baughman RD. Photosensitivity to desoximetasone emollient cream. *Arch Dermatol* 1988; **124:** 1870–1.

Preparations
USP 25: Desoximetasone Cream; Desoximetasone Gel; Desoximetasone Ointment.

Proprietary Preparations (details are given in Part 3)
Aust.: Topisolon; **Belg.:** Topicorte†; **Braz.:** Esperson; **Canad.:** Topicort; **Denm.:** Ibaril; **Fin.:** Ibaril; **Fr.:** Topicorte†; **Ger.:** Topisolon; **Hong Kong:** Esperson; **Irl.:** Topisolon; **Israel:** Desicort; **Ital.:** Flubason; **Neth.:** Ibaril; Topicorte; **Norw.:** Ibaril; **S.Afr.:** Topisolon†; **Singapore:** Topicorte; **Spain:** Flubason; **Swed.:** Ibaril; **Switz.:** Topisolon; **Thai.:** Esperson; Topicorte; **UK:** Stiedex LP; **USA:** Topicort.

Multi-ingredient: Aust.: Topisolon mit Salicylsaure; **Braz.:** Esperson N; **Denm.:** Ibaril med salicylsyre; **Fr.:** Topifram†; **Ger.:** Topisolon; **Norw.:** Ibaril med salicylsyre; **Singapore:** Topifram; **Swed.:** Ibaril med salicylsyra; **Thai.:** Topifram; **UK:** Stiedex.

Desoxycortone Acetate (1075-a)
Desoxycortone Acetate (BANM, rINNM).
Cortin; Decortone Acetate; 11-Deoxycorticosterone Acetate; Deoxycortone Acetate; Desoxycorticosterone Acetate; Desoxycortoni Acetas. 21-Hydroxypregn-4-ene-3,20-dione 21-acetate.
$C_{23}H_{32}O_4 = 372.5$.
CAS — 64-85-7 (desoxycortone); 56-47-3 (desoxycortone acetate).
Pharmacopoeias. In *Eur.* (see p.vi), *Pol.,* and *US.*

Pharmacopoeial description
Ph. Eur.: A white or almost white, crystalline powder or colourless crystals. Practically insoluble in water; sparingly soluble in alcohol; soluble in acetone; freely soluble in dichloromethane; slightly soluble in propylene glycol and in fatty oils. Protect from light.

USP 25: A white or creamy-white, odourless, crystalline powder. Practically insoluble in water; sparingly soluble in alcohol, in acetone, and in dioxan; slightly soluble in vegetable oils. Protect from light.

Desoxycortone Pivalate (1074-k)
Desoxycortone Pivalate (BANM, rINNM).
Deoxycorticosterone Pivalate; Deoxycorticosterone Trimethylacetate; Desoxycorticosterone Pivalate; Desoxycorticosterone Trimethylacetate; Desoxycorticosterone Pivalate; Desoxycorticosterone Trimethylacetate. 21-Hydroxypregn-4-ene-3,20-dione 21-pivalate.
$C_{26}H_{38}O_4 = 414.6$.
CAS — 808-48-0.
Pharmacopoeias. In *US* for veterinary use only.

Pharmacopoeial description
USP 25: Protect from light.

Profile
Desoxycortone is a corticosteroid secreted by the adrenal cortex and has primarily mineralocorticoid activity (p.1039). It has no significant glucocorticoid action.

Desoxycortone, as the acetate or pivalate, has been used in the treatment of adrenocortical insufficiency (p.1046) as an adjunct to cortisone or hydrocortisone. For this purpose, however, fludrocortisone given by mouth is now usually preferred.

Desoxycortone acetate is given by intramuscular injection as an oily solution, in doses of up to 10 mg once or twice daily. The pivalate has also been used, as an intramuscular depot injection every 4 weeks, and desoxycortone acetate has also been given by subcutaneous implant.

Desoxycortone has also been administered as its enantate, phenylpropionate, and sodium hemisuccinate esters.

Preparations
USP 25: Desoxycorticosterone Acetate Injection; Desoxycorticosterone Acetate Pellets.

Proprietary Preparations (details are given in Part 3)
Aust.: Cortiron; **Fr.:** Syncortyl; **Ital.:** Cortiron†; **Switz.:** Cortisteron.

Multi-ingredient: Braz.: Cortobion; **Ital.:** Sinsurrene†.

Dexamethasone (1084-t)

Dexamethasone (BAN, rINN).

Desamethasone; Dexametasone; Dexamethasonum; 9α-Fluoro-16α-methylprednisolone; Hexadecadrol. 9α-Fluoro-11β,17α,21-trihydroxy-16α-methylpregna-1,4-diene-3,20-dione.

$C_{22}H_{29}FO_5 = 392.5$.

CAS — 50-02-2.

ATC — A01AC02; C05AA09; D07AB19; D07XB05; D10AA03; H02AB02; R01AD03; S01BA01; S01CB01; S02BA06; S03BA01.

Pharmacopoeias. In Eur. (see p.vi), Int., Jpn, Pol., and US.

Pharmacopoeial description

Ph. Eur.: A white or almost white, crystalline powder. Practically insoluble in water; sparingly soluble in dehydrated alcohol; slightly soluble in dichloromethane. Protect from light.

USP 25: A white to practically white, odourless, crystalline powder. Practically insoluble in water; sparingly soluble in alcohol, in acetone, in dioxan, and in methyl alcohol; slightly soluble in chloroform; very slightly soluble in ether.

Dexamethasone Acetate (1079-f)

Dexamethasone Acetate (BANM, USAN, rINNM).

Dexamethasoni Acetas. Dexamethasone 21-acetate.

$C_{24}H_{31}FO_6 = 434.5$.

CAS — 1177-87-3 (anhydrous dexamethasone acetate); 55812-90-3 (dexamethasone acetate monohydrate).

Pharmacopoeias. In Chin. and Eur. (see p.vi).

Int. and US allow the anhydrous form or the monohydrate.

Dexamethasone acetate 1.1 mg is approximately equivalent to 1 mg of dexamethasone.

Pharmacopoeial description

Ph. Eur.: A white or almost white, crystalline powder. It shows polymorphism. Practically insoluble in water; freely soluble in alcohol and in acetone; slightly soluble in dichloromethane. Protect from light.

USP 25: It contains one molecule of water of hydration or is anhydrous. A clear, white to off-white, odourless powder. Practically insoluble in water; freely soluble in acetone, in dioxan, and in methyl alcohol.

Dexamethasone Isonicotinate (1080-z)

Dexamethasone Isonicotinate (BANM, rINNM).

Dexamethasone 21-isonicotinate.

$C_{28}H_{32}FNO_6 = 497.6$.

CAS — 2265-64-7.

Dexamethasone isonicotinate 1.3 mg is approximately equivalent to 1 mg of dexamethasone.

Dexamethasone Phosphate (18485-c)

Dexamethasone Phosphate (BANM, rINNM).

Dexamethasone 21-(dihydrogen phosphate).

$C_{22}H_{30}FO_8P = 472.4$.

CAS — 312-93-6.

Dexamethasone phosphate 1.2 mg is approximately equivalent to 1 mg of dexamethasone.

Dexamethasone Sodium Metasulfobenzoate
(1083-a)

Dexamethasone Sodium Metasulfobenzoate (rINNM).

Dexamethasone Sodium Metasulphobenzoate (BANM). Dexamethasone 21-(sodium m-sulphobenzoate).

$C_{29}H_{32}FNaO_9S = 598.6$.

CAS — 3936-02-5.

Dexamethasone sodium metasulfobenzoate 1.5 mg is approximately equivalent to 1 mg of dexamethasone.

Dexamethasone Sodium Phosphate (1078-r)

Dexamethasone Sodium Phosphate (BANM, rINNM).

Dexamethasone Phosphate Sodium; Dexamethasoni Natrii Phosphas; Sodium Dexamethasone Phosphate. Dexamethasone 21-(disodium orthophosphate).

$C_{22}H_{28}FNa_2O_8P = 516.4$.

CAS — 2392-39-4.

NOTE. DSP is a code approved by the BP 2001 for use on single unit doses of eye drops containing dexamethasone sodium phosphate where the individual container may be too small to bear all the appropriate labelling information.

Pharmacopoeias. In Chin., Eur. (see p.vi), Int., and US.

Dexamethasone sodium phosphate 1.3 mg is approximately equivalent to 1 mg of dexamethasone and 1.1 mg of dexamethasone sodium phosphate is approximately equivalent to 1 mg of dexamethasone phosphate.

Pharmacopoeial description

Ph. Eur.: A white or almost white, very hygroscopic, powder. It exhibits polymorphism. Freely soluble in water; slightly soluble in alcohol; practically insoluble in dichloromethane and in ether. A 1% solution in water has a pH of 7.5 to 9.5. Store in airtight containers. Protect from light.

The symbol † denotes a preparation no longer actively marketed

USP 25: A white or slightly yellow, crystalline powder. Is odourless or has a slight odour of alcohol, and is exceedingly hygroscopic. Soluble 1 in 2 of water; slightly soluble in alcohol; insoluble in chloroform and in ether; very slightly soluble in dioxan. pH of a 1% solution in water is between 7.5 and 10.5. Store in airtight containers.

Adverse Effects, Treatment, Withdrawal, and Precautions

As for corticosteroids in general (see p.1039).

Dexamethasone has little or no effect on sodium and water retention.

When applied topically, particularly to large areas, when the skin is broken, or under occlusive dressings, or when given intranasally, corticosteroids may be absorbed in sufficient amounts to cause systemic effects. Prolonged application to the eye of preparations containing corticosteroids has caused raised intra-ocular pressure and reduced visual function.

Effects on the nervous system. Paraesthesia and irritation, most commonly occurring in the anogenital region, have been associated with the intravenous use of dexamethasone sodium phosphate[1] and hydrocortisone sodium phosphate,[2] but not with hydrocortisone sodium succinate.[2] Further comments and discussions on this topic are listed below.[3-5]

Neurological complications have occurred with corticosteroid-induced epidural lipomatosis, see p.1041.

1. Czerwinski AW, et al. Effects of a single, large, intravenous injection of dexamethasone. Clin Pharmacol Ther 1972; **13:** 638–42.
2. Novak E, et al. Anorectal pruritus after intravenous hydrocortisone sodium succinate and sodium phosphate. Clin Pharmacol Ther 1976; **20:** 109–12.
3. Anonymous. Which form of intravenous hydrocortisone. Drug Ther Bull 1979; **17:** 71–2.
4. Thomas VL. More on dexamethasone-induced perineal irritation. N Engl J Med 1986; **314:** 1643.
5. Allan SG, Leonard RCF. Dexamethasone antiemesis and side-effects. Lancet 1986; **i:** 1035.

Neonates. The adverse effects of corticosteroids on the fetus are discussed on p.1042.

Adverse effects noted in premature neonates with bronchopulmonary dysplasia receiving dexamethasone treatment to enable weaning from assisted ventilation have included hypertension,[1-3] often accompanied by bradycardia,[1,2] gastroduodenal perforation,[4,5] ulceration and thinning of the gastric wall,[4] development of a catabolic state,[6] renal calcification,[7] and transient myocardial hypertrophy.[8-10] There is some evidence of a suppressive effect on motor activity and spontaneous movement.[11] It has been postulated that neonatal dexamethasone may both increase[12] and decrease[13] retinopathy of prematurity; its true effect is uncertain.[14]

There is also a concern that longer term development of the child may be adversely affected, although data are scanty.[15,16] However, a meta-analysis[17] has concluded that postnatal use of corticosteroids to treat or prevent bronchopulmonary dysplasia is associated with dramatic increases in the incidence of cerebral palsy and neurodevelopmental impairment, and suggested that such use should be abandoned.

Pulsed administration may reduce the adverse effects but may also reduce efficacy.[18]

1. Ohlsson A, Heyman E. Dexamethasone-induced bradycardia. Lancet 1988; **ii:** 1074.
2. Puntis JWL, et al. Dexamethasone-induced bradycardia. Lancet 1988; **ii:** 1372.
3. Marinelli KA, et al. Effects of dexamethasone on blood pressure in premature infants with bronchopulmonary dysplasia. J Pediatr 1997; **130:** 594–602.
4. Ng PC, et al. Gastroduodenal perforation in preterm babies treated with dexamethasone for bronchopulmonary dysplasia. Arch Dis Child 1991; **66:** 1164–6.
5. Smith H, Sinha S. Gastrointestinal complications associated with dexamethasone treatment. Arch Dis Child 1992; **67:** 667.
6. Macdonald PD, et al. A catabolic state in dexamethasone treatment of bronchopulmonary dysplasia. Arch Dis Child 1990; **65:** 560–1.
7. Kamitsuka MD, Peloquin D. Renal calcification after dexamethasone in infants with bronchopulmonary dysplasia. Lancet 1991; **337:** 626.
8. Werner JC, et al. Hypertrophic cardiomyopathy associated with dexamethasone therapy for bronchopulmonary dysplasia. J Pediatr 1992; **120:** 286–91.
9. Bensky AS, et al. Cardiac effects of dexamethasone in very low birth weight infants. Pediatrics 1996; **97:** 818–21.
10. Skelton R, et al. Cardiac effects of short course dexamethasone in preterm infants. Arch Dis Child 1998; **78:** F133–F137.
11. Bos AF, et al. Qualitative assessment of general movements in high-risk preterm infants with chronic lung-disease requiring dexamethasone therapy. J Pediatr 1998; **132:** 300–6.
12. Batton DG, et al. Severe retinopathy of prematurity and steroid exposure. Pediatrics 1992; **90:** 534–6.
13. Sobel DB, Philip AGS. Prolonged dexamethasone therapy reduces the incidence of cryotherapy for retinopathy of prematurity in infants of less than 1 kilogram birth weight with bronchopulmonary dysplasia. Pediatrics 1992; **90:** 529–33.
14. Ehrenkranz RA. Steroids, chronic lung disease, and retinopathy of prematurity. Pediatrics 1992; **90:** 646–7.
15. Greenough A. Gains and losses from dexamethasone for neonatal chronic lung disease. Lancet 1998; **352:** 835–6.
16. Shinwell ES, et al. Early postnatal dexamethasone treatment and increased incidence of cerebral palsy. Arch Dis Child Fetal Neonatal Ed 2000; **83:** F177–F181.
17. Barrington KJ. The adverse neuro-developmental effects of postnatal steroids in the preterm infant: a systematic review of RCTs. Available at: http//www.biomedcentral.com/1471–2431/1/1
18. Bloomfield FH, et al. Side effects of 2 different dexamethasone courses for preterm infants at risk of chronic lung disease: a randomized trial. J Pediatr 1998; **133:** 395–400.

Interactions

The interactions of corticosteroids in general are described on p.1043.

Antiepileptics. As described on p.361, dexamethasone may decrease or increase plasma concentrations of phenytoin. Like other enzyme-inducing drugs, phenytoin also has the potential to increase the metabolism of dexamethasone.

Pharmacokinetics

For a brief outline of the pharmacokinetics of corticosteroids, see p.1044.

Dexamethasone is readily absorbed from the gastrointestinal tract. Its biological half-life in plasma is about 190 minutes. Binding of dexamethasone to plasma proteins is about 77%, which is less than for most other corticosteroids. Up to 65% of a dose is excreted in urine within 24 hours. Clearance in premature neonates is reported to be proportional to gestational age, with a reduced elimination rate in the most premature infants. It readily crosses the placenta with minimal inactivation.

Uses and Administration

Dexamethasone is a corticosteroid with mainly glucocorticoid activity (p.1039); 750 µg of dexamethasone is equivalent in anti-inflammatory activity to about 5 mg of prednisolone.

It has been used, either in the form of the free alcohol or in one of the esterified forms, in the treatment of conditions for which corticosteroid therapy is indicated (p.1044), except adrenocortical insufficiency for which hydrocortisone with supplementary fludrocortisone is preferred. Its lack of mineralocorticoid properties makes dexamethasone particularly suitable for treating conditions where water retention would be a disadvantage.

For administration by mouth dexamethasone is given in usual doses of 0.5 to 10 mg daily. Dexamethasone is also used by mouth in the dexamethasone suppression tests for the diagnosis of Cushing's syndrome (for further details see under Diagnosis and Testing, below).

For parenteral administration in intensive therapy or in emergencies, the sodium phosphate ester may be given intravenously by injection or infusion or intramuscularly by injection; doses are sometimes expressed in terms of the free alcohol, the phosphate, or the sodium phosphate and confusion has sometimes arisen in the literature because of these variations. Initial doses used, expressed in terms of dexamethasone phosphate, range from about 0.5 to 20 mg daily (about 0.4 to 16.7 mg of dexamethasone). Intravenous doses of the equivalent of 2 to 6 mg of dexamethasone phosphate per kg body-weight given slowly over a minimum period of several minutes have been suggested for the treatment of severe shock. These high doses may be repeated within 2 to 6 hours and this treatment should be continued only until the patient's condition is stable and usually for no longer than 48 to 72 hours. Alternatively, the initial intravenous injection may be followed immediately by the same dose administered by intravenous infusion.

Dexamethasone sodium phosphate is also used in the treatment of cerebral oedema caused by malignancy. An initial intravenous dose of the equivalent of 10 mg of the phosphate is usually given followed by 4 mg intramuscularly every 6 hours; a response is usually obtained after 12 to 24 hours and dosage may be reduced after 2 to 4 days, and gradually discontinued over 5 to 7 days. A much higher dosage schedule has also been suggested for use in acute life-threatening cerebral oedema; initial doses of the equivalent of 50 mg of phosphate intravenously have been given on the first day together with 8 mg intravenously every 2 hours reduced gradually over 7 to 10 days to a maintenance dose of 2 mg two or three times daily.

The sodium phosphate ester is given by intra-articular, intralesional, intramuscular, or soft-tissue injection. For intra-articular injection doses equivalent to 0.8 to 4 mg of dexamethasone phosphate are employed depending upon the size of the joint. For soft-tissue injection doses of 2 to 6 mg are used. Injections are repeated every 3 to 5 days to every 2 to 3 weeks.

Dexamethasone acetate may be given by intramuscular injection in conditions where corticosteroid treatment is indicated but a prompt response of short duration is not required; doses are the equivalent of 8 to 16 mg of dexamethasone, repeated, if necessary, every 1 to 3 weeks. The acetate may also be administered locally by intra-articular or soft-tissue injection in doses equivalent to 4 to 16 mg of dexamethasone, repeated, if necessary, every 1 to 3 weeks, or by intralesional injection in doses equivalent to 0.8 to 1.6 mg.

For ophthalmic disorders or for topical application in the treatment of various skin disorders, either dexamethasone or its esters may be employed; concentrations are often expressed in terms of dexamethasone or dexamethasone phosphate and are commonly 0.05 to 0.1% for eye or ear drops and ointments and 0.1% for topical skin preparations. For recommendations concerning the correct use of corticosteroids on the skin, and a rough guide to the clinical potencies of topical corticosteroids, see p.1045.

Dexamethasone sodium phosphate is also used by inhalation for the management of asthma (p.757) and related bronchospastic disorders unresponsive to other therapy. The initial dose is equivalent to 300 µg of dexamethasone phosphate or about 250 µg of dexamethasone inhaled three or four times daily, slowly reduced according to the patients' response to the minimum amount necessary to control the asthma.

For allergic rhinitis and other allergic or inflammatory nasal conditions (p.407), a nasal spray containing dexamethasone isonicotinate or dexamethasone sodium phosphate is available; the acetate, phosphate, and sodium metasulfobenzoate have also been employed.

Dexamethasone is administered intravenously and orally for the prevention of nausea and vomiting induced by cancer chemotherapy (see below).

Other esters of dexamethasone which have occasionally been used include the hemisuccinate, linoleate, palmitate, pivalate, propionate, sodium succinate, tebutate, and valerate.

The phenpropionate and troxundate esters have been used in veterinary medicine.

Alcohol withdrawal syndrome. Dexamethasone was reported to be effective in a patient with benzodiazepine-resistant delirium tremens[1] and resolved symptoms of alcohol withdrawal syndrome resistant to other treatments in another 110 patients.[2] However, a subsequent small study found no evidence that dexamethasone was effective.[3]

1. Fischer DK, et al. Efficacy of dexamethasone in benzodiazepine-resistant delirium tremens. Lancet 1988; i: 1340–1.
2. Pol S, et al. Dexamethasone for alcohol withdrawal. Ann Intern Med 1991; 114: 705–6.
3. Adinoff B, Pols B. Dexamethasone in the treatment of the alcohol withdrawal syndrome. Am J Drug Alcohol Abuse 1997; 23: 615–22.

Amyloidosis. For mention of the use of dexamethasone in patients with amyloidosis, see p.501.

Blood disorders. High-dose pulsed dexamethasone therapy has been found useful in some patients with idiopathic thrombocytopenic purpura (p.1052), although results have been variable in children.

Cerebral oedema. Corticosteroids, usually dexamethasone, play an important role in the treatment of cerebral oedema in malignancy (see Raised Intracranial Pressure, p.811), and dexamethasone is advocated for the cerebral oedema associated with high-altitude disorders (see below).

Congenital adrenal hyperplasia. Because of its lack of mineralocorticoid properties, dexamethasone has little advantage in the salt-losing form of congenital adrenal hyperplasia (p.1049), in which mineralocorticoid therapy must be given, and its potency means that dose titration to avoid toxicity can be difficult in infants and children, even with the non-salt-losing form. However, it may be useful in adults with forms of the syndrome that do not require mineralocorticoid replacement. It has also been given antenatally to the mother to prevent virilisation of female fetuses.

Diagnosis and testing. CUSHING'S SYNDROME. Dexamethasone has been used to differentiate Cushing's disease (adrenal hyperplasia caused by defects of pituitary origin) from other forms of Cushing's syndrome (caused by ectopic ACTH secretion from non-pituitary tumours or by cortisol secretion from adrenal tumours). The dexamethasone suppression test first proposed by Liddle[1] involved the administration of dexamethasone in low doses of 500 µg four times daily by mouth for 8 doses followed by higher doses of 2 mg again four times daily for 8 doses. In the low-dose tests the urinary excretion of cortisol and 17-hydroxycorticosteroids is suppressed in healthy persons but not in patients and in the high-dose tests the excretion is still not suppressed in those with Cushing's syndrome but is partially suppressed in those with Cushing's disease. Because this test usually involves patients being admitted to hospital for urine collection over a number of days and because false-negative responses are reported to be fairly frequent, more rapid and reliable tests have been sought. Kennedy et al.[2] have used the low-dose test in conjunction with the measurement of serum-cortisol concentrations and the excretion of free cortisol in urine over 24 hours and considered it to be a reliable method for screening for Cushing's syndrome. In the UK a single dose of 1 mg of dexamethasone given at night is often used and is considered sufficient to inhibit corticotropin secretion for 24 hours in most subjects. Another variation of the test has been reported by Tyrrell et al.[3] who administered a single dose of dexamethasone 8 mg at night and measured plasma-cortisol concentrations the next day; again they also concluded this test (known as the overnight high-dose dexamethasone suppression test) to be a practical and reliable alternative for the differential diagnosis of Cushing's syndrome. A recent review of the diagnostic tests used in Cushing's syndrome[4] concluded that, together with measurement of plasma-ACTH concentrations by radio-immunoassay, the overnight high-dose dexamethasone suppression test may become the test of choice for differential diagnosis.

Further variations in the dexamethasone suppression test have included administration of a continuous intravenous infusion of dexamethasone at a rate of 1 mg per hour for 7 hours, with hourly measurement of blood-cortisol concentrations.[5] Initial results indicate that this variation produces a lower number of false-positive diagnoses than the test using oral dexamethasone. Other alternatives are a combined low-dose dexamethasone suppression test and corticotropin-releasing hormone (corticorelin) test,[6] or combination of a dexamethasone suppression test with a metyrapone test.[7]

For a discussion of Cushing's syndrome and its management, see p.1272.

1. Liddle GW. Tests of pituitary-adrenal suppressibility in the diagnosis of Cushing's syndrome. J Clin Endocrinol Metab 1960; 20: 1539–60.
2. Kennedy L, et al. Serum cortisol concentrations during low dose dexamethasone suppression test to screen for Cushing's syndrome. BMJ 1984; 289: 1188–91.
3. Tyrrell JB, et al. An overnight high-dose dexamethasone suppression test for rapid differential diagnosis of Cushing's syndrome. Ann Intern Med 1986; 104: 180–6.
4. Kaye TB, Crapo L. The Cushing syndrome: an update on diagnostic tests. Ann Intern Med 1990; 112: 434–44.
5. Biemond P, et al. Continuous dexamethasone infusion for seven hours in patients with the Cushing syndrome: a superior differential diagnostic test. Ann Intern Med 1990; 112: 738–42.
6. Yanovski JA, et al. Corticotropin-releasing hormone stimulation following low-dose dexamethasone administration: a new test to distinguish Cushing's syndrome from pseudo-Cushing's states. JAMA 1993; 269: 2232–8.
7. Avgerinos PC, et al. The metyrapone and dexamethasone suppression tests for the differential diagnosis of the adrenocorticotropin-dependent Cushing syndrome: a comparison. Ann Intern Med 1994; 121: 318–27.

DEPRESSION. Comments[1] by the Health and Public Policy Committee of the American College of Physicians concerning the dexamethasone suppression test for depression (p.271). The test is based on the premise that endogenously depressed patients have shown pituitary-adrenal axis abnormalities but has been found to have a low sensitivity for detecting depression. It is of unproven value and is not recommended as a screening test.

1. Young M, Schwartz JS. The dexamethasone suppression test for the detection, diagnosis, and management of depression. Ann Intern Med 1984; 100: 307–8.

High-altitude disorders. Dexamethasone is effective in the prevention of symptoms of acute mountain sickness (p.800), for which mild cerebral oedema may be a contributing factor, but it is not generally considered suitable for prophylaxis because of concern about its adverse effects. In the treatment of acute severe mountain sickness, which may involve the development of pulmonary and cerebral oedema, the mandatory treatment is immediate descent, and drug therapy is primarily adjunctive, to facilitate descent or maintain the patient until descent is possible. Under these circumstances dexamethasone and oxygen form the mainstays of treatment.

References.
1. Ferrazzini G, et al. Successful treatment of acute mountain sickness with dexamethasone. BMJ 1987; 294: 1380–2.
2. Ellsworth AJ, et al. A randomized trial of dexamethasone and acetazolamide for acute mountain sickness prophylaxis. Am J Med 1987; 83: 1024–30.
3. Montgomery AB, et al. Effects of dexamethasone on the incidence of acute mountain sickness at two intermediate altitudes. JAMA 1989; 261: 734–6.

4. Levine BD, et al. Dexamethasone in the treatment of acute mountain sickness. N Engl J Med 1989; 321: 1707–13.
5. Keller H-R, et al. Simulated descent v dexamethasone in treatment of acute mountain sickness: a randomised trial. BMJ 1995; 310: 1232–5.
6. Dumont L, et al. Efficacy and harm of pharmacological prevention of acute mountain sickness: quantitative systematic review. BMJ 2000; 321: 267–72.

Hirsutism. Unbound testosterone concentrations were consistently elevated in 32 hirsute women; when concentrations were suppressed to normal by dexamethasone 0.5 to 1 mg at night hirsutism was generally improved or ceased to progress after 8 to 10 months of treatment.[1] Other studies have shown only a modest improvement[2] or no improvement at all[3] in hirsutism when treated with dexamethasone. Addition of dexamethasone to anti-androgen therapy appeared to prolong the duration of remission in a later study.[4]

The mainstay of drug treatment for hirsutism tends to be an anti-androgen such as cyproterone or spironolactone (p.1468). Although low dose corticosteroids can suppress adrenal androgen production, careful consideration of the risks and benefits is advisable, especially since therapy for hirsutism may have to be given long-term.

1. Paulson JD, et al. Free testosterone concentration in serum: elevation is the hallmark of hirsutism. Am J Obstet Gynecol 1977; 128: 851–7.
2. Carmina E, Lobo RA. Peripheral androgen blockade versus glandular androgen suppression in the treatment of hirsutism. Obstet Gynecol 1991; 78: 845.
3. Rittmaster RS, Thompson DL. Effect of leuprolide and dexamethasone on hair growth and hormone levels in hirsute women: the relative importance of the ovary and the adrenal in the pathogenesis of hirsutism. J Clin Endocrinol Metab 1990; 70: 1096–1102.
4. Carmina E, Lobo RA. The addition of dexamethasone to antiandrogen therapy for hirsutism prolongs the duration of remission. Fertil Steril 1998; 69: 1075–9.

Malaria. Corticosteroids, especially dexamethasone, have been used in cerebral malaria (p.428) in the belief that their anti-inflammatory effect would reduce cerebral oedema.[1] However, studies have shown that cerebral oedema does not play a significant role in the pathophysiology of cerebral malaria and, indeed, double-blind studies using both moderate doses (2 mg per kg body-weight) and high doses (11 mg per kg) of dexamethasone intravenously over 48 hours found no reduction in death rates. Thus it is now considered that corticosteroids have no place in the treatment of cerebral malaria.

1. WHO. Practical chemotherapy of malaria: report of a WHO scientific group. WHO Tech Rep Ser 805 1990.

Malignant neoplasms. Dexamethasone has been used in some regimens for the treatment of malignancy, for example in acute lymphoblastic leukaemia (p.484) and multiple myeloma (p.489).

Meningitis. There is some evidence of benefit from the adjunctive use of dexamethasone in bacterial meningitis (p.128), at least in those cases due to Haemophilus influenzae, particularly in reducing deafness. Dexamethasone has been recommended as adjunctive treatment in Haemophilus meningitis, when it should be given with or before the antibacterial. However, the topic is controversial, and it is by no means certain that any benefit exists in other forms of bacterial meningitis.

References.
1. Prasad K, Haines T. Dexamethasone treatment for acute bacterial meningitis: how strong is the evidence for routine use? J Neurol Neurosurg Psychiatry 1995; 59: 31–7.
2. McIntyre PB, et al. Dexamethasone as adjunctive therapy in bacterial meningitis: a meta-analysis of randomized clinical trials since 1988. JAMA 1997; 278: 925–31.

Nausea and vomiting. Dexamethasone has antiemetic properties, particularly against acute and delayed vomiting induced by cancer chemotherapy[1] (p.1206). It may be used alone for prevention of acute symptoms associated with moderately-emetogenic treatment and is combined with a 5-HT$_3$ antagonist for highly-emetogenic treatment. Typical dosage regimens have been dexamethasone 4 to 8 mg by mouth immediately before moderately-emetogenic chemotherapy and 20 mg by intravenous injection for more severely emetogenic chemotherapy. Dexamethasone is the drug of choice for prevention of delayed symptoms, given alone or in combination with other antiemetics. A typical dose is 8 mg twice daily by mouth for 2 to 4 days.

1. Ioannidis JPA, et al. Contribution of dexamethasone to control of chemotherapy-induced nausea and vomiting: a meta-analysis of randomized evidence. J Clin Oncol 2000; 18: 3409–22.

Opportunistic mycobacterial infections. Dexamethasone in doses of 1 to 4 mg daily was associated with weight gain, reduction in fever, and an improved sense of well-being in 5 patients with HIV and disseminated Mycobacterium avium complex infection.[1] Combination antimycobacterial therapy for opportunistic mycobacterial infections (p.131) was also given. Similar results have been noted by others.[2]

1. Wormser GP, et al. Low-dose dexamethasone as adjunctive therapy for disseminated Mycobacterium avium complex infections in AIDS patients. Antimicrob Agents Chemother 1994; 38: 2215–17.
2. Dorman SE, et al. Adjunctive corticosteroid therapy for patients whose treatment for disseminated Mycobacterium avium complex infection has failed. Clin Infect Dis 1998; 26: 682–6.

Respiratory disorders. Corticosteroids such as dexamethasone are given antenatally to mothers at risk of premature delivery in order to hasten fetal lung maturation and help prevent *neonatal respiratory distress syndrome* (p.1055) and *bronchopulmonary dysplasia* (p.1048). Neonatal dexamethasone has been reported to improve pulmonary outcome and assist weaning from mechanical ventilation in infants that have developed bronchopulmonary dysplasia.

Dexamethasone is also one of the drugs of choice for the management of severe *croup* (see p.1049). However, as with other corticosteroids (p.1048) it appears to be of little value in *bronchiolitis*.[1,2]

1. Roosevelt G, *et al.* Dexamethasone in bronchiolitis: a randomised controlled trial. *Lancet* 1996; **348:** 292–5.
2. Klassen TP, *et al.* Dexamethasone in salbutamol-treated inpatients with acute bronchiolitis: a randomized controlled trial. *J Pediatr* 1997; **130:** 191–6.

Retinopathy of prematurity. For a suggestion that antenatal dexamethasone might be helpful in the prophylaxis of retinopathy of prematurity, see p.1395. For mention of the uncertain effect of neonatal dexamethasone on retinopathy of prematurity, see under Adverse Effects above.

Status epilepticus. Dexamethasone is used in some patients with status epilepticus (for example when associated with cerebral neoplasms) as mentioned on p.341.

Preparations

BP 2001: Dexamethasone Tablets;
USP 25: Dexamethasone Acetate Injectable Suspension; Dexamethasone Elixir; Dexamethasone Gel; Dexamethasone Ophthalmic Suspension; Dexamethasone Oral Solution; Dexamethasone Sodium Phosphate Cream; Dexamethasone Sodium Phosphate Inhalation Aerosol; Dexamethasone Sodium Phosphate Injection; Dexamethasone Sodium Phosphate Ophthalmic Ointment; Dexamethasone Sodium Phosphate Ophthalmic Solution; Dexamethasone Tablets; Dexamethasone Topical Aerosol; Neomycin and Polymyxin B Sulfates and Dexamethasone Ophthalmic Ointment; Neomycin and Polymyxin B Sulfates and Dexamethasone Ophthalmic Suspension; Neomycin Sulfate and Dexamethasone Sodium Phosphate Cream; Neomycin Sulfate and Dexamethasone Sodium Phosphate Ophthalmic Ointment; Neomycin Sulfate and Dexamethasone Sodium Phosphate Ophthalmic Solution; Tobramycin and Dexamethasone Ophthalmic Ointment; Tobramycin and Dexamethasone Ophthalmic Suspension.

Proprietary Preparations (details are given in Part 3)
Aust.: Dexabene; Fortecortin; *Austral.:* Decadron†; Dexmethsone; Maxidex; *Belg.:* Aacidexam; Decadron; Maxidex; Oradexon; *Braz.:* Betametagen; Decadron; Decadronal; Dermazon; Dexadermil; Dexaflan; Dexaminor; Maxidex; Minidex; *Canad.:* Decadron; Dexasone; Diodex; Hexadrol; Maxidex; *Denm.:* Decadron; Maxidex; *Fin.:* Decadron; Oftan Dexa; Oradexon; *Fr.:* Auxisone†; Cebedex†; Decadron; Dectancyl; Desocort; Maxidex; Soludecadron†; *Ger.:* afpred-DEXA; Anemul mono†; Auxiloson; Cortidexason; Cortisumman; Decadron Phosphat†; Dexa; Dexa in der Ophtiole†; Dexa Loscon mono; Dexa-Allvoran; Dexa-Brachialin N; dexa-clinit; Dexa-Effekton; Dexa-POS; Dexa-ratiopharm; Dexa-sine; Dexabene; Dexaflam; Dexaflam N; Dexagalen; Dexagel; Dexahexal; Dexamonozon; Dexamonozon N; Fortecortin; Isopto Dex; Lipotalon; Predni-F-Tablinen†; Solutio Cordes Dexa N; Spersadex; Totocortin; Tuttozem N†; *Hong Kong:* Decadron; Dexalocal; Dexasone; Dexmethsone; Limethason; Maxidex; Spersadex; *Irl.:* Decadron; Maxidex; *Israel:* Dexacort; Maxidex; Sterodex; *Ital.:* Decadron; Dermadex; Desalark; Eta Cortilen†; Luxazone; Megacort; Situalin†; Soldesam; Visumetazone; *Jpn:* Limethason; Voalla†; *Mex.:* Alin; Azona; Beamoken A; Cortidex; Cryometasona; Decadron; Decadronal; Decorex; Dexagrin; Dexatam; Dexicar; Dexona; Dibasona; Indarzona-N; Metax; Mexona; Polideltaxin; Reusan; Taprodex; Taxyl; *Neth.:* Decadron; Decadron Depot†; Dexa-POS†; Maxidex†; Oradexon; *Norw.:* Decadron; Isopto Maxidex; Spersadex; *NZ:* Decadron; Maxidex; *Port.:* Decadron; Dexaval; Oradexon; *S.Afr.:* Decadron; Decasone; Maxidex; Oradexon; Spersadex; *Singapore:* Dexaltin; Dexamed; Dexasone; Erladexone; Limethason; Maxidex; Mexasone; *Spain:* Decadran; Fortecortin; Maxidex; *Swed.:* Decadron; Dexacortal; Isopto Maxidex; Opnol; *Switz.:* Decadron; Dexa-Helvacort; Dexacortin; Dexalocal; Fortecortin; Maxidex; Mephasone; Millicortene; Oradexon; Spersadex; *Thai.:* Decadron; Dexa; Dexa-P; Dexacortisone; Dexaltin; Dexasone; Dexon; Dexthasol; Dexton; Oradexon; *UK:* Decadron; Dexsol; Maxidex; *USA:* Aeroseb-Dex; Ak-Dex; Alba Dex†; Dalalone; Decadron; Decaject; Decaspray; Dexacort; Dexameth; Dexasone; Dexone†; Hexadrol; Maxidex; Solurex.

Multi-ingredient: *Aust.:* Ambene; Clinit†; Dexa-Rhinospray†; Dexagenta; Dexasalyl; Doxiproct mit Dexamethason; Endomethazone; Multodrin; Rheumesser; Uromont; *Austral.:* Otodex; Sofradex; Tobispray†; *Belg.:* De Icin; De Icol; Decadron avec Neomycine; Dexa-Rhinospray; Maxitrol; Neodexon†; Percutalgine; Polaronil; Polydexa; Tobradex; *Braz.:* Baycuten; Biamotil-D; Decadron Nasal; Decadron Oftalmico; Dermogen; Dexa-Citoneurin; Dexa-Neuriberi; Dexa-Vastrictol; Dexacloran; Dexacobal; Dexacort; Dexador; Dexadoze; Dexafenicol; Dexagil; Dexalgen; Dexaneurin; Dexavison; Duo-Decadron; Emistin; Fenidex; Gynax-N; Hidrocin; Maxitrol; Neocortin; Oftcor; Otofenicol-D; Rinosbon; Tobradex; Topidexa; Trivagel N; Vagitrin-N; Vibetrat Dexa; *Canad.:* Dioptrol; Maxitrol; NeoDecadron†; Sofracort; Tobradex; *Denm.:* Decadron med Neomycin; Sofradex; Spersadex Comp; *Fin.:* Dexatopic; Maxitrol; Oftan Dexa-Chlora; Otomize; Sofradex; *Fr.:* Auricularum; Cebedexacol; Chibro-Cadron; Corticetine; Dexagrane; Frakidex; Framyxone; Maxidrol; Percutalgine; Polydexa; Polydexa a la Phenylephrine; Ster-Dex; Tobradex; *Ger.:* Baycuten; Chibro-Cadron†; Corti Biciron N; Cortidexason comp; Corto-Tavegil; Dexa Biciron; Dexa Polyspectran N; Dexa-Gentamicin; Dexa-Phlogont L; Dexa-Rhinospray N; Dexa-Siozwo N; Dexacrinin†; Dexamytrex; Dexasalyl†; Dispadex comp; DoloTendin†; Duodexa N; Ell-Cranell; Isopto Max; Lokalison-antimikrobiell Creme N; Magopsor†; Millicortin-Vioform; Nystalocal; Otobacid N; Rheumasit; Rhinoguttae Dexamethasoni cum Naphazolino; Solupen-D; Spersadex Comp; Spersadexolin; Supertendin 2000 N; Supertendin-Depot; Ultra-

Demoplas; Uro-Stilloson; *Hong Kong:* Colircusi Gentadexa; Decadron with Neomycin; Dexa-Polyspectran; Dexasalyl; Dextracin; Maxitrol; Neo-Dex (Improved); Oftalmolosa Cusi de Icol; Sofradex; Spersadex Comp; Spersadexoline; Tobradex; Trabit; *Irl.:* Dexa-Rhinaspray; Dexa-Rhinaspray Duo; Maxitrol; Otomize; Sofradex; *Israel:* Adexone; Auricularum; Desoren; Dethamycin; Dethaphrine; Dex-Otic; Dexamycin; Dexefrin; Maxitrol; Otomize; Polycutan; Tarocidin D; *Ital.:* Antimicotico; Corti-Arscolloid; Desalfa; Desamix Effe; Desamix-Neomicina; Dexoline; Doxiproct Plus; Eta Biocortilen; Eta Biocortilen VC; Fluorobioptal; Kanazone; Lasoproct†; Luxazone Eparina; Nasicortin; Neo-Cortofen; Rinedrone†; Situalin Antibiotico†; Tobradex; Visumetazone Antistaminico; Visumetazone Decongestionante; *Mex.:* Alin Nasal; Alin Oftalmico; Baycuten N; Biodexan; Decadron Con Neomicina; Decadron Con Nistatina; Dexabion; Dexafrin; Dexamicin; Dexsul; Levodexan; Levofenil; Maxitrol; Neobacigrin; Soldrin; Trazidex; *Neth.:* Decadron met neomycine; Dexagenta-POS†; Dexamytrex; Dexatopic†; Maxitrol†; Sofradex; *Norw.:* Maxitrol; Sofradex; Spersadex med kloramfenikol; *NZ:* Maxitrol; Sofradex; Tobradex; *Port.:* Baycuten; Decadron; Dexamytrex; Dexaval A; Dexaval N; Dexaval O; Dexaval V; Frakidex; Gentadexa; Polydexa; *S.Afr.:* Covomycin-D; Maxitrol; Sofradex; Spersadex Comp; Spersadexoline; Tobradex; *Singapore:* Dexamytrex; Dextracin; Maxitrol; Neo-Deca; Neo-Dex (Improved); Polydexa; Sofradex; Spersadex Comp; Spersadexoline; Tobradex; *Spain:* Amplidermis; Broncoformo Muco Dexa; Cloranfe Hemidex; Croygenase; Dalamon; Decadran Neomicina; Dexa Fenic†; Dexa Tavegil; Dexa Vasoc†; Dexafenicol; Dexam Constric; Gentadexa; Hem Anth; Hongosan; Icol; Inzitan; Liquipom Dexa Antib; Liquipom Dexa Const; Liquipom Dexa Gamida; Maxitrol; Neodexa; Neurocatavin Dexa; Neurodavur Plus; Oftalmol Dexa†; Oftalmotrim Dexa; Otix; Percutalin†; Phonal; Resorborina; Rino Dexa; Rinoblanco Dexa Antibio; Sabanotropico; Sedofarin; Talkosona†; Tobradex; Vasodexa; *Swed.:* Decadron cum neomycin; Sofradex; *Switz.:* Antikeloides Creme; Chronocorte; Corticetine; Cresophene; Dexacortin-K; Dexalocal-F; Dexasalyl; Dexolan; Doxiproct Plus; Frakidex; Maxitrol; Nystalocal; Otospray; Pigmanorm; Polydexa; Pulpomixine; Sebo-Psor; Sofradex; Spersadex Comp; Spersadexoline; Tobradex; *Thai.:* Archidex; Cadexcin-N; Decadron with Neomycin; Dex-Otic; Dexacin; Dexamytrex; Dexasil; Dexoph; Dexylin; Eyedex; Maxitrol; Neo-Optal; Opsardex; Percutalgine; Sofradex; Spersadexoline; Tobradex; Trabit; *UK:* Dexa-Rhinaspray Duo; Dexa-Rhinaspray†; Maxitrol; Otomize; Sofradex; Tobradex; *USA:* Ak-Neo-Dex; Ak-Trol; Dexacidin; Dexacine; Dexasporin; Maxitrol; Neo-Dexair†; Neo-Dexameth; NeoDecadron; Neodexasone; Neopolydex; Ocu-Trol; Poly-Dex; Storz-N-D†; Storz-N-P-D†; Tobradex.

Dichlorisone Acetate   (12645-j)

Dichlorisone Acetate (*rINNM*).

Diclorisone Acetate. $9\alpha,11\beta$-Dichloro-17α,21-dihydroxypregna-1,4-diene-3,20-dione 21-acetate.

$C_{23}H_{28}Cl_2O_5 = 455.4$.
CAS — 7008-26-6 (dichlorisone); 79-61-8 (dichlorisone acetate).

Profile

Dichlorisone acetate is a corticosteroid used topically for its glucocorticoid activity (p.1039) in the treatment of various skin disorders. It is usually employed as a cream or ointment containing 0.25 to 1%.

When applied topically, particularly to large areas, when the skin is broken, or under occlusive dressings, corticosteroids may be absorbed in sufficient amounts to cause systemic effects (see p.1039). The effects of topical corticosteroids on the skin are described on p.1041. For recommendations concerning the correct use of corticosteroids on the skin, see p.1045.

Preparations

Proprietary Preparations (details are given in Part 3)
Spain: Dermaren; Dicloderm Forte.

Diflorasone Diacetate   (12651-l)

Diflorasone Diacetate (*BANM, USAN, rINNM*).

U-34865. $6\alpha,9\alpha$-Difluoro-11β,17α,21-trihydroxy-16β-methylpregna-1,4-diene-3,20-dione 17,21-diacetate.

$C_{26}H_{32}F_2O_7 = 494.5$.
CAS — 2557-49-5 (diflorasone); 33564-31-7 (diflorasone diacetate).
Pharmacopoeias. In US.

Pharmacopoeial description

USP 25: A white to pale yellow, crystalline powder. Insoluble in water; soluble in acetone and in methyl alcohol; very slightly soluble in ether; sparingly soluble in ethyl acetate; slightly soluble in toluene. Store in airtight containers.

Profile

Diflorasone diacetate is a corticosteroid used topically for its glucocorticoid activity (p.1039) in the treatment of various skin disorders. It is usually employed as a cream or ointment containing 0.05%.

When applied topically, particularly to large areas, when the skin is broken, or under occlusive dressings, corticosteroids may be absorbed in sufficient amounts to cause systemic effects (p.1039). The effects of topical corticosteroids on the skin are described on p.1041. For recommendations concerning the correct use of corticosteroids on the skin, and a rough guide to the clinical potencies of topical corticosteroids, see p.1045.

Preparations

USP 25: Diflorasone Diacetate Cream; Diflorasone Diacetate Ointment.

Proprietary Preparations (details are given in Part 3)
Canad.: Florone†; *Ger.:* Florone; *Ital.:* Dermaflor; Sterodelta; *Spain:* Murode; Vincosona†; *Swed.:* Soriflor†; *USA:* Florone; Maxiflor; Psorcon.

Diflucortolone Valerate   (1087-f)

Diflucortolone Valerate (*BANM, rINNM*).

$6\alpha,9\alpha$-Difluoro-11β,21-dihydroxy-16α-methylpregna-1,4-diene-3,20-dione 21-valerate.

$C_{27}H_{36}F_2O_5 = 478.6$.
CAS — 2607-06-9 (diflucortolone); 59198-70-8 (diflucortolone valerate); 15845-96-2 (diflucortolone pivalate).

NOTE. Diflucortolone and Diflucortolone Pivalate are *USAN*.
Pharmacopoeias. In Br.

Pharmacopoeial description

BP 2001: A white to creamy white crystalline powder. Practically insoluble in water; freely soluble in dichloromethane and in dioxan; sparingly soluble in ether; slightly soluble in methyl alcohol. Protect from light.

Profile

Diflucortolone valerate is a corticosteroid used topically for its glucocorticoid activity (p.1039) in the treatment of various skin disorders. It is usually employed as a cream or ointment containing 0.1% or 0.3%.

When applied topically, particularly to large areas, when the skin is broken, or under occlusive dressings, corticosteroids may be absorbed in sufficient amounts to cause systemic effects (p.1039). The effects of topical corticosteroids on the skin are described on p.1041. For recommendations concerning the correct use of corticosteroids on the skin, and a rough guide to the clinical potencies of topical corticosteroids, see p.1045.

Preparations

BP 2001: Diflucortolone Cream; Diflucortolone Oily Cream; Diflucortolone Ointment.

Proprietary Preparations (details are given in Part 3)
Aust.: Neriforte; Nerisona; *Belg.:* Nerisona; *Braz.:* Nerisona; *Canad.:* Nerisone; *Denm.:* Nerisona; *Fr.:* Nerisone; *Ger.:* Nerisona; *Hong Kong:* Nerisona; *Israel:* Neriderm; *Ital.:* Cortical; Dermaval; Dervin; Dicortal; Flu-Cortanest; Nerisona; Temetex; *Mex.:* Nerisona; *Neth.:* Nerisona; *NZ:* Nerisona; *Port.:* Nerisona; *S.Afr.:* Nerisone; *Singapore:* Nerisone; *Spain:* Claral; *Switz.:* Nerisona; *UK:* Nerisone.

Multi-ingredient: *Aust.:* Neriquinol; Travocort; *Belg.:* Travocort; *Braz.:* Bi-Nerisona; *Canad.:* Nerisalic; *Fr.:* Nerisalic; Nerisone C; *Ger.:* Nerisona C; Travocort; *Hong Kong:* Nerisone C; Travocort; *Irl.:* Travocort; *Israel:* Isocort; Multiderm; *Ital.:* Corti-Fluoral; Dermaflogil; Dermobios†; Impetex; Nerisona C; Travocort; *Mex.:* Bi-Nerisona; Scheriderm; *NZ:* Nerisone C; *Port.:* Nerisona C; Travocort; *S.Afr.:* Travocort; *Singapore:* Nerisone C; Travocort; *Spain:* Claral Plus; *Switz.:* Travocort; *Thai.:* Travocort.

Difluprednate   (12652-y)

Difluprednate (*USAN, rINN*).

CM-9155; W-6309. $6\alpha,9\alpha$-Difluoro-11β,17α,21-trihydroxypregna-1,4-diene-3,20-dione 21-acetate 17-butyrate.

$C_{27}H_{34}F_2O_7 = 508.6$.
CAS — 23674-86-4.
ATC — D07AC19.

Profile

Difluprednate is a corticosteroid used topically for its glucocorticoid activity (p.1039) in the treatment of various skin disorders. It is usually employed as a cream, gel, or ointment; concentrations used range from 0.02 to 0.05%.

When applied topically, particularly to large areas, when the skin is broken, or under occlusive dressings, corticosteroids may be absorbed in sufficient amounts to cause systemic effects (p.1039). The effects of topical corticosteroids on the skin are described on p.1041. For recommendations concerning the correct use of corticosteroids on the skin, see p.1045.

Preparations

Proprietary Preparations (details are given in Part 3)
Fr.: Epitopic; *Jpn:* Myser.

Fluclorolone Acetonide   (1088-d)

Fluclorolone Acetonide (*BAN, rINN*).

Flucloronide (*USAN*); RS-2252. $9\alpha,11\beta$-Dichloro-6α-fluoro-21-hydroxy-16α,17α-isopropylidenedioxypregna-1,4-diene-3,20-dione.

$C_{24}H_{29}Cl_2FO_5 = 487.4$.
CAS — 3693-39-8.

Profile

Fluclorolone acetonide is a corticosteroid used topically for its glucocorticoid activity (p.1039) in the treatment of various skin disorders. It is usually employed as a cream or ointment containing 0.2%.

When applied topically, particularly to large areas, when the skin is broken, or under occlusive dressings, corticosteroids may be absorbed in sufficient amounts to cause systemic effects (p.1039). The effects of topical corticosteroids on the skin are described on p.1041. For recommendations concerning the correct use of corticosteroids on the skin, and a rough guide to the clinical potencies of topical corticosteroids, see p.1045.

Preparations

Proprietary Preparations (details are given in Part 3)
Spain: Cutanit.

Fludrocortisone Acetate (1089-n)

Fludrocortisone Acetate (BANM, rINNM).
Fludrocortisoni Acetas; 9α-Fluorohydrocortisone 21-Acetate. 9α-Fluoro-11β,17α,21-trihydroxypregn-4-ene-3,20-dione 21-acetate.
$C_{23}H_{31}FO_6 = 422.5$.
CAS — 127-31-1 (fludrocortisone); 514-36-3 (fludrocortisone acetate).
Pharmacopoeias. In *Chin., Eur.* (see p.vi), *Int., Pol.,* and *US.*

Pharmacopoeial description

Ph. Eur.: A white or almost white, crystalline powder. Practically insoluble in water; sparingly soluble in dehydrated alcohol; slightly soluble in ether.

USP 25: White to pale yellow, odourless or practically odourless, hygroscopic, crystals or crystalline powder. Insoluble in water; sparingly soluble in alcohol and in chloroform; slightly soluble in ether. Protect from light.

Adverse Effects, Treatment, Withdrawal, and Precautions

Fludrocortisone acetate has glucocorticoid actions about 10 times as potent as hydrocortisone and mineralocorticoid effects more than 100 times as potent. Adverse effects are mainly those due to mineralocorticoid activity, as described on p.1039.

When applied topically, particularly to large areas, when the skin is broken, or under occlusive dressings, corticosteroids may be absorbed in sufficient amounts to cause systemic effects. Prolonged application to the eye of preparations containing corticosteroids has caused raised intra-ocular pressure and reduced visual function.

Interactions

The interactions of corticosteroids in general are described on p.1043.

Pharmacokinetics

For a brief outline of the pharmacokinetics of corticosteroids, see p.1044.

Fludrocortisone is readily absorbed from the gastrointestinal tract. The plasma half-life is about 3.5 hours or more, but fludrocortisone exhibits a more prolonged biological half-life of 18 to 36 hours.

Uses and Administration

Fludrocortisone is a corticosteroid with glucocorticoid and highly potent mineralocorticoid activity as described under Corticosteroids, p.1039.

Fludrocortisone acetate is given by mouth to provide mineralocorticoid replacement in primary adrenocortical insufficiency (p.1046), together with glucocorticoids. It is used in a dose range of 50 to 300 µg daily.

Fludrocortisone acetate may also be given concomitantly with glucocorticoid therapy in doses of up to 200 µg daily in the salt-losing form of congenital adrenal hyperplasia (p.1049).

It is also given by mouth in the management of severe orthostatic hypotension (see below).

Fludrocortisone acetate is applied topically to the skin, eye, and ear in the treatment of various disorders. It is employed as an ingredient of cream, ointment, gel, or drops, usually in a concentration of 0.1%. For recommendations concerning the correct use of corticosteroids on the skin, see p.1045.

Administration. A study of fludrocortisone requirements in 10 patients with Addison's disease indicated that dosage was often inadequate.[1] Nine were initially on fludrocortisone 50 to 100 µg daily in addition to cortisone or hydrocortisone; 5 were also taking thyroxine [levothyroxine] for an associated autoimmune thyroid disease; one, who had detectable levels of aldosterone, was not initially receiving fludrocortisone. All the patients had evidence of sodium and water depletion and initiation of fludrocortisone 300 µg daily, with downwards adjustments, demonstrated that most patients required 200 µg daily. Two patients elected to remain on 300 µg daily, but in most this dose caused pronounced sodium and water retention. The patient with detectable aldosterone levels required 50 µg daily. Eight of the 10 patients felt better on the higher fludrocortisone doses while 2 felt no change.

1. Smith SJ, *et al.* Evidence that patients with Addison's disease are undertreated with fludrocortisone. *Lancet* 1984; **i:** 11–14.

Neurally mediated hypotension. Fludrocortisone is reported to be one of the standard drugs used in the management of neurally mediated hypotension (see p.805).

Orthostatic hypotension. Orthostatic (postural) hypotension[1-5] is a fall in blood pressure that occurs upon rising abruptly to an erect position, although it may also occur following a period of prolonged standing. Characteristic symptoms include lightheadedness, dizziness, blurred vision, weakness in the limbs, and syncope.

The causes of orthostatic hypotension are wide-ranging and include autonomic dysfunction, such as in the Shy-Drager syndrome, diabetes mellitus, and Parkinson's disease, circulating volume depletion, phaeochromocytoma, and Addison's disease. Orthostatic hypotension may also occur following a period of prolonged bed rest or following meals.

Orthostatic hypotension may result from the adverse effects of a range of drugs, such as antihypertensives, diuretics, tricyclic antidepressants, phenothiazines, and MAOIs.

In mild cases **nonpharmacological treatment** alone may be adequate. This includes increasing salt intake if not contra-indicated, maintaining adequate hydration, the use of elastic stockings to improve venous return and increase cardiac output, and elevating the head of the bed to reduce early morning symptoms. Drug-induced orthostatic hypotension should be treated by withdrawing the agent or by dose reduction.

Pharmacological treatment. No pharmacological treatment is entirely satisfactory: responses and tolerance vary greatly between patients. Fludrocortisone acetate is usually tried first; it increases sodium retention and thus plasma volume. Most reports indicate some response in about 80% of patients, but hypokalaemia, fluid retention, and supine hypertension may limit its use. In patients who fail to respond adequately an NSAID (usually indometacin) may be tried, alone or in combination with fludrocortisone. In patients with overt autonomic failure a beta blocker with some partial agonist activity, such as xamoterol or pindolol, may be tried although they are potentially dangerous.

Sympathomimetics may be useful in some patients with autonomic failure; the direct acting drugs such as phenylephrine or midodrine usually prove more consistently effective than the indirect such as ephedrine, but even so, responses tend to vary with the degree of denervation. Patients with central neurological abnormalities may respond to desmopressin, while drugs such as ergotamine or dihydroergotamine may be useful for resistant disease.

Other drugs that have been tried include metoclopramide, which may be useful for autonomic symptoms in patients with diabetes mellitus, fluoxetine, octreotide, yohimbine, clonidine, and in patients with concurrent anaemia, erythropoietin. Caffeine has been tried in postprandial hypotension but its value in all but the mildest cases is dubious.[5] The use of MAOIs (which given alone can induce orthostatic hypotension) with a sympathomimetic to induce a pressor reaction is controversial. Most of these drugs have potentially serious adverse effects and few are well evaluated.

1. Ahmad RAS, Watson RDS. Treatment of postural hypotension: a review. *Drugs* 1990; **39:** 74–85.
2. Tonkin AL, Wing LMH. Hypotension: assessment and management. *Med J Aust* 1990; **153:** 474–85.
3. Schoenberger JA. Drug-induced orthostatic hypotension. *Drug Safety* 1991; **6:** 402–7.
4. Stumpf JL, Mitrzyk B. Management of orthostatic hypotension. *Am J Hosp Pharm* 1994; **51:** 648–60.
5. Mathias CJ. Orthostatic hypotension. *Prescribers' J* 1995; **35:** 124–32.

Preparations

BP 2001: Fludrocortisone Tablets;
USP 25: Fludrocortisone Acetate Tablets.

Proprietary Preparations (details are given in Part 3)
Aust.: Astonin H; *Austral.:* Florinef; *Braz.:* Florinefe; *Canad.:* Florinef; *Denm.:* Florinef; *Fin.:* Florinef; *Ger.:* Astonin H; *Hong Kong:* Florinef; *Irl.:* Florinef; *Neth.:* Florinef; *Norw.:* Florinef; *NZ:* Florinef; *S.Afr.:* Florinef; *Singapore:* Florinef; *Spain:* Astonin; *Swed.:* Florinef; *Switz.:* Florinef; *Thai.:* Florinef; *UK:* Florinef; *USA:* Florinef.

Multi-ingredient: *Belg.:* Panotile; *Braz.:* Otodol; Panotil; Rinofluimucil; *Fr.:* Panotile; *Ger.:* Panotile N; *Neth.:* Panotile; *Spain:* Fludronef; Panotile; *Switz.:* Panotile.

Flumetasone Pivalate (1091-a)

Flumetasone Pivalate (BANM, rINNM).
Flumethasone Pivalate (USAN); Flumethasone Trimethylacetate; NSC-107680. Flumethasone 21-pivalate.
$C_{27}H_{36}F_2O_6 = 494.6$.
CAS — 2002-29-1.
Pharmacopoeias. In *Eur.* (see p.vi), *Pol.,* and *US.*

Pharmacopoeial description

Ph. Eur.: A white or almost white, crystalline powder. It shows polymorphism. Practically insoluble in water; slightly soluble in alcohol and in dichloromethane; sparingly soluble in acetone. Protect from light.

USP 25: A white to off-white crystalline powder. Insoluble in water; soluble 1 in 89 of alcohol, 1 in 350 of chloroform, and 1 in 2800 of ether; slightly soluble in methyl alcohol; very slightly soluble in dichloromethane. Store in airtight containers. Protect from light.

Profile

Flumetasone pivalate is a corticosteroid used topically for its glucocorticoid activity (p.1039) in the treatment of various skin disorders. It is usually employed as a 0.02% cream, ointment, or lotion. When applied topically, particularly to large areas, when the skin is broken, or under occlusive dressings, corticosteroids may be absorbed in sufficient amounts to cause systemic effects (p.1039). The effects of topical corticosteroids on the skin are described on p.1041. For recommendations concerning the correct use of corticosteroids on the skin, and a rough guide to the clinical potencies of topical corticosteroids, see p.1045.

Flumetasone pivalate is also used in ear drops in a concentration of 0.02% with clioquinol 1%.

Preparations

USP 25: Flumethasone Pivalate Cream.

Proprietary Preparations (details are given in Part 3)
Belg.: Locacortene; *Canad.:* Locacorten†; *Ger.:* Cerson; Locacorten; *Israel:* Locacorten; *Ital.:* Locorten; *Neth.:* Locacorten; *Spain:* Locortene; *Switz.:* Locacorten.

Multi-ingredient: *Aust.:* Locacorten mit Neomycin; Locacorten Tar; Locacorten Vioform; Locasalen; *Austral.:* Locacorten Vioform; *Belg.:* Locacortene Tar; Locacortene Vioforme; Locasalen; *Braz.:* Locorten Neomicina; Locorten Vioformio; Losalen; *Canad.:* Locacorten Vioform; Locasalen†; *Denm.:* Locacorten med Salicylsyre; Locacorten Vioform; *Fin.:* Locacorten Vioform; *Ger.:* Locacorten Vioform; Locasalen; Lorinden T; *Hong Kong:* Locacorten Tar; Locasalen; *Israel:* Locacorten; Locacorten Tar; Locasalen; Topicorten V; Topicorten-Tar; Topisalen; *Ital.:* Locorten; Locorten Tar†; Locorten Vioformio; Losalen; Vasosterone Oto; *Neth.:* Locacorten Vioform; Locasalen; *Norw.:* Locacorten Vioform; Locasalen†; *NZ:* Locacorten Vioform; *Port.:* Locorten Vioformio; Losalen; *S.Afr.:* Locacorten Tar†; Locacorten Vioform; *Singapore:* Locasalen; *Spain:* Locortene Vioformo; Locasalen; *Swed.:* Locacorten Vioform; Locasalen†; *Switz.:* Locacorten Tar†; Locacorten Triclosan†; Locasalen; *Thai.:* Flumasalen; Locasalen; *UK:* Locorten Vioform.

Flunisolide (1092-t)

Flunisolide (BAN, USAN, rINN).
RS-3999; RS-1320 (acetate). 6α-Fluoro-11β,21-dihydroxy-16α,17α-isopropylidenedioxypregna-1,4-diene-3,20-dione.
$C_{24}H_{31}FO_6 = 434.5$.
CAS — 3385-03-3 (flunisolide); 77326-96-6 (flunisolide hemihydrate); 4533-89-5 (flunisolide acetate).
ATC — R01AD04; R03BA03.
Pharmacopoeias. In *US* which specifies the hemihydrate.

Pharmacopoeial description

USP 25: A white to creamy-white crystalline powder. Practically insoluble in water; soluble in acetone; sparingly soluble in chloroform; slightly soluble in methyl alcohol.

Adverse Effects, Treatment, Withdrawal, and Precautions

As for corticosteroids in general (see p.1039).

Interactions

The interactions of corticosteroids in general are described on p.1043.

Pharmacokinetics

For a brief outline of the pharmacokinetics of corticosteroids, see p.1044. Flunisolide is reported to undergo extensive first-pass metabolism, with only 20% of the dose available systemically if it is given by mouth. The major metabolite, 6β-hydroxyflunisolide has some glucocorticoid activity; it has a half-life of about 4 hours. Only small amounts of flunisolide are absorbed following intranasal administration.

◊ References.
1. Chaplin MD, *et al.* Flunisolide metabolism and dynamics of a metabolite. *Clin Pharmacol Ther* 1980; **27:** 402–13.
2. Möllmann H, *et al.* Pharmacokinetic/pharmacodynamic evaluation of systemic effects of flunisolide after inhalation. *J Clin Pharmacol* 1997; **37:** 893–903.

Uses and Administration

Flunisolide is a corticosteroid with glucocorticoid activity used as a nasal spray for the prophylaxis and treatment of allergic rhinitis (p.407). It is used in a usual initial dose of 50 µg into each nostril two or three times daily, subsequently reduced to the lowest dose adequate to control symptoms which may be as little as 25 µg into each nostril daily. Children over 5 years of age may be given 25 µg into each nostril up to three times daily. In the USA a dose of 50 µg into each nostril twice daily has also been permitted in children.

Flunisolide is also used by inhalation from a metered-dose aerosol in the management of asthma (p.757). The usual adult dosage is 500 µg inhaled twice daily. In severe asthma the dosage may be increased but should not exceed a total of 2 mg daily. A dose for children over 5 years of age is 500 µg inhaled twice daily.

Preparations

USP 25: Flunisolide Nasal Solution.

Proprietary Preparations (details are given in Part 3)
Aust.: Pulmilide; Syntaris; *Belg.:* Broncort; Syntaris; *Braz.:* Flunitec; *Canad.:* Bronalide†; Rhinalar; *Denm.:* Flunitec†; Locasyn; *Fr.:* Bronilide; Nasalide; *Ger.:* Inhacort; Syntaris; *Hong Kong:* Rhinalar; *Irl.:* Syntaris; *Israel:* Flunase; *Ital.:* Gibiflu; Lunibron-A; Lunis; Nisolid; Syntaris; *Neth.:* Syntaris; *Norw.:* Flunitec; Lokilan; *Port.:* Paftec; *S.Afr.:* Syntaris†; *Swed.:* Lokilan Nasal†; *Switz.:* Broncort; Syntaris; *UK:* Syntaris; *USA:* AeroBid; Nasalide; Nasarel.

Multi-ingredient: *Ital.:* Plenaer.

Fluocinolone Acetonide   (1093-x)

Fluocinolone Acetonide (BANM, USAN, rINN).

6α,9α-Difluoro-16α-hydroxyprednisolone Acetonide; Fluocinoloni Acetonidum; NSC-92339. 6α,9α-Difluoro-11β,21-dihydroxy-16α,17α-isopropylidenedioxypregna-1,4-diene-3,20-dione.

$C_{24}H_{30}F_2O_6 = 452.5$.
CAS — 67-73-2.
ATC — C05AA10; D07AC04.

Pharmacopoeias. In Eur. (see p.vi), Jpn, and Pol. Br. has a separate monograph for the dihydrate; US allows either the anhydrous form or the dihydrate.

Pharmacopoeial description

Ph. Eur.: A white or almost white, crystalline powder. It exhibits polymorphism. Practically insoluble in water; soluble in dehydrated alcohol and in acetone. Protect from light.

BP 2001: Fluocinolone acetonide dihydrate is a white or almost white, crystalline powder. Practically insoluble in water and in hexane; soluble in dehydrated alcohol; freely soluble in acetone; sparingly soluble in dichloromethane and in methyl alcohol. Protect from light.

USP 25: It is anhydrous or contains two molecules of water of hydration. A white or practically white, odourless, crystalline powder. Insoluble in water; soluble 1 in 45 of alcohol, 1 in 25 of chloroform, and 1 in 350 of ether; soluble in methyl alcohol.

Profile

Fluocinolone acetonide is a corticosteroid used topically for its glucocorticoid activity (p.1039) in the treatment of various skin disorders. It is usually employed as a cream, gel, lotion, ointment, or scalp application; usual concentrations used range from 0.0025 to 0.025%. When applied topically, particularly to large areas, when the skin is broken, or under occlusive dressings, corticosteroids may be absorbed in sufficient amounts to cause systemic effects (p.1039). The effects of topical corticosteroids on the skin are described on p.1041. For recommendations concerning the correct use of corticosteroids on the skin, and a rough guide to the clinical potencies of topical corticosteroids, see p.1045.

Fluocinolone acetonide is also used topically in combination with an antibacterial in the treatment of infective inflammatory eye, ear, and nose disorders.

Formulation. The potency of fluocinolone acetonide varied with the formulation in a study[1] involving different Synalar topical preparations, the gel, ointment, and cream. The cream was the most potent followed by the gel, and then the ointment. A comparison of topical vasoconstrictor activity (used as an index of potency) unexpectedly found that the commercial dilu-

tions of the cream (containing 0.00625% and 0.0025%) were indistinguishable in their effects from the full-strength (0.025%) cream.
1. Gao HY, Li Wan Po A. Topical formulations of fluocinolone acetonide: are creams, gels and ointments bioequivalent and does dilution affect activity? *Eur J Clin Pharmacol* 1994; **46:** 71–5.

Preparations

BP 2001: Fluocinolone Cream; Fluocinolone Ointment;
USP 25: Fluocinolone Acetonide Cream; Fluocinolone Acetonide Ointment; Fluocinolone Acetonide Topical Solution; Neomycin Sulfate and Fluocinolone Acetonide Cream.

Proprietary Preparations (details are given in Part 3)
Aust.: Synalar; *Belg.:* Synalar; *Braz.:* Synalar; *Canad.:* Fluoderm; Synalar; *Denm.:* Synalar; *Fr.:* Synalar†; *Ger.:* Flucinar; Jellin; Jellisoft; *Hong Kong:* Flunolone-V; *Irl.:* Synalar; *Israel:* Dermalar; *Ital.:* Alfa-Fluorone; Alfabios†; Boniderma; Cortamide; Dermobeta; Dermolin; Esacinone; Fluomix Same; Fluovitef; Fluvean; Localyn; Localyn SV; Neoderm Ginecologico†; Omniderm; Sterolone; Ultraderm; *Mex.:* Cremisona; Flucin; Fusalar; Synalar; *Neth.:* Synalar†; *Norw.:* Synalar; *NZ:* Synalar; *Port.:* Oto-Synalar N; Synalar; *S.Afr.:* Cortoderm; Fluoderm†; Synalar; *Singapore:* Flunolone-V; Synalar; *Spain:* Alvadermo Fuerte; Anatopic†; Co Fluocin Fuerte; Cortiespec; Fluocid Forte; Fluocortan; Fluodermo Fuerte; Gelidina; Oxidermiol Fuerte; Synalar; Synalar Rectal Simple; *Swed.:* Synalar; *Switz.:* Synalar; *Thai.:* Fluciderm; Flunolone-V; Supralan; Synalar; *UK:* Synalar; *USA:* Capex; Derma-Smoothe/FS; Fluonid; Flurosyn; Synalar; Synemol.

Multi-ingredient: *Aust.:* Myco-Synalar; Procto-Synalar; Synalar N; *Belg.:* Procto-Synalar; Synalar Bi-Otic; *Braz.:* Elotin; Fluo-Fenicol; Fluo-Vaso; Gotas Ototilan; Histalerg; Neocinolon; Otocort; Otolone; Otomixyn; Otosynalar; *Denm.:* Synalar med Chinoform; *Fr.:* Antibio-Synalar†; Synalar Neomycine†; *Ger.:* Jellin polyvalent; Jellin-Neomycin; Jellisoft-Neomycin; Procto-Jellin; *Hong Kong:* Flunolone; Synco-CFN; *Irl.:* Synalar C; Synalar N; *Ital.:* Alfa-Fluorone; Cortanest Plus; Doricum; Fluomicetina†; Lauromicina; Localyn; Localyn-Neomicina; Mecloderm F; Meclutin; Nefluan; Proctolyn; *Mex.:* Cetoquina Y; Ercal; Fluo Grin; Lasalar-Y; Promibasol-Plus; Synalar C; Synalar N; Synalar Neomicina; Synalar O; Synalar Oftalmico; Vagitrol-V; *Neth.:* Synalar + DBO†; Synalar Bi-Otic; *Norw.:* Synalar med Chinoform; *Port.:* Synalar Rectal; *S.Afr.:* Synalar C; Synalar N; *Singapore:* Flunolone; Synalar C; Synalar N; *Spain:* Abrasone; Alergical; Artrodesmol Extra; Bazalin; Creanolona; Flodermol; Fluo Fenic; Fluo Vasoc; Intradermo Cort Ant Fung; Midacina; Myco-Synalar†; Neo Analsona; Neo-Synalar†; Otomidrin; Poxider†; Synalar Nasal; Synalar Neomicina; Synalar Otico; Synalar Rectal; Synobel; Vinciseptil Otico; *Switz.:* Myco-Synalar; Procto; Procto-Synalar N; Synalar N; *Thai.:* Fluciderm-N; Fluonid-N; Fluonolone; Gental-F; Supralan-N; Synalar N; *UK:* Synalar C; Synalar N.

Fluocinonide   (1094-r)

Fluocinonide (BAN, USAN, rINN).

Fluocinolide; Fluocinolone Acetonide 21-Acetate; NSC-101791. 6α,9α-Difluoro-11β,21-dihydroxy-16α,17α-isopropylidenedioxypregna-1,4-diene-3,20-dione 21-acetate.

$C_{26}H_{32}F_2O_7 = 494.5$.
CAS — 356-12-7.
ATC — C05AA11; D07AC08.

Pharmacopoeias. In Br., Chin., Jpn, and US.

Pharmacopoeial description

BP 2001: A white or almost white, crystalline powder. Practically insoluble in water; slightly soluble in dehydrated alcohol and in chloroform. Protect from light.

USP 25: A white to cream-coloured, crystalline powder having not more than a slight odour. Practically insoluble in water; slightly soluble in alcohol, in methyl alcohol, and in dioxan; sparingly soluble in acetone and in chloroform; very slightly soluble in ether.

Profile

Fluocinonide is a corticosteroid used topically for its glucocorticoid activity (p.1039) in the treatment of various skin disorders. It is usually employed as a cream, gel, lotion, ointment, or scalp application containing 0.05%.

When applied topically, particularly to large areas, when the skin is broken, or under occlusive dressings, corticosteroids may be absorbed in sufficient amounts to cause systemic effects (p.1039). The effects of topical corticosteroids on the skin are described on p.1041. For recommendations concerning the correct use of corticosteroids on the skin, and a rough guide to the clinical potencies of topical corticosteroids, see p.1045.

Preparations

BP 2001: Fluocinonide Cream; Fluocinonide Ointment;
USP 25: Fluocinonide Cream; Fluocinonide Gel; Fluocinonide Ointment; Fluocinonide Topical Solution.

Proprietary Preparations (details are given in Part 3)
Aust.: Topsym; Topsymin F; *Belg.:* Lidex; *Canad.:* Lidemol; Lidex; Lyderm; Lydonide; Tiamol; Topsyn; *Denm.:* Metosyn; *Fr.:* Topsyne†; *Ger.:* Topsym; *Hong Kong:* Novoter; *Irl.:* Metosyn; *Ital.:* Flu-21; Topsyn; *Mex.:* Gelisyn; Topsyn; *Neth.:* Topsyne; *Norw.:* Metosyn; *Singapore:* Metosyn; *Spain:* Cusigel; Klariderm; Novoter; *Switz.:* Korticoid; Topsym; Topsymin; *UK:* Metosyn; *USA:* Fluonex†; Lidex; Vasoderm†.

Multi-ingredient: *Aust.:* Topsym polyvalent; *Canad.:* Trisyn†; *Fr.:* Topsyne Neomycin†; *Ger.:* Topsym polyvalent; *Hong Kong:* Novoter Gentamicina; *Israel:* Comagis; *Mex.:* Topsyn-Y; *Spain:* Novoter Gentamicina; *Switz.:* Korticoid polyvalent; Topsym polyvalent; *UK:* Vipsogal.

Fluocortin Butyl   (12761-a)

Fluocortin Butyl (BAN, USAN, rINNM).

SH-K-203. Butyl 6α-fluoro-11β-hydroxy-16α-methyl-3,20-dioxopregna-1,4-dien-21-oate.

$C_{26}H_{35}FO_5 = 446.6$.
CAS — 33124-50-4 (fluocortin); 41767-29-7 (fluocortin butyl).

Profile

Fluocortin butyl is a corticosteroid which has been used topically for its glucocorticoid activity (p.1039) in the treatment of various skin disorders. It is usually employed as a cream or ointment containing 0.75%. When applied topically, particularly to large areas, when the skin is broken, or under occlusive dressings, or intranasally, corticosteroids may be absorbed in sufficient amounts to cause systemic effects (p.1039). The effects of topical corticosteroids on the skin are described on p.1041. For recommendations concerning the correct use of corticosteroids on the skin, and a rough guide to the clinical potencies of topical corticosteroids, see p.1045.

Fluocortin butyl is also used in the form of a dry powder nasal inhalation for the management of allergic rhinitis (p.407) in usual doses of 0.5 mg inhaled into each nostril 2 to 4 times daily.

Preparations

Proprietary Preparations (details are given in Part 3)
Belg.: Varlane; *Ger.:* Lenen; Vaspit; *Ital.:* Vaspit; *Spain:* Vaspit.
Multi-ingredient: *Ger.:* Bi-Vaspit.

Fluocortolone   (1095-f)

Fluocortolone (BAN, USAN, rINN).

6α-Fluoro-16α-methyl-1-dehydrocorticosterone; SH-742. 6α-Fluoro-11β,21-dihydroxy-16α-methylpregna-1,4-diene-3,20-dione.

$C_{22}H_{29}FO_4 = 376.5$.
CAS — 152-97-6.
ATC — C05AA08; D07AC05; H02AB03.

Fluocortolone Caproate   (1096-d)

Fluocortolone Caproate (USAN, rINNM).

Fluocortolone Hexanoate (BANM); SH-770. Fluocortolone 21-hexanoate.

$C_{28}H_{39}FO_5 = 474.6$.
CAS — 303-40-2.

Pharmacopoeial description

BP 2001: A white or creamy-white, odourless or almost odourless, crystalline powder. It exhibits polymorphism. Practically insoluble in water and in ether; very slightly soluble in alcohol and in methyl alcohol; slightly soluble in acetone and in dioxan; sparingly soluble in chloroform. Protect from light.

Fluocortolone Pivalate   (1097-n)

Fluocortolone Pivalate (BANM, rINNM).

Fluocortolone Trimethylacetate; Fluocortoloni Pivalas. Fluocortolone 21-pivalate.

$C_{27}H_{37}FO_5 = 460.6$.
CAS — 29205-06-9.

Pharmacopoeias. In Eur. (see p.vi).

Pharmacopoeial description

Ph. Eur.: A white or almost white crystalline powder. Practically insoluble in water; sparingly soluble in alcohol; freely soluble in dichloromethane and in dioxan. Protect from light.

Profile

Fluocortolone and its esters are corticosteroids mainly used topically for their glucocorticoid activity (p.1039) in the treatment of various skin disorders. They are usually employed as a cream or ointment; concentrations usually used are 0.25% of the caproate with 0.25% of either the free alcohol or pivalate ester. The pivalate and caproate esters have also been used together in ointments or suppositories for the treatment of anorectal disorders.

When applied topically, particularly to large areas, when the skin is broken, or under occlusive dressings, corticosteroids may be absorbed in sufficient amounts to cause systemic effects (p.1039). The effects of topical corticosteroids on the skin are described on p.1041. For recommendations concerning the correct use of corticosteroids on the skin, and a rough guide to the clinical potencies of topical corticosteroids, see p.1045.

Fluocortolone free alcohol is sometimes given by mouth for its systemic effects in conditions for which corticosteroids are indicated (p.1044), in usual doses of 5 to 100 mg daily.

Preparations

BP 2001: Fluocortolone Cream.

Proprietary Preparations (details are given in Part 3)
Aust.: Omnilan†; Ultralan; *Ger.:* Ultralan; *Hong Kong:* Ultralan; *Israel:* Ultralan; *Ital.:* Ultralan; *Mex.:* Ultralan; *Neth.:* Ultralan; *Spain:* Ultralan M.

Multi-ingredient: *Aust.:* Pilison; Ultralan; Ultraproct; Ultraquinol†; *Austral.:* Ultraproct; *Belg.:* Ultraproct; *Braz.:* Ultraproct; *Denm.:* Doloproct; Doloproct Comp; *Fin.:* Neoproct; *Fr.:* Myco-

Ultralan; Ultralan; Ultraproct; *Ger.:* Doloproct; Ultralan; Ultralan-
crinale†; Ultraproct; *Hong Kong:* Ultraproct; *Irl.:* Ultraproct;
Ital.: Ultralan; Ultraproct; *Mex.:* Ultraproct; *Neth.:* Ultraproct†;
NZ: Ultraproct; *Port.:* Ultraproct; *Swed.:* Ultralanum†; *Switz.:*
Ultralan†; Ultraproct†; *UK:* Ultralanum Plain; Ultraproct.

Fluorometholone   (1098-h)

Fluorometholone *(BAN, rINN)*.

9α-Fluoro-11β,17α-dihydroxy-6α-methylpregna-1,4-diene-
3,20-dione.

$C_{22}H_{29}FO_4 = 376.5$.

CAS — 426-13-1.

*ATC — C05AA06; D07AB06; D07XB04; D10AA01;
S01BA07; S01CB05.*

Pharmacopoeias. In Br., Jpn, and US.

Pharmacopoeial description

BP 2001: A white to yellowish white, crystalline powder. Practically insoluble in water; slightly soluble in dehydrated alcohol and in ether.

USP 25: A white to yellowish-white, odourless, crystalline
powder. Practically insoluble in water; soluble 1 in 200 of alcohol and 1 in 2200 of chloroform; very slightly soluble in ether.
Store in airtight containers. Protect from light.

Fluorometholone Acetate   (14792-a)

Fluorometholone Acetate *(BANM, USAN, rINNM)*.

U-17323. 9α-Fluoro-11β,17α-dihydroxy-6α-methylpregna-1,4-
diene-3,20-dione 17-acetate.

$C_{24}H_{31}FO_5 = 418.5$.

CAS — 3801-06-7.

Fluorometholone acetate 1.1 mg is approximately equivalent to
1 mg of fluorometholone.

Profile

Fluorometholone is a corticosteroid employed for its glucocorticoid activity (p.1039), usually as eye drops containing 0.1%,
in the treatment of allergic and inflammatory conditions of the
eye. Fluorometholone acetate has been used similarly.

Fluorometholone has also been used topically in the treatment
of various skin disorders.

Prolonged application to the eye of preparations containing
corticosteroids has caused raised intra-ocular pressure and reduced visual function. When applied topically, particularly to
large areas, when the skin is broken, or under occlusive dressings, corticosteroids may be absorbed in sufficient amounts to
cause systemic effects (p.1039). The effects of topical corticosteroids on the skin are described on p.1041. For recommendations concerning the correct use of corticosteroids on the skin,
see p.1045.

Preparations

BP 2001: Fluorometholone Eye Drops;
USP 25: Fluorometholone Cream; Fluorometholone Ophthalmic
Suspension; Neomycin Sulfate and Fluorometholone Ointment;
Tobramycin and Fluorometholone Acetate Ophthalmic Suspen-
sion.

Proprietary Preparations (details are given in Part 3)
Aust.: Flarex; *Austral.:* Flarex; Flucon; FML; *Belg.:* Flucon;
FML; *Braz.:* Florate; Flumex; Flumetol; *Canad.:* FML; *Denm.:* Flu-
rolon; *Fin.:* FML Liquifilm; *Fr.:* Flucon; *Ger.:* Efflumidex; Fluor-
opos; Isopto Flucon; *Hong Kong:* Flucon; FML; *Irl.:* FML; *Isra-
el:* Flarex; FML; *Ital.:* Flarex; Fluaton; Flumetol Semplice; *Mex.:*
Flarex; Fluforte; FML; *Neth.:* Flarex†; FML Liquifilm†; *NZ:*
Flarex; Flucon; FML; *Port.:* Flurop; FML Liquifilm; *S.Afr.:* Flu-
con; FML; *Singapore:* FML; *Spain:* FML; Isopto Flucon; *Switz.:*
Flarex; FML; *Thai.:* Flarex; Flu Oph; Flucon; FML; *UK:* FML
Liquifilm; *USA:* Eflone; Flarex; Fluor-Op; FML.

Multi-ingredient: *Braz.:* Flumex-N; *Ger.:* Cibaflam; Efemolin;
Efflumycin; *Hong Kong:* Efemoline; Infectoflam; *Israel:* FML
Neo; *Ital.:* Efemoline; Flumetol; Flumetol Antibiotico; Gentacort;
NZ: Tobrasone; *Port.:* FML Neo; Neo-Preocil; *S.Afr.:* Efemoline;
FML Neo; *Singapore:* Efemoline; Infectoflam; *Spain:* Bexicortil;
Cortisdin Urea; Flugen; Fluorvas; FML Neo; *Switz.:* Efemoline;
FML Neo; Infectoflam; *Thai.:* Efemoline; FML Neo; Infectoflam;
UK: FML Neo Liquifilm†; *USA:* FML-S.

Fluprednidene Acetate   (1100-m)

Fluprednidene Acetate *(BANM, rINNM)*.

Fluprednylidene 21-Acetate. 9α-Fluoro-11β,17α,21-trihydroxy-
16-methylenepregna-1,4-diene-3,20-dione 21-acetate.

$C_{24}H_{29}FO_6 = 432.5$.

*CAS — 2193-87-5 (fluprednidene); 1255-35-2 (flupredni-
dene acetate).*

Profile

Fluprednidene acetate is a corticosteroid used topically for its
glucocorticoid activity (p.1039) in the treatment of various skin
disorders. It is usually employed as a cream, lotion, or ointment
containing 0.1%.

When applied topically, particularly to large areas, when the
skin is broken, or under occlusive dressings, corticosteroids
may be absorbed in sufficient amounts to cause systemic effects (p.1039). The effects of topical corticosteroids on the skin
are described on p.1041. For recommendations concerning the
correct use of corticosteroids on the skin, and a rough guide to
the clinical potencies of topical corticosteroids, see p.1045.

Preparations

Proprietary Preparations (details are given in Part 3)
Aust.: Decoderm; *Belg.:* Decoderm; *Denm.:* Corticoderm; *Ger.:*
Decoderm; *Neth.:* Decoderm; *Norw.:* Corticoderm†; *Spain:* De-
coderm; *Swed.:* Corticoderm; *Switz.:* Decoderm.

Multi-ingredient: *Aust.:* Decoderm compositum; Decoderm trivalent; Sali-Decoderm; *Belg.:* Decoderm Comp; *Braz.:* Pan-
Emecort; *Ger.:* Candio-Hermal Plus; Crinohermal fem neu; Deco-
derm Comp; Decoderm tri; Sali-Decoderm; Vobaderm; *Spain:*
Decoderm Trivalente; *Switz.:* Decoderm bivalent.

Fluprednisolone   (1101-b)

Fluprednisolone *(BAN, USAN, rINN)*.

6α-Fluoroprednisolone; NSC-47439; U-7800. 6α-Fluoro-
11β,17α,21-trihydroxypregna-1,4-diene-3,20-dione.

$C_{21}H_{27}FO_5 = 378.4$.

*CAS — 53-34-9 (fluprednisolone); 23257-44-5 (flupred-
nisolone valerate).*

Profile

Fluprednisolone is a corticosteroid with mainly glucocorticoid
activity (p.1039); 2 mg of fluprednisolone is roughly equivalent in anti-inflammatory activity to 5 mg of prednisolone. It
has been given by mouth in the management of a variety of
conditions requiring systemic glucocorticoid therapy (p.1044).

Preparations

Proprietary Preparations (details are given in Part 3)
Aust.: Isopredon†.

Multi-ingredient: *Braz.:* Rinisone.

Flurandrenolone   (1102-v)

Flurandrenolone *(BAN)*.

Fludroxycortide *(BAN, rINN)*; 33379; Flurandrenolone; 6α-
Fluoro-16α-hydroxyhydrocortisone 16,17-Acetonide; Flurandrenolide *(USAN)*. 6α-Fluoro-11β,21-dihydroxy-16α,17α-iso-
propylidenedioxypregn-4-ene-3,20-dione.

$C_{24}H_{33}FO_6 = 436.5$.

CAS — 1524-88-5.

ATC — D07AC07.

Pharmacopoeias. In US.

Pharmacopoeial description

USP 25: A white to off-white, fluffy, odourless, crystalline
powder. Practically insoluble in water and in ether; soluble 1 in
72 of alcohol, 1 in 10 of chloroform, and 1 in 25 of methyl
alcohol. Store in airtight containers at a temperature not exceeding 8°. Protect from light.

Profile

Flurandrenolone [fludroxycortide] is a corticosteroid used topically for its glucocorticoid activity (p.1039) in the treatment of
various skin disorders. It is usually employed as a cream or
ointment containing 0.0125% or a lotion containing 0.05%. It
is also used as an adhesive polyethylene tape impregnated with
4 µg of flurandrenolone [fludroxycortide] per cm².

When applied topically, particularly to large areas, when the
skin is broken, or under occlusive dressings, corticosteroids
may be absorbed in sufficient amounts to cause systemic effects (p.1039). The effects of topical corticosteroids on the skin
are described on p.1041. For recommendations concerning the
correct use of corticosteroids on the skin, and a rough guide to
the clinical potencies of topical corticosteroids, see p.1045.

Preparations

USP 25: Flurandrenolide Cream; Flurandrenolide Lotion; Fluran-
drenolide Ointment; Flurandrenolide Tape; Neomycin Sulfate and
Flurandrenolide Cream; Neomycin Sulfate and Flurandrenolide
Lotion; Neomycin Sulfate and Flurandrenolide Ointment.

Proprietary Preparations (details are given in Part 3)
Braz.: Drenison; *Canad.:* Drenison†; *Ger.:* Sermaka; *Irl.:* Haelan;
Spain: Drenison†; *UK:* Haelan; *USA:* Cordran.

Multi-ingredient: *Braz.:* Dreniformio; Drenison N; *Hong Kong:*
Drenison N; *Spain:* Drenison Neomicina†.

Fluticasone Propionate   (14742-p)

Fluticasone Propionate *(BANM, USAN, rINNM)*.

CCI-18781. S-Fluoromethyl 6α,9α-difluoro-11β,17α-dihy-
droxy-16α-methyl-3-oxoandrosta-1,4-diene-17β-carbothioate
17-propionate.

$C_{25}H_{31}F_3O_5S = 500.6$.

CAS — 80474-14-2.

Pharmacopoeias. In Br.

Pharmacopoeial description

BP 2001: A white or almost white crystalline powder. Practically insoluble in water; slightly soluble in alcohol; sparingly
soluble in acetone and in dichloromethane; freely soluble in
dimethylformamide.

Adverse Effects, Treatment, Withdrawal, and Precautions

As for corticosteroids in general (see p.1039). Hypersensitivity reactions have occurred. Eosinophilic conditions, including Churg-Strauss syndrome, have
been reported rarely, in most cases following a transfer from oral corticosteroid therapy.

When applied topically, particularly to large areas,
when the skin is broken, or under occlusive dressings,
corticosteroids may be absorbed in sufficient amounts
to cause systemic effects. Inhalation or nasal administration of large amounts of fluticasone propionate
may produce systemic effects also (see below).

Adrenal suppression. Despite the fact that inhaled fluticasone is generally thought to lack systemic effects at therapeutic
doses, a study in 25 healthy subjects[1] indicated that fluticasone
propionate as single inhaled doses of 250, 500, and 1000 µg did
produce a reduction in plasma cortisol, indicating suppression of
the hypothalamic-pituitary-adrenal axis to some degree.
Others have also found evidence of adrenal suppression with
fluticasone,[2-4] particularly at high doses, and the effect may be
more marked with repeated than with single doses.[4-6] Conflicting claims have been made concerning the risk of clinical effects, for example on growth.[7-9]

1. Grahnén A, *et al.* An assessment of the systemic activity of single doses of inhaled fluticasone propionate in healthy volunteers.
Br J Clin Pharmacol 1994; **38:** 521–5.
2. Clark DJ, *et al.* Comparative systemic bioactivity of inhaled
budesonide and fluticasone propionate in asthmatic children. *Br
J Clin Pharmacol* 1996; **42:** 264P.
3. Rohatagi S, *et al.* Dynamic modeling of cortisol reduction after
inhaled administration of fluticasone propionate. *J Clin Pharmacol* 1996; **36:** 938–41.
4. Clark DJ, Lipworth BJ. Adrenal suppression with chronic dosing
of fluticasone propionate compared with budesonide in adult
asthmatic patients. *Thorax* 1997; **52:** 55–8.
5. Lönnebo A, *et al.* An assessment of the systemic effects of single
and repeated doses of inhaled fluticasone propionate and inhaled
budesonide in healthy volunteers. *Eur J Clin Pharmacol* 1996;
49: 459–63.
6. Wilson AM, *et al.* Adrenal suppression with high doses of inhaled fluticasone propionate and triamcinolone acetonide in
healthy voluteers. *Eur J Clin Pharmacol* 1997; **53:** 33–7.
7. Todd G, *et al.* Growth and adrenal suppression in asthmatic children treated with high-dose fluticasone propionate. *Lancet* 1996;
348: 27–9.
8. Whitaker K, *et al.* Effect of fluticasone on growth in children
with asthma. *Lancet* 1996; **348:** 63–4.
9. Cade A, *et al.* High-dose inhaled steroids in asthmatic children.
Lancet 1996; **348:** 819.

Interactions

The interactions of corticosteroids in general are described on p.1043.

Pharmacokinetics

For a brief outline of the pharmacokinetics of corticosteroids, see p.1044.

Fluticasone propionate is poorly absorbed from the
gastrointestinal tract and undergoes extensive first-
pass metabolism; oral bioavailability is reported to be
only about 1%.

◊ References.

1. Falcoz C, *et al.* Oral bioavailability of fluticasone propionate in
healthy subjects. *Br J Clin Pharmacol* 1996; **41:** 459P–460P.
2. Mackie AE, *et al.* Pharmacokinetics of intravenous fluticasone
propionate in healthy subjects. *Br J Clin Pharmacol* 1996; **41:**
539–42.
3. Daley-Yates PT, Baker RC. Systemic bioavailability of fluticasone propionate administered as nasal drops and aqueous nasal
spray formulations. *Br J Clin Pharmacol* 2001; **51:** 103–5.

Uses and Administration

Fluticasone propionate is a corticosteroid with mainly
glucocorticoid activity (p.1039).

Fluticasone propionate is stated to exert a topical effect on the lungs without significant systemic effects
at usual doses, due to its low systemic bioavailability
(but see Adrenal Suppression, above). It is used by
powder or aerosol inhalation for the prophylaxis of
asthma. Initial doses in the UK range from 100 to
250 µg twice daily in mild asthma up to 1000 µg
twice daily in severe asthma, adjusted according to
response. Children over 4 years of age may be given
initial doses of 50 to 100 µg twice daily, increased to
200 µg twice daily if necessary. The drug may also be
given via a nebuliser in severe chronic asthma. Usual
adult doses are 0.5 to 2 mg twice daily.

Fluticasone propionate is also available in some
countries as a powder or aerosol inhalation for the
treatment of chronic obstructive pulmonary disease,
when it is given in doses of 500 µg twice daily.

Fluticasone propionate is administered by nasal spray in the prophylaxis and treatment of allergic rhinitis. The usual dose is 100 µg into each nostril once daily, increased if necessary to 100 µg into each nostril twice daily. Children over 4 years of age may be given half these doses. Fluticasone propionate drops are used in the treatment of nasal polyps. A total dose of 400 µg should be instilled once or twice daily for at least 4 to 6 weeks.

It is applied topically in the treatment of various skin disorders. Creams and ointments containing 0.05% and 0.005% respectively are available. For recommendations concerning the correct use of corticosteroids on the skin, see p.1045.

Asthma. Corticosteroids and beta$_2$-adrenoceptor agonists form the cornerstone of the management of asthma (p.757). Patients requiring only occasional relief from symptoms may be managed with an inhaled short-acting beta$_2$ agonist, and an inhaled corticosteroid such as fluticasone is added if symptomatic relief is needed more than once daily. The dose of inhaled corticosteroid is increased in more severe asthma, often together with the addition of other drugs.

Some references to the use of fluticasone propionate for asthma are given below,[1-6] including one to a study indicating that increasing the dose of inhaled fluticasone did not produce increased benefit.[1]

1. Boe J, et al. High-dose inhaled steroids in asthmatics: moderate efficacy gain and suppression of the hypothalamic-pituitary-adrenal (HPA) axis. Eur Respir J 1994; 7: 2179–84.
2. Fitzgerald D, et al. Fluticasone propionate 750 µg/day versus beclomethasone dipropionate 1500 µg/day: comparison of efficacy and adrenal function in paediatric asthma. Thorax 1998; 53: 656–61.
3. Jarvis B, Faulds D. Inhaled fluticasone propionate: a review of its therapeutic efficacy at dosages ≤ 500 µg/day in adults and adolescents with mild to moderate asthma. Drugs 1999; 57: 769–803.
4. Bisgaard H, et al. The effect of inhaled fluticasone propionate in the treatment of young asthmatic children: a dose comparison study. Am J Respir Crit Care Med 1999; 160: 126–31.
5. Markham A, Jarvis B. Inhaled salmeterol/fluticasone propionate combination: a review of its use in persistent asthma. Drugs 2000; 60: 1207–33.
6. ZuWallack R, et al. Long-term efficacy and safety of fluticasone propionate powder administered once or twice daily via inhaler to patients with moderate asthma. Chest 2000; 118: 303–312.

Chronic obstructive pulmonary disease. For discussion of the value of inhaled corticosteroids in chronic obstructive pulmonary disease, including reference to the use of fluticasone, see p.1049.

Inflammatory bowel disease. Fluticasone propionate, given by mouth, has produced variable results in the treatment of Crohn's disease[1] and ulcerative colitis;[2,3] some benefit was also reported in coeliac disease.[4] The dose was 5 mg four times daily but some consider[2] higher doses necessary.

Corticosteroids with low bioavailability, which might be able to exert topical anti-inflammatory actions on the gut without producing systemic adverse effects, are currently under investigation in the management of inflammatory bowel disease, as discussed on p.1205.

1. Carpani de Kaski M, et al. Fluticasone propionate in Crohn's disease. Gut 1991; 32: 657–61.
2. Hawthorne AB, et al. Double blind trial of oral fluticasone propionate v prednisolone in the treatment of active ulcerative colitis. Gut 1993; 34: 125–8.
3. Angus P, et al. Oral fluticasone propionate in active distal ulcerative colitis. Gut 1992; 33: 711–14.
4. Mitchison HC, et al. A pilot study of fluticasone propionate in untreated coeliac disease. Gut 1991; 32: 260–5.

Nasal polyps. For discussion of the value of intranasal corticosteroids in the treatment of nasal polyps, including reference to the use of fluticasone, see p.1054.

Rhinitis. For a discussion of the management of rhinitis, including the use of corticosteroids, see p.407. Some further references to the use of fluticasone in rhinitis are given below.

1. Wiseman LR, Benfield P. Intranasal fluticasone propionate: a reappraisal of its pharmacology and clinical efficacy in the treatment of rhinitis. Drugs 1997; 53: 885–907.

Preparations

BP 2001: Fluticasone Cream; Fluticasone Ointment.

Proprietary Preparations (details are given in Part 3)
Aust.: Cutivate; Flixonase; Flixotide; *Austral.:* Flixotide; *Belg.:* Cutivate; Flixonase; Flixotide; *Canad.:* Flonase; Flovent; *Denm.:* Cutivat; Flixonase; Flixotide; *Fin.:* Flixonase; Flixotide; *Fr.:* Flixonase; Flixotide; *Ger.:* Atemur; Flutide; Flutivate; *Hong Kong:* Cutivate; Flixonase; Flixotide; *Irl.:* Flixonase; Flixotide; *Israel:* Cutivate; Flixonase; Flixotide; *Ital.:* Flixonase; Flixotide; Fluspiral; *Mex.:* Cutivate; Flixonase; Flixotide; *Neth.:* Cutivate; Flixonase; Flixotide; *Norw.:* Flutide; Flutivate; *NZ:* Flixonase; Flixotide; *Port.:* Asmatil; Asmo-Lavi; Brisovent; Cutivate; Flixotaide; Flutaide; Ubizol; *S.Afr.:* Cutivate; Flixonase; Flixotide; *Singapore:* Cutivate; Flixonase; Flixotide; *Spain:* Cutivate; Drolasona;

Flixonase; Flixotide; Fluinol; Flusonal; Inalacor; Rinosone; Rontilona; Seretide; Trialona; *Swed.:* Flutide; Flutivate; *Switz.:* Axotide; Cutivate; Flutinase; *Thai.:* Flixonase; Flixotide; *UK:* Cutivate; Flixonase; Flixotide; *USA:* Cutivate; Flonase; Flovent.

Multi-ingredient: *Aust.:* Seretide; *Austral.:* Seretide; *Canad.:* Advair; *Denm.:* Seretide; *Fin.:* Seretide; *Ger.:* Viani; *Irl.:* Seretide; *Neth.:* Seretide; *Norw.:* Seretide; *Port.:* Seretaide; *Singapore:* Seretide; *Swed.:* Seretide; *Switz.:* Seretide; *UK:* Seretide; *USA:* Advair.

Formocortal (1103-g)

Formocortal (BAN, USAN, rINN).

Fl-6341; Fluoroformylon. 3-(2-Chloroethoxy)-9α-fluoro-11β,21-dihydroxy-16α,17α-isopropylidenedioxy-20-oxopregna-3,5-diene-6-carbaldehyde 21-acetate.
$C_{29}H_{38}ClFO_8 = 569.1$.
CAS — 2825-60-7.
ATC — S01BA12.

Profile
Formocortal is a corticosteroid that is used for its glucocorticoid activity (see p.1039) in the treatment of inflammatory eye disorders as eye drops and eye ointments containing 0.05%.

Prolonged application to the eye of preparations containing corticosteroids has caused raised intra-ocular pressure and reduced visual function.

Preparations

Proprietary Preparations (details are given in Part 3)
Ital.: Formoftil.

Multi-ingredient: *Ital.:* Formomicin.

Halcinonide (1104-q)

Halcinonide (BAN, USAN, rINN).

Alcinonide; SQ-18566. 21-Chloro-9α-fluoro-11β-hydroxy-16α,17α-isopropylidenedioxypregn-4-ene-3,20-dione.
$C_{24}H_{32}ClFO_5 = 455.0$.
CAS — 3093-35-4.
ATC — D07AD02.
Pharmacopoeias. In Chin. and US.

Pharmacopoeial description

USP 25: A white to off-white, odourless, crystalline powder. Insoluble in water and in hexanes; slightly soluble in alcohol and in ether; soluble in acetone and in chloroform.

Profile
Halcinonide is a corticosteroid used topically for its glucocorticoid activity (p.1039) in the treatment of various skin disorders. It is usually employed as a 0.1% cream, lotion, or ointment.

When applied topically, particularly to large areas, when the skin is broken, or under occlusive dressings, corticosteroids may be absorbed in sufficient amounts to cause systemic effects (p.1039). The effects of topical corticosteroids on the skin are described on p.1041. For recommendations concerning the correct use of corticosteroids on the skin, and a rough guide to the clinical potencies of topical corticosteroids, see p.1045.

Preparations

USP 25: Halcinonide Cream; Halcinonide Ointment; Halcinonide Topical Solution.

Proprietary Preparations (details are given in Part 3)
Aust.: Halog; *Austral.:* Halciderm; *Braz.:* Halog; *Canad.:* Halog; *Fr.:* Halog†; *Ger.:* Halog; *Hong Kong:* Halog; *Ital.:* Halciderm; *Mex.:* Dermalog; *Neth.:* Halciderm†; *Norw.:* Halog; *Spain:* Halog; *Switz.:* Betacortone; *UK:* Halciderm; *USA:* Halog.

Multi-ingredient: *Fr.:* Halog Neomycine†; *Ger.:* Halog Tri; *Ital.:* Anfocort; Halciderm; Halciderm Combi; *Mex.:* Dermalog-C; *Switz.:* Betacortone; Betacortone S.

Halometasone (16830-n)

Halometasone (rINN).

C-48401-Ba; Halomethasone. 2-Chloro-6α,9-difluoro-11β,17,21-trihydroxy-16α-methylpregna-1,4-diene-3,20-dione.
$C_{22}H_{27}ClF_2O_5 = 444.9$.
CAS — 50629-82-8.
ATC — D07AC12.

Profile
Halometasone is a corticosteroid used topically for its glucocorticoid activity (p.1039) in the treatment of various skin disorders. It is usually employed as a cream or ointment containing 0.05% of halometasone monohydrate.

When applied topically, particularly to large areas, when the skin is broken, or under occlusive dressings, corticosteroids may be absorbed in sufficient amounts to cause systemic effects (p.1039). The effects of topical corticosteroids on the skin are described on p.1041. For recommendations concerning the correct use of corticosteroids on the skin, see p.1045.

Preparations

Proprietary Preparations (details are given in Part 3)
Aust.: Sicorten; *Belg.:* Sicorten; *Ger.:* Sicorten; *Hong Kong:* Sicorten; *Israel:* Sicorten; *Neth.:* Sicorten; *Port.:* Sicorten; *Spain:* Sicorten; *Switz.:* Sicorten.

Multi-ingredient: *Ger.:* Sicorten Plus; *Hong Kong:* Sicorten Plus; *Israel:* Sicorten Plus; *Port.:* Sicorten Plus; *Spain:* Sicorten Plus; *Switz.:* Sicorten Plus.

Hydrocortamate Hydrochloride (1105-p)

Hydrocortamate Hydrochloride (rINNM).

Ethamicort; Hydrocortisone Diethylaminoacetate Hydrochloride. 11β,17α,21-Trihydroxypregn-4-ene-3,20-dione 21-diethylaminoacetate.
$C_{27}H_{41}NO_6,HCl = 512.1$.
CAS — 76-47-1 (hydrocortamate); 125-03-1 (hydrocortamate hydrochloride).

Profile
Hydrocortamate hydrochloride is a corticosteroid that has been used topically for its glucocorticoid activity (p.1039) in the treatment of various skin disorders.

Preparations

Proprietary Preparations (details are given in Part 3)
Multi-ingredient: *Ital.:* Cortanest†.

Hydrocortisone (1138-k)

Hydrocortisone (BAN, rINN).

Anti-inflammatory Hormone; Compound F; Cortisol; Hydrocortisonum; 17-Hydroxycorticosterone; NSC-10483. 11β,17α,21-Trihydroxypregn-4-ene-3,20-dione.
$C_{21}H_{30}O_5 = 362.5$.
CAS — 50-23-7.
ATC — A01AC03; A07EA02; C05AA01; D07AA02; D07XA01; H02AB09; S01BA02; S01CB03; S02BA01.
Pharmacopoeias. In Chin., Eur. (see p.vi), Int., Jpn, Pol., and US.

Pharmacopoeial description

Ph. Eur.: A white or almost white, crystalline powder. It shows polymorphism. Practically insoluble in water; sparingly soluble in alcohol and in acetone; slightly soluble in dichloromethane. Protect from light.

USP 25: A white to practically white, odourless, crystalline powder. Very slightly soluble in water and in ether; soluble 1 in 40 of alcohol and 1 in 80 of acetone; slightly soluble in chloroform.

Hydrocortisone Acetate (1107-w)

Hydrocortisone Acetate (BANM, rINNM).

Cortisol Acetate; Hydrocortisoni Acetas. Hydrocortisone 21-acetate.
$C_{23}H_{32}O_6 = 404.5$.
CAS — 50-03-3.

NOTE. HCOR is a code approved by the BP 2001 for use on single unit doses of eye drops containing hydrocortisone acetate where the individual container may be too small to bear all the appropriate labelling information.

Pharmacopoeias. In Chin., Eur. (see p.vi), Int., Jpn, Pol., and US.

Hydrocortisone acetate 112 mg is approximately equivalent to 100 mg of hydrocortisone.

Pharmacopoeial description

Ph. Eur.: A white or almost white, crystalline powder. Practically insoluble in water; slightly soluble in dehydrated alcohol and in dichloromethane. Protect from light.

USP 25: A white to practically white, odourless, crystalline powder. Insoluble in water; soluble 1 in 230 of alcohol and 1 in 200 of chloroform.

Hydrocortisone Butyrate (1108-e)

Hydrocortisone Butyrate (BANM, USAN, rINNM).

Cortisol Butyrate. Hydrocortisone 17α-butyrate.
$C_{25}H_{36}O_6 = 432.5$.
CAS — 13609-67-1.
ATC — D07AB02.
Pharmacopoeias. In Jpn and US.

Hydrocortisone butyrate 119 mg is approximately equivalent to 100 mg of hydrocortisone.

Pharmacopoeial description

USP 25: A white to practically white, practically odourless crystalline powder. Practically insoluble in water; soluble in alcohol, in acetone, and in methyl alcohol; freely soluble in chloroform; slightly soluble in ether.

The symbol † denotes a preparation no longer actively marketed

Hydrocortisone Cipionate (1109-I)

Hydrocortisone Cipionate (BANM, rINNM).

Cortisol Cypionate; Hydrocortisone Cyclopentylpropionate; Hydrocortisone Cypionate. Hydrocortisone 21-(3-cyclopentylpropionate).

$C_{29}H_{42}O_6 = 486.6$.

CAS — 508-99-6.

Hydrocortisone Hydrogen Succinate (1110-v)

Hydrocortisone Hydrogen Succinate (BANM, rINNM).

Cortisol Hemisuccinate; Hydrocortisone Hemisuccinate; Hydrocortisone Succinate; Hydrocortisoni Hydrogenosuccinas. Hydrocortisone 21-(hydrogen succinate).

$C_{25}H_{34}O_8 = 462.5$.

CAS — 2203-97-6 (anhydrous hydrocortisone hydrogen succinate); 83784-20-7 (hydrocortisone hydrogen succinate monohydrate).

Pharmacopoeias. In Eur. (see p.vi) and Jpn. US allows the anhydrous form or the monohydrate.

Hydrocortisone hydrogen succinate 128 mg is approximately equivalent to 100 mg of hydrocortisone.

Pharmacopoeial description

Ph. Eur.: A white or almost white, hygroscopic powder. Practically insoluble in water; freely soluble in dehydrated alcohol and in acetone; dissolves in dilute solutions of alkali carbonates and alkali hydroxides. Store in airtight containers. Protect from light.

USP 25: It contains one molecule of water of hydration or is anhydrous. Store in airtight containers.

Hydrocortisone Sodium Phosphate (1111-g)

Hydrocortisone Sodium Phosphate (BANM, rINNM).

Cortisol Sodium Phosphate. Hydrocortisone 21-(disodium orthophosphate).

$C_{21}H_{29}Na_2O_8P = 486.4$.

CAS — 6000-74-4.

Pharmacopoeias. In Br., Jpn, and US.

Hydrocortisone sodium phosphate 134 mg is approximately equivalent to 100 mg of hydrocortisone.

Pharmacopoeial description

BP 2001: A white or almost white, hygroscopic powder. Freely soluble in water; practically insoluble in dehydrated alcohol and in chloroform. A 0.5% solution in water has a pH of 7.5 to 9.0. Protect from light.

USP 25: A white to light yellow, odourless or practically odourless, exceedingly hygroscopic, powder. Soluble 1 in 1.5 of water; slightly soluble in alcohol; practically insoluble in chloroform, in dioxan, and in ether. Store in airtight containers.

Hydrocortisone Sodium Succinate (1112-q)

Hydrocortisone Sodium Succinate (BANM, rINNM).

Cortisol Sodium Succinate. Hydrocortisone 21-(sodium succinate).

$C_{25}H_{33}NaO_8 = 484.5$.

CAS — 125-04-2.

Pharmacopoeias. In Int., It., Jpn., Pol., and US.

Hydrocortisone sodium succinate 134 mg is approximately equivalent to 100 mg of hydrocortisone.

Pharmacopoeial description

USP 25: A white or nearly white, odourless, hygroscopic, amorphous solid. Very soluble in water and in alcohol; very slightly soluble in acetone; insoluble in chloroform. Store in airtight containers. Protect from light.

Hydrocortisone Valerate (1106-s)

Hydrocortisone Valerate (BANM, USAN, rINNM).

Cortisol Valerate. Hydrocortisone 17-valerate.

$C_{26}H_{38}O_6 = 446.6$.

CAS — 57524-89-7.

Pharmacopoeias. In US.

Hydrocortisone valerate 123 mg is approximately equivalent to 100 mg of hydrocortisone.

Adverse Effects, Treatment, Withdrawal, and Precautions

As for corticosteroids in general (see p.1039).

When applied topically, particularly to large areas, when the skin is broken, or under occlusive dressings, corticosteroids may be absorbed in sufficient amounts to cause systemic effects. Prolonged application to the eye of preparations containing corticosteroids has caused raised intra-ocular pressure and reduced visual function.

Effects on fluid and electrolyte balance. A report of marked hypokalaemia and hypomagnesaemia associated with high dose intravenous hydrocortisone therapy in an alcoholic patient with suspected immune thrombocytopenia.[1] Cardiac arrhythmias developed, and prolonged infusion of magnesium

and potassium was required to restore normal plasma concentrations.

1. Ramsahoye BH, et al. The mineralocorticoid effects of high dose hydrocortisone. BMJ 1995; **310:** 656–7.

Effects on the nervous system. For reports and comments on paraesthesia or perineal irritation associated with hydrocortisone sodium phosphate given intravenously, see p.1041.

Hypersensitivity and anaphylaxis. References to hypersensitivity reactions and anaphylaxis associated with the intravenous administration of hydrocortisone;[1-6] topical application can also result in hypersensitivity.[7]

1. Chan CS, et al. Hydrocortisone-induced anaphylaxis. Med J Aust 1984; **141:** 444–6.
2. Seale JP. Anaphylactoid reaction to hydrocortisone. Med J Aust 1984; **141:** 446.
3. Corallo CE, Sosnin M. Bronchospasm, tachycardia following intravenous hydrocortisone. Aust J Hosp Pharm 1985; **15:** 103–4.
4. Al Mahdy H, Hall M. Anaphylaxis and hydrocortisone. Ann Intern Med 1988; **108:** 487–8.
5. Fulcher DA, Katelaris CH. Anaphylactoid reaction to intravenous hydrocortisone sodium succinate: a case report and literature review. Med J Aust 1991; **154:** 210–14.
6. Kawane H. Anaphylactoid reaction to intravenous hydrocortisone sodium succinate. Med J Aust 1991; **154:** 782.
7. Wilkinson SM, et al. Hydrocortisone: an important cutaneous allergen. Lancet 1991; **337:** 761–2.

Interactions

The interactions of corticosteroids in general are described on p.1043.

Pharmacokinetics

For a brief account of the pharmacokinetics of corticosteroids, see p.1044.

Hydrocortisone is readily absorbed from the gastrointestinal tract and peak blood concentrations are attained in about an hour. The biological half-life is about 100 minutes. It is more than 90% bound to plasma proteins. Following intramuscular injection, the absorption of the water-soluble sodium phosphate and sodium succinate esters is rapid, while absorption of hydrocortisone free alcohol and its lipid-soluble esters is slower. Absorption of hydrocortisone acetate after intra-articular or soft-tissue injection is also slow. Hydrocortisone is absorbed through the skin, particularly in denuded areas.

Hydrocortisone is metabolised in the liver and most body tissues to hydrogenated and degraded forms such as tetrahydrocortisone and tetrahydrocortisol. These are excreted in the urine, mainly conjugated as glucuronides, together with a very small proportion of unchanged hydrocortisone. Hydrocortisone readily crosses the placenta.

Uses and Administration

Hydrocortisone is a corticosteroid with both glucocorticoid and to a lesser extent mineralocorticoid activity (p.1039). As cortisol it is the most important of the predominantly glucocorticoid steroids secreted by the adrenal cortex. Hydrocortisone is used, usually in combination with a more potent mineralocorticoid, for replacement therapy in adrenocortical insufficiency (p.1046). It may also be used for its glucocorticoid properties in other conditions for which corticosteroid therapy is indicated (p.1044) but drugs with fewer mineralocorticoid effects tend to be preferred for the long-term systemic therapy of auto-immune and inflammatory disease.

For administration by mouth hydrocortisone free alcohol is usually used and sometimes the cipionate ester is also employed.

For replacement therapy in acute or chronic adrenocortical insufficiency the normal requirement is 20 or 30 mg daily (usually taken in 2 doses, the larger in the morning and the smaller in the early evening, to mimic the circadian rhythm of the body). Additional sodium chloride may be required if there is defective aldosterone secretion, but mineralocorticoid activity is usually supplemented by fludrocortisone acetate by mouth. Similar regimens have also been used to correct glucocorticoid deficiency in the salt-losing form of congenital adrenal hyperplasia (p.1049).

Hydrocortisone may be given intravenously, by slow injection or infusion, in the form of a water-soluble derivative such as hydrocortisone sodium succinate or hydrocortisone sodium phosphate when a rapid effect

is required in emergencies: such conditions are acute adrenocortical insufficiency caused by Addisonian or post-adrenalectomy crises, by the abrupt accidental withdrawal of therapy in corticosteroid-treated patients, or by the inability of the adrenal glands to cope with increased stress in such patients; certain allergic emergencies such as anaphylaxis; acute severe asthma (status asthmaticus—see also p.757); and shock. The usual dose is the equivalent of 100 to 500 mg of hydrocortisone, repeated 3 or 4 times in 24 hours, according to the severity of the condition and the patient's response. Children up to 1 year of age may be given 25 mg, those aged 1 to 5 years 50 mg, and those aged 6 to 12 years 100 mg. Fluids and electrolytes should be given as necessary to correct any associated metabolic disorder. Similar doses to those specified above may also be given intramuscularly but the response is likely to be less rapid than that observed following intravenous administration. Corticosteroids are considered to be of secondary value in anaphylactic shock because of their relatively slow onset of action, but intravenous hydrocortisone may be a useful adjunct to adrenaline [epinephrine] to prevent further deterioration in severely affected patients.

In patients with adrenal deficiency states supplementary corticosteroid therapy may be necessary during some surgical operations and hydrocortisone sodium succinate or sodium phosphate may be given intramuscularly or intravenously before surgery. Various regimens have been proposed (see also under Surgery, p.1045). In patients taking more than 10 mg of prednisolone or its equivalent by mouth daily, the British National Formulary recommends the following regimen:

- minor surgery under general anaesthesia, either the usual oral corticosteroid dose on the morning of surgery or hydrocortisone 25 to 50 mg (usually as the sodium succinate) intravenously at induction; the usual oral corticosteroid dose is recommended after surgery

- moderate or major surgery, the usual oral corticosteroid dose on the morning of surgery, plus hydrocortisone 25 to 50 mg intravenously at induction, and followed by similar doses of hydrocortisone 3 times daily, for 24 hours after moderate surgery and 48 to 72 hours after major surgery; the usual corticosteroid dose is resumed once hydrocortisone injections are stopped.

For local administration by injection into soft tissues hydrocortisone in the form of the sodium phosphate or sodium succinate esters is usually employed; doses in terms of hydrocortisone are usually 100 to 200 mg. For intra-articular injection hydrocortisone acetate is usually used in doses of 5 to 50 mg depending upon the size of the joint.

For topical application in the treatment of various skin disorders hydrocortisone and the acetate, buteprate, butyrate, and valerate esters are normally employed in creams, ointments, or lotions. Concentrations usually used have ranged from 0.1 to 2.5%. Although it is considered that hydrocortisone has fewer side-effects on the skin and is less liable to cause adrenal suppression than the more potent topical corticosteroids (see p.1045 for a rough guide to the clinical potencies of topical corticosteroids), it should be borne in mind, especially in view of the availability of 'over-the-counter' hydrocortisone preparations in many countries, that this property may be considerably modified both by the type of formulation or vehicle used and by the type of esterification present; other factors that may also influence the degree of absorption include the site of application, use of an occlusive dressing, the degree of skin damage, and the size of the area to which the preparation is applied.

Hydrocortisone or its esters are also available in a variety of other dosage forms including those for ophthalmic, aural, dental, and rectal application, for use in allergic and inflammatory disorders.

Other esters of hydrocortisone which have occasionally been used include the aceponate, glycyrrhetinate, and propionate. Esters such as the aceponate may show modified topical activity.

Preparations

BP 2001: Hydrocortisone Acetate and Neomycin Ear Drops; Hydrocortisone Acetate and Neomycin Eye Drops; Hydrocortisone Acetate and Neomycin Eye Ointment; Hydrocortisone Acetate Cream; Hydrocortisone Acetate Injection; Hydrocortisone Acetate Ointment; Hydrocortisone and Clioquinol Cream; Hydrocortisone and Clioquinol Ointment; Hydrocortisone and Neomycin Cream; Hydrocortisone Cream; Hydrocortisone Ointment; Hydrocortisone Sodium Phosphate Injection; Hydrocortisone Sodium Succinate Injection;

USP 25: Chloramphenicol and Hydrocortisone Acetate for Ophthalmic Suspension; Chloramphenicol, Polymyxin B Sulfate, and Hydrocortisone Acetate Ophthalmic Ointment; Clioquinol and Hydrocortisone Cream; Clioquinol and Hydrocortisone Ointment; Colistin and Neomycin Sulfates and Hydrocortisone Acetate Otic Suspension; Hydrocortisone Acetate Cream; Hydrocortisone Acetate Injectable Suspension; Hydrocortisone Acetate Lotion; Hydrocortisone Acetate Ointment; Hydrocortisone Acetate Ophthalmic Ointment; Hydrocortisone Acetate Ophthalmic Suspension; Hydrocortisone and Acetic Acid Otic Solution; Hydrocortisone Butyrate Cream; Hydrocortisone Cream; Hydrocortisone Gel; Hydrocortisone Injectable Suspension; Hydrocortisone Lotion; Hydrocortisone Ointment; Hydrocortisone Rectal Suspension; Hydrocortisone Sodium Phosphate Injection; Hydrocortisone Sodium Succinate for Injection; Hydrocortisone Tablets; Hydrocortisone Valerate Cream; Neomycin and Polymyxin B Sulfates and Hydrocortisone Acetate Cream; Neomycin and Polymyxin B Sulfates and Hydrocortisone Acetate Ophthalmic Suspension; Neomycin and Polymyxin B Sulfates and Hydrocortisone Ophthalmic Suspension; Neomycin and Polymyxin B Sulfates and Hydrocortisone Otic Solution; Neomycin and Polymyxin B Sulfates and Hydrocortisone Otic Suspension; Neomycin and Polymyxin B Sulfates, Bacitracin Zinc, and Hydrocortisone Acetate Ophthalmic Ointment; Neomycin and Polymyxin B Sulfates, Bacitracin Zinc, and Hydrocortisone Ointment; Neomycin and Polymyxin B Sulfates, Bacitracin Zinc, and Hydrocortisone Ophthalmic Ointment; Neomycin and Polymyxin B Sulfates, Bacitracin, and Hydrocortisone Acetate Ointment; Neomycin and Polymyxin B Sulfates, Bacitracin, and Hydrocortisone Acetate Ophthalmic Ointment; Neomycin and Polymyxin B Sulfates, Gramicidin, and Hydrocortisone Acetate Cream; Neomycin Sulfate and Hydrocortisone Acetate Lotion; Neomycin Sulfate and Hydrocortisone Acetate Ointment; Neomycin Sulfate and Hydrocortisone Acetate Ophthalmic Ointment; Neomycin Sulfate and Hydrocortisone Acetate Ophthalmic Suspension; Neomycin Sulfate and Hydrocortisone Cream; Neomycin Sulfate and Hydrocortisone Ointment; Neomycin Sulfate and Hydrocortisone Otic Suspension; Oxytetracycline Hydrochloride and Hydrocortisone Acetate Ophthalmic Suspension; Oxytetracycline Hydrochloride and Hydrocortisone Ointment; Polymyxin B Sulfate and Hydrocortisone Otic Solution.

Proprietary Preparations (details are given in Part 3)
Aust.: Colifoam; Ekzemsalbe; Hydrocortone; Hydroderm; Locoidon; Schericur; **Austral.:** Colifoam; Cortaid; Cortef; Cortic; Derm-Aid; Egocort; Hycor; Hysone; Nordicort†; Sigmacort; Siguent Hycor; Solu-Cortef; Squibb-HC; **Belg.:** Buccaloxone; Colifoam†; Cortril; Cremicort-H; Locoid; Pannocort; Solu-Cortef; **Braz.:** Berlison; Flebocortid; Nutracort; Solu-Cortef; Stiefcortil; **Canad.:** A-Hydrocort; Aquacort; Barriere-HC; Cortacet; Cortamed; Cortate; Cortef; Cortenema; Corticreme; Cortifoam; Cortiment†; Cortoderm; Emo-Cort; Hycort; Hyderm; Hydrosone; Lanacort†; Novo-Hydrocort; Prevex HC; Rectocort†; Sarna HC; Solu-Cortef; Texacort†; Westcort; **Denm.:** Colifoam; Dermil†; Locoid; Mildison; Solu-Cortef; Uniderm; **Fin.:** Apocort; Bucort; Colifoam; Cortril; Dermacort; Kyypakkaus; Locoid; Mildison; Nutracort; Solu-Cortef; Uniderm; **Fr.:** Colofoam; Dermaspraid; Dermaspray demangeaison; Efficort; Hydracort; Locoid; Mitocortyl; Proctocort; **Ger.:** Alfason; Colifoam; Dermalleg; Dermo Posterisan; Ebenol; Fenistil; Ficortril; Glycocortison; Hydrocort; Hydrocort Mild†; Hydrocutan; Hydrocutan mild; Hydroderm HC; Hydrogalen; Laticort; Latimit†; Munitren H; Pandel; Posterine Corte; ratioAllerg; Remederm HC; Retef; Sagittacortin; Sanatison Mono; Soventol; Systral Hydrocort; velopural; **Hong Kong:** Corticreme; Efficort; Egocort; Hytisone; Rectocort; Solu-Cortef; **Irl.:** Colifoam; Corlan; Cortopin; Dioderm; Hc45; Hydrocortisyl; Hydrocortone; Locoid; Mildison; Solu-Cortef; **Israel:** Colifoam; Cortizone; Hydrocort; Lanacort; Solu-Cortef; **Ital.:** Colifoam; Cortaid; Cortidro; Cortop; Dermirit; Dermocortal; Flebocortid; Foille Insetti; Idracemi; Lanacort; Lenirit; Locoidon; Novocortal; Paro†; Rapicort†; Sintotrat; Solu-Cortef; **Mex.:** Aquanil HC; Fadol; Flebocortid; Flemex; Lacticare-HC; Locoid; Nositrol; Nutracort; Vicortin; Westcort; **Neth.:** Buccaloxone; Hydro-Adreson†; Locoid; Mildison; Solu-Cortef; **Norw.:** Apocortal; Colifoam; Locoid; Mildison; Solu-Cortef; **NZ:** BK HC; Colifoam; Cortaid; Derm-Aid; DP HC; DP Hydrocortisone; Egocort; Locoid; Skincalm; Solu-Cortef; **Port.:** Colifoam; Dermimade Hidrocortisona; Hidalone; Hydrocortisone; Lactisona; Locoid; Pandel; Pandermil; **S.Afr.:** Biocort; Colifoam†; Covocort; Cutaderm; Dilucort; Locoid; Mylocort; Procuta; Skincalm†; Solu-Cortef; Stopitch; **Singapore:** Derm-Aid; Efficort; Egocort; Hydro-Adreson; Solu-Cortef; **Spain:** Actocortina; Aftasone; Ceneo; Derminovag†; Dermosa Hidrocortisona; Hemorrane; Hidroaltesona; Isdinium; Lactisona; Oralsone; Picosyl; Scalpicin Capilar; Schericur; Suniderma; Supralef†; **Swed.:** Amberin†; Colifoam; Ficortril; Locoid; Locoid Crelo; Mildison; Solu-Cortef; Uniderm; **Switz.:** Alfacortone; Colifoam†; Glycocortisone H; Hydrocort; Locoid; Sanadermil; Solu-Cortef; **Thai.:** Hydro-Adreson; Hytisone; Solu-Cortef; **UAE:** Alfacort; **UK:** Colifoam; Corlan; Cortrophin; Dermacort; Dioderm; Efcortelan; Efcortesol; Hc45; Hydrocortisyl; Hydrocortisyl†; Hydrocortone; Jungle Formula Sting Relief Cream; Lanacort; Locoid; Mildison; Solu-Cortef; Zenoxone; **USA:** A-Hydrocort; Acticort; Aeroseb-HC†; Ala-Cort; Anucort-HC; Anusol-HC; Aquanil HC; Bactine; CaldeCort†; Carmol HC; Cetacort; Cort-Dome; CortaGel†; Cortaid; Cortef; Cortef

Feminine Itch; Cortenema; Corticaine; Cortifoam; Cortizone; Delcort†; Dermacort†; Dermarest Dri-Cort; Dermol HC; Dermolate; EarSol-HC; Gynecort; Hemril-HC; Hi-Cor; Hycort; Hydrocortone; HydroSkin; HydroTex; Hytone; Lacticare-HC; Lanacort; Locoid; Massengill Medicated; Maximum Strength Dermarest Dricort†; Maximum Strength KeriCort-10†; Neutrogena T/Scalp; Nutracort; Orabase HCA; Pandel; Penecort; Preparation H Hydrocortisone†; Procort; Proctocort; Proctocream HC; Recort Plus; S-T Cort; Solu-Cortef; Synacort; Tegrin-HC; Texacort; U-Cort†; Westcort.

Multi-ingredient: Aust.: Calmurid HC; Cortison Kemicetin; Daktacort; Ecomytrin-Hydrocortison†; Endomethazone; Hydoftal†; Hydrocortimycin; Hydrodexan; Ichtho-Cortin; Otosporin; Systrason; Terra-Cortril met Gentamicin†; Terra-Cortril mit Polymyxin B-Sulfat†; Terra-Cortril†; Tropoderm; **Austral.:** Chlorocort†; Ciproxin HC; Hydroform; Hydrozole; Proctosedyl; Rectinl HC; Xyloproct; **Belg.:** Alphaderm†; Daktacort; Eoline; Fucidin Hydrocortisone; Onctose a l'Hydrocortisone; Otosporin; Pimafucort; Sulfo-Selenium†; Terra-Cortril†; Xyloproct; **Braz.:** Anusol-HC; Dermilan; Elocort; Furazolon; Gingilone; Hidrocorete; Hipoglos; Hipoglos com Hidrocortisona; Hipoglos Oftalmico; Infladerm; Otosporin; Terra-Cortril; Terra-Cortril com Polimixina B; Vioformio-Hidrocortisona; Xyloproct; **Canad.:** Actinac; Anodan-HC; Anugesic-HC; Anusol; Calmurid HC†; Cipro HC; Cortimyxin; Cortisporin; Diospor HC†; Fucidin H; Hemcort HC; Neo-Cortef; Ophthocort†; Pentamycetin-HC; PMS-Egozinc-HC; Pramox HC; Proctodan-HC; Proctofoam-HC; Proctosone; Proctosone; Rectogel HC; Rivasol HC; Ti-U-Lac HC; Uremol-HC; Vioform-Hydrocortisone; VoSoL HC; **Denm.:** Brentacort; Ciflox; Fucidin-Hydrocortison; Locoidol; Proctosedyl; **Fin.:** Ciproxin-Hydrocortison; Daktacort; Duocort; Fucidin-Hydrocortison; Locoidol; Pantyson; Pimafucort; Proctosedyl; Sibicort; Terra-Cortril; Terra-Cortril P; Trosycort†; Xyloproct; **Fr.:** Anti-Hemorroidaires†; Bacicoline; Cortibiotique; Daktacort†; Dermocalm†; Locoide N; Madecassol Neomycine Hydrocortisone; Onctose Hydrocortisone†; Soframycine Hydrocortisone; **Ger.:** Antipruvit; Calmurid HC; Canesten HC; Corti Jaikal; Corti-Flexiole†; Eksalb; Farco-Tril; Fucidine plus; Hydrodexan; Ichthocortin; Novifort; Nubral 4 HC; Nystaderm comp; Otosporin; Pantocrinale; Pigmanorm; Pimafucort; Poloris HC†; Polyspectran HC; Posterisan forte; Terracortril; Topoderm N; **Hong Kong:** Anusol-HC; Cortiphenol H; Cortison-Kemiceteine; Daktacort; Hemcort HC; Otosporin; Posterisan Forte; Proctosedyl; Proctosone; Protozone; Xyloproct; **Irl.:** Actinac; Alphaderm; Alphosyl HC; Anugesic-HC; Anusol-HC; Calmurid HC; Canesten HC; Daktacort; Eurax-Hydrocortisone; Fucidin H; Gentisone HC; Hydrocal; Locoid C; Neo-Cortef; Nystaform-HC; Otosporin; Perinal; Proctofoam-HC; Proctosedyl; Quinocort; Terra-Cortril; Terra-Cortril Nystatin; Timodine; Vioform-Hydrocortisone; Xyloproct; **Israel:** Alphosyl HC; Benzantine H; Calmurid HC; Daktacort; Epifoam; Fucidin H; Hycocin; Hycomycin; Hydroagisten; Otosporin; Panthisone; Perinal; Proctofoam-HC; Proctosedyl; Proctozorin-N; Xyloproct; **Ital.:** Argisone; Cort-Inal; Cortison Chemicetina; Emorril; Idracemi; Idracemi Eparina; Idrocet; Idroneomicil; Kinogen; Mictasone; Mixotone; Mobilat; Nasomixin; Nevacort; Pomata Midy HC†; Preparazione Antiemorroidaria; Proctidol; Proctofoam-HC; Proctosedyl; Proctosoll; Reumacort; Scalpicin; Sedalen Cort; Sinsurrene†; Vasosterone; Vasosterone Antibiotico; Vasosterone Collirio; Xyloproct; **Mex.:** Cortisporin; Daktacort; Hidropolicin; Soldrin; Sulfa Hidro; Vioformo-Cort; Xyloproct; **Neth.:** Alphacortison†; Bacicoline-B†; Calmurid HC; Daktacort; Otosporin; Pimafucort†; Proctosedyl; Terra-Cortril Gel Steraject met polymyxine-B; Terra-Cortril met polymyxine-B; Terra-Cortril†; Xyloproct; **Norw.:** Daktacort; Fucidin-Hydrocortison; Locoidol; Proctosedyl; Terra-Cortril; Terra-Cortril Polymyxin B; Xyloproct; **NZ:** Coly-Mycin S Otic; Daktacort; Fungocort; Locoid C; Micreme H; Pimafucort; Proctosedyl; Xyloproct; **Port.:** Alphosyl HC; Anucet; Clorcorticil; Corticil T; Cortigripe; Davimicina; Fucidine H; Leuco Hubber†; Locoid C; Otolys†; Otosporin; Pimafucort; **S.Afr.:** Anusol-HC†; Calmurid HC; Chloramex H†; Corti-Flexiole†; Daktacort; Fucidin H; Locoid C†; Manoderm†; Nasomixin; Neoderm; Otoseptil†; Otosporin; Panthisone; Perinal; Proctosedyl; Quinoderm-H†; Terra-Cortril; Viocort; **Singapore:** Canesten HC; Cortaid with Aloe; Daktacort; Decocort; Fucidin H; Otosporin; Proctosedyl; Xyloproct; Zaricort; **Spain:** Aftajuventus; Aftasone B C; Alantomicina Complex†; Anginovag; Antiblef Eczem; Antihemorroidal; Bacisporin; Brentan; Cilinafosal Hidrocort; Cohortan; Cohortan Antibiotico†; Cortenema; Cortison Chemicet Topica; Dermo Hubber; Detraine; Edifaringen; Euraxil Hidrocort; Fucidine H; Grietalgen Hidrocort; Halibut Hidrocortisona; Hemodren Compuesto; Hepro; Hidroc Cloranf; Hidroc Neomic; Leuco Hubber; Milrosina Nistatina; Neo Bacitrin Hidrocortis; Neo Hubber; Neo Visage; Oftalmo; Oto Difusor; Oto Neomicin Calm†; Otosporin; Roberfarin; Terra-Cortril; Tisuderma; Tyroneomicin†; **Swed.:** Calmuril-Hydrokortison†; Chloromycetin Hydrocortison†; Cortimyk; Daktacort; Ecomytrin-Hydrocortison†; Fenuril-Hydrokortison; Fucidin-Hydrocortison; Proctosedyl; Sterosan-Hydrocortisone†; Terracortril; Terracortril med polymyxin B; Xyloproct; **Switz.:** Calmurid HC; Cortifluid N; Cortimycine; Daktacort; Dermacalm-d; Endomethasone†; Fucidin H; Haemocortin; Hydrocortisone comp; Neo-Hydro; Otosporin; Rocanal Permanent Gangrene†; Septomixine; Terracortril; **Thai.:** Antergan; Daktacort; Dermasol; Ladocort; Neo-Hytisone; Otosporin; Proctosedyl; Xyloproct; **UK:** Actinac; Alphaderm; Alphosyl HC; Anugesic-HC; Anusol-HC, Plus HC; Calmurid HC; Canesten HC; Carbo-Cort†; Chloromycetin Hydrocortisone†; Cobadex; Daktacort HC; Econacort; Eurax-Hydrocortisone; Fucidin H; Gentisone HC; Gregoderm; Hydrocal†; Locoid C; Neo-Cortef; Nystaform-HC; Otosporin; Perinal; Proctocream HC†; Proctofoam-HC; Proctosedyl; Quinocort; Tarcortin†; Terra-Cortril; Terra-Cortril Nystatin; Timodine; Uniroid-HC; Uniroid†; Vioform-Hydrocortisone; Xyloproct; **USA:** 1 + 1-F; AA-HC Otic†; Acetasol HC; Ak-Spore HC; Ala-Quin†; Albaform HC†; Analpram-HC; AntibiOtic; Anumed HC; Bacticort†; Chloromycetin Hydrocortisone†; Cipro HC; Coly-Mycin S Otic; Coracin†; Corque; Cortane-B Otic; Cortatrigen; Cortic; Corticaine; Cortimycin; Cortisporin; Cortisporin-TC; Dermtex HC with Aloe; Ear-Eze; Emergent-Ez; Enzone; Epifoam; Fungoid HC; HC Derma-Pax; Hysone; LazerSporin-C; Lida-Mantle-HC; Mantadil†; Neo-Cortef†; Neotricin HC; Octicair; Oti-Med; Otic-Care; Oticin HC†; OtiTricin; Otobiotic; Otocort;

Otomar-HC; Otomycin-HPN; Otosporin; Pedi-Cort V†; Pediotic; Pramosone; Proctofoam-HC; Terra-Cortril; Tri-Otic; UAD-Otic; Vanoxide-HC; VoSoL HC; Vytone; Zone-A; Zoto-HC.

Isoflupredone Acetate (12869-q)

Isoflupredone Acetate (BANM, USAN, rINNM).
9α-Fluoroprednisolone Acetate; U-6013. 9α-Fluoro-11β,17α,21-trihydroxypregna-1,4-diene-3,20-dione 21-acetate.
$C_{23}H_{29}FO_6 = 420.5$.
CAS — 338-95-4 (isoflupredone); 338-98-7 (isoflupredone acetate).

Profile
Isoflupredone acetate is a corticosteroid that has been employed for its topical glucocorticoid activity (p.1039) in allergic rhinitis.
Isoflupredone is also employed in veterinary medicine.

Preparations
Proprietary Preparations (details are given in Part 3)
Multi-ingredient: Belg.: Deltarhinol†; **Israel:** Proaf.

Loteprednol Etabonate (14750-p)

Loteprednol Etabonate (BANM, USAN, rINNM).
CDDD-5604; HGP-1; Loteprednol Ethyl Carbonate; P-5604. (11β,17α)-17-[(Ethoxycarbonyl)oxy]-11-hydroxy-3-oxoandrosta-1,4-diene-17-carboxylic acid chloromethyl ester.
$C_{24}H_{31}ClO_7 = 467.0$.
CAS — 129260-79-3 (loteprednol); 82034-46-6 (loteprednol etabonate).

Profile
Loteprednol etabonate is a corticosteroid used for its glucocorticoid activity (p.1039) in the topical management of inflammatory and allergic disorders of the eye. It is usually employed as eye drops containing 0.2 or 0.5%.
Prolonged application to the eye of preparations containing corticosteroids has caused raised intra-ocular pressure and reduced visual function.

◊ References.
1. Noble S, Goa KL. Loteprednol etabonate: clinical potential in the management of ocular inflammation. *BioDrugs* 1998; **10:** 329–39.

Preparations
Proprietary Preparations (details are given in Part 3)
USA: Alrex; Lotemax.

Medrysone (1113-p)

Medrysone (USAN, pINN).
11β-Hydroxy-6α-methylprogesterone; Medrisona; NSC-63278; U-8471. 11β-Hydroxy-6α-methylpregn-4-ene-3,20-dione.
$C_{22}H_{32}O_3 = 344.5$.
CAS — 2668-66-8.
ATC — S01BA08.

Profile
Medrysone is a corticosteroid employed for its glucocorticoid activity (see p.1039) in the topical treatment of allergic and inflammatory conditions of the eye. It is usually given as 1% eye drops.
Prolonged application to the eye of preparations containing corticosteroids has caused raised intra-ocular pressure and reduced visual function.

Preparations
Proprietary Preparations (details are given in Part 3)
Austral.: HMS Liquifilm; **Ger.:** Ophtocortin†; Spectramedryn; **Neth.:** HMS Liquifilm†; **Port.:** Medrisocil; S.Afr.: HMS†; **Spain:** Liquipom Medrisone; **Switz.:** HMS; **USA:** HMS.
Multi-ingredient: Ital.: Medramil†; **Spain:** Mirantal†.

Meprednisone (1114-s)

Meprednisone (USAN, rINN).
16β-Methylprednisone; NSC-527579; Sch-4358. 17α,21-Dihydroxy-16β-methylpregna-1,4-diene-3,11,20-trione.
$C_{22}H_{28}O_5 = 372.5$.
CAS — 1247-42-3.
ATC — H02AB15.
Pharmacopoeias. In US.

Pharmacopoeial description
USP 25: Store in airtight containers at a temperature not exceeding 40°. Protect from light.

Profile
Meprednisone is a corticosteroid with mainly glucocorticoid activity, as described under Corticosteroids, p.1039. It has been given by mouth as either the free alcohol or the acetate and by injection as the sodium hemisuccinate.

Methylprednisolone (1115-w)

Methylprednisolone (BAN, rINN).

6α-Methylprednisolone; Methylprednisolonum; NSC-19987. 11β,17α,21-Trihydroxy-6α-methylpregna-1,4-diene-3,20-dione.

$C_{22}H_{30}O_5 = 374.5$.

CAS — 83-43-2.

ATC — D07AA01; D10AA02; H02AB04.

Pharmacopoeias. In Eur. (see p.vi), Jpn, and US.

Pharmacopoeial description

Ph. Eur.: A white or almost white, crystalline powder. It shows polymorphism. Practically insoluble in water; sparingly soluble in alcohol; slightly soluble in acetone and in dichloromethane. Protect from light.

USP 25: A white to practically white, odourless, crystalline powder. Practically insoluble in water; soluble 1 in 100 of alcohol, and in 1 in 800 of chloroform and of ether; slightly soluble in acetone; sparingly soluble in dioxan and in methyl alcohol. Store in airtight containers. Protect from light.

Methylprednisolone Acetate (1116-e)

Methylprednisolone Acetate (BANM, rINNM).

Methylprednisoloni Acetas. Methylprednisolone 21-acetate.

$C_{24}H_{32}O_6 = 416.5$.

CAS — 53-36-1.

Pharmacopoeias. In Eur. (see p.vi) and US.

Methylprednisolone acetate 44 mg is approximately equivalent to 40 mg of methylprednisolone.

Pharmacopoeial description

Ph. Eur.: A white or almost white, crystalline powder. Practically insoluble in water; sparingly soluble in alcohol and in acetone; slightly soluble in ether. Protect from light.

USP 25: A white or practically white, odourless, crystalline powder. Soluble 1 in 1500 of water, 1 in 400 of alcohol, 1 in 250 of chloroform, and 1 in 1500 of ether; sparingly soluble in acetone and in methyl alcohol; soluble in dioxan. Store in airtight containers. Protect from light.

Methylprednisolone Hydrogen Succinate

(1117-I)

Methylprednisolone Hydrogen Succinate (BANM, rINNM). Methylprednisolone Hemisuccinate; Methylprednisoloni Hydrogenosuccinas. Methylprednisolone 21-(hydrogen succinate).

$C_{26}H_{34}O_8 = 474.5$.

CAS — 2921-57-5.

Pharmacopoeias. In Eur. (see p.vi) and US.

Methylprednisolone hydrogen succinate 51 mg is approximately equivalent to 40 mg of methylprednisolone.

Pharmacopoeial description

Ph. Eur.: A white or almost white, hygroscopic powder. Practically insoluble in water and in ether; slightly soluble in dehydrated alcohol and in acetone; dissolves in dilute solutions of alkali hydroxides. Store in airtight containers. Protect from light.

USP 25: A white or nearly white, odourless or nearly odourless, hygroscopic solid. Very slightly soluble in water; freely soluble in alcohol; soluble in acetone. Store in airtight containers.

Methylprednisolone Sodium Succinate (1118-y)

Methylprednisolone Sodium Succinate (BANM, rINNM).

Methylprednisolone 21-(sodium succinate).

$C_{26}H_{33}NaO_8 = 496.5$.

CAS — 2375-03-3.

Pharmacopoeias. In US.

Methylprednisolone sodium succinate 53 mg is approximately equivalent to 40 mg of methylprednisolone.

Pharmacopoeial description

USP 25: A white or nearly white, odourless, hygroscopic, amorphous solid. Soluble 1 in 1.5 of water and 1 in 12 of alcohol; very slightly soluble in acetone; insoluble in chloroform and in ether. Store in airtight containers. Protect from light.

Stability. Methylprednisolone sodium succinate injection (Solu-Medrol, USA) was considered to be stable for 7 days when diluted in water for injection and stored in glass vials at 4°. When stored under similar conditions at 22°, it was considered to be stable for 24 hours.[1] The manufacturers state that the prepared solution should be stored at 20 to 25° and used within 48 hours of mixing.

1. Nahata MC, et al. Stability of diluted methylprednisolone sodium succinate injection at two temperatures. Am J Hosp Pharm 1994; 51: 2157–9.

Adverse Effects, Treatment, Withdrawal, and Precautions

As for corticosteroids in general (see p.1039). Rapid intravenous administration of large doses has been associated with cardiovascular collapse.

Methylprednisolone may be slightly less likely than prednisolone to cause sodium and water retention.

When applied topically, particularly to large areas, when the skin is broken, or under occlusive dressings, corticosteroids may be absorbed in sufficient amounts to cause systemic effects.

◊ References to various adverse effects associated with intravenous administration of methylprednisolone in high-dose pulse therapy[1-11] and to adverse effects following intra-articular[12] and intranasal injection.[13] Epidural administration (or more particularly inadvertent intrathecal administration during attempted epidural placement) may be associated with serious adverse effects including arachnoiditis and aseptic meningitis, although the degree of risk is uncertain.[14]

1. Newmark KJ, et al. Acute arthralgia following high-dose intravenous methylprednisolone therapy. Lancet 1974; ii: 229.
2. Bailey RR, Armour P. Acute arthralgia after high-dose intravenous methylprednisolone. Lancet 1974; ii: 1014.
3. Bennett WM, Strong D. Arthralgia after high-dose steroids. Lancet 1975; i: 332.
4. Moses RE, et al. Fatal arrhythmia after pulse methylprednisolone therapy. Ann Intern Med 1981; 95: 781–2.
5. Oto A, et al. Methylprednisolone pulse therapy and peritonitis. Ann Intern Med 1983; 99: 282.
6. Suchman AL, et al. Seizure after pulse therapy with methyl prednisolone. Arthritis Rheum 1983; 26: 117.
7. Ayoub WT, et al. Central nervous system manifestations after pulse therapy for systemic lupus erythematosus. Arthritis Rheum 1983; 26: 809–10.
8. Williams AJ, et al. Disseminated aspergillosis in high dose steroid therapy. Lancet 1983; i: 1222.
9. Barrett DF. Pulse methylprednisolone therapy. Lancet 1983; ii: 800.
10. Baethge BA, Lidsky MD. Intractable hiccups associated with high-dose intravenous methylprednisolone therapy. Ann Intern Med 1986; 104: 58–9.
11. Gardiner PVG, Griffiths ID. Sudden death after treatment with pulsed methylprednisolone. BMJ 1990; 300: 125.
12. Black DM, Filak AT. Hyperglycemia with non-insulin-dependent diabetes following intraarticular steroid injection. J Fam Pract 1989; 28: 462–3.
13. Johns KJ, Chandra SR. Visual loss following intranasal corticosteroid injection. JAMA 1989; 261: 2413.
14. Rodgers PT, Connelly JF. Epidural administration of methylprednisolone for back pain. Am J Hosp Pharm 1994; 51: 2789–90.

Interactions

The interactions of corticosteroids in general are described on p.1043.

Pharmacokinetics

For a brief outline of the pharmacokinetics of corticosteroids, see p.1044.

Methylprednisolone is fairly rapidly distributed following oral administration, with a plasma half-life of 3.5 hours or more. The tissue half-life is reported to range from 18 to 36 hours.

Methylprednisolone acetate is absorbed from joints over a week but is more slowly absorbed following deep intramuscular injection. The sodium succinate ester is rapidly absorbed following intramuscular administration, with peak plasma concentrations obtained in 2 hours.

Methylprednisolone crosses the placenta.

◊ References.

1. Tornatore KM, et al. Repeated assessment of methylprednisolone pharmacokinetics during chronic immunosuppression in renal transplant recipients. Ann Pharmacother 1995; 29: 120–4.
2. Rohatagi S, et al. Pharmacokinetics of methylprednisolone and prednisolone after single and multiple oral administration. J Clin Pharmacol 1997; 37: 916–25.

Uses and Administration

Methylprednisolone is a corticosteroid with mainly glucocorticoid activity, as described under Corticosteroids, p.1039; 4 mg of methylprednisolone is equivalent in anti-inflammatory activity to about 5 mg of prednisolone.

It is used, either in the form of the free alcohol or in one of the esterified forms, in the treatment of conditions for which corticosteroid therapy is indicated (see p.1044) except adrenocortical-deficiency states, for which hydrocortisone with supplementary fludrocortisone is preferred.

For administration by mouth, methylprednisolone is usually given in an initial dosage range of 4 to 48 mg daily but higher initial doses of up to 100 mg or more daily may be used in acute severe disease.

For parenteral administration in intensive or emergency therapy, methylprednisolone sodium succinate may be administered by intramuscular or intravenous injection or by intravenous infusion. The intravenous

route is preferred for its more rapid effect in emergency therapy. The usual initial intramuscular or intravenous dose ranges from the equivalent of 10 to 500 mg of methylprednisolone daily. Large intravenous doses (over 250 mg) should normally be given slowly over at least 30 minutes; doses up to 250 mg should be given over at least 5 minutes. High doses should generally not be given for prolonged periods; emergency treatment should only be given until the patient is stabilised. High doses given intermittently for a limited period have sometimes been known as 'pulse therapy' (see under Administration, below) and in graft rejection (see p.502) up to 1 g has been given daily for up to 3 days. In intensive therapy of acute spinal cord injury (p.1058) initial doses of the equivalent of up to 30 mg per kg body-weight of methylprednisolone have been given by bolus intravenous injection over 15 minutes and followed, after a 45-minute pause, by intravenous infusion of 5.4 mg per kg per hour over 24 hours or longer. For slow intravenous infusion methylprednisolone sodium succinate is dissolved in an appropriate volume of glucose 5% or sodium chloride 0.9% or sodium chloride 0.9% and glucose 5%.

Parenteral doses in children have varied considerably, depending on the condition: a range of 1 to 30 mg of methylprednisolone per kg body-weight daily has been given by the intravenous or intramuscular routes. A total dose of 1 g daily should not normally be exceeded.

Methylprednisolone acetate may be administered by intramuscular injection for a prolonged systemic effect, the dose varying from 40 mg every 2 weeks to 120 mg weekly.

For intra-articular injection and for injection into soft tissues methylprednisolone acetate as an aqueous suspension is employed. The dose by intra-articular injection varies from 4 to 80 mg according to the size of the affected joint. The acetate may also be administered by intralesional injection in doses of 20 to 60 mg.

For use in the treatment of various skin disorders methylprednisolone acetate may be applied topically, usually in concentrations of 0.25 to 1%. The aceponate, which may exhibit modified topical activity, has also been applied as a 0.1% cream or ointment. For recommendations concerning the correct use of corticosteroids on the skin, and a rough guide to the clinical potencies of topical corticosteroids, see p.1045.

Other esters of methylprednisolone which have occasionally been used include the cipionate and the suleptanate.

◊ General references.

1. Cronstein BN. Clinical use of methylprednisolone sodium succinate: a review. Curr Ther Res 1995; 56: 1–15.

Administration. For short-term intensive therapy or in certain emergency situations a technique of corticosteroid administration known as 'pulse therapy' has been employed. Methylprednisolone has often been used in this manner. Typically, high doses of about 1 g intravenously have been given, daily or on alternate days or weekly, for a limited number of doses; the most common regimen appears to be 1 g daily for 3 days.

Blood disorders. Methylprednisolone is one of the corticosteroids that have been used in the management of haemangioma (p.1052) and the Kasabach-Merritt syndrome.[1] There is also a report of benefit from very high-dose therapy in a few patients with refractory red cell aplasia due to Blackfan-Diamond anaemia.[2]

1. Özsoylu Ş, et al. Megadose methylprednisolone therapy for Kasabach-Merritt syndrome. J Pediatr 1996; 129: 947.
2. Bernini JC, et al. High-dose intravenous methylprednisolone therapy for patients with Diamond-Blackfan anemia refractory to conventional doses of prednisone. J Pediatr 1995; 127: 654–9.

IDIOPATHIC THROMBOCYTOPENIC PURPURA. High dose intravenous methylprednisolone may be employed as part of the emergency management of acute idiopathic thrombocytopenic purpura (p.1052), for example when major acute bleeding or intracranial haemorrhage supervene. There is some evidence that methylprednisolone is less effective than normal immunoglobulins in children with the condition. Methylprednisolone has also been used by mouth or intravenously in the management of the chronic form, although prednisolone or prednisone are more frequently used for oral therapy and good controlled trials are scanty.

References.
1. von dem Borne AEGKR, et al. High dose intravenous methyl-prednisolone or high dose intravenous gammaglobulin for au-toimmune thrombocytopenia. BMJ 1988; 296: 249–50.
2. Özsoylu S, et al. Megadose methylprednisolone for chronic idi-opathic thrombocytopenic purpura. Lancet 1990; 336: 1078–9.
3. Akoğlu T, et al. Megadose methylprednisolone pulse therapy in adult idiopathic thrombocytopenic purpura. Lancet 1991; 337: 56.
4. Özsoylu S. Mega-dose methylprednisolone for chronic idiopath-ic thrombocytopenic purpura. Lancet 1991; 337: 1611–12.
5. Rosthøj S, et al. Randomized trial comparing intravenous immu-noglobulin with methylprednisolone pulse therapy in acute idio-pathic thrombocytopenic purpura. Acta Paediatr 1996; 85: 910–15.
6. Alpdoğan Ö, et al. Efficacy of high-dose methylprednisolone as a first-line therapy in adult patients with idiopathic thrombocyto-penic purpura. Br J Haematol 1998; 103: 1061–3.

Rheumatoid arthritis. Methylprednisolone administered in intravenous pulses has been reported[1-7] to be effective in the treatment of rheumatoid arthritis (p.9) including juvenile idio-pathic arthritis. Some studies have shown this treatment to be of greatest benefit when given concomitantly with a disease-modifying antirheumatic drug (DMARD) such as gold,[1,2,4] al-though some showed the addition of methylprednisolone to ex-isting therapy to have no extra benefit.[6] A comparatively low dose of 100 mg was found to be as effective as 1000 mg in one study.[3] Monthly administration of methylprednisolone by deep intramuscular injection was also an effective adjunct to gold therapy.[8]

A preliminary study in children has found intravenous pulses of methylprednisolone 30 mg per kg body-weight to be effective treatment for systemic flares of juvenile idiopathic arthritis.[7]

1. Walters HT, Cawley MID. Combined suppressive drug treatment in severe refractory rheumatoid disease: an analysis of the rela-tive effects of parenteral methylprednisolone, cyclophosphamide and sodium aurothiomalate. Ann Rheum Dis 1988; 47: 924–9.
2. Smith MD, et al. The clinical and immunological effects of pulse methylprednisolone therapy in rheumatoid arthritis I: clinical ef-fects. J Rheumatol 1988; 15: 229–32.
3. Igelhart IW, et al. Intravenous pulsed steroids in rheumatoid ar-thritis: a comparative dose study. J Rheumatol 1990; 17: 159–62.
4. Smith MD, et al. Pulse methylprednisolone therapy in rheuma-toid arthritis: unproved therapy, unjustified therapy, or effective adjunctive treatment? Ann Rheum Dis 1990; 49: 265–7.
5. Kapisinszky N, Keszthelyi B. High dose intravenous methyl-prednisolone pulse therapy in patients with rheumatoid arthritis. Ann Rheum Dis 1990; 49: 567–8.
6. Hansen TM, et al. Double blind placebo controlled trial of pulse treatment with methylprednisolone combined with disease mod-ifying drugs in rheumatoid arthritis. BMJ 1990; 301: 268–70.
7. Adebajo AO, Hall MA. The use of intravenous pulsed methyl-prednisolone in the treatment of systemic-onset juvenile chronic arthritis. Br J Rheumatol 1998; 37: 1240–2.
8. Corkill MM, et al. Intramuscular depot methylprednisolone in-duction of chrysotherapy in rheumatoid arthritis: a 24-week ran-domized controlled trial. Br J Rheumatol 1990; 29: 274–9.

Preparations

BP 2001: Methylprednisolone Acetate Injection; Methylpred-nisolone Tablets;
USP 25: Methylprednisolone Acetate Cream; Methylprednisolo-ne Acetate Injectable Suspension; Methylprednisolone Acetate for Rectal Suspension; Methylprednisolone Sodium Succinate for In-jection; Methylprednisolone Tablets; Neomycin Sulfate and Meth-ylprednisolone Acetate Cream.

Proprietary Preparations (details are given in Part 3)
Aust.: Advantan; Depo-Medrol†; Promedrol†; Solu-Medrol; Ur-bason; **Austral.:** Advantan; Depo-Medrol; Depo-Nisolone; Me-drol; Solu-Medrol; **Belg.:** Advantan; Depo-Medrol; Medrol; Solu-Medrol; **Braz.:** Depo-Medrol; Solu-Medrol; **Canad.:** Depo-Me-drol; Medrol; Solu-Medrol; **Denm.:** Depo-Medrol; Medrol; Solu-Medrol; **Fin.:** Advantan; Depo-Medrol; Me-drol; Solomet; Solu-Medrol; **Fr.:** Depo-Medrol; Medrol; Solu-Medrol; **Ger.:** Advantan; Depo-Medrate; Medrate; Metypred; Me-tysolon; Predni M; Urbason; **Hong Kong:** Advantan; Depo-Me-drol; Solu-Medrol; **Irl.:** Depo-Medrone; Medrone; Solu-Medrone; **Israel:** A-Methapred; Depo-Medrol; Medrol; Solu-Me-drol; Vanderm; **Ital.:** Advantan; Asmacortone; Avancort; Depo-Medrol; Emmetip†; Esametone; Firmacort; Medrol; Metilbeta-sone Solubile; Solu-Medrol; Urbason; **Mex.:** Advantan; Cryosolo-na; Depo-Medrol; Metisona; Prednilem; Radilem; Solsolona; Solu-Medrol; **Neth.:** Depo-Medrol; Medrol†; Solu-Medrol; **Norw.:** Depo-Medrol; Medrol; Solu-Medrol; **NZ:** Advantan; Depo-Medrol; Medrol; Solu-Medrol; **Port.:** Advantan; Depo-Medrol; Medrol; Metilpren; Solu-Medrol; **S.Afr.:** Advantan; Depo-Medrol; Medrol; Metypresol; Solu-Medrol; **Singapore:** Solu-Me-drol; **Spain:** Adventan; Depo Moderin; Solu-Moderin; Urbason; **Swed.:** Depo-Medrol; Medrol; Solu-Medrol; **Switz.:** Advantan; Depo-Medrol; Medrol; Promedrol†; Solu-Medrol; Urbason; **Thai.:** Depo-Medrol; Solu-Medrol; **UK:** Depo-Medrone; Me-drone; Solu-Medrone; **USA:** A-Methapred; Adlone†; D-Med†; depMedalone; Depo-Medrol; Depoject; Depopred; Duralone; M-Prednisol; Medralone; Medrol; Solu-Medrol.

Multi-ingredient: Aust.: Depo-Medrol mit Lidocain†; **Austral.:** Neo-Medrol; **Belg.:** Depo-Medrol + Lidocaine; **Braz.:** Emecort; **Canad.:** Depo-Medrol with Lidocaine; Medrol Acne Lotion; Neo-Medrol Acne; Neo-Medrol Veriderm; **Fin.:** Depo-Medrol cum Lidocain; Neo-Medrol comp; Solomet c bupivacain hydrochlorid; **Hong Kong:** Depo-Medrol with Lidocaine; Neo-Medrol Acne; **Irl.:** Depo-Medrone with Lidocaine; Neo-Medrone†; **Israel:** Depo-Medrol with Lidocaine; Neo-Medrol; **Ital.:** Depo-Medrol + Lidocaina; Medrol Lozione Antiacne; Neo-Medrol Veriderm; **Neth.:** Depo-Medrol + Lidocaine; **Norw.:** Depo-Medrol cum Lidocain; **NZ:** Depo-Medrol with Lidocaine; **Port.:** Depo-Medrol com Lidocaina; **S.Afr.:** Depo-Medrol with Lidocaine; Neo-Medrol; **Singapore:** Neo-Medrol; **Spain:** Moderin Acne; Neo Moder-

in; **Swed.:** Depo-Medrol cum Lidokain; **Switz.:** Depo-Medrol Lidocaine; **Thai.:** Depo-Medrol with Lidocaine; Neo-Medrol; **UK:** Depo-Medrone with Lidocaine.

Mometasone Furoate (11466-m)

Mometasone Furoate (BANM, USAN, rINNM).
Mometasoni Furoas; Sch-32088. 9α,21-Dichloro-11β,17-dihy-droxy-16α-methylpregna-1,4-diene-3,20-dione 17-(2-furoate).
$C_{27}H_{30}Cl_2O_6 = 521.4$.
CAS — 105102-22-5 (mometasone); 83919-23-7 (mometasone furoate).
Pharmacopoeias. In Eur. (see p.vi) and US.

Pharmacopoeial description

Ph. Eur.: A white or almost white powder. Practically insolu-ble in water; slightly soluble in alcohol; freely soluble in ace-tone and in dichloromethane.

USP 25: A white to off-white powder. insoluble in water; sol-uble in acetone and in dichloromethane; sparingly soluble in heptane.

Profile

Mometasone furoate is a corticosteroid used topically for its glucocorticoid activity (see p.1039) in the treatment of various skin disorders. It is usually employed as a cream, ointment, or lotion containing 0.1%.

It is also given as a 0.05% nasal suspension of mometasone furoate monohydrate in the treatment and prophylaxis of the symptoms of allergic rhinitis (p.407); the usual adult dose is the equivalent of 100 μg of mometasone furoate in each nostril once daily, increased if necessary to 200 μg in each nostril dai-ly. Once symptoms are controlled a dose of 50 μg in each nos-tril daily may be effective for maintenance. In the UK, the dose for children aged between 6 and 11 years is the equivalent of 50 μg in each nostril once daily. In the USA, similar doses may be given to treat allergic rhinitis in children from 3 years of age.

Mometasone furoate is under investigation by inhalation for the management of asthma (p.757).

When applied topically, particularly to large areas, when the skin is broken, or under occlusive dressings, or when given in-tranasally, corticosteroids may be absorbed in sufficient amounts to cause systemic effects (see p.1039). The effects of topical corticosteroids on the skin are described on p.1041. For recommendations concerning the correct use of corticosteroids on the skin, see p.1045.

◊ References.
1. Prakash A, Benfield P. Topical mometasone: a review of its phar-macological properties and therapeutic use in the treatment of dermatological disorders. Drugs 1998; 55: 145–63.
2. Onrust SV, Lamb HM. Mometasone furoate: a review of its intra-nasal use in allergic rhinitis. Drugs 1998; 56: 725–45.
3. Meltzer EO, et al. A dose-ranging study of mometasone furoate aqueous nasal spray in children with seasonal allergic rhinitis. J Allergy Clin Immunol 1999; 104: 107–14.
4. Sharpe M, Jarvis B. Inhaled mometasone furoate: a review of its use in adults and adolescents with persistent asthma. Drugs 2001; 61: 1325–50.

Preparations

USP 25: Mometasone Furoate Cream; Mometasone Furoate Oint-ment; Mometasone Furoate Topical Solution.

Proprietary Preparations (details are given in Part 3)
Aust.: Elocon; **Austral.:** AllerMax; Elocon; Nasonex; Novasone; **Belg.:** Elocom; **Braz.:** Elocom; **Canad.:** Elocom; Nasonex; **Denm.:** Elocon; Nasonex; **Fin.:** Elocon; Nasonex; **Fr.:** Nasonex; **Ger.:** Ecural; Nasonex; **Hong Kong:** Elomet; Nasonex; **Irl.:** Elo-con; Nasonex; **Israel:** Elocom; Nasonex; **Ital.:** Altosone; Elocon; Rinelon; **Mex.:** Elomet; Rinelon; **Neth.:** Elocon; Nason-ex; **Norw.:** Elocon; Nasonex; **NZ:** Elocon; Nasonex; **Port.:** Nasom-et; **S.Afr.:** Elica; Elocon; Nasonex; **Singapore:** Elomet; Nasonex; **Spain:** Elica; Elocom; Nasonex; Rinelon; **Swed.:** Elocon; Nason-ex; **Switz.:** Elocom; Nasonex; **Thai.:** Elomet; Nasonex; **UK:** Elo-con; Nasonex; **USA:** Elocon; Nasonex.

Paramethasone Acetate (1119-j)

Paramethasone Acetate (BANM, USAN, rINNM).
6α-Fluoro-16α-methylprednisolone 21-Acetate. 6α-Fluoro-11β,17α,21-trihydroxy-16α-methylpregna-1,4-diene-3,20-di-one 21-acetate.
$C_{24}H_{31}FO_6 = 434.5$.
CAS — 53-33-8 (paramethasone); 1597-82-6 (parametha-sone acetate).
Pharmacopoeias. In Fr. and US.

Pharmacopoeial description

USP 25: A white to creamy-white, fluffy, odourless, crystalline powder. Insoluble in water; soluble 1 in 50 of chloroform and 1 in 40 of methyl alcohol; soluble in ether. Store in airtight con-tainers.

Profile

Paramethasone acetate is a corticosteroid which has been used systemically for its predominantly glucocorticoid activity (p.1039); 2 mg of paramethasone is equivalent in anti-inflam-matory activity to about 5 mg of prednisolone. The disodium phosphate has also been used.

Preparations

USP 25: Parameterhasone Acetate Tablets.

Proprietary Preparations (details are given in Part 3)
Fr.: Dilar†; **Mex.:** Dilar; **Neth.:** Depodillar†; **Spain:** Cortidene.

Multi-ingredient: Mex.: Dilarmine; **Spain:** Triniol†.

Prednicarbate (2367-z)

Prednicarbate (BAN, USAN, rINN).
Hoe-777; Prednicarbatum; S-77-0777. 11β,17,21-Trihydrox-ypregna-1,4-diene-3,20-dione 17-(ethyl carbonate) 21-propi-onate.
$C_{27}H_{36}O_8 = 488.6$.
CAS — 73771-04-7.
ATC — D07AC18.
Pharmacopoeias. In Eur. (see p.vi).

Pharmacopoeial description

Ph. Eur.: A white or almost white, crystalline powder. It shows polymorphism. Practically insoluble in water; freely soluble in alcohol and in acetone; sparingly soluble in propylene glycol. Protect from light.

Profile

Prednicarbate is a corticosteroid used topically for its glucocor-ticoid activity (see p.1039) in the treatment of various skin dis-orders. It has usually been employed as a cream, ointment, or lotion, containing 0.1 to 0.25%.

When applied topically, particularly to large areas, when the skin is broken, or under occlusive dressings, corticosteroids may be absorbed in sufficient amounts to cause systemic ef-fects (see p.1039). The effects of topical corticosteroids on the skin are described on p.1041. For recommendations concern-ing the correct use of corticosteroids on the skin, and a rough guide to the clinical potencies of topical corticosteroids, see p.1045.

◊ References.
1. Schäfer-Korting M, et al. Prednicarbate activity and benefit/risk ratio in relation to other topical glucocorticoids. Clin Pharmacol Ther 1993; 54: 448–56.

Preparations

Proprietary Preparations (details are given in Part 3)
Aust.: Prednitop; **Braz.:** Dermatop; **Ger.:** Dermatop; **Ital.:** Der-matop; **Spain:** Batmen; Peitel; **Switz.:** Prednitop; **Thai.:** Der-matop; **USA:** Dermatop.

Prednisolamate Hydrochloride (1120-q)

Prednisolamate Hydrochloride (BANM, rINNM).
Prednisolone 21-Diethylaminoacetate Hydrochloride. 11β,17α,21-Trihydroxypregna-1,4-diene-3,20-dione 21-di-ethylaminoacetate hydrochloride.
$C_{27}H_{39}NO_6,HCl = 510.1$.
CAS — 5626-34-6 (prednisolamate).

Profile

Prednisolamate hydrochloride has the general properties of prednisolone (see below) and has been used in some countries as a water-soluble form of prednisolone for intravenous injec-tion and as an ointment.

Prednisolone (1129-c)

Prednisolone (BAN, rINN).
1,2-Dehydrohydrocortisone; Deltahydrocortisone; Δ¹-Hydro-cortisone; Metacortandralone; NSC-9120; Prednisolonum. 11β,17α,21-Trihydroxypregna-1,4-diene-3,20-dione.
$C_{21}H_{28}O_5 = 360.4$.
CAS — 50-24-8 (anhydrous prednisolone); 52438-85-4 (prednisolone sesquihydrate).
ATC — A07EA01; C05AA04; D07AA03; D07XA02; H02AB06; R01AD02; S01BA04; S01CB02; S02BA03; S03BA02.
Pharmacopoeias. In Chin., Eur. (see p.vi), Int., Jpn., and Pol. US al-lows the anhydrous form or the sesquihydrate.

Pharmacopoeial description

Ph. Eur.: A white or almost white, hygroscopic, crystalline powder. It shows polymorphism. Very slightly soluble in water; soluble in alcohol and in methyl alcohol; sparingly soluble in acetone; slightly soluble in dichloromethane. Store in airtight containers. Protect from light.

USP 25: It is anhydrous or contains one and one-half mole-cules of water of hydration. A white to practically white, odourless, crystalline powder. Very slightly soluble in water; soluble 1 in 30 of alcohol, 1 in 50 of acetone, and 1 in 180 of chloroform; soluble in dioxan and in methyl alcohol.

The symbol † denotes a preparation no longer actively marketed

Prednisolone Acetate (1122-s)

Prednisolone Acetate (BANM, rINNM).

Prednisoloni Acetas. Prednisolone 21-acetate.

$C_{23}H_{30}O_6 = 402.5$.

CAS — 52-21-1.

Pharmacopoeias. In Chin., Eur. (see p.vi), Int., Jpn, Pol., and US.

Prednisolone acetate 11 mg is approximately equivalent to 10 mg of prednisolone.

Pharmacopoeial description

Ph. Eur.: A white or almost white, crystalline powder. Practically insoluble in water; slightly soluble in alcohol and in dichloromethane. Protect from light.

USP 25: A white to practically white, odourless, crystalline powder. Practically insoluble in water; soluble 1 in 120 of alcohol; slightly soluble in acetone and in chloroform.

Prednisolone Caproate (1123-w)

Prednisolone Caproate (rINNM).

Prednisolone Hexanoate (BANM). Prednisolone 21-hexanoate.

$C_{27}H_{38}O_6 = 458.6$.

Prednisolone caproate 127 mg is approximately equivalent to 100 mg of prednisolone.

Prednisolone Hydrogen Succinate (1128-z)

Prednisolone Hydrogen Succinate (BANM, rINNM).

Prednisolone Hemisuccinate. Prednisolone 21-(hydrogen succinate).

$C_{25}H_{32}O_8 = 460.5$.

CAS — 2920-86-7.

Pharmacopoeias. In Jpn and US.

Prednisolone hydrogen succinate 128 mg is approximately equivalent to 100 mg of prednisolone.

Pharmacopoeial description

USP 25: A fine, creamy-white, practically odourless, powder with friable lumps. Soluble 1 in 4170 of water, 1 in 6.3 of alcohol, 1 in 1064 of chloroform, and 1 in 248 of ether; soluble in acetone. Store in airtight containers.

Prednisolone Metasulfobenzoate Sodium

(1125-l)

Prednisolone Metasulfobenzoate Sodium (rINNM).

Prednisolone Metasulphobenzoate Sodium (BANM); Prednisolone Sodium Metasulphobenzoate; R-812. Prednisolone 21-(sodium m-sulphobenzoate).

$C_{28}H_{31}NaO_9S = 566.6$.

CAS — 630-67-1.

Prednisolone metasulfobenzoate sodium 157 mg is approximately equivalent to 100 mg of prednisolone.

Prednisolone Pivalate (1124-e)

Prednisolone Pivalate (BANM, rINNM).

Prednisolone Trimethylacetate; Prednisoloni Pivalas. Prednisolone 21-pivalate.

$C_{26}H_{36}O_6 = 444.6$.

CAS — 1107-99-9.

Pharmacopoeias. In Eur. (see p.vi) and Pol.

Prednisolone pivalate 123 mg is approximately equivalent to 100 mg of prednisolone.

Pharmacopoeial description

Ph. Eur.: A white, or almost white, crystalline powder. Practically insoluble in water; slightly soluble in alcohol; soluble in dichloromethane. Protect from light.

Prednisolone Sodium Phosphate (1126-y)

Prednisolone Sodium Phosphate (BANM, rINNM).

Prednisoloni Natrii Phosphas. Prednisolone 21-(disodium orthophosphate).

$C_{21}H_{27}Na_2O_8P = 484.4$.

CAS — 125-02-0.

NOTE. PRED is a code approved by the BP 2001 for use on single unit doses of eye drops containing prednisolone sodium phosphate where the individual container may be too small to bear all the appropriate labelling information.

Pharmacopoeias. In Eur. (see p.vi) and US.

Prednisolone sodium phosphate 27 mg is approximately equivalent to 20 mg of prednisolone.

Pharmacopoeial description

Ph. Eur.: A white or almost white, hygroscopic, crystalline powder. Freely soluble in water; very slightly soluble in alcohol. A 5% solution in water has a pH of 7.5 to 9.0. Protect from light.

USP 25: A white or slightly yellow friable granules or powder. Is odourless or has a slight odour. Is slightly hygroscopic. Soluble 1 in 4 of water and 1 in 13 of methyl alcohol; slightly soluble in alcohol and in chloroform; very slightly soluble in acetone and in dioxan. pH of a 1% solution in water is between 7.5 and 10.5. Store in airtight containers.

Prednisolone Sodium Succinate (16319-s)

Prednisolone Sodium Succinate (BANM, rINNM).

Prednisolone Sodium Hemisuccinate. 11β,17α,21-Trihydroxypregna-1,4-diene-3,20-dione 21-(sodium succinate).

$C_{25}H_{31}NaO_8 = 482.5$.

CAS — 1715-33-9.

Pharmacopoeias. US includes Prednisolone Sodium Succinate for Injection.

Prednisolone sodium succinate 134 mg is approximately equivalent to 100 mg of prednisolone.

Pharmacopoeial description

USP 25: Prednisolone Sodium Succinate for Injection is a creamy white powder with friable lumps, having a slight odour.

Prednisolone Steaglate (1127-j)

Prednisolone Steaglate (BAN, rINN).

Prednisolone 21-stearoylglycolate.

$C_{41}H_{64}O_8 = 684.9$.

CAS — 5060-55-9.

Prednisolone steaglate 190 mg is approximately equivalent to 100 mg of prednisolone.

Prednisolone Tebutate (1121-p)

Prednisolone Tebutate (BANM, rINNM).

Prednisolone Butylacetate; Prednisolone 21-tert-Butylacetate; Prednisolone Tertiary-butylacetate. Prednisolone 21-(3,3-dimethylbutyrate).

$C_{27}H_{38}O_6,H_2O = 476.6$.

CAS — 7681-14-3 (anhydrous prednisolone tebutate).

Pharmacopoeias. In US.

Prednisolone tebutate 132 mg is approximately equivalent to 100 mg of prednisolone.

Pharmacopoeial description

USP 25: A white to slightly yellow, hygroscopic, free-flowing powder, which may show some soft lumps. Is odourless or has not more than a moderate characteristic odour. Very slightly soluble in water; sparingly soluble in alcohol and in methyl alcohol; soluble in acetone; freely soluble in chloroform and in dioxan. Store in airtight containers sealed under nitrogen at a temperature not exceeding 8°.

Adverse Effects, Treatment, Withdrawal, and Precautions

As for corticosteroids in general (see p.1039).

Owing to its less pronounced mineralocorticoid activity prednisolone is less likely than cortisone or hydrocortisone to cause sodium retention, electrolyte imbalance, and oedema. Prolonged application to the eye of preparations containing corticosteroids has caused raised intra-ocular pressure and reduced visual function.

Hepatic impairment. Conversion of prednisone to prednisolone has been reported to be impaired in chronic active liver disease.[1,2] However, although plasma-prednisolone concentrations were found to be more predictable after administration of prednisolone than of prednisone to a group of healthy subjects,[3] no difference was noted in patients with chronic active hepatitis, in whom impaired elimination of prednisolone compensated for any impaired conversion of prednisone. A review of the pharmacokinetics of prednisone and prednisolone[4] concluded that fear of inadequate conversion of prednisone into prednisolone was not justified.

1. Powell LW, Axelsen E. Corticosteroids in liver disease: studies on the biological conversion of prednisone to prednisolone and plasma protein binding. *Gut* 1972; **13:** 690–6.
2. Madsbad S, *et al.* Impaired conversion of prednisone to prednisolone in patients with liver cirrhosis. *Gut* 1980; **21:** 52–6.
3. Davis M, *et al.* Prednisone or prednisolone for the treatment of chronic active hepatitis? A comparison of plasma availability. *Br J Clin Pharmacol* 1978; **5:** 501–5.
4. Frey BM, Frey FJ. Clinical pharmacokinetics of prednisone and prednisolone. *Clin Pharmacokinet* 1990; **19:** 126–46.

Inflammatory bowel disease. Symptoms recurred in a patient with Crohn's disease on changing from conventional to enteric-coated tablets of prednisolone.[1] This was not an isolated occurrence in the authors' unit, and it was advocated that only non-enteric-coated prednisolone tablets should be used in Crohn's disease, and that the enteric-coated form be used with caution in any condition characterised by diarrhoea or a rapid transit time.

1. Beattie RM, Walker-Smith JA. Use of enteric coated prednisolone in Crohn's disease. *Arch Dis Child* 1994; **71:** 282.

Interactions

The interactions of corticosteroids in general are described on p.1043.

Pharmacokinetics

For a brief outline of the pharmacokinetics of corticosteroids, see p.1044.

Prednisolone and prednisone are both readily absorbed from the gastrointestinal tract, but whereas prednisolone already exists in a metabolically active form, prednisone must be converted in the liver to its active metabolite, prednisolone. In general, this conversion is rapid so this difference is of little consequence when seen in the light of intersubject variation in the pharmacokinetics of prednisolone itself; bioavailability also depends on the dissolution rates of the tablet formulations. As discussed under Hepatic Impairment, above, the possibility of reduced corticosteroid concentrations following administration of prednisone to patients with liver disease does not seem to be a problem in practice. Following intramuscular administration the sodium phosphate ester of prednisolone is rapidly absorbed whereas the acetate, in the suspension form, is only slowly absorbed.

Peak plasma concentrations of prednisolone are obtained 1 or 2 hours after administration by mouth, and it has a usual plasma half-life of 2 to 4 hours. Its initial absorption, but not its overall bioavailability, is affected by food.

Prednisolone is extensively bound to plasma proteins, although less so than hydrocortisone (cortisol). The volume of distribution, and also the clearance are reported to increase with an increase from low to moderate doses; at very high doses, clearance appears to become saturated.

Prednisolone is excreted in the urine as free and conjugated metabolites, together with an appreciable proportion of unchanged prednisolone. Prednisolone is largely inactivated as it crosses the placenta; small amounts are excreted in breast milk.

Prednisolone has a biological half-life lasting several hours, intermediate between those of hydrocortisone (cortisol) and the longer-acting glucocorticoids, such as dexamethasone. It is this intermediate duration of action which makes it suitable for the alternate-day administration regimens which have been found to reduce the risk of adrenocortical insufficiency, yet provide adequate corticosteroid coverage in some disorders.

◊ General reviews of the pharmacokinetics of prednisolone[1,2] and some references to its pharmacokinetics in healthy subjects[3] and in various disease states.[4-8]

1. Begg EJ, *et al.* The pharmacokinetics of corticosteroid agents. *Med J Aust* 1987; **146:** 37–41.
2. Frey BM, Frey FJ. Clinical pharmacokinetics of prednisone and prednisolone. *Clin Pharmacokinet* 1990; **19:** 126–46.
3. Rohatagi S, *et al.* Pharmacokinetics of methylprednisolone and prednisolone after single and multiple oral administration. *J Clin Pharmacol* 1997; **37:** 916–25.
4. Berghouse LM, *et al.* Plasma prednisolone levels during intravenous therapy in acute colitis. *Gut* 1982; **23:** 980–3.
5. Shaffer JA, *et al.* Absorption of prednisolone in patients with Crohn's disease. *Gut* 1983; **24:** 182–6.
6. Reece PA, *et al.* Prednisolone protein binding in renal transplant patients. *Br J Clin Pharmacol* 1985; **20:** 159–62.
7. Frey FJ, *et al.* Altered metabolism and decreased efficacy of prednisolone and prednisone in patients with hyperthyroidism. *Clin Pharmacol Ther* 1988; **44:** 510–21.
8. Miller PFW, *et al.* Pharmacokinetics of prednisolone in children with nephrosis. *Arch Dis Child* 1990; **65:** 196–200.

Distribution into breast milk. Concentrations of prednisone and prednisolone in breast milk from one lactating woman 120 minutes after prednisone 10 mg by mouth were found to be 26.7 nanograms and 1.6 nanograms per mL respectively.[1] In 7 similar women given a single 5-mg dose of tritium-labelled prednisolone by mouth, a mean of 0.14% of the radioactivity from the dose was recovered per litre of milk during the following 48 to 61 hours.[2]

1. Katz FH, Duncan BE. Entry of prednisone into human milk. *N Engl J Med* 1975; **293:** 1154.
2. McKenzie SA, *et al.* Secretion of prednisolone into breast milk. *Arch Dis Child* 1975; **50:** 894–6.

Uses and Administration

Prednisolone is a corticosteroid with mainly glucocorticoid activity (p.1039); 5 mg of prednisolone is equivalent in anti-inflammatory activity to about 25 mg of cortisone acetate. In general, prednisolone, either in the form of the free alcohol or in one of the esterified forms, is the drug of choice in the UK for conditions in which routine systemic corticosteroid therapy is indicated (see p.1044), except adrenocortical-deficiency states for which hydrocortisone with supplementary fludrocortisone is preferred. The more potent pituitary-suppressant properties of a glucocorticoid such as dexamethasone may, however, be required for the diagnosis and management of conditions associated with adrenal hyperplasia.

For administration by mouth prednisolone is usually used although prednisolone sodium phosphate or prednisolone steaglate are also employed; the usual dose, expressed in terms of prednisolone, is about 5 to 60 mg daily in divided doses, as a single daily dose after breakfast, or as a double dose on alternate days. Alternate-day early-morning dosage regimens produce less suppression of the hypothalamic-pituitary axis but may not always provide adequate control. Enteric-coated tablets of prednisolone are also available (for the view that these should not be employed in patients with inflammatory bowel disease, see above).

For parenteral administration the sodium phosphate ester is normally employed and may be given intravenously by injection or infusion or intramuscularly by injection; doses appear to have been variously expressed in terms of prednisolone, prednisolone phosphate, or prednisolone sodium phosphate but are generally within the range of 4 to 60 mg daily. An aqueous suspension of prednisolone acetate is also used intramuscularly to give a prolonged effect with doses of 25 to 100 mg of the acetate being given once or twice weekly. The sodium succinate ester has also been given parenterally.

For intra-articular injection the acetate, sodium phosphate, and tebutate esters are used. Suggested doses are 5 to 25 mg of prednisolone acetate, 2 to 30 mg of prednisolone phosphate (for the sodium phosphate ester), and 4 to 40 mg of prednisolone tebutate. The sodium phosphate and tebutate esters are also given by intralesional injection and by injection into soft tissue.

Prednisolone acetate and prednisolone sodium phosphate are also used in the topical treatment of allergic and inflammatory conditions of the eyes or ears, usually as drops containing 0.5% or 1%. Prednisolone has also been used topically as the free alcohol and as the hemisuccinate, pivalate, and metasulfobenzoate sodium esters.

For rectal use prednisolone metasulfobenzoate sodium or prednisolone sodium phosphate are often employed. Retention enemas containing the equivalent of 20 mg of prednisolone per 100 mL, rectal foam containing the equivalent of 20 mg of prednisolone per dose, or suppositories containing the equivalent of 5 mg of prednisolone are available. Prednisolone has also been used rectally as the free alcohol and as the acetate and caproate esters.

Other esters of prednisolone which have occasionally been used include the palmitate and sodium tetrahydrophthalate.

Preparations

BP 2001: Enteric-coated Prednisolone Tablets; Prednisolone Enema; Prednisolone Sodium Phosphate Eye Drops; Prednisolone Tablets;
USP 25: Chloramphenicol and Prednisolone Ophthalmic Ointment; Gentamicin and Prednisolone Acetate Ophthalmic Ointment; Neomycin and Polymyxin B Sulfates and Prednisolone Acetate Ophthalmic Suspension; Neomycin Sulfate and Prednisolone Acetate Ointment; Neomycin Sulfate and Prednisolone Acetate Ophthalmic Ointment; Neomycin Sulfate and Prednisolone Sodium Phosphate Ophthalmic Ointment; Neomycin Sulfate, Sulfacetamide Sodium, and Prednisolone Acetate Ophthalmic Ointment; Prednisolone Acetate Injectable Suspension; Prednisolone Acetate Ophthalmic Suspension; Prednisolone Cream; Prednisolone Sodium Phosphate Injection; Prednisolone Sodium Phosphate Ophthalmic Solution; Prednisolone Sodium Succinate for Injection; Prednisolone Syrup; Prednisolone Tablets; Prednisolone Tebutate Injectable Suspension; Sulfacetamide Sodium and Prednisolone Acetate Ophthalmic Ointment; Sulfacetamide Sodium and Prednisolone Acetate Ophthalmic Suspension.

Proprietary Preparations (details are given in Part 3)
Aust.: Aprednislon; Kuhlprednon; Prednihexal; Rectopred; Solu-Dacortin; Ultracortenol; *Australia.:* Deltasolone†; Panafcortelone; Predsol; Redipred; Solone; Sterofrin; *Belg.:* Deltacortril; Pred Forte; Prednicortelone; Solu-Dacortine; *Braz.:* Pred Fort; *Canad.:* Diopred; Inflamase; Ophtho-Tate; Pediapred; Pred Forte; Pred Mild; *Denm.:* Pred-Clysma; Predniment†; Ultracortenol; *Fin.:* Di-Adreson-F; Pred Forte; Predniment; Ultracortenol; *Fr.:* Hydrocortancyl; Solucort; Solupred; *Ger.:* Decapredvil; Decortin H; Dontisolon D; duraprednisolon; hefasolon; Inflanefran; Klismacort; Linola-H N; Linola-H-Fett N; Prectal; Predna-

bene; Predni; Predni H; Predni-Ophtal; Predni-POS; Prednihexal; Prednisolut; Solu-Decortin-H; Ultracortenol; *Hong Kong:* Dhasolone; Di-Adreson-F; Panafcortelone; Pred Forte; Pred Mild; Predenema; Predfoam; Sintisone; Ultracortenol; *Irl.:* Deltacortril; Pred Forte; Pred Mild; Predenema; Predfoam; Prednesol; Predsol; *Israel:* Prelone; Ultracorten H; Ultracortenol; *Ital.:* Meticortelone; Soludacortin; *Mex.:* Delta-Diona; Fisopred; Pred; Prednefrin SF; Sophipren; *Neth.:* Di-Adreson-F; Pred Forte†; Ultracortenol; *Norw.:* Pred-Clysma; Ultracortenol; *NZ:* Pred Forte; Pred Mild; Predsol; Redipred; *Port.:* Frisolona; Lepicortinolo; Predniocil; Sintisone; Solu-Dacortina; *S.Afr.:* Capsoid; Lenisolone; Meticortelone; Pred Mild; Predeltilone†; Predsol; Prelone; *Singapore:* Pred; Walesolone; Xepasone; *Spain:* Dacortin H; Estilsona; Normonsona†; Pred Forte; Solu-Dacortin H†; *Swed.:* Precortalon aquosum; Pred-Clysma; Sintisone†; Ultracortenol; *Switz.:* Corti-Clyss; Hexacortone; Pred Forte; Pred Mild; Predni-Helvacort†; Solu-Dacortine; Spiricort; Ultracortene-H; Ultracortenol; *Thai.:* Di-Adreson-F; Inf-Oph; Opredsone; Polypred; Pred Forte; Pred Mild; Predisole; Prednersone; Predninol; Prenilone; *UAE:* Gupisone; *UK:* Deltacortril; Deltastab; Precortisyl; Pred Forte; Predenema; Predfoam; Prednesol†; Predsol; *USA:* Ak-Pred; Articulose-50†; Delta-Cortef; Econopred; Hydeltra-TBA†; Hydeltrasol; Inflamase; Key-Pred; Key-Pred-SP; Orapred; Pediapred; Pred; Pred Forte; Pred Mild; Pred-Phosphate; Predalone; Predcor; Prednisol; Prelone.

Multi-ingredient: Aust.: Alpicort; Blephamide; Delta-Hadensa; Delta-Tomanol†; Phoscortil; Scheriproct; *Australia.:* Blephamide; Prednefrin; Scheriproct; *Belg.:* Cetapred; Hemosedan; Isopto Cetapred; Predmycin; Scheriproct; Sofrasolone; Viscocort†; *Braz.:* Asmosterona; Colutoide; Dermicin; Fonergin; Isopto Cetapred; Polipred; Predmicin; Prenefrin; Proctium; Reumazine; Rifocort; *Canad.:* Blephamide; Dioptimyd; Metimyd†; Vasocidin; *Fin.:* Scheriproct; Septison; *Fr.:* Colicort; Cortisal; Deliproct; Derinox; Desocort†; Deturgylone; Tergynan†; *Ger.:* Adeptolon†; Alferm†; Alpicort F neu; Alpicort N; Anumedin; Aquapred; Berlicetin-Ohrentropfen; Bismolan H Corti; Blefcon; Blephamide; Corti-Dynexan; Dexa-Phlogont L; Imazol comp; Inflanegent; Leioderm P; Linola-H-compositum N; Linoladiol-H N; Lygal Kopftinktur; NeyChondrin N (Revitorgan-Dilutionen N Nr 68); NeyNormin N (Revitorgan-Dilutionen N Nr 65); NeyTumorin N (Revitorgan-Dilutionen N Nr 66); Prednitracin; Scheriproct; Thesit P; Ultra-Demoplas; Virunguent P; *Hong Kong:* Blephamide; Chlomy-P; Cortison-Kemicetine; Prednitracin; *Irl.:* Scheriproct; *Israel:* Aflumycin; Blephamide; Prednistyle; Threolone; *Ital.:* Bio-Delta Cortilen; Deltamidrina; Dutimelan†; Solprene; *Mex.:* Blefamide SF; Deltamid; Metimyd; Premid; Scheriproct; *Neth.:* Predmycin-P Liquifilm†; *Norw.:* Scheriproct; *NZ:* Blephamide; *Port.:* Anacal; Blifamol; Conjunctilone-S; Flogiftalmina; Meocil; Mobilat†; Neo-Davisolona; Predniderma; Predniftalmina; Scheriproct; Vitasma; *S.Afr.:* Blephamide; Pred G; Scheriproct; *Singapore:* Blephamide; Predmycin-P; *Spain:* Alergical; Antigrietun; Cortivel†; Kanapomada; Lidrone; Nasopomada; Otonina; Poly Pred; Predni Azuleno; Proctium; Rinobanedif; Rinovel; Ruscus; Scheriproct; Teolixir Compositum; *Swed.:* Blefcon†; Metimyd; Scheriproct N; *Switz.:* Alpicort; Alpicort F; Blephamide; Calpred; Derinox; Imacort; Locaseptil-Neo; Mycinopred; Nystacortone; Pred G†; Prednitracin; Premandol; Scheriproct; *Thai.:* Denson; Farakil; Levoptin; Mysolone-N; Neopred; Neozolone; Otosil; Pred Oph; Predex; Predmycin; Prednisil; Prednisil-N; Scheriproct; *UK:* Predsol-N; Scheriproct; *USA:* Ak-Cide; Blephamide; Cetapred; Isopto Cetapred; Metimyd; Optimyd†; Poly-Pred; Pred G; Sulfamide; Sulster†; Vasocidin; Vasocine.

Prednisone (1131-w)

Prednisone (BAN, rINN).

Δ^1-Cortisone; 1,2-Dehydrocortisone; Deltacortisone; Deltadehydrocortisone; Metacortandracin; NSC-10023; Prednisonum. 17α,21-Dihydroxypregna-1,4-diene-3,11,20-trione.
$C_{21}H_{26}O_5 = 358.4$.
CAS — 53-03-2.
ATC — A07EA03; H02AB07.

Pharmacopoeias. In *Eur.* (see p.vi). *US* allows the anhydrous form or the monohydrate.

Pharmacopoeial description

Ph. Eur.: A white or almost white, crystalline powder. It shows polymorphism. Practically insoluble in water; slightly soluble in alcohol and in dichloromethane. Protect from light.

USP 25: It contains one molecule of water of hydration or is anhydrous. A white to practically white, odourless, crystalline powder. Very slightly soluble in water; soluble 1 in 150 of alcohol and 1 in 200 of chloroform; slightly soluble in dioxan and in methyl alcohol.

Prednisone Acetate (1130-s)

Prednisone Acetate (BANM, rINNM).
Prednisone 21-acetate.
$C_{23}H_{28}O_6 = 400.5$.
CAS — 125-10-0.

Pharmacopoeias. In *Chin.* and *Pol.*

Prednisone acetate 11 mg is approximately equivalent to 10 mg of prednisone.

Profile

Prednisone is a biologically inert corticosteroid which is converted to the predominantly glucocorticoid corticosteroid prednisolone in the liver. It has the same chemical relationship to prednisolone as cortisone has to hydrocortisone. The indications and dos-

age of prednisone for oral use are exactly the same as those for prednisolone (see p.1078, and the chapter introduction, p.1044).

In the UK prednisolone has historically been preferred to prednisone, on the grounds that it does not require conversion to the active substance, but in practice this is rarely significant (see Hepatic Impairment, under Prednisolone, p.1078), and in some countries, such as the USA, prednisone is the drug of choice for many of the conditions in which routine systemic corticosteroid therapy is indicated.

Preparations

USP 25: Prednisone Oral Solution; Prednisone Tablets.

Proprietary Preparations (details are given in Part 3)
Austral.: Deltasone†; Panafcort; Sone; *Belg.:* Prednicort; *Braz.:* Meticorten; Predicorten; *Canad.:* Deltasone†; Winpred; *Fr.:* Cortancyl; *Ger.:* Decortin; Predni Tablinen; Rectodelt; *Hong Kong:* Deltasone; *Israel:* Prednitone; *Ital.:* Deltacortene; *Mex.:* Meprosona-F; Meticorten; Ofisolona; Predicor; Prednidib; Promifen; *NZ:* Deltasone; *Port.:* Meticorten; *S.Afr.:* Meticorten; Panafcort; Predeltin; Pulmison; Trolic†; *Spain:* Dacortin; *Swed.:* Deltison; *USA:* Deltasone; Liquid Pred; Meticorten; Orasone†; Panasol-S; Sterapred.

Multi-ingredient: Aust.: Fluorex Plus; Oleomycetin-Prednison; *Canad.:* Metreton; *Ger.:* Oleomycetin-Prednison; *Mex.:* Pre Clor; *Port.:* Ciclobiotico; *Spain:* Coliriocilina Prednisona; Fiacin; Kanafosal Predni; Prednis Neomic.

Prednylidene (1132-e)

Prednylidene (BAN, rINN).

16-Methyleneprednisolone. 11β,17α,21-Trihydroxy-16-methylenepregna-1,4-diene-3,20-dione.
$C_{22}H_{28}O_5 = 372.5$.
CAS — 599-33-7.
ATC — H02AB11.

Profile

Prednylidene is a corticosteroid that has been used for its glucocorticoid activity similarly to prednisolone (see p.1078). It has been given by mouth as the free alcohol and by injection as the diethylaminoacetate hydrochloride.

Preparations

Proprietary Preparations (details are given in Part 3)
Ger.: Decortilen; *Swed.:* Dacortilen†.

Procinonide (6449-m)

Procinonide (USAN, rINN).

RS-2362. (6α,11β,16α)-6,9-Difluoro-11-hydroxy-16,17-[(1-methylethylidene)bis(oxy)]-21-(1-oxopropoxy)-pregna-1,4-diene-3,20-dione.
$C_{27}H_{34}F_2O_7 = 508.6$.
CAS — 58497-00-0.

Profile

Procinonide is a derivative of fluocinolone acetonide (p.1071) that has been applied topically in combination with fluocinonide and ciprocinonide in the management of various skin disorders.

Preparations

Proprietary Preparations (details are given in Part 3)
Multi-ingredient: Canad.: Trisyn†.

Rimexolone (5646-d)

Rimexolone (BAN, USAN, rINN).

Org-6216. 11β-Hydroxy-16α,17α-dimethyl-17β-propionylandrosta-1,4-dien-3-one.
$C_{24}H_{34}O_3 = 370.5$.
CAS — 49697-38-3.
ATC — H02AB12; S01BA13.
Pharmacopoeias. In *US*.

Pharmacopoeial description

USP 25: A white to off-white powder. Freely soluble in chloroform; sparingly soluble in methyl alcohol.

Profile

Rimexolone is a corticosteroid applied topically to the eye for its glucocorticoid activity (see p.1039) in the treatment of inflammatory eye disorders including uveitis (p.1060) and postoperative inflammation. It is used as a 1% suspension.

Prolonged application to the eye of preparations containing corticosteroids has caused raised intra-ocular pressure and reduced visual function.

Preparations

USP 25: Rimexolone Ophthalmic Suspension.

Proprietary Preparations (details are given in Part 3)
Aust.: Vexol; *Belg.:* Vexolon; *Canad.:* Vexol; *Denm.:* Vexol; *Fin.:* Vexol; *Fr.:* Vexol; *Ger.:* Vexol; *Irl.:* Vexol; *Ital.:* Vexol; *Port.:* Vexol; *Spain:* Vexol; *Swed.:* Vexol; *Switz.:* Vexol; *UK:* Vexol; *USA:* Vexol.

The symbol † denotes a preparation no longer actively marketed

Suprarenal Cortex (1133-l)

Suprarenal cortex contains a number of steroid compounds the most active of which are corticosterone, dehydrocorticosterone, hydrocortisone, cortisone, and aldosterone. It has been prepared from the adrenal glands of oxen.

Profile

Suprarenal cortex was formerly used intramuscularly for the treatment of adrenocortical insufficiency but it has been superseded by hydrocortisone and other corticosteroids (see p.1046). Suprarenal cortex is an ingredient of a wide range of preparations, often together with other organ extracts or vitamins, promoted for indications ranging from asthenia to liver disorders.

Preparations

Proprietary Preparations (details are given in Part 3)
Aust.: Cortiglanden; *Fr.:* Cortine Naturelle†; *Spain:* Pleocortex.
Multi-ingredient: *Aust.:* Flexurat; Mobilat; *Belg.:* Cromaton†; Mobilat; *Braz.:* Broncopinol; Suprasten; *Canad.:* Heracline; Revitonus C; *Fin.:* Mobilat; *Ger.:* Arthrodeformat P; Flexurat†; Mobilat; *Hong Kong:* Mobilat; *Singapore:* Mobilat; *Spain:* Movilat; Neurocatavin Dexa; Pleocortex B6; Rubrocortin; *Switz.:* Mobilat†; *Thai.:* Mobilat.

Tixocortol Pivalate (13356-y)

Tixocortol Pivalate (BANM, USAN, rINNM).
JO-1016. 11β,17α-Dihydroxy-21-mercaptopregn-4-ene-3,20-dione 21-pivalate.
$C_{26}H_{38}O_5S = 462.6$.
CAS — 61951-99-3 (tixocortol); 55560-96-8 (tixocortol pivalate).

Profile

Tixocortol pivalate is a corticosteroid with mainly glucocorticoid activity, as described under Corticosteroids, p.1039. It is used as buccal, nasal, throat, and rectal preparations. It is reported to undergo rapid first-pass metabolism, primarily in the liver, and to have minimal systemic effect.

Preparations

Proprietary Preparations (details are given in Part 3)
Belg.: Rhinovalon; *Canad.:* Rectovalone†; *Fr.:* Pivalone; Rectovalone†; *Neth.:* Pivalone†; Rectovalone; *Singapore:* Pivalone; *Spain:* Rectovalone; Tiovalone; *Switz.:* Pivalone.
Multi-ingredient: *Belg.:* Rhinovalon Neomycine; *Fr.:* Dontopivalone†; Oropivalone Bacitracine; Pivalone Neomycine; Thiovalone; *Singapore:* Pivalone Neomycin; *Switz.:* Oro-Pivalone; Pivalone compositum.

Triamcinolone (1134-y)

Triamcinolone (BAN, rINN).
9α-Fluoro-16α-hydroxyprednisolone; Fluoxiprednisolonum. 9α-Fluoro-11β,16α,17α,21-tetrahydroxypregna-1,4-diene-3,20-dione.
$C_{21}H_{27}FO_6 = 394.4$.
CAS — 124-94-7.
ATC — A01AC01; D07AB09; D07XB02; H02AB08; R01AD11; R03BA06; S01BA05.
Pharmacopoeias. In Eur. (see p.vi), Jpn, Pol., and US.

Pharmacopoeial description

Ph. Eur.: A white or almost white, crystalline powder. It shows polymorphism. Practically insoluble in water and in dichloromethane; slightly soluble in methyl alcohol. Protect from light.

USP 25: A white or practically white, odourless, crystalline powder. Very slightly soluble in water, in chloroform, and in ether; slightly soluble in alcohol and in methyl alcohol.

Triamcinolone Acetonide (1137-c)

Triamcinolone Acetonide (BANM, rINNM).
CL-61965 (triamcinolone acetonide sodium phosphate); CL-106359 (triamcinolone acetonide sodium phosphate); Triamcinoloni Acetonidum. 9α-Fluoro-11β,21-dihydroxy-16α,17α-isopropylidenedioxypregna-1,4-diene-3,20-dione.
$C_{24}H_{31}FO_6 = 434.5$.
CAS — 76-25-5 (triamcinolone acetonide); 1997-15-5 (triamcinolone acetonide sodium phosphate); 989-96-8 (triamcinolone acetonide 21-(dihydrogen phosphate)).

NOTE. Triamcinolone Acetonide Sodium Phosphate is USAN.
Pharmacopoeias. In Eur. (see p.vi), Jpn, Pol., and US.
Chin. includes Triamcinolone Acetonide Acetate.

Triamcinolone acetonide 11 mg is approximately equivalent to 10 mg of triamcinolone.

Pharmacopoeial description

Ph. Eur.: A white or almost white, crystalline powder. It shows polymorphism. Practically insoluble in water; sparingly soluble in alcohol; very slightly soluble in ether. Protect from light.

USP 25: A white to cream-coloured crystalline powder, having not more than a slight odour. Practically insoluble in water; sparingly soluble in dehydrated alcohol, in chloroform, and in methyl alcohol.

Triamcinolone Diacetate (1136-z)

Triamcinolone Diacetate (BANM, rINNM).
Triamcinolone 16α,21-diacetate.
$C_{25}H_{31}FO_8 = 478.5$.
CAS — 67-78-7.
Pharmacopoeias. In US.

Triamcinolone diacetate 12 mg is approximately equivalent to 10 mg of triamcinolone.

Pharmacopoeial description

USP 25: A fine, white to off-white, crystalline powder, having not more than a slight odour. Practically insoluble in water; soluble 1 in 13 of alcohol, 1 in 80 of chloroform, and 1 in 40 of methyl alcohol; slightly soluble in ether.

Triamcinolone Hexacetonide (1135-j)

Triamcinolone Hexacetonide (BAN, USAN, rINN).
CL-34433; TATBA; Triamcinolone Acetonide 21-(3,3-Dimethylbutyrate); Triamcinoloni Hexacetonidum. 9α-Fluoro-11β,21-dihydroxy-16α,17α-isopropylidenedioxypregna-1,4-diene-3,20-dione 21-(3,3-dimethylbutyrate).
$C_{30}H_{41}FO_7 = 532.6$.
CAS — 5611-51-8.
Pharmacopoeias. In Eur. (see p.vi) and US.

Triamcinolone hexacetonide 14 mg is approximately equivalent to 10 mg of triamcinolone.

Pharmacopoeial description

Ph. Eur.: A white or almost white, crystalline powder. Practically insoluble in water; sparingly soluble in dehydrated alcohol and in methyl alcohol. Protect from light.

USP 25: A white to cream-coloured powder. Practically insoluble in water; soluble in chloroform; slightly soluble in methyl alcohol.

Adverse Effects, Treatment, Withdrawal, and Precautions

As for corticosteroids in general (see p.1039). High doses of triamcinolone may have a greater tendency to produce proximal myopathy. Its effects on sodium and water retention are less than those of prednisolone.

When applied topically, particularly to large areas, when the skin is broken, or under occlusive dressings, or when given intranasally, corticosteroids may be absorbed in sufficient amounts to cause systemic effects.

Hypersensitivity. Local reactions to topical triamcinolone preparations have been attributed to the content of ethylenediamine.[1,2] However, there have also been reports of anaphylactic shock following intra-articular[3] or intramuscular[4] injection of triamcinolone acetonide.

1. Wright S, Harman RRM. Ethylenediamine and piperazine sensitivity. *BMJ* 1983; **287:** 463–4.
2. Freeman S. Allergy to Kenacomb cream. *Med J Aust* 1986; **145:** 361.
3. Larsson L. Anaphylactic shock after ia administration of triamcinolone acetonide in a 35-year-old female. *Scand J Rheumatol* 1989; **18:** 441–2.
4. Gonzalo FE, *et al.* Anaphylactic shock caused by triamcinolone acetonide. *Ann Pharmacother* 1994; **28:** 1310.

Pharmacokinetics

For a brief outline of the pharmacokinetics of corticosteroids, see p.1044.

Triamcinolone is reported to have a half-life in plasma of about 2 to over 5 hours. It is bound to plasma albumin to a much smaller extent than hydrocortisone.

The acetonide, diacetate, and hexacetonide esters of triamcinolone are only very slowly absorbed from injection sites.

Triamcinolone crosses the placenta.

◊ References to the pharmacokinetics of triamcinolone and its esters.

1. Möllmann H, *et al.* Pharmacokinetics of triamcinolone acetonide and its phosphate ester. *Eur J Clin Pharmacol* 1985; **29:** 85–9.
2. Derendorf H, *et al.* Pharmacokinetics and pharmacodynamics of glucocorticoid suspensions after intra-articular administration. *Clin Pharmacol Ther* 1986; **39:** 313–17.
3. Derendorf H, *et al.* Pharmacokinetics of triamcinolone acetonide after intravenous, oral, and inhaled administration. *J Clin Pharmacol* 1995; **35:** 302–5.

Uses and Administration

Triamcinolone is a corticosteroid with mainly glucocorticoid activity (p.1039); 4 mg of triamcinolone is equivalent in anti-inflammatory activity to about 5 mg of prednisolone. It is used, either in the form of the free alcohol or in one of the esterified forms, in the treatment of conditions for which corticosteroid therapy is indicated (see p.1044), except adrenocortical insufficiency for which hydrocortisone with supplementary fludrocortisone is preferred.

For administration by mouth triamcinolone is used in doses of 4 to 48 mg daily although daily doses over 32 mg are seldom indicated.

For parenteral administration the acetonide or diacetate esters are used in doses of about 40 mg by intramuscular injection. They are usually given as suspensions to provide a prolonged systemic effect. A dose of 40 to 100 mg of the acetonide may provide symptomatic control throughout the pollen season for hay fever sufferers (but see Rhinitis, below); for the diacetate, a 40-mg dose is administered weekly.

For intra-articular injection triamcinolone acetonide, diacetate, and hexacetonide have all been used. Doses for these esters have been in the range of 2.5 to 40 mg, 3 to 48 mg, and 2 to 30 mg respectively, depending upon the size of the joint injected.

For topical application in the treatment of various skin disorders triamcinolone acetonide is used, usually in creams, lotions, or ointments containing 0.1% although concentrations ranging from 0.025 to 0.5% have been employed. Several topical preparations also contain an antimicrobial drug. For recommendations concerning the correct use of corticosteroids on the skin, and a rough guide to the clinical potencies of topical corticosteroids, see p.1045.

Triamcinolone esters are also commonly used by intralesional or intradermal injection in the treatment of some inflammatory skin disorders such as keloids. Suggested doses for the various esters have been: acetonide, 1 to 3 mg per site with no more than 5 mg injected into any one site or not more than 30 mg in total if several sites of injection are used; diacetate, a total of 5 mg in divided doses into small lesions or up to a total of 48 mg in divided doses into large lesions with no more than 12.5 mg injected into any one site or 25 mg injected into any one lesion; hexacetonide, up to 500 µg per square inch (approximately 80 µg per cm²) of affected skin.

Triamcinolone acetonide is also used by inhalation for the control of asthma in a usual dose of about 200 µg by metered-dose inhaler three or four times daily; the dose should not exceed 1600 µg daily.

In the prophylaxis and treatment of allergic rhinitis triamcinolone acetonide may be administered by a nasal spray in a usual initial dose of 2 sprays (110 µg) into each nostril once daily, reduced to 1 spray (55 µg) when control is achieved.

Other esters of triamcinolone which have occasionally been used include the acetonide dipotassium phosphate, acetonide hemisuccinate, aminobenzal benzamidoisobutyrate, and benetonide. Another derivative of triamcinolone, flupamesone has also been used.

Asthma. Intramuscular triamcinolone acetonide has been reported to be more effective than oral low-dose prednisone in controlling exacerbations in patients with severe, chronic, life-threatening asthma,[1] although this conclusion is controversial.[2-7]

Corticosteroids and beta₂-adrenoceptor agonists form the cornerstone of the management of asthma (p.757). Inhaled corticosteroids are added to therapy with a short-acting beta₂ agonist if symptom relief with the latter is needed more than once daily, although corticosteroids with reduced systemic activity are generally preferred to triamcinolone. Systemic corticosteroids are reserved for the most severe cases, and for the management of acute severe asthma attacks (status asthmaticus).

1. Ogirala RG, *et al.* High-dose intramuscular triamcinolone in severe, chronic, life-threatening asthma. *N Engl J Med* 1991; **324:** 589–9. Correction. *ibid.;* 1380.
2. Salmeron S, *et al.* Intramuscular triamcinolone in severe asthma. *N Engl J Med* 1991; **325:** 429–30.
3. Nicholas SS. Intramuscular triamcinolone in severe asthma. *N Engl J Med* 1991; **325:** 430.
4. Kidney JC, *et al.* Intramuscular triamcinolone in severe asthma. *N Engl J Med* 1991; **325:** 430.
5. Capewell S, McLeod DT. Intramuscular triamcinolone in severe asthma. *N Engl J Med* 1991; **325:** 430.
6. Ogirala RG, *et al.* Intramuscular triamcinolone in severe asthma. *N Engl J Med* 1991; **325:** 431.
7. Capewell S, McLeod D. Injected corticosteroids in refractory asthma. *Lancet* 1991; **338:** 1075–6.

Haemangioma. For reference to the use of a mixture of triamcinolone and betamethasone for intralesional injection of haemangioma, see p.1052.

Rhinitis. Triamcinolone is used[1,2] in the management of allergic rhinitis (p.407). However, the use of depot injections of triamcinolone to manage seasonal allergic rhinitis has been deemed unacceptable by some.[3]

1. Jeal W, Faulds D. Triamcinolone acetonide: a review of its pharmacological properties and therapeutic efficacy in the management of allergic rhinitis. *Drugs* 1997; **53:** 257–80.
2. Gawchik SM, Saccar CL. A risk-benefit assessment of intranasal triamcinolone acetonide in allergic rhinitis. *Drug Safety* 2000; **23:** 309–22.
3. Anonymous. Any place for depot triamcinolone in hay fever? *Drug Ther Bull* 1999; **37:** 17–18.

Preparations

BP 2001: Triamcinolone Acetonide Injection; Triamcinolone Cream; Triamcinolone Hexacetonide Injection; Triamcinolone Ointment; Triamcinolone Oromucosal Paste; Triamcinolone Tablets;

USP 25: Neomycin Sulfate and Triamcinolone Acetonide Cream; Neomycin Sulfate and Triamcinolone Acetonide Ophthalmic Ointment; Nystatin and Triamcinolone Acetonide Cream; Nystatin and Triamcinolone Acetonide Ointment; Nystatin, Neomycin Sulfate, Gramicidin, and Triamcinolone Acetonide Cream; Nystatin, Neomycin Sulfate, Gramicidin, and Triamcinolone Acetonide Ointment; Triamcinolone Acetonide Cream; Triamcinolone Acetonide Dental Paste; Triamcinolone Acetonide Injectable Suspension; Triamcinolone Acetonide Lotion; Triamcinolone Acetonide Ointment; Triamcinolone Acetonide Topical Aerosol; Triamcinolone Diacetate Injectable Suspension; Triamcinolone Diacetate Syrup; Triamcinolone Hexacetonide Injectable Suspension; Triamcinolone Tablets.

Proprietary Preparations (details are given in Part 3)
Aust.: Delphicort; Lederspan†; Nasacort; Solu-Volon A; Volon; Volon A; *Austral.:* Aristocort; Kenacort-A; Kenalog in Orabase; Kenalone; Nasacort AQ; *Belg.:* Albicort; Delphi; Kenacort; Kenacort Solubile; Kenacort-A; Ledercort; Lederspan†; *Braz.:* Omcilon A Orabase; *Canad.:* Aristocort; Aristospan; Azmacort; Kenalog; Kenalog in Orabase; Nasacort; Oracort; Scheinpharm Triamcine-A†; Triaderm; *Denm.:* Kenalog; Lederspan†; Nasacort; *Fin.:* Aftab; Kenacort; Lederspan†; Nasacort; *Fr.:* Hexatrione; Kenacort; Nasacort; *Ger.:* Aftab; Arutrin; Berlicort; Delphicort; Delphimix; Extracort; Kenalog; Kortikoid-ratiopharm; Lederlon; Nasacort; Tri-Anemul†; Triam; Triam-Injekt; Triamoral; TriamCreme; Triamgalen; Triamhexal; TriamSalbe; Volon; Volon A; Volonimat; Volonimat N; *Hong Kong:* Aristocort; Denkacort; Dermacort; Kenacort-A; Kenalog in Orabase; Stacort-

A; *Irl.:* Adcortyl; Adcortyl in Orabase; Kenalog; Lederspan†; Nasacort; *Israel:* Adcortyl; Kenalog; Kenalog in Orabase; Oracort; Sterocort; Steronase Aq; *Ital.:* Aftab; Ipercortis; Kenacort-A; Ledercort; Nasacort; *Mex.:* Kenacort; Kenalog Dental; Nasacort; Triamsicort; Zamacort; *Neth.:* Albicort; Delphi; Kenacort-A; Kenacort†; Ledercort; Lederspan†; Nasacort; *Norw.:* Kenacort-T; Lederspan†; Nasacort; *NZ:* Aristocort; Kenacort-A; Kenalog in Orabase; Nasacort; Oracort; *Port.:* Aftach; *S.Afr.:* Kenalog in Orabase; Ledercort; Lederspan; Nasacor; *Singapore:* Kemzid; Kenalog in Orabase; Nasacort; Oramedy; *Spain:* Flutenal; Kenalog Orabase; Ledercort; Nasacort; Proctosteroid; Trigon Depot; *Swed.:* Kenacort-T; Kenacort†; Lederspan†; Nasacort; *Switz.:* Kenacort; Kenacort-A; Kenacort-A Solubile; Ledercort; Nasacort; Triamcort; *Thai.:* Aristocort; Facort; Ftorocort; Generlog; Kanolone; Kela; Kemzid; Kenacort; Kenalog in Orabase; Keno; Nasacort; Oracort; Oral-T; Orcilone; Risto; Shincort; Simacort; Tacinol; Topilone; Tramsilione; Triama; Trilosil; Trim; Trimasone; Unif; Vacinolone; *UK:* Adcortyl; Adcortyl in Orabase; Kenalog; Lederspan†; Nasacort; *USA:* Amcort; Aristocort; Aristospan; Articulose LA†; Atolone; Azmacort; Delta-Tritex; Flutex; Kenacort†; Kenaject; Kenalog; Kenalog in Orabase; Kenonel; Nasacort; Oralone Dental; Tac; Tri-Kort; Tri-Nasal; Triacet; Triam; Triam-A; Triamolone†; Triamonide; Triderm; Trilog; Trilone; Tristoject.

Multi-ingredient: *Aust.:* Aureocort; Ledermix; Mycostatin V; Neo-Delphicort; Pevisone; Steros-Anal; Volon A antibiotikahaltig; Volon A Tinktur; Volon A-Zinklotion; *Austral.:* Aristocomb†; Kenacomb; Otocomb Otic; *Belg.:* Albicort Compositum; Albicort Oticum; Mycolog; Pevisone; Trianal; *Braz.:* Omcilon A; Omcilon AM; *Canad.:* Kenacomb; Triacomb; Viaderm-KC; *Denm.:* Kenacutan; Kenalog Comp; Kenalog Comp med Mycostatin; Kenalog med Salicylsyre; Ledermix; Pevisone; *Fin.:* Aureocort; Kenacort-T comp; Pevisone; *Fr.:* Cidermex; Corticotulle Lumiere; Kenalcol; Localone; Mycolog; Pevisone; *Ger.:* Ampho-Moronal V; Ampho-Moronal V L; Aureodelf; Corticotulle Lumiere; Epipevisone; Extracort Rhin sine; Extracort Tinktur N; Moronal V; mykoproct sine†; Polcortolon TC; Steros-Anal; Ultexiv; Volon A antibiotikahaltig N; Volon A Tinktur N; Volon A-Rhin; Volon A-Schuttelmix; Volonimat Plus N; *Hong Kong:* Anso; Kenacomb; Pevisone; Tri-Gel; Triacomb; Triaformo; Triditol-G; *Irl.:* Audicort; Aureocort; Kenacomb; Ledermix; Oracort E; Pevisone; *Ital.:* Assocort; Aureocort; Dirahist; Kataval; Neo-Audiocort; Pevisone; *Mex.:* Kenacomb; *Neth.:* Albicort Compositum; Kenalog; Mycolog; Trianal; *Norw.:* Kenacort-T comp; Kenacutan; Pevisone; *NZ:* Kenacomb; Kenoid; Port.: Kenacomb; Localone; Pevisone;

S.Afr.: Kenacomb; Ledermix; Pevisone; Trialone; *Singapore:* Ecocort; Kenacomb; Oral-Aid; Pevisone; *Spain:* Aldo Otico; Aldoderma; Anasilpiel; Anso; Cemalyt; Cremsol; Deltasiton†; Flutenal Gentamicina; Flutenal Sali; Interderm; Nesfare Antibiotico; Positon; Trigon Rectal; Trigon Topico; *Swed.:* Kenacombin Novum; Kenacombin†; Kenacort-T comp; Kenacutan; Pevisone; *Switz.:* Kenacort-A; Ledermix; Mycolog; Pevisone; *Thai.:* Dermacombin; Ecoderm; Fungisil-T; KA-Cilone; Kelaplus; Kenacomb; Pevisone; Tara-Plus; Trilosil N; *UAE:* Panderm; *UK:* Adcortyl with Graneodin†; Audicort; Aureocort; Ledermix; Nystadermal†; Pevaryl TC; Tri-Adcortyl; *USA:* Myco-Biotic II; Myco-Triacet II; Mycogen II; Mycolog-II; Myconel; Mytrex; NGT; Tri-Statin II.

Ulobetasol Propionate (12198-q)

Ulobetasol Propionate (rINNM).

BMY-30056; CGP-14458; Halobetasol Propionate (USAN). 21-Chloro-6α,9-difluoro-11β,17-dihydroxy-16β-methylpregna-1,4-diene-3,20-dione 17-propionate.
$C_{25}H_{31}ClF_2O_5 = 485.0$.
CAS — 98651-66-2 (ulobetasol); 66852-54-8 (ulobetasol propionate).

Profile

Ulobetasol propionate is a corticosteroid that is used topically for its glucocorticoid activity (p.1039) in the treatment of various skin disorders. It is usually employed as cream or ointment containing 0.05%.

When applied topically, particularly to large areas, when the skin is broken, or under occlusive dressings, corticosteroids may be absorbed in sufficient amounts to cause systemic effects (p.1039). The effects of topical corticosteroids on the skin are described on p.1041. For recommendations concerning the correct use of corticosteroids on the skin, and a rough guide to the clinical potencies of topical corticosteroids, see p.1045.

Preparations

Proprietary Preparations (details are given in Part 3)
Aust.: Miracorten; *Canad.:* Ultravate; *Switz.:* Miracorten†; *USA:* Ultravate.

The symbol † denotes a preparation no longer actively marketed

Cough Suppressants Expectorants Mucolytics and Nasal Decongestants

This chapter describes drugs that are used mainly as cough suppressants, expectorants, or mucolytics, and also those sympathomimetics primarily used for the relief of nasal congestion. Other drugs used in cough include antihistamines (p.404), bronchodilators (p.757 and p.459), and local anaesthetics (p.1302). Compounds with a demulcent action such as glycerol (p.1616) and sucrose (p.1380) are also used, as are various hydrating inhalations.

Cough suppressants have either a central or a peripheral action on the cough reflex or a combination of both. Centrally acting cough suppressants increase the threshold of the cough centre in the brain to incoming stimuli whereas those acting peripherally decrease the sensitivity of the receptors in the respiratory tract. Some drugs have an indirect peripheral mechanism of action and may alter mucociliary factors, exert a local analgesic or anaesthetic action on the receptors, protect the receptors from irritant stimuli, or act as bronchodilators.

Those centrally acting cough suppressants structurally related to morphine that are included in this chapter, such as dextromethorphan, have little or no analgesic action. Those that also have an important analgesic action, such as codeine or diamorphine, are described in the chapter on Analgesics, p.1.

Expectorants are considered to increase the volume of secretions in the respiratory tract thereby facilitating their removal by ciliary action and coughing. Some, such as small doses of ipecacuanha and squill, ammonium salts, some volatile oils, and various iodide compounds are traditionally believed to achieve this by a reflex irritant effect on the gastric mucosa.

Mucolytics alter the structure of mucus to decrease its viscosity thereby facilitating its removal by ciliary action or expectoration.

Acetylcysteine, carbocisteine, mecysteine, and stepronin all have thiol groups; if this group is free, as in acetylcysteine, it may be substituted for disulfide bonds in mucus and therefore break the mucus chains. However, drugs such as carbocisteine with 'protected' thiol groups cannot act by this mechanism and their exact mode of action is unclear. Thiol groups are also involved in the mechanism of action of some of these drugs when they are used in the treatment of poisoning.

Deoxyribonucleases such as dornase alfa act as mucolytics by hydrolysing the accumulated extracellular DNA from decaying neutrophils that contributes to the viscous respiratory secretions of cystic fibrosis.

Sympathomimetics described in this chapter may be used systemically (e.g. phenylephrine, p.1097) or locally (e.g. naphazoline, p.1095), for their alpha agonist actions to produce vasoconstriction of the nasal mucosa, thus relieving congestion. Others (e.g. ephedrine, p.1090) have both alpha and beta agonist actions. The beta agonist actions confer upon them bronchodilating properties, but they have been superseded as bronchodilators by the more selective beta$_2$ agonists such as salbutamol (p.770). The value of bronchodilators in non-asthmatic cough has not been confirmed.

Cough

Cough is an important physiological protective mechanism, but may also occur as a symptom of an underlying disorder. Treatment of the disorder often alleviates the cough, but there are times when symptomatic treatment is appropriate. The treatment chosen depends on whether the cough is productive or non-productive.

A *non-productive cough* may be considered as serving no useful purpose for the patient. For example, the symptoms of the common cold often include a non-productive cough, and cough suppressants may provide some relief, particularly if given at night. Of the commonly used cough suppressants, pholcodine and dextromethorphan are considered to have fewer adverse effects than co-

deine. However, there is little evidence that these drugs are effective in severe cough. Codeine or similar opioids are not generally recommended as cough suppressants in children, and should be avoided altogether in those under 1 year of age.

A potent cough suppressant such as morphine is needed for the relief of *intractable cough in terminal illness*. The use of such a potent opioid is not otherwise considered appropriate for cough.

A *productive cough* is characterised by the presence of sputum and may be associated with conditions such as chronic bronchitis, bronchiectasis, or cystic fibrosis. Cough suppressants are inappropriate, but expectorants have been used for productive cough on the grounds that increasing the volume of secretions in the respiratory tract facilitates removal by ciliary action and coughing. However, clinical evidence of efficacy is lacking, and many authorities consider expectorants to be of no value other than as a placebo. Commonly used expectorants include ammonium salts, guaifenesin, ipecacuanha, and sodium citrate. Iodides have also been used but there has been concern over their safety for prolonged administration in respiratory disorders and because of their potential for thyroid suppression; in particular, it has been recommended that they should not be given to children, adolescents, pregnant women, or patients with goitre.

Mucolytics have been shown to affect sputum viscosity and structure and patients have reported alleviation of their symptoms, but no consistent improvement has been demonstrated in lung function. Commonly used mucolytics include acetylcysteine, bromhexine, carbocisteine, and mecysteine. Dornase alfa is also available, in particular for patients with cystic fibrosis. In theory mucolytics may disrupt the gastric mucosal barrier and caution has been recommended in patients with a history of peptic ulceration.

Other drugs are also employed in the treatment of cough.

*   *Sedating antihistamines* such as diphenhydramine are frequently employed as cough suppressants in compound preparations. Suggested mechanisms of action have included reduction in cholinergic nerve transmission, or cough suppression as a result of their sedative effects. Antihistamines reduce nasal secretions and may be of value in treating cough caused by postnasal drip, particularly if associated with allergic rhinitis (see p.407). However, they should not be used to treat a productive cough because they may cause formation of viscid mucus plugs. Their sedative effects are a disadvantage for daytime use but may be a short-term advantage for night coughs.
*   *Bronchodilators* such as salbutamol (a beta$_2$ agonist) or ipratropium (an antimuscarinic) alleviate cough associated with bronchospasm. However, they are not generally considered of benefit in other forms of cough, and hence are not recommended for use in non-asthmatic patients.
*   *Demulcents* may be considered as indirect peripherally acting cough suppressants. Their action may involve provision of a protective coating over sensory receptors in the pharynx. Demulcents include glycerol, honey, liquorice, and sucrose syrups.
*   *Hydrating agents* liquefy mucus and also have a demulcent effect. Hydration may be achieved simply by inhaling warm moist air. The addition of substances such as menthol, benzoin, or volatile oils is unlikely to provide any additional benefit but may encourage the use of such inhalations. Inhalation aerosols of water, sodium bicarbonate, sodium chloride, surfactants such as tyloxapol, and proteolytic enzymes such as chymotrypsin and trypsin, have also been used for their reported hydrating or mucolytic effects on respiratory secretions.
*   *Local anaesthetics* such as lignocaine [lidocaine] or bupivacaine have been administered by inhalation in severe intractable cough, including cough caused by malignant neoplasms. Cough suppression is produced by an indirect peripheral action on sensory receptors, but as all protective pulmonary reflexes may be lost and bronchospasm may be induced, such treatment should be used with care. There may also be temporary loss of the swallowing reflex.

Cough and cold preparations containing various combinations of cough suppressants and expectorants, together

with sympathomimetics, antihistamines, or analgesics are available. Some of these combinations such as a cough suppressant and an expectorant are illogical and there is little evidence to support their efficacy. As with many combinations, doses of individual drugs may be inadequate or inappropriate, and the large number of ingredients may expose the patient to unnecessary adverse effects.

References.

1. Fuller RW, Jackson DM. Physiology and treatment of cough. *Thorax* 1990; **45:** 425–30.
2. Pratter MR, *et al.* An algorithmic approach to chronic cough. *Ann Intern Med* 1993; **119:** 977–83.
3. Irwin RS, *et al.* Appropriate use of antitussives and protussives: a practical review. *Drugs* 1993; **46:** 80–91.
4. Irwin RS, *et al.* Managing cough as a defense mechanism and as a symptom: a consensus panel report of the American College of Chest Physicians. *Chest* 1998; **114** (suppl): 133S–181S.
5. Anonymous. Cough medications in children. *Drug Ther Bull* 1999; **37:** 19–21.
6. Irwin RS, Madison JM. The diagnosis and treatment of cough. *N Engl J Med* 2000; **343:** 1715–21.
7. Schroeder K, Fahey T. Over-the-counter medications for acute cough in children and adults in ambulatory settings (updated 18 July 2001). Available in The Cochrane Library; Issue 4. Oxford: Update Software; 2001.

Nasal congestion

Nasal congestion is frequently a symptom of conditions such as rhinitis (p.407), treatment of which can include the use of antihistamines, sympathomimetics, corticosteroids, antimuscarinics, and cromoglicate or nedocromil.

Sympathomimetics are also widely employed as nasal decongestants to provide symptomatic relief of the common cold (p.605). They are used for the vasoconstriction produced by their alpha-adrenergic effects; redistribution of local blood flow reduces oedema of the nasal mucosa, thus improving ventilation, drainage, and nasal stuffiness. Sympathomimetics such as ephedrine, phenylephrine, oxymetazoline, and xylometazoline can be used topically as nasal drops or sprays. Those such as phenylpropanolamine and pseudoephedrine are given by mouth.

Topical use of sympathomimetics has been associated with rebound congestion, particularly if use has been prolonged, as vasodilatation becomes prominent and the effects of vasoconstriction subside. Use is therefore restricted to periods of not more than 7 consecutive days. Administration by mouth is not associated with such rebound congestion, but is more likely to be associated with systemic side-effects and a higher risk of drug interactions. However, a systematic review found no difference in efficacy between oral and topical decongestants from the limited evidence available.[1]

The benefits of *antihistamines* in nasal congestion other than that associated with allergic rhinitis are doubtful, particularly by topical application.

Inhalations of warm moist air are also useful in the treatment of nasal congestion associated with the common cold. As in the case of cough (see above) the addition of substances such as menthol, benzoin, or volatile oils may encourage the use of such inhalations.

1. Taverner D, *et al.* Nasal decongestants for the common cold (updated 18 July 2001). Available in The Cochrane Library; Issue 4. Oxford: Update Software; 2001.

Acetylcysteine (3701-r)

Acetylcysteine (BAN, USAN, rINN).

5052; Acetylcysteinum; NSC-111180. N-Acetyl-L-cysteine.
$C_5H_9NO_3S = 163.2$.
CAS — 616-91-1.
ATC — R05CB01; S01XA08; V03AB23.
Pharmacopoeias. In *Chin.,* Eur. (see p.vi), and US.

Incompatible with some metals, including iron and copper, with rubber, and with oxygen and oxidising substances. Some antibiotics including amphotericin B, ampicillin sodium, erythromycin lactobionate, and some tetracyclines are either physically incompatible with or may be inactivated on mixture with acetylcysteine.

A change in colour of solutions of acetylcysteine to light purple does not indicate significant impairment of safety or efficacy.

Pharmacopoeial description

Ph. Eur.: A white, crystalline powder or colourless crystals. Freely soluble in water and in alcohol; practically insoluble in dichloromethane. A 1% solution in water has a pH of 2.0 to 2.8. Protect from light.

USP 25: A white crystalline powder having a slight acetic odour. Soluble 1 in 5 of water and 1 in 4 of alcohol; practically insoluble in chloroform and in ether. pH of a 1% solution in water is between 2.0 and 2.8. Store in airtight containers.

Acetylcysteine Sodium (15577-t)

$C_5H_8NNaO_3S = 185.2$.
CAS — 19542-74-6.

Adverse Effects

Hypersensitivity reactions have been reported in patients receiving acetylcysteine, including bronchospasm, angioedema, rashes and pruritus; hypotension, or occasionally hypertension, may occur. Other adverse effects reported with acetylcysteine include flushing, nausea and vomiting, fever, syncope, sweating, arthralgia, blurred vision, disturbances of liver function, acidosis, convulsions, and cardiac or respiratory arrest. Haemoptysis, rhinorrhoea, and stomatitis have been associated with inhalation of acetylcysteine.

◊ The most common symptoms of patients experiencing anaphylactoid reactions after the intravenous use of acetylcysteine in the treatment of paracetamol poisoning are rash and pruritus; other features have included flushing, nausea or vomiting, angioedema, tachycardia, bronchospasm, hypotension, and hypertension;[1,2] ECG abnormalities associated with an anaphylactoid reaction have also been reported in a patient.[3] Anaphylactoid reactions to intravenous acetylcysteine appear to be dose-related.[4] One group estimated that when acetylcysteine was administered correctly the frequency of the anaphylactoid response was between 0.3% and 3%, whereas 11 of 15 patients who had received an overdose experienced an anaphylactoid reaction.[5] Intradermal testing and study of plasma-acetylcysteine concentrations in patients who developed reactions to acetylcysteine suggests a 'pseudo-allergic' rather than an immunological reaction,[6,7] although symptoms consistent with a serum sickness-like illness developed following exposure to acetylcysteine in one patient.[8] It has been suggested that generalised reactions to acetylcysteine can be treated with intravenous injection of an antihistamine;[4,9] infusion of acetylcysteine should be temporarily stopped but can usually be restarted at a slower rate without further reaction.

Symptoms following overdosage with acetylcysteine have been more severe. Hypotension appears to be especially prominent;[5] additional symptoms have included respiratory depression, haemolysis, disseminated intravascular coagulation, and renal failure, but some of these may have been due to paracetamol poisoning.[1] Death occurred in 3 patients who received an overdose of acetylcysteine while being treated for paracetamol poisoning,[1,10] but in 2 of them the role of acetylcysteine in this outcome was unclear.

1. Mant TGK, et al. Adverse reactions to acetylcysteine and effects of overdose. BMJ 1984; 289: 217–19.
2. Dawson AH, et al. Adverse reactions to N-acetylcysteine during treatment for paracetamol poisoning. Med J Aust 1989; 150: 329–31.
3. Bonfiglio MF, et al. Anaphylactoid reaction to intravenous acetylcysteine associated with electrocardiographic abnormalities. Ann Pharmacother 1992; 26: 22–5.
4. Bailey B, McGuigan MA. Management of anaphylactoid reactions to intravenous N-acetylcysteine. Ann Emerg Med 1998; 31: 710–15.
5. Sunman W, et al. Anaphylactoid response to intravenous acetylcysteine. Lancet 1992; 339: 1231–2.
6. Bateman DN, et al. Adverse reactions to N-acetylcysteine. Hum Toxicol 1984; 3: 393–8.
7. Donovan JW, et al. Adverse reactions of N-acetylcysteine and their relation to plasma levels. Vet Hum Toxicol 1987; 29: 470.
8. Mohammed S, et al. Serum sickness-like illness associated with N-acetylcysteine therapy. Ann Pharmacother 1994; 28: 285.
9. Bateman DN. Adverse reactions to antidotes. Adverse Drug React Bull 1988; (Dec.): 496–9.
10. Anonymous. Death after N-acetylcysteine. Lancet 1984; i: 1421.

Precautions

Acetylcysteine should be used with caution in asthmatic patients. It should also be used with caution in patients with a history of peptic ulceration, both because drug-induced nausea and vomiting may increase the risk of gastrointestinal haemorrhage in patients predisposed to the condition, and because of a theoretical risk that mucolytics may disrupt the gastric mucosal barrier.

Asthma. Reports of bronchospasm precipitated in two asthmatic patients[1] and severe asthma and respiratory arrest in another[2] after intravenous treatment with acetylcysteine.

1. Ho SW-C, Beilin LJ. Asthma associated with N-acetylcysteine infusion and paracetamol poisoning: report of two cases. BMJ 1983; 287: 876–7.
2. Reynard K, et al. Respiratory arrest after N-acetylcysteine for paracetamol overdose. Lancet 1992; 340: 675.

Hepatic impairment. The total clearance of acetylcysteine in patients with cirrhosis was found to be markedly impaired, and the elimination half-life almost twice that of healthy controls.[1] Since some of the more serious adverse effects of acetylcysteine occur when plasma concentrations are high, the authors considered that increased vigilance for untoward anaphylactoid reactions and other adverse effects was necessary in patients with cirrhosis receiving acetylcysteine, and further studies to determine the optimum dosage regimen in such patients were required.

1. Jones AL, et al. Pharmacokinetics of N-acetylcysteine are altered in patients with chronic liver disease. Aliment Pharmacol Ther 1997; 11: 787–91.

Pharmacokinetics

◊ Acetylcysteine is rapidly absorbed from the gastrointestinal tract and peak plasma concentrations are about 0.5 to 1 hour after oral administration of doses of 200 to 600 mg.[1] Some studies indicate dose-dependent pharmacokinetics with peak concentrations, the time taken to reach peak concentrations, and bioavailability increasing with increasing doses.[2] Acetylcysteine may be present in plasma as the parent compound or as various oxidised metabolites such as N-acetylcystine, N,N-diacetylcystine, and cysteine either free or bound to plasma proteins by labile disulfide bonds or as a fraction incorporated into protein peptide chains.[3] In one study about 50% was in a covalently protein-bound form 4 hours after administration.[4] Oral bioavailability is low and mean values have ranged from 4 to 10% depending on whether total acetylcysteine or just the reduced forms are measured.[4,5] It has been suggested that acetylcysteine's low oral bioavailability may be due to metabolism in the gut wall and first-pass metabolism in the liver.[4,5] Renal clearance may account for about 30% of total body clearance.[5] Following intravenous administration mean terminal half-lives have been calculated to be 1.95 and 5.58 hours for reduced and total acetylcysteine respectively; the terminal half-life of total acetylcysteine was 6.25 hours after oral administration.[4]

For reference to altered pharmacokinetics in patients with hepatic impairment, see above.

1. Holdiness MR. Clinical pharmacokinetics of N-acetylcysteine. Clin Pharmacokinet 1991; 20: 123–34.
2. Borgström L, Kågedal B. Dose dependent pharmacokinetics of N-acetylcysteine after oral dosing to man. Biopharm Drug Dispos 1990; 11: 131–6.
3. De Caro L, et al. Pharmacokinetics and bioavailability of oral acetylcysteine in healthy volunteers. Arzneimittelforschung 1989; 39: 383–6.
4. Olsson B, et al. Pharmacokinetics and bioavailability of reduced and oxidized N-acetylcysteine. Eur J Clin Pharmacol 1988; 34: 77–82.
5. Borgström L, et al. Pharmacokinetics of N-acetylcysteine in man. Eur J Clin Pharmacol 1986; 31: 217–22.

Uses and Administration

Acetylcysteine is a mucolytic that reduces the viscosity of secretions probably by the splitting of disulfide bonds in mucoproteins. This action is greatest at a pH of 7 to 9 and the pH may have been adjusted in commercial preparations with sodium hydroxide. It is sometimes stated that acetylcysteine sodium is used, although the dose is expressed in terms of acetylcysteine.

Acetylcysteine is also able to promote the detoxification of an intermediate paracetamol metabolite, and has a key role in the management of paracetamol overdosage.

Acetylcysteine is used for its **mucolytic** activity in respiratory disorders associated with acute cough. Administration can be by nebulisation of 3 to 5 mL of a 20% solution or 6 to 10 mL of a 10% solution through a face mask or mouthpiece 3 to 4 times daily. If necessary 1 to 10 mL of a 20% solution or 2 to 20 mL of a 10% solution may be given by nebulisation every 2 to 6 hours. It can also be given by direct endotracheal instillation of 1 to 2 mL of a 10 to 20% solution as often as every hour. Mechanical suction of the liquefied secretions may be necessary, and nebulisers containing iron, copper, or rubber components should not be used.

Acetylcysteine has been given by mouth in doses of 200 mg three times daily as granules or effervescent tablets dissolved in water. Children aged up to 2 years may be given 200 mg daily, and those aged 2 to 7 years 200 mg twice daily.

In the treatment of **dry eye** (p.1498) associated with abnormal mucus production, acetylcysteine, usually as a 5% solution with hypromellose, is administered topically 3 to 4 times daily. Higher concentrations have been used in some centres.

Acetylcysteine is given by intravenous infusion or by mouth in the treatment of **paracetamol poisoning**. In the UK acetylcysteine is given intravenously: 150 mg per kg body-weight of acetylcysteine in 200 mL of glucose 5% is given initially over 15 minutes, followed by infusion of 50 mg per kg in 500 mL of glucose 5% over the next 4 hours and then 100 mg per kg in one litre of glucose 5% over the next 16 hours. Sodium chloride 0.9% may be used where glucose 5% is unsuitable. The volume of intravenous fluids should be modified for children. In the USA, acetylcysteine is given by mouth in an initial dose of 140 mg per kg as a 5% solution followed by 70 mg per kg every 4 hours for an additional 17 doses. Acetylcysteine is reported to be most effective when administered within 8 hours of paracetamol overdosage, with the protective effect diminishing after this time. However, later initiation of treatment with acetylcysteine (up to and beyond 24 hours) may still be of benefit (see below).

Aspergillosis. Although not one of the standard therapies discussed on p.372, local instillation of acetylcysteine into the cavity containing the fungus ball has been used to treat aspergilloma.[1] There is some evidence in vitro that acetylcysteine has inhibitory properties against Aspergillus and Fusarium spp.[2]

1. Kauffman CA. Quandary about treatment of aspergillomas persists. Lancet 1996; 347: 1640.
2. De Lucca AJ, et al. N-Acetylcysteine inhibits germination of conidia and growth of Aspergillus spp. and Fusarium spp. Antimicrob Agents Chemother 1996; 40: 1274–6.

Cystic fibrosis. Mucolytics such as acetylcysteine are generally not considered to be effective in treating the pulmonary manifestations of cystic fibrosis (p.117). Some references to the use of acetylcysteine in cystic fibrosis are listed below.[1-3]

Meconium ileus equivalent (bowel obstruction due to abnormally viscid contents of the terminal ileum and right colon[4]) in patients with cystic fibrosis has largely disappeared with the use of pancreatic enzymes but may occur when insufficient doses are given;[5] mild cases may be treated with acetylcysteine.[5] Doses of 10 mL of a 20% solution of acetylcysteine have been given by mouth 4 times daily together with 100 mL of a 10% solution of acetylcysteine administered as an enema up to 4 times daily depending on the degree of the obstruction.[4]

1. Ratjen F, et al. A double-blind placebo controlled trial with oral ambroxol and N-acetylcysteine for mucolytic treatment in cystic fibrosis. Eur J Pediatr 1985; 144: 374–8.
2. Stanfanger G, et al. The clinical effect and the effect on the ciliary motility of oral N-acetylcysteine in patients with cystic fibrosis and primary ciliary dyskinesia. Eur Respir J 1988; 1: 161–7.
3. Duijvestijn YC, Brand PL. Systematic review of N-acetylcysteine in cystic fibrosis. Acta Paediatr 1999; 88: 38–41.
4. Hanly JG, Fitzgerald MX. Meconium ileus equivalent in older patients with cystic fibrosis. BMJ 1983; 286: 1411–13.
5. David TJ. Cystic fibrosis. Arch Dis Child 1990; 65: 152–7.

HIV infection and AIDS. The cysteine-containing peptide glutathione is involved in intracellular defence mechanisms, and it has been shown that low glutathione concentrations are associated with poorer survival in HIV-infected patients.[1] Since acetylcysteine can replenish glutathione, it has been suggested[2,3] that it may have a role in the treatment of AIDS (p.608). In-vitro studies indicate that acetylcysteine can suppress HIV expression,[4,5] and there has been a suggestion from observational data that acetylcysteine supplements can improve survival in HIV-infected individuals.[1] However, an attempt to use acetylcysteine supplementation to reduce the frequency of adverse reactions to co-trimoxazole in HIV-infected patients was not successful.[6]

1. Herzenberg LA, et al. Glutathione deficiency is associated with impaired survival in HIV disease. Proc Natl Acad Sci U S A 1997; 94: 1967–72.
2. Staal FJT, et al. Glutathione deficiency and human immunodeficiency virus infection. Lancet 1992; 339: 909–12.
3. Roederer M, et al. N-Acetylcysteine: potential for AIDS therapy. Pharmacology 1993; 46: 121–9.
4. Roederer M, et al. Cytokine-stimulated human immunodeficiency virus replication is inhibited by N-acetyl-L-cysteine. Proc Natl Acad Sci U S A 1990; 87: 4884–8.
5. Kalebic T, et al. Suppression of human immunodeficiency virus expression in chronically infected monocytic cells by glutathione, glutathione ester, and N-acetylcysteine. Proc Natl Acad Sci U S A 1991; 88: 986–90.
6. Åkerlund B, et al. N-acetylcysteine treatment and the risk of toxic reactions to trimethoprim-sulphamethoxazole in primary Pneumocystis carinii prophylaxis in HIV-infected patients. J Infect 1997; 35: 143–7.

Kidney disorders. Acetylcysteine has been reported to improve kidney function in patients with the hepatorenal syndrome and may offer a potential bridging therapy in such patients awaiting liver transplantation.[1]

1. Holt S, et al. Improvement in renal function in hepatorenal syndrome with N-acetylcysteine. Lancet 1999; 353: 294–5.

Liver disorders. As well as being effective in the management of paracetamol-induced liver damage (see Overdosage, p.71), acetylcysteine has produced beneficial effects in patients with acute liver failure[1] when used alone or in combination with epoprostenol. It may also prevent the development of tissue hypoxia in patients with acute liver failure who are receiving vasopressors.[2] However, intravenous infusion of acetylcysteine has not been shown to be of any benefit when added to therapy in patients undergoing orthotopic liver transplantation.[3,4]

For reference to use in the hepatorenal syndrome, see under Kidney Disorders, above.

1. Harrison PM, et al. Improvement by acetylcysteine of hemodynamics and oxygen transport in fulminant hepatic failure. N Engl J Med 1991; 324: 1852–7.
2. Caraceni P, Van Thiel DH. Acute liver failure. Lancet 1995; 345: 163–9.
3. Bromley PN, et al. Effects of intraoperative N-acetylcysteine in orthotopic liver transplantation. Br J Anaesth 1995; 75: 352–4.
4. Steib A, et al. Does N-acetylcysteine improve hemodynamics and graft function in liver transplantation? Liver Transpl Surg 1998; 4: 152–7.

Myocardial infarction. There is limited evidence suggesting that addition of intravenous acetylcysteine to thrombolytic therapy in patients with acute myocardial infarction (p.805) may be of benefit,[1,2] and would reward further investigation.

1. Arstall MA, et al. N-Acetylcysteine in combination with nitroglycerin and streptokinase for the treatment of evolving acute myocardial infarction: safety and biochemical effects. Circulation 1995; 92: 2855–62.
2. Sochman J, et al. Infarct size limitation: acute N-acetylcysteine defense (ISLAND trial): preliminary analysis and report after the first 30 patients. Clin Cardiol 1996; 19: 94–100.

Nitrate tolerance. Acetylcysteine appears to be able to potentiate the peripheral and coronary effects of glyceryl trinitrate.[1,2] While some studies[3–6] suggest that it can reverse tolerance to nitrates in patients with coronary heart disease or heart failure, others have failed to demonstrate any benefit.[7] There may be a specific subgroup of responders.[6] The various attempts at overcoming nitrate tolerance are discussed on p.898.

1. Horowitz JD, et al. Combined use of nitroglycerin and N-acetylcysteine in the management of unstable angina pectoris. Circulation 1988; 77: 787–94.
2. Elkayam U. Tolerance to organic nitrates: evidence, mechanisms, clinical relevance, and strategies for prevention. Ann Intern Med 1991; 114: 667–77.
3. Packer M, et al. Prevention and reversal of nitrate tolerance in patients with congestive heart failure. N Engl J Med 1987; 317: 799–804.
4. May DC, et al. In vivo induction and reversal of nitroglycerin tolerance in human coronary arteries. N Engl J Med 1987; 317: 805–9.
5. Boesgaard S, et al. Preventive administration of intravenous N-acetylcysteine and development of tolerance to isosorbide dinitrate in patients with angina pectoris. Circulation 1992; 85: 143–9.
6. Pizzulli L, et al. N-acetylcysteine attenuates nitroglycerin tolerance in patients with angina pectoris and normal left ventricular function. Am J Cardiol 1997; 79: 28–33.
7. Hogan JC, et al. Chronic administration of N-acetylcysteine fails to prevent nitrate tolerance in patients with stable angina pectoris. Br J Clin Pharmacol 1990; 30: 573–7.

Poisoning and toxicity. Acetylcysteine has been studied for the potential treatment of many forms of toxicity,[1] but only treatment of acute paracetamol poisoning is widely accepted.

1. Chyka PA, et al. Utility of acetylcysteine in treating poisonings and adverse drug reactions. Drug Safety 2000; 22: 123–48.

CARBON TETRACHLORIDE. The treatment of carbon tetrachloride poisoning is discussed on p.1401. Reports suggest that prompt intravenous therapy with acetylcysteine may help to minimise hepatorenal damage in acute poisoning with carbon tetrachloride.[1,2] It could be used in addition to supportive therapy when the initial dosage regimen should be that used for paracetamol poisoning but as carbon tetrachloride has a much longer half-life than paracetamol, the duration of treatment may need to be increased.[3]

1. Ruprah M, et al. Acute carbon tetrachloride poisoning in 19 patients: implications for diagnosis and treatment. Lancet 1985; i: 1027–9.
2. Mathieson PW, et al. Survival after massive ingestion of carbon tetrachloride treated by intravenous infusion of acetylcysteine. Hum Toxicol 1985; 4: 627–31.
3. Meredith TJ, et al. Diagnosis and treatment of acute poisoning with volatile substances. Hum Toxicol 1989; 8: 277–86.

PARACETAMOL. Acetylcysteine is the antidote of choice for paracetamol overdosage (see p.71). The intravenous route is favoured in the UK, despite possible anaphylactic reaction, mainly because of concerns over the effects of vomiting and activated charcoal on oral absorption.[1] In the USA the oral route is usually used, despite the unpleasant odour and taste of acetylcysteine solutions, with no evident reduction in effect by charcoal.[2]

1. Vale JA, Proudfoot AT. Paracetamol (acetaminophen) poisoning. Lancet 1995; 346: 547–52.
2. Bowden CA, Krenzelok EP. Clinical applications of commonly used contemporary antidotes: a US perspective. Drug Safety 1997; 16: 9–47.

Respiratory disorders. Acetylcysteine has been used as a mucolytic in a variety of respiratory disorders associated with productive cough (p.1082). Although there is controversy over the benefits of mucolytics in treating chronic bronchitis, there is some evidence that they may reduce exacerbations (see p.759).

Repeated bronchoalveolar lavage with heparin and acetylcysteine to remove proteinaceous material in patients with alveolar proteinosis may prolong survival.[1] Administration of acetylcysteine by nebulisation has relieved severe recurrent at-

electasis during mechanical ventilation in premature infants.[2] It has been suggested that intravenous acetylcysteine might also be of use in acute respiratory distress syndrome (ARDS—p.1046),[3] possibly due to its action as a free radical scavenger,[3,4] but controlled studies in established ARDS failed to show benefit.[5,6]

See above for the use of acetylcysteine in the management of cystic fibrosis.

1. Morrison HM, Stockley RA. The many uses of bronchoalveolar lavage. BMJ 1988; 296: 1758.
2. Amir J, et al. Acetylcysteine for severe atelectasis in premature infants. Clin Pharm 1985; 4: 255.
3. Bernard GR. Potential of N-acetylcysteine as treatment for the adult respiratory distress syndrome. Eur Respir J 1990; 3 (suppl 11): 496S–498S.
4. Skolnick A. Inflammation-mediator blockers may be weapons against sepsis syndrome. JAMA 1990; 263: 930–1.
5. Jepsen S, et al. Antioxidant treatment with N-acetylcysteine during adult respiratory distress syndrome: a prospective, randomized, placebo-controlled study. Crit Care Med 1992; 20: 918–23.
6. Domenighetti G, et al. Treatment with N-acetylcysteine during acute respiratory distress syndrome: a randomized, double-blind, placebo-controlled clinical study. J Crit Care 1997; 12: 177–82.

Preparations

BP 2001: Acetylcysteine Injection;
USP 25: Acetylcysteine and Isoproterenol Hydrochloride Inhalation Solution; Acetylcysteine Solution.

Proprietary Preparations (details are given in Part 3)
Aust.: ACC; Aeromuc; Cimelin; Cimexyl; Fluimucil; Husten ACC; Mucobene; Mucomyst; Mucret†; Pulmovent; Siccoral; Solvomed; *Austral.:* Mucomyst; Parvolex; *Belg.:* Lysodrop; Lysomucil; Lysox; Mucolair; Mucolator†; Mucomyst; Pectomucil; *Braz.:* Fluimucil; Fluimucil Solucao Nasal; *Canad.:* Mucomyst; Parvolex; *Denm.:* Granon; Hostop†; Mucolysin; Mucomyst; *Fin.:* Mucomyst; Mucoporetta; *Fr.:* Broncoclar; Codotussyl Expectorant; Exomuc; Fluimucil; Genac; Humex Expectorant; Mucolator; Mucomyst; Mucospire; Solmucol; Tixair; *Ger.:* ACC; Acemuc; Acetabs; Acetyst; Azubronchin; Bisolvon NAC†; Bromuc; Broncho-Fips†; Durabronchal; Fluimucil; Jenacysteine†; Larylin NAC Husten-Loser; Mentopin; Muciteran; Muco Sanigen; Muco-Perasthman N†; Mucocedyl; Mucret; Mykofat; NAC; Optipect†; Pulmicret; Sigamucil; Siran; Stas Akut†; Tamuc†; Tussiverlan; Vitenur; *Hong Kong:* Fluimucil; Mucolator; Parvolex; Solmucol; *Irl.:* Alveolex; Parvolex; *Israel:* Agisolvan; Mucosil; Mucomyst; Siran; *Ital.:* Brunac; Fluimucil; Hidonac; Mucisol; Solmucol; Tirocular; *Mon.:* Euronac; *Neth.:* Bisolbruis; Dampo Mucopect†; Fluimucil; Libronchin; Mucocil; Mucomyst; Norw.: Bronkyl; Mucomyst; *NZ:* Parvolex; *Port.:* Fluimucil; *S.Afr.:* ACC; Parvolex; Solmucol; *Singapore:* Fluimucil; Mucoza; *Spain:* Fluimucil; Locomucil; *Swed.:* Fabrol†; Mucomyst; Viskoferm; *Switz.:* ACC; Acemucol; Bisolapid; Demolibral; Dynamucil; Ecomucyl; Fluimucil, L-Cimexyl; Muco-Mepha; Mucofluid; Mucostop; Neo Expectan†; Robitussin Expectorant; Secresol; Solmucol; *Thai.:* Acetin; Fluci; Fluimucil; Mucil; Mucocil; Mucotic; Mysoven; NAC; *UK:* Parvolex; *USA:* Mucomyst; Mucosil.

Multi-ingredient: *Braz.:* Fluimucil Biotic; Rinofluimucil; *Fr.:* Rhinofluimucil; *Ger.:* Rinofluimucil-S; *Hong Kong:* Rinofluimucil; *Irl.:* Ilube; *Ital.:* Rinofluimucil; *Spain:* Rinofluimucil; *Switz.:* Rinofluimucil; Solmucaine; Solmucalm†; *Thai.:* Fluimucil Antibiotic; *UK:* Ilube.

Acetyldihydrocodeine Hydrochloride (12311-z)

4,5-Epoxy-3-methoxy-9a-methylmorphinan-6-yl acetate hydrochloride.

$C_{20}H_{25}NO_4,HCl = 379.9.$
CAS — 3861-72-1 (acetyldihydrocodeine).

Profile

Acetyldihydrocodeine hydrochloride is an opioid derivative related to dihydrocodeine (p.33). It is used as a centrally acting cough suppressant for non-productive cough (p.1082) and has been given by mouth in a daily dose of 20 to 50 mg; no more than 20 mg should be taken as a single dose.

Preparations

Proprietary Preparations (details are given in Part 3)
Belg.: Acetylcodone.

Adamexine (3900-v)

Adamexine (rINN).

α-(1-Adamantylmethylamino)-4′,6′-dibromo-2-acetotoluidide.
$C_{20}H_{26}Br_2N_2O = 470.2.$
CAS — 54785-02-3.

Profile

Adamexine is a derivative of bromhexine (p.1085) that has been used as a mucolytic in the treatment of respiratory disorders associated with productive cough.

Preparations

Proprietary Preparations (details are given in Part 3)
Spain: Broncostyl†.

Alloclamide Hydrochloride (5603-I)

Alloclamide Hydrochloride (rINNM).
CE-264. 2-Allyloxy-4-chloro-N-(2-diethylaminoethyl)benzamide hydrochloride.
$C_{16}H_{23}ClN_2O_2,HCl = 347.3.$
CAS — 5486-77-1 (alloclamide); 5107-01-7 (alloclamide hydrochloride).

Profile

Alloclamide hydrochloride is a cough suppressant.

Preparations

Proprietary Preparations (details are given in Part 3)
Multi-ingredient: *Spain:* Tuselin Expectorante.

Ambroxol Hydrochloride (16360-w)

Ambroxol Hydrochloride (BANM, rINNM).
Ambroxoli Hydrochloridum; NA-872 (ambroxol). trans-4-(2-Amino-3,5-dibromobenzylamino)cyclohexanol hydrochloride.
$C_{13}H_{18}Br_2N_2O,HCl = 414.6.$
CAS — 18683-91-5 (ambroxol); 15942-05-9 (ambroxol hydrochloride); 23828-92-4 (ambroxol hydrochloride).
Pharmacopoeias. In Eur. (see p.vi).

Pharmacopoeial description

Ph. Eur.: A white or yellowish crystalline powder. Sparingly soluble in water; practically insoluble in dichloromethane; soluble in methyl alcohol. A 1% solution in water has a pH of 4.5 to 6.0. Protect from light.

Profile

Ambroxol is a metabolite of bromhexine (p.1085) and is used similarly as a mucolytic. It is given in a usual daily dose of 60 to 120 mg of the hydrochloride by mouth, in 2 to 3 divided doses. Similar doses have been given by inhalation, injection, or rectally.

Ambroxol acefyllinate has been used similarly.

Adverse effects. HYPERSENSITIVITY. A report[1] of contact allergy to ambroxol, but not bromhexine.

1. Mancuso G, Berdondini RM. Contact allergy to ambroxol. Contact Dermatitis 1989; 20: 154.

Pharmacokinetics. References to pharmacokinetic studies of ambroxol.

1. Hammer R, et al. Speziesvergleich in Pharmakokinetik und Metabolismus von NA 872 Cl Ambroxol bei Ratte, Kaninchen, Hund und Mensch. Arzneimittelforschung 1978; 28: 899–903.
2. Jauch R, et al. Ambroxol, Untersuchungen zum Stoffwechsel beim Menschen und zum quantitativen Nachweis in biologischen Proben. Arzneimittelforschung 1978; 28: 904–11.
3. Vergin H, et al. Untersuchungen zur Pharmakokinetik und Bioäquivalenz unterscheidlicher Darreichungsformen von Ambroxol. Arzneimittelforschung 1985; 35: 1591–5.

Respiratory disorders. Ambroxol has been tried in a variety of respiratory disorders: mixed results[1–3] were obtained when used in chronic bronchitis (p.759); it was ineffective[4] when given to mothers for the prophylaxis of neonatal respiratory distress syndrome (p.1055), although it may be of modest benefit in the early treatment of established disease in infants.[5,6] Inhalation of ambroxol aerosol has also produced beneficial effects in a patient with alveolar proteinosis who refused alveolar lavage.[7]

The management of cough, including the use of mucolytics in productive cough, is discussed on p.1082.

1. Olivieri D, et al. Ambroxol for the prevention of chronic exacerbations: long-term multicenter trial: protective effect of ambroxol against winter semester exacerbations: a double-blind study versus placebo. Respiration 1987; 51 (suppl 1): 42–51.
2. Guyatt GH, et al. A controlled trial of ambroxol in chronic bronchitis. Chest 1987; 92: 618–20.
3. Alcozer G, et al. Prevention of chronic bronchitis exacerbations with ambroxol (Mucosolvan Retard): an open, long-term, multicenter study in 5,635 patients. Respiration 1989; 55 (suppl 1): 84–96.
4. Dani C, et al. Antenatal ambroxol treatment does not prevent the respiratory distress syndrome in premature infants. Eur J Pediatr 1997; 156: 392–3.
5. Wauer RR, et al. Randomized double blind trial of Ambroxol for the treatment of respiratory distress syndrome. Eur J Pediatr 1992; 151: 357–63.
6. Schmalisch G, et al. Changes in pulmonary function in preterm infants recovering from RDS following early treatment with ambroxol: results of a randomized trial. Pediatr Pulmonol 1999; 27: 104–12.
7. Diaz JP, et al. Response to surfactant activator (ambroxol) in alveolar proteinosis. Lancet 1984; i: 1023.

Uricosuric action. A study[1] was carried out in 48 young male healthy volunteers to examine the uricosuric effect of ambroxol. The minimum effective dose for lowering plasma-uric acid concentrations was found to be between 250 mg and 500 mg daily given in 2 divided doses. Although these doses are much higher than those used to treat bronchopulmonary disease, doses as high as 1 g daily were well tolerated.

1. Oosterhuis B, et al. Dose-dependent uricosuric effect of ambroxol. Eur J Clin Pharmacol 1993; 44: 237–41.

Preparations

Proprietary Preparations (details are given in Part 3)
Aust.: Ambrobene; Ambrolan; Broxol; Mucosolvan; Sekretovit; *Belg.:* Surbronc; *Braz.:* Benatoss; Expectuss; Fluibron; Mucibron; Mucolin; Mucosolvan; Surfactil; *Fr.:* Muxol; Surbronc; *Ger.:* Ambril; Ambro; Ambro-Puren; Ambrobeta; Ambrohexal;

Ambrolos; Ambropp; Antussan†; Bisolvon AM†; Bronchopront; Bronchowern; Contac Husten-Trunk†; Dignobroxol†; duramucal; Expit; Farmabroxol†; frenopect; Jenabroxol†; Larylin Husten-Heissgetrank†; Larylin Husten-Loser Pastillen; Larylin Husten-Loser Saft; Lindoxyl; Logomed Husten†; Mibrox; Muco-Aspecton; Muco-Fips†; Muco-Tablinen†; Mucobroxol; Mucophlogat; Mucosolvan; Mucotablin; neo-bronchol; Nymix Mucolytikum†; Padiamuc; Pect Hustenloser; Pulmonal S†; Sigabroxol; stas-Hustenloser; Tusso; **Hong Kong:** Amxol; Bronchopront; Mucosolvan; **Ital.:** Ambromucil; Amobronc; Atus; Broncomnes; Broxol; Fluibron; Fluixol; Lisopulm; Muciclar; Mucobron; Mucosolvan; Secretil; Surfactal; Surfolase; Tauxolo; Viscomucil; **Mex.:** Ambrofur; Broxofar; Broxol; Ebromin; Expeflen; Ital-Ultra; Mucosolvan; Mucovibrol; Mucovibrol T; Muxol; Sekretovit; Septacin; Trimexine; Tunitol-BX; **Port.:** Benflux; Bromax; Bronchopront; Broncoliber; Drenoxol; Fluidox; Hipotosse; Mucosolvan; Surfolase; **Singapore:** Amxol; Bronchopront; Fluibron; Mucosolvan; **Spain:** Ambrolitic; Dinobroxol; Motosol; Mucibron; Mucosan; Naxpa; **Switz.:** Fluibron; Mucabrox; Mucosolvon; **Thai.:** Ambrol; Ambrolytic; Ambrox; Amoxl; Bronchopront; Broncol; Broxol; Broxsa; Max; Medovent; Misovan; Mucodic; Mucolan; Mucolid; Mucomed; Mucosolvan; Mucoxine-F; Musocan; Polibroxol; Posecus; Simusol.

Multi-ingredient: Aust.: Mucospas; Mucotectan; Vibrabron†; **Ger.:** Ambrodoxy; Ambroxol AL comp; Ambroxol comp; Amdox-Puren; Azudoxat comp; Broncho-Euphyllin; Doxam; Doximucol; Doxy Comp; Doxy Lindoxyl; Doxy Plus; Doxy-duramucal; Doxy-Wolff Mucolyt; Doxysolvat; Jenabroxol comp; Mucotectan; Sagittamuc; Sigamuc; Spasmo-Mucosolvan; Terelit; **Mex.:** Acimox-Ex; Aeroflux; Aminoefedrison NF; Brogal Compositum; Brogal-T; Broxofar Compuesto; Broxol Plus; Histiacil; Mucosolvan Compositum; Mucovibrol C; Rombox; Sekretovit Amoxi; Septacin Amoxi; Septacin Ex; **Port.:** Clembroxol; Mucospas; Ventoliber.

Amidefrine Mesilate (2043-a)

Amidefrine Mesilate (rINN).

5190; Amidephrine Mesilate (BANM); Amidephrine Mesylate (USAN); MJ-5190. 3-(1-Hydroxy-2-methylaminoethyl)methanesulphonanilide methanesulphonate.

$C_{10}H_{16}N_2O_3S,CH_4O_3S = 340.4$.

CAS — 3354-67-4 (amidefrine); 1421-68-7 (amidefrine mesilate).

Profile

Amidefrine mesilate is a sympathomimetic with alpha-adrenergic activity similar to that of phenylephrine (p.1097). It is used for its vasoconstrictor properties in the local treatment of nasal congestion.

Preparations

Proprietary Preparations (details are given in Part 3)
Aust.: Fentrinol.

Ammonium Acetate (2003-w)

$CH_3CO_2NH_4 = 77.08$.

CAS — 631-61-8 (ammonium acetate); 8013-61-4 (ammonium acetate solution).

Pharmacopoeias. Br. includes Strong Ammonium Acetate Solution.

Ammonium Bicarbonate (2004-e)

Ammonium Bicarbonate (BAN).

Ammonii Hydrogenocarbonas; E503. Ammonium hydrogen carbonate.

$NH_4HCO_3 = 79.06$.

CAS — 1066-33-7.

Pharmacopoeias. In Eur. (see p.vi).

Pharmacopoeial description

Ph. Eur.: A fine, white, slightly hygroscopic, crystalline powder or white crystals. It volatilises rapidly at 60°; volatilisation takes place slowly at ambient temperatures if slightly moist. It is in a state of equilibrium with ammonium carbamate. Freely soluble in water; practically insoluble in alcohol. Store in airtight containers.

NOTE. The BP 2001 directs that when Ammonium Carbonate is prescribed or demanded Ammonium Bicarbonate shall be dispensed or supplied.

Ammonium Carbonate (2005-l)

Carbonato de Amonio; E503.

CAS — 8000-73-5.

Pharmacopoeias. In Fr. and It. Also in USNF.

Pharmacopoeial description

BP 2001: NOTE. The BP directs that Ammonium Bicarbonate shall be dispensed or supplied when Ammonium Carbonate is prescribed or demanded.

USNF 20: A white powder, or hard, white or translucent masses having a strong odour of ammonia, without empyreuma. It consists of ammonium bicarbonate and ammonium carbamate, in varying proportions. It yields 30 to 34% of NH_3. On exposure to air it loses ammonia and carbon dioxide, becoming opaque, and is finally converted into friable porous lumps or a white powder of ammonium bicarbonate. Soluble 1 in 4 of wa-

ter. It is decomposed by hot water. Its solutions are alkaline to litmus. Store in airtight containers at a temperature not exceeding 30°. Protect from light.

Ammonium Chloride (2006-y)

510; Ammonii Chloridum; Ammonium Chloratum; Cloruro de Amonio; Muriate of Ammonia; Sal Ammoniac.

$NH_4Cl = 53.49$.

CAS — 12125-02-9.

ATC — B05XA04; G04BA01.

NOTE. The food additive number E380 is used for ammonium citrate.

Pharmacopoeias. In Chin., Eur. (see p.vi), Pol., and US.

Each g represents 18.69 mmol of chloride.

Pharmacopoeial description

Ph. Eur.: A white, crystalline powder or colourless crystals. Freely soluble in water.

USP 25: Colourless crystals or white, fine or course, crystalline powder. Is somewhat hygroscopic. Freely soluble in water and in glycerol, and even more so in boiling water; sparingly soluble in alcohol. pH of a 5% solution in water is between 4.6 and 6.0. Store in airtight containers.

Adverse Effects and Treatment

Ammonium salts are irritant to the gastric mucosa and may produce nausea and vomiting particularly in large doses. Large doses of ammonium chloride may cause a profound acidosis and hypokalaemia which should be treated symptomatically. Intravenous administration of ammonium chloride may cause pain and irritation at the site of injection, which may be decreased by slowing the rate of infusion.

Excessive doses of ammonium salts, particularly if administered by rapid intravenous injection, may give rise to hepatic encephalopathy due to the inability of the liver to convert the increased load of ammonium ions to urea.

Precautions

Ammonium salts are contra-indicated in the presence of impaired hepatic or renal function.

Pharmacokinetics

Ammonium chloride is absorbed from the gastrointestinal tract. The ammonium ion is converted into urea in the liver; the anion thus liberated into the blood stream and extracellular fluid causes a metabolic acidosis and decreases the pH of the urine; this is followed by transient diuresis.

Uses and Administration

Ammonium chloride is used as an expectorant in productive cough (p.1082). Other ammonium salts which have been used similarly include the acetate, bicarbonate, camphorate, carbonate, citrate, and glycyrrhizinate.

The administration of ammonium chloride produces a transient diuresis and acidosis. It may be used in the treatment of severe metabolic alkalosis (p.1180). It is administered usually as a 1 to 2% solution by slow intravenous infusion, in a dosage depending on the severity of the alkalosis. A concentrated solution of ammonium chloride may be diluted by sodium chloride injection.

Ammonium chloride may also be used to maintain the urine at an acid pH in the treatment of some urinary-tract disorders, or in forced acid diuresis procedures to aid the excretion of basic drugs, such as amfetamines, in severe cases of overdosage. It is usually given by mouth, often as enteric-coated tablets, in a dose of 1 to 2 g every four to six hours, although 4 g every two hours has been given in forced acid diuresis procedures.

Ammonium chloride has been promoted for self administration as a diuretic, for example in premenstrual water retention; a dose of 1 g three times daily for up to 6 days has been suggested, but such use is generally considered inappropriate.

Preparations

BP 2001: Ammonium Chloride Mixture; Aromatic Ammonia Solution; Aromatic Ammonia Spirit; Strong Ammonium Acetate Solution; White Liniment;
USP 25: Ammonium Chloride Delayed-release Tablets; Ammonium Chloride Injection; Aromatic Ammonia Spirit; Potassium Gluconate, Potassium Citrate, and Ammonium Chloride Oral Solution.

Proprietary Preparations (details are given in Part 3)
Fr.: Chlorammonic; **Jpn:** Glycyron†; Neo-Minophagen C†; **Spain:** Apir Cloruro Amonico; **Switz.:** Chloramon.

Multi-ingredient: numerous preparations are listed in Part 3.

Benproperine (12427-b)

Benproperine (rINN).

ASA-158/5 (benproperine phosphate). 1-[2-(2-Benzylphenoxy)-1-methylethyl]piperidine.

$C_{21}H_{27}NO = 309.4$.

CAS — 2156-27-6.

ATC — R05DB02.

Profile

Benproperine is used as a cough suppressant in non-productive cough (p.1082). It is reported to have a peripheral and central action and has been given by mouth in usual doses of 25 to 50 mg two to four times daily as the embonate or the phosphate.

Preparations

Proprietary Preparations (details are given in Part 3)
Ger.: Tussafug; **Hong Kong:** Cofrel; **Switz.:** Tussafug.

Benzonatate (5605-j)

Benzonatate (BAN, rINN).

Benzononatine; KM-65. 3,6,9,12,15,18,21,24,27-Nonaoxaoctacosyl 4-butylaminobenzoate.

$C_{13}H_{18}NO_2(OCH_2CH_2)_nOCH_3$, where n has an average value of 8.

CAS — 104-31-4 (where n = 8).

ATC — R05DB01.

Pharmacopoeias. In US.

Pharmacopoeial description

USP 25: A clear, pale yellow, viscous liquid having a faint characteristic odour. Soluble 1 in less than 1 of water, of alcohol, of chloroform, and of ether; freely soluble in benzene. Store in airtight containers. Protect from light.

Adverse Effects

Headache, dizziness, gastrointestinal disturbances, nasal congestion, hypersensitivity, pruritus and skin rash have been reported. There may be drowsiness. Benzonatate has local anaesthetic properties and may produce numbness of the mouth, tongue, and pharynx. CNS stimulation and convulsions may occur in overdosage followed by CNS depression.

Uses and Administration

Benzonatate is a cough suppressant used in non-productive cough (p.1082); it is stated to act peripherally. It is related to amethocaine [tetracaine] (p.1305) and has a local anaesthetic action on mucosa. It is given by mouth in a dose of 100 mg three times daily; up to 600 mg daily in divided doses may be given if necessary. Benzonatate is reported to act within about 20 minutes and its effects are reported to last for 3 to 8 hours.

Preparations

USP 25: Benzonatate Capsules.

Proprietary Preparations (details are given in Part 3)
Mex.: Alzomed-F; Beknol; Benzonal; Bloktus; Capsicof; D-Tato; Lemtosid; Novapsyl; Pebegal; Tesalon; Texoven; Tusehli; Tusical; Tusitato; Velpro; **USA:** Tessalon.

Bibenzonium Bromide (5640-k)

Bibenzonium Bromide (BAN, rINN).

Diphenetholine Bromide; ES-132. [2-(1,2-Diphenylethoxy)ethyl]trimethylammonium bromide.

$C_{19}H_{26}BrNO = 364.3$.

CAS — 59866-76-1 (bibenzonium); 15585-70-3 (bibenzonium bromide).

ATC — R05DB12.

Profile

Bibenzonium bromide is a cough suppressant used in non-productive cough (p.1082) which is stated to have a central action. It has been given by mouth in a usual dose of 30 to 60 mg two to three times daily.

Preparations

Proprietary Preparations (details are given in Part 3)
Aust.: Lysbex; **Port.:** Tussis†.

Bromhexine (11273-k)

Bromhexine (BAN, rINN).

Bromexina. 2-Amino-3,5-dibromobenzyl(cyclohexyl)methylamine.

$C_{14}H_{20}Br_2N_2 = 376.1$.

CAS — 3572-43-8.

ATC — R05CB02.

Bromhexine Hydrochloride (2008-z)

Bromhexine Hydrochloride (BANM, USAN, rINNM).

Bromhexini Hydrochloridum; Cloridrato de Bromexina; NA-274.

$C_{14}H_{20}Br_2N_2,HCl = 412.6$.

CAS — 611-75-6.

Pharmacopoeias. In Chin., Eur. (see p.vi), Jpn, and Pol.

Pharmacopoeial description

Ph. Eur.: A white or almost white crystalline powder. Very slightly soluble in water; slightly soluble in alcohol and in dichloromethane. Protect from light.

Adverse Effects

Gastrointestinal side-effects may occur occasionally with bromhexine and a transient rise in serum aminotransferase values has been reported. Other reported adverse effects include headache, dizziness, sweating, and skin rashes. Inhalation of bromhexine has occasionally produced cough or bronchospasm in susceptible subjects.

Precautions

Since mucolytics may disrupt the gastric mucosal barrier bromhexine should be used with care in patients with a history of peptic ulceration. Care is also advisable in asthmatic patients. Clearance of bromhexine or its metabolites may be reduced in patients with severe hepatic or renal impairment.

Pharmacokinetics
Bromhexine hydrochloride is rapidly absorbed from the gastrointestinal tract and undergoes extensive first-pass metabolism in the liver: its oral bioavailability is stated to be only about 20%. It is widely distributed to body tissues. About 85 to 90% of a dose is excreted in the urine mainly as metabolites. Ambroxol (p.1084) is a metabolite of bromhexine. Bromhexine is highly bound to plasma proteins. It has a terminal elimination half-life of up to about 12 hours. Bromhexine crosses the blood-brain barrier and small amounts cross the placenta.

◊ Administration of bromhexine hydrochloride by mouth to healthy subjects produced peak plasma concentrations after about 1 hour.[1] Only small amounts were excreted unchanged in the urine with a half-life of about 6.5 hours.

1. Bechgaard E, Nielsen A. Bioavailability of bromhexine tablets and preliminary pharmacokinetics in humans. *Biopharm Drug Dispos* 1982; **3:** 337–44.

Uses and Administration
Bromhexine is a mucolytic used in the treatment of respiratory disorders associated with productive cough (p.1082). Bromhexine is usually given by mouth in a dose of 8 to 16 mg of the hydrochloride three times daily. It has also been given by deep intramuscular or slow intravenous injection or inhaled as an aerosol solution.

Bromhexine has also been used orally and topically in the treatment of dry eye associated with abnormal mucus production (see below).

Dry eye. Bromhexine has been used orally in the treatment of dry eye (p.1498) in Sjögren's syndrome but results have been conflicting,[1-3] and it appears to have no effect on tear secretion in healthy subjects.[4] It has also been tried topically.

1. Frost-Larsen K, *et al.* Sjögren's syndrome treated with bromhexine: a randomised clinical study. *BMJ* 1978; **1:** 1579–81.
2. Tapper-Jones LM, *et al.* Sjögren's syndrome treated with bromhexine: a reassessment. *BMJ* 1980; **280:** 1356.
3. Prause JU, *et al.* Lacrimal and salivary secretion in Sjögren's syndrome: the effect of systemic treatment with bromhexine. *Acta Ophthalmol (Copenh)* 1984; **62:** 489–97.
4. Avisar R, *et al.* Oral bromhexine has no effect on tear secretion in healthy subjects. *Ann Pharmacother* 1996; **30:** 1498.

Respiratory-tract infection. USE WITH AN ANTIBACTERIAL. Bromhexine has been shown to enhance the penetration of erythromycin into bronchial secretions.[1] Although bromhexine is often administered with other antibiotics as an adjuvant in the treatment of respiratory infections, few controlled studies appear to have been conducted to determine if any additional benefit is obtained. However, among those studies that have been carried out, improved responses have been reported for cefalexin[2] and amoxicillin.[3]

1. Bergogne-Berezin E, *et al.* Etude de l'influence d'un agent mucolytique (bromhexine) sur le passage de l'érythromycine dans les sécrétions bronchiques. *Therapie* 1979; **34:** 705–11.
2. Boraldi F, Palmieri B. Antibiotic and mucolytic therapy in elderly patients with different cases of bronchopulmonary diseases. *Curr Ther Res* 1983; **33:** 686–91.
3. Roa CC, Dantes RB. Clinical effectiveness of a combination of bromhexine and amoxicillin in lower respiratory tract infection: a randomized controlled trial. *Arzneimittelforschung* 1995; **45:** 267–72.

Preparations
Proprietary Preparations (details are given in Part 3)
Aust.: Bisolvon; *Austral.:* Bisolvon Chesty; Bisolvon Sinus; Dur-Elix; Duro-Tuss Mucolytic Cough Liquid; *Belg.:* Bisolvon; Bromex; *Braz.:* Bisolvon; *Denm.:* Bisolvon; Viscolyt; *Fin.:* Bisolvon; Medipekt; Mucovin; *Fr.:* Bisolvon; *Ger.:* Aparsonin N; Bisolvon; Hustentabs; Lubrirhin; Omniapharm; *Hong Kong:* Asthmaxine; Bisolvon; Bromxine; Mucolix; Vasican; *Irl.:* Bisolvon; *Israel:* Movex; Solvex; *Ital.:* Bisolvon; Broncokin; *Mex.:* Bisolvon; Dibroxin; Tesacof; *Neth.:* Bisolvon; Darolan Slijmplossende†; Famel Broomhexine; *Norw.:* Bisolvon; *NZ:* Bisolvon; Dur-Elix; *Port.:* Bisolvon; Lisomucin; Tosseque; *S.Afr.:* Bisolvon; Bronkese; Dur-Elix; *Singapore:* Bisolvon; Bromxine; Broxine; Exolit; Mucosol; Swedol; Vasican; *Spain:* Bisolvon; *Switz.:* Bisolvon; Metasolvens†; Solvolin†; *Thai.:* Asovon; Axistal; Behexine; Bislan; Bromex; Bromoson; Bromso; Bromxin; Bromxine; Bronclear; Disol; Dutross; Exolit; Ida; Mucine; Mucola; Mucoxin; Ohexine; Romulin; Tromadil; *UAE:* Mucolyte.

Multi-ingredient: numerous preparations are listed in Part 3.

Brovanexine Hydrochloride (5170-m)
Brovanexine Hydrochloride (*rINNM*).
4-(Acetyloxy)-N-[2,4-dibromo-6-[(cyclohexylmethylamino)methyl]phenyl]-3-methoxybenzamide monohydrochloride.
$C_{24}H_{29}Br_2ClN_2O_4 = 604.8$.
CAS — 54340-61-3 (brovanexine); 54340-60-2 (brovanexine hydrochloride).

Profile
Brovanexine is a derivative of bromhexine (above) and is given by mouth as the hydrochloride, usually as an adjunct to antibacterials in preparations for the treatment of respiratory-tract infections.

Preparations
Proprietary Preparations (details are given in Part 3)
Braz.: Bronquimucil; *Port.:* Bronquimucil†; Pulmo-San.

Multi-ingredient: *Spain:* Amoxidel Bronquial; Bronquimucil; Eupen Bronquial.

Butamirate Citrate (5606-z)
Butamirate Citrate (*BANM, USAN, rINNM*).
Abbott-36581; Butamyrate Citrate; HH-197. 2-(2-Diethylaminoethoxy)ethyl 2-phenylbutyrate dihydrogen citrate.
$C_{18}H_{29}NO_3,C_6H_8O_7 = 499.6$.
CAS — 18109-80-3 (butamirate); 18109-81-4 (butamirate citrate).

Profile
Butamirate citrate is a cough suppressant used in non-productive cough (p.1082) and stated to have a central action. The usual dose is 20 to 30 mg daily in 3 to 5 divided doses by mouth. Some countries permit up to 90 mg daily in divided doses; modified-release tablets containing 50 mg have been given 2 or 3 times daily.

Preparations
Proprietary Preparations (details are given in Part 3)
Belg.: Quintex; Quintex Pediatrique; Sinecod; *Braz.:* Besedan; *Ital.:* Butiran; Sinecod Tosse Sedativo; *Port.:* Sinecod; *Switz.:* Demotussol; Sinecod; *Thai.:* Sinecod.

Multi-ingredient: *Braz.:* Novotussan; *Switz.:* Hicoseen†.

Butetamate Citrate (2045-x)
Butetamate Citrate (*BANM, rINNM*).
Butethamate Citrate; Butethamate Dihydrogen Citrate. 2-Diethylaminoethyl 2-phenylbutyrate citrate.
$C_{16}H_{25}NO_2,C_6H_8O_7 = 455.5$.
CAS — 14007-64-8 (butetamate); 13900-12-4 (butetamate citrate).

Profile
Butetamate citrate is reported to be an antispasmodic and bronchodilator and has been used alone or in combination with other drugs for the symptomatic treatment of coughs and other associated respiratory-tract disorders.

Preparations
Proprietary Preparations (details are given in Part 3)
Irl.: CAM.

Multi-ingredient: *Aust.:* Coldadolin; Influbene; Panax; *Switz.:* Bronchotussine; Dragees contre la toux no 536.

Calcium Iodide (4573-j)
$CaI_2 = 293.9$.
CAS — 10102-68-8.

Profile
Calcium iodide has been used by mouth in expectorant mixtures. The limitations of iodides as expectorants are discussed on p.1082. The actions of the iodides are discussed under Iodine (p.1522).

Preparations
Proprietary Preparations (details are given in Part 3)
Multi-ingredient: *USA:* Calcidrine; Norisodrine with Calcium Iodide.

Caramiphen Edisilate (18490-y)
Caramiphen Edisilate (*BANM, rINNM*).
Caramiphen Edisylate. 2-Diethylaminoethyl 1-phenylcyclopentane-1-carboxylate ethane-1,2-disulphonate.
$C_{38}H_{60}N_2O_{10}S_2 = 769.0$.
CAS — 77-22-5 (caramiphen); 125-86-0 (caramiphen edisilate); 125-85-9 (caramiphen hydrochloride).

Profile
Caramiphen is a centrally acting cough suppressant used as the edisilate in combination products for coughs (p.1082). Caramiphen was originally used as the hydrochloride similarly to benzhexol [trihexyphenidyl] (p.463) for its antimuscarinic actions.

Preparations
Proprietary Preparations (details are given in Part 3)
Multi-ingredient: *USA:* Ordrine AT Extended-Release†; Rescaps-D SR†; Tuss-Allergine Modified TD†; Tuss-Genade Modified†; Tuss-Ornade†; Tussogest Extended-Release†.

Carbocisteine (577-s)
Carbocisteine (*BAN, rINN*).
AHR-3053; Carbocisteinum; Carbocysteine (*USAN*); LJ-206. S-Carboxymethyl-L-cysteine.
$C_5H_9NO_4S = 179.2$.
CAS — 2387-59-9; 638-23-3 (carbocisteine, L-form).
ATC — R05CB03.
Pharmacopoeias. In Eur. (see p.vi) and Jpn.

The UK manufacturer states that mixture of carbocisteine with pholcodine linctus causes precipitation of carbocisteine from solution but provides no information on whether this incompatibility is with the pholcodine or some component of the formulation used.

Pharmacopoeial description
Ph. Eur.: A white crystalline powder. Practically insoluble in water, in alcohol, and in ether; dissolves in dilute mineral acids and in dilute solutions of alkali hydroxides. A 1% suspension in water has a pH of 2.8 to 3.0. Protect from light.

Carbocisteine Sodium (11293-r)
Carbocisteine Sodium (*BANM, rINNM*).
Carbocysteine Sodium.
CAS — 49673-84-9 (carbocisteine sodium, L-form).

Adverse Effects and Precautions
Nausea and gastric discomfort, gastrointestinal bleeding, and skin rash have occasionally occurred with carbocisteine.

Since mucolytics may disrupt the gastric mucosal barrier carbocisteine should be used with caution in patients with a history of peptic ulceration.

Effects on endocrine function. A report[1] of transient hypothyroidism associated with the administration of carbocisteine in a patient with compromised thyroid function.

1. Wiersinga WM. Antithyroid action of carbocisteine. *BMJ* 1986; **293:** 106.

Pharmacokinetics
Carbocisteine is rapidly and well absorbed from the gastrointestinal tract with peak plasma concentrations occurring 90 to 120 minutes after an oral dose. It appears to penetrate into lung tissue and respiratory mucus. Carbocisteine is excreted in the urine as unchanged drug and metabolites. Acetylation, decarboxylation, and sulfoxidation have been identified as the major metabolic pathways. Sulfoxidation may be governed by genetic polymorphism.

◊ References.
1. Karim EFIA, *et al.* An investigation of the metabolism of S-carboxymethyl-L-cysteine in man using a novel HPLC-ECD method. *Eur J Drug Metab Pharmacokinet* 1988; **13:** 253–6.
2. Brockmoller J, *et al.* Evaluation of proposed sulphoxidation pathways of carbocysteine in man by HPLC quantification. *Eur J Clin Pharmacol* 1991; **40:** 387–92.
3. Steventon GB. Diurnal variation in the metabolism of S-carboxymethyl-L-cysteine in humans. *Drug Metab Dispos* 1999; **27:** 1092–7.

Uses and Administration
Carbocisteine is used for its mucolytic activity in respiratory disorders associated with productive cough (p.1082). It is given by mouth in a dose of 750 mg three times daily, reduced by one-third when a response is obtained. Children aged 2 to 5 years may be given 62.5 to 125 mg four times daily and those aged 6 to 12 years 250 mg three times daily. Carbocisteine is also given by mouth as the sodium or lysine salts.

Chronic obstructive pulmonary disease. The value of mucolytic therapy in bronchitis (p.759) is controversial. Two studies have reported some improvements in lung function in patients with chronic bronchitis given carbocisteine for up to 6 months,[1,2] but it appeared to have no effect on the number of acute exacerbations.[1] However, a later multicentre study (using the lysine salt) did report a reduction in the number of acute exacerbations.[3] Carbocisteine may also produce some beneficial effects on sputum rheology.[2,4]

1. Grillage M, Barnard-Jones K. Long-term oral carbocisteine therapy in patients with chronic bronchitis: a double blind trial with placebo control. *Br J Clin Pract* 1985; **39:** 395–8.
2. Aylward M, *et al.* Clinical evaluation of carbocisteine (Mucolex) in the treatment of patients with chronic bronchitis: a double-blind trial with placebo control. *Clin Trials J* 1985; **22:** 36–44.
3. Allegra L, *et al.* Prevention of acute exacerbations of chronic obstructive bronchitis with carbocisteine lysine salt monohydrate: a multicenter, double-blind, placebo-controlled trial. *Respiration* 1996; **63:** 174–80.
4. Braga PC, *et al.* Identification of subpopulations of bronchitic patients for suitable therapy by a dynamic rheological test. *Int J Clin Pharmacol Res* 1989; **IX:** 175–82.

Preparations

Proprietary Preparations (details are given in Part 3)
Belg.: Bronchathiol; Mucosteine; Pulmoclase†; Rhinathiol Mucolyticum; Romilar Mucolyticum; Siroxyl; **Braz.:** Mucodestrol; Mucofan; Mucoflux; Mucolisil; Mucolitic; Mucotoss; **Fin.:** Pulmoclase; Reodyn; **Fr.:** Actifed Expectorant; Bronchathiol;
Bronchocyst†; Bronchokod; Bronchyteine†; Broncoclar; Broncorinol Expectorant; Bronkirex; Codotussyl Expectorant; Dimotapp Expectorant; Drill Expectorant; Ergix; Fluditec; Fluvic; Hex-
afluid†; Humex Expectorant; Medibronc†; Muciclar;
Mucoplexil†; Mucotrophir; Pectojuvene; Pectosan Expectorant;
Pneumoclar; Rhinathiol; Sirop des Vosges Expectorant; Toclase
Expectorant; Tussilene; **Ger.:** Mucopront; Pectox†; Sedotussin
muco; Transbronchin; **Hong Kong:** Mucodyne; Mucospect; Rhinathiol; Solmux; **Irl.:** Exputex; Mucodyne; Mucogen; Mucolex;
Pulmoclase; Viscolex; **Israel:** Mical; Mucolit; Mucomed; **Ital.:**
Broncomucil; Bronx; Carbocit; Fluifort; Lisil; Lisomucil; Mucocis; Mucojet; Mucolase; Mucotreis; Polimucil; Reomucil; Sinecod
Tosse Fluidificante; Solfomucil†; Solucis; Superthiol; **Mex.:** Loviscol; Mucolin; **Neth.:** Dampo Solvopect; Mucodyne; Pulmoclase; Rami Slijmoplossende; Rhinathiol†; Siroxyl†; **Port.:** Bronquial; Finatux; Mucolex; Mucoral; Pulmoclase; **S.Afr.:** Acuphlem†;
Arcanacysteine†; Betaphlem; Carbo-Syrup†; Carbospect†; Co-
Flem; Corbar M; Dynaphlem†; Flemex; Flemgo; Flemlite; Ilvispect; Lessmusec; Medphlem†; Mucocaps; Mucoflem; Mucoless;
Mucolinct; Mucopan†; Mucopront†; Mucosirop; Mucospect; **Singapore:** Mucopront; Rhinathiol; **Spain:** Actithiol; Anatac; Fluidin
Mucolitico NF; Mucovital; Pectox; Viscoteina; **Switz.:** Mephathi-
ol; Mucogeran; Mucoseptal†; Pectox†; Rhinathiol; Tussantiol;
Thai.: Bocytin; Mucopront; Muflex; Pectox; Rhinathiol; **UK:** Mu-
codyne.
Multi-ingredient: Fr.: Acnaveen; Rhinathiol Promethazine;
Hong Kong: Rhinathiol Promethazine; **Ital.:** Broncofluid; Libexin
Mucolitico; Sebaveen†; **Mex.:** Caltusine; **Port.:** Acnaveen†; Nif-
lux; Sebaveen†; **Singapore:** Rhinathiol Promethazine; **Spain:** Ac-
tithiol Antihist; Amoxtiol; Bronquicisteina; Eduprim Mucolitico;
Pectoral Funk Antitus†; Pectox Ampicilina†; Tilfilin†; Tuselin
Expectorante; **Switz.:** Broncatar; Rhinathiol Promethazine; Trio-
fan.

Clobutinol Hydrochloride   (5609-a)

Clobutinol Hydrochloride (rINNM).
KAT-256. 2-(4-Chlorobenzyl)-3-(dimethylaminomethyl)butan-
2-ol hydrochloride.
$C_{14}H_{22}ClNO,HCl = 292.2.$
CAS — 14860-49-2 (clobutinol); 1215-83-4 (clobutinol hydrochloride).

Profile
Clobutinol hydrochloride is a centrally acting cough suppressant for non-productive cough (p.1082) given by mouth in doses of 40 to 80 mg three times daily; doses of 20 mg have been
given by subcutaneous, intramuscular, or intravenous injection.

Preparations
Proprietary Preparations (details are given in Part 3)
Aust.: Silomat; **Belg.:** Silomat; **Braz.:** Silomat; **Fin.:** Silomat; **Fr.:**
Silomat; **Ger.:** Mentopin Hustenstiller; Nullatuss; Rofatuss; Silo-
mat; stas-Hustenstiller N; Tussamed†; Tussed; **Ital.:** Silomat-
Fher; **Port.:** Silomat; **Singapore:** Silomat; **Thai.:** Silomat.
Multi-ingredient: Braz.: Silomat Plus; **Fr.:** Silomat; **S.Afr.:** Silo-
mat DA; **Swed.:** Silomat Compositum†; **Thai.:** Silomat Composi-
tum; **UAE:** Orcinol.

Clofedanol Hydrochloride   (5608-k)

Clofedanol Hydrochloride (BANM, rINNM).
Chlophedianol Hydrochloride (USAN); SL-501. 2-Chloro-α-(2-
dimethylaminoethyl)benzyl alcohol hydrochloride.
$C_{17}H_{20}ClNO,HCl = 326.3.$
CAS — 791-35-5 (clofedanol); 511-13-7 (clofedanol hydro-
chloride).
Pharmacopoeias. In Jpn.

Profile
Clofedanol hydrochloride is a centrally acting cough suppressant for non-productive cough (p.1082) that has been given by
mouth in doses of 25 to 30 mg three to four times daily.

Preparations
Proprietary Preparations (details are given in Part 3)
Canad.: Ulone; **Hong Kong:** Coldrin; **Singapore:** Coldrin; **Spain:**
Gentos.
Multi-ingredient: Spain: Xibornol Prodes.

Clonazoline Hydrochloride   (14173-j)

Clonazoline Hydrochloride (rINNM).
2-[(4-Chloro-1-naphthyl)methyl]-2-imidazoline hydrochloride.
$C_{14}H_{13}ClN_2,HCl = 281.2.$
CAS — 17692-28-3 (clonazoline); 23593-08-0 (clonazoline hydrochloride).

Profile
Clonazoline hydrochloride is a sympathomimetic with effects
similar to those of naphazoline (p.1095) used for its vasoconstrictor activity in the local treatment of nasal congestion
(p.1082).

Preparations

Proprietary Preparations (details are given in Part 3)
Multi-ingredient: Ital.: Localyn.

Cloperastine Fendizoate   (9885-n)

Cloperastine Fendizoate (rINNM).
Cloperastine Hydroxyphenylbenzoyl Benzoic Acid; Cloperas-
tine Phendizoate.
$C_{20}H_{24}ClNO,C_{20}H_{14}O_4 = 648.2.$
CAS — 85187-37-7.

Cloperastine Hydrochloride   (5610-e)

Cloperastine Hydrochloride (rINNM).
1-{2-[(p-Chloro-α-phenylbenzyl)oxy]ethyl}piperidine hydrochloride.
$C_{20}H_{24}ClNO,HCl = 366.3.$
CAS — 3703-76-2 (cloperastine); 14984-68-0 (cloperastine hydrochloride).
Pharmacopoeias. In Jpn.

Cloperastine fendizoate 177 mg is approximately equivalent to
100 mg of cloperastine hydrochloride.

Profile
Cloperastine is primarily a centrally acting cough suppressant
used for non-productive cough (p.1082). It also has some antihistaminic action. The hydrochloride has been given by mouth
as tablets in usual doses of 10 to 20 mg three times daily. Cloperastine fendizoate is used in oral liquid preparations in equivalent doses.

Preparations
Proprietary Preparations (details are given in Part 3)
Belg.: Novotossil; Sekin; **Braz.:** Seki; **Hong Kong:** Costop; **Ital.:**
Cloel; Clofend; Nitossil; Politosse; Privituss; Quik; Risoltuss†;
Seki; **Jpn:** Hustazol†; **Spain:** Flutox; Sekisan.
Multi-ingredient: Thai.: Hustazol-C.

Cocillana   (2009-c)

Grape Bark; Guapi Bark; Huapi Bark.
CAS — 1398-77-2.
Pharmacopoeias. In Br.

Pharmacopoeial description
BP 2001: The dried bark of *Guarea rusbyi* and closely related
species containing not less than 3.5% of alcohol (60%)-soluble
extractive.

Profile
Cocillana is used as an expectorant similarly to ipecacuanha
(p.1093). It has been used in large doses as an emetic.

Preparations
Proprietary Preparations (details are given in Part 3)
Multi-ingredient: Braz.: Elixir de Marinheiro; **Canad.:** Alsid-
rine; Bronchosyl†; Sirop Cocillana Codeine; **Fin.:** Codesan
Comp; Codesan N; **Hong Kong:** Cocillana Compound; **Ital.:**
Broncosedina; **S.Afr.:** Cocillana Co; Corbar; **Swed.:** Cocillana-
Etyfin.

Coltsfoot   (5612-y)

Coughwort; Farfara; Huflattich; Tussilage.
Pharmacopoeias. Chin. and Swiss include Coltsfoot Flower. A
monograph for Coltsfoot Leaf is included in Aust.

Profile
The leaves and flowers of coltsfoot (*Tussilago farfara*) have
been used for their demulcent and supposed expectorant properties in the treatment of cough and other mild respiratory disorders. However, there has been some concern about potential
hepatotoxicity and carcinogenicity due to the content of pyrrolizidine alkaloids.

◊ In a review[1] of the actions and uses of coltsfoot it was pointed
out that given the potential risks of long-term use or use in
pregnancy, and the availability of other demulcent herbs, the
use of coltsfoot preparations to treat throat irritations can no
longer be considered appropriate.

1. Berry M. Coltsfoot. *Pharm J* 1996; **256:** 234–5.

Preparations
Proprietary Preparations (details are given in Part 3)
Multi-ingredient: Fr.: Mediflor Tisane Pectorale d'Alsace; **UK:**
Antibron.

Creosote   (2010-s)

Creasote; Creosotal (creosote carbonate); Wood Creosote.
CAS — 8021-39-4 (creosote); 8001-59-0 (creosote carbo-
nate).
ATC — R05CA08.
Pharmacopoeias. In Belg. and Jpn.

A liquid consisting of a mixture of guaiacol, cresol, and other
phenols obtained from wood tar. Commercial creosote used for
timber preservation is obtained from coal tar.

Profile
Creosote possesses disinfectant properties and has been used as
an expectorant. It has also been used as the carbonate and as
lactocreosote.
Adverse effects are similar to those of Phenol, p.1152.

Preparations
Proprietary Preparations (details are given in Part 3)
Multi-ingredient: Aust.: Famel cum Codein; Famel cum Ephe-
drin; **Austral.:** Compound Inhalation of Menthol; **Braz.:** Calmante
Creosotado; Rhum Creosotado; **Ital.:** Famel; **Neth.:** Famel; **Port.:**
Creodermol; **Spain:** Dentikrisos; Sanaden Reforzado; **Switz.:**
Famel; **UK:** Catarrh Pastilles; Famel Catarrh & Throat Pastilles†;
Famel Original; Penetrol†; Potter's Catarrh Pastilles.

Dembrexine   (3491-b)

Dembrexine (BAN, rINN).
Dembroxol. trans-4-[(3,5-Dibromosalicyl)amino]cyclohexanol.
$C_{13}H_{17}Br_2NO_2 = 379.1.$
CAS — 83200-09-3 (dembrexine); 52702-51-9 (dembrex-
ine hydrochloride).

Profile
Dembrexine is a mucolytic used as the hydrochloride in veterinary medicine.

Dextromethorphan   (5634-t)

Dextromethorphan (BAN, pINN).
(+)-3-Methoxy-9a-methylmorphinan; (9S,13S,14S)-6,18-Dide-
oxy-7,8-dihydro-3-O-methylmorphine.
$C_{18}H_{25}NO = 271.4.$
CAS — 125-71-3.
ATC — R05DA09.
Pharmacopoeias. In US.

Dextromethorphan 7.3 mg is approximately equivalent to
10 mg of dextromethorphan hydrobromide.
Pharmacopoeial description
USP 25: A practically white to slightly yellow, odourless, crystalline powder. Practically insoluble in water; freely soluble in
chloroform. Store in airtight containers.

Dextromethorphan Hydrobromide   (5613-j)

Dextromethorphan Hydrobromide (BANM, pINNM).
Dextromethorphani Hydrobromidum. Dextromethorphan hydrobromide monohydrate.
$C_{18}H_{25}NO,HBr,H_2O = 370.3.$
CAS — 125-69-9 (anhydrous dextromethorphan hydrobromide); 6700-34-1 (dextromethorphan hydrobromide monohydrate).
Pharmacopoeias. In Eur. (see p.vi), Int., Jpn, and US.

Pharmacopoeial description
Ph. Eur.: An almost white, crystalline powder. Sparingly soluble in water; freely soluble in alcohol; practically insoluble in
ether. Protect from light.

USP 25: Practically white crystals or crystalline powder having a faint odour. Soluble 1 in 65 of water; freely soluble in
alcohol and in chloroform; insoluble in ether. pH of a 1% solution in water is between 5.2 and 6.5. Store in airtight containers.

Adverse Effects and Treatment
Adverse effects with dextromethorphan appear to be
rare and may include dizziness and gastrointestinal
disturbances. Excitation, confusion, and respiratory
depression may occur after overdosage. Dextromethorphan has been subject to abuse, but there is little
evidence of dependence of the morphine type.

◊ General references.
1. Bem JL, Peck R. Dextromethorphan: an overview of safety issues. *Drug Safety* 1992; **7:** 190–9.

Effects on the skin. A report[1] of a fixed-drug reaction in a
patient following ingestion of dextromethorphan 30 mg. Oral
provocation with dextromethorphan produced a positive reaction but the results of topical application tests were negative.
1. Stubb S, Reitamo S. Fixed-drug eruption due to dextromethorphan. *Arch Dermatol* 1990; **126:** 970–1.

Overdosage. There have been reports[1-6] of overdosage or accidental poisoning (usually in children) due to dextromethorphan, including rare fatalities. Naloxone may be effective in
reversing toxicity. Extrapyramidal reactions were seen in a

The symbol † denotes a preparation no longer actively marketed

child who ingested dextromethorphan.[6] Overdosage has also been associated with abuse (see below).

1. Shaul WL, et al. Dextromethorphan toxicity: reversal by naloxone. Pediatrics 1977; 59: 117–19.
2. Katona B, Wason S. Dextromethorphan danger. N Engl J Med 1986; 314: 993.
3. Rammer L, et al. Fatal intoxication by dextromethorphan: a report on two cases. Forensic Sci Int 1988; 37: 233–6.
4. Schneider SM, et al. Dextromethorphan poisoning reversed by naloxone. Am J Emerg Med 1991; 9: 237–8.
5. Pender ES, Parks BR. Toxicity with dextromethorphan-containing preparations: a literature review and report of two additional cases. Pediatr Emerg Care 1991; 7: 163–5.
6. Warden CR, et al. Dystonic reaction associated with dextromethorphan ingestion in a toddler. Pediatr Emerg Care 1997; 13: 214–15.

Precautions

Dextromethorphan should not be given to patients at risk of developing respiratory failure. Caution is needed in patients with a history of asthma and it should not be given during an acute attack.

◊ For doubts about the use of dextromethorphan as an antitussive in children see Cough, under Uses and Administration, below.

Abuse. Reports of abuse of dextromethorphan.

1. Fleming PM. Dependence on dextromethorphan hydrobromide. BMJ 1986; 293: 597.
2. Orrell MW, Campbell PG. Dependence on dextromethorphan hydrobromide. BMJ 1986; 293: 1242–3.
3. Walker J, Yatham LN. Benylin (dextromethorphan) abuse and mania. BMJ 1993; 306: 896.
4. Wolfe TR, Caravati EM. Massive dextromethorphan ingestion and abuse. Am J Emerg Med 1995; 13: 174–6.

Interactions

Severe and sometimes fatal reactions have been reported following administration of dextromethorphan to patients receiving MAOIs. Dextromethorphan is primarily metabolised by the cytochrome P450 isoenzyme CYP2D6; the possibility of interactions with inhibitors of this enzyme, including amiodarone, fluoxetine, haloperidol, paroxetine, propafenone, quinidine, and thioridazine, should be borne in mind.

Antiarrhythmics. *Quinidine* can increase serum concentrations of dextromethorphan markedly, and some patients have experienced symptoms of dextromethorphan toxicity when the two drugs have been used together.[1] *Amiodarone* also appears to be able to increase serum concentrations of dextromethorphan.[2]

1. Zhang Y, et al. Dextromethorphan: enhancing its systemic availability by way of low-dose quinidine-mediated inhibition of cytochrome P4502D6. Clin Pharmacol Ther 1992; 51: 647–55.
2. Funck-Brentano C, et al. Influence of amiodarone on genetically determined drug metabolism in humans. Clin Pharmacol Ther 1991; 50: 259–66.

Antidepressants. A patient receiving *fluoxetine* experienced visual hallucinations after she began taking dextromethorphan.[1] The hallucinations were similar to those she had had 12 years earlier with lysergide. She had previously taken dextromethorphan alone without any adverse reactions. A serotonin syndrome (p.304) has been reported in a patient who took a cold-remedy including dextromethorphan while receiving *paroxetine*.[2]

1. Achamallah NS. Visual hallucinations after combining fluoxetine and dextromethorphan. Am J Psychiatry 1992; 149: 1406.
2. Skop BP, et al. The serotonin syndrome associated with paroxetine, an over-the-counter cold remedy, and vascular disease. Am J Emerg Med 1994; 12: 642–4.

Pharmacokinetics

Dextromethorphan is rapidly absorbed from the gastrointestinal tract. It is metabolised in the liver and excreted in the urine as unchanged dextromethorphan and demethylated metabolites including dextrorphan (p.1603), which has some cough suppressant activity.

◊ The O-demethylation of dextromethorphan and the hydroxylation of debrisoquine are under common polymorphic control, involving the cytochrome P450 isoenzyme CYP2D6, and dextromethorphan has been used as an alternative to debrisoquine for the phenotyping of oxidative metabolism.[1,2] Non-invasive determinations can be made using samples of urine or saliva.[3,4] Dextromethorphan has also been suggested as a tool to investigate N-demethylation, an alternate metabolic pathway for this drug.[5]

1. Belec L, et al. Extensive oxidative metabolism of dextromethorphan in patients with almitrine neuropathy. Br J Clin Pharmacol 1989; 27: 387–90.
2. Streetman DS, et al. Dose dependency of dextromethorphan for cytochrome P450 2D6 (CYP2D6) phenotyping. Clin Pharmacol Ther 1999; 66: 535–41.
3. Hildebrand M, et al. Determination of dextromethorphan metabolizer phenotype in healthy volunteers. Eur J Clin Pharmacol 1989; 36: 315–18.

4. Hou Z-Y, et al. Salivary analysis for determination of dextromethorphan metabolic phenotype. Clin Pharmacol Ther 1991; 49: 410–19.
5. Jones DR, et al. Determination of cytochrome P450 3A4/5 activity in vivo with dextromethorphan N-demethylation. Clin Pharmacol Ther 1996; 60: 374–84.

Uses and Administration

Dextromethorphan hydrobromide is a cough suppressant used for the relief of non-productive cough; it has a central action on the cough centre in the medulla. It is also an antagonist of N-methyl-D-aspartate (NMDA) receptors. Although structurally related to morphine, dextromethorphan has no classical analgesic properties and little sedative activity.

Dextromethorphan hydrobromide is reported to act within half an hour of administration by mouth and to exert an effect for up to 6 hours. It is given by mouth in doses of 10 to 20 mg every 4 hours, or 30 mg every 6 to 8 hours, to a usual maximum of 120 mg in 24 hours. Children aged 6 to 12 years may be given 5 to 10 mg every 4 hours or 15 mg every 6 to 8 hours to a maximum of 60 mg in 24 hours, and children aged 2 to 6 years 2.5 to 5 mg every 4 hours, or 7.5 mg every 6 to 8 hours, to a maximum of 30 mg in 24 hours. (But see also Cough, below.)

Dextromethorphan polistirex (a dextromethorphan and sulfonated diethenylbenzene-ethenylbenzene copolymer complex) is used in modified-release oral preparations. The dosage of dextromethorphan polistirex, expressed as dextromethorphan hydrobromide, is 60 mg every 12 hours; children aged 6 to 12 years may be given 30 mg every 12 hours; children aged 2 to 6 years may be given 15 mg every 12 hours. Dextrorphan (p.1603), the O-demethylated metabolite of dextromethorphan also has cough suppressant properties.

Cough. Equal doses of dextromethorphan hydrobromide and codeine phosphate were of similar efficacy in reducing the frequency of chronic cough (p.1082) in a double-blind crossover study in adults, but dextromethorphan had a greater effect than codeine on cough intensity.[1] However, these drugs were little more effective than placebo in suppressing night-time cough in children.[2,3] The American Academy of Pediatrics has commented[4] that there is no good evidence for the antitussive efficacy of dextromethorphan in children, that dosage guidelines are derived from (possibly inappropriate) extrapolation from effects in adults, and that adverse effects have been reported.

There is also some evidence that genetic polymorphism in the cytochrome P450 isoenzyme CYP2D6, and hence variations in metabolism, may have a significant influence on the antitussive efficacy of dextromethorphan.[5]

1. Matthys H, et al. Dextromethorphan and codeine: objective assessment of antitussive activity in patients with chronic cough. J Int Med Res 1983; 11: 92–100.
2. Gadomski A, Horton L. The need for rational therapeutics in the use of cough and cold medicine in infants. Pediatrics 1992; 89: 774–6.
3. Taylor JA, et al. Efficacy of cough suppressants in children. J Pediatr 1993; 122: 799–802.
4. American Academy of Pediatrics Committee on Drugs. Use of codeine- and dextromethorphan-containing cough remedies in children. Pediatrics 1997; 99: 918–20.
5. Wright CE, et al. CYP2D6 polymorphism and the anti-tussive effect of dextromethorphan in man. Thorax 1997; 52 (suppl 6): A73.

Neurological disorders. Dextromethorphan appears to have anticonvulsant activity and may have neuroprotective effects in cerebral ischaemia.[1] These effects may be related to its activity as an antagonist of N-methyl-D-aspartate (NMDA) receptors or to interaction with σ-receptors. It is being studied in Parkinson's disease for treatment[2] or for management of levodopa-induced dyskinesias,[3] and for its potential protective action in stroke (p.813) and acute brain injury. Dextromethorphan has also been studied for the management of amyotrophic lateral sclerosis (see Motor Neurone Disease, p.1658) but has not been found to be of benefit.[4-6] Its NMDA-antagonist properties are also being investigated for the treatment[7,8] of nonketotic hyperglycinaemia (see under Strychnine, p.1667).

1. Tortella FC, et al. Dextromethorphan and neuromodulation: old drug coughs up new activities. Trends Pharmacol Sci 1989; 10: 501–7.
2. Bonuccelli U, et al. Dextromethorphan and parkinsonism. Lancet 1992; 340: 53.
3. Verhagen Metman L, et al. Dextromethorphan improves levodopa-induced dyskinesias in Parkinson's disease. Neurology 1998; 51: 203–6.
4. Askmark H, et al. A pilot trial of dextromethorphan in amyotrophic lateral sclerosis. J Neurol Neurosurg Psychiatry 1993; 56: 197–200.
5. Blin O, et al. A controlled one-year trial of dextromethorphan in amyotrophic lateral sclerosis. Clin Neuropharmacol 1996; 19: 189–92.

6. Gredal O, et al. A clinical trial of dextromethorphan in amyotrophic lateral sclerosis. Acta Neurol Scand 1997; 96: 8–13.
7. Alemzadeh R, et al. Efficacy of low-dose dextromethorphan in the treatment of nonketotic hyperglycinemia. Pediatrics 1996; 97: 924–6.
8. Hamosh A, et al. Long-term use of high-dose benzoate and dextromethorphan for the treatment of nonketotic hyperglycinemia. J Pediatr 1998; 132: 709–13.

Pain. Dextromethorphan has a potential role in the blockade of pain. It has been investigated[1] in the management of neuropathic pain with promising results in diabetic neuropathy (p.5), although pain was not reduced in postherpetic neuralgia (p.7). However, a review[2] concluded that there are insufficient data to justify the use of dextromethorphan at present in diabetic neuropathy and further well-controlled trials are needed.

Dextromethorphan given pre-operatively and for 48 hours post-operatively at the highest tolerable dose did not reduce postoperative pain (p.4) immediately after oral surgery,[3] but did reduce pain after 48 hours, suggesting that NMDA receptor antagonists such as dextromethorphan might be useful pharmacologic interventions to reduce hyperalgesia or mitigate chronic pain. Dextromethorphan given as an adjunct to analgesics also demonstrated a morphine-sparing effect in adults 48 hours after hysterectomy,[4] but pre-operative administration to adults undergoing laparotomy,[5] or children scheduled for adenotonsillectomy,[6] did not improve postoperative pain at 24 hours.

1. Nelson KA, et al. High-dose oral dextromethorphan versus placebo in painful diabetic neuropathy and postherpetic neuralgia. Neurology 1997; 48: 1212–18.
2. Criner TM, Perdun CS. Dextromethorphan and diabetic neuropathy. Ann Pharmacother 1999; 33: 1221–3.
3. Gordon SM, et al. Antihyperalgesic effect of the N-methyl-D-aspartate receptor antagonist dextromethorphan in the oral surgery model. J Clin Pharmacol 1999; 39: 139–46.
4. Henderson DJ, et al. Perioperative dextromethorphan reduces postoperative pain after hysterectomy. Anesth Analg 1999; 89: 399–402.
5. Grace RF, et al. Preoperative dextromethorphan reduces intraoperative but not postoperative morphine requirements after laparotomy. Anesth Analg 1998; 87: 1135–8.
6. Rose JB, et al. Preoperative oral dextromethorphan does not reduce pain or analgesic consumption in children after adenotonsillectomy. Anesth Analg 1999; 88: 749–53.

Preparations

USP 25: Acetaminophen, Dextromethorphan Hydrobromide, Doxylamine Succinate, and Pseudoephedrine Hydrochloride Oral Solution; Dextromethorphan Hydrobromide Syrup; Guaifenesin, Pseudoephedrine Hydrochloride, and Dextromethorphan Hydrobromide Capsules; Pseudoephedrine Hydrochloride, Carbinoxamine Maleate, and Dextromethorphan Hydrobromide Oral Solution.

Proprietary Preparations (details are given in Part 3)

Aust.: Wick Formel 44; Wick Formel 44 Plus Hustenstiller; *Austral.:* Benadryl for the Family Dry Forte; Bisolvon Dry; Robitussin DX; Strepsils Cough Relief; Tussinol for Dry Coughs; *Belg.:* Akindex†; Benylin Antitussivum†; Bronchosedal; Dexir; Humex; Rhinathiol Antitussivum; Romilar Antitussivum; Touxium†; Tussipect; Tussiphane; Vicks Vaposyrup Antitussif; *Canad.:* Balminil DM; Benylin DM; Broncho-Grippol-DM; Bronchopan DM; Buckley's DM; Calmylin #1; Centratuss DM†; Cough Suppressant Syrup DM; Cough Syrup; Cough Syrup DM; Delsym; DM Cough Syrup; DM Sans Sucre; Drixoral Cough†; Drixoral†; Formula 44; Koffex; Koffex DM; Novahistex DM; Novahistine DM; Pharmilin-DM; Pharminil DM; Robitussin Childrens; Sedatuss DM; Sirop DM; Sucrets Cough Control; Syrup DM; Triaminic Long Lasting DM; Tussin Antitussive; *Denm.:* Dexofan; *Fin.:* Lagun; Resilar; *Fr.:* Akindex; Atuxane†; Bronchytuc†; Capsyl†; Codotussyl Toux Seche; Dexir; Drill toux seche; Ergix; Nodex; Rhinathiol Toux Seche; Sebrane; Tarituxl; Tuxium; Vicks Toux Seche; Vicks Vaposyrup toux seche†; *Ger.:* Arpha Hustensirup; Hustenstiller; NeoTussan; Tuss Hustenstiller; Wick Formel 44 Husten-Stiller; Wick Formel 44 plus Husten-Pastillen S; Wick Kinder Formel 44 Husten-Stiller†; *Hong Kong:* Balminil DM; Pusiran; Robitussin Maximum Strength Cough; Robitussin Pediatric Cough; *Irl.:* Benylin Non-Drowsy Dry Coughs; Delsym; Robitussin Cough Soother; *Israel:* Cough Control Sucrets; Tarodex; *Ital.:* Aricodil; Bechilar; Bronchenolo; Fluprim Tosse†; Formitrol; Metorfan; Sanabronchiol; Tossoral; Tussycalm; Valatux†; Vicks Tosse Pastiglie; Vicks Tosse Sedativo; *Mex.:* Atassol; Athos; Balbek; Bekfan; Bekidiba Dex; Bioquidan; Brocolan; Delsym; Dontuxin; Formula S; Mebran; Megal Simple; Neo-Ulcoid; Neopulmonier; Protan; Romilar; Tartrina; Vimen; *Neth.:* Benylin-Dextromethorfanhydrobromide†; Dampo bij droge hoest; Darolan Hoestprikkeldempende†; Rami-Dextromethorphan; Tosion Retard†; Vicks Vaposiroop; Vicks Vapotab; *NZ:* Strepsils Cough; *Port.:* Akindex†; Rhinathiol Tosse Seca; *S.Afr.:* Benylin Dry Cough; Benylin Solid†; *Singapore:* Pusiran; Tussidex; Tussils; *Spain:* Benylin Antitusivo; Cinfatos; Formulatus; Humex†; Pastillas Dr Andreu; Robitussin DM Antitusivo; Romilar; Siepex; TIP; Tosfriol; Tusitinas; Tusorama; Tussidrill; Valdatos; *Swed.:* Tussidyl; *Switz.:* Bexine; Calmerphan; Calmerphan-L; Calmesine; Dextrocalmine; Emedrin N; Pulmofor; Vicks Formule 44 Calmine; *Thai.:* Cortuss; Dec; Detuss; Dex; Dextroral; Polydex; Pusiran; Tusco; Tussils; *UK:* Benylin Dry Coughs Non-Drowsy; Contac Coughcaps†; Covonia for Children†; Franolyn Sedative; Meltus Cough Control†; Nirolex for Dry Coughs; Robitussin for Dry Coughs; Robitussin Junior; Strepsils Cough; Vicks Vaposyrup for dry coughs; *USA:* Benylin Adult; Benylin DM; Benylin Pediatric; Creo-Terpin; DexAlone; Diabe-Tuss DM; Drixoral Cough†; Hold DM; Pertussin; Robitussin Cough Calmers; Robitussin Pediatric; Scot-Tussin DM Cough Chasers; Silphen DM; St. Joseph Cough Suppressant; Sucrets 4-Hour Cough; Sucrets Cough Control; Suppress; Trocal; Vicks Dry Hacking Cough.

Multi-ingredient: numerous preparations are listed in Part 3.

Dimemorfan Phosphate (5615-c)

Dimemorfan Phosphate (rINNM).

AT-17. (+)-3,9a-Dimethylmorphinan phosphate.

$C_{18}H_{25}N,H_3PO_4 = 353.4$.

CAS — 36309-01-0 (dimemorfan); 36304-84-4 (dimemorfan phosphate).

Pharmacopoeias. In Jpn.

Profile

Dimemorfan phosphate is a centrally acting cough suppressant used for non-productive cough (p.1082). It is given by mouth in doses of 10 to 20 mg three or four times daily.

Preparations

Proprietary Preparations (details are given in Part 3)
Ital.: Gentus†; Tusben; **Jpn:** Astomin†; **Spain:** Dastosin.

Dimethoxanate Hydrochloride (5616-k)

Dimethoxanate Hydrochloride (BANM, rINNM).

2-(2-Dimethylaminoethoxy)ethyl phenothiazine-10-carboxylate hydrochloride.

$C_{19}H_{22}N_2O_3S,HCl = 394.9$.

CAS — 477-93-0 (dimethoxanate); 518-63-8 (dimethoxanate hydrochloride).

Profile

Dimethoxanate hydrochloride is a centrally acting cough suppressant used for non-productive cough (p.1082). It is given by mouth in usual doses of 37.5 mg 3 or 4 times daily.

Preparations

Proprietary Preparations (details are given in Part 3)
Belg.: Cotrane.

Dioxethedrin Hydrochloride (11600-c)

Dioxethedrin Hydrochloride (rINNM).

Dioxethedrine Hydrochloride. α-(1-Ethylaminoethyl)protocatechuyl alcohol hydrochloride.

$C_{11}H_{17}NO_3,HCl = 247.7$.

CAS — 497-75-6 (dioxethedrin).

Profile

Dioxethedrin hydrochloride is a sympathomimetic that has been used with antitussives in preparations intended for the relief of coughs and associated respiratory-tract disorders.

Preparations

Proprietary Preparations (details are given in Part 3)
Multi-ingredient: Fr.: Quintopan Enfant†.

Domiodol (12678-d)

Domiodol (USAN, pINN).

MG-13608. 2-Iodomethyl-1,3-dioxolan-4-ylmethanol.

$C_5H_9IO_3 = 244.0$.

CAS — 61869-07-6.

ATC — R05CB08.

Profile

Domiodol has been used for its mucolytic properties in the relief of productive cough (p.1082).

The actions of the iodides are discussed under Iodine, p.1522.

Preparations

Proprietary Preparations (details are given in Part 3)
Ital.: Mucolitico Maggioni†.

Dornase Alfa (3717-g)

Dornase Alfa (BAN, USAN, rINN).

Deoxyribonuclease; Desoxyribonuclease; DNase I; rhDNase. Deoxyribonuclease I (human recombinant).

$C_{1321}H_{1995}N_{339}O_{396}S_9 = 29249.6$.

CAS — 143831-71-4; 132053-08-8.

ATC — B06AA10; R05CB13.

An enzyme derived from cloned human pancreatic deoxyribonuclease I and having the same amino acid sequence and glycosylation pattern as human deoxyribonuclease I.

Adverse Effects

Common adverse effects with dornase alfa aerosol include pharyngitis, hoarseness of the voice, and chest pain. Occasionally laryngitis, conjunctivitis, and skin rashes and urticaria have been reported. There may be a transient decline in pulmonary function on beginning therapy with dornase alfa.

Uses and Administration

Dornase alfa acts as a mucolytic by hydrolysing DNA that has accumulated in sputum from decaying neu-

The symbol † denotes a preparation no longer actively marketed

trophils. It is used as a nebulised solution in patients with cystic fibrosis; in the UK its indication is limited to patients with a forced vital capacity greater than 40% of predicted value and to patients over 5 years of age, but in the USA it may also be given for advanced disease (FVC less than 40%) and to younger children. The usual dose is 2500 units (2.5 mg) of dornase alfa given once daily via a jet nebuliser. This dose may be given twice daily to patients over 21 years of age.

Bovine deoxyribonuclease has been used similarly. It has also been used topically, often with fibrinolysin (human), as a debriding agent in a variety of inflammatory and infected lesions. Bovine deoxyribonuclease has also been given by injection.

Administration in children. Although in some countries dornase alfa is not recommended for use in children under 5 years of age, a study[1] to assess the delivery of dornase alfa to the lungs of children with cystic fibrosis aged between 3 months and 5 years, showed that the drug was present in the lower airways in comparable amounts to older children. It also appeared to be safe in these younger patients during the 2-week study period.

1. Wagener JS, et al. Aerosol delivery and safety of recombinant human deoxyribonuclease in young children with cystic fibrosis: a bronchoscopic study. J Pediatr 1998; **133:** 486–91.

Asthma. There is a report of the use of dornase alfa to liquefy a mucus plug and relieve an attack of acute severe asthma (p.757) in an 8-year-old child.[1]

1. Greally P. Human recombinant DNase for mucus plugging in status asthmaticus. Lancet 1995; **346:** 1423–4.

Chronic obstructive pulmonary disease. A large phase III study in patients hospitalised for acute exacerbations of chronic bronchitis (p.759) was halted prematurely because of a non-significant trend to increased mortality in patients given dornase alfa.[1]

1. Hudson TJ. Dornase in treatment of chronic bronchitis. Ann Pharmacother 1996; **30:** 674–5.

Cystic fibrosis. There is good evidence that inhalation therapy with dornase alfa can produce modest but useful improvement in lung function in some patients with cystic fibrosis (p.117). Most studies have concentrated on patients with mild or moderate disease (forced vital capacity at least 40% of the predicted value) in whom FEV_1 and forced vital capacity have shown improvements generally of the order of 5 to 10%,[1-3] and in whom more prolonged therapy (24 weeks) has been shown to reduce the risk of exacerbations of respiratory infections, and hence the need for intravenous antibiotic therapy.[3] There is also evidence that benefit may occur in patients with more severe disease.[4] Meta-analysis of these and 3 other studies confirmed the short-term improvement in lung function, but noted that longer-term studies were needed.[5] Studies differ on whether subjective symptoms such as dyspnoea and general well-being are improved by dornase alfa.

Only a minority of patients, perhaps about one-third,[6] benefit from the drug, and at present there is no way of identifying those who will respond other than by a therapeutic trial.[7,8] It is also unclear whether longer-term therapy can alter the underlying pathophysiology of the disease and retard or prevent the progressive decline in lung function (which is in any case low in optimally-treated patients[9,10]), although there are reasons to think that this might be the case.[11-13]

Given the high cost of therapy, which is not entirely recouped by savings in acute care, there has been some controversy about the appropriate use of dornase alfa:[14-17] it seems to be generally felt that it should be reserved for specialist use in cystic fibrosis clinics, but that patients should not be denied a trial where appropriate. Most responders with mild to moderate impairment of lung function will show improvements within 2 weeks, although in more severely affected patients a 6-week trial is advocated.[7,9]

1. Ramsey BW, et al. Efficacy and safety of short-term administration of aerosolized recombinant human deoxyribonuclease in patients with cystic fibrosis. Am Rev Respir Dis 1993; **148:** 145–51.
2. Ranasinha C, et al. Efficacy and safety of short-term administration of aerosolised recombinant human DNase I in adults with stable stage cystic fibrosis. Lancet 1993; **342:** 199–202.
3. Fuchs H, et al. Effect of aerosolized recombinant human DNase on exacerbations of respiratory symptoms and on pulmonary function in patients with cystic fibrosis. N Engl J Med 1994; **331:** 637–42.
4. McCoy K, et al. Effects of 12-week administration of dornase alfa in patients with advanced cystic fibrosis lung disease. Chest 1996; **110:** 889–95.
5. Kearney CE, Wallis CE. Deoxyribonuclease for cystic fibrosis (updated 22 August 2001). Available in the Cochrane Library; Issue 4. Oxford: Update Software; 2001.
6. Davis PB. Evolution of therapy for cystic fibrosis. N Engl J Med 1994; **331:** 672–3.
7. Conway SP, Littlewood JM. rhDNase in cystic fibrosis. Br J Hosp Med 1997; **57:** 371–2.
8. Ledson MJ, et al. Targeting of dornase alpha therapy in adult cystic fibrosis. J R Soc Med 1998; **91:** 360–4.
9. Conway SP. Recombinant human DNase (rhDNase) in cystic fibrosis: is it cost effective? Arch Dis Child 1997; **77:** 1–3.
10. Milla CE. Long term effects of aerosolised rhDNase on pulmonary disease progression in cystic fibrosis. Thorax 1998; **53:** 1014–17.
11. Shah PL, et al. Two years experience with recombinant human DNase I in the treatment of pulmonary disease in cystic fibrosis. Respir Med 1995; **89:** 499–502.
12. Costello CM, et al. Effect of nebulised recombinant human DNase on neutrophil elastase load in cystic fibrosis. Thorax 1996; **51:** 619–23.
13. Johnson CA, et al. Estimating effectiveness in an observational study: a case study of dornase alfa in cystic fibrosis. J Pediatr 1999; **134:** 734–9.
14. Anonymous. Dornase alfa for cystic fibrosis. Drug Ther Bull 1995; **33:** 15–16.
15. Spencer D, Weller P. Dornase-alfa for cystic fibrosis. Lancet 1995; **345:** 1307.
16. Bush A, et al. Dornase alfa for cystic fibrosis. BMJ 1995; **310:** 1533.
17. Robert G, et al. Dornase alfa for cystic fibrosis. BMJ 1995; **311:** 813.

Preparations

Proprietary Preparations (details are given in Part 3)
Aust.: Pulmozyme; **Austral.:** Pulmozyme; **Belg.:** Pulmozyme; **Braz.:** Pulmozyme; **Canad.:** Pulmozyme; **Denm.:** Pulmozyme; **Fin.:** Pulmozyme; **Fr.:** Pulmozyme; **Ger.:** Pulmozyme; **Irl.:** Pulmozyme; **Israel:** Pulmozyme; **Ital.:** Pulmozyme; **Mex.:** Pulmozyme; **Neth.:** Pulmozyme; **Norw.:** Pulmozyme; **NZ:** Pulmozyme; **Port.:** Pulmozyme; **S.Afr.:** Pulmozyme; **Spain:** Pulmozyme; **Swed.:** Pulmozyme; **Switz.:** Pulmozyme; **UK:** Pulmozyme; **USA:** Pulmozyme.

Multi-ingredient: Aust.: Fibrolan; **Austral.:** Elase†; **Braz.:** Cauterex com Gentamicina; Fibrase com Clorafenicol; Gino-Cauterex; Gino-Fibrase; **Canad.:** Elase-Chloromycetin†; Elase†; **Fr.:** Elase; **Ger.:** Fibrolan; **Ital.:** Derinase Plus†; Elase; **Mex.:** Fibrase; Fibrase SA; Ridasa; **Neth.:** Elase; **Spain:** Parkelase Chloromycetin†; Parkelase†; **Switz.:** Fibrolan; **USA:** Elase-Chloromycetin†; Elase†.

Dropropizine (12680-k)

Dropropizine (BAN, rINN).

UCB-1967. 3-(4-Phenylpiperazin-1-yl)propane-1,2-diol.

$C_{13}H_{20}N_2O_2 = 236.3$.

CAS — 17692-31-8.

ATC — R05DB19.

Levodropropizine (5399-n)

Levodropropizine (BAN, rINN).

DF-526; Levdropropizine; Levodropropizinum. The (−)-(S)-isomer of dropropizine.

$C_{13}H_{20}N_2O_2 = 236.3$.

CAS — 99291-25-5.

ATC — R05DB27.

Pharmacopoeias. In Eur. (see p.vi).

Pharmacopoeial description

Ph. Eur.: A white or almost white powder. Slightly soluble in water and in alcohol; freely soluble in dilute acetic acid and in methyl alcohol. A 2.5% solution in water has a pH of 9.2 to 10.2. Protect from light.

Profile

Dropropizine is a cough suppressant reported to have a peripheral action in non-productive cough (p.1082). It is given by mouth in a dose of 30 mg three to four times daily. Levodropropizine, the (−)-(S)-isomer of dropropizine, is claimed to produce fewer CNS effects and is used similarly by mouth in a dose of 60 mg up to three times daily.

◊ References.

1. Catena E, Daffonchio L. Efficacy and tolerability of levodropropizine in adult patients with non-productive cough: comparison with dextromethorphan. Pulm Pharmacol Ther 1997; **10:** 89–96.

Preparations

Proprietary Preparations (details are given in Part 3)
Belg.: Catabex; Levotuss; **Braz.:** Atosson; Eritos; Tussiflex D; Vibral; **Ger.:** Larylin Husten-Stiller; Larylin Hustensirup N†; **Ital.:** Danka; Domutussina; Levotuss; Rapitux; Ribex Tosse; Salvituss; **Mex.:** Troferit; Zyplo; **Port.:** Catabina; **Singapore:** Levopront; **Spain:** Levotuss; Tautoss; Tusofren; **Thai.:** Levopront.

Multi-ingredient: Belg.: Catabex Expectorans; **Braz.:** Notuss; **Fr.:** Catabex†; **Ital.:** Elisir Terpina; Guaiacalcium Complex; Ribexen con Espettorante; Tiocalmina; Tussamag Complex; **Port.:** Catabina Expectorante.

Elecampane (16013-j)

Alant; Aunée; Inula.

Pharmacopoeias. In Chin. (which also includes various other species of Inula) and Fr.

Profile

Elecampane is the root of Inula helenium (Compositae). It has been used in herbal preparations for the treatment of cough for its supposed expectorant and cough suppressant properties. It is also used as a flavouring in foods and alcoholic beverages.

Elecampane contains sesquiterpene lactones including alantolactone (alant camphor; elecampane camphor; inula camphor; helenin), which was formerly employed in the treatment of worm infections, and has also been an ingredient of some cough preparations.

Preparations

Proprietary Preparations (details are given in Part 3)

Multi-ingredient: *Belg.:* Euphon; *Fr.:* Marrubene Codethyline†; Mediflor Tisane Digestive No 3†; Mediflor Tisane Hepatique No 5†; Tisanes de l'Abbe Hamon no 15†; Tossarel†; *Ger.:* Leber-Galle-Tropfen 83; *Switz.:* Boldoflorine†; Hederix; *UK:* Catarrh-eeze; Cough-eeze†; Horehound and Aniseed Cough Mixture; Vegetable Cough Remover.

Ephedra (2054-r)

Ma-huang.

Pharmacopoeias. In Chin., Ger., and Jpn.

Ephedra consists of the dried young branches of *Ephedra sinica*, *E. equisetina*, and *e. gerardiana* (including *E. nebrodensis*) (Ephedraceae), containing not less than 1.25% of alkaloids, calculated as ephedrine. (*Jpn P.* specifies not less than 0.6%). *Chin. P.* also includes Radix Ephedrae, prepared from the roots of *E. sinica* or *E. intermedia*.

Profile

The action of ephedra is due to the presence of ephedrine (p.1090) and pseudoephedrine (p.1099). It has been used chiefly as a source of these alkaloids.

◊ For reference to the adverse effects of herbal products containing ephedra see under Abuse in Ephedrine, below.

Preparations

Proprietary Preparations (details are given in Part 3)

Multi-ingredient: *Canad.:* Herbal Cold Relief; *Ger.:* Cardibisana; Cefedrin N; Repursan ST.

Ephedrine (2055-f)

Ephedrine *(BAN)*.

Efedrina; Ephedrina; (–)-Ephedrine; Ephedrinum. (1R,2S)-2-Methylamino-1-phenylpropan-1-ol.

$C_{10}H_{15}NO = 165.2$.

CAS — 299-42-3 (anhydrous ephedrine); 50906-05-3 (ephedrine hemihydrate).

ATC — R01AA03; R01AB05; R03CA02; S01FB02.

Pharmacopoeias. In Eur. (see p.vi), Int., and US, which have specifications, in either the same monograph or in separate monographs, for anhydrous ephedrine and for ephedrine hemihydrate.

An alkaloid obtained from species of *Ephedra*, or prepared synthetically. It may exist in a hemihydrate form or as the anhydrous substance.

Pharmacopoeial description

Ph. Eur.: Anhydrous Ephedrine is a white, crystalline powder or colourless crystals. Soluble in water; very soluble in alcohol; freely soluble in ether. It melts at about 36°. Protect from light.

Ephedrine Hemihydrate is a white, crystalline powder or colourless crystals. Soluble in water; very soluble in alcohol; freely soluble in ether. It melts at about 42°, determined without previous drying. Protect from light.

USP 25: Ephedrine is anhydrous or contains not more than one-half molecule of water of hydration. It is an unctuous, practically colourless solid or white crystals or granules. It gradually decomposes on exposure to light. M.p. between 33° and 40°, the variability being the result of differences in the moisture content, anhydrous ephedrine having a lower melting-point than the hemihydrate. Soluble 1 in 20 of water and 1 in 0.2 of alcohol; soluble in chloroform and in ether; moderately and slowly soluble in liquid paraffin, the solution becoming turbid if the ephedrine contains more than about 1% of water. Its solutions are alkaline to litmus. Store in airtight containers at a temperature not exceeding 8°. Protect from light.

Ephedrine Hydrochloride (2057-n)

Ephedrine Hydrochloride *(BANM)*.

Ephedrine Hydrochloridum; Ephedrine Chloride; Ephedrini Hydrochloridum; Ephedrinium Chloratum; *l*-Ephedrinum Hydrochloricum.

$C_{10}H_{15}NO,HCl = 201.7$.

CAS — 50-98-6.

Pharmacopoeias. In Chin., Eur. (see p.vi), Int., Jpn, Pol., and US. Eur. also includes the racemic form (racephedrine hydrochloride).

Pharmacopoeial description

Ph. Eur.: A white, crystalline powder or colourless crystals. Freely soluble in water; soluble in alcohol; practically insoluble in ether. It melts at about 219°. Protect from light.

Racemic Ephedrine Hydrochloride is a white, crystalline powder or colourless crystals. Freely soluble in water; soluble in alcohol; practically insoluble in ether. It melts at about 188°. Protect from light.

USP 25: Fine, white, odourless crystals or powder. Soluble 1 in 3 of water and 1 in 14 of alcohol; insoluble in ether. Protect from light.

Ephedrine Sulfate (2058-h)

Ephedrine Sulphate *(BANM)*.

$(C_{10}H_{15}NO)_2,H_2SO_4 = 428.5$.

CAS — 134-72-5.

Pharmacopoeias. In Int. and US.

Pharmacopoeial description

USP 25: Fine, white, odourless crystals or powder. It darkens on exposure to light. Soluble 1 in 1.3 of water and 1 in 90 of alcohol. Protect from light.

Adverse Effects

For the adverse effects of sympathomimetics in general, see under Adrenaline, p.829. The commonest adverse effects of ephedrine are tachycardia, anxiety, restlessness, and insomnia. Tremor, dry mouth, impaired circulation to the extremities, hypertension, and cardiac arrhythmias may also occur.

Ephedrine may be used in labour to maintain blood pressure during spinal anaesthesia but can cause fetal tachycardia.

Paranoid psychosis, delusions, and hallucinations may also follow ephedrine overdosage. Prolonged administration has no cumulative effect, but tolerance with dependence has been reported.

◊ For a discussion of the toxicity reported from the self-administration of ephedrine-containing dietary supplements or herbal stimulants, see under Abuse, below.

Precautions

For the precautions to be observed with sympathomimetics in general, see under Adrenaline, p.830. Ephedrine should be given with care to patients with hyperthyroidism, diabetes mellitus, ischaemic heart disease, hypertension, renal impairment, or angle-closure glaucoma. In patients with prostatic enlargement, ephedrine may increase difficulty with micturition.

Irritability and disturbed sleep have been reported in breast-fed infants.

Abuse. Although illicit use of ephedrine is primarily in the manufacture of street stimulants such as metamfetamine (p.1511), there is increasing evidence of the abuse of ephedrine preparations in some countries,[1] and the public health and social problems associated with its abuse appear to be significant, particularly in certain African countries. Ephedrine is also sold as a street substitute for 'Ecstasy' (Methylenedioxyamfetamine, p.1511).

Adverse effects reported with illicit ephedrine use include cardiovascular toxicity[2,3] and chest pain.[4]

There is controversy over the abuse liability of over-the-counter (OTC) stimulants such as ephedrine:[5] some studies have indicated that ephedrine is, overall, a relatively weak reinforcer whereas others have suggested that the abuse potential may be high. Examination of the characteristics of 5 patients who had been taking ephedrine-containing OTC preparations in high doses for periods ranging from 8 months to 2 years, emphasised the reinforcing and, therefore, addictive potential of ephedrine; similar observations were made for 2 patients who had ingested phenylpropanolamine long term, combined with pseudoephedrine in one of these cases. The authors suggested that, for most people, OTC preparations containing weaker sympathomimetics will not be reinforcing at the recommended doses. However, these cases strengthen the research findings that high-dose use of an OTC stimulant increases its potency, and thus its effects become more like amfetamine (p.1506).

Toxicity has also been reported[6] from the self-administration of ephedrine-containing dietary supplements or herbal stimulants, usually based on ephedra (ma-huang) and marketed for a variety of purposes including weight loss and as an alternative to illegal drugs of abuse.

Not all cases of ephedrine toxicity have arisen as a result of overt abuse but rather because of inadequate labelling of content and dosage instructions on some unlicensed products. In the USA, restrictions upon the ephedrine content of such preparations and appropriate warning labelling have been proposed.[7]

Adverse effects from ingestion of ephedrine-containing OTC preparations, including herbal products (usually in high doses and/or long term) have included coronary artery thrombosis, myocardial infarction, seizures,[8] psychotic reactions,[9] nephrolithiasis,[10,11] and myocarditis;[12] a number of fatalities have been reported. Frank dependence has been reported in female weightlifters following long-term use of high doses.[13]

For a report of urinary calculi developing in a patient who had ingested a preparation containing guaifenesin and ephedrine, see under Guaifenesin, p.1092.

1. WHO. Recommendations from the Expert Committee on Drug Dependence. *WHO Drug Inf* 1998; **12:** 227–9.
2. Cockings JGL, Brown MA. Ephedrine abuse causing acute myocardial infarction. *Med J Aust* 1997; **167:** 199–200.
3. Zahn KA, *et al.* Cardiovascular toxicity after ingestion of "herbal ecstasy" [sic]. *J Emerg Med* 1999; **17:** 289–91.
4. James LP, *et al.* Sympathomimetic drug use in adolescents presenting to a pediatric emergency department with chest pain. *J Toxicol Clin Toxicol* 1998; **36:** 321–8.
5. Tinsley JA, Watkins DD. Over-the-counter stimulants: abuse and addiction. *Mayo Clin Proc* 1998; **73:** 977–82.
6. Haller CA, Benowitz NL. Adverse cardiovascular and central nervous system events associated with dietary supplements containing ephedra alkaloids. *N Engl J Med* 2000; **343:** 1833–8.
7. Anonymous. FDA proposes constraints on ephedrine dietary supplements. *Am J Health-Syst Pharm* 1997; **54:** 1578.
8. Anonymous. Adverse events associated with ephedrine-containing products—Texas, December 1993-September 1995. *JAMA* 1996; **276:** 1711–12.
9. Doyle H, Kargin M. Herbal stimulant containing ephedrine has also caused psychosis. *BMJ* 1996; **313:** 756.
10. Powell T, *et al.* Ma-huang strikes again: ephedrine nephrolithiasis. *Am J Kidney Dis* 1998; **32:** 153–9.
11. Blau JJ. Ephedrine nephrolithiasis associated with chronic ephedrine abuse. *J Urol (Baltimore)* 1998; **160:** 825.
12. Zaacks SM, *et al.* Hypersensitivity myocarditis associated with ephedra use. *J Toxicol Clin Toxicol* 1999; **37:** 485–9.
13. Gruber AJ, Pope HG. Ephedrine abuse among 36 female weightlifters. *Am J Addict* 1998; **7:** 256–61.

Interactions

For the interactions of the sympathomimetics in general, see under Adrenaline, p.830. Administration of ephedrine may cause a hypertensive crisis in patients receiving an MAOI (including an RIMA); the possibility of such an interaction following intranasal use of ephedrine should also be borne in mind. For additional warnings see under Phenelzine (p.305) and Moclobemide (p.299). Ephedrine should be avoided or used with care in patients undergoing anaesthesia with cyclopropane, halothane, or other volatile anaesthetics. An increased risk of arrhythmias may occur if given to patients receiving cardiac glycosides, quinidine, or tricyclic antidepressants, and there is an increased risk of vasoconstrictor or pressor effects in patients receiving ergot alkaloids or oxytocin.

Pharmacokinetics

Ephedrine is readily and completely absorbed from the gastrointestinal tract. It is largely excreted unchanged in the urine, together with small amounts of metabolites produced by hepatic metabolism. Ephedrine has been variously reported to have a plasma half-life ranging from 3 to 6 hours depending on urinary pH; elimination is enhanced and half-life accordingly shorter in acid urine.

◊ References.

1. Welling PG, *et al.* Urinary excretion of ephedrine in man without pH control following oral administration of three commercial ephedrine sulfate preparations. *J Pharm Sci* 1971; **60:** 1629–34.
2. Sever PS, *et al.* The metabolism of (–)-ephedrine in man. *Eur J Clin Pharmacol* 1975; **9:** 193–8.
3. Pickup ME, *et al.* The pharmacokinetics of ephedrine after oral dosage in asthmatics receiving acute and chronic treatment. *Br J Clin Pharmacol* 1976; **3:** 123–34.

Uses and Administration

Ephedrine is a sympathomimetic (see Adrenaline, p.831) with direct and indirect effects on adrenergic receptors. It has alpha- and beta-adrenergic activity and has pronounced stimulating effects on the CNS. It has a more prolonged though less potent action than adrenaline [epinephrine]. In therapeutic doses it raises the blood pressure by increasing cardiac output and also by inducing peripheral vasoconstriction. Tachycardia may occur but is less frequent than with adrenaline [epinephrine]. Ephedrine also causes bronchodilatation, reduces intestinal tone and motility, relaxes the bladder wall while contracting the sphincter muscle but relaxes the detrusor muscle of the bladder and usually reduces the activity of the uterus. It has a stimulant action on the respiratory centre. It dilates the pupil but does not affect the light reflexes. After ephedrine has been used for a short while, tachyphylaxis may develop.

Ephedrine salts are used, either alone or in conjunction with other drugs, in the symptomatic relief of nasal congestion (p.1082). They may be given by mouth or topically as nasal drops or sprays. Ephedrine salts have sometimes been used in motion sickness in conjunction with hyoscine or an antihistamine and have been tried for postoperative nausea and vomiting (p.1206).

Ephedrine salts have been given parenterally to combat a fall in blood pressure during spinal or epidural anaesthesia. Ephedrine is of little value in hypotensive crises due to shock, circulatory collapse, or haemorrhage. It is no longer generally advocated for orthostatic hypotension.

Ephedrine salts have been used as bronchodilators, but more beta$_2$-selective sympathomimetics, such as salbutamol, are now preferred.

Other uses of ephedrine salts include diabetic neuropathic oedema, in which they may provide marked relief. They have also been used in micturition disorders.

Nasal drops or sprays usually contain ephedrine 0.5%; a 0.25% strength may be used for infants and young children. Ephedrine salts can also be given by oral inhalation.

To reverse hypotension induced by spinal or epidural anaesthesia, a solution containing ephedrine hydrochloride 3 mg per mL is given by slow intravenous injection in doses of 3 to 6 mg (or at most 9 mg) repeated every 3 to 4 minutes as required; the maximum total dose is 30 mg. Ephedrine salts have also been given by intramuscular or subcutaneous injection.

A suggested dose in diabetic neuropathic oedema is 30 to 60 mg of ephedrine hydrochloride three times daily by mouth.

Several other salts of ephedrine have been given including the camsilate and the tannate. Racephedrine hydrochloride has also been used.

Micturition disorders. Ephedrine salts have been used in nocturnal enuresis, although other treatments are usually preferred, and have been tried in patients with stress incontinence but the value of such treatment is not clear.

Spinal anaesthesia. Several sympathomimetics such as ephedrine and phenylephrine have been advocated for parenteral use in the correction of hypotension developing during local anaesthesia. The risk of hypotension developing with spinal or epidural block is greater than many other forms of nerve block (see p.1302). Ephedrine has been used[1,2] although not always successfully[3] for the correction of such hypotension. Although it has also been used prophylactically[4] one of the most important ways of minimising the hypotension is by making sure that the patient is adequately hydrated before induction of anaesthesia.

1. Hall PA, et al. Spinal anaesthesia for Caesarean section: comparison of infusions of phenylephrine and ephedrine. Br J Anaesth 1994; **73:** 471–4.
2. Thomas DG, et al. Randomized trial of bolus phenylephrine or ephedrine for maintenance of arterial pressure during spinal anaesthesia for Caesarean section. Br J Anaesth 1996; **76:** 61–5.
3. Critchley LAH, et al. Hypotension during subarachnoid anaesthesia: haemodynamic effects of ephedrine. Br J Anaesth 1995; **74:** 373–8.
4. Sternlo J-E, et al. Prophylactic im ephedrine in bupivacaine spinal anaesthesia. Br J Anaesth 1995; **74:** 517–20.

Preparations

BP 2001: Ephedrine Elixir; Ephedrine Hydrochloride Tablets; Ephedrine Nasal Drops;
USP 25: Ephedrine Sulfate Capsules; Ephedrine Sulfate Injection; Ephedrine Sulfate Nasal Solution; Ephedrine Sulfate Syrup; Theophylline, Ephedrine Hydrochloride, and Phenobarbital Tablets.

Proprietary Preparations (details are given in Part 3)
Mex.: Ephed 20th; Tendrin; **UK:** CAM; **USA:** Kondon's Nasal; Pretz-D; Resp†.

Multi-ingredient: numerous preparations are listed in Part 3.

Eprazinone Hydrochloride (12696-h)

Eprazinone Hydrochloride (rINNM).
CE-746. 3-[4-(β-Ethoxyphenethyl)piperazin-1-yl]-2-methylpropiophenone dihydrochloride.
C$_{24}$H$_{32}$N$_2$O$_2$,2HCl = 453.4.
CAS — 10402-90-1 (eprazinone); 10402-53-6 (eprazinone hydrochloride).

Profile
Eprazinone hydrochloride has been variously described as having mucolytic or expectorant properties (p.1082) as well as a direct relaxant action on bronchial smooth muscle. It is given by mouth in doses of 50 to 100 mg three times daily. It has also been administered rectally.

Effects on the skin. A report[1] of a skin eruption associated with the oral administration of eprazinone.

1. Faber M, et al. Eprazinonexanthem mit subkornealer Pustelbildung. Hautarzt 1984; **35:** 200–3.

Overdosage. Symptoms in two 22-month-old children who received an overdose of 800 mg of eprazinone included somnolence, ataxia, and seizures.[1]

1. Merigot P, et al. Les convulsions avec trois antitussifs dérivés substitués de la pipérazine: (zipéprol, éprazinone, éprozinol). Ann Pediatr (Paris) 1985; **32:** 504–11.

Preparations

Proprietary Preparations (details are given in Part 3)
Aust.: Eftapan†; **Belg.:** Isilung; **Fr.:** Mucitux; **Ger.:** Eftapan.

Multi-ingredient: Aust.: Eftapan Tetra†.

Eprozinol Hydrochloride (12697-m)

Eprozinol Hydrochloride (rINNM).
3-[4-(β-Methoxyphenethyl)piperazin-1-yl]-1-phenylpropan-1-ol dihydrochloride.
C$_{22}$H$_{30}$N$_2$O$_2$,2HCl = 427.4.
CAS — 32665-36-4 (eprozinol).

Profile
Eprozinol hydrochloride is given by mouth in doses of 50 mg three times daily for its mucolytic or expectorant properties.

◊ Convulsions and coma were reported in a 19-year-old patient following administration of eprozinol.[1]

1. Merigot P, et al. Les convulsions avec trois antitussifs dérivés substitués de la pipérazine: (zipéprol, éprazinone, éprozinol). Ann Pediatr (Paris) 1985; **32:** 504–11.

Preparations

Proprietary Preparations (details are given in Part 3)
Fr.: Eupneron.

Erdosteine (2948-y)

Erdosteine (rINN).
(±)-({[(Tetrahydro-2-oxo-3-thienyl)carbamoyl]methyl}thio)acetic acid.
C$_8$H$_{11}$NO$_4$S$_2$ = 249.3.
CAS — 84611-23-4.
ATC — R05CB15.

Profile
Erdosteine is a mucolytic that is used in the treatment of disorders of the respiratory tract characterised by productive cough (p.1082) It is given by mouth in doses of 300 mg twice daily.

◊ Erdosteine has been used in the management of chronic obstructive pulmonary disease[1,2] but the value of mucolytics in this disorder is controversial (see p.759).

1. Dechant KL, Noble S. Erdosteine. Drugs 1996; **52:** 875–81.
2. Marchioni CF, et al. Evaluation of efficacy and safety of erdosteine in patients affected by chronic bronchitis during an infective exacerbation phase and receiving amoxycillin as basic treatment (ECOBES, European Chronic Obstructive Bronchitis Erdosteine Study). Int J Clin Pharmacol Ther 1995; **33:** 612–18.

Preparations

Proprietary Preparations (details are given in Part 3)
Belg.: Mucothera; **Fin.:** Erdopect; **Fr.:** Edirel; Vectrine; **Ital.:** Erdotin; **Mex.:** Dostein; Esteclin; **Switz.:** Mucofor.

Multi-ingredient: Mex.: Esteclin Bac.

Eriodictyon (2012-e)

Mountain Balm; Yerba Santa.
CAS — 8013-08-9.

The dried leaves of Eriodictyon californicum (Hydrophyllaceae).

Profile
Eriodictyon has been used as an expectorant. It has also been used to mask the taste of bitter drugs.

Preparations

Proprietary Preparations (details are given in Part 3)
Multi-ingredient: Ital.: Broncosedina; **USA:** Feminease.

Etafedrine Hydrochloride (2059-m)

Etafedrine Hydrochloride (BANM, USAN, rINNM).
Ethylephedrine Hydrochloride. (−)-2-(Ethylmethylamino)-1-phenylpropan-1-ol hydrochloride.
C$_{12}$H$_{19}$NO,HCl = 229.7.
CAS — 7681-79-0 (etafedrine); 48141-64-6 ((−)-etafedrine); 5591-29-7 (etafedrine hydrochloride).

Profile
Etafedrine hydrochloride is a sympathomimetic related to ephedrine (p.1090). It is used for its bronchodilator effects in combination with other drugs for the relief of cough and associated respiratory-tract disorders.

Preparations

Proprietary Preparations (details are given in Part 3)
Multi-ingredient: Braz.: Bronco-Ped; Broncolex; EMS Expectorante; Revenil; Revenil Dospan; Revenil Expectorante; **Canad.:** Calmydone; Dalmacol; Mercodol with Decapryn; **S.Afr.:** Nethaprin Dospan; Nethaprin Expectorant.

Ethyl Cysteine Hydrochloride (16008-k)

Ethyl L-2-amino-3-mercaptopropionate hydrochloride.
C$_5$H$_{11}$NO$_2$S,HCl = 185.7.
CAS — 3411-58-3 (ethyl cysteine); 868-59-7 (ethyl cysteine hydrochloride).
Pharmacopoeias. In Jpn.

Profile
Ethyl cysteine hydrochloride is a mucolytic used in the treatment of disorders of the respiratory tract associated with productive cough.

Ethyl Orthoformate (5618-t)

Ether de Kay; Triethoxymethane. Triethyl orthoformate.
C$_7$H$_{16}$O$_3$ = 148.2.
CAS — 122-51-0.
Pharmacopoeias. In Fr.

Profile
Ethyl orthoformate is a cough suppressant (see p.1082). It is reported to be a respiratory antispasmodic and has been administered by mouth or rectally.

Preparations

Proprietary Preparations (details are given in Part 3)
Multi-ingredient: Switz.: Rectoquintyl; Rectoquintyl-Promethazine.

Fedrilate (5619-x)

Fedrilate (rINN).
Fedrilatum; UCB-3928. 1-Methyl-3-morpholinopropyl perhydro-4-phenylpyran-4-carboxylate.
C$_{20}$H$_{29}$NO$_4$ = 347.4.
CAS — 23271-74-1.
ATC — R05DB14.

Profile
Fedrilate is a cough suppressant used for non-productive cough (p.1082) which has been given by mouth in doses of 50 mg three to six times daily.

Preparations

Proprietary Preparations (details are given in Part 3)
Braz.: Gotas Binelli; Sedatoss; **S.Afr.:** Corbar S.

Fenoxazoline Hydrochloride (2064-d)

Fenoxazoline Hydrochloride (rINNM).
2-(2-Isopropylphenoxymethyl)-2-imidazoline hydrochloride.
C$_{13}$H$_{18}$N$_2$O,HCl = 254.8.
CAS — 4846-91-7 (fenoxazoline); 21370-21-8 (fenoxazoline hydrochloride).

Profile
Fenoxazoline hydrochloride is a sympathomimetic with effects similar to those of naphazoline (p.1095) used for its vasoconstrictor properties in the symptomatic treatment of nasal congestion (p.1082). It is used topically, usually as a nasal spray containing 0.03 or 0.1%.

Preparations

Proprietary Preparations (details are given in Part 3)
Braz.: Aturgyl; **Port.:** Bisolspray.

Fominoben Hydrochloride (5620-y)

Fominoben Hydrochloride (rINNM).
PB-89. 3′-Chloro-2′-[N-methyl-N-(morpholinocarbonylmethyl)aminomethyl]benzanilide hydrochloride.
C$_{21}$H$_{24}$ClN$_3$O$_3$,HCl = 438.3.
CAS — 18053-31-1 (fominoben); 24600-36-0 (fominoben hydrochloride).

Profile
Fominoben hydrochloride is a centrally acting cough suppressant (see p.1082) which is also reported to have respiratory stimulant properties. It is given in doses of 160 mg up to three times daily by mouth; it has also been given by slow intravenous injection.

Preparations

Proprietary Preparations (details are given in Part 3)
Mex.: Noleptan; **Spain:** Tosifar.

Glaucine (19251-g)

Boldine Dimethyl Ether; DL-832 (dl-glaucine phosphate); dl-Glaucine; MDL-832 (dl-glaucine phosphate). DL-1,2,9,10-Tetramethoxyaporphine.
C$_{21}$H$_{25}$NO$_4$ = 355.4.
CAS — 5630-11-5 (dl-glaucine); 73239-87-9 (dl-glaucine phosphate); 475-81-0 (d-glaucine); 5996-06-5 (d-glaucine hydrobromide).

Profile
Glaucine is a centrally acting cough suppressant used in non-productive cough (p.1082) which has been studied as the phosphate.

d-Glaucine has been used as the hydrobromide and the hydrochloride as a cough suppressant in eastern Europe. It has been obtained from *Glaucium flavum* (Papaveraceae).

◊ References.
1. Redpath JBS, Pleuvry BJ. Double-blind comparison of the respiratory and sedative effects of codeine phosphate and (±)-glaucine phosphate in human volunteers. *Br J Clin Pharmacol* 1982; **14:** 555–8.
2. Rühle KH, *et al.* Objective evaluation of dextromethorphan and glaucine as antitussive agents. *Br J Clin Pharmacol* 1984; **17:** 521–4.
3. Gastpar H, *et al.* Efficacy and tolerability of glaucine as an antitussive agent. *Curr Med Res Opin* 1984; **9:** 21–7.
4. Cortijo J, *et al.* Bronchodilator and anti-inflammatory activities of glaucine: in vitro studies in human airway smooth muscle and polymorphonuclear leukocytes. *Br J Pharmacol* 1999; **127:** 1641–51.

Guacetisal (12801-w)
Guacetisal *(rINN)*.

Acetylsalicylic Acid Guaiacol Ester. *o*-Methoxyphenyl salicylate acetate.

$C_{16}H_{14}O_5 = 286.3.$
CAS — 55482-89-8.
ATC — N02BA14.

Profile
Guacetisal has been used in respiratory disorders as an expectorant (see p.1082). It has also been used as an antipyretic to reduce fever (p.8). It has been administered by mouth and rectally.

Preparations
Proprietary Preparations (details are given in Part 3)
Ital.: Balsacetil†; Broncaspin†; Guaiaspir; Guajabronc†; Prontomucil.

Guaiacol (2016-z)
Guajacol; Methyl Catechol.

CAS — 90-05-1 (guaiacol); 553-17-3 (guaiacol carbonate); 60296-02-8 (calcium guaiacolglycolate); 4112-89-4 (guaiacol phenylacetate).

Pharmacopoeias. In Belg., Fr., and Swiss. Fr. also includes Guaiacol Carbonate.

The main constituent of guaiacol is 2-methoxyphenol, $CH_3O.C_6H_4.OH = 124.1.$

Profile
Guaiacol has disinfectant properties and has been used as an expectorant for productive cough (p.1082).

Adverse effects are similar to those of phenol (p.1152).

A wide range of salts and derivatives of guaiacol have been used similarly including the carbonate, cinnamate, ethylglycolate, calcium and sodium glycolates, phenylacetate, and phenylbutyrate. See also Guaifenesin, p.1092 and Sulfogaiacol, p.1101.

Preparations
Proprietary Preparations (details are given in Part 3)
Ger.: Anastil.

Multi-ingredient: *Belg.:* Baume Dalet†; Eucalyptine Pholcodine Le Brun; *Braz.:* Axol; Canfomenol; Durapen Balsamico; Eucalyptine; Massubal; Transpulmin Balsamo; Transpulmin Supositorio; Tripulmin; Yatropan; *Canad.:* Analgesic Balm; Creo-Rectal; Demo-Cineol; Dentalgar; Gouttes Dentaires; Omni-Tuss; Pastilles Valda†; Sedatuss†; Valda; *Fr.:* Baume Dalet†; Bi-Qui-Nol†; Biocalyptol; Bronchodermine; Bronchorectine au Citral; Campho-Pneumine; Essence Algerienne; Eucalyptine Le Brun†; Gaiarsol; Pulmo Bailly; Pulmoserum; Rectophedrol†; Sirop Boint†; Valda; *Ger.:* Dalet Med Balsam†; *Hong Kong:* Biocalyptol; Valda; *Irl.:* Pulmo Bailly†; Valda; *Ital.:* Eucalyptina†; Fosfoguaiacol; Lactocol; Lipobalsamo; Resina Carbolica Dentilin; *Mex.:* Yadegal Compuesto; *Port.:* Analgil; Valda; *Spain:* Bronco Aseptilex Fuerte; Bronco Aseptilex†; Bronquimar Vit A†; Bronquimar†; Edusan Fte Rectal; Eucalyptospirine; Eucalyptospirine Lact†; Maboterpen†; Pulmo Grey Balsam†; Tos Mai; *Switz.:* Liberol†; Rectoseptal-Neo Pholcodine; Rectoseptal-Neo simple; Spirogel†; *UK:* Dragon Balm; Pulmo Bailly; Valda†; *USA:* Methagual.

Guaietolin (12795-v)
Guaietolin *(rINN)*.

Glycerylguethol; Glyguetol. 3-(2-Ethoxyphenoxy)propane-1,2-diol.

$C_{11}H_{16}O_4 = 212.2.$
CAS — 63834-83-3.

Profile
Guaietolin is an analogue of guaifenesin which is used as an expectorant (see p.1082). It has been given by mouth in doses of 300 to 600 mg two to three times daily.

Preparations
Proprietary Preparations (details are given in Part 3)
Fr.: Guethural.

Guaifenesin (2018-k)
Guaifenesin *(BAN, USAN, rINN)*.

Glyceryl Guaiacolate; Glycerylguayacolum; Guaiacol Glycerol Ether; Guaiacyl Glyceryl Ether; Guaifenesina; Guaifenesinum; Guaiphenesin; Guajacolum Glycerolatum. *(RS)*-3-(2-Methoxyphenoxy)propane-1,2-diol.

$C_{10}H_{14}O_4 = 198.2.$
CAS — 93-14-1.
ATC — R05CA03.

Pharmacopoeias. In Eur. (see p.vi), Jpn, and US.

Pharmacopoeial description
Ph. Eur.: A white or almost white, crystalline powder. Sparingly soluble in water; soluble in alcohol; slightly soluble in ether.

USP 25: A white to slightly grey crystalline powder. May have a slight characteristic odour. Soluble 1 in 60 to 70 of water; soluble in alcohol, in chloroform, and in propylene glycol; sparingly soluble in glycerol. Store in airtight containers.

Adverse Effects and Precautions
Gastrointestinal discomfort, nausea, and vomiting have occasionally been reported with guaifenesin, particularly in very large doses.

Abuse. Urinary calculi have been reported in patients consuming large quantities of over-the-counter preparations containing guaifenesin.[1,2] Spectroscopic analysis[1] revealed that the stones were composed of a calcium salt of beta-(2-methoxyphenoxy)-lactic acid, which is a metabolite of guaifenesin. Small quantities of ephedrine were also present in the stones of one of several patients who had ingested preparations containing a combination of guaifenesin and ephedrine.[2]

1. Pickens CL, *et al.* Abuse of guaifenesin-containing medications generates an excess of a carboxylate salt of beta-(2-methoxyphenoxy)-lactic acid, a guaifenesin metabolite, and results in urolithiasis. *Urology* 1999; **54:** 23–7.
2. Assimos DG, *et al.* Guaifenesin- and ephedrine-induced stones. *J Endourol* 1999; **13:** 665–7.

Porphyria. Guaifenesin is considered to be unsafe in patients with porphyria because it has been shown to be porphyrinogenic in *animals*.

Pharmacokinetics
Guaifenesin is absorbed from the gastrointestinal tract. It is metabolised and then excreted in the urine.

Uses and Administration
Guaifenesin is reported to increase the volume and reduce the viscosity of tenacious sputum and is used as an expectorant for productive cough. It has been given by mouth in doses of 200 to 400 mg every 4 hours. Children aged 6 to 12 years may be given 100 to 200 mg every 4 hours, and children aged 2 to 6 years 50 to 100 mg every 4 hours. It has been used similarly as the calcium salt.

Respiratory disorders. An FDA review of preparations available 'over-the-counter' concluded that guaifenesin was an effective expectorant.[1] The use of expectorants for productive cough is discussed on p.1082.

1. Thomas J. Guaiphenesin—an old drug now found to be effective. *Aust J Pharm* 1990; **71:** 101–3.

Preparations
USP 25: Dyphylline and Guaifenesin Elixir; Dyphylline and Guaifenesin Tablets; Guaifenesin and Codeine Phosphate Syrup; Guaifenesin and Pseudoephedrine Hydrochloride Capsules; Guaifenesin Capsules; Guaifenesin Syrup; Guaifenesin Tablets; Guaifenesin, Pseudoephedrine Hydrochloride, and Dextromethorphan Hydrobromide Capsules; Theophylline and Guaifenesin Capsules; Theophylline and Guaifenesin Oral Solution.

Proprietary Preparations (details are given in Part 3)
Aust.: Guafen; Myoscain; Resyl; Wick Formel 44 Plus Hustenloser; *Austral.:* Lemsip Chesty Cough; Robitussin EX; Robitussin†; *Belg.:* Vicks Vaposyrup Expectorant; *Canad.:* Balminil Expectorant; Benylin-E; Calmylin Expectorant; Cough Syrup Expectorant; Expectorant Cough Formula; Expectorant Cough Syrup; Expectorant Syrup; Koffex Expectorant; Robitussin; Sirop Expectorant; Tussin Expectorant; *Fin.:* Tintus; *Fr.:* Vicks Expectorant; *Ger.:* Fagusan; Gufen N; Nephulon G†; Wick Formel 44 Husten-Loser; Wick Kinder Formel 44 Husten-Loser†; *Hong Kong:* Breacol; Excaugh; Robitussin Expectorant; Uni-Colex; *Irl.:* Robitussin Expectorant; Tixylix Chesty Cough; *Israel:* Bronchocal; Resyl; Robitussin; Vitussin; *Ital.:* Broncovanil; Idropulmina; Resyl; Vicks Tosse Fluidificante; *Mex.:* Formula E; Tukol; *NZ:* Lemsip Chesty Cough; *S.Afr.:* Dimetap Cough Expectorant†; *Singapore:* Robitussin; *Spain:* Fluidin†; Formulaexpec; Lactocol Expectorante†; Robitussin; *Swed.:* Resyl; *Switz.:* Bronchol; Resyl; Vicks Formule 44 Expectine; *Thai.:* Robitussin; Tussa; *UK:* Benylin Childrens Chesty Coughs; Childrens Chesty Cough Syrup; Do-Do Expectorant Linctus†; Expulin Chesty Cough; Famel Expectorant; Hill's Balsam Chesty Cough; Jackson's All Fours; Jacksons Bronchial Balsam; Owbridges for Chesty Coughs; Robitussin for Chesty Coughs; Tixylix Chesty Cough; Vicks Vaposyrup for chesty coughs; *USA:* Anti-Tuss; Breonesin; Diabetic Tussin EX; Duratuss G; Fenesin; Ganidin NR; Gee-Gee; Genatuss; GG-Cen†; Glyate; Glycotuss; Glytuss; Guaifenex G; Guaifenex LA; Guiatuss; Halotussin; Humavent; Humibid; Hytuss; Liquibid; Monafed; Muco-Fen; Muco-Fen-LA;

Mytussin; Naldecon Senior EX; Numobid†; Organidin NR; Pneumomist; Refenesen; Respa-GF; Robitussin; Scot-Tussin Expectorant; Siltussin; Sinumist-SR; Touro Ex; Tusibron; Uni-tussin.

Multi-ingredient: numerous preparations are listed in Part 3.

Guaimesal (1749-r)
Guaimesal *(rINN)*.

(±)-2-(o-Methoxyphenoxy)-2-methyl-1,3-benzodioxan-4-one.
$C_{16}H_{14}O_5 = 286.3.$
CAS — 81674-79-5.

Profile
Guaimesal is reported to have expectorant and antipyretic properties and has been given by mouth in a usual dose of 500 mg two to three times daily as an adjunct in the treatment of respiratory tract disorders. It has also been administered rectally in suppositories.

◊ References.
1. Jager EGH. Double-blind, placebo-controlled clinical evaluation of guaimesal in outpatients. *Clin Ther* 1989; **11:** 341–62.

Preparations
Proprietary Preparations (details are given in Part 3)
Ital.: Bronteril.

Guethol (15580-j)
2-Ethoxyphenol.
$C_8H_{10}O_3 = 138.2.$
CAS — 94-71-3.

Profile
Guethol has been used as the carbonate as an expectorant for productive cough (p.1082) in doses of 170 to 340 mg given 2 or 3 times daily; the nicotinate has also been used in respiratory-tract disorders.

Preparations
Proprietary Preparations (details are given in Part 3)
Fr.: Guethural†.

Multi-ingredient: *Fr.:* Bronchospray†.

Helicidine (13455-c)
Helixinum.

Profile
Helicidine is a mucoglycoprotein from the snail *Helix pomatia* that has been used as a cough suppressant.

◊ References.
1. Pons F, *et al.* L'effect bronchorelaxant de l'helicidine, un extrait d'Helix pomatia, fait intervenir une liberation de prostaglandine E2. *Pathol Biol (Paris)* 1999; **47:** 73–80.

Indanazoline Hydrochloride (11418-a)
Indanazoline Hydrochloride *(rINNM)*.
$C_{12}H_{15}N_3,HCl = 237.7.$
CAS — 56601-85-5.

Profile
Indanazoline is a sympathomimetic with effects similar to those of naphazoline (p.1095). It has been used as the hydrochloride for its vasoconstrictor effect in the management of nasal congestion (p.1082). It has been given as nasal drops or as a nasal spray in a concentration equivalent to indanazoline 0.1%.

Preparations
Proprietary Preparations (details are given in Part 3)
Ger.: Farial.

Iodinated Glycerol (4576-k)
Iodinated Glycerol *(BAN, USAN)*.

Iodopropylidene Glycerol.
$C_6H_{11}IO_3 = 258.1.$
CAS — 5634-39-9.

An isomeric mixture of iodinated dimers of glycerol.

Profile
Iodinated glycerol, a methyl derivative of domiodol (p.1089), has been used as an expectorant. The limitations of iodides as expectorants are discussed under Cough on p.1082. The actions of iodides and iodine compounds are discussed under Iodine p.1522. Prolonged use of iodinated glycerol has been associated with hypothyroidism and severe skin eruptions; gastrointestinal disturbances and hypersensitivity reactions have also occurred. Administration of iodinated glycerol to *animals* has resulted in the development of malignant neoplasms.

Effects on the thyroid gland. There have been reports of thyroid dysfunction (both hyperthyroidism and hypothyroidism) following administration of iodinated glycerol to previously euthyroid patients. It was recommended that baseline thyroid function tests should be carried out before commencing treatment with iodinated glycerol;[1] it should be withdrawn if abnormal results are obtained during use.

1. Gittoes NJL, Franklyn JA. Drug-induced thyroid disorders. *Drug Safety* 1995; **13:** 46–55.

Chronic obstructive pulmonary disease. Studies[1-3] of the use of iodinated glycerol in patients with chronic bronchitis have produced conflicting results. The use of mucolytics or expectorants in chronic obstructive pulmonary disease (p.759) is controversial.

1. Petty TL. The National Mucolytic Study: results of a randomized, double-blind, placebo-controlled study of iodinated glycerol in chronic obstructive bronchitis. *Chest* 1990; **97:** 75–83.
2. Repsher LH. Treatment of stable chronic bronchitis with iodinated glycerol: a double-blind, placebo-controlled trial. *J Clin Pharmacol* 1993; **33:** 856–60.
3. Rubin BK, *et al.* Iodinated glycerol has no effect on pulmonary function, symptom score, or sputum properties in patients with stable chronic bronchitis. *Chest* 1996; **109:** 348–52.

Preparations

Proprietary Preparations (details are given in Part 3)
USA: Iophen; Par Glycerol; R-Gen.
Multi-ingredient: *Ital.:* Golamed Oral; Mucantil†; *Spain:* Mucorama; Mucorama TS; *USA:* Tusso-DM†.

Ipecacuanha (2020-e)

Ipecac; Ipecacuanha Root; Ipecacuanhae Radix.
CAS — 8012-96-2.
ATC — R05CA04; V03AB01.

Pharmacopoeias. In Eur. (see p.vi), Int., Jpn, and US.
Eur., Jpn, and US also include a monograph for Prepared Ipecacuanha (Ipecacuanhae Pulvis Normatus) or a similar standardised form.

Pharmacopoeial description

Ph. Eur.: Ipecacuanha Root consists of the fragmented and dried underground organs of *Cephaelis ipecacuanha* known as Matto Grosso ipecacuanha, or of *C. acuminata* known as Costa Rica ipecacuanha, or a mixture of both species. It contains not less than 2.0% of total alkaloids, calculated as emetine. It has a slight odour. Store in airtight containers. Protect from light.

Prepared Ipecacuanha is ipecacuanha root powder adjusted to an alkaloidal content of 1.9 to 2.1% of total alkaloids, calculated as emetine. Store in airtight containers. Protect from light.

NOTE. The BP 2001 directs that when Ipecacuanha, Ipecacuanha Root, or Powdered Ipecacuanha is prescribed or demanded, Prepared Ipecacuanha shall be dispensed or supplied.

USP 25: The dried rhizome and roots of *Cephaelis acuminata* or of *C. ipecacuanha* (Rubiaceae). It yields not less than 2% of ether-soluble alkaloids of which not less than 90% is emetine and cephaeline; the content of cephaeline varies from an amount equal to, to an amount not more than 2.5 times, that of emetine.

Powdered Ipecac contains 1.9 to 2.1% of ether-soluble alkaloids, with emetine and cephaeline content as for Ipecacuanha. It is pale brown, weak yellow, or light olive-grey powder that should be stored in airtight containers.

Adverse Effects

Large doses of ipecacuanha have an irritant effect on the gastrointestinal tract, and persistent bloody vomiting or bloody diarrhoea may occur. Mucosal erosions of the entire gastrointestinal tract have been reported. The absorption of emetine, which is most likely if vomiting does not occur after the administration of emetic doses of ipecacuanha, may give rise to adverse effects on the heart, such as conduction abnormalities or myocardial infarction. These, combined with dehydration due to vomiting may cause vasomotor collapse followed by death.

There have been several reports of chronic abuse of ipecacuanha to induce vomiting in eating disorders; cardiotoxicity and myopathy have occurred and may be a result of accumulation of emetine.

There have also been several reports of ipecacuanha poisoning due to the unwitting substitution of Ipecac Fluidextract (USP XVI) for Ipecac Syrup (USP 25); the fluidextract was about 14 times the strength of the syrup.

◊ References.

1. Manno BR, Manno JE. Toxicology of ipecac: a review. *Clin Toxicol* 1977; **10:** 221–42.

Hypersensitivity. Allergy, characterised by rhinitis, conjunctivitis, and chest tightness, has occurred due to inhalation of ipecacuanha dust in packers of ipecacuanha tablets.[1]

1. Luczynska CM, *et al.* Occupational allergy due to inhalation of ipecacuanha dust. *Clin Allergy* 1984; **14:** 169–75.

Vomiting. Prolonged vomiting has been reported in 17% of patients given ipecacuanha in the treatment of poisoning and may lead to gastric rupture, Mallory-Weiss tears of the oesoph-

---

agogastric junction, cerebrovascular events, and pneumomediastinum and pneumoperitoneum.[1]

1. Bateman DN. Adverse reactions to antidotes. *Adverse Drug React Bull* 1988; **133:** (Dec.): 496–9.

Treatment of Adverse Effects

After acute overdose of ipecacuanha, activated charcoal is given to delay absorption followed if necessary by gastric lavage. Prolonged vomiting may be controlled by the injection of antiemetics. Fluid and electrolyte imbalance should be corrected and facilities should be available to correct any cardiac effects and subsequent shock.

After the withdrawal of ipecacuanha following chronic abuse, recovery may be prolonged due to the slow elimination of emetine.

Precautions

The use of emetics is now rarely favoured; in particular, ipecacuanha should not be used as an emetic in patients who are unconscious or whose condition otherwise increases the risk of aspiration, nor in patients who have taken substances, such as corrosive compounds or petroleum products, that might be especially dangerous if aspirated. Ipecacuanha should not be given to patients in shock or to those at risk from seizures either as a result of their condition or from compounds, such as strychnine, that have been ingested. Patients with cardiovascular disorders are at risk if ipecacuanha is absorbed.

Abuse. Ipecac Syrup has been abused by patients with eating disorders to induce vomiting.[1] Adverse effects of repeated vomiting, such as metabolic complications, aspiration pneumonitis, parotid enlargement, dental abnormalities, and oesophagitis or haematemesis due to mucosal lacerations (the Mallory-Weiss syndrome) may be observed. Cardiotoxicity may occur and fatalities have been reported including one patient who had ingested 90 to 120 mL of ipecac syrup daily for 3 months.[2] It has been suggested that cardiac effects and myopathy following the prolonged abuse of Ipecac Syrup may be due to the long-term accumulation of emetine[3,4] but some have expressed doubts.[5]

Cardiomyopathy has also been reported in children given ipecacuanha to produce factitious illness (Munchausen's syndrome by proxy);[6,7] fatalities have occurred.

1. Harris RT. Bulimarexia and related serious eating disorders with medical complications. *Ann Intern Med* 1983; **99:** 800–7.
2. Adler AG, *et al.* Death resulting from ipecac syrup poisoning. *JAMA* 1980; **243:** 1927–8.
3. Palmer EP, Guay AT. Reversible myopathy secondary to abuse of ipecac in patients with major eating disorders. *N Engl J Med* 1985; **313:** 1457–9.
4. Pope HG, *et al.* The epidemiology of ipecac abuse. *N Engl J Med* 1986; **314:** 245–6.
5. Isner JM. Effects of ipecac on the heart. *N Engl J Med* 1986; **314:** 1253.
6. Goebel J, *et al.* Cardiomyopathy from ipecac administration in Munchausen syndrome by proxy. *Pediatrics* 1993; **92:** 601–3.
7. Schneider DJ, *et al.* Clinical and pathologic aspects of cardiomyopathy from ipecac administration in Munchausen's syndrome by proxy. *Pediatrics* 1996; **97:** 902–6.

Interactions

The action of ipecacuanha may be delayed or diminished if it is given with or after charcoal; antiemetics may also diminish its effect.

Food. Concomitant administration of milk had been believed to impair the emetic efficacy of ipecacuanha but there was no significant difference in the time to onset of vomiting, the duration of vomiting, or the number of episodes in 250 children who were given ipecac syrup with milk compared with 250 given ipecac syrup with clear fluids.[1]

1. Klein-Schwartz W, *et al.* The effect of milk on ipecac-induced emesis. *J Toxicol Clin Toxicol* 1991; **29:** 505–11.

Uses and Administration

Ipecacuanha is used as an expectorant in productive cough (p.1082) in doses of 0.02 to 0.06 mL of Ipecacuanha Liquid Extract (BP 2001) (about 0.4 to 1.2 mg of total alkaloids) and 0.3 to 1 mL of Ipecac Syrup (USP 25) (about 0.4 to 1.4 mg of total alkaloids).

Ipecacuanha may also be used in larger doses as an emetic (but see below). Vomiting usually occurs within 30 minutes of administration by mouth of an emetic dose due to an irritant effect on the gastrointestinal tract and a central action on the chemoreceptor trigger zone. Doses are usually followed by a copious drink of water or fruit juice; in young children this may be given before the dose. Adults may be given doses of 21 to 42 mg of total alkaloids represented by 15 to

---

30 mL of Paediatric Ipecacuanha Emetic Mixture (BP 2001) or of Ipecac Syrup (USP 25). Children aged 6 months to 1 year may be given 7 to 14 mg of total alkaloids, represented by 5 to 10 mL of Paediatric Ipecacuanha Emetic Mixture (BP 2001) or of Ipecac Syrup (USP 25); older children may be given 21 mg, represented by 15 mL of Paediatric Ipecacuanha Emetic Mixture (BP 2001) or of Ipecac Syrup (USP 25). Doses may be repeated once only after 20 to 30 minutes if emesis has not occurred.

Ipecacuanha (Ipeca) is used in homoeopathic medicine.

Emesis induction in acute poisoning. Standard practice in the management of acute poisoning (p.1000) has varied widely, with different procedures favoured at different times and in different countries. However, measures to reduce absorption of the toxic substance, such as stomach emptying, have often been advocated.

Two techniques of stomach emptying have been very widely employed: gastric lavage; and emesis induction, with ipecacuanha as the emetic of choice. Neither technique is without hazard and the dangers of attempting to empty the stomach have to be balanced against the toxicity of the ingested poison. If the patient presents late or the risk of toxicity is small, then gastric emptying is unnecessary.

Gastric lavage is not recommended in the routine management of poisoned patients[1] because there is little evidence from experimental studies that it improves the clinical outcome and it may cause significant morbidity. It should only be considered if a potentially life-threatening amount of toxic substance has been ingested within the preceding hour. There is significant danger of aspiration of stomach contents associated with the procedure and it should only be attempted in fully conscious patients with good airway protective reflexes, unless other means are undertaken to protect the airway. Gastric lavage is also contra-indicated if corrosive or petroleum products have been ingested. There is also a risk that the procedure may propel stomach contents beyond the pylorus and thus enhance absorption in some cases.[2]

Ipecacuanha has often been advocated for use in children, in whom gastric lavage may be particularly traumatic, although it is also used in adults. However, like gastric lavage, its routine use is not recommended in the management of poisoned patients[3] because there is no clear evidence from clinical studies that it improves the outcome; clinically significant absorption may not be prevented even if it is administered within 1 hour of the ingested poison. It may also delay the administration or reduce the effectiveness of activated charcoal or oral antidotes. Ipecacuanha should not be administered to patients with compromised airway relexes, nor following ingestion of corrosive or petroleum products. In addition it should be avoided in debilitated or elderly patients, or those with medical conditions that may be compromised by induction of emesis. It should generally only be considered if a potentially life-threatening amount of toxic substance has been ingested within the preceding hour, and if gastric lavage or administration of activated charcoal are deemed inappropriate.

Because of the limitations of both methods of gastric emptying, a number of studies has addressed the question of whether either is appropriate. Such studies have indicated that the administration of activated charcoal alone, without gastric emptying, is as effective as a combination of both methods.[4-6]

1. American Academy of Clinical Toxicology, European Association of Poisons Centres and Clinical Toxicologists. Position statement: gastric lavage. *Clin Toxicol* 1997; **35:** 711–19.
2. Saetta JP, *et al.* Gastric emptying procedures in the self-poisoned patient: are we forcing gastric content beyond the pylorus? *J R Soc Med* 1991; **84:** 274–6.
3. American Academy of Clinical Toxicology, European Association of Poisons Centres and Clinical Toxicologists. Position statement: ipecac syrup. *Clin Toxicol* 1997; **35:** 699–709.
4. Albertson TE, *et al.* Superiority of activated charcoal alone compared with ipecac and activated charcoal in the treatment of acute toxic ingestions. *Ann Emerg Med* 1989; **18:** 56–9.
5. Merigian KS, *et al.* Prospective evaluation of gastric emptying in the self-poisoned patient. *Am J Emerg Med* 1990; **8:** 479–83.
6. Pond SM, *et al.* Gastric emptying in acute overdose: a prospective randomised controlled trial. *Med J Aust* 1995; **163:** 345–9.

Preparations

BP 2001: Ipecacuanha Liquid Extract; Paediatric Ipecacuanha Emetic Mixture;
Ph. Eur.: Ipecacuanha Tincture, Standardised;
USP 25: Ipecac Syrup.

Proprietary Preparations (details are given in Part 3)
Aust.: Ipetitrin; *Belg.:* Bromofotyl†; *Fin.:* Ipeca; *Switz.:* Orpec†; *UK:* Fennings Little Healers.
Multi-ingredient: *Belg.:* Folcodex; Phenergan Expectorant†; Solucamphre†; *Braz.:* Expec; Expectomel; Fenergan Expectorante; Iodesin; Iodobec; Ipecol; KI-Expectorante; Melagriao; Pectoss; Pilulas Ross; Tosseina; Xarope Grindelia de Oliveira Junior; *Canad.:* Bronchisaft†; *Fr.:* Elixir Contre La Toux Weleda†; Humex; Sirop Pectoral adulte†; *Hong Kong:* Pectoral; *Irl.:* Ipesil; *Israel:* Doveri; Laxative Comp; Promethazine Expectorant; Prothiazine Expectorant; *Neth.:* Abdijsiroop (Akker-Siroop)†; *Port.:* Fluidin Adulto; Fluidin Antiasmatico; *S.Afr.:* Efcod†; Efcospect†; Expectco†; Linctus Tussi Infans; *Spain:* Alofedina; Buco Regis; Encilaina; Fenergan Expectorante; Pectoral Brum†; Toscal Com-

---

The symbol † denotes a preparation no longer actively marketed

puesto†; Toscal†; Tuselin Expectorante; **Switz.:** Aloinophen†; Bromocod N; Bronchalin†; Bronchofluid†; Cimex Sirop contre la toux†; Demo elixir pectoral N; Demo gouttes contre la toux†; Demo pates pectorales†; Demo sirop contre la toux†; Demotussil†; Gouttes contre la toux "S"; Neo-Codion N; Pastilles pectorales Demo N; Patussol†; Phenergan Expectorant; Sirop antitussif Wyss a base de codeine†; Sirop Wyss contre la toux†; Solucamphre†; Spedro†; Thymodrosin†; **Thai.:** Diolin; **UK:** Allens Dry Tickly Cough; Allens Pine & Honey; Asthma & Catarrh Relief; Bronchial Mixture; Buttercup Syrup (Blackcurrant flavour)†; Buttercup Syrup (Honey and Lemon flavour); Cough-eeze†; ES Bronchial Mixture; Galloway's Cough Syrup; Hill's Balsam Chesty Cough for Children; Hill's Balsam Chesty Cough Pastilles; Hill's Balsam Extra Strong; Honey & Molasses; Jackson's Troublesome Coughs; Kilkof; Liqufruta Cough Medicine†; Lockets Medicated Linctus; Modern Herbals Cough Mixture; Mu-Cron Junior†; Potters Children's Cough Pastilles; Secron; Throaties Family Cough Linctus†; Vegetable Cough Remover; **USA:** Poison Antidote Kit; Quelidrine; Tusquelin†.

Isoaminile   (9888-b)

Isoaminile (BAN, rINN).

4-Dimethylamino-2-isopropyl-2-phenylpentanonitrile.

$C_{16}H_{24}N_2 = 244.4$.
CAS — 77-51-0.
ATC — R05DB04.
Pharmacopoeias. In *Br.*

Pharmacopoeial description

BP 2001: A colourless or slightly yellow, oily liquid with an amine-like odour. Practically insoluble in water; freely soluble in alcohol, in acetone, in chloroform, in ether, and in methyl alcohol; dissolves in dilute acids.

Isoaminile Citrate   (5622-z)

Isoaminile Citrate (BANM, rINNM).

4-Dimethylamino-2-isopropyl-2-phenylvaleronitrile dihydrogen citrate.

$C_{16}H_{24}N_2,C_6H_8O_7 = 436.5$.
CAS — 126-10-3; 28416-66-2.

Profile

Isoaminile is a centrally acting cough suppressant which has actions and uses similar to dextromethorphan hydrobromide (p.1087). Isoaminile has usually been given by mouth as the citrate but the cyclamate has also been used.

Preparations

Proprietary Preparations (details are given in Part 3)
Aust.: Peracon; **Ger.:** Peracon†; **S.Afr.:** Peracon.

Multi-ingredient: **S.Afr.:** Peracon Expectorant.

Letosteine   (12893-q)

Letosteine (pINN).

2-[2-(Ethoxycarbonylmethylthio)ethyl]thiazolidine-4-carboxylic acid.

$C_{10}H_{17}NO_4S_2 = 279.4$.
CAS — 53943-88-7.
ATC — R05CB09.

Profile

Letosteine is a mucolytic that has been used in the treatment of respiratory disorders associated with productive cough (p.1082) in a dose of 50 mg by mouth three times daily.

Preparations

Proprietary Preparations (details are given in Part 3)
Fr.: Viscotiol; **Ital.:** Letofort; Viscotiol; **Spain:** Broluidan.

Levmetamfetamine   (17746-y)

Levmetamfetamine (USAN, rINN).

l-Deoxyephedrine; L-Desoxyephedrine; Lesoxyephedrine; l-Methamphetamine; l-Methylamphetamine. (R)-N,α-Dimethylbenzeneethanamine; (−)-(R)-N,α-Dimethylphenethylamine.

$C_{10}H_{15}N = 149.2$.
CAS — 33817-09-3.
Pharmacopoeias. In *US*.

Pharmacopoeial description

USP 25: A clear, practically colourless, liquid. Store in airtight containers. Protect from light.

Profile

Levmetamfetamine is the *laevo* isomer of metamfetamine (p.1511) and is used topically in the treatment of nasal congestion (p.1082).

Preparations

Proprietary Preparations (details are given in Part 3)
USA: Vicks Vapor Inhaler.

Levopropoxyphene Napsilate   (5623-c)

Levopropoxyphene Napsilate (BANM, rINNM).

29866; Levopropoxyphene Napsylate (USAN). (1R,2S)-1-Benzyl-3-dimethylamino-2-methyl-1-phenylpropyl propionate naphthalene-2-sulphonate monohydrate.

$C_{22}H_{29}NO_2,C_{10}H_8O_3S,H_2O = 565.7$.
CAS — 2338-37-6 (levopropoxyphene); 5714-90-9 (anhydrous levopropoxyphene napsilate); 55557-30-7 (levopropoxyphene napsilate monohydrate).

Profile

Levopropoxyphene napsilate has been used as a centrally acting cough suppressant for non-productive cough (p.1082). Unlike the dextro-isomer, dextropropoxyphene, levopropoxyphene has little or no analgesic activity. It has also been given as the dibudinate.

Marrubium   (11837-j)

Andornkraut; Herba Marrubii; White Horehound.

Pharmacopoeias. In *Aust.* and *Fr.*

Profile

Marrubium is the flower or leaf of *Marrubium vulgare* (Labiatae). It has been used for its supposed expectorant properties in herbal preparations for the treatment of cough. It has also been used as a flavouring.

Preparations

Proprietary Preparations (details are given in Part 3)
Ger.: Angocin Bronchialtropfen.

Multi-ingredient: **Aust.:** Asthmatee; Gallen- und Lebertee; Krautertee Nr 28; Krautertee Nr 7; St Radegunder Leber-Galle-Tee; **Austral.:** Verbascum Complex; **Canad.:** Herbal Throat; Swiss Herb Cough Drops; **Fr.:** Elixir Contre La Toux Weleda†; Marrubene Codethyline†; Tisanes de l'Abbe Hamon no 15†; Tossarel†; **Ital.:** Broncosedina; **Spain:** Stomosan; **Switz.:** Bronchosan; Hederix; **UK:** Allens Chesty Cough; Asthma & Catarrh Relief; Catarrh; Catarrh Tablets; Catarrh-eeze; Chest Mixture; Cough Elixir; Cough-eeze†; Herb and Honey Cough Elixir; Honey & Molasses; Horehound and Aniseed Cough Mixture; Modern Herbals Cough Mixture; Vegetable Cough Remover.

Mecysteine Hydrochloride   (607-f)

Mecysteine Hydrochloride (BANM, rINNM).

Methyl Cysteine Hydrochloride; Methylcysteine Hydrochloride. Methyl L-2-amino-3-mercaptopropionate hydrochloride.

$C_4H_9NO_2S,HCl = 171.6$.
CAS — 2485-62-3 (mecysteine); 18598-63-5 (mecysteine hydrochloride); 5714-80-7 (mecysteine hydrochloride).

Adverse Effects and Precautions

Nausea and heartburn have occasionally been reported. Since mucolytics may disrupt the gastric mucosal barrier mecysteine hydrochloride should be used with caution in patients with a history of peptic ulceration.

Uses and Administration

Mecysteine hydrochloride is used as a mucolytic in respiratory disorders associated with productive cough (p.1082). It is given by mouth in a dose of 100 to 200 mg three or four times daily before meals reduced to 200 mg twice daily after 6 weeks. Children over 5 years of age may be given 100 mg three times daily. It has also been administered by inhalation.

Respiratory disorders. Mecysteine hydrochloride given by mouth has reduced symptoms of cough in patients with chronic bronchitis or other respiratory disorders, but its effect on sputum production and pulmonary function has been variable.[1,2] The use of mucolytics in chronic obstructive pulmonary disease (p.759) is controversial.

1. Aylward M, *et al.* Clinical therapeutic evaluation of methylcysteine hydrochloride in patients with chronic obstructive bronchitis: a balanced double-blind trial with placebo control. *Curr Med Res Opin* 1978; **5:** 461–71.
2. Sahay JN, *et al.* The effect of methyl cysteine (Visclair) in respiratory diseases: a pilot study. *Clin Trials J* 1982; **19:** 137–43.

Preparations

Proprietary Preparations (details are given in Part 3)
Irl.: Visclair; **UK:** Visclair.

Multi-ingredient: **Ital.:** Donatiol.

Menglytate   (11608-n)

Menglytate (rINN).

Menthol Ethylglycolate. p-Menth-3-yl ethoxyacetate.

$C_{14}H_{26}O_3 = 242.4$.
CAS — 579-94-2.

Profile

Menglytate is an ingredient of a number of preparations promoted for the treatment of cough.

Preparations

Proprietary Preparations (details are given in Part 3)

Multi-ingredient: **Aust.:** Expigen; **Ital.:** Coryfin C; Neo Borocillina Balsamica; Neo Borocillina Tosse Compresse; Neo Borocillina Tosse Sciroppo.

Methoxyphenamine Hydrochloride   (2081-n)

Methoxyphenamine Hydrochloride (BANM, rINNM).

Methoxiphenadrin Hydrochloride; Mexyphamine Hydrochloride. 2-Methoxy-N-α-dimethylphenethylamine hydrochloride.

$C_{11}H_{17}NO,HCl = 215.7$.
CAS — 93-30-1 (methoxyphenamine); 5588-10-3 (methoxyphenamine hydrochloride).

Profile

Methoxyphenamine is a sympathomimetic with effects similar to those of ephedrine (p.1090), given by mouth as the hydrochloride. It has been used as a bronchodilator and in combination with other ingredients for the relief of cough and nasal congestion.

Preparations

Proprietary Preparations (details are given in Part 3)

Multi-ingredient: **Belg.:** Orthoxicol; **Braz.:** Cheracap; Sedagripe; **Hong Kong:** Asmeton; **Irl.:** Casacol; **Mex.:** Cheracol; **S.Afr.:** Orthoxicol; **Thai.:** Asmeton.

Methyl Dacisteine   (13491-x)

Methyl Dacisteine (rINNM).

EL-1035 (dacisteine); Methyl Diacetylcysteinate. Methyl N,S-diacetyl-L-cysteinate.

$C_8H_{13}NO_4S = 219.3$.
CAS — 18725-37-6 (dacisteine); 19547-88-7 (methyl dacisteine).

Profile

Like acetylcysteine (p.1082), methyl dacisteine has been used as a mucolytic in respiratory disorders associated with productive cough (p.1082). It has been given by mouth in a dose of 600 mg daily, divided into 3 or 4 doses.

Preparations

Proprietary Preparations (details are given in Part 3)
Fr.: Mucothiol; **Ital.:** Mucothiol.

Methylephedrine Hydrochloride   (2083-m)

Methylephedrine Hydrochloride (BANM).

2-Dimethylamino-1-phenylpropan-1-ol hydrochloride.

$C_{11}H_{17}NO,HCl = 215.7$.
CAS — 552-79-4 ((−)-methylephedrine); 1201-56-5 ((±)-methylephedrine); 38455-90-2 ((−)-methylephedrine hydrochloride); 942-46-1 ((±)-methylephedrine hydrochloride); 18760-80-0 ((±)-methylephedrine hydrochloride).
Pharmacopoeias. Jpn includes the (±)-form, dl-Methylephedrine Hydrochloride.

Profile

Methylephedrine hydrochloride is a sympathomimetic with effects similar to those of ephedrine (p.1090). It has been used as a bronchodilator and is given by mouth in combination preparations for the relief of cough and nasal congestion.

Preparations

Proprietary Preparations (details are given in Part 3)

Multi-ingredient: **Aust.:** Tussoretardin; **S.Afr.:** Ilvico; **Switz.:** Tossamine plus; **Thai.:** Coughmin; Hustazol-C; Methorcon.

Metizoline Hydrochloride   (6183-c)

Metizoline Hydrochloride (BANM, USAN, rINNM).

EX-10-781; Metyzoline Hydrochloride; RMI-10482A. 2-(2-Methylbenzo[b]thienylmethyl)-2-imidazoline hydrochloride.

$C_{13}H_{14}N_2S,HCl = 266.8$.
CAS — 17692-22-7 (metizoline); 5090-37-9 (metizoline hydrochloride).

Profile

Metizoline hydrochloride is a sympathomimetic with effects similar to those of naphazoline (p.1095) used for its vasoconstrictor activity in the treatment of nasal congestion. It is given as a 0.05% nasal spray.

Preparations

Proprietary Preparations (details are given in Part 3)
Ital.: Eunasin†.

Moguisteine (11023-f)

Moguisteine (rINN).

Ethyl (±)-2-[(o-methoxyphenoxy)methyl]-β-oxo-thiazolidine-propionate.

$C_{16}H_{21}NO_5S = 339.4$.

CAS — 119637-67-1.

Profile

Moguisteine has been investigated as a cough suppressant. It is reported to have a peripheral mechanism of action.

◊ References.

1. Aversa C, et al. Clinical trial of the efficacy and safety of moguisteine in patients with cough associated with chronic respiratory diseases. Drugs Exp Clin Res 1993; 19: 273–9.
2. Fasciolo G, et al. Efficacy and safety of moguisteine in comparison with levodropropizine in patients with cough associated with chronic obstructive pulmonary disease, lung cancer, or pulmonary fibrosis. Curr Ther Res 1994; 55: 251–61.
3. Bernareggi A, et al. Stereoselective pharmacokinetics of moguisteine metabolites in healthy subjects. Eur J Drug Metab Pharmacokinet 1995; 20: 263–70.

Morclofone (14231-p)

Morclofone (rINN).

Dimeclofenone; Morclophon. 4'-Chloro-3,5-dimethoxy-4-(2-morpholinoethoxy)benzophenone.

$C_{21}H_{24}ClNO_5 = 405.9$.

CAS — 31848-01-8 (morclofone); 31848-02-9 (morclofone hydrochloride).

ATC — R05DB25.

Profile

Morclofone is a centrally acting cough suppressant used for non-productive cough (p.1082) by mouth in usual doses of 150 mg four to five times daily. It has also been given as the hydrochloride.

Preparations

Proprietary Preparations (details are given in Part 3)

Ital.: Plausitin; *Mex.:* Plausital; *Switz.:* Nitux.

Naphazoline (9504-a)

Naphazoline (BAN, rINN).

2-(1-Naphthylmethyl)-2-imidazoline.

$C_{14}H_{14}N_2 = 210.3$.

CAS — 835-31-4.

ATC — R01AA08; R01AB02; S01GA01.

Naphazoline Hydrochloride (2085-v)

Naphazoline Hydrochloride (BANM, rINNM).

Naphazolini Hydrochloridum.

$C_{14}H_{14}N_2,HCl = 246.7$.

CAS — 550-99-2.

Pharmacopoeias. In Eur. (see p.vi), Jpn, and US.

Pharmacopoeial description

Ph. Eur.: A white or almost white, crystalline powder. Freely soluble in water; soluble in alcohol. Protect from light.

USP 25: A white, odourless, crystalline powder. Freely soluble in water and in alcohol; very slightly soluble in chloroform; practically insoluble in ether. pH of a 1% solution in water is between 5.0 and 6.6. Store in airtight containers. Protect from light.

Naphazoline Nitrate (2086-g)

Naphazoline Nitrate (BANM, rINNM).

Naphazolini Nitras; Naphazolinium Nitricum; Naphthizinum.

$C_{14}H_{14}N_2,HNO_3 = 273.3$.

CAS — 5144-52-5.

Pharmacopoeias. In Eur. (see p.vi), Jpn, and Pol.

Pharmacopoeial description

Ph. Eur.: A white or almost white, crystalline powder. Sparingly soluble in water; soluble in alcohol. A 1% solution in water has a pH of 5.0 to 6.5. Protect from light.

Adverse Effects, Treatment, and Precautions

After local use of naphazoline transient irritation may occur. Rebound congestion may occur after frequent or prolonged use. Systemic effects, including nausea, headache, and dizziness have occurred after local administration. Overdosage or accidental administration by mouth may cause depression of the CNS with marked reduction of body temperature and bradycardia, sweating, drowsiness, and coma, particularly in children; it should be used with great caution, if at all, in infants and young children. Liberation of pigment granules from the iris may occur after ocular administration of naphazoline, especially in high doses to elderly patients. Hypertension may be followed by re-bound hypotension. Treatment of side-effects is symptomatic.

For the adverse effects of sympathomimetics in general, and precautions for their use, see under Adrenaline, p.829.

Effects on the eyes. For mention of conjunctivitis induced by ophthalmic decongestant preparations containing naphazoline, see under Phenylephrine, p.1097.

Interactions

Since naphazoline is absorbed through the nasal mucosa interactions may follow topical application. The *British National Formulary* considers that all sympathomimetic nasal decongestants are liable to cause a hypertensive crisis if used during treatment with an MAOI. For the interactions of sympathomimetics in general, see under Adrenaline, p.830.

Pharmacokinetics

Systemic absorption has been reported following topical application of solutions of naphazoline. It is not used systemically, but it is readily absorbed from the gastrointestinal tract.

Uses and Administration

Naphazoline is a sympathomimetic (see Adrenaline, p.831) with marked alpha-adrenergic activity. It is a vasoconstrictor with a rapid and prolonged action in reducing swelling and congestion when applied to mucous membranes.

Naphazoline and its salts are used for the symptomatic relief of nasal congestion (p.1082). Solutions containing 0.05 to 0.1% of the hydrochloride or the nitrate may be applied topically as nasal drops or a spray usually up to once every 6 hours. Children over 6 years of age have used a preparation containing 0.025%.

Solutions containing up to 0.1% of naphazoline hydrochloride have been instilled into the eye as a conjunctival decongestant (see Conjunctivitis, p.406).

Naphazoline has been used as a vasoconstrictor with local anaesthetics.

Naphazoline acetate has also been used in nasal preparations.

Preparations

USP 25: Naphazoline Hydrochloride Nasal Solution; Naphazoline Hydrochloride Ophthalmic Solution.

Proprietary Preparations (details are given in Part 3)

Aust.: Aconex; Coldan; Isoftal; Privin; Rhinon; Rhinoperd; *Austral.:* Albalon; Clear Eyes; Naphcon; Optazine; *Belg.:* Albalon; Deltarhinol-Mono; Neusinol; Priciasol; Vasocedine; *Braz.:* Narix; Privina; *Canad.:* Ak-Con; Albalon; Allergy Drops; Clear Eyes; Diopticon; Naphcon Forte; Red Away; Rhino-Mex-N†; RO-Naphz†; Vasocon; *Denm.:* Antistina-Privin; *Ger.:* Piniol; Piniol Nasenspray; Privin; Proculin; Rhinex; Vistalbalon†; *Hong Kong:* Albalon; Israel: Naphasal; Naphcon Forte; *Ital.:* Collirio Alfa; Desamin Same; Imidazyl; Imizol†; Iridina Due; Naftazolina; Pupilla; Rinazina; Rino Naftazolina; Video-Mill; Virginiana Gocce Verdi; *Mex.:* Afazol; Alpadinal; Naphacel; Oftazil; *Neth.:* Albalon Liquifilm†; *NZ:* Albalon; Clear Eyes; Naphcon; *Port.:* Murine†; *S.Afr.:* Albalon; Murine Clear Eyes; *Singapore:* Antistin-Privin; *Spain:* Alfa; Miraclar; Privina†; Vasoconstrictor Pensa; *Swed.:* Rimidol; *Switz.:* Albalon; Minha; *Thai.:* Albalon; Naphcon; *UK:* Murine; *USA:* Ak-Con; Albalon; All Clear; Allerest; Allergy Drops; Allersol; Clear Eyes; Comfort Eye Drops; Degest; Nafazair; Napha Forte; Naphcon; Privine; Vasocon.

Multi-ingredient: *Aust.:* Coldistan; Coldophthal; Histophtal†; Luuf-Nasenspray; Ophtaguttal; Rectosan; Rhinodrin; Rhinon; Rhinoperd comp; *Austral.:* Albalon-A; Antistine-Privine; In A Wink; Naphcon-A; Optazine A†; Optrex Medicated; *Belg.:* Deltarhinol†; Diphenhydramine Comfort; Neofenox; Sofraline; Sofrasolone; Zincfrin Antihistaminicum; *Braz.:* Adnax; Albassol; Alergotox Nasal; Angino-Rub; Borato de Sodio; Claril; Colirio Blumen; Colirio Legrand; Colirio Moura Brasil; Colirio Vima; Colyrazul; Conidrin; Dexa-Vastrictol; Fluo-Vaso; Hidrocin; Lerin; Naricin; Naridrin; Naso Instil; Nasopan; Nazobel; Nazobio; Nazotiran; Nitrileno; Nitronasal; Novo Rino; Oftazul; Penetran; Rhinodex; Rhinosept; Rinatrol; Rinisone; Rinocron; Rinozina; Rinozin; Solucao Nasal de Nafazolina; Sorine Adulto; Vastrictol; Visiplex; Visolon; Visual; Zincolok; *Canad.:* Albalon-A Liquifilm; Blue Collyrium†; Collyre Bleu; Cooper AR†; Diopticon A; Naphcon-A; Onrectal; Opcon-A; Rhino-Mex; Vasocon-A; Zincfrin-A; *Denm.:* Sesal; *Fin.:* Antistin-Privin; *Fr.:* Collyre Bleu; Derinox; Frazoline; Soframycine Naphazoline; *Ger.:* Antistin-Privin; Bisrenin†; Combiamid†; Dexa-Siozwo N; Diabenyl-Rhinex; duraultra; Idril sine; Konjunktival Thilo; Oculosan N; Ophtalmin; Ophtocain; Ophtopur-N; Rhinoguttae Dexamethasoni cum Naphazolino; Rhinosovil; Siozwo N; Solupen-D; Stipo; Syncarpin; Tele-Stulln; *Hong Kong:* Konjunktival; Naphcon-A; Oculosan; *Israel:* Alnase; Antistin-Privin; Diphenazol; Nazodin; Nodryl; Optryl; Phenyphrine-Azol; Proaf; *Ital.:* Alfaflor; Antisettico Astringente Sedativo; Antistin-Privina; Citroftalmina VC; Collirio Alfa Antistaminico; Corizzina; Deltarinolo; Fenox†; Fotofil; Ge-nalfa; Idroneomicil; Imidazyl Antistaminico; Indaco; Iristamina; Lucisan; Nafcon A; Oftalmil; Oftalzina; Pupilla Antistaminico; Rinocidina; Rinofomentil; Rinospray†; Rinovit Nube†; Zinc-Imizol; *Mex.:* Afazol Z; Solutina; *NZ:* Albalon-A; Betnesol Aqueous; Clear Eyes ACR; Degest 2; Naphcon-A; Optrex Red-Eye Relief; *Port.:* Alergiftalmina; Gramixina; Naso Prieulina; *S.Afr.:* Albalon-A; Antistin-Privin; Covomycin; Covosan; ENT; Fenox†; Nasdro; Oculosan; Universal Nasal Drops; Wink†; Zincfrin-A†; *Singapore:* Alergiftal; Flucur; Naphcon-A; *Spain:* Alergoftal; Centilux; Clo Zinc†; Cloranfenic Zinc; Coliriocilina Adren Astr; Dexa Vasoc†; Epistaxol; Euboral; Fluo Vasoc; Kanafosal; Kanafosal Predni; Lidrone; Oftalmol Dexa†; Oftalmol Ocular; Ojosbel; Ojosbel Azul; Rinovel; Vasocon Ant; Vasoconstr; Zolina; *Swed.:* Antasten-Privin; *Switz.:* Antistin-Privin; Collyre Alpha; Collyre Bleu Laiter; Derinox; Gouttes nasales N; Oculosan; Optazine†; *Thai.:* Levoptin; Naphcon-A; Oculosan; *UK:* Eye Dew; Optrex Clear Eyes; *USA:* 4-Way Fast Acting; Ak-Con-A†; Antazoline-V; Clear Eyes ACR; Estivin†; Maximum Strength Allergy Drops; Muro's Opcon†; Nafazair A; Naphazole-A†; Naphazoline Plus; Naphcon-A; Naphoptic-A; Ocuhist; Opcon-A; VasoClear; Vaso-Clear A; Vasocon-A.

Used as an adjunct in: *Fr.:* Xylocaine; *Port.:* Anestesico; *Spain:* Anest Compuesto†; Anestesico.

Neltenexine (13828-g)

Neltenexine (rINN).

4',6'-Dibromo-α-[(trans-4-hydroxycyclohexyl)amino]-2-thiophene-carboxy-o-toluidide.

$C_{18}H_{20}Br_2N_2O_2S = 488.2$.

CAS — 99453-84-6.

ATC — R05CB14.

Profile

Neltenexine is a mucolytic that has been used in patients with respiratory disorders associated with productive cough (p.1082). It has been given by mouth as the monohydrate, in usual doses of 37.4 mg three times daily. Neltenexine has also been given rectally as the hydrochloride.

Preparations

Proprietary Preparations (details are given in Part 3)

Ital.: Alveoten; Muco4; Tenoxol.

Nepinalone (13829-q)

Nepinalone (rINN).

(±)-3,4-Dihydro-1-methyl-1-(2-piperidinoethyl)-2(1H)-naphtalenone.

$C_{18}H_{25}NO = 271.4$.

CAS — 22443-11-4.

ATC — R05DB26.

Profile

Nepinalone has been used as the hydrochloride as a cough suppressant in non-productive cough (p.1082). Doses of nepinalone hydrochloride 10 mg have been given three times daily by mouth.

Preparations

Proprietary Preparations (details are given in Part 3)

Ital.: Nepituss; Placatus; Tussolvina.

Nicocodine (10339-e)

Nicocodine (BAN, rINN).

6-Nicotinoylcodeine; 3-O-Methyl-6-O-nicotinoylmorphine.

$C_{24}H_{24}N_2O_4 = 404.5$.

CAS — 3688-66-2.

Profile

Nicocodine is an opioid related to codeine (p.25). It has been used as the hydrochloride for its central cough suppressant effects in non-productive cough (p.1082). Nicocodine hydrochloride is given by mouth in doses of 5 to 7.5 mg up to three times daily.

Preparations

Proprietary Preparations (details are given in Part 3)

Aust.: Tusscodin.

Normethadone Hydrochloride (13033-k)

Normethadone Hydrochloride (BANM, rINNM).

Desmethylmethadone Hydrochloride; Hoechst-10582 (normethadone); Phenyldimazone Hydrochloride. 6-Dimethylamino-4,4-diphenylhexan-3-one hydrochloride.

$C_{20}H_{25}NO,HCl = 331.9$.

CAS — 467-85-6 (normethadone); 847-84-7 (normethadone hydrochloride).

Profile

Normethadone is closely related to methadone (p.53). The hydrochloride is given by mouth as a cough suppressant in non-productive cough.

Preparations

Proprietary Preparations (details are given in Part 3)

Multi-ingredient: *Canad.:* Cophylac.

The symbol † denotes a preparation no longer actively marketed

Noscapine (5625-a)

Noscapine (BAN, rINN).

Narcotine; L-α-Narcotine; Noscapinum; NSC-5366. (3S)-6,7-Dimethoxy-3-[(5R)-5,6,7,8-tetrahydro-4-methoxy-6-methyl-1,3-dioxolo[4,5-g]isoquinolin-5-yl]phthalide.
$C_{22}H_{23}NO_7 = 413.4$.
CAS — 128-62-1.
ATC — R05DA07.

Pharmacopoeias. In Eur. (see p.vi), Int., Jpn, and US.

Noscapine is an alkaloid obtained from opium.

Pharmacopoeial description

Ph. Eur.: A white, crystalline powder or colourless crystals. Practically insoluble in water at 20°, very slightly soluble at 100°; slightly soluble in alcohol and in ether; soluble in acetone; dissolves in strong acids although the base may be precipitated on dilution with water. Protect from light.

USP 25: A fine, white or practically white, crystalline powder. Practically insoluble in water; slightly soluble in alcohol and in ether; soluble in acetone; freely soluble in chloroform.

Noscapine Camsilate (12514-m)

Camphoscapine; Noscapine Camsylate. Noscapine camphor-10-sulphonate.
$C_{22}H_{23}NO_7,C_{10}H_{16}O_4S = 645.7$.
CAS — 25333-79-3.

Noscapine Hydrochloride (5626-t)

Noscapine Hydrochloride (BANM, rINNM).

Narcotine Hydrochloride; Noscapini Hydrochloridum; Noscapinium Chloride.
$C_{22}H_{23}NO_7,HCl,H_2O = 467.9$.
CAS — 912-60-7 (anhydrous noscapine hydrochloride).
Pharmacopoeias. In Eur. (see p.vi) and Int. (both with H_2O); in Jpn (with xH_2O).

Pharmacopoeial description

Ph. Eur.: A white, hygroscopic, crystalline powder or colourless crystals. Freely soluble in water and in alcohol; practically insoluble in ether. Aqueous solutions are faintly acid; the base may be precipitated when the solutions are allowed to stand. A 2% solution in water has a pH of not less than 3.0. Protect from light.

Adverse Effects and Precautions

As for Dextromethorphan, p.1087. Hypersensitivity reactions have been reported.

◊ The UK Committee on Safety of Medicines stood by their recommendation[1] that products containing noscapine should be contra-indicated in women of child-bearing potential (because of potential mutagenic effects[2]), after criticism that the decision was based solely on the results of in-vitro work.[3]
1. Asscher AW, Fowler LK. Papaveretum in women of childbearing potential. BMJ 1991; 303: 648.
2. Committee on Safety of Medicines. Genotoxicity of papaveretum and noscapine. Current Problems 31 1991.
3. Allen S, et al. Papaveretum in women of child bearing potential. BMJ 1991; 303: 647.

Interactions

Noscapine should not be given concomitantly with alcohol or other CNS depressants.

Pharmacokinetics

◊ References to the pharmacokinetics of noscapine.
1. Karlsson MO, et al. Pharmacokinetics of oral noscapine. Eur J Clin Pharmacol 1990; 39: 275–9.
2. Karlsson MO, Dahlstrom B. Serum protein binding of noscapine: influence of a reversible hydrolysis. J Pharm Pharmacol 1990; 42: 140–3.

Uses and Administration

Noscapine is a centrally acting cough suppressant that has actions and uses similar to those of dextromethorphan (p.1088). It is given by mouth in a dose of up to 50 mg three times daily. It has also been given as the camsilate, embonate, and the hydrochloride, and also administered rectally.

Preparations

Proprietary Preparations (details are given in Part 3)
Belg.: Noscaflex; Ger.: Capval; Neth.: Finipect†; Libronchin Prikkelhoest; Roter Noscapect†; S.Afr.: Nitepax; Spain: Tuscalman; Swed.: Nipaxon; Switz.: Tussanil N.

Multi-ingredient: Aust.: Pneumopect; Tuscalman; Belg.: Noscaflex; Rosils; Braz.: Broncotussan; Expectussin; Fin.: Codesan N; Posivil; Fr.: Broncho-Tulisan Eucalyptol†; Tussisedal; Hong Kong: Asmeton; Panadol Cold and Flu; Ital.: Difmetus Compositum; Ribelfan; Tuscalman; Swed.: Spasmofen; Switz.: Brosoline-Rectocaps; Hederix; No Grip†; Noscorex; Spasmosol; Tossamine; Tossamine plus; Tuscalman; Tussanil Compositum; Thai.: Asmeton.

Oxeladin Citrate (5627-x)

Oxeladin Citrate (BANM, rINNM).

2-(2-Diethylaminoethoxy)ethyl 2-ethyl-2-phenylbutyrate dihydrogen citrate.
$C_{20}H_{33}NO_3,C_6H_8O_7 = 527.6$.
CAS — 468-61-1 (oxeladin); 52432-72-1 (oxeladin citrate).

Profile

Oxeladin citrate has been given by mouth as a centrally acting cough suppressant for non-productive cough (p.1082). Doses of up to 40 mg three times daily have been given by mouth.

Preparations

Proprietary Preparations (details are given in Part 3)
Fr.: Paxeladine; Norw.: Pectamol†.

Multi-ingredient: Braz.: Novotussan; Tetrabronco; Tetratoss; Transpulmin Xarope; Tripulmin; Fr.: Paxeladine Noctee†; Ital.: Tussiflex†; Mex.: Fluxedan.

Oxolamine (14838-c)

Oxolamine (rINN).

683-M. 5-[2-(Diethylamino)ethyl]-3-phenyl-1,2,4-oxadiazole.
$C_{14}H_{19}N_3O = 245.3$.
CAS — 959-14-8.
ATC — R05DB07.

Oxolamine Citrate (13067-b)

Oxolamine Citrate (rINNM).

AF-438; SKF-9976.
$C_{14}H_{19}N_3O,C_6H_8O_7 = 437.4$.
CAS — 1949-20-8.

Oxolamine Phosphate (14238-z)

Oxolamine Phosphate (rINNM).
CAS — 1949-19-5.

Profile

Oxolamine is a cough suppressant with a predominantly peripheral action that has been used for non-productive cough (p.1082). It has been given as the citrate or phosphate in usual doses of 100 to 200 mg three times daily. It has also been given as the tannate.

Hallucinations in children have been reported after its use.

◊ References.
1. McEwen J, et al. Hallucinations in children caused by oxolamine citrate. Med J Aust 1989; 150: 449–52.

Preparations

Proprietary Preparations (details are given in Part 3)
Israel: Symphocal; Ital.: Gantrimex; Perebron; Tussibron; Mex.: Bredon; Cideox; Contuxin; Eumol; Exalamin; Fartoxol; Kentosanil; Oxathos; Oxobron; Oxolam; Oxomifer; Oxoquin; Toxal; Tukson; Tusol; Spain: Perebron.

Multi-ingredient: Braz.: Eritrex A; Ital.: Uniplus; Upsa Plus; Mex.: Caltusine; Spain: Bequipecto†; Dimayon†; Pectoral Funk Antitus†.

Oxymetazoline Hydrochloride

(2093-v)

Oxymetazoline Hydrochloride (BANM, USAN, rINN).

H-990; Oxymetazolini Hydrochloridum; Sch-9384.
$C_{16}H_{24}N_2O,HCl = 296.8$.
CAS — 2315-02-8.

Pharmacopoeias. In Eur. (see p.vi) and US.

Pharmacopoeial description

Ph. Eur.: A white or almost white, crystalline powder. Freely soluble in water and in alcohol; practically insoluble in ether.

USP 25: A white to practically white, fine, hygroscopic, crystalline powder. Soluble 1 in 6.7 of water, 1 in 3.6 of alcohol, and 1 in 862 of chloroform; practically insoluble in ether and in benzene. pH of a 5% solution in water is between 4.0 and 6.5. Store in airtight containers.

Adverse Effects and Precautions

As for Naphazoline, p.1095.

After local use of oxymetazoline transient irritation may occur. Rebound congestion may occur after frequent or prolonged nasal use. Systemic effects have occurred after local administration.

Porphyria. Oxymetazoline has been associated with acute attacks of porphyria and is considered unsafe in porphyric patients.

Interactions

Since oxymetazoline is absorbed through the mucosa interactions may follow topical application. The British National Formulary considers that all sympathomimetic nasal decongestants are liable to cause a hypertensive crisis if used during treatment with an MAOI. For the interactions of sympathomimetics in general, see under Adrenaline, p.830.

Uses and Administration

Oxymetazoline is a direct-acting sympathomimetic (see Adrenaline, p.831) with marked alpha-adrenergic activity. It is a vasoconstrictor which reduces swelling and congestion when applied to mucous membranes. It acts within a few minutes and the effect lasts for up to 12 hours. It is used as the hydrochloride for the symptomatic relief of nasal congestion (p.1082). A 0.05% solution of oxymetazoline hydrochloride is applied topically as nasal drops or a spray, usually twice daily to each nostril as required.

A 0.025% solution of oxymetazoline hydrochloride may be instilled into the eye as a conjunctival decongestant (see Conjunctivitis, p.406).

Hypersensitivity. Anaphylactic reactions are usually treated with adrenaline [epinephrine] (p.832), but occasions do arise when it is not always readily available. One patient who had suffered previous reactions to aspirin or ibuprofen that had been treated with corticosteroid and adrenaline [epinephrine] suffered another attack following a dose of ketoprofen.[1] She was able to relieve the symptoms, including the potentially fatal upper airways obstruction, by pumping 12 inhalations of oxymetazoline nasal solution into each nostril.
1. Kim KT, et al. Use of non-prescription decongestant to abort anaphylaxis. Lancet 1993; 341: 439. Correction. ibid.; 704.

Preparations

USP 25: Oxymetazoline Hydrochloride Nasal Solution; Oxymetazoline Hydrochloride Ophthalmic Solution.

Proprietary Preparations (details are given in Part 3)
Aust.: Nasivin; Austral.: Chemists Own Decongestant Nasal Spray; Dimetapp 12 Hour Nasal; Drixine Nasal; Logicin Rapid Relief; Ordov Sinudec; Belg.: Nesivine; Vicks Sinex; Braz.: Afrin; Nasivin; Oxilin; Rino Spray; Canad.: Decongestant Nasal Mist; Dristan; Drixoral; Nafrine; Ocuclear; Vicks Sinex; Visine Workplace; Denm.: Drixin; Iliadin; Nezeril†; Fin.: Dristan; Nezeril; Vicks Sinex; Fr.: Aturgyl; Ger.: Em-eukal Mono; Nasivin gegen Schnupfen; Nasivin Sanft; Nasivinetten gegen Schnupfen; Vistoxyn†; Wick Sinex; Hong Kong: Afrin; Duration; Iliadin; Nezeril; Oxylin; Irl.: Dristan; Vicks Sinex†; Israel: Alrin; Nasivin; Oxylin; Rhinoclir; Ital.: Actifed Nasale; Coricidin; Nasivin†; Oxilin; Rino Calyptol; Mex.: Afrin; Iliadin; Ocuclear; Oxylin; Visine AD; Neth.: Dampo†; Nasivin; Oxylin Liquifilm†; Vicks Sinex; Norw.: Iliadin; Rhinox; NZ: Drixine; Port.: Alerjon; Nasarox; Nasex; Neozine; Oxylin; Rinerge; Robinaz; S.Afr.: Advil NS†; Afrin†; Drixine; Iliadin; Oxylin; Sinustop†; Singapore: Afrin; Iliadin; Oxylin; Spain: Alerfrin; Corilisina; Descongestan; Egarone Oximetazolina†; Humoxal†; Idasal Nebulizador; Inalintra; Nasolina; Nasovalda; Nebulicina; Oftinal; Respibien; Respir; Rinocorin; Rinodif; Utabon; Swed.: Iliadin; Nasin; Nezeril; Zolin; Switz.: Nasivine; Nasivinettes; Vistoxyn; Thai.: Iliadin; Nasil; Oxylin; Oxymet; UAE: Nasivin; UK: Afrazine; Dristan; Sudafed Nasal Spray; Vicks Sinex; USA: 12 Hour Sinarest†; 4-Way Long Lasting; Afrin; Alleerest 12 Hour Nasal; Cheracol Nasal†; Chlorphed-LA; Dristan 12-hr Nasal Decongestant Spray; Dristan Long Lasting; Duramist Plus; Duration; Genasal; Maximum Strength Nasal Decongestant†; Nasal Relief; Nasal Spray; Neo-Synephrine 12 Hour; Nostrilla; NTZ Long Acting Nasal; Ocuclear; Twice-A-Day; Vicks Sinex 12-Hour; Visine LR.

Multi-ingredient: Aust.: Wick Sinex; Austral.: Euky Bear Nasex†; Nasex; Vasylox; Vicks Sinex; Braz.: Narizima Adulto; Fr.: Deturgylone; Sinex†; Ger.: Larylin Nasenspray N†; Israel: Sinaf; Ital.: Nasicortin; Triaminic; Vicks Sinex; S.Afr.: Nazene; Spain: Antirrinum; Egarone; Orto Nasal; Respir Balsamico†; Vicks Spray; Switz.: Vicks Sinex.

Pentoxyverine (11490-m)

Pentoxyverine (BAN, rINN).

Carbetapentane. 2-[2-(Diethylamino)ethoxy]ethyl 1-phenylcyclopentanecarboxylate.
$C_{20}H_{31}NO_3 = 333.5$.
CAS — 77-23-6.
ATC — R05DB05.

Pentoxyverine Citrate (5607-c)

Pentoxyverine Citrate (BANM, rINNM).

Carbetapentane Citrate; Pentoxyverine Hydrogen Citrate; Pentoxyverini Hydrogenocitras; UCB-2543.
$C_{20}H_{31}NO_3,C_6H_8O_7 = 525.6$.
CAS — 23142-01-0.

Pharmacopoeias. In Chin., Eur. (see p.vi), and Jpn.

Pharmacopoeial description

Ph. Eur.: A white or almost white crystalline powder. M.p. about 93°. Freely soluble in water and in methyl alcohol; soluble in alcohol and in dichloromethane; very soluble in glacial acetic acid. A 10% solution in water has a pH of 3.3 to 3.7. Protect from light.

Pentoxyverine Hydrochloride (9884-d)

Pentoxyverine Hydrochloride (BANM).
$C_{20}H_{31}NO_3,HCl = 369.9$.
CAS — 1045-21-2.

Profile

Pentoxyverine is a centrally acting cough suppressant used for non-productive cough (p.1082). Up to 200 mg daily of the citrate has been given by mouth in divided doses. The hydrochloride and the tannate are also given by mouth. The base has been administered rectally.

Preparations

Phenylephrine (9512-a)

Phenylephrine (BAN, rINN).

Fenilefrina; Phenylephrinum; m-Synephrine. (S)-1-(3-Hydroxy-phenyl)-2-methylaminoethanol.
$C_9H_{13}NO_2 = 167.2$.
CAS — 59-42-7.
ATC — C01CA06; R01AA04; R01AB01; R01BA03; S01FB01; S01GA05.

NOTE. Synephrine has been used as a synonym for oxedrine. Care should be taken to avoid confusion between the two compounds.
Pharmacopoeias. In Eur. (see p.vi).

Pharmacopoeial description

Ph. Eur.: A white or almost white crystalline powder. Slightly soluble in water and in alcohol; sparingly soluble in methyl alcohol. It dissolves in dilute mineral acids and in solutions of alkali hydroxides. Store in airtight containers. Protect from light.

Phenylephrine Acid Tartrate (9511-k)

Phenylephrine Bitartrate; Phenylephrine Tartrate (BANM).
$C_9H_{13}NO_2,C_4H_6O_6 = 317.3$.
CAS — 13998-27-1.

Phenylephrine Hydrochloride (2094-g)

Phenylephrine Hydrochloride (BANM, rINNM).
Mesatonum; Metaoxedrini Chloridum; Phenylephrini Hydrochloridum.
$C_9H_{13}NO_2,HCl = 203.7$.
CAS — 61-76-7.

NOTE. PHNL is a code approved by the BP 2001 for use on single unit doses of eye drops containing phenylephrine hydrochloride where the individual container may be too small to bear all the appropriate labelling information. PHNCYC is a similar code approved for eye drops containing phenylephrine hydrochloride and cyclopentolate hydrochloride.
Pharmacopoeias. In Chin., Eur. (see p.vi), Jpn, and US.

Pharmacopoeial description

Ph. Eur.: A white or almost white, crystalline powder. Freely soluble in water and in alcohol.

USP 25: White or practically white, odourless, crystals. Freely soluble in water and in alcohol. Store in airtight containers. Protect from light.

Incompatibility. Phenylephrine is stated to be incompatible with the local anaesthetic butacaine.

Adverse Effects and Precautions

For the adverse effects of sympathomimetics in general, and precautions for their use, see under Adrenaline, p.829. Phenylephrine has a longer duration of action than noradrenaline [norepinephrine] and an excessive vasopressor response may cause a prolonged rise in blood pressure. It induces tachycardia or reflex bradycardia and should therefore be avoided in severe hyperthyroidism and used with caution in severe ischaemic heart disease.

Since phenylephrine is absorbed through the mucosa systemic effects may follow application to the eyes or the nasal mucosa. In particular, phenylephrine 10% eye drops should be avoided or only used with extreme caution in infants and the elderly since they can have powerful systemic effects.

Liberation of pigment granules from the iris may occur after ocular administration of phenylephrine especially in high doses to elderly patients. Ophthalmic solutions of phenylephrine are contra-indicated in patients with angle-closure glaucoma. Corneal clouding may occur if corneal epithelium has been denuded or damaged.

The symbol † denotes a preparation no longer actively marketed

---

Excessive or prolonged use of phenylephrine nasal drops can lead to rebound congestion.

Phenylephrine hydrochloride is irritant and may cause local discomfort at the site of application; extravasation of the injection may even cause local tissue necrosis.

Effects on the cardiovascular system. Systemic side-effects have occurred following the use of phenylephrine eye drops, particularly at a strength of 10%, and after the use of phenylephrine nasal drops.

Hypertension[1] and hypertension with pulmonary oedema[2] have been described in infants after the use of phenylephrine 10% eye drops, and hypertension has occurred in an infant after phenylephrine was also given intranasally with pseudoephedrine orally.[3] The specific problem of eye drops and neonatal blood pressure has also been reviewed.[4] Hypertension with arrhythmias has been reported in an 8-year-old child[5] and in an adult[6] after phenylephrine 10% eye drops had been used. Details have also been published on a series of 32 patients who experienced systemic cardiovascular reactions after the administration of phenylephrine 10% solutions to the eye.[7]

Despite there being some evidence to suggest that the incidence of such reactions is low,[8] there is a reasonable body of opinion that has advocated the use of lower concentrations[1,7] and use with caution in susceptible patients such as those with cardiovascular disorders or the elderly.[7] A reduction in the eye-drop volume has been found to produce adequate mydriasis and may reduce systemic absorption and the risk of adverse cardiovascular effects.[9,10]

1. Borromeo-McGrail V, et al. Systemic hypertension following ocular administration of 10% phenylephrine in the neonate. *Pediatrics* 1973; **51:** 1032–6.
2. Matthews TG, et al. Eye-drop induced hypertension. *Lancet* 1977; **ii:** 827.
3. Saken R, et al. Drug-induced hypertension in infancy. *J Pediatr* 1979; **95:** 1077–9.
4. Anonymous. Babies' blood pressure raised by eye drops. *BMJ* 1974; **1:** 2–3.
5. Vaughan RW. Ventricular arrhythmias after topical vasoconstrictors. *Anesth Analg* 1973; **52:** 161–5.
6. Lai Y-K. Adverse effect of intraoperative phenylephrine 10%: case report. *Br J Ophthalmol* 1989; **73:** 468–9.
7. Fraunfelder FT, Scafidi AF. Possible adverse effects from topical ocular 10% phenylephrine. *Am J Ophthalmol* 1978; **85:** 447–53.
8. Brown MM, et al. Lack of side effects from topically administered 10% phenylephrine eyedrops: a controlled study. *Arch Ophthalmol* 1980; **98:** 487–9.
9. Craig EW, Griffiths PG. Effect on mydriasis of modifying the volume of phenylephrine drops. *Br J Ophthalmol* 1991; **75:** 222–3.
10. Wheatcroft S, et al. Reduction in mydriatic drop size in premature infants. *Br J Ophthalmol* 1993; **77:** 364–5.

Effects on the eyes. Acute and chronic conjunctivitis has been reported[1] following use of over-the-counter ophthalmic decongestant preparations of phenylephrine, naphazoline, or tetryzoline. The conjunctival inflammation took several weeks to resolve in some cases. Dermatoconjunctivitis[2] has also been reported following use of phenylephrine eye drops.

1. Soparkar CN, et al. Acute and chronic conjunctivitis due to over-the-counter ophthalmic decongestants. *Arch Ophthalmol* 1997; **115:** 34–8.
2. Moreno-Ancillo A, et al. Allergic contact reactions due to phenylephrine hydrochloride in eyedrops. *Ann Allergy Asthma Immunol* 1997; **78:** 569–72.

Effects on mental function. Hallucinations and paranoid delusions have been reported[1] in a patient following excessive use of a nasal spray containing phenylephrine 0.5%. Mania has also followed the use of high doses by mouth.[2]

1. Snow SS, et al. Nasal spray 'addiction' and psychosis: a case report. *Br J Psychiatry* 1980; **136:** 297–9.
2. Waters BGH, Lapierre YD. Secondary mania associated with sympathomimetic drug use. *Am J Psychiatry* 1981; **138:** 837–40.

Hypersensitivity. Cross-sensitivity to phenylephrine has been reported in a patient hypersensitive to pseudoephedrine.[1] See also under Effects on the Eyes, above.

1. Buzo-Sanchez G, et al. Stereoisomeric cutaneous hypersensitivity. *Ann Pharmacother* 1997; **31:** 1091.

Interactions

For the interactions of sympathomimetics in general, see under Adrenaline, p.830.

Phenylephrine is less liable than adrenaline [epinephrine] or noradrenaline [norepinephrine] to induce ventricular fibrillation if used as a pressor agent during anaesthesia with inhalational anaesthetics such as cyclopropane and halothane; nevertheless, caution is necessary. Since phenylephrine is absorbed through the mucosa, interactions may also follow topical application, particularly in patients receiving an MAOI (including an RIMA). For additional warnings see under phenelzine (p.305) and moclobemide (p.299).

Cardiovascular drugs. Hypertensive reactions have been reported in a patient stabilised on *debrisoquine* when given phenylephrine by mouth,[1] in patients receiving *reserpine* or *guanethidine* when given phenylephrine eye drops,[2] and a fatal

---

reaction occurred in a patient receiving *propranolol* and *hydrochlorothiazide* also after the instillation of phenylephrine eye drops.[3]

1. Aminu J, et al. Interaction between debrisoquine and phenylephrine. *Lancet* 1970; **ii:** 935–6.
2. Kim JM, et al. Hypertensive reactions to phenylephrine eyedrops in patients with sympathetic denervation. *Am J Ophthalmol* 1978; **85:** 862–8.
3. Cass E, et al. Hazards of phenylephrine topical medication in persons taking propranolol. *Can Med Assoc J* 1979; **120:** 1261–2.

Pharmacokinetics

Phenylephrine has low oral bioavailability owing to irregular absorption and first-pass metabolism by monoamine oxidase in the gut and liver. When injected subcutaneously or intramuscularly it takes 10 to 15 minutes to act; subcutaneous and intramuscular injections are effective for up to about one hour and up to about two hours, respectively. Intravenous injections are effective for about 20 minutes.

Systemic absorption follows topical administration.

Uses and Administration

Phenylephrine hydrochloride is a sympathomimetic (see Adrenaline, p.831) with mainly direct effects on adrenergic receptors. It has predominantly alpha-adrenergic activity and is without significant stimulating effects on the CNS at usual doses. Its pressor activity is weaker than that of noradrenaline [norepinephrine] (p.948) but of longer duration. After injection it produces peripheral vasoconstriction and increased arterial pressure; it also causes reflex bradycardia. It reduces blood flow to the skin and to the kidneys.

Phenylephrine and its salts are most commonly used, either topically or by mouth, for the symptomatic relief of nasal congestion (p.1082). They are frequently included in preparations intended for the relief of cough and cold symptoms. For nasal congestion, a 0.25 to 0.5% solution may be instilled as nasal drops or a spray into each nostril every 4 hours as required, or phenylephrine hydrochloride may be given by mouth in doses of about 5 to 20 mg three or four times daily.

In ophthalmology, phenylephrine hydrochloride is used as a mydriatic (p.460) in concentrations of up to 10%; generally solutions containing 2.5% or 10% are employed but systemic absorption can occur (see Adverse Effects, above) and the 10% strength, in particular, should be used with caution. The mydriatic effect can last several hours. Solutions stronger than 2% may cause intense irritation and a local anaesthetic other than butacaine (which is incompatible) should be instilled into the eye a few minutes beforehand.

Ocular solutions containing lower concentrations (usually 0.12% phenylephrine hydrochloride) are used as a conjunctival decongestant (see Conjunctivitis, p.406).

Phenylephrine has been used parenterally in the treatment of hypotensive states, such as those encountered during circulatory failure or spinal anaesthesia. For hypotension, an initial dose of phenylephrine hydrochloride 2 to 5 mg may be given as a 1% solution subcutaneously or intramuscularly with further doses of 1 to 10 mg if necessary, according to response. A dose of 100 to 500 µg by slow intravenous injection as a 0.1% solution, repeated as necessary after at least 15 minutes, has also been employed. In severe hypotensive states, 10 mg in 500 mL of glucose 5% or sodium chloride 0.9% has been infused intravenously, initially at a rate of up to 180 µg per minute, reduced, according to the response, to 30 to 60 µg per minute. Phenylephrine has also been used in orthostatic hypotension (p.1070).

Phenylephrine hydrochloride has been given by intravenous injection to stop paroxysmal supraventricular tachycardia but other drugs are preferred (see Cardiac Arrhythmias, p.794). The initial dose is usually not greater than 500 µg given as a 0.1% solution with subsequent doses gradually increased up to 1 mg if necessary.

Phenylephrine hydrochloride has been used as a vaso-constrictor with local anaesthetics.

Phenylephrine has also been used as the acid tartrate to prolong the bronchodilator effects of isoprenaline when administered by inhalation. However, isoprenaline is now little used by this route.

Phenylephrine tannate has also been used.

Priapism. For reference to phenylephrine in low dosage and dilute solution being given by intracavernosal injection to reverse priapism, see under Alprostadil, p.1440.

Preparations

BP 2001: Phenylephrine Eye Drops; Phenylephrine Injection;
USP 25: Antipyrine, Benzocaine, and Phenylephrine Hydrochloride Otic Solution; Isoproterenol Hydrochloride and Phenylephrine Bitartrate Inhalation Aerosol; Phenylephrine Hydrochloride Injection; Phenylephrine Hydrochloride Nasal Jelly; Phenylephrine Hydrochloride Nasal Solution; Phenylephrine Hydrochloride Ophthalmic Solution.

Proprietary Preparations (details are given in Part 3)
Aust.: Prefrin Liquifilm; Visadron; *Austral.:* Albalon Relief; Isopto Frin; Neo-Synephrine; Nyal Decongestant; Prefrin; Visopt; *Belg.:* Isopto Frin; Neo-Synephrine; Visadron; *Braz.:* Neo-Sinefrina; *Canad.:* Dionephrine; Mydfrin; Neo-Synephrine; Novahistine; Prefrin; *Fin.:* Oftan Metaoksedrin; *Fr.:* Auristan; Neosynephrine; *Ger.:* Neo-Mydrial; Neosynephrin-POS; Visadron; Vistosan†; *Hong Kong:* Analux; Prefrin; *Irl.:* Isopto Frin; *Israel:* Af-Taf; Efrin; Neo-Synephrine; Prefrin; *Ital.:* Isonefrine; Neo-Synephrine; Ribex Nasale; Visadron; *Mex.:* Lefrine; Weiscalina; *Neth.:* Boradrine†; Visadron†; *NZ:* Albalon Relief; Isopto Frin; Prefrin; *Port.:* Davinefrina; Humoxal†; Neo-Sinefrina; Visadron; *S.Afr.:* Fenox†; I-Glo; Naphensyl; Prefrin; *Singapore:* Analux; Isopto Frin; Mydfrin; Prefrin; *Spain:* ADA; Analux; Boraline; Disneumon Pernasal; Mirazul; Neo Lacrim; Pulverizador Nasal†; Rin Up; Visadron; Vistafrin; *Swed.:* Neo-Synephrine†; *Switz.:* Gouttes nasales; *Thai.:* Centapp; *UK:* Fenox; Isopto Frin; *USA:* AH-chew D; Ak-Dilate; Ak-Nefrin; Alconefrin; Children's Nostril; Eye Drops Extra; Isopto Frin†; Mydfrin; Neo-Synephrine; Neofrin; Nostril; Ocu-Phrin; Phenoptic; Prefrin Liquifilm; Rectacaine; Relief; Rhinall; Ricobid D†; Sinex; Storzfen†.

Multi-ingredient: numerous preparations are listed in Part 3.

Phenylpropanolamine (18492-z)

Phenylpropanolamine *(BAN, rINN)*.

(±)-Norephedrine. (1RS,2SR)-2-Amino-1-phenylpropan-1-ol.
$C_9H_{13}NO = 151.2$.
CAS — 14838-15-4.
ATC — R01BA01.

Phenylpropanolamine Hydrochloride (2095-q)

Phenylpropanolamine Hydrochloride *(BANM, rINNM)*.
Mydriatin; Phenylpropanolamini Hydrochloridum.
$C_9H_{13}NO,HCl = 187.7$.
CAS — 154-41-6.
Pharmacopoeias. In Eur. (see p.vi) and US.
US also includes phenylpropanolamine bitartrate.

Pharmacopoeial description

Ph. Eur.: A white or almost white, crystalline powder. Freely soluble in water and in alcohol; practically insoluble in dichloromethane.

USP 25: A white crystalline powder, having a slight aromatic odour. Soluble 1 in 1.1 of water, 1 in 7.4 of alcohol, and 1 in 4100 of chloroform; insoluble in ether. pH of a 3% solution in water is between 4.2 and 5.5. Store in airtight containers. Protect from light.

Adverse Effects and Precautions
As for Ephedrine, p.1090.

Severe hypertensive episodes have followed phenylpropanolamine ingestion (see below). As with other indirect-acting sympathomimetics, tolerance to the therapeutic effects of phenylpropanolamine has been reported with prolonged administration.

◊ An extensive and detailed review[1] of adverse effects attributed to phenylpropanolamine noted in 1990 that many of the adverse drug reactions reported in Europe described an alteration of mental status whereas those in North America were more often compatible with hypertension. An author suggested that this might be due to a difference in the isomers present in phenylpropanolamine preparations, based on earlier reports that *d*-norpseudoephedrine, the most potent of several isomeric forms as a stimulant of the CNS, was present in European preparations of phenylpropanolamine. However, later investigation suggests that currently the racemic mixture (±)-norephedrine (*d,l*-norephedrine) is the isomeric form present in commercial preparations in both Europe and the USA.[2]

The original review[1] concentrated on North American cases. The majority of products available were decongestants or cough or cold remedies; a small number were promoted as diet aids.

The data suggested that over-the-counter (OTC) products were more likely to be associated with an adverse reaction than a prescription medication; this may be because such OTC products were more likely to be overused and to be considered innocuous by the patient. It was also likely that drug interactions (below) rather than 'true overdosages', were involved in many of the adverse events, particularly as many OTC preparations contain other ingredients. (See also under Abuse of Ephedrine, p.1090, for further discussion about the consequences of use of OTC preparations containing sympathomimetics, including phenylpropanolamine.)

The adverse reactions varied widely ranging from headache and elevated blood pressure to cardiopulmonary arrest, intracranial haemorrhage, and death. Mild reactions included blurred vision, dizziness, anxiety, agitation, tremor, confusion, and hypersensitivity reaction. Severe reactions also included hypertensive crisis with hypertensive encephalopathy, seizures, arrhythmias, psychosis, and acute tubular necrosis. One unifying theme of many of the severe cases was that high blood pressure or symptoms suggestive of this were the presenting feature; an acute, persistent, severe headache was also noted in many cases.

It was pointed out that overall phenylpropanolamine was relatively safe. Although billions of doses were consumed annually, few cases of adverse drug reactions had been reported.

It was believed that certain groups may be at particular risk of adverse reactions to phenylpropanolamine: persons with elevated blood pressure, overweight persons (who are likely to be both hypertensive and to use diet aids), patients with eating disorders (who tend to abuse substances including diet aids), and the elderly (who may be multiple drug takers and likely to be hypertensive and at risk already of a stroke).

Subsequently, following a large case-control study in the USA which found an increased risk of haemorrhagic stroke associated with the use of preparations containing phenylpropanolamine (and in particular in women who used phenylpropanolamine as an appetite suppressant,[3] the FDA took steps to remove phenylpropanolamine from all drug products in the USA and requested that it no longer be marketed. Products containing phenylpropanolamine have also been withdrawn in some other countries. However, this study has been criticised[4,5] on the basis that it provided no evidence of an increased risk with the amount of phenylpropanolamine normally present in decongestant preparations. The UK Committee on Safety of Medicines[6] considered that the evidence of a link between UK products containing phenylpropanolamine and haemorrhagic stroke was weak (phenylpropanolamine is not licensed as an appetite suppressant in the UK and the maximum recommended dose is lower than was recommended in the USA). It was therefore suggested by UK commentators that use of licensed doses, with appropriate precautions, posed no additional risk.[2]

1. Lake CR, *et al.* Adverse drug effects attributed to phenylpropanolamine: a review of 142 case reports. *Am J Med* 1990; **89:** 195–208.
2. Moffatt T, *et al.* Phenylpropanolamine: putting the record straight. *Pharm J* 2000; **265:** 817.
3. Kernan WN, *et al.* Phenylpropanolamine and the risk of hemorrhagic stroke. *N Engl J Med* 2000; **343:** 1826–32.
4. Ernst ME, Hartz A. Phenylpropanolamine and hemorrhagic stroke. *N Engl J Med* 2001; **344:** 1094.
5. Wolowich WR, *et al.* Phenylpropanolamine and hemorrhagic stroke. *N Engl J Med* 2001; **344:** 1094–5.
6. Committee on Safety of Medicines/Medicines Control Agency. Phenylpropanolamine and haemorrhagic stroke. *Current Problems* 2001; **27:** 5–6.

Interactions

For the interactions of sympathomimetics in general, see under Adrenaline, p.830. For a comment that drug interactions were likely to have been involved in many adverse events associated with phenylpropanolamine see under Adverse Effects and Precautions, above. Hypertensive crisis is a particular risk in patients receiving MAOIs.

Amantadine. Severe psychosis has been reported[1] in a woman taking amantadine and phenylpropanolamine together.

1. Stroe AE, *et al.* Psychotic episode related to phenylpropanolamine and amantadine in a healthy female. *Gen Hosp Psychiatry* 1995; **17:** 457–8.

Antipsychotics. A 27-year-old woman with schizophrenia and T-wave abnormality of the heart, who had responded to thioridazine 100 mg daily with procyclidine 2.5 mg twice daily, died from ventricular fibrillation within 2 hours of taking a single dose of a preparation reported to contain chlorpheniramine [chlorphenamine] maleate 4 mg with phenylpropanolamine hydrochloride 50 mg (Contac C), concurrently with thioridazine.[1]

1. Chouinard G, *et al.* Death attributed to ventricular arrhythmia induced by thioridazine in combination with a single Contac C capsule. *Can Med Assoc J* 1978; **119:** 729–31.

Antivirals. Hypertensive crisis has been reported[1] in a patient taking an over-the-counter nasal decongestant preparation containing phenylpropanolamine and clemastine concomitantly with a triple-drug HIV prophylactic regimen 3 days after *stavu-*

dine was substituted for *zidovudine*; the other antivirals in the regimen were *indinavir* and *lamivudine*.

1. Khurana V, *et al.* Hypertensive crisis secondary to phenylpropanolamine interacting with triple-drug therapy for HIV prophylaxis. *Am J Med* 1999; **106:** 118–19.

Bromocriptine. For a report of hypertension and life-threatening complications following concomitant use of phenylpropanolamine and bromocriptine, see p.1166.

NSAIDs. A 27-year-old woman who had been taking D-phenylpropanolamine [sic.] 85 mg daily for some months, experienced severe hypertension when she also took *indometacin* 25 mg. It was considered that the inhibition of prostaglandin synthesis by indometacin might have caused enhancement of the sympathomimetic effect of phenylpropanolamine.[1]

1. Lee KY, *et al.* Severe hypertension after ingestion of an appetite suppressant (phenylpropanolamine) with indomethacin. *Lancet* 1979; **i:** 1110–11.

Pharmacokinetics

Phenylpropanolamine is readily and completely absorbed from the gastrointestinal tract, peak plasma concentrations being achieved about 1 or 2 hours after oral administration. It undergoes some metabolism in the liver, to an active hydroxylated metabolite, but up to 80 to 90% of a dose is excreted unchanged in the urine within 24 hours. The half-life has been reported to be about 3 to 5 hours.

◊ References.

1. Scherzinger SS, *et al.* Steady state pharmacokinetics and dose-proportionality of phenylpropanolamine in healthy subjects. *J Clin Pharmacol* 1990; **30:** 372–7.
2. Simons FER, *et al.* Pharmacokinetics of the orally administered decongestants pseudoephedrine and phenylpropanolamine in children. *J Pediatr* 1996; **129:** 729–34.

Uses and Administration

Phenylpropanolamine is a largely indirect-acting sympathomimetic (see Adrenaline, p.831) with an action similar to that of ephedrine (p.1090) but less active as a CNS stimulant.

Phenylpropanolamine is given by mouth as the hydrochloride for the symptomatic treatment of nasal congestion (p.1082). It is frequently used in combination preparations for the relief of cough and cold symptoms.

In the management of nasal congestion, phenylpropanolamine hydrochloride is given in usual doses of up to 25 mg three or four times daily by mouth; a maximum dose of 150 mg daily is permitted in the USA, but in the UK the Committee on Safety of Medicines recommends that a dose of 100 mg daily should not be exceeded. Modified-release preparations are also available.

Other uses of phenylpropanolamine include the control of urinary incontinence in some patients (see p.459). It has also been given in the management of some forms of priapism (p.927). Phenylpropanolamine has been used to suppress appetite in the management of obesity (p.1505) but the use of stimulants is no longer recommended.

Phenylpropanolamine polistirex (a phenylpropanolamine and sulfonated diethenylbenzene-ethenylbenzene copolymer complex) is also used, as are phenylpropanolamine bitartrate and phenylpropanolamine sulfate.

Preparations

USP 25: Chlorpheniramine Maleate and Phenylpropanolamine Hydrochloride Extended-release Capsules; Chlorpheniramine Maleate and Phenylpropanolamine Hydrochloride Extended-release Tablets; Phenylpropanolamine Hydrochloride Capsules; Phenylpropanolamine Hydrochloride Extended-release Capsules; Phenylpropanolamine Hydrochloride Extended-release Tablets; Phenylpropanolamine Hydrochloride Oral Solution; Phenylpropanolamine Hydrochloride Tablets.

Proprietary Preparations (details are given in Part 3)
Aust.: Kontexin†; *Fin.:* Rinexin; *Ger.:* Fasupond; Recatol mono; *Hong Kong:* Slimomin; *Irl.:* Procol†; *Norw.:* Monydrin†; Rinexin; *S.Afr.:* Restaslim; *Swed.:* Monydrin†; Rinexin; *Switz.:* Capton Diet; Dexatrim†; Kontexin; Merex; *Thai.:* Centapp; Fansia; *UK:* Procol†; *USA:* Acutrim†; Appedrine†; Control†; Dexatrim†; Just One Per Day†; Phenoxine†; Phenyldrine†; Propagest†; Spray-U-Thin†; Stay Trim†; Unitrol†.

Multi-ingredient: numerous preparations are listed in Part 3.

Pholcodine (5602-e)

Pholcodine (BAN, rINN).

Folcodina; Pholcodinum. 3-O-(2-Morpholinoethyl)morphine monohydrate.

$C_{23}H_{30}N_2O_4,H_2O = 416.5$.

CAS — 509-67-1 (anhydrous pholcodine).

ATC — R05DA08.

Pharmacopoeias. In Eur. (see p.vi).

Pharmacopoeial description

Ph. Eur.: A white or almost white crystalline powder or colourless crystals. Sparingly soluble in water; freely soluble in alcohol and in acetone; slightly soluble in ether; dissolves in dilute mineral acids.

Adverse Effects and Precautions

As for Dextromethorphan, p.1087. Constipation or drowsiness have been reported occasionally.

Interactions

Use of pholcodine with alcohol or other CNS depressants may increase the effects on the CNS.

Uses and Administration

Pholcodine is a centrally acting cough suppressant that has actions and uses similar to those of dextromethorphan (p.1088). It is given by mouth in a usual dose of 5 or 10 mg three or four times daily; children over 5 years of age may be given 2.5 to 5 mg three or four times daily and children 1 to 5 years, 2 to 2.5 mg three times daily. The citrate has also been used. Pholcodine polistirex (a pholcodine and sulfonated diethenylbenzene-ethenylbenzene copolymer complex) is used in modified-release preparations.

Preparations

BP 2001: Pholcodine Linctus; Strong Pholcodine Linctus.

Proprietary Preparations (details are given in Part 3)
Austral.: Actuss; Duro-Tuss; Logicin Cough Suppressant; Ordov Dry Tickly Cough; Pholtrate; Tussinol; *Belg.:* Bromofotyl†; *Fin.:* Tuxi; *Fr.:* Codotussyl Toux Seche; Humex; Respilene; Sirop Des Vosges; *Hong Kong:* Duro-Tuss; Uni-Pholco; *Irl.:* Expulin Dry Cough; *Norw.:* Tuxi; *NZ:* Duro-Tuss; Pharmacycare Cough; *S.Afr.:* Pholcolinct; *Singapore:* Duro-Tuss; *UK:* Benylin Childrens Dry Coughs; Evaphol; Expulin Dry Cough; Famel Linctus†; Galenphol; Hill's Balsam Dry Cough; Pavacol-D; Pholcomed†; Tixylix Daytime.

Multi-ingredient: *Austral.:* Difflam Anti-Inflammatory Lozenges with Cough Suppressant; Duro-Tuss Cough Lozenges; Duro-Tuss Decongestant; Duro-Tuss Expectorant; Phensedyl; Tixylix Nightime; *Belg.:* Broncal; Bronchalene; Broncho-pectoralis; Eucalyptine Pholcodine Le Brun; Folcodex; Folex; Pholco-Mereprine; *Fr.:* Biocalyptol; Broncalene; Broncorinol toux seches; Clarix; Denoral; Dimetane; Eucalyptine Pholcodine; Hexapneumine; Isomyrtine; Lyptocodine†; Pholcodyl; Pholcones†; Polery; Pulmosodyl; Quintopan Enfant†; Trophires; *Hong Kong:* Biocalyptol; Denoral; Duro-Tuss Decongestant; Duro-Tuss Expectorant; Hexapneumine; Tixylix Nightime; Tripe P; *Irl.:* Expulin; Expulin Childrens Cough; Tixylix†; *Norw.:* Tuxidrin; *NZ:* Difflam Anti-inflammatory Cough Lozenges; Duro-Tuss Expectorant; Duro-Tuss Lozenges; Phensedyl Dry Family Cough; Tixylix; *S.Afr.:* Bronchistop†; Contra-Coff†; Docsed; Folcofen; Pholtex; Procof; Respinol Compound; Tixylix; *Singapore:* Delix; Duro-Tuss Decongestant; Duro-Tuss Expectorant; Tixylix; *Spain:* Caltoson Balsamico; Trophires; *Switz.:* Pecto-Baby; Phol-Tussil; Phol-Tux; Rectoseptal-Neo Pholcodine; Tussiplex; *UK:* Cold Relief Daytime; Cold Relief Night-Time; Day Cold Comfort; Expulin; Expulin Childrens Cough; Night Cold Comfort; Phensedyl Plus; Tixylix Cough & Cold; Tixylix Night-Time.

Pipazetate Hydrochloride (5629-f)

Pipazetate Hydrochloride (BANM, rINNM).

D-254 (pipazetate); Pipazetate Hydrochloride; Piperestazine Hydrochloride; SKF-70230-A (pipazetate); SQ-15874 (pipazetate). 2-(2-Piperidinoethoxy)ethyl pyrido[3,2-b][1,4]benzothiazine-10-carboxylate hydrochloride.

$C_{21}H_{25}N_3O_3S,HCl = 436.0$.

CAS — 2167-85-3 (pipazetate); 6056-11-7 (pipazetate hydrochloride).

NOTE. Pipazetate is USAN.

Profile

Pipazetate hydrochloride is a centrally acting cough suppressant which also has some peripheral actions in non-productive cough (p.1082). It has been given by mouth, in usual doses of 20 to 40 mg three times daily, and rectally.

Overdosage. A healthy 4-year-old child became somnolent and agitated, with convulsions, followed by coma, after swallowing an unknown number of tablets containing pipazetate; cardiac arrhythmias also developed.[1] Fatal toxicity has also been reported in children.[2,3]

1. da Silva OA, Lopez M. Pipazetate—acute childhood poisoning. Clin Toxicol 1977; 11: 455–8.

2. Bonavita V, et al. Accidental lethal pipazetate poisoning in a child. Z Rechtsmed 1982; 89: 145–8.

3. Soto E, et al. Pipazetate lethality in a baby. Vet Hum Toxicol 1993; 35: 41.

Preparations

Proprietary Preparations (details are given in Part 3)
Aust.: Selvigon; *Braz.:* Selvigon; *Ger.:* Selvigon Hustensaft; *Ital.:* Selvigon; *Mex.:* Selvigon; *Thai.:* Transpulmin.

Poppy Capsule (6260-y)

Dormideiras; Fruit du Pavot; Fruto de Adormidera; Mohnfrucht; Papaveris Capsula; Poppy Heads.

Pharmacopoeias. In Chin.

The dried fruits of *Papaver somniferum* (Papaveraceae), collected before dehiscence has occurred, containing very small amounts of morphine with traces of other opium alkaloids.

Profile

Poppy capsule is mildly sedative and has been used as a liquid extract or syrup in cough mixtures.

Preparations

Proprietary Preparations (details are given in Part 3)
Multi-ingredient: *Belg.:* Tisane Pectorale; Tisane pour Dormir; *Braz.:* Malvodon; Pectoss; *Fr.:* Mediflor Tisane Pectorale d'Alsace.

Prednazoline (15332-r)

Prednazoline (rINN).

Prednisolone-Fenoxazoline Compound. 11β,17α,21-Trihydroxypregna-1,4-diene-3,20-dione 21-(dihydrogen phosphate) compound with 2-(2-isopropylphenoxymethyl)-2-imidazoline.

$C_{21}H_{29}O_8P,C_{13}H_{18}N_2O = 658.7$.

CAS — 6693-90-9.

Profile

Prednazoline has the general properties of prednisolone (p.1077) and of fenoxazoline (p.1091) and has been used locally in the form of a nasal spray in the treatment of pharyngitis, rhinitis, and sinusitis.

Preparations

Proprietary Preparations (details are given in Part 3)
Braz.: Oto-Rinil.

Prenoxdiazine Hydrochloride (5631-c)

Prenoxdiazine Hydrochloride (rINNM).

HK-256; Prenoxdiazin Hydrochloride. 3-(2,2-Diphenylethyl)-5-(2-piperidinoethyl)-1,2,4-oxadiazole hydrochloride.

$C_{23}H_{27}N_3O,HCl = 397.9$.

CAS — 47543-65-7 (prenoxdiazine); 37671-82-2 (prenoxdiazine hibenzate); 982-43-4 (prenoxdiazine hydrochloride).

Profile

Prenoxdiazine hydrochloride is used as a peripherally acting cough suppressant for non-productive cough (p.1082). It has been given by mouth in doses of 100 to 200 mg three or four times daily. Prenoxdiazine hibenzate is also used.

Preparations

Proprietary Preparations (details are given in Part 3)
Switz.: Libexine; Mephatussine; Mephaxine†.

Multi-ingredient: *Ital.:* Broncofluid; Libexin Mucolitico; *Switz.:* Libexine Compositum; Mephatussine Compositum; Mephaxine Compositum†.

Pseudoephedrine (9514-x)

Pseudoephedrine (BAN, rINN).

d-Ψ-Ephedrine; d-Isoephedrine. (+)-(1S,2S)-2-Methylamino-1-phenylpropan-1-ol.

$C_{10}H_{15}NO = 165.2$.

CAS — 90-82-4.

ATC — R01BA02.

An alkaloid obtained from *Ephedra* spp.

Pseudoephedrine Hydrochloride (2098-w)

Pseudoephedrine Hydrochloride (BANM, USAN, rINNM).

$C_{10}H_{15}NO,HCl = 201.7$.

CAS — 345-78-8.

Pharmacopoeias. In Eur. (see p.vi) and US.

Pharmacopoeial description

Ph. Eur.: A white, crystalline powder or colourless crystals. Freely soluble in water and in alcohol; sparingly soluble in dichloromethane. Protect from light.

USP 25: A fine, white to off-white crystalline powder, having a faint characteristic odour. Soluble 1 in 0.5 of water, 1 in 3.6 of alcohol, 1 in 91 of chloroform, and 1 in 7000 of ether. pH of a 5% solution in water is between 4.6 and 6.0. Store in airtight containers. Protect from light.

Pseudoephedrine Sulfate (2099-e)

Pseudoephedrine Sulfate (USAN, rINNM).

Pseudoephedrine Sulphate (BANM); Sch-4855.

$(C_{10}H_{15}NO)_2,H_2SO_4 = 428.5$.

CAS — 7460-12-0.

Pharmacopoeias. In US.

Pharmacopoeial description

USP 25: Odourless, white crystals or crystalline powder. Freely soluble in alcohol. pH of a 5% solution in water is between 5.0 and 6.5. Store in airtight containers. Protect from light.

Adverse Effects and Precautions

As for Ephedrine, p.1090. The commonest adverse effects of pseudoephedrine include tachycardia, anxiety, restlessness, and insomnia; skin rashes and urinary retention have occasionally occurred. Hallucinations have been reported rarely, particularly in children.

◊ In 34 healthy males given pseudoephedrine 120 or 150 mg, as a modified-release preparation, twice daily for 7 days mean plasma concentrations were about 450 and 510 nanograms per mL respectively. Side-effects (dry mouth, anorexia, insomnia, anxiety, tension, restlessness, tachycardia, palpitations) were common; there was some evidence of tachyphylaxis.[1]

1. Dickerson J, et al. Dose tolerance and pharmacokinetic studies of L(+) pseudoephedrine capsules in man. Eur J Clin Pharmacol 1978; 14: 253–9.

Abuse. Acute psychosis and visual and tactile hallucinations have been reported[1] in an 18-year-old male following intravenous misuse of pseudoephedrine hydrochloride.

For reference to toxic effects following long-term use of over-the-counter preparations containing sympathomimetics, including pseudoephedrine, see under Ephedrine, p.1090.

1. Sullivan G. Acute psychosis following intravenous abuse of pseudoephedrine: a case report. J Psychopharmacol 1996; 10: 324–5.

Effects on the gastrointestinal tract. Ischaemic colitis has been reported[1,2] after acute or chronic use of pseudoephedrine in combination cold and allergy preparations.

1. Dowd J, et al. Ischemic colitis associated with pseudoephedrine: four cases. Am J Gastroenterol 1999; 94: 2430–4.

2. Lichtenstein GR, Yee NS. Ischemic colitis associated with decongestant use. Ann Intern Med 2000; 132: 682.

Effects on mental function. Reports[1-5] of adverse mental effects (particularly in children) associated with combination preparations containing pseudoephedrine. See also under Abuse, above.

1. Leighton KM. Paranoid psychosis after abuse of Actifed. BMJ 1982; 284: 789–90.

2. Sankey RJ, et al. Visual hallucinations in children receiving decongestants. BMJ 1984; 288: 1369.

3. Stokes MA. Visual hallucinations in children receiving decongestants. BMJ 1984; 288: 1540.

4. Roberge RJ, et al. Dextromethorphan and pseudoephedrine-induced agitated psychosis and ataxia: case report. J Emerg Med 1999; 17: 285–8.

5. Soutullo CA, et al. Psychosis associated with pseudoephedrine and dextromethorphan. J Am Acad Child Adolesc Psychiatry 1999; 38: 1471–2.

Effects on the skin. Recurrent pseudo-scarlatina has been described in a female patient and attributed, on some occasions at least, to ingestion of pseudoephedrine.[1] Further fixed drug eruptions associated with pseudoephedrine have been reported.[2-4] In one woman, an erythematous macular rash developed 5½ hours after a challenge dose of pseudoephedrine 60 mg by mouth; other symptoms, which mimicked the effects of toxic shock syndrome, included nausea and vomiting, fever, orthostatic hypotension, light-headedness, fatigue, and desquamation of the skin on her palms and soles.[3] However, considering the frequent use of pseudoephedrine in over-the-counter medications, associated drug eruptions generally appear to be rare.[2]

1. Taylor BJ, Duffill MB. Br J Dermatol 1988; 118: 827–9.

2. Camisa C. Fixed drug reactions to pseudoephedrine hydrochloride. Br J Dermatol 1989; 120: 857–8.

3. Cavanah DK, Ballas ZK. Pseudoephedrine reaction presenting as recurrent toxic shock syndrome. Ann Intern Med 1993; 119: 302–3.

4. Hauken M. Fixed drug eruption and pseudoephedrine. Ann Intern Med 1994; 120: 442.

Epileptogenic effect. A report of a child who suffered a generalised seizure after ingesting a large quantity of pseudoephedrine hydrochloride tablets was believed to be the first report of convulsions associated with overdose of a preparation containing the drug as a single ingredient.[1]

1. Clark RF, Curry SC. Pseudoephedrine dangers. Pediatrics 1990; 85: 389–90.

Interactions

As for Ephedrine, p.1090. Pseudoephedrine may cause a hypertensive crisis in patients receiving an MAOI (including an RIMA). For additional warnings see under phenelzine (p.305) and moclobemide (p.299).

The symbol † denotes a preparation no longer actively marketed

Antacids. The absorption rate of pseudoephedrine hydrochloride was increased by the concomitant administration of aluminium hydroxide mixture but was decreased by the administration of kaolin; in the latter case adsorption may have competed with absorption.[1]

1. Lucarotti RL, *et al.* Enhanced pseudoephedrine absorption by concurrent administration of aluminium hydroxide gel in humans. *J Pharm Sci* 1972; **61**: 903–5.

Vaccines. A 21-year-old mildly obese man taking pseudoephedrine in an over-the-counter formulation for weight loss collapsed and died with a core temperature of 42.2° while exercising, shortly after inoculation with *Japanese encephalitis vaccine* and *typhoid vaccine*.[1] The combined effects of the pseudoephedrine, activity, and the pyrogenic action of the vaccines appeared to have contributed to failure of the thermoregulatory system.

1. Franklin QJ. Sudden death after typhoid and Japanese encephalitis vaccination in a young male taking pseudoephedrine. *Milit Med* 1999; **164**: 157–9.

Pharmacokinetics

Pseudoephedrine is readily absorbed from the gastrointestinal tract. It is largely excreted unchanged in the urine together with small amounts of its hepatic metabolite. It has a half-life of about 5 to 8 hours; elimination is enhanced and half-life accordingly shorter in acid urine. Small amounts are distributed into breast milk.

◊ References.

1. Kuntzman RG, *et al.* The influence of urinary pH on the plasma half-life of pseudoephedrine in man and dog and a sensitive assay for its determination in human plasma. *Clin Pharmacol Ther* 1971; **12**: 62–7.
2. Lai CM, *et al.* Urinary excretion of chlorpheniramine and pseudoephedrine in humans. *J Pharm Sci* 1979; **68**: 1243–6.
3. Yacobi A, *et al.* Evaluation of sustained-action chlorpheniramine-pseudoephedrine dosage form in humans. *J Pharm Sci* 1980; **69**: 1077–81.
4. Simons FER, *et al.* Pharmacokinetics of the orally administered decongestants pseudoephedrine and phenylpropanolamine in children. *J Pediatr* 1996; **129**: 729–34.

Breast feeding. A study of concentrations of pseudoephedrine and triprolidine in plasma and breast milk of 3 lactating mothers for up to 48 hours after ingestion of a preparation containing pseudoephedrine hydrochloride 60 mg with triprolidine hydrochloride 2.5 mg. Concentrations of pseudoephedrine in milk were consistently higher than in plasma; the half-life in both fluids was between 4.2 and 7.0 hours. Assuming a generous milk secretion of 500 mL over 12 hours it was calculated that the excreted dose was the equivalent of 250 to 330 μg of pseudoephedrine base, or 0.5 to 0.7% of the dose ingested by the mothers. Triprolidine did not appear to be concentrated in breast milk. The amounts of pseudoephedrine and triprolidine distributed into breast milk were probably not high enough to warrant cessation of breast feeding.[1]

1. Findlay JWA, *et al.* Pseudoephedrine and triprolidine in plasma and breast milk of nursing mothers. *Br J Clin Pharmacol* 1984; **18**: 901–6.

Uses and Administration

Pseudoephedrine is a direct- and indirect-acting sympathomimetic (see Adrenaline, p.831). It is a stereoisomer of ephedrine (p.1090) and has a similar action, but has been stated to have less pressor activity and fewer CNS effects.

Pseudoephedrine and its salts are given by mouth for the symptomatic relief of nasal congestion (p.1082). They are commonly combined with other ingredients in preparations intended for the relief of cough and cold symptoms.

Pseudoephedrine hydrochloride or sulfate are generally given in doses of 60 mg three to four times daily by mouth. Suggested oral doses for children are: 2 to 5 years, 15 mg three or four times daily; 6 to 12 years, 30 mg three or four times daily. Modified-release preparations are also available; a usual adult dose is 120 mg every 12 hours.

Other uses of pseudoephedrine include the control of urinary incontinence (p.459) in some patients. It has also been given in the management of some forms of priapism (p.927).

Pseudoephedrine polistirex (a pseudoephedrine and sulfonated diethenylbenzene-ethenylbenzene copolymer complex) has also been used, as has pseudoephedrine tannate.

Barotrauma. Results from a controlled trial[1] suggest that pseudoephedrine administered to adults at least 30 minutes before flying appears to decrease the incidence of ear pain associated with pressure changes.[1] However, a similar decrease in risk was not noted in children.[2]

1. Jones JS, *et al.* A double-blind comparison between oral pseudoephedrine and topical oxymetazoline in the prevention of barotrauma during air travel. *Am J Emerg Med* 1998; **16**: 262–4.
2. Buchanan BJ, *et al.* Pseudoephedrine and air travel-associated ear pain in children. *Arch Pediatr Adolesc Med* 1999; **153**: 466–8.

Preparations

BP 2001: Pseudoephedrine Tablets;
USP 25: Acetaminophen and Pseudoephedrine Hydrochloride Tablets; Acetaminophen, Dextromethorphan Hydrobromide, Doxylamine Succinate, and Pseudoephedrine Hydrochloride Oral Solution; Acetaminophen, Diphenhydramine Hydrochloride, and Pseudoephedrine Hydrochloride Tablets; Chlorpheniramine Maleate and Pseudoephedrine Hydrochloride Extended-release Capsules; Chlorpheniramine Maleate and Pseudoephedrine Hydrochloride Oral Solution; Dexbrompheniramine Maleate and Pseudoephedrine Sulfate Oral Solution; Diphenhydramine and Pseudoephedrine Capsules; Guaifenesin and Pseudoephedrine Hydrochloride Capsules; Guaifenesin, Pseudoephedrine Hydrochloride, and Dextromethorphan Hydrobromide Capsules; Ibuprofen and Pseudoephedrine Hydrochloride Tablets; Pseudoephedrine Hydrochloride Extended-release Tablets; Pseudoephedrine Hydrochloride Syrup; Pseudoephedrine Hydrochloride Tablets; Pseudoephedrine Hydrochloride, Carbinoxamine Maleate, and Dextromethorphan Hydrobromide Oral Solution; Triprolidine and Pseudoephedrine Hydrochlorides Syrup; Triprolidine and Pseudoephedrine Hydrochlorides Tablets.

Proprietary Preparations (details are given in Part 3)
Austral.: Bisolvon Sinus; Demazin Sinus; Dimetapp Sinus; Logicin Sinus; Orthoxicol Infant†; Sinutab Sinus Relief†; Sudafed Sinus & Nasal Decongestant; Tixylix Daytime†; *Belg.:* Nasa-12; Vasocedine Pseudoefedrine; *Canad.:* Balminil Decongestant; Congest Aid; Congest-Eze; Contac Cold Nondrowsy; Decongestant Tablets; Drixoral ND; Eltor; Maxenal; Nasal & Sinus Relief; Plus Sinus; Pseudofrin; Robidrine; Sudafed Decongestant; Sudodrin†; Tantafed; Triaminic Pediatric Drops; *Fr.:* Drill rhinites; Ephedroides; Rhinalair†; Sudafed; *Hong Kong:* Balminil Decongestant; Sudafed; *Irl.:* Galpseud†; Sudafed†; *Israel:* Otrinol; Sinufed; Tarophed; *Ital.:* Narixan; Sudafed†; *Mex.:* Dofedrin; Dofen; Sudafed; *NZ:* Sudafed 12 Hour Relief; Sudafed for Children; Sudafed Sinus & Nasal Decongestant; Sudomyl; *Port.:* Sudafed; *S.Afr.:* Acunaso; Demazin Decongestant; Drilix; Drixora; Monofed; Sinumed; Sudafed; Symptofed; *Singapore:* Sudafed; *Switz.:* Otrinol; *Thai.:* Pseudno; Sudosian; *UAE:* Sedofan II; *UK:* Bronalin Decongestant; Contac; Decongestant Tablets; Galpseud; Sudafed; *USA:* Afrin; Allermed; Cenafed; Childrens Sudafed Nasal Decongestant; Congestion Relief†; Decofed; Decorin†; DeFed; Dimetapp Decongestant; Dorcol Children's Decongestant; Drixoral Non-Drowsy Formula; Dynafed Pseudo†; Efidac; Genaphed; Halofed; Kid Kare Pediatric Nasal Decongestant; Mini Pseudo; Myfedrine†; PediaCare Infant's Decongestant; Pseudo; Pseudo-Gest; Seudotabs; Silfedrine; Sinustop Pro; Sudafed; Sudex†; Triaminic AM Decongestant Formula; Triaminic Infant Oral Decongestant.

Multi-ingredient: numerous preparations are listed in Part 3.

Senega Root   (2025-c)

Polígala Raíz; Polygalae Radix; Rattlesnake Root; Seneca Snakeroot; Senega.

CAS — 1260-04-4 (polygalic acid).
ATC — R05CA06.

Pharmacopoeias. In *Eur.* (see p.vi) and *Jpn.*
Jpn also describes Powdered Senega Root.

Pharmacopoeial description
Ph. Eur.: The dried and usually fragmented root and root crown of *Polygala senega* or certain closely related species of *Polygala* or a mixture of these. It has a faint, sweet odour, slightly rancid or reminiscent of methyl salicylate. Protect from light and humidity.

Profile
Senega root has been used as an expectorant in preparations given by mouth for respiratory-tract disorders.

Polygala amara is a related species that is used similarly.

Preparations

Proprietary Preparations (details are given in Part 3)
Multi-ingredient: *Aust.:* Anitos; Bronchiplant; Bronchiplant light; Tussimont; *Austral.:* Asa Tones; Nyal Bronchitis; Senagar; Senega and Ammonia; *Belg.:* Tux; *Braz.:* Broncmel; Expectomel; Limao Bravo; Mel Jatahy; Melagriao; Pectal; *Canad.:* Bronchial; Bronchozone†; Sirop Cocillana Codeine; Wampole Bronchial Cough Syrup; *Fr.:* Broncorinol toux seches; Desbly; Neo-Codion; Sirop Pectoral adulte†; *Ger.:* Asthma 6-N; *Hong Kong:* Cocillana Compound; Pectoral; *Port.:* Calmarum; Fluidin Antiasmatico; Fluidin Infantil; Stodal; *Spain:* Broncovital; Combitorax†; Pastillas Pectoral Kely; Pulmofasa; Pulmofasa Antihist; *Swed.:* Cocillana-Etyfin; Senega†; *Switz.:* Bronchocodin†; Bronchofluid†; Expectoran Codein; Foral; Hederix; Liberol Pastilles contre la toux; Liberol Sirop contre la toux; Makatussin; Makatussin forte; Pastilles pectorales formule 541; Patussol†; Pectocalmine; Pectoral N; Phol-Tux; Sirop antitussif Wyss a base de codeine†; Sirop Wyss contre la toux†; *UK:* Antibron; Chest Mixture; ES Bronchial Mixture.

Sobrerol   (13239-p)

Cyclidrol; Sobrerolo. *p*-Menth-6-ene-2,8-diol.
$C_{10}H_{18}O_2 = 170.2$.
CAS — 498-71-5.
ATC — R05CB07.
Pharmacopoeias. In *It.*

Profile
Sobrerol is a mucolytic that has been used in respiratory disorders characterised by productive cough (p.1082). Doses of up to 800 mg have been given by mouth daily in divided doses. Sobrerol has also been given by injection, inhalation, or rectally.

Pharmacokinetics. The pharmacokinetics of sobrerol after oral or intravenous administration has been studied in patients with acute exacerbations of chronic bronchitis.[1] Sobrerol was rapidly absorbed from the gastrointestinal tract and rapidly distributed. Following intravenous and oral administration, 13% and 23% of the dose respectively was excreted in the urine as unchanged drug, glucuronidated sobrerol, and hydrated carvone. Sobrerol was shown to accumulate in bronchial mucus.

1. Braga PC, *et al.* Pharmacokinetics of sobrerol in chronic bronchitis: comparison of serum and bronchial mucus levels. *Eur J Clin Pharmacol* 1983; **24**: 209–15.

Respiratory disorders. References.

1. Bellussi L, *et al.* Evaluation of the efficacy and safety of sobrerol granules in patients suffering from chronic rhinosinusitis. *J Int Med Res* 1990; **18**: 454–9.
2. Azzollini E, *et al.* Sobrerol (Sobrepim®) administered dropwise to children with acute hypersecretory bronchopulmonary disease: a controlled trial v bromhexine. *Clin Trials J* 1990; **27**: 241–9.

Preparations

Proprietary Preparations (details are given in Part 3)
Braz.: Sobrepim; *Hong Kong:* Mucoflux; *Ital.:* Sobrepin; Sopulmin; *Port.:* Broncopulmo; Bronqual; Mucolavi†; *Singapore:* Mucoflux; *Spain:* Sobrepin; *Thai.:* Mucoflux.

Multi-ingredient: *Ital.:* Fluental; *Port.:* Niflux.

Sodium Dibunate   (5632-k)

Sodium Dibunate (BAN, rINN).

L-1633. Sodium 2,6-di-*tert*-butylnaphthalene-1-sulphonate.
$C_{18}H_{23}NaO_3S = 342.4$.
CAS — 14992-59-7 (sodium dibunate).

Profile
Sodium dibunate is a cough suppressant used in non-productive cough (p.1082). It is claimed to have central and peripheral actions and has been given by mouth in usual doses of 30 mg three to four times daily. Chlorcyclizine dibunate (naftoclizine) has also been administered by mouth or rectally.

Preparations

Proprietary Preparations (details are given in Part 3)
Port.: Becantex; *Thai.:* Becantex.

Multi-ingredient: *Belg.:* Becantex; *Braz.:* Becantosse; Beclase; Cessatosse; Coquevit; Glotil; Gotas Nican; Ipecol; Naquinto; Natoss; Pectal; Pinosil; Plactosse; Pulmoverina; Tossefedrin; Tossefin; Tussodina; *Canad.:* Balminil Suppositories; *Ger.:* Cito-Guakalin; Ephepect-Blocker-Pastillen N; *Ital.:* Sedobex†; *Thai.:* Coughmin.

Squill   (2026-k)

Bulbo de Escila; Cebolla Albarrana; Cila; Meerzwiebel; Scilla; Scillae Bulbus; Scille; White Squill.
Pharmacopoeias. In *Br.* and *Ger.*

Pharmacopoeial description
BP 2001: The dried sliced bulb of *Drimia maritima* with the membranous outer scales removed, and containing not less than 68% of alcohol (60%)-soluble extractive. Store at a temperature not exceeding 25° in a dry place.

Indian Squill   (2027-a)

Urginea.
Pharmacopoeias. In *Br.*

Pharmacopoeial description
BP 2001: The bulb of *Drimia indica*, with the outer membranous scales removed, usually sliced and dried. Store at a temperature not exceeding 25° in a dry place.

Adverse Effects, Treatment, and Precautions
The adverse effects of squill and Indian squill in large doses include nausea, vomiting, and diarrhoea. As squill and Indian squill contain cardiac glycosides they can cause similar adverse effects to digoxin (p.870).

Abuse. Reports of cardiac glycoside toxicity and myopathy associated with the abuse of linctuses which have contained opiates and squill.[1-5]

1. Kennedy M. Cardiac glycoside toxicity: an unusual manifestation of drug addiction. *Med J Aust* 1981; **2**: 686–9.
2. Kilpatrick C, *et al.* Myopathy with myasthenic features possibly induced by codeine linctus. *Med J Aust* 1982; **2**: 410.
3. Seow SSW. Abuse of APF linctus codeine and cardiac glycoside toxicity. *Med J Aust* 1984; **140**: 54.

4. Thurston D, Taylor K. Gee's Linctus. *Pharm J* 1984; **233**: 63.
5. Smith W, *et al.* Wenckebach's phenomenon induced by cough linctus. *BMJ* 1986; **292**: 868.

Uses and Administration

Squill and Indian squill are used as expectorants in productive cough (p.1082) and have been given in doses of 30 to 250 mg, as the oxymel, elixir, tincture, or vinegar. Preparations containing squill are used in some countries in the treatment of cardiovascular disorders.

Red squill has been used as a rodenticide (p.1437).

◊ A history[1] of the use of squill.

1. Court WE. Squill – energetic diuretic. *Pharm J* 1985; **235**: 194–7.

Preparations

BP 2001: Squill Liquid Extract; Squill Oxymel.

Proprietary Preparations (details are given in Part 3)
Ger.: Digitalysat Scilla-Digitaloid; Scillase N.

Multi-ingredient: *Austral.:* Nyal Bronchitis; ***Canad.:*** Bronco Asmol; Sirop Cocillana Codeine; ***Ger.:*** Cefascillan; Cor-loges; Cor-Vel N†; Hevert-Entwaeserungs-Tee†; Miroton; Miroton N; Nephrisan P; Raufuncton N; Szillosan forte†; Venopyronum N triplex†; ***Hong Kong:*** Cocillana Compound; ***Irl.:*** Ipesil; ***S.Afr.:*** Cocillana Co; Contra-Coff†; Linctus Tussi Infans; Tusselix†; ***UK:*** Allens Chesty Cough; Balm of Gilead; Bronchial Mixture; Buttercup Syrup; Catarrh Pastilles; Catarrh Tablets; Chest Mixture; Collins Elixir Pastilles†; Covonia Mentholated; ES Bronchial Mixture; Galloway's Cough Syrup; Honey & Molasses; Lobelia Compound; Modern Herbals Cough Mixture; Potters Children's Cough Pastilles; Sanderson's Throat Specific.

Stepronin (980-x)

Stepronin (*rINN*).

2-(α-Thenoylthio)-propionylglycine; Tiofacic. *N*-(2-Mercaptopropionyl)glycine 2-thiophenecarboxylate.

$C_{16}H_{11}NO_4S_2 = 273.3$.
CAS — 72324-18-6 (stepronin); 78126-10-0 (stepronin sodium).
ATC — R05CB11.

Profile

Stepronin has been reported to have mucolytic actions in productive cough (p.1082), and has also been used in the treatment of liver disorders. It is reported to be metabolised to tiopronin (p.1025). Stepronin is mainly used as the sodium and lysinate salts.

Preparations

Proprietary Preparations (details are given in Part 3)
Ital.: Broncoplus†; Masor†; Mucodil†; Tiase†; Tioten†.

Sulfogaiacol (2022-y)

Sulfogaiacol (*rINN*).

Kalium Guajacolsulfonicum; Potassium Guaiacolsulfonate; Potassium Guaiacolsulphonate. Potassium hydroxymethoxybenzenesulphonate hemihydrate.

$C_7H_7KO_5S,\frac{1}{2}H_2O = 251.3$.
CAS — 1321-14-8 (anhydrous sulfogaiacol); 78247-49-1 (sulfogaiacol hemihydrate).
Pharmacopoeias. In *US.* Also in *Aust., Belg., Fr., Jpn, Neth.,* and *Pol.,* none of which specifies hemihydrate.

Pharmacopoeial description

USP 25: Protect from light.

Profile

Sulfogaiacol is used as an expectorant for productive cough (p.1082). Calcium guaiacolsulfonate has been used similarly.

Preparations

Proprietary Preparations (details are given in Part 3)
Aust.: Pectosorin; *Ital.:* Pulmovirolo†; Tioguaialina.

Multi-ingredient: numerous preparations are listed in Part 3.

Telmesteine (14665-e)

Telmesteine (*rINN*).

(–)-3-Ethyl hydrogen (*R*)-3,4-thiazolidinedicarboxylate.

$C_7H_{11}NO_4S = 205.2$.
CAS — 122946-43-4.

Profile

Telmesteine has been used as a mucolytic (p.1082) in the treatment of respiratory-tract disorders in doses of 300 mg two or three times daily.

Preparations

Proprietary Preparations (details are given in Part 3)
Ital.: Muconorm; Reolase.

Terpin Hydrate (2029-x)

Terpin Hydrate (*BANM*).

Terpene Hydrate; Terpinol. *p*-Menthane-1,8-diol monohydrate; 4-Hydroxy-α,α,4-trimethylcyclohexanemethanol monohydrate.

$C_{10}H_{20}O_2,H_2O = 190.3$.
CAS — 80-53-5 (anhydrous terpin); 2451-01-6 (terpin monohydrate).
Pharmacopoeias. In *Fr., Swiss,* and *US.*

Pharmacopoeial description

USP 25: Colourless lustrous crystals or white powder with a slight odour. It effloresces in dry air. Soluble 1 in 200 of water, 1 in 35 of boiling water, 1 in 13 of alcohol, 1 in 3 of boiling alcohol, and 1 in 140 of chloroform and of ether. A hot 1% solution is neutral to litmus. Store in airtight containers.

Stability. If crystals form in terpin hydrate elixir, they may be redissolved by warming the closed container of solution in warm water and then gently shaking it.

Profile

Terpin hydrate has been stated to increase bronchial secretion directly and has been used as an expectorant in productive cough (p.1082). It has been given by mouth in usual doses of 80 mg four to six times daily.

Nausea, vomiting, or abdominal pain may follow the ingestion of terpin hydrate on an empty stomach.

Terpin hydrochloride has also been used.

Preparations

USP 25: Terpin Hydrate and Codeine Elixir; Terpin Hydrate Elixir.

Proprietary Preparations (details are given in Part 3)
Fr.: Pectotussyl; Terpine des Monts-Dore.

Multi-ingredient: *Belg.:* Balsoclase; Tri-Cold†; ***Braz.:*** Cortagrip D; Pyocoline; ***Canad.:*** Pastilles Valda†; Valda; ***Fin.:*** Toclase Expectorant; ***Fr.:*** Bronchorectine au Citral; Bronpax†; Marrubene Codethyline†; Pulmofluide Simple; Pulmoll; Terpine Gonnon; Terpone; Tossarel†; ***Ger.:*** Ozothin; Sedotussin Expectorans†; ***Hong Kong:*** Bendracol; Codoplex; Panadol Cold and Flu; ***Irl.:*** Coldrex†; ***Ital.:*** Elisir Terpina; Neo Borocillina Balsamica; Tionamil; Tussiflex†; ***Neth.:*** Balsoclase Compositum; ***Port.:*** Codoforme; Fluidin Nocturno†; Recto Bronco Tosse†; ***S.Afr.:*** Dykatuss Expectorant†; Tusselix†; ***Spain:*** Pastillas Pectoral Kely; Terponil; ***Switz.:*** Bromocod N; Libexine Compositum; Mephatussine Compositum; Mephaxine Compositum†; Rectoseptal-Neo bismuthe; Rectoseptal-Neo Pholcodine; Rectoseptal-Neo simple; Sedotussin; Spedro†; ***Thai.:*** Antust; D-Coate; Dexpin; Dimophen; Med-Guaiphan; Mila-Tercon; Stocof; Terco-C; Terco-D; ***UK:*** Coldrex†; Original Cabdrivers Expectorant.

Tetryzoline Hydrochloride (2108-t)

Tetryzoline Hydrochloride (*BANM, rINNM*).

Tetrahydrozoline Hydrochloride. 2-(1,2,3,4-Tetrahydro-1-naphthyl)-2-imidazoline hydrochloride.

$C_{13}H_{16}N_2,HCl = 236.7$.
CAS — 84-22-0 (tetryzoline); 522-48-5 (tetryzoline hydrochloride).
Pharmacopoeias. In *US.*

Pharmacopoeial description

USP 25: A white odourless solid. Soluble 1 in 3.5 of water and 1 in 7.5 of alcohol; very slightly soluble in chloroform; practically insoluble in ether. Store in airtight containers.

Profile

Tetryzoline is a sympathomimetic with effects similar to those of naphazoline (p.1095). It is used as the hydrochloride for its vasoconstrictor effect in the symptomatic relief of nasal congestion (p.1082). A 0.1% solution is instilled into each nostril as nasal drops or a spray up to every 4 hours as necessary; it should not be used more often than every 3 hours. Children aged 2 to 6 years of age may be given 2 to 3 drops of a 0.05% solution in each nostril every 4 to 6 hours.

Solutions of tetryzoline hydrochloride containing 0.05% are used as a conjunctival decongestant (see Conjunctivitis, p.406).

Other salts of tetryzoline including the nitrate, phosphate, and sulfate have been used similarly.

Effects on the eyes. For mention of conjunctivitis induced by ophthalmic decongestant preparations containing tetryzoline, see under Phenylephrine, p.1097.

Preparations

USP 25: Tetrahydrozoline Hydrochloride Nasal Solution; Tetrahydrozoline Hydrochloride Ophthalmic Solution.

Proprietary Preparations (details are given in Part 3)
Austral.: Optazine Fresh; Visine; *Belg.:* Visine; *Canad.:* Eye Drops; RO-Eye Drops†; Visine; *Denm.:* Tyzine; *Fin.:* Oftan Starine; Visine†; *Fr.:* Constrilia; *Ger.:* Caltheon; Diabenyl T; Exrhinin; Ophtalmin N; Rhinopront; Tetrilin; Tyzine; Vasopos N; Vidiseptal EDO Sine†; Yxin; *Hong Kong:* Optizoline; *Israel:* Azoline; Stilla; V-Zoline; Visine; *Ital.:* Demetil; Octilia; Stilla Decongestionante; Vasorinil; Visine†; *Mex.:* Ischemol; *Neth.:* Visine†; *NZ:* Visine; *Port.:* Edolzine; Visine; *Singapore:* Octilia; Visine; *Spain:* Vispring; *Switz.:* Rhinopront Top; Tyzine†; Visine;

Thai.: Opsil-A; Visine; *USA:* Eye Drops; Eye-Zine; Eyesine; Geneye Extra; Mallazine; Optigene 3; Soothe†; Tetrasine; Tyzine; Visine Original.

Multi-ingredient: *Austral.:* In A Wink Allergy; Murine Sore Eyes; Visine Advanced Relief; Visine Allergy; Visine Revive; ***Braz.:*** Mirabel; Vislin; Visodin; ***Canad.:*** Collyrium†; Visine Allergy; Visine Moisturizing; ***Ger.:*** Allergopos N; Berberil N; Efemolin; Spersadexolin; Spersalleg; ***Hong Kong:*** Colircusi Gentadexa; Efemoline; Eye Mo 36; Spersadexoline; Spersalleg; ***Israel:*** Visine AC; ***Ital.:*** Biorinil; Cromozil; Dexoline; Efemoline; Eta Biocortilen VC; Flumetol; Ischemol A; Medramil†; Tetramil; Vasosterone; Vasosterone Antibiotico; Vasosterone Collirio; Visublefarite; Visucloben Decongestionante; Visumetazone Antibiotico; Visumetazone Decongestionante; Visumicina; Visustrin; ***Mex.:*** Visine Extra; ***Norw.:*** Spersalleg; ***NZ:*** Revive; ***Port.:*** Gentadexa; Medrivas Antibiotico; Medrivas†; ***S.Afr.:*** Efemoline; Gemini; Oculoforte; Spersadexoline; Spersalleg; ***Singapore:*** Efemoline; Spersadexoline; Spersalleg; Spersalleg; ***Switz.:*** Collypan; Efemoline; Oculosan forte; Spersadexoline; Spersalleg; ***Thai.:*** Antazallerge; Efemoline; Histaoph; Opsa-His; Spersadexoline; Spersalleg; ***USA:*** Advanced Relief Visine; Collyrium Fresh; Geneye AC Allergy†; Murine Plus; Tetrasine Extra; Visine Allergy Relief; Visine Moisturizing.

Thebacon Hydrochloride (6261-j)

Thebacon Hydrochloride (*BANM, rINNM*).

Acethydrocodone Hydrochloride; Acetyldihydrocodeinone Hydrochloride; Dihydrocodeinone Enol Acetate Hydrochloride. 6-*O*-Acetyl-7,8-dihydro-3-*O*-methyl-6,7-didehydromorphine hydrochloride; (–)-(5*R*)-4,5-Epoxy-3-methoxy-9α-methylmorphin-6-en-6-yl acetate hydrochloride.

$C_{20}H_{23}NO_4,HCl = 377.9$.
CAS — 466-90-0 (thebacon); 20236-82-2 (thebacon hydrochloride).

Profile

Thebacon hydrochloride is a centrally acting cough suppressant used for non-productive cough (p.1082). It has actions similar to those of codeine (p.25) but stated to be approximately 4 times more potent. It has been given by mouth in a usual daily dose of 10 mg in divided doses; the maximum daily dose should not exceed 20 mg.

Preparations

Proprietary Preparations (details are given in Part 3)
Belg.: Acedicone.

Tipepidine Hibenzate (13352-s)

Tipepidine Hibenzate (*rINNM*).

AT-327 (tipepidine); CR-662 (tipepidine); Tipepidine Hybenzate. 3-[Di(2-thienyl)methylene]-1-methylpiperidine 2-(4-hydroxybenzoyl)benzoate.

$C_{15}H_{17}NS_2,C_{14}H_{10}O_4 = 517.7$.
CAS — 5169-78-8 (tipepidine); 31139-87-4 (tipepidine hibenzate).
Pharmacopoeias. In *Jpn.*

Tipepidine hibenzate 11.1 mg is approximately equivalent to 10 mg of tipepidine citrate.

Profile

Tipepidine hibenzate is a cough suppressant used for non-productive cough (p.1082) which is claimed also to have an expectorant action. It has been given by mouth as the hibenzate but doses are expressed as the citrate; a usual dose is the equivalent of 20 to 40 mg of the citrate 3 times daily.

Epileptogenic effect. Report[1] of generalised convulsions associated with therapeutic oral doses of tipepidine hibenzate.

1. Cuomo RM. On the possible convulsive activity of an antitussive piperidinic derivative ('tipepidina ibenzato') in man. *Acta Neurol (Napoli)* 1982; **37**: 110–16.

Preparations

Proprietary Preparations (details are given in Part 3)
Jpn: Asverin; *Spain:* Asvelik†.

Tolu Balsam (287-f)

Balsamum Tolutanum; Baume de Tolu.
CAS — 9000-64-0; 8017-09-2.
Pharmacopoeias. In *Eur.* (see p.vi) and *US.*

A balsam obtained from *Myroxylon balsamum* (=*M. toluiferum*) (Leguminosae).

Pharmacopoeial description

Ph. Eur.: Oleoresin obtained from the trunk of *Myroxylon balsamum* and *M. balsamum* var. *pereirae*. It contains 25 to 50% of free or combined acids, expressed as cinnamic acid, calculated with reference to the dried drug. It occurs as a hard, friable, brownish to reddish-brown mass; thin fragments are brownish-yellow when examined against the light. It has an odour reminiscent of vanillin. Practically insoluble in water and in petroleum spirit; very soluble or freely soluble in alcohol. Do not store in powdered form.

USP 25: A balsam obtained from *Myroxylon balsamum* (Leguminosae). It is a brown or yellowish-brown plastic solid trans-

The symbol † denotes a preparation no longer actively marketed

parent in thin layers and brittle when old, dried, or exposed to cold temperatures. It has a pleasant aromatic odour, resembling that of vanilla. Practically insoluble in water and in petroleum spirit; soluble in alcohol, in chloroform, and in ether, sometimes with slight residue or turbidity. Store at a temperature not exceeding 40° in airtight containers.

Profile
Tolu balsam is considered to have very mild antiseptic properties and some expectorant action but is mainly used in the form of a syrup to flavour cough mixtures. However, Tolu Syrup (BP 2001) no longer contains tolu balsam but is based on cinnamic acid (p.1142).

Preparations
BPC 1954: Compound Iodoform Paint;
USP 25: Compound Benzoin Tincture.

Proprietary Preparations (details are given in Part 3)
Belg.: Bromofotyl†.

Multi-ingredient: *Austral.:* Camphor Linctus Compound; *Belg.:* Folcodex; Tux; *Braz.:* Broncofisin; Calmante Creosotado; Codelasa; Expectomel; Frenotosse; Frenotossil; Glycon; Inalobel; Iodetal; Mel Jatahy; Melagriao; Peitoral Angico Pelotense; Pulmoformil; Pulmonix; Yatropan; *Canad.:* Bronco Asmol; Rophelin; *Fr.:* Broncalene Nourisson; Bronpax†; Dinacode; Dinacode avec codeine; Gaiarsol; Hexapneumine; Pastilles Medicinales Vicks; Pastilles Monleon; Pates Pectorales†; Phytotux; Pulmonase†; Pulmosodyl; Sirop Pectoral adulte†; Sirop Pectoral enfant†; Terpine Gonnon†; Theralene Pectoral Nourrisson; Tussipax; *Hong Kong:* Baby Cough with Antihistamine; Hexapneumine; *Ital.:* Stenobronchial; *S.Afr.:* Stodal; Tussi Infans; Tusselix†; *Spain:* Bactopumon; Bronco Sergo; Broncomicin Bals†; Bronquidiazina CR; Maboterpen†; Mentobox†; Pastillas Antisep Garg M; Pectoral Brum†; Pulmofasa; Pulmofasa Antihist; Toscal Compuesto†; Toscal†; Tosdiazina; *Switz.:* Baume; Bronchocodin†; Cimex Sirop contre la toux†; Demo pates pectorales†; Demo sirop contre la toux†; Dinacode N; Euphon N; Ipeca; Neo-Codion N; Pastilles pectorales Demo N; Pectocalmine Junior N; Phol-Tussil; Saintbois nouvelle formule; Sano Tuss; Sirop pectoral DP1†; Sirop pectoral DP2, DP3†; *Thai.:* Baby Cough Syrup; Baby Cough with Antihistamine; *UK:* Allens Chesty Cough; Modern Herbals Cold & Congestion; Sanderson's Throat Specific; *USA:* Vicks Menthol Cough Drops.

Tramazoline Hydrochloride (2109-x)

Tramazoline Hydrochloride *(BANM, USAN, rINNM).*

Tramazolini Hydrochloridum. 2-(5,6,7,8-Tetrahydro-1-naphthylamino)-2-imidazoline hydrochloride.

$C_{13}H_{17}N_3,HCl = 251.8.$

CAS — 1082-57-1 (tramazoline); 3715-90-0 (tramazoline hydrochloride).

Pharmacopoeias. Eur. (see p.vi) includes the monohydrate.

Tramazoline hydrochloride 116.95 μg is approximately equivalent to 100 μg of tramazoline.

Pharmacopoeial description

Ph. Eur.: Tramazoline hydrochloride monohydrate is a white or almost white crystalline powder. Soluble in water and in alcohol. A 5% solution in water has a pH of 4.9 to 6.3.

Profile
Tramazoline hydrochloride is a sympathomimetic with effects similar to those of naphazoline (p.1095). It is used to provide symptomatic relief of nasal congestion (p.1082). It is given as nasal drops or as a metered-dose nasal spray in usual doses (expressed as tramazoline base) of 100 μg 3 or 4 times daily. The dose may be increased to a maximum of 200 μg four times daily if necessary.

Tramazoline hydrochloride has also been used in eye drops as a conjunctival decongestant (see Conjunctivitis, p.406).

Preparations

Proprietary Preparations (details are given in Part 3)
Austral.: Spray-Tish; *Belg.:* Rhinospray; *Ger.:* Biciron; Ellatun; Rhinospray; *Ital.:* Rinogutt Spray-Fher; *Neth.:* Bisolnasal; Rhinospray†; *Port.:* Rhinospray; *Spain:* Rhinospray.

Multi-ingredient: *Aust.:* Dexa-Rhinospray†; Rhinospray Plus; *Austral.:* Tobispray†; *Belg.:* Dexa-Rhinospray; *Ger.:* Dexa Biciron; Dexa-Rhinospray N; Oxy Biciron; Rhinospray Plus; *Irl.:* Dexa-Rhinaspray; Dexa-Rhinaspray Duo; *Ital.:* Rinogutt Antiallergico Spray; Rinogutt Eucalipto-Fher; *Spain:* Rhinospray Antialergico; *UK:* Dexa-Rhinaspray Duo; Dexa-Rhinaspray†.

Tuaminoheptane Sulfate (2112-z)

Tuaminoheptane Sulfate *(rINNM).*
Tuaminoheptane Sulphate *(BANM).*
$(C_7H_{17}N)_2,H_2SO_4 = 328.5.$
CAS — 6411-75-2.

Profile
Tuaminoheptane is a volatile sympathomimetic (see Adrenaline, p.831) that has been used as the sulfate for the symptomatic relief of nasal congestion. Tuaminoheptane has also been employed in the form of the carbonate.

Preparations

Proprietary Preparations (details are given in Part 3)
Multi-ingredient: *Braz.:* Rinofluimucil; *Fr.:* Rhinofluimucil; *Ger.:* Rinofluimucil-S; *Hong Kong:* Rinofluimucil; *Ital.:* Otomicetina†; Rinofluimucil; *Spain:* Rinofluimucil; *Switz.:* Rinofluimucil.

Tymazoline Hydrochloride (2113-c)

Tymazoline Hydrochloride *(BANM).*
2-Thymyloxymethyl-2-imidazoline Hydrochloride. 2-(2-Isopropyl-5-methylphenoxymethyl)-2-imidazoline hydrochloride.
$C_{14}H_{20}N_2O,HCl = 268.8.$
CAS — 24243-97-8 (tymazoline); 28120-03-8 (tymazoline hydrochloride).
Pharmacopoeias. In Pol.

Profile
Tymazoline is a sympathomimetic that has been used as the hydrochloride similarly to naphazoline (p.1095) for its local vasoconstrictor action in the symptomatic relief of nasal congestion (p.1082).

Preparations

Proprietary Preparations (details are given in Part 3)
Fr.: Pernazene†.

Xylometazoline Hydrochloride

(2114-k)

Xylometazoline Hydrochloride *(BANM, rINNM).*
2-(4-*tert*-Butyl-2,6-dimethylbenzyl)-2-imidazoline hydrochloride.
$C_{16}H_{24}N_2,HCl = 280.8.$
CAS — 526-36-3 (xylometazoline); 1218-35-5 (xylometazoline hydrochloride).
Pharmacopoeias. In Eur. (see p.vi), *Pol.,* and *US.*

Pharmacopoeial description

Ph. Eur.: A white or almost white, crystalline powder. Freely soluble in water, in alcohol, and in methyl alcohol; practically insoluble in ether. Protect from light.

USP 25: A white to off-white, odourless, crystalline powder. Soluble 1 in 35 of water; freely soluble in alcohol; sparingly soluble in chloroform; practically insoluble in ether and in benzene. pH of a 5% solution in water is between 5.0 and 6.6. Store in airtight containers. Protect from light.

Adverse Effects and Precautions
As for Naphazoline, p.1095.

Interactions
Since xylometazoline is absorbed through the mucosa interactions may follow topical application. The *British National Formulary* considers that all sympathomimetic nasal decongestants are liable to cause a hypertensive crisis if used during treatment with an MAOI. For the interactions of sympathomimetics in general, see under Adrenaline, p.830.

Uses and Administration
Xylometazoline is a direct-acting sympathomimetic (see Adrenaline, p.831) with marked alpha-adrenergic activity. It is a vasoconstrictor which reduces swelling and congestion when applied to mucous membranes. The effect begins within 5 to 10 minutes of application and lasts for up to 10 hours.
Xylometazoline is used as the hydrochloride for the symptomatic relief of nasal congestion (p.1082). A 0.1% solution of xylometazoline hydrochloride is applied topically as nasal drops or a spray into each nostril two or three times daily. A 0.05% solution is used

once or twice daily for children less than 12 years of age but is not recommended for infants of less than 3 months of age; 1 or 2 drops of the solution are instilled into each nostril.

A 0.05% solution of xylometazoline hydrochloride may be instilled into the eye as a conjunctival decongestant (see Conjunctivitis, p.406).

Preparations
BP 2001: Xylometazoline Nasal Drops;
USP 25: Xylometazoline Hydrochloride Nasal Solution.

Proprietary Preparations (details are given in Part 3)
Aust.: Olynth; Otrivin; *Austral.:* Otrivin; *Belg.:* Nasa Rhinathiol; Otrivine; Rhinidine; *Braz.:* Otrivina; *Canad.:* Certified Decongestant; Decongest; Decongestant Nasal Spray; Decongestant Nose Drops; Otrivin; Vaporisateur Nasal Decongestionnant; *Denm.:* Otrivin; Passagen; Zymelin; *Fin.:* Nasolin; Otrivin; *Ger.:* Balkis; Dorenasin; Gelonasal; Imidin K; Imidin N; Logomed Nasen-Tropfen†; Mentopin Nasenspray; Nasan; Nasengel; Nasengel AL; Nasenspray AL; Nasenspray E; Nasenspray K; Nasentropfen AL; Nasentropfen E; Nasentropfen K; Olynth; Otalgicin; Otriven; Otriven gegen Schnupfen; Rapako xylo; Rhino-stas†; schnupfen endrine; stas Nasentropfen, Nasenspray; ViviRhin S†; Xylo; Xylo-COMOD; *Hong Kong:* Decongest; Otrivin; Xyloma; *Irl.:* Otrivine; *Israel:* Kalaf; Nazalet; Otrivin; Xylovit; *Ital.:* Neo-Rinoleina; Otrivin; Respiro; *Neth.:* Otrivin; Norw.: Otrivin; Zymelin; *NZ:* Otrivine; *Port.:* Otrivina; *S.Afr.:* Otrivin; Sinutab†; *Singapore:* Otrivin; *Spain:* Amidrin; Desconasal†; Otrivin; Rationasal; *Swed.:* Nasoferm; Otrivin; *Switz.:* Nasben; Olynth; Otrivin; Rinosedin; *Thai.:* Otrivine; *UAE:* Xylolin; *UK:* Otradrops; Otraspray; Otrivine; Tixycolds Cold and Allergy; *USA:* Otrivin.

Multi-ingredient: *Aust.:* Lomusol comp†; *Austral.:* Allergy Eyes; Murine Allergy; *Belg.:* Lomusol plus Xylometazoline; *Canad.:* Ophtrivin-A; *Denm.:* Kombicrom; Otrivin Menthol; *Fin.:* Otrivin Menthol; *Ger.:* Lomupren compositum; Nasic; Vividrin comp; *Hong Kong:* Rynacrom Compound; *Irl.:* Otrivine-Antistin; Rynacrom Compound; *Israel:* Aforinol; *Ital.:* Inalar; Nasalemed†; Rinos; Tirrinol†; *NZ:* Otrivine Menthol; Otrivine-Antistin; *Port.:* Rynacrom Composto; *Singapore:* Rynacrom Compound; *Spain:* Rinoblanco Dexa Antibio; *Swed.:* Otrivin Menthol; *Switz.:* Lomusol-X; Muco-Trin; Triofan; *Thai.:* Rynacrom Compound; *UK:* Otrivine-Antistin; Resiston One†; Rynacrom Allergy; Rynacrom Compound.

Zipeprol Hydrochloride (5633-a)
Zipeprol Hydrochloride *(rINNM).*
CERM-3024. α-(α-Methoxybenzyl)-4-(β-methoxyphenethyl)-1-piperazineethanol dihydrochloride.
$C_{23}H_{32}N_2O_3,2HCl = 457.4.$
CAS — 34758-83-3 (zipeprol); 34758-84-4 (zipeprol hydrochloride).

Profile
Zipeprol is a centrally acting cough suppressant which is stated to have a peripheral action on bronchial spasm. It has been given as the hydrochloride. There have been reports of abuse and overdosage producing neurological symptoms.

Abuse and overdosage. Severe neurological symptoms have been reported in young adults following habitual abuse of zipeprol for euphoria. Patients have presented with generalised seizures, followed by coma.[1] One patient who ingested 750 mg of zipeprol [over twice the maximum daily dose] had several opisthotonic crises and developed cerebral oedema.[2] Symptoms of overdosage in children have included restlessness, somnolence, ataxia, choreic movements, forced deviation of the head and eyes, generalised seizures, respiratory depression, and coma.[1,3] Fatalities have been reported.

Dependence and withdrawal symptoms similar to those produced by opioids have been reported.[4] WHO has assessed zipeprol to have a moderate potential for dependence and liability for abuse.[5] Although zipeprol is a weak opioid agonist at high doses its toxicity and hallucinogenic and other psychotropic effects constitute a significant element in its abuse, and the public health and social problems associated with such abuse were considered substantial.

1. Moroni C, *et al.* Overdosage of zipeprol, a non-opioid antitussive agent. *Lancet* 1984; **i:** 45.
2. Perraro F, Beorchia A. Convulsions and cerebral oedema associated with zipeprol abuse. *Lancet* 1984; **i:** 45–6.
3. Merigot P, *et al.* Les convulsions avec trois antitussifs dérivés substitués de la pipérazine (zipéprol, éprazinone, éprozinol). *Ann Pediatr (Paris)* 1985; **32:** 504–11.
4. Mallaret MP, *et al.* Zipeprol: primary dependence in an unaddicted patient. *Ann Pharmacother* 1995; **29:** 540.
5. WHO. WHO expert committee on drug dependence: twenty-ninth report. *WHO Tech Rep Ser 856* 1995.

Preparations

Proprietary Preparations (details are given in Part 3)
Ital.: Zitoxil†; *Mex.:* Respilene; Tusigen; *Port.:* Respiral; *Switz.:* Mirsol†.

Dermatological Drugs

The skin is subject to a very wide range of lesions. Some may be characteristic of specific systemic diseases and fade as the disease regresses. Some are caused by specific local infections and are best treated by the appropriate antimicrobial (see Skin Infections in the chapters Antibacterials, p.140, and Antifungals, p.376). The skin is also subject to damage from environmental hazards. Exposure to solar radiation is associated with malignant neoplasms of the skin (see p.498). Many skin disorders are side-effects of therapeutic and other agents, ranging from mild hypersensitivity to the life-threatening Stevens-Johnson syndrome or toxic epidermal necrolysis (see Drug-induced Skin Reactions, below). There also remains a wide range of skin disorders whose aetiology is poorly understood.

The distribution and morphological description of the skin lesion (its shape, colour, and surface characteristics) are important in the diagnosis of skin disorders. There are many terms used to describe skin lesions:

- abscess–a collection of pus in a cavity
- bulla (or blister)–a fluid-filled circumscribed lesion larger than 0.5 cm in diameter
- comedo–a plug of keratin and sebum in a pilosebaceous follicle
- ecchymosis–an extravasation of blood into the skin
- erythema–red coloration due to vascular dilatation
- fissure–a slit through the whole thickness of the skin
- horn–a thickening of the skin that is taller than it is broad
- keratosis–a horny thickening of the skin
- lichenification–hard, thickened skin with increased markings
- macule–an area of altered colour or texture with no elevation above the surface of the surrounding skin
- nodule–a dome-shaped or spherical-shaped, solid lesion, usually more than 0.5 cm in diameter and depth
- papilloma–a nipple-like mass
- papule–a raised solid lesion, usually less than 0.5 cm in diameter
- petechia–a pinhead-sized macule of blood in the skin
- plaque–a raised, flat-topped, circumscribed lesion, usually larger than 2 cm in diameter but with no substantial depth
- purpura–a macule of blood in the skin, larger than a petechia
- pustule–an accumulation of pus in the skin
- scale–a flat plate or flake of stratum corneum
- stria–a streak-like, linear, atrophic lesion, pink, purple, or white in colour
- telangiectasia–a visible dilatation of small cutaneous blood vessels
- vesicle–a fluid-filled circumscribed lesion less than 0.5 cm in diameter
- wheal–an elevated, white, compressible area of oedema often surrounded by a red flare.

This chapter describes the drugs used in the management of skin disorders and the treatment of some of the commoner conditions. Treatment may include topical and/or systemic drug therapy, although the pharmacology of many of the drugs used in dermatology is poorly understood. Physical methods such as cryotherapy, UV radiation, radiotherapy, and surgery also have a role.

Drugs with a traditional place in the treatment of skin disorders include coal tar, dithranol, ichthammol, and urea, as well as *keratolytics* such as benzoyl peroxide and salicylic acid. *Photosensitisers* such as the psoralen methoxsalen, vitamin D analogues such as calcipotriol, and the vitamin A analogues (retinoids) such as acitretin, isotretinoin, and tretinoin have an important role in certain skin disorders.

Drugs with primarily a *protective* function include calamine, starch, talc, titanium dioxide, and zinc oxide. Some drugs, for example ammonium lactate and sodium pidolate, have *humectant* properties and are used in topical moisturising preparations.

Drugs used to *increase pigmentation* include dihydroxyacetone, methoxsalen, and trioxysalen. Those used to *reduce pigmentation* include hydroquinone, mequinol, and monobenzone. Other substances used to protect against sunlight are described under Sunscreens, below.

For drugs that are applied topically, the vehicle and formulation may be as important as the active drug. Indeed, some cream and ointment bases are used alone for their protective or emollient properties, while adverse effects of topical preparations are sometimes attributed to constituents of the vehicle such as stabilisers and preservatives. The *choice of formulation* depends on the skin condition being treated and the area affected. Lotions and gels are useful for hairy areas. Creams (oil-in-water emulsions) have cooling and emollient effects, are readily absorbed by the skin, and are used for acute and exudative conditions. Ointments (water-in-oil emulsions) are more occlusive than creams and are particularly suitable for chronic dry skin. Pastes (powder incorporated in an ointment basis) are less occlusive than ointments and are useful for their protective properties and for their use on circumscribed lesions. Other less frequently used formulations include applications, collodions, and dusting powders. Typical quantities of preparations required per week for twice daily application to specific areas of an adult are given in Table 1, below.

Table 1. Typical quantities of preparations required per week for twice daily application to an adult.

	Creams and Ointments	Lotions
Face	15 to 30 g	100 mL
Both hands	25 to 50 g	200 mL
Scalp	50 to 100 g	200 mL
Both arms or both legs	100 to 200 g	200 mL
Trunk	400 g	500 mL
Groins and genitalia	15 to 25 g	100 mL

NOTE. These quantities do *not* apply to corticosteroid preparations.

Acne

Acne is a disorder of the pilosebaceous follicle; common features include increased sebum production, follicular keratinisation, colonisation by *Propionibacterium acnes*, and localised inflammation. Mild acne is characterised by open or closed comedones (blackheads and whiteheads), some of the latter developing into inflamed lesions such as papules and pustules. In moderate acne, the papules and pustules are more widespread, and there

may be mild scarring. Severe acne is characterised by the presence of nodular abscesses or cysts in addition to widespread pustules and papules, and may lead to extensive scarring.

The most common form of acne is acne vulgaris. It is common in teenagers and while by their mid-20s the majority of cases have resolved, a few people still require treatment in their 30s and 40s. Skin areas typically affected are the face, shoulders, upper chest, and back. Acne may also occur in late middle age and in the elderly (late onset acne) and in infants (infantile acne). Certain drugs, including androgens, corticosteroids, corticotropin, hormonal contraceptives containing androgenic progestogens such as levonorgestrel, isoniazid, lithium, methoxsalen, and some antiepileptics may produce an acneiform rash, as may substances such as tars, oils, and oily cosmetics.

Treatment aims to reduce the bacterial population of the pilosebaceous follicles, reduce the rate of sebum production, reduce inflammation, and remove the keratinised layer blocking the follicles. Drugs used include keratolytics and antibacterials. If topical preparations are not effective, oral preparations may be required. Response to therapy is commonly slow and long-term treatment is usually necessary.[1-4]

Mild acne is treated topically, in particular with benzoyl peroxide, retinoids, or antibacterials. Abrasives have been used but their effectiveness is doubtful, and preparations based on sulfur or salicylic acid are considered by some to be obsolete; the effectiveness of degreasing agents has also been questioned. Topical corticosteroids, despite their presence in some compound preparations, should not be used.

Benzoyl peroxide has an antimicrobial action and mild keratolytic properties, and both comedones and inflammation generally respond well. It is probably the most widely used first-line drug. Azelaic acid is an alternative to benzoyl peroxide that may cause less local irritation. Both have been used in combination with other topical agents.

Topical retinoids are an alternative to benzoyl peroxide and some dermatologists consider them to be the treatment of choice for mild to moderate comedonal acne. Isotretinoin and tretinoin appear to be equally effective when used topically; tazarotene is a recently-introduced retinoid for topical use and adapalene, a naphthoic acid derivative, may also be used. Topical retinoids and antibacterials may be used together, since antibacterials are more effective for inflammation and retinoids for comedones; retinoids may also be alternated with benzoyl peroxide.

Topical antibacterials may be used particularly for inflammatory acne, following ineffective or poorly tolerated benzoyl peroxide application. Tetracycline, clindamycin, and erythromycin are generally available as solutions for topical use, and appear to be roughly equivalent in efficacy. However, development of resistance by the skin flora is an increasing problem. Combination therapy with benzoyl peroxide and erythromycin may help to prevent the selection of resistant mutants; alternatively, short intervening courses of benzoyl peroxide or azelaic acid during antibacterial therapy may help to eliminate any resistant bacteria that have been selected. It has also been recommended:[5]

- that courses of topical antibacterials be continued for no longer than necessary (although treatment should be used for at least 6 months)
- that the same drug be used if further treatment is required
- that concomitant treatment with different oral and topical drugs or rotation be avoided.

Nicotinamide is also used topically in mild to moderate acne.

Moderate acne is best treated with oral antibacterials. Topical drugs may also be used as adjunctive anticomedonal treatment. Of the oral antibacterials tetracyclines appear to be the drugs of choice. Tetracycline, doxycycline, or oxytetracycline may be used. Minocycline has also been reported to be effective; however, it may cause skin pigmentation and may be associated rarely with immunologically mediated reactions. Alternatives to the tetracyclines include erythromycin and trimethoprim. All oral antibacterials have to be administered for at least 3 months; the maximal response is thought to occur after

3 to 6 months, although in some cases treatment for 2 or more years may be necessary. Again, resistance may be a problem particularly with erythromycin.

Women with moderate acne who also require oral contraception may be treated additionally with a combined oral contraceptive containing a non-androgenic progestogen.

Severe acne is usually treated with oral isotretinoin. Where it cannot be used, high doses of oral antibacterials may be considered. In women with hormonal disturbances, the anti-androgen cyproterone with ethinylestradiol (available as a combination preparation) or a combined (non-androgenic) contraceptive may be effective as adjunctive treatment. Spironolactone used for its anti-androgenic properties has been advocated for women in whom oestrogens are contra-indicated. Colchicine is being investigated in acne resistant to antibacterial treatment.

Topical drugs, particularly antibacterials, described above under mild acne, may be used as adjunctive treatment.

1. Leyden JJ. Therapy for acne vulgaris. *N Engl J Med* 1997; **336:** 1156–62.
2. Livingstone C. Acne. *Pharm J* 1997; **259:** 725–7.
3. Brown SK, Shalita AR. Acne vulgaris. *Lancet* 1998; **351:** 1871–6.
4. Krowchuk DP. Treating acne: a practical guide. *Med Clin North Am* 2000; **84:** 811–28.
5. Eady EA, *et al.* Antibiotic resistant propionibacteria in acne: need for policies to modify antibiotic usage. *BMJ* 1993; **306:** 555–6.

Alopecia

Alopecia (hair loss) has many causes. The most common form, male-pattern alopecia, is androgen-related. Alopecia may also be congenital, be associated with systemic disorders, severe emotional and physical stress, or skin disorders, or be due to nutritional deficiencies. Some drugs may cause alopecia; examples include antineoplastics, beta blockers, diazoxide, heparin, verapamil, and warfarin. In some cases there is destruction of the hair follicles (scarring) resulting in permanent hair loss. If the hair follicles remain intact (nonscarring alopecia) then treatment of the underlying condition or removal of the suspected drug may produce hair regrowth. For a discussion of the management of chemotherapy-induced alopecia, see under Treatment of the Adverse Effects of Antineoplastics, p.480. Drug treatment may be tried in alopecia areata and male-pattern alopecia, although it is often unsuccessful.

Alopecia areata is an auto-immune disorder in which there is a loss of hair in sharply defined areas of skin that normally bear hair. The affected area can vary in size from about 1 cm² to the whole scalp (alopecia totalis) or all body hair (alopecia universalis).

Small or isolated patches of alopecia areata may not need treatment and in many patients hair regrows within a few months. If loss of hair becomes a problem cosmetically, treatment may be offered but is often not totally satisfactory. Several treatment options have been tried.[1,2] Among these are corticosteroids, which may be given topically, by intralesional injection, or in severe progressive cases, by mouth; photochemotherapy with ultraviolet A radiation (PUVA) with either systemic or topical psoralens; topical dithranol; topical minoxidil; and allergic sensitisation with topical diphencyprone.

Male-pattern alopecia (androgenetic alopecia or male-pattern baldness)[2-4] involves recession of the hairline in the frontal region of the scalp or loss of hair at the vertex. It is usually associated with increasing age in men. A similar pattern of hair loss occurs in women with elevated androgen concentrations; hair loss associated with increasing age in women with normal androgen concentrations is usually much more diffuse. Topical minoxidil is more effective in male-pattern alopecia than it is in the areata forms of alopecia, but is still, at best, only modestly effective. Because of the role of androgens in this condition anti-androgens and 5α-reductase inhibitors may also be tried. The 5α-reductase inhibitor finasteride has been shown to be of benefit in men with male-pattern alopecia, but is restricted to use in males.

1. Shapiro J. Alopecia areata: update on therapy. *Dermatol Clin* 1993; **11:** 35–46.
2. Price VH. Treatment of hair loss. *N Engl J Med* 1999; **341:** 964–73.
3. Bergfeld WF. Androgenetic alopecia: an autosomal dominant disorder. *Am J Med* 1995; **98** (suppl 1A): 95S–98S.
4. Sinclair R. Male pattern androgenetic alopecia. *BMJ* 1998; **317:** 865–9.

Burns

Burns may be caused by chemicals or heat. Initial treatment of burns is irrigation with cold water for 10 to 15 minutes. This limits the skin damage in burns caused by heat and removes the causative agent in chemical burns. Sodium bicarbonate solution is then used on acid burns and acetic acid solution on alkaline burns. The extent of a burn injury is described by area and depth. The affected body-surface can be calculated, and the depth of the burn may be classified as superficial (first-degree); partial thickness (second-degree), which may be further classified as superficial or deep partial thickness; or full thickness (third-degree). The major problems associated with burns are hypovolaemic shock, inhalation injury, metabolic abnormalities, and infection.

- After a burn, fluid accumulates rapidly in the wound area due to increased permeability of the microcirculation and this loss of fluid from the circulation may produce hypovolaemic shock (p.813) if burns involve at least 15 to 20% of the body-surface.
- Inhalation injury producing airway oedema is mainly a result of exposure to toxic gases. Endotracheal intubation is required until the oedema subsides. Oxygen therapy is used, and nebulised beta₂ agonists may be given to treat bronchospasm.
- Hypermetabolism and marked catabolism can result from major burn injury. Protein breakdown and loss causes muscle wasting and weakness, impaired wound healing and skin breakdown, and impaired immunity. Other effects of metabolic disturbances include an increase in liver fat and hepatomegaly, osteopenia, tachycardia and increased myocardial oxygen consumption. Enteral feeding (p.1351) to match nutrient requirements is essential for metabolic management. Other treatments that have been tried to reduce net catabolism include the amino acids arginine and glutamine, and drugs with anabolic effects including oxandrolone and human growth hormone (for concerns about the latter use see p.1287).
- Prevention of infection is an important part of burn wound management. Micro-organisms proliferate rapidly in burn wounds, especially those severe enough to impair immune function and sepsis remains the major fatal complication of burns. Burn wounds should be cleansed with normal saline (see Wounds and Ulcers, below). This may be all that is required for very minor burn wounds; a non-adherent dressing, such as paraffin tulle, may be used if necessary. Topical antibacterials, such as sulfadiazine silver, silver nitrate, and mafenide acetate, may be applied as required. Removal of devitalised tissue is also an essential element of management. Infections require aggressive systemic treatment (see under Skin Infections, p.140).

Full thickness burn wounds require skin grafting. This is performed as soon as possible after stabilisation of the patient. Skin grafting may also be considered for deep partial thickness wounds. If the area to be grafted is very extensive, the grafting procedure may have to be in stages (at intervals of about a week) as sufficient autologous skin becomes available. Alternatively, temporary skin substitutes may be used to supplement autologous skin and allow wound closure in one stage.

References

1. Monafo WW. Initial management of burns. *N Engl J Med* 1996; **335:** 1581–6.
2. Clarke J. Burns. *Br Med Bull* 1999; **55:** 885–94.
3. Ramzy PI, *et al.* Thermal injury. *Crit Care Clin* 1999; **15:** 333–52.
4. Demling RH, Seigne P. Metabolic management of patients with severe burns. *World J Surg* 2000; **24:** 673–80.

Darier's disease

Darier's disease (keratosis follicularis) is an uncommon inherited keratinisation disorder (see below) and is characterised by groups of horny papules over the body. These may become irritated and/or infected, exudative, and crusted. Severity varies greatly; mild disease may require the use of emollients only. More severe cases are treated by topical application of keratolytics such as salicylic acid or topical retinoids such as isotretinoin, tretinoin, or tazarotene. Treatment with oral retinoids (acitretin, etretinate, or isotretinoin) may be needed and has been combined with topical retinoids. Ciclosporin and topical fluorouracil have also been tried.

References

1. Burge S. Management of Darier's disease. *Clin Exp Dermatol* 1999; **24:** 53–6.

Dermatitis herpetiformis

Dermatitis herpetiformis is a rare blistering disorder of the subepidermal tissue in which the vesicles and papules are intensely irritant and pruritic. The knees, elbows, buttocks, shoulders, and scalp are areas typically affected. The disease presents usually during early to middle adult life and is a chronic condition, although there may be periods of remission that last several months. In many patients there is also a mild gastrointestinal absorptive defect characterised by gluten hypersensitivity (gluten enteropathy). Skin lesions can be suppressed by dapsone; the sulfonamides sulfamethoxypyridazine or sulfapyridine have been used as alternatives to dapsone.[1,2] A gluten-free diet may improve both gastrointestinal symptoms and the skin disorder.[3]

1. Fine J-D. Management of acquired bullous skin diseases. *N Engl J Med* 1995; **333:** 1475–84.
2. Garioch JJ. Dermatitis herpetiformis and its management. *Prescribers' J* 1996; **36:** 141–5.
3. Garioch JJ, *et al.* 25 years' experience of a gluten-free diet in the treatment of dermatitis herpetiformis. *Br J Dermatol* 1994; **131:** 541–5.

Drug-induced skin reactions

Drugs are a frequent cause of adverse skin reactions. The skin reaction may mimic a spontaneously occurring skin disorder and is therefore included in the differential diagnosis of most skin diseases. Alternatively, the drug may produce quite specific changes. The reaction can develop after the first dose or after a period of sensitisation. Pigmentation changes or effects on hair may take some months to become apparent. Drug-induced nail changes have also been reported.

Reactions range from mild rashes to severe life-threatening reactions including angioedema with urticaria (see below), Stevens-Johnson syndrome, and toxic epidermal necrolysis. Other serious skin reactions include hypersensitivity syndromes, serum sickness, and vasculitis. **Stevens-Johnson syndrome** (see also Erythema Multiforme, below) is a severe, blistering skin reaction also affecting the mucous membranes of the oropharynx, eyes, and genitalia and accompanied sometimes by fever, pain, and malaise. **Toxic epidermal necrolysis** (Lyell's syndrome or scalded skin syndrome) as described below, is a more severe form of the reaction where considerable amounts of the epidermis may be shed. Sulfonamides, carbamazepine, and allopurinol are among the many drugs that have been associated with both these reactions.

Hypersensitivity syndrome is a severe, idiosyncratic reaction which includes rash and fever, and often hepatitis, arthralgias, lymphadenopathy, and haematological abnormalities. It tends to have a relatively late and slow onset. Some antiepileptics and sulfonamides cause this syndrome, as well as allopurinol, dapsone, and gold salts. **Serum sickness** is manifest as rash, fever, arthralgia and arthritis and typically develops 8 to 14 days after administration of serum preparations and vaccines. **Vasculitic reactions** may occur 7 to 21 days after beginning therapy with drugs such as allopurinol, penicillins, and sulfonamides (see Hypersensitivity Vasculitis, p.1052). The vasculitis usually affects small vessels of the lower extremities producing purpura, although it can also affect vessels in the kidney, liver, and gastrointestinal tract, in which case it may be life-threatening.

Maculopapular exanthematic eruptions are probably the most frequent drug-induced skin reaction. Drugs commonly causing these rashes include carbamazepine, chlorpromazine, nitrofurantoin, penicillins, and sulfonamides. **Urticaria** (below) is also frequently drug-induced. **Photosensitivity** rashes where the skin reaction is confined to light-exposed areas may be phototoxic or photoallergic in nature. Phototoxic reactions occur in many patients and are dose-dependent, while photoallergic reactions affect only a few individuals. Amiodarone produces a phototoxic reaction in many patients. Some drugs cause **pigmentary changes** (see Pigmentation Disorders, below). Chlorpromazine can cause both photosensitivity and pigmentary changes. **Acneiform eruptions** may be produced by a number of drugs (see Acne, above). Some drugs produce skin reactions resembling **pemphigus** and **pemphigoid** (see below). Most of the drugs implicated contain a thiol group or metabolism of the drug generates a thiol group. Examples include captopril, penicillamine, penicillins, piroxicam, and rifampicin. **Fixed-drug eruptions** are inflammatory patches that appear at the same sites each time the drug is taken. Numerous drugs may be responsible including dapsone, sulfonamides, and tetracycline.

Drug-induced **nail changes** include onychomadesis, nail fragility, onycholysis, paronychia, pigmentation, and vascular changes. The effect is usually transient and disappears with drug withdrawal. Drugs that have been reported to cause nail changes include antineoplastics, psoralens, retinoids, tetracyclines, and zidovudine.

The majority of drug-induced adverse skin reactions are mild. However, severe reactions necessitate rapid withdrawal of the suspected drug. In some cases, this may mean stopping several drugs. In most cases the skin reaction will be resolved by symptomatic treatment. Readministration of the offending drug may establish whether the skin eruption is drug-induced, although reactions may be more severe and therefore rechallenge should not be performed after a serious reaction.

General references.

1. Smith AG. Important cutaneous adverse drug reactions. *Adverse Drug React Bull* 1994; **167:** 631–4.
2. Roujeau JC, Stern RS. Severe adverse cutaneous reactions to drugs. *N Engl J Med* 1994; **331:** 1272–85.
3. Wolkenstein P, Revuz J. Drug-induced severe skin reactions: incidence, management and prevention. *Drug Safety* 1995; **13:** 56–68.
4. Lee A, Thomson J. Drug-induced skin reactions. *Pharm J* 1999; **262:** 357–62.
5. Piraccini BM, Tosti A. Drug-induced nail disorders: incidence, management and prognosis. *Drug Safety* 1999; **21:** 187–201.

Eczema

Eczema (often used synonymously with dermatitis) refers to a variety of skin conditions characterised by epidermal inflammation and itching. The areas of skin affected vary in the different types of eczema, but the skin lesions share certain common features. In acute eczema the skin is typically red and inflamed with papules, vesicles, and blisters. In chronic eczema the skin may show the same features but be more dry, scaly, pigmented, and thickened. Eczema may be categorised as exogenous (including allergic, irritant, and photosensitivity eczema) or endogenous (such as atopic, discoid/nummular, gravitational, and seborrhoeic eczema), but there may be multiple causes of eczema, both endogenous and exogenous, in an individual patient. Two of the most common forms of eczema are atopic eczema and seborrhoeic dermatitis (below).

Atopic eczema predominantly affects infants and children although adults may also suffer. The skin is itchy and there is a chronic or relapsing dermatitis in which the face and neck and flexures of the elbows and knees are involved most often and are excoriated and lichenified.

General principles for the management of **atopic eczema** may also be applied to other eczematous skin disorders. Cure of atopic eczema is said to be unrealistic, but good control can be achieved with proper management. The British Association of Dermatologists and the Research Unit of the Royal College of Physicians of London have issued guidelines[1] for management of eczema.

First-line treatment.

• Regular bathing using soap substitutes is important to *cleanse and hydrate* the skin; soaps and detergents should be avoided as these remove the natural lipid from the skin. Suitable bath oils should be used to maintain skin hydration. Emollients should be applied liberally to the whole body at least twice daily, especially after bathing, and more frequently throughout the day to hands and face.

• Overt secondary bacterial infections are treated with systemic *antibacterials* (see Skin Infections, p.140). Topical antibacterials are not generally used as they should be restricted to limited areas and patients with eczema often have widespread bacterial infection.

• Topical *corticosteroids* are the mainstay of treatment for atopic eczema. To minimise potential side-effects preparations should not be applied more than twice daily, the minimum strength should be used to control the disease, and the age of patient, site of eczema, and extent of disease should be considered when selecting the appropriate preparation. For most patients with mild to moderate eczema 1% hydrocortisone for periods of one to two weeks is adequate. In adults and older children with severe atopic eczema or a flare-up of mild to moderate eczema more potent preparations may be required for short periods to control the disease. Wet wrap bandaging may be useful especially in younger children. In adults, mild to moderately potent corticosteroids are unlikely to cause systemic or local adverse effects. More potent preparations should be used with caution for short periods only. In general, only 1% hydrocortisone should be used on the face and in flexures as absorption is increased in these areas.

Ointment bases are usually preferred to cream bases since the occlusive effect of ointments produces better penetration of the corticosteroid. Impermeable or semi-impermeable films may sometimes be used on the palms and soles, or on limited very thickened lichenified areas, to enhance absorption.

• *Ichthammol* and *coal tar* preparations are occasionally used. Ichthammol is less irritant than coal tar and may be used as an ointment or paste bandages especially on lichenified areas. Coal tar is used in a variety of topical preparations and may be added to the bath water.

• A sedating *antihistamine* may be used short term for severe pruritus associated with relapse or at night-time if scratching disturbs sleep or occurs while asleep. Large doses may be required in children. Non-sedating antihistamines are ineffective in eczema.

Patients whose eczema fails to respond to these first-line treatments, even under specialist supervision, require further measures.

Second-line treatment. *PUVA*, that is photochemotherapy with psoralen (P) [generally methoxsalen] and ultraviolet A (UVA), and to a lesser extent phototherapy with UVB have been useful in selected patients. However, potential long-term adverse effects such as premature ageing of the skin and skin malignancy need to be considered. There has been much research into the *role of allergens* such as house dust mites and certain food allergens in atopic eczema, although the degree of benefit from measures to eradicate house dust mites is uncertain, and dietary restriction should only be tried in highly motivated patients with eczema that does not respond to conventional treatment.[2]

Third-line treatment. In patients with resistant severe atopic eczema *systemic corticosteroids* may be required for short periods to control the disease and very occasionally they may be necessary for maintenance therapy if all other forms of treatment are unsuccessful. It is especially important to avoid systemic corticosteroids during rapid adolescent growth. Various *other drugs* have been tried in resistant eczema. Azathioprine and ciclosporin may be tried in selected patients. Topical formulations of tacrolimus are used for moderate to severe atopic eczema. Evening primrose oil and borage oil have also been tried although evidence in favour of a useful therapeutic effect is poor. Other drugs at an experimental stage include interferons, mycophenolate mofetil, pimecrolimus (SDZ-ASM-981), and thymopentin. There has been much interest in the use of Chinese herbal medicines, but serious adverse effects have occasionally occurred and although encouraging results have been reported the degree of benefit is still uncertain.[3]

1. McHenry PM, *et al.* Management of atopic eczema. *BMJ* 1995; **310:** 843–7.
2. Charman C. Clinical evidence: atopic eczema. *BMJ* 1999; **318:** 1600–4.
3. Armstrong NC, Ernst E. The treatment of eczema with Chinese herbs: a systematic review of randomized clinical trials. *Br J Clin Pharmacol* 1999; **48:** 262–4.

Epidermolysis bullosa

Epidermolysis bullosa consists of a group of similar congenital disorders characterised by severe blistering of the skin. Sometimes the mucosae, especially of the mouth and oesophagus, are also affected. The blistering may be caused by various structural and metabolic defects and occurs at different levels in the skin in the different forms (simple, junctional, and dystrophic). Blistering can follow even minor trauma or can arise spontaneously. In some patients blistering and scarring can cause marked tissue loss of the affected areas and the most severe forms are fatal in early infancy due to infection of the blisters. Milder forms may be managed by avoiding trauma and keeping blisters clean and dry, but there is no truly effective treatment for the severe forms. High-dose oral corticosteroids may be needed. Phenytoin has been tried, but was unsuccessful in a controlled study. Thalidomide has also been tried.

There is also an acquired form of the disease, epidermolysis bullosa acquisita, and it too is difficult to treat;[1] corticosteroids and immunosuppressants may be tried. Individual patients have responded to high-dose intravenous immunoglobulins or extracorporeal photochemotherapy (oral methoxsalen followed by removal of blood and UV irradiation of leucocytes outside the body before reinfusion).[2,3]

1. Fine J-D. Management of acquired bullous skin diseases. *N Engl J Med* 1995; **333:** 1475–84.

2. Miller JL, *et al.* Remission of severe epidermolysis bullosa acquisita by extracorporeal photochemotherapy. *Br J Dermatol* 1995; **133:** 467–71.
3. Gordon KB, *et al.* Treatment of refractory epidermolysis bullosa acquisita with extracorporeal photochemotherapy. *Br J Dermatol* 1997; **136:** 415–20.

Erythema multiforme

Erythema multiforme is an inflammatory reaction of the skin in which the lesions are maculopapules which may become annular and blister. Areas typically affected are the hands, forearms, elbows, knees, and feet. It is usually associated with a precipitating trigger such as infection (notably herpes simplex infection); it may also be associated with drug use, neoplastic disease, or collagen or inflammatory diseases. In severe forms there is also blistering of the mucous membranes (usually of the mouth). It is unclear whether erythema multiforme with mucosal involvement and the Stevens-Johnson syndrome represent, as some suggest, two distinct clinical entities.[1] Erythema multiforme occurs predominantly after infections, whereas the Stevens-Johnson syndrome is mainly a drug-induced reaction and seems to be part of a spectrum of skin reactions with life-threatening toxic epidermal necrolysis being the more severe form (see Drug-induced Skin Reactions, above).

As erythema multiforme is usually an acute reaction of relatively short duration, symptomatic treatment as for burns (see above) may be all that is required. If severe reactions occur systemic corticosteroids may be considered, although there has been controversy about their value. Erythema multiforme may become a recurrent disorder in some patients and various drugs have been tried for treatment and prophylaxis.[2] Aciclovir, given in short courses or continuously, has been used particularly when herpes simplex infection appeared to be a trigger factor. Other drugs that have been tried for recurrent erythema multiforme include dapsone, hydroxychloroquine, mepacrine, azathioprine, and thalidomide.

1. Assier H, *et al.* Erythema multiforme with mucous membrane involvement and Stevens-Johnson syndrome are clinically different disorders with distinct causes. *Arch Dermatol* 1995; **131:** 539–43.
2. Schofield JK, *et al.* Recurrent erythema multiforme: clinical features and treatment in a large series of patients. *Br J Dermatol* 1993; **128:** 542–5.

Hyperhidrosis

Hyperhidrosis (excessive sweating) can affect the hands, feet, and axillae. No cause can usually be established although it may be secondary to an underlying endocrinological or inflammatory disorder.[1]

Drug therapy should be tried initially but is often ineffective in severe cases. Aluminium salts, such as aluminium chloride or aluminium chlorohydrate in alcoholic solvents applied topically, may be successful in milder forms. Topical antimuscarinics such as diphemanil metilsulfate, glycopyrronium bromide, or hyoscine hydrobromide may also provide some relief. Side-effects of antimuscarinics administered by mouth generally preclude such use, although oral propantheline bromide has been used successfully to control excessive sweating in a few patients with spinal cord injuries. Intradermal injection of botulinum A toxin is used in patients with severe resistant hyperhidrosis; the subcutaneous route has also been tried.[2] Formaldehyde and glutaral solutions have been used topically for hyperhidrosis affecting the feet but are not very effective and are not usually recommended.

When drug therapy fails to provide adequate relief surgery may be attempted.[1,2] Subcutaneous curettage or excision of skin bearing the eccrine glands has been employed but minimally invasive techniques, notably endoscopic transthoracic sympathectomy, are now available; the latter offers a simple and effective management for severe localised upper limb hyperhidrosis.

1. Quraishy MS, Giddings AEB. Treating hyperhidrosis. *BMJ* 1993; **306:** 1221–2.
2. Collin J, Whatling P. Treating hyperhidrosis. *BMJ* 2000; **320:** 1221–2.

Ichthyosis

Ichthyosis is a term used for generalised noninflammatory dry scaling or keratinisation disorders (see below). There are several different forms of ichthyosis and severity and incidence varies. They are generally inherited disorders. Emollients, including urea, are used to provide relief to the dry skin by coating the skin surface with an oily film thus preventing evaporation of water. If scaling is more severe topical keratolytics such as salicylic acid or urea are used. In the severest forms of ichthyosis oral retinoids may be necessary where emollients and topical keratolytics fail to provide adequate relief. Acitretin, etretinate, and isotretinoin have all been used. Topical tazarotene has also been tried. A few patients are reported to have responded to topical calcipotriol.

References.
1. Shwayder T. Ichthyosis in a nutshell. *Pediatr Rev* 1999; **20:** 5–12.

Keratinisation disorders
Keratinisation is the process whereby basal epidermal cells are transformed into dead cells of the stratum corneum from where they are shed. The process takes about fourteen days and shedding normally balances production so that the thickness of the stratum corneum does not alter. Keratinisation disorders (keratoses) are characterised by reduced shedding and the formation of scale at the skin surface. A scale is an aggregate of horn cells that have failed to separate horizontally and hyperkeratosis is an exaggeration of this failure in which there is also a vertical build up on the horn cells. Keratinisation disorders include Darier's disease and ichthyosis (see above). Certain inflammatory skin disorders, such as psoriasis (see below), also show enhanced epidermal proliferation.

Lichen planus
Lichen planus is an inflammatory skin disorder with itchy papular lesions arising usually on the extremities. The nails and oral or buccal mucosa, and rarely the genital mucosa, may also be affected. Its cause is uncertain although sufferers have a higher incidence of auto-immune disease than normal. Some drugs can produce lichenoid reactions; examples include mepacrine, methyldopa, penicillamine, and sodium aurothiomalate.

Evidence for the various treatments that have been tried is mostly scanty.[1,2] In most patients lichen planus remits spontaneously and, if mild and localised, little or no treatment is needed. For more generalised mild disease topical corticosteroids may be useful for relieving pruritus and intralesional corticosteroids can be employed for hypertrophic and hyperkeratotic lesions.[3,4] Mucosal lesions are usually asymptomatic and require no treatment; symptomatic mucosal lesions may be treated with corticosteroid pastes or lozenges. Ciclosporin mouthwashes have been tried for oral mucosal lesions, with variable results. In severe forms systemic therapy may be necessary. Corticosteroids, ciclosporin, and retinoids such as acitretin, etretinate, and isotretinoin have been successfully employed by the oral route. Other treatments tried have included griseofulvin, antimalarials such as chloroquine or hydroxychloroquine, enoxaparin, topical tacrolimus, and oral photochemotherapy with PUVA.

1. Cribier B, *et al.* Treatment of lichen planus: an evidence-based medicine analysis of efficacy. *Arch Dermatol* 1998; **134:** 1521–30.
2. Chan ES-Y, *et al.* Interventions for treating oral lichen planus (updated 30 August 2000). Available in The Cochrane Library; Issue 4. Oxford: Update Software, 2001.
3. Anonymous. Treatment of oral lichen planus. *Lancet* 1990; **336:** 913–14.
4. Oliver GF, Winkelmann RK. Treatment of lichen planus. *Drugs* 1993; **45:** 56–65.

Pemphigus and pemphigoid
Pemphigus and pemphigoid are rare, disabling, and severe or potentially fatal blistering skin diseases. They are distinct disorders although both have an auto-immune basis. There are several types of pemphigus. In pemphigus vulgaris, the most common type, the blistering is intra-epidermal and can occur anywhere on the skin surface or on the mucous membranes. It is a chronic, progressive disorder requiring prolonged treatment. Pemphigoid is also known as bullous pemphigoid and occurs mainly in elderly persons. The blistering is subepidermal and affects the skin but rarely the mucous membranes. Pemphigoid is usually a self-limiting disorder and treatment can often be stopped after a couple of years. Cicatricial pemphigoid (mucous membrane pemphigoid) is a rare form that affects mainly the oral mucosa and conjunctiva, and other mucosae, causing scarring.

The treatment of the blistering in both pemphigus and pemphigoid follows a similar pattern. Wet dressings and general treatment as for burns (see above) are commonly employed. Systemic corticosteroids are given to control the blistering and high doses initially are usually required. The doses suggested have varied enormously; the usual range is equivalent to about 60 to 100 mg daily of prednisolone by mouth although up to 400 mg daily has been suggested. However, there is some controversy about the appropriate corticosteroid dosage for initial therapy, since one study has indicated that the highest doses are associated with a poorer prognosis.[1] Maintenance therapy with corticosteroids at lower oral doses or topically may then follow. Intralesional corticosteroids may be useful for isolated lesions. Blistering of the oral mucous membranes may be treated with corticosteroid lozenges, and dinoprostone has also been reported to be effective.

Various therapies have been used as adjuncts or occasionally as alternatives to treatment with corticosteroids.[2-8] However, due to the rarity of the diseases, few controlled studies have been performed. Immunosuppressive therapy, usually with azathioprine, cyclophosphamide, or methotrexate, may be combined with a corticosteroid to improve disease control and permit a reduction in corticosteroid dosage. Mycophenolate mofetil has been used similarly in small numbers of patients. Systemic gold therapy has also been used. However, it has been suggested that evidence for the steroid-sparing effect of these drugs is lacking, and that they should be reserved for patients who cannot tolerate corticosteroids or in whom corticosteroids are contra-indicated.[3] Ciclosporin has been tried in a few patients with refractory pemphigus, with some apparent benefit, and high-dose intravenous immunoglobulin has been given to permit reduction of corticosteroid therapy to maintenance doses in pemphigus and pemphigoid. Some patients with bullous pemphigoid respond to dapsone. Plasmapheresis (plasma exchange) may be tried in severe, unresponsive pemphigus.

There have also been a number of reports suggesting that a tetracycline (often minocycline) alone or in combination with nicotinamide, may be useful in controlling the lesions of various types of pemphigus and pemphigoid.

1. Mourellou O, *et al.* The treatment of pemphigus vulgaris: experience with 48 patients seen over an 11-year period. *Br J Dermatol* 1995; **133:** 83–7.
2. Fine J-D. Management of acquired bullous skin diseases. *N Engl J Med* 1995; **333:** 1475–84.
3. Bystryn J-C, Steinman NM. The adjuvant therapy of pemphigus: an update. *Arch Dermatol* 1996; **132:** 203–12.
4. Carson PJ, *et al.* Influence of treatment on the clinical course of pemphigus vulgaris. *J Am Acad Dermatol* 1996; **34:** 645–52.
5. Stanley JR. Therapy of pemphigus vulgaris. *Arch Dermatol* 1999; **135:** 76–8.
6. Scully C, *et al.* Pemphigus vulgaris: the manifestations and long-term management of 55 patients with oral lesions. *Br J Dermatol* 1999; **140:** 84–9.
7. Nousari HC, Anhalt GJ. Pemphigus and bullous pemphigoid. *Lancet* 1999; **354:** 667–72.
8. Yancey KB, Egan CA. Pemphigoid: clinical, histologic, immunopathologic, and therapeutic considerations. *JAMA* 2000; **284:** 350–6.

Pigmentation disorders
The pigment melanin is produced in melanocytes in the basal layer of the epidermis. It is a complex polymer synthesised from the amino acid, dihydroxyphenylalanine. Melanin production is under pituitary control but is also influenced by other endocrine secretions.

Decreased pigmentation (hypopigmentation) and excessive pigmentation (hyperpigmentation) can occur and may be either generalised or localised.

Albinism is a rare inherited disorder that can cause generalised **hypopigmentation**. Affected individuals are extremely sensitive to solar irradiation and must use sunscreens regularly.

A common form of localised hypopigmentation is **vitiligo**. Sharply defined areas of depigmentation are seen and may remain localised or spread so that total depigmentation eventually occurs. There is no totally effective treatment, although some therapies may offer a degree of benefit. Oral or topical photochemotherapy with psoralens (PUVA) is currently considered to be the best treatment.[1-3] Topical corticosteroids are sometimes effective at inducing repigmentation.[4] Dihydroxyacetone produces a brown staining of the skin which may be cosmetically acceptable. Experimental drug therapy for re-inducing pigment has included UVA light therapy with either khellin or phenylalanine; oral levamisole, alone or with topical corticosteroids, has also been reported to be of benefit. UVB phototherapy has also been tried.[4] If the vitiligo affects a large proportion of the body (more than 50%), and if PUVA is ineffective at inducing repigmentation, an option is to consider inducing depigmentation in the remaining normal skin in order to match the lighter vitiligous areas. Permanent depigmentation may be induced by monobenzone, but patients must subsequently use topical sunscreens in order to avoid damage caused by solar exposure. Hydroquinone produces less permanent depigmentation; exposure to sunlight reverses the effect and sunscreens are used to maintain the benefit.

Hyperpigmentation can be caused by increased amounts of melanin, or by other substances such as iron in the skin. Generalised hyperpigmentation may be seen in Addison's disease, acanthosis nigricans, and primary haemochromatosis; other causes may include cirrhosis, chronic renal failure, and glycogen storage disease. Darkening of the skin can also occur in patients taking certain drugs due to a deposition of the drug-melanin complex in the skin. Notable examples include amiodarone, minocycline, and phenothiazines. Localised hyperpigmentation is seen in chloasma (melasma) in which there is facial involvement and is encountered most commonly in pregnancy. A number of compounds have been used basically as bleaching agents in hyperpigmentary disorders, and of these hydroquinone has been used most often;[5] monobenzone is not recommended. A beneficial response to topical tretinoin and azelaic acid in patients with chloasma has been described. Laser therapy, or the use of chemical peels, has also been tried.[5]

1. Antoniou C, Katsambas A. Guidelines for the treatment of vitiligo. *Drugs* 1992; **43:** 490–8.
2. British Photodermatology Group. British Photodermatology Group guidelines for PUVA. *Br J Dermatol* 1994; **130:** 246–55.
3. Drake LA, *et al.* Guidelines of care for vitiligo. *J Am Acad Dermatol* 1996; **35:** 620–6.
4. Njoo MD, *et al.* Nonsurgical repigmentation therapies in vitiligo: meta-analysis of the literature. *Arch Dermatol* 1998; **134:** 1532–40.
5. Grimes PE. Melasma: etiologic and therapeutic considerations. *Arch Dermatol* 1995; **131:** 1453–7.

Pruritus
Pruritus (itching) is a common and distressing symptom of many skin disorders but may also be due to systemic causes such as obstructive jaundice, endocrine disease, certain malignancies, and of drug hypersensitivity reactions. The exact pathophysiology of itching is unclear, and different inflammatory mediators may be associated with itching in different disorders; the CNS is also thought to play a role in the perception of itch.

Treatment of the underlying disorder or removal of the offending substance are important, but symptomatic treatment of pruritus may also be necessary. Emollients may be useful where dry skin is a contributory factor, and may be employed for pruritus in otherwise healthy elderly people. Calamine and crotamiton are often used topically, despite some uncertainty about their value, as are preparations containing phenol or agents such as menthol that cause capillary dilatation with a subsequent sensation of cold and analgesia. Local anaesthetics or antihistamines are sometimes included in topical preparations. However, they are only marginally effective for such use and can very occasionally cause sensitisation. Topical capsaicin has also been used and topical corticosteroids may be used to relieve pruritus when there is associated inflammation. Doxepin, a tricyclic antidepressant with very potent antihistaminic activity, has been used topically for the relief of pruritus associated with dermatitis, although its efficacy is questioned by some.

Sedating antihistamines given by mouth are commonly employed to relieve more generalised pruritus and are used to control the severe itching associated with dermatoses such as atopic eczema (see above). Bile-acid binding resins, such as colestyramine, are used to relieve pruritus associated with the deposition in dermal tissue of excess bile acids in patients with partial biliary obstruction or primary biliary cirrhosis. There are reports of cholestatic pruritus also responding to ondansetron. Pruritus caused by obstetric cholestasis has been treated with ursodeoxycholic acid. Central opioid receptors modulate itch and opioid antagonists such as nalmefene have been reported to relieve pruritus. Numerous other drugs including cimetidine and propofol have been of benefit in some patients. PUVA (see under Methoxsalen, p.1120) may be helpful in some pruritic skin conditions including aquagenic pruritus.

Psoriasis
Psoriasis is a chronic inflammatory skin disorder characterised by enhanced epidermal proliferation leading to erythema, scaling, and thickening of the skin. There are several types of psoriasis including guttate, flexural, pustular, and erythrodermic, but chronic plaque psoriasis (psoriasis vulgaris) is the most common form. In chronic plaque psoriasis the areas most commonly affected are the extensor sides of the knees, elbows, and hands, and

the sacrum. There is no cure and treatment is designed to induce a remission or suppress disease to a tolerable level.

The treatment of psoriasis has been the subject of a number of reviews.[1-6]

Topical drugs are the treatment of first choice for chronic plaque psoriasis. Mild conditions may be managed with the use of emollients alone but dithranol, coal tar, or calcipotriol are the usual active treatments for mild to moderate forms. Patients unresponsive to one topical drug may respond to another and alternatives should be tried before considering more aggressive management. Topical drugs are often used in combination.

Although effective, dithranol stains the skin and clothes and as it is irritant careful adjustment of the strength and duration of application needs to be made. It has traditionally been applied overnight in the form of ointments or pastes but newer short-contact regimens and creams are more suitable for home therapy. Coal tar is used either as crude extracts or refined products and although the refined products may be more aesthetically acceptable they may also be less effective. Salicylic acid enhances the rate of loss of surface scale and is included in many combination preparations with dithranol or coal tar. Calcipotriol, a vitamin D analogue, has the advantage of being odourless and nonstaining. Tacalcitol, another vitamin D analogue, and tazarotene, a topical retinoid, have recently been introduced. Maxacalcitol is a vitamin D analogue under investigation.

Topical corticosteroids are also effective but they may lead to dermal atrophy, tachyphylaxis, systemic toxicity, and may precipitate unstable and pustular psoriasis. Although UK dermatologists tend to reserve their use for special circumstances, they are reported to be the most widely used treatment in the USA.[5]

Guttate psoriasis is strongly associated with streptococcal infection and patients may require antimicrobial treatment but firm evidence of a beneficial effect on the skin lesions[7] (or indeed of any intervention for guttate psoriasis[8]) is lacking.

Phototherapy with UVB light is effective used alone for chronic plaque or guttate psoriasis but also enhances the effectiveness of calcipotriol, coal tar, or dithranol. Commercially available sunbeds, which emit UVA light, are not recommended as they are rarely effective and induce skin ageing and fragility.

Psoriasis refractory to topical therapy may respond to **systemic drugs**. Systemic treatment may also be indicated for extensive chronic plaque psoriasis in elderly or infirm patients, for generalised pustular or erythrodermic psoriasis, or for severe psoriatic arthritis (see Spondyloarthropathies, p.10). The administration of oral or topical psoralens such as methoxsalen with UVA light (PUVA) is generally considered to be the systemic treatment of first choice and guidelines for PUVA have been published.[9,10] Psoralens have also been used with UVB light.

Immunosuppressants such as methotrexate are useful for severe refractory psoriasis, the aim of treatment being to bring psoriasis under control, enabling a return to other modes of treatment rather than to induce remission. Ciclosporin is also used in severe refractory psoriasis and may be employed either to induce a remission or in low-dose maintenance therapy to prevent relapse. Tacrolimus is under investigation for both oral and topical use. Retinoids, such as acitretin are effective and combination with PUVA may allow a reduction in doses and associated toxicity for each therapy. Hydroxyurea [hydroxycarbamide] has also been tried.

Many anecdotal reports note improvement of psoriasis when patients are given drug therapy for other concomitant disease. The value of such drugs can be difficult to establish particularly due to the chronic relapsing and recurring nature of psoriasis.

1. Gawkrodger DJ (ed.). Current management of psoriasis. *J Dermatol Treat* 1997; **8:** 27–55.
2. Stern RS. Psoriasis. *Lancet* 1997; **350:** 349–53.
3. Livingstone C. Psoriasis. *Pharm J* 1997; **259:** 890–2.
4. Griffiths CEM. Novel therapeutic approaches to psoriasis. *Hosp Med* 1998; **59:** 539–42.
5. Linden KG, Weinstein GD. Psoriasis: current perspectives with an emphasis on treatment. *Am J Med* 1999; **107:** 595–605.
6. Peters BP, *et al.* Pathophysiology and treatment of psoriasis. *Am J Health-Syst Pharm* 2000; **57:** 645–62.
7. Owen CM, *et al.* Antistreptococcal interventions for guttate and chronic plaque psoriasis (updated 12 February 2001). Available in The Cochrane Library; Issue 4. Oxford: Update Software; 2001.
8. Chalmers RJG, *et al.* Interventions for guttate psoriasis (updated 23 February 2000). Available in The Cochrane Library; Issue 4. Oxford: Update Software; 2001.
9. British Photodermatology Group. British Photodermatology Group guidelines for PUVA. *Br J Dermatol* 1994; **130:** 246–55.
10. Halpern SM, *et al.* Guidelines for topical PUVA: a report of a workshop of the British Photodermatology Group. *Br J Dermatol* 2000; **142:** 22–31.

Pyoderma gangrenosum

Pyoderma gangrenosum is a rare serious ulcerative skin disorder often associated with systemic diseases such as inflammatory bowel disease, rheumatoid arthritis, or myeloproliferative disorders. Initially an acutely inflamed nodule is present which progresses very rapidly to large ulcers. Any area of the body may be involved, but the legs, buttocks, and face are frequent sites.

Treatment essentially consists of cleansing and dressings for the ulcers and appropriate therapy for any underlying disease. When necessary high doses of systemic corticosteroids have been given. There have also been reports in small numbers of patients of benefit with sulfasalazine, dapsone, azathioprine, ciclosporin, tacrolimus, colchicine, and nicotine chewing gum.

A related but less severe form of the disease, superficial granulomatous pyoderma has responded to intralesional or oral corticosteroids.

General references.

1. Callen JP. Pyoderma gangrenosum. *Lancet* 1998; **351:** 581–5.

Rosacea

Rosacea is a chronic inflammatory condition affecting the face; rarely, the trunk and limbs may be affected. Phases of this disorder include flushing episodes, persistent erythema and telangiectasia, a papulopustular phase, and in advanced cases rhinophyma (nasal hypertrophy and deformity).[1,2] The precise cause remains unclear; although the mite, *Demodex folliculorum*,[3] and controversially, *Helicobacter pylori*, have been suggested to play a role, good evidence is lacking.[2]

The inflammatory episodes of rosacea (papules, swelling, and pustules) are responsive to treatment, but the underlying erythema and telangiectasia usually persist. Surgery, sometimes with perioperative isotretinoin, is required for rhinophyma.[1,2] Oral antibacterials are usually effective in controlling papulopustular rosacea. Tetracycline has been most widely used, but doxycycline or erythromycin are suitable alternatives when tetracycline is inappropriate. Long-term treatment is usually necessary. In resistant cases of rosacea, isotretinoin may be tried. Topical antibacterials, in particular metronidazole, provide an effective alternative to oral drugs. Topical metronidazole and clindamycin generally improve the inflammatory episodes of rosacea, although other features may not respond. Topical retinoids or imidazole antifungals such as ketoconazole have also been tried.[2] Topical corticosteroids should not be used since they exacerbate the condition.

1. Rebora A. The red face: rosacea. *Clin Dermatol* 1993; **11:** 225–34.
2. Jansen T, Plewig G. Rosacea: classification and treatment. *J R Soc Med* 1997; **90:** 144–50.
3. Forton F, Seys B. Density of Demodex folliculorum in rosacea: a case-control study using standardized skin-surface biopsy. *Br J Dermatol* 1993; **128:** 650–9.

Seborrhoeic dermatitis

Seborrhoeic dermatitis is a common eczematous skin disorder (see Eczema above) in which erythematous pruritic patches of skin may become either scaly or exudative and crusted. Scaling lesions are the type most commonly observed. In some cases, known as seborrhoeic folliculitis, there may also be follicular papules or pustules. Seborrhoeic dermatitis occurs in regions of the body where sebaceous glands are plentiful, such as the scalp, face, and chest, although the condition is not associated with increased sebum production. The cause of seborrhoeic dermatitis is unknown, although it might be related to overgrowth with *Malassezia ovalis* (*Pityrosporum ovale*), a normal commensal yeast.

Treatment is suppressive rather than curative. Topical preparations containing an imidazole antifungal such as clotrimazole, ketoconazole, or miconazole, usually together with hydrocortisone may be effective and are the main drugs used. If unsuccessful, keratolytics such as salicylic acid or tars may be used. Shampoos containing ketoconazole, pyrithione zinc, or selenium sulfide are commonly used for scalp involvement. Topical lithium succinate has been tried.

Dandruff due to normal shedding of scalp skin (pityriasis capitis) is treated similarly to seborrhoeic dermatitis of the scalp.

Toxic epidermal necrolysis

Toxic epidermal necrolysis (Lyell's syndrome or scalded skin syndrome) is usually a drug-induced skin reaction (above). It has been described as a severe form of Stevens-Johnson syndrome, or as the most severe form of erythema multiforme (above), although these classifications of toxic epidermal necrolysis have been debated. It generally begins with lesions of the mucous membranes of the oropharynx, eyes, and genitalia, and fever and pain. Subsequently, a macular rash, blisters, or diffuse erythema develop, and affected skin may detach irregularly, sometimes in large sheets. Toxic epidermal necrolysis is managed similarly to burns (above), but specific treatments have not been established. The use of systemic corticosteroids is controversial; other treatments that have been tried include plasmapheresis, cyclophosphamide, and ciclosporin.

References.

1. Becker DS. Toxic epidermal necrolysis. *Lancet* 1998; **351:** 1417–20.

Urticaria and angioedema

Urticaria and angioedema are conditions caused by the release of inflammatory mediators from mast cells and basophils. **Urticaria** (also known as nettlerash or hives) is characterised by circumscribed, elevated, erythematous, and usually pruritic areas of oedema (wheals) involving the superficial portion of the dermis. Individual lesions arise suddenly, often within a few minutes, and may last up to 24 hours. In severe, acute urticaria, wheals may cover most of the skin surface. In chronic urticaria (continuous or recurrent lesions over at least 6 weeks) only a few wheals may develop each day. When subcutaneous or submucosal tissues are involved, causing swelling of the eyelids, lips, tongue, larynx, or genitalia, the condition is called **angioedema**.

Although urticaria may be caused by an allergy, it often has a non-allergic mechanism. Urticaria occurs as an adverse effect of many drugs, for example aspirin and many antibacterials. Other types of urticaria include dermographism (linear wheal formation on scratching or stroking) and cholinergic urticaria (evoked by such triggers as exercise, heat, and emotion and characterised by small papulous wheals surrounded by an erythematous flare). In idiopathic anaphylaxis, patients experience attacks of urticaria or angioedema, sometimes with bronchospasm, hypotension, or syncope.[1]

The **management** of urticaria and angioedema has been reviewed.[2-6] Avoidance of unnecessary exposure to known allergens or triggers is of prime importance in the management of urticaria, although in the majority of chronic cases no trigger factor can be found. Severe, acute urticaria or angioedema requires urgent treatment as for anaphylaxis (p.832).

Topical treatment of urticaria is rarely effective except for mild cases. Calamine, menthol, and crotamiton have cooling or antipruritic effects. Topical corticosteroids are of no value; topical antihistamines are not very effective and carry a slight risk of sensitisation.

Most patients with urticaria derive some benefit from oral antihistamines, especially in the relief of pruritus. A non-sedating antihistamine is the first line of treatment. Sedating antihistamines are useful at bedtime. If such antihistamines (H$_1$-antagonists) are only partly successful combination with an H$_2$-antagonist may be tried; cimetidine or ranitidine, administered alone or in combination with an H$_1$-antagonist, have shown benefit in certain types of urticaria, especially those associated with cold or angioedema. The routine use of H$_2$-antagonists in urticaria is controversial, but in practice their addition to conventional treatment can be tried in resistant cases. Little additional benefit has been found with combination therapy in dermographic urticaria.[7]

The tricyclic antidepressant doxepin has H$_1$- and H$_2$-antagonist properties and has sometimes been effective in patients with urticaria.

Addition of a sympathomimetic such as terbutaline or a calcium-channel blocker such as nifedipine has also been suggested for patients unresponsive to treatment with an H$_1$-antagonist alone, but results have varied.

A short course of an oral corticosteroid may be indicated for patients refractory to other measures. A number of other drugs including danazol, stanozolol, dapsone, sulfasalazine, ciclosporin, and leukotriene antagonists, have reportedly produced benefit in limited numbers of patients, but such therapies are largely used empirically.

Patients with frequent attacks of idiopathic anaphylaxis have benefited from prophylaxis with a corticosteroid and antihistamine, sometimes with a beta agonist.[8]

1. Patterson R, Harris KE. Idiopathic anaphylaxis. *Allergy Asthma Proc* 1999; **20:** 311–15.
2. Ormerod AD. Urticaria: recognition, causes, and treatment. *Drugs* 1994; **48:** 717–30.
3. Greaves MW. Chronic urticaria. *N Engl J Med* 1995; **332:** 1767–72.
4. Greaves MW, Sabroe RA. Allergy and the skin: urticaria. *BMJ* 1998; **316:** 1147–50.
5. Greaves M. Management of urticaria. *Hosp Med* 2000; **61:** 463–9.
6. Grattan C, *et al.* Management and diagnostic guidelines for urticaria and angio-oedema. *Br J Dermatol* 2001; **144:** 708–14.
7. Sharpe GR, Shuster S. In dermographic urticaria H$_2$ receptor antagonists have a small but therapeutically irrelevant additional effect compared with H$_1$ antagonists alone. *Br J Dermatol* 1993; **129:** 575–9.
8. Wong S, *et al.* Outcome of prophylactic therapy for idiopathic anaphylaxis. *Ann Intern Med* 1991; **114:** 133–6.

Warts

Warts are caused by human papillomaviruses. The lesions present in several different forms and can affect any skin site although the hands, feet, and anogenital areas are most frequently affected. Plantar warts on the soles of the feet are sometimes called verrucas. Anogenital warts are known as condylomata acuminata. Warts do disappear spontaneously but as they may not do so for months or years patients often seek treatment.

There is no specific antiviral therapy against the human papillomavirus.[1-6] Treatment relies on some form of local tissue destruction. Non-pharmacological techniques include surgical excision, electrocauterisation, or laser therapy. Cryotherapy (tissue freezing) may be performed with liquid nitrogen or solid carbon dioxide. Chemical destruction with acids (acetic acid, lactic acid, nitric acid, salicylic acid, or trichloroacetic acid), silver nitrate, potassium hydroxide, formaldehyde or glutaral, or podophyllum resin or its derivatives (podophyllotoxin) is another option. Podophyllum resin or podophyllotoxin are possibly used more frequently than other forms of drug therapy in anogenital warts. Intralesional injection of cytotoxics such as bleomycin or fluorouracil also destroys the wart and may be employed in severe or resistant cases. Fluorouracil may also be applied topically. Tretinoin has been tried topically for its effect on epidermal growth. Interferons have antiviral, antiproliferative, and immunomodulatory actions and have thus been investigated in the management of warts; some studies, especially those involving intralesional administration, have demonstrated benefit. Imiquimod has recently been introduced for the topical treatment of anogenital warts. Other drugs with immunomodulatory effects, such as cimetidine, have been tried in a few patients. There are also small studies of treatment with diphencyprone, a contact sensitiser, and photodynamic therapy using 5-aminolaevulinic acid.

1. Phelps WC, Alexander KA. Antiviral therapy for human papillomaviruses: rationale and prospects. *Ann Intern Med* 1995; **123:** 368–82.
2. Beutner KR, Ferenczy A. Therapeutic approaches to genital warts. *Am J Med* 1997; **102** (suppl 5A): 28–37.
3. Centers for Disease Control. 1998 Guidelines for treatment of sexually transmitted diseases. *MMWR* 1998; **47** (RR-1): 88–95.
4. Anonymous. Tackling warts on the hands and feet. *Drug Ther Bull* 1998; **36:** 22–4.
5. Verbov J. How to manage warts. *Arch Dis Child* 1999; **80:** 97–9.
6. Sterling JC, *et al.* Guidelines for the management of cutaneous warts. *Br J Dermatol* 2001; **144:** 4–11.

Wounds and ulcers

Wounds (physical injuries of the skin and underlying structures) may be the result of mechanical trauma, burns, or chemical injury. Ulcers are often the result of various underlying disorders. Among the commonest types, *decubitus ulcers* (bedsores, pressure sores) occur in patients with extended immobility when prolonged pressure on the skin over a bony prominence produces localised ischaemia. *Leg ulcers* may result from venous incompetence or be ischaemic in origin, while patients with peripheral neuropathy, such as diabetics or those with leprosy, may develop *neuropathic ulcers* due to repetitive inadvertent injury. Wounds or ulcers may be described as superficial, partial thickness, or full thickness. Superficial wounds are limited to epithelial tissue and heal rapidly by regeneration of epithelial cells. Partial thickness wounds involve the dermis and include some blood vessel damage, and therefore wound repair is a longer process. Full thickness wounds extend to the subcutaneous fat layer at least and healing requires synthesis of new connective tissue.

Healing mechanisms are essentially the same regardless of the cause of the damage:

- immediate haemostatic processes involve formation of a platelet plug and fibrin clot, as described under Haemostasis and Fibrinolysis, p.718
- the early granulation and re-epithelialisation phase takes place up to about 21 days after injury depending on wound size and site. Platelet-derived growth factors stimulate fibroblasts to produce granulation tissue, comprising a collagen matrix well-supplied with capillary vessels, and growth of epidermal cells leading to re-epithelialisation of the wound surface
- during the final dermal repair and remodelling phase the collagen matrix undergoes strengthening and there is a reduction in vascularity. This phase can continue for up to 2 years after injury.

Several factors are important for efficient wound healing. Adequate supplies of nutrients, especially vitamin C and zinc (which are often given as supplements) and oxygen are needed. A good blood supply is thus essential. Clinical infection, either systemic or local, due to contamination by environmental microbes, causes tissue damage and delays healing. The process of wound repair requires many cellular and acellular factors, such as platelets and growth factors, and deficiencies in these may also be responsible for delayed healing. Thus, the patient's age, systemic conditions, concomitant drugs, nutritional status, and congenital deficiencies all influence the rate of healing.

Local **wound management** includes cleansing, removal of exudate, and prevention of microbial contamination. Choice of wound treatment preparation will depend on the size, location, type, and cause of the wound, on the presence of infection, and on the particular stage of healing.

Wound **cleansing** is required to remove any dirt or foreign body and to **remove exudate** and slough (pus and necrotic tissue). This helps to prevent infection and aids healing. Commonly used cleansing solutions are sodium chloride 0.9%, hypochlorite, hydrogen peroxide, povidone-iodine, and chlorhexidine. However, some antiseptics and hypochlorites might be associated with delayed wound healing, especially with prolonged use, as they delay collagen production and cause inflammation. Also, many antiseptics are inactivated by organic material. Sodium chloride solution may be all that is required for routine cleansing of non-infected wounds. Many of the cleansing solutions also help to remove slough. Other wound management preparations more specifically directed at removing slough include dextranomer, hydrogels, hydrocolloids, and enzyme preparations such as a mixture of streptokinase and streptodornase. Dextranomer, hydrogels, and hydrocolloids cause debridement by their occlusive, rehydrating properties. Surgical debridement is a fast and efficient way of removing necrotic tissue. Larval therapy (the use of live sterile maggots of *Lucilia sericata*, the common greenbottle fly) has also been effective for debridement of infected or necrotic wounds, including diabetic foot ulceration. Wounds may produce large volumes of exudate as a result of inflammatory reactions, especially during the first few days. Hydrocolloid and alginate preparations and foam dressings are effective moisture absorbers.

All wounds are colonised by bacteria to some extent and there is no evidence that this superficial **infection** affects healing. However, infection with *Pseudomonas aeruginosa* may delay healing and sulfadiazine silver is used especially in burns. Acetic acid has also been used. Infections are treated systemically if there are indications of clinical infection such as sudden pain, cellulitis, and increased discharge; systemic management of bacterial skin infections is described on p.140.

Wound **dressings** and packing preparations help to protect the wound and provide the correct environment for wound healing. Some also help by absorbing exudate. Superficial wounds usually only require a low-adherent dressing. Alginates may be used for exuding wounds. Traditional dry dressings such as cotton wool, gauze, and lint are not used for partial or full thickness cavity wounds since they shed fibres, adhere to the wound, and cause wound dehydration. Hydrogels, hydrocolloids, polysaccharides, cadexomer-iodine, alginates, and foam dressings are all effective cavity wound preparations.

Activated charcoal is very effective at reducing offensive odours from **malodorous wounds**, as sugar (sucrose) pastes. Sucrose may exert its antibacterial effect by competing for water present in the cells of bacteria. Metroni-

dazole is active against anaerobic bacteria that are associated with the pungent smell and is used topically for deodorising malodorous tumours. Metronidazole is not generally used on wounds because of the risk of inducing resistance but it is sometimes used to deodorise malodorous venous leg ulcers or decubitus ulcers.

In addition to the use of wound preparations, there may be other measures that aid healing of specific wounds or ulcers. Some wounds may require skin grafting. Skin substitutes, and the use of certain cytokines, such as becaplermin and molgramostim, are being investigated in non-healing ulcers and wounds. Measures that aid the return of fluid from the leg, such as flexing the ankles, elevation, and use of compression bandages are beneficial in **venous ulcers**. The bioflavonoids, given orally, may improve venous insufficiency and therefore also aid healing. Systemic drugs that improve the supply of oxygen to tissues, for example oxpentifylline [pentoxifylline], may be useful in ischaemic and venous ulcers. Topical and systemic ketanserin has been investigated in a few patients and may be beneficial in wounds and ulcers where there is impaired blood flow. Vascular surgery may be necessary in the management of some ulcers caused by ischaemia. In **decubitus ulcers**, relief of pressure is the most important measure in management. The management of **burns** and **chemical burns** is described above.

General references.

1. Vohra RK, McCollum CN. Pressure sores. *BMJ* 1994; **309:** 853–7.
2. Douglas WS, Simpson NB. Guidelines for the management of chronic venous leg ulceration: report of a multidisciplinary workshop. *Br J Dermatol* 1995; **132:** 446–52.
3. Smith DM. Pressure ulcers in the nursing home. *Ann Intern Med* 1995; **123:** 433–42.
4. Cooke ED, Nicolaides AN. Management of leg ulcers. *Prescribers' J* 1997; **37:** 61–8.
5. Angle N, Bergan JJ. Chronic venous ulcer. *BMJ* 1997; **314:** 1019–23.
6. Warren K, Bennett G. Wound care. *Prescribers' J* 1998; **38:** 115–22.
7. Grey JE, Harding KG. The chronic non-healing wound: how to make it better. *Hosp Med* 1998; **59:** 557–63.
8. Orlando PL. Pressure ulcer management in the geriatric patient. *Ann Pharmacother* 1998; **32:** 1221–7.
9. Anonymous. Leg ulcers. In: Buxton PK, ed. *ABC of Dermatology.* London: BMJ Publishing Group, 1998: 42–5.
10. Thomas S, *et al.* Maggots are useful in treating infected or necrotic wounds. *BMJ* 1999; **318:** 807–8.
11. Singer AJ, Clark RAF. Cutaneous wound healing. *N Engl J Med* 1999; **341:** 738–46.
12. Morgan DA. Wound management products in the drug tariff. *Pharm J* 1999; **263:** 820–5.
13. London NJM, Donnelly R. ABC of arterial and venous disease: ulcerated lower limb. *BMJ* 2000; **320:** 1589–91.

Abrasive Agents (10099-e)

Aluminium Oxide (12348-v)

Al$_2$O$_3$ = 102.0.
CAS — 1344-28-1.
ATC — D10AX04.
Pharmacopoeias. Eur. (see p.vi) includes Hydrated Aluminium Oxide.

Pharmacopoeial description

Ph. Eur.: Hydrated Aluminium Oxide contains the equivalent of 47 to 60% of Al$_2$O$_3$. A white, amorphous powder. Practically insoluble in water; it dissolves in dilute mineral acids and in solutions of alkali hydroxides. Store in airtight containers at a temperature below 30°.

Pumice (1631-q)

Lapis Pumicis; Pierre Ponce Granulée; Pumex; Pumex Granulatus; Pumice Stone.
CAS — 1332-09-8.
Pharmacopoeias. In Fr. and US.

Pharmacopoeial description

USP 25: Pumice is a substance of volcanic origin consisting chiefly of complex silicates of aluminium, potassium, and sodium. Odourless, very light, hard, rough, porous greyish masses or gritty, greyish powder. It is stable in air. Practically insoluble in water and not attacked by acids. Three grades of powdered pumice are recognised: (1) superfine (=pumice flour)—not less than 97% passes through a No. 200 [US] sieve; (2) fine—not less than 95% passes through a No. 150 sieve and not more than 75% passes through a No. 200 sieve; (3) coarse—not less than 95% passes through a No. 60 sieve and not more than 5% through a No. 200 sieve.

Profile

Abrasive agents such as fused synthetic aluminium oxide or powdered pumice have been used either as adjuncts in the treatment of acne (despite doubts about their value—see p.1103) or for the removal of hard skin. Pumice has also been used as a dental abrasive and as a filtering medium. Other agents used as abrasives for acne include polyethylene granules.

Preparations

Proprietary Preparations (details are given in Part 3)
Austral.: Brasivol; Ionax Scrub; **Canad.:** Brasivol; **Fr.:** Brasivol; Ionax Scrub; **Ger.:** Brasivil; **Hong Kong:** Brasivol; **Irl.:** Brasivol; Ionax Scrub; **Singapore:** Ionax Scrub; **Thai.:** Ionax Scrub; **UK:** Brasivol; Ionax Scrub; **USA:** Brasivol†; Ionax Scrub.

Multi-ingredient: **Canad.:** Pernox; **Ital.:** Neo Zeta-Foot†; **Mex.:** Dermobras; **S.Afr.:** Magagel†; Pedimed; **Switz.:** Cliniderm; **Thai.:** Belcid; **USA:** Pernox; Zanfel.

Acitretin   (19160-m)

Acitretin (BAN, USAN, rINN).

Acitretinum; Etretin; Ro-10-1670; Ro-10-1670/000. (all-trans)-9-(4-Methoxy-2,3,6-trimethylphenyl)-3,7-dimethyl-2,4,6,8-nonatetraenoic acid; (2E,4E,6E,8E)-9-(4-Methoxy-2,3,6-tri-methylphenyl)-3,7-dimethylnona-2,4,6,8-tetraenoic acid.

$C_{21}H_{26}O_3 = 326.4$.
CAS — 55079-83-9.
ATC — D05BB02.

Pharmacopoeias. In Eur. (see p.vi).

Pharmacopoeial description

Ph. Eur.: A yellow or greenish-yellow, crystalline powder. Practically insoluble in water; slightly soluble in alcohol and in acetone; very slightly soluble in cyclohexane; sparingly soluble in tetrahydrofuran. It is sensitive to air, heat, and light, especially in solution. Store at 2° to 8° in airtight containers. Protect from light. It is recommended that the contents of an opened container be used as soon as possible and any unused part be protected by an atmosphere of inert gas.

Adverse Effects and Precautions

As for Isotretinoin, p.1115.

Acitretin has a relatively short half-life, but etretinate, which has a much longer half-life, has been detected in the plasma of some patients receiving acitretin. Recommendations vary slightly in different countries but pregnancy should be avoided for at least 2 to 3 years after treatment has been withdrawn (see also under Pregnancy, below) and patients should not donate blood for at least 1 to 3 years after cessation of therapy. Female patients should avoid alcohol during treatment with acitretin and for 2 months after stopping treatment (see under Interactions, below).

Effects on the musculoskeletal system. For reference to severe myopathy occurring during therapy with acitretin, see under Isotretinoin, p.1116.

Effects on the skin. For mention of the phototoxic potential of acitretin, see under Isotretinoin, p.1116.

Pregnancy. In the UK the manufacturers of acitretin recommend that pregnancy should be avoided for at least 2 years (3 years in the US) after withdrawal of therapy since etretinate, which is teratogenic and has a much longer half-life than acitretin, has been detected in the plasma of some patients receiving acitretin. It has been pointed out that plasma-etretinate concentrations are a poor indication of total body stores; one study[1] has indicated that there may be substantial concentrations of etretinate in the fatty tissues of women who have received acitretin.

1. Sturkenboom MCJM, et al. Inability to detect plasma etretinate and acitretin is a poor predictor of the absence of these teratogens in tissue after stopping acitretin treatment. Br J Clin Pharmacol 1994; **38:** 229–35.

Interactions

As for Isotretinoin, p.1117.

Etretinate has been detected in the plasma of some patients receiving acitretin and acitretin is also a metabolite of etretinate; therefore interactions associated with etretinate (see p.1114) may also apply to acitretin. Concurrent ingestion of acitretin and alcohol has been associated with etretinate formation.

For discussion of the potential interactions of retinoids with hormonal contraceptives, and the effect this might have on contraceptive choice during retinoid treatment, see p.1459.

Pharmacokinetics

Acitretin is absorbed from the gastrointestinal tract and peak plasma concentrations have been obtained 1 to 6 hours after oral administration. Oral bioavailability may be increased by administration with food. Acitretin is highly bound to plasma proteins. It is metabolised to 13-cis-acitretin. Etretinate (p.1114) has also been detected in the plasma of some patients fol-

lowing administration of acitretin. The elimination half-life of acitretin is approximately 2 days but account should always be taken of the fact that the half-life of etretinate is much longer, being about 120 days. Acitretin is excreted in bile and urine.

◊ General references.

1. Larsen FG, et al. Pharmacokinetics and therapeutic efficacy of retinoids in skin diseases. Clin Pharmacokinet 1992; **23:** 42–61.

Renal impairment. The pharmacokinetics of acitretin are reported to be altered in patients with chronic renal failure but neither acitretin nor its 13-cis metabolite are removed by haemodialysis.[1]

1. Stuck AE, et al. Pharmacokinetics of acitretin and its 13-cis metabolite in patients on haemodialysis. Br J Clin Pharmacol 1989; **27:** 301–4.

Uses and Administration

Acitretin is a retinoid. It is a metabolite of etretinate (p.1114). Acitretin is used by mouth in the treatment of severe psoriasis resistant to other forms of therapy and in severe congenital ichthyosis and Darier's disease (keratosis follicularis).

It is given in an initial daily dose of 25 or 30 mg with food for 2 to 4 weeks. The daily dosage is adjusted thereafter according to clinical response and adverse effects; optimal results are usually obtained with 25 to 50 mg given daily for a further 6 to 8 weeks but some patients may require up to 75 mg daily. For the treatment of Darier's disease a starting dose of 10 mg may be appropriate, adjusted thereafter according to response. In Darier's disease and congenital ichthyosis treatment may be required for more than 3 months but a daily dosage of 50 mg should not be exceeded. In the UK, the manufacturer recommends that continuous treatment should not last longer than 6 months for any indication.

Acitretin is not generally considered suitable for use in children, but if deemed necessary a dose of 0.5 mg per kg body-weight daily or occasionally up to 1 mg per kg daily has been suggested, but the maximum daily dose should not exceed 35 mg.

Administration in children. Acitretin is not generally considered suitable for use in children. A review of its use in 29 children with severe inherited disorders of keratinisation[1] reported that acitretin is an effective and safe treatment in children provided that the minimal effective dose is used and that side-effects are carefully monitored.

1. Lacour M, et al. An appraisal of acitretin therapy in children with inherited disorders of keratinization. Br J Dermatol 1996; **134:** 1023–9.

Skin disorders. Acitretin is used alone or with PUVA or UVB in psoriasis[1] (p.1106). Studies have shown that use with PUVA or UVB light may increase efficacy and allow a reduction in the exposure to radiation required. It is also used in keratinisation disorders such as severe forms of ichthyosis[2,3] (p.1105) and Darier's disease (keratosis follicularis)[4] (p.1104). Benefit has been reported in various other skin disorders.[5-12]

1. Gollnick HPM. Oral retinoids—efficacy and toxicity in psoriasis. Br J Dermatol 1996; **135** (suppl 49): 6–17.
2. Bruckner-Tuderman L, et al. Acitretin in the symptomatic therapy for severe recessive X-linked ichthyosis. Arch Dermatol 1988; **124:** 529–32.
3. Steijlen PM, et al. Acitretin in the treatment of lamellar ichthyosis. Br J Dermatol 1994; **130:** 211–14.
4. van Dooren-Greebe RJ, et al. Acitretin monotherapy in Darier's disease. Br J Dermatol 1989; **121:** 375–9.
5. Lassus A, Geiger J-M. Acitretin and etretinate in the treatment of palmoplantar pustulosis: a double-blind comparative trial. Br J Dermatol 1988; **119:** 755–9.
6. Ruzicka T, et al. Efficiency of acitretin in the treatment of cutaneous lupus erythematosus. Arch Dermatol 1988; **124:** 897–902.
7. Laurberg G, et al. Treatment of lichen planus with acitretin: a double-blind, placebo-controlled study in 65 patients. J Am Acad Dermatol 1991; **24:** 434–7.
8. Lucker GPH, et al. Treatment of palmoplantar lichen nitidus with acitretin. Br J Dermatol 1994; **130:** 791–3.
9. Yuan Z-f, et al. Use of acitretin for the skin complications in renal transplant recipients. N Z Med J 1995; **108:** 255–6.
10. McKenna DB, Murphy GM. Skin cancer chemoprophylaxis in renal transplant recipients: 5 years of experience using low-dose acitretin. Br J Dermatol 1999; **140:** 656–60.
11. Kirby B, Watson R. Pityriasis rubra pilaris treated with acitretin and narrow-band ultraviolet B (Re-TL-01). Br J Dermatol 2000; **142:** 376–7.
12. Herbst RA, et al. Combined ultraviolet A1 radiation and acitretin therapy as a treatment option for pityriasis rubra pilaris. Br J Dermatol 2000; **142:** 574–5.

Preparations

Proprietary Preparations (details are given in Part 3)
Aust.: Neotigason; **Austral.:** Neotigason; **Belg.:** Neotigason; **Canad.:** Soriatane; **Denm.:** Neotigason; **Fin.:** Neotigason; **Fr.:** Soriatane; **Ger.:** Neotigason; **Hong Kong:** Neotigason; **Irl.:** Neotigason; **Israel:** Neotigason; **Ital.:** Neotigason; **Neth.:** Neotigason; **Norw.:** Neotigason; **NZ:** Neotigason; **Port.:** Neotigason; **S.Afr.:**

Neotigason; **Singapore:** Neotigason; **Spain:** Neotigason; **Swed.:** Neotigason; **Switz.:** Neotigason; **Thai.:** Neotigason; **UK:** Neotigason; **USA:** Soriatane.

Adapalene   (14937-t)

Adapalene (BAN, USAN, rINN).

CD-271. 6-[3-(1-Adamantyl)-4-methoxyphenyl]-2-naphthoic acid.

$C_{28}H_{28}O_3 = 412.5$.
CAS — 106685-40-9.
ATC — D10AD03.

Adverse Effects

Adapalene is a skin irritant. Topical application may cause transitory stinging and a feeling of warmth at the site of application.

Precautions

As for Tretinoin, p.1126.

Pregnancy. Anophthalmia and agenesis of the optic chiasma were found in a fetus following termination of pregnancy in a woman who had applied adapalene 0.1% topically for the month before pregnancy until 13 weeks' gestation.[1]

1. Autret E, et al. Anophthalmia and agenesis of optic chiasma associated with adapalene gel in early pregnancy. Lancet 1997; **350:** 339.

Uses and Administration

Adapalene is a naphthoic acid derivative and retinoid analogue with actions similar to those of tretinoin (p.1126). Adapalene is used in topical treatment of mild to moderate acne (p.1103) where comedones, papules, and pustules predominate.

Adapalene is applied once daily at night as a 0.1% solution, cream, or gel to skin that has been cleansed and dried. Some patients may require less frequent applications. Other topical preparations that may cause irritation should not be used concurrently. If treatment with topical antibacterials or benzoyl peroxide is required, these should be applied with an interval of 12 hours between application of adapalene.

There may be apparent exacerbations of the acne during early treatment and a therapeutic response may not be evident for 8 to 12 weeks.

◊ References.

1. Brogden RN, Goa KL. Adapalene: a review of its pharmacological properties and clinical potential in the management of mild to moderate acne. Drugs 1997; **53:** 511–19.

Preparations

Proprietary Preparations (details are given in Part 3)
Aust.: Differin; **Austral.:** Differin; **Belg.:** Differin; **Canad.:** Differin; **Denm.:** Redap; **Fin.:** Differin; **Fr.:** Differine; **Ger.:** Differin; **Hong Kong:** Differin; **Irl.:** Differin; **Israel:** Adaferin; **Ital.:** Differin; **Mex.:** Adaferin; **Norw.:** Differin; **NZ:** Differin; **Port.:** Differin; **S.Afr.:** Differin; **Singapore:** Differin; **Spain:** Differine; **Swed.:** Differin; **Switz.:** Differin; **Thai.:** Differin; **UK:** Differin; **USA:** Differin.

Alcloxa   (1591-z)

Alcloxa (USAN, rINN).

ALCA; Aluminium Chlorhydroxyallantoinate; RC-173. Chlorotetrahydroxy[(2-hydroxy-5-oxo-2-imidazolin-4-yl)ureato]dialuminium.

$C_4H_9Al_2ClN_4O_7 = 314.6$.
CAS — 1317-25-5.

Profile

Alcloxa is an astringent and keratolytic related to allantoin (below). It is present in multi-ingredient preparations intended for various skin and gastrointestinal disorders.

Preparations

Proprietary Preparations (details are given in Part 3)
Multi-ingredient: **Austral.:** Z-Acne†; **Fr.:** Ulfon; **Ital.:** Aseptil; **NZ:** Acnederm; **Singapore:** Neo-Medrol; **Thai.:** Neo-Medrol; **UK:** Dermidex.

Aldioxa   (1592-c)

Aldioxa (USAN, rINN).

ALDA; Aluminium Dihydroxyallantoinate; Dihydroxyaluminum Allantoinate; RC-172. Dihydroxy[(2-hydroxy-5-oxo-2-imidazolin-4-yl)ureato]aluminium.

$C_4H_7AlN_4O_5 = 218.1$.
CAS — 5579-81-7.
Pharmacopoeias. In Jpn.

Profile

Aldioxa is an astringent and keratolytic related to allantoin (below). It is present in multi-ingredient preparations intended for various skin and gastrointestinal disorders.

Preparations

Proprietary Preparations (details are given in Part 3)

Multi-ingredient: *Austral.:* ZeaSorb; *Canad.:* ZeaSorb; *Fr.:* Ulfon; ZeaSorb; *Ger.:* ZeaSorb; *Irl.:* ZeaSorb; *Israel:* Aronal Forte; *Ital.:* Rikospray; *Singapore:* ZeaSorb; *Thai.:* ZeaSorb; *UK:* Cetanorm; ZeaSorb.

Allantoin (1593-k)

Allantoin *(BAN, USAN)*.

Glyoxyldiureide. 5-Ureidohydantoin; 5-Ureidoimidazolidine-2,4-dione; 2,5-Dioxoimidazolidin-4-ylurea.

$C_4H_6N_4O_3 = 158.1$.

CAS — 97-59-6.

Pharmacopoeias. In Eur. (see p.vi).

Pharmacopoeial description

Ph. Eur.: A white crystalline powder. Slightly soluble in water; very slightly soluble in alcohol.

Profile

Allantoin is an astringent and keratolytic. It is present in multi-ingredient preparations intended for various skin disorders and is also used for its astringent properties in preparations for the treatment of haemorrhoids and other anorectal disorders.

◊ In the USA the FDA decided that allantoin should be removed from lotions indicated for psoriasis as it was considered to be ineffective.[1]

1. Anonymous. Nonprescription drug review gains momentum. *WHO Drug Inf* 1991; **5:** 62.

Preparations

Proprietary Preparations (details are given in Part 3)
Canad.: Soothex.

Multi-ingredient: *Aust.:* Alphosyl; Contractubex; Rheumex; Riker Silicone-Spray†; Sunsan-Heillotion; Ulcurilen; *Austral.:* Acne & Pimple Gel; Alphosyl; Blistex Medicated Lip Ointment; ER Cream; Hemocane; Macro Natural Vitamin E Cream; Medi Creme; Medi Pulv; Paxyl; SoloSite; Solyptol; VR; *Belg.:* Alphosyl†; *Braz.:* Gargotrat; Senol; Tratoderm; Vitaderme; *Canad.:* Actinac; Alphosyl; Blistex Lip Ointment; Bye Bye Burn†; Le Stick a Levres; Phenoris; Tanac; *Fin.:* Alphosyl; *Fr.:* Alphosyl; Aveenoderm; Cicatryl; Genola; *Ger.:* Alferm†; Brand- und Wund-Gel Eu Rho; Contractubex; Ellsurex; Essaven Tri-Complex; Haemo-Exhirud; Hydro Cordes; Leukona-Wundsalbe; Lipo Cordes; Magopsort†; Poloris; Poloris HC†; Psoriasis-Salbe M†; Retterspitz Gelee†; Retterspitz Heilsalbe†; Ulcurilen N; Wund- und Brand-Gel Eu Rho; *Hong Kong:* Blistex Lip Ointment; Contractubex; Medicreme; Medipulv†; *Irl.:* Actinac; Alphosyl; Alphosyl HC; *Israel:* Alphosyl; Alphosyl HC; Comfrey Plus; Pitrisan; Proctozorin-N; Rekasitin; *Ital.:* Aflogine†; Alphosyle; Angstrom Viso/Labbra Alta Protezione; Balta-Crin Tar; Cerox; Ginoxil Ecoschiuma; Herbatar; Herbatar Plus; Orostick; Sensigel; Xerial; *Mex.:* Antaderm; Dealan; Glossderm; Hipoglos Plus; Sebryl; Sebryl Plus; *NZ:* Egoderm; Egopsoryl TA; Medipulv; *Port.:* Alphosyl; Alphosyl HC; Aveenocream†; Aveenoderm†; Hidratoderme†; Tegrin†; *S.Afr.:* Alphosyl; Arola Rosebalm; Masse; *Singapore:* Egoderm; *Spain:* Alantomicina Complex†; Alantomicina†; Alphosyl; Amplidermis; Antigrietun; Balneogel; Cortenema; Egarone; Hepro; Polaramine Topico; *Swed.:* Alphosyl; *Switz.:* Alphastria; Alphosyl; Alumagall; Contractubex; Demosept; Dolorex Neo†; Gorgonium; Hepathrombine; Keli-med; Lyman; Optrex compresses; Sportium Emgel; Teerol-H†; Unatol; *Thai.:* Opplin; *UK:* Actinac; Alphosyl; Alphosyl HC; Anodesyn; Heelbalm; Modantis; Sunspot; *USA:* Alasulf; Blistex; Blistex Lip Balm; Deltavac; DIT1-2; Dr Dermi-Heal; Herpecin-L; Ionax Astringent; Orabase Lip; Tanac; Tanac Dual Core; Triple Care Protective Cream†.

Aloe Vera (20617-w)

Profile

Aloe vera gel is a mucilaginous preparation obtained from the leaves of *Aloe vera* (=*A. barbadensis*). It does not include the sap of *Aloe vera*, which contains anthraquinones, and should not be confused with aloes (p.1210).

◊ Aloe vera is widely used in cosmetics and toiletries for a reported moisturising and revitalising action. There are also claims for the beneficial and even curative properties of aloe vera gel in the treatment of conditions such as acne, psoriasis, burns, wounds, arthritis, diabetes, hyperlipidaemia, peptic ulcer, and genital herpes.[1,2] Evidence to support these claims is lacking.

1. Marshall JM. Aloe vera gel: what is the evidence? *Pharm J* 1990; **244:** 360–2.
2. Vogler BK, Ernst E. Aloe vera: a systematic review of its clinical effectiveness. *Br J Gen Pract* 1999; **49:** 823–8.

Preparations

Proprietary Preparations (details are given in Part 3)
UK: Forehead-C; *USA:* Dermaide†.

Multi-ingredient: *Austral.:* Aloe Vera Plus; Blistex Aloe & Vitamin E†; *Ital.:* Capso; Ektrofil; Ginoxil Ecoschiuma; *Port.:* Antiacneicos Ac-Sal; Disoderme; Equilibrium Creme Anti-transpirante†; *Singapore:* Cortaid with Aloe; *UK:* Solarcaine; *USA:* Aloe Grande; Dermtex HC with Aloe; Entertainer's Secret; Hawaiian Tropic Cool Aloe with I.C.E.; Hemorid For Women; Maximum Strength Flexall 454; Nasal-Ease; Solarcaine Aloe Extra Burn Re-

---

lief; Stay Moist Lip Conditioner†; Triple Care Cleanser†; Triple Care Protective Cream†; Yeast-Gard Advanced Sensitive Formula†.

Aluminium Chloride (297-n)

Aluminii Chloridum Hexahydricum; Aluminium Chloratum; Aluminum Chloride; Cloreto de Aluminio; Cloruro de Aluminio. Aluminium chloride hexahydrate.

$AlCl_3,6H_2O = 241.4$.

CAS — 7446-70-0 (anhydrous aluminium chloride); 7784-13-6 (aluminium chloride hexahydrate).

ATC — D10AX01.

Pharmacopoeias. In Eur. (see p.vi) and US.

Pharmacopoeial description

Ph. Eur.: A deliquescent, white or slightly yellow, crystalline powder or colourless crystals. Very soluble in water; freely soluble in alcohol; soluble in glycerol. Store in airtight containers.

USP 25: Deliquescent, white or yellowish-white, practically odourless, crystalline powder. Its solutions are acid to litmus. Soluble 1 in 0.9 of water and 1 in 4 alcohol; soluble in glycerol. Store in airtight containers.

Adverse Effects

Aluminium chloride may cause irritation especially if applied to damp skin; this is attributed to the formation of hydrochloric acid.

Uses and Administration

Aluminium chloride has astringent properties and is used in a 20% alcoholic solution as an antiperspirant in the treatment of hyperhidrosis (p.1105). It is applied to dry skin usually at bedtime and is washed off in the morning before the sweat glands are fully active.

◊ References.

1. Scholes KT, *et al.* Axillary hyperhidrosis treated with alcoholic solution of aluminium chloride hexahydrate. *BMJ* 1978; **2:** 84–5.

Preparations

BP 2001: Aluminium Chloride Solution.

Proprietary Preparations (details are given in Part 3)
Austral.: Driclor; Odaban; *Fr.:* Driclor; *Ger.:* Alubron-Saar; Gargarisma zum Gurgeln; Mallebrin Konzentrat; *Hong Kong:* Driclor; *Irl.:* Anhydrol Forte; Driclor; *Israel:* Anhydrol Forte; *Mex.:* Prespir; *NZ:* Hidrosol; *Port.:* Anidrosan; *Singapore:* Driclor; *Switz.:* Etiaxil; Racestyptine; *UK:* Anhydrol Forte; Driclor; Odaban; *USA:* Certain Dri†; Drysol.

Multi-ingredient: *Aust.:* Racestyptin; *Ger.:* Gargarisma†; *Switz.:* Deca†; Racestyptine; *USA:* Stypto-Caine; Xerac AC.

Aluminium Chlorohydrate (298-h)

Aluminium Chlorohydrate; Aluminium Chloride Hydroxide Hydrate; Aluminum Chlorhydroxide; Aluminum Chloride Hydroxide Hydrate; Aluminum Chlorohydrate *(USAN)*; Aluminum Hydroxychloride; Basic Aluminium Chloride.

$Al_2(OH)_5Cl,xH_2O$.

CAS — 1327-41-9 (anhydrous aluminium chlorohydrate).

ATC — D09AA08; M05BX02.

Pharmacopoeias. In US.

US also includes a range of compounds based on aluminium chlorohydrate. These are:

- aluminium dichlorohydrate and sesquichlorohydrate

- the polyethylene glycol (macrogol) complexes and propylene glycol complexes of aluminium chlorohydrex, aluminium dichlorohydrex, and aluminium sesquichlorohydrex

- the tri-, tetra-, penta-, and octachlorohydrates of aluminium zirconium and their respective glycine derivatives

Pharmacopoeial description

USP 25: A 15% w/w solution in water has a pH of 3.0 to 5.0.

Profile

Aluminium chlorohydrate is used similarly to aluminium chloride in hyperhidrosis (p.1105). Single-ingredient products for hyperhidrosis generally have a concentration in the range of 10 to 25%.

Aluminium chlorohydrate is also included in a variety of dermatological preparations for its astringent and antiperspirant properties.

Preparations

Proprietary Preparations (details are given in Part 3)
USP 25: Aluminum Chlorohydrate Solution; Aluminum Dichlorohydrate Solution; Aluminum Sesquichlorohydrate Solution; Aluminum Zirconium Octachlorohydrex Gly Solution; Aluminum Zirconium Pentachlorohydrate Solution; Aluminum Zirconium Pentachlorohydrex Gly Solution; Aluminum Zirconium Tetrachlorohydrate Solution; Aluminum Zirconium Tetrachlorohydrex

---

Gly Solution; Aluminum Zirconium Trichlorohydrate Solution; Aluminum Zirconium Trichlorohydrex Gly Solution.

Proprietary Preparations (details are given in Part 3)
Canad.: Roll-On; Scholl Dry Antiperspirant Foot Spray; *Fr.:* pM; Spirial; *Ger.:* Phosphonorm; Primamed; *Israel:* Aloxan Derma; *Ital.:* Spirial; *Mex.:* Drysol; Skin Dry; *Mon.:* Dermagor; *NZ:* Neat Effect; Neat Feat; Neat One; Neat Touch; *Port.:* Dermagor-Antitranspirante; Lambda; *Switz.:* Alopon; Gelsica; Phosphonorm; Sansudor; *UK:* Chiron Barrier Cream; *USA:* Bromi-Lotion.

Multi-ingredient: *Aust.:* Sulgan 99; *Austral.:* Nappy-Mate; Neo-Medrol; *Canad.:* Athletes Foot Antifungal†; Medrol Acne Lotion; Neo-Medrol Acne; *Fin.:* Neo-Medrol comp; *Ger.:* Ansudor; Epipak; *Hong Kong:* Neo-Medrol Acne; *Irl.:* Neo-Medrone†; *Israel:* Fungimon; Neo-Medrol; Pedisol; *Ital.:* Medrol Lozione Antiacne; *Port.:* Equilibrium Creme Anti-transpirante; *S.Afr.:* Neo-Medrol; *Spain:* Hongosan; Moderin Acne; *USA:* Ostiderm; Pedi-Pro.

Ammonium Lactate (19210-x)

Ammonium Lactate *(USAN)*.

BMS-186091.

$C_3H_9NO_3 = 107.1$.

CAS — 52003-58-4.

Profile

Ammonium lactate is a humectant applied as a cream or lotion containing 12% lactic acid neutralised with ammonium hydroxide. It is used in the treatment of dry scaly conditions of the skin including ichthyosis.

Preparations

Proprietary Preparations (details are given in Part 3)
Canad.: Lac-Hydrin; *Fr.:* Kerapil; Lactagel; *Ital.:* Keratotal; *Mex.:* Lac-Hydrin; *NZ:* Lac-Hydrin; Lanate; *USA:* Amlactin; Lac-Hydrin.

Multi-ingredient: *Fr.:* Ichtyosoft; Keralac Plus; Keraliss 14; Lactar; Zeniac LP Fort; *Ital.:* Alfa Acid; Herbatar Plus; *Port.:* Lactonico.

Azelaic Acid (14036-v)

Azelaic Acid *(USAN, rINN)*.

Anchoic acid; Lepargylic acid; ZK-62498. Nonanedioic acid; Heptane-1,7-dicarboxylic acid.

$C_9H_{16}O_4 = 188.2$.

CAS — 123-99-9.

ATC — D10AX03.

Adverse Effects and Precautions

Topical application of azelaic acid may produce a transient skin irritation that disappears on continued treatment. In a few patients the irritation may persist requiring reduced frequency of application or temporary suspension of treatment. There have been rare reports of hypopigmentation and photosensitivity. Azelaic acid should not be applied to the eyes, mouth, or other mucous membranes.

Uses and Administration

Azelaic acid inhibits the growth of *Propionibacterium* spp. and reduces keratinisation. It is used in the topical treatment of mild to moderate inflammatory acne (p.1103). It has also been tried in hyperpigmentary skin disorders such as melasma, and in malignant melanoma.

In the treatment of acne azelaic acid is applied twice daily for up to 6 months as a 20% cream. Improvement usually occurs within four weeks.

◊ References.

1. Fitton A, Goa KL. Azelaic acid: a review of its pharmacological properties and therapeutic efficacy in acne and hyperpigmentary skin disorders. *Drugs* 1991; **41:** 780–98.
2. Breathnach AS. Melanin hyperpigmentation of skin: melasma, topical treatment with azelaic acid, and other therapies. *Cutis* 1996; **57** (suppl): 36–45.

Preparations

Proprietary Preparations (details are given in Part 3)
Aust.: Skinoren; *Austral.:* Skinoren; *Belg.:* Skinoren; *Braz.:* Azelan; *Denm.:* Skinoren; *Fin.:* Skinoren; *Fr.:* Skinoren; *Ger.:* Skinoren; *Hong Kong:* Skinoren; *Israel:* Skinoderm; *Ital.:* Acnezaic; Azelcream; Neocutis; Skinoren; *Mex.:* Cutacelan; *Norw.:* Skinoren; *Port.:* Skinoren; *S.Afr.:* Skinoren; *Singapore:* Skinoren; *Spain:* Skinoren; Zeliderm; *Swed.:* Skinoren; *Switz.:* Skinoren; *Thai.:* Skinoren; *UK:* Skinoren; *USA:* Azelex; Finevin.

Becaplermin (2718-f)

Becaplermin *(BAN, USAN, rINN)*.

RWJ-60235. Recombinant human platelet-derived growth factor B.

CAS — 165101-51-9.

ATC — D03AX06.

Profile
Becaplermin is a platelet-derived growth factor that enhances the formation of granulation tissue and promotes wound healing (p.1108). Becaplermin is applied topically as a 0.01% gel in the management of neuropathic diabetic skin ulcers (see Diabetic Complications, p.317). It is applied once daily, covered by a moist saline gauze dressing, for up to 20 weeks.

◊ References.
1. Anonymous. Platelet-derived growth factor for diabetic ulcers. *Med Lett Drugs Ther* 1998; **40:** 73–4.
2. Wieman TJ, *et al.* Efficacy and safety of a topical gel formulation of recombinant human platelet-derived growth factor-BB (becaplermin) in patients with chronic neuropathic diabetic ulcers: a phase III randomized placebo-controlled double-blind study. *Diabetes Care* 1998; **21:** 822–7.
3. Smiell JM, *et al.* Efficacy and safety of becaplermin (recombinant human platelet-derived growth factor-BB) in patients with nonhealing, lower extremity diabetic ulcers: a combined analysis of four randomized studies. *Wound Repair Regen* 1999; **7:** 335–46.

Preparations
Proprietary Preparations (details are given in Part 3)
Canad.: Regranex; **Fr.:** Regranex; **Ger.:** Regranex; **Israel:** Regranex; **Mex.:** Regranex; **Singapore:** Regranex; **Swed.:** Regranex; **UK:** Regranex; **USA:** Regranex.

Bentoquatam (5759-s)
Bentoquatam *(USAN)*.
Quaternium 18-bentonite.
CAS — 1340-69-8.

Profile
Bentoquatam, described as an organoclay compound, is a barrier preparation that is applied topically as a 5% lotion to prevent allergic contact dermatitis caused by poison ivy, poison oak, or poison sumac. The lotion is applied in a sufficient quantity to form a visible coating 15 minutes before possible contact with the plants. If continued protection is required the lotion may be re-applied every 4 hours or at any time if the visible coating is removed.

Preparations
Proprietary Preparations (details are given in Part 3)
USA: Ivy Block.

Benzoyl Peroxide (5905-m)
Benzoyl Peroxide *(USAN)*.
Benzoylis Peroxidum; NSC-675. Dibenzoyl peroxide.
$C_{14}H_{10}O_4 = 242.2.$
CAS — 94-36-0 (anhydrous benzoyl peroxide).
ATC — D10AE01.

Pharmacopoeias. In Eur. (see p.vi) and US.

Pharmacopoeial description
Ph. Eur.: Hydrous Benzoyl Peroxide (Benzoylis Peroxidum Cum Aqua) contains not less than 70% and not more than 77% of anhydrous benzoyl peroxide and not less than 20% of water. It rapidly loses water on exposure to air and may explode if the water content is too low. A white amorphous or granular powder. Practically insoluble in water; slightly soluble in alcohol; soluble in acetone; soluble in dichloromethane with separation of water. Store at 2° to 8° in a container that has been treated to reduce static charges and that has a device for the release of excess pressure. Unused material should not be returned to its original container but should be destroyed by the addition of sodium hydroxide solution (10%). Destruction can be considered to be complete if the addition of a crystal of potassium iodide does not result in the release of free iodine after acidification with dilute hydrochloric acid. Protect from light.

USP 25: Hydrous Benzoyl Peroxide contains not less than 65% and not more than 82% of anhydrous benzoyl peroxide with a water content of about 26%. The hydrous form is a white granular powder with a characteristic odour. Sparingly soluble in water and in alcohol; soluble in acetone, in chloroform, and in ether. Store in the original container, treated to reduce static charges. Unused material should not be returned to its original container but should be destroyed by the addition of sodium hydroxide solution (10%). Destruction can be considered to be complete if the addition of a crystal of potassium iodide does not result in the release of free iodine.

◊ CAUTION. *Benzoyl peroxide may explode if subjected to grinding, percussion, or heat. Hydrous benzoyl peroxide containing water to reduce the risk of explosion may still explode if exposed to temperatures higher than 60° or cause fires in the presence of reducing substances.*

Adverse Effects and Precautions
Topical application of benzoyl peroxide may produce skin irritation, particularly on beginning treatment. In some patients the irritation may require reduced frequency of application or temporary suspension of treatment. Skin dryness, peeling, rash, and transient local oedema may also occur. Contact sensitisation

The symbol † denotes a preparation no longer actively marketed

has been reported in some patients using preparations containing benzoyl peroxide. Caution is required when applying it near the eyes, the mouth and other mucous membranes, and to the neck and other sensitive areas. Patients should be alerted to benzoyl peroxide's bleaching property.

Body odour. A report of an unusual unpleasant body odour in a patient attributed to the topical use of benzoyl peroxide.[1]
1. Molberg P. Body odor from topical benzoyl peroxide. *N Engl J Med* 1981; **304:** 1366.

Carcinogenicity. There has been concern at the implications of some *animal* studies showing benzoyl peroxide to possess some tumour-promoting activity.[1] However, a retrospective survey in Canada concluded that there was no indication that the normal use of benzoyl peroxide in the treatment of acne was associated with an increased risk of facial cancer.[2]
1. Jones GRN. Skin cancer: risk to individuals using the tumour promoter benzoyl peroxide for acne treatment. *Hum Toxicol* 1985; **4:** 75–8.
2. Hogan DJ, *et al.* A study of acne treatments as risk factors for skin cancer of the head and neck. *Br J Dermatol* 1991; **125:** 343–8.

Hypersensitivity. When used in the treatment of leg ulcers benzoyl peroxide appears to induce contact hypersensitivity frequently[1] but there is some uncertainty over its sensitising potential when used in the treatment of acne. Like some other acne treatments benzoyl peroxide can produce irritation but this usually resolves on continued use.[2] Patch testing[3,4] in some studies suggests that up to 76% of patients may be hypersensitive to benzoyl peroxide but this does not appear to correlate either with the clinical irritation produced during treatment or with the reported incidence of hypersensitivity.[2,4] In one study 25% of patients were deemed to be hypersensitive from patch testing but only 2 of 44 patients developed clinical hypersensitivity.[4] Another study involving 204 patients with acne found that the incidence of false-positive irritant skin reactions to benzoyl peroxide was about 15% but only 1% of the patients had true allergic reactions to the drug on further testing.[5] However, there has been concern that hypersensitivity to benzoyl peroxide may be mistaken for irritation or worsening of the acne.[3]
1. Vena GA, *et al.* Contact dermatitis to benzoyl peroxide. *Contact Dermatitis* 1982; **8:** 338.
2. Cunliffe WJ, Burke B. Benzoyl peroxide: lack of sensitization. *Acta Derm Venereol (Stockh)* 1982; **62:** 458–9.
3. Leyden JJ, Kligman AM. Contact sensitization to benzoyl peroxide. *Contact Dermatitis* 1977; **3:** 273–5.
4. Rietschel RL, Duncan SH. Benzoyl peroxide reactions in an acne study group. *Contact Dermatitis* 1982; **8:** 323–6.
5. Balato N, *et al.* Acne and allergic contact dermatitis. *Contact Dermatitis* 1996; **34:** 68–9.

Pharmacokinetics
◊ Work *in vitro* and in *animals*[1] suggests that although there is some absorption of benzoyl peroxide following topical application, any absorbed drug appears to be metabolised in the skin to benzoic acid and rapidly excreted in the urine.
1. Yeung D, *et al.* Benzoyl peroxide: percutaneous penetration and metabolic disposition II: effect of concentration. *J Am Acad Dermatol* 1983; **9:** 920–4.

Uses and Administration
Benzoyl peroxide has mild keratolytic properties. Its antimicrobial action is probably due to its oxidising effect and activity has been reported against *Staphylococcus epidermidis* and *Propionibacterium acnes*. It is used mainly in the treatment of acne (below), in topical preparations usually containing 2.5 to 10%, sometimes in conjunction with other antimicrobials. It has been used similarly in the treatment of fungal skin infections such as tinea pedis (p.376) although other drugs are usually preferred. A 20% lotion has been applied every 8 to 12 hours in the treatment of decubitus or stasis ulcers. Strengths are expressed as anhydrous benzoyl peroxide although it is employed in a hydrous form for safety (see Pharmacopoeial Description, above).

Benzoyl peroxide is also used as a bleaching agent in the food industry and as a catalyst in the plastics industry.

Acne. Benzoyl peroxide applied topically in concentrations of up to 10% is probably the most widely used first-line drug in the management of mild acne (p.1103). Early studies in *animals* found benzoyl peroxide to be sebosuppressive[1] but later studies demonstrated that sebum excretion rises during the first few months of treatment,[2,3] probably due to the comedolytic action of benzoyl peroxide, and remains at a stable level thereafter. Benzoyl peroxide has been shown to have a significant inhibitory effect on skin microflora, with reductions in surface and follicular micro-organisms within 48 hours of beginning treatment, but clinical improvement took several more days to appear.[4] Benzoyl peroxide has also been used in combination

therapy with topical erythromycin when it has been reported to be helpful in preventing the selection of antibiotic resistance.[5,6]
1. Gloor M, *et al.* Cytokinetic studies on the sebo-suppressive effect of drugs using the example of benzoyl peroxide. *Arch Dermatol Res* 1980; **267:** 97–9.
2. Cunliffe WJ, *et al.* Topical benzoyl peroxide increases the sebum excretion rate in patients with acne. *Br J Dermatol* 1983; **109:** 577–9.
3. Pierard-Franchimont C, *et al.* Topical benzoyl peroxide increases the sebum excretion rate in acne. *Br J Dermatol* 1984; **110:** 506.
4. Bojar RA, *et al.* The short-term treatment of acne vulgaris with benzoyl peroxide: effects on the surface and follicular cutaneous microflora. *Br J Dermatol* 1994; **131:** 204–8.
5. Eady EA, *et al.* Effects of benzoyl peroxide and erythromycin alone and in combination against antibiotic-sensitive and -resistant skin bacteria from acne patients. *Br J Dermatol* 1994; **131:** 331–6.
6. Eady EA, *et al.* The effects of acne treatment with a combination of benzoyl peroxide and erythromycin on skin carriage of erythromycin-resistant propionibacteria. *Br J Dermatol* 1996; **134:** 107–13.

Preparations
BP 2001: Benzoyl Peroxide Cream; Benzoyl Peroxide Gel; Benzoyl Peroxide Lotion; Potassium Hydroxyquinoline Sulphate and Benzoyl Peroxide Cream;
USP 25: Benzoyl Peroxide Gel; Benzoyl Peroxide Lotion; Erythromycin and Benzoyl Peroxide Topical Gel.

Proprietary Preparations (details are given in Part 3)
Aust.: Akneroxid; Benzaknen; Brevoxyl; PanOxyl; Scherogel; Ultra-Clear-A-Med; **Austral.:** Benzac; Brevoxyl; Clearasil Ultra; Neutrogena Acne Mask; Oxy; PanOxyl; **Belg.:** Akneroxid; Benzac; Pangel; Scherogel; Tinagel; **Braz.:** Acnesan; Benzac; Benzac-AC; Benzagel; **Canad.:** Acetoxyl; Acnomel BP 5†; Benoxyl; Benzac; Benzagel; Clear & Clean Persa; Clearasil B.P. Plus; Dermacne; Dermoxyl; Desquam-X; H₂Oxyl†; Loroxide†; Neutrogena Acne Mask†; Neutrogena On-The-Spot Acne Lotion†; Oxy; Oxyderm; PanOxyl; Solugel; **Denm.:** Basiron; **Fin.:** Basiron; Brevoxyl; PanOxyl; **Fr.:** Brevoxyl; Cutacnyl; Eclaran; Effacne; Pannogel; PanOxyl; **Ger.:** Aknederm Oxid; Aknefug-oxid; Akneroxid; Benzaknen; Benzoyt; Brevoxyl; Cordes BPO; Dercome; Klinoxid; Marduk; Oxy; Oxy Fissan†; PanOxyl; Sanoxit; Scherogel; **Hong Kong:** Acnacyl; Antopar; Benzac-AC; Brevoxyl; Oxy; PanOxyl; **Irl.:** Acnecide; Benoxyl†; Brevoxyl; PanOxyl; **Israel:** Acne Derm; Acne Mask; Benzac-AC; Clearex Cover Up; Oxy; Oxy Sensitive; PanOxyl; **Ital.:** Benoxid; Benzac; Benzomix†; Clearasil Ultra†; Delta 80; PanOxyl; Reloxyl; Scherogel; **Mex.:** Benoxyl; Benzac; Benzaderm; Clearasil Plus; Oxy; PanOxyl; Solugel; **Neth.:** Akneroxid; Benzac; Peauline†; Tinagel†; **Norw.:** Basiron; PanOxyl; **NZ:** Benoxyl; Benzac; Brevoxyl; PanOxyl; **Port.:** Benacne; Benoxygel; Benzac; Eclaran; PanOxyl; **S.Afr.:** Benoxyl; Benzac-AC; PanOxyl; **Singapore:** Acnacyl; Benzac; Brevoxyl; PanOxyl; **Spain:** Aldoacne; Benoxygel; Clearamed; Oxiderma; PanOxyl; Peroxacne; Peroxiben; Solucel; Stop Espinilla Normaderm; **Swed.:** Basiron; Brevoxyl; Clearamed†; Stioxyl; **Switz.:** Acnefuge; Akneroxid; Aknex; Basiron†; Benzac; Desanden; Effacne; Ledoxid Acne†; Lubexyl; PanOxyl; **Thai.:** Benzac; Brevoxyl; PanOxyl; **UK:** Acetoxyl†; Acnecide; Benoxyl; Brevoxyl; Clearasil Max 10; Mediclear; Nericur†; Oxy; PanOxyl; Valderma Active†; **USA:** Ambi 10; Ben-Aqua†; Benoxyl; Benzac; Benzagel; Benzashave; Blemerase; Brevoxyl; Clear By Design; Clearasil; Clinac BPO; Del Aqua; Desquam; Exact; Fostex; Loroxide; Neutrogena Acne Mask; Oxy; PanOxyl; Peroxin; Persa-Gel; Triaz; Vanoxide.

Multi-ingredient: **Aust.:** Acnidazil; **Austral.:** Clearasil Extra Strength†; **Belg.:** Acnidazil†; Benzamycin; **Braz.:** Acnase; Acnosil; **Canad.:** Benzamycin; Persol†; Sulfoxyl; **Denm.:** Acnidazil†; **Ger.:** Acne Plus; Acnidazil†; **Hong Kong:** Benzamycin; **Irl.:** Benzamycin; Quinoderm; **Israel:** Benzamycin; **Ital.:** Acnidazil; Delta 80 Plus; Katoxyn; **Mex.:** Benzamycin; **Neth.:** Acnecure; Acnidazil; **S.Afr.:** Acneclear; Acnidazil; Benzamycine; Quinoderm; Quinoderm-H†; **Singapore:** Benzamycin; **Switz.:** Acne Creme Plus; Acnidazil†; Quinoderm†; **UK:** Acnidazil†; Benzamycin; Quinoderm; Quinoped; **USA:** BenzaClin; Benzamycin; Sulfoxyl; Vanoxide-HC.

Calamine (1598-f)
Prepared Calamine.

Pharmacopoeias. In Br., Chin., Int., and US.

Pharmacopoeial description
BP 2001: Calamine is a basic zinc carbonate coloured with ferric oxide. It is an amorphous, impalpable, pink or reddish-brown powder, the colour depending on the variety and amount of ferric oxide present and the process by which it is incorporated. Practically insoluble in water; it dissolves with effervescence in hydrochloric acid.

USP 25: Calamine is zinc oxide with a small proportion of ferric oxide. A pink, odourless, fine powder. Insoluble in water; practically completely soluble in mineral acids.

Profile
Calamine has mild astringent and antipruritic actions and is used as a dusting powder, cream, lotion, or ointment in a variety of skin conditions although its value is uncertain.

Preparations
BP 2001: Aqueous Calamine Cream; Calamine and Coal Tar Ointment; Calamine Lotion; Calamine Ointment;
USP 25: Calamine Lotion; Phenolated Calamine Lotion.

Proprietary Preparations (details are given in Part 3)
USA: Calamox.

Multi-ingredient: **Austral.:** Animine; Calaband; Caladryl†; Calamine Lotion; Dermalife Plus; Quinaband; **Braz.:** Caladerm; Caladryl; Calamina; Calamina Composta; **Canad.:** Aveeno Anti-Itch; Caladryl; Calamine Antihistamine; Noivy†; **Fr.:** Gel de Calamine; *Hong Kong:* Cadramine-V; Caladryl; Improved Versal; *Irl.:* Caladryl; Hydrocal; RBC; Vasogen; *Israel:* Calamine Lotion; Calatrim; Calatrim cum Sulphur; Kamiltract Baby; *Ital.:* Mavipiu; *Neth.:* Caladryl; *NZ:* Am-O-Lin; Dermalife Plus; Lacto Calamine; Ungvita; *Port.:* Benaderma com Calamina; Caladryl; Pruridermase†; Solpic; *S.Afr.:* Beracal†; Biohist; Caladryl; Calasthetic; Histamed; Lacto Calamine†; Pasta Prura†; *Spain:* Caladryl; Poliglicol Anti Acne; Talco Antihistam Calber; Talquissar†; Talquistina; *Thai.:* Ancamin; Cadinyl; Cadramine; Caladryl; Calanol; Calapro; Caldramine; Lanol; M-D; *UK:* Calaband; Hydrocal†; Lacto Calamine; Quinaband; RBC; Swarm; Vasogen; *USA:* Aveeno Anti-Itch; Caladryl; Calamatum; Calamycin; Dome-Paste; Ivarest; RA Lotion; Resinol; Rhuli Spray.

Calcipotriol (10943-p)

Calcipotriol *(BAN, rINN)*.

Calcipotriene *(USAN)*; MC-903. (5Z,7E,22E,24S)-24-Cyclopropyl-9,10-secochola-5,7,10(19),22-tetraene-1α,3β,24-triol.
$C_{27}H_{40}O_3 = 412.6$.
CAS — 112828-00-9; 112965-21-6.
ATC — D05AX02.

Adverse Effects and Precautions

The most frequent adverse effect associated with calcipotriol is skin irritation and it should not therefore be applied to the facial area. Symptoms may include burning, itching, erythema, and dry skin, but discontinuation of therapy is seldom necessary. Aggravation of psoriasis may occur. Hypercalcaemia that is rapidly reversible on withdrawal has occurred during treatment with calcipotriol and it should not be used in patients with disorders of calcium metabolism. Other adverse effects include skin atrophy and photosensitivity.

Effects on calcium homoeostasis. Calcipotriol is a vitamin D derivative and therefore has the potential to cause hypercalcaemia and hypercalciuria. Up to December 1993, when about 150 000 patients in the UK had been treated with calcipotriol, the UK Committee on Safety of Medicines had received 6 reports of hypercalcaemia and 2 of hypercalciuria.[1] Three of the patients with hypercalcaemia either had used doses in excess of the recommended maximum (see Uses and Administration, below) or had pustular or exfoliative psoriasis. Hypercalcaemia and hypercalciuria were reversible on withdrawal of calcipotriol. A study[2] investigating the effect of calcipotriol on urine calcium excretion found that use of the maximum recommended dose for four weeks produced increased urine calcium excretion, and the authors suggested that patients requiring the maximum dose of calcipotriol should be monitored for hypercalciuria before and during treatment. A review[3] of the effects of vitamin D analogues on calcium homoeostasis concluded that patients with unstable psoriasis are at particular risk of toxicity from calcipotriol and that measurement of urine calcium excretion is a more sensitive indicator of toxicity than serum-calcium concentrations.

1. Committee on Safety of Medicines/Medicines Control Agency. Dovonex ointment (calcipotriol). *Current Problems* 1994; **20:** 3.
2. Berth-Jones J, *et al.* Urine calcium excretion during treatment of psoriasis with topical calcipotriol. *Br J Dermatol* 1993; **129:** 411–14.
3. Bourke JF, *et al.* Vitamin D analogues in psoriasis: effects on systemic calcium homeostasis. *Br J Dermatol* 1996; **135:** 347–54.

Hyperpigmentation. Hyperpigmentation occurred at the site of calcipotriol application in two patients following use with PUVA-bath therapy for psoriasis.[1] The effect persisted for at least 4 months and 5 months in these patients.

1. Gläser R, *et al.* Hyperpigmentation due to topical calcipotriol and photochemotherapy in two psoriatic patients. *Br J Dermatol* 1998; **139:** 148–51.

Uses and Administration

Calcipotriol is a vitamin D_3 derivative. *In vitro* it appears to induce differentiation and to suppress proliferation of keratinocytes.

Calcipotriol is used in a cream or ointment for the management of plaque psoriasis and as a solution in the management of scalp psoriasis; the concentration of calcipotriol used is 0.005%. In adults, applications should be made once or twice daily. No more than 100 g of cream or ointment and no more than 60 mL of scalp solution should be applied in one week. If used in combination the limit is 60 g of cream or ointment together with 30 mL of scalp solution or 30 g of cream or ointment with 60 mL of scalp solution.

In children, the cream or ointment may be applied twice daily. No more than 50 g of cream or ointment should be applied in one week in children aged 6 to 12 years; not more than 75 g per week should be applied in children over 12-years-old.

Skin disorders. Topical drugs are the treatment of first choice for *chronic plaque psoriasis* (p.1106). Calcipotriol, dithranol, and coal tar are commonly used for mild to moderate forms of the disorder. Calcipotriol has been shown to be effective[1,2] and has the advantages of being odourless and nonstaining. Its efficacy in children[3] and during long-term[4] use has also been demonstrated. A study comparing calcipotriol ointment with coal tar for chronic plaque psoriasis[5] found rapid improvement within the first 2 weeks of treatment with calcipotriol, whereas improvement with tar occurred only after 4 weeks. When solutions of calcipotriol and betamethasone were compared for mild to moderate scalp psoriasis,[6] calcipotriol produced a satisfactory response, but betamethasone was more effective and was associated with less irritation of the scalp and face. In a study of patients with nail psoriasis about half received benefit from calcipotriol ointment over a 3 to 5 month treatment period.[7] This result was similar to that found for patients treated with betamethasone and salicylic acid ointment. Combination of calcipotriol with other antipsoriatic drugs may be beneficial; combination with betamethasone was more effective than treatment with calcipotriol alone in one study[8] and in another,[9] addition of calcipotriol to treatment with acitretin improved efficacy. A 2-week course of high-dose calcipotriol (up to 360 g of 0.005% ointment per week) has been used for inpatient treatment of extensive psoriasis, followed by the usual recommended dose (up to 100 g per week) for residual psoriasis.[10] Asymptomatic hypercalcaemia and hypercalciuria occurred in some patients; the monitoring of calcium homoeostasis is mandatory (see Effects on Calcium Homoeostasis, above). Relapse occurred in most patients within one year.

Beneficial results with calcipotriol have also been reported in *pityriasis rubra pilaris*,[11] *congenital ichthyoses*,[12] *acrodermatitis continua of Hallopeau*,[13] and *confluent and reticulated papillomatosis*.[14]

1. Murdoch D, Clissold SP. Calcipotriol: a review of its pharmacological properties and therapeutic use in psoriasis vulgaris. *Drugs* 1992; **43:** 415–29.
2. Ashcroft DM, *et al.* Systematic review of comparative efficacy and tolerability of calcipotriol in treating chronic plaque psoriasis. *BMJ* 2000; **320:** 963–7.
3. Darley CR, *et al.* Safety and efficacy of calcipotriol ointment (Dovonex®) in treating children with psoriasis vulgaris. *Br J Dermatol* 1996; **135:** 390–3.
4. Ellis JP, *et al.* Long-term treatment of chronic plaque psoriasis with calcipotriol ointment in patients unresponsive to short-contact dithranol. *Eur J Clin Res* 1995; **7:** 247–57.
5. Tham SN, *et al.* A comparative study of calcipotriol ointment and tar in chronic plaque psoriasis. *Br J Dermatol* 1994; **131:** 673–7.
6. Klaber MR, *et al.* Comparative effects of calcipotriol solution (50 µg/mL) and betamethasone 17-valerate solution (1 mg/mL) in the treatment of scalp psoriasis. *Br J Dermatol* 1994; **131:** 678–83.
7. Tosti A, *et al.* Calcipotriol ointment in nail psoriasis: a controlled double-blind comparison with betamethasone dipropionate and salicylic acid. *Br J Dermatol* 1998; **139:** 655–9.
8. Ruzicka T, Lorenz B. Comparison of calcipotriol monotherapy and a combination of calcipotriol and betamethasone valerate after 2 weeks' treatment with calcipotriol in the topical therapy of psoriasis vulgaris: a multicentre, double-blind, randomized study. *Br J Dermatol* 1998; **138:** 254–8.
9. van de Kerkhof PCM, *et al.* The effect of addition of calcipotriol ointment (50 µg/g) to acitretin therapy in psoriasis. *Br J Dermatol* 1998; **138:** 84–9.
10. Bleiker TO, *et al.* Long-term outcome of severe chronic plaque psoriasis following treatment with high-dose topical calcipotriol. *Br J Dermatol* 1998; **139:** 285–6.
11. van de Kerkhof PCM, Steijlen PM. Topical treatment of pityriasis rubra pilaris with calcipotriol. *Br J Dermatol* 1994; **130:** 675–8.
12. Lucker GPH, *et al.* Effect of topical calcipotriol on congenital ichthyoses. *Br J Dermatol* 1994; **131:** 546–50.
13. Mozzanica N, Cattaneo A. The clinical effect of topical calcipotriol in acrodermatitis continua of Hallopeau. *Br J Dermatol* 1998; **138:** 556.
14. Güleç AT, Seçkin D. Confluent and reticulated papillomatosis: treatment with topical calcipotriol. *Br J Dermatol* 1999; **141:** 1150–1.

Preparations

Proprietary Preparations (details are given in Part 3)
Aust.: Psorcutan; *Austral.:* Daivonex; *Belg.:* Daivonex; *Braz.:* Daivonex; *Canad.:* Dovonex; *Denm.:* Daivonex; *Fin.:* Daivonex; *Fr.:* Daivonex; *Ger.:* Daivonex; *Hong Kong:* Daivonex; *Irl.:* Dovonex; *Israel:* Daivonex; *Ital.:* Daivonex; Psorcutan; *Mex.:* Daivonex; *Neth.:* Daivonex; *Norw.:* Daivonex; *NZ:* Daivonex; *Port.:* Daivonex; *S.Afr.:* Dovonex; *Singapore:* Daivonex; *Spain:* Daivonex; *Swed.:* Daivonex; *Switz.:* Daivonex; *Thai.:* Daivonex; *UK:* Dovonex; *USA:* Dovonex.

Centella (1600-d)

Centellae Asiaticae Herba; Herba Centellae; Hydrocotyle; Indian Pennywort.
CAS — 18449-41-7 (madecassic acid); 464-92-6 (asiatic acid); 16830-15-2 (asiaticoside).
Pharmacopoeias. In Chin. and Eur. (see p.vi).

It contains madecassic acid, asiatic acid, and asiaticoside.

Pharmacopoeial description

Ph. Eur.: The dried, fragmented aerial parts of *Centella asiatica.* It contains not less than 6% of total triterpenoid derivatives, expressed as asiaticoside, calculated with reference to dried drug. Protect from light.

Profile

Centella has been used topically and by mouth in the management of wounds, ulcers, and keloid scars. Contact dermatitis has been reported.

The names gotu kola, gotu cola, and gota kola are used for *Centella asiatica (=Hydrocotyle asiatica)* in herbal medicine. Centella is also used in homoeopathic medicine.

◊ References.
1. Santucci B, *et al.* Contact dermatitis due to Centelase®. *Contact Dermatitis* 1985; **13:** 39.

Preparations

Proprietary Preparations (details are given in Part 3)
Aust.: Collaven; Madecassol; *Belg.:* Madecassol; *Braz.:* Celumax; *Canad.:* Cothilyne†; *Fr.:* Madecassol; Madecassol Tulgras; *Ital.:* Centellase; *Mex.:* Madecassol; *Neth.:* Madecassol†; *Port.:* Madecassol; *Singapore:* Centellase; Centica; *Spain:* Blastoestimulina; *Switz.:* Madecassol†.

Multi-ingredient: *Austral.:* Extralife Leg-Care; *Fr.:* Calmiphase; Fadiamone; Madecassol Neomycine Hydrocortisone; *Ital.:* Angioton; Centella Complex; Centella Complex C; Centeril H; Emmenoiasi; Fluiven†; Neomyrt Plus; Pik-Gel; Venactive; *Mex.:* Madecassol C; *Mon.:* Akildia; *Port.:* Antiestrias; Equilibrium Creme Anti-transpirante; *Spain:* Blastoestimulina; Cemalyt; Nesfare Antibiotico.

Cerous Nitrate (12550-q)

Cerium Nitrate.
$Ce(NO_3)_3 = 326.1$.
CAS — 10108-73-3.

Profile

Cerous nitrate has been used topically, mainly in conjunction with sulfadiazine silver, in the treatment of burns.

◊ References.
1. Scheidegger D, *et al.* Survival in major burn injuries treated by one bathing in cerium nitrate. *Burns* 1992; **18:** 296–300.
2. Boeckx W, *et al.* Effect of cerium nitrate-silver sulphadiazine on deep dermal burns: a histological hypothesis. *Burns* 1992; **18:** 456–62.
3. Ross DA, *et al.* The use of cerium nitrate-silver sulphadiazine as a topical burns dressing. *Br J Plast Surg* 1993; **46:** 582–4.
4. Koller J, Orsag M. Our experience with the use of cerium sulphadiazine in the treatment of extensive burns. *Acta Chir Plast* 1998; **40:** 73–5.

Preparations

Proprietary Preparations (details are given in Part 3)

Multi-ingredient: *Belg.:* Flammacerium; *Fr.:* Flammacerium; *Israel:* Flammacerium; *Neth.:* Flammacerium; *UK:* Flammacerium.

Crilanomer (2788-y)

Crilanomer *(rINN)*.
Acrylonitrile-starch Copolymer; ZK-94006. A starch polymer with acrylonitrile.
CAS — 37291-07-9.

Profile

Crilanomer is a starch copolymer used as a hydrogel wound dressing in the management of wounds.

Preparations

Proprietary Preparations (details are given in Part 3)
Austral.: Intrasite; *S.Afr.:* Intrasite.

Crotamiton (1603-m)

Crotamiton *(BAN, rINN)*.
Crotam; Crotamitonum. N-Ethyl-N-o-tolylcrotonamide; N-Ethylcrotono-o-toluidide; N-Ethyl-N-(2-methylphenyl)-2-butenamide.
$C_{13}H_{17}NO = 203.3$.
CAS — 483-63-6.
Pharmacopoeias. In Eur. (see p.vi) and US.

Pharmacopoeial description

Ph. Eur.: A colourless or pale yellow oily liquid. It solidifies partly or completely at low temperatures. It is predominantly the (E)-isomer, with not more than 15% of the (Z)-isomer.
Slightly soluble in water; miscible with alcohol. Store in well-filled containers. Protect from light.

USP 25: A colourless to slightly yellowish oil with a faint amine-like odour. It is a mixture of *cis*- and *trans*-isomers. Soluble in alcohol and in methyl alcohol. Store in airtight containers. Protect from light.

Adverse Effects and Precautions

Applied topically, crotamiton occasionally causes irritation. There have been rare reports of hypersensitivity reactions. Crotamiton should not be used in the presence of acute exudative dermatitis. It should not be applied near the eyes, mouth, or other mucous membranes or on excoriated skin.

Ingestion of crotamiton may cause burning and irritation of oral, oesophageal, and gastric mucosa with nausea, vomiting, and abdominal pain.

Overdosage. A report of a 23-year-old woman who developed tonic-clonic seizures requiring treatment with diazepam after ingestion of a crotamiton emulsion.[1] Other hospital treatment included gastric lavage, activated charcoal, and metoclopramide. Crotamiton was detected in serum at a concentration of 34 µg per mL and was also detectable with several metabolites in the urine. Reference was also made to a report of a 2½-month-old child who had developed pallor and cyanosis after excessive dermal application of a crotamiton cream.

1. Meredith TJ, et al. Crotamiton overdose. Hum Exp Toxicol 1990; **9:** 57.

Uses and Administration
Crotamiton is used as an antipruritic (p.1106), although its value is considered uncertain (see below). It is applied as a 10% cream or lotion 2 or 3 times daily; children aged less than 3 years may receive one application daily.

Crotamiton has also been used as an acaricide in the treatment of scabies but other more effective drugs are usually preferred (p.1427). The 10% cream or lotion is applied, after first bathing and drying, to the whole of the body surface below the chin, particular attention being paid to body folds and creases. A second application should be applied 24 hours later but it may need to be used once daily up to a total of 5 days to be effective.

Pruritus. A double-blind study in 31 patients[1] found that 10% crotamiton lotion was no more effective an antipruritic than its vehicle.

1. Smith EB, et al. Crotamiton lotion in pruritus. Int J Dermatol 1984; **23:** 684–5.

Preparations
BP 2001: Crotamiton Cream; Crotamiton Lotion;
USP 25: Crotamiton Cream.

Proprietary Preparations (details are given in Part 3)
Aust.: Eurax; *Austral.:* Eurax; *Belg.:* Eurax; *Canad.:* Eurax; *Fr.:* Eurax; *Ger.:* Crotamitex; Euraxil; *Hong Kong:* Eurax; *Irl.:* Eurax; *Israel:* Eurax; Scabicin; *Ital.:* Eurax; *Mex.:* Eurax; *Norw.:* Eurax; *NZ:* Eurax; *Port.:* Eurax; Scabicin†; *S.Afr.:* Eurax; *Singapore:* Eurax; Moz-Bite; *Spain:* Euraxil; *Switz.:* Eurax; *UK:* Eurax; *USA:* Eurax.

Multi-ingredient: *Fr.:* Acarcid; *Irl.:* Eurax-Hydrocortisone; *Israel:* Duo-Scabil; *Spain:* Euraxil Hidrocort; *UK:* Eurax-Hydrocortisone.

Dextranomer   (1604-b)
Dextranomer *(BAN, rINN)*.
Dextran cross-linked with epichlorohydrin (1-chloro-2,3-epoxypropane); Dextran 2,3-dihydroxypropyl 2-hydroxy-1,3-propanediyl ether.
CAS — 56087-11-7.
ATC — D03AX02.

Precautions
Dextranomer should not be used in deep wounds or cavities from which its removal cannot be assured, nor should it be used on dry wounds. Care should be exercised when paste formulations of dextranomer are used near the eyes.

Spillage may render surfaces very slippery.

◊ Implantation studies in *animals* indicated that entrapment of dextranomer beads in wounds was unlikely to initiate granuloma formation or chronic inflammation.[1] Most beads were apparently unchanged 3 years after implantation.

1. Falk J, Tollerz G. Chronic tissue response to implantation of Debrisan®: an experimental study. Clin Ther 1977; **1:** 185–91.

Uses and Administration
The action of dextranomer depends upon its ability to absorb up to 4 times its weight of fluid, including dissolved and suspended material of molecular weight up to about 5000.

Dextranomer is used for the cleansing of exudative and infected burns (p.1104), wounds and ulcers (p.1108), and for preparation for skin grafting.

The wound is cleansed with sterile water or saline and allowed to remain wet; dextranomer in the form of spherical beads is sprinkled on to a depth of at least 3 to 6 mm and covered with a sterile dressing. Occlusive dressings are not recommended as they may lead to maceration around the wound. The dextranomer can be renewed up to 5 times daily (usually once or twice daily), before the layer has become saturated with exudate; the old layer is washed off with a stream of sterile water or saline before renewal. All dextranomer must be removed before skin grafting. Dextranomer may also be applied as a paste (either ready-made or prepared by mixing 4 parts of the dextranomer beads with 1 part glycerol) or a paste-containing absorbent pad which need only be changed twice daily to every 2 days according to the rate of wound exudation.

Preparations
Proprietary Preparations (details are given in Part 3)
Aust.: Debrisorb; *Belg.:* Debrisan; *Canad.:* Debrisan†; *Fr.:* Debrisan†; *Ger.:* Debrisorb; *Hong Kong:* Debrisan; *Irl.:* Debrisan; *Israel:* Debrisan; *Ital.:* Debrisan; *Mex.:* Debrisan; *Neth.:* Debripad†; *Debrisan†; *S.Afr.:* Debrisan†; *Swed.:* Debrisan†; *Switz.:* Debrisan†; *UK:* Debrisan; *USA:* Debrisan.

Dihydroxyacetone   (1605-v)
DHA; Ketotriose. 1,3-Dihydroxypropan-2-one.
$C_3H_6O_3 = 90.08$.
CAS — 96-26-4.
Pharmacopoeias. In US.

Pharmacopoeial description
USP 25: A white to off-white crystalline powder. The monomeric form is freely soluble in water, in alcohol, and in ether; the dimeric form is freely soluble in water, soluble in alcohol, and sparingly soluble in ether. A 5% solution in water has a pH between 4.0 and 6.0. Store at a temperature of 8° to 15° in airtight containers.

Adverse Effects and Precautions
Skin irritation from dihydroxyacetone occurs rarely; rashes and allergic dermatitis have been reported. Contact with eyes, abraded skin, and clothing should be avoided.

Uses and Administration
Application to the skin of preparations containing dihydroxyacetone slowly produces a brown coloration similar to that caused by exposure to the sun, probably due to a reaction with the amino acids of the skin.

A single application may give rise to a patchy appearance; progressive darkening of the skin results from repeated use until a point is reached when the maximum effect is achieved. If the treatment is stopped the colour starts to fade after about 2 days and disappears completely within 8 to 14 days as the external epidermal cells are lost by normal attrition.

Preparations containing up to 8% (but usually 5%) of dihydroxyacetone have been used to camouflage vitiligo (see Pigmentation Disorders, p.1106) or to produce an artificial suntan. Some preparations include sunscreens since the pigmentation produced gives no protection against sunburn.

Preparations
Proprietary Preparations (details are given in Part 3)
Austral.: Le Tan Fast Extra Dark; Le Tan Fast Self Tan; Vitadye; *USA:* Chromelin Complexion Blender.
Multi-ingredient: *Austral.:* Le Tan Fast Plus; *USA:* QT.

Diphencyprone   (4896-w)
2,3-Diphenylcyclopropenone-1.
$C_{15}H_{10}O = 206.2$.
CAS — 886-38-4.

Profile
Diphencyprone has been applied as a contact sensitiser for the treatment of alopecia. It has also been tried in warts.

Adverse effects. Diphencyprone is considered to lack serious adverse effects but some patients may not be able to tolerate the induced hypersensitivity reaction and there have been reports of generalised urticaria following the use of diphencyprone.[1,2] Allergy to diphencyprone has been reported in medical and nursing staff in spite of taking protective precautions during its application.[3] One patient who received diphencyprone treatment for warts developed a widespread pruritic rash and palpitations due to ventricular extrasystoles.[2] Vitiligo has also been reported in patients treated with diphencyprone[4-6] and it has been suggested that this might be due to unmasking of subclinical vitiligo.[4,5] Erythema multiforme-like eruptions were associated with the topical application of diphencyprone in 3 patients.[7]

1. Tosti A, et al. Contact urticaria during topical immunotherapy. Contact Dermatitis 1989; **21:** 196–7.
2. Lane PR, Hogan DJ. Diphencyprone. J Am Acad Dermatol 1988; **19:** 364–5.
3. Shah M, et al. Hazards in the use of diphencyprone. Br J Dermatol 1996; **134:** 1151–65.
4. Hatzis J, et al. Vitiligo as a reaction to topical treatment with diphencyprone. Dermatologica 1988; **177:** 146–8.
5. Duhra P, Foulds IS. Persistent vitiligo induced by diphencyprone. Br J Dermatol 1990; **123:** 415–16.
6. Henderson CA, Ilchyshyn A. Vitiligo complicating diphencyprone sensitization therapy for alopecia universalis. Br J Dermatol 1995; **133:** 496–7.
7. Perret CM, et al. Erythema multiforme-like eruptions: a rare side effect of topical immunotherapy with diphenylcyclopropenone. Dermatologica 1990; **180:** 5–7.

Alopecia. Diphencyprone has been used with varying degrees of success in the treatment of various forms of alopecia (p.1104) including areata, totalis, and universalis.[1-6] While some workers have achieved good results in adults[1,2,4] and children[5,7] others have obtained little benefit using diphencyprone.[3] Induction of a delayed (type IV) hypersensitivity reaction after application of diphencyprone appears to be an integral part of successful treatment.[8] Sensitisation has been achieved by applying a 2% solution of diphencyprone in acetone to a small area of scalp but this may be repeated if necessary beneath plastic occlusion if adequate sensitisation is not produced.[4] Thereafter, weaker concentrations of 0.01 to 2% are applied and gradually increased in strength to produce erythema and pruritus for 36 hours post-therapy; treatment is repeated weekly. Only one side of the scalp is treated until the optimum concentration is found, in order to prevent a widespread adverse reaction. One group of patients who achieved total regrowth of hair were able to discontinue treatment with diphencyprone for a mean of 15 months without relapse[9] and

another group maintained satisfactory hair growth for a mean follow-up period of 19.8 months.[10]

1. MacDonald Hull S, Norris JF. Diphencyprone in the treatment of long-standing alopecia areata. Br J Dermatol 1988; **119:** 367–74.
2. Monk B, Williams HC. Topical diphencyprone therapy in alopecia totalis. Br J Dermatol 1988; **119** (suppl 33): 16.
3. Ashworth J, et al. Allergic and irritant contact dermatitis compared in the treatment of alopecia totalis and universalis: a comparison of the value of topical diphencyprone and tretinoin gel. Br J Dermatol 1989; **120:** 397–401.
4. MacDonald Hull S, Cunliffe WJ. Successful treatment of alopecia areata using the contact allergen diphencyprone. Br J Dermatol 1991; **124:** 212–13.
5. MacDonald Hull S, et al. Alopecia areata in children: response to treatment with diphencyprone. Br J Dermatol 1991; **125:** 164–8.
6. Hoting E, Boehm A. Therapy of alopecia areata with diphencyprone. Br J Dermatol 1992; **127:** 625–9.
7. Schuttelaar M-L, et al. Alopecia areata in children: treatment with diphencyprone. Br J Dermatol 1996; **135:** 581–5.
8. MacDonald Hull S, et al. Alopecia areata treated with diphencyprone: is an allergic response necessary? Br J Dermatol 1990; **122:** 716–17.
9. van der Steen PHM, et al. Topical immunotherapy for alopecia areata: re-evaluation of 139 cases after an additional follow-up period of 19 months. Dermatology 1992; **184:** 198–201.
10. Gordon PM, et al. Topical diphencyprone for alopecia areata: evaluation of 48 cases after 30 months' follow-up. Br J Dermatol 1996; **134:** 869–71.

Warts. Diphencyprone has been tried in the treatment of recalcitrant warts. The successful treatment of digital or plantar warts in 42 of 60 patients has been described.[1] The patients were initially sensitised with a 2% topical solution of diphencyprone, then the warts treated with solutions ranging from 0.01 to 6%.

1. Buckley DA, et al. Recalcitrant viral warts treated by diphencyprone immunotherapy. Br J Dermatol 1999; **141:** 292–6.

Dipyrithione   (3520-c)
Dipyrithione *(USAN, rINN)*.
OMDS. 2,2'-Dithiodipyridine 1,1'-dioxide.
$C_{10}H_8N_2O_2S_2 = 252.3$.
CAS — 3696-28-4.

Profile
Dipyrithione is reported to have antibacterial and antifungal properties and is included in preparations for the treatment of dandruff.

Preparations
Proprietary Preparations (details are given in Part 3)
Multi-ingredient: *Switz.:* Crimanex.

Dithiosalicylic Acid   (13417-w)
2-Hydroxybenzenecarbodithioic acid.
$C_7H_6OS_2 = 170.3$.
CAS — 527-89-9.

Profile
Dithiosalicylic acid has been used in multi-ingredient preparations used topically for the treatment of acne and seborrhoeic dermatitis.

Preparations
Proprietary Preparations (details are given in Part 3)
Multi-ingredient: *Fr.:* Sacnel†; *Ital.:* Sacnel.

Dithranol   (1606-g)
Dithranol *(BAN, rINN)*.
Anthralin; Dioxyanthranol; Dithranolum. 1,8-Dihydroxyanthrone; 1,8-Dihydroxy-9(10H)-anthracenone.
$C_{14}H_{10}O_3 = 226.2$.
CAS — 1143-38-0 (dithranol); 16203-97-7 (dithranol triacetate).
ATC — D05AC01.
Pharmacopoeias. In Chin., Eur. (see p.vi), and US.

Pharmacopoeial description
Ph. Eur.: A yellow or brownish-yellow, crystalline powder. Practically insoluble in water; slightly soluble in alcohol; sparingly soluble in acetone; soluble in dichloromethane; dissolves in dilute solutions of alkali hydroxides. Protect from light.

USP 25: A yellowish-brown, odourless, crystalline powder. Insoluble in water; slightly soluble in alcohol, in ether, and in glacial acetic acid; soluble in acetone, in chloroform, in benzene, and in solutions of alkali hydroxides. The filtrate from a suspension in water is neutral to litmus. Store at a temperature of 8° to 15° in airtight containers. Protect from light.

◊ CAUTION. *Dithranol is a powerful irritant and should be kept away from the eyes and tender parts of the skin.*

Stability. The stability of dithranol has been studied in a number of bases and vehicles.[1,2] The weaker preparations of dithranol may be less stable.[1] Salicylic acid is included in dithranol preparations as an antioxidant and prevents their discoloration due to the inactivation of dithranol by zinc oxide.[3] However, zinc ox-

---

The symbol † denotes a preparation no longer actively marketed

ide or starch can be omitted from dithranol pastes without loss of effectiveness provided stiffness is maintained.[3] Addition of ascorbic or oxalic acid may improve dithranol's stability in 'Unguentum Merck' but salicylic acid appears to be ineffective.[1] The effect of salicylic acid on the instability of dithranol in yellow soft paraffin is variable[1,2] and its inclusion has been questioned as it can be irritant and percutaneous absorption can be significant.[1] Dithranol is relatively stable in white soft paraffin.[1]

The application of any type of heat and contact with metal spatulas should be avoided during the manufacture of dithranol pastes[4] and if milling facilities are not available dithranol can be incorporated into Lassar's paste by dissolving it first in chloroform.[3]

1. Green PG, *et al.* The stability of dithranol in various bases. *Br J Dermatol* 1985; **113** (suppl 29): 26.
2. Lee RLH. Stability of dithranol (anthralin) in various vehicles. *Aust J Hosp Pharm* 1987; **17**: 254–8.
3. Comaish S, *et al.* Factors affecting the clearance of psoriasis with dithranol (anthralin). *Br J Dermatol* 1971; **84**: 282–9.
4. *PSGB Lab Report P/79/1* 1979.

Adverse Effects and Precautions

Dithranol may cause a burning sensation especially on perilesional skin. Patients with fair skin may be more sensitive than those with dark skin. It is irritant to the eyes and mucous membranes. Use on the face, skin flexures, and genitals should be avoided. Hands should be washed after use.

Dithranol should not be used for acute or pustular psoriasis or on inflamed skin. It stains skin, hair, some fabrics, plastics, and enamel. Staining of bathroom ware may be less of a problem with creams than ointments. Stains on skin and hair disappear on cessation of treatment although such disappearance may be slow.

Uses and Administration

Dithranol is used in the treatment of subacute and chronic psoriasis, usually in one of two ways.

Conventional treatment is commonly started with an ointment or paste containing 0.1% dithranol (0.05% in very fair patients) applied for a few hours; the strength is gradually increased as necessary to 0.5%, occasionally to 1%, and the duration of contact extended to overnight periods or longer. The preparation is sparingly and accurately applied to the lesions only. If, on initial treatment, lesions spread or excessive irritation occurs, the concentration of dithranol or the frequency of application should be reduced; if necessary, treatment should be stopped. After each treatment period the patient should bathe or shower to remove any residual dithranol.

For *short-contact therapy* dithranol is usually applied in a soft basis to the lesions for up to 60 minutes daily, before being washed off. As with conventional treatment the strength used is gradually increased from 0.1 to 2% but strengths up to 5% have been used. Surrounding unaffected skin may be protected by white soft paraffin.

Treatment for psoriasis should be continued until the skin is entirely clear. Intermittent courses may be needed to maintain the response. Treatment schedules often involve coal tar and UV irradiation (preferably UVB) before the application of dithranol (see below). Salicylic acid is included in many topical preparations of dithranol.

A cream containing dithranol triacetate 1% has been used similarly to dithranol in conventional treatment of psoriasis.

Psoriasis. Dithranol used alone or with coal tar, (with or without ultraviolet light), continues to be one of the drugs of first-line treatment for psoriasis (p.1106). It is particularly suited to the treatment of stable chronic plaque psoriasis but unlike coal tar, is irritant to healthy skin and care is required to ensure that it is only applied to lesions. Treatment with dithranol is therefore more feasible when the plaques are large, or few in number. Concomitant use of coal tar may help to reduce the irritant effects of dithranol without affecting efficacy. Traditional treatment with dithranol is time consuming and more suitable for use on hospital inpatients. Dithranol formulated in stiff preparations such as Lassar's paste to minimise spreading to perilesional skin is left on overnight covered with a suitable dressing and washed off the next day. Treatment is usually initiated with a concentration of 0.1% (0.05% in fair-skinned patients) and gradually increased according to the response and irritation produced. Cream formulations may be less effective

but are more suitable for domestic use. Short-contact therapy in which concentrations of up to 5% of dithranol are applied daily for up to 1 hour is more suitable for use on an outpatient basis and there appears to be little reduction in efficacy; irritation and staining may also be reduced.

Dithranol is also used with UVB phototherapy and there have been many modifications of the original Ingram's regimen in which dithranol is applied after bathing in a tar bath and exposure to ultraviolet light. Inpatient stays of up to 3 weeks may be required but long periods of remission can be obtained.

Preparations

BP 2001: Dithranol Cream; Dithranol Ointment; Dithranol Paste;
USP 25: Anthralin Cream; Anthralin Ointment.

Proprietary Preparations (details are given in Part 3)
Aust.: Micanol; *Austral.:* Dithrocream; *Braz.:* Antranol; *Canad.:* Anthraforte; Anthranol; Anthrascalp; Micanol; *Fin.:* Micanol; *Ger.:* Micanol; *Irl.:* Dithrocream; Micanol; *Israel:* Dithrocream; Micanol; *Ital.:* Psoriderm; Timicolid; *Mex.:* Anthranol; *Neth.:* Psoricreme; *Norw.:* Micanol; *Port.:* Desmoline; Micanol; *S.Afr.:* Anthranol†; *Singapore:* Micanol; *Spain:* Anthranol; *Swed.:* Micanol; *Thai.:* Micanol; *UK:* Dithrocream; Micanol; *USA:* Anthra-Derm; Dritho-Scalp; Drithocreme; Micanol.

Multi-ingredient: *Aust.:* Anthraderm; Psoradexan†; *Austral.:* Dithrasal; *Fr.:* Anaxeryl; *Ger.:* Psoradexan; Psoralon MT; *Irl.:* Psoradrate; *Spain:* Lapices Epiderm Metadier; Psorantral; *Switz.:* Psoradexan†; *UK:* Psorin.

Ethyl Lactate   (16638-n)

$C_5H_{10}O_3 = 118.1$.
CAS — 97-64-3.

Profile

Ethyl lactate has been applied topically in the treatment of acne vulgaris. It is reported to lower the pH within the skin thereby exerting a bactericidal effect.

Ethyl lactate is also used in the flavouring of foods.

Etretinate   (1609-s)

Etretinate (BAN, USAN, rINN).
Ro-10-9359. Ethyl 3-methoxy-15-apo-φ-caroten-15-oate; Ethyl (all-trans)-9-(4-methoxy-2,3,6-trimethylphenyl)-3,7-dimethyl-nona-2,4,6,8-tetra-enoate.
$C_{23}H_{30}O_3 = 354.5$.
CAS — 54350-48-0.
ATC — D05BB01.

Adverse Effects and Precautions

As for Isotretinoin, p.1115.

Donation of blood should be avoided for at least 2 years after cessation of treatment. The period of time during which pregnancy must be avoided following cessation of treatment has not been determined; detectable plasma-etretinate concentrations have been reported nearly 3 years after stopping treatment.

◊ In addition to the references cited below under the various headings, further references to the adverse effects of etretinate can be found in Isotretinoin, p.1116, under Effects on the Blood, Eyes, Liver, Musculoskeletal System, Serum Lipids, and the Skin as well as under Vasculitic Syndromes.

Carcinogenicity. A report of 2 patients developing lymphomas while receiving etretinate[1] prompted a report of 3 other malignancies in patients taking etretinate.[2]

1. Woll PJ, *et al.* Lymphoma in patients taking etretinate. *Lancet* 1987; **ii:** 563–4.
2. Harrison PV. Retinoids and malignancy. *Lancet* 1987; **ii:** 801.

Effects on the cardiovascular system. The Italian Ministry of Health recommended[1] that the ECG, blood lipids, and clotting factors should be monitored before, and throughout, treatment with etretinate as there had been rare suspected cases of myocardial ischaemia and infarction.

1. Anonymous. Reports from regulatory agencies: etretinate. *WHO Drug Inf* 1987; **1:** 29.

Effects on the kidneys. A report of impaired renal function associated with etretinate in a patient.[1] It was noted that in manufacturer-sponsored studies the mean serum-creatinine concentration had been raised in patients receiving etretinate.

1. Horber FF, *et al.* Impaired renal function and hypercalcaemia associated with etretinate. *Lancet* 1984; **ii:** 1093.

Oedema. A report of generalised oedema following treatment with etretinate.[1] Five other cases had been reported in the literature and rechallenge in 4 patients had provoked a recurrence.

1. Allan S, Christmas T. Severe edema associated with etretinate. *J Am Acad Dermatol* 1988; **19:** 140.

Interactions

As for Isotretinoin, p.1117.

Methotrexate. The risk of developing hepatotoxicity may be increased by concomitant administration of etretinate and methotrexate (see p.555).

Oral contraceptives. For discussion of the potential interactions of retinoids with hormonal contraceptives, and the effect this might have on contraceptive choice during retinoid treatment, see p.1459.

Warfarin. Etretinate has been reported to reduce the therapeutic efficacy of warfarin (see p.996).

Pharmacokinetics

The mean bioavailability of etretinate is about 40% following oral administration but there is a large interindividual variation. Absorption can be increased by administration with milk or fatty food. Etretinate undergoes significant first-pass metabolism and plasma concentrations of the active carboxylic acid metabolite, acitretin (p.1109), may be detected before those of the parent drug; acitretin may itself be metabolised to etretinate (p.1109). Both etretinate and acitretin are extensively bound to plasma protein. Etretinate appears to accumulate in adipose tissue after repeated dosing and has a prolonged elimination half-life of about 120 days; detectable serum concentrations have been observed up to 3 years after the discontinuation of therapy. Up to 75% of a dose is excreted in the faeces mainly as unchanged drug. Etretinate is also excreted in the urine as metabolites. Etretinate crosses the placenta and is distributed into breast milk.

◊ References.

1. Brazzell RK, Colburn WA. Pharmacokinetics of the retinoids isotretinoin and etretinate. *J Am Acad Dermatol* 1982; **6:** 643–51.
2. Rollman O, Vahlquist A. Retinoid concentrations in skin, serum and adipose tissue of patients treated with etretinate. *Br J Dermatol* 1983; **109:** 439–47.
3. Colburn WA, *et al.* Effect of meals on the kinetics of etretinate. *J Clin Pharmacol* 1985; **25:** 583–9.
4. Lucek RW, Colburn WA. Clinical pharmacokinetics of the retinoids. *Clin Pharmacokinet* 1985; **10:** 38–62.
5. DiGiovanna JJ, *et al.* Etretinate: persistent serum levels after long-term therapy. *Arch Dermatol* 1989; **125:** 246–51.

Uses and Administration

Etretinate is a retinoid and is a derivative of tretinoin (p.1126). It has been given by mouth for the treatment of severe, extensive psoriasis that has not responded to other treatment, especially generalised and palmo-plantar pustular psoriasis. It has also been used in severe congenital ichthyosis, and severe Darier's disease (keratosis follicularis) as well as other disorders of keratinisation. Acitretin (p.1109) is now preferred to etretinate.

Therapy generally starts at a dosage of 0.75 to 1 mg per kg body-weight daily in divided doses by mouth. A maximum dose of 1.5 mg per kg daily should not be exceeded (some sources have suggested a maximum of 75 mg daily). Erythrodermic psoriasis may respond to lower initial doses of 0.25 mg per kg daily, increased at weekly intervals by 0.25 mg per kg daily until optimal response occurs. Following the initial response, generally after 8 to 16 weeks of therapy, maintenance doses of 0.5 to 0.75 mg per kg daily have been given. Therapy should be discontinued once lesions have sufficiently resolved.

Preparations

Proprietary Preparations (details are given in Part 3)
Braz.: Tigason; *Ital.:* Tigason†; *USA:* Tegison†.

Fumaric Acid   (1310-y)

Allomalenic Acid; Boletic Acid; E297. *trans*-Butenedioic acid.
$C_2H_2(CO_2H)_2 = 116.1$.
CAS — 110-17-8 (fumaric acid); 624-49-7 (dimethyl fumarate).
ATC — D05AX01.
Pharmacopoeias. In *Pol.* Also in *USNF.*

Pharmacopoeial description

USNF 20: White, odourless granules or crystalline powder. Slightly soluble in water and in ether; soluble in alcohol; very slightly soluble in chloroform.

Profile

Fumaric acid and some of its derivatives have been used in the treatment of psoriasis and other skin disorders.

Fumaric acid is also used as an acidifier and flavouring agent in foods.

Skin disorders. Fumaric acid, its sodium salts, and derivatives such as dimethyl fumarate, monoethyl fumarate (ethyl hydrogen fumarate), and octil hydrogen fumarate have been used, both topically and systemically, in the treatment of psoriasis (p.1106) and other skin disorders. Dimethyl fumarate appears to be the most active compound given orally but combination with various salts of monoethyl fumarate has been claimed to improve efficacy.[1-5] However, there have been reports of acute renal failure associated with treatment and the German Federal Office of Health has expressed the opinion that the available evidence did not establish the value of fumaric acid derivatives in psoriasis or other skin disorders.[6] Other adverse effects with oral therapy have included disturbances of liver function,[3,7] gastrointestinal effects,[2-4,7,8] and flushing.[2-4,7,8]

1. van Loenen AC, *et al.* Fumaarzuurtherapie: van fictie tot werkelijkheid? *Pharm Weekbl* 1989; **124:** 894–900.
2. Kolbach DN, Nieboer C. Fumaric acid therapy in psoriasis: a long-term retrospective study on the effect of fumaric acid combination (FAC-EC) therapy and dimethyl-fumaric acid ester (DMFAE) monotherapy. *Br J Dermatol* 1990; **123:** 534–5.
3. Nugteren-Huying WM, *et al.* Fumaric acid therapy for psoriasis: a randomized, double-blind, placebo-controlled study. *J Am Acad Dermatol* 1990; **22:** 311–12.
4. Altmeyer PJ, *et al.* Antipsoriatic effect of fumaric acid derivatives: results of a multicenter double-blind study in 100 patients. *J Am Acad Dermatol* 1994; **30:** 977–81.
5. Mrowietz U, *et al.* Treatment of severe psoriasis with fumaric acid esters: scientific background and guidelines for therapeutic use. *Br J Dermatol* 1999; **141:** 424–9.

6. Anonymous. Fumaric acid derivatives and nephrotoxicity. *WHO Drug Inf* 1990; **4:** 28.
7. Nieboer C, *et al.* Systemic therapy with fumaric acid derivates: new possibilities in the treatment of psoriasis. *J Am Acad Dermatol* 1989; **20:** 601–8.
8. Mrowietz U, *et al.* Treatment of psoriasis with fumaric acid esters: results of a prospective multicentre study. *Br J Dermatol* 1998; **138:** 456–60.

Preparations

Proprietary Preparations (details are given in Part 3)
Ger.: Psoriasis-Solution†; Psoriasis-Tabletten†.

Multi-ingredient: *Austral.:* Pro-PS; *Ger.:* Fumaderm; Psoriasis-Bad†; Psoriasis-Salbe M†.

Glycolic Acid (8922-v)

Hydroxyacetic Acid. Hydroxyethanoic acid.
$C_2H_4O_3 = 76.05$.

Profile

Glycolic acid is an organic acid that has been used in topical preparations for hyperpigmentation and photodamaged skin.

Preparations

Proprietary Preparations (details are given in Part 3)
Canad.: Neostrata; Reversa AHA; *Hong Kong:* Glyderm; *Ital.:* Neostrata; Revitalizing; *Mex.:* Glicoderm; Nova Derm; *Singapore:* Glyderm.

Multi-ingredient: *Austral.:* Neostrata; *Canad.:* Dilusol AHA; Neostrata AHA Blemish; Neostrata AHA Daytime; Neostrata AHA Smoothing and Moisturizing; Reversa AHA HQ; Viquin Forte; *Ital.:* Acnesan; Lightening; NeoCeuticals Spot Treatment; Phytic Acid; *Mex.:* Nova Derm; *Port.:* Eutrofic Forte Gel Despigmentante; Hyfac AHA; Ureadin 30; *Singapore:* AHA Skin Lightening Gel.

Hydroquinone (1612-b)

Hydrochinonum; Quinol. 1,4-Benzenediol.
$C_6H_6O_2 = 110.1$.
CAS — 123-31-9.

NOTE. Do not confuse with Hydroquinine (p.1622).
Pharmacopoeias. In Belg. and US.

Pharmacopoeial description

USP 25: Fine white needles which darken on exposure to light and air. Soluble 1 in 17 of water, 1 in 4 of alcohol, 1 in 51 of chloroform, and 1 in 16.5 of ether. Store in airtight containers. Protect from light.

Adverse Effects, Treatment, and Precautions

Topical hydroquinone may cause transient erythema and a mild burning sensation. High concentrations or prolonged use may produce hyperpigmentation especially on areas of skin exposed to sunlight. Occasionally hypersensitivity has occurred and some recommend skin testing before use. Hydroquinone should not be applied to abraded or sunburnt skin. It should not be used to bleach eyelashes or eyebrows and contact with the eyes should be avoided as it may produce staining and corneal opacities. The systemic effects of hydroquinone and their treatment are similar to those of phenol (see p.1152) but tremors and convulsions may also occur.

Effects on the liver. Toxic hepatitis in a radiographer was attributed to occupational exposure to hydroquinone fumes from the developing medium used in the darkroom.[1] However, it has been pointed out[2] that hydroquinone is not volatile under normal conditions of use and that surveillance of 879 people engaged in the manufacture and use of hydroquinone from 1942 to 1990 found no association between toxic hepatitis and hydroquinone exposure.
1. Nowak AK, *et al.* Darkroom hepatitis after exposure to hydroquinone. *Lancet* 1995; **345:** 1187.
2. O'Donaghue JL, *et al.* Hydroquinone and hepatitis. *Lancet* 1995; **346:** 1427–8.

Effects on the skin. The incidence of exogenous ochronosis (blue-black hyperpigmentation) in a survey of black South African patients was found to be 15% in males and 42% in females with 69% of affected individuals admitting to using hydroquinone-containing preparations.[1] This was considered to be more consistent with a toxic side-effect of a drug with a low therapeutic index, rather than an idiosyncratic reaction. The data revealed that even preparations with hydroquinone 2% or less with a sunscreen produced ochronosis. Ochronosis usually became apparent after about 6 months of use and, once established, was probably irreversible. Patients may initially use skin lighteners for cosmetic purposes but once ochronosis develops they may fall into the 'skin lightener trap' as they use other hydroquinone preparations to remove the disfigurement.[1] The problems caused by over-the-counter skin-lightening creams in countries such as the UK have also been highlighted.[2] Reversible brown discoloration of the nails has also been

reported following the use of skin lighteners containing hydroquinone.[3]
1. Hardwick N, *et al.* Exogenous ochronosis: an epidemiological study. *Br J Dermatol* 1989; **120:** 229–38.
2. Williams H. Skin lightening creams containing hydroquinone. *BMJ* 1992; **305:** 903–4.
3. Mann RJ, Harman RRM. Nail staining due to hydroquinone skin-lightening creams. *Br J Dermatol* 1983; **108:** 363–5.

Uses and Administration

Hydroquinone increases melanin excretion from melanocytes and may also prevent its production. Hydroquinone is used topically as a depigmenting agent for the skin in hyperpigmentation conditions (p.1106) such as chloasma (melasma), freckles, and lentigines (small macules that resemble freckles). Concentrations of 2 to 4% are commonly employed; higher concentrations may be very irritant and increase the risk of ochronosis. It may be several weeks before any effect is apparent but depigmentation may last for 2 to 6 months after discontinuation. Application of hydroquinone should be discontinued if there is no improvement after 2 months of treatment. Hydroquinone should be applied twice daily only to intact skin which should be protected from sunlight to reduce repigmentation. Hydroquinone preparations often include a sunscreen or a sunblocking basis.

Hydroquinone is also used as an antioxidant for ether and in photographic developers.

Preparations

USP 25: Hydroquinone Cream; Hydroquinone Topical Solution.

Proprietary Preparations (details are given in Part 3)
Canad.: African Gold; Banishing Cream; Eldopaque; Eldoquin; Esoterica Regular; Esoterica Unscented; Jouvence†; Nadinola; Neostrata HQ; Porcelana; Ultraquin Plain; *Fr.:* Aida; Creme des 3 Fleurs d'Orient; *Hong Kong:* Eldopaque; Eldoquin; Solaquin; *Ital.:* Discromil; Epocler; *Mex.:* Crema Blanca; Eldopaque; Eldoquin; Hidroquin; *NZ:* Eldoquin; Solaquin; *Singapore:* Aida; Eldopaque; Eldoquin; Melanex; Melanox; Solaquin; *UK:* Esoterica†; *USA:* Claripel; Eldopaque; Eldoquin; Esoterica Sensitive Skin and Regular; Lustra; Melanex; Melpaque HP†; Melquin HP†; Neostrata AHA†; Porcelana†; Solaquin.

Multi-ingredient: *Austral.:* Superfade; *Canad.:* Esoterica; Porcelana with Sunscreen; Reversa AHA HQ; Skinicles; Solaquin Forte; Ultraquin; Viquin Forte; *Fr.:* Melanex Duo; *Ger.:* Pigmanorm; *Mex.:* Nova Derm; Solaquin; *Port.:* Eutrofic Forte Gel Despigmentante; Melanex Duo†; *Singapore:* AHA Skin Lightening Gel; High Potency Lightening Serum; *Switz.:* Pigmanorm; *USA:* Ambi Skin Tone; Esoterica Facial and Sunscreen; Nuquin HP†; Porcelana with Sunscreen†; Solaquin Forte; Viquin Forte†.

Ichthammol (1615-q)

Ichthammol (BAN).

Ammonii Sulfogyrodalas; Ammonio Sulfoittiolato; Ammonium Bithiolicum; Ammonium Bitumenosulfonicum; Ammonium Bituminosulphonate; Ammonium Ichthosulphonate; Ammonium Sulfobituminosum; Ammonium Sulpho-Ichthyolate; Bithiolate Ammonique; Bithyol; Bituminol; Ichthammolum; Ichthosulphol; Ichthyol; Ichthyolammonium.
CAS — 8029-68-3.
Pharmacopoeias. In Chin., Eur. (see p.vi), Jpn, Pol., and US.

Light Ammonium Bituminosulfonate (Ammoniumbituminosulfonat Hell) is produced from the light distillate fraction of shale oil.

Ammoniumsulfobitol, an ammonium bituminosulfonate similar to ichthammol but with a low sulfur content, is commercially available as Tumenol Ammonium.

Ichthammol is incompatible with wool alcohols.

Pharmacopoeial description

Ph. Eur.: Ichthammol is a dense blackish-brown liquid. It is obtained by distillation of certain bituminous schists, sulfonation of the distillate, and neutralisation of the product with ammonia. It contains not less than 4.5% and not more than 7.0% of total ammonia, not less than 10.5% of organically combined sulfur, calculated with reference to the dried substance, and not more than 20% of the total sulfur in the form of sulfates.

Miscible with water and with glycerol; slightly soluble in alcohol, in ether, in fatty oils, and in liquid paraffin; forms homogeneous mixtures with wool fat and soft paraffin.

USP 25: Ichthammol is a reddish-brown to brownish-black viscous fluid with a strong characteristic empyreumatic odour. It is obtained by the destructive distillation of a bituminous schist, sulfonation of the distillate, and neutralisation of the product with ammonia. It yields not less than 10.0% of total sulfur and not less than 2.5% of ammonia. Miscible with water, with glycerol, and with fixed oils and fats. Partially soluble in alcohol and in ether.

Profile

Ichthammol has slight bacteriostatic properties and is used in a wide range of topical preparations, for a variety of skin disorders; it has also been used in suppositories for anorectal disor-

ders. Ichthammol is often used with zinc oxide in medicated bandages for chronic lichenified eczema (p.1105). Ichthammol may be slightly irritant to the skin and there have been rare reports of hypersensitivity.

Preparations

BP 2001: Zinc and Ichthammol Cream;
USP 25: Ichthammol Ointment.

Proprietary Preparations (details are given in Part 3)
Aust.: Ichtho-Bad; Ichtholan; Ichtopur; *Austral.:* Egoderm Cream; *Fr.:* Gelictar; *Ger.:* Ichtho-Bad; Ichtholan; Ichtholan spezial; Ichthyol Hochviskose Flussigkeit; Schwarze-Salbe†; Thiobitum; *Hong Kong:* Egoderm Cream; *Switz.:* Ichtho-Bad; Ichtholan.

Multi-ingredient: *Aust.:* Aknemycin compositum; Delta-Hadensa; Hadensa; Ichth-Oestren; Inotyol; *Austral.:* Acnederm; Egoderm Ointment; Icthaband; *Belg.:* Inotyol; Zinc-Ichtyol; *Canad.:* Boil Ease; Ictholin†; *Denm.:* Inotyol; *Fin.:* Hadensa; *Fr.:* Anaxeryl; Gelictar Fort; Inotyol; Oxythyol; Phytolithe; *Ger.:* Aknemycin; Hoemarin Derma; Rheumichthol Bad†; *Hong Kong:* Acnederm; Egoderm Ointment; *Israel:* Aknemycin; Inotyol; *Ital.:* Antiemorroidali; Bal Tart†; Dermatar; Ichthopaste; Inotyol; *Norw.:* Inotyol; *NZ:* Acnederm; Egoderm; *Port.:* Oleoban Composto; Pansebase Composto†; Secpel Composto; *S.Afr.:* Antipeol; *Singapore:* Acnederm; Egoderm; *Spain:* Hadensa; Ictiomen; Lamnotyl; Queratil; *Swed.:* Inotyol; *Switz.:* Aknemycin; Bain extra-doux dermatologique Nouvelle Formule; Furodermal; Furodermil†; Phlogidermil†; Riccomycine†; Riccovitan; *UK:* Antipeol; Ichthopaste; Icthaband; St James Balm; *USA:* Boil Ease; Boyol Salve; Medicone Derma.

Ictasol (6045-g)

Ictasol (USAN).

Ichthyol-Natrium Hell; Light Sodium Bituminosulphonate; Natrium Sulfobituminosum Decoloratum.
$C_{28}H_{36}N_2O_6S_3 = 610.8$.
CAS — 12542-33-5; 1340-06-3.

Sodium bituminosulfonate is obtained by the destructive distillation of certain bituminous schists, sulfonation of the distillate, and neutralisation of the product with sodium hydroxide. Ictasol is a sodium bituminosulfonate produced from the light distillate fraction of shale oil.

Profile

Ictasol has similar properties to ichthammol (above) and is used in a wide range of preparations for a variety of skin disorders.

Preparations

Proprietary Preparations (details are given in Part 3)
Aust.: Ichthraletten; Lavichthol; Solutio Cordes; *Ger.:* Aknichthol Creme; Crino Cordes N; Dermichthol; Ichthoderm; Ichtholan T; Ichthosin; Ichthraletten; Leukichtan N†; Solutio Cordes; *Switz.:* Ichthraletten†.

Multi-ingredient: *Aust.:* Aknichthol; Crino Cordes; Ichthalgan forte; Ichtho-Bellol; Ichtho-Cadmin; Ichtho-Cortin; Leukichtan; Pelvichthol†; *Fr.:* Ichtyosoft; Sebosquam; *Ger.:* Aknederm Neu; Aknichthol N; Ichthalgan; Ichtho-Bellol; Ichtho-Bellol compositum S; Ichthocortin; Ichthoseptal; Pelvichthol N; *Switz.:* Aknichthol N.

Isotretinoin (1616-p)

Isotretinoin (BAN, USAN, rINN).

Isotretinoinum; 13-cis-Retinoic Acid; Ro-4-3780. (13Z)-15-Apo-β-caroten-15-oic acid; (2Z,4E,6E,8E)-3,7-Dimethyl-9-(2,6,6-trimethylcyclohex-1-enyl)nona-2,4,6,8-tetraenoic acid.
$C_{20}H_{28}O_2 = 300.4$.
CAS — 4759-48-2.
ATC — D10AD04; D10BA01.
Pharmacopoeias. In Eur. (see p.vi) and US.

Pharmacopoeial description

Ph. Eur.: A yellow or light orange, crystalline powder. Practically insoluble in water; slightly soluble in alcohol; soluble in dichloromethane. It is sensitive to air, heat, and light, especially in solution. Store in airtight containers at a temperature not exceeding 25°. Protect from light. It is recommended that the contents of an opened container be used as soon as possible and that any unused part be protected by an atmosphere of an inert gas.

USP 25: Yellow crystals. Practically insoluble in water; sparingly soluble in alcohol, in isopropyl alcohol, and in macrogol 400; soluble in chloroform. Store in airtight containers under an atmosphere of an inert gas. Protect from light.

Adverse Effects

The adverse effects of isotretinoin and other oral retinoids are similar to those of vitamin A (see p.1382) and are generally reversible and dose-related. The most common are dryness of the mucous membranes and of the skin with scaling, fragility, and erythema, especially of the face, cheilitis, pruritus, epistaxis, conjunctivitis, dry sore mouth, and palmoplantar exfoliation. Corneal opacities, dry eyes, visual disturbances, skeletal hyperostosis, and musculoskel-

The symbol † denotes a preparation no longer actively marketed

etal symptoms may also occur. Elevation of serum triglycerides, hepatic enzymes, erythrocyte sedimentation rate, and blood glucose have been reported. Pancreatitis may occur, in particular in patients with high triglyceride concentrations. Other effects have included hair thinning (occasionally irreversible), photosensitivity, changes in skin pigmentation, paronychia, gastrointestinal symptoms, jaundice or hepatitis, headache, drowsiness, sweating, mood changes, psychotic symptoms, depression, suicidal behaviour, benign intracranial hypertension, seizures, vasculitis, hypersensitivity reactions including anaphylaxis, and an association with skin infections and an inflammatory bowel syndrome.

Isotretinoin and other retinoids are teratogenic.

When isotretinoin is applied topically the adverse effects are similar to those of tretinoin (see p.1126).

◊ General references.
1. David M, et al. Adverse effects of retinoids. Med Toxicol 1988; 3: 273–88.
2. Keefe M. Adverse reactions profile: retinoids. Prescribers' J 1995; 35: 71–6.

Effects on the blood. Thrombocytopenia has been reported in 2 patients receiving etretinate and in a patient treated with isotretinoin.[1] There has also been a report of agranulocytosis associated with isotretinoin therapy in a 16-year-old boy.[2]
1. Naldi L, et al. Etretinate therapy and thrombocytopenia. Br J Dermatol 1991; 124: 395.
2. Waisman M. Agranulocytosis from isotretinoin. J Am Acad Dermatol 1988; 18: 395–6.

Effects on the eyes. Corneal opacities and papilloedema are among the more serious effects of isotretinoin on the eye but they are usually reversible if therapy is discontinued; papilloedema can result from benign intracranial hypertension[1,2] and patients receiving concomitant treatment with tetracyclines are particularly at risk.[2] Oral retinoids appear to interfere with retinal function[3] and there have been reports of alterations in colour sense,[4] poor night vision, and photophobia.[5] However, a 1-year follow-up failed to find any evidence of ocular toxicity attributable to etretinate in patients who had received long-term treatment and one patient who had toxic optic neuropathy due to methotrexate was able to continue treatment with etretinate.[6] A unilateral subconjunctival haemorrhage occurred during a 16-week course of isotretinoin in a patient being treated for acne.[7]

Ectropion has been associated with etretinate therapy in a patient.[8]
1. Fraunfelder FT, et al. Adverse ocular reactions possibly associated with isotretinoin. Am J Ophthalmol 1985; 100: 534–7.
2. Gibberd B. Drug-induced benign intracranial hypertension. Prescribers' J 1991; 31: 118–21.
3. Brown RD, Grattan CEH. Visual toxicity of synthetic retinoids. Br J Ophthalmol 1989; 73: 286–8.
4. Weber U, et al. Abnormal retinal function associated with long-term etretinate? Lancet 1988; i: 235–6.
5. Weleber RG, et al. Abnormal retinal function associated with isotretinoin therapy for acne. Arch Ophthalmol 1986; 104: 831–7.
6. Pitts JF, et al. Etretinate and visual function: a 1-year follow-up study. Br J Dermatol 1991; 125: 53–5.
7. Azurdia RM, Sharpe GR. Isotretinoin treatment for acne vulgaris and its cutaneous and ocular side-effects. Br J Dermatol 1999; 141: 941.
8. Brenner S, et al. Ectropion: an adverse effect of etretinate therapy for psoriasis. DICP Ann Pharmacother 1990; 24: 1007.

Effects on the liver. Transient slight elevations of serum concentrations of liver enzymes are common with etretinate, but there have been few reports of acute hepatitis[1,2] or cholestatic jaundice.[3] In one patient, acute hepatitis progressed to chronic active hepatitis, despite cessation of etretinate therapy[4] but studies of serial liver biopsies from patients receiving long-term etretinate have failed to show any significant chronic liver damage.[5-7] The manufacturers have reported instances of hepatic fibrosis, necrosis, and/or cirrhosis.

An overview considered that some form of hepatotoxicity may be seen in up to 20% of patients treated with etretinate and significant liver disease in 1%.[8]

Isotretinoin may also cause mild elevations of liver enzymes and the manufacturers state that jaundice and hepatitis have occurred rarely. There is also a report of fatty liver.[9]
1. Foged EK, Jacobsen FK. Side effects due to RO 10-9359 (Tigason). Dermatologica 1982; 164: 395–403.
2. Weiss VC, et al. Hepatotoxic reactions in a patient treated with etretinate. Arch Dermatol 1984; 120: 104–6.
3. Gavish D, et al. Cholestatic jaundice, an unusual side effect of etretinate. J Am Acad Dermatol 1985; 13: 669–70.
4. Weiss VC, et al. Chronic active hepatitis associated with etretinate therapy. Br J Dermatol 1985; 112: 591–7.
5. Glazer SD, et al. Ultrastructural survey and tissue analysis of human livers after a 6-month course of etretinate. J Am Acad Dermatol 1984; 10: 632–8.
6. Foged E, et al. Histologic changes in the liver during etretinate treatment. J Am Acad Dermatol 1984; 11: 580–3.
7. Roenigk HH, et al. Serial liver biopsies in psoriatic patients receiving long-term etretinate. Br J Dermatol 1985; 112: 77–81.

8. Boyd AS. An overview of the retinoids. Am J Med 1989; 86: 568–74.
9. Taylor AEM, Mitchison H. Fatty liver following isotretinoin therapy. Br J Dermatol 1991; 124: 505–6.

Effects on the musculoskeletal system. An ossification disorder resembling diffuse skeletal hyperostosis, with myalgia, arthralgia, and stiffness was first reported in patients who had taken large doses of isotretinoin for prolonged periods.[1] Premature closure of the epiphyses in a child treated with isotretinoin has also been described.[2] A later report found radiographic evidence of extraspinal tendon and ligament calcification in patients who had received long-term therapy with etretinate[3] and there were reports of spinal hyperostosis[4] and one of spinal cord compression.[5] Some were unable to find radiographic skeletal changes after 6 to 18 months of treatment with etretinate[6] but others[7] found that hyperostosis was fairly common in patients taking moderately prolonged therapy and recommended that radiological examinations should be carried out every 12 months in patients taking etretinate. However, there was no clear association between these effects and the total dose or duration of treatment. Another study found evidence of changes after 4 months in patients who had taken isotretinoin 1 mg per kg body-weight daily and recommended that radiological examinations should be made every 6 months in patients receiving isotretinoin for more than a year.[8] However, a further study found that although 12% of patients receiving isotretinoin 500 μg per kg had evidence of hyperostoses this was not clinically significant in any patient.[9] It has been suggested that monitoring beyond the treatment period might be unnecessary as calcifications and hyperostosis in patients who had received isotretinoin for 3 years had neither progressed nor improved 10 to 24 months after the end of treatment; additionally no new hyperostoses had developed during that period.[10] Of 25 patients treated with acitretin for a mean of 5 years one had abnormal calcification thought to be caused by the drug;[11] therapy with acitretin was continued with no further side-effects. The authors recommended radiological examinations after twelve months of treatment and then every second year. A study in 135 patients[12] who had received oral retinoids for a mean of 30 months could establish no relationship between spinal abnormalities and prolonged oral retinoid treatment and the authors suggested that spinal abnormalities only occur sporadically in predisposed patients.

There have been individual reports of hypercalciuria[7] and hypercalcaemia[13-15] associated with oral retinoid therapy. Oral retinoids may also cause muscle damage;[16,17] myositis has been reported with tretinoin[18] and severe myopathy with acitretin.[19]
1. Pittsley RA, Yoder FW. Retinoid hyperostosis: skeletal toxicity associated with long-term administration of 13-cis-retinoic acid for refractory ichthyosis. N Engl J Med 1983; 308: 1012–14.
2. Milstone LM, et al. Premature epiphyseal closure in a child receiving oral 13-cis-retinoic acid. J Am Acad Dermatol 1982; 7: 663–6.
3. DiGiovanna JJ, et al. Extraspinal tendon and ligament calcification associated with long-term therapy with etretinate. N Engl J Med 1986; 315: 1177–82.
4. Archer CB, et al. Spinal hyperostosis and etretinate. Lancet 1987; i: 741.
5. Tfelt-Hansen P, et al. Spinal cord compression after long-term etretinate. Lancet 1989; ii: 325–6.
6. Gilbert M, et al. Lack of skeletal radiographic changes during short-term etretinate therapy for psoriasis. Dermatologica 1986; 172: 160–3.
7. Wilson DJ, et al. Skeletal hyperostosis and extraosseous calcification in patients receiving long-term etretinate (Tigason). Br J Dermatol 1988; 119: 597–607.
8. Török L, et al. Bone-scintigraphic examinations in patients treated with retinoids: a prospective study. Br J Dermatol 1989; 120: 31–6.
9. Carey BM, et al. Skeletal toxicity with isotretinoin therapy: a clinico-radiological evaluation. Br J Dermatol 1988; 119: 609–14.
10. Tangrea JA, et al. Isotretinoin and the axial skeleton. Lancet 1992; 340: 495–6.
11. Mørk N-J, et al. Skeletal side-effects of 5 years' acitretin treatment. Br J Dermatol 1996; 134: 1156–7.
12. Van Dooren-Greebe RJ, et al. Prolonged treatment with oral retinoids in adults: no influence on the frequency and severity of spinal abnormalities. Br J Dermatol 1996; 134: 71–6.
13. Valentic JP, et al. Hypercalcemia associated with oral isotretinoin in the treatment of severe acne. JAMA 1983; 250: 1899–1900.
14. Horber FF, et al. Impaired renal function and hypercalcaemia associated with etretinate. Lancet 1984; ii: 1093.
15. Akiyama H, et al. Hypercalcaemia due to all-trans retinoic acid. Lancet 1992; 339: 308–9.
16. Hodak E, et al. Muscle damage induced by isotretinoin. BMJ 1986; 293: 425–6.
17. David M, et al. Electromyographic abnormalities in patients undergoing long-term therapy with etretinate. J Am Acad Dermatol 1988; 19: 273–5.
18. Miranda N, et al. Myositis with tretinoin. Lancet 1994; 334: 1096.
19. Lister RK, et al. Acitretin-induced myopathy. Br J Dermatol 1996; 134: 989–90.

Effects on the respiratory system. There have been reports of exercise-induced wheezing,[1] eosinophilic pleural effusion,[2] and worsening asthma[3,4] associated with isotretinoin therapy. The USA manufacturers have records of adverse effects on the lung including worsening asthma, recurrent pneumothorax, interstitial fibrosis, and pulmonary granuloma.[5] A study of healthy subjects confirmed that lung function tests could deteriorate after treatment with isotretinoin.[5]
1. Fisher DA. Exercise-induced bronchoconstriction related to isotretinoin therapy. J Am Acad Dermatol 1985; 13: 524.
2. Bunker CB, et al. Isotretinoin and eosinophilic pleural effusion. Lancet 1989; i: 435–6.

3. Sabroe RA, et al. Bronchospasm induced by isotretinoin. BMJ 1996; 312: 886.
4. Kapur N, et al. Exacerbation of asthma by isotretinoin. Br J Dermatol 2000; 142: 388–9.
5. Bunker CB, et al. Isotretinoin and the lung. Br J Dermatol 1991; 125 (suppl 38): 29.

Effects on serum lipids. The oral retinoids induce dose-dependent changes in serum lipids. There can be increases in very-low-density-lipoprotein cholesterol with smaller increases in low-density-lipoprotein cholesterol and reductions in high-density-lipoprotein cholesterol.[1] These effects appear to be unrelated to age or sex. They occur early during treatment and are usually reversible within a few weeks of discontinuation. Overall, the effect of isotretinoin is much greater than that of etretinate. Although the total cholesterol and triglyceride concentrations may remain within normal limits, types IIb and IV hyperlipidaemias are not uncommon among patients receiving oral retinoids. Pancreatitis may be associated with hypertriglyceridaemia in patients treated with isotretinoin.[2]

Retinoids should be used with caution in patients with pre-existing hypertriglyceridaemia or in those at risk of developing hypertriglyceridaemia.[1] Concomitant administration of fish oil containing eicosapentaenoic acid has been reported to attenuate retinoid-induced increases in serum-cholesterol and serum-triglyceride concentrations.[3]
1. Henkin Y, et al. Secondary dyslipidemia: inadvertent effects of drugs in clinical practice. JAMA 1992; 267: 961–8.
2. Flynn WJ, et al. Pancreatitis associated with isotretinoin-induced hypertriglyceridemia. Ann Intern Med 1987; 107: 63.
3. Marsden JR. Effect of dietary fish oil on hyperlipidaemia due to isotretinoin and etretinate. Hum Toxicol 1987; 6: 219–22.

Effects on sexual function. Ejaculatory failure has been reported in 3 men to be associated with isotretinoin treatment.[1] A possible mechanism could be an effect on the goblet cells of the seminal vesicles, an effect similar to the general reduction in body secretions which leads to dry mucous membranes.
1. Coleman R, MacDonald D. Effects of isotretinoin on male reproductive system. Lancet 1994; 344: 198.

Effects on the skin, hair, and nails. Apart from the more common effects of oral retinoids on the skin and hair (see Adverse Effects, above), there have been isolated reports of granulomatous lesions,[1,2] precipitation or exacerbation of erythroderma,[3,4] palmo-plantar eruptions,[5] prurigo-like eruptions,[6] scalp folliculitis,[7] pyoderma gangrenosum,[7,8] palmo-plantar stickiness,[9] curling hair,[10] and chloasma (melasma).[11] There has been a report of fatal toxic epidermal necrolysis associated with etretinate.[12] Acne fulminans has been reported as a complication of isotretinoin treatment[13] although there have also been cases of acne fulminans being treated successfully with isotretinoin.[14] For other reports of acne fulminans and eruptions associated with vasculitic syndromes, see below. Skin erosion following wax depilation has been reported in patients receiving retinoids (see Skin Fragility under Precautions, below).

Oral retinoids have been associated with paronychia and other forms[15] of nail dystrophy.
1. Lane PR, Hogan DJ. Granulomatous lesions appearing during isotretinoin therapy. Can Med Assoc J 1984; 130: 550.
2. Williamson DM, Greenwood R. Multiple pyogenic granulomata occurring during etretinate therapy. Br J Dermatol 1983; 109: 615–17.
3. Wantzin GL, Thomsen K. A new cutaneous side effect of isotretinoin. J Am Acad Dermatol 1985; 13: 665.
4. Levin J, Almeyda J. Erythroderma due to etretinate. Br J Dermatol 1985; 112: 373.
5. David M, et al. Palmoplantar eruption associated with etretinate therapy. Acta Derm Venereol (Stockh) 1986; 66: 87–9.
6. Boer J, Smeenk G. Nodular prurigo-like eruptions induced by etretinate. Br J Dermatol 1987; 116: 271–4.
7. Hughes BR, Cunliffe WJ. Development of folliculitis and pyoderma gangrenosum in association with abdominal pain in a patient following treatment with isotretinoin. Br J Dermatol 1990; 122: 683–7.
8. Gangaram HB, et al. Pyoderma gangrenosum following treatment with isotretinoin. Br J Dermatol 1997; 136: 636–7.
9. Penneys NS, Hernandez D. A sticky problem with etretinate. N Engl J Med 1991; 325: 521.
10. van der Pijl JW, et al. Isotretinoin and azathioprine: a synergy that makes hair curl? Lancet 1996; 348: 622–3.
11. Burke H, Carmichael AJ. Reversible melasma associated with isotretinoin. Br J Dermatol 1996; 135: 862.
12. McIvor A. Fatal toxic epidermal necrolysis associated with etretinate. BMJ 1992; 304: 548.
13. Huston NR, Mules R. Acne fulminans with severe myalgia precipitated by isotretinoin therapy. N Z Med J 1985; 36: 821.
14. Darley CR, et al. Acne fulminans with arthritis in identical twins treated with isotretinoin. J R Soc Med 1984; 77: 328–30.
15. Dharmagunawardena B, Charles-Holmes R. Median canaliform dystrophy following isotretinoin therapy. Br J Dermatol 1997; 137: 658–9.

PHOTOTOXICITY. In vitro photohaemolysis studies demonstrated that tretinoin and isotretinoin have a phototoxic potential while etretinate has none.[1] However, acitretin the major metabolite of etretinate had a phototoxic potential greater than that of tretinoin. The apparently low incidence of photosensitivity suggested that an idiosyncrasy is responsible. Patients should use appropriate photoprotection against UVA and UVB wavebands.
1. Ferguson J, Johnson BE. Photosensitivity due to retinoids: clinical and laboratory studies. Br J Dermatol 1986; 115: 275–83.

Effects on taste. Almost complete loss of taste has been reported in a patient given isotretinoin 600 μg per kg body-weight daily by mouth for 20 weeks.[1] Sense of taste returned about 6 months after isotretinoin was discontinued. Up to September 1994 the UK Committee on Safety of Medicines knew of 5 cases of taste changes, including 4 reports of loss of taste.

1. Halpern SM, *et al.* Loss of taste associated with isotretinoin. *Br J Dermatol* 1996; **134:** 378.

Overdosage. Apart from vague abdominal discomfort there were no other symptoms or significant abnormalities in a 15-year-old who was treated with gastric lavage 1.5 hours after ingestion of 350 mg of isotretinoin.[1] There was a similar outcome in the 2 other cases of isotretinoin overdosage reported in the literature.

1. Hepburn NC. Deliberate self-poisoning with isotretinoin. *Br J Dermatol* 1990; **122:** 840–1.

Vasculitic syndromes. The manufacturer of isotretinoin and etretinate has received isolated reports of vasculitis associated with the use of these oral retinoids; Wegener's granulomatosis has also been reported following the use of isotretinoin.[1,2] The precise mechanism underlying these effects is unknown; in some patients there may have been a direct toxic effect as symptoms developed shortly after the start of treatment, in other patients the onset was long-delayed and in some may have been triggered by the incidental use of antibiotics. Erythema nodosum and acne fulminans associated with circulating immune complexes had previously been reported after the use of isotretinoin.[3]

1. Dwyer JM, *et al.* Vasculitis and retinoids. *Lancet* 1989; **ii:** 494–6.
2. Anonymous. Retinoids and necrotizing vasculitis. *WHO Drug Inf* 1989; **3:** 187.
3. Kellett JK, *et al.* Erythema nodosum and circulating immune complexes in acne fulminans after treatment with isotretinoin. *BMJ* 1985; **290:** 820.

Precautions

Isotretinoin is teratogenic and therefore contra-indicated in pregnant patients. It is advisable for female patients to commence using contraceptive measures one month before starting isotretinoin treatment. Pregnancy should be avoided during treatment and for 1 month after treatment has been withdrawn. Patients receiving isotretinoin should not donate blood during, or for 1 month after cessation of therapy. *Pregnancy or blood donation must be avoided for much longer periods in patients taking acitretin or etretinate.* Isotretinoin is contra-indicated in patients with hepatic and renal impairment, hyperlipidaemias, hypervitaminosis A, and in breast-feeding mothers. Isotretinoin should be used with care in patients with a history of depression and patients receiving isotretinoin should be monitored for signs of depressive illness.

Liver function and fasting blood lipids should be measured at the start of therapy, after the first month, and thereafter as appropriate. Blood glucose should be monitored throughout treatment in patients who either have, or are predisposed to, diabetes mellitus. Some recommend routine radiological evaluation in patients receiving long-term therapy (see under Effects on the Musculoskeletal System, above). Patients may experience a reduced tolerance to contact lenses.

Excessive exposure to sunlight and UV light should be avoided.

When applied topically the precautions described under tretinoin (see p.1126) should be adopted.

Pregnancy. The problem of prescribing oral retinoids to women of child-bearing potential has been discussed.[1,2] Intra-uterine exposure to isotretinoin has caused spontaneous abortion and a characteristic pattern of fetal malformations involving craniofacial, cardiac, thymic, and CNS structures.[3,4] Some infants have also shown subnormal intelligence and other neuropsychological impairments.[5] The risk of malformation appears to be high at all therapeutic doses of isotretinoin even when the duration of exposure is short.[6] Despite warnings on the use of retinoids during pregnancy and the need for adequate contraception in women of child-bearing potential and other strict guidelines on their use, intra-uterine exposure to retinoids has still occurred.[7,8] Isotretinoin has a relatively short half-life and it has been recommended that conception should be avoided for at least one month after the end of treatment. A survey of women who conceived after the use of isotretinoin (64% within one month of discontinuation of treatment) suggested that the incidence of spontaneous abortion or congenital malformations was no greater than in the general population.[9] However, patients taking oral retinoids with longer half-lives must avoid conception for much longer periods; at least 2 years (3 years in the US) is recommended if patients are taking acitretin although the period of time for patients taking etretinate has not been established. Malformations similar to those associated with isotretinoin have been reported in infants conceived within two years of stopping etretinate.[10-12] Unless otherwise contra-indicated, oral combined contraceptives have been recommended as the contraceptive method of choice for women undergoing retinoid treatment.[13] The concomitant use of anoth-

er form of contraception, such as a barrier method, is also recommended.[2,8] For further information on the use of hormonal contraceptives, see p.1459.

1. Mitchell AA. Oral retinoids: what should the prescriber know about their teratogenic hazards among women of child-bearing potential? *Drug Safety* 1992; **7:** 79–85.
2. Chan A, *et al.* Oral retinoids and pregnancy. *Med J Aust* 1996; **165:** 164–7.
3. Lammer EJ, *et al.* Retinoic acid embryopathy. *N Engl J Med* 1985; **313:** 837–41.
4. Rosa F. Isotretinoin dose and teratogenicity. *Lancet* 1987; **ii:** 1154.
5. Adams J. High incidence of intellectual deficits in 5-year-old children exposed to isotretinoin 'in utero'. *Teratology* 1990; **41:** 614.
6. Dai WS, *et al.* Epidemiology of isotretinoin exposure during pregnancy. *J Am Acad Dermatol* 1992; **26:** 599–606.
7. Stern RS. When a uniquely effective drug is teratogenic: the case of isotretinoin. *N Engl J Med* 1989; **320:** 1007–9.
8. Atanackovic G, Koren G. Fetal exposure to oral isotretinoin: failure to comply with the Pregnancy Prevention Program. *Can Med Assoc J* 1999; **160:** 1719–20.
9. Dai WS, *et al.* Safety of pregnancy after discontinuation of isotretinoin. *Arch Dermatol* 1989; **125:** 362–5.
10. Grote W, *et al.* Malformation of fetus conceived 4 months after termination of maternal etretinate treatment. *Lancet* 1985; **i:** 1276.
11. Lammer EJ. Embryopathy in infant conceived one year after termination of maternal etretinate. *Lancet* 1988; **ii:** 1080–1.
12. Geiger J-M, *et al.* Teratogenic risk with etretinate and acitretin treatment. *Dermatology* 1994; **189:** 109–16.
13. Lehucher Ceyrac D, *et al.* Retinoids and contraception. *Dermatology* 1992; **184:** 161–70.

Skin fragility. Wax depilation should be avoided in patients receiving retinoids since they cause increased skin fragility and facial and leg erosions have occurred.[1-3] The UK manufacturers also recommend that wax depilation should be avoided for at least 6 months after isotretinoin treatment because of the risk of scarring and dermatitis, and that aggressive dermabrasion should be avoided for a period of 5 to 6 months after treatment because of the risk of hypertrophic scarring in atypical areas.

1. Egido Romo M. Isotretinoin and wax epilation. *Br J Dermatol* 1991; **124:** 393.
2. Holmes SC, Thomson J. Isotretinoin and skin fragility. *Br J Dermatol* 1995; **132:** 165.
3. Woollons A, Price ML. Roaccutane and wax epilation: a cautionary tale. *Br J Dermatol* 1997; **137:** 839–40.

Interactions

Concomitant use of isotretinoin and vitamin A (including dietary supplements) should be avoided because of additive toxic effects. Tetracyclines should be avoided as their use with isotretinoin has been associated with the development of benign intracranial hypertension.

Carbamazepine. For the effect of isotretinoin on carbamazepine, see p.345.

Oral contraceptives. For discussion of the potential interactions of retinoids with hormonal contraceptives, and the effect this might have on contraceptive choice during retinoid treatment, see p.1459.

Pharmacokinetics

Isotretinoin is absorbed from the gastrointestinal tract and absorption may be increased by administration with food. Minimal systemic absorption occurs following topical administration of isotretinoin. Peak plasma concentrations have been obtained 1 to 4 hours after oral administration. Oral bioavailability is low possibly due to metabolism in the gut wall and first-pass metabolism in the liver. Isotretinoin is highly bound to plasma proteins. It is metabolised in the liver to its major metabolite 4-oxo-isotretinoin; there is also some isomerisation of isotretinoin to tretinoin. Isotretinoin, tretinoin, and their metabolites undergo enterohepatic recycling. The terminal elimination half-life of isotretinoin is 10 to 20 hours, while that of the 4-oxo metabolite may be up to 50 hours; return to physiological levels of retinoids takes about 2 weeks after stopping therapy. Equal amounts of a dose appear in the faeces, mainly as unchanged drug, and in the urine as metabolites.

Isotretinoin crosses the placenta.

◊ References.

1. Colburn WA, *et al.* Food increases the bioavailability of isotretinoin. *J Clin Pharmacol* 1983; **23:** 534–9.
2. Lucek RW, Colburn WA. Clinical pharmacokinetics of the retinoids. *Clin Pharmacokinet* 1985; **10:** 38–62.
3. Kraft JC, *et al.* Embryonic retinoid concentrations after maternal intake of isotretinoin. *N Engl J Med* 1989; **321:** 262.
4. Larsen FG, *et al.* Pharmacokinetics and therapeutic efficacy of retinoids in skin diseases. *Clin Pharmacokinet* 1992; **23:** 42–61.
5. Chen C, *et al.* Negligible systemic absorption of topical isotretinoin cream: implications for teratogenicity. *J Clin Pharmacol* 1997; **37:** 279–84.
6. Nulman I, *et al.* Steady-state pharmacokinetics of isotretinoin and its 4-oxo metabolite: implications for fetal safety. *J Clin Pharmacol* 1998; **38:** 926–30.

Uses and Administration

Isotretinoin is a retinoid. It is the *cis* configuration of tretinoin (p.1126) which is the acid form of vitamin A (p.1382). Isotretinoin is given by mouth for the treatment of severe acne (below) that has not responded to other measures; it is also applied topically in milder forms of acne. It is not indicated for uncomplicated adolescent acne. Isotretinoin has also been tried in a number of other skin disorders and in some forms of neoplastic disease.

In the UK and a number of other countries the initial oral dose of isotretinoin for acne is 500 µg per kg body-weight daily, although in the USA initial doses of up to 1 mg per kg daily are permitted. The dose is given with food once daily or in two divided doses and adjusted if necessary after 4 weeks up to 1 mg per kg daily according to response and side-effects. Patients intolerant to the initial dose may be able to continue treatment at 100 to 200 µg per kg daily. Doses up to 2 mg per kg daily are permitted in the USA and some other countries for patients whose disease is very severe or primarily on the body instead of the face. Acute exacerbation of acne is occasionally seen during the initial period, but usually subsides within 7 to 10 days on continued treatment. Treatment should continue for 12 to 20 weeks or until the total cyst count has decreased by over 70%. Improvement may continue for several months after cessation of treatment; prolonged remissions can occur. It is recommended that repeat courses should not normally be given but occasionally they may be required. However, since acne may continue to improve following discontinuation of isotretinoin, there must be at least a 2-month drug-free period before initiating repeat treatment.

For the topical treatment of acne a gel containing 0.05% of isotretinoin is applied sparingly once or twice daily. A therapeutic response may not be evident for 6 to 8 weeks.

◊ General reviews.

1. Orfanos CE, *et al.* Current use and future potential role of retinoids in dermatology. *Drugs* 1997; **53:** 358–88.

◊ Apart from its established role in the treatment of acne (below), isotretinoin has been used in other skin disorders including the keratinisation disorders Darier's disease[1] (p.1104) and ichthyosis (p.1105); lichen planus (p.1106); rosacea[2] (p.1107); and some malignant neoplasms (below).

1. Burge SM, Buxton PK. Topical isotretinoin in Darier's disease. *Br J Dermatol* 1995; **133:** 924–8.
2. Ertl GA, *et al.* A comparison of the efficacy of topical tretinoin and low-dose oral isotretinoin in rosacea. *Arch Dermatol* 1994; **130:** 319–24.

Acne. The retinoids play an important role in the treatment of acne (p.1103). Severe conglobate and nodulocystic acne unresponsive to other therapy including systemic antibacterials is the main indication for oral isotretinoin therapy. Administration of isotretinoin produces a dose-related reduction in sebum excretion with a subsequent reduction in levels of *Propionibacterium acnes*, inflammation, and cyst formation.[1] A skin reaction with the appearance of papulopustules frequently occurs after 2 to 4 weeks of therapy but this rapidly clears with continued treatment. Although sebum excretion may approach pretreatment levels after discontinuation of therapy most patients remain free of their disease after a single course and long-term remissions lasting months or years have been obtained.[2,3] Men under 25 appear to be more prone to relapse than older men or women.[4] To avoid relapse long-term therapy of up to 5 months' duration is required. Improvement may continue for several months after cessation of therapy and at least 2 months should elapse before determining whether further treatment is necessary. Approximately 10% of patients relapse and may require further treatment with antibacterials; repeat courses of isotretinoin are not usually recommended but may occasionally be required. Use of isotretinoin with antibacterials or anti-androgens does not markedly improve efficacy but if concomitant antibacterial therapy is contemplated then erythromycin is preferred as use with tetracyclines can produce benign intracranial hypertension. Isotretinoin has also been used for the treatment of acne associated with immunosuppressive therapy in transplant recipients.[5,6] Variable results have been obtained when using isotretinoin topically[7,8] and it appears to interact with the epidermis in a different manner to other retinoids.[9]

Although isotretinoin is not licensed for the treatment of prepubertal acne because of the risk of adverse effects including early epiphyseal closure, it has been tried orally in a few children with toddler-age nodulocystic acne.[10]

1. Jones DH. The role and mechanism of action of 13-cis-retinoic acid in the treatment of severe (nodulocystic) acne. *Pharmacol Ther* 1989; **40:** 91–106.

2. Layton AM, et al. Isotretinoin for acne vulgaris—10 years later: a safe and successful treatment. Br J Dermatol 1993; **129:** 292–6.
3. Lehucher-Ceyrac D, Weber-Buisset MJ. Isotretinoin and acne in practice: a prospective analysis of 188 cases over 9 years. Dermatology 1993; **186:** 123–8.
4. Orfanos CE, et al. The retinoids: a review of their clinical pharmacology and therapeutic use. Drugs 1987; **34:** 459–503.
5. Tam M, Cooper A. The use of isotretinoin in a renal transplant patient with acne. Br J Dermatol 1987; **116:** 463.
6. Bunker CB, et al. Isotretinoin treatment of severe acne in post-transplant patients taking cyclosporine. J Am Acad Dermatol 1990; **22:** 693–4.
7. Harms M, et al. Isotretinoin ineffective topically. Lancet 1985; **i:** 398.
8. Chalker DK, et al. Efficacy of topical isotretinoin 0.05% gel in acne vulgaris: results of a multicenter, double-blind investigation. J Am Acad Dermatol 1987; **17:** 251–4.
9. Hirschel-Scholz S, et al. Isotretinoin differs from other synthetic retinoids in its modulation of human cellular retinoic acid binding protein (CRABP). Br J Dermatol 1989; **120:** 639–44.
10. Mengesha YM, Hansen RC. Toddler-age nodulocystic acne. J Pediatr 1999; **134:** 644–8.

Malignant neoplasms. Retinoids including isotretinoin have been studied in the treatment of various neoplastic or preneoplastic disorders. Encouraging results were reported in a pilot study[1] of isotretinoin in juvenile chronic myelogenous leukaemia. [Note that oral tretinoin (p.1127) is used in acute promyelocytic leukaemia.]

Benefit has been noted in patients with T-cell lymphomas, including mycosis fungoides[2-4] (p.489), although in patients with advanced disease[5] treated with isotretinoin rather than acitretin (which had been used in some of the previous successes) no benefit, and even deterioration, occurred. The comment[6] was also made that the two retinoids do not share a similar therapeutic profile.

There is some evidence that retinoids may be useful in preventing the development of cutaneous squamous cell carcinoma in high-risk individuals (p.498) and squamous cell carcinoma of the head and neck (p.494),[7,8] and other neoplasms.[9]

1. Castleberry RP, et al. A pilot study of isotretinoin in the treatment of juvenile chronic myelogenous leukaemia. N Engl J Med 1994; **331:** 1680–4.
2. Thomsen K, et al. Retinoids plus PUVA (RePUVA) and PUVA in mycosis fungoides, plaque stage: a report from the Scandinavian Mycosis Fungoides Group. Acta Derm Venereol (Stockh) 1989; **69:** 536–8.
3. Knobler RM, et al. Treatment of cutaneous T cell lymphoma with a combination of low-dose interferon alfa-2b and retinoids. J Am Acad Dermatol 1991; **24:** 247–52.
4. French LE, et al. Remission of cutaneous T-cell lymphoma with combined calcitriol and acitretin. Lancet 1994; **344:** 686–7.
5. Thomsen K. Cutaneous T-cell lymphoma and calcitriol and isotretinoin treatment. Lancet 1995; **345:** 1583.
6. French LE, Saurat J-H. Treatment of cutaneous T-cell lymphoma by retinoids and calcitriol. Lancet 1995; **346:** 376.
7. Hong WK, et al. Prevention of second primary tumors with isotretinoin in squamous-cell carcinoma of the head and neck. N Engl J Med 1990; **323:** 795–801.
8. Lippman SM, et al. Comparison of low-dose isotretinoin with beta carotene to prevent oral carcinogenesis. N Engl J Med 1993; **328:** 15–20.
9. De Palo G, Formelli F. Risks and benefits of retinoids in the chemoprevention of cancer. Drug Safety 1995; **13:** 245–56.

Preparations

BP 2001: Isotretinoin Capsules; Isotretinoin Gel;
USP 25: Isotretinoin Capsules.

Proprietary Preparations (details are given in Part 3)
Aust.: Roaccutan; *Austral.:* Accure; Isohexal; Isotrex; Oratane; Roaccutane; *Belg.:* Roaccutane; *Braz.:* Roacutan; *Canad.:* Accutane; Isotrex; *Denm.:* Isotrex; Roaccutan; *Fin.:* Roaccutan; *Fr.:* Isotrex; Roaccutane; *Ger.:* Isotrex; Roaccutan; *Hong Kong:* Isotrex; Roaccutane; *Irl.:* Isotrex; Roaccutane; *Israel:* Isotrex; Roaccutane; *Ital.:* Isotrex; Roaccutan; *Mex.:* Isotrex; Roaccutan; *Neth.:* Roaccutane; *NZ:* Isotrex; Oratane; Roaccutane; *Port.:* Isotrex; Roaccutan; *S.Afr.:* Isotrex; Roaccutane; *Singapore:* Isotrex; Nimegen; Roaccutane; *Spain:* Isotrex; Roacutan; *Switz.:* Roaccutane; *Thai.:* Isotrex; Roaccutane; *UK:* Isotrex; Roaccutane; *USA:* Accutane.

Multi-ingredient: *Aust.:* Isotrex; *Fr.:* Antibiotrex; *Ger.:* Isotrexin; *Irl.:* Isotrexin; *Ital.:* Isotrexin; *Port.:* Isotrexin; *Spain:* Isotrex Eritromicina; *UK:* Isotrexin.

Keluamid (13467-x)

Profile
Keluamid has been used in topical preparations for the treatment of seborrhoeic dermatitis and other scaling skin disorders.

Preparations
Proprietary Preparations (details are given in Part 3)
Fr.: Kelual.

Multi-ingredient: *Fr.:* Kelual Zinc; Sabal.

Lithium Succinate (19412-q)

$C_4H_6O_4.xLi.$
$CAS — 16090-09-8.$
$ATC — D11AX04.$

Profile
Lithium succinate is reported to have anti-inflammatory properties and is used as an 8% ointment, usually in combination with zinc sulfate. It is applied twice daily initially in the treat-

ment of seborrhoeic dermatitis (p.1107). It should be used with caution in patients with psoriasis as it may exacerbate their condition.

◊ References.
1. Gould DJ, et al. A double-blind, placebo-controlled, multicenter trial of lithium succinate ointment in the treatment of seborrheic dermatitis. J Am Acad Dermatol 1992; **26:** 452–7.
2. Cuelenaere C, et al. Use of topical lithium succinate in the treatment of seborrhoeic dermatitis. Dermatology 1992; **184:** 194–7.
3. Langtry JA, et al. Topical lithium succinate ointment (Efalith) in the treatment of AIDS-related seborrhoeic dermatitis. Clin Exp Dermatol 1997; **22:** 216–19.

Preparations
Proprietary Preparations (details are given in Part 3)
Multi-ingredient: *Ger.:* Efadermin; *Irl.:* Efalith; *NZ:* Efalith; *Switz.:* Efalith; *UK:* Efalith.

Lonapalene (719-q)

Lonapalene (USAN, rINN).
RS-43179. 6-Chloro-2,3-dimethoxy-1,4-naphthalenediol diacetate.
$C_{16}H_{15}ClO_6 = 338.7.$
$CAS — 91431-42-4.$

Profile
Lonapalene is a 5-lipoxygenase inhibitor studied for the topical treatment of psoriasis.

◊ References.
1. Lassus A, Forsstrom S. A dimethoxynaphthalene derivative (RS-43179 gel) compared with 0.025% fluocinolone acetonide gel in the treatment of psoriasis. Br J Dermatol 1985; **113:** 103–6.
2. Black AK, et al. Pharmacologic and clinical effects of lonapalene (RS 43179), a 5-lipoxygenase inhibitor, in psoriasis. J Invest Dermatol 1990; **95:** 50–4.

Maggots (20342-f)

Sterile Larvae.

Maggots used in wound management are the live sterile larvae of *Lucilia sericata*, the common greenbottle fly.

Profile
Larval therapy (sometimes called biosurgery) may be used for debridement of infected or necrotic wounds (p.1108), including diabetic foot ulcers. The maggots are applied to the surface of the wound and kept in place with dressings for up to 3 days. The maggots are removed with the dressing, and the wound is irrigated with sodium chloride solution; any remaining maggots are removed with forceps.

Maggots should not be applied to wounds that have a tendency to bleed easily, or that communicate with a body cavity or any internal organ. Pain has been reported with larval therapy.

◊ References.
1. Thomas S, et al. Maggots are useful in treating infected or necrotic wounds. BMJ 1999; **318:** 807–8.
2. Courtenay M, et al. Larva therapy in wound management. J R Soc Med 2000; **93:** 72–4.

Preparations
Proprietary Preparations (details are given in Part 3)
UK: LarvE.

Mequinol (1619-e)

Mequinol (USAN, rINN).
BMS-181158; p-Guaiacol; 4-HA; HQMME; Hydroquinone Monomethyl Ether; p-Hydroxyanisole; Hydroxyquinone Methyl Ether. 4-Methoxyphenol.
$C_7H_8O_2 = 124.1.$
$CAS — 150-76-5.$
$ATC — D11AX06.$

Profile
Mequinol is used similarly to hydroquinone (p.1115), in concentrations of up to 20%, in the treatment of hyperpigmentation (see Pigmentation Disorders, p.1106). It has also been investigated in the treatment of melanoma.

Adverse effects. A report of severe reversible irregular hypopigmentation of the hands, arms, neck, and legs in a West Indian woman who applied a bleaching wax containing mequinol for 2 to 3 months to lighten the colour of her skin.[1]
1. Boyle J, Kennedy CTC. British cosmetic regulations inadequate. BMJ 1984; **288:** 1998–9.

Pigmentation disorders. References.
1. Fleischer AB, et al. The combination of 2% 4-hydroxyanisole (mequinol) and 0.01% tretinoin is effective in improving the appearance of solar lentigines and related hyperpigmented lesions in two double-blind multicenter clinical studies. J Am Acad Dermatol 2000; **42:** 459–67.
2. Njoo MD, et al. Depigmentation therapy in vitiligo universalis with topical 4-methoxyphenol and the Q-switched ruby laser. J Am Acad Dermatol 2000; **42:** 760–9.

Preparations
Proprietary Preparations (details are given in Part 3)
Aust.: Leucobasal; *Braz.:* Leucodin; *Fr.:* Any; Clairodermyl†; Creme des 3 Fleurs d'Orient; Leucodinine B; *Spain:* Novo Dermoquinona; *Switz.:* Leucobasal.

Ammoniated Mercury (1620-b)

Aminomercuric Chloride; Hydrargyri Aminochloridum; Hydrargyrum Amidochloratum; Hydrargyrum Ammoniatum; Hydrargyrum Praecipitatum Album; Mercuric Ammonium Chloride; Mercury Amide Chloride; Mercury Aminochloride; White Precipitate.
$NH_2HgCl = 252.1.$
$CAS — 10124-48-8.$

NOTE. 'White Precipitate' has also been used as a name for Precipitated Mercurous Chloride.
Pharmacopoeias. In US.

Pharmacopoeial description
USP 25: A white amorphous powder or pulverulent pieces; odourless. It is stable in air, but darkens on exposure to light. Insoluble in water and in alcohol; readily soluble in warm hydrochloric, nitric, and acetic acids. Protect from light.

Profile
Ammoniated mercury was formerly used topically in the treatment of skin infections and psoriasis but the use of such mercurial preparations is generally deprecated. Frequent or prolonged application to large areas or to broken skin or mucous membranes can cause mercury poisoning (see p.1634) and use on infants has produced acrodynia (pink disease). Ammoniated mercury is also a potent sensitiser and can produce allergic reactions.

◊ Of 60 patients who were found to have nephrotic syndrome, 32 had used skin-lightening creams containing 5 to 10% of ammoniated mercury.[1] Concentrations of mercury in the urine of these patients were up to 250 nanograms per mL compared with a usual upper limit of 80 nanograms per mL. Of 26 patients followed up for up to 2 years, 13 had no remission or response to treatment; 6 of these had used skin lighteners.
1. Barr RD, et al. Nephrotic syndrome in adult Africans in Nairobi. BMJ 1972; **2:** 131–4.

Preparations
Proprietary Preparations (details are given in Part 3)
Multi-ingredient: *USA:* Emersal†; Unguentum Bossi.

Mesulphen (1622-g)

Mesulphen (BAN).
Mesulfen (pINN); Dimethyldiphenylene Disulphide; Dimethylthianthrene. It consists mainly of 2,7-dimethylthianthrene.
$C_{14}H_{12}S_2 = 244.4.$
$CAS — 135-58-0.$
$ATC — D10AB05; P03AA03.$
Pharmacopoeias. In Aust.
Jpn includes thianthol, a mixture of 2,7-dimethylthianthrene and ditolyl disulfide.

Profile
Mesulphen has been used as a parasiticide and antipruritic in a range of skin disorders including acne, scabies, and seborrhoea. Sensitivity to mesulphen has occasionally been reported.

Preparations
Proprietary Preparations (details are given in Part 3)
Ger.: Citemul S; *Switz.:* Soufrol.
Multi-ingredient: *Aust.:* Tineafax†.

Methoxsalen (1623-q)

Methoxsalen (BAN).
Ammoidin; 8-Methoxypsoralen; Metoxaleno; Xanthotoxin. 9-Methoxyfuro[3,2-g]chromen-7-one; 9-Methoxy-7H-furo[3,2-g][1]benzopyran-7-one.
$C_{12}H_8O_4 = 216.2.$
$CAS — 298-81-7.$
$ATC — D05AD02; D05BA02.$
Pharmacopoeias. In Jpn and US.

A constituent of the fruits of *Ammi majus*.

Pharmacopoeial description
USP 25: White to cream-coloured, odourless, fluffy, needle-like crystals. Practically insoluble in water; sparingly soluble in boiling water and in ether; soluble in boiling alcohol, in acetone, in acetic acid, in propylene glycol, and in benzene; freely soluble in chloroform. Protect from light.

Adverse Effects
Methoxsalen given orally commonly causes nausea and less frequently mental effects including insomnia, nervousness, and depression.

Photochemotherapy or PUVA (see under Uses and Administration, below) may cause pruritus and mild transient erythema. Other effects include oedema, dizziness, headache, vesiculation, bulla formation, onycholysis, acneform eruption, and severe skin pain. Overexposure to sunlight or UVA radiation may produce severe burns in patients being treated with psoralens. PUVA can produce premature ageing of the skin. Hypertrichosis and pigmentation alterations of skin or nails have also been reported. PUVA may be associated with an increased risk of malignant neoplasms of the skin.

Carcinogenicity. See under Effects on the Blood and Effects on the Skin, below.

Effects on the blood. There have been isolated reports of leukaemia[1-3] or a preleukaemic condition[4] developing after PUVA therapy.

1. Hansen NE. Development of acute myeloid leukaemia in a patient with psoriasis treated with oral 8-methoxypsoralen and longwave ultraviolet light. *Scand J Haematol* 1979; **22:** 57–60.
2. Sheehan-Dare RA, *et al.* Transformation of myelodysplasia to acute myeloid leukaemia during psoralen photochemotherapy (PUVA) treatment of psoriasis. *Acta Derm Venereol (Stockh)* 1989; **69:** 262–4.
3. Kwong YL, *et al.* Acute myeloid leukemia following psoralen with ultraviolet A therapy: a fluorescence in situ hybridization study. *Cancer Genet Cytogenet* 1997; **99:** 11–13.
4. Wagner J, *et al.* Preleukaemia (haemopoietic dysplasia) developing in a patient with psoriasis treated with 8-methoxypsoralen and ultraviolet light (PUVA) treatment. *Scand J Haematol* 1978; **21:** 299–304.

Effects on the eyes. Free methoxsalen has been detected in the lens of the eye for at least 12 hours after oral administration[1] although it may become integrated into the structure of the lens and cataracts may occur in patients who fail to wear suitable eye protection for 12 to 24 hours after therapy.[2] However, provided that eye protection is used there appears to be no significant dose-dependent increase in the risk of cataract formation, although a higher risk of developing nuclear sclerosis and posterior subcapsular opacities has been noted in patients who have received more than 100 treatments.[3] Other ocular effects include dose-related transient visual-field defects reported in 3 patients receiving PUVA therapy.[4] Psoralens may also increase the sensitivity of the retina to visible light.[5]

1. Lerman S, *et al.* Potential ocular complications from PUVA therapy and their prevention. *J Invest Dermatol* 1980; **74:** 197–9.
2. Woo TY, *et al.* Lenticular psoralen photoproducts and cataracts of a PUVA-treated psoriatic patient. *Arch Dermatol* 1985; **121:** 1307–8.
3. Stern RS, *et al.* Ocular findings in patients treated with PUVA. *J Invest Dermatol* 1985; **85:** 269–73.
4. Fenton DA, Wilkinson JD. Dose-related visual-field defects in patients receiving PUVA therapy. *Lancet* 1983; **i:** 1106.
5. Souêtre E, *et al.* 5-Methoxypsoralen increases the sensitivity of the retina to light in humans. *Eur J Clin Pharmacol* 1989; **36:** 59–61.

Effects on the hair. Hypertrichosis was noticed in 15 of 23 female patients receiving PUVA therapy compared with 2 of 14 patients treated with UVA alone.[1]

1. Rampen FHJ. Hypertrichosis in PUVA-treated patients. *Br J Dermatol* 1983; **109:** 657–60.

Effects on the immune system. PUVA therapy appears to have immunosuppressive effects and inhibits lymphocytes, polymorphonuclear leucocytes, and Langerhans' cells.[1-3] It is capable of inducing antinuclear antibody formation and a syndrome similar to systemic lupus syndrome has developed during treatment.[4,5] An immunological basis has also been suspected for the development of nephrotic syndrome in one patient who received PUVA therapy.[6]
See also Hypersensitivity, below.

1. Farber EM, *et al.* Long-term risks of psoralen and UV-A therapy for psoriasis. *Arch Dermatol* 1983; **119:** 426–31.
2. Morison WL, *et al.* Abnormal lymphocyte function following long-term PUVA therapy for psoriasis. *Br J Dermatol* 1983; **108:** 445–50.
3. Chang A, *et al.* PUVA and UVB inhibit the intra-epidermal accumulation of polymorphonuclear leukocytes. *Br J Dermatol* 1988; **119:** 281–7.
4. Bruze M, *et al.* Fatal connective tissue disease with antinuclear antibodies following PUVA therapy. *Acta Derm Venereol (Stockh)* 1984; **64:** 157–60.
5. Bruze M, Ljunggren B. Antinuclear antibodies appearing during PUVA therapy. *Acta Derm Venereol (Stockh)* 1985; **65:** 31–6.
6. Lam Thuon Mine LTK, *et al.* Nephrotic syndrome after treatment with psoralens and ultraviolet A. *BMJ* 1983; **287:** 94–5.

Effects on the skin. MALIGNANT NEOPLASMS. Squamous cell carcinoma, basal cell carcinoma, keratoacanthoma, actinic keratosis, Bowen's disease, and malignant melanoma have all been reported during or after cessation of PUVA.[1-3] There have been several large long-term follow-up studies to assess the risk of **non-melanoma** skin cancer in patients receiving PUVA therapy. Early studies from Europe found no clear evidence that PUVA was independently carcinogenic but did find that previous treatment with arsenic, methotrexate, or ionising radiation increased the incidence of skin tumours.[4] Studies from the USA have found an increase in the incidence of basal cell carcinoma and squamous cell carcinoma independent of other treatment,[5] which was dose-related in some studies.[6] Male genitalia appeared to be particularly susceptible.[7] It has been suggested that the differences between the findings might be due to the fact that in Europe higher and fewer doses are used and the median total dose employed may be only 29% of that used in the USA.[8] However, more recent studies from northern Europe have also found a dose-related increase in the risk of developing squamous cell carcinomas.[9-11] One small series suggested that about 50% of the recipients of high-dose PUVA went on to develop squamous cell carcinomas or premalignant lesions.[12] While some European workers have findings that confirm the increased susceptibility of the male genitalia[13] others have failed to find any such evidence.[14] A few patients have gone on to develop metastatic disease.[15,16]

There are anecdotal reports of **malignant melanomas** occurring in patients who had received PUVA. A prospective study[17] study in 1380 patients with psoriasis who were first treated with PUVA in 1975 or 1976 found that the risk of melanoma increases about 15 years after the first treatment with PUVA and that the risk was increased especially in patients who had received 250 treatments or more. The authors suggested that long-term PUVA should therefore be used with caution, especially in younger patients. However, a similar follow-up study[11] of 4799 patients treated with PUVA found no increase in the risk for malignant melanoma. Comparing their findings with the earlier study, the authors suggested that the results might differ because one-fifth of their cohort had received bath PUVA in which lower UVA doses are used. The comment has also been made[18] that patients receiving long-term therapy should be followed up carefully and that such therapy should not be used in patients at risk for melanoma.

A study[19] of follow-up data on patients who had received trioxysalen bath PUVA did not find an increase in risk of developing either squamous cell carcinoma or malignant melanoma, but the authors suggested that further study is needed to determine the carcinogenicity of trioxysalen PUVA.

There has also been a suggestion that PUVA may increase the risk of some internal cancers.[10]

1. Reshad H, *et al.* Cutaneous carcinoma in psoriatic patients treated with PUVA. *Br J Dermatol* 1984; **110:** 299–305.
2. Kemmett D, *et al.* Nodular malignant melanoma and multiple squamous cell carcinomas in a patient treated by photochemotherapy for psoriasis. *BMJ* 1984; **289:** 1498.
3. Suurmond D, *et al.* Skin cancer and PUVA maintenance therapy for psoriasis. *Br J Dermatol* 1985; **113:** 485–6.
4. Henseler T, *et al.* Skin tumors in the European PUVA study. *J Am Acad Dermatol* 1987; **16:** 108–16.
5. Forman AB, *et al.* Long-term follow-up of skin cancer in the PUVA-48 cooperative study. *Arch Dermatol* 1989; **125:** 515–19.
6. Stern RS, *et al.* Non-melanoma skin cancer occurring in patients treated with PUVA five to ten years after first treatment. *J Invest Dermatol* 1988; **91:** 120–4.
7. Stern RS, *et al.* Genital tumors among men with psoriasis exposed to psoralens and ultraviolet A radiation (PUVA) and ultraviolet B radiation. *N Engl J Med* 1990; **322:** 1093–7.
8. Moseley H, Ferguson J. Photochemotherapy: a reappraisal of its use in dermatology. *Drugs* 1989; **38:** 822–37.
9. Bruynzeel I, *et al.* 'High single-dose' European PUVA regimen also causes an excess of non-melanoma skin cancer. *Br J Dermatol* 1991; **124:** 49–55.
10. Lindelöf B, *et al.* PUVA and cancer: a large-scale epidemiological study. *Lancet* 1991; **338:** 91–3.
11. Lindelöf B, *et al.* PUVA and cancer risk: the Swedish follow-up study. *Br J Dermatol* 1999; **141:** 108–12.
12. Lever LR, Farr PM. Skin cancers or premalignant lesions occur in half of high-dose PUVA patients. *Br J Dermatol* 1994; **131:** 215–19.
13. Perkins W, *et al.* Cutaneous malignancy in males treated with photochemotherapy. *Lancet* 1990; **336:** 1248.
14. Wolff K, Hönigsmann H. Genital carcinomas in psoriasis patients treated with photochemotherapy. *Lancet* 1991; **337:** 439.
15. Lewis FM, *et al.* Metastatic squamous-cell carcinoma in patient receiving PUVA. *Lancet* 1994; **344:** 1157.
16. Stern RS. Metastatic squamous cell cancer after psoralen photochemotherapy. *Lancet* 1994; **344:** 1644–5.
17. Stern RS, *et al.* Malignant melanoma in patients treated for psoriasis with methoxsalen (psoralen) and ultraviolet A radiation (PUVA). *N Engl J Med* 1997; **336:** 1041–5.
18. Wolff K. Should PUVA be abandoned? *N Engl J Med* 1997; **336:** 1090–1.
19. Hannuksela-Svahn A, *et al.* Trioxsalen bath PUVA did not increase the risk of squamous cell skin carcinoma and cutaneous malignant melanoma in a joint analysis of 944 Swedish and Finnish patients with psoriasis. *Br J Dermatol* 1999; **141:** 497–501.

NON-MALIGNANT SKIN DISORDERS. Toxic pustuloderma, marked by erythema and superficial pustular lesions, has been reported in a patient given PUVA therapy for mycosis fungoides.[1] Another effect sometimes associated with PUVA is severe skin pain;[2,3] the pain may respond to treatment with topical capsaicin.[3]

1. Yip J, *et al.* Toxic pustuloderma due to PUVA treatment. *Br J Dermatol* 1991; **125:** 401–2.
2. Burrows NP, *et al.* PUVA-induced skin pain. *Br J Dermatol* 1993; **129:** 504.
3. Burrows NP, Norris PG. Treatment of PUVA-induced skin pain with capsaicin. *Br J Dermatol* 1994; **131:** 584–5.

Hypersensitivity. Hypersensitivity reactions to methoxsalen and PUVA therapy occur rarely but there have been reports of drug-induced fever,[1] bronchoconstriction,[2] and contact dermatitis.[3]

1. Tóth Kása I, Dobozy A. Drug fever caused by PUVA treatment. *Acta Derm Venereol (Stockh)* 1985; **65:** 557–8.
2. Ramsay B, Marks JM. Bronchoconstriction due to 8-methoxypsoralen. *Br J Dermatol* 1988; **119:** 83–6.
3. Takashima A, *et al.* Allergic contact and photocontact dermatitis due to psoralens in patients with psoriasis treated with topical PUVA. *Br J Dermatol* 1991; **124:** 37–42.

Precautions

Methoxsalen should not be given to patients with diseases associated with light sensitivity such as porphyria, although it is used with care to decrease some patients' sensitivity to sunlight. Other contraindications include aphakia, melanoma or a history of melanoma, and invasive squamous cell carcinoma. It is generally recommended that PUVA therapy should not be used in children. Methoxsalen should be used with caution in patients with hepatic insufficiency. It is recommended that unless specific treatment is required male genitalia should be shielded during PUVA therapy.

Patients should not sunbathe for 24 hours before and 48 hours after PUVA treatment. They should avoid exposure to sun, even through glass or cloud cover for at least 8 hours after methoxsalen ingestion and patients should wear wrap-around UVA absorbing glasses for 24 hours after ingestion. Photosensitivity is more prolonged following topical application and treated skin should be protected from exposure to sunlight for at least 12 to 48 hours. It has been recommended that patients should undergo an ophthalmic examination, and that measurements of anti-nuclear antibody titre and hepatic function be carried out before, and at intervals after, commencing therapy. Patients should also receive regular examinations for signs of premalignant or malignant skin lesions.

Porphyria. Methoxsalen should not be given to patients with porphyria.

Interactions

Methoxsalen should be used with caution with other drugs also known to cause photosensitivity.

Food. Some foods, for example, celery, parsnip, and parsley, contain psoralens and consumption of large quantities may increase the risk of phototoxicity with methoxsalen. A patient[1] who had consumed a large quantity of celery soup the evening before and two hours before undergoing PUVA therapy for atopic eczema developed severe phototoxicity following the treatment which was attributed to the additive effects of methoxsalen and psoralens contained in the celery.

1. Boffa MJ, *et al.* Celery soup causing severe phototoxicity during PUVA therapy. *Br J Dermatol* 1996; **135:** 334.

Phenytoin. Failure of PUVA treatment due to abnormally low serum concentrations of methoxsalen in a patient with epilepsy was probably a result of induction of hepatic enzymes by phenytoin.[1]

1. Staberg B, Hueg B. Interaction between 8-methoxypsoralen and phenytoin. *Acta Derm Venereol (Stockh)* 1985; **65:** 553–5.

Pharmacokinetics

When taken by mouth methoxsalen is well but variably absorbed from the gastrointestinal tract and there is considerable interindividual variation in peak serum concentrations. Depending on the oral formulation used increased photosensitivity is present 1 hour after a dose, reaches a peak at about 1 to 4 hours, and disappears after about 8 hours. Methoxsalen is highly protein bound. It appears to be preferentially taken up by epidermal cells. It also diffuses into the lens of the eye. Methoxsalen is almost completely metabolised. Approximately 95% of a dose is excreted in the urine within 24 hours. Photosensitivity after topical application may persist for several days, reaching a peak after about 2 days.

◊ References.

1. de Wolff FA, Thomas TV. Clinical pharmacokinetics of methoxsalen and other psoralens. *Clin Pharmacokinet* 1986; **11:** 62–75.

Uses and Administration

Methoxsalen, a psoralen, is a photosensitiser markedly increasing skin reactivity to long-wavelength ultraviolet radiation (320 to 400 nm), an effect used in photochemotherapy or PUVA [psoralen (P) and high-intensity long-wavelength UVA irradiation]. In the presence of UVA, methoxsalen bonds with DNA inhibiting DNA synthesis and cell division, and can lead to cell injury. Recovery from the cell injury may be followed by increased melanisation of the epidermis. Methoxsalen may also increase pigmentation by an action on melanocytes.

The symbol † denotes a preparation no longer actively marketed

PUVA is used to treat idiopathic vitiligo and severe, recalcitrant, disabling psoriasis not adequately responsive to conventional topical therapy. It may also be useful in selected cases of atopic eczema and polymorphic light eruptions and may be used in T-cell lymphomas such as mycosis fungoides.

Methoxsalen is given both by mouth and applied topically in PUVA regimens. Differing oral dosage forms of methoxsalen may exhibit significantly varying bioavailabilities and times to onset of photosensitisation. The UVA exposure dose should generally be based on prior measurement of the minimal phototoxic dose although it can be calculated with regard to the skin type of the patient if phototoxic dose testing cannot be carried out.

To repigment **vitiliginous** areas, methoxsalen is given in a dose of up to 600 µg per kg body-weight by mouth 2 to 4 hours before measured periods of exposure to UVA twice a week, at least 48 hours apart. Methoxsalen may also be applied topically to repigment small, well-defined vitiliginous lesions. Preparations containing up to 1% have been used but dilution to 0.1 or 0.01% may be necessary to avoid adverse cutaneous effects. The surrounding skin should be protected by an opaque sunscreen. Some suggest that the treated area should be exposed to UVA immediately after application while others recommend waiting up to 2 hours. After exposure the lesions should be washed and protected from light; protection may be necessary for up to 48 hours or longer. Treatment is repeated usually once weekly. Significant repigmentation may not appear until after 6 to 9 months of treatment.

For the treatment of **psoriasis** a similar schedule is used to that outlined above for vitiligo. A dose of up to about 600 µg per kg by mouth 2 hours before UVA is usually given twice a week although increased frequencies, but with at least 48-hour intervals between doses, have been suggested. If there is no response or only minimal response after the fifteenth PUVA treatment some suggest that the dosage may be increased, once only, by 10 mg for the remainder of the course of treatment. Methoxsalen may also be used topically with UVA exposure for the treatment of psoriasis. For direct application to affected areas of skin a preparation containing approximately 0.15% (or diluted to 0.015% if necessary to avoid adverse cutaneous effects) is applied 15 minutes before UVA exposure. Alternatively the patient may take a whole-body bath for 15 minutes in a methoxsalen solution, followed immediately by UVA exposure. UK guidelines (see also below) suggest a typical concentration of 2.6 mg methoxsalen per litre for such solutions although higher concentrations (up to about 3.7 mg per litre) have been used. Hand and foot soaks may be used to treat only those affected areas; a solution containing methoxsalen 3 mg per litre may be used with the affected areas immersed for 15 minutes followed by a delay of 30 minutes before UVA exposure. Baths or soaks are generally given twice a week.

Psoralen itself has also been used.

Administration. The dose of methoxsalen is usually calculated on the basis of body-weight. This method of dose calculation produces a considerable difference between the doses received by heavy and light patients. A study in 41 patients with psoriasis[1] suggested that using methoxsalen 25 mg per m² body-surface gave more consistent plasma concentrations and may reduce the potential for burning in heavy patients and prevent underdosing in light patients undergoing PUVA therapy.

1. Sakuntabhai A, et al. Calculation of 8-methoxypsoralen dose according to body surface area in PUVA treatment. Br J Dermatol 1995; 133: 919–23.

PUVA. PUVA combines psoralens with ultraviolet A irradiation. The psoralens may be administered directly to the patient, either orally or topically, and the patient is then exposed to UVA. In extracorporeal PUVA (extracorporeal photochemotherapy; photopheresis), an oral dose of psoralen is administered, after which the patient's leucocytes are isolated, exposed to UVA extracorporeally, and then reinfused. In another method of photopheresis that is under investigation, methoxsalen is added directly to leucocytes that have already been removed from the patient. The mixture is then treated with UVA extracorporeally after which it is returned to the patient; the total dose of methoxsalen used by this method is lower than that

used orally. PUVA has been used in a wide range of disorders including skin disorders, mycosis fungoides, and organ and tissue transplant rejection (below).

MYCOSIS FUNGOIDES. PUVA therapy is used in the treatment of the manifestations of cutaneous mycosis fungoides and Sèzary syndrome, two forms of cutaneous T-cell lymphoma (see p.489). Extracorporeal PUVA therapy (photopheresis; see above) has also been used,[1-4] particularly for disease with erythrodermic features.

1. Duvic M, et al. Photopheresis therapy for cutaneous T-cell lymphoma. J Am Acad Dermatol 1996; 35: 573–9.
2. Zic JA, et al. Long-term follow-up of patients with cutaneous T-cell lymphoma treated with extracorporeal photochemotherapy. J Am Acad Dermatol 1996; 35: 935–45.
3. Zic JA, et al. The North American experience with photopheresis. Ther Apher 1999; 3: 50–62.
4. Rubegni P, et al. Extracorporeal photochemotherapy in long-term treatment of early stage cutaneous T-cell lymphoma. Br J Dermatol 2000; 143: 894–6.

ORGAN AND TISSUE TRANSPLANTATION. Extracorporeal PUVA therapy (photopheresis; see above) has been tried in patients with graft-versus-host disease[1,2] and to prevent rejection in cardiac[3] and other solid organ transplantation.[2]

1. Konstantinow A, et al. Chronic graft-versus-host disease: successful treatment with extracorporeal photochemotherapy: a follow-up. Br J Dermatol 1996; 135: 1007–8.
2. Zic JA, et al. The North American experience with photopheresis. Ther Apher 1999; 3: 50–62.
3. Barr ML, et al. Photopheresis for the prevention of rejection in cardiac transplantation. N Engl J Med 1998; 339: 1744–51.

SKIN DISORDERS. PUVA has been used in a wide range of skin disorders and guidelines have been published by the British Photodermatology Group[1,2] which are summarised as follows.

• Indications for PUVA in chronic plaque **psoriasis** include severe extensive psoriasis unresponsive to conventional topical therapies, relapse within 3 to 6 months of successful topical treatment, or patient refusal of topical treatment if UVB phototherapy has failed (see p.1106 for a discussion of the various treatments of psoriasis). Initial UVA exposure should preferably be determined on the basis of prior measurement of the minimal phototoxic dose rather than on the skin type. Increases in UVA irradiation are then calculated as a percentage of previous doses. Methoxsalen in a dose of 600 µg per kg body-weight by mouth given 2 hours before UVA exposure is the widely accepted standard regimen. Alternatively, 5-methoxypsoralen 1.2 mg per kg, again 2 hours before UVA exposure, can be given and appears to be almost free of the adverse reactions such as nausea, pruritus, and erythema induced by methoxsalen. However, until the clinical efficacy of 5-methoxypsoralen has been clearly demonstrated, methoxsalen should remain the psoralen of choice for most clinical situations. Alternatives to oral PUVA are baths or soaks using methoxsalen or trioxysalen. For whole-body bathing a concentration of methoxsalen 2.6 mg per litre is typically utilised with the patient bathing for 15 minutes followed by immediate exposure to UVA. For hand and foot soaks a concentration of methoxsalen 3 mg per litre is used with the affected area immersed for 15 minutes followed by a delay of 30 minutes before UVA exposure. For trioxysalen a concentration of about 330 µg per litre is used for a 15-minute whole-body bath or hand and foot soak followed by immediate UVA exposure for whole-body therapy, or a 30 minute delay before hand and foot UVA exposure. Whole-body baths or hand and foot soaks are given twice each week. Methoxsalen may also be applied topically to the affected areas. A concentration of approximately 0.15% (or 0.015% if erythema occurs) is employed in an emulsion, or 0.005% in an aqueous gel, and applied 15 minutes before UVA exposure. PUVA treatment should be discontinued as soon as clearance is achieved and maintenance PUVA after routine clearance should be avoided. A combination of PUVA with acitretin (300 to 700 µg per kg by mouth) or etretinate (0.5 to 1 mg per kg by mouth) may be considered in patients who have reached 50 treatment sessions or relapsed within 6 months of PUVA. PUVA and methotrexate are effective for severe psoriasis but should be reserved for such cases because of the possible increased risk of skin cancer

• Oral PUVA twice weekly with methoxsalen 600 µg per kg or 5-methoxypsoralen 1.2 mg per kg has been effective in many patients with **vitiligo** (see Pigmentation Disorders, p.1106). If patches are large and well demarcated topical application of methoxsalen 0.15% may be preferable

• In **mycosis fungoides** PUVA is an effective symptomatic treatment for early disease and a useful adjunct for late-stage disease but optimal regimens have not been established (see above)

• PUVA is effective for atopic **eczema** (p.1105) but clearance is less certain than for psoriasis, twice the number of treatments may be needed, and relapse is more frequent. It should therefore be reserved for severe disease unresponsive to conventional treatments. Optimal regimens have not been established

• In **polymorphic light eruptions** PUVA is effective in up to 90% of patients but is only indicated in those who are frequently or severely affected despite the regular use of high-protection broad-spectrum sunscreens. Several arbitrary regimens are in use

• Variable results have also been reported in a variety of other disorders but data has been insufficient to establish precise guidelines. Such disorders include actinic prurigo, alopecia areata, aquagenic pruritus, chronic actinic dermatitis, granuloma annulare, lichen planus, nodular prurigo, pityriasis lichenoides, localised scleroderma, solar urticaria, and urticaria pigmentosa. In most cases relapse occurs in the absence of maintenance therapy and PUVA should usually only be tried as a last resort.

Extracorporeal PUVA has been tried in patients with severe epidermolysis bullosa acquisita,[3,4] and scleroderma.[5]

1. British Photodermatology Group. British Photodermatology Group guidelines for PUVA. Br J Dermatol 1994; 130: 246–55.
2. Halpern SM, et al. Guidelines for topical PUVA: a report of a workshop of the British Photodermatology Group. Br J Dermatol 2000; 142: 22–31.
3. Miller JL, et al. Remission of severe epidermolysis bullosa acquisita induced by extracorporeal photochemotherapy. Br J Dermatol 1995; 133: 467–71.
4. Gordon KB, et al. Treatment of refractory epidermolysis bullosa acquisita with extracorporeal photochemotherapy. Br J Dermatol 1997; 136: 415–20.
5. Zic JA, et al. The North American experience with photopheresis. Ther Apher 1999; 3: 50–62.

Preparations

USP 25: Methoxsalen Capsules; Methoxsalen Topical Solution.

Proprietary Preparations (details are given in Part 3)
Aust.: Oxsoralen; *Austral.:* Oxsoralen; *Belg.:* Mopsoralen; Oxsoralen†; *Canad.:* Oxsoralen; Ultramop; *Denm.:* Geroxalen; *Fr.:* Meladinine; *Ger.:* Meladinine; *Hong Kong:* Oxsoralen; *Irl.:* Deltasoralen; *Israel:* Oxsoralen; *Ital.:* Oxsoralen; *Mex.:* Dermox; Meladinina; Oxsoralen; *Neth.:* Geroxalen; Meladinine; Oxsoralen†; *Norw.:* Geroxalen; *NZ:* Oxsoralen; *S.Afr.:* Oxsoralen; *Singapore:* Oxsoralen; *Spain:* Oxsoralen; *Switz.:* Meladinine; *Thai.:* Meladinine; *UK:* Puvasoralen; *USA:* Oxsoralen; Uvadex.

5-Methoxypsoralen (12944-h)

Bergapten. 4-Methoxy-7H-furo[3,2-g]chromen-7-one.
$C_{12}H_8O_4 = 216.2$.
CAS — 484-20-8.
ATC — D05BA03.

5-Methoxypsoralen is an ingredient of bergamot oil.

Profile
5-Methoxypsoralen is a photosensitiser with actions similar to those of methoxsalen (above). It may be given by mouth in the PUVA therapy (p.1120) of psoriasis and vitiligo.

5-Methoxypsoralen is included in some cosmetic suntan preparations to enhance tanning but because of its potential phototoxicity this is considered unwise by some authorities. Photosensitivity caused by 5-methoxypsoralen is sometimes known as Berloque dermatitis.

◊ References.
1. McNeely W, Goa KL. 5-Methoxypsoralen: a review of its effects in psoriasis and vitiligo. Drugs 1998; 56: 667–90.

Preparations

Proprietary Preparations (details are given in Part 3)
Aust.: Geralen; *Fr.:* Psoraderm 5†; *Switz.:* Psoraderm 5.

Monobenzone (1624-p)

Monobenzone (rINN).
Hydroquinone Monobenzyl Ether. 4-Benzyloxyphenol.
$C_{13}H_{12}O_2 = 200.2$.
CAS — 103-16-2.
Pharmacopoeias. In US.

Pharmacopoeial description
USP 25: Store at a temperature not exceeding 30° in airtight containers. Protect from light.

Adverse Effects and Precautions
Monobenzone may cause skin irritation and sensitisation. In some patients, this may be transient and need not necessitate withdrawal of the drug. In other patients, an eczematous sensitisation may occur. Excessive depigmentation may occur even beyond the areas under treatment and may produce unsightly patches.

Monobenzone can produce permanent depigmentation and should not be used as a substitute for hydroquinone.

Uses and Administration
Monobenzone has actions similar to those of hydroquinone (p.1115) but in some patients it also produces extensive and selective destruction of melanocytes. It is used locally for final, permanent depigmentation of normal skin in extensive vitiligo (see Pigmentation Disorders, p.1106). Monobenzone is not recommended for freckling, chloasma, or hyperpigmentation following skin inflammation or due to photosensitisation following the use of certain perfumes. It has no effect on melanomas or pigmented naevi.

For vitiligo monobenzone is applied in the form of a cream containing up to 20% to the affected parts two or three times daily until a satisfactory response is obtained, and thereafter as necessary, usually about twice weekly. Excessive exposure to sunlight should be avoided during treatment. The results are variable. Depigmentation only becomes apparent when the preformed melanin pigments have been lost with the normal sloughing of the stratum corneum and this may take several months. If, however, no improvement is noted after 4 months, treatment should be abandoned.

Preparations

USP 25: Monobenzone Cream.

Proprietary Preparations (details are given in Part 3)
Canad.: Benoquin; *USA:* Benoquin†.

Motretinide   (12980-g)

Motretinide (USAN, rINN).

Ro-11-1430. (*all-trans*)-N-Ethyl-9-(4-methoxy-2,3,6-trimethyl-phenyl)-3,7-dimethyl-2,4,6,8-nonatetraenamide.
$C_{23}H_{31}NO_2 = 353.5$.
CAS — 56281-36-8.
ATC — D10AD05.

Profile

Motretinide is a retinoid structurally related to acitretin (p.1109). Motretinide is used topically in the treatment of acne (p.1103). It is applied in preparations containing 0.1%.

Preparations

Proprietary Preparations (details are given in Part 3)
Switz.: Tasmaderm.

Piroctone Olamine   (6387-v)

Piroctone Olamine (USAN, rINNM).

1-Hydroxy-4-methyl-6-(2,4,4-trimethylpentyl)-2(1H)-pyridone compound with 2-aminoethanol (1:1).
$C_{14}H_{23}NO_2,C_2H_7NO = 298.4$.
CAS — 50650-76-5 (piroctone); 68890-66-4 (piroctone olamine).

Profile

Piroctone olamine has been used in shampoos for the treatment of dandruff.

Preparations

Proprietary Preparations (details are given in Part 3)
Austral.: Neoceuticals Therapeutic Shampoo; *Fr.:* Cystelle Antipelliculaire; *Irl.:* Saliker; *Ital.:* Olamin P.

Multi-ingredient: *Fr.:* Biolan Tar†; T/Gel; *Ital.:* Shamday Antiforfora; *Port.:* Alpha Septol; Hyfac; Hyfac AHA; Ionil P; Peliphane†; Savorix T; Squaphane.

Podophyllum   (7523-v)

American Mandrake; May Apple Root; Podoph.; Podophyllum Rhizome.
CAS — 568-53-6 (α-peltatin); 518-29-6 (β-peltatin).
Pharmacopoeias. In US.

Pharmacopoeial description

USP 25: The dried rhizomes and roots of *Podophyllum peltatum* (Berberidaceae). It yields not less than 5% of resin. It has a slight odour.

Indian Podophyllum   (7524-g)

Ind. Podoph.; Indian Podophyllum Rhizome.
Pharmacopoeias. Chin. includes a monograph for the fruits only.

The dried fruits or rhizomes and roots of *Podophyllum hexandrum* (=*P. emodi*) (Berberidaceae).

Podophyllum Resin   (7525-q)

Podoph. Resin; Podophylli Resina; Podophyllin.
CAS — 8050-60-0.
Pharmacopoeias. In *Aust., Int., Swiss,* and *US* (all from podophyllum only). In *Br.* from Indian podophyllum.

Pharmacopoeial description

BP 2001: The resin obtained from the rhizomes and roots of *Podophyllum hexandrum* (*P. emodi*). It contains not less than 50% of total aryltetralin lignans, calculated as podophyllotoxin.

An amorphous powder, varying in colour from light brown to greenish-yellow or brownish-grey masses, with a characteristic odour; caustic. On exposure to light or to temperatures above 25° it becomes darker in colour.

Partly soluble in hot water but precipitated again on cooling; partly soluble in chloroform, in ether, and in dilute ammonia solution. Protect from light.

USP 25: The powdered mixture of resins extracted from podophyllum (the rhizomes and roots of *Podophyllum peltatum*) by percolation with alcohol and subsequent precipitation with acidified water. It contains not less than 40% and not more than 50% of hexane-insoluble matter.

An amorphous caustic powder, varying in colour from light brown to greenish-yellow. On exposure to light or to temperatures above 25° it becomes darker in colour.

The symbol † denotes a preparation no longer actively marketed

---

Soluble in alcohol with a slight opalescence; partially soluble in chloroform and in ether. A solution in alcohol is acid to litmus. Store in airtight containers. Protect from light.

◊ CAUTION. *Podophyllum resin is strongly irritant to the skin, eyes, and mucous membranes and requires careful handling.*

Podophyllotoxin   (10037-x)

Podophyllotoxin (BAN).

Podofilox (USAN). (5R,5aR,8aR,9R)-5,5a,6,8,8a,9-Hexahydro-9-hydroxy-5-(3,4,5-trimethoxyphenyl)furo[3′4′:6,7]naph-tho[2,3-d]-1,3-dioxol-6-one.
$C_{22}H_{22}O_8 = 414.4$.
CAS — 518-28-5.
ATC — D06BB04.

Adverse Effects

Podophyllum is very irritant, especially to the eyes and mucous membranes. It can also cause severe systemic toxicity after ingestion or topical application, which is usually reversible but has been fatal. Symptoms of toxicity include nausea, vomiting, abdominal pain, and diarrhoea; there may be thrombocytopenia, leucopenia, renal failure, and hepatotoxicity. Central effects are delayed in onset and prolonged in duration and include acute psychotic reactions, hallucinations, confusion, dizziness, stupor, ataxia, hypotonia, seizures, and coma. EEG changes may persist for several days. Peripheral and autonomic neuropathies develop later and may result in paraesthesias, reduced reflexes, muscle weakness, tachycardia, apnoea, orthostatic hypotension, paralytic ileus, and urinary retention. Neuropathy may improve but full recovery is unusual.

Carcinogenicity. A report of the transformation of a condyloma acuminatum into an invasive squamous cell carcinoma after treatment with podophyllum 25% in alcohol.[1]

1. Svindland HB. Malignant transformation of condyloma acuminatum after treatment with podophyllin. *Eur J Sex Transm Dis* 1984; **1:** 165–7.

Poisoning. Reports and reviews of podophyllum toxicity.[1-7] A few of the cases followed consumption of herbal preparations containing podophyllum or the related plant bajiaolian (*Dysosma pleianthum*). Death has occurred following ingestion of 10 g of podophyllum.

1. Cassidy DE, *et al.* Podophyllum toxicity: a report of a fatal case and a review of the literature. *J Toxicol Clin Toxicol* 1982; **19:** 35–44.
2. Dobb GJ, Edis RH. Coma and neuropathy after ingestion of herbal laxative containing podophyllin. *Med J Aust* 1984; **140:** 495–6.
3. Holdright DR, Jahangiri M. Accidental poisoning with podophyllin. *Hum Exp Toxicol* 1990; **9:** 55–6.
4. Tomczak RL, Hake DH. Near fatal systemic toxicity from local injection of podophyllin for pedal verrucae treatment. *J Foot Surg* 1992; **31:** 36–42.
5. Kao W-F, *et al.* Podophyllotoxin intoxication: toxic effect of bajiaolian in herbal therapeutics. *Hum Exp Toxicol* 1992; **11:** 480–7.
6. Chan TYK, Critchley JAJH. Usage and adverse effects of Chinese herbal medicines. *Hum Exp Toxicol* 1996; **15:** 5–12.
7. Chu CC, *et al.* Sensory neuropathy due to bajiaolian (podophyllotoxin) intoxication. *Eur Neurol* 2000; **44:** 121–3.

Precautions

Podophyllum should not be used during pregnancy or breast feeding or in children.

The risk of systemic toxicity after topical application is increased by the treatment of large areas with excessive amounts for prolonged periods, by the treatment of friable, bleeding, or recently biopsied warts, and by inadvertent application to normal skin or mucous membranes.

Uses and Administration

Podophyllum resin has an antimitotic action and is used principally as a topical treatment for anogenital warts (condylomata acuminata). It is applied as a 15% (Indian podophyllum) or up to a 25% solution (American podophyllum) in alcohol or compound benzoin tincture, left on the warts for 1 to 6 hours, and then washed off. This procedure is carried out once a week and, if unsuccessful after about 6 weeks, an alternative treatment should be tried. A preparation containing podophyllotoxin 0.5% in alcohol or alcoholic gel, or a 0.15% podophyllotoxin cream is used similarly. They are applied twice daily for 3 days but not washed off. Treatment may be repeated at weekly intervals for up to a total of 5 weeks of treatment. Podo-

---

phyllum resin has been used on external genital, perianal, and intra-meatal warts, but should not be used on cervical or urethral warts. Only a small area or number of warts should be treated at any one time. Care must be taken to avoid application to healthy tissue. Podophyllum resin is also used with other keratolytics for the removal of plantar warts.

When taken by mouth podophyllum resin has a drastic purging action and it is highly irritant to the intestinal mucosa and produces violent peristalsis. It has been superseded by less toxic laxatives.

Podophyllum has been used in homoeopathic medicine.

Anogenital warts. Podophyllum preparations are one of the treatment choices for anogenital warts caused by human papillomavirus infection (condylomata acuminata) (p.1108). Paints containing 10% or 25% of podophyllum resin appear to be equally effective for the treatment of external anogenital warts.[1] However, preparations containing podophyllotoxin 0.5%, the major active constituent of podophyllum resin, appear to be initially more effective[2] and unlike podophyllum, may be suitable for self-treatment in both men and women.[3,4]

1. Simmons PD. Podophyllin 10% and 25% in the treatment of anogenital warts: a comparative double-blind study. *Br J Vener Dis* 1981; **57:** 208–9.
2. Anonymous. Painting penile warts. *Drug Ther Bull* 1990; **28:** 63–4.
3. Beutner KR, *et al.* Patient-applied podofilox for treatment of genital warts. *Lancet* 1989; **i:** 831–4.
4. Greenberg MD, *et al.* A double-blind, randomized trial of 0.5% podofilox and placebo for the treatment of genital warts in women. *Obstet Gynecol* 1991; **77:** 735–9.

Preparations

BP 2001: Compound Podophyllin Paint;
USP 25: Podophyllum Resin Topical Solution.

Proprietary Preparations (details are given in Part 3)
Aust.: Condylox; *Austral.:* Condyline; Wartec; *Belg.:* Condyline†; *Canad.:* Condyline; Podofilm; Wartec; *Denm.:* Condyline; Wartec; *Fin.:* Condyline; Wartec; *Fr.:* Condyline; Wartec; *Ger.:* Condylox; Wartec; *Hong Kong:* Podofilm; *Irl.:* Condyline; Warticon; *Israel:* Condyline; *Ital.:* Condyline; Mex.: Condil; Papilo Lisin; Podofilia; *Neth.:* Condyline; *Norw.:* Condyline; Wartec; *NZ:* Condyline; *Port.:* Cholagett; Condyline; *S.Afr.:* Condyline; *Singapore:* Podofilm; *Spain:* Condelone†; Wartec; *Swed.:* Condyline; Wartec; *Switz.:* Condyline; Warix; *UK:* Condyline; Warticon; *USA:* Condylox; Pod-Ben-25; Podocon; Podofin.

Multi-ingredient: *Austral.:* Posalfilin; *Belg.:* Carters†; Sanicolax†; *Braz.:* Steitonit; *Canad.:* Canthacur-PS; Cantharone Plus; *Ger.:* Unguentum lymphaticum; *Hong Kong:* Posalfilin; *Irl.:* Posalfilin; *NZ:* Posalfilin; *S.Afr.:* Posalfilin; *Singapore:* Posalfilin; *Spain:* Alofedina; Laxo Vian†; *UK:* Posalfilin; *USA:* Verrex†.

Polyphloroglucinol Phosphate   (13148-v)

Polyphloroglucin Phosphate. Poly[benzene-1,3,5-triol mono(dihydrogen phosphate)].
$(C_6H_7O_6P)_n$.
CAS — 51202-77-8.

Profile

Polyphloroglucinol phosphate has an inhibitory effect on hyaluronidase and has been applied topically in the treatment of wounds and pruritic skin disorders.

Preparations

Proprietary Preparations (details are given in Part 3)
Aust.: Dealyd.

Polyprenoic Acid   (2035-a)

E-5166; Polyprenic Acid. (*all-E*)-3,7,11,15-Tetramethyl-2,4,6,10,14-hexadecapentaenoic acid.
$C_{20}H_{30}O_2 = 302.5$.
CAS — 81485-25-8.

Profile

Polyprenoic acid is a retinoid that has been tried in psoriasis and keratoderma and is being studied in the treatment of liver cancers.

◊ References.

1. Muto Y, *et al.* Prevention of second primary tumors by an acyclic retinoid, polyprenoic acid, in patients with hepatocellular carcinoma. *N Engl J Med* 1996; **334:** 1561–7.
2. Muto Y, *et al.* Prevention of second primary tumors by an acyclic retinoid in patients with hepatocellular carcinoma. *N Engl J Med* 1999; **340:** 1046–7.

Prezatide Copper Acetate   (16788-z)

Prezatide Copper Acetate (USAN, rINN).

PC-1020 (prezatide copper). Hydrogen [N^2-(N-glycyl-L-histidyl)-L-lysinato][N^2-(N-glycyl-L-histidyl)-L-lysinato(2–)]cuprate(1–) diacetate.
$C_{28}H_{46}CuN_{12}O_8,2C_2H_4O_2 = 862.4$.
CAS — 130120-57-9.

Profile

Prezatide copper acetate is a copper-containing tripeptide that is used as a wound-healing agent and has been investigated in inflammatory bowel disease.

Preparations

Proprietary Preparations (details are given in Part 3)
USA: Iamin Hydrating Gel.

Pyrithione Zinc (1633-s)

Pyrithione Zinc *(BAN, USAN, rINN)*.

Zinc 2-Pyridinethiol 1-Oxide; Zinc Pyridinethione. Bis[1-hydroxypyridine-2(1*H*)-thionato]zinc.
$C_{10}H_8N_2O_2S_2Zn = 317.7$.
CAS — 13463-41-7.

Profile

Pyrithione zinc has bacteriostatic and fungistatic properties. It is used similarly to selenium sulfide (p.1123) in usual concentrations of 1 to 2% in the control of seborrhoeic dermatitis and dandruff (p.1107). It is an ingredient of some proprietary shampoos. It has also been used in the treatment of pityriasis versicolor.

Pyrithione magnesium has also been used.

◊ Peripheral neuritis with paraesthesia and muscle weakness in a patient was associated with the prolonged use of a shampoo containing pyrithione zinc 2%.[1] The muscle weakness had disappeared 3 months after stopping the shampoo and 2 years later the paraesthesia had improved by about 75%.

Studies in *animals* had found signs of neurotoxicity following oral administration of pyrithione zinc but whereas absorption following topical application was found to be 13% for pyrithione sodium it was less than 1% for pyrithione zinc.[2]

1. Beck JE. Zinc pyrithione and peripheral neuritis. *Lancet* 1978; **i**: 444.
2. Parekh CK. Zinc pyrithione and peripheral neuritis. *Lancet* 1978; **i**: 940.

Preparations

Proprietary Preparations (details are given in Part 3)
Aust.: Desquaman; *Austral.:* Dan-Gard; Dandruff Control Pert 2 in 1; *Canad.:* Anti-Dandruff Shampoo; Avant Garde Shampoo; Avon Techniques Anti-Dandruff; Brylcreem Anti-Dandruff; Dan-Gard; Dandruff Treatment Shampoo; Hair & Scalp; Head & Shoulders; Keep Clear Anti-Dandruff Shampoo; Lander Dandruff Control; No-Name Dandruff Treatment†; Out of Africa; Pert Plus; Redken Solve Acid Balance; Satinique Anti-Dandruff; Sebulon; Shaklee Dandruff Control; Shampooing Anti-Pelliculaire; ZNP; ZP 11; *Denm.:* Skaelud; *Fr.:* Hermal†; Provegol; ZNP; *Ger.:* Desquaman N; *Hong Kong:* Hair & Scalp; *Israel:* Desquaman; *Ital.:* Rivescal ZPT; Shampoo SDE Zinc; ZNP; *Mex.:* Skin Cap; ZNP; *Port.:* Desquaman†; ZP Dermil; *Spain:* Zination; *USA:* DHS Zinc; Head & Shoulders; Sebulon†; Skin Cure; Theraplex Z; TVC-2 Dandruff Shampoo†; Zincon; ZNP.

Multi-ingredient: *Austral.:* Fongitar; *Canad.:* Dan-Tar Plus; Multi-Tar Plus; Polytar AF; X-Seb Plus; Z-Plus; *Hong Kong:* Fongitar; Multi-Tar; *Ital.:* Aminotril; Fongitar†; Kevis; Omadine; *NZ:* Fongitar; *Port.:* All Pecium; Alpha Septol; Fongitar; Hyfac; *Singapore:* Fongitar; pHisoHex Reformulated; *Spain:* Zincation Plus; *Switz.:* Crinotar†; Sebo Shampooing; Soufrol ZNP; Squamed; *Thai.:* Fongitar; *UK:* Polytar AF; *USA:* X-Seb Plus.

Pyrogallol (1634-w)

Pyrogallic Acid. Benzene-1,2,3-triol.
$C_6H_6O_3 = 126.1$.
CAS — 87-66-1.
Pharmacopoeias. In Aust., Fr., and Pol.

Profile

Pyrogallol was formerly used topically in the treatment of psoriasis and parasitic skin diseases, but application over large areas or denuded surfaces is dangerous and may produce systemic effects similar to phenol poisoning (see p.1152); methaemoglobinaemia, haemolysis, and kidney damage may also occur.

Pyrogallol stains the skin and hair black.

Preparations

Proprietary Preparations (details are given in Part 3)
USA: Pyrogallic.

Pyroxylin (1636-l)

Pyroxylin *(rINN)*.

Algodão-Polvora; Cellulose Nitrate; Colloxylinum; Fulmicoton; Gossypium Collodium; Kollodiumwolle; Pyroxylinum; Soluble Guncotton.
CAS — 9004-70-0.
Pharmacopoeias. In Aust., Br., Jpn, and US.

Pharmacopoeial description

BP 2001: A nitrated cellulose obtained by the action of a mixture of nitric and sulfuric acids on wood pulp or cotton linters that have been freed from fatty matter. It must be damped with not less than 25% of isopropyl alcohol or of industrial methylated spirit. White or almost white cuboid granules or fibrous material resembling absorbent cotton but harsher to the touch

and more powdery. It is highly flammable. Soluble in acetone and in glacial acetic acid. Store in well-closed containers, loosely packed, protected from light, and at a temperature not exceeding 15°, remote from fire. The container should be suitably designed to disrupt should the internal pressure reach or exceed 1400 kPa. The amount of damping fluid must not be allowed to fall below 25% w/w; should this happen, the material should be either rewetted or used immediately for the preparation of Collodion.

USP 25: Pyroxylin is obtained by the action of a mixture of nitric and sulfuric acids on cotton and consists chiefly of cellulose tetranitrate $(C_{12}H_{16}N_4O_{18})_n$. It occurs as a light yellow, matted mass of filaments resembling raw cotton but harsher to the touch. It is highly flammable. Store loosely packed, protected from light. When kept in well-closed containers and exposed to light, it decomposes with the evolution of nitrous vapours, leaving a carbonaceous residue.

◊ CAUTION. *Dry pyroxylin is explosive and sensitive to ignition by impact or friction and should be handled carefully.*

Profile

Pyroxylin is used in the preparation of collodions which are applied to the skin for the protection of small cuts and abrasions. Collodions are also used as vehicles for the application of drugs when prolonged local action is required.

Preparations

BP 2001: Collodion; Flexible Collodion;
USP 25: Collodion; Flexible Collodion.

Resorcinol (1637-y)

m-Dihydroxybenzene; Dioxybenzolum; Resorcin; Resorcinolum. Benzene-1,3-diol.
$C_6H_6O_2 = 110.1$.
CAS — 108-46-3.
ATC — D10AX02; S01AX06.
Pharmacopoeias. In Chin., Eur. (see p.vi), Pol., and US.

Incompatible with ferric salts.

Pharmacopoeial description

Ph. Eur.: Colourless or slightly pinkish-grey crystals or crystalline powder. M.p. 109° to 112°. It becomes red on exposure to air and light. Very soluble in water and in alcohol; freely soluble in ether. Protect from light.

USP 25: White or practically white, needle-shaped crystals or powder with a faint characteristic odour. M.p. 109° to 111°. It acquires a pink tint on exposure to air and light. Soluble 1 in 1 of water and of alcohol; slightly soluble in chloroform; freely soluble in ether and in glycerol. A 5% solution in water is neutral or acid to litmus. Protect from light.

Resorcinol Monoacetate (1638-j)

Resorcin Acetate. 3-Acetoxyphenol.
$C_8H_8O_3 = 152.1$.
CAS — 102-29-4.
Pharmacopoeias. In US.

Pharmacopoeial description

USP 25: A pale yellow or amber, viscous liquid with a faint characteristic odour. Sparingly soluble in water; soluble in alcohol and in most organic solvents. A saturated solution in water is acid to litmus. Store in airtight containers. Protect from light.

Adverse Effects, Treatment, and Precautions

Resorcinol is a mild irritant and may result in skin sensitisation. It should not be applied to large areas of the body, for prolonged periods, or in high concentrations, especially in children, as it is absorbed through intact skin as well as broken skin and may interfere with thyroid function or produce methaemoglobinaemia. Resorcinol may produce hyperpigmentation in patients with dark skins and may darken light-coloured hair. Systemic toxic effects of resorcinol are similar to those of phenol and are treated similarly (see p.1153) but convulsions may occur more frequently.

◊ Resorcinol could cause green discoloration of the urine.[1]

1. Karlstrand J. The pharmacist and the ostomate. *J Am Pharm Assoc* 1977; **NS17:** 735–8.

Uses and Administration

Resorcinol has keratolytic properties and has been used in topical preparations for the treatment of acne (p.1103) and seborrhoeic skin conditions (p.1107) usually in combination with sulfur, although other treatments are generally preferred.

Resorcinol has also been used in preparations for the treatment of anorectal disorders often complexed with bismuth compounds (see Haemorrhoids, p.1205).

Resorcinol monoacetate has been used similarly but may provide a milder action with a longer duration.

Preparations

BPC 1973: Magenta Paint;
USP 25: Carbol-Fuchsin Topical Solution; Compound Resorcinol Ointment; Resorcinol and Sulfur Lotion.

Proprietary Preparations (details are given in Part 3)
Mex.: Astriderm; *USA:* Castel.

Multi-ingredient: *Aust.:* Apotheker Bauer's Huhneraugentinktur; Wisamt; *Austral.:* Acne & Pimple Gel; Egomycol; Eskamel;

Seborrol; *Belg.:* Synthol†; *Braz.:* Clearasil; Cravo-Espin; Pantevit; *Canad.:* Acne-Aid†; Acnomel; Acnomel Acne Mask; Clearasil Acne Cream; Clearskin 2 Tinted Blemish; Lanacane Medicated Cream; Mazon Medicated Cream; Sebo Concept D/A; Vagisil; *Fr.:* Anaxeryl; Bain de Bouche Lipha; Eau Precieuse; Gelictar Fort; Nestosyl; Osmotol; Synthol; *Ger.:* Jaikal; Wisamt N; *Hong Kong:* Acne-Aid; Seborrol; *Irl.:* Anugesic-HC; Anusol-HC; *Israel:* Acnex; Pitrisan; Vagisil; *Ital.:* Anusol; Blefarolin; Labocaina; Rinantipiol; *NZ:* Egomycol; Lanacane; Seborrol; *Port.:* Edoltar; Resodermil; Squaphane; *S.Afr.:* Anugesic; Anusol-HC†; Rectosan 'A'†; *Singapore:* Acne-Aid; Anusol; *Spain:* Acnisdin; Acnosan; Anti-Acne; Dermomycose Liquido; Milrosina; Poliglicol Anti Acne; Regal†; Resorborina; *Switz.:* Clabin; Euproctol†; Lotio decapans; *Thai.:* Anusol; *UK:* Eskamel; *USA:* Acnomel; Bensulfoid; Bicozene; Castaderm; Dermarest; Fungi-Nail; Heal Aid Plus; R/S Lotion†; RA Lotion; Resinol; Rezamid; Sulforcin; Vagisil; Yeast-Gard Maximum Strength Formula†.

Ro-13-6298 (518-r)

Ethyl *p*-[(*E*)-2-(5,6,7,8-tetrahydro-5,5,8,8-tetramethyl-2-naphthyl)-1-propenyl] benzoate.
$C_{26}H_{32}O_2 = 376.5$.
CAS — 71441-09-3.

Profile

Ro-13-6298 is an arotinoid studied in psoriasis and other keratinisation disorders.

Salicylic Acid (2701-y)

Acido Ortóxibenzoico; Acidum Salicylicum; Salizylsäure. 2-Hydroxybenzoic acid.
$C_7H_6O_3 = 138.1$.
CAS — 69-72-7.
ATC — D01AE12; S01BC08.
Pharmacopoeias. In Chin., Eur. (see p.vi), Int., Jpn, Pol., and US.

Pharmacopoeial description

Ph. Eur.: White or colourless acicular crystals or a white crystalline powder. Slightly soluble in water; freely soluble in alcohol and in ether; sparingly soluble in dichloromethane. Protect from light.

USP 25: White crystals, usually in fine needles or a white, fluffy, crystalline powder. The synthetic form is white and odourless but if prepared from natural methyl salicylate it may have a slightly yellow or pink tint, and a faint, mint-like odour. Soluble 1 in 460 of water, 1 in 15 of boiling water, 1 in 3 of alcohol, 1 in 45 of chloroform, 1 in 3 of ether, and 1 in 135 of benzene.

Adverse Effects and Precautions

Salicylic acid is a mild irritant and application of salicylic acid preparations to the skin may cause dermatitis. Salicylic acid is readily absorbed through the skin and symptoms of acute systemic salicylate poisoning (see Aspirin, p.14) have been reported after excessive application of salicylic acid to large areas of the body; several deaths have occurred, mainly in children. To minimise absorption following topical application salicylic acid should not be used for prolonged periods, in high concentrations, on large areas of the body, or on inflamed or broken skin. Contact with mouth, eyes, and other mucous membranes should be avoided. It should also be used with care on the extremities of patients with impaired peripheral circulation or diabetes.

◊ There has been a report that application of 2% salicylic acid in a cream base before phototherapy delayed or reduced the clearance of psoriatic lesions when compared with the use of the base alone.[1] It was suggested that salicylic acid might have been acting as a photoprotective agent[1] but a later study[2] failed to confirm this. However, emulsifying ointment was found to have such an effect and it was recommended that it should not be used before phototherapy or in phototesting procedures.[2]

1. Kristensen B, Kristensen O. Salicylic acid and ultraviolet B for psoriasis. *Lancet* 1989; **i**: 1109–10.
2. Cox NH, Sharpe G. Emollients, salicylic acid, and ultraviolet erythema. *Lancet* 1990; **335:** 53–4.

Uses and Administration

Salicylic acid has keratolytic properties and is applied topically in the treatment of hyperkeratotic and scaling skin conditions such as dandruff and seborrhoeic dermatitis (p.1107), ichthyosis (p.1105), psoriasis (p.1106), and acne (p.1103). Initially a concentration of about 2% is used, increased to about 6% if necessary, though a wider range of concentrations has been used. It is often used in conjunction with other drugs, notably coal tar.

Preparations containing up to 60% salicylic acid have been used as a caustic for the removal of plantar warts (p.1108), corns, or calluses.

Salicylic acid also possesses fungicidal properties and is used topically in the treatment of dermatophyte skin infections (see p.376).

Preparations

BP 2001: Coal Tar and Salicylic Acid Ointment; Compound Benzoic Acid Ointment; Dithranol Paste; Salicylic Acid Collodion; Salicylic Acid Ointment; Zinc and Salicylic Acid Paste;
BPC 1973: Salicylic Acid and Sulphur Ointment;
USP 25: Benzoic and Salicylic Acids Ointment; Salicylic Acid Collodion; Salicylic Acid Gel; Salicylic Acid Plaster; Salicylic Acid Topical Foam; Zinc Oxide and Salicylic Acid Paste.

Proprietary Preparations (details are given in Part 3)
Aust.: Dermi-cyl Schrunden; Squamasol; *Austral.:* Clear Away; Clearasil Medicated Wipes; Duofilm; Egocappol†; Egozite Cradle Cap; Ionil Scalp Cleanser; Isophyl†; Johnsons Clean & Clear Skin Balancing Moisturiser; Salact†; Sunspot; *Belg.:* Sicombyl; *Braz.:* A Curitybina; Curakalos; Ionil; Ionil Plus; Ionil-T Plus; *Canad.:* Acnex; Anti-Acne Control Formula; Anti-Acne Spot Treatment; Blemish Control; Callus Salve†; Carnation; Clean & Clear Deep Cleaning Astringent; Clean & Clear Invisible Blemish; Clear Away†; Clear Pore†; Clearasil Cleanser; Clearasil Clearstick; Clearasil Pads; Clearskin 2 Medicated Wash; Clearskin 2 Triple Action; Clearskin Cleansing; Clearskin Medicated Wash; Clearskin Overnight Acne Treatment; Compound W; Compound W Plus; Duoforte; Fostex Medicated Cleansing; Freezone; Ionil†; Keralyt; Mosco; Mudd Acne†; Neostrata AHA Astringent Acne; Neutrogena Healthy Scalp Anti-Dandruff; Nova Perfecting Lotion†; Noxema 2-in-1; Occlusal; Off-Ezy; Oil-Free Acne Wash†; Oxy Clean Pore; Oxy Control†; Oxy Deep Pore; Oxy Medicated Pads; Oxy Night Watch†; P & S; Propa PH; Salac; Salseb; Scholl 2-Drop Corn Remedy; Scholl Callus Remover; Scholl Clear Away; Scholl Corn Remover; Scholl Corn Salve†; Scholl Corn, Callus Plaster Preparation†; Scholl One Step; Scholl Wart Remover; Scholl Zino; Sebcur; Soluver; Soluver Plus; Ten-O-Six†; Trans-Plantar; Trans-Ver-Sal; Wart Remover†; X-Seb; *Denm.:* Salicyl; *Fin.:* Diprosalic; *Fr.:* Ciella; Clear Pore; Coricide le Diable; Disques Coricides; Feuille de Saule; Kertyol; Pansements Coricides; Pommade Mo Cochon; S/Gel; Septisol†; Transvercid; Verrucosal†; *Ger.:* Aknefug-liquid; Clabin; Cornina Hornhaut†; Cornina Huhneraugen†; Efasit N†; Gehwol Schalpaste; Guttaplast; Hansaplast Hornhaut-Pflaster; Hansaplast Huhneraugen-Pflaster; Humopin N†; Lygal Kopfsalbe N; Psorimed; Schrundensalbe Dermi-cyl; Sophtal-POS N; Squamasol; Urgo-N Huhneraugenpflaster; Verrucid; *Hong Kong:* Egozite Cradle Cap; Oxy Balance; *Irl.:* Acnisal; Compound W; Freezone; Occlusal; Saliker; Vericaps; *Israel:* Clearex; Salikaren; Scholl Corn/Callous Removers; *Ital.:* Keranon; Neutrogena Anti-Acne; Sebium K2; Trans-Ver-Sal; *Mex.:* Clearasil Pads; Duoplant; Ionil; Ionil Plus; Trans-Ver-Sal; *Neth.:* Formule W; *NZ:* Clear Away; Duofilm; Egozite Cradle Cap; *S.Afr.:* Jiffy Corn Plasters†; *Spain:* Callicida Globodermis; Callicida Gras; Callicida Salve; Callofin; Unguento Morry; Urgocall; Verrupatch; Verruplan; *Swed.:* Salsyvase; *Thai.:* Ionil-T; *UK:* Acnisal; Carnation; Clearasil Dual Action Pads; Clearasil Nightclear; Compound V; Compound W; Freezone†; Occlusal; Pickles Foot Ointment; Scholl Callous Removal; Scholl Corn Removal; Scholl Verucca Removal; SCR; Verruca Treatment; Verrugon; Verucca Removal System; Wartex; *USA:* Clearasil Clearstick; Compound W; DHS Sal†; Dr Scholl's Callus Removers; Dr Scholl's Clear Away; Dr Scholl's Corn Removers; Dr Scholl's Corn/Callus Remover; Dr Scholl's Wart Remover; Duofilm; Duoplant; Fostex Acne Medication Cleansing; Freezone; Gordofilm; Hydrisalic; Ionil; Ionil Plus; Keralyt; Mediplast; MG217 Sal-Acid; Mosco; Occlusal; Off-Ezy; Oxy Night Watch; P & S; Panscol; PropapH; Psor-a-set; Sal-Acid; Sal-Clens†; Sal-Plant; Salac; Salactic Film; Sebucare; Stri-Dex Clear; Trans-Ver-Sal AdultPatch; Trans-Ver-Sal PediaPatch; Trans-Ver-Sal Plantar-Patch; Wart Remover; Wart-Off; X-Seb.

Multi-ingredient: Numerous preparations are listed in Part 3.

Sebacic Acid (13225-h)

Decanedioic acid; Octane-1,8-dicarboxylic acid.
$C_{10}H_{18}O_4 = 202.2.$
$CAS — 111-20-6.$

Profile
Sebacic acid is an emollient included in preparations used to protect damaged skin.

Diisopropyl sebacate ($C_{16}H_{30}O_4 = 286.4$) has been used in skin moisturising preparations.

Selenium Sulfide (1639-z)

Selenii Disulfidum; Selenium Disulphide; Selenium Sulphide.
$SeS_2 = 143.1.$
$CAS — 7488-56-4.$
$ATC — D01AE13.$
Pharmacopoeias. In *Eur.* (see p.vi) and *US.*

Selenium sulfide may discolour metals.

Pharmacopoeial description
Ph. Eur.: A bright orange to reddish-brown powder. Practically insoluble in water.

USP 25: A bright orange to reddish-brown powder with not more than a faint odour. Practically insoluble in water and in organic solvents; soluble 1 in 161 of chloroform and 1 in 1667 of ether.

Adverse Effects and Treatment

Topical application of selenium sulfide can produce irritation of the conjunctiva, scalp, and skin, especially in the genital area and skin folds. Oiliness or dryness of scalp or hair, hair discoloration, and hair loss have been reported.

Selenium sulfide can be highly toxic when taken by mouth. Only traces of selenium sulfide are absorbed through intact skin but prolonged use on broken skin has resulted in systemic toxicity.

Treatment of poisoning is symptomatic.

Systemic toxicity. A woman with excoriated eruptions on her scalp developed weakness, anorexia, abdominal pain, vomiting, tremors, sweating, a metallic taste in her mouth, and a garlic-like smell on her breath after using a shampoo containing selenium sulfide 2 or 3 times weekly for 8 months.[1] All symptoms subsided 10 days after withdrawal of the shampoo.

1. Ransone JW, et al. Selenium sulfide intoxication. *N Engl J Med* 1961; **264:** 384–5.

Precautions

To minimise absorption selenium sulfide should not be applied to mucous membranes, inflamed or broken skin, or to extensive areas of the skin. Contact with the eyes should be avoided.

Selenium sulfide shampoos should not be used within 48 hours of applying hair colours or permanent waving preparations.

Uses and Administration

Selenium sulfide has antifungal and antiseborrhoeic properties. It is used as a shampoo in the treatment of dandruff (pityriasis capitis) and seborrhoeic dermatitis of the scalp (p.1107). Five to 10 mL of a suspension containing 2.5% of selenium sulfide is applied to the wet scalp; the hair is rinsed and the application repeated; the suspension should remain in contact with the scalp for 2 to 3 minutes each time. The hair should be well rinsed after the treatment and all traces of the suspension removed from the hands and nails. Applications are usually made twice weekly for 2 weeks, then once weekly for 2 weeks and then only when necessary. Shampoos containing 1% are also used.

Selenium sulfide is also used as a 2.5% lotion in the treatment of pityriasis versicolor (p.376). The lotion may be applied to the affected areas with a small amount of water and allowed to remain for 10 minutes before thorough rinsing. This procedure is repeated once daily for about 7 to 14 days. Alternatively undiluted 2.5% lotion has been applied at bedtime and washed off in the morning on 3 separate occasions at 3-day intervals.

Selenium sulfide has also been used as an adjunct to the systemic treatment of tinea capitis (see Dermatophytoses under Skin Infections, p.376).

Preparations

BP 2001: Selenium Sulphide Scalp Application;
USP 25: Selenium Sulfide Lotion.

Proprietary Preparations (details are given in Part 3)
Aust.: Selsun; Selukos; *Austral.:* Selsun; *Belg.:* Selsun; *Braz.:* Selsun; *Canad.:* Selsun; Versel; *Denm.:* Selenol; Selsun; *Fin.:* Selsun; Selukos; *Fr.:* Selegel; Selsun; *Ger.:* Selsun; Selukos; *Hong Kong:* Selsun; *Irl.:* Lenium; *Israel:* Sebosel; Selsun; *Ital.:* Selsun Blu; *Neth.:* Selsun-R; *Norw.:* Selsun; *NZ:* Selsun; *Port.:* Selenix; Selsun; *S.Afr.:* Selsun; *Spain:* Abbottselsun; Bioselenium; Caspiselenio; *Swed.:* Selsun; Selukos; *Switz.:* Selsun; *Thai.:* Sebosel; Selsun; *UK:* Lenium†; Selsun; *USA:* Exsel; Head & Shoulders Intensive Treatment; Selsun.

Multi-ingredient: *Belg.:* Sulfo-Selenium†; *Canad.:* Selsun with Provitamin B5; *Ger.:* Ellsurex; *Ital.:* Node Tar†; Selsun Plus; *Spain:* Sebumselen; Sulfiselen; *Switz.:* Ektoselene.

Skin Substitutes (13151-d)

Profile
A variety of biological and semisynthetic materials have been developed for use as temporary dressings in burns, ulcers, and other injuries associated with skin loss. The rationale is to prevent fluid and heat loss, to reduce infection, to protect exposed structures, to reduce pain, and to prepare the site for grafting (see Burns, p.1104).

Denatured porcine and bovine skin, consisting of the dermal and/or epidermal layers, have been used. More recently bioen-gineered human skin equivalents have been produced which more closely mimic human skin, as well as a human, living dermal replacement product.

◊ References.
1. Muhart M, et al. Bioengineered skin. *Lancet* 1997; **350:** 1142.
2. Purdue GF, et al. A multicenter clinical trial of a biosynthetic skin replacement, Dermagraft-TC, compared with cryopreserved human cadaver skin for temporary coverage of excised burn wounds. *J Burn Care Rehabil* 1997; **18:** 52–7.
3. Freedlander E. New forms of skin grafting: from the laboratory to the clinic. *Hosp Med* 1998; **59:** 484–7.
4. Demling RH, DeSanti L. Management of partial thickness facial burns (comparison of topical antibiotics and bio-engineered skin substitutes). *Burns* 1999; **25:** 256–61.
5. Noordenbos J, et al. Safety and efficacy of TransCyte for the treatment of partial-thickness burns. *J Burn Care Rehabil* 1999; **20:** 275–81.
6. Falanga V, Sabolinski M. A bilayered living skin construct (APLIGRAF) accelerates complete closure of hard-to-heal venous ulcers. *Wound Repair Regen* 1999; **7:** 201–7.

Preparations

Proprietary Preparations (details are given in Part 3)
UK: Corethium†; Dermagraft; *USA:* Apligraf; TransCyte.

Sodium Pidolate (13256-s)

Sodium Pidolate (pINNM).
NaPCA; Sodium Pyroglutamate; Sodium Pyrrolidone Carboxylate. Sodium 5-oxopyrrolidine-2-carboxylate.
$C_5H_7NNaO_3 = 152.1.$
$CAS — 28874-51-3$ (DL-sodium pidolate); $54571-67-4$ (L-sodium pidolate).

Profile
Sodium pidolate is used as a humectant. It is applied topically as a cream or lotion, often in multi-ingredient preparations, in the treatment of dry skin disorders.

Preparations

Proprietary Preparations (details are given in Part 3)
UK: Humiderm†.

Multi-ingredient: *Austral.:* Dermadrate; DermaVeen Moisturising; DermaVeen Shower and Bath; Lacticare†; *Canad.:* Lacticare; *Fr.:* Lacticare; *Hong Kong:* Lacticare; *Irl.:* Hydromol; Lacticare; *Ital.:* Angstrom Viso/Labbra Alta Protezione; Detoxergon†; *Mex.:* Lacticare; *Port.:* Hidro-Lact; Hyseke; *Singapore:* Lacticare; *Thai.:* Lacticare; *UK:* Hydromol; Lacticare.

Squaric Acid Dibutylester (3919-c)

Quadratic Acid Dibutylester. The dibutyl ester of 3,4-dihydroxy-3-cyclobutene-1,2-dione; 3,4-Dibutoxy-3-cyclobutene-1,2-dione; .
$C_{12}H_{18}O_4 = 226.3.$
$CAS — 2892-62-8$ (squaric acid dibutylester); $2892-51-5$ (squaric acid).

Profile
Squaric acid dibutylester has been tried similarly to diphencyprone (p.1113) as a contact sensitiser in the treatment of alopecia. It has also been tried in warts.

◊ References.
1. Van der Steen PHM, et al. Topical immunotherapy for alopecia areata: re-evaluation of 139 cases after an additional follow-up period of 19 months. *Dermatology* 1992; **184:** 198–201.
2. Tosti A, et al. Long-term results of topical immunotherapy in children with alopecia totalis or alopecia universalis. *J Am Acad Dermatol* 1996; **35:** 199–201.
3. Micali G, et al. Treatment of alopecia areata with squaric acid dibutylester. *Int J Dermatol* 1996; **35:** 44–7.
4. Lee AN, Mallory SB. Contact immunotherapy with squaric acid dibutylester for the treatment of recalcitrant warts. *J Am Acad Dermatol* 1999; **41:** 595–9.

Sulfur (1643-e)

Azufre; Enxôfre; Schwefel; Soufre; Sulphur.
$S = 32.065.$
$CAS — 7704-34-9.$
$ATC — D10AB02.$
Pharmacopoeias. In *Chin., Eur.* (see p.vi), *Jpn, Pol.,* and *US.* Some have monographs for Precipitated Sulfur (Milk of Sulfur), Sublimed Sulfur (Flowers of Sulfur), or both. Some specify it is only for external use.

Colloidal sulfur has a smaller particle size than either precipitated or sublimed sulfur. It is sulfur in an aqueous medium containing a colloid such as albumin or gelatin.

Pharmacopoeial description
Ph. Eur.: Sulphur for External Use is a yellow powder. The size of most of the particles is not greater than 20 µm and that of almost all the particles is not greater than 40 µm. Practically insoluble in water; soluble in carbon disulfide; slightly soluble in vegetable oils. Protect from light.

USP 25: Precipitated Sulfur is a very fine, pale yellow, odourless, amorphous or microcrystalline powder. Practically insoluble in water; very slightly soluble in alcohol; slowly and usually incompletely soluble 1 in 2 of carbon disulfide; soluble 1 in 100 of olive oil.

Sublimed Sulfur is a fine, yellow, crystalline powder with a faint odour. Practically insoluble in water and in alcohol; sparingly soluble in olive oil.

◊ WARNING. *Sulfur has been used for the illicit preparation of explosives or fireworks; care is required with its supply.*

Adverse Effects and Precautions
Topical application of sulfur can cause skin irritation and dermatitis has been reported following repeated application. Contact with the eyes, mouth, and other mucous membranes should be avoided. Contact with sulfur can discolour certain metals such as silver, and concomitant application of sulfur and topical mercurial compounds can lead to the generation of hydrogen sulfide which has a foul odour and may stain the skin black.

Uses and Administration
Sulfur is a keratolytic, a mild antiseptic, a mild antifungal, and a parasiticide. It has been widely used in lotions, creams, or ointments, usually in combination with other agents, in concentrations of up to 10% in the treatment of acne, dandruff, seborrhoeic conditions, scabies, and superficial fungal infections, although there are more convenient and effective preparations.

Lotions of precipitated sulfur with lead acetate have been used to darken grey hair.

Sulfur was also formerly used as a mild irritant laxative.

Sulfur is used in homoeopathic medicine.

◊ General references.
1. Lin AN, *et al.* Sulfur revisited. *J Am Acad Dermatol* 1988; **18**: 553–8.

Preparations
BPC 1973: Salicylic Acid and Sulphur Ointment;
USP 25: Resorcinol and Sulfur Lotion; Sulfur Ointment.

Proprietary Preparations (details are given in Part 3)
Aust.: Sulfosol†; **Canad.:** Acne Blemish Cream†; Postacne; Pureness Blemish Control; **Ger.:** Schwefel-Diasporal; Sulfopino†; **Ital.:** Acqua di Sirmione; Eudermal Sapone Allo Zolfo pH 5; Nosebo; Veriderm†; **Mex.:** Azuder; **USA:** Acne Lotion 10; Liquimat; Sastid; Sulfoam; Sulmasque.

Multi-ingredient: Numerous preparations are listed in Part 3.

Sulfurated Lime (1645-y)
Calcium Sulphide; Calx Sulphurata; Sulphurated Lime.
CAS — 8028-82-8 (sulfurated lime solution).

Sulfurated lime is a mixture containing calcium sulfate and not less than 50% of calcium sulfide (CaS), prepared by heating calcium sulfate. Sulfurated lime solution (Vleminckx's solution) is an aqueous solution containing calcium polysulfides and calcium thiosulfate prepared by boiling sublimed sulfur with calcium hydroxide in water.

Profile
Sulfurated lime has been used topically as sulfurated lime solution for acne, scabies, seborrhoeic dermatitis, and pustular infections such as boils and carbuncles. A similar solution known as 'lime-sulphur' is used as a fungicide in horticulture.

An impure grade of calcium sulfide (Hepar Sulphuris; Hepar Sulph.) is used in homoeopathic medicine.

NOTE. The titles Hepar Sulfuris and Hepar Sulph are also applied to Sulfurated Potash (see below).

Sulfurated Potash (1646-j)
Foie de Soufre; Hepar Sulfuris; Kalii Sulfidum; Liver of Sulphur; Potassa Sulphurata; Schwefelleber; Sulphurated Potash.
CAS — 39365-88-3.

NOTE. The title Hepar Sulphuris is used in homoeopathic medicine for an impure grade of calcium sulfide—see Sulfurated Lime, above.

Pharmacopoeias. In US.

Incompatible with acids.

Pharmacopoeial description
USP 25: A mixture composed chiefly of potassium polysulfides and potassium thiosulfate, containing not less than 12.8% of sulfur as sulfide. Irregular, liver-brown pieces when freshly made, changing to greenish-yellow. It has an odour of hydrogen sulfide. Soluble 1 in 2 of water, usually leaving a slight residue. Alcohol dissolves only the sulfides. A 10% solution is light brown in colour and alkaline to litmus. Store in small, airtight containers.

Profile
Sulfurated potash has been used in the treatment of acne and other skin disorders usually in the form of a lotion with zinc sulfate.

Sulfurated potash is used in homoeopathic medicine when it is known as Hepar Sulph.

Preparations
USP 25: White Lotion.

Proprietary Preparations (details are given in Part 3)
Ger.: Schwefelbad-Saar.

Multi-ingredient: **Aust.:** Leukona-Sulfomoor-Bad; **Ger.:** Leukona-Sulfomoor-Bad N.

Tacalcitol (15404-r)
Tacalcitol *(BAN, rINN)*.
1α,24-Dihydroxycholecalciferol; 1α,24-Dihydroxyvitamin D$_3$. (+)-(5Z,7E,24R)-9,10-Secocholesta-5,7,10(19)-triene-1α,3β,24-triol monohydrate.
$C_{27}H_{44}O_3,H_2O = 434.7$.
CAS — 57333-96-7 (anhydrous tacalcitol); 93129-94-3 (tacalcitol monohydrate).
ATC — D05AX04.

Adverse Effects and Precautions
As for Calcipotriol, p.1112. Paraesthesia may also occur. Tacalcitol may be applied to the face, but care should be taken to avoid the eyes. Tacalcitol may be degraded by UV radiation (see Uses and Administration, below).

Uses and Administration
Tacalcitol is a vitamin D$_3$ derivative. *In vitro* it appears to induce differentiation and to suppress proliferation of keratinocytes.

Tacalcitol is used as the monohydrate in an ointment for the management of plaque psoriasis (p.1106); the concentration is equivalent to 4 μg of tacalcitol per g (0.0004%) . Applications are made once daily, preferably at bedtime, and no more than 10 g of ointment should be applied each day. Duration of treatment depends on the severity of the lesions; continuous and intermittent treatments for up to 12 months have been used.

Tacalcitol may be degraded by UV radiation and therefore if combined with UV therapy, the radiation should be given in the morning and tacalcitol applied at bedtime.

◊ References.
1. Peters DC, Balfour JA. Tacalcitol. *Drugs* 1997; **54**: 265–71.
2. Gollnick H, Menke T. Current experience with tacalcitol ointment in the treatment of psoriasis. *Curr Med Res Opin* 1998; **14**: 213–18.
3. Harrison PV. Topical tacalcitol treatment for psoriasis. *Hosp Med* 2000; **61**: 402–5.

Preparations
Proprietary Preparations (details are given in Part 3)
Aust.: Curatoderm; **Belg.:** Curatoderm; **Fr.:** Apsor; **Ger.:** Curatoderm; **Israel:** Curatoderm; **Ital.:** Vellutan; **Mex.:** Bonalfa; **Spain:** Bonalfa; **Switz.:** Curatoderm; **UK:** Curatoderm.

Purified Talc (1647-z)
E553(b); Powdered Talc; Purified French Chalk; Talc; Talcum; Talcum Purificatum.
CAS — 14807-96-6.
Pharmacopoeias. In Chin., Eur. (see p.vi), Int., Jpn, Pol., and US.

Pharmacopoeial description
Ph. Eur.: A powdered, selected, natural, hydrated, magnesium silicate. Pure talc has the formula $Mg_3Si_4O_{10}(OH)_2$; it may contain varying amounts of associated minerals. A light, homogeneous, white or almost white powder, greasy and non-abrasive to the touch. It should be free from asbestos. Practically insoluble in water, in alcohol, and in dilute solutions of acids and of alkali hydroxides.

USP 25: A native hydrous magnesium silicate containing a small proportion of aluminium silicate. A very fine, white or greyish-white, unctuous crystalline powder, which adheres readily to the skin, and is free from grittiness.

Adverse Effects and Precautions
Contamination of wounds or body cavities with talc is liable to cause granulomas and it should not be used for dusting surgical gloves.

Inhalation of talc can cause respiratory irritation; prolonged exposure may produce pneumoconiosis.

Talc is liable to be heavily contaminated with bacteria, including *Clostridium tetani*, *Cl. welchii*, and *Bacillus anthracis*. When used in dusting powders or to treat pneumothorax and pleural effusions, it should be sterilised.

Abuse. Pulmonary granulomas occurring after intravenous or intranasal drug abuse have been associated with the presence of talc as a filler in the abused preparations.[1,2]
1. Schwartz IS, Bosken C. Pulmonary vascular talc granulomatosis. *JAMA* 1986; **256**: 2584.
2. Johnson DC, *et al.* Foreign body pulmonary granulomas in an abuser of nasally inhaled drugs. *Pediatrics* 1991; **88**: 159–61.

Carcinogenicity. A review by a working group of the International Agency for Research on Cancer concluded that there was inadequate evidence to confirm whether purified talc was carcinogenic in humans but there was sufficient evidence to confirm that talc containing asbestiform fibres was carcinogenic to man.[1] There have been suggestions of a link between the use of talc and ovarian cancer[2] but although a case-controlled study suggested an approximate doubling of the risk among women after perineal use of talc the working group noted that

information was not available on the asbestos content of the talcs.[1]
1. IARC/WHO. Silica and some silicates. *IARC monographs on the evaluation of the carcinogenic risk of chemicals to humans volume 42* 1987.
2. Longo DL, Young RC. Cosmetic talc and ovarian cancer. *Lancet* 1979; **ii**: 349–51.

Effects on the lungs. Inhalation of talc can cause respiratory irritation. Acute respiratory failure developed in 4 of 338 patients who underwent pleurodesis for benign or malignant effusions using insufflated talc in conjunction with thoracoscopy.[1] Three of the 4 patients died. Talc crystals were found in the bronchoalveolar lavage of all 4 patients and on necropsy of one patient talc crystals were found in almost every organ.

For other effects on the lungs, see under Abuse, above and Infant Skin Care, below.
1. Campos JRM, *et al.* Respiratory failure due to insufflated talc. *Lancet* 1997; **349**: 251–2.

Infant skin care. The routine use of non-medicated powders in the skin care of infants can be hazardous and their use should be discouraged.[1,2] Talc acts as a pulmonary irritant and inhalation of baby-powders by infants has caused severe respiratory difficulties and several deaths have been reported. Careful respiratory monitoring is indicated in children suspected of inhaling talcum powder as the onset of symptoms may be delayed for several hours.[1] There have also been reports of umbilical granulomas resulting from contamination of umbilical stumps with talcum powder used for skin care.[2]
1. Pairaudeau PW, *et al.* Inhalation of baby powder: an unappreciated hazard. *BMJ* 1991; **302**: 1200–1.
2. Sparrow SA, Hallam LA. Talc granulomas. *BMJ* 1991; **303**: 58.

Uses and Administration
Purified talc is used in massage and as a dusting powder to allay irritation and prevent chafing. It is usually mixed with starch, to increase absorption of moisture, and zinc oxide. Talc used in dusting powders or as talc poudrage should be sterilised. Purified talc is used as a lubricant and diluent in making tablets and capsules and to clarify liquids.

Talc may be used as a sclerosant for malignant effusions (p.489) and for recurrent spontaneous pneumothorax.

◊ References.
1. Eselin J, Thompson DF. Talc in the treatment of malignant pleural effusion. *DICP Ann Pharmacother* 1991; **25**: 1187–9.
2. Vaughan LM, Bishop TD. Sterilization of talc USP for intrapleural use. *Ann Pharmacother* 1994; **28**: 1309–10.
3. Kennedy L, Sahn SA. Talc pleurodesis for the treatment of pneumothorax and pleural effusion. *Chest* 1994; **106**: 1215–22.

Preparations
BP 2001: Talc Dusting Powder.

Proprietary Preparations (details are given in Part 3)

Multi-ingredient: **Aust.:** Cutimix; Herposicc; Prurimix; Rombay; **Belg.:** Aloplastine; Baseler Haussalbe†; **Braz.:** Pasta d'Agua; **Canad.:** Bebia†; **Fr.:** Aloplastine; Bebia†; **Israel:** Pedisol; **NZ:** Grans Remedy; **Port.:** Cuidaderma; **Spain:** Amniolina; Ictiomen; Pomada Infantil Vera; Talco Antihistam Calber; Talquis Cusi; Talquissar†; Tegunal; **USA:** ZBT.

Tars and Tar Oils (15703-s)

Birch Tar Oil (1652-l)
Birkenteer; Goudron de Bouleau; Oleum Betulae Albae; Oleum Betulae Empyreumaticum; Oleum Betulae Pyroligneum; Oleum Rusci; Pix Betulae; Pyroleum Betulae.

Birch tar oil is obtained by the destructive distillation of the wood and bark of the silver birch, *Betula verrucosa* (= *B. pendula*; *B. alba*), and the birch, *B. pubescens* (Betulaceae); the distillate is allowed to stand and the oily upper layer separated from the residual tar.

Cade Oil (1595-t)
Alquitrán de Enebro; Goudron de Cade; Juniper Tar; Juniper Tar Oil; Kadeöl; Oleum Cadinum; Oleum Juniperi Empyreumaticum; Pix Cadi; Pix Juniperi; Pix Oxycedri; Pyroleum Juniperi; Pyroleum Oxycedri; Wacholderteer.
Pharmacopoeias. In Swiss and US.

Cade oil contains guaiacol, ethylguaiacol, creosol, and cadinene.

Pharmacopoeial description
USP 25: Juniper Tar is the empyreumatic volatile oil obtained from the woody portions of *Juniperus oxycedrus* (Pinaceae). It is a dark brown, clear, thick liquid with a tarry odour. Very slightly soluble in water; soluble 1 in 9 of alcohol; soluble 1 in 3 of ether leaving only a slight flocculent residue; partially soluble in petroleum spirit; miscible with amyl alcohol, with chloroform, and with glacial acetic acid. Store in airtight containers at a temperature not exceeding 40°. Protect from light.

Coal Tar (1650-w)

Alcatrão Mineral; Alquitrán de Hulla; Brea de Hulla; Crude Coal Tar; Goudron de Houille; Oleum Lithanthracis; Pix Carbon.; Pix Carbonis; Pix Lithanthracis; Pix Mineralis; Pyroleum Lithanthracis; Steinkohlenteer.

Pharmacopoeias. In Aust., Br., Fr., Int., Port., and US.

Incompatible with wool alcohols. Prepared coal tar is commercial coal tar heated at 50° for 1 hour. Alcoholic solutions of coal tar or prepared coal tar prepared with the aid of polysorbate have been referred to as Liquor Picis Carbonis and Liquor Carbonis Detergens.

Pharmacopoeial description

BP 2001: Coal tar is obtained by the destructive distillation of bituminous coal at a temperature of about 1000°. A nearly black, viscous liquid with a strong characteristic penetrating odour. On exposure to air it gradually becomes more viscous. It burns in air with a luminous sooty flame. Slightly soluble in water; partly soluble in absolute alcohol, in chloroform, in ether, and in volatile oils. A saturated solution is alkaline to litmus.

USP 25: Coal tar is obtained by the destructive distillation of bituminous coal at temperatures in the range of 900° to 1100°. It may be processed further either by extraction with alcohol and suitable dispersing agents and maceration times or by fractional distillation with or without the use of suitable organic solvents.

A nearly black, viscous liquid with a characteristic naphthalene-like odour. Slightly soluble in water to which it imparts an alkaline reaction; partially soluble in alcohol, in acetone, in carbon disulfide, in chloroform, in ether, in methyl alcohol, and in petroleum spirit; more soluble in benzene; almost completely soluble in nitrobenzene. Store in airtight containers.

Tar (1648-c)

Alquitrán Vegetal; Brea de Pino; Goudron Végétal; Nadelholzteer; Pine Tar; Pix Abietinarum; Pix Liquida; Pix Pini; Pyroleum Pini; Wood Tar.

NOTE. It is known in commerce as Stockholm tar.
Pharmacopoeias. In Aust. and Br.
Aust. also includes beech tar.

Tar has an acid reaction which it imparts to water when shaken with it, and it may thereby be distinguished from coal tar, which has an alkaline reaction.

When stored for some time tar separates into a layer which is granular in character due to minute crystallisation of catechol, resin acids, etc. and a surface layer of a syrupy consistence.

Pharmacopoeial description

BP 2001: A bituminous liquid obtained from the wood of various trees of the family Pinaceae by destructive distillation. A dark brown or nearly black semi-liquid with a characteristic empyreumatic odour; it is heavier than water. Soluble in alcohol (90%), in chloroform, in ether, and in fixed and volatile oils.

Adverse Effects and Precautions

Tars and tar oils may cause irritation and acne-like eruptions of the skin and should not be applied to inflamed or broken skin. They should be used with caution on the face, skin flexures, or on the genitalia. Hypersensitivity reactions are rare but wood tars are more likely to cause sensitisation than coal tar. However, unlike wood tars, coal tar has a photosensitising action. Preparations of refined tar products appear to be less likely than crude tars to stain the skin, hair, and clothing.

Depending on their composition the systemic effects of tars and tar oils are similar to those for phenol (see p.1152).

Carcinogenicity. Although an increased risk of skin carcinoma was found[1] in 59 patients with psoriasis who had had very high exposures to tar and/or UV radiation, no such evidence was apparent[2] in 260 patients followed for a mean of 20 years and long-term topical tar therapy alone was not associated with an increase in malignancy in 719 patients.[3] Relatively high systemic absorption of polycyclic aromatic hydrocarbons, which are potential carcinogens, has, however, been reported after use of a coal-tar shampoo.[4]

1. Stern RS, *et al.* Skin carcinoma in patients with psoriasis treated with topical tar and artificial ultraviolet radiation. *Lancet* 1980; i: 732–5.
2. Pittelkow MR, *et al.* Skin cancer in patients with psoriasis treated with coal tar. *Arch Dermatol* 1981; **117:** 465–8.
3. Jones SK, *et al.* Further evidence of the safety of tar in the management of psoriasis. *Br J Dermatol* 1985; **113:** 97–101.
4. van Schooten F-J, *et al.* Dermal uptake of polycyclic aromatic hydrocarbons after hairwash with coal-tar shampoo. *Lancet* 1994; **344:** 1505–6.

Extemporaneous preparation. Concern about the possible carcinogenic potential of coal tar (see above) led the Health and Safety Executive in the UK to recommend that chemical gloves, as opposed to disposable surgeon's gloves, should be worn during the extemporaneous preparation of formulations containing coal tar.[1]

1. Anonymous. Chemical protection gloves recommended for coal tar ointments. *Pharm J* 1997; **259:** 757.

Uses and Administration

Tars and tar oils can reduce the thickness of the epidermis. They are antipruritic and may be weakly antiseptic. They are used topically in eczema (p.1105), psoriasis (below), dandruff, seborrhoeic dermatitis (p.1107), and other skin disorders. Coal tar preparations have largely replaced the use of wood tars. Ultraviolet (UVB) light increases the efficacy of coal tar in the treatment of psoriasis.

Some wood tars, including creosote (p.1087) have been used in expectorant preparations. Tar has also been used in homoeopathic medicine.

◊ Following its review of products for safety and efficacy the FDA ruled that cade oil or tar should not be used in nonprescription shampoos[1] and that tar should no longer be included in nonprescription expectorants.[2]

1. Anonymous. Nonprescription drug review gains momentum. *WHO Drug Inf* 1991; **5:** 62.
2. Anonymous. FDA announces standards for nonprescription sleep-aid products and expectorants. *Clin Pharm* 1989; **8:** 388.

Psoriasis. Coal tar has long been employed in the treatment of psoriasis (p.1106) and used alone or with dithranol and/or ultraviolet light it continues to be one of the drugs of first choice. It is particularly suited to the treatment of stable chronic plaque psoriasis. Its mode of action is unknown but it is considered to have antiproliferative and anti-inflammatory activity, producing a reduction in the thickness of viable epidermis. Crude tar preparations are considered to be safe even if rather messy and unpleasant; refined products may be more aesthetically acceptable and less likely to stain skin, hair, and clothing although some consider them to be less effective. Treatments usually start with concentrations equivalent to 0.5 to 1% of crude coal tar with the concentration being increased as necessary every few days up to a maximum of 10%. The higher strength preparations may be required for the management of thicker patches of psoriasis. Coal tar may not clear psoriasis as fast as other agents but extended periods of remission can be obtained with its use. The Goeckerman regimen utilises the enhanced efficacy obtained when coal tar is applied before exposure to ultraviolet (UVB) light. The mechanism for this effect is not known but it does not appear to be due to the photosensitising action of coal tar. In most regimens the coal tar is applied 2 hours before exposure to UVB light. In Ingram's regimen and its modifications the use of coal tar and UVB light is followed by topical treatment with dithranol. It has been suggested that the irritant effects of dithranol treatment are reduced by concomitant treatment with coal tar without loss of efficacy.

References.
1. Rotstein H, Baker C. The treatment of psoriasis. *Med J Aust* 1990; **152:** 153–64.
2. Menter A, Barker JNWN. Psoriasis in practice. *Lancet* 1991; **338:** 231–4.
3. Foreman MI, *et al.* Isoquinoline is a possible anti-psoriatic agent in coal tar. *Br J Dermatol* 1985; **112:** 323–8.
4. Williams REA, *et al.* Workshop of the Research Unit of the Royal College of Physicians of London; Department of Dermatology, University of Glasgow; British Association of Dermatologists. Guidelines for management of patients with psoriasis. *BMJ* 1991; **303:** 829–35.
5. Arnold WP. Tar. *Clin Dermatol* 1997; **15:** 739–44.

Preparations

BP 2001: Calamine and Coal Tar Ointment; Coal Tar and Salicylic Acid Ointment; Coal Tar and Zinc Ointment; Coal Tar Paste; Coal Tar Solution; Strong Coal Tar Solution; Zinc and Coal Tar Paste;
USP 25: Coal Tar Ointment; Coal Tar Topical Solution; Compound Resorcinol Ointment.

Proprietary Preparations (details are given in Part 3)
Aust.: Exorex; **Austral.:** Alpha Keri Tar; Alphosyl; Dermatar†; Formicare Bath†; Formicare Shower†; Formicare Skin Gel†; Formicare Skin Wash†; Ionil-T Plus; Linotar; Neutrogena T/Gel; Psorigel; **Canad.:** Balnetar; Doak-Oil; Estar; Ionil-T Plus†; Ionil-T†; Mazon Medicated Soap; Neutrogena T/Gel†; Pentrax; Psoriasol†; Psorigel†; Robatar; Spectro Tar; Tar Doak†; Target; Tarseb; Tegrin; Tersa-Tar; Zetar; **Denm.:** Basotar; **Fr.:** Caditar; Cosmetar-S†; Ramet Cade; **Ger.:** Basiter; Berniter; Hoepixin Bad N; Pixfix; Tarmed; Teer-Linola-Fett; **Hong Kong:** Pinetarsol; Psorigel; Tersatar; **Irl.:** Baltar; Clinitar; Pentrax; Psoriderm; Psorigel; **Israel:** Alphosyl 2 in 1; Denorex; T/Gel; **Ital.:** Konor; Meditar; Polytar†; Shampoo SDE Tar; Tarmed†; **Mex.:** Ionil-T Plus; Shampoo Tersa-Tar; Tarmed; **Norw.:** Soraderm; **NZ:** Pinetarsol; Psoriacreme; Psorigel; **S.Afr.:** Linotar; Psorigel†; **Singapore:** Pinetarsol; **Spain:** Alphosyl; Piroxgel; Psoriasdin; Tar Isdin Champu; Tarmed; **Switz.:** Teerol†; **Thai.:** Ionil-T; **UK:** Alphosyl 2 in 1; Baltar†; Carbo-Dome; Clinitar; Exorex; Pentrax; Psoriderm; Psorigel†; T/Gel; **USA:** Advanced Formula Tegrin; AquaTar; Balnetar; Creamy Tar; Cutar; DHS Tar; Doctar; Duplex T; Estar; Fototar; Iocon; Ionil-T Plus; MG217 Medicated; Neutrogena T/Derm; Neutrogena T/Gel; Oxipor VHC; Pentrax; Pentrax Gold; Polytar; Protar Protein†; Psorigel; PsoriNail†; Taraphilic; Tegrin; Tegrin Medicated; Theraplex T; Zetar.

Multi-ingredient: Aust.: Alphosyl; Alpicort; Balneum mit Teer; Locacorten Tar; **Austral.:** Alpha Keri Tar; Alphosyl; Eczema Cream; ER Cream; Fongitar; Formicare Skin Relief†; Ionil-T; Neutrogena T/Sal; Pinetarsol; Polytar; Psor-Asist; Sebitar; Tarband; **Belg.:** Alphosyl†; Locacortene Tar; **Braz.:** Codelasa; Dai Natha; Hebrin; Ionil-T; Kabala; **Canad.:** Alphosyl; Boil Ease; Dan-Tar Plus; Denorex; Mazon Medicated Cream; Mazon Medicated Shampoo; Medi-Dan; Multi-Tar Plus; Oxipor; P & S Plus; Polytar; Polytar AF; Sebcur/T; Sebutone; SJ Liniment; Spectro Tar; Sterex; Tardan; Target SA; X-Seb T; X-Seb T Plus; X-Tar; **Fin.:** Alphosyl; **Fr.:** Alphosyl; Biolan Tar†; Coaltar Saponine le Beuf; Cystelle Shampooing Cheveux Gras; Ionax T†; Laccoderme a l'huile de cade; Lactar; Phytolithe; S-Coaltar†; Sebosquam; **Ger.:** Dexacrinit†; Discmigon; Hoepixin N; Lorinden T; Poloris; Poloris HC†; Polytar; Psoriasis-Salbe M†; Psorigerb N; **Hong Kong:** Cocois; Egopsoryl TA; Fongitar; Gelcotar; Ionil-T; Locacorten Tar; Multi-Tar; Polytar; Polytar Plus; Sebitar; **Irl.:** Alphosyl; Alphosyl HC; Balneum with Tar; Capasal; Cocois; Denorex; Gelcotar; Genisol; Ionil-T; Polytar; Polytar Emollient; Polytar Plus†; Pragmatar; **Israel:** Alphosyl; Alphosyl HC; Capasal; CT Ointment; CT Pommade; CT Shampoo; Locacorten Tar; Polytar; Topicorten-Tar†; **Ital.:** Alphosyle; Balta-Crin Tar; Fongitar†; Genisol; Herbatar; Herbatar Plus; Ionil-T†; Locorten Tar†; Node Tar†; Pentrax; Rivescal Tar; Soluzione Composta Alcoolica Saponosa di Coaltar†; **Mex.:** Antaderm; Dariseb; Dealan; Ionil-T; Polytar; Sebryl; Sebryl Plus; **Neth.:** Denorex; Resdan Rx†; **NZ:** Egopsoryl TA; Fongitar; Ionil-T; Polytar; Polytar Emollient; Polytar Plus; Sebitar; **Port.:** Alpha Cade; Alphosyl; Alphosyl HC; Banholeum Composto†; Edoltar; Fongitar; Ionax T†; Squaphane; Sucadermil; Tegrin†; **S.Afr.:** Alphosyl; Locacorten Tar†; Pasta Prura†; Polytar; **Singapore:** Denorex; Egopsoryl TA; Fongitar; Ionil-T; Polytar; Sebitar; Sebutone; **Spain:** Alphosyl; Bazalin; Deltasiton†; Emolytar; Polytar; Quinortar; Tar Isdin Plus; Tarisdin†; Zincation Plus; **Swed.:** Alphosyl; **Switz.:** Alphosyl; Bain extra-doux dermatologique†; Crinotar†; Jonil T†; Locacorten Tar†; Teerol-H†; **Thai.:** Fongitar; Polytar; **UK:** Alphosyl; Alphosyl HC; Balneum with Tar†; Capasal; Carbo-Cort†; Cocois; Coltapaste; Denorex; Gelcosal†; Gelcotar†; Ionil-T; Pixol†; Polytar AF; Polytar Emollient; Polytar Liquid; Polytar Plus; Pragmatar; Psorin; Snowfire; Tarband; Tarcortin†; Varicose Ointment; **USA:** Boil Ease; Denorex; Ionil-T; Medotar; Neutrogena T/Sal; P & S Plus; Sal-Oil-T; Sebex-T; Sebutone†; SLT; Tarlene; Tarsum; Unguentum Bossi; X-Seb T; X-Seb T Plus.

Tazarotene (15710-p)

Tazarotene (BAN, USAN, rINN).
AGN-190168. Ethyl 6-[(4,4-dimethylthiochroman-6-yl)ethynyl]nicotinate.
$C_{21}H_{21}NO_2S = 351.5.$
CAS — 118292-40-3.
ATC — D05AX05.

Adverse Effects and Precautions

As for Tretinoin, p.1126.

Tazarotene is fetotoxic and teratogenic in *animals*. Experience in human pregnancy is very limited.

◊ A 57-year-old man with diabetes and recalcitrant psoriasis on the trunk and limbs developed acute dermatitis[1] in the genital area two weeks after starting treatment with topical tazarotene 0.1%. The affected areas became ulcerated over the next few days. It was suspected that accidental contact with the tazarotene that had been applied to the truncal psoriasis was responsible.

1. Wollina U. Genital ulcers in a psoriasis patient using topical tazarotene. *Br J Dermatol* 1998; **138:** 713–14.

Uses and Administration

Tazarotene is a retinoid used for the topical treatment of mild to moderate acne and plaque psoriasis. Tazarotene is a prodrug that is de-esterified in the skin to its active form, tazarotenic acid. The mode of action of tazarotenic acid in acne and psoriasis is unknown but it appears to modulate cell proliferation and differentiation.

In the treatment of psoriasis, tazarotene is applied as a 0.05% or 0.1% gel once daily in the evening. In the UK tazarotene is licensed for use in patients with psoriasis affecting up to 10% of the body surface; in the USA, it may be used on psoriasis involving up to 20% of the body surface.

In the treatment of acne, tazarotene is applied as a 0.1% gel once daily in the evening.

There may be exacerbation of acne during early treatment or of psoriasis at any time during treatment. The treatment period is usually up to 12 weeks, although tazarotene has been used for up to 12 months in the treatment of psoriasis.

◊ Reviews.
1. Foster RH, *et al.* Tazarotene. *Drugs* 1998; **55:** 705–11.
2. Tang-Liu DD-S, *et al.* Clinical pharmacokinetics and drug metabolism of tazarotene: a novel topical treatment for acne and psoriasis. *Clin Pharmacokinet* 1999; **37:** 273–87.

Skin disorders. Tazarotene is used for the topical treatment of mild to moderate acne (p.1103) and plaque psoriasis[1] (p.1106). Some benefit has been reported in keratinisation disorders such as Darier's disease[2] (p.1104) and congenital ichthyosis[3] (p.1105).

1. Anonymous. Tazarotene—a topical retinoid for psoriasis. *Drug Ther Bull* 1999; **37:** 47–8.
2. Oster-Schmidt C. The treatment of Darier's disease with topical tazarotene. *Br J Dermatol* 1999; **141:** 603–4.
3. Hofmann B, *et al.* Effect of topical tazarotene in the treatment of congenital ichthyosis. *Br J Dermatol* 1999; **141:** 642–6.

Preparations

Proprietary Preparations (details are given in Part 3)
Aust.: Zorac; **Canad.:** Tazorac; **Fin.:** Zorac; **Fr.:** Zorac; **Ger.:** Zorac; **Irl.:** Zorac; **Ital.:** Suretin; Zorac; **S.Afr.:** Zorak; **Spain:** Zorac; **Swed.:** Zorac; **UK:** Zorac; **USA:** Tazorac.

Thioglycollic Acid (15327-n)

Mercaptoacetic acid.
$C_2H_4O_2S = 92.12$.
CAS — 68-11-1.

Calcium Thioglycollate (1599-d)

Calcium Mercaptoacetate. Calcium mercaptoacetate trihydrate.
$C_2H_2CaO_2S,3H_2O = 184.2$.
CAS — 814-71-1.

Profile

Thioglycollic acid is used, usually as the calcium salt, in depilatory preparations. Thioglycollates are also used in hair waving or straightening products together with potassium bromate as the neutraliser. There have been reports of skin reactions associated with the use of thioglycollates.

Tioxolone (1654-j)

Tioxolone (BAN, rINN).
OL-110; Thioxolone. 6-Hydroxy-1,3-benzoxathiol-2-one; 4-Hydroxy-1,3-benzoxathiol-2-one.
$C_7H_4O_3S = 168.2$.
CAS — 4991-65-5.
ATC — D10AB03.
Pharmacopoeias. In Pol.

Profile

Tioxolone has been used topically in the treatment of various skin and scalp disorders.

Preparations

Proprietary Preparations (details are given in Part 3)
Swed.: Camyna†.
Multi-ingredient: Ger.: Loscon.

Titanium Dioxide (1655-z)

CI Pigment White 6; Colour Index No. 77891; E171; Titanii Dioxidum; Titanium Oxide.
$TiO_2 = 79.87$.
CAS — 13463-67-7.
Pharmacopoeias. In Eur. (see p.vi), Jpn, and US.

Pharmacopoeial description

Ph. Eur.: A white or almost white powder. Practically insoluble in water; it does not dissolve in dilute mineral acids but dissolves slowly in hot concentrated sulfuric acid.
USP 25: A white odourless powder. Insoluble in water, in hydrochloric acid, in nitric acid, and in 2N sulfuric acid; dissolves in hot sulfuric acid and in hydrofluoric acid; it is rendered soluble by fusion with potassium bisulfate or with alkali hydroxides or carbonates. A 10% suspension in water is neutral to litmus.

Profile

Titanium dioxide has an action on the skin similar to that of zinc oxide (p.1128) and has similar uses. Titanium peroxide and titanium salicylate are used in combination with titanium dioxide for napkin rash. Titanium dioxide reflects ultraviolet light and is used in sunscreens. It is also an ingredient of some cosmetics. It is used to pigment and opacify hard gelatin capsules and tablet coatings and as a delustring agent for regenerated cellulose and other man-made fibres. Specially purified grades may be used in food colours.

Preparations

BP 2001: Titanium Ointment.
Proprietary Preparations (details are given in Part 3)
Austral.: Sunsense Low Irritant; UV Triplegard Low Allergenic†; UV Triplegard Sensitive Skin; **Canad.:** Baby Block; Life Brand Natural Source†; Marcelle Protective Block; Natural Defense; Neutrogena Sunblocker; Presun; Special Defense Sun Block; Sunblock; True Illusion; **Fr.:** Anthelios T; Uriage Ecran Total Mineral; **Ger.:** Haemo-Exhirud Bufexamac Zapfchen; **Hong Kong:** Sunsense Low Irritant; **Mex.:** Blancaler; **NZ:** Hamilton Sunscreen Quadblock, Water Resistant; **Port.:** Dermagor Ecran Solar; **Singapore:** Sunsense Low Irritant; **UK:** Coppertone Sunstick; **USA:** Hawaiian Tropic Protective Tanning; Neutrogena Chemical-Free; TI Baby Natural; TI Screen Natural.
Multi-ingredient: Numerous preparations are listed in Part 3.

Tretinoin (1656-c)

Tretinoin (BAN, USAN, rINN).
NSC-122758; Retinoic Acid; Tretinoinum; Vitamin A Acid. all-trans-Retinoic acid; 15-Apo-β-caroten-15-oic acid; 3,7-Dimethyl-9-(2,6,6-trimethylcyclohex-1-enyl)nona-2,4,6,8-all-trans-tetraenoic acid.
$C_{20}H_{28}O_2 = 300.4$.
CAS — 302-79-4.
ATC — D10AD01; L01XX14.
Pharmacopoeias. In Eur. (see p.vi) and US.

Pharmacopoeial description

Ph. Eur.: A yellow or light orange crystalline powder. Practically insoluble in water; slightly soluble in alcohol; soluble in dichloromethane. It is sensitive to light, heat, and air, especially in solution. Store in airtight containers at a temperature not exceeding 25°. Protect from light. The contents of an opened container should be used as soon as possible and any unused portion should be protected by an atmosphere of an inert gas.
USP 25: A yellow to light-orange crystalline powder. Insoluble in water; slightly soluble in alcohol and in chloroform. Store in airtight containers, preferably under an atmosphere of an inert gas. Protect from light.

Adverse Effects

Tretinoin is a skin irritant. Topical application may cause transitory stinging and a feeling of warmth and in normal use it produces some erythema and peeling similar to that of mild sunburn. Sensitive individuals may experience oedema, blistering, and crusting of the skin. Excessive application can cause severe erythema, peeling, and discomfort with no increase in efficacy. Photosensitivity may occur. Temporary hypopigmentation and hyperpigmentation have been reported.

Oral administration of tretinoin may produce similar adverse effects to those of isotretinoin (see p.1115). Cardiac arrhythmias may also occur. A potentially life-threatening 'retinoic acid syndrome' (see below) has been described following oral use.

Carcinogenicity. Studies in *mice* suggested that tretinoin could enhance photocarcinogenesis.[1] However, other studies refuted this[2] and evidence indicates that topical tretinoin is not carcinogenic in humans.

1. Epstein JH. Chemicals and photocarcinogenesis. *Australas J Dermatol* 1977; **18:** 57–61.
2. Epstein JH. All-trans-retinoic acid and cutaneous cancers. *J Am Acad Dermatol* 1986; **15:** 772–8.

Effects on the endocrine system. Symptoms typical of the premenstrual syndrome followed by vaginal bleeding in a 64-year-old woman were reported to be associated with the topical application of tretinoin[1] but others doubted a causal relationship.[2]

1. Meurehg CC, Xóchitl Amelio P. Vaginal bleeding and tretinoin cream. *Ann Intern Med* 1990; **113:** 483.
2. Worobec SM, *et al.* Topical tretinoin and vaginal bleeding. *Ann Intern Med* 1991; **114:** 97.

Effects on the musculoskeletal system. For a report of myositis occurring in a patient receiving oral tretinoin, see Isotretinoin, p.1116.

Effects on the nervous system. Oral retinoids may produce neurotoxic adverse effects. Children seem to be particularly sensitive to the CNS effects of tretinoin.[1,2] Neurotoxicity (ataxia, dysarthria, and headache) has been reported in a woman with liver impairment using topical tretinoin 0.025% for acne.[3]

1. Warrell RP, *et al.* Acute promyelocytic leukaemia. *N Engl J Med* 1993; **329:** 177–89.
2. Mahmoud HH, *et al.* Tretinoin toxicity in children with acute promyelocytic leukaemia. *Lancet* 1993; **342:** 1394–5.
3. Bernstein AL, Leventhal-Rochon JL. Neurotoxicity related to the use of topical tretinoin (Retin-A). *Ann Intern Med* 1996; **124:** 227–8.

Retinoic acid syndrome. A syndrome consisting primarily of fever and respiratory distress developed in 9 of 35 cases between 2 and 21 days after starting induction therapy with oral tretinoin for suspected acute promyelocytic leukaemia.[1] Other symptoms included weight gain, oedema of the lower extremities, pleural or pericardial effusions, and episodic hypotension. Symptoms were life-threatening in 5 patients, 3 of whom subsequently died of multi-system failure. Leucocytosis was frequently, although not invariably, associated with development of the syndrome. Experience showed that early treatment with high-dose corticosteroids should be given to these patients irrespective of the leucocyte count.

A review[2] of this syndrome, known as the 'retinoic acid syndrome', reported that it occurs in about 25% of patients with acute promyelocytic leukaemia treated with tretinoin and that the median time to onset is 10 to 12 days after the start of treatment; the severity of the syndrome varies greatly. A high leucocyte count at diagnosis or a rapidly-increasing count on initiation of therapy increase the likelihood of the syndrome occurring. Close monitoring of leucocyte counts and clinical

signs is recommended with the initiation of high-dose intravenous corticosteroids, and possibly the use of antineoplastic drugs, if symptoms appear or the leucocyte count increases rapidly.

A similar syndrome has also been reported in patients with acute promyelocytic leukaemia treated with arsenic trioxide (see p.1582).

1. Frankel SR, *et al.* The "retinoic acid syndrome" in acute promyelocytic leukemia. *Ann Intern Med* 1992; **117:** 292–6.
2. Fenaux P, De Botton S. Retinoic acid syndrome: recognition, prevention and management. *Drug Safety* 1998; **18:** 273–9.

Precautions

Tretinoin is contra-indicated in pregnancy and in breast-feeding mothers.

Contact of tretinoin with the eyes, mouth, or other mucous surfaces should be avoided. It should not be applied to eczematous, sunburnt, or abraded skin and the effects of other topical treatment, especially with keratolytics, should be allowed to subside before topical use of tretinoin. Exposure to UV light and excessive exposure to sunlight should be avoided.

Absorption does not seem to occur to any great extent with topical use. When tretinoin is given by mouth the precautions described under isotretinoin (see p.1117) should be adopted.

◊ The use of depilatory products should be avoided in patients treated with tretinoin. Erosions of the skin occurred in 2 patients after the use of wax depilation on facial areas also being treated topically with tretinoin.[1]

1. Goldberg NS, Zalka AD. Retin-A and wax epilation. *Arch Dermatol* 1989; **125:** 1717.

Pregnancy. Although there have been isolated reports[1-4] of congenital abnormalities in infants born to mothers who used tretinoin 0.05% topically before and during pregnancy, studies involving 215 women[5] and 94 women,[6] respectively showed no increased risk for major congenital disorders in infants who had been exposed in the first trimester.

1. Camera G, Pregliasco P. Ear malformation in baby born to mother using tretinoin cream. *Lancet* 1992; **339:** 687.
2. Lipson AH, *et al.* Multiple congenital defects associated with maternal use of topical tretinoin. *Lancet* 1993; **341:** 1352–3.
3. Navarre-Belhassen C, *et al.* Multiple congenital malformations associated with topical tretinoin. *Ann Pharmacother* 1998; **32:** 505–6.
4. Colley SMJ, *et al.* Topical tretinoin and fetal malformations. *Med J Aust* 1998; **168:** 467.
5. Jick SS, *et al.* First trimester topical tretinoin and congenital disorders. *Lancet* 1993; **341:** 1181–2.
6. Shapiro L, *et al.* Safety of first-trimester exposure to topical tretinoin: prospective cohort study. *Lancet* 1997; **350:** 1143–4.

Interactions

As for Isotretinoin, p.1117.

Tretinoin is metabolised by microsomal liver enzymes therefore there is a potential for interaction between oral tretinoin and inhibitors or inducers of these enzymes.

Minoxidil. Percutaneous absorption of minoxidil is enhanced by tretinoin as a result of increased stratum corneum permeability.[1]

1. Ferry JJ, *et al.* Influence of tretinoin on the percutaneous absorption of minoxidil from an aqueous topical solution. *Clin Pharmacol Ther* 1990; **47:** 439–46.

Pharmacokinetics

Following oral administration tretinoin is well absorbed from the gastrointestinal tract and peak plasma concentrations are obtained after 1 to 2 hours. Oral bioavailability is about 50%. Tretinoin is highly bound to plasma proteins. It undergoes metabolism in the liver. Metabolites include isotretinoin, 4-oxo-trans-retinoic acid, and 4-oxo-cis-retinoic acid. The terminal elimination half-life of tretinoin is 0.5 to 2 hours. Tretinoin is excreted in the bile and the urine.

◊ References.
1. Regazzi MB, *et al.* Clinical pharmacokinetics of tretinoin. *Clin Pharmacokinet* 1997; **32:** 382–402.

Uses and Administration

Tretinoin is a retinoid and is the acid form of vitamin A (p.1382).

Tretinoin is used primarily in the topical treatment of acne vulgaris when comedones, papules, and pustules predominate. It appears to stimulate mitosis and turnover of follicular epithelial cells and reduce their cohesiveness thereby facilitating the extrusion of existing comedones and preventing the formation of new ones. It also appears to have a thinning effect on the stratum corneum. Tretinoin is applied as a cream, gel, or alcoholic solution, usually containing 0.01 to 0.1%. The skin should be cleansed to remove excessive oiliness and dried 15 to 30 minutes before applying tretinoin lightly, once or twice daily according to response and irritation; some patients may require less frequent applications. Other topical preparations (including skin moisturisers) should not be applied at the same time as tretinoin is applied, and caution is required if other local irritants are used concurrently; however, applications of tretinoin can be alternated with applications of benzoyl peroxide with an interval of 12 or 24 hours between each application. There may be apparent exacerbations of the acne during early treatment and a therapeutic response may not be evident for 6 to 8 weeks. When the condition has resolved maintenance therapy should be less frequent.

A preparation containing tretinoin 0.05% is available for the treatment of mottled hyperpigmentation, roughness, and fine wrinkling of photodamaged skin. It is applied once daily at night. Effects may not be seen until about 6 months after starting treatment.

Tretinoin is also used to induce remission in acute promyelocytic leukaemia. A daily dose of 45 mg per m² body-surface is given by mouth in 2 divided doses. Treatment is continued until complete remission occurs or 90 days of treatment have been given.

◊ General reviews.
1. Orfanos CE, *et al.* Current use and future potential role of retinoids in dermatology. *Drugs* 1997; **53**: 358–88.

Malignant neoplasms. Tretinoin differentiation therapy has become the established treatment for acute promyelocytic leukaemia (APL), a subtype of acute myeloid leukaemia (p.485). Tretinoin is effective in APL because the characteristic chromosomal abnormalities result in an abnormal retinoic acid receptor.[1] When given by *mouth*, it has produced complete remissions in more than 90% of patients.[2] However the duration of remission is short unless consolidation, usually with an anthracycline- and cytarabine-based regimen, is given concurrently or subsequently. The combination of tretinoin followed by chemotherapy has been shown to result in improved survival compared with chemotherapy alone.[3,4] Prolonged maintenance therapy including intermittent tretinoin also appears to reduce the rate of relapse.[4] Although benefit has been reported with continuous tretinoin maintenance this is generally considered to lead to resistance.[4] A life-threatening syndrome has developed in some patients who have received oral tretinoin for APL (see under Adverse Effects, above). Children seem particularly sensitive to the adverse effects of oral tretinoin on the CNS (see also under Adverse Effects, above). A lipid-based *intravenous* formulation of tretinoin is under investigation for the treatment of APL.

Tretinoin has also been tried for the *topical* treatment of various neoplastic and related **skin disorders**. Some beneficial effects have been reported in the treatment of actinic keratoses, basal cell carcinoma, metastatic melanoma, and dysplastic naevi.[5-7] It also appears to be of use for the treatment of warts and solar keratoses in organ transplant recipients.[8]

1. Warrell RP, *et al.* Acute promyelocytic leukemia. *N Engl J Med* 1993; **329**: 177–89.
2. Gillis JC, Goa KL. Tretinoin: a review of its pharmacodynamic and pharmacokinetic properties and use in the management of acute promyelocytic leukaemia. *Drugs* 1995; **50**: 897–923.
3. Tallman MS, *et al.* All-trans-retinoic acid in acute promyelocytic leukemia. *N Engl J Med* 1997; **337**: 1021–8.
4. Fenaux P, Degos L. Treatment of acute promyelocytic leukaemia. *Clin Haematol* 1996; **9**: 107–27.
5. Meyskens FL, *et al.* Role of topical tretinoin in melanoma and dysplastic nevi. *J Am Acad Dermatol* 1986; **15**: 822–5.
6. Peck GL. Topical tretinoin in actinic keratosis and basal cell carcinoma. *J Am Acad Dermatol* 1986; **15**: 829–35.
7. Edwards L, Jaffe P. The effect of topical tretinoin on dysplastic nevi: a preliminary trial. *Arch Dermatol* 1990; **126**: 494–9.
8. Euvrard S, *et al.* Topical retinoids for warts and keratoses in transplant recipients. *Lancet* 1992; **340**: 48–9.

Skin disorders. Topical treatment with tretinoin has been tried with varying success in a wide range of cutaneous conditions. Its use in acne (p.1103) is well established. Some benefit has also been reported in rosacea[1] (p.1107), in keratinisation disorders such as Darier's disease (p.1104), in pigmentation disorders (p.1106) such as chloasma,[2] and in some neoplastic disorders (above).

A number of studies suggest that tretinoin can reverse some of the skin changes associated with chronic exposure to sunlight.[3-12] However, the effects seen during treatment are transient and the skin reverts to its pretreatment state once application stops.[13] One study found that several changes taken as indicative of an antiphoto-ageing effect, such as thickening of the skin and epidermis and an increase in the blood supply were not specific to topically applied retinoids and could equally be produced by the use of an abrasive preparation.[14]

1. Ertl GA, *et al.* A comparison of the efficacy of topical tretinoin and low-dose oral isotretinoin in rosacea. *Arch Dermatol* 1994; **130**: 319–24.

2. Griffiths CEM, *et al.* Topical tretinoin (retinoic acid) improves melasma: a vehicle-controlled, clinical trial. *Br J Dermatol* 1993; **129**: 415–21.
3. Weiss JS, *et al.* Topical tretinoin improves photoaged skin: a double-blind vehicle-controlled study. *JAMA* 1988; **259**: 527–32.
4. Leyden JJ, *et al.* Treatment of photodamaged facial skin with topical tretinoin. *J Am Acad Dermatol* 1989; **21**: 638–44.
5. Lever L, *et al.* Topical retinoic acid for treatment of solar damage. *Br J Dermatol* 1990; **122**: 91–8.
6. Berardesca E, *et al.* In vivo tretinoin-induced changes in skin mechanical properties. *Br J Dermatol* 1990; **122**: 525–9.
7. Woodley DT, *et al.* Treatment of photoaged skin with topical tretinoin increases epidermal-dermal anchoring fibrils: a preliminary report. *JAMA* 1990; **263**: 3057–9.
8. Weinstein GD, *et al.* Topical tretinoin for treatment of photodamaged skin: a multicenter study. *Arch Dermatol* 1991; **127**: 659–65.
9. Rafal ES. Topical tretinoin (retinoic acid) treatment for liver spots associated with photodamage. *N Engl J Med* 1992; **326**: 368–74.
10. Griffiths CEM, *et al.* Restoration of collagen formation in photodamaged human skin by tretinoin (retinoic acid). *N Engl J Med* 1993; **329**: 530–5.
11. Popp C, *et al.* Pretreatment of photoaged forearm skin with topical tretinoin accelerates healing of full-thickness wounds. *Br J Dermatol* 1995; **132**: 46–53.
12. Gilchrest BA. A review of skin ageing and its medical therapy. *Br J Dermatol* 1996; **135**: 867–75.
13. Anonymous. Tretinoin for sun-aged skin. *Drug Ther Bull* 1996; **34**: 55–6.
14. Marks R, *et al.* The effects of an abrasive agent on normal skin and on photoaged skin in comparison with topical tretinoin. *Br J Dermatol* 1990; **123**: 457–66.

Preparations

BP 2001: Tretinoin Gel; Tretinoin Solution;
USP 25: Tretinoin Cream; Tretinoin Gel; Tretinoin Topical Solution.

Proprietary Preparations (details are given in Part 3)
Aust.: Airol†; Eudyna; Retin-A; Vesanoid; **Austral.:** Retin-A; Re-Trieve; Stieva-A; Vesanoid; **Belg.:** Retinova; Vesanoid; **Braz.:** Dermoretin; Retin-A; **Canad.:** Rejuva-A; Renova; Retin-A; Retisol-A; Stieva-A; Vesanoid; Vitinoin; **Fin.:** Avitcid; Vesanoid; **Fr.:** Aberel; Effederm; Kerlocal; Ketrel; Locacid; Retacnyl; Retin-A; Retinova; Retitop; Tretinoine Kefrane; Vesanoid; **Ger.:** Airol; Cordes VAS; Epi-Aberel†; Eudyna; Vesanoid; **Hong Kong:** Acta; Alten; Eudyna; Retacnyl; Retin-A; Stieva-A; Vesanoid; **Irl.:** Retin-A; **Israel:** Airol; Locacid; Retavit; Retin-A; Vesanoid; **Ital.:** Airol; Retin-A; Vesanoid; **Mex.:** A-Plex; Airol; Arretin; Eudyna; Ret-A-Pres; Retacnyl; Retin-A; Stieva-A; Tretinon; Vesanoid; **Neth.:** Acid A Vit†; Vesanoid; **Norw.:** Aberela; Vesanoid†; **NZ:** Retin-A; Retinova; Vesanoid; **Port.:** Ketrel; Locacid; Retin-A; Vesanoid; Vitacid; **S.Afr.:** Renova; Retin-A; Vesanoid; **Singapore:** Acta; Airol; Alten; Eudyna; Retacnyl; Retin-A; Stieva-A; Vesanoid; **Spain:** Dermojuventus; Retinova; Retirides; **Swed.:** Aberela; Retinova; Vesanoid†; **Switz.:** Airol; Retin-A; Vesanoid; **Thai.:** Renova; Retacnyl; Retin-A; Stieva-A; Vesanoid; **UK:** Acticin; Retin-A; Retinova; Vesanoid; **USA:** Altinac; Avita; Renova; Retin-A; Vesanoid.

Multi-ingredient: **Aust.:** Keratosis forte; **Canad.:** Stievamycin; **Fin.:** Wicaran; **Fr.:** Antibio-Aberel; Erylik; **Ger.:** Aknemycin Plus; Balisa VAS; Carbamid + VAS; Clinesfar; Pigmanorm; Ureotop + VAS; **Hong Kong:** Dermabaz; **Ital.:** Apsor†; Psorinase; **Spain:** Acnisdin Retinoico; Loderm Retinoico; **Switz.:** Carbamide + VAS; Pigmanorm; Sebo-Psor; Tretinoine†; Verra-med; **UK:** Aknemycin Plus.

Trioxysalen   (1657-k)

Trioxysalen (rINN).
NSC-71047;   4,5′,8-Trimethylpsoralen;   Trioxsalen   (USAN). 2,5,9-Trimethyl-7H-furo[3,2-g][1]benzopyran-7-one.
$C_{14}H_{12}O_3 = 228.2$.
CAS — 3902-71-4.
ATC — D05AD01; D05BA01.
Pharmacopoeias. In US.

Pharmacopoeial description
USP 25: A white to off-white or greyish, odourless, crystalline solid. Practically insoluble in water; soluble 1 in 1150 of alcohol, 1 in 84 of chloroform, 1 in 43 of dichloromethane, and 1 in 100 of methyl isobutyl ketone. Protect from light.

Profile
Trioxysalen, a psoralen, is a photosensitiser used similarly to methoxsalen in photochemotherapy or PUVA therapy (p.1120).

Trioxysalen is used in idiopathic vitiligo to enhance pigmentation or increase the tolerance to sunlight in selected patients. In vitiligo a dose of 10 mg daily is given by mouth 2 to 4 hours before exposure to sunlight or ultraviolet radiation; prolonged therapy may be necessary. To increase tolerance to sunlight a dose of 10 mg daily is given 2 hours before exposure; treatment should not be continued for longer than 14 days.

Trioxysalen may also be used topically in the PUVA treatment of psoriasis.

Preparations

USP 25: Trioxsalen Tablets.

Proprietary Preparations (details are given in Part 3)
Austral.: Trisoralen†; **Canad.:** Trisoralen; **Fin.:** Tripsor; **Hong Kong:** Puvadin; Trisoralen; **Ital.:** Trisoralen†; **S.Afr.:** Trisoralen†; **USA:** Trisoralen.

Triphenyl Antimony Sulfide   (11585-w)

Triphenyl Antimony Sulphide; Triphenylstibinsulfid.
$C_{18}H_{15}SbS = 385.1$.
CAS — 3958-19-8.

Profile
Triphenyl antimony sulfide has been applied topically for the treatment of a range of skin disorders including seborrhoea, acne, eczema, and minor fungal infections.

Urea   (2361-s)

Carbamide; E927b; Ureia; Ureum. Carbonic acid diamide.
$NH_2.CO.NH_2 = 60.06$.
CAS — 57-13-6.
ATC — B05BC02; D02AE01.
Pharmacopoeias. In Chin., Eur. (see p.vi), Jpn, Pol., and US.

Pharmacopoeial description
Ph. Eur.: Transparent, slightly hygroscopic, crystals or a white crystalline powder. Very soluble in water; soluble in alcohol; practically insoluble in dichloromethane.
USP 25: Colourless or white, practically odourless, prismatic crystals, or white crystalline powder or pellets. May gradually develop a slight odour of ammonia on prolonged standing. Soluble 1 in 1.5 of water, 1 in 10 of alcohol, and 1 in 1 of boiling alcohol; practically insoluble in chloroform and in ether. Solutions are neutral to litmus.

◊ *Urea can cause haemolysis when mixed with blood and should never be added to whole blood for transfusion or given through the same set by which blood is being infused.*

Adverse Effects and Precautions
As for Mannitol, p.924.

Urea is reported to be more irritant than mannitol, and intravenous administration may cause venous thrombosis or phlebitis at the site of injection; extravasation may cause sloughing or necrosis. Only large veins should be used for infusion, and urea should not be infused into veins of the lower limbs of elderly subjects. Extreme care is essential to prevent accidental extravasation of urea infusions.

Rapid intravenous injection of solutions of urea can cause haemolysis; the risk is reduced by using glucose or invert sugar solutions as diluent. Urea should not be administered with whole blood.

Topical applications may be irritant to sensitive skin.

Infants and neonates. High plasma-urea concentrations have been reported[1,2] in neonates following topical application of emollient creams containing urea. Since there was no evidence of dehydration[2,3] absorption of urea through the skin was the likely cause. Raised plasma-urea concentrations have been reported[4] in infants with erythematous skin conditions who had not been treated with urea cream and this was attributed to dehydration due to increased insensible water loss through the damaged skin.

1. Beverley DW, Wheeler D. High plasma urea concentrations in collodion babies. *Arch Dis Child* 1986; **61**: 696–8.
2. Oudesluys-Murphy AM, van Leeuwen M. High plasma urea concentrations in collodion babies. *Arch Dis Child* 1987; **62**: 212.
3. Beverley DW, Wheeler D. High plasma urea concentration in babies with lamellar ichthyosis. *Arch Dis Child* 1986; **61**: 1245–6.
4. Garty BZ. High plasma urea concentration in babies with lamellar ichthyosis. *Arch Dis Child* 1986; **61**: 1245.

Pregnancy. There have been reports of women suffering coagulopathy associated with urea administered for termination of pregnancy.[1,2]

1. Grundy MFB, Craven ER. Consumption coagulopathy after intra-amniotic urea. *BMJ* 1976; **2**: 677–8.
2. Burkman RT, *et al.* Coagulopathy with midtrimester induced abortion: association with hyperosmolar urea administration. *Am J Obstet Gynecol* 1977; **127**: 533–6.

Pharmacokinetics
Urea is fairly rapidly absorbed from the gastrointestinal tract but causes gastrointestinal irritation. Urea is distributed into extracellular and intracellular fluids including lymph, bile, CSF, and blood. It is reported to cross the placenta, and penetrate the eye. It is excreted unchanged in the urine.

Uses and Administration
Urea is an osmotic agent similar to mannitol (p.925). It is mainly applied topically in the treatment of ichthyosis and hyperkeratotic skin disorders (p.1105). It has been used intravenously in the treatment of acute increases in intracranial pressure (p.811), due to cerebral oedema, and to decrease intra-ocular pressure in acute glaucoma (p.1413), but has been largely super-

seded by mannitol. Urea has also been given intra-amniotically for the termination of pregnancy (p.1439).

When applied topically urea has hydrating and kera-tolytic properties. In the management of ichthyosis and other dry skin disorders it is applied in creams or lotions containing 5 to 25% urea. A preparation containing 40% may be used for nail destruction.

For the reduction of raised intracranial or intra-ocular pressure, urea is given intravenously, as an infusion of a 30% solution in glucose 5 to 10% or invert sugar 10%, at a rate not exceeding 4 mL per minute, in a dose of 0.5 to 1.5 g per kg body-weight to a maximum of 120 g daily. For children under 2 years a dose of 100 mg per kg has been suggested. Rebound increases in intracranial and intra-ocular pressure may occur after about 12 hours.

Solutions of urea 40 to 50% have been given by intra-amniotic injection for the termination of pregnancy.

Urea labelled with carbon-13 (p.1591) is used in the *in vivo* diagnosis of *Helicobacter pylori* infection (see Peptic Ulcer Disease, p.1208). A single dose of ^{13}C-urea is taken by mouth, and a breath or blood sample taken 30 minutes later. *H. pylori* produces urease which hydrolyses the urea to carbon dioxide and ammonia; therefore, an excess of carbon-13-labelled carbon dioxide in the sample, compared with a base-line sample, indicates infection. Doses of ^{13}C-urea include 75 mg, 100 mg, or 125 mg, depending on the kit being used. Urea labelled with the radionuclide carbon-14 (p.1449) is also used in a urea breath test for *H. pylori* detection.

Preparations

BP 2001: Urea Cream;
USP 25: Urea for Injection.

Proprietary Preparations (details are given in Part 3)
Aust.: Basodexan; Excipial U†; Nubral; *Austral.:* Aquacare-HP; Aquadrate†; Hamilton Dry Skin; Nutraplus; Urecare; Urederm; *Braz.:* Nutraplus; *Canad.:* Calmurid†; Dermaflex; Ti-U-Lac; Ultra Mide; Uree; Uremol; Urisec; Velvelan†; *Fin.:* Fenuril; *Fr.:* Charlieu Topic; Nutraplus; Urecrem; *Ger.:* Balisa; Basodexan; Elacutan; Eucerin Salbe; Hyanit N†; Laceran†; Nubral; Onychomal; Penaderm; Rubio N; Sebexol cum urea; Ureotop; *Hong Kong:* Carmol; Euderm; Nutraplus; Urederm; *Irl.:* Aquadrate; Nutraplus; *Ital.:* Dermal Care; *Mex.:* Derma Keri; Dermoplast; Nutraplus; *Neth.:* Alphadrate†; Calmurid; *NZ:* Aquacare; Nutraplus; *Port.:* Eucerin Pele Seca; Laceran†; Rebladerm; Ureadin 10 and 20; *S.Afr.:* Eulactol; *Singapore:* Nutraplus; Urecare; *Swed.:* Calmuril; Canoderm; Caress; Fenuril; Karbasal; Monilen; *Switz.:* Excipial U; Nutraplus; *UK:* Aquadrate; Nutraplus; *USA:* Aquacare; Atrac-Tain†; Carmol; Gormel; Lanaphilic; Nutraplus; Ultra Mide; Ureacin; Ureaphil.

Multi-ingredient: *Aust.:* Aleot; Calmurid; Calmurid comp; Calmurid HC; Hydrodexan; Ichth-Oestren; Keratosis; Keratosis forte; Mirfulan; Mykozem†; Optiderm; Psoradexan†; *Austral.:* Aussie Tan Skin Moisturiser; Calmurid; Curaderm; Dermadrate; Psor-Asist; SP Cream; *Belg.:* Alphaderm†; Calmurid; *Braz.:* Colpanist; Colpatrin; Donnagel; Oto-Biotic; Sedauric; Tricolpex; Vagi Biotic; *Canad.:* Amino-Cerv; Calmurid HC†; Hydrophil; Ti-U-Lac HC; Uremol-HC; *Denm.:* Mycospor Carbamid†; *Fin.:* Calmuril; Wicaran; Wicarba; Wicnecarb; Wicnevit; *Fr.:* Amycor Onychoset; Charlieu Topicrem; Keratosane; *Ger.:* Balisa VAS; Brand- u. Wundgel-Medice N; Calmurid; Calmurid HC; Carbamid + VAS; Fungidexan; Grune Salbe "Schmidt" N†; Hydrodexan; Kelofibrase; Mirfulan; Mycospor Nagelset; Nubral 4; Nubral 4 HC; Nubral Forte; Oestrugol N; Optiderm; Psoradexan; Psorigerb N; Remederm; Ureata S; Ureotop + VAS; *Irl.:* Alphaderm; Calmurid; Calmurid HC; Psoradrate; *Israel:* Agispor Onychoset; Calmurid; Calmurid HC; Derma-Care; Keratospor; U-Lactin Foot Cream; U-Lactin Forte; *Ital.:* Eudermico; Optiderm; Verunec 3; Xerial; *Mex.:* Mycospor Onicoset; Neth.: Alphacortison†; Calmurid HC; Symbial; *Norw.:* Mycospor Carbamid†; *NZ:* Calmurid; *Port.:* Calmurid; Carmitol; Creme Laser Hidrante; Hidrato-

derme†; Mycospor†; Optiderme†; U Lactin†; Ureadin 10 Plus; Ureadin 30; Ureadin Facial; Ureadin Maos; *S.Afr.:* Calmurid HC; Covacaine; *Singapore:* Topicrem; *Spain:* Cortisdin Urea; Kanapomada; Mycospor Onicoset; *Swed.:* Calmuril-Hydrokortison†; Fenuril-Hydrokortison; Mycosporan Karbamid†; *Switz.:* Acne Gel; Antikeloides Creme; Betacortone; Calmurid; Calmurid HC; Carbamide + VAS; Carbamide Creme; Kerasal; Klyx Magnum; Optiderm; Psoradexan†; Sebo Creme; Sebo-Psor; Squa-med; Tretinoine†; Turexan Capilla; Turexan Lotion; *Thai.:* Gynestin; *UK:* Alphaderm; Antipeol; Balneum Plus; Calmurid; Calmurid HC; Cymex; E45 Itch Relief; Heelbalm; St James Balm; *USA:* Accuzyme; Amino-Cerv; Dayto Sulf†; Panafil; Panafil-White.

Xenysalate Hydrochloride (1658-a)

Xenysalate Hydrochloride (BANM, rINNM).
Biphenamine Hydrochloride (USAN). 2-Diethylaminoethyl 3-phenylsalicylate hydrochloride; 2-Diethylaminoethyl 2-hydroxy-3-phenylbenzoate hydrochloride.
$C_{19}H_{23}NO_3,HCl = 349.9$.
CAS — 3572-52-9 (xenysalate); 5560-62-3 (xenysalate hydrochloride).

Profile

Xenysalate hydrochloride has antibacterial and antifungal properties and has been used for the control of seborrhoeic dermatitis of the scalp.

Preparations

Proprietary Preparations (details are given in Part 3)
Fr.: Sebaklen†.

Zinc Carbonate (1659-t)

Zinc Carbonate (USAN).
$ZnCO_3 = 125.4$.
CAS — 3486-35-9.

Basic Zinc Carbonate (11593-w)

NOTE. The names zinc carbonate, hydrated zinc carbonate, zinc subcarbonate, and zinc carbonate hydroxide have all been applied to basic zinc carbonate of varying composition occurring naturally or produced by the reaction of a soluble zinc salt with sodium carbonate.
Pharmacopoeias. In US.

Pharmacopoeial description

USP 25: Zinc carbonate corresponds to $3Zn(OH)_2.2ZnCO_3$ containing the equivalent of not less than 70% ZnO. Store in airtight containers.

Profile

Zinc carbonate is mildly astringent and protective to the skin and is used topically, mainly in the form of calamine (p.1111), in a variety of skin conditions. In the USA the name calamine is used for zinc oxide (rather than zinc carbonate) with a small proportion of ferric oxide.

Preparations

Proprietary Preparations (details are given in Part 3)
Multi-ingredient: *Fr.:* Pygmal; *Spain:* Neo Visage.

Zinc Oxide (1660-l)

Blanc de Zinc; Flores de Zinc; Zinci Oxidum; Zinci Oxydum; Zincum Oxydatum.
$ZnO = 81.39$.
CAS — 1314-13-2.

NOTE. 'Zinc White' is a commercial form of zinc oxide for use as a pigment.
Pharmacopoeias. In Chin., Eur. (see p.vi), Int., Jpn, Pol., and US.

Black discoloration has been reported when zinc oxide and glycerol are in contact in the presence of light.

Pharmacopoeial description

Ph. Eur.: A white or faintly yellowish-white, soft, amorphous powder, free from gritty particles. Practically insoluble in water and in alcohol; it dissolves in dilute mineral acids.

USP 25: A white or yellowish-white, odourless, amorphous, very fine powder, free from grittiness. It gradually absorbs carbon dioxide from air. Insoluble in water and in alcohol; soluble in dilute acids.

Uses and Administration

Zinc oxide is mildly astringent and is used topically as a soothing and protective application in eczema and slight excoriations, in wounds, and for haemorrhoids. It is also used with coal tar (p.1125) or ichthammol (p.1115) in the treatment of eczema. Zinc oxide reflects ultraviolet radiation and is used in sunscreens.

In the USA the name calamine is used for zinc oxide with a small proportion of ferric oxide.

Zinc oxide is used as the basis for the production of a number of dental cements. Mixed with phosphoric acid it forms a hard material composed largely of zinc phosphate; mixed with clove oil or eugenol, it is used as temporary dental filling.

For further details of zinc and its salts, see p.1398.

Complications of dental use. Solitary aspergillosis of the maxillary sinus in 29 of 30 patients was associated with zinc oxide from overfilled teeth.[1] Treatment consisted of removal of the fungal ball containing the zinc oxide; no antifungal treatment was necessary. Zinc oxide has been shown to accelerate the growth of *Aspergillus fumigatus.*

1. Beck-Mannagetta J, *et al.* Solitary aspergillosis of maxillary sinus, a complication of dental treatment. *Lancet* 1983; **ii:** 1260.

Preparations

BP 2001: Aqueous Calamine Cream; Calamine and Coal Tar Ointment; Calamine Lotion; Coal Tar and Zinc Ointment; Coal Tar Paste; Compound Aluminium Paste; Compound Zinc Paste; Dithranol Paste; Hexachlorophene Dusting Powder; Zinc and Castor Oil Ointment; Zinc and Coal Tar Paste; Zinc and Ichthammol Cream; Zinc and Salicylic Acid Paste; Zinc Cream; Zinc Ointment;
USP 25: Calamine Lotion; Coal Tar Ointment; Compound Resorcinol Ointment; Zinc Oxide and Salicylic Acid Paste; Zinc Oxide Ointment; Zinc Oxide Paste.

Proprietary Preparations (details are given in Part 3)
Austral.: Curash Anti-Rash; Curash Medicated; Prickly Heat Powder; Zinc Cream White; Zincaband; Zink'N'Swim; *Canad.:* Babys Own Ointment; Diaper Rash†; Egozinc; Herisan; Infazinc; Johnson's Diaper Rash; Johnson's Medicated; Neoderm; Pate d'Unna; Prevex Diaper Rash Cream†; Triple Care Cream; Zinaderm; Zincoderm; Zincofax; *Denm.:* Zipzoc; *Fin.:* Zipzoc; *Fr.:* Lanofene†; Oxyplastine; Senophile; *Ger.:* Desitin; Fissan-Zinks-chuttelmixtur; Labiosan; Robuvalen; St. Jakobs-Balsam Mono; Weiche Zinkpaste†; Zinkorell; Zinkpaste; Zinksalbe Dialon; *Hong Kong:* Anuzinc; *Irl.:* Coltapaste; Viscopaste PB7; Zipzoc; *Israel:* Dyprotex; Lotio Zinc; Zinc Lotion; *Ital.:* Delicate Skin; Gelocast; Gelostretch; Milsana; Oz; Triderm Zeta; Varicex; Viscopaste PB7; Zinco All' Acqua; Zincoderm; Zincotape; Zincotex; *Mex.:* Dermo Lassar; Lassarmex; Pasta De Lassar; *Neth.:* Zinkolie; Zinkzalf; *Port.:* Lassadermil; Oleo Dermosina Simples; Zincoderma; *S.Afr.:* Johnson's Baby Nappy Rash Ointment†; Vernleigh Baby Cream; Viscopaste PB7; *Spain:* Anticongestiva; *Swed.:* Zincaband†; Zipzoc Salvstrumpa; *Switz.:* Oxyplastine; Zincream; *Thai.:* Spectraban; *UAE:* Proskin; *UK:* Steripaste; Viscopaste PB7; Zincaband; Zipzoc; *USA:* Borofax; Diaparene Diaper Rash; Flanders Buttocks; Nupercainal.

Multi-ingredient: Numerous preparations are listed in Part 3.

Zinc Phenolsulfonate (17036-g)

Zinc 4-Hydroxybenzenesulphonate. Zinc p-hydroxybenzenesulphonate; Zinc Phenolsulphonate.
$C_{12}H_{10}O_8S_2Zn = 411.7$.
CAS — 127-82-2.

Profile

Zinc phenolsulfonate has astringent properties and has been used in multi-ingredient preparations applied topically for the treatment of a variety of disorders.

Preparations

Proprietary Preparations (details are given in Part 3)
Multi-ingredient: *Austral.:* BFI†; *Braz.:* Lerin; *Ital.:* Antisettico Astringente Sedativo; Citroftalmina; Citroftalmina VC; Oftalmil; *Spain:* Regal†; *Switz.:* Medi-Kord†; *USA:* BFI.

Disinfectants and Preservatives

This chapter describes those antimicrobial agents which are used for chemical methods of disinfection, antisepsis, preservation, and sterilisation. There is some overlap between these procedures and some agents may be used as both disinfectants and preservatives. Iodine (p.1522) is also used for its disinfectant properties.

Definition of terms. There is often confusion between the terms disinfectant and antiseptic.

- The term **disinfectant** is applied to a chemical agent which destroys or inhibits the growth of pathogenic micro-organisms in the non-sporing or vegetative state; disinfectants do not necessarily kill all micro-organisms, but reduce them to a level which is harmful neither to health nor the quality of perishable goods. The term is applicable to agents used to treat inanimate objects and materials and may also be applied to agents used to treat the skin and other body membranes and cavities

- An **antiseptic** is a disinfectant which is used on skin and other living tissues thereby limiting or preventing infection.

- **Sterilisation** is the total removal or destruction of all living micro-organisms; a few disinfectants (such as ethylene oxide) are capable of producing sterility under suitable conditions but, in general, sterility is produced by heat or radiation methods, with filtration being employed for some heat-labile materials. Sterilisation by heating with a bactericide is no longer a recommended practice.

- A **preservative** is one of a number of chemical agents which are included in preparations to prevent deterioration from oxidation (**antioxidants**) or to kill or inhibit the growth of micro-organisms inadvertently introduced during manufacture or use (**antimicrobial preservatives**).

Use of disinfectants. Disinfectants are used in hospitals, industrial establishments, public buildings, on farms, and in the home for control and prevention of infection.

The choice of disinfectant depends on the purpose for which it is used and the likely contaminating organisms. In addition to vegetative bacteria, many common disinfectants could be expected to kill some fungi and lipid-containing viruses. Gram-negative bacteria, mycobacteria, and bacterial spores are generally more resistant to disinfectants, and some disinfectants are less effective against non-lipid enveloped viruses, for example the enteroviruses including polio and coxsackie. Prions are generally resistant to many disinfectants (see Disinfection in Creutzfeldt-Jakob Disease, below). Other factors affecting the effectiveness of disinfectants include the contact time, concentration of the disinfectant, the pH of the system, the number and accessibility of the contaminating micro-organisms, and the presence of interfering substances including lipids, organic matter, rubber and plastics. Aqueous solutions of disinfectants, particularly quaternary ammonium compounds (such as benzalkonium chloride and cetrimide), chlorhexidine, and phenols, may be susceptible to contamination with micro-organisms. To reduce this risk many preparations are provided for clinical use in a sterile form for single use.

Use of preservatives. Antimicrobial preservatives are used in sterile preparations such as eye drops and multidose injections to maintain sterility during use. They may also be added to aqueous injections that cannot be sterilised in their final containers and have to be prepared using aseptic precautions, unless the volume to be injected as a single dose exceeds 15 mL. Antimicrobial preservatives are also used in cosmetics, foods, and non-sterile pharmaceutical products such as oral liquids and creams to prevent microbial spoilage. They should not be used indiscriminately. Preparations that should *not* contain preservatives in-

clude those for injection into the CSF, eye, or heart. Generally, the antimicrobial preservatives that may be added to foods, animal feeding stuffs, and cosmetics are controlled.

Preservatives used as antioxidants may be classified in 3 groups:

- *true antioxidants*, or anti-oxygens, which probably inhibit oxidation by reacting with free radicals blocking the chain reaction. Examples are the alkyl gallates, butylated hydroxyanisole, butylated hydroxytoluene, nordihydroguaiaretic acid, and the tocopherols (see Vitamin E Substances, p.1393).

- *reducing agents* which are substances having a lower redox potential than the drug or adjuvants which they are intended to protect and are therefore more readily oxidised. Reducing agents may act also by reacting with free radicals. Examples are ascorbic acid (p.1389) and the potassium and sodium salts of sulfurous acid (see Sulfites and Sulfur Dioxide)

- *antioxidant synergists* which usually have little antioxidant effect themselves but probably enhance the action of antioxidants in the first group by reacting with heavy-metal ions which catalyse oxidation. Examples of synergists are citric acid (p.1596), edetic acid and its salts (p.1008), lecithin (p.1628) and tartaric acid (p.1669).

◊ General references and guidelines for the use of disinfectants.

1. BMA. *A code of practice for sterilisation of instruments and control of cross-infection.* London: BMA, 1989.
2. Ayliffe GAJ, *et al. Hospital-acquired infection: principles and prevention.* London: Wright, 1990.
3. Ayliffe GAJ, *et al. Chemical disinfection in hospitals.* 2nd ed. London: PHLS, 1993.
4. Rutala WA. APIC guideline for selection and use of disinfectants. *Am J Infect Control* 1996; **24:** 313–42.
5. Russell AD, *et al. Principles and practice of disinfection, preservation, and sterilization.* 3rd ed. Oxford: Blackwell, 1999.
6. DoH. Standard principle for preventing hospital-acquired infections. *J Hosp Infect* 2001; **47** (suppl): S21–S37.

Contact lens care

Wearers of contact lenses are at increased risk of corneal infections. Factors that predispose the cornea to infection include surface abrasions which may occur during normal wear, accidental trauma during insertion of a lens, and anoxia. In addition, the lens may provide a medium for introducing pathogens into the eye, especially if handling, cleaning, and disinfecting procedures are not adhered to. The most common pathogens are bacteria, in particular *Pseudomonas aeruginosa, Serratia marcescens, Staphylococcus aureus, Staph. epidermidis,* and *Streptococcus pneumoniae.* Fungi rarely cause lens-related keratitis, although contamination of soft (hydrogel) lenses has been reported. *Acanthamoeba* can cause rare but serious corneal infections (p.582) mainly associated with soft contact lens wear. These protozoa are resistant to some commonly used disinfection systems and can colonise lens storage cases.

Lens care systems for rigid lenses typically entail cleansing and disinfection stages. Daily cleansing with solutions containing surfactants and sometimes mild abrasives can substantially reduce microbial contamination as well as removing organic material which can compromise the activity of the disinfection stage. Cleansing solutions frequently contain substances which are irritant to the eye and should be removed by rinsing and soaking the lens. Soaking solutions also maintain lens hydration, disinfect the lens, and prevent contamination during storage. Although not intended for introduction into the eye, soaking solutions should be non-irritant. Commonly used disinfectants include benzalkonium chloride and chlorhexidine. Thiomersal is also used but has been associated with a high incidence of hypersensitivity reactions. Wetting or rewetting solutions are used to improve the comfort of the lens and, since they are applied to the eye, must be non-irritant. They commonly contain hypromellose, hyetellose, polyvinyl alcohol, or povidone, although a simple sodium chloride 0.9% solution may be used.

Soft contact lenses contain a high proportion of water and are liable to absorb substances from solution. For this reason some disinfectants, notably benzalkonium chloride, are not suitable for inclusion in solutions for soft lenses. Soft lenses may be disinfected by heating in a suitable unit, usually in isotonic saline solution, but this can shorten the life of the lens by denaturing the polymer or causing deposits of denatured protein, minerals, or

preservatives from the saline solution. Stabilised hydrogen peroxide is suitable for cold disinfection of soft lenses and is particularly useful for preventing *Acanthamoeba* infections. However, it is irritant to the cornea and must be neutralised before the lens is inserted into the eye. Other disinfectants for soft lenses may include chlorhexidine and polihexanide. Cleansers for soft lenses may contain surfactants or enzymes such as papain or pancreatin which remove protein deposits.

Disinfection in Creutzfeldt-Jakob disease

Creutzfeldt-Jakob disease is a transmissible spongiform encephalopathy believed to be caused by infection of the nervous system with prions. The agent causing Creutzfeldt-Jakob disease (CJD) is resistant to many disinfection procedures including dry heat, ultraviolet irradiation, alcohols, ethylene oxide, eusol, formaldehyde, glutaral, hydrogen peroxide, iodine or iodophores, peracetic acid, phenolics, and propiolactone. Although no sterilisation procedure can be guaranteed to be completely effective under all circumstances, the method recommended in the UK[1] is immersion in sodium hypochlorite (providing 20 000 ppm available chlorine) for 1 hour. Alternatives are autoclaving at 134° to 137° for a single cycle of 18 minutes, or 6 successive cycles of 3 minutes each, or immersion in 2M sodium hydroxide for 1 hour; however these methods are not known to be completely effective. Neurosurgical and ophthalmic instruments should be destroyed by incineration if used in patients with confirmed or suspected CJD.

1. Advisory Committee on Dangerous Pathogens, Spongiform Encephalopathy Advisory Committee. *Transmissible spongiform encephalopathy agents: safe working and the prevention of infection.* London, The Stationary Office, 1998. Also available at: http://www.official-documents.co.uk/document/doh/spongiform/report.htm (accessed 27/02/01).

Disinfection of endoscopes

Whenever possible, medical equipment which comes into intimate contact with the body should be heat sterilised, but some equipment, notably endoscopes, will not withstand high temperatures. Low-temperature steam and formaldehyde or ethylene oxide will achieve sterilisation, but may not be practical in a clinical setting. Satisfactory chemical disinfection of endoscopes and other heat-sensitive instruments relies on initial thorough cleansing of the instrument and choice of an appropriate disinfectant which should be rapidly active against a wide range of pathogens including vegetative bacteria, bacterial spores, mycobacteria, and viruses. The disinfectant should not damage the instrument or discolour the optical components, and it should not leave a toxic residue. It is usually necessary to rinse the instrument with sterile water or alcohol after disinfection.[1,2]

Glutaral 2% is commonly used.[1] To achieve sterilisation, immersion in glutaral 2% for 3 hours is necessary, but high-level disinfection, achieved by immersion for 10 to 20 minutes, is usually considered adequate for most endoscopes.[1,3,4] Immersion for a minimum of 20 minutes is required for elimination of tubercle bacilli, but immersion for 4 minutes may be adequate for gastroscopes, except those for use on immunocompromised patients. Specific information relating to HIV and hepatitis viruses is given below.

A disadvantage of glutaral is that it is irritant and may cause sensitisation. In addition, glutaral-resistant strains of *M. chelonae* have been isolated from endoscope disinfecting equipment.[5] Alternative disinfectants include peracetic acid, chlorine dioxide, and superoxidised water.[4] Other alternatives include peroxygen compounds, a quaternary ammonium compound followed by alcohol, succinic dialdehyde, povidone-iodine, and alcohol 70%.[1,4,6,7] However, peracetic acid and chlorine dioxide produce irritant fumes, peroxygen-containing compounds and quaternary ammonium compounds have questionable activity against mycobacteria and viruses, and alcohol and povidone-iodine have a number of practical limitations.[4,8]

1. Ayliffe GAJ, *et al. Chemical disinfection in hospitals.* 2nd ed. London: PHLS, 1993.
2. Ryan CK, Potter GD. Disinfectant colitis: rinse as well as you wash. *J Clin Gastroenterol* 1995; **21:** 6–9.
3. American Society for Gastrointestinal Endoscopy. Reprocessing of flexible gastrointestinal endoscopes. *Gastrointest Endosc* 1996; **43:** 540–6.

4. British Society of Gastroenterology Working Party. Cleaning and disinfection of equipment for gastrointestinal endoscopy. *Gut* 1998; **42**: 585–93.
5. Griffiths PA, *et al.* Glutaraldehyde-resistant Mycobacterium chelonae from endoscope washer disinfectors. *J Appl Microbiol* 1997; **82**: 519–26.
6. Axon ATR, Cotton PB. Endoscopy and infection. *Gut* 1983; **24**: 1064–6.
7. Fraise AP. Disinfection in endoscopy. *Lancet* 1995; **346**: 787–8.
8. Ridgway GL. Decontamination of fibreoptic endoscopes. *J Hosp Infect* 1985; **6**: 363–8.

Disinfection in hepatitis and HIV infection

Hepatitis viruses and HIV are susceptible to heat and the methods recommended for sterilisation of equipment in the UK[1] are conventional procedures using moist or dry heat. Heat-labile articles and surfaces may undergo chemical disinfection but only in the absence of a satisfactory alternative. Although various publications have claimed efficacy against HIV for a wide range of disinfectants and detergents, the evidence for some claims is equivocal.

Fresh aqueous solutions of sodium hypochlorite or sodium dichloroisocyanurate are recommended for general surface disinfection. If contaminated by blood, the concentration must be equivalent to 10 000 ppm of available chlorine. For non-corrosive disinfection of delicate items such as fibreoptic endoscopes, freshly activated alkaline glutaral 2% may be used following thorough washing. If a sterile body cavity will be entered the endoscope must be immersed for a minimum of 3 hours; otherwise a minimum of 30 minutes is sufficient, or 1 hour if the presence of *Mycobacterium tuberculosis* is suspected.

1. DoH. *UK Health Departments guidance for clinical health care workers: protection against infection with blood-borne viruses: recommendations of the expert advisory group on AIDS and the advisory group on hepatitis.* Available at: http://www.doh.gov.uk/chcguid1.htm (accessed 01/03/01).

Disinfection of water

Travellers to regions of the world where water is not disinfected at source should be advised to boil or chemically sterilise water for drinking, cleaning teeth, and washing fruit and vegetables. Chlorine-releasing disinfectants including tosylchloramide sodium, halazone, sodium dichloroisocyanurate, and sodium hypochlorite are commonly used. Iodine-releasing disinfectants such as tetraglycine hydroperiodide or iodine itself are also sometimes used. Organic material suspended in the water may reduce the available halogen concentration, and cloudy water should be filtered or allowed to settle and decanted before treatment. Emergency treatment of drinking water with lemon juice has been suggested during epidemics of waterborne gastro-enteritis.[1] Chlorine-releasing disinfectants are also used for recreational and therapeutic bathing pools, often in combination with ozone.[2]

Legionnaires' disease (p.126) is commonly transmitted via cooling water in air conditioning systems or hot water supplies. Hyperchlorination has been attempted to eradicate the organism from contaminated water sources but has been largely ineffective[3,4] and is no longer recommended. Other disadvantages of using chlorine-based systems at these temperatures and concentrations are corrosion of the plumbing system[4] and the production of potentially carcinogenic byproducts.[5] Effective disinfection can be achieved by raising the water temperature, ultraviolet light, and copper-silver ionisation.

1. D'Aquino M, Teves SA. Lemon juice as a natural biocide for disinfecting drinking water. *Bull Pan Am Health Organ* 1994; **28**: 324–30.
2. Dadswell JV. Managing swimming, spa, and other pools to prevent infection. *Commun Dis Rep* 1996; **6** (review 2): R37–R40.
3. Kurtz JB, *et al.* Legionella pneumophila in cooling water systems: report of a survey of cooling towers in London and a pilot trial of selected biocides. *J Hyg (Camb)* 1982; **88**: 369–81.
4. Helms CM, *et al.* Legionnaires' disease associated with a hospital water system: a five-year progress report on continuous hyperchlorination. *JAMA* 1988; **259**: 2423–7.
5. Morris RD, *et al.* Chlorination, chlorination by-products, and cancer: a meta-analysis. *Am J Public Health* 1992; **82**: 955–63.

Injection site and catheter care

The need to disinfect the skin before injection is controversial.[1] Routine skin preparation of the injection site by swabbing with antiseptic has been reported to be both ineffective and unnecessary.[2,3] Central venous and arterial catheters, however, require the application of strict aseptic technique and injection site antisepsis to reduce the chance of infection.[4] Disinfection of catheter insertion sites with aqueous chlorhexidine 2% has been reported to be associated with fewer local and systemic infections than site preparation with either 10% povidone-iodine solution or 70% isopropyl alcohol,[5] although this

has been challenged.[6] A subsequent study reported lower rates of catheter colonisation and catheter-related infection with an alcoholic solution of chlorhexidine 0.25% and benzalkonium chloride 0.025% than with povidone-iodine 10%.[7] In a study in preterm infants, technique had greater influence on bacterial counts at injection sites than the antiseptic used; chlorhexidine 0.5% in isopropyl alcohol and aqueous povidone-iodine 10% were equally effective, but cleansing with alcoholic chlorhexidine for 30 seconds or for two 10-second periods was more effective than cleansing for 5 or 10 seconds.[8]

The use of catheters impregnated with antiseptics or antibacterials has also been studied.[9] Catheters impregnated with chlorhexidine and sulfadiazine silver do appear to be effective in reducing both catheter colonisation and related blood stream infection in high-risk patients.[9,10] Central venous catheters impregnated with minocycline and rifampicin have been reported to be associated with a lower infection rate than those impregnated with chlorhexidine and sulfadiazine silver.[11]

1. Ayliffe GAJ, *et al. Chemical disinfection in hospitals.* 2nd ed. London: PHLS, 1993.
2. Dann TC. Routine skin preparation before injection: an unnecessary procedure. *Lancet* 1969; **ii**: 96–8.
3. Liauw J, Archer GJ. Swabaholics? *Lancet* 1995; **345**: 1648.
4. Shepherd A, Williams N. Care of long-term central venous catheters. *Br J Hosp Med* 1994; **51**: 598–602.
5. Maki DG, *et al.* Prospective randomised trial of povidone-iodine, alcohol, and chlorhexidine for prevention of infection associated with central venous and arterial catheters. *Lancet* 1991; **338**: 339–43.
6. Segura M, Sitges-Serra A. Intravenous catheter sites and sepsis. *Lancet* 1991; **338**: 1218.
7. Mimoz O, *et al.* Prospective, randomized trial of two antiseptic solutions for prevention of central venous or arterial catheter colonization and infection in intensive care unit patients. *Crit Care Med* 1996; **24**: 1818–23.
8. Malathi I, *et al.* Skin disinfection in preterm infants. *Arch Dis Child* 1993; **69**: 312–16.
9. DoH. Guidelines for preventing infections associated with the insertion and maintenance of central venous catheters. *J Hosp Infect* 2001; **47**(suppl): S47–S67.
10. Veenstra DL, *et al.* Efficacy of antiseptic-impregnated central venous catheters in preventing catheter-related bloodstream infection: a meta-analysis. *JAMA* 1999; **281**: 261–7.
11. Darouiche RO, *et al.* A comparison of two antimicrobial-impregnated central venous catheters. *N Engl J Med* 1999; **340**: 1–8.

Wound disinfection

Antiseptic preparations are widely used to treat or prevent superficial infections, but their usefulness on broken skin and wounds has been questioned.[1] Antiseptic solutions are commonly used to clean wounds (p.1108) but are of doubtful value. Chlorine-releasing antiseptic solutions are generally regarded as irritant and although there is little direct evidence in patients there is concern that they may delay wound healing. Cetrimide,[2] tosylchloramide sodium,[3] hydrogen peroxide 3%,[4] iodophores,[4] and sodium hypochlorite solutions[2] are all reported to be cytotoxic *in vitro* or in *animal* models. Long term or repeated use of these antiseptics for wound toilet should probably be avoided. Chlorhexidine is relatively non-toxic.[2,3]

1. Brown CD, Zitelli JA. A review of topical agents for wounds and methods of wounding: guidelines for wound management. *J Dermatol Surg Oncol* 1993; **19**: 732–7.
2. Thomas S, Hay NP. Wound cleansing. *Pharm J* 1985; **2**: 206.
3. Brennan SS, *et al.* Antiseptic toxicity in wounds healing by secondary intention. *J Hosp Infect* 1986; **8**: 263–7.
4. Lineweaver W, *et al.* Topical antimicrobial toxicity. *Arch Surg* 1985; **120**: 267–70.

Acridine Derivatives (12107-e)

A group of quinoline antimicrobial dyes structurally related to acridine.

Acriflavinium Chloride (2201-c)

Acriflavinium Chloride (rINN).

Acriflavine; Acriflavina Hydrochloride. A mixture of 3,6-diamino-10-methylacridinium chloride hydrochloride and 3,6-diaminoacridine dihydrochloride.

CAS — 8063-24-9; 65589-70-0.
ATC — R02AA13.

NOTE. Distinguish from euflavine (below).

Pharmacopoeias. In Aust. Swiss includes separate monographs for the hydrochloride and the dihydrochloride.

Aminoacridine Hydrochloride (2204-t)

Aminoacridine Hydrochloride (BANM, rINNM).

Aminacrine Hydrochloride (USAN); NSC-7571. 9-Aminoacridine hydrochloride monohydrate.

$C_{13}H_{10}N_2,HCl,H_2O$ = 248.7.
CAS — 90-45-9 (aminoacridine); 134-50-9 (anhydrous aminoacridine hydrochloride).

Ethacridine Lactate (2243-m)

Ethacridine Lactate (BANM, rINNM).

Acrinol; Aethacridinium Lacticum; Ethacridini Lactas; Lactoacridine. 6,9-Diamino-2-ethoxyacridine lactate.

$C_{15}H_{15}N_3O,C_3H_6O_3$ = 343.4.
CAS — 442-16-0 (ethacridine); 1837-57-6 (ethacridine lactate); 6402-23-9 (ethacridine lactate monohydrate).
ATC — B05CA08; D08AA01.

Pharmacopoeias. In Pol.; in Eur. (see p.vi) and Jpn as monohydrate.

Pharmacopoeial description

Ph. Eur.: Ethacridine lactate monohydrate is a yellow crystalline powder. Sparingly soluble in water; very slightly soluble in alcohol; practically insoluble in dichloromethane. A 2% solution in water has a pH of 5.5 to 7.0. Protect from light.

Euflavine (2245-v)

Neutral Acriflavine; Neutroflavin. A mixture of 3,6-diamino-10-methylacridinium chloride and 3,6-diaminoacridine monohydrochloride. The latter is usually present to the extent of between 30 and 40%.
CAS — 68518-47-8.
ATC — D08AA03.

NOTE. Distinguish from acriflavinium chloride (above).

Proflavine Hemisulfate (2271-q)

Proflavine Hemisulphate (pINNM); Neutral Proflavine Sulphate. 3,6-Diaminoacridine sulphate dihydrate.
$(C_{13}H_{11}N_3)_2,H_2SO_4,2H_2O$ = 552.6.
CAS — 92-62-6 (proflavine).

Profile

The acridine derivatives are slow-acting antiseptics. They are bacteriostatic against many Gram-positive bacteria but less effective against Gram-negative bacteria. They are ineffective against spores. Their activity is increased in alkaline solutions and is not reduced by tissue fluids.

The acridine derivatives have been used for the treatment of infected wounds or burns and for skin disinfection, although they have been largely superseded by other antiseptics or suitable antibacterials. Prolonged treatment may delay healing. They have also been used for the local treatment of ear, oropharyngeal, and genito-urinary infections.

Aminoacridine is reported to be non-staining and is used as the hydrochloride as eye drops in the treatment and prophylaxis of superficial eye infections.

Ethacridine lactate is included in some preparations for the treatment of diarrhoea. It has also been given by extra-amniotic injection for the termination of pregnancy (p.1439) but other methods are usually preferred.

Hypersensitivity to acridine derivatives has been reported.

Preparations

BPC 1973: Proflavine Cream.

Proprietary Preparations (details are given in Part 3)
Austral.: Aminopt; *Ger.:* Biseptol simplex†; Metifex; Neochinosol; Panflavin†; Rivanol; Urocridin†; Uroseptol; *Singapore:* Dettol; *Thai.:* Flavinol.

Multi-ingredient: *Aust.:* Dermowund; Tebege-Tannin; Tonexol†; *Austral.:* Medijel; *Braz.:* Acridin; Cezane; Cystex; Nene Dent; Senol; *Fr.:* Chromargon; Pyorex; *Ger.:* Anaesthesin-Rivanol; Nordapanin N; Otolitan N mit Rivanol; Tannacomp; *Hong Kong:* Medijel; *Israel:* Medijel; *S.Afr.:* Achromide; AMS; Daromide; Masse; Vagarsol; *Singapore:* Burnol; Medijel; *Spain:* Antigrietun; Hepro; *Switz.:* Anginol; Flavangin; Haemocortin; Haemolan; Tyrothricin; *Thai.:* Burnol Plus; *UK:* Bonjela†; Medijel; *USA:* Alasulf; Deltavac; DIT1-2.

Alcohol (551-f)

Aethanolum; Alcool; Ethanol; Ethanolum; Ethyl Alcohol.
C_2H_5OH = 46.07.
CAS — 64-17-5.
ATC — V03AB16; V03AZ01.

*Pharmacopoeias. In Chin., Eur. (see p.vi), Int., Jpn, Pol., and US. Various strengths are included and are described in more detail below. Br. includes diluted forms, also discussed below.
In Martindale the term alcohol is used for alcohol 95 or 96% v/v.*

Alcoholic strength is expressed as a percentage by volume of alcohol. It was previously often expressed in terms of *proof spirit*. Proof spirit contained about 57.1% v/v or 49.2% w/w of C_2H_5OH, and was defined as 'that which at the temperature of 51° F weighs exactly twelve-thirteenths of an equal measure of distilled water'. Spirit of such a strength that 100 volumes contained as much ethyl alcohol as 160 volumes of proof spirit was described as '60 OP' (over proof). Spirit of which 100 volumes contained as much alcohol as 40 volumes of proof spirit was described as '60 UP' (under proof). An alternative method of indicating spirit strength was used on the labels of alcoholic beverages in the UK where the strength was given as a number of degrees, proof spirit being taken as 100°. In the USA alcoholic strength is expressed in degrees, the value of which is equal to twice the percentage by volume. Thus 70° proof (old UK system) is equivalent to 40% v/v, and therefore to 80° proof (USA system).

Pharmacopoeial description

Ph. Eur.: Anhydrous Ethanol (Ethanol (BP 2001); Absolute Alcohol; Dehydrated Alcohol) contains not less than 99.5% v/v or 99.2% w/w of C_2H_5OH. A colourless, clear, volatile, flammable, hygroscopic liquid; it burns with a blue, smokeless flame. B.p. about 78°. Miscible with water and with dichloromethane. Protect from light.

Ethanol (96 per cent) contains not less than 95.1% v/v or 92.6% w/w and not more than 96.9% v/v or 95.2% w/w of C_2H_5OH at 20°, and water. A colourless, clear, volatile, flammable, hygroscopic liquid; it burns with a blue, smokeless flame. B.p. about 78°. Miscible with water and with dichloromethane. Protect from light.

BP 2001: Dilute Ethanols includes several dilute alcohols containing between 20 and 90% v/v of C_2H_5OH, and one of these, ethanol (90%), is also known as rectified spirit.

USP 25: Alcohol contains not less than 92.3% w/w or 94.9% v/v and not more than 93.8% w/w or 96.0% v/v of C_2H_5OH at 15.56°. A clear, colourless, mobile, volatile liquid with a characteristic odour and burning taste; readily flammable. B.p. about 78°. Miscible with water and with almost all other organic solvents. Store away from fire in airtight containers.

Dehydrated Alcohol contains not less than 99.5% v/v or 99.2% w/w of C_2H_5OH (sp. gr. not more than 0.7962 at 15.56°). Store away from fire in airtight containers.

USNF 20: Diluted Alcohol contains 48.4 to 49.5% v/v or 41 to 42% w/w of C_2H_5OH. Store away from fire in airtight containers.

Adverse Effects

Adverse effects of alcohol arise chiefly from the intake of alcoholic beverages. The concentration of alcohol in the blood producing a state of intoxication varies between individuals. At low to moderate concentrations alcohol acts as an apparent stimulant; depression of cortical function causes loss of judgement, emotional lability, visual impairment, slurred speech, and ataxia. Hangover effects may include nausea, headache, dizziness, and tremor. Alcohol depresses medullary action; lethargy, amnesia, hypothermia, hypoglycaemia (especially in children), stupor, coma, respiratory depression, cardiomyopathy, hypertension or hypotension, and cardiovascular collapse may occur. The median lethal blood-alcohol concentration is generally estimated to be approximately 400 to 500 mg per 100 mL. Death may occur at lower blood-alcohol concentrations due to inhalation of vomit during unconsciousness.

Chronic excessive consumption of alcohol may cause damage to many organs, particularly the brain and the liver. Brain damage may lead to Wernicke-Korsakoff syndrome. Fat deposits may occur in the liver and there may be a reduction in various blood-cell counts. Nutritional diseases may occur due to inadequate diet. High alcohol consumption has been associated with pancreatitis, and an increased risk of cardiovascular disease, although moderate consumption may have a protective effect against ischaemic heart disease.

Alcohol consumption has also been associated with an increased risk of some types of cancer.

The term 'alcoholism' may be used to denote dependence on alcohol, which is of the barbiturate-alcohol type (see Amobarbital, p.655) and usually involves tolerance to other sedatives and anaesthetics. Following prolonged periods of excessive alcohol consumption, a drop in blood-alcohol concentration may precipitate a withdrawal syndrome characterised by tremor, agitation, feelings of dread, nausea, vomiting, and sweating; hallucinations, seizures, and delirium tremens may also develop.

A fetal alcohol syndrome has been identified in which infants born to some alcoholic mothers have characteristic features and abnormalities. There have been some reports of the syndrome and other adverse effects on the fetus being associated with moderate alcohol intake in pregnancy; it is generally suggested that alcohol is best avoided during pregnancy.

Frequent application of alcohol to the skin produces irritation and dry skin.

The symbol † denotes a preparation no longer actively marketed

◊ Reviews of the adverse effects of alcohol.

1. Adinoff B, *et al.* Acute ethanol poisoning and the ethanol withdrawal syndrome. *Med Toxicol* 1988; **3:** 172–96.
2. Charness ME, *et al.* Ethanol and the nervous system. *N Engl J Med* 1989; **321:** 442–54.
3. Edwards G, Peters TJ, eds. Alcohol and alcohol problems. *Br Med Bull* 1994; **50:** 1–230.
4. Lieber CS. Medical disorders of alcoholism. *N Engl J Med* 1995; **333:** 1058–65.
5. Sherlock S. Alcoholic liver disease. *Lancet* 1995; **345:** 227–9.
6. Cowie MR. Alcohol and the heart. *Br J Hosp Med* 1997; **57:** 457–60.
7. Hills KS, Westaby D. Alcohol and the liver. *Br J Hosp Med* 1997; **57:** 517–21.
8. Scheepers BDM. Alcohol and the brain. *Br J Hosp Med* 1997; **57:** 548–51.
9. Marshall EJ, Alan F. Psychiatric problems associated with alcohol misuse and dependence. *Br J Hosp Med* 1997; **58:** 44–6.
10. O'Connor PG, Schottenfeld RS. Patients with alcohol problems. *N Engl J Med* 1998; **338:** 592–601.
11. Dunn N, Cook CCH. Psychiatric aspects of alcohol misuse. *Hosp Med* 1999; **60:** 169–72.

Effects on the skin. A 70% solution of alcohol, containing povidone-iodine, caused partial thickness chemical burns when held under pressure against the skin of 3 young children.[1] Other adverse effects on the skin reported with the topical application of alcohols have included necrosis occurring following skin cleansing of preterm neonates with methylated spirits[2,3] and haemorrhagic skin necrosis due to the alcohol content of chlorhexidine in spirit used as a disinfectant in umbilical artery catheterisation in preterm infants.[4]

See also Neonates, under Adverse Effects of Isopropyl Alcohol, p.1149.

1. Dickinson JC, Bailey BN. Chemical burns beneath tourniquets. *BMJ* 1988; **297:** 1513.
2. Harpin V, Rutter N. Percutaneous alcohol absorption and skin necrosis in a preterm infant. *Arch Dis Child* 1982; **57:** 477–9.
3. Murch S, Costelloe K. Hyperosmolality related to propylene glycol in an infant. *BMJ* 1990; **301:** 389.
4. Al-Jawad ST. Percutaneous alcohol absorption and skin necrosis in a preterm infant. *Arch Dis Child* 1983; **58:** 395–6.

Treatment of Adverse Effects

In acute poisoning the patient should be kept warm and given supportive and symptomatic care. The use of intravenous infusions of fructose to treat severe alcohol poisoning is not recommended as they may produce metabolic disturbances. Haemodialysis is of value in severe alcoholic poisoning.

The management of the alcohol withdrawal syndrome and long-term abstinence following withdrawal are discussed below.

Alcohol withdrawal and abstinence. The alcohol withdrawal syndrome presents in the early stages as a classical hyperadrenergic state with tremor, tachycardia, sweating, and hypertension. Sometimes this is accompanied by mild disorientation, anxiety, impaired concentration, depression, agitation, and gastrointestinal symptoms. Insomnia, nightmares, and transient hallucinations can also be present. The condition may be self-limiting without the need for therapeutic intervention or it may progress to the severe and potentially fatal condition of delirium tremens (DTs), often characterised by delirium, disorientation, and hallucinations. In some cases generalised tonic-clonic seizures occur within 24 hours of alcohol withdrawal and are followed by delirium tremens.

Withdrawal. The general management of the alcohol withdrawal syndrome has been the subject of many reviews and discussions.[1-13] In most cases symptoms do not require treatment and disappear within a few days but more severe cases may require managed withdrawal from alcohol to avoid complications.

Sedatives are commonly used to reduce the symptoms of alcohol withdrawal and, if administered promptly, can prevent progression to seizures and delirium tremens. *Benzodiazepines* are usually the drugs of first choice. Longer-acting drugs such as chlordiazepoxide or diazepam may be more effective against withdrawal seizures and provide smoother withdrawal while shorter-acting ones such as lorazepam or oxazepam have a smaller risk of producing oversedation and may be more suitable for use in the elderly, and, since they do not rely on hepatic enzymes for their metabolism, for patients with liver disease. Benzodiazepines should be given in short courses only, to prevent the development of dependence. Some advocate that benzodiazepine dosage should be adjusted according to the severity of symptoms with special care being paid to patients with a history of withdrawal seizures, comorbid conditions, or those using sedative or hypnotic medication. This reduces the amount of drug required and the duration of treatment but entails regular monitoring by trained nursing staff. For mild to moderate symptoms standard anxiolytic or muscle-relaxing oral doses of benzodiazepines may be sufficient. For severe symptoms or for the treatment of delirium tremens higher doses and use of the intravenous route may be required. *Clomethiazole* appears to be an effective alternative to the benzodiazepines (but see p.669); although widely used in Europe it is not available in the US. Some centres use phenobarbital but *barbiturates* are generally not recommended for the treatment of alcohol withdrawal syndrome.

Antipsychotics are not usually recommended for use in the control of symptoms of alcohol withdrawal since they do not re-

duce delirium tremens and some may reduce the seizure threshold. However, they might be considered for use as an adjunct in patients requiring treatment of marked agitation or hallucinations.

The generalised tonic-clonic seizures associated with alcohol withdrawal are usually self-limiting and patients who experience only one or two seizures do not usually require any specific treatment beyond continuing therapy with benzodiazepines or clomethiazole. For recurrent seizures or status epilepticus (p.341) diazepam may be given intravenously. Other types of seizure may be associated with head trauma or preexisting seizure disorders (p.338) and should be treated accordingly. Other *antiepileptics* such as carbamazepine have been tried in the treatment of alcohol withdrawal seizures and may be of use as adjuncts in controlling other symptoms of alcohol withdrawal syndrome. As benzodiazepines are effective in preventing withdrawal seizures other prophylactic drugs are not usually indicated.

Beta blockers can reduce symptoms of autonomic overactivity such as tachycardia, hypertension, tremor, and agitation but because they can mask these symptoms of withdrawal and do not prevent the development of more serious complications they should not be used alone. Some beta blockers such as propranolol which penetrate the CNS may produce CNS effects which complicate therapy. The alpha$_2$-adrenoceptor agonist *clonidine* may be of similar benefit as an adjunct.

Other drugs that have been reported to be of benefit in alcohol withdrawal syndrome include nitrous oxide and gamma-hydroxybutyric acid.

It is essential that in all cases of alcohol withdrawal syndrome hypoglycaemia, dehydration, electrolyte disturbances (in particular magnesium), and vitamin deficiencies be corrected. It is usually recommended that all patients should be given thiamine because of their increased risk of developing Wernicke's encephalopathy (p.1385). It should be noted that intravenous administration of glucose solutions before thiamine may precipitate Wernicke's encephalopathy in thiamine-deficient patients. However, hydration should be undertaken with care as alcoholics may be more prone to develop cerebral oedema, the management of which is discussed under Raised Intracranial Pressure on p.811.

Abstinence. Once the initial acute withdrawal of alcohol is achieved treatment may be required to maintain long-term abstinence. Pharmacotherapy should only be used as an adjunct to psychotherapy and supportive care. Drugs used to modify alcohol seeking behaviour either sensitise the patient to alcohol (aversive drugs) or reduce or alleviate the craving for alcohol. The main uses for aversive therapy are *disulfiram* and *calcium carbimide*. A patient who ingests alcohol after taking an adequate dose of one of these drugs will experience a severe and unpleasant reaction (p.1605). However, the deterrent value of aversive drugs, and their potential toxicity, has long been a matter of debate. Such treatment is likely to be of little use unless it is undertaken with the willing cooperation of the patient and is used with psychotherapy, and even then there is no evidence that it has any effect on the long-term course of alcoholism.

Of those drugs which have been reported to reduce alcohol craving *acamprosate* and *naltrexone* have been the most promising as adjuncts for management of alcohol dependence and have been shown to improve abstinence and reduce relapse rates. Whether benefit is maintained long-term after treatment is stopped is unclear. *Other drugs* tried with varying benefit include tiapride, gamma-hydroxybutyric acid, and bromocriptine.

1. McMicken DB, Freedland ES. Alcohol-related seizures: pathophysiology, differential diagnosis, evaluation, and treatment. *Emerg Med Clin North Am* 1994; **12:** 1057–79.
2. Lohr RH. Treatment of alcohol withdrawal in hospitalized patients. *Mayo Clin Proc* 1995; **70:** 777–82.
3. Erstad BL, Cotugno CL. Management of alcohol withdrawal. *Am J Health-Syst Pharm* 1995; **52:** 697–709.
4. Hall W, Zador D. The alcohol withdrawal syndrome. *Lancet* 1997; **349:** 1897–1900.
5. Mayo-Smith MF. American Society of Addiction Medicine Working Group on Pharmacological Management of Alcohol Withdrawal. Pharmacological management of alcohol withdrawal: a meta-analysis and evidence-based practice guideline. *JAMA* 1997; **278:** 144–51.
6. Saitz R, O'Malley SS. Pharmacotherapies for alcohol abuse: withdrawal and treatment. *Med Clin North Am* 1997; **81:** 881–907.
7. O'Connor PG, Schottenfeld RS. Patients with alcohol problems. *N Engl J Med* 1998; **338:** 592–602.
8. Tinsley JA, *et al.* Developments in the treatment of alcoholism. *Mayo Clin Proc* 1998; **73:** 857–63.
9. Schaffer A, Naraiyo CA. Recommended drug treatment strategies for the alcoholic patient. *Drugs* 1998; **56:** 571–85.
10. Naik PC, Brownell LW. Treatment of psychiatric aspects of alcohol misuse. *Hosp Med* 1999; **60:** 173–7.
11. Garbutt JC, *et al.* Pharmacological treatment of alcohol dependence: a review of the evidence. *JAMA* 1999; **281:** 1318–25.
12. Swift RM. Drug therapy for alcohol dependence. *N Engl J Med* 1999; **340:** 1482–90.
13. Kraemer KL, *et al.* Managing alcohol withdrawal in the elderly. *Drugs Aging* 1999; **14:** 409–25.

Precautions

Women and the elderly may be more susceptible to the adverse effects of alcohol ingestion. Alcohol may aggravate peptic ulcer disease or impaired liver function. Ingestion of alcohol during pregnancy or breast feeding is not advisable. Excessive alcohol intake should be avoided, especially in patients with diabetes mellitus or epilepsy. In chronic alcoholics there may be tolerance to the effects of other CNS depressants including general anaesthetics.

All processes requiring judgement and coordination are affected by alcohol and these include the driving of any form of transport and the operating of machinery. It is an offence in many countries for motorists to drive when the blood-alcohol concentration is above a stated value. The alcohol concentration in urine and expired air can be used to estimate the blood-alcohol concentration.

It should be remembered that alcohol may be present in a number of pharmaceutical preparations such as elixirs and mouthwashes, and that children may be particularly susceptible to its hypoglycaemic effects.

Porphyria. Alcohol has been associated with acute attacks of porphyria and is considered unsafe in porphyric patients.

Interactions

Reports of interactions between alcohol and other drugs are not consistent, possibly because acute alcohol intake may inhibit drug metabolism while chronic alcohol intake may enhance the induction of drug-metabolising enzymes in the liver. Alcoholic beverages containing tyramine may cause reactions when taken by patients receiving MAOIs. Alcohol may enhance the acute effects of drugs which depress the CNS, such as hypnotics, antihistamines, opioid analgesics, antiepileptics, antidepressants, antipsychotics, and sedatives. Unpleasant reactions, similar to those occurring with disulfiram (p.1605), may occur when alcohol is taken concomitantly with chlorpropamide, mepacrine, metronidazole and other nitroimidazoles, the nitrofuran derivatives furazolidone and nifuratel, procarbazine, and some cephalosporins.

Alcohol may cause hypoglycaemic reactions in patients receiving sulfonylurea antidiabetics or insulin, and may cause orthostatic hypotension in patients taking drugs with vasodilator action. It may enhance the hypotensive effects of antihypertensives and has also increased the sedative effect of indoramin. Alcohol may increase gastric bleeding caused by analgesics and may have a variable effect on oral anticoagulants. It may decrease the antidiuretic effect of vasopressin.

◊ Interactions involving alcohol have been reviewed.[1-3]

The effects of *paracetamol* poisoning may be exacerbated by prolonged alcohol use (see p.71).

When taken concomitantly with alcohol *verapamil*[4] has been reported to cause an increase in peak blood-alcohol concentrations of approximately 17%. Such an interaction may extend the toxic effects of alcohol and raise its blood concentration above the legal limit for driving.[5] Increased blood-alcohol concentrations have also been reported in patients receiving *cycloserine*.[6]

The existence of an interaction between H$_2$-antagonists and alcohol is controversial and has not been established. While some studies suggest that *cimetidine*[7-9] and *nizatidine*[9] can increase peak blood concentrations of alcohol the effects of *ranitidine*[8,10] have been variable; *famotidine* appears to have no significant effect.[8] Recent studies report that any interaction between H$_2$-antagonists and alcohol is minor and unlikely to be of clinical importance.[11-14]

1. McInnes GT. Interactions that matter: alcohol. *Prescribers' J* 1985; **25:** 87–90.
2. Lieber CS. Interaction of alcohol with other drugs and nutrients: implications for the therapy of alcoholic liver disease. *Drugs* 1990; **40** (suppl 3): 23–44.
3. Fraser AG. Pharmacokinetic interactions between alcohol and other drugs. *Clin Pharmacokinet* 1997; **33:** 79–90.
4. Schumock G, et al. Verapamil inhibits ethanol elimination. *Pharmacotherapy* 1989; **9:** 184–5.
5. Anonymous. Does verapamil increase the effects of alcohol? *Pharm J* 1990; **244:** 14.
6. Glass F, et al. Beobachtungen und untersuchungen über die gemeinsame wirkung von alkohol und D-cycloserin. *Arzneimittelforschung* 1965; **15:** 684–8.
7. Caballeria J, et al. Effects of cimetidine on gastric alcohol dehydrogenase activity and blood ethanol levels. *Gastroenterology* 1989; **96:** 388–92.
8. DiPadova C, et al. Effects of ranitidine on blood alcohol levels after ethanol ingestion: comparison with other H$_2$-receptor antagonists. *JAMA* 1992; **267:** 83–6.
9. Holt S, et al. Evidence for an interaction between alcohol and certain H$_2$ receptor antagonists. *Gut* 1991; **32:** A1220.
10. Toon S, et al. Lack of effect of high dose ranitidine on the postprandial pharmacokinetics of alcohol. *Gut* 1992; **33** (suppl): S10.
11. Raufman J-P, et al. Histamine-2 receptor antagonists do not alter serum ethanol levels in fed, nonalcoholic men. *Ann Intern Med* 1993; **118:** 488–94.
12. Levitt MD. Do histamine-2 receptor antagonists influence the metabolism of ethanol? *Ann Intern Med* 1993; **118:** 564–5.
13. Kleine M-W, Ertl D. Comparative trial in volunteers to investigate possible ethanol-ranitidine interaction. *Ann Pharmacother* 1993; **27:** 841–5.
14. Gugler R. H$_2$-antagonists and alcohol: do they interact? *Drug Safety* 1994; **10:** 271–80.

Pharmacokinetics

Alcohol is rapidly absorbed from the gastrointestinal tract and is distributed throughout the body fluids. It readily crosses the placenta. Alcohol vapour can be absorbed through the lungs. Absorption through intact skin is said to be negligible.

The rate of absorption of alcohol from the gastrointestinal tract may be modified by such factors as the presence of food, the concentration of alcohol, and the period of time during which it is ingested. Some alcohol is reported to be metabolised by the gastric mucosa.

Alcohol is mainly metabolised in the liver; it is converted by alcohol dehydrogenase to acetaldehyde and is then further oxidised to acetate. A hepatic microsomal oxidising system is also involved. About 90 to 98% of alcohol is oxidised and the remainder is excreted unchanged by the kidneys and the lungs. It also appears in breast milk, sweat, and other secretions.

The rate of metabolism may be accelerated following repeated excessive intake and by certain substances including insulin.

◊ The pharmacokinetics of alcohol have been reviewed.[1]
Gastric oxidation of alcohol was reduced in one study[2] in women compared with men leading to women having increased blood-alcohol concentrations, stimulating considerable correspondence. In another study,[3] it was found that only women under the age of 50 years have lower alcohol dehydrogenase activity than men, and that in elderly women the activity was not significantly less than in men. Others[4] considered that acetaldehyde may be more toxic than alcohol and that reduced first-pass metabolism in women may lessen their risk of toxic liver effects. The initial study[2] was also criticised on pharmacokinetic grounds[5,6] and on the basis that men and women display differences in social drinking patterns.[7] In reply the authors refuted some of these criticisms but pointed out that other factors, such as sex-related differences in tissue vulnerability, may contribute to differences in the severity of medical problems related to drinking.[8]

1. Holford NHG. Clinical pharmacokinetics of ethanol. *Clin Pharmacokinet* 1987; **13:** 273–92.
2. Frezza M, et al. High blood alcohol levels in women: the role of decreased gastric alcohol dehydrogenase activity and first-pass metabolism. *N Engl J Med* 1990; **322:** 95–9.
3. Seitz HK, et al. High blood alcohol levels in women. *N Engl J Med* 1990; **323:** 58.
4. Phillips M. High blood alcohol levels in women. *N Engl J Med* 1990; **323:** 58.
5. Sweeney GD. High blood alcohol levels in women. *N Engl J Med* 1990; **323:** 58–9.
6. Zedeck MS. High blood alcohol levels in women. *N Engl J Med* 1990; **323:** 59.
7. York JL. High blood alcohol levels in women. *N Engl J Med* 1990; **323:** 59–60.
8. Frezza M, et al. High blood alcohol levels in women. *N Engl J Med* 1990; **323:** 60–1.

Uses and Administration

Alcohol has bactericidal activity and is used to disinfect skin prior to injection, venepuncture, or surgical procedures. It is also used to disinfect hands and clean surfaces. A concentration of 70%, often as methylated spirits (p.1150), is commonly employed for disinfection. Alcohol should not be used for disinfection of surgical or dental instruments because of its low efficacy against bacterial spores.

Alcohol also has anhidrotic, rubefacient, and astringent and haemostatic properties. It is sometimes used for its skin-cooling properties and to harden the skin. It is an ingredient of several topical preparations used for skin disorders.

Alcohol is widely used as a solvent and preservative in pharmaceutical preparations.

Alcohol may be used as a neurolytic in the management of severe and chronic pain.

Alcohol is given intravenously in the treatment of acute poisoning from ethylene glycol (p.1609) and methyl alcohol (p.1404).

Alcohol is also used in sclerotherapy.

Pain. The neurolytic use of alcohol to produce destructive nerve block (p.3) has produced variable results, and some consider the risk of complications outweighs the benefits. However, alcohol has been injected into the pituitary gland for relief of severe pain of the head and neck;[1,2] doses of 1 mL of absolute alcohol have been used.[1] It may be useful in coeliac plexus block, and has been injected into the muscle sheath to relieve painful muscle spasms in patients with multiple sclerosis.[1] Alcohol 50 to 100% may be used for peripheral or central nerve block in terminally ill patients with pain that does not respond to drug therapy;[3] the block produced by alcohol may occasionally last up to 2 years, even longer than that produced by phenol.

Intrathecal injection of alcohol has also been used for the intractable pain of spasticity (p.1322).

1. Lloyd JW. Use of anaesthesia: the anaesthetist and the pain clinic. *BMJ* 1980; **281:** 432–4.
2. Lipton S. Pain relief in active patients with cancer: the early use of nerve blocks improves the quality of life. *BMJ* 1989; **298:** 37–8.
3. Hardy, PAJ. The role of the pain clinic in the management of the terminally ill. *Br J Hosp Med* 1990; **43:** 142–6.

Sclerotherapy. Alcohol has been used successfully as a sclerosant in a variety of conditions including aldosterone-producing adenoma,[1] parathyroid adenoma,[2] thyroid nodules,[3,4] advanced rectal cancer,[5] hepatocellular carcinoma,[6,7] dysphagia associated with oesophagastric cancer,[8,9] hepatic cyst,[10] and gallbladder obstruction.[11] It has also been used in the sclerotherapy of oesophageal varices[12,13] although the safety of this procedure has been questioned following a report of complications developing in 13 of 17 patients, 2 of whom died.[14] Other conditions in which alcohol has been used include bleeding from ruptured hepatomas[15] and in peptic ulcer disease,[16] and obstructive cardiomyopathies[17] resistant to usual treatment.

Other sclerosants used in oesophageal varices are discussed on p.1637.

1. Mathias CJ, et al. Therapeutic venous infarction of an aldosterone producing adenoma (Conn's tumour). *BMJ* 1984; **288:** 1416–17.
2. Verges B, et al. Percutaneous ethanol injection of parathyroid adenomas in primary hyperparathyroidism. *Lancet* 1991; **337:** 1421–2.
3. Monzani F, et al. Autonomous thyroid nodule and percutaneous ethanol injection. *Lancet* 1991; **337:** 743.
4. Bennedbaek FN, Hegedüs L. Alcohol sclerotherapy for benign solitary solid cold thyroid nodules. *Lancet* 1995; **346:** 1227.
5. Payne-James J, et al. Advanced rectal cancer. *BMJ* 1990; **300:** 746.
6. Sheu J-C, et al. Intratumor injection of absolute ethanol under ultrasound guidance for the treatment of small hepatocellular carcinoma. *Hepatogastroenterology* 1987; **34:** 255–61.
7. Salmi A. Percutaneous alcohol injection of hepatocellular carcinoma. *Ann Intern Med* 1989; **110:** 494.
8. Payne-James JJ, et al. Use of ethanol-induced tumor necrosis to palliate dysphagia in patients with esophagogastric cancer. *Gastrointest Endosc* 1990; **36:** 43–6.
9. Stanners AJ, et al. Alcohol injection for palliation of malignant oesophageal disease. *Lancet* 1993; **341:** 767.
10. Bean WJ, Rodan BA. Hepatic cysts: treatment with alcohol. *Am J Roentg* 1985; **144:** 237–41.
11. Asfar S, et al. Percutaneous sclerosis of gallbladder. *Lancet* 1989; **ii:** 387.
12. Sarin SK, et al. Endoscopic sclerotherapy using absolute alcohol. *Gut* 1985; **26:** 120–4.
13. Hassall E, et al. Sclerotherapy for extrahepatic portal hypertension in childhood. *J Pediatr* 1989; **115:** 69–74.
14. Bhargava DK, et al. Endoscopic sclerotherapy using absolute alcohol. *Gut* 1986; **27:** 1518.
15. Chung SCS, et al. Injection of alcohol to control bleeding from ruptured hepatomas. *BMJ* 1990; **301:** 421.
16. Lin IIJ, et al. Heat probe thermocoagulation and pure alcohol injection in massive peptic ulcer haemorrhage: a prospective, randomised controlled trial. *Gut* 1990; **31:** 753–7.
17. Sigwart U. Non-surgical myocardial reduction for hypertrophic obstructive cardiomyopathy. *Lancet* 1995; **346:** 211–14.

Preparations

USP 25: Alcohol in Dextrose Injection; Rubbing Alcohol.

Proprietary Preparations (details are given in Part 3)
Canad.: Skin So Soft Antibacterial; *Fr.:* Curethyl†; Pharmadose alcool; *Ger.:* AHD 2000; Amphisept E; Desderman†; Fugaten; Manusept HD; Sterillium Virugard; *Spain:* Alcohten; *Switz.:* Amphisept; *USA:* Alcare; Alco-Gel†; Kleen-Handz.

Multi-ingredient: numerous preparations are listed in Part 3.

Alkyl Gallates (12172-x)

Dodecyl Gallate (6645-q)

E312; Lauryl Gallate; Laurylum Gallicum. Dodecyl 3,4,5-trihydroxybenzoate.

$C_{19}H_{30}O_5 = 338.4$.
$CAS — 1166-52-5$.

Pharmacopoeias. In Aust., Br., and Fr.

Pharmacopoeial description

BP 2001: A white or creamy-white, odourless or almost odourless powder. M.p. 96° to 97.5°. Practically insoluble in water; freely soluble in alcohol, in acetone, in ether, and in methyl alcohol; sparingly soluble in arachis oil, in chloroform, and in propylene glycol. Protect from light. Avoid contact with metals.

Ethyl Gallate (6647-s)

Ethyl 3,4,5-trihydroxybenzoate.
$C_9H_{10}O_5 = 198.2$.
CAS — 831-61-8.
Pharmacopoeias. In Br.

Pharmacopoeial description

BP 2001: A white to creamy-white, odourless or almost odourless, crystalline powder. Slightly soluble in water; freely soluble in alcohol and in ether; practically insoluble in arachis oil. Protect from light. Avoid contact with metals.

Octil Gallate (6654-p)

E311; Octyl Gallate. Octyl 3,4,5-trihydroxybenzoate.
$C_{15}H_{22}O_5 = 282.3$.
CAS — 1034-01-1.
Pharmacopoeias. In Br. and Fr.

Pharmacopoeial description

BP 2001: A white or creamy-white, odourless or almost odourless powder. Practically insoluble in water; freely soluble in alcohol, in acetone, in ether, and in propylene glycol; sparingly soluble in arachis oil and in chloroform; very soluble in methyl alcohol. Protect from light. Avoid contact with metals.

Propyl Gallate (6664-w)

E310; Propylis Gallas; Propylum Gallicum. Propyl 3,4,5-trihydroxybenzoate.
$C_{10}H_{12}O_5 = 212.2$.
CAS — 121-79-9.
Pharmacopoeias. In Eur. (see p.vi) and Pol. Also in USNF.

Pharmacopoeial description

Ph. Eur.: A white or almost white, crystalline powder. Very slightly soluble in water; freely soluble in alcohol and in ether; dissolves in dilute solutions of alkali hydroxides. Protect from light.

USNF 20: A white crystalline powder with a slight characteristic odour. Slightly soluble in water; freely soluble in alcohol. Store in airtight containers. Avoid contact with metals. Protect from light.

Adverse Effects and Precautions

The alkyl gallates may cause contact sensitivity and skin reactions.

Effects on the blood. Methaemoglobinaemia associated with the antioxidants (butylated hydroxyanisole, butylated hydroxytoluene, and propyl gallate) used to preserve the oil in a soybean infant feed formula has been reported.[1] Propyl gallate was suspected of being the most likely cause because its chemical structure is similar to pyrogallol, a methaemoglobinaemia inducer.

1. Nitzan M, *et al.* Infantile methemoglobinemia caused by food additives. *Clin Toxicol* 1979; **15:** 273–80.

Uses

The alkyl esters of gallic acid (3,4,5-trihydroxybenzoic acid) have antoxidant properties and are used as preservatives in pharmaceuticals and cosmetics. Alkyl gallates are also used as antoxidants in foods and are useful in preventing deterioration and rancidity of fats and oils. They are used in concentrations of 0.001 to 0.1%.

To improve acceptability and efficacy, the alkyl gallates are frequently used in combination with other antioxidants such as butylated hydroxyanisole or butylated hydroxytoluene and with sequestrants and synergists such as citric acid.

The alkyl gallates have also been reported to have limited antimicrobial activity.

Ambazone (2203-a)

Ambazone (BAN, rINN).
Ambazonum.   4-Amidinohydrazonocyclohexa-1,4-dien-3-one thiosemicarbazone monohydrate.
$C_8H_{11}N_7S,H_2O = 255.3$.
CAS — 539-21-9 (anhydrous ambazone); 6011-12-7 (ambazone monohydrate).
ATC — R02AA01.

Profile

Ambazone is an antiseptic that has been used in the form of lozenges for minor infections of the mouth and pharynx.

Aminoquinuride Hydrochloride (11245-y)

Aminoquinuride Hydrochloride (rINNM).
1,3-Bis(4-amino-2-methyl-6-quinolyl)urea dihydrochloride.
$C_{21}H_{20}N_6O,2HCl = 445.3$.
CAS — 3811-56-1 (aminoquinuride); 5424-37-3 (aminoquinuride hydrochloride).

Profile

Aminoquinuride hydrochloride is an antiseptic that has been used in topical preparations for the treatment of mouth and skin disorders.

The symbol † denotes a preparation no longer actively marketed

Preparations

Proprietary Preparations (details are given in Part 3)
Multi-ingredient: *Aust.:* Herviros; *Ger.:* Herviros; *Hong Kong:* Herviros.

Amylmetacresol (2205-x)

Amylmetacresol (BAN, rINN).
6-Pentyl-*m*-cresol; 5-Methyl-2-pentylphenol.
$C_{12}H_{18}O = 178.3$.
CAS — 1300-94-3.
Pharmacopoeias. In Br.

Pharmacopoeial description

BP 2001: A clear or almost clear liquid or a solid crystalline mass with a characteristic odour, colourless or slightly yellow when freshly prepared; it darkens on keeping. F.p. about 22°. Practically insoluble in water; soluble in alcohol, in ether, and in fixed and volatile oils. Protect from light.

Profile

Amylmetacresol is a phenolic antiseptic used chiefly as an ingredient of lozenges in the treatment of minor infections of the mouth and throat.

Preparations

Proprietary Preparations (details are given in Part 3)
Canad.: Strepsils 1; *Fin.:* Strepsils; *Ital.:* Benagol Collutorio†; *UK:* Antiseptic Throat Lozenges.
Multi-ingredient: *Aust.:* Coldangin; Neo-Angin; *Austral.:* Sore Throat Chewing Gum; Strepsils; Strepsils Anaesthetic†; Strepsils Plus; *Belg.:* Strepsils; Strepsils + Lidocaine; Strepsils Menthol; Strepsils Vit C; *Canad.:* Strepsils; *Denm.:* Strepsils; *Fin.:* Strepsils Menthol; *Fr.:* Strepsils Lidocaine; Strepsils Miel-Citron; Strepsils Vitamine C; Strepsilspray Lidocaine; *Ger.:* Neo-Angin N; *Hong Kong:* Strepsils; *Irl.:* Strepsils; Strepsils Dual Action; Strepsils Vitamin C; *Israel:* Strepsils; Strepsils Plus; Strepsils with Vitamin C; *Ital.:* Benagol; Benagol Mentolo-Eucaliptolo; Benagol Vitamina C; *Neth.:* Strepsils; Strepsils Menthol en Eucalyptus; Strepsils Sinaasappel en Vitamine C; *NZ:* Strepsils; Strepsils Plus Anaesthetic; Strepsils with Vitamin C; *S.Afr.:* Strepsils; Strepsils Eucalyptus Menthol; Strepsils Orange-C; Strepsils Plus; Strepsils Soothing Honey & Lemon; *Singapore:* Floxil; Strepsils; Strepsils Dual Action; *Spain:* Strepsils; Strepsils con Anestesico; Strepsils con Vitamina C; *Swed.:* Strepsils; *Switz.:* Neo-Angin au miel et citron; Neo-Angin avec vitamin C exempt de sucre; Neo-Angin exempt de sucre; *Thai.:* Strepsils Plus Anaesthetic; Strepsils Plus Vit C; Strepsils Sugar Free; *UK:* Antiseptic Lozenges; Antiseptic Throat Lozenges†; Mac; Strepsils; Strepsils Pain Relief Plus; Strepsils with Vitamin C.

Ascorbyl Palmitate (6633-m)

Ascorbylis Palmitas; E304; Vitamin C Palmitate. L-Ascorbic acid 6-hexadecanoate; L-Ascorbic acid 6-palmitate; 3-Oxo-L-gulofuranolactone 6-palmitate.
$C_{22}H_{38}O_7 = 414.5$.
CAS — 137-66-6.
Pharmacopoeias. In Eur. (see p.vi). Also in USNF.

Pharmacopoeial description

Ph. Eur.: A white or yellowish-white powder. Practically insoluble in water; freely soluble in alcohol and in methyl alcohol; practically insoluble in dichloromethane and in fatty oils. Store at 8° to 15° in airtight containers. Protect from light.

USNF 20: A white to yellowish-white powder with a characteristic odour. Very slightly soluble in water, in chloroform, in ether, and in vegetable oils; soluble 1 in 125 of alcohol. Store at 8° to 15° in airtight containers.

Profile

Ascorbyl palmitate is an antioxidant used as a preservative in pharmaceutical products and foods. It is often used in combination with alpha tocopherol (p.1393), and this combination shows marked synergy.

Benzalkonium Chloride (2206-r)

Benzalkonium Chloride (BAN, rINN).
Benzalconio Cloruro; Benzalkonii Chloridum; Benzalkonium Chloratum; Cloreto de Benzalconio.
CAS — 8001-54-5.
Pharmacopoeias. In Eur. (see p.vi), Int., Jpn, and Pol. Also in USNF.
Some pharmacopoeias also have a monograph for Benzalkonium Chloride Solution.
Chin. includes benzalkonium bromide.

Incompatible with soaps and other anionic surfactants, citrates, iodides, nitrates, permanganates, salicylates, silver salts, and tartrates. Incompatibilities have been demonstrated with ingredients of some commercial rubber mixes or plastics. Incompatibilities have also been reported with other substances including aluminium, cotton dressings, fluorescein sodium, hydrogen peroxide, kaolin, hydrous wool fat, and some sulfonamides.

Pharmacopoeial description

Ph. Eur.: A mixture of alkylbenzyldimethylammonium chlorides, the alkyl groups having chain lengths of C_8 to C_{18}. It contains not less than 95% and not more than 104% of alkylbenzyldimethylammonium chlorides, calculated as $C_{22}H_{40}ClN$ with reference to the anhydrous substance.

A white or yellowish-white powder, or gelatinous yellowish-white pieces, hygroscopic and soapy to the touch. It forms a clear molten mass on heating. It contains not more than 10% of water. Very soluble in water and in alcohol. An aqueous solution froths copiously when shaken.

USNF 20: A mixture of alkylbenzyldimethylammonium chlorides of the general formula $[C_6H_5.CH_2.N(CH_3)_2.R]Cl$, in which R represents a mixture of the alkyls having chain lengths from C_8 to C_{16}. It contains not less than 40% of the $C_{12}H_{25}$ compound, calculated on the anhydrous substance, not less than 20% of the $C_{14}H_{29}$ compound, and not less than 70% of the 2 compounds together.

A white or yellowish-white, thick gel, or gelatinous pieces with a mild aromatic odour. It contains not more than 15% of water. Very soluble in water and in alcohol; the anhydrous form is soluble 1 in 100 of ether and 1 in 6 of benzene. A solution in water is usually slightly alkaline and foams strongly when shaken. Store in airtight containers.

Adverse Effects, Treatment, and Precautions

As for Cetrimide, p.1137.

Catheters and cannulas. For reference to benzalkonium chloride used in the manufacturing process of heparin-bonded catheters interfering with determination of serum concentrations of sodium and potassium, see under Precautions for Heparin, p.903.

Effects on the eyes. Benzalkonium chloride is one of the most disruptive ophthalmic additives to the stability of the lipid film and to corneal epithelial membranes; it has been shown to be toxic to the eyes of *rabbits* but less so to the eyes of humans.[1] Toxicity experiments have tended to be carried out using relatively high concentrations of benzalkonium chloride[2] but deleterious effects on the tear film and corneoconjunctival surface have been noted in patients receiving regular long-term treatment for glaucoma with eye drops preserved with benzalkonium chloride in usual concentrations.[3,4] However, the use of preservatives in eye drops should generally be avoided and the formulation of such preparations in single-dose containers is desirable.[1,2] Benzalkonium chloride is not suitable for use in solutions employed in storing and washing hydrophilic soft contact lenses, as it can bind to the lenses and may later produce ocular toxicity when the lenses are worn.[5]

1. Burstein NL. The effects of topical drugs and preservatives on the tears and corneal epithelium in dry eye. *Trans Ophthalmol Soc U K* 1985; **104:** 402–9.
2. Burstein NL. Corneal cytotoxicity of topically applied drugs, vehicles and preservatives. *Surv Ophthalmol* 1980; **25:** 15–30.
3. Herreras JM, *et al.* Ocular surface alteration after long-term treatment with an antiglaucomatous drug. *Ophthalmology* 1992; **99:** 1082–8.
4. Kuppens EVMJ, *et al.* Effect of timolol with and without preservative on the basal tear turnover in glaucoma. *Br J Ophthalmol* 1995; **79:** 339–42.
5. Gasset AR. Benzalkonium chloride toxicity to the human cornea. *Am J Ophthalmol* 1977; **84:** 169–71.

Effects on the respiratory tract. A hypersensitivity reaction in a patient to benzalkonium chloride used as a preservative in nose drops was confirmed by challenge which produced nasal congestion and irritation of the eyes and throat lasting 48 hours.[1] Benzalkonium chloride used as a preservative in nebulised solutions of anti-asthma drugs has been reported to cause dose-related bronchoconstriction especially in asthmatic patients[2] and has been associated with the precipitation of respiratory arrest in a patient.[3]

1. Hillerdal G. Adverse reaction to locally applied preservatives in nose drops. *ORL J Otorhinolaryngol Relat Spec* 1985; **47:** 278–9.
2. Committee on Drugs, American Academy of Pediatrics. "Inactive" ingredients in pharmaceutical products: update. *Pediatrics* 1997; **99:** 268–78.
3. Boucher M, *et al.* Possible association of benzalkonium chloride in nebulizer solutions with respiratory arrest. *Ann Pharmacother* 1992; **26:** 772–4.

Uses and Administration

Benzalkonium chloride is a quaternary ammonium antiseptic and disinfectant with actions and uses similar to those of the other cationic surfactants (see Cetrimide, p.1137). It is also used as an antimicrobial preservative for pharmaceutical products. Benzalkonium bromide and benzalkonium saccharinate have also been used.

Solutions of benzalkonium chloride 0.01 to 0.1% are used for cleansing skin, mucous membranes, and wounds. More dilute solutions of 0.005% are suitable for irrigation of deep wounds. A 0.02 to 0.05% solution has been used as a vaginal douche. An aqueous solution containing 0.005 to 0.02% has been used for irrigation of the bladder and urethra and a 0.0025 to 0.005% solution for retention lavage of the bladder.

Creams containing benzalkonium chloride are used in the treatment of napkin rash and other dermatoses.

A 0.2 to 0.5% solution has been used as a shampoo in seborrhoeic dermatitis.

Lozenges containing benzalkonium chloride are used for the treatment of superficial infections of the mouth and throat.

A 0.005 to 0.02% solution of benzalkonium chloride is used as a preservative for some eye drops. It is not suitable for eye drops containing local anaesthetics as it accelerates their dehydrating effect. Because some rubbers are incompatible with benzalkonium chloride silicone rubber teats should be used on eye drop containers unless the suitability has been established. Benzalkonium chloride is used for disinfecting rigid contact lenses (p.1129) but is unsuitable as a preservative in solutions for washing and storing hydrophilic soft contact lenses (see also Effects on the Eyes, above).

Benzalkonium chloride is also used as a spermicide.

Solutions of 0.13% are used for disinfection and storage of surgical instruments, sometimes with the addition of sodium nitrite to inhibit rust.

Action. The antibacterial effect of benzalkonium chloride 0.003% was enhanced by 0.175% of benzyl alcohol, phenylpropanol, or phenethyl alcohol.[1] For the use of phenethyl alcohol with benzalkonium chloride as a preservative for ophthalmic solutions, see Phenethyl Alcohol, p.1152.

1. Richards RME, McBride RJ. Enhancement of benzalkonium chloride and chlorhexidine acetate activity against Pseudomonas aeruginosa by aromatic alcohols. *J Pharm Sci* 1973; **62**: 2035–7.

Catheter-related sepsis. Benzalkonium chloride has been investigated[1,2] for incorporation into catheters to reduce catheter-related sepsis (p.1130).

1. Tebbs SE, Elliott TSJ. A novel, antimicrobial central venous catheter impregnated with benzalkonium chloride. *J Antimicrob Chemother* 1993; **31**: 261–71.
2. Moss HA, *et al.* A central venous catheter coated with benzalkonium chloride for the prevention of catheter-related microbial colonization. *Eur J Anaesthesiol* 2000; **17**: 680–7.

Preparations

USNF 20: Benzalkonium Chloride Solution.

Proprietary Preparations (details are given in Part 3)
Austral.: Bepanthen; Cetal Concentrate†; Dettol Fresh; *Belg.:* Cedium; Pansteryl†; *Braz.:* Fluimucil Solucao Nasal; Ionax Scrub; Merthiolate; *Canad.:* Antiseptic Skin Cream; Arkonsol; Zephiran; *Fr.:* Comprimes Gynecologiques Pharmatex†; Flexogyne; Humex; Pharmatex; Sparaplaie; *Ger.:* Baktonium; Laudamonium; Lysoform Killavon; Quartamon Med; Rheila Stringiet N†; Sagrotan Med†; *Irl.:* Roccal; *Israel:* Pharmatex; *Ital.:* Alfa C; Bluesteril; Ceroxmed Steril†; Citrosil; Citrosil Fazzoletto; Citrosil Sapoplus; Citrosil Spray; Citrosteril Deterferri; Colli; Collirium Geymonat; Contusil; Detergil; Di-Mill; Diseptil; Disintyl; Display; Distasil; Disteril; Eso Deterferri; Eso Ferri; Esoform Deterferri†; Esosan; Germicidin; Germozero Plus; Geyderm; Helis; Hygienist Pavimenti e Piastrelle; Iridina Light; Lacribase; Lozione Vittoria; Neo-Desogen; Norica; Polisan; Sanaform; Sangen Medical; Saquat; Sguardi; Sincosan†; Sirigen; Steramin; Steramina G; Sterilix†; Stilla Delicato; Streptosil L PMC; Video-Light; Zefirol; *Mex.:* Merthiolate; *NZ:* Dettol Fresh; *Port.:* Pharmatex; *S.Afr.:* Oraldettes†; *Spain:* Armil; Benzalc†; Crema Contracepti Lanzas; Mini Ovulo Lanzas; Novamina; *Thai.:* Pose-Bac; Zephirol; *UK:* Bradosol; Dettol Antiseptic Wash; Dettol Fresh; Roccal; Zensyls†; *USA:* Bacti-Cleanse; Benza; Mycocide NS; Ony-Clear; Zephiran.

Multi-ingredient: *Aust.:* Aleot; Cutasept; Dequonal; Dermaspray; Dr Schmidgall Halsweh; Nasimild; Tonsicur; Tyrothricin comp; *Austral.:* Clean Skin Face Wash; Gum-Ese; Mycil; Oilatum Plus; Paxyl; Solyptol; TAGG; Virasolve; *Belg.:* Akinspray; Dermaspray; *Braz.:* Belagin; Cetrilan; Colpanist; Colpistin; Colpist MT; Colpistar; Colpistatin; Dinill; Donnagel; Drapolene; Ginestatin; Ginometrim; Lacrima; Nestosyl; Pomada Minancora; Rhinodex; Rinosoro; Rinotil; Sorine Adulto; Sorine Infantil; Soronal; Vagi Biotic; Visolon†; *Canad.:* Aseptone Quat; Bactine; Family Medicated First Aid Treatment; Medi-Dan; Medi-Quik; Orajel Mouth Aid; Protectaid; Sporex; Tanac; *Fr.:* Acarcid; Biseptine; Dermaspray; Dermobacter; Euvanol†; Frekaderm†; Humex; Kenalcol; Mercryl; Pharmatex; Rhinofluimucil; *Ger.:* Baccalin; Bacillocid rasant; Bacillocid Spezial; Baktobod; Baktobod N†; Cutasept; Dequonal; Dorithricin Original; Dynexan A; Freka-Derm; Freka-Sept 80; Gingicain D; Hexaquart L; Hexaquart S; Incidin Extra; Incidin extra N; Incidin perfekt; Incidur Spray; Indulfan plus†; Kohrsolin FF; Lysetol Med; Mikrobac; Neo-Angin†; Quatohex; Sekusept Extra N; Sekusept forte; Septolit; Skinman Soft; Terralin; Thesit; Ultrasol-F; Ultrasol-S†; *Hong Kong:* Dermojela; Drapolene; Oilatum Plus; Protectaid; Virasolve; *Irl.:* Conotrane; Drapolene; Emulsiderm; Mycil; Oilatum Junior Flare-up; Torbetol; *Israel:* Emulsiderm; Garonsept; *Ital.:* Agena†; Agipiu; Alfa-Fluorone; AZ 15 Gengidentifricio; Barrycidal; Benzogen Ferri; Betaform Habitat; Cedril Strumenti†; Cedril†; Cepacol†; Cerox; Citrosil Alcolico Azzu; Citrosil Alcolico Bruno; Citrosil Alcolico Incolore; Citrosil Nubesan; Citrosteril Impronte; Citrosteril Pronto; Citrosteril Strumenti; Collyria; Conta-Lens Wetting; Dentaton Antisettico; Emoplast†; Eso Ferri Alcolico; Eso Ferri Alcolico Plus; Eso S 80; Esoalcolico Incolore; Esoform 92; Esoform Alcolico; Esoform Ferri Alcolico†; Esoform Ferri†; Esosan Pronto; Hamamilla; Herbe; Incidin Spezial; Indulfan; Linea F; Lycia Luminique; Mediplus; Neo-Emocicatrol;

Neomedil; Odongi; Oradyne-Z†; Otazul†; Pupilla Light; Rexichlor; Sangen Casa; Sekusept Extra N; Silvana; Simp; Simpottantacinque; Sterosan; Tirs; Zincometil; *Mex.:* Glossderm; *Mon.:* Akila spray†; *NZ:* Oilatum Plus; *S.Afr.:* Oilatum Plus; *Singapore:* Dettol; Drapolene; Oilatum Plus; *Spain:* Aftajuventus; Alcohcan; Alcohol Benzalconio; Alcohol CL Benz; Alcohol Potenciado; Alcohol Reforzado; Alcopac Reforzado; Avril; Curine; Dermo H Infantil; Desinvag; Egarone; Ginejuvent; Gradin Del D Andreu; Hemostatico Antisep Asen†; Lindemil; Odamida; Otogen Calmante; Pental Forte; Phonal; Pomada Heridas; Resorborina; Sebumselen; Talkosona†; Topicaina; Tulgrasum Cicatrizante; Vaselatum; *Switz.:* Dequonal; Frekaderm; Jonil T††; *Thai.:* Drapolene; Gynoco; Napilene; Nystin; Oilatum Plus; Sanaco; *UK:* Beechams Throat-Plus; Bumps 'n Falls; Cetanorm; Conotrane; Dermol; Dettol; Drapolene; Emulsiderm; Germolene; Germoloids; Medi-Tissue; Mycil; Neo; Oilatum Junior Flare-up; Oilatum Plus; Protectaid; Sunspot; Tegador; *USA:* Bactine Antiseptic; Cetylcide II; Medi-Quik; Orajel Mouth Aid; Oxyzal; Tanac; Tanac Dual Care; Vagi-Gard Medicated Cream; Yeast-Gard Advanced Sensitive Formula†; Zonite.

Benzethonium Chloride (2207-f)

Benzethonium Chloride *(BAN, rINN)*.

Benzethonii Chloridum; Diisobutylphenoxyethoxyethyldimethylbenzylammonium chloride. Benzyldimethyl(2-{2-[4-(1,1,3,3-tetramethylbutyl)phenoxy]ethoxy}ethyl)ammonium chloride.

$C_{27}H_{42}ClNO_2 = 448.1$.
CAS — 121-54-0.
Pharmacopoeias. In *Eur.* (see p.vi), *Jpn,* and *US.*

Incompatible with soaps and other anionic surfactants.

Pharmacopoeial description

Ph. Eur.: A white or yellowish-white powder. Very soluble in water and in alcohol; freely soluble in dichloromethane. An aqueous solution froths copiously when shaken. Protect from light.

USP 25: White crystals with a mild odour. Soluble 1 in less than 1 of water, of alcohol, and of chloroform, and 1 in 6000 of ether. A 1% solution in water is slightly alkaline to litmus. Store in airtight containers. Protect from light.

Profile

Benzethonium chloride is a quaternary ammonium antiseptic with actions and uses similar to those of other cationic surfactants (see Cetrimide, p.1137). It has also been used as a vaginal spermicide.

◊ Benzethonium chloride produced mild skin irritation at a concentration of 5% but not lower, was not considered to be a sensitiser, and was considered to be safe at a concentration of 0.5% in cosmetics applied to the skin and at a maximum concentration of 0.02% in cosmetics used in the eye area.[1]

1. The Expert Panel of the American College of Toxicology. Final report on the safety assessment of benzethonium chloride and methylbenzethonium chloride. *J Am Coll Toxicol* 1985; **4**: 65–106.

Preparations

USP 25: Benzethonium Chloride Tincture; Benzethonium Chloride Topical Solution.

Proprietary Preparations (details are given in Part 3)
Canad.: Skin Cleanser & Deodorizer; *Ital.:* Ribex Gola†; *S.Afr.:* Johnson's Antiseptic Powder†.

Multi-ingredient: *Austral.:* Summers Eve Feminine; *Belg.:* Neo-Golaseptine; *Braz.:* Acitra; Andolba; Hipodex; Otosulf; *Canad.:* Antiseptic Skin Cream; Buro Derm†; Buro-Sol; Dermoplast†; MRX; Protecto; Skin Shield†; VoSoL; VoSoL HC; *Ger.:* Brand- u. Wundgel-Medice N; *Hong Kong:* Cemaquin; *Ital.:* Barrycidal; Borossigeno Plus Stomatologico†; Cedril Strumenti†; Cedril†; Neo Topico Giusto†; Sangen Casa; *NZ:* VoSoL; *Spain:* Alcohol Poten; Eupnol; Halibut; Halibut Hidrocortisona; Isdinex; Tegunal; *Switz.:* Angidine; Rhinocure Simplex†; Rhinocure†; Tyrocombine; Tyrothricin + Gramicidine; *Thai.:* Iwazin; *USA:* AA-HC Otic†; Acetasol; Acetasol HC; Aerocaine; Aerotherm; Americaine First Aid; Skin Shield; Triple Care Cleanser†; Vagisil; VoSoL; VoSoL HC.

Benzoates (11730-m)

Benzoic Acid (6634-b)

Acidum Benzoicum; Benzoesäure; Dracylic Acid; E210.
$C_6H_5.CO_2H = 122.1$.
CAS — 65-85-0.
Pharmacopoeias. In *Chin., Eur.* (see p.vi), *Int., Jpn, Pol.,* and *US.*

Incompatibilities are described under Sodium Benzoate, below.

Pharmacopoeial description

Ph. Eur.: A white, crystalline powder or colourless crystals, odourless or with a very slight characteristic odour. Slightly soluble in water; soluble in boiling water; freely soluble in alcohol, in ether, and in fatty oils. M.p. 121° to 124°.

USP 25: White crystals, scales, or needles, with a slight characteristic odour. Soluble 1 in 300 of water, 1 in 3 of alcohol, 1 in 5 of chloroform, and 1 in 3 of ether; freely volatile in steam. Congealing range 121° to 123°.

Sodium Benzoate (6666-I)

E211; Natrii Benzoas; Natrium Benzoicum; Sodii Benzoas.
$C_6H_5.CO_2Na = 144.1$.
CAS — 532-32-1.
Pharmacopoeias. In *Chin., Eur.* (see p.vi), *Jpn,* and *Pol.* Also in *US-NF.*

Benzoic acid and its salts are incompatible with quaternary compounds, calcium salts, ferric salts, and salts of heavy metals. Their activity is also diminished by nonionic surfactants or due to absorption by kaolin. They are relatively inactive above a pH of about 5.

Pharmacopoeial description

Ph. Eur.: A white, slightly hygroscopic, crystalline or granular powder or flakes. Freely soluble in water; sparingly soluble in alcohol (90% v/v).

USNF 20: A white, odourless or practically odourless, granular or crystalline powder. Soluble 1 in 2 of water, 1 in 75 of alcohol, and 1 in 50 of alcohol 90%.

Adverse Effects and Precautions

The benzoates can cause hypersensitivity reactions, but there have also been reports of non-immunological contact urticaria. The acid can be irritant to skin, eyes, and mucous membranes.

Infants given large doses of sodium benzoate have suffered vomiting. Symptoms of overdosage reported in this group have been restricted to vomiting and irritability.

Premature infants have been reported to be at risk of metabolic acidosis and kernicterus.

Hypersensitivity. Respiratory reactions to benzoates may occur, especially in patients susceptible to aspirin-induced asthma.[1,2] Urticarial reactions have also been associated with these compounds,[3,4] though at a lower incidence[5] and they can be non-immunological.[6] However, these reports have to be balanced against a controlled study[7] that showed no difference in the incidence of urticaria or atopic symptoms between patients given benzoic acid and those given lactose placebo.

Anaphylactoid reactions have been reported in two patients.[8,9] Erythema multiforme has been observed in several patients.[10]

1. Rosenhall L. Evaluation of intolerance to analgesics, preservatives and food colorants with challenge tests. *Eur J Respir Dis* 1982; **63:** 410–19.
2. Settipane GA. Aspirin and allergic diseases: a review. *Am J Med* 1983; **74** (suppl): 102–9.
3. Michaëlsson G, Juhlin L. Urticaria induced by preservatives and dye additives in food and drugs. *Br J Dermatol* 1973; **88:** 525–32.
4. Warin RP, Smith RJ. Challenge test battery in chronic urticaria. *Br J Dermatol* 1976; **94:** 401–6.
5. Wüthrich B, Fabro L. Acetylsalicylsäure-und lebensmitteladditiva-intoleranz bei urtikaria, asthma bronchiale und chronischer rhinopathie. *Schweiz Med Wochenschr* 1981; **III:** 1445–50.
6. Nethercott JR, *et al.* Airborne contact urticaria due to sodium benzoate in a pharmaceutical manufacturing plant. *J Occup Med* 1984; **26:** 734–6.
7. Lahti A, Hannuksela M. Is Benzoic acid really harmful in cases of atopy and urticaria? *Lancet* 1981; **ii:** 1055.
8. Moneret-Vautrin DA, *et al.* Anaphylactoid reaction to general anaesthesia: a case of intolerance to sodium benzoate. *Anaesth Intensive Care* 1982; **10:** 156–7.
9. Michils A, *et al.* Anaphylaxis with sodium benzoate. *Lancet* 1991; **337:** 1424–5.
10. Lewis MAO, *et al.* Recurrent erythema multiforme: a possible role of foodstuffs. *Br Dent J* 1989; **166:** 371–3.

Neonates. Serious metabolic disturbances in premature neonates given intravenous fluids with benzyl alcohol as a preservative have been attributed to the accumulation of the benzoic acid metabolite of the benzyl alcohol (see p.1135). This risk led to the recommendation that Caffeine and Sodium Benzoate Injection (USP), which has been given as a respiratory stimulant, should not be used in neonates.[1]

Benzoates can also displace bound bilirubin from albumin putting neonates at risk of kernicterus.[2] However, sodium benzoate has been tried in the treatment of some neonatal metabolic disorders (see Uses and Administration, below).

1. Edwards RC, Voegeli CJ. Inadvisability of using caffeine and sodium benzoate in neonates. *Am J Hosp Pharm* 1984; **41:** 658.
2. Schiff D, *et al.* Fixed drug combinations and the displacement of bilirubin from albumin. *Pediatrics* 1971; **48:** 139–41.

Pharmacokinetics

The benzoates are absorbed from the gastrointestinal tract and conjugated with glycine in the liver to form hippuric acid which is rapidly excreted in the urine.

Neonates. References.
1. Green TP, *et al.* Disposition of sodium benzoate in newborn infants with hyperammonemia. *J Pediatr* 1983; **102:** 785–90.

Uses and Administration

Benzoates have antibacterial and antifungal properties. Their antimicrobial activity is due to the undissociated benzoic acid and is therefore pH-dependent. They are relatively inactive above a pH of about 5.

They are used as preservatives in pharmaceutical formulations including oral preparations; benzoic acid and sodium benzoate are typically employed in concentrations of up to 0.2% and 0.5%, respectively. They are used as preservatives in foods, (and are also present naturally in some foods), and at similar concentrations in cosmetics.

Benzoic acid 6% with salicylic acid 3%, as Compound Benzoic Acid Ointment (BP 2001) (Whitfield's Ointment) has a long history of use as an antifungal (see Skin Infections, p.376). Benzoic acid has also been employed in desloughing preparations and has been given as a urinary antiseptic.

An injection of caffeine and sodium benzoate has been used as a CNS stimulant, but see above for a caution against its use in neonates.

Sodium benzoate is used as part of the treatment of hyperammonaemia that occurs in inborn errors of the urea cycle. It has also been reported to be effective in reducing plasma-glycine concentrations in nonketotic hyperglycinaemia (p.1667), although it may not be effective in preventing mental retardation.

Sodium benzoate is a common ingredient of cough preparations.

Hyperammonaemia. The dose of sodium benzoate used for treatment of hyperammonaemia (p.1354) has generally been 250 mg per kg body-weight daily by intravenous infusion.[1-3]

1. Maestri NE, et al. Long-term survival of patients with argininosuccinate synthetase deficiency. J Pediatr 1995; 127: 929–35.
2. Maestri NE, et al. Long-term treatment of girls with ornithine transcarbamylase deficiency. N Engl J Med 1996; 335: 855–9.
3. Zammarchi E, et al. Neonatal onset of hyperornithinemia-hyperammonemia-homocitrullinuria syndrome with favorable outcome. J Pediatr 1997; 131: 440–3.

Preparations

BP 2001: Benzoic Acid Solution; Compound Benzoic Acid Ointment; Tolu-flavour Solution;
USP 25: Benzoic and Salicylic Acids Ointment; Caffeine and Sodium Benzoate Injection.

Proprietary Preparations (details are given in Part 3)
Mex.: Colufase; *USA:* Drazoic†.

Multi-ingredient: *Aust.:* Acerbine; Aplexil; Bisolvotin†; Expigen; Mycopol; *Austral.:* Egomycol; Mycozol†; Whitfields (Benzoic Acid Compound) Ointment; *Belg.:* Bronchobel; Colimax; Kamfeine; Normogastryl†; Pholco-Mereprine; Rectoplexil; Toplexil; Tux; *Braz.:* Bronquidex; Bronquiogen; Cessatosse; Codelasa; Colagolen; Dermicon; Dermofytol; Dermycose; Eaca Balsamico; Efedronal; Expec; Frenotosse; Gotas Nican; Iodermol; Iodesin; Iodobec; Ipecol; KI-Expectorante; Limao Bravo; Locao Mancha Branca; Mel Jatahy; Micocid; Micofim; Micotiazol; Micotissim; Micoz; Natoss; Pectoss; Peitoral Angico Pelotense; Penetro; Pinosil; Plactosse; Po Antisseptico; Psiu; Pulmoverina; Tolusil; Toplexil; Tosseina; Traqueobron; Tussodina; Tuzo; Xarope de Caraguata + Bromoformio; Xarope de Limao Bravo; Xarope Peitoral de Ameixa Composto; Xarope Sao Joao; Xarope Valda; *Canad.:* Mouthrinse†; MRX; Plax; Sea Breeze†; *Denm.:* Pectyl; Throat; *Fr.:* Asthmalgine†; Broncalene; Broncalene Nourisson; Broncorinol toux seches; Bronpax†; Codotussyl Maux de Gorge; Dermacide; Dimetane; Dinacode; Dinacode avec codeine; Ephydion; Germose; Glyco-Thymoline; Gynescal†; Marrubene Codethyline†; Neo-Codion; Ozothine; Paregorique; Passedyl; Pneumaseptic†; Pulmocod; Pulmofluide Simple; Pulmonase†; Pulmosodyl; Quintopan; Rhinamide; Silomat; Sirop Pectoral adulte†; Sirop Pectoral enfant†; Tossarel†; *Israel:* Oxacatin; Phytoderm Compositum; Pitrisan; Toplexil; Tussophedrine; Whitfield Plus; *Ital.:* Borocaina; Dentinale; Neo Borocillina; Sedobex†; Sedocalcio; Tiocosol; Tionamil; *Neth.:* Toplexil; *NZ:* Egomycol; Listerine; *Port.:* Broncodiazina; Bronquiasmol; Calmarum; Codeisan†; Codoforme; Diacol; Drenoflux†; Fluidin Adulto; Fluidin Antiasmatico; Fluidin Infantil; Lactucol; Micaveen†; *S.Afr.:* Aserbine; *Singapore:* Whitfield; *Spain:* Acerbiol; Bronco Sergo; Broncoformo Muco Dexa; Broncomicin Bals†; Broncovital; Bronquidiazina CR; Bronquimar; Etermol Antitusivo; Maboterpen†; Mentobox†; Neumopectolina; Pastillas Pectoral Kely; Pazbronquial; Pectoral Brum†; Pulmo Menal; Pulmofasa; Pulmofasa Antihist; Tos Mai; *Switz.:* Acerbine; Bronchalin†; Bronchocodin†; Demo pates pectorales†; Dinacode N; Foral; Nasobol; Nican; Phol-Tussil; Phol-Tux; Saintbois nouvelle formule; Sirop pectoral DP1†; Sirop pectoral DP2, DP3†; Spedro†; Toplexil; *UK:* Antiseptic Throat Pastilles†; Aserbine; Eczema Ointment; Hemocane; Melissin; Sanderson's Throat Specific; Toepedo; *USA:* Atrosept; Bensal HP; Cystex; Dolsed; Feminique; Prosed/DS; Summers Eve Disposable; Trac Tabs 2X; UAA; Ucephan; Uridon Modified; Urised.

Benzododecinium Bromide (2208-d)

Benzyldodecyldimethylammonium bromide.
$C_{21}H_{38}BrN = 384.4$.
CAS — 10328-35-5 (benzododecinium); 7281-04-1 (benzododecinium bromide); 139-07-1 (benzododecinium chloride).

NOTE. Benzododecinium Chloride is *rINN*.
Pharmacopoeias. In Fr.

The symbol † denotes a preparation no longer actively marketed

---

Profile

Benzododecinium bromide is a quaternary ammonium antiseptic with properties similar to those of other cationic surfactants (see Cetrimide, p.1137). It is used in mouthwashes and nasal sprays and solutions for the treatment of minor infections. It is also used as a spermicide. Benzododecinium chloride has also been used.

Preparations

Proprietary Preparations (details are given in Part 3)
Fr.: Rhinedrine.

Multi-ingredient: *Fr.:* Fluorhinose; Genola; Prorhinel; Sedacollyre; *Ger.:* Prorhinel†; *Ital.:* Larilon; *Switz.:* Kemerhinose; Prorhinel.

Benzoxonium Chloride (11594-e)

Benzoxonium Chloride (rINN).
Benzyldodecylbis(2-hydroxyethyl)ammonium chloride.
$C_{23}H_{42}ClNO_2 = 400.0$.
CAS — 19379-90-9.
ATC — A01AB14; D08AJ05.

Profile

Benzoxonium chloride is a quaternary ammonium antiseptic used for disinfection of the skin and mucous membranes. It is also used for instrument disinfection.

Preparations

Proprietary Preparations (details are given in Part 3)
Belg.: Orofar; *Ital.:* Bactofen; Bialcol; Sinecod Bocca†.

Multi-ingredient: *Belg.:* Orofar Lidocaine; *Ger.:* Lemocin Flexibels; Loscon; *Israel:* Vita-Merfen NF; *Port.:* Orofar; *Spain:* Cohortan; Cohortan Antibiotico†; *Switz.:* Merfen; Orofar; Vita-Merfen; *Thai.:* Orofar.

Benzyl Alcohol (554-h)

Benzyl Alcohol (rINN).
Alcohol Benzylicus; Alcool Benzylique; Benzenemethanol; Phenylcarbinol; Phenylmethanol.
$C_6H_5.CH_2OH = 108.1$.
CAS — 100-51-6.

Pharmacopoeias. In Eur. (see p.vi), Int., Jpn, and Pol. Also in USNF.

Benzyl alcohol oxidises to produce benzaldehyde and benzoic acid and oxidation may take place slowly on exposure to air. Benzaldehyde may also be produced on autoclaving.

Benzyl alcohol is incompatible with oxidising agents and strong acids. The antimicrobial activity may be reduced by nonionic surfactants and benzyl alcohol may be lost from solutions stored in polyethylene containers.

Pharmacopoeial description

Ph. Eur.: A clear colourless, oily liquid. Soluble in water; miscible with alcohol, and with fatty and essential oils. Store under nitrogen in airtight containers at a temperature of 2° to 8°. Protect from light.

USNF 20: A clear, colourless, oily liquid. Sparingly soluble in water; freely soluble in alcohol (50%); miscible with alcohol, with chloroform, and with ether. It is neutral to litmus. Store in airtight containers. Protect from light.

Adverse Effects and Precautions

There have been a few reports of hypersensitivity reactions to benzyl alcohol when used as a preservative.

The pure alcohol is irritant and requires handling with care; ingestion or inhalation can cause nausea, vomiting, diarrhoea, headache, vertigo, and CNS depression. However, concentrations of benzyl alcohol normally used for preservation are not associated with such effects.

There have been some instances of neurotoxic effects in patients given intrathecal injections that contained benzyl alcohol.

A fatal toxic syndrome in premature infants was attributed to benzyl alcohol present as a preservative in solutions used to flush intravenous catheters. This has led to restriction on the use of benzyl alcohol in neonates and young children, see below.

Effects on the lungs. Severe bronchitis and haemoptysis was reported in a patient with obstructive pulmonary disease who, over a period of 2 years, had inhaled salbutamol nebuliser solution diluted with a bacteriostatic sodium chloride solution containing benzyl alcohol.[1]

1. Reynolds RD. Nebulizer bronchitis induced by bacteriostatic saline. JAMA 1990; 264: 35.

Effects on the nervous system. Rapid development of flaccid areflexic paraplegia, total anaesthesia below the groin, and radicular abdominal pain occurred in a 64-year-old man fol-

---

lowing a lumbar intrathecal injection of cytarabine which contained 1.5% benzyl alcohol.[1] The patient recovered fully after 100 mL of CSF was replaced with sodium chloride 0.9% and 40 mg of methylprednisolone. Intrathecal injections of cytarabine dissolved in sterile distilled water before and after the episode of paraplegia caused no neurologic symptoms. On reviewing 20 other cases of paraparesis associated with methotrexate or cytarabine intrathecal injections, benzyl alcohol had been used as a preservative in 7. Of the 7, 4 developed neurotoxicity immediately; in the other 3 it did not develop until 6 to 48 hours after administration. The duration varied. One patient did not improve, one made a partial recovery, a third took 6 weeks to recover, another took 5 days; yet 2 patients recovered within 1½ to 2½ hours while the final patient experienced only transient effects.

1. Hahn AF, et al. Paraparesis following intrathecal chemotherapy. Neurology 1983; 33: 1032–8.

Hypersensitivity. Some reports of hypersensitivity reactions to benzyl alcohol.

1. Grant JA, et al. Unsuspected benzyl alcohol hypersensitivity. N Engl J Med 1982; 306: 108.
2. Shmunes E. Allergic dermatitis to benzyl alcohol in an injectable solution. Arch Dermatol 1984; 120: 1200–1.
3. Wilson JP, et al. Parenteral benzyl alcohol-induced hypersensitivity reaction. Drug Intell Clin Pharm 1986; 20: 689–91.

Neonates. During 1981 and 1982 reports were published from 2 centres in the USA[1-3] of 20 deaths in low-birth-weight neonates attributed to the use of benzyl alcohol as a preservative in solutions used to flush their umbilical catheters and in some cases also to dilute their medication. The neonates suffered a toxic syndrome whose features included metabolic acidosis, symptoms of progressive encephalopathy, intracranial haemorrhage, and respiratory depression with gasping.

These deaths prompted the FDA[4] to recommend that benzyl alcohol should not be used in such flushing solutions; sodium chloride injection (0.9%) without preservative should be used instead. The FDA has also advised against the use of benzyl alcohol or any preservative in fluids being used for the dilution or reconstitution of medicines for the newborn.

Those reporting the deaths[2,3] considered that the toxic syndrome could have been caused by the accumulation of the benzoic acid metabolite of benzyl alcohol, which could not be handled effectively by the immature liver; given the very low weight of the neonates they would have been receiving a high dose of benzyl alcohol. In commenting on the problem, the American Academy of Pediatrics[5] agreed that the FDA's warning was warranted, but pointed out that there was no evidence from controlled studies to confirm that benzyl alcohol was responsible.

1. Gershanik JJ, et al. The gasping syndrome: benzyl alcohol (BA) poisoning? Clin Res 1981; 29: 895A.
2. Brown WJ, et al. Fatal benzyl alcohol poisoning in a neonatal intensive care unit. Lancet 1982; i: 1250.
3. Gershanik J, et al. The gasping syndrome and benzyl alcohol poisoning. N Engl J Med 1982; 307: 1384–8.
4. Anonymous. Benzyl alcohol may be toxic to newborns. FDA Drug Bull 1982; 12: 10–11.
5. American Academy of Pediatrics. Benzyl alcohol: toxic agent in neonatal use. Pediatrics 1983; 72: 356–7.

Pharmacokinetics

Benzyl alcohol is metabolised to benzoic acid. This is conjugated with glycine in the liver to form hippuric acid which is excreted in the urine. Benzaldehyde and benzoic acid are degradation products *in vitro*.

Uses

Benzyl alcohol is used as an antimicrobial preservative. It is bacteriostatic mainly against Gram-positive organisms and some fungi. It is used in a range of pharmaceutical preparations in concentrations up to 2%. Concentrations of 5% or more are employed when it is used as a solubiliser. Benzyl alcohol is used as a preservative in foods and cosmetics. It is also used as a disinfectant at a concentration of 10%.

In addition to its antiseptic properties, diluted benzyl alcohol possesses weak local anaesthetic and antipruritic activity and this is the reason for its inclusion in some preparations.

Preparations

Proprietary Preparations (details are given in Part 3)
Canad.: Babys Own Teething Gel; Zilactin.

Multi-ingredient: *Aust.:* Dermaspray; *Austral.:* Coso; Soothe'n Heal; *Belg.:* Dermaspray; *Canad.:* Foille†; *Denm.:* Doloproct Comp; *Fr.:* Biseptine; Codotussyl Maux de Gorge; Dermaspray; Pastilles Medicinales Vicks; *Ger.:* Spitacid; *Irl.:* Sudocrem†; *Israel:* Otomycin; *Ital.:* Borocaina; Foille; Foille Sole; *Port.:* Friax†; *Spain:* Acerbiol; Pastillas Antisep Garg M; *UK:* Sudocrem; *USA:* Anusol; Cepacol Throat; Florida Sunburn Relief†; Itch-X; MouthKote O/R; Rhuli Gel; Step 2†; Super Ivy Dry; TiSol; Topic.

Biclotymol (16535-k)

Biclotymol (rINN).

2,2'-Methylenebis(6-chlorothymole).

$C_{21}H_{26}Cl_2O_2 = 381.3$.

CAS — 15686-33-6.

Profile

Biclotymol is a phenolic antiseptic that is used in lozenges and sprays for mouth and throat infections. It is also an ingredient of cough preparations.

Preparations

Proprietary Preparations (details are given in Part 3)
Fr.: Hexadreps†; Hexaspray; Humex; *Hong Kong:* Hexaspray.
Multi-ingredient: *Fr.:* Hexalyse; Hexapneumine; *Hong Kong:* Hexalyse; Hexapneumine.

Brilliant Green (2211-a)

CI Basic Green 1; Colour Index No. 42040; Diamond Green G; Emerald Green; Ethyl Green; Malachite Green G; Solid Green; Viride Nitens. 4-(4-Diethylaminobenzhydrylidene)cyclohexa-2,5-dien-1-ylidenediethylammonium hydrogen sulphate.

$C_{27}H_{34}N_2O_4S = 482.6$.

CAS — 633-03-4.

NOTE. The name Emerald Green has also been used to denote copper acetoarsenite.

Profile

Brilliant green is a triphenylmethane antiseptic dye with actions similar to those of methylrosanilinium chloride (p.1151). Its activity is greatly reduced in the presence of serum.

A gel containing brilliant green 0.5% with lactic acid was formerly used in the treatment of skin ulcers.

An alcoholic solution of brilliant green 0.5% and methylrosanilinium chloride 0.5% (Bonney's Blue) was formerly used for disinfecting the skin, but concern at evidence of *animal* carcinogenicity with methylrosanilinium chloride has led to the decline of such paints. A solution of the two disinfectants has been used for marking incisions prior to surgery.

There have been occasional reports of sensitivity to brilliant green.

Adverse effects. For a report of necrotic skin reactions following application of a 1% solution of brilliant green to stripped skin, see under the Adverse Effects of Methylrosanilinium Chloride, p.1150.

Bromchlorophen (11596-y)

Bromchlorophene; Bromochlorophane. 2,2'-Methylenebis[6-bromo-4-chlorophenol].

$C_{13}H_8Br_2Cl_2O_2 = 426.9$.

CAS — 15435-29-7.

Profile

Bromchlorophen is a halogenated bisphenol antiseptic more active against Gram-positive than Gram-negative bacteria. It is used for disinfection of the hands and skin.

Preparations

Proprietary Preparations (details are given in Part 3)
Multi-ingredient: *Ger.:* Dibromol.

Bromsalans (2289-k)

CAS — 55830-61-0.

A series of brominated salicylanilides which possess antimicrobial activity.

Dibromsalan (2290-w)

Dibromsalan (USAN, pINN).

NSC-20527. 4',5-Dibromosalicylanilide; 5-Bromo-N-(4-bromophenyl)-2-hydroxybenzamide.

$C_{13}H_9Br_2NO_2 = 371.0$.

CAS — 87-12-7.

Metabromsalan (2291-e)

Metabromsalan (USAN, pINN).

NSC-526280. 3,5-Dibromosalicylanilide; 3,5-Dibromo-2-hydroxy-N-phenylbenzamide.

$C_{13}H_9Br_2NO_2 = 371.0$.

CAS — 2577-72-2.

Tribromsalan (2213-x)

Tribromsalan (BAN, USAN, rINN).

ET-394; NSC-20526; TBS. 3,4',5-Tribromosalicylanilide; 3,5-Dibromo-N-(4-bromophenyl)-2-hydroxybenzamide.

$C_{13}H_8Br_3NO_2 = 449.9$.

CAS — 87-10-5.

Profile

Bromsalans have antibacterial and antifungal activity and have been used in medicated soaps, but there have been many reports of photosensitivity arising from this use.

Preparations

Proprietary Preparations (details are given in Part 3)
Ital.: Bergamon Sapone.

Bronopol (6636-g)

Bronopol (BAN, rINN).

2-Bromo-2-nitropropane-1,3-diol.

$C_3H_6BrNO_4 = 200.0$.

CAS — 52-51-7.

Pharmacopoeias. In Br. and Pol.

Incompatibilities. Activity can be diminished by sodium metabisulfite, sodium thiosulfate, cysteine hydrochloride, and compounds with a thiol group. Increases in temperature affect stability as do increases in pH above 8. Incompatibility with unprotected aluminium affects packaging.

Pharmacopoeial description

BP 2001: White or almost white crystals or crystalline powder, odourless or almost odourless. Freely soluble in water and in alcohol; slightly soluble in glycerol and in liquid paraffin. A 1% solution in water has a pH of 5.0 to 7.0. Protect from light.

◊ Creams and shampoos containing bronopol 0.01% as a preservative were found to contain free nitrite and, as a result of amines present in the preparations, nitrosamines.[1] It was recommended that nitrosamine formation could be reduced in preparations containing amines and bronopol by limiting the bronopol concentration to 0.01% and inclusion of alpha tocopherol 0.2% or butylated hydroxytoluene 0.05%.

1. Dunnett PC, Telling GM. Study of the fate of bronopol and the effects of antioxidants on N-nitrosamine formation in shampoos and skin creams. *Int J Cosmet Sci* 1984; **6**: 241–7.

Adverse Effects

Bronopol may be irritant when applied topically.

Pharmacokinetics

Bronopol is absorbed following topical administration.

Uses

Bronopol is active against a wide range of bacteria, including *Pseudomonas aeruginosa*, but is less active against moulds and yeasts. Bronopol is used as a preservative in shampoos, cosmetics, and both topical and oral pharmaceutical preparations; concentrations in pharmaceutical preparations range from 0.01 to 0.1%, with the usual concentration being 0.02%.

Butylated Hydroxyanisole (6638-p)

Butylated Hydroxyanisole (BAN).

BHA; Butilidrossianisolo; Butylhydroxyanisolum; E320. 2-tert-Butyl-4-methoxyphenol; 2-(1,1-dimethylethyl)-4-methoxyphenol.

$C_{11}H_{16}O_2 = 180.2$.

CAS — 25013-16-5.

Pharmacopoeias. In Eur. (see p.vi), Int., and Pol. Also in USNF.

Incompatible with oxidising agents and ferric salts. Traces of metals can cause loss of activity.

Pharmacopoeial description

Ph. Eur.: A white, yellowish, or slightly pinkish, crystalline powder. It contains not more than 10% of 3-(1,1-dimethylethyl)-4-methoxyphenol. Practically insoluble in water; freely soluble in alcohol and in fatty oils; very soluble in dichloromethane; it dissolves in dilute solutions of alkali hydroxides. Protect from light.

USNF 20: A white, or slightly yellow, waxy solid with a faint characteristic odour. Insoluble in water; soluble 1 in 4 of alcohol, 1 in 2 of chloroform, and 1 in 1.2 of ether; freely soluble in propylene glycol.

Adverse Effects

Butylated hydroxyanisole can be irritant to the eyes, skin, and mucous membranes and can cause depigmentation. There are reports of delayed (type IV) hypersensitivity reactions and non-immunogenic skin reactions.

Effects on the blood. For a report of methaemoglobinaemia associated with the antioxidants (butylated hydroxyanisole, butylated hydroxytoluene, and propyl gallate) used to preserve the oil in a soybean infant feed, see under Adverse Effects in Alkyl Gallates (p.1133).

Pharmacokinetics

Butylated hydroxyanisole is absorbed from the gastrointestinal tract, then metabolised and conjugated, and excreted in the urine; less than 1% is excreted in the urine as unchanged drug within 24 hours of ingestion.

Uses

Butylated hydroxyanisole is an antioxidant with some antimicrobial activity. It is used as a preservative in cosmetics and foods as well as pharmaceutical preparations, particularly to delay or prevent oxidative rancidity of fats and oils in concentrations of up to 0.02%; higher concentrations have been used for essential oils. It is also used to prevent the loss of activity of oil-soluble vitamins.

Commercial supplies of butylated hydroxyanisole employed in food technology consist of mixtures of the 2-tert and 3-tert isomers.

To improve efficacy, butylated hydroxyanisole is frequently used in combination with other antioxidants such as butylated hydroxytoluene or an alkyl gallate and with sequestrants or synergists such as citric acid.

Use in food. In the UK the Food Advisory Committee has recommended that the use of butylated hydroxyanisole and butylated hydroxytoluene should no longer be permitted as additives for infant formulas as they are no longer required for the economic manufacture of vitamin A and vitamin A esters.[1]

1. MAFF. Food Advisory Committee: report on the review of the use of additives in foods specially prepared for infants and young children. *FdAC/REP/12.* London: HMSO, 1992.

Butylated Hydroxytoluene (6639-s)

Butylated Hydroxytoluene (BAN).

BHT; Butylhydroxitoluenum; Butylhydroxytoluene; E321. 2,6-Di-tert-butyl-p-cresol.

$C_{15}H_{24}O = 220.4$.

CAS — 128-37-0.

Pharmacopoeias. In Eur. (see p.vi), Int., and Pol. Also in USNF.

Incompatible with oxidising agents and ferric salts. Traces of metals can cause loss of activity.

Pharmacopoeial description

Ph. Eur.: A white or yellowish-white, crystalline powder. F.p. 69° to 70°. Practically insoluble in water; freely soluble in alcohol and in vegetable oils; very soluble in acetone and in ether.

USNF 20: A white crystalline solid with a faint characteristic odour. Insoluble in water and in propylene glycol; soluble 1 in 4 of alcohol and 1 in 1.1 of chloroform and of ether.

Adverse Effects

As for Butylated Hydroxyanisole, p.1136.

Poisoning. A 22-year-old woman experienced severe epigastric cramping, nausea and vomiting, and generalised weakness, followed by dizziness, confusion, and a brief loss of consciousness after ingesting 4 g of butylated hydroxytoluene. She recovered following conservative treatment which was given 2 days later. The antioxidant had been taken as an unauthorised remedy for genital herpes simplex.[1]

1. Shlian DM, Goldstone J. Toxicity of butylated hydroxytoluene. *N Engl J Med* 1986; **314**: 648–9.

Effects on the blood. For a report of methaemoglobinaemia associated with the antioxidants (butylated hydroxyanisole, butylated hydroxytoluene, and propyl gallate) used to preserve the oil in a soybean infant feed formula, see under Adverse Effects in Alkyl Gallates, p.1133.

Pharmacokinetics

Butylated hydroxytoluene is readily absorbed from the gastrointestinal tract. It is excreted in the urine mainly as glucuronide conjugates of oxidation products.

Uses

Butylated hydroxytoluene is an antioxidant with uses similar to those of Butylated Hydroxyanisole, p.1136.

Cadexomer-Iodine (15334-d)

Cadexomer-Iodine (BAN).

Cadexomer Iodine (USAN). 2-Hydroxymethylene cross-linked (1→4)-α-D-glucan carboxymethyl ether containing iodine.

CAS — 94820-09-4.

ATC — D03AX01.

Adverse Effects and Precautions

As for Povidone-Iodine, p.1155. Some patients have experienced stinging and erythema following application of cadexomer-iodine to their ulcers. Free iodine is released during exposure of cadexomer-iodine preparations to wound exudate and absorption of iodine may occur. Prolonged treatment with cadexomer-iodine should be used with caution in patients with thyroid disorders.

Uses and Administration

Cadexomer-iodine, like povidone-iodine (p.1155), is an iodophore that releases iodine. It is used for its absorbent and antiseptic properties in the management of venous leg ulcers and pressure sores. It is applied as a powder, ointment, or paste containing iodine 0.9%; sufficient powder or ointment should be applied to form a layer about 3 mm thick. Treatment should not usually be continued for more than 3 months.

Preparations

Proprietary Preparations (details are given in Part 3)
Aust.: Iodosorb; *Canad.:* Iodosorb; *Denm.:* Iodosorb; *Fin.:* Iodosorb; *Ger.:* Iodosorb†; *Irl.:* Iodoflex; *Ital.:* Iodosorb; *Spain:* Iodosorb; *Swed.:* Iodosorb; *Switz.:* Iodosorb; *UK:* Iodoflex; Iodosorb.

Cetalkonium Chloride (2214-r)

Cetalkonium Chloride (BAN, USAN, rINN).
NSC-32942. Benzylhexadecyldimethylammonium chloride.
$C_{25}H_{46}CIN = 396.1$.
CAS — 122-18-9.

Profile
Cetalkonium chloride is a quaternary ammonium antiseptic with actions and uses similar to those of other cationic surfactants (see Cetrimide, p.1137). It is used in a variety of topical preparations in the treatment of minor infections of the mouth and throat. It has also been used in the treatment of eye infections. Cetalkonium bromide has also been used.

Preparations
Proprietary Preparations (details are given in Part 3)
Multi-ingredient: Aust.: Mundisal; **Austral.:** Bonjela; **Braz.:** Pondicilina; **Canad.:** Bionet; Emercol; **Fr.:** Pansoral; **Ger.:** Mundisal; **Hong Kong:** Bonjela; **Irl.:** Bonjela; **Israel:** Bonjela; **NZ:** Bonjela; **Port.:** Bucagel; **S.Afr.:** AAA; Bonjela; **Singapore:** Bonjela; **Switz.:** Deca†; Mundisal; Pansoral†; **Thai.:** Bonjela; **UK:** Bonjela; **USA:** Babee.

Cethexonium Bromide (2215-f)

Hexadecyl(2-hydroxycyclohexyl)dimethylammonium bromide.
$C_{24}H_{50}BrNO = 448.6$.
CAS — 6810-42-0 (cethexonium); 1794-74-7 (cethexonium bromide); 58703-78-9 (cethexonium chloride).

NOTE. Cethexonium Chloride is rINN.

Profile
Cethexonium bromide is a quaternary ammonium antiseptic with properties similar to those of other cationic surfactants (see Cetrimide, p.1137). It is used in preparations for the local treatment of minor infections of the eye, nose, and throat.

Preparations
Proprietary Preparations (details are given in Part 3)
Fr.: Biocidan.

Multi-ingredient: Fr.: Biocidan.

Cetrimide (2216-d)

Cetrimide (BAN, rINN).
Cetrimidum.
CAS — 1119-97-7 (trimethyltetradecylammonium bromide); 1119-94-4 (dodecyltrimethylammonium bromide); 8044-71-1 (cetrimide).
ATC — D08AJ04; D11AC01.

NOTE. The name cetrimonium bromide was often formerly applied to cetrimide. Cetrimonium bromide is hexadecyltrimethylammonium bromide.

Pharmacopoeias. In Eur. (see p.vi) and Int.

Incompatible with soaps and other anionic surfactants, bentonite, iodine, phenylmercuric nitrate, and alkali hydroxides. Aqueous solutions react with metals. The antimicrobial activity of quaternary ammonium compounds may be diminished through absorption, or through combination with organic matter, or by reducing pH.

Pharmacopoeial description

Ph. Eur.: Cetrimide consists of trimethyltetradecylammonium bromide and may contain smaller amounts of dodecyltrimethylammonium bromide and hexadecyltrimethylammonium bromide (= cetrimonium bromide, p.1137). A white or almost white, voluminous, free-flowing powder. Freely soluble in water and in alcohol; practically insoluble in ether. A 2.0% solution in water froths copiously when shaken.

BP 2001: Strong Cetrimide Solution is an aqueous solution of cetrimide. It contains 20 to 40% w/v of cetrimide, calculated as $C_{17}H_{38}BrN$ and up to 10% alcohol or isopropyl alcohol, or both; alcohol may be replaced by industrial methylated spirit. It may be perfumed and may contain colouring matter. Store at a temperature above 15°.

Adverse Effects and Treatment
At the concentrations used on the skin, solutions of cetrimide and other quaternary compounds do not generally cause irritation, but some patients become hypersensitive to cetrimide after repeated applications. Cetrimide powder is reported to be irritant. There have been rare reports of burns with concentrated solutions of cetrimide.

If ingested, cetrimide and other quaternary ammonium compounds cause nausea and vomiting; strong solutions may cause oesophageal damage and necrosis. They have depolarising muscle relaxant properties and toxic symptoms include dyspnoea and cyanosis due to paralysis of the respiratory muscles, possibly leading to asphyxia. Depression of the CNS (sometimes preceded by excitement and convulsions), hy-

potension, coma, and death may also occur. Accidental intra-uterine or intravenous administration may cause haemolysis.

Treatment of poisoning is symptomatic; demulcents may be given if necessary but emesis should be avoided, particularly if concentrated solutions have been ingested. Lavage may be considered if the patient presents within an hour of ingestion and if no burns are present in the mouth. CNS stimulants and cholinesterase inhibitors are reported not to reverse paralysis due to cetrimide intoxication although sympathomimetics have been tried. Corticosteroids may reduce oropharyngeal oedema.

Effects following cyst irrigation. Adverse effects following irrigation with cetrimide solutions in the treatment of hydatid cysts have included chemical peritonitis,[1] methaemoglobinaemia with cyanosis,[2] and metabolic acidosis.[3]

1. Gilchrist DS. Chemical peritonitis after cetrimide washout in hydatid-cyst surgery. Lancet 1979; **ii:** 1374.
2. Baraka A, et al. Cetrimide-induced methaemoglobinaemia after surgical excision of hydatid cyst. Lancet 1980; **ii:** 88–9.
3. Momblano P, et al. Metabolic acidosis induced by cetrimonium bromide. Lancet 1984; **ii:** 1045.

Poisoning. The fatal dose of quaternary ammonium compounds was estimated to be 1 to 3 g.[1]

1. Arena JM. Poisonings and other health hazards associated with use of detergents. JAMA 1964; **190:** 56–8.

Precautions
Prolonged and repeated applications of cetrimide to the skin are inadvisable as hypersensitivity may occur. Contact with the eyes, brain, meninges, and middle ear should be avoided. Cetrimide should not be used in body cavities or as an enema.

Quaternary ammonium compounds are not reliable agents for sterilising surgical instruments and heat-labile articles.

Solutions of quaternary ammonium compounds should not be used for disinfection of soft contact lenses.

Aqueous solutions of cetrimide or other quaternary ammonium disinfectants may be susceptible to contamination with micro-organisms. To reduce this risk, a sterilised preparation should be used or, where necessary, solutions must be freshly prepared at the recommended concentration and appropriate measures should be taken to prevent contamination during storage or dilution.

Handling. Cetrimide powder is irritant; it has been recommended that the nose and mouth should be protected by a mask when working with the powder[1] and eyes should be protected by goggles.

1. Jacobs JY. Work hazards from drug handling. Pharm J 1984; **233:** 195–6.

Uses and Administration
Cetrimide is a quaternary ammonium antiseptic with actions and uses typical of cationic surfactants. These surfactants dissociate in aqueous solution into a relatively large and complex cation, which is responsible for the surface activity, and a smaller inactive anion. In addition to emulsifying and detergent properties, quaternary ammonium compounds have bactericidal activity against Gram-positive and, at a higher concentration, against some Gram-negative bacteria. Some *Pseudomonas* spp. are particularly resistant as are strains of *Mycobacterium tuberculosis*. They are ineffective against bacterial spores, have variable antifungal activity, and are effective against some viruses.

Quaternary ammonium compounds are most effective in neutral or slightly alkaline solution and their bactericidal activity is appreciably reduced in acid media; their activity is enhanced by alcohols.

Like other quaternary ammonium compounds, notably benzalkonium chloride, cetrimide has been employed for cleansing skin, wounds (but see under Wound Disinfection, p.1130), and burns. For these purposes it has been used as a 0.1 to 1.0% aqueous solution, generally prepared by dilution of a more concentrated solution, or as a cream containing 0.5%.

However, a mixture of cetrimide with chlorhexidine (p.1138) has often been preferred to cetrimide alone. This combination is also used in a lotion for acne (p.1103).

Solutions containing up to 10% of cetrimide have been used as shampoos to remove the scales in seborrhoeic dermatitis (p.1107).

Cetrimide solution 0.5 or 1% has been used as a scolicide to irrigate hydatid cysts during surgery (see Echinococcosis, p.92) but systemic adverse effects have been reported (see above).

Cetrimide and benzalkonium chloride are also used as preservatives in cosmetics and pharmaceutical formulations including eye drops and in disinfecting solutions for hard contact lenses; neither compound should be used for disinfection of soft contact lenses.

Cetrimide is also present in some emulsifying preparations such as Cetrimide Emulsifying Ointment (BP 2001).

Preparations
BP 2001: Cetrimide Cream; Cetrimide Emulsifying Ointment; Cetrimide Solution.

Proprietary Preparations (details are given in Part 3)
Austral.: Acnederm Wash; **Canad.:** Resdan†; Savlon†; **Fr.:** Cetavlon; Septisept; **Irl.:** Cetavlex; Vesagex; **Israel:** Capillon; **Ital.:** Germozero Hospital†; **Neth.:** Cetavlon; **Port.:** Cetavlex; **S.Afr.:** Cetavlon; Wound-A-Sept; **Singapore:** Acnederm Wash; Cetavlex; **Spain:** Cetavlon; **UK:** Bactrian; Bansor; Cetavlex; Cradocap; Medi-Prep; Medicaid; Vesagex.

Multi-ingredient: Aust.: Lemocin; Xylonor; **Austral.:** Cetal Instrument Disinfectant†; Cross Prep†; Curacleanse; Dermocaine; Dimethicream; Formicare Skin Relief†; Hamilton Skin Repair; Hibicet; Medi Creme; Microshield Antiseptic; Pro-PS; Savlon Antiseptic; Soov Bite; Soov Burn; Soov Cream; **Belg.:** Lemocin; **Braz.:** Cetrilan; **Canad.:** Savlodil; Savlon; **Fr.:** Broncorinol rhinites; Buccawalter; Rectoquotane; **Hong Kong:** Borraginol-N; Drapolene; Hamilton Skin Repair; Hibicet Hospital Concentrate; Medicreme; Soov Bite; Tri-Gel; **Irl.:** Ceanel; Drapolene; Hibicet; RBC; Savlon; Siopel; Torbetol; **Israel:** Cetrin; Dermaor; Savior; Septacare; Tisept; Travasept; **Ital.:** Baxidin; Cetrexidin; Cetrisan; Cuprosodio; Farviceti; Hibicet; Hibizene; Iketoncid; Panseptil; Steridol; **Neth.:** Hibicet concentraat; Hibicet verdunning; **NZ:** Acnederm Wash; Dermocaine; Hibicet; Karicare Barrier Cream; Medicreme; Savlon; **Port.:** Friax†; Savlon; **S.Afr.:** Benzet; Bronchistop†; Burnocaine; Ceanel†; Hibicet; Medituss; Orocaine; Savlon; Siopel; Trochain; Virobis; **Singapore:** Burnol; Drapolene; Hibicet Hospital Concentrate; Savlon; Soov Bite; Soov Cream; **Spain:** Lidrone; **Thai.:** Bacard; Burnol Plus; Drapolene; Hibicet; Inhibac; Napilene; Septine; Septone; **UK:** Ceanel; Cetanorm; Cymex; Dermidex; Drapolene; Hibicet; Lypsyl Cold Sore Gel; Modantis; Neo; Quinoderm Antibacterial Face Wash; RBC; Savlon Concentrated Antiseptic; Savlon Cream; Siopel; Steripod Chlorhexidine Gluconate with Cetrimide; Tisept; Torbetol; Travasept; **USA:** Scadan.

Cetrimonium Bromide (16343-s)

Cetrimonium Bromide (rINN).
Cetyltrimethylammonium Bromide; CTAB. Hexadecyltrimethylammonium bromide.
$C_{19}H_{42}BrN = 364.4$.
CAS — 57-09-0 (cetrimonium bromide); 6899-10-1 (cetrimonium); 112-02-7 (cetrimonium chloride).

NOTE. Cetrimonium Chloride is BAN.
The name cetrimonium bromide was formerly applied to cetrimide.

Profile
Cetrimonium bromide is a quaternary ammonium antiseptic with actions and uses similar to those of other cationic surfactants (see Cetrimide, p.1137). Cetrimonium chloride and cetrimonium tosilate are also used.

Preparations
Proprietary Preparations (details are given in Part 3)
Belg.: Aseptiderm; **Braz.:** Tiracaspa; **Ital.:** Golaval; Neo-Intol†; Senol; **Switz.:** Turisan.

Multi-ingredient: Aust.: Xylestesin; **Belg.:** Cetavlex; HAC; Hacdil-S; **Braz.:** Amigdalol; Drapolene; Leucocida; **Canad.:** Bye Bye Burn†; Clearasil Sensitive Skin Cleanser†; **Fr.:** Eryteal; Nostril; **Ger.:** Lemocin; Xylestesin Pumpspray; **Ital.:** Aflogine†; Golamixin; Leucorsan†; Xylonor; **Spain:** Diformilitricina; Hongosan; Topicaina; Xylonor; **Switz.:** Desitur; Largal ultra†; Lemocin; Septivon N; Turexan Capilla; Xylestesin; Xylonor.

Cetyldimethylethylammonium Bromide
(18468-z)

Ethylhexadecyldimethylammonium bromide.
$C_{20}H_{44}BrN = 378.5$.

Profile
Cetyldimethylethylammonium bromide is a quaternary ammonium disinfectant with properties similar to those of other cati-

onic surfactants (see Cetrimide, p.1137). It has been used for the disinfection of instruments and hard surfaces.

Cetylpyridinium Chloride (2217-n)

Cetylpyridinium Chloride (BAN, rINN).

Cetylpyridinii Chloridum. 1-Hexadecylpyridinium chloride monohydrate.

$C_{21}H_{38}ClN,H_2O = 358.0$.

CAS — 7773-52-6 (cetylpyridinium); 123-03-5 (anhydrous cetylpyridinium chloride); 6004-24-6 (cetylpyridinium chloride, monohydrate).

Pharmacopoeias. In Eur. (see p.vi) and US.

Incompatible with soaps and other anionic surfactants.

Pharmacopoeial description

Ph. Eur.: A white powder, slightly soapy to the touch. Soluble in water, frothing copiously when shaken; soluble in alcohol; very slightly soluble in ether.

USP 25: A white powder with a slight characteristic odour. Soluble 1 in 4.5 of water and of chloroform, and 1 in 2.5 of alcohol; slightly soluble in ether and in benzene.

Profile

Cetylpyridinium chloride is a quaternary pyridinium antiseptic with actions and uses similar to those of other cationic surfactants (see Cetrimide, p.1137). It is used chiefly as lozenges or solutions for the treatment of minor infections of the mouth and throat. It is also used topically for the treatment of skin and eye infections.

Preparations

USP 25: Cetylpyridinium Chloride Lozenges; Cetylpyridinium Chloride Topical Solution.

Proprietary Preparations (details are given in Part 3)

Aust.: Dobendan; Halset; *Austral.:* Cepacol Antibacterial; Cepacol Mint; Cepacol Regular; Lemsip Lozenges; *Braz.:* Gargocetil; *Canad.:* Cepacol; Emereze Plus; Mouthwash; Rince Bouche Antiseptique; Throat Lozenges; *Fr.:* Cetylyre; Novoptine; *Ger.:* Dobendan; Frubizin; *Hong Kong:* Cepacol; *Irl.:* Merocets; *Israel:* Gargaron; *Ital.:* Alsol†; Bat; Borocaina Gola; Bronchenolo; Cetilsan; Exil; Farin Gola; Geyderm Sepsi; Golacetin; Herbagola; Johnson's Penaten Crema Disinfettante; Neo Coricidin Gola; Neo Formitrol; Ragaden; Sterinet; Stomygen; *Mex.:* Cepadyne; *Norw.:* Pyrisept; *NZ:* Cepacol; Lemsip Throat Lozenges; *Port.:* Septoral; *S.Afr.:* Cepacol; Denti Gum C†; Universal Throat Lollies; *Singapore:* Cepacol; *Spain:* Angifonil; *Thai.:* Cepacol; Orasept; *UK:* Merocets; Search†; *USA:* Cepacol Mouthwash; Scope.

Multi-ingredient: *Aust.:* Coldistan; Dentinox; Focusan†; Paididont; Riker Silicone-Spray†; Tetesept; Tyrosolvin†; *Austral.:* Actifed Anaesthetic†; Cepacaine; Cepacol Anaesthetic; Cepacol Cough and Sore Throat; Difflam Anti-Inflammatory Lozenges; Difflam Anti-Inflammatory Lozenges with Cough Suppressant; Difflam Mouth Gel; Duro-Tuss Cough Lozenges; Gentlees; *Braz.:* Alergotox Pastilhas; Cetildrops; Dentalivo; Eucament; Fenotricin; Filogargan; Forsalil; Gargotrat; Limao Bravo com Vitamina C; Malvol; Malvona; Pondicilina; Psiu; Tonsildrops; Xarope Valda; Xarope Vick; *Canad.:* Balminil Lozenges; Cepacol Citrus; Cepacol with Fluoride; Emercol; Emercreme No 4; Green Antiseptic Mouthwash & Gargle; Kank-A; Mouthrinse†; Mouthwash & Gargle†; Mouthwash Mint/Peppermint†; Oral Plan; Oral-B Anti-Bacterial with Fluoride; Scope; Throat Lozenges; *Fin.:* Bafucin; *Fr.:* Alodont; Broncorinol maux de gorge; *Ger.:* Bioget; Brand- und Wund-Gel Eu Rho; Broncho-Tyrosolvetten; Dolo-Dobendan; Dori; Em-eukal; Em-eukal forte; Frubienzym; Frubizin Forte; Imposit N; Nordathricin N; Psilo-Balsam N†; stas Halsschmerz-Tabletten; Tonsilase dolo†; Trachiform; Tussipect†; Tyrosolvetten; Tyrosolvetten-C; Tyrosur; Wick Sulagil; Wund- und Brand-Gel Eu Rho; *Hong Kong:* Dentinox Teething Gel; Pharynx; *Irl.:* AAA†; Anbesol; Listermint with Fluoride†; Merocaine; Vicks Original Cough Syrup for Chesty Coughs†; *Israel:* Cepadont; Kank-A; *Ital.:* Bo-Gum†; Cepral†; Delta 80 Plus; Ginvapast; Neo Cepacol Collutorio†; Neo Cepacol Pastiglie; Neo-Stomygen; Oral-B Collutorio per la Protezione di Denti e Gengive; Oraseptic Gola; Orosanyl; Ridiodent; Rikospray; Rinosil†; *Mex.:* Mentalgina; *Neth.:* Agre-Gola; *Norw.:* Aselli; *NZ:* Cepacaine; Cepacol Anaesthetic; Cepacol Cough; Difflam Anti-inflammatory Antibacterial Lozenges; Difflam Anti-inflammatory Cough Lozenges; Difflam Mouth Gel; Duro-Tuss Lozenges; Lenactin; *Port.:* Biofluor Sensitive; Dropcina; Mebocaina; *S.Afr.:* Cepacaine; Cepacol; Cepacol Cough Discs; Cetoxol†; Colphen; Denti Gum CF†; Medi-Keel A; Vagarsol; *Singapore:* Dentinox Teething Gel; Difflam Mouth Gel; Pharynx; *Spain:* Alcohocel; Alcohol Cetil; Alcohol Sanit Cune; Babysiton†; Capota†; Dequadin Complex; Farmalcohol; Noquemat†; Pastillas Antisep Garg L; Pastillas Antisep Garg M; Silidermil; Vicks Formula 44; Xylonibsa†; *Swed.:* Bafucin; *Switz.:* Alodont nouvelle formule; Angina MCC; Flavangin; Hextriletten; Lidazon; Mebucaine; Nasex; Neo-Angin Lido; Novomint N†; Otothricinol; Vicks Formel 44†; *Thai.:* Sentril; Sore Mouth Gel; *UAE:* B-Cool; *UK:* Adult Meltus for Chesty Coughs & Catarrh; Allens Dry Tickly Cough; Anbesol; Calgel; De Witt's Lozenges; Dentinox Teething Gel; Kilkof; Listermint; Listermint with Fluoride; Macleans Mouthguard; Meltus Expectorant; Merocaine; Merocet†; Merocets Plus; Oragard; Rinstead; Rinstead Teething Gel; Vicks Expectorant†; Woodwards Teething Gel; *USA:* Cepacol Anesthetic; Cepacol Maximum Strength Sore Throat; Cepacol Regular Strength; Cepacol Throat; Cylex; Massengill Disposable; MouthKote O/R; MouthKote P/R; Orajel Mouth Aid.

Chlorhexidine (12118-j)

Chlorhexidine (BAN, rINN).

CAS — 55-56-1.

ATC — A01AB03; B05CA02; D08AC02; D09AA12; R02AA05; S01AX09; S02AA09; S03AA04.

Chlorhexidine Acetate (2220-t)

Chlorhexidine Acetate (BANM, rINNM).

Chlorhexidine Diacetate; Chlorhexidini Diacetas. 1,1'-Hexamethylenebis[5-(4-chlorophenyl)biguanide] diacetate.

$C_{22}H_{30}Cl_2N_{10},2C_2H_4O_2 = 625.6$.

CAS — 56-95-1.

Pharmacopoeias. In Chin., Eur. (see p.vi), Int., and Pol.

Stability and incompatibilities are discussed under Chlorhexidine Hydrochloride, below.

Pharmacopoeial description

Ph. Eur.: A white or almost white, microcrystalline powder. Sparingly soluble in water; soluble in alcohol; slightly soluble in glycerol and in propylene glycol.

Chlorhexidine Gluconate (2221-x)

Chlorhexidine Gluconate (BANM, USAN, rINNM).

Chlorhexidine Digluconate. 1,1'-Hexamethylenebis[5-(4-chlorophenyl)biguanide] digluconate.

$C_{22}H_{30}Cl_2N_{10},2C_6H_{12}O_7 = 897.8$.

CAS — 18472-51-0.

Pharmacopoeias. Eur. (see p.vi), Pol., and US include a solution which contains 19 to 21% of chlorhexidine gluconate.

NOTE. Commercial 5% concentrate contains a nonionic surfactant to prevent precipitation on dilution with hard water and is not suitable for use in body cavities or for disinfection of instruments containing cemented glass components; dilutions of the 20% concentrate should be used for this purpose. Dilutions of commercial concentrated solutions may be sterilised by autoclaving.

Stability and incompatibilities are discussed under Chlorhexidine Hydrochloride, below.

Pharmacopoeial description

Ph. Eur.: Chlorhexidine Digluconate Solution is an aqueous solution which contains not less than 190 g per litre and not more than 210 g per litre of chlorhexidine gluconate. An almost colourless or pale-yellowish liquid. Miscible with water; soluble in alcohol and in acetone. A 5% v/v dilution in water has a pH of 5.5 to 7.0. Protect from light.

USP 25: Chlorhexidine Gluconate Solution is an aqueous solution which contains not less than 19% and not more than 21% of chlorhexidine gluconate. An almost colourless or pale yellow, clear liquid. Miscible with water and with glacial acetic acid; miscible with five times its volume of dehydrated alcohol and with three times its volume of acetone; further addition of dehydrated alcohol or of acetone yields a white turbidity. A 5% v/v dilution in water has a pH of 5.5 to 7.0. Protect from light.

Chlorhexidine Hydrochloride (2222-r)

Chlorhexidine Hydrochloride (BANM, USAN, rINNM).

AY-5312; Chlorhexidine Dihydrochloride; Chlorhexidini Dihydrochloridum. 1,1'-Hexamethylenebis[5-(4-chlorophenyl)biguanide] dihydrochloride.

$C_{22}H_{30}Cl_2N_{10},2HCl = 578.4$.

CAS — 3697-42-5.

Pharmacopoeias. In Eur. (see p.vi), Int., and Jpn.

Pharmacopoeial description

Ph. Eur.: A white or almost white, crystalline powder. Sparingly soluble in water and in propylene glycol; very slightly soluble in alcohol.

Incompatibility. Chlorhexidine salts are incompatible with soaps and other anionic materials. Activity may be reduced in the presence of suspending agents such as alginates and tragacanth, insoluble powders such as kaolin, and insoluble compounds of calcium, magnesium, and zinc. Chlorhexidine acetate is incompatible with potassium iodide. At a concentration of 0.05%, chlorhexidine salts are incompatible with borates, bicarbonates, carbonates, chlorides, citrates, nitrates, phosphates, and sulfates, forming salts of low solubility which may precipitate out of solution. At dilutions of 0.01% or more, these salts are generally soluble. Insoluble salts may form in hard water. Chlorhexidine salts are inactivated by cork.

References to incompatibilities of chlorhexidine with suspending agents and insoluble solids.[1-3]

1. McCarthy TJ. The influence of insoluble powders on preservatives in solution. *J Mond Pharm* 1969; **12**: 321–8.
2. Yousef RT, et al. Effect of some pharmaceutical materials on the bactericidal activities of preservatives. *Can J Pharm Sci* 1973; **8**: 54–6.
3. McCarthy TJ, Myburgh JA. The effect of tragacanth gel on preservative activity. *Pharm Weekbl* 1974; **109**: 265–8.

Stability. Chlorhexidine and its salts are stable at normal storage temperatures but when heated may decompose with the production of trace amounts of 4-chloroaniline. Chlorhexidine hydrochloride is less readily decomposed than chlorhexidine

acetate and may be heated at 150° for 1 hour without appreciable production of 4-chloroaniline. Aqueous solutions of chlorhexidine salts decompose with the formation of trace amounts of 4-chloroaniline. This decomposition is increased by heating and alkaline pH.

Washing precautions. Fabrics which have been in contact with chlorhexidine solution may develop a brown stain if bleached with a hypochlorite. A peroxide bleach may be used instead.

Adverse Effects and Treatment

Skin sensitivity to chlorhexidine has occasionally been reported. Strong solutions may cause irritation of the conjunctiva and other sensitive tissues. The use of chlorhexidine dental gel and mouthwash has been associated with reversible discoloration of the tongue, teeth, and silicate or composite restorations. Transient taste disturbances and a burning sensation of the tongue may occur on initial use. Oral desquamation and occasional parotid gland swelling have been reported with the mouthwash. If desquamation occurs, 50% dilution of the mouthwash with water and less vigorous rinsing may allow continued use.

The main consequence of ingestion is mucosal irritation and systemic toxicity is rare (see Poisoning, below). Haemolysis has been reported following accidental intravenous administration. Gastric lavage with demulcents has been suggested following acute ingestion.

Effects on the eyes. Report of 4 cases of corneal damage due to contact with chlorhexidine gluconate, that was being used for pre-operative preparation of facial skin.[1]

1. Tabor E, et al. Corneal damage due to eye contact with chlorhexidine gluconate. *JAMA* 1989; **261**: 557–8.

Effects on the nose. Temporary hyposmia (reduced sense of smell) in some patients after transsphenoidal pituitary adenoma operation was assumed to be caused by pre-operative disinfection of the nasal cavity with chlorhexidine gluconate solution.[1]

1. Yamagishi M, et al. Impairment of olfactory epithelium treated with chlorhexidine digluconate (Hibitane). *Pract Otol* 1985; **78**: 399–409.

Hypersensitivity. Severe hypersensitivity reactions including anaphylactic shock have been reported following topical applications of chlorhexidine,[1-4] and from the use of chlorhexidine-containing lubricants for urinary catheterisation or cystoscopy.[5] There is concern that similar reactions may occur with chlorhexidine-impregnated medical devices including intravenous catheters and implanted surgical mesh.[6] Occupational asthma has been attributed to an alcoholic chlorhexidine spray.[7]

1. Cheung J, O'Leary JJ. Allergic reaction to chlorhexidine in an anaesthetised patient. *Anaesth Intensive Care* 1985; **13**: 429–39.
2. Okano M, et al. Anaphylactic symptoms due to chlorhexidine gluconate. *Arch Dermatol* 1989; **125**: 50–2.
3. Evans RJ. Acute anaphylaxis due to topical chlorhexidine acetate. *BMJ* 1992; **304**: 686.
4. Chisholm DG, et al. Intranasal chlorhexidine resulting in an anaphylactic circulatory arrest. *BMJ* 1997; **315**: 785.
5. Visser LE, et al. Anafylaxie door chloorhexidine na cystoscopie of urethrale catheterisatie. *Ned Tijdschr Geneeskd* 1994; **138**: 778–80.
6. Anonymous. Hypersensitivity to chlorhexidine-impregnated medical devices. *JAMA* 1998; **279**: 1684.
7. Waclawski ER, et al. Occupational asthma in nurses caused by chlorhexidine and alcohol aerosols. *BMJ* 1989; **298**: 929–30.

Poisoning. Reports of adverse effects following ingestion of chlorhexidine salts include a neonate who developed multiple episodes of cyanosis and bradycardia;[1] the infant's mother had sprayed chlorhexidine onto her breasts to prevent mastitis. In contrast an 89-year-old woman only experienced mild giddiness, unusual laughter, and an increased appetite after mistakenly drinking 30 mL of a solution containing chlorhexidine gluconate 4% and isopropyl alcohol 4%.[2] There has also been a report of a patient who developed gastritis after ingesting a pre-operative skin preparation containing chlorhexidine gluconate 4% after using it as a mouthwash.[3] Another subject experienced much more serious effects in a suicide attempt after drinking about 150 mL of chlorhexidine gluconate solution, corresponding to about 30 g of the pure substance.[4] Besides pharyngeal oedema and necrotic oesophageal lesions, the patient had very high aminotransferase concentrations which rose to 30 times normal 5 days after ingestion and were still 8 times normal one week later. After one month the serum aspartate aminotransferase was returning to normal while the serum alanine aminotransferase was still 3 times normal. Six months after ingestion the aminotransferase levels were normal. A liver biopsy performed soon after the peak in aminotransferase levels showed diffuse fatty degeneration and lobular hepatitis suggesting that chlorhexidine was absorbed from the gastrointestinal tract in a concentration high enough to produce liver necrosis.

1. Quinn MW, Bini RM. Bradycardia associated with chlorhexidine spray. *Arch Dis Child* 1989; **64**: 892–3.
2. Emerson D, Pierce C. A case of a single ingestion of 4% Hibiclens. *Vet Hum Toxicol* 1988; **30**: 583.

3. Roche S, *et al.* Chlorhexidine-induced gastritis. *Postgrad Med J* 1991; **67:** 210–11.
4. Massano G, *et al.* Striking aminotransferase rise after chlorhexidine self-poisoning. *Lancet* 1982; **i:** 289.

Precautions

Since chlorhexidine is irritant it is recommended that it should not be used on the brain, meninges, middle ear, or other sensitive tissues. Contact with the eye should be avoided except for dilute solutions expressly for use in the eyes. Chlorhexidine may be adsorbed by some soft contact lenses and cause eye irritation, although it may be suitable for use with others (see Contact Lens Care, p.1129). Syringes and needles that have been immersed in chlorhexidine solutions should be thoroughly rinsed with sterile water or saline before use.

Aqueous solutions of chlorhexidine salts may be susceptible to contamination with micro-organisms. To reduce this risk, a sterilised preparation should be used or, where necessary, solutions must be freshly prepared at the recommended concentration and appropriate measures should be taken to prevent contamination during storage or dilution.

Aqueous solutions of chlorhexidine used for instrument storage should contain sodium nitrite 0.1% to inhibit metal corrosion, and should be changed every 7 days.

Contamination. *Ralstonia pickettii* (*Burkholderia pickettii*; *Pseudomonas pickettii*) septicaemia developed in 6 patients following the use of aqueous chlorhexidine 0.05%, prepared with contaminated twice-distilled water, for skin disinfection prior to venepuncture and it was considered that unsterilised 0.05% solutions should not be used for such skin preparation.[1] Positive blood cultures of *Burkholderia cepacia* (*Pseudomonas cepacia*) were found in 2 patients following inappropriate use of a chlorhexidine handwash for the same purpose.[2] Further studies showed that the handwash supported pseudomonal growth only when diluted.[3]

1. Kahan A, *et al.* Is chlorhexidine an essential drug? *Lancet* 1984; **ii:** 759–60.
2. Gosden PE, Norman P. Pseudobacteraemia associated with contaminated skin cleansing agent. *Lancet* 1985; **ii** 671–2.
3. Norman P, *et al.* Pseudobacteraemia associated with contaminated skin cleansing agent. *Lancet* 1986; **i:** 209.

Neonates. Haemorrhagic skin necrosis associated with umbilical artery catheterisation in extremely preterm infants was attributed to damage by the alcohol from the use of chlorhexidine 0.5% in spirit 70% as a disinfectant.[1]

For reference to the percutaneous absorption of chlorhexidine following topical use in neonates and infants, see Pharmacokinetics, below.

1. Rutter N. Percutaneous alcohol absorption and skin necrosis in a preterm infant. *Arch Dis Child* 1983; **58:** 396.

Oral hygiene. As toothpastes may contain anionic surfactants such as sodium laurilsulfate, which are incompatible with chlorhexidine, it has been recommended that at least 30 minutes should be allowed to elapse between the use of toothpaste and oral chlorhexidine preparations.[1]

1. Barkvoll P, *et al.* Interaction between chlorhexidine digluconate and sodium lauryl sulfate in vivo. *J Clin Periodontol* 1989; **16:** 593–5.

Pharmacokinetics

Chlorhexidine is poorly absorbed from the gastrointestinal tract and skin.

Neonates. Occasional reports of the percutaneous absorption of chlorhexidine in neonates and infants include a study in which chlorhexidine was detected in low concentrations in the venous blood of 5 of 24 infants after washing them with a preparation containing chlorhexidine gluconate 4% (Hibiscrub); no adverse effects were observed.[1] Low concentrations have been found in the venous blood of neonates following the topical use of a powder containing chlorhexidine 1%.[2] Percutaneous absorption of chlorhexidine was reported in preterm neonates (but not full-term infants) treated with chlorhexidine 1% in alcohol for neonatal cord care; no such absorption occurred when a dusting powder containing chlorhexidine 1% and zinc oxide 3% was used.[3]

1. Cowen J, *et al.* Absorption of chlorhexidine from the intact skin of newborn infants. *Arch Dis Child* 1979; **54:** 379–83.
2. Alder VG, *et al.* Comparison of hexachlorophane and chlorhexidine powders in prevention of neonatal infection. *Arch Dis Child* 1980; **55:** 277–80.
3. Aggett PJ, *et al.* Percutaneous absorption of chlorhexidine in neonatal cord care. *Arch Dis Child* 1981; **56:** 878–91.

Uses and Administration

Chlorhexidine is a bisbiguanide antiseptic and disinfectant which is bactericidal or bacteriostatic against a wide range of Gram-positive and Gram-negative bacteria. It is more effective against Gram-positive

than Gram-negative bacteria, and some species of *Pseudomonas* and *Proteus* have low susceptibility. It is relatively ineffective against mycobacteria. Chlorhexidine inhibits some viruses and is active against some fungi. It is inactive against bacterial spores at room temperature. Chlorhexidine is most active at a neutral or slightly acid pH. Combinations of chlorhexidine with cetrimide (p.1137) or in alcoholic solution are used to enhance the efficacy.

Chlorhexidine is formulated as lotions, washes, and creams for disinfection and cleansing of skin and wounds (p.1108), and as oral gels, sprays, and mouthwashes for mouth infections including candidiasis and to reduce dental plaque accumulation. It has also been used in combination with neomycin to eliminate nasal carriage of staphylococci (p.140) and for disinfection of some contact lenses (but see Precautions, above). It has been suggested for use for the treatment of Acanthamoeba keratitis in combination with propamidine isetionate and in spermicides to prevent transmission of HIV infection (p.610).

For pre-operative skin disinfection and hand-washing, chlorhexidine is used as a 0.5% solution of the acetate or gluconate in alcohol (70%) or as a 2 or 4% detergent solution of the gluconate. For disinfection of wounds, burns, or other skin damage or disorders chlorhexidine is used as a 0.05% aqueous solution of the acetate or gluconate, as a tulle dressing impregnated with chlorhexidine acetate 0.5%, or as a cream or powder containing chlorhexidine acetate or gluconate 1%. Preparations containing chlorhexidine acetate or gluconate 0.015% and cetrimide 0.15% are also used for cleansing and disinfection of skin and wounds. In obstetrics, chlorhexidine gluconate is used as a 0.05% aqueous solution or a 1% cream. The cream is also used as a barrier against bacterial hand infection.

Chlorhexidine gluconate is used in a 1% dental gel, 0.2% oral spray, and 0.1 to 0.2% mouthwash for the prevention of plaque and the prevention and treatment of gingivitis and in the treatment of oral candidiasis. A slow-release formulation for insertion into periodontal pockets is also available.

A 0.02% solution may be used as a bladder irrigation in some urinary-tract infections. A gel containing 0.25% chlorhexidine gluconate solution and lignocaine [lidocaine] hydrochloride has been used in catheterisation and cystoscopy.

For the emergency disinfection of clean instruments a 2-minute immersion in chlorhexidine acetate or gluconate 0.5% in alcohol (70%) is used; for the storage and disinfection of clean instruments a 30-minute immersion in a 0.05% aqueous solution containing 0.1% sodium nitrite to inhibit metal corrosion is used.

As an antimicrobial preservative, chlorhexidine is used at a concentration of 0.01% of the acetate or gluconate in eye drops. Solutions containing 0.002 to 0.006% of chlorhexidine gluconate have also been used for disinfection of hydrophilic contact lenses.

Acanthamoeba infections. As discussed on p.582, the optimal antiamoebic therapy for *Acanthamoeba* keratitis has yet to be determined. Propamidine isetionate is commonly used, usually in combinations including a biguanide. Chlorhexidine gluconate 0.02% with propamidine isetionate 0.1% has been suggested.[1] However, concern has been expressed over the possible toxicity of chlorhexidine at this concentration on the cornea.[2]

Chlorhexidine is also an effective disinfectant against *Acanthamoeba* cysts and most bacteria found in contact lens storage cases.[1]

Chlorhexidine has also been used to treat skin lesions associated with disseminated *Acanthamoeba* infection[3] as an adjunct to systemic therapy (see p.582).

1. Seal DV. Acanthamoeba keratitis. *BMJ* 1994; **308:** 1116–17.
2. Elder MJ, Dart JKG. Chemotherapy for acanthamoeba keratitis. *Lancet* 1995; **345:** 791–2.
3. Slater CA, *et al.* Brief report: successful treatment of disseminated Acanthamoeba infection in an immunocompromised patient. *N Engl J Med* 1994; **331:** 85–7.

Contraception. Bisbiguanides of the chlorhexidine type are reported to have the ability to diffuse into cervical mucus and render it impenetrable to sperm at concentrations as low as 1 mg per mL.[1] Higher concentrations of chlorhexidine structurally modify the mucus, producing a barrier to both the entry of sperm and chlorhexidine. The potency[1] of chlorhexidine in in-

hibiting sperm motility *in vitro* is identical to that of nonoxinol 9, but unlike spermicides containing nonoxinol 9, which tend to trickle out, the clearance of chlorhexidine from the vagina is delayed.[2] Chlorhexidine also has potential for reducing transmission of HIV infection as it does not disrupt the vaginal epithelium and has activity *in vitro* against the HIV virus in low concentrations.[2]

For a review of contraception, including the view that spermicides are not a particularly effective method unless combined with other means of contraception, see p.1460.

1. Pearson RM. Update on vaginal spermicides. *Pharm J* 1985; **234:** 686–7.
2. Anonymous. Multipurpose spermicides. *Lancet* 1992; **340:** 211–13.

Disinfection. Viable bacterial counts on the hands were reduced by a mean of 97.9% by the application of chlorhexidine gluconate 0.5% in alcohol 95%.[1] The reduction was not so substantial with a 0.5% chlorhexidine aqueous solution (65.1% reduction in bacterial count) or a 4% detergent solution (86.7%). Hand disinfection with chlorhexidine gluconate 4% appeared to be more effective than the use of isopropyl alcohol 60% and soap in preventing nosocomial infections in a study conducted in intensive care units but this may have been partly due to better compliance with hand-washing instructions when using chlorhexidine.[2] In another study,[3] pre-operative total body bathing with a 4% detergent did not decrease the risk of wound infection in patients compared with bathing in detergent alone. Chlorhexidine 1% nasal cream failed to control an epidemic of meticillin-resistant *Staphylococcus aureus* in a neurosurgical ward[4] and handwashing with chlorhexidine soap failed to control an outbreak of infection with *Staph. aureus* resistant to meticillin and gentamicin in a neonatal intensive care unit.[5] The organisms were subsequently eradicated by the use of nasal mupirocin and hexachlorophene handwashing, respectively.

1. Lowbury EJL, *et al.* Preoperative disinfection of surgeons' hands: use of alcoholic solutions and effects of gloves on skin flora. *BMJ* 1974; **4:** 369–72.
2. Doebbeling BN, *et al.* Comparative efficacy of alternative hand-washing agents in reducing nosocomial infections in intensive care units. *N Engl J Med* 1992; **327:** 88–93.
3. The European Working Party on Control of Hospital Infections. A comparison of the effects of preoperative whole-body bathing with detergent alone and with detergent containing chlorhexidine gluconate on the frequency of wound infections after clean surgery. *J Hosp Infect* 1988; **11:** 310–20.
4. Duckworth G. New method for typing Staphylococcus aureus resistant to meticillin. *BMJ* 1986; **293:** 885.
5. Reboli AC, *et al.* Epidemic meticillin-gentamicin-resistant Staphylococcus aureus in a neonatal intensive care unit. *Am J Dis Child* 1989; **143:** 34–9.

INJECTION SITE AND CATHETER CARE. See p.1130.

Endocarditis. Antiseptics applied immediately before dental procedures may reduce postextraction bacteraemia. Chlorhexidine mouthwash or gel may be used as an adjunct to antibacterial prophylaxis in dental patients at risk of bacterial endocarditis.[1,2] The protective cover required for such patients is discussed in detail on p.119.

1. Dajani AS, *et al.* Prevention of bacterial endocarditis: recommendations by the American Heart Association. *JAMA* 1997; **277:** 1794–1801.
2. Simmons NA, *et al.* Antibiotic prophylaxis and infective endocarditis. *Lancet* 1992; **339:** 1292–3.

Mouth disorders. Chlorhexidine mouthwashes, sprays, and gels are used to prevent accumulation of dental plaque (see Mouth Infections, p.130). Studies have generally shown chlorhexidine mouthwash 0.1% to 0.2% used 2 or 3 times daily to be effective in reducing plaque accumulation and gingivitis,[1-4] and to be superior to other disinfectant mouthwashes.[5] Its effect against subgingival plaque bacteria is enhanced by phenoxyethanol.[6] However, a 1% gel used nightly as a toothpaste was not more effective than placebo in reducing gingivitis in children.[7] Other studies have shown that chlorhexidine reduces gingivitis by 60 to 90% but its use is limited by its unpleasant taste and staining properties; special circumstances in which chlorhexidine is helpful include management of acute gingivitis, control of periodontal involvement in immunocompromised patients, and promotion of healing after periodontal treatment.[8]

Chlorhexidine gluconate may be useful in controlling secondary bacterial infections of aphthous ulcers (see Mouth Ulceration, p.1206). Local application of chlorhexidine has been reported to reduce the incidence[9] and duration and severity[10] of recurrent ulcers, although one study showed no benefit compared with placebo.[11]

Chlorhexidine may be a useful adjunct to antifungal treatment of oral candidiasis[12] (p.372).

For the need for a delay when using chlorhexidine with other oral hygiene preparations, see under Precautions, above.

1. Flötra L, *et al.* A 4-month study on the effect of chlorhexidine mouth washes on 50 soldiers. *Scand J Dent Res* 1972; **80:** 10–17.
2. O'Neil TCA, Figures KH. The effects of chlorhexidine and mechanical methods of plaque control on the recurrence of gingival hyperplasia in young patients taking phenytoin. *Br Dent J* 1982; **152:** 130–3.
3. de la Rosa M, *et al.* The use of chlorhexidine in the management of gingivitis in children. *J Periodontol* 1988; **59:** 387–9.
4. O'Neil TCA. The use of chlorhexidine mouthwash in the control of gingival inflammation. *Br Dent J* 1976; **141:** 276–80.
5. Breex M, *et al.* Efficacy of Listerine, Meridol and chlorhexidine mouthrinses on plaque, gingivitis and plaque bacteria vitality. *J Clin Periodontol* 1990; **17:** 292–7.

The symbol † denotes a preparation no longer actively marketed

6. Wilson M, *et al.* Effect of phenoxyethanol, chlorhexidine and their combination on subgingival plaque bacteria. *J Antimicrob Chemother* 1990; **25:** 921–9.
7. Hoyos DF, *et al.* The effect of chlorhexidine gel on plaque and gingivitis in children. *Br Dent J* 1977; **142:** 366–9.
8. Greene JC, *et al.* Preventive dentistry II: periodontal diseases, malocclusion, trauma, and oral cancer. *JAMA* 1990; **263:** 421–5.
9. Hunter L, Addy M. Chlorhexidine gluconate mouthwash in the management of minor aphthous ulceration. *Br Dent J* 1987; **162:** 106–10.
10. Addy M, *et al.* Management of recurrent aphthous ulceration: a trial of chlorhexidine gluconate gel. *Br Dent J* 1976; **141:** 118–20.
11. Matthews RW, *et al.* Clinical evaluation of benzydamine, chlorhexidine, and placebo mouthwashes in the management of recurrent aphthous stomatitis. *Oral Surg Oral Med Oral Pathol* 1987; **63:** 189–91.
12. WHO. *WHO model prescribing information: drugs used in skin diseases.* Geneva: WHO, 1997.

Obstetric use. Cleansing of the birth canal with chlorhexidine gluconate 0.25% has not been shown to reduce perinatal transmission of HIV except when membranes were ruptured for more than 4 hours before delivery,[1] although it has been reported to reduce neonatal morbidity and mortality from other neonatal infections in Africa.[2] In Swedish hospitals, flushing the vagina every 6 hours during labour with chlorhexidine acetate 0.2% reduced the incidence of transmission of group B streptococci but a reduction in neonatal morbidity was not demonstrated.[3,4] Comparable results have been reported with the use of chlorhexidine gluconate 1% obstetric cream at each examination during labour.[5]

1. Biggar RJ, *et al.* Perinatal intervention trial in Africa: effect of a birth canal cleansing intervention to prevent HIV transmission. *Lancet* 1996; **347:** 1647–50.
2. Taha TE, *et al.* Effect of cleansing the birth canal with antiseptic solution on maternal and newborn morbidity and mortality in Malawi: clinical trial. *BMJ* 1997; **315:** 216–20.
3. Burman LG, *et al.* Prevention of excess neonatal morbidity associated with group B streptococci by vaginal chlorhexidine disinfection during labour. *Lancet* 1992; **340:** 65–9.
4. Burman LG, Tullus K. Vaginal chlorhexidine disinfection during labour. *Lancet* 1992; **340:** 791–2.
5. Lindemann R, *et al.* Vaginal chlorhexidine disinfection during labour. *Lancet* 1992; **340:** 792.

Peritoneal dialysis. The addition of chlorhexidine to ambulatory dialysis fluid containing high concentrations of chloride ions was not recommended as precipitation of chlorhexidine was likely.[1] In contrast, lavage with aqueous solutions of chlorhexidine had been shown to be both acceptable and very effective for controlling peritoneal sepsis.

1. Denton GW. Chlorhexidine: a WHO essential drug. *Lancet* 1984; **ii:** 517.

Urinary-tract infection. Chlorhexidine solutions have been used in the management of catheter-related bladder infections and for urinary catheter maintenance. Twice-daily bladder irrigation with chlorhexidine acetate 0.02% did not produce a reduction in urinary bacterial counts in geriatric patients with indwelling catheters, and there was a tendency for overgrowth of *Proteus* spp. in patients given chlorhexidine.[1] In patients undergoing prostatectomy, intermittent pre-operative bladder irrigation with chlorhexidine gluconate 0.05% reduced the incidence of bacteraemia and severe wound infection although urinary infections were eradicated in only 3 of the 13 patients treated.[2] Addition of chlorhexidine to catheter drainage bags was not shown to reduce the frequency of urinary infections[3] but infection rates were reduced by combining this technique with the use of a catheter lubricant containing chlorhexidine, disinfection of the urethral meatus, and aseptic nursing procedures.[4] The use of lubricating gel containing chlorhexidine did not reduce the risk of urinary-tract infections associated with short-term catheterisation.[5]

The treatment of urinary-tract infections is discussed on p.146.

1. Davies AJ, *et al.* Does instillation of chlorhexidine into the bladder of catheterized geriatric patients help reduce bacteriuria? *J Hosp Infect* 1987; **9:** 72–5.
2. Adesanya AA, *et al.* The use of intermittent chlorhexidine bladder irrigation in the prevention of post-prostatectomy infective complications. *Int Urol Nephrol* 1993; **25:** 359–67.
3. Gillespie WA, *et al.* Does the addition of disinfectant to urine drainage bags prevent infection in catheterised patients? *Lancet* 1983; **i:** 1037–9.
4. Southampton Infection Control Team. Evaluation of aseptic techniques and chlorhexidine on the rate of catheter-associated urinary-tract infection. *Lancet* 1982; **i:** 89–91.
5. Schiøtz HA. Antiseptic catheter gel and urinary tract infection after short-term postoperative catheterization in women. *Arch Gynecol Obstet* 1996; **258:** 97–100.

Preparations

BP 2001: Chlorhexidine Irrigation Solution; Chlorhexidine Mouthwash; Lidocaine and Chlorhexidine Gel;
USP 25: Chlorhexidine Gluconate Oral Rinse.

Proprietary Preparations (details are given in Part 3)
Aust.: Angisan†; Chlorhexamed; Hexidin; Hibident; Kleenocid; Plak Out; Vitawund; *Austral.:* Anti-Plaque Chewing Gum; Bactigras; Bush Formula; Catheter Preparation; CX Powder†; Clorhexitulle; Hexol; Hibiclens; Hibitane; Microshield 2, 4, 5, and 20; Novaclens†; Novacol†; Novatane†; Periogard Chlorohex; Plaqacide; Savacol Mouth and Throat Rinse; Trisdine†; *Belg.:* Astrexine; Corsodyl; Hibident†; Hibidil; Hibiguard; Hibiscrub; Hibitane; Mefren Solution; Mefren Pastilles; Pixidin; Sterilon; Uro-Tainer; *Braz.:* Hibitane; *Canad.:* Bactigras; Baxedin†; Chlorhexsepti†; Hibidil; Hibitane; Oro-Clense; Peridex; Rouhex-G; Spectro Gram; Stanhexidine; *Denm.:* Hibitane; *Fin.:* Corsodyl; Hibiscrub; Klorhexol; Travahex; *Fr.:* Bucasept; Collunovar; Corsodyl; D-Seb; Diaseptyl; Dosiseptine; Elgydium; Elugel; Exoseptoplix; Hibidil;

Hibiscrub; Hibisprint; Hibitane; Lysofon; Merfene; Pareox; Plurexid; Prexidine; Septeal; *Ger.:* Bactigras; Cathejell S; Chlorhexamed; CHX Dental Gel; Cidegol C; Corsodyl; Frubilurgyl; Gurgellosung Chauvin; Hansamed Spray; Lemocin CX; Mentopin Gurgellosung†; Nur 1 Tropfen Chlorhexidin; Periogard Chlorohex; *Hong Kong:* Bactigras; Corsodyl; Hexol; Hibiscrub; Hibitane; Hydrex; *Irl.:* Corsodyl; Hibiscrub; Hibitane; Hydrex; Rotersept†; *Israel:* Alcoxidine; Bactoscrub; Bactosept; Corsodyl; Medident; Medipe; Perio Chip; Periodentix; Septal; Septalone; Septol; Tarodent; Uniscrub; Unisept; *Ital.:* Benodent CLX; Broxodin; Clorexident†; Clorosan; Contact†; Corsodyl; D-Seb; Dempol; Dentosan Clorexidina; Dentosan Parodontale; Eburos; Effetre; Ekuba; Esoform Mani; Germozero Hospital†; Golasan; Golasol; Hibiscrub; Lenil; Lenixil†; Lyasin†; N32 Collutorio; Neomercurochromo; Neoxene; Neoxinal; Odontoxina; Oralsan; Periogard Chlorohex; Plak; Plak Out; Sanoral; Triseptil; Vaxidina†; *Mex.:* Hibiscrub; *Neth.:* Corsodyl; Hibident†; Hibigel†; Hibiscrub; Hibitane; Roter Keel†; Sterilon; Urogliss-S; *Norw.:* Corsodyl; Hexidin†; Hibiscrub; Hibitane; *NZ:* Hibiclens; Hibitane; Port.: Chlorohex†; Corsodyl; Dialens; Hibiscrub; Hibitane; Periogard Chlorohex†; Plak Out; *S.Afr.:* Bactigras; Hibidil; Hibiscrub; Hibitane; Orosept; *Singapore:* Chlorohex; Hibiscrub; Hibitane; *Spain:* Antisept; Clorxil; Cristalcrom; Cristalmina; Curafil; Cuvefilm; Deratin; Hibimax; Hibiscrub; Menalmina; Odol Med Dental†; Septisan; Sterilon†; *Swed.:* Cervitec; Corsodyl; Descutan; Hibiscrub; Hibitane; *Switz.:* Chlorhexamed; Chlorohex; Collunovar†; Corsodyl; Dentohexine; Hibidil; Hibiscrub; Hibitane; Lifo-Scrub; *Thai.:* Bacard Antiseptic; Bactigras; C-20; Desmanol G; Hexene; Hexide; Hexol; Hibiscrub; Hibitane; Hidine; Hydrex; *UK:* Acriflex; Bactigras; Cepton; Chlorasept; Chlorohex; Chlorhexitulle†; Corsodyl; CX Powder; Elgydium; Hibiscrub; Hibitane; Hydrex; Periochip; pHiso-MED; Savlon Wound Wash; Serotulle; Spotoway; Sterets Unisept; Sterexidine; Steripod Chlorhexidine Gluconate; Uniscrub; Uriflex C; *USA:* Betasept; Biopatch†; Dyna-Hex; Exidine; Hibiclens; Hibistat; Peridex; Periochip; Periogard.

Multi-ingredient: *Aust.:* Bepanthen Plus; Cathejell; Cathejell mit Lidocain; Dermaspray; Endosgel; Hermasept†; Instillagel; Salbei-Halspastillen; Uromont; Vitawund; *Austral.:* Body Lotion; Cetal Instrument Disinfectant†; Cleansing Lotion; Cross Prep†; Curacleanse; Difflam-C; Egomycol; Hemocane; Hexidin†; Hibicet; Hibicol; Hibitane; Medi Creme; Medi Pulv; Microshield Antiseptic; Microshield Handrub; Microshield Tincture; Mycil; Nasalate; Oralife Peppermint; Paraderm Plus; Pro-PS; Savlon Antiseptic; Silvazine; Soov Cream; Xylocaine Jelly with Chlorhexidine; *Belg.:* Angiocine; Cetavlex; Dermaspray; HAC; Hacdil-S; Hibitane; Medica; Neo-Cutigenol; Neo-Golaseptine; Nestosyl; Sedasept; Vita-Mefren; *Braz.:* Flex-Care; Topidexa; *Canad.:* Clearasil Sensitive Skin Cleanser†; Flamazine C; Ic-Gel; Savlodil; Savlon; Spectro Tar; *Denm.:* Hexokain; Instillagel; Xylocain Klorhexidin; *Fin.:* Citanest; Dexatopic; Duocort; Sibicort; Toncils; *Fr.:* Amygdol; Antalyre; Aphtoral; Biseptine; Cantalene; Chlorispray; Collunosol†; Collupressine; Collustan; Cyteal; Dacryne; Dacryoseptil; Dermaspray; Dermobacter; Desocort†; Dontopivalone†; Drill; Eludril; Isodril†; Lysofon; Mercryl; Nostril; Parodium; Posine; Sophtal; Spitaderm; Thiovalone; Visiodose; *Ger.:* Cathejell; Desmanol; Endosgel; Hermalind; Hexoraletten N; Instillagel; Nystalocal; Skinman Intensiv†; Skinsept F; Skinsept mucosa; Trachisan; Uro-Stilloson; *Hong Kong:* Difflam-C; Hibicet Hospital Concentrate; Hibisol; Instillagel; Medicreme; Medipulv; Norgotin; *Irl.:* Alltracel S; Germolene First Aid; Hibicet; Hibisol; Mycil; Naseptin; Nystaform; Nystaform-HC; Savlon; *Israel:* Bepanthen Plus; Cathejell; Cetrin; Dermaor; Hexidin; Instillagel; Savior; Septacare; Septadine; Sterets H; Tisept; Travasept; Vita-Merfen NF; *Ital.:* Anadermin; Baxidin; Benodent; Cetrexidin; Cetrisan; Citrosteril Pronto; Clorexan; Clorexan Ferri; Clorexident Ortodontico†; Dentaton Antisettico; Dentosan Azione Intensiva; Dentosan Mese; Dentosan Placca & Carie; Eso Ferri Plus; Eso S 80; Esoform Maniferri†; Esosan Pronto; Farvicett; Handexin; Hibicet; Hibisept; Jalovis†; Larilon; Levaknel†; Medical Pic; Neo-Destomygen; Panseptil; PR 100-Cloressidina; Rexichlor; Simp; Simpottantacinque; Spitaderm; Steridol; Videorelax; *Mon.:* Akila mains et peau†; *Neth.:* Dexatopic†; Hibicet concentraat; Hibicet verdunning; Hibisol; Urogliss; *Norw.:* Bacimycin; Citanest; *NZ:* Acnederm Wash; Difflam-C; Egomycol; Hibicet; Medicreme; Medipulv; Oralife Peppermint; Savlon; Silvazine; Xylocaine with Chlorhexidine; *Port.:* Bepanthene; Bepanthene Plus; Biofluor; Cyteal; Drill; Eludril; Hibitane; Savlon; *S.Afr.:* Andolex-C; Burnocaine; Dermoswab†; Hibicet; Naseptin; Orochlor; Savlon; *Singapore:* Cyteal; Difflam-C; Eludril; Hibicet Hospital Concentrate; Hibisol; Oral-Aid; Savlon; Silvazine; Soov Cream; Trachisan; *Spain:* Angileptol; Antirrinum; Bucodrin; Bucometasana; Bucospray; Cloraseptic; Drill; Eludril; Faringesic; Garydol; Hibitane; Mastiol; Menalcol; Salvesept; *Swed.:* Instillagel; *Switz.:* Adro-derm; Antebor N; Bepanthene Plus; Cathejell-N†; Collu-Blache; Collunosol-N; Demosept; Eludril; Endosgel†; Eubucal; Galamila; Gleitmittel; Hibital; Instillagel†; Kamillosan†; Lidohex†; Merfen; Neo-Urtisan†; Nystacortone; Nystalocal; Rexophtal; Rhinipan†; Secalan†; Trachisan†; Vita-Hexin; Vita-Merfen; *Thai.:* Bacard; Cathejell with Lidocaine; Hibicet; Hibimax; Sepdine; Septone; *UK:* Cathejell with Lidocaine; Clearasil Medicated Lotion; Dermol; Eludril; Germolene; Germoloids; Hibicet; Hibisol; Instillagel; Medi-Swab H; Medi-Wipe; Mycil; Naseptin; Nystaform; Nystaform-HC; Primahex; Quinoderm Antibacterial Face Wash; Savlon Concentrated Antiseptic; Savlon Cream; Sterets H; Steripod Chlorhexidine Gluconate with Cetrimide; Tisept; Torbetol; Travasept; Xylocaine Antiseptic; *USA:* BactoShield.

Chlorinated Lime (2223-f)

Bleaching Powder; Cal Clorada; Calcaria Chlorata; Calcii Hypochloris; Calcium Hypochlorite; Calcium Hypochlorosum; Calx Chlorata; Calx Chlorinata; Chloride of Lime; Chlorkalk; Chlorure de Chaux; Cloruro de Cal.

CAS — 7778-54-3.

Pharmacopoeias. In *Br.*, *Chin.*, *Jpn*, and *Swiss.*

Pharmacopoeial description

BP 2001: A dull white powder with a characteristic odour, containing not less than 30.0% w/w of 'available chlorine'. It becomes moist and gradually decomposes on exposure to air, carbon dioxide being absorbed and chlorine evolved. Partly soluble in water and in alcohol.

Adverse Effects, Treatment, and Precautions
As for Sodium Hypochlorite, p.1156.

Uses and Administration
Chlorinated lime is a disinfectant and antiseptic with the general properties of chlorine (p.1140).

Its action is rapid but brief, the 'available chlorine' soon being exhausted by combination with organic material. It is used to disinfect faeces, urine, and other organic material, and as a cleansing agent for lavatories, drains, and effluents.

Chlorinated lime is used in the preparation of Surgical Chlorinated Soda Solution (BPC 1973) (Dakin's Solution) which has been employed as a wound disinfectant, and Chlorinated Lime and Boric Acid Solution (BP 1993), (Eusol), which has been used as a disinfectant lotion and wet dressing, sometimes with equal parts of liquid paraffin. However, such solutions are irritant when applied undiluted, and are no longer recommended for use in this way. In addition, there is some evidence that such chlorine-releasing solutions may delay wound healing (see Disinfection, Wounds under Uses and Administration of Chlorine, p.1141).

Preparations

BPC 1973: Surgical Chlorinated Soda Solution;
BP 1993: Chlorinated Lime and Boric Acid Solution.

Chlorine (2224-d)

925; 926 (chlorine dioxide).
$Cl_2 = 70.906$.
CAS — 7782-50-5.

A greenish-yellow gas with a suffocating odour; commonly available as a pressurised liquid.

Adverse Effects and Treatment

Chlorine gas is irritant and corrosive producing inflammation, burns, and necrosis. Inhalation may result in coughing, choking, headache, dyspnoea, dizziness, expectoration of frothy white sputum (which may be blood stained), a burning chest pain, and nausea. Bronchospasm, laryngeal oedema, acute pulmonary oedema with cyanosis, and hypoxia may occur. There may be vomiting and development of acidosis. Death may result from hypoxia.

Some of the toxicity of chlorine may be due to its dissolution in tissue water to produce hydrochloric acid and hypochlorite. Following exposure to chlorine, conjunctivitis may require a topical anaesthetic and frequent irrigations of water or saline. Respiratory distress should be treated with inhalations of humidified oxygen and bronchodilators; mechanical ventilation may be required. Corticosteroids have been given in an attempt to minimise pulmonary damage. Acidosis may require the intravenous use of sodium bicarbonate or other suitable alkalising agent.

◊ Experience gained from 186 cases of acute chlorine exposure indicated that medical support was required for only a short time even when exposure was repeated;[1] late sequelae were not observed, even in patients with abnormal respiratory function tests or blood gases on admission. Another report on 76 children with chlorine poisoning revealed that the longest period of hospitalisation was 12 hours.[2] There have been reports of deliberate inhalation of chlorine,[3,4] in one instance for pleasure,[3] leading to severe adverse effects. Some individuals may be unduly insensitive to chlorine-induced irritation and workers should be warned that concentrations of chlorine which can be tolerated for short periods without undue discomfort can still cause serious injury which may not be immediately apparent.[4]

1. Barret L, Faure J. Chlorine poisoning. *Lancet* 1984; **i:** 561–2.
2. Fleta J, *et al.* Intoxication of 76 children by chlorine gas. *Hum Toxicol* 1986; **5:** 99–100.
3. Rafferty P. Voluntary chlorine inhalation: a new form of self-abuse? *BMJ* 1980; **281:** 1178–9.
4. Dewhurst F. Voluntary chlorine inhalation. *BMJ* 1981; **282:** 565–6.

Effects on the eyes. Eye examinations performed on 50 subjects immediately before and after swimming in a chlorinated pool (chlorine range 1.0 to 1.5 ppm) showed that 68% had symptoms of corneal oedema and 94% had corneal epithelial erosions. No subject experienced a measurable decrease in visual acuity.[1]

1. Haag JR, Gieser RG. Effects of swimming pool water on the cornea. *JAMA* 1983; **249:** 2507–8.

Precautions

The antimicrobial activity of chlorine disinfectants is diminished by the presence of organic material and by increasing pH. Hypochlorite solutions may delay wound healing (see Disinfection: Wounds under Uses and Administration, below).

Uses and Administration

Chlorine is a disinfectant with a rapid potent brief bactericidal action. It is capable of killing most bacteria, and some fungi, yeasts, algae, viruses, and protozoa. It is slowly active against spores.

It is used as liquid chlorine for the treatment of water (p.1130), but for most other purposes it is used in the form of hypochlorites, organic and inorganic chloramines, chlorinated hydantoins, chlorinated isocyanurates, and similar oxidising compounds capable of releasing chlorine. In the presence of water these compounds produce hypochlorous acid (HOCl) and hypochlorite ion (OCl⁻) and it is generally considered that the lethal action on organisms is due to chlorination of cell protein or enzyme systems by nonionised hypochlorous acid, although the hypochlorite ion may also contribute.

The activity of most of the compounds decreases with increase of pH, the activity of solutions of pH 4 to 7 being greater than those of higher pH values. However, stability is usually greater at an alkaline pH.

The potency of chlorine disinfectants is expressed in terms of **available chlorine**. This is based on the concept of chlorine gas (Cl_2) as the reference substance. Two atoms of chlorine ($2 \times Cl$) yield in water only one molecule of hypochlorous acid (on which activity is based), while hypochlorites and chloramines yield one molecule of hypochlorous acid for each atom of chlorine as shown in the following equations:

$$Cl_2 + H_2O \leftrightarrow HOCl + H^+ + Cl^-$$

$$NaOCl + H_2O \leftrightarrow HOCl + NaOH$$

Thus the assayed chlorine in such compounds has to be multiplied by 2 to produce 'available chlorine'. The term 'active chlorine' has been used confusingly for either 'available chlorine' (Cl_2) or 'combined chlorine' (Cl).

Because they have relatively low residual toxicity, chlorine compounds are useful for the disinfection of relatively clean impervious surfaces, such as babies' feeding bottles, baths, and food and dairy equipment. A concentration of 100 to 300 ppm of 'available chlorine' is used; a detergent may be added to ensure wetting of the surface. Solutions containing 1000 ppm 'available chlorine' are recommended for minor surface contamination and as part of general good hygiene practice. Solutions containing 10 000 ppm 'available chlorine' are used to disinfect surfaces contaminated with spilled blood or body fluids; this strength is effective against viruses including human immunodeficiency virus (HIV) and hepatitis B virus (p.1130). A concentration providing 20 000 ppm 'available chlorine' is used for material from patients with Creutzfeldt-Jakob disease (p.1129).

On a large scale, chlorine gas is used to disinfect public water supplies. On a smaller scale, the use of chlorine compounds is more convenient and sodium hypochlorite, tosylchloramide sodium, chlorinated lime, chlorine dioxide, or halazone are used. After satisfying the chlorine demand (the amount of chlorine needed to react with organic matter and other substances), a free-residual content of 0.2 to 0.4 ppm 'available chlorine' should be maintained, though more is required for alkaline waters with a pH of 9 or more. For the disinfection of potentially contaminated water a concentration of 1 ppm is recommended. Excessive residual chlorine may be removed by adding a little citric acid or sodium thiosulfate.

For use in small swimming pools, sodium or calcium hypochlorite may be added daily to maintain a free-residual 'available chlorine' concentration of 1 to 3 ppm. Tosylchloramide sodium, chlorinated lime, and the isocyanurates (see Sodium Dichloroisocyanu-

rate, p.1156) may also be used. To minimise irritation of the eyes, maintain disinfectant activity, prevent precipitation of salts, and prevent metal corrosion, a pH of 7.2 to 7.8 should be maintained.

Solutions of chlorine-releasing compounds are also used in wound desloughing and disinfection (but see below).

Disinfection. INSTRUMENTS. Chlorine dioxide solutions have been assessed as an alternative to glutaral for the disinfection of endoscopes (p.1129). They were reported to be rapidly sporicidal, but their compatibility with endoscope and processing components had yet to be determined.[1] Needles and syringes should not usually be sterilised chemically. However, use of full-strength domestic bleach (approximately 5% sodium hypochlorite, about 2% of 'available chlorine') was reported to be effective for the cleaning by intravenous drug users of needles and syringes as a last resort in the absence of sterile equipment; a 30-second contact time was required.[2,3] A 1 in 10 dilution of bleach was not effective after 5 minutes' exposure.[3]

1. Fraise AP. Disinfection in endoscopy. *Lancet* 1995; **346**: 787–8.
2. Donoghoe MC, Power R. Household bleach as disinfectant for use by injecting drug users. *Lancet* 1993; **341**: 1658.
3. Watters JK, *et al.* Household bleach as disinfectant for use by injecting drug users. *Lancet* 1993; **342**: 742–3.

WORMS. Sodium hypochlorite in aqueous solution at a concentration of 3.75% (or greater) is an effective ovicide for *Echinococcus* and may be used on hard surfaces, glassware, and sinks.[1]

1. Craig PS, Macpherson CNL. Sodium hypochlorite as an ovicide for Echinococcus. *Ann Trop Med Parasitol* 1988; **82**: 211–13.

WOUNDS. Hypochlorite solutions are now generally considered to be too irritant for use in the management of wounds (p.1108). Studies suggest that they may delay wound healing if repeatedly applied to open wounds.[1,2] It has been suggested that they may still be of use in debriding burns or necrotic chronic wounds,[3] but any benefit that might be seen from the desloughing of necrotic tissue might be produced by damage of the superficial cell layer leading to separation[4] or from tissue hydration produced by wet dressing packs.[5]

See also p.1130.

1. Thomas S, Hay NP. Wound healing. *Pharm J* 1985; **235**: 206.
2. Lineweaver W, *et al.* Topical antimicrobial toxicity. *Arch Surg* 1985; **120**: 267–70.
3. Leaper DJ. Eusol. *BMJ* 1992; **304**: 930–1.
4. Anonymous. Local applications to wounds—I: cleansers, antibacterials, debriders. *Drug Ther Bull* 1991; **29**: 93–5.
5. Thomas S. Milton and the treatment of burns. *Pharm J* 1986; **236**: 128–9.

Chloroacetamide (18953-v)

Chloracetamide. 2-Chloroacetamide.
$C_2H_4ClNO = 93.51$.
CAS — 79-07-2.

Profile
Chloroacetamide is a preservative that has been used in topical pharmaceutical preparations and cosmetics.

N-(3-Chloroallyl)hexaminium Chloride (5579-v)

Quaternium-15. 1-(3-Chloroallyl)-3,5,7-triaza-1-azoniaadamantane chloride.
$C_9H_{16}Cl_2N_4 = 251.2$.
CAS — 4080-31-3.

Profile
N-(3-Chloroallyl)hexaminium chloride is an antimicrobial preservative used in pharmaceutical preparations and cosmetics. Skin reactions have been reported.

Chlorobutanol (6640-h)

Chlorobutanol (BAN, rINN).

Acetone-Chloroforme; Alcohol Trichlorisobutylicus; Chlorbutanol; Chlorbutanolum; Chlorbutol; Chloretone; Chlorobutanolum; Trichlorbutanolum. 1,1,1-Trichloro-2-methylpropan-2-ol.
$C_4H_7Cl_3O = 177.5$.
CAS — 57-15-8 (anhydrous chlorobutanol); 6001-64-5 (chlorobutanol hemihydrate).
ATC — A04AD04.
Pharmacopoeias. Eur. (see p.vi), *Int.,* and *USNF* allow either the anhydrous form or the hemihydrate; *Eur.* includes them as separate monographs. *Chin.* specifies the hemihydrate. *Jpn* permits up to 6% of water.

Pharmacopoeial description
Ph. Eur.: A white crystalline powder or colourless crystals. It sublimes readily. The hemihydrate melts at about 78° and the anhydrous form at about 95°. Slightly soluble in water; very soluble in alcohol and in ether; soluble in glycerol (85%). Store at 8° to 15° in airtight containers.

USNF 20: Colourless or white crystals with a characteristic, somewhat camphoraceous odour. It melts at about 76° for the

hemihydrate and about 95° for the anhydrous form. Soluble 1 in 125 of water, 1 in 1 of alcohol, and 1 in 10 of glycerol; freely soluble in chloroform, in ether, and in volatile oils. Store in airtight containers.

Incompatibilities. The activity of chlorobutanol can be adversely affected by the presence of other compounds as well as by the packaging material. There may be sorption onto substances like magnesium trisilicate, bentonite, carmellose,[1] polyethylene,[2,3] or polyhydroxy-ethylmethacrylate that has been used in soft contact lenses.[4] Increasing heat[2,3] or pH[5,6] can reduce stability and activity.

1. Yousef RT, *et al.* Effect of some pharmaceutical materials on the bactericidal activities of preservatives. *Can J Pharm Sci* 1973; **8**: 54–6.
2. Friesen WT, Plein EM. The antibacterial stability of chlorobutanol stored in polyethylene bottles. *Am J Hosp Pharm* 1971; **28**: 507–12.
3. Holdsworth DG, *et al.* Fate of chlorbutol during storage in polyethylene dropper containers and simulated patient use. *J Clin Hosp Pharm* 1984; **9**: 29–39.
4. Richardson NE, *et al.* The interaction of preservatives with polyhydroxy-ethylmethacrylate (polyHEMA). *J Pharm Pharmacol* 1978; **30**: 469–75.
5. Nair AD, Lach JL. The kinetics of degradation of chlorobutanol. *J Am Pharm Assoc (Sci)* 1959; **48**: 390–5.
6. Patwa NV, Huyck CL. Stability of chlorobutanol. *J Am Pharm Assoc* 1966; **NS6**: 372–3.

Adverse Effects
Acute poisoning with chlorobutanol may produce CNS depression with weakness, loss of consciousness, and depressed respiration. Delayed (type IV) hypersensitivity reactions have been reported rarely.

Effects on the cardiovascular system. Rapid falls in arterial blood pressure were observed following injections of heparin with chlorobutanol in patients undergoing coronary bypass.[1] No fall in blood pressure was seen in patients who received preservative-free heparin injection.

1. Bowler GMR, *et al.* Sharp fall in blood pressure after injection of heparin containing chlorbutol. *Lancet* 1986; **i**: 848–9.

Effects on mental function. The sedative effects of chlorobutanol have been reported to be a problem in a patient dependent on large doses (0.9 to 1.5 g daily with salicylamide 1.8 to 3.0 g daily)[1] and in another patient given high doses of morphine in an infusion preserved with chlorobutanol.[2]

1. Borody T, *et al.* Chlorbutol toxicity and dependence. *Med J Aust* 1979; **i**: 288.
2. DeChristoforo R, *et al.* High-dose morphine infusion complicated by chlorobutanol-induced somnolence. *Ann Intern Med* 1983; **98**: 335–6.

Hypersensitivity. A delayed, cellular type of hypersensitivity reaction to chlorobutanol used to preserve heparin injection following subcutaneous injection has been reported.[1] Pruritus from intranasal desmopressin has been reported as due to the chlorobutanol preservative.[2]

1. Dux S, *et al.* Hypersensitivity reaction to chlorbutanol-preserved heparin. *Lancet* 1981; **i**: 149.
2. Itabashi A, *et al.* Hypersensitivity to chlorobutanol in DDAVP solution. *Lancet* 1982; **i**: 108.

Uses and Administration
Chlorobutanol has antibacterial and antifungal properties and it is used at a concentration of 0.5% as a preservative in injections and in eye drops as well as cosmetics.

Chlorobutanol has been used as a mild sedative and local analgesic but other compounds are preferred. It has been used in preparations for inflammatory and painful conditions of the ear and oropharynx.

Preparations
Proprietary Preparations (details are given in Part 3)
Port.: Vizoptal.

Multi-ingredient: Aust.: Aleot; DDD; Nautisan†; **Austral.:** Cerumol; **Belg.:** Givalex; **Braz.:** Angino-Rub; Auritricin; Colirio Helios; Lavolho; Nazobio; Providex; Visogenol; **Canad.:** Aurisan; Balminil Nasal Ointment; Cerumol; Gouttes pour Mal d'Orreilles; Oralgar; Outgro†; **Fr.:** Alodont; Angispray†; Balsamorhinol; Eludril; Givalex; **Ger.:** Givalex; **Hong Kong:** Cerumol†; Cerumol†; Karvol; Monphytol†; **Irl.:** Cerumol†; Karvol; Monphytol†; **Israel:** Cepadont; Cerumol; Dentin; Karvol; Pitrisan; **Ital.:** Fialetta Odontalgica Dr Knapp; **Port.:** Eludril; Otoceril; **S.Afr.:** Cerumol; Karvol; **Singapore:** Cerumol; Eludril; Karvol; **Spain:** Claraseptic; Eludril; Otocerum; **Switz.:** Alodont nouvelle formule; Cerumonol; Demo baume†; Dental-Phenjoca†; Eludril; Spirogel†; **Thai.:** Opplin; Optal; **UK:** Aezodent; Cerumol; Cetanorm; DDD; Dermidex; Eludril; Frador; Karvol; Monphytol; **USA:** Outgro.

Chlorocresol (2226-h)

Chlorocresol (USAN, rINN).

Chlorkresolum; Parachlorometacresol; PCMC. *p*-Chloro-*m*-cresol; 4-Chloro-3-methylphenol.
$C_7H_7ClO = 142.6$.
CAS — 59-50-7.

Pharmacopoeias. In Eur. (see p.vi) and *Int.* Also in *USNF.*

The antimicrobial activity of chlorocresol may be diminished through incompatibility (see below), through adsorption, through increasing pH, or through combination with organic matter (including oils and fats) or nonionic surfactants.

Pharmacopoeial description

Ph. Eur.: A white or almost white, crystalline powder or compacted crystalline masses supplied as pellets or colourless or white crystals. M.p. 64° to 67°. Slightly soluble in water; very soluble in alcohol; freely soluble in ether and in fatty oils. It dissolves in solutions of alkali hydroxides. Protect from light.

USNF 20: Colourless or practically colourless crystals or crystalline powder with a characteristic nontarry odour; it is volatile in steam. M.p. 63° to 66°. Soluble 1 in 260 of water; more soluble in hot water; soluble 1 in 0.4 of alcohol; soluble in ether, in terpenes, in fixed oils, and in solutions of alkali hydroxides. Store in airtight containers. Protect from light.

Incompatibilities. Chlorocresol has long been recognised to be incompatible with a range of compounds including: codeine phosphate, diamorphine hydrochloride, papaveretum, quinine hydrochloride,[1] methylcellulose,[2] and nonionic surfactants such as cetomacrogol 1000[3] and polysorbate 80.[4]

1. McEwan JS, Macmorran GH. The compatibility of some bactericides. *Pharm J* 1947; **158:** 260–2.
2. Harris WA. The inactivation of cationic antiseptics by bentonite suspensions. *Australas J Pharm* 1961; **42:** 583–8.
3. *PSGB Lab Report P/70/15* 1970.
4. Yousef RT, *et al.* Effect of some pharmaceutical materials on the bactericidal activities of preservatives. *Can J Pharm Sci* 1973; **8:** 54–6.

Adverse Effects, Treatment, and Precautions

As for Phenol, p.1152.

Chlorocresol is less toxic than phenol. Sensitisation reactions may follow application to the skin and hypersensitivity has occurred following systemic administration of injections containing chlorocresol as a preservative.

Uses and Administration

Chlorocresol is a potent chlorinated phenolic disinfectant and antiseptic. It has bactericidal activity against Gram-positive and Gram-negative bacteria and is effective against fungi but has little activity against bacterial spores except at high temperatures. It is more active in acid than in alkaline solution.

Chlorocresol is used in various preparations for disinfection of the skin and wounds. It is also used as a preservative in cosmetics and in creams and other preparations for external use which contain water.

Chlorocresol is used as a preservative in aqueous injections issued in multidose containers. It may also be added to aqueous preparations that cannot be sterilised in their final containers and have to be prepared using aseptic precautions. Concentrations of 0.1% have generally been used. Injections prepared with chlorocresol should not be injected into the CSF, the eye, or the heart. Also such injections should generally not be administered in volumes greater than 15 mL. Sterilisation by heating with a bactericide such as chlorocresol in no longer a recommended practice.

Preparations

BPC 1973: Proflavine Cream.

Proprietary Preparations (details are given in Part 3)
UK: Wright's Vaporizing Fluid.

Multi-ingredient: *Aust.:* Ulcurilen; *Austral.:* Curatin; Soothe'n Heal; *Fr.:* Cicatryl; Cyteal; *Ger.:* Bacillotox†; Bomix; Grotanat; Helipur; Ulcurilen N; *Irl.:* Anbesol; Valderma; *Ital.:* Helipur; Hygienist; *Port.:* Cyteal; *Singapore:* Cyteal; *Spain:* Fungusol; *UK:* Anbesol; Cymex; Valderma.

Chlorothymol   (2227-m)

Monochlorothymol. 6-Chlorothymol; 4-Chloro-2-isopropyl-5-methylphenol.
$C_{10}H_{13}ClO = 184.7$.
CAS — 89-68-9.

Profile

Chlorothymol is a chlorinated phenolic antiseptic used as an ingredient of preparations for hand and skin disinfection and topical treatment of fungal infections. It has also been used in preparations for anorectal disorders, cold symptoms, and mouth disorders.

Preparations

Proprietary Preparations (details are given in Part 3)
Ital.: Pioral Pasta.

Multi-ingredient: *Ital.:* Labocaina; Traumicid; Vagisil; *Neth.:* Rhinocaps†.

Chloroxylenol   (2228-b)

Chloroxylenol *(BAN, USAN, rINN)*.
Parachlorometaxylenol; PCMX. 4-Chloro-3,5-xylenol; 4-Chloro-3,5-dimethylphenol.
$C_8H_9ClO = 156.6$.
CAS — 88-04-0.
ATC — D08AE05.
Pharmacopoeias. In Br. and US.

Incompatibility has been reported with nonionic surfactants and methylcellulose. The antimicrobial activity of chloroxylenol may be diminished through combination with organic matter.

Pharmacopoeial description

BP 2001: White or cream crystals or crystalline powder with a characteristic odour; volatile in steam. Very slightly soluble in water; freely soluble in alcohol; soluble in ether, in terpenes, in fixed oils, and in solutions of alkali hydroxides.

USP 25: White crystals or crystalline powder with a characteristic odour; volatile in steam. Very slightly soluble in water; freely soluble in alcohol, in ether, in terpenes, in fixed oils, and in solutions of alkali hydroxides.

Adverse Effects and Precautions

Chloroxylenol in the recommended dilutions is generally non-irritant but skin sensitivity has occurred. There have been isolated reports of poisoning.

Aqueous solutions of chloroxylenol may be susceptible to contamination with micro-organisms. To reduce this risk, solutions must be freshly prepared at the recommended concentration and appropriate measures should be taken to prevent contamination during storage or dilution.

◊ Reports of fatal[1] or severe[2,3] self-poisoning with chloroxylenol solution.

1. Meek D, *et al.* Fatal self-poisoning with Dettol. *Postgrad Med J* 1977; **53:** 229–31.
2. Joubert P, *et al.* Severe Dettol (chloroxylenol and terpineol) poisoning. *BMJ* 1978; **1:** 890.
3. Chan TYK, *et al.* Chemical gastro-oesophagitis, upper gastrointestinal haemorrhage and gastroscopic findings following Dettol poisoning. *Hum Exp Toxicol* 1995; **14:** 18–19.

Uses and Administration

Chloroxylenol is a chlorinated phenolic antiseptic which is bactericidal against most Gram-positive bacteria but less active against staphylococci and Gram-negative bacteria, and is often inactive against *Pseudomonas* spp. Its activity against *Ps. aeruginosa* appears to be increased by the addition of edetic acid. It is inactive against bacterial spores.

Chloroxylenol Solution (BP 2001) is used for skin and wound disinfection, and chloroxylenol is used in a variety of other topical formulations.

Preparations

BP 2001: Chloroxylenol Solution.

Proprietary Preparations (details are given in Part 3)
Austral.: Dettol Classic; *Belg.:* Dettol; *Canad.:* Antiseptic Ointment; *Hong Kong:* Dettol; *Ital.:* Neomercurochromo; *NZ:* Dettol; *S.Afr.:* Dettol; *Singapore:* Dettol; *Thai.:* Dettol; *UK:* Dettol; Prinsyl; *USA:* PramOtic.

Multi-ingredient: *Aust.:* Dolothricin†; *Austral.:* Dettol Cream; Solyptol; ZeaSorb; *Canad.:* Acne-Aid†; Iba-Cide†; ZeaSorb; *Ger.:* Bacillotox†; Gehwol Fungizid; ZeaSorb; *Hong Kong:* Acne-Aid; Dettol; *Irl.:* Dettol; ZeaSorb; *Israel:* Gargol; Hemo; Rexitol; *Ital.:* Foille; Foille Sole; Vironox; *NZ:* Dettol; *S.Afr.:* Dettol Antiseptic; Respisniffers; *Singapore:* Acne-Aid; Dettol; ZeaSorb; *Thai.:* Dettol; Johnson's Baby Prickly Heat Powder; ZeaSorb; *UK:* Dettol; Rinstead; Skintex; TCP; Waxwane; ZeaSorb; *USA:* Calamycin; Comfortine; Cortane-B Otic; Cortic; Dermacoat; Foille; Fungi-Nail; Gordochom; Lobana Peri-Garde; Otomar-HC; Pedi-Pro; Tri-Otic; Triple Care Extra Protective Cream†; Unguentine Plus; Zoto-HC.

Cinnamic Acid   (6641-m)

Cinnamylic Acid. *trans*-3-Phenylpropenoic acid.
$C_6H_5.CH{:}CH.CO_2H = 148.2$.
CAS — 621-82-9.
Pharmacopoeias. In Br.

Pharmacopoeial description

BP 2001: Colourless crystals with a faint balsamic odour. Very slightly soluble in water; freely soluble in alcohol; soluble in chloroform and in ether.

Profile

Cinnamic acid has preservative properties. It is used with benzoic acid and other substances to simulate the flavour of tolu.

Preparations

BP 2001: Tolu-flavour Solution.

Proprietary Preparations (details are given in Part 3)

Multi-ingredient: *Switz.:* Spirogel†; *UK:* Hemocane; Sanderson's Throat Specific.

Clorindanol   (3423-z)

Clorindanol *(rINN)*.
Chlorindanol *(USAN)*; NSC-158565. 7-Chloro-4-indanol; 7-Chloro-2,3-dihydro-1H-inden-4-ol.
$C_9H_9ClO = 168.6$.
CAS — 145-94-8.

Profile

Clorindanol is reported to have antiseptic and spermicidal properties.

Clorophene   (2230-r)

Clorophene *(USAN)*.
Clorofene *(pINN)*; Clorfene; NSC-59989; Septiphene. 2-Benzyl-4-chlorophenol.
$C_{13}H_{11}ClO = 218.7$.
CAS — 120-32-1.

Profile

Clorophene is a chlorinated phenolic antiseptic stated to be active against a wide range of bacteria, fungi, protozoa, and viruses. It is used as a skin disinfectant and for surface and instrument disinfection. Clorophene sodium has also been used.

Preparations

Proprietary Preparations (details are given in Part 3)

Multi-ingredient: *Belg.:* Neo-Sabenyl; *Canad.:* Aseptone 1; Aseptone 2; Aseptone 5; *Fr.:* Frekaderm†; *Ger.:* Bacillotox†; Bomix; Freka-Derm; Freka-Sept 80; Grotanat; Helipur; *Ital.:* Helipur; Hygienist; *Switz.:* Frekaderm.

Cresol   (2231-f)

Cresolum Crudum; Cresylic Acid; Kresolum Venale; Tricresol; Trikresolum. Methylphenol.
$C_7H_8O = 108.1$.
CAS — 1319-77-3; 95-48-7 (o-cresol); 108-39-4 (m-cresol); 106-44-5 (p-cresol).
Pharmacopoeias. In Aust., Br., Chin., Fr., It., and Jpn. Also in USNF.

NOTE. Some grades of mixed cresols may be equivalent to Tar Acids (p.1158).

Pharmacopoeial description

BP 2001: It is a mixture of cresols and other phenols obtained from coal tar. An almost colourless to pale brownish-yellow liquid, becoming darker with age or on exposure to light, with an odour resembling that of phenol but more tarry. Almost completely soluble 1 in 50 of water; freely soluble in alcohol, in ether, in chloroform, and in fixed and volatile oils. Protect from light.

USNF 20: A colourless, yellowish to brownish-yellow, or pinkish, highly refractive liquid, becoming darker with age or on exposure to light, with a phenol-like, sometimes empyreumatic odour. It consists of a mixture of cresol isomers obtained from coal tar or petroleum. Sparingly soluble in water, usually forming a cloudy solution; miscible with alcohol, with ether, and with glycerol; dissolves in solutions of fixed alkali hydroxides. A saturated solution in water is neutral or slightly acid to litmus. Store in airtight containers. Protect from light.

Profile

Cresol is a disinfectant with a similar action to phenol (p.1153); suitable precautions should be taken to prevent absorption through the skin.

It has been used as Cresol and Soap Solution (BP 1968) (Lysol) as a general disinfectant but it has been largely superseded by other, less irritant, phenolic disinfectants. Cresol has been used in dentistry, alone or in combination with formaldehyde, but is caustic to the skin and unsuitable for skin and wound disinfection. The cresols have been widely used in disinfectants for domestic and hospital use. Cresol is also used as an antimicrobial preservative in parenteral pharmaceutical preparations and in some topical formulations.

Poisoning. References to poisoning with cresol solutions.

1. Côté M-A, *et al.* Acute Heinz-body anaemia due to severe cresol poisoning: successful treatment with erythrocytapheresis. *Can Med Assoc J* 1984; **130:** 1319–22.
2. Wu ML, *et al.* Concentrated cresol intoxication. *Vet Hum Toxicol* 1998; **40:** 341–3.

Preparations

Proprietary Preparations (details are given in Part 3)
Ital.: Creolina.

Multi-ingredient: *Austral.:* Formo-Cresol Mitis; *Canad.:* Gernel; *Fr.:* Eau Precieuse; *Spain:* Empapol; Neodesfila; Tifell; *USA:* Cresylate.

Dehydroacetic Acid   (6642-b)

Methylacetopyronone. 3-Acetyl-6-methyl-2H-pyran-2,4(3H)-dione (keto form); 3-Acetyl-4-hydroxy-6-methyl-2H-pyran-2-one (enol form).
$C_8H_8O_4 = 168.1$.
CAS — 520-45-6 (keto form); 771-03-9 (enol form).

Sodium Dehydroacetate   (6668-j)

The sodium salt of 3-acetyl-6-methyl-2H-pyran-2,4(3H)-dione.
$C_8H_7NaO_4 = 190.1$.
CAS — 4418-26-2.
Pharmacopoeias. In USNF.

Incompatibilities. Activity may be reduced by alkaline pH or interaction with nonionic surfactants.

Pharmacopoeial description

USNF 20: A white or practically white, odourless powder. Freely soluble in water, in glycerol, and in propylene glycol.

Profile
Dehydroacetic acid and sodium dehydroacetate have some antifungal activity and have been used in the preservation of cosmetics.

Dequalinium Chloride   (2234-h)

Dequalinium Chloride (BAN, rINN).

BAQD-10; Decalinium Chloride; Decaminum; Dequalinii Chloridum. N,N-Decamethylenebis(4-amino-2-methylquinolinium chloride).

$C_{30}H_{40}Cl_2N_4 = 527.6$.

CAS — 6707-58-0 (dequalinium); 522-51-0 (dequalinium chloride); 4028-98-2 (dequalinium acetate); 16022-70-1 (dequalinium salicylate).

Pharmacopoeias. In Eur. (see p.vi).

Incompatible with soaps and other anionic surfactants, with phenol, and with chlorocresol.

Pharmacopoeial description
Ph. Eur.: A white or yellowish-white, hygroscopic powder. Slightly soluble in water and in alcohol. Store in airtight containers.

Profile
Dequalinium chloride is a bisquaternary quinolinium antiseptic, bactericidal against many Gram-positive and Gram-negative bacteria, and effective against fungi. It is mainly used in the form of lozenges in the treatment of minor infections of the mouth and throat. It has been applied topically in the treatment of skin and vaginal infections.

Dequalinium salicylate and undecenoate have also been used.

Preparations
Proprietary Preparations (details are given in Part 3)
Aust.: Dequadin; Dequavagyn; Evazol; Sorot; Tonsillot; **Belg.:** Anginol; **Canad.:** Dequadin; **Ger.:** Efisol S; Evazol; Fluomycin N; Gurgellosung-ratiopharm; Maltyl; Soor-Gel†; Sorot; **Hong Kong:** Delin; Dequadin; Roxine; **Irl.:** Dequadin; Labosept†; **Ital.:** Dequadin; Dequosangola; Faringina; Goladin; Osangin; Pumilsan; **Mex.:** Decatylen; **Neth.:** Gargilon; **NZ:** Dequadin; **S.Afr.:** Dequadin; **Singapore:** SP Troches; **Spain:** Dequadin; **Switz.:** Decatylene; Pastilles pour la gorge no 535; **Thai.:** Dequa/Delin; Dequadin; V Day Lozenges; **UK:** Dequadin; Labosept; Mac Sugar Free.

Multi-ingredient: Aust.: Dequafungan; Dequalinetten; Dequonal; Eucillin; Fluorex Plus; Tetesept; **Belg.:** Anginol-Lidocaine; Bucco-Spray; Buccosan; Dequalid; Dequalinium†; Laryngarsol; **Fin.:** Septison; **Fr.:** Humex Kinaldine; Oroseptol Lysozyme; Oroseptol†; **Ger.:** Bakteriostat "Herbrand"†; Corti-Dynexan; Dementhasin†; Dequonal; Ephepect-Blocker-Pastillen N; Inspirol Halsschmerztabletten; Jasimenth CN; Mycatox; Neo-Pyodron; Otolitan N farblos; stas Halsschmerz-Tabletten; Wick Sulagil; **Hong Kong:** Decatylen; Deq; Quadezyme; **Irl.:** Dequacaine; **Israel:** Dequasept; **Ital.:** Lisomucil Gola; Rinospray†; Transpulmina Gola; Tririnol†; **Norw.:** Apolar med dekvalon; **Port.:** Anginova; Medifon; **S.Afr.:** Dequadin Mouth Paint; Dequamed; **Singapore:** Decatylen; Deq; **Spain:** Anginovag; Dequadin Complex; Roberfarin; Sedofarin; **Switz.:** Anginova Nouvelle formule; Arbid-top; Decasept N; Decatylene Neo; Dequonal; Gramipan; Neo-Bucosin; Rhinipan†; Tyroqualine; **Thai.:** Deq; Detoch; Sentril; **UK:** Dequacaine.

Dibrompropamidine Isetionate   (2236-b)

Dibrompropamidine Isetionate (BANM, rINNM).

Dibromopropamidine Isethionate. 3,3′-Dibromo-4,4′-trimethylenedioxydibenzamidine bis(2-hydroxyethanesulphonate).

$C_{17}H_{18}Br_2N_4O_2,2C_2H_6O_4S = 722.4$.

CAS — 496-00-4 (dibrompropamidine); 614-87-9 (dibrompropamidine isetionate).

Pharmacopoeias. In Br.

Pharmacopoeial description
BP 2001: A white or almost white, odourless or almost odourless, crystalline powder. Freely soluble in water; sparingly soluble in alcohol; practically insoluble in chloroform, in ether, in fixed oils, and in liquid paraffin; soluble in glycerol. A 5% solution has a pH of 5.0 to 7.0.

Profile
Dibrompropamidine isetionate is an aromatic diamidine antiseptic similar to propamidine (p.1155). It is bactericidal against Gram-positive bacteria but is less active against Gram-negative bacteria and spore-forming organisms. It also has antifungal properties. It is available as topical preparations for the local treatment of minor eye and skin infections.

Preparations
Proprietary Preparations (details are given in Part 3)
Austral.: Brolene; Brulidine; **Hong Kong:** Brulidine; **Irl.:** Brolene; Brulidine; **Norw.:** Brulidine; **NZ:** Brolene; Brulidine; **UK:** Brolene; Brulidine; Golden Eye Ointment; Pickles Antiseptic Cream.

Multi-ingredient: S.Afr.: Phenergan†; **UK:** Healthy Feet; No-Sor Nose Balm; Soleze; Swarm.

Dichlordimethylhydantoin   (2237-v)

1,3-Dichloro-5,5-dimethylhydantoin; 1,3-Dichloro-5,5-dimethylimidazolidine-2,4-dione.

$C_5H_6Cl_2N_2O_2 = 197.0$.

CAS — 118-52-5.

It contains about 72% w/w of 'available chlorine' (see p.1141).

Profile
Dichlordimethylhydantoin is a disinfectant used as a source of chlorine, for sterilising food and dairy equipment and as a bleach.

Bromochlorodimethylhydantoin ($C_5H_6N_2O_2BrCl = 241.5$) is a closely related bromine-releasing compound used for the disinfection of swimming-pool water.

Dichlorobenzyl Alcohol   (2238-g)

Dichlorophenylcarbinol. 2,4-Dichlorobenzyl alcohol.

$C_7H_6Cl_2O = 177.0$.

CAS — 1777-82-8.

ATC — R02AA03.

Profile
Dichlorobenzyl alcohol is an antiseptic used chiefly as an ingredient of lozenges in the treatment of minor infections of the mouth and throat.

Preparations
Proprietary Preparations (details are given in Part 3)
Fin.: Strepsils; **Ital.:** Neo Borocillina Collutorio; Neo Borocillina Spray.

Multi-ingredient: Aust.: Coldangin; Neo-Angin; Sulgan 99; **Austral.:** Actifed Anaesthetic†; Ayrton's Antiseptic; Logicin Rapid Relief; Sore Throat Chewing Gum; Strepsils; Strepsils Anaesthetic†; Strepsils Plus; **Belg.:** Neofenox; Strepsils; Strepsils + Lidocaine; Strepsils Menthol; Strepsils Vit C; **Canad.:** Strepsils; **Denm.:** Strepsils; **Fin.:** Bafucin; Strepsils Menthol; **Fr.:** Strepsils; Strepsils Lidocaine; Strepsils Miel-Citron; Strepsils Vitamine C; Strepsilspray Lidocaine; **Ger.:** Neo-Angin N; **Hong Kong:** Strepsils; **Irl.:** Strepsils; Strepsils Dual Action; Strepsils Vitamin C; **Israel:** Strepsils; Strepsils Plus; Strepsils with Vitamin C; **Ital.:** Arscolloid; Benagol; Benagol Mentolo-Eucaliptolo; Benagol Vitamina C; Bio-Arscolloid; Corti-Arscolloid; Neo Borocillina; Neo Borocillina Balsamica; Neo Borocillina C; Neo Borocillina Tosse Compresse; Oraseptic Gola; **Neth.:** Strepsils; Strepsils Menthol en Eucalyptus; Strepsils Sinaasappel en Vitamine C; **NZ:** Strepsils; Strepsils Plus Anaesthetic; Strepsils with Vitamin C; **Port.:** Dropcina; **S.Afr.:** Strepsils; Strepsils Eucalyptus Menthol; Strepsils Orange-C; Strepsils Plus; Strepsils Soothing Honey & Lemon; **Singapore:** Floxil; Strepsils; Strepsils Dual Action; **Spain:** Strepsils; Strepsils con Anestesico; Strepsils con Vitamina C; **Swed.:** Bafucin; Strepsils; **Switz.:** Demosept; Hextriletten; Lidazon; Neo-Angin au miel et citron; Neo-Angin avec vitamin C exempt de sucre; Neo-Angin exempt de sucre; Sulgan; **Thai.:** Strepsils Plus Anaesthetic; Strepsils Plus Vit C; Strepsils Sugar Free; **UK:** Antiseptic Throat Lozenges†; Strepsils; Strepsils Pain Relief Plus; Strepsils with Vitamin C.

Didecyldimethylammonium Chloride   (11329-k)

N-Decyl-N,N-demethyl-1-decanaminium chloride.

$C_{22}H_{48}ClN = 362.1$.

ATC — D08AJ06.

Profile
Didecyldimethylammonium chloride is a quaternary ammonium disinfectant used in preparations for disinfection of the skin and mucous membranes. It is also used to disinfect instruments and surfaces.

Preparations
Proprietary Preparations (details are given in Part 3)
Multi-ingredient: Fr.: Amphosept BV†; Aniospray; Bacterianos D; Chlorispray; Hexanios G+R; Sanytol; Ultrasep†; **Ger.:** Baccalin; Bacillol rasant; Desoform; Freka-Nol; Fugisept; Gercid forte; Gigasept AF; Gigasept Med; Hexaquart L; Hexaquart plus; Hexaquart S; Kohrsolin FF; Lysetol V; Lysoformin 3000; Lysoformin spezial; Melsept SF; Melsitt; Quatohex; Teta Extra; **Ital.:** Cedril Strumenti†; Cedril†; Melsept SF.

Dodicin   (11358-f)

Dodicin (BAN).

Dodecyldi(aminoethyl) glycine. 3,6,9-Triazahenicosanoic acid.

$C_{18}H_{39}N_3O_2 = 329.5$.

CAS — 6843-97-6 (dodicin); 59079-49-1 (dodicin sodium); 18205-85-1 (dodicin hydrochloride).

Profile
Dodicin is an ampholytic surfactant with bactericidal and fungicidal properties. It is also active against some viruses. It has been used mainly for surface disinfection. The hydrochloride has also been used.

Domiphen Bromide   (2242-h)

Domiphen Bromide (BAN, USAN, rINN).

NSC-39415; PDDB; Phenododecinium Bromide. Dodecyldimethyl-2-phenoxyethylammonium bromide.

$C_{22}H_{40}BrNO = 414.5$.

CAS — 13900-14-6 (domiphen); 538-71-6 (domiphen bromide).

Pharmacopoeias. In Br. and Chin.

Incompatible with soaps and other anionic surfactants.

Pharmacopoeial description
BP 2001: Colourless or faintly yellow, crystalline flakes. Freely soluble in water and in alcohol; soluble in acetone.

Profile
Domiphen bromide is a quaternary ammonium antiseptic with actions and uses similar to those of other cationic surfactants (see Cetrimide, p.1137). Preparations containing domiphen bromide are used in the treatment of minor infections of the mouth and throat.

Preparations
Proprietary Preparations (details are given in Part 3)
Canad.: Antiseptic Pastilles; Bronchodex Pastilles; Oraseptic; **Ital.:** Bradoral; **Port.:** Neobradoral.

Multi-ingredient: Aust.: Bepanthen; Bradosol; **Canad.:** Mouthwash & Gargle†; Mouthwash Mint/Peppermint†; Nupercainal; Scope; **Fr.:** Fluoselgine; **Ital.:** Golamed Oral; Inalar; Nasalemed†; **UK:** Bradosol Plus.

Ethoxyquin   (6646-p)

6-Ethoxy-1,2-dihydro-2,2,4-trimethylquinoline.

$C_{14}H_{19}NO = 217.3$.

CAS — 91-53-2.

Profile
Ethoxyquin has been used as an antoxidant for the prevention of common scald of apples and pears during storage and as an additive to animal feeds. Concern has been expressed over the toxicity of ethoxyquin and its residues on foodstuffs and its use is limited or restricted in some countries.

Ethylene Oxide   (2244-b)

Oxirane.

$C_2H_4O = 44.05$.

CAS — 75-21-8.

A colourless flammable gas at room temperature and atmospheric pressure.

CAUTION. *Mixtures of ethylene oxide with oxygen or air are explosive but the risk can be reduced by the addition of carbon dioxide or fluorocarbons.*

Adverse Effects and Precautions
Ethylene oxide irritates the eyes and respiratory tract and may also cause nausea and vomiting, diarrhoea, headache, vertigo, CNS depression, dyspnoea, and pulmonary oedema. Liver and kidney damage and haemolysis may occur. Fatalities have occurred. Excessive exposure of the skin to liquid or solution causes burns, blistering, irritation, and dermatitis; percutaneous absorption may lead to systemic effects.

Many materials including plastics and rubber adsorb ethylene oxide. If such materials are being sterilised with ethylene oxide all traces of the gas must be removed before the materials can be used; removal may be by ventilation or more active means. Hypersensitivity reactions, including anaphylaxis, have been associated with ethylene oxide-contaminated materials. Ethylene oxide may also react with materials being sterilised to produce substances such as ethylene chlorohydrin (with chloride) or ethylene glycol (with water); these may contribute to any toxicity.

Pharmaceutical manufacturers within the European Union have been advised to use ethylene oxide only when there is no alternative. Ethylene oxide has been shown to have carcinogenic and mutagenic properties and there is evidence of increased risk of neoplasms following occupational exposure.

Carcinogenicity. Exposure of workers to ethylene oxide has been associated with the development of lymphatic and haematopoietic cancer. However, epidemiological studies have not consistently shown an excess of cases among workers exposed to ethylene oxide, and excesses that have been seen have been small[1-4] although a trend towards increased risk related to cumulative exposure has been reported.[2,4]

1. Hogstedt C, et al. Epidemiologic support for ethylene oxide as a cancer-causing agent. JAMA 1986; **255:** 1575–8.

2. Steenland K, *et al.* Mortality among workers exposed to ethylene oxide. *N Engl J Med* 1991; **324:** 1402–7.
3. Hagmar L, *et al.* An epidemiological study of cancer risk among workers exposed to ethylene oxide using hemoglobin adducts to validate environmental exposure assessments. *Int Arch Occup Environ Health* 1991; **63:** 271–7.
4. Stayner L, *et al.* Exposure-response analysis of cancer mortality in a cohort of workers exposed to ethylene oxide. *Am J Epidemiol* 1993; **138:** 787–98.

Effects on the nervous system. Four men exposed to ethylene oxide at a concentration of greater than 700 ppm developed neurological disorders. One experienced headaches, nausea, vomiting, and lethargy followed by major motor seizures. The others experienced headaches, limb numbness and weakness, increased fatigue, trouble with memory and thought processes, and slurred speech. Three also developed cataracts, and one required bilateral cataract extractions.[1]

1. Jay WM, *et al.* Possible relationship of ethylene oxide exposure to cataract formation. *Am J Ophthalmol* 1982; **93:** 727–32.

Hypersensitivity. Anaphylactoid reactions in dialysis patients have resulted from the use of dialysis equipment sterilised with ethylene oxide.[1-3] There have also been reports of hypersensitivity[4] and anaphylactoid[5] reactions in plateletpheresis donors caused by residues of ethylene oxide in components of apheresis kits. The most common adverse reactions reported have been dyspnoea, wheezing, urticaria, flushing, headache, and hypotension, but acute severe bronchospasm, circulatory collapse, cardiac arrest, and death have also occurred. It was noted[6] that where severe, sometimes fatal, anaphylactoid reactions have occurred at the beginning of dialysis, ethylene oxide has almost universally been implicated, although exposure to cuprammonium cellulose (cuprophane) dialysis membranes may also have been involved.

It has been reported that there may be an increased risk of ethylene oxide-induced anaphylactic shock in children undergoing surgery for spina bifida.[7] Such children might be at increased risk of sensitisation and anaphylaxis, and came into frequent contact with ethylene oxide through multiple operations and catheterisations.

Occupational asthma and contact dermatitis have been attributed to residual ethylene oxide in surgical gloves.[8]

1. Bommer J, *et al.* Anaphylactoid reactions in dialysis patients: role of ethylene-oxide. *Lancet* 1985; **i:** 1382–5.
2. Rumpf KW, *et al.* Association of ethylene-oxide-induced IgE antibodies with symptoms in dialysis patients. *Lancet* 1985; **ii:** 1385–7.
3. Röckel A, *et al.* Ethylene oxide hypersensitivity in dialysis patients. *Lancet* 1986; **i:** 382–3.
4. Leitman SF, *et al.* Allergic reactions in healthy plateletpheresis donors caused by sensitization to ethylene oxide gas. *N Engl J Med* 1986; **315:** 1192–6.
5. Muylle L, *et al.* Anaphylactoid reaction in platelet-pheresis donor with IgE antibodies to ethylene oxide. *Lancet* 1986; **ii:** 1225.
6. Nicholls A. Ethylene oxide and anaphylaxis during haemodialysis. *BMJ* 1986; **292:** 1221–2.
7. Moneret-Vautrin DA, *et al.* High risk of anaphylactic shock during surgery for spina bifida. *Lancet* 1990; **335:** 865–6.
8. Verraes S, Michel O. Occupational asthma induced by ethylene oxide. *Lancet* 1995; **346:** 1434–5.

Pregnancy. A study[1] of female hospital sterilising staff in all general hospitals in Finland showed that the incidence of spontaneous abortion (analysed according to employment at the time of conception and corrected for maternal age, parity, decade of pregnancy, smoking, and consumption of alcohol and coffee) was significantly increased in those exposed to ethylene oxide during pregnancy compared with those not so exposed. This study provoked criticism,[2,3] and the authors conceded that the study was not large enough to compare abortion rates and known ethylene oxide concentrations.[4]

1. Hemminki K, *et al.* Spontaneous abortions in hospital staff engaged in sterilising instruments with chemical agents. *BMJ* 1982; **285:** 1461–3.
2. Gordon JE, Meinhardt TJ. Spontaneous abortions in hospital sterilising staff. *BMJ* 1983; **286:** 1976.
3. Austin SG. Spontaneous abortions in hospital sterilising staff. *BMJ* 1983; **286:** 1976.
4. Hemminki K, *et al.* Spontaneous abortions in hospital sterilising staff. *BMJ* 1983; **286:** 1976–7.

Pharmacokinetics

Ethylene oxide gas is rapidly absorbed through the lungs and distributed throughout the body. Percutaneous absorption can occur from aqueous solutions. It is rapidly metabolised by hydrolysis or conjugation with glutathione.

Uses

Ethylene oxide is a bactericidal and fungicidal gaseous disinfectant which is effective against most micro-organisms, including viruses. It is also sporicidal. It is used for the gaseous sterilisation of heat-labile pharmaceutical and surgical materials that cannot be sterilised by other means.

Ethylene oxide forms explosive mixtures with air; this may be overcome by using mixtures containing 10% ethylene oxide in carbon dioxide, or by removing at least 95% of the air from the apparatus before admitting either ethylene oxide or a mixture of 90%

ethylene oxide in carbon dioxide. Alternatively, non-flammable mixtures of dichlorodifluoromethane and trichlorofluoromethane with 9 to 12% w/w of ethylene oxide have been employed, but restrictions on the release of fluorocarbons or CFCs limit their use.

Effective sterilisation by ethylene oxide depends on exposure time, temperature, humidity, the amount and type of microbial contamination, and the partial pressure of the ethylene oxide in the exposure chamber. The material being sterilised must be permeable to ethylene oxide if occluded micro-organisms are present. The bactericidal action is accelerated by increase of temperature; a temperature of about 55° can be used for most thermolabile materials.

Moisture is essential for sterilisation by ethylene oxide. In practice, dry micro-organisms need to be rehydrated before ethylene oxide can be effective; humidification is normally carried out under vacuum prior to introduction of ethylene oxide. Relative humidities of 40 to 60% are used. Control of physical factors does not assure sterility, and the process should be monitored usually by employing standardised suspensions of aerobic spores such as those of *Bacillus subtilis* var. *niger*.

Formaldehyde Solution (2246-g)

Formaldehydi Solutio.

NOTE. The names formalin and formol have been used for formaldehyde solution but in some countries Formalin is a trade mark.

Pharmacopoeias. In *Eur.* (see p.vi), *Jpn,* and *US.*

Incompatibilities. Formaldehyde reacts with protein and this may diminish its antimicrobial activity.

Pharmacopoeial description

Ph. Eur.: Formaldehyde Solution (35 per cent) contains 34.5 to 38.0% w/w of CH_2O (= 30.03) with methyl alcohol as a stabiliser. It is a clear, colourless, liquid. Miscible with water and with alcohol. It may be cloudy after storage. Store at a temperature between 15° and 25°. Protect from light.

USP 25: Formaldehyde Solution contains not less than 36.5% or 37.0% w/w (depending on the packaging) of CH_2O with methyl alcohol added to prevent polymerisation. It is a clear, colourless, or practically colourless liquid with a pungent, irritating odour. Miscible with water and with alcohol. Store at a temperature above 15° in airtight containers. It may become cloudy on standing due to the separation of paraformaldehyde, especially if the solution is kept in a cold place; the cloudiness disappears on warming.

◊ NOTE. Formaldehyde solution is sometimes known simply as formaldehyde and this has led to confusion in interpreting the strength and the form in which formaldehyde is being used. In practice formaldehyde is available as formaldehyde solution which is diluted before use, the percentage strength being expressed in terms of formaldehyde solution rather than formaldehyde (CH_2O). For example, in the UK, formaldehyde solution 3% consists of 3 volumes of Formaldehyde Solution (Ph. Eur.) diluted to 100 volumes with water and thus contains 1.04 to 1.14% w/w of formaldehyde (CH_2O); it is *not* prepared by diluting Formaldehyde Solution (Ph. Eur.) to arrive at a solution containing 3% w/w of formaldehyde (CH_2O).

Adverse Effects and Precautions

Concentrated formaldehyde solutions applied to the skin cause whitening and hardening. Contact dermatitis and sensitivity reactions have occurred after the use of conventional concentrations and after contact with residual formaldehyde in resins.

Ingestion of formaldehyde solution causes intense pain, with inflammation, ulceration, and necrosis of mucous membranes. There may be vomiting, haematemesis, blood-stained diarrhoea, haematuria, and anuria; metabolic acidosis, vertigo, convulsions, loss of consciousness, and circulatory failure may occur. Death has occurred after the ingestion of the equivalent of about 30 mL of formaldehyde solution. If the patient survives 48 hours, recovery is probable. Formaldehyde vapour is irritant to the eyes, nose, and upper respiratory tract, and may cause coughing, dysphagia, spasm and oedema of the larynx, bronchitis, pneumonia, and rarely, pulmonary oedema. Asthma has been reported after repeated exposure.

◊ General references.
1. Health and Safety Executive. Formaldehyde. *Toxicity Review 2.* London: HMSO, 1981.
2. Formaldehyde. *Environmental Health Criteria 89.* Geneva: WHO, 1989.
3. Formaldehyde health and safety guide. *IPCS Health and Safety Guide 57.* Geneva: WHO, 1991.

Carcinogenicity. There is controversy as to the risk formaldehyde presents as a carcinogen. Studies on the occupational exposure of medical personnel[1] and industrial workers[2-4] to formaldehyde have generally concluded that although the risk is small or non-existent, the possibility that formaldehyde is a human carcinogen cannot be excluded. Reanalyses of such studies have led to different interpretations of the results, with some workers concluding that the risk of cancer from formaldehyde is greater than originally thought,[5-7] while others maintain that the risk is small,[8] and that follow-up of large cohorts exposed to high concentrations for long periods is required to detect such a risk.[9] In the USA, regulatory authorities consider formaldehyde to be a probable human carcinogen.[10]

1. Kreiger N. Formaldehyde and nasal cancer mortality. *Can Med Assoc J* 1983; **128:** 248–9.
2. Acheson ED, *et al.* Formaldehyde in the British chemical industry. *Lancet* 1984; **i:** 611–16.
3. Acheson ED, *et al.* Formaldehyde process workers and lung cancer. *Lancet* 1984; **i:** 1066–7.
4. Gérin M, *et al.* Cancer risks due to occupational exposure to formaldehyde: results of a multi-site case-control study in Montreal. *Int J Cancer* 1989; **44:** 53–8.
5. Sterling T, Arundel A. Formaldehyde and lung cancer. *Lancet* 1985; **ii:** 1366.
6. Infante PF, Schneiderman MA. Formaldehyde, lung cancer, and bronchitis. *Lancet* 1986; **i:** 436–7.
7. Sterling TD, Weinkam JJ. Reanalysis of lung cancer mortality in a National Cancer Institute study on mortality among industrial workers exposed to formaldehyde. *J Occup Med* 1988; **30:** 895–901.
8. Gardner MJ, *et al.* Formaldehyde and lung cancer. *Lancet* 1985; **ii:** 1366–7.
9. Gardner MJ, *et al.* Formaldehyde, lung cancer, and bronchitis. *Lancet* 1986; **i:** 437–8.
10. Council on Scientific Affairs of the American Medical Association. Formaldehyde. *JAMA* 1989; **261:** 1183–7.

Effects on the blood. Haemolysis during chronic haemodialysis was due to formaldehyde eluted from filters.[1]

1. Orringer EP, Mattern WD. Formaldehyde-induced hemolysis during chronic hemodialysis. *N Engl J Med* 1976; **294:** 1416–20.

Effects on the urinary tract. Adverse effects of intravesical instillation of formaldehyde solutions in the treatment of haemorrhagic cystitis have included dysuria, suprapubic pain, ureteric and bladder fibrosis, hydronephrosis, vesicoureteral reflux, and fatal acute renal failure.[1] Intraperitoneal spillage through a fistula, leading to adverse systemic effects, has also occurred.[2] See also Haemorrhagic Cystitis under Uses, below.

There has also been a report[3] of 4 patients exposed to high levels of atmospheric formaldehyde who developed membranous nephropathy, suggesting that there may be genetic susceptibility for this effect.

1. Melekos M, Lalos J. Intravesical instillation of formalin and its complications. *Urology* 1983; **21:** 331–2.
2. Capen CV, *et al.* Intraperitoneal spillage of formalin after intravesical instillation. *Urology* 1982; **19:** 599–601.
3. Breysse P, *et al.* Membranous nephropathy and formaldehyde exposure. *Ann Intern Med* 1994; **120:** 396–7.

Hypersensitivity. Hypersensitivity to formaldehyde has had several manifestations. Effects on the skin have included acute exacerbation of eczema after injection of hepatitis B vaccine, containing up to 20 μg of formaldehyde per mL.[1] In another case, formaldehyde sensitivity was characterised by pruritus, burning, and redness within minutes of exposure to sunlight.[2] Painful, enlarged, and haemorrhagic gingival margins occurred following the use of a toothpaste containing a solution of formaldehyde.[3] There is conflicting evidence of the respiratory effects of formaldehyde: although a low concentration has been reported not to trigger an asthma attack in patients with severe bronchial hyperresponsiveness,[4] occupational asthma has been documented.[5] More severe manifestations of hypersensitivity include 7 cases of shock of possible toxic or anaphylactic aetiology, which occurred after the use of formaldehyde solutions during surgical removal of hydatid cysts.[6]

For mention of an allergic response to root canal paste containing paraformaldehyde, see p.1152.

1. Ring J. Exacerbation of eczema by formalin-containing hepatitis B vaccine in formaldehyde-allergic patients. *Lancet* 1986; **ii:** 522–3.
2. Shelley WB. Immediate sunburn-like reaction in a patient with formaldehyde photosensitivity. *Arch Dermatol* 1982; **118:** 117–18.
3. Laws IM. Toothpaste formulations. *Br Dent J* 1984; **156:** 240.
4. Harving H, *et al.* Low concentrations of formaldehyde in bronchial asthma: a study of exposure under controlled conditions. *BMJ* 1986; **293:** 310.
5. Heard BE. Low concentrations of formaldehyde in bronchial asthma. *BMJ* 1986; **293:** 821.
6. Galland MC, *et al.* Risques thérapeutiques de l'utilisation des solutions de formol dans le traitement chirurgical des kystes hydatiques du foie. *Therapie* 1980; **35:** 443–6.

Treatment of Adverse Effects

Contaminated skin should be washed with soap and water. After ingestion water, milk, charcoal, and/or demulcents should be given; gastric lavage and emesis should be avoided. Assisted ventilation may be required and shock should be alleviated appropriately. Acidosis, resulting from metabolism of formaldehyde to formic acid, may require the intravenous administration of sodium bicarbonate or sodium lactate. The use of haemodialysis has been suggested.

Uses and Administration

Formaldehyde solution is a bactericidal disinfectant also effective against fungi and many viruses. It is slowly effective against bacterial spores but its sporicidal effect is greatly increased by increase in temperature.

Formaldehyde solution is usually used diluted and it is important to note that the strength of preparations is given in terms of the content of formaldehyde solution and not in terms of the final concentration of formaldehyde (see NOTE, above).

Formaldehyde solution is used in the disinfection of blankets and bedding and in the disinfection of the membranes in dialysis equipment. It is important to ensure that there are no traces of formaldehyde on any equipment before it is used. Formaldehyde solution is also used in combination with succinic dialdehyde for instrument disinfection.

When applied to the unbroken skin, formaldehyde solution hardens the epidermis, renders it tough and whitish, and produces a local anaesthetic effect. Formaldehyde solution 3% v/v has been used for the treatment of warts on the palms of the hands and soles of the feet. Sweating of the feet may be treated by the application of formaldehyde solution in glycerol or alcohol but such applications are liable to produce sensitisation reactions and other treatments are regarded as more effective (see Hyperhidrosis, p.1105).

After surgical removal of hydatid cysts, diluted formaldehyde solution has been used for irrigating the cavities to destroy scolices but other larvicides are preferred (see Echinococcosis, p.92). It is generally too irritant for use on mucous membranes but it has been used in mouthwashes and pastes as an antiseptic and hardening agent for the gums. In dentistry it has been used in endodontic treatment.

Formaldehyde solution in concentrations of up to 10% v/v in saline is used as a preservative for pathological specimens. It is not suitable for preserving urine for subsequent examination. Formaldehyde solution has been used for the inactivation of viruses in vaccine production.

Formaldehyde gas has little penetrating power and readily polymerises and condenses on surfaces and its effectiveness depends on it dissolving in a film of moisture before acting on micro-organisms; in practice a relative humidity of 80 to 90% is necessary. Formaldehyde gas is used for the disinfection of rooms and cabinets. The gas may be produced from 500 mL of undiluted formaldehyde solution by boiling with 1 litre of water or by addition of potassium permanganate or by heating a formaldehyde-containing solid such as paraformaldehyde (p.1152). Formaldehyde gas is used in combination with low-temperature steam for the sterilisation of heat-sensitive items.

Other compounds which are thought to act by releasing formaldehyde include noxytiolin (p.1151) and methenamine (p.223).

Haemorrhagic cystitis. Formaldehyde has been used for local therapy of haemorrhagic cystitis although there has been debate about the most appropriate regimen. The Fair regimen[1] for the intravesical administration of formaldehyde solution in haemorrhagic cystitis involves passive irrigation of the bladder with 500 to 1000 mL of formaldehyde solution 1% v/v for a total of 10 minutes, the bladder subsequently being emptied and washed out with one litre of distilled water. Stronger concentrations of formaldehyde solution and other methods can be used if bleeding does not stop.[2] In a review of 118 patients treated with solutions of formaldehyde for intractable haematuria, the authors felt that this was probably the most effective treatment, but also probably the most dangerous.[3] More concentrated instillations, containing formaldehyde solution 5 to 10% seem to be generally viewed as unnecessary, and associated with an increased risk of complications which militates against their use.[4-7] Instillation of intravesical alum (p.1577) has successfully controlled bleeding without complications and has been reported[7] to be a safe and effective treatment for

intractable bladder bleeding; the authors considered that it should replace formaldehyde solution, no matter how dilute. Instillation of prostaglandins such as alprostadil (p.1440) or carboprost trometamol (p.1441) has also been used.

1. Fair WR. Formalin in the treatment of massive bladder hemorrhage: techniques, results, and complications. *Urology* 1974; **3:** 573–6.
2. Anonymous. Haemorrhagic cystitis after radiotherapy. *Lancet* 1987; **i:** 304–6.
3. Godec CJ, Gleich P. Intractable hematuria and formalin. *J Urol (Baltimore)* 1983; **130:** 688–91.
4. Bullock N, Whitaker RH. Massive bladder haemorrhage. *BMJ* 1985; **291:** 1522–3.
5. Donahue LA, Frank IN. Intravesical formalin for haemorrhagic cystitis: analysis of therapy. *J Urol (Baltimore)* 1989; **141:** 809–12.
6. Murray JA, *et al.* Massive bladder haemorrhage. *BMJ* 1986; **292:** 57.
7. Smith PJB, *et al.* Massive bladder haemorrhage. *BMJ* 1986; **292:** 412.

Warts. Formaldehyde solution 3% v/v has been applied for the treatment of warts (p.1108), in conjunction with the removal of scale and dead tissue by scraping.[1] However, in another study the efficacy of formaldehyde solution was no better than the use of an inert agent.[2]

1. Vickers CFH. Treatment of plantar warts in children. *BMJ* 1961; **2:** 743–5.
2. Anderson I, Shirreffs E. The treatment of plantar warts. *Br J Dermatol* 1963; **75:** 29–32.

Preparations

Proprietary Preparations (details are given in Part 3)
Braz.: Emoform; **Fr.:** Emoform†; **Ger.:** Lysoform; **Irl.:** Veracur†; **Spain:** Diformil; **UK:** Emoform†; Veracur; **USA:** Formadon; Formalyde; Lazerformaldehyde.

Multi-ingredient: Austral.: Formo-Cresol Mitis; **Canad.:** British Army Foot Powder; Duoplant; Sporex; **Fr.:** Aniospray; Bacterianos D; Chlorispray; Ephydrol; Incidine; Parodium; Pipiol; Veybirol-Tyrothyricine; **Ger.:** Aseptisol; Buraton 10 F; Desoform; Gigasept; Gigasept FF; Incidin perfekt; Incidin Spezial; Indulfan plus†; Lysetol V; Lysoformin; Melsept; Melsitt; Minutil; Pfefferminz-Lysoform†; Prontocid N; Sekusept forte; Sekusept forte S; Sporcid; Ultrasol-F; Ultrasol-S†; **Ital.:** Melsept; **Spain:** Diformiltricina; Sudosin; Tifell; Viberol Tirotricina; **UK:** Tegodor.

Glutaral (2248-p)

Glutaral *(USAN, rINN).*

Glutaraldehyde; Glutaric Dialdehyde; Pentanedial. Pentane-1,5-dial.

$C_5H_8O_2 = 100.1.$

$CAS — 111-30-8.$

Pharmacopoeias. Solutions of glutaral are included in *Br., Chin.,* and *US.* A solution is also in *USNF.*

Pharmacopoeial description

BP 2001: Strong Glutaral Solution contains 47 to 53% w/w of glutaral. Store at a temperature not exceeding 15°.

USP 25: Glutaral Concentrate contains 50 to 52% w/w of glutaral and has a pH between 3.7 and 4.5. Store at a temperature not exceeding 40° in airtight containers. Protect from light.

USNF 20: Glutaral Disinfectant Solution has a pH between 2.7 and 3.7. Store at a temperature not exceeding 40° in airtight containers. Protect from light.

Adverse Effects

As for Formaldehyde Solution, p.1144.

◊ In a brief review[1] of the occupational hazards of glutaral it was noted that several studies showed adverse effects, including nausea, headache, airway obstruction, asthma, rhinitis, eye irritation, and dermatitis, occurring among medical personnel exposed to glutaral, generally at concentrations below the recommended limits. Skin reactions were due to hypersensitivity or a direct irritant effect. It was concluded that, when using glutaral, workers should take suitable precautions to protect the skin and should avoid inhaling the vapour.

The risk of occupational exposure to glutaral vapour may be higher in warm climates.[2]

There has also been a report of accidental ocular contact with glutaral due to leakage of glutaral solution retained in an anaesthesia mask; moderate chemical conjunctivitis ensued.[3]

1. Burge PS. Occupational risks of glutaraldehyde. *BMJ* 1989; **299:** 342.
2. Mwaniki DL, Guthua SW. Occupational exposure to glutaraldehyde in tropical climates. *Lancet* 1992; **340:** 1476–7.
3. Murray WJ, Ruddy MP. Toxic eye injury during induction of anaesthesia. *South Med J* 1985; **78:** 1012–13.

Effects on the gastrointestinal tract. Insufficient rinsing of a glutaral 2% solution from flexible sigmoidoscopes after disinfection appeared to be responsible for an outbreak of fever and gastrointestinal symptoms including abdominal cramps, bloody diarrhoea, and nausea and vomiting in patients undergoing sigmoidoscopy.[1]

1. Durante L, *et al.* Investigation of an outbreak of bloody diarrhea: association with endoscopic cleaning solution and demonstration of lesions in an animal model. *Am J Med* 1992; **92:** 476–80.

Uses and Administration

Glutaral is a bactericidal disinfectant which is rapidly effective against Gram-positive and Gram-negative bacteria. It is also effective against *Mycobacterium tuberculosis*, some fungi, and viruses, including hepatitis B virus and HIV, and is slowly effective against bacterial spores. Aqueous solutions show optimum activity between pH 7.5 and 8.5; such solutions are chemically stable for about 14 days. Solutions at lower pH values are more stable.

A 2% aqueous solution buffered to a pH of about 8 (activated glutaral; alkaline glutaral) is used for the sterilisation of endoscopic and dental instruments, rubber or plastic equipment, and for other equipment which cannot be sterilised by heat. Glutaral is non-corrosive towards most materials. Complete immersion in the solution for 10 to 20 minutes is sufficient for rapid disinfection of thoroughly cleansed instruments but exposure for up to 10 hours may be necessary for sterilisation. For further details, see Disinfection of Endoscopes, p.1129, and Disinfection in Hepatitis and HIV Infection, p.1130.

A 10% solution is applied twice daily for the treatment of warts (p.1108); a 5% solution and a 10% gel have also been used. Glutaral should not be used for facial or anogenital warts. Glutaral has also been used topically for treating hyperhidrosis of the palms and soles, although other agents are generally preferred (see p.1105).

Preparations

BP 2001: Glutaraldehyde Solution; Strong Glutaraldehyde Solution;
USNF 20: Glutaral Disinfectant Solution;
USP 25: Glutaral Concentrate.

Proprietary Preparations (details are given in Part 3)
Austral.: Diswart; Glutarall†; **Braz.:** Braudeide; **Canad.:** Sonacide†; **Fr.:** Cidex; Endosporine; Sekucid; Steranios; Verutal; **Ger.:** Cidex; Korsolex-Endo-Disinfectant; Sekumatic FD; **Irl.:** Glutarol; Verucasep†; **Ital.:** Asporin 2†; Cidex†; Citrosteril Sterilferri; Diba; Eso Cem; Eso H1, HP, and HP1; Esoxid; Ferriseptil; H1; Sporacid; Sporex; Sporicidin; **NZ:** Zenicide; **Switz.:** Glutarol†; **Thai.:** Glutarin; Mycidal; Pose-Dex; Totacide; **UK:** ASEP; Cidex; Glutarol; Verucasep†; **USA:** Cetylcide-G; Cidex.

Multi-ingredient: Fr.: Aniospray; Bacterianos D; Chlorispray; Incidine; Ultrasep†; **Ger.:** Aerodesin; Aseptisol; Bacillocid rasant; Bacillocid Spezial; Bacillol plus; Baktobod; Buraton 10 F; Desoform; Helipur H plus; Helipur H plus N; Incidin perfekt; Incidin Spezial; Incidur; Incidur Spray; Indulfan plus†; Kohrsolin; Kohrsolin FF; Kohrsolin iD; Korsolex basic; Korsolex FF†; Lysetol FF; Lysetol V; Lysoformin; Lysoformin 3000; Melsept; Melsept SF; Melsitt; Minutil; Prontocid N; Sekucid konz; Sekusept Extra N; Sekusept forte; Sekusept forte S; Sporcid; Ultrasol-F; Ultrasol-S†; **Ital.:** Asporin 0.5†; Citrosteril Impronte; Diaril; Eso Din; Esoform 92; Iketoncid; Incidin Spezial; Melsept; Melsept SF; Sekucid; Sekugerm†; Sekumatic D; Sekusept Extra N; **Mon.:** Akila spray†; **UK:** Tegodor.

Glyoxal (11603-t)

Ethanedial; Oxalaldehyde. 1,2-Ethanedione.

$C_2H_2O_2 = 58.04.$

$CAS — 107-22-2.$

Profile

Glyoxal is an aldehyde used for the disinfection of surfaces and of medical and surgical instruments.

Preparations

Proprietary Preparations (details are given in Part 3)
Multi-ingredient: Fr.: Aniospray; Bacterianos D; Incidine; **Ger.:** Antifect†; Baktobod; Baktobod N†; Buraton 10 F; Desoform; Freka-Nol; Fugisept; Helipur H plus; Incidin perfekt; Incidin Spezial; Incidur; Indulfan plus†; Lysoformin 3000; Meliseptol; Melsept; Melsept SF; Minutil; Pursept A†; Sekusept forte; Ultrasol-F; Ultrasol-S†; **Ital.:** Incidin Spezial; Indulfan; Melsept; Melsept SF; Melsept Spray†; Sekugerm†.

Halazone (2249-s)

Halazone *(rINN).*

Pantocide. 4-(Dichlorosulphamoyl)benzoic acid.

$C_7H_5Cl_2NO_4S = 270.1.$

$CAS — 80-13-7.$

Pharmacopoeias. In *Pol.* and *US.*

It contains about 52% of 'available chlorine' (see p.1141).

Pharmacopoeial description

USP 25: A white crystalline powder with a characteristic odour of chlorine. Soluble 1 in more than 1000 of water and of chloroform, 1 in 140 of alcohol, and 1 in more than 2000 of ether; soluble in glacial acetic acid. It dissolves in solutions of alkali hydroxides and carbonates with the formation of a salt. Store in airtight containers. Protect from light.

The symbol † denotes a preparation no longer actively marketed

Profile

Halazone is a disinfectant with the general properties of chlorine (p.1140) in aqueous solution and is used for the disinfection of drinking water (p.1130). One tablet containing 4 mg of halazone, stabilised with sodium carbonate and sodium chloride, may be sufficient to treat about 1 litre of water in about 30 minutes to 1 hour. The taste of residual chlorine may be removed by adding sodium thiosulfate.

Preparations

USP 25: Halazone Tablets for Solution.

Proprietary Preparations (details are given in Part 3)
Ital.: Clordispenser; Steridrolo a rapida idrolisi; *Port.:* Speton†.

Multi-ingredient: *Spain:* Cloritines.

Hexachlorophene (2250-h)

Hexachlorophene *(BAN, rINN)*.

G-11; Hexachlorophane. 2,2′-Methylenebis(3,4,6-trichlorophenol).

$C_{13}H_6Cl_6O_2 = 406.9$.

CAS — 70-30-4.

ATC — D08AE01.

Pharmacopoeias. In Aust., Br., and US.

Incompatibilities. The activity of hexachlorophene may be reduced in the presence of blood or other organic material. It retains some activity in the presence of soap.

Pharmacopoeial description

BP 2001: A white or pale buff, odourless or almost odourless, crystalline powder. Practically insoluble in water; freely soluble in alcohol; very soluble in acetone and in ether. It dissolves in dilute solutions of alkali hydroxides. Protect from light.

USP 25: A white or light tan, crystalline powder which is odourless or has a slight phenolic odour. Insoluble in water; freely soluble in alcohol, in acetone, and in ether; soluble in chloroform and in dilute solutions of fixed alkali hydroxides. Store in airtight containers. Protect from light.

◊ Hexachlorophene's activity has been reported[1] to be reduced by alkaline media and by nonionic surfactants such as polysorbate 80. It is extremely sensitive to iron, and to avoid discoloration due to traces of this metal in hexachlorophene detergent solutions, it is advisable to incorporate a sequestrant such as disodium edetate.[2]

1. Walter G, Gump W. Effect of pH on hexachlorophene. *Soap Chem Spec* 1963; **39:** 55–6.
2. Bell M. Hexachlorophene-based skin cleansers. *Specialities* 1965; **1:** 16–18.

Adverse Effects and Treatment

Following ingestion, anorexia, nausea, vomiting, diarrhoea, abdominal cramps, dehydration, shock, and confusion may occur. Convulsions and death may follow. CNS stimulation, convulsions, and death have also occurred after absorption of hexachlorophene from burns and damaged skin. There have been reports showing that hexachlorophene can be absorbed through the skin of infants in amounts sufficient to produce spongy lesions of the brain, sometimes fatal.

Photosensitivity and skin sensitisation have occasionally occurred after repeated use of hexachlorophene.

Treatment of adverse effects is as for Phenol, p.1153.

Effects on the respiratory system. Asthma developed in a 43-year-old nurse after long-term exposure to hexachlorophene powder.[1]

1. Nagy L, Orosz M. Occupational asthma due to hexachlorophene. *Thorax* 1984; **39:** 630–1.

Precautions

Hexachlorophene should not be applied to mucous membranes, large areas of skin, or to burnt, damaged, or denuded skin and should not be used vaginally, applied under occlusive dressings, or applied to areas affected by dermatoses. It should be used with caution on infants, especially premature and low birthweight neonates. Its use is advised against in pregnancy.

Preparations of hexachlorophene are liable to contamination, especially with Gram-negative bacteria.

Neonates. Spongiform encephalopathy has occurred in neonates who have been treated topically with hexachlorophene.[1] Neonates with a birth-weight of 1.4 kg or less appear to be most susceptible, whereas those weighing over 2 kg were not considered to be at risk.[1,2] Also most of the reports have involved hexachlorophene applied in a concentration of 3%. This concentration appears to be used in some areas for the control of neonatal staphylococcal infection when other measures are not

effective; in the UK the concentration that is now used for this purpose is 0.33%.

1. Anonymous. Hexachlorophene today. *Lancet* 1982; **i:** 87–8.
2. Plueckhahn VD, Collins RB. Hexachlorophene emulsions and antiseptic skin care of newborn infants. *Med J Aust* 1976; **1:** 815–19.

Pregnancy. Hexachlorophene is absorbed from the skin and crosses the placenta, but whether it has produced teratogenic effects is subject to debate.[1,2] However, it is considered best to avoid its use during pregnancy.

1. Halling H. Suspected link between exposure to hexachlorophene and malformed infants. *Ann N Y Acad Sci* 1979; **320:** 426–35.
2. Baltzar B, *et al.* Pregnancy outcome among women working in Swedish hospitals. *N Engl J Med* 1979; **300:** 627–8.

Pharmacokinetics

Hexachlorophene is absorbed from the gastrointestinal tract after accidental ingestion, and through intact and denuded skin. Percutaneous absorption may be significant in premature infants and through damaged skin. Hexachlorophene crosses the placenta.

Uses and Administration

Hexachlorophene is a chlorinated bisphenol antiseptic with a bacteriostatic action against Gram-positive organisms, but much less effective against Gram-negative organisms. It is most active at pH 5 to 6.

Hexachlorophene is mainly used in soaps and creams in a concentration of 0.23 to 3% and is an ingredient of various preparations used for skin disorders. After repeated use of these preparations for several days there is a marked diminution of the bacterial flora due to accumulation of hexachlorophene in the skin. This residual effect is rapidly lost after washing with unmedicated soap or alcohol.

A preparation containing 3% is used for the disinfection of the hands of surgeons and other health-care personnel. Thorough rinsing is recommended before drying. Hexachlorophene may be applied as a 0.33% dusting powder to the umbilical cord stump for the control of staphylococcal infection in the newborn. However, care is necessary when using hexachlorophene in neonates (see above).

Hexachlorophene sodium has also been used.

Disinfection. Eradication of an outbreak of infection with meticillin-resistant *Staphylococcus aureus* in a neonatal intensive care unit was achieved by use of hexachlorophene soap for hand washing. Previous infection-control measures including the use of chlorhexidine had failed.[1] For a discussion of staphylococcal infections and their treatment, see p.140.

1. Reboli AC, *et al.* Epidemic meticillin-gentamicin-resistant Staphylococcus aureus in a neonatal intensive care unit. *Am J Dis Child* 1989; **143:** 34–9.

Preparations

BP 2001: Hexachlorophene Dusting Powder;
USP 25: Hexachlorophene Cleansing Emulsion; Hexachlorophene Liquid Soap.

Proprietary Preparations (details are given in Part 3)
Canad.: Hexaphenyl†; Sapoderm†; *Ger.:* Aknefug simplex; *S.Afr.:* Lotocreme†; *Spain:* Jabon Antiseptico Asens†; *UK:* Dermalex†; Ster-Zac; *USA:* pHisoHex; Septisol.

Multi-ingredient: *Belg.:* Hemosedan; *Braz.:* Lindanoxil; Micosan; *Canad.:* pHisoHex; *Fr.:* Acnestrol†; *Ger.:* Aknefug-Emulsion; *Irl.:* Torbetol; *Israel:* Acnex; *Port.:* Anacal; *Spain:* Cresophene; Neo Visage; Solarcaine; *Switz.:* Acerbine; *Thai.:* Cibis.

Hexamidine Isetionate (2251-m)

Hexamidine Isetionate *(BANM, rINNM)*.

Hexamidine Diisetionate; Hexamidine Isethionate; Hexamidini Diisetionas. 4,4′-(Hexamethylenedioxy)dibenzamidine bis(2-hydroxyethanesulphonate).

$C_{20}H_{26}N_4O_2,2C_2H_6O_4S = 606.7$.

CAS — 3811-75-4 (hexamidine); 659-40-5 (hexamidine isetionate).

NOTE. The name Hexamidinum has also been used for primidone.

Pharmacopoeias. In Eur. (see p.vi).

Pharmacopoeial description

Ph. Eur.: A white or slightly yellow hygroscopic powder. Sparingly soluble in water; slightly soluble in alcohol; practically insoluble in dichloromethane. Store in airtight containers.

Profile

Hexamidine isetionate has antibacterial and antifungal properties and is available in a variety of preparations for the local treatment of minor infections.

Acanthamoeba keratitis. Hexamidine was suggested[1] as a possible alternative to propamidine for the treatment of *Acanthamoeba* keratitis (p.582).

1. Perrine D, *et al.* Amoebicidal efficiencies of various diamidines against two strains of Acanthamoeba polyphaga. *Antimicrob Agents Chemother* 1995; **39:** 339–42.

Preparations

Proprietary Preparations (details are given in Part 3)
Belg.: Hexomedine; Ophtamedine†; *Fr.:* Desomedine; Hexaseptine; Hexomedine; *Ger.:* Hexomedin N; Laryngomedin N; *Hong Kong:* Desomedine; *Neth.:* Hexomedine†; *Singapore:* Desomedine; *Spain:* Hexomedin; *Switz.:* Desomedine; Hexomedine†.

Multi-ingredient: *Austral.:* Medi Creme; Medi Pulv; *Belg.:* Colludol; Pulvo 47; *Braz.:* Hexomedine; *Fr.:* Amygdospray†; Aurigoutte; Colludol; Cyteal; Hexo-Imotryl†; Hexomedine; Oromedine; Oroseptol†; Otomide; Pulvo 47; Solutricine Maux de Gorge; *Ger.:* Imazol; Imazol comp; Pulvo; *Hong Kong:* Medicreme; Medipulv; *NZ:* Medicreme; Medipulv; *Port.:* Cyteal; *Singapore:* Cyteal; *Spain:* Tantum; *Switz.:* Imacort; Imazol; *Thai.:* Pulvo 47.

Hexetidine (2587-b)

Hexetidine *(BAN, rINN)*.

Hexetidine. 5-Amino-1,3-bis(2-ethylhexyl)hexahydro-5-methylpyrimidine.

$C_{21}H_{45}N_3 = 339.6$.

CAS — 141-94-6.

ATC — A01AB12.

Pharmacopoeias. In Eur. (see p.vi).

Pharmacopoeial description

Ph. Eur.: An oily, colourless or slightly yellow liquid. Very slightly soluble in water; very soluble in alcohol, in acetone, and in dichloromethane. It dissolves in dilute mineral acids. Protect from light.

Adverse Effects

Allergic contact dermatitis and alterations in taste and smell have occasionally been reported.

Uses and Administration

Hexetidine is a bactericidal and fungicidal antiseptic. It is used for minor infections of mucous membranes, and in particular as a 0.1% mouthwash for local infections and oral hygiene.

Mouth ulceration. A mouthwash containing 0.1% hexetidine was no more effective than placebo in the management of patients with aphthous ulceration (p.1206) and provided no additional benefits to oral hygiene or gingival health.[1]

1. Chadwick B, *et al.* Hexetidine mouthrinse in the management of minor aphthous ulceration and as an adjunct to oral hygiene. *Br Dent J* 1991; **171:** 83–7.

Preparations

Proprietary Preparations (details are given in Part 3)
Aust.: Gurfix; Hexatin; Hexoral; Isozid-H; Kleenosept; *Belg.:* Hextril; *Canad.:* Steri/Sol; *Fr.:* Collu-Hextril; Hextril; *Ger.:* Doreperol N; Hexoral; Stas Gurgellosung†; Vagi-Hex; *Hong Kong:* Bactidol; *Irl.:* Oraldene; *Ital.:* Oraseptic; *Neth.:* Hextril; *NZ:* Sterisol; *Port.:* Collu-Hextril; Hexifluor; Hextril; *S.Afr.:* Oraldine; *Singapore:* Bactidol; *Spain:* Oraldine; Oralspray; *Switz.:* Drossadin; Hexigel†; Hextril; Vagi-Hex; *UK:* Oraldene.

Multi-ingredient: *Aust.:* Neo-Angin; *Belg.:* Givalex; *Fr.:* Angispray†; Givalex; Nifluril†; *Ger.:* Anginasin N; De-menthasin†; Givalex; Neo-Angin†; *Hong Kong:* Anso; *Port.:* Nifluril†; *Spain:* Abrasone Rectal; Anso; Mentamida.

Hexylresorcinol (782-j)

Hexylresorcinol *(BAN)*.

Esilresorcina; Hexylresorc; Hexylresorcinolum. 4-Hexylbenzene-1,3-diol.

$C_{12}H_{18}O_2 = 194.3$.

CAS — 136-77-6.

ATC — R02AA12.

Pharmacopoeias. In Eur. (see p.vi) and US.

Incompatible with alkalis and oxidising agents.

Pharmacopoeial description

Ph. Eur.: A colourless, yellowish or reddish crystalline powder or needles, turning brownish-pink on exposure to light or air. It exhibits polymorphism. M.p. 66° to 68°; melting may occur at about 60° followed by solidification and a second melting at 66° to 68°. Very slightly soluble in water; freely soluble in alcohol and in dichloromethane. Store in airtight containers. Protect from light.

USP 25: M.p. 62° to 67°. Store in airtight containers. Protect from light.

Profile

Hexylresorcinol is a phenolic antiseptic which is used topically for the treatment of minor infections of the skin and mucous membranes, and in the form of lozenges for the treatment of sore throat. It is also used in vaginal spermicidal preparations.

High concentrations of hexylresorcinol are irritant and corrosive to skin and mucous membranes. Alcoholic solutions are vesicant.

It was formerly used as an anthelmintic.

Preparations

USP 25: Hexylresorcinol Lozenges.

Proprietary Preparations (details are given in Part 3)
Austral.: Nyal Medithroat Anaesthetic Lozenges; Strepsils Extra; *Canad.:* Antiseptic Throat Lozenges; Bradosol; Bronchodex Pastilles Antiseptiques; Soothe Aid; Sucrets Extra Strength; Throat Lozenges; *Israel:* Sucrets; *UK:* Benylin Sore Throat Lozenge; Lemsip Sore Throat; Mac Dual Action; Strepsils Extra; TCP; *USA:* ST 37; Sucrets Sore Throat.
Multi-ingredient: *Braz.:* Andriodermol; *Fr.:* Genola; *Ger.:* Hexamon; Mycatox; *Ital.:* Golamed Due; *UK:* Beechams Throat-Plus.

Hydrogen Peroxide (13871-s)

Hydrogenii Peroxidum.
$H_2O_2 = 34.01$.
CAS — 7722-84-1.
ATC — A01AB02; D08AX01; S02AA06.

Aqueous solutions of hydrogen peroxide gradually decompose on standing and if allowed to become alkaline. Decomposition is increased by light, agitation, and heat. Incompatibility may also produce decomposition. Hydrogen peroxide solutions are **incompatible** with reducing agents, including organic matter and oxidisable substances, and with some metals, metallic salts, alkalis, iodides, permanganates, and other stronger oxidising agents. Solutions are comparatively stable in the presence of a slight excess of acid. Strong solutions are considered to be more stable than weak solutions.

Solutions of hydrogen peroxide should be stored in airtight containers at 15° to 30° (but see Hydrogen Peroxide Solution (30 per cent), below). Solutions should not be stored for long periods. Those not containing a stabiliser should be stored at a temperature not exceeding 15°. Protect from light.

Hydrogen Peroxide Solution (3 per cent)
(5901-f)

Dilute Hydrogen Peroxide Solution; Hydrogen Peroxide Solution (10-volume); Hydrogen Peroxide Topical Solution; Oxydol.

Pharmacopoeias. In Chin., Eur. (see p.vi), Jpn, Pol., and US.

Pharmacopoeial description
Ph. Eur.: A clear colourless liquid containing 2.5% w/w to 3.5% w/w of H_2O_2 corresponding to about 10 times its volume of oxygen. It decomposes in contact with oxidisable organic matter and with certain metals and if allowed to become alkali. It may contain a suitable stabilising agent. Solutions not containing a stabilising agent should be stored at a temperature below 15°. Protect from light.
The **BP 2001** directs that when Hydrogen Peroxide is prescribed or demanded, Hydrogen Peroxide Solution (6 per cent) be dispensed or supplied.
USP 25: Hydrogen Peroxide Topical Solution contains 2.5 to 3.5% w/v of H_2O_2. It may contain up to 0.05% of a suitable preservative or preservatives. Store in airtight containers at a temperature between 15° and 30°. Protect from light.

Hydrogen Peroxide Solution (6 per cent)
(5902-d)

Hydrog. Perox. Soln; Hydrogen Dioxide Solution; Hydrogen Peroxide Solution; Hydrogen Peroxide Solution (20-volume); Liq. Perox.; Liquor Hydrogenii Peroxidi; Solución de Bióxido de Hidrogeno; Soluté Officinal d'Eau Oxygénée; Wasserstoffsuperoxydlösung.

Pharmacopoeias. In Br.

Pharmacopoeial description
BP 2001: A clear colourless aqueous liquid containing 5.0% w/w to 7.0% w/v of H_2O_2 corresponding to about 20 times its volume of available oxygen. It decomposes in contact with oxidisable organic matter and with certain metals and if allowed to become alkali. It may contain a suitable stabilising agent. It should not be stored for long periods. Solutions not containing a stabilising agent should be stored at a temperature below 15°. Protect from light.
The BP directs that when Hydrogen Peroxide is prescribed or demanded, Hydrogen Peroxide Solution (6 per cent) be dispensed or supplied.

Hydrogen Peroxide Solution (27 per cent)
(5903-n)

Hydrogenii Peroxidum; Perossido D'Idrogeno Soluzione; Solutio Hydrogenii Peroxydati; Strong Hydrog. Perox. Soln; Strong Hydrogen Peroxide Solution.

Pharmacopoeias. In Aust. and It.

A clear, colourless aqueous solution containing 26 to 28% w/w of H_2O_2, corresponding to about 100 times its volume of available oxygen. It may contain a suitable stabilising agent.
The **BP 2001** directs that when Hydrogen Peroxide is prescribed or demanded, Hydrogen Peroxide Solution (6 per cent) be dispensed or supplied.

The symbol † denotes a preparation no longer actively marketed

Hydrogen Peroxide Solution (30 per cent)
(5904-h)

Hydrogen Peroxide Concentrate; Hydrogen Peroxide Solution (100-volume).

Pharmacopoeias. In Chin., Eur. (see p.vi), and Pol. US specifies 29 to 32%.

Pharmacopoeial description
Ph. Eur.: A clear colourless liquid containing 29.0 w/w to 31.0% w/w of H_2O_2 corresponding to about 110 times its volume of available oxygen. It decomposes in contact with oxidisable organic matter and with certain metals and if allowed to become alkali. It may contain a suitable stabilising agent. Solutions not containing a stabilising agent should be stored at a temperature below 15°. Protect from light.
The **BP 2001** directs that when Hydrogen Peroxide is prescribed or demanded, Hydrogen Peroxide Solution (6 per cent) be dispensed or supplied.
USP 25: Hydrogen Peroxide Concentrate is a clear, colourless liquid containing 29 to 32% w/w of H_2O_2. It may contain up to 0.05% of a suitable preservative or preservatives. It is acid to litmus. It slowly decomposes and is affected by light. Store in partially-filled containers having a small vent in the closure, at a temperature of 8° to 15°.

Adverse Effects and Precautions

Strong solutions of hydrogen peroxide produce irritating 'burns' on the skin and mucous membranes with a white eschar, but the pain disappears in about an hour. Continued use of hydrogen peroxide as a mouthwash may cause reversible hypertrophy of the papillae of the tongue.

It is dangerous to inject or instil hydrogen peroxide into closed body cavities from which the released oxygen has no free exit. Colonic lavage with solutions of hydrogen peroxide has been followed by gas embolism, rupture of the colon, proctitis, ulcerative colitis, and gangrene of the intestine.

Closed body cavities. Liberation of oxygen during the use of hydrogen peroxide in surgical procedures has resulted in oxygen embolism and local emphysema.[1-3] Gas embolism has also been reported after accidental ingestion of hydrogen peroxide solution.[4] Local damage to the colonic and rectal mucosa has followed the use of hydrogen peroxide 3% as an enema[5] and from residual hydrogen peroxide following disinfection of endoscopes.[6]
1. Sleigh JW, Linter SPK. Hazards of hydrogen peroxide. *BMJ* 1985; 291: 1706.
2. Saïssy JM, *et al.* Risques de l'irrigation au peroxyde d'hydrogène en chirurgie de guerre. *Ann Fr Anesth Reanim* 1994; 13: 749–53.
3. Konrad C, *et al.* Pulmonary embolism and hydrogen peroxide. *Can J Anaesth* 1997; 44: 338–9.
4. Rackoff WR, Merton DF. Gas embolism after ingestion of hydrogen peroxide. *Pediatrics* 1990; 85: 593–4.
5. Auroux J, *et al.* Rectocolite aiguë iatrogène après lavement à l'eau oxygénée. *Rev Geriatr* 1997; 22: 21–4.
6. Ryan CK, Potter GD. Disinfectant colitis: rinse as well as you wash. *J Clin Gastroenterol* 1995; 21: 6–9.

Effects on the eyes. Hydrogen peroxide, in a concentration as low as 50 ppm, caused damage to human corneal epithelial cells *in vitro*; concentrations of 70 to 100 ppm caused cell death within minutes.[1]
1. Tripathi BJ, Tripathi RC. Hydrogen peroxide damage to human corneal epithelial cells in vitro: implications for contact lens disinfection systems. *Arch Ophthalmol* 1989; 107: 1516–19.

Effects on the mouth. Use of hydrogen peroxide 3% as a mouthwash has been reported to cause mouth ulceration.[1]
1. Rees TD, Orth CF. Oral ulcerations with use of hydrogen peroxide. *J Periodontol* 1986; 57: 689–92.

Intravascular administration. Intravenous administration of hydrogen peroxide solutions as unconventional therapy for AIDS or cancer has resulted in severe acute haemolysis.[1,2] Haemolysis was also reported following contamination of haemodialysis fluid with hydrogen peroxide.[3]
1. Jordan KS, *et al.* A 39-year-old man with acute hemolytic crisis secondary to intravenous injection of hydrogen peroxide. *J Emerg Nurs* 1991; 17: 8–10.
2. Hirschtick RE, *et al.* Death from an unconventional therapy for AIDS. *Ann Intern Med* 1994; 120: 694.
3. Gordon SM, *et al.* Hemolysis associated with hydrogen peroxide at a pediatric dialysis center. *Am J Nephrol* 1990; 10: 123–7.

Uses and Administration

Hydrogen peroxide is an oxidising agent used as an antiseptic, disinfectant, and deodorant. It has weak antibacterial activity and is also effective against viruses, including HIV. It also has a mild haemostatic action. It owes its antiseptic action to its ready release of oxygen when applied to tissues, but the effect lasts only as long as the oxygen is being released and is of short duration; in addition the antimicrobial effect of the liberated oxygen is reduced in the presence of organic matter. The mechanical effect of effervescence is probably more useful for wound cleansing than the antimicrobial action (but see p.1130).

Hydrogen peroxide solutions are used to cleanse wounds and ulcers in concentrations of up to 6%; creams containing 1% or 1.5% stabilised hydrogen peroxide are also used. Although hydrogen peroxide alone is not considered effective on intact skin, it is used in combination with other antiseptics for the disinfection of hands, skin, and mucous membranes. Injection into closed body cavities is dangerous (see above). Adhering and blood-soaked dressings may be released by the application of a solution of hydrogen peroxide.

A 1.5% solution of hydrogen peroxide has been used as a mouthwash in the treatment of acute stomatitis and as a deodorant gargle. A suitable solution can be prepared by diluting 15 mL of hydrogen peroxide 6% in half a tumblerful of warm water. An oral gel has also been used.

Hydrogen peroxide ear drops have been used for the removal of wax. Such ear drops were prepared by diluting a 6% solution of hydrogen peroxide with 3 parts of water preferably just before use.

Hydrogen peroxide 3% is used for disinfecting soft contact lenses.

Immersion for 30 minutes in hydrogen peroxide 6% has been suggested for disinfecting cleaned equipment.

For bleaching hair and delicate fabrics hydrogen peroxide 6% should be diluted with an equal volume of water.

Strong solutions (27 per cent and 30 per cent) of hydrogen peroxide are used for the preparation of weaker solutions and should not be applied to tissues undiluted.

Hydrogen peroxide and other peroxides have many industrial uses as bleaching and oxidising agents.

Disinfection. CONTACT LENSES. Hydrogen peroxide 3% is particularly useful for disinfecting soft contact lenses (p.1129) and lens storage cases since it is effective against *Acanthamoeba* spp. However, it is irritant to the cornea (see Effects on the Eyes, above) and requires inactivating with sodium pyruvate, catalase, or sodium thiosulfate before the lenses are used.

DIALYSIS EQUIPMENT. A disinfectant containing hydrogen peroxide and peracetic acid (Renalin) was not completely effective in killing *Mycobacterium chelonae* in high-flux dialysers. This possibly led to infection of 5 dialysis patients.[1] For a report of haemolysis following inadvertent contamination of dialysis fluid with hydrogen peroxide, see Intravascular Administration, under Adverse Effects and Precautions, above.
1. Lowry PW, *et al.* Mycobacterium chelonae infection among patients receiving high-flux dialysis in a hemodialysis clinic in California. *J Infect Dis* 1990; 161: 85–90.

ENDOSCOPES. Peroxygen compounds have been suggested for disinfection of endoscopes as an alternative to glutaral (p.1129). Hydrogen peroxide solution 3% is fully effective against oocysts of *Cryptosporidium* and immersion for 30 minutes at room temperature has been recommended.[1] However, it has been pointed out that hydrogen peroxide damages external surfaces, particularly rubbers and plastics of the insertion tubes, and thus is not ideal for such purposes.[2] Other peroxygen-containing compounds have been assessed for disinfecting endoscopes but their activity against enteroviruses and mycobacteria may be inadequate.[3,4] Residual hydrogen peroxide solution can cause mucosal damage (see Closed Body Cavities, under Adverse Effects, above) and endoscopes should be thoroughly rinsed before use.
1. Casemore DP, *et al.* Cleaning and disinfection of equipment for gastrointestinal flexible endoscopy: interim recommendations of a working party of the British Society of Gastroenterology. *Gut* 1989; 30: 1156.
2. Weller IVD, *et al.* Reply. *Gut* 1989; 30: 1156–7.
3. Tyler R, *et al.* Virucidal activity of disinfectants: studies with the poliovirus. *J Hosp Infect* 1990; 15: 339–45.
4. Broadley SJ, *et al.* Antimycobacterial activity of 'Virkon'. *J Hosp Infect* 1993; 23: 189–97.

Mouth ulceration and infection. The use of antiseptic mouthwashes may be helpful in the management of mouth ulcers (p.1206), although the use of hydrogen peroxide 3% is not advisable. However, application of a 1.5% solution to individual ulcers in combination with a topical corticosteroid may be useful. For oral candidal infections, specific antifungals are recommended (see p.372), and a hydrogen peroxide denture cleaner was not effective in either preventing re-infection or in reducing mucosal inflammation in a study of 49 patients.[1] See also Adverse Effects on the Mouth, above.
1. Walker DM, *et al.* The treatment of denture-induced stomatitis: evaluation of two agents. *Br Dent J* 1981; 151: 416–19.

Preparations

BP 2001: Hydrogen Peroxide Mouthwash;
USP 25: Hydrogen Peroxide Topical Solution.

Proprietary Preparations (details are given in Part 3)
Aust.: Aosept; Austrosept; Hioxyl; Lensan A; Lensept; Les Yeux 1; Persol†; Titmus Losung 1; **Austral.:** Aosept; Focus Care One Step; Soft Mate Consept 1†; **Belg.:** Crystacide; **Braz.:** Oxysept; **Canad.:** Aosept; Consept Step 1; **Denm.:** Brintoverilte; Microcid; **Fr.:** Dosoxygenee; **Ger.:** Crystacide; Hioxyl; **Israel.:** Crystacide; **NZ:** Aosept; Focus Care One Step; **Spain:** Ahecan; Crystacide; Oximen; **Swed.:** Microcid; **UK:** Crystacide; Hioxyl; Peroxyl; **USA:** Oxysept; Peroxyl.

Multi-ingredient: Aust.: Omnicare†; Oxy-Care; Oxysept Comfort†; Oxysept†; Septicon; Soft Mate Consept 1; **Austral.:** Omnicare 1 Step; Oxysept; **Canad.:** UltraCare; **Fr.:** Spitaderm; **Ger.:** Oxysept Comfort†; Oxysept†; Peresal; Skinsept F; Skinsept mucosa; **Israel:** Omnicare; Oxysept; **Ital.:** Esoform 7 mc; Esoform 70 mc; Peresal; Spitaderm; **Mon.:** Akila mains et peau†; **NZ:** Omnicare 1 Step; Oxysept; **USA:** Aosept; Lensept†; MiraSept; Renalin Dialyzer Reprocessing Concentrate†; Soft Mate Consept; UltraCare.

Hydroxybenzoates (11734-q)

Parabens.

Benzyl Hydroxybenzoate (6635-v)

Benzyl Parahydroxybenzoate; Benzylparaben. Benzyl 4-hydroxybenzoate.
$C_{14}H_{12}O_3 = 228.2$.
CAS — 94-18-8.
Pharmacopoeias. In *Br.* and *Int.*

Incompatibilities are described under Sodium Propyl Hydroxybenzoate, below.

Pharmacopoeial description

BP 2001: A white to creamy-white, odourless or almost odourless, crystalline powder. Practically insoluble in water; freely soluble in alcohol and in ether. It dissolves in solutions of alkali hydroxides. M.p. about 112°.

Butyl Hydroxybenzoate (6637-q)

Butyl Parahydroxybenzoate; Butylis Parahydroxybenzoas; Butylis Paraoxybenzoas; Butylparaben. Butyl 4-hydroxybenzoate.
$C_{11}H_{14}O_3 = 194.2$.
CAS — 94-26-8.
Pharmacopoeias. In *Eur.* (see p.vi) and *Jpn.* Also in *USNF.*

Incompatibilities are described under Sodium Propyl Hydroxybenzoate, below.

Pharmacopoeial description

Ph. Eur.: Colourless crystals or a white or almost white crystalline powder. Very slightly soluble in water; freely soluble in alcohol and in methyl alcohol. M.p. 68° to 71°.

USNF 20: Small colourless crystals or a white powder. Very slightly soluble in water and in glycerol; freely soluble in alcohol, in acetone, in ether, and in propylene glycol. M.p. 68° to 72°.

Ethyl Hydroxybenzoate (6648-w)

Aethylum Hydroxybenzoicum; E214; Ethyl Parahydroxybenzoate; Ethylis Parahydroxybenzoas; Ethylis Paraoxybenzoas; Ethylparaben. Ethyl 4-hydroxybenzoate.
$C_9H_{10}O_3 = 166.2$.
CAS — 120-47-8.
ATC — D01AE10.
Pharmacopoeias. In *Chin., Eur.* (p.vi), *Int., Jpn.,* and *Pol.* Also in *USNF.*

Incompatibilities are described under Sodium Propyl Hydroxybenzoate, below.

Pharmacopoeial description

Ph. Eur.: Colourless crystals or a white or almost white crystalline powder. Very slightly soluble in water; freely soluble in alcohol and in methyl alcohol. M.p. 115° to 118°.

USNF 20: Small colourless crystals or a white powder. Slightly soluble in water and in glycerol; freely soluble in alcohol, in acetone, in ether, and in propylene glycol. M.p. 115° to 118°.

Methyl Hydroxybenzoate (6651-v)

E218; Metingin; Methyl Parahydroxybenzoate; Methylis Oxybenzoas; Methylis Parahydroxybenzoas; Methylis Paraoxybenzoas; Methylparaben (USAN); Metilparabeno. Methyl 4-hydroxybenzoate.
$C_8H_8O_3 = 152.1$.
CAS — 99-76-3.
Pharmacopoeias. In *Eur.* (see p.vi), *Int., Jpn.,* and *Pol.* Also in *USNF.*

Incompatibilities are described under Sodium Propyl Hydroxybenzoate, below.

Pharmacopoeial description

Ph. Eur.: Colourless crystals or a white crystalline powder. Very slightly soluble in water; freely soluble in alcohol and in methyl alcohol. M.p. 125° to 128°.

USNF 20: Colourless crystals or a white crystalline powder. Soluble 1 in 400 of water, 1 in 50 of water at 80°, 1 in 3 of alcohol, and 1 in 10 of ether; freely soluble in methyl alcohol. M.p. 125° to 128°.

Propyl Hydroxybenzoate (6665-e)

E216; Propagin; Propyl Parahydroxybenzoate; Propylis Oxybenzoas; Propylis Parahydroxybenzoas; Propylis Paraoxibenzoas; Propylparaben (USAN). Propyl 4-hydroxybenzoate.
$C_{10}H_{12}O_3 = 180.2$.
CAS — 94-13-3.
Pharmacopoeias. In *Eur.* (see p.vi), *Int., Jpn,* and *Pol.* Also in *USNF.*

Incompatibilities are described under Sodium Propyl Hydroxybenzoate, below.

Pharmacopoeial description

Ph. Eur.: A white crystalline powder. Very slightly soluble in water; freely soluble in alcohol and in methyl alcohol. M.p. 96° to 99°.

USNF 20: Small colourless crystals or a white powder. Soluble 1 in 2500 of water, 1 in 400 of boiling water, 1 in 1.5 of alcohol, and 1 in 3 of ether. M.p. 95° to 98°.

Sodium Butyl Hydroxybenzoate (6667-y)

Sodium Butyl Parahydroxybenzoate; Sodium Butylparaben.
$C_{11}H_{13}NaO_3 = 216.2$.
CAS — 36457-20-2.
Pharmacopoeias. In *Br.*

Incompatibilities are described under Sodium Propyl Hydroxybenzoate, below.

Pharmacopoeial description

BP 2001: A white, odourless or almost odourless, hygroscopic powder. Freely soluble in water and in alcohol. A 0.1% solution in water has a pH of 9.5 to 10.5.

Sodium Methyl Hydroxybenzoate (6674-l)

E219; Methylis Parahydroxybenzoas Natricum; Methylparaben Sodium (USAN); Sodium Methyl Parahydroxybenzoate; Sodium Methylparaben; Soluble Methyl Hydroxybenzoate.
$C_8H_7NaO_3 = 174.1$.
CAS — 5026-62-0.
Pharmacopoeias. In *Eur.* (see p.vi). Also in *USNF.*

Incompatibilities are described under Sodium Propyl Hydroxybenzoate, below.

Pharmacopoeial description

Ph. Eur.: A white crystalline powder. Freely soluble in water; sparingly soluble in alcohol; practically insoluble in dichloromethane. A 0.1% solution in water has a pH of 9.5 to 10.5.

USNF 20: A white, hygroscopic, powder. Freely soluble in water; sparingly soluble in alcohol; insoluble in fixed oils. A 0.1% solution in water has a pH of 9.5 to 10.5. Store in airtight containers.

Sodium Propyl Hydroxybenzoate (6676-j)

E217; Propylis Parahydroxybenzoas Natricum; Propylparaben Sodium (USAN); Sodium Propyl Parahydroxybenzoate; Sodium Propylparaben; Soluble Propyl Hydroxybenzoate.
$C_{10}H_{11}NaO_3 = 202.2$.
CAS — 35285-69-9.
Pharmacopoeias. In *Eur.* (see p.vi). Also in *USNF.*

Pharmacopoeial description

Ph. Eur.: A white crystalline powder. Freely soluble in water; sparingly soluble in alcohol; practically insoluble in dichloromethane. A 0.1% solution in water has a pH of 9.5 to 10.5.

USNF 20: A white, hygroscopic, odourless powder. Freely soluble in water; sparingly soluble in alcohol; insoluble in fixed oils. A 0.1% solution in water has a pH of 9.5 to 10.5. Store in airtight containers.

Incompatibilities. The activity of hydroxybenzoates can be adversely affected by the presence of other excipients or active ingredients. There may be adsorption onto substances like magnesium trisilicate, aluminium magnesium silicate, talc, polysorbate 80,[1,2] carmellose sodium,[3] or plastics.[4] Nonionic surfactants can reduce hydroxybenzoate activity,[5] as may essential oils.[6] Other incompatibilities that have been reported include atropine,[7] iron,[4] sorbitol,[8] weak alkalis,[4] and strong acids.[4] Syrup preserved with hydroxybenzoates is incompatible with a range of compounds.[9,10] Methyl hydroxybenzoate 0.1% was reported[11] to be a poor preservative in insulin preparations, especially soluble insulin preparations. Increasing heat or pH can reduce stability and activity;[12] freeze-drying may also lead to a loss of activity.[13]

1. Yousef RT, *et al.* Effect of some pharmaceutical materials on the bactericidal activities of preservatives. *Can J Pharm Sci* 1973; **8:** 54–6.
2. Allwood MC. The adsorption of esters of p-hydroxybenzoic acid by magnesium trisilicate. *Int J Pharmaceutics* 1982; **11:** 101–7.
3. Fawcett JP, *et al.* Binding of parabens to sodium carboxymethylcellulose in oral liquid formulations. *Aust J Hosp Pharm* 1996; **26:** 552–4.
4. Rieger MM. Methylparaben. In: Kibbe AH, ed. *Handbook of pharmaceutical excipients.* 3rd ed. Washington and London: American Pharmaceutical Association and The Pharmaceutical Press, 2000: 340–4.

5. Yamaguchi M, *et al.* Antimicrobial activity of butylparaben in relation to its solubilization by nonionic surfactants. *J Soc Cosmet Chem* 1982; **33:** 297–307.
6. Chemburkar PB, Joslin RS. Effect of flavoring oils on preservative concentrations in oral liquid dosage forms. *J Pharm Sci* 1975; **64:** 414–17.
7. Deeks T. Oral atropine sulphate mixtures. *Pharm J* 1983; **230:** 481.
8. Runesson B, Gustavii K. Stability of parabens in the presence of polyols. *Acta Pharm Suec* 1986; **23:** 151–62.
9. *PSGB Lab Report P/79/2* 1979.
10. *PSGB Lab Report P/80/1* 1980.
11. Allwood MC. The effectiveness of preservatives in insulin injections. *Pharm J* 1982; **229:** 340.
12. Sunderland VB, Watts DW. Kinetics of the degradation of methyl, ethyl and n-propyl 4-hydroxybenzoate esters in aqueous solution. *Int J Pharmaceutics* 1984; **19:** 1–15.
13. Flora KP, *et al.* The loss of paraben preservatives during freeze drying. *J Pharm Pharmacol* 1980; **32:** 577–80.

Adverse Effects and Precautions

Hypersensitivity reactions occur with the hydroxybenzoates. Generally these are of the delayed type, appearing as contact dermatitis. Immediate reactions with urticaria and bronchospasm have occurred rarely.

Hypersensitivity. Immediate hypersensitivity reactions have been reported following the injection of preparations containing hydroxybenzoates.[1,2] Delayed contact dermatitis occurs more frequently, usually after topical application but has also occurred after oral administration of an ester or of p-hydroxybenzoic acid.[3-5] The North American Contact Dermatitis Group[6] provided an incidence of 3%, while another review[7] of a large number of patients gave an incidence of 2.2%. However, subjects with healthy skin exposed to hydroxybenzoates, for example in cosmetics, are considered to have a much lower incidence of reactions.[8] Unusually, patients who have reacted to a hydroxybenzoate with a contact dermatitis appear to be able to apply that preservative to another unaffected site and yet not suffer a reaction; this has been termed the 'paraben paradox'.[9] Hypersensitivity reactions have occurred in patients given local anaesthetics containing hydroxybenzoates[1,10] and cross-sensitivity between the two groups of drugs has been proposed.[1]

1. Aldrete JA, Johnson DA. Allergy to local anaesthetics. *JAMA* 1969; **207:** 356–7.
2. Nagel JA, *et al.* Paraben allergy. *JAMA* 1977; **237:** 1594–5.
3. Michäelsson G, Juhlin L. Urticaria induced by preservatives and dye additives in food and drugs. *Br J Dermatol* 1973; **88:** 525–32.
4. Warin RP, Smith RJ. Challenge test battery in chronic urticaria. *Br J Dermatol* 1976; **94:** 401–6.
5. Kaminer Y, *et al.* Delayed hypersensitivity reaction to orally administered methylparaben. *Clin Pharm* 1982; **1:** 469–70.
6. North American Contact Dermatitis Group. Epidemiology of contact dermatitis in North America 1972. *Arch Dermatol* 1973; **108:** 537–40.
7. Moore J. Final report on the safety assessment of methylparaben, ethylparaben, propylparaben, and butylparaben. *J Am Coll Toxicol* 1984; **3:** 147–209.
8. Fisher AA. Cosmetic dermatitis. Part I: reactions to some commonly used preservatives. *Cutis* 1980; **26:** 136–7, 141–2, 147–8.
9. Fisher AA. Cortaid cream dermatitis and the "paraben paradox". *J Am Acad Dermatol* 1982; **6:** 116–7.
10. Lederman DA, *et al.* An unusual skin reaction following local anesthetic injection: review of the literature and report of four cases. *Oral Surg* 1980; **49:** 28–33.

Neonates. An *in-vitro* study on serum from neonates with hyperbilirubinaemia indicated that methyl hydroxybenzoate at a concentration of 200 µg per mL of serum increased the concentration of free unconjugated bilirubin and interfered with the binding of bilirubin to serum proteins. Methyl hydroxybenzoate was present in an injection of gentamicin sulfate at a concentration of 1.3 to 1.8 mg per mL. Neither gentamicin nor propyl hydroxybenzoate had a significant effect on bilirubin.[1]

1. Loria CJ, *et al.* Effect of antibiotic formulations in serum protein: bilirubin interaction of newborn infants. *J Pediatr* 1976; **89:** 479–82.

Pharmacokinetics

Neonates. Following intramuscular injection, methyl hydroxybenzoate present in an injectable preparation of gentamicin was excreted in the urine of preterm infants to a variable extent and mainly in the conjugated form.[1] p-Hydroxybenzoic acid was detected as a metabolite. The injection contained 3.6 mg of methyl hydroxybenzoate, 400 µg of propyl hydroxybenzoate, and 80 mg of gentamicin. Propyl hydroxybenzoate was also detected in the urine samples.

1. Hindmarsh KW, *et al.* Urinary excretion of methylparaben and its metabolites in preterm infants. *J Pharm Sci* 1983; **72:** 1039–41.

Uses

The hydroxybenzoate preservatives (parabens) are alkyl esters of p-hydroxybenzoic acid with antibacterial and antifungal properties. They are active over a broad pH range (4 to 8), though are generally more active in acidic solutions. Activity increases with increasing alkyl chain length but aqueous solubility decreases, although this may be overcome by employing the more soluble sodium salts as long as the pH of the preparation is not increased. Activity may also be increased by combining two hydroxybenzoates with short alkyl chains. Another way of increasing activity is to use a hydroxybenzoate with propylene glycol.

Hydroxybenzoates are used as preservatives in pharmaceutical preparations in usual concentrations of up to 0.25%. Methyl hydroxybenzoate and propyl hydroxybenzoate are used together in some preparations. There have been reports of the hydroxybenzoates not being satisfactory preservatives for ophthalmic preparations because of their relative lack of efficacy against some Gram-negative bacteria, particularly *Pseudomonas aeruginosa*. The hydroxybenzoate preservatives are widely used in cosmetics and are also used for food preservation.

Hydroxybenzoates are also used for treating skin infections.

Preparations

Proprietary Preparations (details are given in Part 3)
Fr.: Nisapulvol; Nisaseptol; Nisasol.

Multi-ingredient: *Austral.:* Mycoderm; *Braz.:* Pelmic; *Ger.:* Trachitol†; *UK:* Brushtox.

Imidurea (18353-b)

N,N''-Methylenebis{*N'*-[3-(hydroxymethyl)-2,5-dioxo-4-imidazolidinyl]urea}.
$C_{11}H_{16}N_8O_8 = 388.3$.
CAS — 39236-46-9.
Pharmacopoeias. In *USNF.*

Pharmacopoeial description

USNF 20: A white odourless powder. Soluble in water and in glycerol; sparingly soluble in propylene glycol; insoluble in most organic solvents. A 1% solution in water has a pH of 6.0 to 7.5. Store in airtight containers.

Profile

Imidurea is used as an antimicrobial preservative in topical pharmaceutical and cosmetic preparations.

Iodoform (4577-a)

Tri-iodomethane.
$CHI_3 = 393.7$.
CAS — 75-47-8.
Pharmacopoeias. In *Aust., It., Jpn,* and *US.*

Pharmacopoeial description

USP 25: A lustrous greenish-yellow powder or lustrous crystals. It is slightly volatile at ordinary temperatures and distils slowly with steam. It decomposes at high temperatures emitting vapours of iodine. Practically insoluble in water; sparingly soluble in alcohol, in glycerol, and in olive oil; soluble in boiling alcohol; freely soluble in chloroform and in ether. Store in airtight containers at a temperature not exceeding 40°. Protect from light.

Profile

Iodoform slowly releases iodine (p.1522) when applied to the tissues and is used for its mild antiseptic action. Bismuth Subnitrate and Iodoform Paste (BPC 1954) (BIPP) has been applied to wounds and abscesses. Sterile gauze impregnated with the paste has also been used for packing cavities after oral and otorhinological surgery.

Adverse effects on the nervous system. Encephalopathy has been associated with the use of bismuth subnitrate and iodoform paste for the packing of wound cavities after surgery to the head and neck,[1] although there is some debate as to whether the bismuth or the iodoform component is responsible.[1,2] However, encephalopathy has been reported after application of iodoform gauze without bismuth.[3,4]

1. Wilson APR. The dangers of BIPP. *Lancet* 1994; **344:** 1313–14.
2. Farrell RWR. Dangers of bismuth iodoform paraffin paste. *Lancet* 1994; **344:** 1637–8.
3. Roy P-M, *et al.* Dangers of bismuth iodoform paraffin paste. *Lancet* 1994; **344:** 1708.
4. Yamasaki K, *et al.* Delirium and a subclavian abscess. *Lancet* 1997; **350:** 1294.

Preparations

BPC 1954: Bismuth Subnitrate and Iodoform Paste; Compound Iodoform Paint.

Proprietary Preparations (details are given in Part 3)
Ger.: Jodoform.

Multi-ingredient: *Spain:* Alvogil; *Switz.:* Alvogyl; Pate Iodoforme du Prof Dr Walkhoff†; *UK:* OxBipp.

Isopropyl Alcohol (555-m)

Alcohol Isopropylicus; Dimethyl Carbinol; Isopropanol; 2-Propanol; Secondary Propyl Alcohol. Propan-2-ol.
$(CH_3)_2CHOH = 60.10$.
CAS — 67-63-0.
ATC — D08AX05.
Pharmacopoeias. In *Eur.* (see p.vi), *Int., Jpn, Pol.,* and *US.*

Pharmacopoeial description

Ph. Eur.: A clear colourless liquid. Miscible with water, with alcohol, and with ether. Protect from light.

USP 25: A transparent, colourless, mobile, volatile, flammable liquid with a characteristic odour. Miscible with water, with alcohol, with chloroform, and with ether. Store in airtight containers remote from heat.

Adverse Effects, Treatment, and Precautions

Isopropyl alcohol is considered to be more toxic than ethyl alcohol (p.1131), and the symptoms of intoxication appear to be similar, except that isopropyl alcohol has no initial euphoric action and gastritis, haemorrhage, pain, nausea, and vomiting are more prominent. The lethal dose by mouth is reported to be about 120 to 240 mL; however, toxic symptoms may be produced by as little as 20 mL. Ketoacidosis and ketonuria commonly occur due to the presence of the major metabolite, acetone, in the circulation. Inhalation of isopropyl alcohol vapour has been reported to produce coma.

Application of isopropyl alcohol to the skin may cause dryness and irritation; suitable precautions should be taken to prevent absorption through the skin.

Treatment of adverse effects is as for Alcohol, p.1131.

◊ General references.
1. 2-Propanol. *Environmental Health Criteria 103.* Geneva: WHO, 1990.

Neonates. Reports of chemical skin burns caused by the topical application of isopropyl alcohol in premature infants.[1,2]
1. Schick JB, Milstein JM. Burn hazard of isopropyl alcohol in the neonate. *Pediatrics* 1981; **68:** 587–8.
2. Weintraub Z, Iancu TC. Isopropyl alcohol burns. *Pediatrics* 1982; **69:** 506.

Rectal absorption. A report of intoxication and raised serum-creatinine concentrations due to absorption of isopropyl alcohol following its use as a rectal douche.[1]
1. Barnett JM, *et al.* Intoxication after an isopropyl alcohol enema. *Ann Intern Med* 1990; **113:** 638–9.

Pharmacokinetics

Isopropyl alcohol is readily absorbed from the gastrointestinal tract but there appears to be little absorption through intact skin. The vapour may be absorbed through the lungs. Isopropyl alcohol is metabolised more slowly than ethyl alcohol and about 15% of an ingested dose is metabolised to acetone.

◊ For a report of rectal absorption of isopropyl alcohol, see above.

Uses and Administration

Isopropyl alcohol is an antiseptic with bactericidal properties similar to those of alcohol (p.1132). It is used for pre-operative skin cleansing in concentrations of about 60 to 70%, and is an ingredient of preparations used for disinfection of hands and surfaces. Its marked degreasing properties may limit its usefulness in preparations used repeatedly. It is also used as a solvent, especially in cosmetics and perfumes, and as a vehicle for other disinfectant compounds.

Propyl alcohol (p.1155) is also used as an antiseptic.

Preparations

USP 25: Azeotropic Isopropyl Alcohol; Isopropyl Rubbing Alcohol.

Proprietary Preparations (details are given in Part 3)
Austral.: Clearasil Daily Face Wash; *Canad.:* Alcojel; Alko Isol; Duonalc; Friction Rub; *Switz.:* Avitracid; Mundisept; *UK:* Alcowipe; Medi-Swab; Sterets; Steriwipe.

Multi-ingredient: numerous preparations are listed in Part 3.

Isothiazolinones (9492-q)

Methylchloroisothiazolinone (10323-m)

5-Chloro-2-methyl-3(2*H*)-isothiazolone; 5-Chloro-2-methyl-4-isothiazolin-3-one.
CAS — 26172-55-4.

Methylisothiazolinone (5495-n)

2-Methyl-3(2*H*)-isothiazolone; 2-Methyl-4-isothiazolin-3-one.
CAS — 2682-20-4.

Profile

A mixture of isothiazolinones consisting of methylchloroisothiazolinone and methylisothiazolinone in a ratio of approximately 3:1 is used as a preservative in industry and in cosmetic products. The mixture is often referred to as Kathon CG, one of its proprietary names.

Isothiazolinones may cause contact dermatitis and local irritation.

Hypersensitivity. There have been several reports of allergic contact dermatitis arising from the use of isothiazolinones in cosmetics.[1-4] One review[4] lists incidences ranging from 0.4 to 8.4% and considers that the risks are reduced when these preservatives are used in 'rinse-off' preparations such as shampoos at low concentrations. Irritant reactions can also occur,[1,3] and occupational asthma has been reported.[5]

1. Björkner B, *et al.* Contact allergy to the preservative Kathon CG. *Contact Dermatitis* 1986; **14:** 85–90.
2. De Groot AC, Bos JD. Preservatives in the European standard series for epicutaneous testing. *Br J Dermatol* 1987; **116:** 289–92.
3. Fransway AF. Sensitivity to Kathon CG: findings in 365 consecutive patients. *Contact Dermatitis* 1988; **19:** 342–7.
4. De Groot AC, Herxheimer A. Isothiazolinone preservative: cause of a continuing epidemic of cosmetic dermatitis. *Lancet* 1989; **i:** 314–16.
5. Bourke SJ, *et al.* Occupational asthma in an isothiazolinone manufacturing plant. *Thorax* 1997; **52:** 746–8.

Preparations

Proprietary Preparations (details are given in Part 3)
Multi-ingredient: *Switz.:* Saltrates.

Magenta (2254-g)

Aniline Red; Basic Fuchsin; Basic Magenta; CI Basic Violet 14; Colour Index No. 42510; Fuchsine.
CAS — 569-61-9 (pararosaniline hydrochloride); 632-99-5 (rosaniline hydrochloride).
Pharmacopoeias. In *US.*

A mixture of the hydrochlorides of pararosaniline {4-[(4-aminophenyl)(4-iminocyclohexa-2,5-dien-1-ylidene)-methyl]aniline} and rosaniline {4-[(4-aminophenyl)(4-iminocyclohexa-2,5-dien-1-ylidene)methyl]-2-methylaniline}.

Pharmacopoeial description

USP 25: A mixture of rosaniline and pararosaniline hydrochlorides. It contains the equivalent of not less than 88% of rosaniline hydrochloride ($C_{20}H_{20}ClN_3$), calculated on the dried basis. A dark green powder or greenish glistening crystalline fragments with a bronze-like lustre and not more than a faint odour. Soluble in water, in alcohol, and in amyl alcohol; insoluble in ether.

Profile

Magenta is a triphenylmethane antiseptic dye effective against Gram-positive bacteria and some fungi. Magenta Paint (BPC 1973) (Castellani's Paint) was formerly used in the treatment of superficial dermatophytoses (see Skin Infections, p.376).

Decolorised magenta solution (Schiff reagent) is used as a test for the presence of aldehydes.

Concerns about possible carcinogenicity have restricted the use of magenta.

◊ The handling of magenta was not thought to induce carcinogenesis but its actual manufacture may produce tumours.[1] Magenta was also considered to be unsafe for use in food.[2]
1. Glashan RW. Changes in compensation for occupationally induced bladder cancer. *BMJ* 1984; **288:** 1181–2.
2. FAO/WHO. Specifications for the identity and purity of food additives and their toxicological evaluation: food colours and some antimicrobials and antioxidants: eighth report of the joint FAO/WHO expert committee on food additives. *WHO Tech Rep Ser 309* 1965.

Preparations

BPC 1973: Magenta Paint;
USP 25: Carbol-Fuchsin Topical Solution.

Proprietary Preparations (details are given in Part 3)
Multi-ingredient: *Braz.:* Fungol.

Magnesium Peroxide (5906-b)

Magnesii Peroxidum; Magnesium Perhydrolum.
CAS — 1335-26-8; 14452-57-4.
ATC — A02AA03; A06AD03.
Pharmacopoeias. In *Eur.* (see p.vi).

Pharmacopoeial description

Ph. Eur.: A mixture of magnesium peroxide and magnesium oxide. It contains not less than 22% and not more than 28% of MgO_2. A white or slightly yellow, amorphous, light powder. Practically insoluble in water and in alcohol; dissolves in mineral acids. Protect from light.

Profile

Magnesium peroxide is used as an antiseptic. It is also an ingredient of preparations for gastrointestinal disorders.

Preparations

Proprietary Preparations (details are given in Part 3)
Aust.: Ozovit; **Ger.:** Ozovit.
Multi-ingredient: Fr.: Ektogan†; **Israel:** Digestif-Ara; **Ital.:** Carbonesia; Ektogan; **Switz.:** Magenpulver Hafter.

Malachite Green   (2255-q)

Aniline Green; China Green; CI Basic Green 4; Colour Index No. 42000; Diamond Green B; Viride Malachitum. [4-(4-Dimethylaminobenzhydrylidene)cyclohexa-2,5-dienylidene]dimethylammonium chloride.
CAS — 569-64-2.

Profile

Malachite green is a triphenylmethane antiseptic dye with actions similar to those of brilliant green (p.1136). It has been used for skin disinfection.

Mecetronium Etilsulfate   (3820-v)

Mecetronium Etilsulfate (BAN, rINN).
Mecetronium Ethylsulfate (USAN); Mecetronium Ethylsulphate. Ethylhexadecyldimethylammonium ethyl sulphate.
$C_{22}H_{49}NO_4S = 423.7$.
CAS — 3006-10-8.

Profile

Mecetronium etilsulfate is a quaternary ammonium antiseptic with actions and uses similar to those of other cationic surfactants (see Cetrimide, p.1137). It is active against bacteria, including mycobacteria, fungi, and viruses, including hepatitis B virus. It is used in alcoholic solution for disinfection of the skin and hard surfaces.

Preparations

Proprietary Preparations (details are given in Part 3)
Multi-ingredient: Aust.: Sterillium; **Fr.:** Sterillium; **Ger.:** Bacillol; Sterillium.

Merbromin   (2256-p)

Merbromin (rINN).
Disodium 2,7-dibromo-4-hydroxymercurifluorescein; Mercuresceéine Sodique; Mercurochrome; Mercurodibromofluorescein. The disodium salt of [2,7-dibromo-9-(2-carboxyphenyl)-6-hydroxy-3-oxo-3H-xanthen-5-yl]hydroxymercury.
$C_{20}H_8Br_2HgNa_2O_6 = 750.7$.
CAS — 129-16-8.
ATC — D08AK04.

NOTE. The use of the name Merbromin is limited; in some countries it is a trade-mark.
Pharmacopoeias. In Fr., It., and Jpn.

Incompatible with acids, most alkaloidal salts, many local anaesthetics, metals, and sulfides. Activity may be reduced in the presence of organic material.

Adverse Effects, Treatment, and Precautions
As for Mercury, p.1634.

◊ Reports of merbromin toxicity have included contact dermatitis[1] and epidermal cell toxicity.[2] A fatality has occurred following transcutaneous absorption of merbromin during treatment of infected omphalocele (umbilical hernia)[3,4] and death due to shock, with aplastic anaemia, has followed application to surgical wounds and decubitus areas.[5] Anaphylaxis has also occurred.[6] Extensive absorption following ingestion has also been reported.[7]

1. Camarasa G. Contact dermatitis from mercurochrome. *Contact Dermatitis* 1976; **2:** 120.
2. Anonymous. Topical antiseptics and antibiotics. *Med Lett Drugs Ther* 1977; **19:** 83–4.
3. Yeh T-F, *et al.* Mercury poisoning from mercurochrome therapy of infected omphalocele. *Lancet* 1978; **i:** 210.
4. Yeh TF, *et al.* Mercury poisoning from mercurochrome therapy of an infected omphalocele. *Clin Toxicol* 1978; **13:** 463–7.
5. Slee PHTJ, *et al.* A case of Merbromin (mercurochrome) intoxication possibly resulting in aplastic anemia. *Acta Med Scand* 1979; **205:** 463–6.
6. Galindo PA, *et al.* Mercurochrome allergy: immediate and delayed hypersensitivity. *Allergy* 1997; **52:** 1138–41.
7. Magarey JA. Absorption of mercurochrome. *Lancet* 1993; **342:** 1424.

Uses and Administration

Merbromin is a mercurial antiseptic that has been used for disinfection of skin and wounds.

Preparations

Proprietary Preparations (details are given in Part 3)
Belg.: Medichrom; **Braz.:** Mercurio Cromo; Mercuro Cromo; **Fr.:** Pharmadose mercuresceine; Soluchrom; **Ger.:** Mercuchrom; **Mex.:** Erthiol; **S.Afr.:** Spraychrome; **Spain:** Cinfacromin; Cromer Orto; Logacron; Mercromina; Mercurin; Mercurobromo; Mercutina Brota; Pintacrom†; Super Cromer Orto.
Multi-ingredient: S.Afr.: Achromide; AMS; Daromide; Ung Vernleigh; **Spain:** Argentocromo; Mercrotona.

Mercurobutol   (13488-h)

Mercurobutol (rINN).
L-542. 4-tert-Butyl-2-chloro-mercuriphenol.
$C_{10}H_{13}ClHgO = 385.3$.
CAS — 498-73-7.
Pharmacopoeias. In Fr.

Profile

Mercurobutol is an organic mercurial antiseptic with antifungal properties. It has been used in the treatment of infections of the skin and mucous membranes.

Preparations

Proprietary Preparations (details are given in Part 3)
Spain: Mercryl Lauryle.

Methylated Spirits   (557-v)

CAS — 8013-52-3 (ethyl alcohol-methyl alcohol mixture; industrial methylated spirit).

Three classes of methylated spirits are listed under the Methylated Spirits Regulations, 1987 (SI 1987: No. 2009): industrial methylated spirits, mineralised methylated spirits, and denatured ethanol (denatured alcohol).

Industrial Methylated Spirits is defined as 95 parts by volume of spirits mixed with wood naphtha (mostly methyl alcohol—p.1404) 5 parts by volume. Mineralised methylated spirits is spirits mixed with wood naphtha 9.5 parts by volume and crude pyridine 0.5 parts by volume, and to every 2000 litres of this mixture is added 7.5 litres of mineral naphtha (petroleum oil) and 3 g of synthetic organic dyestuff (methyl violet). This is the only variety that may be sold in Great Britain for general use. Denatured ethanol is 999 parts by volume of spirits (of a strength not less than 85%) mixed with 1 part by volume of tertiary butyl alcohol, and to this mixture is added Bitrex (denatonium benzoate) 10 mg per litre.

As Industrial Methylated Spirit may contain small amounts of acetone it should not be used for the preparation of iodine solutions, since an irritating compound is formed by reaction between iodine and acetone; for such preparations Industrial Methylated Spirit (Ketone-free) should be used.

Pharmacopoeial description

BP 2001: Industrial Methylated Spirit (Industrial Methylated Spirits; IMS) is a mixture of 19 volumes of ethyl alcohol of an appropriate strength with 1 volume of approved wood naphtha. Two strengths are available containing 99% and 95% v/v alcohol (also known as 74 OP and 66 OP respectively). It is a colourless, clear, mobile, volatile liquid with an odour which is spirituous and of wood naphtha. B.p. is about 78°.

Industrial Methylated Spirit (Ketone-free) is a mixture of the same strength as Industrial Methylated Spirit, but is substantially free from ketones, containing not more than the equivalent of 500 ppm of acetone.

Adverse Effects

As for Alcohol, p.1131, and Methyl Alcohol, p.1404. Adverse effects are due chiefly to consumption of methylated spirits rather than its topical use as a disinfectant.

Uses and Administration

Industrial methylated spirit, in a concentration of about 70%, is the usual form in which alcohol (p.1130) is used for disinfection. It is applied externally for its astringent action, but mucous membranes and excoriated skin surfaces must be protected. It may be used for skin preparation before injection.

Methylated spirits may be used in the form of Surgical Spirit (BP 2001), a mixture of methyl salicylate (0.5% v/v), diethyl phthalate (2% v/v), and castor oil (2.5% v/v) in industrial methylated spirit.

Preparations

BP 2001: Surgical Spirit.

Methylbenzethonium Chloride   (2258-w)

Methylbenzethonium Chloride (BAN, rINN).
Benzyldimethyl-2-{2-[4-(1,1,3,3-tetramethylbutyl)-o-tolyloxy]ethoxy}ethylammonium chloride monohydrate.
$C_{28}H_{44}ClNO_2,H_2O = 480.1$.
CAS — 25155-18-4 (anhydrous methylbenzethonium chloride); 1320-44-1 (methylbenzethonium chloride monohydrate).
Pharmacopoeias. In US.

Pharmacopoeial description

USP 25: White hygroscopic crystals with a mild odour. Soluble 1 in 0.8 of water, 1 in 0.9 of alcohol, 1 in more than 10 000 of chloroform, and 1 in 0.7 of ether. Solutions are neutral or slightly alkaline to litmus. Store in airtight containers.

Profile

Methylbenzethonium chloride is a quaternary ammonium disinfectant and antiseptic with actions and uses similar to those of other cationic surfactants (see Cetrimide, p.1137). It is used topically for minor infections or irritation of the skin.

Leishmaniasis. Topical treatment of cutaneous leishmaniasis (p.584) with methylbenzethonium chloride 5 or 12% and paromomycin sulfate has produced a promising response.

Preparations

USP 25: Methylbenzethonium Chloride Lotion; Methylbenzethonium Chloride Ointment; Methylbenzethonium Chloride Topical Powder.

Proprietary Preparations (details are given in Part 3)
Ital.: Benzibel†; **USA:** Puri-Clens†.
Multi-ingredient: Israel: Leshcutan; **Ital.:** Traumicid; **USA:** Acnotex; Dermasept Antifungal; Drytex; Finac; Orasept.

Methylrosanilinium Chloride   (2232-d)

Methylrosanilinium Chloride (rINN).
CI Basic Violet 3; Colour Index No. 42555; Crystal Violet; Gentian Violet; Hexamethylpararosaniline Chloride; Kristallviolett; Methylrosaniline Chloride; Pyoctaninum Caeruleum; Viola Crystallina. 4-[4,4′Bis(dimethylamino)benzhydrylidene]cyclohexa-2,5-dien-1-ylidenedimethylammonium chloride.
$C_{25}H_{30}ClN_3 = 408.0$.
CAS — 548-62-9.
Pharmacopoeias. In Chin., Fr., and US.
Aust. and Jpn include mixtures of hexamethylpararosaniline hydrochloride with the tetramethyl- and pentamethyl- compounds.
The name methyl violet—CI Basic Violet 1; Colour Index No. 42535—has been used as a synonym for methylrosanilinium chloride, but is applied to a mixture of the hydrochlorides of the higher methylated pararosanilines consisting principally of the tetramethyl-, pentamethyl-, and hexamethyl- compounds.

Pharmacopoeial description

USP 25: A dark green powder or greenish, glistening pieces with a metallic lustre, and with not more than a faint odour. Sparingly soluble in water; soluble 1 in 10 of alcohol and 1 in 15 of glycerol; soluble in chloroform; insoluble in ether.

Incompatibility. The antimicrobial activity of methylrosanilinium chloride may be diminished through incompatibilities, decreasing pH, or through combination with organic matter.

The antibacterial activity of methylrosanilinium chloride was inhibited in suspensions of bentonite with which it formed a stable complex.[1]

1. Harris WA. The inactivation of cationic antiseptics by bentonite suspensions. *Australas J Pharm* 1961; **42:** 583–8.

Adverse Effects and Precautions

Topical application of methylrosanilinium chloride can produce irritation and ulceration of mucous membranes. Ingestion of methylrosanilinium chloride during prolonged or frequent treatment for oral candidiasis has resulted in oesophagitis, laryngitis, and tracheitis; ingestion may also cause nausea, vomiting, diarrhoea, and abdominal pain. In the UK it is recommended that methylrosanilinium chloride should not be applied to mucous membranes or open wounds. Contact with the eyes or broken skin should be avoided. Methylrosanilinium chloride may stain skin and clothing.

Animal carcinogenicity has restricted its use.

Carcinogenicity. Methylrosanilinium chloride has been shown *in vitro* to be capable of interacting with DNA of living cells,[1] and has demonstrable carcinogenicity in *mice*.[2]

1. Rosenkranz HS, Carr HS. Possible hazard in use of gentian violet. *BMJ* 1971; **3:** 702–3.
2. MAFF Food Advisory Committee. Final report on the review of the Colouring Matter in Food Regulations 1973: FdAC/REP/4. London: HMSO, 1987.

Effects on the skin and mucous membranes. Necrotic skin reactions have been reported following the use of topical 1% aqueous solutions of methylrosanilinium chloride;[1] areas affected include the submammary folds, gluteal fold, genitalia, and toe-webs. Similar reactions were observed in 2 patients following use of 1% methylrosanilinium chloride or brilliant green on stripped skin.[1] Oral ulceration developed in all of 6 neonates treated with aqueous methylrosanilinium chloride 0.5 or 1% for oral candidiasis.[2]

In the UK it is recommended that methylrosanilinium chloride should not be applied to mucous membranes or open wounds.

1. Björnberg A, Mobacken H. Necrotic skin reactions caused by 1% gentian violet and brilliant green. *Acta Derm Venereol (Stockh)* 1972; **52:** 55–60.
2. Horsfield P, *et al.* Oral irritation with gentian violet. *BMJ* 1976; **2:** 529.

Effects on the urinary tract. Severe haemorrhagic cystitis rapidly occurred in a 32-year-old woman after accidental injection through the urethra of a solution of methylrosanilinium chloride 1% and alcohol 2%.[1] Severe cystitis was also reported following instillation into the bladder of a solution containing methylrosanilinium chloride and brilliant green 1:1 (Bonney's blue).[2]

1. Walsh C, Walsh A. Haemorrhagic cystitis due to gentian violet. *BMJ* 1986; **293:** 732.
2. Christmas TJ, *et al.* Bonney's blue. *Lancet* 1988; **ii:** 459–60.

Porphyria. Methylrosanilinium chloride has been associated with acute attacks of porphyria and is considered unsafe in porphyric patients.

Uses and Administration

Methylrosanilinium chloride is a triphenylmethane antiseptic dye effective against some Gram-positive bacteria, particularly *Staphylococcus* spp., and some pathogenic fungi such as *Candida* spp. It is much less active against Gram-negative bacteria and ineffective against acid-fast bacteria and bacterial spores. Its activity increases as pH increases.

Methylrosanilinium chloride has been applied topically as a 0.25 to 2.0% aqueous solution or as a cream for the treatment of bacterial and fungal infections, but in the UK its use is now restricted to application to unbroken skin because of concern over *animal* carcinogenicity. However, it has been used as a 0.5% solution with brilliant green 0.5% (Bonney's blue) for skin marking prior to surgery.

In the UK, methylrosanilinium chloride is no longer permitted for use in foods.

Trypanosomiasis. Methylrosanilinium chloride is used in some countries to prevent the transmission of American trypanosomiasis (p.587) by blood transfusion.[1] In areas where the proportion of blood donors seropositive for *Trypanosoma cruzi* is high, emergency blood supplies positive for *T. cruzi* can be made safe[2] by the addition of methylrosanilinium chloride 125 mg per 500 mL of blood and storing it for 24 hours at 4°; it appears to work for most but not all strains of *T. cruzi in vitro*.[1] There is no evidence that methylrosanilinium chloride at such doses produces any side-effects apart from transient blue staining of the skin and mucosa.[2] It has been suggested that addition of sodium ascorbate can markedly reduce the amount of methylrosanilinium chloride required.[3]

1. Gutteridge WE. Existing chemotherapy and its limitations. *Br Med Bull* 1985; **41:** 162–8.
2. WHO. Control of Chagas disease: report of a WHO expert committee. *WHO Tech Rep Ser 811* 1991.
3. Chagas' Disease. In: *Tropical diseases: progress in research, 1989–1990.* Tenth programme report of the UNDP/World Bank/WHO Special Programme for Research and Training in Tropical Diseases (TDR). Geneva: WHO, 1991: 69–77.

Preparations

USP 25: Gentian Violet Cream; Gentian Violet Topical Solution.

Proprietary Preparations (details are given in Part 3)
Spain: Vigencial.

Multi-ingredient: *Braz.:* Vulgix; *Fr.:* Antiseptique-Calmante; *Ital.:* Violgen.

Miripirium Chloride (2260-b)

Miripirium Chloride *(rINN)*.

Myristyl-gamma-picolinium Chloride. 4-Methyl-1-tetradecylpyridinium chloride.

$C_{20}H_{36}ClN = 326.0$.
CAS — 7631-49-4 (miripirium); 2748-88-1 (miripirium chloride).

Profile

Miripirium chloride is used as an antimicrobial preservative in some pharmaceutical products.

Hypersensitivity. Two patients displayed delayed hypersensitivity reactions to retrobulbar injection of methylprednisolone acetate suspension (Depo-Medrol).[1] Intradermal testing confirmed sensitivity to methylprednisolone and to miripirium chloride, included as a preservative in the formulation.

1. Mathias CGT, Robertson DB. Delayed hypersensitivity to a corticosteroid suspension containing methylprednisolone. *Arch Dermatol* 1985; **121:** 258–61.

Miristalkonium Chloride (2259-e)

Miristalkonium Chloride *(BAN, rINN)*.

Myristylbenzalkonium Chloride. Benzyldimethyltetradecylammonium chloride.

$C_{23}H_{42}ClN = 368.0$.
CAS — 139-08-2.

Profile

Miristalkonium chloride is a quaternary ammonium antiseptic with actions and uses similar to those of other cationic surfactants (see Cetrimide, p.1137). It is used in creams and lotions for disinfection of the skin and has been an ingredient of sprays used for treatment of minor infections of the mouth and throat. It is also used as a vaginal spermicide.

Preparations

Proprietary Preparations (details are given in Part 3)
Fr.: Alpagelle.

Multi-ingredient: *Fr.:* Sterlane; *Ital.:* Eburdent F.

Monalazone Disodium (12972-g)

Monalazone Disodium *(rINN)*.

Disodium 4-(*N*-chlorosulphamoyl)benzoate.

$C_7H_4ClNNa_2O_4S = 279.6$.
CAS — 61477-95-0.

Profile

Monalazone disodium is an antiseptic closely related structurally to halazone (p.1145) and has been used as a vaginal disinfectant and spermicide.

Monothioglycerol (6652-g)

α-Monothioglycerol; Thioglycerol. 3-Mercaptopropane-1,2-diol.

$C_3H_8O_2S = 108.2$.
CAS — 96-27-5.
Pharmacopoeias. In USNF.

Pharmacopoeial description
USNF 20: A colourless or pale yellow, viscous, hygroscopic liquid with a slight odour of sulfide. Freely soluble in water; miscible with alcohol; insoluble in ether. A 10% solution in water has a pH of 3.5 to 7.0. Store in airtight containers.

Profile

Monothioglycerol is used as an antioxidant preservative in pharmaceutical preparations. It has some antimicrobial activity.

Nitromersol (2261-v)

5-Methyl-2-nitro-7-oxa-8-mercurabicyclo[4.2.0]octa-1,3,5-triene.

$C_7H_5HgNO_3 = 351.7$.
CAS — 133-58-4.
Pharmacopoeias. In US.

Incompatible with metals and sulfides. Its antimicrobial activity may be diminished in the presence of organic material.

Pharmacopoeial description
USP 25: A brownish-yellow to yellow odourless powder or granules. Very slightly soluble in water, in alcohol, in acetone, and in ether; soluble in solutions of alkalis and of ammonia with the formation of salts. Store in airtight containers. Protect from light.

Adverse Effects, Treatment, and Precautions
As for Mercury, p.1634.

Nitromersol occasionally gives rise to hypersensitivity reactions.

Uses and Administration
Nitromersol is a mercurial antiseptic effective against some bacteria. It is not effective against spores or acid-fast bacteria. It has been used for superficial skin infections and for disinfection of the skin prior to surgical treatment.

Preparations

USP 25: Nitromersol Topical Solution.

Proprietary Preparations (details are given in Part 3)
Multi-ingredient: *Austral.:* Butesin Picrate; Cold Sore Balm; Dental Ointment†; *NZ:* Cold Sore Balm.

Nordihydroguaiaretic Acid (6653-q)

NDGA. 4,4′-(2,3-Dimethyltetramethylene)bis(benzene-1,2-diol).

$C_{18}H_{22}O_4 = 302.4$.
CAS — 500-38-9.

Profile

Nordihydroguaiaretic acid has been used as an antioxidant preservative. Allergic contact dermatitis has been reported.

Noxytiolin (2262-g)

Noxytiolin *(BAN, rINN)*.

Noxythiolin. 1-Hydroxymethyl-3-methyl-2-thiourea.

$C_3H_8N_2OS = 120.2$.
CAS — 15599-39-0.
ATC — B05CA07.

Adverse Effects
When given initially by irrigation for the treatment of the purulent infected bladder there may be an intense reaction with a burning sensation and the passage of large fibrin clumps. Administration of a local anaesthetic such as amethocaine [tetracaine] hydrochloride with noxytiolin may control the pain.

Breath odour. A pervasive sweet breath odour characteristic of decaying vegetables has been noted in patients treated with peritoneal dialysis fluid containing noxytiolin.[1] The odour was attributed to unidentified sulfur metabolites.

1. Stewart WK, Fleming LW. Use your nose. *Lancet* 1983; **i:** 426.

Uses and Administration
Noxytiolin is an antiseptic with wide antibacterial and antifungal actions. It may act by slowly releasing formaldehyde in solution.

For instillation into, or irrigation of, the peritoneal cavity or other body cavities, a 0.5 to 2.5% solution is used. Solutions of noxytiolin should be warmed to 37° prior to instillation or irrigation. Treatment is usually for 3 to 7 days, modified or repeated thereafter as required. The normal total daily amount used in adults should not exceed 5 g for instillation or 10 g for continuous irrigation.

Action. Although noxytiolin has generally been thought to act, at least in part, by slowly releasing formaldehyde into solution it has been reported[1] that much smaller amounts are released than have previously been thought and that the antimicrobial effects of noxytiolin solutions cannot be attributed solely to the presence of formaldehyde. There is evidence *in vitro* that noxytiolin might reduce the adherence of microorganisms to epithelial surfaces.[2]

1. Gorman SP, *et al.* Formaldehyde release from noxythiolin solutions. *Pharm J* 1984; **234:** 62–3.
2. Anderson L, *et al.* Clinical implications of the microbial anti-adherence properties of noxythiolin. *J Pharm Pharmacol* 1985; **37** (suppl): 64P.

Infections of the pleural cavity. Three patients with pleural empyema or pneumonectomy space infection were treated by irrigation of the cavity with noxytiolin 1% in normal saline for 3 hours, followed by drainage for 1 hour, the cycle being repeated 4-hourly. Infection was eradicated within 21 days in all 3 patients.[1]

1. Rosenfeldt FL, *et al.* Comparison between irrigation and conventional treatment for empyema and pneumonectomy space infection. *Thorax* 1981; **36:** 272–7.

Preparations

Proprietary Preparations (details are given in Part 3)
Fr.: Noxyflex; *Irl.:* Noxyflex S; *UK:* Noxyflex S.

Octafonium Chloride (2263-q)

Octafonium Chloride *(BAN, rINN)*.

Octafonium Chloride; Phenoctide. Benzyldiethyl-2-[4-(1,1,3,3-tetramethylbutyl)phenoxy]ethylammonium chloride monohydrate.

$C_{27}H_{42}ClNO,H_2O = 450.1$.
CAS — 15687-40-8; 78-05-7 (both anhydrous octafonium chloride).

Profile

Octafonium chloride is a quaternary ammonium antiseptic with actions and uses similar to those of other cationic surfactants (see Cetrimide, p.1137). It is used in topical preparations for skin disinfection.

Preparations

Proprietary Preparations (details are given in Part 3)
Multi-ingredient: *Irl.:* Germolene; *UK:* Germolene.

Octenidine Hydrochloride (19599-e)

Octenidine Hydrochloride *(BANM, USAN, rINNM)*.

Win-41464 (octenidine); Win-41464-2 (octenidine hydrochloride); Win-41464-6 (octenidine saccharin). 1,1′,4,4′-Tetrahydro-N,N′-dioctyl-1,1′-decamethylenedi-(4-pyridylideneamine) dihydrochloride.

$C_{36}H_{62}N_4,2HCl = 623.8$.
CAS — 71251-02-0 (octenidine); 70775-75-6 (octenidine hydrochloride).

NOTE. Octenidine Saccharin is *USAN*.

Profile

Octenidine hydrochloride is a bispyridine bactericidal antiseptic with some antiviral and antifungal activity. It has been used for skin and mucous membrane disinfection.

Preparations

Proprietary Preparations (details are given in Part 3)

Multi-ingredient: *Aust.:* Octenisept; *Ger.:* Neo Kodan; Octenisept; *Switz.:* Octenisept.

Orthophenylphenol (6661-q)

2-Biphenylol; E231; E232 (sodium-o-phenylphenol); 2-Hydroxybiphenyl; o-Hydroxydiphenyl.

$C_{12}H_{10}O = 170.2$.

CAS — 90-43-7.

Profile

Orthophenylphenol is a phenolic disinfectant with antimicrobial properties similar to those of chloroxylenol (p.1142). It is used for disinfection of skin, hands, instruments, and hard surfaces. It also has many industrial uses as a preservative for a wide range of materials, particularly against moulds and rots. Sodium-o-phenylphenol has been used similarly.

Preparations

Proprietary Preparations (details are given in Part 3)

Ger.: Amocid; Manusept; *Ital.:* Citrosteril Aspiratori; Crescom; Esofenol 60; Germozero Plus; Helix I; Neo Esoformolo; Vcanalare; *Switz.:* Manusept.

Multi-ingredient: *Canad.:* Aseptone 1; Aseptone 2; Aseptone 5; *Fr.:* Frekadermϯ; *Ger.:* Bacillotoxϯ; Bomix; Desderman N; Freka-Derm; Freka-Sept 80; Grotanat; Helipur; Incidin Extra; Kodan Tinktur Forte; Primasept Med; *Ital.:* Diaril; Esofenol Ferri; Helipur; Hygienist; Sangen Casa; *Switz.:* Frekaderm; Stellisept.

Oxychlorosene (2264-p)

Oxychlorosene *(USAN)*.

Monoxychlorosene.

$C_{20}H_{34}O_3S$,HOCl = 407.0.

CAS — 8031-14-9 (oxychlorosene); 52906-84-0 (oxychlorosene sodium).

NOTE. Oxychlorosene Sodium is *USAN*.

The hypochlorous acid complex of a mixture of the phenyl sulfonate derivatives of aliphatic hydrocarbons.

Profile

Oxychlorosene is a chlorine-releasing antiseptic with the general properties of chlorine (p.1140).

A 0.4% solution of the sodium salt of oxychlorosene has been used for cleansing wounds (although chlorine-releasing antiseptics are generally regarded as too irritant for this purpose—see Disinfection, Wounds, under Uses and Administration of Chlorine, p.1141) and pre-operative skin preparation; a 0.1% or 0.2% solution has been used in urological and ophthalmological disinfection.

Preparations

Proprietary Preparations (details are given in Part 3)

Canad.: Clorpactinϯ; *USA:* Clorpactin WCS-90.

Parachlorophenol (2265-s)

4-Chlorophenol.

$C_6H_5ClO = 128.6$.

CAS — 106-48-9.

Pharmacopoeias. In *Aust., Swiss,* and *US. US* also includes camphorated parachlorophenol.

Pharmacopoeial description

USP 25: Parachlorophenol consists of white or pink crystals with a characteristic phenolic odour. M.p. about 42°; congealing temperature between 42° and 44°. Sparingly soluble in water and in liquid paraffin; very soluble in alcohol, in chloroform, in ether, in glycerol, and in fixed and volatile oils; soluble in soft paraffin. A 1% solution in water is acid to litmus. Store in airtight containers. Protect from light.

Camphorated parachlorophenol contains not less than 33% and not more than 37% of parachlorophenol and not less than 63% and not more than 67% of camphor, with the sum of the percentages of parachlorophenol and camphor not less than 97% and not more than 103%. Store in airtight containers. Protect from light.

Profile

Parachlorophenol is a chlorinated phenolic disinfectant and antiseptic with similar properties to phenol (p.1152). Camphorated parachlorophenol has been used in dentistry in the treatment of infected root canals.

Preparations

USP 25: Camphorated Parachlorophenol.

Proprietary Preparations (details are given in Part 3)

Multi-ingredient: *Ital.:* Esofenol Ferri; *Spain:* Cresophene; *Switz.:* Cresophene; Pate Iodoforme du Prof Dr Walkhoffϯ; Solution ChKM du Prof Dr Walkhoffϯ.

Paraformaldehyde (2266-w)

Paraform; Paraformic Aldehyde; Polymerised Formaldehyde; Polyoxymethylene; Trioxyméthylène.

$(CH_2O)_n$.

CAS — 30525-89-4.

Pharmacopoeias. In *Aust., Jpn,* and *Swiss.*

Adverse Effects, Treatment, and Precautions

As for Formaldehyde Solution, p.1144. There have been reports of allergic reactions and nerve damage associated with the dental use of paraformaldehyde as a root canal sealant; it should not extrude beyond the apex.

Uses and Administration

Paraformaldehyde is a disinfectant and antiseptic with the properties and uses of formaldehyde (p.1145) and is used as a source of formaldehyde. For disinfecting rooms it has been vapourised by heating. Tablets prepared for disinfecting rooms by vaporisation should be coloured by the addition of a suitable blue dye.

Paraformaldehyde has been used in lozenges for the treatment of minor throat infections. In dentistry, it has been used as an obtundent for sensitive dentine and as an antiseptic in mummifying pastes and for root canals.

Preparations

Proprietary Preparations (details are given in Part 3)

Multi-ingredient: *Aust.:* Umadrenϯ; *Austral.:* Gartech; *Fr.:* Gynescalϯ; *Ital.:* Esoform 7 mc; Esoform 70 mc; *Switz.:* Asphaline; Caustinerf forte; Rocanal Permanent Gangreneϯ; Rocanal Permanent Vitalϯ.

Peracetic Acid (13094-q)

Acetyl Hydroperoxide; Peroxyacetic Acid.

$C_2H_4O_3 = 76.05$.

CAS — 79-21-0.

Profile

Peracetic acid is a strong oxidising disinfectant which is corrosive to the skin. It is active against many micro-organisms including bacteria, spores, fungi, and viruses. It is used for disinfecting medical equipment including dialysers and endoscopes. It is used in the food industry and for disinfecting sewage sludge, and has been used as a spray for sterilisation of laboratories.

◊ Peracetic acid has been used to disinfect endoscopes;[1,2] it is a possible alternative to glutaral (see p.1129).

For use of peracetic acid with hydrogen peroxide in the disinfection of dialysis equipment, see under Hydrogen Peroxide, p.1147.

1. Bradley CR, *et al.* Evaluation of the Steris system 1 peracetic acid endoscope processor. *J Hosp Infect* 1995; **29:** 143–51.
2. Middleton AM, *et al.* Disinfection of bronchoscopes, contaminated in vitro with Mycobacterium tuberculosis, Mycobacterium avium-intracellulare and Mycobacterium chelonae in sputum, using stabilized, buffered peracetic acid solution ('Nu-Cidex'). *J Hosp Infect* 1997; **37:** 137–43.

Preparations

Proprietary Preparations (details are given in Part 3)

Multi-ingredient: *Ger.:* Peresal; *Ital.:* Peresal; *USA:* Renalin Dialyzer Reprocessing Concentrateϯ.

Phenethyl Alcohol (6656-w)

Phenethyl Alcohol *(BAN)*.

Benzyl Carbinol; Phenethanolum; Phenylethyl alcohol. 2-Phenylethanol.

$C_6H_5.CH_2.CH_2OH = 122.2$.

CAS — 60-12-8.

Pharmacopoeias. In *Pol.* and *US.*

Incompatible with oxidising agents and proteins. Activity may be reduced by nonionic surfactants or by adsorption onto low density polyethylene containers.

Pharmacopoeial description

USP 25: A colourless liquid with a rose-like odour. Soluble 1 in 60 of water, 1 in less than 1 of alcohol, of chloroform, of ether, of benzyl benzoate, and of diethyl phthalate, and 1 in 2 of alcohol 50%; very soluble in glycerol, in propylene glycol, and in fixed oils; slightly soluble in liquid paraffin. Store in airtight containers in a cool, dry place. Protect from light.

Profile

Phenethyl alcohol is more active against Gram-negative than Gram-positive bacteria. It is used as a preservative in ophthalmic and parenteral solutions at a concentration of 0.25 to 0.5%, in conjunction with another bactericide, and up to 1% in topical preparations. It is also used as an antiseptic in topical products in concentrations of up to 7.5%. It is also used as a component of flavouring essences and perfumes.

Phenethyl alcohol may cause eye irritation.

◊ Antimicrobial activity may be enhanced by the addition of phenethyl alcohol to solutions preserved with benzalkonium chloride, chlorhexidine acetate, phenylmercuric nitrate, chlorocresol, or chlorobutanol.[1]

1. Richards RME, McBride RJ. The preservation of ophthalmic solutions with antibacterial combinations. *J Pharm Pharmacol* 1972; **24:** 145–8.

Preparations

Proprietary Preparations (details are given in Part 3)

Multi-ingredient: *Austral.:* Sebirinse; *Ger.:* Imazol; *Irl.:* Ceanel; *NZ:* Sebirinse; *S.Afr.:* Ceanelϯ; *UK:* Ceanel.

Phenol (2268-l)

Carbolic Acid; Fenol; Phenolum; Phenyl Hydrate; Phenylic Acid. Hydroxybenzene.

$C_6H_5.OH = 94.11$.

CAS — 108-95-2.

ATC — C05BB05; D08AE03; N01BX03.

Pharmacopoeias. In *Chin., Eur.* (see p.vi), *Jpn, Pol.,* and *US. Aust., Br., Swiss,* and *US* also include a monograph for Liquefied Phenol.

Incompatible with alkaline salts and nonionic surfactants. The antimicrobial activity of phenol may be diminished through increasing pH or through combination with blood and other organic matter.

Phenol should not be used to preserve preparations that are to be freeze-dried.

Pharmacopoeial description

BP 2001: Liquefied Phenol is an aqueous mixture containing phenol 77.0 to 81.5% w/w in purified water. A colourless to faintly coloured, caustic liquid with a characteristic and not tarry odour. Soluble in water; miscible with alcohol, with ether, and with glycerol. Protect from light. It may congeal or deposit crystals if stored at a temperature below 4°. It should be completely melted before use.

When phenol is to be mixed with collodion, fixed oils, or paraffins, melted phenol should be used, and not Liquefied Phenol.

Ph. Eur.: Phenol consists of colourless or faintly pink or faintly yellow deliquescent crystals or crystalline masses. F.p. not less than 39.5°. Soluble in water; very soluble in alcohol, in dichloromethane, and in glycerol. Store in airtight containers. Protect from light.

USP 25: Phenol consists of colourless to light pink, interlaced or separate, needle-shaped crystals, or a white to light pink crystalline mass, with a characteristic odour. It gradually darkens on exposure to light and air. Soluble 1 in 15 of water; very soluble in alcohol, in chloroform, in ether, in glycerol, and in fixed and volatile oils; soluble 1 in 70 of liquid paraffin. A solution of 1 g in 15 mL water is clear and is neutral or acid to litmus. Store in airtight containers. Protect from light.

Liquefied Phenol is maintained in a liquid condition by the presence of about 10% of water; it contains not less than 89% by weight of phenol. It may contain a suitable stabiliser. A colourless to pink liquid which may develop a red tint upon exposure to air or light, and with a characteristic, somewhat aromatic odour. Miscible with alcohol, with ether, and with glycerol. Store in airtight glass containers. Protect from light.

When phenol is to be mixed with a fixed oil, liquid paraffin, or white soft paraffin, crystalline Phenol and not Liquefied Phenol should be used.

Adverse Effects

When ingested, phenol causes extensive local corrosion, with pain, nausea, vomiting, sweating, and diarrhoea. Excitation may occur initially but it is quickly followed by unconsciousness. There is depression of the CNS, with cardiac arrhythmias, and circulatory and respiratory failure which may lead to death. Acidosis may develop and occasionally there is haemolysis and methaemoglobinaemia with cyanosis. The urine may become dark brown or green. Pulmonary oedema and myocardial damage may develop, and damage to the liver and kidneys may lead to organ failure.

Severe or fatal poisoning may occur from the absorption of phenol from unbroken skin or wounds and suitable precautions should be taken to prevent absorption. Applied to skin, phenol causes blanching and corrosion, sometimes with little pain. Aqueous solutions as dilute as 10% may be corrosive.

Toxic symptoms may also arise through absorption of phenol vapour by the skin or lungs. Phenol throat spray may cause local oedema.

Cresols and other phenolic substances have similar effects.

Effects on the heart. A 10-year-old boy developed life-threatening premature ventricular complexes during the application of a solution of phenol 40% and croton oil 0.8% in hexachlorophene soap and water for chemical peeling of a giant hairy naevus.[1] Cardiac arrhythmias have been reported following the use of phenol for chemical face peeling.[2] They were also observed in 3 of 16 children who received phenol 5% as a neurolytic.[3]

1. Warner MA, Harper JV. Cardiac dysrhythmias associated with chemical peeling with phenol. *Anesthesiology* 1985; **62:** 366–7.
2. Botta SA, *et al.* Cardiac arrhythmias in phenol face peeling: a suggested protocol for prevention. *Aesthetic Plast Surg* 1988; **12:** 115–17.
3. Morrison JE, *et al.* Phenol motor point blocks in children: plasma concentrations and cardiac dysrhythmias. *Anesthesiology* 1991; **75:** 359–62.

Effects on the kidneys. A 41-year-old man developed acute renal failure due to cutaneous absorption of phenol after falling into a shallow vat of industrial solvent containing 40% phenol in dichloromethane. No ingestion occurred. Other symptoms included 50% body-surface burns, cold extremities, nausea, vomiting, and respiratory distress. The patient required haemodialysis for 3 weeks; some abnormalities of renal function remained one year later.[1]

1. Foxall PJD, *et al.* Acute renal failure following accidental cutaneous absorption of phenol: application of NMR urinalysis to monitor the disease process. *Hum Toxicol* 1989; **9:** 491–6.

Effects on sexual function. A report[1] of 3 patients who developed urinary symptoms and impotence which lasted up to one year after each receiving phenol 5% in arachis oil sclerotherapy for haemorrhoids.

1. Bullock N. Impotence after sclerotherapy of haemorrhoids: case reports. *BMJ* 1997; **314:** 419.

Effects on the throat. Acute life-threatening epiglottitis occurred in a 49-year-old woman following the use of a throat spray containing the equivalent of 1.4% phenol. The reaction may have been anaphylactic or due to a direct toxic effect of the spray.[1] The UK Committee on Safety of Medicines[2] reported in 1990 that it had received 4 reports (probably including the one detailed above) of oedema of the epiglottis and/or larynx leading to respiratory difficulties. While the incidence was rare, the effects were severe; one patient died and 2 survived only after emergency hospital treatment.

1. Ho S-L, Hollinrake K. Acute epiglottitis and Chloraseptic. *BMJ* 1989; **298:** 1584.
2. Committee on Safety of Medicines. Chloraseptic throat spray and oedema of the epiglottis and larynx. *Current Problems 28* 1990.

Treatment of Adverse Effects

If phenol has been swallowed, activated charcoal may be useful. Some sources suggest the cautious use of gastric lavage although this is generally inappropriate following ingestion of corrosive substances.

If phenol has been spilled on the skin removal of contaminated clothing and excess phenol should be followed by washing of the skin with glycerol or, alternatively, with copious amounts of water. Macrogol 300 and vegetable oils have also been used.

Contamination of the eyes should be treated by flooding with water only for at least ten minutes.

The patient should be kept warm and given supportive treatment. Intravenous sodium bicarbonate should be given where there is metabolic acidosis.

Precautions

Solutions containing phenol should not be applied to large areas of skin or large wounds since sufficient phenol may be absorbed to give rise to toxic symptoms. Phenol should not be used as a throat spray in patients with epiglottitis, or in children aged under 6 years.

Pharmacokinetics

Phenol is absorbed from the gastrointestinal tract and through skin and mucous membranes. It is metabolised to phenylglucuronide and phenyl sulfate, and small amounts are oxidised to catechol and quinol which are mainly conjugated. The metabolites are excreted in the urine; on oxidation to quinones they may tint the urine dark brown or green.

Uses and Administration

Phenol is an antiseptic and disinfectant effective against vegetative Gram-positive and Gram-negative bacteria, mycobacteria, and some fungi, but only very slowly effective against spores. It is also active against certain viruses. Phenol is more active in acid solution.

Aqueous solutions up to 1% are bacteriostatic while stronger solutions are bactericidal.

A 0.5 to 1% solution has been used for its local anaesthetic effect to relieve itching.

The symbol † denotes a preparation no longer actively marketed

A 1.4% solution is used for pain or irritation of the mouth and throat. Weak concentrations have also been used topically for disinfection. A 5% solution has been used as a disinfectant for excreta.

Oily Phenol Injection (BP 2001), up to 10 mL, has been injected into the tissues around internal haemorrhoids as an analgesic sclerosing agent, but alternative procedures may be preferred. Aqueous phenol has also been used as a sclerosant in the treatment of hydroceles.

Solutions of phenol in glycerol have been administered intrathecally for the alleviation of spasticity (p.1322) or injected intrathecally or into soft-tissue structures for the treatment of chronic low back pain. Other types of severe intractable pain may be relieved by injecting aqueous phenol close to motor nerves. Aqueous phenol has been used for chemical sympathectomy in peripheral vascular disorders and for the treatment of urinary incontinence.

Liquefied phenol has been used in the treatment of ingrowing toenails.

Chemical face peeling. References to the use of phenol in chemical face peeling.[1,2] For a report of adverse cardiac effects associated with phenol being used for skin peeling, see Effects on the Heart under Adverse Effects, above.

1. Baker TJ, *et al.* Chemical face peeling for facial wrinkling. *JAMA* 1974; **228:** 898–9.
2. Ariagno RP, Briggs DR. Chemexfoliation as an adjunct to facial rejuvenation. *Trans Am Acad Ophthalmol Otolaryngol* 1975; **80:** 536–9.

Haemorrhoids. Sclerotherapy with oily phenol injection has been used[1] to treat haemorrhoids (p.1205). The technique for preventing mucosal prolapse is to inject small volumes (about 2 or 3 mL) of a 5% solution of phenol in arachis oil into the submucous space above each of the 3 principal haemorrhoids. Rather than causing the haemorrhoidal veins to thrombose, the injection works by producing submucosal fibrosis, fixing the mucosa to the underlying muscle. Other techniques for mucosal fixation such as rubber band ligation or perhaps infra-red coagulation are more effective and associated with fewer complications.[2-5]

1. Alexander-Williams J. The management of piles. *BMJ* 1982; **285:** 1137–9.
2. Gartell PC, *et al.* A randomised clinical trial to compare rubber band ligation with phenol injection in the treatment of haemorrhoids. *Gut* 1984; **25:** A563.
3. Ambrose NS, *et al.* Prospective randomised trial of injection therapy against photocoagulation therapy in first and second degree haemorrhoids. *Gut* 1984; **25:** A563–4.
4. Johanson JF, Rimm A. Optimal nonsurgical treatment of hemorrhoids: a comparative analysis of infrared coagulation, rubber band ligation, and injection sclerotherapy. *Am J Gastroenterol* 1992; **87:** 1601–6.
5. MacRae HM, McLeod RS. Comparison of hemorrhoidal treatment modalities: a meta-analysis. *Dis Colon Rectum* 1995; **38:** 687–94.

Ingrowing toenails. Liquefied phenol ablation has been performed as an alternative to surgical avulsion in the treatment of ingrowing toenails.[1-5] Cauterisation with phenol 88% has also been successfully used to treat ingrowing toenails and onychogryphosis.[6]

1. Shepherdson A. Nail matrix phenolization: a preferred alternative to surgical excision. *Practitioner* 1977; **219:** 725–8.
2. Cameron PF. Ingrowing toenails: an evaluation of two treatments. *BMJ* 1981; **283:** 821–2.
3. Morkane AJ, *et al.* Segmental phenolization of ingrowing toenails: a randomized controlled study. *Br J Surg* 1984; **71:** 526–7.
4. Sykes PA, Kerr R. Treatment of ingrowing toenails by surgeons and chiropodists. *BMJ* 1988; **297:** 335–6.
5. Leahy AL, *et al.* Ingrowing toenails: improving treatment. *Surgery* 1990; **107:** 566–7.
6. Andrew T, Wallace WA. Nail bed ablation—excise or cauterise? A controlled study. *BMJ* 1979; **1:** 1539.

Pain. The neurolytic use of phenol to produce destructive nerve block (p.3) has produced variable results, and some consider the risk of complications outweighs the benefits.

Spasmodic torticollis. Intramuscular phenol was reported[1] to have produced improvement in 2 adult patients with moderately severe spasmodic torticollis (p.1326) who had not responded adequately to intramuscular injections of botulinum A toxin. Response was maintained by re-injection every 6 months.

1. Massey JM. Treatment of spasmodic torticollis with intramuscular phenol injection. *J Neurol Neurosurg Psychiatry* 1995; **58:** 258–9.

Urinary incontinence. Although injection of phenol into the pelvic plexus to produce partial denervation has been used in the management of severe intractable urge incontinence, its use has been largely abandoned. Some patients, especially those with detrusor hyperreflexia, have derived benefit[1,2] but overall efficacy can be poor and benefits short-lived.[3]

1. Ewing R, *et al.* Subtrigonal phenol injection therapy for incontinence in female patients with multiple sclerosis. *Lancet* 1983; **i:** 1304–5.

2. Blackford HN, *et al.* Results of transvesical infiltration of the pelvic plexuses with phenol in 116 patients. *Br J Urol* 1984; **56:** 647–9.
3. Rosenbaum TP, *et al.* Trans-trigonal phenol failed the test of time. *Br J Urol* 1990; **66:** 164–9.

Preparations

BP 2001: Aqueous Phenol Injection; Liquefied Phenol; Oily Phenol Injection; Phenol and Glycerol Injection;
BPC 1973: Magenta Paint;
USP 25: Carbol-Fuchsin Topical Solution; Liquefied Phenol; Phenolated Calamine Lotion.

Proprietary Preparations (details are given in Part 3)
Austral.: Summers Eve Disposable; **Canad.:** Chloraseptic Sore Throat Spray; P & S; **Irl.:** Vicks Chloraseptic†; **S.Afr.:** Medi-Keel A; Septosol; **USA:** Cheracol Sore Throat; P & S; Phenaseptic; Ulcerease; Vicks Children's Chloraseptic; Vicks Chloraseptic.

Multi-ingredient: numerous preparations are listed in Part 3.

Phenoxyethanol (6657-e)

Ethyleneglycol Monophenylether; Phenoxyaethanol; Phenoxyethanolum; β-Phenoxyethyl Alcohol. 2-Phenoxyethanol.
$C_8H_{10}O_2 = 138.2.$
CAS — 122-99-6.
Pharmacopoeias. In *Eur.* (see p.vi).

Incompatibilities. The activity of phenoxyethanol may be reduced by interaction with nonionic surfactants and possibly by adsorption onto polyvinyl chloride.

Pharmacopoeial description

Ph. Eur.: A colourless slightly viscous liquid. Slightly soluble in water, in arachis oil and in olive oil; miscible with alcohol, with acetone, and with glycerol.

Profile

Phenoxyethanol is effective against strains of *Pseudomonas aeruginosa* but less so against other Gram-negative and Gram-positive bacteria. It has been used as a preservative in cosmetics and topical pharmaceuticals at a concentration of 0.5 to 1%. It is often used in combination with other preservatives, commonly hydroxybenzoates, to obtain a wider spectrum of antimicrobial activity.

Phenoxyethanol is used in concentrations of about 2% as an antiseptic for minor infections of skin, wounds, and mucous membranes. Aqueous solutions may be prepared by shaking the phenoxyethanol with hot water until dissolved, then adjusting to final volume when cool. Preparation of the solution can be aided by propylene glycol.

Phenoxypropanol and chlorophenoxyethanol are related compounds used in topical preparations.

Preparations

Proprietary Preparations (details are given in Part 3)
Canad.: Lanohex; **Hong Kong:** Lanohex; **Irl.:** Biactol Antibacterial Facewash†; **UK:** Biactol Liquid; Clearasil Medicated Face Wash.

Multi-ingredient: **Aust.:** Octenisept; **Austral.:** Dermocaine; **Belg.:** Solubeol; **Ger.:** Gigasept AF; Gigasept Med; Lysetol Med; Octenisept; Terralin; **Ital.:** Fitostimoline; Florigien; **Mex.:** Fitoestimulina; Italdermol; **NZ:** Dermocaine; **S.Afr.:** Tantol Skin Cleanser†; **Switz.:** Octenisept.

Phenoxyisopropanol (20592-k)

Phenoxyisopropyl Alcohol. 1-phenoxypropan-2-ol.
$C_9H_{12}O_2 = 152.2.$
CAS — 770-35-4.

Profile

Phenoxyisopropanol is used as a preservative and as an antiseptic in preparations for the treatment of acne, insect bites and minor abrasions to the skin.

Preparations

Proprietary Preparations (details are given in Part 3)
Austral.: Clearasil Daily Face Wash.

Multi-ingredient: **Hong Kong:** Soov Bite.

Phenylmercuric Salts (12171-t)

Phenylmercuric Acetate (6658-I)

Phenylhydrargyri Acetas; PMA. (Acetato)phenylmercury.
$C_8H_8HgO_2 = 336.7.$
CAS — 62-38-4.
Pharmacopoeias. In *Aust.*, *Fr.*, and *Pol.* Also in *USNF.*

Incompatibilities are described under Phenylmercuric Nitrate, below.

Pharmacopoeial description

USNF 20: A white to creamy-white, odourless, crystalline powder or small white prisms or leaflets. Soluble 1 in 180 of water, 1 in 225 of alcohol, 1 in 6.8 of chloroform, and 1 in 200 of ether; soluble in acetone. Store in airtight containers. Protect from light.

Phenylmercuric Borate (6659-y)

Phenylmercuric Borate (rINN).

Hydrargyrum Phenyloboricum; Phenomerborum; Phenylhydrargyri Boras.

C_6H_5HgOH, $C_6H_5HgOB(OH)_2 = 633.2$ or C_6H_5HgOH, $C_6H_5HgBO_2 = 615.2$.

CAS — 8017-88-7 ($C_{12}H_{13}BHg_2O_4$); 6273-99-0 ($C_{12}H_{11}BHg_2O_3$); 102-98-7 ($C_6H_7BHgO_3$).

ATC — D08AK02.

Pharmacopoeias. In Eur. (see p.vi) and Pol.

Incompatibilities are described under Phenylmercuric Nitrate, below.

Pharmacopoeial description

Ph. Eur.: A compound consisting of equimolecular proportions of phenylmercuric orthoborate and phenylmercuric hydroxide ($C_{12}H_{13}BHg_2O_4$) or of the dehydrated form (metaborate, $C_{12}H_{11}BHg_2O_3$) or a mixture of the two compounds. Colourless shiny crystals or a white or slightly yellowish crystalline powder. Slightly soluble in water and in alcohol. Protect from light.

Phenylmercuric Nitrate (6660-g)

Basic Phenylmercury Nitrate; Phenylhydrargyri Nitras; PMN. Nitratophenylmercury.

$C_6H_5HgOH,C_6H_5HgNO_3 = 634.4$.

CAS — 8003-05-2 ($C_6H_5HgOH,C_6H_5HgNO_3$); 55-68-5 ($C_6H_5HgNO_3$).

ATC — D09AA04.

Pharmacopoeias. In Eur. (see p.vi), Int., and Pol. Also in USNF.

Pharmacopoeial description

Ph. Eur.: A mixture of phenylmercuric nitrate and phenylmercuric hydroxide. A white or pale yellow powder. Very slightly soluble in water and in alcohol; slightly soluble in hot water; dissolves in glycerol and in fatty oils. Protect from light.

USNF 20: A mixture of phenylmercuric nitrate and phenylmercuric hydroxide. A white crystalline powder. Soluble 1 in 600 of water; slightly soluble in alcohol and in glycerol; more soluble in the presence of nitric acid or alkali hydroxides. A saturated solution in water is acid to litmus. Store in airtight containers. Protect from light.

Incompatibilities. The activity of phenylmercuric salts may be reduced by interaction with compounds such as kaolin, magnesium trisilicate, starch, and talc.[1,2] Disodium edetate and sodium thiosulfate can also produce inactivation.[3] Sodium metabisulfite can lead to precipitation,[3] or chemical destruction,[4] but it can also produce increased activity.[3] Other incompatibilities include bromides, iodides (chlorides to a lesser extent), metals, and ammonia and its salts.[5] There can be adsorption onto rubber and some plastics[5,6] although sorption by low density polyethylene can be inhibited by phosphate ions.[7] Some filters, though not membrane filters, used for sterilisation removed considerable amounts of phenylmercuric nitrate from solution.[8] The pH may also affect activity.[9]

1. Yousef RT, et al. Effect of some pharmaceutical materials on the bactericidal activities of preservatives. Can J Pharm Sci 1973; 8: 54–6.
2. Horn NR, et al. Interactions between powder suspensions and selected quaternary ammonium and organomercurial preservatives. Cosmet Toilet 1980; 95: 69–73.
3. Richards RME, Reary JME. Changes in antibacterial activity of thiomersal and PMN on autoclaving with certain adjuvants. J Pharm Pharmacol 1972; 24 (suppl): 84P–89P.
4. Collins AJ, et al. Incompatibility of phenylmercuric acetate with sodium metabisulphite in eye drop formulations. J Pharm Pharmacol 1985; 37 (suppl): 123P.
5. Weller PJ. Phenylmercuric nitrate. In: Kibbe AH, ed. Handbook of pharmaceutical excipients. 3rd ed. Washington and London: American Pharmaceutical Association and The Pharmaceutical Press, 2000: 379–82.
6. Aspinall JA, et al. The effect of low density polyethylene containers on some hospital-manufactured eyedrop formulations. J Clin Hosp Pharm 1980; 5: 21–9.
7. Aspinall JE, et al. The effect of low density polyethylene containers on some hospital-manufactured eyedrop formulations II. Inhibition of the sorption of phenylmercuric acetate. J Clin Hosp Pharm 1983; 8: 233–40.
8. Naido NT, et al. Preservative loss from ophthalmic solutions during filtration sterilisation. Aust J Pharm Sci 1972; NS1: 16–18.
9. Wessels JMC, Adema DMM. Some data on the relationship between fungicidal protection and pH. In: Walters AH, Elphick JJ, eds. Biodeterioration of materials. Amsterdam: Elsevier, 1968: 517–23.

Adverse Effects and Precautions

While the adverse effects of inorganic mercury (p.1634) should be taken into account when considering the adverse effects of phenylmercuric compounds, there is little evidence of systemic toxicity arising from their use. They are irritant to the skin and may give rise to erythema and blistering. Hypersensitivity reactions have been reported. Topical application to eyes has been associated with mercurialentis and atypical band keratopathy; prolonged use of eye drops containing phenylmercuric preservatives is not recommended.

Effects on the eyes. References to primary atypical band keratopathy and pigmentation of the anterior capsule of the lens (mercurialentis) associated with the prolonged use of eye drops containing phenylmercuric preservative.

1. Kennedy RE, et al. Further observations on atypical band keratopathy in glaucoma patients. Trans Am Ophthalmol Soc 1974; 72: 107–22.
2. Garron LK, et al. A clinical pathologic study of mercurialentis medicamentosus. Trans Am Ophthalmol Soc 1976; 74: 295–320.
3. Brazier DJ, Hitchings RA. Atypical band keratopathy following long-term pilocarpine treatment. Br J Ophthalmol 1989; 73: 294–6.

Uses

Phenylmercuric salts have antibacterial and antifungal properties. They are primarily bacteriostatic compounds although they also have a slow bactericidal action. Their activity has been reported to be pH dependent.

Phenylmercuric compounds are used as preservatives in cosmetic, ophthalmic, or pharmaceutical preparations and as antiseptics. They have also been used as spermicides.

When employed as a preservative in eye drops, a concentration of 0.002% is usually used; in injection solutions, the concentration is usually 0.001%.

Preparations

Proprietary Preparations (details are given in Part 3)
Ger.: Soklinal†; **Israel:** Clean-N-Soak.
Multi-ingredient: USA: Hem-Prep.

Picloxydine (2269-y)

Picloxydine (BAN, rINN).

1,1'-[Piperazine-1,4-diylbis(formimidoyl)]bis[3-(4-chlorophenyl)guanidine].

$C_{20}H_{24}Cl_2N_{10} = 475.4$.

CAS — 5636-92-0.

ATC — S01AX16.

Profile

Picloxydine is a biguanide disinfectant with properties similar to those of chlorhexidine (p.1138). It has been used in eye drops as the dihydrochloride for the treatment of superficial infections of the eye. It has also been used as a surface disinfectant in combination with quaternary ammonium compounds.

Preparations

Proprietary Preparations (details are given in Part 3)
Fr.: Vitabact; **Switz.:** Vitabact.

Polihexanide (13146-m)

Polihexanide (BAN, rINN).

ICI-9073; Polyhexamethylene Biguanide Hydrochloride; Polyhexanide. Poly(1-hexamethylenebiguanide hydrochloride).

$(C_8H_{17}N_5,HCl)_n$.

CAS — 32289-58-0.

ATC — D08AC05.

Profile

Polihexanide has antibacterial and antiamoebic activity. It is used as a surface disinfectant and for disinfecting soft contact lenses (p.1129). It has been tried in the treatment of Acanthamoeba keratitis (p.582).

Preparations

Proprietary Preparations (details are given in Part 3)
Switz.: Lavasept.
Multi-ingredient: Fr.: Ampholysine Plus; Hexanios G+R; Instruzyme; Novospray; **Ger.:** Complete†; Teta Extra; Teta-S; **Israel:** Complete All-In-One.

Polynoxylin (2270-g)

Polynoxylin (BAN, rINN).

Poly{[bis(hydroxymethyl)ureylene]methylene}.

$(C_4H_8N_2O_3)_n$.

CAS — 9011-05-6.

ATC — A01AB05; D01AE05.

Profile

Polynoxylin is a condensation product of formaldehyde and urea. It is an antiseptic with antibacterial and antifungal actions and, like noxytiolin (p.1151), may act by the release of formaldehyde. It is used topically for the local treatment of minor infections, usually at a concentration of 10%.

Preparations

Proprietary Preparations (details are given in Part 3)
Aust.: Anaflex†; **Austral.:** Ponoxylan†; **NZ:** Ponoxylan; **Singapore:** Anaflex; **UK:** Anaflex.

Potassium Nitrate (13155-b)

E252; Kalii Nitras; Kalium Nitricum; Nitre; Saltpetre.

$KNO_3 = 101.1$.

CAS — 7757-79-1.

Pharmacopoeias. In Eur. (see p.vi), Pol., and US.

Pharmacopoeial description

Ph. Eur.: Colourless crystals or a white crystalline powder. Freely soluble in water; very soluble in boiling water; practically insoluble in alcohol.

USP 25: Colourless crystals or a white crystalline powder. Freely soluble in water; very soluble in boiling water; practically insoluble in alcohol; soluble in glycerol. Store in airtight containers.

◊ CAUTION. Potassium nitrate has been used for the illicit preparation of explosives or fireworks; care is required with its supply.

◊ The name saltpetre has been used as a generic term for a number of potassium- and sodium-based preservatives used in food manufacture. For a report of poisoning when a mixture of sodium nitrate and sodium nitrite was supplied for saltpetre, see p.1156.

Adverse Effects

After ingestion potassium nitrate may be reduced to nitrite in the gastrointestinal tract by the action of bacteria and ingestion of large amounts can therefore cause methaemoglobinaemia. Gastrointestinal disturbances, vertigo, headache, flushing of the skin, hypotension, irregular pulse, cyanosis, convulsions, and collapse may occur. The toxic dose varies greatly; 15 g may prove fatal but much larger doses have been taken without serious effects. Poisoning has frequently been reported in infants given water from wells contaminated with nitrates.

Nitrites are precursors of nitrosamines, which are animal carcinogens, but a realtionship with human cancer has not been established.

◊ Concern has been expressed regarding the concentrations of nitrates and nitrites in the public drinking water supply. In the UK a maximum nitrate concentration of 50 mg per litre and a maximum nitrite concentration of 0.1 mg per litre have been set for drinking water.[1]

1. MAFF. Nitrate, nitrite and N-nitroso compounds in food: second report. Food Surveillance Paper 32. London: HMSO, 1992.

Uses and Administration

Potassium nitrate is used as a preservative in foods. It is also included in dentrifices to reduce the pain of hypersensitive teeth. When taken by mouth in dilute solution, it acts as a diuretic and was formerly used for this purpose.

Preparations

USP 25: Potassium Nitrate Solution.

Proprietary Preparations (details are given in Part 3)
USA: Denquel; Mint Sensodyne†.
Multi-ingredient: Austral.: Mackenzies Menthoids†; Oral-B Sensitive; Thermodent†; **Belg.:** Escouflaire†; **Braz.:** Pilulas De Witt's; **Canad.:** Sensodyne-F; **Ital.:** Dentosan Sensibile; **Port.:** Biofluor Sensible; **Switz.:** Grafco batonnets de bois; **UK:** Avoca; **USA:** Sensitivity Protection Crest; Sensodyne-F.

Potassium Permanganate (5907-v)

Kalii Permanganas; Kalium Hypermanganicum; Kalium Permanganicum; Pot. Permang.

$KMnO_4 = 158.0$.

CAS — 7722-64-7.

ATC — D08AX06; V03AB18.

Pharmacopoeias. In Chin., Eur. (see p.vi), Jpn, Pol., and US.

Incompatible with iodides, reducing agents, and most organic substances.

Pharmacopoeial description

Ph. Eur.: Dark purple or almost black crystals or a dark purple or brownish-black granular powder, usually with a metallic lustre. It decomposes in contact with certain organic substances. Soluble in cold water and freely soluble in boiling water.

USP 25: Dark purple crystals, almost opaque by transmitted light and with a blue metallic lustre by reflected light; its colour is sometimes modified by a dark bronze-like appearance. Soluble 1 in 15 of water and 1 in 3.5 of boiling water.

◊ CAUTION. Potassium permanganate may be explosive if it is brought into contact with organic or other readily oxidisable substances. It has been used for the illicit preparation of fireworks; care is required with its supply.

Adverse Effects and Treatment

The crystals and concentrated solutions of potassium permanganate are caustic and even fairly dilute solutions are irritant to tissues and stain skin brown.

Symptoms of poisoning following ingestion of potassium permanganate should be treated symptomatically; they include nausea, vomiting of a brownish-coloured material, corrosion, oedema, and brown coloration of the buccal mucosa, gastrointestinal haemorrhage, liver and kidney damage, and cardiovascular depression. The fatal dose is probably about 5 to 10 g and death may occur up to 1 month from the time of poisoning.

The insertion into the vagina of potassium permanganate for its supposed abortifacient action causes corrosive burns, severe vaginal haemorrhage, and perforation of the vaginal wall, leading to peritonitis. Vascular collapse may occur.

◊ Case reports of adverse effects following ingestion of potassium permanganate.

1. Mahomedy MC, *et al.* Methaemoglobinaemia following treatment dispensed by witch doctors: two cases of potassium permanganate poisoning. *Anaesthesia* 1975; **30**: 190–3.
2. Kochhar R, *et al.* Potassium permanganate induced oesophageal stricture. *Hum Toxicol* 1986; **5**: 393–4.
3. Southwood T, *et al.* Ingestion of potassium permanganate crystals by a three-year-old boy. *Med J Aust* 1987; **146**: 639–40.
4. Middleton SJ, *et al.* Haemorrhagic pancreatitis—a cause of death in severe potassium permanganate poisoning. *Postgrad Med J* 1990; **66**: 657–8.
5. Young RJ, *et al.* Fatal acute hepatorenal failure following potassium permanganate ingestion. *Hum Exp Toxicol* 1996; **15**: 259–61.
6. Ong KL, *et al.* Potassium permanganate poisoning—a rare cause of fatal self poisoning. *J Accid Emerg Med* 1997; **14**: 43–5.
7. Lifshitz M, *et al.* Fatal potassium permanganate intoxication in an infant. *J Toxicol Clin Toxicol* 1999; **37**: 801–2.

Uses and Administration
Potassium permanganate possesses oxidising properties which in turn confer disinfectant and deodorising properties. It is also astringent. Though bactericidal *in vitro* its clinical value as a bactericide is minimised by its rapid reduction in the presence of body fluids.

Solutions are used as cleansing applications to wounds, ulcers, or abscesses and as wet dressings and in baths in eczematous conditions and acute dermatoses especially where there is secondary infection. It is often prepared as a concentrated 0.1% solution in water to be diluted 1 in 10 before use to provide a 0.01% (1 in 10 000) solution. Solutions have also been used in bromhidrosis, in mycotic infections such as athlete's foot, and in poison ivy dermatitis.

Potassium permanganate is added to formaldehyde solution to produce formaldehyde vapour for the disinfection of rooms and cabinets (see p.1145).

Preparations
Proprietary Preparations (details are given in Part 3)
UK: Permitabs.

Povidone-Iodine (4580-y)

Povidone-Iodine (BAN).
Iodinated Povidone; Polyvidone-Iodine; Polyvinylpyrrolidone-Iodine Complex; Povidonum Iodinatum; PVP-Iodine.
CAS — 25655-41-8.
ATC — D08AG02; D09AA09; D11AC06; G01AX11; R02AA15.
Pharmacopoeias. In *Chin., Eur.* (see p.vi), *Jpn,* and *US.*

Pharmacopoeial description
Ph. Eur.: A complex of iodine with povidone containing 9 to 12% of available iodine calculated on the dried basis. Yellowish-brown or reddish-brown amorphous powder. It loses not more than 8% of its weight on drying. Soluble in water and in alcohol; practically insoluble in acetone. A 10% solution in water has a pH of 1.5 to 5.0. Protect from light.

USP 25: A complex of iodine with povidone containing 9 to 12% of available iodine calculated on the dried basis. A yellowish-brown to reddish-brown amorphous powder with a slight characteristic odour. It loses not more than 8% of its weight on drying. Soluble in water and in alcohol; practically insoluble in acetone, in carbon tetrachloride, in chloroform, in ether, and in petroleum spirit. Its solutions are acid to litmus. Store in airtight containers.

Incompatibilities. Antimicrobial activity may be reduced at high pH.

Dermatological reactions, described as second- and third-degree burns, were observed in 4 patients in whom wounds were covered with a povidone-iodine soaked bandage secured to the skin by compound benzoin tincture. It was suggested that an interaction had occurred resulting in a more acidic pH.[1]

A mixture of povidone-iodine solution and hydrogen peroxide [brown bubbly] has caused explosions.[2]

1. Schillaci LJ, *et al.* Reduced pH associated with mixture of povidone-iodine and compound tincture of benzoin. *Am J Hosp Pharm* 1983; **40**: 1694–5.
2. Dannenberg E, Peebles J. Betadine-hydrogen peroxide irrigation solution incompatibility. *Am J Hosp Pharm* 1978; **35**: 525.

Adverse Effects and Precautions
Povidone-iodine can cause hypersensitivity reactions and irritation of the skin and mucous membranes, although severe reactions are rare and povidone-iodine is considered to be less irritant than iodine.

The application of povidone-iodine to severe burns or to large areas otherwise denuded of skin may produce the systemic adverse effects associated with iodine (p.1522) such as metabolic acidosis, hypernatraemia, and impairment of renal function. Hyperthyroidism or hypothyroidism may occur following ingestion of large quantities. Hypothyroidism has occurred in neo-

nates both as a result of absorption of iodine from povidone-iodine applied to the neonate and also to the mother during pregnancy or breast feeding.

Regular or prolonged use should be avoided in patients with thyroid disorders or those receiving lithium therapy.

Acidosis. There have been a number of reports of acidosis in patients whose burns were treated topically with povidone-iodine.[1,2] Fatal metabolic acidosis[3] and seizures[4] have been reported following mediastinal irrigation with povidone-iodine.

1. Pietsch J, Meakins JL. Complications of povidone-iodine absorption in topically treated burn patients. *Lancet* 1976; **i:** 280–2.
2. Scoggin C, *et al.* Hypernatraemia and acidosis in association with topical treatment of burns. *Lancet* 1977; **i:** 959.
3. Glick PL, *et al.* Iodine toxicity in a patient treated by continuous povidone-iodine mediastinal irrigation. *Ann Thorac Surg* 1985; **39**: 478–80.
4. Zec N, *et al.* Seizures in a patient treated with continuous povidone-iodine mediastinal irrigation. *N Engl J Med* 1992; **326**: 1784.

Hypersensitivity. Anaphylaxis was associated with vaginal application of povidone-iodine solution.[1]

1. Waran KD, Munsick RA. Anaphylaxis from povidone-iodine. *Lancet* 1995; **345**: 1506.

Neonates. Hypothyroidism has been reported in premature and very low birth-weight infants following the use of povidone-iodine for routine antisepsis,[1,2] and hyperthyroidism in a full-term infant following mediastinal lavage.[3] Perinatal vaginal use of povidone-iodine may also cause neonatal thyroid dysfunction.[4]

1. Parravicini E, *et al.* Iodine, thyroid function, and very low birth weight infants. *Pediatrics* 1996; **98**: 730–4.
2. Linder N, *et al.* Topical iodine-containing antiseptics and subclinical hypothyroidism in preterm infants. *J Pediatr* 1997; **131**: 434–9.
3. Bryant WP, Zimmerman D. Iodine-induced hyperthyroidism in a newborn. *Pediatrics* 1995; **95**: 434–6. Correction. *ibid.*; **96**: 779.
4. l'Allemand D, *et al.* Iodine-induced alterations of thyroid function in newborn infants after prenatal and perinatal exposure to povidone iodine. *J Pediatr* 1997; **102**: 935–8.

Uses and Administration
Povidone-iodine is an iodophore which is used as a disinfectant and antiseptic mainly for the treatment of contaminated wounds and pre-operative preparation of the skin and mucous membranes as well as for the disinfection of equipment.

Iodophores are loose complexes of iodine and carrier polymers. Solutions of povidone-iodine gradually release iodine to exert an effect against bacteria, fungi, viruses, protozoa, cysts, and spores; povidone-iodine is thus less potent than preparations containing free iodine but it is less toxic.

A wide variety of topical formulations is available, the majority containing about 4 to 10% of povidone-iodine; a 1% mouthwash has been used for oral infections including candidiasis and topical powders containing 0.5 to 5% povidone-iodine have been tried in the treatment and prevention of wound infection. For vaginal application povidone-iodine has also been used as pessaries containing 200 mg.

Preparations
BP 2001: Povidone-Iodine Mouthwash; Povidone-Iodine Solution;
USP 25: Povidone-Iodine Cleansing Solution; Povidone-Iodine Ointment; Povidone-Iodine Topical Aerosol; Povidone-Iodine Topical Solution.

Proprietary Preparations (details are given in Part 3)
Aust.: Betaisodona; Betasan; Betaseptic; Braunol; Braunovidon; Wundesin; *Austral.:* Betadine; EDP-Evans Dermal Powder; Isodine; Microshield PVP; Microshield PVP-S; Minidine; Novadine†; Nyal Medithroat Gargle; Savlon Antiseptic; Viodine; Viraban†; *Belg.:* Braunol; Iodex Buccal; Iodex Dermique; Iso-Betadine; *Braz.:* Braunoderm; Braunol; Povid-Derme; Prepcare; Silvedine; *Canad.:* Betadine; Massengill Medicated†; Proviodine†; *Fin.:* Betadine; *Fr.:* Betadine; Poliodine; *Ger.:* Betaisodona; Braunol; Braunovidon; Freka-cid; Inadine; Jodobac; Logomed Desinfektions-Salbe†; Polydona; Polysept; Sepso J; SP Betaisodona†; Traumasept; *Hong Kong:* Betadine; Pevidine; Providine; Videne; *Irl.:* Betadine; Braunol†; Braunosan†; Braunovidon†; Inadine; *Israel:* Betadine; Iodiflor; Iodo-Vit; Massengill Medicated; Polydine; Yodon; *Ital.:* Betadine; Betaseptic; Braunol; Destrobac; Eso-Jod 100 500; Esoform Jod 35 and 75; Evadermin; Gammadin; Garze Disinfettanti alla Pomata Betadine; Golasept; Inadine; Iododocid; Iodosteril; Iodoten; Iodocur; Jodogard; Oftasteril; Paniodal; Paniodine; Poviderm; *Jpn:* Isodine†; *Mex.:* Isodine; Yodacua; Yodine; *Neth.:* Betadine; Biocil; Viodine; *Port.:* Betadine; Cromoseptil Plus; Dinasepte†; Isodine; Septil; *S.Afr.:* Betadine; Dermadine; Podine; Septadine; Septisooth; *Singapore:* Summers Eve Medicated; *Spain:* Betadine; Betatul; Braunoderm; Braunol; Iodina; Kaput†; Orto Dermo P; Sanoyodo; Solucionic†; Topionic; *Swed.:* Inadine†; *Switz.:* Betadine; Braunol; Braunosan; Braunosan H Plus; Braunovidon; Destrobac; Jodoplex; Rocanal Imediat†; *Thai.:* Annadine; Bernadine; Betadine; Cavodine; Isodine; P-Vidine; Povadine; Sepfadine; Septidine; Videne; *UK:* Betadine; Brush Off; Inadine; Savlon Dry; Videne; *USA:* ACU-dyne; Aerodine; Betadine; Biodine; Efodine; Femidine†; Iodex; Mal-

lisol†; Massengill Medicated; Minidyne; Operand; Polydine; Povidex†; Summers Eve Medicated; Yeast-Gard Medicated†.
Multi-ingredient: *Aust.:* Braunoderm; *Austral.:* Microshield PVP Plus; Novasrub†; *Belg.:* Braunoderm; *Canad.:* Metadyne; *Ger.:* Betaseptic; Braunoderm; *Irl.:* Braunoderm†; *Ital.:* Braunoderm; Jodieci; *Switz.:* Betaseptic; Braunoderm; Jodobac; *UK:* Codella; *USA:* Anbesol; Orasol; ProTech.

Propamidine Isetionate (2272-p)

Propamidine Isetionate (BANM, rINNM).
M&B-782; Propamidine Isethionate. 4,4′-Trimethylenedioxydibenzamidine bis(2-hydroxyethanesulphonate).
$C_{17}H_{20}N_4O_2,2C_2H_6O_4S = 564.6.$
CAS — 104-32-5 (propamidine); 140-63-6 (propamidine isetionate).

Profile
Propamidine isetionate is an aromatic diamidine antiseptic which is active against Gram-positive bacteria, but less active against Gram-negative bacteria and spore-forming organisms. It also has antifungal properties and is active against *Acanthamoeba*. Ophthalmic solutions containing 0.1% of propamidine isetionate are used for the treatment of conjunctivitis and blepharitis.

Acanthamoeba keratitis. The optimal regimen for the treatment of *Acanthamoeba* keratitis (p.582) has yet to be determined. Propamidine isetionate 0.1% is commonly used, usually in conjunction with neomycin[1,2] or a neomycin-polymyxin-gramicidin combination,[3] plus chlorhexidine gluconate,[4] or polihexanide.[5] However, reported resistance of some strains of *Acanthamoeba* to propamidine has prompted the suggestion that it should be replaced by another diamidine such as hexamidine.[6]

1. Wright P, *et al.* Acanthamoeba keratitis successfully treated medically. *Br J Ophthalmol* 1985; **69**: 778–82.
2. Varga JH, *et al.* Combined treatment of Acanthamoeba keratitis with propamidine, neomycin, and polyhexamethylene biguanide. *Am J Ophthalmol* 1993; **115**: 466–70.
3. Moore MB, McCulley JP. Acanthamoeba keratitis associated with contact lenses: six consecutive cases of successful management. *Br J Ophthalmol* 1989; **73**: 271–5.
4. Seal DV. Chlorhexidine or polyhexamethylene biguanide for acanthamoeba keratitis. *Lancet* 1995; **345**: 136.
5. Kilvington S. Chemotherapy for acanthamoeba keratitis. *Lancet* 1995; **345**: 792.
6. Perrine D, *et al.* Amoebicidal efficiencies of various diamidines against two strains of Acanthamoeba polyphaga. *Antimicrob Agents Chemother* 1995; **39**: 339–42.

Preparations
Proprietary Preparations (details are given in Part 3)
Austral.: Brolene; *Irl.:* Brolene; *NZ:* Brolene; *S.Afr.:* Brolene; *UK:* Brolene; Golden Eye Drops.

Propiolactone (2273-s)

Propiolactone (BAN, USAN, rINN).
BPL; NSC-21626; 2-Oxetanone; Propanolide; β-Propiolactone. Propiono-3-lactone.
$C_3H_4O_2 = 72.06.$
CAS — 57-57-8.

Profile
Propiolactone vapour is an irritant, mutagenic, possibly carcinogenic disinfectant which is very active against most microorganisms including viruses. It is rather less effective against bacterial spores.

Propiolactone vapour has been used for the gaseous sterilisation of pharmaceutical and surgical materials and for disinfecting large enclosed areas. It has low penetrating power. Propiolactone liquid has also been used.

Propyl Alcohol (561-n)

Normal Propyl Alcohol; Primary Propyl Alcohol; Propanol; Propanolum. Propan-1-ol.
$CH_3.CH_2.CH_2OH = 60.10.$
CAS — 71-23-8.
ATC — D08AX03.

Adverse Effects and Treatment
As for Alcohol, p.1131; propyl alcohol is considered more toxic.

◊ References.

1. 1-Propanol. *Environmental Health Criteria 102.* Geneva: WHO, 1990.

Uses and Administration
Propyl alcohol, an antiseptic with properties similar to those of alcohol (p.1132), is used in preparations for disinfection of the hands, skin, surfaces, and instruments.

Isopropyl alcohol (p.1149) is also used as an antiseptic.

Preparations
Proprietary Preparations (details are given in Part 3)
Multi-ingredient: *Aust.:* Marcocid; Sterillium; *Fr.:* Sterillium; *Ger.:* Aerodesin; Antifect†; Bacillol; Bacillol AF; Bacillol plus; Desmanol; Freka-Steril; Hospisept; Incidin; Incidur Spray; Kodan Tinktur Forte; Meliseptol; Mikrozid; Neo Kodan; Primasept Med;

Sagrosept; Softa Man; Sterillium; *Ital.:* Softa Man; *Mon.:* Akila mains et peau†; Akila spray†; *Switz.:* Adro-derm; Jodobac; Orosept†.

Ritiometan (2979-x)

Ritiometan (*rINN*).
(Methylidynetrithio)triacetic acid.
$C_7H_{10}O_6S_3 = 286.3$.
CAS — 34914-39-1.
ATC — R01AX05.

Profile
Ritiometan has been used as the magnesium salt in an aerosol preparation for the treatment of infections of the nose and throat.

Preparations
Proprietary Preparations (details are given in Part 3)
Fr.: Necyrane.

Scarlet Red (2274-w)

Biebrich Scarlet R Medicinal; CI Solvent Red 24; Colour Index No. 26105; Fat Ponceau R; Rubrum Scarlatinum; Scharlachrot; Sudan IV. 1-[4-(o-Tolylazo)-o-tolylazo]naphth-2-ol.
$C_{24}H_{20}N_4O = 380.4$.
CAS — 85-83-6.
Pharmacopoeias. In Aust.

Profile
Scarlet red is an antiseptic dye which has been used topically. It can be irritant.

Sodium Azide (16985-x)

$N_3Na = 65.01$.
CAS — 26628-22-8.

Adverse Effects and Precautions
Acute poisoning with sodium azide may cause nausea and vomiting, diarrhoea, life-threatening hypotension, tachycardia, convulsions, and severe headache. Fatalities have been reported. Solutions containing sodium azide must not be disposed of into drain pipelines containing copper, lead or brass since highly explosive heavy metal azides may be produced.

◊ References to acute poisoning with sodium azide.
1. Edmonds OP, Bourne MS. Sodium azide poisoning in five laboratory technicians. *Br J Ind Med* 1982; **39:** 308–9.
2. Klein-Schwartz W, *et al.* Three fatal sodium azide poisonings. *Med Toxicol Adverse Drug Exp* 1989; **4:** 219–27.
3. Anonymous. Sodium azide contamination of hemodialysis water supplies. *JAMA* 1989; **261:** 2603.

Uses
Sodium azide has been used as an antimicrobial preservative in laboratory reagents, serum samples, and dialysis equipment.

Sodium Diacetate (6669-z)

E262. Sodium hydrogen diacetate.
$CH_3COONa, CH_3COOH(+xH_2O)$.
CAS — 126-96-5 (anhydrous sodium diacetate).

Profile
Sodium diacetate is used as a preservative in foods, particularly as an inhibitor of moulds and rope-forming micro-organisms in bread.

Sodium Dichloroisocyanurate (2276-l)

Sodium Dichloro-s-triazinetrione; Sodium Troclosene. 1,3-Dichloro-1,3,5-triazine-2,4,6(1H,3H,5H)-trione sodium.
$C_3Cl_2N_3NaO_3 = 219.9$.
CAS — 2893-78-9.

It contains about 65% of 'available chlorine' (see p.1141).

Profile
Sodium dichloroisocyanurate is a disinfectant with the general properties of chlorine (p.1140) and sodium hypochlorite (p.1156) but it remains active as pH increases from 6 to 10 and is reported to be less susceptible to inactivation by organic material. It is used for disinfecting hard surfaces (see Disinfection in Hepatitis and HIV Infection, p.1130), babies' feeding bottles, and food and dairy equipment, for treating water (p.1130), for soft contact lens care (p.1129) and in various commercial bleach detergents and scouring powders as a relatively stable source of chlorine.
Dichloroisocyanuric acid ($C_3HCl_2N_3O_3 = 198.0$), potassium dichloroisocyanurate (potassium troclosene; troclosene potassium, $C_3Cl_2KN_3O_3 = 236.1$), and trichloroisocyanuric acid (symclosene, $C_3Cl_3N_3O_3 = 232.4$) are similarly used.

Preparations
Proprietary Preparations (details are given in Part 3)
Aust.: Polyrinse Desinfektionssystem; *Austral.:* Milton Anti-Bacterial; Puritabs; Softab†; *Fr.:* Milton; Polycare; Solusteril†; *Hong Kong:* Actichlor; *Irl.:* Aquatabs†; Klorsept†; Milton†; Sterinova†; *Israel:* Klor-De; Klorsept; Taharmayim; Taharsept; Tahartaf;

Ital.: Dialster; Presept†; *Mex.:* Aquatabs; *NZ:* Softab; *UK:* Milton; Presept.
Multi-ingredient: *Irl.:* Klor-Kleen†.

Sodium Formaldehyde Sulfoxylate (6671-s)

Sodium Formaldehyde Sulphoxylate. Sodium hydroxymethanesulphinate dihydrate.
$CH_3NaO_3S, 2H_2O = 154.1$.
CAS — 149-44-0 (anhydrous sodium formaldehyde sulfoxylate); 6035-47-8 (sodium formaldehyde sulfoxylate, dihydrate).
Pharmacopoeias. In Pol. Also in USNF.

Pharmacopoeial description
USNF 20: White crystals or hard white masses with the characteristic odour of garlic. Soluble in 3.4 of water, 1 in 510 of alcohol, 1 in 175 of chloroform, and 1 in 180 of ether; slightly soluble in benzene. A 2% solution in water has a pH of 9.5 to 10.5. Store at 15° to 30°. Protect from light.

Profile
Sodium formaldehyde sulfoxylate is an antioxidant used as a preservative in pharmaceuticals. It has been used in the treatment of acute mercury poisoning (p.1634).

Sodium Hypochlorite (2277-y)

$NaOCl, 5H_2O = 164.5$.
CAS — 7681-52-9.
ATC — D08AX07.

Pharmacopoeias. Br., Fr., Jpn, Port., and US include sodium hypochlorite solutions.

Sodium hypochlorite pentahydrate contains about 43% of 'available chlorine' (see p.1141); anhydrous sodium hypochlorite contains about 95%.

Incompatibilities. The antimicrobial activity of hypochlorites is rapidly diminished in the presence of organic material; it is also pH dependent being greater in acid pH although hypochlorites are more stable at alkaline pH.

Pharmacopoeial description
BP 2001: Dilute Sodium Hypochlorite Solution contains 1% of available chlorine. Store away from acids at a temperature not exceeding 20°. Protect from light.
Strong Sodium Hypochlorite Solution contains not less than 8% of available chlorine. It should be diluted before use. Store away from acids at a temperature not exceeding 20°. Protect from light.
USP 25: Sodium Hypochlorite Solution contains not less than 4% and not more than 6% w/w of anhydrous sodium hypochlorite. It is not suitable for application to wounds. Store in airtight containers. Protect from light.
Sodium Hypochlorite Topical Solution contains 0.025% sodium hypochlorite. Store in airtight containers. Protect from light.

◊ CAUTION. *Sodium hypochlorite solutions should not be mixed with solutions of strong acids or ammonia; the subsequent reactions release chlorine gas and tosylchloramide sodium gas, respectively.*

Stability. The stability of sodium hypochlorite solutions increases with pH, solutions of pH 10 or more being most stable.[1] Stability studies have shown that solutions providing 0.04 to 0.12% 'available chlorine' stored in amber glass bottles at room temperature could carry a 23-month expiry date.[2]
1. Bloomfield SF, Sizer TJ. Eusol BPC and other hypochlorite formulations used in hospitals. *Pharm J* 1985; **235:** 153–5 and 157.
2. Fabian TM, Walker SE. Stability of sodium hypochlorite solutions. *Am J Hosp Pharm* 1982; **39:** 1016–17.

Adverse Effects
Hypochlorite solutions release hypochlorous acid upon contact with gastric juice and acids, and ingestion causes irritation and corrosion of mucous membranes with pain and vomiting, oedema of the pharynx and larynx, and, rarely, perforation of the oesophagus and stomach. A fall in blood pressure, delirium, and coma may occur. Inhalation of hypochlorous fumes causes coughing and choking and may cause severe respiratory tract irritation and pulmonary oedema. Hypochlorite solutions may be irritating to the skin.

◊ A patient who accidentally received an intravenous infusion of 150 mL of a 1% solution of sodium hypochlorite experienced a slow heart rate, mild hypotension, and increased respiratory rate. The slow heart rate persisted for 3 days but other parameters returned to normal after symptomatic treatment.[1]
1. Marroni M, Menichetti F. Accidental intravenous infusion of sodium hypochlorite. *DICP Ann Pharmacother* 1991; **25:** 1008–9.

◊ For comment on the adverse effects of hypochlorite solutions on wound healing, see Disinfection: Wounds under Uses and Administration of Chlorine, p.1141.

Effects on the blood. An acute haemolytic crisis was reported in a child who had swum for about 4 hours in an indoor pool containing very high concentrations of sodium hypochlorite.[1] The child was subsequently found to have glucose-6-phosphate dehydrogenase deficiency.
1. Ong SJ, Kearney B. Local swimming pool and G-6-PD deficiency. *Med J Aust* 1994; **161:** 226–7.

Treatment of Adverse Effects
If sodium hypochlorite solution is ingested, water, milk, or other demulcents should be given; opinion over the use of antacids is divided. Sodium thiosulfate 1 to 2.5% solution has been used but is of questionable value. Gastric lavage may be considered if a large amount has been ingested within the previous hour and there is no evidence of corrosive oesophagitis or gastritis. If spilled on skin, washing with copious amounts of water is recommended.

Precautions
Topically applied hypochlorites may dissolve blood clots and cause bleeding.

Uses and Administration
Sodium hypochlorite is a disinfectant and antiseptic with the brief and rapid actions of chlorine (see p.1141). Powders and solutions are commonly used for the rapid disinfection of hard surfaces (see Disinfection in Creutzfeldt-Jakob Disease, p.1129 and in Hepatitis and HIV Infection, p.1130), food and dairy equipment, babies' feeding bottles, excreta, and water (p.1130). Solutions for use as domestic bleaches contain about 5% of hypochlorite. Only diluted solutions containing up to 0.5% of 'available chlorine' are suitable for use on the skin and in wounds (but see Wound Disinfection, p.1130).
Solutions of hypochlorites used as disinfectants have included Labarraque's Solution containing sodium hypochlorite with an alkali, and Eau de Javel, containing sodium or potassium hypochlorite.

Preparations
BP 2001: Dilute Sodium Hypochlorite Solution; Strong Sodium Hypochlorite Solution;
USP 25: Sodium Hypochlorite Solution; Sodium Hypochlorite Topical Solution.
Proprietary Preparations (details are given in Part 3)
Austral.: Milton Anti-Bacterial; *Belg.:* Dakincooper; *Braz.:* Colix; Milton; *Canad.:* Hygeol; *Fr.:* Dakin; Milton; *Ger.:* Maranon H; *Irl.:* Hypercidin; Milton†; *Israel:* Chlorasol; *Ital.:* Amukine Med; Milton; Naclon; *UK:* Chlorasol; Milton.
Multi-ingredient: *Fr.:* Amukine; *Mex.:* Amuchina.

Sodium Nitrate (13254-q)

E251; Natrii Nitras; Natrium Nitricum.
$NaNO_3 = 84.99$.
CAS — 7631-99-4.
NOTE. Crude sodium nitrate is known as Chile Saltpetre.
Pharmacopoeias. In Pol.

◊ CAUTION. *Sodium nitrate has been used for the illicit preparation of explosives or fireworks; care is required with its supply.*

Profile
Sodium nitrate has similar actions to potassium nitrate (p.1154) and is used as a preservative in foods, particularly in meat products.
Crude sodium nitrate is used as a fertiliser.

Poisoning. Cyanosis and methaemoglobinaemia has been reported[1] in 3 patients after eating sausages which had been preserved mistakenly with a mixture of sodium nitrate and sodium nitrite rather than with potassium nitrate (saltpetre). The name saltpetre is used as a generic term for a number of potassium- or sodium-based preservatives used in food manufacture.
1. Kennedy N, *et al.* Faulty sausage production causing methaemoglobinaemia. *Arch Dis Child* 1997; **76:** 367–8.

Sodium Perborate (5908-g)

Natrii Perboras; Sod. Perbor.
$NaBO_2, H_2O_2, 3H_2O = 153.9$.
CAS — 7632-04-4 (anhydrous sodium perborate); 10042-91-4 (sodium perborate hydrate).
ATC — A01AB19.
NOTE. Sodium Perborate Monohydrate is USAN.
Pharmacopoeias. In Eur. (see p.vi).

Pharmacopoeial description
Ph. Eur.: Colourless prismatic crystals or a white powder, stable in crystalline form. Sparingly soluble in water, with slow

decomposition. It dissolves in dilute mineral acids. Store in air-tight containers.

Adverse Effects

Frequent use of toothpowders containing sodium perborate may cause blistering and oedema. Hypertrophy of the papillae of the tongue has also been reported. The effects of swallowed sodium perborate are similar to those of boric acid (p.1586).

Uses and Administration

Sodium perborate is a mild disinfectant and deodorant. It readily releases oxygen in contact with oxidisable matter and has been used in aqueous solutions for purposes similar to weak solutions of hydrogen peroxide.

Sodium perborate has also been used, with calcium carbonate, as a toothpowder. A freshly prepared solution is used as a mouthwash.

The less soluble $NaBO_2,H_2O_2$ known as sodium perborate monohydrate is used similarly.

Preparations

Proprietary Preparations (details are given in Part 3)
Canad.: Amosan; **Irl.:** Bocasan†; **Ital.:** Kavosan; Sekusept N; **UK:** Bocasan; **USA:** Amosan.

Multi-ingredient: **Austral.:** Amosan; **Belg.:** Sulfaryl†; **Braz.:** Angino Tricin; **Fr.:** Bactident; Hydralin; **Ger.:** Sekusept; **Ital.:** Borossigeno Plus Stomatologico†; **Port.:** Dentolamina†; **Switz.:** Saltrates Rodell; **USA:** Trichotine.

Sorbates (12173-r)

Potassium Sorbate (6663-s)

E202; Kalii Sorbas. Potassium (E,E)-hexa-2,4-dienoate.
$C_6H_7KO_2 = 150.2$.
CAS — 590-00-1; 24634-61-5;.
Pharmacopoeias. In Eur. (see p.vi). Also in USNF.

Incompatibility is discussed under Sorbic Acid, below.

Pharmacopoeial description

Ph. Eur.: White or almost white granules or powder. Very soluble in water; slightly soluble in alcohol. Protect from light.

USNF 20: White crystals or powder with a characteristic odour. Soluble 1 in 4.5 of water, 1 in 35 of alcohol, and 1 in more than 1000 of chloroform and of ether. Store in airtight containers at a temperature not exceeding 40°. Protect from light.

Sorbic Acid (6679-k)

Acidum Sorbicum; E200. (E,E)-Hexa-2,4-dienoic acid.
$C_6H_8O_2 = 112.1$.
CAS — 22500-92-1.
Pharmacopoeias. In Eur. (see p.vi) and Pol. Also in USNF.

Pharmacopoeial description

Ph. Eur.: A white or almost white, crystalline powder. Slightly soluble in water; freely soluble in alcohol and in ether. Protect from light.

USNF 20: A free-flowing white crystalline powder with a characteristic odour. Soluble 1 in 1000 of water, 1 in 10 of alcohol, 1 in 8 of dehydrated alcohol, 1 in 15 of chloroform, 1 in 30 of ether, 1 in 8 of methyl alcohol, and 1 in 19 of propylene glycol. Store in airtight containers at a temperature not exceeding 40°. Protect from light.

Incompatibility. Sorbic acid can be inactivated by oxidation and to some extent by nonionic surfactants and plastics. Activity of the sorbates may be reduced by increases in pH.[1]

1. Beasley M. Sorbic acid. In: Kibbe AH, ed. *Handbook of pharmaceutical excipients.* 3rd ed. Washington and London: American Pharmaceutical Association and The Pharmaceutical Press, 2000: 508–10.

Adverse Effects and Precautions

The sorbates can be irritant and have caused contact dermatitis.

Hypersensitivity. References to allergic-type skin reactions[1] and non-allergic irritant-type reactions[2,3] with potassium sorbate or sorbic acid.

1. Saihan EM, Harman RRM. Contact sensitivity to sorbic acid in 'Unguentum Merck'. *Br J Dermatol* 1978; **99:** 583–4.
2. Soschin D, Leyden JJ. Sorbic acid-induced erythema and edema. *J Am Acad Dermatol* 1986; **14:** 234–41.
3. Fisher AA. Erythema limited to the face due to sorbic acid. *Cutis* 1987; **40:** 395–7.

Uses

Potassium sorbate and sorbic acid possess antifungal, and to a lesser extent antibacterial, activity. They are relatively ineffective above a pH of about 6. They are used as preservatives in pharmaceutical preparations in concentrations of up to 0.2%, in enteral formulas, foods, and in cosmetic preparations.

Preparations

Proprietary Preparations (details are given in Part 3)
Multi-ingredient: **Aust.:** Onycho Phytex; Phytex; **Austral.:** CapriVate; **Ger.:** Klysma Sorbit; **Ital.:** Bo-Gum†; Évasen Dischetti; **Mex.:** Adapettes; **UK:** Relaxit; **USA:** Feminique.

Sozoiodol Sodium (11613-r)

Sozoiodole Sodium. Sodium 2,6-diiodophenol-4-sulphonate.
$C_6H_3I_2NaO_4S = 447.9$.
CAS — 554-71-2 (sozoiodolic acid); 515-44-6 (anhydrous sozoiodol sodium).

Sozoiodol Zinc (11614-f)

Sozoiodole Zinc. Zinc di(2,6-diiodophenol-4-sulphonate).
$C_{12}H_6I_4O_8S_2Zn = 915.3$.
CAS — 547-41-1 (anhydrous sozoiodol zinc).

Profile

Sozoiodol contains iodine and the sodium and zinc salts have been used for their disinfectant properties.

Preparations

Proprietary Preparations (details are given in Part 3)
Multi-ingredient: **Switz.:** Euproctol†.

Sulfites and Sulfur Dioxide (12174-f)

Potassium Bisulfite (16966-k)

E228; Potassium Bisulphite; Potassium Hydrogen Sulphite.
$KHSO_3 = 120.2$.
CAS — 7773-03-7.

Potassium Metabisulfite (6662-p)

Dipotassium Pyrosulphite; E224; Potassium Metabisulphite; Potassium Pyrosulphite.
$K_2S_2O_5 = 222.3$.
CAS — 16731-55-8.
Pharmacopoeias. In Fr. Also in USNF.

Incompatibility is discussed under Sulfur Dioxide, below.

Pharmacopoeial description

USNF 20: White or colourless, free-flowing crystals, crystalline powder, or granules, usually with an odour of sulfur dioxide. Gradually oxidises in air to the sulfate. Soluble in water; insoluble in alcohol. Its solutions are acid to litmus. Store in well-filled airtight containers at a temperature not exceeding 40°.

Sodium Bisulfite (9880-t)

E222; Sodium Bisulphite; Sodium Hydrogen Sulphite.
$NaHSO_3 = 104.1$.
CAS — 7631-90-5.
Pharmacopoeias. In Jpn which has Sodium Bisulfite, described as consisting of the acid sulfite ($NaHSO_3 = 104.1$) and the metabisulfite in varying proportions.

Sodium Metabisulfite (6673-e)

Disodium Pyrosulphite; E223; Natrii Disulfis; Natrii Metabisulfis; Sodium Disulphite; Sodium Metabisulphite; Sodium Pyrosulphite.
$Na_2S_2O_5 = 190.1$.
CAS — 7681-57-4.
Pharmacopoeias. In Chin., Eur. (see p.vi), Jpn, and Pol. Also in USNF.

Incompatibility is discussed under Sulfur Dioxide, below.

Pharmacopoeial description

Ph. Eur.: Colourless crystals or a white or almost white crystalline powder. Freely soluble in water; slightly soluble in alcohol. A 5% solution in water has a pH of 3.5 to 5.0. Protect from light.

USNF 20: White crystals or a white to yellowish crystalline powder with an odour of sulfur dioxide. Freely soluble in water and in glycerol; slightly soluble in alcohol. Store in well-filled airtight containers at a temperature not exceeding 40°.

Sodium Sulfite (6678-c)

Anhydrous Sodium Sulphite; E221; Exsiccated Sodium Sulphite; Natrii Sulfis Anhydricus; Natrii Sulfis Siccatus; Natrii Sulphis; Sodium Sulphite.
$Na_2SO_3 = 126.0$.
CAS — 7757-83-7.
Pharmacopoeias. In Eur. (see p.vi), Jpn, and Pol. Eur. and Pol. also include Sodium Sulfite Heptahydrate.

Incompatibility is discussed under Sulfur Dioxide, below.

Pharmacopoeial description

Ph. Eur.: A white powder (anhydrous) or colourless crystals (heptahydrate). Freely soluble in water; very slightly soluble in alcohol. Anhydrous sodium sulfite should be stored in airtight containers.

Sulfur Dioxide (6680-w)

E220; Sulphur Dioxide.
$SO_2 = 64.06$.
CAS — 7446-09-5.
Pharmacopoeias. In USNF.

Pharmacopoeial description

USNF 20: A colourless non-flammable gas with a strong suffocating odour characteristic of burning sulfur. It condenses readily under pressure to a colourless liquid that boils at −10° and has a wt per mL of about 1.5 g. Soluble 36 in 1 of water and 114 in 1 of alcohol by vol. at 20° and standard pressure. Soluble in chloroform and in ether. Store in cylinders. It is usually packaged under pressure in liquid form.

Incompatibilities. Sulfite antioxidants can react with sympathomimetics such as adrenaline [epinephrine] leading to their inactivation.[1] Measures need to be taken to prevent such a reaction if sulfites have to be used. Cisplatin is another compound that can be inactivated.[2] Phenylmercuric nitrate may be inactivated or its activity enhanced.[3,4] Sulfites are reported to react with chloramphenicol.[1] Hydrogen peroxide generation has been reported on exposure to light of amino acid solutions containing sulfites.[5] When used in foods there can be a noticeable taste and a reduction in thiamine content.[6] Stability is affected by air and moisture,[7] and there is decomposition at very low pH.[7] There can be adsorption on to rubber closures.[8]

1. Higuchi T, Schroeter LC. Reactivity of bisulfite with a number of pharmaceuticals. *J Am Pharm Assoc (Sci)* 1959; **48:** 535–40.
2. Garren KW, Repta AJ. Incompatibility of cisplatin and Reglan Injectable. *Int J Pharmaceutics* 1985; **24:** 91–9.
3. Richards RME, Reary JME. Changes in antibacterial activity of thiomersal and PMN on autoclaving with certain adjuvants. *J Pharm Pharmacol* 1972; **24** (suppl): 84P–89P.
4. Collins AJ, *et al.* Incompatibility of phenylmercuric acetate with sodium metabisulphite in eye drop formulations. *J Pharm Pharmacol* 1985; **37** (suppl): 123P.
5. Brawley V, *et al.* Effect of sodium metabisulfite on hydrogen peroxide production in light-exposed pediatric parenteral amino acid solutions. *Am J Health-Syst Pharm* 1998; **55:** 1288–92.
6. FAO/WHO. Evaluation of the toxicity of a number of antimicrobials and antioxidants: sixth report of the joint FAO/WHO expert committee on food additives. *WHO Tech Rep Ser 228* 1962.
7. Stewart JT. Sodium metabisulfite. In: Kibbe AH, ed. *Handbook of pharmaceutical excipients.* 3rd ed. Washington and London: American Pharmaceutical Association and The Pharmaceutical Press, 2000: 490–2.
8. Schroeter LC. Sulfurous acid salts as pharmaceutical antioxidants. *J Pharm Sci* 1961; **50:** 891–901.

Adverse Effects and Precautions

Gastric irritation due to liberation of sulfurous acid can follow ingestion of sodium metabisulfite and other sulfites. Large doses of sulfites may cause gastrointestinal upsets, respiratory or circulatory failure, and CNS disturbances.

Concentrated solutions of salts of sulfurous acid are irritant to skin and mucous membranes.

Sulfur dioxide is highly irritant to the eyes, skin, and mucous membranes. Inhalation results in irritation of the respiratory tract which may lead to bronchoconstriction and pulmonary oedema; very high concentrations may cause respiratory arrest and asphyxia. Contact with liquid sulfur dioxide results in acid burns.

Allergic reactions including anaphylaxis and deaths have been reported.

Hypersensitivity. Hypersensitivity reactions including bronchospasm, anaphylaxis, and some deaths have occurred in subjects, especially those with a history of asthma or atopic allergy, exposed to sulfites used as preservatives in foods.[1] These reactions have led to restrictions by the FDA on such use.[2] There have been case reports of reactions to sulfites in drugs;[3-7] such reports are considered to be few in number and the FDA has not extended the restriction on sulfites in foods to apply to their use in drugs since it was felt that in certain medications there was no suitable alternative to a sulfite.[2] It was even accepted that adrenaline [epinephrine] recommended for use in treating allergic reactions could itself contain sulfite and that its presence should not preclude use of the adrenaline [epinephrine] preparation even in sulfite-sensitive patients.[2]

1. Anonymous. Sulfites in drugs and food. *Med Lett Drugs Ther* 1986; **28:** 74–5.
2. Anonymous. Warning for prescription drugs containing sulfites. *FDA Drug Bull* 1987; **17:** 2–3.
3. Baker GJ, *et al.* Bronchospasm induced by metabisulphite-containing foods and drugs. *Med J Aust* 1981; **ii:** 614–17.
4. Twarog FJ, Leung DYM. Anaphylaxis to a component of isoetharine (sodium bisulfite). *JAMA* 1982; **248:** 2030–1.
5. Koepke JW, *et al.* Dose-dependent bronchospasm from sulfites in isoethatine. *JAMA* 1984; **251:** 2982–3.
6. Mikolich DJ, McCloskey WW. Suspected gentamicin allergy could be sulfite sensitivity. *Clin Pharm* 1988; **7:** 269.
7. Deziel-Evans LM, Hussey WC. Possible sulfite sensitivity with gentamicin infusion. *DICP Ann Pharmacother* 1989; **23:** 1032–3.

Pharmacokinetics

Sulfites and metabisulfites are oxidised in the body to sulfate and excreted in the urine. Any sulfurous acid or sulfur dioxide is also converted to sulfate.

The symbol † denotes a preparation no longer actively marketed

Uses

Sulfur dioxide and the sulfites which produce sulfur dioxide and sulfurous acid are strong reducing agents and are used as antoxidants. Concentrations of the sulfites in pharmaceutical preparations have ranged from 0.01 to 1.0%. At higher concentrations and preferably at an acid pH sulfur dioxide and the sulfites exhibit antimicrobial activity.

Sulfur dioxide and the sulfites are used in the food industry as antoxidants, antimicrobial preservatives, and anti-browning agents. They are used in wine making where tabletted sodium metabisulfite is commonly known as Campden Tablets. Concentrations of sulfites above 500 ppm impart a noticeable unpleasant taste to preparations. There is concern at the risk of severe allergic reactions arising from the use of sulfites in foods (see Hypersensitivity, above).

Preparations

Proprietary Preparations (details are given in Part 3)
Multi-ingredient: *Switz.:* Schwefelbad Dr Klopfer†.

Tar Acids (2279-z)

Tar acids are phenolic substances derived from the distillation of coal tar or petroleum fractions. The lowest boiling fraction of coal tar, distilling at 188° to 205°, consists of mixed cresol isomers. The middle fraction, known as 'cresylic acids', distils at 205° to 230° and consists of cresols and xylenols. The 'high-boiling tar acids', distilling at 230° to 290°, consist mainly of alkyl homologues of phenol, with naphthalenes and other hydrocarbons. Cresol is described on p.1142.

Black Fluids are homogeneous solutions of coal-tar acids, or similar acids derived from petroleum, or any mixture of these, with or without hydrocarbons and with a suitable emulsifying agent. **White Fluids** are finely dispersed emulsions of coal-tar acids, or similar acids derived from petroleum, or any mixture of these, with or without hydrocarbons. **Modified Black Fluids** and **Modified White Fluids** may contain, as an addition, any other active ingredients, but if these are used, the type and amount must be disclosed, if required.

Adverse Effects and Treatment
As for Phenol, p.1152.

Tar acids are generally very irritant and corrosive to the skin, even when diluted to concentrations used for disinfection.

Poisoning. A report of fatal self-poisoning in a 59-year-old man following the ingestion of approximately 250 mL of a xylenol-containing disinfectant (Stericol Hospital Disinfectant).[1]

1. Watson ID, *et al.* Fatal xylenol self-poisoning. *Postgrad Med J* 1986; **62:** 411–12.

Uses

Tar acids are phenolic disinfectants used in the preparation of a range of fluids of varied activity used for household and general disinfection purposes.

Hydrocarbons are often used to enhance the activity of the tar acids in disinfectant fluids; they also help to reduce crystallisation of phenols.

Preparations

Proprietary Preparations (details are given in Part 3)
UK: Clearsol; Cresolox; Printol; Sterilite; Sudol.

Tertiary Butylhydroquinone (9873-x)

TBHQ. 2-*tert*-butylhydroquinone.
$C_{10}H_{14}O_2 = 166.2$.
CAS — 1948-33-0.

Profile
Tertiary butylhydroquinone is an antoxidant preservative used in foods. It has some antimicrobial activity.

Tetrabromocresol (16356-j)

3,4,5,6-Tetrabromo-*o*-cresol.
$C_7H_4Br_4O = 423.7$.

Profile
Tetrabromocresol is a brominated phenolic antiseptic. It is used for hand disinfection and is applied topically for the treatment of fungal infections of the skin.

Preparations
Proprietary Preparations (details are given in Part 3)
Multi-ingredient: *Austral.:* Pedoz; *Ger.:* Gehwol Fungizid.

Tetraglycine Hydroperiodide (17597-c)

$C_{16}H_{42}I_7N_8O_{16} = 1490.9$.
CAS — 7097-60-1.

Profile
Tetraglycine hydroperiodide is an iodine-based disinfectant used in the treatment of drinking water (p.1130).

Preparations
Proprietary Preparations (details are given in Part 3)
USA: Potable Aqua†.

Thiomersal (2281-s)

Thiomersal (*BAN, rINN*).
Mercurothiolate; Mercurothiolate Sodique; Sodium Ethyl Mercurithiosalicylate; Thimerosal; Thimerosalate; Thiomersalum. Sodium (2-carboxyphenylthio)ethylmercury.
$C_9H_9HgNaO_2S = 404.8$.
CAS — 54-64-8.
ATC — D08AK06.
Pharmacopoeias. In *Eur.* (see p.vi), *Pol.*, and *US.*

Pharmacopoeial description
Ph. Eur.: A white or almost white crystalline powder. Freely soluble in water; sparingly soluble or soluble in alcohol; practically insoluble in dichloromethane. An 8% solution in water has a pH of 6.0 to 8.0. Protect from light.

USP 25: A light cream-coloured crystalline powder with a slight characteristic odour. Soluble 1 in 1 of water and 1 in 12 of alcohol; practically insoluble in ether. A 1% solution in water has a pH of about 6.7. Store in airtight containers. Protect from light.

Incompatibility. Incompatible with acids, metal ions, and iodine. It forms precipitates with many alkaloids. The rate of oxidation of thiomersal in solution is greatly increased by traces of copper ions. In slightly acid solution thiomersal may be precipitated as the corresponding acid which undergoes slow decomposition with the formation of insoluble products. The activity of thiomersal may also be reduced by boric acid, edetic acid, or sodium thiosulfate or the presence of blood or organic matter. Thiomersal may be adsorbed by plastic or rubber packaging materials.

References to incompatibilities.
1. Richards RME, Reary JME. Changes in antibacterial activity of thiomersal and PMN on autoclaving with certain adjuvants. *J Pharm Pharmacol* 1972; **24** (suppl): 84P–89P.
2. Reader MJ. Influence of isotonic agents on the stability of thiomersal in ophthalmic formulations. *J Pharm Sci* 1984; **73:** 840–1.
3. Morton DJ. EDTA reduces antimicrobial efficacy of thiomersal. *Int J Pharmaceutics* 1985; **23:** 357–8.

Adverse Effects, Treatment, and Precautions
As for Mercury, p.1634.

Hypersensitivity reactions occasionally occur. Allergic conjunctivitis has been reported.

Appropriate measures should be taken to prevent contamination of thiomersal preparations during storage or dilution.

◊ Serious adverse effects have followed parenteral and topical use of thiomersal. Six poisonings (5 fatal) resulted from the use of 1000 times the normal concentration of thiomersal in a preparation of chloramphenicol for intramuscular injection.[1] Thiomersal used in topical antiseptic preparations was found to be toxic to epidermal cells.[2] Following the death of 10 of 13 children as a result of treatment of omphaloceles (umbilical hernia) with a tincture of thiomersal, it was recommended that organic mercurial disinfectants be heavily restricted or withdrawn from hospital use as absorption occurred readily through intact membranes.[3]

1. Axton JHM. Six cases of poisoning after a parenteral organic mercurial compound (Merthiolate). *Postgrad Med J* 1972; **48:** 417–21.
2. Anonymous. Topical antiseptics and antibiotics: organic mercurials. *Med Lett Drugs Ther* 1977; **19:** 83.
3. Fagan DG, *et al.* Organ mercury levels in infants with omphaloceles treated with organic mercurial antiseptic. *Arch Dis Child* 1977; **52:** 962–4.

Hypersensitivity. The safety of thiomersal as a preservative for vaccines, eye and nose drops, and contact lens solutions has been questioned.[1] There have been reports of severe reactions to vaccines preserved with thiomersal,[2,3] and the regulatory authorities in both Europe[4] and the USA[5] have issued statements recommending that the use of thiomersal in vaccines be phased out. Delayed hypersensitivity reactions have been associated with the use of thiomersal in contact lens solutions.[6] In one clinic, 7 of 116 patients with chronic blepharitis, who had never worn contact lenses, were found to be already sensitised to thiomersal.[1] Furthermore there has been an isolated report of acute laryngeal obstruction in a patient previously sensitised to thiomersal who used a throat spray preserved with thiomersal.[7] False positive reactions to old tuberculin have also been attributed to the presence of thiomersal.[8]

1. Seal D, *et al.* The case against thiomersal. *Lancet* 1991; **338:** 316–16.
2. Cox NH, Morley WN. Vaccination reactions and thiomersal. *BMJ* 1987; **294:** 250.
3. Noel I, *et al.* Hypersensitivity to thiomersal in hepatitis B vaccine. *Lancet* 1991; **338:** 705.

4. European Agency for the Evaluation of Medicinal Products (EMEA). EMEA public statement on thiomersal containing medicinal products. EMEA publication no. 20962/99. Full Version: http://www.emea.eu.int/pdfs/human/press/pus/2096299EN.pdf (accessed 07/12/01).
5. American Academy of Pediatrics, United States Public Health Service. Thimerosal in vaccines: a joint statement of the American Academy of Pediatrics and the Public Health Service. *MMWR* 1999; **48:** 563–5.
6. Wilson LA, *et al.* Delayed hypersensitivity to thiomersal in soft contact lens wearers. *Ophthalmology* 1981; **88:** 804–9.
7. Maibach H. Acute laryngeal obstruction presumed secondary to thiomersal (merthiolate) delayed hypersensitivity. *Contact Dermatitis* 1975; **1:** 221–2.
8. Hansson H, Möller H. Intracutaneous test reactions to tuberculin containing merthiolate as a preservative. *Scand J Infect Dis* 1971; **3:** 169–72.

Interactions

◊ Nine patients using a contact lens solution containing 0.004% thiomersal developed varying degrees of ocular irritation after taking oral *tetracyclines* concurrently. Exposure to either the tetracyclines or thiomersal alone did not cause the response.[1]

1. Crook TG, Freeman JJ. Reactions induced by the concurrent use of thimerosal and tetracycline. *Am J Optom Physiol Opt* 1983; **60:** 759–61.

Uses and Administration

Thiomersal is a bacteriostatic and fungistatic mercurial antiseptic that has been applied topically usually in a concentration of 0.1%.

Thiomersal, 0.001 to 0.02%, is used as a preservative in biological and pharmaceutical products. It has also been used to preserve solutions used in the care of contact lenses (p.1129).

Preparations
USP 25: Thimerosal Tincture; Thimerosal Topical Aerosol; Thimerosal Topical Solution.

Proprietary Preparations (details are given in Part 3)
Braz.: Curativ; *Fr.:* Vitaseptol; *Israel:* LC-65; *Mex.:* Mercural; Septicol; *S.Afr.:* Merthiolate; *Thai.:* Merthiolate; *USA:* Aeroaid; Mersol.

Multi-ingredient: *Austral.:* Hexidin†; *Braz.:* Cauterex com Gentamicina; Flex-Care; Herpesine; Nazotiran; Rinocron; *Fr.:* Collyrex; Dermachrome; *Israel:* Cleaner No 4; Hexidin; *Spain:* Deltacina; Proskin; Tintu. Mertiolato Asens†.

Thymol (2282-w)

Acido Timico; Isopropilmetacresol; Thymolum; Timol. 2-Isopropyl-5-methylphenol.
$C_{10}H_{14}O = 150.2$.
CAS — 89-83-8.
Pharmacopoeias. In *Eur.* (see p.vi), *Jpn*, and *Pol.* Also in *USNF.*

Incompatibilities. The antimicrobial activity of thymol is diminished through combination with protein.

Pharmacopoeial description
Ph. Eur.: Colourless crystals. The melting range is 48° to 52°. Very slightly soluble in water; very soluble in alcohol and in ether; freely soluble in volatile and in fixed oils; sparingly soluble in glycerol; dissolves in dilute solutions of alkali hydroxides. Protect from light.

USNF 20: Colourless, often large, crystals or a white crystalline powder with an aromatic thyme-like odour. The melting range is 48° to 51°; when melted it remains liquid at a considerably lower temperature. Soluble 1 in 1000 of water, 1 in 1 of alcohol and of chloroform, 1 in 1.5 of ether, and 1 in 2 of olive oil; soluble in glacial acetic acid and in fixed and volatile oils. Store in airtight containers. Protect from light.

Adverse Effects, Treatment, and Precautions
As for Phenol, p.1152.

When ingested, thymol is less toxic than phenol. It is irritant to the gastric mucosa. Fats and alcohol increase absorption and aggravate the toxic symptoms.

Appropriate measures should be taken to avoid contamination of thymol preparations during storage or dilution.

Hypersensitivity. Contact allergy to a heparinoid cream was due to an allergen formed by the reaction between thymol and the degradation products of a triazine derivative, both present as preservatives.[1]

1. Smeenk G, *et al.* Contact allergy to a reaction product in Hirudoid cream: an example of compound allergy. *Br J Dermatol* 1987; **116:** 223–31.

Uses and Administration

Thymol is a phenolic antiseptic with antibacterial and antifungal activity. It is more powerful than phenol but its use is limited by its low solubility in water, irritancy, and susceptibility to protein.

Thymol is used chiefly as a deodorant in mouthwashes and gargles such as Compound Thymol Glycerin (BP 1988), an aqueous mixture of thymol 0.05% and glycerol 10% with colouring and flavouring, which may be used undiluted or, alternatively, diluted with about 3 times its volume of warm water before use. Thymol has been used topically in the treatment of skin disorders and is also inhaled, with other volatile substances, for colds, coughs, and associated respiratory disorders.

Thymol (0.01%) is added as an antoxidant to halothane, trichloroethylene, and tetrachloroethylene.

Thymol iodide is used in preparations for dental hygiene.

Preparations

Proprietary Preparations (details are given in Part 3)
Ger.: Medophyll; *Switz.:* Intrasol†; *Thai.:* Flavinol.

Multi-ingredient: *Aust.:* Alpicort; Criniton; DDD; Kinder Luuf; Linobion-Globuli; Linobion-Salbenstift; Luuf Balsam; Pe-Ce; Recessan†; Resol; Spasmo Claim; Thrombocid; Wick Vaporub; *Austral.:* BFI†; Gartech; Logicin Chest Rub; SM-33; Thymol Mouthwash Red; *Belg.:* Balsoclase; Borostyrol; Dentophar; Perubore; Vicks Vaporub; *Braz.:* Anestesiol; Axol; Boralina; Cutisanol; Friccex; Frixodon; Gyrol; Higienex; Lenidor; Mentolatun; Passaja; Pomalgex; Tabletes Valda; Vick Vaporub; *Canad.:* Antiseptic Mouthwash; Boil Ease; Buckley's White Rub; Carboseptol; Listerine; Mouthwash Antiseptic & Gargle; Nasal Jelly; Pastilles Valda†; Thermo-Gel; Valda; Vap Air†; Vaporisateur Medicamente; Vaporizing Ointment; *Fin.:* Vicks Vaporub; *Fr.:* Borostyrol; Glyco-Thymoline; Pastilles Medicinales Vicks; Perubore; Valda; Vicks Vaporub; *Ger.:* Alferm†; Criniton; Customed†; DDD†; Denosol; Em-eukal; Kamistad; Nasentropfen-ratiopharm; Oestrugol N; Parodontal F5 med; Pulmotin-N; Pumilen-N†; Retterspitz Ausserlich†; Retterspitz Gelee†; Retterspitz Heilsalbe†; Retterspitz Quick†; Salviathymol N; Sedotussin Expectorans†; Thrombocid; *Hong Kong:* Kamistad; Valda; *Irl.:* Karvol; Listerine†; Valda; *Israel:* Gargol; Garonsept; Karvol; Pronaestin; Rectozorin; *Ital.:* Eucalipto Composto; Florigien; Pinselina Dr. Knapp; Resina Carbolica Dentilin; Rinos; Rinostil; Salonpas; *Neth.:* Vicks Vaporub; *NZ:* Listerine; Solucol; Vicks Vaporub; *Port.:* Edoltar; Freimax; Listerine; Thrombocid; Valda; *S.Afr.:* Karvol; *Singapore:* Kamistad; Karvol; *Spain:* Cloroboral; Co Bucal; Contusin; Kneipp Balsamo; Mentobox; Pastillas Antisep Garg M; Piorlis; Pomada Balsamica†; Sudosin; Thrombocid; Vicks Vaporub; *Swed.:* Vicks Vaporub; *Switz.:* Adrectal†; Asphaline; Borostyrol N; Butaparin; Cresophene; Dental-Phenjoca†; Ederphyt; Endomethasone†; Furodermal; Huile analgesique "Polar-Bar"; Perubore; Rapura; Roliwol†; Sedasept; Sedotussin; Spirogel†; Thrombocid; Tumarol; Vicks Vaporub N; *Thai.:* Burnol Plus; Kamistad; Stopain; *UK:* Boots Vapour Rub; DDD; Dragon Balm; Eftab; Karvol; Listerine Antiseptic Mouthwash; No-Sor Vapour Rub; Potter's Catarrh Pastilles; Valda†; *USA:* BFI; Boil Ease; Cool-Mint Listerine; FreshBurst Listerine; Listerine; Massengill; Vicks Menthol Cough Drops; Zonite.

Toloconium Metilsulfate (13361-w)

Toloconium Metilsulfate (*rINN*).

Toloconium Methylsulphate. Trimethyl[1-(p-tolyl)dodecyl]ammonium methylsulphate.
$C_{23}H_{43}NO_4S = 429.7$.
CAS — 552-92-1.

Profile
Toloconium metilsulfate is a quaternary ammonium antiseptic that has been used for disinfection of skin, mucous membranes, and surgical instruments.

Preparations

Proprietary Preparations (details are given in Part 3)
Ital.: Desogen†.

Tosylchloramide Sodium (2218-h)

Tosylchloramide Sodium (*BAN, rINN*).

Chloramidum; Chloramine; Chloramine T; Chloraminum; Cloramina; Mianin; Natrium Sulfaminochloratum; Tosylchloramidum Natricum. Sodium N-chlorotoluene-p-sulphonimidate trihydrate.
$C_7H_7ClNNaO_2S,3H_2O = 281.7$.
CAS — 127-65-1 (anhydrous).
ATC — D08AX04.

NOTE. The name Chloramin has been applied to a preparation of chlorpheniramine [chlorphenamine] maleate.
Pharmacopoeias. In *Eur.* (see p.vi). *Pol.* includes tosylchloramide sodium B.

It contains about 25% w/w of 'available chlorine' (see p.1141).

Pharmacopoeial description
Ph. Eur.: A white or slightly yellow, crystalline powder. Freely soluble in water; soluble in alcohol; practically insoluble in ether. A 5% solution in water has a pH of 8.0 to 10.0. Store in airtight containers at a temperature of 8° to 15°. Protect from light.

Adverse Effects and Treatment
Vomiting, cyanosis, circulatory collapse, frothing at the mouth, and respiratory failure can occur within a few minutes of tosylchloramide sodium ingestion. Fatalities have occurred. Tosylchloramide sodium in tap water has caused methaemoglobinaemia and haemolysis in patients undergoing dialysis. Bronchospasm has occurred after inhalation.

Treatment of adverse effects is similar to that for Sodium Hypochlorite, p.1156.

◊ Shortness of breath progressing to pneumonitis requiring emergency tracheostomy occurred in a previously healthy 53-year-old woman who used a mixture of household ammonia and bleach for cleaning purposes.[1] It was considered that inhalation of tosylchloramide sodium gas produced by reaction of the two cleaning products had caused the lung damage.

1. Tanen DA, *et al.* Severe lung injury after exposure to chloramine gas from household cleaners. *N Engl J Med* 1999; **341:** 848–9.

Uses and Administration
Tosylchloramide sodium is an organic chlorine-releasing compound with the general properties of chlorine (p.1140). It is stable at an alkaline pH although it is much more active in acid media. It is more slowly active than hypochlorite solutions.

Tosylchloramide sodium is used for the treatment of minor wound infections and as a skin and hard surface disinfectant. It is also used for the treatment of drinking water (p.1130). It was formerly used as a spermicide.

Tosylchloramide sodium B (chlorogenium; sodium N-chlorobenzenesulphonimidate sesquihydrate) has been used similarly to tosylchloramide sodium.

Preparations

Proprietary Preparations (details are given in Part 3)
Belg.: Chlorazol; Dercusan; *Fr.:* Hydroclonazone; *Ger.:* Clorina; Trichlorol; *Ital.:* Cloromi-T†; Dermedal; Disinclor; Euclorina; Germozero; Minachlor; Ottoclor†; Steridrolo; *Spain:* Clorina.

Triclocarban (2286-j)

Triclocarban (*USAN, rINN*).

NSC-72005; TCC; 3,4,4'-Trichlorocarbanilide. 1-(4-Chlorophenyl)-3-(3,4-dichlorophenyl)urea.
$C_{13}H_9Cl_3N_2O = 315.6$.
CAS — 101-20-2.

Adverse Effects and Precautions
When subjected to prolonged high temperatures triclocarban can decompose to form toxic chloroanilines, which can be absorbed through the skin and cause methaemoglobinaemia. Mild photosensitivity has been seen in patch testing.

Uses and Administration
Triclocarban is an anilide antiseptic. It is bacteriostatic against Gram-positive organisms in high dilutions but is less effective against Gram-negative organisms and some fungi. It is used in antiperspirants and soaps for disinfection of skin and mucous membranes.

Preparations

Proprietary Preparations (details are given in Part 3)
Braz.: Derso TCC; *Fr.:* Cutisan; Nobacter†; Solubacter; *Irl.:* Valderma; *Ital.:* Citrosil Sapone; Sangen Sapone Disinfettante; *Port.:* Solubacter; *UK:* Valderma; *USA:* Cuticura.

Multi-ingredient: *Braz.:* Soapex; *Fr.:* Septivon; Septosan; *Ger.:* Ansudor; *Spain:* Cusiter†; *Switz.:* Septivon N.

Triclosan (2287-z)

Triclosan (*BAN, USAN, rINN*).

CH-3565; Cloxifenol. 5-Chloro-2-(2,4-dichlorophenoxy)phenol; 2,4,4'-Trichloro-2'-hydroxydiphenyl ether.
$C_{12}H_7Cl_3O_2 = 289.5$.
CAS — 3380-34-5.
ATC — D08AE04; D09AA06.
Pharmacopoeias. In *US*.

Pharmacopoeial description
USP 25: A fine whitish crystalline powder. M.p. about 57°. Practically insoluble in water; soluble in alcohol, in acetone, and in methyl alcohol; slightly soluble in petroleum spirit. Store in airtight containers. Protect from light.

Profile
Triclosan is a chlorinated bisphenol antiseptic, effective against Gram-positive and most Gram-negative bacteria but with variable or poor activity against *Pseudomonas* spp. It is also active against fungi. It is used in soaps, creams and solutions in concentrations of up to 2% for disinfection of the hands and wounds and for disinfection of the skin prior to surgery, injections, or venepuncture. It is also used in oral hygiene products and in preparations for acne. There have been isolated reports of contact dermatitis.

◊ Reports of control of meticillin-resistant *Staphylococcus aureus* (MRSA) infection in surgical units involving handwashing and bathing with triclosan.[1-3] Triclosan resistance has been reported.[4,5]

1. Bartzokas CA, *et al.* Control and eradication of methicillin-resistant Staphylococcus aureus on a surgical unit. *N Engl J Med* 1984; **311:** 1422–5.
2. Bartzokas CA. Eradication of resistant Staphylococcus aureus on a surgical unit. *N Engl J Med* 1985; **312:** 858–9.
3. Brady LM, *et al.* Successful control of endemic MRSA in a cardiothoracic surgical unit. *Med J Aust* 1990; **152:** 240–5.
4. Cookson BD, *et al.* Transferable resistance to triclosan in MRSA. *Lancet* 1991; **337:** 1548–9.
5. Sasatsu M, *et al.* Triclosan-resistant Staphylococcus aureus. *Lancet* 1993; **341:** 756. Correction. *ibid.* **342:** 248.

Preparations

Proprietary Preparations (details are given in Part 3)
Austral.: Bioband; Dettol Liquid Wash; Gamophen; Johnsons Clean & Clear Facial Cleansing Bar; Johnsons Clean & Clear Foaming Facial Wash; Liquid Soap Pre-Op; Microshield Clean; Neutrogena Acne Skin Cleanser; Novaderm†; Oxy Skin Wash; pHisoHex Face Wash; Sapoderm; Softwash†; Solyptol; *Belg.:* Dettol Liquid Wash; *Braz.:* Fisohex; Proderm; *Canad.:* Adasept; Clean & Clear Foaming Cleanser; Clearasil Face Wash; Clearskin Medicated Cleanser; Oxy Daily Facial Cleanser Regular; Oxy Gentle; Oxy Medicated Soap; Promani†; Skin So Soft Antibacterial; Tersaseptic; *Hong Kong:* Oxy Daily Wash; pHisoHex Cleanser; Prewash; *Israel:* Dermax; *Ital.:* Dermo-Steril†; Geroderm; Ippi Verde; Irgaman; Lactacyd Antibatterico; Till; *Mex.:* Clearasil Jabon; Clearasil Wash Antiseptico; *NZ:* Dalacin T Prewash; Oxy Daily Skin Wash; *S.Afr.:* Acneclear; *Switz.:* Cliniderm; Lipo Sol; Procoutol; Shampooing extra-doux; *UK:* Aquasept; Clearasil Medicated Moisturiser; Clearasil Soap; Gamophen; Oxy Facial Wash; Ster-Zac; *USA:* Ambi 10; Clearasil Daily Face Wash; Oxy Medicated Soap; Septi-Soft; Septisol; Stri-Dex Antibacterial Cleansing; Stri-Dex Face Wash.

Multi-ingredient: *Austral.:* Burnaid First Aid Burn Gel; Clearasil Acne Treatment Cream; Clearasil Medicated Foam†; Dettol Cream; Microshield PVP Plus; Novasrub†; Oilatum Plus; Z-Acne†; *Braz.:* Clearasil; Cravo-Espin; Soapex; Tratoderm; *Canad.:* Adasept; Oral Plan; Solarcaine; Tersac; *Fin.:* Wicne; Wicnecarb; Wicnelact; Wicnevit; *Fr.:* Clinogel; Sanytol; Septosan; *Ger.:* Rutisept extra; Sicorten Plus; *Hong Kong:* Dettol; Oilatum Plus; Sicorten Plus; Solarcaine; *Irl.:* Dettol; Oilatum Junior Flare-Up; *Israel:* Pedisol; Sicorten Plus; *Ital.:* Aknicare; Solarcaine; AZ Protezione Viso/Labbra Alta Protezione; AZ Protezione Completa; AZ Protezione Gengive; Dopo Pik; Geroderm Zolfo; Levaknel†; Plax; Steril Zeta; *Mex.:* Dermobras; Sebryl Plus; *NZ:* Dettol; Oilatum Plus; *Port.:* Aknicare; Antiacneicos Ac-Sal; Disoderme; Lambda; Sicorten Plus; *S.Afr.:* Dettol Antiseptic; Oilatum Plus; Tantol Skin Cleanser†; *Singapore:* Dettol; Oilatum Plus; pHisoHex Reformulated; *Spain:* Anti-Acne; Doctodermis; Poliglicol Anti Acne; Sicorten Plus; Vaselatum; *Switz.:* Acne Creme; Acne Gel; Acne Lotion; Antebor N; Keroderm; Locacorten Triclosan†; Pixor Stick Anti-acne N; Saltrates; Sebo Creme; Sebo Shampooing; Sicorten Plus; Sulgan; Teerol-H†; Tretinoine†; Turexan Emulsion; *Thai.:* Dettol; Oilatum Plus; *UK:* Actibrush†; Clearasil Treatment Cream; Dentyl pH; Dettol; Germolene; Manusept; Oilatum Junior Flare-up; Oilatum Plus; Oxy Clean Facial Scrub; Oxy Cleanser; Oxy Dots; Oxy Duo Pads; Sensodyne-F; Solarcaine; TCP; *USA:* Clearasil Antibacterial; Oxy ResiDon't†; Solarcaine.

Urea Hydrogen Peroxide (5910-d)

Carbamide Peroxide; Hydroperite; Urea Peroxide.
$NH_2.CO.NH_2,H_2O_2 = 94.07$.
CAS — 124-43-6.
Pharmacopoeias. In *US*.

Pharmacopoeial description
USP 25: Store in airtight containers at a temperature not exceeding 40°. Protect from light.

Profile
Urea hydrogen peroxide consists of hydrogen peroxide and urea in equimolecular proportions. It is used for the extemporaneous preparation of hydrogen peroxide. It has been employed for infections of the ear, mouth, skin, and mucous membranes and for softening ear wax.

Preparations

USP 25: Carbamide Peroxide Topical Solution.

Proprietary Preparations (details are given in Part 3)
Austral.: Ear Clear; *Braz.:* Aceratun; *Canad.:* Murine; *Ger.:* Elawox; *Irl.:* Exterol; *Israel:* Exterol; *Ital.:* Debrox; Dermoxyl; Ginoxil; *Mex.:* Amosan; *UK:* Exterol; Otex; *USA:* Auraphene-B; Auro; Debrox; ERO; Gly-Oxide; Mollifene; Murine; Orajel Perioseptic; Proxigel.

Zinc Peroxide (5912-h)

CAS — 1314-22-3.

Profile
The action of zinc peroxide is similar to that of hydrogen peroxide (p.1147). Applied locally it has been used for disinfecting and deodorising burns, wounds and various ulcers and lesions.

Preparations

Proprietary Preparations (details are given in Part 3)
Canad.: Neoderm.

Multi-ingredient: *Braz.:* Anaseptil; *Fr.:* Bioxyol; Ektogan†; *Ital.:* Ektogan.

Dopaminergics

Dopamine is a key neurotransmitter in the CNS; in particular, striatal dopamine depletion is associated with the clinical condition of parkinsonism. Dopamine also inhibits prolactin release from the pituitary and is believed to be the prolactin-release inhibiting factor (PRIF or PIF); its deficiency here is associated with conditions characterised by hyperprolactinaemia.

Accordingly, drugs which replenish central dopamine or which themselves can act as stimulants of dopamine receptors (dopamine agonists), may alleviate the symptoms of parkinsonism (see below), hyperprolactinaemia (p.1274), and related disorders.

At least 5 subtypes of dopamine receptor are thought to exist: D_1 receptors appear to stimulate adenylate cyclase activity; D_2 receptors activate various systems and inhibit adenylate cyclase activity; D_3, D_4, and D_5 receptors have been less well studied. D_2 receptors have been implicated in the pathophysiology of parkinsonism and schizophrenia.

Dopaminergics, or drugs that enhance their actions, described in this chapter include:

- levodopa, which is converted by decarboxylation into dopamine in the body, and which, unlike dopamine itself, can penetrate the blood-brain barrier and supply a source of dopamine to the brain
- the peripheral dopa-decarboxylase inhibitors, benserazide and carbidopa, which have no antiparkinsonian action of their own but increase the availability of levodopa
- apomorphine, which is structurally related to dopamine and acts as a dopamine agonist
- the adamantanamines, amantadine and memantine, which may augment dopaminergic activity
- the ergot derivatives, bromocriptine, cabergoline, lisuride, and pergolide, which act as dopamine agonists
- various other non-ergot dopamine agonists, such as piribedil, pramipexole, quinagolide, and ropinirole
- the specific monoamine oxidase type B inhibitor, selegiline, which enhances the action of dopamine and levodopa
- the catechol-O-methyltransferase inhibitors (COMT-inhibitors), entacapone and tolcapone, which enhance the action of levodopa.

Parkinsonism

The syndrome of parkinsonism is characterised by tremor, rigidity, akinesia or bradykinesia, and loss of postural reflexes. It may be classified into primary (idiopathic) parkinsonism, usually referred to as Parkinson's disease (formerly paralysis agitans); secondary (acquired) parkinsonism, including postencephalitic parkinsonism, drug-induced parkinsonism, and symptoms associated with manganese poisoning; and 'parkinsonism-plus' syndromes where parkinsonism is a feature of other degenerative diseases of the CNS, such as progressive supranuclear palsy and multiple system atrophy. 'Arteriosclerotic parkinsonism' has been used to describe parkinsonism associated with cerebrovascular disease although this may be confusing since vascular brain damage is not a cause of Parkinson's disease. The term parkinsonism is often used for the idiopathic form, that is, Parkinson's disease.

In parkinsonism there is reduced dopamine activity in the brain. Parkinson's disease and postencephalitic parkinsonism have been attributed primarily to depletion of striatal dopamine in the basal ganglia as a result of the loss of neurones in the substantia nigra. Striatal dopamine deficiency results in loss of the normal functional balance between dopaminergic and cholinergic activity and treatment aims to increase the former and/or decrease the latter.

The cause of Parkinson's disease is not established although environmental and genetic factors superimposed on a background of neuronal loss related to ageing has been postulated. Great interest was aroused by the discovery that MPTP (1-methyl-4-phenyl-1,2,3,6-tetrahy-dropyridine), a contaminant of an illicitly produced pethidine analogue MPPP (1-methyl-4-phenyl-4-propionoxypiperidine), caused irreversible parkinsonism which had a pathology similar to that of Parkinson's disease and likewise responded to treatment with levodopa. *Animal* studies revealed that MPTP was converted by monoamine oxidase B to the neurotoxic methylphenylpyridinium ion which was selectively concentrated in dopaminergic neurones in the substantia nigra. Of those biochemical mechanisms proposed as possibly being involved in the pathogenesis of Parkinson's disease the most prominent has been the oxidant stress hypothesis. Proponents of this theory have postulated that free radicals produced during normal metabolism of dopamine in the brain by monoamine oxidase B might be neurotoxic to dopaminergic neurones in the substantia nigra. This has led to concern that administration of levodopa, by increasing the supply of dopamine, might therefore exacerbate neurodegeneration and hasten the progression of Parkinson's disease but compelling evidence of such an effect is lacking.

Drug-induced parkinsonism can arise from depletion of presynaptic dopamine, as with reserpine and tetrabenazine, or from blockade of postsynaptic dopamine receptors in the striatum, as by antipsychotics and some antiemetics such as metoclopramide. It is generally reversible on drug withdrawal or dose reduction and may sometimes disappear gradually despite continuous drug therapy. Although the use of levodopa to overcome antipsychotic-induced blockade of dopamine receptors might appear rational, it has generally been reported to be ineffective or to increase psychiatric symptoms. For a discussion of the treatment of drug-induced parkinsonism see under Extrapyramidal Disorders in Adverse Effects of Chlorpromazine, p.662.

There is no cure for Parkinson's disease. Although the possibility of using drug therapy to slow neurodegeneration is being investigated, no drug so far has a proven neuroprotective effect. Treatment is palliative and symptomatic and consists mainly of drug therapy supplemented when necessary with physical treatment such as physiotherapy and speech therapy. Surgery is occasionally used and there is growing interest in the use of transplantation and in electrical devices for the control of tremor.

Drugs used in Parkinson's disease. Drug therapy consists largely of the use of dopaminergics or antimuscarinics in an attempt to restore the normal balance between dopaminergic and cholinergic activity. Dopaminergics may act by direct replacement of dopamine, by delaying the metabolism of endogenous dopamine, by stimulation of dopamine receptors directly, or by enhancement of release of endogenous dopamine. Drugs with differing actions are often used together to achieve optimum control of symptoms.

- *Levodopa* is converted by decarboxylation into dopamine and, unlike dopamine, can penetrate the blood-brain barrier hence supplying a source of dopamine to the brain. Levodopa is usually given with a peripheral dopa-decarboxylase inhibitor such as *benserazide* or *carbidopa*. These drugs are unable to penetrate the blood-brain barrier and therefore prevent only extracerebral conversion of levodopa to dopamine. This allows effective concentrations of dopamine to be achieved in the brain with lower doses of levodopa and also reduces unwanted effects such as nausea and vomiting and cardiovascular effects associated with peripheral formation of dopamine.
The majority of patients respond initially to levodopa and its use has improved the quality and duration of life. However, after 2 or more years, benefit is reduced as the disease progresses and late complications emerge. Apart from dyskinesias and psychiatric effects, a major problem with long-term levodopa treatment is the appearance of fluctuations in mobility, the two predominant forms being 'end-of-dose' deterioration ('wearing-off' effect) and the 'on-off' phenomenon (see Complications of Treatment, below). Thus, although it is generally agreed that levodopa, given with a peripheral dopa-decarboxylase inhibitor such as carbidopa or benserazide, is currently the most effective treatment for Parkinson's disease, views differ as to the best time to start treatment and the dosage to employ in order to limit the long-term complications. Those who consider that these long-term effects reflect severity of the disease favour the early use of levodopa, whereas those implicating cumulative exposure to levodopa advocate later use. Catechol-O-methyltransferase (COMT) inhibitors, such as *entacapone* and *tolcapone*, are selective and reversible inhibitors of catechol-O-methyltransferase (COMT), with mainly peripheral actions. They are given as adjunctive therapy to patients experiencing fluctuations in disability related to levodopa and dopa-decarboxylase inhibitor combinations. When levodopa is administered concurrently with a peripheral dopa-decarboxylase inhibitor, O-methylation becomes the predominant form of metabolism of levodopa; co-administration of a peripheral COMT inhibitor can thus extend the duration and effect of levodopa in the brain, and allow a reduction in the dose and frequency of administration of levodopa. They therefore can help to stabilise patients, especially those experiencing 'end-of-dose' deterioration.

- *Selegiline* is a selective inhibitor of monoamine oxidase type B, an enzyme involved in the metabolism of dopamine in the brain. Used with levodopa in severe parkinsonism it has a dose-sparing effect and is of use in patients experiencing fluctuations in mobility. Although early treatment with selegiline may delay the need for levodopa there is no evidence that it has a favourable effect on the long-term course of the disease. Whether any benefit obtained is due to a symptomatic or neuroprotective effect is unclear. Used alone, selegiline produces few side-effects but when used with levodopa it can provoke or worsen dyskinesias or psychiatric symptoms and doubts have been expressed on the safety of long-term use.

- *Bromocriptine* and similar dopamine agonists such as *cabergoline*, *lisuride*, *pergolide*, *pramipexole*, and *ropinirole* act by direct stimulation of remaining postsynaptic dopamine receptors. Some neurologists use dopamine agonists early in treatment in an attempt to delay therapy with levodopa but as their efficacy often decreases after a few years others reserve them for adjunctive use when levodopa is no longer effective alone or cannot be tolerated. They are sometimes useful in reducing 'off' periods with levodopa and in ameliorating fluctuations in mobility in the later stages of the disease. *Apomorphine* is a potent dopamine agonist, but must be given parenterally and with an antiemetic. Although this restricts its use, it has a role in stabilising patients who suffer unpredictable 'on-off' effects. It is also used in the differential diagnosis of parkinsonism syndromes.

- *Antimuscarinics* are considered to have a weak antiparkinsonian effect compared with levodopa. They may reduce tremor but have little effect on bradykinesia. They may be of use alone or with other drugs in the initial treatment of patients with mild symptoms, especially when tremor is pronounced, or later as an adjunct to levodopa such as in patients with refractory tremor or dystonias. Antimuscarinic side-effects occur frequently and can limit their use. However, some side-effects can ameliorate complications associated with Parkinson's disease; dry mouth may be an advantage in patients with sialorrhoea. There appear to be no important differences in the efficacy of antimuscarinics for Parkinson's disease but some patients may tolerate one drug better than another. Those commonly used for Parkinson's disease include *benzhexol [trihexyphenidyl]*, *benzatropine*, *orphenadrine*, and *procyclidine*.

- *Amantadine* is a weak dopamine agonist with some antimuscarinic activity although its activity as an antagonist of N-methyl-D-aspartate may also have a beneficial effect in Parkinson's disease. It has mild antiparkinsonian effects compared with levodopa but is relatively free from side-effects. It can improve bradykinesia as well as tremor and rigidity but only a small proportion of patients derive much benefit. It is used similarly to antimuscarinics in early disease when symptoms are mild, but tolerance to its effects can occur rapidly.

Choice and implementation of drug treatment. There is no consensus on when to initiate treatment with *levodopa* or whether to use other drugs before levodopa. Many neurologists delay initial treatment with levodopa as they believe early use may increase the likelihood of problems such as dyskinesias and fluctuations in mobility and may accelerate the loss of dopaminergic neurones. If symptoms are mild, drug therapy may not be required in the early stages of the disease. Some have initiated treatment with *selegiline* immediately, but there have been doubts over whether it has a neuroprotective effect, as postulated, and also over long-term safety. When symptoms become troublesome but are still relatively mild *amantadine* or an *antimuscarinic* may be started; antimuscarinics are useful when tremor predominates but are generally more suitable for younger patients. As the disease progresses some neurologists may advocate a trial of a *dopamine agonist* in an attempt to delay the introduction of levodopa. For most patients treatment with levodopa eventually becomes necessary.

The usual practice is to start with small doses of levodopa, together with a peripheral dopa-decarboxylase inhibitor, and increase slowly to a dose which reduces disability to an acceptable level. Variations in response and diminishing effectiveness over the years necessitate careful adjustment of the size and form of the dose and the schedule of administration.

Complications of treatment. Fluctuations in mobility have been reported in more than half of patients on levodopa after 5 years of therapy. They generally proceed through predictable **'end-of-dose'** deterioration to the **'on-off'** phenomenon with marked very sudden swings from mobility to immobility. The cause of the fluctuations is not known, but multiple factors including desensitisation of dopamine receptors, interference with the response to dopamine by other levodopa metabolites such as 3-*O*-methyldopa, fluctuating plasma concentrations, and erratic transport of levodopa from blood to the brain have been suggested. It appears that as the disease progresses the capacity of the nigrostriatal dopaminergic system to synthesise and store dopamine, and to act as a buffer in maintaining dopamine brain concentrations, declines. Dopamine concentrations therefore become more dependent on levodopa administration and the pattern of response will come to reflect more closely the rise and fall in levodopa concentrations. Eventually the effect of various factors which produce even small changes in plasma concentrations of levodopa will progressively become more pronounced.

Approaches to the management of 'end-of-dose' fluctuations include more frequent administration of smaller doses and the use of modified-release preparations. Addition of selegiline or partial replacement of levodopa with a dopamine agonist with a more prolonged action are also used.

Various attempts have been made to overcome the 'on-off' phenomenon. Those speculating that long-term treatment results in altered dopamine receptor sensitivity have used controlled withdrawal of levodopa for short periods ('drug holidays') but it is a dangerous procedure of doubtful value and no longer recommended.

Others have linked the 'on-off' phenomenon to variable plasma concentrations although, since transfer of levodopa into the brain involves active transport mechanisms, concentrations in plasma may not necessarily reflect those in the brain. Continuous intravenous infusion of levodopa has been shown to reduce fluctuations in mobility which suggests that dopamine receptors are still sensitive but this is not practical for day-to-day management. However, there is evidence that some patients may benefit from modified-release formulations of levodopa with a peripheral dopa-decarboxylase inhibitor. As levodopa competes with amino acids for uptake into the brain, attempts to lessen fluctuations in dopamine brain concentrations have included taking levodopa on an empty stomach and also delaying most of a day's protein consumption until the evening. Addition of selegiline or a dopamine agonist may also help to reduce 'on-off' phenomena. If fluctuations remain a problem subcutaneous apomorphine is often effective.

Other complications of treatment with levodopa may include **dyskinesia** which may respond to dosage adjustment or partial replacement of levodopa with a dopamine agonist. Some patients with Parkinson's disease may experience **severe pain** and **dystonia** and it has been considered that measures to increase 'on' periods will reduce or eliminate pain in most patients.

Patients with Parkinson's disease can suffer from a range of **psychiatric effects** due to the adverse effects of drug therapy and to disease progression. It has been recommended that if patients develop psychotic reactions the use of antiparkinsonian drugs should be manipulated before resorting to the use of antipsychotics. Although antipsychotics are usually contra-indicated because they can exacerbate parkinsonism, atypical antipsychotics such as clozapine have been tried—see Disturbed Behav-

iour, p.650. **Nausea and vomiting** induced by dopaminergics may be minimised by introducing the drug gradually and administering the dose with food, but if this is ineffective or apomorphine is being used these effects can be controlled by the antiemetic domperidone. Domperidone does not readily cross the blood-brain barrier and therefore acts mainly as a peripheral dopamine antagonist. Tolerance to the nausea usually develops after a few weeks and domperidone may then be withdrawn.

References.
1. Marsden CD. Parkinson's disease. *Lancet* 1990; **335:** 948–52.
2. Clough CG. Parkinson's disease: management. *Lancet* 1991; **337:** 1324–7.
3. Marsden CD. Parkinson's disease. *Postgrad Med J* 1992; **68:** 538–43.
4. Calne DB. Treatment of Parkinson's disease. *N Engl J Med* 1993; **329:** 1021–7.
5. Montastruc JL, *et al.* Current status of dopamine agonists in Parkinson's disease management. *Drugs* 1993; **46:** 384–93.
6. Mizuno Y, *et al.* Potential of neuroprotective therapy in Parkinson's disease. *CNS Drugs* 1994; **1:** 45–56.
7. Bodagh IYO, Robertson DRC. A risk-benefit assessment of drugs used in the management of Parkinson's disease. *Drug Safety* 1994; **11:** 94–103.
8. Mizuno Y, *et al.* Practical guidelines for the drug treatment of Parkinson's disease. *CNS Drugs* 1994; **1:** 410–26.
9. Quinn N. Drug treatment of Parkinson's disease. *BMJ* 1995; **310:** 575–9.
10. Harder S, *et al.* Concentration-effect relationship of levodopa in patients with Parkinson's disease. *Clin Pharmacokinet* 1995; **29:** 243–56.
11. Giron LT, Koller WC. Methods of managing levodopa-induced dyskinesias. *Drug Safety* 1996; **14:** 365–74.
12. Ahlskog JE. Treatment of early Parkinson's disease: are complicated strategies justified? *Mayo Clin Proc* 1996; **71:** 659–70.
13. Mendis T, *et al.* Drug-induced psychosis in Parkinson's disease: a review of management. *CNS Drugs* 1996; **5:** 166–74.
14. Hughes AJ. Drug treatment of Parkinson's disease in the 1990s. *Drugs* 1997; **53:** 195–205.
15. Gottwald MD, *et al.* New pharmacotherapy for Parkinson's disease. *Ann Pharmacother* 1997; **31:** 1205–17.
16. Lang AE, Lozano AM. Parkinson's disease. *N Engl J Med* 1998; **339:** 1044–53 and 1130–43.
17. Bhatia K, *et al.* Guidelines for the management of Parkinson's disease. *Hosp Med* 1998; **59:** 469–80.
18. Ahlskog JE. Medical treatment of later-stage motor problems of Parkinson disease. *Mayo Clin Proc* 1999; **74:** 1239–54.
19. Anonymous. Developments in the treatment of Parkinson's disease. *Drug Ther Bull* 1999; **37:** 36–40.
20. Olanow CW, *et al.* An algorithm (decision tree) for the management of Parkinson's disease (2001): treatment guidelines. *Neurology* 2001; **56** (suppl 5): S1–S88.

Amantadine Hydrochloride (9852-z)

Amantadine Hydrochloride *(BANM, USAN, pINNM)*.

1-Adamantanamine Hydrochloride; Amantadini Hydrochloridum; EXP-105-1; NSC-83653. Tricyclo[3.3.1.1^{3,7}]dec-1-ylamine hydrochloride.

$C_{10}H_{17}N,HCl = 187.7$.

CAS — 768-94-5 (amantadine); 665-66-7 (amantadine hydrochloride).

Pharmacopoeias. In Chin., Eur. (see p.vi), Jpn, and US.

Pharmacopoeial description

Ph. Eur.: A white or almost white crystalline powder. It sublimes on heating. Freely soluble in water and in alcohol; practically insoluble in ether.

USP 25: A white or practically white crystalline powder. Soluble 1 in 2.5 of water, 1 in 5.1 of alcohol, 1 in 18 of chloroform, and 1 in 70 of macrogol 400. pH of a 20% solution in water is between 3.0 and 5.5.

Amantadine Sulfate (4542-q)

Amantadine Sulphate.

$(C_{10}H_{17}N)_2,SO_4 = 398.6$.

CAS — 31377-23-8.

Adverse Effects

Most side-effects associated with amantadine therapy appear to be dose-related and relatively mild; some resemble those of antimuscarinic drugs. They may be reversed by withdrawing therapy but many resolve despite continuation.

Livedo reticularis, sometimes associated with ankle oedema, is quite common in patients given amantadine long-term. Mild CNS effects such as nervousness, inability to concentrate, dizziness, insomnia, nightmares, headache, and changes in mood may occur. Psychotic reactions, hallucinations, and confusion have been reported, especially in the elderly, patients with impaired renal function, and those also receiving antimuscarinic drugs.

Other side-effects reported have included orthostatic hypotension, urinary retention, slurred speech, ataxia, lethargy, nausea, anorexia, vomiting, dry mouth, constipation, skin rash, diaphoresis, photosensitisation,

and blurred vision. There have been isolated reports of congestive heart failure, palpitations, leucopenia, neutropenia, facial dyskinesias, oculogyric episodes, and convulsions.

Effects on the cardiovascular system. Congestive heart failure has been associated with amantadine;[1] in this report the patient had been receiving combined treatment with amantadine, levodopa, and orphenadrine for 4 years. Others have considered that while amantadine sometimes causes ankle oedema, an association between amantadine and heart failure is not proven.[2] Livedo reticularis, a mottled blue discoloration of the skin due to prominence of the normal pattern of venous drainage, has been reported[2] to occur in about 50% of all elderly patients given amantadine 100 to 300 mg daily for 2 to 6 weeks and was associated with oedema in 5 to 10%. Both livedo and oedema have usually been confined to the legs and may result from the catecholamine-releasing action of amantadine in certain vascular beds; the oedema was unlikely to be due to heart failure. Angina, dyspnoea, pulmonary congestion, or distension of neck veins has also been reported[2] in 4 of 89 parkinsonian patients treated with amantadine; only 2 of these 4 had had ankle oedema before heart failure developed. No patient had been observed in whom heart failure seemed due directly to amantadine.

See also under Overdosage, below.
1. Vale JA, Maclean KS. Amantadine-induced heart-failure. *Lancet* 1977; **i:** 548.
2. Parkes JD, *et al.* Amantadine-induced heart-failure. *Lancet* 1977; **i:** 904.

Effects on electrolytes. For a report of a patient who developed hyponatraemia when given amantadine or levodopa, see under Effects on Kidney Function in Levodopa, p.1170.

Effects on the eyes. Superficial punctate keratitis and corneal abrasion with loss of visual acuity was observed in both eyes of a 64-year-old man about 3 weeks after starting treatment with amantadine 100 mg daily.[1] Symptoms resolved on discontinuation of amantadine but recurred when re-treatment with amantadine was attempted.
1. Nogaki H, Morimatsu M. Superficial punctate keratitis and corneal abrasion due to amantadine hydrochloride. *J Neurol* 1993; **240:** 388–9.

Effects on mental function. It has been suggested[1] that the ability of amantadine and memantine to cause psychotic disturbances in patients with Parkinson's disease might be related to their action as *N*-methyl-D-aspartate antagonists.
1. Riederer P, *et al.* Pharmacotoxic psychosis after memantine in Parkinson's disease. *Lancet* 1991; **338:** 1022–3.

Effects on the nervous system. Peripheral sensory motor neuropathy secondary to long-term (8 years) administration of amantadine has been reported[1] in a 48-year-old woman with parkinsonism. Trophic skin ulcers, paraesthesias, and distal weakness resolved on discontinuation of amantadine.
1. Shulman LM, *et al.* Amantadine-induced peripheral neuropathy. *Neurology* 1999; **53:** 1862–5.

Overdosage. A patient with postencephalitic parkinsonism who had taken an estimated 2.8 g of amantadine hydrochloride in a suicide attempt suffered an acute toxic psychosis with disorientation, visual hallucinations, and aggressive behaviour.[1] Convulsions did not occur, possibly because he had been receiving phenytoin which was continued. The patient was treated with hydration and chlorpromazine and recovered in 4 days.

A 2-year-old child who had ingested 600 mg of amantadine hydrochloride developed symptoms of acute toxicity, including agitation and dystonic posturing, despite emesis with 'syrup of ipecac'.[2] She responded immediately to a trial of physostigmine 500 µg intravenously, repeated after 10 minutes. Her pupils remained moderately dilated until about 20 hours after the ingestion; thereafter she made a full recovery.

Cardiac arrest developed 4 hours after a 37-year-old woman ingested 2.5 g of amantadine hydrochloride and was treated successfully.[3] However, ventricular arrhythmias, including torsade de pointes, continued over the ensuing 48 hours and may have been exacerbated by administration of isoprenaline and dopamine. The patient was subsequently stabilised with lignocaine [lidocaine] by intravenous infusion, but died of respiratory failure 10 days after admission.
1. Fahn S, *et al.* Acute toxic psychosis from suicidal overdosage of amantadine. *Arch Neurol* 1971; **25:** 45–8.
2. Berkowitz CD. Treatment of acute amantadine toxicity with physostigmine. *J Pediatr* 1979; **95:** 144–5.
3. Sartori M, *et al.* Torsade de pointe: malignant cardiac arrhythmia induced by amantadine poisoning. *Am J Med* 1984; **77:** 388–91.

Precautions

Amantadine is usually contra-indicated in severe renal disease and in patients with a history of epilepsy or other seizure disorders or gastric ulceration. It should be used with caution in patients with cardiovascular or liver disease, impaired renal function, recurrent eczema, or psychosis. Care should be taken in all elderly patients, who may be more sensitive to antimuscarinic effects, and in whom renal clearance is likely to be reduced.

Amantadine should not be used during pregnancy; toxicity has been reported in *animal* studies. It is also distributed into breast milk and the manufacturer has reported that adverse effects have occurred in infants being breast fed by mothers taking amantadine.

In common with other drugs having antimuscarinic properties amantadine may cause blurred vision or impair alertness; patients so affected should not drive or operate machinery. Treatment with amantadine should not be stopped abruptly in parkinsonian patients since they may experience a sudden marked clinical deterioration. There have been isolated reports of neuroleptic malignant syndrome associated with abrupt withdrawal of amantadine, especially in patients receiving concomitant treatment with antipsychotics.

Antiviral resistance. See under Influenza in Uses and Administration, below.

Pregnancy. A complex cardiovascular lesion occurred in an infant whose mother had taken amantadine hydrochloride 100 mg daily during the first 3 months of pregnancy.[1] Amantadine has been reported to be embryotoxic and teratogenic in *rats* given high doses[1] and it is recommended that it should not be used in pregnancy.[2]

1. Nora JJ, *et al.* Cardiovascular maldevelopment associated with maternal exposure to amantadine. *Lancet* 1975; ii: 607.
2. Anonymous. Safety of antimicrobial drugs in pregnancy. *Med Lett Drugs Ther* 1985; 27: 93–5.

Renal impairment. Evidence of extremely limited excretion of amantadine was found in 12 patients who were either anephric or had negligible renal function, and who received a single dose of 100 mg of amantadine hydrochloride.[1] Only small amounts were removed by dialysis. It was suggested that amantadine should be given with caution to patients requiring maintenance haemodialysis. It should be remembered that a single dose may provide adequate plasma concentrations for many days.[1] Dosage regimens based on creatinine clearance[2] or fixed doses at extended intervals[3] have been published. However both regimens have been criticised, and a conservative approach to amantadine dosage in these patients recommended.[4] The need for caution in using amantadine in patients with renal impairment is highlighted by a report of a patient with end-stage renal disease who progressed from delirium to coma after receiving amantadine 100 mg twice daily for 3 days.[5]

1. Soung L-S, *et al.* Amantadine hydrochloride pharmacokinetics in hemodialysis patients. *Ann Intern Med* 1980; 93: 46–9.
2. Horadam VW, *et al.* Pharmacokinetics of amantadine hydrochloride in subjects with normal and impaired renal function. *Ann Intern Med* 1981; 94: 454–8.
3. Wu MJ, *et al.* Amantadine hydrochloride pharmacokinetics in patients with impaired renal function. *Clin Nephrol* 1982; 17: 19–23.
4. Aoki FY, Sitar DS. Clinical pharmacokinetics of amantadine hydrochloride. *Clin Pharmacokinet* 1988; 14: 35–51.
5. Macchio GJ, *et al.* Amantadine-induced coma. *Arch Phys Med Rehabil* 1993; 74: 1119–20.

Withdrawal. Neuroleptic malignant syndrome occurred in a patient being treated for heat stroke when all his medication, including antipsychotics and amantadine, was withdrawn.[1] It is suggested that dopamine agonists should not be discontinued in patients with hyperpyrexia at risk from this syndrome.

1. Simpson DM, Davis GC. Case report of neuroleptic malignant syndrome associated with withdrawal from amantadine. *Am J Psychiatry* 1984; 141: 796–7.

Interactions

Amantadine may enhance the adverse effects of antimuscarinics and the dose of these drugs should be reduced when amantadine is given concomitantly; side-effects of levodopa may also be exacerbated.

The manufacturer recommends that amantadine should be used with caution in patients receiving drugs with CNS stimulant properties. The rate of excretion of amantadine may be reduced by drugs that raise urinary pH.

Antiarrhythmics. Quinine and quinidine have been reported to reduce the renal clearance of amantadine in healthy male, but not female, subjects.[1] Patients taking these drugs concomitantly should be observed for signs of amantadine toxicity.

1. Gaudry SE, *et al.* Gender and age as factors in the inhibition of renal clearance of amantadine by quinine and quinidine. *Clin Pharmacol Ther* 1993; 54: 23–7.

Antimalarials. See under Antiarrhythmics, above.

Diuretics. A patient with Parkinson's disease, previously stabilised on amantadine hydrochloride 300 mg daily, developed symptoms of amantadine toxicity, including ataxia, myoclonus, and confusion, 7 days after starting treatment with a preparation containing triamterene and hydrochlorothiazide (Dyazide).[1] It was postulated that the effect was due to reduction of the tubular secretion of amantadine.

1. Wilson TW, Rajput AH. Amantadine-Dyazide interaction. *Can Med Assoc J* 1983; 129: 974–5.

MAOIs. Hypertension occurred about 48 hours after starting treatment with phenelzine sulfate in a patient already receiving amantadine.[1]

1. Jack RA, Daniel DG. Possible interaction between phenelzine and amantadine. *Arch Gen Psychiatry* 1984; 41: 726.

Pharmacokinetics

Amantadine hydrochloride is readily absorbed from the gastrointestinal tract; peak concentrations in the plasma appear within about 4 hours. It is mainly excreted unchanged in the urine by glomerular filtration and tubular secretion although small amounts of an acetylated metabolite have also been detected in urine; the plasma elimination half-life is reported to be about 11 to 15 hours in patients with normal renal function but is significantly prolonged in the elderly and in patients with renal impairment. The rate of elimination may be increased by acidification of the urine. Amantadine crosses the placenta and the blood-brain barrier. It is also distributed into breast milk. Plasma protein binding is reported to be about 67%.

◊ References.
1. Aoki FY, Sitar DS. Clinical pharmacokinetics of amantadine hydrochloride. *Clin Pharmacokinet* 1988; 14: 35–51.

Uses and Administration

Amantadine is a weak dopamine agonist with some antimuscarinic activity; it is also an antagonist of *N*-methyl-D-aspartate receptors. Amantadine has mild antiparkinsonian activity and is used in the management of parkinsonism, mainly in early disease when symptoms are mild. It may improve bradykinesia, rigidity, and tremor but tolerance can develop.

Amantadine is also an antiviral that inhibits replication of influenza type A virus. Variable activity has been reported *in vitro* against other viruses. It is used prophylactically against infection with influenza type A virus and to ameliorate symptoms when administered during the early stages of infection.

Amantadine has also been used in the management of herpes zoster.

Amantadine is usually given by mouth as the hydrochloride and the doses below are expressed in terms of the hydrochloride.

In parkinsonism, treatment is usually started with 100 mg daily and is increased to 100 mg twice daily after a week or more. Doses of up to 400 mg daily have occasionally been used, but this dose should not be exceeded. The lowest effective dose should be used in patients over 65 years of age because of the potential for reduced renal clearance in this age group. Withdrawal of amantadine treatment for parkinsonism should be gradual to avoid exacerbating the condition; the manufacturers suggest decreasing the dose by half at weekly intervals.

In the treatment of influenza A 100 mg is usually given daily for about 5 days. For the prophylaxis of influenza A the same dose is given for as long as protection from infection is required, which may be for about 6 weeks. If amantadine is being given in conjunction with influenza vaccination then it is usually only given for up to 3 weeks after vaccination. A daily dose of less than 100 mg or 100 mg given at intervals greater than one day has been recommended for patients over 65 years of age.

In herpes zoster, treatment with 100 mg twice daily may be given for 14 days; if pain persists treatment may be continued for a further 14 days.

The dosage of amantadine should be reduced in patients with renal impairment.

Amantadine sulfate has been used similarly to the hydrochloride; it has been given by mouth or by intravenous infusion.

Administration. Amantadine sulfate has been used successfully in doses of up to 600 mg daily by intravenous infusion in the management of akinetic crisis in patients with Parkinson's disease.[1]

1. Gadoth N, *et al.* I.V. amantadine sulfate for extrapyramidal crisis. *Clin Pharm* 1985; 4: 146.

Extrapyramidal disorders. Amantadine has been used as an alternative to antimuscarinics[1] in the short-term management

of drug-induced extrapyramidal symptoms (p.662). However the development of tolerance has limited its usefulness. See also Parkinsonism, below.

1. König P, *et al.* Amantadine versus biperiden: a double-blind study of treatment efficacy in neuroleptic extrapyramidal movement disorders. *Neuropsychobiology* 1996; 33: 80–4.

Hiccup. Amantadine[1] has been reported to have produced beneficial results in patients with intractable hiccups (p.667).

1. Askenasy JJM, *et al.* Persistent hiccup cured by amantadine. *N Engl J Med* 1988; 318: 711.

Influenza. Amantadine is used similarly to rimantadine (p.640) in the prophylaxis and symptomatic treatment of influenza A (p.611); the two are equally effective, but amantadine is associated with more adverse effects.[1] It can reduce the duration of influenza A symptoms when given within 48 hours of the onset of symptoms and may be considered for treatment in high-risk individuals.[2] Treatment and prophylaxis failures may be due to the rapid emergence of drug-resistant viruses.[3] Some authorities recommend that to reduce the risk of resistance emerging, amantadine should not be used for both prophylaxis and treatment of influenza A in the same household. Vaccination is usually the method of choice for prophylaxis of influenza but amantadine may be indicated in addition to vaccination in certain individuals or when vaccination is contra-indicated.

1. Jefferson TO, *et al.* Amantadine and rimantadine for preventing and treating influenza A in adults (updated 18 July 2001). Available in The Cochrane Library; Issue 4. Oxford: Update Software, 2001.
2. Nicholson KG, Wiselka MJ. Amantadine for influenza A. *BMJ* 1991; 302: 425–6.
3. Belshe RB, *et al.* Resistance of influenza A virus to amantadine and rimantadine: results of one decade of surveillance. *J Infect Dis* 1989; 159: 430–5.

Multiple sclerosis. Amantadine may help to alleviate fatigue[1,2] associated with multiple sclerosis (p.633).

1. Kemp BA, Gora ML. Amantadine and fatigue of multiple sclerosis. *Ann Pharmacother* 1993; 27: 893–5.
2. Krupp LB, *et al.* Fatigue therapy in multiple sclerosis: results of a double-blind, randomized, parallel trial of amantadine, pemoline and placebo. *Neurology* 1995; 45: 1956–61.

Neuroleptic malignant syndrome. Amantadine has been tried[1-3] in the treatment of the neuroleptic malignant syndrome (p.662).

1. McCarron MM, *et al.* A case of neuroleptic malignant syndrome successfully treated with amantadine. *J Clin Psychiatry* 1982; 43: 381–2.
2. Amdurski S, *et al.* A therapeutic trial of amantadine in haloperidol-induced malignant neuroleptic syndrome. *Curr Ther Res* 1983; 33: 225–9.
3. Woo J, *et al.* Neuroleptic malignant syndrome successfully treated with amantadine. *Postgrad Med J* 1986; 62: 809–10.

Parkinsonism. Amantadine's mechanism of action in parkinsonism (p.1160) is unclear but may be due to its antimuscarinic activity and alterations in dopamine release and reuptake. It has also been suggested that amantadine's action as a non-competitive antagonist of *N*-methyl-D-aspartate may have a beneficial effect.[1,2] It has mild antiparkinsonian activity compared with levodopa but is relatively free from side-effects. It can improve bradykinesia as well as tremor and rigidity and is used in a similar manner to antimuscarinics mainly in the treatment of patients with early Parkinson's disease when symptoms are mild. However few patients obtain much benefit and tolerance to its effects can occur. The manufacturers suggest that the effectiveness of amantadine may be prolonged by withdrawing it for 3 to 4 weeks, continuing with existing antiparkinsonian therapy or initiating low dose levodopa treatment if clinically necessary in the meantime.

1. Laing P. Stroke treatment. *Lancet* 1991; 337: 1601.
2. Greenamyre JT, O'Brien CF. N-Methyl-D-aspartate antagonists in the treatment of Parkinson's disease. *Arch Neurol* 1991; 48: 977–81.

Withdrawal syndromes. COCAINE. Despite some earlier promising results more recent studies[1,2] have failed to confirm the value of amantadine in the management of the symptoms of cocaine withdrawal (p.1310). Any benefit appeared to decline after a few weeks of treatment.

1. Kosten TR, *et al.* Pharmacotherapy for cocaine-abusing methadone-maintained patients using amantadine or desipramine. *Arch Gen Psychiatry* 1992; 49: 894–8.
2. Kampman K, *et al.* Amantadine in the early treatment of cocaine dependence: a double-blind, placebo-controlled trial. *Drug Alcohol Depend* 1996; 41: 25–33.

Preparations

BP 2001: Amantadine Capsules; Amantadine Oral Solution;
USP 25: Amantadine Hydrochloride Capsules; Amantadine Hydrochloride Syrup.

Proprietary Preparations (details are given in Part 3)
Aust.: Hofcomant; PK-Merz; Virucid; **Austral.:** Symmetrel; **Belg.:** Amantan; Mantadix†; **Braz.:** Mantidan; **Canad.:** Endantadine; Symmetrel; **Denm.:** Virofral†; **Fin.:** Atarin; **Fr.:** Mantadix; **Ger.:** Adekin; Aman; Amanta; Amantagamma; Amixx; Cerebramed; Grippin-Merz†; InfectoFlu; Infex; PK-Merz; tregor; Viregyt†; **Hong Kong:** PK-Merz; Symmetrel; **Irl.:** Symmetrel; **Israel:** A-Parkin; Paritrel; PK-Merz; Symmetrel; **Ital.:** Mantadan; **Mex.:** Padiken; **Neth.:** Symmetrel; **NZ:** Symmetrel; **Port.:** Parkadina; Profil; **S.Afr.:** Antadine†; **Singapore:** Symmetrel; **Swed.:** Virofral; **Switz.:** PK-Merz; Symmetrel; **UK:** Lysovir; Symmetrel; **USA:** Symmetrel.

Multi-ingredient: **Mex.:** Antiflu-Des.

Apomorphine Hydrochloride (4543-p)

Apomorphine Hydrochloride (BANM).

Apomorphini Hydrochloridum. 6aβ-Aporphine-10,11-diol hydrochloride hemihydrate; (R)-10,11-Dihydroxy-6a-aporphine hydrochloride hemihydrate; (6aR)-5,6,6a,7-Tetrahydro-6-methyl-4H-dibenzo[de,g]quinoline-10,11-diol hydrochloride hemihydrate.

$C_{17}H_{17}NO_2,HCl,\frac{1}{2}H_2O = 312.8$.

CAS — 58-00-4 (apomorphine); 314-19-2 (anhydrous apomorphine hydrochloride); 41372-20-7 (apomorphine hydrochloride, hemihydrate).

Pharmacopoeias. In Chin., Eur. (see p.vi), Pol., and US.

Aqueous solutions decompose on storage and should not be used if they turn green or brown or contain a precipitate.

Pharmacopoeial description

Ph. Eur.: White or faintly yellow to green-tinged greyish crystals or crystalline powder, the green tinge becoming more pronounced on exposure to air and light. Sparingly soluble in water and in alcohol; very slightly soluble in ether. A 1% solution in water has a pH of 4.0 to 5.0. Store in airtight containers. Protect from light.

USP 25: Odourless, minute white or greyish-white, glistening crystals or white powder. It gradually acquires a green colour on exposure to light and air. Soluble 1 in 50 of water and 1 in 20 of water at 80°; soluble 1 in 50 of alcohol; very slightly soluble in ether and in chloroform. Its solutions are neutral to litmus. Store in small, airtight containers. Containers from which it is to be taken for immediate use in compounding prescriptions contain no more than 350 mg. Protect from light.

Adverse Effects

Treatment of parkinsonism. Apomorphine usually produces nausea and vomiting when given in therapeutic doses but these effects can be controlled by treatment with domperidone. Apomorphine may induce dyskinesias during 'on' periods in patients with parkinsonism and these may be severe enough to require discontinuation of therapy; postural instability and falls may also be a problem. Transient sedation can be common during the first few weeks of treatment. Transient postural hypotension may also occur infrequently. Apomorphine can produce neuropsychiatric disturbances including increasing cognitive impairment, personality changes, confusion, and visual hallucinations. Signs of CNS stimulation including euphoria, lightheadedness, restlessness, tremor, tachycardia, and tachypnoea occur less frequently. Increased salivation and perspiration have also been reported. Eosinophilia has occurred rarely. The use of apomorphine with levodopa may cause haemolytic anaemia and treatment may need to be discontinued if this cannot be satisfactorily controlled through dosage adjustment. Induration, nodule formation, and panniculitis, sometimes leading to ulceration often develops at the site of subcutaneous injection.

Management of erectile dysfunction. The most common adverse effects have been nausea, headache, and dizziness. Other effects reported include yawning, rhinitis, pharyngitis, somnolence, infection, pain, increased cough, flushing, taste disturbances, and sweating. Fainting and syncope have also occurred.

Overdosage with apomorphine can produce persistent vomiting, respiratory depression, bradycardia, hypotension, and coma; death may occur.

Akinesia. A 60-year-old man who was being investigated for parkinsonian symptoms became totally immobile and mute 15 minutes after receiving apomorphine 4 mg subcutaneously.[1] He remained conscious but was drowsy and sweating. Similar profound akinesia occurred on rechallenge with 2- and 6-mg doses. A diagnosis of probable nigrostriatal degeneration was made as the patient had previously shown no improvement after administration of levodopa but the mechanism of the idiosyncratic reaction to apomorphine was unclear.

1. Jenkins JR, Pearce JMS. Paradoxical akinetic response to apomorphine in parkinsonism. *J Neurol Neurosurg Psychiatry* 1992; **55:** 414–15.

Effects on the heart. A 67-year-old man developed palpitations with cold perspiration and chest pain, in addition to asthenia, salivation, nausea and vomiting, 5 minutes after receiving 3 mg apomorphine subcutaneously. An ECG demonstrated atrial fibrillation with a ventricular frequency of 140 beats per minute.[1]

1. Stocchi F, et al. Transient atrial fibrillation after subcutaneous apomorphine bolus. *Mov Disord* 1996; **11:** 584–5.

The symbol † denotes a preparation no longer actively marketed

Effects on mental function. Severe confusion, hallucinations, and acute psychosis were reported in 4 of 6 parkinsonian patients given subcutaneous apomorphine.[1] Three of the 4 had previously experienced mental disturbances while receiving lisuride. However, other studies failed to note effects on mental function in parkinsonian patients given apomorphine[2,3] and it has been suggested that the risk of psychosis in patients with no history of confusion or hallucinations is low.[3] The UK manufacturer notes that apomorphine has been reported both to exacerbate and to improve neuropsychiatric disturbances in patients with parkinsonism.

1. Ruggieri S, et al. Side-effects of subcutaneous apomorphine in Parkinson's disease. *Lancet* 1989; **i:** 566.
2. Stibe CMH, et al. Subcutaneous apomorphine in parkinsonian on-off oscillations. *Lancet* 1988; **i:** 403–6.
3. Poewe W, et al. Side-effects of subcutaneous apomorphine in Parkinson's disease. *Lancet* 1989; **i:** 1084–5.

Hypersensitivity. Allergic reactions including contact dermatitis, severe rhinitis, and respiratory distress have been reported in 2 workers who came into contact with apomorphine powder.[1] Contact allergy has also been reported in a patient who developed a swollen nose and lips after intranasal use of apomorphine.[2] Skin testing in all these cases[1,2] gave a positive reaction to apomorphine. Biopsy of subcutaneous nodules, which develop at the site of injection in most patients using apomorphine subcutaneously, has not been able to clarify what type of reaction was responsible for the development of panniculitis.[3] Although the nodules may slowly resolve the sites are often unsuitable for reuse as absorption from them is unpredictable; concern has been expressed that this may limit long-term use of apomorphine.[3]

1. Dahlquist I. Allergic reactions to apomorphine. *Contact Dermatitis* 1977; **3:** 349–50.
2. van Laar T, et al. Nasolabiale allergische reactie op intranasale toediening van apomorfine bij de ziekte van Parkinson. *Ned Tijdschr Geneeskd* 1992; **136** (suppl 47): 26–7.
3. Acland KM, et al. Panniculitis in association with apomorphine infusion. *Br J Dermatol* 1998; **138:** 480–2.

Oedema. A report of severe reversible oedema of the lower limbs in a patient receiving subcutaneous apomorphine.[1] Oedema recurred when apomorphine was reintroduced, but to a lesser extent.

1. Vermersch P. Severe oedema after subcutaneous apomorphine in Parkinson's disease. *Lancet* 1989; **ii:** 802.

Stomatitis. Stomatitis, severe enough to warrant discontinuation of treatment, occurred in 4 of 8 patients after 2 to 6 months of therapy with sublingual apomorphine.[1]

1. Montastruc JL, et al. Sublingual apomorphine in Parkinson's disease: a clinical and pharmacokinetic study. *Clin Neuropharmacol* 1991; **14:** 432–7.

Treatment of Adverse Effects

Domperidone is usually given to control nausea and vomiting when apomorphine is used in the management of Parkinson's disease; pretreatment with domperidone for at least 2 days is advised before starting treatment with apomorphine. Usually domperidone can be withdrawn gradually over several weeks to 6 months although some patients may need to continue treatment indefinitely.

In overdosage an opioid antagonist such as naloxone has been given to treat excessive vomiting and CNS and respiratory depression.

◊ References.
1. Bonuccelli U, et al. Naloxone partly counteracts apomorphine side effects. *Clin Neuropharmacol* 1991; **14:** 442–9.

Precautions

Apomorphine should not be given to patients with respiratory or CNS depression, hypersensitivity to opioids, neuropsychiatric problems, or dementia. It is not suitable for use in parkinsonian patients who have an 'on' response to levodopa marred by severe dyskinesia, hypotonia, or psychiatric effects.

The cardiovascular risks of sexual activity should be considered before beginning therapy with apomorphine for erectile dysfunction; in some patients sexual activity may be inadvisable. Apomorphine should be used with caution in patients with anatomical penile deformity.

It should be used with caution in patients prone to nausea and vomiting or when vomiting is likely to pose a risk. Apomorphine should also be used with care in patients with pulmonary, cardiovascular, or endocrine disease or with renal or hepatic impairment. Extra care is needed during initiation of treatment in elderly or debilitated patients and in those with a history of postural hypotension. In the management of parkinsonism periodic monitoring of hepatic, renal, haematopoietic, and cardiovascular function

has been advised and it is recommended that patients receiving apomorphine and levodopa together should be screened for haemolytic anaemia before starting treatment and then every 6 months.

Patients who develop anaemia, or those who have continuing confusion, or hallucinations during treatment with apomorphine require observation and dosage adjustment under specialist supervision; treatment may need to be discontinued.

Patients who experience dizziness, lightheadedness, or syncope should not drive or operate hazardous machinery.

Local subcutaneous reactions can sometimes be reduced by using sodium chloride 0.9% to dilute injection solutions, by rotating injection sites, and possibly by use of ultrasound in areas of nodularity and induration.

Interactions

Apomorphine should be used with caution in patients receiving antihypertensives or organic nitrates as it may potentiate their hypotensive effects. The therapeutic effects of apomorphine may be antagonised by antipsychotics and other drugs that act as CNS dopamine inhibitors. The effect of apomorphine is possibly enhanced by entacapone.

Pharmacokinetics

Apomorphine is well absorbed following subcutaneous administration but undergoes extensive first-pass hepatic metabolism when given by mouth and oral bioavailability is low. However, it is readily absorbed following sublingual administration and peak plasma concentrations are achieved in about 40 to 60 minutes; bioavailability is reported to be about 17 to 18% compared with subcutaneous administration. Apomorphine is about 90% bound to plasma proteins.

Apomorphine is extensively metabolised in the liver by conjugation with glucuronic acid or sulfate. It is also demethylated to produce norapomorphine. Most of a dose is excreted in urine, mainly as metabolites.

◊ References.
1. Neef C, van Laar T. Pharmacokinetic-pharmacodynamic relationships of apomorphine in patients with Parkinson's disease. *Clin Pharmacokinet* 1999; **37:** 257–71.

Uses and Administration

Apomorphine is a morphine derivative with structural similarities to dopamine. It is a potent dopamine D_1- and D_2-receptor agonist used in the diagnosis and management of parkinsonism, especially in the control of the 'on-off' effect. It is also used in the management of erectile dysfunction.

The optimal dose of apomorphine in the management of 'off' periods in **parkinsonism** should be established individually under specialist care. At least 2 days of pretreatment with the antiemetic domperidone is advised before administration of apomorphine. After withholding antiparkinsonian therapy overnight to provoke an 'off' period, test doses of apomorphine hydrochloride ranging from 1.5 to 7 mg or occasionally 10 mg are given subcutaneously at intervals of 40 minutes in an increasing regimen to determine the lowest dose producing a response. Once the patient's normal antiparkinsonian therapy is re-established, this dose of apomorphine hydrochloride is given at the first signs of an 'off' period. The dose and frequency of administration is further adjusted according to response; patients typically require 3 to 30 mg daily in divided doses but individual injections should not be greater than 10 mg. Patients who require more than 10 injections per day or those whose overall control of symptoms remains unsatisfactory with intermittent injections may benefit from continuous subcutaneous infusion. The infusion is started at a rate of 1 mg per hour and this may be increased in steps of 0.5 mg per hour at intervals of not less than 4 hours up to a maximum rate of 4 mg per hour. It is advised that infusions should only be given during waking hours and that the infusion site should be changed every 12 hours; 24-hour infusions are not advised unless there are severe night-time symptoms. Patients usually need to supplement the infusion with intermittent bolus injections but the recommended maximum total daily dose given by infusion and/or injection is 100 mg.

In the management of **erectile dysfunction** the usual initial dose is 2 mg taken sublingually about 20 minutes before sexual activity. A dose of 3 mg may be used on subsequent occasions if necessary but a minimum of 8 hours should be allowed between doses. The maximum dose should be limited to 2 mg in patients with severe renal impairment.

Apomorphine stimulates the chemoreceptor trigger zone in the brain and can produce emesis within a few minutes of administration. However the use of apomorphine for the induction of emesis in poisoning is considered dangerous owing to the risk of inducing protracted vomiting and shock and is not recommended.

Erectile dysfunction. Apomorphine is among a wide range of drugs that has been used in the management of erectile dysfunction (p.1663) with some beneficial results. It has been given subcutaneously[1] or by sublingual administration.[2,3]

1. Segraves RT, et al. Effect of apomorphine on penile tumescence in men with psychogenic impotence. J Urol (Baltimore) 1991; **145:** 1174–5.
2. Heaton JPW, et al. Recovery of erectile function by the oral administration of apomorphine. Urology 1995; **45:** 200–6.
3. Dula E, et al. Efficacy and safety of fixed-dose and dose-optimization regimens of sublingual apomorphine versus placebo in men with erectile dysfunction. Urology 2000; **56:** 130–5.

Parkinsonism. Although apomorphine has produced benefit in Parkinson's disease (p.1160) when given orally, the high doses required to overcome extensive first-pass hepatic metabolism (up to 1.4 g daily in one study[1]), were associated with uraemia. The use of apomorphine in Parkinson's disease has therefore been limited by the need for parenteral administration. The current main use of apomorphine in Parkinson's disease is for the stabilisation of patients with 'on-off' fluctuations unresponsive to other dopamine agonists. It is usually given subcutaneously either by injection or infusion but a review[2] of the use of apomorphine in Parkinson's disease also discusses studies of rectal, sublingual, and intranasal administration. Of these, the intranasal route was considered to be the most promising alternative route.

1. Cotzias GC, et al. Treatment of Parkinson's disease with apomorphines. N Engl J Med 1976; **294:** 567–72.
2. Corboy DL, et al. Apomorphine for motor fluctuations and freezing in Parkinson's disease. Ann Pharmacother 1995; **29:** 282–8.

DIAGNOSIS. There have been a number of reports of the use of subcutaneous apomorphine in the differential diagnosis of parkinsonian syndromes, to distinguish forms responsive to dopaminergics, such as idiopathic Parkinson's disease, from other parkinsonian syndromes such as Wilson's disease, corticobasal degeneration, and diffuse Lewy body dementia, which are unresponsive to, or made worse by, dopaminergics.[1-4] Some consider that oral challenge with levodopa is still the best test of dopaminergic responsiveness[5] but testing with apomorphine has proved of value in re-assessing patients who have become less responsive to levodopa.[1,4] In most cases testing has involved administration of a series of increasing doses of subcutaneous apomorphine hydrochloride, usually starting with 1 mg and increasing up to about 5 mg or until central adverse effects supervene; the patient's motor function is assessed at various times after each dose and a suitable interval allowed between doses. Patients should be pretreated with domperidone before the test to prevent nausea and vomiting.

1. Barker R, et al. Subcutaneous apomorphine as a diagnostic test for dopaminergic responsiveness in parkinsonian syndromes. Lancet 1989; **i:** 675.
2. Oertel WH, et al. Apomorphine test for dopaminergic responsiveness. Lancet 1989; **i:** 1262–3.
3. Frankel JP, et al. Use of apomorphine to test for dopamine responsiveness in Wilson's disease. Lancet 1989; **ii:** 801–2.
4. Hughes AJ, et al. Apomorphine test to predict dopaminergic responsiveness in parkinsonian syndromes. Lancet 1990; **336:** 32–4.
5. Steiger MJ, Quinn NP. Levodopa challenge test in Parkinson's disease. Lancet 1992; **339:** 751–2.

Preparations

USP 25: Apomorphine Hydrochloride Tablets.

Proprietary Preparations (details are given in Part 3)

Austral.: Apomine; *Fr.:* Apokinon; *Ital.:* Apofin; *Neth.:* Britaject; *NZ:* Apomine; *UK:* APO-go; Britaject; Uprima.

Benserazide Hydrochloride (4544-s)

Benserazide Hydrochloride (BANM, rINNM).

Benserazidi Hydrochloridum; Ro-4-4602 (benserazide); Serazide Hydrochloride. DL-Serine 2-(2,3,4-trihydroxybenzyl)hydrazide hydrochloride; 2-Amino-3-hydroxy-2'-(2,3,4-trihydroxybenzyl)propionohydrazide hydrochloride.

$C_{10}H_{15}N_3O_5$,HCl = 293.7.

CAS — 322-35-0 (benserazide); 14919-77-8 (benserazide hydrochloride); 14046-64-1 (benserazide hydrochloride).

NOTE. Benserazide is *USAN*.
Compounded preparations of benserazide hydrochloride may be represented by the following names:

* Co-beneldopa *(BAN)*—benserazide 1 part and levodopa 4 parts (w/w).

Pharmacopoeias. In *Chin., Eur.* (see p.vi), and *Jpn.*

Benserazide hydrochloride 28.5 mg is approximately equivalent to 25 mg of benserazide.

Pharmacopoeial description

Ph. Eur.: A white or yellowish-white or orange-white crystalline powder. It shows polymorphism. Freely soluble in water; very slightly soluble in dehydrated alcohol; practically insoluble in acetone. A 1% solution in water has a pH of 4.0 to 5.0. Protect from light.

Solubility. Benserazide is unstable in a neutral, alkaline, or strongly acidic medium.[1]

1. Schwartz DE, Brandt R. Pharmacokinetic and metabolic studies of the decarboxylase inhibitor benserazide in animals and man. Arzneimittelforschung 1978; **28:** 302–7.

Adverse Effects and Precautions

◊ Developmental abnormalities of the *rat* skeleton have been reported with benserazide by Theiss and Schärer,[1] but Ziegler *et al.* found no evidence of any disorder involving bone metabolism in man.[2] Nevertheless the manufacturers have recommended that benserazide should not be given to patients under 25 years of age or to pregnant women.

1. Theiss E, Schärer K. Toxicity of L-dopa and a decarboxylase inhibitor in animal experiments. In: de Ajuriaguerra J, Gauthier G, eds. Monoamines Noyaux Gris Centraux et Syndrome de Parkinson. Geneva: Georg, 1971: 497–504.
2. Ziegler WH, et al. Toxicity of L-dopa and a dopa decarboxylase inhibitor in humans. In: de Ajuriaguerra J, Gauthier G, eds. Monoamines Noyaux Gris Centraux et Syndrome de Parkinson. Geneva: Georg, 1971: 505–16.

Pharmacokinetics

◊ Pharmacokinetic and metabolic studies of benserazide in *animals* and man.[1,2] Following oral administration to parkinsonian patients benserazide was rapidly absorbed to the extent of about 58%, simultaneous administration of levodopa tending to increase this slightly. It was rapidly excreted in the urine in the form of metabolites, mostly within the first 6 hours; 85% of urinary excretion had occurred within 12 hours. Benserazide is predominantly metabolised in the gut and appears to protect levodopa against decarboxylation primarily in the gut, but also in the rest of the organism, mainly by way of its metabolite trihydroxybenzylhydrazine. Benserazide did not cross the blood-brain barrier in *rats*.

1. Schwartz DE, et al. Pharmacokinetics of the decarboxylase benserazide in man: Its tissue distribution in the rat. Eur J Clin Pharmacol 1974; **7:** 39–45.
2. Schwartz DE, Brandt R. Pharmacokinetic and metabolic studies of the decarboxylase inhibitor benserazide in animals and man. Arzneimittelforschung 1978; **28:** 302–7.

Uses and Administration

Benserazide hydrochloride is a peripheral dopa-decarboxylase inhibitor with actions similar to those of carbidopa (p.1168) and is used similarly as an adjunct to levodopa in the treatment of parkinsonism (p.1160). For details of administration and dosage, see Levodopa, p.1172.

◊ References.

1. Dingemanse J, et al. Pharmacodynamics of benserazide assessed by its effects on endogenous and exogenous levodopa pharmacokinetics. Br J Clin Pharmacol 1997; **44:** 41–8.

Preparations

BP 2001: Co-beneldopa Capsules; Dispersible Co-beneldopa Tablets.

Proprietary Preparations (details are given in Part 3)

Multi-ingredient: *Aust.:* Madopar; *Austral.:* Madopar; *Belg.:* Prolopa; *Braz.:* Prolopa; *Canad.:* Prolopa; *Denm.:* Madopar; *Fin.:* Aktipar; Madopar; *Fr.:* Modopar; *Ger.:* Levodopa comp B; Levopar; Madopar; *Hong Kong:* Madopar; *Irl.:* Madopar; *Israel:* Levopar Plus; *Ital.:* Madopar; *Mex.:* Madopar; *Neth.:* Madopar; *Norw.:* Madopar; *NZ:* Madopar; *Port.:* Madopar; *S.Afr.:* Madopar; *Singapore:* Madopar; *Spain:* Madopar; *Swed.:* Madopark; *Switz.:* Madopar; *Thai.:* Madopar; *UK:* Madopar.

Bromocriptine Mesilate (4546-e)

Bromocriptine Mesilate (BANM, rINNM).

Bromocriptine Mesylate (USAN); Bromocriptine Methanesulphonate; Bromocriptini Mesilas; Bromocryptine Mesylate; 2-Bromo-α-ergocryptine Mesylate; 2-Bromoergocryptine Monomethanesulfonate; CB-154 (bromocriptine). (5'S)-2-Bromo-12'-hydroxy-2'-(1-methylethyl)-5'-(2-methylpropyl)-ergotaman-3',6',18-trione methanesulphonate.

$C_{32}H_{40}BrN_5O_5,CH_4O_3S = 750.7.$

CAS — 25614-03-3 (bromocriptine); 22260-51-1 (bromocriptine mesilate).

Pharmacopoeias. In *Eur.* (see p.vi), *Jpn,* and *US.*

Bromocriptine mesilate 2.87 mg is approximately equivalent to 2.5 mg of bromocriptine.

Pharmacopoeial description

Ph. Eur.: A white or slightly coloured fine crystalline powder. Practically insoluble in water; soluble in alcohol; sparingly soluble in dichloromethane; freely soluble in methyl alcohol. A 1% solution in a mixture of 2 parts methyl alcohol to 8 of water has a pH of 3.1 to 3.8. Store in airtight containers at a temperature not exceeding −15°. Protect from light.

USP 25: A white or slightly coloured fine crystalline powder; odourless or having a weak characteristic odour. Store in airtight containers at a temperature not exceeding 8°. Protect from light.

Adverse Effects

Nausea is the most common side-effect at the beginning of treatment with bromocriptine, but vomiting, dizziness, and orthostatic hypotension may also occur. Syncope has followed initial doses of bromocriptine.

Side-effects are generally dose-related and may therefore be more frequent with the higher doses that have been used in the treatment of parkinsonism and acromegaly. Reduction of the dosage of bromocriptine, followed in a few days by a more gradual increase, may alleviate many side-effects. Nausea may be diminished by taking bromocriptine with food.

Bromocriptine is a vasoconstrictor; digital vasospasm, induced by cold, and leg cramps have been reported. Other cardiovascular effects have included erythromelalgia, prolonged severe hypotension, arrhythmias, and exacerbation of angina. Very rarely hypertension, myocardial infarction, seizures or stroke (both sometimes preceded by severe headache or visual disturbances), and mental disorders have been reported in postpartum women given bromocriptine.

The use of ergot derivatives such as bromocriptine has been associated with retroperitoneal fibrosis, pleural thickening and effusions, and pericarditis and pericardial effusions.

Other side-effects reported include headache, nasal congestion, drowsiness, dry mouth, constipation, diarrhoea, and altered liver-function tests. Dyskinesias and psychomotor excitation have occurred in patients suffering from parkinsonism. Gastrointestinal bleeding has been reported in acromegalic patients. Psychosis, with hallucinations, delusions, and confusion, occurs particularly when high doses are used to treat parkinsonism, but has also been reported with low doses.

◊ In 27 published studies of bromocriptine in the treatment of Parkinson's disease, 217 of the 790 patients given bromocriptine had adverse effects.[1] Mental changes were noted in 90 patients, dyskinesia in 20, orthostatic hypotension in 40, and gastrointestinal effects in 40. The fewest adverse effects (9%) occurred with low-dose bromocriptine, more occurred with high-dose bromocriptine (27%) or with low-dose bromocriptine with levodopa (26%), and the most occurred with high-dose bromocriptine and levodopa (32%). However, those on high doses had more advanced disease and might be more susceptible to mental changes and dyskinesias.

An analysis by the manufacturer of published reports on patients treated with bromocriptine for 1 to 10 years concluded that in general, side-effects noted were no different from those associated with short-term treatment.[2]

1. Lieberman AN, Goldstein M. Bromocriptine in Parkinson disease. Pharmacol Rev 1985; **37:** 217–27.
2. Weil C. The safety of bromocriptine in long-term use: a review of the literature. Curr Med Res Opin 1986; **10:** 25–51.

Effects on the blood. Severe leucopenia and mild thrombocytopenia developed in a 23-year-old woman after treatment with bromocriptine 7.5 to 10 mg daily for about 3 months.[1]

1. Giampietro O, et al. Severe leukopenia and mild thrombocytopenia after chronic bromocriptine (CB-154) administration. Am J Med Sci 1981; 281: 169–72.

Effects on the cardiovascular system. An early reviewer noted that asymptomatic hypotension occurred in many subjects given bromocriptine.[1] However, faintness and dizziness, sometimes accompanied by nausea and vomiting, were common at the start of treatment with bromocriptine and these symptoms rather than an anaphylactic type of reaction were likely to account for the collapse that occurred in a few sensitive patients. Two of 53 patients with Parkinson's disease fainted after an initial dose of 1.25 or 2.5 mg, but the exact incidence of shock-like syndromes was difficult to assess; the manufacturers had stated that 22 of over 10 000 subjects given bromocriptine had had hypotension and collapse, mainly at the start of treatment. It was essential to warn all patients starting treatment of the possibility of fainting. The initial dose should not exceed 1.25 to 2.5 mg and should be taken with food and in bed. If fainting did occur recovery was usually rapid and spontaneous. Tolerance to side-effects such as hypotension and nausea might develop rapidly.

Hypertension, seizures, stroke, and myocardial infarction have been associated with bromocriptine therapy, notably in postpartum women.[2-4] A study involving 1813 women suggested that the risk of postpartum hypertension was increased in women who experienced pregnancy-induced hypertension and that this risk was further increased in those who took bromocriptine for suppression of lactation.[5] A case-controlled study[6] involving 43 of the women who had had postpartum seizures while taking bromocriptine found that while the initial risk of seizures appeared to be lower in patients taking bromocriptine there was a small positive association with seizures occurring more than 72 hours after delivery.

Although a causal relationship between the use of bromocriptine and these adverse effects in postpartum women has not been established the manufacturer recommends that bromocriptine should not be used postpartum or in the puerperium in women with high blood pressure, coronary artery disease, or symptoms or history of serious mental disorders. It is also recommended that when bromocriptine is used in postpartum women blood pressure should be carefully monitored, especially during the first few days and if hypertension, unremitting headache, or signs of CNS toxicity develop treatment should be discontinued immediately.

1. Parkes D. Side effects of bromocriptine. N Engl J Med 1980; 302: 749–50.
2. Anonymous. Postpartum hypertension, seizures, strokes reported with bromocriptine. FDA Drug Bull 1984; 14: 3.
3. Ruch A, Duhring JL. Postpartum myocardial infarction in a patient receiving bromocriptine. Obstet Gynecol 1989; 74: 448–51.
4. Larrazet F, et al. Possible bromocriptine-induced myocardial infarction. Ann Intern Med 1993; 118: 199–200.
5. Watson DL, et al. Bromocriptine mesylate for lactation suppression: a risk for postpartum hypertension? Obstet Gynecol 1989; 74: 573–6.
6. Rothman KJ, et al. Bromocriptine and puerperal seizures. Epidemiology 1990; 1: 232–8.

Effects on the ears. Audiometric evidence of bilateral sensorineural hearing loss was reported in 3 patients receiving bromocriptine 15 or 20 mg daily for chronic hepatic encephalopathy.[1] Hearing improved when the dose was reduced to 10 mg daily.

1. Lanthier PL, et al. Bromocriptine-associated ototoxicity. J Laryngol Otol 1984; 98: 399–404.

Effects on electrolytes. There have been isolated reports of severe hyponatraemia associated with the use of bromocriptine.[1,2]

1. Marshall AW, et al. Bromocriptine-associated hyponatraemia in cirrhosis. BMJ 1982; 285: 1534–5.
2. Damase-Michel C, et al. Hyponatraemia in a patient treated with bromocriptine. Drug Invest 1993; 5: 285–7.

Effects on the eyes. Blurred vision and diplopia has been reported in several patients receiving bromocriptine.[1] There is a report of reversible myopia developing in a patient with hyperprolactinaemia given bromocriptine.[2]

In a patient with progressive visual loss due to compression of the optic chiasm by a large pituitary tumour, administration of bromocriptine caused total visual loss within hours.[3] Vision slowly returned to normal when the patient was placed in the supine position; the most likely cause of the visual loss was thought to be orthostatic hypotension with resultant decrease in perfusion pressure to the visual system.

Bromocriptine has been reported to cause visual cortical disturbances.[4] In some cases blurred vision and transient cortical blindness have preceded seizures and strokes.

1. Calne DB, et al. Long-term treatment of parkinsonism with bromocriptine. Lancet 1978; i: 735–7.
2. Manor RS, et al. Myopia during bromocriptine treatment. Lancet 1981; i: 102.
3. Couldwell WT, Weiss MH. Visual loss associated with bromocriptine. Lancet 1992; 340: 1410–11.
4. Lane RJM, Routledge PA. Drug-induced neurological disorders. Drugs 1983; 26: 124–47.

Effects on mental function. Psychotic reactions to high doses of bromocriptine are well known in patients with parkinsonism.[1] However, mania has been associated with the use of

bromocriptine post partum[2,3] and it has been stated that psychological symptoms may occur with doses of only 2.5 to 5 mg daily.[4] It was also noted that, unlike the relatively mild and transient symptoms associated with levodopa, bromocriptine produces a severe psychosis in which the patient is violent and aggressive, suffering from intense delusions which are often hostile and violent; complete withdrawal of bromocriptine may still leave a residue of severe psychotic illness persisting for 1 to 3 weeks. Psychosis associated with low doses of bromocriptine has often occurred in patients with a history of psychotic illness or disturbances in behaviour and mood prior to treatment.[5-7] Drug-related psychotic reactions have also been reported in patients with no psychiatric history;[8,9] 8 of 600 patients given bromocriptine or lisuride for the treatment of acromegaly or prolactinoma developed symptoms including anxiety, depression, auditory hallucinations, delusions, hyperactivity, disinhibition, euphoria, and insomnia and 4 had received doses only previously associated with psychosis in susceptible patients.[9] For reports of daytime somnolence occurring in patients receiving dopamine agonists including bromocriptine, see under Levodopa, p.1170.

1. Calne DB, et al. Long-term treatment of parkinsonism with bromocriptine. Lancet 1978; i: 735–7.
2. Vlissides DN, et al. Bromocriptine-induced mania? BMJ 1978; 1: 510.
3. Brook NM, Cookson IB. Bromocriptine-induced mania? BMJ 1978; 1: 790.
4. Pearce I, Pearce JMS. Bromocriptine in parkinsonism. BMJ 1978; 1: 1402–4.
5. Pearson KC. Mental disorders from low-dose bromocriptine. N Engl J Med 1981; 305: 173.
6. Le Feuvre CM, et al. Bromocriptine-induced psychosis in acromegaly. BMJ 1982; 285: 1315.
7. Procter AW, et al. Bromocriptine induced psychosis in acromegaly. BMJ 1983; 286: 50. Correction. ibid.; 311.
8. Einarson TR, Turchet EN. Psychotic reaction to low-dose bromocriptine. Clin Pharm 1983; 2: 273–4.
9. Turner TH, et al. Psychotic reactions during treatment of pituitary tumours with dopamine agonists. BMJ 1984; 289: 1101–3.

Effects on the nervous system. A report of 2 cases of cerebrospinal-fluid rhinorrhoea associated with the use of bromocriptine following partial surgical resection of prolactinoma.[1]

For reference to seizures associated with the use of bromocriptine in postpartum women, see under Effects on the Cardiovascular System, above.

1. Baskin DS, Wilson CB. CSF rhinorrhea after bromocriptine for prolactinoma. N Engl J Med 1982; 306: 178.

Effects on the respiratory tract. Interstitial lung disease, with dyspnoea, chest pain, cough, and pulmonary fibrosis was reported in a patient following administration of relatively high doses of bromocriptine (62 mg daily) for Parkinson's disease.[1] Respiratory symptoms largely resolved on withdrawal of the drug, although functional respiratory changes and moderate dyspnoea persisted after 6 months. A review of the literature revealed a number of other reports of pleuro-pulmonary fibrosis associated with relatively high doses of bromocriptine. Although the incidence of this effect did not seem to be high, similar cases continue to be reported.[2,3]

1. Vergeret J, et al. Fibrose pleuro-pulmonaire et bromocriptine. Sem Hop Paris 1984; 60: 741–4.
2. Kinnunen E, Viljanen A. Pleuropulmonary involvement during bromocriptine treatment. Chest 1988; 94: 1034–6.
3. Macak IA, et al. Bromocriptine-induced pulmonary disease. Can J Hosp Pharm 1991; 44: 37–8, xxiv.

Effects on sexual function. Severe hypersexuality has been reported in a middle-aged man receiving bromocriptine and levodopa for Parkinson's disease.[1] About 3 years after the onset of hypersexuality he developed paranoid-hallucinatory psychoses which subsided on the reduction of dosage. It was apparent that addictive abuse of dopaminergic drugs had occurred. Clitoral tumescence and increased libido has been noted in a woman receiving bromocriptine to suppress lactation[2] but there has been a report of sexual dissatisfaction and decreased libido in 3 women receiving bromocriptine for hyperprolactinaemia.[3]

1. Vogel HP, Schiffter R. Hypersexuality—a complication of dopaminergic therapy in Parkinson's disease. Pharmacopsychiatry 1983; 16: 107–10.
2. Blin O, et al. Painful clitoral tumescence during bromocriptine therapy. Lancet 1991; 337: 1231–2.
3. Saleh AK, Moussa MAA. Sexual dysfunction in women due to bromocriptine. BMJ 1984; 289: 228.

Effects on the urinary tract. Constant dribbling urinary incontinence developed in a woman receiving bromocriptine 2.5 mg daily for a recurrent pituitary growth; symptoms resolved on discontinuing the drug and recurred on rechallenge.[1] Bromocriptine has been shown to have two effects, one on the bladder outflow tract and one on the detrusor muscle, that could predispose to urinary incontinence.[2]

1. Sandyk R, Gillman MA. Urinary incontinence in patient on long-term bromocriptine. Lancet 1983; ii: 1260–1.
2. Caine M. Bromocriptine and urinary incontinence. Lancet 1984; i: 228.

Hypersensitivity. A report of an allergic reaction due to bromocriptine in a 26-year-old woman being treated for a prolactin-secreting microadenoma.[1] The patient reacted similarly to lisuride and treatment was continued with quinagolide.

1. Merola B, et al. Allergy to ergot-derived dopamine agonists. Lancet 1992; 339: 620.

Oedema. Oedema poorly responsive to diuretics has been reported[1] in a patient given bromocriptine as part of treatment for prolactinoma. The oedema improved on substitution of pergolide but worsened with higher doses. Oedema resolved when treatment was changed to quinagolide. The reaction was considered to be idiosyncratic since enquiries by the author of the report had revealed only one similar case.

1. Blackard WG. Edema—an infrequently recognized complication of bromocriptine and other ergot dopaminergic drugs. Am J Med 1993; 94: 445.

Overdosage. The most striking symptom in two children aged 2 and 2½ years who accidentally ingested an estimated 25 and 7.5 mg of bromocriptine respectively, was lethargy with altered mental status.[1] The first child vomited and became sleepy. On admission he was markedly lethargic, but combative when disturbed, and also had hypotension, shallow breathing, dilated pupils, and hyperreflexic lower extremities. Nasogastric lavage was promptly performed and activated charcoal and then magnesium citrate administered. Blood pressure and ECG were monitored and glucose and sodium chloride solution infused. The other child vomited, became lethargic, and had dilated pupils. Ipecacuanha was administered and activated charcoal followed by magnesium citrate given by nasogastric tube. Both children recovered completely.

1. Vermund SH, et al. Accidental bromocriptine ingestion in childhood. J Pediatr 1984; 105: 838–40.

Withdrawal syndromes. Transient galactorrhoea and hyperprolactinaemia occurred in a young woman after withdrawal of bromocriptine therapy for Parkinson's disease.[1] It was suggested the effects were due to a rebound phenomenon. There has been a report of hyperthermia following withdrawal of treatment with levodopa/carbidopa and bromocriptine.[2]

1. Pentland B, Sawers JSA. Galactorrhoea after withdrawal of bromocriptine. BMJ 1980; 281: 716.
2. Figà-Talamanca L, et al. Hyperthermia after discontinuance of levodopa and bromocriptine therapy: impaired dopamine receptors a possible cause. Neurology 1985; 35: 258–61.

Precautions

Patients with hyperprolactinaemia should be investigated for the possibility of a pituitary tumour before treatment with bromocriptine. Annual gynaecological examinations (or every 6 months for postmenopausal women) are recommended. Treatment of women with hyperprolactinaemic amenorrhoea results in ovulation; such patients should be advised to use contraceptive measures other than an oral contraceptive. Acromegalic patients should be checked for symptoms of peptic ulceration before therapy and should immediately report symptoms of gastrointestinal discomfort during therapy.

Bromocriptine should be given with caution to patients with cardiovascular disease, Raynaud's syndrome, or a history of psychotic disorders. It is contra-indicated in patients with hypersensitivity to bromocriptine or other ergot alkaloids.

Bromocriptine is contra-indicated in patients with hypertensive disorders during pregnancy, or with hypertension postpartum or in the puerperium. It should not be used postpartum or in the puerperium in women with coronary artery disease or serious mental disorders. Blood pressure should be monitored carefully, especially during the first few days in postpartum women. Particular caution is necessary in patients who are receiving or who have recently received drugs which can alter blood pressure; concomitant administration of ergot alkaloids during the puerperium is not recommended. Treatment in postpartum women should be discontinued immediately if hypertension, unremitting headache, or signs of CNS toxicity develop.

Hypotensive reactions may be disturbing in some patients during the first few days of treatment. Patients who drive or operate machinery should be warned of the possibility of dizziness and fainting during the first few days of treatment.

Patients on long-term, high-dose therapy should be monitored for signs of retroperitoneal fibrosis and bromocriptine withdrawn if fibrotic changes are diagnosed or suspected.

Porphyria. Bromocriptine is considered to be unsafe in patients with porphyria because it has been shown to be porphyrinogenic in in-vitro systems.

Pregnancy. Details of various surveys of the effect of the use of bromocriptine during pregnancy have been published by the manufacturer.[1,2] The first survey was based on spontaneous reporting of all pregnancies between 1973 and 1980 in women who had taken bromocriptine after conception.[1] Information was obtained on 1410 pregnancies in 1335 women, the majority of whom had been treated for hyperprolactinaemic conditions, while in 256 pregnancies pituitary tumours and acromegaly were the primary diagnosis. Bromocriptine was generally taken at some time in the first 8 weeks after conception, the mean duration of treatment being 21 days. In 4 patients bromocriptine was not prescribed until late in pregnancy and in 9 with acromegaly and pituitary microadenoma it was taken continuously throughout gestation. There were 157 (11.1%) spontaneous abortions, 12 (0.9%) extrauterine pregnancies, 2 patients with 3 hydatidiform moles (0.2%), and an incidence of twin pregnancies of 1.8%. Major congenital abnormalities were detected in 12 (1%) infants at birth and minor abnormalities in 31 (2.5%). A second survey,[2] which consisted of formal monitoring of the use of bromocriptine at 33 clinics between 1979 and 1980, collected data on a further 743 pregnancies in 668 women and had similar findings. The incidence rates reported in these surveys were comparable with those quoted for normal populations and the data indicate that the use of bromocriptine in the treatment of women with infertility is not associated with an increased risk of abortion, multiple pregnancy, or congenital abnormalities. Furthermore, follow-up, for up to 9 years, of 546 children exposed to bromocriptine *in utero* found no evidence that bromocriptine had any adverse effect on postnatal development.[2] Nevertheless, since the risk of abortion is not increased by interruption of treatment, it is still recommended that bromocriptine therapy be stopped as soon as pregnancy is confirmed unless there is a definite indication for its continuation.

See also Pregnancy under Hyperprolactinaemia and Prolactinomas, below.

1. Turkalj I, *et al.* Surveillance of bromocriptine in pregnancy. *JAMA* 1982; **247:** 1589–91.
2. Krupp P, Monka C. Bromocriptine in pregnancy: safety aspects. *Klin Wochenschr* 1987; **65:** 823–7.

Interactions

Dopamine antagonists such as the phenothiazines, butyrophenones, thioxanthenes, and metoclopramide (but see below) might be expected to reduce the prolactin-lowering and the antiparkinsonian effect of bromocriptine. Domperidone might reduce the prolactin-lowering effect. Concomitant administration of octreotide and bromocriptine increases the bioavailability of bromocriptine.

Alcohol. Alcohol intolerance has been noted in 5 of 73 patients receiving bromocriptine 10 to 60 mg daily for the treatment of acromegaly.[1] Two patients who experienced gastrointestinal side-effects while taking low doses of bromocriptine had a marked reduction in their symptoms and were able to tolerate higher doses when they refrained completely from alcohol.[2]

1. Wass JAH, *et al.* Long-term treatment of acromegaly with bromocriptine. *BMJ* 1977; **1:** 875–8.
2. Ayres J, Maisey MN. Alcohol increases bromocriptine's side effects. *N Engl J Med* 1980; **302:** 806.

Antibacterials. Drowsiness, dystonia, choreoathetoid dyskinesias, and visual hallucinations occurred when *josamycin* was given to a patient receiving bromocriptine.[1]

The systemic bioavailability of a single oral dose of bromocriptine 5 mg was markedly increased in 5 healthy subjects following treatment with *erythromycin estolate* 250 mg four times daily for 4 days;[2] clearance of bromocriptine decreased by 70.6% and peak plasma concentrations of bromocriptine were more than 4 times higher than following the same dose before erythromycin administration.

1. Montastruc JL, Rascol A. Traitement de la maladie de Parkinson par doses élevées de bromocriptine: interaction possible avec la josamycine. *Presse Med* 1984; **13:** 2267–8.
2. Nelson MV, *et al.* Pharmacokinetic evaluation of erythromycin and caffeine administered with bromocriptine in normal subjects. *Clin Pharmacol Ther* 1990; **47:** 166.

Antifungals. The response to bromocriptine was blocked in a patient who was also receiving *griseofulvin*.[1]

1. Schwinn G, *et al.* Metabolic and clinical studies on patients with acromegaly treated with bromocriptine over 22 months. *Eur J Clin Invest* 1977; **7:** 101–7.

Antipsychotics. Serum concentrations of prolactin rose and visual fields deteriorated following administration of *thioridazine* to a 40-year-old man receiving bromocriptine therapy for a large prolactinoma.[1]

For a discussion of the effect of bromocriptine on patients receiving antipsychotics, see under Antiparkinsonian Drugs in Chlorpromazine on p.665.

1. Robbins RJ, *et al.* Interactions between thioridazine and bromocriptine in a patient with a prolactin-secreting pituitary adenoma. *Am J Med* 1984; **76:** 921–3.

Metoclopramide. As noted in Interactions, above, there are theoretical reasons to suppose that dopamine antagonists might reduce the effects of bromocriptine. However, an early study[1] in 10 patients with Parkinson's disease given single doses of bromocriptine 12.5 to 100 mg found that pretreatment with metoclopramide 60 mg had no consistent effect upon plasma

concentrations of bromocriptine or growth hormone and no consistent effect upon clinical response.

1. Price P, *et al.* Plasma bromocriptine levels, clinical and growth hormone responses in parkinsonism. *Br J Clin Pharmacol* 1978; **6:** 303–9.

Sympathomimetics. There have been isolated reports[1,2] of severe hypertension, with headache and life-threatening complications, in patients receiving bromocriptine concomitantly with *isometheptene mucate* or *phenylpropanolamine*.

1. Kulig K, *et al.* Bromocriptine-associated headache: possible life-threatening sympathomimetic interaction. *Obstet Gynecol* 1991; **78:** 941–3.
2. Chan JCN, *et al.* Postpartum hypertension, bromocriptine and phenylpropanolamine. *Drug Invest* 1994; **8:** 254–6.

Pharmacokinetics

Only about 30% of an oral dose of bromocriptine is absorbed from the gastrointestinal tract and, owing to extensive first-pass metabolism, the bioavailability is only about 6%. It is metabolised in the liver, mainly by hydrolysis to lysergic acid and peptides, and excreted chiefly in faeces via the bile, with small amounts in urine. It has been reported to be 90 to 96% bound to serum albumin *in vitro*.

◊ In a study involving 10 patients with Parkinson's disease, single doses of bromocriptine 12.5, 25, 50, and 100 mg resulted in very variable peak plasma concentrations ranging from 1.3 to 5.3, 1.4 to 3.5, 2.6 to 19.7, and 6.5 to 24.6 nanograms per mL respectively, 30 to 210 minutes (mean 102 minutes) after dosage.[1] After 4 hours plasma concentrations were about 75% of the peak values. Clinical improvement was evident within 30 to 90 minutes of a dose with peak effect at about 130 minutes and in most patients improvement persisted throughout the 4-hour study period. Peak clinical response, peak fall in blood pressure, and peak rise in plasma concentrations of growth hormone occurred about 30, 60, and 70 minutes respectively after peak plasma-bromocriptine concentrations but there was no significant relationship between them. There was however a significant relationship between plasma concentrations and concurrent changes in clinical response compared with pretreatment scores. Dyskinesias occurred within 90 to 180 minutes of dosage in 5 of 10 patients.

Bromocriptine is well absorbed from standard oral tablets placed in the vagina and plasma concentrations sufficient to lower plasma prolactin concentrations have been achieved using this route.[2,3]

1. Price P, *et al.* Plasma bromocriptine levels, clinical and growth hormone responses in parkinsonism. *Br J Clin Pharmacol* 1978; **6:** 303–9.
2. Vermesh M, *et al.* Vaginal bromocriptine: pharmacology and effect on serum prolactin in normal women. *Obstet Gynecol* 1988; **72:** 693–8.
3. Katz E, *et al.* Successful treatment of a prolactin-producing pituitary macroadenoma with intravaginal bromocriptine mesylate: a novel approach to intolerance of oral therapy. *Obstet Gynecol* 1989; **73:** 517–20.

Uses and Administration

Bromocriptine, an ergot derivative (p.1608), is a dopamine D$_2$-agonist. It inhibits the secretion of prolactin (p.1295) from the anterior pituitary and is used in the treatment of prolactinoma and in endocrinological disorders associated with hyperprolactinaemia, including amenorrhoea, galactorrhoea, hypogonadism, and infertility in both men and women. Bromocriptine is also used to suppress puerperal lactation for medical reasons; it is not recommended for the routine suppression of physiological lactation or for the treatment of postpartum breast pain and engorgement that may be adequately relieved with simple analgesics and breast support. Growth-hormone secretion may be suppressed by bromocriptine in some patients with acromegaly. Because of its dopaminergic activity bromocriptine is also used in the management of Parkinson's disease.

Bromocriptine is usually administered by mouth as the mesilate; doses are expressed in terms of the base. It should be taken with food.

For the prevention of puerperal lactation bromocriptine 2.5 mg is given on the day of delivery followed by 2.5 mg twice daily for 14 days. The risk of hypotension and, more rarely, hypertension must be borne in mind and it has been recommended that bromocriptine should not be given until at least 4 hours after delivery. For the suppression of established lactation it is given in a dose of 2.5 mg daily for 2 to 3 days subsequently increased to 2.5 mg twice daily for 14 days.

For the treatment of other conditions the dose of bromocriptine is usually increased gradually. In the UK,

typically, an initial dose of 1 to 1.25 mg at night is given, increased to 2 to 2.5 mg at night after 2 to 3 days, and subsequently increased by 1 mg at intervals of 2 to 3 days to a dose of 2.5 mg twice daily, or more if necessary. In the USA, increments of 2.5 mg are used, usually at intervals of 3 to 7 days.

In the treatment of hypogonadism and galactorrhoea syndromes and infertility bromocriptine is introduced gradually as described above. Most of the patients with hyperprolactinaemia respond to 7.5 mg daily but up to 30 mg daily may be required. In patients known to have prolactinomas the dose is increased gradually up to 5 mg every 6 hours but occasionally patients may require up to 30 mg daily. Infertile patients without raised serum concentrations of prolactin are usually given 2.5 mg twice daily.

In cyclical benign breast and menstrual disorders bromocriptine is introduced gradually up to a usual dosage of 2.5 mg twice daily.

Bromocriptine may be used as an adjunct to surgery and radiotherapy to reduce growth-hormone concentrations in plasma in acromegalic patients. It is introduced gradually up to a dose of 2.5 mg twice daily and may then be increased further by 2.5 mg every 2 to 3 days if necessary up to 5 mg every 6 hours, according to response.

In Parkinson's disease bromocriptine has been used alone, although it is usually given as an adjunct to levodopa treatment. It should be introduced gradually and during this period patients already receiving levodopa can have their levodopa dosage decreased gradually until an optimal response is achieved. A suggested initial dose is 1 to 1.25 mg of bromocriptine at night during week 1, increased to 2 to 2.5 mg at night for week 2, 2.5 mg twice daily for week 3, and for week 4, 2.5 mg three times daily; the dose may be increased thereafter by 2.5 mg every 3 to 14 days depending on response. Most patients require doses within the range of 10 to 40 mg daily.

Bromocriptine mesilate has also been given intramuscularly as a depot injection for disorders associated with hyperprolactinaemia.

Acromegaly. Dopaminergics can produce a paradoxical reduction in growth hormone secretion and bromocriptine has been used in acromegaly (p.1271) as adjunctive therapy to surgery and/or radiotherapy to reduce circulating growth hormone levels. While it is less effective than octreotide, it can be given orally and is therefore more convenient to administer.

Cushing's syndrome. There have been occasional reports of benefit with the use of bromocriptine in the treatment of Cushing's syndrome (p.1272). Atkinson *et al.*[1] reported that remission of ACTH-dependent Cushing's syndrome was maintained for 6 years by bromocriptine 2.5 mg twice daily in a patient who had initially received pituitary irradiation. However, in a later review Atkinson reported that they had recently found that bromocriptine did not effectively reduce ACTH secretion following bilateral adrenalectomy.[2]

1. Atkinson AB, *et al.* Six year remission of ACTH-dependent Cushing's syndrome using bromocriptine. *Postgrad Med J* 1985; **61:** 239–42.
2. Atkinson AB. The treatment of Cushing's syndrome. *Clin Endocrinol (Oxf)* 1991; **34:** 507–13.

Hyperprolactinaemia and prolactinomas. Prolactinomas (prolactin-secreting pituitary adenomas) are among the commonest causes of hyperprolactinaemia. Raised serum-prolactin concentrations may result in reduced gonadotrophin production, which in turn may suppress gonadal function. Consequences may include oligomenorrhoea or amenorrhoea, and infertility in either sex. Galactorrhoea may also result from high prolactin levels and can occur in men as well as women.

Dopamine is the major inhibitory factor in the hypothalamus and directly inhibits the secretion of prolactin. Bromocriptine, a dopamine agonist, has been the first choice of treatment in many centres for the treatment of hyperprolactinaemia secondary to a prolactinoma although cabergoline is now preferred by some. Bromocriptine is extremely effective in controlling elevated circulating prolactin concentrations and restoring gonadal function; although it is rarely curative, it may produce considerable shrinkage of the adenoma.[1-5]

The sensitivity of hyperprolactinaemia to bromocriptine therapy can vary considerably between patients and this is reflected in the wide range of oral doses required to reduce prolactin concentrations to normal levels. Although methods such as initiating therapy with gradually increasing doses can minimise adverse effects it has been reported that about 5 to 10% of patients are unable to tolerate bromocriptine by mouth;[6] various other routes of administration have therefore been investigated. Bromocriptine is well absorbed from standard oral tablets placed in the vagina and appears to be both effective in lowering prolactin concentrations and well tolerated when given by this route.[7] However, limitations are considered to be the relatively short duration of action and the relatively low dose that can be administered.[6] Of the various injectable depot formulations that have been tried, one preparation given intramuscularly in a dose of 50 to 250 mg monthly has been found to be effective and well tolerated in long-term studies;[8,9] it is reported to be used in some centres to initiate treatment for macroprolactinomas.[6]

For discussions of the management of hyperprolactinaemia and associated disorders see p.1274 (hyperprolactinaemia), p.1272 (amenorrhoea), p.1274 (hypogonadism), p.1663 (erectile dysfunction), and p.1275 (infertility).

1. Prescott RWG, et al. Hyperprolactinaemia in men—response to bromocriptine therapy. *Lancet* 1982; **i:** 245–8.
2. Hancock KW, et al. Long term suppression of prolactin concentrations after bromocriptine induced regression of pituitary prolactinomas. *BMJ* 1985; **290:** 117–8.
3. Grossman A, Besser GM. Prolactinomas. *BMJ* 1985; **290:** 182–4.
4. Liuzzi A, et al. Low doses of dopamine agonists in the long-term treatment of macroprolactinomas. *N Engl J Med* 1985; **313:** 656–9.
5. Ho KY, Thorner MO. Therapeutic applications of bromocriptine in endocrine and neurological diseases. *Drugs* 1988; **36:** 67–82.
6. Ciccarelli E, Camanni F. Diagnosis and drug therapy of prolactinoma. *Drugs* 1996; **51:** 954–65.
7. Ginsburg J, et al. Vaginal bromocriptine. *Lancet* 1991; **338:** 1205–6.
8. Ciccarelli E, et al. Long term therapy of patients with macroprolactinoma using repeatable injectable bromocriptine. *J Clin Endocrinol Metab* 1993; **76:** 484–8.
9. Ciccarelli E, et al. Double blind randomized study using oral or injectable bromocriptine in patients with hyperprolactinaemia. *Clin Endocrinol (Oxf)* 1994; **40:** 193–8.

PREGNANCY. Pregnancy and the hyperprolactinaemic woman has been discussed.[1] The continuous administration of bromocriptine throughout pregnancy has been advocated in women with macroadenomas, but the effects on the developing fetus are unknown and such therapy cannot be recommended. However, existing information is reassuring and discovery of pregnancy at an advanced stage in a woman taking bromocriptine does not justify therapeutic abortion. If symptomatic tumour enlargement occurs during pregnancy reinstitution of bromocriptine is probably less harmful to the mother and child than surgery.

See also under Precautions, above.

1. Molitch ME. Pregnancy and the hyperprolactinemic woman. *N Engl J Med* 1985; **312:** 1364–70.

Lactation inhibition. Because of its effects on prolactin, bromocriptine is a potent suppressor of lactation and has been widely used for the prevention of lactation in women who choose not to breast feed postpartum. However, bromocriptine has been associated with severe adverse effects in some women, and its use to suppress a physiological state has been criticised (see p.1276). Consequently, the manufacturers in a number of countries recommend that bromocriptine should only be used to suppress puerperal lactation for medical reasons; it is also not recommended for the treatment of postpartum breast pain and engorgement that may be adequately relieved with simple analgesics and breast support.

Mastalgia. Since mastalgia (p.1470) can improve spontaneously, treatment should rarely be considered unless pain has been present for about 6 months. Bromocriptine is one of the drugs that may be used to treat mastalgia.[1,2] It may improve symptoms in up to about 50% of patients with cyclical mastalgia, but is less effective in the non-cyclical form.[3,4] Adverse effects can be severe in some patients.

1. Gateley CA, Mansel RE. Management of the painful and nodular breast. *Br Med Bull* 1991; **47:** 284–94.
2. Anonymous. Cyclical breast pain—what works and what doesn't. *Drug Ther Bull* 1992; **30:** 1–3.
3. Pye JK, et al. Clinical experience of drug treatments for mastalgia. *Lancet* 1985; **ii:** 373–7.
4. Mansel RE, Dogliotti L. European multicentre trial of bromocriptine in cyclical mastalgia. *Lancet* 1990; **335:** 190–3.

Neuroleptic malignant syndrome. Bromocriptine has been used in doses of up to 30 mg daily,[1-5] usually alone or with dantrolene, in the treatment of neuroleptic malignant syndrome (p.662) although some workers have not found it to be of use.[6]

1. Mueller PS, et al. Neuroleptic malignant syndrome: successful treatment with bromocriptine. *JAMA* 1983; **249:** 386–8.
2. Dhib-Jalbut S, et al. Treatment of the neuroleptic malignant syndrome with bromocriptine. *JAMA* 1983; **250:** 484–5.
3. Clarke CE, et al. Clinical spectrum of neuroleptic malignant syndrome. *Lancet* 1988; **ii:** 969–70.
4. Guerrero RM, Shifrar KA. Diagnosis and treatment of neuroleptic malignant syndrome. *Clin Pharm* 1988; **7:** 697–701.
5. Lo TCM, et al. Neuroleptic malignant syndrome: another medical cause of acute abdomen. *Postgrad Med J* 1989; **65:** 653–5.
6. Rosebush PI, et al. The treatment of neuroleptic malignant syndrome: are dantrolene and bromocriptine useful adjuncts to supportive care? *Br J Psychiatry* 1991; **159:** 709–12.

Parkinsonism. While some neurologists use dopamine agonists such as bromocriptine early in the treatment of parkinsonism (p.1160) in an attempt to delay therapy with levodopa, others reserve them for adjunctive use when levodopa is no longer effective alone or cannot be tolerated. They are sometimes use-

ful in reducing 'off' periods with levodopa and in ameliorating other fluctuations of mobility in the later stage of the disease.

References.

1. Temlett JA, et al. Adjunctive therapy with bromocriptine in Parkinson's disease. *S Afr Med J* 1990; **78:** 680–5.
2. Hely MA, et al. The Sydney Multicentre Study of Parkinson's disease: a randomised, prospective five year study comparing low dose bromocriptine with low dose levodopa-carbidopa. *J Neurol Neurosurg Psychiatry* 1994; **57:** 903–10.
3. Montastruc JL, et al. A randomised controlled study comparing bromocriptine to which levodopa was later added, with levodopa alone in previously untreated patients with Parkinson's disease: a five year follow up. *J Neurol Neurosurg Psychiatry* 1994; **57:** 1034–8.
4. Giménez-Roldán S, et al. Early combination of bromocriptine and levodopa in Parkinson's disease: a prospective randomized study of two parallel groups over a total follow-up period of 44 months including an initial 8-month double-blind stage. *Clin Neuropharmacol* 1997; **20:** 67–76.
5. Ogawa N, et al. Nationwide multicenter prospective study on the long-term effects of bromocriptine for Parkinson's disease: final report of a ten-year follow-up. *Eur Neurol* 1997; **38** (suppl 2): 37–49.
6. Ramaker C, van Hilten JJ. Bromocriptine versus levodopa in early Parkinson's disease (updated 22 February 2000). Available in The Cochrane Library; Issue 4. Oxford: Update Software; 2001.

Polycystic ovary syndrome. Bromocriptine has been tried in women with the polycystic ovary syndrome (p.1276) who have mild basal hyperprolactinaemia without evidence of a pituitary tumour.

Restless legs syndrome. The aetiology of restless legs syndrome (see under Parasomnias, p.653) is obscure and treatment has largely been empirical. Bromocriptine showed some benefit in one small study.[1]

1. Walters AS, et al. A double-blind randomized crossover trial of bromocriptine and placebo in restless legs syndrome. *Ann Neurol* 1988; **24:** 455–8.

Withdrawal syndromes. ALCOHOL. Studies of the efficacy of bromocriptine as an aid in the maintenance of abstinence from alcohol (p.1131) have yielded conflicting results.[1-4] However, it has been suggested[3] that response to bromocriptine might be linked to a specific genotype of the D_2 dopamine receptor.

1. Dongier M, et al. Bromocriptine in the treatment of alcohol dependence. *Alcohol Clin Exp Res* 1991; **15:** 970–7.
2. Naranjo CA, et al. Long-acting bromocriptine (B) does not reduce relapse in alcoholics. *Clin Pharmacol Ther* 1995; **57:** 161.
3. Lawford BR, et al. Bromocriptine in the treatment of alcoholics with the D_2 dopamine receptor A1 allele. *Nat Med* 1995; **1:** 337–41.
4. Powell BJ, et al. A double-blind, placebo-controlled study of nortriptyline and bromocriptine in male alcoholics subtyped by comorbid psychiatric disorders. *Alcohol Clin Exp Res* 1995; **19:** 462–8.

Preparations

BP 2001: Bromocriptine Capsules; Bromocriptine Tablets;
USP 25: Bromocriptine Mesylate Capsules; Bromocriptine Mesylate Tablets.

Proprietary Preparations (details are given in Part 3)
Aust.: Broman; Bromed; Cehapark†; Parlodel; Umprel; **Austral.:** Bromohexal; Bromolactin; Kripton; Parlodel; **Belg.:** Parlodel; **Braz.:** Bagren; Parlodel; **Canad.:** Parlodel; **Denm.:** Bromergon; Bromopar; Parlodel; **Fin.:** Parlodel; **Fr.:** Bromo-Kin; **Ger.:** Bromocrel; kirim; kirim gyn; Pravidel; **Hong Kong:** Bromtine; Medocriptine; Parlodel; Serocryptin; Zolac; **Irl.:** Parlodel; **Israel:** Parilac; **Ital.:** Parlodel; **Jpn:** Parlodel†; **Mex.:** Crilem; Cryocriptina; Inovapar; Kriptiser; Lactess; Mesiken; Parlodel; Serocryptin; **Neth.:** Parlodel; **Norw.:** Parlodel; **NZ:** Parlodel; **Port.:** Parlodel; **S.Afr.:** Parlodel; Serocryptin; Suplac; **Spain:** Parlodel; **Swed.:** Pravidel; **Switz.:** Parlodel; Serocryptin; Suplac; **Thai.:** Bromergon; Parlodel; Serocryptin; Suplac; **UAE:** Antiprotin; **UK:** Parlodel; **USA:** Parlodel.

Budipine (1967-p)

Budipine (rINN).

1-tert-Butyl-4,4-diphenylpiperidine.
$C_{21}H_{27}N = 293.4$.
CAS — 57982-78-2.
ATC — N04BX03.

Profile

Budipine is a phenylpiperidine derivative used as adjunctive therapy in the treatment of parkinsonism. It is given by mouth as the hydrochloride in daily doses up to 60 mg.

◊ References.

1. Spieker S, et al. Tremorlytic activity of budipine: a quantitative study with long-term tremor recordings. *Clin Neuropharmacol* 1995; **18:** 266–72.
2. Groen H, et al. A study to investigate the pharmacokinetics and metabolism of budipine after administration of a single oral dose of [^{14}C]-B757-01 to six healthy volunteers. *Br J Clin Pharmacol* 1999; **48:** 771P–772P.
3. Malsch U, et al. Monotherapie der Parkinsonschen Erkrankung mit Budipin: ein randomisierter Doppelblindvergleich mit Amantadin. *Fortschr Neurol Psychiatr* 2001; **69:** 86–9.

Preparations

Proprietary Preparations (details are given in Part 3)
Ger.: Parkinsan.

Cabergoline (2841-h)

Cabergoline (BAN, USAN, rINN).
FCE-21336. 1-[(6-Allylergolin-8β-yl)carbonyl]-1-[3-(dimethylamino)propyl]-3-ethylurea; (8R)-6-Allyl-N-[3-(dimethylamino)propyl]-N-(ethylcarbamoyl)ergoline-8-carboxamide.
$C_{26}H_{37}N_5O_2 = 451.6$.
CAS — 81409-90-7.
ATC — G02CB03; N04BC06.

Adverse Effects and Precautions

As for Bromocriptine, p.1164, although patients unable to tolerate bromocriptine may tolerate cabergoline (and *vice versa*).

The manufacturer recommends that conception should be avoided for at least one month after treatment.

Effects on the respiratory system. Report[1] of a patient who developed pleuropulmonary disease 16 months after starting treatment with cabergoline. The patient had previously received bromocriptine for 10 years and had had a normal chest X-ray at the time of transfer to treatment with cabergoline. In another report, two cases of pleural effusion/pulmonary fibrosis, occurring after 10 to 11 months of treatment, were described.[2] One patient had modest pre-treatment lung alterations attributed to previous bromocriptine treatment. Withdrawal was associated with improvement in both cases. Congestive heart failure secondary to constrictive pericarditis, and severe pleuropulmonary fibrosis that resulted in persistent dyspnoea have also been reported in a patient receiving cabergoline.[3]

1. Bhatt MH, et al. Pleuropulmonary disease associated with dopamine agonist therapy. *Ann Neurol* 1991; **30:** 613–16.
2. Geminiani G, et al. Cabergoline in Parkinson's disease complicated by motor fluctuations. *Mov Disord* 1996; **11:** 495–500.
3. Ling LH, et al. Constrictive pericarditis and pleuropulmonary disease linked to ergot dopamine agonist therapy (cabergoline) for Parkinson's disease. *Mayo Clin Proc* 1999; **74:** 371–5.

Oedema. Three cases of lower limb oedema following chronic treatment with cabergoline have been reported.[1] In one case the oedema was severe enough to necessitate withdrawal of therapy.

1. Geminiani G, et al. Cabergoline in Parkinson's disease complicated by motor fluctuations. *Mov Disord* 1996; **11:** 495–500.

Interactions

As for Bromocriptine, p.1166.

Pharmacokinetics

Cabergoline is absorbed from the gastrointestinal tract and extensively metabolised to several metabolites, which do not appear to contribute to its pharmacological activity. Plasma protein binding has been estimated to be about 40%. Cabergoline is mainly eliminated via the faeces; a small proportion is excreted in the urine.

◊ Pharmacokinetic studies of cabergoline have been hampered by lack of an assay method sensitive enough to detect plasma concentrations of cabergoline following therapeutic doses. However, the plasma elimination half-life of cabergoline has been estimated indirectly to be 63 to 68 hours in healthy volunteers and 79 to 115 hours in patients with hyperprolactinaemia.[1]

1. Rains CP, et al. Cabergoline: a review of its pharmacological properties and therapeutic potential in the treatment of hyperprolactinaemia and inhibition of lactation. *Drugs* 1995; **49:** 255–79.

Uses and Administration

Cabergoline, an ergot derivative, is a dopamine D_2-agonist with actions and uses similar to those of bromocriptine (p.1166). It is a potent and long-lasting inhibitor of prolactin secretion used in the management of disorders associated with hyperprolactinaemia. It is also used to suppress puerperal lactation for medical reasons; it is not recommended for the routine suppression of physiological lactation or for the treatment of postpartum breast pain and engorgement that may be adequately relieved with simple analgesics and breast support. Cabergoline is also used in the management of Parkinson's disease.

Cabergoline is administered by mouth and should be taken with food.

To inhibit physiological lactation, cabergoline is given as a single 1-mg dose on the first day postpartum. For suppression of established lactation, the dose is 250 μg every 12 hours for 2 days. In the treatment of disorders associated with hyperprolactinaemia, the initial dose of cabergoline is 500 μg per week. The dose is then increased at monthly intervals by 500 μg per week according to response. The weekly dose may be administered on a single occasion or divided into 2 doses on separate days; doses over 1 mg should be given as divided doses. The usual dose is 1 mg per week but up to 4.5 mg has been used.

In Parkinson's disease, cabergoline is used as an adjunct in patients experiencing 'on-off' fluctuations in control with levodopa treatment alone. It should be introduced gradually and during this period the dose of levodopa may be reduced gradually until an optimal response is achieved. A suggested initial dose of cabergoline is 1 mg as a single daily dose given with meals. The dose may be increased in increments of 0.5 or 1 mg at intervals of 7 or 14 days. The recommended therapeutic dose range is 2 to 6 mg daily.

◊ General references.
1. Rains CP, et al. Cabergoline: a review of its pharmacological properties and therapeutic potential in the treatment of hyperprolactinaemia and inhibition of lactation. *Drugs* 1995; **49:** 255–79.

Acromegaly. Dopamine agonists have been used in acromegaly (p.1271) as adjuvants to surgery or radiotherapy to reduce circulating growth hormone concentrations, although they are less effective than the somatostatin analogue octreotide. However, a small study comparing cabergoline with depot bromocriptine and quinagolide failed to find evidence of its effectiveness (see p.1176).

Hyperprolactinaemia and prolactinomas. Dopamine agonists are widely used for the treatment of hyperprolactinaemia secondary to a prolactinoma (see p.1274). Although bromocriptine has been the first choice for this indication, some now prefer cabergoline,[1] which appears to be more effective and better tolerated.[2]

Further references.[3-9]

1. Webster J. A comparative review of the tolerability profiles of dopamine agonists in the treatment of hyperprolactinaemia and inhibition of lactation. *Drug Safety* 1996; **14:** 228–38. Correction. *ibid.,* 342.
2. Pascal-Vigneron V, et al. Aménorrhée hyperprolactinémique: traitement par cabergoline versus bromocriptine. *Presse Med* 1995; **24:** 753–7.
3. Falsetti L, et al. Cabergoline treatment in hyperprolactinaemic women. *J Obstet Gynaecol* 1991; **11:** 68–71.
4. Webster J, et al. Dose-dependent suppression of serum prolactin by cabergoline in hyperprolactinaemia: a placebo controlled, double blind, multicentre study. *Clin Endocrinol (Oxf)* 1992; **37:** 534–41.
5. Ferrari C, et al. Cabergoline in the long-term therapy of hyperprolactinemic disorders. *Acta Endocrinol (Copenh)* 1992; **126:** 489–94.
6. Webster J, et al. The efficacy and tolerability of long-term cabergoline therapy in hyperprolactinaemic disorders: an open, uncontrolled, multicentre study. *Clin Endocrinol (Oxf)* 1993; **39:** 323–9.
7. Webster J, et al. A comparison of cabergoline and bromocriptine in the treatment of hyperprolactinemic amenorrhea. *N Engl J Med* 1994; **331:** 904–9.
8. Verhelst J, et al. Cabergoline in the treatment of hyperprolactinaemia: a study in 455 patients. *J Clin Endocrinol Metab* 1999; **84:** 2518–22.
9. Colao A, et al. Macroprolactinoma shrinkage during cabergoline treatment is greater in naive patients than in patients pretreated with other dopamine agonists: a prospective study in 110 patients. *J Clin Endocrinol Metab* 2000; **85:** 2247–52.

Lactation inhibition. A single 1-mg dose of cabergoline was found to be as effective as bromocriptine 2.5 mg given twice daily for 14 days for preventing puerperal lactation in a double-blind multicentre study involving 272 women.[1] It has been suggested that cabergoline would be a better choice than bromocriptine for lactation inhibition.[2] However, as discussed on p.1276, the routine use of dopaminergics such as bromocriptine or cabergoline is not recommended for the suppression of physiological lactation.

1. European Multicentre Study Group for Cabergoline in Lactation Inhibition. Single dose cabergoline versus bromocriptine in inhibition of puerperal lactation: randomised, double blind, multicentre study. *BMJ* 1991; **302:** 1367–71.
2. Webster J. A comparative review of the tolerability profiles of dopamine agonists in the treatment of hyperprolactinaemia and inhibition of lactation. *Drug Safety* 1996; **14:** 228–38. Correction. *ibid.;* 342.

Parasomnias. The aetiology of *restless legs syndrome* is obscure and treatment has been largely empirical (p.653). Results from a 12-week open label pilot study[1] in 9 patients with idiopathic restless legs syndrome given cabergoline following insufficient response to levodopa therapy were promising; doses of cabergoline ranged from 1 to 4 mg.

1. Stiasny K, et al. Treatment of idiopathic restless legs syndrome (RLS) with the D2-agonist cabergoline—an open clinical trial. *Sleep* 2000; **23:** 349–54.

Parkinsonism. Cabergoline is used as a long-acting dopamine agonist in Parkinson's disease (p.1160). While some neurologists use dopamine agonists early in treatment in an attempt to delay therapy with levodopa others reserve their use for when levodopa is no longer effective or cannot be tolerated. They are sometimes useful in reducing 'off' periods with levo-

dopa and in ameliorating other fluctuations of mobility in the later stages of the disease.

References.
1. Inzelberg R, et al. Double-blind comparison of cabergoline and bromocriptine in Parkinson's disease patients with motor fluctuations. *Neurology* 1996; **47:** 785–8.
2. Geminiani G, et al. Cabergoline in Parkinson's disease complicated by motor fluctuations. *Mov Disord* 1996; **11:** 495–500.
3. Hutton JT, et al. Multicenter, placebo-controlled trial of cabergoline taken once daily in the treatment of Parkinson's disease. *Neurology* 1996; **46:** 1062–5.
4. Marsden CD. Clinical experience with cabergoline in patients with advanced Parkinson's disease treated with levodopa. *Drugs* 1998; **55** (suppl 1): 17–22.
5. Rinne UK, et al. Early treatment of Parkinson's disease with cabergoline delays the onset of motor complications: results of a double-blind levodopa controlled trial. *Drugs* 1998; **55** (suppl 1): 23–30.
6. Clarke CE, Deane KH. Cabergoline for levodopa-induced complications in Parkinson's disease (updated 17 November 2000). Available in The Cochrane Library; Issue 4. Oxford: Update Software; 2001.
7. Clarke CE, Deane KH. Cabergoline versus bromocriptine for levodopa-induced complications in Parkinson's disease (updated 17 November 2000). Available in The Cochrane Library; Issue 4. Oxford: Update Software; 2001.

Preparations

Proprietary Preparations (details are given in Part 3)
Aust.: Dostinex; *Austral.:* Cabaser; Dostinex; *Belg.:* Dostinex; Sostilar; *Denm.:* Cabaser; Dostinex; *Fin.:* Cabaser; Dostinex; *Fr.:* Dostinex; *Ger.:* Cabaseril; *Irl.:* Dostinex; *Israel:* Dostinex; *Ital.:* Dostinex; *Neth.:* Dostinex; *Norw.:* Cabaser; Dostinex; *NZ:* Dostinex; *Port.:* Dostinex; *S.Afr.:* Dostinex; *Singapore:* Dostinex; *Spain:* Dostinex; *Swed.:* Cabaser; Dostinex; *Switz.:* Cabaser; Dostinex; *UK:* Cabaser; Dostinex; *USA:* Dostinex.

Carbidopa (4547-I)

Carbidopa *(BAN, USAN, rINN).*

Carbidopum; α-Methyldopa Hydrazine; MK-486. (+)-2-(3,4-Dihydroxybenzyl)-2-hydrazinopropionic acid monohydrate; (−)-L-α-Hydrazino-3,4-dihydroxy-α-methylhydrocinnamic acid monohydrate.
$C_{10}H_{14}N_2O_4,H_2O = 244.2.$
CAS — 28860-95-9 (anhydrous); 38821-49-7 (monohydrate).

NOTE. The synonym MK-485 has been used for the racemic mixture.
Compounded preparations of carbidopa and levodopa may be represented by the following names:

- Co-careldopa *x/y (BAN)*—where *x* and *y* are the strengths in milligrams of carbidopa and levodopa respectively
- Co-careldopa *(USP 25)*—carbidopa and levodopa.

Pharmacopoeias. In *Eur.* (see p.vi), *Int., Jpn,* and *US.*

Pharmacopoeial description

Ph. Eur.: A white or yellowish-white powder. Slightly soluble in water; very slightly soluble in alcohol; practically insoluble in dichloromethane; dissolves in dilute solutions of mineral acids. Protect from light.

USP 25: A white to creamy-white, odourless or practically odourless powder. Slightly soluble in water and in methyl alcohol; practically insoluble in alcohol, in acetone, in chloroform, and in ether; freely soluble in 3N hydrochloric acid. Protect from light.

Adverse Effects

Hypersensitivity. Henoch-Schönlein purpura which developed in a 68-year-old patient being treated for Parkinson's disease appeared to be due to either carbidopa or an excipient of the preparation containing the carbidopa (Sinemet).[1]

1. Niedermaier G, Briner V. Henoch-Schönlein syndrome induced by carbidopa/levodopa. *Lancet* 1997; **349:** 1071–2.

Pharmacokinetics

Carbidopa is rapidly but incompletely absorbed from the gastrointestinal tract. It is rapidly excreted in the urine both unchanged and in the form of metabolites. It does not cross the blood-brain barrier. In *rats,* carbidopa has been reported to cross the placenta and to be distributed into breast milk.

Uses and Administration

Carbidopa is a peripheral dopa-decarboxylase inhibitor with little or no pharmacological activity when given alone in usual doses. It inhibits the peripheral decarboxylation of levodopa to dopamine and as, unlike levodopa, it does not cross the blood-brain barrier, effective brain concentrations of dopamine are produced with lower doses of levodopa. At the same time reduced peripheral formation of dopamine reduces peripheral side-effects, notably nausea and vomiting, and cardiac arrhythmias, although the dyskinesias and adverse mental effects associated with levodopa therapy tend to develop earlier. Contrary to its effect in patients on levodopa alone, pyridoxine does not inhibit the response to levodopa in patients also receiving a peripheral dopa-decarboxylase inhibitor.

In the treatment of parkinsonism carbidopa is given with levodopa to enable a lower dosage of the latter to be used and a more rapid response to be obtained, and to decrease side-ef-

fects. For details of administration and dosage, see Levodopa, p.1172.
Carbidopa also inhibits the peripheral decarboxylation of the serotonin precursor oxitriptan (p.302).

◊ General references.
1. Pinder RM, et al. Levodopa and decarboxylase inhibitors: a review of their clinical pharmacology and use in the treatment of parkinsonism. *Drugs* 1976; **11:** 329–77.
2. Boshes B. Sinemet and the treatment of parkinsonism. *Ann Intern Med* 1981; **94:** 364–70.

Preparations

BP 2001: Co-careldopa Tablets;
USP 25: Carbidopa and Levodopa Tablets.

Proprietary Preparations (details are given in Part 3)
USA: Lodosyn.

Multi-ingredient: *Aust.:* Sinemet; *Austral.:* Kinson; Sinacarb; Sinemet; *Belg.:* Sinemet; *Braz.:* Cronomet; Levocarb; Sinemet; *Canad.:* Apo-Levocarb; Nu-Levocarb; Sinemet; *Denm.:* Sinemet; *Fin.:* Kardopal; Sinemet; *Fr.:* Sinemet; *Ger.:* Isicom; Levocarb-GRY; Levodopa comp C; Nacom; Striaton; *Hong Kong:* Apo-Levocarb; Sinemet; *Irl.:* Half Sinemet; Sinemet; *Israel:* Dopicar; Sinemet; *Ital.:* Sinemet; *Mex.:* Lemdopa; Racovel; Sinemet; *Neth.:* Sinemet; *Norw.:* Sinemet; *NZ:* Apo-Levocarb; Sindopa; Sinemet; *Port.:* Sinemet; *S.Afr.:* Carbilev; Sinemet; *Singapore:* Sinemet; *Spain:* Sinemet; *Swed.:* Sinemet; *Switz.:* Sinemet; *Thai.:* Levomed; Sinemet; Syndopa; *UK:* Half Sinemet; Sinemet; *USA:* Atamet; Sinemet.

Droxidopa (3676-y)

Droxidopa *(rINN).*
L-*threo*-3,4-Dihydroxyphenylserine. (−)-*threo*-3-(3,4-Dihydroxyphenyl)-L-serine.
$C_9H_{11}NO_5 = 213.2.$
CAS — 23651-95-8.

Profile

Droxidopa is a precursor of noradrenaline that is used in the treatment of parkinsonism and some forms of orthostatic hypotension. The racemic form (DL-*threo*-3,4-dihydroxyphenylserine) has been studied for similar uses.

◊ References.
1. Iida N, et al. Treatment of dialysis-induced hypotension with L-threo-3, 4-dihydroxyphenylserine. *Nephrol Dial Transplant* 1994; **9:** 1130–5.

Preparations

Proprietary Preparations (details are given in Part 3)
Jpn: Dops.

Entacapone (15430-d)

Entacapone *(BAN, USAN, rINN).*
OR-611. (E)-α-Cyano-N,N-diethyl-3,4-dihydroxy-5-nitrocinnamamide; (E)-2-Cyano-3-(3,4-dihydroxy-5-nitrophenyl)-N,N-diethylacrylamide.
$C_{14}H_{15}N_3O_5 = 305.3.$
CAS — 130929-57-6.
ATC — N04BX02.

Adverse Effects

The most frequent adverse effects produced by entacapone relate to increased dopaminergic activity and occur most commonly at the start of treatment; reduction of the levodopa dosage may reduce the severity and frequency of such effects. Adverse effects may include nausea, vomiting, abdominal pain, constipation, diarrhoea, dry mouth, and dyskinesias. A decrease in haemoglobin has been observed in some patients treated for more than 6 months. Increases in liver enzyme values have been reported rarely. Entacapone may produce a harmless reddish-brown discoloration of the urine.

Precautions

Entacapone is contra-indicated in patients with phaeochromocytoma and in patients with a previous history of neuroleptic malignant syndrome or nontraumatic rhabdomyolysis. It should be avoided in patients with hepatic impairment, and given with caution to patients with biliary obstruction. Use with levodopa may cause dizziness and orthostatic hypotension; if affected patients should not drive or operate machinery. Treatment with entacapone should not be stopped abruptly; when necessary withdrawal should be made gradually, increasing the dose of levodopa as required.

Interactions

Entacapone should be used with caution or not at all in patients receiving drugs metabolised by catechol-O-methyltransferase (COMT) including adrenaline [epinephrine], apomorphine, dobutamine, dopamine, isoprenaline, methyldopa, noradrenaline [norepinephrine], and rimiterol.

Entacapone may aggravate levodopa-induced orthostatic hypotension and should be used cautiously in patients who are taking other drugs which may cause orthostatic hypotension.

Entacapone may form chelates with iron preparations in the gastrointestinal tract; the two drugs should be taken at least 2 to 3 hours apart.

Pharmacokinetics

There are large intra- and interindividual variations in the absorption of entacapone. Peak plasma concentrations are achieved about one hour after oral administration. Entacapone undergoes extensive first-pass metabolism and oral bioavailability is about 35%. Absorption is not affected significantly by food. Entacapone is extensively bound to plasma proteins. It is eliminated mainly in the faeces with about 10 to 20% being excreted in the urine, mainly as glucuronide conjugates.

◊ Entacapone is rapidly absorbed from the gastrointestinal tract and bioavailability following oral administration has been reported to range from 29 to 46%. It does not cross the blood-brain barrier. Over half of a dose appears in the faeces with smaller amounts being excreted in the urine as glucuronides of entacapone and its (Z)-isomer. Elimination half-lives of about 1.6 to 3.4 hours have been reported for entacapone.

References.
1. Wikberg T, *et al.* Identification of major metabolites of the catechol-*O*-methyltransferase inhibitor entacapone in rats and humans. *Drug Metab Dispos* 1993; **21:** 81–92.
2. Keränen T, *et al.* Inhibition of soluble catechol-O-methyltransferase and single-dose pharmacokinetics after oral and intravenous administration of entacapone. *Eur J Clin Pharmacol* 1994; **46:** 151–7.

Uses and Administration

Entacapone is a selective, reversible, peripheral inhibitor of catechol-*O*-methyltransferase (COMT) an enzyme involved in the metabolism of dopamine and levodopa. It is used as an adjunct to combination preparations of levodopa and dopa-decarboxylase inhibitors, in patients with Parkinson's disease and 'end-of-dose' motor fluctuations who cannot be stabilised on levodopa combinations alone. Entacapone is given by mouth in a dosage of 200 mg at the same time as each dose of levodopa with dopa-decarboxylase inhibitor, up to a maximum of 200 mg ten times daily. It is often necessary to gradually reduce the dosage of levodopa by about 10 to 30% within the first few weeks after starting treatment with entacapone.

Parkinsonism. Entacapone is a selective and reversible inhibitor of catechol-*O*-methyltransferase (COMT), with mainly peripheral actions. It is given as adjunctive therapy to patients with Parkinson's disease (p.1160) experiencing fluctuations in disability related to levodopa and dopa-decarboxylase inhibitor combinations. When levodopa is administered concurrently with a peripheral dopa-decarboxylase inhibitor, *O*-methylation then becomes the predominant form of metabolism of levodopa; therefore co-administration of a peripheral COMT inhibitor such as entacapone potentially extends the duration and effect of levodopa in the brain, and consequently allows a reduction in the dose and frequency of administration of levodopa.

References.
1. Nutt JG. Catechol-O-methyltransferase inhibitors for treatment of Parkinson's disease. *Lancet* 1998; **351:** 1221–2.
2. Ruottinen HM, Rinne UK. A double-blind pharmacokinetic and clinical dose-response study of entacapone as an adjuvant to levodopa therapy in advanced Parkinson's disease. *Clin Neuropharmacol* 1996; **19:** 283–96.
3. Parkinson Study Group. Entacapone improves motor fluctuations in levodopa-treated Parkinson's disease patients. *Ann Neurol* 1997; **42:** 747–55.
4. Rinne UK, *et al.* Entacapone enhances the response to levodopa in parkinsonian patients with motor fluctuations. *Neurology* 1998; **51:** 1309–14.
5. Holm KJ, Spencer CM. Entacapone: a review of its use in Parkinson's disease. *Drugs* 1999; **58:** 159–177.
6. Anonymous. Entacapone for Parkinson's disease. *Med Lett Drugs Ther* 2000; **42:** 7–8.
7. Chong BS, Mersfelder TL. Entacapone. *Ann Pharmacother* 2000; **34:** 1056–65.

Preparations

Proprietary Preparations (details are given in Part 3)
Aust.: Comtan; *Austral.:* Comtan; *Belg.:* Comtan; *Denm.:* Comtess; *Fin.:* Comtess; *Fr.:* Comtan; *Ger.:* Comtess; *Irl.:* Comtess; *Ital.:* Comtan; *Neth.:* Comtan; *Norw.:* Comtess; *NZ:* Comtan; *Port.:* Comtan; *S.Afr.:* Comtan; *Singapore:* Comtan; *Spain:* Comtan; *Swed.:* Comtess; *Switz.:* Comtan; *Thai.:* Comtan; *UK:* Comtess; *USA:* Comtan.

Lazabemide (15902-c)

Lazabemide (BAN, USAN, rINN).

Ro-19-6327; Ro-19-6327/000. N-(2-Aminoethyl)-5-chloropicolinamide.

$C_8H_{10}ClN_3O = 199.6$.

CAS — 103878-84-8 (lazabemide); 103878-83-7 (lazabemide hydrochloride).

Profile

Lazabemide is a reversible inhibitor of monoamine oxidase type B that was investigated in the management of parkinsonism, but development was discontinued when clinical trials highlighted a risk of severe hepatotoxicity.

Levodopa (4541-g)

Levodopa *(BAN, USAN, rINN).*

Dihydroxyphenylalanine; L-Dopa; 3-Hydroxy-L-tyrosine; Laevo-dopa; Levodopum. (–)-3-(3,4-Dihydroxyphenyl)-L-alanine.

$C_9H_{11}NO_4 = 197.2$.

CAS — 59-92-7.

ATC — N04BA01.

NOTE. Compounded preparations of levodopa may be represented by the following names:

- Co-beneldopa *(BAN)*—benserazide 1 part and levodopa 4 parts (w/w)
- Co-careldopa *x/y (BAN)*—where *x* and *y* are the strengths in milligrams of carbidopa and levodopa respectively
- Co-careldopa *(USP 25)*—carbidopa and levodopa.

Pharmacopoeias. In Chin., Eur. (see p.vi), *Int., Jpn,* and *US.*

Pharmacopoeial description

Ph. Eur.: A white or slightly cream-coloured, crystalline powder. Slightly soluble in water; freely soluble in 1M hydrochloric acid but sparingly soluble in 0.1M hydrochloric acid; practically insoluble in alcohol, and in ether. A 1% suspension in water has a pH of 4.5 to 7.0. Protect from light.

USP 25: A white to off-white, odourless, crystalline powder. In the presence of moisture, it is rapidly oxidised by atmospheric oxygen and darkens. Slightly soluble in water; freely soluble in 3N hydrochloric acid; insoluble in alcohol. Store in a dry place in airtight containers at a temperature not exceeding 40°. Protect from light.

Stability. A warning that extemporaneously prepared oral liquid dosage forms may be unstable and manufacturers' formulations should be used where possible.[1] An extemporary formula is available for levodopa syrup. Water dispersible formulations of levodopa with benserazide are available in some countries but a method that can be used by patients to prepare daily solutions of levodopa with carbidopa has been suggested by Giron and Koller.[2] One litre of a solution in potable water may be prepared with ten crushed standard tablets of levodopa 100 mg with carbidopa 25 mg and 2 g of ascorbic acid added to stabilise the levodopa.

1. Walls TJ, *et al.* Problems with inactivation of drugs used in Parkinson's disease. *BMJ* 1985; **290:** 444–5.
2. Giron LT, Koller WC. Methods of managing levodopa-induced dyskinesias. *Drug Safety* 1996; **14:** 365–74.

Adverse Effects

Gastrointestinal effects, notably nausea, vomiting, and anorexia are common early in treatment with levodopa, particularly if the dosage is increased too rapidly. Gastrointestinal bleeding has been reported in patients with a history of peptic ulcer disease.

The commonest cardiovascular effect is orthostatic hypotension, which is usually asymptomatic, but may be associated with faintness and dizziness. Cardiac arrhythmias have been reported and hypertension has occasionally occurred.

Psychiatric symptoms occur in a high proportion of patients, especially the elderly, and include agitation, anxiety, euphoria, nightmares, and insomnia, or sometimes drowsiness and depression. More serious effects, usually requiring a reduction in dosage or withdrawal of levodopa, include aggression, paranoid delusions, hallucinations, delirium, severe depression, with or without suicidal behaviour, and unmasking of psychoses. Psychotic reactions are more likely in patients with postencephalitic parkinsonism or a history of mental disorders.

Abnormal involuntary movements or dyskinesias are the most serious dose-limiting adverse effects of levodopa and are very common at the optimum dose required to control parkinsonism; their frequency increases with duration of treatment. Involuntary movements of the face, tongue, lips, and jaw often appear first and those of the trunk and extremities later. Severe generalised choreoathetoid and dystonic movements may occur after prolonged administration. Muscle twitching and blepharospasm may be early signs of excessive dosage. Exaggerated respiratory movements and exacerbated oculogyric crises have been reported in patients with postencephalitic parkinsonism. Re-emergence of bradykinesia and akinesia, in the form of 'end-of-dose' deterioration and the 'on-off' phenomenon, in patients with parkinsonism is a complication of long-term treatment, but may be due to progression of the disease rather than to levodopa (see also under Parkinsonism, p.1160).

A positive response to the direct Coombs' test may occur, usually without evidence of haemolysis although auto-immune haemolytic anaemia has occasionally been reported. Transient leucopenia has occurred rarely. The effects of levodopa on liver and kidney function are generally slight. Levodopa may cause discoloration of the urine; reddish at first then darkening on standing. Other body fluids may also be discoloured.

Some of the adverse effects reported may not be attributable directly to levodopa, but rather to the concomitant use of antimuscarinics, to increased mobility, or to the unmasking of underlying conditions as parkinsonism improves. Concomitant administration of a peripheral dopa-decarboxylase inhibitor may reduce the severity of peripheral symptoms such as gastrointestinal and cardiovascular effects, but central effects such as dyskinesias and mental disturbances may occur earlier in treatment.

◊ The major adverse effects of levodopa are dyskinesia in 75% of patients and psychiatric disturbances in 25%.[1] Nausea and vomiting in 40 to 50% gradually regress and hypotension in 25 to 30% is generally asymptomatic. Other adverse effects include cardiac arrhythmias, particularly atrial and ventricular ectopic beats and less commonly atrial flutter and fibrillation; palpitations and flushing often accompanied by excessive sweating; hypertension; polyuria, incontinence, and urinary retention, although antimuscarinic drugs often contribute to problems with micturition; and dark coloration of the urine and saliva. Rare adverse effects include abdominal pain, constipation, and diarrhoea; mydriasis, blurred vision, diplopia, and precipitation of glaucoma; headache; stridor; tachypnoea; and paraesthesias.

1. Calne DB, Reid JL. Antiparkinsonian drugs: pharmacological and therapeutic aspects. *Drugs* 1972; **4:** 49–74.

Abnormal coloration. Black pigmentation of ribs cartilage has been noted at necropsy in patients treated with levodopa.[1,2] Abnormal pigmentation is generally not seen at other sites[2] but there have been isolated reports[2,3] of patients who also had pigmentation of the intervertebral discs. Although the pigmentation appears to be irreversible it was considered to be probably harmless.[2] It has been suggested that the pigmentation was due to deposition of dihydroxyphenylalanine (DOPA) in the cartilage.[1] It is known that DOPA will readily auto-oxidise *in vitro* in the presence of oxygen to a black pigment and this can also happen *in vivo* since black urine is a well known side-effect of levodopa therapy. Dark sweat and pigmentation of the skin and teeth are also side-effects known to the manufacturers of levodopa.
See also Effects on the Skin and Hair, below.

1. Connolly CE, *et al.* Black cartilage associated with levodopa. *Lancet* 1986; **i:** 690.
2. Rausing A, Rosén U. Black cartilage after therapy with levodopa and methyldopa. *Arch Pathol Lab Med* 1994; **118:** 531–5.
3. Keen CE. *BMJ* 1998; **316:** 240.

Dysgeusia. A change in taste sensation was reported[1] in one study by 23 of 514 patients treated with levodopa in association with a peripheral dopa-decarboxylase inhibitor; 2 of the 23 had total loss of taste initially. The altered taste was often described as insipid, metallic, or plastic, was first observed 3 to 32 weeks after beginning treatment, and lasted for 2 to 40 weeks. In an earlier report 22 of 100 patients receiving levodopa alone had experienced changes in taste.[2]

1. Siegfried J, Zumstein H. Changes in taste under L-DOPA therapy. *Z Neurol* 1971; **200:** 345–8.
2. Barbeau A. L-DOPA therapy: past, present and future. *Ariz Med* 1970; **27:** 1–4.

Effects on the blood. Reports of effects of levodopa on the blood are mostly confined to individual case reports. One study in 365 patients, receiving levodopa in a mean daily dosage of 4.04 g, found that 32 developed a positive direct Coombs' test, the majority after between 3 and 12 months of therapy, but none developed haemolytic anaemia.[1] However, occasional cases of auto-immune haemolytic anaemia have been reported;[2-4] in one case dosage reduction and concurrent administration of a peripheral dopa-decarboxylase inhibitor largely abolished haemolysis,[3] but in another report haemolysis recurred on re-institution of levodopa with carbidopa and required corticosteroid treatment.[4] A case of severe acute non-haemolytic anaemia related to levodopa therapy has also been reported.[5]

Although levodopa is widely stated to produce leucopenia in some patients, there are few published reports. However transient minor decreases in total leucocyte counts were reported in 3 of a group of 80 patients receiving levodopa.[6]

There is also a report of severe thrombocytopenia in a patient who had received levodopa for 3 years;[7] the condition was apparently an auto-immune response and responded to prednisone therapy.

1. Joseph C. Occurrence of positive Coombs test in patients treated with levodopa. *N Engl J Med* 1972; **286:** 1401–2.
2. Territo MC, *et al.* Autoimmune hemolytic anemia due to levodopa therapy. *JAMA* 1973; **226:** 1347–8.
3. Lindström FD, *et al.* Dose-related levodopa-induced haemolytic anaemia. *Ann Intern Med* 1977; **86:** 298–300.

---

4. Bernstein RM. Reversible haemolytic anaemia after levodopa-carbidopa. *BMJ* 1979; **1:** 1461–2.
5. Alkalay I, Zipoli T. Levodopa-induced acute non-hemolytic anemia. *Ann Allergy* 1977; **39:** 191.
6. Barbeau A. L-Dopa therapy in Parkinson's disease: a critical review of nine years' experience. *Can Med Assoc J* 1969; **101:** 791–800.
7. Wanamaker WM, *et al.* Thrombocytopenia associated with long-term levodopa therapy. *JAMA* 1976; **235:** 2217–19.

Effects on the cardiovascular system. There have been conflicting reports on the effects of peripheral dopa-decarboxylase inhibitors on orthostatic hypotension attributed to levodopa therapy. Calne *et al.*[1] found supine and erect systolic blood pressure to be significantly higher in parkinsonian patients given levodopa in association with carbidopa than in those receiving levodopa alone and suggested that the peripheral actions of dopamine contribute to levodopa-induced hypotension. However, Leibowitz and Lieberman[2] found no change in the incidence and degree of orthostatic hypotension after levodopa in association with carbidopa and, similarly, no difference in the frequency of ventricular arrhythmias.

See also Effects on Kidney Function, below and Cardiovascular Disorders, under Precautions, below.

1. Calne DB, *et al.* Action of L-α-methyldopahydrazine on the blood pressure of patients receiving levodopa. *Br J Pharmacol* 1972; **44:** 162–4
2. Leibowitz M, Lieberman A. Comparison of dopa decarboxylase inhibitor (carbidopa) combined with levodopa and levodopa alone on the cardiovascular system of patients with Parkinson's disease. *Neurology* 1975; **25:** 917–21.

Effects on electrolytes. See under Effects on Kidney Function, below.

Effects on the endocrine system. Single doses of levodopa cause an increase in plasma concentrations of glucose, insulin, and glucagon, as well as of growth hormone, when given to healthy subjects[1] and there has been concern over the potential endocrine effects of levodopa therapy in patients with Parkinson's disease.[2] A study of carbohydrate metabolism in 24 patients with Parkinson's disease indicated that these patients had abnormally low rates of glucose utilisation when untreated, apparently due to impaired insulin release, and this was not altered when levodopa therapy was given.[3] However, a similar study completed by 19 patients[2] noted increased impairment of glucose utilisation following levodopa therapy for 1 year with a delayed hypersecretion of insulin in response to a glucose load similar to the metabolic changes of acromegaly. It was considered that patients receiving levodopa for parkinsonism should be monitored for evidence of diabetes mellitus or frank acromegaly.[2]

Postmenopausal bleeding occurred in varying degrees in 12 of 47 women treated with levodopa.[4] In one case bleeding was severe enough to warrant interrupting treatment and subsequent dosage reduction.

1. Rayfield EJ, *et al.* L-Dopa stimulation of glucagon secretion in man. *N Engl J Med* 1975; **293:** 589–91.
2. Sirtori CR, *et al.* Metabolic responses to acute and chronic L-dopa administration in patients with parkinsonism. *N Engl J Med* 1972; **287:** 729–33.
3. Van Woert MH, Mueller PS. Glucose, insulin, and free fatty acid metabolism in Parkinson's disease treated with levodopa. *Clin Pharmacol Ther* 1971; **12:** 360–7.
4. Wajsbort J. Post-menopause bleeding after L-dopa. *N Engl J Med* 1972; **286:** 784.

Effects on the eyes. Both miosis[1] and mydriasis[2] have been reported with levodopa.

For a report of the exacerbation of oculogyric crises by levodopa, see under Extrapyramidal Effects, below.

1. Spiers ASD, *et al.* Miosis during L-dopa therapy. *BMJ* 1970; **2:** 639–40.
2. Weintraub MI, *et al.* Pupillary effects of levodopa therapy: development of anisocoria in latent Horner's syndrome. *N Engl J Med* 1970; **283:** 120–3.

Effects on the gastrointestinal tract. Although gastrointestinal bleeding has more commonly been reported in patients with a history of peptic ulceration there is a rare report[1] of acute melaena and non-specific gastritis associated with levodopa therapy in a 56-year-old man without any previous evidence of a gastric disorder.

See also Dysgeusia, above.

1. Riddoch D. Gastritis and L-dopa. *BMJ* 1972; **1:** 53–4.

Effects on kidney function. Administration of levodopa 1 to 2 g to 7 patients with idiopathic or postencephalitic Parkinson's disease produced significant increments in renal plasma flow, glomerular filtration rate, and sodium and potassium excretion.[1] It was considered that the natriuretic effects could contribute to the orthostatic hypotension commonly noted in patients receiving levodopa. There is a report of a patient who developed hyponatraemia when treated with levodopa with carbidopa.[2] The patient had previously had a similar reaction when given amantadine. On each occasion symptoms disappeared when dopaminergic medication was withdrawn and recurred on rechallenge. Inappropriate secretion of antidiuretic hormone was suggested as a possible mechanism.

Levodopa has also been reported to have a kaliuretic effect, resulting in hypokalaemia, in some parkinsonian patients;[3] the effect could be prevented by concomitant administration of a peripheral dopa-decarboxylase inhibitor.

1. Finlay GD, *et al.* Augmentation of sodium and potassium excretion, glomerular filtration rate and renal plasma flow by levodopa. *N Engl J Med* 1971; **284:** 865–70.

2. Lammers GJ, Roos RAC. Hyponatraemia due to amantadine hydrochloride and L-dopa/carbidopa. *Lancet* 1993; **342:** 439.
3. Granérus A-K, *et al.* Kaliuretic effect of L-dopa treatment in parkinsonian patients. *Acta Med Scand* 1977; **201:** 291–7.

Effects on mental function. Psychiatric complications were the single commonest reason for stopping levodopa treatment in a follow-up study of 178 patients with idiopathic Parkinson's disease, 81 of whom were still taking levodopa after 6 years.[1] Within 2 years levodopa was withdrawn because of toxic confusional states (21 patients), paranoid psychosis (6), unipolar depression (2), and mania (1). The incidence of visual hallucinations increased as treatment continued but, as with toxic confusional states, patients generally improved when levodopa was withdrawn. Before treatment 40 patients had suffered severe depression and levodopa produced sustained improvement in only 2. After 6 years, 20 of the 81 patients remaining were moderately or severely depressed and were rarely improved by withdrawal or reduction in dosage of levodopa. Increasing dementia affected 26 of the 81 patients after 6 years; withdrawal of levodopa in 5 failed to improve cognitive disabilities, but increased parkinsonism.

Another study[2] reported that 141 of 400 patients being treated for Parkinson's disease developed mental disorders. In this study certain acute states, particularly anxiety, on-off hallucinations, and fits of delirium were linked to treatment with levodopa, whereas dementia and depression were not.

Sleep-related complaints have occurred and were reported by 74 of 100 patients with Parkinson's disease.[3] All 74 were on levodopa and the prevalence of symptoms increased with the duration of treatment. Symptoms included insomnia, excessive daytime somnolence, altered dream phenomena, nocturnal vocalisation, involuntary myoclonic movements, and rarely, sleep walking. Sleep fragmentation, which includes insomnia and somnolence, was the most common symptom overall. It has been suggested[4] that in patients with mild to moderate disease levodopa and dopamine agonists could cause sleep disruption. However, these drugs produce beneficial effects on nocturnal disabilities in patients with more severe disease. Reports[5-8] of daytime somnolence with various other dopamine agonists, including bromocriptine, lisuride, pergolide, piribedil, pramipexole, and ropinirole, suggest that this may be a class effect of dopaminergic antiparkinsonian therapy.

1. Shaw KM, *et al.* The impact of treatment with levodopa on Parkinson's disease. *Q J Med* 1980; **49:** 283–93.
2. Rondot P, *et al.* Mental disorders in Parkinson's disease after treatment with L-dopa. *Adv Neurol* 1984; **40:** 259–69.
3. Nausieda PA, *et al.* Psychiatric complications of levodopa therapy of Parkinson's disease. *Adv Neurol* 1984; **40:** 271–7.
4. van Hilten B, *et al.* Sleep disruption in Parkinson's disease: assessment by continuous activity monitoring. *Arch Neurol* 1994; **51:** 922–8.
5. Frucht S, *et al.* Falling asleep at the wheel: motor vehicle mishaps in persons taking pramipexole and ropinirole. *Neurology* 1999; **52:** 1908–10.
6. Schapira AHV. Sleep attacks (sleep episodes) with pergolide. *Lancet* 2000; **355:** 1332–3.
7. Ferreira JJ, *et al.* Sleep attacks and Parkinson's disease treatment. *Lancet* 2000; **355:** 1333–4.
8. Pirker W, Happe S. Sleep attacks in Parkinson's disease. *Lancet* 2000; **356:** 597–8.

Effects on respiration. Respiratory crises, including attacks of gasping, panting, sniffing, puffing, and breath-holding, occurred in 12 of 25 patients with postencephalitic parkinsonism during treatment with levodopa.[1] A further 8 developed respiratory and phonatory tics, including sudden deep breaths, yawns, coughs, giggles, sighing, grunting, and moaning. All 20 patients also suffered tachypnoea, bradypnoea, and asymmetrical movement of both sides of the chest, paradoxical diaphragmatic movements, and reversal of inspiratory and expiratory phases. The induction of respiratory crises may be prompt or greatly delayed; 3 patients only developed crises after more than 9 months of treatment with levodopa. Crises were readily precipitated by psychophysiological arousals such as rage and exertion. Most of the patients who developed marked respiratory disorders had shown slight irregularities of respiratory rhythm, rate, and force before receiving levodopa.

In another report a distressing dose-related irregularity in the rate and depth of breathing occurred when a patient with Parkinson's disease was given levodopa with benserazide.[2] The respiratory abnormality was completely suppressed by concomitant administration of tiapride, with no reduction in the beneficial effect of levodopa.

1. Sacks OW, *et al.* Side-effects of L-dopa in postencephalitic parkinsonism. *Lancet* 1970; **i:** 1006.
2. De Keyser J, Vincken W. L-Dopa-induced respiratory disturbance in Parkinson's disease suppressed by tiapride. *Neurology* 1985; **35:** 235–7.

Effects on sexual function. An increase in libido, over and above the effects of improved mobility and well-being, has been reported in parkinsonian patients receiving levodopa. One group of workers noted increased libido but no improvement in sexual performance in 4 of 80 patients[1] while another group reported a moderate increase in sexual interest in 4 of 7 male patients.[2] Reports of extreme hypersexuality are rare and include one patient receiving levodopa and bromocriptine who may have been abusing the drugs.[3] Hypersexual behaviour and hypergenitalism has also been reported in a pre-pubertal boy given levodopa for behaviour disturbances.[4]

1. Barbeau A. L-Dopa therapy in Parkinson's disease: a critical review of nine years' experience. *Can Med Assoc J* 1969; **101:** 791–9.

2. Brown E, *et al.* Sexual function and affect in parkinsonian men treated with L-dopa. *Am J Psychiatry* 1978; **135:** 1552–5.
3. Vogel HP, Schiffter R. Hypersexuality—a complication of dopaminergic therapy in Parkinson's disease. *Pharmacopsychiatry* 1983; **16:** 107–10.
4. Korten JJ, *et al.* Undesirable prepubertal effects of levodopa. *JAMA* 1973; **226:** 355.

Effects on the skin and hair. Two women who were given levodopa, up to 3 g daily, developed diffuse alopecia in addition to other adverse effects.[1] Repigmentation of hair has occurred in a white-bearded man after being treated with levodopa 1.5 g daily for 8 months.[2] Vitiligo has been reported[3] in a patient with Parkinson's disease following addition of tolcapone to his levodopa/carbidopa regimen. The development of vitiligo was attributed to the increase in plasma-levodopa concentrations brought about by concomitant tolcapone administration.

See also Melanoma, under Precautions, below.

1. Marshall A, Williams MJ. Alopecia and levodopa. *BMJ* 1971; **2:** 47.
2. Grainger KM. Pigmentation in Parkinson's disease treated with levodopa. *Lancet* 1973; **i:** 97–8.
3. Sabaté M, *et al.* Vitiligo associated with tolcapone and levodopa in a patient with Parkinson's disease. *Ann Pharmacother* 1999; **33:** 1228–9.

Extrapyramidal effects. Choreiform movements were the major dose-limiting complication of long-term treatment with levodopa in a follow-up study of 178 patients with idiopathic Parkinson's disease, 81 of whom were still taking levodopa after 6 years.[1] Dyskinesias usually appeared in the first year and became more severe and generalised with time. Certain distinctive patterns of involuntary movement occurred as follows: peak-dose movements affected 65 of the 81 patients and were dose-related. Movements were usually choreic, affecting the face and limbs, but dystonic and ballistic movements were also seen; characteristically they began 20 to 90 minutes after an oral dose and lasted from 10 minutes to 4 hours with a tendency to be more severe mid-way through the interdose period; biphasic movements presenting as 2 distinct episodes of chorea or dystonia within each interdose period occurred in only 3 patients; early morning and 'end-of-dose' dystonia was present in 15 patients after 6 years of treatment with levodopa, but rarely developed during the first 3 years; nocturnal myoclonus occurred in 12 patients. The frequency, intensity, and complexity of spontaneous fluctuations in performance were greatly enhanced by long-term levodopa therapy. Two clinically distinct types of fluctuation, 'end-of-dose' deterioration and the 'on-off' phenomenon, were related to treatment. 'End-of-dose' deterioration or the 'wearing-off' effect affected 52 patients after 6 years of treatment and was characterised by progressive reduction in the duration of benefit from each dose together with a gradual return of nocturnal and early morning disability in some patients. The 'on-off' phenomenon affected 14 patients who experienced completely unpredictable swings from relative mobility, usually accompanied by involuntary movements, to periods of profound bradykinesia and hypotonia. In addition, 'freezing episodes' and abrupt falls became increasingly common and affected 50 patients after 6 years compared with 33 before therapy.

1. Shaw KM, *et al.* The impact of treatment with levodopa on Parkinson's disease. *Q J Med* 1980; **49:** 283–93.

OCULOGYRIC CRISIS. After initial remission, oculogyric crises in 5 of 25 patients with postencephalitic parkinsonism recurred and were subsequently severely exacerbated during treatment with levodopa.[1] One patient, who previously had not had oculogyric crises, developed severe crises in the fourth month of therapy with levodopa. During these crises forced gaze deviation was always accompanied by severe neurological and mental symptoms, some of which were scarcely tolerable.

1. Sacks OW, Kohl M. L-Dopa and oculogyric crises. *Lancet* 1970; **ii:** 215–16.

Gout. There have been reports of elevated serum uric acid concentrations in patients receiving levodopa, but some of these are of doubtful significance since levodopa has been shown to give falsely-elevated uric acid concentrations in colorimetric methods.[1] However, hyperuricaemia as measured by more specific methods,[2,3] with a few cases of overt gout,[2,3] has also been reported.

1. Cawein MJ, Hewins J. False rise in serum uric acid after L-dopa. *N Engl J Med* 1969; **281:** 1489–90.
2. Honda H, Gindin RA. Gout while receiving levodopa for parkinsonism. *JAMA* 1972; **219:** 55–7.
3. Calne DB, Fermaglich J. Gout induced by L-dopa and decarboxylase inhibitors. *Postgrad Med J* 1976; **52:** 232–3.

Hypersensitivity. Reports of hypersensitivity reactions to levodopa have included a vasculitis characterised by neuromyopathy, periarteriolitis with eosinophilia,[1] and a lupus-like auto-immune syndrome.[2]

1. Wolf S, *et al.* Neuromyopathy and periarteriolitis in a patient receiving levodopa. *Arch Intern Med* 1976; **136:** 1055–7.
2. Massarotti G, *et al.* Lupus-like autoimmune syndrome after levodopa and benserazide. *BMJ* 1979; **2:** 553.

Overdosage. Adverse effects following ingestion of 80 to 100 g of levodopa over a 12-hour period by a parkinsonian patient included hypertension initially, followed by hypotension of a few hours' duration, sinus tachycardia, and symptomatic postural hypotension for more than a week.[1] Marked confusion, agitation, insomnia, and restlessness were the most prominent clinical symptoms and did not disappear completely for over a week; severe anorexia and insomnia persisted for 2 to 3 weeks. After the overdose the patient had virtually no signs of parkinsonism and received no levodopa or antimuscarinic medication for 6 days; rigidity and akinesia began to recur on the fourth day.

1. Hoehn MM, Rutledge CO. Acute overdose with levodopa: clinical and biochemical consequences. *Neurology* 1975; **25**: 792–4.

Withdrawal syndromes. There are several reports implicating the withdrawal of levodopa in the development of a syndrome resembling the neuroleptic malignant syndrome,[1-4] characterised by fever, muscle rigidity, profuse sweating, tachycardia, tachypnoea, and elevated muscle enzyme values.[1] Several fatalities have occurred.[1,2] It has been suggested that the neuroleptic malignant syndrome is associated with blockade of dopamine receptors in the striatum, leading to increased rigidity and heat production, and in the hypothalamus, resulting in impaired thermoregulation[5] and it seems reasonable that withdrawal of levodopa might have a similar effect in patients with depleted central dopamine concentrations. Thus, the use of a 'drug holiday' to manage fluctuations in response to levodopa (see under Parkinsonism, p.1160) is no longer recommended.

Fever, extrapyramidal symptoms and raised creatine kinase concentrations, resembling a very mild form of the neuroleptic malignant syndrome, have also been reported in parkinsonian patients exposed to stress such as dehydration or infection but without any change in medication.[6]

1. Friedman JH, *et al.* A neuroleptic malignantlike syndrome due to levodopa therapy withdrawal. *JAMA* 1985; **254**: 2792–5.
2. Sechi GP, *et al.* Fatal hyperpyrexia after withdrawal of levodopa. *Neurology* 1984; **34**: 249–51.
3. Figà-Talamanca L, *et al.* Hyperthermia after discontinuance of levodopa and bromocriptine therapy: impaired dopamine receptors a possible cause. *Neurology* 1985; **35**: 258–61.
4. Gibb WRG, Griffith DNW. Levodopa withdrawal syndrome identical to neuroleptic malignant syndrome. *Postgrad Med J* 1986; **62**: 59–60.
5. Henderson VW, Wooten GF. Neuroleptic malignant syndrome: a pathogenetic role for dopamine receptor blockade? *Neurology* 1981; **31**: 132–7.
6. Mezaki T, *et al.* Benign type of malignant syndrome. *Lancet* 1989; **i**: 49–50.

Treatment of Adverse Effects

Reduction in dosage reverses most of the side-effects of levodopa. Nausea and vomiting may be diminished by increasing the dose of levodopa gradually, and/or by taking with or after meals, although taking levodopa on a full stomach may lead to lower plasma concentrations. Gastrointestinal effects may also be reduced by giving an antiemetic such as cyclizine hydrochloride or domperidone but not a phenothiazine (see Antipsychotics, under Interactions, below). Administration with a peripheral dopa-decarboxylase inhibitor reduces peripheral but not central side-effects. Orthostatic hypotension may respond to the use of elastic stockings.

If acute overdosage occurs the stomach should be emptied by lavage and supportive measures instituted. Pyridoxine may reverse some effects of levodopa (see under Interactions, below) but its value in overdosage has not been established; it does not reverse the effects of levodopa given with a peripheral dopa-decarboxylase inhibitor.

Nausea and vomiting. For reference to the use of domperidone in the management of nausea and vomiting associated with levodopa in patients with Parkinson's disease, see under Uses and Administration of Domperidone, p.1224.

Psychosis. Atypical antipsychotics such as clozapine (p.673) have been tried in the management of psychosis occurring as a complication of parkinsonism and of drugs like levodopa used in its treatment.

Precautions

Levodopa is contra-indicated in patients with angle-closure glaucoma and should be used with caution in open-angle glaucoma. Caution is also required in patients with cardiovascular disease, pulmonary disease, endocrine disorders, psychiatric disturbances, osteomalacia, or a history of peptic ulceration. Periodic evaluations of hepatic, psychiatric, haematological, renal, and cardiovascular functions have been advised.

Since an association between levodopa and activation of malignant melanoma has been suspected (although not confirmed), it is generally recommended that levodopa should not be given to patients with (or with a history of) the disease or with skin disorders suggestive of it.

Parkinsonian patients who benefit from levodopa therapy should be warned to resume normal activities gradually to avoid the risk of injury. Treatment with levodopa should not be stopped abruptly.

Levodopa inhibits prolactin secretion and may therefore interfere with lactation.

Food interferes with the absorption of levodopa, though levodopa is usually given with or immediately after meals to reduce nausea and vomiting. However, patients experiencing the 'on-off' phenomenon may benefit from administration on an empty stomach (see under Parkinsonism, p.1160).

Abuse. Several cases of abuse of levodopa in patients with Parkinson's disease have been reported.[1,2] Patients had progressively increased the dosage of levodopa to obtain psychotropic effects such as euphoria despite accompanying dystonia and other extrapyramidal adverse effects. Discontinuation often led to craving, drug-seeking behaviour, and mood disturbances such as depression, features resembling a psychological dependence syndrome.

1. Nausieda PA. Sinemet "abusers". *Clin Neuropharmacol* 1985; **8**: 318–27.
2. Soyka M, Huppert D. L-dopa abuse in a patient with former alcoholism. *Br J Addict* 1992; **87**: 117–18.

Cardiovascular disorders. A high incidence of cardiovascular side-effects was reported in early studies of levodopa, although both Parkinson's disease and heart disease are common in the elderly and adverse cardiac effects of levodopa may be less prevalent than was first thought. A study in 40 patients[1] concluded that, apart from those with severe postural hypotension or unstable coronary disease, levodopa may be used safely in parkinsonian patients with heart disease. Others[2] noted that levodopa and bromocriptine cause cardiac arrhythmias in less than 1% of all patients, the incidence for levodopa in association with a peripheral dopa-decarboxylase inhibitor being lower still. Nevertheless, caution is advised in patients with cardiovascular disease.

1. Jenkins RB, *et al.* Levodopa therapy of patients with parkinsonism and heart disease. *BMJ* 1972; **3**: 512–14.
2. Parkes JD, *et al.* Amantadine-induced heart failure. *Lancet* 1977; **i**: 904.

Diabetes mellitus. For reference to concern over the potential of levodopa to impair glucose utilisation, see Effects on the Endocrine System under Adverse Effects, above.

Melanoma. There has been concern over the effects of levodopa on melanoma in view of the ability of malignant melanoma cells to convert levodopa to melanin and isolated reports of melanoma developing or being exacerbated during levodopa therapy continue to appear.[1] However, in a survey of 1099 patients with primary cutaneous malignant melanoma only one had taken levodopa.[2] It was concluded that levodopa therapy is not an important factor in the induction of malignant melanoma. Furthermore, administration of levodopa in daily doses of up to 4 g with carbidopa to 17 patients with metastatic melanoma failed to provide any evidence that levodopa accelerated the progression of the disease.[3] A review[4] of these and later reports concluded that the purported link between levodopa and malignant melanoma was tenuous.

For a report of antineoplastic chemotherapy used for the treatment of melanoma reducing the efficacy of levodopa, see under Interactions, below.

1. Haider SA, Thaller VT. Lid melanoma and parkinsonism. *Br J Ophthalmol* 1992; **76**: 246–7.
2. Sober AJ, Wick MM. Levodopa therapy and malignant melanoma. *JAMA* 1978; **240**: 554–5.
3. Gurney H, *et al.* The use of L-dopa and carbidopa in metastatic malignant melanoma. *J Invest Dermatol* 1991; **96**: 85–7.
4. Siple JF, *et al.* Levodopa therapy and the risk of malignant melanoma. *Ann Pharmacother* 2000; **34**: 382–5.

Pregnancy. Levodopa alone and with carbidopa has been associated with fetal abnormalities in *animals* given high doses; no teratogenic effect has been noted with carbidopa alone. However, 2 women with parkinsonism who received levodopa with carbidopa or levodopa alone throughout their pregnancies gave birth to normal infants.[1]

1. Cook DG, Klawans HL. Levodopa during pregnancy. *Clin Neuropharmacol* 1985; **8**: 93–5.

Withdrawal. For adverse effects associated with withdrawal of levodopa, see under Adverse Effects, above.

Interactions

The therapeutic or adverse effects of levodopa may be affected by interactions with a variety of drugs. Mechanisms may include effects on catecholamine metabolising enzymes, neurotransmitters, or receptor sites, effects on the endocrine system, and effects on gastrointestinal absorption. Drugs which modify gastric emptying may affect the absorption of levodopa.

Antibacterials. A study[1] in 7 healthy subjects showed that administration of *spiramycin* with levodopa and carbidopa re-

sulted in reduced plasma-levodopa concentrations and an increase in its peripheral metabolism.

A hypertensive reaction and severe tremor occurred when *isoniazid* was given to a patient receiving levodopa;[2] it was not certain whether isoniazid was acting as an MAOI.

1. Brion N, *et al.* Effect of a macrolide (spiramycin) on the pharmacokinetics of L-dopa and carbidopa in healthy volunteers. *Clin Neuropharmacol* 1992; **15**: 229–35.
2. Morgan JP. Isoniazid and levodopa. *Ann Intern Med* 1980; **92**: 434.

Antidepressants. BUPROPION. Caution has been advised with bupropion because of reports of a higher incidence of adverse effects during concomitant use with levodopa.

MAOIS. Administration of levodopa with non-specific MAOIs such as *phenelzine*, *pargyline*, *nialamide*, or *tranylcypromine* may cause dangerous hypertension;[1-4] it is recommended that levodopa should not be given within at least 14 days of stopping an MAOI. Teychenne *et al.*[5] found that hypertensive reactions to levodopa with *tranylcypromine* were inhibited by carbidopa, but the manufacturers of preparations containing levodopa with carbidopa or benserazide still contra-indicate the concomitant use of MAOIs. There has also been a warning that hypertensive crises may occur if levodopa is used with *moclobemide*, a monoamine oxidase type A inhibitor. *Selegiline*, a monoamine oxidase type B inhibitor, is used to enhance the antiparkinsonian effect of levodopa, see p.1178.

1. Hunter KR, *et al.* Monoamine oxidase inhibitors and L-dopa. *BMJ* 1970; **3**: 388.
2. Hodge JV. Use of monoamine oxidase inhibitors. *Lancet* 1965; **i**: 764–5.
3. Friend DG, *et al.* The action of L-dihydroxyphenylalanine in patients receiving nialamide. *Clin Pharmacol Ther* 1965; **6**: 362–6.
4. Sharpe J, *et al.* Idiopathic orthostatic hypotension treated with levodopa and MAO inhibitor: a preliminary report. *Can Med Assoc J* 1972; **107**: 296–300.
5. Teychenne PF, *et al.* Interactions of levodopa with inhibitors of monoamine oxidase and L-aromatic amino acid decarboxylase. *Clin Pharmacol Ther* 1975; **18**: 273–7.

TRICYCLIC ANTIDEPRESSANTS. Although tricyclic antidepressants have been used safely with levodopa[1] hypertensive crises have occurred in patients receiving *amitriptyline* or *imipramine* and levodopa with carbidopa.[2,3] Imipramine has been reported to impair the rate of levodopa absorption,[4] presumably due to its antimuscarinic properties (for the effect of antimuscarinics on the absorption of levodopa, see below).

1. Hunter KR, *et al.* Use of levodopa with other drugs. *Lancet* 1970; **ii**: 1283–5.
2. Rampton DS. Hypertensive crisis in a patient given Sinemet, metoclopramide, and amitriptyline. *BMJ* 1977; **2**: 607–8.
3. Edwards M. Adverse interaction of levodopa with tricyclic antidepressants. *Practitioner* 1982; **226**: 1447–8.
4. Morgan JP, *et al.* Imipramine-mediated interference with levodopa absorption from the gastrointestinal tract in man. *Neurology* 1975; **25**: 1029–34.

TRYPTOPHAN. See Amino Acids under Nutritional Agents, below.

Antiepileptics. *Phenytoin* has been shown to diminish the therapeutic effect of levodopa in patients with parkinsonism or chronic manganese poisoning.[1] The mechanism of the interaction was considered uncertain.

1. Mendez JS. Diphenylhydantoin: blocking of levodopa effects. *Arch Neurol* 1975; **32**: 44–6.

Antihypertensives. Concurrent administration of levodopa with *guanethidine* may cause increased hypotension.[1] *Clonidine* has been reported to inhibit the therapeutic effect of levodopa, possibly by stimulating central alpha-adrenoceptors.[2] *Methyldopa* and levodopa may enhance each other's therapeutic or adverse effects, although there has been mention of the inhibitory effect of methyldopa on the therapeutic response to levodopa.[3,4]

1. Hunter KR, *et al.* Use of levodopa with other drugs. *Lancet* 1970; **ii**: 1283–5.
2. Shoulson I, Chase TN. Clonidine and the anti-parkinsonian response to L-dopa or piribedil. *Neuropharmacology* 1976; **15**: 25–7.
3. Cotzias GC, *et al.* L-Dopa in Parkinson's syndrome. *N Engl J Med* 1969; **281**: 272.
4. Kofman O. Treatment of Parkinson's disease with L-dopa: a current appraisal. *Can Med Assoc J* 1971; **104**: 483–7.

Antimuscarinics. Antimuscarinic antiparkinsonian drugs may enhance the therapeutic effects of levodopa but by delaying gastric emptying they may reduce its absorption.[1]

1. Algeri S, *et al.* Effect of anticholinergic drugs on gastro-intestinal absorption of L-dopa in rats and in man. *Eur J Pharmacol* 1976; **35**: 293–9.

Antineoplastics. A patient with Parkinson's disease noted[1] that the efficacy of levodopa was reduced each time he received *dacarbazine* for the treatment of melanoma. As serum-dopamine concentrations were unchanged it was suggested[1] that dacarbazine might compete with levodopa at the blood-brain barrier.

1. Merello M, *et al.* Impaired levodopa response in Parkinson's disease during melanoma therapy. *Clin Neuropharmacol* 1992; **15**: 69–74.

Antipsychotics. The therapeutic effects of levodopa may be diminished by CNS dopamine inhibitors including phenothiazine derivatives[1] such as *prochlorperazine*.[2] Butyrophenones such as *haloperidol* and thioxanthenes such as *flupentixol* might be expected to have a similar effect due to their antidopaminergic properties.

1. Yahr MD, Duvoisin RC. Drug therapy of parkinsonism. *N Engl J Med* 1972; **287:** 20–4.
2. Duvoisin RC. Diphenidol for levodopa induced nausea and vomiting. *JAMA* 1972; **221:** 1408.

Anxiolytics. Reversible deterioration of parkinsonism has been reported in patients receiving levodopa who were given *benzodiazepines* such as *diazepam*,[1,2] *nitrazepam*[1] (although the evidence was equivocal), or *chlordiazepoxide*.[3] In one case parkinsonian symptoms resolved without alteration in the medication.[1]

1. Hunter KR, *et al.* Use of levodopa with other drugs. *Lancet* 1970; **ii:** 1283–5.
2. Wodak J, *et al.* Review of 12 months' treatment with L-dopa in Parkinson's disease, with remarks on unusual side effects. *Med J Aust* 1972; **2:** 1277–82.
3. Yosselson-Superstine S, Lipman AG. Chlordiazepoxide interaction with levodopa. *Ann Intern Med* 1982; **96:** 259–60.

Baclofen. Adverse effects including hallucinations, confusion, headache, and nausea and worsening of symptoms have been reported[1,2] in patients with Parkinson's disease taking levodopa when given baclofen.

1. Skausig OB, Korsgaard S. Hallucinations and baclofen. *Lancet* 1977; **i:** 1258.
2. Lees AJ, *et al.* Baclofen in Parkinson's disease. *J Neurol Neurosurg Psychiatry* 1978; **41:** 707–8.

Gastrointestinal drugs. ANTACIDS. Some studies have suggested that administration of an antacid before a dose of levodopa enhances the absorption of levodopa, apparently by enhancing gastric emptying and reducing metabolism of levodopa in the stomach.[1,2] This was particularly marked in one case report in a patient with prolonged gastric emptying time.[1] However, another study in 8 patients with presumably normal gastric motility, only 3 of whom had Parkinson's disease, found no significant increase in overall absorption of levodopa when given with an antacid although there was some evidence of increased absorption in one or two of the patients.[3]

1. Rivera-Calimlim L, *et al.* L-Dopa treatment failure: explanation and correction. *BMJ* 1970; **4:** 93–4.
2. Pocelinko R, *et al.* The effect of an antacid on the absorption and metabolism of levodopa. *Clin Pharmacol Ther* 1972; **13:** 149.
3. Leon AS, Spiegel HE. The effect of antacid administration on the absorption and metabolism of levodopa. *J Clin Pharmacol* 1972; **12:** 263–7.

ANTIEMETICS. *Metoclopramide* accelerates gastric emptying and has been reported to increase the rate of levodopa absorption.[1] The importance of timing has been noted[2] since levodopa delayed gastric emptying and metoclopramide antagonised this effect. *Domperidone* has been reported to increase the bioavailability of levodopa slightly.[3]

1. Morris JGL, *et al.* Plasma dopa concentrations after different preparations of levodopa in normal subjects. *Br J Clin Pharmacol* 1971; **3:** 983–90.
2. Berkowitz DM, McCallum RW. Interaction of levodopa and metoclopramide on gastric emptying. *Clin Pharmacol Ther* 1980; **27:** 414–20.
3. Shindler JS, *et al.* Domperidone and levodopa in Parkinson's disease. *Br J Clin Pharmacol* 1984; **18:** 959–62.

PROKINETICS. Maximum plasma concentrations of levodopa are increased by concomitant administration of *cisapride*.[1]

See also Metoclopramide and Domperidone, under Antiemetics, above.

1. Neira WD, *et al.* The effects of cisapride on plasma L-dopa levels and the clinical response in Parkinson's disease. *Mov Disord* 1995; **10:** 66–70.

General anaesthetics. The general anaesthetics *cyclopropane* and *halothane* lower the threshold for ventricular arrhythmias to sympathomimetic amines, including dopamine, and should probably not be used within 6 to 8 hours of the administration of levodopa.[1,2] Although other general anaesthetics are now usually preferred, it was suggested that in any case, levodopa could safely be used before surgery when given with a peripheral dopa-decarboxylase inhibitor.[3]

1. Goldberg LI, Whitsett TL. Cardiovascular effects of levodopa. *Clin Pharmacol Ther* 1971; **12:** 376–82.
2. Bianchine JR, Sunyapridakul L. Interactions between levodopa and other drugs: significance in the treatment of Parkinson's disease. *Drugs* 1973; **6:** 364–88.
3. Anonymous. Surgery and long-term medication. *Drug Ther Bull* 1984; **22:** 73–6.

Nutritional agents. AMINO ACIDS. Daniel *et al.* reported that transport of levodopa into the brain is subject to competition from chemically related L-amino acids, especially the other aromatic amino acids *phenylalanine, tyrosine, tryptophan*, and *histidine*.[1] Later, Nutt *et al.* demonstrated that a high-protein diet or the large neutral amino acids phenylalanine, *leucine*, or *isoleucine* reduced the therapeutic effect of levodopa given by intravenous infusion to parkinsonian patients and concluded that alterations in the absorption and transport of levodopa may contribute to the fluctuating responses seen in Parkinson's disease, the so-called 'on-off' phenomenon[2] (see also under Parkinsonism, p.1160). Other reported interactions with amino acids include *methionine*-antagonism of the therapeutic effect of levodopa in parkinsonism[3] and *tryptophan*-reduced blood concentrations of levodopa.[4]

1. Daniel PM, *et al.* Do changes in blood levels of other aromatic aminoacids influence levodopa therapy? *Lancet* 1976; **i:** 95.
2. Nutt JG, *et al.* The "on-off" phenomenon in Parkinson's disease: relation to levodopa absorption and transport. *N Engl J Med* 1984; **310:** 483–8.

3. Pearce LA, Waterbury LD. L-methionine: a possible levodopa antagonist. *Neurology* 1974; **24:** 640–1.
4. Weitbrecht W-U, Weigel K. Der Einfluß von L-Tryptophan auf die L-Dopa-Resorption. *Dtsch Med Wochenschr* 1976; **101:** 20–2.

IRON SALTS. Levodopa forms complexes with iron salts and administration with ferrous sulfate has reduced bioavailability of levodopa by about 50% in healthy subjects.[1] Administration of ferrous sulfate to 9 patients with Parkinson's disease receiving levodopa with carbidopa reduced the area under the curve by 30% and greater than 75% for levodopa and carbidopa respectively. Although this was associated with deterioration in some patients' disability the average reduction in efficacy of therapy did not achieve statistical significance.[2]

1. Campbell NRC, Hasinoff BB. Iron supplements: a common cause of drug interactions. *Br J Clin Pharmacol* 1991; **31:** 251–5.
2. Campbell NRC, *et al.* Sinemet-ferrous sulphate interaction in patients with Parkinson's disease. *Br J Clin Pharmacol* 1990; **30:** 599–605.

PYRIDOXINE. The enzyme responsible for the decarboxylation of levodopa, L-amino acid decarboxylase, is dependent on pyridoxine and pyridoxine supplements have been reported to enhance the peripheral metabolism of levodopa to dopamine leaving less available to cross the blood-brain barrier for central conversion to dopamine;[1-4] pyridoxine therefore inhibits the action of levodopa but this can be stopped by concurrent administration of a peripheral dopa-decarboxylase inhibitor.[3,4]

1. Carter AB. Pyridoxine and parkinsonism. *BMJ* 1973; **4:** 236.
2. Leon AS. Pyridoxine antagonism of levodopa in parkinsonism. *JAMA* 1971; **218:** 1924–7.
3. Cotzias GC, Papavasiliou PS. Blocking the negative effects of pyridoxine on patients receiving levodopa. *JAMA* 1971; **215:** 1504–5.
4. Yahr MD, Duvoisin RC. Pyridoxine, levodopa, and L-α-methyldopa hydrazine regimen in parkinsonism. *JAMA* 1971; **216:** 2141.

Papaverine. Antagonism of the beneficial effects of levodopa in parkinsonism has been reported when patients were also given papaverine,[1,2] and it was recommended that the combination should be avoided.

1. Duvoisin RC. Antagonism of levodopa by papaverine. *JAMA* 1975; **231:** 845.
2. Posner DM. Antagonism of levodopa by papaverine. *JAMA* 1975; **233:** 768.

Penicillamine. Isolated case reports suggest that penicillamine increases plasma-levodopa concentrations.[1]

1. Mizuta E, *et al.* Effect of D-penicillamine on pharmacokinetics of levodopa in Parkinson's disease. *Clin Neuropharmacol* 1993; **16:** 448–50.

Sympathomimetics. It has been suggested that sympathomimetics such as *adrenaline [epinephrine]* or *isoprenaline* may enhance the cardiac side-effects of levodopa.[1]

1. Goldberg LI, Whitsett TL. Cardiovascular effects of levodopa. *Clin Pharmacol Ther* 1971; **12:** 376–82.

Pharmacokinetics

Levodopa is rapidly absorbed from the gastrointestinal tract by an active transport system. Most absorption takes place in the small intestine; absorption is very limited from the stomach, and since decarboxylation may take place in the stomach wall, delays in gastric emptying may reduce the amount of levodopa available for absorption.

Levodopa is rapidly decarboxylated by the enzyme aromatic L-amino acid decarboxylase, mostly in the gut, liver, and kidney, to dopamine, which is metabolised in turn, principally to dihydroxyphenylacetic acid (DOPAC) and homovanillic acid (HVA). Other routes of metabolism include *O*-methylation, transamination, and oxidation, producing a variety of minor metabolites including noradrenaline and 3-*O*-methyldopa; the latter may accumulate in the CNS due to its relatively long half-life. The plasma half-life of levodopa itself is reported to be about 1 to 3 hours.

Unlike dopamine, levodopa is actively transported across the blood-brain barrier, but because of the extent of peripheral decarboxylation very little is available to enter the CNS unless it is given in association with a peripheral dopa-decarboxylase inhibitor. In the presence of a peripheral dopa-decarboxylase inhibitor the major route of metabolism of levodopa becomes the formation of 3-*O*-methyldopa by the enzyme catechol-*O*-methyltransferase.

About 80% of an oral dose of levodopa is excreted in the urine within 24 hours, mostly as dihydroxyphenylacetic and homovanillic acids. Only small amounts of levodopa are excreted unchanged in the faeces.

◊ General references.

1. Nutt JG, Fellman JH. Pharmacokinetics of levodopa. *Clin Neuropharmacol* 1984; **7:** 35–49.
2. Cedarbaum JM. Clinical pharmacokinetics of anti-parkinsonian drugs. *Clin Pharmacokinet* 1987; **13:** 141–78.
3. Robertson DRC, *et al.* The effect of age on the pharmacokinetics of levodopa administered alone and in the presence of carbidopa. *Br J Clin Pharmacol* 1989; **28:** 61–9.
4. Robertson DRC, *et al.* The influence of levodopa on gastric emptying in man. *Br J Clin Pharmacol* 1990; **29:** 47–53.

Uses and Administration

Levodopa, a naturally occurring amino acid, is the immediate precursor of the neurotransmitter dopamine. The actions of levodopa are mainly those of dopamine (p.881).

Unlike dopamine, levodopa can readily enter the CNS and is used in the treatment of conditions, such as Parkinson's disease, which are associated with depletion of dopamine in the brain. Levodopa is rapidly decarboxylated so that very little unchanged drug is available to cross the blood-brain barrier for central conversion into dopamine. Consequently levodopa is usually given together with a peripheral dopa-decarboxylase inhibitor such as benserazide (p.1164) or carbidopa (p.1168) to increase the proportion of levodopa that can enter the brain. This enables the dosage of levodopa to be reduced and may diminish peripheral side-effects, such as nausea and vomiting and cardiac arrhythmias, by blocking the peripheral production of dopamine. It may also provide a more rapid response at the start of therapy.

The majority of patients with Parkinson's disease benefit from levodopa therapy, but after 2 or more years improvement in disability is gradually lost as the disease progresses and fluctuations in mobility emerge. Postencephalitic parkinsonism responds to levodopa, but a higher incidence of side-effects has been reported than in the idiopathic form so smaller doses are generally used. Levodopa has also been used to control the neurological symptoms of chronic manganese poisoning, which resemble those of parkinsonism. It should not be used in antipsychotic-induced parkinsonism.

Levodopa has an effect on pituitary function as a result of its conversion to dopamine. It may enhance growth-hormone secretion and has been used diagnostically as a provocative test for growth-hormone deficiency. Levodopa also inhibits prolactin secretion.

Response to levodopa varies considerably between patients. **Treatment of parkinsonism** should commence with small doses increased gradually, ideally to a dose which improves mobility without incurring side-effects. Levodopa should be taken with or after meals, although in later disease, it may be preferable to administer on an empty stomach (see Precautions, above). Once established, maintenance doses may need to be reduced as the patient ages. When given **without a peripheral dopa-decarboxylase inhibitor** (which is rare) a suggested initial dose is 125 mg twice daily by mouth increased gradually every 3 to 7 days, according to response, to up to 8 g daily in divided doses. The intervals between doses should be adjusted to meet individual needs; many patients find 4 or 5 divided doses daily to be satisfactory although some may require smaller, more frequent doses in order to control fluctuations in mobility. Maximum improvement may take up to 6 months or longer to occur.

When given **with a peripheral dopa-decarboxylase inhibitor** lower doses of levodopa are employed. As high central dopamine concentrations can be achieved more quickly, both beneficial and adverse effects tend to occur more rapidly than with levodopa alone and patients should be monitored carefully. In those already receiving levodopa the drug should be discontinued and benserazide or carbidopa with levodopa started on the following day or after 24 hours if the patient was receiving a modified-release preparation of levodopa.

Benserazide hydrochloride is usually given with levodopa in the ratio of 1 part of benserazide base to

4 parts of levodopa (co-beneldopa) and the doses for co-beneldopa that follow are expressed in terms of the levodopa component.

- An initial dose for *patients not previously treated with levodopa* is levodopa 50 mg three or four times daily by mouth increased gradually in increments of levodopa 100 mg once or twice weekly, according to response. For some elderly patients, an initial dose of levodopa 50 mg once or twice daily, increased by 50 mg every third or fourth day, may be suitable. If the disease is at an advanced stage, the initial starting dose may be increased to levodopa 100 mg three times daily. Maintenance doses usually lie within the range of levodopa 400 to 800 mg daily in divided doses, although most patients require no more than 600 mg daily. If optimal improvement has not been achieved after several weeks at the average dose, further increases may be made with caution; it is rarely necessary to give more than 1 g of levodopa daily.

- The initial dose of levodopa given with benserazide in *patients previously treated with levodopa* should be about 10 to 15% of the dose previously being taken, thus levodopa 300 mg would be appropriate for a patient previously taking levodopa 2 g daily. For *patients previously treated with other levodopa/dopa-decarboxylase inhibitor combinations* an initial dose is levodopa 50 mg given three or four times daily.

- Modified-release capsules containing benserazide 25 mg with levodopa 100 mg are available to reduce fluctuations in response to conventional preparations. For *patients not already receiving levodopa* the initial dose is one capsule three times daily adjusted every 2 to 3 days according to response; it is recommended that initial dosages should not exceed 600 mg of levodopa daily. For *patients already receiving a conventional preparation* of levodopa with benserazide, initially one capsule should be substituted for every 100 mg of levodopa and should be given at the same dosage frequency as before; increases in dosage can then be made every 2 to 3 days according to response. An average of 50% more levodopa may be required compared with previous therapy and titration may take up to 4 weeks. *Supplementary doses* of a conventional preparation of benserazide with levodopa may also be required with the first morning dose.

Carbidopa is usually given with levodopa (co-careldopa) as tablets in the ratio of 1 to 4 or 1 to 10, which allows dosage adjustments of either drug for individual patients. Doses of carbidopa are expressed in terms of the anhydrous base. Full inhibition of peripheral dopa-decarboxylase is reported to be achieved by 70 to 100 mg of carbidopa daily.

- A suggested initial dose for *patients not previously treated with levodopa* is carbidopa 25 mg with levodopa 100 mg three times daily by mouth, increased gradually, in increments of carbidopa 12.5 mg with levodopa 50 mg or carbidopa 25 mg with levodopa 100 mg every day or on alternate days, as necessary. The usual maintenance dosage range is carbidopa 75 to 200 mg with levodopa 0.75 to 2 g daily in divided doses. Carbidopa doses greater than 200 mg daily are not generally exceeded.

- The initial dose of levodopa given with carbidopa in *patients previously treated with levodopa* should be about 20 to 25% of the dose previously being taken, thus for patients taking less than 1.5 g of levodopa daily a suggested initial dose is carbidopa 25 mg with levodopa 100 mg given three or four times daily; a suggested initial dose for patients taking more than 1.5 g of levodopa daily is carbidopa 25 mg with levodopa 250 mg given three or four times daily.

- Modified-release tablets containing carbidopa with levodopa in the ratio of 1 to 4 are available to reduce fluctuations in response to conventional preparations. For *patients not already receiving levo-*

dopa therapy, or for those currently receiving levodopa alone, the initial dose is carbidopa 50 mg with levodopa 200 mg twice daily adjusted according to response at intervals of not less than 3 days. It is recommended that for patients who are not already receiving levodopa initial dosages should not exceed 600 mg of levodopa daily. For *patients already receiving a conventional preparation* of carbidopa with levodopa, the initial dose of the modified-release preparation should provide a similar amount of levodopa per day, but the dosing intervals should be prolonged and are normally between 4 to 12 hours. The initial substitution dose of the modified-release preparation should provide not more than 10% more levodopa than was previously given for doses of levodopa greater than 900 mg daily. Doses and intervals may then be altered according to clinical response, allowing at least 3 days between adjustments. Up to 30% more levodopa may be required in the modified-release preparation than was previously administered in the conventional preparation. Average maintenance doses of modified-release preparations lie within the range of carbidopa 100 mg with levodopa 400 mg to carbidopa 400 mg with levodopa 1.6 g. *Supplementary doses* of a conventional preparation of carbidopa with levodopa may be required in some patients.

Chorea. Levodopa usually exacerbates Huntington's disease. It was formerly used as a diagnostic agent to attempt to identify presymptomatic patients at risk of developing Huntington's chorea by provoking chorea. However, this practice has been abandoned, partly because of the distress caused, and also because of false negative results.[1] More accurate non-provocative testing based on genetic markers for the disease is now feasible (see p.650).

1. Marsden CD. Basal ganglia disease. *Lancet* 1982; **ii:** 1141–6.

Drug-induced extrapyramidal disorders. The management of drug-induced extrapyramidal disorders is discussed under the Adverse Effects of Chlorpromazine on p.662. Although the use of dopamine agonists, especially levodopa, to overcome antipsychotic-induced blockade of dopamine receptors might appear rational, levodopa has generally been reported to be ineffective or to increase psychiatric symptoms.

Dysphagia. Results of a small study[1] have suggested that levodopa may improve the impaired swallowing reflex in patients with basal ganglia infarctions and thereby help to prevent aspiration pneumonia.

1. Kobayashi H, *et al.* Levodopa and swallowing reflex. *Lancet* 1996; **348:** 1320–1.

Dystonias. Dystonias and their management have been reviewed.[1-3] A dystonia is a syndrome of sustained muscle contractions, frequently causing twisting and repetitive movements or abnormal postures; it may also have additional myoclonic or tremulous components. Typically it starts as a focal dystonia localised in one part of the body and to begin with may appear only during a specific motor act (action dystonia). If the syndrome is progressive the dystonias may become apparent at rest and spread first to more than one part of the body (segmental dystonia) and may eventually affect most or all of the body (generalised dystonia). Progression of the dystonia appears to be related to age of onset. Dystonia beginning in childhood usually starts in the legs and progresses to become segmental or generalised, whereas in adults the dystonia usually starts in other parts of the body and rarely becomes generalised. Examples of focal dystonias are blepharospasm (affecting the eye and surrounding facial muscles), writer's cramp (hand and arm), spasmodic torticollis (neck), spasmodic dysphonia, or dystonic dysphagia (larynx or pharynx), and leg dystonias. Some dystonias may be associated with metabolic disorders such as Wilson's disease or Lesch-Nyhan syndrome; with neurological disorders such as Huntington's disease; or with other causes including head trauma, manganese or carbon disulfide toxicity, or the side-effects of antipsychotics or antiparkinsonian drugs. However, in the majority of cases the disease is idiopathic.

There are no cures for most types of dystonia, but symptomatic relief is possible in many patients. It has been suggested that all children and adolescents presenting with dystonia, particularly starting in the legs, should first be given a trial with levodopa.[2] A suggested regimen is to gradually build up to a dose of levodopa 200 mg with carbidopa 50 mg given three times daily and to maintain this dose for three months; if there is no useful response in this period the drug is withdrawn. Where there is benefit it is usually dramatic and is sustained as long as the drug is taken, which may be more than 10 years in some cases, in general without the long-term problems associated with levodopa for parkinsonism (see p.1160).

In children and adolescents who fail to respond to levodopa an antimuscarinic such as benzhexol [trihexyphenidyl] is second

choice. Side-effects are minimised by starting with a low dose which is then gradually increased. General experience indicates that about half of all children and adolescents benefit from antimuscarinics; adults tolerate the drug less well and only about a fifth of adult patients with focal dystonia benefit.

In patients who do not respond to levodopa or high-dose antimuscarinics other drugs may be used. Many benefit from benzodiazepines such as diazepam; a few have responded to baclofen or carbamazepine. Antipsychotics are sometimes useful but carry the risk of inducing tardive dyskinesia. Tetrabenazine carries less risk of tardive dyskinesia but may induce depression. In very severe dystonia combination therapy may be required: tetrabenazine with pimozide and benzhexol [trihexyphenidyl] is sometimes effective.

The response in patients with adult onset focal dystonia is usually poor. However, the use of botulinum A toxin can produce relief in blepharospasm, spasmodic torticollis, and spasmodic dysphonia, and is under investigation for writer's cramp and other occupational dystonias. Local injections into the affected muscles produce weakness over the next week or so, thereby reducing or abolishing dystonic spasms. The effect lasts some 2 to 4 months.

Further details of the management of blepharospasm and spasmodic torticollis can be found under Botulinum Toxins on p.1325. For a discussion of the management of antipsychotic-induced dystonic reactions, see under Extrapyramidal Disorders in the Adverse Effects of Chlorpromazine on p.662.

1. Anonymous. Dystonia: underdiagnosed and undertreated? *Drug Ther Bull* 1988; **26:** 33–6.
2. Marsden CD, Quinn NP. The dystonias. *BMJ* 1990; **300:** 139–44.
3. Williams A. Consensus statement for the management of focal dystonias. *Br J Hosp Med* 1993; **50:** 655–9.

Neuroleptic malignant syndrome. There have been isolated reports[1-4] that levodopa used alone or with bromocriptine has been successful in the treatment of patients with neuroleptic malignant syndrome (p.662). However, bromocriptine is usually preferred when a dopaminergic is required for the treatment of this condition.

1. Knezevic W, *et al.* Neuroleptic malignant syndrome. *Med J Aust* 1984; **140:** 28–30.
2. Clarke CE, *et al.* Clinical spectrum of neuroleptic malignant syndrome. *Lancet* 1988; **ii:** 969–70.
3. Lo TCN, *et al.* Neuroleptic malignant syndrome: another medical cause of acute abdomen. *Postgrad Med J* 1989; **65:** 653–5.
4. Shoop SA, Cernek PK. Carbidopa/levodopa in the treatment of neuroleptic malignant syndrome. *Ann Pharmacother* 1997; **31:** 119.

Parasomnias. The aetiology of *restless legs syndrome* and *periodic limb movements in sleep* is obscure and treatment has been largely empirical (p.653). Few of the treatments tried in these often co-existent disorders have been studied in a controlled manner but small controlled studies[1-6] have reported beneficial effects such as improved sleep quality and reduced leg movements from levodopa used with a peripheral dopa-decarboxylase inhibitor. Most patients received a bedtime dose of 50 to 200 mg of levodopa with possible additional doses during the night.

Levodopa has also been reported to have been of benefit in a study of 10 patients with *sleep bruxism*.[7]

1. von Scheele C. Levodopa in restless legs. *Lancet* 1986; **ii:** 426–7.
2. Brodeur C, *et al.* Treatment of restless legs syndrome and periodic movements during sleep with L-dopa: a double-blind controlled study. *Neurology* 1988; **38:** 1845–8.
3. Kaplan PW, *et al.* A double-blind, placebo-controlled study of the treatment of periodic limb movements in sleep using carbidopa/levodopa and propoxyphene. *Sleep* 1993; **16:** 717–23.
4. Trenkwalder C, *et al.* L-dopa therapy of uremic and idiopathic restless legs syndrome: a double-blind crossover trial. *Sleep* 1995; **18:** 681–8.
5. Beneš H, *et al.* Rapid onset of action of levodopa in restless legs syndrome: a double-blind, randomized, multicenter, crossover trial. *Sleep* 1999; **22:** 1073–81.
6. Janzen L, *et al.* An overview of levodopa in the management of restless legs syndrome in a dialysis population: pharmacokinetics, clinical trials, and complications of therapy. *Ann Pharmacother* 1999; **33:** 86–92.
7. Lobbezoo F, *et al.* The effect of the catecholamine precursor L-dopa on sleep bruxism: a controlled clinical trial. *Mov Disord* 1997; **12:** 73–8.

Parkinsonism. Levodopa is the mainstay in the treatment of Parkinson's disease (p.1160) but opinion varies on when it should be used in the course of the disease. Most patients respond to levodopa initially but after a few years benefit may be reduced. There may be problems with dyskinesias and psychiatric effects and fluctuations in mobility necessitating careful dosage adjustment or the use of adjunctive drugs. Levodopa is generally administered concurrently with a peripheral dopa-decarboxylase inhibitor, but co-administration of a peripheral catechol-*O*-methyltransferase (COMT) inhibitor may also be necessary for patients experiencing fluctuations in disability related to levodopa and dopa-decarboxylase inhibitor combinations. Those who consider that long-term complications reflect the progressing severity of the disease favour early use of levodopa, whereas those who regard them as being due to cumulative exposure to levodopa advocate later use. The various methods used for the pharmacokinetic optimisation of levodopa administration as Parkinson's disease progresses include timing of administration, the use of modified-release formulations, oral solutions (but see Stability, p.1169) and dispersible formulations for immediate absorption, the timing of food intake, and the use of other drugs to increase the absorption of levodopa.

References.
1. Giron LT, Koller WC. Methods of managing levodopa-induced dyskinesias. *Drug Safety* 1996; **14:** 365–74.
2. Contin M, *et al.* Pharmacokinetic optimisation in the treatment of Parkinson's disease. *Clin Pharmacokinet* 1996; **30:** 463–81.
3. Murer MG, *et al.* Levodopa in Parkinson's disease: neurotoxicity laid to rest? *Drug Safety* 1999; **21:** 339–52.

Pituitary and hypothalamic disorders. DIAGNOSIS AND TESTING. Diminished growth-hormone reserve is one of the earliest functional abnormalities in anterior pituitary failure and, since dopamine is believed to stimulate growth-hormone secretion, the administration of levodopa has been used as a provocative test for the diagnosis of growth-hormone deficiency.[1,2] Levodopa 500 mg has been given by mouth after an overnight fast and serum concentrations of growth hormone measured hourly at 0 to 3 hours; children may be given 10 mg per kg body-weight to a maximum of 500 mg. Transient nausea, vomiting, vertigo, and hypotension may occur and the patient should be kept recumbent during the test. A normal response is an increase in serum concentration of growth hormone of more than 5 nanograms per mL or to a level of more than 10 nanograms per mL, although 10 to 15% of normal subjects may not respond. However, there is some dispute as to whether stimulated growth hormone secretion tests are superior to measurements of circulating somatomedins in detecting growth hormone deficiency.[3-5] For a discussion of the management of growth retardation, including the problems of accurate diagnosis, see p.1273.

1. Abboud CF. Laboratory diagnosis of hypopituitarism. *Mayo Clin Proc* 1986; **61:** 35–48.
2. Müller EE, *et al.* Involvement of brain catecholamines and acetylcholine in growth hormone deficiency states: pathophysiological, diagnostic and therapeutic implications. *Drugs* 1991; **41:** 161–77.
3. Hoffman DM, *et al.* Diagnosis of growth-hormone deficiency in adults. *Lancet* 1994; **343:** 1064–8. Correction. *ibid.,* **344:** 206.
4. de Boer H, *et al.* Diagnosis of growth hormone deficiency in adults. *Lancet* 1994; **343:** 1645–6.
5. Rosenfeld RG, *et al.* Diagnostic controversy: the diagnosis of childhood growth hormone deficiency revisited. *J Clin Endocrinol Metab* 1995; **80:** 1532–40.

Tourette's syndrome. Levodopa has been studied in the management of Tourette's syndrome (see Tics, p.650). A small pilot study[1] has produced encouraging results.

1. Black KJ, *et al.* Response to levodopa challenge in Tourette syndrome. *Mov Disord* 2000; **15:** 1194–8.

Preparations

BP 2001: Co-beneldopa Capsules; Co-careldopa Tablets; Dispersible Co-beneldopa Tablets; Levodopa Capsules; Levodopa Tablets;
USP 25: Carbidopa and Levodopa Tablets; Levodopa Capsules; Levodopa Tablets.

Proprietary Preparations (details are given in Part 3)
Aust.: Ceredopa†; **Ger.:** Dopaflex; **Ital.:** Levomet; **Neth.:** Eldopal†; **S.Afr.:** Larodopa†; **UK:** Larodopa; **USA:** Dopar; Larodopa.

Multi-ingredient: Aust.: Madopar; Sinemet; **Austral.:** Kinson; Madopar; Sinacarb; Sinemet; **Belg.:** Prolopa; Sinemet; **Braz.:** Cronomet; Levocarb; Prolopa; Sinemet; **Canad.:** Apo-Levocarb; Nu-Levocarb; Prolopa; Sinemet; **Denm.:** Madopar; Sinemet; **Fin.:** Aktipar; Kardopal; Madopar; Sinemet; **Fr.:** Modopar; Sinemet; **Ger.:** Isicom; Levocarb-GRY; Levodopa comp B; Levodopa comp C; Levopar; Madopar; Nacom; NeyDop N (Revitorgan-Dilutionen N Nr 97); PK-Levo; Striaton; **Hong Kong:** Apo-Levocarb; Madopar; Sinemet; **Irl.:** Half Sinemet; Madopar; Sinemet; **Israel:** Dopicar; Levopar Plus; Sinemet; **Ital.:** Madopar; Sinemet; **Mex.:** Lemdopa; Madopar; Racovel; Sinemet; **Neth.:** Madopar; Sinemet; **Norw.:** Madopar; Sinemet; **NZ:** Apo-Levocarb; Madopar; Sindopa; Sinemet; **Port.:** Madopar; Sinemet; **S.Afr.:** Carbilev; Madopar; Sinemet; **Singapore:** Madopar; Sinemet; **Spain:** Madopar; Sinemet; **Swed.:** Madopark; Sinemet; **Switz.:** Madopar; Sinemet; **Thai.:** Levomed; Madopar; Syndopa; **UK:** Half Sinemet; Madopar; Sinemet; **USA:** Atamet; Sinemet.

Lisuride Maleate (1510-r)

Lisuride Maleate (BANM, rINNM).
Lysuride Maleate; Methylergol Carbamide Maleate. 3-(9,10-Didehydro-6-methylergolin-8α-yl),1,1-diethylurea hydrogen maleate; 8-Decarboxamido-8-(3,3-diethylureido)-D-lysergamide maleate.
$C_{20}H_{26}N_4O,C_4H_4O_4 = 454.5$.
CAS — 18016-80-3 (lisuride); 19875-60-6 (lisuride maleate).

Adverse Effects and Precautions

As for Bromocriptine, p.1164. Infusion of lisuride in parkinsonian patients has been associated with severe psychiatric adverse effects.

Effects on mental function. For reports of daytime somnolence occurring in patients receiving dopamine agonists including lisuride, see Effects on Mental Function, under Adverse Effects of Levodopa, p.1170.

Effects on the respiratory tract. A report[1] of a woman with Parkinson's disease who developed bilateral pleural effu-

sions after taking lisuride 4 mg daily for about 17 months. Her condition improved on discontinuation of lisuride.

1. Bhatt MH, *et al.* Pleuropulmonary disease associated with dopamine agonist therapy. *Ann Neurol* 1991; **30:** 613–16.

Porphyria. Lisuride maleate is considered to be unsafe in patients with porphyria because it has been shown to be porphyrinogenic in *animals*.

Interactions

As for Bromocriptine, p.1166.

Pharmacokinetics

◊ Plasma concentrations varied widely following a single oral dose of lisuride maleate 300 µg in 11 patients with Parkinson's disease.[1] Absorption was rapid and the mean plasma elimination half-life was 2.2 hours. Only a mean of 0.05% of the dose was excreted unchanged in the urine in 24 hours. The mean oral bioavailability of lisuride maleate has been reported[2] to be 10% after a 100-µg dose and 22% after a 300-µg dose.
A single dose of lisuride 25 µg given by intravenous, intramuscular, or subcutaneous injection reduced plasma-prolactin concentrations by up to 60% in 11 of 12 healthy subjects, the effect lasting for about 10 hours.[3] Plasma concentrations after intravenous administration fell in 2 phases with half-lives of 14 minutes and 1.5 hours respectively. Peak plasma concentrations following subcutaneous and intramuscular injection were obtained after 12 and 15 minutes respectively.

1. Burns RS, *et al.* Disposition of oral lisuride in Parkinson's disease. *Clin Pharmacol Ther* 1984; **35:** 548–56.
2. Hümpel M, *et al.* Radioimmunoassay of plasma lisuride in man following intravenous and oral administration of lisuride hydrogen maleate; effect on plasma prolactin level. *Eur J Clin Pharmacol* 1981; **20:** 47–51.
3. Krause W, *et al.* The pharmacokinetics and pharmacodynamics of lisuride in healthy volunteers after intravenous, intramuscular, and subcutaneous injection. *Eur J Clin Pharmacol* 1991; **40:** 399–403.

Uses and Administration

Lisuride maleate, an ergot derivative, is a dopamine D_2-agonist with actions and uses similar to those of bromocriptine (p.1164). It is also reported to have serotonergic activity. It is used similarly in the management of Parkinson's disease and has been used in disorders associated with hyperprolactinaemia. It is also used to suppress puerperal lactation for medical reasons; it is not recommended for the routine suppression of physiological lactation or for the treatment of postpartum breast pain and engorgement that may be adequately relieved with simple analgesics and breast support. Lisuride has been used in some countries for the treatment of acromegaly.

In the management of Parkinson's disease lisuride maleate has been given alone or added to treatment in patients experiencing 'on-off' fluctuations in control with levodopa. It is normally given by mouth; doses should be taken with food. Initially 200 µg is taken at bedtime and additional doses of 200 µg may be added, at intervals of a week, first at midday and then in the morning; further increases are made, until an optimum response is obtained, by adding 200 µg each week using the same sequence of increases, starting with the bedtime dose; dosage should not normally exceed 5 mg daily in divided doses.

Lisuride maleate has also been given for the prophylaxis of migraine in some countries in usual doses of up to 25 µg three times daily.

Acromegaly. Dopaminergics can produce a paradoxical reduction in growth hormone secretion and may be used in the treatment of acromegaly as adjunctive therapy to surgery and/or radiotherapy to reduce circulating growth hormone levels, although they are less effective than octreotide (p.1271). While bromocriptine has been the main dopamine agonist used, lisuride has been used in some countries.

Hyperprolactinaemia and prolactinomas. Dopamine agonists have been widely used for the treatment of hyperprolactinaemia secondary to a prolactinoma (p.1274). Lisuride has been used as an alternative to bromocriptine. There is a report of plasma-prolactin concentrations being reduced to normal in 4 female patients with macroprolactinomas given lisuride 400 to 800 µg daily for 2 years.[1] Subsequent dosage reduction in 3 was followed by a rise in prolactin values. In the fourth patient prolactin remained in the normal range when the dose was progressively reduced from 400 to 50 µg daily, although complete withdrawal was followed by an increase in prolactin concentration within 3 months.

Vaginal administration of lisuride is being studied in an attempt to avoid adverse effects associated with oral therapy. In a study[2] involving 40 women with hyperprolactinaemia a 200-µg standard oral tablet placed in the vagina at night produced a similar

reduction in prolactin concentrations to that obtained with 400 µg taken orally and was better tolerated.

1. Liuzzi A, *et al.* Low doses of dopamine agonists in the long-term treatment of macroprolactinomas. *N Engl J Med* 1985; **313:** 656–9.
2. Tasdemir M, *et al.* Vaginal lisuride for hyperprolactinaemia. *Lancet* 1995; **346:** 1362.

Lactation inhibition. Lisuride is used in some countries for the prevention of puerperal lactation (p.1276). However, the routine use of dopaminergics is not recommended for the suppression of physiological lactation.

References.
1. Venturini PL, *et al.* Effects of lisuride and bromocriptine on inhibition of lactation and on serum prolactin levels: comparative double-blind study. *Eur J Obstet Gynecol Reprod Biol* 1981; **11:** 395–400.

Migraine. Although lisuride has been used in some countries for the prophylaxis of migraine (p.449) it is not usually considered to be the drug of choice or even one of the main alternatives.

Parkinsonism. While some neurologists use dopamine agonists such as lisuride early in the treatment of parkinsonism (p.1160) in an attempt to delay therapy with levodopa others reserve them for adjunctive use when levodopa is no longer effective alone or cannot be tolerated. They are sometimes useful in reducing 'off' periods with levodopa and in ameliorating other fluctuations in mobility in the later stages of the disease.

References.
1. Rinne UK. Lisuride, a dopamine agonist in the treatment of early Parkinson's disease. *Neurology* 1989; **39:** 336–9.
2. Clarke CE, Speller JM. Lisuride for levodopa-induced complications in Parkinson's disease (updated 24 July 2001). Available in The Cochrane Library; Issue 4. Oxford: Update Software; 2001.
3. Clarke CE, Speller JM. Lisuride versus bromocriptine for levodopa-induced complications in Parkinson's disease (updated 24 July 2001). Available in The Cochrane Library; Issue 4. Oxford: Update Software; 2001.

ADMINISTRATION. Lisuride has been of benefit when administered by continuous intravenous or subcutaneous infusion in patients experiencing fluctuations in mobility with levodopa therapy[1-3] but severe psychiatric effects have been associated with the use of these routes.[3]

1. Obeso JA, *et al.* Intravenous lisuride corrects oscillations of motor performance in Parkinson's disease. *Ann Neurol* 1986; **19:** 31–5.
2. Obeso JA, *et al.* Lisuride infusion pump: a device for the treatment of motor fluctuations in Parkinson's disease. *Lancet* 1986; **i:** 467–70.
3. Critchley P, *et al.* Psychosis and the lisuride pump. *Lancet* 1986; **i:** 349.

Preparations

Proprietary Preparations (details are given in Part 3)
Aust.: Dopergin; Prolacam; **Braz.:** Dopergin; **Fr.:** Arolac; Dopergin; **Ger.:** Cuvalit; Dopergin; **Israel:** Dopergin; **Ital.:** Dopergin; **Mex.:** Dopergin; **Neth.:** Dopergin; **NZ:** Dopergin; **Spain:** Dopergin; **Switz.:** Dopergin; **Thai.:** Dopergin; **UK:** Revanil.

Memantine Hydrochloride (11453-r)

Memantine Hydrochloride (BANM, rINNM).
1-Amino-3,5-dimethyladamantane Hydrochloride; D-145 (memantine); 3,5-Dimethyl-1-adamantanamine hydrochloride; DMAA (memantine). 3,5-Dimethyltricyclo[3.3.1.1.^{3,7}]decan-1-amine hydrochloride.
$C_{12}H_{21}N,HCl = 215.8$.
CAS — 19982-08-2 (memantine).

Profile

Memantine is a derivative of amantadine (p.1161) and is likewise an antagonist of *N*-methyl-D-aspartate receptors. It has been given as the hydrochloride in the treatment of parkinsonism (p.1160) and central spasticity (p.1322), and has also been used in dementia (p.1412), brain injury, or comatose states. It is given by mouth in usual doses of up to 30 mg of the hydrochloride daily in divided doses.

Memantine hydrochloride is also given by slow intravenous injection for cerebral spasticity.

Memantine is also under investigation in the treatment of glaucoma and peripheral neuropathy.

◊ References.
1. Ditzler K. Efficacy and tolerability of memantine in patients with dementia syndrome: a double-blind, placebo controlled trial. *Arzneimittelforschung* 1991; **41:** 773–80.
2. Görtelmeyer R, Erbler H. Memantine in the treatment of mild to moderate dementia syndrome: a double-blind placebo-controlled study. *Arzneimittelforschung* 1992; **42:** 904–13.
3. Winblad B, Portis N. Memantine in severe dementia: results of the ⁹m-best study (benefit and efficacy in severely demented patients during treatment with memantine). *Int J Geriatr Psychiatry* 1999; **14:** 135–46.
4. Jain KK. Evaluation of memantine for neuroprotection in dementia. *Expert Opin Invest Drugs* 2000; **9:** 1397–1406.

Preparations

Proprietary Preparations (details are given in Part 3)
Ger.: Akatinol.

Metergoline (1511-f)

Metergoline (BAN, rINN).

FI-6337; MCE; Methergoline. Benzyl (8S,10S)-(1,6-dimethyler-golin-8-ylmethyl)carbamate.

$C_{25}H_{29}N_3O_2 = 403.5$.
CAS — 17692-51-2.
ATC — G02CB05.

Profile
Metergoline, an ergot derivative, is a dopamine agonist with actions and uses similar to those of bromocriptine (p.1164). It is also a serotonin antagonist. Metergoline has been used similarly to bromocriptine in disorders associated with hyperprolactinaemia and to inhibit lactation. In some countries it has also been used in the prophylaxis of migraine and other vascular headaches.

Hyperprolactinaemia and prolactinomas. Dopamine agonists have been widely used for the treatment of hyperprolactinaemia secondary to a prolactinoma (p.1274). There is a report of metergoline being tried in patients intolerant of bromocriptine.[1] In this report metergoline lowered plasma-prolactin concentrations, although not to normal, in 3 men and 8 women with hyperprolactinaemia. Galactorrhoea was abolished and/or a regular menstrual cycle established in 5 of the women. Prolactin concentrations and symptoms were unchanged in 3 further women with normoprolactinaemic galactorrhoea. Initial doses of 2 mg daily were increased over 2 weeks to 4 mg three times daily and at monthly re-assessment the dose was increased up to 24 mg daily in divided doses, according to response.

1. Casson IF, et al. Intolerance of bromocriptine: is metergoline a satisfactory alternative? BMJ 1985; 290: 1783–4.

Lactation inhibition. Metergoline has been tried for the prevention of puerperal lactation (p.1276) in doses of 8 to 12 mg daily for 5 days.[1,2] However the routine use of dopaminergics is not recommended for the suppression of physiological lactation.

1. Delitala G, et al. Metergoline in the inhibition of puerperal lactation. BMJ 1977; 1: 744–6.
2. Crosignani PG, et al. Suppression of puerperal lactation by metergoline. Obstet Gynecol 1978; 51: 113–15.

Migraine. Although metergoline has been used in some countries for the prophylaxis of migraine (p.449) it is not usually considered to be the drug of choice or even one of the main alternatives.

Preparations
Proprietary Preparations (details are given in Part 3)
Ger.: Liserdol; *Hong Kong:* Liserdol; *Ital.:* Liserdol; *S.Afr.:* Liserdol†; *Singapore:* Liserdol; *Switz.:* Liserdol.

Pergolide Mesilate (13095-p)

Pergolide Mesilate (BANM, rINN).

LY-127809; Pergolide Mesylate (USAN); Pergolidi Mesilas. 8β-Methylthiomethyl-6-propylergoline methanesulphonate; Methyl (8R,10R)-6-propylergolin-8-ylmethyl sulphide methanesulphonate.

$C_{19}H_{26}N_2S,CH_4O_3S = 410.6$.
CAS — 66104-22-1 (pergolide); 66104-23-2 (pergolide mesilate).

Pharmacopoeias. In Eur. (see p.vi).

Pharmacopoeial description

Ph. Eur.: A white or almost white crystalline powder. Slightly soluble in water, in alcohol, and in dichloromethane; very slightly soluble in acetone; sparingly soluble in methyl alcohol. Protect from light.

Adverse Effects and Precautions
As for Bromocriptine, p.1164. Other reported adverse effects include rash and fever and abnormal liver function tests. Abrupt withdrawal of pergolide may precipitate hallucinations and confusion, and withdrawal should be undertaken gradually.

An increased incidence of uterine neoplasms has been reported in *rodents* given high doses of pergolide mesilate.

Effects on mental function. For reports of daytime somnolence occurring in patients receiving dopamine agonists including pergolide, see Effects on Mental Function, under Adverse Effects of Levodopa, p.1170.

Interactions
As for Bromocriptine, p.1166.

Pharmacokinetics
Pergolide mesilate is absorbed from the gastrointestinal tract. It is reported to be about 90% bound to plasma proteins. It is excreted mainly in the urine in the form of metabolites.

The symbol † denotes a preparation no longer actively marketed

Uses and Administration
Pergolide mesilate, an ergot derivative, is a dopamine agonist with actions and uses similar to those of bromocriptine (p.1166), but in contrast to bromocriptine (a dopamine D_2-agonist) it also has agonist properties at D_1 and D_3 receptors. Pergolide is used in the management of Parkinson's disease as monotherapy, or as an adjunct to levodopa therapy to reduce 'end-of-dose' or 'on-off' fluctuations in response. Pergolide is administered by mouth as the mesilate with doses expressed as the base.

For administration as *monotherapy* an initial dose of 50 μg pergolide is given on the first evening of therapy. The dose is thereafter gradually increased: 50 μg twice daily is taken on days 2 to 4, then increased by 100 to 250 μg daily every 3 to 4 days, given in 3 divided doses, up to a daily dose of 1.5 mg at day 28. After day 30, the dose should be increased further by a maximum of 250 μg twice a week until an optimum response is achieved. Usual maintenance doses are 2.1 to 2.5 mg daily. The daily dose is usually given in 3 divided doses.

For administration as *adjunctive therapy* with levodopa, pergolide should be introduced gradually and during this period patients already receiving levodopa can have their levodopa dosage decreased gradually until an optimum response is achieved. The initial dose of pergolide is 50 μg daily for the first 2 days, increased gradually by 100 or 150 μg every third day over the next 12 days of therapy. Further increases of 250 μg may then be made every third day until an optimum response is achieved. A usual maintenance dose is 3 mg daily. The daily dose is usually given in 3 divided doses.

Acromegaly. Dopaminergics can produce a paradoxical reduction of growth hormone secretion and may be used in the treatment of acromegaly as adjunctive therapy to surgery and/or radiotherapy to reduce circulating growth hormone levels, although they are less effective than octreotide (p.1271). While bromocriptine has been the main dopamine agonist used pergolide has also been tried.[1]

1. Kleinberg DL, et al. Pergolide for the treatment of pituitary tumors secreting prolactin or growth hormone. N Engl J Med 1983; 309: 704–9.

Hyperprolactinaemia and prolactinomas. Dopamine agonists are widely used for the treatment of hyperprolactinaemia secondary to a prolactinoma (p.1274). Pergolide has been suggested as an alternative to bromocriptine in this condition. Studies[1-3] of pergolide mesilate in patients with hyperprolactinaemia indicate that single doses reduce serum-prolactin concentrations for more than 24 hours. In most patients, the effective daily dose was between 50 and 150 μg daily. Adverse effects were similar to those seen with bromocriptine, although some patients who could not take bromocriptine were able to tolerate pergolide (and *vice versa*). Pergolide reportedly lost favour for this indication following reports of an increased incidence of uterine neoplasms in *rodents* receiving high doses. However, the manufacturers point out that no cases of uterine malignancies have to date been reported in humans receiving pergolide. The long-term outcome of treatment of macroprolactinomas with pergolide has been examined in 23 patients,[4] and efficacy and relative safety of pergolide was demonstrated after an average of 27 months (range: 9 to 64 months) treatment.

1. Franks S, et al. Treatment of hyperprolactinaemia with pergolide mesylate: acute effects and preliminary evaluation of long-term treatment. Lancet 1981; ii: 659–61.
2. Franks S, et al. Effectiveness of pergolide mesylate in long-term treatment of hyperprolactinaemia. BMJ 1983; 286: 1177–9.
3. Kleinberg DL, et al. Pergolide for the treatment of pituitary tumors secreting prolactin or growth hormone. N Engl J Med 1983; 309: 704–9.
4. Freda PU, et al. Long-term treatment of prolactin-secreting macroadenomas with pergolide. J Clin Endocrinol Metab 2000; 85: 8–13.

Parkinsonism. While some neurologists use dopamine agonists such as pergolide early in the treatment of parkinsonism (p.1160) in an attempt to delay therapy with levodopa, others reserve them for adjunctive use when levodopa is no longer effective alone or cannot be tolerated. They are sometimes useful in reducing 'off' periods with levodopa and in ameliorating other fluctuations in mobility in the later stages of the disease. Pergolide has a relatively long duration of action compared with other dopamine agonists commonly used. Although the duration of the clinical antiparkinsonian effect of pergolide remains to be determined, studies suggest it is of the order of 5 to 8 hours. Depending on the dose used the response to other dop-

amine agonists in late parkinsonism is 1 to 4 hours for levodopa, 2 to 4 hours for lisuride, and 4 to 6 hours for bromocriptine.

References.

1. Anonymous. Pergolide (Celance)—a third dopamine agonist. Drug Ther Bull 1991; 29: 79.
2. Markham A, Benfield P. Pergolide: a review of its pharmacology and therapeutic use in Parkinson's disease. CNS Drugs 1997; 7: 328–40.
3. Barone P, et al. Pergolide monotherapy in the treatment of early PD: a randomized, controlled study. Neurology 1999; 53: 573–9.
4. Clarke CE, Speller JM. Pergolide for levodopa-induced complications in Parkinson's disease (updated 24 July 2001). Available in The Cochrane Library, Issue 4. Oxford: Update Software; 2001.
5. Clarke CE, Speller JM. Pergolide versus bromocriptine for levodopa-induced motor complications in Parkinson's disease (updated 24 July 2001). Available in The Cochrane Library, Issue 4. Oxford: Update Software; 2001.

Restless legs syndrome. The aetiology of restless legs syndrome (see under Parasomnias, p.653) is obscure and treatment has largely been empirical. Pergolide has produced some benefit in small studies.[1-4]

1. Silber MH, et al. Pergolide in the management of restless legs syndrome: an extended study. Sleep 1997; 20: 878–82.
2. Winkelmann J, et al. Treatment of restless legs syndrome with pergolide—an open clinical trial. Mov Disord 1998; 13: 566–9.
3. Earley CJ, et al. Randomized, double-blind, placebo-controlled trial of pergolide in restless legs syndrome. Neurology 1998; 51: 1599–1602.
4. Wetter TC, et al.. A randomized controlled study of pergolide in patients with restless legs syndrome. Neurology 1999; 52: 944–50.

Tourette's syndrome. Pergolide has been studied in the management of Tourette's syndrome (see Tics, p.650). A preliminary study[1] has produced encouraging results, subsequently confirmed by a placebo-controlled trial in 24 children aged 7 to 17 years.[2]

1. Lipinski JF, et al. Dopamine agonist treatment of Tourette disorder in children: results of an open-label trial of pergolide. Mov Disord 1997; 12: 402–7.
2. Gilbert DL, et al. Tourette's syndrome improvement with pergolide in a randomized, double-blind, crossover trial. Neurology 2000; 54: 1310–15.

Preparations
Proprietary Preparations (details are given in Part 3)
Aust.: Permax; *Austral.:* Permax; *Belg.:* Permax; *Braz.:* Celance; *Canad.:* Permax; *Denm.:* Permax; *Fin.:* Permax; *Fr.:* Celance; *Ger.:* Parkotil; *Hong Kong:* Celance; *Irl.:* Celance; *Ital.:* Nopar; *Mex.:* Permax; *Neth.:* Permax; *NZ:* Permax; *Port.:* Permax; *S.Afr.:* Permax; *Singapore:* Celance; *Spain:* Pharken; *Switz.:* Permax; *Thai.:* Celance; *UK:* Celance; *USA:* Permax.

Piribedil (4551-p)

Piribedil (rINN).

ET-495; EU-4200. 2-(4-Piperonylpiperazin-1-yl)pyrimidine.

$C_{16}H_{18}N_4O_2 = 298.3$.
CAS — 3605-01-4.
ATC — C04AX13.

Profile
Piribedil is a non-ergot dopamine agonist that has been given by mouth in the treatment of parkinsonism and in circulatory disorders. Piribedil mesilate has been given by injection for circulatory disorders.

Adverse effects reported include nausea and vomiting, dizziness, hallucinations, confusion, drowsiness, hypothermia, dyskinesias, and occasional changes in liver function.

When used as monotherapy in Parkinson's disease a usual daily dose of piribedil is 150 to 250 mg given by mouth in divided doses; a daily dose of 80 to 140 mg may be suitable when used as an adjunct to levodopa.

Effects on mental function. For reports of daytime somnolence occurring in patients receiving dopamine agonists including piribedil, see Effects on Mental Function, under Adverse Effects of Levodopa, p.1170.

Parkinsonism. The antiparkinsonian actions of piribedil have been discussed briefly in a review[1] of the status of dopamine agonists in the management of Parkinson's disease (p.1160). Piribedil is a dopamine D_2-agonist while its metabolite is reported to act on D_1 receptors. It has been mainly used as an adjunct to levodopa therapy and appears to act more on tremor than on other symptoms of Parkinson's disease, although it was noted that most of the evidence for this came from uncontrolled studies.

1. Montastruc JL, et al. Current status of dopamine agonists in Parkinson's disease management. Drugs 1993; 46: 384–93.

Preparations
Proprietary Preparations (details are given in Part 3)
Braz.: Trivastal; *Fr.:* Trivastal; *Ger.:* Trivastal; *Ital.:* Trivastan; *Port.:* Trivastal; *Singapore:* Trivastal; *Thai.:* Trivastal.

Pramipexole Hydrochloride (19970-j)

Pramipexole Hydrochloride (BANM, rINNM).
PNU-98528-E; Pramipexole Dihydrochloride (USAN); SND-919-CL-2Y (pramipexole hydrochloride); SUD-919Y (pramipexole). (S)-2-Amino-4,5,6,7-tetrahydro-6-(propylamino)benzothiazole dihydrochloride monohydrate.
$C_{10}H_{17}N_3S,2HCl, H_2O = 302.3$.
CAS — 104632-26-0 (pramipexole); 104632-25-9 (anhydrous pramipexole hydrochloride); 191217-81-9 (pramipexole hydrochloride monohydrate).

Pramipexole 87.37 µg is approximately equivalent to 125 µg of pramipexole dihydrochloride monohydrate.

Adverse Effects and Precautions

As for Bromocriptine, p.1164.

Sudden onset of sleep, with or without any prior feeling of drowsiness, has been rarely reported and can occur at any time during treatment (see below). Patients should not drive or undertake other potentially hazardous activities such as operating machinery. A reduction in dosage or withdrawal of pramipexole will, in most cases, alleviate the problem. (As with other dopaminergic agonists, abrupt discontinuation of pramipexole therapy may lead to development of the neuroleptic malignant syndrome.)

Pramipexole should be administered with caution to patients with renal impairment and reduced doses are recommended.

Ophthalmological monitoring is recommended at regular intervals or if vision abnormalities occur.

Effects on mental function. Pramipexole has been associated with attacks of sudden onset of sleep. The UK manufacturer has reported that the incidence of daytime somnolence is increased at daily doses of pramipexole hydrochloride higher than 1.5 mg. A retrospective analysis[1] of data to evaluate the incidence and nature of somnolence experienced by patients receiving pramipexole in clinical trials showed that for patients with moderate or severe somnolence, the onset of worst-reported somnolence occurred at a mean dose of around 4.0 mg (range: 0.75 to 4.5 mg).

For further reports of daytime somnolence occurring in patients receiving dopamine agonists including pramipexole, see Effects on Mental Function, under Adverse Effects of Levodopa, p.1170.

1. Hauser RA, et al. Pramipexole-induced somnolence and episodes of daytime sleep. Mov Disord 2000; 15: 658–63.

Interactions

As for Bromocriptine, p.1166. Cimetidine or probenecid are reported to reduce the renal clearance of pramipexole.

Caution is advised when other sedating drugs or alcohol are used with pramipexole because of possible additive effects and the risk of precipitating sudden onset of sleep (see above).

◊ References.
1. Wright CE, et al. Influence of probenecid and cimetidine on pramipexole pharmacokinetics. Clin Pharmacol Ther 1996; 59: 183.

Pharmacokinetics

Pramipexole is readily absorbed from the gastrointestinal tract and peak plasma concentrations have been reached within about 2 hours in fasting patients and in about 3 hours when given with food. Oral bioavailability is reported to be about 90%. Pramipexole is widely distributed throughout the body and its protein binding is low. Metabolism is minimal and more than 90% of a dose is excreted via renal tubular secretion unchanged into the urine. Elimination half-lives of 8 to 12 hours have been reported.

◊ References.
1. Wright CE, et al. Steady-state pharmacokinetic properties of pramipexole in healthy volunteers. J Clin Pharmacol 1997; 37: 520–5.

Uses and Administration

Pramipexole is a non-ergot dopamine agonist with actions similar to those of bromocriptine (p.1166). It is used similarly in the management of Parkinson's disease (p.1160) as an adjunct to levodopa therapy to reduce 'end-of-dose' or 'on-off' fluctuations in response. Pramipexole is administered by mouth as the hydrochloride; doses have been described in terms of the hydrochloride (as below) or of the base. The dose of pramipexole should be increased gradually and the dose of levodopa gradually reduced during the dose-titration and maintenance phases until an optimum response is achieved.

The initial dose of pramipexole hydrochloride is 125 µg given three times daily increased to 250 µg three times daily in the second week and then to 500 µg three times daily in the third week according to response. Thereafter the daily dose may be increased if necessary by 750 µg at weekly intervals to a maximum of 4.5 mg daily. The dosage should be reduced in patients with renal impairment (see below).

If it is necessary to discontinue pramipexole therapy, it should be withdrawn gradually. The UK manufacturer suggests tapering off the dose of pramipexole hydrochloride at a rate of 750 µg daily until a daily dose of 750 µg has been reached; thereafter, the dose should be reduced by 375 µg daily.

Administration in renal impairment. The elimination of pramipexole is dependent on renal function and the dosage of pramipexole should therefore be reduced in patients with renal impairment. The following dosage schedule has been suggested by the UK manufacturers for initiation of therapy: for patients with a creatinine clearance (CC) between 20 and 50 mL per minute the initial daily dose of pramipexole hydrochloride is 125 µg given twice daily. In patients with a CC of less than 20 mL per minute a single daily dose of 125 µg may be used. If renal function declines during maintenance therapy it is recommended that the daily dose of pramipexole should be reduced by the same percentage as the decline in CC.

Parasomnias. The aetiology of restless legs syndrome (p.653) is obscure and treatment has largely been empirical. Pramipexole has produced some benefit in small studies.[1,2]

1. Lin S-C, et al. Effect of pramipexole in treatment of resistant restless legs syndrome. Mayo Clin Proc 1998; 73: 497–500.
2. Montplaisir J, et al. Restless legs syndrome improved by pramipexole: a double-blind randomized trial. Neurology 1999; 52: 938–43.

Parkinsonism. Pramipexole is a dopamine agonist used in the treatment of Parkinson's disease (p.1160) as an adjunct to levodopa therapy to reduce 'off' periods with levodopa and ameliorate other fluctuations of mobility in the later stages of the disease. It has also been studied as monotherapy early in the course of the disease in an attempt to delay therapy with levodopa.

References.
1. Parkinson Study Group. Safety and efficacy of pramipexole in early Parkinson disease: a randomized dose-ranging study. JAMA 1997; 278: 125–30.
2. Lieberman A, et al. Clinical evaluation of pramipexole in advanced Parkinson's disease: results of a double-blind, placebo-controlled, parallel-group study. Neurology 1997; 49: 162–8.
3. Shannon KM, et al. Efficacy of pramipexole, a novel dopamine agonist, as monotherapy in mild to moderate Parkinson's disease. Neurology 1997; 49: 724–8.
4. Guttman M. International Pramipexole-Bromocriptine Study Group. Double-blind comparison of pramipexole and bromocriptine treatment with placebo in advanced Parkinson's disease. Neurology 1997; 49: 1060–5.
5. Parkinson Study Group. Pramipexole vs levodopa as initial treatment for Parkinson disease: a randomized controlled trial. JAMA 2000; 284: 1931–8.
6. Clarke CE, et al. Pramipexole for levodopa-induced complications in Parkinson's disease (updated 24 July 2001). Available in The Cochrane Library; Issue 4. Oxford: Update Software; 2001.
7. Clarke CE, et al. Pramipexole versus bromocriptine for levodopa-induced complications in Parkinson's disease (updated 24 July 2001). Available in The Cochrane Library; Issue 4. Oxford: Update Software; 2001.

Schizophrenia. Beneficial results have been reported in a preliminary trial[1] of pramipexole as an adjunct to haloperidol in the treatment of schizophrenia (p.651).

1. Kasper S, et al. Pramipexole as adjunct to haloperidol in schizophrenia: safety and efficacy. Eur Neuropsychopharmacol 1997; 7: 65–70.

Preparations

Proprietary Preparations (details are given in Part 3)
Canad.: Mirapex; **Denm.:** Sifrol; **Fin.:** Sifrol; **Ger.:** Sifrol; **Irl.:** Mirapexin; **Ital.:** Mirapexin; **Neth.:** Sifrol; **Norw.:** Sifrol; **Spain:** Mirapexin; **Swed.:** Sifrol; **Switz.:** Sifrol; **UK:** Mirapexin; **USA:** Mirapex.

Quinagolide Hydrochloride (17700-f)

Quinagolide Hydrochloride (BANM, rINNM).
CV-205-502 (quinagolide); SD2-CV-205-502 (quinagolide). (±)-N,N-Diethyl-N'-[(3R*,4aR*,10aS*)-1,2,3,4,4a,5,10,10a-octahydro-6-hydroxy-1-propylbenzo[g]quinolin-3-yl]sulfamide hydrochloride.
$C_{20}H_{33}N_3O_3S,HCl = 432.0$.
CAS — 87056-78-8 (quinagolide); 94424-50-7 (quinagolide hydrochloride).

Adverse Effects and Precautions

As for Bromocriptine, p.1164, although some patients unable to tolerate bromocriptine may tolerate quinagolide (and vice versa).

Interactions

As for Bromocriptine, p.1166.

Pharmacokinetics

Quinagolide is rapidly absorbed from the gastrointestinal tract and undergoes extensive first-pass metabolism to the N-desethyl analogue which is biologically active and the N,N-didesethyl analogue. Approximately equal amounts of a dose appear in the urine and the faeces; it is excreted in the urine as sulfate or glucuronide conjugates of quinagolide and its metabolites and in the faeces as the unconjugated forms. Protein binding has been reported to be about 90%. The elimination half-life of quinagolide at steady state is about 17 hours.

Uses and Administration

Quinagolide is a non-ergot dopamine D_2-agonist that has actions and uses similar to those of bromocriptine (p.1166). It is used as the hydrochloride in the treatment of disorders associated with hyperprolactinaemia.

Quinagolide hydrochloride is given in single daily doses with food at bedtime; doses are expressed in terms of the base. The initial dose is 25 µg daily for 3 days increasing thereafter at 3-day intervals in steps of 25 µg until the optimal response is achieved, which is usually within the range of 75 to 150 µg daily. If doses greater than 300 µg daily are required, increases should be made in steps of 75 to 150 µg daily at intervals of not less than 4 weeks.

Quinagolide has also been investigated in the treatment of acromegaly, lactation inhibition, and Parkinson's disease.

Acromegaly. Dopaminergics can produce a paradoxical reduction in growth hormone secretion and may be used in the treatment of acromegaly as adjunctive therapy to surgery and/or radiotherapy to reduce circulating growth hormone levels, although they are less effective than octreotide (see p.1271). Bromocriptine has been the main dopamine agonist used, but quinagolide has been tried and results of an open study[1] in which quinagolide was administered to 17 patients with acromegaly suggest that quinagolide has a more prolonged effect on suppression of growth hormone secretion than bromocriptine. However, it was ineffective in bromocriptine-resistant patients. In another study involving 34 patients, quinagolide was more effective than either cabergoline or a depot preparation of bromocriptine in normalising circulating growth hormone and insulin-like growth factor.[2]

1. Chiodini PG, et al. CV 205-502 in acromegaly. Acta Endocrinol (Copenh) 1993; 128: 389–93.
2. Colao A, et al. Effect of different dopaminergic agents in the treatment of acromegaly. J Clin Endocrinol Metab 1997; 82: 518–23.

Hyperprolactinaemia and prolactinomas. Dopamine agonists are widely used for the treatment of hyperprolactinaemia secondary to a prolactinoma (see p.1274). Quinagolide has been tried as an alternative in patients unresponsive to or intolerant of bromocriptine.

References.
1. Vance ML, et al. Treatment of prolactin-secreting pituitary macroadenomas with the long-acting non-ergot dopamine agonist CV 205-502. Ann Intern Med 1990; 112: 668–73.
2. Shoham Z, et al. CV 205-502—effectiveness, tolerability, and safety over 24-month study. Fertil Steril 1991; 55: 501–6.
3. Rasmussen C, et al. Clinical response and prolactin concentration in hyperprolactinemic women during and after treatment for 24 months with the new dopamine agonist, CV 205-502. Acta Endocrinol (Copenh) 1991; 125: 170–6.
4. Verhelst JA, et al. Acute and long-term effects of once-daily oral bromocriptine and a new long-acting non-ergot dopamine agonist, quinagolide, in the treatment of hyperprolactinaemia: a double-blind study. Acta Endocrinol (Copenh) 1991; 125: 385–91.
5. van der Heijden PFM, et al. CV205-502, a new dopamine agonist, versus bromocriptine in the treatment of hyperprolactinaemia. Eur J Obstet Gynecol Reprod Biol 1991; 40: 111–18.
6. Vilar L, Burke CW. Quinagolide efficacy and tolerability in hyperprolactinaemic patients who are resistant to or intolerant of bromocriptine. Clin Endocrinol (Oxf) 1994; 41: 821–6.
7. Rohmer V, et al. Efficacy of quinagolide in resistance to dopamine agonists: results of a multicenter study. Ann Endocrinol (Paris) 2000; 61: 411–17.

Lactation inhibition. A small preliminary study[1] has suggested that quinagolide is of similar efficacy to bromocriptine for prevention of puerperal lactation. However, the routine use of dopaminergics is not recommended for the suppression of physiological lactation (see p.1276).

1. van der Heijden PFM, *et al.* Lactation inhibition by the dopamine agonist CV 205-502. *Br J Obstet Gynaecol* 1991; **98:** 270–6.

Preparations

Proprietary Preparations (details are given in Part 3)
Aust.: Norprolac; **Fin.:** Norprolac; **Fr.:** Norprolac; **Ger.:** Norprolac; **Hong Kong:** Norprolac; **Israel:** Norprolac; **Mex.:** Norprolac; **Neth.:** Norprolac; **Norw.:** Norprolac; **S.Afr.:** Norprolac; **Spain:** Norprolac; **Swed.:** Norprolac; **Switz.:** Norprolac; **UK:** Norprolac.

Ropinirole Hydrochloride (17393-b)

Ropinirole Hydrochloride *(BANM, USAN, pINNM).*
SKF-101468 (ropinirole); SKF-0101468-A (ropinirole hydrochloride). 4-[2-(Dipropylamino)ethyl]-2-indolinone hydrochloride.
$C_{16}H_{24}N_2O,HCl = 296.8$.
CAS — 91374-21-9 (ropinirole); 91374-20-8 (ropinirole hydrochloride).

Adverse Effects and Precautions

As for Bromocriptine, p.1164. It should not be used in patients with hepatic or severe renal impairment.

Sudden onset of sleep, with or without any prior feeling of drowsiness, has been rarely reported and can occur at any time during treatment. Patients should not drive or undertake other potentially hazardous activities such as operating machinery. A reduction in dosage or withdrawal of ropinirole will, in most cases, alleviate the problem.

As with other dopaminergic agonists, ropinirole therapy should not be discontinued abruptly.

Effects on mental function. For reports of daytime somnolence occurring in patients receiving dopamine agonists including ropinirole, see Effects on Mental Function, under Adverse Effects of Levodopa, p.1170.

Interactions

Since it is a dopamine agonist, ropinirole may share some of the pharmacological interactions of bromocriptine, p.1166. In addition, high doses of oestrogens can increase plasma concentrations of ropinirole and dosage adjustments may be necessary if oestrogen therapy is started or withdrawn during treatment with ropinirole. Ropinirole is metabolised by the cytochrome P450 isoenzyme CYP1A2 and there is therefore the potential for interactions between ropinirole and other drugs that are metabolised similarly or are enzyme inducers.

Caution is advised when other sedating drugs or alcohol are used with ropinirole because of possible additive effects and the risk of precipitating sudden onset of sleep (see above).

Pharmacokinetics

Ropinirole is rapidly absorbed from the gastrointestinal tract and mean peak plasma concentrations have been achieved 1.5 hours after oral administration; the rate of absorption, but not the extent, may be reduced if taken with food. Bioavailability is reported to be about 50%. Plasma protein binding of ropinirole is low (10 to 40%).

Ropinirole is metabolised primarily by the cytochrome P450 isoenzyme CYP1A2 and excreted in the urine as metabolites. A mean elimination half-life of about 6 hours has been reported for ropinirole.

◊ References.
1. Brefel C, *et al.* Effect of food on the pharmacokinetics of ropinirole in parkinsonian patients. *Br J Clin Pharmacol* 1998; **45:** 412–15.
2. Hubble J, *et al.* Linear pharmacokinetic behavior of ropinirole during multiple dosing in patients with Parkinson's disease. *J Clin Pharmacol* 2000; **40:** 641–6.
3. Kaye CM, Nicholls B. Clinical pharmacokinetics of ropinirole. *Clin Pharmacokinet* 2000; **39:** 243–54.

Uses and Administration

Ropinirole is a non-ergot dopamine D_2-agonist with similar actions to those of bromocriptine (p.1166). It is given by mouth as the hydrochloride in the management of Parkinson's disease, either alone or as an adjunct to levodopa; doses are expressed in terms of the base. It should be introduced gradually and during this period patients already receiving levodopa can

have their levodopa dosage decreased gradually until an optimal response is achieved. The concurrent dose of levodopa may be reduced by about 20%. The daily dosage of ropinirole should be given in three divided doses, preferably with food. The initial daily dose of ropinirole is 750 µg increased at weekly intervals in steps of 750 µg daily until the optimal response is achieved, which is usually within the range of 3 to 9 mg daily, although higher doses may be required if used with levodopa. If doses greater than 3 mg daily are required the weekly increments may be made in steps of up to 3 mg. The daily dosage should not exceed 24 mg.

If it is necessary to discontinue ropinirole therapy, it should be withdrawn gradually by reducing the number of daily doses over the period of one week.

◊ Reviews.
1. Tulloch IF. Pharmacologic profile of ropinirole: a nonergoline dopamine agonist. *Neurology* 1997; **49** (suppl 1): S58–S62.

Parkinsonism. While some neurologists use dopamine agonists such as ropinirole early in the treatment of parkinsonism (p.1160) in an attempt to delay therapy with levodopa others reserve them for adjunctive use when levodopa is no longer effective alone or cannot be tolerated. They are sometimes useful in reducing 'off' periods with levodopa and in ameliorating other fluctuations of mobility in the later stage of the disease. References.
1. Rascol O, *et al.* A placebo-controlled study of ropinirole a new D₂ agonist, in the treatment of motor fluctuations of L-DOPA-treated parkinsonian patients. *Adv Neurol* 1996; **69:** 531–4.
2. Adler CH, *et al.* The Ropinirole Study Group. Ropinirole for the treatment of early Parkinson's disease. *Neurology* 1997; **49:** 393–9.
3. Rascol O, *et al.* Ropinirole in the treatment of early Parkinson's disease: a 6-month interim report of a 5-year levodopa-controlled study. *Mov Disord* 1998; **13:** 39–45.
4. Korczyn AD, *et al.* A 3-year randomized trial of ropinirole and bromocriptine in early Parkinson's disease. *Neurology* 1999; **53:** 364–70.
5. Matheson AJ, Spencer CM. Ropinirole: a review of its use in the management of Parkinson's disease. *Drugs* 2000; **60:** 115–37.
6. Clarke CE, Deane KHO. Ropinirole for levodopa-induced complications in Parkinson's disease (updated 13 November 2000). Available in The Cochrane Library; Issue 4. Oxford: Update Software; 2001.
7. Clarke CE, Deane KHO. Ropinirole versus bromocriptine for levodopa-induced complications in Parkinson's disease (updated 12 July 2001). Available in The Cochrane Library: Issue 4. Oxford: Update Software; 2001.

Restless legs syndrome. The aetiology of restless legs syndrome (see under Parasomnias, p.653) is obscure and treatment has largely been empirical. Ropinirole showed some benefit in a small study.¹
1. Ondo W. Ropinirole for restless legs syndrome. *Mov Disord* 1999; **14:** 138–40.

Preparations

Proprietary Preparations (details are given in Part 3)
Aust.: Requip; **Belg.:** Requip; **Canad.:** Requip; **Denm.:** Requip; **Fr.:** Requip; **Ger.:** Requip; **Hong Kong:** Requip; **Irl.:** Requip; **Israel:** Requip; **Ital.:** Requip; **Neth.:** Requip; **Norw.:** Requip; **Port.:** Requip; **Spain:** Requip; **Swed.:** Requip; **Switz.:** Requip; **UK:** Requip; **USA:** Requip.

Selegiline Hydrochloride (13228-v)

Selegiline Hydrochloride *(BANM, USAN, rINNM).*
Deprenyl; L-Deprenyl; Selegilini Hydrochloridum. (−)-(R)-N,α-Dimethyl-N-(prop-2-ynyl)phenethylamine hydrochloride; (R)-Methyl(α-methylphenethyl)prop-2-ynylamine hydrochloride.
$C_{13}H_{17}N,HCl = 223.7$.
CAS — 14611-51-9 (selegiline); 2079-54-1 (selegiline hydrochloride); 14611-52-0 (selegiline hydrochloride).
Pharmacopoeias. In Eur. (see p.vi) and US.

Pharmacopoeial description

Ph. Eur.: A white or almost white, crystalline powder. Freely soluble in water and in methyl alcohol; slightly soluble in acetone. A 2% solution in water has a pH of 3.5 to 4.5. Protect from light.

USP 25: A white, odourless crystalline powder. Freely soluble in water, in chloroform, and in methyl alcohol. Store in airtight containers. Protect from light.

Adverse Effects

Selegiline is often given as an adjunct to levodopa therapy and many of the adverse effects reported may be attributed to enhanced levodopa activity; dosage of levodopa may have to be reduced. However, most reported adverse effects, with the possible exception of increased dyskinesias and cardiac arrhythmias, have also been seen with selegiline monotherapy. Adverse effects have included hypotension, chest pain, nausea,

vomiting, constipation, diarrhoea, confusion, headache, tremor, vertigo, dizziness, psychosis, depression, hallucinations, agitation, dry mouth, stomatitis, sore throat, difficulty in micturition, skin reactions, back pain, muscle cramps, joint pain, myopathy, and increased dyskinesias. The amfetamine metabolites of selegiline may cause insomnia and abnormal dreams; evening doses should be avoided. Transient increases in liver enzymes have been reported. Mouth ulcers may occur with the oral lyophilisate (Zelapar, UK).

Since the selectivity of selegiline is lost at higher doses, signs and symptoms of overdosage may resemble those of non-selective MAOIs such as phenelzine (see p.303).

◊ For reference to a study which observed an increased mortality rate in patients with Parkinson's disease taking selegiline and levodopa compared with those taking levodopa alone, see under Parkinsonism in Uses and Administration, below.

Effects on carbohydrate metabolism. Profound hypoglycaemia developed in a 70-year-old man after selegiline was added to his existing medication for Parkinson's disease.¹ Hypoglycaemia was accompanied by hyperinsulinaemia and resolved 1 week after discontinuation of selegiline.
1. Rowland MJ, *et al.* Hypoglycemia caused by selegiline, an antiparkinsonian drug: can such side effects be predicted? *J Clin Pharmacol* 1994; **34:** 80–5.

Precautions

Selegiline should be used with caution in patients with a history of peptic ulceration and avoided in those with active ulceration. It should also be used with caution in uncontrolled hypertension, arrhythmias, angina, or psychosis.

◊ Investigation¹ of the autonomic effects of selegiline as a potential cause of the unexpected mortality observed in one study² in patients with Parkinson's disease receiving selegiline and levodopa (see Parkinsonism, below) suggested that the risk of orthostatic hypotension with this combination had been underestimated. It was considered prudent to withdraw selegiline from those with symptomatic orthostatic hypotension or concomitant cardiovascular or cerebrovascular disease. For those without symptomatic morbidity, but a greater than 20 mmHg fall in blood pressure on standing for 2 minutes, gradual withdrawal of selegiline with a concomitant retitration of levodopa dosage should be considered.
1. Churchyard A, *et al.* Autonomic effects of selegiline: possible cardiovascular toxicity in Parkinson's disease. *J Neurol Neurosurg Psychiatry* 1997; **63:** 228–34.
2. Parkinson's Disease Research Group of the United Kingdom. Comparison of therapeutic effects and mortality data of levodopa and levodopa combined with selegiline in patients with early, mild Parkinson's disease. *BMJ* 1995; **311:** 1602–7.

Interactions

Selegiline is less likely than non-selective MAOIs, such as phenelzine, to interact with tyramine in food; such hypertensive reactions have been reported rarely at usual doses but the manufacturer has warned that its selectivity is lost at higher doses and it must be assumed that selegiline can usually only be used safely without dietary restrictions at doses of up to 10 mg daily. For dietary restrictions applicable to patients taking MAOIs, see p.305.

Even when given in therapeutic doses life-threatening interactions can occur between selegiline and pethidine. Serious reactions, sometimes fatal, have also been reported when selegiline has been used with tricyclic antidepressants or selective serotonin reuptake inhibitors (SSRIs). The manufacturer recommends that 14 days should elapse between discontinuation of selegiline and starting treatment with tricyclic antidepressants or SSRIs. Conversely, selegiline should not be given to patients who have recently received these antidepressants; at least 5 weeks should elapse between discontinuing fluoxetine and starting treatment with selegiline.

Selegiline is contra-indicated in patients receiving serotonin agonists such as sumatriptan.

◊ Although selegiline (a selective inhibitor of monoamine oxidase type B) is less likely than non-selective MAOIs to interact with tyramine in food, like other MAOIs it can produce life-threatening reactions when given with *pethidine*.¹ The US manufacturers (Somerset, USA) have stated that there has been a report of hypertensive crisis in a patient taking recommended doses of selegiline and *ephedrine*.

Although there have been studies in which patients with parkinsonism[2] have received selegiline with *SSRIs* such as fluoxetine[2] or paroxetine[3] (apparently without any problems) there have been reports of reactions[4-6] such as shivering and sweating, hypertension, hyperactivity, and ataxia occurring when selegiline and fluoxetine have been given together. The FDA noted[7] that reactions similar to those between SSRIs and non-selective MAOIs had also been reported in patients taking selegiline with paroxetine or sertraline.

Severe reactions, sometimes fatal, have also occurred in patients taking selegiline and *tricyclic antidepressants*.[7] For a report of serotonin syndrome developing when *venlafaxine* was given after selegiline (despite a drug-free period) see p.313.

There has been a report[8] of a patient receiving the non-selective MAOI *iproniazid* who experienced severe orthostatic hypotension when given selegiline. A study[9] of selegiline and the reversible MAOI *moclobemide* administered concomitantly to healthy subjects showed that the two drugs together markedly increased the pressor response to tyramine compared with the effects of each drug used alone. The authors concluded that dietary restriction of tyramine-containing foods would be necessary if these two drugs were to be used together.

A hypertensive reaction following low-dose dopamine infusion has been reported[10] in a 75-year-old patient receiving a daily dose of 10 mg of selegiline for Parkinson's disease. The authors suggest that this may indicate a non-specific action of selegiline at usual doses on peripheral monoamine oxidase inhibitor type-A.

1. Zornberg GL, *et al.* Severe adverse interaction between pethidine and selegiline. *Lancet* 1991; **337:** 246. Correction. *ibid.*; 440.
2. Waters CH. Fluoxetine and selegiline—lack of significant interaction. *Can J Neurol Sci* 1994; **21:** 259–61.
3. Toyama SC, Iacono RP. Is it safe to combine a selective serotonin reuptake inhibitor with selegiline? *Ann Pharmacother* 1994; **28:** 405–6.
4. Suchowersky O, de Vries JD. Interaction of fluoxetine and selegiline. *Can J Psychiatry* 1990; **35:** 571–2.
5. Jermain DM, *et al.* Potential fluoxetine-selegiline interaction. *Ann Pharmacother* 1992; **26:** 1300.
6. Montastruc JL, *et al.* Pseudophaeochromocytoma in parkinsonian patient treated with fluoxetine plus selegiline. *Lancet* 1993; **341:** 555.
7. Anonymous. Eldepryl and antidepressant interaction. *FDA Med Bull* 1995; **25** (Feb.): 6.
8. Pare CMB, *et al.* Attempts to attenuate the 'cheese effect': combined drug therapy in depressive illness. *J Affect Disord* 1985; **9:** 137–41.
9. Korn A, *et al.* Tyramine pressor sensitivity in healthy subjects during concomitant treatment with moclobemide and selegiline. *Eur J Clin Pharmacol* 1996; **49:** 273–8.
10. Rose LM, *et al.* A hypertensive reaction induced by concurrent use of selegiline and dopamine. *Ann Pharmacother* 2000; **34:** 1020–4.

Oral contraceptives. The total area under the curve for selegiline given in single doses of 5 to 40 mg was raised 10- to 20-fold in 4 women who were using oral hormonal contraceptives when compared with 4 women receiving no concomitant medication.[1] It was suggested that concomitant use of selegiline and oral hormonal contraceptives should be avoided or the dosage of selegiline reduced.

1. Laine K, *et al.* Dose linearity study of selegiline pharmacokinetics after oral administration: evidence for strong drug interaction with female sex steroids. *Br J Clin Pharmacol* 1999; **47:** 249–54.

Pharmacokinetics

Selegiline is readily absorbed from the gastrointestinal tract from conventional preparations and crosses the blood-brain barrier. It undergoes extensive first-pass metabolism in the liver to produce at least 5 metabolites, including *l*-(–)-desmethylselegiline (norselegiline), *l*-(–)-*N*-methylamfetamine and *l*-(–)-amfetamine. Concentrations of selegiline metabolites are greatly reduced following administration of the oral lyophilisate preparation, the majority of which undergoes absorption through the buccal mucosa. It is excreted as metabolites mainly in the urine and approximately 15% appears in the faeces.

◊ References.
1. Heinonen EH, *et al.* Pharmacokinetic aspects of l-deprenyl (selegiline) and its metabolites. *Clin Pharmacol Ther* 1994; **56:** 742–9.
2. Mahmood I, *et al.* Clinical pharmacokinetics and pharmacodynamics of selegiline: an update. *Clin Pharmacokinet* 1997; **33:** 91–102.

Uses and Administration

Selegiline is an irreversible selective inhibitor of monoamine oxidase type B, an enzyme involved in the metabolic degradation of dopamine in the brain. It enhances the effects of levodopa and is used in Parkinson's disease as an adjunct to levodopa therapy, usually when fluctuations in mobility have become a problem, but see Parkinsonism, below. Selegiline may also be given alone in early Parkinsonism disease in an attempt to delay the need for levodopa therapy.

Selegiline hydrochloride is given by mouth as conventional preparations such as tablets or oral liquid, or as oral lyophilisate tablets (Zelapar, UK). The dose of the conventional preparations is 10 mg daily, either as a single dose in the morning or in 2 divided doses of 5 mg at breakfast and lunchtime. The initial dose of the oral lyophilisate tablets is 1.25 mg daily at least 5 minutes before breakfast; patients already receiving 10 mg of conventional preparations can be transferred to 1.25 mg of the oral lyophilisate. Addition of selegiline to levodopa therapy may enable the dosage of levodopa to be reduced by about 10 to 50%. To avoid initial confusion and agitation, particularly in the elderly, it may be appropriate for the conventional preparations to start treatment with a dose of 2.5 mg daily.

Other conditions in which selegiline has been tried include dementia and depression.

◊ Some references to the actions of selegiline.
1. Youdim MBH, Finberg JPM. Pharmacological actions of l-deprenyl (selegiline) and other selective monoamine oxidase B inhibitors. *Clin Pharmacol Ther* 1994; **56:** 725–33.
2. Lange KW, *et al.* Biochemical actions of l-deprenyl (selegiline). *Clin Pharmacol Ther* 1994; **56:** 734–41.

Dementia. The hypothesis that neurodegeneration in Alzheimer's disease (p.1412) might be due to free radical formation has led to drugs such as selegiline being tried as antioxidant therapy. However, the value of selegiline in Alzheimer's disease remains unclear.

Double-blind studies[1,2] indicate that selegiline 10 mg daily may produce beneficial effects in patients with Alzheimer's disease but it has been suggested that improvements in mood and cognitive function may be due to a reduction in tension and depression.[3] A 15-month study in Alzheimers's patients with mild cognitive impairment showed selegiline 10 mg daily to have little effect,[4] although the authors pointed out that those with more severe dementia have shown more response in other studies. The conclusion of a later study[5] that selegiline 10 mg daily slowed progression in patients with moderate disease has been criticised[6] on the grounds that any effect was only evident after statistical adjustment to the original analysis. A meta-analysis[7] that examined the effects of selegiline concluded that the evidence for a beneficial effect of selegiline on patients with Alzheimer's disease was promising, but that there was not yet enough evidence to recommend its routine use in practice.

1. Piccinin GL, *et al.* Neuropsychological effects of L-deprenyl in Alzheimer's type dementia. *Clin Neuropharmacol* 1990; **13:** 147–63.
2. Mangoni A, *et al.* Effects of a MAO-B inhibitor in the treatment of Alzheimer disease. *Eur Neurol* 1991; **31:** 100–107.
3. Anonymous. Drugs for Alzheimer's disease. *Drug Ther Bull* 1990; **28:** 42–4.
4. Burke WJ, *et al.* L-Deprenyl in the treatment of mild dementia of the Alzheimer type: results of a 15-month trial. *J Am Geriatr Soc* 1993; **41:** 1219–25.
5. Sano M, *et al.* A controlled trial of selegiline, alpha-tocopherol, or both as treatment for Alzheimer's disease. *N Engl J Med* 1997; **336:** 1216–22.
6. Pincus MM. Alpha-tocopherol and Alzheimer's disease. *N Engl J Med* 1997; **337:** 572.
7. Birks J, Flicker L. Selegiline for Alzheimer's disease (updated 30 May 2001). Available in The Cochrane Library; Issue 4. Oxford: Update Software; 2001.

Depression. Selegiline is a selective inhibitor of monoamine oxidase type B and there are reports of it producing improvement in depression.[1-3] However at the dosage level usually required to produce an antidepressant effect the specificity of selegiline is reported to be lost and it has been suggested that the efficacy of selegiline as an antidepressant might depend on inhibition of monoamine oxidase A rather than inhibition of monoamine oxidase B alone. Such a loss of specificity would mean that patients taking selegiline for depression would need to observe the dietary restrictions applicable to non-selective MAOIs.

1. Mendlewicz J, Youdim MBH. L-Deprenil, a selective monoamine oxidase type B inhibitor, in the treatment of depression: a double-blind evaluation. *Br J Psychiatry* 1983; **142:** 508–11
2. Mann JJ, *et al.* A controlled study of the antidepressant efficacy and side-effects of (–)-deprenyl. *Arch Gen Psychiatry* 1989; **46:** 45–50.
3. Sunderland T, *et al.* High-dose selegiline in treatment-resistant older depressive patients. *Arch Gen Psychiatry* 1994; **51:** 607–15.

Narcoleptic syndrome. Small controlled studies[1,2] have suggested that selegiline 20 to 40 mg daily has a beneficial effect on symptoms of narcolepsy and cataplexy (p.1505); at such a dosage a low-tyramine diet is considered necessary.

1. Hublin C, *et al.* Selegiline in the treatment of narcolepsy. *Neurology* 1994; **44:** 2095–2101.
2. Mayer G, *et al.* Selegeline [sic] hydrochloride in narcolepsy: a double-blind, placebo-controlled study. *Clin Neuropharmacol* 1995; **18:** 306–19.

Parkinsonism. As a selective monoamine oxidase type B inhibitor, selegiline reduces the metabolism of dopamine and thereby enhances its actions. It reduces levodopa's 'end-of-dose' effect and has a dose-sparing effect. Some have used it in an attempt to delay the need for levodopa. It has been postulat-

ed that progression of Parkinson's disease (p.1160) might be due to free radicals, generated during the metabolism of dopamine, having a cytotoxic effect on dopaminergic neurones in the substantia nigra. It has been suggested that selegiline might therefore slow disease progression by reducing the formation of free radicals generated by oxidation of dopamine by monoamine oxidase type B. In one large early study,[1] the DATATOP study, selegiline monotherapy delayed the need to start levodopa in patients with early Parkinson's disease. These findings were corroborated by other smaller studies.[2,3] There has been much debate over whether the benefit was due to a neuroprotective or symptomatic effect. Re-analysis of the DATATOP data by independent workers[4,5] and findings of other studies[6] support a symptomatic effect. Subsequent studies involving DATATOP patients have also been consistent with a symptomatic effect; any benefit produced by selegiline appeared to be less pronounced as the duration of treatment increased[7] and was lost completely long-term.[8,9] A later study[10] designed to minimise any symptomatic effect has cast doubt on whether the delay in progression of the signs and symptoms of Parkinson's disease obtained with selegiline is entirely due to a symptomatic effect.

Studies of the addition of levodopa to selegiline therapy[6,11,12] indicate that selegiline permits a modest reduction in the dosage requirements of levodopa. An interim analysis of a study of the early addition of selegiline to levodopa has also suggested that selegiline might stabilise the long-term daily levodopa dosage.[13]

However, the use of selegiline in Parkinson's disease has been questioned after one UK study[11] found an unexpected increase in mortality in patients taking levodopa with selegiline compared with those taking levodopa alone. No difference in mortality had been detected at the 3-year follow-up[14] but after an average follow-up of 5.6 years[11] mortality was 60% higher in the group receiving selegiline. The study has been criticised on many grounds including the fact that mortality was very high in both arms of the study[15] and has been the subject of much debate.[16,17] The authors of the study[11] had stated that they would advise the study patients to withdraw selegiline therapy. Analysis of follow-up data[18] until the selegiline arm of the study was terminated (average 6.8 years) found an excess mortality of about 35%, a figure calculated[19] to be no longer significant. However, because of the premature termination of the study such results were considered[20] to be biased. Whether any excess in mortality is causally related to selegiline is still unclear. Some consider that changes in prescribing practice based on this study are not warranted.[16] Others[20] have made a cautious recommendation not to start combination treatment in patients with newly diagnosed Parkinson's disease but consider that there is little evidence to advise patients who have been using selegiline with levodopa for years without problem to change their treatment. An evaluation of mortality among patients taking antiparkinsonian drugs (using the UK General Practice Research Database) provided evidence against there being substantial excess mortality associated with the use of selegiline.[21] These results are supported by a meta-analysis[23] of 5 randomised, double-blind trials which found no increase in mortality associated with selegiline treatment regardless of concurrent levodopa. Furthermore, increased mortality was not observed in patients in the original DATATOP trial[1] after an average follow-up time of 8.2 years. However, it was noted that the delay of disability observed in the early phase of selegiline therapy[1,7] was not associated with longer life during follow-up.[22]

1. The Parkinson Study Group. Effect of deprenyl on the progression of disability in early Parkinson's disease. *N Engl J Med* 1989; **321:** 1364–71.
2. Tetrud JW, Langston JW. The effect of deprenyl (selegiline) on the natural history of Parkinson's disease. *Science* 1989; **245:** 519–22.
3. Allain H, *et al.* Selegiline in de novo parkinsonian patients: the French selegiline multicenter trial (FSMT). *Acta Neurol Scand* 1991; **84** (suppl 136): 73–8.
4. Schulzer M, *et al.* The antiparkinson efficacy of deprenyl derives from transient improvement that is likely to be symptomatic. *Ann Neurol* 1992; **32:** 795–8.
5. Ward CD. Does selegiline delay progression of Parkinson's disease? A critical re-evaluation of the DATATOP study. *J Neurol Neurosurg Psychiatry* 1994; **57:** 217–20.
6. Brannan T, Yahr MD. Comparative study of selegiline plus L-dopa–carbidopa versus L-dopa–carbidopa alone in the treatment of Parkinson's disease. *Ann Neurol* 1995; **37:** 95–8.
7. The Parkinson Study Group. Effects of tocopherol and deprenyl on the progression of disability in early Parkinson's disease. *N Engl J Med* 1993; **328:** 176–83.
8. Parkinson Study Group. Impact of deprenyl and tocopherol treatment on Parkinson's disease in DATATOP subjects not requiring levodopa. *Ann Neurol* 1996; **39:** 29–36.
9. Parkinson Study Group. Impact of deprenyl and tocopherol treatment on Parkinson's disease in DATATOP patients requiring levodopa. *Ann Neurol* 1996; **39:** 37–45.
10. Olanow CW, *et al.* The effect of deprenyl and levodopa on the progression of Parkinson's disease. *Ann Neurol* 1996; **38:** 771–7.
11. Parkinson's Disease Research Group of the United Kingdom. Comparison of therapeutic effects and mortality data of levodopa and levodopa combined with selegiline in patients with early, mild Parkinson's disease. *BMJ* 1995; **311:** 1602–7.
12. Myllylä VV, *et al.* Early selegiline therapy reduces levodopa dose requirement in Parkinson's disease. *Acta Neurol Scand* 1995; **91:** 177–82.
13. Larsen JP, Boas J. Norwegian-Danish Study Group. The effects of early selegiline therapy on long-term treatment and parkinsonian disability: an interim analysis of a Norwegian-Danish 5-year study. *Mov Disord* 1997; **12:** 175–82.

14. Parkinson's Disease Research Group in the United Kingdom. Comparisons of the therapeutic effects of levodopa, levodopa and selegiline, and bromocriptine in patients with early, mild Parkinson's disease: three year interim report. *BMJ* 1993; **307:** 467–72.
15. Olanow CW, *et al.* Patients taking selegiline may have received more levodopa than necessary. *BMJ* 1996; **312:** 702–3.
16. Ahlskog JE. Treatment of early Parkinson's disease: are complicated strategies justified? *Mayo Clin Proc* 1996; **71:** 659–70.
17. Mizuno Y, Kondo T. Mortality associated with selegiline in Parkinson's disease: what do the available data mean? *Drug Safety* 1997; **16:** 289–94.
18. Ben-Shlomo Y, *et al.* Investigation by Parkinson's Disease Research Group of United Kingdom into excess mortality seen with combined levodopa and selegiline treatment in patients with early, mild Parkinson's disease: further results of randomised trial and confidential inquiry. *BMJ* 1998; **316:** 1191–6.
19. Abrams KR. Monitoring randomised controlled trials. *BMJ* 1998; **316:** 1183–4.
20. Breteler MMB. Selegiline, or the problem of early termination of clinical trials. *BMJ* 1998; **316:** 1182–3.
21. Thorogood M, *et al.* Mortality in people taking selegiline: observational study. *BMJ* 1998; **317:** 252–4.
22. The Parkinson Study Group. Mortality in DATATOP: A multicenter trial in early Parkinson's disease. *Ann Neurol* 1998; **43:** 318–25.
23. Olanow CW, *et al.* Effect of selegiline on mortality in patients with Parkinson's disease: a meta-analysis. *Neurology* 1998; **51:** 825–30.

Preparations

BP 2001: Selegiline Oral Solution; Selegiline Tablets;
USP 25: Selegiline Hydrochloride Tablets.

Proprietary Preparations (details are given in Part 3)
Aust.: Amboneural; Cognitiv†; Jumex; Regepar; *Austral.:* Eldepryl; Selgene; *Belg.:* Eldepryl; *Braz.:* Deprilan; Elepril; Jumexil; Niar; *Canad.:* Eldepryl; *Denm.:* Eldepryl; Tremorex; *Fin.:* Eldepryl; *Fr.:* Deprenyl; *Ger.:* Amindan; Antiparkin; Deprenyl†; MA-Otil; Movergan; Selegam; Selemerck; Selepark; Selgimed; *Hong Kong:* Jumex; Selegos; *Irl.:* Clondepryl; Eldepryl; *Israel:* Apomex; Jumex; *Ital.:* Egibren; Jumex; Seledat; Selpar†; *Mex.:* Niar; *Neth.:* Eldepryl; *Norw.:* Eldepryl; *NZ:* Eldepryl; Selgene; *Port.:* Jumex; *S.Afr.:* Eldepryl; *Singapore:* Elegelin; Jumex; Selegos; *Spain:* Plurimen; *Swed.:* Eldepryl; *Switz.:* Jumexal; Regepar; Selecim; *Thai.:* Julab; Jumex; Kinline; Sefmex; Selgene; Seline; *UK:* Centrapryl†; Eldepryl; Stilline†; Vivapryl†; Zelapar; *USA:* Atapryl; Carbex; Eldepryl.

Talipexole Hydrochloride (2990-z)

Talipexole Hydrochloride (*rINNM*).

Alefexole Hydrochloride; B-HT-920. 6-Allyl-2-amino-5,6,7,8-tetrahydro-4*H*-thiazolo[4,5-*d*]azepine dihydrochloride.
$C_{10}H_{15}N_3S,2HCl$ = 282.2.
CAS — 101626-70-4 (talipexole); 36085-73-1 (talipexole hydrochloride).

Profile

Talipexole hydrochloride is a dopamine D_2-agonist that is used in the management of parkinsonism in usual doses of 1.2 to 3.6 mg daily, in divided doses by mouth. It is also under investigation in the treatment of schizophrenia.

◊ References.
1. Mizuno Y, *et al.* Preliminary study of B-HT 920, a novel dopamine agonist, for the treatment of Parkinson's disease. *Drug Invest* 1993; **5:** 186–92.
2. Ohmori T, *et al.* B-HT 920, a dopamine D2 agonist, in the treatment of negative symptoms of chronic schizophrenia. *Biol Psychiatry* 1993; **33:** 687–93.

Preparations

Proprietary Preparations (details are given in Part 3)
Jpn: Domin.

Terguride (3639-p)

Terguride (*rINN*).

1,1-Diethyl-3-(6-methylergolin-8α-yl) urea.
$C_{20}H_{28}N_4O$ = 340.5.
CAS — 37686-84-3.

Profile

Terguride, an ergot derivative, is a partial dopamine agonist with general properties similar to those of bromocriptine (p.1164). It is used in the treatment of disorders related to hyperprolactinaemia. It is also being investigated in the management of parkinsonism.

◊ References.
1. Krause W, *et al.* Pharmacokinetics and endocrine effects of terguride in healthy subjects. *Eur J Clin Pharmacol* 1990; **38:** 609–15.
2. Baronti F, *et al.* Partial dopamine agonist therapy of levodopa-induced dyskinesias. *Neurology* 1992; **42:** 1241–3.

Tolcapone (15928-m)

Tolcapone (*BAN, USAN, rINN*).

Ro-40-7592. 3,4-Dihydroxy-4'-methyl-5-nitrobenzophenone; 3,4-Dihydroxy-5-nitrophenyl(4-methylphenyl)methanone.
$C_{14}H_{11}NO_5$ = 273.2.
CAS — 134308-13-7.
ATC — N04BX01.

Adverse Effects

The most common adverse effects associated with tolcapone are diarrhoea, nausea, anorexia, dyskinesia, orthostatic hypotension, hallucinations, and sleep disorders. Diarrhoea may be severe enough to warrant discontinuation. Increases in liver enzyme values have occurred and hepatitis, sometimes fatal, has been reported. Tolcapone and its metabolites can produce a yellow intensification in the colour of urine.

Effects on the liver. The UK Committee on Safety of Medicines had noted[1] that, following a report[2] in September 1998 of fatal acute hepatic failure associated with tolcapone the European Committee for Proprietary Medicinal Products had reviewed all reports of hepatic injury with tolcapone. There had been 10 reports of serious hepatic adverse reactions since tolcapone was marketed in October 1997, which included 7 reports of hepatitis, 3 of which had a fatal outcome. Serious hepatic reactions occurred unpredictably and their development was not always predicted by liver function monitoring. Consequently, in Europe, tolcapone is voluntarily withdrawn by the manufacturers in November 1998.
1. Committee on Safety of Medicines/Medicines Control Agency. Withdrawal of tolcapone (Tasmar). *Current Problems* 1999; **25:** 2.
2. Assal F, *et al.* Tolcapone and fulminant hepatitis. *Lancet* 1998; **352:** 958.

Effects on the skin. For reference to the development of vitiligo in a patient following addition of tolcapone to levodopa/carbidopa treatment, see under Levodopa, p.1170.

Precautions

Tolcapone should not be given to patients with hepatic impairment or raised liver enzymes values. Liver enzyme levels should be monitored when starting treatment with tolcapone and then every 2 weeks for the first year of therapy, every 4 weeks for the next 6 months, and then every 8 weeks thereafter. If the dose is to be increased to 200 mg three times daily liver enzyme monitoring should take place before increasing the dose and then re-initiated at the frequency above. Tolcapone should be discontinued if liver enzyme levels exceed the upper limit of normal or if signs or symptoms suggestive of the onset of hepatic failure occur. Tolcapone should not be reintroduced to patients who have developed evidence of hepatic injury while receiving tolcapone. Tolcapone should be administered with caution to patients with severe renal impairment.

Tolcapone is contra-indicated in patients with a previous history of nontraumatic rhabdomyolysis or symptoms of hyperpyrexia and confusion possibly related to the neuroleptic malignant syndrome. Use with levodopa may cause dizziness and orthostatic hypotension; if affected patients should not drive or operate machinery.

Abrupt withdrawal of tolcapone or dose reduction should be avoided.

Elderly. A report of confusion in 3 elderly patients with severe Parkinson's disease associated with addition of tolcapone to antiparkinsonian therapy.[1] It was suggested that a starting dose of tolcapone 100 mg daily might be more suitable in frail patients with severe disease. It was noted[2] that a reduction in levodopa dosage is generally recommended when tolcapone is given to patients such as these, who were receiving 500 to 600 mg of levodopa daily.
1. Henry C, Wilson JA. Catechol-O-methyltransferase inhibitors in Parkinson's disease. *Lancet* 1998; **351:** 1965–6.
2. Harper J, Vieira B. Catechol-O-methyltransferase inhibitors in Parkinson's disease. *Lancet* 1998; **352:** 578.

Interactions

Tolcapone may influence the pharmacokinetics of drugs metabolised by catechol-*O*-methyltransferase; concomitant administration should be undertaken with care. Increased concentrations of benserazide and its active metabolite have been reported during concomitant administration. The manufacturer advises that non-selective MAOIs should not be used with tolcapone.

Pharmacokinetics

Tolcapone is rapidly absorbed from the gastrointestinal tract and maximum plasma concentrations have been obtained within 2 hours of administration by mouth; food delays and decreases the absorption. Absolute bioavailability is reported to be about 65%. Tolcapone is more than 99% bound to plasma proteins and is not widely distributed into body tissues. It is extensively metabolised, mainly by conjugation to the inactive glucuronide, but methylation by catechol-*O*-methyltransferase to 3-*O*-methyltolcapone and metabolism by cytochrome P450 isoenzymes also occurs. About 60% of a dose is excreted in the urine with the remainder appearing in the faeces. The elimination half-life has been reported to be about 2 hours. The clearance of unbound tolcapone may be reduced by 50% in patients with moderate cirrhotic liver disorders.

◊ References.
1. Dingemanse J, *et al.* Integrated pharmacokinetics and pharmacodynamics of the novel catechol-O-methyltransferase inhibitor tolcapone during first administration to humans. *Clin Pharmacol Ther* 1995; **57:** 508–17.
2. Jorga KM, *et al.* Effect of liver impairment on the pharmacokinetics of tolcapone and its metabolites. *Clin Pharmacol Ther* 1998; **63:** 646–54.

Uses and Administration

Tolcapone is a peripheral inhibitor of catechol-*O*-methyltransferase (COMT), an enzyme involved in the metabolism of dopamine and levodopa. It has been used as an adjunct to levodopa and dopa-decarboxylase inhibitor combinations in the management of Parkinson's disease for patients who cannot be stabilised on these levodopa combinations or for those who experience 'end-of-dose' deterioration. Because of the risk of serious hepatotoxicity the FDA in the USA restricted its use to when other adjunctive therapy was ineffective or contra-indicated. In Europe, tolcapone was withdrawn from the market in November 1998.

The usual recommended dosage of tolcapone is 100 mg given three times daily; up to a maximum of 200 mg three times daily may be considered if the clinical benefit justifies the increased risk of hepatotoxicity. The first dose of the day should be taken at the same time as the levodopa preparation. Most patients already taking more than 600 mg of levodopa daily will require a reduction in their dosage of levodopa.

Tolcapone should be withdrawn gradually if a substantial clinical benefit is not obtained within the first 3 weeks of treatment; abrupt withdrawal or dose reduction should be avoided.

Parkinsonism. Tolcapone is a reversible peripheral inhibitor of catechol-*O*-methyltransferase (COMT), an enzyme involved in the metabolism of levodopa and dopamine.[1] It appears to differ from entacapone (p.1168) by being a more potent COMT inhibitor in the periphery and by penetrating into the brain (although the significance of any central effects of COMT inhibition are not known).[1] When given to patients with Parkinson's disease (p.1160) and levodopa-related fluctuations in disability or 'end-of-dose' effects, it has prolonged the clinical benefit obtained with levodopa and allowed the total daily dosage of levodopa to be reduced.[2,3] Benefit has also been reported[4] when added to levodopa therapy in patients with stable Parkinson's disease.
1. Nutt JG. Catechol-O-methyltransferase inhibitors for treatment of Parkinson's disease. *Lancet* 1998; **351:** 1221–2.
2. Kurth MC, *et al.* Tolcapone improves motor function and reduces levodopa requirement in patients with Parkinson's disease experiencing motor fluctuations: a multicenter, double-blind, randomized, placebo-controlled trial. *Neurology* 1997; **48:** 81–7.
3. Rajput AH, *et al.* Tolcapone improves motor function in parkinsonian patients with the "wearing-off" phenomenon: a double-blind placebo-controlled, multicenter trial. *Neurology* 1997; **49:** 1066–71.
4. Waters CH, *et al.* Tolcapone Stable Study Group. Tolcapone in stable Parkinson's disease: efficacy and safety of long-term treatment. *Neurology* 1997; **49:** 665–71.

Preparations

Proprietary Preparations (details are given in Part 3)
Aust.: Tasmar; *Denm.:* Tasmar†; *Hong Kong:* Tasmar; *Irl.:* Tasmar†; *Mex.:* Tasmar; *Norw.:* Tasmar; *NZ:* Tasmar; *S.Afr.:* Tasmar; *Singapore:* Tasmar; *Swed.:* Tasmar†; *Switz.:* Tasmar; *Thai.:* Tasmar; *UK:* Tasmar†; *USA:* Tasmar.

Electrolytes

Electrolytes are used to correct disturbances in fluid and electrolyte homoeostasis or acid-base balance and to re-establish osmotic equilibrium of specific ions. The osmotic effects of solutions may be expressed in terms of osmolality which is defined as the 'molal' concentration in moles (or osmoles) per kg of solvent, or in terms of osmolarity which is the 'molar' concentration in moles (or osmoles) per litre of solution. In clinical practice, solute concentrations are measured per litre of solution and are expressed as millimoles (mmol) per litre or sometimes as milliequivalents (mEq) per litre. Milliequivalents are converted to millimoles by dividing by the valency of the ion. Positively charged ions are known as *cations* and include calcium, magnesium, potassium, and sodium ions. Negatively charged ions are known as *anions* and include bicarbonate, chloride, and phosphate ions. The ions principally involved in fluid and electrolyte homoeostasis and acid-base balance are sodium, chloride, bicarbonate, and potassium. Calcium, phosphate, and magnesium have a central role in the formation of bone mineral.

Acid-base Balance

Within the body, acid is mostly produced during cellular respiration in the form of carbon dioxide. Small amounts of various non-volatile acids are generated via metabolism, including lactic acid, uric acid, keto acids, and some inorganic acids such as sulfuric and phosphoric acids. However, for normal tissue function, the pH of the body needs to be held within a narrow range. The pH of arterial blood is normally maintained between about 7.38 and 7.42 by means of compensatory respiratory, renal, and buffering mechanisms.

The most important buffer system in the extracellular fluid is the bicarbonate-carbonic acid system. Bicarbonate and hydrogen ions are in equilibrium with carbonic acid which is in turn in equilibrium with carbon dioxide in the body fluid, as expressed by:

$$H^+ + HCO_3^- \leftrightarrow H_2CO_3 \leftrightarrow CO_2 + H_2O$$

A normal plasma-bicarbonate concentration in adults is in the range of 20 to 30 mmol per litre and arterial partial pressure of carbon dioxide (P_aCO_2) is normally 4.7 to 5.7 kPa (31 to 43 mmHg).

Ultimately, excess acid must be removed from the body and base regenerated. P_aCO_2 is under respiratory control with carbon dioxide being excreted by the lungs. Plasma-bicarbonate concentrations are regulated by the kidneys, where bicarbonate is actively regenerated or reabsorbed. Organic acids such as lactic acid may be eliminated by metabolism; and other non-volatile acids, such as the inorganic acids of phosphate and sulfate, are excreted via the kidneys with simultaneous regeneration of bicarbonate.

The relationship between plasma pH, P_aCO_2, and bicarbonate is defined by the Henderson-Hasselbalch equation which is used to assess acid-base balance. For clinical purposes, this equation becomes

$$pH = pK_{CO_2} + \log\left(\frac{C_{HCO_3}}{\alpha \times P_aCO_2}\right)$$

where pH is the plasma pH, pK_{CO_2} is the carbonic acid dissociation constant (6.1), C_{HCO_3} is the plasma-bicarbonate concentration, α is a value representing carbon dioxide solubility, and P_aCO_2 is the arterial partial pressure of carbon dioxide. Disorders of acid-base balance may be due to a change in plasma-bicarbonate concentrations (metabolic) or to a change in P_aCO_2 (respiratory), although mixed disorders do occur.

The 4 major acid-base disturbances are:

• metabolic acidosis—a decrease in the plasma-bicarbonate concentration
• metabolic alkalosis—an increase in the plasma-bicarbonate concentration
• respiratory acidosis—hypoventilation and a raised P_aCO_2
• respiratory alkalosis—hyperventilation and a reduced P_aCO_2

A further measure that may provide useful information in the assessment of metabolic acidosis is the plasma anion gap. This is the difference in ionic charge between the principal plasma cation (sodium) and anions (chloride and bicarbonate), and provides an estimation of unmeasured serum anions, which include inorganic and organic acids.

◊ References.
1. Gluck SL. Acid-base. *Lancet* 1998; **352:** 474–9.
2. Hood VL, Tannen RL. Protection of acid-base balance by pH regulation of acid production. *N Engl J Med* 1998; **339:** 819–26.

Metabolic acidosis. Metabolic acidosis, characterised by a low plasma-bicarbonate concentration and a tendency towards a fall in arterial pH, is the most frequent acid-base abnormality.

Metabolic acidosis with a normal anion gap is usually caused by excessive losses of bicarbonate from the gastrointestinal tract (as in severe diarrhoeas) or failure of the kidneys to reabsorb or regenerate adequate bicarbonate (as in the renal tubular acidoses). Ingestion of acidifying salts such as ammonium chloride, which generate hydrochloric acid, can also result in this type of acidosis. Metabolic acidosis characterised by an increased anion gap is often due to a reduction in the renal excretion of inorganic acids such as phosphates and sulfates as in renal failure (uraemic acidosis), or to the net accumulation of organic acids as, for example, in lactic acidosis or diabetic ketoacidosis.

Metabolic acidosis is diagnosed and monitored by measurement of serum electrolytes, arterial pH, and P_aCO_2. There is often hyperventilation with reduced cardiac function, constriction of peripheral veins, inhibition of the hepatic metabolism of lactate, and impairment of consciousness.

The main aim of **treatment** is to manage any underlying disorder, and in some cases this will be sufficient to enable the body's homoeostatic mechanisms to correct the acid-base imbalance. The advantages of more active treatment of the acidosis must be balanced against the risks, including over-alkalinisation, and in consequence such therapy tends to be reserved for more persistent or severe cases.

The usual alkalinising agent is sodium bicarbonate. It may be given by mouth to replace bicarbonate losses in various chronic metabolic acidoses such as uraemic acidosis or renal tubular acidosis. Potassium bicarbonate may be preferred if the acidosis is associated with potassium deficiency. Potassium citrate and sodium citrate have also been used. More severe and acute cases (particularly where arterial pH is below 7.1) may require intravenous sodium bicarbonate therapy. Intravenous sodium bicarbonate has a role in acute metabolic acidoses attributable to severe renal failure, severe secretory diarrhoeas, and renal tubular acidosis. Although hypertonic solutions have been used, for example, in patients with circulatory overload, roughly isotonic bicarbonate solutions are otherwise preferred; arterial pH and plasma bicarbonate should be raised a little at a time and the patient's response monitored.

Although the role of bicarbonate is accepted in the forms of metabolic acidosis mentioned, its use in the treatment of metabolic acidosis with concomitant tissue hypoxia, particularly lactic acidosis, is controversial.[1,2] The administration of bicarbonate generates carbon dioxide which, if not appropriately eliminated, due to poor tissue perfusion or impaired ventilation or both, diffuses rapidly into the cells exacerbating intracellular acidosis. In addition, in metabolic acidosis associated with organic acids such as lactic acid, there is a risk of over-alkalinisation due to the metabolism of the acid after correction of the arterial pH.

For similar reasons, the use of sodium bicarbonate in advanced cardiac life support (p.790) is no longer routine, although current guidelines permit consideration of its use to correct acidosis if the resuscitation effort is prolonged.

The role of bicarbonate in the management of diabetic ketoacidosis is also limited, although it may be appropriate in certain situations—see Diabetic Emergencies, p.318.

Because of concerns about the effects of bicarbonate other agents have been investigated for the treatment of metabolic acidosis, including trometamol (THAM) and sodium dichloroacetate.[1,2] Alkalinising agents that have to be metabolised to bicarbonate before they have an effect, such as sodium lactate, are not generally used as many patients with acute acidosis have impaired metabolic activity, particularly of lactate.

Peritoneal dialysis, haemodialysis, or haemofiltration is required for refractory metabolic acidosis associated with acute renal failure (p.1184).

1. Arieff AI. Indications for use of bicarbonate in patients with metabolic acidosis. *Br J Anaesth* 1991; **67:** 165–77.
2. Adrogué HJ, Madias NE. Management of life-threatening acid-base disorders. *N Engl J Med* 1998; **338:** 26–34. Correction. *ibid.* 1999; **340:** 247.

Metabolic alkalosis. Metabolic alkalosis with an increased plasma-bicarbonate concentration and a sustained elevation in arterial pH results from excessive renal reabsorption and/or regeneration of bicarbonate. It is commonly seen with volume contraction (chloride depletion), potassium depletion, or mineralocorticoid excess, and may occur with excessive alkali intake as in the milk-alkali syndrome. If the metabolic alkalosis is severe, cardiac arrhythmias and hypoventilation may develop and there can be symptoms of concomitant hypokalaemia such as muscle weakness.

Treatment is generally aimed at the underlying disturbances.[1] Correcting volume depletion by administration of a chloride salt often obviates the need for other treatment; sodium chloride is normally used. However, potassium chloride may also be required if there is potassium depletion, particularly if this is severe. Rarely, direct acidification by the administration of ammonium chloride, dilute hydrochloric acid, or acidifying salts such as lysine hydrochloride or arginine hydrochloride may be required if the alkalosis is severe.

1. Adrogué HJ, Madias NE. Management of life-threatening acid-base disorders. *N Engl J Med* 1998; **338:** 107–11.

Calcium Homoeostasis

The adult body contains about 1.2 kg of calcium, of which approximately 99% is incorporated into the skeleton where its primary role is structural. The remaining 1% is found in body tissues and fluids and is essential for normal nerve conduction, muscle activity, and blood coagulation.

The concentration of calcium in plasma is normally kept within a narrow range (total calcium about 2.15 to 2.60 mmol per litre) by homoeostatic mechanisms involving parathyroid hormone, calcitonin, and vitamin D. Normally about 47% of calcium in plasma is in the ionised physiologically active form (giving a usual range of about 1.00 to 1.25 mmol per litre), about 6% is complexed with anions such as phosphate or citrate, and the remainder is bound to proteins, principally albumin. If the plasma-albumin concentration is raised (as in dehydration) or reduced (as is common in malignancy) it will affect the proportion of ionised calcium. Thus, the total plasma-calcium concentration is commonly adjusted for plasma albumin.

Hypercalcaemia. Hypercalcaemia, an increase in plasma-calcium concentration above the normal range, is most commonly due to primary hyperparathyroidism or malignant disease.[1,2] Less common causes of hypercalcaemia include vitamin D intoxication, granulomatous diseases such as sarcoidosis, familial benign hypercalcaemia, renal failure, thyrotoxicosis, and excess calcium carbonate ingestion (milk-alkali syndrome).[1,2]

Mild asymptomatic hypercalcaemia is often associated with a plasma-concentration elevated above the normal but below 3.00 mmol per litre. Severe symptomatic hypercalcaemia is broadly correlated with a plasma-calcium concentration of more than 3.50 mmol per litre.

Symptoms of hypercalcaemia include thirst, polyuria, anorexia, constipation, muscle weakness, fatigue, and confusion. In severe cases, there may be nausea and vomiting; cardiac arrhythmias may develop but are rare. Extreme hypercalcaemia may result in coma and death. Chronic hypercalcaemia can lead to interstitial nephritis and calcium renal calculi.

Mild asymptomatic hypercalcaemia does not require specific **treatment** and is best corrected by increasing oral fluid intake and treating any identified underlying disease. Patients with severe hypercalcaemia and/or significant symptoms require immediate therapy to reduce plasma-calcium concentrations independent of the cause.[2,3] The first step is rehydration with intravenous sodium chloride 0.9% to restore the intravascular volume and to promote calcium diuresis. Frusemide [furosemide] or other loop diuretics may assist in promoting the renal excretion of calcium but only in the presence of adequate volume expansion and control of other electrolyte losses. Large doses, for example 80 to 100 mg of frusemide [furosemide] administered intravenously every one to two hours, may be required. Thiazide diuretics should be avoided as they increase the renal tubular reabsorption of calcium. Peritoneal dialysis or haemodialysis with calcium-free dialysate should be considered in patients with renal failure for whom urinary excretion of calcium is inadequate. In life-threatening hypercalcaemia, more specific immediate therapy is generally required in addition to saline.[2,3] Most experience has been gained in the treatment of hypercalcaemia of malignancy (see below) using drugs that inhibit bone resorption such as bisphosphonates. Calcitonins are useful as they have a rapid onset of action. However, their effect is moderate and generally short-lived, and drugs with a more sustained effect may also be required. Corticosteroids have been used to prolong the efficacy of calcitonin. Intravenous phosphates have been used to rapidly lower plasma-calcium concentrations but can cause soft tissue calcification resulting in serious adverse effects such as irreversible renal damage and hypotension, and are best avoided. Another drug that has been used for the emergency treatment of hypercalcaemia is trisodium edetate.

Choice of subsequent therapy is likely to depend on the specific cause.

1. Heath D. Hypercalcaemia. *Prescribers' J* 1999; **39:** 234–41.
2. Bushinsky DA, Monk RD. Calcium. *Lancet* 1998; **352:** 306–11.
3. Bilezikian JP. Management of acute hypercalcaemia. *N Engl J Med* 1992; **326:** 1196–1203.

HYPERCALCAEMIA OF MALIGNANCY. About 10% of patients with cancer develop hypercalcaemia of malignancy, which is typically severe and progressive.[1-4] The condition is generally thought to be due to either the production of parathyroid hormone-related protein by a tumour (humoral hypercalcaemia of malignancy) or to the release of bone-resorbing factors (osteoclast-activating factors), which include cytokines such as tumour necrosis factor, growth factors, and interleukin-1, from the site of bone metastases (local osteolytic hypercalcaemia of malignancy). Humoral hypercalcaemia is frequently associated with squamous cell carcinomas of the lung and head and neck whereas local osteolytic hypercalcaemia tends to occur with breast cancer or myeloma.[2,5]

The bisphosphonate pamidronate has been widely used and is considered by many to be the drug of choice[1-5] for **treating** hypercalcaemia once the patient has been adequately rehydrated (see Hypercalcaemia, above). It is given as a single dose or in divided doses over 2 to 4 days, adjusted according to initial plasma-calcium concentrations, by slow intravenous infusion. Although it may be

24 to 48 hours before calcium concentrations start to decrease, the effects can last for 20 to 30 days; regular infusions at intervals of 2 to 3 weeks can be given to maintain normocalcaemia. Clodronate has also been given, administered by intravenous infusion and then by mouth or by intermittent infusion. Etidronate, administered by intravenous infusion on 3 successive days, has been found to reduce hypercalcaemia but has been reported to be less effective than pamidronate[6] and to have a shorter duration of action. Subsequent oral therapy with daily doses of etidronate can prolong the period of normocalcaemia but may cause osteomalacia. There is some evidence that the bisphosphonates may be less effective for humoral than for osteolytic hypercalcaemia.[7]

Plicamycin, a cytotoxic antibiotic with particular activity against osteoclasts, has been used to obtain a rapid (within 24 hours) and sustained reduction in plasma-calcium concentrations in severe hypercalcaemia. However, it is highly toxic and safer drugs such as the bisphosphonates and calcitonins are generally preferred. Gallium nitrate also inhibits bone resorption; initial studies in patients with hypercalcaemia associated with malignancy have indicated beneficial effects but clinical experience is limited; again, the bisphosphonates are likely to be preferred.[3,4]

Corticosteroids are useful in hypercalcaemia associated with corticosteroid-sensitive haematological malignancies such as lymphoma or myeloma. In addition they may be useful to overcome renal tubular resistance to calcitonin[8] but otherwise are not usually effective.[9] There have been individual reports of beneficial results using somatostatin analogues such as octreotide for the treatment of hypercalcaemia of malignancy.

1. Anonymous. Treating cancer-associated hypercalcaemia. *Drug Ther Bull* 1990; **28:** 85–7.
2. Hall TG, Schaiff RAB. Update on the medical treatment of hypercalcaemia of malignancy. *Clin Pharm* 1993; **12:** 117–25.
3. Chisholm MA, *et al.* Acute management of cancer-related hypercalcemia. *Ann Pharmacother* 1996; **30:** 507–13.
4. Watters J, *et al.* The management of malignant hypercalcaemia. *Drugs* 1996; **52:** 837–48.
5. Mundy GR, Guise TA. Hypercalcemia of malignancy. *Am J Med* 1997; **103:** 134–45.
6. Ralston SH, *et al.* Comparison of three intravenous bisphosphonates in cancer-associated hypercalcaemia. *Lancet* 1989; **ii:** 1180–82.
7. Gurney H, *et al.* Parathyroid hormone-related protein and response to pamidronate in tumour-induced hypercalcaemia. *Lancet* 1993; **341:** 1611–13.
8. Hosking DJ, *et al.* Potentiation of calcitonin by corticosteroids during the treatment of the hypercalcaemia of malignancy. *Eur J Clin Pharmacol* 1990; **38:** 37–41.
9. Percival RC, *et al.* Role of glucocorticoids in management of malignant hypercalcaemia. *BMJ* 1984; **389:** 287.

HYPERPARATHYROIDISM. Excess secretion of parathyroid hormone in primary hyperparathyroidism is characterised by hypercalcaemia, which is most frequently asymptomatic, and by hypophosphataemia. Oral phosphates have been used to control hypercalcaemia, and oral bisphosphonates are being investigated. However, in the long term, hypercalcaemia associated with primary hyperparathyroidism appears to be best managed by parathyroidectomy (p.746). Symptomatic hypocalcaemia may occur after surgery, requiring short-term treatment with calcium supplements and vitamin D.

VITAMIN D-MEDIATED HYPERCALCAEMIA. Hypercalcaemia can occur because of increased gastrointestinal absorption of calcium mediated by the active metabolite of vitamin D, 1,25-dihydroxycholecalciferol (calcitriol). This may be a feature of diseases associated with increased vitamin D sensitivity or increased vitamin D production, or may occur due to excess vitamin D administration. For example, granulomatous diseases such as sarcoidosis (p.1058) are associated with unregulated production of 1,25-dihydroxycholecalciferol. Hypercalcaemia due to vitamin D is most commonly seen in patients with renal failure receiving vitamin D analogues such as ergocalciferol.

Treatment of severe hypercalcaemia requires prompt rehydration regardless of the cause (see Hypercalcaemia, above). Where hypercalcaemia is due to vitamin D administration, the vitamin D analogue should be discontinued until normocalcaemia is achieved. Corticosteroids effectively reduce gastrointestinal absorption of calcium, and these may be used intravenously as adjuncts to rehydration in severe hypercalcaemia, and orally for milder hypercalcaemia or longer term therapy. Oral sodium cellulose phosphate, which binds calcium in the gastrointestinal tract, and a low-calcium diet may also be considered. Oral chloroquine or hydroxychloroquine have been used in hypercalcaemia associated with sarcoidosis. Ke-

toconazole may be useful as an alternative to corticosteroids.

References.

1. Adams JS. Vitamin D metabolite-mediated hypercalcemia. *Endocrinol Metab Clin North Am* 1989; **18:** 765–78.
2. Yavuz H. Familiar drugs for the treatment of hypercalcemia. *J Pediatr* 1998; **133:** 311.

Hypocalcaemia. Hypocalcaemia, a decrease in plasma-calcium concentration below the normal range, may be due to impaired or reduced absorption of calcium from the gastrointestinal tract as with vitamin D deficiency disorders (see Osteomalacia, p.744) and chronic renal failure (see Renal Osteodystrophy, p.746). Alternatively, it may be due to deficient parathyroid hormone secretion and/or action as in hypoparathyroidism (p.747) and hypomagnesaemia (see below). Excessive phosphate administration is also a cause of hypocalcaemia (see Hyperphosphataemia, below). Rarely, hypocalcaemia may follow repeated infusions of citrate ions, for example, during transfusions utilising citrated blood, as the citrate complexes with the calcium ion. Respiratory alkalosis due to hyperventilation can also lead to depression of ionised plasma-calcium concentrations.

Where symptoms of hypocalcaemia occur, they are typically associated with increased neuromuscular excitability; paraesthesias can occur and in more severe cases, carpopedal spasm, muscle cramps, tetany, and convulsions may develop.[1-3] Other symptoms include ECG changes and mental disturbances such as irritability and depression. Prolonged hypocalcaemia can lead to dental defects, cataract formation, and in children can result in mental retardation.

In patients with hypocalcaemia due to an underlying disease, long-term management should be aimed at **treating** this disease. Vitamin D supplements are widely used to enhance calcium absorption and correct vitamin D deficiency disorders and hypoparathyroidism. Oral supplements of calcium salts are often also given. Acute hypocalcaemia or hypocalcaemic tetany require emergency treatment with calcium salts given intravenously.

1. Lebowitz MR, Moses AM. Hypocalcemia. *Semin Nephrol* 1992; **12:** 146–58.
2. Reber PM, Heath H. Hypocalcemic emergencies. *Med Clin North Am* 1995; **79:** 93–106.
3. Bushinsky DA, Monk RD. Calcium. *Lancet* 1998; **352:** 306–11.

Magnesium Homoeostasis

Magnesium is an essential body cation which is involved in numerous enzymatic reactions and physiological processes including energy transfer and storage, skeletal development, nerve conduction, and muscle contraction. Over half of the magnesium in the body is found in bone, about 40% is present in muscle and soft tissue, and only about 1% is present in the extracellular fluid. A normal concentration for magnesium in plasma is from about 0.7 to 1.0 mmol per litre.

Magnesium homoeostasis appears to be primarily regulated by the kidney where magnesium is extensively reabsorbed. Bone may act as a magnesium reservoir to reduce plasma-magnesium fluctuations. Magnesium is actively absorbed from the gastrointestinal tract and this is enhanced to some extent by 1,25-dihydroxycholecalciferol (calcitriol).

Hypermagnesaemia. Hypermagnesaemia is an increase in the plasma concentration of magnesium above the normal range, as may follow excessive parenteral administration of salts such as magnesium sulfate. Hypermagnesaemia due to oral magnesium intake is uncommon as the kidneys are able to excrete a relatively large magnesium load. However, it may occur in patients with impaired renal function taking large amounts of magnesium, for example, in antacids or laxatives.

Symptoms of hypermagnesaemia include nausea, vomiting, CNS and respiratory depression, hyporeflexia, muscle weakness, and cardiovascular effects including peripheral vasodilatation, hypotension, bradycardia, and cardiac arrest.

Treatment of mild hypermagnesaemia is usually limited to restricting magnesium intake. In severe hypermagnesaemia, ventilatory and circulatory support may be required. Slow intravenous administration of 10 to 20 mL of calcium gluconate 10% is recommended to reverse the effects on cardiovascular and respiratory systems. If renal function is normal, adequate fluids should be given to promote renal magnesium clearance. This may be increased by the use of frusemide [furosemide]. Haemodialysis using a magnesium-free dialysis solution effectively removes magnesium, and this may be necessary in patients with renal impairment, or for whom other methods prove ineffective.

Hypomagnesaemia. Hypomagnesaemia, a plasma-magnesium concentration below the normal range, may result from a reduced magnesium intake as in dietary deficiency or malabsorption syndromes. Alternatively, it may be due to excessive magnesium loss either via the kidney because of inadequate reabsorption or more often from the gut, for example, during chronic diarrhoea. Drugs that may cause renal magnesium wasting include aminoglycosides, cisplatin (see Effects on Electrolytes, p.525), and diuretics.

Hypomagnesaemia is closely associated with other electrolyte disturbances, especially hypocalcaemia (see above) and hypokalaemia (see below), and rarely occurs alone. Specific symptoms are therefore difficult to determine but may include anorexia, nausea, weakness, neuromuscular dysfunction such as tetany, tremor, and muscle fasciculations, and rarely seizures. Cardiac arrhythmias may occur, but the relative contribution of hypomagnesaemia and hypokalaemia to these is uncertain.

Magnesium salts can be given by mouth for the **treatment** of chronic or asymptomatic magnesium deficiency.[1,2] Parenteral therapy may be preferred in patients with poor gastrointestinal absorption of magnesium or who are unable to tolerate oral supplements (usually because they cause diarrhoea); magnesium sulfate can be given by intravenous or intramuscular injection. In acute symptomatic hypomagnesaemia, rapid replacement therapy with intravenous magnesium salts may be necessary. Renal function and plasma-magnesium concentrations should be monitored.

1. Whang R, et al. Magnesium homeostasis and clinical disorders of magnesium deficiency. Ann Pharmacother 1994; 28: 220–6.
2. Weisinger JR, Bellorín-Font E. Magnesium and phosphorus. Lancet 1998; 352: 391–6.

Phosphate Homoeostasis

Phosphate is an essential bone mineral; about 80% of phosphorus in an adult body is incorporated into the skeleton as a calcium salt where it is required to give rigidity. The remainder is present in the soft tissues and is involved in several metabolic and enzymatic reactions including energy storage and transfer.

Phosphate exists in body fluids mainly as the divalent HPO_4^{2-} ion (about 80%) or monovalent $H_2PO_4^-$ ion (about 20%). Phosphate measurements are usually expressed as inorganic phosphorus to avoid confusion with the anion content. A normal range for phosphorus in plasma in adults is about 0.85 to 1.45 mmol per litre, but as only a small proportion of body phosphate is found in the extracellular fluid, plasma-phosphorus levels may not always reflect total body stores or predict replacement needs.

Phosphate concentrations in plasma are primarily regulated by renal excretion; parathyroid hormone reduces the renal tubular reabsorption of phosphate. Intestinal absorption of phosphate is enhanced by the vitamin D metabolite, 1,25-hydroxycholecalciferol.

Hyperphosphataemia. Hyperphosphataemia, an abnormally raised plasma-phosphorus concentration, is usually associated with renal failure and may lead to renal osteodystrophy (p.746). Hyperphosphataemia may also be a consequence of release of phosphate from cells; this may occur in conditions of cell breakdown such as in haemolysis or rhabdomyolysis, during chemotherapy when it may be part of the tumour lysis syndrome, or as a result of acidoses. Hypoparathyroidism may also lead to hyperphosphataemia due to decreased levels of parathyroid hormone (see p.747). Other causes include excessive phosphate administration during treatment of hypophosphataemia, overuse of phosphate enemas or oral phosphate bowel preparations, and excessive vitamin D intake.

Hyperphosphataemic symptoms include those of associated hypocalcaemia (see above). Complexation with calcium may lead to metastatic calcification.

The **treatment** of hyperphosphataemia[1] usually involves control of the relevant underlying condition, and the use of low-phosphate diets, and if necessary oral phosphate-binding agents, such as calcium acetate or carbonate or aluminium hydroxide. Sevelamer, a polymer capable of binding phosphate, may also be given. Haemodialysis

has been used to correct hyperphosphataemia due to oral phosphate administration in renal failure.

1. Weisinger JR, Bellorín-Font E. Magnesium and phosphorus. Lancet 1998; 352: 391–6.

Hypophosphataemia. Hypophosphataemia, a reduction in plasma-phosphorus concentrations below the normal range, may be due to insufficient absorption of phosphate or increased renal clearance as in primary hyperparathyroidism, vitamin D deficiency, or X-linked familial hypophosphataemia. An increased cell uptake of phosphate can also result in hypophosphataemia, as for example, in chronic respiratory alkalosis and related disorders including alcoholism, hepatic failure, and septicaemia. As phosphate is widely available in most foods, dietary deficiency is rare though it may occur in infants of low birth-weight fed exclusively on human breast milk (see Rickets of Prematurity, p.1194). The absorption of phosphate from the gastrointestinal tract can be reduced if phosphate-binding antacids are taken in large amounts. Hypophosphataemia is usually asymptomatic but clinical symptoms become apparent when plasma-phosphorus concentrations fall below 0.3 mmol per litre.[1-3] Symptoms include neuromuscular dysfunction such as muscle weakness and paraesthesias, convulsions, cardiomyopathy, respiratory failure, and haematological abnormalities. Prolonged hypophosphataemia can result in rickets or osteomalacia (p.744).

Treatment of hypophosphataemia primarily involves correction of any underlying disease. Milk or oral phosphate supplements may be appropriate if a phosphate deficiency is identified or in certain disorders such as X-linked hypophosphataemic rickets. Intravenous phosphate administration may be required for severe hypophosphataemia, but this should be used cautiously to avoid hypocalcaemia and metastatic calcification.[2,3] Consideration should be given to correcting concomitant electrolyte disturbances such as hypomagnesaemia.

1. Larner AJ. Clinical applicability of inorganic phosphate measurements. Br J Hosp Med 1992; 48: 748–53.
2. Lloyd CW, Johnson CE. Management of hypophosphatemia. Clin Pharm 1988; 7: 123–8.
3. Weisinger JR, Bellorín-Font E. Magnesium and phosphorus. Lancet 1998; 352: 391–6.

Potassium Homoeostasis

Potassium is predominantly an intracellular cation, primarily found in muscle; only about 2% is present in the extracellular fluid. It is essential for numerous metabolic and physiological processes including nerve conduction, muscle contraction, and acid-base regulation. A normal concentration of potassium in plasma is about 3.5 to 5.0 mmol per litre, but factors influencing transfer between intracellular and extracellular fluids such as acid-base disturbances can distort the relationship between plasma concentrations and total body stores. The body content of potassium is primarily regulated by renal glomerular filtration and tubular secretion. Aldosterone enhances the renal secretion of potassium and several other factors such as sodium excretion, dietary potassium intake, and plasma pH can modulate the excretion of potassium by the kidney. Insulin, beta$_2$ agonists, and aldosterone, and increases in plasma pH, can promote the cellular uptake of potassium. The passage of potassium into the cells and retention against the concentration gradient requires active transport via the Na^+/K^+ ATPase enzyme.

Hyperkalaemia. Hyperkalaemia, an abnormally raised plasma-potassium concentration, can occur if the potassium intake is increased, if the renal excretion decreases as in renal failure or adrenocortical insufficiency, or if there is a sudden efflux of potassium from the intracellular stores, for example, in acidosis or cell destruction due to tissue trauma, burns, haemolysis, or rhabdomyolysis. Hyperkalaemia may also be induced by drugs such as the potassium-sparing diuretics, ciclosporin, tacrolimus, NSAIDs, or ACE inhibitors.[1] Usually the renal mechanisms for potassium excretion adapt readily to an increased potassium load and hyperkalaemia due to increased dietary intake is rare unless renal function is also impaired.

Hyperkalaemia predominantly results in disruption of cardiac function, but skeletal muscle function may also be affected. Symptoms include ECG abnormalities, ventricular arrhythmias, cardiac arrest, and also neuromuscular dysfunction such as muscle weakness and paralysis.[2-5]

Treatment involves the administration of calcium to counteract the negative effects of hyperkalaemia on cardiac excitability, the use of agents such as insulin or sodium bicarbonate to promote the transfer of potassium from the extracellular to the intracellar fluid compartment, and enhanced potassium excretion with exchange resins or dialysis.[2-5] The methods employed depend largely on the severity of the hyperkalaemia and critically, any associated ECG changes. Hyperkalaemia associated with a plasma concentration of potassium above 6.0 to 7.0 mmol per litre or with ECG changes is usually considered a medical emergency.

If cardiac manifestations of hyperkalaemia are present, then first-line therapy should be with a calcium salt given intravenously; typically 10 to 20 mL of calcium gluconate 10% is given by slow intravenous injection, the dosage being titrated and adjusted based on ECG improvement.

Calcium will not, however, reduce the plasma-potassium concentration. In moderate to severe hyperkalaemia, insulin, together with glucose to prevent hypoglycaemia, may be given intravenously in order to reduce the potassium concentration by stimulating the uptake of potassium by cells. Insulin is given as a rapid-acting soluble insulin and typical doses are 5 to 15 units with 50 mL of glucose 50% given slowly over 5 to 15 minutes. Doses may need to be repeated as necessary. Alternatively or additionally, sodium bicarbonate may be used to correct acidosis and promote cellular uptake of potassium; usual doses are in the order of 50 to 100 mL of a 4.2% solution (equivalent to 25 to 50 mmol) given intravenously.

The beta$_2$ agonist, salbutamol, administered intravenously or by a nebuliser, has also been found to enhance the cellular uptake of potassium and reduce plasma-potassium concentrations.[2,4,6] However, its effect may be inconsistent,[6] and some clinicians prefer to avoid beta$_2$ agonists because of fears that large doses may induce cardiac arrhythmias.[7]

After the plasma-potassium concentration has been reduced in the immediate term by enhancing cellular potassium uptake, treatments are often required that will remove excess potassium from the body over the longer term. Cation exchange resins such as calcium or sodium polystyrene sulfonate can be given orally or rectally and, after about 1 to 2 hours, will begin to remove potassium from the body. Haemodialysis removes potassium from the body very effectively and is particularly useful in patients with acute renal failure, hypervolaemia, hypernatraemia, or severe hyperkalaemia. Peritoneal dialysis is effective in some patients.

1. Perazella MA. Drug-induced hyperkalemia: old culprits and new offenders. Am J Med 2000; 109: 307–14.
2. Anonymous. Hyperkalaemia—silent and deadly. Lancet 1989; i: 1240.
3. Saxena K. Clinical features and management of poisoning due to potassium chloride. Med Toxicol Adverse Drug Exp 1989; 4: 429–43.
4. Anonymous. Potassium disorders and cardiac arrhythmias. Drug Ther Bull 1991; 29: 73–5.
5. Vaughan RS. Potassium in the perioperative period. Br J Anaesth 1991; 67: 194–200.
6. Wong S-L, Maltz HC. Albuterol for the treatment of hyperkalemia. Ann Pharmacother 1999; 33: 103–6.
7. Halperin ML, Kamel KS. Potassium. Lancet 1998; 352: 135–40.

HYPERKALAEMIC PERIODIC PARALYSIS. Hyperkalaemic periodic paralysis is an inherited disorder in which sudden increases in plasma-potassium concentrations cause muscle paralysis. An acute attack may require intravenous calcium gluconate and insulin with glucose (see above). Inhalation of a beta$_2$ agonist such as salbutamol has been used to treat or abort attacks.[1,2] Diuretics such as acetazolamide or the thiazides are used prophylactically to reduce the frequency of attacks.

1. Wang P, Clausen T. Treatment of attacks in hyperkalaemic familial periodic paralysis by inhalation of salbutamol. Lancet 1976; i: 221–3.
2. Hanna MG, et al. Salbutamol treatment in a patient with hyperkalaemic periodic paralysis due to a mutation in the skeletal muscle sodium channel gene (SCN4A). J Neurol Neurosurg Psychiatry 1998; 65: 248–50.

Hypokalaemia. Chronic hypokalaemia, a prolonged reduction of the plasma concentration of potassium, usually indicates a reduction in total body potassium. It may result from an inadequate intake, or gastrointestinal losses, for example in patients with secretory diarrhoeas, or from excessive renal losses as in hyperaldosteronism, Cushing's syndrome, or chronic metabolic alkalosis. Thiazides or loop diuretics increase urinary-potassium losses. Other drugs, notably corticosteroids and some antibacterials such as gentamicin, also have this effect. Hypokalaemia can also be caused by an increased cellular uptake of potassium rather than excess body losses. This may occur with drugs such as beta$_2$ agonists or xanthines, during insulin therapy, acute alkalosis, or possibly be induced by catecholamines after myocardial infarction. Hypokalaemia secondary to hypomagnesaemia (see above) can occur.

Hypokalaemia results in neuromuscular disturbances ranging from muscle weakness to paralysis and respiratory insufficiency and can also cause rhabdomyolysis, ECG abnormalities, and ileus. Chronic hypokalaemia may lead to renal tubular damage (hypokalaemic nephropathy). Hypokalaemia increases the risk of digoxin toxicity.

Treatment involves correcting any underlying disorder and replacement therapy with potassium salts. Oral potassium supplements are generally preferred but in severe hypokalaemia associated with cardiac arrhythmias, paralysis or diabetic ketoacidosis, parenteral therapy may be necessary. Potassium salts, usually potassium chloride, may be given by intravenous infusion but must be administered slowly to avoid causing hyperkalaemia and associated cardiac toxicity; plasma-potassium concentrations should be closely monitored and ECG monitoring may be required. The choice of salt for oral potassium replacement depends on co-existing acid-base and electrolyte disturbances. Potassium chloride is generally the drug of choice for the treatment of hypokalaemia in patients with metabolic alkalosis with hypochloraemia, whereas a salt such as the bicarbonate may be preferred in patients with hyperchloraemic acidosis as in some renal tubular acidoses. Hypokalaemia secondary to hypomagnesaemia requires magnesium replacement therapy.

References.

1. Anonymous. Potassium disorders and cardiac arrhythmias. *Drug Ther Bull* 1991; **29:** 73–5.
2. Vaughan RS. Potassium in the perioperative period. *Br J Anaesth* 1991; **67:** 194–200.
3. Halperin ML, Kamel KS. Potassium. *Lancet* 1998; **352:** 135–40.
4. Gennari FJ. Hypokalaemia. *N Engl J Med* 1998; **339:** 451–8.
5. Cohn JN, *et al.* New guidelines for potassium replacement in clinical practice: a contemporary review by the National Council on Potassium in Clinical Practice. *Arch Intern Med* 2000; **160:** 2429–36.

BARTTER'S SYNDROME. Bartter's syndrome is a set of closely related disorders thought to result from inherited defects in ion transport in various sections of the renal tubule.[1] Patients exhibit hyperplasia of the juxtaglomerular cells, hypokalaemia and metabolic alkalosis, and excess aldosterone, prostaglandin, and renin production. Symptoms are primarily those of the hypokalaemia, including muscle weakness; polyuria and enuresis, and growth retardation in children, can occur. In contrast to other hyperreninaemic states, patients do not have hypertension or oedema.

Treatment rarely completely corrects hypokalaemia. Potassium supplementation may be given, while a cyclo-oxygenase inhibitor such as indometacin,[2,3] or an ACE inhibitor such as captopril,[4,5] can produce benefit. Spironolactone and propranolol have also been tried.[5] Magnesium sulfate may be given by depot injection if there is hypomagnesaemia.[5]

1. Guay-Woodford LM. Bartter syndrome: unraveling the pathophysiologic enigma. *Am J Med* 1998; **105:** 151–61.
2. Littlewood JM, *et al.* Treatment of childhood Bartter's syndrome with indomethacin. *Lancet* 1976; **ii:** 795.
3. Craig JC, Falk MC. Indomethacin for renal impairment in neonatal Bartter's syndrome. *Lancet* 1996; **347:** 550.
4. Jest P, *et al.* Angiotensin-converting enzyme inhibition as a therapeutic principle in Bartter's syndrome. *Eur J Clin Pharmacol* 1991; **41:** 303–5.
5. Crowe P, *et al.* Bartter's syndrome in two generations of an Irish family. *Postgrad Med J* 1993; **69:** 791–6.

DIURETIC-INDUCED HYPOKALAEMIA. Reduced potassium concentrations may result from the use of potassium-losing diuretics, particularly thiazides and loop diuretics. Clinically significant hypokalaemia is unlikely at the doses used in hypertension and the routine use of potassium supplements is no longer recommended. However, the concomitant administration of a potassium-sparing diuretic such as amiloride or, less usually, a potassium supplement may be necessary in patients at risk of hypokalaemia (see also Hydrochlorothiazide, Effects on Electrolyte Balance, p.908).

HYPOKALAEMIC PERIODIC PARALYSIS. Hypokalaemic periodic paralysis is an inherited disorder in which episodes of hypokalaemia with muscle weakness or paralysis appear to be associated with a shift in potassium from the extracellular to the intracellular fluid. Acute attacks are treated with potassium, given orally or intravenously.

Prophylaxis with acetazolamide has been found to reduce the frequency and severity of attacks.[1,2]

1. Griggs RC, *et al.* Acetazolamide treatment of hypokalemic periodic paralysis: prevention of attacks and improvement of persistent weakness. *Ann Intern Med* 1970; **73:** 39–48.
2. Ahlawat SK, Sachdev A. Hypokalaemic paralysis. *Postgrad Med J* 1999; **75:** 193–7.

Sodium Homoeostasis

Sodium is the principal cation in the extracellular fluid and is responsible for the maintenance of the extracellular fluid volume and osmolality. In addition, sodium is also involved in nerve conduction, muscle contraction, acid-base balance, and cell nutrient uptake. A normal concentration of sodium in plasma would be expected to be within 135 to 145 mmol per litre.

Sodium homoeostasis is complex and closely associated with fluid balance. The osmolality and volume of the extracellular fluid are tightly regulated. Small changes in osmolality (plasma-sodium concentrations) are corrected by alteration of extracellular volume. This balance of plasma osmolality is achieved by the secretion or suppression of antidiuretic hormone (ADH; vasopressin), which primarily controls water excretion by the kidney. A tendency towards hyponatraemia suppresses ADH secretion and promotes renal loss of water; an increase in ADH secretion increases water reabsorption by the renal distal tubules. Changes in extracellular volume will also affect ADH release independently of osmolality. In addition, changes in extracellular volume result in modulation of the renal excretion of sodium.

Total body sodium content is regulated by renal sodium excretion, which can vary widely depending on dietary intake. Various mechanisms are involved in controlling renal sodium excretion including the renin-angiotensin system, glomerular filtration rate, and natriuretic factors. A reduction in extracellular fluid volume leads to the production of angiotensin II which stimulates the secretion of aldosterone. Aldosterone promotes the reabsorption of sodium ions by the distal tubules. There may be significant effects on sodium homoeostasis if adrenal insufficiency or mineralocorticoid excess disturb this mechanism.

Hypernatraemia. Hypernatraemia is an abnormal rise in the plasma-sodium concentration with a simultaneous rise in plasma osmolality. It is generally associated with volume depletion when water intake is less than water losses through renal or extrarenal routes. The causes include impaired thirst, as in coma or essential hypernatraemia, osmotic diuresis (solute diuresis), as in diabetic ketoacidosis (see Diabetic Emergencies, p.318) or after mannitol administration, and excessive water losses, either from the kidney, as in diabetes insipidus (p.1273), or extrarenally, for example, because of excessive sweating or diarrhoea.

Hypernatraemia can also occur following excessive oral sodium intake (but this is uncommon) and after inappropriate use of intravenous sodium chloride.

The clinical manifestations of hypernatraemia are caused by the effect of increased plasma osmolality on the brain and include somnolence, confusion, respiratory paralysis, and coma. CNS symptoms are more severe when hypernatraemia develops rapidly. In the presence of volume depletion, other symptoms such as hypotension, tachycardia, and various symptoms of circulatory insufficiency may occur concomitantly. A high volume of dilute urine is seen in patients with abnormal renal water conservation, whereas a low volume of concentrated urine is expected in patients with impaired thirst or excessive extrarenal water loss.

Treatment of hypernatraemia usually requires water replacement, and oral administration of water may be sufficient for some patients. In more severe conditions, glucose 5% may be given by slow intravenous infusion. Alternatively, some recommend the use of sodium chloride 0.9%. Care is required as too rapid correction can induce cerebral oedema, particularly in chronic conditions.

If the total body sodium is too high, loop diuretics may be used to increase sodium excretion with fluid losses being replaced by an infusion of glucose 5% and potassium chloride. It has also been suggested that dialysis may be necessary if there is significant renal impairment, if the patient is moribund, or if the serum-sodium concentration is greater than 200 mmol per litre.

Hyponatraemia. Hyponatraemia, an abnormal fall in the plasma-sodium concentration, usually with a simultaneous fall in the plasma osmolality, is a frequent electrolyte disturbance that occurs with many different diseases including heart failure, cirrhosis, adrenocortical insufficiency, hyperglycaemia, and AIDS.

The kidney is able to conserve sodium and sodium depletion due to low salt intake is rare. Sodium depletion may occur if there are abnormal losses, either from the gut as a consequence of repeated diarrhoea and/or vomiting or from the kidney, for example, due to various renal disorders or the overuse of diuretics (see under Hydrochlorothiazide, Effects on Electrolyte Balance, p.908).

The most common cause of hyponatraemia is dilution. This may result from excessive fluid intake, for example, due to the ingestion of large volumes of water in patients with primary polydipsia (psychogenic polydipsia). More frequently, however, it is a result of reduced water excretion, for example in impaired renal function or the syndrome of inappropriate secretion of antidiuretic hormone (SIADH—p.1277). Postoperative hyponatraemia is a frequent complication which may be exacerbated by the inappropriate intravenous administration of hypotonic, or even isotonic,[1] fluids.

Hyponatraemia due to sodium depletion in the presence of volume contraction may cause postural hypotension and circulatory insufficiency. Dilutional hyponatraemia can be asymptomatic but headache, confusion, nausea, vomiting, somnolence, and weakness may occur. If severe, cerebral oedema is present, and respiratory arrest, convulsions, and coma may ensue. CNS symptoms are more common when the condition is acute.

Therapy is guided by the rate of development and degree of hyponatraemia, accompanying symptoms, and the state of water balance, and should also take into account the underlying cause. Mild asymptomatic hyponatraemia does not usually require specific therapy. Chronic mild to moderate sodium depletion, such as occurs in salt-losing bowel or renal disease, may be treated with oral sodium chloride supplements while ensuring adequate fluid intake.

When there is substantial volume depletion, volume replacement is necessary and intravenous sodium chloride 0.9% is often used.

Chronic dilutional hyponatraemia, which is often asymptomatic, can generally be managed by correcting the underlying disease; water restriction may also be necessary and drugs that interfere with the action of ADH such as demeclocycline or lithium carbonate may be useful in SIADH.[2,3] Frusemide [furosemide] plus oral sodium chloride supplements have also been used.

Acute symptomatic hyponatraemia (water intoxication) is generally associated with plasma-sodium concentrations below 120 mmol per litre and requires more aggressive therapy. This involves giving hypertonic or isotonic sodium chloride intravenously, often with a loop diuretic such as frusemide [furosemide], especially if fluid overload is likely to be a problem.[2,3] The aim is to render the patient asymptomatic with a plasma-sodium concentration of 120 to 130 mmol per litre; the plasma-sodium concentration should not be corrected to normal values nor should hypernatraemia be allowed to develop.[2,3] Plasma-sodium concentrations and the total-body-water volume should be monitored throughout.

A rare neurological syndrome known as central pontine myelinolysis (osmotic demyelination) has been associated with the over-rapid correction of symptomatic hyponatraemia, particularly if the condition is well established, and it has been recommended that the plasma-sodium concentration should be increased at a rate not exceeding 0.5 mmol per litre per hour[4,5] in these patients, though the best correction rate is debatable.[3,6] Some have suggested an initial prompt increase in plasma sodium of about 10% or 10 mmol per litre, followed by correction at a rate not exceeding 1.0 to 1.5 mmol per litre per hour or 15 mmol per litre per 24 hours.[7] However, the association of hyponatraemia with central pontine myelinolysis is controversial and some authorities do not consider the rate of correction to be a factor in hyponatraemic brain injury.[3]

1. Steele A, *et al.* Postoperative hyponatremia despite near-isotonic saline infusion: a phenomenon of desalination. *Ann Intern Med* 1997; **126:** 20–5.
2. Swales JD. Management of hyponatraemia. *Br J Anaesth* 1991; **67:** 146–53.
3. Arieff AI. Management of hyponatraemia. *BMJ* 1993; **307:** 305–8.

4. Cluitmans FHM, Meinders AE. Management of severe hyponatremia: rapid or slow correction? *Am J Med* 1990; **88**: 161–6.
5. Laureno R, Karp BI. Myelinolysis after correction of hyponatremia. *Ann Intern Med* 1997; **126**: 57–62.
6. Stems RH. The treatment of hyponatremia: first, do no harm. *Am J Med* 1990; **88**: 557–60.
7. Kumar S, Berl T. Sodium. *Lancet* 1998; **352**: 220–8.

Dialysis Solutions (3276-x)

Pharmacopoeias. In *Eur.* (see p.vi), which includes separate monographs for solutions for haemodialysis, haemofiltration and haemodiafiltration, and peritoneal dialysis.

Dialysis and filtration solutions are solutions of electrolytes formulated in concentrations similar to those of extracellular fluid or plasma. They always contain sodium and chloride and bicarbonate or a bicarbonate precursor. In addition, they often contain calcium and magnesium, and rarely potassium. Glucose may be added as an osmotic agent. These solutions allow the removal of water and metabolites and the replacement of electrolytes.

In *haemodialysis*, the exchange of ions between the solution and the patient's blood is made across a semi-permeable membrane, primarily by diffusion. Excess fluid is removed by ultrafiltration achieved by a pressure gradient. Membranes are either derived from cellulose (e.g. cuprophane) or are synthetic. Bicarbonate rather than a bicarbonate precursor is increasingly preferred as the bicarbonate source in haemodialysis since the problems of precipitation of calcium and magnesium have been overcome by changes in dialysis technique. Acetate is still used in some dialysers, but is thought to have vasodilator and cardiodepressant actions, and may not be converted to bicarbonate fast enough for high-flux haemodialysis or in patients with liver disease. Haemodialysis solutions are provided in a sterile concentrated form for dilution with water before use; this water need not be sterile.

In *peritoneal dialysis*, the exchange is made across the membranes of the peritoneal cavity primarily by diffusion. Excess fluid is removed by ultrafiltration achieved by the use of osmotic agents such as glucose. The problems of calcium bicarbonate precipitation have not yet been overcome, and lactate is generally used as the bicarbonate precursor. Peritoneal dialysis solutions must be sterile and apyrogenic.

In *haemofiltration*, blood is filtered rather than dialysed. Metabolites are removed by convective transport, and excess water by hydrostatic ultrafiltration. Fluid and electrolytes are replaced by direct intravenous infusion of haemofiltration solution. Most haemofiltration solutions use acetate as the bicarbonate source. Haemofiltration solutions must be sterile and apyrogenic.

Adverse Effects

Adverse effects occurring during *haemodialysis* include nausea, vomiting, hypotension, muscle cramps, and air embolus. Effects related to vascular access include infection, thrombosis, and haemorrhage. Adverse effects occurring during *haemofiltration* are similar to those for haemodialysis.

The most common adverse effects associated with *peritoneal dialysis* include peritonitis, hernias, hyperglycaemia, protein malnutrition, and catheter complications.

Long-term complications in dialysed patients, some of which may relate to renal failure itself, include haemodialysis-related amyloidosis, acquired cystic kidney disease, and accelerated atherosclerosis. Dialysis dementia is a special hazard of aluminium overload. Long-term peritoneal dialysis results in progressive structural changes to the peritoneal membrane ultimately resulting in dialysis failure.

Aluminium overload. Accumulation of aluminium in patients on dialysis may result in dialysis dementia, anaemia, and aluminium-related bone disease (see also p.1577). Sources of aluminium include the water used for preparation of dialysis fluids and aluminium-containing phosphate binders used in treating renal osteodystrophy (p.746). It is therefore important that water used for the preparation of dialysis fluids has a low aluminium concentration; Ph. Eur. specifies a limit of aluminium of 10 μg per litre. Non-aluminium-containing phosphate binders such as calcium acetate or calcium carbonate may be preferred for long-term therapy. Aluminium overload in patients on dialysis has been treated with desferrioxamine (p.1005).

Copper toxicity. Liver and haematological toxicity has occurred as a result of absorption of copper from dialysis fluids (p.1358).

Haemodialysis-induced cramp. Muscle cramps commonly occur during haemodialysis procedures, and are often associated with hypotension as a result of inappropriate volume removal. In addition, they may be exacerbated by cellulose-derived membranes or the use of acetate as a bicarbonate precursor. Sodium chloride tablets (p.1196), intravenous sodium chloride 0.9%, intravenous hypertonic glucose (p.1365), and quinine (p.448) have been used in the prevention or treatment of haemodialysis-induced cramp.

Hypersensitivity. For anaphylactic reactions associated with the use of ethylene oxide for the disinfection of dialysis equipment, see p.1144.

Infections. Patients undergoing haemodialysis are at risk of infections from microbial contamination of dialysis fluid, and from inadequate care of vascular access sites. Maximum microbial counts and limits for endotoxins have been specified for water used in dialysis fluids. Bicarbonate-based dialysis solutions are more susceptible to microbial growth than acetate-based solutions.

Peritonitis is common in patients receiving peritoneal dialysis. The risk of infection may be minimised by using disconnect systems, good aseptic technique, and by good care of catheters. Treatment of bacterial peritonitis requires intraperitoneal administration of antibacterials, which are usually added to the dialysis fluid (see p.134).

Dialysis equipment should be regularly disinfected with agents such as formaldehyde (p.1145) or ethylene oxide (p.1144), but for mention of ethylene oxide anaphylactoid reactions, see p.1144.

Metabolic complications. The high concentrations of glucose in peritoneal dialysis solutions required to form an osmotic gradient can lead to weight gain, hyperglycaemia, hyperlipidaemia, and increased protein loss. Alternative osmotic agents such as icodextrin (p.1359) can be used, and amino acid-based solutions are being investigated.

Precautions

Peritoneal dialysis is not appropriate for patients with abdominal sepsis, previous abdominal surgery, or severe inflammatory bowel disease.

Haemodialysis should be used with caution in patients with unstable cardiovascular disease or active bleeding. During haemodialysis and haemofiltration, heparin (see Extracorporeal Circulation, p.905) or epoprostenol (Uses, p.1444) are required to prevent clotting of the blood in the extracorporeal circuit.

Dialysis solutions should be warmed to body temperature with dry heat because wet heat carries a risk of microbial contamination.

Interactions

The effects of dialysis and filtration procedures on drug concentrations in the body can be complex. More drug may be removed by one dialysis technique than another. In general, drugs of low molecular weight, high water solubility, low volume of distribution, low protein binding, and high renal clearance are most extensively removed by dialysis. For example, aminoglycosides are extensively removed by dialysis procedures, and extra doses may be needed to replace losses, usually guided by serum-drug concentrations. Specific drug dosage adjustments for dialysis procedures may be used where these are known. For drugs where the effect of dialysis is unknown, it is usual to give maintenance doses after dialysis. Dialysis has been used to remove some drugs in the treatment of overdosage (see below).

Dialysis-induced changes in fluids and electrolytes have the potential to alter the effects of some drugs. For example, hypokalaemia predisposes to digoxin toxicity.

In patients undergoing peritoneal dialysis, drugs such as insulin and antibacterials may be added to the dialysis fluid. Consideration should be given to the possibility of adsorption of drugs onto the PVC bags.

◊ References.
1. Aronson JK. The principles of prescribing in renal failure. *Prescribers' J* 1992; **32**: 220–31.
2. Bennett WM, *et al.* *Drug Prescribing in renal failure: dosing guidelines for adults.* 3rd ed. Philadelphia: American College of Physicians, 1994.
3. Cotterill S. Antimicrobial prescribing in patients on haemofiltration. *J Antimicrob Chemother* 1995; **36**: 773–80.

Uses and Administration

Dialysis and filtration procedures are used in renal failure to correct electrolyte imbalance, correct fluid overload, and remove metabolites. They also have a limited role in the treatment of overdosage and poisoning. The two main techniques are haemodialysis and peritoneal dialysis; haemofiltration is used less frequently. The choice of technique will depend on the condition to be treated, the clinical state of the patient, patient preference, and availability.

Haemodialysis is more efficient than peritoneal dialysis at clearing small molecules such as urea, whereas peritoneal dialysis may be better at clearing larger molecules. Haemodialysis is considered to be less physiological as it alternates periods of high clearance with periods of no clearance.

Haemodialysis is usually performed intermittently (often 3 times a week); a typical session takes 3 to 5 hours. More recently high-flux dialysers have been developed which have reduced the time required for dialysis sessions.

Peritoneal dialysis may be performed continuously or intermittently. Continuous ambulatory peritoneal dialysis (CAPD) is the most commonly used technique. Patients remain mobile, except during exchanges, and can carry out the procedure themselves. There is always dialysis solution in the peritoneal cavity, and this is drained and replaced 3 to 5 times a day. Continuous cycle peritoneal dialysis (CCPD) is similar, except that exchanges are carried out automatically overnight, and patients do not have to carry out any exchanges during the day. Intermittent peritoneal dialysis (IPD) requires the patient to be connected to a dialysis machine for 12 to 24 hours 2 to 4 times a week. During this time, dialysis solution is pumped into and out of the peritoneal cavity, with a dwell time of about 10 to 20 minutes.

Haemofiltration is usually performed as a continuous technique and, as it is not portable, its principal use is in intensive care units. It may also be used intermittently as an adjunct to haemodialysis in patients with excess fluid weight gain. Continuous arteriovenous or venovenous haemodiafiltration (CAVHD or CVVHD) combines dialysis and filtration by perfusing the filtrate side of the haemofiltration membrane with peritoneal dialysis fluid.

Assessing serum concentrations of urea or creatinine before the next dialysis session is not a good measure of the adequacy of the dialysis, so various other measures have been developed including the urea reduction ratio and urea kinetic modelling. The use of such measures is more established for haemodialysis than for peritoneal dialysis.

◊ References.
1. Zucchelli P, Santoro A. How to achieve optimal correction of acidosis in end-stage renal failure patients. *Blood Purif* 1995; **13**: 375–84.
2. Carlsen DB, Wild ST. Grams to milliequivalents: a concise guide to adjusting hemodialysate composition. *Adv Ren Replace Ther* 1996; **3**: 261–5.
3. Passlick-Deetjen J, Kirchgessner J. Bicarbonate: the alternative buffer for peritoneal dialysis. *Perit Dial Int* 1996; **16** (suppl 1): S109–S113.
4. Pastan S, Bailey J. Dialysis therapy. *N Engl J Med* 1998; **338**: 1428–37.
5. Ifudu O. Care of patients undergoing hemodialysis. *N Engl J Med* 1998; **339**: 1054–62.
6. Mallick NP, Gokal R. Haemodialysis. *Lancet* 1999; **353**: 737–42.
7. Gokal R, Mallick NP. Peritoneal dialysis. *Lancet* 1999; **353**: 823–8.

Acute renal failure. Acute renal failure is characterised by a rapid decline in kidney function, and has a variety of causes.[1-5] It is often classified by origin as *prerenal* (e.g. due to hypovolaemia such as that associated with shock, burns, or dehydration; congestive heart failure; or renal artery obstruction), *renal* (such as acute tubular necrosis or interstitial nephritis of various causes, including nephrotoxic drugs and infections), or *postrenal* (acute urinary tract obstruction). The prognosis depends on the underlying disease, which should be identified and treated if possible, but the mortality may still be as high as 60%, particularly in patients who become oliguric, and after surgery or trauma. Management is essentially supportive in the hope that renal function will recover. Complications of acute renal failure include extracellular volume overload and hyponatraemia, hyperkalaemia, metabolic acidosis, hyperphosphataemia and hypocalcaemia. Those complications requiring urgent treatment, often including the use of dialysis, are severe hyperkalaemia (p.1182), pulmonary oedema, pericarditis, and severe metabolic acidosis (p.1180). The use of dialysis before clinical signs of uraemia is a matter of debate since it does not appear to hasten recovery *per se*,[1] but all save the shortest episodes of acute renal failure will require some form of renal replacement therapy with dialysis or filtration. Intermittent haemodialysis and peritoneal dialysis are both used, but the newer haemofiltration techniques have theoretical advantages in terms of volume control and cardiovascular stability, and are increasingly preferred.[2,6,7]

Numerous drugs have been tried in attempts to attenuate renal injury or hasten recovery in patients with acute tubular necrosis due to ischaemia or nephrotoxins.[1,5] These include drugs to increase renal blood flow (e.g. low-dose dopamine, atrial natriuretic peptide, or prostaglandins), drugs to increase urine flow and protect the epithelial cells (mannitol and loop diuretics, calcium-channel blockers), or the use of chelating agents or antidotes against specific nephrotoxins. Consistent clinical benefit has not, however, been demonstrated.

Acute renal failure is reversible in about 95% of patients who survive the complications. A few patients who survive acute renal failure will require long-term dialysis or renal transplantation (p.503).

1. Brady HR, Singer GG. Acute renal failure. *Lancet* 1995; **346:** 1533–40.
2. Morgan AG. The management of acute renal failure. *Br J Hosp Med* 1996; **55:** 167–70.
3. Evans JHC. Acute renal failure in children. *Br J Hosp Med* 1994; **52:** 159–61.
4. Klahr S, Miller SB. Acute oliguria. *N Engl J Med* 1998; **338:** 671–5.
5. Dishart MK, Kellum JA. An evaluation of pharmacological strategies for the prevention and treatment of acute renal failure. *Drugs* 2000; **59:** 79–91.
6. McCarthy JT. Renal replacement therapy in acute renal failure. *Curr Opin Nephrol Hypertens* 1996; **5:** 480–4.
7. Joy MS, *et al.* A primer on continuous renal replacement therapy for critically ill patients. *Ann Pharmacother* 1998; **32:** 362–75.

Chronic renal failure. Chronic renal failure is the irreversible, usually progressive, loss of renal function that eventually results in end-stage renal disease (ESRD) and the need for renal replacement therapy (dialysis or renal transplantation). The rate of decline in renal function is generally constant for each patient and is usually monitored by measuring serum-creatinine concentrations as an indirect index of the glomerular filtration rate (GFR). In its early stages when the patient is asymptomatic, progressive loss of renal function is described as diminished renal reserve or chronic renal insufficiency. When the limits of renal reserve have been exceeded and symptoms become apparent, it is termed chronic renal failure or overt renal failure. When renal function is diminished to such an extent that life is no longer sustainable (GFR less than 5 mL per minute), the condition is termed ESRD or uraemia. Many diseases can lead to ESRD, the most common being diabetes (p.317), glomerulonephritis (p.1051), and hypertension (p.802).

The management of patients with chronic renal failure prior to ESRD involves measures to conserve renal function and compensate for renal insufficiency. Methods to slow the progression of renal failure include the treatment of hypertension, reduction of proteinuria with dietary protein restriction (p.1351) or in some cases ACE inhibitors (p.824), or both, and the reduction of hyperlipidaemia (p.800). Anaemia (p.732) and renal osteodystrophy (p.746) often require active treatment. Nephrotoxic drugs, including NSAIDs, should be avoided.

The choice between haemodialysis, peritoneal dialysis, and organ transplantation is considered, and the patient prepared, before it is actually required. In patients for whom transplantation is the preferred option, dialysis may still be required while waiting for a kidney. Kidney transplantation is discussed on p.503. There are differences between countries in the choice of dialysis technique for patients with ESRD. For example, incentre haemodialysis is used in about 80% of patients in the USA, whereas CAPD is used in over 50% of patients in the UK. Overall survival appears to be similar between the 2 techniques, but more patients on CAPD will eventually require a change to another dialysis method because of treatment failure.

Unlike renal transplant patients, dialysis patients still require replacement therapy with hormones that are usually produced by the kidney. Thus, recombinant erythropoietin and hydroxylated vitamin D analogues are commonly administered.

References.
1. Klahr S. Chronic renal failure: management. *Lancet* 1991; **338:** 423–7.
2. Gokal R, Mallick N. Continuous ambulatory peritoneal dialysis. *Prescribers' J* 1992; **32:** 251–6.
3. NIH. Morbidity and mortality of dialysis. *NIH Consens Statement* 1993; **11:** 1–33.
4. The Renal Association. *Treatment of adult patients with renal failure: recommended standards and audit measures.* London: Royal College of Physicians of London, 1995.

The symbol † denotes a preparation no longer actively marketed

5. Friedman AL. Etiology, pathophysiology, diagnosis, and management of chronic renal failure in children. *Curr Opin Pediatr* 1996; **8:** 148–51.
6. Steinman TI. Kidney protection: how to prevent or delay chronic renal failure. *Geriatrics* 1996; **51:** 28–35.
7. Walker R. General management of end stage renal disease. *BMJ* 1997; **315:** 1429–32.

Electrolyte disturbances. Haemodialysis with magnesium-free dialysis solution has been used to remove magnesium from the body in severe hypermagnesaemia (p.1181). Similarly, haemodialysis, and sometimes peritoneal dialysis, has been used in treating hypercalcaemia (p.1181), hyperkalaemia (p.1182), hypernatraemia (p.1183), and hyperphosphataemia (p.1182).

Overdosage and poisoning. Haemodialysis, or less often peritoneal dialysis, can be used to remove some substances from the body after overdosage or poisoning. Substances most readily removed have a low molecular weight, low volume of distribution, low protein binding, high water solubility, and high renal clearance. Examples of agents for which haemodialysis may have a role in the treatment of severe overdosage include alcohol (p.1131), ethylene glycol (p.1609), methyl alcohol (p.1404), lithium (p.293), and salicylates such as aspirin (p.14). Dialysis may be particularly important when poisoning with these agents is complicated by renal failure.

Preparations

Ph. Eur.: Solutions for Haemodialysis; Solutions for Haemofiltration and for Haemodiafiltration; Solutions for Peritoneal Dialysis.

Proprietary Preparations (details are given in Part 3)

Aust.: Acetat-Haemodialyse; Dianeal; HAMFL; Hamofiltrasol; Peritofundin; **Austral.:** Dianeal; **Braz.:** HD; Peritofundin; Solurin; **Canad.:** Nutrineal PD4; **Denm.:** Bicbag; Dianeal; Extraneal; Gambrosol; Hemosol Bicar; Gambrosol; Lockolys; Nutrineal PD4; Physioneal; **Fin.:** Dianeal; Extraneal; Gambrosol; Lockolys; **Fr.:** Dialysol Acide; Dialysol Bicarbonate; Dialytan H; DPCA 2†; **Israel:** CAPD; D-204; D-248; D-300; D-326; Dialine; Dianeal; G-204; G-248; Nutrineal PD4; **Ital.:** Nutrineal PD2 and PD4; **Mex.:** Solucion DP; **Port.:** Dianeal†; Nutrineal†; Peritofundinas; Renofundina; **Spain:** CAPD; Dialisol; Dianeal; Extraneal; Gambrosol; Hemofiltracion E2 and E3; Hemofiltracion E4 and E5; Hemofiltracion HF 01; Hemofiltracion HF 02; Hemofiltracion HF 11 and HF 23; Nutrineal PD4; Peritoflex; **Swed.:** Altracart II†; BiCart†; Bicbag†; Biorenal†; Biosol A†; Biosol B†; CAPD/DPCA; Dianeal; Dicalys 11; Dicalys 17; Duolys A†; Duolys B†; Extraneal; Gambrolys†; Gambrosol; Haemovex 4; Haemovex 8; Hemofiltrasol; Hemofiltrationslosning 401; Hemoset A; Hemoset A glucos; Hemosol B0; HF-BIC35+HF-EL010; HF-BIC35+HF-EL210; Nutrineal PD4; Schiwalys Hemofiltration; Sterilys B 84†; **Switz.:** Clear-Flex Formula 13, 15, 55, 62, 91, AA, AB, AC†; Dianeal; DPCA; Extraneal; Gambrosol; HF; Nutrineal PD4; SK-F, BIC-F; **Thai.:** Dialyte; **UK:** Dianeal; Nutrineal PD4; **USA:** Dialyte.

Oral Rehydration Solutions (3277-r)

Oral rehydration solutions have 4 main constituents:

• electrolytes—typically sodium chloride and potassium chloride

• a bicarbonate source to correct or prevent metabolic acidosis, such as sodium bicarbonate or sodium citrate

• water to replace fluid losses

• a carbohydrate source to maximise absorption of fluid and electrolytes—typically glucose, although cereal-based formulations may also be used.

They are most commonly available as oral powders (oral rehydration salts) that are reconstituted with water before use, but effervescent tablets and ready-to-use oral solutions are also available.

The composition of oral rehydration solutions varies, particularly in sodium content. For example, in the UK the sodium content of oral rehydration solutions ranges from 50 to 60 mmol per litre, whereas the original WHO formulation contains 90 mmol of sodium per litre. The total osmolarity of the solution should be slightly hypotonic (about 250 mmol per litre) to prevent the possible induction of osmotic diarrhoea. For discussion of modified formulations of oral rehydration solutions in the treatment of diarrhoea, including the use of cereal-based and low osmolarity preparations, see oral rehydration therapy under Diarrhoea on p.1203.

◊ References.

1. Booth I, *et al.* Recommendations for composition of oral rehydration solutions for the children of Europe: report of an ESPGAN working group. *J Pediatr Gastroenterol Nutr* 1992; **14:** 113–15.

2. Fontaine O, *et al.* Rice-based oral rehydration solution for treating diarrhoea (updated 28 February 2001). Available in The Cochrane Library: Issue 4. Oxford: Update Software; 2001.

3. Kim Y, *et al.* Reduced osmolarity oral rehydration solution for treating dehydration caused by acute diarrhoea in children (updated 28 February 2001). Available in The Cochrane Library: Issue 4. Oxford: Update Software; 2001.

Adverse Effects

Vomiting can occur after administration of oral rehydration solution, and may be an indication that it was administered too quickly. If vomiting occurs, administration should be halted for 10 minutes then resumed in smaller, more frequent, amounts.

The risk of hypernatraemia or overhydration after administration of oral rehydration solutions is low in patients with normal renal function. Overdosage of oral rehydration solutions in patients with renal impairment may lead to hypernatraemia and hyperkalaemia.

Precautions

Oral rehydration salts or effervescent tablets should be reconstituted only with water and at the volume stated. Fresh drinking water is generally appropriate, but freshly boiled and cooled water is preferred when the solution is for infants or when drinking water is not available. The solution should not be boiled after it is prepared. Other ingredients such as sugar should not be added. Unused solution should be stored in a refrigerator and discarded within 24 hours of preparation.

Oral rehydration solutions are not appropriate for patients with gastrointestinal obstruction, oliguric or anuric renal failure, or when parenteral rehydration therapy is indicated as in severe dehydration or intractable vomiting.

Uses and Administration

Oral rehydration solutions are used for oral replacement of electrolytes and fluids in patients with dehydration, particularly that associated with acute diarrhoea of various aetiologies (p.1203).

The dosage of oral rehydration solutions should be tailored to the individual based on body-weight and the stage and severity of the condition. The initial aim of treatment is to rehydrate the patient, and, subsequently, to maintain hydration by replacing any further losses due to continuing diarrhoea and vomiting and normal losses from respiration, sweating, and urination. Initial rehydration should be rapid, over 3 to 4 hours, unless the patient is hypernatraemic, in which case rehydration over 12 hours is appropriate.

For adults, a usual dose of 200 to 400 mL of oral rehydration solution for every loose motion has been suggested. The dosage for children is 200 mL for every loose motion, and for infants is 1 to 1.5 times their usual feed volume. Normal feeding can continue after the initial fluid deficit has been corrected. Breast feeding should continue between administrations of oral rehydration solution.

Preparations

BP 2001: Oral Rehydration Salts;
USP 25: Oral Rehydration Salts;
WHO/UNICEF: Oral Rehydration Salts.

Proprietary Preparations (details are given in Part 3)

Aust.: Elotrans†; Eloverlan; Milupa GES; Normhydral; Normolyt; Oralpadon†; **Austral.:** Gastrolyte; Gastrolyte-R; Hydralyte; Pedialyte; Repalyte; **Braz.:** Dietasal; Emidrat; Golac; H-Sal; Hidrabene; Hidrafix; Hidrafix 90; Hidrolyte; Hidroral; Hydroplus; Isolyte P 45 E 90; Pedialyte; Pedialyte 90; Phosphocalcina Iodada; Reafix; Rehidrat; Sindrat; Wassertrat; **Canad.:** Enfalac Lytren; Gastrolyte; Lytren; Lytren RHS; Pedialyte; Pediatric Electrolyte; Rehydralyte; **Denm.:** Revolyt; **Fin.:** Osmosal; **Fr.:** Adiaril; Alhydrate; Caril; Carogil; GES 45; Hydrigoz; Lytren; Picolite; **Ger.:** D-Iso; Elotrans; InfectoDyspept; Isolyt†; Oralpadon; Saltadol; Santalyt; **Hong Kong:** Gastrolyte-R; GES 45; Pedialyte; **Irl.:** Dioralyte; Electrolade; Rapolyte; Rehidrat; **Israel:** Hydran; Orset; Rehidrat; **Ital.:** Alhydrate; Dicodral; Milupa GES; Pedialyte; Reidrax; Sodioral with Inulina; Sodioral†; Soluzione Darrow; **Mex.:** Electrolit; Electrolit Pediatrico; **Neth.:** Dioralyte; Dioralyte Rice; **Norw.:** Gem; **NZ:** Gastrolyte; Pedialyte; **Port.:** Dioralyte; Redrate; **S.Afr.:** Darrow-Liq; Darrowped†; Electrona; Electropak; Enterolyte; Hemapep†; Hydrol; Kaostatex; Pectolin†; Pectrolyte; Rehidrat; **Singapore:** GES 45; **Spain:** Bebesales; Didrica; Huberlitren†; Oral Rehidr Sal Farmasur; Oralesper; Reemplazante Intesti†; Sueroral; Sueroral Hiposodico; **Switz.:** Elotrans; GES 45; Normolytoral; Oralpadon†; **Thai.:** Infanolyte; Oreda; Osaline; Pedialyte; Rehydralyte;

Servidrat; *UK:* Diocalm Replenish†; Dioralyte; Dioralyte Effervescent; Dioralyte Relief; Electrolade; Entrocalm Replace; Rehidrat; Replavite; *USA:* Infalyte; Kao Lectrolyte†; Naturalyte; Pedialyte; Rehydralyte; Resol.

Bicarbonate (3269-r)

Bicarbonate is an alkalinising agent administered as bicarbonate-containing salts (sodium or potassium bicarbonate) or bicarbonate-producing salts (acetate, citrate, or lactate salts). Allowance should be made for the effect of the cation. Bicarbonate-producing or bicarbonate-containing solutions have been reported to be **incompatible** with a wide range of drugs. In many cases this incompatibility is a function of the alkaline nature of the bicarbonate solution. Precipitation of insoluble carbonates may occur, as may production of gaseous carbon dioxide when the bicarbonate ion is reduced by acidic solutions.

Potassium Bicarbonate (1178-h)

E501; Kalii Hydrogenocarbonas; Monopotassium Carbonate; Potassium Hydrogen Carbonate.
$KHCO_3 = 100.1$.
CAS — 298-14-6.
Pharmacopoeias. In *Eur.* (see p.vi), *Pol.,* and *US.*

Each g of potassium bicarbonate represents approximately 10 mmol of potassium and of bicarbonate. Potassium bicarbonate 2.56 g is approximately equivalent to 1 g of potassium.

Pharmacopoeial description
Ph. Eur.: A white, crystalline powder or colourless crystals. Freely soluble in water; practically insoluble in alcohol. When heated in the dry state or in solution, it is gradually converted to potassium carbonate. A freshly prepared 5% solution in water has a pH of not more than 8.6.

USP 25: Colourless, odourless, transparent monoclinic prisms or white granular powder. Freely soluble in water; practically insoluble in alcohol. Its solutions are neutral or alkaline to phenolphthalein.

Potassium Citrate (1180-t)

E332; Kalii Citras; Tripotassium Citrate. Tripotassium 2-hydroxypropane-1,2,3-tricarboxylate monohydrate.
$C_6H_5K_3O_7,H_2O = 324.4$.
CAS — 866-84-2 (anhydrous potassium citrate); 6100-05-6 (potassium citrate monohydrate).
ATC — A12BA02.
Pharmacopoeias. In *Chin., Eur.* (see p.vi), *Int.,* and *US.*

Each g of potassium citrate (anhydrous) represents approximately 9.8 mmol of potassium and 3.26 mmol of citrate. Each g of potassium citrate (monohydrate) represents approximately 9.3 mmol of potassium and 3.08 mmol of citrate. Potassium citrate (monohydrate) 2.77 g is approximately equivalent to 1 g of potassium.

Pharmacopoeial description
Ph. Eur.: Transparent, hygroscopic crystals or a white granular powder. Very soluble in water; practically insoluble in alcohol. Store in airtight containers.

USP 25: Transparent crystals or a white granular powder. It is odourless and is deliquescent in moist air. Soluble 1 in 1 of water and 1 in 2.5 of glycerol; almost insoluble in alcohol. Store in airtight containers.

Sodium Acetate (1189-v)

E262; Natrii Acetas; Natrium Aceticum.
$CH_3.CO_2Na,3H_2O = 136.1$.
CAS — 127-09-3 (anhydrous sodium acetate); 6131-90-4 (sodium acetate trihydrate).
ATC — B05XA08.
Pharmacopoeias. In *Eur.* (see p.vi), *Jpn, Pol.,* and *US.*
US also allows the anhydrous form.

Each g of sodium acetate (anhydrous) represents approximately 12.2 mmol of sodium and of acetate. Each g of sodium acetate (trihydrate) represents approximately 7.3 mmol of sodium and of acetate. Sodium acetate (anhydrous) 3.57 g is approximately equivalent to 1 g of sodium. Sodium acetate (trihydrate) 5.92 g is approximately equivalent to 1 g of sodium.

Pharmacopoeial description
Ph. Eur.: Colourless crystals. Very soluble in water; soluble in alcohol. A 5% solution in water has a pH of 7.5 to 9.0. Store in airtight containers.

USP 25: It contains three molecules of water of hydration or is anhydrous. Colourless, transparent crystals, or a white, granular crystalline powder, or white flakes. It is odourless or has a faint acetous odour. It is efflorescent in warm dry air. Soluble 1 in 0.8 of water, 1 in 0.6 of boiling water, and 1 in 19 of alcohol. pH of a solution in water containing the equivalent of 3% of anhydrous sodium acetate is between 7.5 and 9.2. Store in airtight containers.

Sodium Acid Citrate (1192-d)

Disodium Hydrogen Citrate; E331; Natrium Citricum Acidum.
$C_6H_6Na_2O_7,1\frac{1}{2}H_2O = 263.1$.
CAS — 144-33-2.
Pharmacopoeias. In *Br.*

Each g of sodium acid citrate (sesquihydrate) represents approximately 7.6 mmol of sodium and 3.8 mmol of citrate. Sodium acid citrate (sesquihydrate) 5.72 g is approximately equivalent to 1 g of sodium.

Pharmacopoeial description
BP 2001: A white, odourless or almost odourless, powder. Freely soluble in water; practically insoluble in alcohol. A 3% solution in water has a pH of 4.9 to 5.2.

Sodium Bicarbonate (1190-r)

Baking Soda; E500; Monosodium Carbonate; Natrii Bicarbonas; Natrii Hydrogenocarbonas; Sal de Vichy; Sodium Acid Carbonate; Sodium Hydrogen Carbonate.
$NaHCO_3 = 84.01$.
CAS — 144-55-8.
ATC — B05CB04; B05XA02.
Pharmacopoeias. In *Chin., Eur.* (see p.vi), *Int., Jpn, Pol.,* and *US.*

Each g of sodium bicarbonate (anhydrous) represents approximately 11.9 mmol of sodium and of bicarbonate. Sodium bicarbonate 3.65 g is approximately equivalent to 1 g of sodium.

Pharmacopoeial description
Ph. Eur.: A white, crystalline powder. Soluble in water; practically insoluble in alcohol. The pH of a freshly prepared 5% solution in water is not more than 8.6. When heated in the dry state or in solution, it gradually changes into sodium carbonate.

USP 25: A white crystalline powder that slowly decomposes in moist air. Soluble 1 in 12 of water; insoluble in alcohol. Its solutions, when freshly prepared with cold water, without shaking, are alkaline to litmus; alkalinity increases on standing, agitation, or heating.

Sodium Citrate (1193-n)

E331; Natrii Citras; Trisodium Citrate. Trisodium 2-hydroxypropane-1,2,3-tricarboxylate dihydrate.
$C_6H_5Na_3O_7,2H_2O = 294.1$.
CAS — 68-04-2 (anhydrous sodium citrate); 6132-04-3 (sodium citrate dihydrate).
ATC — B05CB02.
Pharmacopoeias. In *Chin., Eur.* (see p.vi), *Int., Jpn,* and *Pol.*
Int. and *US* specify anhydrous or dihydrate.

Each g of sodium citrate (anhydrous) represents approximately 11.6 mmol of sodium and 3.9 mmol of citrate. Each g of sodium citrate (dihydrate) represents approximately 10.2 mmol of sodium and 3.4 mmol of citrate. Sodium citrate (anhydrous) 3.74 g is approximately equivalent to 1 g of sodium. Sodium citrate (dihydrate) 4.26 g is approximately equivalent to 1 g of sodium.

Sterilised solutions when stored may cause separation of particles from glass containers and solutions containing such particles must not be used.

Pharmacopoeial description
Ph. Eur.: A white, crystalline powder or white, granular crystals; slightly deliquescent in moist air. Freely soluble in water; practically insoluble in alcohol. Store in airtight containers.

USP 25: It is anhydrous or contains two molecules of water of hydration. Colourless crystals, or a white crystalline powder. The hydrous form is soluble 1 in 1.5 of water and 1 in 0.6 of boiling water; insoluble in alcohol. Store in airtight containers.

Sodium Lactate (1194-h)

E325. Sodium 2-hydroxypropionate.
$C_3H_5NaO_3 = 112.1$.
CAS — 72-17-3.
Pharmacopoeias. Chin., Eur. (see p.vi), and *US* include preparations of sodium lactate.

Each g of sodium lactate (anhydrous) represents approximately 8.9 mmol of sodium and of lactate. Sodium lactate (anhydrous) 4.88 g is approximately equivalent to 1 g of sodium.

Pharmacopoeial description
Ph. Eur.: Sodium Lactate Solution contains a minimum of 50% w/w of sodium lactate and is a mixture of the two enantiomers in approximately equal proportions. Sodium (S)-Lactate Solution contains a minimum of 50% w/w of sodium lactate, not less than 95% of which is the (S)-enantiomer. The solutions are clear, colourless, slightly syrupy liquids. Miscible with water and with alcohol. pH 6.5 to 9.0.

USP 25: Sodium Lactate Solution is an aqueous solution containing at least 50% sodium lactate. A clear, colourless or practically colourless, slightly viscous liquid, odourless or having a slight, not unpleasant, odour. Miscible with water. pH between 5.0 and 9.0. Store in airtight containers.

Adverse Effects and Treatment

Excessive administration of bicarbonate or bicarbonate-forming compounds may lead to hypokalaemia and metabolic alkalosis, especially in patients with impaired renal function. Symptoms include mood changes, tiredness, shortness of breath, muscle weakness, and irregular heartbeat. Muscle hypertonicity, twitching, and tetany may develop, especially in hypocalcaemic patients. Treatment of metabolic alkalosis associated with bicarbonate overdose consists mainly of appropriate correction of fluid and electrolyte balance. Replacement of calcium, chloride, and potassium ions may be of particular importance.

Excessive doses of *sodium salts* may also lead to sodium overloading and hyperosmolality (see Adverse Effects of Sodium, p.1196). Administration of sodium bicarbonate by mouth can cause stomach cramps, belching, and flatulence. Extravasation of irritant hypertonic sodium bicarbonate solutions resulting in local tissue necrosis has been reported following intravenous administration.

Excessive doses of *potassium salts* may lead to hyperkalaemia (see Adverse Effects of Potassium, p.1195). Oral administration of potassium salts can cause gastrointestinal adverse effects, and tablet formulations may cause contact irritation due to high local concentrations of potassium.

Excessive oral administration of *citrate salts* may have a laxative effect.

Effects on the gastrointestinal tract. In addition to minor gastrointestinal effects (see above), spontaneous rupture of the stomach, although an exceedingly rare event, has been reported on several occasions following ingestion of sodium bicarbonate. The bicarbonate was believed to have resulted in the rapid production of enough carbon dioxide to rupture a stomach already distended with food.[1]
1. Mastrangelo MR, Moore EW. Spontaneous rupture of the stomach in a healthy adult man after sodium bicarbonate ingestion. *Ann Intern Med* 1984; **101:** 649.

Effects on mental state. Lactate infusions have been reported to induce feelings of anxiety, especially in patients with anxiety states, and have been used as a pharmacological model in the evaluation of mechanisms involved in clinical anxiety.[1] There has also been a report[2] of a patient receiving oral lactate (as calcium lactate) who was suffering from panic disorder associated with agoraphobia; when lactate was discontinued, the patient reported a reduction in panic intensity without a decrease in the frequency of attacks.
1. Lader M, Bruce M. States of anxiety and their induction by drugs. *Br J Clin Pharmacol* 1986; **22:** 251–61.
2. Robinson D, *et al.* Possible oral lactate exacerbation of panic disorder. *Ann Pharmacother* 1995; **29:** 539–40.

Epileptogenic effect. Alkalosis may precipitate seizures; however, absence seizures have also been reported to be associated with sodium bicarbonate administration in a child in whom the serum pH was normal.[1]
1. Reif S, *et al.* Absence seizures associated with bicarbonate therapy and normal serum pH. *JAMA* 1989; **262:** 1328–9.

Precautions

It is generally recommended that bicarbonate or bicarbonate-forming compounds should not be given to patients with metabolic or respiratory alkalosis, hypocalcaemia, or hypochlorhydria. During treatment of acidosis, frequent monitoring of serum-electrolyte concentrations and acid-base status is essential.

Sodium-containing salts should be administered extremely cautiously to patients with heart failure, oedema, renal impairment, hypertension, eclampsia, or aldosteronism (see Sodium, p.1196).

Potassium-containing salts should be administered with considerable care to patients with renal or adrenocortical insufficiency, cardiac disease, or other conditions that may predispose to hyperkalaemia (see Potassium, p.1195).

Abuse. High doses of bicarbonate have been taken by athletes to enhance performance in endurance sports by buffering hydrogen ions produced in conjunction with lactic acid.[1] Bicarbonates have also been used to alkalinise the urine and prolong the half-life of basic drugs, notably sympathomimetics and stimulants, thereby avoiding detection; however, such a practice may enhance toxicity.
1. Kennedy M. Drugs and athletes—an update. *Adverse Drug React Bull* 1994; (Dec): 639–42.

Interactions

The effect of oral bicarbonate or bicarbonate-forming compounds in raising intra-gastric pH may reduce or increase the rate and/or extent of absorption of a number of drugs (see also Antacids, p.1201). Alkalinisation of the urine leads to increased renal clearance of acidic drugs such as salicylates and barbiturates. Conversely, it prolongs the half-life of basic drugs and may result in toxicity (see also under Abuse, above).

Sodium bicarbonate enhances lithium excretion. The concomitant use of *potassium-containing salts* with drugs that increase serum-potassium concentrations such as ACE inhibitors and potassium-sparing diuretics should generally be avoided (p.1195). *Citrate salts* taken by mouth can enhance the absorption of aluminium from the gastrointestinal tract (see p.1211 under Adverse Effects of Aluminium Hydroxide). Patients with impaired renal function are particularly susceptible to aluminium accumulation and citrate-containing oral preparations, including many effervescent or dispersible tablets, are best avoided by patients with renal failure taking aluminium-containing compounds.

Pharmacokinetics

Administration of bicarbonate, such as sodium bicarbonate, by mouth causes neutralisation of gastric acid with the production of carbon dioxide. Bicarbonate not involved in that reaction is absorbed and in the absence of a deficit of bicarbonate in the plasma, bicarbonate ions are excreted in the urine, which is rendered alkaline, and there is an accompanying diuresis.

Acetates such as potassium acetate and sodium acetate, citrates such as potassium citrate, sodium acid citrate, and sodium citrate, and lactates such as sodium lactate are metabolised, after absorption, to bicarbonate.

Uses and Administration

Bicarbonate-providing salts are alkalinising agents used for a variety of purposes including the correction of metabolic acidosis, alkalinisation of the urine, and as antacids.

When an alkalinising agent is indicated for treating acute or chronic **metabolic acidosis** (p.1180), sodium bicarbonate is usually used. In conditions when acute metabolic acidosis is associated with tissue hypoxia, such as *cardiac arrest* and *lactic acidosis*, the role of such alkalinising agents is controversial (see p.1180, and for guidelines on advanced cardiac life support, p.790). Sodium lactate has been given as an alternative to sodium bicarbonate in acute metabolic acidosis, but is no longer recommended because of the risk of precipitating lactic acidosis. In *chronic hyperchloraemic acidosis* associated with potassium deficiency, potassium bicarbonate may be preferred to sodium bicarbonate. The citrate salts of potassium or sodium have also been used as alternatives to sodium bicarbonate in treating chronic metabolic acidosis resulting from *renal disorders*. Sodium bicarbonate, lactate and acetate, and potassium acetate are used as bicarbonate sources in *dialysis fluids* (p.1184).

The dose of bicarbonate required for the treatment of acidotic states must be calculated on an individual basis, and is dependent on the acid-base balance and electrolyte status of the patient. In the treatment of chronic acidosis bicarbonate has been given by mouth and doses providing 57 mmol (4.8 g sodium bicarbonate) or more daily may be required. In severe acidosis, sodium bicarbonate has been given intravenously by continuous infusion usually as a 1.26% (150 mmol per litre) solution or by slow intravenous injection of a stronger (hypertonic) solution of up to 8.4% (1000 mmol per litre) sodium bicarbonate (but see the discussion on metabolic acidosis, p.1180). For the correction of acidosis during advanced cardiac life support procedures, doses of 50 mmol of sodium bicarbonate (50 mL of an 8.4% solution) may be given intravenously to adults. Frequent monitoring of serum-electrolyte concentrations and acid-base status is essential during treatment of acidosis.

Sodium bicarbonate may be used in the management of **hyperkalaemia** (p.1182) to promote the intracellu-

The symbol † denotes a preparation no longer actively marketed

lar uptake of potassium and correct associated acidosis.

Sodium bicarbonate, sodium citrate, and potassium citrate cause **alkalinisation of the urine**. They may therefore be given to relieve discomfort in mild *urinary-tract infections* (p.146) and to prevent the development of uric-acid renal calculi in the initial stages of *uricosuric* therapy for hyperuricaemia in chronic gout (for example, see Probenecid, p.401). In both cases, they are administered with a liberal fluid intake, usually by mouth, in divided doses of up to about 10 g daily. Sodium bicarbonate has also been used with a diuretic in the treatment of *acute poisoning* from weakly acidic drugs to enhance their excretion, but this process, which is known as 'forced alkaline diuresis', is generally no longer recommended.

When given by mouth, sodium bicarbonate and potassium bicarbonate neutralise acid secretions in the gastrointestinal tract and sodium bicarbonate in particular is therefore frequently included in **antacid** preparations (p.1201). To relieve *dyspepsia* doses of about 1 to 5 g of sodium bicarbonate in water have been taken when required. Sodium citrate has been widely used as a 'clear' (non-particulate) antacid, usually with an H₂-antagonist, for the *prophylaxis of acid aspiration* associated with anaesthesia (p.1202). Sodium bicarbonate is also used in various preparations for *double-contrast radiography* where production of gas (carbon dioxide) in the gastrointestinal tract is necessary. Similarly, solutions containing sodium bicarbonate or citrate have been used to treat acute *oesophageal impaction*.

Sodium bicarbonate and sodium or potassium citrate are used as buffering or alkalinising agents in *pharmaceutical formulation*. Sodium bicarbonate and anhydrous sodium citrate are used in effervescent tablet formulations.

Individual salts also have **other specific uses**. A 5% solution of sodium bicarbonate can be administered as ear drops to soften and remove *ear wax*. Sodium bicarbonate injection has been used to treat *extravasation of anthracycline antineoplastics* (p.480) although as mentioned in Adverse Effects, above, hypertonic solutions may themselves cause necrosis.

Sodium citrate has anti-clotting properties and is employed, as sodium acid citrate, with other agents in solutions for the anticoagulation and preservation of blood for *transfusion* purposes. Similarly, sodium citrate 3% irrigation may be useful for the dissolution of *blood clots in the bladder* as an alternative to sodium chloride 0.9%. Enemas containing sodium citrate are given rectally as *osmotic laxatives*. Sodium citrate is also a common ingredient in *cough* mixtures.

Eye disorders. Sodium citrate eye drops have been employed in the management of certain ocular injuries. It has been suggested that corneal epithelial defects due to chemical weapon injuries and lasting for more than one week or accompanied by limbal ischaemia require intensive topical therapy with eye drops of sodium citrate 10% and of potassium ascorbate 10%. Such therapy is said to prevent late corneal melting and to permit the continuation of local corticosteroid therapy as necessary.[1] The two types of eye drops are given in alternate doses and are believed to act by mopping up free oxygen radicals after chemical burns.[2]

Sodium bicarbonate is also used in the management of blepharitis, an inflammation of the margin of the eyelids that may be caused by a variety of conditions. It may be allergic in nature or associated with seborrhoea of the scalp. Infection of the eyelids can produce ulcerative blepharitis, a condition characterised by the formation of yellow crusts which may glue the eyelashes together. Parasites occasionally cause blepharitis. The condition is first treated by cleaning the eyes and eyelids with sodium bicarbonate solution or a suitable bland eye lotion; simple eye ointment or diluted baby shampoo can also be used to soften crusts to aid removal. If an infection is present, antibacterials may be required (p.121). Long-term management consists of daily cleansing of the lid margins with a bland eye lotion.

1. Wright P. Injuries due to chemical weapons. *BMJ* 1991; **302**: 239.
2. Anonymous. Citrate/ascorbate eye-drops for chemical weapons injuries. *Pharm J* 1991; **246**: 145.

Osteoporosis. Potassium bicarbonate administered by mouth in a dose of 1 to 2 mmol per kg body-weight daily for 18 days in 18 postmenopausal women was found to improve calcium

and phosphorus balance, reduce bone resorption and increase its formation.[1] However, elderly subjects with renal impairment might be at risk of hyperkalaemia with the doses used and long-term studies would be required before this emerged as an effective treatment or preventative strategy for postmenopausal osteoporosis (p.745).[2]

1. Sebastian A, *et al.* Improved mineral balance and skeletal metabolism in postmenopausal women treated with potassium bicarbonate. *N Engl J Med* 1994; **330**: 1776–81.
2. Sebastian A, Morris RC. Improved mineral balance and skeletal metabolism in postmenopausal women treated with potassium bicarbonate. *N Engl J Med* 1994; **331**: 279.

Renal calculi. Citrate forms soluble complexes with calcium, thereby reducing urinary saturation of stone-forming calcium salts. Potassium citrate has a hypocalciuric effect when given by mouth, probably due to enhanced renal calcium absorption. Urinary calcium excretion is unaffected by sodium citrate, since the alkali-mediated hypocalciuric effect is offset by a sodium-linked calciuresis.[1] An uncontrolled study has demonstrated that potassium citrate may be beneficial in reducing the rate of stone formation in patients with hypocitraturia.[2] As mentioned in Uses above, sodium bicarbonate or sodium or potassium citrate may also be used for their alkalinising action, as an adjunct to a liberal fluid intake, to prevent development of uric-acid renal calculi during uricosuric therapy.

Other causes of renal calculi and their treatment are discussed on p.910.

Urinary alkalinisation with sodium bicarbonate, sodium citrate, or potassium citrate may be useful in the management of cystine stone formation in patients with cystinuria (p.1019).

1. Anonymous. Citrate for calcium nephrolithiasis. *Lancet* 1986; **i**: 955.
2. Pak CYC, Fuller C. Idiopathic hypocitraturic calcium-oxalate nephrolithiasis successfully treated with potassium citrate. *Ann Intern Med* 1986; **104**: 33–7.

Preparations

BP 2001: Alkaline Gentian Mixture; Aromatic Magnesium Carbonate Mixture; Compound Magnesium Trisilicate Oral Powder; Compound Sodium Bicarbonate Tablets; Compound Sodium Chloride Mouthwash; Kaolin and Morphine Mixture; Kaolin Mixture; Magnesium Trisilicate Mixture; Potassium Citrate Mixture; Sodium Bicarbonate Ear Drops; Sodium Bicarbonate Eye Lotion; Sodium Bicarbonate Intravenous Infusion; Sodium Citrate Eye Drops; Sodium Citrate Irrigation Solution; Sodium Citrate Tablets; Sodium Lactate Intravenous Infusion;
BPC 1968: Effervescent Potassium Tablets;
Ph. Eur.: Anticoagulant Acid-Citrate-Glucose Solutions (ACD); Anticoagulant Citrate-Phosphate-Glucose Solution (CPD);
USP 25: Anticoagulant Citrate Dextrose Solution; Anticoagulant Citrate Phosphate Dextrose Adenine Solution; Anticoagulant Citrate Phosphate Dextrose Solution; Anticoagulant Sodium Citrate Solution; Half-strength Lactated Ringer's and Dextrose Injection; Lactated Ringer's and Dextrose Injection; Lactated Ringer's Injection; Magnesium Carbonate and Sodium Bicarbonate for Oral Suspension; Potassium and Sodium Bicarbonates and Citric Acid Effervescent Tablets for Oral Solution; Potassium Bicarbonate and Potassium Chloride Effervescent Tablets for Oral Solution; Potassium Bicarbonate and Potassium Chloride for Effervescent Oral Solution; Potassium Bicarbonate Effervescent Tablets for Oral Solution; Potassium Chloride in Lactated Ringer's and Dextrose Injection; Potassium Chloride, Potassium Bicarbonate, and Potassium Citrate Effervescent Tablets for Oral Solution; Potassium Citrate And Citric Acid Oral Solution; Potassium Citrate Extended-release Tablets; Potassium Gluconate and Potassium Citrate Oral Solution; Potassium Gluconate, Potassium Citrate, and Ammonium Chloride Oral Solution; Sodium Acetate Injection; Sodium Acetate Solution; Sodium Bicarbonate Injection; Sodium Bicarbonate Oral Powder; Sodium Bicarbonate Tablets; Sodium Citrate and Citric Acid Oral Solution; Sodium Lactate Injection; Sodium Lactate Solution; Tricitrates Oral Solution; Trikates Oral Solution.

Proprietary Preparations (details are given in Part 3)
Aust.: Bullrich Salz; *Austral.:* Chlorvescent; Sodibic; Urocit-K; *Canad.:* Brioschi; Eno; K-Lyte; Polycitra-K; *Fr.:* Soludial; *Ger.:* Alkala T; Kalitrans; Kohlensaurebad Bastian; Nephrotrans; *Irl.:* Cystopurin; *Israel:* Babic; *Ital.:* Citrosodina; Kation†; *Mex.:* Betsol Z; Bicarnat; Debonal; *Norw.:* Kajos; *Port.:* Acalka; *S.Afr.:* Nitrocit; *Singapore:* Urocit-K; *Spain:* Acalka; Plurisalina; *Swed.:* Kajos; *Switz.:* Nephrotrans; *UK:* Canesten Oasis; Cystemme; Cystitis Relief; Cystocalm; Cystofem; Cystoleve; Cystopurin; *USA:* Bell/ans; Citra pH; K + Care; K-Lyte; Neut; Urocit-K.

Multi-ingredient: numerous preparations are listed in Part 3.

Calcium (1151-j)

Ca = 40.078.

Calcium is a cation administered as various calcium-containing salts. Calcium salts have been reported to be **incompatible** with a wide range of drugs. Complexes may form resulting in the formation of a precipitate.

Calcium Acetate (1152-z)

E263.
$C_4H_6CaO_4 = 158.2$.
CAS — 62-54-4.
Pharmacopoeias. In Br. and US.

Each g of calcium acetate (anhydrous) represents approximately 6.3 mmol of calcium. Calcium acetate (anhydrous) 3.95 g is approximately equivalent to 1 g of calcium.

Pharmacopoeial description

BP 2001: A white, hygroscopic, odourless or almost odourless, powder. Freely soluble in water; slightly soluble in alcohol. A 5% solution in water has a pH of 7.2 to 8.2.

USP 25: A white, odourless or almost odourless, hygroscopic, crystalline powder. It decomposes to calcium carbonate and acetone when heated to above 160°. Freely soluble in water; slightly soluble in methyl alcohol; practically insoluble in dehydrated alcohol, in acetone, and in benzene. A 5% solution in water has a pH of 6.3 to 9.6. Store in airtight containers.

Calcium Chloride (1154-k)

Calcii Chloridum; Calcium Chloratum; Calcium Chloride Dihydrate; Cloreto de Cálcio; Cloruro de Calcio; E509.
$CaCl_2,2H_2O = 147.0$.
CAS — 10043-52-4 (anhydrous calcium chloride); 7774-34-7 (calcium chloride hexahydrate); 10035-04-8 (calcium chloride dihydrate).
ATC — A12AA07; B05XA07; G04BA03.
Pharmacopoeias. In *Chin., Eur.* (see p.vi), *Jpn,* and *US. Eur.* also specifies the hexahydrate. *Pol.* only specifies the hexahydrate.

Each g of calcium chloride (dihydrate) represents approximately 6.8 mmol of calcium and 13.6 mmol of chloride. Calcium chloride (dihydrate) 3.67 g is approximately equivalent to 1 g of calcium.

Each g of calcium chloride (hexahydrate) represents approximately 4.56 mmol of calcium and 9.13 mmol of chloride. Calcium chloride (hexahydrate) 5.47 g is approximately equivalent to 1 g of calcium.

Pharmacopoeial description

Ph. Eur.: The dihydrate is a white, hygroscopic, crystalline powder. Freely soluble in water; soluble in alcohol.
The hexahydrate is a white, crystalline mass or colourless crystals. Very soluble in water; freely soluble in alcohol. F.p. about 29°.

USP 25: White, hard, odourless fragments or granules. Is deliquescent. Soluble 1 in 0.7 of water, 1 in 0.2 of boiling water, 1 in 4 of alcohol, and 1 in 2 of boiling alcohol. A pH of a 5% solution in water is between 4.5 and 9.2. Store in airtight containers.

Calcium Citrate (3275-t)

Tricalcium Citrate. Tricalcium 2-hydroxypropane-1,2,3-tricarboxylate tetrahydrate.
$C_{12}H_{10}Ca_3O_{14},4H_2O = 570.5$.
CAS — 5785-44-4.
Pharmacopoeias. In *Aust.* and *US.*

Each g of calcium citrate (tetrahydrate) represents approximately 5.3 mmol of calcium and 3.5 mmol of citrate. Calcium citrate (tetrahydrate) 4.74 g is approximately equivalent to 1 g of calcium.

Pharmacopoeial description

USP 25: A white, odourless, crystalline powder. Slightly soluble in water; insoluble in alcohol; freely soluble in diluted 3N hydrochloric acid and in diluted 2N nitric acid.

Calcium Glubionate (1156-t)

Calcium Glubionate (USAN, rINN). Calcium Glubionate Lactobionate Monohydrate; Calcium Gluconogalactogluconate Monohydrate. Calcium D-gluconate lactobionate monohydrate.
$(C_{12}H_{21}O_{12},C_6H_{11}O_7)Ca,H_2O = 610.5$.
CAS — 31959-85-0 (anhydrous calcium glubionate); 12569-38-9 (calcium glubionate monohydrate).
ATC — A12AA02.
Pharmacopoeias. US includes Calcium Glubionate Syrup.

Each g of calcium glubionate (monohydrate) represents approximately 1.6 mmol of calcium. Calcium glubionate (monohydrate) 15.2 g is approximately equivalent to 1 g of calcium.

Calcium Gluceptate (1157-x)

Calcium Glucoheptonate (pINN); Calcii Glucoheptonas.
$C_{14}H_{26}CaO_{16} = 490.4$.
CAS — 17140-60-2 (anhydrous calcium gluceptate); 29039-00-7 (anhydrous calcium gluceptate).
ATC — A12AA10.
Pharmacopoeias. In *Eur.* (see p.vi). *US* allows anhydrous or with varying amounts of water of hydration.

Each g of calcium gluceptate (anhydrous) represents approximately 2 mmol of calcium. Calcium gluceptate (anhydrous) 12.2 g is approximately equivalent to 1 g of calcium.

Pharmacopoeial description

Ph. Eur.: Calcium Glucoheptonate is a mixture in variable proportions of calcium di(D-*glycero*-D-*gulo*-heptonate) and calcium di(D-*glycero*-D-*ido*-heptonate). A white or very slightly yellow, hygroscopic, amorphous powder. Practically insoluble in alcohol and in acetone. A 10% solution in water has a pH of 6.0 to 8.0. Store in airtight containers.

USP 25: It is anhydrous or contains varying amounts of water of hydration. It consists of the calcium salt of the alpha-epimer of glucoheptonic acid or of a mixture of the alpha and beta epimers of glucoheptonic acid. A white to faintly yellow amorphous powder. It is stable in air, but the hydrous forms may lose part of their water of hydration on standing. Freely soluble in water; insoluble in alcohol and in many other organic solvents. pH of a 10% solution in water is between 6.0 and 8.0.

Calcium Gluconate (1158-r)

Calcii Gluconas; Calcium Glyconate; E578. Calcium D-gluconate monohydrate.
$C_{12}H_{22}CaO_{14},H_2O = 448.4$.
CAS — 299-28-5 (anhydrous calcium gluconate); 18016-24-5 (calcium gluconate monohydrate).
ATC — A12AA03; D11AX03.
Pharmacopoeias. In *Chin., Eur.* (see p.vi), *Int., Jpn,* and *Pol.* Also in *US* as the anhydrous or the monohydrate form.
Calcium borogluconate is included in *Aust.* and as an injection in *BP(Vet).*

Each g of calcium gluconate (monohydrate) represents approximately 2.2 mmol of calcium. Calcium gluconate (monohydrate) 11.2 g is approximately equivalent to 1 g of calcium.

Pharmacopoeial description

Ph. Eur.: A white, crystalline or granular, powder. Sparingly soluble in water; freely soluble in boiling water.

USP 25: It is anhydrous or contains one molecule of water of hydration. White, odourless, crystalline granules or powder. Slowly soluble 1 in 30 of water; soluble 1 in 5 of boiling water; insoluble in alcohol. Its solutions are neutral to litmus.

Calcium Glycerophosphate (1931-t)

Calcii Glycerophosphas; Calcium Glycerinophosphate.
$C_3H_7CaO_6P(+xH_2O) = 210.1$ (anhydrous).
CAS — 27214-00-2 (anhydrous calcium glycerophosphate).
Pharmacopoeias. In *Eur.* (see p.vi).

Each g of calcium glycerophosphate (anhydrous) represents approximately 4.8 mmol of calcium. Calcium glycerophosphate (anhydrous) 5.24 g is approximately equivalent to 1 g of calcium.

Pharmacopoeial description

Ph. Eur.: A mixture in variable proportions of calcium (*RS*)-2,3-dihydroxypropyl phosphate and of calcium 2-hydroxy-1-(hydroxymethyl)ethyl phosphate, which may be hydrated. It contains not less than 18.6% and not more than 19.4% of calcium, calculated with reference to the dried substance. A white hygroscopic powder. Sparingly soluble in water; practically insoluble in alcohol. It loses not more than 12% of its weight on drying.

Calcium Hydrogen Phosphate (1159-f)

Calcii et Hydrogenii Phosphas; Calcii Hydrogenophosphas; Calcium Hydrophosphoricum; Calcium Monohydrogen Phosphate; Dibasic Calcium Phosphate; Dicalcium Orthophosphate; Dicalcium Phosphate; E341. Calcium hydrogen orthophosphate dihydrate.
$CaHPO_4,2H_2O = 172.1$.
CAS — 7757-93-9 (anhydrous calcium hydrogen phosphate); 7789-77-7 (calcium hydrogen phosphate dihydrate).
Pharmacopoeias. In *Eur.* (see p.vi), *Jpn, Pol.,* and *US,* which include specifications for the anhydrous substance, the dihydrate form, or both.

Each g of calcium hydrogen phosphate (dihydrate) represents approximately 5.8 mmol of calcium and of phosphate. Calcium hydrogen phosphate (dihydrate) 4.29 g is approximately equivalent to 1 g of calcium.

Pharmacopoeial description

Ph. Eur.: The anhydrous substance is a white crystalline powder or colourless crystals. Practically insoluble in water and in alcohol; dissolves in dilute hydrochloric acid and in dilute nitric acid.
The dihydrate is a white, crystalline powder. Practically insoluble in cold water and in alcohol; dissolves in dilute hydrochloric acid and in dilute nitric acid.

USP 25: It is anhydrous or contains two molecules of water of hydration. A white, odourless, powder. Practically insoluble in water; insoluble in alcohol; soluble in 3N hydrochloric acid and in 2N nitric acid.

Calcium Lactate (1160-z)

Calcii Lactas; E327. Calcium 2-hydroxypropionate.
$C_6H_{10}CaO_6,xH_2O = 218.2$ (anhydrous); 308.3 (pentahydrate); 272.3 (trihydrate).
CAS — 814-80-2 (anhydrous calcium lactate); 41372-22-9 (hydrated calcium lactate); 5743-47-5 (calcium lactate pentahydrate); 63690-56-2 (calcium lactate trihydrate).
ATC — A12AA05.
Pharmacopoeias. In *Chin., Eur.* (see p.vi), *Jpn, Pol.,* and *US. Eur.* has separate monographs for the pentahydrate and the trihydrate. *Port.* also includes the hexahydrate. *US* allows anhydrous or hydrous forms.

Each g of calcium lactate (trihydrate) represents approximately 3.7 mmol of calcium. Each g of calcium lactate (pentahydrate) represents approximately 3.2 mmol of calcium. Calcium lactate (pentahydrate) 7.7 g and calcium lactate (trihydrate) 6.8 g are approximately equivalent to 1 g of calcium.

Pharmacopoeial description

Ph. Eur.: The trihydrate is a white or almost white, crystalline or granular powder. Soluble in water; freely soluble in boiling water; very slightly soluble in alcohol.
The pentahydrate is a white or almost white, slightly efflorescent, crystalline or granular powder. Soluble in water; freely soluble in boiling water; very slightly soluble in alcohol.

USP 25: White, practically odourless, granules or powder. The pentahydrate is somewhat efflorescent and at 120° becomes anhydrous. The pentahydrate is soluble 1 in 20 of water and practically insoluble in alcohol. Store in airtight containers.

Calcium Lactate Gluconate (16157-q)

$Ca_5(C_3H_5O_3)_6,(C_6H_{11}O_7)_4,2H_2O = 1551.4$.
ATC — A12AA06.

Each g of calcium lactate gluconate (dihydrate) represents approximately 3.2 mmol of calcium. Calcium lactate gluconate (dihydrate) 7.74 g is approximately equivalent to 1 g of calcium.

Calcium Lactobionate (16158-p)

Calcium Lactobionate Dihydrate. Calcium 4-O-β-D-galactopyranosyl-D-gluconate dihydrate.
$C_{24}H_{42}CaO_{24},2H_2O = 790.7$.
CAS — 110638-68-1.
Pharmacopoeias. In *US.*

Each g of calcium lactobionate (dihydrate) represents approximately 1.3 mmol of calcium. Calcium lactobionate (dihydrate) 19.7 g is approximately equivalent to 1 g of calcium.

Pharmacopoeial description

USP 25: pH of a 5% solution in water is between 5.4 and 7.4.

Calcium Levulinate (1161-c)

Calcium Levulinate (BAN). Calcii Levulinas; Calcium Laevulate; Calcium Laevulinate; Lévulinate Calcique. Calcium 4-oxovalerate dihydrate.
$C_{10}H_{14}CaO_6,2H_2O = 306.3$.
CAS — 591-64-0 (anhydrous calcium levulinate); 5743-49-7 (calcium levulinate dihydrate).
ATC — A12AA30.
Pharmacopoeias. In *Eur.* (see p.vi) and *US.*

Each g of calcium levulinate (dihydrate) represents approximately 3.3 mmol of calcium. Calcium levulinate (dihydrate) 7.64 g is approximately equivalent to 1 g of calcium.

Pharmacopoeial description

Ph. Eur.: A white or almost white, crystalline powder. Freely soluble in water; very slightly soluble in alcohol; practically insoluble in dichloromethane. A 10% solution in water has a pH of 6.8 to 7.8. Protect from light.

USP 25: A white crystalline or amorphous powder, having a faint odour suggestive of burnt sugar. Freely soluble in water; slightly soluble in alcohol; insoluble in chloroform and in ether. pH of a 10% solution in water is between 7.0 and 8.5.

Calcium Phosphate (1162-k)

Calcium Orthophosphate; E341; Fosfato Tricalcico; Phosphate Tertiaire de Calcium; Precipitated Calcium Phosphate; Tribasic Calcium Phosphate; Tricalcii Phosphas; Tricalcium Phosphate.
CAS — 7758-87-4 (tricalcium diorthophosphate); 12167-74-7 (calcium hydroxide phosphate).
ATC — A12AA01.
Pharmacopoeias. In *Eur.* (see p.vi) and *Pol.* Also in *USNF.*

Calcium phosphate is not a clearly defined chemical entity but is a mixture of calcium phosphates that has been most frequently described as tricalcium diorthophosphate, $Ca_3(PO_4)_2$ =310.2, or calcium hydroxide phosphate, $Ca_5(OH)(PO_4)_3$ =502.3.

Pharmacopoeial description

Ph. Eur.: It consists of a mixture of calcium phosphates and contains 35 to 40% of Ca. A white or almost white powder. Practically insoluble in water; dissolves in dilute hydrochloric acid and in dilute nitric acid.

USNF 20: It consists of a variable mixture of calcium phosphates having the approximate composition $10CaO.3P_2O_5.H_2O$. It contains not less than 34% and not more than 40% of calcium. A white, odourless, powder. Practically insoluble in water; insoluble in alcohol; readily soluble in 3N hydrochloric acid and in 2N nitric acid.

Calcium Pidolate (12511-d)

Calcium Pidolate (pINNM). Calcium Pyroglutamate. Calcium 5-oxopyrrolidine-2-carboxylate.
$Ca(C_5H_6NO_3)_2 = 296.3$.
CAS — 31377-05-6.

Each g of calcium pidolate (anhydrous) represents approximately 3.4 mmol of calcium. Calcium pidolate (anhydrous) 7.39 g is approximately equivalent to 1 g of calcium.

Calcium Silicate (683-e)

E552.

CAS — 1344-95-2; 10101-39-0 (calcium metasilicate); 10034-77-2 (calcium diorthosilicate); 12168-85-3 (calcium trisilicate).

ATC — A02AC02.

Pharmacopoeias. In USNF.

A naturally occurring mineral, the most common forms being calcium metasilicate ($CaSiO_3$ = 116.2), calcium diorthosilicate (Ca_2SiO_4 = 172.2), and calcium trisilicate (Ca_3SiO_5 = 228.3). It is usually found in hydrated forms containing various amounts of water of crystallisation. Commercial calcium silicate is prepared synthetically.

Pharmacopoeial description

USNF 20: A compound of calcium oxide and silicon dioxide containing not less than 4% of CaO and not less than 45% of SiO_2. A white to off-white free-flowing powder. Insoluble in water; with mineral acids it forms a gel. A 5% aqueous suspension has a pH of 8.4 to 10.2.

Calcium Sodium Lactate (1164-t)

$2C_3H_5NaO_3,(C_3H_5O_3)_2Ca,4H_2O$ = 514.4.

Pharmacopoeias. In Br.

Each g of calcium sodium lactate (tetrahydrate) represents approximately 1.9 mmol of calcium and 3.9 mmol of sodium and of lactate. Calcium sodium lactate (tetrahydrate) 12.8 g is approximately equivalent to 1 g of calcium.

Pharmacopoeial description

BP 2001: A white deliquescent powder or granules with a slight characteristic odour. Soluble in water and in boiling alcohol; practically insoluble in ether.

Adverse Effects and Treatment

Administration of some calcium salts by mouth can cause gastrointestinal irritation; calcium chloride is generally considered to be the most irritant of the commonly used calcium salts.

Injection of calcium salts can also produce irritation and in particular intramuscular or subcutaneous injection can cause local reactions including sloughing or necrosis of the skin; solutions of calcium chloride are extremely irritant and should not be injected intramuscularly or subcutaneously. Soft-tissue calcification has also followed the use of calcium salts parenterally.

Excessive amounts of calcium salts may lead to hypercalcaemia. This complication is usually associated with parenteral administration, but can occur after oral administration, usually in patients with renal failure or who are taking vitamin D concurrently. Symptoms of hypercalcaemia may include anorexia, nausea, vomiting, constipation, abdominal pain, muscle weakness, mental disturbances, polydipsia, polyuria, nephrocalcinosis, renal calculi, and, in severe cases, cardiac arrhythmias and coma. Too rapid intravenous injection of calcium salts may also lead to many of the symptoms of hypercalcaemia as well as a chalky taste, hot flushes, and peripheral vasodilatation. Mild asymptomatic hypercalcaemia will usually resolve on stopping administration of calcium and other contributory drugs such as vitamin D (see also Vitamin D-mediated Hypercalcaemia, p.1181). If hypercalcaemia is severe, urgent treatment is required as outlined on p.1181.

Precautions

Solutions of calcium salts, particularly calcium chloride, are irritant, and care should be taken to prevent extravasation during intravenous injection. Calcium salts should be given cautiously to patients with impaired renal function, or diseases associated with hypercalcaemia such as sarcoidosis and some malignancies. In addition, they should generally be avoided in patients with calcium renal calculi, or a history of renal calculi. Calcium chloride, because of its acidifying nature, is unsuitable for the treatment of hypocalcaemia caused by renal insufficiency or in patients with respiratory acidosis or failure.

Plasma-calcium concentrations should be monitored closely in patients with renal insufficiency and during parenteral administration and if large doses of vitamin D are used concurrently.

The symbol † denotes a preparation no longer actively marketed

Interactions

Hypercalcaemia has occurred when calcium salts are coadministered with thiazide diuretics or vitamin D. Vitamin D increases the gastrointestinal absorption of calcium and thiazide diuretics decrease its urinary excretion. Plasma-calcium concentrations should be monitored in patients receiving the drugs together.

Bran decreases the gastrointestinal absorption of calcium, and may therefore decrease the efficacy of calcium supplements. Corticosteroids also reduce calcium absorption.

Calcium enhances the effects of digitalis glycosides on the heart and may precipitate digitalis intoxication; parenteral calcium therapy is best avoided in patients receiving cardiac glycosides. Citrate salts increase the absorption of aluminium from the gastrointestinal tract (see under Adverse Effects of Aluminium Hydroxide, p.1211), therefore patients with renal failure taking aluminium phosphate should avoid taking calcium citrate. Calcium salts reduce the absorption of a number of other drugs such as bisphosphonates, fluoride, some fluoroquinolones, and tetracyclines; administration should be separated by at least 3 hours.

Pharmacokinetics

Calcium is absorbed predominantly from the small intestine by active transport and passive diffusion. About one-third of ingested calcium is absorbed although this can vary depending upon dietary factors and the state of the small intestine; also absorption is increased in calcium deficiency and during periods of high physiological requirement such as during childhood or pregnancy and lactation. 1,25-Dihydroxycholecalciferol (calcitriol), a metabolite of vitamin D, enhances the active phase of absorption.

Excess calcium is predominantly excreted renally. Unabsorbed calcium is eliminated in the faeces, together with that secreted in the bile and pancreatic juice. Minor amounts are lost in the sweat, skin, hair, and nails. Calcium crosses the placenta and is distributed into breast milk.

Human Requirements

Calcium is the most abundant mineral in the body and is an essential body electrolyte. However, defining individual calcium requirements has proved difficult and guidelines vary widely by country and culture. Some authorities have adopted a factorial approach. For example, in the UK the dietary reference value (DRV) represents the apparent calcium requirements of healthy people under the prevailing dietary circumstances. The amount of calcium absorbed varies according to several factors including the requirements of the body, but is normally only about 30 to 40% of the dietary intake.

The richest dietary sources of calcium are milk and milk products. Significant amounts can also be consumed in green leafy vegetables, fortified flour, and hard water.

◊ In the UK dietary reference values (DRV—see p.1352) have been published for calcium.[1] In the USA recommended dietary allowances (RDA) had been set,[2] and have recently been replaced by dietary reference intakes (see p.1352).[3] In the UK estimated average requirement (EAR) for adults is 525 mg (13.1 mmol) daily and the reference nutrient intake (RNI) for adults is 700 mg (17.5 mmol); these figures are based on a mean absorption of calcium of 30% from mixed diets. In the USA the traditional RDA was 800 mg daily for adults aged over 25 years; this figure was based on an absorption rate of 40%. Under the new dietary reference intakes, adequate intakes (AI) for calcium have been set, which are higher in some age groups than the previous RDAs.[3] For adults aged up to 50 years the AI is 1 g daily, and for those aged 51 years or older, it is 1.2 g daily.[3] The tolerable upper intake is considered to be 2.5 g daily.[3]

1. DoH. Dietary reference values for food energy and nutrients for the United Kingdom: report of the panel on dietary reference values of the committee on medical aspects of food policy. *Report on health and social subjects 41.* London: HMSO, 1991.
2. Subcommittee on the tenth edition of the RDAs, Food and Nutrition Board, Commission on Life Sciences, National Research Council. *Recommended dietary allowances.* 10th ed. Washington, DC: National Academy Press, 1989.
3. Standing Committee on the Scientific Evaluation of Dietary Reference Intakes of the Food and Nutrition Board. *Dietary Reference Intakes for calcium, phosphorus, magnesium, vitamin D, and fluoride.* Washington, DC: National Academy Press, 1999.

Uses and Administration

Calcium salts are used in the management of **hypocalcaemia** (p.1181) and **calcium deficiency states** resulting from dietary deficiency or ageing (see also Osteoporosis, p.745). Doses may be expressed in terms of mmol or mEq of calcium, mass (mg) of calcium, or mass of calcium salt (for comparative purposes, see Table 1, below).

In simple deficiency states calcium salts may be given by mouth, usually in doses of 10 to 50 mmol (400 mg to 2 g) of calcium daily adjusted to the individual patient's requirements.

In severe acute hypocalcaemia or hypocalcaemic tetany parenteral administration is necessary, generally by slow intravenous injection or continuous infusion of calcium chloride or calcium gluconate (see also Administration, below). A typical dose is 2.25 mmol of calcium by slow intravenous injection, either repeated as required, or followed by continuous intravenous infusion of about 9 mmol daily. 2.25 mmol of calcium is provided by 10 mL of calcium gluconate 10%. Calcium gluceptate and calcium glycerophosphate with calcium lactate have been given by the intramuscular route; the chloride and gluconate are unsuitable for this route because of their irritancy. The intravenous route is used in children.

Intravenous calcium salts are also used to reverse the toxic cardiac effects of potassium in the emergency treatment of severe **hyperkalaemia** (p.1182), and as an antidote to magnesium in severe **hypermagnesaemia** (p.1181). For these indications, 2.25 to 4.5 mmol of calcium (10 to 20 mL of calcium gluconate 10%) is commonly used.

Individual calcium salts have specific uses. Calcium carbonate (p.1215) or acetate are effective phosphate binders and are given by mouth to reduce phosphate absorption from the gut in patients with **hyperphosphataemia**; this is particularly relevant to patients with chronic renal failure in order to prevent the development of renal osteodystrophy (p.746). The initial dose of calcium carbonate is 2.5 g daily titrated to a maximum of 17 g daily. The initial dose of calcium acetate is 3 or 4 g daily; most patients require 6 to 12 g daily.

Calcium carbonate and calcium silicate, administered by mouth, are used for their **antacid** properties (p.1201).

Table 1. Some calcium salts and their calcium content.

Calcium salt	Calcium content per g		
	mg	mmol	mEq
Calcium acetate (anhydrous)	253	6.3	12.6
Calcium carbonate	400	10.0	20.0
Calcium chloride (dihydrate)	273	6.8	13.6
Calcium citrate (tetrahydrate)	211	5.3	10.5
Calcium glubionate (monohydrate)	66	1.6	3.3
Calcium gluceptate (anhydrous)	82	2.0	4.1
Calcium gluconate (monohydrate)	89	2.2	4.5
Calcium glycerophosphate (anhydrous)	191	4.8	9.5
Calcium lactate (anhydrous)	184	4.6	9.2
Calcium lactate (trihydrate)	147	3.7	7.3
Calcium lactate (pentahydrate)	130	3.2	6.5
Calcium lactate gluconate (dihydrate)	129	3.2	6.4
Calcium lactobionate (dihydrate)	51	1.3	2.5
Calcium levulinate (anhydrous)	131	3.3	6.5
Calcium hydrogen phosphate (dihydrate)	233	5.8	11.6
Calcium phosphate [$10CaO.3P_2O_5.H_2O$]	399	10.0	19.9
Calcium pidolate (anhydrous)	135	3.4	6.7
Calcium silicate [$CaSiO_3$]	345	8.6	17.2
Calcium sodium lactate (tetrahydrate)	78	1.9	3.9

Some of the calcium salts discussed here also have *pharmaceutical uses* as diluents in capsules and tablets, buffers and dissolution aids in dispersible tablets, disintegrant and anticaking agents, and as a basis or abrasive in dental preparations.

Calcium phosphate (Calcarea Phosphorica; Calc. Phos.) is used in homoeopathic medicine.

Administration. Some think that calcium chloride should be preferred to calcium gluconate for parenteral preparations,[1,2] because retention of the chloride is greater and more predictable than of the gluconate, and results in a more predictable increase in extracellular ionised calcium concentration. However, calcium chloride is considered to be the most irritant of the calcium salts in general use (see Adverse Effects, above).

Calcium gluconate has been administered by the intraperitoneal route[3] for the treatment of chronic hypocalcaemia after parathyroidectomy in a patient undergoing continuous ambulatory peritoneal dialysis, resulting in improved systemic bioavailability compared with oral and intravenous administration.

1. Worthley LIG, Phillips PJ. Intravenous calcium salts. *Lancet* 1980; **ii:** 149.
2. Broner CW, *et al.* A prospective, randomized, double-blind comparison of calcium chloride and calcium gluconate therapies for hypocalcemia in critically ill children. *J Pediatr* 1990; **117:** 986–9.
3. Stamatakis MK, Seth SK. Treatment of chronic hypocalcemia with intraperitoneal calcium. *Am J Health-Syst Pharm* 1995; **52:** 201–3.

Bites and stings. Calcium gluconate 10% solution has been administered intravenously as an alternative to the use of conventional muscle relaxants for the management of pain and muscle spasm associated with neurotoxic spider envenomation (p.1564). Mention has been made of such use of calcium in the management of *Latrodectus mactans* (black widow spider) envenomation.[1] Although the precise mechanism of action of calcium in the alleviation of neuromuscular symptoms is unknown it is believed to be due to the replenishment of calcium stores in the sarcoplasmic reticulum of muscle depleted by stimulation.

1. Binder LS. Acute arthropod envenomation: incidence, clinical features and management. *Med Toxicol Adverse Drug Exp* 1989; **4:** 163–73.

Bone disease. Calcium is essential for the development and maintenance of normal bone, and calcium salts may be indicated in the treatment of some bone disorders associated with calcium deficiency, such as certain types of osteomalacia and rickets (p.744). Doses of 1 to 3 g of calcium daily are used in osteomalacia.

Oral calcium supplements can also be used as an adjunct in the management of osteoporosis (p.745) and corticosteroid-induced osteoporosis (see Effects on Bones and Joints, under Corticosteroids, p.1040).

Cramps. Calcium salts are one of a number of interventions that have been tried in the management of cramps (see Muscle Spasm, p.1322). Although evidence for these interventions is mostly lacking, a small systematic review did conclude that oral calcium was possibly of benefit for leg cramps during pregnancy.[1]

1. Young GL, Jewell D. Interventions for leg cramps in pregnancy (updated 22 February 2000). Available in The Cochrane Library; Issue 4. Oxford: Update Software; 2001.

Diagnosis of insulinoma. Calcium stimulates the release of insulin from insulinomas. Consequently, intra-arterial calcium gluconate has been investigated in the diagnosis and localisation of insulinomas, but its value is uncertain.[1,2]

1. Doppman JL, *et al.* Localization of insulinomas to regions of the pancreas by intra-arterial stimulation with calcium. *Ann Intern Med* 1995; **123:** 269–73.
2. Abernethy LJ, *et al.* Intra-arterial calcium stimulation test in the investigation of hyperinsulinaemic hypoglycaemia. *Arch Dis Child* 1998; **78:** 359–63.

Fluoride toxicity. Inorganic fluoride is corrosive to skin and mucous membranes and acute intoxication disrupts many physiological systems; severe burns and profound hypocalcaemia may ensue. Absorption of the fluoride can be prevented by conversion to an insoluble form such as calcium fluoride and thus irrigation of skin (or gastric lavage as appropriate) with lime water, milk, or a 1% solution of calcium gluconate is recommended. Immediate treatment should also consist of 10 mL of calcium gluconate 10% intravenously repeated after one hour; 30 mL should be given if tetany is present. In the short term affected skin and tissue should be injected with a 10% solution of calcium gluconate at a dose of 0.5 mL per cm^2 and burnt skin treated with a calcium gluconate 2.5% gel.[1]

See also under Hydrofluoric Acid, p.1621.

1. McIvor ME. Acute fluoride toxicity: pathophysiology and management. *Drug Safety* 1990; **5:** 79–85.

Hypertension. Meta-analyses suggest that calcium supplementation results in a small reduction in systolic, but not diastolic, blood pressure.[1,2] The effect was too small to support the use of calcium supplementation for preventing or treating hypertension (p.802), but the authors of one analysis considered it possible that calcium supplementation might have beneficial effects on blood pressure in those with an inadequate intake.[2]

1. Allender PS, *et al.* Dietary calcium and blood pressure: a meta-analysis of randomized clinical trials. *Ann Intern Med* 1996; **124:** 825–31.
2. Bucher HC, *et al.* Effects of dietary calcium supplementation on blood pressure: a meta-analysis of randomized controlled trials. *JAMA* 1996; **275:** 1016–22.

PREGNANCY. Despite an earlier meta-analysis[1] which concluded that calcium supplementation during pregnancy reduced systolic and diastolic blood pressure and the incidence of pre-eclampsia and hypertension, results from a double-blind, placebo-controlled trial in a total of 4589 women indicated that calcium supplementation during normal pregnancy did not prevent pre-eclampsia, pregnancy-associated hypertension without pre-eclampsia, and a number of other related disorders.[2] The inclusion criteria for the meta-analysis have been criticised.[3] However, subsequent systematic reviews also concluded that calcium supplementation reduced hypertension and pre-eclampsia in pregnant women, although the benefit was most pronounced in women at high risk of hypertension or in communities with low dietary calcium intake.[4,5]

For discussions of hypertension in pregnancy and eclampsia and pre-eclampsia, see p.802 and p.341, respectively.

1. Bucher HC, *et al.* Effect of calcium supplementation on pregnancy-induced hypertension and preeclampsia: a meta-analysis of randomized controlled trials. *JAMA* 1996; **275:** 1113–17. Correction. *ibid.*; **276:** 1388.
2. Levine RJ, *et al.* Trial of calcium to prevent preeclampsia. *N Engl J Med* 1997; **337:** 69–76.
3. Various. Effects of calcium supplementation on pregnancy-induced hypertension. *JAMA* 1996; **276:** 1386–7.
4. DerSimonian R, Levine RJ. Resolving discrepancies between a meta-analysis and a subsequent large controlled trial. *JAMA* 1999; **282:** 664–70.
5. Atallah AN, *et al.* Calcium supplementation during pregnancy for preventing hypertensive disorders and related problems (updated 14 June 2001). Available in The Cochrane Library; Issue 4. Oxford: Update Software; 2001.

Malignant neoplasms. There is some evidence that calcium supplements may modestly reduce the risk of recurrent colorectal adenomas.[1,2]

1. Baron JA, *et al.* Calcium supplements for the prevention of colorectal adenomas. *N Engl J Med* 1999; **340:** 101–7.
2. Bonithon-Kopp C, *et al.* Calcium and fibre supplementation in prevention of colorectal adenoma recurrence: a randomised intervention trial. *Lancet* 2000; **356:** 1300–6.

Premenstrual syndrome. Calcium supplementation was effective in relieving the luteal phase symptoms of premenstrual syndrome (p.1475) in 1 study.[1] A review of this and other studies suggested that calcium supplementation at a dose of 1.2 to 1.6 g per day should be considered in patients with premenstrual syndrome.[2]

1. Thys-Jacobs S, *et al.* Calcium carbonate and the premenstrual syndrome: effects on premenstrual and menstrual symptoms. *Am J Obstet Gynecol* 1998; **179:** 444–52.
2. Ward MW, Holimon TD. Calcium treatment for premenstrual syndrome. *Ann Pharmacother* 1999; **33:** 1356–8.

Preparations

BP 2001: Calcium and Ergocalciferol Tablets; Calcium Chloride Injection; Calcium Gluconate Injection; Calcium Gluconate Tablets; Calcium Lactate Tablets; Effervescent Calcium Gluconate Tablets;
BPC 1973: Calcium with Vitamin D Tablets;
USP 25: Aluminum Sulfate and Calcium Acetate Tablets for Topical Solution; Calcium Acetate Tablets; Calcium Chloride Injection; Calcium Glubionate Syrup; Calcium Gluceptate Injection; Calcium Gluconate Injection; Calcium Gluconate Tablets; Calcium Lactate Tablets; Calcium Levulinate Injection; Calcium with Vitamin D Tablets; Dibasic Calcium Phosphate Tablets; Half-strength Lactated Ringer's and Dextrose Injection; Lactated Ringer's and Dextrose Injection; Lactated Ringer's Injection; Potassium Chloride in Lactated Ringer's and Dextrose Injection.

Proprietary Preparations (details are given in Part 3)
Aust.: Calcilin; Calcium Fresenius; Calcium Novartis; *Austral.:* Celloids CP 57; Nephrex; Sandocal; *Belg.:* Calcium-Sandoz; *Braz.:* Calcium-Sandoz; Calcium-Sandoz F; Solucalcine; *Canad.:* Cal Gel†; Calais; Calcimax†; Calcium-Rougier; Calcium-Sandoz; *Denm.:* Calcium-Sandoz; *Fin.:* Calcium-Sandoz; Phos-Ex; *Fr.:* Calcium Corbiere†; Calcium-Sandoz; Glucalcium; Ostram; Sandocal; *Ger.:* Calcipot†; Calcitrat; Calcium Freesenius; Calcium-Sandoz; Cerasorb; Eubiolac; RMS; *Hong Kong:* Calcium-Sandoz; Citracal; Gluco-Calcium; Mega-Cal; Nephrex; *Irl.:* Calcium-Sandoz; Sandocal; *Israel:* Calcium-Sandoz; *Ital.:* Calcetat; Calcium-Sandoz; Rubrocalcium†; *Mex.:* Calcium-Sandoz; Calcival; Ostram; Rical; *Neth.:* Calcium-Sandoz; Norw.: Calcium-Sandoz; Phos-Ex; *NZ:* Calcium-Sandoz; *Port.:* Calcigenol; Calcium-Sandoz; Sandocal; *S.Afr.:* Calcium-Sandoz; Kalci-300; *Singapore:* Calcium-Sandoz; Citracal; Hydrofluoric Acid Antidote; Os-Cal; *Spain:* Calbion†; Calcio 20 Emulsion; Calcium-Sandoz; Calcium-Sandoz Forte; Ibercal; Ostram; Royen; Tepox Cal; *Swed.:* Calcium-Sandoz; Ostram; Phos-Ex; *Switz.:* Calcium-Sandoz; *Thai.:* Calcibon; Calcium Unison; Calcium-Sandoz; Calsorp; Caltrate; Lo-P-Caps; *UK:* Calcium-Sandoz; Ostram; Phos-Ex; Sandocal; *USA:* Cal-Citrate; Cal-Lac; Calphron; Citracal; Neo-Calglucon†; PhosLo; Posture; Prelief†.

Multi-ingredient: numerous preparations are listed in Part 3.

Used as an adjunct in: *Swed.:* Deltison.

Magnesium (1170-k)

Mg = 24.305.

Magnesium is a cation administered as various magnesium-containing salts. Magnesium salts have been reported to be **incompatible** with a wide range of drugs.

Magnesium Acetate (1171-a)

$C_4H_6MgO_4,4H_2O = 214.5$.
CAS — 142-72-3 (anhydrous magnesium acetate); 16674-78-5 (magnesium acetate tetrahydrate).
Pharmacopoeias. In Br.

Each g of magnesium acetate (tetrahydrate) represents approximately 4.7 mmol of magnesium and the equivalent of bicarbonate. Magnesium acetate (tetrahydrate) 8.83 g is approximately equivalent to 1 g of magnesium.

Pharmacopoeial description

BP 2001: Odourless or almost odourless colourless crystals or a white crystalline powder. Freely soluble in water and in alcohol. A 5% solution in water has a pH of 7.5 to 8.5.

Magnesium Ascorbate (12907-x)

$(C_6H_7O_6)_2Mg = 374.5$.
CAS — 15431-40-0.

Each g of magnesium ascorbate (anhydrous) represents approximately 2.7 mmol of magnesium. Magnesium ascorbate (anhydrous) 15.4 g is approximately equivalent to 1 g of magnesium.

Magnesium Aspartate (600-z)

Magnesium aminosuccinate tetrahydrate.
$C_8H_{12}MgN_2O_8,4H_2O = 360.6$.
CAS — 7018-07-7.
ATC — A12CC05.
Pharmacopoeias. In Ger. Eur. (see p.vi) includes the dihydrate form of the (S)-aspartate.

Each g of magnesium aspartate (tetrahydrate) represents approximately 2.8 mmol of magnesium. Magnesium aspartate (tetrahydrate) 14.8 g is approximately equivalent to 1 g of magnesium.

Pharmacopoeial description

Ph. Eur.: The dihydrate is a white, crystalline powder or colourless crystals. Freely soluble in water. A 2.5% solution in water has a pH of 6.0 to 8.0.

Magnesium Chloride (1172-t)

Chlorure de Magnésium Cristallisé; Cloreto de Magnésio; E511; Magnesii Chloridum Hexahydricum; Magnesium Chloratum; Magnesium Chloride Hexahydrate.
$MgCl_2,6H_2O = 203.3$.
CAS — 7786-30-3 (anhydrous magnesium chloride); 7791-18-6 (magnesium chloride hexahydrate).
ATC — A12CC01; B05XA11.
Pharmacopoeias. In Eur. (see p.vi), which also includes Magnesium Chloride 4.5-Hydrate, Pol., and US.

Each g of magnesium chloride (hexahydrate) represents approximately 4.9 mmol of magnesium and 9.8 mmol of chloride. Magnesium chloride (hexahydrate) 8.36 g is approximately equivalent to 1 g of magnesium.

Pharmacopoeial description

Ph. Eur.: The 4.5-hydrate is a white or almost white, hygroscopic, granular powder. Very soluble in water; freely soluble in alcohol. Store in airtight containers.

The hexahydrate is described as colourless, hygroscopic crystals. Very soluble in water; freely soluble in alcohol. Store in airtight containers.

USP 25: Colourless, odourless, deliquescent flakes or crystals, which lose water when heated to 100° and lose hydrochloric acid when heated to 110°. Very soluble in water; freely soluble in alcohol. pH of a 5% solution in water is between 4.5 and 7.0. Store in airtight containers.

Magnesium Gluceptate (12909-f)

Magnesium Glucoheptonate.
$C_{14}H_{26}MgO_{16} = 474.7$.

Each g of magnesium gluceptate (anhydrous) represents approximately 2.1 mmol of magnesium. Magnesium gluceptate (anhydrous) 19.5 g is approximately equivalent to 1 g of magnesium.

Magnesium Gluconate (1203-w)

Magnesium D-gluconate hydrate.
$C_{12}H_{22}MgO_{14} (+xH_2O) = 414.6$ (anhydrous).
CAS — 3632-91-5 (anhydrous magnesium gluconate); 59625-89-7 (magnesium gluconate dihydrate).
ATC — A12CC03.
Pharmacopoeias. In US which allows either anhydrous or the dihydrate.

Each g of magnesium gluconate (anhydrous) represents approximately 2.4 mmol of magnesium. Magnesium gluconate (anhydrous) 17.1 g is approximately equivalent to 1 g of magnesium.

Pharmacopoeial description

USP 25: Colourless crystals or a white powder or granules. Is odourless. Freely soluble in water; very slightly soluble in alcohol; insoluble in ether. pH of a 5% solution in water is between 6.0 and 7.8.

Magnesium Glycerophosphate (1938-m)

Magnesii Glycerophosphas; Magnesium Glycerinophosphate.

$C_3H_7MgO_6P(+xH_2O) = 194.4$ (anhydrous).

CAS — 927-20-8 (anhydrous magnesium glycerophosphate).

Pharmacopoeias. In Eur. (see p.vi).

Each g of magnesium glycerophosphate (anhydrous) represents approximately 5.1 mmol of magnesium. Magnesium glycerophosphate (anhydrous) 8 g is approximately equivalent to 1 g of magnesium.

Pharmacopoeial description

Ph. Eur.: A mixture, in variable proportions, of magnesium (R,S)-2,3-dihydroxypropyl phosphate and magnesium 2-hydroxy-1-(hydroxymethyl)ethyl phosphate. It may be hydrated. A white, hygroscopic powder. Practically insoluble in alcohol; dissolves in dilute solutions of acids. Store in airtight containers.

Magnesium Lactate (12911-c)

Magnesium 2-hydroxypropionate.

$C_6H_{10}MgO_6 = 202.4$.

CAS — 18917-93-6.

ATC — A12CC06.

Each g of magnesium lactate (anhydrous) represents approximately 4.9 mmol of magnesium. Magnesium lactate (anhydrous) 8.33 g is approximately equivalent to 1 g of magnesium.

Magnesium Phosphate (703-f)

Tribasic Magnesium Phosphate; Trimagnesium Phosphate.

$Mg_3(PO_4)_2,5H_2O = 352.9$.

CAS — 7757-87-1 (anhydrous magnesium phosphate); 10233-87-1 (magnesium phosphate pentahydrate).

ATC — B05XA10.

Pharmacopoeias. In US.

Ger. includes Dibasic Magnesium Phosphate Trihydrate (Magnesium Hydrogen Phosphate Trihydrate).

Each g of magnesium phosphate (pentahydrate) represents approximately 8.5 mmol of magnesium and 5.7 mmol of phosphate. Magnesium phosphate (pentahydrate) 4.84 g is approximately equivalent to 1 g of magnesium.

Pharmacopoeial description

USP 25: A white, odourless, powder. Almost insoluble in water; readily soluble in dilute mineral acids.

Magnesium Pidolate (12912-k)

Magnesium Pidolate (pINNM).

Magnesii Pidolas; Magnesium Pyroglutamate. Magnesium 5-oxopyrrolidine-2-carboxylate.

$(C_5H_6NO_3)_2Mg = 280.5$.

CAS — 62003-27-4.

ATC — A12CC08.

Pharmacopoeias. In Eur. (see p.vi).

Each g of magnesium pidolate (anhydrous) represents approximately 3.6 mmol of magnesium. Magnesium pidolate (anhydrous) 11.5 g is approximately equivalent to 1 g of magnesium.

Pharmacopoeial description

Ph. Eur.: An amorphous, white or almost white, hygroscopic powder. Very soluble in water; practically insoluble in dichloromethane; soluble in methyl alcohol. A 10% solution in water has a pH of 5.5 to 7.0. Store in airtight containers.

Magnesium Sulfate (1174-r)

518; Epsom Salts; Magnesii Sulfas; Magnesium Sulfuricum Heptahydricum; Magnesium Sulphate; Sal Amarum; Sel Anglais; Sel de Sedlitz.

$MgSO_4,7H_2O = 246.5$.

CAS — 7487-88-9 (anhydrous magnesium sulfate); 10034-99-8 (magnesium sulfate heptahydrate).

ATC — A06AD04; A12CC02; B05XA05; D11AX05; V04CC02.

Pharmacopoeias. In Chin., Eur. (see p.vi), Jpn, Pol., and US.

US allows the dried form, the monohydrate, or the heptahydrate form.

Dried Magnesium Sulphate (Dried Epsom Salts) is included in *Aust., Br.,* and *Pol.*

Each g of magnesium sulfate (heptahydrate) represents approximately 4.1 mmol of magnesium. Magnesium sulfate (heptahydrate) 10.1 g is approximately equivalent to 1 g of magnesium.

The symbol † denotes a preparation no longer actively marketed

Pharmacopoeial description

Ph. Eur.: A white, crystalline powder or brilliant, colourless crystals. Freely soluble in water; very soluble in boiling water; practically insoluble in alcohol.

NOTE. The BP 2001 specifies that when magnesium sulfate is prescribed or demanded, Magnesium Sulphate Heptahydrate shall be dispensed or supplied.

BP 2001: Dried magnesium sulfate is a white odourless or almost odourless powder, prepared by drying magnesium sulfate (heptahydrate) at 100° until it has lost about 25% of its weight; it contains 62 to 70% of $MgSO_4$. Freely soluble in water; more rapidly soluble in hot water.

USP 25: It is the dried form, monohydrate, or the heptahydrate. Small, colourless crystals, usually needle-like. It effloresces in warm dry air. Soluble 1 in 0.8 of water and 1 in 0.5 of boiling water; freely but slowly soluble 1 in 1 of glycerol; sparingly soluble in alcohol. pH of a 5% solution in water is between 5.0 and 9.2.

Adverse Effects

Excessive parenteral administration of magnesium salts leads to the development of hypermagnesaemia, important signs of which are loss of deep tendon reflexes and respiratory depression, both due to neuromuscular blockade. Other symptoms of hypermagnesaemia may include nausea, vomiting, flushing of the skin, thirst, hypotension due to peripheral vasodilatation, drowsiness, confusion, slurred speech, double vision, muscle weakness, bradycardia, coma, and cardiac arrest.

Hypermagnesaemia is uncommon after oral administration of magnesium salts except in the presence of renal impairment. Ingestion of magnesium salts may cause gastrointestinal irritation and watery diarrhoea.

Effects on the gastrointestinal tract. Although oral magnesium salts stimulate peristalsis, paralytic ileus has occurred in a woman receiving an intravenous infusion of magnesium sulfate for premature labour; magnesium concentrations were within the normal range.[1] See also Pregnancy, under Precautions, below.

1. Hill WC, *et al.* Maternal paralytic ileus as a complication of magnesium sulfate tocolysis. *Am J Perinatol* 1985; **2:** 47–8.

Hypersensitivity. Hypersensitivity reactions characterised by urticaria were described in 2 women after receiving magnesium sulfate intravenously.[1]

1. Thorp JM, *et al.* Hypersensitivity to magnesium sulfate. *Am J Obstet Gynecol* 1989; **161:** 889–90.

Treatment of Adverse Effects

The management of hypermagnesaemia is reviewed on p.1181.

◊ A patient with hypermagnesaemia of a degree that is normally fatal was successfully treated using assisted ventilation, calcium chloride administered intravenously, and forced diuresis with mannitol infusions.[1]

1. Bohman VR, Cotton DB. Supralethal magnesemia with patient survival. *Obstet Gynecol* 1990; **76:** 984–6.

Precautions

Parenteral magnesium salts should generally be avoided in patients with heart block or severe renal impairment. They should be used with caution in less severe degrees of renal impairment and in patients with myasthenia gravis. Patients should be monitored for clinical signs of excess magnesium (see Adverse Effects, above), particularly when being treated for conditions not associated with hypomagnesaemia such as eclampsia. An intravenous preparation of a calcium salt should be available in case of toxicity. When used for hypomagnesaemia, serum-magnesium concentrations should be monitored.

Magnesium crosses the placenta. When used in pregnant women, fetal heart rate should be monitored and administration within 2 hours of delivery should be avoided.

Oral magnesium salts should be used cautiously in patients with impaired renal function. Administration with food may decrease the incidence of diarrhoea. Chronic diarrhoea due to long-term administration may result in electrolyte imbalance.

Hepatic disorders. Severe hypermagnesaemia and hypercalcaemia developed in 2 patients with hepatic encephalopathy following the administration of magnesium sulfate enemas; both patients died, one during and one after asystole. It was recommended that patients with liver disease who might develop renal impairment, or in whom renal failure is established, should not be prescribed enemas containing magnesium for

treatment of hepatic encephalopathy as serious magnesium toxicity can occur, which may contribute to death.[1]

1. Collinson PO, Burroughs AK. Severe hypermagnesaemia due to magnesium sulphate enemas in patients with hepatic coma. *BMJ* 1986; **293:** 1013–14.

Pregnancy. The meconium-plug syndrome (abdominal distention and failure to pass meconium) has been described in 2 neonates who were hypermagnesaemic after their mothers had received magnesium sulfate for eclampsia.[1] It was believed that the hypermagnesaemia may have depressed the function of intestinal smooth muscle. See also Effects on the Gastrointestinal Tract, above.

In a study in 12 women with pre-eclampsia there was a decrease in short-term fetal heart rate variability when women were administered intravenous magnesium sulfate; however, although variability is considered a sign of fetal well-being the decrease was considered clinically insignificant.[2]

1. Sokal MM, *et al.* Neonatal hypermagnesemia and the meconium-plug syndrome. *N Engl J Med* 1972; **286:** 823–5.
2. Atkinson MW, *et al.* The relation between magnesium sulfate therapy and fetal heart rate variability. *Obstet Gynecol* 1994; **83:** 967–70.

Interactions

Parenteral administration of magnesium sulfate potentiates the effects of competitive and depolarising neuromuscular blockers (p.1335). The neuromuscular blocking effects of parenteral magnesium and aminoglycoside antibacterials may be additive. Similarly, parenteral magnesium sulfate and nifedipine have been reported to have additive effects (p.943).

Oral magnesium salts decrease the absorption of tetracyclines and bisphosphonates, and administration should be separated by a number of hours.

Pharmacokinetics

Approximately one third to one half of magnesium is absorbed from the small intestine following oral administration and even soluble magnesium salts are generally very slowly absorbed. The fraction of magnesium absorbed increases if magnesium intake decreases. In plasma, about 25 to 30% of magnesium is protein bound. Parenterally administered magnesium salts are excreted mainly in the urine, and orally administered magnesium salts are eliminated in the urine (absorbed fraction) and the faeces (unabsorbed fraction). Small amounts are distributed into breast milk. Magnesium crosses the placenta.

Human Requirements

Magnesium is the second most abundant cation in intracellular fluid and is an essential body electrolyte which is a cofactor in numerous enzyme systems.

The body is very efficient at maintaining magnesium concentrations by regulating absorption and renal excretion, and symptoms of deficiency are rare. It is therefore difficult to establish a daily requirement.

Foods rich in magnesium include nuts, unmilled grains, and green vegetables.

◊ In the United Kingdom dietary reference values (DRV—see p.1352)[1] and in the United States recommended daily allowances (RDA)[2] have been published for magnesium. In the UK the estimated average requirement (EAR) is 200 mg (or 8.2 mmol) daily for adult females and 250 mg (or 10.3 mmol) daily for adult males; the reference nutrient intake (RNI) is 270 mg (or 10.9 mmol) daily for adult females and 300 mg (or 12.3 mmol) daily for adult males; no increment is recommended during pregnancy but an increment of 50 mg (or 2.1 mmol) daily in the RNI is advised during lactation. In the USA under the new dietary reference intakes an EAR of 330 to 350 mg daily has been set in adult males and 255 to 265 mg daily in adult females; the corresponding RDAs are 400 to 420 mg and 310 to 320 mg daily.[2] An increase in RDA to 350 to 360 mg is recommended during pregnancy but the standard RDA is considered adequate during lactation. In the USA a tolerable upper intake level of 350 mg daily has been set for adults.[2]

1. DoH. Dietary reference values for food energy and nutrients for the United Kingdom: report of the panel on dietary reference values of the committee on medical aspects of food policy. *Report on health and social subjects 41.* London: HMSO, 1991.
2. Standing Committee on the Scientific Evaluation of Dietary Reference Intakes of the Food and Nutrition Board. *Dietary Reference Intakes for calcium, phosphorus, magnesium, vitamin D, and fluoride.* Washington, DC: National Academy Press, 1999.

Uses and Administration

Magnesium salts have a variety of actions and uses. Many are given as a source of magnesium ions in the treatment of **magnesium deficiency and hypomagnesaemia** (p.1182). Doses may be expressed in terms of mmol or mEq of magnesium, mass (mg) of magnesium, or mass of magnesium salt (for comparative purposes, see Table 2, below).

In simple deficiency states magnesium salts may be given by mouth in doses of up to 50 mmol of magnesium daily adjusted according to individual requirements. Salts that are, or have been, employed include magnesium aspartate, magnesium chloride, magnesium gluceptate, magnesium gluconate, magnesium glycerophosphate, magnesium lactate, magnesium levulinate, magnesium orotate, and magnesium pidolate. In acute or severe hypomagnesaemia, magnesium may be given parenterally, usually as the chloride or sulfate. A suggested regimen is to administer 35 to 75 mmol of magnesium by slow intravenous infusion (in glucose 5%) on the first day followed by 25 mmol daily until the hypomagnesaemia is corrected; up to a total of 160 mmol may be required. Alternatively, magnesium sulfate has been given by intramuscular or slow intravenous injection. Careful monitoring of plasma-magnesium and other electrolyte concentrations is essential. Doses should be reduced in renal impairment. Other salts which are, or have been, used parenterally include magnesium acetate, magnesium ascorbate, magnesium aspartate hydrochloride, magnesium levulinate, and magnesium pidolate.

Several magnesium salts such as the carbonate, hydroxide, oxide, and trisilicate are widely used for their **antacid** properties (p.1201). Magnesium salts also act as **osmotic laxatives** (see Constipation, p.1202); the salts generally used for this purpose are magnesium sulfate (an oral dose of 5 to 10 g in 250 mL of water being administered for rapid bowel evacuation) and magnesium hydroxide (p.1233).

Parenterally administered magnesium sulfate has some specific uses. It is used for the emergency treatment of some **arrhythmias** such as torsade de pointes (p.794) and those associated with hypokalaemia (p.1182). The usual dose is 2 g of magnesium sulfate (8 mmol of magnesium) administered intravenously over 10 to 15 minutes and repeated once if necessary.

Parenteral magnesium sulfate is also used for the prevention of recurrent seizures in pregnant women with **eclampsia** (see below). A variety of dosage regimens have been used and debate continues as to which is most appropriate. Typically an intravenous loading dose of 4 g of magnesium sulfate (16 mmol of magnesium) is administered over 5 to 10 minutes. This is then followed by either an infusion of 1 g (4 mmol magnesium) per hour or deep intramuscular administration of 5 g (20 mmol magnesium) into each buttock then 5 g intramuscularly every 4 hours for at least 24 hours after the last seizure. Should seizures recur under either regimen, then an additional intravenous dose of 2 to 4 g can be administered. It is essential to monitor for signs of hypermagnesaemia, and to stop magnesium administration should this occur. Doses should be reduced in renal impairment.

Table 2. Some magnesium salts and their magnesium content.

Magnesium salt	Magnesium content per g		
	mg	mmol	mEq
Magnesium acetate (tetrahydrate)	113	4.7	9.3
Magnesium ascorbate (anhydrous)	65	2.7	5.3
Magnesium aspartate (tetrahydrate)	67	2.8	5.5
Magnesium chloride (hexahydrate)	120	4.9	9.8
Magnesium gluceptate (anhydrous)	51	2.1	4.2
Magnesium gluconate (anhydrous)	59	2.4	4.8
Magnesium glycerophosphate (anhydrous)	125	5.1	10.3
Magnesium lactate (anhydrous)	120	4.9	9.9
Magnesium phosphate (pentahydrate)	207	8.5	17.0
Magnesium pidolate (anhydrous)	87	3.6	7.1
Magnesium sulfate (heptahydrate)	99	4.1	8.1

The use of magnesium sulfate in **acute myocardial infarction** and **premature labour** is discussed below.

Dried magnesium sulfate has been used in the form of Magnesium Sulphate Paste (BP 2001) as an application to inflammatory skin conditions such as boils and carbuncles, but prolonged or repeated use may damage the surrounding skin.

◊ General references.
1. McLean RM. Magnesium and its therapeutic uses: a review. *Am J Med* 1994; **96:** 63–76.
2. Fawcett WJ, *et al.* Magnesium: physiology and pharmacology. *Br J Anaesth* 1999; **83:** 302–20.

Anaesthesia. Magnesium sulfate has been used to prevent the undesirable haemodynamic response sometimes associated with intubation (p.1331).

Eclampsia and pre-eclampsia. For many years magnesium sulfate has been the preferred treatment in the USA for seizures associated with **eclampsia** (p.341) and studies and systematic reviews have shown it to be more effective than phenytoin,[1-4] diazepam,[2,5] or lytic cocktail,[6] as well as causing fewer adverse effects.

A commentary[7] on 2 of these studies thought that magnesium sulfate offered considerable advantages. It produced a rapid effect and did not cause sedation in the mother or the infant. It was also considered to have a wide safety margin with the added security of calcium gluconate being an easily available antidote should overdose occur. Subsequent meta-analysis[8] and systematic review[4-6] has reinforced this favourable view. Thus many in the UK now consider magnesium sulfate to be the preferred drug for the treatment of eclampsia.

Magnesium sulfate may also be used for prophylaxis in **pre-eclampsia,** but some uncertainty remains about the degree of benefit; nonetheless, it appears to be more effective than phenytoin.[8,9] (For a recent study that raised some concerns about the effects of *early* use of magnesium sulfate on the fetus, see Premature Labour, below.)

1. Dommisse J. Phenytoin sodium and magnesium sulphate in the management of eclampsia. *Br J Obstet Gynaecol* 1990; **97:** 104–9.
2. The Eclampsia Trial Collaborative Group. Which anticonvulsant for women with eclampsia: evidence from the Collaborative Eclampsia Trial. *Lancet* 1995; **345:** 1455–63. Correction. *ibid.*; **346:** 258.
3. Lucas MJ, *et al.* A comparison of magnesium sulfate with phenytoin for the prevention of eclampsia. *N Engl J Med* 1995; **333:** 201–5.
4. Duley L, Henderson-Smart D. Magnesium sulphate versus phenytoin for eclampsia (updated 4 July 2000). Available in The Cochrane Library; Issue 4. Oxford: Update Software; 2001.
5. Duley L, Henderson-Smart D. Magnesium sulphate versus diazepam for eclampsia (updated 5 November 1999). Available in The Cochrane Library; Issue 4. Oxford: Update Software; 2001.
6. Duley L, Gulmezoglu AM. Magnesium sulphate versus lytic cocktail for eclampsia (updated 27 November 2000). Available in The Cochrane Library; Issue 4. Oxford: Update Software; 2001.
7. Saunders N, Hammersley B. Magnesium for eclampsia. *Lancet* 1995; **346:** 788–9.
8. Chien PFW, *et al.* Magnesium sulphate in the treatment of eclampsia and pre-eclampsia: an overview of the evidence from randomised trials. *Br J Obstet Gynaecol* 1996; **103:** 1085–91.
9. Duley L, *et al.* Anticonvulsants for women with pre-eclampsia (updated 28 October 1999). Available in The Cochrane Library; Issue 4. Oxford: Update Software; 2001.

Hypokalaemia. Potassium and magnesium homoeostasis are linked, and hypokalaemia with increased urine potassium excretion may occur in patients with hypomagnesaemia. In this situation, correction of potassium deficit usually requires concomitant magnesium administration. Administration of magnesium sulfate at doses greater than those required to correct hypomagnesaemia has been associated with greater improvements in potassium balance than doses just sufficient to correct hypomagnesaemia.[1]

1. Hamill-Ruth RJ, McGory R. Magnesium repletion and its effect on potassium homeostasis in critically ill adults: results of a double-blind, randomized, controlled trial. *Crit Care Med* 1996; **24:** 38–45.

Migraine. Low magnesium concentrations are thought to be important in the pathogenesis of migraine (p.449), but the precise role of magnesium supplementation in the disorder remains to be determined.[1] In 1 double-blind study,[2] 24 mmol magnesium daily (in the form of magnesium citrate) reduced the incidence of migraine headache by 42% compared with a reduction of 16% with placebo. However, in a similar study,[3] 20 mmol magnesium daily (in the form of magnesium aspartate hydrochloride) was no more effective than placebo in producing a 50% reduction in migraine frequency or intensity. Intravenous magnesium sulfate has been tried for the treatment of migraine attack.[1]

1. Mauskop A, Altura BM. Role of magnesium in the pathogenesis and treatment of migraines. *Clin Neurosci* 1998; **5:** 24–7.
2. Peikert A, *et al.* Prophylaxis of migraine with oral magnesium: results from a prospective, multi-center, placebo-controlled and double-blind randomized study. *Cephalalgia* 1996; **16:** 257–63.
3. Pfaffenrath V, *et al.* Magnesium in the prophylaxis of migraine: a double-blind placebo-controlled study. *Cephalalgia* 1996; **16:** 436–40.

Myocardial infarction. Magnesium has an important physiological role in maintaining the ion balance in muscle including the myocardium. Administration of magnesium might have an antiarrhythmic effect and might protect the myocardium against reperfusion injury including myocardial stunning (delayed recovery of myocardial contractility function). Intravenous magnesium salts have been used for cardiac arrhythmias and in an overview of studies in patients with suspected myocardial infarction their administration, generally within 12 hours of the onset of chest pain, had reduced mortality.[1] The beneficial effect on mortality appeared to be confirmed by the LIMIT-2 study[2] in which 8 mmol of magnesium was given by intravenous injection before thrombolysis and followed by a maintenance infusion of 65 mmol over the following 24 hours. Benefit was confirmed at follow-up an average of 2.7 years later;[3] however, there was no evidence of an antiarrhythmic effect. These beneficial effects were not borne out by the larger ISIS-4 study,[4] and although there were slight differences in the magnesium regimen and its timing which might have played a part in these contradictory results, at present the routine use of magnesium in myocardial infarction (p.805) cannot be recommended.

Patients with acute myocardial infarction may have magnesium deficiency and long-term treatment with oral magnesium has been tried, but in one study was associated with an increased risk of adverse cardiac events and could not be recommended for secondary prevention.[5]

1. Teo KK, *et al.* Effects of intravenous magnesium in suspected acute myocardial infarction: overview of randomised trials. *BMJ* 1991; **303:** 1499–1503.
2. Woods KL, *et al.* Intravenous magnesium sulphate in suspected acute myocardial infarction: results of the second Leicester Intravenous Magnesium Intervention Trial (LIMIT-2). *Lancet* 1992; **339:** 1553–8.
3. Woods KL, Fletcher S. Long-term outcome after intravenous magnesium sulphate in suspected acute myocardial infarction: the second Leicester Intravenous Magnesium Intervention Trial (LIMIT-2). *Lancet* 1994; **343:** 816–19.
4. Fourth International Study of Infarct Survival Collaborative Group. ISIS–4: a randomised factorial trial assessing early oral captopril, oral mononitrate, and intravenous magnesium sulphate in 58 050 patients with suspected acute myocardial infarction. *Lancet* 1995; **345:** 669–85.
5. Galløe AM, *et al.* Influence of oral magnesium supplementation on cardiac events among survivors of an acute myocardial infarction. *BMJ* 1993; **307:** 585–7.

Porphyria. Magnesium sulfate is one of the drugs that has been used for seizure prophylaxis in patients with porphyria (p.342) who continue to experience convulsions while in remission.

Premature labour. Magnesium sulfate has been given intravenously to suppress initial uterine contractions in the management of premature labour[1-6] and has been found to possess similar efficacy to beta$_2$ agonists (see Salbutamol, p.773). Other magnesium salts have also sometimes been given by mouth. Retrospective observational studies have also found a lower incidence of cerebral palsy in children with birth-weights of less than 1500 g when mothers were treated with magnesium sulfate for pre-eclampsia, eclampsia or premature labour.[7,8] However, increased total paediatric mortality was noted in an interim analysis of a trial of antenatal magnesium sulfate in preterm labour,[9] and the trial was subsequently discontinued. Although they considered the safety of magnesium sulfate well established in gestation at term, the authors cautioned against the use of magnesium sulfate in very preterm labour. A subsequent retrospective study by the same group found that magnesium sulfate was associated with perinatal mortality in low birth-weight offspring, particularly when doses of more than 48 g were used.[10] The authors of these studies have commented[11] on other results which supported the hypothesis that magnesium exposure increased the risk of infant death.

1. Martin RW, *et al.* Comparison of oral ritodrine and magnesium gluconate for ambulatory tocolysis. *Am J Obstet Gynecol* 1988; **158:** 1440–3.
2. Weiner CP, *et al.* The therapeutic efficacy and cost-effectiveness of aggressive tocolysis for premature labor associated with premature rupture of the membranes. *Am J Obstet Gynecol* 1988; **159:** 216–22.
3. Wilkins IA, *et al.* Efficacy and side effects of magnesium sulfate and ritodrine as tocolytic agents. *Am J Obstet Gynecol* 1988; **159:** 685–9.
4. Ridgway LE, *et al.* A prospective randomized comparison of oral terbutaline and magnesium oxide for the maintenance of tocolysis. *Am J Obstet Gynecol* 1990; **163:** 879–82.
5. Dudley D, *et al.* Long-term tocolysis with intravenous magnesium sulfate. *Obstet Gynecol* 1989; **73:** 373–8.
6. Amon E, *et al.* Tocolysis with advanced cervical dilatation. *Obstet Gynecol* 2000; **95:** 358–62.
7. Nelson KB, Grether JK. Can magnesium sulfate reduce the risk of cerebral palsy in very low birthweight infants? *Pediatrics* 1995; **95:** 263–9.
8. Schendel DE, *et al.* Prenatal magnesium sulfate exposure and the risk for cerebral palsy or mental retardation among very low-birth-weight children aged 3 to 5 years. *JAMA* 1996; **276:** 1805–10.
9. Mittendorf R, *et al.* Is tocolytic magnesium sulphate associated with increased total paediatric mortality? *Lancet* 1997; **350:** 1517–18.
10. Scudiero R, *et al.* Perinatal death and tocolytic magnesium sulfate. *Obstet Gynecol* 2000; **96:** 178–82.
11. Mittendorf R, *et al.* If tocolytic magnesium sulfate is associated with excess total pediatric mortality, what is its impact? *Obstet Gynecol* 1998; **92:** 308–11.

Pulmonary hypertension of the newborn. Preliminary studies have suggested that intravenous magnesium sulfate may be effective in treating persistent pulmonary hypertension of the newborn, as mentioned on p.810.

Respiratory disorders. Magnesium sulfate, administered intravenously over 20 minutes in doses of 1.2 g to patients with acute exacerbations of chronic obstructive pulmonary disease (p.759) who had received inhaled salbutamol, appeared to have moderate efficacy.[1]

Infusion of magnesium has been reported to be of benefit in some patients with acute asthma (p.757), but results have been conflicting;[2-4] a meta-analysis of these and other studies concluded that its routine use was not justified, but that it may benefit some patients with severe exacerbations.[5] Inhalation of magnesium has also been tried.[6]

1. Skorodin MS, et al. Magnesium sulfate in exacerbations of chronic obstructive pulmonary disease. Arch Intern Med 1995; **155:** 496–500.
2. Skobeloff EM, et al. Intravenous magnesium sulfate for the treatment of acute asthma in the emergency department. JAMA 1989; **262:** 1210–13.
3. Green SM, Rothrack SG. Intravenous magnesium for acute asthma: failure to decrease emergency treatment duration or need for hospitalization. Ann Emerg Med 1992; **21:** 260–5.
4. Ciarallo L, et al. Intravenous magnesium therapy for moderate to severe pediatric asthma: results of a randomized, placebo-controlled trial. J Pediatr 1996; **129:** 809–14.
5. Rowe BH, et al. Magnesium sulfate for treating exacerbations of acute asthma in the emergency department (updated 30 July 2001). Available in The Cochrane Library; Issue 4. Oxford: Update Software; 2001.
6. Mangat HS, et al. Nebulized magnesium sulphate versus nebulized salbutamol in acute bronchial asthma: a clinical trial. Eur Respir J 1998; **12:** 341–4.

Preparations

BP 2001: Magnesium Chloride Injection; Magnesium Sulphate Injection; Magnesium Sulphate Mixture; Magnesium Sulphate Paste;
USP 25: Magnesium Gluconate Tablets; Magnesium Sulfate in Dextrose Injection; Magnesium Sulfate Injection.

Proprietary Preparations (details are given in Part 3)
Aust.: Cormagnesin; Emgecard; FX Passage; Magnesium Diasporal; Magvital; Mg 5-Longoral; Solumag; Ultra-Mag; **Austral.:** Celloids MP 65; Magmin; **Belg.:** Magnespasmyl; Ultra-Mag; **Braz.:** Pidomag; **Canad.:** Mag 2†; Maglucate; Magnolex; Magnorol; Slow-Mag; **Fr.:** Efimag; Ionimag; Mag 2; Magnespasmyl; Magnogene; Megamag; Solumag; Spasmag; Top-Mag; **Ger.:** Basti-Mag; Cormagnesin; FX Passage; Magium; Magnaspart; Magnerot A†; magnerot Classic; Magnesiocard; Magnesium Diasporal; Magnesium Tonil; Magnesorot; Magnorbin†; Magtrom†; metamagnesol; Mg 5-Granulat; Mg 5-Longoral; Mg 5-Sulfat; Mgnor†; Nourymag; Power Orot; **Ital.:** Actimag; Mag 2; Solumag; **Mex.:** Magnefusin; **Mon.:** Oromag; **Port.:** Magnesiocard; Magnesona; Magnespasmil; Magnoral; **S.Afr.:** Magnesit; Slow-Mag; **Spain:** Actimag; Mag 2†; Magnesioboi; Sulmetin; **Switz.:** Mag 2; Mag-Min; Magnesiocard; Magnesium Biomed; Magnesium Vital; Magnespasmyl; Magnogene; Magvital†; Mg 5-Granoral; Mg 5-Longoral; Mg 5-Oraleff; Mg 5-Sulfat; Solmag; **USA:** Almora; Mag-G; Mag-SR; Mag-Tab SR; Magonate; Magtrate; Slow-Mag.

Multi-ingredient: numerous preparations are listed in Part 3.

Phosphate   (2898-t)

Phosphate is an anion administered as various potassium or sodium salts. Phosphates are **incompatible** with calcium salts; the mixing of calcium and phosphate salts can lead to the formation of insoluble calcium-phosphate precipitates. Incompatibility has also been reported with magnesium salts.

Monobasic Potassium Phosphate   (1183-f)

E340; Kalii Dihydrogenophosphas; Monopotassium Phosphate; Potassium Acid Phosphate; Potassium Biphosphate; Potassium Dihydrogen Phosphate. Potassium dihydrogen orthophosphate.
$KH_2PO_4 = 136.1$.
CAS — 7778-77-0.

Pharmacopoeias. In Eur. (see p.vi). Also in USNF.

Each g of monobasic potassium phosphate represents approximately 7.3 mmol of potassium and of phosphate.

Pharmacopoeial description
Ph. Eur.: A white, crystalline powder or colourless crystals. Freely soluble in water; practically insoluble in alcohol. A 5% solution in water has a pH of 4.2 to 4.5.
USNF 20: Colourless crystals or a white granular or crystalline powder. Is odourless. Freely soluble in water; practically insoluble in alcohol. pH of a 1% solution in water is about 4.5. Store in airtight containers.

Dibasic Potassium Phosphate   (1184-d)

Dikalii Phosphas; Dipotassium Hydrogen Phosphate; Dipotassium Phosphate; E340; Potassium Phosphate. Dipotassium hydrogen orthophosphate.
$K_2HPO_4 = 174.2$.
CAS — 7758-11-4.

Pharmacopoeias. In Eur. (see p.vi) and US.

Each g of dibasic potassium phosphate represents approximately 11.5 mmol of potassium and 5.7 mmol of phosphate.

The symbol † denotes a preparation no longer actively marketed

Pharmacopoeial description
Ph. Eur.: A very hygroscopic, white powder or colourless crystals. Very soluble in water; very slightly soluble in alcohol. Store in airtight containers.
USP 25: Colourless or white, somewhat hygroscopic, granular powder. Freely soluble in water; very slightly soluble in alcohol. pH of a 5% solution in water is between 8.5 and 9.6.

Monobasic Sodium Phosphate   (1195-m)

E339; Natrii Dihydrogenophosphas; Natrium Phosphoricum Monobasicum; Sodium Acid Phosphate; Sodium Biphosphate; Sodium Dihydrogen Phosphate. Sodium dihydrogen orthophosphate.
NaH_2PO_4,xH_2O.
CAS — 7558-80-7 (anhydrous monobasic sodium phosphate); 10049-21-5 (monobasic sodium phosphate monohydrate); 13472-35-0 (monobasic sodium phosphate dihydrate); 10028-24-7 (monobasic sodium phosphate dihydrate).
Pharmacopoeias. In Eur. (see p.vi) and Pol. (with 2H_2O); in Chin. (with 1H_2O). Br. also includes monographs for the anhydrous and monohydrate forms. US permits the anhydrous, monohydrate, and dihydrate forms.

Each g of monobasic sodium phosphate (anhydrous) represents approximately 8.3 mmol of sodium and of phosphate. Each g of monobasic sodium phosphate (monohydrate) represents approximately 7.2 mmol of sodium and of phosphate. Each g of monobasic sodium phosphate (dihydrate) represents approximately 6.4 mmol of sodium and of phosphate.

Pharmacopoeial description
Ph. Eur.: The dihydrate is a white powder or colourless crystals. Very soluble in water; very slightly soluble in alcohol. A 5% solution in water has a pH of 4.2 to 4.5.
BP 2001: The anhydrous substance is described as white, slightly deliquescent, crystals or granules. Very soluble in water; very slightly soluble in alcohol. A 5% solution in water has a pH of 4.2 to 4.5.
The monohydrate is a white powder or colourless crystals. Very soluble in water; very slightly soluble in alcohol. A 5% solution in water has a pH of 4.2 to 4.5.
USP 25: It contains one or two molecules of water of hydration, or is anhydrous. Colourless crystals or white crystalline powder. Is odourless and is slightly deliquescent. Freely soluble in water; practically insoluble in alcohol. Its solutions are acid to litmus and effervesce with sodium carbonate. pH of a 5% solution in water of the monohydrate form is between 4.1 and 4.5.

Dibasic Sodium Phosphate   (1196-b)

Dinatrii Phosphas; Disodium Hydrogen Phosphate; Disodium Phosphate; E339; Natrii Phosphas; Sodium Phosphate. Disodium hydrogen orthophosphate.
Na_2HPO_4.
CAS — 7558-79-4 (anhydrous dibasic sodium phosphate); 10028-24-7 (dibasic sodium phosphate dihydrate); 7782-85-6 (dibasic sodium phosphate heptahydrate); 10039-32-4 (dibasic sodium phosphate dodecahydrate).
ATC — A06AG01; V10XX01 (^{32}P).
Pharmacopoeias. In Eur. (see p.vi), Jpn, Pol., and US. The pharmacopoeias may specify one or more states of hydration; monographs and specifications can be found for the anhydrous form (Na_2HPO_4 =142.0), the dihydrate ($Na_2HPO_4,2H_2O$ =178.0), the heptahydrate ($Na_2HPO_4,7H_2O$ =268.1), and the dodecahydrate ($Na_2HPO_4,12H_2O$ =358.1), although not necessarily all will be found in any one pharmacopoeia.

Each g of dibasic sodium phosphate (anhydrous) represents approximately 14.1 mmol of sodium and 7.0 mmol of phosphate. Each g of dibasic sodium phosphate (dihydrate) represents approximately 11.2 mmol of sodium and 5.6 mmol of phosphate. Each g of dibasic sodium phosphate (heptahydrate) represents approximately 7.5 mmol of sodium and 3.7 mmol of phosphate. Each g of dibasic sodium phosphate (dodecahydrate) represents approximately 5.6 mmol of sodium and 2.8 mmol of phosphate.

Pharmacopoeial description
Ph. Eur.: The anhydrous form is a white, hygroscopic powder. Soluble in water; practically insoluble in alcohol. Store in airtight containers.
The dihydrate is a white or almost white powder or colourless crystals. Soluble in water; practically insoluble in alcohol.
The dodecahydrate is described as colourless, transparent, very efflorescent crystals. Very soluble in water; practically insoluble in alcohol.
USP 25: It is dried, or contains one, two, seven, or twelve molecules of water of hydration.
The dried substance is a white powder that readily absorbs moisture. It is soluble 1 in 8 of water; insoluble in alcohol.
The heptahydrate is a colourless or white, granular or caked salt that effloresces in warm, dry air. It is freely soluble in water; very slightly soluble in alcohol. Its solutions are alkaline to phenolphthalein, a 0.1M solution having a pH of about 9.
Store all forms in airtight containers.

Tribasic Sodium Phosphate   (14285-f)

E339; Trisodium Orthophosphate; Trisodium Phosphate.
$Na_3PO_4 = 163.9$.
CAS — 7601-54-9.

Each g of tribasic sodium phosphate (anhydrous) represents approximately 18.3 mmol of sodium and 6.1 mmol of phosphate.

Adverse Effects and Treatment

Excessive administration of intravenous phosphate causes hyperphosphataemia, particularly in patients with renal failure. Hyperphosphataemia leads in turn to hypocalcaemia, which may be severe, and to ectopic calcification, particularly in patients with initial hypercalcaemia. Tissue calcification may cause hypotension and organ damage and result in acute renal failure. Hyperphosphataemia, hypocalcaemia, and tissue calcification are rare after oral or rectal phosphate administration (but see also Effects on Electrolytes, below).

Adverse effects that may occur with the use of oral phosphates include nausea, vomiting, diarrhoea, and abdominal pain. When oral phosphates are being used for indications other than their laxative effects, diarrhoea may necessitate a reduction in dosage. When administered rectally for bowel evacuation, sodium phosphates may cause local irritation.

Phosphates are administered as the potassium or sodium salts or both; therefore, additional electrolyte disturbances that may be expected on excessive administration include hyperkalaemia, and hypernatraemia and dehydration.

Treatment of adverse effects involves withdrawal of phosphate, general supportive measures, and correction of serum-electrolyte concentrations, especially calcium. Measures to remove excess phosphate such as oral phosphate binders and haemodialysis may be required (see also Hyperphosphataemia, p.1182).

Effects on electrolytes. Although less common than after intravenous therapy, hyperphosphataemia, accompanied by hypocalcaemia or other severe electrolyte disturbances and resulting in tetany[1,2] and even death,[2] has been reported on a number of occasions following the use of phosphate enemas. Similar effects have also been reported with the use of oral phosphate laxatives.[3,4] Infants or children,[2,5] and those with renal impairment,[1,4] have often been the subjects of these adverse effects. Soft tissue calcification appears to occur rarely with oral phosphate, but nephrocalcinosis has been reported in children with hypophosphataemic rickets treated with calcitriol and phosphate supplements, and was found to be associated with the phosphate dose.[6]

1. Haskell LP. Hypocalcaemic tetany induced by hypertonic-phosphate enema. Lancet 1985; **ii:** 1433.
2. Martin RR, et al. Fatal poisoning from sodium phosphate enema: case report and experimental study. JAMA 1987; **257:** 2190–2.
3. Peixoto Filho AJ, Lassman MN. Severe hyperphosphatemia induced by a phosphate-containing oral laxative. Ann Pharmacother 1994; **30:** 141–3.
4. Adverse Drug Reactions Advisory Committee. Electrolyte disturbances with oral phosphate bowel preparations. Aust Adverse Drug React Bull 1997; **16:** 2.
5. McCabe M, et al. Phosphate enemas in childhood: cause for concern. BMJ 1991; **302:** 1074.
6. Verge CF, et al. Effects of therapy in X-linked hypophosphatemic rickets. N Engl J Med 1991; **325:** 1843–8.

Local toxicity. Rectal gangrene has been associated with the use of phosphate enemas in elderly patients and was believed to be due to a direct necrotising effect of the phosphate on the rectum.[1]

1. Sweeney JL, et al. Rectal gangrene: a complication of phosphate enema. Med J Aust 1986; **144:** 374–5.

Precautions

Phosphates should not generally be given to patients with severely impaired renal function. They should be avoided in patients who may have low serum-calcium concentrations, as these may decrease further, and in patients with infected phosphate renal calculi. Potassium phosphates should be avoided in patients with hyperkalaemia and sodium phosphates should generally be avoided in patients with congestive heart failure, hypertension, and oedema. Serum electrolytes and renal function should be monitored during therapy, particularly if phosphates are given parenterally.

Oral or rectal sodium phosphate preparations for bowel evacuation should not be used in patients with gastrointestinal obstruction, inflammatory bowel disease, and conditions where there is likely to be increased colonic absorption. They should be used cautiously in elderly and debilitated patients, and in those with pre-existing electrolyte disturbances.

Interactions
Oral phosphate supplements should not be administered concomitantly with aluminium, calcium, or magnesium salts as these will bind phosphate and reduce its absorption. Vitamin D increases the gastrointestinal absorption of phosphates and therefore increases the potential for hyperphosphataemia.

Hyperphosphataemia, hypocalcaemia, and hypernatraemia are more likely to occur with phosphate enemas or oral laxatives if these are administered to patients receiving diuretics or other drugs that may affect serum electrolytes. The risk of ectopic calcification may be increased by concurrent use of calcium supplements or calcium-containing antacids.

The risk of hyperkalaemia is increased if potassium phosphates are coadministered with drugs that can increase serum-potassium concentrations.

Pharmacokinetics
Approximately two-thirds of ingested phosphate is absorbed from the gastrointestinal tract. Excess phosphate is predominantly excreted in the urine, the remainder being excreted in the faeces.

◊ References.
1. Larson JE, *et al.* Laxative phosphate poisoning: pharmacokinetics of serum phosphorus. *Hum Toxicol* 1986; **5:** 45–9.

Human Requirements
Phosphorus requirements are usually regarded as equal to those of calcium.

Most foods contain adequate amounts of phosphate, particularly meat and dairy products, hence deficiency is virtually unknown except in certain disease states, in patients receiving total parenteral nutrition, or in those who have received phosphate-binding agents for prolonged periods; for further details see under Hypophosphataemia, p.1182.

◊ In the UK dietary reference values (DRV—see p.1352)[1] and in the USA dietary reference intakes including recommended dietary allowances (RDA)[2] have been published for phosphorus. In the UK the reference nutrient intake (RNI) for adults is approximately 550 mg (17.5 mmol) daily; no additional amount is recommended for pregnancy although an additional amount of about 440 mg (14.3 mmol) daily is advised during lactation. In the USA the RDA is 1250 mg daily for those aged 9 to 18 years and 700 mg daily in adults; no increase in RDA is recommended during pregnancy and lactation. A tolerable upper intake level of 4 g daily has been set in adults aged up to 70 years; in those older than 70 a maximum of 3 g daily is recommended.[2]

1. DoH. Dietary reference values for food energy and nutrients for the United Kingdom: report of the panel on dietary reference values of the committee on medical aspects of food policy. *Report on health and social subjects 41.* London: HMSO, 1991.
2. Standing Committee on the Scientific Evaluation of Dietary Reference Intakes of the Food and Nutrition Board. *Dietary Reference Intakes for calcium, phosphorus, magnesium, vitamin D, and fluoride.* Washington, DC: National Academy Press, 1999.

Uses and Administration
Phosphates are used in the management of **hypophosphataemia** caused by phosphate deficiency or hypophosphataemic states (p.1182). Doses of up to 100 mmol of phosphate daily may be given by mouth. The intravenous route is seldom necessary, but a dose of up to 9 mmol of phosphate as monobasic potassium phosphate may be given over 12 hours and repeated every 12 hours as necessary for severe hypophosphataemia (see also below). Plasma-electrolyte concentrations, especially phosphate and calcium, and renal function should be carefully monitored. Reduced doses may be necessary in patients with impaired renal function. Phosphate supplements are used in total parenteral nutrition regimens; typical daily requirements are 20 to 30 mmol of phosphate.

Phosphates act as mild osmotic **laxatives** (p.1201) when administered by mouth as dilute solutions or by the rectal route. Phosphate enemas or concentrated oral solutions are used for bowel cleansing prior to surgery or endoscopy procedures. Preparations typically combine monobasic and dibasic sodium phosphates but the composition and dosage do vary slightly. Phosphate enemas act within 2 to 5 minutes,

whereas the oral solutions act within 30 minutes to 6 hours.

Phosphates also have **other uses**. They lower the pH of urine and have been given as adjuncts to urinary antimicrobials that depend on an acid urine for their activity. Phosphates have also been used for the prophylaxis of calcium renal calculi; the phosphates reduce urinary excretion of calcium thus preventing calcium deposition. A suggested dose for both uses is 7.4 mmol of phosphate four times daily by mouth.

Butafosfan (1-butylamino-1-methylethylphosphinic acid) and the sodium salt of toldimfos (4-dimethylamino-*O*-tolylphosphinic acid) are used as phosphorus sources in veterinary medicine.

Hypercalcaemia. Intravenous phosphates have been used to lower plasma-calcium concentrations in hypercalcaemic emergencies (p.1181), but because of their potential to cause serious adverse effects other drugs are now preferred. Oral phosphates may be used to prevent gastrointestinal absorption of calcium in the treatment of hypercalcaemia. The dose in adults is up to 100 mmol phosphate daily adjusted according to response.

Hypophosphataemia. Phosphate salts are given in the management of hypophosphataemia when a phosphate deficiency is identified, as discussed in Uses and Administration, above. Intravenous phosphates are associated with serious adverse effects if hypophosphataemia is over-corrected, and the rise in serum-phosphorus concentration cannot be predicted from a given dose. Consequently, it has been recommended that intravenous phosphate be used cautiously in the treatment of severe hypophosphataemia.[1-4] However, some advocate a more aggressive fixed-dose regimen in critically ill patients.[5]

1. Vannatta JB, *et al.* Efficacy of intravenous phosphorus therapy in the severely hypophosphatemic patient. *Arch Intern Med* 1981; **141:** 885–7.
2. Anonymous. Treatment of severe hypophosphatemia. *Lancet* 1981; **ii:** 734.
3. Lloyd CW, Johnson CE. Management of hypophosphatemia. *Clin Pharm* 1988; **7:** 123–8.
4. Coyle S, *et al.* Treatment of hypophosphataemia. *Lancet* 1992; **340:** 977.
5. Perreault MM, *et al.* Efficacy and safety of intravenous phosphate replacement in critically ill patients. *Ann Pharmacother* 1997; **31:** 683–8.

Osteomalacia. Vitamin D deficiency, or its abnormal metabolism, is the most usual cause of osteomalacia and rickets (p.744); however, phosphate depletion may also contribute, and phosphate supplementation may be given as appropriate. A suggested dose for vitamin-D-resistant hypophosphataemic osteomalacia in adults is 65 to 100 mmol phosphate daily, and for vitamin D-resistant rickets in children is 32 to 48 mmol phosphate daily.

RICKETS OF PREMATURITY. Dietary deficiency of phosphorus is unusual, but can occur in small premature infants fed exclusively on human breast milk. The phosphate intake in these infants appears to be inadequate to meet the needs of bone mineralisation, and hypophosphataemic rickets can develop. It has been proposed that this condition, variably called metabolic bone disease of prematurity, or rickets of prematurity, could be prevented by giving phosphorus supplements to very low-birth-weight babies (less than about 1000 g) fed on breast milk alone.[1] A suggested regimen is to add 10 to 15 mg of phosphorus per 100 mL of feed (as buffered sodium phosphate) until the infant reached 2000 g. Concomitant calcium and vitamin D supplementation are also recommended.[1] A placebo-controlled study[2] in infants weighing less than 1250 g at birth confirmed that phosphate supplements (50 mg daily) could prevent the development of the bone defects of rickets of prematurity.

1. Brooke OG, Lucas A. Metabolic bone disease in preterm infants. *Arch Dis Child* 1985; **60:** 682–5.
2. Holland PC, *et al.* Prenatal deficiency of phosphate, phosphate supplementation, and rickets in very-low-birthweight infants. *Lancet* 1990; **335:** 697–701. Correction. *ibid.* 1408–9.

Preparations
BP 2001: Phosphates Enema;
Ph. Eur.: Anticoagulant Citrate-Phosphate-Glucose Solution (CPD);
USP 25: Anticoagulant Citrate Phosphate Dextrose Adenine Solution; Anticoagulant Citrate Phosphate Dextrose Solution; Potassium Phosphates Injection; Sodium Phosphates Injection; Sodium Phosphates Oral Solution; Sodium Phosphates Rectal Solution.

Proprietary Preparations (details are given in Part 3)
Aust.: Fleet Phospho-Soda; Relaxyl; **Austral.:** Celloids PP 85; Celloids SP 96; Kwikprep; Phosphoprep; **Belg.:** Fleet Phospho-Soda; **Canad.:** Fleet Phospho-Soda; **Fin.:** K-Fosforsteril; **Fr.:** Fleet Phospho-Soda; **Ger.:** Fleet Phospho-Soda; **Hong Kong:** Fleet Phospho-Soda; **Neth.:** Fleet Klysma†; **NZ:** Fleet Phosphate Enema; Phospho-Soda; **Singapore:** Fleet Phospho-Soda; **Spain:** Clisma Bieffe Medital; Fosfosoda; **Swed.:** Phosphoral; **UK:** Fleet Phospho-Soda; New Era Calm & Clear†; **USA:** Fleet Phospho-Soda; K-Phos Original; Visicol.

Multi-ingredient: Aust.: Clysmol; Klysma Salinisch†; Precacol†; Reducto; **Austral.:** Bio-Chromium; Cal Alkyline; Celloid Compounds Magcal Plus; Celloid Compounds Sodical Plus; Duo Celloids PPIP; Duo Celloids PPMP; Duo Celloids SPCF; Duo Celloids SPCP; Duo Celloids SPIP; Duo Celloids SPMP; Duo Celloids SPPC; Duo Celloids SPPP; Duo Celloids SPPS; Duo Celloids SPS; Duo Celloids SPSS; Fleet Phospho-Soda; Fleet Ready-

to-Use; Gingo A; Ginkgo Plus Herbal Plus Formula 10; Lifesystem Herbal Plus Formula 11 Ginkgo; Lifesystem Herbal Plus Formula 2 Valerian; Magcal Plus†; Magnesium Plus; ML 20; Phosphate-Sandoz; Potasi; Sodical Plus†; Travad; Valerian Plus Herbal Plus Formula 12; **Belg.:** Fleet Enema; Lavement au Phosphate; Normogastryl†; Practo-Clyss; Prepacol; **Braz.:** Digestron; Fleet Enema; Phosfo Enema; **Canad.:** Enemol; Fleet Enema; Gent-L-Tip; Normo Gastryl; Phosphate-Novartis; Phosphates; PMS-Phosphates†; **Denm.:** Fleet; Phosphoral; **Fin.:** Phosphoral; **Fr.:** Azym; Bactident; Digedryl; Gastrilax†; Hepargitol; Normacol Lavement; Normogastryl; Oxyboldine; Phosphocholine; Phosphoneuros; Phosphore-Sandoz†; Prefagyl; Prepacol; Soker†; **Ger.:** Isogutt; Klistier; Klysma Salinisch; Lecicarbon; Practo-Clyss; Prepacol; Reducto-spezial; **Hong Kong:** Fleet Enema; **Irl.:** Fleet; Fletchers Phosphate Enema; Phosphate-Sandoz†; **Israel:** Calciless; Fleet Enema; Soffodex; **Ital.:** Clisflex; Clisma Evacuante†; Clisma Fleet; Clisma-Lax; Enemac; Fosfo-Soda Fleet; Non Acid†; Phospho-Lax; Ra-Cliss; **Mex.:** Fleet; **Neth.:** Colex; **Norw.:** Phosphoral; **NZ:** Phosphate-Sandoz; **S.Afr.:** Colo-Prep; Lenolax; Phosphate-Sandoz; Sabax Fosenema; **Singapore:** Fleet Enema; **Spain:** Acetuber; Alcalinos Gelos; Boldosal; Darmen Salt; Enema Casen; Eupeptina; Lebersal; Normogastryl; **Switz.:** Colophos; Freka-Clyss; Lecicarbon; Normogastryl; Practo-Clyss; Reducto-special†; **Thai.:** Swiff; Uni-Ma; **UK:** Carbalax; Fleet Ready-to-Use; Fletchers Phosphate Enema; Juno Junipah; Phosphate-Sandoz; Salivix; **USA:** Fleet Enema; K-Phos MF; K-Phos Neutral; K-Phos No.2; Neutra-Phos; Neutra-Phos-K; Summers Eve Post-Menstrual; Urimar-T; Urimax; Uro-Phosphate; Urogesic Blue; Uroqid-Acid.

# Potassium (1176-d)
K = 39.0983.

Potassium salts covered in this section are those principally given as a source of potassium ions, but consideration should also be given to the effect of the anion. Phosphate salts of potassium are covered under Phosphate, p.1193, and the bicarbonate and citrate salts under Bicarbonate, p.1186.

Potassium Acetate (1177-n)
E261; Kalii Acetas.
$CH_3.CO_2K = 98.14$.
CAS — 127-08-2.
Pharmacopoeias. In *Eur.* (see p.vi), *Pol.*, and *US*.

Each g of potassium acetate (anhydrous) represents approximately 10.2 mmol of potassium. Potassium acetate (anhydrous) 2.51 g is approximately equivalent to 1 g of potassium.
Pharmacopoeial description
Ph. Eur.: Deliquescent white, crystalline powder or colourless crystals. Very soluble in water; freely soluble in alcohol. A 5% solution in water has a pH of 7.5 to 9.0. Protect from moisture.
USP 25: Colourless, monoclinic crystals, or a white crystalline powder. It is odourless or has a faint acetous odour. Deliquesces on exposure to moist air. Soluble 1 in 0.5 of water, 1 in 0.2 of boiling water, and 1 in 3 of alcohol. pH of a 5% solution in water is between 7.5 and 8.5. Store in airtight containers.

Potassium Chloride (1179-m)
Cloreto de Potássio; E508; Kalii Chloridum; Kalium Chloratum.
KCl = 74.55.
CAS — 7447-40-7.
ATC — A12BA01; B05XA01.
Pharmacopoeias. In *Chin., Eur.* (see p.vi), *Int., Jpn, Pol.,* and *US*.

Each g of potassium chloride represents approximately 13.4 mmol of potassium. Potassium chloride 1.91 g is approximately equivalent to 1 g of potassium.
Pharmacopoeial description
Ph. Eur.: A white, crystalline powder or colourless crystals. Freely soluble in water; practically insoluble in dehydrated alcohol.
USP 25: Colourless, elongated, prismatic, or cubical crystals, or a white, granular powder. Is odourless. Soluble 1 in 2.8 of water, and 1 in 2 of boiling water; insoluble in alcohol. Its solutions are neutral to litmus.

Potassium Gluconate (1181-x)
E577. Potassium D-gluconate.
$CH_2OH.[CH(OH)]_4.CO_2K = 234.2$.
CAS — 299-27-4 (anhydrous potassium gluconate); 35398-15-3 (potassium gluconate monohydrate).
ATC — A12BA05.
Pharmacopoeias. In *Fr.*
US permits anhydrous or the monohydrate.

Each g of potassium gluconate (anhydrous) represents approximately 4.3 mmol of potassium. Each g of potassium gluconate (monohydrate) represents approximately 4 mmol of potassium. Potassium gluconate (anhydrous) 5.99 g and potassium gluconate (monohydrate) 6.45 g are each approximately equivalent to 1 g of potassium.
Pharmacopoeial description
USP 25: It is anhydrous or contains one molecule of water of hydration. A white or yellowish-white, odourless, crystalline powder or granules. Soluble 1 in 3 of water; practically insoluble in dehydrated alcohol, in chloroform, in ether, and in benzene. Its solutions are slightly acid to litmus. Store in airtight containers.

Potassium Sulfate (1185-n)

E515; Kalium Sulfuricum; Potassii Sulphas; Potassium Sulphate; Tartarus Vitriolatus.
$K_2SO_4 = 174.3$.
CAS — 7778-80-5.
Pharmacopoeias. In Aust., Jpn, and Swiss.

Each g of potassium sulfate represents approximately 11.5 mmol of potassium. Potassium sulfate 2.23 g is approximately equivalent to 1 g of potassium.

Potassium Tartrate (1187-m)

E336.
$C_4H_4K_2O_6, \frac{1}{2}H_2O = 235.3$.
CAS — 921-53-9 (anhydrous potassium tartrate).

Each g of potassium tartrate (hemihydrate) represents approximately 8.5 mmol of potassium. Potassium tartrate (hemihydrate) 3.00 g is approximately equivalent to 1 g of potassium.

Adverse Effects

Excessive administration of potassium may lead to the development of hyperkalaemia, especially in patients with renal impairment. Symptoms include paraesthesia of the extremities, muscle weakness, paralysis, cardiac arrhythmias, heart block, cardiac arrest, and mental confusion. Cardiac toxicity is of particular concern after intravenous administration.

Pain or phlebitis may occur during intravenous administration via the peripheral route, particularly at higher concentrations.

Nausea, vomiting, diarrhoea, and abdominal cramps may occur following oral administration of potassium salts. There have been numerous reports of gastrointestinal ulceration, sometimes with haemorrhage and perforation or with the late formation of strictures, after the use of enteric-coated tablets of potassium chloride. Ulceration has also occurred after the use of sustained-release tablets.

Treatment of Adverse Effects

The treatment of hyperkalaemia discussed on p.1182 also applies when hyperkalaemia occurs during potassium therapy. However, in mild hyperkalaemia that has developed on long-term treatment, discontinuation of the potassium supplement and other drugs that may increase plasma-potassium concentrations, and avoidance of foods with a high potassium content may be sufficient to correct the hyperkalaemia.

In cases of acute oral overdosage of potassium supplements, the stomach should be emptied by gastric lavage in addition to the measures described on p.1182.

Precautions

Potassium salts should be administered with considerable care to patients with cardiac disease or conditions predisposing to hyperkalaemia such as renal or adrenocortical insufficiency, acute dehydration, or extensive tissue destruction as occurs with severe burns. Excessive use of potassium-containing salt substitutes or potassium supplements may lead to accumulation of potassium especially in patients with renal insufficiency. Regular monitoring of clinical status, serum electrolytes, and the ECG is advisable in patients receiving potassium therapy, particularly those with cardiac or renal impairment.

Liquid or effervescent preparations are preferred to solid dosage forms for oral administration; use of the former, with or after food, may reduce gastric irritation. Solid oral dosage forms of potassium salts should not be given to patients with gastrointestinal ulceration or obstruction. They should be given with care to patients in whom passage through the gastrointestinal tract may be delayed, as in pregnant patients. Treatment should be discontinued if severe nausea, vomiting, or abdominal distress develops.

Potassium chloride should not be used in patients with hyperchloraemia.

Direct injection of potassium chloride concentrates without appropriate dilution may cause instant death. For the view that glucose-containing solutions should not be used for the initial intravenous administration of potassium in hypokalaemia see Administration, below.

Interactions

Potassium supplements should be used with caution, if at all, in patients receiving drugs that increase serum-potassium concentrations. These include potassium-sparing diuretics, ACE inhibitors, and ciclosporin, and drugs that contain potassium such as the potassium salts of penicillin. Similarly, the concomitant use of potassium-containing salt substitutes for flavouring food should be avoided. Antimuscarinics delay gastric emptying and consequently may increase the risk of gastrointestinal adverse effects in patients receiving solid oral dosage forms of potassium.

Pharmacokinetics

Potassium salts other than the phosphate, sulfate, and tartrate are generally readily absorbed from the gastrointestinal tract. Potassium is excreted mainly by the kidneys; it is secreted in the distal tubules in exchange for sodium or hydrogen ions. The capacity of the kidneys to conserve potassium is poor and some urinary excretion of potassium continues even when there is severe depletion. Some potassium is excreted in the faeces and small amounts may also be excreted in sweat.

Human Requirements

Potassium is an essential body electrolyte. However, requirements are difficult to determine and have been estimated from the amount accumulated during growth and reported urinary and faecal excretion.

Over 90% of dietary potassium is absorbed from the gastrointestinal tract. Potassium is particularly abundant in vegetables, potatoes, and fruit.

◊ In the UK dietary reference values (DRV—see p.1352)[1] have been estimated for potassium. The reference nutrient intake (RNI) for adults is 3.5 g (90 mmol) daily. In the USA, no recommended dietary allowance (RDA) has been established for potassium. However a daily intake of 1.6 to 2 g (40 to 50 mmol) is considered adequate for adults.

1. DoH. Dietary reference values for food energy and nutrients for the United Kingdom: report of the panel on dietary reference values of the committee on medical aspects of food policy. *Report on health and social subjects 41.* London: HMSO, 1991.

Uses and Administration

Potassium salts in this section are used for the prevention and treatment of potassium depletion and/or **hypokalaemia** (p.1182) and have been used in the prevention of **diuretic-induced hypokalaemia** (see Hydrochlorothiazide, Effects on Electrolyte Balance, p.908). Doses may be expressed in terms of mmol or mEq of potassium, mass (mg) of potassium, or mass of potassium salt (for comparative purposes see Table 3, below). Treatment should be monitored by plasma-potassium estimations because of the risk of inducing hyperkalaemia, especially where there is renal impairment.

Potassium chloride is probably the most commonly used potassium salt; this is because hypochloraemic alkalosis, which is often associated with hypokalaemia, can be corrected by the chloride ions. An alkalinising salt such as potassium acetate, potassium bi-

Table 3. Some potassium salts and their potassium content.

Potassium salt	Potassium content per g		
	mg	mmol	mEq
Potassium acetate (anhydrous)	398	10.2	10.2
Potassium bicarbonate	391	10.0	10.0
Potassium chloride	524	13.4	13.4
Potassium citrate (anhydrous)	383	9.8	9.8
Potassium citrate (monohydrate)	361	9.3	9.3
Potassium gluconate (anhydrous)	167	4.3	4.3
Potassium gluconate (monohydrate)	155	4.0	4.0
Potassium sulfate (anhydrous)	449	11.5	11.5
Potassium tartrate (hemihydrate)	332	8.5	8.5

carbonate, or potassium citrate may be preferable if a metabolic acidosis, such as occurs in renal tubular acidosis, accompanies the hypokalaemia (see p.1180). Other salts that are or have been employed in the management of potassium deficiency include potassium ascorbate, potassium aspartate, potassium benzoate, potassium gluceptate, potassium gluconate and potassium tartrate. Typical doses for the prevention of hypokalaemia may be up to 50 mmol daily and similar doses may be adequate in mild potassium deficiency. However, higher doses may be needed in more severe deficiency. Patients with renal impairment should receive correspondingly lower doses. Oral treatment is used for prophylaxis and is also suitable for treating most cases of hypokalaemia. Potassium salts by mouth are more irritating than the corresponding sodium salts; they should be taken with or after meals with plenty of fluid and liquid preparations are preferable.

Intravenous administration of a potassium salt may be required in severe acute hypokalaemia. This is normally carried out by infusing a solution containing 20 mmol of potassium in 500 mL over 2 to 3 hours under ECG control. A recommended maximum dose is 2 to 3 mmol of potassium per kg body-weight in 24 hours. Higher concentrations have been given when an infusion pump has been employed (see Administration below). Adequate urine flow must be ensured and careful monitoring of plasma-potassium and other electrolyte concentrations is essential. Potassium chloride is the salt most commonly employed and solutions intended for intravenous use that are in a concentrated form (such as 1.5 or 2 mmol per mL) *must* be diluted to the appropriate concentration before administration. There should be careful and thorough mixing when adding concentrated potassium chloride solutions to infusion fluids. Potassium chloride is also available as premixed infusions with sodium chloride and/or glucose containing 10 to 40 mmol of potassium per litre (but see also Administration, below). Potassium acetate is also given intravenously.

Amongst **other uses**, the phosphate, sulfate, and tartrate salts of potassium have been given by mouth as osmotic laxatives (p.1201).

Some potassium salts are used as sodium-free condiments when sodium intake must be restricted.

Potassium chloride is sometimes used as a capsule and tablet diluent.

Administration. The standard concentration and rate of administration of potassium chloride for infusion is discussed in Uses and Administration, above. However, higher concentrations (200 or 300 mmol per litre) and faster infusion rates have been used, via an infusion pump, for cases of severe symptomatic hypokalaemia, especially with fluid overload.[1,2]

There has been controversy regarding the preferred route of administration of these higher concentrations of potassium chloride.[1] The central route avoids the problems of pain and phlebitis when potassium is given peripherally. However, it has been suggested that high concentrations of potassium administered centrally may carry a greater risk of cardiac toxicity if the infusion is carried directly to the heart. Use of lignocaine [lidocaine] has improved tolerability of peripheral administration of potassium chloride.[2]

Intravenous potassium is usually given in sodium chloride and/or glucose infusion. However, it has been pointed out that glucose administration can reduce serum-potassium concentrations, and that glucose-free solutions should be used for the initial intravenous administration of potassium in hypokalaemia.[3]

1. Kruse JA, Carlson RW. Rapid correction of hypokalemia using concentrated intravenous potassium chloride infusions. *Arch Intern Med* 1990; **150:** 613–17.
2. Pucino F, *et al.* Patient tolerance to intravenous potassium chloride with and without lidocaine. *Drug Intell Clin Pharm* 1988; **22:** 676–9.
3. Agarwal A, Wingo CS. Treatment of hypokalaemia. *N Engl J Med* 1999; **340:** 154–5.

Diabetic ketoacidosis. As discussed under Diabetic Emergencies on p.318, potassium replacement is given in diabetic ketoacidosis to restore total body stores of potassium and thereby prevent the hypokalaemia induced by the administration of insulin.

Hypertension. A meta-analysis[1] has reported that potassium supplementation results in reductions of both systolic and diastolic blood pressure. The size of the effect in hypertensive patients was sufficiently great to suggest a possible role in the treatment of hypertension (p.802); effects in normotensive sub-

The symbol † denotes a preparation no longer actively marketed

jects were less marked but consistent with a role for potassium supplementation in preventing hypertension.

1. Whelton PK, *et al.* Effects of oral potassium on blood pressure: meta-analysis of randomized controlled clinical trials. *JAMA* 1997; **277:** 1624–32.

Myocardial infarction. There is some evidence to suggest that a glucose, insulin, and potassium infusion may be beneficial in acute myocardial infarction (see p.331).

Termination of pregnancy. Solutions of potassium chloride are used to reduce fetal numbers in multifetal pregnancies[1,2] by abolishing the fetal cardiac activity. The solution is injected into the thorax of the fetus without affecting the others which are allowed to continue to term.

1. Wapner RJ, *et al.* Selective reduction of multifetal pregnancies. *Lancet* 1990; **335:** 90–3.
2. Berkowitz RL. The current status of multifetal pregnancy reduction. *Am J Obstet Gynecol* 1996; **174:** 1265–72.

Preparations

BP 1973: Strong Potassium Chloride Solution;
BP 2001: Bumetanide and Slow Potassium Tablets; Effervescent Potassium Chloride Tablets; Potassium Chloride and Glucose Intravenous Infusion; Potassium Chloride and Sodium Chloride Intravenous Infusion; Potassium Chloride, Sodium Chloride and Glucose Intravenous Infusion; Slow Potassium Chloride Tablets; Sterile Potassium Chloride Concentrate;
USP 25: Half-strength Lactated Ringer's and Dextrose Injection; Lactated Ringer's and Dextrose Injection; Lactated Ringer's Injection; Potassium Acetate Injection; Potassium Bicarbonate and Potassium Chloride Effervescent Tablets for Oral Solution; Potassium Bicarbonate and Potassium Chloride for Effervescent Oral Solution; Potassium Chloride Extended-release Capsules; Potassium Chloride Extended-release Tablets; Potassium Chloride for Injection Concentrate; Potassium Chloride for Oral Solution; Potassium Chloride in Dextrose and Sodium Chloride Injection; Potassium Chloride in Dextrose Injection; Potassium Chloride in Lactated Ringer's and Dextrose Injection; Potassium Chloride in Sodium Chloride Injection; Potassium Chloride Oral Solution; Potassium Chloride, Potassium Bicarbonate, and Potassium Citrate Effervescent Tablets for Oral Solution; Potassium Gluconate and Potassium Chloride for Oral Solution; Potassium Gluconate and Potassium Chloride Oral Solution; Potassium Gluconate and Potassium Citrate Oral Solution; Potassium Gluconate Elixir; Potassium Gluconate Tablets; Potassium Gluconate, Potassium Citrate, and Ammonium Chloride Oral Solution; Trikates Oral Solution.

Proprietary Preparations (details are given in Part 3)
Aust.: KCl-retard; Micro-Kalium; Rekawan; *Austral.:* Celloids PC 73; Celloids PS 29; Chlorvescent; KSR; Slow-K; Span-K; *Belg.:* Chloropotassuril; Kalium Durettes; Ultra-K; *Braz.:* Slow-K; *Canad.:* Apo-K; K-10; K-Dur; K-Lor; K-Lyte/Cl; Kalium Durules†; Kaochlor; Kaon; Micro-K; Potassium-Rougier; Roychlor; Slow-K; *Denm.:* Kaleorid; Kalinorm†; *Fin.:* Durekal; Kalinorm; Kalisol; Kalisteril; Kalium Duretter; *Fr.:* Diffu-K; Kaleorid; Nati-K; *Ger.:* Kalinor-retard P; Kalitrans retard†; Kalium-Duriles; KCl-retard; Rekawan; *Hong Kong:* Addi-K; Apo-K; Kalium; KSR; Slow-K; Span-K; *Irl.:* Kay-Cee-L; Slow-K; *Israel:* Slow-K; *Ital.:* K-Flebo; Kadalex; Lento-Kalium; *Mex.:* Ceposil; Clor-K-Zaf; K-Dur; Kaliolite; Kelefusin; Potasoral; *Neth.:* Kalium Durettes; Slow-K; *Norw.:* Kaleorid; Kalinorm; *NZ:* Chlorvescent; K-SR; Slow-K; Span-K; *S.Afr.:* Micro-K†; Plenish-K; Slow-K; Swiss-Kal SR; *Singapore:* Addi-K; Kalium Durules; KSR; *Spain:* Boi K; Boi K Aspartico; Potasion; *Swed.:* K-MIC†; Kaleorid; Kalitabs; Kalium Duretter; Kalium Retard; *Switz.:* Kaliglutol; Plus Kalium retard; *Thai.:* Addi-K; Enpott; Potassride; *UK:* Kay-Cee-L; Slow-K; *USA:* Cena-K; Gen-K; K + 10; K + 8; K-Dur; K-G Elixir; K-Lease; K-Lor; K-Lyte/Cl; K-Norm; K-Tab; Kaochlor; Kaon; Kaon-Cl; Kay Ciel; Kaylixir†; Klor-Con; Klorvess; Klotrix; Micro-K; Potasalan; Rum-K; Slow-K; Ten-K.

Multi-ingredient: numerous preparations are listed in Part 3.

Sodium   (1188-b)

Na = 22.98977.

Sodium chloride is the principal sodium salt used as a source of sodium ions. Sodium salts used chiefly as sources of bicarbonate ions, such as the acetate, bicarbonate, citrate, and lactate, are covered under Bicarbonate, p.1186. Phosphate salts of sodium are covered under Phosphate, p.1193.

Sodium Chloride   (1191-f)

Chlorure de Sodium; Cloreto de Sódio; Natrii Chloridum; Salt.
NaCl = 58.44.
CAS — 7647-14-5.
ATC — A12CA01; B05CB01; B05XA03.

NOTE. An aqueous solution of sodium chloride 0.9% is often known as physiological saline.
SALINE is a code approved by the BP 2001 for use on single unit doses of eye drops containing sodium chloride 0.9% where the individual container may be too small to bear all the appropriate labelling information. HECL is a similar code approved for hyetellose and sodium chloride eye drops.
Pharmacopoeias. In *Chin., Eur.* (see p.vi), *Int., Jpn, Pol.,* and *US.*

Each g of sodium chloride represents approximately 17.1 mmol of sodium and of chloride. Sodium chloride 2.54 g is approximately equivalent to 1 g of sodium.

A 0.9% solution in water is iso-osmotic, and thus in most cases isotonic with serum and lachrymal secretions.

Solutions of some sodium salts, including sodium chloride, when stored, may cause separation of solid particles from glass

containers and solutions containing such particles must not be used.

Pharmacopoeial description
Ph. Eur.: A white, crystalline powder or colourless crystals or white pearls. Freely soluble in water; practically insoluble in dehydrated alcohol.

USP 25: Colourless cubic crystals or white crystalline powder. Soluble 1 in 2.8 of water, 1 in 2.7 of boiling water, and 1 in 10 of glycerol; slightly soluble in alcohol.

Adverse Effects

Adverse effects of sodium salts are attributable to electrolyte imbalances from excess sodium; there may also be effects due to the specific anion.

Retention of excess sodium in the body usually occurs when there is defective renal sodium excretion. This leads to the accumulation of extracellular fluid to maintain normal plasma osmolality, which may result in pulmonary and peripheral oedema and their consequent effects.

Hypernatraemia (a rise in plasma osmolality) is usually associated with inadequate water intake, or excessive water losses (see p.1183). It rarely occurs after therapeutic doses of sodium chloride, but has occurred with the use of hypertonic saline for induction of emesis or for gastric lavage and after errors in the formulation of infant feeds. Hypernatraemia may also occur after inappropriate intravenous administration of hypertonic saline.

The most serious effect of hypernatraemia is dehydration of the brain which causes somnolence and confusion progressing to convulsions, coma, respiratory failure, and death. Other symptoms include thirst, reduced salivation and lachrymation, fever, tachycardia, hypertension, headache, dizziness, restlessness, irritability, and weakness.

Gastrointestinal effects associated with acute oral ingestion of hypertonic solutions or excessive amounts of sodium chloride include nausea, vomiting, diarrhoea, and abdominal cramps.

Excessive administration of chloride salts may cause a loss of bicarbonate with an acidifying effect.

Intra-amniotic injection of hypertonic solutions of sodium chloride, which has been used for abortion induction, has been associated with serious adverse effects including disseminated intravascular coagulation, renal necrosis, cervical and uterine lesions, haemorrhage, pulmonary embolism, pneumonia, and death.

◊ General references.
1. Moder KG, Hurley DL. Fatal hypernatremia from exogenous salt intake: report of a case and review of the literature. *Mayo Clin Proc* 1990; **65:** 1587–94.

Treatment of Adverse Effects

In patients with mild sodium excess, oral administration of water and restriction of sodium intake is sufficient. However, in the event of recent acute oral overdose of sodium chloride, induction of emesis or gastric lavage should be carried out along with general symptomatic and supportive treatment. Serum-sodium concentrations should be measured, and if severe hypernatraemia is present this should be treated (see p.1183).

Precautions

Sodium salts should be administered with caution to patients with hypertension, heart failure, peripheral or pulmonary oedema, impaired renal function, pre-eclampsia, or other conditions associated with sodium retention.

When sodium supplements are given by mouth, adequate water intake should be maintained. Sustained-release tablets should not be administered to patients with gastrointestinal disorders associated with strictures or diverticula because of the risk of obstruction.

Pharmacokinetics

Sodium chloride is well absorbed from the gastrointestinal tract. Excess sodium is predominantly excreted by the kidney, and small amounts are lost in the faeces and sweat.

Human Requirements

The body contains about 4 mol (92 g) of sodium of which about one-third is found in the skeleton and approximately half is present in the extracellular fluid.

The body can adapt to a wide range of intakes by adjustment of renal excretion through physical and hormonal factors. Loss through the skin is significant only if excessive sweating occurs. Sodium requirements may be increased with exercise or exposure to high ambient temperatures in the short term, until the body adjusts.

Sodium is widely available in foods and is also added as salt during processing, cooking, and at the table. Dietary deficiency of sodium is therefore extremely rare and more concern has been expressed that current intakes are excessive. Restriction of sodium intake, by limiting the amount of culinary salt consumed, may be a useful aid in the management of some patients with hypertension (p.802).

◊ In the UK dietary reference values (DRV—see p.1352)[1] have been published for sodium. The reference nutrient intake (RNI) for adults is 1.6 g of sodium (70 mmol) daily, which is about 4 g of sodium chloride. In the USA, it has been recommended that daily intakes of sodium be limited to 2.4 g (6 g of sodium chloride) or less.[2] Dietary intake is often in excess of these recommendations, and may be a factor in essential hypertension,[3] and osteoporosis.[4]

1. DoH. Dietary reference values for food energy and nutrients for the United Kingdom: report of the panel on dietary reference values of the committee on medical aspects of food policy. *Report on health and social subjects 41.* London: HMSO, 1991.
2. Subcommittee on the tenth edition of the RDAs, Food and Nutrition Board, Commission on Life Sciences, National Research Council. *Recommended dietary allowances.* 10th ed. Washington, DC: National Academy Press, 1989.
3. Midgley JP, *et al.* Effect of reduced dietary sodium on blood pressure: a meta-analysis of randomized controlled trials. *JAMA* 1996; **275:** 1590–7.
4. Devine A, *et al.* A longitudinal study of the effect of sodium and calcium intakes on regional bone density in postmenopausal women. *Am J Clin Nutr* 1995; **62:** 740–5.

Uses and Administration

Sodium chloride is used in the management of deficiencies of sodium and chloride ions in salt-losing conditions (see Hyponatraemia, p.1183). Sodium chloride solutions are used as a source of sodium chloride and water for hydration. Doses may be expressed in terms of mEq or mmol of sodium, mass (mg) of sodium, or mass of sodium salt. For comparative purposes, see Table 4, below.

A typical oral replacement dose of sodium chloride in **chronic salt-losing conditions** is about 2.4 to 4.8 g (about 40 to 80 mmol of sodium) daily as a modified-release preparation, accompanied by a suitable fluid intake; doses of up to 12 g daily may be necessary in severe cases. Oral supplements are also used for the prevention of muscle cramps during routine haemodialysis; a suggested dose is about 6 to 10 g of a modified-release preparation per dialysis session.

Glucose facilitates the absorption of sodium from the gastrointestinal tract, and solutions containing sodium chloride and glucose usually with additional electrolytes (see p.1185) are used for oral rehydration in acute diarrhoea (p.1203).

The concentration and dosage of sodium chloride solutions for intravenous use is determined by several factors including the age, weight, and clinical condi-

Table 4. Some sodium salts and their sodium content.

Sodium salt	Sodium content per g		
	mg	mmol	mEq
Sodium acetate (anhydrous)	280	12.2	12.2
Sodium acetate (trihydrate)	169	7.3	7.3
Sodium acid citrate	175	7.6	7.6
Sodium bicarbonate	274	11.9	11.9
Sodium chloride	394	17.1	17.1
Sodium citrate (anhydrous)	267	11.6	11.6
Sodium citrate (dihydrate)	235	10.2	10.2
Sodium lactate	205	8.9	8.9

tion of the patient and in particular the patients' hydration state. Serum-electrolyte concentrations should be carefully monitored.

In severe sodium depletion, 2 to 3 litres of sodium chloride 0.9% (isotonic; iso-osmotic) may be given over 2 to 3 hours and thereafter at a slower rate. If there is combined water and sodium depletion a 1 to 1 mixture of sodium chloride 0.9% and glucose 5% may be appropriate. Although hypertonic sodium chloride solutions may be used in certain patients with severe acute dilutional hyponatraemia, over-rapid correction may have severe neurological adverse effects—see p.1183. Solutions containing 1.8 to 5% are available.

In **hypernatraemia** with volume depletion (p.1183), sodium chloride 0.9% may be used to maintain plasma-sodium concentrations with expanding fluid volume. Sodium chloride 0.9% (or rarely, in marked hypernatraemia, 0.45%) is used for fluid replacement in diabetic ketoacidosis (see Diabetic Emergencies, p.318).

Among its **other uses**, sodium chloride solution 0.9%, being isotonic, is a useful fluid for sterile irrigations, for example, of the eye or bladder, and general skin or wound cleansing. The 0.9% concentration is also widely used as a vehicle or diluent for the parenteral administration of other drugs. Nasal drops of sodium chloride 0.9% are used to relieve nasal congestion. A mouthwash containing sodium chloride is also available for oral hygiene.

Sodium chloride solutions should *not* be used to induce emesis; this practice is dangerous and deaths from resulting hypernatraemia have been reported.

Sodium chloride (Natrium muriaticum; Nat. Mur.) is used in homoeopathic medicine. It is also sometimes used as an excipient in capsules and tablets.

Catheters and cannulas. For reference to sodium chloride 0.9% being used to maintain the patency of catheters and cannulas, and to its equivalent efficacy to heparin, see Catheters and Cannulas under Uses and Administration of Heparin, p.904.

Termination of pregnancy. Trans-abdominal intra-amniotic instillation of sodium chloride 20% (maximum volume 200 to 250 mL) has been used for the termination of second-trimester pregnancy. However, serious adverse effects have occurred (see above), and other methods are generally preferred (p.1439).

Preparations

BP 2001: Compound Sodium Chloride Mouthwash; Potassium Chloride and Sodium Chloride Intravenous Infusion; Potassium Chloride, Sodium Chloride and Glucose Intravenous Infusion; Sodium Chloride and Glucose Intravenous Infusion; Sodium Chloride Eye Drops; Sodium Chloride Eye Lotion; Sodium Chloride Intravenous Infusion; Sodium Chloride Irrigation Solution; Sodium Chloride Solution; Sodium Chloride Tablets;
USP 25: Bacteriostatic Sodium Chloride Injection; Dextrose and Sodium Chloride Injection; Fructose and Sodium Chloride Injection; Half-strength Lactated Ringer's and Dextrose Injection; Inulin in Sodium Chloride Injection; Lactated Ringer's and Dextrose Injection; Lactated Ringer's Injection; Mannitol in Sodium Chloride Injection; Potassium Chloride in Dextrose and Sodium Chloride Injection; Potassium Chloride in Lactated Ringer's and Dextrose Injection; Potassium Chloride in Sodium Chloride Injection; Sodium Chloride and Dextrose Tablets; Sodium Chloride Inhalation Solution; Sodium Chloride Injection; Sodium Chloride Irrigation; Sodium Chloride Ophthalmic Ointment; Sodium Chloride Ophthalmic Solution; Sodium Chloride Tablets; Sodium Chloride Tablets for Solution.

Proprietary Preparations (details are given in Part 3)

Aust.: Otrisal; Polyrinse-Aufnahmelosung; Uro-Pract; *Austral.:* Bausch & Lomb Saline Plus†; Bausch & Lomb Sensitive Eyes Saline; Fess; Lens Plus; Narium; Slow-Sodium; Softwear; *Belg.:* Naaprep; Physiologica; Physiorhine; *Braz.:* Fisiologico; Fluimucil Solucao Nasal; Narisoro; Nasoflux; Nesoro; Rinoben; Rinoflux; *Canad.:* Certified Nasal; EFA Steri; Lens Plus Buffered Saline Solution; Muro 128; Physium; Safeway Nasal; Salinex; Softwear; Thalaris; *Denm.:* Viskose ojendraber; *Fin.:* Natrosteril; *Fr.:* Aequalyre; Aquarhine; Erjean; Irriclens; Larmabak; Larmes Artificielles; Physiologica; Physiomer; Physiosoin; Polyrinse; Selgine; Serophy†; Unilarm; Uro 3000†; Versol; Vesirig; *Ger.:* Adsorbonac; Freka-Drainjet; Isogutt akut; Isotone Kochsalz; Olynth salin; Otrisal; Rhinomer; Rhinospray Atlantik; Tetrisal; Uro-Pract N†; *Hong Kong:* Adsorbonac; Atomic Enema; Larmabak; *Irl.:* Slow-Sodium; *Israel:* Baby AF; Clean-AF; Drossanose; Normasol; Uro-Tainer; *Ital.:* Adsorbonac; Hydrabak; Libenar; Naribel; Physiomer; *Mex.:* Corni Limp; Hiperton; *NZ:* Hydrocare Preserved Saline; Narium; *Port.:* Rhinomer; Sterimar; *Singapore:* Adsorbonac; Larmabak; *Spain:* Antiedema; Apir Clorurado; Apiroflex Clorurado; Estericlean; Fisiologica; Fisiologico; Fisiologico Bieffe M; Fisiologico Braun; Fisiologico Farmacelsia; Fisiologico Mein; Fisiologico Vitulia; Flebobag Fisio; Fleboplast Fisio; Lavaflac; Libenar†; Liberanas; Meinvenil Fisiologico; Plast Apyr Fisio Irrigac†; Plast Apyr Fisiologico; Respitol; Solucion Fisio; Suero Fisiologico; *Swed.:* Lisal†; Tresal†; *Switz.:* Naaprep; Nasben soft; Nose Fresh; Physiologica; Physiosoin; Rhinomer; Serophy; Triomer; *UK:* Askina; Irriclens; Labmist; Normasol; Rhinomer; Slow-Sodium; Sterac; Sterijet†; Steripod Blue; Uriflex S; Uro-Tainer M; *USA:* Adsorbonac; Afrin Moisturizing Saline Mist; Ak-NaCl; Ayr Saline; Breathe Free; Broncho Saline; Dristan Saline Spray; HuMist Nasal Mist; Irigate†; Marlin Salt System; Muro 128; Muroptic; NaSal; Nasal Moist; Normaline; Ocean; Pretz; Salinex; SeaMist; Soft Rinse 250†; Your Choice.

Multi-ingredient: numerous preparations are listed in Part 3.

Gases

This chapter includes monographs on gases with medical or pharmaceutical uses and applications (such as oxygen, carbon dioxide, helium, and nitrogen) as well as those where the medical interest lies primarily in management of their toxicity or adverse effects (such as carbon monoxide or hydrogen sulfide). Also included are some compressed and liquefied gases used as refrigerants and aerosol propellants. Nitric oxide gas is used in bronchopulmonary disorders and is discussed in Cardiovascular Drugs (p.947). Other gases with medical uses can be found in Disinfectants and Preservatives (p.1129) and General Anaesthetics (p.1255).

Refrigerants and Aerosol Propellants

A number of compressed and liquefied gases are used as refrigerants and as aerosol propellants; these include nitrogen, nitrous oxide, carbon dioxide, propane, and the butanes. Chlorofluorocarbons (CFCs) were widely used but because of environmental hazards their general use has been severely restricted and they are being phased out in medicine and pharmacy. Hydrogenated chlorofluorocarbons (hydrochlorofluorocarbons) and nonchlorinated fluorocarbons (hydrofluorocarbons) are being developed as alternatives, although neither are devoid of environmental effects.

The evaporation of halogenated hydrocarbon propellants produces an intense cold that numbs the tissues, and they have been used as topical analgesics (p.4).

Refrigerants and aerosol propellants have been subject to deliberate abuse. Inhalation of high concentrations of halogenated hydrocarbons for their euphoriant effect may result in CNS depression, cardiac arrhythmias, respiratory depression, and death. Propane and butane can act as simple asphyxiants. Heat can cause the decomposition of halogenated hydrocarbons into irritant and toxic gases such as hydrogen chloride and phosgene.

◊ Reviews have covered the toxicity and adverse effects that may occur as a consequence of the deliberate abuse of aerosol propellants[1-3] as well as the hazards associated with occupational exposure.[4] Further references relevant to the toxicity of individual gases are given in the monographs.

1. Volatile substance abuse—an overview. *Hum Toxicol* 1989; **8:** 255–344.
2. Ashton CH. Solvent abuse. *BMJ* 1990; **300:** 1356–6.
3. Anderson HR. Increase in deaths from deliberate inhalation of fuel gases and pressurised aerosols. *BMJ* 1990; **301:** 41.
4. Matthews G. Toxic gases. *Postgrad Med J* 1989; **65:** 224–32.

Bromochlorodifluoromethane (18869-s)

$CBrClF_2 = 165.4$.

Profile
Bromochlorodifluoromethane has been employed as a fire-extinguishing agent.

◊ Reports of toxicity following the misuse or abuse of fire extinguishers containing bromochlorodifluoromethane.[1,2]

1. Steadman C, *et al.* Abuse of fire-extinguishing agent and sudden death in adolescents. *Med J Aust* 1984; **141:** 115–17.
2. Lerman Y, *et al.* Fatal accidental inhalation of bromochlorodifluoromethane (Halon 1211). *Hum Exp Toxicol* 1991; **10:** 125–8.

Butane (18361-b)

n-Butane; E942.
$C_4H_{10} = 58.12$.
CAS — 106-97-8.

Pharmacopoeias. In USNF.

It is supplied compressed in metal cylinders which should be stored in a cool place free from materials of a flammable nature.

Pharmacopoeial description
USNF 20: A colourless gas. It is highly flammable and explosive. Store in airtight cylinders at a temperature not exceeding 40°.

Profile
Butane is used as an aerosol propellant (above). It is widely used as a fuel.

◊ Reports of toxicity associated with the abuse of butane.[1-3]

1. Gunn J, *et al.* Butane sniffing causing ventricular fibrillation. *Lancet* 1989; **i:** 617.
2. Siegel E, Wason S. Sudden death caused by inhalation of butane and propane. *N Engl J Med* 1990; **323:** 1638.
3. Roberts MJD, *et al.* Asystole following butane gas inhalation. *Br J Hosp Med* 1990; **44:** 294.

Carbon Dioxide (5202-a)

Carbonei Dioxidum; Carbonei Dioxydum; Carbonic Acid Gas; Carbonic Anhydride; E290.
$CO_2 = 44.01$.
CAS — 124-38-9.

Pharmacopoeias. In Chin., Eur. (see p.vi), Jpn, and US.

It is supplied liquefied under pressure in metal cylinders. National standards are usually in operation for the labelling and marking of such cylinders. It is about 1½ times as heavy as air.

Pharmacopoeial description
Ph. Eur.: A colourless gas. Soluble 1 in about 1 of water by volume at 20° and at a pressure of 101 kpA. Store liquefied under pressure in suitable containers.

USP 25: A colourless, odourless gas. Its solutions are acid to litmus. One volume dissolves in about 1 volume of water. Store in cylinders.

Adverse Effects
Above a concentration of 6%, carbon dioxide gives rise to headache, dizziness, confusion, palpitations, hypertension, dyspnoea, increased depth and rate of respiration, and CNS depression. Concentrations of about 20% and higher produce convulsions and loss of consciousness; inhalation of 50% carbon dioxide is reported to produce central effects similar to anaesthetics. The inhalation of high concentrations may produce respiratory acidosis.

Abrupt withdrawal of carbon dioxide after prolonged inhalation commonly produces pallor, hypotension, dizziness, severe headache, and nausea or vomiting.

Skin contact with solid carbon dioxide may cause frostbite.

Uses and Administration
Carbon dioxide has been added to the oxygen in certain types of pump oxygenators to maintain the carbon dioxide content of the blood.

Although carbon dioxide stimulates respiration, it is seldom used for this purpose. Treatment of carbon monoxide poisoning with carbon dioxide/oxygen mixtures is discouraged due to the risk of respiratory acidosis.

Inhalation of carbon dioxide has been tried for relief of intractable hiccup (p.667). Carbonated vehicles are useful for masking the unpleasant taste of some medicinal preparations.

Solid carbon dioxide, or 'dry ice' has a temperature of −80° and has been used to treat warts (p.1108) and naevi by cryotherapy.

Carbon dioxide may be used as the insufflating gas for laparoscopy and as a contrast agent in radiography (p.1030).

Preparations
Proprietary Preparations (details are given in Part 3)
Multi-ingredient: *Ger.:* Ensinger Schiller-Quelle Heilwasser.

Carbon Monoxide (12525-g)

$CO = 28.01$.
CAS — 630-08-0.

A colourless, odourless, tasteless, highly flammable gas.

Adverse Effects
Carbon monoxide is produced by incomplete combustion of organic materials and is highly toxic when inhaled; infants, small children, and elderly people are particularly susceptible. Although the number of cases of poisoning in countries like the UK has fallen as the availability of coal gas has declined and as changes have been made to motor vehicles to improve their exhaust fumes, carbon monoxide is still a major cause of poisoning. Common sources of carbon monoxide include poorly maintained and ventilated heating systems and improperly burnt fuel in domestic fires.

When inhaled, carbon monoxide combines with haemoglobin in the blood to form carboxyhaemoglobin which is unable to transport oxygen; the symptoms of carbon monoxide poisoning are largely due to anoxia. The skin and tissues turn a classic cherry red in patients poisoned with carbon monoxide although this is seen most often after death.

The symptoms of carbon monoxide poisoning are varied and depend on the degree and duration of exposure. Unconsciousness may occur suddenly but is commonly preceded by headache, dizziness, weakness, nausea, and vomiting, which may be misdiagnosed as a viral illness or food poisoning. Other symptoms may include skin lesions, excessive sweating, pyrexia, increased respiration, mental dullness and confusion, visual disturbances, convulsions, hypotension, tachycardia or other cardiac arrhythmias, myocardial ischaemia, and possibly myocardial infarction. Death may result from respiratory failure, pulmonary oedema, cardiovascular failure, or cerebral damage. The lethal concentration of carboxyhaemoglobin in the blood is about 50% or more. Concentrations over 1000 ppm of carbon monoxide in inspired air may be fatal in 1 hour. Neurological and psychiatric sequelae may develop some weeks later in the survivors of severe poisoning and therefore a prolonged follow-up of such patients is advised; symptoms include memory impairment, apathy, mutism, irritability, personality change, gait disturbance, and urinary and faecal incontinence. Chronic carbon monoxide exposure may present as a non-specific illness with headache, nausea, and flu-like symptoms.

◊ General references.

1. Carbon Monoxide. *Environmental Health Criteria 13.* Geneva: WHO, 1979.
2. Meredith T, Vale A. Carbon monoxide poisoning. *BMJ* 1988; **296:** 77–9.
3. Crawford R, *et al.* Carbon monoxide poisoning in the home: recognition and treatment. *BMJ* 1990; **301:** 977–9.
4. Ernst A, Zibrak JD. Carbon monoxide poisoning. *N Engl J Med* 1998; **339:** 1603–8.

Treatment of Adverse Effects
The patient should be removed from the contaminated atmosphere and an effective airway established. Oxygen (100%) should be given until blood carboxyhaemoglobin concentration has fallen below dangerous levels (usually 5%). Management is then usually symptomatic and supportive with attention being given to the possible need to treat or correct any cardiovascular disorders, metabolic acidosis, or cerebral oedema. Hyperbaric oxygen therapy may be considered in pregnant patients or in severe poisoning (if the patient is, or has been, unconscious; if the carboxyhaemoglobin concentration exceeds 20%; or if there are neurological symptoms or cardiac complications) but is of unproven benefit (see below) and its use is controversial.

◊ References.

1. Anonymous. Treatment of carbon monoxide poisoning. *Drug Ther Bull* 1988; **26:** 77–9.
2. Ely EW, *et al.* Warehouse workers' headache: emergency evaluation and management of 30 patients with carbon monoxide poisoning. *Am J Med* 1995; **98:** 145–55.

Hyperbaric oxygen. The use of hyperbaric oxygen therapy in the management of carbon monoxide poisoning is controversial. Administration of hyperbaric oxygen is of theoretical benefit since it increases the rate at which carboxyhaemoglobin dissociates, and beneficial results have been reported in patients with carbon monoxide poisoning.[1,2] Its use has therefore been widely recommended, particularly in patients with severe poisoning. However, the availability of hyperbaric oxygen administration is limited, and it remains unclear which patients should receive therapy. A controlled trial[3] comparing hyperbaric oxygen with normobaric oxygen (at higher levels than commonly used) in patients with severe poisoning found no benefit from hyperbaric oxygen and its place in therapy has therefore been questioned. Nevertheless, the study has been criticised[4,5] and some consider that the use of hyperbaric oxygen should still be considered. Hyperbaric oxygen has been successfully used in pregnant patients with carbon monoxide poisoning[6] and its use should possibly be considered earlier in pregnant patients due to the risks to the fetus from hypoxia.

1. Gorman DF. Problems and pitfalls in the use of hyperbaric oxygen for the treatment of poisoned patients. *Med Toxicol Adverse Drug Exp* 1989; **4:** 393–9.
2. Hawkins M, *et al.* Severe carbon monoxide poisoning: outcome after hyperbaric oxygen therapy. *Br J Anaesth* 2000; **84:** 584–6.
3. Scheinkestel CD, *et al.* Hyperbaric or normobaric oxygen for acute carbon monoxide poisoning: a randomised controlled clinical trial. *Med J Aust* 1999; **170:** 203–10.
4. Moon RE, DeLong E. Hyperbaric oxygen for carbon monoxide poisoning. *Med J Aust* 1999; **170:** 197–9.
5. Weaver LK. Hyperbaric oxygen in carbon monoxide poisoning. *BMJ* 1999; **319:** 1083–4.
6. Van Hoesen KB, *et al.* Should hyperbaric oxygen be used to treat the pregnant patient for acute carbon monoxide poisoning: a case report and literature review. *JAMA* 1989; **261:** 1039–43. Correction. *ibid.* 1990; **263:** 2750.

Uses
Carbon monoxide has been used in low concentrations as a tracer gas in measurements of lung function. Carbon monoxide labelled with carbon-11 may also be employed to assess the blood volume.

Chlorofluorocarbons   (10497-h)

CFCs.

Cryofluorane   (5207-d)

Cryofluorane (rlNN).

CFC-114; Dichlorotetrafluoroethane; Propellant 114; Refrigerant 114; Tetrafluorodichloroethane. 1,2-Dichloro-1,1,2,2-tetrafluoroethane.

$C_2Cl_2F_4 = 170.9$.

CAS — 76-14-2.

Pharmacopoeias. In *USNF*.

It is supplied under compression in metal cylinders.

Pharmacopoeial description

USNF 20: A clear, colourless gas having a faint ethereal odour. Store in airtight cylinders at a temperature not exceeding 40°.

Dichlorodifluoromethane   (5206-f)

CFC-12; Difluorodichloromethane; Propellant 12; Refrigerant 12.

$CCl_2F_2 = 120.9$.

CAS — 75-71-8.

Pharmacopoeias. In *USNF*.

It is supplied under compression in metal cylinders.

Pharmacopoeial description

USNF 20: A clear, colourless gas having a faint ethereal odour. Store in airtight cylinders at a temperature not exceeding 40°.

Trichlorofluoromethane   (5208-n)

CFC-11; Fluorotrichloromethane; Propellant 11; Refrigerant 11; Trichloromonofluoromethane.

$CCl_3F = 137.4$.

CAS — 75-69-4.

Pharmacopoeias. In *USNF*.

It is a gas above 24°. It is usually supplied under compression in metal cylinders.

Pharmacopoeial description

USNF 20: A clear, colourless gas having a faint ethereal odour. Store in airtight cylinders at a temperature not exceeding 40°.

Profile

Chlorofluorocarbons are used as refrigerants and as aerosol propellants (p.1198). They may also be used as a spray for topical anaesthesia, the intense cold produced by the rapid evaporation of the spray making the tissues insensitive.

Preparations

Proprietary Preparations (details are given in Part 3)

Aust.: Pharmaethyl; *Ger.:* Provotest†; *USA:* Gebauer "114" Spray†.

Multi-ingredient: *Austral.:* Derm-Freeze; *Fr.:* Dynacold†; *USA:* Aerofreeze; Fluori-Methane; Fluro-Ethyl.

Dimethyl Ether   (6963-r)

Dimethyl Oxide; Methoxymethane; Oxybismethane.

$C_2H_6O = 46.07$.

CAS — 115-10-6.

Profile

Dimethyl ether is used as a refrigerant, aerosol propellant (p.1198), and topical anaesthetic.

Preparations

Proprietary Preparations (details are given in Part 3)

Multi-ingredient: *Austral.:* Histofreezer; *Fr.:* Histofreezer; *UK:* PR Freeze Spray; Ralgex Freeze Spray; Wartner.

Helium   (5203-t)

E939.

$He = 4.002602$.

CAS — 7440-59-7.

Pharmacopoeias. In *US*.

It is usually supplied under compression in metal cylinders. National standards are usually in operation for the labelling and marking of such cylinders.

Pharmacopoeial description

USP 25: A colourless, odourless, tasteless gas which is not combustible and does not support combustion. Very slightly soluble in water. Store in cylinders.

Profile

As helium is less dense than nitrogen, breathing a mixture of 80% helium and 20% oxygen requires less effort than breathing air. Thus mixtures containing the desired concentration of oxygen ('Heliox') have been used in patients with respiratory disorders. Due to the low solubility of helium, mixtures of helium and oxygen are used by divers or others working under high pressure to prevent the development of decompression sickness

The symbol † denotes a preparation no longer actively marketed

(caisson disease); they are preferred to compressed air since they do not cause nitrogen narcosis. Helium has been employed in pulmonary function testing.

Breathing helium increases vocal pitch and causes voice distortion.

Hydrochlorofluorocarbons   (10495-d)

HCFCs.

Chlorodifluoroethane   (17661-p)

Propellant 142b; Refrigerant 142b. 1-Chloro-1,1-difluoroethane.

$C_2H_3ClF_2 = 100.5$.

CAS — 75-68-3.

Chlorodifluoromethane   (17662-s)

Propellant 22; Refrigerant 22.

$CHClF_2 = 86.47$.

CAS — 75-45-6.

Profile

Hydrochlorofluorocarbons are used as refrigerants and as aerosol propellants (p.1198).

Hydrofluorocarbons   (10513-s)

Fluorocarbons; HFAs; HFCs; Hydrofluroalkanes.

Difluoroethane   (17663-w)

Ethylene Fluoride; HFC-152a; Propellant 152a; Refrigerant 152a. 1,1-Difluoroethane.

$C_2H_4F_2 = 66.05$.

CAS — 75-37-6.

Norflurane   (15021-g)

Norflurane (BAN, USAN, rlNN).

Fluorocarbon 134a; GR-106642X; HFA-134a; HFC-134a; Propellant 134a; Refrigerant 134a. 1,1,1,2-Tetrafluoroethane.

$C_2H_2F_4 = 102.0$.

CAS — 811-97-2.

Profile

Hydrofluorocarbons are used as refrigerants and as aerosol propellants (p.1198). As they are nonchlorinated fluorocarbons, it is believed that they will have a less detrimental effect on the environment than the chlorinated fluorocarbons.

◊ References.

1. Denyer LH, *et al.* GR106642X, a non-chlorinated propellant for use in metered-dose inhalers: safety, tolerability and pharmacokinetics in healthy volunteers. *Br J Clin Pharmacol* 1994; **38:** 509P.
2. Taggart SCO, *et al.* GR106642X: a new, non-ozone depleting propellant for inhalers. *BMJ* 1995; **310:** 1639–40.

Hydrogen Sulfide   (12832-k)

Hydrogen Sulphide; Sulphuretted Hydrogen.

$H_2S = 34.08$.

CAS — 7783-06-4.

A colourless flammable gas with a characteristic odour.

Adverse Effects

Hydrogen sulfide is a common industrial hazard and is encountered in such places as chemical works, mines, sewage works, and stores of decomposing protein. Concentrations of 0.1 to 0.2% in the atmosphere may be fatal in a few minutes. At concentrations of about 0.005% and above hydrogen sulfide causes anosmia and its unpleasant odour is no longer detectable. Pulmonary irritation, oedema, and respiratory failure usually occur after acute poisoning; prolonged exposure to low concentrations may give rise to severe conjunctivitis with photophobia and corneal opacity, irritation of the respiratory tract, cough, nausea, vomiting and diarrhoea, pharyngitis, headache, dizziness, and lassitude. There are some similarities to poisoning with cyanides.

◊ General references.

1. Hydrogen Sulfide. *Environmental Health Criteria 19.* Geneva: WHO, 1981.

Treatment of Adverse Effects

In poisoning with hydrogen sulfide the patient should be removed from the contaminated atmosphere and an effective airway established. Inhalation of amyl nitrite or parenteral therapy with sodium nitrite have been suggested since the methaemoglobin produced may bind sulfide. Some authorities have advocated oxygen by mask or hyperbaric oxygen therapy. The conjunctival sacs should be carefully washed out if eye irritation is severe. Management is then usually symptomatic and supportive.

◊ References.

1. Gorman DF. Problems and pitfalls in the use of hyperbaric oxygen for the treatment of poisoned patients. *Med Toxicol Adverse Drug Exp* 1989; **4:** 393–9.

Uses

Hydrogen sulfide is widely employed in many industrial processes.

Isobutane   (18352-m)

E942; 2-Methylpropane.

$C_4H_{10} = 58.12$.

Pharmacopoeias. In *USNF*.

It is usually supplied under compression in metal cylinders.

Pharmacopoeial description

USNF 20: A colourless gas. It is highly flammable and explosive. Store in airtight cylinders at a temperature not exceeding 40°.

Profile

Isobutane is used as an aerosol propellant (p.1198).

Nitrogen   (5204-x)

Azote; E941; Nitrogenium.

$N_2 = 28.0134$.

CAS — 7727-37-9.

Pharmacopoeias. In *Eur.* (see p.vi) and *Jpn*.

USNF has two monographs: Nitrogen (not less than 99% by volume of N_2) and Nitrogen 97 Percent (not less than 97% by volume of N_2).

It is usually supplied under compression in metal cylinders. National standards are usually in operation for the labelling and marking of such cylinders.

Pharmacopoeial description

Ph. Eur.: A colourless, odourless gas. Soluble 1 in about 62 of water and 1 in about 10 of alcohol by volume at 20° and at a pressure of 101 kPA. Store as a compressed gas or a liquid in appropriate containers.

USNF 20: A colourless, odourless, tasteless gas. It is non-flammable and does not support combustion. Soluble 1 in about 65 of water v/v and 1 in about 9 of alcohol v/v at 20° and at a pressure of 760 mmHg. Store in cylinders.

Adverse Effects

Nitrogen narcosis has been reported from nitrogen breathed at high pressure as in deep-water diving. Under high pressure, nitrogen dissolves in blood and lipid. If decompression is too rapid, nitrogen effervesces from body stores producing gas emboli and leading to the syndrome of decompression sickness. Skin contact with liquid nitrogen causes frostbite or burns.

◊ References.

1. Roblin P, *et al.* Liquid nitrogen injury: a case report. *Burns* 1997; **23:** 638–40.
2. Kernbach-Wighton G, *et al.* Clinical and morphological aspects of death due to liquid nitrogen. *Int J Legal Med* 1998; **111:** 191–5.
3. Koplewitz BZ, *et al.* Gastric perforation attributable to liquid nitrogen ingestion. *Pediatrics* 2000; **105:** 121–3.

Uses and Administration

Nitrogen is used as a diluent for pure oxygen or other active gases and as an inert gas to replace air in containers holding oxidisable substances. Liquid nitrogen is used as a cryotherapeutic agent for the removal of warts (p.1108) and for preservation of tissues and organisms.

Oxygen   (5201-k)

E948; Ossigeno; Oxygenium; Sauerstoff.

$O_2 = 31.9988$.

CAS — 7782-44-7.

Pharmacopoeias. In *Chin., Eur.* (see p.vi), *Jpn,* and *US*.

US also includes Oxygen 93 Percent (90 to 96% by volume of O_2).

Eur. also includes Medicinal Air. *US* also includes Medical Air.

Oxygen intended for aviation or mountain rescue must have a sufficiently low moisture content to avoid blocking of valves by freezing.

Oxygen is usually supplied under compression in metal cylinders. National standards are usually in operation for the labelling and marking of such cylinders.

Pharmacopoeial description

Ph. Eur.: Oxygen is a colourless, odourless gas. Soluble 1 in about 32 of water by volume at 20° and at a pressure of 101 kPA. Store as a compressed gas or liquid in appropriate containers.

Medicinal Air is compressed ambient air containing not less than 20.4% and not more than 21.4% of oxygen. A colourless, odourless gas. Soluble 1 in about 50 of water by volume at 20° and at a pressure of 101 kPA. Store as a gas in suitable containers.

USP 25: A colourless, odourless, tasteless gas that supports combustion more energetically than does air. Soluble 1 in about

32 of water v/v and 1 in about 7 of alcohol v/v at 20° and at a pressure of 760 mmHg. Store in cylinders or in a pressurised storage tank.

Medical Air is a natural or synthetic mixture of gases consisting largely of nitrogen and oxygen. It contains not less than 19.5% and not more than 23.5% of oxygen. Store in cylinders or in a low pressure collecting tank.

Adverse Effects

Oxygen toxicity depends upon both the inspired pressure (a function of concentration and barometric pressure) and the duration of exposure, the safe duration decreasing as the pressure increases. At lower pressures of up to 2 atmospheres absolute, pulmonary toxicity occurs before CNS toxicity; at higher pressures, the reverse applies. Symptoms of pulmonary toxicity include a decrease in vital capacity, cough, and substernal distress. Symptoms of CNS toxicity include nausea, mood changes, vertigo, twitching, convulsions, and loss of consciousness.

◊ In a review of hyperbaric oxygen therapy[1] the following were mentioned as potential complications: barotrauma (ear or sinus trauma, tympanic membrane rupture, or rarely pneumothorax or air embolism); oxygen toxicity (CNS toxicity or pulmonary toxicity); and reversible visual changes.

1. Grim PS, et al. Hyperbaric oxygen therapy. JAMA 1990; 263: 2216–20.

Retinopathy of prematurity. In the 1940s and 1950s an epidemic of retinopathy of prematurity, affecting perhaps 10 000 babies, was believed to have been caused by excessive administration of oxygen to the neonates. This resulted in the use of oxygen being reduced or curtailed and the incidence of the condition fell dramatically. However, in the 1970s and later an unexpected resurgence of retinopathy of prematurity occurred (probably *not* due to excessive oxygen administration). It is now believed that oxygen plays only a minor part and that retinopathy of prematurity is a multifactorial condition that affects the most immature and sick children.[1,2] The increased incidence may reflect the improved survival of these very premature neonates. A study[3] of supplemental oxygen in infants with pre-threshold retinopathy of prematurity suggested that therapy was safe, but a beneficial effect could not be confirmed.

1. Anonymous. Retinopathy of prematurity. Lancet 1991; 337: 83–4.
2. Holmström G. Retinopathy of prematurity. BMJ 1993; 307: 694–5.
3. The STOP-ROP Multicenter Study Group. Supplemental therapeutic oxygen for prethreshold retinopathy of prematurity (STOP-ROP), a randomized, controlled trial. I: Primary outcomes. Pediatrics 2000; 105: 295–310.

Precautions

Any fire or spark is highly dangerous in the presence of increased oxygen concentrations especially when oxygen is used under pressure.

Metal cylinders containing oxygen should be fitted with a reducing valve by which the rate of flow can be controlled. It is important that the reducing valve should be free from all traces of oil or grease, as otherwise a violent explosion may occur. Combustible material soaked in liquid oxygen is potentially explosive and the low temperature of liquid oxygen may cause unsuitable equipment to become brittle and crack. Liquid oxygen should not be allowed to come into contact with the skin as it produces severe 'cold burns'.

High concentrations of oxygen should be avoided in patients whose respiration is dependent upon hypoxic drive, otherwise carbon dioxide retention and respiratory depression may ensue.

Uses and Administration

Oxygen is given by inhalation to correct hypoxaemia in conditions causing respiratory failure (below) and in conditions where the oxygen content of the air breathed is inadequate such as in high-altitude disorders (p.800). Oxygen is of value in the treatment of poisoning with a number of substances, including carbon monoxide (p.1198), cyanides (p.1433), and dichloromethane (p.1402). It provides enhanced oxygenation in inhalation injury. Oxygen is also given by inhalation to subjects working in pressurised spaces and to divers to reduce the concentration of nitrogen inhaled. It is used as a diluent of volatile and gaseous anaesthetics.

Oxygen is usually administered by means of nasal prongs or via a face mask; these can usually deliver concentrations of up to 60%. Tight-fitting anaesthetic-type masks, or delivery via an endotracheal tube or oxygen tent can provide higher concentrations of up to 100%. Face masks are commonly employed for domiciliary oxygen therapy when flow rates are 2 or 4 litres per minute. Oxygen is commonly supplied compressed in metal cylinders although oxygen concentrators produce oxygen-enriched air and are useful for domiciliary therapy, especially in patients using large quantities of oxygen. Oxygen may also be supplied at low temperature in insulated containers as liquid oxygen.

In respiratory failure in conditions not usually associated with retention of carbon dioxide, such as pneumonia, pulmonary oedema, or fibrosing alveolitis, oxygen should be administered in high concentrations (usually 40 to 100%). Concentrations of 40 to 60% should be used in acute severe asthma even though carbon dioxide retention may have increased as the patient's condition deteriorated. High concentrations of oxygen should always be reduced as soon as possible to the lowest concentra-

tion needed to correct hypoxaemia in order to prevent development of any associated oxygen toxicity, including increased carbon dioxide retention. High concentrations of oxygen should be administered in carbon monoxide poisoning and, in selected patients, treatment with hyperbaric oxygen considered.

In respiratory failure associated with chronic obstructive pulmonary disease (conditions such as chronic bronchitis and emphysema) oxygen is usually administered to initially give an inspired concentration of up to 28%. High concentrations are to be avoided as they may enhance carbon dioxide retention and narcosis.

Oxygen at a pressure greater than 1 atmosphere absolute, i.e. hyperbaric oxygen therapy (below), is administered by enclosing the patient in a special high-pressure chamber. It may be used in carbon monoxide poisoning, as an adjunct in the treatment of severe anaerobic infections, especially gas gangrene, and for the treatment of decompression sickness and gas emboli.

◊ General references.

1. Naylor-Shepherd MF, et al. Oxygen homeostasis: theory, measurement, and therapeutic implications. DICP Ann Pharmacother 1990; 24: 1195–1203.
2. Gribbin HR. Management of respiratory failure. Br J Hosp Med 1993; 49: 461–77.
3. Tarpy SP, Celli BR. Long-term oxygen therapy. N Engl J Med 1995; 333: 710–14.
4. Bateman NT, Leach RM. ABC of oxygen: acute oxygen therapy. BMJ 1998; 317: 798–801.
5. Rees PJ, Dudley F. ABC of oxygen: oxygen therapy in chronic lung disease. BMJ 1998; 317: 871–4.
6. Rees PJ, Dudley F. ABC of oxygen: provision of oxygen at home. BMJ 1998; 317: 935–8.
7. Treacher DF, Leach RM. ABC of oxygen: oxygen transport: basic principles. BMJ 1998; 317: 1302–6.
8. Leach RM, Treacher DF. ABC of oxygen: oxygen transport: tissue hypoxia. BMJ 1998; 317: 1370–3.

Cluster headache. Inhalation of 100% oxygen can provide rapid and effective treatment of cluster headache attacks (p.449) but practical difficulties associated with its use result in other drugs being preferred.

References.

1. Fogan L. Treatment of cluster headache: a double-blind comparison of oxygen v air inhalation. Arch Neurol 1985; 42: 362–3.

Hyperbaric oxygen therapy. The use of hyperbaric oxygen therapy, which involves the intermittent inhalation of 100% oxygen under a pressure of greater than 1 atmosphere, has been the subject of reviews.[1-3] In the 1960s hyperbaric therapy was used for disorders such as *myocardial infarction, stroke, senility,* and *cancer* but clinical studies and experience have shown little benefit and enthusiasm has since waned. Hyperbaric oxygen therapy has also been tried in *multiple sclerosis* but there is little evidence of benefit. There are, however, other disorders for which the evidence supporting the efficacy of hyperbaric oxygen is much stronger.

Hyperbaric oxygen is a safe and effective primary therapy for *decompression sickness* and *air or gas embolism*. The effect is achieved through the mechanical reduction in bubble size in the blood brought about by an increase in ambient pressure; the increased oxygenation of blood due to the additional pressure employed for these conditions (often 6 rather than 2 or 3 atmospheres) is also beneficial.

The role of hyperbaric oxygen therapy in *carbon monoxide poisoning* is unclear but it should be considered in selected patients (see p.1198). Its mechanism of action is not fully understood; it increases the rate at which carboxyhaemoglobin concentrations decline, increases intracellular delivery of oxygen, and may also reduce lipid peroxidation and thus spare neuronal cell membranes.

Hyperbaric oxygen is employed as adjunctive therapy in *clostridial infections (gas gangrene)* (p.121). Early treatment appears to reduce systemic toxic reactions (probably by inhibiting the production of alpha toxin by the anaerobic bacteria, *Clostridium*) thus enabling patients to tolerate surgery more readily; additionally there is a clearer demarcation of viable and nonviable tissue. *Necrotising fasciitis* (p.130) is another infection in which hyperbaric oxygen therapy may be useful.

There is some evidence that hyperbaric oxygen may be useful in other types of *wounds*. In an *acute crush injury* therapy may reduce oedema via vasoconstriction and reverse ischaemia by increased oxygen delivery. In *problem wounds*, including venous ulcers, therapy may increase the tissue oxygen tension and stimulate angioneogenesis but it is emphasised that it is adjunctive therapy and not a replacement for meticulous local care. Other wounds in which therapy may be beneficial include thermal burns and compromised skin grafts and flaps. The management of burns and wounds is described on p.1104 and p.1108, respectively.

Radiation therapy can damage normal adjacent tissue resulting in tissue hypoxia and eventual cell death. Hyperbaric oxygen therapy appears to aid in salvaging such tissue by stimulating angionogenesis in marginally viable tissue and has been demonstrated to be beneficial in osteoradionecrosis, radiation-induced cystitis,[4] and other radiation-damaged soft tissue.

1. Grim PS, et al. Hyperbaric oxygen therapy. JAMA 1990; 263: 2216–20.
2. Tibbles PM, Edelsberg JS. Hyperbaric-oxygen therapy. N Engl J Med 1996; 334: 1642–8.

3. Leach RM, et al. ABC of oxygen: hyperbaric oxygen therapy. BMJ 1998; 317: 1140–3.
4. Bevers RFM, et al. Hyperbaric oxygen treatment for haemorrhagic radiation cystitis. Lancet 1995; 346: 803–5.

Respiratory failure. Respiratory failure occurs when the arterial plasma partial pressure of oxygen (P_aO_2) and of carbon dioxide (P_aCO_2) cannot be maintained within normal physiological limits.[1] Respiratory failure can be classified into 2 types both of which are characterised by a low P_aO_2 (hypoxaemia). However, in type I the P_aCO_2 is normal or low whereas in type II, referred to as ventilatory failure, P_aCO_2 is raised (hypercapnia). Some conditions, for example asthma, can produce either type of respiratory failure.

Management of respiratory failure primarily involves administration of oxygen to reverse hypoxaemia, and specific therapy for any underlying condition. Respiratory stimulants may be considered in some situations.

In type I respiratory failure oxygen is administered in high concentrations. Nasal prongs and certain face masks can provide concentrations of up to 60% but if concentrations higher than this are needed then tight-fitting anaesthetic-type masks or methods of delivery such as by endotracheal intubation have to be employed.

In type II respiratory failure both high and low concentrations are used according to need.

Patients with *acute severe asthma* (p.757) should usually be given oxygen at high concentrations of 40 to 60%. Low controlled concentrations of oxygen (beginning with about 24 to 28%) are used in the management of respiratory failure in patients with chronic respiratory disorders such as *chronic obstructive pulmonary disease* (p.759) the aim being to improve hypoxaemia without increasing hypercapnia and respiratory acidosis. Patients with exacerbations of chronic ventilatory failure already have an increased central drive to the respiratory muscles and therefore respiratory stimulants such as doxapram have a limited role but may be indicated for short-term use if hypercapnia worsens as a result of the administration of oxygen. Respiratory stimulants may be considered in the management of *postanaesthetic hypoventilation*. Although naloxone can reverse respiratory depression caused by opioid analgesics careful dosage adjustment is required as it can also abolish analgesia. Specific antagonists such as naloxone and flumazenil are also used to treat hypoventilation associated with opioid and benzodiazepine overdosage, respectively. If oxygen therapy fails to raise P_aO_2 in respiratory failure and there is worsening hypercapnia and respiratory acidosis the use of artificial ventilation should be considered.

Severe respiratory failure in *neonates* may result from various disorders. Administration of surfactant or inhaled nitric oxide may be of benefit in some cases but extracorporeal membrane oxygenation (ECMO), where blood is removed from the neonate, oxygenated, and re-injected in a continuous circuit that also removes carbon dioxide, may be required.[2] ECMO has also been used in older children and in adults,[3] but is less well established.

1. Gribbin HR. Management of respiratory failure. Br J Hosp Med 1993; 49: 461–77.
2. Barrington KJ, Finer NN. Care of near term infants with respiratory failure. BMJ 1997; 315: 1215–18.
3. Peek GJ, et al. Extracorporeal membrane oxygenation: potential for adults and children? Hosp Med 1998; 59: 304–8.

Preparations

Proprietary Preparations (details are given in Part 3)

Multi-ingredient: UK: Entonox; Equanox.

Propane   (16196-j)

Dimethylmethane; E942; Propyl Hydride.

$C_3H_8 = 44.10$.

CAS — 74-98-6.

Pharmacopoeias. In USNF.

It is usually supplied under compression in metal cylinders which should be stored in a cool place free from materials of a flammable nature.

Pharmacopoeial description

USNF 20: A colourless gas. It is highly flammable and explosive. Store in airtight cylinders at a temperature not exceeding 40°.

Profile

Propane is used as a refrigerant and as an aerosol propellant (p.1198). It is also widely used as a fuel.

◊ Reports of toxicity associated with the abuse or misuse of propane.[1,2]

1. James NK, Moss ALH. Cold injury from liquid propane. BMJ 1989; 299: 950–1.
2. Siegel E, Wason S. Sudden death caused by inhalation of butane and propane. N Engl J Med 1990; 323: 1638.

Preparations

Proprietary Preparations (details are given in Part 3)

Multi-ingredient: Austral.: Histofreezer; Fr.: Histofreezer; UK: Wartner.

Gastrointestinal Drugs

This chapter describes the principal drugs used in the treatment of gastrointestinal disorders, and the choice of treatment for some of the main disorders.

Gastrointestinal Drug Groups

Antacids

Antacids are basic compounds which neutralise hydrochloric acid in the gastric secretions. They are used in the symptomatic management of gastrointestinal disorders associated with gastric hyperacidity such as dyspepsia, gastro-oesophageal reflux disease, and peptic ulcer disease (see below).

Antacids do not reduce the volume of hydrochloric acid secreted and elevation of the gastric pH may actually promote an increase in acid and pepsin secretion. However, this is usually minor and short-lived except after large doses of calcium carbonate. Antacids are normally given between meals and at bedtime when symptoms of gastric hyperacidity usually occur; the presence of food in the stomach can prolong the neutralising activity. Some calculate doses as mEq or mmol of acid-neutralising capacity, but the relationship between neutralising capacity and beneficial effect is not straightforward. Other factors, including formulation (liquid preparations are more effective than solids) and duration of action (relatively insoluble antacids are longer acting) are also important.

Aluminium salts tend to produce constipation and to delay gastric emptying, while magnesium salts have the reverse effect; a combination of the two may reduce adverse gastrointestinal effects. Another advantage of combined antacid formulations is that a slow-acting antacid such as aluminium hydroxide may be combined with a more rapidly acting drug such as magnesium hydroxide to improve the onset and duration of effect. Alternatively, complexes containing both aluminium and magnesium may be used, such as almasilate, hydrotalcite, and magaldrate. Other drugs that may be combined with antacid formulations include simeticone, which acts as a defoaming agent to reduce excess gas in the stomach, and alginates, which form a gel or foam on the surface of the stomach contents thereby impeding reflux and protecting the oesophageal mucosa from acid attack.

Calcium carbonate and sodium bicarbonate are both rapidly acting but have disadvantages: calcium carbonate is usually reserved for short-term treatment because of the risks of rebound acid secretion and metabolic alkalosis, while sodium bicarbonate is absorbed and is contra-indicated in patients who must control sodium intake (e.g. in heart failure, hypertension, renal failure, cirrhosis, or pregnancy).

Antacids may interact with numerous other drugs, affecting the rate and extent of their absorption, and in some cases their renal elimination. Changes in gastric pH affect the dissolution of other drugs, and together with altered gastric emptying can markedly influence absorption. Aluminium compounds in particular are noted for their propensity to adsorb other drugs and to form insoluble complexes that are not absorbed. Antacids that alter urinary pH will affect renal clearance of drugs that are weak acids or bases. Several mechanisms may play a part in any particular interaction. Interactions can be minimised by giving antacids and other medication 2 to 3 hours apart.

Antacids in this chapter include aluminium salts, magnesium salts, and calcium carbonate. For sodium bicarbonate, see p.1186.

Described in this chapter are

Aceglutamide Aluminium, p.1209	Basic Aluminium Carbonate, p.1210
Alexitol Sodium, p.1209	Bismuth Compounds, p.1213
Almagate, p.1209	Calcium Carbonate, p.1215
Almasilate, p.1210	Dihydroxyaluminum Sodium Carbonate, p.1222
Aloglutamol, p.1210	Hydrotalcite, p.1228
Aluminium Glycinate, p.1210	Magaldrate, p.1232
Aluminium Hydroxide, p.1210	Magnesium Carbonate, p.1232
Aluminium Hydroxide-Magnesium Carbonate Co-dried Gel, p.1211	Magnesium Hydroxide, p.1233
Aluminium Phosphate, p.1211	Magnesium Oxide, p.1233
Aluminium Sodium Silicate, p.1211	Magnesium Trisilicate, p.1233

Antidiarrhoeals

Antidiarrhoeals are used as adjuncts in the symptomatic treatment of diarrhoea (see below), although the main aim in the management of *acute* diarrhoea is the correction of fluid and electrolyte depletion with rehydration therapy; this is especially important in infants and young children and antidiarrhoeals are not generally recommended for this age group. Their use is also limited in *chronic* diarrhoea since treatment aimed at the underlying disorder will often alleviate the diarrhoea.

Described in this chapter are drugs which reduce intestinal motility such as the opioid analogues diphenoxylate and loperamide, and adsorbents such as attapulgite and kaolin. Bulking agents (which include bran and ispaghula) have also been used for diarrhoea and for adjusting faecal consistency in patients with colostomies.

Described in this chapter are

Albumin Tannate, p.1209	Ispaghula, p.1229
Attapulgite, p.1212	Kaolin, p.1229
Bismuth Compounds, p.1213	Lidamidine, p.1231
Bran, p.1214	Loperamide, p.1231
Chalk, p.1216	Racecadotril, p.1245
Difenoxin, p.1222	Zaldaride, p.1254
Diphenoxylate, p.1222	

Antiemetics

Antiemetics are a diverse group of drugs used to treat or prevent nausea and vomiting, including that associated with cancer therapy, anaesthesia, and motion sickness (see below).

The choice of drug depends partly on the cause of nausea and vomiting. For example, hyoscine or an antihistamine are used in motion sickness whereas dopamine antagonists (such as metoclopramide and domperidone) and 5-HT_3 antagonists (such as ondansetron) are ineffective. Conversely, nausea and vomiting associated with cancer chemotherapy is often hard to control and special regimens have been devised including the use of metoclopramide in high doses, dexamethasone, and, more recently, the 5-HT_3 antagonists.

Described in this chapter are

Alizapride, p.1209	Ginger, p.1227
Azasetron, p.1212	Granisetron, p.1227
Bromopride, p.1215	Itopride, p.1229
Cerium Oxalate, p.1216	Metoclopramide, p.1235
Clebopride Malate, p.1221	Metopimazine, p.1237
Difenidol, p.1222	Nabilone, p.1237
Dolasetron, p.1223	Ondansetron, p.1241
Domperidone, p.1224	Ramosetron, p.1245
Dronabinol, p.1224	Tropisetron, p.1253

Antisecretory drugs

Antisecretory drugs are used in the treatment and prophylaxis of peptic ulcer disease (below); some are also employed in other disorders associated with gastric hyperacidity such as gastro-oesophageal reflux disease and dyspepsia (below). They may be divided into:

- *Histamine H_2-receptor antagonists* (H_2-antagonists), which act by blocking histamine H_2-receptors on gastric parietal cells, thereby antagonising the normal stimulatory effect of endogenous histamine on gastric acid production. Those described in this chapter include cimetidine, famotidine, nizatidine, and ranitidine.

- *Proton pump inhibitors*, which act by blocking the enzyme system responsible for active transport of protons into the gastrointestinal lumen, namely the hydrogen/potassium adenosine triphosphatase (H^+/K^+ ATPase) of the gastric parietal cell, also known as the 'proton pump'. Those described in this chapter include lansoprazole, omeprazole, pantoprazole, and rabeprazole.

- *Selective antimuscarinics*, which block cholinergic stimulation of gastric acid production with fewer adverse effects than standard antimuscarinics (p.459), but have already largely been superseded. Pirenzepine (p.472) is an example.

- *Prostaglandin analogues*, which inhibit gastric acid secretion by a direct action on the parietal cell and may also inhibit gastrin release and possess cytoprotective properties. Misoprostol (p.1446) is an example.

Described in this chapter are

Cimetidine, p.1216	Omeprazole, p.1239
Ebrotidine, p.1225	Pantoprazole, p.1243
Esomeprazole, p.1225	Rabeprazole, p.1245
Famotidine, p.1225	Ranitidine, p.1245
Lansoprazole, p.1230	Roxatidine, p.1248
Niperotidine, p.1238	Urogastrone, p.1254
Nizatidine, p.1238	

Laxatives

Laxatives (purgatives or cathartics) promote defaecation and are used in the treatment of constipation (below) and for bowel evacuation before investigational procedures, such as endoscopy or radiological examination, or before surgery.

Laxatives are frequently employed for self-medication and may sometimes be abused. Abuse of laxatives is a well-known phenomenon that may occasionally lead to toxicity.

Laxatives may be classified according to their mode of action. There is, however, a degree of overlap between the various groups and in some cases the precise mechanisms of action are not fully understood. Many traditionally used laxatives have fallen from use owing to the violence of their action or their adverse effect profile.

- *Bulk laxatives* (bulk-forming laxatives or bulking agents) cause retention of fluid and an increase in faecal mass resulting in stimulation of peristalsis. Owing to their hydrophilic nature, bulk laxatives may also be used to control diarrhoea and to regulate the consistency of effluent in colostomy patients. Those described in this chapter include bran, ispaghula, and sterculia.

- *Stimulant laxatives* (contact laxatives) act by directly stimulating nerve endings in the colonic mucosa, thereby increasing intestinal motility. It is this group of laxatives which is most commonly associated with abuse. Those described in this chapter include bisacodyl, cascara, phenolphthalein, senna, and sodium picosulfate.

- *Osmotic laxatives* act by increasing intestinal osmotic pressure thereby promoting retention of fluid within the bowel. Those described in this chapter include saline laxatives such as magnesium citrate, magnesium hydroxide, and sodium sulfate (for magnesium sulfate and sodium phosphate see p.1191 and p.1193 respectively). Lactulose may also be classified as an osmotic laxative because its breakdown products exert a similar effect. Also included in this group are the hyperosmotic laxatives such as glycerol (p.1616) and sorbitol (p.1377), and the macrogols (p.1630).

- *Faecal softeners* (emollient laxatives) are claimed to act by decreasing surface tension and increasing penetration of intestinal fluid into the faecal mass. Those described in this chapter include docusate (which is also believed to have a stimulant action).

For the lubricant laxative liquid paraffin see p.1407.

Mucosal protectants

Cytoprotective drugs (mucosal protectants) play a role in the management of peptic ulcer disease (below). They may be divided into:

- *Chelates or complexes*, which coat the gastric mucosa preferentially at sites of ulceration by forming an adherent complex with proteins. Those described in this chapter include sucralfate and tripotassium dicitratobismuthate (which also has an antibacterial role in regimens aimed at eradicating *Helicobacter pylori*).
- *Miscellaneous drugs* include liquorice and its derivatives, such as carbenoxolone, which may act by stimulating the synthesis of protective mucus.

Prokinetic drugs

Prokinetic drugs stimulate the motility of the gastrointestinal tract. Gastrointestinal smooth muscle exhibits intrinsic motor activity which is modified by autonomic innervation, local reflexes, and gastrointestinal hormones. This activity produces peristaltic waves, which move the gut contents from stomach to anus, and segmentations, which encourage digestion. Prokinetic drugs may act at various points within this complex system to enhance gastrointestinal movement. Those described in this chapter include metoclopramide, cisapride, and domperidone. Other drugs with prokinetic properties include parasympathomimetics such as bethanechol (p.1415) or neostigmine (p.1420), and the macrolide antibiotic erythromycin (p.201).

Management of Gastrointestinal Disorders

The management of some gastrointestinal disorders is discussed below.

Aspiration syndromes

Regurgitation and aspiration of gastric contents (Mendelson's syndrome) is an important cause of morbidity and mortality associated with anaesthesia, especially in obstetrics and in emergency surgery. Chemical pneumonitis and respiratory distress result from the acid aspiration, the risk of which is increased by the drugs given as adjuncts to anaesthesia such as opioid analgesics and atropine.

Apart from good anaesthetic technique, including a prohibition on oral intake before elective procedures, efforts to **prevent** or reduce the problem have focussed mainly on increasing the pH of gastric contents to above 2.5, and in reducing gastric volume. However, there is little evidence to show that reduced gastric acidity or volume is associated with decreased morbidity or mortality in pa-

tients who have aspirated gastric contents,[1] and some do not recommend the routine pre-operative use of pharmacological prophylaxis in patients undergoing elective surgery with no apparent increased risk for pulmonary aspiration.[1]

The *H2-antagonists* decrease gastric acid secretion and may decrease gastric fluid volume. However, they do not affect the pH of fluid already in the stomach; they must therefore be given some time before anaesthesia which limits their value in emergency procedures. Cimetidine is considered effective in most patients, although where more prolonged reduction of acidity is required H2-antagonists with a longer duration of action such as ranitidine or famotidine may be preferred. Nizatidine has the advantage of a relatively rapid onset of action.[2] The *proton pump inhibitors*, have also been tried, but results have been variable. Combination with a prokinetic drug may produce better results.[3]

Because of the lack of effect of antisecretory drugs on the pH of existing gastric fluid they may be combined with *antacids* to neutralise gastric acidity. Although magnesium trisilicate has been extensively used[4] without apparent problems particulate antacids are potentially toxic to the lung, which is why soluble antacids such as sodium citrate have been widely used. An effervescent formulation of sodium citrate with cimetidine has been reported to raise gastric pH above 2.5 in more than 98% of patients undergoing caesarean section.[5]

A third component of prophylactic regimens for acid aspiration may be use of a *prokinetic drug* such as metoclopramide. These increase gastric emptying and thereby decrease the volume of stomach contents, and also increase pressure at the lower oesophageal sphincter. The ability of metoclopramide to reverse the effects of opioids on gastric emptying appears to depend on the route of administration: 10 mg given intravenously after opioid analgesia is reported to be effective in promoting gastric emptying, whereas the same dose intramuscularly is not.[6]

If aspiration occurs, pulmonary damage may result within seconds; **treatment** has included removal of any particulate matter, and measures to maintain the airway and ensure adequate oxygenation. Corticosteroids have been used but are no longer considered helpful.[7]

1. American Society of Anesthesiologists Task Force on Preoperative Fasting. Practice guidelines for preoperative fasting and the use of pharmacologic agents to reduce the risk of pulmonary aspiration: application to healthy patients undergoing elective procedures. *Anesthesiology* 1999; **90:** 896–905.
2. Popat MT, *et al.* Comparison of the effects of oral nizatidine and ranitidine on gastric volume and pH in patients undergoing gynaecological laparoscopy. *Anaesthesia* 1991; **46:** 816–19.
3. Orr DA, *et al.* Effects of omeprazole, with and without metoclopramide, in elective obstetric anaesthesia. *Anaesthesia* 1993; **48:** 114–19.
4. Sweeney BL, Wright I. The use of antacids as a prophylaxis against Mendelson's syndrome in the United Kingdom: a survey. *Anaesthesia* 1986; **41:** 419–22.
5. Ormezzano X, *et al.* Aspiration pneumonitis prophylaxis in obstetric anaesthesia: comparison of effervescent cimetidine–sodium citrate mixture and sodium citrate. *Br J Anaesth* 1990; **64:** 503–6.
6. McNeill MJ, *et al.* Effect of iv metoclopramide on gastric emptying after opioid premedication. *Br J Anaesth* 1990; **64:** 450–2.
7. Ryan DW. Pulmonary aspiration: high dose steroids should be abandoned. *BMJ* 1984; **289:** 51.

Constipation

The pattern of normal defaecation is extremely variable.[1] Constipation may be considered to occur if there is a change in that pattern with 2 or more of the following features: a reduced frequency of defaecation, a hardening of the stool, straining on defaecation, or a feeling of incomplete evacuation.[2,3] It is of serious clinical concern when faecal impaction is likely. Constipation can be a symptom of a range of disorders or of drug toxicity[4] and the necessary attention to these underlying causes can resolve it. Constipation can also reflect a change in lifestyle.

An increase in fibre intake, preferably through a high-fibre diet, will help to relieve constipation in the majority of patients[5] without the need for laxatives. Laxatives are often taken unnecessarily and their regular use can lead to problems of abuse, but when dietary modification is difficult or unacceptable a *bulk laxative* may be appropriate.[5,6] The choice of bulk laxative includes bran, ispaghula, methylcellulose and related compounds, psyllium, or sterculia. Bulk laxatives generally have an effect after 1 to 3 days and are of particular value in those with small hard stools; a gradual increase in dose is advisable to avoid flatulence and distention.[1] They may not be the first choice for elderly patients who are frail or immobile

since the resulting soft faeces may result in faecal incontinence.[2,7]

If constipation fails to respond to an increase in fibre intake or use of a bulk laxative, other laxatives should be considered, the choice depending on the clinical condition.[1] For short-term treatment a *stimulant laxative* may be given. Many traditional stimulant laxatives have fallen from use due to adverse effects, and their prolonged use or abuse may irreversibly damage colonic nerves and muscles.[1,6] Provided appropriate stimulant laxatives are used infrequently and at the minimal effective dose, however, they are unlikely to cause significant harm.[6] Commonly used stimulant laxatives include anthraquinone-containing drugs such as senna, and diphenylmethane derivatives such as bisacodyl or sodium picosulfate. Stimulant laxatives have a more rapid onset of action than bulk laxatives, usually proving effective within 6 to 12 hours.[1] Combined preparations are also available, and a combination of senna and fibre has been found to be more effective than lactulose in elderly patients with chronic constipation.[8]

Osmotic laxatives such as magnesium hydroxide and magnesium sulfate have a very rapid action and are also useful for short-term treatment, but the resultant watery stool, urgency, and occasional incontinence may limit their value.[6] Lactulose and sorbitol have a similar, but slower, action, and may be useful for chronic constipation when a bulk-forming agent is unsuitable.[1] Macrogol 3350 or 4000 is also used as an osmotic laxative.

Other laxatives include surfactants such as docusates which are relatively ineffective alone but are often combined with a stimulant laxative,[1] and may be of value in patients with haemorrhoids or anal fissures, or those in whom straining is potentially hazardous (such as the elderly or those with existing cardiovascular disease). Liquid paraffin is no longer recommended owing to its adverse effects, which include anal seepage and the risks of granulomatous disease of the gastrointestinal tract or of lipoid pneumonia on aspiration.[1]

Rectal administration of laxatives using enemas or suppositories is appropriate in patients requiring rapid relief from constipation. Enemas, which usually combine osmotic and stimulant laxatives, are generally easier for patients to retain than suppositories.[1] Phosphate enemas should be used with caution in patients with renal impairment because of the risks of absorption of significant amounts of phosphate.[1] Glycerol may be administered rectally as suppositories to promote faecal evacuation, and usually acts within 15 to 30 minutes; its action is probably due to an osmotic effect although it may have additional stimulant, lubricating, or faecal-softening properties. Bisacodyl suppositories also have a rapid stimulant effect on the bowel.[1]

Faecal impaction is the inability to pass a hard collection of stool, and may result in overflow diarrhoea. Faecal impaction should be treated with a laxative enema and/or manual disimpaction.[1-4] Oral laxatives should not be used because of the risk of colonic perforation.[2] When all stool has been cleared, it is important to institute measures, often including regular laxatives, to prevent constipation and recurrent impaction.[2,3]

1. Bateman DN. Management of constipation. *Prescribers' J* 1991; **31:** 7–15.
2. Romero Y, *et al.* Constipation and fecal incontinence in the elderly population. *Mayo Clin Proc* 1996; **71:** 81–92.
3. Prather CM, Ortiz-Camacho CP. Evaluation and treatment of constipation and fecal impaction in adults. *Mayo Clin Proc* 1998; **73:** 881–7.
4. Moriarty KJ, Irving MH. Constipation. *BMJ* 1992; **304:** 1237–40.
5. Taylor R. Management of constipation 1: high fibre diets work. *BMJ* 1990; **300:** 1063–4.
6. Spiller R. Management of constipation 2: when fibre fails. *BMJ* 1990; **300:** 1064–5.
7. Ardron ME, Main ANH. Management of constipation. *BMJ* 1990; **300:** 1400.
8. Passmore AP, *et al.* Chronic constipation in long stay elderly patients: a comparison of lactulose and a senna-fibre combination. *BMJ* 1993; **307:** 769–71.

Decreased gastrointestinal motility

Decreased gastrointestinal motility may occur in any part of the gastrointestinal tract, with symptoms depending on the site. It is of varying aetiology and often secondary to some other disorder, such as infection, metabolic or electrolyte disturbance (for example in gastroparesis due to diabetic neuropathy—see also p.317), or insult to the gastrointestinal tract (for example, paralytic or adynamic ileus is frequently a consequence of abdominal surgery and is a serious adverse effect of some drugs).

Acute loss of gastrointestinal motility is often self-limiting once the underlying cause has been treated. Provided the ability of gastrointestinal smooth muscle to contract has not been lost, however, prokinetic drugs such as metoclopramide, or domperidone, or erythromycin, or drugs capable of stimulating functional contraction including parasympathomimetics such as neostigmine or bethanechol, may be employed.

Drugs are less successful in chronic conditions such as chronic intestinal pseudo-obstruction where neuromuscular function of the gastrointestinal tract has some intrinsic abnormality.

References.

1. Malagelada J-R, Distrutti E. Management of gastrointestinal motility disorders: a practical guide to drug selection and appropriate ancillary measures. *Drugs* 1996; **52:** 494–506.
2. Luckas M, Buckett W. Acute colonic pseudo-obstruction in the obstetric patient. *Br J Hosp Med* 1997; **57:** 378–81.
3. Mann SD, *et al.* Clinical characteristics of chronic idiopathic intestinal pseudo-obstruction in adults. *Gut* 1997; **41:** 675–81.
4. Laine L. Management of acute colonic pseudo-obstruction. *N Engl J Med* 1999; **341:** 192–3.

Diarrhoea

Diarrhoea is characterised by liquid stools and increased stool weight and frequency of defaecation. Although diarrhoea is commonly associated with infection (see Gastro-enteritis, p.121), it may also result from the accumulation of nonabsorbed osmotically active solutes in the gastrointestinal lumen, such as in lactase deficiency, or from the gastrointestinal effects of secretory stimuli, other than the enterotoxins from an infection. It may also occur when intestinal motility or morphology is altered.

Acute diarrhoea may lead to excessive water and electrolyte loss and dehydration, and is potentially life-threatening in infants; frail and elderly patients are also at risk. Severe dehydration associated with acute diarrhoea (greater than 10% loss of body-weight), requires *intravenous rehydration therapy* preferably with Ringer's lactate solution.[1,2] Intravenous therapy is also needed for patients who are unable to drink. Otherwise, *oral rehydration therapy* to correct fluid and electrolyte depletion forms the basis of treatment for acute diarrhoea[1-6] and an oral rehydration solution containing essential electrolytes (sodium, potassium, chloride, and bicarbonate or citrate) and glucose is indicated regardless of the age of the patient or the cause of the diarrhoea. A rehydration phase, which involves the replenishment of fluid and electrolytes lost through the diarrhoea, is followed by a maintenance phase to replace continuing losses. Oral rehydration therapy does not stop diarrhoea, which usually continues for a limited period. Oral rehydration therapy may need to be modified if the diarrhoea is associated with malnutrition.[7] (Malnourished children may also benefit from zinc supplementation in acute diarrhoea—see p.1399; vitamin A supplementation may also be important in reducing mortality—see p.1383.) The rationale[4] for the composition of oral rehydration solutions is that glucose promotes the active transport of electrolytes, the absorption of which theoretically increases in efficiency as the ratio of carbohydrate to sodium approaches 1:1. WHO recommends a solution containing 90 mmol sodium per litre and 111 mmol of glucose per litre; this type of preparation is used predominantly in developing countries where diarrhoeas are commonly bacterial in origin. Once initial rehydration has been achieved extra water may be added to the preparation to make a solution containing about 60 mmol of sodium per litre for maintenance. In developed countries viral diarrhoeas, which are associated with less electrolyte loss, are more common. Commercial preparations available in the UK therefore usually provide 50 to 60 mmol of sodium per litre and 90 to 111 mmol of glucose per litre; the total osmolarity is slightly hypotonic (about 250 mmol per litre) to prevent possible induction of osmotic diarrhoea.[8] There is now evidence from studies and metaanalyses to suggest that solutions of reduced sodium content and osmolarity may be preferable to conventional WHO solutions, even in developing countries.[9-12] Other areas of debate include the necessity for inclusion of citrate or bicarbonate,[8] and whether cereal-based rather than glucose-based rehydration solutions would be preferable.[13-16] There is considerable evidence that cereal-based solutions tend to produce more rapid resolution of diarrhoea, although one study has suggested that the reduction in stool output is temporary,[17] and another found that a glucose-based solution was equally effective when combined with early re-introduction of feeding.[14] In 1994, a review of clinical trials concluded that a rice-based rehydration solution should be recommended for patients with cholera, but that there was no reason to change from WHO's glucose-based formulation for children with non-cholera diarrhoea,[18] a view confirmed by a recent meta-analysis.[19]

Home remedies[1,2] which have been used for oral rehydration include coconut water, rice water, soups, weak tea, and solutions of various salts and sugars; these may be of value when more conventional oral rehydration solutions are unavailable. The use of cordials and soft drinks with low pH and high osmolality, however, may exacerbate diarrhoea and infant deaths have been associated with their use for rehydration.[20]

Oral rehydration therapy should be combined with *dietary measures*, particularly in children, to avoid malnutrition owing to low food intake during the illness, and as mentioned above, may need to be modified if the diarrhoea is associated with malnutrition. Breast feeding should be continued throughout rehydration therapy.[8,20,21] In the case of cows' milk formula feeds dilution has been advocated because of the possibility of lactose intolerance[22] but is usually not necessary.[23,24] Withholding food during diarrhoea in both adults and children is not recommended:[1,11] feeding may decrease stool output and shorten the duration of diarrhoea.[6]

Oral rehydration therapy prevents dehydration, but does not necessarily shorten the duration of the diarrhoea, and patients therefore frequently desire the symptomatic relief provided by *drug therapy*. Use of such therapy should be balanced against the risk that it may distract from the need for oral rehydration therapy and may have undesirable side-effects. WHO considers that antidiarrhoeal drug therapy is of limited value for acute infectious diarrhoea, does not reduce fluid and electrolyte loss, may delay the expulsion of causative micro-organisms, and should never be used in children.[25] Nevertheless, short courses of antidiarrhoeals are occasionally used if symptoms are causing considerable discomfort.[26] The main groups of antidiarrhoeal drugs are adsorbents such as attapulgite, kaolin, and pectin, and drugs that reduce intestinal motility such as diphenoxylate, loperamide, and codeine. Bulk laxatives such as methylcellulose have also been used for symptomatic treatment because of their absorptive capacity. Bismuth salicylate is another compound used in diarrhoea and is favoured in the USA when antidiarrhoeal therapy is deemed desirable.[26] The calmodulin inhibitor zaldaride has also been investigated.

Antibacterial and antiprotozoal drugs have been used for infective diarrhoeas, including the prophylaxis and treatment of travellers' diarrhoea (see Gastro-enteritis, p.121 and p.583), but their overuse encourages the development of resistance. Prophylactic use should be reserved for adults who are not in good health spending up to 3 weeks in areas where clean food and water cannot be obtained, or when it is important that travel is not interrupted. Vaccines are being developed for the prevention of rotaviral diarrhoeas (p.1562).

Chronic diarrhoea may be associated with underlying disease and therefore symptomatic relief is less appropriate than treatment of the disease itself. For example, colestyramine will reduce the diarrhoea associated with bile acid malabsorption. Where the disease process responsible for chronic diarrhoea cannot be satisfactorily suppressed, however, symptomatic relief may be appropriate, for example in diabetic diarrhoea (see p.317).

1. WHO. *The management and prevention of diarrhoea: practical guidelines.* 3rd ed. Geneva: WHO, 1993.
2. Sack DA. Use of oral rehydration therapy in acute watery diarrhoea: a practical guide. *Drugs* 1991; **41:** 566–73.
3. WHO Diarrhoeal Diseases Control Programme/Fédération Internationale Pharmaceutique. *The treatment of acute diarrhoea: information for pharmacists.* Geneva: (WHO/CDD/SER/87.11).
4. Avery ME, Snyder JD. Oral therapy for acute diarrhea: the underused simple solution. *N Engl J Med* 1990; **323:** 891–4.
5. Balistreri WF. Oral rehydration in acute infantile diarrhoea. *Am J Med* 1990; **88** (suppl 6A): 30S–33S.
6. American Academy of Pediatrics. Practice parameter: the management of acute gastroenteritis in young children. *Pediatrics* 1996; **97:** 424–35.
7. Golden MHN, Briend A. Treatment of malnutrition in refugee camps. *Lancet* 1993; **342:** 360.
8. Murphy MS. Guidelines for managing acute gastroenteritis based on a systematic review of published research. *Arch Dis Child* 1998; **79:** 279–84.
9. International Study Group on Reduced-osmolarity ORS Solutions. Multicentre evaluation of reduced-osmolarity oral rehydration salts solution. *Lancet* 1995; **345:** 282–5.
10. Santosham M, *et al.* A double-blind clinical trial comparing World Health Organization oral rehydration solution with a reduced osmolarity solution containing equal amounts of sodium and glucose. *J Pediatr* 1996; **128:** 45–51.
11. Alam NH, *et al.* Efficacy and safety of oral rehydration solution with reduced osmolarity in adults with cholera: a randomised double-blind clinical trial. *Lancet* 1999; **354:** 296–9.
12. Kim Y, *et al.* Reduced osmolarity oral rehydration solution for treating dehydration caused by acute diarrhoea in children (updated 28 February 2001). Available in The Cochrane Library; Issue 3. Oxford: Update Software; 2001.
13. Gore SM, *et al.* Impact of rice-based oral rehydration solution on stool output and duration of diarrhoea: metaanalysis of 13 clinical trials. *BMJ* 1992; **304:** 287–91.
14. Fayad IM, *et al.* Comparative efficacy of rice-based and glucose-based oral rehydration salts plus early reintroduction of food. *Lancet* 1993; **342:** 772–5.
15. Bang A. Towards better rehydration. *Lancet* 1993; **342:** 755–6.
16. Islam A, *et al.* Is rice-based oral rehydration therapy effective in young infants? *Arch Dis Child* 1994; **71:** 19–23.
17. Molina S, *et al.* Clinical trial of glucose-oral rehydration solution (ORS), rice dextrin-ORS, and rice flour-ORS for the management of children with acute diarrhea and mild or moderate dehydration. *Pediatrics* 1995; **95:** 191–7.
18. Bhan MK, *et al.* Clinical trials of improved oral rehydration salt formulations: a review. *Bull WHO* 1994; **72:** 945–55.
19. Fontaine O, *et al.* Rice-based oral rehydration solution for treating diarrhoea (updated 28 February 2001). Available in The Cochrane Library; Issue 3. Oxford: Update Software; 2001.
20. Elliott EJ. Viral diarrhoeas in childhood. *BMJ* 1992; **305:** 1111–12.
21. Jelliffe DB, Jelliffe EFP. *Dietary management of young children with acute diarrhoea.* 2nd ed. Geneva: WHO, 1991.
22. Kleinman RE. We have the solution: now what's the problem? *Pediatrics* 1992; **90:** 113–15.
23. Chew F, *et al.* Is dilution of cows' milk formula necessary for dietary management of acute diarrhoea in infants aged less than 6 months? *Lancet* 1993; **341:** 194–7.
24. Duggan C, Nurko S. 'Feeding the gut': the scientific basis for continued enteral nutrition during acute diarrhea. *J Pediatr* 1997; **131:** 801–8.
25. WHO. *The rational use of drugs in the management of acute diarrhoea in children.* Geneva: WHO, 1990.
26. Aranda-Michel J, Giannella RA. Acute diarrhea: a practical review. *Am J Med* 1999; **106:** 670–6.

Diverticular disease

Diverticula are small hernias or pouches of mucosa which develop through the muscular wall of the gut (especially the colon) or other hollow organs; they increase in prevalence with increasing age. Diverticular disease (the presence of colonic diverticula) is usually asymptomatic, but may be associated with symptoms of abdominal pain and altered bowel habit (diverticulosis). Occasionally there may be severe life-threatening complications such as inflammation and necrosis of diverticula (diverticulitis), perforation, fistula formation, obstruction, or haemorrhage.

In uncomplicated diverticular disease, treatment is with a high-fibre diet, gradually supplemented if necessary with a bulk laxative such as bran or ispaghula, to ease constipation, but such supplements may not relieve the other symptoms of diverticular disease. Antispasmodics such as antimuscarinics or mebeverine may be useful in relieving pain due to muscle spasm.

Diverticulitis requires treatment with broad-spectrum antibacterials and fluid support; analgesia may be needed for severe pain. If peritonitis or abscess develops, surgical intervention may be necessary. Surgical resection is usually considered when fistula, perforation, or obstruction are present.

References.

1. Jones DJ. Diverticular disease. *BMJ* 1992; **304:** 1435–7.
2. Cook TA, Mortensen NJM. Diverticular disease of the colon. *Prescribers' J* 1997; **37:** 213–19.
3. Ferzoco LB, *et al.* Acute diverticulitis. *N Engl J Med* 1998; **338:** 1521–6.

Dumping syndrome

The word dumping in this context is used to describe the unnaturally rapid transport of gastric contents to the small intestine. The dumping syndrome is an important cause of morbidity following gastrointestinal surgery, and is thought to be due to the destruction of normal regulatory mechanisms in the upper gastrointestinal tract.[1,2] Early dumping begins within 10 to 30 minutes of the ingestion of a meal (typically, symptoms are precipitated by hyperosmolar, carbohydrate-rich food) and comprises gastrointestinal symptoms (fullness, abdominal pain, nausea and vomiting, explosive diarrhoea) and vasomotor symptoms (sweating, weakness, dizziness, flushing, and palpitations). The effects are thought to be due to fluid shifts from the intravascular space to the bowel lumen. Some patients experience late dumping, 1 to 4 hours after a meal, which comprises only the vasomotor symptoms and appears to be due to reactive hypoglycaemia following high carbohydrate concentrations in the small intestine.

The mainstays of therapy are dietary modifications, taking small frequent meals low in carbohydrate, followed by liquids 30 minutes later. Attempts to slow or reduce carbohydrate absorption have involved the use of dietary fibre (guar gum or pectin) or α-glucosidase inhibitors such as acarbose; acarbose and pectin have also been tried in combination.[3] However, such agents may themselves cause gastrointestinal disturbances and they do not seem to be helpful in most patients.[2] More recently, beneficial results with somatostatin have led to the use of its longer-acting analogue, octreotide.[2,4] Octreotide substantially reduces the symptoms of both early and late dumping, probably by slowing gastric emptying and by inhibiting the release of gastrointestinal mediators (peptide hormones such as neurotensin), and prevents hyperinsulinaemia and subsequent reactive hypoglycaemia. It may be given up to 2 hours before a meal.

In the minority of patients who do not respond to medical therapy surgery may be required.[1,2]

1. Eagon JC, et al. Postgastrectomy syndromes. Surg Clin North Am 1992; 72: 445–65.
2. Carvajal SH, Mulvihill SJ. Postgastrectomy syndromes: dumping and diarrhea. Gastroenterol Clin North Am 1994; 23: 261–79.
3. Speth PAJ, et al. Effect of acarbose, pectin, a combination of acarbose with pectin, and placebo on postprandial reactive hypoglycaemia after gastric surgery. Gut 1983; 24: 799–802.
4. Li-Ling J, Irving M. Therapeutic value of octreotide for patients with severe dumping syndrome—a review of randomised controlled trials. Postgrad Med J 2001; 77: 441–2.

Dyspepsia

Dyspepsia, also commonly known as indigestion, is a frequent but ill-defined disorder primarily associated with epigastric discomfort or pain. It may be a symptom of specific diseases such as peptic ulcer disease, gastro-oesophageal reflux disease, gastric carcinoma, chronic pancreatitis, or gallstones. However, in many patients there is no identifiable systemic disease, in which case it is known as non-ulcer dyspepsia or functional dyspepsia.

A number of reviews and recommendations have addressed the subject of dyspepsia,[1-5] but despite the frequency with which the disorder occurs, definitive treatment guidelines have yet to be established. The initial management of non-ulcer dyspepsia usually includes advice to avoid alcohol, smoking, and aggravating foods, and to eat small regular meals to aid digestion. Results of studies of drugs for non-ulcer dyspepsia have been variable and difficult to evaluate since the condition tends to be self-limiting, and there is often a large placebo response.

Drugs to suppress gastric acid such as antacids or histamine H2-antagonists are commonly tried. Antacids may give some symptomatic relief, and are widely used for self-medication. Similarly, H2-antagonists are often tried, especially for symptoms of reflux, although studies in non-ulcer dyspepsia have been largely disappointing. Most authorities consider that a short course of drug therapy may be given to younger patients (under 40 to 45 years of age) lacking obvious symptoms of organic disease before any investigation needs to be performed. However, the use of H2-antagonists can mask the symptoms of gastric carcinoma, and in older patients who are at greater risk, early investigation may be desirable.

Alternatively, prokinetic drugs such as metoclopramide may be given, particularly if an underlying gastrointestinal motility disorder is suspected. Meta-analysis has suggested that prokinetic therapy may be more effective than an H2-antagonist in non-ulcer dyspepsia.[6] Other approaches to drug therapy include the use of an insoluble bismuth salt, and the administration of antimuscarinics to relieve spasm. It is not clear whether Helicobacter pylori plays any role in the pathology of non-ulcer dyspepsia, but eradication in H. pylori-positive patients has been suggested on the grounds that it will benefit patients with undiagnosed peptic ulcer disease and reduce the need for endoscopy.[3] An analysis of five H. pylori-eradication trials suggested a modest improvement in symptoms in patients with non-ulcer dyspepsia.[7] Although a subsequent study found no evidence of benefit from H. pylori eradication,[8] others have suggested that response to omeprazole may be greater in H. pylori-positive patients.[9] Meta-analyses have come to opposite conclusions regarding the benefits of eradication.[10,11]

1. Holtmann G, Talley NJ. Functional dyspepsia: current treatment recommendations. Drugs 1993; 45: 918–30.
2. Whitaker MJ, et al. Controversy and consensus in the management of upper gastrointestinal disease in primary care. Int J Clin Pract 1997; 51: 239–43.
3. Agréus L, Talley N. Challenges in managing dyspepsia in general practice. BMJ 1997; 315: 1284–8.
4. Fisher RS, Parkman HP. Management of nonulcer dyspepsia. N Engl J Med 1998; 339: 1376–81.
5. Locke GR. Nonulcer dyspepsia: what it is and what it is not. Mayo Clin Proc 1999; 74: 1011–15.
6. Finney JS, et al. Meta-analysis of antisecretory and gastrokinetic compounds in functional dyspepsia. J Clin Gastroenterol 1998; 26: 312–20.
7. Jaakkimainen RL, et al. Is Helicobacter pylori associated with non-ulcer dyspepsia and will eradication improve symptoms? A meta-analysis. BMJ 1999; 319: 1040–4.

8. Talley NJ, et al. Absence of benefit of eradicating Helicobacter pylori in patients with nonulcer dyspepsia. N Engl J Med 1999; 341: 1106–11.
9. Blum AL, et al. Short course acid suppressive treatment for patients with functional dyspepsia: results depend on Helicobacter pylori status. Gut 2000; 47: 473–80.
10. Moayyedi P, et al. Eradication of Helicobacter pylori for non-ulcer dyspepsia (updated 21 November 2000). Available in The Cochrane Library; Issue 3. Oxford: Update Software; 2001.
11. Laine L, et al. Therapy for Helicobacter pylori in patients with nonulcer dyspepsia: a meta-analysis of randomized, controlled trials. Ann Intern Med 2001; 134: 361–9.

Gastrointestinal spasm

Pain or discomfort of the gastrointestinal tract may be associated with spasm of the smooth muscle of the gut; such pain and spasm may be associated with the irritable bowel syndrome (below), dyspepsia (above), or diverticular disease (above). Antispasmodic drugs have traditionally been used in patients thought to have gastrointestinal spasm, and have mainly been of two types: antimuscarinics such as dicyclomine [dicycloverine], and direct smooth muscle relaxants such as mebeverine; use of antimuscarinics, in particular, has tended to be limited by concern about their adverse effects.

Colic is a general term used to describe spasmodic or griping pain, usually of the viscera, and when not otherwise qualified is often understood to refer to pain in the gastrointestinal tract. Infant colic is common in the first few months of childhood,[1] and tends to be managed by nonpharmacological measures and assessment of the feeding technique. Elimination of cows' milk protein appears to be of benefit, but use of a low-lactose formula is not.[1] There is no evidence to support the use of tilactase to aid lactose digestion. Traditional remedies such as gripe water, which contains essential oils of dill or fennel and is mildly carminative, are of dubious efficacy. Antimuscarinic antispasmodics, although effective[1] may be associated with adverse effects, and are no longer considered appropriate. Simeticone suspension, given before feeds, is commonly used, but has been found to be no better than a placebo.[2] It has been reported that sucrose, given as a 12% solution, improves infant colic.[3]

1. Lucassen PLBJ, et al. Effectiveness of treatments for infantile colic: systematic review. BMJ 1998; 316: 1563–9.
2. Metcalf TJ, et al. Simethicone in the treatment of infant colic: a randomized, placebo-controlled, multicenter trial. Pediatrics 1994; 94: 29–34.
3. Markestad T. Use of sucrose as a treatment for infant colic. Arch Dis Child 1997; 76: 356–8.

Gastro-oesophageal reflux disease

Gastro-oesophageal reflux disease results from the reflux of gastric or duodenal contents into the oesophagus. Symptoms include heartburn, acid regurgitation, and dysphagia (difficulty in swallowing); oesophageal inflammation and ulceration (reflux oesophagitis), and stricture formation may occur. Protracted reflux over several years can lead to the development of Barrett's oesophagus (columnar epithelial metaplasia) which is a risk factor for malignancy.

In the management of gastro-oesophageal reflux disease, lifestyle measures including avoidance of alcohol and aggravating foods such as chocolate and coffee can reduce symptoms.[1-5] Raising the head of the bed for patients with nocturnal symptoms,[4] and avoiding lying down within 2 to 3 hours of a meal may be useful.[1,3] Cessation of smoking does not appear to alter reflux symptoms.[4] Withdrawing drugs that reduce gastro-oesophageal sphincter tone and hence exacerbate reflux may be considered:[3] such drugs include theophylline, and antimuscarinics.

Antacids are used for mild disease and as adjuncts to other therapies. Alginate-containing antacids are said to form an alkaline 'raft' that floats on the surface of the stomach contents to impede reflux and protect the oesophageal mucosa; they are more effective than simple antacids for symptomatic relief.[3]

Should more vigorous therapy be needed suppression of gastric acid secretion is a likely next step. In the first instance, particularly in patients with mild oesophagitis, this may be with a histamine H2-antagonist such as cimetidine or ranitidine.[1,2] Although H2-antagonists have been found to relieve symptoms and reduce antacid consumption, rates of oesophageal healing depend on the severity of the disease and duration of therapy. There do not appear to be useful gains in efficacy from doubling the standard dose of H2-antagonists,[4] but use of divided doses may possibly be of additional benefit.[4,5] Alternatively, a prokinetic drug such as metoclopramide may improve gastro-oesophageal sphincter function and accelerate gastric emptying. These appear to be as effective as H2-

antagonists. The combination of an H2-antagonist and cisapride may be more effective than either drug alone.[4] However, concern over the risk of cardiotoxicity and potential for serious interactions with cisapride has led to severe restrictions on its use.

A better alternative for resistant disease, or for initial therapy in patients with moderate or severe disease, may be treatment with a proton pump inhibitor such as omeprazole or lansoprazole. Proton pump inhibitors are more effective than H2-antagonists in terms of both rate and extent of reduction in symptoms and healing of oesophagitis.[6] Consequently, some advocate the use of proton pump inhibitors as first-line drugs even in mild disease, using a step-down approach after successful therapy.[4]

In patients with mild disease, a trial of withdrawal of drug therapy is appropriate after successful initial drug therapy.[4] Short courses of therapy as and when symptoms demand (intermittent treatment) may be effective in uncomplicated disease.[7] However, in patients with severe oesophagitis, long-term maintenance therapy is likely to be required.[4] Maintenance with H2-antagonists has generally been disappointing although some patients respond. A proton pump inhibitor is more effective. Another approach is to use a combination for maintenance and in one study omeprazole with cisapride provided more effective maintenance than ranitidine or cisapride alone or in combination.[8] Again, however, cisapride is now unlikely to be used in practice because of the risks.

Eradication of Helicobacter pylori infection does not heal or prevent relapse of gastro-oesophageal reflux disease.[4] However, eradication of H. pylori has been suggested on the basis that treatment with proton pump inhibitors is associated with worsening of gastritis in H. pylori-infected patients. Conversely, epidemiological evidence suggests that H. pylori infection protects against gastro-oesophageal reflux disease.[9]

In patients who have a poor response to drug therapy, or in those with complications such as oesophageal stricture or ulceration, surgery to re-establish gastro-oesophageal competence may be considered.[4] Elimination of acid reflux by surgery or proton pump inhibitors has at best modest effects on metaplasia in Barrett's oesophagus.[10] Consequently combining acid suppression with thermal ablation or photodynamic therapy (5-aminolaevulinic acid or porfimer) is being investigated.[10]

In infants, gastro-oesophageal reflux is common but usually resolves spontaneously with increasing age and requires no treatment. Occasionally, it may be associated with complications such as failure to thrive, oesophagitis, and pulmonary symptoms of acid regurgitation but may be managed by upright positioning and the use of thickened foods; drug therapy is controversial. It has been suggested that where drug therapy is needed, an alginate-antacid combination may be appropriate initially, and if necessary cisapride to improve gastric motility.[11] Some favour the combination of cisapride with an antisecretory drug.[12] However, the risk of cardiotoxicity makes the use of cisapride in infants extremely problematic (see p.1220).

Gastro-oesophageal reflux is commonly encountered during normal pregnancy, and is generally managed by lifestyle and dietary modifications.[13] If drug therapy is required, nonsystemically absorbed antacids and sucralfate should be tried first. If these are ineffective, ranitidine may be tried.[13] Proton pump inhibitors are not recommended during pregnancy; if one must be used for severe or intractable symptoms lansoprazole may be considered.[13]

1. Klinkenberg-Knol EC, et al. Pharmacological management of gastro-oesophageal reflux. Drugs 1995; 49: 695–710.
2. Anonymous. The medical management of gastro-oesophageal reflux. Drug Ther Bull 1996; 34: 1–4.
3. Galmiche JP, et al. Treatment of gastro-oesophageal reflux disease in adults. BMJ 1998; 316: 1720–3.
4. Dent J, et al. An evidence-based appraisal of reflux disease management—the Genval Workshop Report. Gut 1999; 44 (Suppl 2): S1–S16.
5. De Vault KR, et al. Updated guidelines for the diagnosis and treatment of gastroesophageal reflux disease. Am J Gastroenterol 1999; 94: 1434–42.
6. Chiba N, et al. Speed of healing and symptom relief in grade II to IV gastroesophageal reflux disease: a meta-analysis. Gastroenterology 1997; 112: 1798–810.
7. Bardhan KD, et al. Symptomatic gastro-oesophageal reflux disease: double blind controlled study of intermittent treatment with omeprazole or ranitidine. BMJ 1999; 318: 502–7.
8. Vigneri S, et al. A comparison of five maintenance therapies for reflux esophagitis. N Engl J Med 1995; 333: 1106–10.
9. Labenz J, Malfertheiner P. Helicobacter pylori in gastro-oesophageal reflux disease: causal agent, independent or protective factor? Gut 1997; 41: 277–80.
10. Cameron AJ. Management of Barrett's esophagus. Mayo Clin Proc 1998; 73: 457–61.

11. Anonymous. Managing childhood gastro-oesophageal reflux. *Drug Ther Bull* 1997; **35:** 77–80.
12. Faubion WA, Zein NN. Gastroesophageal reflux in infants and children. *Mayo Clin Proc* 1998; **73:** 166–73.
13. Broussard CN, Richter JE. Treating gastro-oesophageal reflux disease during pregnancy and lactation: what are the safest therapy options? *Drug Safety* 1998; **19:** 325–37.

Haemorrhoids

Haemorrhoids ('piles') are venous swellings of the tissues around the anus: those above the dentate line (the point where the modified skin of the outer anal canal becomes gut epithelium), which usually protrude into the anal canal, are termed internal haemorrhoids, while those below this point are called external haemorrhoids. Due to internal pressure, internal haemorrhoids tend to congest, bleed, and eventually prolapse; with external haemorrhoids painful thrombosis may develop.

Initial treatment of internal haemorrhoids involves a high-fibre diet and avoidance of straining at stool, so bulk laxatives and faecal softeners may be indicated. Small bleeding haemorrhoids may be injected with a sclerosing agent such as oily phenol injection, but rubber band ligation, or perhaps a technique such as infra-red coagulation, is more effective and associated with fewer complications.[1,2] More severe and prolonged prolapse generally requires surgery. Surgical excision to remove the clot is used for thrombosed external haemorrhoids.

An enormous range of mainly topical drug treatments is available for symptomatic relief, but in many cases their value is at best unproven.

Topical preparations are usually made up in a lubricating or emollient base. Local anaesthetics may be included to relieve pain, and corticosteroids may be used where infection is not present: preparations containing either group of drugs are intended only for short-term use. Inclusion of antibacterials is thought to be of little value and may encourage the development of resistant organisms. Some preparations include heparinoids. Other agents frequently included for their soothing properties include various bismuth salts, zinc oxide, hamamelis, resorcinol, and peru balsam.

Bioflavonoids and various derivatives of aesculus may also be included in topical preparations; they have also been given systemically in some countries as have some other compounds such as calcium dobesilate and tribenoside, presumably for their supposed action on venous capillary walls.

Other agents which have been employed in the treatment of haemorrhoids include pilewort (ficaria) and combinations of yeast extract with shark-liver oil.

1. Johanson JF, Rimm A. Optimal nonsurgical treatment of hemorrhoids: a comparative analysis of infrared coagulation, rubber band ligation, and injection sclerotherapy. *Am J Gastroenterol* 1992; **87:** 1601–6.
2. MacRae HM, McLeod RS. Comparison of hemorrhoidal treatment modalities: a meta-analysis. *Dis Colon Rectum* 1995; **38:** 687–94.

Hepatic encephalopathy

Hepatic encephalopathy (portal systemic encephalopathy) is a metabolically related dysfunction of the brain associated with abnormalities of liver function. It may be acute, as in patients with fulminant hepatic failure, or chronic, with acute episodes precipitated by some triggering factor, as in patients with cirrhosis or other chronic liver disease.

Treatment is aimed at identifying any precipitating factor and correcting it, decreasing the production and absorption of ammonia in the gut, and increasing metabolism of ammonia in the tissues. Precipitating factors include infection, increased protein load due to gastrointestinal haemorrhage or high protein intake, alcohol abuse, electrolyte imbalance, and certain drugs (notably anxiolytics, hypnotics, and diuretics).

Restriction of dietary protein intake is a mainstay of short-term treatment, but in the long-term, care must be taken to provide adequate protein to avoid malnutrition. A daily protein intake of 0.5 to 1.5 g per kg body-weight has been recommended.[1] There is some evidence that vegetable protein is better tolerated than animal protein.[2] The administration of branched-chain amino acids (valine, isoleucine, and leucine) by infusion or as dietary supplements may facilitate adequate protein intake in some patients.[1,2] Supplementation with ornithine aspartate has been used to increase metabolic conversion of ammonia to urea and glutamine.[2] Sodium benzoate has also been tried.[2]

Active drug treatment is generally initiated with bowel cleansing by means of a magnesium sulfate enema, espe-cially if the patient is constipated. Lactulose is subsequently the treatment of choice in many cases, particularly in the elderly, the constipated, and those with renal impairment. It reduces colonic pH and absorption of ammonia and aromatic amino acids. The lactulose analogue lactitol is also effective,[3] and is reportedly more palatable than lactulose. Alternatively, locally active antibacterials have been given to reduce the urease-producing bacteria. Neomycin is the traditional drug but adverse effects such as ototoxicity and nephrotoxicity may be a problem, particularly if used long-term. Metronidazole is also used,[2] and rifaximin has been tried. A combination of lactulose and neomycin[2] or metronidazole has been tried in patients who fail to respond to single-drug therapy. Another approach which has been tried, apparently with some success, in low grade chronic recurrent encephalopathy, is the oral ingestion of *Enterococcus faecium* SF68, in an attempt to produce a more favourable bowel flora.[4] *Helicobacter pylori* is a urease-producing organism, but the relevance of *H. pylori* infection to hepatic encephalopathy is unclear.[5]

Investigational therapy has also attempted to affect cerebral function directly. Flumazenil, a benzodiazepine antagonist, has been tried (on the basis of the suspected role of endogenous benzodiazepine-like agonists[6]) but improvements have been modest.[2] Liver transplantation (p.504) is the ultimate therapy for end-stage cirrhosis, acute liver failure, or patients with severe refractory hepatic encephalopathy.[2]

1. Plauth M, *et al.* ESPEN guidelines for nutrition in liver disease and transplantation. *Clin Nutr* 1997; **16:** 43–55.
2. Riordan SM, Williams R. Treatment of hepatic encephalopathy. *N Engl J Med* 1997; **337:** 473–9.
3. Cammà C, *et al.* Lactitol in treatment of chronic hepatic encephalopathy: a meta-analysis. *Dig Dis Sci* 1993; **38:** 916–22.
4. Loguercio C, *et al.* Long-term effects of Enterococcus faecium SF68 versus lactulose in the treatment of patients with cirrhosis and grade 1-2 hepatic encephalopathy. *J Hepatol* 1995; **23:** 39–46.
5. Taylor-Robinson SD, *et al.* Helicobacter pylori, ammonia and the brain. *Gut* 1997; **40:** 805–6.
6. Basile AS, *et al.* The pathogenesis and treatment of hepatic encephalopathy: evidence for the involvement of benzodiazepine receptor ligands. *Pharmacol Rev* 1991; **43:** 27–71.

Inflammatory bowel disease

Inflammatory bowel disease covers chronic non-specific inflammatory conditions of the gastrointestinal tract, of which the two major forms are **Crohn's disease** and **ulcerative colitis.**

Crohn's disease is characterised by thickened areas of the gastrointestinal wall, with inflammation extending through all layers, deep ulceration and fissuring of the mucosa, and the presence of granulomas; affected areas may occur in any part of the gastrointestinal tract, interspersed with areas of relatively normal tissue; the terminal ileum is frequently involved. Symptoms depend on the site of disease but may include abdominal pain, diarrhoea, fever, weight loss, and rectal bleeding. Extra-intestinal manifestations may include joint inflammation, skin lesions, mouth ulcers, and liver disorders.

In ulcerative colitis, disease is confined to the colon and rectum, inflammation is superficial but continuous over the affected area, and granulomas are rare. In mild disease, the rectum alone may be affected (proctitis); in severe disease, ulceration is extensive and much of the mucosa may be lost, with an increased risk of toxic dilatation of the colon, a potentially life-threatening complication. Symptoms include diarrhoea and rectal bleeding. The extra-intestinal manifestations are similar to those of Crohn's disease.

Although there are important differences between Crohn's disease and ulcerative colitis which affect their management, the broad principles of treatment, and the drugs used, are similar.[1-7] A corticosteroid is generally the first choice in active disease, dosage and route varying with disease site and severity. The aminosalicylate derivatives may be used to treat mild active disease, but are of particular value for maintenance treatment of ulcerative colitis; the role of maintenance treatment in Crohn's disease is less well established. Immunosuppressant therapy may be helpful in chronic active disease. For Crohn's disease an elemental diet (see p.1350) may have some value in active disease, but diet plays a lesser role in ulcerative colitis.

Active disease.

The major group of drugs used to induce remission in moderate to severe *active ulcerative colitis* and *Crohn's disease* (including ileal disease) is the **corticosteroids**. Oral prednisolone or prednisone is often used; in the most severe cases hydrocortisone or methylprednisolone may be given intravenously. Dosage is high initially, and is reduced gradually as symptoms improve, but adverse effects remain a problem, hence the interest in poorly absorbed or rapidly metabolised corticosteroids such as beclometasone, budesonide, or tixocortol. Oral budesonide is effective in inducing remission in Crohn's disease,[8-11] and is probably comparable in effect to conventional corticosteroids;[11] although some suggest that it may be slightly less effective,[10] adverse effects are reduced. It appears to be more effective than the 5-aminosalicylate mesalazine in inducing remission of Crohn's disease affecting the ileum and/or colon.[12]

In patients with disease confined to the *distal colon* or *rectum*, local topical therapy may be appropriate. Suppositories of prednisolone or mesalazine may be suitable in *mild proctitis*. However, *proctocolitis* involving more of the distal colon is usually treated with enemas of corticosteroids or of mesalazine. Meta-analysis has suggested that rectal mesalazine is more effective than rectal corticosteroids in the management of distal ulcerative colitis.[13] Combined oral and rectal mesalazine may be more effective for ulcerative colitis than either alone.[14,15] Systemic corticosteroids are reserved for patients who fail to respond to topical therapy.

Oral sulfasalazine, a **5-aminosalicylate** derivative (5-aminosalicylic acid linked to sulfapyridine), is of value in producing remission of mild ulcerative colitis and in Crohn's disease affecting the colon, but has produced equivocal results in Crohn's ileitis.[16-18]

The discovery that 5-aminosalicylate was the active component of sulfasalazine led to the development of numerous derivatives, including mesalazine (5-aminosalicylic acid itself in slow-release or enteric-coated form), olsalazine (2 molecules of 5-aminosalicylic acid joined by an azo bond), and a variety of forms in which the active moiety was joined to inert carriers, such as balsalazide. All the above have been shown to be effective in *active ulcerative colitis*, and may be better tolerated than sulfasalazine, since many of the latter's adverse effects are due to its sulfonamide portion. However, in patients who can tolerate sulfasalazine, the newer drugs have no clinical advantage for remission induction.[18] Nevertheless, the risk of adverse effects on starting treatment with sulfasalazine has led to increasing use of the newer derivatives.

Other drugs used in active inflammatory bowel disease include **immunosuppressants**. The majority of studies have been with azathioprine, or its metabolite mercaptopurine. Because they have a slow onset of action (months) their use in acute disease is limited, but they are of benefit in remission induction in patients with chronically active disease, particularly corticosteroid-resistant or corticosteroid-dependent disease. Low-dose methotrexate also appears to be useful in active Crohn's disease, and probably in ulcerative colitis. Conversely, ciclosporin has not generally proved useful in chronically active inflammatory bowel disease but may have some value in the short-term treatment of acute severe ulcerative colitis. Infliximab, the monoclonal antibody to tumour necrosis factor, is effective in active Crohn's disease refractory to other treatments, especially in fistulising Crohn's disease. Thalidomide, a tumour necrosis factor inhibitor, has also been tried in Crohn's disease with some benefit,[19] but another such inhibitor, oxpentifylline [pentoxifylline], was ineffective.[20]

Metronidazole is useful in *perineal Crohn's disease* and may be used in colonic Crohn's disease. It is usually given for 3 months. Ciprofloxacin is an alternative, and has also been given with metronidazole,[21] although the combination is not very well tolerated. Antibacterials do not have a role in ulcerative colitis, except for infection prophylaxis in severe attacks.

A wide variety of **other drugs** are or have been tried in inflammatory bowel disease, including immunoglobulins, some interleukins, interferons, ICAM-antisense oligonucleotides, short-chain fatty acids, heparin, factor XI-II, omega-3 triglycerides (fish oils), and aminosalicylic acid (4-aminosalicylic acid as opposed to 5-aminosalicylic acid). Nicotine has been tried, based on the observation that ulcerative colitis is rare in smokers. Studies have suggested that nicotine, supplied via transdermal patch, may have benefit in active disease, although it is ineffective for maintenance.[22] Rectal and oral formulations of nicotine are under investigation. Correction of nutritional deficiencies may be necessary in severe disease. In Crohn's disease, enteral feeding, often with an elemental diet is effective in inducing remission (p.1350), but corticosteroids are more effective.[23] Elemental diets are useful in children and those unable to tolerate corticosteroids.

Maintenance of remission.

Treatment in patients who achieve remission depends on disease type. The 5-aminosalicylates are of value in the maintenance of remission in *ulcerative colitis* and are widely used for this purpose; sulfasalazine may be more effective than other aminosalicylates. One study found that treatment with non-pathogenic *Escherichia coli* was equivalent to mesalazine in maintaining remission in ulcerative colitis.[25] Maintenance therapy for *Crohn's disease* is less well established.[26,27] Aminosalicylate maintenance is less effective in Crohn's disease than ulcerative colitis, but may still be considered, particularly to reduce postsurgical recurrence;[28] most studies have used mesalazine. Metronidazole may also reduce postsurgical recurrence. It is generally agreed that conventional corticosteroids have no role in the maintenance of remission of either ulcerative colitis or Crohn's disease,[29] although there is limited evidence that budesonide may modestly prolong the time to relapse in patients with Crohn's disease.[30,31] Azathioprine and mercaptopurine are used for maintenance treatment in Crohn's disease. Once the disease has been in remission for 4 years it may be possible to withdraw therapy.[32] Ciclosporin has not proved effective in maintaining remission of Crohn's disease. There has been interest in the possible role of *Mycobacterium paratuberculosis* in Crohn's disease, but there is currently insufficient evidence to support the use of antituberculous therapy for maintenance therapy.[33] A controlled diet, excluding foods that precipitated symptoms, has been reported to maintain remission in patients with Crohn's disease brought to remission by an elemental diet.[34] Unlike patients with ulcerative colitis (see above) those with Crohn's disease may have an increased risk of relapse if they smoke and should be particularly encouraged to stop.

Surgery.

In patients with ulcerative colitis in whom medical therapy is inadequate surgical colectomy is curative, and may avoid the risks of long-term corticosteroid therapy and the increased risk of bowel cancer to which patients with inflammatory bowel disease are subject. Formation of an ileoanal pouch, which acts as a reservoir for the ileal contents, avoids the necessity for a standard ileostomy and maintains a degree of continence in suitable patients. Curative surgery is not possible in Crohn's disease, since recurrence elsewhere in the gut is almost inevitable, but resection of the affected area becomes necessary in many patients during the course of their illness.

1. Hanauer SB. Inflammatory bowel disease. *N Engl J Med* 1996; **334:** 841–8.
2. Gross V, *et al.* Low dose oral pH modified release budesonide for maintenance of steroid induced remission in Crohn's disease. *Gut* 1998; **42:** 493–6.
3. Kornbluth A, Sachar DB. Ulcerative colitis practice guidelines in adults. *Am J Gastroenterol* 1997; **92:** 204–11.
4. Rampton DS. Ulcerative colitis. *Prescribers' J* 1997; **37:** 220–31.
5. Rhodes JM. Crohn's disease. *Prescribers' J* 1997; **37:** 232–42.
6. Stein RB, Hanauer SB. Medical therapy for inflammatory bowel disease. *Gastroenterol Clin North Am* 1999; **28:** 297–321.
7. Rampton DS. Management of Crohn's disease. *BMJ* 1999; **319:** 1480–85.
8. Greenberg GR, *et al.* Oral budesonide for active Crohn's disease. *N Engl J Med* 1994; **331:** 836–41.
9. Rutgeerts P, *et al.* A comparison of budesonide with prednisolone for active Crohn's disease. *N Engl J Med* 1994; **331:** 842–5.
10. Anonymous. Controlled-release budesonide in Crohn's disease. *Drug Ther Bull* 1997; **35:** 30–1.
11. Campieri M, *et al.* Oral budesonide is as effective as oral prednisolone in active Crohn's disease. *Gut* 1997; **41:** 209–14.
12. Thomsen OØ, *et al.* A comparison of budesonide and mesalamine for active Crohn's disease. *N Engl J Med* 1998; **339:** 370–4.
13. Marshall JK, Irvine EJ. Rectal corticosteroids versus alternative treatments in ulcerative colitis: a meta-analysis. *Gut* 1997; **40:** 775–81.
14. d'Albasio G, *et al.* Combined therapy with 5-aminosalicylic acid tablets and enemas for maintaining remission in ulcerative colitis: a randomized double-blind study. *Am J Gastroenterol* 1997; **92:** 1143–7.
15. Safdi M, *et al.* A double-blind comparison of oral versus rectal mesalamine versus combination therapy in the treatment of distal ulcerative colitis. *Am J Gastroenterol* 1997; **92:** 1867–71.
16. Summers RW, *et al.* National cooperative Crohn's disease study: results of drug treatment. *Gastroenterology* 1979; **77:** 847–69.
17. Malchow H, *et al.* European cooperative Crohn's disease study (ECCDS): results of drug treatment. *Gastroenterology* 1984; **86:** 249–66.
18. Sutherland LR, *et al.* Oral 5-aminosalicylic acid for inducing remission in ulcerative colitis (updated 24 September 1999). Available in The Cochrane Library; Issue 3. Oxford: Update Software; 2001.
19. Sands BE, Podolsky DK. New life in a sleeper: thalidomide and Crohn's disease. *Gastroenterology* 1999; **117:** 1485–98.
20. Bauditz J, *et al.* Treatment with tumour necrosis factor inhibitor oxpentifylline does not improve corticosteroid dependent chronic active Crohn's disease. *Gut* 1997; **40:** 470–4.
21. Prantera C, *et al.* An antibiotic regimen for the treatment of active Crohn's disease: a randomized, controlled clinical trial of metronidazole plus ciprofloxacin. *Am J Gastroenterol* 1996; **91:** 328–32.
22. Guslandi M. Nicotine treatment for ulcerative colitis. *Br J Clin Pharmacol* 1999; **48:** 481–4.
23. Zachos M, *et al.* Enteral nutritional therapy for inducing remission of Crohn's disease (updated 25 May 2001). Available in The Cochrane Library; Issue 3. Oxford: Update Software; 2001.
24. Sutherland L, *et al.* Oral 5-aminosalicylic acid for maintaining remission in ulcerative colitis (updated 23 November 1998). Available in The Cochrane Library; Issue 3. Oxford: Update Software; 2001.
25. Rembacken BJ, *et al.* Non-pathogenic Escherichia coli versus mesalazine for the treatment of ulcerative colitis: a randomised trial. *Lancet* 1999; **354:** 635–9.
26. Stark ME, Tremaine WJ. Maintenance of symptomatic remission in patients with Crohn's disease. *Mayo Clin Proc* 1993; **68:** 1183–90.
27. Greenberger NJ, Miner PB. Is maintenance therapy effective in Crohn's disease? *Lancet* 1994; **344:** 900–1.
28. Cammà C, *et al.* Mesalamine in the maintenance treatment of Crohn's disease: a meta-analysis adjusted for confounding variables. *Gastroenterology* 1997; **113:** 1465–73.
29. Steinhart AH, *et al.* Corticosteroids for maintaining remission of Crohn's disease (updated 30 May 2001). Available in The Cochrane Library; Issue 3. Oxford: Update Software; 2001.
30. Löfberg R, *et al.* Budesonide prolongs time to relapse in ileal and ileocaecal Crohn's disease: a placebo controlled one year study. *Gut* 1996; **39:** 82–6.
31. Greenberg GR, *et al.* Oral budesonide as maintenance treatment for Crohn's disease: a placebo-controlled, dose-ranging study. *Gastroenterology* 1996; **110:** 45–51.
32. Bouhnik Y, *et al.* Long-term follow-up of patients with Crohn's disease treated with azathioprine or 6-mercaptopurine. *Lancet* 1996; **347:** 215–19.
33. Borgaonkar M, *et al.* Anti-tuberculous therapy for maintaining remission of Crohn's disease (updated 24 February 1999). Available in The Cochrane Library; Issue 3. Oxford: Update Software; 2001.
34. Riordan AM, *et al.* Treatment of active Crohn's disease by exclusion diet: East Anglian Multicentre Controlled Trial. *Lancet* 1993; **342:** 1131–4.

Irritable bowel syndrome

Irritable bowel syndrome is a functional gastrointestinal disorder of abdominal pain and altered bowel habit; pain is characteristically relieved by defaecation and may be associated with increase or decrease in stool frequency. There may be abdominal bloating. The value of drug therapy is difficult to demonstrate, given the heterogeneity of symptoms and the high rate of response to placebo.[1] Primary treatment comprises counselling and when necessary dietary modification; short-term drug therapy may bring some benefit if directed at individual symptoms,[1-6] as follows:

• in patients in whom *diarrhoea* is predominant, loperamide may be considered; it is preferred to other opioid antidiarrhoeal drugs because it does not pass the blood-brain barrier. Alternatively, colestyramine may be of benefit

• in *constipation-predominant* forms of the syndrome bran or ispaghula should be tried to increase dietary fibre. Fibre supplementation should be gradual to avoid bloating. Nevertheless, a proportion of patients are intolerant of bran, which will exacerbate symptoms such as abdominal distension and pain. An osmotic laxative or stool softener may be added in patients who fail to respond to fibre, but stimulant laxatives should be avoided

• in patients with *abdominal pain*, 'as-needed' antispasmodics or antimuscarinics may be tried. These should be taken before meals if abdominal pain occurs principally after eating. Examples include dicyclomine [dicycloverine], hyoscine, mebeverine, alverine, and peppermint oil. Antidepressants are also effective. Analgesic use needs to be minimised

• patients whose symptoms are associated with mild or masked *depression* may obtain benefit from antidepressant therapy; a depressed patient with increased bowel frequency and abdominal pain may benefit from a tricyclic antidepressant, which slows intestinal transit. It has been suggested that patients with constipation may be better treated with an SSRI.

Many other drugs have been tried in the irritable bowel syndrome, including cromoglicate, leuprorelin, and naloxone, with variable results.[1,7] Newer approaches being investigated are cholecystokinin antagonists (loxiglumide), kappa opioid agonists (fedotozine), somatostatin analogues (octreotide), 5-HT$_4$ agonists (tegaserod), and 5-HT$_3$ antagonists (such as the now withdrawn alosetron).[7,8]

1. Lynn RB, Friedman LS. Irritable bowel syndrome. *N Engl J Med* 1993; **329:** 1940–5.
2. Farthing MJG. Irritable bowel, irritable body, or irritable brain? *BMJ* 1995; **310:** 171–5.
3. Maxwell PR, *et al.* Irritable bowel syndrome. *Lancet* 1997; **350:** 1691–5.
4. Malcolm A, Kellow JE. Irritable bowel syndrome. *Med J Aust* 1998; **169:** 274–9.
5. Camilleri M. Review article: clinical evidence to support current therapies of irritable bowel syndrome. *Aliment Pharmacol Ther* 1999; **13** (suppl. 2): 48–53.
6. Jones J, *et al.* British Society of Gastroenterology guidelines for the management of the irritable bowel syndrome. *Gut* 2000; **47** (suppl 2): ii1–ii19.
7. Farthing MJG. New drugs in the management of the irritable bowel syndrome. *Drugs* 1998; **56:** 11–21.
8. Horwitz BJ, Fisher RS. The irritable bowel syndrome. *N Engl J Med* 2001; **344:** 1846–50.

Mouth ulceration

Recurrent ulceration of the oral mucosa is usually idiopathic and self-limiting and is known as recurrent aphthous stomatitis or recurrent aphthous ulceration. However, oral ulcers (canker sores) may also be caused by mechanical trauma, nutritional deficiencies (particularly iron, folic acid, or vitamin B_{12}), drug reactions, or underlying disease such as Behçet's syndrome (p.1047).

Management includes identifying any underlying disease or nutritional deficiency and treating these as appropriate. Usually no underlying cause can be found, and treatment is purely symptomatic including topical anti-inflammatories, local anaesthetics, antiseptics, astringents, or antihistamines. The value of many of these drugs in reducing symptoms remains anecdotal, and no treatments have yet been proven to reduce the incidence of recurrences.

Where ulceration is due to minor trauma frequent use of a warm saline or compound thymol glycerin mouthwash may be all that is required to relieve discomfort and swelling. Alternatively, pain relief may be obtained with local anaesthetics or analgesics, but their effectiveness in oral ulceration is limited by their relatively short duration of action when applied topically. Salicylates are widely used, mainly as choline salicylate gel, although they themselves have the potential for local irritation and ulceration. Benzydamine spray or mouthwash may also be helpful. Lignocaine [lidocaine], as a gel or lozenges, may be of value in pain that has not responded to other measures. Topical corticosteroids are probably the most effective symptomatic treatment for recurrent aphthous stomatitis. Pellets or lozenges of hydrocortisone are allowed to dissolve next to an ulcer, or triamcinolone in an oral paste formulation may be used, although the paste may sometimes be difficult to apply. Mouthwash formulations have been employed particularly when ulceration is widespread in the mouth and a dexamethasone mouthwash has been used effectively. The healing properties of carbenoxolone have also been employed as a gel or mouthwash, and the mast-cell stabilising agent amlexanox is also used as an oral paste.

Mechanical protection may be provided by a paste or powder of carmellose sodium, although application may be difficult.

Use of an antiseptic mouthwash such as chlorhexidine or povidone-iodine may be helpful, since secondary bacterial infection can delay healing. Chlorhexidine is also available as a gel. Tetracyclines, used as mouthwashes, reportedly reduce ulcer pain and duration, but their potential for adverse effects if swallowed must be borne in mind. Use of hydrogen peroxide 3% is inadvisable, as it can cause ulceration, but application of a 1.5% solution to individual ulcers in combination with a topical corticosteroid may be helpful in producing resolution.

A wide variety of other drugs have been tried in aphthous ulceration. Sucralfate may be of benefit. Drugs such as levamisole and thalidomide, although possibly beneficial, are unlikely to be suitable in most cases because of their adverse effects, although thalidomide is used, for example, for aphthous stomatitis in patients with AIDS. Oxpentifylline [pentoxifylline], which, like thalidomide, inhibits tumour necrosis factor production, has been used in patients with minor recurrent aphthous ulceration. Systemic corticosteroids are generally reserved for cases with severe underlying disease.

References.

1. Burgess JA, *et al.* Pharmacological management of recurrent oral mucosal ulceration. *Drugs* 1990; **39:** 54–65.
2. Fischman SL. Oral ulcerations. *Semin Dermatol* 1994; **13:** 74–7.
3. Woo SB, Sonis ST. Recurrent aphthous ulcers: a review of diagnosis and treatment. *J Am Dent Assoc* 1996; **127:** 1202–13.
4. Porter SR, *et al.* Recurrent aphthous stomatitis. *Crit Rev Oral Biol Med* 1998; **9:** 306–21.

Nausea and vomiting

Vomiting follows stimulation of the vomiting centre in the medulla of the brain, and closely associated with this centre is the chemoreceptor trigger zone (CTZ) which is sensitive to many drugs and to certain metabolic disturbances. Stimulation of the vomiting centre also occurs following actions on other areas such as the vestibular apparatus of the ear in motion sickness, the cerebral cortex in psychogenic vomiting, and multiple peripheral receptors. In adults vomiting is almost invariably preceded by a sensation of nausea.

As well as being a symptom of gastrointestinal disease, nausea and vomiting occurs in many conditions including motion sickness, other vestibular disorders such as Ménière's disease, and migraine; it is common in early pregnancy.

Nausea and vomiting are side-effects of numerous drugs, but may be a particular problem with antineoplastics, anaesthetics, opioid analgesics, and the dopaminergic antiparkinsonian drugs levodopa and bromocriptine. It is also a side-effect of radiotherapy.

In situations where it can be anticipated, such as motion sickness, surgery, and cancer therapy, antiemetic drugs are given prophylactically, but if this fails they may need to be given therapeutically. Vomiting of unknown origin should ideally not be treated until the underlying cause has been found. If vomiting is prolonged, dehydration, hypokalaemia, and alkalosis may occur and replacement of fluid and electrolytes may be necessary, especially in young children and the elderly.

Cancer chemotherapy. Nausea and vomiting are common adverse effects of cancer chemotherapy and for many patients represent a major drawback to treatment. Once experienced, anticipatory vomiting may occur at the sight of medical staff or a needle and this problem may be severe enough in some cases to hinder or prevent further treatment.

Antineoplastic or cytotoxic drugs may induce vomiting by both a central action on the chemoreceptor trigger zone and a peripheral action on the gastrointestinal tract. The cerebral cortex is probably responsible for anticipatory vomiting. Mechanisms involving 5-HT$_3$-receptors are important in the pathogenesis of *acute cisplatin-associated vomiting*, whereas different mechanisms are probably involved in *delayed emesis*.

The emetic potential of antineoplastics varies in terms of severity and incidence. Vomiting may be *very severe* with cisplatin, dacarbazine, dactinomycin, mustine [chlormethine], high-dose cyclophosphamide, and streptozocin, and occurs in most patients. *Moderate* vomiting is likely with the taxanes, doxorubicin, more modest doses of cyclophosphamide, and high-dose methotrexate, while vinca alkaloids, fluorouracil, lower doses of methotrexate, chlorambucil, bleomycin, and etoposide have *low* emetogenic potential. Emetogenicity may depend to some extent on the dose, route, and schedule of administration. Some combination therapy has resulted in a higher incidence of vomiting than would be expected from the constituents.

The *onset and duration* of vomiting also varies from drug to drug. After cisplatin the onset may be between 4 and 8 hours following a dose, while the duration may be up to 48 hours or occasionally even longer; a persistent feeling of nausea, and sometimes vomiting, lasting for several days may also occur. After mustine [chlormethine], vomiting may begin within a half to 2 hours, whereas after cyclophosphamide there may be a latent interval of 9 to 18 hours, but in both cases vomiting is generally less prolonged than with cisplatin. *Acute emesis* (that occurring within 24 hours of chemotherapy) has generally been easier to control than *delayed emesis* (that occurring more than 24 hours after chemotherapy) or *anticipatory emesis*.

MANAGEMENT. Guidelines for the management of nausea and vomiting associated with chemotherapy have been produced.[1-3] It is important that effective antiemetic prophylaxis is given from the first course of chemotherapy, to avoid subsequent problems with anticipatory vomiting. With the antiemetic drugs now available it should be possible to control *acute emesis*; *delayed emesis* is more resistant. A variety of drugs has been used in antiemetic regimens including:

• dopamine antagonists such as metoclopramide, domperidone, and some phenothiazines
• corticosteroids such as dexamethasone
• 5-HT$_3$ antagonists such as ondansetron
• cannabinoids such as nabilone
• benzodiazepines such as lorazepam
• antihistamines such as diphenhydramine.

The choice depends on the emetogenicity of the cancer chemotherapy regimen, as well as factors such as the age of the patient.

For prophylaxis of *acute emesis* associated with *highly emetogenic chemotherapy*, 5-HT$_3$ antagonists are used, often combined with dexamethasone. At equipotent doses, granisetron, ondansetron, dolasetron, and tropisetron are effective and equally safe.[1-3] High-dose metoclopramide was formerly used, but frequently caused extrapyramidal adverse effects particularly in patients under 30 years of age; diphenhydramine was used to reduce these effects. For prophylaxis of *acute emesis* associated with *moderately emetogenic chemotherapy*, dexamethasone alone is preferred. No routine prophylactic antiemetic needs to be given for chemotherapy of low emetic risk; however, as-needed or prophylactic use of prochlorperazine, domperidone, or metoclopramide is common. Lorazepam may be used for its amnestic, sedative, and anxiolytic effects as an adjunct to antiemetics when *anticipatory emesis* is a problem. Good control of acute emesis is important in preventing delayed emesis. In addition, for prophylaxis of *delayed emesis*, dexamethasone alone or combined with oral metoclopramide or perhaps a 5-HT$_3$ antagonist or prochlorperazine, is used. Cannabinoids such as dronabinol and nabilone have been used for chemotherapy-induced nausea and vomiting, usually as second-line drugs. Neurokinin-1 (NK$_1$) receptor antagonists are being investigated for control of acute and delayed cisplatin-induced emesis in combination with a 5-HT$_3$ antagonist and dexamethasone.[4]

Motion sickness has been described as a normal reaction to stimuli that occur during passive transportation and to which the individual is not adapted. The term embraces all forms of travel sickness including sea sickness, car sickness, train sickness, and air sickness. It is a type of vertigo in which autonomic symptoms predominate, therefore signs and symptoms include pallor, sweating, increased salivation, yawning, malaise, and hyperventilation.

MANAGEMENT. The aim is to *prevent* motion sickness and antiemetics are more effective if given prophylactically before nausea and vomiting has developed. The principal drugs used are the antimuscarinic hyoscine and some of the centrally acting antihistamines.[5] Antiemetic drugs *not* effective against motion sickness include metoclopramide, domperidone, chlorpromazine, and 5-HT$_3$ antagonists. Ginger has been tried.

For short-term protection against motion sickness hyoscine hydrobromide by mouth is often the drug of choice. It is taken about 30 minutes before a journey followed by further doses every 6 hours if necessary. Transdermal administration of hyoscine markedly prolongs the duration of action, but the patches need to be applied to the skin several hours before travelling.

Antihistamines may be slightly less effective than hyoscine against motion sickness, but are often better tolerated. They are usually given by mouth and include cinnarizine, cyclizine, dimenhydrinate, meclozine, and promethazine; all have similar efficacy, but differ in onset and duration of action and in the extent of side-effects such as drowsiness. Their antimuscarinic properties may contribute to their effects. Non-sedating antihistamines (e.g. astemizole and terfenadine) penetrate poorly into the CNS and do not appear to be effective against motion sickness.

Once motion sickness has developed gastric motility is inhibited and it may be preferable to administer antiemetics intramuscularly rather than by mouth. In one study promethazine was preferred to hyoscine for intramuscular use because of its longer duration of action.[6]

Palliative care. Nausea and vomiting are common in terminal illness, and may be prolonged. There are various causes, and more than one cause may occur in the same patient. They include unpalatable or excess food, gastric irritation or delayed emptying, constipation or intestinal obstruction, renal failure, increased intracranial pressure, hypercalcaemia, infection, and treatments such as chemotherapy (see above), radiotherapy (see below), opioid analgesics, NSAIDs, or corticosteroids.[7,8]

MANAGEMENT. Nausea and vomiting can often be *reduced* by treatment of associated symptoms such as pain, anxiety, and cough. Non-drug measures include appropriate diet and avoidance of unpleasant odours, adequate fluid intake, and regular mouth care. Drugs used for *prevention and treatment* are selected depending on the cause of nausea and vomiting. These include haloperidol, phenothiazines, antihistamines such as cyclizine and hydroxyzine, the antimuscarinic hyoscine, prokinetics such as metoclopramide and domperidone, 5-HT$_3$ antagonists such as ondansetron and granisetron, corticosteroids

such as dexamethasone, benzodiazepines, and cannabinoids. Although antiemetic treatments are given orally, patients with severe vomiting will require drug administration by other routes such as subcutaneous infusion.[7,8] Octreotide may be helpful to reduce intestinal secretions and vomiting.

Postoperative nausea and vomiting is a common and distressing side-effect of anaesthesia and surgery; it may sometimes be more of a problem than pain, especially in day-case surgery.[9-11] The incidence depends on many factors, including the type of anaesthetic, the type and duration of operation, and the sex of the patient (women are more at risk than men). Patients with a history of postoperative vomiting or of motion sickness may be more susceptible.

MANAGEMENT. The aim is prevention and most studies have been directed at this rather than treatment. Routine antiemetic prophylaxis is not necessary in all surgical patients.[2,9,11,12] Widely used drugs for the *prevention and treatment* of postoperative nausea and vomiting include dopamine antagonists such as metoclopramide, droperidol, and some phenothiazines; 5-HT$_3$ antagonists such as ondansetron; and antihistamines (including phenothiazine antihistamines such as promethazine). In a meta-analysis[13] of studies comparing ondansetron, droperidol, and metoclopramide for *prophylaxis*, ondansetron and droperidol were more effective than metoclopramide for preventing vomiting, and droperidol was more effective than metoclopramide for preventing nausea. In an analysis[14] of studies comparing metoclopramide with placebo it was concluded that metoclopramide was not an effective antiemetic in the doses currently used in anaesthesia, and that doses are likely to be too low. When intravenous ondansetron was compared with phenothiazines for prevention of nausea and vomiting after surgery, it was equivalent to intravenous perphenazine in 1 study,[15] and less effective than intramuscular prochlorperazine in another.[16] In the *treatment* of established nausea and vomiting, ondansetron was no different to droperidol[17] and at least as effective as metoclopramide,[17,18] with an overall efficacy of only about 25% greater than placebo.[17] There are fewer studies of combined antiemetic regimens for preventing and treating nausea and vomiting after surgery, but combinations of drugs from different classes may be used for high-risk situations.[11,12] Ondansetron or granisetron combined with dexamethasone is reportedly more effective than the 5-HT$_3$-receptor antagonist alone.[19] Ondansetron has also been combined with droperidol for the prophylaxis of postoperative emesis.[20]

Other drugs that have been tried include transdermal hyoscine,[21] clonidine,[21] ginger,[22,23] and ephedrine.[24,25] The use of propofol for maintenance anaesthesia may be associated with a reduction in risk of postoperative nausea and vomiting (see p.1267). Some nonpharmacological techniques to prevent postoperative nausea and vomiting may be effective in adults.[11,26]

Pregnancy. Nausea and vomiting or 'morning sickness' is common in the first trimester of pregnancy, but is generally mild and does not require drug therapy. Dietary modification such as eating small frequent carbohydrate meals often helps. There is also some evidence that pyridoxine can reduce nausea in pregnancy.[27] On rare occasions short-term treatment with an antihistamine such as promethazine may be required if vomiting is severe. For reference to the controversy that has surrounded the risk to the fetus of antiemetic therapy during pregnancy, see under the Precautions of Antihistamines, p.405. Persistent vomiting and severe nausea may progress to *hyperemesis gravidarum* if adequate hydration cannot be maintained; the condition occurs in up to 1% of pregnancies.[28] Management of hyperemesis includes hospitalisation for intravenous fluid and electrolyte replacement, and this is usually sufficient. Routine thiamine supplementation, by mouth if tolerated otherwise parenterally, has been recommended to reduce the risk of Wernicke's encephalopathy[28,29] (p.1385), although there is some dissent from this view.[30] If hyperemesis fails to respond to rehydration, antiemetics should be used; options include domperidone, phenothiazines, and antihistamines.[28] There is some evidence that hyperemesis unresponsive to conventional therapy may respond to oral prednisolone or intravenous hydrocortisone.[28] There have also been anecdotal reports of ondansetron being used successfully in life-threatening hyperemesis gravidarum unresponsive to conventional treatment,[31] although a double-blind pilot study found it to be no more effective than promethazine.[32]

Radiotherapy. The risk of emesis with radiotherapy varies with the treatment administered, particularly the area of the body irradiated. However, emetic risk, and recommendations for use of antiemetics, are less clearly defined than in the situation of chemotherapy-induced nausea and vomiting.[2,3] Total body irradiation is considered to have high emetogenic potential, but is not a common treatment. It has been suggested that a prophylactic 5-HT$_3$ antagonist should be given before each fraction, perhaps combined with a corticosteroid. For radiotherapy of intermediate emetogenic risk, such as that to the abdomen, prophylactic antiemetics may also be considered; options are dopamine antagonists (metoclopramide, domperidone) or 5-HT$_3$ antagonists. For radiotherapy of low emetogenic potential, treatment on an as-needed only basis has been suggested.[3]

1. Fauser AA, *et al.* Guidelines for anti-emetic therapy: acute emesis. *Eur J Cancer* 1999; **35:** 361–70.
2. American Society of Health-System Pharmacists. ASHP therapeutic guidelines on the pharmacologic management of nausea and vomiting in adult and pediatric patients receiving chemotherapy or radiation therapy or undergoing surgery. *Am J Health-Syst Pharm* 1999; **56:** 729–64.
3. Gralla RJ, *et al.* Recommendations for the use of antiemetics: evidence-based, clinical practice guidelines. *J Clin Oncol* 1999; **17:** 2971–94. Correction. *ibid.* 2000; **18:** 3064.
4. Navari RM, *et al.* Reduction of cisplatin-induced emesis by a selective neurokinin-1-receptor antagonist. *N Engl J Med* 1999; **340:** 190–5.
5. Gahlinger PM. Motion sickness: how to help your patients avoid travel travail. *Postgrad Med* 1999; **106:** 177–84.
6. Wood CD, *et al.* Effectiveness and duration of intramuscular antimotion sickness medications. *J Clin Pharmacol* 1992; **32:** 1008–12.
7. WHO. Nausea and vomiting. In: *Symptom relief in terminal illness.* Geneva: WHO, 1998.
8. Baines MJ. ABC of palliative care: nausea, vomiting, and intestinal obstruction. *BMJ* 1997; **315:** 1148–50.
9. Watcha MF, White PF. Postoperative nausea and vomiting: its etiology, treatment, and prevention. *Anesthesiology* 1992; **77:** 162–84.
10. Sung Y-F. Risks and benefits of drugs used in the management of postoperative nausea and vomiting. *Drug Safety* 1996; **14:** 181–97.
11. Kovac AL. Prevention and treatment of postoperative nausea and vomiting. *Drugs* 2000; **59:** 213–43.
12. Rose JB, Watcha MF. Postoperative nausea and vomiting in paediatric patients. *Br J Anaesth* 1999; **83:** 104–17.
13. Domino KB, *et al.* Comparative efficacy and safety of ondansetron, droperidol, and metoclopramide for preventing postoperative nausea and vomiting: a meta-analysis. *Anesth Analg* 1999; **88:** 1370–9.
14. Henzi I, *et al.* Metoclopramide in the prevention of postoperative nausea and vomiting: a quantitative systematic review of randomized, placebo-controlled studies. *Br J Anaesth* 1999; **83:** 761–71.
15. Desilva PHDP, *et al.* The efficacy of prophylactic ondansetron, droperidol, perphenazine, and metoclopramide in the prevention of nausea and vomiting after major gynecologic surgery. *Anesth Analg* 1995; **81:** 139–43.
16. Chen JJ, *et al.* Efficacy of ondansetron and prochlorperazine for the prevention of postoperative nausea and vomiting after total hip replacement or total knee replacement procedures: a randomized, double-blind, comparative trial. *Arch Intern Med* 1998; **158:** 2124–8.
17. Tramèr MR, *et al.* A quantitative systematic review of ondansetron in treatment of established postoperative nausea and vomiting. *BMJ* 1997; **314:** 1088–92.
18. Diemunsch P, *et al.* Ondansetron compared with metoclopramide in the treatment of established postoperative nausea and vomiting. *Br J Anaesth* 1997; **79:** 322–6.
19. Henzi I, *et al.* Dexamethasone for the prevention of postoperative nausea and vomiting: a quantitative systematic review. *Anesth Analg* 2000; **90:** 186–94.
20. Koivuranta M, *et al.* The anti-emetic efficacy of a combination of ondansetron and droperidol. *Anaesthesia* 1997; **52:** 863–8.
21. Mikawa K, *et al.* Oral clonidine premedication reduces vomiting in children after strabismus surgery. *Can J Anaesth* 1995; **42:** 977–81.
22. Phillips S, *et al.* Zingiber officinale (ginger)—an antiemetic for day case surgery. *Anaesthesia* 1993; **48:** 715–17.
23. Arfeen Z, *et al.* A double-blind randomized controlled trial of ginger for the prevention of postoperative nausea and vomiting. *Anaesth Intensive Care* 1995; **23:** 449–52.
24. Rothenberg DM, *et al.* Efficacy of ephedrine in the prevention of postoperative nausea and vomiting. *Anesth Analg* 1991; **72:** 58–61.
25. Liu Y-C, *et al.* Comparison of antiemetic effect among ephedrine, droperidol and metoclopramide in pediatric inguinal hernioplasty. *Acta Anaesthesiol Sin* 1992; **32:** 37–42.
26. Lee A, *et al.* The use of nonpharmacologic techniques to prevent postoperative nausea and vomiting: a meta-analysis. *Anesth Analg* 1999; **88:** 1362–9.
27. Vutyavanich T, *et al.* Pyridoxine for nausea and vomiting of pregnancy: a randomized, double-blind, placebo-controlled trial. *Am J Obstet Gynecol* 1995; **173:** 881–4.
28. Nelson-Piercy C. Treatment of nausea and vomiting in pregnancy: when should it be treated and what can be safely taken? *Drug Safety* 1998; **19:** 155–64.
29. Child TJ. Management of hyperemesis in pregnant women. *Lancet* 1999; **353:** 325.
30. Dickson MJ. Management of hyperemesis in pregnant women. *Lancet* 1999; **353:** 325.
31. World MJ. Ondansetron and hyperemesis gravidarum. *Lancet* 1993; **341:** 185.
32. Sullivan CA, *et al.* A pilot study of intravenous ondansetron for hyperemesis gravidarum. *Am J Obstet Gynecol* 1996; **174:** 1565–8.

Oesophageal motility disorders

Oesophageal disorders, many due to disturbances in oesophageal motility, may produce non-cardiac chest pain, similar to that of angina pectoris, from which they must be differentiated.

Achalasia is obstruction caused by failure of the lower oesophageal sphincter to relax and permit passage of food into the stomach. It is accompanied by dilatation and abnormal peristalsis in the oesophagus, which becomes a reservoir for the unassimilated matter; symptoms include dysphagia and sometimes pain. The treatment of choice is mechanical dilatation of the sphincter or, if necessary, surgery. Laparoscopic techniques have reduced the risks associated with surgery, and this may become the preferred treatment. Taking isosorbide dinitrate or nifedipine prior to eating results in some improvement in achalasia, but these drugs have a role only as a temporary measure, or when other options are not suitable. More recently, injection of botulinum toxin into the lower oesophageal sphincter has been found to be effective, but remission in the long-term is better with mechanical dilatation than botulinum toxin. Therefore, it has been recommended that botulinum toxin be reserved for patients thought to be at risk from mechanical dilatation or surgery.

Oesophageal spasm, although frequently asymptomatic, can produce dysphagia and pain. Drug treatment of diffuse oesophageal spasm, or its variant 'nutcracker oesophagus' which is characterised by high amplitude peristalsis in the oesophagus, is often ineffective. Antimuscarinics, nitrates, and calcium-channel blockers have been tried in an attempt to relax the smooth muscle, but results are often disappointing; experience with nifedipine in patients with nutcracker oesophagus suggests that decrease in oesophageal pressure may not correlate with reduction in pain. As with achalasia, minimally invasive surgery is effective for these conditions, and is likely to be preferred.

Reviews.

1. Vaezi MF, Richter JE. Current therapies for achalasia: comparison and efficacy. *J Clin Gastroenterol* 1998; **27:** 21–35.
2. Spiess AE, Kahrilas PJ. Treating achalasia: from whalebone to laparoscope. *JAMA* 1998; **280:** 638–42.
3. Patti MG, Way LW. Evaluation and treatment of primary esophageal motility disorders. *West J Med* 1997; **166:** 263–9.

Peptic ulcer disease

Peptic ulceration is a common condition consisting of a distinct break in the gastrointestinal mucosa, usually of the stomach or duodenum. Duodenal ulcers are rarely malignant but gastric ulcers are more commonly associated with malignancy.

The aetiology of peptic ulcer disease is probably multifactorial but the bacterium *Helicobacter pylori* plays an important role. Abnormalities of normal mucosal defence mechanisms and, in the case of gastric ulcer, reflux of duodenal contents into the stomach or delayed gastric emptying may also be involved. Other factors include emotional stress, smoking, alcohol, and drugs such as NSAIDs or corticosteroids.

Peptic ulcer disease usually presents as dyspeptic pain, sometimes associated with nausea, vomiting, anorexia, heartburn, or bloating. Patients may develop complications such as bleeding, obstruction, or perforation.

Certain simple measures such as bed rest, dietary modification, and cessation of smoking, may accelerate ulcer healing, but these play an adjuvant role, and the basis of treatment is pharmacological. Treatment is aimed at eradicating *H. pylori* with antibacterials and neutralising or inhibiting acid activity with antisecretory drugs, and a number of guidelines are available.[1-4] Surgical treatment is employed in patients with acute complications such as perforation, haemorrhage, obstruction, or pyloric stenosis, or in patients with recurrent or intractable ulcer disease, or where there is suspicion of malignancy.

Anti-Helicobacter therapy. The presence of *H. pylori* should usually be confirmed before therapy to eradicate the infection is started. The urea breath test is the most widely used method to test for *H. pylori*, but may produce false-negatives if used soon after treatment with proton pump inhibitors (see under Omeprazole, p.1240) or antibacterials. The best eradication regimen has not yet been established, and the number of regimens being tried is large.[5-7] The most widely used regimens comprise so-called **'triple therapy'** with a proton pump inhibitor and two antibacterials. The initial choice of antibacterial is normally between clarithromycin, a nitroimidazole (metronidazole or tinidazole), and amoxicillin, and depends on the likelihood of metronidazole or clarithromy-

cin resistance. In the UK, the *British National Formulary* recommends a regimen containing amoxicillin and clarithromycin for initial therapy, and one with amoxicillin and metronidazole if this fails. Ranitidine bismuth citrate may replace the proton pump inhibitor. Other regimens, including those combining clarithromycin and metronidazole are considered best used in specialist settings. Therapy is usually given for 7 to 14 days with the drugs given twice daily. Two-week triple therapy regimens are associated with high eradication rates, but adverse effects are common and compliance is a problem, so consensus favours the shorter 7-day course. Such regimens can produce eradication of *H. pylori* in over 80 to 90% of patients. Two-week triple therapy with a bismuth compound and 2 antibacterials (metronidazole and tetracycline) was formerly used, but is not as effective as proton pump inhibitor-based regimens.[5] Two-week **dual therapy** of omeprazole with amoxicillin or clarithromycin has also been used, but although less complex than triple therapy, it is also less effective. Two-week **quadruple therapy** in which omeprazole is added to a conventional bismuth-based triple therapy regimen may have a role in refractory *H. pylori* infection.[8] Although continuation of acid suppressive therapy for 4 to 8 weeks after eradication of *H. pylori* is often recommended to promote healing, some consider this unwarranted except for large or complicated lesions.[9] The recurrence rate of duodenal or gastric ulcers after successful eradication of *H. pylori* has generally been reported to be low (about 4 to 8%),[10] but in one analysis a 6-month recurrence rate of 20% was reported.[11]

Before the advent of *H. pylori* eradication therapy, drug treatment of gastric and duodenal ulcers relied mainly on antisecretory therapy. Four to 8 weeks of H$_2$-antagonist or proton pump inhibitor therapy was required for ulcer healing. Because of the high incidence of relapse, these drugs were then often given as maintenance therapy. Numerous other drugs were formerly used in peptic ulcer disease before the development of H$_2$-antagonists and proton pump inhibitors, including antacids, antimuscarinics such as pirenzepine, and mucosal protectants such as sucralfate.

NSAID-induced ulceration. The ulcerogenic effects of NSAIDs have been attributed to inhibition of prostaglandin synthesis and of mucosal cell proliferation and the ulcers they cause may differ from non-iatrogenic ulcers in their pathology and prognosis.[12,13] In particular, they are not directly related to *H. pylori* infection.[14] If peptic ulceration develops during treatment with an NSAID the drug should be withdrawn if possible. If this can be done, the ulcer may be treated with an antisecretory drug such as an H$_2$-antagonist or proton pump inhibitor given for 4 to 8 weeks. If NSAIDS have to be continued, *treatment* is with antisecretory drugs or the prostaglandin analogue misoprostol.[12,13] Ulcers tend to heal more slowly with H$_2$-antagonists if NSAIDs are continued, whereas the rate of ulcer healing with proton pump inhibitors appears not to be affected. There is also some evidence that omeprazole is more effective at healing NSAID-associated ulceration than misoprostol.[15] Patients at high risk of NSAID-associated gastrointestinal complications, including those with a history of these events, should receive *prophylactic therapy*.[12,13] Options for prophylaxis include misoprostol, H$_2$-antagonists, and proton pump inhibitors. Full-dose H$_2$-antagonists prevent NSAID-associated duodenal ulceration, but appear to be less effective in preventing gastric ulceration. In one study high-dose famotidine prevented both gastric and duodenal ulcers,[16] but the definition of ulcer in this study has been queried.[13] After healing of NSAID-associated ulceration, omeprazole prophylaxis was more effective than ranitidine,[17] and was more effective and better tolerated than misoprostol.[15] It is not clear whether eradication of *H. pylori* infection reduces the occurrence of NSAID-induced ulcer,[18,19] and despite a European guideline indicating that eradication should be considered in planned or existing NSAID therapy[2] some doubt the benefits of such a policy.[20] Treatment to eradicate infection only in patients with a history of peptic ulcer has been suggested.[12]

Stress ulceration may occur in the stomach or the duodenum following major physical trauma such as burns or surgery, or after severe sepsis or illness. H$_2$-antagonists and sucralfate are widely used for the prevention of stress ulceration in high-risk patients in intensive care units.[21,22] Pirenzepine is used in a few countries, and some[21] prefer it in neurosurgical patients and those with head trauma. H$_2$-antagonists may be given by mouth, nasogastric tube, or by intermittent or continuous intravenous administration. It has been suggested that the rise in gastric pH which results from such use may predispose patients to nosocomial pneumonia due to bacterial overgrowth in the stomach and retrograde colonisation of the pharynx. Sucralfate does not increase gastric pH, and meta-analysis has indicated that it may be as effective as an H_2-antagonist in reducing bleeding, and is associated with lower rates of pneumonia and mortality.[23] The findings of a subsequent large randomised study[24] by the same authors were at odds with those of this meta-analysis, suggesting that intravenous ranitidine was more effective than sucralfate administered orally or via nasogastric tube in reducing clinically significant gastrointestinal bleeding. Moreover, there was no difference in rate of ventilator-associated mortality between ranitidine and sucralfate recipients. A further meta-analysis[25] has in turn raised doubts about the efficacy of ranitidine; no significant benefit was found for ranitidine, compared with placebo, in the prevention of bleeding. One clinical guideline suggests that, given the conflicting evidence, the choice between antacids, H_2-antagonists, and sucralfate be made on an institutional basis.[22]

Bleeding ulcer. Peptic ulceration is responsible for about 50% of all cases of upper gastrointestinal bleeding. Although many patients cease to bleed without a specific intervention, the condition is potentially life-threatening and in severe cases prompt resuscitation with intravenous fluids and blood may be required. Endoscopic therapy has substantially improved management of patients with severe bleeding or at high risk of rebleeding.[26,27] Endoscopic treatments include local injection therapy with adrenaline [epinephrine] or sclerosants such as alcohol, and thermal therapy with lasers or electrocoagulation. Injection therapy tends to be preferred. Combining injection and thermal therapies, or using 2 injection agents has not been conclusively proven to be better than single therapies. Investigational injection therapies include a fibrin glue,[28] and thrombin.[29] If endoscopic treatments fail to stop bleeding, or rebleeding occurs, further endoscopic therapy may be considered, but otherwise patients require surgery.

There is little evidence that treatment with H_2-antagonists[30] is useful in the acute management of bleeding, although some consider that there is evidence of benefit for omeprazole;[31] evidence of value for tranexamic acid or somatostatin is ambiguous.[27] However, once haemorrhage has been controlled, long-term treatment with an antisecretory drug to promote healing and reduce the risk of rebleeding is often given, particularly in frail and elderly patients. Eradication of *H. pylori* is generally recommended, using an appropriate regimen.[26]

1. Soll AH. Medical treatment of peptic ulcer disease: practice guidelines. *JAMA* 1996; **275:** 622–9.
2. The European Helicobacter Pylori Study Group. Current European concepts in the management of Helicobacter pylori infection: the Maastricht consensus report. *Gut* 1997; **41:** 8–13.
3. Peura D. The report of the Digestive Health Initiative International Update Conference on Helicobacter pylori. *Gastroenterology* 1997; **113:** S4–S8.
4. Hunt RH, *et al.* Canadian Helicobacter pylori Consensus Conference update: infections in adults. *Can J Gastroenterol* 1999; **13:** 213–17.
5. Unge P, Berstad A. Pooled analysis of anti-Helicobacter pylori treatment regimens. *Scand J Gastroenterol* 1996; **31** (suppl 220): 27–40.
6. Penston JG, McColl KEL. Eradication of Helicobacter pylori: an objective assessment of current therapies. *Br J Clin Pharmacol* 1997; **43:** 223–43.
7. Huang J-Q, Hunt RH. The importance of clarithromycin dose in the management of Helicobacter pylori infection: a meta-analysis of triple therapies with a proton pump inhibitor, clarithromycin and amoxycillin or metronidazole. *Aliment Pharmacol Ther* 1999; **13:** 719–29.
8. Peitz U, *et al.* A practical approach to patients with refractory Helicobacter pylori infection, or who are re-infected after standard therapy. *Drugs* 1999; **57:** 905–20.
9. Treiber G, Lambert JR. The impact of Helicobacter pylori eradication on peptic ulcer healing. *Am J Gastroenterol* 1998; **93:** 1080–4.
10. Hopkins RJ, *et al.* Relationship between Helicobacter pylori eradication and reduced duodenal and gastric ulcer recurrence: a review. *Gastroenterology* 1996; **110:** 1244–52.
11. Laine L, *et al.* Has the impact of Helicobacter pylori therapy on ulcer recurrence in the United States been overstated? A meta-analysis of rigorously designed trials. *Am J Gastroenterol* 1998; **93:** 1409–15.
12. Wolfe MM, *et al.* Gastrointestinal toxicity of nonsteroidal antiinflammatory drugs. *N Engl J Med* 1999; **340:** 1888–99.
13. La Corte R, *et al.* Prophylaxis and treatment of NSAID-induced gastroduodenal disorders. *Drug Safety* 1999; **20:** 527–43.
14. Barkin J. The relationship between Helicobacter pylori and nonsteroidal anti-inflammatory drugs. *Am J Med* 1998; **105** (suppl 5A): 22S–27S.
15. Hawkey CJ, *et al.* Omeprazole compared with misoprostol for ulcers associated with nonsteroidal antiinflammatory drugs. *N Engl J Med* 1998; **338:** 727–34.
16. Taha AS, *et al.* Famotidine for the prevention of gastric and duodenal ulcers caused by nonsteroidal antiinflammatory drugs. *N Engl J Med* 1996; **334:** 1435–9.

17. Yeomans ND, *et al.* A comparison of omeprazole with ranitidine for ulcers associated with nonsteroidal antiinflammatory drugs. *N Engl J Med* 1998; **338:** 719–26.
18. Chan FKL, *et al.* Randomised trial of eradication of Helicobacter pylori before non-steroidal anti-inflammatory drug therapy to prevent peptic ulcers. *Lancet* 1997; **350:** 975–9.
19. Hawkey CJ, *et al.* Randomised controlled trial of Helicobacter pylori eradication in patients on non-steroidal anti-inflammatory drugs: HELP NSAIDs study. *Lancet* 1998; **352:** 1016–21. Correction. *ibid.;* 1634.
20. Hawkey CJ, *et al.* Helicobacter pylori, NSAIDs, and peptic ulcers. *Lancet* 1998; **351:** 61.
21. Tryba M, Cook D. Current guidelines on stress ulcer prophylaxis. *Drugs* 1997; **54:** 581–96.
22. ASHP Commission on Therapeutics. ASHP therapeutic guidelines on stress ulcer prophylaxis. *Am J Health-Syst Pharm* 1999; **56:** 347–79.
23. Cook DJ, *et al.* Stress ulcer prophylaxis in critically ill patients: resolving discordant meta-analyses. *JAMA* 1996; **275:** 308–14.
24. Cook D, *et al.* A comparison of sucralfate and ranitidine for the prevention of upper gastrointestinal bleeding in patients requiring mechanical ventilation. *N Engl J Med* 1998; **338:** 791–7.
25. Messori A, *et al.* Bleeding and pneumonia in intensive care patients given ranitidine and sucralfate for prevention of stress ulcer: meta-analysis of randomised controlled trials. *BMJ* 2000; **321:** 1103–6.
26. Laine L, Peterson WL. Bleeding peptic ulcer. *N Engl J Med* 1994; **331:** 717–27.
27. Villanueva C, Balanzó J. A practical guide to the management of bleeding ulcers. *Drugs* 1997; **53:** 389–403.
28. Rutgeerts P, *et al.* Randomised trial of single and repeated fibrin glue compared with injection of polidocanol in treatment of bleeding peptic ulcer. *Lancet* 1997; **350:** 692–6.
29. Kubba AK, *et al.* Endoscopic injection for bleeding peptic ulcer: a comparison of adrenaline alone with adrenaline plus human thrombin. *Gastroenterology* 1996; **111:** 623–8.
30. Peterson WL, Cook DJ. Antisecretory therapy for bleeding peptic ulcer. *JAMA* 1998; **280:** 877–8.
31. Erstad BL. Proton-pump inhibitors for acute peptic ulcer bleeding. *Ann Pharmacother* 2001; **35:** 730–40.

Zollinger-Ellison syndrome

Zollinger-Ellison syndrome is a rare disorder characterised by the presence of a gastrin-producing tumour (gastrinoma), which leads to hypersecretion of gastric acid and consequent peptic ulcer disease (often with complications such as perforation or bleeding), diarrhoea, or malabsorption. Gastrinomas usually occur in the non-beta islet cells of the pancreas or in the duodenal wall. Up to two-thirds are malignant. About 20 to 25% of cases are seen in patients with multiple endocrine neoplasia type 1 (MEN-1) syndrome.

Initial treatment is aimed at controlling the hypersecretion of gastric acid with an antisecretory drug. Giving enough medication just to control symptoms is not considered adequate, and it is important that acid secretion is reduced below 10 mmol per hour. Intravenous H_2-antagonists or proton pump inhibitors may be required initially. Once the symptoms have been controlled the tumour can be investigated for surgical removal. When complete removal is not possible then antisecretory therapy is continued indefinitely. A proton pump inhibitor is the drug of choice; it profoundly reduces acid secretion with once- or twice-daily administration, although relatively high doses are required compared with those used in other conditions. An H_2-antagonist such as cimetidine or ranitidine may be used as an alternative to omeprazole, and, as with omeprazole, daily doses are higher than those used for other conditions; they are given in 3 or 4 divided doses. The somatostatin analogue octreotide can be used to reduce serum gastrin, but has to be given subcutaneously, and is not well tolerated.

Parietal cell vagotomy may be performed to reduce acid secretion if the tumour is not found, to allow lower doses of antisecretory drugs to be used.

References.

1. Maton PN. Zollinger-Ellison syndrome: recognition and management of acid hypersecretion. *Drugs* 1996; **52:** 33–44.
2. Qureshi W, Rashid S. Zollinger-Ellison syndrome: improved treatment options for this complex disorder. *Postgrad Med* 1998; **104:** 155–164.

Aceglutamide Aluminium (12307-t)

Aceglutamide Aluminium *(rINNM)*.

Aceglutamide Aluminum *(USAN)*; KW-110. Pentakis (N^2-acetyl-L-glutaminato)tetrahydroxytrialuminium.

$C_{35}H_{59}Al_3N_{10}O_{24} = 1084.8$.
CAS — 12607-92-0.

Profile

Aceglutamide aluminium, a complex of aceglutamide with aluminium hydroxide, is an antacid with general properties similar to those of aluminium hydroxide (p.1210). It is given by mouth in usual doses of 700 mg three or four times daily.

Preparations

Proprietary Preparations (details are given in Part 3)
Jpn: Glumal; *Spain:* Glumal†.

Albumin Tannate (293-x)

Albutannin; Tannin Albuminate.
CAS — 9006-52-4.
ATC — A07XA01.
Pharmacopoeias. In Aust. and Jpn.

Profile

Albumin tannate, a compound of tannin with albumin, is given by mouth for its astringent properties in the treatment of diarrhoea (p.1203). It is stated to liberate tannic acid (p.1669) in the gastrointestinal tract.

Preparations

Proprietary Preparations (details are given in Part 3)
Aust.: Tannalbin; *Austral.:* Tannalbin†; *Ger.:* Tannalbin; *Neth.:* Entosorbine-N; Tannalbin; Tendosimol†; *Port.:* Tanalbina; *Spain:* Cunticina.

Multi-ingredient: *Aust.:* Neoplex; *Belg.:* Tanalone; *Fin.:* Tannopon; *Ger.:* Tannacomp; *Spain:* Demusin; Salitanol Estreptomicina.

Alexitol Sodium (712-d)

Alexitol Sodium *(BAN, rINN)*.
Sodium poly(hydroxyaluminium) carbonate-hexitol complex.
CAS — 66813-51-2.

Profile

Alexitol sodium is an antacid with general properties similar to those of aluminium hydroxide (p.1210). It is given in doses of 360 to 720 mg by mouth.

Preparations

Proprietary Preparations (details are given in Part 3)
Hong Kong: Actal; *Irl.:* Actal; *S.Afr.:* Actan; *Singapore:* Actal; *Thai.:* Actal; *UK:* Actal.

Multi-ingredient: *UK:* Magnatol†.

Alizapride Hydrochloride (16020-y)

Alizapride Hydrochloride *(rINNM)*.
N-(1-Allyl-2-pyrrolidinylmethyl)-6-methoxy-1H-benzotriazole-5-carboxamide hydrochloride.
$C_{16}H_{21}N_5O_2,HCl = 351.8$.
CAS — 59338-93-1 (alizapride); 59338-87-3 (alizapride hydrochloride).

Alizapride 50 mg is approximately equivalent to alizapride hydrochloride 55.8 mg.

Adverse Effects and Precautions

As for Metoclopramide, (see p.1235).

Pharmacokinetics

Alizapride is well absorbed from the gastrointestinal tract. It is mainly excreted unchanged in the urine and has an elimination half-life of about 3 hours.

Uses and Administration

Alizapride hydrochloride is a substituted benzamide similar to metoclopramide (p.1236), which is used to control nausea and vomiting (p.1206) associated with a variety of disorders. Alizapride hydrochloride is given in usual doses equivalent to 100 to 300 mg of alizapride daily in divided doses by mouth; children have been given 5 mg per kg body-weight daily. It is also given by intravenous or intramuscular injection in doses equivalent to 50 to 200 mg of alizapride daily.

For patients receiving cancer chemotherapy usual daily doses equivalent to alizapride 2 to 5 mg per kg body-weight have been administered intravenously or intramuscularly in 2 divided doses, one 30 minutes before and one 4 to 8 hours after cytotoxic drug administration. For highly emetic cytotoxic regimens requiring doses above 5 mg of alizapride per kg it may be given by intravenous infusion over 15 minutes every 2 hours for 5 doses, starting 30 minutes before cytotoxic administration. It has been recommended that the total dose given with a course of chemotherapy does not exceed 4.5 g.

Preparations

Proprietary Preparations (details are given in Part 3)
Belg.: Litican; *Braz.:* Superan; *Fr.:* Plitican; *Ger.:* Vergentan; *Hong Kong:* Plitican; *Ital.:* Limican; Nausilen†; *Neth.:* Litican†; *Port.:* Plitican†; *Switz.:* Plitican.

Almagate (19021-z)

Almagate *(BAN, USAN, rINN)*.
LAS-3876. Aluminium trimagnesium carbonate heptahydroxide dihydrate.
$AlMg_3(CO_3)(OH)_7,2H_2O = 315.0$.
CAS — 66827-12-1 (almagate); 72526-11-5 (anhydrous almagate).
ATC — A02AD03.

Profile

Almagate is a hydrated aluminium-magnesium hydroxycarbonate. It is an antacid with general properties similar to those of aluminium hydroxide (p.1210) and magnesium carbonate (p.1232). It is given in doses of 1 to 1.5 g by mouth.

Preparations

Proprietary Preparations (details are given in Part 3)
Spain: Almax; Deprece; Obetine.

Almasilate (15333-f)

Almasilate (BAN, rINN).
Aluminium Magnesium Silicate Hydrate; Magnesium Aluminosilicate Hydrate; Magnesium Aluminum Silicate Hydrate.
$Al_2O_3.MgO.2SiO_2,xH_2O = 262.4$ (anhydrous).
CAS — 71205-22-6; 50958-44-6.
ATC — A02AD05.

Profile
Almasilate is an artificial form of aluminium magnesium silicate hydrate. It is an antacid (p.1201) that is given in doses of up to about 1 g by mouth.

A hydrated native aluminium magnesium silicate (p.1499) is used as a suspending, thickening, and stabilising agent in pharmaceutical preparations. Attapulgite (p.1212) is another native form.

Preparations

Proprietary Preparations (details are given in Part 3)
Aust.: Gelusil; *Ger.:* Gelusil; Lac 4 n†; Megalac; Simagel; *Spain:* Alubifar; Sinegastrin; *Switz.:* Gelusil.

Multi-ingredient: *Aust.:* Gastripan†; *Ger.:* Gelusil-Lac; Neo-Pyodron; Ultilac N; *Spain:* Dolcopin; *Switz.:* Gelusil-Lac.

Aloes (7501-f)

Acibar.
CAS — 8001-97-6; 67479-27-0 (aloe gum).
NOTE. Do not confuse with Aloe vera (p.1110).
Pharmacopoeias. In *Chin., Eur.* (see p.vi), *Jpn,* and *US.*

The residue obtained by evaporating the juice of the leaves of various species of *Aloe* (Liliaceae).

Pharmacopoeial description
Ph. Eur.: Barbados Aloes (Curaçao aloes) is obtained from *Aloe barbadensis* (= *A. vera*) and contains not less than 28% of hydroxyanthracene derivatives, calculated as anhydrous barbaloin.

Cape Aloes (Aloe capensis) is obtained mainly from *Aloe ferox* and its hybrids and contains not less than 18% of hydroxyanthracene derivatives, calculated as anhydrous barbaloin.

Barbados aloes is dark brown masses, slightly shiny or opaque with a conchoidal fracture, or a brown powder. Cape aloes is similar, but tinged with green. Barbados and Cape aloes are partly soluble in boiling water, soluble in hot alcohol, and practically insoluble in ether. Store in airtight containers. Protect from light.

USP 25: The dried latex of the leaves of *Aloe barbadensis* (= *A. vera*) known in commerce as Curaçao Aloe, or of *A. ferox* and its hybrids, known in commerce as Cape Aloe. It yields not less than 50% of water-soluble extractive. It has a characteristic, somewhat sour and disagreeable, odour. Curaçao Aloe is brownish-black, opaque masses with a fractured, uneven, waxy, and somewhat resinous surface. Cape Aloe is dusty to dark brown irregular masses, the surfaces of which are often covered with a yellowish powder. Its fracture is smooth and glassy.

Adverse Effects and Precautions
As for Senna, p.1248, although aloes has a more drastic and irritant action.

Uses and Administration
Aloes is an anthraquinone stimulant laxative (p.1201) but other less toxic laxatives are generally preferred.

It has also been used in homoeopathic medicine.

Preparations

BP 2001: Compound Benzoin Tincture;
Ph. Eur.: Standardised Aloes Dry Extract;
USP 25: Compound Benzoin Tincture.

Proprietary Preparations (details are given in Part 3)
Fr.: Contre-Coups de l'Abbe Perdrigeon; Vulcase; *Ger.:* Aristo L†; Dr Janssens Teebohnen; Krauterlax A; Rheogen; *Switz.:* Elixir Rebleuten†.

Multi-ingredient: *Aust.:* Abfuhrdragees; Abfuhrdragees mild; Aristochol; Artin; Dragees Neunzehn; Euflat†; Pserhofer's; Schwedenjorg mild†; Spasmo Gallosanol†; *Austral.:* Herbal Cleanse; Lexat; Peritone; Proacid†; Psor-Asist; Vitaglow Herbal Laxative†; *Belg.:* Carters†; Grains de Vals; *Braz.:* Camomila; *Canad.:* Extra Strong Formula 12; Laxative; Natures Remedy; *Fr.:* Ideolaxyl; Opobyl; Petites Pilules Carters; Pilules Dupuis†; Spark†; Tonilax; *Ger.:* Aristochol; Befelka-Tinktur†; Chol-Kugeletten Neu; Cholhepan N; Eupond†; Montana; Pascoletten N; Plantoletten†; Redaxa Lax†; Reducelle†; Schwedentrunk mit Ginseng†; Schwedentrunk†; Spasmo Gallo Sanol N†; *Hong Kong:* Rheogen; *Israel:* Laxative Comp; *Ital.:* Crisolax†; Cura†; Frerichs Maldifassi; Grani di Vals; Neutrogena Anti-Acne; Pillole Fattori; *Port.:* Emopads; *Spain:* Cinaro Bilina†; Crislaxo; Cynaro Bilina; Laxante Sanatorium; Nico Hepatocyn; Opobyl; Pildoras Zeninas; *Switz.:* Adistop Lax†; Ajaka†; Aloinophen†; Dragees laxatives no 510†; Kneipp Woerisettes†; Opobyl†; Padma-Lax; Physiolax†; Phytolax; PhyLaxin; Tavolax†; *UK:* Cleansing Herb Tablets; Dual-Lax Normal Strength; Gerard House Gladlax;

Laxative Tablets; Natural Herb Tablets; Out-of-Sorts; Sure-Lax (Herbal); *USA:* Diaparene Corn Starch; Natures Remedy; Vagisil.

Aloglutamol (12343-d)

2-Amino-2-hydroxymethylpropane-1,3-diol gluconate dihydroxyaluminate.
$C_{10}H_{24}AINO_{12} = 377.3$.
ATC — A02AB06.

Profile
Aloglutamol has been used as an antacid (p.1201).

Preparations

Proprietary Preparations (details are given in Part 3)
Mex.: Sabro; *Spain:* Pyreses†.

Aloin (7502-d)

Aloin (BAN).
Alloin.
CAS — 5133-19-7; 8015-61-0; 1415-73-2 (barbaloin).

Aloin is a crystalline substance obtained from aloes (see above). It consists of *C*-glycosides such as barbaloin.

Profile
Aloin is an anthraquinone stimulant laxative. Like aloes it is very irritant and other less toxic laxatives are generally preferred. Aloin is used as a flavouring agent.

Preparations

Proprietary Preparations (details are given in Part 3)
UK: Beechams Pills†; Calsalettes.

Multi-ingredient: *Austral.:* Ford Pills; *Belg.:* Sanicolax†; *Braz.:* Pilulas Ross; *Canad.:* Aid-Lax†; Alsiline†; Bicholate; Laxa†; Thunas Bilettes†; Triolax†; *Irl.:* Alophen†; *Israel:* Laxative Comp; *Ital.:* Boldina He; Cuscutine; Grani di Vals; *Mex.:* Redotex NF; *Spain:* Alofedina; Laxante Bescansa Aloico; Takata; *Switz.:* Ajaka†; Carter Petites Pilules†; *UK:* Alophen; Carters†; Dual-Lax Extra Strong; Modern Herbals Laxative.

Alosetron (10697-w)

Alosetron (BAN, rINN).
GR-68755X. 2,3,4,5-Tetrahydro-5-methyl-2-[(5-methylimidazol-4-yl)methyl]-1H-pyrido[4,3-b]indol-1-one.
$C_{17}H_{18}N_4O = 294.4$.
CAS — 122852-42-0.

Profile
Alosetron is a 5-HT$_3$-receptor antagonist with general properties similar to those of ondansetron (p.1241). It has been used as the hydrochloride in the treatment of irritable bowel syndrome (p.1206) in women whose predominant bowel symptom is diarrhoea; effectiveness in men has not been established. However following reports of severe constipation or ischaemic colitis in patients receiving alosetron the manufacturers (*Glaxo Wellcome, USA*) withdrew the drug from the market.

Alosetron has also been investigated for schizophrenia and other mental disorders.

◊ References.
1. Camilleri M, *et al.* Improvement in pain and bowel function in female irritable bowel patients with alosetron, a 5-HT3 receptor antagonist. *Aliment Pharmacol Ther* 1999; **13:** 1149–59.
2. Bardhan KD, *et al.* A double-blind, randomized, placebo-controlled dose ranging study to evaluate the efficacy of alosetron in the treatment of irritable bowel syndrome. *Aliment Pharmacol Ther* 2000; **14:** 23–34.
3. Camilleri M, *et al.* Efficacy and safety of alosetron in women with irritable bowel syndrome: a randomised, placebo-controlled trial. *Lancet* 2000; **355:** 1035–40.
4. Camilleri M, *et al.* A randomized controlled clinical trial of the serotonin type 3 receptor antagonist alosetron in women with diarrhea-predominant irritable bowel syndrome. *Arch Intern Med* 2001; **161:** 1733–40.

Preparations

Proprietary Preparations (details are given in Part 3)
USA: Lotronex†.

Basic Aluminium Carbonate (9518-n)

Aluminium Hydroxycarbonate; Basic Aluminum Carbonate (USAN).

A combination of aluminium hydroxide and aluminium carbonate.

Profile
Basic aluminium carbonate gel is an antacid with general properties similar to those of aluminium hydroxide (below). Doses are given in terms of the equivalent amount of aluminium hydroxide; a dose equivalent to about 1 g of aluminium hydroxide is usually taken.

Basic aluminium carbonate may also be given by mouth as a phosphate binder in the treatment of hyperphosphataemia. For a discussion of the choice of phosphate binders, see Renal Osteodystrophy, p.746.

Preparations

Proprietary Preparations (details are given in Part 3)
Fr.: Lithiagel†; *USA:* Basaljel.

Multi-ingredient: *Fr.:* Dextoma.

Aluminium Glycinate (671-q)

Basic Aluminium Aminoacetate; Dihydroxyaluminum Aminoacetate. (Glycinato-N,O)dihydroxyaluminium hydrate.
$C_2H_6AINO_4(+xH_2O) = 135.1$ (anhydrous).
CAS — 13682-92-3 (anhydrous aluminium glycinate); 41354-48-7 (aluminium glycinate hydrate).
ATC — A02AB07.
Pharmacopoeias. In *Br.* and *US.*

Pharmacopoeial description
BP 2001: A white or almost white, odourless or almost odourless, powder. It contains 34.5 to 38.5% of Al_2O_3 calculated on the dried substance, and not more than 12% loss of weight on drying. Practically insoluble in water and in organic solvents; it dissolves in dilute mineral acids and in aqueous solutions of alkali hydroxides. A 4% suspension in water has a pH of 6.5 to 7.5.
USP 25: A white, odourless, powder. It may contain small amounts of aluminium oxide and aminoacetic acid. It loses not more than 14.5% of its weight on drying. Insoluble in water and in organic solvents; soluble in dilute mineral acids and in solutions of fixed alkalis. A 4% suspension in water has a pH of 6.5 to 7.5.

Profile
Aluminium glycinate is an antacid with general properties similar to those of aluminium hydroxide (below). It has been given in doses of up to 1 g by mouth.

Preparations

USP 25: Dihydroxyaluminum Aminoacetate Magma.

Proprietary Preparations (details are given in Part 3)
Multi-ingredient: *Aust.:* Acidrine; Gastripan†; *Belg.:* Acidrine; Alucid; Normacidine†; *Braz.:* Betazon; *Denm.:* Alminox; *Fr.:* Acidrine; Gastralgine†; *Ger.:* Acidrine; *Ital.:* Acidrine; Gastrostop†; Digestinas Super†; Gastroglutal; Jorkil†; Meteoril; Natrocitral; Secrepat.

Used as an adjunct in: *Aust.:* Ambene N; Indobene; *Braz.:* Reumix; Somalgin; *Canad.:* Bufferin; *Ger.:* Indomet-ratiopharm m; *Hong Kong:* Trabit; *Ital.:* Aspirina 03 and 05; *Switz.:* Bonidon; *USA:* Buffex.

Aluminium Hydroxide (673-s)

Aluminii Oxidum Hydricum; Aluminum Hydroxide; Wasserhaltiges Aluminiumoxid.
CAS — 21645-51-2 [$Al(OH)_3$].
ATC — A02AB01.
NOTE. Compounded preparations of aluminium hydroxide may be represented by the following names:
- Co-magaldrox *x/y* (BAN)—where *x* and *y* are the strengths in milligrams of magnesium hydroxide and aluminium hydroxide respectively.
Pharmacopoeias. In *Chin., Eur.* (see p.vi), *Int., Jpn, Pol.,* and *US.*

Pharmacopoeial description
Ph. Eur.: Hydrated Aluminium Oxide (Dried Aluminium Hydroxide (BP 2001)) contains the equivalent of 47 to 60% Al_2O_3. It is a white amorphous powder. Practically insoluble in water; it dissolves in dilute mineral acids and in solutions of alkali hydroxides. Store in airtight containers at a temperature not exceeding 30°.
USP 25: Aluminum Hydroxide Gel is a suspension of amorphous aluminium hydroxide in which there is a partial substitution of carbonate for hydroxide. It is a white viscous suspension from which small amounts of clear liquid may separate on standing. It has a pH of between 5.5 and 8.0. Store in airtight containers. Avoid freezing.
Dried Aluminum Hydroxide Gel is an amorphous form of aluminium hydroxide in which there is a partial substitution of carbonate for hydroxide. It contains the equivalent of not less than 76.5% of $Al(OH)_3$ and may contain varying quantities of basic aluminium carbonate and bicarbonate. The labelling requirements states that 1 g of dried aluminum hydroxide gel is equivalent to 765 mg of $Al(OH)_3$. It is a white, odourless, tasteless, amorphous powder. Insoluble in water and in alcohol; soluble in dilute mineral acids and in solutions of fixed alkali hydroxides. A 4% aqueous dispersion has a pH of not more than 10.0. Store in airtight containers.
Algeldrate (USAN, pINN) is defined as a hydrated aluminium hydroxide with the general formula of $Al(OH)_3.xH_2O$.

Adverse Effects and Precautions
Aluminium hydroxide, like other aluminium compounds, is astringent and may cause constipation; large doses can cause intestinal obstruction.

Excessive doses, or even normal doses in patients with low-phosphate diets, may lead to phosphate depletion accompanied by increased bone resorption and hypercalciuria with the risk of osteomalacia.

Aluminium salts are not, in general, well absorbed from the gastrointestinal tract, and systemic effects are therefore rare in patients with normal renal function. However, care is necessary in patients with chronic renal impairment: osteomalacia or adynamic bone disease, encephalopathy, dementia, and microcytic anaemia have been associated with aluminium accumulation in such patients given large doses of aluminium hydroxide as a phosphate-binding agent. Similar adverse effects have also been associated with the aluminium content of dialysis fluids.

Aluminium hydroxide used as an adjuvant in adsorbed vaccines has been associated with the formation of granulomas.

◊ References to aluminium toxicity in dialysis patients and the possible association between aluminium ingestion and Alzheimer's disease are included under Aluminium (see p.1578). Aluminium accumulation does not generally appear to be significant in patients with normal renal function taking therapeutic doses of aluminium-containing antacids, and there is little evidence that such antacids are a risk factor for Alzheimer's disease.[1] Elevated plasma-aluminium concentrations have been reported in infants with normal renal function given aluminium-containing antacids but there were no obvious signs of toxicity.[2] However, aluminium accumulation resulting in osteomalacia or encephalopathy with seizures and dementia has been reported in children with renal failure treated with aluminium-containing phosphate binders.[3-7] Aluminium-containing antacids should therefore be used with caution in patients with chronic renal failure, especially in children.

Oral citrate salts increase the absorption of aluminium from the gastrointestinal tract[8] and patients with renal failure taking aluminium compounds should avoid citrate-containing preparations, which include many effervescent or dispersible tablets.[9,10] Ascorbic acid has also been reported to enhance aluminium absorption.[11]

1. Flaten TP, et al. Mortality from dementia among gastroduodenal ulcer patients. J Epidemiol Community Health 1991; 45: 203–6.
2. Tsou VM, et al. Elevated plasma aluminum levels in normal infants receiving antacids containing aluminum. Pediatrics 1991; 87: 148–51.
3. Pedersen S, Nathan E. Water treatment and dialysis dementia. Lancet 1982; ii: 1107.
4. Griswold WR, et al. Accumulation of aluminum in a nondialyzed uremic child receiving aluminum hydroxide. Pediatrics 1983; 71: 56–8.
5. Randall ME. Aluminium toxicity in an infant not on dialysis. Lancet 1983; i: 1327–8.
6. Sedman AB, et al. Encephalopathy in childhood secondary to aluminum toxicity. J Pediatr 1984; 105: 836–8.
7. Andreoli SP, et al. Aluminum intoxication from aluminum-containing phosphate binders in children with azotemia not undergoing dialysis. N Engl J Med 1984; 310: 1079–84.
8. Walker JA, et al. The effect of oral bases on enteral aluminum absorption. Arch Intern Med 1990; 150: 2037–9.
9. Mees EJD, Basçi A. Citric acid in calcium effervescent tablets may favour aluminium intoxication. Nephron 1991; 59: 322.
10. Main J, Ward MK. Potentiation of aluminium absorption by effervescent analgesic tablets in a haemodialysis patient. BMJ 1992; 304: 1686.
11. Domingo JL, et al. Effect of ascorbic acid on gastrointestinal aluminium absorption. Lancet 1992; 338: 1467.

Porphyria. Aluminium hydroxide is considered to be unsafe in patients with porphyria because it has been shown to be porphyrinogenic in *animals*.

Interactions

As outlined on p.1201, aluminium compounds used as antacids interact with many other drugs, both by alterations in gastric pH and emptying, and by direct adsorption and formation of complexes that are not absorbed. Interactions can be minimised by giving the aluminium compound and any other medication 2 to 3 hours apart. The absorption of aluminium from the gastrointestinal tract may be enhanced if aluminium compounds are taken concomitantly with citrates or ascorbic acid (see above).

Pharmacokinetics

Aluminium hydroxide, given by mouth, slowly reacts with the hydrochloric acid in the stomach to form soluble aluminium chloride, some of which is absorbed. The presence of food or other factors which decrease gastric emptying prolongs the availability of aluminium hydroxide to react and may increase the amount of aluminium chloride formed. About 0.1 to 0.5 mg of the cation is reported to be absorbed from standard daily doses of an aluminium-containing antacid, leading to about a doubling of usual aluminium concentrations in the plasma of patients with normal renal function.

Absorbed aluminium is eliminated in the urine, and patients with renal failure are therefore at particular risk of accumulation (especially in bone and the CNS), and aluminium toxicity.

The aluminium compounds remaining in the gastrointestinal tract, which account for most of a dose, form insoluble, poorly absorbed aluminium salts in the intestines including hydroxides, carbonates, phosphates and fatty acid derivatives, which are excreted in the faeces.

Uses and Administration

Aluminium hydroxide is used as an antacid (p.1201). It is given in doses of up to about 1 g by mouth. In order to reduce the constipating effects, aluminium hydroxide is often given in association with a magnesium-containing antacid, such as magnesium oxide or magnesium hydroxide.

Aluminium hydroxide binds phosphate in the gastrointestinal tract to form insoluble complexes and reduces phosphate absorption. It is thus used to treat hyperphosphataemia in patients with chronic renal failure (see Renal Osteodystrophy, p.746). With this use the dose must be adjusted to the individual patient's requirement but up to about 10 g daily by mouth may be given in divided doses.

Aluminium hydroxide is also used as an adjuvant in adsorbed vaccines.

Polymyositis and dermatomyositis. Corticosteroids form the basis of the management of polymyositis (p.1057) but the calcinosis that may occur in dermatomyositis does not always respond well. Aluminium hydroxide 1.68 to 2.24 g daily produced clinical improvement with complete clearing of most calcified nodules after 1 year in a patient with calcinosis cutis complicating juvenile dermatomyositis.[1] The calcified masses are made up of hydroxyapatite and amorphous calcium phosphate and reduction in phosphate absorption by aluminium hydroxide probably helped to reverse their formation. Subsequent cases[2,3] have also reported benefit from aluminium hydroxide treatment in the management of calcinosis.

1. Wang W-J, et al. Calcinosis cutis in juvenile dermatomyositis: remarkable response to aluminium hydroxide therapy. Arch Dermatol 1988; 124: 1721–2.
2. Nakagawa T, Takaiwa T. Calcinosis cutis in juvenile dermatomyositis responsive to aluminium hydroxide treatment. J Dermatol 1993; 20: 558–60.
3. Wananukul S, et al. Calcinosis cutis presenting years before other clinical manifestations of juvenile dermatomyositis: report of two cases. Australas J Dermatol 1997; 38: 202–5.

Preparations

BP 2001: Aluminium Hydroxide Oral Suspension; Aluminium Hydroxide Tablets; Co-magaldrox Oral Suspension; Co-magaldrox Tablets; Compound Magnesium Trisilicate Tablets;
USP 25: Alumina and Magnesia Oral Suspension; Alumina and Magnesia Tablets; Alumina and Magnesium Carbonate Oral Suspension; Alumina and Magnesium Carbonate Tablets; Alumina and Magnesium Trisilicate Oral Suspension; Alumina and Magnesium Trisilicate Tablets; Alumina, Magnesia, and Calcium Carbonate Oral Suspension; Alumina, Magnesia, and Calcium Carbonate Tablets; Alumina, Magnesia, and Simethicone Oral Suspension; Alumina, Magnesia, and Simethicone Tablets; Alumina, Magnesia, Calcium Carbonate, and Simethicone Tablets; Alumina, Magnesium Carbonate, and Magnesium Oxide Tablets; Aluminum Hydroxide Gel; Aspirin, Alumina, and Magnesia Tablets; Aspirin, Alumina, and Magnesium Oxide Tablets; Dried Aluminum Hydroxide Gel; Dried Aluminum Hydroxide Gel Capsules; Dried Aluminum Hydroxide Gel Tablets.

Proprietary Preparations (details are given in Part 3)
Aust.: Anti-Phosphat; *Austral.:* Alu-Tab; Amphojel†; *Braz.:* Aldrox; Anacidron-H; Fluagel; Mylanta Plus; Natusgel; No-Acid; Pepsamar; *Canad.:* Alu-Tab; Alugel; Amphojel; Basaljel; *Ger.:* Aludrox; Antacidum OPT†; Anti-Phosphat; Gastrocaps A; *Hong Kong:* Alu-Tab; *Irl.:* Aludrox; *Israel:* Alu-Cap; *Ital.:* Diplogel†; Polisilon; *Mex.:* Galcdexan; Magnalum; *NZ:* Alutabs; Amphojel; *Port.:* Almigastrico; Gelumina; Pepsamar; *S.Afr.:* Acidex; Alukon†; Amphojel; *Singapore:* Alu-Tab; *Spain:* Alugel; Dialume; Pepsamar; *Switz.:* Anti-Phosphate; Gastracol; *UK:* Alu-Cap; Aludrox; *USA:* ALternaGEL; Alu-Cap; Alu-Tab; Amphojel; Dialume; Nephrox.

Multi-ingredient: numerous preparations are listed in Part 3.

Aluminium Hydroxide-Magnesium Carbonate Co-dried Gel (674-w)

F-MA 11.

A co-precipitate of aluminium hydroxide and magnesium carbonate dried to contain a proportion of water for antacid activity.

Profile
Aluminium hydroxide-magnesium carbonate co-dried gel is an antacid with general properties similar to those of aluminium hydroxide (above) and magnesium carbonate (p.1232). It is given in doses of about 400 to 800 mg by mouth.

Preparations

Proprietary Preparations (details are given in Part 3)
Denm.: Link; *Fin.:* Link; PeeHoo; *Norw.:* Link; *Swed.:* Link; *UK:* Dijex; Gastrils†.

Multi-ingredient: *Austral.:* Algicon†; *Belg.:* Barexal; Gastropulgite†; Nozid; Regla pH Forte; Syngel; *Braz.:* Acidex; Algicote; Andursil; *Canad.:* Amphojel Plus†; Diovol; Diovol Plus; Gastrinol; Gastrocalm; Thunas Hyperacidity Tablets; *Fin.:* PH maxi; *Fr.:* Gastropulgite; *Ger.:* Colina Spezial; Duovolrinetten N; Gastropulgit; *Hong Kong:* Diovol Plus; Simeco; Veragel; *Irl.:* Algicon; *Israel:* Silain; *Mex.:* Algicon; Ditopax; Ditopax-F; *Neth.:* Algicon; Regla pH; Rigoletten; *Norw.:* Algicon†; *Port.:* Di-Gel Forte; *S.Afr.:* Tacid-4†; *Singapore:* Simeco; Tocid; Veragel DMS; *Spain:* Acylene; *Switz.:* Anacidol; Andursil; Combacid; Gastropulgite; Refluxine; Regla pH†; *Thai.:* Defomil; Diovol; Kremil-S; Machto; Simeco; Veragel; *UK:* Algicon; Aludrox; Simeco; *USA:* Maalox Heartburn Relief.

Used as an adjunct in: Braz.: Superhist.

Aluminium Phosphate (676-l)

Aluminii Phosphas; Aluminum Phosphate.
CAS — 7784-30-7 (AlPO$_4$).
ATC — A02AB03.
*Pharmacopoeias. In Pol.
Eur. (see p.vi) includes Hydrated Aluminium Phosphate. US includes Aluminum Phosphate Gel.*

Pharmacopoeial description
Ph. Eur.: Hydrated Aluminium Phosphate (Dried Aluminium Phosphate BP 2001) is a white or almost white powder. Very slightly soluble in water; practically insoluble in alcohol. It dissolves in dilute solutions of alkali hydroxides and mineral acids. A 4% suspension in water has a pH of 5.5 to 7.2. Store in airtight containers.

USP 25: Aluminum Phosphate Gel is a 4 to 5% suspension of aluminium phosphate (AlPO$_4$) in water and has a pH of 6.0 to 7.2. It is a white viscous suspension from which small amounts of water separate on standing. Store in airtight containers.

Profile
Aluminium phosphate is an antacid with general properties similar to those of aluminium hydroxide (p.1210), but it does not produce phosphate depletion.

Aluminium phosphate is also used as an adjuvant in adsorbed vaccines.

Preparations
USP 25: Aluminum Phosphate Gel.

Proprietary Preparations (details are given in Part 3)
Aust.: Phosphalugel; *Belg.:* Phosphalugel; *Fr.:* Phosphalugel; *Ger.:* Phosphalugel; *Ital.:* Fosfalugel; *Port.:* Phosphalugel; *Spain:* Fosfalumina†; *Switz.:* Phosphalugel.
Multi-ingredient: *Aust.:* Phoscortil; *Fr.:* Isudrine; Moxydar.

Aluminium Sodium Silicate (677-y)

E554; Sodium Aluminium Silicate; Sodium Aluminosilicate; Sodium Silicoaluminate.
CAS — 1344-00-9.

Profile
Aluminium sodium silicate is an antacid with general properties similar to those of aluminium hydroxide (p.1210). Aluminium silicate has been used similarly. They are also used as food additives.

Preparations
Proprietary Preparations (details are given in Part 3)
Fr.: Sulfuryl.

Multi-ingredient: *Aust.:* Diphlogen; *Belg.:* Mucal†; *Braz.:* Colestase; Diteutrin; *Fr.:* Anti-H; Cerat Inalterable; Mucal†; Sulfuryl; *Ger.:* Enelbin-Paste N; Mucal†; Sulfredox; *Port.:* Gastroplex†; Mucal; *Spain:* Doctogaster†; *Switz.:* TRI-OM; *Thai.:* Ulgastrin.

Alverine Citrate (5226-m)

Alverine Citrate *(BANM, USAN, rINNM).*
Dipropyline Citrate; Phenpropamine Citrate. *N*-Ethyl-3,3'-diphenyldipropylamine citrate.
$C_{20}H_{27}N,C_6H_8O_7 = 473.6.$
CAS — 150-59-4 (alverine); 5560-59-8 (alverine citrate).

Alverine citrate 67.3 mg is approximately equivalent to 40 mg of alverine.

Adverse Effects and Precautions
Nausea, headache, pruritus, rash, and dizziness have been reported. Allergic reactions, including anaphylaxis, have also occurred. Alverine is contra-indicated in patients with intestinal obstruction or paralytic ileus.

Pharmacokinetics
Alverine is absorbed from the gastrointestinal tract following oral administration and is rapidly metabolised to an active metabolite, peak plasma concentrations of which occur 1 to 1.5 hours after an oral dose. Further metabolism to inactive metabolites occurs; metabolites are excreted in the urine by active renal secretion.

Uses and Administration

Alverine is an antispasmodic that acts directly on intestinal and uterine smooth muscle. It is used for the relief of smooth muscle spasm in the treatment of gastrointestinal disorders such as irritable bowel syndrome (p.1206). It is also used in the treatment of dysmenorrhoea (p.6).

Alverine is given by mouth as the citrate in doses of 60 to 120 mg one to three times daily or by suppository as the base in doses of 80 mg two or three times daily.

Preparations

Proprietary Preparations (details are given in Part 3)
Belg.: Spasmine; *Fr.:* Spasmaverine; *Hong Kong:* Profenil; Spasmonal; *Irl.:* Spasmonal; *Singapore:* Spasmonal; *Thai.:* Spasmonal; *UK:* Relaxyl; Spasmonal.

Multi-ingredient: *Austral.:* Alvercol; *Belg.:* Normacol Antispasmodique; *Fr.:* Hepatoum; Meteospasmyl; Schoum; Spasmaverine; *Hong Kong:* Alvercol; Meteospasmyl; *Irl.:* Alvercol; *S.Afr.:* Alvercol; *Singapore:* Meteospasmyl; *UK:* Spasmonal Fibre.

Attapulgite (679-z)

CAS — 1337-76-4; 12174-11-7.
ATC — A07BC04.
Pharmacopoeias. In *Br.* Activated Attapulgite is included in *Br., It.,* and *US.* Colloidal Activated Attapulgite is included in *US.*

Pharmacopoeial description

BP 2001: Attapulgite is a purified native hydrated aluminium magnesium silicate essentially consisting of the clay mineral palygorskite. Activated Attapulgite is attapulgite that has been carefully heated to increase its adsorptive capacity. A light, cream or buff, very fine powder, free or almost free from gritty particles. A 5% suspension in water has a pH of 7.0 to 9.5.

USP 25: Activated Attapulgite is processed native aluminium magnesium silicate which has been carefully heated. It is a cream-coloured, micronised, nonswelling powder, free from gritty particles. Insoluble in water.

Colloidal Activated Attapulgite is native aluminium magnesium silicate which has been purified. It is a cream-coloured, micronised, nonswelling powder, free from gritty particles. Insoluble in water. A 10% suspension in water has a pH of 7.0 to 9.5. Another native aluminium magnesium silicate is described on p.1499.

Profile

Attapulgite is highly adsorbent and is used in a wide range of products including fertilisers, pesticides, and pharmaceuticals. Activated attapulgite is an adsorbent antidiarrhoeal used as an adjunct in the management of diarrhoea (p.1203) in a daily dose of up to 9 g by mouth in divided doses.

Preparations

Proprietary Preparations (details are given in Part 3)
Belg.: Actapulgite; *Canad.:* Fowlers; Kaopectate; *Fr.:* Actapulgite; Norgagil†; *Hong Kong:* New Diatabs; *Switz.:* Actapulgite; *Thai.:* Atta; Entox-P; *UAE:* Kaptin II; *USA:* Children's Kaopectate; Diasorb; Donnagel; K-Pek; Kaopectate Advanced Formula; Kaopectate Maximum Strength; Rheaban Maximum Strength.

Multi-ingredient: *Austral.:* Diarcalm†; Diareze; *Belg.:* Gastropulgite†; Mucipulgite; *Braz.:* Atacoly; Diapool; Diazol; Dientrin; Duoctrin Enterico; Entercal; Enterocler; Enteropen; Fluocal com Pectina; Linadin; Magnostase; *Canad.:* Diban; Donnagel-PG; *Fr.:* Gastropulgite; Mucipulgite; *Ger.:* Gastropulgit; *Irl.:* Diocalm†; *Ital.:* Streptomagma; *S.Afr.:* Kantrexil; *Spain:* Terpalate†; *Switz.:* Gastropulgite; Mucipulgite; *Thai.:* Attafur; *UK:* Diocalm Dual Action; Entrotabs.

Azasetron Hydrochloride (17071-s)

Azasetron Hydrochloride (rINNM).
Nazasetron Hydrochloride; Y-25130. (±)-6-Chloro-3,4-dihydro-4-methyl-3-oxo-N-3-quinuclidinyl-2H-1,4-benzoxazine-8-carboxamide hydrochloride.
$C_{17}H_{20}ClN_3O_3,HCl = 386.3$.
CAS — 123040-69-7 (azasetron); 141922-90-9 (azasetron hydrochloride).

Profile

Azasetron hydrochloride is a 5-HT₃-receptor antagonist with general properties similar to those of ondansetron (p.1241). It is used as an antiemetic in the management of nausea and vomiting induced by cytotoxic therapy, in a usual dose of 10 mg given once daily by mouth or intravenously.

Preparations

Proprietary Preparations (details are given in Part 3)
Jpn: Serotone.

Balsalazide Sodium (18555-j)

Balsalazide Sodium (BANM, rINNM).
Balsalazide Disodium (USAN); Balsalazine Disodium; BX-661A. 5-[4-(2-Carboxyethylcarbamoyl)phenylazo]salicylic acid, disodium salt, dihydrate.
$C_{17}H_{13}N_3Na_2O_6,2H_2O = 437.3$.
CAS — 80573-04-2 (balsalazide); 150399-21-6 (balsalazide disodium dihydrate).

Adverse Effects and Precautions

As for Mesalazine, p.1234. If a blood dyscrasia is suspected treatment should be stopped immediately and a blood count performed. Patients or their carers should be told how to recognise signs of blood toxicity and should be advised to seek immediate medical attention if symptoms such as fever, sore throat, mouth ulcers, bruising, or bleeding develop. Balsalazide should not be used in patients with severe hepatic impairment or moderate or severe renal impairment; care is required in those with lesser degrees of hepatic or renal impairment, and in asthma, bleeding disorders, or active peptic ulcer disease.

Hypersensitivity. A case of acute pericarditis, cholestasis, and vasculitis resulting from hypersensitivity to balsalazide has been reported.[1] The authors noted similarities to mesalazine-associated pericarditis and lupus-like syndrome (see Effects on the Cardiovascular System, p.1234).

1. Adhiyaman V, *et al.* Hypersensitivity reaction to balsalazide. *BMJ* 2001; **323:** 489.

Pharmacokinetics

The absorption of intact balsalazide from the gastrointestinal tract is negligible. It is split by bacteria in the colon to 5-aminosalicylic acid (mesalazine), which is active, and 4-aminobenzoylalanine, which is considered to be an inert carrier. About 25% of the released mesalazine is absorbed and acetylated, as described under mesalazine (p.1235). A small proportion of 4-aminobenzoylalanine is absorbed and acetylated on first pass through the liver. The acetylated metabolites are excreted in the urine.

Uses and Administration

Balsalazide consists of mesalazine linked to 4-aminobenzoylalanine via an azo bond. This bond is broken by colonic bacteria releasing the active mesalazine (p.1235). Balsalazide sodium is given by mouth in the treatment of mild to moderate active ulcerative colitis (p.1205), in a dose of 2.25 g three times daily until remission or for up to 12 weeks. For maintenance of remission of ulcerative colitis a dose of 1.5 g twice daily is recommended, adjusted as necessary up to 6 g daily.

◊ General references.
1. Prakash A, Spencer CM. Balsalazide. *Drugs* 1998; **56:** 83–9.

Preparations

Proprietary Preparations (details are given in Part 3)
Denm.: Premid; *UK:* Colazide; *USA:* Colazal.

Multi-ingredient: *Swed.:* Colazid.

Benexate Hydrochloride (3666-e)

Benexate Hydrochloride (rINNM).
Benzyl salicylate *trans*-4-(guanidinomethyl)cyclohexanecarboxylate hydrochloride.
$C_{23}H_{27}N_3O_4,HCl = 445.9$.
CAS — 78718-52-2 (benexate); 78718-25-9 (benexate hydrochloride).

Profile

Benexate hydrochloride has been used in the management of peptic ulcer disease. It has been given by mouth as the clathrate with β-cyclodextrin, benexate betadex.

Bisacodyl (7503-n)

Bisacodyl (BAN, rINN).
Bisacodylum. 4,4′-(2-Pyridylmethylene)di(phenyl acetate).
$C_{22}H_{19}NO_4 = 361.4$.
CAS — 603-50-9 (bisacodyl); 1336-29-4 (bisacodyl tannex).
ATC — A06AB02; A06AG02.

NOTE. Bisacodyl Tannex is USAN.
Pharmacopoeias. In *Eur.* (see p.vi), *Jpn, Pol.,* and *US.*

Pharmacopoeial description

Ph. Eur.: A white or almost white crystalline powder. Practically insoluble in water; sparingly soluble in alcohol; soluble in acetone; slightly soluble in ether. It dissolves in dilute mineral acids. Protect from light.

USP 25: A white to off-white crystalline powder. Practically insoluble in water; soluble in benzene; soluble 1 in 210 of alcohol, 1 in 2.5 of chloroform, and 1 in 275 of ether; sparingly soluble in methyl alcohol.

◊ CAUTION. *Avoid inhalation of the powder and contact with eyes, skin, and mucous membranes.*

Adverse Effects

Bisacodyl and other stimulant laxatives may cause abdominal discomfort such as colic or cramps. Prolonged use or overdosage can result in diarrhoea with excessive loss of water and electrolytes, particularly potassium; there is also the possibility of developing an atonic non-functioning colon. When administered rectally bisacodyl sometimes causes irritation and repeated use may cause proctitis or sloughing of the epithelium. To avoid gastric irritation bisacodyl tablets are enteric-coated.

Precautions

As with other laxatives, prolonged use should be avoided. Bisacodyl should not be given to patients with intestinal obstruction or acute abdominal conditions such as appendicitis; care should also be taken in patients with inflammatory bowel disease. It should not be used in patients with severe dehydration. The suppositories should preferably be avoided in patients with anal fissures, proctitis, or ulcerated haemorrhoids.

Pharmacokinetics

Following administration of bisacodyl by mouth or rectally, it is converted to the active desacetyl metabolite bis(p-hydroxyphenyl)pyridyl-2-methane by intestinal and bacterial enzymes. Absorption from the gastrointestinal tract is minimal with enteric-coated tablets or suppositories; the small amount absorbed is excreted in the urine as the glucuronide. Bisacodyl is mainly excreted in the faeces.

Uses and Administration

Bisacodyl is a diphenylmethane stimulant laxative (p.1201) used for the treatment of constipation (p.1202) and for bowel evacuation before investigational procedures or surgery. Its action is mainly in the large intestine and it is usually effective within 6 to 12 hours following administration by mouth and within 15 to 60 minutes following rectal administration. Bisacodyl tablets should be swallowed whole and should not be taken within one hour of milk or antacids.

For constipation, bisacodyl is given in usual doses of 5 to 10 mg daily as enteric-coated tablets administered at night or 10 mg as a suppository or enema administered in the morning. Doses of 10 to 20 mg are given by mouth for complete bowel evacuation, followed by 10 mg as a suppository the next morning.

Children under 10 years of age may be given 5 mg rectally in the morning for constipation; those over 4 years may alternatively be given 5 mg by mouth at night. For bowel evacuation the dose is 5 mg by mouth the night before and 5 mg rectally the morning of the procedure. Children over 10 years of age may be given doses similar to those for adults.

Bisacodyl has been administered with a barium sulfate enema before radiographic examination of the colon. A complex of bisacodyl with tannic acid (bisacodyl tannex) is generally used in a dose equivalent to 1.5 to 3 mg of bisacodyl dissolved in 1 litre of barium sulfate suspension. The total dose for one procedure should not exceed 4.5 mg of bisacodyl and no more than 6 mg should be administered in 72 hours.

Preparations

BP 2001: Bisacodyl Suppositories; Bisacodyl Tablets;
USP 25: Bisacodyl Delayed-release Tablets; Bisacodyl Rectal Suspension; Bisacodyl Suppositories.

Proprietary Preparations (details are given in Part 3)
Aust.: Dulcolax; Laxbene; *Austral.:* Bisalax; Durolax; Fleet Laxative; *Belg.:* Dulcolax; Horton†; Mucinum; Purgo-Pil; *Braz.:* Dislax; Dulcolax; *Canad.:* Bisacolax; Carters Little Pills; Correctol; Dulcolax; Feen-A-Mint; Soflax EX; *Denm.:* Dulcolax; Perilax; Toilax; *Fin.:* Metalax; Toilax; *Fr.:* Contalax; Dulcolax; *Ger.:* Agaroletten; Bekunis Bisacodyl; Bisco-Zitron; Darmol Bisacodyl; Drix N; Dulcolax; Florisan N†; Laxagetten; Laxanin N; Laxansratiopharm; Laxbene; Laxbene N; Laxoberal Bisa; Laxysat Burger; Mandrolax†; Marienbader Pillen N; Mediolax; Pyrilax; Rhabarex B†; Stadalax; Tempolax; Tirgon N; Vinco Forte†; Vinco-Abfuhr-Perlen; *Hong Kong:* Correctol; Dulcolax; *Irl.:* Dulcolax;

Toilax; *Israel:* Contalax; Laxadin; *Ital.:* Alaxa; Confetto CM; Dulcolax; Normalene; Verecolene CM; *Mex.:* Dulcolan; *Neth.:* Dulcolax; Nourilax†; Zwitsalax/N†; *Norw.:* Dulcolax; Toilax; *NZ:* Dulcolax; *Port.:* Dulcolax; *S.Afr.:* Capolax†; Dulcolax; Megalax; *Singapore:* Dulcolax; *Spain:* Dulco Laxo; Medesup†; *Swed.:* Dulcolax; Toilax; *Switz.:* Demolaxin; Dulcolax; Ercolax†; Muxol; Prontolax; Tavolax nouvelle formule; *Thai.:* Dulcolax; Emulax; Gencolax; Kadolax; Laxcodyl; Vacolax; *UAE:* Laxocodyl; *UK:* Biolax; Dulcolax; *USA:* Bisac-Evac†; Bisco-Lax†; Clysodrast†; Correctol; Dulcagen†; Dulcolax; Evac-Q-Kwik Suppository; Evac-Q-Tabs; Feen-A-Mint; Fleet Bisacodyl; Fleet Laxative.

Multi-ingredient: *Aust.:* Laxbene; Prepacol†; Purgazen; Purigoa; *Austral.:* Coloxyl; Durolax X-Pack; Go Kit; Go Kit Plus; *Belg.:* Prepacol; Softene; *Braz.:* Humectol; *Canad.:* Bicholate; Evac-Q-Kwik†; Extra Strong Formula 12; Fruitatives; Royvac Kit; *Fr.:* Pilules Dupuis†; Prepacol; *Ger.:* Potsilo; Prepacol; *NZ:* Coloxyl; *Port.:* Bekunis†; *Spain:* Bekunis Complex; Boldolaxin; *Switz.:* Aloinophen†; Bekunis; Drix†; Tavolax†; *Thai.:* Bisolax; UK: Nylax†; *USA:* Dulcolax Bowel Prep Kit†; Fleet Prep Kit No. 1; Fleet Prep Kit No. 2; Fleet Prep Kit No. 3; Fleet Prep Kit No. 4†; Fleet Prep Kit No. 5†; Fleet Prep Kit No. 6†; Tridrate Bowel Evacuant Kit†; X-Prep Bowel Evacuant Kit-1; X-Prep Bowel Evacuant Kit-2.

Bismuth Compounds (17157-z)

Bismuth compounds have been used for their astringent and antidiarrhoeal properties in a variety of gastrointestinal disorders, and have been applied topically in skin disorders and anorectal disorders such as haemorrhoids. Certain salts are active against *Helicobacter pylori* and are used in the treatment of peptic ulcer disease.

Bismuth Aluminate (5268-y)
Bismuth Aluminate *(USAN)*.
Aluminum Bismuth Oxide.
$Bi_2(Al_2O_4)_3,10H_2O = 952.0$.
CAS — 12284-76-3 (anhydrous bismuth aluminate).
Pharmacopoeias. In Fr.

Bismuth Citrate (14763-y)
CAS — 813-93-4.
Pharmacopoeias. In US.

Pharmacopoeial description
USP 25: A white, amorphous or crystalline powder. Insoluble in water and in alcohol; soluble in dilute ammonia solution and in solutions of alkali citrates. Store at a temperature not exceeding 40° in airtight containers. Protect from light.

Bismuth Oxide (5271-p)
Bismuth Trioxide.
$Bi_2O_3 = 466.0$.
CAS — 1304-76-3.

Bismuth Salicylate (5275-l)
Basic Bismuth Salicylate; Bismuth Oxysalicylate; Bismuth Subsalicylate *(USAN)*; Bismuthi Subsalicylas.
$C_7H_5BiO_4 = 362.1$.
CAS — 14882-18-9.
Pharmacopoeias. In Eur. (see p.vi) and US.

Pharmacopoeial description
Ph. Eur.: It contains not less than 57% and not more than 60% of Bi, calculated with reference to the dried substance. A white powder. Practically insoluble in water and in alcohol; dissolves in mineral acids with decomposition. Protect from light.
USP 25: A basic salt corresponding to $C_7H_5BiO_4 = 362.1$ and containing not less than 56.0% and not more than 59.4% of Bi and not less than 36.5% and not more than 39.3% of total salicylates. It is a fine, odourless, white to off-white microcrystalline powder. Practically insoluble in water, in alcohol, and in ether. It reacts with alkalis and mineral acids. Store in airtight containers. Protect from light.

Bismuth Subcarbonate (5279-c)
Bismuth Subcarbonate *(USAN)*.
Basic Bismuth Carbonate; Basisches Wismutkarbonat; Bism. Carb.; Bismuth Carbonate; Bismuth Oxycarbonate; Bismuthi Subcarbonas; Bismutylum Carbonicum; Carbonato de Bismutila.
CAS — 5892-10-4 (anhydrous bismuth subcarbonate); 5798-45-8 (bismuth subcarbonate hemihydrate).
Pharmacopoeias. In Chin., Eur. (see p.vi), and US.

Pharmacopoeial description
Ph. Eur.: A white or almost white powder. Practically insoluble in water, in alcohol, and in ether. It dissolves in mineral acids with effervescence. Protect from light.
USP 25: A white or almost white powder. Practically insoluble in water, in alcohol, and in ether; dissolves in dilute acids with effervescence. Protect from light.

The symbol † denotes a preparation no longer actively marketed

Bismuth Subgallate (5280-s)
Bismuth Subgallate *(USAN)*.
Basic Bismuth Gallate; Basisches Wismutgallat; Bism. Subgall.; Bismuth Oxygallate; Bismuthi Subgallas.
$C_7H_5BiO_6 = 394.1$.
CAS — 99-26-3.
Pharmacopoeias. In Eur. (see p.vi), Jpn, Pol., and US.

Pharmacopoeial description
Ph. Eur.: It contains not less than 48% and not more than 51% of Bi, calculated with reference to the dried substance. A yellow powder. Practically insoluble in water and in alcohol; dissolves in mineral acids with decomposition and in alkali hydroxides, producing a reddish-brown liquid. Protect from light.
USP 25: A basic salt containing 52 to 57% of Bi_2O_3 when dried at 105° for 3 hours. It is an odourless amorphous bright yellow powder. Practically insoluble in water, in alcohol, in chloroform, and in ether; insoluble in very dilute mineral acids; dissolves readily with decomposition in warm, moderately dilute hydrochloric, nitric, or sulfuric acids; readily dissolves in solutions of alkali hydroxides to form a clear yellow liquid which rapidly becomes deep red. Store in airtight containers. Protect from light.

Bismuth Subnitrate (5281-w)
Basic Bismuth Nitrate; Basisches Wismutnitrat; Bism. Subnit.; Bismuth Hydroxide Nitrate Oxide; Bismuth Nitrate, Heavy; Bismuth Oxynitrate; Bismuth (Sous-Nitrate de) Lourd; Bismuthi Subnitras; Bismuthyl Nitrate; Magistery of Bismuth; Nitrato de Bismutilo; Subazotato de Bismuto; White Bismuth.
$Bi_5O(OH)_9(NO_3)_4 = 1462.0$.
CAS — 1304-85-4.
ATC — A02BX12.
Pharmacopoeias. In Eur. (see p.vi), Jpn, Pol., and US.
Fr. also includes Bismuth (Sous-Nitrate de) Léger (Bismuthi Subnitras Levis) which is described as a variable mixture of bismuth hydroxide, carbonate, and subnitrate.

Pharmacopoeial description
Ph. Eur.: It contains not less than 71% and not more than 74% of Bi, calculated with reference to the dried substance. A white powder. Practically insoluble in water and in alcohol; dissolves in mineral acids with decomposition.
USP 25: A basic salt containing not less than 79% of Bi_2O_3 calculated on the dried basis. It is a white, slightly hygroscopic powder. Practically insoluble in water and in alcohol; readily dissolves in nitric and hydrochloric acids.

Tripotassium Dicitratobismuthate (3778-t)
Colloidal Bismuth Subcitrate.
CAS — 57644-54-9.

Adverse Effects, Treatment, and Precautions
The bismuth compounds listed above are insoluble or very poorly soluble, and bismuth toxicity does not appear to be common with them if they are used for limited periods. However, excessive or prolonged dosage may produce symptoms of bismuth poisoning, and for this reason long-term systemic therapy is not recommended. Reversible encephalopathy (see below) was once a problem in some countries, notably France and Australia; bone and joint toxicity had also occurred, sometimes associated with the encephalopathy. This led to restrictions on the use of bismuth salts and a virtual disappearance of these toxic effects.

Nausea and vomiting have been reported. Darkening or blackening of the faeces and tongue may occur due to conversion to bismuth sulfide in the gastrointestinal tract.

The effects of *acute bismuth intoxication* include gastrointestinal disturbances, skin reactions, stomatitis, and discoloration of mucous membranes; a characteristic blue line may appear on the gums. There may be renal failure and liver damage.

Other adverse effects may not be related to the bismuth content. With bismuth subnitrate given orally there is a risk of the nitrate being reduced in the intestines to nitrite and the development of methaemoglobinaemia. Absorption of salicylate occurs following the administration of bismuth salicylate by mouth and therefore the adverse effects, treatment of adverse effects, and precautions of aspirin (p.14) should be considered.

Gastric lavage should be considered following overdosage; activated charcoal by mouth and the use of a chelating agent such as dimercaprol or unithiol have

been recommended (see also Overdosage, below). Renal function should be monitored for 10 days following acute overdosage.

Bismuth compounds should not be given to patients with moderate to severe renal impairment.

Encephalopathy. Reviews[1,2] and reports[3-10] of bismuth encephalopathy. Many of the original reports implicated bismuth subgallate or subnitrate, in most but not all cases at high doses or for prolonged periods; toxicity has also occurred with other salts.[6-9] Patients receiving the subcitrate (480 mg daily) or the subnitrate (1.8 g daily) for 8 weeks in the treatment of *Helicobacter pylori* infection, showed no evidence of neurological changes compared with a control group.[11]

1. Winship KA. Toxicity of bismuth salts. *Adverse Drug React Acute Poisoning Rev* 1983; **2:** 103–21.
2. Slikkerveer A, de Wolff FA. Pharmacokinetics and toxicity of bismuth compounds. *Med Toxicol Adverse Drug Exp* 1989; **4:** 303–23.
3. Morrow AW. Request for reports: adverse reactions with bismuth subgallate. *Med J Aust* 1973; **1:** 912.
4. Martin-Bouyer G. Intoxications par les sels de bismuth administrés par voie orale: enquête épidémiologique. *Therapie* 1976; **31:** 683–702.
5. Stahl JP, et al. Encéphalites au sel insoluble de bismuth: toujours d'actualité. *Nouv Presse Med* 1982; **11:** 3856.
6. Hasking GJ, Duggan JM. Encephalopathy from bismuth subsalicylate. *Med J Aust* 1982; **2:** 167.
7. Weller MPI. Neuropsychiatric symptoms following bismuth intoxication. *Postgrad Med J* 1988; **64:** 308–10.
8. Mendelowitz PC, et al. Bismuth absorption and myoclonic encephalopathy during bismuth subsalicylate therapy. *Ann Intern Med* 1990; **112:** 140–1.
9. Playford RJ, et al. Bismuth induced encephalopathy caused by tri potassium dicitrato bismuthate in a patient with chronic renal failure. *Gut* 1990; **31:** 359–60.
10. Von Bose MJ, Zaudig M. Encephalopathy resembling Creutzfeldt-Jakob disease following oral, prescribed doses of bismuth nitrate. *Br J Psychiatry* 1991; **158:** 278–80.
11. Noach LA, et al. Bismuth salts and neurotoxicity: a randomised, single-blind and controlled study. *Hum Exp Toxicol* 1995; **14:** 349–55.

FOLLOWING TOPICAL APPLICATION. Encephalopathy has been associated with the use of bismuth iodoform paraffin paste (BIPP) for the packing of wound cavities after surgery to the head and neck, although there is some debate as to whether the bismuth or the iodoform component is responsible—see p.1149.

Overdosage. Bismuth salicylate or tripotassium dicitratobismuthate in recommended doses are rarely associated with serious adverse effects but there are reports of renal failure,[1-4] encephalopathy,[5-7] and neurotoxicity[1] following acute[1,4,6] or chronic[5,7] overdose. Bismuth has been detected in the blood, urine, stools, and kidneys of these patients; a blood concentration of 1.6 µg per mL was found 4 hours after a dose of 9.6 g.[2]

The optimal treatment of bismuth overdosage is unknown. Gastric lavage, purgation, and hydration should be considered, even if the patient presents late, as bismuth may be absorbed from the colon.[1,2] Chelating agents may be effective; unithiol has been reported to increase the renal clearance of bismuth with a reduction in the blood concentration.[5] Haemodialysis may be necessary[1-3] but whether this hastens tissue clearance is uncertain.

Prolonged ingestion of bismuth salicylate in excessive doses by an elderly diabetic was associated with hearing disturbances, vertigo, acid-base abnormalities and mild clotting disturbances.[8] The toxicity was thought to be due to the salicylate component of the drug.

1. Hudson M, et al. Reversible toxicity in poisoning with colloidal bismuth subcitrate. *BMJ* 1989; **299:** 159.
2. Taylor EG, Klenerman P. Acute renal failure after colloidal bismuth subcitrate overdose. *Lancet* 1990; **335:** 670–1.
3. Huwez F, et al. Acute renal failure after overdose of colloidal bismuth subcitrate. *Lancet* 1992; **340:** 1298.
4. Akpolat I, et al. Acute renal failure due to overdose of colloidal bismuth. *Nephrol Dial Transplant* 1996; **11:** 1890–8.
5. Playford RJ, et al. Bismuth induced encephalopathy caused by tri potassium dicitrato bismuthate in a patient with chronic renal failure. *Gut* 1990; **31:** 359–60.
6. Hasking GJ, Duggan JM. Encephalopathy from bismuth subsalicylate. *Med J Aust* 1982; **2:** 167.
7. Mendelowitz PC, et al. Bismuth absorption and myoclonic encephalopathy during bismuth subsalicylate therapy. *Ann Intern Med* 1990; **112:** 140–1.
8. Vernace MA, et al. Chronic salicylate toxicity due to consumption of over-the-counter bismuth subsalicylate. *Am J Med* 1994; **97:** 308–9.

Interactions
Bismuth salts given by mouth reduce the absorption of tetracyclines, possibly by chelation or by reducing tetracycline solubility as a result of increasing the gastric pH. This interaction can be minimised by separating doses of the two drugs by a couple of hours. The clinical significance of this interaction to the use of bismuth salts for peptic ulcer disease is unclear; tripotassium dicitratobismuthate or bismuth salicylate have been given at the same time as tetracycline as part of triple therapy for the eradication of *Helicobacter pylori*.

Antisecretory drugs. Pretreatment with *omeprazole* resulted in about a threefold increase in absorption of bismuth from tripotassium dicitratobismuthate in 6 healthy subjects.[1] The mean peak plasma concentration of bismuth following a single dose of 240 mg of tripotassium dicitratobismuthate was increased from 36.7 to 86.7 nanograms per mL after omeprazole administration, suggesting an increased risk of toxicity from combined therapy. The mechanism was thought to be the increase in gastric pH produced by the antisecretory drug as similar results had been reported with *ranitidine*.[2] However, the clinical significance of these interactions to the use of antisecretory drugs with bismuth compounds for eradication of *Helicobacter pylori* is unclear; bismuth compounds have been combined with proton pump inhibitors or H_2 antagonists in short-term regimens as part of triple or quadruple therapy.

1. Treiber G, *et al.* Omeprazole-induced increase in the absorption of bismuth from tripotassium dicitrato bismuthate. *Clin Pharmacol Ther* 1994; **55:** 486–91.
2. Nwokolo. CU, *et al.* The effect of histamine H_2-receptor blockade on bismuth absorption from three ulcer-healing compounds. *Gastroenterology* 1991; **101:** 889–94.

Pharmacokinetics

Poorly soluble bismuth compounds are largely converted to insoluble bismuth oxide, hydroxide, and oxychloride in the acidic environment of the stomach. Most of the bismuth compounds included in this monograph are thus only slightly absorbed. Increased gastric pH may increase bismuth absorption—see under Interactions, above. Unabsorbed bismuth is excreted in the faeces. Absorbed bismuth is distributed throughout body tissues, including bone, and is slowly excreted in the urine and bile. It has a plasma half-life of about 5 days and continues to be excreted for about 12 weeks after stopping therapy.

◊ References.
1. Nwokolo CU, *et al.* The absorption of bismuth from oral doses of tripotassium dicitrato bismuthate. *Aliment Pharmacol Ther* 1989; **3:** 29–39.
2. Froomes PRA, *et al.* Absorption and elimination of bismuth from oral doses of tripotassium dicitrato bismuthate. *Eur J Clin Pharmacol* 1989; **37:** 533–6.
3. Lacey LF, *et al.* Comparative pharmacokinetics of bismuth from ranitidine bismuth citrate (GR122311X), a novel anti-ulcerant and tripotassium dicitrato bismuthate (TDB). *Eur J Clin Pharmacol* 1994; **47:** 177–80.

Uses and Administration

Some insoluble salts of bismuth are given by mouth for their supposed antacid action and for their mildly astringent action in various gastrointestinal disorders, including diarrhoea (p.1203) and dyspepsia (p.1204). Such salts include the aluminate, salicylate, subcarbonate, and subnitrate. Bismuth salicylate, which is given as an antidiarrhoeal and weak antacid in doses up to about 4 g daily in divided doses, possesses in addition the properties of the salicylates.

Tripotassium dicitratobismuthate is used as a mucosal protectant for the treatment of peptic ulcer disease (p.1208). It is active against *Helicobacter pylori* and has been used as triple therapy (with metronidazole and either tetracycline or amoxicillin) to eradicate this organism and thereby prevent relapse of duodenal ulcer. Bismuth salicylate is also active against *H. pylori* and has been used similarly.

The usual dose of tripotassium dicitratobismuthate in benign gastric and duodenal ulceration is 240 mg twice daily, or 120 mg four times daily by mouth taken before food. Treatment is for a period of 4 weeks, extended to 8 weeks if necessary. Maintenance therapy with tripotassium dicitratobismuthate is not recommended although treatment may be repeated after a drug-free interval of one month. When used as part of triple therapy the usual dose of tripotassium dicitratobismuthate is 120 mg four times daily and the treatment period is usually 2 weeks. The usual dose of bismuth salicylate as part of triple therapy is 525 mg four times daily for 2 weeks. Appropriate antisecretory treatment with a histamine H_2-antagonist or a proton pump inhibitor may also be added to these regimens.

A complex of bismuth citrate with ranitidine, ranitidine bismuth citrate (p.1247), is also used in the treatment of peptic ulcer disease.

Some insoluble salts of bismuth have been used topically in the treatment of skin disorders, wounds, and burns. Some have been used as ingredients of ointments or suppositories (sometimes containing more than one bismuth salt) in the treatment of haemorrhoids and other anorectal disorders (p.1205). Bismuth compounds that have been used topically and/or rectally include the oxide, subgallate, and subnitrate; bismuth resorcinol compounds have also been used. For the use of bismuth subnitrate and iodoform paste as a wound dressing, see Iodoform, p.1149.

Numerous other salts and compounds of bismuth have been promoted for various therapeutic purposes. Glycobiarsol was formerly used by mouth as an amoebicide.

Bismuth (Bismuthum) is used in homoeopathic medicine.

Preparations

BPC 1954: Bismuth Subnitrate and Iodoform Paste;
USP 25: Compound Resorcinol Ointment; Milk of Bismuth.

Proprietary Preparations (details are given in Part 3)
Austral.: De-Nol; **Belg.:** De-Nol†; **Braz.:** Peptulan; Ulcerosol; **Canad.:** Bismed; Bismylate; Neo-Laryngobis; Pepto-Bismol; Personel; Pink Bismuth Rose; **Fr.:** Amygdorectol; **Ger.:** Angass S; Dermatol; Haemo-Exhirud Bufexamac Zapfchen; Jatrox†; Katulcin-R; Noemin N; Telen; Ulcolind Wismut†; Ulgastrin Bis†; Ulkowis; **Hong Kong:** Anuzinc; De-Nol; **Irl.:** De-Nol; De-Noltab; **Israel:** De-Nol; Kalbeten; **Ital.:** De-Nol; **Mex.:** Biselic; Bismofarma; Bismopepsin; Pepto-Bismol; Sucrato; **Neth.:** De-Nol; **Norw.:** De-Nol†; **NZ:** De-Nol; **Port.:** De-Nol; **S.Afr.:** De-Nol; Ulcerone; **Spain:** Gastrodenol; Helol†; Rectamigdol; **Switz.:** Amygdorectol; Bismuth Tulasne; De-Nol; **Thai.:** De-Nol; **UK:** De-Nol†; De-Noltab; Pepto-Bismol; **USA:** Bismatrol; Devrom; Pepto-Bismol; Pink Biscoat†; Stomax†.

Multi-ingredient: Austral.: BFI†; Helidac; Roter†; **Belg.:** Amazyl†; Baseler Haussalbe†; Gastrofilm; Procto-Synalar; Rectovasol; **Braz.:** Anusol-HC; Bisuisan; Claudemor; Cutisanol; Magnesia Bisurada; Neoseptil; Neutracido; Salicilato de Bismuto Composto; Senophile; **Canad.:** Bismed†; Bismutal; Eczema Ointment†; Onrectal; Pepto-Bismol; Thunas Pile; **Denm.:** Xylocain Comp; **Fin.:** Tannopon; **Fr.:** Anoreine; Anusol; Bi-Qui-Nol†; Bismurectol; Cutiphile; Paps; Pholcones Bismuth; **Ger.:** Angass; Anisan; Anusept†; Bismofalk; Bismolan; Bismolan H Corti; Bisrenin†; Bufeproct†; Combustin Heilsalbe; Duoventrin; Eulatin N; Eulatin NN; Faktu akut; Friosmin N; Haemomac†; Hamo-ratiopharm; Hamoagil plus; Karaya Bismuth; Katulcin-Rupha†; Logomed Hamorrhoiden†; Mastu S; Nervogastrol; Pascomag; Proctoparf; Sagittaproct; Sagittaproct S; Siozwo N; Spasmo-Nervogastrol; Tamposit N; Varitan N; Ventricon N; Vit-u-pept; Wismut comp; **Hong Kong:** Anusol; Anusol-HC; Biscasil; Bismofalk; Mastu S; Rowatanal; **Irl.:** Anugesic-HC; Anusol; Anusol-HC; Rowatanal; **Israel:** Anusol; Contra Combustiones; Hemo; Rectozorin; Rekiv; **Ital.:** Antiemorroidali; Anusol; **Mex.:** Ercal; Heliton; **Neth.:** Anusol; Caved-S†; Roter†; Theranal; Zwitsanal†; **Norw.:** Biserirte Magnesia†; **Port.:** Claudemor; Gastroplex†; Servetinal; Synalar Rectal; **S.Afr.:** Anugesic; Anusol; Anusol-HC†; Arola Rosebalm; Biskapect; Chloropect; Collodyne†; Dyrosol; Enterodyne; Kantrexil; Peter Pote's†; Rectosan 'A'†; Roter†; **Singapore:** Anusol; Rowatanal; **Spain:** Grietalgen; Grietalgen Hidrocort; Hemodren Compuesto; Metagliz Bismutico†; Nasopomada; Pomada Infantil Vera; Roter Complex†; Sabanotropico; Stomosan; Sualyn†; Synalar Rectal; Tanogastrin Calber; Talkosona†; Talquissar†; **Swed.:** Cavedess†; **Switz.:** Anusol†; Bismorectal; Cicafissan; Fissan; Furodermal; Furodermil†; Haemocortin; Haemolan; Magenpulver Hafter; Magentabletten Hafter; Rectoseptal-Neo bismuthe; **Thai.:** Anusol; Biodan; Roter; Ulgastrin; **UK:** Anusol-HC; Anusol; Anusol-HC, Plus HC; Bisma-Rex; Caved-S†; Hemocane; Moorland; OxBipp; Stomach Mixture; **USA:** A-Caine†; Anumed; Anumed HC; BFI; Calmol; Helidac; Hem-Prep; Hemril; K-C; Kao-Paverin; Kaodene Non-Narcotic; Mammol; Rectagene II†; Rectagene Medicated Rectal Balm; Wyanoids†.

Bisoxatin Acetate (12446-q)

Bisoxatin Acetate (BANM, USAN, rINNM).
Bisoxatin Diacetate; Wy-8138. 2,2-Bis(4-hydroxyphenyl)-1,4-benzoxazin-3(2H,4H)-one diacetate.
$C_{24}H_{19}NO_6 = 417.4$.
CAS — 17692-24-9 (bisoxatin); 14008-48-1 (bisoxatin acetate).

Profile

Bisoxatin acetate is a stimulant laxative that has been used in the treatment of constipation (p.1202) in doses of 120 to 180 mg by mouth daily at bedtime.

Preparations

Proprietary Preparations (details are given in Part 3)
Belg.: Wylaxine†.

Bran (681-s)

Crusca; Farelo; Kleie; Salvado; Son.
Pharmacopoeias. US includes Wheat Bran.

The fibrous outer layers of cereal grains. It contains celluloses, polysaccharides or hemicelluloses, protein, fat, minerals, and moisture and may contain part of the germ or embryo. Bran provides water-insoluble fibre and, depending on the source, may also provide water-soluble fibre (see also below). It comprises about 12% of the weight of the grain and is a byproduct of flour milling. It is available in various grades.

Pharmacopoeial description

USP 25: Wheat Bran is defined as the outer fraction of the cereal grain (comprising the pericarp, seed coat (testa), nucellar tissue, and aleurone layer) derived from *Triticum aestivum*, *T. compactum*, *T. durum*, or other common einkorn and emmer wheat cultivars. It is obtained by milling and processing the whole wheat grain, and is available in a variety of particle sizes depending on the degree of milling. It contains not less than 36% of dietary fibre. It is a light tan powder having a characteristic aroma. Practically insoluble in cold water and in alcohol.

Adverse Effects

Large quantities of bran may temporarily increase flatulence and abdominal distension, and intestinal obstruction may occur rarely.

Diarrhoea. A report of diarrhoea induced by a dramatic increase in fibre intake. Reduction of dietary fibre led to a return to normal bowel habit in 2 to 3 days.[1]
1. Saibil F. Diarrhea due to fiber overload. *N Engl J Med* 1989; **320:** 599.

Intestinal obstruction. Intestinal obstruction associated with excessive bran intake has been reported.[1-3]
1. Allen-Mersh T, De Jode LR. Is bran useful in diverticular disease? *BMJ* 1982; **284:** 740.
2. Cooper SG, Tracey EJ. Small-bowel obstruction caused by oat-bran bezoar. *N Engl J Med* 1989; **320:** 1148–9.
3. Miller DL, *et al.* Small-bowel obstruction from bran cereal. *JAMA* 1990; **263:** 813–14.

Precautions

Bran is contra-indicated in patients with intestinal obstruction or with undiagnosed abdominal symptoms. There is a particular risk of intestinal or oesophageal obstruction if bulk laxatives are swallowed dry; they should be taken with sufficient fluid and should not be taken immediately before going to bed. Wheat bran should be avoided in gluten enteropathies and coeliac disease.

Interactions

Bran may reduce the absorption of some drugs when given concomitantly by mouth. Interference with iron, zinc, and calcium absorption has been reported; calcium phosphate may be added to bran to neutralise phytic acid, which can contribute to such interference.

Uses and Administration

The main use of bran is as a bulk laxative and source of dietary fibre in the management of disorders of the gastrointestinal tract such as constipation (p.1202), especially in diverticular disease (p.1203) and the irritable bowel syndrome (p.1206). It should always be taken with plenty of fluid.

Bran is used as the basis for some breakfast cereals.

Dietary role. There is no precise definition for the complex mixture of substances known as dietary fibre. It has been defined as plant polysaccharides and lignin resistant to hydrolysis by the digestive enzymes of humans but this covers many substances other than cell-wall and related polysaccharides. Non-starch polysaccharides are the major component of the plant cell wall and are used as an index of dietary fibre. They comprise water-soluble fibres such as pectins, gums, and mucilages and water-insoluble fibres such as cellulose. Wheat, maize, and rice contain mainly insoluble non-starch polysaccharides whereas oats, barley, and rye have a significant proportion of soluble fibres.

In the United Kingdom dietary reference values (DRV) have been published for non-starch polysaccharides.[1] In the UK it is proposed that adult diets should contain an average for the population of 18 g daily (individual range 12 to 24 g daily) non-starch polysaccharide from a variety of foods whose constituents contain it as a naturally integrated component. Children should receive proportionately less non-starch polysaccharide according to body size. No evidence exists for benefit of intakes of non-starch polysaccharide in excess of 32 g daily, and therefore there is no advantage in exceeding this amount.
1. DOH. Dietary reference values for food energy and nutrients for the United Kingdom: report of the panel on dietary reference values of the committee on medical aspects of food policy. *Report on health and social subjects 41.* London: HMSO, 1991.

Disease prevention. Diseases such as colorectal cancer, ischaemic heart disease, diabetes mellitus, and obesity are common in affluent developed countries but occur rarely in rural Africa. This difference in disease patterns has been linked to the low fibre intake in developed countries compared with rural Africans. However, there are many other differences in diet and lifestyle, such as a lower intake of fat, protein, and sugar in rural Africans and less exposure to toxins and pollutants, any of which could contribute to the difference. The excessive consumption of energy-rich foods may be more to blame for diseases of affluence than is deficiency of dietary fibre.[1] Furthermore, there is some concern that the use of fibre supplements is not entirely without harmful effects: it has been pointed out that fermentable fibre substrates can stimulate cell proliferation in the colon.[2] However the role of cell proliferation as a marker for the development of colonic cancer is questioned by some authors.[3] Results from the Nurses' Health Study, a large prospective cohort study, have in any case failed to support any reduction in risk of colon cancer associated with a high intake of dietary fibre.[4] Controlled trials of the effect of dietary intervention, over three to four years, on the recurrence rate of colorectal adenomas have been reported. Neither a high fibre diet based on wheat bran cereal supplements,[5] nor a diet of low fat, high fibre foods, fruit and vegetables,[6] were found to reduce the recurrence of colorectal adenomas. However, although adenomas are precursors of colorectal cancer, most adenomas do not develop into cancer, and so the relevance of these study results for the prevention of colorectal cancer is unclear.[7]

1. Anonymous. The bran wagon. *Lancet* 1987; **i**: 782–3.
2. Wasan HS, Goodlad RA. Fibre-supplemented foods may damage your health. *Lancet* 1996; **348**: 319–20.
3. Hill MJ, Leeds AR. Fibre and colorectal cancer. *Lancet* 1996; **348**: 957.
4. Fuchs CS, *et al.* Dietary fibre and the risk of colorectal cancer and adenoma in women. *N Engl J Med* 1999; **340**: 169–76.
5. Alberts DS, *et al.* Lack of effect of a high-fiber cereal supplement on the recurrence of colorectal adenomas. *N Engl J Med* 2000; **342**: 1156–62.
6. Schatzkin A, *et al.* Lack of effect of a low-fat, high-fiber diet on the recurrence of colorectal adenomas. *N Engl J Med* 2000; **342**: 1149–55.
7. Byers T. Diet, colorectal adenomas, and colorectal cancer. *N Engl J Med* 2000; **342**: 1206–7.

Preparations

Proprietary Preparations (details are given in Part 3)
Braz.: Dietoman; Fibrocol; Trifibra Mix; *Canad.*: Fibyrax†; *Fr.*: Celluson; Doses-O-Son; Infibran; *Irl.*: Trifyba; *Ital.*: Crusken; *Port.*: Infibran; *Swed.*: Fibertabletter†; *Switz.*: Fibion; *UK*: Trifyba.

Multi-ingredient: *Aust.*: Herbelax; *Austral.*: Fibyrax; Neo-Trim Fibre; Prochol; Proslender; *Ital.*: Crusken; Dialibra†; Ecofibra; Fibrovit; Levoplus; Melaprugna; Plurilac; Resource Benefiber; *Mex.*: Psilumax.

Bromopride (12454-q)

Bromopride *(rINN)*.
CM-8252; VAL-13081. 4-Amino-5-bromo-*N*-(2-diethylaminoethyl)-*o*-anisamide.
$C_{14}H_{22}BrN_3O_2$ = 344.2.
CAS — 4093-35-0.
ATC — A03FA04.

Profile
Bromopride is a substituted benzamide similar to metoclopramide (p.1235), used in a variety of gastrointestinal disorders including nausea and vomiting (p.1206) and motility disorders. It is given in a usual dose of 20 to 60 mg daily by mouth in divided doses, or 10 to 20 mg daily by intramuscular or intravenous injection. The hydrochloride has also been used.

Preparations
Proprietary Preparations (details are given in Part 3)
Braz.: Digecap; Digerex; Digesan; Digestina; Digeston; Plamet; Pridecil; *Ger.*: Cascapride; *Ital.*: Opridan†; Valopride.

Multi-ingredient: *Braz.*: Digecap-Zimatico; Enziprid; Normopride Enzimatico; Primeral; *Port.*: Modulanzime.

Buckthorn (7504-h)

Bacca Spinae Cervinae; Espino Cerval; Kreuzdorn; Nerprun.
Pharmacopoeias. In *Fr.* and *Ger.*

The dried ripe fruit of buckthorn, *Rhamnus cathartica* (Rhamnaceae). The bark is occasionally used.

Profile
Buckthorn is an anthraquinone stimulant laxative.

Preparations
Proprietary Preparations (details are given in Part 3)
Ger.: Laxysat mono†.

Multi-ingredient: *Austral.*: Neo-Cleanse; *Canad.*: Floralaxative†; *Ger.*: Salus Abfuhr-Tee Nr. 2†; *UK*: Lion Cleansing Herbs.

Calcium Carbonate (682-w)

Calcii Carbonas; Creta Preparada; E170; Precipitated Calcium Carbonate; Precipitated Chalk.
$CaCO_3$ = 100.1.
CAS — 471-34-1.
ATC — A02AC01; A12AA04.
Pharmacopoeias. In *Eur.* (see p.vi), *Int*, *Jpn, Pol.*, and *US*.

Pharmacopoeial description
Ph. Eur.: A white powder. Practically insoluble in water.
USP 25: A fine, white, odourless, microcrystalline powder. Practically insoluble in water; its solubility in water is increased by the presence of carbon dioxide or ammonium salts

The symbol † denotes a preparation no longer actively marketed

---

although the presence of any alkali hydroxide reduces its solubility; insoluble in alcohol; dissolves with effervescence in acetic acid, in hydrochloric acid, and in nitric acid.

Adverse Effects, Treatment, and Precautions
Calcium carbonate may occasionally cause constipation. Flatulence from released carbon dioxide may occur in some patients. High doses or prolonged use may lead to gastric hypersecretion and acid rebound. Like other calcium salts (see p.1189), calcium carbonate can cause hypercalcaemia, particularly in patients with renal impairment or after high doses. Alkalosis (p.1180) may also occur as a result of the carbonate anion. There have been rare reports of the milk-alkali syndrome, see below, and tissue calcification.

For precautions to be observed with the use of calcium carbonate, see Calcium, p.1189.

Milk-alkali syndrome. The milk-alkali syndrome of hypercalcaemia, alkalosis and renal impairment was first identified in the 1920s and may still occur in patients who ingest large amounts of calcium and absorbable alkali.[1] Metastatic calcification can develop.[2] For reference to thiazide diuretics increasing the risk of the milk-alkali syndrome in patients taking moderately large doses of calcium carbonate, see p.909.

1. Orwoll ES. The milk-alkali syndrome: current concepts. *Ann Intern Med* 1982; **97**: 242–8.
2. Duthie JS, *et al.* Milk-alkali syndrome with metastatic calcification. *Am J Med* 1995; **99**: 102–3.

Interactions
As for other calcium salts, p.1189.

As outlined on p.1201 antacids, including calcium salts, interact with many other drugs both by alterations in gastric pH and emptying, and by formation of complexes that are not absorbed. Interactions can be minimised by giving calcium carbonate and any other medication 2 to 3 hours apart.

Pharmacokinetics
Calcium carbonate is converted to calcium chloride by gastric acid. Some of the calcium is absorbed from the intestines and the unabsorbed portion is excreted in the faeces, as described for other calcium salts, p.1189.

Uses and Administration
Calcium carbonate is used as an antacid (p.1201), usually in doses of up to about 1.5 g by mouth. It is often given in association with other antacids, especially magnesium-containing antacids.

Calcium carbonate is also used as a calcium supplement in deficiency states and as an adjunct in the management of osteoporosis, as described under Calcium, p.1189.

Calcium carbonate binds phosphate in the gastrointestinal tract to form insoluble complexes and reduces phosphate absorption. It is used to treat hyperphosphataemia in patients with chronic renal failure (see Renal Osteodystrophy, p.746). For this purpose, initial doses of 2.5 g daily by mouth have been given, increased to up to 17 g daily.

A preparation of a native calcium carbonate (Calcarea Carbonica; Calc. Carb.) is used in homoeopathic medicine.

Calcium carbonate is also used as a food additive.

Preparations
BP 2001: Calcium and Colecalciferol Tablets; Chewable Calcium Carbonate Tablets;
USP 25: Alumina, Magnesia, and Calcium Carbonate Oral Suspension; Alumina, Magnesia, and Calcium Carbonate Tablets; Alumina, Magnesia, Calcium Carbonate, and Simethicone Tablets; Aluminum Subacetate Topical Solution; Calcium and Magnesium Carbonates Oral Suspension; Calcium and Magnesium Carbonates Tablets; Calcium Carbonate and Magnesia Tablets; Calcium Carbonate Lozenges; Calcium Carbonate Oral Suspension; Calcium Carbonate Tablets; Calcium Carbonate, Magnesia, and Simethicone Tablets.

Proprietary Preparations (details are given in Part 3)
Aust.: Dreisacarb; Kalzonorm; Tetesept Calcium; *Austral.*: Andrews Tums Antacid; Cal-Sup; Caltrate; Sandocal; Titralac; *Belg.*: Cacit; Calci-Chew; Calcium-Sandoz; Steocar; *Braz.*: Calcium-Sandoz F; Tums; *Canad.*: Apo-Cal; Cal-500; Calcite; Calcium Oyster Shell; Calcium-Sandoz; Calsan; Caltrate; Hi Potency Cal; Maalox Quick Dissolve; Neo Cal; Nu-Cal; Os-Cal; Prevencal†; Titralac†; Tums; *Denm.*: Calcium-Sandoz; *Fin.*: Calcichew; Cal-

---

cium-Sandoz; Kalcidon; Kalcipos; Maxi-Calsor; *Fr.*: Cacit; Calcidia; Calcidose; Calciprat; Calcium-Sandoz; Calperos; Calprimum; Caltrate; Densical; Densical vitamine D₃; Eucalcic; Fixical; Perical; Sandocal; *Ger.*: Basti-Cal; Calcedon†; Calcilos; Calcimagon; Calcitridin; Calcium AL; Calcium beta; Calcium Dago; Calcium Heumann; Calcium Hexal; Calcium Stada; Calcium Verla; Calcium von CT; Calcium-dura; Calcium-Sandoz; CC-Nefro; Dreisacarb; Frubiase Calcium; Loscalcon; Ospur Ca; Vivural; *Hong Kong:* Calcichew; Calcium-Sandoz; Caltrate; Os-Cal; Titralac; *Irl.*: Cacit; Calcichew; Remegel†; Rennie Rap-Eze; Rowarolan; Sandocal; Setlers Tums; *Israel:* Calci-Rav; Calcimore; Calcium-Sandoz; Caltrate; Tums; *Ital.*: Biocalcium; Cacit; Cal-Car; Calciodie; Calciomed; Calciopiu; Calcium-Sandoz; Calma; Carbo; Carbosint; Carbotop; Citracal; Effercal; Fervical; Metocal; Recal; Remegel†; Savecal; Top Calcium; *Mex.*: Calcifar; Calcium-Sandoz; Calsan; Caltrate; Osteomin; *Mon.*: Orocal; *Neth.*: Cacit; Calci-Chew; Calcium-Sandoz; *Norw.*: Calcium-Sandoz; Titralac; *NZ:* Cal-Sup; Calcium-Sandoz; Caltrate; Oscal; Osteo; Titralac; *Port.*: Calcioral; Calcium-Sandoz; Sandocal; *S.Afr.*: Calcium-Sandoz; Caltrate; Titralac; *Singapore:* Cal-Sup; Calcium-Sandoz; Caltrate; *Spain:* Calcium-Sandoz Forte; Caosina; Carbocal; Cimascal; Densical; Fortical; Mastical; Natecal; Swed.: Calcitugg; Calcium-Sandoz; Kalcidon; Kalcipos; Kalcitena; *Switz.*: Calcium-Sandoz; Calperos; Calsan; Fixateur phospho-calcique; Maxi-calc; *Thai.*: Bo-Ne-Ca; Calcanate; Calcium 625; Calcium-Sandoz; Caltab; Prima-Cal; *UK*: Adcal; Cacit; Calcette†; Calcichew; Calcidrink; Citrical†; Rap-eze; Remegel; Rennie Gold†; Sandocal; Sea-Cal; Setlers; Titralac; Tums; *USA*: Alka-Mints; Alkets; Amitone; Antacid; Cal Carb-HD†; Cal-Guard†; Cal-Plus; Calci-Chew; Calci-Mix; Calciday; Caltrate; Caltrate Jr.; Chooz; Dicarbosil†; Equilet; Gencalc; Maalox Antacid; Maalox Quick Dissolve; Mallamint; Mylanta; Nephro-Calci; Os-Cal; Oysco; Oyst-Cal; Oyster Shell Calcium; Oystercal; Surpass; Titralac Extra Strength; Tums.

Multi-ingredient: numerous preparations are listed in Part 3.

Carbenoxolone Sodium (685-y)

Carbenoxolone Sodium *(BANM, USAN, rINNM)*.
Disodium Enoxolone Succinate. 3β-(3-Carboxypropionyloxy)-11-oxo-olean-12-en-30-oic acid, Disodium Salt.
$C_{34}H_{48}Na_2O_7$ = 614.7.
CAS — 5697-56-3 (carbenoxolone); 7421-40-1 (carbenoxolone disodium).
Pharmacopoeias. In *Br.* and *Chin.*

Pharmacopoeial description
BP 2001: A white or pale cream-coloured, hygroscopic powder. Freely soluble in water; sparingly soluble in alcohol; practically insoluble in chloroform and in ether. A 10% solution in water has a pH of 8.0 to 9.2.

◊ CAUTION. *Carbenoxolone sodium powder is irritant to nasal membranes.*

Adverse Effects
Carbenoxolone sodium has mineralocorticoid-like effects and ingestion may produce sodium and water retention and hypokalaemia. This may cause or exacerbate hypertension, heart failure, oedema, alkalosis, and muscle weakness and damage. If hypokalaemia is prolonged, renal impairment can occur.

◊ Muscle weakness,[1-5] muscle necrosis,[4] myopathy,[1] hypertension,[2] headache,[2] cardiac failure,[2] mental confusion,[4] areflexia,[3] renal tubular dysfunction,[5] and acute tubular necrosis[4] have all been associated with carbenoxolone-induced hypokalaemia. Carbenoxolone-induced hypertension may have precipitated the onset of fatal polyarteritis in a patient predisposed to this condition.[6]

1. Fyfe T, *et al.* Myopathy and hypokalaemia in carbenoxolone therapy. *BMJ* 1969; **3**: 476.
2. Davies GJ, *et al.* Complications of carbenoxolone therapy. *BMJ* 1974; **3**: 400–2.
3. Royston A, Prout BJ. Carbenoxolone-induced hypokalaemia simulating Guillain-Barré syndrome. *BMJ* 1976; **2**: 150–1.
4. Descamps C, *et al.* Rhabdomyolysis and acute tubular necrosis associated with carbenoxolone and diuretic treatment. *BMJ* 1977; **1**: 272.
5. Dickinson RJ, Swaminathan R. Total body potassium depletion and renal tubular dysfunction following carbenoxolone therapy. *Postgrad Med J* 1978; **54**: 836–7.
6. Sloan J, Weaver JA. A case of polyarteritis developing after carbenoxolone therapy. *Ir Med J* 1968; **1**: 505–7.

Precautions
Systemic use of carbenoxolone sodium is contra-indicated in patients with hypokalaemia, in pregnancy, in the elderly, and in children. It should be used with caution, if at all, in patients with cardiac disease, hypertension, or impaired hepatic or renal function.

Interactions
Because of the risk of toxicity, carbenoxolone should not be taken with digitalis glycosides unless serum-electrolyte concentrations are measured at weekly intervals and measures are taken to avoid hypokalaemia.

Although amiloride or spironolactone relieve sodium and water retention, they antagonise the healing properties of systemic carbenoxolone and should not be used concomitantly. The hypokalaemia associated with diuretics may be exacerbated by carbenoxolone.

Pharmacokinetics
Carbenoxolone sodium is absorbed from the gastrointestinal tract, mainly from the stomach. It is highly bound to plasma proteins. Carbenoxolone is chiefly excreted in the faeces via the bile. It appears to undergo enterohepatic circulation.

Uses and Administration

Carbenoxolone sodium is a synthetic derivative of glycyr-rhizinic acid (see Liquorice, p.1231) that was formerly used as a mucosal protectant in peptic ulcer disease (p.1208) and may be given in gastro-oesophageal reflux disease (p.1204). The suggested dosage of carbenoxolone sodium in gastro-oesophageal reflux disease is 20 mg three times daily by mouth and 40 mg at night for 6 to 12 weeks, as a preparation also containing antacids and alginic acid.

Carbenoxolone sodium is one of many topical treatments for the symptomatic management of mouth ulceration (p.1206). It is used as a 2% gel or as a 1% mouthwash.

Preparations

Proprietary Preparations (details are given in Part 3)
Aust.: Rowadermat; **Austral.:** Bioral; **Hong Kong:** Herpesan; **Irl.:** Bioral†; Carbosan; **S.Afr.:** Bioral†; **Singapore:** Herpesan; **Spain:** Sanodin; **UK:** Bioplex; Bioral.

Multi-ingredient: Irl.: Pyrogastrone; **UK:** Pyrogastrone.

Casanthranol (7505-m)

Casanthranol (USAN).
CAS — 8024-48-4.
Pharmacopoeias. In US.

Pharmacopoeial description

USP 25: Casanthranol is obtained from cascara. It contains not less than 20% of total hydroxyanthracene derivatives calculated on the dried basis, of which not less than 80% consists of cascarosides, both calculated as cascaroside A.

It is a light tan to brown, amorphous, hygroscopic powder. Freely soluble in water with some residue; partially soluble in methyl alcohol and in hot isopropyl alcohol; practically insoluble in acetone. Store in airtight containers at a temperature not exceeding 30°. Protect from light.

Profile

Casanthranol is an anthraquinone stimulant laxative with general properties similar to those of senna (p.1248). It is given in usual doses of 30 to 60 mg daily by mouth, together with a faecal softener. In severe cases a dose of 90 mg daily, or 60 mg twice daily, may be given.

Preparations

Proprietary Preparations (details are given in Part 3)
Belg.: Cascalax.

Multi-ingredient: Canad.: Peri-Colace; **Hong Kong:** Softon Plus; **Spain:** Laxvital; **USA:** Black-Draught; D-S-S Plus†; Diocto-K Plus†; Dioctolose Plus†; Disanthrol†; Disolan Forte†; Docusoft Plus; DSMC Plus†; Genasoft Plus Softgels; Laxative & Stool Softener; Peri-Colace; Peri-Dos Softgels; Pro-Sof Plus†; Regulace†; Silace-C; Soflax Overnight†.

Cascara (7506-b)

Cascara Sagrada; Cascararinde; Chittem Bark; Rhamni Purshianae Cortex; Rhamni Purshiani Cortex; Sacred Bark.
CAS — 8047-21-4; 8015-89-2 (cascara sagrada extract).
ATC — A06AB07.
Pharmacopoeias. In Eur. (see p.vi) and US.

Pharmacopoeial description

Ph. Eur.: The dried, whole or fragmented bark of *Rhamnus purshianus* (=*Frangula purshiana*). It contains not less than 8.0% of hydroxyanthracene glycosides of which not less than 60% consists of cascarosides, both expressed as cascaroside A ($C_{27}H_{32}O_{14}$ = 580.5). and calculated with reference to the dried drug. Protect from light.

USP 25: The dried bark of *Rhamnus purshianus* (Rhamnaceae). It contains not less than 7% of total hydroxyanthracene derivatives calculated on the dried basis, of which not less than 60% consists of cascarosides, both calculated as cascaroside A. It has a distinct odour.

Profile

Cascara is an anthraquinone stimulant laxative with general properties similar to those of senna (p.1248). It has been used in the treatment of constipation in doses equivalent to up to about 20 to 70 mg of total hydroxyanthracene derivatives daily by mouth.

Preparations

BP 2001: Cascara Dry Extract; Cascara Tablets;
USP 25: Aromatic Cascara Fluidextract; Cascara Sagrada Extract; Cascara Sagrada Fluidextract; Cascara Tablets.

Proprietary Preparations (details are given in Part 3)
Canad.: Le 500 D; **Fr.:** Peristaltine; **Ger.:** Legapas mono; **Ital.:** Bonlax†; Colamint†; Sagrada-Lax; **Port.:** Laxolen; Mucinum; **Switz.:** Legapas†; **USA:** LBC-LAX†.

Multi-ingredient: Aust.: Cascara-Salax; Dragees Neunzehn; Silberne; **Austral.:** Peritone; Plantago Complex†; Vitaglow Herbal Laxative†; **Belg.:** Grains de Vals; Vethoine; **Braz.:** Boldobeba; Boldopeptan; Chofranina; Dioctosal; Enterotonus; Epagogo; Eparema; Epatovis; Fideine; Figadosan; Gotas Hepaticas; Hepato-Flux; Hepavirmo; Licor de Cacau; Metionina Composta; Pilulas De Witt's; Prisoventril; Purgoleite; Solvobil†; Ventre Livre; **Canad.:** Aid-Lax†; Alsilax†; Alsiline†; Bicholate; Caroid†; Cholasyn; Cholasyn II; Control; Doulax; Extra Strong Formula 1†; Herbal Laxative; Herbalax; Herbalax Forte†; Herbolax; Herborex; Lapidar; Laxa†; Laxaco; Laxative; Le 100 B†; Mucinum; Natures

Remedy; Phytolax†; Thunas Bilettes†; Thunas Laxative; Triolax†; Vesilax†; **Denm.:** Cosylan†; **Fr.:** Aromabyl†; Dragees Fuca; Dragees Vegetales Rex; Ducase†; Grains de Vals; Imegul; Mucinum a l'Extrait de Cascara; Spevin; **Ger.:** Cascara-Salax†; Legapas comp†; Reducelle†; **Hong Kong:** Mucinum Cascara; **Ital.:** Amaro Medicinale; Amaro Padil; Bitteridina; Certobil†; Coladren; Confetti Lassativi CM; Confetti Lassativi†; Crisolax†; Critichol; Depurativo; Digelax; Dis-Cinil Complex; Eparema; Eparema-Levul; Eupatol; Fave di Fuca; Grani di Vals; Hepasil Composto; Hepatos; Hepatos B12; Lassatina; Magisbile; Mepalax; Neo-Heparbil†; Pillole Fattori; Raboldo; Reolina†; Schias-Amaro Medicinale; Sintobil†; Solvobil; Vadolax; Vegebyl†; Verecolene Complesso†; **Norw.:** Cosylan; **Port.:** Caroid; **S.Afr.:** Veracolate; **Spain:** Crislaxo; Laxante Derly; Laxo Vian†; Lipograsil; Menabil Complex; Nico Hepatocyn; Pildoras Zeninas; **Swed.:** Cosylan†; Emulax; **Switz.:** Cascara-Salax†; Fuca†; Grains de Vals; Lapidar 10†; Laxativum Nouvelle Formule†; Padma-Lax; Tavolax†; **Thai.:** Flatulence Gastulence; Hemolax; Veracolate; **UK:** Cleansing Herb Tablets; Dual-Lax Extra Strong; Dual-Lax Normal Strength; Laxative Tablets; Modern Herbals Laxative; Modern Herbals Pile; Natural Herb Tablets; Out-of-Sorts; Pileabs; Piletabs; Pilewort Compound; Rhuaka; Skin Eruptions Mixture; **USA:** Concentrated Milk of Magnesia-Cascara; Herbal Laxative†; Natures Remedy; Veracolate†.

Cassia Pulp (7507-v)

The evaporated aqueous extract of crushed ripe cassia fruits (cassia pods), *Cassia fistula* (Leguminosae).

Profile

Cassia pulp is a mild anthraquinone stimulant laxative with general properties similar to those of senna (p.1248).

Preparations

Proprietary Preparations (details are given in Part 3)
Multi-ingredient: Braz.: Fitolax; Florlax; Frutalax; Frutarine; Laxan; Laxarine; Laxtam; Novolax; Tamaril; Tamarine; Tamarix; **Ital.:** Tamarine; **Mex.:** Naturetti; **Spain:** Pruina; **Switz.:** Tamarine†.

Cerium Oxalate (12549-j)

CAS — 139-42-4 (anhydrous cerous oxalate).
ATC — A04AD02.

NOTE. The chemically defined substance $Ce_2(C_2O_4)_3$ is cerous oxalate.
Pharmacopoeias. In Aust.

Profile

Cerium oxalate is used as an antiemetic.

Preparations

Proprietary Preparations (details are given in Part 3)
Multi-ingredient: Spain: Novonausin.

Cetraxate Hydrochloride (15314-t)

Cetraxate Hydrochloride (USAN, rINNM).
DV-1006. 4-(2-Carboxyethyl)phenyl tranexamate hydrochloride; 4-(2-Carboxyethyl)phenyl *trans*-4-aminomethylcyclohexanecarboxylate hydrochloride.
$C_{17}H_{23}NO_4,HCl$ = 341.8.
CAS — 34675-84-8 (cetraxate); 27724-96-5 (cetraxate hydrochloride).
Pharmacopoeias. In Jpn.

Profile

Cetraxate hydrochloride is stated to be a mucosal protectant with actions on gastric microcirculation as well as prostaglandin synthesis and kallikrein. It is used in the treatment of gastritis and peptic ulcer disease (p.1208) in doses of 600 to 800 mg daily.

Preparations

Proprietary Preparations (details are given in Part 3)
Hong Kong: Neuer; **Jpn:** Neuer.

Chalk (713-n)

Prepared Chalk.
$CaCO_3$ = 100.1.
CAS — 13397-25-6.
Pharmacopoeias. In Br.

Pharmacopoeial description

BP 2001: A native form of calcium carbonate freed from most of its impurities by elutriation and dried. It consists of the calcareous shells and detritus of various foraminifera and contains not less than 97.0% and not more than 100.5% of $CaCO_3$, calculated with reference to the dried substance.

White or greyish-white, odourless or almost odourless, amorphous, earthy, small friable masses, usually conical in form, or in powder. Practically insoluble in water; slightly soluble in water containing carbon dioxide; it absorbs water readily.

Profile

Chalk has been used as an adsorbent antidiarrhoeal. Calcium carbonate (precipitated chalk) is used as an antacid, calcium supplement, and phosphate binder, see p.1215.

Preparations

BP 2001: Compound Magnesium Trisilicate Oral Powder.

Cimetidine (6117-g)

Cimetidine (BAN, USAN, rINN).
Cimetidinum; SKF-92334. 2-Cyano-1-methyl-3-[2-(5-methylimidazol-4-ylmethylthio)ethyl]guanidine.
$C_{10}H_{16}N_6S$ = 252.3.
CAS — 51481-61-9 (cimetidine); 70059-30-2 (cimetidine hydrochloride).
ATC — A02BA01.

NOTE. Cimetidine Hydrochloride is USAN.
Pharmacopoeias. In Chin., Eur. (see p.vi), Int., Jpn, Pol., and US. Eur. and US also include cimetidine hydrochloride ($C_{10}H_{16}N_6S,HCl$ = 288.8).

Cimetidine 100 mg is approximately equivalent to cimetidine hydrochloride 114.4 mg.

Pharmacopoeial description

Ph. Eur.: A white or almost white, polymorphic powder. Slightly soluble in water; soluble in alcohol; practically insoluble in dichloromethane and in ether. It dissolves in dilute mineral acids. Store in airtight containers. Protect from light.

USP 25: A white to off-white crystalline powder, odourless or with a slight mercaptan odour. Slightly soluble in water and in chloroform; soluble in alcohol and in macrogol 400; practically insoluble in ether; sparingly soluble in isopropyl alcohol; freely soluble in methyl alcohol. Store in airtight containers. Protect from light.

Adverse Effects

Adverse reactions to cimetidine and other histamine H_2-antagonists are generally infrequent. The commonest side-effects reported have been diarrhoea and other gastrointestinal disturbances, dizziness, tiredness, headache, and rashes.

Altered liver function tests have occurred and there have been rare reports of hepatotoxicity. Reversible confusional states, especially in the elderly or in seriously ill patients such as those with renal failure, have occasionally occurred. Other adverse effects which have been reported rarely are hypersensitivity reactions and fever, arthralgia and myalgia, blood disorders including agranulocytosis and thrombocytopenia, acute pancreatitis, and cardiovascular disorders including bradycardia and heart block.

Cimetidine has a weak anti-androgenic effect and gynaecomastia and impotence have also occasionally occurred in men receiving relatively high doses for conditions such as the Zollinger-Ellison syndrome.

◊ In a meta-analysis of 24 double-blind placebo-controlled studies,[1] the incidence of adverse effects with cimetidine was not significantly different from placebo. The most common adverse effects reported by patients taking cimetidine who were followed up for at least one year[2,3] were diarrhoea, headache, fatigue, skin rash or pruritus, and gynaecomastia. The incidence of adverse effects was dose-related and decreased with length of treatment.[3] No fatal adverse effect of cimetidine could be found in a mortality survey involving 9928 patients taking cimetidine and 9351 controls;[4] although the mortality rate was higher in the cimetidine patients, this was explained by the presence of underlying disease (known or unknown) before starting cimetidine treatment and the use of cimetidine to counter adverse gastric effects of other drugs. Follow-up of 9377 of these cimetidine-treated patients for a further 3 years[5] still revealed no fatal disorder attributable to cimetidine treatment and a steady fall in the excess death rate in cimetidine users was observed with increasing length of follow-up; by the fourth year there was little difference between the observed and expected death rate. Cimetidine still appeared to be safe after 10 years of follow-up.[6]

1. Richter JM, *et al.* Cimetidine and adverse reactions: a meta-analysis of randomized clinical trials of short-term therapy. *Am J Med* 1989; 87: 278–84.
2. Colin-Jones DG, *et al.* Post-marketing surveillance of the safety of cimetidine : twelve-month morbidity report. *Q J Med* 1985; 54: 253–68.
3. Bardhan KD, *et al.* Safety of longterm cimetidine (CIM) treatment: the view from one centre. *Gut* 1990; 31: A599.
4. Colin-Jones DG, *et al.* Postmarketing surveillance of the safety of cimetidine: 12 month mortality report. *BMJ* 1983; 286: 1713–16.
5. Colin-Jones DG, *et al.* Postmarketing surveillance of the safety of cimetidine: mortality during second, third, and fourth years of follow up. *BMJ* 1985; 291: 1084–8.
6. Colin-Jones DG, *et al.* Postmarketing surveillance of the safety of cimetidine: 10 year mortality report. *Gut* 1992; 33: 1280–4.

Carcinogenicity. An association between H_2-antagonists and gastric cancer was proposed following individual case reports, the finding of tumours in long-term high-dose *animal* studies, and the possibility that nitrites and nitroso compounds may be produced, but seemed to be of little clinical relevance.[1,2] The excess risk of gastric cancer reported in patients taking cimetidine[3-6] or ranitidine[6] decreases with time and there is no evidence for any long-term persistence of the effect.[6] The increased risk may be explained by misdiagnosis and inappropriate cimetidine treatment of existing malignancy.[3-5] An apparently protective effect has been observed for H_2-antagonist use starting 10 or more years before diagnosis of gastric cancer.[6]

The observed excess risk for cancers of the respiratory system is probably related to smoking, since this is causally related to both peptic ulcer and lung cancer and the excess risk does not decline with time.[3-5]

1. Penston J, Wormsley KG. H_2-receptor antagonists and gastric cancer. *Med Toxicol* 1986; **1:** 163–8.
2. Møller H, *et al.* Use of cimetidine and other peptic ulcer drugs in Denmark 1977–1990 with analysis of the risk of gastric cancer among cimetidine users. *Gut* 1992; **33:** 1166–9.
3. Colin-Jones DG, *et al.* Postmarketing surveillance of the safety of cimetidine: 12 month mortality report. *BMJ* 1983; **286:** 1713–16.
4. Colin-Jones DG, *et al.* Postmarketing surveillance of the safety of cimetidine: mortality during second, third, and fourth years of follow up. *BMJ* 1985; **291:** 1084–8.
5. Møller H, *et al.* Cancer occurrence in a cohort of patients treated with cimetidine. *Gut* 1989; **30:** 1558–62.
6. La Vecchia C, *et al.* Histamine-2-receptor antagonists and gastric cancer risk. *Lancet* 1990; **336:** 355–7.

Effects on the blood. A review[1] in 1988 noted that leucopenia, thrombocytopenia, and pancytopenia have all been reported with cimetidine and ranitidine, with neutropenia and agranulocytosis occurring most often. There were also isolated reports of haemolytic anaemia and leucocytosis associated with cimetidine therapy. The overall incidence of cimetidine-associated blood cytopenia was estimated as 2.3 per 100 000 treated patients; the incidence for ranitidine was less and although there were reports with famotidine the incidence had not been determined. A subsequent case-control study,[2] concluded that the risk of hospitalisation due to neutropenia in patients receiving a six-week course of cimetidine was no more than 1 in 116 000, while agranulocytosis did not occur in more than 1 in 573 000 patients.

A review[3] of the safety profile of famotidine noted that as of May 1992 there had been 60 reports of serious blood dyscrasias in patients receiving famotidine, of which 22 were considered possibly related to drug therapy (6 cases of pancytopenia or bone marrow depression, 5 of thrombocytopenia, 4 of leucopenia, 3 of combined leucopenia and thrombocytopenia, and 3 of agranulocytosis).

1. Aymard J-P, *et al.* Haematological adverse effects of histamine H_2-receptor antagonists. *Med Toxicol* 1988; **3:** 430–48.
2. Strom BL, *et al.* Is cimetidine associated with neutropenia? *Am J Med* 1995; **99:** 282–90.
3. Howden CW, Tytgat GNJ. The tolerability and safety profile of famotidine. *Clin Ther* 1996; **18:** 36–54.

Effects on the cardiovascular system. Bradycardia,[1-4] atrioventricular block,[5,6] tachycardia,[7] and hypotension[4,8] have been reported during cimetidine treatment given by mouth and by intravenous injection or infusion. Although there are studies in patients[9] and healthy subjects[10,11] that have found no significant cardiovascular effects associated with cimetidine treatment, it is likely that a small proportion of patients are more susceptible to the cardiovascular effects of cimetidine. Caution is recommended if the drug is given intravenously to patients with cardiovascular disease (see Precautions, below).

See also under Overdosage, below.

1. Jefferys DB, Vale JA. Cimetidine and bradycardia. *Lancet* 1978; **i:** 828.
2. Ligumsky M, *et al.* Cimetidine and arrhythmia suppression. *Ann Intern Med* 1978; **89:** 1008–9.
3. Tanner LA, Arrowsmith JB. Bradycardia and H_2 antagonists. *Ann Intern Med* 1988; **109:** 434–5.
4. Drea EJ, *et al.* Cimetidine-associated adverse reaction. *DICP Ann Pharmacother* 1990; **24:** 581–3.
5. Tordjman T, *et al.* Complete atrioventricular block and long-term cimetidine therapy. *Arch Intern Med* 1984; **144:** 861.
6. Ishizaki M, *et al.* First-degree atrioventricular block induced by oral cimetidine. *Lancet* 1987; **i:** 225–6.
7. Dickey W, Symington M. Broad-complex tachycardia after intravenous cimetidine. *Lancet* 1987; **i:** 99–100.
8. Mahon WA, Kolton M. Hypotension after intravenous cimetidine. *Lancet* 1978; **i:** 828.
9. Jackson G, Upward JW. Cimetidine, ranitidine, and heart rate. *Lancet* 1982; **ii:** 265.
10. Hughes DG, *et al.* Cardiovascular effects of H_2-receptor antagonists. *J Clin Pharmacol* 1989; **29:** 472–7.
11. Hilleman DE, *et al.* Impact of chronic oral H_2-antagonist therapy on left ventricular systolic function and exercise capacity. *J Clin Pharmacol* 1992; **32:** 1033–7.

Effects on the endocrine system. Cimetidine has dose-related mild anti-androgenic properties and reduced sperm counts and raised serum-prolactin concentrations have been reported in men during cimetidine treatment[1] as have gynaecomastia, breast tenderness, and impotence.[2] Those symptoms resolved following withdrawal of cimetidine,[1,2] reduction of the dose,[2] or transfer to ranitidine.[2]

A study by the Boston Collaborative Drug Surveillance Program, using data from 81 535 men in the UK, found that cimetidine was associated with an incidence of 3.29 cases of gynaecomastia per 1000 person years, representing a relative risk 7.2 times greater than that of non-users.[3] The period at highest risk seemed to be between the seventh and twelfth month after starting treatment, and the occurrence was related to dose, with most of the risk associated with doses over 1 g daily. This large

study found no significant risk of gynaecomastia with ranitidine or omeprazole. However, there have been isolated reports of gynaecomastia or impotence with ranitidine (p.1245), nizatidine (p.1238), and famotidine (p.1226).

1. Wang C, *et al.* Effect of cimetidine on gonadal function in man. *Br J Clin Pharmacol* 1982; **13:** 791–4.
2. Jensen RT, *et al.* Cimetidine-induced impotence and breast changes in patients with gastric hypersecretory states. *N Engl J Med* 1983; **308:** 883–7.
3. García Rodríguez LA, Jick H. Risk of gynaecomastia associated with cimetidine, omeprazole, and other antiulcer drugs. *BMJ* 1994; **308:** 503–6. Correction. *ibid.*; 819.

Effects on the eyes. Ocular pain, blurred vision, and a rise in intra-ocular pressure occurred in a patient with chronic glaucoma during treatment with cimetidine; ocular symptoms associated with raised intra-ocular pressure subsequently developed during treatment with ranitidine.[1] However, a study suggested that cimetidine had no effect on intra-ocular pressure.[2] A cohort study involving 140 128 patients receiving anti-ulcer therapy, 68 504 of whom received cimetidine, found no evidence that any of the drugs were associated with a major increased risk of vascular or inflammatory disorders of the eye.[3]

1. Dobrilla G, *et al.* Exacerbation of glaucoma associated with both cimetidine and ranitidine *Lancet* 1982; **i:** 1078.
2. Feldman F, Cohen MM. Intraocular pressure and H_2 receptor antagonists. *Lancet* 1982; **i:** 1359.
3. García Rodríguez LA, *et al.* A cohort study of the ocular safety of anti-ulcer drugs. *Br J Clin Pharmacol* 1996; **42:** 213–16.

Effects on the kidneys. Up to the end of 1981 the manufacturers of cimetidine were aware of 20 patients who may have had interstitial nephritis out of an estimated total of 20 million cimetidine-treated patients. On the assumption that only 10% of these adverse effects have been reported, which is a figure consistent with that suggested for a voluntary reporting system, the incidence would be around 1 in 100 000 treated patients. The interstitial nephritis related to cimetidine use has always been reversed on cessation of therapy.[1]

1. Rowley-Jones D, Flind AC. Cimetidine-induced renal failure. *BMJ* 1982; **285:** 1422–3.

Effects on the liver. A cohort study[1] involving 108 891 patients who had received cimetidine, ranitidine, famotidine, or omeprazole between 1990 and 1993, found 33 cases meeting the authors' definition of clinically serious liver injury (cholestatic in 8 cases, hepatocellular in 15 and mixed in 10), most of whom presented with jaundice. Of these cases of liver injury, 12 were among current users of cimetidine, compared with 5 among users of ranitidine and 1 omeprazole user. It was estimated that the incidence of hepatotoxicity among patients using cimetidine was 2.3 cases per 10 000 users, and the adjusted relative risk was 5.5 times that of non-users. The relative risk for use of ranitidine or omeprazole was calculated at 1.7 and 2.1 respectively. The risk with cimetidine was greatest at high doses (800 mg daily or above) and at the beginning of therapy. For reports of liver damage with famotidine, see p.1226.

1. García Rodríguez LA, *et al.* The risk of acute liver injury associated with cimetidine and other acid-suppressing anti-ulcer drugs. *Br J Clin Pharmacol* 1997; **43:** 183–8.

Effects on the nervous system. Cimetidine has been associated with a number of adverse neurological effects including confusion,[1-8] bizarre behaviour,[9] reversible brain stem syndrome (with ataxia, dysarthria, visual impairment, deafness, and paraesthesia),[10] coma,[8,11] convulsions,[7] encephalopathy,[12] visual hallucinations,[9,13,14] paranoia,[5] chorea,[15,16] myopathy,[17] and neuropathy.[18,19] These reactions occur mainly in patients who are elderly, critically ill, or with impaired renal or hepatic function, in whom there may be increased penetration of the blood-brain barrier by cimetidine. Single-dose studies in young healthy subjects[20] have found no adverse changes in performance, central nervous function, or subjective assessment of mood after administration of cimetidine 200 or 400 mg by mouth.

There is no clear evidence that cimetidine is a more frequent cause of CNS reactions than ranitidine, famotidine, or nizatidine.[21]

1. Robinson TJ, Mulligan TO. Cimetidine and mental confusion. *Lancet* 1977; **ii:** 719.
2. Spears JB. Cimetidine and mental confusion. *Am J Hosp Pharm* 1978; **35:** 1035.
3. Wood CA, *et al.* Cimetidine and mental confusion. *JAMA* 1978; **239:** 2550–1.
4. McMillen MA, *et al.* Cimetidine and mental confusion. *N Engl J Med* 1978; **298:** 284–5.
5. Kinnell HG, Webb A. Confusion associated with cimetidine. *BMJ* 1979; **ii:** 1438.
6. Mogelnicki SR, *et al.* Physostigmine reversal of cimetidine-induced mental confusion. *JAMA* 1979; **241:** 826–7.
7. Edmonds ME, *et al.* Cimetidine: does neurotoxicity occur? Report of three cases. *J R Soc Med* 1979; **72:** 172–5.
8. Sonnenblick M, *et al.* Neurological and psychiatric side effects of cimetidine—report of 3 cases with review of the literature. *Postgrad Med J* 1982; **58:** 415–18.
9. Papp KA, Curtis RM. Cimetidine-induced psychosis in a 14-year-old girl. *Can Med Assoc J* 1984; **131:** 1081–4.
10. Cumming WJK, Foster JB. Cimetidine-induced brainstem dysfunction. *Lancet* 1978; **i:** 1096.
11. Levine ML. Cimetidine-induced coma in cirrhosis of the liver. *JAMA* 1978; **240:** 1238.
12. Niv Y, *et al.* Cimetidine and encephalopathy. *Ann Intern Med* 1986; **105:** 977.
13. Agarwal SK. Cimetidine and visual hallucinations. *JAMA* 1978; **240:** 214.
14. Rushton AR. Pseudohypoparathyroidism, cimetidine, and neurologic toxicity. *Ann Intern Med* 1983; **98:** 677.

15. Kushner MJ. Chorea and cimetidine. *Ann Intern Med* 1982; **96:** 126.
16. Lehmann AB. Reversible chorea due to ranitidine and cimetidine. *Lancet* 1988; **ii:** 158.
17. Feest TG, Read DJ. Myopathy associated with cimetidine? *BMJ* 1980; **281:** 1284–5.
18. Walls TJ, *et al.* Motor neuropathy associated with cimetidine. *BMJ* 1980; **281:** 974–5.
19. Atkinson AB, *et al.* Neurological dysfunction in two patients receiving captopril and cimetidine. *Lancet* 1980; **ii:** 36–7.
20. Nicholson AN, Stone BM. The H_2-antagonists, cimetidine and ranitidine : studies on performance. *Eur J Clin Pharmacol* 1984; **26:** 579–82.
21. Cantú TG, Korek JS. Central nervous system reactions to histamine-2 receptor blockers. *Ann Intern Med* 1991; **114:** 1027–34.

Effects on the skin. Widespread erythrosis-like lesions in a 36-year-old man were probably induced by cimetidine.[1] There has been a report[2] of a skin eruption clinically consistent with erythema annulare centrifugum developing in a patient after 6 months of treatment with cimetidine; the eruption resolved after withdrawal of cimetidine and reappeared on rechallenge. The condition had not recurred during therapy with ranitidine. Erythema multiforme eruptions occurred after both cimetidine and famotidine administration in one patient (see p.1226). There have been reports of the Stevens-Johnson syndrome during cimetidine treatment in patients with a history of hypersensitivity to penicillin[3] or sulfonamides,[4] and a report of toxic epidermal necrolysis.[5]

Urticarial vasculitis[6] and alopecia[7] have also been associated with cimetidine treatment.

1. Angelini G, *et al.* Cimetidine and erythrosis-like lesions. *BMJ* 1979; **i:** 1147–8.
2. Merrett AC, *et al.* Cimetidine-induced erythema annulare centrifugum: no cross-sensitivity with ranitidine. *BMJ* 1981; **283:** 698.
3. Ahmed AH, *et al.* Stevens-Johnson syndrome during treatment with cimetidine. *Lancet* 1978; **ii:** 433.
4. Guan R, Yeo PPB. Stevens-Johnson syndrome: was it cimetidine? *Aust N Z J Med* 1983; **13:** 182.
5. Tidwell BH, *et al.* Cimetidine-induced toxic epidermal necrolysis. *Am J Health-Syst Pharm* 1998; **55:** 163–4.
6. Mitchell GG, *et al.* Cimetidine-induced cutaneous vasculitis. *Am J Med* 1983; **75:** 875–6.
7. Khalsa JH, *et al.* Cimetidine-associated alopecia. *Int J Dermatol* 1983; **22:** 202–4.

Fever. Reports of febrile reactions associated with cimetidine. Fever has also been reported with famotidine (p.1226) and ranitidine (p.1246).

1. Ramboer C. Drug fever with cimetidine. *Lancet* 1978; **i:** 330–1.
2. McLoughlin JC, *et al.* Cimetidine fever. *Lancet* 1978; **ii:** 499–500.
3. Corbett CL, Holdsworth CD. Fever, abdominal pain, and leucopenia during treatment with cimetidine. *BMJ* 1978; **i:** 753–4.
4. Landolfo K, *et al.* Cimetidine-induced fever. *Can Med Assoc J* 1984; **130:** 1580.

Hypersensitivity. Facial oedema,[1] laryngospasm,[1] pruritus,[2,3] rash,[2,3] angioedema[3] and anaphylaxis[4] have been reported in patients receiving cimetidine by mouth or intravenously.

See also under Effects on the Skin, above.

1. Delaunois L. Hypersensitivity to cimetidine. *N Engl J Med* 1979; **300:** 1216.
2. Hadfield WA. Cimetidine and giant urticaria. *Ann Intern Med* 1979; **91:** 128–9.
3. Sandhu BS, Requena R. Hypersensitivity to cimetidine. *Ann Intern Med* 1982; **97:** 138.
4. Knapp AB, *et al.* Cimetidine-induced anaphylaxis. *Ann Intern Med* 1982; **97:** 374–5.

Infection. Treatment with H_2-antagonists may predispose patients to salmonella infection, probably because the decrease in gastric acidity reduces the gastric killing of ingested organisms.[1] The greatest increase in risk was seen in patients over 65 years of age. There are conflicting data on whether the use of H_2-antagonists for prophylaxis of stress ulcers in critically ill patients increases the risk for pneumonia (see under Peptic Ulcer Disease, p.1208).

1. Neal KR, *et al.* Recent treatment with H_2 antagonists and antibiotics and gastric surgery as risk factors for salmonella infection. *BMJ* 1994; **308:** 176.

Overdosage. No serious toxic effects were noted in reports[1-3] of overdosage in patients who took cimetidine 5.2 to 20 g (including one patient who took about 12 g daily for 5 days[1]), despite resultant plasma concentrations of up to 57 μg per mL (peak plasma concentration after a 200-mg dose is reported to be 1 μg per mL). However, an overdose of about 12 g produced high pulse rate, dilated pupils, speech disturbances, agitation and disorientation in one patient[4] who had chronic schizophrenia and was also taking trifluoperazine and hydroxyzine.[5] Also, fatal bradycardia has been reported after overdosage with an unknown amount of cimetidine and diazepam.[6] In a review of 881 cases of cimetidine overdose, excluding cases where several drugs were taken, it was concluded that the toxicity of cimetidine after acute overdose was very low.[7] No symptoms were observed in 79% of cases, which included ingestions of up to 15 g of cimetidine, and only 3 patients had moderate clinical manifestations (dizziness and bradycardia; CNS depression; vomiting). No patients had major medical outcomes and there were no fatalities. Gastric emptying was performed in 34% of cases.

Emptying the stomach, for example by gastric lavage, has been employed in overdosage, provided that not more than 4 hours have elapsed since ingestion of the drug, but supportive measures and symptomatic treatment alone may be adequate.

The symbol † denotes a preparation no longer actively marketed

Forced diuresis does not appear to enhance the excretion of cimetidine from the body, and is not recommended.[3]

1. Gill GV. Cimetidine overdose. *Lancet* 1978; i: 99.
2. Illingworth RN, Jarvie DR. Absence of toxicity in cimetidine overdosage. *BMJ* 1979; i: 453–4.
3. Meredith TJ, Volans GN. Management of cimetidine overdose. *Lancet* 1979; ii: 1367.
4. Nelson PG. Cimetidine and mental confusion. *Lancet* 1977; ii: 928.
5. Wilson JB. Cimetidine overdosage. *BMJ* 1979; i: 955.
6. Hiss J, et al. Fatal bradycardia after intentional overdose of cimetidine and diazepam. *Lancet* 1982; ii: 982.
7. Krenzelok EP, et al. Cimetidine toxicity: an assessment of 881 cases. *Ann Emerg Med* 1987; 1: 1217–21.

Precautions

Before giving cimetidine or other histamine H₂-antagonists to patients with gastric ulcers the possibility of malignancy should be considered since these drugs may mask symptoms and delay diagnosis. They should be given in reduced dosage to patients with impaired renal function.

Intravenous injections of cimetidine should be given slowly and intravenous infusion is preferred, particularly for high doses and in patients with cardiovascular impairment.

Breast feeding. See under Distribution into Breast Milk, below.

Burns. The clearance of cimetidine has been reported to be increased in burn patients, with the increase correlating to the size of the burn.[1] Despite another study which reported a decreased renal clearance (but an increased non-renal clearance) early in the evolution of burn injury,[2] it has been recommended that the dosage of cimetidine be increased in patients with burns, depending on the extent of injury. A requirement for increased dosage has also been noted in paediatric burns patients.[3]

1. Martyn JAJ, et al. Increased cimetidine clearance in burn patients. *JAMA* 1985; 253: 1288–91.
2. Ziemniak JA, et al. Cimetidine kinetics during resuscitation from burn shock. *Clin Pharmacol Ther* 1984; 36: 228–33.
3. Martyn JAJ, et al. Alteration by burn injury of the pharmacokinetics and pharmacodynamics of cimetidine in children. *Eur J Clin Pharmacol* 1989; 36: 361–7.

Helicobacter pylori testing. In one study, 2 of 11 patients with *Helicobacter pylori* infection had false-negative urea breath tests while receiving high dose ranitidine (600 mg daily). The breath test became positive again within 5 days of stopping therapy. The manufacturers of the breath test recommend it should not be performed within 4 weeks of stopping antisecretory drug therapy.

1. Chey WD, et al. Lansoprazole and ranitidine affect the accuracy of the ¹⁴C-urea breath test by a pH-dependent mechanism. *Am J Gastroenterol* 1997; 92: 446–50.

Hepatic impairment. The bioavailability of cimetidine may be increased in patients with cirrhosis[1,2] and a dosage reduction of up to 40% has been suggested in patients with portal systemic encephalopathy.[3]

An increased resistance to H₂-receptor antagonists has been reported in patients with cirrhosis, see Ranitidine, p.1246.

1. Gugler R, et al. Altered disposition and availability of cimetidine in liver cirrhotic patients. *Br J Clin Pharmacol* 1982; 14: 421–30.
2. Cello JP, Øie S. Cimetidine disposition in patients with Laennec's cirrhosis during multiple dosing therapy. *Eur J Clin Pharmacol* 1983; 25: 223–9.
3. Ziemniak JA, et al. Hepatic encephalopathy and altered cimetidine kinetics. *Clin Pharmacol Ther* 1983; 34: 375–82.

Porphyria. Cimetidine is considered to be unsafe in patients with porphyria although there is conflicting experimental evidence of porphyrinogenicity.

For reference to clinical and biochemical improvement in porphyric patients receiving cimetidine, see below.

Renal impairment. The clearance of cimetidine is reduced in renal impairment and dosage reduction is recommended (see Uses and Administration, below).

Interactions

Cimetidine and other H₂-antagonists can reduce the absorption of drugs such as ketoconazole, and possibly itraconazole, whose absorption is dependent on an acid gastric pH.

Cimetidine may inhibit the hepatic metabolism of many drugs by binding to cytochrome P450 isoenzymes, notably CYP1A2, CYP2C9, CYP2D6, and CYP3A4. Although many such interactions have been demonstrated, only a few are considered clinically significant, notably those with phenytoin, theophylline, lignocaine [lidocaine], and oral anticoagulants. Avoidance of the combination, or a reduction in the dosage of these drugs may be required.

◊ Cimetidine can affect a wide range of drugs[1-4] but these interactions are of clinical significance for only a small number of

drugs, particularly those which have a narrow therapeutic index where the risk of toxicity may necessitate adjustment of dosage. The majority of interactions are due to binding of cimetidine to cytochrome P450 isoenzymes in the liver with subsequent inhibition of microsomal oxidative metabolism and increased bioavailability or plasma concentrations of drugs metabolised by these enzymes. A few interactions are due to competition for renal tubular secretion. Other mechanisms of interaction such as changes in hepatic blood flow play only a minor role.

Significant or potentially significant interactions have occurred with lignocaine [lidocaine] (p.1314), procainamide (p.961), biguanide antidiabetics (p.320), antiepileptics such as phenytoin (p.361) and carbamazepine (p.345), ciclosporin (p.522), nifedipine (p.943), pethidine (p.68), theophylline (p.781), tricyclic antidepressants such as amitriptyline (p.277), warfarin and other oral anticoagulants (p.996), zalcitabine (p.644), and zolmitriptan (p.458). Combinations of these drugs and cimetidine should be avoided or used with caution, with monitoring of effects or plasma-drug concentrations and reductions in dosage as appropriate.

Famotidine, nizatidine, and ranitidine do not inhibit cytochrome P450, and the potential for drug interactions is therefore reduced.

1. Penston J, Wormsley KG. Adverse reactions and interactions with H₂-receptor antagonists. *Med Toxicol* 1986; i: 192–216.
2. Somogyi A, Muirhead M. Pharmacokinetic interactions of cimetidine 1987. *Clin Pharmacokinet* 1987; 12: 321–66.
3. Smith SR, Kendall MJ. Ranitidine versus cimetidine: a comparison of their potential to cause clinically important drug interactions. *Clin Pharmacokinet* 1988; 15: 44–56.
4. Shinn AF. Clinical relevance of cimetidine drug interactions. *Drug Safety* 1992; 7: 245–67.

Alcohol. Any interaction between H₂-antagonists and alcohol is generally thought unlikely to be clinically significant (see p.1132).

Antacids. Single-dose studies of the interaction between cimetidine and antacids[1] have shown reduced bioavailability of cimetidine as well as no interaction. The neutralising capacity of the antacid appears to be a factor in determining whether an interaction occurs and a dose with less than 50 mmol neutralising capacity will have little, if any, effect on cimetidine absorption. There is no evidence that the therapeutic efficacy of cimetidine is reduced and with long-term use of the combination the bioavailability of cimetidine is unlikely to be reduced.

1. Gugler R, Allgayer H. Effects of antacids on the clinical pharmacokinetics of drugs: an update. *Clin Pharmacokinet* 1990; 18: 210–19.

Antimuscarinics. The antimuscarinic *propantheline* delays gastric emptying and reduces intestinal motility and has been reported to reduce the bioavailability of cimetidine.[1]

1. Kanto J, et al. The effect of metoclopramide and propantheline on the gastrointestinal absorption of cimetidine. *Br J Clin Pharmacol* 1981; 11: 629–31.

Prokinetic drugs. *Metoclopramide* may reduce the bioavailability of cimetidine possibly due to reduction of gastrointestinal transit time.[1-3] A similar interaction has been reported between cimetidine and the prokinetic drug *cisapride*.[4] The clinical significance of this interaction is questionable since such combinations may be clinically effective.

1. Gugler R, et al. Impaired cimetidine absorption due to antacids and metoclopramide. *Eur J Clin Pharmacol* 1981; 20: 225–8.
2. Kanto J, et al. The effect of metoclopramide and propantheline on the gastrointestinal absorption of cimetidine. *Br J Clin Pharmacol* 1981; 11: 629–31.
3. Barzaghi N, et al. Effects on cimetidine bioavailability of metoclopramide and antacids given two hours apart. *Eur J Clin Pharmacol* 1989; 37: 409–10.
4. Kirch W, et al. Cisapride-cimetidine interactions; enhanced cisapride bioavailability and accelerated cimetidine absorption. *Ther Drug Monit* 1989; 11: 411–14.

Sucralfate. The manufacturers of the mucosal protectant sucralfate state that it has been shown to reduce the bioavailability of cimetidine and other H₂ antagonists, presumably due to binding in the gastrointestinal tract. The effect can be avoided by separating doses of the two drugs by 2 hours, but it is not clear whether the interaction has a clinical significance.

Pharmacokinetics

Cimetidine is readily absorbed from the gastrointestinal tract and peak plasma concentrations are obtained about an hour after administration on an empty stomach; a second peak may be seen after about 3 hours. Food delays the rate and may slightly decrease the extent of absorption, with the peak plasma concentration occurring after about 2 hours.

The bioavailability of cimetidine following oral administration is about 60 to 70%. Cimetidine is widely distributed and has a volume of distribution of about 1 litre per kg and is weakly bound, about 20%, to plasma proteins. The elimination half-life from plasma is about 2 hours and is increased in renal impairment. Cimetidine is partially metabolised in the liver to the sulfoxide and to hydroxymethylcimetidine. Approximately 50% of an oral dose, and 75% of an

intravenous dose, is excreted unchanged in the urine in 24 hours. Cimetidine crosses the placental barrier and is distributed into breast milk.

◊ Reviews.

1. Somogyi A, Gugler R. Clinical pharmacokinetics of cimetidine. *Clin Pharmacokinet* 1983; 8: 463–95.
2. Lin JH. Pharmacokinetic and pharmacodynamic properties of histamine H₂-receptor antagonists: relationship between intrinsic potency and effective plasma concentrations. *Clin Pharmacokinet* 1991; 20: 218–36.
3. Gladziwa U, Klotz U. Pharmacokinetics and pharmacodynamics of H₂-receptor antagonists in patients with renal insufficiency. *Clin Pharmacokinet* 1993; 24: 319–32.

Children. Renal function is limited in the first few months of life and half-lives of 1.1 to 3.7 hours have been reported for cimetidine in neonates.[1-3] A dosage regimen for neonates based on renal function has been suggested[1] with 15 to 20 mg per kg body-weight daily for full-term neonates, but with lower doses for premature neonates and those with renal dysfunction. However, a dose of 5 to 7 mg per kg may be sufficient to suppress gastric acid secretion in neonates.[3]

In older infants and children maturation of renal function is complete and the clearance of cimetidine is increased compared with that in adults while younger children show higher clearance values than older children. A typical dosage regimen for children is 30 mg per kg daily, in 3 or 4 divided doses.[4] However, even this dose might not produce optimal control of gastric acid.[5]

1. Ziemniak JA, et al. The pharmacokinetics and metabolism of cimetidine in neonates. *Dev Pharmacol Ther* 1984; 7: 30–8.
2. Lloyd CW, et al. The pharmacokinetics of cimetidine and metabolites in a neonate. *Drug Intell Clin Pharm* 1985; 19: 203–5.
3. Stile IL, et al. Pharmacokinetic evaluation of cimetidine in newborn infants. *Clin Ther* 1985; 7: 361–4.
4. Somogyi A, et al. Cimetidine pharmacokinetics and dosage requirements in children. *Eur J Pediatr* 1985; 144: 72–6.
5. Lambert J, et al. Efficacy of cimetidine for gastric acid suppression in pediatric patients. *J Pediatr* 1992; 120: 474–8.

Distribution into breast milk. In the UK manufacturers advise that mothers receiving cimetidine avoid breast feeding. Cimetidine is reported to be actively transported into breast milk, resulting in a milk:serum ratio 5.5 times higher than that expected with passive diffusion.[1] In one case, where cimetidine was detected in the milk of a nursing mother in concentrations higher than in her plasma, it was calculated[2] that the maximum amount of cimetidine that an infant could ingest assuming an intake of about 1 litre of milk daily and fed at the time of peak concentrations would be about 6 mg. However, the Committee on Drugs of the American Academy of Pediatrics has pointed out that there was no evidence of signs or symptoms attributable to the drug in the infant in this case,[3] despite 6 months of breast feeding, and cimetidine has been classified by that body as usually compatible with breast feeding.[4]

1. Oo CY, et al. Active transport of cimetidine into human milk. *Clin Pharmacol Ther* 1995; 58: 548–55.
2. Somogyi A, Gugler R. Cimetidine excretion into breast milk. *Br J Clin Pharmacol* 1979; 7: 627–9.
3. Berlin CM. Cimetidine and breast-feeding. *Pediatrics* 1991; 88: 1294.
4. American Academy of Pediatrics Committee on Drugs. The transfer of drugs and other chemicals into human milk. *Pediatrics* 2001; 108: 776–89.

Uses and Administration

Cimetidine is a histamine H₂-antagonist and inhibits actions of histamine mediated by H₂-receptors such as gastric acid secretion and pepsin output. It is used where inhibition of gastric acid secretion may be beneficial, as in peptic ulcer disease, including stress ulceration (p.1208), gastro-oesophageal reflux disease (p.1204), selected cases of persistent dyspepsia (p.1204), pathological hypersecretory states such as the Zollinger-Ellison syndrome (p.1209), and in patients at risk of acid aspiration (p.1202) during general anaesthesia or child birth. Cimetidine may also be used to reduce malabsorption and fluid loss in patients with the short bowel syndrome and to reduce the degradation of enzyme supplements given to patients with pancreatic insufficiency.

Cimetidine may be given by mouth, by the nasogastric route, or parenterally by the intravenous or intramuscular routes; the total daily dose by any route should not normally exceed 2.4 g. Although some formulations are prepared as the hydrochloride, strengths and doses are expressed in terms of the base.

SPECIFIC DISEASE DOSES.

In the management of benign **gastric** and **duodenal ulceration** a single daily dose of 800 mg by mouth at bedtime is recommended which should be given initially for at least 4 weeks in the case of duodenal, and for at least 6 weeks in the case of gastric, ulcers. Where appropriate a maintenance dose of 400 mg may then be given once daily at bedtime, or twice daily in the morning and at bedtime. Other regimens have also been used for treatment and maintenance.

In **gastro-oesophageal reflux disease** the recommended dose is 400 mg by mouth four times daily (with meals and at bedtime), or 800 mg twice daily, for 4 to 8 weeks. In pathological hypersecretory conditions, such as the **Zollinger-Ellison syndrome**, a dose of 300 or 400 mg by mouth four times daily is normally used, although sometimes higher doses may be necessary.

Doses of 200 to 400 mg by mouth, by nasogastric administration, or parenterally (200 mg only for direct intravenous injection) every 4 to 6 hours are recommended for the management of patients at risk from **stress ulceration** of the upper gastrointestinal tract. In patients at risk of developing the **acid aspiration syndrome**, a dose of 400 mg by mouth may be given 90 to 120 minutes before the induction of anaesthesia, or at the start of labour (in obstetric practice), and doses of up to 400 mg (by the parenteral route if appropriate, see below) may be repeated at intervals of 4 hours if required.

Doses of up to 200 mg four times daily have been taken for non-ulcer **dyspepsia**; 100 mg at night has been used in the prophylaxis of nocturnal heart burn.

To reduce the degradation of pancreatic enzyme supplements, patients with **pancreatic insufficiency**, as in cystic fibrosis (p.117), may be given cimetidine 800 to 1600 mg daily by mouth in 4 divided doses, 60 to 90 minutes before meals.

PARENTERAL ADMINISTRATION.

In the UK, the usual dose of cimetidine by intravenous injection is 200 mg which should be given slowly over at least 5 minutes and may be repeated every 4 to 6 hours. If a larger dose is required, or if the patient has cardiovascular impairment, intravenous infusion is recommended. For an intermittent intravenous infusion the recommended dose is 200 to 400 mg every 4 to 6 hours if necessary. For a continuous intravenous infusion the recommended rate is 50 to 100 mg per hour. The usual intramuscular dose is 200 mg which may be repeated at intervals of 4 to 6 hours. In the USA, dosage recommendations for parenteral administration are 300 mg every 6 to 8 hours by intramuscular injection or by slow intravenous injection over at least 5 minutes. The same dosage may be given by intermittent intravenous infusion over 15 to 20 minutes; for continuous intravenous infusion the recommended rate is 37.5 mg per hour, which may be preceded by 150 mg as an intravenous loading dose. However, a rate of 50 mg per hour is recommended for prevention of stress ulceration.

CHILDREN'S DOSES.

For **children** over one year of age 25 to 30 mg per kg body-weight daily may be given in divided doses, by mouth or parenterally. Under 1 year of age, 20 mg per kg daily in divided doses has been used (see also under Pharmacokinetics, above).

DOSAGE IN RENAL OR HEPATIC IMPAIRMENT.

The dosage of cimetidine should be reduced in patients with **impaired renal function**; suggested doses according to creatinine clearance are: creatinine clearance of 0 to 15 mL per minute, 200 mg twice daily; 15 to 30 mL per minute, 200 mg three times daily; 30 to 50 mL per minute, 200 mg four times daily; over 50 mL per minute, normal dosage. Cimetidine is removed by haemodialysis, but not significantly removed by peritoneal dialysis. Dosage reduction may be required in some patients with hepatic impairment—see Precautions, above.

Dapsone toxicity. Cimetidine might reduce the haemolysis and methaemoglobinaemia associated with dapsone. References supporting this suggestion are given under Dapsone on p.197.

Diagnostic use. Cimetidine blocks renal tubular secretion of creatinine and has been used experimentally to improve the accuracy of estimations of glomerular filtration rate from creatinine clearance in patients with renal disease.[1] Best results were

The symbol † denotes a preparation no longer actively marketed

achieved with a bolus dose of 1.2 g and the use of such a high dose was questioned.[2]

1. van Acker BAC, et al. Creatinine clearance during cimetidine administration for measurement of glomerular filtration rate. Lancet 1992; 340: 1326–9.
2. Agarwal R. Creatinine clearance with cimetidine for measurement of GFR. Lancet 1993; 341: 188.

Echinococcosis. Cimetidine has been given with albendazole to increase its effect (by inhibiting its metabolism) in the treatment of echinococcosis (p.92).

Immunomodulation. Studies in *mice* and humans have shown that H_2-antagonists have an immunoregulatory effect.[1] T-lymphocyte suppressor cells have histamine H_2 receptors and cimetidine has been reported to reduce their activity, thus enhancing immune response.[1,2] There is also some evidence that it enhances cellular immunity, notably natural killer cell activity.[3] This discovery has led to the investigation of cimetidine in a number of disorders associated with alteration of the immune response including eosinophilic fasciitis, herpesvirus infections, mucocutaneous candidiasis,[4] hypogammaglobulinaemia,[5] and various malignancies.[1]

1. Kumar A. Cimetidine: an immunomodulator. DICP Ann Pharmacother 1990; 24: 289–95.
2. Snyman JR, et al. Cimetidine as modulator of the cell-mediated immune response in vivo using the tuberculin skin test as parameter. Br J Clin Pharmacol 1990; 29: 257–60.
3. Katoh J, et al. Cimetidine and immunoreactivity. Lancet 1996; 348: 404–5.
4. Polizzi B, et al. Successful treatment with cimetidine and zinc sulphate in chronic mucocutaneous candidiasis. Am J Med Sci 1996; 311: 189–90.
5. White WB, Ballow M. Modulation of suppressor-cell activity by cimetidine in patients with common variable hypogammaglobulinemia. N Engl J Med 1985; 312: 198–202.

EOSINOPHILIC FASCIITIS. Eosinophilic fasciitis is a scleroderma-like syndrome of inflammation of the muscle fascia and associated eosinophilia and hypergammaglobulinaemia. Although it responds well to corticosteroid therapy in most cases, cimetidine has also been tried. The effect of cimetidine on eosinophilic fasciitis is unpredictable with both remission[1-4] and lack of response[5,6] having been reported in a few patients.

1. Solomon G, et al. Eosinophilic fasciitis responsive to cimetidine. Ann Intern Med 1982; 97: 547–9.
2. Laso FJ, et al. Cimetidine and eosinophilic fasciitis. Ann Intern Med 1983; 98: 1026.
3. Garcia-Morteo O, et al. Cimetidine and eosinophilic fasciitis. Ann Intern Med 1984; 100: 318–19.
4. Farrell AM, et al. Eosinophilic fasciitis associated with autoimmune thyroid disease and myelodysplasia treated with pulsed methylprednisolone and antihistamines. Br J Dermatol 1999; 140: 1185–7.
5. Loftin EB. Cimetidine and eosinophilic fasciitis. Ann Intern Med 1983; 98: 111–12.
6. Herson S, et al. Cimetidine in eosinophilic fasciitis. Ann Intern Med 1990; 113: 412–13.

HERPESVIRUS AND PAPILLOMAVIRUS INFECTIONS. Although there have been numerous isolated and anecdotal reports of a beneficial response to cimetidine in patients with infections due to various *herpesviruses* (p.606), including genital herpes simplex,[1] infectious mononucleosis,[2,3] and herpes zoster[4-7] some of these reports have been criticised[8,9] mainly on the grounds that the majority of cases of herpes zoster will resolve within 2 to 3 weeks whether any treatment is given or not. Also, a double-blind placebo-controlled study involving 63 patients with herpes zoster[10] found no evidence that cimetidine relieved the pain or accelerated the rate of healing of lesions.

There are reports[11] of benefit from the use of cimetidine in patients with *viral warts* (p.1108), but controlled studies have failed to show significant benefit.[12,13]

1. Wakefield D. Cimetidine in recurrent genital herpes simplex infection. Aust J Med 1984; 101: 882.
2. Goldstein JA. Cimetidine and mononucleosis. Ann Intern Med 1983; 99: 410–11.
3. Goldstein JA. Cimetidine, ranitidine, and Epstein-Barr virus infection. Ann Intern Med 1986; 105: 139.
4. Hayne ST, Mercer JB. Herpes zoster: treatment with cimetidine. Can Med Assoc J 1983; 129: 1284–5.
5. Shandera R. Treatment of herpes zoster with cimetidine. Can Med Assoc J 1984; 131: 279.
6. Mavligit GM, Talpaz M. Cimetidine for herpes zoster. N Engl J Med 1984; 310: 318–19.
7. Arnot RS. Herpes zoster and cimetidine. Med J Aust 1984; 141: 903.
8. Tyrrell DL. Course of herpes zoster. Can Med Assoc J 1984; 130: 1109.
9. Giles KE. Herpes zoster and cimetidine. Med J Aust 1985; 142: 283.
10. Levy DW, et al. Cimetidine in the treatment of herpes zoster. J R Coll Physicians Lond 1985; 19: 96–8.
11. Glass AT, et al. Cimetidine therapy for recalcitrant warts in adults. Arch Dermatol 1996; 132: 680–2.
12. Karabulut AA, et al. Is cimetidine effective for nongenital warts: a double-blind, placebo-controlled study. Arch Dermatol 1997; 133: 533–4.
13. Rogers CJ, et al. Cimetidine therapy for recalcitrant warts in adults: is it any better than placebo? J Am Acad Dermatol 1999; 41: 123–7.

MALIGNANT NEOPLASMS. Because of its immunomodulatory effects cimetidine has been tried, with some reported benefit,[1-3] as an adjuvant in the management of a variety of malignant neoplasms such as those of the gastrointestinal tract (see p.493). However, a large randomised study[4] failed to show any benefit for cimetidine compared with placebo in gastric cancer.

A similar study with ranitidine also failed to show any significant benefit.[5]

1. Tønnesen H, et al. Effect of cimetidine on survival after gastric cancer. Lancet 1988; ii: 990–2.
2. Adams WJ, Morris DL. Short-course cimetidine and survival with colorectal cancer. Lancet 1994; 344: 1768–9.
3. Matsumoto S. Cimetidine and survival with colorectal cancer. Lancet 1995; 346: 115.
4. Langman MJS, et al. Prospective, double-blind, placebo-controlled randomized trial of cimetidine in gastric cancer. Br J Cancer 1999; 81: 1356–62.
5. Primrose JN, et al. A prospective randomised controlled study of the use of ranitidine in patients with gastric cancer. Gut 1998; 42: 17–19.

Mastocytosis. Cimetidine, alone or in combination with an antihistamine (histamine H_1-antagonist), has been reported to relieve gastrointestinal symptoms,[1,2] pruritus, and urticaria[3,4] in patients with mastocytosis (p.775).

1. Hirschowitz BI, Groarke JF. Effect of cimetidine on gastric hypersecretion and diarrhea in systemic mastocytosis. Ann Intern Med 1979; 90: 769–71.
2. Linde R, et al. Combination H1 and H2 receptor antagonist therapy in mastocytosis. Ann Intern Med 1980; 92: 716.
3. Simon RA. Treatment of systemic mastocytosis. N Engl J Med 1980; 302: 231.
4. Frieri M, et al. Comparison of the therapeutic efficacy of cromolyn sodium with that of combined chlorpheniramine and cimetidine in systemic mastocytosis: results of a double-blind clinical trial. Am J Med 1985; 78: 9–14.

Paracetamol toxicity. It has been suggested that cimetidine might be of use in the treatment of paracetamol poisoning (see p.71) because of its inhibition of the cytochrome P450 system. However, there is no current evidence to support the claims of benefit made in some anecdotal reports.[1]

1. Kaufenberg AJ, Shepherd MF. Role of cimetidine in the treatment of acetaminophen poisoning. Am J Health-Syst Pharm 1998; 55: 1516–19.

Porphyria. There are reports[1,2] of patients with acute intermittent porphyria (p.1011) showing clinical and biochemical improvement during treatment with cimetidine. Cimetidine is, however, considered to be unsafe in patients with porphyria (see above).

1. Baccino E, et al. Cimetidine in the treatment of acute intermittent porphyria. JAMA 1989; 262: 3000.
2. Horie Y, et al. Clinical usefulness of cimetidine treatment for acute relapse in intermittent porphyria. Clin Chim Acta 1995; 234: 171–5.

Skin disorders. Cimetidine has been used alone[1-8] and in combination with an antihistamine (H_1-antagonist)[5,8,9] in various skin disorders. H_2-antagonists such as cimetidine and ranitidine have produced improvement in certain types of *urticaria* (p.1107), especially those associated with cold or angioedema. Their routine use in urticaria is controversial, but in practice their addition to conventional treatment can be tried in resistant cases.[10-12] Little additional benefit has been found with combination therapy in dermographic urticaria.[13] Although they may act by antagonism of H_2-receptors on cutaneous blood vessels, other mechanisms of action may be involved.[8] Patients with *pruritus* (p.1106) of various causes may also respond to H_2-antagonists,[1,2,6,7,9] but studies in larger groups of patients have demonstrated no benefit.[3-5,14]

1. Easton P, Galbraith PR. Cimetidine treatment of pruritus in polycythemia vera. N Engl J Med 1978; 299: 1134.
2. Hess CE. Cimetidine for the treatment of pruritus. N Engl J Med 1979; 300: 370.
3. Harrison AR, et al. Pruritus, cimetidine and polycythemia. N Engl J Med 1979; 300: 433–4.
4. Scott GL, Horton RJ. Pruritus, cimetidine and polycythemia. N Engl J Med 1979; 300: 434. Correction. ibid.; 936.
5. Zappacosta AR, Hauss D. Cimetidine doesn't help pruritus of uremia. N Engl J Med 1979; 300: 1280.
6. Schapira DV, Bennett JM. Cimetidine for pruritus. Lancet 1979; i: 726–7.
7. Aymard JP, et al. Cimetidine for pruritus in Hodgkin's disease. BMJ 1980; 280: 151–2.
8. Theoharides TC. Histamine2 (H_2)-receptor antagonists in the treatment of urticaria. Drugs 1989; 37: 345–55.
9. Deutsch PH. Dermatographism treated with hydroxyzine and cimetidine and ranitidine. Ann Intern Med 1984; 101: 569.
10. Advenier C, Queille-Roussel C. Rational use of antihistamines in allergic dermatological conditions. Drugs 1989; 38: 634–44.
11. Ormerod AD. Urticaria: recognition, causes, and treatment. Drugs 1994; 48: 717–30.
12. Greaves MW. Chronic urticaria. N Engl J Med 1995; 332: 1767–72.
13. Sharpe GR, Shuster S. In dermographic urticaria H_2 receptor antagonists have a small but therapeutically irrelevant additional effect compared with H_1 antagonists alone. Br J Dermatol 1993; 129: 575–9.
14. Raisch DW, et al. Evaluation of a non-food and drug administration-approved use of cimetidine: treatment of pruritus resulting from epidural morphine analgesia. DICP Ann Pharmacother 1991; 25: 716–2.

Preparations

BP 2001: Cimetidine Injection; Cimetidine Oral Solution; Cimetidine Oral Suspension; Cimetidine Tablets;
USP 25: Cimetidine in Sodium Chloride Injection; Cimetidine Injection; Cimetidine Tablets.

Proprietary Preparations (details are given in Part 3)
Aust.: Cimetag; Neutromed; Neutronorm; Sodexx; Ulcometin; Ulcostad; *Austral.:* Cimehexal; Cimetimax†; Magicul; Sigmetadine; Tagamet; *Belg.:* Nuardin; Tagamet; *Braz.:* Cimetidan; Cimetil; Cimetin; Cimex; Climatidine; Duomet; Gastrodine; Laveran; Stomakon; Stomet; Tagamet; Ulcedine; Ulcedor; Ulcenon; Ulceracid; Ulcerase; Ulcimet; Ulcitag; Ulgastrin; Up Mep; Zagastrol; *Canad.:* Novo-Cimetine; Nu-Cimet; Peptol; Tagamet; *Denm.:* Aciloc; Acinil; Cimecodan; Hocimin; Metinet†; Novamet; Tag-

amet; *Fin.*: Cimex; *Fr.*: Stomedine; Tagamet; *Ger.*: Altramet; Azucimet; Cime; Cimebeta; Cimehexal; Cimemerck†; Cimephil†; Cimet; CimLich; Ciuk†; Contracid†; duraH2; Gastroprotect; H 2 Blocker; Jenametidin†; Sigacimet; Tagagel†; Tagamet; Ulcolind H₂; Ulcubloc; Ulkusal†; *Hong Kong*: Altramet; Cementin; Cimeta; Cimulcer; Citidine; Gastidine; Megadin; Neutronorm; Pallia; Syncomet; Tagadine; Tagamet; Ultec; *Irl.*: Cedine; Cimagen; Cimeldine; Dyspamet; Galenamet; Geramet; Pinamet; Tagamet; *Israel*: Cemidin; Cimetag; Cimi; Tagamet; *Ital.*: Biomag; Brumetidina; Citimid†; Dina; Eureceptor; Gastromet†; Neo Gastrausil†; Notul; Stomet; Tagamet; Tametin†; Temic; Ulcedin; Ulcestop; Ulcodina; Ulcomedina; Ulis; Vagolisal†; *Mex.*: Alcatex; Antil; Asaurex; Beamat; Blocan; Cimebec; Cimetase; Columina; Dimetigal; Gastrodina; Gastrolem; Inesfay; Novamet; Procimeti; Sinegastrin; Tagamet; Ulcerim; Ulogen; Ulserral; Zimerol; Zymerol; *Neth.*: Tagamet; *Norw.*: Acinil; Cimal; Cimetid; Gastrobitan†; Tagamet; *NZ*: Cytine; Duomet; Tagamet; *Port.*: Cim; Evicer; Tagamet; *S.Afr.*: Aci-Med; Acidown†; Cimlok; Cinadine; Cymi†; Duomet; Hexamet; Lenamet; Secadine; Sonsuur; Tagamet; Ulcim; Ulmet†; *Singapore*: Cementin; Cimulcer; Citidine; Erlmetin; Tagamet; Xepamet; *Spain*: Ali Veg; Fremet; Gastro H2; Mansal; Tagamet; *Swed.*: Aciloc; Acinil; Tagamet; *Switz.*: Malimed; Tagamet; *Thai.*: Alserine; Cencamet; Cidine; Cigamet; Cimag; Cimet-P; Cimidine; Cimulcer; Citidine; CMD; Duotric; Gastrodin; Histodil; Iwamet; Med-Gastramet; Milamet; Peptica; Pondarmett; Pose-CM; Rinadine; Servicimet; Siamidine; Simaglen; Simex; Tagamet; Ulcedine; Ulcemet; Ulcimet; *UAE*: Cimetag; *UK*: Acid-Eze; Acilok; Dyspamet; Galenamet; Peptimax; Phimetin†; Tagamet; Ultec; Zita; *USA*: Tagamet.

Multi-ingredient: *Aust.*: Cimetalgin†; *Irl.*: Algitec; *Neth.*: Aciflux; *UK*: Algitec†; Tagamet Dual Action†.

Cinitapride (11133-v)

Cinitapride (*rINN*).
4-Amino-*N*-[1-(3-cyclohexen-1-ylmethyl)-4-piperidyl]-2-ethoxy-5-nitrobenzamide.
$C_{21}H_{30}N_4O_4 = 402.5$.
$CAS — 66564-14-5$.

Profile
Cinitapride is a substituted benzamide used for its prokinetic properties. It is given by mouth as the acid tartrate in doses of 1 mg three times daily before meals in the management of gastroparesis and gastro-oesophageal reflux disease (p.1204).

Preparations
Proprietary Preparations (details are given in Part 3)
Spain: Blaston; Cidine.

Cisapride (16581-d)

Cisapride (*BAN, USAN, rINN*).
Cisapridum; R-51619. cis-4-Amino-5-chloro-*N*-{1-[3-(4-fluorophenoxy)propyl]-3-methoxy-4-piperidyl}-2-methoxybenzamide monohydrate.
$C_{23}H_{29}ClFN_3O_4,H_2O = 484.0$.
$CAS — 81098-60-4$ (anhydrous cisapride).
ATC — A03FA02.

Pharmacopoeias. In Eur. (see p.vi) and Pol. Eur. also includes cisapride tartrate.

Cisapride monohydrate 10.39 mg is approximately equivalent to 10 mg of anhydrous cisapride.

Pharmacopoeial description
Ph. Eur.: A white or almost white powder; it exhibits polymorphism. Practically insoluble in water; soluble in dichloromethane; freely soluble in dimethylformamide; sparingly soluble in methyl alcohol. Protect from light.

Adverse Effects
The most commonly reported side-effects with cisapride are gastrointestinal disturbances including abdominal cramps, borborygmi, and diarrhoea. Headache and lightheadedness may also occur. Hypersensitivity (including rash, pruritus, and bronchospasm), convulsions, extrapyramidal effects, and increased urinary frequency, have occasionally been reported. Cases of arrhythmia, including ventricular tachycardia, ventricular fibrillation, torsade de pointes, and QT interval prolongation have occurred rarely, fatalities have resulted, and have led to severe restrictions on its use (see Effects on the Heart, below). There have been a few cases of disturbances in liver function among patients receiving cisapride.

◊ A comparison of data from prescription-event monitoring in over 13 000 recipients of cisapride and from a further 9726 recipients involved in a controlled study showed that diarrhoea, in about 2 to 4% of patients, was the commonest adverse effect reported.[1] Other relatively common adverse effects were headache, abdominal pain, nausea and vomiting, and constipation, all in around 1 to 1.5% of patients. There were 46 reports in the prescription-event monitoring data of increased urinary frequency (plus a further 20 among the controlled study patients), and 5 reports of arrhythmias.

1. Wager E, *et al.* A comparison of two cohort studies evaluating the safety of cisapride: prescription-event monitoring and a large phase IV study. *Eur J Clin Pharmacol* 1997; **52**: 87–94.

Effects on the heart. Seven reports[1] of cardiac effects associated with cisapride were submitted to the WHO Programme for International Drug Monitoring between 1989 and 1991. They included palpitations in 4, tachycardia and hypertension in 1, and extrasystole in 2. Subsequent reports have implicated

cisapride in the development of prolonged QT interval and torsade de pointes or ventricular fibrillation or both.[2,3] By December 1999 the FDA had received 341 reports of heart rhythm abnormalities associated with cisapride use, including 80 reports of deaths. Most patients were either receiving other drugs known to impair cisapride metabolism (see Interactions, below) or had other factors predisposing to arrhythmias. In the light of earlier reports of cardiac effects and of evidence for a direct effect of cisapride on the heart at therapeutic concentrations in 1998 the UK Committee on Safety of Medicines (CSM) **contra-indicated**[2] the use of cisapride in patients receiving drugs that could impair cisapride metabolism or that prolong the QT interval, as well as in patients with a history of QT interval prolongation, ventricular arrhythmia, or torsade de pointes, or other risk factors for arrhythmia (see Precautions, below). Neonates[4] (especially of low gestational age[5]) are vulnerable to cisapride-induced QT interval prolongation, and the CSM also specifically contra-indicated use in premature neonates[2] and noted that there were insufficient data to support use in children up to the age of 12. Other studies have also noted a prolongation of QT interval in children.[6,7] However, some commentators have questioned the general contra-indication in prematurity,[8] and one retrospective analysis estimated the rate of serious adverse events such as arrhythmia in premature newborns to be less than 1 in 11 000, excluding those cases related to concurrent treatment with a contra-indicated drug or to overdose.[9] Conversely, other commentators emphasise the lack of objective evidence for benefit for cisapride in most paediatric indications.[10] The European Society of Paediatric Gastroenterology, Hepatology and Nutrition has published recommendations on the use of cisapride in paediatric gastro-oesophageal reflux disease,[11] including that the total daily dose of cisapride should rarely exceed 0.8 mg per kg body-weight, and that ECG monitoring should be performed before and after 3 days of treatment in certain groups such as premature infants.

The use of cisapride has also been the subject of warnings and restrictions in other countries. In the USA, prescribing information was amended in January 2000 to recommend that all patients should receive an ECG before beginning cisapride therapy and extending the contra-indications to use; the drug was subsequently **withdrawn** from general supply, remaining available only in severely restricted cases. In July 2000 cisapride was also withdrawn completely from the UK market, pending a Europe-wide review of its risks and benefits.[12]

1. Olsson S, Edwards IR. Tachycardia during cisapride treatment. *BMJ* 1992; **305**: 748–9.
2. Committee on Safety of Medicines/Medicines Control Agency. Cisapride (Prepulsid): risk of arrhythmias. *Current Problems* 1998; **24**: 11.
3. Wysowski DK, Bacsanyi J. Cisapride and fatal arrhythmia. *N Engl J Med* 1996; **335**: 290–1.
4. Bernardini S, *et al.* Effect of cisapride on QTc interval in neonates. *Arch Dis Child* 1997; **77**: F241–3.
5. Dubin A, *et al.* Cisapride associated with QTc prolongation in very low birth weight preterm infants. *Pediatrics* 2001; **107**: 1313–16.
6. Hill SL, *et al.* Proarrhythmia associated with cisapride in children. *Pediatrics* 1998; **101**: 1053–6.
7. Khongphatthanayothin A, *et al.* Effects of cisapride on QT interval in children. *J Pediatr* 1998; **133**: 51–6.
8. Lander A, Desai A. The risks and benefits of cisapride in premature neonates, infants, and children. *Arch Dis Child* 1998; **79**: 469–71.
9. Ward RM, *et al.* Cisapride: a survey of the frequency of use and adverse events in premature newborns. *Pediatrics* 1999; **103**: 469–72.
10. Cairns P. The risks and benefits of cisapride. *Arch Dis Child* 1999; **80**: 493.
11. Vandenplas Y, *et al.* The role of cisapride in the treatment of pediatric gastroesophageal reflux: the European Society of Paediatric Gastroenterology, Hepatology and Nutrition. *J Pediatr Gastroenterol Nutr* 1999; **28**: 518–28.
12. Committee on Safety of Medicines/Medicines Control Agency. Cisapride (Prepulsid) withdrawn. *Current Problems* 2000; **26**: 9–10.

Effects on the respiratory system. Chest tightness, wheezing, and a fall in peak flow rate occurred in a patient with severe brittle asthma following administration of cisapride 10 mg.[1] Four other cases of bronchospasm associated with cisapride use have been discussed in a subsequent report;[2] in 2 of these cases symptoms resolved on withdrawal and recurred on rechallenge.

1. Nolan P, *et al.* Cisapride and brittle asthma. *Lancet* 1990; **336**: 1443.
2. Pillans P. Bronchospasm associated with cisapride. *BMJ* 1995; **311**: 1472.

Effects on the urinary tract. There had been 12 cases of urinary disturbances associated with use of cisapride[1] reported to the Australian Adverse Drug Reactions Advisory Committee between March 1991 and July 1993. Five reports were of urinary incontinence, 8 involved frequency, and individual reports involved cystitis, hesitancy, and urinary retention. The majority of the cases involved women, and most patients were elderly.

1. Boyd IW, Rohan AP. Urinary disorders associated with cisapride. *Med J Aust* 1994; **160**: 579–80.

Precautions
Cisapride should not be used when stimulation of muscular contractions might adversely affect gastrointestinal conditions as in gastrointestinal haemorrhage, obstruction, perforation, or immediately after surgery. Cisapride is contra-indicated in any patient receiving potent inhibitors of the cytochrome P450 isoenzyme CYP3A4 such as macrolide antibiotics, azole anti-

fungals, HIV-protease inhibitors, or nefazodone (see also under Interactions, below). It is also contra-indicated in those taking other drugs that predispose to electrolyte disturbances or that prolong the QT interval, and in those with a personal or family history of QT interval prolongation or a previous history of ventricular arrhythmia or torsade de pointes. Furthermore, it should not be given to those with other risk factors for arrhythmia including clinically significant heart disease, uncorrected electrolyte disturbances (particularly hypokalaemia and hypomagnesaemia), and renal or respiratory failure. Use is also contra-indicated in premature infants for up to 3 months after birth.

Cisapride should be used with caution and in reduced doses in patients with hepatic or renal impairment.

Care should be taken not to exceed the recommended dose.

Interactions
Cisapride is metabolised by the cytochrome P450 isoenzyme CYP3A4. Concomitant administration of drugs that significantly inhibit this enzyme is contra-indicated as it may result in increased plasma concentrations of cisapride and hence a greater risk of QT interval prolongation and ventricular arrhythmias. Examples of such drugs include the azole antifungals ketoconazole, fluconazole, itraconazole, and miconazole; the macrolide antibacterials troleandomycin, erythromycin, and clarithromycin; the non-nucleoside reverse transcriptase inhibitors delavirdine and efavirenz; and the HIV-protease inhibitors indinavir and ritonavir. Nefazodone may interact similarly. Cisapride should not be used in patients receiving other medication known to prolong the QT interval, including quinine or halofantrine, terfenadine, astemizole, certain antiarrhythmics such as amiodarone or quinidine, some antidepressants such as amitriptyline, phenothiazine antipsychotics, and sertindole. Cimetidine may enhance cisapride bioavailability. Grapefruit juice also increases the bioavailability of cisapride and concomitant use should be avoided. In addition, drugs such as potassium-wasting diuretics, or insulin in acute settings, can result in altered electrolyte balance, and concomitant use with cisapride may also increase the risk of arrhythmias.

Antimuscarinics and possibly opioid analgesics may antagonise the gastrointestinal effects of cisapride. Because cisapride increases intestinal motility it may affect the absorption of other drugs, either diminishing absorption from the stomach or enhancing absorption from the small intestine. Prothrombin times may be increased in some patients receiving oral anticoagulants, and the effects of alcohol and some other CNS depressants may be enhanced.

◊ Reviews.
1. Bedford TA, Rowbotham DJ. Cisapride: drug interactions of clinical significance. *Drug Safety* 1996; **15**: 167–75.
2. Michalets EL, Williams CR. Drug interactions with cisapride: clinical implications. *Clin Pharmacokinet* 1999; **39**: 49–75.

Antidepressants. It has been pointed out[1] that a number of antidepressants, including *fluoxetine, fluvoxamine, nefazodone,* and *sertraline* all appear to markedly inhibit cytochrome P450 isoenzyme CYP3A4, and therefore might interact with cisapride. See also above.

1. Caley CF. Cisapride interaction with antidepressants. *Ann Pharmacother* 1996; **30**: 684.

Antimicrobials. Of 57 cases of prolonged QT interval or torsade de pointes reported to the US FDA as of April 1996 in patients receiving cisapride, 32 (56%) were also receiving azole antifungals *(fluconazole, itraconazole, ketoconazole,* or *miconazole)* or macrolide antibacterials *(erythromycin* or *clarithromycin)*.[1] Subsequently, concurrent administration of cisapride and clarithromycin has been shown to prolong the QT interval in healthy volunteers,[2] and further cases of torsade de pointes[3,4] and QT prolongation with syncope[5] have been reported in patients receiving the combination. A case of torsade de pointes in a patient receiving erythromycin and cisapride has also been reported.[6] There is a theoretical possibility of a serious interaction with *quinupristin/dalfopristin*. Similar interactions could also be anticipated with *non-nucleoside reverse transcriptase inhibitor antiretrovirals* and *HIV-protease inhibitors*.

1. Wysowski DK, Bacsanyi J. Cisapride and fatal arrhythmia. *N Engl J Med* 1996; **335**: 290–1.
2. van Haarst AD, *et al.* The influence of cisapride and clarithromycin on QT intervals in healthy volunteers. *Clin Pharmacol Ther* 1998; **64**: 542–6.
3. Mekkarie MA. Torsade de pointes in two chronic renal failure patients treated with cisapride and clarithromycin. *Am J Kidney Dis* 1997; **30**: 437–9.
4. Piquette RK. Torsade de pointes induced by cisapride/clarithromycin interaction. *Ann Pharmacother* 1999; **33**: 22–6.
5. Seals Gray V. Syncopal episodes associated with cisapride and concurrent drugs. *Ann Pharmacother* 1998; **32**: 648–51.
6. Tierney MG, *et al.* Potential cisapride-erythromycin interaction. *Can J Clin Pharmacol* 1997; **4**: 82–4.

Calcium-channel blockers. Near syncope and a prolonged QT interval occurred in a patient treated with cisapride and diltiazem.[1] Diltiazem may have inhibited the metabolism of cisapride.

1. Thomas AR, *et al.* Prolongation of the QT interval related to cisapride-diltiazem interaction. *Pharmacotherapy* 1998; **18**: 381–5.

Grapefruit juice. Grapefruit juice increased the oral bioavailability of cisapride, with large interindividual variation, in healthy volunteers.[1,2] The manufacturer advises that the combination be avoided.

1. Gross AS, *et al.* Influence of grapefruit juice on cisapride pharmacokinetics. *Clin Pharmacol Ther* 1999; **65:** 395–401.
2. Kivistö KT, *et al.* Repeated consumption of grapefruit juice considerably increases plasma concentrations of cisapride. *Clin Pharmacol Ther* 1999; **66:** 448–53.

H₂-antagonists. *Cimetidine*[1] but not *ranitidine*[2] has been reported to enhance the bioavailability of oral cisapride, possibly by inhibition of cisapride metabolism (cimetidine is an inhibitor of the cytochrome P450 isoenzyme CYP3A4). Cisapride conversely increases the rate of absorption and decreases the oral bioavailability of both cimetidine[1] and ranitidine (see p.1246).

1. Kirch W, *et al.* Cisapride-cimetidine interaction: enhanced cisapride bioavailability and accelerated cimetidine absorption. *Ther Drug Monit* 1989; **11:** 411–14.
2. Rowbotham DJ, *et al.* Effect of single doses of cisapride and ranitidine administered simultaneously on plasma concentrations of cisapride and ranitidine. *Br J Anaesth* 1991; **67:** 302–305.

Pharmacokinetics

Cisapride is readily absorbed from the gastrointestinal tract, with peak plasma concentrations achieved 1 to 2 hours after a dose by mouth. It undergoes extensive first-pass metabolism in the liver and gut wall, resulting in an absolute bioavailability of 35 to 40%. The main metabolic pathways are oxidative *N*-dealkylation by the cytochrome P450 isoenzyme CYP3A4, producing the major metabolite norcisapride, and aromatic hydroxylation. More than 90% of a dose is excreted as metabolites in the urine and faeces in approximately equal amounts. A small amount is distributed into breast milk. The elimination half-life is about 10 hours. Cisapride is about 98% bound to plasma proteins.

◊ References.
1. Hofmeyr GJ, Sonnendecker EWW. Secretion of the gastrokinetic agent cisapride in human milk. *Eur J Clin Pharmacol* 1986; **30:** 735–6.
2. Meuldermans W, *et al.* Excretion and biotransformation of cisapride in dogs and humans after oral administration. *Drug Metab Dispos* 1988; **16:** 403–9.
3. Hedner T, *et al.* Comparative bioavailability of a cisapride suppository and tablet formulation in healthy volunteers. *Eur J Clin Pharmacol* 1990; **38:** 629–31.
4. Zhou H, *et al.* Pharmacokinetic profile of cisapride 20 mg after once- and twice-daily dosing. *Clin Ther* 1998; **20:** 292–8.
5. Preechagoon Y, *et al.* Population pharmacokinetics of enterally administered cisapride in young infants with gastro-oesophageal reflux disease. *Br J Clin Pharmacol* 1999; **48:** 688–93.

Uses and Administration

Cisapride is a substituted benzamide used for its prokinetic properties. It stimulates gastrointestinal motility, probably by increasing the release of acetylcholine in the gut wall at the level of the myenteric plexus, increases the resting tone of the lower oesophageal sphincter, and increases the amplitude of lower oesophageal contractions. Gastric emptying is accelerated and the mouth-to-caecum transit time is reduced. Colonic peristalsis is also increased which decreases colonic transit time. Cisapride apparently lacks antidopaminergic effects (unlike metoclopramide, p.1235, to which it is chemically related) or direct parasympathomimetic activity and it does not affect prolactin release or gastric secretion. It is reported to be an agonist at serotonin-4 (5-HT₄) receptors.

Cisapride has been used mainly in the treatment of gastro-oesophageal reflux disease (p.1204), in disorders associated with decreased gastric motility (below), and in non-ulcer dyspepsia. However, as mentioned under Effects on the Heart, above, its use is severely restricted by its propensity to cause cardiac arrhythmias, and it has been withdrawn completely in the UK.

Cisapride is given as the monohydrate, but doses are calculated in terms of the anhydrous substance. It is taken by mouth 15 or 30 minutes before a meal and at bedtime, if necessary.

For **dyspepsia**, 10 mg has been given 3 times daily, usually for 4 weeks. In patients with **decreased gastrointestinal motility**, 10 mg has been given 3 or 4 times daily, initially for 6 weeks. For **gastro-oesophageal reflux disease** 10 mg has been given 3 or 4 times daily; alternatively, 20 mg twice daily may be given. The usual course has been 12 weeks. In the USA, doses of up to 20 mg four times daily were permitted, although the drug has since been withdrawn there from general use. A dose of 10 mg twice daily or 20 mg at night has been given for maintenance treatment; the maintenance dose might be increased to 20 mg twice daily if oesophageal lesions were initially very severe.

In patients with impaired hepatic function the initial dose should be half the usual dose, followed by adjustment depending on clinical response. Where renal impairment is not considered to contra-indicate the use of cisapride, a similar reduction in initial dose has been recommended.

◊ Reviews.
1. Barone JA, *et al.* Cisapride: a gastrointestinal prokinetic drug. *Ann Pharmacother* 1994; **28:** 488–500.
2. Wiseman LR, Faulds D. Cisapride: an updated review of its pharmacology and therapeutic efficacy as a prokinetic agent in gastrointestinal motility disorders. *Drugs* 1999; **47:** 116–52.

Decreased gastrointestinal motility. Some benefit has been reported from the use of cisapride in patients with chronic

intestinal pseudo-obstruction[1-3] and also in the acute form.[4,5] For a general discussion of decreased gastrointestinal motility and its treatment, see p.1202. Cisapride has also been used in diabetic gastroparesis (below).

1. Camilleri M, *et al.* Impaired transit of chyme in chronic intestinal pseudoobstruction: correction by cisapride. *Gastroenterology* 1986; **91:** 619–26.
2. Puntis JWL, *et al.* Cisapride in neonatal short gut. *Lancet* 1986; **ii:** 108–9.
3. Coombs RC, Booth IW. Small intestinal motor activity response to cisapride in children with dysmotility syndromes. *Gut* 1989; **30:** A1473.
4. Vantrappen G. Acute colonic pseudo-obstruction. *Lancet* 1993; **341:** 152–3.
5. Lander A, *et al.* Cisapride reduces neonatal postoperative ileus: randomised placebo controlled trial. *Arch Dis Child* 1997; **77:** F119–22.

Diabetes mellitus. Cisapride has been used as an alternative to metoclopramide in the management of diabetic gastroparesis. For a discussion of diabetic complications, and their management, see p.317.

References.
1. Chang CS, *et al.* Effect of cisapride on gastric dysrhythmia and emptying of indigestible solids in type-II diabetic patients. *Scand J Gastroenterol* 1998; **33:** 600–4.
2. Stacher G, *et al.* Cisapride versus placebo for 8 weeks on glycemic control and gastric emptying in insulin-dependent diabetes: a double blind cross-over trial. *J Clin Endocrinol Metab* 1999; **84:** 2357–62.

Preparations

Proprietary Preparations (details are given in Part 3)
Aust.: Prepulsid; Pulsitil; ***Austral.:*** Prepulsid; ***Belg.:*** Cyprid; Prepulsid; ***Braz.:*** Cispride; Enteropride; Pangest; Prepulsid; ***Canad.:*** Prepulsid; ***Denm.:*** Prepulsid; ***Fin.:*** Prepulsid; ***Fr.:*** Prepulsid; ***Ger.:*** Alimix; Propulsin; ***Hong Kong:*** Prepulsid; ***Irl.:*** Prepulsid; ***Israel:*** Prepulsid; ***Ital.:*** Alimix; Cipril; Prepulsid; ***Mex.:*** Enteropride; Kinestase; Prepulsid; Sapriken; Unamol; ***Neth.:*** Prepulsid; ***Norw.:*** Prepulsid; ***NZ:*** Prepulsid; ***Port.:*** Prepulsid; ***S.Afr.:*** Prepulsid; ***Singapore:*** Prepulsid; ***Spain:*** Arcasin; Fisiogastrol; Kelosal; Kinet; Prepulsid; Trautil; ***Swed.:*** Prepulsid; ***Switz.:*** Prepulsid; ***Thai.:*** Cipasid; Cipride; Cisapin; Metison; Palcid; Prepulsid; Pri-De-Sid; ***UAE:*** Prokinate; ***UK:*** Alimix†; Prepulsid†; ***USA:*** Propulsid†.

Clebopride Malate (14171-l)

Clebopride Malate *(BANM, rINNM)*.

LAS-9273 (clebopride). 4-Amino-*N*-(1-benzyl-4-piperidyl)-5-chloro-o-anisamide malate.
$C_{20}H_{24}ClN_3O_2,C_4H_6O_5 = 508.0$.
CAS — 55905-53-8 (clebopride); 57645-91-7 (clebopride malate).

NOTE. Clebopride is *USAN*.
Pharmacopoeias. In Eur. (see p.vi).

Clebopride malate 679 µg is approximately equivalent to clebopride 500 µg.

Pharmacopoeial description

Ph. Eur.: A white or almost white, crystalline powder. Sparingly soluble in water and in methyl alcohol; slightly soluble in dehydrated alcohol; practically insoluble in dichloromethane. The pH of a 1% solution in water is 3.8 to 4.2. Protect from light.

Profile

Clebopride is a substituted benzamide similar to metoclopramide (p.1235), that is used for its antiemetic and prokinetic actions in nausea and vomiting (p.1206) and various other gastrointestinal disorders.

Clebopride malate is given in a usual dose equivalent to clebopride 0.5 mg by mouth three times daily before meals or 0.5 to 1 mg by intramuscular or intravenous injection for acute symptoms. A dose equivalent to clebopride 15 to 20 µg per kg bodyweight daily has been recommended for children.

Preparations

Proprietary Preparations (details are given in Part 3)
Ital.: Motilex; ***Port.:*** Clebofex; Clebutec; ***Spain:*** Clanzol†; Cleboril; Madurase†.

Multi-ingredient: ***Spain:*** Clanzoflat; Flatoril.

Colocynth (7508-g)

Bitter Apple; Bitter Cucumber; Colocynth Pulp; Colocynthis; Coloquinte; Coloquintidas; Koloquinthen.

NOTE. The synonym Bitter Apple has also been applied to the fruits of *Solanum incanum*.

The dried pulp of the fruit of *Citrullus colocynthis* (Cucurbitaceae).

Profile

Colocynth has a drastic purgative and irritant action. It has been superseded by less toxic laxatives. Colocynth is used in homoeopathic medicine.

Croton Oil (7509-q)

Oleum Crotonis; Oleum Tiglii.

CAS — 8001-28-3.

Pharmacopoeias. Chin. includes fruits of Croton tiglium.

An oil expressed from the seeds of *Croton tiglium* (Euphorbiaceae).

Profile

Croton oil has such a violent purgative action that it should not be used as a laxative. Externally, it is a powerful counter-irritant and vesicant. It is used in homoeopathic medicine. Croton oil contains phorbol esters, which are carcinogenic.

Preparations

Proprietary Preparations (details are given in Part 3)
Multi-ingredient: ***Canad.:*** Rheumalan.

Dantron (7510-d)

Dantron *(BAN, rINN)*.

Antrapurol; Chrysazin; Danthron; Dianthon; Dioxyanthrachinonum. 1,8-Dihydroxyanthraquinone.
$C_{14}H_8O_4 = 240.2$.
CAS — 117-10-2.
ATC — A06AB03.

NOTE. Compounded preparations of dantron may be represented by the following names:

- Co-danthramer *x/y (BAN)*—where *x* and *y* are the strengths in milligrams of dantron and poloxamer respectively
- Co-danthrusate *(BAN)*—dantron 5 parts and docusate sodium 6 parts (w/w).

Pharmacopoeias. In Aust., Br., and Neth.

Pharmacopoeial description

BP 2001: An orange, odourless or almost odourless, crystalline powder. Practically insoluble in water; very slightly soluble in alcohol; soluble in chloroform; slightly soluble in ether; dissolves in solutions of alkali hydroxides.

Adverse Effects and Precautions

As for Senna, p.1248. Dantron may colour the urine pink or red. Discoloration and superficial sloughing of perianal skin can occur after prolonged contact, therefore dantron should not be used in infants wearing nappies (diapers) and should be used with caution in incontinent patients. The mucosa of the large intestine may be discoloured with prolonged use or high dosage.

In *rodents*, dantron has been associated with the development of intestinal and liver tumours. Consequently, its use has been restricted, see below.

◊ References to adverse effects occurring with dantron-containing laxatives include individual cases of leucopenia with liver damage,[1] greyish-blue skin discoloration,[2] and orange vaginal discharge.[3] There has also been a report of intestinal sarcoma in an 18-year-old girl with a history of prolonged use of a dantron-containing laxative.[4] In May 2000 the UK Committee on Safety of Medicines restricted the use of dantron to terminally ill patients on the grounds that pre-clinical evidence had increased and dantron was now established as a potential human carcinogen.[5]

1. Tolman KG, *et al.* Possible hepatotoxicity of Doxidan. *Ann Intern Med* 1976; **84:** 290–2.
2. Darke CS, Cooper RG. Unusual case of skin discoloration. *BMJ* 1978; **1:** 1188–9.
3. Greer IA. Orange periods. *BMJ* 1984; **289:** 323.
4. Patel PM, *et al.* Anthraquinone laxatives and human cancer: an association in one case. *Postgrad Med J* 1989; **65:** 216–17.
5. Committee on Safety of Medicines/Medicine Control Agency. Danthron restricted to constipation in the terminally ill. *Current Problems* 2000; **26:** 4.

Pharmacokinetics

Dantron is metabolised by bacteria in the colon. Dantron or its metabolites are absorbed from the gastrointestinal tract, as indicated by discoloration of urine in some patients. Dantron or its metabolites are excreted in the faeces and the urine, and also in other secretions including breast milk.

Uses and Administration

Dantron is an anthraquinone stimulant laxative, but unlike senna (p.1248), it is not a glycoside. It is given by mouth to treat constipation (p.1202) and is effective within 6 to 12 hours. However, because of concern over *rodent* carcinogenicity it has been withdrawn in some countries, and its use restricted in others. In the UK it may be used only in terminally ill patients.

Dantron is given in doses of 25 to 75 mg when given with poloxamer 188 (p.1347) as co-danthramer, and in doses of 50 to 150 mg when given with docusate sodium (p.1223) as co-danthrusate. Doses are usually given at bedtime. Children have been given dantron 12.5 to 25 mg as co-danthramer or, in those aged 6 to 12 years, 50 mg as co-danthrusate.

The symbol † denotes a preparation no longer actively marketed

Preparations

BP 2001: Co-danthrusate Capsules.
Proprietary Preparations (details are given in Part 3)
Multi-ingredient: *Braz.*: Perlax; *Canad.*: Doss†; Regulex-D†; *Irl.*: Ailax; Codalax; Cotron; *Mex.*: Modaton; *NZ*: Codalax; *S.Afr.*: Norilax†; *UK*: Ailax; Capsuvac; Codalax; Danlax; Normax.

Difenidol Hydrochloride (6543-n)

Difenidol Hydrochloride *(BANM, rINNM)*.
Diphenidol Hydrochloride *(USAN)*; SKF-478 (difenidol); SKF-478-A; SKF-478-J (difenidol embonate). 1,1-Diphenyl-4-piperidinobutan-1-ol hydrochloride.
$C_{21}H_{27}NO,HCl = 345.9$.
CAS — 972-02-1 (difenidol); 3254-89-5 (difenidol hydrochloride); 26363-46-2 (difenidol embonate).
Pharmacopoeias. In Chin. and Jpn.

Profile
Difenidol hydrochloride is an antiemetic which probably acts through the chemoreceptor trigger zone. It is claimed to control vertigo by means of a specific effect on the vestibular apparatus. Difenidol also has a weak peripheral antimuscarinic action. It has been used in the treatment of some forms of nausea and vomiting (p.1206) such as those associated with surgery, radiotherapy, and cancer chemotherapy. It has also been used for the symptomatic treatment of vertigo, nausea and vomiting due to Ménière's disease, and other labyrinthine disturbances (p.408).
It has been given in doses equivalent to 25 to 50 mg of difenidol by mouth every 4 hours as required. Difenidol hydrochloride has also been given parenterally.

Preparations
Proprietary Preparations (details are given in Part 3)
Braz.: Vontrol; *Hong Kong*: Cephadol; *Jpn*: Cephadol; *Mex.*: Dicavin; Hemetiken; Laudefen; Nautrol; Normavom; Normitrol; Serratol; Vernausin; Vontrol; *Singapore*: Cephadol; *Thai.*: Cephadol.

Difenoxin Hydrochloride (6220-v)

Difenoxin Hydrochloride *(BANM, rINNM)*.
Difenoxylic Acid Hydrochloride; Diphenoxylic Acid Hydrochloride; McN-JR-15403-11 (difenoxin); R-15403. 1-(3-Cyano-3,3-diphenylpropyl)-4-phenylpiperidine-4-carboxylic acid hydrochloride.
$C_{28}H_{28}N_2O_2,HCl = 461.0$.
CAS — 28782-42-5 (difenoxin); 35607-36-4 (difenoxin hydrochloride).
NOTE. Difenoxin is *USAN*.

Profile
Difenoxin is the principal active metabolite of diphenoxylate (p.1222) and has similar actions and uses. It is given by mouth as the hydrochloride, but doses are in terms of the base.
In the treatment of diarrhoea (p.1203), the usual dose in adults is the equivalent of difenoxin 2 mg initially, followed by 1 mg after each loose stool or every 3 to 4 hours as required, up to a maximum of 8 mg daily.
Preparations of difenoxin usually contain subclinical amounts of atropine sulfate in an attempt to discourage abuse.

Preparations
Proprietary Preparations (details are given in Part 3)
Switz.: Lyspafen†; *USA*: Motofen.

Dihydroxyaluminum Sodium Carbonate (689-k)

Aluminium Sodium Carbonate Hydroxide; Carbaldrate; Dihydroxyaluminium Sodium Carbonate. Sodium (carbonato)dihydroxyaluminate(1-).
$CH_2AlNaO_5 = 144.0$.
CAS — 12011-77-7; 16482-55-6.
Pharmacopoeias. In US.

Pharmacopoeial description
USP 25: A fine white odourless powder. It loses not more than 14.5% of its weight on drying. Practically insoluble in water and in organic solvents; soluble in dilute mineral acids with the evolution of carbon dioxide. A 4% suspension in water has a pH of 9.9 to 10.2. Store in airtight containers.

Profile
Dihydroxyaluminum sodium carbonate is an antacid with general properties similar to aluminium hydroxide (p.1210) that is given in doses of about 300 to 600 mg by mouth.

Preparations
USP 25: Dihydroxyaluminum Sodium Carbonate Tablets.
Proprietary Preparations (details are given in Part 3)
Aust.: Antacidum; *Denm.*: Noacid; *Ger.*: Kompensan; *Port.*: Kompensan; *Switz.*: Kompensan.
Multi-ingredient: *Ger.*: Kompensan-S; *Port.*: Kompensan-S.

Diisopromine Hydrochloride (3719-p)

Diisopromine Hydrochloride *(rINNM)*.
Di-isopromine Hydrochloride. NN-Di-isopropyl-3,3-diphenylpropylamine hydrochloride.
$C_{21}H_{29}N,HCl = 331.9$.
CAS — 5966-41-6 (diisopromine); 24358-65-4 (diisopromine hydrochloride).

Profile
Diisopromine hydrochloride is an antispasmodic used with sorbitol in various gastrointestinal disorders.

Preparations
Proprietary Preparations (details are given in Part 3)
Multi-ingredient: *Belg.*: Bilagol†; *Braz.*: Biliflux; *Fr.*: Megabyl†; *S.Afr.*: Agofell.

Diphenoxylate Hydrochloride

(6223-p)

Diphenoxylate Hydrochloride *(BANM, rINNM)*.
Diphenoxylati Hydrochloridum; R-1132. Ethyl 1-(3-cyano-3,3-diphenylpropyl)-4-phenylpiperidine-4-carboxylate hydrochloride.
$C_{30}H_{32}N_2O_2,HCl = 489.0$.
CAS — 915-30-0 (diphenoxylate); 3810-80-8 (diphenoxylate hydrochloride).
NOTE. Compounded preparations of diphenoxylate hydrochloride may be represented by the following names:

• Co-phenotrope *(BAN)*—diphenoxylate hydrochloride 100 parts and atropine sulfate 1 part (w/w).
Pharmacopoeias. In Chin., Eur. (see p.vi), Int., and US.

Pharmacopoeial description
Ph. Eur.: A white or almost white, crystalline powder. Very slightly soluble in water; sparingly soluble in alcohol; freely soluble in dichloromethane; practically insoluble in ether. Protect from light.
USP 25: A white odourless crystalline powder. Slightly soluble in water and in isopropyl alcohol; sparingly soluble in alcohol and in acetone; freely soluble in chloroform; practically insoluble in ether and in petroleum spirit; soluble in methyl alcohol. A saturated solution in water has a pH of about 3.3.

Dependence and Withdrawal
Preparations of diphenoxylate usually contain subclinical amounts of atropine sulfate in an attempt to discourage abuse. Short-term administration of diphenoxylate with atropine in the recommended dosage carries a negligible risk of dependence, although prolonged use or use of high doses may produce dependence of the morphine type (see p.66).

Adverse Effects and Treatment
Diphenoxylate is related to the opioid analgesics (p.67), and its adverse effects and their treatment are similar, particularly in overdosage. Reported side-effects include: gastrointestinal effects such as anorexia, nausea and vomiting, abdominal distension or discomfort, paralytic ileus, toxic megacolon, and pancreatitis; nervous system effects such as headache, drowsiness, dizziness, restlessness, euphoria, depression, numbness of the extremities; and hypersensitivity reactions including angioedema, urticaria, pruritus, and swelling of the gums. Signs of overdosage may be delayed and patients should be observed for at least 48 hours after an overdose. Young children are particularly susceptible to the effects of overdosage.
The presence of subclinical doses of atropine sulfate in preparations containing diphenoxylate may give rise to the side-effects of atropine in susceptible individuals or in overdosage—see Atropine Sulfate, p.461.

Precautions
Diphenoxylate hydrochloride should be avoided in patients with jaundice, intestinal obstruction, antibiotic-associated colitis, or diarrhoea associated with enterotoxin-producing bacteria, and should be used with caution in patients with hepatic dysfunction. It should also be used with caution in young children because of a greater variability of response in this age group, and is not generally recommended for use in infants. Patients with inflammatory bowel disease receiving diphenoxylate should be carefully observed

for signs of toxic megacolon and diphenoxylate discontinued promptly should abdominal distention occur.

Interactions
Because of the structural relationship of diphenoxylate to pethidine there is a theoretical risk of hypertensive crisis if diphenoxylate is given concomitantly with MAOIs. Diphenoxylate may potentiate the effects of other CNS depressants such as alcohol, barbiturates, and some anxiolytics.

Pharmacokinetics
Diphenoxylate hydrochloride is well absorbed from the gastrointestinal tract. It is rapidly and extensively metabolised in the liver principally to diphenoxylic acid (difenoxin, p.1222) which has antidiarrhoeal activity; other metabolites include hydroxydiphenoxylic acid. It is excreted mainly as metabolites and their conjugates in the faeces; lesser amounts are excreted in urine. It may be distributed into breast milk.

Uses and Administration
Diphenoxylate hydrochloride is a synthetic derivative of pethidine with little or no analgesic activity; it reduces intestinal motility and is used in the symptomatic treatment of acute and chronic diarrhoea (p.1203). It may also be used to reduce the frequency and fluidity of the stools in patients with colostomies or ileostomies.
In acute diarrhoea the usual initial dose for adults is 10 mg by mouth followed by 5 mg every six hours, later reduced as the diarrhoea is controlled. In the UK diphenoxylate hydrochloride is not recommended for children under 4 years of age. Suggested initial doses for children are: 4 to 8 years, 2.5 mg three times daily; 9 to 12 years, 2.5 mg four times daily; over 12 years, 5 mg three times daily. In the USA diphenoxylate is not recommended for children under the age of 2 years and an initial dose of 0.3 to 0.4 mg per kg bodyweight (up to an effective maximum of 10 mg) daily in 4 divided doses is suggested for children aged 2 to 12 years. (For the view that antidiarrhoeal drugs should not be used at all in children, see p.1203.)
Similar initial doses are used for chronic diarrhoea, and subsequently reduced as necessary. If clinical improvement is not observed after 10 days' treatment with the maximum daily dose of 20 mg (in adults) further administration is unlikely to result in any benefit.
Preparations of diphenoxylate usually contain subclinical amounts of atropine sulfate in an attempt to discourage abuse.

Substance dependence. Diphenoxylate may be useful[1] in the symptomatic management of diarrhoea associated with opioid withdrawal syndromes (p.66).

1. DOH. *Drug misuse and dependence: guidelines on clinical management.* London: HMSO, 1999.

Preparations
USP 25: Diphenoxylate Hydrochloride and Atropine Sulfate Oral Solution; Diphenoxylate Hydrochloride and Atropine Sulfate Tablets.

Proprietary Preparations (details are given in Part 3)
Austral.: Lofenoxal; Lomotil; *Belg.*: Reasect†; *Braz.*: Lomotil; *Canad.*: Lomotil; *Denm.*: Retardin; *Fr.*: Diarsed; *Ger.*: Reasect†; *Hong Kong*: Dhamotil; Lomotil; *Irl.*: Lomotil; *Ital.*: Reasect†; *Mex.*: Lomotil; *NZ*: Diastop; Lomotil; *Port.*: Lomotil†; *S.Afr.*: Eldox; Lomotil; *Singapore*: Dhamotil; Erlotyl; Lomotil; Remodil; *Switz.*: Reasec; *Thai.*: Dilomil; Ditropine; Lomotil; *UAE*: Intard; *UK*: Diarphen†; Lomotil; Lotharin; Tropergen; *USA*: Logen; Lomotil; Lonox.

Multi-ingredient: *Braz.*: Colestase; Magnostase.

Docusates (17137-e)

Docusate Calcium (6018-m)

Docusate Calcium *(USAN)*.
Dioctyl Calcium Sulfosuccinate; Dioctyl Calcium Sulphosuccinate. Calcium 1,4-bis(2-ethylhexyl) sulphosuccinate.
$C_{40}H_{74}CaO_{14}S_2 = 883.2$.
CAS — 128-49-4.
Pharmacopoeias. In US.

Pharmacopoeial description

USP 25: A white amorphous solid with the characteristic odour of octil alcohol. Soluble 1 in 3300 of water; very soluble in alcohol, in macrogol 400, and in maize oil.

Docusate Potassium (6019-b)

Docusate Potassium (USAN).

Dioctyl Potassium Sulfosuccinate; Dioctyl Potassium Sulphosuccinate. Potassium 1,4-bis(2-ethylhexyl) sulphosuccinate.

$C_{20}H_{37}KO_7S = 460.7$.

CAS — 7491-09-0.

Pharmacopoeias. In US.

Pharmacopoeial description

USP 25: A white amorphous solid with a characteristic odour suggestive of octil alcohol. Sparingly soluble in water; soluble in alcohol and in glycerol; very soluble in petroleum spirit.

Docusate Sodium (6020-x)

Docusate Sodium (BAN, USAN, rINN).

Dioctyl Sodium Sulfosuccinate; Dioctyl Sodium Sulphosuccinate; Docusatum Natricum; DSS; Sodium Dioctyl Sulphosuccinate. Sodium 1,4-bis(2-ethylhexyl) sulphosuccinate.

$C_{20}H_{37}NaO_7S = 444.6$.

CAS — 577-11-7.

ATC — A06AA02.

NOTE. Compounded preparations of docusate sodium may be represented by the following names:

- Co-danthrusate (BAN)—docusate sodium 6 parts and dantron 5 parts.

Pharmacopoeias. In Eur. (see p.vi) and US.

Pharmacopoeial description

Ph. Eur.: White or almost white, hygroscopic, waxy masses or flakes. Sparingly soluble in water; freely soluble in alcohol and in dichloromethane. Store in airtight containers.

USP 25: A white wax-like plastic solid with a characteristic odour suggestive of octil alcohol. Slowly soluble 1 in 70 of water; freely soluble in alcohol and in glycerol; very soluble in petroleum spirit.

Adverse Effects and Precautions

Adverse effects occur rarely with docusates; diarrhoea, nausea, abdominal cramps, and skin rash have been reported. Anorectal pain or bleeding have occasionally occurred following rectal administration.

Like all laxatives, docusates should not be administered when intestinal obstruction or undiagnosed abdominal symptoms are present; prolonged use should be avoided. Docusate sodium should not be administered rectally to patients with haemorrhoids or anal fissures.

Docusate sodium should not be used to soften ear wax when the ear is inflamed or the ear drum perforated.

Pregnancy. Hypomagnesaemia, manifested by jitteriness, in a neonate was considered to be secondary to maternal hypomagnesaemia caused by the use of docusate sodium by the mother during pregnancy.[1]

1. Schindler AM. Isolated neonatal hypomagnesaemia associated with maternal overuse of stool softener. Lancet 1984; ii: 822.

Interactions

Docusates may enhance the gastrointestinal uptake of other drugs, such as liquid paraffin (which should not be given concomitantly). Dosage of anthraquinone laxatives may need to be reduced if given together with docusates. It has also been suggested that concomitant administration of docusates and aspirin increases the incidence of adverse effects on the gastrointestinal mucosa.

Pharmacokinetics

Docusate salts are absorbed from the gastrointestinal tract and excreted in bile. Docusate sodium is also distributed into breast milk.

Uses and Administration

Docusates are administered as the calcium or sodium salt and are used as laxatives in the management of constipation (p.1202). They are also used as adjuncts for bowel evacuation before abdominal radiological procedures. Docusate potassium has also been used.

Docusates are anionic surfactants which have been considered to act primarily by increasing the penetration of fluid into the faeces, but may also have other effects on intestinal fluid secretion, and probably act both as stimulants and as faecal softening agents.

The symbol † denotes a preparation no longer actively marketed

The usual daily dose by mouth of docusate calcium is 240 mg. Docusate sodium is given in usual doses of 50 to 300 mg daily in divided doses by mouth, although doses of up to 500 mg daily may be used. Suggested doses for children have been up to 120 mg daily. The effect is usually seen within 12 to 72 hours. It is also given rectally as an enema in doses of 120 to 200 mg; the effect is usually seen in 5 to 20 minutes. Docusate sodium is also used in combination with anthraquinone stimulant laxatives such as casanthranol (p.1216), dantron (p.1221), and senna (p.1248).

Docusate sodium is used for softening wax in the ear as ear drops containing 0.5 or 5%.

Docusate sodium and other docusate salts are widely used as anionic surfactants in pharmaceutical formulations.

Ear wax removal. Cerumen or ear wax is a normal secretion of the ceruminous glands present in the lining of the external auditory canal. Excessive accumulation or impaction of ear wax may decrease hearing acuity, and may also produce tinnitus and otalgia.

Syringing of the external auditory canal with warm water is the favoured method for removing wax from the ear; a suitable dispersing agent may be given as ear drops for 7 days beforehand.[1] Such agents may also be used alone for self-medication. Traditionally a fixed oil such as olive oil or almond oil has been favoured;[1] other dispersing agents that have been reported as effective include docusates,[2] peroxides such as hydrogen peroxide or urea hydrogen peroxide,[3] choline salicylate,[4] and an oily solution of paradichlorobenzene and chlorobutanol.[4] Glycerol and sodium bicarbonate solution have also been used. However, a comparative study in vitro of the efficacy of various wax dispersing agents found the most effective to be water, which had originally been included as a control.[5]

1. Sharp JF, et al. Ear wax removal: a survey of current practice. BMJ 1990; **301**: 1251–3.
2. Chen DA, Caparosa RJ. A nonprescription cerumenolytic. Am J Otol 1991; **12**: 475–6.
3. Fahmey S, Whitefield M. Multicentre clinical trial of Exterol as a cerumenolytic. Br J Clin Pract 1982; **36**: 197–204.
4. Drummer DS, et al. A single-blind, randomized study to compare the efficacy of two ear drop preparations ('Audax' and 'Cerumol') in the softening of ear wax. Curr Med Res Opin 1992; **13**: 26–30.
5. Andaz C, Whittet HB. An in vitro study to determine efficacy of different wax-dispersing agents. ORL J Otorhinolaryngol Relat Spec 1993; **55**: 97–9.

Preparations

BP 2001: Co-danthrusate Capsules; Compound Docusate Enema; Docusate Capsules; Docusate Oral Solution; Docusate Tablets; Paediatric Docusate Oral Solution;
USP 25: Docusate Calcium Capsules; Docusate Potassium Capsules; Docusate Sodium Capsules; Docusate Sodium Solution; Docusate Sodium Syrup; Docusate Sodium Tablets; Ferrous Fumarate and Docusate Sodium Extended-release Tablets.

Proprietary Preparations (details are given in Part 3)

Austral.: Coloxyl; Waxsol; **Belg.:** Norgalax; **Canad.:** Calax; Colace; Colax-C†; Colax-S†; Correctol Stool Softener; Dioctyl; Doxate-C†; Doxate-S†; Ex-Lax Stool Softener; Laxagel; Regulex; Selax; Silace; Soflax; Surfak; **Fr.:** Jamylene; Norgalax; **Ger.:** Norgalax†; Otitex; Otowaxol; Fruitatives; **Hong Kong:** Hisof; Norgalax; Softon; Waxsol; **Irl.:** Fletchers Enemette; Norgalax; Waxsol; **Israel:** Docusoft; **Mex.:** Correctol; **Neth.:** Norgalax; **NZ:** Coloxyl; Waxsol; **S.Afr.:** Waxsol NF; **Singapore:** Norgalax; Waxsol; **Spain:** Dama-Lax; Tirolaxo†; **Switz.:** Norgalax; **Thai.:** Cusate; Dewax; Pedoc; Waxsol; **UK:** Clear Ear; Dioctyl; Docusol; Fletchers Enemette; Molcer; Norgalax; Waxsol; **USA:** Colace; Correctol Extra Gentle†; D-S-S; DC Softgels; Dialose†; Diocto-K†; Dioeze†; Disonate†; Docusoft; DOK; DOS Softgel; Ex-Lax Stool Softener; Kasoff†; Modane Soft; Pro-Cal-Sof†; Regulax SS; Regutol†; Silace; Soflax Fleet†; Sulfalax Calcium†; Surfak.

Multi-ingredient: Aust.: Purigoa; Yal; **Austral.:** Coloxyl; Coloxyl with Senna; Rectalad; Sennesoft; **Belg.:** Laxavit; Softene; **Braz.:** Dioctosal; Humectol; Ventre Livre; **Canad.:** Calcium Docuphen†; Doss†; Doxidan†; Ex-Lax Light†; Fruitatives; Peri-Colace; Phillips Gelcaps†; Regulex-D†; Senokot-S; **Denm.:** Glyoktyl; Klyx; **Fin.:** Klyx; **Fr.:** Neo-Boldolaxine†; **Ger.:** Norgalax Miniklistier; Potsilo; Yal; **Hong Kong:** Softon Plus; **Israel:** Migraleve; **Ital.:** Macrolax; Sorbiclis; **Mex.:** Clyss-Go; **Norw.:** Klyx; **NZ:** Coloxyl; Coloxyl with Senna; **Port.:** Clyss-Go; **S.Afr.:** Norilax†; **Spain:** Boldolaxin; Laxvital; Migraleve; **Swed.:** Emulax; Klyx; **Switz.:** Elle-care; Klyx Magnum; Tavolax†; Yal; **Thai.:** Bisolax; Hemorhin; **UK:** Capsuvac; Normax; **USA:** Colax†; D-S-S Plus†; Dialose Plus†; Diocto-K Plus†; Dioctolose Plus†; Disanthrol†; Disolan Forte†; Disolan†; Disoplex†; Docucal-P†; Docusoft Plus; Doxidan; DSMC Plus†; Ex-Lax Extra Gentle Pills†; Feen-a-mint Pills†; Femilax†; Genasoft Plus Softgels; Gentlax S†; Laxative & Stool Softener; Modane Plus†; Peri-Colace; Peri-Dos Softgels; Phillips' Laxative Gelcaps†; Phillips' Laxcaps†; Pro-Sof Plus†; Regulace†; Senokot-S; Silace-C; Soflax Overnight†; Therevac Plus; Therevac SB; Unilax†; X-Prep Bowel Evacuant Kit-1.

Used as an adjunct in: **Hong Kong:** Ferosof; **Spain:** Glutaferro; **USA:** Anemagen OB; Ferocyl†; Ferro-Dok; Ferro-Sequels†; Hem Fc; Hemaspan; Natal Extra; Nephron FA; TriHEMIC.

Dolasetron Mesilate (13692-g)

Dolasetron Mesilate (BANM, rINNM).

Dolasetron Mesylate (USAN); MDL-73147EF (dolasetron or dolasetron mesilate). (6R,8r,9aS)-3-Oxoperhydro-2H-2,6-methanoquinolizin-8-yl indole-3-carboxylate methanesulphonate.

$C_{19}H_{20}N_2O_3,CH_4O_3S = 420.5$.

CAS — 115956-12-2 (dolasetron); 115956-13-3 (dolasetron mesilate).

Adverse Effects and Precautions

As for Ondansetron, p.1241. Diarrhoea and abdominal pain may also occur. Various ECG changes have been noted with dolasetron. Dolasetron should be administered with caution to patients who have or may develop prolongation of the QT interval, or other alterations in cardiac conduction intervals. No dosage reduction is considered necessary in renal or hepatic impairment, despite possible reductions in clearance.

Effects on the cardiovascular system. References.

1. Benedict CR, et al. Single-blind study of the effects of intravenous dolasetron mesylate versus ondansetron on electrocardiographic parameters in normal volunteers. J Cardiovasc Pharmacol 1996; **28**: 53–9.

Interactions

Plasma concentrations of hydrodolasetron, the active metabolite of dolasetron, are increased by cimetidine and atenolol and decreased by rifampicin. Dolasetron should be used with caution in patients taking drugs that prolong the QT interval.

Pharmacokinetics

Dolasetron administered by mouth and intravenously is rapidly converted to the active metabolite hydrodolasetron by carbonyl reductase, a ubiquitous enzyme. Peak plasma concentrations of hydrodolasetron occur 1 hour after oral, and 0.6 hours after intravenous, dolasetron administration. The apparent oral bioavailability of dolasetron determined as hydrodolasetron is about 75%. It has a mean elimination half-life of about 7 to 8 hours.

Some hydrodolasetron is metabolised by cytochrome P450 isoenzymes CYP2D6 and CYP3A, while about 50 to 60% is eliminated unchanged in the urine. Two thirds of a dose of dolasetron is recovered in the urine and one third in the faeces.

Clearance of hydrodolasetron is increased in children, but is not altered in the elderly. Clearance is reduced in severe hepatic and severe renal impairment.

◊ References.

1. Lerman J, et al. Pharmacokinetics of the active metabolite (MDL 74,156) of dolasetron mesylate after oral or intravenous administration to anesthetized children. Clin Pharmacol Ther 1996; **60**: 485–92.
2. Dempsey E, et al. Pharmacokinetics of single intravenous and oral doses of dolasetron mesylate in healthy elderly volunteers. J Clin Pharmacol 1996; **36**: 903–10.
3. Stubbs K, et al. Pharmacokinetics of dolasetron after oral and intravenous administration of dolasetron mesylate in healthy volunteers and patients with hepatic dysfunction. J Clin Pharmacol 1997; **37**: 926–36.
4. Dimmitt DC, et al. Pharmacokinetics of oral and intravenous dolasetron mesylate in patients with renal impairment. J Clin Pharmacol 1998; **38**: 798–806.
5. Dimmitt DC, et al. Effect of infusion rate on the pharmacokinetics and tolerance of intravenous dolasetron mesylate. Ann Pharmacother 1998; **32**: 39–44.

Uses and Administration

Dolasetron is a 5-HT$_3$-receptor antagonist with antiemetic actions similar to those of ondansetron (see p.1242). It is used as the mesilate in the prevention of nausea and vomiting (p.1206) associated with chemotherapy, and in the prevention and treatment of postoperative nausea and vomiting.

For prevention of acute nausea and vomiting associated with chemotherapy dolasetron mesilate may be given by mouth in a dose of 100 mg within 1 hour before treatment. Alternatively it may be given in a dose of 1.8 mg per kg body-weight, or 100 mg, by intravenous injection at a rate of up to 100 mg over 30 seconds about 30 minutes before chemotherapy; the same dose may be diluted to 50 mL with a suitable infusion solution and given intravenously over up to 15 minutes. Another regimen has involved treatment with 200 mg of dolasetron mesilate by mouth 1 hour before chemotherapy, followed by a further 200 mg once daily for up to 7 days to prevent delayed nausea and vomiting.

When given for the prophylaxis of postoperative nausea and vomiting a recommended dose is 100 mg of dolasetron mesilate by mouth within 2 hours before surgery, or 12.5 mg intravenously approximately 15 minutes before the end of anaesthesia. The same intravenous dose may be given to treat established postoperative nausea and vomiting.

Children may be given dolasetron mesilate 1.8 mg per kg orally (within 1 hour before chemotherapy) or intravenously (about 30 minutes before chemotherapy), up to a maximum dose of 100 mg, to prevent acute chemotherapy-induced nausea and vomiting. For postoperative nausea and vomiting 1.2 mg per kg by mouth, up to a maximum of 100 mg, may be given within 2 hours before surgery, or 0.35 mg per kg, up to a maximum of 12.5 mg, may be given intravenously 15 minutes before the end of anaesthesia. The same intravenous dose may be given to treat established postoperative nausea and vomiting.

◊ Reviews.
1. Balfour JA, Goa KL. Dolasetron: a review of its pharmacology and therapeutic potential in the management of nausea and vomiting induced by chemotherapy, radiotherapy or surgery. *Drugs* 1997; **54:** 273–98.
2. Dolasetron for prevention of nausea and vomiting due to cancer chemotherapy. *Med Lett Drug Ther* 1998; **40:** 53–4.

Preparations

Proprietary Preparations (details are given in Part 3)
Aust.: Anzemet; *Austral.:* Anzemet; *Canad.:* Anzemet; *Fr.:* Anzemet; *Ger.:* Anemet; *Ital.:* Anzemet; *Mex.:* Anzemet; *S.Afr.:* Zamanon; *USA:* Anzemet.

Domperidone (6544-h)

Domperidone *(BAN, USAN, rINN)*.
Domperidonum; R-33812. 5-Chloro-1-{1-[3-(2-oxobenzimidazolin-1-yl)propyl]-4-piperidyl}benzimidazolin-2-one.
$C_{22}H_{24}ClN_5O_2 = 425.9$.
CAS — 57808-66-9.
ATC — A03FA03.
Pharmacopoeias. In *Eur.* (see p.vi).

Pharmacopoeial description
Ph. Eur.: A white or almost white powder. Practically insoluble in water; slightly soluble in alcohol and in methyl alcohol; soluble in dimethylformamide. Protect from light.

Domperidone Maleate (18227-r)

Domperidone Maleate *(BANM, rINNM)*.
Domperidoni Maleas.
$C_{22}H_{24}ClN_5O_2,C_4H_4O_4 = 542.0$.
CAS — 99497-03-7.
Pharmacopoeias. In *Eur.* (see p.vi).

Domperidone maleate 12.73 mg is approximately equivalent to 10 mg domperidone.

Pharmacopoeial description
Ph. Eur.: A white or almost white powder; it exhibits polymorphism. Very slightly soluble in water and in alcohol; sparingly soluble in dimethylformamide; slightly soluble in methyl alcohol. Protect from light.

Adverse Effects

Plasma-prolactin concentrations may be increased which may lead to galactorrhoea or gynaecomastia. There have been reports of reduced libido, and rashes and other allergic reactions. Domperidone does not readily cross the blood-brain barrier and the incidence of central effects such as extrapyramidal reactions or drowsiness may be lower than with metoclopramide (p.1235); however, there have been reports of dystonic reactions.

Domperidone by injection has been associated with convulsions, arrhythmias, and cardiac arrest. Fatalities have restricted administration by this route.

Effects on the cardiovascular system. Sudden death has occurred in cancer patients given domperidone intravenously in high doses.[1-3] Four cancer patients experienced cardiac arrest following high intravenous doses[4] and 2 of 4 similar patients experienced ventricular arrhythmias.[5] Following such reports the manufacturers withdrew the injection from general use in the UK.
1. Joss RA, *et al.* Sudden death in cancer patient on high-dose domperidone. *Lancet* 1982; **i:** 1019.
2. Giaccone G, *et al.* Two sudden deaths during prophylactic antiemetic treatment with high doses of domperidone and methylprednisolone. *Lancet* 1984; **ii:** 1336–7.
3. Weaving A, *et al.* Seizures after antiemetic treatment with high dose domperidone: report of four cases. *BMJ* 1984; **288:** 1728.
4. Roussak JB, *et al.* Cardiac arrest after treatment with intravenous domperidone. *BMJ* 1984; **289:** 1579.
5. Osborne RJ, *et al.* Cardiotoxicity of intravenous domperidone. *Lancet* 1985; **ii:** 385.

Effects on the endocrine system. Reports of galactorrhoea with gynaecomastia[1] or mastalgia[2,3] generally associated with raised serum-prolactin concentrations. Gynaecomastia without galactorrhoea has also been reported.[4]
1. Van der Steen M, *et al.* Gynaecomastia in a male infant given domperidone. *Lancet* 1982; **ii:** 884–5.
2. Cann PA, *et al.* Galactorrhoea as side effect of domperidone. *BMJ* 1983; **286:** 1395–6.
3. Cann PA, *et al.* Oral domperidone: double blind comparison with placebo in irritable bowel syndrome. *Gut* 1983; **24:** 1135–40.
4. Keating JP, Rees M. Gynaecomastia after long-term administration of domperidone. *Postgrad Med J* 1991; **67:** 401–2.

Extrapyramidal effects. Reports of extrapyramidal symptoms, including acute dystonic reactions, in individual patients given domperidone.
1. Sol P, *et al.* Extrapyramidal reactions due to domperidone. *Lancet* 1980; **ii:** 802.
2. Debontridder O. Extrapyramidal reactions due to domperidone. *Lancet* 1980; **ii:** 802. Correction, *ibid.*; 1259.
3. Casteels-Van Daele M, *et al.* Refusal of further cancer chemotherapy due to antiemetic drug. *Lancet* 1984; **i:** 57.

Precautions

Domperidone is not recommended for chronic administration or for the routine prophylaxis of postoperative nausea and vomiting. Domperidone should be used with great caution if given intravenously, because of the risk of arrhythmias, especially in patients predisposed to cardiac arrhythmias or hypokalaemia.

Interactions

Similarly to other dopamine antagonists (see Metoclopramide, p.1236), there is a theoretical potential that domperidone may antagonise the hypoprolactinaemic effect of drugs such as bromocriptine. In addition, the prokinetic effects of domperidone may alter the absorption of some drugs. Opioid analgesics and antimuscarinics may antagonise the prokinetic effects of domperidone.

Pharmacokinetics

The systemic bioavailability of domperidone is only about 15% in fasting subjects given a dose by mouth, although this is increased when domperidone is given after food. The low bioavailability is thought to be due to first-pass hepatic and intestinal metabolism. The bioavailability of rectal domperidone is similar to that following oral administration, although peak plasma concentrations are only achieved after about an hour, compared with 30 minutes after a dose by mouth.

Domperidone is more than 90% bound to plasma protein, and has a terminal elimination half-life of about 7.5 hours. It is chiefly cleared from the blood by extensive metabolism. About 30% of an oral dose is excreted in urine within 24 hours, almost entirely as metabolites; the remainder of a dose is excreted in faeces over several days, about 10% as unchanged drug. It does not readily cross the blood-brain barrier.

Small amounts of domperidone are distributed into breast milk, reaching concentrations about one-quarter of those in maternal serum.

Uses and Administration

Domperidone is a dopamine antagonist with actions and uses similar to those of metoclopramide (p.1236). It is used as an antiemetic for the short-term treatment of nausea and vomiting of various aetiologies (p.1206), including that associated with cancer therapy, and nausea and vomiting associated with levodopa or bromocriptine therapy for parkinsonism (see below). It is not considered suitable for chronic nausea and vomiting, nor for the routine prophylaxis of postoperative vomiting.

Domperidone is also used for its prokinetic actions in dyspepsia (p.1204) and has been tried in diabetic gastroparesis (see Diabetic Complications, p.317). It is given with paracetamol in the symptomatic treatment of migraine (p.449).

Domperidone is used as the maleate in tablet preparations and as the base in suppositories and the oral suspension; doses are expressed in terms of the base.

For the acute treatment of nausea and vomiting it is administered in doses of 10 to 20 mg by mouth or 30 to 60 mg rectally every 4 to 8 hours. In the treatment of nausea and vomiting in parkinsonian patients, therapy may be continued for a maximum of 12 weeks. In children doses of 200 to 400 µg per kg body-weight may be given by mouth every 4 to 8 hours. The maximum daily dose rectally in children is 120 mg for those weighing 35.5 to 45 kg; 90 mg, 25.5 to 35 kg; 60 mg, 15.5 to 25 kg; and 30 mg, 10 to 15 kg. Use in children is restricted in the UK to nausea and vomiting following cytotoxics or radiotherapy.

For the symptomatic treatment of non-ulcer dyspepsia, adults may receive up to 10 to 20 mg by mouth 3 times daily before meals and at night, depending on clinical response. A course of treatment should not exceed 12 weeks. In migraine a dose of 20 mg by mouth may be taken up to every 4 hours, in combination with paracetamol, as required, up to a maximum of 4 doses in 24 hours.

Domperidone has been administered parenterally, but such administration has been associated with severe adverse effects (see above).

◊ Reviews.
1. Prakash A, Wagstaff AJ. Domperidone: a review of its use in diabetic gastropathy. *Drugs* 1998; **56:** 429–45.
2. Barone JA. Domperidone: a peripherally acting dopamine₂-receptor antagonist. *Ann Pharmacother* 1999; **33:** 429–40.

Parkinsonism. Domperidone is used to control gastrointestinal effects of dopaminergic drugs given in the management of parkinsonism (p.1160). It may be of use in those patients who experience peripheral effects with levodopa despite the use of peripheral dopa-decarboxylase inhibitors and for patients using dopamine agonists such as bromocriptine or apomorphine since peripheral dopa-decarboxylase inhibitors are ineffective for preventing the peripheral effects of these drugs. Although domperidone does not readily cross the blood-brain barrier there have been isolated reports of extrapyramidal effects associated with its use (see above). Consequently there has been concern over its potential to produce central effects and some consider that domperidone should only be used in patients with parkinsonism when safer antiemetic measures have failed.[1,2] However this view has been contested both by the manufacturers and other workers.[3,4] In a subsequent review of the use of domperidone in Parkinson's disease Parkes[5] considered that domperidone might produce central blockade of the therapeutic effects of levodopa if given at a high oral dosage such as 120 mg daily for prolonged periods but also noted that such high doses were rarely required to control levodopa-induced vomiting. In the UK, domperidone is limited to a maximum of 12 weeks' treatment in nausea and vomiting induced by antiparkinsonian treatment.
1. Leeser J, Bateman DN. Domperidone. *BMJ* 1985; **290:** 241.
2. Bateman DN. Domperidone. *BMJ* 1985; **290:** 1079.
3. Lake-Bakaar G, Cameron HA. Domperidone. *BMJ* 1985; **290:** 241–2.
4. Critchley P, *et al.* Domperidone. *BMJ* 1985; **290:** 788.
5. Parkes JD. Domperidone and Parkinson's disease. *Clin Neuropharmacol* 1986; **9:** 517–32.

Preparations

BP 2001: Domperidone Tablets.

Proprietary Preparations (details are given in Part 3)
Aust.: Motilium; *Austral.:* Motilium; *Belg.:* Motilium; *Braz.:* Motilium; Peridal; Pleiadon; *Canad.:* Motilidone; Motilium; *Denm.:* Motilium; *Fr.:* Motilium; Peridys; *Ger.:* Motilium; Motilium; *Irl.:* Motilium; *Israel:* Motilium; *Ital.:* Digestivo Giuliani; Fobidon; Gastronorm; Mod†; Motilium; Peridon; *Mex.:* Emiken; Motilium; Seronex; *Neth.:* Gastrocure; Motilium; *NZ:* Motilium; *Port.:* Cinet; Mogasinte; Motilium; Nordonil†; Remotil; *S.Afr.:* Motilium; *Singapore:* Dompenyl; Mirax; Motilium; *Spain:* Motilium; Nauzelin; *Switz.:* Motilium; *Thai.:* Costi; Dany; Dolium; Domerdon; Domidone; Domilium; Domperdone; Donum; Mirax; Mocydone; Modomed; Molax; Moticon; Motidom; Motilium; Ninlium; Peptomet; Poselium; *UK:* Motilium.

Multi-ingredient: *Belg.:* Touristil; *UK:* Domperamol.

Dronabinol (3780-y)

Dronabinol *(USAN, rINN)*.
NSC-134454; Δ⁹-Tetrahydrocannabinol; Δ⁹-THC. (6aR,10aR)-6a,7,8,10a-Tetrahydro-6,6,9-trimethyl-3-pentyl-6H-dibenzo[b,d]pyran-1-ol.
$C_{21}H_{30}O_2 = 314.5$.
CAS — 1972-08-3.
Pharmacopoeias. In *US*.

Pharmacopoeial description
USP 25: Store at a temperature between 8° and 15° in airtight glass containers in an inert atmosphere. Protect from light.

Adverse Effects and Precautions

As for Nabilone, p.1237. The most frequent adverse effects of dronabinol include abdominal pain, nausea and vomiting, dizziness, euphoria, paranoid reactions, and somnolence.

◊ The abuse liability of dronabinol was rated as being substantially lower than that of cannabis.[1]
1. WHO. WHO expert committee on drug dependence: twenty-seventh report. *WHO Tech Rep Ser* 808 1991.

Pharmacokinetics

Following oral administration dronabinol is slowly and erratically absorbed from the gastrointestinal tract; the bioavailability of an oral dose is about 10 to 20%, due to extensive first-pass metabolism. Peak plasma concentrations of dronabinol and its 11-hydroxy metabolite are achieved about 2 to 3 hours after a dose by mouth. It is widely distributed and is extensively protein bound, with a volume of distribution of approximately 10 litres per kg.

Dronabinol is extensively metabolised; the primary metabolite, 11-hydroxydronabinol is also active, and has an elimination half-life of 15 to 18 hours. The 11-hydroxy metabolite is converted to other, more polar and acidic compounds which are excreted in faeces via the bile, and in the urine. About 50% of an oral dose is recovered in faeces within 72 hours and 10 to 15% in urine. Many of the metabolites have relatively prolonged half-lives of 25 to 36 hours, and accumulation may occur with repeated administration.

Dronabinol is found in breast milk, and should be avoided, where possible, in nursing mothers.

Uses and Administration
Dronabinol, the major psychoactive constituent of cannabis (p.1590), has antiemetic properties and is used for the control of nausea and vomiting associated with cancer chemotherapy (p.1206) in patients who have failed to respond adequately to conventional antiemetics.

The usual initial dose of dronabinol by mouth is 5 mg per m^2 body-surface given 1 to 3 hours before the first dose of the antineoplastic drug with subsequent doses being given every 2 to 4 hours after chemotherapy to a maximum of 4 to 6 doses daily. If necessary, the dose may be increased by increments of 2.5 mg per m^2 to a maximum dose of 15 mg per m^2 if adverse effects permit.

Dronabinol also has appetite-stimulant effects and is used in the treatment of anorexia associated with weight loss in patients with AIDS. For this purpose 2.5 mg may be taken twice daily by mouth, before lunch and supper, reduced to a single 2.5-mg dose in the evening in patients who tolerate the drug poorly. If necessary, and if adverse effects permit, doses may also be increased up to 20 mg daily in divided doses.

◊ General references.
1. Voth EA, Schwartz RH. Medicinal applications of delta-9-tetrahydrocannabinol and marijuana. *Ann Intern Med* 1997; **126**: 791–8.
2. Williamson EM, Evans FJ. Cannabinoids in clinical practice. *Drugs* 2000; **60**: 1303–14.

HIV-associated wasting and diarrhoea. Dronabinol is used for the management of anorexia in patients with HIV-associated wasting and diarrhoea (p.610). However, although dronabinol may stimulate appetite and prevent weight loss,[1] it does not appear to produce significant weight gain, and may produce less benefit than megestrol acetate.[2]
1. Beal JE, *et al.* Dronabinol as a treatment for anorexia associated with weight loss in patients with AIDS. *J Pain Symptom Manage* 1995; **10**: 89–97.
2. Timpone JG, *et al.* The safety and pharmacokinetics of single-agent and combination therapy with megestrol acetate and dronabinol for the treatment of HIV wasting syndrome. *AIDS Res Hum Retroviruses* 1997; **13**: 305–15.

Preparations
USP 25: Dronabinol Capsules.

Proprietary Preparations (details are given in Part 3)
Canad.: Marinol; **Israel:** Ronabin; **S.Afr.:** Elevat†; **USA:** Marinol.

Ebrotidine   (3677-j)
Ebrotidine *(rINN)*.
p-Bromo-*N*-[({2-[({2-[(diaminomethylene)amino]-4-thiazolyl}methyl)thio]ethyl}amino)methylene]benzenesulfonamide.
$C_{14}H_{17}BrN_6O_2S_3 = 477.4$.
CAS — 100981-43-9.

Profile
Ebrotidine is a histamine H$_2$-antagonist with general properties similar to those of cimetidine (p.1216), but which also has cytoprotective actions. It has been used in peptic ulcer disease. Serious liver damage has been reported.

◊ References.
1. Patel SS, Wilde MI. Ebrotidine. *Drugs* 1996; **51**: 974–80.
2. Various. Ebrotidine: a new generation H$_2$-receptor antagonist and gastroprotective agent. *Arzneimittelforschung* 1997; **47**: 427–590.
3. Andrade RJ, *et al.* Acute liver injury associated with the use of ebrotidine, a new H$_2$-receptor antagonist. *J Hepatol* 1999; **31**: 641–6.

Preparations
Proprietary Preparations (details are given in Part 3)
Spain: Ebrocit†.

Ecabet Sodium   (15272-h)
Ecabet Sodium *(rINNM)*.
12-Sulphodehydroabietic Acid, Monosodium Salt; TA-2711. 13-Isopropyl-12-sulphopodocarpa-8,11,13-trien-15-oic acid pentahydrate, sodium salt.
$C_{20}H_{27}NaO_5S,5H_2O = 492.6$.
CAS — 33159-27-2 (ecabet); 86408-72-2 (ecabet sodium).

Profile
Ecabet sodium is a cytoprotective drug used in the treatment of peptic ulcer disease (p.1208). The suggested dose is 1 g of ecabet sodium by mouth twice daily.

◊ References.
1. Shibata K, *et al.* Bactericidal activity of a new antiulcer agent, ecabet sodium, against Helicobacter pylori under acidic conditions. *Antimicrob Agents Chemother* 1995; **39**: 1295–9.
2. Ohkusa T, *et al.* Prospective evaluation of a new anti-ulcer agent, ecabet sodium, for the treatment of Helicobacter pylori infection. *Aliment Pharmacol Ther* 1998; **12**: 457–61.

Preparations
Proprietary Preparations (details are given in Part 3)
Jpn: Gastrom.

Enoxolone Aluminium   (14505-a)
Enoxolone Aluminium *(BANM, rINNM)*.
Aluminium Glycyrrhetate; Aluminium Glycyrrhetinate; Enoxolone Aluminum. 3β-Hydroxy-11-oxo-olean-12-en-30-oic acid, aluminium salt.
$(C_{30}H_{46}O_4)_3 \cdot Al = 1439.0$.
CAS — 4598-66-7.

Profile
Enoxolone aluminium is an analogue of carbenoxolone (p.1215) that has been used in preparations for the treatment of peptic ulcer disease and other gastrointestinal disorders.

Preparations
Proprietary Preparations (details are given in Part 3)
Multi-ingredient: **Spain:** Gastroalgine; Terpalate†.

Esomeprazole Magnesium   (20570-e)
Esomeprazole Magnesium *(BANM, USAN, rINNM)*.
H199/18 (esomeprazole); Perprazole (esomeprazole). 5-Methoxy-2-{(S)-[(4-methoxy-3,5-dimethyl-2-pyridyl)methyl]sulfinyl}benzimidazole magnesium (2:1) trihydrate.
$C_{34}H_{36}MgN_6O_6S_2,3H_2O = 767.2$.
CAS — 217087-09-7 (esomeprazole magnesium); 119141-88-7 (esomeprazole).

Adverse Effects and Precautions
As for Omeprazole, p.1239.

Interactions
As for Omeprazole, p.1240.

◊ References.
1. Andersson T, *et al.* Drug interaction studies with esomeprazole, the (S)-isomer of omeprazole. *Clin Pharmacokinet* 2001; **40**: 523–37.

Pharmacokinetics
Esomeprazole is rapidly absorbed following oral administration, with peak plasma levels occurring after approximately 1 to 2 hours. It is acid labile and an enteric-coated formulation has been developed. Bioavailability of esomeprazole increases with both dose and repeated administration to about 68 and 89% for doses of 20 and 40 mg respectively. Food delays and decreases the absorption of esomeprazole, but this does not significantly change its effect on intragastric acidity. Esomeprazole is about 97% bound to plasma proteins. It is extensively metabolised in the liver by the cytochrome P450 isoenzyme CYP2C19 to hydroxy and desmethyl metabolites, which have no effect on gastric acid secretion. The remainder is metabolised by the cytochrome P450 isoenzyme CYP3A4 to esomeprazole sulfone. With repeated administration, there is a decrease in first-pass metabolism and systemic clearance, probably caused by an inhibition of the CYP2C19 isoenzyme. However, there is no accumulation during once daily administration. The plasma elimination half-life is about 1.3 hours. Almost 80% of an oral dose is eliminated as metabolites in the urine, the remainder in the faeces.

◊ References.
1. Andersson T, *et al.* Pharmacokinetic studies with esomeprazole, the (S)-isomer of omeprazole. *Clin Pharmacokinet* 2001; **40**: 411–26.

Uses and Administration
Esomeprazole is the *S*-isomer of the proton pump inhibitor omeprazole (p.1239). It is given as the magnesium salt for the treatment of peptic ulcer disease (p.1208) and gastro-oesophageal reflux disease (p.1204) but doses are calculated in terms of esomeprazole. Usual doses for peptic ulcer disease, as a component of a triple therapy regimen with amoxicillin and clarithromycin, are the equivalent of 20 mg esomeprazole by mouth twice daily for 7 days, or 40 mg once daily for 10 days. In the UK the dose for treatment of severe (erosive) gastro-oesophageal reflux disease is 40 mg once daily for 4 weeks, extended for a further 4 weeks if necessary; in the USA, where doses of 20 to 40 mg are permitted for initial treatment, a further 4 to 8 weeks of treatment may be considered for patients who do not heal after 4 to 8 weeks. For maintenance, or for symptomatic disease without erosive oesophagitis, doses equivalent to 20 mg of esomeprazole daily may be used in both countries. For patients with severe hepatic impairment the maximum dose is 20 mg.

◊ General references.
1. Spencer CM, Faulds D. Esomeprazole. *Drugs* 2000; **60**: 321–9.
2. Maton PN, *et al.* Safety and efficacy of long term esomeprazole therapy in patients with healed erosive oesophagitis. *Drug Safety* 2001; **24**: 625–35.

Preparations
Proprietary Preparations (details are given in Part 3)
Austral.: Nexium; **Irl.:** Nexium; **Swed.:** Nexium; **UK:** Nexium; **USA:** Nexium.

Euonymus   (7511-n)
Fusain Noir Pourpré; Spindle Tree Bark; Wahoo Bark.

The dried root-bark of *Euonymus atropurpureus* (=*Evonymus atropurpurea*) (Celastraceae).

Profile
Euonymus is reported to have laxative, choleretic, and diuretic activity.

Preparations
Proprietary Preparations (details are given in Part 3)
Multi-ingredient: **Fr.:** Jecopeptol; **Port.:** Solucao Stago; **UK:** GB Tablets; Indigestion Mixture.

Famotidine   (16598-s)
Famotidine *(BAN, USAN, rINN)*.
Famotidinum; L-643341; MK-208; YM-11170. 3-[2-[(Diaminomethyleneamino)thiazol-4-ylmethylthio]-*N*-sulphamoylpropionamidine.
$C_8H_{15}N_7O_2S_3 = 337.4$.
CAS — 76824-35-6.
ATC — A02BA03.

Pharmacopoeias. In *Eur.* (see p.vi), *Jpn, Pol.,* and *US.*

Pharmacopoeial description
Ph. Eur.: A white or yellowish-white, crystalline powder or crystals. Very slightly soluble in water and in dehydrated alcohol; freely soluble in dimethylformamide and in glacial acetic acid; practically insoluble in ether and in ethyl acetate; slightly soluble in methyl alcohol. It dissolves in dilute mineral acids. Protect from light.
USP 25: A white to pale yellowish-white crystalline powder. Very slightly soluble in water; practically insoluble in alcohol, in acetone, in chloroform, in ether, and in ethyl acetate; freely soluble in dimethylformamide and in glacial acetic acid; slightly soluble in methyl alcohol. Protect from light.

Adverse Effects
As for Cimetidine, p.1216. However, unlike cimetidine, famotidine is reported to have little or no anti-androgenic effect, although there are isolated reports of gynaecomastia and impotence.

◊ General references.
1. Howden CW, Tytgat GNJ. The tolerability and safety profile of famotidine. *Clin Ther* 1996; **18**: 36–54.

Effects on the blood. For reports of blood dyscrasias, some serious, occurring with famotidine, see under Cimetidine p.1217.

The symbol † denotes a preparation no longer actively marketed

Effects on the cardiovascular system. Famotidine 40 mg daily by mouth reduced cardiac output and stroke volume, measured by noninvasive techniques, compared with placebo, cimetidine, or ranitidine in healthy subjects.[1] Similar effects observed in another study[2] were delayed by pretreatment with ranitidine. However, other workers have found that oral famotidine had no effect on exercise capacity or left ventricular systolic function in healthy subjects,[3] and that famotidine 20 mg intravenously had no effect on any of the haemodynamic parameters measured in 11 critically ill patients.[4] As with other H₂-antagonists (p.1217), bradycardia and atrioventricular block have been reported with famotidine.[5]

1. Hinrichsen H, et al. Hemodynamic effects of different H₂-receptor antagonists. Clin Pharmacol Ther 1990; 48: 302–8.
2. Mescheder A, et al. Changes in the effects of nizatidine and famotidine on cardiac performance after pretreatment with ranitidine. Eur J Clin Pharmacol 1993; 45: 151–6.
3. Hillermann DE, et al. Impact of chronic oral H₂-antagonist therapy of left ventricular systolic function and exercise capacity. J Clin Pharmacol 1992; 32: 1033–7.
4. Heiselman DE, et al. Hemodynamic status during famotidine infusion. DICP Ann Pharmacother 1990; 24: 1163–5.
5. Schoenwald PK, et al. Complete atrioventricular block and cardiac arrest following intravenous famotidine administration. Anesthesiology 1999; 90: 623–6.

Effects on the endocrine system. Hyperprolactinaemia and breast engorgement occurred in a woman during the fourth month of treatment with famotidine 80 mg daily;[1] she had by mistake been given twice the usual maximum dose. Recovery occurred when famotidine was withdrawn. Transient hyperprolactinaemia and galactorrhoea have also been reported in a woman after standard doses (40 mg daily) of famotidine.[2] There have been a few instances of impotence.[3]

1. Delpre G, et al. Hyperprolactinaemia during famotidine therapy. Lancet 1993; 342: 868.
2. Güven K. Hyperprolactinemia and galactorrhea with standard-dose famotidine therapy. Ann Pharmacother 1995; 29: 788.
3. Kassianos GC. Impotence and nizatidine. Lancet 1989; i: 963.

Effects on the liver. Mixed hepatocellular jaundice[1] and acute hepatitis[2] have been associated with famotidine administration; in the latter case the patient subsequently experienced a recurrence when given cimetidine.

1. Ament PW, et al. Famotidine-induced mixed hepatocellular jaundice. Ann Pharmacother 1994; 28: 40–2.
2. Hashimoto F, et al. Hepatitis following treatments with famotidine and then cimetidine. Ann Pharmacother 1994; 28: 37–9.

Effects on the nervous system. Similarly to other H₂-antagonists (p.1217), CNS reactions have occurred with famotidine, particularly in the elderly and those with renal failure.[1-3] In 1 report,[1] convulsions and mental deterioration in 2 elderly patients with renal failure were associated with grossly elevated plasma and cerebrospinal fluid concentrations of the drug; symptoms resolved within 3 days of withdrawing famotidine.

1. Yoshimoto K, et al. Famotidine-associated central nervous system reactions and plasma and cerebrospinal drug concentrations in neurosurgical patients with renal failure. Clin Pharmacol Ther 1994; 55: 693–700.
2. Catalano G, et al. Famotidine-associated delirium: a series of six cases. Psychosomatics 1996; 37: 349–55.
3. Odeh M, Oliven A. Central nervous system reactions associated with famotidine: report of five cases. J Clin Gastroenterol 1998; 27: 253–4.

Effects on the skin. Toxic epidermal necrolysis or erythema multiforme have been reported following administration of famotidine;[1,2] the second patient had a recurrence after use of cimetidine.

1. Brunner M, et al. Toxic epidermal necrolysis (Lyell syndrome) following famotidine administration. Br J Dermatol 1995; 133: 814–15.
2. Horiuchi Y, Ikezawa K. Famotidine-induced erythema multiforme: cross-sensitivity with cimetidine. Ann Intern Med 1999; 131: 795.

Fever. Famotidine 20 mg intravenously every 12 hours was associated with hyperpyrexia in a patient with facial and cranial trauma.[1] Rectal temperature in the 24 hours after starting famotidine was 40.5° and remained elevated for the 5 days of famotidine treatment, despite administration of antipyretics. Withdrawal of famotidine resulted in a return to normal temperature within 24 hours.

1. Norwood J, et al. Famotidine and hyperpyrexia. Ann Intern Med 1990; 112: 632.

Precautions

As for Cimetidine, p.1218.

Hepatic impairment. For a report of increased resistance to H₂-antagonists in patients with liver cirrhosis, see Ranitidine, p.1246.

Renal impairment. In patients with renal impairment, famotidine clearance is reduced and the elimination half-life increased, resulting in increased serum-drug concentrations and in some cases clinical sequelae (see Effects on the Nervous System, above). The half-life of famotidine in healthy subjects is about 3 hours, but in patients with a creatinine clearance less than 38 mL per minute[1] or those with end-stage renal disease[2] it has been reported to be 19.3 hours and 27.2 hours respectively. A 50% reduction in the dose of famotidine in patients with renal impairment has therefore been recommended. However, it may not be sufficient to adjust the dose only on the basis of

creatinine clearance since famotidine is partly eliminated by tubular secretion which may also be diminished.[1]

Haemodialysis does not effectively remove famotidine from the systemic circulation. The proportion removed depends on the type of membrane used; with a high flux polysulfone membrane about 16% is reported to be removed, but only 6% with a cuprophan membrane.[2] Continuous ambulatory peritoneal dialysis is reported to remove about 5% of a dose.[2] Continuous haemofiltration may remove about 16% of a dose;[2] intermittent haemofiltration is reported to remove about 4%[3] or 8%.[2] Dosage supplements of famotidine are not required during or after dialysis or filtration procedures.

1. Inotsume N, et al. Pharmacokinetics of famotidine in elderly patients with and without renal insufficiency and in healthy young volunteers. Eur J Clin Pharmacol 1989; 36: 517–20.
2. Gladziwa U, et al. Pharmacokinetics and dynamics of famotidine in patients with renal failure. Br J Clin Pharmacol 1988; 26: 315–21.
3. Saima S, et al. Hemofiltrability of H₂-receptor antagonist, famotidine, in renal failure patients. J Clin Pharmacol 1990; 30: 159–62.

Interactions

Unlike cimetidine (see p.1218) famotidine does not inhibit cytochrome P450, and therefore is considered to have little effect on the metabolism of other drugs. However, like other H₂-antagonists its effects on gastric pH may affect the absorption of some other drugs.

Antacids. Concurrent administration of famotidine 40 mg and a 10 mL dose of antacid containing 800 mg aluminium hydroxide with 800 mg magnesium hydroxide,[1] resulted in a decrease in the bioavailability of famotidine which was considered clinically insignificant. Concurrent administration of famotidine 40 mg and a 30 mL dose of the same antacid resulted in a greater reduction in the absorption of famotidine from the gastrointestinal tract, but the interaction could be minimised by separating ingestion by 2 hours.[2]

1. Lin JH, et al. Effects of antacids and food on absorption of famotidine. Br J Clin Pharmacol 1987; 24: 551–3.
2. Barzaghi N, et al. Impaired bioavailability of famotidine given concurrently with a potent antacid. J Clin Pharmacol 1989; 29: 670–2.

Probenecid. Probenecid in a total dose of 1500 mg had a significant effect on the pharmacokinetics of famotidine 20 mg in 8 healthy subjects.[1] The maximum serum concentration of famotidine and the area under the concentration/time curve were significantly increased and renal clearance significantly reduced. These effects were explained by inhibition of the renal tubular secretion of famotidine by probenecid.

1. Inotsume N, et al. The inhibitory effect of probenecid on renal excretion of famotidine in young, healthy volunteers. J Clin Pharmacol 1990; 30: 50–6.

Theophylline. Although famotidine is considered not to interfere with the metabolism of other drugs there is a report of a clinically significant interaction with theophylline—see p.781.

Pharmacokinetics

Famotidine is readily but incompletely absorbed from the gastrointestinal tract with peak concentrations in plasma occurring 1 to 3 hours after administration by mouth. The bioavailability of famotidine following oral administration is about 40 to 45% and is not significantly affected by the presence of food.

The elimination half-life from plasma is reported to be about 3 hours and is prolonged in renal impairment. Famotidine is weakly bound, about 15 to 20%, to plasma proteins. A small proportion of famotidine is metabolised in the liver to famotidine S-oxide. Approximately 25 to 30% of an oral dose, and 65 to 70% of an intravenous dose, is excreted unchanged in the urine in 24 hours, primarily by active tubular secretion. Famotidine is also found in breast milk.

◊ Reviews.
1. Echizen H, Ishizaki T. Clinical pharmacokinetics of famotidine. Clin Pharmacokinet 1991; 21: 178–94.

Children. Famotidine 300 μg per kg body-weight intravenously was given to 10 children aged 2 to 7 years, after cardiac surgery and before extubation, to prevent aspiration.[1] This dose (equivalent to about 20 mg in adults) induced a rise in the intragastric pH within 1 hour of administration and the pH remained above 3.5 for about 9 hours. The mean elimination half-life was 3.3 hours, similar to the value in healthy adults and it was considered that doses in children need therefore only be adjusted according to body-weight and renal function. This conclusion was supported by a review of 8 studies in children over 1 year of age.[2] Conversely, in infants aged 5 to 19 days, the mean elimination half-life was prolonged (10.5 hours) secondary to reduced renal clearance.[3]

1. Kraus G, et al. Famotidine: pharmacokinetic properties and suppression of acid secretion in paediatric patients following cardiac surgery. Clin Pharmacokinet 1990; 18: 77–81.

2. James LP, Kearns GL. Pharmacokinetics and pharmacodynamics of famotidine in paediatric patients. Clin Pharmacokinet 1996; 31: 103–10.
3. James LP, et al. Pharmacokinetics and pharmacodynamics of famotidine in infants. J Clin Pharmacol 1998; 38: 1089–95. Correction. ibid. 2000; 40: 1298.

Distribution into breast milk. The peak concentration of famotidine in breast milk which occurred in 8 lactating women 6 hours after an oral dose of 40 mg was similar to the peak plasma concentration which occurred 2 hours after the dose.[1]

1. Courtney TP, et al. Excretion of famotidine in breast milk. Br J Clin Pharmacol 1988; 26: 639P.

Enterohepatic recirculation. Some individuals exhibit a second peak in the plasma concentration of famotidine which could be due to enterohepatic recirculation. However, a maximum of 0.43% of a dose of famotidine was excreted in the bile of 2 patients following single doses of 20 mg intravenously or 40 mg by mouth indicating that significant recirculation had not occurred.[1]

1. Klotz U, Walker S. Biliary excretion of H₂-receptor antagonists. Eur J Clin Pharmacol 1990; 39: 91–2.

Uses and Administration

Famotidine is a histamine H₂-antagonist with actions and uses similar to those of cimetidine (see p.1218).

Famotidine may be given by mouth or parenterally by the intravenous route.

In the management of benign **gastric** and **duodenal ulceration** (p.1208) the dose is 40 mg daily by mouth at bedtime, for 4 to 8 weeks. A dose of 20 mg twice daily has also been given. A maintenance dose of 20 mg at bedtime may be given to prevent recurrence of duodenal ulceration. In **gastro-oesophageal reflux disease** (p.1204) the recommended dose is 20 mg by mouth twice daily for 6 to 12 weeks, or up to 40 mg twice daily if there is oesophageal ulceration. A maintenance dose of 20 mg twice daily may be given to prevent recurrence. For the short-term symptomatic relief of heartburn or non-ulcer **dyspepsia** (p.1204) a dose of 10 mg up to twice daily is suggested. In the **Zollinger-Ellison syndrome** (p.1209) the initial dose by mouth is 20 mg every 6 hours, increased as necessary; doses up to 800 mg daily have been employed.

The usual dose of famotidine by the intravenous route is 20 mg and may be given by injection over at least 2 minutes or as an infusion over 15 to 30 minutes; the dose may be repeated every 12 hours.

The dosage of famotidine should be reduced in patients with impaired renal function. In the UK, a 50% reduction is suggested for patients whose creatinine clearance is less than 10 mL per minute; in the USA this reduction is recommended in all those with creatinine clearance less than 50 mL per minute. Alternatively, the dosage interval may be prolonged to 36 to 48 hours.

◊ Reviews.
1. Berardi RR, et al. Comparison of famotidine with cimetidine and ranitidine. Clin Pharm 1988; 7: 271–84.
2. Langtry HD, et al. Famotidine: an updated review of its pharmacodynamic and pharmacokinetic properties, and therapeutic use in peptic ulcer disease and other allied diseases. Drugs 1989; 38: 551–90.

Administration. Although famotidine is most usually given as a film-coated tablet an alternative wafer formulation, designed to dissolve on the tongue without the need for water, has also been developed.[1]

Parenteral formulations of famotidine are also available in some countries. Although the manufacturers recommend that intravenous injections be given over at least 2 minutes, a study which compared rapid intravenous injection (over up to 1 minute) with slow intravenous infusion found both to be safe.[2] Continuous infusion has however been reported by others[3] to be more effective in the prevention of stress ulceration than bolus injection.

1. Schwartz JI, et al. Novel oral medication delivery system for famotidine. J Clin Pharmacol 1995; 35: 362–7.
2. Fish DN. Safety and cost of rapid iv injection of famotidine in critically ill patients. Am J Health-Syst Pharm 1995; 52: 1889–94.
3. Baghaie AA, et al. Comparison of the effect of intermittent administration and continuous infusion of famotidine on gastric pH in critically ill patients: results of a prospective, randomized, crossover study. Crit Care Med 1995; 23: 687–91.

Schizophrenia. There are reports of improvement in schizophrenic symptoms (p.651) in patients given famotidine.[1-4]

1. Kaminsky R, et al. Effect of famotidine on deficit symptoms of schizophrenia. Lancet 1990; 335: 1351–2.
2. Rosse RB, et al. Famotidine adjunctive pharmacotherapy of schizophrenia: a case report. Clin Neuropharmacol 1995; 18: 369–74.

3. Rosse RB, *et al.* An open-label study of the therapeutic efficacy of high-dose famotidine adjuvant pharmacotherapy in schizophrenia: preliminary evidence for treatment efficacy. *Clin Neuropharmacol* 1996; **19:** 341–8.
4. Martinez MC. Famotidine in the management of schizophrenia. *Ann Pharmacother* 1999; **33:** 742–7.

Preparations

BP 2001: Famotidine Tablets;
USP 25: Famotidine Tablets.

Proprietary Preparations (details are given in Part 3)
Aust.: Pepcidine; Ulcusan; *Austral.:* Amfamox; Pepcid; Pepcidine; *Belg.:* Pepcidine; *Braz.:* Famodine; Famoset; Famox; *Canad.:* Acid Control; Acid Halt; Maalox H_2 Acid Controller; Pepcid; Peptic Guard; Ulcidine; *Denm.:* Pepcidin; *Fin.:* Pepcid; Pepcidin; *Fr.:* Pepcidac; Pepdine; *Ger.:* Ganor; Pepcid; Pepdul; *Hong Kong:* Actidine; Famodine; Famopsin; Famox; Gastrodomina; Pepcid; Pepcidine; Pepzan; Quamatel; Servipep; Ulceran; *Irl.:* Pepcid; *Israel:* Apogastine; Famo; Gastro; Rogasti; *Ital.:* Famodil; Gastridin; Motiax; *Jpn:* Gaster; *Mex.:* Amofat; Durater; Famoxal; Farmotex; Fawodin; Pepcidine; Sertidine; Sigafam; Ultidin; *Neth.:* Pepcid; Pepcidin; *Norw.:* Famotal; Pepcid; Pepcidin; *NZ:* Famox; Pepcid; Pepcidine; Pepzan; *Port.:* Dinul†; Dipsin; Fatidin; Gastopride†; Gastrifam; Mensoma; Nulceran; Pepcidina; *S.Afr.:* Pepcid; *Singapore:* Famoc; Famocid; Famopsin; Famotin; Famox; Motidine; Pepcidine; Pepzan; Servipep; Ulceran; *Spain:* Brolin; Confobos; Cronol; Digervin; Dispromil; Eviantrina; Fagastril; Famulcer; Fanosin; Fanox; Gastrion; Gastrodomina; Gastropen; Ingastri; Invigan; Muclox†; Nos; Nulcerin; Pepcid; Rubacina; Tairal; Tameran; Tamin; Tipodex; Ulcetrax; Ulgarine; Vagostal; *Swed.:* Pepcid; Pepcidin; *Switz.:* Pepcid; Pepcidine; *Thai.:* Fadine; Famoc; Famocid; Famonox; Famopsin; Famotin; Fasidine; Motidine; Pepcidine; Pepcine; Pepfamin; Peptoci; Pepzan; Servipep; Ulceran; Ulcofam; Ulfamet; *UAE:* Famotec; *UK:* Pepcid; Ultra Heartburn Relief; *USA:* Mylanta AR Acid Reducer; Pepcid.

Multi-ingredient: *Fr.:* Pepcidduo; *UK:* Pepcidtwo; *USA:* Pepcid Complete.

Fedotozine (13790-p)

Fedotozine (*rINN*).

(+)-(R)-α-Ethyl-N,N-dimethyl-α-{[(3,4,5-trimethoxybenzyl)oxy]methyl}benzylamine.
$C_{22}H_{31}NO_4 = 373.5$.
CAS — 123618-00-8.

Profile

Fedotozine is a peripherally acting selective agonist of opioid κ-receptors which is under investigation in dyspepsia and the irritable bowel syndrome.

◊ References.
1. Fraitag B, *et al.* Double-blind dose-response multicenter comparison of fedotozine and placebo in treatment of nonulcer dyspepsia. *Dig Dis Sci* 1994; **39:** 1072–7.
2. Read NW, *et al.* Efficacy and safety of the peripheral kappa agonist fedotozine versus placebo in the treatment of functional dyspepsia. *Gut* 1997; **41:** 664–8.
3. Delvaux M, *et al.* The kappa agonist fedotozine relieves hypersensitivity to colonic distention in patients with irritable bowel syndrome. *Gastroenterology* 1999; **116:** 38–45.

Fig (7512-h)

Carica; Ficus.

Pharmacopoeias. In *Br.* and *Swiss.*

Pharmacopoeial description

BP 2001: The sun-dried succulent fruit of *Ficus carica* containing not less than 60.0% of water-soluble extractive. Store in a dry place.

Profile

Fig is a mild laxative and demulcent used medicinally as a syrup, usually with other laxatives.

Preparations

Proprietary Preparations (details are given in Part 3)
Multi-ingredient: *Aust.:* Frugelletten; Herbelax; Neda Fruchtewurfel; Sinolax-Milder; *Braz.:* Limao Bravo; *Denm.:* Figen; *Ger.:* florabio Mann-Feigen-Sirup mit Senna; *Switz.:* Agarol Soft; Dragees aux figues avec du sene; Pursana; Valverde Dragees laxatives; Valverde Sirop laxatif; *UK:* Califig.

Frangula Bark (7513-m)

Alder Buckthorn Bark; Amieiro Negro; Bourdaine; Faulbaumrinde; Frangulae Cortex; Rhamni Frangulae Cortex.
CAS — 8057-57-6 (frangula extract).
Pharmacopoeias. In *Eur.* (see p.vi) and *Pol.*

Pharmacopoeial description

Ph. Eur.: The dried, whole or fragmented bark of the stems and branches of *Rhamnus frangula* (=*Frangula alnus*). It contains not less than 7.0% of glucofrangulins, expressed as glucofrangulin A ($C_{27}H_{30}O_{14} = 578.5$) and calculated with reference to the dried drug. Protect from light.

Profile

Frangula bark is an anthraquinone stimulant laxative with actions and uses similar to those of senna (p.1248).
It is also used in homoeopathic medicine.

Preparations

Ph. Eur.: Standardised Frangula Bark Dry Extract.

Proprietary Preparations (details are given in Part 3)
Ger.: Eupond-F†; *Switz.:* Emodella†; *UK:* Heath & Heather Inner Fresh Tablets.

Multi-ingredient: *Aust.:* Abdomilon; Abfuhrdragees mild; Abfuhrtee; Artin; Dr Ernst Richter's Abfuhrtee; Dr Ernst Richter's Abfuhrtee-tassen-fertig; Dr. Ernst Richter's Abfuhrtee-Filterbeutel; Dragees Neunzehn; Gallesyn; Laxalpin; Laxolind†; May-Cur-Tee; Planta Lax; Pserhofer's; Sigman-Haustropfen; St Bonifatius-Tee; *Austral.:* Granocol; Herb-a-Lax; Normacol Plus; Roter†; *Belg.:* Grains de Vals; Normacol Plus; Tisane Antibiliaire et Stomachique; Tisane Contre la Tension; Tisane Depurative "les 12 Plantes"; Tisane Purgative; *Canad.:* Constipation; Extra Strong Formula 12; Herbalax; Lapidar; *Denm.:* Ferroplex-frangula; *Fr.:* Boldoflorine; Bronpax†; Depuratif des Alpes; Dragees Fuca; Dragees Vegetales Rex; Mediflor Tisane Antirhumatismale No 2†; Mediflor Tisane Circulation du Sang No 12†; Mucinum†; Normacol a la Bourdaine; Pilules Dupuis†; Santane C_6; Sirop Pectoral enfant†; Spark†; Tisane des Familles; Tisane Grande Chartreuse; Tisane Mexicaine†; Tisane Touraine†; Tisanes de l'Abbe Hamon no 17†; Tisanes de l'Abbe Hamon no 3; Tonilax; *Ger.:* Eupond†; Floradix Maskam†; Heumann Abfuhrtee Solubilax N; Hevertolax duo; *Hong Kong:* Hepatofalk; Normacol Plus; *Irl.:* Normacol Plus; *Israel:* Encypalmed; Rekiv; *Ital.:* Crisolax†; Fave di Fuca; Fitodorf Alghe Marine; Frangulina; Ginolax†; Hepasil Composto; Lactolas; Neo-Heparbil†; Sintobil†; Tisana Arnaldi†; Verecolene Complesso†; *Mex.:* Normacol; *Neth.:* Roter†; *NZ:* Granocol; Normacol Plus; *Port.:* Normacol Plus; *S.Afr.:* Normacol Plus; Roter†; *Singapore:* Normacol Plus; *Spain:* Caved-S†; Doctogaster†; Jarabe Manzanas Siken; Normacol Forte; Rabro†; Roter Complex†; *Switz.:* Adistop Lax†; Boldoflorine†; Caved-S†; Colosan plus; Drix†; Fuca†; Lapidar 10; Lapidar 10 plus†; Lapidar 10†; Lapidar 14†; Linoforce; Normacol (avec bourdaine); Optilax†; Padma-Lax; Phytolax; PhytoLaxin; The laxatif Solubilax†; Tisane laxative; *Thai.:* Roter; *UK:* Herbulax; Lustys Herbalene; Normacol Plus.

Gefarnate (690-w)

Gefarnate (*BAN, rINN*).

DA-688; Geranyl Farnesylacetate. A mixture of stereoisomers of 3,7-dimethylocta-2,6-dienyl 5,9,13-trimethyltetradeca-4,8,12-trienoate.
$C_{27}H_{44}O_2 = 400.6$.
CAS — 51-77-4.
ATC — A02BX07.

Profile

Gefarnate is a cytoprotective that has been used by mouth in the treatment of peptic ulcer disease and gastritis.

Preparations

Proprietary Preparations (details are given in Part 3)
Jpn: Gefanil†.

Ginger (4653-j)

Gengibre; Gingembre; Ingwer; Zingib.; Zingiber; Zingiberis Rhizoma.

Pharmacopoeias. In *Chin.*, *Eur.* (see p.vi), and *Jpn.* Also in *USNF.*

Pharmacopoeial description

Ph. Eur.: The dried, whole or cut rhizome of *Zingiber officinale*, with the cork removed, either completely or from the wide flat surfaces only. Whole or cut, it contains not less than 1.5% of essential oil, calculated with reference to the anhydrous drug. It has a characteristic aromatic odour. Protect from light.

USNF 20: The scraped or unscraped rhizome of *Zingiber officinale* (Zingiberaceae), known in commerce as unbleached ginger. It contains not less than 4.5% of alcohol-soluble extractive and not less than 10% of water-soluble extractive. Protect from light and moisture.

Profile

Ginger has carminative properties. It is used as a flavouring agent and has been tried for the prophylaxis of motion sickness and postoperative nausea and vomiting (p.1206).

It is also used in homoeopathic medicine.

Nausea and vomiting. References.
1. Grøntved A, Hentzer E. Vertigo-reducing effect of ginger root: a controlled clinical study. *ORL J Otorhinolaryngol Relat Spec* 1986; **48:** 282–6.
2. Bone ME, *et al.* Ginger root—a new antiemetic: the effect of ginger root on postoperative nausea and vomiting after major gynaecological surgery. *Anaesthesia* 1990; **45:** 669–71.
3. Stewart JJ, *et al.* Effects of ginger on motion sickness susceptibility and gastric function. *Pharmacology* 1991; **42:** 111–20.
4. Phillips S, *et al.* Zingiber officinale (ginger)—an antiemetic for day case surgery. *Anaesthesia* 1993; **48:** 715–17.
5. Arfeen Z, *et al.* A double-blind randomized controlled trial of ginger for the prevention of postoperative nausea and vomiting. *Anaesth Intensive Care* 1995; **23:** 449–52.
6. Ernst E, Pittler MH. Efficacy of ginger for nausea and vomiting: a systematic review of randomized clinical trials. *Br J Anaesth* 2000; **84:** 367–71.

Preparations

BP 2001: Aromatic Cardamom Tincture; Strong Ginger Tincture; Weak Ginger Tincture;
USNF 20: Ginger Tincture.

Proprietary Preparations (details are given in Part 3)
Aust.: Zintona; *Austral.:* Travacalm Natural; *Ger.:* Zintona; *Hong Kong:* Zinaxin; *Singapore:* Zinaxin; *Switz.:* Zintona; *Thai.:* Zinaxin; *UK:* Travel Sickness; Travellers; Zinaxin.

Multi-ingredient: *Aust.:* Mariazeller; Sanvita Magen; *Austral.:* Bioglan Ginger-Vite Forte; Bioglan Psylli-Mucil Plus; Cal Alkyline; Digestive Aid; Extralife Arthri-Care; Feminine Herbal Complex; Ginkgo Plus Herbal Plus Formula 10; Herbal Cleanse; Herbal Digestive Formula; Lifesystem Herbal Plus Formula 11 Ginkgo; PC Regulax; Peritone; PMS Support; PMT Complex; Travelaide; Vitaglow Herbal Laxative†; *Braz.:* Catuaba; Catuama; Geripan; Pulmoiodo; Tussifen; *Canad.:* Chase Kolik Gripe Water; *Ger.:* Fovysat; Gastrosecur; Imbak; JuViton; Presselin Dyspeptikum; Unex Amarum; *Hong Kong:* GI; *Ital.:* Cura†; Donalg; *Singapore:* Artrex; *Switz.:* Padma-Lax; *Thai.:* Carmicide; Flatulence Gastulence; Papytazyme; *UK:* Digestive; Herbal Booster; HRI Golden Seal Digestive; Indigestion Relief; Neo; Super Mega B+C; Travel-Caps; Wind & Dyspepsia Relief.

Granisetron Hydrochloride (15846-n)

Granisetron Hydrochloride (*BANM, USAN, rINNM*).

BRL-43694A. 1-Methyl-N-(9-methyl-9-azabicyclo[3.3.1]non-3-yl)-1H-indazole-3-carboxamide hydrochloride.
$C_{18}H_{24}N_4O$, HCl = 348.9.

CAS — 109889-09-0 (granisetron); 107007-99-8 (granisetron hydrochloride).

Granisetron hydrochloride 1.1 mg is approximately equivalent to 1 mg of granisetron base.

Adverse Effects and Precautions

As for Ondansetron, p.1241.

◊ The manufacturer has reported an increased incidence of hepatic neoplasms in *rodents* given very high doses of granisetron for prolonged periods, although the relevance of these results to the clinical situation is undetermined. Although mutagenicity and genotoxicity have not been seen in some tests, others have reported an increased incidence of polyploidy or unscheduled DNA synthesis in exposed cells.

Pharmacokinetics

Granisetron is absorbed following administration by mouth, with peak plasma concentrations occurring about 2 hours after a dose. Oral bioavailability is about 60% as a result of first-pass hepatic metabolism. It has a large volume of distribution of around 3 litres per kg; plasma protein binding is about 65%. The pharmacokinetics of granisetron exhibit considerable interindividual variation, and the elimination half-life is reported to be around 3 to 4 hours in healthy subjects but about 9 to 12 hours in cancer patients. It is metabolised in the liver, primarily by 7-hydroxylation, with less than 20% of a dose recovered unchanged in urine, the remainder being excreted in faeces and urine as metabolites. Granisetron clearance is not affected by renal impairment, but is lower in the elderly and in patients with hepatic impairment.

Uses and Administration

Granisetron is a 5-HT₃-receptor antagonist with an antiemetic action similar to that of ondansetron (p.1242). It is used in the management of nausea and vomiting induced by cytotoxic chemotherapy and radiotherapy and for the prevention and treatment of postoperative nausea and vomiting (p.1206). Granisetron is administered as the hydrochloride, but doses are expressed in terms of the base.

For acute **nausea and vomiting** associated with **chemotherapy** granisetron is used in *prevention* and *treatment* in similar doses.

• In the UK, a dose equivalent to 3 mg of granisetron is diluted to a volume of 20 to 50 mL with a suitable infusion solution and given intravenously over 5 minutes before the start of chemotherapy; alternatively this dose may be administered in 15 mL of infusion solution and given as a bolus over not less than 30 seconds. The dose may be repeated up to twice in 24 hours; doses should be administered at least 10 minutes apart and a total daily dose of 9 mg should not be exceeded. The efficacy of granisetron may be enhanced by the use of dexamethasone. The

---

The symbol † denotes a preparation no longer actively marketed

recommended dose by mouth is 1 to 2 mg within one hour before therapy begins, then 2 mg daily as a single dose or in 2 divided doses.

- In children, intravenous infusion of 40 µg per kg body-weight, up to a maximum total dose of 3 mg, has been recommended, dissolved in 10 to 30 mL of infusion fluid and given over 5 minutes. This dose may be repeated once within 24 hours, but at least 10 minutes after the original infusion. Alternatively, children may be given 20 µg per kg (up to 1 mg) twice daily by mouth for up to 5 days during therapy; the first dose should be administered within 1 hour of the start of chemotherapy.
- In the USA, lower intravenous doses of the equivalent of 10 µg of granisetron per kg are recommended in both adults and children over 2 years of age, beginning within 30 minutes before chemotherapy. Doses by mouth are the same as those described above.

For the *prevention* of nausea and vomiting associated with **radiotherapy** the recommended adult dosage is 2 mg daily by mouth taken within 1 hour of irradiation. It has also been given intravenously.

For the *prevention* of **postoperative** nausea and vomiting 1 mg is diluted to 5 mL and administered by intravenous injection over 30 seconds. Administration should be completed prior to induction of anaesthesia. The same dose may be given up to twice daily for the *treatment* of established postoperative nausea and vomiting.

◊ References.
1. Anonymous. Granisetron to prevent vomiting after cancer chemotherapy. *Med Lett Drugs Ther* 1994; **36:** 61–2.
2. Yarker YE, McTavish D. Granisetron: an update of its therapeutic use in nausea and vomiting induced by antineoplastic therapy. *Drugs* 1994; **48:** 761–93.
3. Adams VR, Valley AW. Granisetron: the second serotonin-receptor antagonist. *Ann Pharmacother* 1995; **29:** 1240–51. Correction. *ibid.* 1996; **30:** 1043.

Preparations

Proprietary Preparations (details are given in Part 3)
Aust.: Kytril; *Belg.:* Kytril; *Braz.:* Kytril; *Canad.:* Kytril; *Denm.:* Kytril; *Fin.:* Kytril; *Fr.:* Kytril; *Ger.:* Kevatril; *Hong Kong:* Kytril; *Irl.:* Kytril; *Israel:* Kytril; Setron; *Ital.:* Kytril; *Mex.:* Kytril; *Neth.:* Kytril; *Norw.:* Kytril; *Port.:* Kytril; *S.Afr.:* Kytril; *Singapore:* Kytril; *Spain:* Kytril; *Swed.:* Kytril; *Switz.:* Kytril; *Thai.:* Kytril; *UK:* Kytril; *USA:* Kytril.

Hydrotalcite (691-e)

Hydrotalcite (BAN, rINN).
Aluminium magnesium carbonate hydroxide hydrate.
$Mg_6Al_2(OH)_{16}CO_3,4H_2O = 604.0.$
CAS — 12304-65-3.
ATC — A02AD04.

NOTE. Compounded preparations of hydrotalcite may be represented by the following names:
- Co-simalcite *x/y* (BAN)—where *x* and *y* are the strengths in milligrams of simeticone and hydrotalcite respectively.

Pharmacopoeias. In Br.

Pharmacopoeial description
BP 2001: A hydrated form of an aluminium magnesium basic carbonate corresponding to the formula $Al_2Mg_6(OH)_{16}CO_3,4H_2O.$ It contains not less than 15.3% and not more than 18.7% of Al_2O_3 and not less than 36.0% and not more than 44.0% of MgO. The ratio of Al_2O_3 to MgO is not less than 0.40 and not more than 0.45. A white or almost white, free-flowing, granular powder. Practically insoluble in water; it dissolves in dilute mineral acids with slight effervescence. A 4% suspension in water has a pH of 8.0 to 10.0.

Profile
Hydrotalcite is an antacid (see p.1201) that is given in doses of up to about 1 g by mouth.

Preparations
BP 2001: Hydrotalcite Tablets.

Proprietary Preparations (details are given in Part 3)
Aust.: Talcid; *Fr.:* Ultacite†; *Ger.:* Ancid; Megalac; Talcid; Talidat; *Irl.:* Altacite†; *Mex.:* Talcid; *Neth.:* Ultacit; *S.Afr.:* Altacite†; *Spain:* Hidralmat; Talcid; Talidat; *Swed.:* Altacet†; Talcid†; *UK:* Actal; Altacite†.

Multi-ingredient: *Hong Kong:* GI; *Irl.:* Altacite Plus†; *UK:* Altacite Plus.

Infliximab (9898-g)

Infliximab (BAN, rINN).
cA2; CenTNF.
CAS — 170277-31-3.
ATC — L04AA12.

Store at a temperature of 2° to 8°.

Adverse Effects, Treatment, and Precautions
Infliximab may cause acute infusion reactions during or within 1 to 2 hours of administration, particularly with the first or second dose. Symptoms include fever, chills, pruritus, urticaria, dyspnoea, chest pain, and hypertension or hypotension. Mild reactions may respond to a reduced rate of infusion or a temporary interruption. If reactions are more severe, discontinuation of therapy should be considered. Pretreatment with paracetamol and antihistamines may be considered. Infliximab should only be given where facilities for resuscitation are available. Delayed reactions have occurred 3 to 12 days after infusion, including myalgia, arthralgia, fever, and rash (see below).

Other, common, adverse effects include nausea and vomiting, abdominal pain, diarrhoea, fatigue, dizziness, headache, and back pain.

Infections are also common in patients treated with infliximab, and most often affect the upper respiratory tract and the urinary tract. Infliximab has been associated rarely with the development of serious opportunistic infections, and onset or re-activation of tuberculosis (see below). Infliximab should be avoided in patients with severe infection, including active tuberculosis and opportunistic infections, and should be discontinued if these develop. It should also be used with care in those with a history of recurrent infections. Patients should be evaluated for latent and active tuberculosis before beginning therapy; if evidence of latent tuberculosis is found the risks and benefits of treatment should be considered carefully and chemoprophylaxis should be given. Patients should be instructed to seek medical advice if symptoms suggestive of tuberculosis (such as persistent cough, weight loss, or low grade fever) occur. Patients should be monitored for signs of infection for 6 months after treatment.

Antibodies to infliximab (human antichimeric antibodies) may develop, and are associated with an increased incidence of hypersensitivity reactions. Antinuclear antibodies and anti-double-stranded-DNA antibodies have also developed. A lupus-like syndrome has occurred rarely; treatment should be discontinued if it develops. Infliximab should be avoided in patients with a history of hypersensitivity to the drug or other murine proteins. Caution is required if infliximab therapy is repeated after a prolonged period (see below).

Infliximab has been associated in rare cases with clinical or radiological worsening of demyelinating disorders such as multiple sclerosis or optic neuritis; care is required in prescribing it to patients with such disorders or symptoms suggestive of their onset.

Delayed reactions. Ten of 40 patients re-treated with infliximab after a 2 to 4 year period without treatment experienced delayed hypersensitivity reactions, of which 6 were considered serious. None of the patients had experienced infusion-related adverse effects with their original infliximab treatment. Adverse reactions developed in 9 of the 23 patients who had received a liquid formulation no longer available, and in 1 of the 17 patients who received the marketed formulation, leading to speculation that the formulation may have been a contributing factor.

Infection. There have been spontaneous reports of onset or re-activation of *tuberculosis* in patients treated with infliximab, including cases of miliary tuberculosis and unusual extrapulmonary disease.[1] The UK Committee on Safety of Medicines noted in February 2001 that there had been 28 such reports worldwide. The US manufacturers subsequently reported (in October 2001) that other serious opportunistic infections, including histoplasmosis, listeriosis, and pneumocystosis had occurred, and had led to some deaths; the number of reported cases of tuberculosis had risen to 84.[2] The majority of patients also had a history of treatment with immunosuppressants including corticosteroids but inhibition of tumour necrosis factor may af-

fect normal immune responses and predispose patients to opportunistic infections.
1. Committee on Safety of Medicines/Medicines Control Agency. Infliximab (Remicade) and tuberculosis. *Current Problems* 2001; **27:** 7.
2. Schaible TF [Centocor, Inc.]. Important drug warning. Available at: http://www.fda.gov/medwatch/safety/2001/remicadeTB_deardoc.pdf

Interactions
It is recommended that live vaccines are not given concurrently with infliximab as the effect of infliximab on the efficacy of vaccination or the risk of infection transmission is unknown.

Pharmacokinetics
Infliximab shows linear pharmacokinetics. It is distributed primarily in the vascular compartment and has a terminal elimination half-life of 8 to 9.5 days. After a single dose of 5 mg per kg body-weight, infliximab was detected in serum for 8 weeks.

Uses and Administration
Infliximab is a chimeric monoclonal antibody to tumour necrosis factor α. It is used in the treatment of refractory Crohn's disease (p.1205), and in the treatment of rheumatoid arthritis (p.9) in combination with methotrexate. Infliximab is given by intravenous infusion over a period of not less than 2 hours.

In severe active Crohn's disease, a single dose of 5 mg per kg body-weight is given. In fistulising Crohn's disease, the dose is 5 mg per kg repeated at 2 and 6 weeks. If signs and symptoms of Crohn's disease recur within 14 weeks of the last infusion, infliximab may be readministered.

In rheumatoid arthritis, the dose is 3 mg per kg repeated at 2 and 6 weeks then every 8 weeks thereafter.

◊ References.
1. Onrust SV, Lamb HM. Infliximab: a review of its use in Crohn's disease and rheumatoid arthritis. *BioDrugs* 1998; **10:** 397–422.
2. Anonymous. Infliximab (Remicade) for Crohn's disease. *Med Lett Drug Ther* 1999; **41:** 19–20.
3. Present DH, *et al.* Infliximab for the treatment of fistulas in patients with Crohn's disease. *N Engl J Med* 1999; **340:** 1398–405.
4. Maini R, *et al.* Infliximab (chimeric anti-tumour necrosis factor α monoclonal antibody) versus placebo in rheumatoid arthritis patients receiving concomitant methotrexate: a randomised phase III trial. *Lancet* 1999; **354:** 1932–9.
5. Lipsky PE, *et al.* Infliximab and methotrexate in the treatment of rheumatoid arthritis. *N Engl J Med* 2000; **343:** 1594–1602.
6. Markham A, Lamb HM. Infliximab: a review of its use in the management of rheumatoid arthritis. *Drugs* 2000; **59:** 1341–59.
7. Anonymous. Etanercept and infliximab for rheumatoid arthritis. *Drug Ther Bull* 2001; **39:** 49–52.

Preparations
Proprietary Preparations (details are given in Part 3)
Denm.: Remicade; *Fin.:* Remicade; *Fr.:* Remicade; *Ger.:* Remicade; *Irl.:* Remicade; *Ital.:* Remicade; *Neth.:* Remicade; *Port.:* Remicade; *Spain:* Remicade; *Swed.:* Remicade; *UK:* Remicade; *USA:* Remicade.

Ipomoea (7514-b)
Ipomoea Root; Mexican Scammony Root; Orizaba Jalap Root; Scammony Root.

The dried root of *Ipomoea orizabensis* (Convolvulaceae).

Ipomoea Resin (7515-v)
Mexican Scammony Resin; Scammony Resin.
CAS — 9000-34-4.

A mixture of glycosidal resins obtained from ipomoea.

Profile
Ipomoea resin has a drastic purgative and irritant action. It has been superseded by less toxic laxatives.

Preparations
Proprietary Preparations (details are given in Part 3)
Multi-ingredient: *Fr.:* Mucinum†.

Irsogladine Maleate (19528-t)
Irsogladine Maleate (rINNM).
MN-1695. 2,4-Diamino-6-(2,5-dichlorophenyl)-S-triazine maleate.
$C_9H_7Cl_2N_5.C_4H_4O_4 = 372.2.$
CAS — 57381-26-7 (irsogladine); 84504-69-8 (irsogladine maleate).

Profile
Irsogladine maleate is a cytoprotective drug that is used in the

treatment of peptic ulcer disease (p.1208) in a usual dose of 4 mg daily by mouth.

Preparations

Proprietary Preparations (details are given in Part 3)
Jpn: Gaslon N.

Ispaghula   (5440-s)

Pharmacopoeias. In *Eur.* (see p.vi) under the titles of Ispaghula Husk and Ispaghula Seed. Also in *US* under the titles of Psyllium Husk and Plantago Seed.

Pharmacopoeial description

Ph. Eur.: Ispaghula Husk consists of the episperm and collapsed adjacent layers removed from the seeds of *Plantago ovata* (=*P. ispaghula*). The powdered drug loses not more than 12.0% of its weight on drying. Protect from light.

Ispaghula Seed consists of the dried ripe seeds of *Plantago ovata* (=*P. ispaghula*). The powdered drug loses not more than 10.0% of its weight on drying. Protect from light.

USP 25: Psyllium Husk is the cleaned, dried seed coat (epidermis), in whole or in powdered form, separated by winnowing and threshing from the seeds of *Plantago ovata* (known in commerce as Blond Psyllium, Indian Psyllium, Indian Plantago, or Ispaghula), or from *Plantago psyllium*, or from *Plantago indica* (*P. arenaria*) known in commerce as Spanish or French Psyllium.

Plantago Seed is the cleaned, dried, ripe seed of *Plantago ovata*, or of *Plantago psyllium*, or of *Plantago indica* (*P. arenaria*).

Psyllium Seed   (5452-y)

Flea Seed; Psyllii Semen.

Pharmacopoeias. In *Eur.* (see p.vi) and *Pol.* Also in *US* under the title of Plantago Seed.

Pharmacopoeial description

Ph. Eur.: The ripe, whole, dry seeds of *Plantago afra* (*P. psyllium*) or *Plantago indica* (*P. arenaria*). It loses not more than 14.0% of its weight on drying. Protect from light and moisture.

USP 25: Plantago Seed is the cleaned, dried, ripe seed of *Plantago ovata*, or of *Plantago psyllium*, or of *Plantago indica* (*P. arenaria*) (see also Ispaghula, above).

Adverse Effects and Precautions

Large quantities of ispaghula and other bulk laxatives may temporarily increase flatulence and abdominal distension; hypersensitivity reactions have been reported. There is a risk of intestinal or oesophageal obstruction and faecal impaction, especially if such compounds are swallowed dry. Therefore, they should always be taken with sufficient fluid and should not be taken immediately before going to bed. They should be avoided by patients who have difficulty swallowing.

Bulk laxatives should not be given to patients with pre-existing faecal impaction, intestinal obstruction, or colonic atony.

Hypersensitivity. Hypersensitivity reactions associated with the ingestion or inhalation of ispaghula or psyllium have been reported;[1-6] symptoms have included rhinitis, urticaria, bronchospasm, and anaphylactic shock. In most patients, sensitisation was thought to have occurred during occupational exposure.

1. Busse WW, Schoenwetter WF. Asthma from psyllium in laxative manufacture. *Ann Intern Med* 1975; **83:** 361–2.
2. Gross R. Acute bronchospasm associated with inhalation of psyllium hydrophilic mucilloid. *JAMA* 1979; **241:** 1573–4.
3. Suhonen R, *et al.* Anaphylactic shock due to ingestion of psyllium laxative. *Allergy* 1983; **38:** 363–5.
4. Zaloga GP, *et al.* Anaphylaxis following psyllium ingestion. *J Allergy Clin Immunol* 1984; **74:** 79–80.
5. Kaplan MJ. Anaphylactic reaction to "Heartwise". *N Engl J Med* 1990; **323:** 1072–3.
6. Lantner RR, *et al.* Anaphylaxis following ingestion of a psyllium-containing cereal. *JAMA* 1990; **264:** 2534–6.

Interactions

There is a possibility that ispaghula may reduce or delay gastrointestinal absorption of other drugs given concomitantly.

Lithium. For reference to ispaghula possibly reducing the absorption of lithium, see Gastrointestinal Drugs, p.295.

Uses and Administration

Ispaghula seed, ispaghula husk, and psyllium seed are bulk laxatives (p.1201). They absorb water in the gastrointestinal tract to form a mucilaginous mass which increases the volume of faeces and hence promotes peristalsis. They are used in the treatment of constipation (p.1202), especially in diverticular disease

(p.1203) and irritable bowel syndrome (p.1206), and when excessive straining at stool must be avoided, for example following anorectal surgery or in the management of haemorrhoids. The ability to absorb water and increase faecal mass means that they may also be used in the management of diarrhoea (p.1203) and for adjusting faecal consistency in patients with colostomies.

The usual dose is about 3.5 g one to three times daily by mouth although higher doses have been given. It should be taken dispersed in at least 150 mL water or fruit juice immediately after mixing. The full effect may not be achieved for up to 3 days.

Ispaghula is also given for mild to moderate hypercholesterolaemia as an adjunct to a lipid-lowering diet. The recommended dose is about 3.5 to 5.25 g in at least 150 mL water twice daily by mouth.

Hyperlipidaemias. Preparations of ispaghula have been reported[1,2] to lower serum-cholesterol concentrations in patients with mild to moderate hypercholesterolaemia. They have also been given in combination with reduced doses of a bile-acid binding resin in the treatment of hyperlipidaemia,[3] which is reported to be effective and better tolerated than full doses of the resin alone. However, ispaghula or psyllium should be regarded as adjuncts to dietary modification rather than substitutes for it. For a discussion of the hyperlipidaemias and their management, see p.800.

1. Anderson JW, *et al.* Cholesterol-lowering effect of psyllium hydrophilic mucilloid for hypercholesterolemic men. *Arch Intern Med* 1988; **148:** 292–6.
2. Bell LP, *et al.* Cholesterol-lowering effects of psyllium hydrophilic mucilloid: adjunct therapy to a prudent diet for patients with mild to moderate hypercholesterolemia. *JAMA* 1989; **261:** 3419–23.
3. Spence JD, *et al.* Combination therapy with colestipol and psyllium mucilloid in patients with hyperlipidemia. *Ann Intern Med* 1995; **123:** 493–9.

Preparations

BP 2001: Ispaghula Husk Effervescent Granules; Ispaghula Husk Granules; Ispaghula Husk Oral Powder;
USP 25: Psyllium Hydrophilic Mucilloid for Oral Suspension.

Proprietary Preparations (details are given in Part 3)
Aust.: Agiocur; Agiolind†; Laxans; Metamucil; Pascomucil; *Austral.:* Agiofibe; Ford Fibre; Fybogel; Metamucil; Mucilax; Natural Fibre; *Belg.:* Colofiber; Fybogel; Metamucil†; Mucivital; *Braz.:* Metamucil; *Canad.:* Fibrepur†; Floralax†; Karacil†; Laxagel; Laxucil; Metamucil; Mucilloid†; Natural Source Laxative; Naturcil†; Novo-Mucilax; Prodiem Plain; *Denm.:* Vi-Siblin; *Fin.:* Agiocur; Laxamucil; Vi-Siblin; *Fr.:* Mucivital; Phytofibre†; Spagulax; Transilane; *Ger.:* Agiocur; Agiolax Ballast; Bekunis Leicht†; Flosa; Flosine; Kneipp Abfuhr Herbagran; Laxiplant Soft; Metamucil; Mucofalk; Pascomucil; Plantocur; *Hong Kong:* Agiocur; Fybogel; Metamucil; Mucofalk; Vitalax; *Irl.:* Fybogel; Regulan; *Israel:* Agiocur; Metamucil; Planten; *Ital.:* Fibrolax; Mucivital; Planten; *Mex.:* Agiofibra; Fibromucil; Fybogel; Hormolax; Konsyl; Laxen; Metabyn; Metamucil; Novagon; Pygosal; Tagozzard; *Mon.:* Psylia; *Neth.:* Metamucil; Volcolon; *Norw.:* Lunelax; Vi-Siblin; *NZ:* Isogel; Konsyl; Metamucil; Mucilax; *Port.:* Agiocur; Bekunis Fibra†; Metamucil†; Mucofalk; *S.Afr.:* Agiobulk; Fybogel; Metamucil; *Singapore:* Fybogel; Isogel; Metamucil; Mucilin; Mucofalk; *Spain:* Biopasal Fibra; Cenat; Fibramucil; Fybogel†; Laxisoft; Metamucil; Plantaben; *Swed.:* Lunelax; Metamucil†; Vi-Siblin; *Switz.:* Agiolax mite; Bekunis Plantago Granule†; Colosoft; Dulconatur†; Konsyl; Laxiplant Soft; Metamucil; Mucilar; Valverde regulateur du transit intestinal granules; *Thai.:* Agiocur; Fybogel; Metamucil; Mucilin; Mucofalk; *UK:* Fibre Plus; Fybogel; Fybozest; Isogel; Ispagel; Konsyl; Regulan; *USA:* Alramucil Instant Mix†; Alramucil†; Effer-Syllium†; Fiberall; Hydrocil Instant; Konsyl; Konsyl-D; Maalox Daily Fiber†; Metamucil; Modane Bulk; Mylanta Natural Fiber; Perdiem Fiber†; Reguloid; Restore†; Serutan; Siblin†; Syllact; V-Lax†.

Multi-ingredient: *Aust.:* Abbiofort; Agiolax; Effersyllium; *Austral.:* Agiolax; Bioglan Psylli-Mucil Plus; Enterocare; Herb-a-Lax; Herbal Cleanse; Herbal Laxative†; Nucolox; PC Regulax; Plantago Complex†; *Belg.:* Agiolax; Braz.:* Agiolax; Plantax; Prompt; *Canad.:* Prodiem Plus; *Fin.:* Agiolax; *Fr.:* Agiolax; Imegul; Parapsyllium†; Spagulax au Citrate de Potassium; Spagulax au Sorbitol; *Ger.:* Agiolax; Kneipplax N†; *Hong Kong:* Agiolax; *Irl.:* Fybogel Mebeverine; *Israel:* Agiolax; *Ital.:* Agiolax; Fibrolax Complex; Ginolax†; *Mex.:* Agiolax; Psilumax; *Neth.:* Agiolax; *Port.:* Agiolax; *S.Afr.:* Agiolax; *Singapore:* Fybogel Mebeverine; *Spain:* Agiolax; *Swed.:* Lunelax comp†; Vi-Siblin S; *Switz.:* Agiolax; Bronchalin†; Laxiplant cum Senna†; Mucilar Avena; *Thai.:* Agiolax; *UK:* Fybogel Mebeverine; Lion Cleansing Herbs; Lipolest; Manevac; *USA:* Perdiem; Syllamalt†.

Itopride Hydrochloride   (15899-j)

Itopride Hydrochloride *(rINNM)*.
HC-803. *N*-{*p*-[2-(Dimethylamino)ethoxy]benzyl}veratramide hydrochloride.
$C_{20}H_{26}N_2O_4,HCl = 394.9$.
CAS — 122898-67-3 (itopride).

Profile

Itopride hydrochloride is a substituted benzamide with general properties similar to those of metoclopramide (p.1235) that has been used by mouth for its prokinetic and antiemetic actions.

Preparations

Proprietary Preparations (details are given in Part 3)
Jpn: Ganaton.

Jalap   (7516-g)

Jalap Root; Jalap Tuber; Jalapa; Jalapenwurzel; Vera Cruz Jalap.
Pharmacopoeias. In *Aust.*

The dried tubercles of *Ipomoea purga* (=*Exogonium purga*) (Convolvulaceae).

Jalap Resin   (7517-q)

Jalapenharz.
CAS — 9000-35-5.
Pharmacopoeias. In *Aust.*

A mixture of glycosidal resins obtained by extraction of jalap with alcohol.

Profile

Jalap resin has a drastic purgative and irritant action. It has been superseded by less toxic laxatives.

Kaolin   (694-j)

Bolus Alba; E559; Weisser Ton.
CAS — 1332-58-7.
ATC — A07BC02.
Pharmacopoeias. In *Chin.*, *Eur.* (see p.vi), *Int.*, *Jpn*, and *US*. Some pharmacopoeias do not differentiate between the heavy and light varieties.

Pharmacopoeial description

Ph. Eur.: Heavy kaolin is a purified, natural, hydrated aluminium silicate of variable composition. It is a fine, white or greyish-white, unctuous powder. Practically insoluble in water and in organic solvents.

BP 2001: Light Kaolin is a native hydrated aluminium silicate, freed from most of its impurities by elutriation, and dried. It contains a suitable dispersing agent. It is a light, white, odourless or almost odourless, unctuous powder free from gritty particles. Practically insoluble in water and in mineral acids.

Light Kaolin (Natural) is Light Kaolin which does not contain a dispersing agent. It is a light, white, odourless or almost odourless, unctuous powder free from gritty particles. Practically insoluble in water and in mineral acids.

NOTE. The BP 2001 directs that when Kaolin or Light Kaolin is prescribed or demanded, Light Kaolin must be dispensed or supplied unless it is ascertained that Light Kaolin (Natural) is required.

USP 25: Kaolin is a native hydrated aluminium silicate, powdered and freed from gritty particles by elutriation. It is a soft, white or yellowish-white powder or lumps with an earthy or clay-like taste, and when moistened with water assumes a darker colour and develops a marked clay-like odour. Insoluble in water, in cold dilute acids, and in solutions of alkali hydroxides.

Profile

Light kaolin and light kaolin (natural) are adsorbent antidiarrhoeal agents that have been used as adjuncts to rehydration therapy in the management of diarrhoea (p.1203). They may be taken by mouth in doses of about 2 to 6 g every four hours as required. Kaolin is often given in combination with other antidiarrhoeals, especially pectin.

Kaolin can form insoluble complexes with a number of other drugs in the gastrointestinal tract and reduce their absorption; concomitant oral administration should be avoided.

Externally, light kaolin is used as a dusting powder. Kaolin is liable to be heavily contaminated with bacteria, and when used in dusting powders, it should be sterilised.

Heavy kaolin is used in the preparation of kaolin poultice, which is applied topically with the intention of reducing inflammation and alleviating pain (see Rubefacients and Topical Analgesia, p.4).

Light kaolin is also used as a food additive.

Preparations

BP 2001: Kaolin and Morphine Mixture; Kaolin Mixture; Kaolin Poultice.

Proprietary Preparations (details are given in Part 3)
Ital.: Kao-Pront†; *UK:* Childrens Diarrhoea Mixture; Entrocalm.

Multi-ingredient: *Austral.:* De Witts Antacid; Diarcalm; Donnagel; Kaomagma; Kaomagma with Pectin; Kaopectate; *Belg.:* Alopate; Kaopectate; Neutroses; *Braz.:* Atalin; Digastril; Eviprostat; Kal Sept; Kaomagma; Kaopectate; Kaopectin; Neutracido; Pectalin; Pectimax; Plexo Enterin; *Canad.:* Bebia†; Diarex; Donnagel-PG; *Fr.:* Anti-H; Antiphlogistine; Bebia†; Gastropax; Gelogastrine†; Kaobrol; Kaologeais; Kaomuth; Karayal; Neutroses; *Ger.:* Kaoprompt-H; rohasal; *Hong Kong:* Uni-Kaotin; *Irl.:* Kaopectate; *Israel:* Digestif-Ara; Kaopectin; Kapectin Forte; Zincod; *Ital.:* Carbotiol†; Katoxyn; Magnesia Bisurata†; Neo Zeta-Foot†; Neutrose S Pellegrino; Streptomagma; *Mex.:* Colfur; Coralzul; Dibapec Compuesto; Farpectol; Fuzotyl; Kaomycin; Kaopectate; Tapzol; Tapzol Con Neomicina; Treda; *S.Afr.:* Betapect; Bipectinol; Biskapect; Chloropect; Collodyne†; Diastat†; Enterolyte; Gastropect; Kao; Kaoneo†; Kaopectin; Kaostatex; Neopec†; Pectikon; Pectin-K; Pectolin†; Pectrolyte; *Switz.:* Cicafissan; Fissan; Kaopectate; Neo-Decongestine; Neutroses; Padma-Lax; *Thai.:* Alkamine; Antacil; Coccila; Di-Su-Frone; Difuran; Diolin; Disento; Disento PF; Droximag; Furasian; Furopectin; Kaopectal; Kaopectal-N; Kaopectate; Med-Kafuzone; *UAE:* Kaptin; *UK:* Codella; Collis Browne's; De Witt's Antacid; Enterosan†; Junior Kao-C†; Kaodene; Kaopectate†; KLN; Moorland; Opazimes; *USA.:* K-C; Kao-Paverin; Kao-Spen; Kaodene Non-Narcotic; Mexsana.

Lactitol (19392-t)

Lactitol *(BAN, rINN).*
E966; β-Galactosido-sorbitol; Lactit; Lactobiosit; Lactositol. 4-*O*-(β-D-Galactopyranosyl)-D-glucitol.
$C_{12}H_{24}O_{11} = 344.3$.
CAS — 585-86-4.
ATC — A06AD12.
Pharmacopoeias. In *USNF. Eur.* (see p.vi) includes the monohydrate.

Lactitol monohydrate 1.05 g is approximately equivalent to 1 g of anhydrous lactitol. Lactitol dihydrate 1.10 g is approximately equivalent to 1 g of anhydrous lactitol.

Pharmacopoeial description

Ph. Eur.: Lactitol monohydrate is a white crystalline powder. Very soluble in water; slightly soluble in alcohol; practically insoluble in dichloromethane.

USNF 20: Lactitol may be the anhydrous form, the monohydrate, or the dihydrate.

Profile

Lactitol is a disaccharide analogue of lactulose (below) and has similar actions and uses.

Lactitol monohydrate is used as an oral powder in the management of hepatic encephalopathy (p.1205) and in constipation (p.1202).

In the treatment of hepatic encephalopathy, lactitol monohydrate is given in usual doses of 500 to 700 mg per kg bodyweight daily by mouth in 3 divided doses at meal times. The dose is subsequently adjusted to produce 2 soft stools daily.

In the treatment of constipation, lactitol monohydrate is given in an initial dose of 20 g daily by mouth as a single dose with the morning or evening meal, subsequently adjusted to produce one stool daily. A dose of 10 g daily may be sufficient for many patients.

Doses should be mixed with food or liquid, and 1 to 2 glasses of liquid should be drunk with the meal.

Lactitol is a permitted sweetener in foods.

Preparations

Proprietary Preparations (details are given in Part 3)
Aust.: Importal; Portolac; Pselac; *Belg.:* Importal; Portolac; *Denm.:* Importal; *Fin.:* Importal; Lalax; *Fr.:* Importal; *Ger.:* Importal; Neda Lactose Intolerance; *Israel:* Importal; *Ital.:* Portolac; *Jpn.:* Portolac; *Neth.:* Importal; *Norw.:* Importal; *NZ:* Importal; *Port.:* Importal; *S.Afr.:* Importal†; *Spain:* Emportal; Oponaf; *Swed.:* Importal; *Switz.:* Importal; *Thai.:* Importal.

Multi-ingredient: *Fr.:* Fucafibres†; *Ital.:* Levoplus.

Lactulose (7519-s)

Lactulose *(BAN, USAN, rINN).*
Lactulosum. 4-*O*-β-D-Galactopyranosyl-D-fructose.
$C_{12}H_{22}O_{11} = 342.3$.
CAS — 4618-18-2.
ATC — A06AD11.
Pharmacopoeias. In *Eur.* (see p.vi) and *Jpn. US* only contains specifications for lactulose in solution and concentrate.

Pharmacopoeial description

Ph. Eur.: A white or almost white, crystalline powder. Freely soluble in water; sparingly soluble in methyl alcohol; practically insoluble in toluene.

Liquid lactulose is an aqueous solution of lactulose. It contains not less than 62.0% w/v of lactulose; it may contain lesser amounts of other sugars including lactose, epilactose, galactose, tagatose, and fructose. It may contain a suitable antimicrobial preservative. It is a clear, colourless or pale brownish-yellow, viscous liquid. Miscible with water. It may be a supersaturated solution or may contain crystals which disappear on heating.

USP 25: Lactulose Concentrate is a colourless to amber syrupy liquid which may exhibit some precipitation and darkening on standing. Miscible with water. Store in airtight containers preferably at a temperature between 2° and 30°.

Adverse Effects

Lactulose may cause abdominal discomfort associated with flatulence or cramps. Nausea and vomiting have occasionally been reported following high doses. Some consider the taste to be unpleasant. Prolonged use or excessive dosage may result in diarrhoea with excessive loss of water and electrolytes, particularly potassium. Hypernatraemia has been reported.

Precautions

Lactulose should not be given to patients with intestinal obstruction. It should not be used in patients on a low galactose diet and care should be taken in patients with lactose intolerance or in diabetic patients because of the presence of some free galactose and lactose.

◊ Severe lactic acidosis developed in a patient with adynamic ileus who was being given lactulose for hepatic encephalopathy.[1]

1. Mann NS, *et al.* Lactulose and severe lactic acidosis. *Ann Intern Med* 1985; **103:** 637.

Pharmacokinetics

Following administration by mouth, lactulose passes essentially unchanged into the large intestine where it is metabolised by saccharolytic bacteria with the formation of simple organic acids, mainly lactic acid and small amounts of acetic and formic acids. The small amount of absorbed lactulose is subsequently excreted unchanged in the urine.

Uses and Administration

Lactulose is a synthetic disaccharide osmotic laxative (p.1201) used in the treatment of constipation (p.1202) and in hepatic encephalopathy (p.1205). Lactulose is broken down by colonic bacteria mainly into lactic acid. This exerts a local osmotic effect in the colon resulting in increased faecal bulk and stimulation of peristalsis. It may take up to 48 hours before an effect is obtained. When larger doses are given for hepatic encephalopathy the pH in the colon is reduced significantly and the absorption of ammonium ions and other toxic nitrogenous compounds is decreased, leading to a fall in blood-ammonia concentration and an improvement in mental function.

Lactulose is usually administered as a solution containing approximately 3.35 g of lactulose per 5 mL together with other sugars such as galactose and lactose; an oral powder formulation is also available in some countries. In the treatment of **constipation**, the usual initial dose is 10 to 20 g (15 to 30 mL) given daily by mouth in a single dose or in 2 divided doses; doses up to 40 g (60 mL) daily have been given. The dose is gradually adjusted according to the patient's needs. Children aged 5 to 10 years may be given initial doses of 10 mL twice daily; 1 to 5 years, 5 mL twice daily; under 1 year, 2.5 mL twice daily.

In **hepatic encephalopathy**, 60 to 100 g (90 to 150 mL) is given daily by mouth in 3 divided doses. The dose is subsequently adjusted to produce 2 or 3 soft stools each day. Lactulose solution 300 mL mixed with 700 mL of water or sodium chloride 0.9% has been used as a retention enema; the enema is retained for 30 to 60 minutes, repeated every 4 to 6 hours until the patient is able to take oral medication.

◊ References.

1. Clausen MR, Mortensen PB. Lactulose, disaccharides and colonic flora: clinical consequences. *Drugs* 1997; **53:** 930–42.

Diagnosis and testing. THE SUGAR ABSORPTION TEST. In healthy individuals lactulose is largely unabsorbed from the gastrointestinal tract, but in, for example, coeliac disease (p.1350) there is increased permeability to disaccharides such as lactulose and a paradoxical decrease in the absorption of monosaccharides. This led to the development of the differential sugar absorption test in which 2 sugars are given simultaneously by mouth and the urinary recovery of each is determined; mannitol is commonly used as the monosaccharide component and lactulose as the disaccharide. Alternatives include mannitol plus cellobiose and rhamnose plus lactulose. This absorption test is useful in the investigation of intestinal disease.[1]

THE LACTULOSE BREATH TEST (hydrogen breath test). Lactulose is converted by bacteria in the large bowel to short chain fatty acids with the production of small quantities of hydrogen gas. The hydrogen is rapidly absorbed and is exhaled in the breath and measurement of its production is used to measure orocaecal transit time and carbohydrate malabsorption. However, even small doses of lactulose shortens transit time which may limit the value of this test.[2]

1. Uil JJ, *et al.* Clinical implications of the sugar absorption test: intestinal permeability test to assess mucosal barrier function. *Scand J Gastroenterol* 1997; **223** (suppl): 70–8.
2. Miller MA, *et al.* Comparison of scintigraphy and lactulose breath hydrogen test for assessment of orocecal transit: lactulose accelerates small bowel transit. *Dig Dis Sci* 1997; **42:** 10–18.

Preparations

BP 2001: Lactulose Oral Powder;
Ph. Eur.: Liquid Lactulose;
USP 25: Lactulose Solution.

Proprietary Preparations (details are given in Part 3)
Aust.: Bifiteral; Duphalac; Eugalac†; Floralac; Laevolac; *Austral.:* Actilax; Duphalac; Lac-Dol; *Belg.:* Bifiteral; Certalac; Duphalac; *Braz.:* Farlac; Lactulona; *Canad.:* Acilac; Cephulac†; Chronulac†; Comalose-R; Duphalac; Gen-Lac; Laxilose; Laxulax; *Denm.:* Danilax; *Fin.:* Duphalac; Levolac; Loraga; *Fr.:* Duphalac; Fitaxal†; Laxaron; *Ger.:* Bifinorma; Bifiteral; Eugalac; Hepa-Merz Lact; Hepaticum-Lac-Medice; Kattwilact; Lactocur; Lactofalk; Lactuflor; Lactuverlan; Laevilac S; Laxomundin†; Mandrolax Lactu†; Medilet; Natulax†; Tulotract; *Hong Kong:* Danilax; Duphalac; *Irl.:* Dulax; Duphalac; Gerelax; Laxose; *Israel:* Avilac; Sirolax; *Ital.:* Biolac EPS; Dia-Colon; Duphalac; Epalat EPS; Epalfen; Idrolac; Lactoger; Lactyl; Laevolac; Lassifar; Lattulac; Lis; Normase; Osmolac; Sintolatt; Verelait; *Jpn.:* Monilac; *Mex.:* Lactulax; Regulact; *Neth.:* Duphalac; Legendal; *Norw.:* Duphalac; Levolac; *NZ:* Duphalac; Laevolac; *Port.:* Colsanac; Duphalac; Laevolac; *S.Afr.:* Duphalac; Lacson; Laevolac†; Laxette; *Singapore:* Duphalac; Spain: Belmalax; Duolax; Duphalac; Gatinar†; *Swed.:* Betulac†; Duphalac; Laktipex; Loraga; *Switz.:* Duphalac; Gatinar; Laevolac; Legendal; Rudolac; *Thai.:* Duphalac; Hepalac; *UAE:* Soflax; *UK:* Duphalac; Lactugal; Laxose†; Lemlax; Regulose; *USA.:* Cephulac; Cholac; Chronulac; Constilac; Constulose; Duphalac; Enulose; Evalose†; Heptalac†; Kristalose.

Multi-ingredient: *Fr.:* Melaxose; Transulose; *Ger.:* Eugalan Topfer forte; Eugalan Topfer forte LC; *Ital.:* Dimalosio; Lacomannan; Lactolas; Levoplus; Naturalass.

Lansoprazole (9499-j)

Lansoprazole *(BAN, USAN, rINN).*
A-65006; AG-1749. 2-({3-Methyl-4-(2,2,2-trifluoroethoxy)-2-pyridyl}methyl} sulphinylbenzimidazole.
$C_{16}H_{14}F_3N_3O_2S = 369.4$.
CAS — 103577-45-3.
ATC — A02BC03.

Adverse Effects and Precautions

As for Omeprazole, p.1239.

◊ Reviews.

1. Freston JW, *et al.* Safety profile of lansoprazole: the US clinical trial experience. *Drug Safety* 1999; **20:** 195–205.

Effects on the gastrointestinal tract. Glossitis (associated in some cases with black tongue or stomatitis) has been reported in a few patients taking lansoprazole as part of a triple therapy regimen for *Helicobacter pylori* elimination in peptic ulcer disease.[1] Discoloured tongue has been reported in a patient taking lansoprazole alone.[2]

An increase in gastritis was observed in patients infected with *Helicobacter pylori* when treated with long term lansoprazole therapy.[3] For further discussion of the link between *H. pylori*, gastritis, and proton pump inhibitor use, see Gastrointestinal Tumours, p.1239.

1. Greco S, *et al.* Glossitis, stomatitis, and black tongue with lansoprazole plus clarithromycin and other antibiotics. *Ann Pharmacother* 1997; **31:** 1548.
2. Scully C. Discoloured tongue: a new cause? *Br J Dermatol* 2001; **144:** 1293–4.
3. Berstad AE, *et al.* Helicobacter pylori gastritis and epithelial cell proliferation in patients with reflux oesophagitis after treatment with lansoprazole. *Gut* 1997; **41:** 740–7.

Effects on the skin. For mention of skin reactions to lansoprazole, see p.1239.

Musculoskeletal effects. For reference to a case of eosinophilia and myalgia related to lansoprazole therapy, see p.1240.

Interactions

As for Omeprazole, p.1240. Antacids and sucralfate may reduce the bioavailability of lansoprazole, and should not be taken within 1 hour of a dose of lansoprazole.

◊ For reference to a lack of effect of lansoprazole on diazepam, see Gastrointestinal Drugs, p.678, and for a clinically insignificant effect on theophylline clearance, see p.781. For reference to glossitis occurring when lansoprazole was used with some antibacterials, see Effects on the Gastrointestinal Tract, above.

Pharmacokinetics

Lansoprazole is rapidly absorbed after oral administration, with peak plasma concentrations achieved about 1.5 hours after a dose by mouth. Bioavailability is reported to be 80% or more even with the first dose, although the drug must be given in an enteric-coated form since lansoprazole is unstable at acid pH. It is extensively metabolised in the liver primarily by cytochrome P450 isoenzyme CYP2C19 to form 5-hydroxyl-lansoprazole and by CYP3A to form lansoprazole sulfone. Metabolites are excreted primarily in faeces via the bile; only about 15 to 30% of a dose is excreted in urine. The plasma elimination half-life is around 1 to 2 hours but the duration of action is much longer. Lansoprazole is about 97% bound to plasma protein. Clearance is decreased in elderly patients, and in liver disease.

◊ References.
1. Hussein Z, *et al.* Age-related differences in the pharmacokinetics and pharmacodynamics of lansoprazole. *Br J Clin Pharmacol* 1993; **36:** 391–8.
2. Flouvat B, *et al.* Single and multiple dose pharmacokinetics of lansoprazole in elderly subjects. *Br J Clin Pharmacol* 1993; **36:** 467–9.
3. Delhotal-Landes B, *et al.* Pharmacokinetics of lansoprazole in patients with renal or liver disease of varying severity. *Eur J Clin Pharmacol* 1993; **45:** 367–71.
4. Delhotal Landes B, *et al.* Clinical pharmacokinetics of lansoprazole. *Clin Pharmacokinet* 1995; **28:** 458–70.
5. Karol MD, *et al.* Lansoprazole pharmacokinetics in subjects with various degrees of kidney function. *Clin Pharmacol Ther* 1997; **61:** 450–8.

Metabolism. As for omeprazole (p.1241), the cytochrome P450 isoenzyme CYP2C19 (*S*-mephenytoin hydroxylase) is involved in the hydroxylation of lansoprazole, and individuals who are deficient in this enzyme are poor metabolisers of lansoprazole.

References.
1. Pearce RE, *et al.* Identification of the human P450 enzymes involved in lansoprazole metabolism. *J Pharmacol Exp Ther* 1996; **277:** 805–16.
2. Sohn DR, *et al.* Metabolic disposition of lansoprazole in relation to the S-mephenytoin 4'-hydroxylation phenotype status. *Clin Pharmacol Ther* 1997; **61:** 574–82.

Uses and Administration

Lansoprazole is a proton pump inhibitor with actions and uses similar to those of omeprazole (p.1241). It is used in the treatment of peptic ulcer disease and in other conditions where inhibition of gastric acid secretion may be beneficial.

Lansoprazole is given by mouth as capsules or suspension containing enteric-coated granules. Once daily regimens are taken before food in the morning.

For the relief of acid-related **dyspepsia** (p.1204) intermittent courses of lansoprazole may be given in doses of 15 or 30 mg once daily, for 2 to 4 weeks.

In the treatment of **gastro-oesophageal reflux disease** (p.1204) the dose is 30 mg once daily for 4 to 8 weeks; thereafter maintenance therapy can be continued with 15 or 30 mg once daily according to response.

Lansoprazole is given for the treatment of **peptic ulcer disease** (p.1208) in doses of 30 mg once daily. Treatment is continued for 4 weeks for duodenal and 8 weeks for gastric ulcer. In the USA a dose of 15 mg daily for 4 weeks is recommended for duodenal ulcer. When appropriate, 15 mg daily may be used as maintenance therapy for the prevention of relapse of duodenal ulcer. Lansoprazole may be combined with antibacterials in one-week **triple therapy** regimens for the eradication of *Helicobacter pylori.* Effective regimens include lansoprazole 30 mg twice daily combined with clarithromycin 500 mg twice daily and either amoxicillin 1 g twice daily or metronidazole 400 mg twice daily; lansoprazole, amoxicillin, and metronidazole has also been used. In patients with **NSAID-associated ulceration** a dose of 15 or 30 mg daily for 4 to 8 weeks is recommended; the same dose may be used as prophylaxis for patients who require continued NSAID treatment.

In the treatment of pathological hypersecretory states such as the **Zollinger-Ellison syndrome** (p.1209) the initial dose is 60 mg daily, adjusted as required. Doses of up to 90 mg twice daily have been used. Daily doses greater than 120 mg should be given in divided doses.

DOSAGE IN HEPATIC IMPAIRMENT.

Care is required in patients with severe hepatic impairment, and doses should not exceed 30 mg daily.

◊ General references. For general reviews of proton pump inhibitors, see Omeprazole, p.1241.
1. Barradell LB, *et al.* Lansoprazole: a review of its pharmacodynamic and pharmacokinetic properties and its therapeutic efficacy in acid-related disorders. *Drugs* 1992; **44:** 225–50.
2. Spencer CM, Faulds D. Lansoprazole: a reappraisal of its pharmacodynamic and pharmacokinetic properties, and its therapeutic efficacy in acid-related disorders. *Drugs* 1994; **48:** 404–30.
3. Anonymous. Lansoprazole–another proton pump inhibitor. *Drug Ther Bull* 1995; **33:** 36–7.

4. Anonymous. Lansoprazole. *Med Lett Drugs Ther* 1995; **37:** 63–4.
5. Blum RA. Lansoprazole and omeprazole in the treatment of acid peptic disorders. *Am J Health-Syst Pharm* 1996; **53:** 1401–15.
6. Garnett WR. Lansoprazole: a proton pump inhibitor. *Ann Pharmacother* 1996; **30:** 1425–36.
7. Langtry HD, Wilde MI. Lansoprazole: an update of its pharmacological properties and clinical efficacy in the management of acid-related disorders. *Drugs* 1997; **54:** 473–500.

Administration. Lansoprazole capsules should be swallowed whole and not crushed or chewed. Lansoprazole granules for oral suspension should be reconstituted in a little water and swallowed immediately. Where the suspension formulation is not available, the contents of the capsules (enteric-coated granules) can be sprinkled on apple sauce or mixed with a little fruit juice and swallowed.

Preparations

Proprietary Preparations (details are given in Part 3)
Aust.: Agopton; *Austral.:* Zoton; *Belg.:* Dakar; *Braz.:* Ilsatec; Ogastro; *Canad.:* Prevacid; *Denm.:* Lanzo; *Fin.:* Lanzo; *Fr.:* Lanzor; Ogast; *Ger.:* Agopton; Lanzor; *Hong Kong:* Takepron; *Irl.:* Zoton; *Israel:* Zoton; *Ital.:* Lansox; Limpidex; Zoton; *Jpn:* Takepron; *Mex.:* Ilsatec; Ogastro; Ulpax; *Neth.:* Prezal; *Norw.:* Lanzo; *NZ:* Zoton; *Port.:* Ogasto; *S.Afr.:* Lanzor; *Singapore:* Prevacid; *Spain:* Bamalite; Estomil; Monolitum; Opiren; Pro Ulco; *Swed.:* Lanzo; *Switz.:* Agopton; *Thai.:* Prevacid; *UAE:* Lanfast; *UK:* Zoton; *USA:* Prevacid.

Multi-ingredient: *Canad.:* Hp-Pac; *Fin.:* Helipak A; Helipak K; Helipak T; *UK:* Heliclear; HeliMet; *USA:* Prevpac.

Lidamidine Hydrochloride (16875-j)

Lidamidine Hydrochloride (USAN, rINNM).
WHR-1142A.   N-(2,6-Dimethylphenyl)-N'-[imino(methylamino)methyl]urea hydrochloride.
$C_{11}H_{16}N_4O,HCl = 256.7.$
CAS — 66871-56-5 (lidamidine); 65009-35-0 (lidamidine hydrochloride).

Profile

Lidamidine hydrochloride is an alpha$_2$-adrenergic receptor stimulant used for the management of diarrhoea.

Preparations

Proprietary Preparations (details are given in Part 3)
Mex.: Idealid; Supra.

Liquorice (2021-l)

Alcaçuz; Glycyrrhiza; Licorice; Liquiritiae Radix; Liquorice Root; Orozuz; Raiz de Regaliz; Süssholzwurzel.

Pharmacopoeias. In *Chin.*, *Eur.* (see p.vi), *Jpn*, and *Pol.* Many allow peeled or unpeeled liquorice. Also in *USNF*, which also includes Powdered Licorice and Powdered Licorice Extract. *Br.* and *Ger.* also include Ammonium Glycyrrhizinate (Ammonium Dihydrogen Glycyrrhizinate) $(C_{42}H_{65}NO_{16} = 840.0).$

The dried rhizome and roots of *Glycyrrhiza glabra* var. *typica* are known in commerce as Spanish Liquorice, those of *G. glabra* var. *glandulifera* as Russian Liquorice, and those of *G. glabra* var. β-*violacea* as Persian Liquorice.

Pharmacopoeial description

Ph. Eur.: Liquorice Root consists of the dried unpeeled or peeled, whole or cut root and stolons of *Glycyrrhiza glabra* containing not less than 4% of glycyrrhizinic acid. Protect from light.

USNF 20: Licorice consists of the roots, rhizomes, and stolons of *Glycyrrhiza glabra* or *G. uralensis.* It contains not less than 2.5% of glycyrrhizinic acid, calculated on the dried basis. Store in a cool, dry place.

Adverse Effects

Liquorice has mineralocorticoid-like actions manifesting as sodium and water retention and hypokalaemia (see below). Deglycyrrhizinised liquorice is not usually associated with such adverse effects.

Effects on fluid and electrolyte homoeostasis. Mineralocorticoid effects have been reported following excessive ingestion of liquorice. The liquorice may be ingested in confectionery, soft drinks, medicines, or by chewing tobacco. Adverse effects reported include hypokalaemia,[1-14] hypertension,[1,2,6,9,14] congestive heart failure,[1] arrhythmias,[13,15] fatal cardiac arrest,[10] headache,[1] muscle weakness,[1,6,9,13] myopathy,[3,7,8] myoglobinuria,[5] paralysis,[5,11] hyperprolactinaemia,[4] and amenorrhoea.[4] The effects are thought to be due to inhibition of 11-β-hydroxysteroid dehydrogenase (cortisol oxidase) by glycyrrhetinic acid, (a metabolite produced by the hydrolysis of glycyrrhizinic acid), resulting in increased concentrations of cortisol in the body.[12,16-18]
1. Chamberlain TJ. Licorice poisoning, pseudoaldosteronism, and heart failure. *JAMA* 1970; **213:** 1343.
2. Wash LK, Bernard JD. Licorice-induced pseudoaldosteronism. *Am J Hosp Pharm* 1975; **32:** 73–4.
3. Bannister B, *et al.* Cardiac arrest due to liquorice-induced hypokalaemia. *BMJ* 1977; **2:** 738–9.
4. Werner S, *et al.* Hyperprolactinaemia and liquorice. *Lancet* 1979; **i:** 319.
5. Cumming AMM, *et al.* Severe hypokalaemia with paralysis induced by small doses of liquorice. *Postgrad Med J* 1980; **56:** 526–9.

6. Blachley JD, Knochel JP. Tobacco chewer's hypokalemia: licorice revisited. *N Engl J Med* 1980; **302:** 784–5.
7. Lai F, *et al.* Licorice, snuff, and hypokalemia. *N Engl J Med* 1980; **303:** 463.
8. Nightingale S, *et al.* Anorexia nervosa, liquorice and hypokalaemic myopathy. *Postgrad Med J* 1981; **57:** 577–9.
9. Cereda JM, *et al.* Liquorice intoxication caused by alcohol-free pastis. *Lancet* 1983; **i:** 1442.
10. Haberer JP, *et al.* Severe hypokalaemia secondary to overindulgence in alcohol-free "pastis". *Lancet* 1984; **i:** 575–6.
11. Nielsen I, Pedersen RS. Life-threatening hypokalaemia caused by liquorice ingestion. *Lancet* 1984; **i:** 1305.
12. Farese RV, *et al.* Licorice-induced hypermineralocorticoidism. *N Engl J Med* 1991; **325:** 1223–7.
13. Bauchart J-J, *et al.* Alcohol-free pastis and hypokalaemia. *Lancet* 1995; **346:** 1701.
14. de Klerk GJ, *et al.* Hypokalaemia and hypertension associated with use of liquorice flavoured chewing gum. *BMJ* 1997; **314:** 731–2.
15. Eriksson JW, *et al.* Life-threatening ventricular tachycardia due to liquorice-induced hypokalaemia. *J Intern Med* 1999; **245:** 307–10.
16. Edwards CRW. Lessons from licorice. *N Engl J Med* 1991; **325:** 1242–3.
17. Teelucksingh S, *et al.* Liquorice. *Lancet* 1991; **337:** 1549.
18. Walker BR, Edwards CR. Licorice-induced hypertension and syndromes of apparent mineralocorticoid excess. *Endocrinol Metab Clin North Am* 1994; **23:** 359–77.

Uses and Administration

Liquorice is used as a flavouring and sweetening agent. It has demulcent and expectorant properties and has been used in cough preparations. It has ulcer-healing properties which may result from stimulation of mucus synthesis. It also has mild anti-inflammatory and mineralocorticoid properties associated with the presence of glycyrrhizinic acid and its metabolite glycyrrhetinic acid, which is an inhibitor of cortisol metabolism. Liquorice may also possess some antispasmodic and laxative properties.

Deglycyrrhizinised liquorice has a reduced mineralocorticoid activity and has been used, usually in combination with antacids, for the treatment of peptic ulcer disease (p.1208). Ammonium glycyrrhizinate is used as a sweetener.

Preparations

Ph. Eur.: Liquorice Ethanolic Liquid Extract, Standardised.

Proprietary Preparations (details are given in Part 3)
Fr.: Trio D; *Ger.:* Fichtensirup N; Lakriment Neu; Suczulen mono; Ulgastrin Neu; *Jpn:* Glycyron†; Neo-Minophagen C†.

Multi-ingredient: numerous preparations are listed in Part 3.

Loperamide Hydrochloride (5235-b)

Loperamide Hydrochloride (BANM, USAN, rINNM).
Loperamidi Hydrochloridum; R-18553. 4-(4-*p*-Chlorophenyl-4-hydroxypiperidino)-NN-dimethyl-2,2-diphenylbutyramide hydrochloride.
$C_{29}H_{33}ClN_2O_2,HCl = 513.5.$
CAS — 53179-11-6 (loperamide); 34552-83-5 (loperamide hydrochloride).

Pharmacopoeias. In *Eur.* (see p.vi), *Int.*, and *US.*

Pharmacopoeial description

Ph. Eur.: A white or almost white powder. Slightly soluble in water; soluble in alcohol; freely soluble in methyl alcohol. Protect from light.

USP 25: A white to slightly yellow powder. Slightly soluble in water and in dilute acids; freely soluble in chloroform, in isopropyl alcohol, and in methyl alcohol.

Adverse Effects and Treatment

Abdominal pain or bloating, nausea, constipation, dry mouth, dizziness, fatigue, and hypersensitivity reactions including skin rashes have been reported. Loperamide hydrochloride has been associated with paralytic ileus, particularly in infants and young children, and deaths have been reported. Depression of the CNS, to which children may be more sensitive, may be seen in overdosage, and naloxone hydrochloride (see p.1015) has been recommended for its treatment.

◊ Some references to loperamide toxicity covering toxic megacolon[1,2] and severe effects in young children including coma,[3] paralytic ileus with death,[4] and delirium.[5]
1. Brown JW. Toxic megacolon associated with loperamide therapy. *JAMA* 1979; **241:** 501–2.
2. Walley T, Milson D. Loperamide related toxic megacolon in Clostridium difficile colitis. *Postgrad Med J* 1990; **66:** 582.
3. Minton NA, Smith PGD. Loperamide toxicity in a child after a single dose. *BMJ* 1987; **294:** 1383.
4. Bhutta TI, Tahir KI. Loperamide poisoning in children. *Lancet* 1990; **335:** 363.
5. Schwartz RH, Rodriquez WJ. Toxic delirium possibly caused by loperamide. *J Pediatr* 1991; **118:** 656–7.

Precautions

Loperamide should not be used when inhibition of peristalsis is to be avoided, in particular where ileus or constipation occur, and should be avoided in patients with abdominal distension, acute inflammatory bowel disease, or antibiotic-associated colitis. Loperamide should not be used alone in patients with dysentery.

Loperamide should be used with caution in patients with hepatic dysfunction because of its considerable first-pass metabolism in the liver. It should also be used with caution in young children because of a greater variability of response in this age group; it is not recommended for use in infants (see Uses and Administration, below).

Interactions

Co-trimoxazole. Concomitant administration with co-trimoxazole increases the bioavailability of loperamide,[1] apparently by inhibiting its first-pass metabolism.

1. Kamali F, Huang ML. Increased systemic availability of loperamide after oral administration of loperamide and loperamide oxide with cotrimoxazole. *Br J Clin Pharmacol* 1996; **41:** 125–8.

Pharmacokinetics

About 40% of a dose of loperamide is reported to be absorbed from the gastrointestinal tract to undergo first-pass metabolism in the liver and excretion in the faeces via the bile as inactive conjugate; there is slight urinary excretion. Little intact drug reaches the systemic circulation. The elimination half-life is reported to be about 10 hours.

Uses and Administration

Loperamide hydrochloride is a synthetic opioid analogue which inhibits gut motility and may also reduce gastrointestinal secretions. It is given by mouth as an antidiarrhoeal drug as an adjunct in the management of acute and chronic diarrhoeas and may also be used in the management of colostomies or ileostomies to reduce the volume of discharge.

In acute diarrhoea the usual initial dose for adults is 4 mg followed by 2 mg after each loose stool to a maximum of 16 mg daily; the usual daily dose is 6 to 8 mg. In the UK, loperamide hydrochloride is not recommended for children under 4 years of age. Suggested doses for older children are: 4 to 8 years, 1 mg three or four times daily for up to 3 days; 9 to 12 years, 2 mg four times daily for up to 5 days. In the USA, loperamide is not recommended for children under the age of 2 years and an initial dose of 1 mg three times daily is suggested for children aged 2 to 5 years. (For restrictions on the use of loperamide in children and the view that antidiarrhoeal drugs should not be used at all in children, see Diarrhoea, below.)

In chronic diarrhoea the usual initial dose for adults is 4 to 8 mg daily in divided doses subsequently adjusted as necessary; doses of 16 mg daily should not be exceeded. If no improvement has been observed after treatment with 16 mg daily for at least 10 days, further administration is unlikely to be of benefit.

Loperamide has also been given as the prodrug, loperamide oxide, which is converted to loperamide in the gastrointestinal tract. It has been given for acute diarrhoea in doses of 2 to 4 mg initially followed by 1 mg after each loose stool, to a maximum of 8 mg daily.

Diarrhoea. The mainstay of treatment for acute diarrhoea (p.1203) is rehydration therapy. Antidiarrhoeals like loperamide have a limited role for symptomatic relief in adults with acute diarrhoea, but WHO does not recommend the use of *any* antidiarrhoeal drug in children with diarrhoea. There have been problems regarding the use of antidiarrhoeals such as loperamide in young children in developing countries. Manufacturers have considered that a lower age limit is acceptable in those countries than is recommended in the UK or USA; even that lower limit is not always observed in practice and there have been reports of serious toxicity in very young children.[1] In response to such reports the manufacturers withdrew concentrated drops of loperamide worldwide and the syrup from countries where the WHO had a programme for control of diarrhoeal diseases, but tablets and capsules remain available.[2] In some countries the use of antidiarrhoeals is now restricted by law.

1. Bhutta TI, Tahir KI. Loperamide poisoning in children. *Lancet* 1990; **335:** 363.
2. Gussin RZ. Withdrawal of loperamide drops. *Lancet* 1990; **335:** 1603–4.

◊ References to the use of *loperamide oxide* in diarrhoea.
1. Van Den Eynden B, *et al.* New approaches to the treatment of patients with acute, nonspecific diarrhoea: a comparison of the effects of loperamide and loperamide oxide. *Curr Ther Res* 1995; **56:** 1132–41.
2. Hughes IW, *et al.* First-line treatment in acute non-dysenteric diarrhoea: clinical comparison of loperamide oxide, loperamide and placebo. *Br J Clin Pract* 1995; **49:** 181–5.
3. van Outryve M, Toussaint J. Loperamide oxide for the treatment of chronic diarrhoea in Crohn's disease. *J Int Med Res* 1995; **23:** 335–41.

Preparations

BP 2001: Loperamide Capsules;
USP 25: Loperamide Hydrochloride Capsules; Loperamide Hydrochloride Tablets.

Proprietary Preparations (details are given in Part 3)
Aust.: Arestal; Enterobene; Imodium; *Austral.:* Gastro-Stop; Imodium; *Belg.:* Ercestopyl; Imodium; Toriac†; *Braz.:* Closecs; Diarresec; Enteronorm; Imosec; Obstar; *Canad.:* Anti-Diarrheal; Diahalt; Diarr-Eze; Diarrhea Relief; Imodium; Loperacap; *Denm.:* Imodium; Propiden; Travello; *Fin.:* Imocur; Imodium; Lopex; *Fr.:* Altocel; Antidiar; Arestal; Celkalm; Diaretyl; Dyspagon; Ercestop; Imodium; Imossel; Indiaral; Lodiarid; Lopelin†; Nabutil; Nimaz; Peracel†; *Ger.:* Aperamid†; Azuperamid; Boxolip; D-Stop†; duralopid; Endiaron; Imodium; Logomed Durchfall-Kapseln†; Lop-Dia; Lopalind; Lopedium; Loperamerck†; Loperhoe; Lopetrans†; Mandros Diarstop†; Metifex-L; Sanifug; *Hong Kong:* Imodium; Loperax; Loperium; Lopermide; Reximide; *Irl.:* Arret; Diarrest RF; Imodium; *Israel:* Imodium; Kamidex; Loperid; Loperium; Stopit; *Ital.:* Dissenten; Imodium; Lodis†; Lopemid; Loperyl†; Ramidox; Tebloc; *Mex.:* Cryoperacid; Imodium; Pramidal; Raxamida; Raxedin; Top-Dal; *Neth.:* Arestal; Diacure; Imodium; *Norw.:* Imodium; Travello; *NZ:* Dicap; Imodium; *Port.:* Imodium; *S.Afr.:* Betaperamide; Gastron; Imodium; Lenide-T; Lopedium; Loperastat; Loperol; Norimode; Prodium; *Singapore:* Colodium; IMD; Imodium; Lorpa; Vacontil; *Spain:* Elissan; Fortasec; Imodium; Imosec; Loperan; Loperkey; Orulop†; Protector; Salvacolina NF; Taguinol; *Swed.:* Dimor; Imodium; Primodium; Travello; *Switz.:* Binaldan; Imodium; Lopimed; *Thai.:* Diarent; Diarodil; Entermid; Imodium; Impelium; Impore; Lomide; Lomy; Lopamine; Lopela; Lopercin; Lopredium; Loperia; Lopermide; Operium; Perasian; SBOB; Vacontil; *UK:* Arret; Diah-Limit; Diareze; Diasorb; Diocalm Ultra; Diocaps; Entrocalm; Imodium; Lodiar†; LoperaGen; Norimode; Normaloe; *USA:* Imodium; Kaopectate II; Maalox Anti-Diarrheal; Neo-Diaral; Pepto Diarrhea Control.

Multi-ingredient: *Austral.:* Imodium Advanced; *Canad.:* Imodium Advanced; *Fr.:* Imosselduo; *Ger.:* Imodium plus; *Neth.:* Diacure Plus; *NZ:* Imodium Advanced; *S.Afr.:* Imodium Plus; *Spain:* Imodium Plus; *Switz.:* Imodium Plus; *UK:* Imodium Plus; *USA:* Imodium Advanced; Kao-Paverin.

Loxiglumide (3692-y)

Loxiglumide (rINN).
CR-1505.   (±)-4-(3,4-Dichlorobenzamido)-*N*-(3-methoxypropyl)-*N*-pentylglutaramic acid.
$C_{21}H_{30}Cl_2N_2O_5 = 461.4$.
CAS — 107097-80-3.

Profile

Loxiglumide is a specific cholecystokinin antagonist related to proglumide (see p.1244), and has been investigated in biliary and gastrointestinal dyskinesias, constipation and irritable bowel syndrome, and pancreatitis.
The R-isomer of loxiglumide, dexloxiglumide is also under investigation for irritable bowel syndrome.

◊ References.
1. Meyer BM, *et al.* Role of cholecystokinin in regulation of gastrointestinal motor functions. *Lancet* 1989; **ii:** 12–15.
2. Beglinger C, *et al.* Treatment of biliary colic with loxiglumide. *Lancet* 1989; **ii:** 167.
3. Setnikar I, *et al.* Pharmacokinetics and tolerance of repeated oral doses of loxiglumide. *Arzneimittelforschung* 1989; **39:** 1454–9.
4. Meier R, *et al.* Therapeutic effects of loxiglumide, a cholecystokinin antagonist, on chronic constipation in elderly patients: a prospective, randomized, double-blind, controlled trial. *J Gastrointest Mot* 1993; **5:** 129–35.
5. Lieverse RJ, *et al.* Effects of somatostatin and loxiglumide on gallbladder motility. *Eur J Clin Pharmacol* 1995; **47:** 489–92.

Magaldrate (695-z)

Magaldrate (BAN, USAN, rINN).
Aluminum Magnesium Hydroxide Sulfate; AY-5710; Magaldratum.
$Al_5Mg_{10}(OH)_{31}(SO_4)_2,xH_2O = 1097.3$ (anhydrous).
CAS — 74978-16-8.
ATC — A02AD02.

NOTE. Magaldrate was formerly described as Aluminium Magnesium Hydroxide ($AlMg_2(OH)_7$ monohydrate, CAS—1317-26-6).

Pharmacopoeias. In *Eur.* (see p.vi) and *US*.

Pharmacopoeial description

Ph. Eur.: A combination of aluminium and magnesium hydroxides (see p.1210 and p.1233 respectively) and sulfates. It contains the equivalent of 90 to 105% of $Al_5Mg_{10}(OH)_{31}(SO_4)_2$, calculated with reference to the dried substance. A white or almost white crystalline powder. Practically insoluble in water and in alcohol; soluble in dilute mineral acids. It loses between 10 and 20% of its weight on drying at 200° for 4 hours.

USP 25: A combination of aluminium and magnesium hydroxides and sulfates. It contains the equivalent of 90 to 105% of $Al_5Mg_{10}(SO_4)_2$, calculated on the dried basis. A white odourless crystalline powder. Insoluble in water and in alcohol; soluble in dilute solutions of mineral acids. It loses between 10 and 20% of its weight on drying at 200° for 4 hours.

Profile

Magaldrate is an antacid (see p.1201) that is given in doses of up to about 2 g by mouth.

Preparations

BP 2001: Magaldrate Oral Suspension;
USP 25: Magaldrate and Simethicone Oral Suspension; Magaldrate and Simethicone Tablets; Magaldrate Oral Suspension; Magaldrate Tablets.

Proprietary Preparations (details are given in Part 3)
Aust.: Riopan; *Belg.:* Gastricalm; Riopan; *Braz.:* Riopan; Selanac; *Canad.:* Riopan; *Fr.:* Riopan; *Ger.:* Gastrimagal†; Gastripan; Gastrostad†; Glysan; Hevert-Mag; Logomed Magen†; Magalphil†; Magasan†; Magastron; Magmed†; Marax; ProWohl†; Riopan; Simaphil; *Ital.:* Riopan; *Neth.:* Riopan; *Port.:* Riopan; *S.Afr.:* Gastrobon†; Riopone†; *Spain:* Bemolan; Gastromol; Magion; Minoton; *Switz.:* Riopan; *UK:* Dynese; *USA:* Iosopan; Riopan.

Multi-ingredient: *Austral.:* Mylanta Heartburn Relief; *Braz.:* Riopan Plus; *Canad.:* Riopan Plus; *Hong Kong:* Nilcid-MPS; *Mex.:* Nilcid; Riopan; *Spain:* Compagel; *UK:* Bisodol Heartburn Relief; *USA:* Iosopan Plus; Lowsium Plus; Riopan Plus.

Magnesium Carbonate (698-a)

E504; Magnesii Subcarbonas.
CAS — 546-93-0 (anhydrous magnesium carbonate); 23389-33-5 (hydrated normal magnesium carbonate); 39409-82-0 (hydrated basic magnesium carbonate).
ATC — A02AA01; A06AD01.

Pharmacopoeias. In *Chin., Eur.* (see p.vi), *Jpn, Pol.,* and *US.* Some pharmacopoeias include a single monograph which permits both the light and heavy varieties while some have 2 separate monographs for the 2 varieties.

Pharmacopoeial description

Ph. Eur.: Heavy Magnesium Carbonate and Light Magnesium Carbonate are hydrated basic magnesium carbonates containing the equivalent of 40 to 45% of MgO. Both are white powders and are practically insoluble in water but dissolve in dilute acids with strong effervescence. For the heavy variety 15 g occupies a volume of about 30 mL and for the light variety 15 g occupies a volume of about 180 mL.

USP 25: A basic hydrated magnesium carbonate or a normal hydrated magnesium carbonate containing the equivalent of 40.0 to 43.5% of MgO. It is an odourless, bulky white powder or light, white, friable masses. Practically insoluble in water; insoluble in alcohol; dissolves in dilute acids with effervescence.

Profile

Magnesium carbonate is an antacid with general properties similar to those of magnesium hydroxide (below) that is given in doses of up to about 500 mg by mouth. When administered by mouth, it reacts with gastric acid to form soluble magnesium chloride and carbon dioxide in the stomach; the carbon dioxide may cause flatulence and eructation. Magnesium carbonate is often given in conjunction with aluminium-containing antacids such as aluminium hydroxide which counteract its laxative effect.

Magnesium carbonate may be used as a magnesium supplement. It is also used as a food additive.

Preparations

BP 2001: Aromatic Magnesium Carbonate Mixture; Compound Magnesium Trisilicate Oral Powder; Kaolin Mixture; Magnesium Sulphate Mixture; Magnesium Trisilicate Mixture;
USP 25: Alumina and Magnesium Carbonate Oral Suspension; Alumina and Magnesium Carbonate Tablets; Alumina, Magnesium Carbonate, and Magnesium Oxide Tablets; Calcium and Magnesium Carbonates Oral Suspension; Calcium and Magnesium Carbonates Tablets; Magnesium Carbonate and Citric Acid for Oral Solution; Magnesium Carbonate and Sodium Bicarbonate for Oral Suspension; Magnesium Citrate Oral Solution.

Proprietary Preparations (details are given in Part 3)
Aust.: Tetesept Magnesium; *Belg.:* Magnezyme; *Canad.:* Cepasium†; *Fr.:* Mag 2; Magnosol; *Ger.:* Palmicol; *Ital.:* Magnofit; *USA:* Mag-Carb.

Multi-ingredient: numerous preparations are listed in Part 3.

Magnesium Citrate (1173-x)

$C_{12}H_{10}Mg_3O_{14} = 451.1$.
CAS — 3344-18-1.
ATC — A12CC04; B05CB03.
Pharmacopoeias. In *US*.

Pharmacopoeial description

USP 25: A 5% suspension in water has a pH of 5.0 to 9.0. Store in airtight containers.

Profile

Magnesium citrate is an osmotic laxative (p.1201) used as a bowel evacuant prior to investigational procedures or surgery of the colon. For one UK product (*Citramag*), an aqueous solution containing 17.7 g of magnesium citrate is prepared from a sachet containing magnesium carbonate and anhydrous citric acid by mixing with 200 mL of hot water. After the solution has cooled, one dose is taken by mouth at 8 a.m. the day before the procedure, and a second dose between 2 and 4 p.m. Dosages with other preparations have ranged from about 11 to 25 g of magnesium citrate. A high fluid intake and low residue diet are needed in conjunction with such bowel preparation. It is also used in combination with sodium picosulfate p.1249.

Magnesium citrate is also used as a magnesium supplement in doses of up to about 1.9 g daily by mouth.

For the general properties of magnesium salts, see p.1190.

Migraine. For mention of the use of magnesium supplementation, including magnesium citrate, for the prophylaxis of migraine, see p.1192.

Preparations
USP 25: Magnesium Citrate for Oral Solution.

Proprietary Preparations (details are given in Part 3)
Aust.: Magnesium Diasporal; *Austral.:* Mag Cit Prep; *Canad.:* Citro-Mag; *Ger.:* Magnesium Diasporal; Magnesium Tonil N; Magnorell; Presselin Heilozon P; *Hong Kong:* Citro-Mag; *Mon.:* Oromag; *Switz.:* Magnesium Biomed; Magnesium Diasporal; *UK:* Citramag; *USA:* Evac-Q-Mag.

Multi-ingredient: *Aust.:* Biovital Weissdorn; Magnofit; *Austral.:* Go Kit; Go Kit Plus; *Belg.:* Carbobel; *Canad.:* Evac-Q-Kwik†; Royvac Kit; *Fr.:* Citrocholine; *Ger.:* Acidovert; Lithurex; Magnerot N†; *Irl.:* Picolax; *Spain:* Salmagne; *UK:* Picolax; Porosis D; *USA:* Fleet Prep Kit No. 4†; Fleet Prep Kit No. 5†; Fleet Prep Kit No. 6†; Tridrate Bowel Evacuant Kit†.

Magnesium Hydroxide (699-t)

E528; Magnesii Hydroxidum; Magnesium Hydrate.
Mg(OH)$_2$ = 58.32.
CAS — 1309-42-8.
ATC — A02AA04; G04BX01.

NOTE. Compounded preparations of magnesium hydroxide may be represented by the following names:
• Co-magaldrox *x/y* (*BAN*)—where *x* and *y* are the strengths in milligrams of magnesium hydroxide and aluminium hydroxide respectively.

Pharmacopoeias. In Eur. (see p.vi), Int., and US.

Pharmacopoeial description
Ph. Eur.: A fine white amorphous powder. Practically insoluble in water; dissolves in dilute acids. A solution in water is alkaline to phenolphthalein.
USP 25: A bulky white powder. Practically insoluble in water, in alcohol, in chloroform, and in ether; soluble in dilute acids. Store in airtight containers.

Adverse Effects, Treatment, and Precautions
As for magnesium salts in general, see p.1191. Magnesium hydroxide may cause diarrhoea, an effect that is dose-dependent. Hypermagnesaemia may occur, usually in patients with impaired renal function.

◊ Reports of hypermagnesaemia in infants given magnesium-containing antacids,[1,2] and in a patient with normal renal function but bowel obstruction.[3]

1. Brand JM, Greer FR. Hypermagnesemia and intestinal perforation following antacid administration in a premature infant. *Pediatrics* 1990; **85:** 121–4.
2. Alison LH, Bulugahapitiya D. Laxative induced magnesium poisoning in a 6 week old infant. *BMJ* 1990; **300:** 125.
3. Laughlin SA, McKinney PE. Antacid-induced hypermagnesemia in a patient with normal renal function and bowel obstruction. *Ann Pharmacother* 1998; **32:** 312–15.

Interactions
As outlined on p.1201, antacids, including magnesium salts, interact with many other drugs both by alterations in gastric pH and emptying, and by formation of complexes that are not absorbed. Interactions can be minimised by giving the antacid and any other medications 2 to 3 hours apart.

Pharmacokinetics
Magnesium hydroxide, given by mouth, reacts relatively rapidly with hydrochloric acid in the stomach to form magnesium chloride and water. About 30 to 50% of the magnesium ions are absorbed from the small intestine, as described for Magnesium Salts, p.1191.

Uses and Administration
Magnesium hydroxide is an antacid (see p.1201) that is given in doses of up to about 1 g by mouth. It is

often given in conjunction with aluminium-containing antacids such as aluminium hydroxide which counteract its laxative effect.

Magnesium hydroxide is also given as an osmotic laxative (p.1201) in doses of up to about 5 g by mouth.

Magnesium hydroxide has also been used as a food additive and as a magnesium supplement in deficiency states.

Preparations
BP 2001: Co-magaldrox Oral Suspension; Co-magaldrox Tablets; Liquid Paraffin and Magnesium Hydroxide Oral Emulsion; Magnesium Hydroxide Mixture;
USP 25: Alumina and Magnesia Oral Suspension; Alumina and Magnesia Tablets; Alumina, Magnesia, and Calcium Carbonate Oral Suspension; Alumina, Magnesia, and Calcium Carbonate Tablets; Alumina, Magnesia, and Simethicone Oral Suspension; Alumina, Magnesia, and Simethicone Tablets; Alumina, Magnesia, Calcium Carbonate, and Simethicone Tablets; Aspirin, Alumina, and Magnesia Tablets; Calcium Carbonate and Magnesia Tablets; Calcium Carbonate, Magnesia, and Simethicone Tablets; Magnesia Tablets; Magnesium Hydroxide Paste; Milk of Magnesia.

Proprietary Preparations (details are given in Part 3)
Braz.: Leite de Magnesia de Phillips; Leite de Magnesia Honfar; Magnesia Fluida; Mylanta Plus; *Canad.:* Phillips' Milk of Magnesia; *Denm.:* Magnesia; *Fin.:* Emgesan; Magnesiamaito; *Fr.:* Carbonex; Chlorumagene†; Magnesie S Pellegrino; *Irl.:* Milk of Magnesia; *Israel:* Magnesia S Pellegrino; *Ital.:* Citrato Espresso S. Pellegrino; Magnesia S Pellegrino; Magnesia Volta; *Port.:* Leite de Magnesia; *S.Afr.:* Deopens; *Spain:* Crema de Magnesia; Magnesia; Magnesia san Pellegrino; *Swed.:* Emgesan; *Switz.:* Chlorumagene; Magnesia S Pellegrino; *UK:* Milk of Magnesia; *USA:* Phillips' Chewable; Phillips' Milk of Magnesia.

Multi-ingredient: numerous preparations are listed in Part 3.

Magnesium Oxide (702-r)

E530; Magnesii Oxidum.
MgO = 40.30.
CAS — 1309-48-4.
ATC — A02AA02; A06AD02.

Pharmacopoeias. In Chin., Eur. (see p.vi), Int., Jpn, Pol., and US. Some pharmacopoeias include a single monograph which permits both the light and heavy varieties while some have 2 separate monographs for the 2 varieties.

Pharmacopoeial description
Ph. Eur.: Heavy Magnesium Oxide and Light Magnesium Oxide are fine white powders and are practically insoluble in water yielding solutions that are alkaline to phenolphthalein. Both heavy and light magnesium oxide dissolve in dilute acids with at most slight effervescence. For the heavy variety 15 g occupies a volume of about 30 mL and for the light variety 15 g occupies a volume of about 150 mL.

USP 25: Magnesium Oxide is either the heavy or light variety. Heavy magnesium oxide is a relatively dense white powder with 5 g occupying a volume of about 10 to 20 mL. Light magnesium oxide is a very bulky white powder with 5 g occupying a volume of about 40 to 50 mL. Both varieties are practically insoluble in water; insoluble in alcohol; soluble in dilute acids. Store in airtight containers.

Profile
Magnesium oxide is an antacid with general properties similar to those of magnesium hydroxide (above). It is given in usual doses of about 400 mg by mouth. It is often given in conjunction with aluminium-containing antacids such as aluminium hydroxide which counteract its laxative effect.

Magnesium oxide has been employed for its osmotic laxative properties in bowel preparation; doses of 3.5 g by mouth are given for this purpose, combined with bisacodyl or sodium picosulfate.

Magnesium oxide is also used as a magnesium supplement in deficiency states in doses of up to 800 mg (20 mmol) daily by mouth. It is also used as a food additive.

Preparations
USP 25: Alumina, Magnesium Carbonate, and Magnesium Oxide Tablets; Aromatic Cascara Fluidextract; Aspirin, Alumina, and Magnesium Oxide Tablets; Citric Acid, Magnesium Oxide, and Sodium Carbonate Irrigation; Magnesium Oxide Capsules; Magnesium Oxide Tablets.

Proprietary Preparations (details are given in Part 3)
Aust.: Magnofit; Magnonorm; *Denm.:* Salilax; *Fr.:* Magnosol; Magocean; *Ger.:* Dystomin M†; Magium; Magnesium Diasporal; Magnetrans forte; *S.Afr.:* Solumag; *Swed.:* Salilax; *Thai.:* Magoral; *USA:* Mag-200; Mag-Ox; Maox; Uro-Mag.

Multi-ingredient: numerous preparations are listed in Part 3.

Magnesium Trisilicate (704-d)

E553(a); Magnesii Trisilicas.
CAS — 14987-04-3 (anhydrous magnesium trisilicate); 39365-87-2 (magnesium trisilicate hydrate).

NOTE. Magnesium trisilicate is regarded as a type of magnesium silicate. The code 553(a) seems to have been applied to both.
Pharmacopoeias. In Chin., Eur. (see p.vi), Jpn, and US.

A hydrated magnesium silicate.
Pharmacopoeial description
Ph. Eur.: Has variable composition corresponding approximately to the formula Mg$_2$Si$_3$O$_8$,xH$_2$O containing not less than 29% of magnesium oxide and not less than the equivalent of 65% of silicon dioxide, both calculated with reference to the ignited substance. A white powder. Practically insoluble in water and in alcohol.

USP 25: A compound of magnesium oxide and silicon dioxide with varying proportions of water. It contains not less than 20% of magnesium oxide and not less than 45% of silicon dioxide. A fine, white, odourless, powder, free from grittiness. Insoluble in water and in alcohol. It is readily decomposed by mineral acids.

Profile
Magnesium trisilicate is an antacid with general properties similar to those of magnesium hydroxide (p.1233). It is given in doses of up to about 2 g by mouth. When given by mouth it reacts more slowly with hydrochloric acid in the stomach than magnesium hydroxide. Magnesium trisilicate is often given in conjunction with aluminium-containing antacids such as aluminium hydroxide which counteract its laxative effect.
Magnesium trisilicate is also used as a food additive.

Effects on the kidneys. A 68-year-old man with a history of renal calculus passed a 300-mg stone which was found to consist chiefly of silica.[1] He had been taking the equivalent of 2 g of magnesium trisilicate daily for many years.

1. Joekes AM, *et al.* Multiple renal silica calculi. *BMJ* 1973; **1:** 146–7.

Preparations
BP 2001: Compound Magnesium Trisilicate Oral Powder; Compound Magnesium Trisilicate Tablets; Magnesium Trisilicate Mixture;
USP 25: Alumina and Magnesium Trisilicate Oral Suspension; Alumina and Magnesium Trisilicate Tablets; Magnesium Trisilicate Tablets.

Proprietary Preparations (details are given in Part 3)
Ger.: Solitab†; *Spain:* Mabosil†; Silimag.

Multi-ingredient: numerous preparations are listed in Part 3.

Manna (604-t)

Manne en Larmes.
Pharmacopoeias. In Aust. It. permits other Fraxinus species.

The dried exudation from the bark of the European flowering ash, *Fraxinus ornus* (Oleaceae), containing about 40 to 60% of mannitol (p.924).

Profile
Manna has been used as an osmotic laxative.

Preparations
Proprietary Preparations (details are given in Part 3)
Multi-ingredient: *Aust.:* Krauterdoktor Entschlackungs-Elixier; Sinolax-Milder; St Radegunder Entschlackungs-Elixier; *Ger.:* florabio Mann-Feigen-Sirup mit Senna; Infi-tract N; Schwedentrunk mit Ginseng†; Schwedentrunk†; *Ital.:* Certobil†.

Mebeverine Hydrochloride (5236-v)

Mebeverine Hydrochloride (BANM, USAN, rINNM).
CSAG-144. 4-[Ethyl(4-methoxy-α-methylphenethyl)amino]butyl veratrate hydrochloride.
C$_{25}$H$_{35}$NO$_5$,HCl = 466.0.
CAS — 3625-06-7 (mebeverine); 2753-45-9 (mebeverine hydrochloride).
Pharmacopoeias. In Br.

Pharmacopoeial description
BP 2001: A white or almost white crystalline powder. Very soluble in water; freely soluble in alcohol; practically insoluble in ether. A 2% solution in water has a pH of 4.5 to 6.5. Store in airtight containers at a temperature not exceeding 30°. Protect from light.

Adverse Effects and Precautions
Although adverse effects appear rare, gastrointestinal disturbances, dizziness, headache, insomnia, anorexia, and decreased heart rate have been reported in patients receiving mebeverine. Mebeverine should be avoided in patients with paralytic ileus. Based on theoretical concerns, it should be used with care in patients with marked hepatic or renal impairment, and those with cardiac disorders such as heart block.

◊ A 24-year-old man with cystic fibrosis, prescribed mebeverine hydrochloride for lower abdominal pain and constipation, was found to have a perforated stercoral ulcer with generalised peritonitis.[1] It was suggested that mebeverine produced colonic stasis which predisposed the patient to ulceration,[1] but the manufacturers[2] considered that the concomitant development of constipation and distal intestinal syndrome (meconium ileus equivalent) in this patient precipitated the development of stercoral ulceration. It was recommended[1] that antispasmodics such as mebeverine should not be used for the symptomatic treatment of distal intestinal syndrome in cystic fibrosis.

1. Hassan W, Keaney N. Mebeverine-induced perforated colon in distal intestinal syndrome of cystic fibrosis. *Lancet* 1990; **335:** 1225.
2. Whitehead AM. Perforation of colon in distal intestinal syndrome of cystic fibrosis. *Lancet* 1990; **336:** 446.

Porphyria. Mebeverine hydrochloride is considered to be unsafe in patients with porphyria because it has been shown to be porphyrinogenic in *in-vitro* systems.

Pharmacokinetics
Mebeverine is absorbed after administration by mouth, with peak plasma concentrations occurring in 1 to 3 hours. It is 75% bound to albumin in plasma. Mebeverine is completely metabolised by hydrolysis to veratric acid and mebeverine alcohol, the latter of which may then be conjugated. The metabolites are excreted in the urine.

Uses and Administration
Mebeverine hydrochloride is an antispasmodic with a direct action on the smooth muscle of the gastrointestinal tract. It is used in conditions such as irritable bowel syndrome (p.1206) in doses of 135 mg three times daily by mouth before meals, or 100 mg three or four times daily. A modified-release preparation is also available, taken as 200 mg twice daily. The embonate is also used in a dose equivalent to 150 mg of the hydrochloride three times daily.

Preparations
BP 2001: Mebeverine Tablets.

Proprietary Preparations (details are given in Part 3)
Aust.: Colofac; *Austral.:* Colese; Colofac; *Belg.:* Duspatalin; Spasmoval; *Denm.:* Duspatalin; *Fr.:* Colopriv; Duspatalin; Spasmopriv; *Ger.:* Duspatal; Mebemerck; *Hong Kong:* Duspatalin; *Irl.:* Colofac; *Israel:* Colotal; *Ital.:* Duspatal; *Neth.:* Duspatal; *NZ:* Colofac; *Port.:* Duspatal; *S.Afr.:* Bevispas; Colofac; *Singapore:* Duspatalin; Mebetin; *Spain:* Duspatalin; *Switz.:* Duspatalin; *Thai.:* Colofac; Menosor; *UK:* Colofac; Equilon; Fomac†; IBS Relief.

Multi-ingredient: *Irl.:* Fybogel Mebeverine; *Singapore:* Fybogel Mebeverine; *UK:* Fybogel Mebeverine.

Mesalazine   (16887-a)

Mesalazine *(BAN, rINN).*

5-Aminosalicylic Acid; 5-ASA; Fisalamine; Mesalamine *(USAN).* 5-Amino-2-salicylic acid.
$C_7H_7NO_3 = 153.1.$
CAS — 89-57-6.
ATC — A07EC02.

NOTE. Distinguish from 4-aminosalicylic acid (Aminosalicylic Acid, p.148) which is used in the treatment of tuberculosis.
Pharmacopoeias. In Belg. and US.

Pharmacopoeial description
USP 25: Light tan to pink needle-shaped crystals, odourless or with a slight characteristic odour. The colour may darken on exposure to air. Slightly soluble in water; very slightly soluble in dehydrated alcohol, in acetone, and in methyl alcohol; practically insoluble in butyl alcohol, in chloroform, in dichloromethane, in ether, in ethyl acetate, in *n*-hexane, and in propyl alcohol; soluble in dilute hydrochloric acid and in dilute alkali hydroxides. A 2.5% suspension in water has a pH of 3.5 to 4.5. Store in airtight containers. Protect from light.

Adverse Effects and Precautions
Mesalazine may cause headache and gastrointestinal disturbances, such as nausea, diarrhoea, and abdominal pain. Hypersensitivity reactions may occasionally occur. Some patients may experience exacerbation of symptoms of colitis. There are some reports of myocarditis, pericarditis, pancreatitis, interstitial nephritis, nephrotic syndrome, allergic lung reaction, increased liver enzyme values, hepatitis, lupus-like syndrome, alopecia, myalgia, and arthralgia. Blood disorders reported rarely include aplastic anaemia, agranulocytosis, leucopenia, neutropenia, thrombocytopenia, and methaemoglobinaemia.

Mesalazine should not be given to patients with severely impaired renal or hepatic function or salicylate hypersensitivity. It should be used with caution in the elderly, and in mild to moderate renal or hepatic impairment, active peptic ulceration, or sulfasalazine allergy.

If a blood dyscrasia is suspected treatment should be stopped immediately and a blood count performed.

Patients or their carers should be told how to recognise signs of blood toxicity and should be advised to seek immediate medical attention if symptoms such as fever, sore throat, mouth ulcers, bruising, or bleeding develop. It has been recommended that renal function be monitored during therapy but see Effects on the Kidneys, below.

◊ Many of the adverse effects associated with sulfasalazine therapy have been attributed to the sulfapyridine moiety and most patients unable to tolerate sulfasalazine because of hypersensitivity or adverse reactions can be transferred to mesalazine without adverse effects occurring.[1-4] However, a small number of patients also experience adverse effects while taking mesalazine and these are often very similar to those seen with sulfasalazine.[1-4] They may include nausea, abdominal discomfort or pain, exacerbation of diarrhoea, headache, fever, and rashes. Mesalazine is not associated with sulfasalazine's adverse effects on sperm.

Mesalazine therapy should be initiated cautiously in patients with a history of sulfasalazine hypersensitivity and it should be withdrawn if signs of sensitivity develop or if there is diarrhoea or rectal bleeding. It has been suggested[2] that patients with a history of sulfasalazine hypersensitivity should be given test doses of mesalazine before starting a full course.

1. Dew MJ, et al. Treatment of ulcerative colitis with oral 5-aminosalicylic acid in patients unable to take sulphasalazine. *Lancet* 1983; **ii:** 801.
2. Campieri M, et al. 5-Aminosalicylic acid as rectal enema in ulcerative colitis patients unable to take sulphasalazine. *Lancet* 1984; **i:** 403.
3. Donald IP, Wilkinson SP. The value of 5-aminosalicylic acid in inflammatory bowel disease for patients intolerant or allergic to sulphasalazine. *Postgrad Med J* 1985; **61:** 1047–8.
4. Rao SS, et al. Clinical experience of the tolerance of mesalazine and olsalazine in patients intolerant of sulphasalazine. *Scand J Gastroenterol* 1987; **22:** 332–6.

Breast feeding. The concentrations of mesalazine in maternal plasma and breast milk in a lactating woman taking 500 mg three times daily, were 410 and 110 nanograms per mL respectively.[1] Although it was considered that the amount of mesalazine excreted in breast milk was small and that it was safe during breast feeding,[2,3] maternal use of mesalazine 500 mg suppositories twice daily has been associated with watery diarrhoea in a breast-fed infant.[2]

1. Jenss H, et al. 5-Aminosalicylic acid and its metabolite in breast milk during lactation. *Am J Gastroenterol* 1990; **85:** 331.
2. Nelis GF. Diarrhoea due to 5-aminosalicylic acid in breast milk. *Lancet* 1989; **i:** 383.
3. Klotz U, Harings-Kaim A. Negligible excretion of 5-aminosalicylic acid in breast milk. *Lancet* 1993; **342:** 618–19.

Effects on the blood. Although uncommon, mesalazine-associated adverse effects on the blood have been reported, including thrombocytopenia,[1] neutropenia,[2] fatal aplastic anaemia,[3] and pancytopenia.[4] In July 1995 the UK Committee on Safety of Medicines stated that it had been notified of 49 haematological reactions suspected of being associated with mesalazine,[5] including 5 reports of aplastic anaemia, 1 of agranulocytosis, 11 of leucopenia, and 17 of thrombocytopenia. There had been 3 fatalities. They recommended a blood count and immediate withdrawal of the drug if a dyscrasia was suspected. Antilymphocyte immunoglobulin has been used in the management of mesalazine-associated aplastic anaemia.[6]

1. Daneshmend TK. Mesalazine-associated thrombocytopenia. *Lancet* 1991; **337:** 1297–8.
2. Wyatt S, et al. Filgrastim for mesalazine-associated neutropenia. *Lancet* 1993; **341:** 1476.
3. Abboudi ZH, et al. Fatal aplastic anaemia after mesalazine. *Lancet* 1994; **343:** 542.
4. Kotanagi H, et al. Pancytopenia associated with 5-aminosalicylic acid use in a patient with Crohn's disease. *J Gastroenterol* 1998; **33:** 571–4.
5. Committee on Safety of Medicines/Medicines Control Agency. Blood dyscrasias and mesalazine. *Current Problems* 1995; **21:** 5–6.
6. Laidlaw ST, Reilly JT. Antilymphocyte globulin for mesalazine-associated aplastic anaemia. *Lancet* 1994; **343:** 981–2.

Effects on the cardiovascular system. Myocarditis associated with chest pain and ECG abnormalities has been reported[1,2] in 2 patients taking mesalazine; 1 patient died in cardiogenic shock.[2] It was suggested that mesalazine or sulfasalazine should be replaced by glucocorticoids if cardiac symptoms arise during treatment.[2] Pericarditis[3,4] together with fever, rash, dyspnoea, pleural and pericardial effusions, and arthritis, has also been described, and is considered to constitute a drug-induced lupus-like syndrome.

1. Agnholt J, et al. Cardiac hypersensitivity to 5-aminosalicylic acid. *Lancet* 1989; **i:** 1135.
2. Kristensen KS, et al. Fatal myocarditis associated with mesalazine. *Lancet* 1990; **335:** 605.
3. Dent MT, et al. Mesalazine induced lupus-like syndrome. *BMJ* 1992; **305:** 159.
4. Lim AG, Hine KR. Fever, vasculitic rash, arthritis, pericarditis, and pericardial effusion after mesalazine. *BMJ* 1994; **308:** 113.

Effects on the hair. For a report of accelerated hair loss from the scalp in 2 patients receiving mesalazine enemas, see under Sulfasalazine, p.1252.

Effects on the kidneys. The risk of nephrotoxicity may be low for mesalazine and the related compounds sulfasalazine and olsalazine.[1] Even so, adverse effects on the kidneys have

occurred and between February 1988 and December 1990 the UK Committee on Safety of Medicines[2] received 9 reports of serious nephrotoxic reactions associated with the use of Asacol, a modified-release mesalazine preparation. The reactions included 4 cases of interstitial nephritis, 3 of severe renal failure, and 2 cases of nephrotic syndrome. A subsequent case report[3] indicated that by September 1998 the number of such reports for mesalazine totalled 104, including 35 cases of interstitial nephritis. The authors considered that monitoring of renal function was required in patients receiving mesalazine. A protocol for such monitoring has been suggested,[4] with serum creatinine being estimated before treatment, then monthly for 3 months, 3-monthly for 9 months, 6-monthly thereafter and annually after 5 years of treatment; however, the *British National Formulary* considers the practical value of such monitoring unproven. The nephrotic syndrome[5] and interstitial nephritis[6] have also been reported with sulfasalazine.

1. Anonymous. Choosing an oral 5-aminosalicylic acid preparation for ulcerative colitis. *Drug Ther Bull* 1992; **30:** 50–2.
2. Committee on Safety of Medicines. Nephrotoxicity associated with mesalazine (Asacol). *Current Problems 30* 1990.
3. Popoola J, et al. Late onset interstitial nephritis associated with mesalazine treatment. *BMJ* 1998; **317:** 795–7.
4. Corrigan G, Stevens PE. Review article: interstitial nephritis associated with the use of mesalazine in inflammatory bowel disease. *Aliment Pharmacol Ther* 2000; **14:** 1–6.
5. Barbour VM, Williams PF. Nephrotic syndrome associated with sulphasalazine. *BMJ* 1990; **301:** 818.
6. Dwarakanath AD, et al. Sulphasalazine induced renal failure. *Gut* 1992; **33:** 1006–1007.

Effects on the liver. A case of chronic hepatitis and liver fibrosis have been reported after prolonged mesalazine administration.[1] The authors considered that mesalazine should be discontinued when liver dysfunction occurred.

1. Deltenre P, et al. Mesalazine (5-aminosalicylic acid) induced chronic hepatitis. *Gut* 1999; **44:** 886–8.

Effects on the nervous system. Peripheral neuropathy,[1] mainly affecting the legs, has occurred during mesalazine treatment. The symptoms resolved on discontinuing the drug. Mononeuritis multiplex was part of the presentation of an eosinophilic reaction attributed to mesalazine in an asthmatic patient;[2] Churg-Strauss syndrome developed after withdrawal of mesalazine, but the patient subsequently recovered without sequelae.

1. Woodward DK. Peripheral neuropathy and mesalazine. *BMJ* 1989; **299:** 1224.
2. Morice AH, et al. Mesalazine activation of eosinophil. *Lancet* 1997; **350:** 1105.

Effects on the pancreas. Reports of pancreatitis, with abdominal pain and raised serum amylase activity, in 2 patients taking mesalazine.[1,2] The reaction was confirmed by rechallenge in both patients and symptoms resolved on withdrawal of mesalazine. The UK Committee on Safety of Medicines had received 15 reports[3] of pancreatitis associated with mesalazine therapy at February 1994.

1. Sachedina B, et al. Acute pancreatitis due to 5-aminosalicylate. *Ann Intern Med* 1989; **110:** 490–2.
2. Deprez P, et al. Pancreatitis induced by 5-aminosalicylic acid. *Lancet* 1989; **ii:** 445–6.
3. Committee on Safety of Medicines. Drug-induced pancreatitis. *Current Problems* 1994; **20:** 2–3.

Effects on the respiratory system. Pulmonary complications occur rarely with sulfasalazine (see p.1252). It is not known which component of sulfasalazine is responsible although, following a report of alveolitis in a patient with ulcerative colitis given mesalazine,[1] it was concluded that both sulfasalazine and 5-aminosalicylate (mesalazine) could induce hypersensitivity lung disease. Similar cases have since been reported,[2-4] and pulmonary symptoms may also manifest as part of a broader lupus-like syndrome (see Effects on the Cardiovascular System, above).

1. Welte T, et al. Mesalazine alveolitis. *Lancet* 1991; **338:** 1273. Correction *ibid.* 1992; **339:** 70.
2. Honeybourne D. Mesalazine toxicity. *BMJ* 1994; **308:** 533–4.
3. Pascual-Lledó JF, et al. Interstitial pneumonitis due to mesalamine. *Ann Pharmacother* 1997; **31:** 499.
4. Sesin GP, et al. Mesalamine-associated pleural effusion with pulmonary infiltration. *Am J Health-Syst Pharm* 1998; **55:** 2304–5.

Lupus. For reports of lupus-like syndrome occurring with mesalazine, see Effects on the Cardiovascular System, above.

Pregnancy. Renal insufficiency in a neonate whose mother received mesalazine 2 to 4 g daily by mouth during the second trimester of pregnancy was suggested to be due to the drug,[1] although the proposed mechanism, inhibition of prostaglandin synthesis in the neonatal kidney, has been questioned.[2] A subsequent case-control study[3] found that use of oral mesalazine in 165 pregnant women with inflammatory bowel disease was not associated with a greater incidence of malformations. However, women treated with mesalazine were more likely to have preterm deliveries and newborns with decreased birth-weights, although the disease may have been a factor in this finding. A commentator on this study,[4] considered that active inflammatory bowel disease was a greater risk to pregnancy than drug treatment. In a further cohort of 123 pregnancies,[5] oral mesalazine at doses of 3 g daily or less did not increase the risk of fetal malformations or affect pregnancy outcome. The researchers concluded that further information was required on doses higher than 3 g daily. In another study,[6] all of 19 pregnancies in women receiving rectal mesalazine were full-term with no fetal abnormalities. For a discussion of sulfasalazine in pregnancy, see p.1252.

1. Colombel J-F, et al. Renal insufficiency in infant: side-effect of prenatal exposure to mesalazine? Lancet 1994; 344: 620–1.
2. Marteau P, Devaux CB. Mesalazine during pregnancy. Lancet 1994; 344: 1708–9.
3. Diav-Citrin O, et al. The safety of mesalamine in human pregnancy: a prospective controlled cohort study. Gastroenterology 1998; 114: 23–8.
4. Sachar D. Exposure to mesalamine during pregnancy increased preterm deliveries (but not birth defects) and decreased birth weight. Gut 1998; 43: 316.
5. Marteau P, et al. Foetal outcome in women with inflammatory bowel disease treated during pregnancy with oral mesalazine microgranules. Aliment Pharmacol Ther 1998; 12: 1101–8.
6. Bell CM, Habal FM. Safety of topical 5-aminosalicylic acid in pregnancy. Am J Gastroenterol 1997; 92: 2201–2.

Interactions

Preparations formulated to release mesalazine in the colon should not be given with drugs such as lactulose that lower pH as they may prevent the release of mesalazine (but see Gastrointestinal Drugs below).

Anticoagulants. For reference to a case of mesalazine reducing the effect of *warfarin*, see Gastrointestinal Drugs, p.996.

Antineoplastics. For mention of 5-aminosalicylates such as mesalazine inhibiting the metabolism of thiopurine antineoplastics, and increasing their toxicity, see Mercaptopurine, p.552.

Gastrointestinal drugs. Although it has been suggested that *lactulose* could delay the intestinal release of mesalazine from modified release preparation, 1 study found no evidence that lactulose co-administration influenced the release or disposition of mesalazine.[1] Similarly, *omeprazole* did not appear to increase the likelihood of premature mesalazine release.

1. Hussain FN, et al. Mesalazine release from a pH dependent formulation: effects of omeprazole and lactulose co-administration. Br J Clin Pharmacol 1998; 46: 173–5.

Pharmacokinetics

Following oral administration of conventional formulations, mesalazine would be extensively absorbed from the upper gastrointestinal tract, with little of the drug reaching the colon. Oral preparations are therefore generally formulated to release the drug in the terminal ileum and colon, where it is thought to exert a mainly local action. The specific release characteristics differ somewhat between formulations and this, together with interindividual variation, makes comparison of pharmacokinetic data between studies difficult. Some 20 to 50% of an oral dose is thought to be lost to absorption in healthy subjects, but absorption is lower in patients with active inflammatory bowel disease. Absorption from rectal dosage forms has also varied widely, with factors such as the dose, the formulation, and the pH also playing a role, but mean absorption of around 10 to 20% of a rectal dose has been reported in several studies.

The absorbed portion of mesalazine is almost completely acetylated in the gut wall and in the liver to acetyl-5-aminosalicylic acid. The rate of acetylation, and hence the concentration of parent drug and metabolite in the systemic circulation, is independent of the acetylator status. The acetylated metabolite is excreted mainly in urine by tubular secretion, together with traces of the parent compound; a clearance of about 3 to 4 mL per minute per kg has been reported for the former.

The elimination half-life of mesalazine is reported to be about 1 hour and it is 40 to 50% bound to plasma proteins; the acetylated metabolite has a half-life of up to 10 hours and is about 80% bound to plasma proteins.

Only negligible quantities of mesalazine cross the placenta. Amounts distributed into breast milk are very small.

◊ Reviews.
1. Klotz U. Clinical pharmacokinetics of sulphasalazine, its metabolites and other prodrugs of 5-aminosalicylic acid. Clin Pharmacokinet 1985; 10: 285–302.
2. De Vos M. Clinical pharmacokinetics of slow release mesalazine. Clin Pharmacokinet 2000; 39: 85–97.

Uses and Administration

Mesalazine is an anti-inflammatory drug structurally related to the salicylates and active in inflammatory bowel disease (p.1205); it is considered to be the active moiety of sulfasalazine (p.1251). Its mode of ac-

tion is uncertain, but may be due, at least in part, to its ability to inhibit local prostaglandin and leukotriene synthesis in the gastrointestinal mucosa.

Mesalazine is given by mouth or rectally in the treatment of *acute attacks* of mild to moderate acute ulcerative colitis or the *maintenance of remission* of ulcerative colitis or Crohn's disease. An oral dose of 400 mg of mesalazine is theoretically equivalent to 1 g of sulfasalazine.

There are several differently formulated oral preparations of mesalazine available, and dosage recommendations vary. Recommended doses for some UK preparations are as follows:

- *Asacol* tablets (SmithKline Beecham, UK); acute attack, initially 2.4 g daily in divided doses; maintenance of remission, 1.2 to 2.4 g daily in divided doses.

- *Pentasa Slow Release* tablets (Ferring, UK); acute attack, initially up to 4 g daily in 2 or 3 divided doses; maintenance of remission, adjusted individually from an initial dose of 1.5 g daily in 2 or 3 divided doses

- *Pentasa Slow Release* granules (Ferring, UK); acute attack, initially, up to 4 g daily in 2 to 4 divided doses; maintenance of remission, 2 g daily in 2 divided doses

- *Salofalk* tablets (Cortecs, UK); acute attack, initially 1.5 g daily in 3 divided doses; maintenance of remission, 0.75 to 1.5 g daily in divided doses.

When given rectally, the suggested dose is 0.75 to 3 g daily as suppositories. In the UK, 1 or 2 g is also given daily as an enema formulation, but in the USA an enema containing 4 g of mesalazine has been given.

◊ General references.
1. Clemett D, Markham A. Prolonged-release mesalazine: a review of its therapeutic potential in ulcerative colitis and Crohn's disease. Drugs 2000; 59: 929–56.

Administration. Because the release characteristics of different formulations of mesalazine vary, they should not be regarded as interchangeable.[1] This applies even to those formulations where the dosage is apparently similar.[2]

1. Forbes A, Chadwick C. Mesalazine preparations. Lancet 1997; 350: 1329.
2. Benbow AG, Gould I. Mesalazine preparations. Lancet 1998; 351: 68.

Preparations

USP 25: Mesalamine Delayed-Release Tablets; Mesalamine Extended-Release Capsules; Mesalamine Rectal Suspension.

Proprietary Preparations (details are given in Part 3)
Aust.: Claversal; Pentasa; Salofalk; *Austral.:* Mesasal; *Belg.:* Asacol; Claversal; Colitofalk; Pentasa; *Braz.:* Asalit; *Canad.:* Asacol; Mesasal; Pentasa; Quintasa; Salofalk; *Denm.:* Asacol; Mesasal; Pentasa; *Fin.:* Asacol; Pentasa; *Fr.:* Fivasa; Pentasa; Rowasa; *Ger.:* Asacolitin; Claversal; Pentasa; Salofalk; *Hong Kong:* Asacol; Pentasa; Salofalk; *Irl.:* Asacolon; Pentasa; Salofalk; *Israel:* Asacol; Pentasa; Rafassal; *Ital.:* Asacol; Asalex; Claversal; Enterasin; Mesaflor; Pentacol; Pentasa; Salofalk; Xalazin; *Jpn:* Pentasa; *Mex.:* Salofalk; *Neth.:* Asacol; Pentasa; Salofalk; *Norw.:* Asacol; Mesasal; Pentasa; *NZ:* Asacol; Pentasa; *Port.:* Asacol; Claversal; Pentasa; Salofalk; *S.Afr.:* Asacol; Pentasa; *Singapore:* Asacol; Mesacol; Pentasa; Salofalk; *Spain:* Claversal; Lixacol; Quintasa; *Swed.:* Asacol; Mesasal; Pentasa; *Switz.:* Asacol; Asazine; Pentasa; Salofalk; *Thai.:* Asacol; Mesacol; Salofalk; *UK:* Asacol; Coltec†; Pentasa; Salofalk; *USA:* Asacol; Pentasa; Rowasa.

Metoclopramide Hydrochloride

(6541-f)

Metoclopramide Hydrochloride *(BANM, USAN, rINNM).*
AHR-3070-C; DEL-1267; Metoclopramidi Hydrochloridum; MK-745. 4-Amino-5-chloro-*N*-(2-diethylaminoethyl)-2-methoxybenzamide hydrochloride monohydrate.
$C_{14}H_{22}ClN_3O_2,HCl,H_2O = 354.3$.

CAS — 364-62-5 (metoclopramide); 7232-21-5 (anhydrous metoclopramide hydrochloride); 54143-57-6 (metoclopramide hydrochloride monohydrate); 2576-84-3 (anhydrous metoclopramide dihydrochloride).

Pharmacopoeias. In Eur. (see p.vi), Int., Pol., and US.
Chin., Eur., and Jpn include anhydrous metoclopramide.

Metoclopramide hydrochloride 10.5 mg is approximately equivalent to 10.0 mg of the anhydrous substance which is approximately equivalent to 8.9 mg of the anhydrous base.

Pharmacopoeial description

Ph. Eur.: A white or almost white, crystalline powder or crystals. Very soluble in water; freely soluble in alcohol; sparingly soluble in dichloromethane; practically insoluble in ether. A 10% solution in water has a pH of 4.5 to 6.0. Protect from light.

USP 25: A white or practically white, odourless or practically odourless, crystalline powder. Very soluble in water; freely soluble in alcohol; sparingly soluble in chloroform; practically insoluble in ether. Store in airtight containers. Protect from light.

Incompatibilities. Proprietary preparations of metoclopramide hydrochloride are stated to be incompatible with cephalosporins, chloramphenicol sodium, and sodium bicarbonate.

Cisplatin, cyclophosphamide, and doxorubicin hydrochloride are stated to be compatible with metoclopramide hydrochloride but compatibility is dependent upon factors such as the particular formulation, drug concentration, and temperature.

Adverse Effects

Metoclopramide is a dopamine antagonist and may cause extrapyramidal symptoms which usually occur as acute dystonic reactions; these are more common in children and young adults, especially if female, and at daily doses above 500 µg per kg body-weight. Parkinsonism and tardive dyskinesia have occasionally occurred, usually during prolonged treatment in elderly patients.

Other adverse effects include restlessness, drowsiness, and diarrhoea. Hypotension, hypertension, dizziness, headache, and depression may occur and there are isolated reports of blood disorders, hypersensitivity reactions (rash, bronchospasm), and neuroleptic malignant syndrome. Disorders of cardiac conduction have been reported with intravenous metoclopramide.

Metoclopramide stimulates prolactin secretion and may cause galactorrhoea or related disorders. Transient increases in plasma-aldosterone concentrations have been reported.

Effects on the blood. A report[1] of agranulocytosis associated with administration of metoclopramide on 2 separate occasions. Both episodes resolved within 2 to 3 weeks of withdrawing metoclopramide. Methaemoglobinaemia[2] has also been reported.

1. Harvey RL, Luzar MJ. Metoclopramide-induced agranulocytosis. Ann Intern Med 1988; 108: 214–15.
2. Grant SCD, et al. Methaemoglobinaemia produced by metoclopramide in an adult. Eur J Clin Pharmacol 1994; 47: 89.

Effects on the cardiovascular system. Reports of hypotension,[1] hypertension,[2,3] and supraventricular tachycardia[4] associated with metoclopramide. Bradycardia followed by total heart block,[5] and sinus arrest,[6] have also been reported.

1. Park GR. Hypotension following metoclopramide administration during hypotensive anaesthesia for intracranial aneurysm. Br J Anaesth 1978; 50: 1268–9.
2. Sheridan C, et al. Transient hypertension after high doses of metoclopramide. N Engl J Med 1982; 307: 1346.
3. Filibeck DJ, et al. Metoclopramide-induced hypertensive crisis. Clin Pharm 1984; 3: 548–9.
4. Bevacqua BK. Supraventricular tachycardia associated with postpartum metoclopramide administration. Anesthesiology 1988; 68: 124–5.
5. Midttun M, Øberg B. Total heart block after intravenous metoclopramide. Lancet 1994; 343: 182–3.
6. Malkoff MD, et al. Sinus arrest after administration of intravenous metoclopramide. Ann Pharmacother 1995; 29: 381–3.

Effects on the endocrine system. ALDOSTERONISM. Metoclopramide has been reported to increase plasma-aldosterone concentrations in healthy individuals[1] and in patients with liver cirrhosis and ascites associated with secondary hyperaldosteronism.[2] Increased plasma aldosterone following metoclopramide administration has also been associated with the development of oedema in a patient with congestive heart failure.[3] The metoclopramide-induced aldosterone response was blunted by prior administration of neostigmine.[1]

1. Sommers DK, et al. Effect of neostigmine on metoclopramide-induced aldosterone secretion in man. Eur J Clin Pharmacol 1989; 36: 411–13.
2. Mazzacca G, et al. Metoclopramide and secondary hyperaldosteronism. Ann Intern Med 1983; 98: 1024–5.
3. Zumoff B. Metoclopramide and edema. Ann Intern Med 1983; 98: 557.

HYPERPROLACTINAEMIA. Hyperprolactinaemia, galactorrhoea, and pituitary adenoma occurred in a 49-year-old woman with reflux oesophagitis who had received metoclopramide for 3 months.[1] Her plasma-prolactin concentrations fell to normal and her symptoms resolved over 4 months following withdrawal of metoclopramide. The pituitary tumour was considered to be incidental to, and not caused by, metoclopramide therapy.

1. Cooper BT, et al. Galactorrhoea, hyperprolactinaemia, and pituitary adenoma presenting during metoclopramide therapy. Postgrad Med J 1982; 58: 314–15.

Effects on mental state. There are isolated reports of dose-related delirium, depression, and uncontrollable crying in patients treated with metoclopramide in doses of 40 to 80 mg daily.[1-3] Symptoms resolved on reducing the dose or withdrawing metoclopramide and tolerance could be achieved by gradually increasing the dose.

Insomnia, with or without daytime drowsiness, has also been reported in patients taking metoclopramide 40 mg daily.[4]

1. Bottner RK, Tullio CJ. Metoclopramide and depression. Ann Intern Med 1985; 103: 482.
2. Adams CD. Metoclopramide and depression. Ann Intern Med 1985; 103: 960.

3. Fishbain DA, Rogers A. Delirium secondary to metoclopramide hydrochloride. *J Clin Psychopharmacol* 1987; **7**: 281–2.

4. Saxe TG. Metoclopramide side effects. *Ann Intern Med* 1983; **98**: 674.

Extrapyramidal effects. The Adverse Reactions Register of the UK Committee on Safety of Medicines for the years 1967-82 contained 479 reports of extrapyramidal reactions in which metoclopramide was the suspected drug: 455 were for dystonic-dyskinetic reactions, 20 for parkinsonism, and 4 for tardive dyskinesia.[1]

Acute **dystonic-dyskinetic** reactions occur most commonly in children and young adults[1-3] and about 70% of reactions are in females;[1,3] a substantial proportion of reactions are associated with doses in excess of those recommended by the manufacturers.[1,3,4] Symptoms reported include oculogyric crisis,[4,5] opisthotonus,[6] torticollis,[5,7] trismus,[5,7] a tetanus-like reaction,[8] and blue coloration of the tongue;[6] akathisia following the preoperative use of metoclopramide with droperidol has been reported.[9] The effects usually occur within 72 hours of starting treatment[1] but have been reported within 30 minutes of receiving metoclopramide.[4] They may occur in patients who have previously received metoclopramide without complications[5,8,9] and may be precipitated by other drugs. Although generally self-limiting, deaths have occurred.[1,5] The reactions are readily reversed by an antihistamine such as diphenhydramine,[7] or an antimuscarinic such as benzatropine;[4,6] prophylactic use of diphenhydramine has been suggested for patients with a history of extrapyramidal reactions and in those less than 30 years of age.[7,8]

Metoclopramide-associated **parkinsonism** is thought to occur less commonly than the acute dystonias and is seen predominantly in older patients. Symptoms usually appear several months after starting metoclopramide, but may occur within days or not for several years. Withdrawal of metoclopramide usually results in resolution of symptoms, although it may take several months.[1] A study has suggested that metoclopramide-induced parkinsonism (misdiagnosed as idiopathic Parkinson's disease) may be more common in the elderly than generally realised.[10]

Tardive dyskinesia may rarely be associated with metoclopramide administration. The reaction is usually confined to elderly patients following prolonged oral use,[11,12] but it has been reported after short-term high-dose parenteral use as an antiemetic in cancer chemotherapy,[13] and a case has been reported in an 8-year-old child treated with metoclopramide for gastro-oesophageal reflux disease in usual doses.[14] The average duration of treatment before the onset of symptoms was 14 months (range 4 to 44 months) in a report of 11 cases[12] and 26 months (range 8 to 60 months) in a report of 12 cases;[15] some patients did not experience symptoms until after withdrawal of metoclopramide. Tardive dyskinesia is potentially irreversible and its management is difficult.[15] Some patients improve after withdrawal of metoclopramide but symptoms persisting during follow-up periods of up to 3 years have been reported[11,12] The emphasis must be on prevention hence the recommendation that metoclopramide should not be prescribed for the long-term treatment of minor symptoms, especially in elderly patients.[15]

1. Bateman DN, *et al.* Extrapyramidal reactions with metoclopramide. *BMJ* 1985; **291**: 930–1.
2. Anonymous. Measuring therapeutic risk. *Lancet* 1989; **ii**: 139–40.
3. Adverse Drug Reactions Advisory Committee. Metoclopramide—choose the dose carefully. *Aust Adverse Drug React Bull* 1990; Feb.
4. Tait P, *et al.* Metoclopramide side effects in children. *Med J Aust* 1990; **152**: 387.
5. Pollera CF, *et al.* Sudden death after acute dystonic reaction to high-dose metoclopramide. *Lancet* 1984; **ii**: 460–1.
6. Alroe C, Bowen P. Metoclopramide and prochlorperazine: "the blue-tongue sign". *Med J Aust* 1989; **150**: 724–5.
7. Kris MG, *et al.* Extrapyramidal reactions with high-dose metoclopramide. *N Engl J Med* 1983; **309**: 433–4.
8. Della Valle R, *et al.* Metoclopramide-induced tetanus-like dystonic reaction. *Clin Pharm* 1985; **4**: 102–3.
9. Barnes TRE, *et al.* Acute akathisia after oral droperidol and metoclopramide preoperative medication. *Lancet* 1982; **ii**: 48–9.
10. Avorn J, *et al.* Increased incidence of levodopa therapy following metoclopramide use. *JAMA* 1995; **274**: 1780–2.
11. Grimes JD, *et al.* Long-term follow-up of tardive dyskinesia due to metoclopramide. *Lancet* 1982; **ii**: 563.
12. Wiholm B-E, *et al.* Tardive dyskinesia associated with metoclopramide. *BMJ* 1984; **288**: 545–7.
13. Breitbart W. Tardive dyskinesia associated with high-dose intravenous metoclopramide. *N Engl J Med* 1986; **315**: 518.
14. Putnam PE, *et al.* Tardive dyskinesia associated with use of metoclopramide in a child. *J Pediatr* 1992; **121**: 983–5.
15. Orme ML'E, Tallis RC. Metoclopramide and tardive dyskinesia in the elderly. *BMJ* 1984; **289**: 397–8.

Neuroleptic malignant syndrome. Neuroleptic malignant syndrome has occurred very rarely with metoclopramide. In a report of a case with a fatal outcome, it was noted that 17 additional cases had been published in the years 1978 to 1998, three of which resulted in death.[1] Metoclopramide should be stopped immediately if the syndrome occurs, and the patient treated urgently with bromocriptine.

1. Nonino F, Campomori A. Neuroleptic malignant syndrome associated with metoclopramide. *Ann Pharmacother* 1999; **33**: 644–5.

Precautions

Metoclopramide should not be used when stimulation of muscular contractions might adversely affect gastrointestinal conditions as in gastrointestinal haemorrhage, obstruction, perforation, or immediately after surgery. There have been reports of hypertensive crises in patients with phaeochromocytoma given metoclopramide, thus its use is not recommended in such patients.

Children, young patients, and the elderly should be treated with care as they are at increased risk of extrapyramidal reactions; in the UK, use of metoclopramide is restricted in patients under 20 years (see Uses and Administration, below). Patients on prolonged therapy should be reviewed regularly. Care should also be taken when metoclopramide is administered to patients with renal impairment, epilepsy, Parkinson's disease, or a history of depression.

Metoclopramide may cause drowsiness or impaired reactions; patients so affected should not drive or operate machinery.

Hepatic impairment. The UK manufacturers recommend that the dose of metoclopramide should be reduced in patients with clinically significant hepatic impairment, although the US manufacturers note that it has been used safely in some patients with advanced liver disease and make no such recommendation. Decreases in clearance and increases in half-life and area under the plasma concentration-time curve have been reported in patients with cirrhosis given metoclopramide.[1,2]

1. Hellstern A, *et al.* Absolute bioavailability of metoclopramide given orally or by enema in patients with normal liver function or with cirrhosis of the liver. *Arzneimittelforschung* 1987; **37**: 733–6.
2. Magueur E, *et al.* Pharmacokinetics of metoclopramide in patients with liver cirrhosis. *Br J Clin Pharmacol* 1991; **31**: 185–7.

Porphyria. Metoclopramide has been associated with acute attacks of porphyria and is considered to be unsafe in porphyric patients, although there is conflicting evidence of porphyrinogenicity, and indeed some have used it successfully in the management of acute attacks.[1]

1. Elder GH, *et al.* Metoclopramide and acute porphyria. *Lancet* 1997; **350**: 1104.

Renal impairment. Total clearance of metoclopramide is significantly reduced in patients with renal impairment[1-3] and the elimination half-life is prolonged to up to 19 hours.[2] This may be due to impaired metabolism[1,2] or to an alteration in enterohepatic circulation of metoclopramide.[1] Accumulation of metoclopramide could therefore occur in renal impairment with a possible increased risk of side-effects. Dosage reductions of at least 50% have therefore been recommended in patients with moderate to severe renal impairment.[1,2]

Patients undergoing haemodialysis do not require dosage supplements since relatively little metoclopramide is cleared by this process.[2,3]

1. Bateman DN, *et al.* The pharmacokinetics of single doses of metoclopramide in renal failure. *Eur J Clin Pharmacol* 1981; **19**: 437–41.
2. Lehmann CR, *et al.* Metoclopramide kinetics in patients with impaired renal function and clearance by haemodialysis. *Clin Pharmacol Ther* 1985; **37**: 284–9.
3. Wright MR, *et al.* Effect of haemodialysis on metoclopramide kinetics in patients with severe renal failure. *Br J Clin Pharmacol* 1988; **26**: 474–7.

Interactions

Caution should be observed when using metoclopramide in patients taking other drugs that can also cause extrapyramidal reactions, such as the phenothiazines. Increased toxicity may occur if metoclopramide is used in patients receiving lithium, and caution is advisable with other centrally active drugs such as antiepileptics. Antimuscarinics and opioid analgesics antagonise the gastrointestinal effects of metoclopramide.

The absorption of other drugs may be affected by metoclopramide; it may either diminish absorption from the stomach (as with digoxin) or enhance absorption from the small intestine (for example, with ciclosporin or paracetamol). It inhibits serum cholinesterase and may prolong neuromuscular blockade produced by suxamethonium (see p.1342) and mivacurium (p.1338). Metoclopramide may also increase prolactin blood concentrations and therefore interfere with drugs which have a hypoprolactinaemic effect such as bromocriptine (but see p.1166). It has been suggested that it should not be given to patients receiving MAOIs.

Carbamazepine. For a report of neurotoxicity associated with administration of metoclopramide and carbamazepine, see p.345.

Hydroxyzine. Acute anxiety, rigidity, generalised tremor, opisthotonus, and hypertension developed in a 20-year-old man after administration of metoclopramide 10 mg intravenously and hydroxyzine 100 mg intramuscularly.[1] The side-effects occurred 30 minutes after hydroxyzine administration and it was suggested that hydroxyzine potentiated the onset of the reaction.

1. Fouilladieu JL, *et al.* Possible potentiation by hydroxyzine of metoclopramide's undesirable side effects. *Anesth Analg* 1985; **64**: 1227–8.

Pharmacokinetics

Metoclopramide is rapidly and almost completely absorbed from the gastrointestinal tract following a dose by mouth, although conditions such as vomiting or impaired gastric motility may reduce absorption. However, it undergoes hepatic first-pass metabolism, which varies considerably between subjects, and hence absolute bioavailability and plasma concentrations are subject to wide interindividual variation. On average, the bioavailability of oral metoclopramide is about 75%, but it varies between about 30 and 100%. Peak plasma concentrations of metoclopramide occur about 1 to 2 hours after an oral dose. Bioavailability is equally variable following rectal or intranasal administration, although it may be somewhat better if the drug is given intramuscularly.

Metoclopramide is widely distributed in the body, with an apparent volume of distribution of about 3.5 litres per kg. It readily crosses the blood-brain barrier into the CNS. It also freely crosses the placenta, and has been reported to attain concentrations in fetal plasma about 60 to 70% of those in maternal plasma. Concentrations higher than those in maternal plasma may be reached in the breast milk of lactating mothers, particularly in the early puerperium, although concentrations decrease somewhat in the late puerperium.

Elimination of metoclopramide is biphasic, with a terminal elimination half-life of about 4 to 6 hours, although this may be prolonged in renal impairment, with consequent elevation of plasma concentrations. It is excreted in the urine, about 85% of a dose being eliminated in 72 hours, 20 to 30% as unchanged metoclopramide and the remainder as sulfate or glucuronide conjugates, or as metabolites. About 5% of a dose is excreted in faeces via the bile.

Uses and Administration

Metoclopramide hydrochloride is a substituted benzamide used for its prokinetic and antiemetic properties. It stimulates the motility of the upper gastrointestinal tract without affecting gastric, biliary, or pancreatic secretion and increases gastric peristalsis, leading to accelerated gastric emptying. Duodenal peristalsis is also increased which decreases intestinal transit time. The resting tone of the gastro-oesophageal sphincter is increased and the pyloric sphincter is relaxed. Metoclopramide possesses parasympathomimetic activity as well as being a dopamine-receptor antagonist with a direct effect on the chemoreceptor trigger zone. It may have serotonin-receptor (5-HT$_3$) antagonist properties.

Metoclopramide is used in disorders of decreased gastrointestinal motility (p.1202) such as gastroparesis or ileus; in gastro-oesophageal reflux disease (p.1204) and dyspepsia (p.1204); and in nausea and vomiting (p.1206) associated with various gastrointestinal disorders, with migraine, following surgery, and with cancer therapy. Metoclopramide is of no value in the prevention or treatment of motion sickness. It may be used to stimulate gastric emptying during radiographic examinations, to facilitate intubation of the small bowel, and in the management of aspiration syndromes (p.1202).

It is usually given as the hydrochloride monohydrate with doses expressed as the anhydrous hydrochloride. In the USA the strength of preparations of the hydrochloride monohydrate is usually expressed in terms of the base. For most purposes the total daily dose should not exceed 500 µg per kg body-weight; dosage reduction is recommended in renal and perhaps hepatic impairment (see Precautions, above). In the UK, the recommended dose by mouth, intramuscularly, or by slow intravenous injection, is 10 mg (expressed as anhydrous metoclopramide hydrochloride) three times daily. In the USA the recommended dose is 10 to 15 mg (expressed as the base) up to four times daily. Single doses should be considered where appropriate and single doses of 10 to 20 mg (expressed as anhydrous base or anhydrous hydrochloride) have been used.

In the UK the use of metoclopramide is restricted in patients under 20 years of age to severe intractable vomiting of known cause, chemotherapy- or radiotherapy-induced vomiting, as an aid to gastrointestinal intubation, and in premedication. Suggested doses for those aged 15 to 19 years are 10 mg three times daily for those weighing 60 kg and over and 5 mg three times daily for those weighing 30 to 59 kg; 9 to 14 years (30 kg and over), 5 mg three times daily; 5 to 9 years (20 to 29 kg), 2.5 mg three times daily; 3 to 5 years (15 to 19 kg), 2 mg two or three times daily; 1 to 3 years (10 to 14 kg), 1 mg two or three times daily; and under 1 year (up to 10 kg) 1 mg twice daily. Where body-weight is below that specified for a given age group, the dose should reflect the weight rather than the age, so that a lower dose is chosen.

An intranasal formulation of metoclopramide is available in some countries.

The base, the dihydrochloride, and the glycyrrhizinate have also been used.

Metoclopramide has been investigated as a radiosensitiser in patients undergoing radiotherapy for malignant neoplasms.

High-dose therapy. High doses of metoclopramide have been employed in the treatment of the nausea and vomiting associated with cancer chemotherapy often in combination with other agents such as dexamethasone. The loading dose of metoclopramide given before cancer therapy is 2 to 4 mg per kg body-weight administered as a continuous intravenous infusion over 15 to 20 minutes and is followed by a maintenance dose of 3 to 5 mg per kg, again as a continuous intravenous infusion, administered over 8 to 12 hours. Alternatively, initial doses of up to 2 mg per kg by intravenous infusion over at least 15 minutes may be given before cancer therapy and repeated every 2 or 3 hours. The total dosage by either continuous or intermittent infusion should not normally exceed 10 mg per kg in 24 hours.

Administration. INTRANASAL. References.
1. Ormrod D, Goa KL. Intranasal metoclopramide. *Drugs* 1999; **58**: 315–22. Commentaries. *ibid.*; 323–4.

Hiccup. Metoclopramide has been used with chlorpromazine in protocols for the management of intractable hiccup. For a discussion of hiccup and its management see p.667.

Lactation induction. Metoclopramide has been used for its dopamine antagonist properties to stimulate lactation in women who wish to breast feed and in whom mechanical stimulation of the nipple alone is inadequate. Doses of 10 mg three times daily have been used for this purpose, but should be viewed as adjunctive to mechanical methods and the duration of therapy should probably be limited to 7 to 14 days.[1] Young women are at increased risk of extrapyramidal effects from metoclopramide—see under Adverse Effects, above. There has also been concern about the presence of the drug in breast milk. For a discussion of lactation inhibition and induction, see p.1276.
1. Anderson PO, Valdés V. Increasing breast milk supply. *Clin Pharm* 1993; **12**: 479–80.

Migraine. Metoclopramide is used in the treatment of migraine (p.449) to alleviate nausea and vomiting and gastric stasis, which commonly develop as a migraine attack progresses and can lead to poor absorption of oral antimigraine preparations. It may also be given to counteract nausea and vomiting from the use of ergotamine. Metoclopramide is included in some combination analgesic preparations for the treatment of acute attacks of migraine. In one study lysine aspirin with metoclopramide was as effective as sumatriptan in the treatment of migraine.[1]

Metoclopramide given intravenously can relieve the pain of migraine attacks;[2,3] this effect may be related to its action as a dopamine antagonist and may be worth trying in patients who require parenteral treatment and do not respond to sumatriptan or dihydroergotamine.
1. Tfelt-Hansen P, *et al.* The effectiveness of combined oral lysine acetylsalicylate and metoclopramide compared with oral sumatriptan for migraine. *Lancet* 1995; **346**: 923–6.
2. Tek DS, *et al.* A prospective, double-blind study of metoclopramide hydrochloride for the control of migraine in the emergency department. *Ann Emerg Med* 1990; **19**: 1083–7.
3. Ellis GL, *et al.* The efficacy of metoclopramide in the treatment of migraine. *Ann Emerg Med* 1993; **22**: 191–5.

Orthostatic hypotension. Metoclopramide has been tried in the management of some patients with orthostatic hypotension, as mentioned on p.1070.

Variceal haemorrhage. Metoclopramide 20 mg intravenously controlled bleeding from oesophageal varices within 15 minutes in 10 of 11 patients compared with 4 of 11 patients given placebo; all patients were treated by sclerotherapy.[1] Lower oesophageal sphincter pressure is increased by metoclopramide, thus reducing blood flow to varices and achieving haemostasis; another study[2] found a combination of metoclopramide and intravenous glyceryl trinitrate to be more effective than glyceryl trinitrate alone in reducing intravariceal pressure.

For a discussion of variceal haemorrhage and its management, see p.1637.
1. Hosking SW, *et al.* Pharmacological constriction of the lower oesophageal sphincter: a simple method of arresting variceal haemorrhage. *Gut* 1988; **29**: 1098–1102.
2. Sarin SK, Saraya A. Effects of intravenous nitroglycerin and nitroglycerin and metoclopramide on intravariceal pressure: a double blind, randomized study. *Am J Gastroenterol* 1995; **90**: 48–53.

Preparations

BP 2001: Metoclopramide Injection; Metoclopramide Oral Solution; Metoclopramide Tablets;
USP 25: Metoclopramide Injection; Metoclopramide Oral Solution; Metoclopramide Tablets.

Proprietary Preparations (details are given in Part 3)
Aust.: Gastro-Timelets; Gastronerton; Gastrosil; Metogastron; Nausigon; Paspertin; Pertin†; **Austral.:** Maxolon; Pramin; **Belg.:** Dibertil; Primperan; **Braz.:** Citroplus; Dart; Emetic; Estomaplus; Eucil; No-Vomit; Plamin; Plasil; Vomix; Vonil; **Canad.:** Apo-Metoclop; Maxeran; Reglan; **Denm.:** Emperal; Gastro-Timelets; Primperan; **Fin.:** Metopram; Primperan; **Fr.:** Anausin; Primperan; **Ger.:** Cerucal; duraMCP; Gastro-Timelets; Gastronerton; Gastrosil; Gastrotranquil; Hyrin; MCP; Paspertin; Primperan; **Hong Kong:** Apo-Metoclop; Maxolon; Metocyl; Primperan; **Irl.:** Antimet; Gastrobid Continus; Maxolon; Metocyl; Primperan†; **Israel:** Pramin; **Ital.:** Citroplus; Clopan; Plasil; Pramidin; Randum; Viscal†; **Mex.:** Biopram; Carnotprim; Cirulan; Clorimet Z; Meclomid; Plasil; Pramilem; Pramotil; Propace; Vonifin; **Mon.:** Prokinyl; **Neth.:** Primperan†; **Norw.:** Afipran; Primperan; **NZ:** Maxolon; Metamide; **Port.:** Metoclan; Primperan; Reglan; **S.Afr.:** Acumet†; Ametic; Betaclopramide; Clinamide†; Clopamon; Contromet; Dynamide†; Gastrocolon†; Gastrotat†; Maxolon; Metalon; Metcon†; Perinorm; Primperan†; Prostal; Setin; **Singapore:** Maril; Maxolon; Metocyl; Metolon; Primperan; **Spain:** Metagliz; Primperan; **Swed.:** Primperan; **Switz.:** Gastro-Timelets†; Gastrosil; Paspertin; Primperan; **Thai.:** Elitan; Emetal; Gensil; H-Peran; Hawkperan; Maril; Meramide; Met-Sil; Metoclor; Metono; Nausil; Plasil; Vasil; **UAE:** Premosan; **UK:** Gastrobid Continus; Gastroflux; Gastromax†; Maxolon; Mygdalon; Parmid; Primperan; **USA:** Clopra; Intensol†; Maxolon; Octamide; Reclomide; Reglan.

Multi-ingredient: Aust.: Ceolat Compositum; Paspertase; **Belg.:** Migpriv; **Braz.:** Cefalium; Diagrin; Digeplus; Digest; Dramavit; Essen; Estac; Plagon; Plasil Enzimatico; Plasonil; Sintozima; Vominil; Vomistop; Vonil Enzimatico; Vopax; **Denm.:** Migpriv; **Fin.:** Migpriv; **Fr.:** Cephalgan; Migpriv; Primperoxane†; **Ger.:** Migraeflux MCP; Migrane-Neuridal; Migranerton; Paspertase; **Irl.:** Paramax; **Ital.:** Ede†; Geffer; Migpriv; Migraprim; **Mex.:** Digenor Plus; Espaven MD; Plasil Enzimatico; Pramigel; **Neth.:** Migrafin; **NZ:** Paramax; **Spain:** Aero Plus; Aeroflat; Anti Anorex Triple; Edym Sedante†; Gastro Gobens; Hepadigest†; Jorkil†; Liberbil†; Metagliz Bismutico†; Novo Aerofil Sedante; Paidozim; Primperan Complex†; Salcemetic; Starlep; Sualyn†; Surifarm; Suxidina; **Swed.:** Migpriv; **Switz.:** Migpriv; **UK:** Migramax; Migravess†; Paramax.

Metopimazine (6545-m)

Metopimazine (BAN, USAN, rINN).
EXP-999; RP-9965. 1-[3-(2-Methylsulphonylphenothiazin-10-yl)propyl]piperidine-4-carboxamide.
$C_{22}H_{27}N_3O_3S_2 = 445.6$.
CAS — 14008-44-7.
ATC — A04AD05.
Pharmacopoeias. In Fr.

Profile

Metopimazine, a phenothiazine dopamine antagonist, is an antiemetic with general properties similar to those of chlorpromazine (p.660). It is used in the treatment of nausea and vomiting, including that associated with cancer chemotherapy (p.1206). It is given in usual doses of 15 to 30 mg daily by mouth, in 2 or 3 divided doses; similar doses have been given by rectum. It has also been given by injection in a dose of 10 to 20 mg daily, usually intramuscularly but occasionally by the intravenous route.

Preparations

Proprietary Preparations (details are given in Part 3)
Belg.: Vogalene; **Denm.:** Vogalene; **Fr.:** Vogalene; **Israel:** Vogalene.

Mosapride Citrate (3261-y)

Mosapride Citrate (rINNM).
AS-4370; Rimopride Citrate. (±)-4-Amino-5-chloro-2-ethoxy-N-{[4-(p-fluorobenzyl)-2-morpholinyl]methyl}benzamide citrate dihydrate.
$C_{21}H_{25}ClFN_3O_3,C_6H_8O_7,2H_2O = 650.0$.
CAS — 112885-41-3 (mosapride); 112885-42-4 (mosapride citrate).

Profile

Mosapride citrate is a substituted benzamide used for its prokinetic properties. It is reported to be an agonist at 5-HT$_4$ receptors, increasing acetylcholine release and stimulating gastrointestinal motility (see also Cisapride, p.1221), as well as having 5-HT$_3$ antagonist properties. It is given by mouth as the citrate dihydrate, but doses are expressed as the anhydrous citrate, and are 5 mg three times daily before or after meals.

◊ References.
1. Sakashita M, *et al.* Pharmacokinetics of the gastrokinetic agent mosapride citrate after single and multiple oral administrations in healthy subjects. *Arzneimittelforschung* 1993; **43**: 867–72.
2. Ruth M, *et al.* The effect of mosapride, a novel prokinetic, on acid reflux variables in patients with gastro-oesophageal reflux disease. *Aliment Pharmacol Ther* 1998; **12**: 35–40.

Preparations

Proprietary Preparations (details are given in Part 3)
Jpn: Gasmotin.

Nabilone (843-e)

Nabilone (BAN, USAN, rINN).
Compound 109514; Lilly-109514. (±)-(6aR,10aR)-3-(1,1-Dimethylheptyl)-6a,7,8,9,10,10a-hexahydro-1-hydroxy-6,6-dimethyl-6H-benzo[c]chromen-9-one.
$C_{24}H_{36}O_3 = 372.5$.
CAS — 51022-71-0.

Adverse Effects

Nabilone may produce adverse effects similar to those of cannabis (see p.1590). The most common side-effect is reported to be drowsiness; other neurological side-effects have included confusion, disorientation, dizziness, euphoria, dysphoria, hallucinations, psychosis, depression, headache, decreased concentration, blurred vision, sleep disturbances, decreased coordination, and tremors. Adverse cardiovascular reactions that have occurred are postural hypotension and tachycardia. Dry mouth, decreased appetite, and abdominal cramp have also been reported.

Precautions

Nabilone is extensively metabolised and largely excreted in bile, and therefore is not recommended in patients with severe liver impairment. It should be administered cautiously to patients with a history of psychosis or depression, or those with hypertension or heart disease.

Because of the possibility of CNS depression patients should be warned not to drive or operate machinery.

The possibility of dependence similar to that of cannabis should be borne in mind.

Interactions

Nabilone has been shown to have an additive CNS depressant effect when given with alcohol, diazepam, or other CNS depressants.

Pharmacokinetics

Nabilone is well absorbed from the gastrointestinal tract and is rapidly and extensively metabolised; one or more of the metabolites may be active. The major excretory pathway is the biliary system; about 65% of a dose is excreted in the faeces and about 20% in the urine. The elimination half-life of nabilone is about 2 hours, but the half-life of its combined metabolites is about 35 hours after a dose by mouth.

◊ References.
1. Rubin A, *et al.* Physiologic disposition of nabilone, a cannabinol derivative, in man. *Clin Pharmacol Ther* 1977; **22**: 85–91.

The symbol † denotes a preparation no longer actively marketed

Uses and Administration

Nabilone, a synthetic cannabinoid with antiemetic and anxiolytic properties, is used for the control of nausea and vomiting associated with cancer chemotherapy in patients who have failed to respond adequately to conventional antiemetics (p.1206).

The usual dose for adults is 1 mg twice daily by mouth initially, increased to 2 mg twice daily if necessary. The first dose should be given the evening before initiation of chemotherapy with the second dose of nabilone being given 1 to 3 hours before the first dose of the antineoplastic. Nabilone may be given throughout each cycle of chemotherapy and for 48 hours after the last dose of chemotherapy, if required. The dose of nabilone should not exceed 6 mg daily.

Multiple sclerosis. There is a report of reduction in spasticity and nocturia, and improvement in mood and well-being, in a patient with multiple sclerosis (p.633) who received nabilone 1 mg every second day.[1] Given that there are also anecdotal reports of improvement in symptoms in patients with multiple sclerosis who took cannabis, it was suggested that synthetic cannabinoids might be worthy of study in the treatment of spasticity.

1. Martyn CN, et al. Nabilone in the treatment of multiple sclerosis. Lancet 1995; 345: 579.

Preparations

Proprietary Preparations (details are given in Part 3)
Canad.: Cesamet; **Irl.:** Cesamet; **UK:** Cesamet.

Niperotidine Hydrochloride (2874-e)

Niperotidine Hydrochloride (rINNM).
Piperonyl Ranitidine Hydrochloride. N-[2-({5-[(Dimethylamino)methyl]furfuryl}thio)ethyl]-2-nitro-N'-piperonyl-1,1-ethenediamine hydrochloride.
$C_{20}H_{26}N_4O_5S,HCl = 471.0$.
CAS — 84845-75-0 (niperotidine).

Profile

Niperotidine hydrochloride is a histamine H_2-receptor antagonist with general properties similar to those of cimetidine (p.1216). Severe hepatic disorders have occurred in patients receiving niperotidine.

◊ References.
1. Gasbarrini G, et al. Acute liver injury related to the use of niperotidine. J Hepatol 1997; 27: 583–6.

Nizatidine (12003-m)

Nizatidine (BAN, USAN, rINN).
LY-139037; Nizatidinum. 4-[2-(1-Methylamino-2-nitrovinylamino)ethylthiomethyl]thiazol-2-ylmethyl(dimethyl)amine;   N-[2-(2-Dimethylaminomethylthiazol-4-ylmethylthio)ethyl]-N'-methyl-2-nitrovinylidenediamine.
$C_{12}H_{21}N_5O_2S_2 = 331.5$.
CAS — 76963-41-2.
ATC — A02BA04.
Pharmacopoeias. In Eur. (see p.vi) and US.

Pharmacopoeial description

Ph. Eur.: An almost white or slightly brownish, crystalline powder. Sparingly soluble in water; soluble in methyl alcohol. A 1% solution in water has a pH of 8.5 to 10.0.

USP 25: An off-white to buff crystalline solid. Sparingly soluble in water; freely soluble in chloroform; soluble in methyl alcohol. Store in airtight containers. Protect from light.

Adverse Effects

As for Cimetidine, p.1216. Some patients taking nizatidine may experience excessive sweating and urticaria; anaemia may also occur.

Nizatidine is considered to have little or no anti-androgenic activity although there are isolated reports of gynaecomastia and impotence.

Effects on the cardiovascular system. Nizatidine has been reported to reduce heart rate in healthy subjects,[1,2] an effect that was not seen when they were pretreated with ranitidine[1] or also given the antimuscarinic pirenzepine.[2] As with other H_2-antagonists (see Cimetidine, p.1217), tachycardia, bradycardia, postural hypotension and syncope have been reported rarely with rapid intravenous injection of nizatidine.

1. Mescheder A, et al. Changes in the effects of nizatidine and famotidine on cardiac performance after pretreatment with ranitidine. Eur J Clin Pharmacol 1993; 45: 151–6.
2. Hinrichsen H, et al. Dose-dependent heart rate reducing effect of nizatidine, a histamine H_2-receptor antagonist. Br J Clin Pharmacol 1993; 35: 461–6.

Effects on the endocrine system. A report of reversible impotence in a patient taking nizatidine 300 mg at night.[1]
1. Kassianos GC. Impotence and nizatidine. Lancet 1989; i: 963.

Effects on the skin. Similarly to cimetidine (p.1217), vasculitis has been reported with nizatidine.[1] Exfoliative dermatitis has also occurred.
1. Suh J-G, et al. Leukocytoclastic vasculitis associated with nizatidine therapy. Am J Med 1997; 102: 216–17.

Precautions

As for Cimetidine, p.1218.

Interactions

Unlike cimetidine (p.1218) nizatidine does not inhibit cytochrome P450, and therefore is considered to have little effect on the metabolism of other drugs. However, like other H_2-antagonists its effects on gastric pH may affect the absorption of some other drugs.

Pharmacokinetics

Nizatidine is readily and almost completely absorbed from the gastrointestinal tract. The bioavailability of nizatidine following oral administration exceeds 70% and may be slightly increased by the presence of food. It is widely distributed and is approximately 35% bound to plasma proteins.

The elimination half-life of nizatidine is 1 to 2 hours and is prolonged in renal impairment. Nizatidine is partly metabolised in the liver: nizatidine N-2-oxide, nizatidine S-oxide, and N-2-monodesmethylnizatidine have been identified, the latter having about 60% of the activity of nizatidine.

More than 90% of a dose of nizatidine is excreted in the urine, in part by active tubular secretion, within 12 hours, about 60% as unchanged drug. Less than 6% is excreted in the faeces. Nizatidine is distributed into breast milk.

◊ Reviews.
1. Callaghan JT, et al. A pharmacokinetic profile of nizatidine in man. Scand J Gastroenterol 1987; 22 (suppl 136): 9–17.

Distribution into breast milk. About 0.1% of an oral dose of nizatidine was secreted in breast milk in a study in lactating women.[1] The milk to serum ratio varied (from 1:1 to 4.9:1) with the time of samples.
1. Obermeyer BD, et al. Secretion of nizatidine into human breast milk after single and multiple doses. Clin Pharmacol Ther 1990; 47: 724–30.

Uses and Administration

Nizatidine is a histamine H_2-antagonist with actions and uses similar to those of cimetidine (see p.1218). It is given by mouth and by intravenous infusion.

In the management of benign **gastric** and **duodenal ulceration** (p.1208) a single daily dose of nizatidine 300 mg by mouth at night is recommended, which should be given initially for 4 weeks and may be extended to 8 weeks if necessary; alternatively 150 mg may be given twice daily in the morning and evening. Where appropriate a maintenance dose of 150 mg daily may be given at night. In patients who are unsuited to receive oral therapy nizatidine may be given on a short-term basis by continuous intravenous infusion of 10 mg per hour; alternatively 100 mg may be diluted in 50 mL of infusion fluid and be given over 15 minutes, three times daily. The total intravenous dose should not exceed 480 mg daily.

In **gastro-oesophageal reflux disease** (p.1204) a dose of 150 to 300 mg twice daily by mouth is recommended for up to 12 weeks.

For the short-term symptomatic relief of **dyspepsia** a dose of 75 mg, repeated if necessary up to a maximum of 150 mg daily may be taken by mouth for up to 14 days.

The dosage of nizatidine should be reduced in patients with **impaired renal function**. In those with creatinine clearance of 20 to 50 mL per minute, doses should be reduced by 50%, or where the standard dose would be 150 mg, given on alternate days. If creatinine clearance is less than 20 mL per minute, doses are reduced by 75%, or where the standard dose would be 150 mg, given every third day.

◊ Reviews.
1. Price AH, Brogden RN. Nizatidine: a preliminary review of its pharmacodynamic and pharmacokinetic properties, and its therapeutic use in peptic ulcer disease. Drugs 1988; 36: 521–39.

Preparations

USP 25: Nizatidine Capsules.

Proprietary Preparations (details are given in Part 3)
Aust.: Ulxit; **Austral.:** Tazac; **Belg.:** Panaxid; **Braz.:** Axid; **Canad.:** Axid; **Denm.:** Nizax; **Fin.:** Nizax; **Fr.:** Nizaxid; **Ger.:** Gastrax; Nizax; **Hong Kong:** Axid; **Irl.:** Axid; **Ital.:** Cronizat; Nizax; Zanizal; **Mex.:** Axid; **Neth.:** Axid; Naxidine; **Port.:** Nizaxid; **S.Afr.:** Antizid; Axid†; **Spain:** Distaxid; Ulcosal; **Swed.:** Nizax; **Switz.:** Calmaxid; **Thai.:** Axid; **UK:** Axid; Zinga; **USA:** Axid.

Olsalazine Sodium (16608-a)

Olsalazine Sodium (BANM, USAN, rINNM).
Azodisal Sodium; CI Mordant Yellow 5; CI No. 14130; CJ-91B; Olsalazinum Natricum; Sodium Azodisalicylate. Disodium 5,5'-azodisalicylate.
$C_{14}H_8N_2Na_2O_6 = 346.2$.
CAS — 6054-98-4.
Pharmacopoeias. In Eur. (see p.vi).

Pharmacopoeial description

Ph. Eur.: A yellow, fine, crystalline powder; it exhibits polymorphism. Sparingly soluble in water; soluble in dimethyl sulfoxide; very slightly soluble in methyl alcohol.

Adverse Effects and Precautions

As for Mesalazine, p.1234. The most common adverse effects associated with olsalazine sodium are diarrhoea, arthralgia, and skin rashes. Diarrhoea may be watery in some patients; it may resolve with dosage reduction but can be severe enough to require withdrawal of treatment. Diarrhoea is less likely if the drug is taken after meals. There have been a few reports of blood dyscrasias. If a blood dyscrasia is suspected treatment should be stopped immediately and a blood count performed. Patients or their carers should be told how to recognise signs of blood toxicity and should be advised to seek immediate medical attention if symptoms such as fever, sore throat, mouth ulcers, bruising, or bleeding develop.

◊ In an open study[1] of olsalazine 1 g daily by mouth involving 160 patients with active ulcerative colitis and a history of sulfasalazine intolerance, 103 (64.4%) patients experienced no side-effects; 29 patients reported only minor side-effects: gastrointestinal disturbances in 22 patients, transient skin rash in 3, and headache, increased salivation, cough, and irritability each in one patient. The most common side-effect was frequent loose stools which affected 25 patients, 20 of whom had to discontinue treatment. This side-effect occurred early in treatment, within 10 hours of the first dose in 13 patients. Severe diarrhoea was more frequent in patients with widespread disease, but the incidence of diarrhoea did not correlate with disease severity.

A subsequent study[2] in healthy subjects has shown that olsalazine has a significant inhibitory effect on water and electrolyte absorption in the small intestine, which may account, at least in part, for the induction of diarrhoea. Patients with extensive colitis have reduced colonic absorptive function and may be less able to assimilate the increased colonic inflow volumes.

1. Sandberg-Gertzén H, et al. Azodisal sodium in the treatment of ulcerative colitis: a study of tolerance and relapse-prevention properties. Gastroenterology 1986; 90: 1024–30.
2. Raimundo AH, et al. Effects of olsalazine and sulphasalazine on jejunal and ileal water and electrolyte absorption in normal human subjects. Gut 1991; 32: 270–4.

Effects on the blood. As of July 1995, the UK Committee on Safety of Medicines had received 4 reports of blood dyscrasias associated with olsalazine, none of them fatal.[1] It was recommended that a blood count be performed and the drug stopped immediately if there was suspicion of a dyscrasia. See also under Mesalazine, p.1234.
1. Committee on Safety of Medicines/Medicines Control Agency. Blood dyscrasias and mesalazine. Current Problems 1995; 21: 5–6.

Effects on the kidneys. A report of nephrotoxicity, characterised by interstitial nephritis, associated with the use of olsalazine.[1] Symptoms resolved on discontinuation of the drug. See also under Mesalazine, p.1234.
1. Wilcox GM, et al. Nephrotoxicity associated with olsalazine. Am J Med 1996; 100: 238–40.

Interactions

Antineoplastics. For mention of 5-aminosalicylates such as olsalazine inhibiting the metabolism of thiopurine antineoplastics, and increasing their toxicity, see Mercaptopurine, p.552.

Pharmacokinetics

Very little of an oral dose of olsalazine is absorbed via the upper gastrointestinal tract, and almost the entire dose reaches its site of action in the colon intact. It is broken down by the colonic bacterial flora into 2 molecules of 5-aminosalicylic acid (mesalazine). Some mesalazine is absorbed and acetylated (see p.1235) but systemic concentrations of mesalazine and its metabolite are lower than after comparable doses of mesalazine by mouth, perhaps because there is less release of mesalazine in the small intestine, where absorption is better. Mesalazine concentrations in the colon following a dose of olsalazine are stated to be about 1000 times greater than systemic concentrations.

The small amounts (1 to 2% of the dose or less) of intact olsalazine which are absorbed are excreted mainly in urine; the elimination half-life after an intravenous dose has been calculated at about 1 hour. Some olsalazine is metabolised by sulfate conjugation in the liver: the elimination half-life of the metabolite is reported to be about 7 days.

◊ References.
1. Ryde EM. Pharmacokinetic aspects of drugs targeted for the colon, with special reference to olsalazine. *Acta Pharm Suec* 1988; **25:** 327–8.
2. Laursen LS, *et al.* Disposition of 5-aminosalicylic acid by olsalazine and three mesalazine preparations in patients with ulcerative colitis: comparison of intraluminal colonic concentrations, serum values, and urinary excretion. *Gut* 1990; **31:** 1271–6.

Uses and Administration
Olsalazine consists of two molecules of mesalazine (p.1234) linked with an azo bond. It is activated in the colon where the active mesalazine is released. It is used as the sodium salt in the management of acute mild ulcerative colitis and for the maintenance of remission (see Inflammatory Bowel Disease, p.1205). The usual initial dose is 1 g by mouth daily in divided doses and this is gradually increased, if necessary, over one week, to a maximum dose of 3 g daily. The usual dose for the maintenance of remission is 500 mg twice daily. Doses should be taken after meals and a single dose should not exceed 1 g.

◊ References.
1. Anonymous. Olsalazine—a further choice in ulcerative colitis. *Drug Ther Bull* 1990; **28:** 57–8.
2. Anonymous. Olsalazine for ulcerative colitis. *Med Lett Drugs Ther* 1990; **32:** 105–6.
3. Wadworth AN, Fitton A. Olsalazine: a review of its pharmacodynamic and pharmacokinetic properties, and therapeutic potential in inflammatory bowel disease. *Drugs* 1991; **41:** 647–64.

Preparations
Proprietary Preparations (details are given in Part 3)
Aust.: Dipentum; *Austral.:* Dipentum; *Canad.:* Dipentum; *Denm.:* Dipentum; *Fin.:* Dipentum; *Fr.:* Dipentum; *Ger.:* Dipentum; *Hong Kong:* Dipentum; *Irl.:* Dipentum; *Israel:* Dipentum; *Ital.:* Dipentum; *Neth.:* Dipentum; *Norw.:* Dipentum; *NZ:* Dipentum; *S.Afr.:* Dipentum; *Spain:* Rasal; *Swed.:* Dipentum; *Switz.:* Dipentum; *UK:* Dipentum; *USA:* Dipentum.

Omeprazole (16938-y)

Omeprazole *(BAN, USAN, rINN)*.
H-168/68; Omeprazolum. *(RS)*-5-Methoxy-2-(4-methoxy-3,5-dimethyl-2-pyridylmethylsulphinyl)benzimidazole.
$C_{17}H_{19}N_3O_3S = 345.4$.
CAS — 73590-58-6.
ATC — A02BC01.
Pharmacopoeias. In *Eur.* (see p.vi) and *US.*

Pharmacopoeial description
Ph. Eur.: A white or almost white powder. Very slightly soluble in water; sparingly soluble in alcohol and in methyl alcohol; soluble in dichloromethane. It dissolves in dilute solutions of alkali hydroxides. Store in airtight containers at a temperature between 2° and 8°. Protect from light.

USP 25: A white to off-white powder. Very slightly soluble in water; sparingly soluble in alcohol and in methyl alcohol; soluble in dichloromethane. Store in airtight containers at a temperature not exceeding 8°. Protect from moisture.

Omeprazole Magnesium (19975-t)

Omeprazole Magnesium *(BANM, USAN, rINNM)*.
$C_{34}H_{36}MgN_6O_6S_2 = 713.1$.
CAS — 95382-33-5.

Omeprazole magnesium 10.32 mg is approximately equivalent to 10 mg of omeprazole.

Omeprazole Sodium (15383-s)

Omeprazole Sodium *(BANM, USAN, rINNM)*.
$C_{17}H_{18}N_3NaO_3S = 367.4$.
CAS — 95510-70-6.
Pharmacopoeias. In *Eur.* (see p.vi).

Omeprazole sodium 10.64 mg is approximately equivalent to 10 mg omeprazole.

Pharmacopoeial description
Ph. Eur.: A white or almost white, hygroscopic powder. Freely soluble in water and in alcohol; very slightly soluble in dichloromethane; soluble in propylene glycol. The pH of a 2% solution in water is 10.3 to 11.3. Store in airtight containers. Protect from light.

Adverse Effects
Adverse effects reported most frequently with omeprazole and other proton pump inhibitors have been headache, diarrhoea, and skin rashes; they have sometimes been severe enough to require discontinuation of treatment. Other effects include pruritus, dizziness, fatigue, constipation, nausea and vomiting, flatulence, abdominal pain, arthralgia and myalgia, urticaria, and dry mouth. Isolated cases of photosensitivity, bullous eruption, erythema multiforme, angioedema, and anaphylaxis have been reported. Effects on the CNS include occasional insomnia, somnolence, and vertigo; reversible confusional states, agitation, depression, and hallucinations have occurred in severely ill patients. Raised liver enzymes, and isolated cases of hepatitis, jaundice, and hepatic encephalopathy, have been reported. Other adverse effects reported rarely or in isolated cases include paraesthesia, blurred vision, alopecia, stomatitis, taste disturbances, peripheral oedema, hyponatraemia, blood disorders (including agranulocytosis, leucopenia, and thrombocytopenia), and interstitial nephritis.

Proton pump inhibitors may increase the risk of gastrointestinal infections because of their acid suppressive effects.

Early toxicological studies identified carcinoid-like tumours of the gastric mucosa in *rats* given very high doses of omeprazole over long periods; this is reviewed in more detail under Gastrointestinal Tumours, below.

Effects on the blood. There have been rare cases of leucopenia, agranulocytosis, thrombocytopenia, and pancytopenia, with omeprazole and other proton pump inhibitors.
References.
1. Holt TL, *et al.* Neutropenia associated with omeprazole. *Med J Aust* 1999; **170:** 141–2.

Effects on the endocrine system. Up to December 1991, WHO had received 30 reports of impotence or gynaecomastia which might have been due to omeprazole;[1] of these reports 15 were of impotence, 13 of gynaecomastia in men, and 2 of breast enlargement in women. For reference to a case-control study showing no statistical link between gynaecomastia and omeprazole, see under Cimetidine, p.1217.
1. Lindquist M, Edwards IR. Endocrine adverse effects of omeprazole. *BMJ* 1992; **305:** 451–2.

Effects on the eyes. Visual disturbances associated with the use of omeprazole have included 6 cases of irreversible blindness or visual impairment in severely ill patients given the drug intravenously, and 13 cases of visual disturbances associated with oral use.[1] As a result of concern about these effects the availability of intravenous omeprazole was restricted in Germany; however, the consensus appears to be that a causal link has not been established between omeprazole and these ocular effects. Suggestions that visual (and also auditory[2]) impairment could follow drug-induced vasculitis[2-4] appear to be contentious.[1,5-7] A cohort study involving 140 128 patients receiving antisecretory therapy, 33 988 of whom received omeprazole, found no evidence that any of the drugs used was associated with a major increase in risk of vascular or inflammatory disorders of the eye;[8] however, the statistical power of this study was not high.[9]
1. Creutzfeldt WC, Blum AL. Safety of omeprazole. *Lancet* 1994; **343:** 1098.
2. Schönhöfer PS. Intravenous omeprazole and blindness. *Lancet* 1994; **343:** 665.
3. Schönhöfer PS. Safety of omeprazole and lansoprazole. *Lancet* 1994; **343:** 1369–70.
4. Schönhöfer PS, *et al.* Ocular damage associated with proton pump inhibitors. *BMJ* 1997; **314:** 1805.
5. Colin-Jones D. Safety of omeprazole and lansoprazole. *Lancet* 1994; **343:** 1369.
6. Lessell S. Omeprazole and ocular damage. *BMJ* 1998; **316:** 67.
7. Sachs G. Omeprazole and ocular damage. *BMJ* 1998; **316:** 67–8.
8. García Rodríguez LA, *et al.* A cohort study of the ocular safety of anti-ulcer drugs. *Br J Clin Pharmacol* 1996; **42:** 213–16.
9. Merlo J, Ranstam J. Ocular safety of anti-ulcer drugs. *Br J Clin Pharmacol* 1997; **43:** 449.

Effects on the kidneys. Acute interstitial nephritis developed in 2 elderly patients receiving omeprazole for the treatment of gastro-oesophageal reflux disease.[1,2] Following discontinuation, renal function improved rapidly in 1, but recurred upon rechallenge,[1] while in the other renal function remained

severely affected for several months.[2] It was postulated that this adverse effect might have an allergic mechanism.[2] In these cases interstitial nephritis was associated with rash and eosinophilia; however, a further 2 cases of acute interstitial nephritis associated with omeprazole therapy in elderly patients[3,4] did not exhibit these symptoms. In another report, associated rash without eosinophiluria was seen.[5]
1. Ruffenach SJ, *et al.* Acute interstitial nephritis due to omeprazole. *Am J Med* 1992; **93:** 472–3.
2. Christensen PB, *et al.* Renal failure after omeprazole. *Lancet* 1993; **341:** 55.
3. Assouad M, *et al.* Recurrent acute interstitial nephritis on rechallenge with omeprazole. *Lancet* 1994; **344:** 549.
4. Jones B, *et al.* Acute interstitial nephritis due to omeprazole. *Lancet* 1994; **344:** 1017–18.
5. Kuiper JJ. Omeprazole-induced acute interstitial nephritis. *Am J Med* 1993; **95:** 248.

Effects on the liver. Raised liver enzymes have occurred with omeprazole and other proton pump inhibitors, and there have been isolated cases of hepatotoxicity. For a study suggesting a relatively low incidence of acute liver injury in patients receiving omeprazole see Cimetidine, p.1217.
References.
1. Jochem V, *et al.* Fulminant hepatic failure related to omeprazole. *Am J Gastroenterol* 1992; **87:** 523–5.
2. Kourg SI, *et al.* Omeprazole and the development of acute hepatitis. *Eur J Emerg Med* 1998; **5:** 467–9.

Effects on the nervous system. A report of ataxia in a patient receiving omeprazole;[1] symptoms resolved on discontinuing the drug.
1. Varona L, *et al.* Gait ataxia during omeprazole therapy. *Ann Pharmacother* 1996; **30:** 192.

Effects on the skin. An extensive blistering erythematous skin rash in an elderly woman given omeprazole[1] was characteristic of acute disseminated epidermal necrosis. The UK Committee on Safety of Medicines (CSM) had received 223 reports of cutaneous reactions to omeprazole up to August 1992, including 6 of erythema multiforme, but none of this severity. Other severe reactions that have subsequently been reported include a toxic bullous skin reaction,[2] exfoliative dermatitis,[3,4] erythema multiforme,[4] and toxic erythema.[4] One patient developed exfoliative dermatitis with both omeprazole and lansoprazole.[4] The authors of this report noted that by January 1998 a total of 1296 skin reactions to omeprazole, 500 to lansoprazole, and 44 to pantoprazole, had been reported to the CSM. Most were non-specific rashes, pruritus, urticaria, erythematous rashes, and photosensitive eruptions. A lichenoid reaction that occurred in a patient during omeprazole treatment cleared after ceasing the drug, but recurred during treatment with both lansoprazole and pantoprazole.[5]

For a report of urticaria and angioedema possibly associated with the formulation of omeprazole see Hypersensitivity, below. For the association of rash with interstitial nephritis, see Effects on the Kidneys, above.
1. Cox NH. Acute disseminated epidermal necrosis due to omeprazole. *Lancet* 1992; **340:** 857.
2. Stenier C, *et al.* Bullous skin reaction induced by omeprazole. *Br J Dermatol* 1995; **133:** 343–4.
3. Epelde Gonzalo FD, *et al.* Exfoliative dermatitis related to omeprazole. *Ann Pharmacother* 1995; **29:** 82–3.
4. Cockayne SE, *et al.* Severe erythrodermic reactions to the proton pump inhibitors omeprazole and lansoprazole. *Br J Dermatol* 1999; **141:** 173–5.
5. Bong JL, *et al.* Lichenoid drug eruption with proton pump inhibitors. *BMJ* 2000; **320:** 283.

Gastrointestinal tumours. Early toxicological studies in *rats* given high doses of omeprazole over 2 years identified carcinoid tumours of the gastric mucosa associated with complete block of gastric acid secretion leading to *hypergastrinaemia and hyperplasia of enterochromaffin-like cells.*[1] This has been the main issue concerning the safety of omeprazole and other proton pump inhibitors and initially led to restrictions in use and duration of treatment. Glaxo developed a new test to detect genotoxicity of antisecretory drugs which indicated that a genotoxic effect of omeprazole could not be discounted.[2] This study was heavily criticised; more established genotoxicity tests have been reported to be negative for omeprazole,[3-5] and other groups have not been able to replicate the findings with the new test.[6] The lowest doses at which Glaxo found a genotoxic effect of omeprazole were 10 to 20 mg per kg bodyweight[2] and the clinical significance of their results was questioned.[3] Long-term studies of omeprazole in patients with Zollinger-Ellison syndrome have found no increase in fasting serum-gastrin concentrations and no evidence of gastric carcinoid tumours.[7,8] For mention of the risk of proton pump inhibitors delaying the diagnosis of gastric carcinoma, see under Precautions, below. Hypergastrinaemia can occur with both short- and long-term omeprazole therapy,[9] and may be higher in patients with *Helicobacter pylori* infection.[10] Patients who had *H. pylori* eradicated before long-term omeprazole treatment had lower gastrin concentrations than those who did not, since *H. pylori* eradication reduced the pretreatment gastrin concentrations.[11]

H. pylori is also a cause of *atrophic gastritis*, another risk factor for stomach cancer, and one study found that omeprazole increased the risk of atrophic gastritis in *H. pylori*-positive patients with gastro-oesophageal reflux disease.[12] However, the results of this study require confirmation since it was nonrandomised and retrospective. Nevertheless, some have suggested that it may be appropriate to eradicate *H. pylori* before long-term treatment with a proton pump inhibitor.[11,12] Conversely, there is some evidence that *H. pylori* may be protective in gastro-oesophageal reflux disease.[13]

There has been a report of *gastric polyps* developing in 3 of 8 patients after receiving omeprazole 20 or 40 mg daily for one year.[14] In a subsequent report it was noted that these omeprazole-induced fundic gland polyps had remained asymptomatic and non-malignant for up to five years after their onset.[15]

Further long-term studies of omeprazole may be needed before a realistic risk assessment can be made.

1. Ekman L, *et al.* Toxicological studies on omeprazole. *Scand J Gastroenterol* 1985; **20** (suppl 108): 53–69.
2. Burlinson B, *et al.* Genotoxicity studies of gastric acid inhibiting drugs. *Lancet* 1990; **335**: 419.
3. Ekman L, *et al.* Genotoxicity studies of gastric acid inhibiting drugs. *Lancet* 1990; **335**: 419–20.
4. Wright NA, Goodlad RA. Omeprazole and genotoxicity. *Lancet* 1990; **335**: 909–10.
5. Helander HF, *et al.* Omeprazole and genotoxicity. *Lancet* 1990; **335**: 910–11.
6. Goodlad RA. Acid suppression and claims of genotoxicity: what have we learned? *Drug Safety* 1994; **10**: 413–19.
7. Lloyd-Davies KA, *et al.* Omeprazole in the treatment of Zollinger-Ellison syndrome: a 4-year international study. *Aliment Pharmacol Ther* 1988; **2**: 13–32.
8. Maton PN, *et al.* Long-term efficacy and safety of omeprazole in patients with Zollinger-Ellison syndrome: a prospective study. *Gastroenterology* 1989; **97**: 827–36.
9. Koop H, *et al.* Serum gastrin levels during long-term omeprazole treatment. *Aliment Pharmacol Ther* 1990; **4**: 131–8.
10. Sanduleanu S, *et al.* Serum gastrin and chromogranin A during medium- and long-term acid suppressive therapy: a case-control study. *Aliment Pharmacol Ther* 1999; **13**: 145–53.
11. El-Nujumi A, *et al.* Eradicating Helicobacter pylori reduces hypergastrinaemia during long term omeprazole treatment. *Gut* 1998; **42**: 159–65.
12. Kuipers EJ, *et al.* Atrophic gastritis and Helicobacter pylori infection in patients with reflux esophagitis treated with omeprazole or fundoplication. *N Engl J Med* 1996; **334**: 1018–22.
13. Labenz J, Malfertheiner P. Helicobacter pylori in gastro-oesophageal reflux disease: causal agent, independent or protective factor? *Gut* 1997; **41**: 277–80.
14. Graham JR. Gastric polyposis: onset during long-term therapy with omeprazole. *Med J Aust* 1992; **157**: 287–8.
15. Graham JR. Gastric acne: omeprazole-induced fundic gland polyposis. *Med J Aust* 1998; **168**: 93.

Hypersensitivity. Cases of anaphylactic reactions following treatment with omeprazole, lansoprazole, and pantoprazole, have been reported in the literature and to WHO.[1]

Urticaria, facial angioedema, and bronchospasm in a patient given omeprazole capsules did not recur when the patient was given omeprazole granules and the reaction might have been precipitated by the ingredients of the capsule shell.[2]

See also under Effects on the Kidney, above, and Musculoskeletal Effects, below.

1. Natsch S, *et al.* Anaphylactic reactions to proton-pump inhibitors. *Ann Pharmacother* 2000; **34**: 474–6.
2. Haeney MR. Angio-oedema and urticaria associated with omeprazole. *BMJ* 1992; **305**: 870.

Infection. Oesophageal candidiasis occurred in 2 elderly patients receiving omeprazole but was successfully treated with antifungal therapy. It was postulated that gastric acid secretion and a degree of physiological reflux of acid into the oesophagus might normally play a protective role in preventing candidal infection.[1] The profound reduction in acid secretion produced by omeprazole may also predispose to gastrointestinal infection; there is some evidence for an increased risk of campylobacter infection,[2] as well as a report of recurrent salmonella infection.[3]

1. Larner AJ, Lendrum R. Oesophageal candidiasis after omeprazole therapy. *Gut* 1992; **33**: 860–1.
2. Neal KR, *et al.* Omeprazole as a risk factor for campylobacter gastroenteritis: case-control study. *BMJ* 1996; **312**: 414–15.
3. Wingate DL. Acid reduction and recurrent enteritis. *Lancet* 1990; **335**: 222.

Lupus syndrome. For a report of drug-induced lupus syndrome associated with omeprazole therapy, see Musculoskeletal Effects, below.

Malabsorption. Omeprazole has been reported to result in a substantial reduction in cyanocobalamin (vitamin B_{12}) absorption,[1] probably related to the increase in gastric pH, and indicating a potential risk of vitamin deficiency with long-term therapy.[2] Fat malabsorption, secondary to increased deconjugation of bile acids caused by bacterial overgrowth in the jejunum, has also been reported with omeprazole treatment.[3]

1. Marcuard SP, *et al.* Omeprazole therapy causes malabsorption of cyanocobalamin (vitamin B_{12}). *Ann Intern Med* 1994; **120**: 211–15.
2. Termanini B, *et al.* Effect of long-term gastric acid suppressive therapy on serum vitamin B_{12} levels in patients with Zollinger-Ellison syndrome. *Am J Med* 1998; **104**: 422–30.
3. Shindo K, *et al.* Omeprazole induces altered bile acid metabolism. *Gut* 1998; **42**: 266–71.

Musculoskeletal effects. Progressive muscular weakness suggestive of *myopathy* developed in a 78-year-old patient given omeprazole.[1] After 4 weeks of treatment the patient required assistance in walking and rising from squatting. Weakness resolved on withdrawal of the drug, but returned on rechallenge.

A report of 5 cases of *arthralgia*, sometimes associated with swelling of the affected joints, in patients receiving omeprazole,[2] also noted that some reported cases of omeprazole-associated headache were accompanied by arthralgia or *myalgia*.[2] In another case[3] arthralgia in a patient with a hereditary myopathy receiving omeprazole appeared to represent one aspect of a

drug-induced *lupus* syndrome, being accompanied by malaise, fever, Raynaud's phenomenon, raised antinuclear antibody titres, and anticardiolipin and antihistone antibodies. Symptoms resolved on withdrawal of the drug.

A case of eosinophilia and myalgia related to lansoprazole treatment has been reported.[4]

There has also been a report of 2 cases of acute *gout* associated with omeprazole;[5] in one patient symptoms, which resolved on withdrawal, recurred on rechallenge. However, case control studies have failed to show an increased risk of polyarthralgia[6] or gout[7] associated with omeprazole use.

1. Garrote FJ, *et al.* Subacute myopathy during omeprazole therapy. *Lancet* 1992; **340**: 672.
2. Beutler M, *et al.* Arthralgias and omeprazole. *BMJ* 1994; **309**: 1620.
3. Sivakumar K, Dalakas MC. Autoimmune syndrome induced by omeprazole. *Lancet* 1994; **344**: 619–20.
4. Smith JD, *et al.* Possible lansoprazole-induced eosinophilic syndrome. *Ann Pharmacother* 1998; **32**: 196–200.
5. Kraus A, Flores-Suárez LF. Acute gout associated with omeprazole. *Lancet* 1995; **345**: 461–2.
6. Meier CR, Jick H. Omeprazole, H_2 blockers, and polyarthralgia: case-control study. *BMJ* 1997; **315**: 1283.
7. Meier CR, Jick H. Omeprazole, other antiulcer drugs and newly diagnosed gout. *Br J Clin Pharmacol* 1997; **44**: 175–8.

Overdosage. A report of 2 cases of overdosage with omeprazole.[1] The major clinical features were drowsiness, headache (possibly due to a metabolite), and tachycardia. Both patients recovered uneventfully without specific treatment.

1. Ferner RE, Allison TR. Omeprazole overdose. *Hum Exp Toxicol* 1993; **12**: 541–2.

Precautions

Before giving omeprazole or other proton pump inhibitors to patients with gastric ulcers the possibility of malignancy should be considered since these drugs may mask symptoms and delay diagnosis. Omeprazole and other proton pump inhibitors should be used with caution in hepatic impairment.

Gastric carcinoma. Proton pump inhibitors relieve dyspeptic symptoms associated with gastric carcinoma and can therefore delay its diagnosis. In addition, there is some evidence that they may also endoscopically 'heal' early gastric carcinoma so that the diagnosis is missed.[1] Consequently, some commentators recommend that proton pump inhibitors should not be prescribed for symptom control prior to endoscopy in patients at risk for gastric carcinoma.[2]

1. Wayman J, *et al.* The response of early gastric cancer to proton-pump inhibitors. *N Engl J Med* 1998; **338**: 1924–5.
2. Griffin SM, Raimes SA. Proton pump inhibitors may mask early gastric cancer: dyspeptic patients over 45 should undergo endoscopy before these drugs are started. *BMJ* 1998; **317**: 1606–7.

Helicobacter infection. Treatment with proton pump inhibitors may cause false-negative results in the urea breath test for *Helicobacter pylori* infection. In one study in patients with *H. pylori* infection, 4 weeks treatment with lansoprazole 30 mg daily caused 33% of patients to have negative urea breath tests.[1] The breath test became positive again in all patients within 2 weeks of stopping lansoprazole therapy. In a similar study, 52% of patients had negative urea breath tests for *H. pylori* while receiving omeprazole 20 mg daily, and the breath test became positive again in all patients within 2 to 6 days of stopping treatment.[2] The manufacturers of the urea breath test for *H. pylori* recommend that it should not be performed within 4 weeks of treatment with an antisecretory drug.

For a discussion of the link between proton pump inhibitors, *H. pylori*, and gastritis, see under Gastrointestinal Tumours above.

1. Laine L, *et al.* Effect of proton pump inhibitor therapy on diagnostic testing for Helicobacter pylori. *Ann Intern Med* 1998; **129**: 547–50.
2. Connor SJ, *et al.* The effect of dosing with omeprazole on the accuracy of the ^{13}C-urea breath test in Helicobacter pylori-infected subjects. *Aliment Pharmacol Ther* 1999; **13**: 1287–93.

Hepatic impairment. In patients with cirrhosis an increase in omeprazole bioavailability, and elimination half-life has been reported.[1] For dosage adjustment in hepatic impairment see Uses and Administration, below.

1. Andersson T, *et al.* Pharmacokinetics of [^{14}C]omeprazole in patients with liver cirrhosis. *Clin Pharmacokinet* 1993; **24**: 71–8.

Pregnancy. Proton pump inhibitors are not generally licensed for use during pregnancy, although in a case-control study in 113 women who had taken omeprazole during pregnancy,[1] the incidence of major malformations in neonates exposed to omeprazole during the first trimester (5.1%) was not significantly different to that in neonates exposed to H_2-antagonists (3.1%) or non-teratogens (3%). For the suggestion that lansoprazole might be considered if a proton pump inhibitor must be given during pregnancy, see Gastro-oesophageal Reflux Disease, p.1204.

1. Lalkin A, *et al.* The safety of omeprazole during pregnancy: a multicentre prospective controlled study. *Am J Obstet Gynecol* 1998; **179**: 727–30.

Interactions

Omeprazole and other proton pump inhibitors are metabolised by the cytochrome P450 system, primarily by isoenzyme CYP2C19, and may alter the me-

tabolism of some other drugs metabolised by these enzymes. Omeprazole may prolong the elimination of diazepam, phenytoin, and warfarin (but see below). Omeprazole and other proton pump inhibitors can reduce the absorption of drugs such as ketoconazole, and possibly itraconazole, whose absorption is dependent on an acid gastric pH.

◊ Omeprazole is metabolised primarily by the cytochrome P450 isoenzyme CYP2C19 (see Metabolism, below) and therefore may interact with diazepam (see under Gastrointestinal Drugs, p.678). Some metabolism of phenytoin (see p.361), tolbutamide, and the R-enantiomer of warfarin (see p.996) also takes place by CYP2C19, but the effects seen have been minor.[1] Although some induction of CYP1A2, which metabolises caffeine and theophylline (p.781), has been reported this does not appear to be clinically significant.[2] Omeprazole does not appear to have a significant effect on CYP3A4, which is an important cytochrome for drug metabolism.[1,3] (For a study *in vitro* suggesting that omeprazole affected CYP3A4 metabolism of tacrolimus, see p.570.)

For reference to the possibility of enhanced digoxin absorption with omeprazole, see p.872. For a study suggesting that omeprazole reduces the absorption of cyanocobalamin, see Malabsorption, above. For reference to elevated serum concentrations of methotrexate during concomitant use with omeprazole, see p.555.

1. Andersson T. Pharmacokinetics, metabolism and interactions of acid pump inhibitors: focus on omeprazole, lansoprazole and pantoprazole. *Clin Pharmacokinet* 1996; **31**: 9–28.
2. Rizzo N, *et al.* Omeprazole and lansoprazole are not inducers of cytochrome P4501A2 under conventional therapeutic conditions. *Eur J Clin Pharmacol* 1996; **49**: 491–5.
3. Tateishi T, *et al.* Omeprazole does not affect measured CYP3A4 activity using the erythromycin breath test. *Br J Clin Pharmacol* 1995; **40**: 411–12.

Clarithromycin. Studies in healthy subjects have indicated that concurrent administration of omeprazole and clarithromycin results in an approximate 30% increase in peak plasma concentrations of omeprazole, and an increase in its mean half-life from 1.2 to 1.6 hours.[1] At the same time, plasma concentrations of clarithromycin were also modestly increased, as were local concentrations in gastric tissue and mucus.[1] Clarithromycin inhibits[2] the metabolism of omeprazole mediated by the cytochrome P450 isoenzyme CYP3A4. The interaction may contribute to the benefits of combined therapy for *Helicobacter pylori* infection.

1. Gustavson LE, *et al.* Effect of omeprazole on concentrations of clarithromycin in plasma and gastric tissue at steady state. *Antimicrob Agents Chemother* 1995; **39**: 2078–83.
2. Furuta T, *et al.* Effects of clarithromycin on the metabolism of omeprazole in relation to CYP2C19 genotype status in humans. *Clin Pharmacol Ther* 1999; **66**: 265–74.

Pharmacokinetics

Omeprazole is rapidly but variably absorbed following oral administration. Absorption is not affected by food. Omeprazole is acid-labile and pharmacokinetics may vary between the various formulations developed to improve oral bioavailability. The absorption of omeprazole also appears to be dose-dependent; increasing the dosage above 40 mg has been reported to increase the plasma concentrations in a non-linear fashion because of saturable first-pass hepatic metabolism. In addition, absorption is higher after long-term administration.

Bioavailability of omeprazole may be increased in elderly patients, in some ethnic groups such as Chinese, and in patients with impaired hepatic function, but is not markedly affected in patients with renal impairment.

Following absorption, omeprazole is almost completely metabolised in the liver, primarily by the cytochrome P450 isoenzyme CYP2C19 to form hydroxyomeprazole, and to a small extent by CYP3A to form omeprazole sulfone. The metabolites are inactive, and are excreted mostly in the urine and to a lesser extent in bile. The elimination half-life from plasma is reported to be about 0.5 to 3 hours. Omeprazole is highly bound (about 95%) to plasma proteins.

◊ References.

1. Andersson T, *et al.* Pharmacokinetics of various single intravenous and oral doses of omeprazole. *Eur J Clin Pharmacol* 1990; **39**: 195–7.
2. Andersson T, Regårdh C-G. Pharmacokinetics of omeprazole and metabolites following single intravenous and oral doses of 40 and 80 mg. *Drug Invest* 1990; **2**: 255–63.
3. Ching MS, *et al.* Oral bioavailability of omeprazole before and after chronic therapy in patients with duodenal ulcer. *Br J Clin Pharmacol* 1991; **31**: 166–70.
4. Landahl S, *et al.* Pharmacokinetic study of omeprazole in elderly healthy volunteers. *Clin Pharmacokinet* 1992; **23**: 469–76.

5. Andersson T, *et al.* Pharmacokinetics of [^{14}C]omeprazole in patients with liver cirrhosis. *Clin Pharmacokinet* 1993; **24:** 71–8.
6. Jacqz-Aigrain E, *et al.* Pharmacokinetics of intravenous omeprazole in children. *Eur J Clin Pharmacol* 1994; **47:** 181–5.

Metabolism. The major enzyme involved in omeprazole metabolism is cytochrome P450 isoenzyme CYP2C19. This enzyme is polymorphically expressed, and individuals who are deficient in the enzyme are poor metabolisers of omeprazole. This occurs in about 3% of Caucasians and 15% of Chinese, Japanese, and Koreans. These individuals have markedly higher plasma concentrations of omeprazole, and they may require dosage adjustment. Some omeprazole is metabolised by CYP3A to form omeprazole sulfone and hydroxy-omeprazole, and some by CYP2D6 to form desmethylomeprazole.

References.

1. Andersson T, *et al.* Identification of human liver cytochrome P450 isoforms mediating omeprazole metabolism. *Br J Clin Pharmacol* 1993; **36:** 521–30.
2. Caraco Y, *et al.* Ethnic and genetic determinants of omeprazole disposition and effect. *Clin Pharmacol Ther* 1996; **60:** 157–67.
3. Karam WG, *et al.* Human CYP2C19 is a major omeprazole 5-hydroxylase, as demonstrated with recombinant cytochrome P450 enzymes. *Drug Metab Dispos* 1996; **24:** 1081–7.

Uses and Administration

Omeprazole is a proton pump inhibitor. It inhibits secretion of gastric acid by irreversibly blocking the enzyme system of hydrogen/potassium adenosine triphosphatase (H$^+$/K$^+$ ATPase), the 'proton pump' of the gastric parietal cell. It is used in conditions where inhibition of gastric acid secretion may be beneficial, including aspiration syndromes (p.1202), dyspepsia (p.1204), gastro-oesophageal reflux disease (p.1204), peptic ulcer disease (p.1208), and the Zollinger-Ellison syndrome (p.1209).

Esomeprazole (p.1225), an isomer of omeprazole, is also used.

Omeprazole may be given by mouth as the base or magnesium salt, or intravenously as the sodium salt. Doses are expressed in terms of the base.

For the relief of acid-related **dyspepsia** omeprazole is given in usual doses of 10 or 20 mg daily by mouth for 2 to 4 weeks.

The usual dose for the treatment of **gastro-oesophageal reflux disease** is 20 mg by mouth once daily for 4 weeks, followed by a further 4 to 8 weeks if not fully healed. In refractory oesophagitis, a dose of 40 mg daily may be used. Maintenance therapy after healing of oesophagitis is 20 mg once daily, and for acid reflux is 10 mg daily. In children, doses in the range 0.7 to 1.4 mg per kg body-weight daily, up to a maximum daily dose of 40 mg, have been given for 4 to 12 weeks.

In the management of **peptic ulcer disease** a single daily dose of 20 mg by mouth, or 40 mg in severe cases, is given. Treatment is continued for 4 weeks for duodenal ulcer and 8 weeks for gastric ulcer. Where appropriate, a dose of 10 to 20 mg once daily may be given for maintenance.

For the eradication of *Helicobacter pylori* in peptic ulceration omeprazole may be combined with antibacterials in dual or triple therapy. Effective **triple therapy** regimens include omeprazole 20 mg twice daily combined with: amoxicillin 500 mg and metronidazole 400 mg, both three times daily; clarithromycin 500 mg and metronidazole 400 mg (or tinidazole 500 mg) both twice daily; or with amoxicillin 1 g and clarithromycin 500 mg both twice daily. These regimens are given for 1 week. **Dual therapy** regimens such as omeprazole 40 mg daily with either amoxicillin 750 mg to 1 g twice daily or clarithromycin 500 mg three times daily, are less effective and must be given for 2 weeks. Omeprazole alone may be continued for a further 2 to 8 weeks.

Doses of 20 mg daily are used in the treatment of **NSAID-associated ulceration**; a dose of 20 mg daily may also be used for prophylaxis in patients with a previous history of gastroduodenal lesions who require continued NSAID treatment.

The initial recommended dosage for patients with the **Zollinger-Ellison syndrome** is 60 mg by mouth once daily, adjusted as required. The majority of patients are effectively controlled by doses in the range 20 to 120 mg daily, but doses up to 120 mg three times

daily have been used. Daily doses above 80 mg should be administered in divided doses (usually 2).

Omeprazole is also used for the prophylaxis of **acid aspiration** during general anaesthesia, in a dose of 40 mg the evening before surgery and a further 40 mg two to six hours before the procedure.

DOSAGE IN HEPATIC IMPAIRMENT.

Consideration should be given to reducing the dose of omeprazole in patients with impaired hepatic function. In the UK, a maximum daily dose of 20 mg is recommended for patients with impaired hepatic function. In the USA, it is recommended that dose adjustment should be considered, particularly where maintenance treatment is required.

PARENTERAL DOSAGE.

In patients who are unsuited to receive oral therapy omeprazole sodium may be given on a short-term basis by intravenous infusion, in a usual dose equivalent to 40 mg of the base over a period of 20 to 30 minutes in 100 mL of sodium chloride 0.9% or glucose 5%. It has also been given by slow intravenous injection. Higher intravenous doses have been given to patients with Zollinger-Ellison syndrome.

◊ General reviews.

1. Richardson P, *et al.* Proton pump inhibitors: pharmacology and rationale for use in gastrointestinal disorders. *Drugs* 1998; **56:** 307–35.
2. Langtry HD, Wilde MI. Omeprazole: a review of its use in Helicobacter pylori infection, gastro-oesophageal reflux disease and peptic ulcers induced by nonsteroidal anti-inflammatory drugs. *Drugs* 1998; **56:** 447–86.
3. Berardi RR, Welage LS. Proton-pump inhibitors in acid-related diseases. *Am J Health-Syst Pharm* 1998; **55:** 2289–98.
4. Brown GJE, Yeomans ND. Prevention of the gastrointestinal adverse effects of nonsteroidal anti-inflammatory drugs: the role of proton pump inhibitors. *Drug Safety* 1999; **21:** 503–12.

Administration. Omeprazole is given by mouth as tablets or capsules containing enteric-coated pellets or granules which should be swallowed whole and not crushed or chewed. In patients with swallowing difficulties the manufacturers generally recommend that the tablet be dispersed in water, fruit juice, or yogurt before swallowing. Similarly the contents of the capsules can be mixed with a little fruit juice or yogurt and swallowed.

Asthma. Gastro-oesophageal reflux has been suggested as a potential exacerbating factor for asthma (p.757), and acid suppressive therapy with omeprazole has been reported to reduce asthma symptoms in some[1] but not other[2] studies. A meta-analysis of acid suppressive therapy concluded it was not effective in improving asthma symptoms in patients with gastro-oesophageal reflux,[3] and the link between reflux and asthma symptoms has been disputed.[4]

1. Harding SM, *et al.* Asthma and gastroesophageal reflux: acid suppressive therapy improves asthma outcome. *Am J Med* 1996; **100:** 395–405.
2. Ford GA, *et al.* Omeprazole in the treatment of asthmatics with nocturnal symptoms and gastro-oesophageal reflux: a placebo-controlled cross-over trial. *Postgrad Med J* 1994; **70:** 350–4.
3. Gibson PG, *et al.* Interventions for gastro-oesophageal reflux in treating adults and children with asthma (updated 12 July 1999). Available in The Cochrane Library; Issue 4. Oxford: Update Software; 1999.
4. Field SK. A critical review of the studies of the effects of simulated or real gastroesophageal reflux on pulmonary function in asthmatic adults. *Chest* 1999; **115:** 848–56.

Inflammatory bowel disease. There are a few reports[1,2] of responses to omeprazole 20 mg daily in patients with inflammatory bowel disease (p.1205). Combination of omeprazole with mesalazine has also been tried.[2]

1. Heinzow U, Schlegelberger T. Omeprazole in ulcerative colitis. *Lancet* 1994; **343:** 477.
2. Dickinson JB. Is omeprazole helpful in inflammatory bowel disease? *J Clin Gastroenterol* 1994; **18:** 317–19.

Scleroderma. Gastro-oesophageal reflux is one of the gastrointestinal manifestations of systemic sclerosis, and proton pump inhibitors such as omeprazole play a major role in the management of such gastrointestinal disease.[1] For a discussion of the broader management of the condition see p.505.

1. Williamson DJ. Update on scleroderma. *Med J Aust* 1995; **162:** 599–601.

Preparations

Proprietary Preparations (details are given in Part 3)
Aust.: Antra; Losec; *Austral.:* Acimax; Losec; Maxor; *Belg.:* Logastric; Losec; *Braz.:* Gaspiren; Gastrium; Losec; Omep; Omeprasec; Peprazol; Ulconar; Victrix; *Canad.:* Losec; *Denm.:* Losec; *Fin.:* Losec; *Fr.:* Mopral; Zoltum; *Ger.:* Antra; Gastroloc†; Ombeta; Ome-nerton; Ome-Puren; Omep; *Hong Kong:* Losec; *Irl.:* Losec; *Israel:* Losec; Omepradex; *Ital.:* Antra; Losec; Mepral; Omeprazen; *Jpn:* Omepral; *Mex.:* Inhibitron; Losec; Olexin; Osiren; Ozoken; Plazolit; Prazidec; Prazolit; Ulsen; *Neth.:* Losec; *Norw.:* Losec; *NZ:* Losec; *Port.:* Gasec; Losec; Mepraz; Ometon; Omezolan; Prazentol; Proclor; Proton; *S.Afr.:* Losec; *Singapore:* Losec; *Spain:* Audazol; Aulcer; Belmazol; Ceprandal; Elgam; Emeproton; Gastrimut; Indurgan; Losec; Miol; Mopral; Norpramin; Nuclosina; Omapren; Ompranyt; Parizac; Pepticum;

Prysma; Sanamidol; Secrepina; Ulceral; Ulcesep; Ulcometion; Zimor; *Swed.:* Losec; *Switz.:* Antra; Antramups; *Thai.:* Airomet; Desec; Dosate; Gomec; Gomec; Losec; Madiprazole; Metsec; Miracid; O-Sid; OMP; Oprazole; Peptizole; Ulprazole; Zefxon; *UAE:* Risek; *UK:* Losec; *USA:* Prilosec.

Multi-ingredient: *Austral.:* Klacid HP 7; Losec Helicopak; Losec Hp 7; *Canad.:* Losec 1-2-3 A; Losec 1-2-3 M; *Fin.:* Losec Heliara; *NZ:* Helicosec; Klacid HP7; Losec Hp7; *S.Afr.:* Losec 20 Triple.

Ondansetron   (10033-c)

Ondansetron *(BAN, rINN)*.

GR-38032. (±)-1,2,3,9-Tetrahydro-9-methyl-3-(2-methylimidazol-1-ylmethyl)-carbazol-4(9H)-one.

$C_{18}H_{19}N_3O = 293.4$.

CAS — 99614-02-5; 116002-70-1.

ATC — A04AA01.

Ondansetron Hydrochloride   (3149-y)

Ondansetron Hydrochloride *(BANM, USAN, rINNM)*.

GR-38032F.

$C_{18}H_{19}N_3O,HCl,2H_2O = 365.9$.

CAS — 103639-04-9.

Pharmacopoeias. In US.

Ondansetron hydrochloride 1.25 mg is approximately equivalent to 1 mg of ondansetron base.

Pharmacopoeial description

USP 25: A white to off-white powder. Sparingly soluble in water and in alcohol; very slightly soluble in acetone, in chloroform, and in ethyl acetate; slightly soluble in dichloromethane and in isopropyl alcohol; soluble in methyl alcohol. Store in airtight containers. Protect from light.

Incompatibility. Ondansetron hydrochloride and dexamethasone sodium phosphate were not compatible when high concentrations were combined in polypropylene syringes.[1] Lower concentrations (up to 640 µg per mL of ondansetron and 400 µg per mL of dexamethasone phosphate) were stable in 50 mL containers of infusion fluid for 30 days under refrigeration. Compatibility has been reported for 24 hours in plastic syringes at 4° or 23° with a variety of other drugs,[2] and with several antineoplastics (cytarabine, dacarbazine, doxorubicin, etoposide, or methotrexate) in PVC infusion bags for 48 hours at room temperature.[3]

1. Hagan RL, *et al.* Stability of ondansetron hydrochloride and dexamethasone sodium phosphate in infusion bags and syringes for 32 days. *Am J Health-Syst Pharm* 1996; **53:** 1431–5.
2. Stewart JT, *et al.* Stability of ondansetron hydrochloride and 12 medications in plastic syringes. *Am J Health-Syst Pharm* 1998; **55:** 2630–4.
3. Stewart JT, *et al.* Stability of ondansetron hydrochloride and five antineoplastic medications. *Am J Health-Syst Pharm* 1996; **53:** 1297–1300.

Adverse Effects and Precautions

Ondansetron and other 5-HT$_3$-receptor antagonists may cause headache, a sensation of flushing or warmth, and constipation. A transient rise in liver enzymes has occasionally occurred. There have been rare reports of immediate hypersensitivity reactions, including anaphylaxis. Chest pain, hypotension, tachycardia, and bradycardia have been reported rarely. Dizziness and transient visual disturbances such as blurred vision have been reported during rapid intravenous administration.

5-HT$_3$-receptor antagonists should generally not be used in patients who have had a hypersensitivity reaction to a member of this drug class. They should be used with care in patients with signs of subacute intestinal obstruction or ileus. Ondansetron should be given in reduced doses to patients with moderate to severe hepatic impairment.

Effects on the cardiovascular system. Chest pain and/or cardiac arrhythmias that might have been associated with ondansetron were reported[1] in 4 patients, 2 of whom died. In 3 subsequent patients who developed severe chest or anginal pain, treatment with ondansetron was discontinued. The manufacturers (Glaxo) had at that time no evidence of a causal relationship between ondansetron and episodes of chest pain and cardiac abnormalities.[2] Administration of ondansetron 32 mg intravenously over 15 minutes produced no clinically important cardiovascular changes in a study in 12 healthy subjects.[3]

1. Ballard HS, *et al.* Ondansetron and chest pain. *Lancet* 1992; **340:** 1107.
2. Palmer JBD, Greenstreet YL. Ondansetron and chest pain. *Lancet* 1992; **340:** 1410.
3. Boike SC, *et al.* Cardiovascular effects of i.v. granisetron at two administration rates and of ondansetron in healthy adults. *Am J Health-Syst Pharm* 1997; **54:** 1172–6.

Effects on the liver. Although disturbances in liver enzyme values have been reported in patients receiving ondansetron, more severe symptoms of liver disorder appear to be very rare; however, there is a report of severe jaundice associated with ondansetron as an antiemetic for chemotherapy.[1] Symptoms did not recur when the patient was given granisetron.

1. Verrill M, Judson I. Jaundice with ondansetron. *Lancet* 1994; **344**: 190–1.

Effects on the nervous system. Tonic-clonic movements and frothing at the mouth occurred in a patient 90 minutes after an infusion of ondansetron;[1] the patient responded to diazepam intravenously. The manufacturers have observed 10 patients who developed *seizures* during initial clinical studies, but considered that, unlike this case, all these patients had predisposing factors. Seizures have also been reported occasionally in patients receiving other 5-HT$_3$ receptor antagonists. *Extrapyramidal reactions* in patients receiving ondansetron as part of a chemotherapy regimen[2,3] and for post-operative nausea and vomiting[4] have also been reported.

1. Sargent AI, *et al.* Seizure associated with ondansetron. *Clin Pharm* 1993; **12**: 613–15.
2. Krstenansky PM, *et al.* Extrapyramidal reaction caused by ondansetron. *Ann Pharmacother* 1994; **28**: 280.
3. Mathews HG, Tancil CG. Extrapyramidal reaction caused by ondansetron. *Ann Pharmacother* 1996; **30**: 196.
4. Stonell C. An extrapyramidal reaction to ondansetron. *Br J Anaesth* 1998; **81**: 658.

Hypersensitivity. Anaphylactoid reactions have been reported in patients receiving ondansetron injection. The FDA stated in October 1993 that it had received 24 reports of such reactions,[1] mostly occurring after the first ondansetron dose of the second or third chemotherapy cycle, and characterised by urticaria, angioedema, hypotension, bronchospasm, and dyspnoea. In a subsequent report, 2 patients in whom a mild hypersensitivity reaction had occurred following one 5-HT$_3$-receptor antagonist developed a more severe reaction after exposure to a second drug of the same class.[2] In the first case severe acute asthma, cyanosis, and loss of consciousness developed after ondansetron in a patient who had previously experienced an asthmatic reaction after tropisetron. The second patient had developed pruritus after a tropisetron injection and urticaria after ondansetron, and subsequently developed anaphylactic shock 5 minutes after a further dose of tropisetron. It was recommended that another 5-HT$_3$-receptor antagonist should not be given as a replacement to patients who developed a hypersensitivity reaction to a drug of this class.

1. Chen M, *et al.* Anaphylactoid-anaphylactic reactions associated with ondansetron. *Ann Intern Med* 1993; **119**: 862.
2. Kataja V, de Bruijn KM. Hypersensitivity reactions associated with 5-hydroxytryptamine$_3$-receptor antagonists: a class effect? *Lancet* 1996; **347**: 584–5.

Interactions

Antibacterials. *Rifampicin* pretreatment reduced the area under the plasma concentration-time curve of oral ondansetron by 65% and of intravenous ondansetron by 48% in healthy volunteers.[1] Concomitant use of rifampicin, or other potent inducers of cytochrome P450 isoenzyme CYP3A4, with ondansetron may reduce antiemetic efficacy.

1. Villikka K, *et al.* The effect of rifampin on the pharmacokinetics of oral and intravenous ondansetron. *Clin Pharmacol Ther* 1999; **65**: 377–81.

Antineoplastics. For mention of retrospective studies suggesting a change of pharmacokinetic parameters of high-dose cyclophosphamide and cisplatin when administered with an ondansetron-containing antiemetic regimen, see Gastrointestinal Drugs, p.528.

Pharmacokinetics

Following oral administration, ondansetron is rapidly absorbed with peak plasma concentrations being reported about 1.5 to 2 hours after an oral dose of 8 mg. The absolute bioavailability is about 60%, due mainly to hepatic first-pass metabolism. It is extensively distributed in the body; results *in vitro* suggest that about 70 to 75% of the drug in plasma is protein bound. It is cleared from the systemic circulation predominantly by hepatic metabolism through multiple enzymatic pathways, with less than 5% of a dose being excreted in urine unchanged: clearances of around 6 mL per minute per kg have been reported in young, healthy subjects. In elderly subjects, bioavailability may be somewhat higher (65%) and clearance lower (4 to 5 mL per minute per kg), presumably due to reduced hepatic metabolism. The terminal elimination half-life is about 3 hours in younger subjects, prolonged to about 5 hours in the elderly and in those with renal impairment. These differences are not considered sufficient to warrant dosage adjustment; however, in patients with severe hepatic impairment, in whom bioavailability may approach 100% and clearance is markedly slowed, with elimination half-lives of 15 to 32 hours, dosage restriction is advisable (see Administration in Hepatic Impairment, below). Children

also have reduced clearance, which is age-related; use of weight-based doses compensates for this change.

◊ References.
1. Roila F, Del Favero A. Ondansetron clinical pharmacokinetics. *Clin Pharmacokinet* 1995; **29**: 95–109.
2. Figg WD, *et al.* Pharmacokinetics of ondansetron in patients with hepatic insufficiency. *J Clin Pharmacol* 1996; **36**: 206–15.

Uses and Administration

Ondansetron is a 5-HT$_3$-receptor antagonist with antiemetic activity. It is used in the management of **nausea and vomiting** induced by cytotoxic chemotherapy and radiotherapy. It is also used for the prevention and treatment of postoperative nausea and vomiting. For the treatment of nausea and vomiting, and the important role of 5-HT$_3$-receptor antagonists, see p.1206.

Ondansetron is given by intramuscular or slow intravenous injection as the hydrochloride, by mouth as the hydrochloride or base, or rectally as the base. Doses are expressed in terms of the base.

For *highly emetogenic chemotherapy* the following dose schedules appear to be equally effective in preventing acute emesis:

• a single dose of 8 mg by slow intravenous or intramuscular injection immediately before treatment, *or*

• 8 mg by slow intravenous or intramuscular injection immediately before treatment, either followed by a continuous intravenous infusion of 1 mg per hour for up to 24 hours, or by a further two doses of 8 mg two to four hours apart, *or*

• a single dose of 32 mg given by intravenous infusion over at least 15 minutes immediately before treatment, *or*

• a 16-mg suppository rectally, given 1 to 2 hours before treatment.

The efficacy of ondansetron in highly emetogenic chemotherapy may be enhanced by intravenous administration of dexamethasone sodium phosphate 20 mg before chemotherapy. To protect against delayed emesis, ondansetron 8 mg orally twice daily, or 16 mg rectally once daily, for up to 5 days after the end of a course of chemotherapy, may be given.

For preventing acute emesis with *less emetogenic chemotherapy* and *radiotherapy*:

• 8 mg may be given as a slow intravenous or intramuscular injection immediately before treatment, *or*

• 16 mg rectally can be given 1 to 2 hours before treatment, *or*

• 8 mg can be given by mouth 1 to 2 hours before treatment followed by 8 mg 12 hours later.

To protect against delayed emesis these regimens are followed by 8 mg by mouth twice daily, or 16 mg rectally once daily, for up to 5 days after the end of a course of chemotherapy.

For children a recommended dose is 5 mg per m^2 body-surface intravenously immediately before chemotherapy, followed by 4 mg orally 12 hours later. A dose of 4 mg orally twice daily may be continued for up to 5 days after the end of chemotherapy.

To *prevent postoperative nausea and vomiting* adults may be given:

• 16 mg by mouth an hour before anaesthesia, *or*

• 8 mg by mouth an hour before anaesthesia followed by 2 further doses of 8 mg at 8-hour intervals, *or*

• a single dose of 4 mg by intramuscular or slow intravenous injection at induction of anaesthesia.

For the *treatment of postoperative nausea and vomiting* a single 4-mg dose by intramuscular or slow intravenous injection is recommended.

Children aged 2 years and over may be given 0.1 mg per kg body-weight by slow intravenous injection, up to a maximum dose of 4 mg, both for the prevention and treatment of postoperative nausea and vomiting.

DOSAGE IN HEPATIC IMPAIRMENT.

In patients with moderate or severe hepatic impairment the manufacturers have recommended that the

total daily dose of ondansetron should not exceed 8 mg (see below).

◊ Reviews.
1. Milne RJ, Heel RC. Ondansetron: therapeutic use as an antiemetic. *Drugs* 1991; **41**: 574–95.
2. Chaffee BJ, Tankanow RM. Ondansetron—the first of a new class of antiemetic agents. *Clin Pharm* 1991; **10**: 430–6.
3. Markham A, Sorkin EM. Ondansetron: an update of its therapeutic use in chemotherapy-induced and postoperative nausea and vomiting. *Drugs* 1993; **45**: 931–52.
4. McQueen KD, Milton JD. Multicenter postmarketing surveillance of ondansetron therapy in pediatric patients. *Ann Pharmacother* 1994; **28**: 85–92.
5. Cooke CE, Mehra IV. Oral ondansetron for preventing nausea and vomiting. *Am J Hosp Pharm* 1994; **51**: 762–71.
6. Wilde MI, Markham A. Ondansetron: a review of its pharmacology and preliminary clinical findings in novel applications. *Drugs* 1996; **52**: 773–94.
7. Perez EA. A risk-benefit assessment of serotonin 5-HT$_3$ receptor antagonists in antineoplastic therapy-induced emesis. *Drug Safety* 1998; **18**: 43–56.
8. Gregory RE, Ettinger DS. 5-HT$_3$ receptor antagonists for the prevention of chemotherapy-induced nausea and vomiting: a comparison of their pharmacology and clinical efficacy. *Drugs* 1998; **55**: 173–89.

Administration. A report[1] of the successful use of ondansetron by continuous subcutaneous infusion to control intractable nausea and vomiting. Despite concern about the low pH of ondansetron injection there was no problem with the skin at the infusion site.

1. Mulvenna PM, Regnard CFB. Subcutaneous ondansetron. *Lancet* 1992; **339**: 1059.

Administration in hepatic impairment. The manufacturers recommend that the dose of ondansetron should not exceed 8 mg daily in patients with moderate or severe hepatic impairment. When this dose was given intravenously to patients with various degrees of impairment it was found that in those who were severely impaired there was an increase in the area under the plasma concentration/time curve and in the terminal plasma half-life, and a decrease in plasma clearance.[1] The authors of this study, some of whom worked for the manufacturers, considered that ondansetron should be restricted to once daily dosage in severe hepatic impairment.

1. Blake JC, *et al.* The pharmacokinetics of intravenous ondansetron in patients with hepatic impairment. *Br J Clin Pharmacol* 1993; **35**: 441–3.

Pain. Preliminary results from a small crossover study[1] indicated that ondansetron was more effective than paracetamol in relieving the pain of fibromyalgia, a chronic disorder that responds poorly to conventional analgesics.

1. Hrycaj P, *et al.* Pathogenetic aspects of responsiveness to ondansetron (5-hydroxytryptamine type 3 receptor antagonist) in patients with primary fibromyalgia syndrome—a preliminary study. *J Rheumatol* 1996; **23**: 1418–23.

Pruritus. There are several case reports of cholestatic pruritus (p.1106) responding to intravenous or oral ondansetron.[1,2] In a randomised double-blind trial ondansetron 8 mg three times daily by mouth produced a modest reduction in pruritus compared with placebo in patients with chronic liver disease.[3] Ondansetron has also been reported to be of benefit in pruritus due to renal failure[4] and possibly in opioid-induced pruritus.[5]

1. Schwörer H, Ramadri G. Improvement of cholestatic pruritus by ondansetron. *Lancet* 1993; **341**: 1471.
2. Raderer M, *et al.* Ondansetron for pruritus due to cholestasis. *N Engl J Med* 1994; **330**: 1540.
3. Müller C, *et al.* Treatment of pruritus in chronic liver disease with the 5-hydroxytryptamine receptor type 3 antagonist ondansetron: a randomized, placebo-controlled, double-blind cross-over trial. *Eur J Gastroenterol Hepatol* 1998; **10**: 865–70.
4. Balaskas EV, *et al.* Histamine and serotonin in uremic pruritus: effect of ondansetron in CAPD-pruritic patients. *Nephron* 1998; **78**: 395–402.
5. Kyriakides K, *et al.* Management of opioid-induced pruritus: a role for 5-HT$_3$ antagonists? *Br J Anaesth* 1999; **82**: 439–41.

Psychiatric disorders. Ondansetron has been tried experimentally in a number of psychiatric disorders including schizophrenia[1] and psychosis in patients with parkinsonism.[2] It is also reported to be under investigation in the management of panic attacks (p.649). For the more conventional management of schizophrenia and parkinsonism see p.651 and p.1160 respectively.

1. White A, *et al.* Ondansetron in the treatment of schizophrenia. *Lancet* 1991; **337**: 1173.
2. Zoldan J, *et al.* Psychosis in advanced Parkinson's disease: treatment with ondansetron, a 5-HT$_3$ receptor antagonist. *Neurology* 1995; **45**: 1305–8.

Substance dependence. Ondansetron is being studied in the management of alcohol dependence (p.1131). However, in one study[1] a significant reduction in alcohol consumption was found only in lighter drinkers after subgroup analysis. Another study[2] found a reduction in alcohol consumption by patients with early-onset alcoholism (onset before age 25) who took ondansetron compared with placebo. No such effect was seen, however, in patients with late-onset alcoholism.

1. Sellers EM, *et al.* Clinical efficacy of the 5-HT$_3$ antagonist ondansetron in alcohol abuse and dependence. *Alcohol Clin Exp Res* 1994; **18**: 879–85.
2. Johnson BA, *et al.* Ondansetron for reduction of drinking among biologically predisposed alcoholic patients. *JAMA* 2000; **284**: 963–71.

Preparations

USP 25: Ondansetron Injection.

Proprietary Preparations (details are given in Part 3)
Aust.: Zofran; *Austral.:* Zofran; *Belg.:* Zofran; *Braz.:* Modifical; Zofran; *Canad.:* Zofran; *Denm.:* Zofran; *Fin.:* Zofran; *Fr.:* Zophren; *Ger.:* Zofran; *Hong Kong:* Zofran; *Irl.:* Zofran; *Israel:* Zofran; *Ital.:* Zofran; *Mex.:* Zofran; *Neth.:* Zofran; *Norw.:* Zofran; *NZ:* Zofran; *Port.:* Zofran; *S.Afr.:* Zofran; *Singapore:* Zofran; *Spain:* Fixca; Helmine; Yatrox; Zofran; *Swed.:* Zofran; *Switz.:* Zofran; *Thai.:* Onsia; Vomitran; Zetron; Zofran; *UK:* Zofran; *USA:* Zofran.

Oxyphenisatine   (7520-h)

Oxyphenisatine *(BAN, rINN)*.

Dihydroxyphenylisatin; Oxyphenisatin. 3,3-Bis(4-hydroxyphenyl)indolin-2-one.
$C_{20}H_{15}NO_3 = 317.3$.
CAS — 125-13-3.

Oxyphenisatine Acetate   (7521-m)

Oxyphenisatine Acetate *(rINNM)*.

Acetphenolisatin; Bisatin; Diacetoxydiphenylisatin; Diacetyldiphenolisatin; Diasatin; Diphesatin; Isaphenin; NSC-59687; Oxyphenisatin Acetate *(USAN)*; Oxyphenisatin Diacetate; Oxyphenisatine Diacetate *(BANM)*; Phenlaxine.
$C_{24}H_{19}NO_5 = 401.4$.
CAS — 115-33-3.
ATC — A06AB01.
Pharmacopoeias. In Pol.

Profile

Oxyphenisatine is a stimulant laxative that has been used by mouth and as an enema. Liver damage has occurred, usually after prolonged use by mouth, and has led to it being withdrawn in some countries.

◊ References.
1. Reynolds TB, *et al.* Chronic active and lupoid hepatitis caused by a laxative, oxyphenisatin. *N Engl J Med* 1971; **285:** 813–20.
2. Gjone E, Stave R. Liver disease associated with a "non-constipating" iron preparation. *Lancet* 1973; **i:** 421–2.
3. Kotha P, *et al.* Liver damage induced by oxyphenisatin. *BMJ* 1980; **281:** 1530.

Preparations

Proprietary Preparations (details are given in Part 3)
UK: Veripaque†.

Pantoprazole   (13840-h)

Pantoprazole *(BAN, USAN, rINN)*.

BY-1023; SKF-96022. 5-Difluoromethoxybenzimidazol-2-yl 3,4-dimethoxy-2-pyridylmethyl sulphoxide.
$C_{16}H_{15}F_2N_3O_4S = 383.4$.
CAS — 102625-70-7 (pantoprazole); 138786-67-1 (pantoprazole sodium).
ATC — A02BC02.

Pantoprazole sodium sesquihydrate ($C_{16}H_{14}F_2N_3NaO_4S, 1\frac{1}{2}$-$H_2O = 432.4$) 11.28 mg is approximately equivalent to 10 mg pantoprazole.

Adverse Effects and Precautions

As for Omeprazole, p.1239. Dosage may need to be reduced in severe liver impairment; liver function should be monitored regularly.

Interactions

As for Omeprazole, p.1240.

◊ For reference to a lack of effect of pantoprazole on diazepam, see Gastrointestinal Drugs, p.678, for a lack of effect on theophylline, see p.781, and for a lack of effect on warfarin, see p.996.

Pharmacokinetics

Peak plasma-pantoprazole concentrations are achieved about 2 to 2.5 hours after a dose by mouth. The oral bioavailability is about 77% with the enteric-coated tablet formulation, and does not vary after single or multiple doses. Pantoprazole is highly bound to plasma proteins (98%). It is extensively metabolised in the liver, primarily by the cytochrome P450 isoenzyme CYP2C19, to desmethylpantoprazole; small amounts are also metabolised by CYP3A4, CYP2D6, and CYP2C9. Metabolites are excreted principally (about 80%) in the urine, with the remainder being excreted in bile. The terminal elimination half-life is about 1 hour, and is prolonged in hepatic impairment; the half-life in patients with cirrhosis was 3 to 6 hours.

The symbol † denotes a preparation no longer actively marketed

◊ References.
1. Pue MA, *et al.* Pharmacokinetics of pantoprazole following single intravenous and oral administration to healthy male subjects. *Eur J Clin Pharmacol* 1993; **44:** 575–8.

Uses and Administration

Pantoprazole is a proton pump inhibitor with actions and uses similar to those of omeprazole (p.1241). It is given as the sodium salt but doses are calculated in terms of the base. Once-daily doses should be taken in the morning.

In the treatment of **gastro-oesophageal reflux disease** (p.1204), the usual dose by mouth is 20 to 40 mg once daily for 4 weeks, increased to 8 weeks if necessary; in the USA, up to 16 weeks' therapy is permitted for healing of erosive oesophagitis. For maintenance therapy, treatment can be continued with 20 to 40 mg daily.

The usual dose for the treatment of **peptic ulcer disease** (p.1208) is 40 mg once daily. Treatment is usually given for 2 to 4 weeks for duodenal ulceration, or 4 to 8 weeks for benign gastric ulceration. For the eradication of *Helicobacter pylori* pantoprazole may be combined with two antibacterials in a 1-week **triple therapy** regimen. Effective regimens include pantoprazole 40 mg twice daily combined with clarithromycin 500 mg twice daily and either amoxicillin 1 g twice daily or metronidazole 400 mg twice daily.

Pantoprazole may also be given intravenously, as the sodium salt, in recommended doses of 40 mg daily given over 2 to 15 minutes.

DOSAGE IN HEPATIC IMPAIRMENT.

Dosage may need to be reduced in severe hepatic impairment, or doses given only on alternate days. A maximum dose of 20 mg daily, or 40 mg on alternate days, has been suggested.

◊ Reviews.
1. Fitton A, Wiseman L. Pantoprazole: a review of its pharmacological properties and therapeutic use in acid-related disorders. *Drugs* 1996; **51:** 460–82.
2. Anonymous. Pantoprazole—a third proton pump inhibitor. *Drug Ther Bull* 1997; **35:** 93–4.
3. Poole P. Pantoprazole. *Am J Health-Syst Pharm* 2001; **58:** 999–1008.

Preparations

Proprietary Preparations (details are given in Part 3)
Aust.: Pantoloc; Zurcal; *Austral.:* Somac; *Belg.:* Pantozol; Zurcale; *Braz.:* Pantozol; Zurcal; *Canad.:* Panto; Pantoloc; *Denm.:* Pantoloc; *Fin.:* Somac; *Fr.:* Eupantol; Inipomp; *Ger.:* Pantozol; Pantozol-Rifun; Rifun; *Hong Kong:* Pantoloc; *Irl.:* Protium; *Israel:* Controloc; *Ital.:* Pantecta; Pantopan; Pantor; Peptazol; *Mex.:* Pantozol; Zurcal; *Neth.:* Pantozol; *Norw.:* Somac; *NZ:* Somac; *Port.:* Apton; Pantoc; Zurcal; *S.Afr.:* Controloc; Pantoloc; *Singapore:* Controloc; *Spain:* Anagastra; Pantecta; Pantocarm; Ulcotenal; *Swed.:* Pantoloc; *Switz.:* Pantozol; Zurcal; *UK:* Protium; *USA:* Protonix.

Multi-ingredient: *Neth.:* PantoPAC.

Pentaerythritol   (13090-m)

Tetramethylolmethane.   2,2-Bis(hydroxymethyl)propane-1,3-diol.
$C_5H_{12}O_4 = 136.1$.
CAS — 115-77-5.

Profile

Pentaerythritol is an osmotic laxative used in the treatment of constipation (p.1202) in doses of 5 to 15 g daily.

Preparations

Proprietary Preparations (details are given in Part 3)
Fr.: Auxitrans.

Peppermint Leaf   (4690-t)

Black Mint; Hoja de Menta; Hortelã-Pimenta; Menth. Pip.; Mentha Piperita; Menthae Piperitae Folium; Menthe Poivrée; Peppermint; Pfefferminzblätter; White Mint.

Pharmacopoeias. In Eur. (see p.vi) and Pol. Also in USNF.
Chin specifies *M. haplocalyx.* Jpn specifies *M. arvensis var. piperascens.*

Pharmacopoeial description

Ph. Eur.: The whole or cut dried leaves of *Mentha × piperita,* containing not less than 1.2% v/w of essential oil if whole, or not less than 0.9% v/w if cut. It has a characteristic and penetrating odour and a characteristic aromatic taste. Protect from light.
USNF 20: The dried leaf and flowering top of *Mentha piperita* (Labiatae). It has an aromatic, characteristic odour and a pungent taste, and produces a cooling sensation in the mouth.

Peppermint Oil   (4691-x)

Essence de Menthe Poivrée; Essência de Hortelã-Pimenta; Menthae Piperitae Aetheroleum; Ol. Menth. Pip.; Oleum Menthae Piperitae; Pfefferminzöl.
CAS — 8006-90-4.

Pharmacopoeias. In Eur. (see p.vi) and Pol. Also in USNF.
Oleum Menthae (*Chin. P.*) is from *M. haplocalyx.* Mentha Oil (*Jpn P.*) is from *M. arvensis var piperascens.*

Pharmacopoeial description

Ph. Eur.: It is obtained by steam distillation from the fresh overground parts of the flowering plant of *Mentha × piperita.* It contains 30.0 to 55.0% menthol, 14.0 to 32.0% menthone, and 2.8 to 10.0% menthyl acetate, 3.5 to 14.0% eucalyptol, 1.5 to 10.0% isomenthone, 1.0 to 9.0% menthofuran, 1.0 to 5.0% limonene, not more than 4.0% pulegone, and not more than 1.0% carvone; the ratio of eucalyptol content to limonene content is greater than two.

It is a colourless, pale yellow, or pale greenish-yellow liquid with a characteristic odour and taste followed by a sensation of cold. Miscible with alcohol, with dichloromethane, and with ether. Store in well-filled, airtight containers. Protect from light and heat.
USNF 20: The volatile oil distilled with steam from the fresh overground parts of the flowering plant *Mentha piperita* (Labiatae), rectified by distillation, and neither partially nor wholly dementholised. It yields not less than 5% of esters calculated as menthyl acetate and not less than 50% of total menthol, free and as esters.

It is a colourless or pale yellow liquid with a strong, penetrating, characteristic odour and a pungent taste, followed by a sensation of cold when air is drawn into the mouth. Soluble 1 in 3 of alcohol (70%) with not more than slight opalescence. Store in airtight containers at a temperature not exceeding 40°.

Storage. The Pharmaceutical Society's Department of Pharmaceutical Sciences found that PVC bottles softened and distorted fairly rapidly in the presence of peppermint oil, which should not be stored or dispensed in such bottles.[1]
1. Department of Pharmaceutical Sciences of the Pharmaceutical Society of Great Britain. Plastic medicine bottles of rigid PVC. *Pharm J* 1973; **210:** 100.

Adverse Effects and Precautions

Peppermint oil can be irritant and may rarely cause hypersensitivity reactions. Reported reactions include erythematous skin rash, headache, bradycardia, muscle tremor, and ataxia. Heartburn has also been reported.

Effects on the cardiovascular system. Idiopathic atrial fibrillation occurred in 2 patients addicted to 'peppermints'. Normal rhythm was restored when peppermint-sucking ceased.[1]
1. Thomas JG. Peppermint fibrillation. *Lancet* 1962; **i:** 222.

Hypersensitivity. Exacerbation of asthma, with wheezing and dyspnoea, associated with the use of paste-based toothpastes containing peppermint or wintergreen as a flavouring.[1]
1. Spurlock BW, Dailey TM. Shortness of (fresh) breath—toothpaste-induced bronchospasm. *N Engl J Med* 1990; **323:** 1845–6.

Interactions

Adverse effects may be more likely if peppermint oil is taken in conjunction with alcohol. Enteric-coated capsules containing peppermint oil should not be taken immediately after food or with antacids.

Uses and Administration

Peppermint oil is an aromatic carminative which relaxes gastrointestinal smooth muscle and relieves flatulence and colic. Enteric-coated capsules containing peppermint oil are used for the relief of symptoms of the irritable bowel syndrome or gastrointestinal spasm secondary to other disorders. Usual doses are 0.2 mL three times daily by mouth, (increased to 0.4 mL three times daily if necessary) for up to 2 to 3 months. The capsules should be taken half to one hour before food and swallowed whole, not chewed.

Peppermint oil is also used as a flavour and with other volatile agents in preparations for respiratory-tract disorders.

Peppermint leaf, the source of the oil, has also been used for its carminative and flavouring properties.

Gastrointestinal disorders. Menthol, the major constituent of peppermint oil, has properties similar to those of calcium-channel blockers on smooth muscle such as that in the human gut.[1-3] A review[4] of randomised studies of peppermint oil in irritable bowel syndrome (p.1206) concluded that there was some evidence of its benefit but that further studies were required.

The relaxant effect of peppermint oil on the gastrointestinal tract has been used to reduce colonic spasm during endoscopy by injecting the oil or a diluted suspension of the oil along the biopsy channel of the colonoscope.[5] Addition of peppermint oil to barium enema has also been tried and appears to reduce spasm and reduce the need for intravenous antispasmodics.[6]
1. Taylor BA, *et al.* Inhibitory effect of peppermint oil on gastrointestinal smooth muscle. *Gut* 1983; **24:** A992.
2. Taylor BA, *et al.* Inhibitory effect of peppermint oil and menthol on human isolated colic. *Gut* 1984; **25:** A1168–9.
3. Taylor BA, *et al.* Calcium antagonist activity of menthol on gastrointestinal smooth muscle. *Br J Clin Pharmacol* 1985; **20:** 293P–4P.

4. Pittler MH, Ernst E. Peppermint oil for irritable bowel syndrome: a critical review and metaanalysis. *Am J Gastroenterol* 1998; **93**: 1131–5.
5. Leicester RJ, Hunt RH. Peppermint oil to reduce colonic spasm during endoscopy. *Lancet* 1982; **ii**: 989.
6. Sparks MJW, *et al.* Does peppermint oil relieve spasm during barium enema? *Br J Radiol* 1995; **68**: 841–3.

Preparations

BP 2001: Concentrated Peppermint Emulsion; Gastro-resistant Peppermint Oil Capsules; Peppermint Spirit;
USNF 20: Peppermint Water;
USP 25: Peppermint Spirit.

Proprietary Preparations (details are given in Part 3)
Aust.: Colpermin; Dr Fischer's Minzol†; Japomin; *Austral.:* Mintec; *Canad.:* Colpermin†; *Ger.:* Carminetum; Chiana; China-Oel; Cholaktol; Euminz; Inspirol Heilpflanzenol; Leukona-Mintol†; Mentacur; Ni-No-Fluid N†; spasmo gall sanol mint; SX Mentha; *Hong Kong:* Colpermin; *Irl.:* Colpermin; *Ital.:* Carmint; *NZ:* Colpermin; *Port.:* Cholagutt; Colominte; *Switz.:* Colpermin; *Thai.:* Colpermin; *UK:* Colpermin; Equilon Herbal; Kiminto; Mintec; Obbekjaers.

Multi-ingredient: numerous preparations are listed in Part 3.

Phenolphthalein (7522-b)

Phenolphthalein *(BAN, rINN)*.
Dihydroxyphthalophenone; Fenolftaleina; Phenolphtaleinum; Phenolphthaleinum. 3,3-Bis(4-hydroxyphenyl)phthalide.
$C_{20}H_{14}O_4 = 318.3$.
CAS — 77-09-8.
ATC — A06AB04.
Pharmacopoeias. In *Chin.* and *Eur.* (see p.vi).

Pharmacopoeial description

Ph. Eur.: A white or almost white powder. Practically insoluble in water; soluble in alcohol. Protect from light.

Adverse Effects and Precautions

As for Bisacodyl, p.1212. Hypersensitivity reactions, usually as skin rashes or eruptions, have occurred with phenolphthalein. Phenolphthalein may cause pink discoloration of alkaline urine.

Tumours have occurred in *rats* and *mice* given very high doses of phenolphthalein; there does not appear to be evidence of carcinogenicity in humans, but phenolphthalein-containing products have been withdrawn in a number of countries because of concerns about long-term safety.

Effects on the skin. Reports of skin reactions associated with phenolphthalein include fixed drug eruptions,[1,2] erythema multiforme reactions,[1,3] and toxic epidermal necrolysis.[4,5]

1. Baer RL, Harris H. Types of cutaneous reactions to drugs. *JAMA* 1967; **202**: 710–13.
2. Savin JA. Current causes of fixed drug eruptions. *Br J Dermatol* 1970; **83**: 546–9.
3. Shelley WB, *et al.* Demonstration of intercellular immunofluorescence and epidermal hysteresis in bullous fixed drug eruption due to phenolphthalein. *Br J Dermatol* 1972; **86**: 118–25.
4. Kar PK, *et al.* Toxic epidermal necrolysis in a patient induced by phenolphthalein. *J Indian Med Assoc* 1986; **84**: 189–93.
5. Artymowicz RJ, *et al.* Phenolphthalein-induced toxic epidermal necrolysis. *Ann Pharmacother* 1997; **31**: 1157–9.

Overdosage. The most likely consequence of phenolphthalein overdosage is excessive purgation, which may require fluid and electrolyte replacement. However, a possible association with acute pancreatitis occurred in a 34-year-old man who inadvertently ingested phenolphthalein 2 g. There was complete recovery with no sequelae from the pancreatitis.[1] Widespread organ failure with disseminated intravascular coagulation, massive liver damage, pulmonary oedema, renal failure, and myocardial damage in a second patient[2] were attributed to self-poisoning with an unknown quantity of phenolphthalein-containing laxative, although the diagnosis was problematic. The patient died despite intensive support.

1. Lambrianides AL, Rosin RD. Acute pancreatitis complicating excessive intake of phenolphthalein. *Postgrad Med J* 1984; **60**: 491–2.
2. Sidhu PS, *et al.* Fatal phenolphthalein poisoning with fulminant hepatic failure and disseminated intravascular coagulation. *Hum Toxicol* 1989; **8**: 381–4.

Pharmacokinetics

Up to 15% of phenolphthalein given by mouth is subsequently excreted in the urine. Enterohepatic circulation occurs and the glucuronide is excreted in the bile. Elimination may take several days.

Uses and Administration

Phenolphthalein is a diphenylmethane stimulant laxative which has been used for the treatment of constipation (p.1202) and for bowel evacuation before investigational procedures or surgery. It has been withdrawn in many countries because of concern over its carcinogenic potential following reports of tumours in *rodents.*

It has been administered in pills or tablets, and as an emulsion with liquid paraffin. It was usually given in a dose of 30 to 200 mg taken at bedtime; doses of 270 mg daily should not be exceeded.

Yellow phenolphthalein, an impure form, has been used similarly.

Preparations

Proprietary Preparations (details are given in Part 3)
Austral.: Figsen†; Laxettes; *Belg.:* Caolax†; *Canad.:* Espotabs†; Neo-Prunex†; *Fr.:* Purganol†; *Hong Kong:* Regulim; *Israel:* Easylax; *Ital.:* Confetto†; Euchessina†; Purgestol†; *S.Afr.:* Laxicaps P; *Singapore:* Regulim; *Spain:* Laxen Busto; Purgante†; Sure Lax; *Switz.:* Euchessina; Reguletts†; *Thai.:* Purmolax; Regulim; *UK:* Bonomint; Brooklax; Reguletts†; Sure-Lax†; *USA:* Alophen Pills†; Espotabs†; Evac-U-Gen†; Evac-U-Lax†; Fletchers Childrens Laxative†; Lax Pills†; Laxative Pills†; Medilax†; Modane†; Phenolax†; Prulet†.

Multi-ingredient: *Aust.:* Abfuhrdragees; *Austral.:* Ford Pills; Mackenzies Menthoids†; *Belg.:* Agarol†; Grains de Vals; Sanicolax†; *Braz.:* Agarol; Dioctosal; Emagrex; Esbelt; Esbeltrat; Fideine; Lacto-Purga; Macroten; Magroton; Normagrin; Obesidex; Obesifran; Prisoventril; Purgoleite; *Canad.:* Agarol†; Aid-Lax†; Alsiline†; Calcium Docuphen†; Caroid†; Doulax†; Doxidan†; Evac-Q-Kwik†; Ex-Lax Light†; Herbalax Forte†; Laxa†; Laxarol†; Le 100 B†; Phillips Gelcaps†; Phytolax†; Thunas Bilettes†; Triolax†; Vesilax†; *Fr.:* Mucinum†; *Ger.:* Obstinol†; Vencipon N; *Hong Kong:* Codoplex†; *Irl.:* Agarol†; Alophen†; Petrolagar No. 2†; Petrolagar with Phenolphthalein; *Israel:* Laxative; Laxative Comp; *Ital.:* Agarbil†; Agarol†; Bilagar†; Confetti Lassativi†; Confetto Complex†; Crisolax†; Ormobyl†; Reolina†; Rim†; Verecolene Complesso†; *Neth.:* Agarol†; Byl; Caroid; *S.Afr.:* Agarol; Dietaid†; Laxicaps†; Redupon; Veracolate; *Spain:* Agarol†; Alofedina; Laxante Bescansa; Laxante Bescansa Aloico; Laxo Vian†; Lipograsil; Mahiou; Takata; *Switz.:* Agarol†; Carter Petites Pilules†; Falqui†; Paragar; Paragol; *Thai.:* Agarol; Emulax; Veracolate; Zenda; *UK:* Agarol; Alophen; Carters†; Fam-Lax; Juno Junipah; Kest; Nylax†; *USA:* Agoral; Colax†; Dialose Plus†; Disolan†; Docucal-P†; Doxidan; Ex-Lax Extra Gentle Pills†; Feen-a-mint Pills†; Femilax†; Kondremul with Phenolphthalein†; Modane Plus†; Phillips' Laxative Gelcaps†; Phillips' Laxcaps†; Unilax†; Veracolate†.

Plaunotol (2366-j)

Plaunotol *(rINN)*.
CS-684. (2Z,6E)-2-[(3E)-4,8-Dimethyl-3,7-nonadienyl]-6-methyl-2,6-octadiene-1,8-diol.
$C_{20}H_{34}O_2 = 306.5$.
CAS — 64218-02-6.

Profile

Plaunotol is a complex aliphatic alcohol extracted from the Thai medicinal plant plau-noi (*Croton sublyratus* (Euphorbiaceae)). It is reported to possess cytoprotective properties and is used in the treatment of gastritis and peptic ulcer disease in a dose of 240 mg daily by mouth.

Preparations

Proprietary Preparations (details are given in Part 3)
Jpn: Kelnac; *Thai.:* Kelnac.

Polaprezinc (15917-d)

Polaprezinc *(rINN)*.
Z-103. catena-Poly{zinc-μ-[β-alanyl-L-histidinato(2-)-N,N^N,O:N^τ]}.
$(C_9H_{12}N_4O_3Zn)_n$.
CAS — 107667-60-7.

Profile

Polaprezinc is a cytoprotective agent used in the treatment of peptic ulcer disease.

◊ **References.**

1. Kashimura H, *et al.* Polaprezinc, a mucosal protective agent, in combination with lansoprazole, amoxycillin and clarithromycin increases the cure rate of Helicobacter pylori infection. *Aliment Pharmacol Ther* 1999; **13**: 483–7.

Polycarbophil (11505-k)

Polycarbophil *(BAN, rINN)*.
CAS — 9003-97-8.
Pharmacopoeias. In *US.*

Pharmacopoeial description

USP 25: Polyacrylic acid cross-linked with divinyl glycol. White to creamy-white granules, with a characteristic, esterlike odour. Swells in water to a range of volumes, depending primarily on the pH. Insoluble in water, in common organic solvents, and in dilute acids and alkalis. A 1% mixture in water has a pH of not more than 4.0. Store in airtight containers.

Polycarbophil Calcium (5008-c)

Polycarbophil Calcium *(BANM, rINNM)*.
AHR-3260B; Calcium Polycarbophil *(USAN)*; Polycarbophilum Calcii; WI-140.
CAS — 126040-58-2.
ATC — A06AC08.
Pharmacopoeias. In *US.*

Pharmacopoeial description

USP 25: A white to creamy-white powder. Insoluble in water, in common organic solvents, and in dilute acids and alkalis. It loses not more than 10% of its weight on drying and contains not less than 18% and not more than 22% of calcium, calculated on the dried basis. Store in airtight containers.

Adverse Effects and Precautions

As for Ispaghula, p.1229. Polycarbophil calcium releases calcium ions in the gastrointestinal tract and should be avoided by patients who must restrict their calcium intake.

There is a risk of intestinal or oesophageal obstruction and faecal impaction, especially if such bulk laxatives are swallowed dry. Therefore, they should always be taken with sufficient fluid and should not be taken immediately before going to bed. They should be avoided by patients who have difficulty swallowing.

Interactions

The calcium component of polycarbophil calcium may reduce the absorption of tetracyclines from the gastrointestinal tract; it should be taken at least 1 hour before or 2 hours after the antibiotic.

Uses and Administration

Polycarbophil calcium has similar properties to ispaghula (p.1229) and is used as a bulk laxative and for adjusting faecal consistency. Following ingestion calcium ions are replaced by hydrogen ions from gastric acid and the resultant polycarbophil exerts a hydrophilic effect in the intestines.

It is given by mouth in a usual dose equivalent to 1 g of polycarbophil up to four times daily, as necessary. Doses should be taken with at least 250 mL of water.

Polycarbophil is used topically as a vaginal moisturiser and as an ocular lubricant.

◊ *Reviews.*

1. Danhof IE. Pharmacology, toxicology, clinical efficacy, and adverse effects of calcium polycarbophil, an enteral hydrosorptive agent. *Pharmacotherapy* 1982; **2**: 18–28.

Preparations

Proprietary Preparations (details are given in Part 3)
Austral.: Replens; *Belg.:* Replens; *Canad.:* Replens; *Israel:* Fibercon; *Ital.:* Modula; Pursennid Fibra†; Replens; *Mex.:* Fibercon; *Port.:* Replens; *S.Afr.:* Replens; *Spain:* Replens; *Swed.:* Replens; *USA:* Equalactin; Fiber-Lax; Fiberall†; Fibercon; FiberNorm; Konsyl Fiber†; Mitrolan; Replens.

Multi-ingredient: *Ital.:* Ormobyl CM; Pursennid Complex†; *USA:* Aquasite.

Potassium Acid Tartrate (1186-h)

E336; Kalii Hydrogenotartras; Kalium Hydrotartaricum; Potassium Bitartrate *(USAN)*; Potassium Hydrogen Tartrate; Purified Cream of Tartar; Tartarus Depuratus; Weinstein.
$C_4H_5KO_6 = 188.2$.
CAS — 868-14-4.
Pharmacopoeias. In *Eur.* (see p.vi) and *US.*

Pharmacopoeial description

Ph. Eur.: A white crystalline powder or colourless crystals. Slightly soluble in water; practically insoluble in alcohol. It dissolves in dilute solutions of mineral acids and alkali hydroxides.
USP 25: Colourless or slightly opaque crystals or a white, crystalline powder. Slightly soluble in water; soluble in boiling water; very slightly soluble in alcohol. A saturated solution is acid to litmus. Store in airtight containers.

Profile

Potassium acid tartrate is given with sodium bicarbonate as a suppository for the treatment of constipation (p.1202) and for bowel evacuation before investigational procedures or surgery. Carbon dioxide gas is produced in the rectum which stimulates defaecation within 10 to 30 minutes.

Potassium acid tartrate is used as a food additive and pharmaceutical aid.

Potassium acid tartrate has been used as an ingredient of preparations for potassium supplementation, although other potassium salts are usually preferred. For the general properties of potassium salts, see p.1194.

Preparations

BPC 1968: Effervescent Potassium Tablets.
Proprietary Preparations (details are given in Part 3)
Multi-ingredient: *Aust.:* Lecicarbon; *Ital.:* Potassium; *Mon.:* Eductyl; *Swed.:* Relaxit; *Thai.:* Circanetten; *USA:* Ceo-Two; Evac-Q-Sert†.

Proglumide (705-n)

Proglumide *(BAN, USAN, rINN)*.
CR-242; W-5219; Xylamide. (±)-4-Benzamido-N,N-dipropylglutaramic acid.
$C_{18}H_{26}N_2O_4 = 334.4$.
CAS — 6620-60-6.
ATC — A02BX06.
Pharmacopoeias. In *Jpn.*

Profile

Proglumide is a cholecystokinin antagonist with an inhibitory effect on gastric secretion. It is used in the treatment of peptic ulcer disease (p.1208) and other gastrointestinal disorders in usual doses of 400 mg three or four times daily by mouth before meals.

Preparations

Proprietary Preparations (details are given in Part 3)
Aust.: Milid; *Ger.:* Milid; *Hong Kong:* Milid; *Ital.:* Milid; *Port.:* Milid; *Thai.:* Milid.

Prune (7526-p)

Ameixa; Prunus.

The dried ripe fruits of *Prunus domestica* and some other species of *Prunus* (Rosaceae).

Profile
Prune has laxative and demulcent properties.

Preparations
Proprietary Preparations (details are given in Part 3)
Multi-ingredient: *Austral.:* Neo-Cleanse; Prolax; *Braz.:* Lumbriquil; Xarope Peitoral de Ameixa Composto; *Canad.:* Fruitatives; *Spain:* Jarabe Manzanas Siken; *Switz.:* Falqui†.

Rabeprazole Sodium (19369-x)

Rabeprazole Sodium (*BANM, USAN, rINNM*).
E-3810; LY-307640; Sodium Pariprazole. 2-({[4-(3-Methoxypropoxy)-3-methyl-2-pyridyl]methyl}sulfinyl)-1*H*-benzimidazole sodium.
$C_{18}H_{20}N_3NaO_3S = 381.4$.
CAS — 117976-89-3 (rabeprazole); 117976-90-6 (rabeprazole sodium).

Adverse Effects and Precautions
As for Omeprazole, p.1239.

Interactions
As for Omeprazole, p.1240. In healthy subjects, clinically significant interactions with diazepam, phenytoin, theophylline, or warfarin have not been demonstrated.

Pharmacokinetics
Peak plasma-rabeprazole concentrations are reached approximately 3.5 hours after a dose by mouth. The oral bioavailability is about 52% with the enteric-coated tablet formulation, because of first-pass metabolism, and does not appear to vary after single or repeated doses. Rabeprazole is highly bound to plasma proteins (97%). It is extensively metabolised in the liver by cytochrome P450 isoenzymes CYP2C19 and CYP3A4 to the thioether, thioether carboxylic acid, sulfone, and desmethylthioether. Metabolites are excreted principally in the urine (about 90%) with the remainder in the faeces. The plasma half-life is about 1 hour, increased two to threefold in hepatic impairment, 1.6 times in CYP2C19 slow metabolisers (see also Omeprazole, p.1241), and by 30% in the elderly.

◊ References.
1. Yasuda S, *et al.* Comparison of the kinetic disposition and metabolism of E3810, a new proton pump inhibitor, and omeprazole in relation to S-mephenytoin 4-hydroxylation status. *Clin Pharmacol Ther* 1995; **58:** 143–54.
2. Keane WF, *et al.* Rabeprazole: pharmacokinetics and tolerability in patients with stable, end-stage renal failure. *J Clin Pharmacol* 1999; **39:** 927–33.

Uses and Administration
Rabeprazole is a proton pump inhibitor with actions and uses similar to those of omeprazole (p.1241). It is given by mouth as rabeprazole sodium in the form of enteric-coated tablets. It is normally taken before food in the morning.

In the treatment of severe (erosive or ulcerative) **gastro-oesophageal reflux disease** (p.1204), the usual dose is 20 mg once daily for 4 to 8 weeks; in the USA, a further 8-week course is permitted for healing of erosive oesophagitis. Thereafter, maintenance therapy can be continued with 10 or 20 mg daily depending on the response. For symptomatic disease without erosive or ulcerative oesophagitis a dose of 10 mg may be given once daily for 4 weeks.

For the treatment of active **peptic ulcer disease** (p.1208), 20 mg daily is given for 4 to 8 weeks for duodenal ulcer and 6 to 12 weeks for gastric ulcer. For the eradication of *Helicobacter pylori* rabeprazole may be combined with two antibacterials in a 1-week

triple therapy regimen. Effective regimens include rabeprazole sodium 20 mg twice daily combined with clarithromycin 500 mg twice daily and either amoxicillin 1 g twice daily or metronidazole 400 mg twice daily.

For **Zollinger-Ellison Syndrome** (p.1209), the starting dose is 60 mg daily, adjusted according to response.

◊ Reviews.
1. Prakash A, Faulds D. Rabeprazole. *Drugs* 1998; **55:** 261–7.
2. Anonymous. Rabeprazole. *Med Lett Drug Ther* 1999; **41:** 110–12.
3. Langtry HD, Markham A. Rabeprazole: a review of its use in acid-related gastrointestinal disorders. *Drugs* 1999; **58:** 725–42.

Preparations
Proprietary Preparations (details are given in Part 3)
Aust.: Pariet; *Denm.:* Pariet; *Fin.:* Pariet; *Fr.:* Pariet; *Ger.:* Pariet; *Irl.:* Pariet; *Ital.:* Pariet; *Jpn:* Pariet; *Mex.:* Pariet; *Neth.:* Pariet; *Port.:* Pariet; *S.Afr.:* Pariet; *Spain:* Pariet; *Swed.:* Pariet; *Thai.:* Pariet; *UK:* Pariet; *USA:* Aciphex.

Racecadotril (14912-w)

Racecadotril (*rINN*).
Acetorphan. (±)-N-{2-[(Acetylthio)methyl]-1-oxo-3-phenylpropyl}glycine phenylmethyl ester; N-[(R,S)-3-acetylthio-2-benzylpropanoyl]glycine benzyl ester; (±)-N-[α-(Mercaptomethyl)hydrocinnamoyl]glycine benzyl ester acetate.
$C_{21}H_{23}NO_4S = 385.5$.
CAS — 81110-73-8.
ATC — A07XA04.

Profile
Racecadotril is an enkephalinase inhibitor given by mouth in doses of 100 mg three times daily before meals for the symptomatic management of acute diarrhoea (p.1203).
The S-form of racecadotril (sinorphan, ecadotril—see Natriuretic Peptides, p.938) has been investigated for hypertension and heart failure.

◊ References.
1. Baumer P, *et al.* Effects of acetorphan, an enkephalinase inhibitor, on experimental and acute diarrhoea. *Gut* 1992; **33:** 753–8.
2. Roge J, *et al.* The enkephalinase inhibitor, acetorphan, in acute diarrhoea: a double-blind, controlled clinical trial versus Loperamide. *Scand J Gastroenterol* 1993; **28:** 352–4.
3. Beaugerie L, *et al.* Treatment of refractory diarrhoea in AIDS with acetorphan and octreotide: a randomized crossover study. *Eur J Gastroenterol Hepatol* 1996; **8:** 485–9.
4. Salazar-Lindo E, *et al.* Racecadotril in the treatment of acute watery diarrhea in children. *N Engl J Med* 2000; **343:** 463–7.
5. Matheson AJ, Noble S. Racecadotril. *Drugs* 2000; **59:** 829–35.

Preparations
Proprietary Preparations (details are given in Part 3)
Fr.: Tiorfan.

Ramosetron Hydrochloride (20338-m)

Ramosetron Hydrochloride (*rINNM*).
YM-060. (−)-(R)-1-Methylindol-3-yl 4,5,6,7-tetrahydro-5-benzimidazolyl ketone hydrochloride.
$C_{17}H_{17}N_3O,HCl = 315.8$.
CAS — 132036-88-5 (ramosetron); 132907-72-3 (ramosetron hydrochloride).

Profile
Ramosetron hydrochloride is a 5-HT$_3$-receptor antagonist with general properties similar to those of ondansetron (p.1241). It is given for its antiemetic properties in the management of nausea and vomiting induced by cancer chemotherapy in usual doses of 300 μg once daily intravenously, or 100 μg once daily by mouth. It has also been tried in irritable bowel syndrome.

Preparations
Proprietary Preparations (details are given in Part 3)
Jpn: Nasea.

Ranitidine Hydrochloride (6162-e)

Ranitidine Hydrochloride (*BANM, rINNM*).
AH-19065; Ranitidini Hydrochloridum. NN-Dimethyl-5-[2-(1-methylamino-2-nitrovinylamino)ethylthiomethyl]furfurylamine hydrochloride.
$C_{13}H_{22}N_4O_3S,HCl = 350.9$.
CAS — 66357-35-5 (ranitidine); 66357-59-3 (ranitidine hydrochloride).

NOTE. Ranitidine is *USAN*.
Pharmacopoeias. In *Chin.*, *Eur.* (see p.vi), and *US*.

Ranitidine hydrochloride 111.6 mg is approximately equivalent to 100 mg of ranitidine.

Pharmacopoeial description
Ph. Eur.: A white or pale yellow, crystalline powder. It exhibits polymorphism. Freely soluble in water and in methyl alcohol;

sparingly soluble in dehydrated alcohol; very slightly soluble in dichloromethane; A 1% solution in water has a pH of 4.5 to 6.0. Store in airtight containers. Protect from light.

USP 25: A white to pale yellow, practically odourless, crystalline powder. It is sensitive to light and to moisture. Very soluble in water; moderately soluble in alcohol; sparingly soluble in chloroform. A 1% solution in water has a pH of 4.5 to 6.0. Store in airtight containers. Protect from light.

Stability and incompatibility. References.
1. Chilvers MR, Lysne JM. Visual compatibility of ranitidine hydrochloride with commonly used critical-care medications. *Am J Hosp Pharm* 1989; **46:** 2057–8.
2. Wohlford JG, *et al.* More information on the visual compatibility of hetastarch with injectable critical-care drugs. *Am J Hosp Pharm* 1990; **47:** 297–8.
3. Williams MF, *et al.* In vitro evaluation of the stability of ranitidine hydrochloride in total parenteral nutrition mixtures. *Am J Hosp Pharm* 1990; **47:** 1574–9.
4. Galante LJ, *et al.* Stability of ranitidine hydrochloride at dilute concentration in intravenous infusion fluids at room temperature. *Am J Hosp Pharm* 1990; **47:** 1580–4.
5. Galante LJ, *et al.* Stability of ranitidine hydrochloride with eight medications in intravenous admixtures. *Am J Hosp Pharm* 1990; **47:** 1606–10.
6. Stewart JT, *et al.* Stability of ranitidine in intravenous admixtures stored frozen, refrigerated, and at room temperature. *Am J Hosp Pharm* 1990; **47:** 2043–6.
7. Montoro JB, Pou L. Comment on stability of ranitidine hydrochloride in total nutrient admixtures. *Am J Hosp Pharm* 1991; **48:** 2384.
8. Stewart JT, *et al.* Stability of ranitidine hydrochloride and seven medications. *Am J Hosp Pharm* 1994; **51:** 1802–7.
9. Crowther RS, *et al.* In vitro stability of ranitidine hydrochloride in enteral nutrient formulas. *Ann Pharmacother* 1995; **29:** 859–62.

Adverse Effects
As for Cimetidine, p.1216. Unlike cimetidine, ranitidine has little or no anti-androgenic effect, despite isolated reports of gynaecomastia and impotence.

◊ General references.
1. Wormsley KG. Safety profile of ranitidine: a review. *Drugs* 1993; **46:** 976–85.

Carcinogenicity. For a discussion of the possible association between histamine H$_2$-antagonists and cancer, including mention of a study with ranitidine, see Cimetidine, p.1216.

Effects on the blood. For a discussion of the adverse haematological effects of H$_2$-antagonists, see Cimetidine, p.1217.

Effects on the cardiovascular system. Similarly to cimetidine (p.1217), bradycardia,[1,2] atrioventricular block,[2] and cardiac arrest[3] have been reported rarely during ranitidine therapy. A positive inotropic effect, without significant changes in heart rate or blood pressure, has also been reported in healthy subjects[4] and pretreatment with ranitidine has blocked the cardiac depressant effects seen in some subjects given famotidine or nizatidine.[5] Although studies in critically ill patients[6] and healthy subjects[7,8] have found no adverse haemodynamic effects associated with ranitidine, it is likely that a small proportion of patients are more susceptible to the cardiovascular effects of ranitidine. Caution is recommended when ranitidine is given intravenously, particularly in patients with cardiovascular disease.
1. Johnson WS, Miller DR. Ranitidine and bradycardia. *Ann Intern Med* 1988; **108:** 493.
2. Tanner LA, Arrowsmith JB. Bradycardia and H$_2$ antagonists. *Ann Intern Med* 1988; **109:** 434–5.
3. Hart AM. Cardiac arrest associated with ranitidine. *BMJ* 1989; **299:** 519.
4. Meyer EC, *et al.* Inotropic effects of ranitidine. *Eur J Clin Pharmacol* 1990; **39:** 301–3.
5. Mescheder A, *et al.* Changes in the effects of nizatidine and famotidine on cardiac performance after pretreatment with ranitidine. *Eur J Clin Pharmacol* 1993; **45:** 151–6.
6. Vohra SB, *et al.* The haemodynamic effects of ranitidine injected centrally in optimally resuscitated patients. *Br J Hosp Med* 1989; **42:** 149.
7. Hughes DG, *et al.* Cardiovascular effects of H$_2$-receptor antagonists. *J Clin Pharmacol* 1989; **29:** 472–7.
8. Hilleman DE, *et al.* Impact of chronic oral H$_2$-antagonist therapy on left ventricular systolic function and exercise capacity. *J Clin Pharmacol* 1992; **32:** 1033–7.

Effects on the endocrine system. Unlike cimetidine (p.1217), ranitidine does not bind to androgen receptors and has little, if any, anti-androgenic effect. Studies in males taking ranitidine for the management of duodenal ulcer[1,2] reported no significant changes in the plasma concentrations of testosterone, luteinising hormone, follicle-stimulating hormone, or prolactin after up to 2 years of treatment; no significant changes in sperm concentration, motility, or morphology were noted.[1] There have been isolated reports of gynaecomastia,[3] loss of libido,[4] and impotence[5] associated with ranitidine, but in 9 patients with cimetidine-induced breast changes and impotence, transfer to ranitidine resulted in resolution of these symptoms.[6]
1. Wang C, *et al.* Ranitidine does not affect gonadal function in man. *Br J Clin Pharmacol* 1983; **16:** 430–2.
2. Knigge U, *et al.* Plasma concentrations of pituitary and peripheral hormones during ranitidine treatment for two years in men with duodenal ulcer. *Eur J Clin Pharmacol* 1989; **37:** 305–7.
3. Tosi S, Cagnoli M. Painful gynaecomastia with ranitidine. *Lancet* 1983; **i:** 160.
4. Smith RN, Elsdon-Dew RW. Alleged impotence with ranitidine. *Lancet* 1983; **ii:** 798.

The symbol † denotes a preparation no longer actively marketed

1246 Gastrointestinal Drugs

5. Kassianos GC. Impotence and nizatidine. *Lancet* 1989; **i:** 963.
6. Jensen RT, *et al.* Cimetidine-induced impotence and breast changes in patients with gastric hypersecretory states. *N Engl J Med* 1983; **308:** 883–7.

Effects on the eyes. For a report of an increase in intra-ocular pressure associated with ranitidine, see under Cimetidine, p.1217. A cohort study involving 140 128 patients receiving anti-ulcer therapy, 70 389 of whom received ranitidine, found no evidence that any of the drugs studied were associated with a major increased risk of vascular or inflammatory disorders of the eye.[1]

For reference to loss of colour vision in a child receiving ranitidine see under Effects on the Nervous System, below.

1. García Rodríguez LA, *et al.* A cohort study of the ocular safety of anti-ulcer drugs. *Br J Clin Pharmacol* 1996; **42:** 213–16.

Effects on the liver. There have been some case reports of ranitidine hepatotoxicity.[1] The increase in relative risk seen in a large cohort study involving 108 891 patients receiving antisecretory therapy was less for ranitidine (1.7:1) than for cimetidine (see p.1217).

1. Souza Lima MA. Ranitidine and hepatic injury. *Ann Intern Med* 1986; **105:** 140.

Effects on the nervous system. Ranitidine has been associated with adverse neurological effects including confusion,[1-8] loss of colour vision,[4] aggressiveness,[2,4,6] lethargy,[8] somnolence,[8] disorientation,[8] depression,[8] hallucinations,[1,7-9] and severe headache.[10] As with cimetidine (p.1218) these reactions occur mainly in the elderly, the severely ill, or patients with renal or hepatic impairment. Single-dose studies in young healthy subjects have found no adverse changes in performance, CNS function, or subjective assessment of mood after administration of ranitidine 150 or 300 mg by mouth.[11]

1. Hughes JD, *et al.* Mental confusion associated with ranitidine. *Med J Aust* 1983; **2:** 12–13.
2. Silverstone PH. Ranitidine and confusion. *Lancet* 1984; **i:** 1071.
3. Epstein CM. Ranitidine and confusion. *Lancet* 1984; **i:** 1071.
4. De Giacomo C, *et al.* Ranitidine and loss of colour vision in a child. *Lancet* 1984; **ii:** 47.
5. Mani RB, *et al.* H₂-receptor blockers and mental confusion. *Lancet* 1984; **ii:** 98.
6. Mandal SK. Psychiatric side effects of ranitidine. *Br J Clin Pract* 1986; **40:** 260.
7. MacDermott AJ, *et al.* Acute confusional episodes during treatment with ranitidine. *BMJ* 1987; **294:** 1616.
8. Slugg PH, *et al.* Ranitidine pharmacokinetics and adverse central nervous system reactions. *Arch Intern Med* 1992; **152:** 2325–9.
9. Price W, *et al.* Ranitidine-associated hallucinations. *Eur J Clin Pharmacol* 1985; **29:** 375–6.
10. Epstein CM. Ranitidine. *N Engl J Med* 1984; **310:** 1602.
11. Nicholson AN, Stone BM. The H₂-antagonists, cimetidine and ranitidine: studies on performance. *Eur J Clin Pharmacol* 1984; **26:** 579–82.

Effects on the skin. A report of vasculitic rash occurring in three patients undergoing ranitidine therapy.[1] In each case the rash cleared following withdrawal of the drug.

See also under Hypersensitivity, below, and also Cimetidine, p.1217.

1. Haboubi N, Asquith P. Rash mediated by immune complexes associated with ranitidine treatment. *BMJ* 1988; **296:** 897.

Fever. A report[1] of pyrexia associated with ranitidine. Apart from raised temperature the patient was otherwise well; fever resolved on discontinuation and recurred on rechallenge with ranitidine.

1. Kavanagh GM, *et al.* Ranitidine fever. *Lancet* 1993; **341:** 1422.

Hypersensitivity. Respiratory stridor and an urticarial rash occurred in a patient shortly after taking the first dose of ranitidine;[1] the symptoms responded to adrenaline [epinephrine] subcutaneously.

1. Brayko CM. Ranitidine. *N Engl J Med* 1984; **310:** 1601–2.

Meningitis. Aseptic meningitis developed on 3 occasions following administration of ranitidine to a 30-year-old man.[1] In each case symptoms resolved rapidly on withdrawal of the drug.

1. Durand JM, *et al.* Ranitidine and aseptic meningitis. *BMJ* 1996; **312:** 886. Correction. *ibid.;* 1392.

Precautions

As for Cimetidine, p.1218.

Helicobacter pylori testing. For reference to the effect of ranitidine on the urea breath test for *Helicobacter pylori*, see p.1218.

Hepatic impairment. Sixteen of 27 patients with cirrhosis of the liver and indications for treatment with an H₂-antagonist (peptic ulcer, gastritis, or reflux oesophagitis) failed to respond to ranitidine 300 mg compared with 6 failures from 32 patients without cirrhosis. Famotidine 40 mg was given to 10 of the cirrhotic nonresponders and 8 still exhibited no response; 7 of these patients were given cimetidine 800 mg and only 1 responded. In the control group, all 3 patients given famotidine did not respond and only 1 responded when given cimetidine. It was concluded that the incidence of non-response to H₂-antagonists is increased in patients with liver cirrhosis but no explanation could be given for this effect.[1] Interestingly there is

an earlier report of patients with cirrhosis demonstrating increased bioavailability and decreased clearance of ranitidine.[2]

1. Walker S, *et al.* Frequent non-response to histamine H₂-receptor antagonists in cirrhotics. *Gut* 1989; **30:** 1105–9.
2. Young CJ, *et al.* Effects of cirrhosis and ageing on the elimination and bioavailability of ranitidine. *Gut* 1982; **23:** 819–23.

Porphyria. Ranitidine is considered to be unsafe in patients with porphyria although there is conflicting experimental evidence of porphyrinogenicity.

Renal impairment. A study in patients with varying degrees of renal impairment[1] found that the mean terminal half-life of ranitidine was increased from 2.09 hours in subjects with normal renal function to between 4.23 and 8.45 hours in patients with renal impairment, the degree of prolongation being proportional to the degree of impairment as measured by glomerular filtration rate. As a result of these findings it was recommended that the dose of ranitidine should be halved in patients with a glomerular filtration rate of 20 mL per minute or less. Ranitidine 150 mg daily provided adequate serum concentrations without excessive accumulation in 20 patients undergoing regular haemodialysis.[2] The serum-ranitidine concentrations fell by about 50% during a 4-hour haemodialysis session but less than 3% of the administered dose was removed and supplemental doses after dialysis were considered unnecessary.

1. Dixon JS, *et al.* The effect of renal function on the pharmacokinetics of ranitidine. *Eur J Clin Pharmacol* 1994; **46:** 167–71.
2. Comstock TJ, *et al.* Ranitidine accumulation in patients undergoing chronic hemodialysis. *J Clin Pharmacol* 1988; **28:** 1081–5.

Interactions

Unlike cimetidine (p.1218) ranitidine does not seem to affect cytochrome P450 to any great extent, and therefore is considered to have little effect on the metabolism of other drugs. However, like other H₂-antagonists its effects on gastric pH may alter the absorption of some other drugs.

◊ A review comparing the drug interactions of ranitidine with those of cimetidine.[1]

1. Smith SR, Kendall MJ. Ranitidine versus cimetidine: a comparison of their potential to cause clinically important drug interactions. *Clin Pharmacokinet* 1988; **15:** 44–56.

Cisapride. Peak plasma concentrations of ranitidine were achieved significantly more rapidly in 12 healthy subjects who took cisapride concomitantly.[1] The clinical significance is questionable and such combinations have been used clinically, although the use of cisapride is now restricted in most countries.

1. Rowbotham DJ, *et al.* Effect of single doses of cisapride and ranitidine administered simultaneously on plasma concentrations of cisapride and ranitidine. *Br J Anaesth* 1991; **67:** 302–305.

Pharmacokinetics

Ranitidine is readily absorbed from the gastrointestinal tract with peak concentrations in plasma occurring about 2 to 3 hours after administration by mouth. Food does not significantly impair absorption. The bioavailability of ranitidine following oral administration is about 50%. Ranitidine is rapidly absorbed following intramuscular injection, with peak plasma concentrations occurring in about 15 minutes. It is weakly bound, about 15%, to plasma proteins.

The elimination half-life is about 2 to 3 hours and is increased in renal impairment. A small proportion of ranitidine is metabolised in the liver to the N-oxide, the S-oxide, and desmethylranitidine; the N-oxide is the major metabolite but accounts for only about 4 to 6% of a dose. Approximately 30% of an oral dose and 70% of an intravenous dose is excreted unchanged in the urine in 24 hours, primarily by active tubular secretion; there is some excretion in the faeces. Ranitidine crosses the placental barrier and is distributed into breast milk.

Distribution into breast milk. Pharmacokinetic study in a lactating mother given multiple doses of ranitidine showed higher concentrations in breast milk than in serum; the minimum milk concentration occurred between 1 and 2 hours after maternal drug administration, and the highest concentration was towards the end of the 12-hour dosing interval.[1] The dose that would be ingested by the infant could not be reliably estimated because of the variable milk to serum ratio.

1. Kearns GL, *et al.* Appearance of ranitidine in breast milk following multiple dosing. *Clin Pharm* 1985; **4:** 322–4.

Enterohepatic recycling. Some individuals exhibit a second peak in the plasma concentration of ranitidine which could be due to enterohepatic recirculation. However, only 0.7 to 2.6% and 0.3 to 1.0% of a dose of ranitidine was excreted into the bile of 3 patients in 24 hours following 50 mg intravenously or 300 mg by mouth indicating that significant recirculation did not occur.[1]

1. Klotz U, Walker S. Biliary excretion of H₂-receptor antagonists. *Eur J Clin Pharmacol* 1990; **39:** 91–2.

Neonates. Renal function is limited in the first month of life, and reduced clearance of ranitidine would be expected. Blood samples taken from 27 full-term neonates given a single intravenous dose of ranitidine 2.4 mg per kg body-weight revealed the following pharmacokinetic data: elimination half-life, 3.45 hours; total volume of distribution, 1.52 litres per kg; total plasma clearance, 5.02 mL per kg per minute.[1] None of the infants had renal or hepatic impairment. In another study,[2] an elimination half-life of 6.61 hours was found in 13 full-term neonates administered ranitidine 2 mg per kg. See also Administration in Children, below.

1. Fontana M, *et al.* Ranitidine pharmacokinetics in newborn infants. *Arch Dis Child* 1993; **68:** 602–3.
2. Wells TG, *et al.* Pharmacokinetics and pharmacodynamics of ranitidine in neonates treated with extracorporeal membrane oxygenation. *J Clin Pharmacol* 1998; **38:** 402–7.

Uses and Administration

Ranitidine is a histamine H₂-antagonist with actions and uses similar to those of cimetidine (p.1218).

Ranitidine may be given by mouth or parenterally by the intravenous or intramuscular routes. Although most preparations contain ranitidine hydrochloride, strengths and doses are expressed in terms of the base.

In the management of benign **gastric** and **duodenal ulceration** (p.1208) a single daily dose of 300 mg by mouth at bedtime or 150 mg twice daily (in the morning and at bedtime) is given initially for at least 4 weeks. A dose of 300 mg twice daily may also be used. Where appropriate a maintenance dose of 150 mg daily may be given at bedtime. Ranitidine 150 mg twice daily may be given during therapy with NSAIDs for prophylaxis against duodenal ulceration. A suggested dose for the treatment of peptic ulcer in children is 2 to 4 mg per kg body-weight twice daily to a maximum of 300 mg in 24 hours.

For duodenal ulcer associated with *Helicobacter pylori* infection ranitidine in a usual dose of 300 mg once daily or 150 mg twice daily by mouth may be given as part of triple therapy in combination with amoxicillin 750 mg and metronidazole 500 mg, both three times daily, for 2 weeks. Therapy with ranitidine should then be continued for a further 2 weeks.

In **gastro-oesophageal reflux disease** (p.1204) the dose is 150 mg twice daily by mouth or 300 mg at bedtime for up to 8 weeks or, if required, 12 weeks. This may be increased to 150 mg four times daily for up to 12 weeks in severe cases. In pathological hypersecretory conditions, such as the **Zollinger-Ellison syndrome**, (p.1209) the initial oral dose is usually 150 mg twice or three times daily and may be increased if necessary; doses of up to 6 g daily have been employed. Alternatively, an intravenous infusion may be given, initially at a rate of 1 mg per kg body-weight per hour; the rate may be increased by increments of 0.5 mg per kg per hour, beginning after 4 hours, if required.

For the management of patients at risk from **stress ulceration** of the upper gastrointestinal tract parenteral therapy may be employed in the form of slow intravenous injection of a 50-mg priming dose followed by a continuous intravenous infusion of 125 to 250 µg per kg body-weight per hour. Doses of 150 mg twice daily by mouth may be given once oral feeding is resumed.

In patients at risk of developing the **acid aspiration syndrome** (p.1202) during general anaesthesia, a dose of 150 mg by mouth may be given 2 hours before the induction of anaesthesia and preferably also 150 mg the previous evening. Alternatively a dose of 50 mg may be given by intramuscular or slow intravenous injection 45 to 60 minutes before the induction of anaesthesia. In obstetric patients at the start of labour a dose of 150 mg by mouth may be given and may be repeated at intervals of 6 hours if required.

In patients with chronic episodic **dyspepsia** (p.1204), a dose of 150 mg twice daily by mouth for up to 6 weeks may be given. For the short-term symptomatic relief of dyspepsia a dose of 75 mg, repeated if necessary up to a maximum of 4 doses daily, may be taken. Treatment should be restricted to a maximum of 2 weeks' continuous use at one time.

PARENTERAL DOSAGE.

The usual dose of ranitidine by intramuscular or intravenous injection is 50 mg which may be repeated every 6 to 8 hours; the intravenous injection should be given slowly over not less than 2 minutes and should be diluted to contain 50 mg in 20 mL. For an intermittent intravenous infusion the recommended dose in the UK is 25 mg per hour given for 2 hours which may be repeated every 6 to 8 hours. A rate of 6.25 mg per hour has been suggested for continuous intravenous infusion although higher rates may be employed for conditions such as Zollinger-Ellison syndrome or in patients at risk from stress ulceration (see above).

DOSAGE IN RENAL IMPAIRMENT.

The dosage of ranitidine should be reduced in patients with severely impaired renal function (see also under Precautions, above); in the UK the suggested doses for those with severe renal impairment are 150 mg daily by mouth or 25 mg for parenteral administration.

Administration in children. The disposition of ranitidine in children is not significantly different from that in young adults and a dose of 2 mg per kg body-weight (approximately equal to an adult dose of 150 mg) by mouth has been used for the prevention of acid aspiration in children undergoing surgery.[1] A study in premature infants being treated with dexamethasone for bronchopulmonary dysplasia found that infusion of ranitidine 62.5 μg per kg per hour was sufficient to raise and maintain gastric pH above 4 to help protect against gastrointestinal bleeding and perforation.[2] Another study found 500 μg per kg twice daily to be sufficient for preterm infants, but that 1.5 mg per kg three times daily was needed for full-term infants.[3] A minimum dosage of 3 mg per kg daily was suggested for stress ulcer prophylaxis in older infants and children.[4]

1. Christensen S, et al. Effects of ranitidine and metoclopramide on gastric fluid pH and volume in children. Br J Anaesth 1990; 65: 456–60.
2. Kelly EJ, et al. The effect of intravenous ranitidine on the intragastric pH of preterm infants receiving dexamethasone. Arch Dis Child 1993; 69: 37–9.
3. Kuusela A-L. Long term gastric pH monitoring for determining optimal dose of ranitidine for critically ill preterm and term neonates. Arch Dis Child Fetal Neonatal Ed 1998; 78: F151–F153.
4. Harrison AM, et al. Gastric pH control in critically ill children receiving intravenous ranitidine. Crit Care Med 1998; 26: 1433–6.

Cystic fibrosis. A comparative study involving 29 patients with cystic fibrosis (p.117) found that ranitidine was more effective than cisapride in improving dyspeptic symptoms and gastric emptying and distension.[1] Antisecretory drugs are also used in this condition to decrease the inactivation of orally administered pancreatic enzymes.

1. Cucchiara S, et al. Ultrasound measurement of gastric emptying time in patients with cystic fibrosis and effect of ranitidine on delayed gastric emptying. J Pediatr 1996; 128: 485–8.

Immunomodulation. Like cimetidine (see p.1219), ranitidine has been proposed to have immunoregulatory effects. However, ranitidine 300 mg twice daily had no effect on absolute CD4 cell counts or plasma HIV RNA in patients with HIV infection in a placebo-controlled trial.[1] Similarly, ranitidine had no significant benefit in patients with gastric cancer (see Malignant Neoplasms, p.1219).

1. Bartlett JA, et al. A placebo-controlled trial of ranitidine in patients with early human immunodeficiency virus infection. J Infect Dis 1998; 177: 231–4.

Skin disorders. As with cimetidine (p.1219), ranitidine has been tried in various skin disorders. Ranitidine 300 mg twice daily by mouth has been reported to be of benefit as an adjuvant to local treatment with corticosteroids and a moisturising ointment in patients with atopic dermatitis.[1] There are reports of improvements in psoriasis (p.1106) following administration of ranitidine,[2-4] although this is a field that is notoriously difficult to evaluate because of the chronic relapsing and remitting nature of the disease, and others have failed to show benefit.[5]

1. Veien NK, et al. Ranitidine treatment of hand eczema in patients with atopic dermatitis: a double-blind placebo-controlled trial. J Am Acad Dermatol 1995; 32: 1056–7.
2. Witkamp L, et al. An open prospective clinical trial with systemic ranitidine in the treatment of psoriasis. J Am Acad Dermatol 1993; 28: 778–81.
3. Smith KC. Ranitidine useful in the management of psoriasis in a patient with acquired immunodeficiency syndrome. Int J Dermatol 1994; 33: 220–1.
4. Kristensen JK, et al. Systemic high-dose ranitidine in the treatment of psoriasis: an open prospective clinical trial. Br J Dermatol 1995; 133: 905–8.
5. Çetin L, et al. High-dose ranitidine is ineffective in the treatment of psoriasis. Br J Dermatol 1997; 137: 1021–2.

The symbol † denotes a preparation no longer actively marketed

Preparations

BP 2001: Ranitidine Injection; Ranitidine Oral Solution; Ranitidine Tablets;
USP 25: Ranitidine in Sodium Chloride Injection; Ranitidine Injection; Ranitidine Oral Solution; Ranitidine Tablets.

Proprietary Preparations (details are given in Part 3)
Aust.: Digestosan; Ulsal; Zantac; *Austral.:* Ausran; Rani 2; Ranihexal; Ranoxyl; Zantac; *Belg.:* Ranic; Zantac; *Braz.:* Antagon; Antak; Antanidina; Label; Logat; Radan; Ranidin; Ranitil; Regalil; Ulcoren; Zadine; Zylium; *Canad.:* Novo-Ranidine; Nu-Ranit; Peptic Relief; Zantac; *Denm.:* Aducin; Kuracid; Kuracidon; Ranikur; Zantac; *Fin.:* Esofex; Ranicur; Ranil; Ranimex; Ranixal; Zantac; *Fr.:* Azantac; Raniplex; Ulcirex; Zidac; *Ger.:* Azuranit; Ran Lich; Rani; Rani-nerton; Raniberl; Ranibeta; Ranibloc; Ranicux; Ranidura T; Ranimerck; Raniprotect; Ranitic; Sostril; Ulcolind Rani†; Zantic; *Hong Kong:* Simetac; Syntidine; Zantac; *Irl.:* Gertac; Ranitic; Ranopine; Xanomel; Zandine; Zantac; *Israel:* Apozan; Zandex; Zantab; Zantac; *Ital.:* Raniben; Ranibloc; Ranidil; Trigger†; Ulcex; Zantac; *Mex.:* Acloral; Alter-H₂; Alvidina; Anistal; Apoprin; Avintac; Azantac; Cauteridol; Credaxol; Danitin; Dinaxin; Galidrin; Gastrec; Gasyran; Iqfadina; Katalem; Microdit; Microtid; Neugal; Radyn; Ranepal; Ranifarma; Ranifur; Ranisen; Ranulin; Ranzil; Raudil; Redacid; Serranit; Serviradine; Sinhcloran; Sirani; Suronit; Ulcedin; Ulkodin; Ulsaven; Ultran; Zerandin; *Neth.:* Zantac; *Norw.:* Noktone; Ranacid†; Zantac; *NZ:* Zanidin; Zantac; *Port.:* Gastridina; Gastrolav; Gastrulcer; Pep-Rani; Peptab; Peptifar; Quardin; Ran; Ranitine; Stacer; Ulcecur; Ulcerol; Zantac; *S.Afr.:* Histak; RaniHexal; Ranteen; Ulcaid; Zantac; *Singapore:* Gastran; Zantac; Zendhin; Zoran; *Spain:* Alquen; Coralen; Denulcer; Fagus; Lake; Meticel; Quantor; Ran H2; Ranidin; Ranilonga; Ranivel; Ranix; Ranuar; Rubiulcer; Tanidina; Terposen; Toriol; Zantac; *Swed.:* Artonil; Inside; Rani-Q; Zantac; *Switz.:* Ranimed; Ulcidine; Zantic; *Thai.:* Aciloc; Histac; Radine; Ranicid; Ranidine; Ratic; Ratica; Xanidine; Zanamet; Zantac; Zantidon; *UAE:* Rantag; *UK:* Indigestion Relief; Ranaps†; Ranitic; Rantec; Zaedoc; Zantac; *USA:* Zantac.

Ranitidine Bismuth Citrate   (15497-t)

Ranitidine Bismuth Citrate (BAN, USAN).
A complex of ranitidine and bismuth citrate; GR-122311X; Ranitidine Bismutrex. N-[2-({5-[(Dimethylamino)methyl]furfuryl}thio)-ethyl]-N'-methyl-2-nitro-1,1-ethenediamine, compound with bismuth(3+) citrate (1:1).
$C_{13}H_{22}N_4O_3S,C_6H_5BiO_7 = 712.5$.
CAS — 128345-62-0.
ATC — A02BA07.

Adverse Effects and Precautions

Ranitidine bismuth citrate would be expected to combine the adverse effects of both bismuth compounds (p.1213) and ranitidine (p.1245). Blackening of the tongue and faeces is common, and gastrointestinal disturbances, headache, mild anaemia, and altered liver enzyme values have been reported. Rarely, hypersensitivity reactions (including anaphylaxis), have occurred.

Ranitidine bismuth citrate should not be given to patients with moderate to severe renal impairment. It is not suitable for long-term or maintenance therapy because of the risk of bismuth accumulation. As with other antisecretory drugs, the possibility of malignancy should be considered when giving ranitidine bismuth citrate to patients with gastric ulcers since the drug may mask symptoms and delay diagnosis.

Interactions

Ranitidine bismuth citrate would be expected to have the interactions of bismuth compounds (p.1213), and ranitidine (p.1246).

Pharmacokinetics

Following oral administration, ranitidine bismuth citrate dissociates into its ranitidine and bismuth components in the stomach. For the pharmacokinetics of ranitidine, see p.1246, and for those of bismuth, see p.1214.

◊ References.
1. Lacey LF, et al. Comparative pharmacokinetics of bismuth from ranitidine bismuth citrate (GR122311X), a novel anti-ulcerant and tripotassium dicitrato bismuthate (TDB). Eur J Clin Pharmacol 1994; 47: 177–80.
2. Koch KM, et al. Pharmacokinetics of bismuth and ranitidine following single doses of ranitidine bismuth citrate. Br J Clin Pharmacol 1996; 42: 201–5.
3. Koch KM, et al. Pharmacokinetics of bismuth and ranitidine following multiple doses of ranitidine bismuth citrate. Br J Clin Pharmacol 1996; 42: 207–11.

Uses and Administration

Ranitidine bismuth citrate is a complex of ranitidine with bismuth and citrate, which releases ranitidine and bismuth in the gastrointestinal tract and therefore possesses both the actions of the bismuth compounds (p.1214) and of ranitidine (p.1246). It is used in the management of peptic ulcer disease (p.1208), and may be given in combination with antibacterials for the eradication of *Helicobacter pylori* infection and the prevention of relapse of duodenal ulcer.

Doses are 400 mg twice daily by mouth; treatment is usually given for 4 to 8 weeks for duodenal ulceration and for 8 weeks for benign gastric ulceration. Ranitidine bismuth citrate should not be used for maintenance therapy, and a maximum of 16 weeks of treatment (two 8-week courses or four 4-week courses) may be given in a 12-month period. For duodenal ulceration where *H. pylori* infection is present, ranitidine bismuth citrate may be given as part of a 7-day triple therapy regimen, typically combined with any two of clarithromycin 500 mg twice daily, amoxicillin 1 g twice daily, or metronidazole 400 mg twice daily. Alternatively, a 14-day dual therapy regimen of ranitidine bismuth citrate combined with clarithromycin 500 mg two or three times daily may be given. In both regimens ranitidine bismuth citrate alone may be continued to a total of 28 days.

◊ References.
1. Bardhan KD, et al. GR122311X (ranitidine bismuth citrate), a new drug for the treatment of duodenal ulcer. Aliment Pharmacol Ther 1995; 9: 497–506.
2. Peterson WL, et al. Ranitidine bismuth citrate plus clarithromycin is effective for healing duodenal ulcers, eradicating H.pylori and reducing ulcer recurrence. Aliment Pharmacol Ther 1996; 10: 251–61.
3. Anonymous. Pylorid, H.pylori and peptic ulcer. Drug Ther Bull 1996; 34: 69–70.
4. van der Wouden EJ, et al. One-week triple therapy with ranitidine bismuth citrate, clarithromycin and metronidazole versus two-week dual therapy with ranitidine bismuth citrate and clarithromycin for Helicobacter pylori infection: a randomized, clinical trial. Am J Gastroenterol 1998; 93: 1228–31.

Preparations

Proprietary Preparations (details are given in Part 3)
Aust.: Helirad; Pylorisin; *Belg.:* Pylorid; *Canad.:* Pylorid; *Denm.:* Pylorid; *Fin.:* Pylorid; *Hong Kong:* Pylorid; *Irl.:* Pylorid; *Ital.:* Elicodil; Pylorid; *Mex.:* Azanplus; *Neth.:* Pylorid; *Norw.:* Pylorid; *Port.:* Gastrimuto; Pylorid; *Singapore:* Pylorid; *Spain:* Pylorid; *Switz.:* Pylorid; *Thai.:* Pylorid; *UK:* Pylorid; *USA:* Tritec.

Multi-ingredient: *Austral.:* Pylorid-KA.

Rebamipide   (11045-v)

Rebamipide (rINN).
(±)-α-(p-Chlorobenzamido)-1,2-dihydro-2-oxo-4-quinolinepropionic acid.
$C_{19}H_{15}CIN_2O_4 = 370.8$.
CAS — 90098-04-7; 111911-87-6.

Profile

Rebamipide is stated to possess cytoprotective properties and is used in the treatment of peptic ulcer disease (p.1208) and gastritis in usual doses of 100 mg by mouth three times daily.

Preparations

Proprietary Preparations (details are given in Part 3)
Jpn: Mucosta.

Renzapride   (3382-f)

Renzapride (BAN, rINN).
BRL-24924A (renzapride hydrochloride). (±)-endo-4-Amino-N-(1-azabicyclo[3.3.1]non-4-yl)-5-chloro-o-anisamide.
$C_{16}H_{22}CIN_3O_2 = 323.8$.
CAS — 88721-77-1; 112727-80-7.

Profile

Renzapride is a substituted benzamide with prokinetic actions on gastrointestinal motility. It also has 5-HT₄ agonist and 5-HT₃ antagonist activity. It has been investigated, mainly as the hydrochloride, in the management of gastrointestinal disorders.

◊ References.
1. Robertson CS, et al. A double-blind dose ranging study of BRL 24924 and metoclopramide on lower oesophageal sphincter pressure in healthy volunteers. Br J Clin Pharmacol 1989; 28: 323–7.
2. Mackie A, et al. BRL 24924, a novel prokinetic agent, potentially valuable in diabetic gastroparesis. Gut 1989; 30: A1489.
3. Staniforth DH, Pennick M. Human pharmacology of renzapride: a new gastrokinetic benzamide without dopamine antagonist properties. Eur J Clin Pharmacol 1990; 38: 161–4.
4. Mackie ADR, et al. The effects of renzapride, a novel prokinetic agent, in diabetic gastroparesis. Aliment Pharmacol Ther 1991; 5: 135–42.

Rhubarb (7527-s)

Chinese Rhubarb; Rabarbaro; Rhabarber; Rhei Radix; Rhei Rhizoma; Rheum; Rhubarb Rhizome; Ruibarbo.

Pharmacopoeias. In *Chin., Eur.* (see p.vi), *Jpn,* and *Pol. Chin.* and *Jpn* also permit *R. tanguticum,* and *Jpn* also permits *R. coreanum.*

Indian rhubarb (Himalayan rhubarb) consists of the dried rhizome and roots of *Rheum emodi, R. webbianum,* or some other related species of *Rheum.*

Rhapontic rhubarb (Chinese rhapontica) consists of the dried rhizomes of *R. rhaponticum.* It may occur as an adulterant of rhubarb, and pharmacopoeias specify a test to confirm its absence. Garden rhubarb, of which the leaf-stalks are used as food, is derived from *R. rhaponticum.*

Pharmacopoeial description

Ph. Eur.: The whole or cut, dried underground parts of *Rheum palmatum* or of *R. officinale* or of hybrids of these two species or of a mixture. The underground parts are often divided; the stem and most of the bark with the rootlets are removed. It contains not less than 2.2% of hydroxyanthracene derivatives, expressed as rhein ($C_{15}H_8O_6 = 284.2$), calculated with reference to the dried drug. Protect from light.

Adverse Effects and Precautions

As for Senna, p.1248.

Uses and Administration

Rhubarb is an anthraquinone stimulant laxative used similarly to senna (p.1248). It also exerts an astringent action due to the presence of gallic acid derivatives and tannins.

It is used in homoeopathic medicine when it is known as Rheum.

Preparations

BP 2001: Compound Rhubarb Tincture.

Proprietary Preparations (details are given in Part 3)
Ger.: Phytoestrol N.

Multi-ingredient: *Aust.:* Abdomilon; Abfuhrtee; Eucarbon; Novocholin; Pyralvex; Silberne; St Bonifatius-Tee; *Austral.:* Betaine Digestive Aid; Hamamelis Complex; Neo-Cleanse; Plantago Complex†; Pyralvex; SM-33 Adult Formula; *Belg.:* Eucarbon; Pyralvex; *Braz.:* Bisuisan; Boldopeptan; Camomila; Epagogo; Eparema; Epatovis; Fargestium; Fideine; Figadosan; Funchicorea; Gotas Hepaticas; Puersan; Steitonit; *Canad.:* Extra Strong Formula 12; Gasmol†; Herbal Laxative; Herbalax; Herbolax; *Fr.:* Depuratum; Parodium; Pyralvex; Tisanes de l'Abbe Hamon no 17†; *Ger.:* Floradix Maskam†; Montana; Plantoletten†; Pyralvex; Redaxa Lax†; *Hong Kong:* Hepatofalk; Rheogen; *Irl.:* Pyralvex; *Israel:* Encypalmed; Eucarbon; Novicarbon; *Ital.:* Amaro Medicinale; Caramelle alle Erbe Digestive; Carbondifer; Certobil†; Colax; Confetti Lassativi†; Confetto Complex†; Crisolax†; Critichol; Depurativo; Digelax; Dis-Cinil Complex; Eparema; Eparema-Levul; Eupatol; Fitodorf Alghe Marine; Fitodorf Rabarbaro; Frerichs Maldifassi; Hepasil Composto; Lactolas; Lassatina; Magisbile; Mepalax; Neo-Heparbil†; Ormobyl†; Pillole Fattori; Pyralvex; Rabarbaroni; Raboldo; Reolina†; Schias-Amaro Medicinale; Tisana Arnaldi†; Tisana Cisbey†; Vegebyl†; Verecolene Complesso†; *Neth.:* Pyralvex; *Port.:* Pyralvex; *S.Afr.:* Pyralvex; Rubilax; *Singapore:* Pyralvex; *Spain:* Crislaxo; Laxante Bescansa Aloico; Menabil Complex; Pildoras Ferrug Sanatori; Pyralvex; Sol Schoum; *Switz.:* Dragees laxatives no 510†; Eucarbon†; Optilax†; Padma-Lax; Pyralvex; *UK:* Acidosis; Digestive; Fam-Lax; Fam-Lax Senna; HRI Golden Seal Digestive; Liminate; Pegina; Pyralvex; Rhuaka; Stomach Mixture; Wind & Dyspepsia Relief; *USA:* Black-Draught.

Roxatidine Acetate Hydrochloride (2430-g)

Roxatidine Acetate Hydrochloride (BANM, USAN, rINNM).

Hoe-062 (roxatidine); Hoe-760 (roxatidine acetate hydrochloride); TZU-0460 (roxatidine acetate hydrochloride). N-{3-[(α-Piperidino-m-tolyl)oxy]propyl}glycolamide acetate monohydrochloride.

$C_{17}H_{26}N_2O_3,C_2H_2O,HCl = 384.9$.

CAS — 97900-88-4 (roxatidine); 78628-28-1 (roxatidine acetate); 93793-83-0 (roxatidine acetate hydrochloride).

Adverse Effects and Precautions

As for Cimetidine, p.1216.

Renal impairment. Preliminary results in 6 patients with chronic renal failure and creatinine clearance less than 20 mL per minute indicated that administration of the recommended dose of roxatidine acetate hydrochloride, 75 mg every other day, was inadequate to maintain gastric pH above 4 for more than 6 hours. Subsequent study in 8 patients showed that a dose of 75 mg daily was well tolerated and effective.[1]

1. Gladziwa U, *et al.* Pharmacokinetics and pharmacodynamics of roxatidine in patients with renal insufficiency. *Br J Clin Pharmacol* 1995; **39:** 161–7.

Interactions

Unlike cimetidine (p.1218) roxatidine does not appear to affect cytochrome P450, and therefore is considered to have little effect on the metabolism of other drugs. However, like other H_2-antagonists its effects on gastric pH may alter the absorption of some other drugs.

Pharmacokinetics

Roxatidine acetate hydrochloride is rapidly and almost completely absorbed from the gastrointestinal tract with peak concentrations in plasma occurring about 1 to 3 hours after administration by mouth. It is rapidly hydrolysed to the active desacetyl metabolite, roxatidine, by esterases in the liver, small intestine, and serum.

Over 90% of a dose is excreted in the urine as roxatidine and other metabolites. The elimination half-life of roxatidine is about 6 hours and is prolonged in renal impairment.

Small amounts of roxatidine have been reported to be distributed into breast milk.

Uses and Administration

Roxatidine acetate hydrochloride is an H_2-antagonist with actions and uses similar to those of cimetidine (p.1216). It is given by mouth.

In the management of peptic ulcer disease the dose is 150 mg at bedtime or 75 mg twice daily for 4 to 8 weeks. Where appropriate a maintenance dose of 75 mg at bedtime may be given to prevent the recurrence of duodenal ulcers. In gastro-oesophageal reflux disease the recommended dose is 75 mg twice daily.

The dosage should be reduced in patients with renal impairment. Suggested doses for patients on acute therapy are: creatinine clearance of 20 to 50 mL per minute, 75 mg at bedtime; creatinine clearance of less than 20 mL per minute, 75 mg every 2 days (but see above).

◊ Reviews.
1. Murdoch D. Roxatidine acetate: a review of its pharmacodynamic and pharmacokinetic properties, and its therapeutic potential in peptic ulcer disease and related disorders. *Drugs* 1991; **42:** 240–60.

Preparations

Proprietary Preparations (details are given in Part 3)
Aust.: Roxane; *Ger.:* Roxit; *Ital.:* Gastralgin; Neo H2; Roxit; *Jpn:* Altat; *Neth.:* Roxit; *S.Afr.:* Roxit†; *Singapore:* Roxane; *Spain:* Roxiwas; Sarilen; Zarocs.

Senna (7530-b)

CAS — 8013-11-4 (senna); 81-27-6 (sennoside A); 128-57-4 (sennoside B); 52730-36-6 (sennoside A, calcium salt); 52730-37-7 (sennoside B, calcium salt).

Pharmacopoeias. Senna fruit, from Alexandrian and Tinnevelly senna is included in *Eur.* (see p.vi) and *Int.* Senna leaf, from Alexandrian or Tinnevelly senna or both, is included in *Eur., Int., Jpn,* and *US. US* also includes Sennosides.

In commerce senna obtained from *Cassia senna* (=*C. acutifolia*) (Leguminosae) is known as Alexandrian senna or Khartoum senna and that from *Cassia angustifolia* (Leguminosae) as Tinnevelly senna.

Pharmacopoeial description

Ph. Eur.: Alexandrian senna pods consist of the dried fruit of *Cassia senna* (*Cassia acutifolia*) containing not less than 3.4% of hydroxyanthracene glycosides, calculated as sennoside B ($C_{42}H_{38}O_{20} = 862.7$) with reference to the dried drug. Protect from light and moisture.

Tinnevelly senna pods consist of the dried fruit of *Cassia angustifolia* containing not less than 2.2% of hydroxyanthracene glycosides, calculated as sennoside B ($C_{42}H_{38}O_{20} = 862.7$) with reference to the dried drug. Protect from light and moisture.

Senna leaf consists of the dried leaflets of *Cassia senna* (=*Cassia acutifolia*), known as Alexandrian or Khartoum senna, or *Cassia angustifolia,* known as Tinnevelly senna, or a mixture of the two species. It contains not less than 2.5% of hydroxyanthracene glycosides, calculated as sennoside B ($C_{42}H_{38}O_{20} = 862.7$) with reference to the dried drug. Protect from light and moisture.

USP 25: Senna consists of the dried leaflet of *Cassia acutifolia* or *Cassia angustifolia.*

Sennosides is a partially purified natural complex of anthraquinone glucosides found in senna, isolated from *Cassia acutifolia* or *Cassia angustifolia* as calcium salts. It is a brownish powder. Soluble 1 in 35 of water, 1 in 2100 of alcohol, 1 in 3700 of chloroform, and 1 in 6100 of ether. A 10% solution in water has a pH of 6.3 to 7.3.

Adverse Effects

Senna may cause mild abdominal discomfort such as colic or cramps. Prolonged use or overdosage can result in diarrhoea with excessive loss of water and electrolytes, particularly potassium; there is also the possibility of developing an atonic non-functioning colon. Anthraquinone derivatives may colour the urine yellowish-brown at acid pH, and red at alkaline pH. Reversible melanosis coli has been reported following chronic use.

Abuse. Prolonged use or abuse of senna laxatives has been associated with reversible finger clubbing,[1-4] hypokalaemia[3] and tetany,[1] hypertrophic osteoarthropathy,[4] intermittent urinary excretion of aspartylglucosamine,[2] hypogammaglobulinaemia,[3] reversible cachexia,[3] and hepatitis.[5]

1. Prior J, White I. Tetany and clubbing in patient who ingested large quantities of senna. *Lancet* 1978; **ii:** 947.
2. Malmquist J, *et al.* Finger clubbing and aspartylglucosamine excretion in a laxative-abusing patient. *Postgrad Med J* 1980; **56:** 862–4.
3. Levine D, *et al.* Purgative abuse associated with reversible cachexia, hypogammaglobulinaemia, and finger clubbing. *Lancet* 1981; **i:** 919–20.
4. Armstrong RD, *et al.* Hypertrophic osteoarthropathy and purgative abuse. *BMJ* 1981; **282:** 1836.
5. Beuers U, *et al.* Hepatitis after chronic abuse of senna. *Lancet* 1991; **337:** 372–3.

Hypersensitivity. Hypersensitivity reactions manifesting as asthma and rhinoconjunctivitis have been reported in those manufacturing[1] or dispensing[2] senna products. However, a study of 125 workers involved in the manufacture of laxatives found only 4 cases of occupational asthma, although sensitisation to senna or ispaghula dust was present in 18 and 9 of the workers respectively, and other airway, eye, and skin symptoms were relatively frequent.[3]

1. Helin T, Mäkinen-Kiljunen S. Occupational asthma and rhinoconjunctivitis caused by senna. *Allergy* 1996; **51:** 181–4.
2. Baggaley P. A shared allergy. *Pharm J* 1997; **259:** 724.
3. Marks GB, *et al.* Asthma and allergy associated with occupational exposure to ispaghula and senna products in a pharmaceutical work force. *Am Rev Respir Dis* 1991; **144:** 1065–9.

Precautions

Senna should not be given to patients with intestinal obstruction; care should also be taken in patients with inflammatory bowel disease. Prolonged use should generally be avoided.

Although anthraquinone derivatives may be distributed into the milk of lactating mothers, following normal dosage the concentration is thought to be insufficient to affect the nursing infant. Nonetheless the *British National Formulary* states that anthraquinones (and particularly cascara and dantron) should be avoided in women who are breast feeding.

◊ Colonic perforation with faecal peritonitis,[1,2] in one case fatal,[1] has been reported following the use of a senna preparation containing total sennosides 142 mg for bowel preparation prior to barium enema. In 1985, the strength of the UK preparation was halved to contain 72 mg of total sennosides; it was subsequently discontinued, although a similar preparation, at the higher strength, remains available in some countries. To reduce the risk of colonic perforation, patients with suspected stricture, inflammatory bowel disease, or impending obstruction should not receive a bowel stimulant.[2]

1. Galloway D, *et al.* Faecal peritonitis after laxative preparation for barium enema. *BMJ* 1982; **284:** 472.
2. Cave-Bigley D. Faecal peritonitis after laxative preparation for barium enema. *BMJ* 1982; **284:** 740.

Pharmacokinetics

There is some absorption of anthraquinone laxatives following administration by mouth. Absorbed anthraquinones are metabolised in the liver. Unabsorbed senna is hydrolysed in the colon by bacteria to release the active free anthraquinones. Anthraquinones are excreted in urine and faeces and distributed into breast milk.

Uses and Administration

Senna is an anthraquinone stimulant laxative (p.1201) which is used to treat constipation (p.1202) and for bowel evacuation before investigational procedures or surgery. The active anthraquinones are liberated into the colon from the sennoside glycosides by colonic bacteria and an effect usually occurs within 6 to 12 hours of administration by mouth.

For constipation senna is usually administered as tablets, granules, or syrup. It has also been administered rectally as suppositories. In the UK, doses of senna preparations are usually expressed in terms of total sennosides calculated as sennoside B. The usual adult dose is 15 to 30 mg given by mouth as a single dose at bedtime. Children over 6 years of age have been given one-half the adult dose, and those aged 2 to 6 years one-quarter the adult dose. In the USA, the usual adult dose is 12 to 50 mg, expressed in terms of total sennosides.

For bowel evacuation before investigational procedures, a dose of 130 mg of sennosides may be given as a liquid preparation by mouth on the day before the examination. A dose of 72 mg was formerly given in the UK, see under Precautions, above.

The purified sennosides (sennosides A and B), and their calcium salts (calcium sennoside A and calcium sennoside B) are used similarly to senna.

Senna is used in homoeopathic medicine.

Preparations

BP 2001: Senna Liquid Extract; Senna Tablets; Standardised Senna Granules;
Ph. Eur.: Standardised Senna Leaf Dry Extract;
USP 25: Senna Fluidextract; Senna Syrup; Sennosides Tablets.

Proprietary Preparations (details are given in Part 3)
Aust.: Bekunis; Carilax; Colonorm; Darmol; Dragees Neunzehn Senna; Tara Abfuhrsirup; X-Prep; *Austral.:* Bekunis Herbal Tea; Bekunis Instant; Laxettes; Sennetabs; Senokot; *Belg.:* Darlin; Midro; Prunasine; Senokot; Transix; *Canad.:* Castoria†; Ex-Lax; Glysennid; Herbal Laxative; Laxative Pills; Senokot; Senolax†; X-Prep; *Denm.:* Pursennid; *Fin.:* Exprep; Pursennid; Sennapur; *Fr.:* Senokot; X-Prep; *Ger.:* Abfuhrtee N; Bekunis Instant; Bekunis-Krautertee N; Depuran N; Drix Abfuhr-Dragees†; Hermes Drix Abfuhr-Tee†; Hevertolax Phyto†; JuLax S†; Kneipp Abfuhr Tee N; Kneipp Worisetten S; Krauterlax-S†; Liquidepur; Maskam Krauter-Tee†; Midro Abfuhr; Midro Tee; Neda Fruchtewurfel; Ramend; Regulax N; X-Prep; *Hong Kong:* Senokot; *Irl.:* Bekunis†; California Syrup of Figs†; Senokot; *Israel:* Bekunis; Florilax; Jungborn; Laxikal Forte; X-Prep; *Ital.:* Falquilax; Tisana Kelemata; X-Prep; *Mex.:* Lagenbach; Senokot; *Neth.:* Sennocol; X-Praep; *Norw.:* Senokot; *NZ:* Senokot; *Port.:* Bekunis†; Pursennid; X-Prep; *S.Afr.:* Depuran; Senokot; Silaxon; X-Prep; *Singapore:* Senokot; *Spain:* Depuran; Justelax; Laxante Olan; Laxante Salud; X-Prep; *Swed.:* Pursennid; *Switz.:* Darmol; Demodon N; X-Prep; *Thai.:* Senokot; *UAE:* Senokot; *UK:* Ex-Lax; Nylax with Senna; Senlax; Senokot; *USA:* Black-Draught; Dosaflex; Dosalax†; Dr Caldwell Senna Laxative†; Ex-Lax; Ex-Lax Gentle Nature†; Fletchers Castoria; Gentlax†; Maximum Relief Ex-Lax; Senexon; Senna-Gen; Sennatural†; Senokot; Senokotxtra; Senolax†; X-Prep.

Multi-ingredient: *Aust.:* Abfuhrtee; Abfuhrtee EF-EM-ES; Agiolax; Dr Ernst Richter's Abfuhrtee; Dr Ernst Richter's Abfuhrteetassen-fertig; Dr. Ernst Richter's Abfuhrtee-Filterbeutel; Entschlackender Abfuhrtee; Eucarbon; Frugelletten; Herbelax; Illings Bozner Maycur-Tee; Joghurt Milkitten†; Laxalpin; Laxolind†; May-Cur-Tee; Midro Tee; Neda Fruchtewurfel; Planta Lax; Pursennid; Sigman-Haustropfen; St Bonifatius-Tee; The Chambard-Tee; *Austral.:* Agiolax; Coloxyl with Senna; Herb-a-Lax; Herbal Laxative†; Neo-Cleanse; Peritone; Prolax; Sennesoft; Vitaglow Herbal Laxative†; *Belg.:* Agiolax; Eucarbon; Manceau†; Solucamphre†; Tamarine; Tisane Antibiliaire et Stomachique; Tisane Depurative "les 12 Plantes"; Tisane pour le Foie; Tisane Purgative; Tux; *Braz.:* Agiolax; Circanetten; Fitolax; Florlax; Frutalax; Frutarine; Laxan; Laxarine; Laxtam; Novolax; Plantax; Prompt; Steitonit; Tamaril; Tamarine; Tamarix; *Canad.:* Cennlacs†; Cholasyn; Cholasyn II; Constipation; Control; Doulax; Extra Strong Formula 12; Floralaxative†; Herbal Laxative; Herbalax; Herbolax; Lapidar; Laxaco; Mucinum; Prodiem Plus; Senokot-S; Thunas Laxative; *Denm.:* Figen; *Fin.:* Agiolax; *Fr.:* Actisane Constipation Occasionnelle†; Agiolax; Boldoflorine; Depuratif des Alpes; Grains de Vals; Herbesan; Herbesan Instantane; Ideolaxyl; Laxasan†; Mediflor Tisane Contre la Constipation Passagere No 7†; Mediflor Tisane Hepatique No 5†; Modane; Mucinum a l'Extrait de Cascara; Mucinum†; Neo-Boldolaxine†; Obeflorine; Pursennide; Santane G; Tamarine; Tisane Clairo†; Tisane des Familles; Tisane Grande Chartreuse; Tisane Mexicaine†; Tisane Touraine†; Vegelax; *Ger.:* Agiolax; Alasenn; Dralinsa†; Floradix Maskam†; Heumann Abfuhrtee Solubilax N; Hevertolax duo; Kneipplax N†; Montana; Presseln Stoffwechsel-Tee Hapeka 225 N; Ramend Krauter; Salus Abfuhr-Tee Nr. 2†; Schwedentrunk mit Ginseng†; Schwedentrunk†; Sirmia Abfuhrkapseln†; *Hong Kong:* Agiolax; Mucinum Cascara; *Irl.:* Pripsen; *Israel:* Agiolax; Eucarbon; Jungborn; Lido Tea; Midro-Tea; Novicarbon; Pursennid; *Ital.:* Agiolax; Carbondifer; Colax; Confetti Lassativi CM; Cura†; Cuscutine; Depurativo; Fibrolax Complex; Fitolinea; Florerbe Lassativa; Lactolas; Lassatina; Midro; Ormobyl CM; Ortisan; Pursennid; Pursennid Complex†; Senna-Specie Composta; Tamarine; Tisana Arnaldi†; Tisana Kelemata; *Mex.:* Agiolax; Naturetti; *Neth.:* Agiolax; *Norw.:* Pursennid; *NZ:* Coloxyl with Senna; *Port.:* Agiolax; Bekunis†; Midro; Xarope de Macas Rainetas; *S.Afr.:* Agiolax; Rubilax; *Spain:* Agiolax; Bekunis Complex; Crislaxo; Diolaxil; Jarabe Manceau; Jarabe Manzanas Siken; Laxante Derly; Laxante Sanatorium; Modane; Pruina; Puntual; Puntualex; Pursennid†; Vegetalin; *Swed.:* Lunelax comp†; *Switz.:* Adistop Lax†; Agiolax; Bekunis; Boldoflorine†; Capsules laxatives Nattermann Nr. 13†; Dragees aux figues avec du sene; Drix†; Eucarbon†; Grains de Vals; Lapidar 10; Lapidar 10 plus†; Lapidar 10†; Lapidar 14†; Laxativum Nouvelle Formule†; Laxiplant cum Senna†; Laxomild†; Linforce; Optilax†; PhytoLaxin; Pursennide; Tamarine†; Tavolax†; The Brioni; The Franklin†; The laxatif Solubilax†; Tisane laxative; Tisane laxative H nouvelle formulation; Tisane laxative Natterman no 13 instant†; Tisane laxative Natterman no 13†; Valverde Dragees laxatives; Valverde Sirop laxatif; *Thai.:* Agiolax; Circanetten; *UK:* Athera; Califig; Clairo Tea; Cleansing Herb Tablets; Dual-Lax Extra Strong; Dual-Lax Normal Strength; Fam-Lax Senna; Kas-Bah; Laxadoron; Laxative Tablets; Liminate; Lion Cleansing Herbs; Lustys Herbalene; Manevac; Modern Herbals Laxative; Modern Herbals Menopause; Natural Herb Tablets; Nylax†; Out-of-Sorts; Pilewort Compound; Pripsen; Rhuaka; Skin Cleansing; Tabritis; *USA:* Black-Draught; Gentlax S†; Herbal Laxative†; Perdiem; Senokot-S; X-Prep Bowel Evacuant Kit-1; X-Prep Bowel Evacuant Kit-2.

Simeticone (6427-x)

Simeticone *(BAN, rINN)*.

Activated Dimethicone; Activated Dimethylpolysiloxane; Antifoam A; Antifoam AF; Simeticone *(USAN)*; Simeticonum.
CAS — 8050-81-5.

NOTE. Compounded preparations of simeticone may be represented by the following names:

- Co-simalcite *x/y (BAN)*—where *x* and *y* are the strengths in milligrams of simeticone and hydrotalcite respectively.

Pharmacopoeias. In *Eur.* (see p.vi) and *US.*

A mixture of liquid dimeticones containing finely divided silicon dioxide to enhance the defoaming properties of the silicone.

Pharmacopoeial description

Ph. Eur.: Simeticone is prepared by incorporation of 4 to 7% silica into poly(dimethylsiloxane) with a degree of polymerisation between 20 and 400. It contains 90.5 to 99.0% of poly(dimethylsiloxane). It is a greyish-white, opalescent, viscous liquid. Practically insoluble in water and in methyl alcohol; very slightly soluble to practically insoluble in dehydrated alcohol; partly miscible with dichloromethane, with ethyl acetate, with methyl ethyl ketone, and with toluene.

USP 25: A mixture of fully methylated linear siloxane polymers containing repeating units of the formula $[-(CH_3)_2SiO-]_n$, stabilised with trimethylsiloxy end-blocking units of the formula $[(CH_3)_3SiO-]$, and silicon dioxide. It contains not less than 90.5% and not more than 99% of polydimethylsiloxane and not less than 4% and not more than 7% of silicon dioxide. A translucent, grey, viscous fluid. Insoluble in water, in alcohol, and in dehydrated alcohol; the liquid phase is soluble 1 in 10 of chloroform, of ether, and of benzene, leaving a residue of silicon dioxide. Store in airtight containers.

Profile

Simeticone lowers surface tension and when administered by mouth causes bubbles of gas in the gastrointestinal tract to coalesce, thus aiding their dispersion.

It is promoted for the relief of flatulence and abdominal discomfort due to excess gastrointestinal gas in disorders such as dyspepsia (p.1204) and gastro-oesophageal reflux disease (p.1204). Doses of 125 to 250 mg three or four times daily have been given. For many gastrointestinal disorders, it is given in conjunction with an antacid.

Doses of 20 to 40 mg of simeticone have been given with feeds to relieve colic in infants (see Gastrointestinal Spasm, p.1204).

Simeticone is also used as a defoaming agent in radiography or endoscopy of the gastrointestinal tract.

◊ A brief review of the use of simeticone for gastrointestinal symptoms concluded that although it was commonly prescribed in combination with an antacid, there was no good evidence that it provided additional benefit. When used alone it probably helped to relieve minor postoperative and postprandial symptoms and it was a useful aid in upper gastrointestinal endoscopy.[1] However, some considered there was no convincing evidence that it was effective for the treatment of eructation, flatulence, or other signs or symptoms of excess gastrointestinal gas.[2]

1. Anonymous. Dimethicone for gastrointestinal symptoms? *Drug Ther Bull* 1986; **24:** 21–2.
2. Anonymous. Simeticone for gastrointestinal gas. *Med Lett Drugs Ther* 1996; **38:** 57–8.

Preparations

BP 2001: Simeticone for Oral Use;
USP 25: Alumina, Magnesia, and Simethicone Oral Suspension; Alumina, Magnesia, Calcium Carbonate, and Simethicone Tablets; Alumina, Magnesia, Calcium Carbonate, and Simethicone Tablets; Calcium Carbonate, Magnesia, and Simethicone Tablets; Magaldrate and Simethicone Oral Suspension; Magaldrate and Simethicone Tablets; Simethicone Capsules; Simethicone Emulsion; Simethicone Oral Suspension; Simethicone Tablets.

Proprietary Preparations (details are given in Part 3)
Aust.: Disflatyl; Lefaxin; SAB Simplex; *Austral.:* Degas Infant Drops; Infacol; Medefoam-2; Phazyme†; *Belg.:* Polysilon; *Braz.:* Anflat; Finigas; Gastroflat; Mylanta Plus; Silidron; *Canad.:* Babys Own Infant Drops; Gas-X; Maalox GRF†; Ovol; Phazyme; Siligaz; *Denm.:* Aeropax; Ceolat; Minifom†; Mylicon; *Fin.:* Ceolat; Cuplaton; Disflatyl; Minifom; *Fr.:* Siligaz; *Ger.:* Absorber HFV; Aegrosan; Busala†; Ceolat; Elugan; Elugan N; Endo-Paractol; Espumisan; Ilio-Funkton; Lefax; Meteosan; SAB Simplex; *Hong Kong:* Disflatyl; Gasteel; Infacol; Ovol; *Irl.:* Infacol; *Israel:* Simicol; *Ital.:* Mylicon; Polisilon; *Mex.:* Espaven Pediatrico; Liberan; *Neth.:* Carboticon†; Ceolat; *Norw.:* Ceolat; Minifom; Siloxan; *NZ:* Infacol; Medefoam; *Port.:* Aero-Om; *S.Afr.:* Telament; *Singapore:* Cuplaton; Infacol; *Spain:* Aero Red; Disflatyl; Enterosilicona; Pergastric†; Phazyme; *Swed.:* Ceolat†; Minifom; *Switz.:* Aeropax†; Disflatyl; Flatulex; Lefax; Polysilane; SAB Simplex†; Sili-Met-San; *Thai.:* Air-X; Babcon; Disflatyl; Gas-X; Gastyl; Mylom; Ovol; Semeth; Simcone; Simecon; *UAE:* Salinal; *UK:* Asilone Windcheaters; Dentinox Colic Drops; Infacol; Setlers Wind-eze; Woodwards Colic Drops; *USA:* Colicon; Degas; Extra Strength Mintox Plus; Flatulex; Gas Relief; Gas-X; Maalox Anti-Gas; Major-Con; Mylanta Gas; Mylicon; Phazyme; SonoRx.

Multi-ingredient: numerous preparations are listed in Part 3.

Sodium Picosulfate (7533-q)

Sodium Picosulfate *(BAN, rINN)*.

DA-1773; LA-391; Natrii Picosulfas; Picosulphol; Sodium Picosulphate. Disodium 4,4'-(2-pyridylmethylene)di(phenyl sulphate).
$C_{18}H_{13}NNa_2O_8S_2 = 481.4$.
CAS — 10040-45-6.
ATC — A06AB08.

Pharmacopoeias. Eur. (see p.vi) and Jpn contain the monohydrate.

Pharmacopoeial description

Ph. Eur.: A white or almost white, crystalline powder. Freely soluble in water; slightly soluble in alcohol; practically insoluble in ether.

Adverse Effects and Precautions

As for Bisacodyl, p.1212.

Bowel evacuation. Sodium picosulfate with magnesium citrate was considered a safe and effective bowel cleansing agent in adults[1] and children[2] with inflammatory bowel disease. They tolerated the preparation as well as patients with other colonic disorders with no adverse effect on their disease symptoms. Patients should be kept well hydrated (it may be appropriate to carry out bowel preparation in hospital in frail or elderly patients to avoid the risks of over- or underhydration[3,4]), and this procedure should not be used in suspected toxic dilatation of the colon.

1. McDonagh AJG, *et al.* Safety of Picolax (sodium picosulphate-magnesium citrate) in inflammatory bowel disease. *BMJ* 1989; **299:** 776–7.
2. Evans M, *et al.* Safety of Picolax in inflammatory bowel disease. *BMJ* 1989; **299:** 1101–2.
3. Lewis M, *et al.* Bowel preparation at home in elderly people. *BMJ* 1997; **314:** 74.
4. Hanning CD. Bowel preparation at home in elderly people. *BMJ* 1997; **314:** 74.

Pharmacokinetics

Like bisacodyl (p.1212), sodium picosulfate is metabolised by colonic bacteria to the active compound bis(*p*-hydroxyphenyl)pyridyl-2-methane.

Uses and Administration

Sodium picosulfate is a stimulant laxative related to bisacodyl (p.1212) used for the treatment of constipation (p.1202) and for evacuation of the colon before investigational procedures or surgery. When taken by mouth it stimulates bowel movements following metabolism by colonic bacteria. It is usually effective within 6 to 12 hours although when used with magnesium citrate for bowel evacuation an effect may be seen within 3 hours.

For constipation it is given by mouth as a single dose of 5 to 10 mg, usually at bedtime. Doses of 2.5 to 5 mg have been given to children aged 4 to 10 years. Children aged less than 4 years have received 250 μg per kg body-weight.

For bowel evacuation, a dose of sodium picosulfate 10 mg with magnesium citrate (p.1232) is given in the morning and again in the afternoon of the day before examination. Doses are reduced in children.

Preparations

BP 2001: Sodium Picosulfate Oral Powder.

Proprietary Preparations (details are given in Part 3)
Aust.: Agaffin; Guttalax; *Austral.:* Durolax SP; *Belg.:* Dulcolax Picosulphate; Fructines; Guttalax; Laxoberon; Obstilax†; Picolaxine; *Braz.:* Diltin; Dulcolax Liquid; Guttalax; *Denm.:* Laxoberal; Picolon; *Fin.:* Laxoberon; *Fr.:* Fructines; *Ger.:* Abfuhrtropfen; Agiolax Pico; AgioPico Plus; Darmol; Darmol Pico; Dulcolax NP; Laxoberal; Mandrolax Pico†; Midro Pico; Regulax Picosulfat; *Hong Kong:* Sur-Lax; *Irl.:* Laxoberal; *Ital.:* Euchessina CM; Falquigut; Gocce Antonetto†; Gocce Lassative Aicardi; Guttalax; *Mex.:* Anara; Laxoberon; *Neth.:* Dulcodruppels; Laxoberon; *Port.:* Guttalax; *Singapore:* Sur-Lax; *Spain:* Contumax; Elimin; Evacuol; Gutalax; Laxonol; Lubrilax; Skilax; *Swed.:* Laxoberal; *Switz.:* Fructines nouvelle formule; Guttalax; Laxoberon; *UK:* Dulcolax Liquid; Laxoberal.

Multi-ingredient: *Austral.:* Colonprep; Picolax; Picoprep; *Belg.:* Picolax de Vichy†; *Irl.:* Picolax; *Israel:* Pico-Salax; *Norw.:* Pico-Salax†; *Spain:* Emuliquen Laxante; *Swed.:* Pico-Salax†; *Switz.:* Laxasan; Pico-Salax†; *UK:* Picolax.

The symbol † denotes a preparation no longer actively marketed

Sodium Potassium Tartrate (1198-g)

E337; Kalii Natrii Tartras; Kalium Natrium Tartaricum; Potassium Sodium Tartrate; Rochelle Salt; Seignette Salt; Sodii et Potassii Tartras; Tartarus Natronatus.
$C_4H_4KNaO_6,4H_2O = 282.2.$
CAS — 304-59-6 (anhydrous sodium potassium tartrate); 6381-59-5 (sodium potassium tartrate tetrahydrate); 6100-16-9 (sodium potassium tartrate tetrahydrate).
Pharmacopoeias. In Eur. (see p.vi) and US.

Pharmacopoeial description

Ph. Eur.: A white crystalline powder or colourless transparent crystals. Very soluble in water; practically insoluble in alcohol.
USP 25: Colourless crystals or a white, crystalline powder, with a cooling, saline taste. It effloresces slightly in warm dry air, the crystals often being coated with a white powder. Soluble 1 in 1 of water; practically insoluble in alcohol. Store in airtight containers.

Profile

Sodium potassium tartrate has been used, in doses of 8 to 16 g, as an osmotic laxative (p.1201). It is also used as a food additive.
For the general properties of potassium salts, see p.1194, and of sodium salts, see p.1196.

Preparations

BPC 1973: Compound Effervescent Powder.
Proprietary Preparations (details are given in Part 3)
Multi-ingredient: *Aust.:* Laxalpin; *Fr.:* Romarene; *UK:* Jaaps Health Salt.

Anhydrous Sodium Sulfate (1200-q)

Anhydrous Sodium Sulphate; Dried Sodium Sulphate; Exsiccated Sodium Sulphate; Natrii Sulfas Anhydricus; Natrium Sulfuricum Siccatum.
$Na_2SO_4 = 142.0.$
CAS — 7757-82-6.
Pharmacopoeias. In Chin., Eur. (see p.vi), Int., and Pol.
US includes a single monograph for both the anhydrous form and the decahydrate.

Pharmacopoeial description

Ph. Eur.: A white, hygroscopic powder. Freely soluble in water.

Sodium Sulfate (1199-q)

E514; Glauber's Salt; Natrii Sulfas Decahydricus; Natrii Sulphas; Natrium Sulfuricum Crystallisatum; Sodium Sulphate; Sodium Sulphate Decahydrate.
$Na_2SO_4,10H_2O = 322.2.$
CAS — 7727-73-3 (sodium sulfate decahydrate).
ATC — A06AD13; A12CA02.
Pharmacopoeias. In Chin., Eur. (see p.vi), Int., and Pol.
US includes a single monograph for both the anhydrous form and the decahydrate.

Pharmacopoeial description

Ph. Eur.: A white, crystalline powder or colourless, transparent crystals. Freely soluble in water; practically insoluble in alcohol. It partly dissolves in its own water of crystallisation at about 33°. It loses between 52.0 and 57.0% of its weight on drying.
USP 25: Sodium sulfate contains 10 molecules of water of hydration or is anhydrous. The decahydrate loses between 51 and 57% of its weight on drying and the anhydrous form loses not more than 0.5% of its weight. Large, colourless, odourless, transparent crystals or a granular powder. It effloresces rapidly in air, liquefies in its water of hydration at about 33°, and loses all of its water of hydration at about 100°. Freely soluble in water; insoluble in alcohol; soluble in glycerol. Store in airtight containers, preferably at a temperature not exceeding 30°.

Profile

Sodium sulfate is an osmotic laxative (p.1201). It is given by mouth in a usual dose of 5 to 10 g daily. It is also given in dilute solution with a high molecular weight macrogol for prompt bowel evacuation before investigational procedures or surgery (see Macrogols, p.1630).
Sodium sulfate is also used as a diluent for colours in foods.
For the general properties of sodium salts, see p.1196.

Preparations

USP 25: Sodium Sulfate Injection.
Proprietary Preparations (details are given in Part 3)
Austral.: Celloids SS 69; *UK:* Fynnon Salt.
Multi-ingredient: *Austral.:* Duo Celloids SPSS; Duo Celloids SSMP; Duo Celloids SSPC; Duo Celloids SSS; Iron Compound; Liv-Detox; Silybum Complex; *Belg.:* Kruschels†; *Braz.:* Argyrophedrine; Visual; *Canad.:* Normo Gastryl; *Fr.:* Actisoufre; Azym; Digedryl; Gastrilax†; Hepargitol; Jecobiase; Normogastryl; Oxyboldine; Prefagyl; *Ital.:* Argirofedrina; Carbotiol†; *Spain:* Boldosal; Darmen Salt; Digestovital; Leberetic; Lebersal; Normogastryl; Salcedol; *Switz.:* Drix†; Normogastryl; Padma-Lax; Thiourbrol; *Thai.:* Ulgastrin; *UK:* Juno Junipah; New Era Zief†; *USA:* Triv.

Sodium Tartrate (1201-p)

E335 (sodium tartrate or monosodium tartrate).
$C_2H_4O_2(CO_2Na)_2,2H_2O = 230.1.$
CAS — 868-18-8 (anhydrous sodium tartrate); 6106-24-7 (sodium tartrate dihydrate).

Profile

Sodium tartrate has been used as an osmotic laxative. It is used as a food additive.
For the general properties of sodium salts, see p.1196.

Preparations

Proprietary Preparations (details are given in Part 3)
Multi-ingredient: *Port.:* Dentolamina†; Sais Zitos†.

Sterculia (5461-j)

E416; Indian Tragacanth; Karaya; Karaya Gum; Sterculia Gum.
CAS — 9000-36-6.
ATC — A06AC03.
Pharmacopoeias. In Br. and Fr.

Pharmacopoeial description

BP 2001: Sterculia is the gum obtained from *Sterculia urens* and other species of *Sterculia*. Irregular or vermiform pieces, greyish-white with a brown or pink tinge, with an odour resembling that of acetic acid. It contains not less than 14.0% of volatile acid (or not less than 10.0% if supplied in powdered form), calculated as acetic acid. Sparingly soluble in water, but swells into a homogeneous, adhesive, gelatinous mass; practically insoluble in alcohol. Store at a temperature not exceeding 25°.

Adverse Effects and Precautions

As for Ispaghula, p.1229. There is a risk of intestinal or oesophageal obstruction and faecal impaction, especially if such compounds are swallowed dry. Therefore they should always be taken with sufficient fluid and should not be taken immediately before going to bed. They should be avoided by patients who have difficulty swallowing.

Uses and Administration

Sterculia is used similarly to ispaghula (p.1229) as a bulk laxative and for adjusting faecal consistency. It has also been used as an aid to appetite control in the management of obesity (p.1505) but there is little evidence of efficacy. It is usually taken in the form of granules by mouth once or twice daily after meals. The granules are washed down without chewing with plenty of water. They may also be sprinkled onto and taken with yogurt.
Sterculia is used topically in the form of a paste or powder as a skin protector and filler in the fitting of ileostomy and colostomy appliances. It has also been used in dental fixative powders, and as an emulsifier and stabiliser in foods.

Preparations

BP 2001: Sterculia Granules.
Proprietary Preparations (details are given in Part 3)
Austral.: Hollister Karaya Paste†; Normafibe; *Belg.:* Calox†; Normacol; *Canad.:* Normacol; *Fr.:* Enteromucilage†; Inolaxine; Norgagil†; Normacol; Prefine; *Ger.:* Decorpa; Granamon; *Hong Kong:* Inolaxine; Normacol; *Irl.:* Normacol; *Ital.:* Normacol; *Neth.:* Normacol; *NZ:* Normacol; *S.Afr.:* Normacol; *Singapore:* Normacol; *Swed.:* Inolaxol; *Switz.:* Colosan mite; Inolaxine; Normacol; *UK:* Normacol; Prefil†.
Multi-ingredient: *Austral.:* Alvercol; Enterocare; Granocol; Normacol Plus; *Belg.:* Normacol Antispasmodique; Normacol Plus; *Braz.:* Formitonicum; *Fr.:* Kaologeais; Karayal; Normacol a la Bourdaine; Poly-Karaya; *Ger.:* Karaya Bismuth; *Hong Kong:* Alvercol; Normacol Plus; *Irl.:* Alvercol; Normacol Plus; *NZ:* Granocol; Normacol Plus; *Port.:* Normacol Plus; *S.Afr.:* Alvercol; Normacol Plus; *Singapore:* Normacol Plus; *Spain:* Normacol Forte; *Switz.:* Colosan plus; Normacol (avec bourdaine); Poly-Karaya; *UK:* Normacol Plus; Spasmonal Fibre.

Sucralfate (707-m)

Sucralfate (BAN, USAN, rINN).
Sucrose hydrogen sulphate basic aluminium salt; Sucrose octakis(hydrogen sulphate) aluminium complex; β-D-Fructofuranosyl-α-D-glucopyranoside octakis (hydrogen sulphate) aluminium complex.
$C_{12}H_mAl_{16}O_nS_8.$
CAS — 54182-58-0.
ATC — A02BX02.
Pharmacopoeias. In Chin., Jpn, and US.

Pharmacopoeial description

USP 25: The hydrous basic aluminium salt of sucrose octasulfate. Store in airtight containers.

Adverse Effects and Precautions

Constipation is the most frequently reported adverse effect of sucralfate although diarrhoea, nausea, or gastric discomfort may also occur. Dry mouth, dizziness, drowsiness, headache, vertigo, back pain, skin rashes, and hypersensitivity reactions such as pruritus have been reported.

Great caution is needed in patients with renal impairment (below) as absorption and accumulation of aluminium may cause adverse effects.

Bezoar formation. As of March 1999, the UK Committee on Safety of Medicines was aware of 7 reports worldwide of bezoar formation associated with sucralfate use in intensive care patients.[1] It advised caution in the use of sucralfate in seriously ill patients because of the risks of bezoar formation and intestinal obstruction.[1] Patients with delayed gastric emptying or receiving concomitant enteral feeds may be at increased risk.
1. Committee on Safety of Medicines/Medicines Control Agency. Bezoar formation with sulcralfate [sic] (Antepsin). *Current Problems* 1999; **25:** 6.

Renal impairment. Sucralfate under acid conditions can release aluminium ions which may be absorbed systemically. Significant increases in the urinary excretion of aluminium have been observed in healthy subjects given sucralfate 4 g daily,[1,2] reflecting gastrointestinal absorption of aluminium; aluminium concentrations in serum and urine were significantly higher in patients with chronic renal insufficiency than in subjects with normal renal function.[3] Aluminium toxicity in patients with normal renal function receiving sucralfate would not be expected, but seizures, muscle weakness, bone pain,[1] and severe aluminium encephalopathy[4] have been reported in patients with end-stage renal disease requiring dialysis. Sucralfate should be used with caution in patients with renal impairment, especially if other aluminium-containing agents are also taken.
1. Robertson JA, *et al.* Sucralfate, intestinal aluminium absorption, and aluminium toxicity in a patient on dialysis. *Ann Intern Med* 1989; **111:** 179–81.
2. Allain P, *et al.* Plasma and urine aluminium concentrations in healthy subjects after administration of sucralfate. *Br J Clin Pharmacol* 1990; **29:** 391–5.
3. Burgess E, *et al.* Aluminum absorption and excretion following sucralfate therapy in chronic renal insufficiency. *Am J Med* 1992; **92:** 471–5.
4. Withers DJ, *et al.* Encephalopathy in patient taking aluminium-containing agents, including sucralfate. *Lancet* 1989; **ii:** 674.

Interactions

Sucralfate may interfere with the absorption of other drugs and it has been suggested that there should be an interval of 2 hours between the administration of sucralfate and other concurrent non-antacid medication. Some of the drugs reported to be affected by sucralfate include cimetidine, ranitidine, digoxin, ketoconazole, phenytoin, fluoroquinolone antibacterials, tetracycline, quinidine, theophylline, thyroxine [levothyroxine], and possibly warfarin. The recommended interval between sucralfate and antacids is 30 minutes. An interval of 1 hour should elapse between sucralfate administration and enteral feeding.

Pharmacokinetics

Sucralfate is only slightly absorbed from the gastrointestinal tract following oral administration. However, there can be some release of aluminium ions and of sucrose sulfate and small quantities of sucrose sulfate may be absorbed and excreted, primarily in the urine; some absorption of aluminium may also occur (see Renal Impairment, above).

Uses and Administration

Sucralfate is a cytoprotective drug which, under acid gastrointestinal conditions, forms an adherent complex with proteins which coats the gastric mucosa and is reported to have a special affinity for ulcer sites. It also inhibits the action of pepsin and adsorbs bile salts.

Sucralfate is used in the treatment of peptic ulcer disease (p.1208) and chronic gastritis. It is given by mouth and should be taken on an empty stomach before meals and at bedtime. The usual dose is 1 g four times daily or 2 g twice daily for 4 to 8 weeks; if necessary the dose may be increased to a maximum of 8 g daily. If longer-term therapy is required sucralfate may be administered for up to 12 weeks. Where appropriate a maintenance dose of 1 g twice daily may be given to prevent the recurrence of duodenal ulcers.

For prophylaxis of stress ulceration the usual dose of sucralfate is 1 g six times daily; a dose of 8 g daily should not be exceeded.

Gastrointestinal bleeding. Sucralfate is an effective drug for the prophylaxis and management of stress-induced gastrointestinal bleeding in severely ill patients, and may reduce the risk of late-onset pneumonia compared with an H_2-antagonist.[1] For further discussion of stress ulceration and bleeding, including the use of sucralfate, see under Peptic Ulcer Disease, p.1208. There is also some evidence from another study[2] that sucralfate reduces gastrointestinal bleeding associated with NSAID administration, although it does not prevent drug-induced gastric erosion.

1. Prod'hom G, et al. Nosocomial pneumonia in mechanically ventilated patients receiving antacid, ranitidine, or sucralfate as prophylaxis for stress ulcer: a randomized controlled trial. *Ann Intern Med* 1994; **120:** 653–62.
2. Hudson N, et al. Effect of sucralfate on aspirin induced mucosal injury and impaired haemostasis in humans. *Gut* 1997; **41:** 19–23.

Gastro-oesophageal reflux disease. Although sucralfate has been tried for gastro-oesophageal reflux disease (p.1204) the results of studies have been inconsistent.[1-3]

1. Orlando RC. Sucralfate therapy and reflux esophagitis: an overview. *Am J Med* 1991; **91** (suppl 2A); 123S–124S.
2. Klinkenberg-Knol EC, et al. Pharmacological management of gastro-oesophageal reflux disease. *Drugs* 1995; **49:** 695–710.
3. Simon B, et al. Sucralfate gel versus placebo in patients with non-erosive gastro-oesophageal reflux disease. *Aliment Pharmacol Ther* 1996; **10:** 441–6.

Mouth ulceration. Sucralfate has been investigated as a mouth rinse in the treatment and prophylaxis of stomatitis induced by cancer chemotherapy[1-3] although evidence of benefit for any drug is ambiguous (see Mucositis, p.480). One study[2] in 40 patients found a significant reduction in symptoms among 23 evaluable patients given sucralfate prophylactically. Seven patients withdrew due to aggravation of chemotherapy-induced nausea. It was suggested that to overcome this problem, the suspension should have a neutral taste, should not be swallowed after rinsing, and that rinsing should not be commenced until nausea had ceased.

Sucralfate has also been reported to be of benefit in patients with recurrent aphthous stomatitis (mouth ulceration—p.1206). A study involving 21 such patients over 2 years found that topical application of sucralfate suspension 4 times daily was superior to treatment with an antacid (aluminium hydroxide with magnesium hydroxide) or placebo.[4]

1. Pfeiffer P, et al. A prospective pilot study on the effect of sucralfate mouth-swishing in reducing stomatitis during radiotherapy of the oral cavity. *Acta Oncol* 1990; **29:** 471–3.
2. Pfeiffer P, et al. Effect of prophylactic sucralfate suspension on stomatitis induced by cancer chemotherapy: a randomized, double-blind cross-over study. *Acta Oncol* 1990; **29:** 171–3.
3. Allison RR, et al. Symptomatic acute mucositis can be minimized or prophylaxed [sic] by the combination of sucralfate and fluconazole. *Cancer Invest* 1995; **13:** 16–22.
4. Rattan J, et al. Sucralfate suspension as a treatment of recurrent aphthous stomatitis. *J Intern Med* 1994; **236:** 341–3.

Skin ulceration. Sucralfate has reportedly been applied topically with some success to treat bleeding skin ulcers (p.1108) associated with malignancy,[1] and to promote the healing of venous stasis ulcers.[2] It has been suggested that sucralfate promotes angiogenesis by binding to, and preventing degradation of, basic fibroblast growth factor (bFGF).[2]

1. Regnard CFB. Control of bleeding in advanced cancer. *Lancet* 1991; **337:** 974.
2. Tsakayannis D, et al. Sucralfate and chronic venous stasis ulcers. *Lancet* 1994; **343:** 424–5.

Preparations

USP 25: Sucralfate Tablets.

Proprietary Preparations (details are given in Part 3)

Aust.: Sucralan; Sucralbene; Sucralstad; Sucramed; Ulcogant; *Austral.:* Carafate; SCF†; Ulcyte; *Belg.:* Ulcogant; *Braz.:* Antepsin; *Canad.:* Novo-Sucralate; Sulcrate; *Denm.:* Antepsin; Hexagastron; *Fin.:* Alsucral; Antepsin; *Fr.:* Keal; Ulcar; *Ger.:* Sucrabest†; Sucraphil; Ulcogant; *Hong Kong:* Sucari; Ulsanic; *Irl.:* Antepsin; *Israel:* Ulsanic; *Ital.:* Antepsin; Citogel; Crafilm; Gastrogel; Ipagastril; Sucrager; Sucral; Sucralfin; Sucramal; Sucrate; Sucroral; Sugar; Sugast; Suril; Ulcrast; Zenodian; *Jpn.:* Ulcerlmin; *Neth.:* Ulcogant; *Norw.:* Antepsin; *NZ:* Carafate; *Port.:* Calfate; Sucralum; Ulcermin; *S.Afr.:* Cralsanic†; Ulcefate†; Ulcetab†; Ulcetic†; Ulsanic; *Singapore:* Ulcertec; *Spain:* Gastrail†; Tiblex†; Ulcufato†; Urbal; *Swed.:* Andapsin; Succosa†; *Switz.:* Gastrogel; Ulcogant; *Thai.:* Sucralen; Sucral; Sucrate; Ulsanic; *UAE:* Sucralose; *UK:* Antepsin; *USA:* Carafate.

Used as an adjunct in: *Ital.:* Ketodol.

Sulfasalazine (4951-n)

Sulfasalazine (BAN, USAN, rINN).

Salazosulfapyridine; Salicylazosulfapyridine; Sulfasalazinum; Sulphasalazine. 4-Hydroxy-4′-(2-pyridylsulphamoyl)azobenzene-3-carboxylic acid.

$C_{18}H_{14}N_4O_5S = 398.4$.

CAS — 599-79-1.

ATC — A07EC01.

Pharmacopoeias. In Eur. (see p.vi), Int., Jpn, and US.

Pharmacopoeial description

Ph. Eur.: A bright yellow or brownish-yellow, fine powder. Practically insoluble in water and in dichloromethane; very slightly soluble in alcohol; dissolves in dilute solutions of alkali hydroxides. Protect from light.

USP 25: A fine odourless bright yellow or brownish-yellow powder. Practically insoluble in water, in chloroform, in ether, and in benzene; soluble 1 in 2900 of alcohol, and 1 in 1500 of methyl alcohol; soluble in aqueous solutions of alkali hydroxides. Store in airtight containers. Protect from light.

The symbol † denotes a preparation no longer actively marketed

---

Adverse Effects and Precautions

Since sulfasalazine is metabolised to sulfapyridine and 5-aminosalicylic acid (mesalazine), its adverse effects and precautions are similar to those of sulfonamides (see Sulfamethoxazole, p.254) and of mesalazine (p.1234). Many adverse effects have been attributed to the sulfapyridine moiety and appear to be more common if serum-sulfapyridine concentrations are greater than 50 μg per mL, if the daily dose of sulfasalazine is 4 g or more, or in slow acetylators of sulfapyridine.

The most commonly reported adverse effects include nausea and vomiting, abdominal discomfort, headache, fever, and skin rash.

Adverse effects can be broadly divided into 2 groups. The first is dose-related, dependent on acetylator phenotype, and largely predictable; this group includes nausea and vomiting, headache, haemolytic anaemia, and methaemoglobinaemia. The second group are the hypersensitivity reactions which are essentially unpredictable and usually occur at the start of treatment; this group includes skin rash, aplastic anaemia, hepatic and pulmonary dysfunction, and auto-immune haemolysis.

Oligospermia, reversible on withdrawal of sulfasalazine, has also been reported. Administration of sulfasalazine may result in yellow-orange discoloration of skin, urine, and other body fluids. Some soft contact lenses may be stained.

Sulfasalazine should not be given to patients with a history of sensitivity to sulfonamides or salicylates. Use in children under 2 years of age is contra-indicated because of the risk of kernicterus.

Blood counts should be performed at the start of therapy and at least once a month for a minimum of the first 3 months of treatment. If a blood dyscrasia is suspected treatment should be stopped immediately and a blood count performed. Patients or their carers should be told how to recognise signs of blood toxicity and should be advised to seek immediate medical attention if symptoms such as fever, sore throat, mouth ulcers, bruising or bleeding develop. Care is advisable in patients with glucose 6-phosphate dehydrogenase deficiency because of the risk of haemolytic anaemia.

Sulfasalazine should be used with caution in hepatic or renal impairment. Liver function tests should be carried out at monthly intervals for the first 3 months of treatment. Periodic monitoring of kidney function has also been recommended, but the *British National Formulary* considers the practical value of such monitoring unproven.

◊ Reviews of the adverse effects associated with the administration of sulfasalazine in patients with inflammatory bowel disease[1] and rheumatoid arthritis.[2,3] The type and incidence of adverse effects appear to be similar in both groups of patients.[2] Although most reactions are minor and patients may continue therapy at the same or reduced dosage, some patients discontinue treatment because of adverse effects and in these cases a hyposensitisation regimen may be considered.[1,4,5] Hyposensitisation should not be attempted in patients with a history of a serious adverse effect such as agranulocytosis, toxic epidermal necrolysis, erythema multiforme, frank haemolysis, or a severe hypersensitivity reaction.[1,4,5] An alternative to hyposensitisation in patients with inflammatory bowel disease who cannot tolerate sulfasalazine, is to try a drug that supplies the active 5-aminosalicylic acid component without sulfapyridine as the latter is thought to be responsible for many of the adverse effects. Examples include mesalazine and olsalazine; however, some patients still experience hypersensitivity, see under Mesalazine, p.1234.

1. Taffet SL, Das KM. Sulfasalazine: adverse effects and desensitization. *Dig Dis Sci* 1983; **28:** 833–42.
2. Amos RS, et al. Sulphasalazine for rheumatoid arthritis: toxicity in 774 patients monitored for one to 11 years. *BMJ* 1986; **293:** 420–3.
3. Farr M, et al. Side effect profile of 200 patients with inflammatory arthritides treated with sulphasalazine. *Drugs* 1986; **32** (suppl 1): 49–53.
4. Purdy BH, et al. Desensitization for sulfasalazine skin rash. *Ann Intern Med* 1984; **100:** 512–14.
5. Bax DE, Amos RS. Sulphasalazine in rheumatoid arthritis: desensitising the patient with a skin rash. *Ann Rheum Dis* 1986; **45:** 139–40.

Breast feeding. Small amounts of sulfasalazine and its sulfapyridine metabolites are excreted in breast milk; the concentrations of sulfasalazine and total sulfapyridine may be up to 30% and 50% of maternal serum concentrations.[1] Bloody diarrhoea in a breast-fed infant whose mother was taking sulfasalazine 3 g daily has been reported.[2] The mother was a slow acetylator with a relatively high blood concentration of sulfapyridine which contributed to the appearance of the drug in the infant's blood. However, continued treatment with sulfasalazine can generally be recommended to breast-feeding mothers of healthy infants.[3]

1. Khan AKA, Truelove SC. Placental and mammary transfer of sulphasalazine. *BMJ* 1979; **2:** 1553.
2. Branski D, et al. Bloody diarrhoea—a possible complication of sulfasalazine transferred through human breast milk. *J Pediatr Gastroenterol Nutr* 1986; **5:** 316–17.
3. Peppercorn MA. Sulfasalazine and related new drugs. *J Clin Pharmacol* 1987; **27:** 260–5.

Effects on the blood. Blood disorders constitute 19% of all reactions reported with sulfasalazine.[1] As of June 1993 the UK Committee on Safety of Medicines was aware of 191 reports of neutropenia, leucopenia, or agranulocytosis (22 fatal), 44 reports of bone marrow depression or aplastic anaemia (13 fatal) and 30 reports of thrombocytopenia (1 fatal).[1]

Although blood dyscrasias were initially thought to be caused by the sulfapyridine moiety, subsequent experience has shown that the aminosalicylates can also cause haematological reactions (see Mesalazine, p.1234). The risk of blood dyscrasias with sulfasalazine has been estimated at 0.6 per 1000 in those given the drug for inflammatory bowel disease, but approximately 10 times greater in patients receiving sulfasalazine for rheumatoid arthritis.[2]

Sulfasalazine inhibits folic acid absorption, interferes with its metabolism, and can increase folic acid requirements through haemolysis of red blood cells.[3,4] These effects are not usually significant in patients with inflammatory bowel disease unless there are additional factors causing folate deficiency such as intercurrent illness or an exacerbation of bowel disease.[3,4] However, clinical folate deficiency with macrocytosis, megaloblastic anaemia, or pancytopenia has been reported rarely.[3,4] Macrocytic anaemia associated with sulfasalazine may occur more commonly in patients with rheumatoid arthritis; it was found in 7 of 50 patients within 3 to 4 months of starting treatment with sulfasalazine.[5] The effects of sulfasalazine on folic acid metabolism appear to be dose-related and respond to withdrawal or dosage reduction, and folic acid supplements;[3-5] intravenous folinic acid may sometimes be needed.[4] Although the effects may be potentially serious, they are not a contra-indication to continuing sulfasalazine treatment.[4,5]

Patients with a history of leucopenia associated with administration of gold for rheumatoid arthritis should not be given sulfasalazine since a similar reaction may occur.[6]

1. Committee on Safety of Medicines/Medicines Control Agency. Sulphasalazine and fatal blood dyscrasias. *Current Problems* 1993; **19:** 6.
2. Committee on Safety of Medicines/Medicines Control Agency. Blood dyscrasias and mesalazine. *Current Problems* 1995; **21:** 5–6.
3. Swinson CM, et al. Role of sulphasalazine in the aetiology of folate deficiency in ulcerative colitis. *Gut* 1981; **22:** 456–61.
4. Logan ECM, et al. Sulphasalazine associated pancytopenia may be caused by acute folate deficiency. *Gut* 1986; **27:** 868–72.
5. Prouse PJ, et al. Macrocytic anaemia in patients treated with sulphasalazine for rheumatoid arthritis. *BMJ* 1986; **293:** 1407.
6. Bliddal H, et al. Gold-induced leucopenia may predict a similar adverse reaction to sulphasalazine. *Lancet* 1987; **i:** 390.

Effects on the cardiovascular system. Reports include Raynaud's syndrome with sulfasalazine[1] and myocarditis with sulfasalazine and with mesalazine.[2] Myocarditis leading to fatal cardiogenic shock has been reported in a patient receiving mesalazine and it has been recommended that sulfasalazine or mesalazine should be replaced by glucocorticoids if cardiac symptoms arise.[3]

1. Reid J, et al. Raynaud's phenomenon induced by sulphasalazine. *Postgrad Med J* 1980; **56:** 106–7.
2. Agnholt J, et al. Cardiac hypersensitivity to 5-aminosalicylic acid. *Lancet* 1989; **i:** 1135.
3. Kristensen KS. Fatal myocarditis associated with mesalazine. *Lancet* 1990; **335:** 605.

Effects on fertility. Although successful pregnancies have been reported in the partners of men taking sulfasalazine,[1,2] male infertility is a well recognised complication of sulfasalazine treatment. Untreated inflammatory bowel disease is not associated with abnormal seminal quality or infertility, but oligospermia, reduced sperm motility, and an increase in morphological abnormalities are seen after treatment with sulfasalazine which may lead to infertility.[1-4] Oligospermia has been reported in 86% of men with inflammatory bowel disease treated with sulfasalazine.[1] Seminal characteristics and fertility return to normal within 2 to 3 months of withdrawing sulfasalazine and successful pregnancies have been reported following withdrawal.[1-3] The mechanism involved is thought to be a direct toxic effect on immature and developing spermatozoa, possibly due to the sulfapyridine moiety.[2-4] Improvement in seminal characteristics and successful pregnancies have been reported following substitution of mesalazine[4,5] or balsalazide[6] for sulfasalazine in patients with ulcerative colitis.

1. Birnie GG, et al. Incidence of sulphasalazine-induced male infertility. *Gut* 1981; **22:** 452–5.
2. Riley SA, et al. Sulphasalazine induced seminal abnormalities in ulcerative colitis: results of mesalazine substitution. *Gut* 1987; **28:** 1008–12.
3. Toovey S, et al. Sulphasalazine and male infertility: reversibility and possible mechanism. *Gut* 1981; **22:** 445–51.

4. Ó'Moráin C, et al. Reversible male infertility due to sulphasala-zine: studies in man and rat. *Gut* 1984; **25:** 1078–84.
5. Cann PA, Holdsworth CD. Reversal of male infertility on chang-ing treatment from sulphasalazine to 5-aminosalicylic acid. *Lan-cet* 1984; **i:** 1119.
6. McIntyre PB, Lennard-Jones JE. Reversal with balsalazide of in-fertility caused by sulphasalazine. *BMJ* 1984; **288:** 1652–3.

Effects on the gastrointestinal tract. Sulfasalazine-in-duced exacerbations of ulcerative colitis have been reported[1,2] and are probably caused by the salicylate moiety rather than sulfapyridine.[3] Other reported effects include a dose-related metallic taste[4] and intestinal villous atrophy.[5]

1. Schwartz AG, et al. Sulfasalazine-induced exacerbation of ulcer-ative colitis. *N Engl J Med* 1982; **306:** 409–12.
2. Ring FA, et al. Sulfasalazine-induced colitis complicating idio-pathic ulcerative colitis. *Can Med Assoc J* 1984; **131:** 43–5.
3. Shanahan F, Targan S. Sulfasalazine and salicylate-induced ex-acerbation of ulcerative colitis. *N Engl J Med* 1987; **317:** 455.
4. Ogburn RM. Sulfamethazine-related dysgeusia. *JAMA* 1979; **241:** 837.
5. Smith MA, et al. Angioimmunoblastic lymphadenopathy, sul-phasalazine exposure and villous atrophy. *Postgrad Med J* 1985; **61:** 337–8.

Effects on the hair. Alopecia occurred on 2 occasions[1] after starting sulfasalazine 2 or 3 g daily in a patient with ulcerative colitis. On both occasions normal hair growth returned after treatment was stopped, and the patient was later successfully desensitised. However, alopecia which developed in another patient during sulfasalazine treatment did not recur on rechal-lenge.[2] In this case postpartum alopecia was considered to be the cause and these authors doubted whether sulfasalazine causes alopecia at all. Hair loss has been reported in 2 patients receiving mesalazine enemas.[3] However, remission of alopecia universalis has been reported during sulfasalazine treatment of rheumatoid arthritis.[4]

1. Breen EG, Donnelly S. Alopecia associated with sulphasalazine (Salazopyrin). *BMJ* 1986; **292:** 802.
2. Fich A, Eliakim R. Does sulfasalazine induce alopecia? *J Clin Gastroenterol* 1988; **10:** 466.
3. Kutty PK, et al. Hair loss and 5-aminosalicylic acid enemas. *Ann Intern Med* 1982; **97:** 785–6.
4. Jawad ASM, Scott DGI. Remission of alopecia universalis dur-ing sulphasalazine treatment for rheumatoid arthritis. *BMJ* 1989; **298:** 675.

Effects on the kidneys. For reports of nephrotic syndrome and of interstitial nephritis associated with sulfasalazine treat-ment, see under Adverse Effects of Mesalazine, p.1234.

Effects on the pancreas. The UK Committee on Safety of Medicines had received 6 reports of pancreatitis associated with sulfasalazine as of February 1994.[1] There had been further reports associated with mesalazine (see p.1234).

1. Committee on Safety of Medicines/Medicines Control Agency. Drug-induced pancreatitis. *Current Problems* 1994; **20:** 2–3.

Effects on the respiratory system. Sulfasalazine-induced pulmonary complications are reported rarely. Most reports in-clude dyspnoea, cough, pulmonary infiltrates, fever, and eosi-nophilia, usually developing in the first few months of treat-ment although they may occur after several years.[1,2] Symptoms are generally readily reversible on withdrawal of sulfasalazine, although death due to fibrosing alveolitis has been reported.[1] These effects have also occurred with mesalazine, p.1234; they have been reported in patients with a history of sensitivity to salicylates, sulfonamides, or with no known sensitivity to these drugs.[1,2]

1. Wang KK, et al. Pulmonary infiltrates and eosinophilia associat-ed with sulfasalazine. *Mayo Clin Proc* 1984; **59:** 343–6.
2. Jordan A, Cowan RE. Reversible pulmonary disease and eosi-nophilia associated with sulphasalazine. *J R Soc Med* 1988; **81:** 233–5.

Lupus. A study in 11 patients with sulfasalazine-induced lupus found that induction of disease was more likely in patients who were slow acetylators of sulfapyridine, and who had HLA hap-lotypes associated with idiopathic systemic lupus erythemato-sus (SLE).[1] Furthermore, the risk of developing persistent SLE and lupus nephritis increased with duration of treatment and cumulative dose of sulfasalazine. Lupus-like syndrome has also occurred with mesalazine, see Effects on the Cardiovas-cular System, p.1234.

1. Gunnarsson I, et al. Predisposing factors in sulphasalazine-in-duced systemic lupus erythematosus. *Br J Rheumatol* 1997; **36:** 1089–94.

Porphyria. Sulfasalazine has been associated with acute at-tacks of porphyria and is considered unsafe in porphyric pa-tients.

Pregnancy. Sulfasalazine and its sulfapyridine metabolites readily cross the placenta resulting in similar concentrations in the cord serum and maternal serum at delivery.[1,2] The concen-tration of the 5-aminosalicylic acid component of sulfasalazine in both cord serum and maternal serum is negligible.[1] There have been isolated reports of congenital abnormalities associ-ated with administration of sulfasalazine during pregnancy in-cluding coarctation of the aorta with a ventricular septal de-fect,[3,4] and genito-urinary disorders.[4] There is also a theoretical risk of kernicterus in the neonate if sulfasalazine is given close to delivery (see p.254). However, given the concentrations of sulfasalazine and its metabolites found in cord blood the risk of kernicterus from maternal administration is considered mini-mal.[2] There have been many successful and uncomplicated pregnancies during treatment with sulfasalazine and the gener-al consensus favours continuing sulfasalazine throughout preg-

nancy when indicated.[1,3-6] (See also Mesalazine, p.1234.) The minimum effective dose should be used and since sulfasalazine may precipitate folate deficiency (see Effects on the Blood, above), folic acid supplements are recommended.[7]

1. Khan AKA, Truelove SC. Placental and mammary transfer of sulphasalazine. *BMJ* 1979; **2:** 1553.
2. Järnerot G, et al. Placental transfer of sulphasalazine and sulp-hapyridine and some of its metabolites. *Scand J Gastroenterol* 1981; **16:** 693–7.
3. Hoo JJ, et al. Possible teratogenicity of sulfasalazine. *N Engl J Med* 1988; **318:** 1128.
4. Newman NM, Correy JF. Possible teratogenicity of sulphasala-zine. *Med J Aust* 1983; **1:** 528–9.
5. Peppercorn MA. Sulfasalazine and related new drugs. *J Clin Pharmacol* 1987; **27:** 260–5.
6. Korelitz BI. Commentary: observations on sulfasalazine in Crohn's disease and ulcerative colitis. *J Clin Pharmacol* 1987; **27:** 265–6.
7. Byron MA. Treatment of rheumatic diseases. *BMJ* 1987; **294:** 236–8.

Interactions

Concurrent administration of sulfasalazine with anti-bacterial therapy may reduce conversion of sulfasala-zine to its active metabolite (see below).

Sulfasalazine has been reported to interfere with the absorption of digoxin (p.872) or folic acid (see Ef-fects on the Blood, above) from the gastrointestinal tract.

Antibacterials. Since sulfasalazine depends for its effects on release of 5-aminosalicylic acid by bacterial metabolism in the gut, any drug which reduces the intestinal microflora may re-duce the production of active metabolite. Evidence for this has been seen in patients given *rifampicin* and *ethambutol*,[1] or sub-jects given *ampicillin*,[2] concurrently with sulfasalazine. How-ever, a decrease in clinical effect does not seem to have been demonstrated.

1. Shaffer JL, Houston JB. The effect of rifampicin on sulphapyri-dine plasma concentrations following sulphasalazine administra-tion. *Br J Clin Pharmacol* 1985; **19:** 526–8.
2. Houston JB, et al. Azo reduction of sulphasalazine in healthy volunteers. *Br J Clin Pharmacol* 1982; **14:** 395–8.

Antineoplastics. For mention of 5-aminosalicylates such as sulfasalazine inhibiting the metabolism of thiopurine antineo-plastics, and increasing their toxicity, see Mercaptopurine, p.552.

Pharmacokinetics

Following oral administration up to about 15% of a dose of sulfasalazine is absorbed from the small intes-tine, although some of this is subsequently returned to the intestine in bile via enterohepatic circulation. The great majority of the dose reaches the colon where the azo bond is cleaved by the action of the intestinal flo-ra, producing sulfapyridine and 5-aminosalicylic acid (mesalazine). Results in patients who have undergone colectomy suggest that between 60 and 90% of the total dose is metabolised in this way, but the degree of metabolism depends both on the activity of the intes-tinal flora and the speed of intestinal transit; colonic metabolism is reduced in patients with diarrhoea (for example, in active inflammatory bowel disease).

The small amount of intact sulfasalazine which is ab-sorbed is extensively protein bound and subsequently excreted unchanged in urine. It crosses the placenta and is found in breast milk.

Following cleavage of the sulfasalazine molecule about 60 to 80% of available sulfapyridine is ab-sorbed and undergoes extensive metabolism by acetylation, hydroxylation, and glucuronidation. Peak steady-state concentrations of sulfapyridine are higher in slow acetylators than fast acetylators after similar doses and the former are 2 to 3 times more likely to experience adverse effects. Some 60% of the original dose of sulfasalazine is excreted in urine as sulfapyridine and its metabolites. Like sulfasalazine, absorbed sulfapyridine crosses the placenta and is found in breast milk.

The 5-aminosalicylic acid (5-ASA) moiety is much less well absorbed. Of the approximately one-third of liberated 5-ASA which is absorbed, almost all is acetylated and is excreted in urine. For further details of the pharmacokinetics of 5-aminosalicylic acid see under Mesalazine, p.1235.

◊ Reviews.
1. Klotz U. Clinical pharmacokinetics of sulphasalazine, its metab-olites and other prodrugs of 5-aminosalicylic acid. *Clin Pharma-cokinet* 1985; **10:** 285–302.

Uses and Administration

Sulfasalazine is a compound of a sulfonamide, sul-fapyridine, with 5-aminosalicylic acid (mesalazine). Its activity is generally considered to lie in the 5-ami-nosalicylic acid moiety, which is released in the colon by bacterial metabolism, although intact sulfasalazine has some anti-inflammatory properties in its own right.

In inflammatory bowel disease (p.1205) it is used alone or as an adjunct to corticosteroids in the treat-ment of active ulcerative colitis and is effective in maintaining remission. Sulfasalazine may also be ef-fective in the treatment of active Crohn's disease, par-ticularly of the colon, but it does not appear to be of value in maintaining remissions. Sulfasalazine is also used as a disease modifying drug in the treatment of severe or progressive rheumatoid arthritis (below).

In **inflammatory bowel disease** the usual initial adult dose of sulfasalazine is 1 to 2 g by mouth 4 times dai-ly in the UK, although doses over 4 g daily are asso-ciated with an increased risk of toxicity. In the USA, therefore, the usual dose is 1 g given 3 or 4 times dai-ly, and an initial dose of 500 mg every 6 to 12 hours may be recommended to lessen gastrointestinal adver-se effects. Enteric-coated tablets are also claimed to reduce the incidence of adverse gastrointestinal ef-fects. The overnight interval between doses should not exceed 8 hours. On remission the dose in patients with ulcerative colitis is gradually reduced to 2 g or less daily and then generally continued indefinitely. For children 2 years of age or older doses should be proportional to body-weight; initially 40 to 60 mg per kg body-weight may be given daily in divided doses reduced to 20 to 30 mg per kg daily for the mainte-nance of remission.

Sulfasalazine is also given rectally, as suppositories, in an adult dose of 0.5 to 1 g night and morning, either alone or as an adjunct to treatment by mouth; it may also be given by enema in a dose of 3 g at bedtime.

In adult **rheumatoid arthritis** treatment is usually commenced with a dose of 500 mg daily by mouth, as enteric-coated tablets, for the first week; dosage is then increased by 500 mg each week to a maximum of 3 g daily given in 2 to 4 divided doses. Sulfasala-zine can also be used for polyarticular juvenile rheu-matoid arthritis in children aged 6 years and older who have not responded adequately to salicylates or other NSAIDs. A dose of 30 to 50 mg per kg daily is given in two divided doses, to a maximum of 2 g daily. To reduce adverse gastrointestinal effects, an enteric-coated tablet is used and the initial dose should be a quarter to a third of the planned mainte-nance; it is then increased weekly to reach the main-tenance dose after one month.

Collagenous colitis. Collagenous colitis is a rare condition which presents as persistent watery diarrhoea and is associated with a thickened band of collagen immediately below the sur-face epithelium of the colonic mucosa. Treatment is largely symptomatic.[1-3] A suggested approach from analysis of data from 163 patients was to try antidiarrhoeal therapy with lopera-mide initially, and then sulfasalazine if this was ineffective.[2] In unresponsive patients colestyramine, prednisolone, antibacteri-als such as metronidazole, or mepacrine, or an immunosup-pressant such as methotrexate, might all be tried. Mesalazine and olsalazine seemed to be less effective than sulfasalazine,[2] although they may be useful where sulfasalazine is not tolerat-ed.[2,4]

1. Rams H, et al. Collagenous colitis. *Ann Intern Med* 1987; **106:** 108–13.
2. Bohr J, et al. Collagenous colitis: a retrospective study of clinical presentation and treatment in 163 patients. *Gut* 1996; **39:** 846–51.
3. Weldon M. A useful collagenous colitis registry. *Lancet* 1997; **349:** 1410–11.
4. O'Mahony S, et al. Coeliac disease and collagenous colitis. *Post-grad Med J* 1990; **66:** 238–41.

Multiple sclerosis. Sulfasalazine did not prevent the progres-sion of disability in patients with multiple sclerosis (p.633) in a large 3-year double-blind study.[1] The authors concluded that the drug has no role in the management of the disease.

1. Noseworthy JH, et al. The Mayo Clinic-Canadian cooperative trial of sulfasalazine in active multiple sclerosis. *Neurology* 1998; **51:** 1342–52.

Psoriasis. In a double-blind placebo-controlled study involv-ing 50 patients with moderate to severe plaque-type psoriasis (p.1106), sulfasalazine 3 to 4 g daily produced a significantly greater clinical improvement than placebo after 4 weeks of treatment with a further improvement at 8 weeks.[1]

See also Psoriatic Arthritis, below.

1. Gupta AK, et al. Sulfasalazine improves psoriasis: a double-blind analysis. Arch Dermatol 1990; **126:** 487–93.

Rheumatoid arthritis. Sulfasalazine is considered to be a useful disease-modifying antirheumatic drug (DMARD) in the treatment of rheumatoid arthritis (p.9). Meta-analyses[1,2] of generally short-term comparative studies suggest that sulfasalazine is roughly comparable in efficacy to methotrexate, intramuscular gold (sodium aurothiomalate), and penicillamine, and some rheumatologists now use it as one of the DMARDs of first choice.[3] In an open study[4] of 200 patients with rheumatoid arthritis who were randomly allocated to treatment with sulfasalazine or auranofin, 31% of the sulfasalazine recipients were still taking the drug after 5 years compared with 15% of auranofin recipients. Improvement over baseline was still significant at 5 years for those patients receiving sulfasalazine but not in those treated with auranofin. Combination treatment with sulfasalazine plus methotrexate and hydroxychloroquine has been reported to be more effective than methotrexate alone or sulfasalazine with hydroxychloroquine.[5]

1. Felson DT, et al. The comparative efficacy and toxicity of second-line drugs in rheumatoid arthritis. Arthritis Rheum 1990; **33:** 1449–61.
2. Capell HA, et al. Second line (disease modifying) treatment in rheumatoid arthritis: which drug for which patient? Ann Rheum Dis 1993; **52:** 423–8.
3. Rains CP, et al. Sulfasalazine: a review of its pharmacological properties and therapeutic efficacy in the treatment of rheumatoid arthritis. Drugs 1995; **50:** 137–56.
4. McEntegart A, et al. Sulfasalazine has a better efficacy/toxicity profile than auranofin—evidence from a 5 year prospective, randomized trial. J Rheumatol 1996; **23:** 1887–90.
5. O'Dell JR, et al. Treatment of rheumatoid arthritis with methotrexate alone, sulfasalazine and hydroxychloroquine, or a combination of all three medications. N Engl J Med 1996; **334:** 1287–91.

JUVENILE IDIOPATHIC ARTHRITIS. Juvenile idiopathic arthritis (p.9) is generally managed similarly to rheumatoid arthritis, but there is limited experience with the use of some antirheumatic drugs in children. Sulfasalazine has produced significant improvement in open studies of patients with juvenile chronic arthritis.[1] Beneficial results were also reported in a controlled study of 69 patients with juvenile chronic arthritis of articular onset who received either sulfasalazine or placebo for 24 weeks.[2] The dose of sulfasalazine used was 50 mg per kg bodyweight daily, starting with one-quarter of the total dose and increased weekly by increments of one-quarter of the total dose. Improvements in some, but not all, disease severity scores and laboratory tests were greater for sulfasalazine than placebo. Adverse effects were also more frequent in the sulfasalazine group, and included gastrointestinal disturbances, skin rashes, headache, elevated liver enzyme concentrations, leucopenia, and hypoimmunoglobulinaemia.

1. Imundo LF, Jacobs JC. Sulfasalazine therapy for juvenile rheumatoid arthritis. J Rheumatol 1996; **23:** 360–6.
2. van Rossum MAJ, et al. Sulfasalazine in the treatment of juvenile chronic arthritis: a randomized, double-blind, placebo-controlled, multicenter study. Arthritis Rheum 1998; **41:** 808–16.

Spondyloarthropathies. ANKYLOSING SPONDYLITIS. Sulfasalazine has been found to be effective[1] in the treatment of active ankylosing spondylitis (p.10), but there is evidence that it is more useful in the treatment of peripheral articular manifestations than in the management of chronic long-standing disease.[2,3] The active moiety appears to be sulfapyridine rather than mesalazine.[4]

1. Ferraz MB, et al. Meta-analysis of sulfasalazine in ankylosing spondylitis. J Rheumatol 1990; **17:** 1482–6.
2. Clegg DO, et al. Comparison of sulfasalazine and placebo in the treatment of ankylosing spondylitis: a Department of Veterans Affairs Cooperative study. Arthritis Rheum 1996; **39:** 2004–12.
3. Clegg DO, et al. Comparison of sulfasalazine and placebo for the treatment of axial and peripheral articular manifestations of the seronegative spondylarthropathies: a Department of Veterans Affairs cooperative study. Arthritis Rheum 1999; **42:** 2325–9.
4. Taggart A, et al. Which is the active moiety of sulfasalazine in ankylosing spondylitis? A randomized, controlled study. Arthritis Rheum 1996; **39:** 1400–5.

PSORIATIC ARTHRITIS. A meta-analysis[1] of interventions for psoriatic arthritis (see p.10) concluded that sulfasalazine was of only two drugs with well demonstrated published efficacy in psoriatic arthritis (the other being high-dose parenteral methotrexate).

See also under Psoriasis, above.

1. Jones G, et al. Interventions for treating psoriatic arthritis (updated 30 August 2000). Available in The Cochrane Library, Issue 3. Oxford: Update Software; 2001.

Preparations

BP 2001: Sulfasalazine Tablets;
USP 25: Sulfasalazine Delayed-release Tablets; Sulfasalazine Tablets.

Proprietary Preparations (details are given in Part 3)
Aust.: Colo-Pleon; Salazopyrin; **Austral.:** Pyralin; Salazopyrin; **Belg.:** Salazopyrine; **Braz.:** Aculfin; Azulfin; **Canad.:** Salazopyrin; SAS; Salazopyrin; **Denm.:** Salazopyrin; **Fin.:** Salazopyrine; **Fr.:** Salazopyrine; **Ger.:** Azulfidine; Colo-Pleon; Pleon RA; **Hong Kong:** Salazopyrin; **Irl.:** Salazopyrin; **Israel:** Salazopyrin; **Ital.:** Salazopyrin; **Neth.:** Salazopyrine; **Norw.:** Salazopyrin; **NZ:** Salazopyrin; **Port.:** Salazopirina; **S.Afr.:** Salazopyrin; **Singapore:**

The symbol † denotes a preparation no longer actively marketed

Salazopyrin; **Spain:** Salazopyrina; **Swed.:** Salazopyrin; **Switz.:** Salazopyrin; **Thai.:** Salazopyrin; Saridine; **UK:** Salazopyrin; Sulazine; Ucine†; **USA:** Azulfidine.

Sulglicotide   (13282-e)

Sulglicotide (BAN, rINN).
Sulglycotide.
CAS — 54182-59-1.
ATC — A02BX08.

Profile
Sulglicotide is a sulfated glycopeptide with cytoprotective properties extracted from pig duodenum. It is used in the treatment of peptic ulcer disease (p.1208) and other gastrointestinal disorders in a usual dose of 600 mg daily by mouth.

◊ References.

1. Luminari M, et al. Effectiveness of sulglycotide treatment for active chronic superficial gastritis. Acta Ther 1988; **14:** 45–54.
2. Psilogenis M, et al. A multicenter double-blind study of sulglycotide versus sucralfate in nonulcer dyspepsia. Int J Clin Pharmacol Ther Toxicol 1990; **28:** 369–74.
3. Bianchi Porro G, et al. Sulglycotide in the prevention of nonsteroidal anti-inflammatory drug-induced gastroduodenal mucosal injury: a controlled double-blind, double-dummy, randomized endoscopic study versus placebo in rheumatic patients. Scand J Gastroenterol 1993; **28:** 875–8.
4. De Conca V, et al. Effect of sulglycotide in the prevention of duodenal ulcer relapse. Eur J Gastroenterol Hepatol 1995; **7:** 25–8.

Preparations

Proprietary Preparations (details are given in Part 3)
Ital.: Gliptide.

Tamarind   (7534-p)

West Indian Tamarind.

The fruits of *Tamarindus indica* (Leguminosae) freed from the brittle outer part of the pericarp and preserved with sugar or syrup. Contains tartaric, citric, and malic acid and their salts.

Profile
Tamarind is used as a laxative in combination with senna.

Preparations

Proprietary Preparations (details are given in Part 3)
Multi-ingredient: Aust.: Frugelletten; Neda Fruchtewurfel; **Belg.:** Tamarine; **Braz.:** Fitolax; Florlax; Frutalax; Frutarine; Laxan; Laxarine; Laxtam; Novolax; Tamaril; Tamarine; Tamarix; **Fr.:** Actisane Constipation Occasionnelle†; Delabarre; Laxasan†; Tamarine; **Ital.:** Ortisan; Tamarine; **Mex.:** Naturetti; **Spain:** Dentomicin; Pruina; **Switz.:** Tamarine†.

Tegaserod Maleate   (19887-t)

Tegaserod Maleate (BANM, rINNM).
SDZ-HTF-919. 1-{[(5-Methoxyindol-3-yl)methylene]amino}-3-pentylguanidine maleate.
$C_{16}H_{23}N_5O,C_4H_4O_4$ = 417.5.
CAS — 145158-71-0 (tegaserod); 189188-57-6 (tegaserod maleate).
NOTE. Tegaserod is USAN.

Profile
Tegaserod maleate is a partial agonist at $5\text{-}HT_4$ receptors and has prokinetic properties. It is used for irritable bowel syndrome, particularly the constipation-predominant form.

◊ References.

1. Scott LJ, Perry CM. Tegaserod. Drugs 1999; **58:** 491–8.

Teprenone   (17004-r)

Teprenone (rINN).
E-671; Geranylgeranylacetone (5E, 9E,13E isomer). 6,10,14,18-Tetramethyl-5,9,13,17-nonadecatetraen-2-one, mixture of (5E,9E,13E) and (5Z,9E,13E) isomers.
$C_{23}H_{38}O$ = 330.5.
CAS — 6809-52-5 (teprenone); 3796-63-2 (5E,9E,13E isomer); 3796-64-3 (5Z,9E,13E isomer).

Profile
Teprenone is a cytoprotective drug which is used in the treatment of gastritis and peptic ulcer disease (p.1208) in a usual dose of 50 mg three times daily by mouth.

Preparations

Proprietary Preparations (details are given in Part 3)
Jpn.: Selbex; **Thai.:** Selbex.

Tropisetron   (20534-q)

Tropisetron (BAN, rINN).
1αH,5αH-Tropan-3α-yl indole-3-carboxylate.
$C_{17}H_{20}N_2O_2$ = 284.4.
CAS — 89565-68-4.
ATC — A04AA03.

Tropisetron Hydrochloride   (3089-k)

Tropisetron Hydrochloride (BANM, rINNM).
ICS-205-930.
$C_{17}H_{20}N_2O_2,HCl$ = 320.8.
CAS — 105826-92-4.

Adverse Effects and Precautions
As for Ondansetron, p.1241. Dizziness, fatigue, abdominal pain, and diarrhoea may also occur. Visual hallucinations, and an increase in blood pressure in patients with pre-existing hypertension, have been noted at high repeated doses. ECG changes such as prolongation of QT interval have been noted with high-dose intravenous tropisetron. The drug should therefore be used with caution in patients with cardiac rhythm or conduction disturbances. The manufacturers have warned that care should be taken when driving or operating machinery.

◊ Adverse effects reported with tropisetron include headache and mild sedation.[1] There have been reports of fever requiring drug withdrawal;[2,3] one patient[3] also experienced mild hypotension, macular rash, joint aches, and cervical lymphadenopathy.

The manufacturer has reported an increased incidence of hepatic neoplasms in male *mice* given high doses of tropisetron but it is suggested that these effects are both species and sex specific.

1. Leibundgut U, Lancranjan I. First results with ICS 205-930 (5-HT₃ receptor antagonist) in prevention of chemotherapy-induced emesis. Lancet 1987; **i:** 1198.
2. Anderson JV, et al. Remission of symptoms in carcinoid syndrome with a new 5-hydroxytryptamine M receptor antagonist. BMJ 1987; **294:** 1129.
3. Coupe M. Adverse reaction to 5-HT₃ antagonist ICS 205930. Lancet 1987; **i:** 1494.

Interactions
Drugs that induce or inhibit hepatic enzymes may affect plasma concentrations of tropisetron. The manufacturer considers that any changes are usually unlikely to be of clinical relevance with the recommended doses.

Tropisetron should be used with caution with antiarrhythmics, beta blockers, or drugs likely to prolong the QT interval.

Pharmacokinetics
Tropisetron is well absorbed following oral administration. Peak plasma concentrations are achieved within 3 hours. Absolute bioavailability depends on the dose since first-pass metabolism is saturable. It is 71% bound to plasma proteins. Tropisetron is metabolised by hydroxylation and conjugation, and metabolites are excreted mainly in the urine with a small amount in the faeces. The cytochrome P450 isoenzyme CYP2D6 is involved in tropisetron metabolism, and shows genetic polymorphism. The elimination half-life is about 8 hours in extensive metabolisers and up to 45 hours in poor metabolisers. Clearance is also reduced in patients with renal impairment.

Uses and Administration
Tropisetron hydrochloride is a $5\text{-}HT_3$-receptor antagonist with an antiemetic action similar to that of ondansetron (p.1242). It is used in the prevention of nausea and vomiting induced by cytotoxic therapy and in the treatment and prevention of postoperative nausea and vomiting (p.1206).

Tropisetron is given by slow intravenous injection or infusion, as the hydrochloride or by mouth as the base; doses are calculated in terms of tropisetron base.

For the *prophylaxis* of acute **nausea and vomiting** associated with cytotoxic **chemotherapy** a single dose of 5 mg may be given by slow intravenous injection or infusion on the day of treatment, shortly before chemotherapy. Subsequent doses of 5 mg daily are given by mouth, at least one hour before food, for a further 5 days. Children over 2 years of age may be given 200 µg per kg body-weight (maximum dose 5 mg) by intravenous injection over at least 1 minute, or by infusion, before chemotherapy. In children weighing less than 25 kg the same dose may be given intravenously once daily for up to a further 4 days as required. In those weighing more than 25 kg, a dose of 5 mg may be given orally once daily for up to a further 5 days; if oral administration is not possible the same dose may be given intravenously.

For the *treatment* of **postoperative** nausea and vomiting in adults 2 mg may be given by slow intravenous injection, or by infusion, within 2 hours of the end of anaesthesia. For *prophylaxis*, the same dose may be given shortly before induction of anaesthesia.

◊ References.

1. van Oosterom AT, Bainco AR. First international symposium on tropisetron. *Drugs* 1992; **43** (suppl 3): 1–44.

2. Lee CR, *et al.* Tropisetron: a review of its pharmacodynamic and pharmacokinetic properties, and therapeutic potential as an antiemetic. *Drugs* 1993; **46**: 925–43.

3. Simpson K, *et al.* Tropisetron: an update of its use in the prevention of chemotherapy-induced nausea and vomiting. *Drugs* 2000; **59**: 1297–1315.

Anxiety disorders. A dose-dependent anxiolytic effect was reported for tropisetron when studied in patients with generalised anxiety,[1] but clinical evidence for the benefit of 5HT$_3$-receptor antagonists in anxiety disorders is lacking.[2]

1. Lecrubier Y, *et al.* A randomized double-blind placebo-controlled study of tropisetron in the treatment of outpatients with generalized anxiety disorder. *Psychopharmacology (Berl)* 1993; **112**: 129–33.

2. Greenshaw AJ, Silverstone PH. The non-antiemetic uses of serotonin 5-HT$_3$ receptor antagonists: clinical pharmacology and therapeutic applications. *Drugs* 1997; **53**: 20–39.

Preparations

Proprietary Preparations (details are given in Part 3)

Aust.: Navoban; *Austral.:* Navoban; *Belg.:* Novaban; *Braz.:* Navoban; *Denm.:* Navoban; *Fin.:* Navoban; *Fr.:* Navoban; *Ger.:* Navoban; *Hong Kong:* Navoban; *Irl.:* Navoban; *Israel:* Navoban; *Ital.:* Navoban; *Jpn:* Navoban; *Mex.:* Navoban; *Neth.:* Novaban; *Norw.:* Navoban; *NZ:* Navoban; *Port.:* Navoban; *S.Afr.:* Navoban; *Spain:* Navoban; *Swed.:* Navoban; *Switz.:* Navoban; *Thai.:* Navoban; *UK:* Navoban.

Troxipide   (2471-z)

Troxipide *(rINN)*.

(±)-3,4,5-Trimethoxy-*N*-3-piperidylbenzamide.

$C_{15}H_{22}N_2O_4 = 294.3$.

CAS — 30751-05-4.

ATC — A02BX11.

Profile

Troxipide is used for its cytoprotective properties in the treatment of gastritis and peptic ulcer disease (p.1208) in a usual dose of 300 mg daily by mouth.

Preparations

Proprietary Preparations (details are given in Part 3)

Jpn: Aplace.

Urogastrone   (709-v)

Anthelone; EGF-URO; Epidermal Growth Factor; Uroanthelone; Uroenterone.

CAS — 9010-53-1.

A polypeptide first isolated from human urine. Two forms have been identified, β and γ urogastrone. The β form consists of 53 amino acids and is distinguishable from the γ form by an additional terminal arginine residue. The β form is reported to be identical to human epidermal growth factor and this term is widely used in the literature.

Uses

Urogastrone inhibits gastric acid secretion and has been tried in the treatment of peptic ulcer disease and other gastrointestinal disorders but its rapid destruction in the stomach has limited its clinical use.

It is a potent stimulator of cellular proliferation and has also been used as an aid to wound healing.

◊ Reviews[1,2] of epidermal growth factor (EGF) and transforming growth factor (TGF).

1. Burgess AW. Epidermal growth factor and transforming growth factor α. *Br Med Bull* 1989; **45**: 401–24.

2. Miyazawa K. Role of epidermal growth factor in obstetrics and gynecology. *Obstet Gynecol* 1992; **79**: 1032–40.

Gastrointestinal disorders. Intravenous infusion of urogastrone 250 nanograms per kg body-weight over 1 hour has been reported[1,2] to reduce the secretion of gastric acid in patients with duodenal ulcer (p.1208) or the Zollinger-Ellison syndrome (p.1209). Ulcer pain was relieved 30 to 60 minutes after the start of the infusion.[2] A dose of 100 nanograms per kg per hour by intravenous infusion has been used with partial success in an infant with microvillous atrophy[3] and was apparently beneficial in an infant with necrotising enteritis.[4]

1. Koffman CG, *et al.* Effect of urogastrone on gastric secretion and serum gastrin concentration in patients with duodenal ulceration. *Gut* 1982; **23**: 951–6.

2. Elder JB, *et al.* Effect of urogastrone in the Zollinger-Ellison syndrome. *Lancet* 1975; **ii**: 424–7.

3. Walker-Smith JA, *et al.* Intravenous epidermal growth factor/urogastrone increases small-intestinal cell proliferation in congenital microvillous atrophy. *Lancet* 1985; **ii**: 1239–40.

4. Sullivan PB, *et al.* Epidermal growth factor in necrotising enteritis. *Lancet* 1991; **338**: 53–4.

Wound healing. The effect on the rate of wound healing (p.1108) of a cream containing sulfadiazine silver plus recombinant human epidermal growth factor (10 µg per mL) was compared with sulfadiazine silver alone in 12 patients each requiring skin grafts at 2 donor sites.[1] The cream containing epidermal growth factor accelerated the rate of epidermal regeneration in all patients and reduced the average time to 100% healing by about 1.5 days. Patients were followed up for a maximum of 1 year after cessation of therapy and no complications or clinical evidence of neoplasia at the healed donor sites occurred.

In contrast, recombinant human epidermal growth factor as an ophthalmic solution containing 30 or 100 µg per mL was investigated in patients who had undergone keratoplasty, but the weaker solution had no effect on the rate of re-epithelialisation, and the more concentrated one was actually associated with slower healing.[2]

1. Brown GL, *et al.* Enhancement of wound healing by topical treatment with epidermal growth factor. *N Engl J Med* 1989; **321**: 76–9.

2. Dellaert MMMJ, *et al.* Influence of topical human epidermal growth factor on postkeratoplasty re-epithelialisation. *Br J Ophthalmol* 1997; **81**: 391–5.

Zaldaride   (15934-n)

Zaldaride *(rINN)*.

CGS-9343B (zaldaride maleate). (±)-1-{1-[(4-Methyl-4*H*,6*H*-pyrrolo[1,2-*a*][4,1]benzoxazepin-4-yl)methyl]-4-piperidyl}-2-benzimidazolinone.

$C_{26}H_{28}N_4O_2 = 428.5$.

CAS — 109826-26-8 (zaldaride); 109826-27-9 (zaldaride maleate).

Profile

Zaldaride is a calmodulin antagonist that has been investigated as the maleate for the treatment of diarrhoea.

Diarrhoea. Studies in patients with travellers' diarrhoea have indicated that zaldaride in doses of 20 mg by mouth as the maleate four times daily is an effective antidiarrhoeal.[1,2] It was somewhat less effective then loperamide when given without a loading dose,[2] but a regimen of 40 mg initially, followed by 20 mg approximately every 6 hours was as effective as loperamide 4 mg initially followed by 2 mg after each unformed stool.[3] Although antidiarrhoeal drugs may be given for symptom control in adults, the mainstay of therapy for acute diarrhoea should still be fluid and electrolyte replacement as discussed on p.1203.

1. DuPont HL, *et al.* Zaldaride maleate, an intestinal calmodulin inhibitor, in the therapy of travelers' diarrhea. *Gastroenterology* 1993; **104**: 709–15.

2. Okhuysen PC, *et al.* Zaldaride maleate (a new calmodulin antagonist) versus loperamide in the treatment of traveler's diarrhea: randomized, placebo-controlled trial. *Clin Infect Dis* 1995; **21**: 341–4.

3. Silberschmidt G, *et al.* Treatment of travellers' diarrhoea: zaldaride compared with loperamide and placebo. *Eur J Gastroenterol Hepatol* 1995; **7**: 871–5.

General Anaesthetics

This chapter includes drugs used for the induction and maintenance of general anaesthesia. General anaesthetics are administered either by inhalation or by intravenous or occasionally intramuscular injection (see below).

Injectable	Inhalational
Barbiturate	*Halogenated*
Methohexital	Chloroform
Thiamylal	Desflurane
Thiopental	Enflurane
Miscellaneous	Halothane
Alfadolone	Isoflurane
Alfaxolone	Methoxyflurane
Eltanolone	Sevoflurane
Etomidate	Trichloroethylene
Ketamine	*Miscellaneous*
Propanidid	Cyclopropane
Propofol	Anaesthetic Ether
Sodium Oxybate	Nitrous Oxide
Tiletamine	Xenon

Adverse Effects of General Anaesthetics

Adverse effects that may be associated with general anaesthesia include involuntary muscle movements, hiccup, coughing, bronchospasm, laryngospasm, hypotension, cardiac arrhythmias, respiratory depression, mild hypothermia, and postoperative nausea and vomiting.

Malignant hyperthermia (malignant hyperpyrexia—see p.1329) is a rare but potentially fatal complication of general anaesthesia that may be induced by inhalational anaesthetics (mainly halogenated hydrocarbons).

Sensitisation of the myocardium to beta-adrenergic stimulation occurs with some anaesthetics.

There has been concern over the possible danger to anaesthetists, dentists, and other personnel from exposure to volatile anaesthetics.

◊ General references.
1. Derrington MC, Smith G. A review of studies of anaesthetic risk, morbidity and mortality. *Br J Anaesth* 1987; **59**: 815–33.
2. Davies CJ, *et al.* Delayed adverse reactions to drugs used in anaesthesia. *Adverse Drug React Bull* 1995 (Apr.): 647–50.
3. Klafta JM, *et al.* Neurological and psychiatric adverse effects of anaesthetics: epidemiology and treatment. *Drug Safety* 1995; **13**: 281–95.
4. Fee JPH, Thompson GH. Comparative tolerability profiles of the inhaled anaesthetics. *Drug Safety* 1997; **16**: 157–70.

◊ Following general anaesthesia many patients will experience drowsiness and impaired mental performance for at least 24 hours. Nausea with or without vomiting occurs in 20 to 40% of postanaesthetic patients; nausea may last for 2 days but vomiting seldom persists beyond the first day. Other adverse effects include anorexia, malaise, fatigue, dizziness, and headache; these have been reported in 6 to 12% of patients. Delirium has been noted in at least 10% of elderly general surgical patients and in up to 50% of elderly patients undergoing hip fracture repair. Sore throat is frequent in patients who have been intubated or have had a throat pack inserted. Dry mouth as a result of premedication can add to the patient's discomfort. Manipulations for the maintenance of a clear airway may result in postoperative jaw pain. Muscle pain, typically involving the neck, shoulders, and upper abdomen, may occur if the neuromuscular blocker suxamethonium has been given. It is usually worse on the second postoperative day and may last up to six days. Shoulder ache after laparoscopy resolves after 24 hours; it is due to accumulation of carbon dioxide under the diaphragm. Backache is common after epidural or spinal anaesthesia. Urinary retention may follow regional block, cystoscopic or gynaecological surgery, or when there is prostatism.

References.
1. Kalmanovitch DVA, Simmons P. Post-anaesthetic complications in the home. *Prescribers' J* 1988; **28**: 124–31.
2. Anonymous. Nausea and vomiting after general anaesthesia. *Lancet* 1989; **i:** 651–2.
3. Anonymous. Following up day case anaesthesia in general practice. *Drug Ther Bull* 1990; **28**: 81–2.
4. Rowbotham DJ, Smith G, eds. Postoperative nausea and vomiting. *Br J Anaesth* 1992; **69** (suppl 1): 1S–68S.

5. O'Keeffe ST, NíChonchubhair Á. Postoperative delirium in the elderly. *Br J Anaesth* 1994; **73**: 673–87.
6. Marcantonio ER, *et al.* A clinical prediction rule for delirium after elective noncardiac surgery. *JAMA* 1994; **271**: 134–9.

Hypersensitivity. Type I hypersensitivity reactions have occurred with general anaesthetics.[1] In most patients the release of histamine and other mediators such as prostaglandins and leukotrienes is of no clinical importance but in a few susceptible individuals anaphylaxis may result. Numerous factors to identify those at risk have been proposed over the years along with suggested modifications for anaesthetic management. Of the drugs used in anaesthesia, neuromuscular blockers are associated with the highest incidence of anaphylaxis; the most commonly implicated is reported to be suxamethonium, followed by alcuronium[2] (see under the Adverse Effects of Suxamethonium, p.1341). It has been suggested[3] that routine prophylaxis with histamine H[1]- and histamine H[2]-antagonists should be considered as part of anaesthetic management but others[2] thought it better to avoid the use of combinations such as thiopental, suxamethonium, and alcuronium that are well known to cause histamine release.

1. McKinnon RP, Wildsmith JAW. Histaminoid reactions in anaesthesia. *Br J Anaesth* 1995; **74**: 217–28.
2. O'Connor B, Edwards ND. Reactions to gelatin plasma expanders. *Lancet* 1994; **344**: 328.
3. Lorenz W, *et al.* Incidence and clinical importance of perioperative histamine release: randomised study of volume loading and antihistamines after induction of anaesthesia. *Lancet* 1994; **343**: 933–40.

Nausea and vomiting. For a discussion on postoperative nausea and vomiting and its management, see p.1206.

Shivering and its treatment. Postoperative shivering, also referred to as spontaneous postanaesthetic tremor, can occur in up to 65% of patients recovering from general anaesthesia;[1] its aetiology and relationship to thermoregulation is unclear.[1,2] Postoperative shivering may be part of a more generalised neurological disturbance associated with anaesthesia.[2] It also occurs following regional anaesthesia, especially when given epidurally, but this is probably produced by different mechanisms.[2] Muscular activity during shivering greatly increases metabolic rate, oxygen consumption, and cardiac output and may cause complications in patients with cardiac or respiratory disorders. It can also strain surgical sutures, raise intra-ocular pressure, and impede haemodynamic monitoring.

Although the relationship between postoperative shivering, body temperature, and heat loss is unclear, patients may respond to warming their environment and the use of blankets.[1,2] Postoperative shivering may sometimes be an appropriate thermoregulatory response to a low body temperature,[2] and it is important before starting therapy to check the patient's temperature and take suitable steps to avoid hypothermia.[1]

Numerous drugs have been tried for the management of postoperative shivering including the central and respiratory stimulant doxapram[3-5] and the opioid analgesic pethidine.[4] Reviews have discussed[1,2] a number of other opioids that have been tried including morphine, butorphanol, fentanyl, and sufentanil but studies suggest that not all opioids are effective or that some may only be effective when given epidurally. However, this may be due to the use of insufficient doses rather than a true difference between opioids.[6] Tramadol has also been tried.[7] Neuromuscular blockers have been used after cardiac surgery in order to reduce cardiovascular stress.[8] Vecuronium might be preferable to pancuronium as it does not increase myocardial work and may be associated with fewer complications.[9] However, as profound neuromuscular block is required to inhibit shivering, repeated or higher doses of vecuronium might be required to prevent recurrence. Other drugs that have been investigated include clonidine,[10-12] ketanserin,[10] and ketamine.[13]

1. Crossley AWA. Postoperative shivering. *Br J Hosp Med* 1993; **49**: 204–8.
2. Anonymous. Perioperative shivering. *Lancet* 1991; **338**: 547–8.
3. Fry ENS. Muscle spasticity. *Anaesthesia* 1990; **45**: 67–8.
4. Sarma V, Fry ENS. Doxapram after general anaesthesia: its role in stopping shivering during recovery. *Anaesthesia* 1991; **46**: 460–1.
5. Singh P, *et al.* Double-blind comparison between doxapram and pethidine in the treatment of postanaesthetic shivering. *Br J Anaesth* 1993; **71**: 685–8.
6. Alfonsi P, *et al.* Fentanyl, as pethidine, inhibits post anaesthetic shivering. *Br J Anaesth* 1993; **70** (suppl 1): 38.
7. De Witte J, *et al.* Tramadol for treatment of shivering after general anaesthesia. *Br J Anaesth* 1996; **76** (suppl 2): 91–2.
8. Cruise C, *et al.* Comparison of meperidine and pancuronium for the treatment of shivering after cardiac surgery. *Can J Anaesth* 1992; **39**: 563–8.
9. Dupuis J-Y, *et al.* Pancuronium or vecuronium for treatment of shivering after cardiac surgery. *Anesth Analg* 1994; **79**: 472–81.
10. Joris J, *et al.* Clonidine and ketanserin both are effective treatment for postanaesthetic shivering. *Anesthesiology* 1993; **79**: 532–9.
11. Steinfath M, *et al.* Clonidine administered intraoperatively prevents postoperative shivering. *Br J Clin Pharmacol* 1995; **39**: 580P–581P.
12. Vanderstappen I, *et al.* The effect of prophylactic clonidine on postoperative shivering. *Anaesthesia* 1996; **51**: 351–5.
13. Sharma DR, Thakur JR. Ketamine and shivering. *Anaesthesia* 1990; **45**: 252–3.

Precautions for General Anaesthetics

Patients with impaired function of the adrenal cortex, for example, those who are being treated, or have recently been treated, with corticosteroids, may experience hypotension with the stress of anaesthesia. Treatment with corticosteroids, pre-operatively and postoperatively, may be necessary. Patients taking other long-term medication such as aspirin, oral anticoagulants, oestrogens, MAOIs and lithium, may require a change in dosage or cessation of therapy before major elective surgery.

Patients with chronic diseases such as diabetes or hypertension may require adjustment to their therapy prior to anaesthesia. Anaesthetics should be used with caution in patients with cardiac, respiratory, renal, or hepatic impairment and care may be needed in elderly or obese patients.

Patients should not undertake hazardous tasks such as driving for at least 24 hours after a general anaesthetic; alcohol should also be avoided.

Intraoperative awareness. The use of neuromuscular blockers has enabled anaesthetic doses to be reduced. However, lack of a reliable method for detecting conscious awareness in patients with complete neuromuscular block has resulted in paralysed patients who have received inadequate anaesthesia being aware during surgery.[1,2] Recommendations to control this problem include premedication with sedative or amnesic drugs, the use of sufficient doses of intravenous induction anaesthetics, the use of effective analgesic techniques during surgery, and, in particular, adequate concentrations of inspired anaesthetic gas. However, even patients given lorazepam or opioids may have some recall and there is no certain way to avoid awareness in paralysed patients. One commentator[3] considered that the routine use of neuromuscular blockers during surgery should be re-assessed since modern anaesthetics and analgesics could provide good operating conditions without paralysis for most major surgical procedures.

1. Brighouse DI, Norman J. To wake in fright. *BMJ* 1992; **304**: 1327–8.
2. Jones JG. Memory of intraoperative events. *BMJ* 1994; **309**: 967–8.
3. Ponte J. Neuromuscular blockers during general anaesthesia. *BMJ* 1995; **310**: 1218–19.

Interactions of General Anaesthetics

Sensitisation of the myocardium to beta-adrenergic stimulation occurs with some anaesthetics and ventricular fibrillation may occur if *sympathomimetics* such as adrenaline [epinephrine] and isoprenaline are administered concomitantly. Enhanced hypotensive effects may result when anaesthetics are given with *ACE inhibitors, tricyclic antidepressants* (which may also increase the risk of arrhythmias), *MAOIs* (see also p.304), *antihypertensives, antipsychotics,* or *beta blockers.* The effects of *competitive neuromuscular blockers* may be increased by inhalational anaesthetics. The concurrent use of anaesthetics with other *CNS depressant drugs* such as those used for premedication may produce synergistic effects on the CNS and, in some cases, a smaller dose of general anaesthetic should be given.

◊ Reviews.
1. Wood M. Pharmacokinetic drug interactions in anaesthetic practice. *Clin Pharmacokinet* 1991; **21**: 285–307.
2. Ransom ES, Mueller RA. Safety considerations in the use of drug combinations during general anaesthesia. *Drug Safety* 1997; **16**: 88–103.

Uses of General Anaesthetics

General anaesthetics depress the CNS and cause loss of consciousness associated with an inability to perceive pain. An ideal anaesthetic would produce unconsciousness, analgesia, and muscle relaxation suitable for all surgical procedures and would be metabolically inert and rapidly eliminated. No anaesthetic fulfils all these requirements in safe concentrations and it is customary to employ a number of drugs to achieve the required conditions while minimising the risk of toxicity.

The activity of any anaesthetic is dependent on its ability to reach the brain. With inhalational anaesthetics there has to be a transfer from the alveolar space to the blood, then to the brain; recovery is a function of the removal of the anaesthetic from the brain. With injectable anaesthetics their activity is similarly dependent on their ability to penetrate the blood/brain barrier and recovery in turn is governed by their redistribution and excretion. The potency of inhalational anaesthetics is often expressed in terms of *minimum alveolar concentrations*, known as MAC values. The MAC of an anaesthetic is the concentration at 1 atmosphere that will produce immobility in 50% of subjects exposed to a noxious stimulus. Values given under the individual monographs are based on use without nitrous oxide as the latter can reduce the MAC. Other factors including age, body temperature, and concurrent medication such as opioid analgesics can also affect MAC values.

Anaesthesia. Many drugs are involved in achieving and maintaining conditions suitable for surgery. Conventional general anaesthesia may be divided into a number of stages including:

• premedication
• induction
• muscle relaxation and intubation
• maintenance
• analgesia
• reversal

A brief outline of the drugs typically used in each stage follows.

For **premedication**, benzodiazepines and various phenothiazines such as promethazine or trimeprazine [alimemazine] may be given to sedate and relieve *anxiety* in apprehensive patients. Butyrophenones such as droperidol have also been used. The benzodiazepines have useful amnesic and muscle-relaxant properties and short-acting oral analogues are common in current regimens. The phenothiazines and butyrophenones are rarely used now although their antiemetic actions may be useful to control *postoperative vomiting* (see p.1206). Cloral hydrate is still used in some countries for pre-operative sedation. The use of barbiturates has largely ceased. For sedation of children the oral route is often preferred to injections, or the rectal route may be used in exceptional circumstances.

Antimuscarinics such as atropine, glycopyrronium, and hyoscine may be given to inhibit excessive *bronchial* and *salivary secretions* induced by intubation and some anaesthetics, although such use is less common nowadays. Antimuscarinics are also given as premedicants to reduce the intra-operative bradycardia and hypotension induced by drugs such as suxamethonium, halothane, or propofol or following vagal stimulation. Hyoscine also provides some degree of amnesia.

Opioids, including morphine and its derivatives, papaveretum and pethidine, have been widely used before surgery to reduce anxiety, smooth induction of anaesthesia, reduce overall anaesthetic requirements, and provide pain relief during and after surgery. The routine use of opioids as premedicants is now rare and their use generally restricted to patients already in pain. However, they continue to find a role at induction (below).

Patients may also be given drugs that reduce the danger from regurgitation and *aspiration* of gastric contents (see under Aspiration Syndromes, p.1202), such as the histamine H$_2$-antagonists, cimetidine and ranitidine, and the proton pump inhibitor, omeprazole. Cardiovascular drugs may be required during surgery to control *blood pressure* and counteract *arrhythmias*.

The aim of **induction** is to produce anaesthesia rapidly and smoothly. Induction may be achieved with intravenous or inhalational anaesthetics but intravenous induction may be more pleasant for the patient. Intravenous drugs used include the barbiturate thiopental, the benzodiazepine midazolam, and other anaesthetics such as etomidate, propofol, or ketamine. Small doses of short-acting opioids, for example alfentanil, fentanyl, or remifentanil, given before or at induction allow the use of smaller induction doses of some drugs used for anaesthesia, and this technique is particularly suitable for poor-risk patients.

Following induction, **muscle relaxation** with a rapidly acting neuromuscular blocker such as suxamethonium facilitates **intubation** of the patient. Longer acting neuromuscular blockers may then be administered to allow procedures such as abdominal surgery to be carried out under lighter anaesthesia. For more detail, see Anaesthesia, p.1331.

Maintenance of anaesthesia may be achieved with an inhalational anaesthetic, an intravenous anaesthetic, or an intravenous opioid, either alone or in combination.

Opioid analgesics may also be given for **analgesia** as supplements during general anaesthesia (see also Balanced Anaesthesia, under Anaesthetic Techniques, below). Long-acting opioids such as morphine or papaveretum are avoided because of problems with postoperative respiratory depression. The short-acting opioids fentanyl and its congeners alfentanil and sufentanil appear to produce fewer circulatory changes and may be preferred to other opioids, especially in cardiovascular surgery; remifentanil may be valuable for its very short duration of action. Various combinations of analgesic techniques, including the use of pre-emptive analgesia, are used or are being investigated for the management of surgical pain (see Postoperative Analgesia, p.4).

At the end of surgery drugs are sometimes administered to accelerate recovery by **reversal** of the effects of the various agents used during anaesthesia. The *neuromuscular block* produced by competitive neuromuscular blockers may be reversed with anticholinesterases such as neostigmine and edrophonium but concomitant administration of atropine or glycopyrronium is required to prevent bradycardia and other muscarinic actions developing. The opioid antagonist naloxone has been given to reverse opioid-induced *respiratory depression*. However, it may antagonise the analgesic effects of the opioids in the control of postoperative pain and the increasing use of short-acting intravenous opioid analgesics should reduce the need for its use. Flumazenil is a benzodiazepine antagonist that is used to reverse the *central sedative effects* of benzodiazepines in anaesthetic procedures.

ANAESTHETIC TECHNIQUES. A balanced combination of drugs with different actions is often used to provide the various components of general anaesthesia including unconsciousness, muscle relaxation, and analgesia. This technique, termed **balanced anaesthesia**, has been reported to minimise intra-operative cardiovascular depression, to facilitate a rapid return of consciousness, and to have a low incidence of postoperative adverse effects such as nausea and vomiting, and excitation. Typically an opioid is given before or with induction and anaesthesia is induced using nitrous oxide and an intravenous barbiturate such as thiopental. The opioid is then given in small incremental doses to achieve and maintain adequate analgesia during surgery. Opioid analgesics commonly used in this technique include morphine, fentanyl, sufentanil, and alfentanil; buprenorphine and nalbuphine have also been used.

In **total intravenous anaesthesia** (TIVA), induction and maintenance of anaesthesia is achieved with one or more anaesthetics given intravenously. This allows a high inspired oxygen concentrations in situations where hypoxaemia may otherwise occur, and is advantageous in surgery where delivery of inhaled anaesthetic may be difficult (for example in bronchoscopy). Combinations used in TIVA include propofol with alfentanil or fentanyl, and midazolam with alfentanil. Neuromuscular blockers are given to produce muscle relaxation but there can be difficulty in assessing the depth of anaesthesia in patients who are paralysed for mechanical ventilation, and there have been reports of awareness during surgery (see also under Intraoperative Awareness in Precautions, above).

Use of a neuroleptic together with an opioid analgesic produces an altered state of consciousness known as **neuroleptanalgesia** in which the patient is calm and indifferent to the surroundings yet is responsive to commands. The technique has been used for diagnostic or therapeutic procedures such as minor surgery, endoscopy, and changing dressings. Neuroleptanalgesia can be converted to **neuroleptanaesthesia** by the concurrent administration of nitrous oxide in oxygen; a muscle relaxant may also be included. Neuroleptanaesthesia is particularly useful if the patient's cooperation is required, as consciousness soon returns once the nitrous oxide is discontinued. The neuroleptic most commonly employed was droperidol and it was usually used with fentanyl although other opioids have also been employed. These techniques are now in decline, having largely evolved into **conscious sedation** techniques employing newer drugs.

Ketamine used alone can produce a state of **dissociative anaesthesia** similar to that of neuroleptanalgesia in which the patient may appear to be awake but is unconscious. Marked analgesia and amnesia are produced, but there may be an increase in muscle tone and emergence reactions. Dissociative anaesthesia is considered suitable

for use in various diagnostic procedures, dressing changes, and in minor surgery not requiring muscle relaxation. Techniques employing **local anaesthetics** are discussed on p.1304.

Alfadolone Acetate (3102-r)

Alfadolone Acetate (BANM, rINNM).
Alphadolone Acetate; GR-2/1574. 3α,21-Dihydroxy-5α-pregnane-11,20-dione 21-acetate.
$C_{23}H_{34}O_5 = 390.5$.
CAS — 14107-37-0 (alfadolone); 23930-37-2 (alfadolone acetate).
Pharmacopoeias. In *BP(Vet)*.

Pharmacopoeial description

BP(Vet) 2001: A white to creamy white powder. Practically insoluble in water and in petroleum spirit; soluble in alcohol; freely soluble in chloroform.

Profile

Alfadolone acetate has been used to enhance the solubility of alfaxalone (below). It possesses some anaesthetic properties and is considered to be about half as potent as alfaxalone.

Alfaxalone (3103-f)

Alfaxalone (BAN, rINN).
Alphaxalone; GR-2/234. 3α-Hydroxy-5α-pregnane-11,20-dione.
$C_{21}H_{32}O_3 = 332.5$.
CAS — 23930-19-0.
ATC — N01AX05.
Pharmacopoeias. In *BP(Vet)*.

Pharmacopoeial description

BP(Vet) 2001: A white to creamy white powder. Practically insoluble in water and in petroleum spirit; soluble in alcohol; freely soluble in chloroform.

Profile

Alfaxalone was formerly used in combination with alfadolone acetate (above) ['Althesin'], as an intravenous anaesthetic for induction and maintenance of general anaesthesia.

Adverse reactions associated with polyethoxylated castor oil (present as a vehicle) led to the general withdrawal of alfaxalone with alfadolone acetate from human use. It is still used in veterinary medicine.

Porphyria. Alfaxalone: alfadolone has been associated with acute attacks of porphyria and is considered unsafe in porphyric patients.

Chloroform (3104-d)

Chloroformium Anaesthesicum; Chloroformum; Chloroformum pro Narcosi. Trichloromethane.
$CHCl_3 = 119.4$.
CAS — 67-66-3.
ATC — N01AB02.
Pharmacopoeias. In *Aust., Belg., Br.,* and *Chin.*
Some pharmacopoeias include a grade of chloroform, with less stringent standards, which may be used in oral preparations but which must not be used as an anaesthetic.

Not flammable. The addition of the small percentage of alcohol greatly retards the gradual oxidation which occurs when chloroform is exposed to air and light, and which results in its becoming contaminated with the very poisonous carbonyl chloride (phosgene) and with chlorine; the alcohol also serves to decompose any carbonyl chloride that may have been formed.

Pharmacopoeial description

BP 2001: A colourless volatile liquid with a characteristic odour. Not more than 5.0% v/v distils below 60° and the remainder distils at 60° to 62°. It contains 1.0 to 2.0% v/v of ethyl alcohol; amylene 50 μg per mL is permitted as an alternative to ethyl alcohol.

Slightly soluble in water; miscible with dehydrated alcohol, with ether, with fixed and volatile oils, and with most other organic solvents. Store in containers with glass stoppers or other suitable closures. Protect from light. The label should state whether it contains ethyl alcohol or amylene.

◊ CAUTION. *Suitable precautions should be taken to avoid skin contact with chloroform as it can penetrate skin and produce systemic toxicity. Care should be taken not to vaporise chloroform in the presence of a flame because of the production of toxic gases.*

Stability. From a study[1] of chloroform losses from chloroform water and from 6 typical BPC mixtures under various conditions of storage the following shelf-lives were recommended: chloroform solutions and non-sedimented mixtures could be stored in well-closed well-filled containers for 2 months at ambient temperatures; when stored in partially-filled containers periodically opened the shelf-life is not to exceed 2 weeks; sedimented mixtures could be stored for 2 months in well-closed well-filled containers, but because loss of chloroform could be expected in containers periodically opened such mixtures should be prepared as required or packed in their final containers; for chloroform-containing mixtures in the home a shelf-life of 2 weeks was suggested.

1. Lynch M, *et al.* Chloroform as a preservative in aqueous systems: losses under "in-use" conditions and antimicrobial effectiveness. *Pharm J* 1977; **219**: 507–10.

Storage. It has been recommended[1] that PVC bottles should not be used for storing or dispensing Chloroform and Morphine Tincture, aqueous mixtures containing more than 5% thereof, mixtures or dispersions in which chloroform was present in excess of its aqueous solubility, aqueous mixtures containing chloroform and high concentrations of electrolytes, or Chloroform Water (BP) or mixtures containing it if the period of use would exceed 6 weeks.

1. Anonymous. Plastics medicine bottles of rigid PVC. *Pharm J* 1973; **210**: 100.

Adverse Effects and Precautions

Chloroform depresses respiration and produces hypotension. Cardiac output is reduced and arrhythmias may develop. Poisoning may therefore lead to respiratory depression and cardiac arrest. Delayed hepatotoxic and nephrotoxic reactions may occur 6 to 24 hours after a dose; symptoms may include abdominal pain, vomiting, and, at a later stage, jaundice.

Liquid chloroform is irritant to the skin and mucous membranes and may cause burns if spilt on them.

In the UK medicinal products are limited to a chloroform content of not more than 0.5% (w/w or v/v as appropriate) of chloroform. Exceptions include supply by a doctor or dentist, or in accordance with his prescription, to a particular patient, and supply for anaesthetic purposes.

In the USA the FDA have banned the use of chloroform in medicines and cosmetics, because of reported carcinogenicity in *animals*. It has also been withdrawn from systemic use in other countries.

The sale within or import into England and Wales and Scotland of food containing any added chloroform is prohibited.

See also Adverse Effects and Precautions for General Anaesthetics, p.1255.

Porphyria. Chloroform has been associated with acute attacks of porphyria and is considered unsafe in porphyric patients.

Uses and Administration

Chloroform is a volatile halogenated anaesthetic administered by inhalation but because of its toxicity it is seldom used now in general anaesthesia.

Chloroform is used as a carminative and as a flavouring agent and preservative. For these purposes it is usually employed as Chloroform Spirit (BP 2001) or Chloroform Water (BP 2001) but doubts have been cast on the safety of the long-term use of chloroform in mixtures.

Externally, chloroform has a rubefacient action.

Chloroform is also used as a solvent.

◊ An historical review of the use of chloroform in clinical anaesthesia.[1]

1. Payne JP. Chloroform in clinical anaesthesia. *Br J Anaesth* 1981; **53**: 11S–15S.

Preparations

BP 2001: Chloroform and Morphine Tincture; Chloroform Spirit; Chloroform Water; Double-strength Chloroform Water.

Proprietary Preparations (details are given in Part 3)

Multi-ingredient: *Belg.:* Baume Dalet†; Dentophar; Dolpyc†; *Braz.:* Algidente; *Fr.:* Baume Dalet†; Dolpyc†; Lao-Dal†.

Cyclopropane (3105-n)

Cyclopropane *(rINN)*.

Trimethylene.

$C_3H_6 = 42.08$.

CAS — 75-19-4.

Pharmacopoeias. In Aust. and US.

It is supplied compressed in metal cylinders. National standards are usually in operation for the labelling and marking of such cylinders.

Pharmacopoeial description

USP 25: A colourless highly flammable gas with a characteristic odour and pungent taste. Freely soluble in alcohol; soluble in fixed oils. One volume dissolves in about 2.7 volumes of water at 15°.

◊ caution. *Mixtures of cyclopropane with oxygen or air at certain concentrations are explosive. Cyclopropane should not be used in the presence of an open flame or of any electrical apparatus liable to produce a spark. Precautions should be taken against the production of static electrical discharge.*

Adverse Effects and Precautions

Cyclopropane depresses respiration to a greater extent than many other anaesthetics. Laryngospasm, cardiac arrhythmias, or hepatic injury may occur. Cyclopropane increases the sensitivity of the heart to sympathomimetic amines. Malignant hyperthermia has also been reported. Postoperative nausea, vomiting, and headache are frequent.

The symbol † denotes a preparation no longer actively marketed

Cyclopropane should be used with caution in patients with bronchial asthma and cardiovascular disorders. Premedication with atropine may be advisable to reduce vagal tone.

See also Adverse Effects and Precautions for General Anaesthetics, p.1255.

Abuse. A report following-on from a nationwide survey in the USA of four deaths from abuse of volatile anaesthetics in operating rooms.[1] Two of the deaths were attributed to cyclopropane.

1. Bass M. Abuse of inhalation anesthetics. *JAMA* 1984; **251**: 604.

Malignant hyperthermia. A case of malignant hyperthermia associated with cyclopropane.[1]

1. Lips FJ, *et al.* Malignant hyperthermia triggered by cyclopropane during cesarean section. *Anesthesiology* 1982; **56**: 144–6.

Interactions

Care is advised if adrenaline [epinephrine] or other sympathomimetics are given during cyclopropane anaesthesia. Potentiation of competitive neuromuscular blockers occurs after cyclopropane administration.

See also Interactions for General Anaesthetics, p.1255.

Uses and Administration

Cyclopropane is an anaesthetic administered by inhalation. It has a minimum alveolar concentration (MAC) value (see p.1255) of 9.2%. It has been used for analgesia and induction and maintenance of general anaesthesia. It produces skeletal muscle relaxation, is non-irritant, and induction and recovery are rapid. Because of the risk of explosion, the usual method of administration has been by means of a closed circuit.

Desflurane (11789-f)

Desflurane *(USAN, rINN)*.

I-653. (±)-2-Difluoromethyl 1,2,2,2-tetrafluoroethyl ether.

$C_3H_2F_6O = 168.0$.

CAS — 57041-67-5.

ATC — N01AB07.

Pharmacopoeias. In US.

Pharmacopoeial description

USP 25: Store in airtight containers. Protect from light.

Adverse Effects

As with other halogenated anaesthetics, respiratory depression, hypotension, and arrhythmias may occur. Desflurane may rarely precipitate malignant hyperthermia in susceptible individuals. Desflurane appears to sensitise the myocardium to sympathomimetics to a lesser extent than halothane or enflurane. Nausea and vomiting have been reported in the postoperative period.

Desflurane is irritant to the airways and may provoke breath holding, apnoea, coughing, increased salivation, and laryngospasm.

See also Adverse Effects of General Anaesthetics, p.1255.

Effects on the blood. The development of carboxyhaemoglobinaemia in patients anaesthetised with volatile anaesthetics is discussed under Precautions, below.

Effects on the cardiovascular system. A review[1] of *animal* and human studies concluded that the cardiorespiratory effects of desflurane were similar to those of isoflurane but that there might be better control of arterial pressure with desflurane during stressful stimuli. One study[2] in patients undergoing coronary artery bypass surgery demonstrated that a state of haemodynamic stability suitable for patients at risk of myocardial ischaemia could be maintained when desflurane was supplemented with the opioid analgesic fentanyl.

1. Warltier DC, Pagel PS. Cardiovascular and respiratory actions of desflurane: is desflurane different from isoflurane? *Anesth Analg* 1992; **75**: S17–S31.
2. Parsons RS, *et al.* Comparison of desflurane and fentanyl-based anaesthetic techniques for coronary artery bypass surgery. *Br J Anaesth* 1994; **72**: 430–8.

Effects on the liver. Although considered to be less hepatotoxic than some other halogenated anaesthetics (see under Adverse Effects of Halothane, p.1260), delayed hepatotoxicity has occurred in a 65-year-old woman following maintenance anaesthesia involving desflurane.[1] She had received halothane on two previous occasions which may have caused sensitisation. Investigation of hepatocellular integrity (by measuring glutathione transferase alpha) in 30 women who had received desflurane indicated a mild subclinical disturbance.[2]

1. Martin JL, *et al.* Hepatotoxicity after desflurane anesthesia. *Anesthesiology* 1995; **83**: 1125–9.
2. Tiainen P, *et al.* Changes in hepatocellular integrity during and after desflurane or isoflurane anaesthesia in patients undergoing breast surgery. *Br J Anaesth* 1998; **80**: 87–9.

Effects on the respiratory tract. The irritant effect of desflurane on the lungs limits its role in the induction of anaesthe-

sia, especially in children. Pre-operative use of nebulised lignocaine [lidocaine] 4% failed to alleviate the response.[1]

1. Bunting HE, *et al.* Effect of nebulized lignocaine on airway irritation and haemodynamic changes during induction of anaesthesia with desflurane. *Br J Anaesth* 1995; **75**: 631–3.

Precautions

Desflurane is not recommended for induction of anaesthesia in paediatric patients because of its irritant effects (see Adverse Effects, above). As with other halogenated anaesthetics, patients with known or suspected susceptibility to malignant hyperthermia should not be anaesthetised with desflurane. Desflurane may increase CSF pressure and should therefore be used with caution in patients with, or at risk from, raised intracranial pressure.

In order to minimise the risk of developing elevated carboxyhaemoglobin levels carbon dioxide absorbents in anaesthetic apparatus should not be allowed to dry out when delivering volatile anaesthetics such as desflurane.

See also Precautions for General Anaesthetics, p.1255.

Carbon dioxide absorbents. Significant carboxyhaemoglobinaemia may develop rarely during anaesthesia with volatile anaesthetics given by circle breathing systems containing carbon dioxide absorbents.[1] The effect is only seen when the absorbent has become excessively dried out. The use of barium hydroxide lime (which is not available in the UK) as an absorbent produces more carbon monoxide than soda lime, particularly at low water content. No cases of this complication had been reported to date in the UK.

1. Committee on Safety of Medicines/Medicines Control Agency. Safety issues in anaesthesia: volatile anaesthetic agents and carboxyhaemoglobinaemia. *Current Problems* 1997; **23**: 7.

Interactions

The effects of competitive neuromuscular blockers such as atracurium are enhanced by desflurane (see p.1335). Lower doses of desflurane are required in those receiving opioids, benzodiazepines or other sedatives. Care is advised if adrenaline [epinephrine] or other sympathomimetics are given to patients during desflurane anaesthesia.

See also Interactions of General Anaesthetics, p.1255.

◊ References.

1. Dale O. Drug interactions in anaesthesia: focus on desflurane and sevoflurane. *Bailliéres Clin Anaesthesiol* 1995; **9**: 105–17.

Pharmacokinetics

Desflurane has a low blood/gas partition coefficient and following inhalation its absorption, distribution, and elimination are reported to be more rapid than for other halogenated anaesthetics such as isoflurane or halothane. It is excreted mainly unchanged through the lungs. A small amount diffuses through the skin. About 0.02% of administered desflurane is metabolised in the liver and trichloroacetic acid has been detected in the serum and urine of patients given desflurane.

◊ References.

1. Caldwell JE. Desflurane clinical pharmacokinetics and pharmacodynamics. *Clin Pharmacokinet* 1994; **27**: 6–18.

Uses and Administration

Desflurane is a volatile halogenated anaesthetic administered by inhalation. It is structurally similar to isoflurane and has anaesthetic actions similar to those of halothane (p.1260). Desflurane has a minimum alveolar concentration (MAC) value (see p.1255) ranging from about 6% in the elderly to about 11% in infants. It is non-flammable and non-explosive in clinical concentrations but, because of its low boiling-point, it must be delivered by a special vaporiser, preferably within a closed circuit system.

Desflurane is used for induction and maintenance of general anaesthesia (p.1256), but because of its pungency is not recommended for induction in children. Concentrations of 4 to 11% v/v have been used for induction and usually produce surgical anaesthesia in 2 to 4 minutes. Concentrations of 2 to 6% v/v with nitrous oxide or 2.5 to 8.5% v/v in oxygen or oxygen-enriched air may be used to maintain anaesthesia.

Higher concentrations of desflurane have been used but it is important to ensure adequate oxygenation; concentrations in excess of 17% v/v are not recommended. Concentrations of 1 to 4% v/v in oxygen and nitrous oxide have been used in patients with chronic renal or hepatic impairment and during renal transplantation surgery.

As with other volatile halogenated anaesthetics supplemental neuromuscular blockers may be required. Recovery from anaesthesia is reported to be more rapid than with other halogenated anaesthetics.

◊ The characteristics of desflurane have been discussed in a number of reviews.[1-3] Its advantages are considered to include rapid induction and emergence from anaesthesia, and minimal metabolism makes end-organ toxicity unlikely. Emergence from anaesthesia and recovery of psychomotor and cognitive skills with desflurane is more rapid than after anaesthesia with other halogenated volatile anaesthetics such as isoflurane and possibly than after the intravenous anaesthetic propofol. This is considered to be of particular advantage for outpatient treatment, but studies so far have found no difference in time to discharge with desflurane or other general anaesthetics. Furthermore, the incidence of nausea and vomiting with desflurane is significantly greater than after the use of propofol. Desflurane's pungency may also limit its use for induction.

1. Jones RM. Desflurane and sevoflurane: inhalation anaesthetics for this decade? *Br J Anaesth* 1990; **65:** 527–36.
2. Caldwell JE. Desflurane clinical pharmacokinetics and pharmacodynamics. *Clin Pharmacokinet* 1994; **27:** 6–18.
3. Patel SS, Goa KL. Desflurane: a review of its pharmacodynamic and pharmacokinetic properties and its efficacy in general anaesthesia. *Drugs* 1995; **50:** 742–67.

Preparations

Proprietary Preparations (details are given in Part 3)
Aust.: Suprane; *Austral.:* Suprane; *Belg.:* Suprane; *Canad.:* Suprane; *Denm.:* Suprane; *Fin.:* Suprane; *Ger.:* Suprane; *Irl.:* Suprane; *Israel:* Sulorane; *Ital.:* Suprane; *Mex.:* Suprane; *Neth.:* Suprane; *Norw.:* Suprane†; *NZ:* Suprane; *S.Afr.:* Suprane; *Singapore:* Suprane; *Spain:* Suprane; *Swed.:* Suprane; *Switz.:* Suprane; *UK:* Suprane; *USA:* Suprane.

Eltanolone (15431-n)

Eltanolone (rINN).

Pregnanolone; ZK-4915. 3α-Hydroxy-5β-pregnan-20-one.
$C_{21}H_{34}O_2 = 318.5$.
CAS — 128-20-1.

Profile

Eltanolone, a naturally occurring metabolite of progesterone (p.1488), has been studied for use as an intravenous anaesthetic. It is insoluble in water and has been administered as an emulsion containing soya oil and egg phospholipids.

◊ References.
1. Sear JW. Eltanolone: 50 years on and still looking for steroid hypnotic agents! *Eur J Anaesthesiol* 1998; **15:** 129–32.

Enflurane (3106-h)

Enflurane (BAN, USAN, rINN).

Anaesthetic Compound No. 347; Compound 347; Methylflurether; NSC-115944. 2-Chloro-1,1,2 trifluoroethyl difluoromethyl ether; 2-Chloro-1-(difluoromethoxy)-1,1,2-trifluoroethane.

$C_3H_2ClF_5O = 184.5$.
CAS — 13838-16-9.
ATC — N01AB04.

Pharmacopoeias. In Jpn and US.

Pharmacopoeial description

USP 25: A clear colourless volatile liquid having a mild sweet odour. Non-flammable. Distilling range 55.5° to 57.5°. Slightly soluble in water; miscible with organic solvents, with fats, and with oils. Store in airtight containers at a temperature not exceeding 40°. Protect from light.

Adverse Effects

As with other halogenated anaesthetics, respiratory depression, hypotension, and arrhythmias have been reported although the incidence of arrhythmias is lower with enflurane than with halothane. It sensitises the myocardium to sympathomimetics to a lesser extent then halothane. Compared with halothane, enflurane has a stimulant effect on the CNS and convulsions may occur when concentrations of enflurane are high or hypocapnia is present. Malignant hyperthermia has also been reported. Asthma and bronchospasm may occur. There have been reports of elevated serum-fluoride concentrations although resulting renal damage appears to be rare. There have been

changes in measurements of hepatic enzymes and a number of reports of liver damage. Shivering, nausea, and vomiting have been reported in the postoperative period.

See also Adverse Effects of General Anaesthetics, p.1255.

Effects on the blood. The development of carboxyhaemoglobinaemia in patients anaesthetised with volatile anaesthetics is discussed under Precautions, below.

Effects on the kidneys. The nephrotoxicity of volatile anaesthetics has been reviewed.[1] Although enflurane released inorganic fluoride it appeared to be safe in patients with normal renal function. It had also been given to patients with mild to moderate renal impairment without any further deterioration. There was an increase in serum-fluoride concentrations when enflurane was administered to a group of patients who had been receiving isoniazid, but there was no change in kidney function. Pretreatment of patients with a single dose of disulfiram before anaesthesia was found to produce a consistent and almost complete inhibition of enflurane metabolism as shown by substantial reductions in plasma-fluoride concentrations and urinary excretion of fluoride.[2]

1. Mazze RI. Nephrotoxicity of fluorinated anaesthetic agents. *Clin Anaesthesiol* 1983; **1:** 469–83.
2. Kharasch ED, *et al.* Clinical enflurane metabolism by cytochrome P450 2E1. *Clin Pharmacol Ther* 1994; **55:** 434–40.

Effects on the liver. A review[1] of 58 cases of suspected enflurane hepatitis considered enflurane to be the likely cause of the liver damage in 24. There was biochemical evidence of liver damage in 23 of these cases. Histology reports were available for 15 patients and all showed some degree of hepatocellular necrosis and degeneration.

While the incidence of liver damage from enflurane seemed to be lower than from halothane, the character of the injury was similar.

Another review[2] of the same cases plus an additional 30 (88 in all) came to different conclusions; the main author was a consultant to the manufacturer of enflurane. Of the 88 patients with suspected enflurane hepatitis, 30 were rejected because of insufficient evidence and 43 were considered to have other factors known to produce liver injury. This left 15 possible cases of enflurane hepatitis compared with the 24 identified by the first review. While agreeing that in the rare patient unexplained liver damage follows enflurane anaesthesia, it was considered that the incidence was too small to suggest an association. No consistent histological pattern was identified in this study.

See also under Adverse Effects in Halothane, p.1260.

1. Lewis JH, *et al.* Enflurane hepatotoxicity: a clinicopathologic study of 24 cases. *Ann Intern Med* 1983; **98:** 984–92.
2. Eger EI, *et al.* Is enflurane hepatotoxic? *Anesth Analg* 1986; **65:** 21–30.

Effects on respiration. Overall, enflurane is considered to produce more respiratory depression than halothane or isoflurane.[1,2]

1. Quail AW. Modern inhalation anaesthetic agents: a review of halothane, isoflurane and enflurane. *Med J Aust* 1989; **150:** 95–102.
2. Merrett KL, Jones RM. Inhalational anaesthetic agents. *Br J Hosp Med* 1994; **52:** 260–3.

Precautions

Enflurane should be used with caution in patients with convulsive disorders. High concentrations of enflurane may cause uterine relaxation. In order to minimise the risk of developing elevated carboxyhaemoglobin levels, carbon dioxide absorbents in anaesthetic apparatus should not be allowed to dry out when delivering volatile anaesthetics such as enflurane.

As with other halogenated anaesthetics, patients with known or suspected susceptibility to malignant hyperthermia should not be anaesthetised with enflurane.

See also Precautions for General Anaesthetics, p.1255.

Abuse. Report[1] of a fatality in a 29-year-old student nurse anaesthetist who had applied enflurane to the herpes simplex lesions of her lower lip. She was found with an empty 250 mL bottle of enflurane.

1. Lingenfelter RW. Fatal misuse of enflurane. *Anesthesiology* 1981; **55:** 603.

Carbon dioxide absorbents. Significant carboxyhaemoglobinaemia may develop rarely during anaesthesia with volatile anaesthetics given by circle breathing systems containing carbon dioxide absorbents.[1] The effect is only seen when the absorbent has become excessively dried out. The use of barium hydroxide lime (which is not available in the UK) as an absorbent produces more carbon monoxide than soda lime, particularly at low water content. No cases of this complication had been reported to date in the UK.

1. Committee on Safety of Medicines/Medicines Control Agency. Safety issues in anaesthesia: volatile anaesthetic agents and carboxyhaemoglobinaemia. *Current Problems* 1997; **23:** 7.

Porphyria. Enflurane is considered to be unsafe in patients with porphyria because it has been shown to be porphyrinogenic in *animals*.

Interactions

Care is advised if adrenaline [epinephrine] or other sympathomimetics are given to patients during enflurane anaesthesia. The effects of competitive neuromuscular blockers such as atracurium are enhanced by enflurane (see p.1335).

See also Interactions of General Anaesthetics, p.1255.

Antibacterials. For the effects of *isoniazid* on enflurane defluorination, see Effects on the Kidneys under Adverse Effects, above.

Antidepressants. It appeared likely that the enflurane-induced seizure activity observed in 2 patients could have been enhanced by *amitriptyline*.[1] It may be advisable to avoid the use of enflurane in patients requiring tricyclic antidepressants, especially when the patient has a history of seizures or when hyperventilation or high enflurane concentrations are a desired part of the anaesthetic technique.

1. Sprague DH, Wolf S. Enflurane seizures in patients taking amitriptyline. *Anesth Analg* 1982; **61:** 67–8.

Disulfiram. For the effect of disulfiram on the metabolism of enflurane, see Effects on the Kidneys under Adverse Effects, above.

Pharmacokinetics

Enflurane is absorbed on inhalation. The blood/gas partition coefficient is low. It is mostly excreted unchanged through the lungs. Up to 10% of administered enflurane is metabolised in the liver, mainly to inorganic fluoride.

◊ Reviews.
1. Dale O, Brown BR. Clinical pharmacokinetics of the inhalational anaesthetics. *Clin Pharmacokinet* 1987; **12:** 145–67.

Uses and Administration

Enflurane is a volatile halogenated anaesthetic administered by inhalation. It is an isomer of isoflurane. It has anaesthetic actions similar to those of halothane (p.1260). Enflurane has a minimum alveolar concentration (MAC) value (see p.1255) ranging from 1.7% in middle age to 2.5% in children. Enflurane is administered using a calibrated vaporiser for induction and maintenance of general anaesthesia (p.1256); it is also used in subanaesthetic doses to provide analgesia in obstetrics and other painful procedures.

To avoid CNS excitement a short-acting barbiturate or other intravenous induction agent is recommended before the inhalation of enflurane. Anaesthesia is induced starting at an enflurane concentration of 0.4% v/v in air, oxygen, or nitrous oxide-oxygen mixtures and increasing by increments of 0.5% v/v every few breaths to a maximum of 4.5%. Anaesthesia may be maintained with a concentration of 0.5 to 3.0% v/v of enflurane in nitrous oxide-oxygen; a concentration of 3.0% v/v should not be exceeded during spontaneous respiration. Although enflurane is reported to possess muscle relaxant properties, neuromuscular blockers may nevertheless be required. Postoperative analgesia may be necessary.

◊ Reviews.
1. Quail AW. Modern inhalational anaesthetic agents: a review of halothane, isoflurane and enflurane. *Med J Aust* 1989; **150:** 95–102.

Pain. Enflurane is used in subanaesthetic doses to provide analgesia in obstetrics and other painful procedures although a study[1] was unable to confirm that it had an analgesic effect at subanaesthetic concentrations.

1. Tomi K, *et al.* Alterations in pain threshold and psychomotor response associated with subanaesthetic concentrations of inhalation anaesthetics in humans. *Br J Anaesth* 1993; **70:** 684–6.

Preparations

Proprietary Preparations (details are given in Part 3)
Aust.: Ethrane; *Austral.:* Alyrane; Ethrane; *Belg.:* Alyrane; Ethrane†; *Braz.:* Etrane; *Canad.:* Ethrane; *Denm.:* Alyrane†; Efrane; *Fin.:* Efrane; *Ger.:* Ethrane; *Hong Kong:* Ethrane; *Irl.:* Ethrane; *Israel:* Alyrane; Ethrane; *Mex.:* Enfran; Enlirane; Ethrane; *Neth.:* Alyrane; Ethrane; *Norw.:* Efrane; *S.Afr.:* Alyrane; Ethrane; *Swed.:* Alyrane†; Efrane; *Switz.:* Ethrane; *UK:* Alyrane; *USA:* Ethrane.

Anaesthetic Ether (3107-m)

Aether ad Narcosin; Aether Anaestheticus; Aether pro Narcosi; Aether Purissimus; Diethyl Ether; Éter Purissimo; Ether; Ether Anesthesicus.

$(C_2H_5)_2O = 74.12$.

CAS — 60-29-7.

ATC — N01AA01.

Pharmacopoeias. In Chin., Eur. (see p.vi), Int., Jpn, Pol., and US.

The label should state that it is suitable for use as an anaesthetic.

Pharmacopoeial description

Ph. Eur.: Anaesthetic ether is diethyl ether to which an appropriate quantity of a non-volatile antoxidant may have been added. It contains not more than 2 g per litre of water. A clear, colourless, volatile, highly flammable, and very mobile liquid. Distillation range 34° to 35°.

Soluble 1 in 15 of water; miscible with alcohol and with fatty oils. Store at a temperature of 8° to 15° in airtight containers. Protect from light. Ether remaining in a partly used container may deteriorate rapidly. The label should state the name and concentration of any added non-volatile antoxidant.

USP 25: Ether consists of 96 to 98% of $C_4H_{10}O$, the remainder consisting of alcohol and water. Ether for anaesthetic use contains not more than 0.2% of water. It is a colourless, mobile, highly flammable, highly volatile liquid, having a characteristic sweet, pungent odour. It is slowly oxidised by the action of air and light, with the formation of peroxides. Its vapour, when mixed with air and ignited, may explode. B.p. about 35°.

Soluble 1 in 12 of water; miscible with alcohol, with chloroform, with dichloromethane, with petroleum spirit, with benzene, and with fixed and volatile oils; soluble in hydrochloric acid. Store in partly-filled, airtight containers, remote from fire and at a temperature not exceeding 40°. Protect from light. Ether to be used for anaesthesia must be preserved in airtight containers of not more than 3 kg capacity and is not to be used for anaesthesia if it has been removed from the original container longer than 24 hours.

◊ CAUTION. *Ether is very volatile and flammable and mixtures of its vapour with oxygen, nitrous oxide, or air at certain concentrations are explosive. It should not be used in the presence of an open flame or any electrical apparatus liable to produce a spark. Precautions should be taken against the production of static electrical discharge.*

Storage. The Pharmaceutical Society's Department of Pharmaceutical Sciences found that free ether, even in low concentrations, caused softening of PVC bottles and was associated with loss by permeation.[1]

1. Anonymous. Plastics medicine bottles of rigid PVC. *Pharm J* 1973; **210:** 100.

Adverse Effects

Ether has an irritant action on the mucous membrane of the respiratory tract; it stimulates salivation and increases bronchial secretion. Laryngeal spasm may occur. Ether causes vasodilatation which may lead to a severe fall in blood pressure and it reduces blood flow to the kidneys; it also increases capillary bleeding. The bleeding time is unchanged but the prothrombin time may be prolonged. Ether may cause malignant hyperthermia in certain individuals. Alterations in kidney and liver function have been reported. Convulsions occasionally occur. Hyperglycaemia due to gluconeogenesis has been noted.

Recovery is slow from prolonged ether anaesthesia and postoperative vomiting commonly occurs. Acute overdosage of ether is characterised by respiratory failure and cardiac arrest.

Dependence on ether or ether vapour has been reported. Prolonged contact with ether spilt on any tissue produces necrosis.

See also Adverse Effects of General Anaesthetics, p.1255.

Precautions

Ether anaesthesia is contra-indicated in patients with diabetes mellitus, impaired kidney function, raised CSF pressure, and severe liver disease. Its use is not advisable in hot and humid conditions in patients with fever as convulsions are liable to occur, particularly in children and in patients who have been given atropine.

See also Precautions for General Anaesthetics, p.1255.

Interactions

Ether enhances the action of competitive neuromuscular blockers to a greater degree than most other anaesthetics. Potentiation of the arrhythmogenic effect of sympathomimetics, including adrenaline [epinephrine], by ether is less than that seen with other inhalational anaesthetics.

See also Interactions of General Anaesthetics, p.1255.

Uses and Administration

Ether is an anaesthetic administered by inhalation. It has a minimum alveolar concentration (MAC) value (see p.1255) of 1.92%. Ether is still used in some countries for the induction and maintenance of general anaesthesia although it has been replaced in many other countries by the halogenated anaesthetics. It possesses a respiratory stimulant effect in all but the deepest planes of anaesthesia. Ether also possesses analgesic and muscle relaxant properties. Premedication with an anti-

The symbol † denotes a preparation no longer actively marketed

---

muscarinic such as atropine is necessary to reduce salivary and bronchial secretions.

Solvent ether is described on p.1403.

Etomidate (3110-r)

Etomidate (BAN, USAN, rINN).

Etomidatum; R-16659; R-26490 (etomidate sulfate). R-(+)-Ethyl 1-(α-methylbenzyl)imidazole-5-carboxylate.

$C_{14}H_{16}N_2O_2 = 244.3$.

CAS — 33125-97-2.

ATC — N01AX07.

Pharmacopoeias. In Eur. (see p.vi).

Pharmacopoeial description

Ph. Eur.: A white or almost white powder. M.p. about 68°. Very slightly soluble in water; freely soluble in alcohol and in dichloromethane. Protect from light.

Adverse Effects and Precautions

Excitatory phenomena (especially involuntary myoclonic muscle movements, which are sometimes severe) are common following injection of etomidate, but may be reduced by the prior administration of an opioid analgesic. Pain on injection may be reduced by giving it into a large vein in the arm rather than into the hand, or, again, by premedication with an opioid analgesic. Convulsions may occur in unpremedicated patients. Hypersensitivity reactions including anaphylaxis have been reported. Etomidate is associated with less hypotension than other drugs commonly used for induction.

Because etomidate inhibits adrenocortical function during maintenance anaesthesia (see below) its use is limited to induction of anaesthesia. In addition it should not be used in patients whose adrenocortical function is already reduced or at risk of being reduced.

Etomidate should be used with care in the elderly, who may be more prone to cardiac depression; lower doses may be required.

See also Adverse Effects and Precautions for General Anaesthetics, p.1255.

Effects on the endocrine system. Etomidate used for sedation in an intensive care unit was implicated in an increase in mortality.[1] The UK Committee on Safety of Medicines agreed that etomidate could cause a significant fall in circulating plasma-cortisol concentrations, unresponsive to corticotropin stimulation.[2] As a result of this effect, use of etomidate is restricted to induction of anaesthesia. The manufacturers advise that the postoperative rise in serum-cortisol concentration, which has been observed after thiopental induction, is delayed for about 3 to 6 hours when etomidate is used for induction.

A study comparing the effects of etomidate with those of methohexital on the adrenocortical function of neonates borne by mothers who received these agents for induction of anaesthesia before caesarean section indicated that there was no evidence to preclude the use of etomidate in such patients. However, regardless of which anaesthetic agent was used, early feeding was recommended to avoid neonatal hypoglycaemia.[3]

1. Ledingham IM, Watt I. Influence of sedation on mortality in critically ill multiple trauma patients. *Lancet* 1983; **i:** 1270.
2. Goldberg A. Etomidate. *Lancet* 1983; **ii:** 60.
3. Crozier TA, *et al.* Effects of etomidate on the adrenocortical and metabolic adaptation of the neonate. *Br J Anaesth* 1993; **70:** 47–53.

Hypersensitivity. Reactions involving immediate widespread cutaneous flushing or urticaria attributed to etomidate have been described.[1] There have also been reports[2,3] of anaphylactic reactions following injection of etomidate.

1. Watkins J. Etomidate: an 'immunologically safe' anaesthetic agent. *Anaesthesia* 1983; **38** (suppl): 34–8.
2. Sold M, Rothhammer A. Lebensbedrohliche anaphylaktoide reaktion nach etomidat. *Anaesthesist* 1985; **34:** 208–10.
3. Krumholz W, *et al.* Ein fall von anaphylaktoider reaktion nach gabe von etomidat. *Anaesthesist* 1984; **33:** 161–2.

Porphyria. Etomidate is considered to be unsafe in patients with porphyria because it has been shown to be porphyrinogenic in *animals.*

Interactions

A reduced dose of etomidate may be necessary in patients who have received antipsychotics, sedatives, or opioids. The hypnotic effect of etomidate has been potentiated by other sedative drugs.

See also Interactions of General Anaesthetics, p.1255.

Calcium-channel blockers. Prolonged anaesthesia and Cheyne-Stokes respiration following etomidate injection has been reported in 2 patients given concomitant treatment with *verapamil.*[1]

1. Moore CA, *et al.* Potentiation of etomidate anesthesia by verapamil: a report of two cases. *Hosp Pharm* 1989; **24:** 24–5.

General anaesthetics. For a report of synergy between *propofol* and etomidate, see p.1266.

Pharmacokinetics

After injection, etomidate is rapidly redistributed from the CNS to other body tissues, and undergoes rapid metabolism in the liver and plasma. Pharmacokinetics are complex and have been described by both 2- and 3-compartment models. Etomidate is about 76% bound to plasma protein. It is mainly excreted in the urine, but some is excreted in the bile. It may cross the placenta and is distributed into breast milk.

◊ References.

1. Swerdlow BN, Holley FO. Intravenous anaesthetic agents: pharmacokinetic-pharmacodynamic relationships. *Clin Pharmacokinet* 1987; **12:** 79–110.
2. Esener Z, *et al.* Thiopentone and etomidate concentrations in maternal and umbilical plasma, and in colostrum. *Br J Anaesth* 1992; **69:** 586–8.

Uses and Administration

Etomidate is an intravenous anaesthetic administered for the induction of general anaesthesia (p.1256). Anaesthesia is rapidly induced and may last for 6 to 10 minutes with a single usual dose. Recovery is usually rapid without hangover effect. Etomidate has no analgesic activity.

For the induction of anaesthesia, the usual dose is 300 µg of etomidate per kg body-weight given slowly, preferably into a large vein in the arm. An initial dose of 150 to 200 µg per kg is recommended in the elderly, subsequently adjusted according to effects. Children may require up to 30% more than the standard adult dose. Opioid analgesics as premedication reduce myoclonic muscle movements and injection site pain. A neuromuscular blocker is necessary if intubation is required.

Administration in the elderly. One study[1] in elderly patients has demonstrated that although reducing the rate of intravenous administration of etomidate reduces the speed of induction, the dosage required is also reduced. Administration of etomidate 0.2% solution at a rate of 10 mg per minute induced anaesthesia in a mean of 89.6 seconds and required a mean dose of 0.11 mg per kg body-weight. Corresponding values for an administration rate of 40 mg per minute were 47.7 seconds and 0.26 mg per kg respectively.

1. Berthoud MC, *et al.* Comparison of infusion rates of three i.v. anaesthetic agents for induction in elderly patients. *Br J Anaesth* 1993; **70:** 423–7.

Anaesthesia. Etomidate might be useful for induction if rapid tracheal intubation is required with a competitive neuromuscular blocker as it has been shown to reduce the time to onset of block with vecuronium.[1]

1. Gill RS, Scott RPF. Etomidate shortens the onset time of neuromuscular block. *Br J Anaesth* 1992; **69:** 444–6.

Status epilepticus. Anaesthesia in conjunction with assisted ventilation may be instituted to control refractory tonic-clonic status epilepticus (p.341). A short-acting barbiturate such as thiopental is usually used, but other anaesthetics including etomidate have also been tried[1] for intractable convulsive status epilepticus. However, like a number of other anaesthetics there have been reports of seizures associated with its use in anaesthesia, especially in patients with epilepsy.

1. Yeoman P, *et al.* Etomidate infusions for the control of refractory status epilepticus. *Intensive Care Med* 1989; **15:** 255–9.

Preparations

Proprietary Preparations (details are given in Part 3)
Aust.: Hypnomidate; *Belg.:* Hypnomidate; *Braz.:* Hypnomidate; *Fr.:* Hypnomidate; *Ger.:* Hypnomidate; Radenarcon; *Mex.:* Hypnomidate; *Neth.:* Hypnomidate; *S.Afr.:* Hypnomidate; *Spain:* Hypnomidate; *Switz.:* Hypnomidate†; *UK:* Hypnomidate; *USA:* Amidate.

Halothane (3101-x)

Halothane (BAN, rINN).

Alotano; Halothanum; Phthorothanum. (RS)-2-Bromo-2-chloro-1,1,1-trifluoroethane.

$CHBrCl.CF_3 = 197.4$.

CAS — 151-67-7.

ATC — N01AB01.

Pharmacopoeias. In Chin., Eur. (see p.vi), Int., Jpn, Pol., and US.

In the presence of moisture it reacts with many metals. Rubber and some plastics deteriorate when in contact with halothane vapour or liquid.

Halothane contains 0.01% w/w of thymol as a stabiliser; some commercial preparations may also contain up to 0.00025% w/w of ammonia. Thymol does not volatilise with halothane and therefore accumulates in the vaporiser. It may give a yellow colour to any remaining liquid; halothane that has discoloured should be discarded.

Pharmacopoeial description

Ph. Eur.: A clear, colourless, mobile, dense, non-flammable liquid. Distillation range 49° to 51°. Slightly soluble in water; miscible with dehydrated alcohol, with ether, and with trichloroethylene. Halothane contains 0.01% w/w of thymol. Store at a temperature not greater than 25° in airtight containers. Protect from light.

USP 25: A colourless, mobile, non-flammable, heavy liquid having a characteristic odour resembling that of chloroform. It contains not less than 0.008% and not more than 0.012% of thymol, by weight, as a stabiliser. It should contain not more than 0.03% of water. Distillation range 49° to 51°.

Slightly soluble in water; miscible with alcohol, with chloroform, with ether, and with fixed oils. Store in airtight containers at a temperature not greater than 40°. Protect from light. Dispense only in the original container.

Adverse Effects

As with other halogenated anaesthetics, halothane has a depressant action on the cardiovascular system and reduces blood pressure; signs of overdosage are bradycardia and profound hypotension. It is also a respiratory depressant and can cause cardiac arrhythmias; there have been instances of cardiac arrest. The sensitivity of the heart to sympathomimetic amines is increased.

Adverse effects on the liver have limited its use in recent years (see below); these effects range from liver dysfunction to hepatitis and necrosis and are more frequent following repeated use.

Halothane can produce nausea, vomiting, and shivering. Malignant hyperthermia has been reported.

See also Adverse Effects of General Anaesthetics, p.1255.

Effects on the cardiovascular system. The incidence of cardiac arrhythmias is higher with halothane than with enflurane or isoflurane; also the arrhythmogenic threshold with injected adrenaline [epinephrine] is lower with halothane than isoflurane or enflurane.

Effects on the kidneys. Renal failure has been reported following halothane anaesthesia,[1,2] sometimes with concurrent liver failure.[2]

1. Cotton JR, et al. Acute renal failure following halothane anesthesia. Arch Pathol Lab Med 1976; 100: 628–9.
2. Gelman ML, Lichtenstein NS. Halothane-induced nephrotoxicity. Urology 1981; 17: 323–7.

Effects on the liver. Liver damage has been recognised as an adverse effect of halothane for many years.[1-3]

Two types of hepatotoxicity are recognised; in the first there is a minor disturbance in liver function shown by increases in liver enzyme values (**type I**); this may occur in up to 30% of patients given halothane,[4] or more if activity is measured by glutathione S-transferase rather than serum aminotransferase.[5] Subsequent re-exposure to halothane is not necessarily associated with liver damage.[2,6]

The second type of hepatotoxicity, which is rarer, involves massive liver cell necrosis (**type II**); reported incidences[2] range from 1 in 2500 to 1 in 36 000. Type II liver toxicity is characterised by several clinical features: non-specific gastrointestinal upset, delayed pyrexia, jaundice, eosinophilia, serum autoantibodies, rash, and arthralgia.[1,3] Biochemical tests of liver function show changes typical of hepatocellular damage; histological features are typified by centrilobular necrosis.[1] Several **risk factors** for development of serious toxicity have become apparent;[1-3] they include repeated exposure, previous adverse reactions to halothane (jaundice, pyrexia), female gender, obesity, middle age, genetic predisposition, enzyme induction, and a history of drug allergy.

The **causes** of halothane hepatotoxicity have been debated. Type I reactions may result from toxic products of halothane metabolism, possibly influenced by genetic factors or from an imbalance between hepatic oxygen supply and demand. Changes in cellular calcium homoeostasis may also be involved. Type II reactions are most likely immune-mediated.[1,2] It has been suggested[4] that metabolism of halothane produces a reactive metabolite which binds covalently to proteins in the endoplasmic reticulum of hepatocytes. In susceptible patients it is believed that these metabolite-modified proteins provoke an immune response which is responsible for the liver damage. Recent findings[7,8] have implicated the cytochrome P450 isoenzyme CYP2E1 as having a major role in the metabolism of halothane and patients with high levels of this isoenzyme may be

predisposed to developing immune-medicated liver damage following halothane exposure.

The Committee on Safety of Medicines,[9] after receiving 84 further reports of hepatotoxicity in the UK between 1978 and 1985, issued the following **guidelines** on **precautions** to be taken before using halothane:

- a careful anaesthetic history should be taken to determine previous exposure and previous reactions to halothane
- repeated exposure to halothane within a period of at least 3 months should be avoided unless there are overriding clinical circumstances. An opinion has been expressed that the 3-month interval between exposures would be unlikely to prevent hepatotoxicity[2]
- a history of unexplained jaundice or pyrexia in a patient following previous exposure to halothane is an absolute contra-indication to its future use in that patient.

These guidelines were reiterated in 1997 after the CSM were notified of a further 15 cases of acute liver failure all requiring transplantation.[10]

The problem of patients sensitised to halothane who require **subsequent anaesthesia** with a volatile anaesthetic has been discussed.[4] Although the incidence of hepatotoxicity produced by *enflurane* appears to be less than with halothane it is of a similar nature and there have been reports of several patients who apparently had cross-sensitivity to both. Hepatotoxicity with *isoflurane* appears to be rare and it was suggested that for the majority of patients sensitised to halothane, isoflurane would be likely to be free from hepatotoxic effects. However, there has been a report[11] of a patient who had had two previous exposures to isoflurane and subsequently developed liver function abnormalities after receiving halothane. Hepatotoxicity with *desflurane* (see p.1257) might also be associated with sensitisation to halothane.

1. Ray DC, Drummond GB. Halothane hepatitis. Br J Anaesth 1991; 67: 84–99.
2. Neuberger JM. Halothane and hepatitis: incidence, predisposing factors and exposure guidelines. Drug Safety 1990; 5: 28–38.
3. Rosenak D, et al. Halothane and liver damage. Postgrad Med J 1989; 65: 129–35.
4. Kenna JG, Neuberger JM. Immunopathogenesis and treatment of halothane hepatitis. Clin Immunother 1995; 3: 108–24.
5. Allan LG, et al. Hepatic glutathione S-transferase release after halothane anaesthesia: open randomised comparison with isoflurane. Lancet 1987; i: 771–4.
6. Neuberger J, Williams R. Halothane anaesthesia and liver damage. BMJ 1984; 289: 1136–9.
7. Kharasch ED, et al. Identification of the enzyme responsible for oxidative halothane metabolism: implications for prevention of halothane hepatitis. Lancet 1996; 347: 1367–71.
8. Kenna JC, et al. Formation of the C[F]3CO-protein antigens implicated in the pathogenesis of halothane hepatitis is catalyzed in human liver microsomes in vitro by CYP 2E1. Br J Clin Pharmacol 1997; 43: 209.
9. Committee on Safety of Medicines. Halothane hepatotoxicity. Current Problems 18 1986.
10. Committee on Safety of Medicines/Medicines Control Agency. Safety issues in anaesthesia: reminder: hepatotoxicity with halothane. Current Problems 1997; 23: 7.
11. Slayter KL, et al. Halothane hepatitis in a renal transplant patient previously exposed to isoflurane. Ann Pharmacother 1993; 27: 101.

Precautions

The risk of halothane hepatitis led the UK Committee on Safety of Medicines to issue guidelines on its use (see Effects on the Liver, under Adverse Effects, above). It is also recommended that patients be informed of any reactions and that this be done in addition to the updating of the patients' medical records.

Halothane reduces uterine muscle tone during pregnancy and generally its use is not recommended in obstetrics because of the increased risk of postpartum haemorrhage.

Premedication with atropine has been recommended to reduce vagal tone and to prevent bradycardia and severe hypotension.

Allowance may need to be made for any increase in CSF pressure or in cerebral blood flow. Halothane should be used with caution in patients with phaeochromocytoma.

As with other halogenated anaesthetics, patients with known or suspected susceptibility to malignant hyperthermia should not be anaesthetised with halothane.

See also Precautions for General Anaesthetics, p.1255.

Abuse. A brief review[1] of abuse of volatile anaesthetics found that of 14 patients who had ingested or sniffed halothane 10 had died. Another patient who had injected halothane intravenously also died. There has also been another report[2] of fatalities resulting from acute pulmonary oedema after intravenous injection of halothane.

1. Yamashita M, et al. Illicit use of modern volatile anaesthetics. Can Anaesth Soc J 1984; 31: 76–9.
2. Berman P, Tattersal M. Self-poisoning with intravenous halothane. Lancet 1982; i: 340.

Porphyria. Halothane has been associated with acute attacks of porphyria and is considered unsafe in porphyric patients.

Interactions

Adrenaline [epinephrine] and most other sympathomimetics, and theophylline should be avoided during halothane anaesthesia since they can produce cardiac arrhythmias; the risk of arrhythmias is also increased if halothane is used in patients receiving dopaminergics. The effects of competitive neuromuscular blockers such as atracurium, and of ganglion blockers such as pentolonium, pempidine, and trimetaphan are enhanced by halothane and if required they should be given in reduced dosage. Morphine increases the depressant effects of halothane on respiration. Chlorpromazine also enhances the respiratory depressant effect of halothane. The effects of both ergometrine and oxytocin on the parturient uterus are diminished by halothane.

See also Interactions of General Anaesthetics, p.1255.

Antiepileptics. For a case of *phenytoin* intoxication associated with halothane anaesthesia, see p.359.

Benzodiazepines. *Midazolam* has been reported to potentiate the anaesthetic action of halothane.[1]

1. Inagaki Y, et al. Anesthetic interaction between midazolam and halothane in humans. Anesth Analg 1993; 76: 613–17.

Neuromuscular blockers. For the potentiation of the neuromuscular blockade of neuromuscular blockers such as atracurium by halothane, see p.1335. For increased toxicity during halothane anaesthesia, see suxamethonium p.1342.

Trichloroethane. A report[1] of 2 patients showing evidence of chronic cardiac toxicity following repeated exposure to trichloroethane. In both cases there was circumstantial evidence of a deterioration after routine anaesthetic use of halothane.

1. McLeod AA, et al. Chronic cardiac toxicity after inhalation of 1,1,1-trichloroethane. BMJ 1987; 294: 727–9.

Xanthines. For references to increased cardiotoxicity in patients taking *theophylline* when anaesthetised with halothane, see p.782.

Pharmacokinetics

Halothane is absorbed on inhalation. It has a relatively low solubility in blood and is more soluble in the neutral fats of adipose tissue than in the phospholipids of brain cells. Up to 80% of administered halothane is excreted unchanged through the lungs. Up to 20% is metabolised by the liver by oxidative and, under hypoxic conditions, reductive pathways. Urinary metabolites include trifluoroacetic acid and bromide and chloride salts (oxidative pathway) and fluoride salts (reductive pathway). Halothane diffuses across the placenta and has been detected in breast milk.

◊ Reviews.

1. Dale O, Brown BR. Clinical pharmacokinetics of the inhalational anaesthetics. Clin Pharmacokinet 1987; 12: 145–67.

Uses and Administration

Halothane is a volatile halogenated anaesthetic administered by inhalation. It has a minimum alveolar concentration (MAC) value (see p.1255) ranging from 0.64% in the elderly to 1.08% in infants. It is non-flammable and is not explosive when mixed with oxygen at normal atmospheric pressure. It is not irritant to the skin and mucous membranes and does not produce necrosis when spilt on tissues. It suppresses salivary, bronchial, and gastric secretions and dilates the bronchioles.

Halothane is used for the induction and maintenance of general anaesthesia (p.1256) and is given using a calibrated vaporiser to provide close control over the concentration of inhaled vapour.

Anaesthesia may be induced with 2 to 4% v/v of halothane in oxygen or mixtures of nitrous oxide and oxygen; induction may also be started at a concentration of 0.5% v/v and increased gradually to the required level. For induction in children a concentration of 1.5 to 2% v/v has been used. It takes up to about 5 minutes to attain surgical anaesthesia and halothane produces little or no excitement in the induction period. The more usual practice is to induce anaesthesia with an intravenous agent. Anaesthesia is maintained with concentrations of 0.5 to 2% v/v depending on the flow rate used; the lower concentration is usually suitable for the elderly.

Adequate muscle relaxation is only achieved with deep anaesthesia so a neuromuscular blocker is given to increase muscular relaxation if necessary.

◊ Reviews.
1. Quail AW. Modern inhalational anaesthetic agents: a review of halothane, isoflurane and enflurane. *Med J Aust* 1989; **150:** 95–102.

Preparations

Proprietary Preparations (details are given in Part 3)
Aust.: Fluothane; *Austral.:* Fluothane; *Belg.:* Fluothane; *Braz.:* Fluothane; *Fr.:* Fluothane; *Ger.:* Fluothane; *Hong Kong:* Fluothane; *Irl.:* Fluothane; *Israel:* Fluothane; *Ital.:* Fluothane; *Mex.:* Fluothane; *Neth.:* Fluothane; *Norw.:* Fluothane†; *NZ:* Fluothane; *Port.:* Fluothane; *S.Afr.:* Fluothane; *Spain:* Fluothane; *Swed.:* Fluothane; *Switz.:* Fluothane; *Thai.:* Fluothane†; *USA:* Fluothane.

Isoflurane (3113-n)

Isoflurane (BAN, USAN, rINN).

Compound 469; Isofluranum. 1-Chloro-2,2,2-trifluoroethyl difluoromethyl ether; 2-Chloro-2-(difluoromethoxy)-1,1,1-trifluoroethane.

$C_3H_2ClF_5O = 184.5$.
CAS — 26675-46-7.
ATC — N01AB06.

Pharmacopoeias. In Eur. (see p.vi) and US.

Pharmacopoeial description

Ph. Eur.: A clear, colourless, mobile, heavy liquid. B.p. about 48°. It is non-flammable. Practically insoluble in water; miscible with dehydrated alcohol and with trichloroethylene. Store in airtight containers. Protect from light.

USP 25: A clear, colourless, volatile liquid having a slight odour. B.p. about 49°. Insoluble in water; miscible with common organic solvents and with fats and oils. Store in airtight containers.

Adverse Effects

As with other halogenated anaesthetics, respiratory depression, hypotension, arrhythmias, and malignant hyperthermia have been reported. Isoflurane differs from halothane and enflurane in that it produces less cardiac depression than either drug and heart rate may be increased. Also isoflurane sensitises the myocardium to sympathomimetics to a lesser extent than halothane and enflurane. The incidence of cardiac arrhythmias is lower with isoflurane than with halothane. Shivering, nausea, and vomiting have been reported in the postoperative period.

Induction with isoflurane is not as smooth as with halothane and this may be connected with its pungency; breath holding, coughing, and laryngospasm may occur.

See also Adverse Effects of General Anaesthetics, p.1255.

◊ A comparison[1] of isoflurane and halothane for outpatient dental anaesthesia in children considered that isoflurane would produce fewer arrhythmias than halothane, but that the ease of induction and the quality of anaesthesia was inferior to that with halothane. Others[2] also found a higher incidence of coughing, salivation, and laryngospasm with isoflurane than halothane, but felt that it could be used as an alternative.

Further information on the adverse effects profile of isoflurane can be obtained from the report and commentaries on an extensive multicentre study of patients undergoing anaesthesia with this agent.[3,4]

1. Cattermole RW, *et al.* Isoflurane and halothane for outpatient dental anaesthesia in children. *Br J Anaesth* 1986; **58:** 385–9.
2. McAteer PM, *et al.* Comparison of isoflurane and halothane in outpatient paediatric dental anaesthesia. *Br J Anaesth* 1986; **58:** 390–3.
3. Forrest JB, *et al.* A multi-centre clinical evaluation of isoflurane. *Can Anaesth Soc J* 1982; **29** (suppl): S1–S69.
4. Levy WJ. Clinical anaesthesia with isoflurane: a review of the multicentre study. *Br J Anaesth* 1984; **56:** 101S–112S.

Effects on the blood. The development of carboxyhaemoglobinaemia in patients anaesthetised with volatile anaesthetics is discussed under Precautions, below.

Effects on the cardiovascular system. Isoflurane is considered to produce less cardiovascular depression than halothane. However, results of a study[1] by one group of workers suggest that while this may be true for young patients, in elderly patients isoflurane appears to have a cardiac depressant effect similar to that of halothane.

1. McKinney MS, *et al.* Cardiovascular effects of isoflurane and halothane in young and elderly adult patients. *Br J Anaesth* 1993; **71:** 696–701.

CEREBRAL BLOOD FLOW. Autoregulation of cerebral blood flow appears to be impaired at higher concentrations of isoflurane. A study[1] in healthy subjects found that increasing isoflurane anaesthesia from a concentration of 1 to 2 MAC increased cerebral blood flow and reduced cerebral oxygen metabolism.

1. Olsen KS, *et al.* Effect of 1 or 2 MAC isoflurane with or without ketanserin on cerebral blood flow autoregulation in man. *Br J Anaesth* 1994; **72:** 66–71.

CORONARY CIRCULATION. Halothane, enflurane, and isoflurane decrease coronary perfusion pressure, coronary blood flow, ventricular function, and myocardial oxygen demand. Halothane and enflurane have a variable effect on coronary vascular resistance, but isoflurane dilates coronary vessels.[1] There has been concern over the potential of isoflurane to produce coronary steal and whether this effect is detrimental in patients with ischaemic heart disease.[2] However, despite conflicting results of individual studies[3-6] a review[7] concluded that isoflurane could be used safely even in high-risk patients with coronary artery disease provided that blood pressure and heart rate were maintained close to baseline concentrations.

1. Quail AW. Modern inhalational anaesthetic agents: a review of halothane, isoflurane and enflurane. *Med J Aust* 1989; **150:** 95–102.
2. Stoelting RK. Anesthesiology. *JAMA* 1991; **265:** 3103–5.
3. Buffington CW, *et al.* The prevalence of steal-prone coronary anatomy in patients with coronary artery disease: an analysis of the coronary artery surgery study registry. *Anesthesiology* 1988; **69:** 721–7.
4. Inoue K, *et al.* Does isoflurane lead to a higher incidence of myocardial infarction and perioperative death than enflurane in coronary artery surgery? A clinical study of 1178 patients. *Anesth Analg* 1990; **71:** 469–74.
5. Slogoff S, *et al.* Steal-prone coronary anatomy and myocardial ischemia associated with four primary anesthetic agents in humans. *Anesth Analg* 1991; **72:** 22–7.
6. Stühmeier KD, *et al.* Isoflurane does not increase the incidence of intraoperative myocardial ischaemia compared with halothane during vascular surgery. *Br J Anaesth* 1992; **69:** 602–6.
7. Hogue CW, *et al.* Anesthetic-induced myocardial ischemia: the isoflurane-coronary steal controversy. *Coron Artery Dis* 1993; **4:** 413–19.

Effects on the kidneys. See under Metabolism in Pharmacokinetics, below.

Effects on the liver. Of 45 cases of isoflurane-associated hepatotoxicity reported to the FDA between 1981 and 1984 there was some other cause for the liver damage in 29. While isoflurane might have been one of the causes of the damage in the other 16 cases, there was not a reasonable likelihood of an association between isoflurane and postoperative liver impairment.[1] A subsequent case report of hepatic necrosis and death following surgery was possibly attributable to isoflurane.[2]

See also under the Adverse Effects of Halothane, p.1260.

1. Stoelting RK, *et al.* Hepatic dysfunction after isoflurane anesthesia. *Anesth Analg* 1987; **66:** 147–53.
2. Carrigan TW, Straughen WJ. A report of hepatic necrosis and death following isoflurane anesthesia. *Anesthesiology* 1987; **67:** 581–3.

Effects on the nervous system. Seizures associated with induction of anaesthesia with isoflurane have been reported in patients without known neurological abnormalities and not undergoing neurosurgery.[1,2] However, data from a retrospective analysis of patients undergoing intracranial surgery indicated that when convulsions occurred postoperatively in these conditions, it was the neurosurgical procedures rather than the anaesthetics that were responsible.[3]

See also under Status Epilepticus in Uses, below.

1. Poulton TJ, Ellingson RJ. Seizure associated with induction of anesthesia with isoflurane. *Anesthesiology* 1984; **61:** 471–6.
2. Hymes JA. Seizure activity during isoflurane anesthesia. *Anesth Analg* 1985; **64:** 367–8.
3. Christys AR, *et al.* Retrospective study of early postoperative convulsions after intracranial surgery with isoflurane or enflurane anaesthesia. *Br J Anaesth* 1989; **62:** 624–7.

Effects on the respiratory tract. A study[1] conducted mainly in adults found that humidification of anaesthetic mixtures containing isoflurane could reduce respiratory complications such as coughing, laryngospasm, and breath-holding that were usually associated with the use of isoflurane for induction. However, a similar study[2] in children failed to confirm these findings.

1. van Heerden PV, *et al.* Effect of humidification on inhalation induction with isoflurane. *Br J Anaesth* 1990; **64:** 235–7.
2. McAuliffe GL, *et al.* Effect of humidification on inhalation induction with isoflurane in children. *Br J Anaesth* 1994; **73:** 587–9.

Effects on the skin. There have been rare reports of contact dermatitis to isoflurane in anaesthetists.[1,2]

1. Caraffini S, *et al.* Isoflurane: an uncommon cause of occupational airborne contact dermatitis. *Contact Dermatitis* 1998; **38:** 286.
2. Muncaster A, *et al.* Allergic contact dermatitis to isoflurane. *Br J Dermatol* 1999; **141:** (suppl 55): 96–7.

Precautions

As with other halogenated anaesthetics, patients with known or suspected susceptibility to malignant hyperthermia should not be anaesthetised with isoflurane. It has been reported to increase the cerebrospinal pressure and should be used with caution in patients with raised intracranial pressure. Isoflurane relaxes the uterine muscle. In order to minimise the

risk of developing elevated carboxyhaemoglobin levels, carbon dioxide absorbents in anaesthetic apparatus should not be allowed to dry out when delivering volatile anaesthetics such as isoflurane.

See also Precautions for General Anaesthetics, p.1255.

Carbon dioxide absorbents. Significant carboxyhaemoglobinaemia may develop rarely during anaesthesia with volatile anaesthetics given by circle breathing systems containing carbon dioxide absorbents.[1] The effect is only seen when the absorbent has become excessively dried out. The use of barium hydroxide lime (which is not available in the UK) as an absorbent produces more carbon monoxide than soda lime, particularly at low water content. No cases of this complication had been reported to date in the UK.

1. Committee on Safety of Medicines/Medicines Control Agency. Safety issues in anaesthesia: volatile anesthetic agents and carboxyhaemoglobinaemia. *Current Problems* 1997; **23:** 7.

Porphyria. Isoflurane is considered to be unsafe in patients with porphyria because it has been shown to be porphyrinogenic in *animals*.

Interactions

The effects of competitive neuromuscular blockers such as atracurium are enhanced by isoflurane (see p.1335). Care is advised if adrenaline [epinephrine] and other sympathomimetics are given during isoflurane anaesthesia.

See also Interactions of General Anaesthetics, p.1255.

General anaesthetics. For a report that isoflurane increases serum concentrations of *propofol*, see p.1266.

Pharmacokinetics

Isoflurane is absorbed on inhalation. The blood/gas partition coefficient is lower than that of enflurane or halothane. It is mostly excreted unchanged through the lungs. About 0.2% of administered isoflurane is metabolised mainly to inorganic fluoride.

◊ Reviews.
1. Dale O, Brown BR. Clinical pharmacokinetics of the inhalational anaesthetics. *Clin Pharmacokinet* 1987; **12:** 145–67.

Metabolism. In 26 patients sedated with isoflurane for 24 hours, plasma fluoride ion concentration increased from a mean of 4.03 nanomol per mL to 13.57 nanomol per mL in 12 hours after stopping sedation.[1] These fluoride concentrations were considered to be too low to cause clinical renal dysfunction. In 30 patients sedated with isoflurane for up to 127 hours (mean duration was 36 hours), mean plasma fluoride ion concentration increased to 20.01 nanomol per mL during sedation and continued rising for 16 hours after discontinuing isoflurane to a maximum mean concentration of 25.34 nanomol per mL;[2] thereafter, levels gradually declined to normal values by the fifth day. Despite the increased plasma fluoride ion concentrations, no biochemical or clinical evidence of deterioration in renal function was found. Administration of isoflurane for 34 days to a patient with tetanus who required sedation to facilitate mechanical ventilation resulted in sustained fluoride ion concentrations of 50 nanomol per mL and a peak concentration of 87 nanomol per mL.[3] Although such concentrations are considered to be potentially nephrotoxic no clinical effect on renal function was found.

1. Kong KL, *et al.* Isoflurane sedation for patients undergoing mechanical ventilation: metabolism to inorganic fluoride and renal effects. *Br J Anaesth* 1990; **64:** 159–62.
2. Spencer EM, *et al.* Plasma inorganic fluoride concentrations during and after prolonged (>24h) isoflurane sedation: effect on renal function. *Anesth Analg* 1991; **73:** 731–7.
3. Stevens JJWM, *et al.* Prolonged use of isoflurane in a patient with tetanus. *Br J Anaesth* 1993; **70:** 107–109.

Uses and Administration

Isoflurane is a volatile halogenated anaesthetic administered by inhalation. It is an isomer of enflurane and has anaesthetic actions similar to those of halothane (p.1260). Isoflurane has a minimum alveolar concentration (MAC) value (see p.1255) ranging from 1.05% in the elderly to 1.87% in infants. It is employed in the induction and maintenance of general anaesthesia (p.1256) although induction is more often carried out using an intravenous anaesthetic. Isoflurane is also used in subanaesthetic doses to provide analgesia in obstetrics and other painful procedures.

Isoflurane is administered using a calibrated vaporiser. If it is used for induction then it is given with oxygen or oxygen and nitrous oxide and induction should start with an isoflurane concentration of 0.5% v/v increased to 1.5 to 3% v/v which generally produces surgical anaesthesia within 10 minutes. Its pungency may limit the rate of induction. Anaesthesia may be maintained with a concentration of 1 to 2.5% v/v with oxygen and nitrous oxide; 1.5 to 3.5% v/v may be required if used only with oxygen. Isoflurane 0.5 to 0.75% v/v with oxygen and nitrous oxide is suitable to maintain anaesthesia for caesarean section. Although isoflurane is reported to possess muscle relaxant properties, neuromuscular blockers may nevertheless be required. Recovery is rapid.

◊ Reviews.
1. Quail AW. Modern inhalational anaesthetic agents: a review of halothane, isoflurane and enflurane. *Med J Aust* 1989; **150:** 95–102.

Anaesthesia. CAESAREAN SECTION. Isoflurane 0.8% v/v has been found to be a suitable supplement to nitrous oxide-oxygen anaesthesia for patients undergoing caesarean section.[1] It has been suggested[2] that an overpressure technique might be of use to further reduce awareness in such patients. Administration of isoflurane at a concentration of 2% v/v for 5 minutes followed by concentrations of 1.5% v/v for the next 5 minutes and 0.8% v/v thereafter produced higher arterial concentrations of isoflurane in patients undergoing caesarean section than when it was given at a concentration of 1% v/v throughout.[2]

1. Dwyer R, *et al.* Uptake of halothane and isoflurane by mother and baby during Caesarean section. *Br J Anaesth* 1995; **74:** 379–83.
2. McCrirrick A, *et al.* Overpressure isoflurane at Caesarean section: a study of arterial isoflurane concentrations. *Br J Anaesth* 1994; **72:** 122–4.

Pain. Isoflurane is used in subanaesthetic doses to provide analgesia in obstetrics and other painful procedures but studies[1,2] have been unable to confirm that it had an analgesic effect at subanaesthetic concentrations. The use of isoflurane 0.2 or 0.25% v/v in a mixture of nitrous oxide 50% v/v and oxygen 50% v/v has been studied.[3,4]

1. Tomi K, *et al.* Alterations in pain threshold and psychomotor response associated with subanaesthetic concentrations of inhalation anaesthetics in humans. *Br J Anaesth* 1993; **70:** 684–6.
2. Roth D, *et al.* Analgesic effect in humans of subanaesthetic isoflurane concentrations evaluated by evoked potentials. *Br J Anaesth* 1996; **76:** 38–42.
3. Wee MYK, *et al.* Isoflurane in labour. *Anaesthesia* 1993; **48:** 369–72.
4. Bryden FM, *et al.* Isoflurane for removal of chest drains after cardiac surgery. *Br J Anaesth* 1994; **73:** 712P–713P.

Sedation. INTENSIVE CARE. The various drugs used to provide sedation in intensive care are discussed on p.652. Isoflurane is not usually considered for such a purpose but in a comparative 24-hour study[1] in 60 patients requiring mechanical ventilation, isoflurane 0.1 to 0.6% v/v in an air-oxygen mixture produced satisfactory sedation for a greater proportion of time than did the continuous infusion of midazolam 0.01 to 0.20 mg per kg body-weight per hour. Patients given isoflurane also recovered more rapidly. Isoflurane has also been used successfully for sedation over 5 days in a 3-year-old infant who required ventilation for pneumonia, a complication of the child's myasthenia gravis.[2] However, there has been some concern over high plasma fluoride concentrations following prolonged use of isoflurane (see under Metabolism in Pharmacokinetics, above).

1. Kong KL, *et al.* Isoflurane compared with midazolam for sedation in the intensive care unit. *BMJ* 1989; **298:** 1277–80.
2. McBeth C, Watkins TGL. Isoflurane for sedation in a case of congenital myasthenia gravis. *Br J Anaesth* 1996; **77:** 672–4.

Status epilepticus. Anaesthesia in conjunction with assisted ventilation may be instituted to control refractory tonic-clonic status epilepticus (p.341). A short-acting barbiturate such as thiopental is usually used. Despite rare reports of seizures associated with the use of isoflurane in anaesthetic procedures (see under Adverse Effects, above) concentrations of 0.5 to 1% v/v have been used successfully in isolated patients[1,2] to control refractory convulsive status epilepticus. Although some[3] consider that isoflurane-induced coma may be more easy to control than barbiturate-induced coma, the use of isoflurane may be limited by the need for special anaesthetic equipment and continuous EEG monitoring.

1. Meeke RI, *et al.* Isoflurane for the management of status epilepticus. *DICP Ann Pharmacother* 1989; **23:** 579–81.
2. Hilz MJ, *et al.* Isoflurane anaesthesia in the treatment of convulsive status epilepticus. *J Neurol* 1992; **239:** 135–7.
3. Bauer J, Elger CE. Management of status epilepticus in adults. *CNS Drugs* 1994; **1:** 26–44.

Preparations

Proprietary Preparations (details are given in Part 3)
Aust.: Forane; *Austral.:* AErrane; Forthane; *Belg.:* AErrane; Forene; *Braz.:* Forane; *Canad.:* Forane; *Denm.:* Forene; *Fin.:* Forene; *Ger.:* Forene; *Hong Kong:* Forene; *Irl.:* AErrane; Forene; *Israel:* AErrane; Forene; *Ital.:* Forane; *Mex.:* Forane; Lisorane; Sofloran; *Neth.:* AErrane; Forene; *Norw.:* Forene; *NZ:* AErrane; Forene; *S.Afr.:* Forene; Isofor†; *Singapore:* Forane; *Spain:* AErrane; Forane; *Swed.:* Forene; *Switz.:* Forene; *Thai.:* AErrane; Forane; *UK:* AErrane; Isoflurane; *USA:* Forane.

Ketamine Hydrochloride (3114-h)

Ketamine Hydrochloride (BANM, USAN, rINNM).
CI-581; CL-369; CN-52372-2; Ketamini Hydrochloridum. (±)-2-(2-Chlorophenyl)-2-methylaminocyclohexanone hydrochloride.
$C_{13}H_{16}ClNO,HCl = 274.2$.
CAS — 6740-88-1 (ketamine); 1867-66-9 (ketamine hydrochloride).
Pharmacopoeias. In Chin., Eur. (see p.vi), Int., Jpn, and US.

Ketamine hydrochloride 1.15 mg is approximately equivalent to 1 mg of ketamine base.
Incompatible with soluble barbiturates. The US manufacturer has recommended that when concomitant administration of diazepam and ketamine is required they should be given separately and not mixed in the same giving equipment.

Pharmacopoeial description
Ph. Eur.: A white crystalline powder. Freely soluble in water and in methyl alcohol; soluble in alcohol. A 10% solution in water has a pH of 3.5 to 4.1. Protect from light.
USP 25: A white crystalline powder having a slight characteristic odour. Soluble 1 in 4 of water, 1 in 14 of alcohol, 1 in 60 of dehydrated alcohol and of chloroform, and 1 in 6 of methyl alcohol; practically insoluble in ether. pH of a 10% solution in water is between 3.5 and 4.1.

Adverse Effects

Emergence reactions are common during recovery from ketamine anaesthesia and include vivid often unpleasant dreams, confusion, hallucinations, and irrational behaviour. Children and elderly patients appear to be less sensitive. Patients may also experience increased muscle tone, sometimes resembling seizures. Blood pressure and heart rate may be temporarily increased by ketamine; hypotension, arrhythmias, and bradycardia have occurred rarely.

Respiration may be depressed following rapid intravenous injection or with high doses. Apnoea and laryngospasm have occurred. Diplopia and nystagmus may occur. Nausea and vomiting, lachrymation, hypersalivation, and raised intra-ocular and CSF pressure have also been reported. Transient skin rashes and pain at the site of injection may occur.

See also Adverse Effects of General Anaesthetics, p.1255.

Effects on the cardiovascular system. Ketamine has been advocated by some for maintaining or increasing cardiovascular performance in selected patients during induction of anaesthesia as it may increase blood pressure and heart rate.[1] However, there have been reports of reduced cardiac and pulmonary performance in severely ill patients[1] and of arrhythmias.[2] Some of the cardiovascular reactions of ketamine may be attenuated by premedication with diazepam[2] or clonidine.[3]

1. Waxman K, *et al.* Cardiovascular effects of anesthetic induction with ketamine. *Anesth Analg* 1980; **59:** 355–8.
2. Cabbabe EB, Behbahani PM. Cardiovascular reactions associated with the use of ketamine and epinephrine in plastic surgery. *Ann Plast Surg* 1985; **15:** 50–2.
3. Tanaka M, Nishikawa T. Oral clonidine premedication attenuates the hypertensive response to ketamine. *Br J Anaesth* 1994; **73:** 758–62.

Effects on the liver. Changes in serum-enzyme levels have occurred following ketamine in an initial dose of 1 mg per kg followed by continuous infusion as a 0.1% solution.[1]

1. Dundee JW, *et al.* Changes in serum enzyme levels following ketamine infusions. *Anaesthesia* 1980; **35:** 12–16.

Effects on mental state. Mental disturbances following ketamine anaesthesia may vary in incidence from less than 5% to greater than 30%.[1] See also Abuse, below.

1. White PF, *et al.* Ketamine—its pharmacology and therapeutic uses. *Anesthesiology* 1982; **56:** 119–36.

Effects on the skin. Harlequin-like colour skin changes were reported[1] in a 9-month-old boy during anaesthesia with ketamine 15 mg.

1. Wagner DL, Sewell AD. Harlequin color change in an infant during anesthesia. *Anesthesiology* 1985; **62:** 695.

Malignant hyperthermia. Malignant hyperthermia has been reported in a patient given ketamine.[1]

1. Rasore-Quartino A, *et al.* Forma atipica di ipertermia maligna: osservazione di un caso da ketamina. *Pathologica* 1985; **77:** 609–17.

Precautions

Ketamine is contra-indicated in patients in whom elevation of blood pressure would be a serious hazard including those with hypertension or a history of cerebrovascular accident. Cardiac function should be monitored in patients found to have hypertension or cardiac decompensation. Ketamine should be used with caution in patients with elevated CSF pressure.

It can raise intra-ocular pressure and should not be used in the presence of eye injury or increased intraocular pressure.
Ketamine does not reliably suppress pharyngeal and laryngeal reflexes and mechanical stimulation of the pharynx should be avoided unless a muscle relaxant is used.

The use of ketamine should be avoided in patients prone to hallucinations or psychotic disorders. Verbal, tactile, and visual stimuli should be kept to a minimum during recovery in an attempt to reduce the risk of emergence reactions.

See also Precautions for General Anaesthetics, p.1255.

Abuse. Health care workers in the USA were alerted to the dangers associated with the abuse of ketamine as long ago as 1979.[1] Similar concern has been voiced more recently in the UK[2] over the abuse of ketamine at social gatherings where it has been taken intranasally or orally under the names of 'vitamin K', 'super K', or 'special K'. Ketamine produces a state of psychological dissociation resulting in hallucinations and out of body or near death experiences. It can induce a state of helplessness in which the user loses awareness of the environment and this together with severe loss of coordination and pronounced analgesia can put the user at great risk. Furthermore, some users experience a state in which they are unconcerned about whether they live or die. Ketamine has the potential for compulsive repeated use and there have been reports of users self-injecting ketamine several times a day for prolonged periods. There has been a report[3] of an acute dystonic reaction in a 20-year old man following self-administration of ketamine intravenously.
Some[2] suggest that patients seeking medical attention are best placed in a quiet darkened room to recover with diazepam being given for unresponsive panic attacks while others advocate that such patients should be admitted to an intensive care unit for close monitoring.[4]

1. Anonymous. Ketamine abuse. *FDA Drug Bull* 1979; **9:** 24.
2. Jansen KLR. Non-medical use of ketamine. *BMJ* 1993; **306:** 601–2.
3. Felser JM, Orban DJ. Dystonic reaction after ketamine abuse. *Ann Emerg Med* 1982; **11:** 673–5.
4. Gill PA. Non-medical use of ketamine. *BMJ* 1993; **306:** 1340.

Interactions

Inhalational anaesthetics, such as ether and halothane, and other cerebral depressants may prolong the effect of ketamine and delay recovery. Prolonged recovery has also occurred when barbiturates and/or opioids have been given concomitantly with ketamine. It has been recommended that ketamine should not be used in combination with ergometrine.

See also Interactions of General Anaesthetics, p.1255.

◊ For the enhancement of the effect of *tubocurarine* or *atracurium* by ketamine, see p.1335. For a reference to increased cardiovascular adverse effects with *thyroid drugs*, see p.1528. For a reference to seizures and tachycardia attributed to an interaction between ketamine and *theophylline*, see p.782.

Pharmacokinetics

After intravenous bolus administration, ketamine shows a bi- or triexponential pattern of elimination. The alpha phase lasts about 45 minutes with a half-life of 10 to 15 minutes. This first phase, which represents ketamine's anaesthetic action, is terminated by redistribution from the CNS to peripheral tissues and hepatic biotransformation to an active metabolite norketamine. Other metabolic pathways include hydroxylation of the cyclohexone ring and conjugation with glucuronic acid. The beta phase half-life is about 2.5 hours. Ketamine is excreted mainly in the urine as metabolites. It crosses the placenta.

◊ References.
1. Clements JA, Nimmo WS. Pharmacokinetics and analgesic effect of ketamine in man. *Br J Anaesth* 1981; **53:** 27–30.
2. Grant IS, *et al.* Pharmacokinetics and analgesic effects of IM and oral ketamine. *Br J Anaesth* 1981; **53:** 805–9.
3. Nimmo WS. The pharmacokinetics of ketamine in children. *Br J Clin Pharmacol* 1982; **14:** 144P.
4. Geisslinger G, *et al.* Pharmacokinetics and pharmacodynamics of ketamine enantiomers in surgical patients using a stereoselective analytical method. *Br J Anaesth* 1993; **70:** 666–71.
5. Malinovsky J-M, *et al.* Ketamine and norketamine plasma concentrations after iv, nasal and rectal administration in children. *Br J Anaesth* 1996; **77:** 203–7.

Uses and Administration

Ketamine is an anaesthetic administered by intravenous injection, intravenous infusion, or intramuscular injection. It produces dissociative anaesthesia characterised by a trance-like state, amnesia, and marked analgesia which may persist into the recovery period. There is often an increase in muscle tone and the patient's eyes may remain open for all or part of the period of anaesthesia. Ketamine is used in general anaesthesia for diagnostic or short surgical operations that do not require skeletal muscle relaxation, for the induction of anaesthesia to be maintained with other drugs, and as a supplementary anaesthetic (see p.1256). It also has good analgesic properties in subanaesthetic doses. It is considered to be of particular value in children requiring frequent repeated anaesthesia. Recovery is relatively slow.

Ketamine is administered as the hydrochloride but doses are expressed in terms of the equivalent amount of base. For induction the dose given by *intravenous injection* may range from 1 to 4.5 mg of ketamine per kg body-weight; a dose of 2 mg of ketamine per kg given intravenously over 60 seconds usually produces surgical anaesthesia within 30 seconds of the end of the injection and lasting for 5 to 10 minutes. The initial *intramuscular* dose may range from 6.5 to 13 mg of ketamine per kg; an intramuscular dose of 10 mg of ketamine per kg usually produces surgical anaesthesia within 3 to 4 minutes lasting for 12 to 25 minutes. For diagnostic or other procedures not involving intense pain an initial intramuscular dose of 4 mg of ketamine per kg has been used. Additional doses may be given for maintenance. For induction by *intravenous infusion* a total dose of 0.5 to 2 mg of ketamine per kg is usually given at an appropriate infusion rate. Maintenance is achieved with 10 to 45 µg per kg per minute, the infusion rate being adjusted according to response.

Administration should be preceded by atropine or another suitable antimuscarinic. Diazepam or another benzodiazepine may be given before surgery or as an adjunct to ketamine to reduce the incidence of emergence reactions.

◊ Reviews.
1. Hirota K, Lambert DG. Ketamine: its mechanism(s) of action and unusual clinical uses. *Br J Anaesth* 1996; **77:** 441–4.

Administration. Although ketamine hydrochloride is usually given intravenously or intramuscularly, oral[1,2] and rectal[3] administration has been used successfully in children. Intranasal administration of ketamine has also been reported.[4] Unfortunately the onset of sedation with these three routes is too slow for emergency procedures and therefore a jet-injector of ketamine was developed[5] to provide non-traumatic, painless, and rapid anaesthesia in children.
1. Tobias JD, *et al.* Oral ketamine premedication to alleviate the distress of invasive procedures in pediatric oncology patients. *Pediatrics* 1992; **90:** 537–41.
2. Gutstein HB, *et al.* Oral ketamine preanesthetic medication in children. *Anesthesiology* 1992; **76:** 28–33.
3. Lökken P, *et al.* Conscious sedation by rectal administration of midazolam or midazolam plus ketamine as alternatives to general anesthesia for dental treatment of uncooperative children. *Scand J Dent Res* 1994; **102:** 274–80.
4. Louon A, *et al.* Sedation with nasal ketamine and midazolam for cryotherapy in retinopathy of prematurity. *Br J Ophthalmol* 1993; **77:** 529–30.
5. Zsigmond EK, *et al.* A new route, jet-injection for anesthetic induction in children—ketamine dose-range finding studies. *Int J Clin Pharmacol Ther* 1996; **34:** 84–8.

Nonketotic hyperglycinaemia. Ketamine was tried in combination with strychnine in a newborn infant with severe nonketotic hyperglycinaemia (p.1667) and resulted in neurological improvement, although motor development remained unsatisfactory.[1] It was thought that ketamine might act by blocking N-methyl-D-aspartate (NMDA) receptors, which are activated in the CNS by glycine.
1. Tegtmeyer-Metadorf H, *et al.* Ketamine and strychnine treatment of an infant with nonketotic hyperglycinaemia. *Eur J Pediatr* 1995; **154:** 649–53.

Pain. For a discussion of pain and its management, see p.2. Ketamine has been used for its analgesic action[1-10] and may be of value in neuropathic or other pain unresponsive to opioid analgesics. (For mention of its use for outpatient procedures in children, see p.3.) Subcutaneous, intramuscular, intravenous, epidural, intrathecal, and oral administration have all been tried.
1. Naguib M, *et al.* Epidural ketamine for postoperative analgesia. *Can Anaesth Soc J* 1986; **33:** 16–21.
2. Oshima E, *et al.* Continuous subcutaneous injection of ketamine for cancer pain. *Can J Anaesth* 1990; **32:** 385–6.
3. Laird D, Lovel T. Paradoxical pain. *Lancet* 1993; **341:** 241.

The symbol † denotes a preparation no longer actively marketed

---

4. Bhattacharya A, *et al.* Subcutaneous infusion of ketamine and morphine for relief of postoperative pain: a double-blind comparative study. *Ann Acad Med Singapore* 1994; **23:** 456–9.
5. Wong C-S, *et al.* Ketamine potentiates analgesic effect of morphine in postoperative epidural pain control. *Reg Anesth* 1996; **21:** 534–41.
6. Gurhani A, *et al.* Analgesia for acute musculoskeletal trauma: low-dose subcutaneous infusion of ketamine. *Anaesth Intensive Care* 1996; **24:** 32–6.
7. Semple D, *et al.* The optimal dose of ketamine for caudal epidural blockade in children. *Anaesthesia* 1996; **51:** 1170–2.
8. Chen E, *et al.* Treatment of phantom limb pain in the early postoperative period by ketamine. *Analgesia* 1996; **2:** 125–8.
9. Nikolajsen L, *et al.* The effect of ketamine on phantom pain: a central neuropathic disorder maintained by peripheral input. *Pain* 1996; **67:** 69–77.
10. Kennedy RM, *et al.* Comparison of fentanyl/midazolam with ketamine/midazolam for pediatric orthopedic emergencies. *Pediatrics* 1998; **102:** 956–63.

Preparations

BP 2001: Ketamine Injection;
USP 25: Ketamine Hydrochloride Injection.

Proprietary Preparations (details are given in Part 3)
Aust.: Ketalar; Ketanest; *Austral.:* Ketalar; *Belg.:* Ketalar; *Braz.:* Ketalar; *Canad.:* Ketalar; *Denm.:* Ketalar; *Fin.:* Ketalar; Ketanest; *Fr.:* Ketalar; *Ger.:* Ketanest; Velonarcon; *Hong Kong:* Ketalar; *Irl.:* Ketalar; *Israel:* Ketalar; *Ital.:* Ketalar; *Mex.:* Ketalin; Ketina; *Neth.:* Ketalar; Ketanest; *Norw.:* Ketalar; *NZ:* Ketalar; *S.Afr.:* Brevinaze; Ketalar†; *Spain:* Ketolar; *Swed.:* Ketalar; *Switz.:* Ketalar; *Thai.:* Calypsol; Ketalar; *UK:* Ketalar; *USA:* Ketalar.

Methohexital   (3115-m)

Methohexital *(BAN, rINN)*.

Methohexitone. (±)-5-Allyl-1-methyl-5-(1-methylpent-2-ynyl)barbituric acid; 1-Methyl-5-(1-methyl-2-pentynyl)-5-(2-propenyl)-2,4,6(1*H*,3*H*,5*H*)-pyrimidinetrione.
$C_{14}H_{18}N_2O_3$ = 262.3.
CAS — 151-83-7; 18652-93-2.
ATC — N01AF01; N05CA15.
Pharmacopoeias. In US.

Pharmacopoeial description

USP 25: A white to faintly yellowish-white crystalline odourless powder. M.p. 92° to 96° but the range between beginning and end of melting does not exceed 3°. Very slightly soluble in water; slightly soluble in alcohol, in chloroform, and in dilute alkalis.

Methohexital Sodium   (3116-b)

Methohexital Sodium *(BANM, rINNM)*.
Compound 25398; Enallynymalnatrium; Methohexitone Sodium.
$C_{14}H_{17}N_2NaO_3$ = 284.3.
CAS — 309-36-4; 22151-68-4; 60634-69-7.
Pharmacopoeias. Br. includes Methohexital Injection; US includes Methohexital Sodium for Injection.

Solutions of methohexital sodium are incompatible with acidic substances including a number of antibiotics, antipsychotics, neuromuscular blockers, antimuscarinics, and analgesics. Compounds commonly listed as incompatible include atropine sulfate, pethidine hydrochloride, metocurine iodide, fentanyl citrate, morphine sulfate, pentazocine lactate, silicones, suxamethonium chloride, tubocurarine chloride, and compound sodium lactate injection. Only preservative-free diluents should be used to reconstitute methohexital sodium; precipitation may occur if a diluent containing a bacteriostatic agent is used.
Solutions in Water for Injections are stable for at least 6 weeks at room temperature; however reconstituted solutions should be stored no longer than 24 hours as they contain no bacteriostatic agent. Solutions in glucose or sodium chloride injections are stable only for about 24 hours.

Pharmacopoeial description

BP 2001: Methohexital Sodium for Injection is a sterile mixture of 100 parts by weight of the a-form of methohexital sodium and 6 parts by weight of dried sodium carbonate included as a buffer. It may also contain auxiliary substances. A 5% solution in water has a pH of 10.6 to 11.6.
USP 25: Methohexital Sodium for Injection is a freeze-dried sterile mixture of methohexital sodium and anhydrous sodium carbonate as a buffer, prepared from an aqueous solution of methohexital, sodium hydroxide, and sodium carbonate. It is a white to off-white, essentially odourless, hygroscopic powder. pH of a 5% solution in water is between 10.6 to 11.6.

Adverse Effects and Precautions

As for Thiopental Sodium, p.1269.

Excitatory phenomena are more common and induction less smooth with methohexital than with thiopental. Methohexital should be used with caution, if at all, in patients with a history of epilepsy.

See also Adverse Effects and Precautions for General Anaesthetics, p.1255.

◊ In a study of 4379 administrations of methohexital to 2722 dental patients the total dose ranged from 20 mg to 560 mg (with a mean of 151 mg), and the duration of treatment was 8 to 32 minutes.[1] The most frequent complication was restlessness (in 292 cases) and was not prevented by diazepam. Respiratory complications occurred in 214 administrations and uncontrollable crying during recovery after 73 administrations. Pain along the vein was recorded in 45 cases, with 5 patients developing thrombophlebitis. In 22 administrations jactitations were observed and allergic reactions occurred in 10 administrations.
1. McDonald D. Methohexitone in dentistry. *Aust Dent J* 1980; **25:** 335–42.

Effects on the nervous system. Two case reports of seizures induced by methohexital in children with seizure disorders.[1] Seizures are considered a rare adverse effect of methohexital. In 48 000 patients given methohexital, only 3 developed clonic-type seizures.[2]
A case of a tonic-clonic seizure possibly due to an interaction between paroxetine and methohexital is discussed below.
1. Rockoff MA, Goudsouzian NG. Seizures induced by methohexital. *Anesthesiology* 1981; **54:** 333–5.
2. Metriyakool K. Seizures induced by methohexital. *Anesthesiology* 1981; **55:** 718.

Pain on injection. Methohexital is associated with severe pain particularly if veins on the back of the hands are used. The incidence of pain on injection may be reduced by using a forearm vein or by pre-injection with lignocaine [lidocaine].

Porphyria. Methohexitone is considered to be unsafe in patients with porphyria because it has been shown to be porphyrinogenic in *animals*.

Rebound anaesthesia. Rebound of anaesthesia with abolition of reflexes and depression of respiration occurred in a 6-year-old boy[1] 100 minutes after anorectal induction with 27.6 mg per kg body-weight methohexital.
1. Kaiser H, Al-Rafai S. Wie sicher ist die rektale Narkoseeinleitung mit Methohexital in der Kinderanaesthesie? *Anaesthesist* 1985; **34:** 359–60.

Interactions

As for Thiopental Sodium, p.1269.

Antidepressants. A 42-year-old woman[1] suffered a generalised tonic-clonic seizure immediately after being anaesthetised with methohexital for the last in a series of six electroconvulsive therapies. She had been receiving *paroxetine* throughout the series. A previous course, without concurrent paroxetine, had been uneventful.
1. Folkerts H. Spontaneous seizure after concurrent use of methohexital anesthesia for electroconvulsive therapy and paroxetine: a case report. *J Nerv Ment Dis* 1995; **183:** 115–16.

Pharmacokinetics

Methohexital is less lipid soluble than thiopental but when administered intravenously as the sodium salt concentrations sufficient to produce anaesthesia are attained in the brain within 30 seconds. Methohexital is also absorbed when given rectally, producing an effect within about 5 to 11 minutes. Recovery from anaesthesia occurs quickly as a result of rapid metabolism and redistribution into other body tissues. Methohexital does not appear to concentrate in fatty tissues to the same extent as other barbiturate anaesthetics. Protein binding has been reported to be about 73%. Methohexital is rapidly metabolised in the liver through demethylation and oxidation. The terminal half-life ranges from 1.5 to 6 hours. Methohexital diffuses across the placenta and has been detected in breast milk.

◊ References.
1. Swerdlow BN, Holley FO. Intravenous anaesthetic agents: pharmacokinetic-pharmacodynamic relationships. *Clin Pharmacokinet* 1987; **12:** 79–110.
2. Le Normand Y, *et al.* Pharmacokinetics and haemodynamic effects of prolonged methohexital infusion. *Br J Clin Pharmacol* 1988; **26:** 589–94.
3. Redke F, *et al.* Pharmacokinetics and clinical experience of 20-h infusions of methohexitone in intensive care patients with postoperative pyrexia. *Br J Anaesth* 1991; **66:** 53–9.
4. van Hoogdalem EJ, *et al.* Pharmacokinetics of rectal drug administration, part I: general considerations and clinical applications of centrally acting drugs. *Clin Pharmacokinet* 1991; **21:** 11–26.
5. Borgatta L, *et al.* Clinical significance of methohexital, meperidine, and diazepam in breast milk. *J Clin Pharmacol* 1997; **37:** 186–92.

Uses and Administration

Methohexital is a short-acting barbiturate anaesthetic which has actions similar to those of thiopental (p.1269) but it is about 2 to 3 times more potent. It is administered as the sodium salt and has similar uses to thiopental in anaesthesia. Induction of anaesthesia is less smooth than with thiopental and there may be excitatory phenomena. It has a shorter duration of action than thiopental and recovery after an induction dose occurs within 5 to 7 minutes although drowsiness may persist for some time.

As with other barbiturate anaesthetics the dose of methohexital required varies greatly according to the state of the patient and the nature of other drugs being used concurrently (see under Precautions of Thiopental, p.1269, and Interactions of Thiopental, p.1269, for further details). Methohexital sodium is usually given intravenously as a 1% solution. Higher concentrations may markedly increase the incidence of adverse effects. A typical dose for induction of anaesthesia is 50 to 120 mg administered at a rate of approximately 10 mg (1 mL of a 1% solution) every 5 seconds. Doses in children range from 1 to 2 mg per kg body-weight. For the maintenance of general anaesthesia methohexital sodium may be given in doses of 20 to 40 mg every 4 to 7 minutes as required or it may be administered as a 0.2% solution by continuous intravenous infusion.

Administration in the elderly. It is usually recommended that the dosage of barbiturate anaesthetics is reduced in the elderly. One study[1] in elderly patients has demonstrated that although reducing the rate of intravenous administration reduces the speed of induction, the dosage required is also reduced. Administration of methohexital sodium 0.5% at a rate of 25 mg per minute induced anaesthesia in a mean of 83.8 seconds and required a mean dose of 0.56 mg per kg body-weight. Corresponding values for an administration rate of 100 mg per minute were 43.6 seconds and 1 mg per kg respectively.

1. Berthoud MC, *et al.* Comparison of infusion rates of three i.v. anaesthetic agents for induction in elderly patients. *Br J Anaesth* 1993; **70:** 423–7.

Dental sedation. Some anaesthetics are used as sedatives in dental procedures (see p.652). Methohexital has been tried for patient-controlled sedation in oral surgery under local anaesthesia.[1] In a group of 42 patients, results with 2.5 mg of methohexital compared favourably with those obtained in patients receiving 5 mg of propofol on demand, although patients in the methohexital group experienced a greater degree of postoperative drowsiness.

1. Hamid SK, *et al.* Comparison of patient-controlled sedation with either methohexitone or propofol. *Br J Anaesth* 1996; **77:** 727–30.

Preparations

USP 25: Methohexital Sodium for Injection.

Proprietary Preparations (details are given in Part 3)
Aust.: Brietal; *Austral.:* Brietal; *Canad.:* Brietal; *Denm.:* Brietal†; *Ger.:* Brevimytal; *Irl.:* Brietal; *Israel:* Brietal; *Neth.:* Brietal; *Norw.:* Brietal†; *NZ:* Brietal; *S.Afr.:* Brietal; *Singapore:* Brietal; *Swed.:* Brietal; *Switz.:* Brietal; *UK:* Brietal†; *USA:* Brevital.

Methoxyflurane (3117-v)

Methoxyflurane *(BAN, USAN, rINN)*.
NSC-110432. 2,2-Dichloro-1,1-difluoro-1-methoxyethane; 2,2-Dichloro-1,1-difluoroethyl methyl ether.
$C_3H_4Cl_2F_2O = 165.0$.
CAS — 76-38-0.
ATC — N01AB03.
Pharmacopoeias. In *US*.

Pharmacopoeial description

USP 25: A clear, practically colourless, mobile liquid having a characteristic odour. It may contain a suitable stabiliser. B.p. about 105°. Soluble 1 in 500 of water; miscible with alcohol, with acetone, with chloroform, with ether, and with fixed oils. Store in airtight containers at a temperature not exceeding 40°. Protect from light.

Adverse Effects

As with other halogenated anaesthetics respiratory depression, hypotension, and malignant hyperthermia have been reported. Methoxyflurane sensitises the myocardium to sympathomimetics to a lesser extent than halothane; arrhythmias appear to be rare.

Methoxyflurane impairs renal function in a dose-related manner due to the effect of the released fluoride on the distal tubule and may cause polyuric or oliguric renal failure, oxaluria being a prominent feature. Nephrotoxicity is greater with methoxyflurane than with other halogenated anaesthetics because of its slower metabolism over several days resulting in prolonged production of fluoride ions and metabolism to other potentially nephrotoxic substances.

There have also been occasional reports of hepatic dysfunction, jaundice, and fatal hepatic necrosis. Headache has been reported by some patients. Cardiac arrest, gastrointestinal side-effects, delirium, and prolonged postoperative somnolence have been observed.

See also Adverse Effects of General Anaesthetics, p.1255.

Precautions

The use of methoxyflurane is limited because of its potential to cause renal toxicity. It should not be used to achieve deep anaesthesia or for surgical procedures expected to last longer than 4 hours. Methoxyflurane is contra-indicated in the presence of renal impairment. Renal function and urine output should be monitored during anaesthesia. As with other halogenated anaesthetics it is advisable not to administer methoxyflurane to patients who have shown signs of liver damage or fever after previous anaesthesia involving halogenated anaesthetics. Patients with known, or suspected, susceptibility to malignant hyperthermia should not be anaesthetised with methoxyflurane. Allowance may need to be made for any increase in CSF pressure or in cerebral blood flow.

There is significant absorption of methoxyflurane by the rubber and soda lime in anaesthetic circuits. Polyvinyl chloride plastics are partially soluble in methoxyflurane.

See also Precautions for General Anaesthetics, p.1255.

Abuse. A 27-year-old nurse suffered from progressive renal disease and painful diffuse and multifocal periostitis which had developed as a probable consequence of intermittent self-exposure to methoxyflurane possibly over a 9-year period.[1] There has also been a report[2] of hepatitis in a 39-year-old physician who repeatedly self-administered subanaesthetic concentrations of methoxyflurane for insomnia. Inhalation of about 2 mL of methoxyflurane had occurred once or twice almost every day for six weeks. A 125 mL bottle of methoxyflurane had been consumed in approximately one month.

1. Klemmer PJ, Hadler NM. Subacute fluorosis: a consequence of abuse of an organofluoride anesthetic. *Ann Intern Med* 1978; **89:** 607–11.

2. Okuno T, *et al.* Hepatitis due to repeated inhalation of methoxyflurane in subanaesthetic concentrations. *Can Anaesth Soc J* 1985; **32:** 53–5.

Porphyria. Methoxyflurane is considered to be unsafe in patients with porphyria because it has been shown to be porphyrinogenic in *animals* or *in-vitro* systems.

Interactions

Care is advised if adrenaline [epinephrine] or other sympathomimetics are given to patients during methoxyflurane anaesthesia. The effects of competitive neuromuscular blockers are enhanced by methoxyflurane. The chronic use of hepatic enzyme-inducing drugs may enhance the metabolism of methoxyflurane thereby increasing the risk of nephrotoxicity. Concurrent use of nephrotoxic drugs with methoxyflurane should be avoided.

See also Interactions of General Anaesthetics, p.1255.

Pharmacokinetics

Methoxyflurane is absorbed on inhalation. The blood/gas partition coefficient is high. Methoxyflurane is metabolised to a greater extent than other inhalational anaesthetics. About 50 to 70% of absorbed methoxyflurane undergoes metabolism in the liver to free fluoride, oxalic acid, difluoromethoxyacetic acid, and dichloroacetic acid. Methoxyflurane is very soluble in adipose tissue and excretion may be slow. Peak plasma concentrations of fluoride occur 2 to 4 days after administration. Methoxyflurane crosses the placenta.

Uses and Administration

Methoxyflurane is a volatile halogenated anaesthetic administered by inhalation. It has a minimum alveolar concentration (MAC) value (see p.1255) of 0.16%. In recommended concentrations it is non-flammable and not explosive when mixed with oxygen. Methoxyflurane possesses good analgesic properties. It does not produce appreciable skeletal muscle relaxation at the concentrations used. Methoxyflurane does not relax the uterus and has little effect on uterine contractions during labour. It is used in subanaesthetic doses to provide analgesia for painful procedures. In anaesthetic doses, it has been used mainly for maintenance of general anaesthesia (p.1256). Use is restricted by its nephrotoxicity.

Concentrations of 0.3 to 0.8% v/v are used to provide analgesia in a variety of situations. The recommended maximum dose for analgesia is 6 mL of liquid per day or 15 mL per patient.

Because of its low vapour pressure, induction of general anaesthesia with methoxyflurane is slow and when it is to be used anaesthesia is usually induced with an intravenous anaesthetic. For maintenance, a concentration of up to 2% v/v methoxyflurane in at least 50% v/v nitrous oxide and oxygen should be given for not more than 5 minutes and then progressively reduced to the lowest concentration that will maintain adequate anaesthesia. The production of deep anaesthesia with methoxyflurane is not recommended, and a maximum of 4 hours exposure to a concentration of 0.25% v/v or the equivalent total dosage is suggested. Recovery may be prolonged.

Preparations

Proprietary Preparations (details are given in Part 3)

Austral.: Penthrane†.

Nitrous Oxide (3119-q)

Azoto Protossido; Dinitrogen Oxide; Dinitrogenii Oxidum; Distickstoffmonoxid; E942; Laughing Gas; Nitrogen Monoxide; Nitrogenii Monoxidum; Nitrogenii Oxidum; Nitrogenium Oxydulatum; Oxyde Nitreux; Oxydum Nitrosum; Protoxyde d'Azote; Stickoxydul.
$N_2O = 44.01$.
CAS — 10024-97-2.
ATC — N01AX13.
Pharmacopoeias. In *Chin., Eur.* (see p.vi), *Jpn,* and *US.*

It supports combustion.

It is supplied compressed in metal cylinders. National standards are usually in operation for the labelling and marking of such cylinders.

Pharmacopoeial description

Ph. Eur.: A colourless gas. One vol. measured at a pressure of 101 kPa dissolves, at 20°, in about 1.5 vol. of water. Store liquefied under pressure in suitable containers complying with the legal regulations.

USP 25: A colourless gas, without appreciable odour or taste. One litre at 0° and at a pressure of 760 mmHg weighs about 1.97 g. One volume dissolves in about 1.4 volumes of water at 20° and at a pressure of 760 mmHg; freely soluble in alcohol; soluble in ether and in oils.

Storage. Cylinders containing 50% nitrous oxide and 50% oxygen should be protected from the cold to prevent separation of the gases. Cylinders exposed to temperatures lower than −7° should be rolled at room temperature to ensure mixing or alternatively stored horizontally for 24 hours at a temperature of not less than 10°.

Adverse Effects

The main complications following the use of nitrous oxide are those due to varying degrees of hypoxia. Prolonged administration has been followed by megaloblastic anaemia and peripheral neuropathy. Depression of white cell formation may also occur. There is a risk of increased pressure and volume from the diffusion of nitrous oxide into air-containing cavities. Malignant hyperthermia has been reported rarely.

See also Adverse Effects of General Anaesthetics, p.1255.

◊ Reviews.

1. Brodsky JB, Cohen EN. Adverse effects of nitrous oxide. *Med Toxicol* 1986; **1:** 362–74.

Effects on the blood. Nitrous oxide interacts with vitamin B_{12}. This blocks the transmethylation reaction for which vitamin B_{12} is a coenzyme and results in depletion of methionine and tetrahydrofolate. Metabolic consequences have been attributed to depletion of either or both. Interference by nitrous oxide with DNA synthesis prevents production of both leucocytes and red blood cells by the bone marrow. Megaloblastic changes in bone marrow and impaired granulocyte production are found in patients exposed to anaesthetic concentrations of nitrous oxide for 24 hours. In patients with normal bone marrow, stores of mature granulocytes will normally be adequate to prevent leucopenia during exposure for up to 3 days; in patients exposed to nitrous oxide for longer periods of time, leucopenia will develop and exposure for 4 days or longer can result in agranulocytosis. In general, healthy surgical patients can be given nitrous oxide for up to 24 hours without harm. In situations where nitrous oxide is used for more than 24 hours, folinic acid 30 mg twice daily has been given to protect the haematopoietic system. Repeat exposure to nitrous oxide at intervals of less than 3 days will have a cumulative effect on DNA synthesis and megaloblastic marrow changes have been reported following multiple short-term exposure.[1] Depletion of methionine has been implicated in the neurological deficit (see below) seen mainly after chronic use of nitrous oxide. It may also account for the fetotoxicity observed in *rats*, see below.

1. Nunn JF. Clinical aspects of the interaction between nitrous oxide and vitamin B_{12}. *Br J Anaesth* 1987; **59:** 3–13.

Effects on the nervous system. Neurological disorders (mainly myeloneuropathies and neuropathies) have occurred in persons who chronically abuse nitrous oxide. Similar effects have been noted after repeated administration of nitrous oxide in hospitalised patients. These neurological effects are considered to be due to nitrous oxide-induced methionine deficiency (see Effects on the Blood, above).

In patients with undiagnosed subclinical deficiency of vitamin B_{12} (a coenzyme involved in methionine synthesis) neurological manifestations, including those consistent with subacute combined degeneration of the spinal cord, have occurred following a single exposure to nitrous oxide for anaesthesia.[1,2]

1. Schilling RF. Is nitrous oxide a dangerous anesthetic for vitamin B_{12}-deficient subjects? *JAMA* 1986; **255:** 1605–6.
2. Nestor PJ, Stark RJ. Vitamin B_{12} myeloneuropathy precipitated by nitrous oxide anaesthesia. *Med J Aust* 1996; **165:** 174.

Malignant hyperthermia. An 11-year-old girl whose father had died from malignant hyperthermia after anaesthesia developed hyperthermia after anaesthesia with nitrous oxide and oxygen.[1]

1. Ellis FR, *et al*. Malignant hyperpyrexia induced by nitrous oxide and treated with dexamethasone. *BMJ* 1974; **4**: 270–1.

Precautions

Hypoxic anaesthesia is dangerous and nitrous oxide should always be administered with at least 20 to 30% oxygen. Nitrous oxide diffuses into gas-filled body cavities and care is essential when using it in patients at risk from such diffusion such as those with abdominal distension, occlusion of the middle ear, pneumothorax, or similar cavities in the pericardium or peritoneum. Care is also required in patients during or after air encephalography. Oxygen should be administered during emergence from prolonged anaesthesia with nitrous oxide to prevent diffusion hypoxia where the alveolar oxygen concentration is diminished. See also Precautions for General Anaesthetics, p.1255. In addition to the above precautions, mixtures of equal parts of nitrous oxide and oxygen should not be employed for analgesia in patients with head injuries with impairment of consciousness, maxillofacial injuries, decompression sickness, or those heavily sedated.

Nitrous oxide has been subject to abuse.

Driving. A slight but quantified impairment in driving ability was found up to 30 minutes following 15 minutes' inhalation of nitrous oxide/oxygen mixtures.[1]

1. Moyes DG, *et al*. Driving after anaesthetics. *BMJ* 1979; **1**: 1425.

Epidural anaesthesia. Nitrous oxide diffuses into gas-filled body cavities and can increase the size of any air bubbles injected into the epidural space to determine placement of the needle in epidural anaesthesia.[1] This could result in uneven spread of the local anaesthetic and produce inadequate analgesia. The volume of air injected should be limited or another technique used to determine placement of the needle if nitrous oxide is to be given subsequently.

1. Stevens R, *et al*. Fate of extradural air bubbles during inhalation of nitrous oxide. *Br J Anaesth* 1994; **72**: 482P–483P.

Hazard to user. A scavenging system and effective ventilation may be necessary to control the nitrous oxide pollution that can occur when this gas is used for analgesia or anaesthesia. Risk areas include, in addition to operating theatres, delivery rooms and dental surgeries.[1-3] Occupational exposure can lead to serious toxicity with bone-marrow and neurological impairment.[2,3] Reduced fertility has been reported in female dental workers exposed to high concentrations of nitrous oxide;[4] such women also appear to have a higher rate of spontaneous abortion.[5] It has been suggested that nitrous oxide can also affect male fertility;[6] in one study a dose-related increase in the incidence of spontaneous abortion was found in the wives of men with occupational exposure to nitrous oxide.[7]

1. Munley AJ, *et al*. Exposure of midwives to nitrous oxide in four hospitals. *BMJ* 1986; **293**: 1063–4. Correction. *ibid*.: 1280.
2. Sweeney B, *et al*. Toxicity of bone marrow in dentists exposed to nitrous oxide. *BMJ* 1985; **291**: 567–9.
3. Brodsky JB, *et al*. Exposure to nitrous oxide and neurologic disease among dental professionals. *Anesth Analg* 1981; **60**: 297–301.
4. Rowland AS, *et al*. Reduced fertility among women employed as dental assistants exposed to high levels of nitrous oxide. *N Engl J Med* 1992; **327**: 993–7.
5. Rowland AS, *et al*. Nitrous oxide and fertility. *N Engl J Med* 1993; **328**: 284.
6. Brodsky JB. Nitrous oxide and fertility. *N Engl J Med* 1993; **328**: 284–5.
7. Cohen EN, *et al*. Occupational disease in dentistry and chronic exposure to trace anesthetic gases. *J Am Dent Assoc* 1980; **101**: 21–31.

Pregnancy. Nitrous oxide is fetotoxic in *rats*.[1] However, retrospective reviews,[2] and individual case reports[3] have not shown nitrous oxide anaesthesia to be fetotoxic in humans. See also under Hazard to User, above.

1. Lane GA, *et al*. Anesthetics as teratogens: nitrous oxide is fetotoxic, xenon is not. *Science* 1980; **210**: 899–901.
2. Aldridge LM, Tunstall ME. Nitrous oxide and the fetus: a review and the results of a retrospective study of 175 cases of anaesthesia for insertion of Shirodkar suture. *Br J Anaesth* 1986; **58**: 1348–56.
3. Park GR, *et al*. Normal pregnancy following nitrous oxide exposure in the first trimester. *Br J Anaesth* 1986; **58**: 576–7.

Vitamin B₁₂ deficiency. For reports of neurological dysfunction associated with the use of nitrous oxide in patients with undiagnosed subclinical vitamin B_{12} deficiency, see Effects on the Nervous System, above.

Interactions

The concurrent administration of nitrous oxide with an inhalational anaesthetic accelerates the uptake of the latter from the lungs. This phenomenon is known as the *second gas effect*. It is due to the disproportion-

ate absorption of nitrous oxide into the blood resulting in an increased alveolar concentration of the second gas.

The use of high doses of opioids such as fentanyl with nitrous oxide may result in a drop in heart rate and cardiac output.

See also Interactions for General Anaesthetics, p.1255.

Methotrexate. Combined use of nitrous oxide and methotrexate may increase the side-effects of methotrexate therapy, see p.555.

Pharmacokinetics

Nitrous oxide is rapidly absorbed on inhalation. The blood/gas partition coefficient is low and most of the inhaled nitrous oxide is rapidly eliminated unchanged through the lungs though small amounts diffuse through the skin.

◊ Reviews of the pharmacokinetics of nitrous oxide.

1. Dale O, Brown BR. Clinical pharmacokinetics of the inhalational anaesthetics. *Clin Pharmacokinet* 1987; **12**: 145–67.

Uses and Administration

Nitrous oxide is an anaesthetic administered by inhalation. It is a weak anaesthetic with a minimum alveolar concentration (MAC) value (see p.1255) of 110%. It has strong analgesic properties, but produces little muscle relaxation. Nitrous oxide must be administered with air or oxygen, otherwise hypoxia will occur although mixtures with air are rarely used now, oxygen being preferred.

Nitrous oxide with oxygen may be used in the induction and maintenance of general anaesthesia (p.1256). However, it is now mainly employed as an adjuvant to other inhalational anaesthetics, permitting them to be used at significantly lower concentrations. It is also used, with oxygen, in subanaesthetic concentrations for analgesia and sedation in emergency care and obstetric and other painful procedures, including dental procedures (see p.652).

Induction of anaesthesia may be carried out using a mixture containing about 70% nitrous oxide with 30% v/v of oxygen; similar or more dilute mixtures may be used for maintenance. Recovery is usually rapid from nitrous oxide anaesthesia.

Nitrous oxide 25 to 50% v/v with oxygen is used for analgesia; cylinders containing premixed nitrous oxide 50% v/v and oxygen 50% v/v are available in some countries.

Alcohol withdrawal syndrome. The symptoms of acute alcohol withdrawal (p.1131) are usually managed with benzodiazepines but nitrous oxide has been reported[1] to reduce symptoms when tried in alcohol withdrawal. In mild to moderate cases a single administration of up to 20 minutes' duration of a nitrous oxide-oxygen mixture in analgesic doses has been employed.

1. Gillman MA, Lichtigfeld FJ. Analgesic nitrous oxide for alcohol withdrawal: a critical appraisal after 10 years' use. *Postgrad Med J* 1990; **66**: 543–6.

Pain. Nitrous oxide with oxygen is used to provide analgesia and sedation during dental procedures. A mixture of nitrous oxide 50% v/v and oxygen 50% v/v can provide good analgesia without loss of consciousness and is suitable for self-administration. It is used for short procedures such as dressing changes,[1,2] for pain relief during childbirth,[3] in the management of postoperative pain,[1] as an aid to postoperative physiotherapy, and for acute pain in emergency situations such as in ambulances. Continuous inhalation of nitrous oxide-oxygen has been tried for periods longer than 24 hours in the management of pain in terminal cancer.[4] However, such a practice is not usually otherwise recommended[1] as it may result in megaloblastic bone-marrow changes.

1. Hull CJ. Control of pain in the perioperative period. *Br Med Bull* 1988; **44**: 341–56.
2. Gaukroger PB. Pediatric analgesia: which drug, which dose? *Drugs* 1991; **41**: 52–9.
3. Brownridge P. Treatment options for the relief of pain during childbirth. *Drugs* 1991; **41**: 69–80.
4. Fosburg MT, Crone RK. Nitrous oxide analgesia for refractory pain in the terminally ill. *JAMA* 1983; **250**: 511–13.

Preparations

Proprietary Preparations (details are given in Part 3)

Multi-ingredient: UK: Entonox; Equanox.

Propanidid (3120-d)

Propanidid (BAN, USAN, rINN).

Bayer-1420; FBA-1420; TH-2180; WH-5668. Propyl 4-diethyl-carbamoylmethoxy-3-methoxyphenylacetate.

$C_{18}H_{27}NO_5 = 337.4$.

CAS — 1421-14-3.

ATC — N01AX04.

Pharmacopoeias. In Pol.

Profile

Propanidid has been used as an intravenous anaesthetic for rapid induction and for maintenance of general anaesthesia of short duration.

Commercial preparations of propanidid were provided as a liquid in polyethoxylated castor oil. Anaphylactoid reactions associated with the vehicle led to the general withdrawal of propanidid from use.

Porphyria. Propanidid is considered to be unsafe in patients with porphyria although there is conflicting experimental evidence of porphyrinogenicity.

Preparations

Proprietary Preparations (details are given in Part 3)

Mex.: Inductol; Panitol.

Propofol (12677-f)

Propofol (BAN, USAN, rINN).

Disoprofol; ICI-35868; Propofolum. 2,6-Di-isopropylphenol; 2,6-Bis(1-methylethyl)phenol.

$C_{12}H_{18}O = 178.3$.

CAS — 2078-54-8.

ATC — N01AX10.

Pharmacopoeias. In Eur. (see p.vi).

Pharmacopoeial description

Ph. Eur.: A colourless or very light yellow, clear liquid. Very slightly soluble in water; miscible with hexane and with methyl alcohol. Store under an inert gas. Protect from light.

Adverse Effects

Early studies with propofol employed a preparation formulated with polyethoxylated castor oil. Because of anaphylactoid reactions the preparation was reformulated with a vehicle of soya oil and purified egg phosphatide. Adverse effects with this preparation include pain on injection especially if the injection is into a small vein. Local pain may be reduced by injection into a large vein or by injection of intravenous lignocaine [lidocaine]. Apnoea may be frequent; apnoea lasting longer than 60 seconds has been reported to occur in 12% of patients. Cardiovascular effects include a reduction in blood pressure and bradycardia. There have been reports of convulsions and involuntary movements. Fever has occurred. Discoloration of urine has been reported following prolonged use. Anaphylactic-like reactions have been reported. Nausea, vomiting, and headache may occur during recovery.

Children who have received propofol for prolonged sedation have suffered severe reactions and there have been fatalities, see below.

See also Adverse Effects of General Anaesthetics, p.1255.

◊ In May 1989 the UK Committee on Safety of Medicines commented on the 268 reports of adverse reactions to propofol that it had received since propofol was introduced to the UK market, during which period about 2 million patients had been anaesthetised with the drug. Among these reports there were 37 describing seizures (13 of these were in known epileptics), 16 involuntary movements, 10 opisthotonus, 32 anaphylactic reactions, and 13 cardiac arrests. There were also 8 reports of delayed recovery.[1] In 1992 the CSM pointed to the risk of delayed convulsions with propofol and its particular importance for day-case surgery.[2] While the incidence of convulsions was low (170 reports), 31% of the reports described the convulsions as delayed.

In June 1992 the CSM commented on the dangers of propofol for the **sedation of children** in intensive care,[3] a use for which it is contra-indicated in the UK. (This prohibition does not apply to its use for the sedation of ventilated adults—but see below—or to propofol's use as an anaesthetic in children.) The CSM reported that there had been 66 reports worldwide of serious adverse effects in children sedated with propofol and some fatalities had ensued. The children had suffered neurological, cardiac, and renal disorders, hyperlipidaemia, hepatomegaly, and metabolic acidosis. Five deaths had been reported to the CSM. These 5 children[4] were aged 4 weeks to 6 years and doses of propofol ranged from 4 to 10.7 mg per kg body-weight per hour. They developed metabolic acidosis, bradyarrhythmia, and progressive myocardial failure resistant to treatment. The

---

The symbol † denotes a preparation no longer actively marketed

latter has been reported by others to be significantly associated with the use of long-term, **high-dose** propofol infusions.[5] Similar adverse effects resulting in fatalities have also been reported in **adult** patients with head injuries who received high doses of propofol infusion (greater than 5 mg per kg per hour) for long-term sedation.[6] The CSM subsequently reminded prescribers that the recommended dose range for sedation (up to 4 mg per kg per hour) should not be exceeded.[7]

1. Committee on Safety of Medicines. Propofol—convulsions, anaphylaxis and delayed recovery from anaesthesia. *Current Problems 26* 1989.
2. Committee on Safety of Medicines. Propofol and delayed convulsions. *Current Problems 35* 1992.
3. Committee on Safety of Medicines. Serious adverse effects and fatalities in children associated with the use of propofol (Diprivan) for sedation. *Current Problems 34* 1992.
4. Parke TJ, *et al.* Metabolic acidosis and fatal myocardial failure after propofol infusion in children: five case reports. *BMJ* 1992; **305:** 613–16.
5. Bray RJ. Propofol infusion syndrome in children. *Paediatr Anaesth* 1998; **8:** 491–9.
6. Cremer OL, *et al.* Long-term propofol infusion and cardiac failure in adult head-injured patients. *Lancet* 2001; **357:** 117–18.
7. Committee on Safety of Medicines/Medicines Control Agency. Long term, high dose propofol (Diprivan) infusion. *Current Problems* 2001; **27:** 6.

Effects on the cardiovascular system. The main effect of propofol on the cardiovascular system is a fall in both systolic and diastolic blood pressure of 20 to 30%. The compensatory tachycardia seen after a fall in arterial pressure with other intravenous anaesthetics is not usually seen with propofol. Propofol can also decrease systemic vascular resistance, cardiac output, myocardial blood flow, and myocardial oxygen consumption. Bradycardia can occur even in those premedicated with antimuscarinics and can occasionally be profound with asystole developing.[1] Despite these cardiodepressant effects propofol in doses of 1.5 to 2.5 mg per kg body-weight does not generally cause unacceptable haemodynamic changes in patients with a healthy cardiovascular system although concern has been expressed regarding its safety in cardiac surgical patients.[2]

Patients (especially children) who have received propofol for continuous sedation in intensive care units have suffered adverse cardiac reactions with bradyarrhythmia, progressive myocardial failure, and death—see above.

1. Tramèr MR, *et al.* Propofol and bradycardia: causation, frequency and severity. *Br J Anaesth* 1997; **78:** 642–51.
2. Ginsberg R, Lippmann M. Haemodynamic effects of propofol. *Br J Anaesth* 1994; **72:** 370–1.

Effects on lipids. Prolonged administration of propofol may be associated with increases in serum triglycerides. In one patient this was believed to have been the cause of necrotising pancreatitis.[1]

1. Metkus AP, *et al.* A firefighter with pancreatitis. *Lancet* 1996; **348:** 1702.

Effects on mental function. There have been anecdotal reports[1] of disinhibited behaviour or sexually orientated hallucinations associated with the use of propofol, but a study using subanaesthetic doses found no evidence that propofol produced euphoria or other mood changes.[2]

1. Canaday BR. Amorous, disinhibited behaviour associated with propofol. *Clin Pharm* 1993; **12:** 449–51.
2. Whitehead C, *et al.* The subjective effects of low-dose propofol. *Br J Anaesth* 1994; **72** (suppl 1): 89.

Effects on the nervous system. See under Precautions, below.

Effects on respiration. See under Precautions, below.

Hypersensitivity. Anaphylactic reactions associated with polyethoxylated castor oil used in propofol preparations had prompted a change to the use of soya oil and egg phosphatide in the formulation. One group of workers have reported a patient who experienced anaphylactic shock when given the reformulated emulsion.[1]

1. Laxenaire MC, *et al.* Anaphylactic shock due to propofol. *Lancet* 1988; **ii:** 739–40.

Infection. Between June 1990 and February 1993 62 cases of postsurgical infections identified in 7 hospitals in the USA were attributed to improper handling of propofol.[1] The infusion was not prepared aseptically and the syringes used in the infusion pumps were reused for several patients. Propofol is formulated as a soybean fat emulsion and the injection contains no antimicrobial preservative although, in the USA, the formulation now contains the microbial-retarding agent, disodium edetate (see under Administration, below). However, either formulation still has the potential to support microbial growth. The UK and USA manufacturers now warn of the importance of aseptic technique in the preparation and administration of propofol. Microbial multiplication did not appear to be clinically significant when propofol infusions were prepared and administered using conventional aseptic techniques.[2]

1. Bennett SN, *et al.* Postoperative infections traced to contamination of an intravenous anesthetic, propofol. *N Engl J Med* 1995; **333:** 147–54.
2. Farrington M, *et al.* Do infusions of midazolam and propofol pose an infection risk to critically ill patients? *Br J Anaesth* 1994; **72:** 415–17.

Malignant hyperthermia. From an *in-vitro* study it was concluded that propofol does not trigger malignant hyperthermia.[1] There is a report of the administration of propofol to 19 patients

considered susceptible to malignant hyperthermia; none of the patients showed signs of malignant hyperthermia.[2]

1. Denborough M, Hopkinson KC. Propofol and malignant hyperpyrexia. *Lancet* 1988; **i:** 191.
2. Harrison GG. Propofol in malignant hyperthermia. *Lancet* 1991; **337:** 503.

Pain on injection. The manufacturers have suggested the use of lignocaine [lidocaine] to reduce the pain associated with injection of propofol; alternatively, the larger veins in the forearm and antecubital fossa can be used. Studies indicate that alfentanil[1] and metoclopramide[2] might also be effective. It has been suggested[3] that the analgesic action of lignocaine [lidocaine] and possibly metoclopramide is due to a pH-lowering effect, rather than to a local anaesthetic action, permitting more propofol to exist in the oily phase of the emulsion. Propofol concentrated in the aqueous phase is believed to be responsible for the pain on injection. However, iontophoretically applied lignocaine [lidocaine] has also been found to be effective.[4]

1. Fletcher JE, *et al.* Pretreatment with alfentanil reduces pain caused by propofol. *Br J Anaesth* 1994; **72:** 342–4.
2. Ganta R, Fee JPH. Pain on injection of propofol: comparison of lignocaine with metoclopramide. *Br J Anaesth* 1992; **69:** 316–17.
3. Eriksson M, *et al.* Effect of lignocaine and pH on propofol-induced pain. *Br J Anaesth* 1997; **78:** 502–6.
4. Sadler PJ, *et al.* Iontophoretically applied lidocaine reduces pain on propofol injection. *Br J Anaesth* 1999; **82:** 432–4.

Urine discoloration. A case report of dark green urine in a 16-year-old during a prolonged infusion of propofol.[1]

1. Bodenham A, *et al.* Propofol infusion and green urine. *Lancet* 1987; **ii:** 740.

Precautions

Propofol should not be given to patients known to be allergic to it. Propofol should be administered with caution to patients with hypovolaemia, epilepsy, lipid metabolism disorders, and the elderly. Since there have been reports of delayed convulsions associated with the use of propofol it is recommended that special care should be taken when propofol is used for day-case surgery. When used in patients with increased intracranial pressure it should be administered slowly to avoid a substantial decrease in mean arterial pressure and a resultant decrease in cerebral perfusion pressure. It is also recommended that propofol should not be used with ECT. Premedication with an antimuscarinic may be advisable since propofol does not cause vagal inhibition.

Propofol is used to provide continuous sedation for ventilated adult patients under intensive care. Account should be taken of increasing the patient's lipid load. If the duration of sedation is in excess of 3 days, lipid concentrations should be monitored. Children aged 16 years or less should not be sedated in this manner with propofol (see under Adverse Effects, above). Propofol is not recommended for use in obstetrics including caesarean section. See also Precautions for General Anaesthetics, p.1255.

For the need for aseptic handling of propofol see Administration, below.

CNS effects. Epileptic activity was seen[1] on the EEGs of 3 patients given propofol and it was suggested that it might be useful in ECT, but others[2,3] found that the duration of seizures was less with propofol anaesthesia than with methohexital anaesthesia. It has been suggested that propofol should not be used with ECT[4] and this is the advice of the manufacturer.

One group of workers considers that abnormal movements induced by propofol are not associated with cortical seizure activity.[5,6] They appear to be more frequent with low doses of propofol and can be abolished in children by increasing the induction dose of propofol from 3 to 5 mg per kg body-weight.[6]

1. Hodkinson BP, *et al.* Propofol and the electroencephalogram. *Lancet* 1987; **ii:** 1518.
2. Simpson KH, *et al.* Seizure duration after methohexitone or propofol for induction of anaesthesia for electroconvulsive therapy (ECT). *Br J Anaesth* 1987; **59:** 1323P–4P.
3. Rampton AJ, *et al.* Propofol and electroconvulsive therapy. *Lancet* 1988; **i:** 296–7.
4. Anonymous. Addendum: propofol better avoided with ECT at present. *Drug Ther Bull* 1990; **28:** 72.
5. Borgeat A, *et al.* Spontaneous excitatory movements during recovery from propofol anaesthesia in an infant: EEG evaluation. *Br J Anaesth* 1993; **70:** 459–61.
6. Borgeat A, *et al.* Propofol and epilepsy: time to clarify. *Anesth Analg* 1994; **78:** 198–9.

Impaired respiration. The manufacturer has stated[1] that some patients who have received propofol for sedation in regional anaesthesia have experienced bradypnoea or hypoxaemia, or both. A reduction in oxygen saturation has also been noted in other patients sedated for endoscopy.[2] The manufacturer therefore recommends that oxygen saturation should be

monitored in all such patients and that oxygen supplementation should be readily available.

1. Arnold BDC. Sedation with propofol during regional anaesthesia. *Br J Anaesth* 1993; **70:** 112.
2. Patterson KW, *et al.* Propofol sedation for outpatient upper gastrointestinal endoscopy: comparison with midazolam. *Br J Anaesth* 1991; **67:** 108–11.

Interactions

The concurrent administration of propofol with other CNS depressants including those used in premedication may increase the sedative, anaesthetic, and cardiorespiratory depressant effects of propofol. It is recommended that propofol is administered after opioids so that the dose of propofol can be carefully titrated against the response. The dosage of propofol should be reduced if given with nitrous oxide or halogenated anaesthetics. Although propofol does not potentiate the effects of neuromuscular blockers, bradycardia and asystole have occurred after administration of propofol with atracurium or suxamethonium (but see under Adverse Effects, above for the effects of propofol itself on the cardiovascular system).

See also Interactions of General Anaesthetics, p.1255.

◊ In one study mean blood concentrations of propofol were higher in patients pretreated with *fentanyl* compared with patients maintained only on nitrous oxide.[1] However, others[2] were unable to confirm this interaction. Concomitant administration of *halothane* or *isoflurane* has also been reported to increase serum concentrations of propofol.[3] Propofol and *midazolam* have been reported to act synergistically.[4–6] Synergy has also been reported between propofol and *etomidate*.[7] A reduction in the amount of propofol required to provide adequate hypnosis[8] or sedation[9] has been reported after the administration of *bupivacaine*[8] or *lignocaine [lidocaine]*.[8,9] Premedication with *clonidine* has been reported[10] to reduce intraoperative requirements of propofol and the dose of propofol required for induction is reduced in patients given *metoclopramide*.[11]

1. Cockshott ID, *et al.* Pharmacokinetics of propofol in female patients. *Br J Anaesth* 1987; **59:** 1103–10.
2. Dixon J, *et al.* Study of the possible interaction between fentanyl and propofol using a computer-controlled infusion of propofol. *Br J Anaesth* 1990; **64:** 142–7.
3. Grundmann U, *et al.* Propofol and volatile anaesthetics. *Br J Anaesth* 1994; **72** (suppl 1): 88.
4. Short TG, Chui PT. Propofol and midazolam act synergistically in combination. *Br J Anaesth* 1991; **67:** 539–45.
5. McClune S, *et al.* Synergistic interaction between midazolam and propofol. *Br J Anaesth* 1992; **69:** 240–5.
6. Teh J, *et al.* Pharmacokinetic interactions between midazolam and propofol: an infusion study. *Br J Anaesth* 1994; **72:** 62–5.
7. Drummond GB, Cairns DT. Do propofol and etomidate interact kinetically during induction of anaesthesia? *Br J Anaesth* 1994; **73:** 272P.
8. Ben-Shlomo I, *et al.* Hypnotic effect of iv propofol is enhanced by im administration of either lignocaine or bupivacaine. *Br J Anaesth* 1997; **78:** 375–7.
9. Mallick A, *et al.* Local anaesthesia to the airway reduces sedation requirements in patients undergoing artificial ventilation. *Br J Anaesth* 1996; **77:** 731–4.
10. Guglielminotti J, *et al.* Effects of premedication on dose requirements for propofol: comparison of clonidine and hydroxyzine. *Br J Anaesth* 1998; **80:** 733–6.
11. Page VJ, Chhipa JH. Metoclopramide reduces the induction dose of propofol. *Acta Anaesthesiol Scand* 1997; **41:** 256–9.

Pharmacokinetics

The pharmacokinetics of propofol are best described by a 3-compartment model. After a single bolus dose, two distribution phases are seen. The first phase has a half-life of 2 to 4 minutes. This is followed by a slow distribution phase with a half-life of 30 to 60 minutes. Significant metabolism of propofol occurs during the second phase. The termination of anaesthetic effect after a single intravenous bolus or maintenance infusion is due to extensive redistribution from the brain to other tissues and to metabolic clearance. Propofol is over 95% bound to plasma proteins. It undergoes extensive hepatic metabolism to conjugates which are eliminated in the urine. The terminal half-life ranges from 3 to 12 hours; with prolonged use, the terminal half-life may be longer. The pharmacokinetics of propofol do not appear to be altered by gender, chronic hepatic cirrhosis, or chronic renal impairment. Propofol crosses the placental barrier and is distributed into breast milk.

◊ References.

1. Saint-Maurice C, *et al.* Pharmacokinetics of propofol in young children after a single dose. *Br J Anaesth* 1989; **63:** 667–70.
2. Kanto J, Gepts E. Pharmacokinetic implications for the clinical use of propofol. *Clin Pharmacokinet* 1989; **17:** 308–26.
3. Gin T, *et al.* Pharmacokinetics of propofol in women undergoing elective caesarean section. *Br J Anaesth* 1990; **64:** 148–53.
4. Servin F, *et al.* Pharmacokinetics of propofol infusions in patients with cirrhosis. *Br J Anaesth* 1990; **65:** 177–83.

5. Jones RDM, *et al*. Pharmacokinetics of propofol in children. *Br J Anaesth* 1990; **65:** 661–7.
6. Morgan DJ, *et al*. Pharmacokinetics of propofol when given by intravenous infusion. *Br J Clin Pharmacol* 1990; **30:** 144–8.
7. Gin T, *et al*. Disposition of propofol at caesarean section and in the postpartum period. *Br J Anaesth* 1991; **67:** 49–53.
8. Bailie GR, *et al*. Pharmacokinetics of propofol during and after long term continuous infusion for maintenance of sedation in ICU patients. *Br J Anaesth* 1992; **68:** 486–91.
9. Altmayer P, *et al*. Propofol binding in human blood. *Br J Anaesth* 1994; **72** (suppl 1): 86.
10. Oei-Lim VLB, *et al*. Pharmacokinetics of propofol during conscious sedation using target-controlled infusion in anxious patients undergoing dental treatment. *Br J Anaesth* 1998; **80:** 324–31.

Uses and Administration

Propofol is a short-acting anaesthetic given intravenously for the induction and maintenance of general anaesthesia (p.1256). It is also used for sedation (p.652) in adult patients undergoing diagnostic procedures, in those undergoing surgery in conjunction with local or regional anaesthesia, and in ventilated adult patients under intensive care. When used for anaesthesia, induction is rapid, as is recovery. Propofol has no analgesic activity and supplementary analgesia may be required.

Propofol is available as a 1 or 2% emulsion. The 1% emulsion may be given by intravenous injection or infusion, but the 2% emulsion is for infusion only. Infusions and injections should be prepared using aseptic techniques, see under Administration, below.

Induction of **anaesthesia** is generally carried out by giving propofol by injection or infusion at a rate of 40 mg every 10 seconds; a rate of 20 mg every 10 seconds may be used in high-risk patients including elderly, neurosurgical, and debilitated patients. Most *adults* under 55 years of age will be anaesthetised by a dose of 1.5 to 2.5 mg per kg body-weight; high-risk patients usually require a dose of 1 to 1.5 mg per kg. When used for maintenance propofol is infused at a rate of between 4 to 12 mg per kg per hour (or 3 to 6 mg per kg per hour for elderly and debilitated patients); alternatively intermittent bolus injections of 20 to 50 mg may be given; rapid administration of bolus doses should be avoided in high-risk patients.

A novel delivery system is also available for the induction and maintenance of anaesthesia in adults. The Diprifusor target-controlled infusion system allows the speed of induction and depth of anaesthesia to be controlled by specifying target blood concentrations of propofol. Initial target concentrations for induction range from 4 to 8 μg per mL for patients under 55 years of age; lower initial target concentrations should be used in older and debilitated patients and should be increased gradually thereafter in steps of 0.5 to 1 μg per mL at intervals of 1 minute to achieve a gradual induction of anaesthesia. Target concentrations for maintenance are 3 to 6 μg per mL.

Children over 3 years of age can be given a dose of 2.5 to 3.5 mg per kg for induction adjusted as necessary; a dose of 9 to 15 mg per kg per hour by intravenous infusion or intermittent bolus injections is suitable for maintenance. In the UK propofol is also licensed for induction of anaesthesia in children 1 month to 3 years of age; it is recommended that the dose should be adjusted for age and/or weight and administered slowly until the onset of anaesthesia. In the USA, children 2 months to 3 years of age may receive propofol for maintenance of anaesthesia; doses are similar to those used in children aged 3 years and over.

For **sedation** in diagnostic and surgical procedures in *adults* an initial infusion of 6 to 9 mg per kg per hour may be given for 3 to 5 minutes; alternatively 0.5 to 1 mg per kg may be injected slowly over 1 to 5 minutes. An infusion of 1.5 to 4.5 mg per kg per hour may be used for maintenance of sedation. High-risk patients usually require a 20% reduction in the maintenance dose.

For the sedation of ventilated adults propofol can be given by intravenous infusion in a dose of 0.3 to 4 mg per kg per hour. If the duration of sedation is in excess of 3 days, lipid concentrations should be monitored.

The symbol † denotes a preparation no longer actively marketed

---

Propofol is contra-indicated for sedation in *children* aged 16 years or less.

◊ Reviews.
1. Langley MS, Heel RC. Propofol: a review of its pharmacodynamic and pharmacokinetic properties and use as an intravenous anaesthetic. *Drugs* 1988; **35:** 334–72.
2. Larijani GE, *et al*. Clinical pharmacology of propofol: an intravenous anesthetic agent. *DICP Ann Pharmacother* 1989; **23:** 743–9.
3. Bryson HM, *et al*. Propofol: an update of its use in anaesthesia and conscious sedation. *Drugs* 1995; **50:** 513–59.
4. Fulton B, Sorkin EM. Propofol: an overview of its pharmacology and a review of its clinical efficacy in intensive care sedation. *Drugs* 1995; **50:** 636–57.

Administration. Propofol is formulated as an oil in water emulsion for injection. Strict aseptic techniques must be maintained when handling propofol as, in some countries including the UK, the parenteral product contains no antimicrobial preservatives and the vehicle can support rapid growth of microorganisms. Aseptic techniques must also be applied to formulations, such as those available in the USA, that contain the microbial-retarding agent disodium edetate as microbial growth is still possible. An emulsion containing 1% of propofol may be diluted with glucose 5% immediately before administration but it should not be diluted to a concentration of less than 2 mg per mL. An emulsion containing 2% of propofol should not be diluted. The use of a 5-micron filter needle to withdraw propofol emulsion from an ampoule does not cause significant loss of drug.[1] A reduction in concentration of propofol can occur when the diluted emulsion is run through polyvinyl chloride intravenous tubing.[1] Propofol 1% or 2% may be administered into a running intravenous infusion through a Y-site close to the injection site and under these circumstances it is compatible with glucose 5%, sodium chloride 0.9%, and glucose with sodium chloride intravenous solutions.

1. Bailey LC, *et al*. Effect of syringe filter and I.V. administration set on delivery of propofol emulsion. *Am J Hosp Pharm* 1991; **48:** 2627–30.

Nausea and vomiting. It is commonly believed that propofol is associated with less postoperative nausea and vomiting than some other anaesthetics.[1,2] However, a review[3] concluded that any reduction in nausea and vomiting when using propofol anaesthesia may be short term and clinically relevant only for maintenance anaesthesia in procedures with an inherent risk of nausea and vomiting.

There are also reports[4-8] indicating that propofol may have some intrinsic antiemetic action when used in sub-hypnotic doses although a study[9] of the effect of sedative and non-sedative (sub-hypnotic) doses against apomorphine-induced vomiting has suggested that any antiemetic effect is probably due to sedation.

1. McCollum JSC, *et al*. The antiemetic action of propofol. *Anaesthesia* 1988; **43:** 239–40.
2. Woodward WM, *et al*. Comparison of post-operative nausea and vomiting after thiopentone/isoflurane or propofol infusion for 'bat-ear' correction in children. *Br J Anaesth* 1994; **72** (suppl 1): 92.
3. Tramèr M, *et al*. Propofol anaesthesia and postoperative nausea and vomiting: quantitative systematic review of randomized controlled studies. *Br J Anaesth* 1997; **78:** 247–55.
4. Borgeat A, *et al*. Adjuvant propofol for refractory cisplatin-associated nausea and vomiting. *Lancet* 1992; **340:** 679–80.
5. Törn K, *et al*. Effects of sub-hypnotic doses of propofol on the side effects of intrathecal morphine. *Br J Anaesth* 1994; **73:** 411–12.
6. Borgeat A, *et al*. Adjuvant propofol enables better control of nausea and emesis secondary to chemotherapy for breast cancer. *Can J Anaesth* 1994; **41:** 1117–19.
7. Ewalenko P, *et al*. Antiemetic effect of subhypnotic doses of propofol after thyroidectomy. *Br J Anaesth* 1996; **77:** 463–7.
8. Gan TJ, *et al*. Determination of plasma concentrations of propofol associated with 50% reduction in postoperative nausea. *Anesthesiology* 1997; **87:** 779–84.
9. Thörn S-E, *et al*. Propofol effects upon apomorphine induced vomiting. *Br J Anaesth* 1994; **72** (suppl 1): 90.

Pruritus. Propofol is one of many drugs that have been tried in the management of pruritus (p.1106). Sub-hypnotic doses of propofol appear to have an antipruritic action. It has been found to be effective in the treatment and prophylaxis of pruritus associated with epidural and intrathecal morphine[1,2] and appears to be able to relieve cholestasis-associated pruritus.[3] It has been suggested that propofol might act by suppression of the spinal transmission of pruritic signals.

1. Borgeat A, *et al*. Subhypnotic doses of propofol relieve pruritus induced by epidural and intrathecal morphine. *Anesthesiology* 1992; **76:** 510–12.
2. Törn K, *et al*. Effects of sub-hypnotic doses of propofol on the side effects of intrathecal morphine. *Br J Anaesth* 1994; **73:** 411–12.
3. Borgeat A, *et al*. Subhypnotic doses of propofol relieve pruritus associated with liver disease. *Gastroenterology* 1993; **104:** 244–7.

Status epilepticus. Anaesthesia in conjunction with assisted ventilation may be instituted to control refractory tonic-clonic status epilepticus (p.341). A short-acting barbiturate such as thiopental is usually used. Propofol is also used[1,2] although good controlled studies of its effectiveness are lacking, and it has caused seizures when used in anaesthesia (see under Precautions, above). It should be given with caution to patients with epilepsy. It has a rapid onset of action and its effects are maintained while the infusion is maintained; recovery is rapid

---

on discontinuation. However, the risks of respiratory and cerebral depression, as well as of lipid overload with prolonged therapy, should be borne in mind. It may induce involuntary movements and care is required to distinguish these from seizures. One suggested regimen for management[2] is an initial intravenous bolus of 2 mg per kg body-weight which can be repeated if seizures continue. This may be followed by an infusion of 5 to 10 mg per kg per hour guided by EEG monitoring. The dose should be gradually reduced and the infusion tapered 12 hours after seizure activity is halted. Lower doses should be used in the elderly. A study[3] comparing propofol with high-dose barbiturates in patients with refractory status epilepticus concluded that recurrent seizures were common when propofol infusions were suddenly discontinued but not when the infusions were gradually tapered.

1. Brown LA, Levin GM. Role of propofol in refractory status epilepticus. *Ann Pharmacother* 1998; **32:** 1053–9.
2. Shorvon S. Tonic clonic status epilepticus. *J Neurol Neurosurg Psychiatry* 1993; **56:** 125–34.
3. Stecker MM, *et al*. Treatment of refractory status epilepticus with propofol: clinical and pharmacokinetic findings. *Epilepsia* 1998; **39:** 18–26.

Preparations

Proprietary Preparations (details are given in Part 3)
Aust.: Diprivan; *Austral.:* Diprivan; *Belg.:* Diprivan; *Braz.:* Diprivan; *Canad.:* Diprivan; *Denm.:* Diprivan; Recofol†; *Fin.:* Diprivan; Recofol; *Fr.:* Diprivan; *Ger.:* Disoprivan; Klimofol; *Hong Kong:* Diprivan; *Irl.:* Diprivan; *Israel:* Diprivan; Diprofol; Recofol; *Ital.:* Diprivan; *Mex.:* Diprivan; Fresofol; Recofol; *Neth.:* Diprivan; *Norw.:* Diprivan; Recofol; *NZ:* Diprivan; *Port.:* Diprivan; Recofol; *S.Afr.:* Diprivan; *Singapore:* Diprivan; Pofol; Recofol; *Spain:* Diprivan; Ivofol; Recofol; *Swed.:* Diprivan; Recofol; *Switz.:* Ansiven; Disoprivan; Recofol; *Thai.:* Diprivan; *UK:* Diprivan; *USA:* Diprivan.

Sevoflurane (13234-m)

Sevoflurane *(BAN, USAN, rINN)*.

BAX-3084; MR-654. Fluoromethyl 2,2,2-trifluoro-1-(trifluoromethyl)ethyl ether; 1,1,1,3,3,3-Hexafluoro-2-(fluoromethoxy)-propane.

$C_4H_3F_7O = 200.1$.

CAS — 28523-86-6.

ATC — N01AB08.

Adverse Effects

As with other halogenated anaesthetics sevoflurane may cause cardiorespiratory depression, hypotension, and malignant hyperthermia. However, the effects of sevoflurane on heart rate have only been seen at higher concentrations and it appears to have little effect on heart rhythm in comparison to other halogenated anaesthetics. Sevoflurane appears to sensitise the myocardium to sympathomimetics to a lesser extent than halothane or enflurane. Other effects seen with sevoflurane include agitation, especially in children, laryngospasm, and increased cough and salivation. Acute renal failure has also been noted. Shivering, nausea, and vomiting have been reported in the postoperative period.

See also Adverse Effects of General Anaesthetics, p.1255.

Effects on the cardiovascular system. The cardiovascular effects of sevoflurane are similar to those of isoflurane (see p.1261) but it does not produce coronary steal. Also sevoflurane produces less tachycardia than isoflurane suggesting that it may be preferable in those predisposed to myocardial ischaemia.

Effects on the kidneys. Investigations[1] of the nephrotoxic potential of sevoflurane have found no evidence of renal function impairment despite peak plasma-fluoride ion concentrations greater than 50 nanomol per mL (a level considered to be nephrotoxic) being recorded in some patients at the end of sevoflurane anaesthesia.[2] The lack of renal toxicity with sevoflurane may be due to low concentrations of intrarenally generated fluoride ions;[3] in comparison, methoxyflurane defluorination in the kidney is much greater and may contribute to its known nephrotoxicity.

Compound A, formed by the breakdown of sevoflurane by carbon dioxide absorbents (see under Precautions, below), is nephrotoxic in *rats*.[1] However, studies in humans undergoing sevoflurane anaesthesia have detected no renal impairment postoperatively even when compound A was detected in the anaesthetic circuits.

1. Malan TP. Sevoflurane and renal function. *Anesth Analg* 1995; **81:** S39–S45.
2. Kobayashi Y, *et al*. Serum and urinary inorganic fluoride concentrations after prolonged inhalation of sevoflurane in humans. *Anesth Analg* 1992; **74:** 753–7.
3. Kharasch ED, *et al*. Human kidney methoxyflurane and sevoflurane metabolism: intrarenal fluoride production as a possible mechanism of methoxyflurane nephrotoxicity. *Anesthesiology* 1995; **82:** 689–99.

Effects on the liver. There have been signs of hepatotoxicity in *animal* studies but in studies in humans, markers for hepatocellular dysfunction were no greater following sevoflurane anaesthesia than those after isoflurane.[1] Also the metabolism of sevoflurane differs from other halogenated anaesthetics in such a way that metabolites implicated in liver toxicity are not formed (see Pharmacokinetics, below).

1. Darling JR, *et al.* Comparison of the effects of sevoflurane with those of isoflurane on hepatic glutathione-S-transferase concentrations after body surface surgery. *Br J Anaesth* 1994; **73:** 268P.

Effects on the nervous system. Clonic and tonic seizure-like movements of the extremities have been reported[1] in a child during induction of anaesthesia using sevoflurane. It was considered that this might have been a result of seizure activity in the CNS or due to myoclonus of the extremities.

1. Adachi M, *et al.* Seizure-like movements during induction of anaesthesia with sevoflurane. *Br J Anaesth* 1992; **68:** 214–15.

Precautions

As with other halogenated anaesthetics, patients with known or suspected susceptibility to malignant hyperthermia should not be anaesthetised with sevoflurane. Although the effects of sevoflurane on cerebral pressure is minimal in normal patients, safety in those with raised intracranial pressure has not been established and therefore sevoflurane should be used with caution.

See also Precautions for General Anaesthetics, p.1255.

Carbon dioxide absorbents. The breakdown of sevoflurane by carbon dioxide absorbents (such as soda lime) results in the formation of pentafluoroisopropenyl fluoromethyl ether (PIFE; compound A), and trace amounts of pentafluoromethoxy isopropyl fluoromethyl ether (PMFE; Compound B). Compound A has been shown to be nephrotoxic in *rats* (see under Effects on the kidneys, above). Even during short exposure times, as required for induction of anaesthesia, use of moist soda lime is important to minimise sevoflurane degradation, which is aggravated by a high potassium hydroxide content of the soda lime.[1]

The manufacturers state that increased amounts of compound A may be formed if barium hydroxide lime is used as a carbon dioxide absorbent rather than soda lime.

1. Funk W, *et al.* Dry soda lime markedly degrades sevoflurane during simulated inhalation induction. *Br J Anaesth* 1999; **82:** 193–8.

Interactions

Care is advised if adrenaline [epinephrine] or other sympathomimetics are given during sevoflurane anaesthesia. The effects of competitive neuromuscular blockers such as atracurium are enhanced by sevoflurane (see p.1335). The metabolism, and hence toxicity, of sevoflurane may be increased by drugs or compounds that induce cytochrome P450 isoenzyme CYP2E1 including isoniazid and alcohol.

See also Interactions of General Anaesthetics, p.1255.

◊ References.
1. Dale O. Drug interactions in anaesthesia: focus on desflurane and sevoflurane. *Baillieres Clin Anaesthesiol* 1995; **9:** 105–17.

Pharmacokinetics

Sevoflurane is absorbed on inhalation. The blood/gas partition coefficient is low. Up to 5% of the absorbed dose of sevoflurane is metabolised in the liver by the cytochrome P450 isoenzyme CYP2E1 and defluorinated to its major metabolites hexafluoroisopropanol (HFIP), inorganic fluoride, and carbon dioxide. HFIP is rapidly conjugated with glucuronic acid and eliminated in the urine. Sevoflurane crosses the placenta.

◊ References.
1. Behne M, *et al.* Clinical Pharmacokinetics of sevoflurane. *Clin Pharmacokinet* 1999; **36:** 13–26.

Uses and Administration

Sevoflurane is a volatile halogenated anaesthetic administered by inhalation. It has a minimum alveolar concentration (MAC) value (see p.1255) ranging from 1.4% in the elderly to 3.3% in neonates. It is employed for the induction and maintenance of general anaesthesia (p.1256). It is non-flammable. Sevoflurane has a nonpungent odour and does not cause respiratory irritation. It also has muscle relaxant properties which may be sufficient for some surgical procedures to be performed without a neuro-

muscular blocker. However, it possesses no analgesic properties.

Sevoflurane is administered using a calibrated vaporiser. For induction, sevoflurane is given in concentrations of up to 5% v/v in adults, with oxygen or oxygen and nitrous oxide. Concentrations of up to 7% v/v may be used in children. A short-acting barbiturate or other intravenous induction agent may be given before inhaling sevoflurane. Induction with sevoflurane is rapid (surgical anaesthesia in less than 2 minutes) and smooth because of its nonpungent odour. Maintenance of anaesthesia is achieved with a concentration of 0.5 to 3% v/v with or without nitrous oxide.

◊ Reviews.
1. Patel SS, Goa KL. Sevoflurane: a review of its pharmacodynamic and pharmacokinetic properties and its clinical use in general anaesthesia. *Drugs* 1996; **51:** 658–700.
2. Smith I, *et al.* Sevoflurane—a long-awaited volatile anaesthetic. *Br J Anaesth* 1996; **76:** 435–45.
3. Grounds RM, Newman PJ. Sevoflurane. *Br J Hosp Med* 1997; **57:** 43–6.

Preparations

Proprietary Preparations (details are given in Part 3)
Aust.: Sevorane; *Austral.:* Sevorane; *Belg.:* Sevorane; *Canad.:* Sevorane; *Denm.:* Sevorane; *Fin.:* Sevorane; *Fr.:* Sevorane; *Ger.:* Sevorane; *Hong Kong:* Sevorane; *Irl.:* Sevorane; *Israel:* Sevorane; *Ital.:* Sevorane; *Mex.:* Sevorane; *Neth.:* Sevorane; *Norw.:* Sevorane; *NZ:* Ultane; *S.Afr.:* Ultane; *Singapore:* Sevorane; *Spain:* Sevorane; *Swed.:* Sevorane; *Switz.:* Sevorane; *Thai.:* Sevorane; *USA:* Ultane.

Sodium Oxybate (3121-n)

Sodium Oxybate *(USAN)*.
NSC-84223; Sodium Gamma-hydroxybutyrate; Wy-3478. Sodium 4-hydroxybutyrate.
$C_4H_7NaO_3 = 126.1$.
CAS — 502-85-2.
Pharmacopoeias. In *Chin.*

Adverse Effects

When used in general anaesthesia side-effects with sodium oxybate include abnormal muscle movements during the induction period and nausea and vomiting. Occasional emergence delirium has been reported. Bradycardia frequently occurs. Respiration may be slowed and hypokalaemia has been reported.

Patients receiving sodium oxybate orally for the management of narcolepsy may experience dizziness, lightheadedness, and confusion; gastrointestinal effects and enuresis occur occasionally.

See also Adverse Effects of General Anaesthetics, p.1255.

Effects on electrolyte balance. A report of severe metabolic disorders occurring during therapy with sodium oxybate and tetracosactide in 4 patients with severe head injuries.[1] The disorders consisted of hypernatraemia, hypokalaemia, and metabolic acidosis.

1. Béal JL, *et al.* Troubles métaboliques induits par l'association gamma-hydroxy butyrate de sodium et tétracosactide chez le traumatisé crânien. *Thérapie* 1983; **38:** 569–71.

Precautions

Sodium oxybate should not be given to patients with severe hypertension, bradycardia, conditions associated with defects of cardiac conduction, epilepsy, eclampsia, renal impairment, or alcohol abuse.

See also Precautions for General Anaesthetics, p.1255.

Abuse. Reports[1] of acute poisoning with sodium oxybate following illicit use led the FDA in the USA to issue warnings[2] about its potential for abuse. It is usually supplied illicitly as the sodium salt under a variety of names including GHB or GBH, gamma-hydroxybutyrate, liquid ecstasy, liquid X, sodium oxybutyrate, and somatomax PM and has been promoted for body building, weight loss, as a psychedelic substance, and as a sleep aid. Adverse effects include vomiting, drowsiness, amnesia, hypotonia, vertigo, respiratory depression, and involuntary movements. Seizure-like activity, bradycardia, hypotension, and respiratory arrest have also been reported. Resolution of symptoms occurs spontaneously over 2 to 96 hours. However, some patients have required hospitalisation and respiratory support and deaths have been reported in both the UK[3] and USA.[4] Severity of symptoms depends on the dose of sodium oxybate and the presence of other drugs such as alcohol, benzodiazepines, cannabis, or amfetamines. Prolonged use of large doses may lead to a withdrawal syndrome on discontinuation.[5]

There is also a report of CNS depression following ingestion of a chemical derivative, gamma-butyrolactone (GBL).[6]

1. Centers for Disease Control. Multistate outbreak of poisonings associated with illicit use of gamma hydroxy butyrate. *JAMA* 1991; **265:** 447–8.
2. Food and Drug Administration. Warning about GHB. *JAMA* 1991; **265:** 1802.

3. Anonymous. GBH death indicates increasing problem. *Pharm J* 1996; **256:** 441.
4. Centers for Disease Control. Gamma hydroxy butyrate use—New York and Texas, 1995–1996. *JAMA* 1997; **277:** 1511.
5. Galloway GP, *et al.* Physical dependence on sodium oxybate. *Lancet* 1994; **343:** 57.
6. LoVecchio F, *et al.* Butyrolactone-induced central nervous system depression after ingestion of RenewTrient, a "dietary supplement" *N Engl J Med* 1998; **339:** 847–8.

Porphyria. Sodium oxybate is considered to be unsafe in patients with porphyria because it has been shown to be porphyrinogenic in *animals* or *in-vitro* systems.

Interactions

Sodium oxybate enhances the effects of opioid analgesics and competitive neuromuscular blockers. The action of sodium oxybate may be potentiated by benzodiazepines or antipsychotics.

See also Interactions of General Anaesthetics, p.1255.

Pharmacokinetics

Following oral administration sodium oxybate is absorbed from the gastrointestinal tract and rapidly metabolised in the liver to carbon dioxide and water. In one study the mean values for the terminal half-life ranged from 20 to 23 minutes. It crosses the blood-brain barrier and the placental barrier.

◊ References.
1. Palatini P, *et al.* Dose-dependent absorption and elimination of gamma-hydroxybutyric acid in healthy volunteers. *Eur J Clin Pharmacol* 1993; **45:** 353–6.
2. Scharf MB, *et al.* Pharmacokinetics of gammahydroxybutyrate (GHB) in narcoleptic patients. *Sleep* 1998; **21:** 507–14.

Uses and Administration

Sodium oxybate has hypnotic properties and, in its endogenous form, Gamma-hydroxybutyrate (a catabolite of gamma-aminobutyric acid), increases dopamine concentrations in the brain. It is given intravenously to produce general anaesthesia (p.1256) usually in conjunction with an opioid analgesic and a neuroleptic. Skeletal muscle relaxants may also be necessary. Sodium oxybate given orally is being investigated for use in narcolepsy.

In general anaesthesia a solution of sodium oxybate equivalent to 20% of the acid is administered slowly by intravenous injection, usually in a dose of 60 mg per kg body-weight; further smaller doses may be required in long procedures. In children up to 100 mg per kg may be necessary.

Alcohol withdrawal syndrome. Gamma-hydroxybutyric acid has been reported[1] to be effective in reducing symptoms of alcohol withdrawal (p.1131) and to be of use as an aid in the maintenance of abstinence.[2,3] However, following reports of CNS toxicity associated with abuse of gamma-hydroxybutyric acid its role in the treatment of substance abuse disorders appears questionable.[4]

1. Gallimberti L, *et al.* Gamma-hydroxybutyric acid for treatment of alcohol withdrawal syndrome. *Lancet* 1989; **ii:** 787–9.
2. Gallimberti L, *et al.* Gamma-hydroxybutyric acid in the treatment of alcohol dependence: a double blind study. *Alcohol Clin Exp Res* 1992; **16:** 673–6.
3. Addolorato G, *et al.* Maintaining abstinence from alcohol with γ-hydroxybutyric acid. *Lancet* 1998; **351:** 38.
4. Quinn DI, *et al.* Pharmacokinetic and pharmacodynamic principles of illicit drug use and treatment of illicit drug users. *Clin Pharmacokinet* 1997; **33:** 344–400.

Narcoleptic syndrome. Sodium oxybate[1-3] given at night has been reported to improve symptoms of patients with narcoleptic syndrome (p.1505) treated with stimulants during the day.

For reference to the pharmacokinetics of sodium oxybate in narcoleptic patients, see above.

1. Scharf MB, *et al.* The effects and effectiveness of γ-hydroxybutyrate in patients with narcolepsy. *J Clin Psychiatry* 1985; **46:** 222–5.
2. Mamelak M, *et al.* Treatment of narcolepsy with γ-hydroxybutyrate: a review of clinical and sleep laboratory findings. *Sleep* 1986; **9:** 285–9.
3. Scrima L, *et al.* Efficacy of gamma-hydroxybutyrate versus placebo in treating narcolepsy-cataplexy: double-blind subjective measures. *Biol Psychiatry* 1989; **26:** 331–43.

Preparations

Proprietary Preparations (details are given in Part 3)
Fr.: Gamma-OH; *Ger.:* Somsanit; *Ital.:* Alcover.

Thiamylal Sodium (3122-h)

Sodium 5-allyl-5-(1-methylbutyl)-2-thiobarbiturate.
$C_{12}H_{17}N_2NaO_2S = 276.3$.
CAS — 77-27-0 (thiamylal); 337-47-3 (thiamylal sodium).
Pharmacopoeias. In *Jpn.*

Profile

Thiamylal sodium is a short-acting intravenous barbiturate anaesthetic. It is possibly slightly more potent than thiopental sodium (p.1269) and has similar actions and uses. It has been used for the production of complete anaesthesia of short duration, for the induction of general anaesthesia, or for inducing a hypnotic state.

Thiopental Sodium (3124-b)

Thiopental Sodium (BANM, rINN).

Natrium Isopentylaethylthiobarbituricum (cum Natrio Carbonico); Penthiobarbital Sodique; Soluble Thiopentone; Thiomebumalnatrium cum Natrii Carbonate; Thiopental Sodium and Sodium Carbonate; Thiopentalum Natricum; Thiopentalum Natricum et Natrii Carbonas; Thiopentobarbitalum Solubile; Thiopentone Sodium; Tiopentol Sódico. Sodium 5-ethyl-5-(1-methylbutyl)-2-thiobarbiturate.

$C_{11}H_{17}N_2NaO_2S = 264.3.$

CAS — 76-75-5 (thiopental); 71-73-8 (thiopental sodium).

NOTE. The name thiobarbital has been applied to thiopental and has also been used to describe a barbiturate of different composition.

Pharmacopoeias. In Chin., Eur. (see p.vi), Int., Jpn, and US. Some include thiopental sodium with, some without, anhydrous sodium carbonate; some only include a sterile mixture for injection.

Solutions of thiopental sodium are incompatible with acidic and oxidising substances including some antibiotics, neuromuscular blockers and analgesics. Compounds commonly listed as incompatible include amikacin sulfate, benzylpenicillin salts, cefapirin sodium, codeine phosphate, ephedrine sulfate, fentanyl citrate, glycopyrronium bromide, morphine sulfate, pentazocine lactate, prochlorperazine edisilate, suxamethonium salts, and tubocurarine chloride. Solutions decompose on standing and precipitation occurs on boiling.

Pharmacopoeial description

Ph. Eur.: A yellowish-white hygroscopic powder. Thiopental Sodium and Sodium Carbonate (Ph. Eur.) contains 84 to 87% thiopental and 10.2 to 11.2% sodium. Freely soluble in water; partly soluble in dehydrated alcohol; practically insoluble in ether. Store in airtight containers. Protect from light.

USP 25: A white to off-white crystalline powder, or yellowish-white to pale greenish-yellow hygroscopic powder. May have a disagreeable odour. Its solutions are alkaline to litmus, decompose on standing, and on boiling, precipitation occurs. Soluble in water and in alcohol; insoluble in ether, in petroleum spirit, and in benzene. Store in airtight containers.

◊ Loss of thiopental in PVC and cellulose propionate delivery systems has been reported,[1,2] but in another study,[3] no loss of potency was noted.

1. Kowaluk EA, et al. Interactions between drugs and polyvinyl chloride infusion bags. Am J Hosp Pharm 1981; **38:** 1308–14.
2. Kowaluk EA, et al. Interactions between drugs and intravenous delivery systems. Am J Hosp Pharm 1982; **39:** 460–7.
3. Martens HJ, et al. Sorption of various drugs in polyvinyl chloride, glass, and polyethylene-lined infusion containers. Am J Hosp Pharm 1990; **47:** 369–73.

Adverse Effects and Treatment

As for Phenobarbital, p.355.

Excitatory phenomena such as coughing, hiccuping, sneezing, and muscle twitching or jerking may occur with any of the barbiturate anaesthetics, particularly during induction, but they occur more frequently with methohexital than with thiopental. Laryngeal spasm or bronchospasm may also occur during induction. The intravenous injection of concentrated solutions of thiopental sodium such as 5% may result in thrombophlebitis. Extravasation of barbiturate anaesthetics may cause tissue necrosis. Intra-arterial injection causes severe arterial spasm with burning pain and may cause prolonged blanching of the forearm and hand and gangrene of digits. Hypersensitivity reactions have been reported. Barbiturate anaesthetics can cause respiratory depression. They depress cardiac output and often cause an initial fall in blood pressure, and overdosage may result in circulatory failure. Postoperative vomiting is infrequent but shivering may occur and there may be persistent drowsiness, confusion, and amnesia. Headache has also been reported.

See also under Adverse Effects of General Anaesthetics, p.1255.

Hypersensitivity. Anaphylactic reactions to thiopental have been reported[1,2] although such reactions are rare. There has also been a report of haemolytic anaemia and renal failure in association with the development of an anti-thiopental antibody in a patient who had undergone general anaesthesia induced by thiopental.[3]

1. Westacott P, et al. Anaphylactic reaction to thiopentone: a case report. Can Anaesth Soc J 1984; **31:** 434–8.
2. Moneret-Vautrin DA, et al. Simultaneous anaphylaxis to thiopentone and a neuromuscular blocker: a study of two cases. Br J Anaesth 1990; **64:** 743–5.
3. Habibi B, et al. Thiopental-related immune hemolytic anemia and renal failure: specific involvement of red-cell antigen I. N Engl J Med 1985; **312:** 353–5. Correction. ibid.: 1136.

The symbol † denotes a preparation no longer actively marketed

Intra-arterial injection. Accidental intra-arterial injection of thiopental sodium produces severe arterial spasm with intense burning pain. Anaesthesia, paresis, paralysis, and gangrene may occur. Therapy has concentrated on dilution of injected thiopental, prevention and treatment of arterial spasm, prophylaxis of thrombosis, thrombectomy and other measures to sustain good blood flow. There has been a report[1] of the successful use of urokinase intra-arterially in the management of one patient accidentally given thiopental intra-arterially.

1. Vangerven M, et al. A new therapeutic approach to accidental intra-arterial injection of thiopentone. Br J Anaesth 1989; **62:** 98–100.

Precautions

Barbiturate anaesthetics are contra-indicated when there is dyspnoea or respiratory obstruction such as in acute severe asthma or when maintenance of an airway cannot be guaranteed.

Barbiturate anaesthetics should be used with caution in shock and dehydration, hypovolaemia, severe anaemia, hyperkalaemia, toxaemia, myasthenia gravis, myxoedema and other metabolic disorders, or in severe renal disease. Caution is also required in patients with cardiovascular disease, muscular dystrophies, adrenocortical insufficiency, or with increased intracranial pressure. Reduced doses are required in the elderly and in severe hepatic disease.

See also Precautions for General Anaesthetics, p.1255.

Porphyria. Barbiturates including thiopental sodium have been associated with acute attacks of porphyria and are considered unsafe in porphyric patients.

Interactions

Difficulty may be experienced in producing anaesthesia with the usual dose of barbiturate anaesthetics in patients accustomed to taking alcohol or other CNS depressants; additional anaesthetics may be necessary. Care is required when anaesthetising patients being treated with phenothiazine antipsychotics since there may be increased hypotension. Some phenothiazines, especially promethazine, may increase the incidence of excitatory phenomena produced by barbiturate anaesthetics; cyclizine may possibly have a similar effect. Opioid analgesics can potentiate the respiratory depressant effect of barbiturate anaesthetics and the dose of the anaesthetic may need to be reduced. Concomitant administration of nitrous oxide greatly reduces the dose of barbiturate anaesthetics required for anaesthesia. Reduced doses of thiopental may be required in patients receiving sulfafurazole.

See also Interactions of General Anaesthetics, p.1255.

Antidepressants. Potentiation of barbiturate anaesthesia may be expected in patients receiving tricyclic antidepressants or MAOIs (see under Anaesthesia in Precautions for Amitriptyline, p.275 and for Phenelzine, p.304, respectively).

Antipsychotics. For mention of the effect of droperidol on thiopental see under Gastrointestinal Drugs, below.

Aspirin. Pretreatment with aspirin, a highly protein-bound drug, has been shown to potentiate thiopental anaesthesia.[1]

1. Dundee JW, et al. Aspirin and probenecid pretreatment influences the potency of thiopentone and the onset of action of midazolam. Eur J Anaesthesiol 1986; **3:** 247–51.

Gastrointestinal drugs. Concomitant treatment with metoclopramide profoundly reduced the dose of thiopental required to produce hypnosis in female patients; droperidol had a similar effect.[1]

1. Mehta D, et al. Metoclopramide decreases thiopental hypnotic requirement. Anesth Analg 1993; **77:** 784–7.

Probenecid. Pretreatment with probenecid, a highly protein-bound drug, has been shown to potentiate thiopental anaesthesia.[1]

1. Dundee JW, et al. Aspirin and probenecid pretreatment influences the potency of thiopentone and the onset of action of midazolam. Eur J Anaesthesiol 1986; **3:** 247–51.

Pharmacokinetics

Thiopental is highly lipid soluble and when it is administered intravenously as the sodium salt, concentrations sufficient to produce unconsciousness are achieved in the brain within 30 seconds. Onset of action occurs within 8 to 10 minutes when thiopental sodium is given rectally but absorption may be unpredictable if a suspension rather than a solution is used.

Recovery from anaesthesia is also rapid due to redistribution to other tissues, particularly fat. About 80% of thiopental may be bound to plasma proteins, although reports show a wide range of figures. Thiopental is metabolised almost entirely in the liver, but as it is only released slowly from lipid stores this occurs at a very slow rate.

It is mostly metabolised to inactive metabolites but a small amount is desulfurated to pentobarbital. Repeated or continuous administration can lead to accumulation of thiopental in fatty tissue and this can result in prolonged anaesthesia and respiratory and cardiovascular depression. Elimination of thiopental following bolus injection can be described by a triexponential curve. The terminal elimination half-life has been reported to be 10 to 12 hours in adults and about 6 hours in children. However, values of 26 to 28 hours have been reported in obese patients and pregnant patients at term. Thiopental readily diffuses across the placenta and is distributed into breast milk.

◊ References.

1. Gaspari F, et al. Elimination kinetics of thiopentone in mothers and their newborn infants. Eur J Clin Pharmacol 1985; **28:** 321–5.
2. Swerdlow BN, Holley FO. Intravenous anaesthetic agents: pharmacokinetic-pharmacodynamic relationships. Clin Pharmacokinet 1987; **12:** 79–110.
3. Esener Z, et al. Thiopentone and etomidate concentrations in maternal and umbilical plasma, and in colostrum. Br J Anaesth 1992; **69:** 586–8.
4. Gedney JA, Ghosh S. Pharmacokinetics of analgesics, sedatives and anaesthetic agents during cardiopulmonary bypass. Br J Anaesth 1995; **75:** 344–51.

Uses and Administration

Thiopental is a short-acting barbiturate anaesthetic. It is given intravenously, usually for the induction of general anaesthesia (p.1256), but may be used as the sole anaesthetic to maintain anaesthesia for short procedures with minimal painful stimuli. It is also used in anaesthesia as a supplement to other anaesthetics, as a hypnotic in balanced anaesthesia, and, when given rectally, for basal anaesthesia or basal narcosis. Thiopental sodium may also be used intravenously in the control of refractory tonic-clonic status epilepticus and in neurosurgical patients to reduce increased intracranial pressure.

Thiopental does not usually produce excitation and induction of anaesthesia is usually smooth. It has poor muscle relaxant properties and a muscle relaxant must be administered before intubation is attempted. Thiopental also has poor analgesic properties and small doses may even lower the pain threshold. Recovery from an induction dose may occur within 10 to 30 minutes although drowsiness may persist for some time.

In anaesthesia, the dosage of thiopental varies greatly according to the state of the patient and the nature of other drugs being used concurrently (see under Precautions above and Interactions above for further details). Thiopental is usually administered intravenously as the sodium salt as a 2.5% solution but a 5% solution is occasionally used. A typical dose for inducing anaesthesia is 100 to 150 mg injected over 10 to 15 seconds, repeated after 30 to 60 seconds according to response. Some prefer to initiate induction with a test dose of 25 to 75 mg. The UK manufacturer recommends that the total dosage used in pregnant patients should not exceed 250 mg. Children's doses range from 2 to 7 mg per kg body-weight. When thiopental is used as the sole anaesthetic, anaesthesia can be maintained by repeat doses as needed or by continuous intravenous infusion of a 0.2 or 0.4% solution.

To reduce elevations of intracranial pressure in neurological patients intermittent bolus injections of 1.5 to 3 mg per kg body-weight may be given if adequate ventilation is provided (but see also Cerebrovascular Disorders, below).

A suggested dose in refractory tonic-clonic status epilepticus is 50 to 125 mg intravenously (see also under Status Epilepticus, below).

Recovery is usually rapid after moderate doses, but the patient may remain sleepy or confused for several hours. Large doses, repeated smaller doses, or continuous administration may markedly delay recovery.

◊ References.
1. Russo H, Bressolle F. Pharmacodynamics and pharmacokinetics of thiopental. *Clin Pharmacokinet* 1998; **35:** 95–134.

Administration in the elderly. It is usually recommended that the dosage of barbiturate anaesthetics is reduced in the elderly. One study[1] in elderly patients has demonstrated that although reducing the rate of intravenous administration reduces the speed of induction, the dosage required is also reduced. Administration of thiopental sodium 2.5% solution at a rate of 125 mg per minute induced anaesthesia in a mean of 90.8 seconds and required a mean dose of 2.8 mg per kg body-weight. Corresponding values for an administration rate of 500 mg per minute were 40.8 seconds and 5 mg per kg respectively.
1. Berthoud MC, *et al.* Comparison of infusion rates of three i.v. anaesthetic agents for induction in elderly patients. *Br J Anaesth* 1993; **70:** 423–7.

Anaesthesia. Some of the adverse effects of the neuromuscular blocker suxamethonium may be reduced when thiopental is used as part of the anaesthetic regimen. For a suggestion that thiopental may help to counteract the rise in intra-ocular pressure associated with the use of suxamethonium for intubation, see under Anaesthesia, p.1331. For reports that thiopental reduces the adverse effects of suxamethonium on muscles, see under Effects on the Muscles in the Adverse Effects of Suxamethonium, p.1340.

Cerebrovascular disorders. Barbiturates are considered to be suitable anaesthetics for use in patients with or at risk of raised intracranial pressure. Barbiturate-induced coma (commonly with pentobarbital or thiopental) has been used, both therapeutically and prophylactically, to protect the brain from ischaemia resulting from neurological insults including head injury, stroke, Reye's syndrome, and hepatic encephalopathy.[1-3] Rationale includes the ability of barbiturates to reduce intracranial pressure and to reduce metabolic demands of cerebral tissues. Although thiopental protected patients against the neuropsychiatric complications of cardiopulmonary bypass,[4] the Brain Resuscitation Clinical Trial I Study Group[5] found no cerebral benefit from thiopental in comatose survivors of cardiac arrest. Nor did others[6] observe any benefit from thiopental-induced coma in infants with severe birth asphyxia. A review in 1989 considered that there was no convincing evidence of improvement in neurological outcome to justify the risks of the procedure in conditions causing global ischaemia, although administration of barbiturates without necessarily inducing coma might have a limited role in reduction of raised intracranial pressure refractory to other therapy. Use of barbiturates in the setting of regional cerebral ischaemia, including use during cardiopulmonary bypass to prevent focal neurological complications, remained controversial.[1] For a discussion of the treatment of raised intracranial pressure, including a mention of the use of barbiturates, see p.811.
1. Rogers MC, Kirsch JR. Current concepts in brain resuscitation. *JAMA* 1989; **261:** 3143–7.
2. Lyons MK, Meyer FB. Cerebrospinal fluid physiology and the management of increased intracranial pressure. *Mayo Clin Proc* 1990; **65:** 684–707.
3. Woster PS, LeBlanc KL. Management of elevated intracranial pressure. *Clin Pharm* 1990; **9:** 762–72.
4. Nussmeier NA, *et al.* Neuropsychiatric complications after cardiopulmonary bypass: cerebral protection by a barbiturate. *Anesthesiology* 1986; **64:** 165–70.
5. Abramson NS, *et al.* Randomized clinical study of thiopental loading in comatose survivors of cardiac arrest. *N Engl J Med* 1986; **314:** 397–403.
6. Eyre JA, Wilkinson AR. Thiopentone induced coma after severe birth asphyxia. *Arch Dis Child* 1986; **61:** 1084–9.

Status epilepticus. Anaesthesia in conjunction with assisted ventilation may be instituted to control refractory tonic-clonic status epilepticus (p.341). A short-acting barbiturate such as thiopental is usually used. A loading dose of 5 mg per kg body-weight given intravenously has been suggested.[1] This may be followed after 30 minutes by an infusion given at a rate of 1 to 3 mg per kg per hour adjusted to maintain a maximum blood concentration of 60 to 100 μg per mL.[1] It has been recommended that administration should be continued for at least 12 hours after seizure activity has ceased and then slowly discontinued.[2]
1. O'Brien MD. Management of major status epilepticus in adults. *BMJ* 1990; **301:** 918.
2. Bauer J, Elger CE. Management of status epilepticus in adults. *CNS Drugs* 1994; **1:** 26–44.

Preparations

BP 2001: Thiopental Injection;
USP 25: Thiopental Sodium for Injection.

Proprietary Preparations (details are given in Part 3)
Austral.: Pentothal; *Belg.:* Nesdonal†; Pentothal; *Braz.:* Thionembutal; *Canad.:* Pentothal; *Denm.:* Pentothal; *Fin.:* Pentothal; *Ger.:* Trapanal; *Hong Kong:* Intraval Sodium; Pentothal; *Irl.:* Intraval Sodium; *Israel:* Pentothal; *Ital.:* Farmotal; Pentothal; *Mex.:* Inductal; Pensoditol; Pentothal; Sodipental; *Neth.:* Nesdonal; Pentothal; *Norw.:* Pentothal; *NZ:* Intraval; Pentothal; *S.Afr.:* Intraval Sodium†; Sandothal†; *Singapore:* Pentothal; *Spain:* Pentothal; Tiobarbital; *Swed.:* Pentothal; *Switz.:* Pentothal; *Thai.:* Intraval Sodium; Pentothal; *UK:* Intraval Sodium†; *USA:* Pentothal.

Tiletamine Hydrochloride (13344-s)

Tiletamine Hydrochloride *(BANM, USAN, rINNM)*.
Cl-634; CL-399; CN-54521-2. 2-Ethylamino-2-(2-thienyl)cyclohexanone hydrochloride.
$C_{12}H_{17}NOS,HCl = 259.8$.
CAS — 14176-49-9 *(tiletamine);* 14176-50-2 *(tiletamine hydrochloride).*
Pharmacopoeias. In US for veterinary use only.

Pharmacopoeial description

USP 25: A white to off-white crystalline powder. Freely soluble in water; slightly soluble in chloroform; practically insoluble in ether; soluble in methyl alcohol; freely soluble in 0.1N hydrochloric acid. pH of a 10% solution in water is between 3.0 and 5.0. Store in airtight containers.

Profile

Tiletamine has similar properties to ketamine (p.1262). It is used as the hydrochloride with zolazepam (p.712) for general anaesthesia in veterinary medicine.

Trichloroethylene (3126-g)

Trichlorethylene *(rINN)*.
Trichlorethylene; Trichlorethylenum; Trichloroethene; Trichloroethylenum.
$CHCl:CCl_2 = 131.4$.
CAS — 79-01-6.
ATC — N01AB05.

Trichloroethylene is non-flammable. Trichloroethylene used for anaesthetic purposes contains thymol 0.01% w/v as a stabiliser and is coloured blue for identification.

Adverse Effects and Precautions

Trichloroethylene increases the rate and decreases the depth of respiration and may be followed by apnoea. The sensitivity of the heart to beta-adrenergic activity may increase, possibly with ventricular arrhythmias.

Acute exposure to trichloroethylene may be followed by dizziness, lightheadedness, lethargy, nausea, and vomiting; hepatic and renal dysfunction may follow. Fatalities have occurred, although temporary unconsciousness is a more common manifestation.

Chronic poisoning may result in visual disturbances, intolerance to alcohol as manifested by transient redness of the face and neck (degreasers' or trichloroethylene flush), impairment of performance, hearing defects, neuralgia and mild liver dysfunction. Prolonged contact with trichloroethylene can cause dermatitis, eczema, burns, and conjunctivitis.

Dependence has been reported in medical personnel and factory workers who regularly inhale trichloroethylene vapour.

If trichloroethylene is used as an anaesthetic it should not be used in closed-circuit apparatus since there is a reaction with soda lime to produce a toxic end product that may cause cranial nerve paralysis and possibly death.

See also Adverse Effects and Precautions for General Anaesthetics, p.1255.

◊ Reviews of the toxicity of trichloroethylene.
1. Health and Safety Executive. Trichloroethylene. *Toxicity Review* 6. London: HMSO, 1982.
2. Davidson IWF, Beliles RP. Consideration of the target organ toxicity of trichloroethylene in terms of metabolite toxicity and pharmacokinetics. *Drug Metab Rev* 1991; **23:** 493–599.

Abuse. Toxicity associated with inhalation of volatile substances including trichloroethylene has been reviewed.[1,2] Trichloroethylene can damage the kidney, liver, heart, and lung. However, in young healthy subjects, organ toxicity becomes apparent only with intensive and protracted abuse of volatile substances.
1. Marjot R, McLeod AA. Chronic non-neurological toxicity from volatile substance abuse. *Hum Toxicol* 1989; **8:** 301–6.
2. Anonymous. Solvent abuse: little progress after 20 years. *BMJ* 1990; **300:** 135–6.

Carcinogenicity. The use of trichloroethylene in foods, drugs, and cosmetics was banned by the FDA following studies demonstrating that hepatocellular carcinomas could be induced in *mice* by chronic exposure to very high doses. However, similar effects have not been found in *rats* and larger species and several epidemiologic studies have failed to demonstrate an increased incidence of liver tumours, total mortality or mortality due to cancer in workers exposed to trichloroethylene. Suggestions that the carcinogenicity of trichloroethylene is due to one of its intermediate metabolites, cloral hydrate, have raised concern over the continuing use of cloral hydrate as a medicine. For further details, see p.670.

Effects on the liver. References[1,2] to hepatotoxicity following occupational exposure to trichloroethylene. See also under Carcinogenicity, above.
1. McCunney RJ. Diverse manifestations of trichloroethylene. *Br J Ind Med* 1988; **45:** 122–6.
2. Schattner A, Malnick SDH. Anicteric hepatitis and uveitis in a worker exposed to trichloroethylene. *Postgrad Med J* 1990; **66:** 730–1.

Effects on the skin. A report[1] of scleroderma in 3 patients occupationally exposed to trichloroethylene and, in 2 cases, also to trichloroethane.
1. Flindt-Hansen H, Isager H. Scleroderma after occupational exposure to trichloroethylene and trichloroethane. *Acta Derm Venereol (Stockh)* 1987; **67:** 263–4.

Interactions

The arrhythmogenic effects of trichloroethylene may be potentiated by the concurrent use of sympathomimetics such as adrenaline [epinephrine]. Alcohol consumption after chronic exposure to trichloroethylene may result in a reddening of the skin (see under Adverse Effects and Precautions, above).
See also Interactions of General Anaesthetics, p.1255.

Pharmacokinetics

Trichloroethylene is rapidly absorbed by inhalation and ingestion. Percutaneous absorption can occur. Some of the inhaled trichloroethylene is slowly eliminated through the lungs; trichloroethylene is metabolised primarily in the liver, cloral hydrate (see p.669) being the first stable major metabolite formed; most is then metabolised to trichloroethanol and trichloroacetic acid which are excreted in the urine. The latter may be used as an indicator of industrial exposure. Trichloroethylene diffuses across the placenta.

Uses and Administration

Trichloroethylene is a volatile halogenated anaesthetic administered by inhalation. It has been used in some countries for the maintenance of light anaesthesia (p.1256) but it has weak anaesthetic properties compared to other halogenated anaesthetics and poor muscle relaxant activity. It has also been used to supplement anaesthesia with nitrous oxide-oxygen or halothane. Trichloroethylene is a potent analgesic and has been used in subanaesthetic concentrations to provide analgesia for obstetrics, emergency management of trauma, and other acutely painful procedures.

Trichloroethylene is used in industry as a solvent for oils and fats, for degreasing metals, and for dry cleaning. It has also been used in typewriter correction fluids but is no longer included in most brands.

Preparations

Proprietary Preparations (details are given in Part 3)
Multi-ingredient: *Spain:* Talgo Odontalgico†.

Xenon (13865-e)

$Xe = 131.293$.

Profile

Xenon is a non-explosive gas. A mixture of 70% v/v xenon and 30% v/v oxygen has been tried as a general anaesthetic.

◊ References.
1. Lachmann B, *et al.* Safety and efficacy of xenon in routine use as an inhalational anaesthetic. *Lancet* 1990; **335:** 1413–15.
2. Yagi M, *et al.* Analgesic and hypnotic effects of subanaesthetic concentrations of xenon in human volunteers: comparison with nitrous oxide. *Br J Anaesth* 1995; **74:** 670–3.
3. Goto T, *et al.* Emergence times from xenon anaesthesia are independent of the duration of anaesthesia. *Br J Anaesth* 1997; **79:** 595–9.

Hypothalamic and Pituitary Hormones

The pituitary gland or hypophysis in humans is composed of the adenohypophysis, which is the anterior lobe, and the neurohypophysis, which comprises the posterior lobe and the neural stalk, above which lies the hypothalamus. The anterior lobe is linked to the hypothalamus by a portal vascular system but there is no vascular link between the posterior lobe and the hypothalamus.

The hormones secreted by the anterior lobe of the **pituitary**, each by its own specialised cells, are: adrenocorticotrophic hormone (ACTH; corticotropin); the gonadotrophic hormones (gonadotrophins), follicle-stimulating hormone and luteinising hormone; growth hormone (somatropin); lactogenic hormone (prolactin); and thyroid-stimulating hormone (thyrotrophin). In some mammals, but apparently not in humans, the pituitary also secretes melanocyte-stimulating hormone.

Oxytocin and antidiuretic hormone (ADH; vasopressin) are synthesised in the **hypothalamus**. They become associated with carrier proteins, neurophysins, and are then transported down nerve fibres to the posterior pituitary where they are stored until required. The release of oxytocin and vasopressin appears to be controlled mainly by nervous reflex responses.

The secretion of anterior pituitary hormones, in which the hypothalamus plays a major part, is regulated by a complex interaction between stimulatory and inhibitory neural and hormonal influences. A stylised representation of the hypothalamic-pituitary-endocrine axis is depicted in Figure 1, below. The hypothalamus produces transmitter substances which regulate pituitary secretion. These substances are secreted by hypothalamic neurones called neuroendocrine transducers, and stored in the median eminence of the hypothalamus. On receipt of an appropriate stimulus they are released into the blood of the hypophyseal portal system which carries them to the anterior pituitary. Conventionally these substances are known as factors until their structure and function is reasonably well established, when they may be referred to as hormones.

Hypothalamic releasing factors or hormones stimulate release of anterior pituitary hormones into the systemic circulation. Growth hormone is under a system of double regulation, since the hypothalamus secretes a release-inhibiting hormone (somatostatin) as well as growth hormone-releasing hormone (somatorelin). For others, secretion of the releasing factor is controlled by feedback mechanisms involving target organ hormones, pituitary hormones, and perhaps the hypothalamic hormones themselves as well as by excitatory and inhibitory impulses from different parts of the brain.

The major groups of hypothalamic and pituitary hormones and their analogues described in this chapter are summarised in Table 1, p.1272.

Use of Hypothalamic and Pituitary Hormones

A number of disorders associated with hypothalamic or pituitary dysfunction are discussed below. Some other endocrine disorders which may be due to dysfunction of the hypothalamic-pituitary-endocrine axes include adrenocortical insufficiency (p.1046), and hyperthyroidism (p.1519) or hypothyroidism (p.1520), as well as some of the disorders discussed in the chapter on Sex Hormones (p.1452).

Acromegaly and gigantism

Acromegaly and gigantism are syndromes of excess growth hormone secretion, usually associated with a secretory pituitary adenoma (somatropinoma).[1-3]

Excessive growth hormone secretion in childhood, while the epiphyses of the long bones are open, results in **gigantism**, with a proportional growth spurt and skeletal enlargement. Subsequently skeletal deformities develop, including kyphosis and deformity of the chest wall, as a consequence of osteoporosis. Puberty, with the increase in sex hormone secretion which leads to epiphyseal fusion, may be delayed by concomitant hypogonadism, leading to attainment of an even greater ultimate height. If growth hormone excess persists into adulthood, features of acromegaly may be superimposed on gigantism.

When excess growth hormone secretion develops first in adulthood the condition is known as **acromegaly**. Signs and symptoms tend to develop slowly and may be missed, sometimes for years. Growth hormone concentrations, and hence those of insulin-like growth factor I (IGF-I), which is produced in the liver in response to growth hormone, are elevated, sometimes markedly. The facial features become coarser, the jaw enlarges (prognathism), and hands and feet become enlarged. Peripheral neuropathy and carpal tunnel syndrome due to nerve entrapment, arthropathy, osteoarthritis, and muscle weakness, abnormal glucose tolerance, hypertension and left ventricular hypertrophy are all common, as is nodular goitre. Daytime somnolence may occur due to sleep apnoea. Acromegalics have an increased mortality if left untreated, largely due to cardiovascular disease.

Treatment. The biochemical goal of treatment is to normalise growth hormone and IGF-I concentrations. Although mean 24-hour growth hormone concentrations of less than 2.5 µg per litre have been used to define diagnosis and cure[2] more sensitive assays have changed the criteria.[3] In patients with acromegaly, growth hormone concentrations are not suppressed during oral glucose tolerance testing, and this measurement of growth hormone is used both diagnostically and to assess treatment efficacy. A concentration of less than 2 µg per litre has been used to define successful therapy,[1-3] and more recently concentrations below 1 µg per litre have been suggested.[4] Random IGF-I concentrations should be reduced to normal for age and sex.[4]

As for most pituitary tumours, **surgery** is the mainstay of treatment. The success rate depends on surgical expertise and the size and extension of the mass, with success rates higher for microadenomas (about 70 to 80%) than macroadenomas (less than 50%) depending on criteria.[1-4] In elderly patients with macroadenomas, where surgery may carry considerable risks, drug therapy with octreotide (see below) may be a better option.[2] It is not yet clear whether any form of treatment to reduce growth hormone concentrations reduces mortality from cardiorespiratory or neoplastic disease in patients with acromegaly.[2]

Tumour regression induced by **radiotherapy** is a possible alternative to surgery where the latter cannot be performed, or more often is used in patients in whom surgical treatment has failed to lower growth hormone

Figure 1. A stylised representation of the hypothalamic-pituitary-endocrine axis.

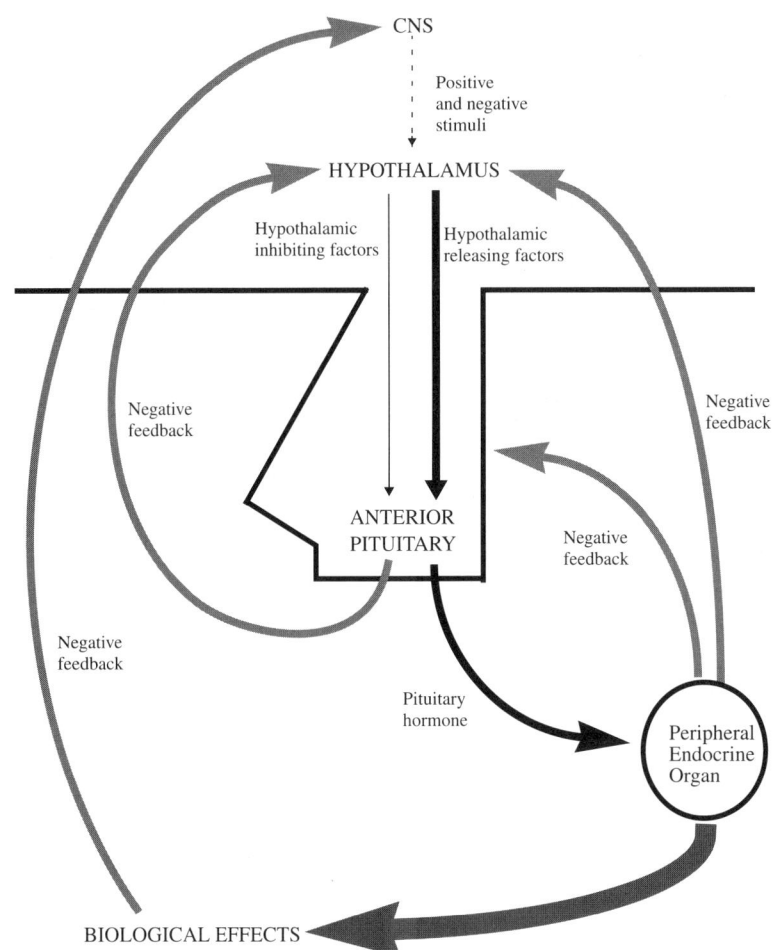

concentrations to acceptable levels.[1,2] Although it reduces growth hormone concentrations in about 90% of patients and prevents recurrence of tumour in 99%, its effects are slow and it often produces hypopituitarism. Some consider these to be disadvantages and prefer to use drug treatment for management of tumours that persist after surgery.[3] Since it may take several years for growth hormone concentrations to fall, drug therapy is also given until the effects of radiation therapy are satisfactory.[1-3]

Drug therapy for acromegaly is indicated for patients who refuse surgery, are at increased risk from surgery, have active disease after surgery, or are awaiting the effects of radiotherapy. Somatostatin analogues reduce growth hormone secretion in about 95% of patients, normalise IGF-I in about 65%, and produce modest tumour shrinkage.[1-3] Growth hormone levels below 2 μg per litre have been found in about 40% of patients treated with octreotide.[1,3] Reduction in growth hormone concentrations using octreotide has been shown to produce reduction of left ventricular hypertrophy.[5] Octreotide is generally given by injection, which, together with its short half-life limits its usefulness. There is some suggestion that continuous subcutaneous infusion may be more effective in acromegaly than intermittent injection,[6] but good controlled studies are lacking. A sustained-release intramuscular injection of octreotide is reportedly as effective as the shorter-acting preparation in historical comparisons,[7] and is undoubtedly more convenient. Another analogue of somatostatin, lanreotide, is also available in sustained-release formulation, and appears to be effective in acromegaly,[8,9] with results roughly comparable to those seen with octreotide, although the two do not appear to have been compared directly in a randomised study. Dopaminergic drugs, particularly bromocriptine, can produce a paradoxical reduction in growth hormone secretion in some patients with acromegaly, providing symptomatic relief. However, bromocriptine produces acceptable suppression of growth hormone secretion in only about 20% of patients and normalises IGF-I in even fewer.[3] Another dopaminergic, quinagolide, has been reported to produce better results than a depot preparation of bromocriptine, or cabergoline.[10] Pegvisomant is a growth hormone-receptor antagonist under investigation for the treatment of acromegaly.

1. Newman CB. Acromegaly. *Curr Ther Endocrinol Metab* 1997; **6:** 47–51.
2. Colao A, Lombardi G. Growth-hormone and prolactin excess. *Lancet* 1998; **352:** 1455–61.
3. Melmed S, *et al.* Current treatment guidelines for acromegaly. *J Clin Endocrinol Metab* 1998; **83:** 2646–52.
4. Giustina A, *et al.* Criteria for cure of acromegaly: a consensus statement. *J Clin Endocrinol Metab* 2000; **85:** 526–9.
5. Lim MJ, *et al.* Rapid reduction of left ventricular hypertrophy in acromegaly after suppression of growth hormone hypersecretion. *Ann Intern Med* 1992; **117:** 719–26.
6. Harris AG, *et al.* Continuous versus intermittent subcutaneous infusion of octreotide in the treatment of acromegaly. *J Clin Pharmacol* 1995; **35:** 59–71.
7. Gillis JC, *et al.* Octreotide long-acting release (LAR): a review of its pharmacological properties and therapeutic use in the management of acromegaly. *Drugs* 1997; **53:** 681–99.
8. Boucekkine C, *et al.* Traitement de l'acromégalie par un nouvel analogue de la somatostatine, le lanréotide à action prolongée. *Ann Endocrinol (Paris)* 1994; **55:** 261–9.
9. Caron P, *et al.* Three year follow-up of acromegalic patients treated with intramuscular slow-release lanreotide. *J Clin Endocrinol Metab* 1997; **82:** 18–22.
10. Colao A, *et al.* Effect of different dopaminergic agents in the treatment of acromegaly. *J Clin Endocrinol Metab* 1997; **82:** 518–23.

Amenorrhoea

Amenorrhoea is the absence of menstruation: a break in menstruation of 6 months or more is considered pathological in an adult woman who is not pregnant, lactating, or menopausal. Amenorrhoea occurring from the time of puberty is known as primary, while amenorrhoea developing later in life is referred to as secondary. Pathological amenorrhoea is usually associated with infertility (see also below). Hirsutism (p.1468) may also be present.

The causes of amenorrhoea (or oligomenorrhoea—infrequent and erratic periods) are most often ovarian or hypothalamic/pituitary in origin. Ovarian causes include failure of normal gonadal development, as in Turner's syndrome (below); premature ovarian failure including that due to trauma, drugs, radiotherapy, or autoimmunity; and conditions such as the polycystic ovary syndrome (below). Hypothalamic or pituitary causes include reduced production of gonadotrophins due to inadequate nutrition, excessive exercise, or pituitary trauma (see also Hypogonadism, below); or excess prolactin production (see Hyperprolactinaemia, below). Other causes, including adrenal disorders, thyroid disorders, abnormalities of the vagina or uterus, or testicular feminisation, may be found rarely.

The management of amenorrhoea essentially involves the identification of any underlying disorder and its correction, if possible. When the cause cannot be corrected, oestrogen replacement therapy, usually in the form of an oral contraceptive, is appropriate to minimise the consequences of long-term oestrogen deficiency.

References.
1. Crosignani PG, Vegetti W. A practical guide to the diagnosis and management of amenorrhoea. *Drugs* 1996; **52:** 671–81.
2. McIver B, *et al.* Evaluation and management of amenorrhea. *Mayo Clin Proc* 1997; **72:** 1161–9.
3. Baird DT. Amenorrhoea. *Lancet* 1997; **350:** 275–9.

Cryptorchidism

The testes are formed within the abdomen and subsequently descend the inguinal canal to the scrotum. Failure of the testes to descend (cryptorchidism) occurs in about 3 to 6% of newborn males but in many the testes descend during the first year of life decreasing the prevalence to about 1%. In children with cryptorchidism, pathological testicular damage has been noted by the age of 2 years, which may result in subsequent infertility;[1,2] cryptorchidism also significantly increases the risk of testicular cancer. Abnormalities of the testes and anatomical abnormalities such as inguinal hernia may contribute to maldescent, and both primary testicular disease and gonadotrophin deficiency may be associated with cryptorchidism. For discussions of Hypogonadism and Infertility, see below. Cryptorchidism should be distinguished from retractile testes in which the testes develop normally and for which treatment is usually not required.[1]

If sterility is to be avoided, treatment should be carried out preferably before 18 months of age.[2] Surgery remains the treatment with the best success rate but in most clinics boys are referred for surgery only after the failure of hormonal therapy.[3] Meta-analysis[4] suggests that gonadorelin, and probably chorionic gonadotrophin, are more effective than placebo in the treatment of cryptorchidism with a success rate of about 20% overall, although this may be considerably lower when care is taken to exclude retractile testes. The lower the position of the undescended testis, the more likely benefit from hormonal therapy appears to be.[4-6] Results may perhaps be improved by combined therapy with gonadorelin and chorionic gonadotrophin.[5] Chorionic gonadotrophin may also be useful as an adjuvant before surgery, in order to cause a nonpalpable testis to become palpable;[7] however, changes suggestive of inflammation in the testis have been reported following such treatment.[6]

1. Palmer JM. The undescended testicle. *Endocrinol Metab Clin North Am* 1991; **20:** 231–40.
2. Cilento BG, *et al.* Cryptorchidism and testicular torsion. *Pediatr Clin North Am* 1993; **40:** 1133–49.
3. Müller J, Skakkebaek NE. Cryptorchidism. *Curr Ther Endocrinol Metab* 1997; **6:** 363–6.
4. Pyörälä S, *et al.* A review and meta-analysis of hormonal treatment of cryptorchidism. *J Clin Endocrinol Metab* 1995; **80:** 2795–9.
5. Nane I, *et al.* Primary gonadotropin releasing hormone and adjunctive human chorionic gonadotropin treatment in cryptorchidism: a clinical trial. *Urology* 1997; **49:** 108–11.
6. Kaleva M, *et al.* Treatment with human chorionic gonadotrophin for cryptorchidism: clinical and histological effects. *Int J Androl* 1996; **19:** 293–8.
7. Polascik TJ, *et al.* Reappraisal of the role of human chorionic gonadotropin in the diagnosis and treatment of the nonpalpable testis: a 10 year-old experience. *J Urol (Baltimore)* 1996; **156:** 804–6.

Cushing's syndrome

Cushing's syndrome is the result of a chronic excess of glucocorticoids. It is commonly divided into those forms independent of adrenocorticotrophic hormone (ACTH; corticotropin) secretion (either due to an adrenal tumour secreting cortisol, or to administration of exogenous corticosteroids) and those which are ACTH-dependent (caused by excessive ACTH secretion from a pituitary adenoma—Cushing's disease proper, pituitary hyperplasia, or an ectopic ACTH-secreting tumour elsewhere—usually bronchus or lung cancer). About two-thirds of all cases are due to Cushing's disease, which is 8 times more common in women than men.

Symptoms may develop insidiously over several years and include obesity, particularly of the trunk, rounding of the face, atrophy of the skin leading to striae, poor wound healing, muscle weakness, osteoporosis, hypertension, diabetes mellitus, and depression and other psychological disturbances. Hypokalaemia is rare in Cushing's disease but common in other forms of the syndrome. Women may experience hirsutism due to adrenal androgen secretion, and both sexes may develop hypogonadism and loss of libido.

Diagnosis of Cushing's syndrome may be problematic since no test is wholly reliable.[1-3] Where there is suspicion, measurement of urinary cortisol and an overnight low dose dexamethasone suppression test may be carried out, and if either of these is abnormal, further measurement of urinary and blood cortisol, plasma electrolytes and ACTH, and high dose dexamethasone suppression testing may be required. For further discussion of the dexamethasone suppression test, see p.1068. Radiological examination can be important in detecting tumours.[3] Administration of corticorelin may be useful in differentiating between a pituitary, adrenal, or ectopic origin of the disease,[4,5] although sampling of central (petrosal) venous blood may be required[3] (see also p.1280). A diagnostic role has also been suggested for octreotide.[6]

Appropriate **treatment** depends on accurate identification of the cause of the syndrome.[7] The usual treatment in Cushing's disease is transsphenoidal resection of the tumour, which when carried out by an experienced surgeon produces a successful response in the great majority of patients.[3,7] If pituitary surgery fails, bilateral adrenalectomy may be considered (although this has some risks including that of Nelson's syndrome due to hyperactivity of residual pituitary tumour). Patients who undergo such surgery require corticosteroid replacement therapy for life.[7] Pituitary radiotherapy is slower than surgery to take effect, produces a lower remission rate, and is more like-

Table 1. Hypothalamic and pituitary hormones.

Antidiuretic hormones	*Oxytocic hormones*
Argipressin	Carbetocin
Lypressin	Demoxytocin
Desmopressin	Oxytocin
Felypressin	Powdered Pituitary,
Ornipressin	Posterior Lobe
Terlipressin	
Powdered Pituitary,	*Oxytocin antagonists*
Posterior Lobe	Atosiban
Vasopressin	
Corticotrophic hormones	*Somatotrophic hormones*
Corticotropin	Mecasermin
Tetracosactide	Somatrem
	Somatropin
Corticotrophic releasing	
hormone	*Somatotrophic hormone*
Corticorelin	*receptor antagonists*
	Pegvisomant
	Somatotrophic releasing
	hormones
	Sermorelin
	Somatorelin
	Somatotrophic release
	inhibitors
	Lanreotide
	Octreotide
	Somatostatin
	Vapreotide
Gonadotrophic hormones	*Thyrotrophic hormones*
Choriogonadotropin Alfa	Thyrotropin
Chorionic Gonadotrophin	Thyrotropin Alfa
Follicle-stimulating	
Hormone	*Thyrotrophic releasing*
Follitropin Alfa	*hormones*
Follitropin Beta	Posatirelin
Luteinising Hormone	Protirelin
Lutropin Alfa	Taltirelin
Menotrophin	
Urofollitropin	
Gonadotrophic releasing	
hormones	
Buserelin	
Deslorelin	
Gonadorelin	
Goserelin	
Histrelin	
Leuprorelin	
Nafarelin	
Triptorelin	
Gonadotrophic releasing	
hormone antagonists	
Abarelix	
Cetrorelix	
Ganirelix	
Lactotrophic hormones	
Prolactin	

ly to produce hypopituitarism.[7] It is thus rarely used as first-line therapy in Cushing's disease. However, excellent results have been reported from the use of pituitary radiotherapy, together with ketoconazole until symptoms regressed, in patients who failed to respond to pituitary surgery,[8] and this may be an alternative to adrenalectomy. Surgery is also the treatment of choice for a resectable adrenal tumour or ectopic ACTH-secreting tumour; even where there is metastasis it may be useful in moderating symptoms.

A number of drugs have been used in patients with Cushing's disease, but their role appears to be mainly adjuvant.[3] Drugs aimed at reducing ACTH secretion do not seem to be of much value, and reports of benefit with bromocriptine[9] or cyproheptadine[10] have not been confirmed[7]. There is some evidence that sodium valproate may further reduce cortisol secretion when combined with metyrapone.[11] Drugs which inhibit adrenal secretion are more effective.[7] Metyrapone inhibits cortisol synthesis and has been used before surgery,[7] to reduce symptoms and improve wound healing. Metyrapone may also have a role in patients treated with pituitary irradiation, the effects of which are slow to manifest.[3] Aminoglutethimide has been used similarly to metyrapone, but its use appears to be in decline. Mitotane can be effective in controlling symptoms but is poorly tolerated.[7] Other inhibitors of steroid synthesis such as trilostane and ketoconazole have also been tried.[3,7] Ketoconazole has been reported to normalise cortisol secretion and relieve symptoms in a number of patients.[12]

In patients with the ectopic ACTH syndrome in whom surgery is unsuitable or ineffective, chemotherapy aimed at the primary tumour is the treatment of choice but is likely to be only palliative. Metyrapone has been widely used, and ketoconazole has also proved effective in relieving symptoms.[13] Other drugs which have been tried include mifepristone,[14-16] octreotide,[6,17] and trilostane.

Surgery is the preferred treatment for an adrenal tumour but, although this is usually curative for adrenal adenoma, it is less successful for adrenal carcinoma and in these patients mitotane is widely employed after surgery and can prolong remission.[3,7] Metyrapone,[7] aminoglutethimide,[7] and ketoconazole[18] can also be given to control steroid hypersecretion.

In patients who are successfully treated for Cushing's syndrome adrenocortical replacement therapy (see p.1046) is usually required until the hypothalamic-pituitary-adrenal axis recovers normal function, a process which may take many months.

1. Orth DN. Differential diagnosis of Cushing's syndrome. *N Engl J Med* 1991; **325:** 957–9.
2. Sheaves R. Adrenal profiles. *Br J Hosp Med* 1994; **51:** 357–60.
3. Orth DN. Cushing's syndrome, *N Engl J Med* 1995; **332:** 791–803.
4. Kaye TB, Crapo L. The Cushing syndrome: an update on diagnostic tests. *Ann Intern Med* 1990; **112:** 434–44.
5. Anonymous. CRH test in the 1990s. *Lancet* 1990; **336:** 1416.
6. Woodhouse NJY, *et al.* Acute and long-term effects of octreotide in patients with ACTH-dependent Cushing's syndrome. *Am J Med* 1993; **95:** 305–8.
7. Atkinson AB. The treatment of Cushing's syndrome. *Clin Endocrinol (Oxf)* 1991; **34:** 507–13.
8. Estrada J, *et al.* The long-term outcome of pituitary irradiation after unsuccessful transsphenoidal surgery in Cushing's disease. *N Engl J Med* 1997; **336:** 172–7.
9. Atkinson AB, *et al.* Six year remission of ACTH-dependent Cushing's syndrome using bromocriptine. *Postgrad Med J* 1985; **61:** 239–42.
10. Marek J, *et al.* Cyproheptadine in Cushing's syndrome. *Lancet* 1977; **ii:** 653–4.
11. Nussey SS, *et al.* The combined use of sodium valproate and metyrapone in the treatment of Cushing's syndrome. *Clin Endocrinol (Oxf)* 1988; **28:** 373–80.
12. Angeli A, Frairia R. Ketoconazole therapy in Cushing's disease. *Lancet* 1985; **i:** 821.
13. Shepherd FA, *et al.* Ketoconazole: use in the treatment of ectopic adrenocorticotrophic hormone production and Cushing's syndrome in small-cell lung cancer. *Arch Intern Med* 1985; **145:** 863–4.
14. Nieman LK, *et al.* Successful treatment of Cushing's syndrome with the glucocorticoid antagonist RU 486. *J Clin Endocrinol Metab* 1985; **61:** 536–40.
15. van der Lely A-J, *et al.* Rapid reversal of acute psychosis in the Cushing syndrome with the cortisol-receptor antagonist mifepristone (RU 486). *Ann Intern Med* 1991; **114:** 143–4.
16. Sartor O, Cutler GB. Mifepristone: treatment of Cushing's syndrome. *Clin Obstet Gynecol* 1996; **39:** 506–10.
17. de Herder WW, Lamberts SWJ. Is there a role for somatostatin and its analogs in Cushing's syndrome. *Metabolism* 1996; **45:** 83–5.
18. Contreras P, *et al.* Regression of metastatic adrenal carcinoma during palliative ketoconazole treatment. *Lancet* 1985; **ii:** 151–2.

Delayed puberty

Puberty in boys usually begins between the ages of 9 and 14 years; in girls pubertal development starts about 2 years earlier than in boys and 95% of normal girls in the UK experience menstruation by 15 years of age. Delay beyond these norms should lead to investigation to try and eliminate the possibility of an underlying organic disorder. In addition to the various causes of hypogonadism (see below), some of which may be difficult to diagnose, severe systemic illness such as asthma or diabetes, or hypothyroidism, may cause delay in sexual maturation. Where no apparent cause can be found a family history of delayed maturation may suggest constitutional delayed puberty, in which normal pubertal development can eventually be expected.

Where pubertal delay is secondary to some other condition appropriate management of the precipitating cause is required. In constitutional delayed puberty small doses of oestrogens in girls, or androgens (such as oxandrolone or a testosterone ester) in boys, may be given to promote growth and sexual development if psychological problems are apparent. Care is required as overly aggressive therapy with sex hormones may lead to premature closure of the epiphyses and compromise final adult height. Treatment should be interrupted periodically to see if spontaneous pubertal development has begun. The use of chorionic gonadotrophin or a gonadorelin analogue has no advantage in such patients, although they have a role in hypogonadotrophic hypogonadism, which may be difficult to distinguish from constitutional delay.

Diabetes insipidus

Diabetes insipidus deprives the kidney of its capacity to produce a concentrated urine, resulting in the passage of large volumes of dilute urine (polyuria) and excessive thirst (polydipsia). Patients generally have moderately raised serum-sodium concentrations but are prone to more severe hypernatraemia (p.1183) when fluid is restricted.

The syndrome of diabetes insipidus is caused either by a deficiency in secretion of antidiuretic hormone (ADH; vasopressin) from the posterior pituitary gland (cranial, pituitary, or neurogenic diabetes insipidus), or by a failure in activity of secreted ADH on renal tubules (nephrogenic diabetes insipidus). Cranial diabetes insipidus is most commonly idiopathic (although it is now increasingly suspected to have an auto-immune basis) or occurs following surgery or trauma when it may be temporary. More rarely, it results from neoplasms, infections, or infiltrations of the CNS, or forms part of the familial DID-MOAD syndrome (diabetes insipidus, diabetes mellitus, optic atrophy, and deafness). Nephrogenic diabetes insipidus may occur as a familial X-linked recessive disorder in male infants, but is more often secondary to hypercalcaemia, hypokalaemia, or drug therapy (including lithium salts, foscarnet, clozapine, and demeclocycline).

The mainstay of diagnosis of diabetes insipidus is measurement of serum and urine osmolality, urine specific gravity, and serum-sodium concentration. If these are found to be normal a formal water deprivation test may be performed in conjunction with careful monitoring of urine volume, osmolality, and body-weight. The test should be discontinued if more than 3 litres of urine is passed or 3% of total body-weight is lost, although this is in any case virtually diagnostic of diabetes insipidus. A dose of ADH in the form of desmopressin is then given to test renal responsiveness—prompt urine concentration is indicative of cranial diabetes insipidus, while failure indicates the nephrogenic form.

Cranial diabetes insipidus is usually treated by replacement therapy with ADH in the form of intranasal desmopressin, although tablets are now also available and may be preferred in children; desmopressin has greater antidiuretic efficacy and considerably less vasoconstrictor activity than lypressin or vasopressin itself.

Nephrogenic diabetes insipidus is by definition unresponsive to ADH therapy and water replacement tends to be the mainstay of treatment. Thiazide diuretics, notably hydrochlorothiazide, are given to patients with nephrogenic diabetes insipidus in conjunction with some restriction of sodium intake; the resultant mild sodium depletion enhances proximal renal tubular sodium and water resorption. The co-administration of amiloride has been reported to have an additive effect while also preventing hypokalaemia.

Other drugs have also been tried in the management of diabetes insipidus. Chlorpropamide stimulates ADH secretion and augments the activity of residual ADH in patients with partial cranial disease and as in nephrogenic disease the thiazides may be useful. Clofibrate and carbamazepine have also been found to promote ADH secretion in these patients. Indometacin and other prostaglandin synthetase inhibitors decrease urine volume in all types of the condition, and the biguanides such as metformin also have this effect in patients with hypokalaemic diabetes insipidus. Combination of indometacin with a thiazide and desmopressin has been investigated.

References.

1. Seckl JR, Dunger DB. Diabetes insipidus: current treatment recommendations. *Drugs* 1992; **44:** 216–24.
2. Knoers N, Monnens LAH. Nephrogenic diabetes insipidus: clinical symptoms, pathogenesis, genetics and treatment. *Pediatr Nephrol* 1992; **6:** 476–82.
3. Singer I, *et al.* The management of diabetes insipidus in adults. *Arch Intern Med* 1997; **157:** 1293–1301.
4. Baylis PH, Cheetham T. Diabetes insipidus. *Arch Dis Child* 1998; **79:** 84–9.
5. Bendz H, Aurell M. Drug-induced diabetes insipidus. *Drug Safety* 1999; **21:** 449–56.

Endometriosis

Gonadorelin analogues are employed in the management of endometriosis (see p.1469) but the need for long-term therapy to prevent recurrence limits their value because of the risk of osteoporosis, and they tend to be reserved for patients unable to tolerate therapy with danazol or progestogens.

Growth retardation

Stature follows a normal (bell-shaped) distribution within the population and there may be some difficulty in deciding at what point short stature becomes abnormal; to some extent this is determined by cultural as well as physiological norms. However, certain disorders are associated with well-defined deficiencies of growth which may be severe enough to warrant the description dwarfism. Some forms are associated with disorders of bone or cartilage growth (skeletal dysplasias), and many of these result additionally in disproportionate growth, as in the short-limbs and large head characteristic of achondroplasia. Other important causes of dwarfism include inadequate production of growth hormone (idiopathic growth hormone deficiency), either alone (isolated growth hormone deficiency) or combined with other pituitary hormone deficiencies as part of hypopituitarism; resistance to circulating growth hormone, as in Laron-type dwarfism, where there is a mutation of the growth hormone receptor; or defects in somatomedin synthesis. Some other endocrine causes of short stature include hypothyroidism, Cushing's syndrome, and Turner's syndrome. Severe chronic disease in childhood such as asthma, chronic renal failure, or liver disorders can result in some growth retardation as can inadequate nutrition due to malabsorption syndromes such as coeliac disease.

Endocrine causes of growth retardation are significant because they may generally be treatable by appropriate replacement therapy. Isolated growth hormone deficiency, or growth hormone and gonadotrophin deficiencies, are the commonest congenital forms of hypopituitarism. The deficiency is rarely complete, and since most children with short stature will not have growth hormone deficiency care is required in its diagnosis. Although provocative growth hormone tests, which use non-physiological means to stimulate growth hormone secretion, have long been considered the gold standard for diagnosis of growth hormone deficiency they have a number of limitations and some consider measurement of circulating somatomedins (insulin-like growth factors; IGFs) or their binding proteins to be more useful.[1] Different assays may give different results, and it has been advised that therapeutic decisions should not be based solely on the results of growth hormone tests.[2]

In children with confirmed growth hormone deficiency replacement therapy is appropriate, and is given with subcutaneous injections of synthetic human growth hormone (somatropin) or its methionyl analogue (somatrem). Treatment improves bone density and growth velocity.[3-6] The greatest increase in the latter occurs in the first year of treatment, and subsequently declines,[3] perhaps due to downregulation of the growth hormone receptor; intermittent[7] or pulsatile[8] administration do not appear to have any advantage in this regard. The extent of the benefit in terms of increase in final height is unclear. A cohort study of French children registered to receive growth hormone between 1973 and 1993 suggested that the eventual outcome was not as good as expected, and treated individuals remained short.[9] However, others are of the opinion that many growth-hormone deficient children achieve their genetic height potential with replacement therapy, and that most attain adult heights significantly greater than untreated children.[2] Increasing the dose or the frequency of administration may improve outcome[10] but the most important prognostic factor is age. For optimum results, treatment should be started as early as possible.[3,9-11] Somatorelin (growth hormone-releasing hormone) or its analogue sermorelin have also been tried to boost growth hormone secretion in patients with growth hormone deficiency,[12-14] and improved growth rates have been reported in some children. Another peptide analogue, pralmorelin is also under investigation.[15] There is a report that the effects of releasing hormone can be enhanced by concomitant use of a beta blocker.[16]

In patients with Laron dwarfism, conventional growth hormone therapy is ineffective because of defects in the growth hormone receptors. However, replacement therapy with mecasermin, the recombinant form of insulin-like growth factor-I, may be of substantial benefit in the treatment of this disorder.[17]

Benefit has been reported from growth hormone therapy in children with chronic renal failure,[18-20] in girls with Turner's syndrome, (but see below), and in young children (6 months to 3 years of age) with Down's syndrome,[21] all of which are associated with marked growth retardation. However, the use of growth hormone in short stature other than that due to indisputable growth hormone deficiency, including these disorders, is controversial. Many commentators see such interventions as essentially cosmetic. The treatment of short stature for which no underlying disorder can be identified, in particular, poses problems as the risks and also the benefits in terms of final height are uncertain.[22-26] Guidelines for paediatric endocrinologists issued in the USA[2] suggest that therapy is justifiable in renal insufficiency and in Turner's syndrome, but that evidence of benefit is lacking for other growth disorders including non-growth hormone deficient short stature and growth retardation associated with Down's syndrome. It was considered that growth hormone should not be given to children with constitutional delay of growth.

Although sex hormones have effects on growth they may also cause premature closure of the epiphyses when given to prepubertal or pubertal children, and this has limited their use. Nonetheless, anabolic drugs such as testosterone,[27] oxandrolone[28] and fluoxymesterone[29] have been used in boys with constitutional delay of growth associated with delayed puberty (see also above) and oestrogens such as ethinylestradiol have been reported to increase growth rate in some girls, for example those with Turner's syndrome.[30]

A number of other drugs have been investigated in growth retardation. Clonidine, which can promote growth hormone-releasing hormone release, has been given to children with growth hormone deficiency as well as to short children without proven deficiency, but results have been contradictory and largely unsatisfactory.[31-33] A possible association of growth with zinc or vitamin A has led to preliminary studies of the benefits of supplementation with these agents.[34,35] Gonadorelin analogues have also been given in combination with growth hormone to short girls without growth hormone deficiency, in an attempt to slow bone maturation and delay puberty, thereby improving adult height.[36]

1. Rosenfeld RG, et al. Diagnostic controversy: the diagnosis of childhood growth hormone deficiency revisited. J Clin Endocrinol Metab 1995; 80: 1532–40.
2. Drug and Therapeutics Committee, Lawson Wilkins Pediatric Endocrine Society. Guidelines for the use of growth hormone in children with short stature. J Pediatr 1995; 127: 857–67.
3. Milner RDG, et al. Experience with human growth hormone in Great Britain: the report of the MRC working party. Clin Endocrinol (Oxf) 1979; 11: 15–38.
4. Clayton PE, et al. Growth hormone state after completion of treatment with growth hormone. Arch Dis Child 1987; 62: 222–6.
5. Leiper AD, et al. Growth in children treated for acute lymphoblastic leukaemia. Lancet 1988; i: 943.
6. Saggese G, et al. Effects of long-term treatment with growth hormone on bone and mineral metabolism in children with growth hormone deficiency. J Pediatr 1993; 122: 37–45.
7. Hakeem V, et al. Intermittent versus continuous administration of growth hormone treatment. Arch Dis Child 1993; 68: 783–4.
8. Smith PJ, et al. Single dose and pulsatile treatment with human growth hormone in growth hormone deficiency. Arch Dis Child 1987; 62: 849–51.
9. Coste J, et al. Long term results of growth hormone treatment in France in children of short stature: population, register based study. BMJ 1997; 315: 708–13.
10. Blethen SL, et al. Factors predicting the response to growth hormone (GH) therapy in prepubertal children with GH deficiency. J Clin Endocrinol Metab 1993; 76: 574–9.
11. Smith PJ, et al. Contribution of dose and frequency of administration to the therapeutic effect of growth hormone. Arch Dis Child 1988; 63: 491–4.
12. Wit JM, et al. Short-term effect on growth of two doses of GRF 1-44 in children with growth hormone deficiency: comparison with growth induced by methionyl-GH administration. Horm Res 1987; 27: 181–9.
13. Ross RJM, et al. Treatment of growth hormone deficiency with growth-hormone-releasing hormone. Lancet 1987; i: 5–8.
14. Smith PJ, Brook CGD. Growth hormone releasing hormone or growth hormone treatment in growth hormone insufficiency? Arch Dis Child 1988; 63: 629–34.
15. Mericq V, et al. Effects of eight months treatment with graded doses of a growth hormone (GH)-releasing peptide in GH-deficient children. J Clin Endocrinol Metab 1998; 83: 2355–60.
16. Cassorla F, et al. The effects of β-1-adrenergic blockade on the growth response to growth hormone (GH)-releasing hormone therapy in GH-deficient children. J Clin Endocrinol Metab 1995; 80: 2997–3001.
17. Laron Z. Somatomedin-1 (insulin-like growth factor-I) in clinical use: facts and potential. Drugs 1993; 45: 1–8.
18. Hokken-Koelega ACS, et al. Placebo-controlled, double-blind, cross-over trial of growth hormone treatment in prepubertal children with chronic renal failure. Lancet 1991; 338: 585–90.
19. Fine RN, et al. Growth after recombinant human growth hormone treatment in children with chronic renal failure: report of a multicenter randomized double-blind placebo-controlled study. J Pediatr 1994; 124: 374–82.
20. Fine RN. Growth retardation in children with chronic renal insufficiency. Nephron 1997; 76: 125–9.
21. Annerén G, et al. Normalized growth velocity in children with Down's syndrome during growth hormone therapy. J Intellect Disabil Res 1993; 37: 381–7.
22. Lantos J, et al. Ethical issues in growth hormone therapy. JAMA 1989; 261: 1020–4.
23. Walker JM, et al. Treatment of short normal children with growth hormone—a cautionary tale? Lancet 1990; 336: 1331–4.
24. Bierich JR, et al. Constitutional delay of growth and adolescence: results of short-term and long-term treatment with GH. Acta Endocrinol (Copenh) 1992; 127: 392–6.
25. Hindmarsh PC, Brook CGD. Final height of short normal children treated with growth hormone. Lancet 1996; 348: 13–16.
26. Kawai M, et al. Unfavorable effects of growth hormone therapy on the final height of boys with short stature not caused by growth hormone deficiency. J Pediatr 1997; 130: 205–9.
27. Brown DC, et al. A double blind, placebo controlled study of the effects of low dose testosterone undecanoate on the growth of small for age, prepubertal boys. Arch Dis Child 1995; 73: 131–5.
28. Stanhope R, et al. Double blind placebo controlled trial of low dose oxandrolone in the treatment of boys with constitutional delay of growth and puberty. Arch Dis Child 1988; 63: 501–5.
29. Strickland AL. Long-term results of treatment with low-dose fluoxymesterone in constitutional delay of growth and puberty and in genetic short stature. Pediatrics 1993; 91: 716–20.
30. Ross JL, et al. A preliminary study of the effect of estrogen dose on growth in Turner's syndrome. N Engl J Med 1983; 309: 1104–6.
31. Pintor C, et al. Clonidine treatment for short stature. Lancet 1987; i: 1226–30.
32. Pescovitz OH, Tan E. Lack of benefit of clonidine treatment for short stature in a double-blind, placebo-controlled trial. Lancet 1988; ii: 874–7.
33. Allen DB. Effects of nightly clonidine administration on growth velocity in short children without growth hormone deficiency: a double-blind, placebo-controlled study. J Pediatr 1993; 122: 32–6.
34. Nakamura T, et al. Mild to moderate zinc deficiency in short children: effect of zinc supplementation on linear growth velocity. J Pediatr 1993; 123: 65–9.
35. Evain-Brion D, et al. Vitamin A deficiency and nocturnal growth hormone secretion in short children. Lancet 1994; 343: 87–8.
36. Saggese G, et al. Combination treatment with growth hormone and gonadotropin-releasing hormone analogs in short normal girls. J Pediatr 1995; 126: 468–73.

Hyperprolactinaemia

Hyperprolactinaemia is a condition of elevated circulating prolactin concentrations. It occurs for physiological reasons in pregnancy or following mechanical stimulation of the nipple, as in suckling. However, hyperprolactinaemia may also be induced pharmacologically as an adverse effect of drugs that inhibit dopaminergic function such as antipsychotics and metoclopramide; other drugs causing hyperprolactinaemia include opioid analgesics, methyldopa, oestrogens, SSRIs, and verapamil. Furthermore, pathological hyperprolactinaemia may be associated with prolactin-secreting pituitary adenomas (prolactinomas), damage to the pituitary stalk or hypothalamus (including that caused by non-secreting tumours), or trauma to the chest wall; it may also be associated with disorders such as Cushing's syndrome or hypothyroidism. Prolactinomas are amongst the commonest pathological causes, and so-called idiopathic hyperprolactinaemia, in which no apparent cause is found, may in fact represent undetected microadenoma.

The consequences of hyperprolactinaemia include suppression of ovarian function in women, leading to erratic cycles or amenorrhoea, and infertility (see also above and below); in men, in whom the condition is less common, reduced gonadotrophin production leads to testosterone deficiency, diminished libido, and impotence. Both sexes may develop unwanted milk flow (galactorrhoea), although this depends on the concomitant presence of oestrogens; men may rarely develop gynaecomastia (p.1470) due to the change in oestrogen/androgen balance.

Management of hyperprolactinaemia depends on its cause. Pathological hyperprolactinaemia must be distinguished from physiological, and where it is secondary to another disease this should be managed appropriately; any drug thought likely to be causative should be withdrawn if possible. Some patients are asymptomatic, or are untroubled by their symptoms; whether such patients should be treated has been a matter of some controversy, although the risk of osteoporosis in women with prolonged suppression of ovarian function has been cited as a reason for such treatment.[1]

In many cases hyperprolactinaemia will be secondary to a prolactinoma. These are generally classified as microadenomas (less than 10 mm in size) or macroadenomas (over 10 mm in size); macroadenomas are often associated with prolactin concentrations more than 10 times the normal upper limit and their rapid expansion may result in visual defects and headache. Initially a course of treatment with a dopamine agonist such as bromocriptine, while rarely curative, is extremely effective in controlling hyperprolactinaemia and restoring gonadal function.[2-4] Surgical removal is now rarely indicated, although transsphenoidal decompression may be necessary for macroadenomas despite bromocriptine therapy, and ultimately radiotherapy may also be required.

The most extensively used dopamine agonist has been bromocriptine. Bromocriptine therapy may produce considerable shrinkage of the tumour, although macroadenomas in particular can re-expand, sometimes rapidly, if treatment is stopped, so compliance is important. In microadenomas, however, remission can occur and there is a case for periodic discontinuation after 1 to 2 years of therapy to see if normoprolactinaemia is maintained.[5] The short half-life and the adverse effects of bromocriptine may pose problems, although depot formulations can minimise these. Combination of oral prednisolone with intramuscular depot injection of bromocriptine has been reported to produce a reduced incidence of adverse effects.[6] If a woman becomes pregnant bromocriptine is usually discontinued, although this may pose problems in women with macroadenoma: if symptomatic enlargement of the tumour occurs during pregnancy re-institution of bromocriptine is probably the least harmful option.[7]

More recently a number of alternative dopaminergic drugs have become available, including cabergoline, lisuride, metergoline, quinagolide, and terguride. All of these can suppress prolactin secretion, but it is not clear whether most of them offer much advantage over bromocriptine. Quinagolide appears to be of similar efficacy,[8,9] but may possibly be useful in patients intolerant of or unresponsive to other drugs.[10] However, cabergoline appears to be both more effective than bromocriptine[11,12] (and probably quinagolide[13]), and better tolerated, and as a result some centres now reportedly use it as first-line treatment in many hyperprolactinaemic patients,[14] although bromocriptine may still be favoured (because of greater experience) in women who wish to become pregnant.

1. Klibanski A, Greenspan SL. Increase in bone mass after treatment of hyperprolactinemic amenorrhea. N Engl J Med 1986; 315: 542–6.
2. Ciccarelli E, Camanni F. Diagnosis and drug therapy of prolactinoma. Drugs 1996; 51: 954–65.
3. Andrews DW. Pituitary adenomas. Curr Opin Oncol 1997; 9: 55–60.
4. Molitch ME, et al. Therapeutic controversy: management of prolactinomas. J Clin Endocrinol Metab 1997; 82: 996–1000.
5. Hancock KW, et al. Long term suppression of prolactin concentrations after bromocriptine induced regression of pituitary prolactinomas. BMJ 1985; 290: 117–18.
6. Jenkins PJ, et al. Oral prednisolone supplement abolishes the acute adverse effects following initiation of depot bromocriptine therapy. Clin Endocrinol (Oxf) 1996; 45: 141–5.
7. Molitch ME. Pregnancy and the hyperprolactinemic woman. N Engl J Med 1985; 312: 1364–70.
8. Verhelst JA, et al. Acute and long-term effects of once-daily oral bromocriptine and a new long-acting non-ergot dopamine agonist, quinagolide, in the treatment of hyperprolactinaemia: a double-blind study. Acta Endocrinol (Copenh) 1991; 125: 385–91.
9. van der Heijden PFM, et al. CV205-502, a new dopamine agonist, versus bromocriptine in the treatment of hyperprolactinaemia. Eur J Obstet Gynecol Reprod Biol 1991; 40: 111–18.
10. Vilar L, Burke CW. Quinagolide efficacy and tolerability in hyperprolactinaemic patients who are resistant to or intolerant of bromocriptine. Clin Endocrinol (Oxf) 1994; 41: 821–6.
11. Webster J, et al. A comparison of cabergoline and bromocriptine in the treatment of hyperprolactinemic amenorrhea. N Engl J Med 1994; 331: 904–9.
12. Pascal-Vigneron V, et al. Aménorrhée hyperprolactinémique: traitement par cabergoline versus bromocriptine. Presse Med 1995; 24: 753–7.
13. Giusti M, et al. A cross-over study with the two novel dopaminergic drugs cabergoline and quinagolide in hyperprolactinemic patients. J Endocrinol Invest 1994; 17: 51–7.
14. Webster J. A comparative review of the tolerability profiles of dopamine agonists in the treatment of hyperprolactinaemia and inhibition of lactation. Drug Safety 1996; 14: 228–38. Correction. ibid; 342.

Hypogonadism

Hypogonadism (decreased or absent gonadal function) may occur in both men and women, and may be either primary, due to some dysfunction of the gonads themselves, or secondary, due to hypopituitarism or some other cause of decreased gonadotrophic stimulation.

Causes of ovarian dysfunction are discussed under Ovarian Dysfunction, below. Primary testicular dysfunction may be due to congenital disorders such as Klinefelter's syndrome (associated with an XXY chromosome constitution); the effects of chemotherapy, radiotherapy, infections (particularly mumps), or trauma; and a few other conditions such as testicular degeneration.

Secondary hypogonadism may be due to general hypopituitarism, or to a specific deficiency of gonadotrophin production, or gonadorelin production. Kallmann's syndrome is a congenital disorder of hypogonadotrophic hypogonadism due to gonadorelin deficiency associated with anosmia or hyposmia. The causes of pituitary or hypothalamic failure include neoplasms, trauma, or infiltrative granulomatous diseases such as tuberculosis. Gonadotrophin production may also be suppressed by various drugs (notably exogenous sex steroids and continuous, rather than pulsatile, administration of gonadorelin analogues), by weight loss or inadequate nutrition, by excessive exercise, by severe systemic illness, and by hyperprolactinaemia (see above).

The fundamental treatment for primary hypogonadism is replacement therapy with sex hormones to produce appropriate sexual development and activity and counteract effects such as osteoporosis, but fertility cannot usually be restored. In prepubertal children, the induction of secondary sexual characteristics must be balanced against a possible reduction in final height due to stimulation of premature closure of the bone epiphyses. Women may be given an oestrogen with a progestogen (for a discussion on the management of ovarian dysfunction, see below) and men are treated with androgens, often in the form of a long-acting testosterone ester such as the cipionate or enantate given intramuscularly. The transdermal administration of testosterone is also effective.

The cause of secondary hypogonadism should be determined and managed appropriately if possible. In some cases this may be adequate to restore gonadal function but in other cases sex hormone replacement therapy as in primary hypogonadism will be required. Where there is no fundamental defect in gonadal function the possibility of using a gonadotrophic hormone or stimulating the release of gonadotrophins also exists. In general, however, such therapy is often reserved for patients desiring restoration of fertility, since it is inconvenient and expensive. For a discussion on the management of infertility including the use of agents such as clomifene, gonadotrophins, and the pulsatile administration of gonadorelin and its analogues in men and women with hypogonadism, see under Infertility, below.

Infertility

Although about one couple in 6 may experience sufficient difficulty in conceiving children to seek medical help, most are subfertile rather than infertile, and may eventually conceive, with or without treatment. A number of possible treatments are available, but which is used depends upon the cause of the problem. Reduced fertility may have its origins in the male or the female partner or may be due to a combination of factors from both.[1-7]

The most obvious cause of infertility is a failure of either ovulation in the female or spermatogenesis in the male. Such failures may be due to damage or abnormal formation of the gonads, a failure of hypothalamic/pituitary stimulation, abnormal feedback as in the polycystic ovary syndrome, or suppression of gonadal function as in hyperprolactinaemia. These conditions and their management are briefly discussed under Hypogonadism (above), Ovarian Dysfunction (below), Polycystic Ovary Syndrome (below), and Hyperprolactinaemia (above).

The first-line treatment for anovulatory infertility in women (the primary problem in about 25 to 30% of infertile couples[1]) is clomifene. This has been reported to produce ovulation in up to 70% of anovulatory women,[1,2] or to increase the odds of ovulation more than 6 times in those with oligomenorrhoea,[8] although amenorrhoeic women are claimed to respond less well.[2] Because of concerns about a possibly increased risk of ovarian cancer (see p.1466) it has been suggested that no more than 6 cycles of clomifene therapy should be given: 3 cycles of treatment at increasing doses are generally enough to tell if the patient will ovulate.[1,2] Combination of clomifene with a mid-cycle injection of chorionic gonadotrophin has also been tried,[2] with variable results.[9,10] Tamoxifen is a possible alternative in those who cannot

tolerate clomifene,[11,12] and may be useful where abnormalities of cervical mucus contribute to infertility.

In anovulatory women who fail to respond to clomifene there is a choice of second-line therapy. Direct administration of gonadotrophins with follicle-stimulating activity, such as human menopausal gonadotrophins or recombinant human follicle-stimulating hormone,[13,14] may be appropriate in hypogonadotrophic women with low oestrogen levels, and can be effective even in others.

The risks of ovarian hyperstimulation and multiple pregnancies are considerable however, and close monitoring is mandatory, using ovarian ultrasound to assess follicle development.[1,2] Once one to three follicles are sufficiently mature, chorionic gonadotrophin is given to induce ovulation, and thereafter for luteal support. Aggregate pregnancy rates of about 10 to 25% per cycle have been reported with such treatment.[1] Combination of gonadotrophin treatment with intra-uterine insemination may be more effective than either method alone.[15] Women with polycystic ovary syndrome (see below) respond less well to gonadotrophins than hypogonadotrophic patients,[1,2] and are at greater risk of the ovarian hyperstimulation syndrome.[2]

The other alternative in those who fail to respond to clomifene is pulsatile administration of gonadorelin (gonadotrophin-releasing hormone) or its analogues. It is primarily indicated in women with hypothalamic causes of anovulation, in whom pregnancy rates approaching 30% per cycle have been stated to occur,[1,2] and again is less effective in women with polycystic ovary syndrome than in hypogonadotrophic patients. However, the risks of ovarian hyperstimulation and multiple pregnancy are lower than with direct administration of gonadotrophins, and gonadorelin therapy is considered by commentators to be the preferred therapy in anovulatory women with hypergonadotrophic amenorrhoea.[1]

Where anovulation is secondary to hyperprolactinaemia treatment with bromocriptine can restore fertility (see Hyperprolactinaemia, above). The use of bromocriptine in infertility of unknown cause does not seem to be justified.[1]

Producing a response in men with impaired sperm production can be difficult.[3-6,16] In men with hypogonadotrophic hypogonadism replacement therapy with a substance with luteinising hormone activity, such as chorionic gonadotrophin, is given to stimulate spermatogenesis and is followed if necessary by an agent such as menopausal gonadotrophins with follicle-stimulating and luteinising activity.[5,17] Treatment must often be continued for 12 months or more to permit development and maturation of spermatozoa, but 70% of these men have shown some degree of spermatogenesis with this therapy.[4] Once initiated, spermatogenesis may be maintained with chorionic gonadotrophin therapy alone. Pulsatile administration of gonadorelin may restore gonadotrophin secretion and correct infertility in men with hypogonadotrophic hypogonadism in whom the pituitary-gonadal axis is intact, such as those with Kallmann's syndrome.[18,19] Again, 12 months' therapy or more may be required.[4]

In idiopathic oligospermia, results of drug therapy have been disappointing, including trials with gonadorelin, and with testolactone and mesterolone; testosterone rebound therapy (in which high doses are given to suppress endogenous pituitary function, and then abruptly stopped, in the hope of provoking a rebound) is not recommended.[5] The anti-oestrogens, clomifene and tamoxifen have both been used in sub-fertile men,[5,6] but with little convincing evidence of benefit.

Where infertility is due to obstruction or inflammation of the fallopian tubes in the woman or the ductal system in the man treatment may be difficult, and the return of normal fertility unlikely. Microsurgical techniques may offer hope for a return of patency, but many patients will require in-vitro fertilisation in order to conceive. Where infection is the cause, appropriate anti-infective agents may be useful.[3,4] (See also under Pelvic Inflammatory Disease, p.133.) Autoantibodies to spermatozoa in some men may interfere with sperm motility; immunosuppression with corticosteroids (prednisolone[20] or methylprednisolone[21]) has been associated with successful pregnancy in such cases, but the usual risks of corticosteroid therapy apply and must be balanced against the equivocal evidence of benefit.[4,6]

Endometriosis (p.1469) is another important cause of infertility in women, although the reason for the association is not fully understood. Medical treatment of endo-

metriosis does not enhance fertility, although conservative surgery may do so.[7]

A variety of other drugs has been employed, on a more or less empirical basis, in the management of infertility. Such drugs include NSAIDs, guaifenesin to improve cervical mucus quality, kallidinogenase because of its supposed role in male genital-tract function, and oxpentifylline [pentoxifylline] to increase sperm count and motility. Growth hormone or one of its analogues has been used as an adjunct to ovarian stimulation with gonadotrophins.

Where other methods fail, assisted reproduction may be considered, including in-vitro fertilisation or gamete or zygote intrafallopian transfer.[1,2,4,6] In particular, intracytoplasmic sperm injection has reportedly revolutionised the treatment of male factor infertility.[16] Gonadotrophins with or without clomifene, together with a gonadorelin analogue to desensitise the pituitary, are used to stimulate follicular maturation and ovulation so that the ova can be collected. So called 'long protocols' in which gonadorelin agonists are started in the midluteal phase of the menstrual cycle or earlier and are maintained until chorionic gonadotrophin is given, appear to give better results than short ('flare-up') or ultrashort regimens, in which gonadorelin agonists are given for less time.[22-25] One study has suggested that results may be better if nafarelin is used rather than leuprorelin.[26] There is also some evidence that higher pregnancy rates are achieved with the use of recombinant follicle-stimulating hormone rather than urofollitropin or human menopausal gonadotrophins for ovarian stimulation.[27] Gonadorelin (gonadotrophin-releasing hormone) antagonists such as cetrorelix have been used as an alternative to gonadorelin analogues for pituitary desensitisation.[28]

1. Collins JA, Hughes EG. Pharmacological interventions for the induction of ovulation. Drugs 1995; 50: 480–94.
2. Hamilton M. Treatment of infertility: anovulatory infertility in women. Prescribers' J 1996; 36: 46–54.
3. Skakkebaek NE, et al. Pathogenesis and management of male infertility. Lancet 1994; 343: 1473–9.
4. Wu FC-W. Treatment of infertility: infertility in men. Prescribers' J 1996; 36: 55–61.
5. Howards SS. Treatment of male infertility. N Engl J Med 1995; 332: 312–17.
6. Wardle PG. Treatment of male infertility. Prescribers' J 1990; 30: 124–30.
7. Templeton A. Infertility and the establishment of pregnancy—overview. Br Med Bull 2000; 56: 577–87.
8. Hughes E, et al. Clomiphene citrate for ovulation induction in women with oligo-amenorrhoea (updated 29 May 2001). Available in The Cochrane Library; Issue 3. Oxford: Update Software; 2001.
9. Nash LD. The treatment of luteal phase dysfunction with clomiphene citrate and human chorionic gonadotrophin (HCG). Infertility 1982; 5: 87–104.
10. Fisch P, et al. Unexplained infertility: evaluation of treatment with clomiphene citrate and human chorionic gonadotropin. Fertil Steril 1989; 51: 828–33.
11. Messinis IE, Nillius SJ. Comparison between tamoxifen and clomiphene for induction of ovulation. Acta Obstet Gynecol Scand 1982; 61: 377–9.
12. Roumen FJME, et al. Treatment of infertile women with a deficient postcoital test with two antiestrogens: clomiphene and tamoxifen. Fertil Steril 1984; 41: 237–43.
13. Chuong CJ, et al. Successful pregnancy after treatment with recombinant human follicle stimulating hormone. Lancet 1993; 341: 1101.
14. Hornnes P, et al. Recombinant human follicle-stimulating hormone treatment leads to normal follicular growth, estradiol secretion, and pregnancy in a World Health Organization group II anovulatory woman. Fertil Steril 1993; 60: 724–6.
15. Guzick DS, et al. Efficacy of superovulation and intrauterine insemination in the treatment of infertility. N Engl J Med 1999; 340: 177–83.
16. Lewis-Jones DI, Gazvani MR. Male infertility: modern management and prognosis. Br J Hosp Med 1997; 58: 271–6.
17. Finkel DM, et al. Stimulation of spermatogenesis by gonadotropins in men with hypogonadotropic hypogonadism. N Engl J Med 1985; 313: 651–5.
18. Shargil AA. Treatment of idiopathic hypogonadotropic hypogonadism in men with luteinizing hormone-releasing hormone: a comparison of treatment with daily injections and with the pulsatile infusion pump. Fertil Steril 1987; 47: 492–501.
19. Crowley WF, Whitcomb RW. Gonadotropin-releasing hormone deficiency in men: diagnosis and treatment with exogenous gonadotropin-releasing hormone. Am J Obstet Gynecol 1990; 163: 1752–8.
20. Hendry WF, et al. Comparison of prednisolone and placebo in subfertile men with antibodies to spermatozoa. Lancet 1990; 335: 85–8.
21. Shulman JF, Shulman S. Methylprednisolone treatment of immunologic infertility in the male. Fertil Steril 1982; 38: 591–9.
22. Urbancsek J, Witthaus E. Midluteal buserelin is superior to early follicular phase buserelin in combined gonadotropin-releasing hormone analog and gonadotropin stimulation in in vitro fertilization. Fertil Steril 1996; 65: 966–71.
23. Tan S-L, et al. Cumulative conception and live-birth rates after in vitro fertilization with and without the use of long, short, and ultrashort regimens of the gonadotropin-releasing hormone agonist buserelin. Am J Obstet Gynecol 1994; 171: 513–20.
24. Filicori M, et al. Different gonadotropin and leuprorelin ovulation induction regimens markedly affect follicular fluid hormone levels and follicullogenesis. Fertil Steril 1996; 65: 387–93.
25. Daya S. Gonadotrophin-releasing hormone agonist protocols for pituitary desensitization in in vitro fertilization and gamete intrafallopian transfer cycles (updated 28 May 2001). Available in The Cochrane Library; Issue 3. Oxford: Update Software; 2001.

26. Martin MC, *et al.* The choice of a gonadotropin-releasing hormone analog influences outcome of in vitro fertilization treatment. *Am J Obstet Gynecol* 1994; **170:** 1629–34.
27. Out HJ, *et al.* Recombinant follicle stimulating hormone (follitropin beta, Puregon) yields higher pregnancy rates in in vitro fertilization than urinary gonadotropins. *Fertil Steril* 1997; **68:** 138–42.
28. Olivennes F, *et al.* The use of a GnRH antagonist (Cetrorelix) in a single dose protocol in IVF-embryo transfer: a dose finding study of 3 versus 2 mg. *Hum Reprod* 1998; **13:** 2411–14.

Lactation inhibition and induction

Lactation is the physiological secretion of milk post partum. Milk production by the breast is induced by prolactin while oxytocin promotes milk ejection into the milk ducts; both prolactin and oxytocin secretion are stimulated by suckling.

Lactation inhibition. The breast engorgement with consequent discomfort and galactorrhoea triggered by prolactin secretion post partum can be problematic in women who choose not to breast feed or are unable to do so. Nonsteroidal or synthetic oestrogens were historically employed to suppress lactation in such women, but this use is now considered inappropriate because of an increased risk of thromboembolism. Bromocriptine is a potent inhibitor of prolactin secretion: it has been given post partum in short treatment courses (about 14 days) to suppress lactation,[1,2] and is more effective than an oestrogen for this purpose.[2] However, bromocriptine is a potent drug which has also been associated with severe adverse effects in some women receiving it, and its use for lactation suppression is no longer advocated in a number of countries. Other dopaminergics with similar actions such as cabergoline, lisuride, metergoline, and quinagolide have also been used to suppress lactation. Although one commentator has suggested that cabergoline, which is generally better tolerated than bromocriptine, may be a better choice for lactation inhibition,[3] the same general objections as for bromocriptine apply to all these drugs. Non-pharmacological methods, such as the avoidance of nipple stimulation, and if necessary the use of mild analgesics, are generally to be preferred.

Lactation induction. Drug therapy has sometimes been used to help stimulate lactation, although mechanical stimulation of the nipple remains the primary method.[4] Dopamine antagonists, of which metoclopramide has been the most widely used, can produce modest increases in breast milk production but carry a risk of adverse effects including dystonias. If used, such therapy should be limited to one or two weeks; there has also been some concern about the presence of these drugs in breast milk.[4,5] Domperidone has also been reported to increase milk production,[6] and may cause fewer adverse central effects than metoclopramide. Protirelin has been given intranasally to stimulate lactation by increasing serum prolactin concentrations, but is expensive, and a suitable commercial preparation is unavailable.[4] The use of oxytocin nasal spray to promote milk ejection is not recommended, as mothers may become dependent upon its action.[4]

1. Duchesne C, Leke R. Bromocriptine mesylate for prevention of postpartum lactation. *Obstet Gynecol* 1981; **57:** 464–7.
2. Walker S, *et al.* Controlled trial of bromocriptine, quinoestrol, and placebo in suppression of puerperal lactation. *Lancet* 1975; **ii:** 842–5.
3. Webster J. A comparative review of the tolerability profiles of dopamine agonists in the treatment of hyperprolactinaemia and inhibition of lactation. *Drug Safety* 1996; **14:** 228–38. Correction. *ibid;* 342.
4. Anderson PO, Valdés V. Increasing breast milk supply. *Clin Pharm* 1992; **12:** 479–80.
5. Kauppila A, *et al.* Metoclopramide and breast feeding: transfer into milk and the newborn. *Eur J Clin Pharmacol* 1983; **25:** 819–23.
6. da Silva OP, *et al.* Effect of domperidone on milk production in mothers of premature newborns: a randomized, double-blind, placebo-controlled trial. *Can Med Assoc J* 2001; **164:** 17–21.

Ovarian dysfunction

Primary ovarian dysfunction may be due to failure of the ovaries to form normally, as in Turner's syndrome (see below), or their degeneration before puberty; there may be premature failure, effectively an early menopause, due to low initial follicle numbers or to destruction of follicles by autoantibodies, chemotherapy, radiotherapy, infection, or trauma; or there may be some other condition such as the polycystic ovary syndrome (see below). Alternatively, ovarian dysfunction can be secondary to decreased gonadotrophic stimulation which may occur with weight loss or due to a defect in the hypothalamic/pituitary axis (see also under Hypogonadism, above).

Primary dysfunction is often associated with high concentrations of circulating gonadotrophins, whereas in hy-

pothalamic or pituitary dysfunction the gonadotrophin concentrations are of course low.

Women with primary ovarian dysfunction generally require sex hormone replacement therapy. Conception is rarely possible in such women. In women with chronic anovulation secondary to gonadotrophin deficiency due to hypothalamic or pituitary dysfunction, ovulation may be induced with clomifene, gonadotrophins, or the pulsatile administration of gonadorelin (see under Infertility, above).

Polycystic ovary syndrome. The polycystic ovary syndrome comprises enlargement of the ovaries with multiple follicular cysts and a thickened, whitish, capsule; there is persistent elevation of serum luteinising hormone concentrations, with a tendency to increased androgen and oestrogen concentrations. Women typically present with erratic menstruation, hirsutism, and obesity, although not all these features may be present; fertility is also often impaired. There is often some degree of associated hyperinsulinaemia with insulin resistance, and increased risk of developing hyperlipidaemia, hypertension, and ischaemic heart disease.[1]

Management is essentially symptomatic. Patients should be encouraged to lose weight if obese; weight loss alone may be sufficient to improve menstrual regularity, hirsutism, and fertility. Clinical commentators suggest that symptoms of hyperandrogenism can be treated with an anti-androgen such as cyproterone acetate or spironolactone together with an oestrogen or a combined contraceptive pill;[2-5] flutamide has also been employed as an anti-androgen in these patients (see also the discussion of the management of hirsutism, p.1468). In women who do not desire pregnancy, a low-dose oral contraceptive is also the recommended means of treating amenorrhoea or oligomenorrhoea.[3,4] An alternative is the cyclic administration of a progestogen which lacks androgenic properties, in order to induce withdrawal bleeding (anovular women who do not receive hormonal treatment may be at increased risk of endometrial cancer).[3-5]

In patients who wish to conceive clomifene citrate is the initial treatment of choice to induce ovulation, but although ovulation may be induced in up to 80% of cases, pregnancy rates are only about half this figure.[4] In patients who do not respond to clomifene, a human menopausal gonadotrophin with follicle-stimulating activity may be tried followed by chorionic gonadotrophin (see also under Infertility, above). Human gonadotrophins such as urofollitropin or the recently developed recombinant follicle-stimulating hormone, which both lack luteinising hormone activity, may be preferable[6] as patients with polycystic ovary syndrome already have raised luteinising hormone concentrations. The use of pulsatile gonadorelin and its analogues in patients with polycystic ovary syndrome appears to be less effective than in hypogonadotrophic hypogonadism (see Infertility, above) and is held to be contra-indicated by some manufacturers. However, pretreatment with a gonadorelin analogue given continuously for 8 weeks, to suppress gonadotrophin production, before the pulsatile administration of gonadorelin, has produced improved ovulation and pregnancy rates.[7] Patients must be monitored carefully during any therapy to induce ovulation, as women with polycystic ovaries are more prone to multiple follicle development and ovarian hyperstimulation;[2] a low-dose regimen of follicle stimulating hormone has been reported to reduce this risk.[6,8]

It has been suggested that hyperinsulinism may play a pathogenetic role in stimulating ovarian androgen production in polycystic ovary syndrome;[9] some small studies have reported an improvement in hyperandrogenism[10,11] and in subsequent fertility[10] associated with metformin treatment although others have reported negligible benefit.[12] Treatment with metformin has also been reported to improve the ovulatory response to clomifene, as well as increasing the rate of spontaneous ovulation.[13]

Occasional reports have suggested some benefit from octreotide[14] and bromocriptine[15] in normalising the hormonal environment; the latter is most likely to be useful in women with associated hyperprolactinaemia—see above.

An alternative to drug therapy is the use of laparoscopic ovarian diathermy, which appears to be as effective as gonadotrophin therapy in inducing ovulation in women resistant to clomifene.[16]

1. Lobo RA, Carmina E. The importance of diagnosing the polycystic ovary syndrome. *Ann Intern Med* 2000; **132:** 989–93.

2. White MC, Turner EI. Polycystic ovary syndrome 2: diagnosis and management. *Br J Hosp Med* 1994; **51:** 349–52. Correction. *ibid.;* **52:** 122.
3. Franks S. Polycystic ovary syndrome. *N Engl J Med* 1995; **333:** 853–61. Correction. *ibid;* 1435.
4. Harrington DJ, Balen AH. Polycystic ovary syndrome: aetiology and management. *Br J Hosp Med* 1996; **56:** 17–20.
5. Anonymous. Tackling polycystic ovary syndrome. *Drug Ther Bull* 2001; **39:** 1–5.
6. Shoham Z, *et al.* Polycystic ovarian syndrome: safety and effectiveness of stepwise and low-dose administration of purified follicle-stimulating hormone. *Fertil Steril* 1991; **55:** 1051–6.
7. Filicori M, *et al.* Polycystic ovary syndrome: abnormalities and management with pulsatile gonadotropin-releasing hormone and gonadotropin-releasing hormone analogs. *Am J Obstet Gynecol* 1992; **163:** 1737–42.
8. White DM, *et al.* Induction of ovulation with low-dose gonadotropins in polycystic ovary syndrome: an analysis of 109 pregnancies in 225 women. *J Clin Endocrinol Metab* 1996; **81:** 3821–4.
9. Utiger RD. Insulin and the polycystic ovary syndrome. *N Engl J Med* 1996; **335:** 657–8.
10. Velazquez EM, *et al.* Metformin therapy in polycystic ovary syndrome reduces hyperinsulinemia, insulin resistance, hyperandrogenemia, and systolic blood pressure, while facilitating normal menses and pregnancy. *Metabolism* 1994; **43:** 647–54.
11. Nestler JE, Jakubowicz DJ. Decreases in ovarian cytochrome P450c17α activity and serum free testosterone after reduction of insulin secretion in polycystic ovary syndrome. *N Engl J Med* 1996; **335:** 617–23.
12. Ehrmann DA, *et al.* Effects of metformin on insulin secretion, insulin action, and ovarian steroidogenesis in women with polycystic ovary syndrome. *J Clin Endocrinol Metab* 1997; **82:** 524–30.
13. Nestler JE, *et al.* Effects of metformin on spontaneous and clomiphene-induced ovulation in the polycystic ovary syndrome. *N Engl J Med* 1998; **338:** 1876–80.
14. Prelević GM, *et al.* Inhibitory effect of Sandostatin on secretion of luteinising hormone and ovarian steroids in polycystic ovary syndrome. *Lancet* 1990; **336:** 900–3.
15. Pehrson JJ, *et al.* Bromocriptine, sex steroid metabolism, and menstrual patterns in the polycystic ovary syndrome. *Ann Intern Med* 1986; **105:** 129–30.
16. Gadir AA. Ovarian electrocautery versus human menopausal gonadotrophins and pure follicle stimulating hormone therapy in the treatment of patients with polycystic ovarian disease. *Clin Endocrinol (Oxf)* 1990; **33:** 585–92.

Turner's syndrome. Turner's syndrome is a congenital disorder associated with the absence of an X or Y chromosome, resulting in an individual with only a single X chromosome who is female in phenotype but in whom the ovaries do not develop. In addition to this gonadal dysgenesis, which results in infertility and primary amenorrhoea, various physical abnormalities may be present including short stature, a short webbed neck and characteristic facial appearance, shield-like chest, multiple naevi, and certain renal and cardiovascular abnormalities. Hypothyroidism and glucose intolerance may occur.

As with other forms of ovarian failure, HRT with oestrogen and intermittent progestogen is indicated in women with Turner's syndrome, in order to produce sexual maturation and the development of secondary sexual characteristics as well as to avoid complications such as osteoporosis. Clinical opinion has generally been that therapy should begin with low doses of oestrogen in girls of prepubertal age, gradually increasing the dose to promote slow development of secondary sexual characteristics and eventual breakthrough bleeding, at which point a cyclic progestogen should be added to oestrogen maintenance.[1-3] In the UK ethinylestradiol has been widely used in girls with Turner's syndrome, but commentators in both the UK and the US suggest that this is inappropriate,[1,2] and that replacement should be with a natural oestrogen such as estradiol, in suitably modest doses. (Good comparative studies of these options are lacking.[4]) Application of a transdermal estradiol patch may be a convenient way to achieve oestrogen replacement in these women, although during adolescence oestrogen requirements are greater than those in normal menopausal women, for whom most transdermal formulations have been developed.[2] Oral contraceptives have been used for maintenance in adult women with Turner's syndrome (again often containing ethinylestradiol)[1] but it has been suggested that these supply too high a dose of oestrogen.[2]

A minority of patients with Turner's syndrome have some residual ovarian function, and there are a few reports of pregnancy in such patients.[2] In women without ovaries it may be possible to maintain pregnancy by appropriate endocrine replacement following implantation of a fertilised donor egg.

Short stature is the most common clinical manifestation of Turner's syndrome. Therapy with growth hormone has been widely tried,[5-11] but there is considerable debate about the extent of the benefit in terms of final height. Results from 622 girls enrolled in the National Cooperative Growth Study[8] suggested a mean height gain of 6.4 ± 4.9 cm, and it has been suggested[3] that a final height of 150 cm is an achievable goal for most patients. Growth hormone therapy during childhood and adolescence may also be important in maximising bone mass and reducing the risk of osteoporosis.[12] Although it is generally recommended that oestrogen replacement be delayed where growth promotion is a priority,[3] optimal oestrogen replacement therapy may also be important in maximising final height.[13] In a comparison[14] of the introduction of conjugated oestrogen therapy at 12 or 15 years of age, the combination of growth hormone and oestrogen initially stimulated growth velocity and bone maturation more than growth hormone alone, but subsequently declined after about 2 years. Patients who received growth hormone for a longer period before the initiation of oestrogen therapy attained greater adult height, a finding also noted in another study;[15] it was suggested that early use of growth hormone could allow oestrogen therapy to be begun at a more appropriate, younger age without compromising final height. Combination of growth hormone with a non-aromatisable anabolic steroid such as oxandrolone is recommended as an option if therapy is begun late.[3]

Adult women with Turner's syndrome require multidisciplinary management including cardiovascular monitoring, psychological support, and a programme of prevention for diabetes, osteoporosis, and hypertension.[3]

1. Masters KW. Treatment of Turner's syndrome—a concern. *Lancet* 1996; **348**: 681–2.
2. Saenger P. Turner's syndrome. *N Engl J Med* 1996; **335**: 1749–54.
3. Saenger P, *et al.* Recommendations for the diagnosis and management of Turner syndrome. *J Clin Endocrinol Metab* 2001; **86**: 3061–9.
4. Conway GS, *et al.* Treatment of Turner's syndrome. *Lancet* 1996; **348**: 1590–1.
5. Rongen-Westerlaken C, *et al.* Methionyl human growth hormone in Turner's syndrome. *Arch Dis Child* 1988; **63**: 1211–17.
6. Takano K, *et al.* Turner's syndrome: treatment of 203 patients with recombinant human growth hormone for one year: a multicentre study. *Acta Endocrinol (Copenh)* 1989; **120**: 559–68.
7. Rosenfeld RG, *et al.* Growth hormone therapy of Turner's syndrome: beneficial effect on adult height. *J Pediatr* 1998; **132**: 319–24.
8. Plotnick L, *et al.* Growth hormone treatment of girls with Turner syndrome: the National Cooperative Growth Study experience. *Pediatrics* 1998; **102**: 479–81.
9. Van den Broeck J, *et al.* Final height after long-term growth hormone treatment in Turner syndrome. *J Pediatr* 1995; **127**: 729–35.
10. Taback SP, *et al.* Does growth-hormone supplementation affect adult height in Turner's syndrome? *Lancet* 1996; **348**: 25–7.
11. Dacou-Voutetakis C, *et al.* The growth pattern and final height of girls with Turner syndrome with and without human growth hormone treatment. *Pediatrics* 1998; **101**: 663–8.
12. Rubin K. Turner syndrome and osteoporosis: mechanisms and prognosis. *Pediatrics* 1998; **102** (suppl): 481–5.
13. Rosenfield RL, *et al.* Optimizing estrogen replacement treatment in Turner syndrome. *Pediatrics* 1998; **102** (suppl): 486–8.
14. Chernausek SD, *et al.* Growth hormone therapy of Turner syndrome: the impact of age of estrogen replacement on final height. *J Clin Endocrinol Metab* 2000; **85**: 2439–45.
15. Reiter EO, *et al.* Early initiation of growth hormone treatment allows age-appropriate estrogen use in Turner's syndrome. *J Clin Endocrinol Metab* 2001; **86**: 1936–41.

Precocious puberty

Precocious puberty is commonly understood to mean the development of secondary sexual characteristics before the age of 8 years in girls or 9 years in boys; it is four to five times more common in girls. However, the age limit used to define precocious puberty in girls has been questioned.[1] Recent data from the United States suggests that puberty is occurring earlier in girls, at age 7 years for white girls, and 6 years for African-American girls. Precocious puberty is either central, due to premature activation of the hypothalamic-pituitary-gonadal axis, or peripheral, due to secretion of extrapituitary gonadotrophins or gonadal steroids independent of gonadorelin secretion from the hypothalamus or pituitary gonadotrophins. In many cases the cause is not apparent, and they are classified as idiopathic. A small proportion of cases are due to tumours. Central precocious puberty may be caused by CNS lesions secondary to diseases such as encephalitis, meningitis, or granuloma, or head trauma. Peripheral precocious puberty can be associated with congenital or familial syndromes such as McCune-Albright syndrome or familial testotoxicosis (familial male precocious puberty). Congenital adrenal hyperplasia (see p.1049) can also produce premature sexual development in boys and virilisation in girls.

Apart from early sexual maturation and the associated emotional distress, the chief clinical consequence of precocious puberty is short stature as an adult, due to premature closure of the epiphyses under the influence of sex steroids.[2-4]

Gonadorelin analogues have replaced drugs such as medroxyprogesterone acetate (which suppressed secondary sexual characteristics but were often ineffective in preventing epiphyseal fusion) as the treatment of choice in central precocious puberty.[3,4] The continuous rather than

pulsatile administration of gonadorelin can paradoxically suppress gonadotrophin secretion by desensitisation and down regulation of pituitary receptors. Although originally given daily, by subcutaneous injection or nasal insufflation, intramuscular depot preparations[5,6] are more convenient, and are now more widely used.[4] Treatment with gonadorelin analogues suppresses sexual development and also skeletal maturation and most studies have reported an improvement in final height.[3,7] However, the treatment of girls with borderline early puberty (between 6 and 8 years of age) has been questioned, as studies suggest that most will reach adult height within the normal range without treatment.[1] Such girls with idiopathic slowly progressing puberty, and no evidence of advanced bone age, may not require gonadorelin therapy, but should be monitored for an onset of rapid pubertal development.[1,8] Children with concomitant growth hormone deficiency (for example after cranial irradiation) may need additional therapy with somatropin or its analogues for maximum benefit.[9] Discontinuation of treatment should be individualised on the basis of final height potential and the patient and family's wishes.[4]

In the peripheral forms of precocious puberty the gonadorelin analogues are ineffective.[3] Any underlying condition such as a gonadal or adrenal neoplasm should be sought and treated appropriately. Otherwise, therapy is aimed at suppressing premature sexual maturation. Medroxyprogesterone acetate retains some usefulness in these conditions,[3] while the aromatase inhibitor testolactone has been used with some success to block oestrogen biosynthesis in girls with the McCune-Albright syndrome to treat the associated precocious puberty.[10,11] Although ineffective when given alone, testolactone was reported to be of benefit when combined with the antiandrogen, spironolactone, in boys with testotoxicosis;[12] a reduction in the rate of bone maturation was reported. Response diminished with long-term treatment, but could be restored by the addition of a gonadorelin analogue, deslorelin, to therapy.[13]

Other drugs with anti-androgenic properties such as cyproterone acetate[4] or ketoconazole[14] have also been tried in boys with precocious puberty, but the use of the former is no longer considered appropriate.

1. Kaplowitz PB, *et al.* Reexamination of the age limit for defining when puberty is precocious in girls in the United States: implications for evaluation and treatment. *Pediatrics* 1999; **104**: 936–41.
2. Anonymous. Precocious puberty. *Lancet* 1991; **337**: 1194–5.
3. Wheeler MD, Styne DM. Drug treatment in precocious puberty. *Drugs* 1991; **41**: 717–28.
4. Merke DP, Cutler GB. Evaluation and management of precocious puberty. *Arch Dis Child* 1996; **75**: 269–71.
5. Neely EK, *et al.* Two-year results of treatment with depot leuprolide acetate for central precocious puberty. *J Pediatr* 1992; **121**: 634–40.
6. Paterson WF, *et al.* Efficacy of Zoladex LA (goserelin) in the treatment of girls with central precocious or early puberty. *Arch Dis Child* 1998; **79**: 323–7.
7. Paul D, *et al.* Long term effect of gonadotropin-releasing hormone agonist therapy on final and near-final height in 26 children with true precocious puberty treated at a median age of less than 5 years. *J Clin Endocrinol Metab* 1995; **80**: 546–51.
8. Léger J, *et al.* Do all girls with apparent idiopathic precocious puberty require gonadotropin-releasing hormone agonist treatment? *J Pediatr* 2000; **137**: 819–25.
9. Cara JF, *et al.* Height prognosis of children with true precocious puberty and growth hormone deficiency: effect of combination therapy with gonadotropin releasing hormone agonist and growth hormone. *J Pediatr* 1992; **120**: 709–15.
10. Feuillan PP, *et al.* Treatment of precocious puberty in the McCune-Albright syndrome with the aromatase inhibitor testolactone. *N Engl J Med* 1986; **315**: 1115–19.
11. Feuillan PP, *et al.* Long term testolactone therapy for precocious puberty in girls with the McCune-Albright syndrome. *J Clin Endocrinol Metab* 1993; **77**: 647–51.
12. Laue L, *et al.* Treatment of familial male precocious puberty with spironolactone and testolactone. *N Engl J Med* 1989; **320**: 496–502.
13. Laue L, *et al.* Treatment of familial male precocious puberty with spironolactone, testolactone, and deslorelin. *J Clin Endocrinol Metab* 1993; **76**: 151–5.
14. Holland FJ, *et al.* Ketoconazole in the management of precocious puberty not responsive to LHRH-analogue therapy. *N Engl J Med* 1985; **312**: 1023–8. Correction. *ibid.*; 1652.

Premenstrual syndrome

Gonadorelin analogues have been used to treat patients with severe symptoms attributable to the premenstrual syndrome (p.1475), together with 'add-back' therapy with oestrogen plus progestogen to prevent the symptoms of oestrogen deficiency.

Syndrome of inappropriate ADH secretion

In some patients secretion of antidiuretic hormone (ADH; vasopressin) occurs despite hypotonicity of the extracellular fluid and normal or raised fluid volume, and such patients are said to have the syndrome of inappropriate ADH secretion (SIADH). With severe water ex-

cess, the resultant hyponatraemia may result in symptoms ranging from lassitude or headache to profound neurological symptoms such as confusion, convulsions, or coma. Some patients may experience inappropriate thirst as well as ADH secretion, thus exacerbating their condition. For a discussion of sodium homoeostasis and dilutional hyponatraemia, see p.1183.

Conditions which may precipitate SIADH include CNS disorders, infections such as encephalitis and meningitis, head trauma, porphyria, or pulmonary diseases such as tuberculosis and pneumonia. ADH may also be secreted ectopically from a variety of malignancies, most commonly from small-cell bronchial carcinoma. Alternatively, SIADH may be drug-induced; drugs associated with the condition include carbamazepine, chlorpropamide, cytotoxic drugs such as cyclophosphamide and the vinca alkaloids, oxytocin, some antipsychotics, and tricyclic antidepressants.

Diagnosis of SIADH is initially prompted by the presence of hyponatraemia and corresponding plasma hypoosmolality with or without neurological symptoms. Hypervolaemia, persistent excess sodium excretion, lack of oedema, and normality of both renal and adrenal function are confirmatory.

Mild degrees of water excess are frequently asymptomatic and may not require specific therapy, but patients with SIADH often have a more severe disorder and initially treatment is best aimed at the underlying cause. If such treatment is not possible or if symptoms persist, water restriction may be considered. However, fluid restriction is an unpleasant form of treatment, particularly for patients who retain inappropriate thirst, and may not be tolerable. In these patients demeclocycline may be given to antagonise the effect of ADH on the renal tubules. Lithium has been given as an alternative, and phenytoin has been used occasionally to inhibit pituitary ADH secretion. Diuretics such as frusemide [furosemide] (in conjunction with oral sodium chloride) have also been tried in an attempt to optimise diuresis while retaining sodium. In patients with life-threatening severe acute water intoxication (see Hyponatraemia, p.1183), treatment initially involves cautious improvement of the profound hyponatraemia with intravenous infusion of hypertonic (up to 5%) or isotonic sodium chloride often with concurrent frusemide [furosemide] or other loop diuretic to avoid volume expansion. Dexamethasone has been used to treat associated cerebral oedema but its effectiveness is unclear.

References.
1. Miyagawa CI. The pharmacologic management of the syndrome of inappropriate secretion of antidiuretic hormone. *Drug Intell Clin Pharm* 1986; **20**: 527–31.
2. Kinzie BJ. Management of the syndrome of inappropriate secretion of antidiuretic hormone. *Clin Pharm* 1987; **6**: 625–33.
3. Kovacs L, Robertson GL. Syndrome of inappropriate antidiuresis. *Endocrinol Metab Clin North Am* 1992; **21**: 859–75.

Abarelix (10219-m)

Abarelix (USAN, rINN).

PPI-149; R-3827. N-Acetyl-3-(2-naphthyl)-D-alanyl-4-chloro-D-phenylalanyl-3-(3-pyridyl)-D-alanyl-L-seryl-N-methyl-L-tyrosyl-D-asparaginyl-L-leucyl-N^6-isopropyl-L-lysyl-L-prolyl-D-alaninamide.

$C_{72}H_{95}ClN_{14}O_{14} = 1416.1$.
CAS — 183552-38-7.

Profile

Like cetrorelix (p.1279), abarelix is a gonadorelin (gonadotrophin-releasing hormone) antagonist. It is under investigation for the treatment of endometriosis and to reduce testosterone concentrations in the hormonal therapy of prostate cancer.

◊ References.
1. Tomera K, *et al.* The gonadotropin-releasing hormone antagonist abarelix depot versus luteinizing hormone releasing hormone agonists leuprolide or goserelin: initial results of endocrinological and biochemical efficacies in patients with prostate cancer. *J Urol (Baltimore)* 2001; **165**: 1585–9.

Atosiban (9359-h)

Atosiban (BAN, USAN, rINN).

ORF-22164; RWJ-22164. 1-(3-Mercaptopropionic acid)-2-[3-(p-ethoxyphenyl)-D-alanine]-4-L-threonine-8-L-ornithineoxytocin; [1-(3-Sulfanylpropanoyl),2-(4-O-ethyltyrosine),4-L-threonine-8-L-ornithine]oxytocin.

$C_{43}H_{67}N_{11}O_{12}S_2 = 994.2$.
CAS — 90779-69-4.

Adverse Effects and Precautions

Adverse effects reported in women receiving atosiban for premature labour include nausea and vomiting, headache, dizziness, flushes, tachycardia, hypotension, and hyperglycaemia. Atosiban should not be used where continuation of pregnancy is hazardous to mother or fetus, including where gestational age is below 24 or over 33 weeks, in eclampsia or severe pre-eclampsia, intra-uterine growth retardation and abnormal fetal heart rate, suspected intra-uterine infection, placenta praevia, or abruptio placentae. Monitoring of uterine contractions and fetal heart rate is recommended during administration, and blood loss should be monitored after delivery.

Although there has been some concern about fetal exposure, the manufacturers report that no specific adverse effects on the newborn have been reported.

Pharmacokinetics

In women in premature labour, atosiban reaches steady-state plasma concentrations within one hour of the start of infusion, and has a terminal half-life of 1.7 hours after ceasing infusion. Atosiban is 46 to 48% bound to plasma proteins, and crosses the placenta. It is metabolised to an active metabolite, which is excreted in the urine, and is distributed into breast milk.

Uses and Administration

Atosiban is a peptide analogue of oxytocin (p.1294) but with oxytocin antagonist properties. It is used as a tocolytic in the management of premature labour. Atosiban is given intravenously as the acetate, but doses are expressed in terms of the base. An initial bolus dose equivalent to atosiban 6.75 mg is given by intravenous injection (as a solution containing 7.5 mg per mL) over one minute. This is immediately followed by a continuous infusion of 300 μg per minute for 3 hours, then 100 μg per minute for up to 45 hours, as a solution containing 750 μg per mL. The total duration of treatment should not exceed 48 hours, and the total dose should not exceed 330 mg.

◊ References.
1. Valenzuela GJ, *et al.* Placental passage of the oxytocin antagonist atosiban. *Am J Obstet Gynecol* 1995; **172:** 1304–6.
2. Goodwin TM, *et al.* Dose ranging study of the oxytocin antagonist atosiban in the treatment of preterm labor. *Obstet Gynecol* 1996; **88:** 331–6.
3. Romero R, *et al.* An oxytocin receptor antagonist (atosiban) in the treatment of preterm labor: a randomized, double-blind, placebo-controlled trial with tocolytic rescue. *Am J Obstet Gynecol* 2000; **182:** 1173–83.
4. Valenzuela GJ, *et al.* Maintenance treatment of preterm labor with the oxytocin antagonist atosiban: the Atosiban PTL-098 Study Group. *Am J Obstet Gynecol* 2000; **182:** 1184–90.
5. Moutquin JM, *et al.* Double-blind, randomized, controlled trial of atosiban and ritodrine in the treatment of preterm labor: a multicenter effectiveness and safety study. *Am J Obstet Gynecol* 2000; **182:** 1191–9.
6. The Worldwide Atosiban versus Beta-agonists Study Group. Effectiveness and safety of the oxytocin antagonist atosiban versus beta-adrenergic agonists in the treatment of preterm labour. *Br J Obstet Gynaecol* 2001; **108:** 133–42.
7. The European Atosiban Study Group. The oxytocin antagonist atosiban versus the beta-agonist terbutaline in the treatment of preterm labor: a randomized, double-blind, controlled study. *Acta Obstet Gynecol Scand* 2001; **80:** 413–22.

Preparations

Proprietary Preparations (details are given in Part 3)
Denm.: Tractocile; **Fin.:** Tractocile; **Irl.:** Tractocile; **UK:** Tractocile.

Buserelin Acetate (14039-p)

Buserelin Acetate (BANM, USAN, rINNM).
Hoe-766; S74-6766 (buserelin); D-Ser (Bu^t)^6 Pro^9 NEt LHRH acetate. (6-O-tert-Butyl-D-serine)-des-10-glycinamidegonadorelin ethylamide acetate; 5-Oxo-L-prolyl-L-histidyl-L-tryptophyl-L-seryl-L-tyrosyl-O-tert-butyl-D-seryl-L-leucyl-L-arginyl-N-ethyl-L-prolinamide acetate.
$C_{60}H_{86}N_{16}O_{13},C_2H_4O_2 = 1299.5$.
CAS — 57982-77-1 (buserelin); 68630-75-1 (buserelin acetate).

Pharmacopoeias. Eur. (see p.vi) includes Buserelin.

105 μg of buserelin acetate is approximately equivalent to 100 μg of buserelin.

Pharmacopoeial description

Ph. Eur.: Buserelin (Buserelinum) is a white or slightly yellowish hygroscopic powder. Sparingly soluble in water and in dilute acids. Store at 2° to 8°. Protect from light and moisture.

Adverse Effects and Precautions

As for Gonadorelin, p.1284.

Effects on the bones. In a study[1] involving 46 patients with symptomatic locally advanced or metastatic prostate cancer, buserelin or triptorelin in various doses produced objective improvement in 26 of 35 given buserelin and 8 of 11 given triptorelin. However 17 of 32 patients who had bone pain at the start of treatment had an increase in bone pain which resolved after the first week; one patient who had no initial bone pain developed such pain on receiving the gonadorelin analogue. Additional symptoms to increased bone pain included lymphoedema in 4, increased serum-creatinine concentration in 1, and one patient who developed signs of compression of the spinal cord with complete sphincter dysfunction and weakness in the legs.

To prevent adverse effects arising from the initial increase in circulating testosterone, cyproterone acetate has been given for 3 days before and for 1 week after initiation of gonadorelin analogue therapy.[2] Another anti-androgen, nilutamide, has been given with buserelin for a similar purpose.[3]
Bone loss has been reported in premenopausal women given buserelin for endometriosis.[4,5]

1. Waxman J, *et al.* Importance of early tumour exacerbation in patients treated with long acting analogues of gonadotrophin releasing hormone for advanced prostatic cancer. *BMJ* 1985; **291:** 1387–8.
2. Waxman J. Early tumour exacerbation in patients treated with long acting analogues of gonadotrophin releasing hormones. *BMJ* 1986; **292:** 58.
3. Kuhn J-M, *et al.* Prevention of the transient adverse effects of a gonadotropin-releasing hormone analogue (buserelin) in metastatic prostatic carcinoma by administration of an antiandrogen (nilutamide). *N Engl J Med* 1989; **321:** 413–18.
4. Matta WH, *et al.* Hypogonadism induced by luteinising hormone releasing hormone agonist analogues: effects on bone density in premenopausal women. *BMJ* 1987; **294:** 1523–4.
5. Devogelaer J-P, *et al.* LHRH analogues and bone loss. *Lancet* 1987; **i:** 1498.

Effects on the cardiovascular system. Hypertension in one patient associated with buserelin acetate.[1]

1. Barrett JFR, Dalton ME. Hypertension in association with buserelin. *BMJ* 1987; **294:** 1101.

Interactions
As for Gonadorelin, p.1284.

Pharmacokinetics

Buserelin is completely absorbed following subcutaneous injection, with peak plasma concentrations occurring about 1 hour after a dose. It accumulates in liver and kidneys as well as in the anterior pituitary. It is metabolised by tissue peptidases and is excreted in urine and bile as unchanged drug and metabolites. The half-life after injection is stated to be about 80 minutes.

Uses and Administration

Buserelin acetate is an analogue of gonadorelin (see p.1284) with similar properties. It is used for the suppression of testosterone in the treatment of malignant neoplasms of the prostate; it is also used in the treatment of endometriosis and as an adjunct to ovulation induction with gonadotrophins in the treatment of infertility. It has also been used in precocious puberty and has been tried in the treatment of uterine fibroids (see below).

In advanced prostatic carcinoma treatment is started with the equivalent of 500 μg of buserelin being injected subcutaneously every 8 hours for 7 days. On the eighth day treatment is changed to the nasal route with 100 μg of buserelin being sprayed into each nostril 6 times daily (usually before and after meals). An acceptable response should be achieved within 4 to 6 weeks. Since there is an initial increase in circulating testosterone, an anti-androgen such as cyproterone acetate may be given for at least 3 days before beginning buserelin therapy, and continued for at least 3 weeks, to avoid the risk of a disease flare.

In endometriosis the equivalent of 150 μg of buserelin is sprayed into each nostril three times daily. The usual duration of therapy is 6 months which should not be exceeded.

In infertility, pituitary desensitisation before ovulation induction with gonadotrophins is achieved with the equivalent of 150 μg of buserelin being given intranasally four times daily, beginning either in the early follicular phase (day 1) or midluteal phase (day 21) of the menstrual cycle. Alternatively, the equivalent of 200 to 500 μg of buserelin may be given daily as a subcutaneous injection. Therapy should be continued until pituitary downregulation occurs, which normally takes 1 to 3 weeks; if necessary 300 μg four times daily intranasally, or 500 μg twice daily subcutaneously may be given. Gonadotrophin treatment is then added to buserelin therapy until an appropriate stage of follicular development, when both are withdrawn and chorionic gonadotrophin is given to induce ovulation.

◊ General reviews of buserelin.
1. Brogden RN, *et al.* Buserelin: a review of its pharmacodynamic and pharmacokinetic properties, and clinical profile. *Drugs* 1990; **39:** 399–437.

Endometriosis. Gonadorelin analogues such as buserelin have a role in the management of endometriosis (p.1469), but the need for long-term therapy limits their value because of the risk of osteoporosis; 'add-back' therapy with concomitant hormone replacement is being investigated.

References.
1. Lemay A, *et al.* Efficacy of intranasal or subcutaneous luteinizing hormone-releasing hormone agonist inhibition of ovarian function in the treatment of endometriosis. *Am J Obstet Gynecol* 1988; **158:** 233–6.
2. Donnez J, *et al.* Administration of nasal buserelin as compared with subcutaneous buserelin implant for endometriosis. *Fertil Steril* 1989; **52:** 27–30.
3. Nieto A, *et al.* Long term follow-up of endometriosis after two different therapies (gestrinone and buserelin). *Clin Exp Obstet Gynecol* 1996; **23:** 198–204.
4. Regidor P-A, *et al.* Long-term follow-up on the treatment of endometriosis with the GnRH-agonist buserelin acetate. *Eur J Obstet Gynecol Reprod Biol* 1997; **73:** 153–60.
5. Takeuchi H, *et al.* A prospective randomized study comparing endocrinological and clinical effects of two types of GnRH agonists in cases of uterine leiomyomas or endometriosis. *J Obstet Gynaecol Res* 2000; **26:** 325–31.

Fibroids. Like other gonadorelin analogues (see also p.1285) buserelin has been used to reduce the volume of uterine fibroids.

References.
1. Maheux R, *et al.* Use of intranasal luteinizing hormone-releasing hormone agonist in uterine leiomyomas. *Fertil Steril* 1987; **47:** 229–31.
2. Matta WHM, *et al.* Long-term follow-up of patients with uterine fibroids after treatment with the LHRH agonist buserelin. *Br J Obstet Gynaecol* 1989; **96:** 200–6.
3. Fedele L, *et al.* Intranasal buserelin versus surgery in the treatment of uterine leiomyomata: long-term follow-up. *Eur J Obstet Gynecol Reprod Biol* 1991; **38:** 53–7.
4. Ueki M, *et al.* Endocrinological and histological changes after treatment of uterine leiomyomas with danazol or buserelin. *J Obstet Gynaecol* 1995; **21:** 1–7.

Infertility. Buserelin is given with gonadotrophic hormone therapy for induction of ovulation and as an aid to improving *in-vitro* fertilisation procedures. Buserelin with gonadotrophic hormones has been found to result in pregnancies in women previously unresponsive to clomifene citrate,[1,2] although there may be a greater risk of multiple births.[3]
The regimens used in *in-vitro* fertilisation may be characterised as long, in which the gonadorelin analogue is given for 2 weeks or more; short, in which it is given for about 8 to 10 days of the menstrual cycle; and ultrashort, where it is given for 3 days only. A comparative study of such regimens found that the best results in all age groups were consistently associated with the long buserelin protocol.[4] The timing of buserelin administration may also be important. Starting buserelin in the midluteal phase of the cycle has been reported to produce more rapid pituitary down regulation and higher pregnancy rates from *in-vitro* fertilisation than when buserelin was begun in the early follicular phase.[5]
For a general discussion of the management of infertility, see p.1275.

1. Armitage M, *et al.* Successful treatment of infertility due to polycystic ovary disease using a combination of luteinising hormone releasing hormone agonist and low dosage menotrophin. *BMJ* 1987; **295:** 96.
2. Owen EJ, *et al.* The use of a short regimen of buserelin, a gonadotrophin-releasing hormone agonist, and human menopausal gonadotrophin in assisted conception cycles. *Hum Reprod* 1989; **4:** 749–53.
3. Rutherford AJ, *et al.* Improvement of in vitro fertilisation after treatment with buserelin, an agonist of luteinising hormone releasing hormone. *BMJ* 1988; **296:** 1765–8.
4. Tan S-L, *et al.* Cumulative conception and live-birth rates after in vitro fertilization with and without the use of long, short, and ultrashort regimens of the gonadotrophin-releasing hormone agonist buserelin. *Am J Obstet Gynecol* 1994; **171:** 513–20.
5. Urbancsek J, Witthaus E. Midluteal buserelin is superior to early follicular phase buserelin in combined gonadotropin-releasing hormone analog and gonadotropin stimulation in in vitro fertilization. *Fertil Steril* 1996; **65:** 966–71.

Malignant neoplasms. The long-term use of buserelin in men decreases the testicular concentration of testosterone. For this reason it is used in the treatment of prostatic cancer (p.497), which is androgen-dependent.[1-6] Gonadorelin analogues are an effective alternative to orchidectomy, sometimes combined with an anti-androgen for enhanced effect, and play a major role in the management of advanced, incurable disease.
Other reports of malignant neoplasms treated with buserelin include its use in metastatic breast cancer[7,8] and meningioma.[9] For further discussion of these malignant neoplasms and their management, see p.491.

1. Waxman JH, *et al.* Treatment with gonadotrophin releasing hormone analogue in advanced prostatic cancer. *BMJ* 1983; **286:** 1309–12.
2. Lock MTWT, *et al.* Long-term effects of buserelin on plasma testosterone and luteinising hormone concentrations. *Lancet* 1985; **i:** 1236–7.
3. Volmer MC, *et al.* Lung metastases of prostate carcinoma cleared by intranasal GRH analogue. *Lancet* 1985; **i:** 1507.
4. Klign JGM, *et al.* Combined treatment with buserelin and cyproterone acetate in metastatic prostatic carcinoma. *Lancet* 1985; **ii:** 493.
5. Labrie F, *et al.* Combined treatment with flutamide and surgical or medical (LHRH agonist) castration in metastatic prostatic cancer. *Lancet* 1986; **i:** 48–9.
6. Waxman J, *et al.* A pharmacological evaluation of a new 3-month depot preparation of buserelin for prostatic cancer. *Cancer Chemother Pharmacol* 1989; **25:** 219–20.

7. Klijn JGM, de Jong FH. Treatment with a luteinising-hormone-releasing-hormone analogue (buserelin) in premenopausal patients with metastatic breast cancer. *Lancet* 1982; **i:** 1213–16.
8. Falkson G, Falkson HC. CAF and nasal buserelin in the treatment of premenopausal women with metastatic breast cancer. *Eur J Cancer Clin Oncol* 1989; **25:** 737–41.
9. van Seters AP, *et al.* Symptomatic relief of meningioma by buserelin maintenance therapy. *Lancet* 1989; **i:** 564–5.

Porphyria. Buserelin given with medroxyprogesterone acetate suppressed cyclic and premenstrual exacerbations of porphyria (p.1011) in 2 patients. Doses used were 300 µg buserelin intranasally in the evenings of days 1 to 21 of the menstrual cycle and 10 mg medroxyprogesterone acetate daily by mouth from day 12 to 21. Both patients were free from porphyric attacks during the reported 11 months of treatment.[1]

1. Bargetzi MJ, *et al.* Premenstrual exacerbations in hepatic porphyria: prevention by intermittent administration of an LH-RH agonist in combination with a gestagen. *JAMA* 1989; **261:** 864.

Precocious puberty. The gonadorelin analogues have largely replaced other treatments in the management of central precocious puberty (p.1277). For some references to the use of buserelin in precocious puberty, see below.

1. Drop SLS, *et al.* The effect of treatment with an LH-RH agonist (buserelin) on gonadal activity growth and bone maturation in children with central precocious puberty. *Eur J Pediatr* 1987; **146:** 272–8.
2. Cacciari E, *et al.* Long-term follow-up and final height in girls with central precocious puberty treated with luteinizing hormone-releasing hormone analogue nasal spray. *Arch Pediatr Adolesc Med* 1994; **148:** 1194–9.
3. Juul A, *et al.* Serum insulin-like growth factor I (IGF-I) and IGF-binding protein 3 levels are increased in central precocious puberty: effects of two different treatment regimens with gonadotropin-releasing hormone agonists, without or in combination with an antiandrogen (cyproterone acetate). *J Clin Endocrinol Metab* 1995; **80:** 3059–67.
4. Bertelloni S, *et al.* Effect of central precocious puberty and gonadotropin-releasing hormone analogue treatment on peak bone mass and final height in females. *Eur J Pediatr* 1998; **157:** 363–7.

Premenstrual syndrome. For reference to the use of buserelin or other gonadorelin analogues with HRT to prevent menopausal symptoms in women unresponsive to other drug treatment, see under Gonadorelin, p.1285.

Preparations

Proprietary Preparations (details are given in Part 3)
Aust.: Suprecur; Suprefact; *Belg.:* Suprefact; *Braz.:* Suprefact; *Canad.:* Suprefact; *Denm.:* Suprecur; Suprefact; *Fin.:* Suprecur; Suprefact; *Fr.:* Bigonist; Suprefact; *Ger.:* Profact; Suprecur; *Hong Kong:* Suprecur; Suprefact; *Irl.:* Suprecur; Suprefact; *Israel:* Suprefact; *Ital.:* Suprefact; *Neth.:* Suprecur; Suprefact; *Norw.:* Suprecur; Suprefact; *NZ:* Suprefact; *Port.:* Suprefact; *S.Afr.:* Suprecur†; Suprefact; *Singapore:* Suprecur; Suprefact; *Spain:* Suprecur†; Suprefact; *Swed.:* Suprecur; Suprefact; *Switz.:* Suprefact; *Thai.:* Suprefact; *UK:* Suprecur; Suprefact.

Carbetocin   (4825-a)

Carbetocin (BAN, rINN).

2,1-Desamino-4,1-desthio-$O^{4,2}$-methyl[1-homocysteine]oxytocin; 1-Butyric acid-2-[3-(*p*-methoxyphenyl)-L-alanine]oxytocin.
$C_{45}H_{69}N_{11}O_{12}S = 988.2$.
CAS — 37025-55-1.

Profile
Carbetocin is a synthetic analogue of oxytocin (p.1294) reported to have a longer duration of action. For the prevention of uterine atony and excessive bleeding following caesarian section a single dose of 100 µg may be given by intravenous injection after delivery. It should not be given before delivery.

◊ References.
1. Sweeney G, *et al.* Pharmacokinetics of carbetocin, a long-acting oxytocin analogue, in nonpregnant women. *Curr Ther Res* 1990; **47:** 528–40.
2. Hunter DJS, *et al.* Effect of carbetocin, a long-acting oxytocin analog on the postpartum uterus. *Clin Pharmacol Ther* 1992; **52:** 60–7.
3. Silcox J, *et al.* Transfer of carbetocin into human breast milk. *Obstet Gynecol* 1993; **82:** 456–9.
4. Dansereau J, *et al.* Double-blind comparison of carbetocin versus oxytocin in prevention of uterine atony after cesarean section. *Am J Obstet Gynecol* 1999; **180:** 670–6.

Preparations
Proprietary Preparations (details are given in Part 3)
Canad.: Duratocin; *UK:* Lonactene.

Cetrorelix   (15264-h)

Cetrorelix (BAN, rINN).

D-20761 (cetrorelix acetate); NS-75A (cetrorelix acetate); SB-75; SB-075. *N*-Acetyl-3-(2-naphthyl)-D-alanyl-*p*-chloro-D-phenylalanyl-3-(3-pyridyl)-D-alanyl-L-seryl-L-tyrosyl-N^5-carbamoyl-D-ornithyl-L-leucyl-L-arginyl-L-prolyl-D-alaninamide.
$C_{70}H_{92}ClN_{17}O_{14} = 1431.0$.
CAS — 120287-85-6 (cetrorelix); 145672-81-7 (cetrorelix acetate).
ATC — H01CC02.

NOTE. Cetrorelix Acetate is *USAN.*

The symbol † denotes a preparation no longer actively marketed

Adverse Effects and Precautions
Transient reactions at the injection site, including erythema, irritation, and swelling, may occur. Systemic hypersensitivity reactions have been reported rarely.
Cetrorelix should not be used in patients with moderate to severe renal or hepatic impairment.

Uses and Administration
Cetrorelix is a gonadorelin (gonadotrophin-releasing hormone) antagonist used as a component of ovarian stimulation regimens for assisted reproduction in infertility (p.1275). It has also been tried in benign prostatic hyperplasia and malignant neoplasms of the prostate, and for uterine fibroids. Cetrorelix is given by subcutaneous injection as the acetate; an intramuscular depot formulation containing cetrorelix embonate is reported to be under development. For assisted reproduction, doses of cetrorelix acetate equivalent to cetrorelix (p.1275) may be given either in the morning beginning on day 5 or 6 of ovarian stimulation or in the evening beginning on day 5, and continued until ovulation induction; alternatively a single dose equivalent to 3 mg of cetrorelix may be given on day 7.

◊ References.
1. Albano C, *et al.* Comparison of different doses of gonadotropin-releasing hormone antagonist cetrorelix during controlled ovarian hyperstimulation. *Fertil Steril* 1997; **67:** 917–22.
2. Gonzalez-Barcena D, *et al.* Treatment of uterine leiomyomas with luteinizing hormone-releasing hormone antagonist cetrorelix. *Hum Reprod* 1997; **12:** 2028–35.
3. Comaru-Schally AM, *et al.* Efficacy and safety of luteinizing hormone-releasing hormone antagonist cetrorelix in the treatment of symptomatic benign prostatic hyperplasia. *J Clin Endocrinol Metab* 1998; **83:** 3826–31.
4. Felberbaum RE, *et al.* Treatment of uterine fibroids with a slow-release formulation of the gonadotrophin releasing hormone antagonist cetrorelix. *Hum Reprod* 1998; **13:** 1660–8.
5. Duijkers IJ, *et al.* Single and multiple dose pharmacokinetics of the gonadotrophin-releasing hormone antagonist cetrorelix in healthy female volunteers. *Hum Reprod* 1998; **13:** 2392–8.
6. Olivennes F, *et al.* The use of a GnRH antagonist (cetrorelix) in a single dose protocol in IVF-embryo transfer: a dose finding study of 3 versus 2 mg. *Hum Reprod* 1998; **13:** 2411–14.

Preparations
Proprietary Preparations (details are given in Part 3)
Aust.: Cetrotide; *Austral.:* Cetrotide; *Belg.:* Cetrotide; *Denm.:* Cetrotide; *Fin.:* Cetrotide; *Fr.:* Cetrotide; *Ger.:* Cetrotide; *Ital.:* Cetrotide; *Neth.:* Cetrotide; *Port.:* Cetrotide; *Swed.:* Cetrotide; *UK:* Cetrotide; *USA:* Cetrotide.

Chorionic Gonadotrophin   (5927-s)

Chorionic Gonadotrophin (BAN, rINN).

CG; Choriogonadotrophin; Chorionic Gonadotropin; Gonadotrophinum Chorionicum; HCG; hCG; Human Chorionic Gonadotrophin; Pregnancy-urine Hormone; PU.
CAS — 9002-61-3.
ATC — G03GA01.

Pharmacopoeias. In Chin., Eur. (see p.vi), Jpn, and US.

Pharmacopoeial description
Ph. Eur.: A dry preparation of placental glycoproteins extracted from the urine of pregnant women. The potency is not less than 2500 units per mg. A white to yellowish-white, amorphous powder. Soluble in water. Store at 2° to 8° in airtight containers. Protect from light.
USP 25: A gonad-stimulating polypeptide hormone obtained from the urine of pregnant women. It has a potency of not less than 1500 USP units per mg. A white or practically white, amorphous powder. Freely soluble in water. Store in airtight containers at 2° to 8°.

Choriogonadotropin Alfa   (5548-r)

Choriogonadotropin Alfa (BAN, USAN, rINN).
CAS — 177073-44-8 (choriogonadotropin alfa); 56832-30-5 (α subunit); 56832-34-9 (β subunit).

Adverse Effects and Precautions
Side-effects that have been reported include headache, tiredness, changes in mood, depression, restlessness, oedema, (especially in males), and pain on injection. Treatment for cryptorchidism may produce precocious puberty. Gynaecomastia has been reported. Ovarian hyperstimulation may occur, with marked ovarian enlargement or cyst formation, acute abdominal pain, ascites, pleural effusion, hypovolaemia, shock, and thromboembolic disorders in severe cases.
Chorionic gonadotrophin should be given with care to patients in whom androgen-induced fluid retention might be a hazard as in asthma, epilepsy, migraine, or cardiovascular disorders, including hypertension, or renal disorders. Hypersensitivity reactions may occur and it is recommended that patients suspected to be susceptible should be given skin tests before treatment. It should not be given to patients with disorders that might be exacerbated by androgen release such as carcinoma of the prostate or precocious puberty.

Pharmacokinetics
Following intramuscular administration peak concentrations of chorionic gonadotrophin occur about 6 hours after a dose. It is distributed primarily to the gonads. Blood concentrations decline in a biphasic manner, with half-lives of about 6 to 11 hours and 23 to 38 hours, respectively. About 10 to 12% of an intramuscular dose is excreted in urine within 24 hours.
Following subcutaneous administration, choriogonadotropin alfa has a bioavailability of about 40%. It is metabolised and excreted similarly to chorionic gonadotrophin.

Uses and Administration
Chorionic gonadotrophin is a hormone produced by the placenta and obtained from the urine of pregnant women. Its effects are predominantly those of the gonadotrophin, luteinising hormone (p.1290), which is responsible for triggering ovulation and formation of the corpus luteum in women, and stimulates the production of testosterone by the testes in men. Choriogonadotropin alfa is a recombinant form of chorionic gonadotrophin.

Chorionic gonadotrophin is given to women with anovulatory infertility due to absent or low concentrations of gonadotrophins, to induce ovulation after follicular development has been stimulated with follicle-stimulating hormone or human menopausal gonadotrophins. A single dose of 5000 to 10 000 units of chorionic gonadotrophin is given by intramuscular injection to mimic the midcycle peak of luteinising hormone which normally stimulates ovulation. Up to 3 repeat injections of up to 5000 units each may be given within the following 9 days to prevent insufficiency of the corpus luteum. Chorionic gonadotrophin is also given in conjunction with menotrophin and sometimes also clomifene citrate as an adjunct to *in-vitro* fertilisation procedures and other assisted conception techniques involving superovulation and oocyte collection.

Choriogonadotropin alfa is used similarly to induce ovulation in the treatment of anovulatory infertility, or as an adjunct to *in-vitro* fertilisation procedures and other assisted conception techniques. A single dose of 250 µg is given, by subcutaneous injection, when optimal stimulation of follicular growth is achieved.

In males, chorionic gonadotrophin has been used in the treatment of prepubertal cryptorchidism. Regimens vary widely, but doses usually range from 500 to 4000 units three times weekly by intramuscular injection.

Chorionic gonadotrophin is also given for male infertility associated with hypogonadotrophic hypogonadism. Again, there is considerable variation in the dosage regimen, and doses have varied from 500 to 4000 units two to three times weekly by intramuscular injection. An agent with follicle-stimulating activity such as menotrophin is often added to enable normal spermatogenesis.

In the treatment of delayed puberty associated with hypogonadism in males, an initial dose of chorionic gonadotrophin 500 to 1500 units is given twice weekly by intramuscular injection; the dose should be titrated against plasma-testosterone concentration.

Chorionic gonadotrophin has also been administered by subcutaneous injection.

Cryptorchidism. Although surgery remains the treatment with the best success rate in cryptorchidism it is often reserved for boys who do not respond to a trial of hormonal therapy (see p.1272). Gonadorelin or chorionic gonadotrophin appear to be of some benefit, although only a minority of cases will respond;[1] they may be given in combination.[2] Chorionic gonadotrophin is also used as an adjuvant to surgery, to render the testes palpable.[3]

1. Pyörälä S, *et al.* A review and meta-analysis of hormonal treatment of cryptorchidism. *J Clin Endocrinol Metab* 1995; **80:** 2795–9.

2. Nane I, *et al.* Primary gonadotropin releasing hormone and adjunctive human chorionic gonadotropin treatment in cryptorchidism: a clinical trial. *Urology* 1997; **49:** 108–11.
3. Polascik TJ, *et al.* Reappraisal of the role of human chorionic gonadotropin in the diagnosis and treatment of the nonpalpable testis: a 10-year experience. *J Urol (Baltimore)* 1996; **156:** 804–6.

Delayed puberty. Use of chorionic gonadotrophin may be appropriate in boys with delayed puberty due to hypogonadotrophic hypogonadism (p.1273).

Infertility. In women with anovulatory infertility chorionic gonadotrophin and choriogonadotropin alfa can be used to provoke ovulation and provide luteal support once maturation of a suitable number of follicles has been stimulated by other means. They are used similarly in the various protocols for assisted reproduction. In men with hypogonadotrophic hypogonadism chorionic gonadotrophin is employed to stimulate and maintain spermatogenesis. The management of male and female infertility, including the role of chorionic gonadotrophin, is discussed on p.1275.

Malignant neoplasms. Control of Kaposi's sarcoma (p.501) has been reported in a few patients given high-dose intramuscular chorionic gonadotrophin, but regrowth occurred when dosage was reduced or withdrawn.[1] Another study, using lower doses, was discontinued due to toxicity and lack of benefit,[2] but others have confirmed benefit following intralesional injection.[3] There is some suggestion that preparations vary in their activity against the tumour, and that it is not chorionic gonadotrophin itself, but some impurity, (perhaps a ribonuclease[4]) which is the active principle.[3,5,6]
Chorionic gonadotrophin is also reported to be under investigation in the treatment of acute myeloid leukaemias (p.485).

1. Harris PJ. Treatment of Kaposi's sarcoma and other manifestations of AIDS with human chorionic gonadotropin. *Lancet* 1995; **346:** 118–19.
2. Bower M, *et al.* Human chorionic gonadotropin for AIDS-related Kaposi's sarcoma. *Lancet* 1995; **346:** 642.
3. Gill PS, *et al.* The effects of preparations of human chorionic gonadotropin on AIDS-related Kaposi's sarcoma. *N Engl J Med* 1996; **335:** 1261–9. Correction. *ibid.* 1997; **336:** 1115.
4. Griffiths SJ, *et al.* Ribonuclease inhibits Kaposi's sarcoma. *Nature* 1997; **390:** 568.
5. Gill PS, *et al.* Intralesional human chorionic gonadotropin for Kaposi's sarcoma. *N Engl J Med* 1997; **336:** 1188.
6. von Overbeck J, *et al.* Human chorionic gonadotropin for AIDS-related Kaposi's sarcoma. *Lancet* 1995; **346:** 642–3.

Obesity. A meta-analysis[1] involving 24 trials concluded that there was no evidence that chorionic gonadotrophin was effective in the treatment of obesity (p.1505).

1. Lijesen GKS, *et al.* The effect of human chorionic gonadotropin (HCG) in the treatment of obesity by means of the Simeons therapy: a criteria-based meta-analysis. *Br J Clin Pharmacol* 1995; **40:** 237–43.

Preparations

BP 2001: Chorionic Gonadotrophin Injection;
USP 25: Chorionic Gonadotropin for Injection.

Proprietary Preparations (details are given in Part 3)
Aust.: Pregnyl; Profasi; *Austral.:* APL; Pregnyl; Profasi; *Belg.:* Pregnyl; *Braz.:* Pregnyl; *Canad.:* APL; Pregnyl; Profasi HP; *Denm.:* Pregnyl; Profasi; *Fin.:* Pregnyl; Profasi; *Ger.:* Choragon; Predalon; Pregnesin; Primogonyl; *Hong Kong:* Choriomon; Pregnyl; Profasi; *Irl.:* Choragon; Gonadotraphon LH; Pregnyl; Profasi; *Israel:* Chorigon; Pregnyl; *Ital.:* Gonasi HP; Profasi HP; *Mex.:* Gonadotropyl C; Gonaplex; Gonasone; Pregnyl; Profasi; *Neth.:* Pregnyl; Profasi; *Norw.:* Pregnyl; Profasi; *NZ:* Pregnyl; Profasi; *Port.:* Pregnyl; Profasi HP; *S.Afr.:* APL; Pregnyl; Profasi; *Singapore:* Pregnyl; Profasi; *Spain:* Physex†; Pregnyl†; Profasi HP; *Swed.:* Pregnyl; Profasi; *Switz.:* Choriomon; Pregnyl; Profasi; *Thai.:* Pregnyl; Profasi; *UK:* Choragon; Gonadotraphon LH†; Ovitrelle; Pregnyl; Profasi; *USA:* APL; Chorex; Choron; Gonic; Novarel; Ovidrel; Pregnyl; Profasi.

Multi-ingredient: *Ger.:* AntiFocal N; NeyNormin N (Revitorgan-Dilutionen N Nr 65); *Mex.:* Gonakor.

Corticorelin (16592-m)

Corticorelin (*rINN*).

Corticoliberin; Corticotrophin-releasing Hormone; Corticotropin-releasing Factor; CRF; CRH.
$C_{208}H_{344}N_{60}O_{63}S_2$ (human) = 4757.5 (human).
ATC — V04CD04.

A polypeptide isolated from the hypothalamus.

Adverse Effects

Flushing of the face and mild dyspnoea may follow injection of corticorelin; hypotension has been reported, especially following large doses.

◊ Loss of consciousness, lasting for 10 seconds to 5 minutes, occurred in 3 patients, two of whom had Cushing's disease and one who had secondary adrenal insufficiency, following intravenous injection of corticorelin 200 μg.[1] The 2 patients with Cushing's disease had a slight accompanying fall in blood pressure. In a fourth patient, receiving corticosteroid and thyroid hormone replacement therapy, injection of corticorelin was associated with a sharp fall in systolic blood pressure and subsequent asystole. These serious side-effects were not noted by others[2,3] and were variously attributed to impurities,[2] high dosage,[2] vasovagal syncope,[3] or to the fact that the corticorelin used in the study was of ovine rather than human origin.[3] The authors of the original study[1] have since stated[4] that lowering of the dose from 200 μg administered intravenously over 10 seconds to 100 μg over 60 seconds had stopped serious adverse effects but that ovine corticorelin was still preferred because of its longer duration of action and lower incidence of hypotensive adverse effects. There has, however, been a further report of chest pain accompanied by a fall in blood pressure in a patient receiving corticorelin at a dose of 100 μg.[5]

1. Hermus A, *et al.* Serious reactions to corticotropin-releasing factor. *Lancet* 1983; **i:** 776.
2. Schulte HM, *et al.* Safety of corticotropin-releasing factor. *Lancet* 1983; **i:** 1222.
3. Oppermann D. Safety of human and ovine corticotropin-releasing hormone. *Lancet* 1986; **ii:** 1031–2.
4. Hermus ARMM, *et al.* Safety of human and ovine corticotropin-releasing hormone. *Lancet* 1986; **ii:** 1032–3.
5. Paloma VC, *et al.* Chest pain after intravenous corticotropin-releasing hormone. *Lancet* 1989; **i:** 222.

Uses and Administration

Corticorelin is a hypothalamic releasing hormone that stimulates the release of corticotropin (p.1280) from the anterior pituitary. It is used in the differential diagnosis of Cushing's syndrome (p.1272) and other adrenal disorders. Doses of 100 μg, or of 1 μg per kg body-weight, as the triflutate derivative, have been given by intravenous injection; higher doses have been given but may be associated with an increased risk of adverse effects (see above).

It is also under investigation in other disorders including shock, respiratory distress syndrome and asthma, rheumatoid arthritis, and cerebral and pulmonary oedema.

Administration. Corticorelin was well absorbed following subcutaneous injection and had a calculated bioavailability of about 60 to 70%; absorption was slower with high doses, suggesting that it may be a saturable process. Given the preservation of bioactivity, the subcutaneous route was considered an attractive alternative to intravenous administration.[1]

1. Angst MS, *et al.* Pharmacokinetics, cortisol release, and hemodynamics after intravenous and subcutaneous injection of human corticotropin-releasing factor in humans. *Clin Pharmacol Ther* 1998; **64:** 499–510.

Diagnosis and testing. The role of corticorelin as a diagnostic agent has been reviewed.[1-5] It is considered effective in the differential diagnosis of adrenal disorders including Cushing's syndrome (p.1272). Patients with pituitary Cushing's syndrome have an exaggerated increase in plasma-corticotropin and plasma-cortisol concentrations in response to corticorelin, whereas those with adrenal or ectopic syndrome have no response.[6-8] The corticorelin stimulation test is of comparable diagnostic efficacy to the dexamethasone suppression test,[9,10] although false results have been obtained with both tests.[9] The corticorelin stimulation test is considered somewhat unreliable if the disease is due to low-grade secretion of corticotropin by small tumours.[4,7,8] A combination of the dexamethasone and corticorelin tests is reportedly more accurate than either alone.[1,10,11]

1. Chrousos GP, *et al.* Clinical applications of corticotropin-releasing factor. *Ann Intern Med* 1985; **102:** 344–58.
2. Taylor AL, Fishman LM. Corticotropin-releasing hormone. *N Engl J Med* 1988; **319:** 213–22.
3. Kaye TB, Crapo L. The Cushing syndrome: an update on diagnostic tests. *Ann Intern Med* 1990; **112:** 434–44.
4. Daughaday WH. Clinical applications of corticotropin releasing hormone. *Mayo Clin Proc* 1990; **65:** 1026–8.
5. Anonymous. CRH test in the 1990s. *Lancet* 1990; **336:** 1416.
6. Chrousos GP, *et al.* The corticotropin-releasing factor stimulation test: an aid in the evaluation of patients with Cushing's syndrome. *N Engl J Med* 1984; **310:** 622–6.
7. Sebastian JP, *et al.* CRH test. *Lancet* 1991; **337:** 233.
8. McCarthy MI, *et al.* CRH test. *Lancet* 1991; **337:** 233–4.
9. Hermus AR, *et al.* The corticotropin-releasing-hormone test versus the high-dose dexamethasone test in the differential diagnosis of Cushing's syndrome. *Lancet* 1986; **ii:** 540–4.
10. Nieman LK, *et al.* The ovine corticotropin-releasing hormone stimulation test and the dexamethasone suppression test in the differential diagnosis of Cushing's syndrome. *Ann Intern Med* 1986; **105:** 862–7.
11. Yanovski JA, *et al.* Corticotropin-releasing hormone stimulation following low-dose dexamethasone administration: a new test to distinguish Cushing's syndrome from pseudo-Cushing's states. *JAMA* 1993; **269:** 2232–8.

Preparations

Proprietary Preparations (details are given in Part 3)
Aust.: CRH; *Ger.:* CRH; *Neth.:* Corticobist†; CRH; *USA:* Acthrel.

Corticotropin (1461-v)

Corticotropin (*BAN, rINN*).

ACTH; Adrenocorticotrophic Hormone; Adrenocorticotrophin; Corticotrophin; Corticotropinum.
CAS — 9002-60-2 (corticotropin); 9050-75-3 (corticotropin zinc hydroxide); 8049-55-6 (corticotropin zinc hydroxide).
ATC — H01AA01.

Pharmacopoeias. In *Eur.* (see p.vi). *US* includes only as preparations for injection.

Pharmacopoeial description

Ph. Eur.: Corticotropin is a substance obtained from the anterior lobe of the pituitary gland of pigs and contains the corticotrophic peptide that increases the rate at which corticoid hormones are secreted by the adrenal gland. The potency is not less than 70 units per mg. A white or almost white hygroscopic powder or flakes. A 1% solution in water is clear or not more than slightly opalescent. A 1% solution in water has a pH of 3.0 to 5.0. Store at a temperature not exceeding 25°. Protect from light.

Units

5 units of porcine corticotropin for bioassay are contained in approximately 50 μg (with lactose 5 mg) in one ampoule of the third International Standard (1962).

Adverse Effects

Corticotropin stimulates the adrenals to produce cortisol (hydrocortisone) and mineralocorticoids; it therefore has the potential to produce similar adverse glucocorticoid and mineralocorticoid effects to those of the corticosteroids (see p.1039). In particular, its mineralocorticoid properties may produce marked sodium and water retention; considerable potassium loss may also occur.

Corticotropin can induce sensitisation, and severe hypersensitivity reactions, including anaphylaxis, may occur.

Whereas corticosteroids replace endogenous cortisol (hydrocortisone) and thereby induce adrenal atrophy, corticotropin's stimulant effect induces hypertrophy. Withdrawal of corticotropin may therefore be easier than withdrawal of corticosteroids; nevertheless, the ability of the hypothalamic-pituitary-adrenal axis to respond to stress is still reduced, and abrupt withdrawal of corticotropin may result in symptoms of hypopituitarism (see Withdrawal, below).

◊ Reports of the adverse effects observed in children given corticotropin for infantile spasms.

1. Riikonen R, Donner M. ACTH therapy in infantile spasms: side effects. *Arch Dis Child* 1980; **55:** 664–72.
2. Hanefeld F, *et al.* Renal and pancreatic calcification during treatment of infantile spasms with ACTH. *Lancet* 1984; **i:** 901.
3. Riikonen R, *et al.* Disturbed calcium and phosphate homeostasis during treatment with ACTH of infantile spasms. *Arch Dis Child* 1986; **61:** 671–6.
4. Perheentupa J, *et al.* Adrenocortical hyporesponsiveness after treatment with ACTH of infantile spasms. *Arch Dis Child* 1986; **61:** 750–3.

Withdrawal

Corticotropin administration may depress the pituitary adrenal axis. Abrupt withdrawal of corticotropin may therefore produce adrenocortical and pituitary unresponsiveness, and therapy should be stopped gradually. See also Withdrawal under Corticosteroids, p.1041.

Precautions

As for Corticosteroids, p.1042.

Phaeochromocytoma. A hypertensive crisis following intravenous administration of tetracosactide resulted in the discovery of an adrenaline-secreting phaeochromocytoma in a patient.[1] It was suggested that caution should be observed when using corticotropin in patients with postural hypotension in whom the diagnosis of phaeochromocytoma has not been excluded.

1. Jan T, *et al.* Epinephrine-producing pheochromocytoma with hypertensive crisis after corticotropin injection. *Am J Med* 1990; **89:** 824–5.

Interactions

Interactions seen with corticotropin are liable to be similar to those with corticosteroids (p.1043).

Uses and Administration

Corticotropin is a naturally occurring hormone of the anterior lobe of the pituitary gland. It induces hyperplasia and increase in weight of the adrenal glands and the secretion of adrenocortical hormones, especially cortisol (hydrocortisone), some mineralocorticoids, such as corticosterone, and, to a lesser extent, androgens. It has little effect on aldosterone secretion which proceeds independently.

Secretion of corticotropin by the functioning pituitary gland is controlled by the release of corticorelin from the hypothalamus and is also regulated by a negative feedback mechanism involving concentrations of circulating glucocorticoids. Conditions of stress may also stimulate secretion.

Corticotropin may be used diagnostically to investigate adrenocortical insufficiency. It has also been used therapeutically in most of the conditions (with the exception of the adrenal deficiency states and adrenocortical overactivity) for which systemic corticosteroid therapy is indicated (p.1044). Such use is now fairly limited. However, corticotropin is used in certain neurological disorders such as infantile spasms and multiple sclerosis. The synthetic polypeptide tetracosactide (p.1298), which has the same amino-acid sequence as the first 24 residues of human corticotropin, may be used as an alternative. Tosactide is another polypeptide analogue of corticotropin; it has the same sequence as the first 28 residues.

Corticotropin has been available for injection in two forms. One form is a plain injection that may be administered by the subcutaneous, intramuscular, or intravenous routes. The other form includes the long-acting depot preparations in which the viscosity is increased by the addition of gelatin or in which corticotropin is combined with zinc hydroxide. The gelatin-containing depot preparation is administered subcutaneously or intramuscularly, the zinc hydroxide-containing depot preparation is administered intramuscularly; neither should be given intravenously. Individual responses to therapeutic corticotropin vary considerably and doses must be adjusted accordingly.

For diagnostic purposes the corticotropin test is based on the measurement of plasma-cortisol concentrations before and after injection. The plain preparation is used in doses of 10 to 25 units in 500 mL of glucose 5% infused intravenously over 8 hours.

For therapeutic purposes typical initial doses for the plain type of injection have been up to 20 units four times daily by the subcutaneous or intramuscular routes, and for the depot preparations about 20 to 80 units every 24 to 72 hours by the subcutaneous route (for the gelatin-containing preparation) or the intramuscular route (for both types of depot preparation). As soon as possible the dosage should be reduced gradually to the minimum necessary to control symptoms.

Epilepsy. The use of corticotropin in the management of infantile spasms is referred to under Corticosteroids, p.1050.
References.
1. Hrachovy RA, *et al.* High-dose, long-duration versus low-dose, short-duration corticotropin therapy for infantile spasms. *J Pediatr* 1994; **124**: 803–6.
2. Baram TZ, *et al.* High-dose corticotropin (ACTH) versus prednisone for infantile spasms: a prospective, randomized, blinded study. *Pediatrics* 1996; **97**: 375–9.

Multiple sclerosis. Short-term courses of corticotropin have been used to speed recovery from acute exacerbations of multiple sclerosis (p.633) but corticosteroids, usually methylprednisolone, are now preferred.

Post-dural puncture headache. There are anecdotal reports of the relief of post-dural puncture headache by corticotropin (or tetracosactide),[1,2] although, as discussed on p.1303, in many cases patients respond to conservative measures.
1. Collier BB. Treatment for postdural puncture headache. *Br J Anaesth* 1994; **72**: 366–7.
2. Foster P. ACTH treatment for post-lumbar puncture headache. *Br J Anaesth* 1994; **73**: 429.

Preparations

USP 25: Corticotropin for Injection; Corticotropin Injection; Corticotropin Zinc Hydroxide Injectable Suspension; Repository Corticotropin Injection.

Proprietary Preparations (details are given in Part 3)
Austral.: Acthar†; *Irl.:* Acthar; *S.Afr.:* Acthar†; *UK:* Acthar; *USA:* Acthar.

Demoxytocin   (12630-q)

Demoxytocin (*rINN*).
Deamino-oxytocin; Desamino-oxytocin; ODA-914. 1-(3-Mercaptopropionic acid)-oxytocin.
$C_{43}H_{65}N_{11}O_{12}S_2 = 992.2$.
CAS — 113-78-0.
ATC — H01BB01.

Profile
Demoxytocin is a synthetic analogue of oxytocin (p.1294) and has similar properties. It is given as buccal tablets, for the induction of labour (p.1438), in doses of 50 units every half-hour until a normal contraction rhythm is established, when the dose should be reduced to 25 units every half hour. Dosage should

not exceed a maximum of 500 units. For the augmentation of labour, 25 units or 50 units if necessary every half-hour has been recommended. Twenty-five or 50 units may be given 5 to 10 minutes before nursing to stimulate milk ejection, although it is generally recommended that oxytocics should not be used for this purpose, see p.1276.

Preparations
Proprietary Preparations (details are given in Part 3)
Ital.: Demopart; Sandopart†.

Deslorelin   (10811-t)

Deslorelin (*BAN, USAN, rINN*).
D-Trp   LHRH-PEA. 5-Oxo-L-prolyl-L-histidyl-L-tryptophyl-L-seryl-L-tyrosyl-D-tryptophyl-L-leucyl-L-arginyl-N-ethyl-L-prolinamide.
$C_{64}H_{83}N_{17}O_{12} = 1282.5$.
CAS — 57773-65-6.

Profile
Deslorelin is an analogue of gonadorelin (p.1283) investigated in the treatment of precocious puberty and for prostate cancer; it has also been tried in endometriosis.

◊ References.
1. Labrie F, *et al.* Long term treatment with luteinising hormone releasing hormone agonists and maintenance of serum testosterone to castration concentrations. *BMJ* 1985; **291**: 369–70.
2. Pescovitz OH, *et al.* NIH experience with precocious puberty: diagnostic subgroups and response to short term luteinizing hormone releasing hormone analog therapy. *J Pediatr* 1986; **108**: 47–54.
3. Comite F, *et al.* Luteinizing hormone releasing hormone analogue therapy for central precocious puberty: long-term effect on somatic growth, bone maturation, and predicted height. *JAMA* 1986; **255**: 2613–16.
4. Manasco PK, *et al.* Six-year results of luteinizing hormone releasing hormone (LHRH) agonist treatment in children with LHRH-dependent precocious puberty. *J Pediatr* 1989; **115**: 105–8.
5. Anonymous. Deslorelin: D-Trp-LHRH-PEA, LHRH agonist analogue, Somagard. *Drugs R D* 1999; **2**: 420–2.

Desmopressin   (5922-b)

Desmopressin (*BAN, rINN*).
DDAVP; Desmopressinum. 1-(3-Mercaptopropionic acid)-8-D-arginine-vasopressin; [1-Deamino,8-D-arginine]vasopressin.
$C_{46}H_{64}N_{14}O_{12}S_2 = 1069.2$.
CAS — 16679-58-6.
ATC — H01BA02.
Pharmacopoeias. In *Eur.* (see p.vi).

Pharmacopoeial description
Ph. Eur.: A white fluffy powder. Soluble in water, in alcohol, and in glacial acetic acid. Store at 2° to 8°. Protect from light and moisture.

Desmopressin Acetate   (5923-v)

Desmopressin Acetate (*BANM, USAN, rINNM*).
$C_{46}H_{64}N_{14}O_{12}S_2,C_2H_4O_2,3H_2O = 1183.3$.
CAS — 62288-83-9 (anhydrous desmopressin acetate); 62357-86-2 (desmopressin acetate trihydrate).

Units
27 units of desmopressin are contained in approximately 27 µg of desmopressin (with 5 mg of human albumin and citric acid) in one ampoule of the first International Standard (1980).

Adverse Effects and Precautions
Adverse effects with desmopressin include headache, nausea, and mild abdominal cramps; there may be pain and swelling at the site of injection. With large intravenous doses hypotension, with tachycardia and facial flushing, may occur; some patients may experience an increase in blood pressure. Occasionally there may be cerebral or coronary thrombosis. Hypersensitivity reactions have also occurred. The antidiuretic action of desmopressin may produce water intoxication and hyponatraemia, occasionally leading to convulsions. Nasal administration may cause local irritation, congestion, and epistaxis.

Precautions to be observed during the administration of desmopressin are similar to those for vasopressin (see p.1300). It should not be used in patients with type IIB von Willebrand's disease, in whom the release of clotting factors may lead to platelet aggregation and thrombocytopenia. When desmopressin is used diagnostically, or for the treatment of enuresis, the fluid intake should be limited to a minimum and

only to satisfy thirst for 8 hours following administration (see also Effects on Electrolytes, below).

Effects on the cardiovascular system. Facial flushing and warmth following intravenous desmopressin reflect a vasodilator action[1] or may be due to an opioid mechanism in the CNS.[2] A drop in diastolic blood pressure of about 14 mmHg and an increase in heart rate of 20 beats per minute are the rule during intravenous infusion of desmopressin in doses of 400 nanograms per kg body-weight or more.[1] The hypotensive effects of desmopressin were responsible for a serious reaction, involving cyanosis and dyspnoea, in a 21-month-old child with cyanotic heart disease.[3] Thrombosis (including myocardial infarction)[4-6] and cerebral infarction[7] have been associated rarely with the use of intravenous desmopressin.
Manufacturers also warn of the possibility of an increase in blood pressure.
1. Brommer EJP, *et al.* Desmopressin and hypotension. *Ann Intern Med* 1985; **103**: 962.
2. Pigache RM. Facial flushing induced by vasopressin-like peptides lacking pressor activity. *J Clin Pharmacol* 1984; **17**: 369–71.
3. Israels SJ, Kobrinsky NL. Serious reaction to desmopressin in a child with cyanotic heart disease. *N Engl J Med* 1989; **320**: 1563–4.
4. Anonymous. Desmopressin and arterial thrombosis. *Lancet* 1989; **i**: 938–9.
5. Mannucci PM, Lusher JM. Desmopressin and thrombosis. *Lancet* 1989; **ii**: 675–6.
6. Hartmann S, Reinhart W. Fatal complication of desmopressin. *Lancet* 1995; **345**: 1302–3. Correction. *ibid.*; 1648.
7. Grunwald Z, Sather SDC. Intraoperative cerebral infarction after desmopressin administration in infant with end-stage renal disease. *Lancet* 1995; **345**: 1364–5.

Effects on electrolytes. There have been a number of reports of seizures due to hyponatraemia and water intoxication following intranasal[1-7] or intravenous[8] desmopressin. The UK Committee on Safety of Medicines noted in March 1996 that it had received reports of hyponatraemic convulsions in 21 children and 3 adults receiving desmopressin (which it somewhat inaccurately described as vasopressin).[9] It was recommended that when this drug was used to treat primary nocturnal enuresis the risks of concomitant hyponatraemia should be minimised by
• avoiding concomitant use of drugs, such as *tricyclic antidepressants*, that increase endogenous ADH secretion
• keeping to the recommended starting dose
• avoiding excessive fluid intake, including during swimming
• stopping treatment temporarily if vomiting or diarrhoea occurred, to allow recovery of normal fluid and electrolyte balance.
Some have suggested that serum sodium concentrations be measured 24 to 48 hours, 1 week, and 1 month after starting treatment with desmopressin.[7]
1. Simmonds EJ, *et al.* Convulsions and coma after intranasal desmopressin in cystic fibrosis. *BMJ* 1988; **297**: 1614.
2. Salvatoni A, *et al.* Hyponatraemia during desmopressin acetate treatment in hypothyroidism. *J Pediatr* 1990; **116**: 835–6.
3. Davis RC, *et al.* Nocturnal enuresis. *Lancet* 1992; **340**: 1550.
4. Hamed M, *et al.* Hyponatraemic convulsion associated with desmopressin and imipramine treatment. *BMJ* 1993; **306**: 1169.
5. Hourihane J, Salisbury AJ. Use caution in prescribing desmopressin for nocturnal enuresis. *BMJ* 1993; **306**: 1545.
6. Robson WLM, Leung AKC. Hyponatraemia following desmopressin. *BMJ* 1993; **307**: 64–5.
7. Odeh M, Oliven A. Coma and seizures due to severe hyponatremia and water intoxication in an adult with intranasal desmopressin therapy for nocturnal enuresis. *J Clin Pharmacol* 2001; **41**: 582–4.
8. Shepherd LL, *et al.* Hyponatremia and seizures after intravenous administration of desmopressin acetate for surgical hemostasis. *J Pediatr* 1989; **114**: 470–2.
9. Committee on Safety of Medicines/Medicines Control Agency. Hyponatraemic convulsions in patients with enuresis treated with vasopressin. *Current Problems* 1996; **22**: 4.

Effects on mental function. Paranoid psychosis occurred after desmopressin therapy in a patient with Alzheimer's dementia.[1]
1. Collins GB, *et al.* Paranoid psychosis after DDAVP therapy for Alzheimer's dementia. *Lancet* 1981; **ii**: 808.

Tolerance. In 3 uraemic patients desmopressin infusion produced an initial shortening of the bleeding time but following repeated infusions this response was reduced and there was even some increase in baseline bleeding times.[1] Two infusions of desmopressin 300 nanograms per kg body-weight in one day appear to induce a near maximum response; different treatment is required subsequently.
1. Canavese C, *et al.* Reduced response of uraemic bleeding time to repeated doses of desmopressin. *Lancet* 1985; **i**: 867–8.

Interactions
As for Vasopressin, p.1300. See also under Effects on Electrolytes, above.

Pharmacokinetics
Desmopressin is absorbed from the nasal mucosa with a bioavailability of 10 to 20%. Following oral administration it is largely destroyed in the gastrointestinal tract but sufficient is absorbed following high

doses to produce therapeutic effects. When given intravenously desmopressin exhibits biphasic pharmacokinetics, with half-lives of about 8 minutes and 75 minutes for the 2 phases respectively.

◊ References.
1. Fjellestad-Paulsen A, et al. Pharmacokinetics of 1-deamino-8-D-arginine vasopressin after various routes of administration in healthy volunteers. Clin Endocrinol (Oxf) 1993; 38: 177–82.
2. Lam KSL, et al. Pharmacokinetics, pharmacodynamics, long-term efficacy and safety of oral 1-deamino-8-D-arginine vasopressin in adult patients with central diabetes insipidus. Br J Clin Pharmacol 1996; 42: 379–85.

Uses and Administration

Desmopressin is a synthetic analogue of vasopressin (p.1300). It has greater antidiuretic activity and a more prolonged action than vasopressin or lypressin. It also stimulates factor VIII and plasminogen activator activity in the blood, but has little pressor activity.

Desmopressin is used in the diagnosis and treatment of cranial diabetes insipidus, and in the treatment of nocturnal enuresis and tests of renal function. It is also used in the management of mild or moderate haemophilia and type I von Willebrand's disease, and in tests of fibrinolytic response.

It is given as the acetate, by mouth, as a solution intranasally, and by injection. The intranasal dose is approximately ten times that required intravenously and the oral dose about ten times greater than the intranasal dose.

In the control of **cranial diabetes insipidus**, desmopressin acetate is given by mouth to adults and children in usual initial doses of 100 μg three times daily. Doses may be adjusted according to response, with maintenance doses usually between 100 and 200 μg three times daily though total doses of between 100 μg and 1200 μg daily have been used. It may also be used intranasally in usual doses of 10 to 40 μg of desmopressin acetate daily as a single dose or in divided doses; children aged 3 months to 12 years may be given 5 to 30 μg intranasally daily. It may also be given subcutaneously, intramuscularly, or intravenously in a dose of 1 to 4 μg daily; a dose from 0.4 μg may be used for children and infants.

A single intranasal dose of 20 μg or 2 μg subcutaneously or intramuscularly has been given to adults and children in the diagnosis of diabetes insipidus. Doses of 10 to 40 μg intranasally or 2 μg by injection have been used to test renal function.

In the management of **primary nocturnal enuresis**, children aged 5 years and older (preferably over 7 years) and adults are given desmopressin acetate in usual doses of 200 to 400 μg by mouth or 20 to 40 μg intranasally at bedtime. The need for continued treatment should be reassessed after 3 months by withdrawing desmopressin for at least 1 week. For the control of **nocturia** in adults with multiple sclerosis 10 to 20 μg intranasally at bedtime is recommended (but see Urinary Incontinence, below).

Desmopressin acetate is given by intravenous infusion to boost concentrations of factor VIII before surgical procedures in patients with mild to moderate **haemophilia** or **type I von Willebrand's disease**. The usual dose for adults and children is 0.3 or 0.4 μg (300 or 400 nanograms) per kg body-weight by slow intravenous infusion over 15 to 30 minutes just before surgery. It may be used similarly to treat spontaneous or trauma-induced bleeding episodes in these patients. It is also given intranasally in doses of 150 μg (in patients weighing less than 50 kg) or 300 μg.

For **testing of fibrinolytic response** desmopressin acetate may be given to adults and children by intravenous infusion in doses of 0.4 μg per kg over 20 minutes; a sample of venous blood is taken 20 minutes after completing the infusion and tested for fibrinolytic activity on fibrin plates.

Diabetes insipidus. Desmopressin is the usual treatment for cranial diabetes insipidus (p.1273).

Haemorrhagic disorders. Desmopressin is used in the management of patients with mild haemophilia A, carriers of haemophilia with low factor VIII concentrations, and patients with

von Willebrand's disease, as discussed on p.721. Intravenous injection of desmopressin may be followed by tranexamic acid to inhibit the enhanced fibrinolytic activity.[1] The resultant three- to fivefold increase in all factor VIII activities should be sufficient to allow minor surgery, providing the basal concentration of the most deficient factor VIII activity is 7% or more. With higher basal factor VIII concentrations, more major surgery such as cholecystectomy or thoracotomy may be possible. Desmopressin can also be given intranasally but the factor VIII response is less predictable than with injection. The use of desmopressin as an alternative to blood products has been recommended whenever possible in the treatment of these disorders, as a precaution against infection with HIV.[2] The references listed below give further information on the use of desmopressin in haemophilia and/or von Willebrand's disease.[3-8]

Bleeding due to liver disease has been controlled by desmopressin,[9,10] as has that associated with uraemia[11-14] (but for a report of tolerance to the effects of repeated doses of desmopressin in uraemic patients, see under Adverse Effects and Precautions, above), and there are reports of bleeding being controlled in other disorders such as telangiectasia,[15] and platelet storage deficiency,[16] and in patients with acquired antibodies to factor VIII.[17] See also Variceal Haemorrhage, in Vasopressin (p.1301) and Terlipressin (p.1298).

Desmopressin has been tried in surgical procedures with conflicting results.[18-21] A meta-analysis, which mainly included trials in cardiac surgery, found no evidence that desmopressin reduces perioperative blood transfusion in patients who do not have congenital bleeding disorders.[22] It has been suggested that desmopressin may only be useful in patients with inadequate haemostatic mechanisms undergoing cardiac surgery[23] and that its usefulness in non-cardiac surgery needs further study.[24] A possible role for desmopressin has been proposed in the control of surgical bleeding in patients whose religious beliefs preclude the use of blood products.[25] It has been reported to be effective in postoperative aspirin-related bleeding that was previously unresponsive to administration of clotting factors,[26] and may be helpful for the prevention of excessive blood loss in patients who have received aspirin within 7 days of cardiac bypass surgery.[27]

1. Anonymous. DDAVP in haemophilia and von Willebrand's disease. Lancet 1983; ii: 774–5.
2. Jones P. HIV infection and haemophilia. Arch Dis Child 1991; 66: 364–8.
3. Anonymous. Desmopressin for hemophilia and other coagulation disorders. Med Lett Drugs Ther 1984; 26: 82.
4. Kobrinsky NL, et al. Shortening of bleeding time by 1-deamino-8-D-arginine vasopressin in various bleeding disorders. Lancet 1984; i: 1145–8.
5. de la Fuente B, et al. Response of patients with mild and moderate hemophilia A and von Willebrand's disease to treatment with desmopressin. Ann Intern Med 1985; 103: 6–14.
6. Vicente V, et al. Intranasal desmopressin in mild hemophilia A. Ann Intern Med 1985; 103: 807–8.
7. Prince S. An alternative to blood product therapy for dental extractions in the mild to moderate haemophiliac patient. Br Dent J 1987; 162: 256–7.
8. Rose EH, Aledort LM. Nasal spray desmopressin (DDAVP) for mild hemophilia A and von Willebrand disease. Ann Intern Med 1991; 114: 563–8.
9. Burroughs AK, et al. Desmopressin and bleeding time in patients with cirrhosis. BMJ 1985; 291: 1377–81.
10. Rak K, et al. Desmopressin and bleeding time in patients with cirrhosis. BMJ 1986; 292: 138.
11. Mannucci PM, et al. Deamino-8-D-arginine vasopressin shortens the bleeding time in uremia. N Engl J Med 1983; 308: 8–12.
12. Shapiro MD, Kelleher SP. Intranasal deamino-8-D-arginine vasopressin shortens the bleeding time in uremia. Am J Nephrol 1984; 4: 260–1.
13. Viganò GL, et al. Subcutaneous desmopressin (DDAVP) shortens the bleeding time in uremia. Am J Hematol 1989; 31: 32–5.
14. Jacquot C, et al. Addition of desmopressin to recombinant human erythropoietin in treatment of haemostatic defect of uraemia. Lancet 1988; i: 420.
15. Quitt M, et al. The effect of desmopressin on massive gastrointestinal bleeding in hereditary telangiectasia unresponsive to treatment with cryoprecipitate. Arch Intern Med 1990; 150: 1744–6.
16. Nieuwenhuis HK, Sixma JJ. 1-Desamino-8-D-arginine vasopressin (desmopressin) shortens the bleeding time in storage pool deficiency. Ann Intern Med 1988; 108: 65–7.
17. Naorose-Abidi SM, et al. Desmopressin therapy in patients with acquired factor VIII inhibitors. Lancet 1988; i: 366.
18. Salzman EW, et al. Treatment with desmopressin acetate to reduce blood loss after cardiac surgery: a double-blind randomized trial. N Engl J Med 1986; 314: 1402–6.
19. Kobrinsky NL, et al. 1-Desamino-8-D-arginine vasopressin (desmopressin) decreases operative blood loss in patients having Harrington rod spinal fusion surgery: a randomized, double-blinded, controlled trial. Ann Intern Med 1987; 107: 446–50. Correction. ibid. 1988; 108: 496.
20. Hackmann T, et al. A trial of desmopressin (1-desamino-8-D-arginine vasopressin) to reduce blood loss in uncomplicated cardiac surgery. N Engl J Med 1989; 321: 1437–43.
21. Cattaneo M, Mannucci PM. Desmopressin and blood loss after cardiac surgery. Lancet 1993; 342: 812.
22. Henry DA, et al. Desmopressin for minimising perioperative allogeneic blood transfusion (updated 26 February 2001). Available in The Cochrane Library; Issue 3. Oxford: Update Software; 2001.
23. Salzman EW. Desmopressin and surgical hemostasis. N Engl J Med 1990; 322: 1085.
24. Anonymous. Can drugs reduce surgical blood loss? Lancet 1988; i: 155–6.
25. Martens PR. Desmopressin and Jehovah's witness. Lancet 1989; i: 1322.

26. Chard RB, et al. Use of desmopressin in the management of aspirin-related and intractable haemorrhage after cardiopulmonary bypass. Aust N Z J Surg 1990; 60: 125–8.
27. Sheridan DP, et al. Use of desmopressin acetate to reduce blood transfusion requirements during cardiac surgery in patients with acetylsalicylic-acid-induced platelet dysfunction. Can J Surg 1994; 37: 33–6.

Nocturnal enuresis. Desmopressin is one of the main drugs used as an alternative or adjunct to nonpharmacological methods for the treatment of nocturnal enuresis in children (p.459). Secretion of vasopressin during the night in normal individuals reduces urine output and it has been suggested that nocturnal enuresis in some children might be due to impaired nocturnal secretion of vasopressin. However, a recent study[1] found no difference in nocturnal vasopressin levels or urine production in enuretic and non-enuretic children, but did find that children with nocturnal enuresis required a greater output of vasopressin to regulate plasma osmolality; other evidence has suggested that developmental delay in 2 separate areas of the CNS is involved.[2] Nonetheless, it has been shown that administration of the synthetic vasopressin analogue, desmopressin, at night can be effective in the short-term control of nocturnal enuresis[3] and many now consider it to be the drug of choice in terms of safety. However, a meta-analysis suggested that benefit might not be sustained once the drug was discontinued.[4] It should not be given where enuresis is due to polydipsia as desmopressin may provoke water intoxication and convulsions due to hyponatraemia. For precautions to be observed when desmopressin is used to treat enuresis see under Effects on Electrolytes, above.

1. Eggert P, Kühn B. Antidiuretic hormone regulation in patients with primary nocturnal enuresis. Arch Dis Child 1995; 73: 508–11.
2. Koff SA. Cure of nocturnal enuresis: why isn't desmopressin very effective? Pediatr Nephrol 1996; 10: 667–70.
3. Moffat MEK, et al. Desmopressin acetate and nocturnal enuresis: how much do we know? Pediatrics 1993; 92: 420–5.
4. Glazener CMA, Evans JHC. Desmopressin for nocturnal enuresis in children (updated 23 May 2001). Available in The Cochrane Library; Issue 3. Oxford: Update Software; 2001.

Orthostatic hypotension. The first drug tried in patients with orthostatic hypotension (p.1070) who cannot be managed by nonpharmacological methods is usually fludrocortisone, but desmopressin is sometimes useful in patients with central neurological abnormalities.[1]

1. Mathias CJ, et al. The effect of desmopressin on nocturnal polyuria, overnight weight loss, and morning postural hypotension in patients with autonomic failure. BMJ 1986; 293: 353–4.

Post-dural puncture headache. Desmopressin acetate has been given to adults in a dose of 4 μg subcutaneously or intramuscularly for the treatment or prophylaxis of headache due to lumbar puncture, repeated if necessary after 24 hours. However, results have generally been disappointing and as mentioned on p.1303 many patients respond to conservative treatment.

References.
1. Durward WF, Harrington H. Headache after lumbar puncture. Lancet 1976; ii: 1403–4.
2. Widerlöv E, Lindström L. DDAVP and headache after lumbar puncture. Lancet 1979; i: 548.
3. Hansen PE, Hansen JH. DDAVP, a synthetic analogue of vasopressin, in prevention of headache after lumbar puncture and lumbar pneumoencephalography. Acta Neurol Scand 1979; 60: 183–8.
4. Cowan JMA, et al. DDAVP in the prevention of headache after lumbar puncture. BMJ 1980; 280: 224.

Renal colic. Intranasal desmopressin is being studied[1] in the management of the pain of acute renal colic (p.5).
1. Zabihi N, Teichman JMH. Dealing with the pain of renal colic. Lancet 2001; 358: 437–8.

Renal-function testing. Desmopressin was equally effective by the intranasal or intramuscular routes in a dose of 40 μg or 2 μg respectively in assessment of the urine-concentrating capacity of the kidneys.[1] It was noted that urine-concentrating ability decreased with advancing age.[2] Experience in 32 adults suggested that desmopressin was as effective as vasopressin tannate for assessing renal function and that a suitable dose was 40 μg intranasally at 8 a.m. after overnight water deprivation.[3] It was also suggested that desmopressin be used routinely by the intranasal route and that it be administered by the intramuscular route to check results if technical difficulties arose.[4] Intramuscular desmopressin 4 μg was found suitable for assessing renal function in sedentary subjects or hospital inpatients[5] and intranasal desmopressin 40 μg was useful in early diagnosis of renal dysfunction caused by chronic abuse of analgesics.[6] In lithium-treated patients a test of urine osmolality using desmopressin before and after 14 hours of total fluid deprivation was a safe, convenient, and reliable means of estimating renal concentrating capacity.[7]

1. Monson JP, Richards P. Desmopressin urine concentration test. BMJ 1978; 1: 24.
2. Monson JP, Richards P. Age and urine concentration after desmopressin. BMJ 1978; 1: 1054–5.
3. Delin K, et al. Urinary concentration test with desmopressin. BMJ 1978; 1: 757–8.
4. Delin K, et al. Assessment of renal concentrating ability. BMJ 1979; 1: 888–9.
5. Curtis JR, Donovan BA. Assessment of renal concentrating ability. BMJ 1979; 1: 304–5.
6. Wambach G, et al. Detection of renal impairment in cases of chronic abuse of analgesics by administration of desamino-D-arginine vasopressin. Arzneimittelforschung 1989; 39: 387–90.
7. Asplund K, et al. DDAVP test in assessment of renal function during lithium therapy. Lancet 1979; i: 491.

Urinary incontinence. Desmopressin given intranasally appeared to be effective in reducing voiding frequency/incontinence when studied in 26 patients with multiple sclerosis whose bladder dysfunction had previously been unresponsive to antimuscarinic therapy.[1] However a review of studies using desmopressin to treat nocturia in patients with multiple sclerosis cast doubt on the clinical relevance of the limited reductions achieved in voiding frequency.[2]

1. Fredrikson S. Nasal spray desmopressin treatment of bladder dysfunction in patients with multiple sclerosis. *Acta Neurol Scand* 1996; **94:** 31–4.
2. Ferreira E, Letwin SR. Desmopressin for nocturia and enuresis associated with multiple sclerosis. *Ann Pharmacother* 1998; **32:** 114–16.

Preparations

BP 2001: Desmopressin Injection; Desmopressin Intranasal Solution.

Proprietary Preparations (details are given in Part 3)
Aust.: Minirin; Octostim; ***Austral.:*** Minirin; Octostim; ***Belg.:*** Minirin; Octostim; ***Braz.:*** DDAVP; ***Canad.:*** DDAVP; Octostim; ***Denm.:*** Minirin; Octostim; ***Fin.:*** Minirin; Octostim; ***Fr.:*** Minirin; Octim; ***Ger.:*** DDAVP; Desmogalen; Minirin; ***Hong Kong:*** Minirin; Octostim; ***Irl.:*** Desmospray; Desmotabs; ***Israel:*** Minirin; Octostim; ***Ital.:*** Emosint; Minirin/DDAVP; ***Mex.:*** DDAVP; Minirin; ***Neth.:*** Minirin; Octostim; ***Norw.:*** Minirin; Octostim; ***NZ:*** Minirin; Octostim; ***Port.:*** DDAVP; Desmospray; ***S.Afr.:*** DDAVP; ***Singapore:*** Minirin; Octostim; ***Spain:*** Minurin; Octostim; ***Swed.:*** Minirin; Octostim; ***Switz.:*** Minirin; Nocutil; Octostim; ***Thai.:*** Minirin; Octostim; ***UK:*** DDAVP; Desmospray; Desmotabs; Nocutil; ***USA:*** DDAVP; Stimate.

Felypressin   (5924-g)

Felypressin *(BAN, USAN, rINN).*

Phelypressine; PLV2. [2-Phenylalanine,8-lysine]vasopressin; Cys-Phe-Phe-Gln-Asn-Cys-Pro-Lys-Gly-NH₂.
$C_{46}H_{65}N_{13}O_{11}S_2 = 1040.2.$
CAS — 56-59-7.

Profile
Felypressin is a synthetic analogue of vasopressin (p.1300) with similar actions. Its antidiuretic effects are less than those of vasopressin. It is used as a vasoconstrictor in local anaesthetic injections for dental use when sympathomimetics should be avoided. It is also an ingredient of preparations used in the treatment of pain and inflammation of the mouth.

Preparations
Proprietary Preparations (details are given in Part 3)
Multi-ingredient: *Fr.:* Collupressine.

Used as an adjunct in: ***Austral.:*** Citanest Dental; ***Braz.:*** Citanest; Citocaina; ***Denm.:*** Citanest Octapressin; ***Fin.:*** Citanest Octapressin; ***Ger.:*** Xylonest; ***Irl.:*** Citanest with Octapressin; ***Ital.:*** Citanest con Octapressin; ***Mex.:*** Citanest Octapressin; ***Neth.:*** Citanest Octapressin; ***Norw.:*** Citanest Octapressin; ***NZ:*** Citanest Octapressin; ***Port.:*** Citanest Octapressin†; ***S.Afr.:*** Citanest Octopressin†; ***Spain:*** Citanest Octapressin; ***Swed.:*** Citanest Octapressin; ***Switz.:*** Xylonest-Octapressin; ***UK:*** Citanest with Octapressin.

Follicle-stimulating Hormone

(15579-r)

FSH.

Follitropin Alfa   (17626-v)

Follitropin Alfa *(BAN, rINN).*

$C_{437}H_{682}N_{122}O_{134}S_{13}$ (α-subunit) = 10206;
$C_{538}H_{833}N_{145}O_{171}S_{13}$ (β-subunit) = 12485.
CAS — 9002-68-0 (follitropin alfa); 56832-30-5 (α-subunit); 110909-60-9 (β-subunit); 146479-72-3 (follitropin alfa).
ATC — G03GA05.

Follitropin Beta   (5037-r)

Follitropin Beta *(BAN, rINN).*

Org-32489.
$C_{437}H_{682}N_{122}O_{134}S_{13}$ (α-subunit) = 10206;
$C_{538}H_{833}N_{145}O_{171}S_{13}$ (β-subunit) = 12485.
CAS — 169108-34-3 (follitropin beta); 150490-84-9 (follitropin beta); 56832-30-5 (α-subunit); 110909-60-9 (β-subunit).
ATC — G03GA06.

Units

80 units of human pituitary follicle-stimulating hormone are contained in approximately 4.17 µg (with 5 mg of mannitol and 1 mg human serum albumin) in one ampoule of the first International Standard (1986).

138 units of recombinant human follicle-stimulating hormone are contained in one ampoule of the first International Standard (1995).

The symbol † denotes a preparation no longer actively marketed

Adverse Effects and Precautions
As for Human Menopausal Gonadotrophins, p.1288.

Spongiform encephalopathies. In a few countries, gonadotrophins derived from cadaver pituitary glands have been used in the treatment of infertility, and a small number of patients are reported to have acquired Creutzfeldt-Jakob disease from such preparations.[1] However, most countries have preferred to use gonadotrophins derived from urine,[1] and these in their turn are being replaced with recombinant products;[2] such preparations do not carry the risk of transmitting the disease.

1. Healy DL, Evans J. Creutzfeldt-Jakob disease after pituitary gonadotrophins. *BMJ* 1993; **307:** 517–18.
2. Eshkol A, Page ML. Human gonadotrophin preparations. *BMJ* 1994; **308:** 789.

Pharmacokinetics
Follitropins alfa and beta are slowly absorbed following subcutaneous or intramuscular injection, with an absolute bioavailability of about 70 to 80%. Peak plasma concentrations of follitropin beta have been stated to occur about 12 hours after subcutaneous or intramuscular injection. Accumulation occurs with repeated doses, reaching a steady state within 3 to 4 days. Follitropins are slowly eliminated from the body, with a terminal half-life ranging from 12 to 70 hours. About one-eighth of a dose of follitropin alfa is reported to be excreted in the urine.

◊ References.

1. Karlsson MO, *et al.* The population pharmacokinetics of recombinant- and urinary-human follicle stimulating hormone in women. *Br J Clin Pharmacol* 1998; **45:** 13–20.

Uses and Administration
Follicle-stimulating hormone is secreted by the anterior lobe of the pituitary gland, together with another gonadotrophin, luteinising hormone (p.1290).

These gonadotrophins stimulate the normal functioning of the gonads and the secretion of sex hormones in both men and women. In women, follicle-stimulating hormone stimulates the development and maturation of the follicles and ova; in men it has a role in spermatogenesis.

Recombinant human follicle-stimulating hormones (follitropins alfa or beta) are used in the treatment of female infertility due to anovulation, in women who have not responded to treatment with clomifene. Follitropins are also used for the stimulation of spermatogenesis in the management of male infertility caused by hypogonadotrophic hypogonadism (see Infertility, p.1275).

The dosage and schedule of treatment for female infertility must be determined according to the needs of each patient; it is usual to monitor response by studying the patient's urinary oestrogen excretion or by ultrasonic visualisation of follicles or both. Treatment is usually begun with 75 to 150 units daily by subcutaneous or intramuscular injection for 7 or 14 days; if there is no response, dosage is increased at 7- or 14-day intervals until an adequate but not excessive response is achieved. Treatment is then stopped and followed after 1 or 2 days by a single dose of chorionic gonadotrophin 5000 to 10 000 units to induce ovulation. In menstruating patients treatment should be started within the first 7 days of the menstrual cycle. It has been suggested by the UK manufacturers of follitropin alfa that a daily dose of 225 units is the usual maximum, and that if a patient fails to respond adequately after 4 weeks of treatment that cycle should be abandoned and the patient should subsequently begin the next cycle at a higher starting dose.

Follitropins are also employed as part of *in-vitro* fertilisation or other assisted reproductive technologies. For this purpose doses of 150 to 225 units daily are generally given, for at least 4 days, commencing on the second or third day of the menstrual cycle. Thereafter the dose may be adjusted individually based on ovarian response to a usual maximum of about 450 units; adequate follicular development generally occurs within about 5 to 10 days of treatment. Pituitary downregulation with a gonadorelin analogue may be employed in conjunction with follitropin ther-

apy, in which case the gonadorelin analogue is generally begun about 2 weeks before follitropin, and the 2 are then continued concomitantly until follicular development is adequate. A single dose of up to 10 000 units of chorionic gonadotrophin is then given to induce final follicular maturation and oocyte retrieval performed about 35 hours later.

Follitropins are used for the stimulation of spermatogenesis in the management of male infertility caused by hypogonadotrophic hypogonadism. Before starting follitropin therapy, chorionic gonadotrophin is given to raise serum testosterone concentrations to the normal range, which may take 3 to 6 months. A dose of follitropin alfa 150 units subcutaneously three times weekly is then used, with continued chorionic gonadotrophin; doses of follitropin alfa up to 300 units three times weekly may be required. Treatment is continued for at least 4 months, and more than 18 months' treatment may be needed. A dose of follitropin beta 75 units daily or two or three times weekly has been used similarly.

Other substances with follicle-stimulating activity are used similarly: these include human menopausal gonadotrophins (p.1288), which have both luteinising and follicle-stimulating activity, and urofollitropin (p.1299).

Preparations

Proprietary Preparations (details are given in Part 3)
Aust.: Gonal-F; Puregon; ***Austral.:*** Gonal-F; Puregon; ***Belg.:*** Puregon; ***Canad.:*** Gonal-F; Puregon; ***Denm.:*** Gonal-F; Puregon; ***Fin.:*** Gonal-F; Puregon; ***Fr.:*** Gonal-F; Puregon; ***Ger.:*** Gonal-F; Puregon; ***Hong Kong:*** Gonal-F; Puregon; ***Irl.:*** Gonal-F; Puregon; ***Israel:*** Gonal-F; Puregon; ***Ital.:*** Gonal-F; Puregon; ***Mex.:*** Gonal-F; Puregon; ***Neth.:*** Gonal-F; Puregon; ***Norw.:*** Gonal-F; Puregon; ***NZ:*** Gonal-F; Puregon; ***Port.:*** Gonal-F; Puregon; ***Singapore:*** Gonal-F; Puregon; ***Spain:*** Gonal-F; Puregon; ***Swed.:*** Gonal-F; Puregon; ***Switz.:*** Gonal-F; Puregon; ***Thai.:*** Gonal-F; Puregon; ***UK:*** Gonal-F; Puregon; ***USA:*** Follistim; Gonal-F.

Ganirelix Acetate   (15424-h)

Ganirelix Acetate *(BANM, USAN, rINNM).*

RS-26306.
$C_{80}H_{113}ClN_{18}O_{13},2C_2H_4O_2 = 1690.4.$
CAS — 124904-93-4 (ganirelix); 129311-55-3 (ganirelix acetate).

Adverse Effects and Precautions
As for Cetrorelix, p.1279.

Uses and Administration
Like cetrorelix (p.1279), ganirelix is a gonadorelin (gonadotrophin-releasing hormone) antagonist. It is used as the acetate as a component of ovarian stimulation regimens for assisted reproduction in infertility (p.1275). Ganirelix acetate is given by subcutaneous injection for the prevention of premature luteinising hormone surges in women undergoing controlled ovarian hyperstimulation for assisted reproduction techniques. In the UK a dose equivalent to ganirelix 250 µg is given once daily, starting on day 6 of ovarian stimulation and continued until ovulation induction. In the USA a dose of ganirelix acetate 250 µg is used similarly.

◊ References.

1. The Ganirelix Dose-finding Study Group. A double-blind, randomized, dose-finding study to assess the efficacy of the gonadotrophin-releasing hormone antagonist ganirelix (Org 37462) to prevent premature luteinizing hormone surges in women undergoing ovarian stimulation with recombinant follicle stimulating hormone (Puregon). *Hum Reprod* 1998; **13:** 3023–31.
2. Gillies PS, *et al.* Ganirelix. *Drugs* 2000; **59:** 107–11.

Preparations

Proprietary Preparations (details are given in Part 3)
UK: Orgalutran; *USA:* Antagon.

Gonadorelin   (5925-q)

Gonadorelin *(BAN, rINN).*

Follicle Stimulating Hormone-releasing Factor; GnRH; Gonadoliberin; Gonadorelinum; Gonadotrophin-releasing Hormone; Hoe-471; LH/FSH-RF; LH/FSH-RH; LH-RF; LH-RH; Luliberin; Luteinising Hormone-releasing Factor. 5-Oxo-L-prolyl-L-histidyl-L-tryptophyl-L-seryl-L-tyrosylglycyl-L-leucyl-L-arginyl-L-prolylglycinamide.
$C_{55}H_{75}N_{17}O_{13} = 1182.3.$
CAS — 33515-09-2;.
ATC — H01CA01; V04CM01.
Pharmacopoeias. In Fr. and Neth.

Gonadorelin Acetate (11392-n)

Gonadorelin Acetate (BANM, USAN, rINNM).
Abbott-41070.
$C_{55}H_{75}N_{17}O_{13}, xC_2H_4O_2, yH_2O$.
CAS — 34973-08-5 (anhydrous gonadorelin diacetate);
52699-48-6 (gonadorelin diacetate tetrahydrate);.
Pharmacopoeias. In Eur. (see p.vi).

Pharmacopoeial description

Ph. Eur.: The acetate form of a hypothalamic peptide that stimulates the release of follicle-stimulating hormone and luteinising hormone from the pituitary gland. It is obtained by chemical synthesis. A white or slightly yellowish powder; soluble in water and in 1% v/v glacial acetic acid; sparingly soluble in methyl alcohol. Store in airtight containers at a temperature of 2° to 8°. Protect from light.

Gonadorelin Hydrochloride (18465-l)

Gonadorelin Hydrochloride (BANM, USAN, rINNM).
AY-24031.
$C_{55}H_{75}N_{17}O_{13}, 2HCl = 1255.2$.
CAS — 51952-41-1.
Pharmacopoeias. In Br. and US.

Pharmacopoeial description

BP 2001: The chloride form of a hypothalamic peptide that stimulates the release of follicle-stimulating hormone and luteinising hormone from the pituitary gland. It is obtained by synthesis. A white or slightly yellowish-white powder; soluble in water and in 1% v/v glacial acetic acid; sparingly soluble in methyl alcohol. Store at a temperature of 2° to 8°. Protect from light and moisture.

USP 25: A synthetic polypeptide hormone having the property of stimulating the release of the luteinising hormone from the hypothalamus. It is extremely hygroscopic. Protect from exposure to moisture and store in airtight well-sealed containers, in a desiccator.

Units

31 units of gonadorelin for bioassay are contained in approximately 50 µg of gonadorelin acetate (with lactose 2.5 mg and human plasma albumin 0.5 mg) in one ampoule of the first International Reference Preparation (1980).

Adverse Effects

Gonadorelin and its analogues are generally well tolerated but may cause gastrointestinal adverse effects, usually nausea and abdominal pain or discomfort. There may be headache or lightheadedness, and an increase in menstrual bleeding. Continued therapy with gonadorelin analogues results in paradoxical suppression of the pituitary gonadal axis; in premenopausal women this may produce menopausal symptoms, including vaginal dryness, hot flushes, and loss of libido. If sufficiently prolonged the suppression of circulating oestrogens may lead to osteoporosis. In men, hot flushes and sexual dysfunction have occurred. Breast swelling and tenderness in men have been reported infrequently with gonadorelin analogues. Other adverse effects reportedly associated with gonadorelin analogue therapy, and presumably related to changes in the hormonal milieu, include mood changes, nervousness, palpitations, acne and dry skin, alterations in liver function tests and blood lipids, decreased glucose tolerance, and changes in scalp and body hair. Ovarian hyperstimulation (as seen with chorionic gonadotrophin, p.1279), although rare, has occurred in women given gonadorelin.

Reactions or pain may occur at the site of injection with rash (local or generalised), thrombophlebitis, swelling, or pruritus. Hypersensitivity reactions, including bronchospasm and anaphylaxis, have been reported.

Other effects may be a consequence of the particular use of gonadorelin or its analogues. Tumour flare, due to an initial surge in testosterone concentrations, has been reported in the initial stages of treatment for cancer of the prostate and concomitant anti-androgen therapy may be given prophylactically. Flare may manifest as an increase in bone pain; occasionally there has been spinal cord compression, or a worsening of urinary-tract symptoms with haematuria and urinary obstruction. Acute degeneration of submucous fibroids with severe bleeding has been reported following use of leuprorelin. An initial increase in signs and symptoms has also been reported in women

with breast cancer receiving gonadorelin analogues; hypercalcaemia has occurred in those with metastatic disease.

Hypersensitivity. Acquired hypersensitivity led to an anaphylactic reaction following intravenous administration of gonadorelin to a man who had been receiving pulsatile subcutaneous gonadorelin therapy for 10 weeks.[1]

1. Potashnik G, et al. Anaphylactic reaction to gonadotropin-releasing hormone. N Engl J Med 1993; 328: 815.

Osteoporosis. Long-term use of a gonadorelin analogue results in oestrogen deficiency-associated osteoporosis. Various drugs have been investigated for their ability to reduce this effect including parathyroid hormone,[1,2] or 'add-back' therapy with tibolone[3] or oestrogen plus progestogen.

1. Finkelstein JS, et al. Parathyroid hormone for the prevention of bone loss induced by estrogen deficiency. N Engl J Med 1994; 331: 1618–23.
2. Finkelstein JS, et al. Prevention of estrogen deficiency-related bone loss with human parathyroid hormone-(1-34): a randomized controlled trial. JAMA 1998; 280: 1067–73.
3. Lindsay PC, et al. The effect of add-back treatment with tibolone (Livial) on patients treated with the gonadotropin-releasing hormone agonist triptorelin (Decapeptyl). Fertil Steril 1996; 65: 342–8.

Precautions

Gonadorelin or its analogues should not generally be used in patients with pituitary adenoma as haemorrhagic infarction (pituitary apoplexy) has sometimes occurred. It is also recommended that patients with weight-related amenorrhoea should not receive these drugs until their weight is corrected. While it has been recommended by at least one manufacturer that gonadorelin should not be used in women with polycystic ovary disease or with endometriotic cysts, gonadorelin and its analogues have produced improvement in polycystic disease and in uterine fibroids, and gonadorelin analogues have been used with benefit in endometriosis. Gonadorelin or its analogues should be discontinued if the patient becomes pregnant. Contraceptive measures should be taken to protect against unwanted ovulation. Men at risk from tumour flare should be carefully monitored in the first month of therapy.

Interactions

Drugs affecting pituitary secretion of gonadotrophins may alter the response to gonadorelin or its analogues; other hormonal therapy and corticosteroids can affect the response. Spironolactone and levodopa can stimulate gonadotrophins while phenothiazines, dopamine antagonists, digoxin, and sex hormones can inhibit gonadotrophin secretion.

Pharmacokinetics

Gonadorelin is poorly absorbed from the gastrointestinal tract. It has a terminal plasma half-life of only 10 to 40 minutes after intravenous injection. It is hydrolysed in the plasma and excreted in the urine as inactive metabolites.

Gonadorelin analogues are absorbed following oral, intramuscular, intranasal, or rectal administration and have a longer half-life.

Uses and Administration

Gonadorelin is a synthetic form of hypothalamic gonadotrophin-releasing hormone. It stimulates the synthesis and release of follicle-stimulating hormone and, in particular, luteinising hormone in the anterior lobe of the pituitary. The secretion of endogenous gonadotrophin-releasing hormone is pulsatile and is controlled by several factors including circulating sex hormones. Gonadotrophic hormones (gonadotrophins), released from the pituitary gland in response to gonadorelin, stimulate secretion of sex hormones from the gonads. A single dose of gonadorelin or one of its analogues has the effect of increasing circulating sex hormones; continued administration leads to down-regulation of gonadorelin-receptor synthesis in the pituitary and results in a paradoxical reduction in sex-hormone secretion.

Gonadorelin is used in the diagnosis of hypothalamic-pituitary-gonadal dysfunction. Assessment is usually based on the response to a dose of gonadorelin of 100 µg by intravenous or subcutaneous injection. In

females, where possible, it should be given early in the follicular stage of the menstrual cycle.

Gonadorelin is also used in the treatment of amenorrhoea and infertility associated with hypogonadotrophic hypogonadism and multifollicular ovaries. Weight-related amenorrhoea should have been corrected by diet. Treatment in such conditions is based on an intermittent pulse pump providing 5 to 20 µg over one minute every 90 minutes for up to 6 months or until conception.

Gonadorelin, or more usually its analogues such as buserelin, goserelin, leuprorelin, nafarelin, and triptorelin (which are more potent and have a longer duration of action) are used in cryptorchidism, malignant neoplasms (especially of the prostate), and in delayed and precocious puberty.

Gonadorelin is sometimes used as the hydrochloride or acetate.

◊ Reviews of gonadorelin and its analogues.

1. Fraser HM, Waxman J. Gonadotrophin releasing hormone analogues for gynaecological disorders and infertility. BMJ 1989; 298: 475–6.
2. Conn PM, Crowley WF. Gonadotropin-releasing hormone and its analogues. N Engl J Med 1991; 324: 93–103.

Benign prostatic hyperplasia. The gonadorelin analogues have been tried in the management of benign prostatic hyperplasia (p.1477) but are considered unsatisfactory for indefinite use. See also under Leuprorelin Acetate, p.1290, and Nafarelin Acetate, p.1291.

Cryptorchidism. Whether gonadorelin or its analogues have a role in the management of cryptorchidism is a matter of debate; surgery remains the treatment with the best success rate, but hormonal therapy, with gonadorelin or chorionic gonadotrophin or both, is widely employed (see p.1272). Some references to the use of gonadorelin in cryptorchidism, with variable results, are listed below.[1-5] Meta-analysis has suggested a success rate of about 20% overall, although this may be reduced when care is taken to exclude retractile testes.[6]

1. Illig R, et al. Treatment of cryptorchidism by intranasal synthetic luteinising-hormone releasing hormone: results of a collaborative double-blind study. Lancet 1977; ii: 518–20.
2. Klidjian AM, et al. Luteinising hormone releasing hormone for incomplete descent of the testis. Arch Dis Child 1985; 60: 568–71.
3. Witjes JA, et al. Use of luteinizing-hormone-releasing hormone nasal spray in the treatment of cryptorchidism: is there still an indication: a clinical study in 78 boys with 103 undescended testicles. Eur Urol 1990; 17: 226–8.
4. Rajfer J, et al. Hormonal therapy of cryptorchidism: a randomized, double-blind study comparing human chorionic gonadotropin and gonadotropin-releasing hormone. N Engl J Med 1986; 314: 466–70.
5. de Muinck Keizer-Schrama SMPF, et al. Double-blind, placebo-controlled study of luteinising-hormone-releasing-hormone nasal spray in treatment of undescended testes. Lancet 1986; i: 876–80.
6. Pyörälä S, et al. A review and meta-analysis of hormonal treatment of cryptorchidism. J Clin Endocrinol Metab 1995; 80: 2795–9.

Delayed and precocious puberty. For mention of the use of gonadorelin or its analogues in delayed and precocious puberty, see p.1273 and p.1277 respectively. Benefit in delayed puberty is most likely in those cases where it is secondary to hypogonadism (see p.1274).

Diagnosis of hypothalamic and pituitary dysfunction. References to gonadorelin in the diagnosis of hypothalamic-pituitary-gonadal dysfunction[1-6] including one[5] suggesting its abandonment on the grounds that it offered no help in classifying patients with amenorrhoea or determining the therapeutic potential of treatment with gonadorelin.

1. Mortimer CH, et al. Luteinising hormone and follicle stimulating hormone-releasing hormone test in patients with hypothalamic-pituitary-gonadal dysfunction. BMJ 1973; 4: 73–7.
2. Yoshimoto Y, et al. Restoration of normal pituitary gonadotropin reserve by administration of luteinizing-hormone-releasing hormone in patients with hypogonadotropic hypogonadism. N Engl J Med 1975; 292: 242–5.
3. Sagel J, et al. The role of luteinizing hormone-releasing hormone in the diagnosis of constitutional delayed puberty. Postgrad Med J 1975; 51: 611–14.
4. Ginsburg J, et al. Use of clomiphene and luteinizing hormone/follicle stimulating hormone-releasing hormone in investigation of ovulatory failure. BMJ 1975; 3: 130–3.
5. Adulwahid NA, et al. Diagnostic tests with luteinising hormone releasing hormone should be abandoned. BMJ 1985; 291: 1471–2.
6. Eckert KL, et al. A single-sample, subcutaneous gonadotropin-releasing hormone test for central precocious puberty. Pediatrics 1996; 97: 517–19.

Disturbed behaviour. For mention of the use of triptorelin in men with paraphilias, see p.1299.

Endometriosis. Gonadorelin analogues are effective in the management of endometriosis (p.1469), but the need for long-term therapy to prevent recurrence limits their value, because of the risk of osteoporosis. 'Add-back' therapy with concomitant hormone replacement may be given in an attempt to reduce bone mineral density loss and vasomotor symptoms.

Some references to gonadorelin analogues in endometriosis are listed below. For further references, see Buserelin Acetate, p.1278, Goserelin Acetate, p.1285, Leuprorelin Acetate, p.1290, and Nafarelin Acetate, p.1291.

1. Gargiulo AR, Hornstein MD. The role of GnRH agonists plus add-back therapy in the treatment of endometriosis. *Semin Reprod Endocrinol* 1997; **15:** 273–84.
2. Hemmings R. Combined treatment of endometriosis: GnRH agonists and laparoscopic surgery. *J Reprod Med* 1998; **43** (suppl 3): 316–20.
3. Pickersgill A. GnRH agonists and add-back therapy: is there a perfect combination? *Br J Obstet Gynaecol* 1998; **105:** 475–85.
4. Surrey ES. Add-back therapy and gonadotropin-releasing hormone agonists in the treatment of patients with endometriosis: can a consensus be reached? *Fertil Steril* 1999; **71:** 420–4.
5. Prentice A, *et al.* Gonadotrophin-releasing hormone analogues for pain associated with endometriosis (updated 29 May 2001). Available in The Cochrane Library; Issue 3. Oxford: Update Software; 2001.

Fibroids. Uterine fibroids (leiomyomas) are benign tumours of uterine smooth muscle.[1,2] They are found in about 25% of women, most of whom are aged in their 30s or 40s when the condition becomes symptomatic. Fibroids may give rise to menstrual problems, particularly menorrhagia, pelvic discomfort, infertility, and miscarriage. Although small fibroids may not require treatment, the management of symptomatic fibroids has traditionally been surgical. However, because fibroids are oestrogen responsive, gonadorelin analogues have also been tried as medical treatment for their ability to induce a hypogonadotrophic hypogonadal state. These drugs produce a significant reduction in uterine and fibroid volume, and amenorrhoea, but when treatment stops uterine and fibroid volume tend to return to pretreatment values. The hypoestrogenism produced during treatment also causes menopausal symptoms such as hot flushes and vaginal dryness, and bone loss may occur. The administration of oestrogens or progestogens, once the uterine fibroid size has significantly reduced, has been tried in order to counteract these side-effects.[3] Subcutaneous administration of long-acting depot preparations of gonadorelin or its analogues appear to be the preferred method of administration and it is considered that this treatment is a valuable pre-operative adjunct to surgery, simplifying the procedure by reducing uterine and fibroid volume and intra-operative blood loss, as well as correcting pre-operative iron-deficiency anaemia.[4] However, concern has been expressed that the use of gonadorelin analogues for treating fibroids may complicate the differentiation of benign and malignant growths.[5]

For further references to gonadorelin analogues being used in the treatment of fibroids, see Buserelin Acetate, p.1278, Goserelin Acetate, p.1286, Leuprorelin Acetate, p.1290, Nafarelin Acetate, p.1291, and Triptorelin, p.1299.

1. Al-Taher H, Farquharson RG. Management of uterine fibroids. *Br J Hosp Med* 1993; **50:** 133–6.
2. Stewart EA. Uterine fibroids. *Lancet* 2001; **357:** 293–8.
3. Friedman AJ, *et al.* Efficacy and safety considerations in women with uterine leiomyomas treated with gonadotropin-releasing hormone agonists: the estrogen threshold hypothesis. *Am J Obstet Gynecol* 1990; **163:** 1114–19.
4. Lethaby A, *et al.* Pre-operative GnRH analogue therapy before hysterectomy or myomectomy for uterine fibroids (updated 26 February 2001). Available in The Cochrane Library; Issue 3. Oxford: Update Software; 2001.
5. Meyer WR, *et al.* Unsuspected leiomyosarcoma: treatment with a gonadotropin-releasing hormone analogue. *Obstet Gynecol* 1990; **75** (suppl): 529–32.

Growth retardation. The use of a gonadorelin analogue to delay precocious puberty may improve the final height of children with the disorder. However, the use of a gonadorelin analogue with growth hormone in short but otherwise normal children is controversial—see under Triptorelin, p.1299.

Hirsutism. For reference to the use of gonadorelin analogues such as leuprorelin in the treatment of hirsutism, see p.1290.

Infertility. Gonadorelin and its analogues are used in the management of infertility related to hypogonadotrophic hypogonadism in both women and men (p.1275). Some further references are given below. See also under Buserelin Acetate, p.1278, Leuprorelin Acetate, p.1290, and Nafarelin Acetate, p.1291.

1. Lingle L, Hart LL. Gonadotropin-releasing hormone in infertility. *DICP Ann Pharmacother* 1989; **23:** 246–8.
2. Thomas AK, *et al.* Induction of ovulation with subcutaneous pulsatile gonadotropin-releasing hormone: correlation with body weight and other parameters. *Fertil Steril* 1989; **51:** 786–90.
3. Homburg R, *et al.* One hundred pregnancies after treatment with pulsatile luteinising hormone releasing hormone to induce ovulation. *BMJ* 1989; **298:** 809–12.
4. Kovacs GT, *et al.* Induction of ovulation with gonadotrophin-releasing hormone—life-table analysis of 50 courses of treatment. *Med J Aust* 1989; **151:** 21–6.
5. Santoro N. Efficacy and safety of intravenous pulsatile gonadotropin-releasing hormone: Lutrepulse for injection. *Am J Obstet Gynecol* 1990; **163:** 1759–64.
6. Nachtigall LB, *et al.* Adult-onset idiopathic hypogonadotropic hypogonadism–a treatable form of male infertility. *N Engl J Med* 1997; **336:** 410–15.

Malignant neoplasms. Gonadorelin analogues are used in the treatment of prostatic cancer (p.497) where they provide an alternative to orchidectomy in the management of advanced disease. They are also being investigated for ovarian ablation in premenopausal women with breast cancer (p.491) and have been tried in neoplasms of the endometrium (p.493), ovary

(p.496), and pancreas (p.497) where their use is much less well established.

Analogues used include buserelin (p.1278), goserelin (p.1286), leuprorelin (p.1290), and triptorelin (p.1299).

Mastalgia. Gonadorelin analogues such as goserelin may be effective in severe refractory mastalgia (see p.1470).

Polycystic ovary syndrome. Gonadorelin and its analogues have been tried in polycystic ovary syndrome (p.1276) even though they are contra-indicated in this condition by some manufacturers. Pulsatile gonadorelin achieves a higher ovulatory rate in women with multifollicular ovaries than in those with large polycystic ovaries, and the incidences of early miscarriage and abortion are higher in those with polycystic ovaries. Nonetheless there is a suggestion that addition of gonadorelin analogues to gonadotrophin stimulation results in better pregnancy rates in women with polycystic ovaries than do gonadotrophins alone.[1] Ovulation rate can be improved by pretreatment with a gonadorelin analogue for 8 weeks before using gonadorelin; 38% of patients achieved pregnancy in one study using this technique.[2] The rate of spontaneous abortion was also decreased from 50 to 38% after administration.

1. Nugent D, *et al.* Gonadotrophin therapy for ovulation induction in subfertility associated with polycystic ovary syndrome (updated 28 May 2001). Available in The Cochrane Library; Issue 3. Oxford: Update Software; 2001.
2. Filicori M, *et al.* Polycystic ovary syndrome: abnormalities and management with pulsatile gonadotropin-releasing hormone and gonadotropin-releasing hormone analogs. *Am J Obstet Gynecol* 1990; **163:** 1737–42.

Porphyria. For mention of the use of buserelin in a regimen to suppress cyclic premenstrual exacerbations of acute porphyria, see p.1279.

Premenstrual syndrome. In women in whom other drug treatments for premenstrual syndrome (p.1475) are ineffective, use of a gonadorelin analogue, usually with HRT to prevent menopausal symptoms, may be considered. Short-term therapy (3 months) has been used to confirm the diagnosis of premenstrual syndrome, or to predict the response to bilateral oophorectomy when this is being considered. Some references to the use of gonadorelin analogues in premenstrual syndrome are given below.[1-4]

1. Mortola JF, *et al.* Successful treatment of severe premenstrual syndrome by combined use of gonadotropin-releasing hormone agonist and estrogen/progestin. *J Clin Endocrinol Metab* 1991; **72:** 252A–F.
2. Hussain SY, *et al.* Buserelin in premenstrual syndrome. *Gynecol Endocrinol* 1992; **6:** 57–64.
3. Mortola JF. Applications of gonadotropin-releasing hormone analogues in the treatment of premenstrual syndrome. *Clin Obstet Gynecol* 1993; **36:** 753–63.
4. Mezrow G, *et al.* Depot leuprolide acetate with estrogen and progestin add-back for long-term treatment of premenstrual syndrome. *Fertil Steril* 1994; **62:** 932–7.

Preparations

BP 2001: Gonadorelin Injection;
USP 25: Gonadorelin for Injection.

Proprietary Preparations (details are given in Part 3)
Aust.: Kryptocur; Lutrelef; Relefact LH-RH; **Austral.:** HRF; **Belg.:** HRF; Kryptocur†; **Braz.:** HRF; Relisorm L; **Canad.:** Factrel; Lutrepulse; Relisorm†; **Fr.:** Lutrelef; Stimu-LH; **Ger.:** Kryptocur; Lutrelef; Relefact LH-RH; **Hong Kong:** Relisorm L; **Irl.:** HRF; Relefact LH-RH†; **Israel:** Lutrelef; Relefact LH-RH; **Ital.:** Kryptocur; Lutrelef; **Mex.:** Relisorm L; **Neth.:** Cryptocur; HRF; Lutrelef; Relefact LH-RH; **NZ:** HRF; **S.Afr.:** HRF†; **Spain:** Luforan; **Swed.:** Lutrelef; **Switz.:** Kryptocur; Lutrelef; Relisorm L; **UK:** Fertiral†; HRF; Relefact LH-RH†; **USA:** Factrel; Lutrepulse†.

Goserelin Acetate (16845-p)

Goserelin Acetate (BANM, rINNM).

ICI-118630 (goserelin); D-Ser (Buᵗ)[6] Azgly[10]-LHRH Acetate. 3-[5-Oxo-L-prolyl-L-histidyl-L-tryptophyl-L-seryl-L-tyrosyl-(3-O-tert-butyl)-D-seryl-L-leucyl-L-arginyl-L-prolyl]carbazamide acetate.

$C_{59}H_{84}N_{18}O_{14}, C_2H_4O_2 = 1329.5.$

CAS — 65807-02-5 (goserelin).

NOTE. Goserelin is *USAN*.

10.5 mg of goserelin acetate is approximately equivalent to 10 mg of goserelin.

Adverse Effects and Precautions

As for Gonadorelin, p.1284. Some women may experience vaginal bleeding during initial therapy, which normally resolves spontaneously. Arthralgia and paraesthesias have been reported.

Pituitary apoplexy. A report of pituitary apoplexy (a clinical syndrome caused by haemorrhage and infarction of a pituitary adenoma) in an elderly patient with a symptomless pituitary adenoma who was given goserelin for advanced prostate cancer.[1] The patient developed headache, vomiting, visual disturbances, gradual impairment of consciousness, intermittent fe-

ver, and progressive hyponatraemia. Symptoms responded to prednisolone replacement therapy.

1. Ando S, *et al.* Pituitary apoplexy after goserelin. *Lancet* 1995; **345:** 458.

Pharmacokinetics

Goserelin is almost completely absorbed following subcutaneous injection, and has a serum elimination half-life of 2 to 4 hours, which may be increased in patients with impaired renal function. More than 90% of a dose is excreted in urine, as unchanged drug and metabolites.

◊ Reviews.
1. Cockshott ID. Clinical pharmacokinetics of goserelin. *Clin Pharmacokinet* 2000; **39:** 27–48.

Uses and Administration

Goserelin acetate is an analogue of gonadorelin (see p.1284) with similar properties. It is used for the suppression of gonadal sex hormone production in the treatment of malignant neoplasms of the prostate, in breast cancer in pre- and peri-menopausal women, and in the management of endometriosis and uterine fibroids. It is also given before surgery for endometrial reduction and as an adjunct to ovulation induction with gonadotrophins in the treatment of infertility.

Goserelin acetate is available as depot preparations; with one such preparation a dose equivalent to 3.6 mg of goserelin injected subcutaneously into the anterior abdominal wall provides effective suppression of oestradiol or testosterone for 28 days. A full response should be achieved by the end of this period and treatment is continued with repeated doses at 28-day intervals; in endometriosis, therapy is given for up to 6 months while in women with anaemia as a result of uterine fibroids it is continued, with concomitant iron supplementation, for up to 3 months before surgery. In men with prostate cancer preparations supplying the equivalent of 10.8 mg of goserelin, given every 12 weeks, may also be employed.

In the treatment of prostatic cancer an anti-androgen such as cyproterone acetate may be given for several days before beginning goserelin therapy and continued for at least 3 weeks, to avoid the risk of a disease flare.

Regimens for oocyte collection for *in-vitro* fertilisation employ gonadorelin analogues for pituitary desensitisation before ovulation induction with gonadotrophins. The equivalent of 3.6 mg of goserelin is given as a subcutaneous depot injection and serum-oestradiol concentrations monitored until they decline to levels similar to those in the early follicular phase, a process which usually takes 7 to 21 days. Once downregulation occurs gonadotrophin (follicle stimulating) therapy is begun until an appropriate stage of follicular development, when it is withdrawn and chorionic gonadotrophin is given to induce ovulation.

Goserelin has also been given in other sex-hormone-related conditions.

◊ Reviews of goserelin.
1. Chrisp P, Goa KL. Goserelin: a review of its pharmacodynamic and pharmacokinetic properties, and clinical use in sex hormone-related conditions. *Drugs* 1991; **41:** 254–88.
2. Perry CM, Brogden RN. Goserelin: a review of its pharmacodynamic and pharmacokinetic properties, and therapeutic use in benign gynaecological disorders. *Drugs* 1996; **51:** 319–46.

Endometriosis. Gonadorelin analogues such as goserelin are effective in the management of endometriosis (p.1469), but the need for long-term therapy to prevent recurrence limits their value because of the risk of osteoporosis. 'Add-back' therapy, with concomitant hormone replacement, may be given in an attempt to reduce bone mineral density loss and vasomotor symptoms in women receiving goserelin.
References.
1. Shaw RW, *et al.* An open randomized comparative study of the effect of goserelin depot and danazol in the treatment of endometriosis. *Fertil Steril* 1992; **58:** 265–72.
2. Schlaff WD. Extending the treatment boundaries: Zoladex and add-back. *Int J Gynaecol Obstet* 1999; **64** (suppl 1): S25–S31.
3. Franke HR, *et al.* Gonadotropin-releasing hormone agonist plus "add-back" hormone replacement therapy for treatment of endometriosis: a prospective, randomized, placebo-controlled, double-blind trial. *Fertil Steril* 2000; **74:** 534–9.
4. Pierce SJ, *et al.* Long-term use of gonadotropin-releasing hormone analogs and hormone replacement therapy in the management of endometriosis: a randomized trial with a 6-year follow-up. *Fertil Steril* 2000; **74:** 964–8.

Fibroids. Gonadorelin analogues such as goserelin have been tried as an adjunct or an alternative to surgery in the treatment of uterine fibroids (p.1285) although there has been some concern that this might complicate the diagnosis of malignancy. Some further references are listed below.

1. Lumsden MA, *et al.* Goserelin therapy before surgery for uterine fibroids. *Lancet* 1987; **i:** 36–7.
2. Lumsden MA, *et al.* Treatment with the gonadotrophin releasing hormone-agonist goserelin before hysterectomy for uterine fibroids. *Br J Obstet Gynaecol* 1994; **101:** 438–42.
3. Benagiano G, *et al.* Zoladex (goserelin acetate) and the anemic patient: results of a multicenter fibroid study. *Fertil Steril* 1996; **66:** 223–9.

Malignant neoplasms. Goserelin is effective in the treatment of prostate cancer (p.497). It has produced a response similar to that of orchidectomy (surgical removal of the testes) in patients with metastatic prostate cancer.[1] Goserelin has been combined with an anti-androgen such as flutamide to provide maximum androgen blockade, but this appears to produce modest additional benefits at most. There is some evidence that adjuvant therapy with goserelin may improve survival in patients with locally advanced prostate cancer when combined with radiotherapy.[2]

Goserelin may also be used as hormonal therapy in premenopausal women with advanced breast cancer (p.491), either alone[3,4] or combined with tamoxifen,[5] and is said to be as effective as oophorectomy.[4] It is also used as an alternative to chemotherapy in pre- or peri-menopausal women with oestrogen receptor positive early breast cancer.

1. Seidenfeld J, *et al.* Single-therapy androgen suppression in men with advanced prostate cancer: a systematic review and meta-analysis. *Ann Intern Med* 2000; **132:** 566–77.
2. Bolla M, *et al.* Improved survival in patients with locally advanced prostrate cancer treated with radiotherapy and goserelin. *N Engl J Med* 1997; **337:** 295–300.
3. Dixon AR, *et al.* Goserelin (Zoladex) in premenopausal advanced breast cancer: duration of response and survival. *Br J Cancer* 1990; **62:** 868–70.
4. Bajetta E, *et al.* Goserelin in premenopausal advanced breast cancer: clinical and endocrine evaluation of responsive patients. *Oncology* 1994; **51:** 262–9.
5. Jonat W, *et al.* A randomised study to compare the effect of the luteinising hormone releasing hormone (LHRH) analogue goserelin with or without tamoxifen in pre- and perimenopausal patients with advanced breast cancer. *Eur J Cancer* 1995; **31A:** 137–42.

Mastalgia. For reference to the use of goserelin in mastalgia, see under Danazol, p.1470.

Preparations

Proprietary Preparations (details are given in Part 3)
Aust.: Zoladex; *Austral.:* Zoladex; *Belg.:* Zoladex; *Braz.:* Zoladex; *Canad.:* Zoladex; *Denm.:* Zoladex; *Fin.:* Zoladex; *Fr.:* Zoladex; *Ger.:* Zoladex; *Hong Kong:* Zoladex; *Irl.:* Zoladex; *Israel:* Zoladex; *Ital.:* Zoladex; *Mex.:* Zoladex; *Neth.:* Zoladex; *Norw.:* Zoladex; *NZ:* Zoladex; *Port.:* Zoladex; *S.Afr.:* Zoladex; *Singapore:* Zoladex; *Spain:* Zoladex; *Swed.:* Zoladex; *Switz.:* Zoladex; *Thai.:* Zoladex; *UK:* Zoladex; *USA:* Zoladex.

Growth Hormone (3882-t)

Growth Hormone (*BAN*).
GH; Phyone; Somatotrophin; Somatotropin; STH.
CAS — 9002-72-6.

Somatrem (12012-b)

Somatrem (*BAN, USAN, pINN*).
Met-HGH; Methionyl Human Growth Hormone.
$C_{995}H_{1537}N_{263}O_{301}S_8 = 22\,256$.
CAS — 82030-87-3.
ATC — H01AC02.

Somatrem is an analogue of somatropin containing an additional (methionyl) amino-acid residue. It may be produced in bacteria from recombinant DNA. Sometribove (*BAN*) is methionyl bovine growth hormone, sometripor (*BAN*) is methionyl porcine growth hormone, and somidobove (*BAN*) is synthetic bovine growth hormone.

Somatropin (5933-q)

Somatropin (*BAN, USAN, rINN*).
CB-311; HGH; Human Growth Hormone; LY-137998.
$C_{990}H_{1528}N_{262}O_{300}S_7 = 22\,125$.
CAS — 12629-01-5.
ATC — H01AC01.

Pharmacopoeias. In Eur. (see p.vi), which also includes Somatropin Bulk Solution.

Somatropin is synthetic human growth hormone having the normal structure of the major (22K) component of natural human pituitary growth hormone. It consists of a single polypeptide chain of 191 amino acids with disulfide linkages between positions 53 and 165 and between 182 and 189. For labelling purposes, the name may carry in parentheses an approved code in lower case letters indicative of the method of production: (epr) indicates production by enzymatic conversion of a precursor produced by a bacterium genetically modified by recombinant DNA technology; (rbe) indicates production from bacteria genetically modified by recombinant DNA technology;

(rmc) indicates production from genetically engineered and transformed mammalian (mouse) cells.

Pharmacopoeial description
Ph. Eur.: Somatropin is a protein having the structure (191 amino acid residues) of the major component of growth hormone produced by the human pituitary. A white or almost white powder, containing not less than 2.5 units per mg. Store at 2° to 8° in airtight containers.
Somatropin Bulk Solution is a clear or slightly turbid, colourless solution. It may contain buffer salts and other auxiliary substances. Store at −20° in airtight containers. Avoid repeated freezing and thawing.

Units

4.4 units of human growth hormone (somatropin) are contained in 1.75 mg of freeze-dried purified human growth hormone, with 20 mg of glycine, 2 mg of mannitol, 2 mg of lactose, and 2 mg of sodium bicarbonate, in one ampoule of the first International Standard (1987).

The first International Standard for Somatropin (1994) has a defined content of 2 mg of protein per ampoule, with a specific activity of 3 units per mg of protein. Commercial preparations vary somewhat in the number of units per mg.

◊ References.
1. WHO. WHO Expert Committee on biological standardization: forty-fourth report. *WHO Tech Rep Ser 848* 1994.
2. WHO. WHO Expert Committee on biological standardization: forty-fifth report *WHO Tech Rep Ser 858* 1995.

Adverse Effects and Precautions

Antibodies to growth hormone have been formed in some patients but these rarely seem to affect growth. There may be redness, itching, lumps, or lipoatrophy at the site of injection. Transient dose-related fluid retention with peripheral oedema has occurred; headache, muscle and joint pain, and cases of benign intracranial hypertension have been reported. Although growth hormone has diabetogenic effects, high acute dosage has been associated with hypoglycaemia.

Growth hormone therapy is contra-indicated in patients with active neoplasms or intracranial lesions and should be discontinued if evidence of tumour growth develops. Growth hormones should not be used for growth promotion in patients with closed epiphyses. Because of the diabetogenic effect of growth hormone it should be given with care to patients with diabetes mellitus; adjustment of antidiabetic therapy may be necessary. Hypothyroidism may develop during treatment, and may result in suboptimal response. For the suggestion that growth hormone should not be used to treat acute catabolic states, as in patients with severe burns or who are otherwise critically ill, see Burns, under Uses and Administration, below.

Benign intracranial hypertension. Benign intracranial hypertension (pseudotumor cerebri) had occurred[1] in 22 children and 1 adult given growth hormone treatment between 1986 and 1993. Eight further cases were identified in a subsequent report[2] in 1995. Three patients treated with mecasermin also developed benign intracranial hypertension. Symptoms such as headache and papilloedema resolved when treatment was stopped. In a report of another case[3] it was pointed out that diagnosis may be complicated by the not infrequent occurrence of headache in patients receiving growth hormone; these normally resolved spontaneously.

1. Malozowski S, *et al.* Growth hormone, insulin-like growth factor I, and benign intracranial hypertension. *N Engl J Med* 1993; **329:** 665–6.
2. Malozowski S, *et al.* Benign intracranial hypertension in children with growth hormone deficiency treated with growth hormone. *J Pediatr* 1995; **126:** 996–9.
3. Price DA, *et al.* Benign intracranial hypertension induced by growth hormone treatment. *Lancet* 1995; **345:** 458–9.

Carcinogenicity. Despite fears to the contrary, studies in children given growth hormone after cranial irradiation for brain tumours or CNS leukaemia have found no evidence that therapy with growth hormone increased the relapse rate.[1-3] Nevertheless, 5 cases of acute leukaemia have been reported among patients in Japan treated with growth hormones, a 9.4-fold increase over the expected incidence,[4] and other cases have been reported subsequently.[5,6] An international workshop convened in 1988 to review known leukaemia cases in patients treated with growth hormones in Europe, North America, Japan, and Australia since 1959 found the observed incidence of leukaemia in growth-hormone-treated patients to represent a twofold increase over the expected rate.[7] After a careful review of the data it was concluded that there may be a small increase in leukaemia incidence associated with growth hormone treatment of growth-hormone-deficient patients, but that it was not clear that

this was actually attributable to growth hormone. A later study involving 6284 patients treated with growth hormone between 1963 and 1985 in the USA confirmed an increase of about 2.5-fold in the incidence of leukaemia in this population, but noted that many of the patients had other risk factors for leukaemia.[8] It has been suggested that growth hormone deficiency is itself a risk factor for leukaemia and that perhaps this, rather than growth hormone treatment, is related to the increased incidence of leukaemia in these patients.[9] If there is any risk it is relatively small, and in view of the essential nature of growth hormone therapy in growth hormone-deficient children it was considered inappropriate and unwise to withhold it.[7]

Further reports of malignancies associated with growth hormone therapy include two children with Bloom's syndrome (a rare chromosomal disorder affecting DNA replication), one of whom developed B-cell non-Hodgkin's lymphoma and the other stem-cell leukaemia.[10]

1. Clayton PE, *et al.* Does growth hormone cause relapse of brain tumours? *Lancet* 1987; **i:** 711–13.
2. Ogilvy-Stuart AL, *et al.* Growth hormone and tumour recurrence. *BMJ* 1992; **304:** 1601–5.
3. Packer RJ, *et al.* Growth hormone replacement therapy in children with medulloblastoma: use and effect on tumor control. *J Clin Oncol* 2001; **19:** 480–7.
4. Watanabe S, *et al.* Leukaemia in patients treated with growth hormone. *Lancet* 1988; **i:** 1159.
5. Delemarre-Van de Waal HA, *et al.* Leukaemia in patients treated with growth hormone. *Lancet* 1988; **i:** 1159.
6. Watanabe S, *et al.* Leukemia and other malignancies among GH users. *J Pediatr Endocrinol* 1993; **6:** 99–108.
7. Fisher DA, *et al.* Leukaemia in patients treated with growth hormone. *Lancet* 1988; **i:** 1159–60.
8. Fradkin JE, *et al.* Risk of leukemia after treatment with pituitary growth hormone. *JAMA* 1993; **270:** 2829–32.
9. Rapaport R, *et al.* Relationship of growth hormone deficiency and leukemia. *J Pediatr* 1995; **126:** 759–61.
10. Brock PR, *et al.* Malignant disease in Bloom's syndrome children treated with growth hormone. *Lancet* 1991; **337:** 1345–6.

Creutzfeldt-Jakob disease. Reports in 1985 of a small number of deaths from Creutzfeldt-Jakob disease in patients under 40 years of age who had received growth hormone extracted from human pituitary glands resulted in the suspension of the distribution of pituitary-derived growth hormone by the licensing authorities in a number of countries, including Australia, Canada, the Netherlands, the UK, and the USA.[1-5] Preparations of non-pituitary-derived growth hormone are now available that are free from contamination with Creutzfeldt-Jakob agent. However, because of the long incubation period of the disease, cases are still being reported in patients who had received pituitary-derived growth hormone years previously.[6-9]

1. Brown P, *et al.* Potential epidemic of Creutzfeldt-Jakob disease from human growth hormone therapy. *N Engl J Med* 1985; **313:** 728–33. Correction. *ibid.*; 967.
2. Powell-Jackson J, *et al.* Creutzfeldt-Jakob disease after administration of human growth hormone. *Lancet* 1985; **ii:** 244–6.
3. Anonymous. Human growth hormone distribution discontinued. *FDA Drug Bull* 1985; **15:** 17–18.
4. Lazarus L. Suspension of the Australian human pituitary hormone programme. *Med J Aust* 1985; **143:** 57–9.
5. Bannister BA, McCormick A. Creutzfeldt-Jakob disease with reference to the safety of pituitary growth hormone. *J Infect* 1987; **14:** 7–12.
6. Fradkin JE, *et al.* Creutzfeldt-Jakob disease in pituitary growth hormone recipients in the United States. *JAMA* 1991; **265:** 880–4.
7. Buchanan CR, *et al.* Mortality, neoplasia, and Creutzfeldt-Jakob disease in patients treated with human pituitary growth hormone in the United Kingdom. *BMJ* 1991; **302:** 824–8.
8. Billette de Villemeur T, *et al.* Creutzfeldt-Jakob disease in children treated with growth hormone. *Lancet* 1991; **337:** 864–5.
9. Macario ME, *et al.* Pituitary growth hormone and Creutzfeldt-Jakob disease. *BMJ* 1991; **302:** 1149.

Effects on carbohydrate metabolism. Symptomatic diabetes mellitus developed in a child given somatropin for familial short stature.[1] In another case[2] nonketotic hyperglycaemia developed within weeks of beginning growth hormone therapy in a 22-month-old child, leading to convulsions and metabolic acidosis; the patient died despite correction of the hyperglycaemia.

A retrospective analysis[3] of data from a pharmacoepidemiological survey of children treated with growth hormone found a higher incidence of type 2 diabetes, compared with that found in untreated children. The researchers speculated that growth hormone treatment might precipitate the onset of type 2 diabetes in predisposed patients, and proposed that patients with risk factors for diabetes, including Turner's syndrome, Prader-Willi syndrome, or intra-uterine growth retardation, be monitored.

1. Botero D, *et al.* Symptomatic non-insulin-dependent diabetes mellitus during therapy with recombinant human growth hormone. *J Pediatr* 1993; **123:** 590–2.
2. Garg AK, Hyperglycemia during replacement growth hormone therapy. *J Pediatr* 1994; **125:** 329.
3. Cutfield WS, *et al.* Incidence of diabetes mellitus and impaired glucose tolerance in children and adolescents receiving growth-hormone treatment. *Lancet* 2000; **355:** 610–13.

Effects on immune function. Growth hormone is generally considered to interact with the immune system although there is a lack of evidence that this is clinically significant.[1,2] There has been a report of acute renal transplant rejection in 2 children receiving treatment for growth retardation with somatropin.[3] In both children renal function of the transplant was stable for several years before somatropin was started, and growth hormone therapy had continued for some months before rejection occurred. It was suggested that during the first months of growth hormone therapy in transplant recipients, immunosuppressive therapy should be increased and transplant function carefully monitored.

1. Church JA, *et al.* Immune functions in children treated with bio-synthetic growth hormone. *J Pediatr* 1989; **115:** 420–3.
2. Rapaport R, Oleske J. Immune function during growth hormone therapy. *J Pediatr* 1990; **116:** 669–70.
3. Tydén G, *et al.* Acute renal graft rejection after treatment with human growth hormone. *Lancet* 1990; **336:** 1455–6.

Effects on skeletal muscle. A report of mild inflammatory myositis, with myalgia and muscle weakness, in 2 patients receiving growth hormone therapy.[1] It was suggested that the effect might be due to *m*-cresol used as a preservative in the preparation.

1. Yordam N. Myositis associated with growth hormone therapy. *J Pediatr* 1994; **125:** 671.

Gynaecomastia. A report of 22 cases of prepubertal gynaecomastia diagnosed during growth hormone treatment.[1]

1. Malozowski S, Stadel BV. Prepubertal gynecomastia during growth hormone therapy. *J Pediatr* 1995; **126:** 659–61.

Hypersensitivity. Generalised urticaria in a patient given somatropin was overcome by a desensitisation regimen.[1] The patient was subsequently maintained uneventfully on daily injections of somatropin.

1. Walker SB, *et al.* Systemic reaction to human growth hormone treated with acute desensitization. *Pediatrics* 1992; **90:** 108–9.

Iron deficiency. The view has been expressed[1] that given the increased production of haemoglobin and the prevalence of iron deficiency in patients treated with growth hormone, supplementation with iron should be considered in patients receiving growth hormone treatment.

1. Vihervuori E, *et al.* Increases in hemoglobin concentration and iron needs in response to growth hormone treatment. *J Pediatr* 1994; **125:** 242–5.

Pancreatitis. A report of acute pancreatitis in a patient with pseudohypoparathyroidism and growth hormone deficiency following the institution of growth hormone treatment.[1] Ten further cases of acute pancreatitis associated with growth hormone treatment had been reported to the FDA at the time of writing.

1. Malozowski S, *et al.* Acute pancreatitis associated with growth hormone therapy for short stature. *N Engl J Med* 1995; **332:** 401–2.

Interactions

High doses of corticosteroids may inhibit the growth promoting effects of growth hormone.

Pharmacokinetics

Somatropin is well absorbed after subcutaneous or intramuscular injection with a bioavailability varying from about 60 to 80%; peak serum concentrations may not be achieved for several hours. After intravenous injection it has a half-life of about 20 to 30 minutes but after subcutaneous or intramuscular administration serum concentrations decline with a half-life of 3 to 5 hours, due to more prolonged release from the injection site. It is metabolised in the liver and kidneys and excreted in bile.

◊ A study of the pharmacokinetics of somatropin following transdermal jet injection in healthy subjects suggested that absorption was more rapid and peak serum concentration higher than after conventional subcutaneous injection of the same dose.[1] However this did not seem to result in any difference in the total amount absorbed, nor in the biological effect of the drug.

1. Verhagen A, *et al.* Pharmacokinetics and pharmacodynamics of a single dose of recombinant human growth hormone after subcutaneous administration by jet-injection: comparison with conventional needle-injection. *Eur J Clin Pharmacol* 1995; **49:** 69–72.

Uses and Administration

Somatropin is synthetic human growth hormone and somatrem its methionyl analogue.

Growth hormone is an anabolic hormone secreted by the anterior lobe of the pituitary, varying in size and amino-acid sequence between animal species. It promotes growth of skeletal, muscular, and other tissues, stimulates protein anabolism, and affects fat and mineral metabolism. The hormone has a diabetogenic action on carbohydrate metabolism. Secretion is pulsatile and dependent on neural and hormonal influences including a hypothalamic release-inhibiting hormone (see Somatostatin, p.1297), and a hypothalamic releasing hormone (see Somatorelin, p.1297). Sleep, hypoglycaemia, and physical or emotional stress result in increased secretion of growth hormone. The effects of growth hormone on skeletal growth are mediated by the somatomedins (see p.1296).

The symbol † denotes a preparation no longer actively marketed

Somatropin or somatrem is given to children with open epiphyses for the treatment of short stature due to growth hormone deficiency (pituitary dwarfism) following assessment of pituitary function. Somatropin is also used in children with some other forms of growth retardation, for example in Turner's syndrome or that due to chronic renal insufficiency. In Prader-Willi syndrome, somatropin is given to improve growth and body composition. In adults, somatropin is given for confirmed growth hormone deficiency. It is also used in the management of wasting or cachexia associated with AIDS.

Doses should be individualised for each patient. Manufacturers vary somewhat in their estimates of the number of units per mg for somatropin and although some countries specify labelling in mg, others require labelling in units or both. Somatrem may be given in doses similar to those of somatropin.

In children with growth hormone deficiency, the usual daily dose in the UK is 25 to 35 µg per kg body-weight by subcutaneous injection (0.07 to 0.1 units per kg), or 0.7 to 1 mg per m^2 body-surface (2 to 3 units per m^2). Similar doses are used in other countries, by subcutaneous or intramuscular injection, and the total weekly dose may be divided into 3, 6, or 7 doses. A suspension of somatropin for subcutaneous depot injection is also available, given in a dose of 1.5 mg per kg on the same day of each month. Alternatively, the dose can be given as 0.75 mg per kg twice monthly (for example, on days 1 and 15 of each month).

In Turner's syndrome (gonadal dysgenesis) higher doses are used, such as a subcutaneous daily dose of 45 to 50 µg per kg (0.14 units per kg), or 1.4 mg per m^2 (4.3 units per m^2). Similar doses may be employed in children with growth retardation due to chronic renal insufficiency.

In children with Prader-Willi syndrome, a daily dose of about 35 µg per kg, or 1 mg per m^2, is given subcutaneously; daily doses should not exceed 2.7 mg.

In adults with growth hormone deficiency lower doses are recommended. The initial dose is about 6 µg per kg (0.018 units per kg) subcutaneously daily. The dose can then be gradually increased according to patient response, to a usual maximum of 12 µg per kg daily, although doses up to 25 µg per kg daily have been used for patients younger than 35 years of age. Dosage requirements may decline with increasing age.

In the treatment of HIV-associated wasting or cachexia somatropin is given is doses of 0.1 mg per kg daily by subcutaneous injection at bedtime.

Administration in adults. Growth hormone continues to be secreted in adult life, although secretion and activity gradually decline with increasing age, and it appears to play a role in maintaining skeletal and lean body-mass amongst other things. In adults with growth hormone deficiency (usually secondary to pituitary adenoma or its treatment) replacement therapy with growth hormone is reported to improve bone mineral density, decrease fat mass and increase lean body-mass, resting metabolic rate, and in some cases improve feelings of well being.[1-8] However, one recent study in adults with growth hormone deficiency found that growth hormone therapy was not associated with an improvement in quality of life.[9] Doses need to be lower than in children.[1,2]

Less well established is the use of growth hormone in otherwise healthy elderly patients.[10-13] Considerable controversy has attended suggestions that growth hormone therapy may retard or reverse some of the metabolic effects of ageing, and there is some concern that these patients may be at increased risk of adverse effects: in one small study 6 of 12 healthy elderly subjects given growth hormone therapy withdrew due to symptoms of carpal tunnel syndrome, fluid retention, or arthralgia.[12]

Other uses for growth hormone in adult patients are discussed below.

1. Powrie J, *et al.* Growth hormone replacement therapy for growth hormone-deficient adults. *Drugs* 1995; **49:** 656–63.
2. Shalet SM. Growth hormone deficiency and replacement in adults. *BMJ* 1996; **313:** 314.
3. Salomon F, *et al.* The effects of treatment with recombinant human growth hormone on body composition and metabolism in adults with growth hormone deficiency. *N Engl J Med* 1989; **321:** 1797–1803.

4. Jørgensen JOL, *et al.* Beneficial effects of growth hormone treatment in GH-deficient adults. *Lancet* 1989; **i:** 1221–5.
5. Whitehead HM, *et al.* Growth hormone treatment of adults with growth hormone deficiency: effect on fat and carbohydrate metabolism. *Diabetes* 1990; **39** (suppl 1): 298.
6. Baum HBA, *et al.* Effects of physiologic growth hormone therapy on bone density and body composition in patients with adult-onset growth hormone deficiency: a randomized, placebo-controlled trial. *Ann Intern Med* 1996; **125:** 883–90.
7. Cuneo RC, *et al.* The Australian multicenter trial of growth hormone (GH) treatment in GH-deficient adults. *J Clin Endocrinol Metab* 1998; **83:** 107–116.
8. Vance ML, Mauras N. Growth hormone therapy in adults and children. *N Engl J Med* 1999; **341:** 1206–16.
9. Baum HBA, *et al.* Effects of physiological growth hormone (GH) therapy on cognition and quality of life in patients with adult-onset GH deficiency. *J Clin Endocrinol Metab* 1998; **83:** 3184–9.
10. Rudman D, *et al.* Effects of human growth hormone in men over 60 years old. *N Engl J Med* 1990; **323:** 1–6.
11. Marcus R, *et al.* Effects of short term administration of recombinant human growth hormone to elderly people. *J Clin Endocrinol Metab* 1990; **70:** 519–27.
12. Yarasheski KE, Zachwieja JJ. Growth hormone therapy for the elderly: the fountain of youth proves toxic. *JAMA* 1993; **270:** 1694.
13. Papadakis MA, *et al.* Growth hormone replacement in healthy older men improves body composition but not functional ability. *Ann Intern Med* 1996; **124:** 708–16.

Burns. In children with severe burns requiring skin grafts, somatropin 200 µg per kg body-weight daily by intramuscular injection reduced donor-site healing times and hospitalisation times; subcutaneous somatropin 100 µg per kg daily was ineffective.[1] Treatment also subsequently ameliorates burn-induced growth delays in such children.[2] However, the manufacturers have recommended that somatropin should not be used to treat acute catabolic states in critically ill and burn patients, as there is some evidence in adults that mortality may be increased.[3] The management of burns is described on p.1104.

1. Herndon DN, *et al.* Effects of recombinant human growth hormone on donor-site healing in severely burned children. *Ann Surg* 1990; **212:** 424–9.
2. Low JFA, *et al.* Effect of growth hormone on growth delay in burned children: a 3-year follow-up study. *Lancet* 1999; **354:** 1789.
3. Takala J, *et al.* Increased mortality associated with growth hormone treatment in critically ill adults. *N Engl J Med* 1999; **341:** 785–92.

Cachexia. Treatment with subcutaneous growth hormone has been reported[1-3] to reverse weight loss and improve body wasting in subjects with HIV disease (p.610). Dosage may be important: most studies have used doses of around 100 µg per kg body-weight, but a study using lower doses, alone or combined with mecasermin, reported only modest improvement.[4] Mecasermin alone was of uncertain value.

Growth hormone therapy has also been reported to improve metabolic indicators of malnutrition when given together with parenteral nutrition to patients undergoing haemodialysis.[5]

1. Krentz AJ, *et al.* Anthropometric, metabolic, and immunological effects of recombinant human growth hormone in AIDS and AIDS-related complex. *J Acquir Immune Defic Syndr* 1993; **6:** 245–51.
2. Mulligan K, *et al.* Anabolic effects of recombinant human growth hormone in patients with wasting associated with human immunodeficiency virus infection. *J Clin Endocrinol Metab* 1993; **77:** 956–62.
3. Schambelan M, *et al.* Recombinant human growth hormone in patients with HIV-associated wasting: a randomized, placebo-controlled trial. *Ann Intern Med* 1996; **125:** 873–82.
4. Waters D, *et al.* Recombinant human growth hormone, insulin-like growth factor 1, and combination therapy in AIDS-associated wasting: a randomized, double-blind, placebo-controlled trial. *Ann Intern Med* 1996; **125:** 865–72.
5. Schulman G, *et al.* The effects of recombinant human growth hormone and intradialytic parenteral nutrition in malnourished haemodialysis patients. *Am J Kidney Dis* 1993; **21:** 527–34.

Cardiomyopathies. Administration of growth hormone for 12 weeks to patients with heart failure secondary to dilated cardiomyopathy (p.796) produced an increase in left-ventricular mass but no improvement in clinical status.[1]

1. Osterziel KJ, *et al.* Randomised, double-blind, placebo-controlled trial of human recombinant growth hormone in patients with chronic heart failure due to dilated cardiomyopathy. *Lancet* 1998; **351:** 1233–7.

Fibromyalgia. Symptomatic improvement was reported after several months in a study of daily subcutaneous growth hormone injection in women with fibromyalgia,[1] a painful form of soft-tissue rheumatism (p.10), and low levels of insulin-like growth factor I (IGF-I).

1. Bennett RM, *et al.* A randomized, double-blind, placebo-controlled study of growth hormone in the treatment of fibromyalgia. *Am J Med* 1998; **104:** 227–31.

Growth retardation. For a discussion of the management of growth retardation, including the role of growth hormone, see p.1273. Where growth retardation is associated with growth hormone deficiency, replacement therapy is an appropriate treatment,[1] and significantly improves growth velocity, although there are some doubts about the extent of the benefit in terms of final height. The use of growth hormone in children with short stature but without clinical growth hormone deficiency is, however, controversial and of unproven efficacy. Guidelines[2] issued in the USA in 1995 considered the use of growth hormone unproven other than in growth hormone deficiency and probably Turner's syndrome (but see p.1276) and chronic renal insufficiency.

1. GH Research Society. Consensus guidelines for the diagnosis and treatment of growth hormone (GH) deficiency in childhood and adolescence: summary statement of the GH Research Society. *J Clin Endocrinol Metab* 2000; **85:** 3990–3.
2. Drug and Therapeutics Committee, Lawson Wilkins Pediatric Endocrine Society. Guidelines for the use of growth hormone in children with short stature. *J Pediatr* 1995; **127:** 857–67.

Infertility. Studies[1,2] have found that somatropin sensitises the ovary to stimulation by gonadotrophins and it has been suggested that it may have a role in the management of female infertility in patients resistant to conventional ovarian stimulation, although not in those with no previous history of poor stimulation.[3] However, some workers have found it of little value.[4] Growth hormone has also been tried similarly to enhance spermatogenesis in infertile men unresponsive to conventional therapy.[5,6]

For a discussion of infertility and the more usual drugs used in its management, see p.1275.

1. Homburg R, *et al.* Cotreatment with human growth hormone and gonadotrophins for induction of ovulation: a controlled clinical trial. *Fertil Steril* 1990; **53:** 254–60.
2. Yoshimura Y, *et al.* Effects of growth hormone on follicle growth, oocyte maturation, and ovarian steroidogenesis. *Fertil Steril* 1993; **59:** 917–23.
3. Kotarba D, *et al.* Growth hormone for in vitro fertilization (updated 28 May 2001). Available in The Cochrane Library; Issue 3. Oxford: Update Software; 2001.
4. Levron J, *et al.* No beneficial effects of human growth hormone therapy in normal ovulatory patients with a poor ovarian response to gonadotropins. *Gynecol Obstet Invest* 1993; **35:** 65–8.
5. Shoham Z, *et al.* Cotreatment with growth hormone for induction of spermatogenesis in patients with hypogonadotrophic hypogonadism. *Fertil Steril* 1992; **57:** 1044–51.
6. Ovesen PG. *et al.* Vaeksthormonbehandling af maend med nedsat saedkvalitet. *Ugeskr Laeger* 1990; **160:** 176–80.

Osteogenesis imperfecta. For reference to possible benefit from growth hormone therapy in patients with osteogenesis imperfecta, see p.744.

Osteomalacia. As mentioned on p.744, there has been some interest in the use of growth hormone in children with hypophosphataemic rickets.

Prader-Willi Syndrome. Growth hormone treatment may be of benefit in the management of Prader-Willi syndrome (p.1506).
References.

1. Lindgren AC, *et al.* Five years of growth hormone treatment in children with Prader-Willi syndrome. *Acta Paediatr Suppl* 1999; **433:** 109–11.
2. Myers SE, *et al.* Physical effects of growth hormone treatment in children with Prader-Willi syndrome. *Acta Paediatr Suppl* 1999; **433:** 112–14.
3. Carrel AL, *et al.* Growth hormone improves body composition, fat utilization, physical strength and agility, and growth in Prader-Willi syndrome: a controlled study. *J Pediatr* 1999; **134:** 215–21.
4. Myers SE, *et al.* Sustained benefit after 2 years of growth hormone on body composition, fat utilization, physical strength and agility, and growth in Prader-Willi syndrome. *J Pediatr* 2000; **137:** 42–9.

Veterinary and agricultural use. Bovine growth hormone or bovine somatotrophin (bovine somatotropin; BST) can increase milk yield. Some references to the debate on the safety of this practice follow.

1. Anonymous. Bovine somatotropin and human health. *Lancet* 1988; **ii:** 376.
2. Davis C. Safety of bovine somatotropin. *Lancet* 1988; **ii:** 629.
3. Brunner E. Safety of bovine somatotropin. *Lancet* 1988; **ii:** 629.
4. Daughaday WH, Barbano DM. Bovine somatotropin supplementation of dairy cows: is the milk safe? *JAMA* 1990; **264:** 1003–5. Correction. *ibid.* 1991; **265:** 1393.
5. Mepham TB. Bovine somatotrophin and public health. *BMJ* 1991; **302:** 483–4.
6. Kronfeld DS. Bovine somatotropin. *JAMA* 1991; **265:** 1389.
7. Daughaday WH, Barbano DM. Bovine somatotropin. *JAMA* 1991; **265:** 1389–90.
8. Morris K. Bovine somatotrophin—who's crying over spilt milk? *Lancet* 1999; **353:** 306.

Preparations

BP 2001: Somatropin Injection.

Proprietary Preparations (details are given in Part 3)
Aust.: Genotropin; Humatrope; Norditropin; Saizen; **Austral.:** Genotropin; Humatro-Pen; Humatrope; Norditropin; Saizen; **Belg.:** Genotonorm; Humatrope; Norditropin; Zomacton; **Braz.:** Genotropin; Humatrope; Norditropin; Saizen; **Canad.:** Humatrope; Nutropin; Protropin; Saizen; Serostim; **Denm.:** Genotropin; Humatrope; Norditropin; Zomacton; **Fin.:** Genotropin; Humatrope; Norditropin; Saizen; Zomacton; **Fr.:** Genotonorm; Maxomat; Norditropine; Saizen; Umatrope; Zomacton; **Ger.:** Genotropin; Humatrope; Norditropin; Saizen; Zomacton; **Hong Kong:** Genotropin; Humatrope; Norditropin; Saizen; Zomacton; **Irl.:** Genotropin; Humatrope; Norditropin; Saizen; Zomacton; **Israel:** Bio-Tropin; Genotropin; Humatrope; Norditropin; Saizen; Zomacton; **Ital.:** Genotropin; Humatrope; Norditropin; Saizen; Zomacton; **Mex.:** Bio-Tropin; Cryo-Tropin; Genotropin; Humatrope; Norditropin; Saizen; **Neth.:** Genotropin; Humatrope; Norditropin; Zomacton; **Norw.:** Genotropin; Humatrope; Norditropin; Saizen; **NZ:** Genotropin; Humatrope; Saizen; **Port.:** Genotropin; Humatrope; Norditropin; Saizen; Zomacton; **S.Afr.:** Genotropin; Humatrope; Norditropin; Saizen; **Singapore:** Genotropin; Humatrope; Norditropin; Saizen; Scitropin; Serostim; **Spain:** Genotonorm; Humatrope; Norditropin; Saizen; Zomacton; **Swed.:** Genotropin; Humatrope; Norditropin; Saizen;

Zomacton; *Switz.:* Genotropin; Humatrope; Norditropine; Saizen; *UK:* Genotropin; Humatrope; Norditropin; Saizen; Zomacton; *USA:* Genotropin; Humatrope; Norditropin; Nutropin; Protropin; Saizen; Serostim.

Histrelin Acetate (15849-b)

Histrelin Acetate (rlNNM).

ORF-17070 (histrelin); RWJ-17070 (histrelin). 5-Oxo-L-prolyl-L-histidyl-L-tryptophyl-L-seryl-L-tyrosyl-N^τ-benzyl-D-histidyl-L-luecyl-L-arginyl-N-ethyl-L-prolinamide acetate.

CAS — 76712-82-8 (histrelin).

Adverse Effects and Precautions
As for Gonadorelin, p.1284.

Uses and Administration
Histrelin is an analogue of gonadorelin (p.1284) with similar properties. It is used for the suppression of gonadal sex hormone production in children with central precocious puberty (p.1277). It is given by subcutaneous injection as the acetate, in usual doses equivalent to 10 μg of histrelin per kg body-weight daily.

It has been investigated in various other disorders, including malignant neoplasms of the prostate (p.497) and disorders related to the menstrual cycle. It is also under investigation in the treatment of acute intermittent porphyria.

◊ References.

1. Anderson KE, *et al.* A gonadotropin releasing hormone analogue prevents cyclical attacks of porphyria. *Arch Intern Med* 1990; **150:** 1469–74.
2. Mortola JF, *et al.* Successful treatment of severe premenstrual syndrome by combined use of gonadotropin-releasing hormone agonist and estrogen/progestin. *J Clin Endocrinol Metab* 1991; **72:** 252A–F.
3. Barradell LB, McTavish D. Histrelin: a review of its pharmacological properties and therapeutic role in central precocious puberty. *Drugs* 1993; **45:** 570–88.
4. Cheung AP, Chang RJ. Pituitary responsiveness to gonadotrophin-releasing hormone agonist stimulation: a dose-response comparison of luteinizing hormone/follicle-stimulating hormone secretion in women with polycystic ovary syndrome and normal women. *Hum Reprod* 1995; **10:** 1054–9.
5. Feuillan PP, *et al.* Reproductive axis after discontinuation of gonadotropin-releasing hormone analog treatment of girls with precocious puberty: long term follow-up comparing girls with hypothalamic hamartoma to those with idiopathic precocious puberty. *J Clin Endocrinol Metab* 1999; **84:** 44–9.
6. Chertin B, *et al.* An implant releasing the gonadotropin hormone-releasing hormone agonist histrelin maintains medical castration for up to 30 months in metastatic prostate cancer. *J Urol (Baltimore)* 2000; **163:** 838–44.

Preparations

Proprietary Preparations (details are given in Part 3)
USA: Supprelin.

Human Menopausal Gonadotrophins (17585-l)

Human Menopausal Gonadotrophins (BAN).
HMG; Org-31338; Urogonadotrophin.

A purified extract of human postmenopausal urine containing follicle-stimulating hormone (FSH) and luteinising hormone (LH); the relative *in-vivo* activity is expressed as a ratio. Human menopausal gonadotrophins with a ratio of FSH:LH of 1:1 are known as menotrophin (see below).

Menotrophin (5930-b)

Menotrophin (BAN).
Menotropins (USAN); Menotropinum.
CAS — 9002-68-0.
Pharmacopoeias. In Aust., Belg., Br., It., Neth., Port., and US.

Pharmacopoeial description
BP 2001: A dry preparation containing glycoprotein gonadotrophins possessing follicle-stimulating and luteinising activities. It contains not less than 40 units of follicle-stimulating hormone activity per mg. The ratio of units of luteinising hormone activity to units of follicle-stimulating hormone activity is approximately 1. The preparation is exclusively or predominantly of pituitary origin and obtained from the urine of post-menopausal women but, when necessary, chorionic gonadotrophin obtained from the urine of pregnant women may be added to achieve the above ratio. An almost white or slightly yellow powder. Soluble in water. Store in airtight containers. Protect from light.

USP 25: An extract of human postmenopausal urine containing both follicle-stimulating hormone and luteinising hormone. It has a potency of not less than 40 USP follicle-stimulating hormone units and not less than 40 USP luteinising hormone units per mg. The ratio of units is approximately 1. Chorionic Gonadotropin obtained from the urine of pregnant women may be

added to achieve this ratio. Not more than 30% of the luteinising hormone activity is contributed by Chorionic Gonadotropin. Store in airtight containers at 2° to 8°.

Units
54 units of follicle-stimulating hormone and 46 units of luteinising hormone are contained in one ampoule of the third International Standard (1993).

Adverse Effects
Human menopausal gonadotrophins may cause dose-related ovarian hyperstimulation varying from mild ovarian enlargement and abdominal discomfort to severe hyperstimulation with marked ovarian enlargement or cyst formation, acute abdominal pain, ascites, pleural effusion, hypovolaemia, shock and thromboembolic disorders. Rupture of ovarian cysts and intraperitoneal haemorrhage has occurred, usually after pelvic examination. Fatalities have been reported.

Hypersensitivity reactions and local reactions at the injection site may occur. Nausea and vomiting, joint pains and fever have been reported; gynaecomastia, acne, and weight gain have occurred in men.

◊ Ovarian hyperstimulation syndrome occurring with human menopausal gonadotrophins treatment in 4 women progressed to acute adnexal torsion[1] and in another became severe and was accompanied by deep-vein thrombosis.[2]

1. Kemmann E, *et al.* Adnexal torsion in menotropin-induced pregnancies. *Obstet Gynecol* 1990; **76:** 403–6.
2. Kaaja R, *et al.* Severe ovarian hyperstimulation syndrome and deep venous thrombosis. *Lancet* 1989; **ii:** 1043.

Precautions
Human menopausal gonadotrophins should not be given to pregnant patients. Use should be avoided in patients with abnormal genital bleeding, hormone sensitive malignancies such as those of the breast, uterus, prostate, ovaries or testes, or ovarian cysts or enlargement not caused by the polycystic ovary syndrome. Pituitary or hypothalamic lesions, adrenal or thyroid disorders, and hyperprolactinaemia should be treated appropriately to exclude them as causes of infertility before attempting therapy with human menopausal gonadotrophins. Patients who experience ovarian enlargement are at risk of rupture; pelvic examinations should be avoided or carried out with care and the recommendation has been made that sexual intercourse should be avoided while there is such a risk.

There is a risk of multiple births.

Interactions
In women who show evidence of excessive ovarian stimulation while receiving human menopausal gonadotrophins the administration of drugs with luteinising-hormone (LH) activity increases the risk of ovarian hyperstimulation syndrome.

Uses and Administration
Human menopausal gonadotrophins possess both follicle-stimulating hormone (FSH) activity (see p.1283) and luteinising hormone (LH) activity (see p.1290).

Human menopausal gonadotrophins are used in the treatment of male and female infertility due to hypogonadism. In anovulatory infertility unresponsive to clomifene, human menopausal gonadotrophins are administered to induce follicular maturation and are followed by treatment with chorionic gonadotrophin to stimulate ovulation and corpus luteum formation, a topic discussed further on p.1275. In women with polycystic ovary syndrome a gonadorelin analogue may be given beforehand to suppress pituitary gonadotrophin production (see p.1276).

The dosage and schedule of treatment for female infertility must be determined according to the needs of each patient; it is usual to monitor response by studying the patient's urinary oestrogen excretion or by ultrasonic visualisation of follicles, or both. Human menopausal gonadotrophins may be given daily by intramuscular or subcutaneous injection to provide a dose of 75 to 150 units of FSH and gradually adjusted if necessary until an adequate response is achieved.

Treatment is then stopped and followed after 1 or 2 days by single doses of chorionic gonadotrophin 5000 to 10 000 units (see p.1279). In menstruating patients treatment should be started within the first 7 days of the menstrual cycle. In the UK it has been suggested that the treatment course should be abandoned if no response is seen in 3 weeks although in the US the manufacturers recommend that an individual course should not exceed 12 days. This course may be repeated at least twice more if necessary.

An alternative schedule is to give three equal doses by intramuscular or subcutaneous injection, each providing 225 to 375 units of FSH on alternate days followed by chorionic gonadotrophin one week after the first dose.

In *in-vitro* fertilisation procedures or other assisted conception techniques human menopausal gonadotrophins are used in conjunction with chorionic gonadotrophin and sometimes also clomifene citrate or a gonadorelin analogue. Stimulation of follicular growth is produced by human menopausal gonadotrophins given by intramuscular or subcutaneous injection, in a dose providing 75 to 300 units of FSH daily, usually beginning on the 2nd or 3rd day of the menstrual cycle. An example of a combined regimen involves clomifene citrate 100 mg on days 2 to 6, with human menopausal gonadotrophins beginning on day 5 in a dose providing 150 to 225 units of FSH daily. Treatment is continued until an adequate response is obtained and the final injection of human menopausal gonadotrophins is followed 1 to 2 days later with up to 10 000 units of chorionic gonadotrophin. Oocyte retrieval is carried out about 32 to 36 hours later.

In men with infertility due to hypogonadotrophic hypogonadism (see Infertility, p.1274), spermatogenesis is stimulated with chorionic gonadotrophin and then human menopausal gonadotrophins are added in a dose of 75 or 150 units of FSH two or three times weekly by intramuscular or subcutaneous injection. Treatment should be continued for at least 3 or 4 months.

Infertility. Anecdotal reports suggest that human menopausal gonadotrophins may be more effective than urofollitropin in treating anovulatory infertility,[1] perhaps because the luteinising hormone content plays some role in follicular development. A meta-analysis has also found that urinary derived gonadotrophins had no advantage over traditional human menopausal gonadotrophin preparations.[2] However, in contrast, others have found the use of a pure recombinant follicle-stimulating hormone to be associated with higher pregnancy rates than human menopausal gonadotrophins when employed in regimens for *in-vitro* fertilisation.[3,4]

For a discussion of infertility and its management, including the role of human menopausal gonadotrophins, see p.1275.

1. Vine S, *et al.* Human gonadotrophin preparations. *BMJ* 1994; **308:** 1509–10.
2. Nugent D, *et al.* Gonadotrophin therapy for ovulation induction in subfertility associated with polycystic ovary syndrome (updated 28 May 2001). Available in The Cochrane Library, Issue 3. Oxford: Update Software; 2001.
3. Out HJ, *et al.* Recombinant follicle-stimulating hormone (follitropin beta, Puregon) yields higher pregnancy rates in in vitro fertilization than urinary gonadotropins. *Fertil Steril* 1997; **68:** 138–42.
4. Daya S. Follicle-stimulating hormone and human menopausal gonadotropin for ovarian stimulation in assisted reproduction cycles (updated 28 May 2001). Available in The Cochrane Library; Issue 3. Oxford: Update Software; 2001.

Preparations

BP 2001: Menotrophin Injection;
USP 25: Menotropins for Injection.

Proprietary Preparations (details are given in Part 3)
Aust.: Humegon; Pergonal†; *Austral.:* Humegon; *Belg.:* Humegon; Menogon; *Braz.:* Humegon; Pergonal; *Canad.:* Humegon; Pergonal; *Denm.:* Menogon; *Fin.:* Menogon; *Fr.:* Humegon†; Menogon; Neo-Pergonal†; *Ger.:* Humegon; Menogon; Pergonal; *Hong Kong:* Humegon; Menogon; Pergonal; *Irl.:* Humegon; Menogon; Pergonal; *Israel:* Humegon; Menogon; Pergonal; *Ital.:* Humegon; Menogon; Pergogreen†; *Mex.:* HMG Massone; Humegon; *Neth.:* Humegon†; Menogon; Pergonal†; *Norw.:* Humegon†; Pergonal†; *Port.:* Humegon†; *S.Afr.:* Humegon; Pergonal; *Singapore:* Humegon; Menogon; Pergonal; *Spain:* HMG; Menogon; Pergonal; *Swed.:* Humegon†; Pergogreen†; Pergonal†; *Switz.:* Humegon; Merional; Pergogreen; Pergonal; *Thai.:* Humegon; Pergonal; *UK:* Humegon†; Menogon; Menopur; Normegon†; Pergonal†; *USA:* Humegon; Pergonal; Repronex.

Lanreotide Acetate (17187-r)

Lanreotide Acetate *(BANM, USAN, rINNM)*.
BIM-23014C. 3-(2-Naphthyl)-D-alanyl-L-cysteinyl-L-tyrosyl-D-tryptophyl-L-lysyl-L-valyl-L-cysteinyl-L-threoninamide cyclic (2→7)-disulfide acetate.
$C_{54}H_{69}N_{11}O_{10}S_2,x(C_2H_4O_2)$.
CAS — 108736-35-2 (lanreotide); 127984-74-1 (lanreotide acetate).

Adverse Effects and Precautions
As for Octreotide Acetate, p.1291.

Interactions
As for Octreotide Acetate, p.1291.

Pharmacokinetics
Following intramuscular administration of sustained-release lanreotide an initial rapid liberation of the drug is followed by more prolonged release with an apparent half-life of about 5 days. The absolute bioavailability is stated to be about 50%.

Uses and Administration
Lanreotide is a somatostatin analogue with similar properties to those of octreotide (p.1292). It is given, as a long-acting intramuscular depot injection, in the treatment of acromegaly (see p.1271), as well as in the management of carcinoid syndrome (p.483).

Lanreotide is given as the acetate. The usual dose, in both acromegaly and the carcinoid syndrome, is the equivalent of 30 mg of lanreotide by intramuscular depot injection every 14 days, increased if necessary to 30 mg every 7 to 10 days.

Lanreotide has been tried for the prevention of restenosis in coronary blood vessels following angioplasty (see Reperfusion and Revascularisation Procedures, p.812).

◊ References.
1. Heron I, *et al.* Pharmacokinetics and efficacy of a long-acting formulation of the new somatostatin analog BIM 23014 in patients with acromegaly. *J Clin Endocrinol Metab* 1993; **76:** 721–7.
2. Boucekkine C, *et al.* Traitement de l'acromégalie par un nouvel analogue de la somatostatine, le lanréotide à action prolongée. *Ann Endocrinol (Paris)* 1994; **55:** 261–9.
3. Emanuelsson H, *et al.* Long-term effects of angiopeptin treatment in coronary angioplasty: reduction in clinical events but not angiographic restenosis. *Circulation* 1995; **91:** 1689–96.
4. Eriksson B, *et al.* The use of new somatostatin analogues, lanreotide and octastatin, in neuroendocrine gastro-intestinal tumours. *Digestion* 1996; **57** (suppl 1): 77–80.
5. Caron P, *et al.* Three year follow-up of acromegalic patients treated with intramuscular slow-release lanreotide. *J Clin Endocrinol Metab* 1997; **82:** 18–22.
6. Wymenga ANM, *et al.* Efficacy and safety of prolonged-release lanreotide in patients with gastrointestinal neuroendocrine tumors and hormone-related symptoms. *J Clin Oncol* 1999; **17:** 1111–17.
7. Baldelli R, *et al.* Two-year follow-up of acromegalic patients treated with slow release lanreotide (30 mg). *J Clin Endocrinol Metab* 2000; **85:** 4099–4103.

Preparations

Proprietary Preparations (details are given in Part 3)
Aust.: Somatuline; *Belg.:* Somatuline; *Fin.:* Somatuline; *Fr.:* Somatuline; *Hong Kong:* Somatuline; *Irl.:* Somatuline; *Ital.:* Ipstyl; *Norw.:* Ipstyl; *Port.:* Somatulina; *Spain:* Somatulina; *UK:* Somatuline.

Leuprorelin Acetate (12895-s)

Leuprorelin Acetate *(BANM, rINNM)*.
Abbott-43818; Leuprolide Acetate *(USAN)*; TAP-144. 5-Oxo-L-prolyl-L-histidyl-L-tryptophyl-L-seryl-L-tyrosyl-D-leucyl-L-leucyl-L-arginyl-*N*-ethyl-L-prolinamide acetate.
$C_{59}H_{84}N_{16}O_{12},C_2H_4O_2 = 1269.5$.
CAS — 53714-56-0 (leuprorelin); 74381-53-6 (leuprorelin acetate).
Pharmacopoeias. Eur. (see p.vi) includes a monograph for Leuprorelin.

Pharmacopoeial description

Ph. Eur.: Leuprorelin (Leuprorelinum) is a synthetic nonapeptide analogue of the hypothalamic peptide gonadorelin. It is obtained by chemical synthesis and is available as an acetate. A white or almost white, hygroscopic, powder. Store in airtight containers at a temperature not exceeding 30°. Protect from light.

Adverse Effects and Precautions

As for Gonadorelin, p.1284. Thrombocytopenia and leucopenia have been reported rarely.

Benign intracranial hypertension. A report of increased intracranial pressure associated with leuprorelin treatment in one patient.[1]
1. Arber N, *et al.* Pseudotumor cerebri associated with leuprorelin acetate. *Lancet* 1990; **335:** 668.

Effects on the eyes. Leuprorelin may be associated with blurred vision, usually lasting 1 to 2 hours after injection, but in rare instances longer.[1] Haemorrhage or occlusion of intra-

ocular blood vessels, ocular pain, and lid oedema have also been reported but the association is less well established.
1. Fraunfelder FT, Edwards R. Possible ocular adverse effects associated with leuprolide injections. *JAMA* 1995; **273:** 773–4.

Hypersensitivity. A report of recurrent anaphylaxis in a patient given a depot injection of leuprorelin acetate, requiring both acute and chronic management.[1]
1. Letterie GS, *et al.* Recurrent anaphylaxis to a depot form of GnRH analogue. *Obstet Gynecol* 1991; **78:** 943–6.

Local reactions. Local reactions, including erythema, pain, induration, and sterile abscess are particularly associated with depot injections of gonadorelin analogues such as leuprorelin and triptorelin;[1-4] they may also occur with subcutaneous daily injection.[1] It has been suggested that the depot vehicle, a lactic acid-glycolic acid copolymer, may be responsible for many, although not all, such reactions.[1-4] Reactions are claimed to be more prevalent in children than in adults;[4] an incidence of about 5% of patients has been suggested. Reactions are apparently idiosyncratic, and may occur at any time during therapy, may be intermittent, or may never recur.[4]
1. Manasco PK, *et al.* Local reactions to depot leuprolide therapy for central precocious puberty. *J Pediatr* 1993; **123:** 334–5.
2. Neely EK, *et al.* Local reactions to depot leuprolide therapy for central precocious puberty. *J Pediatr* 1993; **123:** 335.
3. Tonini G, *et al.* Local reactions to luteinizing hormone releasing hormone analog therapy. *J Pediatr* 1995; **126:** 159.
4. Neely EK, *et al.* Local reactions to luteinizing hormone releasing hormone analog therapy. *J Pediatr* 1995; **126:** 159–60.

Interactions
As for Gonadorelin, p.1284.

Pharmacokinetics

Leuprorelin acetate is not active when given orally but is well absorbed following subcutaneous or intramuscular injection. Following parenteral administration it has an elimination half-life of about 3 hours.

◊ References.
1. Sennello LT, *et al.* Single-dose pharmacokinetics of leuprolide in humans following intravenous and subcutaneous administration. *J Pharm Sci* 1986; **75:** 158–60.

Uses and Administration

Leuprorelin acetate is an analogue of gonadorelin (see p.1284) with similar properties. Continuous administration is used for the suppression of gonadal sex hormone production in the treatment of malignant neoplasms of the prostate, in central precocious puberty, and in the management of endometriosis and uterine fibroids. It is also given before uterine surgery for endometrial reduction, and may be used in the treatment of breast cancer in premenopausal women.

In the management of advanced prostate cancer, leuprorelin acetate may be given by subcutaneous injection in a usual single daily dose of 1 mg. It is also given subcutaneously or intramuscularly as depot preparations but the dosage and route of administration of these may differ between countries. In the UK, 3.75 mg may be given once a month, by subcutaneous or intramuscular injection, or 11.25 mg may be given subcutaneously every 3 months. In the USA, however, the dose administered is 7.5 mg monthly, 22.5 mg every 3 months, or 30 mg every 4 months, and the preparation is given intramuscularly. A nonbiodegradable titanium alloy implant is also available, which is inserted subcutaneously into the inner part of the upper arm. It contains 72 mg of leuprorelin acetate and delivers the drug at a controlled rate of 120 µg daily. After 12 months it must be removed, but can be replaced by another implant to continue therapy. An anti-androgen such as cyproterone acetate may be given for several days before beginning leuprorelin therapy and continued for about 3 weeks, to avoid the risk of a disease flare.

For the management of endometriosis and uterine fibroids, leuprorelin acetate 3.75 mg monthly may be given as a single depot injection, intramuscularly or subcutaneously. Alternatively, 11.25 mg may be given as an intramuscular depot every 3 months. Treatment is initiated during the first 5 days of the menstrual cycle, and may be continued for up to 6 months for endometriosis, while in women with anaemia due to uterine fibroids it is continued, with concomitant iron supplementation, usually for up to 3 months. As preparation for uterine surgery a single 3.75 mg depot injection may be given 5 to 6 weeks before the procedure.

In the management of central precocious puberty leuprorelin acetate has been given by intramuscular depot injection in a dose of 0.3 mg per kg body-weight every 4 weeks, adjusted according to response. Doses of 50 µg per kg daily by subcutaneous injection, adjusted according to response, have also been used.

Leuprorelin acetate has also been given in other sex-hormone-related disorders and has been tried in some gastrointestinal disorders such as irritable bowel syndrome (p.1206).

◊ General references.
1. Plosker GL, Brogden RN. Leuprorelin: a review of its pharmacology and therapeutic use in prostatic cancer, endometriosis and other sex hormone-related disorders. *Drugs* 1994; **48:** 930–67.

Benign prostatic hyperplasia. For a discussion of the management of benign prostatic hyperplasia, including mention of the use of gonadorelin analogues and the view that they are unsatisfactory for indefinite therapy, see p.1477.

References to the use of leuprorelin.
1. Gabrilove JL, *et al.* Effect of long-acting gonadotropin-releasing hormone analog (leuprolide) therapy on prostatic size and symptoms in 15 men with benign prostatic hypertrophy. *J Clin Endocrinol Metab* 1989; **69:** 629–32.
2. Eri LM, Tveter KJ. A prospective, placebo-controlled study of the luteinising hormone-releasing hormone agonist leuprolide as treatment for patients with benign prostatic hyperplasia. *J Urol (Baltimore)* 1993; **150:** 359–64.
3. Eri LM, Tveter KJ. Safety, side effects and patient acceptance of the luteinising hormone releasing hormone agonist leuprolide in treatment of benign prostatic hyperplasia. *J Urol (Baltimore)* 1994; **152:** 448–52.
4. Eri LM, *et al.* Effects on the endocrine system of long-term treatment with the luteinizing hormone-releasing hormone agonist leuprolide in patients with benign prostatic hyperplasia. *Scand J Clin Lab Invest* 1996; **56:** 319–25.

Endometriosis. Gonadorelin analogues are effective in the management of endometriosis (p.1469) but the need for long-term therapy to prevent recurrence limits their value because of the risk of osteoporosis; 'add-back' therapy, with concomitant hormone replacement, is being investigated.

References to the use of leuprorelin.
1. Hornstein MD, *et al.* Leuprolide acetate depot and hormonal add-back in endometriosis: a 12-month study. *Obstet Gynecol* 1998; **91:** 16–24.
2. Ling FW. Randomized controlled trial of depot leuprolide in patients with chronic pelvic pain and clinically suspected endometriosis. *Obstet Gynecol* 1999; **93:** 51–8.
3. Takeuchi H, *et al.* A prospective randomized study comparing endocrinological and clinical effects of two types of GnRH agonists in cases of uterine leiomyomata and endometriosis. *J Obstet Gynaecol Res* 2000; **26:** 325–31.

Fibroids. Gonadorelin analogues may be of some benefit as an adjunct or alternative to surgery in women with uterine fibroids—see p.1285, although there has been some concern that this might complicate the diagnosis of malignancy.

References to the use of leuprorelin.
1. Friedman AJ. Treatment of leiomyomata with intranasal or subcutaneous leuprolide, a gonadotropin-releasing hormone agonist. *Fertil Steril* 1987; **48:** 560–4.
2. Friedman AJ, *et al.* Treatment of leiomyomata uteri with leuprolide acetate depot: a double-blind, placebo-controlled, multicenter study. *Obstet Gynecol* 1991; **77:** 720–5.
3. Friedman AJ, *et al.* Long-term medical therapy for leiomyomata uteri: a prospective, randomized study of leuprolide acetate depot plus either oestrogen-progestin or progestin 'add-back' for 2 years. *Hum Reprod* 1994; **9:** 1618–25.
4. Zullo F, *et al.* A prospective randomized study to evaluate leuprolide acetate treatment before laparoscopic myomectomy: efficacy and ultrasonographic predictors. *Am J Obstet Gynecol* 1998; **178:** 108–112.
5. Scialli AR, Levi AJ. Intermittent leuprolide acetate for the nonsurgical management of women with leiomyomata uteri. *Fertil Steril* 2000; **74:** 540–6.

Hirsutism. The mainstay of drug treatment for hirsutism (p.1468) has been an anti-androgen, usually cyproterone acetate or spironolactone. Although gonadorelin analogues have been used, and are effective, they must be given parenterally or nasally and may produce menopausal effects, notably osteoporosis.

References to the use of leuprorelin.
1. Rittmaster RS, Thompson DL. Effect of leuprolide and dexamethasone on hair growth and hormone levels in hirsute women: the relative importance of the ovary and the adrenal in the pathogenesis of hirsutism. *J Clin Endocrinol Metab* 1990; **70:** 1096–1102.
2. Elkind-Hirsch KE, *et al.* Combination gonadotropin-releasing hormone agonist and oral contraceptive therapy improves treatment of hirsute women with ovarian hyperandrogenism. *Fertil Steril* 1995; **63:** 970–8.

Infertility. Gonadorelin analogues are used in the treatment of infertility—see p.1275. References to the use of leuprorelin.
1. Stone BA, *et al.* Gonadotrophin and estradiol levels during ovarian stimulation in women treated with leuprolide acetate. *Obstet Gynecol* 1989; **73:** 990–5.
2. Sathanandan M, *et al.* Adjuvant leuprolide in normal, abnormal, and poor responders to controlled ovarian hyperstimulation for in vitro fertilization/gamete intrafallopian transfer. *Fertil Steril* 1989; **51:** 998–1006.
3. Filicori M, *et al.* Different gonadotropin and leuprorelin ovulation induction regimens markedly affect follicular fluid hormone levels and folliculogenesis. *Fertil Steril* 1996; **65:** 387–93.

Malignant neoplasms. Gonadorelin analogues are used as an alternative to orchidectomy in the management of advanced malignant neoplasms of the prostate (p.497). Such therapy is as effective as orchidectomy in prolonging survival;[1] combination of leuprorelin or other gonadorelin analogues with nonsteroidal anti-androgens to produce maximal androgen blockade produces only modest additional benefit.[2] Leuprorelin also suppresses oestrogen concentrations to values within the postmenopausal range[3] in premenopausal women with breast cancer (p.491).

There are also reports of endometrial cancer (p.493),[4] and ovarian cancer (p.496)[5] responding to leuprorelin, but the role of the gonadorelin analogues in these conditions is much less well established.
1. Seidenfeld J, *et al.* Single-therapy androgen suppression in men with advanced prostate cancer: a systematic review and meta-analysis. *Ann Intern Med* 2000; **132:** 566–77.
2. Prostate Cancer Trialists' Collaborative Group. Maximum androgen blockade in advanced prostate cancer: an overview of the randomised trials. *Lancet* 2000; **355:** 1491–8.
3. Dowsett M, *et al.* A dose-comparative endocrine-clinical study of leuprorelin in premenopausal breast cancer patients. *Br J Cancer* 1990; **62:** 834–7.
4. Gallagher CJ, *et al.* A new treatment for endometrial cancer with gonadotrophin releasing-hormone analogue. *Br J Obstet Gynaecol* 1991; **98:** 1037–41.
5. Bruckner HW, Motwani BT. Treatment of advanced refractory ovarian carcinoma with a gonadotropin-releasing hormone analogue. *Am J Obstet Gynecol* 1989; **161:** 1216–18.

Precocious puberty. The gonadorelin analogues have replaced other agents as the drugs of choice for the treatment of central precocious puberty (p.1277).

References to the use of leuprorelin.
1. Lee PA, *et al.* Effects of leuprolide in the treatment of central precocious puberty. *J Pediatr* 1989; **114:** 321–4.
2. Kappy M, *et al.* Suppression of gonadotropin secretion by a long-acting gonadotropin-releasing hormone analog (leuprolide acetate, Lupron depot) in children with precocious puberty. *J Clin Endocrinol Metab* 1989; **69:** 1087–9.
3. Neely EK, *et al.* Two-year results of treatment with depot leuprolide acetate for central precocious puberty. *J Pediatr* 1992; **121:** 634–40.
4. Clemons RD, *et al.* Long-term effectiveness of depot gonadotropin-releasing hormone analogue in the treatment of children with central precocious puberty. *Am J Dis Child* 1993; **147:** 653–7.
5. Carel JC, *et al.* Treatment of central precocious puberty with depot leuprorelin. *Eur J Endocrinol* 1995; **132:** 699–704.

Premenstrual syndrome. For reference to the use of leuprorelin or other gonadorelin analogues with HRT to prevent menopausal symptoms in women unresponsive to other drug therapy, see under Gonadorelin, p.1285.

Preparations

Proprietary Preparations (details are given in Part 3)
Aust.: Enantone; Trenantone; *Austral.:* Lucrin; *Belg.:* Lucrin; *Braz.:* Lupron; *Canad.:* Lupron; *Denm.:* Enanton; Procren; *Fin.:* Enanton; Procren; *Fr.:* Enantone; Lucrin; *Ger.:* Carcinil†; Enantone; Enantone-Gyn; Trenantone; Uno-Enantone; *Hong Kong:* Enantone; Lucrin; *Irl.:* Prostap; *Israel:* Lucrin; *Ital.:* Enantone; *Jpn:* Leuplin; *Mex.:* Lucrin; *Neth.:* Lucrin; *Norw.:* Enanton; Procren; *NZ:* Lucrin; *Port.:* Lucrin; *S.Afr.:* Lucrin; *Singapore:* Lucrin; *Spain:* Ginecrin; Procrin; *Swed.:* Enanton; Procren; *Switz.:* Lucrin; *Thai.:* Enantone; *UK:* Prostap; *USA:* Lupron; Viadur.

Luteinising Hormone (5931-v)

Human Interstitial-cell-stimulating Hormone; ICSH; LH; Lutropin.

CAS — 9002-67-9; 39341-83-8 (human).

Lutropin Alfa (17637-p)

Lutropin Alfa (BAN, rINN).

CAS — 152923-57-4 (lutropin alfa); 56832-30-5 (α subunit); 53664-53-2 (βsubunit).

Units

35 units of human pituitary luteinising hormone are contained in approximately 5.8 µg (with 1 mg of human albumin, 5 mg of mannitol, and 1 mg of sodium chloride) in one ampoule of the second International Standard (1988).

10 units of the alpha subunit of human pituitary luteinising hormone are contained in approximately 10 µg (with 0.5 mg of human albumin, 2.5 mg of lactose, and 45 µg of sodium chloride) in one ampoule of the first International Standard (1984).

10 units of the beta subunit of human pituitary luteinising hormone are contained in 10 µg (with 0.5 mg of human albumin, 2.5 mg of lactose, and 45 µg of sodium chloride) in one ampoule of the first International Standard (1984).

Uses and Administration

Luteinising hormone (LH; interstitial-cell-stimulating hormone; ICSH) is a gonadotrophin secreted by the anterior lobe of the pituitary together with another gonadotrophin, follicle-stimulating hormone (FSH) (p.1283).

These gonadotrophins stimulate the normal functioning of the gonads and the secretion of sex hormones in both men and women. In women, follicle-stimulating hormone stimulates the development and maturation of the follicles and ova. As the follicle develops it produces oestrogen in increasing amounts which at mid-cycle stimulates the release of LH. This causes

rupture of the follicle with ovulation and converts the follicle into the corpus luteum which secretes progesterone. In men, luteinising hormone stimulates the interstitial cells of the testis to secrete testosterone, which in turn has a direct effect on the seminiferous tubules.

Gonadotrophic substances with luteinising or follicle-stimulating activity or both are used in the treatment of infertility (p.1275), chiefly in females but also in males. Such substances include chorionic gonadotrophin (p.1279) which possesses LH activity and human menopausal gonadotrophins (p.1288) which possess both LH and FSH activity.

Lutropin alfa is a recombinant human luteinising hormone (rechLH) used to induce ovulation in women with severe deficiency of luteinising and follicle-stimulating hormones, in combination with a preparation with follicle-stimulating activity. A recommended regimen uses initial doses of 75 units of lutropin alfa daily by subcutaneous injection, adjusted according to the individual response at intervals of 7 to 14 days.

◊ References.
1. DeCherney AH, Naftolin F. Recombinant DNA-derived human luteinizing hormone: basic science rapidly applied to clinical medicine. *JAMA* 1988; **259:** 3313–14.
2. Simon JA, *et al.* Characterization of recombinant DNA derived-human luteinizing hormone in vitro and in vivo: efficacy in ovulation induction and corpus luteum support. *JAMA* 1988; **259:** 3290–5.
3. Hull M, *et al.* Recombinant human luteinising hormone: an effective new gonadotropin preparation. *Lancet* 1994; **344:** 334–5.
4. Imthurn B, *et al.* Recombinant human luteinising hormone to mimic mid-cycle LH surge. *Lancet* 1996; **348:** 332–3.
5. Agrawal R, *et al.* Pregnancy after treatment with three recombinant gonadotrophins. *Lancet* 1997; **349:** 29–30.
6. The European Recombinant LH Study Group. Human recombinant luteinising hormone is as effective as, but safer than, urinary human chorionic gonadotrophin in inducing final follicular maturation and ovulation in in vitro fertilization procedures: results of a multicenter double-blind study. *J Clin Endocrinol Metab* 2001; **86:** 2607–18.

Preparations

Proprietary Preparations (details are given in Part 3)
UK: Luveris.

Melanocyte-stimulating Hormone (5936-w)

B Hormone; Chromatophore Hormone; Intermedin; Melanotropin; MSH; Pigment Hormone.

CAS — 9002-79-3.

Profile

Melanocyte-stimulating hormone is a polypeptide isolated from the pars intermedia of the pituitary of fish and amphibia which causes dispersal of melanin granules in the skin of fish and amphibia and allows adaptation to the environment.

In adult humans, the pituitary gland lacks a distinct intermediate lobe, and the pituitary is not thought to secrete melanocyte-stimulating hormone (MSH) directly. However, the precursor molecule, pro-opiomelanocortin, is cleaved in the pituitary into corticotropin (p.1280), the glycoprotein β-lipotrophin (β-LPH), and an amino-terminal peptide. Subsequent processing in other tissues, such as the brain and gastrointestinal tract, may yield three forms of MSH, α-MSH (via corticotropin cleavage), β-MSH, and γ-MSH. The presence and function of these melanocyte-stimulating hormones in man are uncertain. A receptor analogous to that in amphibians is apparently lacking in humans; effects on skin pigmentation emanating from the pituitary are primarily mediated by corticotropin.

Release of melanocyte-stimulating hormone is inhibited in animals by melanostatin; there is also evidence for a hypothalamic releasing factor (MRF).

Melanocyte-stimulating hormone is under investigation, as α-MSH, in the prevention and treatment of ischaemic intrinsic acute renal failure.

◊ Alpha melanocyte-stimulating hormone (α-MSH) has neurotrophic actions during development and has been investigated for its potential in promoting recovery of nerve function after injury.[1]
1. Choo V. Healing with recovery of function. *Lancet* 1993; **342:** 673.

Melanostatin (5937-e)

Intermedin-inhibiting Factor; Melanocyte-stimulating-hormone-release-inhibiting Factor; Melanotropin Release-inhibiting Factor; MIF. Pro-Leu-Gly-NH₂.

CAS — 9083-38-9.

Profile

Melanostatin is a tripeptide obtained from the hypothalamus which inhibits the release of melanocyte-stimulating hormone (see above) in animals. However, there is little evidence of its activity in man. It has been tried in the treatment of depression and parkinsonism but with little benefit.

Nafarelin Acetate (16907-g)

Nafarelin Acetate (BANM, USAN, rINNM).

D-Nal(2)⁶-LHRH acetate hydrate; RS-94991298. 5-Oxo-L-pro-lyl-L-histidyl-L-tryptophyl-L-seryl-L-tyrosyl-3-(2-naphthyl)-D-ala-nyl-L-leucyl-L-arginyl-L-prolylglycinamide acetate hydrate.

$C_{66}H_{83}N_{17}O_{13},xC_2H_4O_2,yH_2O$.

CAS — 76932-56-4 (nafarelin); 86220-42-0 (nafarelin acetate).

Adverse Effects and Precautions

As for Gonadorelin, p.1284.

Effects on electrolytes. A report of severe hyperkalaemia in a woman receiving nafarelin therapy for uterine fibroids.[1] Despite serum potassium greater than 10 mmol per litre she had no symptoms and the electrocardiogram was normal. Hyperkalaemia resolved without treatment following discontinuation of nafarelin.

1. Hata T, et al. Severe hyperkalaemia with nafarelin. Lancet 1996; **347:** 333.

Interactions

As for Gonadorelin, p.1284.

Pharmacokinetics

Nafarelin is rapidly absorbed following intranasal administration with peak plasma concentrations achieved within 20 minutes of a dose, although bioavailability is only about 3%. The plasma half-life is about 3 to 4 hours. Nafarelin is metabolised by peptidases in the body; following subcutaneous administration it is excreted in urine, as metabolites and a small amount of unchanged drug, and in the faeces.

Uses and Administration

Nafarelin acetate is an analogue of gonadorelin (see p.1284) with similar properties. It is used in the treatment of endometriosis and central precocious puberty, and as an adjunct to ovulation induction with gonadotrophins in the treatment of infertility.

For endometriosis it is given in usual doses equivalent to 200 μg of nafarelin twice daily intranasally, doubled after 2 months if amenorrhoea has not occurred. Treatment should begin on days 2 to 4 of the menstrual cycle, and may be continued for up to 6 months.

For central precocious puberty the usual dose is the equivalent of nafarelin 800 μg intranasally (400 μg in each nostril) twice daily. If adequate suppression is not achieved at this dose it may be increased to 600 μg three times daily in alternate nostrils.

Regimens for oocyte collection for in-vitro fertilisation employ gonadorelin analogues for pituitary desensitisation before ovulation induction with gonadotrophins; the equivalent of 400 μg of nafarelin is given intranasally twice daily, beginning either in the early follicular phase (day 2) or midluteal phase (day 21) of the menstrual cycle. Therapy should be continued until downregulation is achieved; if this does not occur within 12 weeks therapy should be withdrawn. Once downregulation occurs gonadotrophin treatment is added to nafarelin therapy until an appropriate stage of follicular development, when both are withdrawn and chorionic gonadotrophin is given to induce ovulation.

Nafarelin has also been given in other sex hormone-related conditions.

Benign prostatic hyperplasia. For a discussion of the management of benign prostatic hyperplasia, including mention of the use of gonadorelin analogues and the view that they are unsatisfactory for indefinite therapy, see p.1477.

Prostate size decreased by a mean of 24.2% in 9 men treated for benign prostatic hyperplasia for 6 months with nafarelin acetate 400 μg daily subcutaneously.[1] Six months after the end of treatment, prostate size approached that of pretreatment values.

1. Peters CA, Walsh PC. The effect of nafarelin acetate, a luteinising-hormone-releasing hormone agonist, on benign prostatic hyperplasia. N Engl J Med 1987; **317:** 599–604.

Endometriosis. Gonadorelin analogues are effective in the management of endometriosis (p.1469), but the need for long-term therapy to prevent recurrence limits their value because of the risk of osteoporosis; 'add-back' therapy, with concomitant hormone replacement, is under investigation.

References to the use of nafarelin.

1. Schriock E, et al. Treatment of endometriosis with a potent agonist of gonadotrophin-releasing hormone (nafarelin). Fertil Steril 1985; **44:** 583–8.

2. Henzl MR, et al. Administration of nasal nafarelin as compared with oral danazol for endometriosis: a multicenter double-blind comparative clinical trial. N Engl J Med 1988; **318:** 485–9.
3. Burry KA. Nafarelin in the management of endometriosis: quality of life assessment. Am J Obstet Gynecol 1992; **166:** 735–9.
4. Hornstein MD, et al. Retreatment with nafarelin for recurrent endometriosis symptoms: efficacy, safety, and bone mineral density. Fertil Steril 1997; **67:** 1013–18.

Fibroids. Gonadorelin analogues have been tried as an adjunct or alternative to surgery in the treatment of uterine fibroids (see p.1285), although there has been some concern that this might complicate the diagnosis of malignancy.

References to the use of nafarelin.

1. Minaguchi H, et al. Clinical use of nafarelin in the treatment of leiomyomas: a review of the literature. J Reprod Med 2000; **45:** 481–9.

Infertility. Gonadorelin analogues are used in the treatment of infertility (p.1275). As well as being used directly they are employed in regimens to induce superovulation to enable ova collection and in-vitro fertilisation, and use of nafarelin has been reported to produce a higher rate of successful pregnancies than leuprorelin in one in-vitro fertilisation programme.[1]

1. Martin MC, et al. The choice of a gonadotropin-releasing hormone analog influences outcome of in vitro fertilization treatment. Am J Obstet Gynecol 1994; **170:** 1629–34.

Precocious puberty. Nafarelin preserved adult height potential in girls with idiopathic precocious puberty (p.1277) having a poor initial height prognosis.[1] However, reviewers have noted that results from earlier studies into other features of precocious puberty have been equivocal.[2]

1. Kreiter M, et al. Preserving adult height potential in girls with idiopathic true precocious puberty. J Pediatr 1990; **117:** 364–70.
2. Chrisp P, Goa KL. Nafarelin: a review of its pharmacodynamic and pharmacokinetic properties, and clinical potential in sex hormone-related conditions. Drugs 1990; **39:** 523–51.

Preparations

Proprietary Preparations (details are given in Part 3)

Austral.: Synarel; **Belg.:** Synarel; **Canad.:** Synarel; **Denm.:** Synarela; **Fin.:** Synarela; **Fr.:** Synarel; **Ger.:** Synarela; **Hong Kong:** Synarel; **Irl.:** Synarel; **Israel:** Synarel; **Mex.:** Synarel; **Neth.:** Synarel; **Norw.:** Synarela; **NZ:** Synarel; **S.Afr.:** Synarel; **Spain:** Synarel; **Swed.:** Synarela; **Switz.:** Synrelina; **UK:** Synarel; **USA:** Synarel.

Octreotide Acetate (16932-q)

Octreotide Acetate (BANM, USAN, rINNM).

SMS-201-995 (octreotide). 2-(D-Phenylalanyl-L-cystyl-L-phenylalanyl-D-tryptophyl-L-lysyl-L-threonyl-L-cystyl)-(2R,3R)-butane-1,3-diol acetate; D-Phenylalanyl-L-cysteinyl-L-phenylalanyl-D-tryptophyl-L-lysyl-L-threonyl-N-[(1R,2R)-2-hydroxy-1-(hydroxymethyl)propyl]-L-cysteinamide cyclic (2→7) disulphide acetate.

$C_{49}H_{66}N_{10}O_{10}S_2,xC_2H_4O_2 = 1019.2$ (octreotide).

CAS — 83150-76-9 (octreotide); 79517-01-4 (octreotide acetate).

Incompatibility. Apparent loss of insulin has been reported from a total parenteral nutrient solution containing octreotide; there may be an incompatibility.[1] Also the manufacturers have suggested that octreotide might be adsorbed onto plastics. However, a solution containing octreotide 200 μg per mL as the acetate was reported to be stable at 5° or −20° for up to 60 days when stored in polypropylene syringes.[2]

1. Rosen GH. Potential incompatibility of insulin and octreotide in total parenteral nutrient solutions. Am J Hosp Pharm 1989; **46:** 1128.
2. Ripley RG, et al. Stability of octreotide acetate in polypropylene syringes at 5 and −20°C. Am J Health-Syst Pharm 1995; **52:** 1910–11.

Adverse Effects and Precautions

There may be a transient local reaction at the site of injection of octreotide. Systemic side-effects are mainly gastrointestinal and may include anorexia, nausea, vomiting, diarrhoea and steatorrhoea, abdominal discomfort, and flatulence. Administration between meals or at bedtime may reduce these gastrointestinal effects.

Gallstones may develop on long-term therapy; there have been isolated reports of hepatic dysfunction and of biliary colic associated with drug withdrawal. Checks should be made for gallstones before prolonged therapy and at 6- to 12-month intervals during treatment. Hypoglycaemia may occur, especially in patients with insulinomas, but there is also a risk of hyperglycaemia or impaired glucose tolerance. Thyroid function should be monitored during octreotide therapy because of the possibility of hypothyroidism. Pituitary tumours that secrete growth hormone can expand during treatment, causing serious complications; patients should be monitored for signs of tumour expansion, such as visual field defects. Cardiac

rhythm should be monitored during intravenous administration of octreotide. Doses may need to be adjusted in patients with end-stage renal failure, in whom the clearance of octreotide is reduced.

Effects on the biliary tract. Octreotide has an inhibitory effect on gallbladder motility accounting for the development of gallstones and biliary colic.[1-8]

1. McKnight JA, et al. Changes in glucose tolerance and development of gall stones during high dose treatment with octreotide for acromegaly. BMJ 1989; **299:** 604–5.
2. Ho KY, et al. Therapeutic efficacy of the somatostatin analog SMS 201-995 (octreotide) in acromegaly: effects of dose and frequency and long-term safety. Ann Intern Med 1990; **112:** 173–81.
3. Bigg-Wither GW, et al. Effects of long term octreotide on gall stone formation and gall bladder function. BMJ 1992; **304:** 1611–12.
4. Redfern JS, Fortuner WJ. Octreotide-associated biliary tract dysfunction and gallstone formation: pathophysiology and management. Am J Gastroenterol 1995; **90:** 1042–52.
5. Tauber JP, et al. The impact of continuous subcutaneous infusion of octreotide on gallstone formation in acromegalic patients. J Clin Endocrinol Metab 1995; **80:** 3262–6.
6. Hussaini SH, et al. Roles of gall bladder emptying and intestinal transit in the pathogenesis of octreotide induced gall bladder stones. Gut 1996; **38:** 775–83.
7. Trendle MC, et al. Incidence and morbidity of cholelithiasis in patients receiving chronic octreotide for metastatic carcinoid and malignant islet cell tumors. Cancer 1997; **79:** 830–4.
8. Moschetta A, et al. Severe impairment of postprandial cholecystokinin release and gall-bladder emptying and high risk of gallstone formation in acromegalic patients during Sandostatin LAR. Aliment Pharmacol Ther 2001; **15:** 181–5.

Effects on carbohydrate metabolism. Changes in glucose tolerance were observed over 12 months in patients treated with octreotide 600 to 1500 μg daily subcutaneously for acromegaly.[1] Of 3 patients with normal glucose tolerance initially, one remained normal, one developed impaired glucose tolerance, and one became diabetic. Of 4 with impaired glucose tolerance initially, 2 remained unchanged, one became diabetic, and the other returned to normal. There has been a report of deterioration in glucose tolerance leading to death from diabetic ketoacidosis occurring after cessation of octreotide treatment in a patient with acromegaly and insulin-resistant diabetes mellitus.[2]

See also Diabetes Mellitus and Hyperinsulinism under Uses and Administration, below.

1. McKnight JA, et al. Changes in glucose tolerance and development of gall stones during high dose treatment with octreotide for acromegaly. BMJ 1989; **299:** 604–5.
2. Abrahamson MJ. Death from diabetic ketoacidosis after cessation of octreotide in acromegaly. Lancet 1990; **336:** 318–19.

Effects on the hair. Diffuse loss of scalp hair has been reported in 4 of 7 women who received octreotide; after withdrawal of octreotide in 3 of the women there was a complete recovery of scalp hair.[1]

1. Jönsson A, Manhem P. Octreotide and loss of scalp hair. Ann Intern Med 1991; **115:** 913.

Effects on the liver. A report of hepatitis occurring during treatment of an acromegalic patient with octreotide 300 μg daily subcutaneously.[1] Liver enzyme values returned to normal within 2 months of withdrawing octreotide.

1. Arosio M, et al. Acute hepatitis after treatment of acromegaly with octreotide. Lancet 1988; **ii:** 1498.

Effects on the pancreas. Reports of pancreatitis associated with octreotide.[1-3] It has been suggested that octreotide-induced pancreatitis may result from spasm of the sphincter of Oddi, resulting in retention of activated pancreatic enzymes due to outflow obstruction.[3]

1. Frederich A, et al. Acute pancreatitis after short-term octreotide. Lancet 1991; **338:** 52–3.
2. Sadoul J-L, et al. Acute pancreatitis following octreotide withdrawal. Am J Med 1991; **90:** 763–4.
3. Bodemar G, Hjortswang H. Octreotide-induced pancreatitis: an effect of increased contractility of Oddi sphincter. Lancet 1996; **348:** 1668–9.

Interactions

Octreotide has been associated with alterations in nutrient absorption and there is a theoretical possibility that it may affect the absorption of orally administered drugs. Patients receiving insulin or oral hypoglycaemic drugs may require dose adjustments of these agents if octreotide is given concomitantly. The bioavailability of bromocriptine is increased by administration with octreotide. It has been suggested that dosage of beta blockers, calcium-channel blockers, or agents to control fluid and electrolyte balance may also need to be adjusted.

Ciclosporin. For a reference to octreotide reducing serum concentrations of ciclosporin, see p.522.

Pharmacokinetics

Octreotide is rapidly absorbed following subcutaneous injection, with peak plasma concentrations reached about 25 to 30 minutes after a dose, and is distributed to body tissues. It is said to exhibit non-linear pharmacokinetics, with reduced clearance at high doses. Octreotide is removed from the body with a plasma elimination half-life of approximately 1.5 hours; half-life is prolonged in elderly patients and in renal failure. About a third of a dose is excreted unchanged in the urine.

Uses and Administration

Octreotide is an octapeptide analogue of somatostatin (p.1297) with similar properties but a longer duration of action.

It is used as the acetate in the symptomatic management of carcinoid tumours and other secretory neoplasms such as VIPomas and glucagonomas. Octreotide acetate is also used in the treatment of acromegaly and the prevention of complications following pancreatic surgery, and has been investigated in the treatment of a variety of other disorders including variceal haemorrhage, HIV-associated diarrhoea, and the dumping syndrome.

In the management of **secretory neoplasms** octreotide acetate is given subcutaneously in an initial dose equivalent to 50 µg of octreotide once or twice daily gradually increased, according to response, to up to 600 µg daily in 2 to 4 divided doses. Higher doses have been used.

Where a rapid response is required, the initial dose may be given by the intravenous route. In the UK the manufacturers state that it should be diluted not less than 1 in 1 or not more than 1 in 9 in sodium chloride 0.9%, but in the USA the manufacturers permit the use of the undiluted solution as an intravenous bolus in emergencies; alternatively the dose may be given by intermittent infusion over 15 to 30 minutes, diluted in 50 to 200 mL of sodium chloride 0.9% or glucose 5%.

Once control has been established maintenance therapy with a depot preparation may be possible; initially 20 mg by intramuscular injection every 4 weeks is suggested. Subcutaneous injection with a rapid-acting preparation should be continued for 2 weeks after the first depot injection to provide symptomatic cover, and may be added to therapy when necessary thereafter. Maintenance doses of the depot preparation may be adjusted after 3 months to between 10 and 30 mg every 4 weeks, as necessary.

In **acromegaly**, the usual dose is the equivalent of 100 to 200 µg of octreotide three times daily by subcutaneous injection. In the USA it is suggested that dosage begin with 50 µg three times daily in order to minimise gastrointestinal disturbance. Once control has been established maintenance therapy with a depot preparation is possible; an initial dose equivalent to 20 mg of octreotide given intramuscularly once a month has been recommended for patients with acromegaly, adjusted after 3 months to between 10 and 30 mg monthly.

For the prevention of complications following **pancreatic surgery** the equivalent of 100 µg of octreotide may be given three times daily by subcutaneous injection of a rapid-acting preparation; treatment is given for 7 consecutive days, beginning at least 1 hour before laparotomy on the day of operation.

◊ General reviews of octreotide.
1. Mosdell KW, Visconti JA. Emerging indications for octreotide therapy, part 1. *Am J Hosp Pharm* 1994; **51:** 1184–92.
2. Mosdell KW, Visconti JA. Emerging indications for octreotide therapy, part 2. *Am J Hosp Pharm* 1994; **51:** 1317–30.
3. Bloom SR, O'Shea D. Octreotide. *Prescribers' J* 1996; **36:** 120–4.
4. Lamberts SWJ, *et al.* Octreotide. *N Engl J Med* 1996; **334:** 246–54.

Acromegaly. Although surgery remains the most important method of treatment, octreotide may be useful in the management of acromegaly (p.1271) particularly in the frail and elderly patient, since it can reduce growth hormone concentrations and tumour size, and may improve cardiovascular parameters.[1-6] Continuous subcutaneous infusion may be more effective than intermittent injection.[7] Sustained-release octreotide also appears to be of value.[8]
1. Chanson P, *et al.* Cardiovascular effects of the somatostatin analog octreotide in acromegaly. *Ann Intern Med* 1990; **113:** 921–5.

2. Ho KY, *et al.* Therapeutic efficacy of the somatostatin analog SMS 201-995 (octreotide) in acromegaly: effects of dose and frequency and long-term safety. *Ann Intern Med* 1990; **112:** 173–81.
3. Vance ML, Harris AG. Long-term treatment of 189 acromegalic patients with the somatostatin analog octreotide: results of the International Multicenter Acromegaly Study Group. *Arch Intern Med* 1991; **151:** 1573–8.
4. Ezzat S, *et al.* Octreotide treatment of acromegaly: a randomized, multicenter study. *Ann Intern Med* 1992; **117:** 711–18.
5. Acromegaly Therapy Consensus Development Panel. Consensus statement: benefits versus risks of medical therapy for acromegaly. *Am J Med* 1994; **97:** 468–73.
6. van der Lely AJ, *et al.* A risk-benefit assessment of octreotide in the treatment of acromegaly. *Drug Safety* 1997; **17:** 317–24.
7. Harris AG, *et al.* Continuous versus intermittent subcutaneous infusion of octreotide in the treatment of acromegaly. *J Clin Pharmacol* 1995; **35:** 59–71.
8. Gillis JC, *et al.* Octreotide long-acting release (LAR): a review of its pharmacological properties and therapeutic use in the management of acromegaly. *Drugs* 1997; **53:** 681–99.

Carcinoid syndrome and other secretory neoplasms. For a discussion of carcinoid tumours and other secretory neoplasms, including reference to the important role of octreotide, see p.483.

Cardiovascular disorders. There have been reports of benefit from octreotide in patients with postprandial hypotension and orthostatic hypotension associated with autonomic neuropathy.[1-3] It is one of many drugs that have been tried in orthostatic hypotension (see p.1070). Octreotide has also produced rapid and sustained cardiac improvement in patients with acromegaly.[4,5] (See also above.) Promising results have also been reported in patients with primary hypertrophic cardiomyopathy.[6,7]
1. Hoeldtke RD, *et al.* Treatment of autonomic neuropathy with a somatostatin analogue SMS-201-995. *Lancet* 1986; **ii:** 602–5.
2. Hoeldtke RD, Israel BC. Treatment of orthostatic hypotension with octreotide. *J Clin Endocrinol Metab* 1989; **68:** 1051–9.
3. Woo J, *et al.* Treatment of severe orthostatic hypotension with the somatostatin analogue octreotide. *Aust N Z J Med* 1990; **20:** 822–3.
4. Chanson P, *et al.* Cardiovascular effects of the somatostatin analog octreotide in acromegaly. *Ann Intern Med* 1990; **113:** 921–5.
5. Colao A, *et al.* Is the acromegalic cardiomyopathy reversible? Effect of 5-year normalization of growth hormone and insulin-like growth factor I levels on cardiac performance. *J Clin Endocrinol Metab* 2001; **86:** 1551–7.
6. Günal AI, *et al.* Short term reduction of left ventricular mass in primary hypertrophic cardiomyopathy by octreotide injections. *Heart* 1996; **76:** 418–21.
7. Demirtas E, *et al.* Effects of octreotide in patients with hypertrophic obstructive cardiomyopathy. *Jpn Heart J* 1998; **39:** 173–81.

Cushing's syndrome. It has been suggested[1] that octreotide may be useful in the diagnosis, and possibly the treatment, of Cushing's syndrome (p.1272).
1. Woodhouse NJY, *et al.* Acute and long-term effects of octreotide in patients with ACTH-dependent Cushing's syndrome. *Am J Med* 1993; **95:** 305–8.

Diabetes mellitus. Although octreotide has been reported to impair glucose tolerance, and even precipitate frank diabetes (see Effects on Carbohydrate Metabolism, under Adverse Effects, above), its variable effects on blood glucose and insulin have led to investigations[1-3] of its possible benefits in diabetes mellitus (p.315). There is also some suggestion that it may be of benefit in the treatment or prevention of diabetic nephropathy[4] and retinopathy.[5] Benefit has been reported from the use of octreotide in patients with diabetic diarrhoea—see Gastrointestinal Disorders, below.
1. Rios MS, *et al.* Somatostatin analog SMS 201-995 and insulin needs in insulin-dependent diabetic patients studied by means of an artificial pancreas. *J Clin Endocrinol Metab* 1986; **63:** 1071–4.
2. Hadjidakis DJ, *et al.* The effects of the somatostatin analogue SMS 201-995 on carbohydrate homeostasis of insulin-dependent diabetics as assessed by the artificial endocrine pancreas. *Diabetes Res Clin Pract* 1988; **5:** 91–8.
3. Candrina R, Giustina G. Effect of a new long-acting somatostatin analogue (SMS 201-995) on glycemic and hormonal profiles in insulin-treated type II diabetic patients. *J Endocrinol Invest* 1988; **11:** 501–7.
4. Serri O, *et al.* Somatostatin analogue, octreotide, reduces increased glomerular filtration rate and kidney size in insulin-dependent diabetes. *JAMA* 1991; **265:** 888–92.
5. Grant MB, *et al.* The efficacy of octreotide in the therapy of severe nonproliferative and early proliferative diabetic retinopathy: a randomized controlled trial. *Diabetes Care* 2000; **23:** 504–9.

Diagnosis and testing. Radiolabelled octreotide or derivatives such as pentetreotide may be used successfully to visualise various malignant neoplasms which express somatostatin receptors.[1-6] Somatostatin receptor scintigraphy is the most sensitive method for imaging lesions in patients with Zollinger-Ellison syndrome.[6]

Octreotide may also have a role in the diagnosis of Cushing's syndrome, a topic discussed in more detail on p.1272.
1. Krenning EP, *et al.* Localisation of endocrine-related tumours with radioiodinated analogue of somatostatin. *Lancet* 1989; **i:** 242–4.
2. Lamberts SWJ, *et al.* Somatostatin-receptor imaging in the localization of endocrine tumors. *N Engl J Med* 1990; **323:** 1246–9.
3. van Eijck CHJ, *et al.* Somatostatin-receptor scintigraphy in primary breast cancer. *Lancet* 1994; **343:** 640–3.
4. McCready VR, Hickish TF. Somatostatin imaging function. *Lancet* 1994; **343:** 617.

5. Dominioni L, *et al.* Localisation of carcinoid tumour with radiolabelled octreotide and intraoperative gamma detection. *Lancet* 1994; **344:** 1783.
6. Gibril F, *et al.* Somatostatin receptor scintigraphy: its sensitivity compared with that of other imaging methods in detecting primary and metastatic gastrinomas: a prospective study. *Ann Intern Med* 1996; **125:** 26–34.

Eye disorders. A report of response to octreotide in a patient with bilateral cystoid macular oedema, a refractory form of retinal oedema.[1] The problem recurred when octreotide was twice discontinued and each time responded to resumption of octreotide injections.
1. Kuijpers RWAM, *et al.* Treatment of cystoid macular edema with octreotide. *N Engl J Med* 1998; **338:** 624–6.

Gastrointestinal disorders. Somatostatin inhibits gastric and intestinal secretion and the production of various active substances in the gastrointestinal tract. It also reduces splanchnic arterial blood flow and portal and gastric mucosal blood flow. These properties are made use of, usually in the form of octreotide, in the management of a number of gastrointestinal disorders. Octreotide is used cautiously in the treatment of carcinoid syndrome arising from **endocrine tumours** (see Carcinoid Tumours, p.483).

The antisecretory properties of octreotide have been of benefit in patients with **diarrhoea** associated with a variety of conditions including AIDS,[1-4] amyloidosis,[5] diabetes mellitus,[6-8] microvillous atrophy,[9] bone-marrow transplantation,[10] and enterocolitis induced by gold therapy.[11] Octreotide has also been used to reduce the output from postoperative small-bowel fistulae[12] and may be useful in decreasing faecal mass or jejunal efflux in patients with the short-bowel syndrome and jejunostomies or ileostomies.[13,14] Octreotide therapy resulted in closure of small bowel fistulae in almost 80% of patients in one study[12] and in accelerated healing of pancreatic cutaneous fistulae.[15,16]

There have been mixed results with octreotide in the treatment of **gastrointestinal bleeding**. Although a large multicentre study[17] showed that octreotide had no benefit compared with placebo in the management of bleeding upper gastrointestinal ulcers, a later meta-analysis suggested there might be some benefit.[18] Octreotide is used to control acute **variceal haemorrhage** (p.1637). It appears to be as effective as balloon tamponade,[19] and there is some evidence that it is as effective as sclerotherapy.[20] Two large controlled studies have suggested that combination of octreotide with endoscopic ligation[21] or sclerotherapy[22] reduces the risk of rebleeding. A subsequent meta-analysis[23] of trials comparing octreotide with other therapies for the control of acute variceal bleeding came to similar conclusions, and also found octreotide treatment to be more effective and associated with fewer major complications than vasopressin or terlipressin. However, there was no evidence of mortality benefit associated with octreotide use. Octreotide has also produced some benefit (combined with regular sclerotherapy), in the long-term management of patients with cirrhotic portal hypertension.[24]

Other gastrointestinal disorders in which octreotide might be useful include **dumping syndrome**[25,26] (further discussed on p.1203), reactive (or postprandial) **hypoglycaemia**,[27,28] **protein-losing enteropathy** associated with intestinal lymphangiectasia,[29] prevention of **NSAID-induced gastric injury**,[30] and **vomiting** secondary to bowel obstruction in patients terminally ill with cancer.[31,32]
1. Cook DJ, *et al.* Somatostatin treatment for cryptosporidial diarrhea in a patient with the acquired immunodeficiency syndrome (AIDS). *Ann Intern Med* 1988; **108:** 708–9.
2. Robinson EN, Fogel R. SMS 201-995, a somatostatin analogue and diarrhea in the acquired immunodeficiency syndrome (AIDS). *Ann Intern Med* 1988; **109:** 680–1.
3. Clotet B, *et al.* Efficacy of the somatostatin analogue (SMS-201-995), Sandostatin, for cryptosporidial diarrhoea in patients with AIDS. *AIDS* 1989; **3:** 857–8.
4. Kim-Sing A, *et al.* Palliative high-dose octreotide in a case of severe AIDS-related diarrhea. *Ann Pharmacother* 1994; **28:** 806–7.
5. O'Connor CR, O'Dorisio TM. Amyloidosis, diarrhea, and a somatostatin analogue. *Ann Intern Med* 1989; **110:** 665–6.
6. Tsai S-T, *et al.* Diabetic diarrhea and somatostatin. *Ann Intern Med* 1986; **104:** 894.
7. Michaels PE, Cameron RB. Octreotide is cost-effective therapy in diabetic diarrhea. *Arch Intern Med* 1991; **151:** 2469.
8. Mourad FH, *et al.* Effective treatment of diabetic diarrhoea with somatostatin analogue, octreotide. *Gut* 1992; **33:** 1578–80.
9. Couper RTL, *et al.* Clinical response to the long acting somatostatin analogue SMS 201-995 in a child with congenital microvillus atrophy. *Gut* 1989; **30:** 1020–4.
10. Crouch MA, *et al.* Octreotide acetate in refractory bone marrow transplant-associated diarrhea. *Ann Pharmacother* 1996; **30:** 331–6.
11. Dorta G, *et al.* Treatment of gold-induced enteritis with octreotide. *Lancet* 1993; **342:** 179.
12. Nubiola-Calonge P, *et al.* Blind evaluation of the effect of octreotide (SMS 201-995), a somatostatin analogue, on small-bowel fistula output. *Lancet* 1987; **ii:** 672–4.
13. Ladefoged K, *et al.* Effect of a long acting somatostatin analogue SMS 201-995 on jejunostomy effluents in patients with severe short bowel syndrome. *Gut* 1989; **30:** 943–9.
14. Nightingale JMD, *et al.* Jejunal efflux in short bowel syndrome. *Lancet* 1990; **336:** 765–8.
15. Prinz RA, *et al.* Treatment of pancreatic cutaneous fistulas with a somatostatin analog. *Am J Surg* 1988; **155:** 36–42.
16. Heij HA, *et al.* A comparison of the effects of two somatostatin analogues in a patient with an external pancreatic fistula. *Pancreas* 1986; **1:** 188–90.
17. Christiansen J, *et al.* Placebo-controlled trial with the somatostatin analogue SMS 201-995 in peptic ulcer bleeding. *Gastroenterology* 1989; **97:** 568–74.

18. Imperiale TF, Birgisson S. Somatostatin or octreotide compared with H₂ antagonists and placebo in the management of acute nonvariceal upper gastrointestinal hemorrhage: a meta-analysis. *Ann Intern Med* 1997; **127:** 1062–71. Correction. *ibid.* 1998; **128:** 245.
19. O'Donnell LJD, Farthing MJG. Octreotide and bleeding oesophageal varices. *Lancet* 1989; **ii:** 1276.
20. Jenkins SA, *et al.* A multicentre randomised trial comparing octreotide and injection sclerotherapy in the management and outcome of acute variceal haemorrhage. *Gut* 1997; **41:** 526–33.
21. Sung JJY, *et al.* Prospective randomised study of effect of octreotide on rebleeding from oesophageal varices after endoscopic ligation. *Lancet* 1995; **346:** 1666–9.
22. Besson I, *et al.* Sclerotherapy with or without octreotide for acute variceal bleeding. *N Engl J Med* 1995; **333:** 555–60.
23. Corley DA, *et al.* Octreotide for acute esophageal variceal bleeding: a meta-analysis. *Gastroenterology* 2001; **120:** 946–54.
24. Jenkins SA, *et al.* Randomised trial of octreotide for long term management of cirrhosis after variceal haemorrhage. *BMJ* 1997; **315:** 1338–41.
25. Hopman WPM, *et al.* Treatment of the dumping syndrome with the somatostatin analogue SMS 201-995. *Ann Surg* 1988; **207:** 155–9.
26. Farthing MJA. Octreotide in dumping and short bowel syndromes. *Digestion* 1993; **54** (suppl 1): 47–52.
27. D'Cruz DP, *et al.* Long-term symptomatic relief of postprandial hypoglycaemia following gastric surgery with a somatostatin analogue. *Postgrad Med J* 1989; **65:** 116–17.
28. Lehnert H, *et al.* Treatment of severe reactive hypoglycemia with a somatostatin analogue (SMS 201-995). *Arch Intern Med* 1990; **150:** 2401–2.
29. Bac DJ, *et al.* Octreotide for protein-losing enteropathy with intestinal lymphangiectasia. *Lancet* 1995; **345:** 1639.
30. Scheiman JM, *et al.* Reduction of non-steroidal anti-inflammatory drug induced gastric injury and leucocyte endothelial adhesion by octreotide. *Gut* 1997; **40:** 720–5.
31. Khoo D, *et al.* control of emesis in bowel obstruction in terminally ill patients. *Lancet* 1992; **339:** 375–6.
32. Crawford R, Quigley C. Octreotide. *Prescribers' J* 1996; **36:** 231–2.

Hypercalcaemia. There have been individual reports of hypercalcaemia associated with raised plasma concentrations of parathyroid hormone-related protein (humoral hypercalcaemia of malignancy—p.1181) being successfully controlled with octreotide in patients with malignant pancreatic endocrine tumours[1,2] and adrenal phaeochromocytoma.[3] In two of these patients,[2,3] hypercalcaemia had previously been resistant to treatment with bisphosphonates. Octreotide also resolved hypercalcaemia occurring in a patient with VIPoma and vasoactive intestinal peptide concentrations declined.[4]

1. Wynick D, *et al.* Treatment of a malignant pancreatic endocrine tumour secreting parathyroid hormone related protein. *BMJ* 1990; **300:** 1314–15.
2. Dodwell D, *et al.* Treatment of a pancreatic tumour secreting parathyroid hormone related protein. *BMJ* 1990; **300:** 1653.
3. Harrison M, *et al.* Somatostatin analogue treatment for malignant hypercalcaemia. *BMJ* 1990; **300:** 1313–14. Correction. *ibid.* 1990; **301:** 97 [dosage error].
4. Venkatesh S, *et al.* Somatostatin analogue: use in the treatment of vipoma with hypercalcaemia. *Am J Med* 1989; **87:** 356–7.

Hyperinsulinism. As well as reactive hypoglycaemia (see Gastrointestinal Disorders, above), octreotide has been used to control inappropriate insulin secretion, both in the short-term and long-term, in children with hypoglycaemia of infancy,[1-4] or nesidioblastosis.[5-7] It has also been used to treat a patient with hyperinsulinaemia induced by quinine.[8] For mention of investigations of octreotide for the reverse effect, see Diabetes Mellitus, above.

1. Kirk JMW, *et al.* Somatostatin analogue in short term management of hyperinsulinism. *Arch Dis Child* 1988; **63:** 1493–4.
2. DeClue TJ, *et al.* Linear growth during long-term treatment with somatostatin analog (SMS 201-995) for persistent hyperinsulinemic hypoglycemia of infancy. *J Pediatr* 1990; **116:** 747–50.
3. Thornton PS, *et al.* Short- and long-term use of octreotide in the treatment of congenital hyperinsulinism. *J Pediatr* 1993; **123:** 637–43.
4. Aynsley-Green A, *et al.* Practical management of hyperinsulinism in infancy. *Arch Dis Child Fetal Neonatal Ed* 2000; **82:** F98–F107.
5. Hindmarsh P, Brook CGD. Short-term management of nesidioblastosis using the somatostatin analogue SMS 201-995. *N Engl J Med* 1987; **316:** 221–2.
6. Delemarre-van de Waal HA, *et al.* Long-term treatment of an infant with nesidioblastosis using a somatostatin analogue. *N Engl J Med* 1987; **316:** 222–3.
7. Behrens R, *et al.* Unusual course of neonatal hyperinsulinaemic hypoglycaemia (nesidioblastosis). *Arch Dis Child* 1998; **78:** F156.
8. Phillips RE, *et al.* Effectiveness of SMS 201-995, a synthetic, long-acting somatostatin analogue, in treatment of quinine-induced hyperinsulinaemia. *Lancet* 1986; **i:** 713–16.

Infertility. Octreotide reduced circulating insulin and luteinising hormone concentrations and lowered androgen production in women with polycystic ovary syndrome.[1,2] This should assist in the development of ovulatory cycles. However, a small placebo-controlled study in women with infertility associated with polycystic ovary syndrome and clomifene resistance did not find octreotide to be of value in reversing the latter,[3] although some evidence suggested it might reduce the risk of ovarian hyperstimulation.

There has been a report of a pregnancy occurring in a previously infertile woman, resistant to clomifene, who was treated with octreotide for acromegaly.[4] The neonate had no malformations and developed normally.

1. Prelevic GM, *et al.* Inhibitory effect of Sandostatin on secretion of luteinising hormone and ovarian steroids in polycystic ovary syndrome. *Lancet* 1990; **336:** 900–3.
2. Prelevic GM, *et al.* The effects of the somatostatin analogue octreotide on ovulatory performance in women with polycystic ovaries. *Hum Reprod* 1995; **10:** 28–32.

3. Morris RS, *et al.* Octreotide is not useful for clomiphene citrate resistance in patients with polycystic ovary syndrome but may reduce the likelihood of ovarian hyperstimulation syndrome. *Fertil Steril* 1999; **71:** 452–6.
4. Landolt AM, *et al.* Successful pregnancy in a previously infertile woman treated with SMS-201-995 for acromegaly. *N Engl J Med* 1989; **320:** 671–2.

Malignant neoplasms. See under Carcinoid Syndrome, above. For mention of the use of octreotide to treat vomiting associated with malignant gastrointestinal obstruction see Gastrointestinal Disorders, above. Octreotide has also proved of benefit in bone pain due to metastatic gastrinoma (see Pain, below). An unconventional regimen employing octreotide or somatostatin with melatonin, bromocriptine, and a solution of retinoids (the Di Bella regimen) was investigated in patients with a variety of advanced malignancies and found to be ineffective.[1,2]

1. Italian Study Group for the Di Bella Multitherapy Trials. Evaluation of an unconventional cancer treatment (the Di Bella multitherapy): results of phase II trials in Italy. *BMJ* 1999; **318:** 224–8.
2. Buiatti E, *et al.* Results from a historical survey of the survival of cancer patients given Di Bella multitherapy. *Cancer* 1999; **86:** 2143–9.

HEPATOCELLULAR CARCINOMA. In a study in 58 patients with advanced hepatocellular carcinoma treatment with octreotide was associated with prolongation of survival compared with no treatment.[1]

1. Kouroumalis E, *et al.* Treatment of hepatocellular carcinoma with octreotide: a randomised controlled study. *Gut* 1998; **42:** 442–7.

MENINGIOMA. Octreotide suppressed severe headaches associated with meningioma in a patient;[1] doses were increased to 500 μg three times daily subcutaneously because of tolerance. The patient was able to discontinue octreotide following subsequent surgical removal of the tumour. It was also thought that octreotide had had a beneficial effect on the meningioma size.

1. Rünzi MW, *et al.* Successful treatment of meningioma with octreotide. *Lancet* 1989; **i:** 1074.

THYMOMA. A patient with thymoma and pure red cell aplasia, in whom corticosteroids alone failed to control anaemia, experienced complete remission following treatment with octreotide and prednisone, and subsequently remained well on long-term maintenance therapy with octreotide 500 μg twice daily and prednisone 200 μg per kg body-weight daily.[1]

1. Palmieri G, *et al.* Successful treatment of a patient with a thymoma and pure red-cell aplasia with octreotide and prednisone. *N Engl J Med* 1997; **336:** 263–5.

Nesidioblastosis. For reference to the use of octreotide in nesidioblastosis, see Hyperinsulinism, above.

Pain. Octreotide 120 to 480 μg daily was administered by continuous intrathecal infusion to 5 patients with cancer pain that had been poorly controlled by opioid analgesics.[1] All patients obtained good pain relief, 3 reporting pain to be totally absent. Sustained decrease in incapacitating bone pain has also been reported in a patient with skeletal metastasis of a gastrinoma who was given subcutaneous octreotide 100 μg three times daily.[2] The pain of hypertrophic pulmonary osteoarthropathy (a paraneoplastic syndrome of periostitis, arthropathy, and gynaecomastia seen particularly with squamous cell lung cancer) has also been reported to respond to octreotide.[3] However, a controlled study of octreotide in cancer pain found that it was no better than placebo in most patients.[4] (General guidelines for the management of cancer pain are discussed on p.5.) Octreotide has also been reported to ease headache associated with meningioma (above), and pituitary adenoma (see below).

1. Penn RD, *et al.* Intrathecal octreotide for cancer pain. *Lancet* 1990; **335:** 738.
2. Burgess JR, *et al.* Effective control of bone pain by octreotide in a patient with metastatic gastrinoma. *Med J Aust* 1996; **164:** 725–7.
3. Johnson SA, *et al.* Treatment of resistant pain in hypertrophic pulmonary osteoarthropathy with subcutaneous octreotide. *Thorax* 1997; **52:** 298–9.
4. De Conno F, *et al.* Subcutaneous octreotide in the treatment of pain in advanced cancer patients. *J Pain Symptom Manage* 1994; **9:** 34–8.

Pancreatic disorders. Octreotide has been tried in the treatment of acute pancreatitis, but was found to be ineffective.[1] For reference to the use of octreotide in the treatment of pancreatic endocrine tumours, see under Carcinoid Tumours (p.483); for its use in pancreatic fistulae, see Gastrointestinal Disorders, above.

1. Uhl W, *et al.* A randomised, double blind, multicentre trial of octreotide in moderate to severe acute pancreatitis. *Gut* 1999; **45:** 97–104.

Pituitary adenoma. Pituitary adenomas, which may be responsible for conditions such as acromegaly (p.1271), or hyperprolactinaemia (p.1274), may respond to therapy with octreotide by shrinkage of the tumour and an improvement in symptoms such as headaches and visual disturbances or reduction in the secretion of active hormones, or both.

References.

1. Williams G, *et al.* Analgesic effect of somatostatin analogue (octreotide) in headache associated with pituitary tumours. *BMJ* 1987; **295:** 247–8.
2. Orme SM, *et al.* Shrinkage of thyrotrophin secreting pituitary adenoma treated with octreotide. *Postgrad Med J* 1991; **67:** 466–8.

3. Donckier J, *et al.* Shrinkage of inoperable adenomas in cavernous sinus with high-dose octreotide. *Lancet* 1993; **342:** 301.
4. Chanson P, *et al.* Octreotide therapy for thyroid-stimulating hormone-secreting pituitary adenomas: a follow-up of 52 patients. *Ann Intern Med* 1993; **119:** 236–40.
5. Thapar K, *et al.* Antiproliferative effect of the somatostatin analogue octreotide on growth hormone-producing pituitary tumors: results of a multicenter randomized trial. *Mayo Clin Proc* 1997; **72:** 893–900.

Pretibial myxoedema. Pretibial myxoedema (deposition of glycosaminoglycans in the subcutaneous tissue of the shins) is associated with Graves' disease (see Hyperthyroidism, p.1519). There are reports of apparent benefit from the use of octreotide for this condition. In one case,[1] octreotide given for 6 months following surgical removal of the myxoedematous tissue may have prevented its recurrence. In another,[2] octreotide injected intralesionally was reported to improve and control the condition.

1. Derrick EK, *et al.* Successful surgical treatment of severe pretibial myxoedema. *Br J Dermatol* 1995; **133:** 317–18.
2. Shinohara M, *et al.* Refractory pretibial myxoedema with response to intralesional insulin-like growth factor 1 antagonist (octreotide): downregulation of hyaluronic acid production by the lesional fibroblasts. *Br J Dermatol* 2000; **143:** 1083–6.

Raised intracranial pressure. For a reference to octreotide being tried in benign intracranial hypertension, see p.811.

Sleep apnoea. There have been reports of improvement in the severity of sleep apnoea in acromegalic patients treated with octreotide.[1,2]

1. Grunstein RR, *et al.* Effect of octreotide, a somatostatin analog, on sleep apnea in patients with acromegaly. *Ann Intern Med* 1994; **121:** 478–83.
2. Buyse B, *et al.* Relief of sleep apnoea after treatment of acromegaly: report of three cases and review of the literature. *Eur Respir J* 1997; **10:** 1401–4.

Preparations

Proprietary Preparations (details are given in Part 3)
Aust.: Sandostatin; *Austral.:* Sandostatin; *Belg.:* Sandostatine; *Braz.:* Sandostatin; *Canad.:* Sandostatin; *Denm.:* Sandostatin; *Fin.:* Sandostatin; *Fr.:* Sandostatine; *Ger.:* Sandostatin; *Hong Kong:* Sandostatin; *Irl.:* Sandostatin; *Israel:* Sandostatin; *Ital.:* Longastatina; Samilstin; *Mex.:* Sandostatina; *Neth.:* Sandostatine; *Norw.:* Sandostatin; *NZ:* Sandostatin; *Port.:* Sandostatina; *S.Afr.:* Sandostatin; *Singapore:* Sandostatin; *Spain:* Sandostatin; *Swed.:* Sandostatin; *Switz.:* Sandostatine; *Thai.:* Sandostatin; *UK:* Sandostatin; *USA:* Sandostatin.

Ornipressin (5938-I)

Ornipressin (rINN).

[8-Ornithine]-vasopressin.

$C_{45}H_{63}N_{13}O_{12}S_2 = 1042.2.$

CAS — 3397-23-7.

ATC — H01BA05.

Profile

Ornipressin is a synthetic derivative of vasopressin (p.1300) with similar actions. It is reported to be a strong vasoconstrictor with only weak antidiuretic properties and is used to reduce bleeding during surgery. A solution containing up to 5 units in 20 to 60 mL of sodium chloride 0.9% is infiltrated into the area involved. Ornipressin is also used for bleeding oesophageal varices (p.1637). For this purpose it has been given by intravenous infusion: a dose of 20 units over 20 minutes, diluted in 100 mL of sodium chloride 0.9% has been suggested. Continuous infusion over 24 or 48 hours has also been advocated.

◊ References.

1. Kam PC, Tay TM. The pharmacology of ornipressin (POR-8): a local vasoconstrictor used in surgery. *Eur J Anaesthesiol* 1998; **15:** 133–9.
2. De Kock M, *et al.* Ornipressin (Por 8): an efficient alternative to counteract hypotension during combined general/epidural anesthesia. *Anesth Analg* 2000; **90:** 1301–7.

Adverse effects. Acute pulmonary oedema occurred in a patient following infiltration of ornipressin (12 units in 40 mL isotonic saline) as a local vasoconstrictor during surgery.[1] It was suggested that no more than 0.1 unit per kg body-weight should be administered in this manner.

1. Borgeat A, *et al.* Acute pulmonary oedema following administration of ornithine-8-vasopressin. *Br J Anaesth* 1990; **65:** 548–51.

Hepatorenal syndrome. Ornipressin has been found to be of benefit[1-3] in the hepatorenal syndrome, a form of renal insufficiency associated with cirrhosis of the liver, and thought to be due to severe renal vasoconstriction secondary to systemic arterial vasodilatation. However, caution in its use has been urged[2] because of the risk of ischaemic complications.

1. Lenz K, *et al.* Ornipressin in the treatment of functional renal failure in decompensated liver cirrhosis: effects on renal hemodynamics and atrial natriuretic factor. *Gastroenterology* 1991; **101:** 1060–7.
2. Guevara M, *et al.* Reversibility of hepatorenal syndrome by prolonged administration of ornipressin and plasma volume expansion. *Hepatology* 1998; **27:** 35–41.
3. Gülberg V, *et al.* Long-term therapy and retreatment of hepatorenal syndrome type 1 with ornipressin and dopamine. *Hepatology* 1999; **30:** 870–5.

Preparations

Proprietary Preparations (details are given in Part 3)
Aust.: POR 8; *Austral.:* POR 8; *Ger.:* POR 8†; *NZ:* POR 8; *S.Afr.:* POR 8; *Switz.:* POR 8.

Oxytocin (5940-g)

Oxytocin (BAN, rINN).

Alpha-hypophamine; Oxytocinum. Cys-Tyr-Ile-Gln-Asn-Cys-Pro-Leu-Gly-NH$_2$ cyclic (1→6) disulphide; [2-Leucine,7-isoleucine]vasopressin.

$C_{43}H_{66}N_{12}O_{12}S_2 = 1007.2$.

CAS — 50-56-6.

ATC — H01BB02.

Pharmacopoeias. In Chin., Eur. (see p.vi), Jpn, and US, as oxytocin, a bulk solution, a nasal solution, or injection, or more than one of these.

Pharmacopoeial description

Ph. Eur.: Oxytocin is a cyclic nonapeptide having the structure of the hormone produced by the posterior lobe of the pituitary that stimulates contraction of the uterus and milk ejection in receptive mammals. It is obtained by chemical synthesis and is available in the freeze-dried form as an acetate. A white or almost white, hygroscopic powder. Very soluble in water and in dilute solutions of dehydrated alcohol and of acetic acid. A 2% solution in water has a pH of 3.0 to 6.0. Store at 2° to 8° in airtight containers. Protect from light.

Oxytocin Bulk Solution is a solution of oxytocin with a concentration of not less than 250 μg of oxytocin per mL. It may contain a suitable antimicrobial preservative. A clear colourless liquid with a pH of 3.0 to 5.0. Store at 2° to 8°. Protect from light.

USP 25: A nonapeptide hormone having the property of causing the contraction of uterine smooth muscle and of the myoepithelial cells within the mammary glands. It is prepared by synthesis or obtained from the posterior lobe of the pituitary of healthy domestic animals used for food by man. Its oxytocic activity is not less than 400 USP units per mg. Store in airtight containers at 2° to 8°.

Units

12.5 units of oxytocin for bioassay are contained in approximately 21.4 μg of synthetic peptide (with human albumin 5 mg) in one ampoule of the fourth International Standard (1978).

Adverse Effects

Administration of oxytocin in high doses or to those hypersensitive to it may cause violent uterine contractions leading to uterine rupture and extensive laceration of the soft tissues, fetal bradycardia, fetal arrhythmias, and fetal asphyxiation, and perhaps fetal or maternal death.

Maternal deaths from severe hypertension and subarachnoid haemorrhage have occurred. Postpartum haemorrhage and fatal afibrinogenaemia have been reported but may be due to obstetric complications. Water retention leading to hyponatraemia and intoxication, with pulmonary oedema, convulsions, coma, and even death may occur, especially when oxytocin is given intravenously over prolonged periods. Vasopressin-like activity (see p.1300) is more likely to occur with oxytocin of natural origin but may occur even with the synthetic peptide.

Anaphylactic and other hypersensitivity reactions, cardiac arrhythmias, pelvic haematomas, and nausea and vomiting may occur. Rapid intravenous injection has produced acute transient hypotension, together with flushing and reflex tachycardia.

There are reports of neonatal jaundice and retinal haemorrhage associated with the use of oxytocin in the management of labour. Adverse effects following the intranasal administration of oxytocin have included nasal irritation, rhinorrhoea, lachrymation, uterine bleeding, and violent uterine contractions.

◊ In a 1988 comment on the misuse of oxytocin in labour,[1] it was observed that statements on the management of labour were often misinterpreted as meaning that all labouring women who failed to make adequate progress in terms of cervical dilatation should be given oxytocin. This was only true if poor progress was due to poor uterine action, and would be dangerous where there was disproportion; the decision to use oxytocin required careful assessment by an experienced obstetrician. In the previous 2 years the authors had seen one case of fractured pelvis, 2 of ruptured uterus, and 7 of cerebral palsy from fetal hypoxia, all of which were thought to be due to the ill-advised use of oxytocin to augment labour.

For reference to haemorrhage and to neonatal hyperbilirubinaemia occurring after an oxytocin challenge test, see under Uses and Administration, below.

1. Taylor RW, Taylor M. Misuse of oxytocin in labour. Lancet 1988; i: 352.

Neonatal jaundice. Analysis of neonatal jaundice in 12 461 single births confirmed a higher incidence in offspring of mothers given oxytocin, independent of gestational age at birth, sex, race, epidural analgesia, method of delivery, and birth-weight, each of which was also associated with jaundice.[1] In a total of 90 infants born to mothers after oxytocin-induced labour in 2 studies,[2,3] haematological disturbances were noted. These included erythrocyte fragility or reduction in erythrocyte deformability, hyponatraemia, hypo-osmolality, and an increase in serum-bilirubin concentration. Glucose injection, used as a vehicle for oxytocin may have further aggravated these changes.[3]

See also under Oxytocin Challenge Test in Uses and Administration, below.

1. Friedman L, et al. Factors influencing the incidence of neonatal jaundice. BMJ 1978; 1: 1235–7.
2. Buchan PC. Pathogenesis of neonatal hyperbilirubinaemia after induction of labour with oxytocin. BMJ 1979; 2: 1255–7.
3. Singhi S, Singh M. Pathogenesis of oxytocin-induced neonatal hyperbilirubinaemia. Arch Dis Child 1979; 54: 400–2.

Water intoxication. Oxytocin-induced water intoxication is most likely to arise as a result of prolonged attempts to empty the uterus in missed abortion or mid-trimester termination of pregnancy, but it has also been described after oxytocin infusion in other conditions including induction of labour.[1] Irrespective of the oxytocin concentration, patients in virtually all the reported cases have received more than 3.5 litres of infused fluid. Convulsions and somnolence associated with hyponatraemia have also been reported in a patient who was drinking more than 5 litres of herbal tea daily while using intranasal oxytocin 8 times a day or more.[2]

Another factor contributing to hyponatraemia is the antidiuretic effect of the pethidine and morphine commonly used for analgesia with oxytocin infusions. Water intoxication usually presents with fits and loss of consciousness but in some cases there may be preceding signs such as raised venous pressure, bounding pulse, and tachycardia. Diagnosis is confirmed by profound hyponatraemia; the mechanism appears to be more complex than simply haemodilution by the infused water. Treatment consists of controlling convulsions and maintaining an airway; oxytocin infusion should be stopped and isotonic, or even hypertonic, saline may be infused. Diuresis may then be assisted with frusemide [furosemide]. The prime objective, however, should be prevention; no patient should receive more than 3 litres of fluid containing oxytocin, and a careful fluid balance record is essential.[3]

1. Feeney JG. Water intoxication and oxytocin. BMJ 1982; 285: 243.
2. Mayer-Hubner B. Pseudotumour cerebri from intranasal oxytocin and excessive fluid intake. Lancet 1996; 347: 623.

Precautions

Oxytocin should not be given where spontaneous labour or vaginal delivery are liable to harm either the mother or the fetus. This includes significant cephalopelvic disproportion or unfavourable presentation of the fetus, placenta praevia or vasa praevia, cord presentation or prolapse, mechanical obstruction to delivery, fetal distress or hypertonic uterine contractions. It should not be used where there is a predisposition to uterine rupture, as in multiple pregnancy or high parity, polyhydramnios, or the presence of a uterine scar from previous caesarean section. Oxytocin should not be employed for prolonged periods in resistant uterine inertia, severe pre-eclampsia, or severe cardiovascular disorders.

When given for induction or enhancement of labour particular care is needed in borderline cephalopelvic disproportion, less severe degrees of cardiovascular disease, and in patients over 35 years of age or with other risk factors. Careful monitoring of fetal heart rate and uterine motility is essential so that dosage of oxytocin can be adjusted to individual response; the drug should be given by intravenous infusion, preferably by means of a syringe pump. Infusion should be discontinued immediately if fetal distress or uterine hyperactivity occur.

Over-vigorous labour should be avoided in cases of fetal death in utero, or where there is meconium-stained amniotic fluid, because there is a risk of amniotic fluid embolism.

The risk of water intoxication should be borne in mind, particularly when high doses of oxytocin are administered over a long time. Infusion volumes should be kept low, and in such circumstances an electrolyte-based infusion fluid should be used rather than glucose solution. Fluid intake by mouth should be restricted and a fluid balance chart maintained; serum electrolytes should be measured if electrolyte imbalance is suspected.

Oxytocin challenge test. For the suggestion that oxytocin challenge testing should be employed with caution in women whose offspring might be at risk of hyperbilirubinaemia, see under Uses and Administration, below.

Interactions

Oxytocin may enhance the vasopressor effects of sympathomimetics.

Pharmacokinetics

Oxytocin undergoes enzymatic destruction in the gastrointestinal tract but it is rapidly absorbed from the mucous membranes when administered buccally or intranasally. It is metabolised by the liver and kidneys with a plasma half-life of only a few minutes. Only small amounts are excreted unchanged in the urine.

◊ References.

1. Seitchik J, et al. Oxytocin augmentation of dysfunctional labor IV: oxytocin pharmacokinetics. Am J Obstet Gynecol 1984; 150: 225–8.

Uses and Administration

Oxytocin is a cyclic nonapeptide secreted by the hypothalamus and stored in the posterior lobe of the pituitary gland. It may be prepared from the gland of mammals or by synthesis.

Oxytocin causes contraction of the uterus, the effect increasing with the duration of pregnancy due to proliferation of oxytocin receptors. Small doses increase the tone and amplitude of the uterine contractions; large or repeated doses result in tetany. Oxytocin also stimulates the smooth muscle associated with the secretory epithelium of the lactating breast causing the ejection of milk but having no direct effect on milk secretion. It has a weak antidiuretic action.

Oxytocin is used for the induction and augmentation of labour, to control postpartum bleeding and uterine hypotonicity in the third stage of labour, and to promote lactation in cases of faulty milk ejection. It is also used in missed abortions, but other measures may be preferred.

For the **induction** or **augmentation of labour** oxytocin may be given by slow intravenous infusion preferably by means of an infusion pump. A solution containing 5 units in 500 mL of a physiological electrolyte solution such as sodium chloride 0.9% has been recommended but more concentrated solutions may be given via infusion pump, and current UK guidelines suggest 10 or 30 units in 500 mL of diluent. Infusion is begun at a recommended initial rate of 1 to 2 milliunits per minute and then gradually increased at intervals of at least 30 minutes, until a maximum of 3 or 4 contractions are occurring every 10 minutes. A rate of up to 6 milliunits per minute is reported to produce plasma oxytocin concentrations comparable to those in natural labour, and 12 milliunits per minute is usually the most that is needed but doses of up to 20 milliunits or more per minute may be required. UK guidelines suggest that 32 milliunits per minute should not be exceeded, and no more than a total of 5 units should be given in 1 day. Fetal heart rate and uterine contractions should be monitored continuously. Once labour is progressing, oxytocin infusion may be gradually withdrawn.

For the treatment and prevention of **postpartum haemorrhage** oxytocin may be given by slow intravenous injection in a dose of 5 units; this may be followed in severe cases by intravenous infusion of 5 to 20 units (the British National Formulary suggests up to 30 units) in 500 mL of a suitable non-hydrating diluent. An alternative for the prophylaxis of postpartum haemorrhage in the routine management of the third stage of labour is the intramuscular injection of oxytocin 5 units with ergometrine maleate 500 μg with or after delivery of the baby's shoulders. In the USA a dose of 10 units of oxytocin, by intravenous infusion at a rate of 20 to 40 milliunits per minute, or as an intramuscular injection, has been recommended for treatment of postpartum haemorrhage.

In **missed abortion** a suggested dose in the UK is 5 units by slow intravenous injection, followed if necessary by intravenous infusion at a rate of 20 to 40 milliunits per minute or higher.

Oxytocin nasal spray is used to facilitate **lactation**; the usual dose is one spray into one or both nostrils 2 to 3 minutes before suckling. However, there is a danger that the mother may become dependent upon its action and such usage is not generally recommended (see p.1276).

Oxytocin citrate has been given in the form of a buccal tablet to induce labour; however, absorption is irregular following buccal administration and this route has been superseded by intravenous infusion.

An **oxytocin challenge test** has been used to evaluate fetal distress in pregnant patients at high-risk.

Synthetic derivatives of oxytocin such as demoxytocin (see p.1281) have been used similarly.

Labour induction and augmentation. Oxytocin infusions have proved to be one of the most successful agents for induction and augmentation of labour, as discussed on p.1438. There have been numerous studies on the dosage of oxytocin required to induce or augment labour,[1-9] which increasingly favour low-dose regimens, starting at infusion rates of 1 milliunit per minute or less. UK guidelines favour a starting dose of 1 to 2 milliunits per minute, increased at intervals of 30 minutes, and titrated against contractions.[10] However, it has been pointed out that no one regimen has been clearly proved superior.[11]

1. Seitchik J, Castillo M. Oxytocin augmentation of dysfunctional labor I: clinical data. *Am J Obstet Gynecol* 1982; **144:** 899–905.
2. Seitchik J, Castillo M. Oxytocin augmentation of dysfunctional labor III: multiparous patients. *Am J Obstet Gynecol* 1983; **145:** 777–80.
3. Seitchik J, *et al.* Oxytocin augmentation of dysfunctional labor V: an alternative oxytocin regimen. *Am J Obstet Gynecol* 1985; **151:** 757–61.
4. Wein P. Efficacy of different starting doses of oxytocin for induction of labor. *Obstet Gynecol* 1989; **74:** 863–8.
5. Blakemore KJ, *et al.* A prospective comparison of hourly and quarter-hourly oxytocin dose increase intervals for the induction of labor at term. *Obstet Gynecol* 1990; **75:** 757–61.
6. Mercer B, *et al.* Labor induction with continuous low-dose oxytocin infusion: a randomized trial. *Obstet Gynecol* 1991; **77:** 659–63.
7. Akoury HA, *et al.* Oxytocin augmentation of labour and perinatal outcome in nulliparas. *Obstet Gynecol* 1991; **78:** 227–30.
8. Satin AJ, *et al.* High versus low-dose oxytocin for labor stimulation. *Obstet Gynecol* 1992; **80:** 111–16.
9. Merrill DC, Zlatnik FJ. Randomized, double-masked comparison of oxytocin dosage in induction and augmentation of labor. *Obstet Gynecol* 1999; **94:** 455–63.
10. Royal College of Obstetricians and Gynaecologists. Induction of labour: evidence-based clinical guideline number 9 (issued June 2001). Available at: http://www.nice.org.uk/pdf/inductionoflabourrcogrep.pdf (accessed 12/09/01).
11. Xenakis EM-J, Piper JM. Chemotherapeutic induction of labour: a rational approach. *Drugs* 1997; **54:** 61–8.

Oxytocin challenge test. The oxytocin challenge test (OCT) is designed to detect placental insufficiency, and identify fetuses at risk of still-birth or complications during labour. In a study, it was performed on 399 occasions in 305 women with pregnancies at risk and a gestational age of 36 weeks or more.[1] Oxytocin 1 milliunit per minute was given by infusion pump and increased every 5 to 10 minutes until a contraction rate of 3 per 10 minutes was achieved. Less than 10% of late or variable decelerations of fetal heart rate (FHR) was judged negative; 10 to 29% was judged equivocal; and 30% or more was judged positive. The finding of a positive or equivocal response to the OCT was considered a prediction of decelerations of the FHR during parturition, though the type of risk might vary. After 100 OCTs in 90 pregnant women considered at risk[2] it was concluded that a negative result is a reliable test of fetal wellbeing which should encourage obstetricians to await spontaneous onset of labour in preference to intervention. However, there have been reports of fetal death occurring despite a negative response to the OCT.[3-5] Adverse effects associated with the OCT have included haemorrhage occurring in a patient after the second of two tests (the patient was found to have a major placenta praevia)[6] and neonatal hyperbilirubinaemia.[7] The latter effect led to the suggestion that the OCT should be used with caution in women whose babies might be at risk from hyperbilirubinaemia.

1. Schulman H, *et al.* Quantitative analysis in the oxytocin challenge test. *Am J Obstet Gynecol* 1977; **129:** 239–44.
2. Sellappah S, Wagman H. Oxytocin challenge test as an out patient procedure. *Br J Clin Pract* 1984; **38:** 255–8.
3. Marcum RG. False negative oxytocin challenge test. *Am J Obstet Gynecol* 1977; **127:** 894.
4. Lorenz RP, Pagano JS. A case of intrauterine fetal death after a negative oxytocin challenge test. *Am J Obstet Gynecol* 1978; **130:** 232.
5. Dittman R, Belcher J. False-negative oxytocin challenge test. *N Engl J Med* 1978; **298:** 56.
6. Ng KH, Wong WP. Risk of haemorrhage in oxytocin stress test. *BMJ* 1976; **2:** 698–9.
7. Peleg D, Goldman JA. Oxytocin challenge test and neonatal hyperbilirubinaemia. *Lancet* 1976; **ii:** 1026.

Postpartum haemorrhage. Oxytocin is used for the prophylaxis and treatment of postpartum haemorrhage (p.1607). In the active management of the third stage of labour, the combination of oxytocin and ergometrine may be associated with a small reduction in the risk of postpartum haemorrhage com-

The symbol † denotes a preparation no longer actively marketed

pared with oxytocin alone, but a higher incidence of nausea, vomiting, and hypertension.

Retained placenta. Oxytocin injected into the vein of the umbilical cord has been used to assist the removal of retained placenta. A meta-analysis[1] of 12 studies found evidence that oxytocin reduced the incidence of manual removal of the retained placenta, although there was no apparent benefit in terms of other measures including blood loss, curettage, and infection. The removal of the placenta is important to allow contraction of the myometrium and prevention of excessive blood loss, and is one reason for the use of oxytocin in the active management of the third stage of labour, as discussed under Postpartum Haemorrhage—see above and on p.1607.

1. Carroli G, Bergel E. Umbilical vein injection for management of retained placenta (updated 25 May 2000). Available in The Cochrane Library; Issue 3. Oxford: Update Software; 2001.

Preparations

BP 2001: Ergometrine and Oxytocin Injection; Oxytocin Injection;
USP 25: Oxytocin Injection; Oxytocin Nasal Solution.

Proprietary Preparations (details are given in Part 3)
Aust.: Pitocin†; Syntocinon; **Austral.:** Syntocinon; **Belg.:** Syntocinon; **Braz.:** Orastina; Syntocinon; **Denm.:** Syntocinon; **Fin.:** Syntocinon; **Fr.:** Syntocinon; **Ger.:** Orasthin; Syntocinon; **Hong Kong:** Syntocinon; **Irl.:** Syntocinon; **Israel:** Partocon; Syntocinon; **Ital.:** Syntocinon; **Mex.:** Oxitopisa; Syntocinon; Xitocin; **Neth.:** Piton-S†; Syntocinon; **Norw.:** Pitocin; Syntocinon; **NZ:** Syntocinon; **Port.:** Syntocinon; **S.Afr.:** Syntocinon; **Singapore:** Syntocinon; **Spain:** Syntocinon; **Swed.:** Partocon†; Syntocinon; **Switz.:** Syntocinon; **Thai.:** Syntocinon; **UK:** Syntocinon; **USA:** Pitocin; Syntocinon†.

Multi-ingredient: Austral.: Syntometrine; **Ger.:** Syntometrin; **Hong Kong:** Syntometrine; **Irl.:** Syntometrine; **Israel:** Syntometrine; **NZ:** Syntometrine; **S.Afr.:** Syntometrine; **UK:** Syntometrine.

Pegvisomant (10744-n)

Pegvisomant *(USAN, rINN)*.
B2036-PEG.

Profile
Pegvisomant is a growth hormone-receptor antagonist. It is under investigation for the treatment of acromegaly.

◊ References.

1. Trainer PJ, *et al.* Treatment of acromegaly with the growth hormone-receptor antagonist pegvisomant. *N Engl J Med* 2000; **342:** 1171–7.
2. Herman-Bonert VS, *et al.* Growth hormone receptor antagonist therapy in acromegalic patients resistant to somatostatin analogs. *J Clin Endocrinol Metab* 2000; **85:** 2958–61.
3. van der Lely AJ, *et al.* Control of tumor size and disease activity during cotreatment with octreotide and the growth hormone receptor antagonist pegvisomant in an acromegalic patient. *J Clin Endocrinol Metab* 2001; **86:** 478–81.

Posatirelin (10389-r)

Posatirelin *(rINN)*.
(2S)-N-[(1S)-1-[[(2S)-2-Carbamoyl-1-pyrrolidinyl]carbonyl]-3-methylbutyl]-6-oxopipecolamide.
$C_{17}H_{28}N_4O_4 = 352.4$.
CAS — 78664-73-0.

Profile
Posatirelin is an analogue of protirelin (p.1295). It is claimed to have beneficial effects on CNS function, and has been investigated in the management of dementia of various causes.

◊ References.

1. Parnetti L, *et al.* Posatirelin for the treatment of late-onset Alzheimer's disease: a double-blind multicentre study vs citicoline and ascorbic acid. *Acta Neurol Scand* 1995; **92:** 135–40.
2. Parnetti L, *et al.* Posatirelin in the treatment of vascular dementia: a double-blind multicentre study vs placebo. *Acta Neurol Scand* 1996; **93:** 456–63.
3. Reboldi G, *et al.* Pharmacokinetic profile and endocrine effects of posatirelin treatment in healthy elderly subjects. *J Clin Pharmacol* 1996; **36:** 823–31.

Powdered Pituitary (Posterior Lobe) (5943-s)

Hypophysis Cerebri Pars Posterior; Hypophysis Sicca; Ipofisi Posteriore; Pituitarium Posterius Pulveratum; Pituitary; Posterior Pituitary.

NOTE. Pituitary Extract (Posterior) is *BAN*.

Pharmacopoeias. In *Aust.* which specifies not less than 1 unit of oxytocic activity per mg.

A preparation from the posterior lobes of mammalian pituitary bodies.

Adverse Effects, Treatment, and Precautions
Similar to those for oxytocin (p.1294) and for vasopressin (p.1300). Hypersensitivity reactions, including anaphylaxis, have occasionally been reported.

Uses and Administration
Powdered pituitary (posterior lobe) has oxytocic, pressor, antidiuretic, and hyperglycaemic actions and has generally been

replaced by compounds or preparations with more specific actions such as oxytocin (p.1294) and desmopressin (p.1282).

It has been included as an ingredient of a number of preparations of combined tissue extracts promoted as tonics or for a variety of non-endocrine disorders.

Preparations
Proprietary Preparations (details are given in Part 3)
Spain: Acetuber†.

Prolactin (5944-w)

Galactin; Lactogen; Lactogenic Hormone; Lactotropin; LMTH; LTH; Luteomammotropic Hormone; Luteotrophic Hormone; Luteotropin; Mammotropin.
CAS — 9002-62-4; 12585-34-1 (sheep); 56832-36-1 (ox); 9046-05-3 (pig).

Profile
Prolactin is a water-soluble protein from the anterior pituitary; it is structurally related to growth hormone (p.1286). In *animals*, prolactin has a wide variety of actions and is involved in reproduction, parental care, feeding of the young, electrolyte balance, and growth and development. In humans it has a definite role in inducing milk production; oxytocin (p.1294) stimulates milk ejection. Relatively high concentrations of prolactin have been found in amniotic fluid. Placental lactogen has been shown to have prolactin-like activity. Prolactin secretion is stimulated by suckling and, for a few months after delivery, it has an inhibitory effect on the ovaries, acting as a natural contraceptive.

The hypothalamus can both stimulate and inhibit prolactin secretion by the anterior pituitary; the inhibitory influence is predominant and is mediated through a dopaminergic system. Dopamine binds to the lactotrope D_2 receptor to inhibit prolactin synthesis and release. Noradrenaline and gamma-aminobutyric acid are also inhibitory as are dopaminergic drugs such as bromocriptine. Although protirelin (below) has prolactin-releasing activity, there is evidence for the existence of a separate hypothalamic releasing factor (PRF). Prolactin secretion may also be stimulated by methyldopa, metoclopramide, reserpine, opioid analgesics, and phenothiazine or butyrophenone antipsychotics.

Hyperprolactinaemia, which is associated with a variety of other endocrine disorders, is discussed on p.1274.

Prolactin has been given by intramuscular injection in the management of lactation disorders and some forms of menstrual disturbance.

Protirelin (5945-e)

Protirelin *(BAN, USAN, rINN)*.
Abbott-38579; Lopremone; Protirelinum; Synthetic TRH; Thyrotrophin-releasing Hormone; Thyrotropin-releasing Hormone; TRF; TRH. L-Pyroglutamyl-L-histidyl-L-prolinamide; 1-[N-(5-Oxo-L-prolyl)-L-histidyl]-L-prolinamide; Glu-His-Pro-NH₂.
$C_{16}H_{22}N_6O_4 = 362.4$.
CAS — 24305-27-9.
ATC — V04CJ02.

Pharmacopoeias. In *Eur.* (see p.vi) and *Jpn*, which also includes the tartrate.

Pharmacopoeial description
Ph. Eur.: A synthetic tripeptide with the same sequence of amino acids as the natural hypothalamic neurohormone, that stimulates the release and synthesis of thyrotrophin. A white or yellowish-white hygroscopic powder. Very soluble in water; freely soluble in methyl alcohol. Store at a temperature of 2° to 8°. Protect from light and moisture.

Adverse Effects
Protirelin given by intravenous injection may cause headache, nausea, a desire to micturate, flushing, dizziness, and a strange taste. These effects have been attributed to contraction of smooth muscles by the bolus injection. Hypertension and an increased pulse rate, or hypotension, have occasionally been reported as have a few cases of amaurosis and convulsions.

Amaurosis. Of 4 patients with pituitary tumours who developed severe headache after protirelin injection, one also developed amaurosis, apparently associated with pituitary apoplexy.[1] Visual acuity improved after surgery.

1. Drury PL, *et al.* Transient amaurosis and headache after thyrotropin releasing hormone. *Lancet* 1982; **i:** 218–19.

Effects on the cardiovascular system. Increased blood pressure has been reported in women given protirelin antenatally,[1,2] and the view has been expressed that although the magnitude of the change is unlikely to be clinically significant in normotensive women, a much greater rise seen in pre-eclamptic women was severe enough to increase the risk of cerebral haemorrhage.[2]

1. ACTOBAT Study Group. Australian collaborative trial of antenatal thyrotropin-releasing hormone (ACTOBAT) for prevention of neonatal respiratory disease. *Lancet* 1995; **345:** 877–82.
2. Peek MJ, *et al.* Hypertensive effect of antenatal thyrotropin-releasing hormone in pre-eclampsia. *Lancet* 1995; **345:** 793. Correction. *ibid.*; 1124.

Effects on the CNS. Adverse effects reported following injection of 400 μg of protirelin included unconsciousness, hypotension, and convulsions.[1] In another patient with a history of convulsions, injection of 500 μg of protirelin induced epileptic seizures.[2]

1. Dolva LØ, *et al.* Side effects of thyrotropin releasing hormone. *BMJ* 1983; **287:** 532.
2. Maeda K, Tanimoto K. Epileptic seizures induced by thyrotropin releasing hormone. *Lancet* 1981; **i:** 1058–9.

Effects on the respiratory system. A report of bronchospasm in an asthmatic boy given protirelin intravenously.[1]
For the suggestion that protirelin may provoke bronchospasm in patients with motor neurone disease, see under Precautions, below.

1. McFadden RG, *et al.* TRH and bronchospasm. *Lancet* 1981; **ii:** 758–9.

Effect on sexual function. On questioning, 7 of 16 women reported a sensation of mild vaginal sexual arousal occurring 1 to 3 minutes after intravenous injection of protirelin.[1] Four women also experienced urinary sensations, and 3 described an urge to urinate with no sexual component.

1. Blum M, Pulini M. Vaginal sensations after injection of thyrotropin releasing hormone. *Lancet* 1980; **ii:** 43.

Pituitary apoplexy. A report of pituitary apoplexy following combined testing of anterior pituitary function in a patient with a pituitary tumour.[1] Of the drugs given, protirelin was thought most likely to have an aetiological role.
See also Amaurosis, above.

1. Chapman AJ, *et al.* Pituitary apoplexy after combined test of anterior pituitary function. *BMJ* 1985; **291:** 26.

Precautions

Protirelin should be given with care to patients with ischaemic heart disease, obstructive airways disease, or severe hypopituitarism. Administration of protirelin while the patient is lying down may reduce the incidence of hypotension.

Eclampsia. For the suggestion that the hypertensive effects of protirelin increase the risk of cerebral haemorrhage in pre-eclamptic women, see Effects on the Cardiovascular System under Adverse Effects, above.

Motor neurone disease. In some patients with amyotrophic lateral sclerosis intravenous injection of protirelin resulted in acute bronchospasm.[1] Five of 25 patients experienced falls in FEV_1 of more than 20%; in 2, a 15% decrease in arterial-oxygen pressure occurred. Patients with sclerosis and weakened respiratory muscles should be warned of this potential side-effect.

1. Braun SR, *et al.* Pulmonary effects of thyrotropin-releasing hormone in amyotrophic lateral sclerosis. *Lancet* 1984; **ii** 529–30.

Interactions

◊ Drugs influencing the response to protirelin have been reviewed.[1] The secretion of thyrotrophin appears to be modulated by dopaminergic and noradrenergic pathways at both the hypothalamic and pituitary level. Dopamine and bromocriptine have depressed the response to protirelin; levodopa is a powerful depressant. Partial depression has been reported after the administration of chlorpromazine, thioridazine, and phentolamine, all of which have alpha-receptor blocking properties. Beta-receptors do not appear to be involved in the thyrotrophin response to protirelin whereas the antiserotonin drug, cyproheptadine, has an inhibitory effect. Aspirin and corticosteroids with predominantly glucocorticoid activity have also depressed the response. An enhanced response to protirelin has been seen after the administration of theophylline. Oestrogens may also increase the response in men but not usually in women; when combined with a progestogen a slightly depressed response has been reported.
Other drugs reported to depress the response to protirelin include lithium[2] and ranitidine.[3]

1. Lamberg B-A, Gordin A. Abnormalities of thyrotrophin secretion and clinical implications of the thyrotrophin releasing hormone stimulation test. *Ann Clin Res* 1978; **10:** 171–83.
2. Lauridsen UB, *et al.* Lithium and the pituitary-thyroid axis in normal subjects. *J Clin Endocrinol Metab* 1974; **39:** 383–5.
3. Tarditi E, *et al.* Impaired TSH response to TRH after intravenous ranitidine in man. *Experientia* 1983; **39:** 109–10.

Uses and Administration

Protirelin is a hypothalamic releasing hormone which stimulates the release of thyrotrophin (p.1298) from the anterior lobe of the pituitary. It also has prolactin-releasing activity. It may be obtained by synthesis.

Protirelin may be used in the assessment of the hypothalamic-pituitary-thyroid axis in the diagnosis of mild hyperthyroidism (p.1519) or hypothyroidism (p.1520), and ophthalmic Graves' disease, although in many cases immunoassays for thyroid-stimulating hormone are now preferred. The response to protirelin may be used for differentiating between primary and secondary hypothyroidism but care is required in interpreting the results of the test and it should not be used alone in establishing the diagnosis. Protirelin is given with gonadorelin (p.1284) in the assessment of anterior pituitary function.

Protirelin is given intravenously usually in doses of 200 to 500 μg. A suggested intravenous dose in children is 1 μg per kg body-weight in the UK, but in the USA a dose of 7 μg per kg has been recommended.

Protirelin has been investigated in the treatment of neurological diseases, and in the prevention of neonatal respiratory distress syndrome, but results have been variable.

Protirelin tartrate has been given in the treatment of neurological disorders.

Lactation induction. Intranasal protirelin has been tried for stimulation of lactation (p.1276) but there is no suitable commercial preparation, and in any case mechanical stimulation is preferable to drug treatment.

Neonatal respiratory distress syndrome. The regulation of fetal lung development is under multihormonal control and thyroid hormones appear to stimulate pulmonary maturation. However, the thyroid hormones and thyrotrophin do not cross the placenta sufficiently for them to be employed for prenatal treatment in premature labour where neonatal respiratory distress syndrome (p.1055) may develop, and therefore therapy with protirelin has been investigated.[1] Protirelin has been given with corticosteroids to the mother and some beneficial effects have been noted.[1] One study using protirelin 400 μg every 8 hours for 4 doses indicated that antenatal protirelin reduced the incidence of chronic lung disease when given with corticosteroids but did not affect the incidence of respiratory distress syndrome.[2] However, 2 large multicentre studies had found that addition of protirelin to corticosteroid treatment had no beneficial effects on outcome compared with corticosteroids only;[3,4] in fact, in the earlier of these studies,[3] respiratory distress syndrome and the need for ventilation were greater in the offspring of mothers given protirelin. Subsequent follow-up appeared to confirm the disadvantages of protirelin in this cohort;[5] however the unexpected conclusions of this study aroused some controversy.[6-8] The second study noted no difference in outcome in the 2 groups of infants.[4]

1. de Zegher F, *et al.* Prenatal treatment with thyrotrophin releasing hormone to prevent neonatal respiratory distress. *Arch Dis Child* 1992; **67:** 450–4.
2. Ballard RA, *et al.* Respiratory disease in very-low-birthweight infants after prenatal thyrotropin-releasing hormone and glucocorticoid. *Lancet* 1992; **339:** 510–5.
3. ACTOBAT Study Group. Australian collaborative trial of antenatal thyrotropin-releasing hormone (ACTOBAT) for prevention of neonatal respiratory disease. *Lancet* 1995; **345:** 877–82.
4. Ballard RA, *et al.* Antenatal thyrotropin-releasing hormone to prevent lung disease in preterm infants. *N Engl J Med* 1998; **338:** 493–8.
5. Crowther CA, *et al.* Australian collaborative trial of antenatal thyrotropin-releasing hormone: adverse effects at 12-month follow-up. *Pediatrics* 1997; **99:** 311–17.
6. Ballard RA, *et al.* Thyrotropin-releasing hormone for prevention of neonatal respiratory disease. *Lancet* 1995; **345:** 1572.
7. Moya FR, Maturana A. Thyrotropin-releasing hormone for prevention of neonatal respiratory disease. *Lancet* 1995; **345:** 1572–3.
8. McCormick MC. The credibility of the ACTOBAT follow-up study. *Pediatrics* 1997; **99:** 476–8.

Neurological disorders. Reports of the use of protirelin in various neurological disorders.

1. Bonuccelli U, *et al.* Oral thyrotropin-releasing hormone treatment in inherited ataxias. *Clin Neuropharmacol* 1988; **11:** 520–8.
2. Filla A, *et al.* Sperimentazione cronica del TRH per via intramuscolare nelle degenerazioni spino-cerebellari: studio in doppio cieco cross-over su 30 soggetti. *Riv Neurol* 1989; **59:** 83–8.
3. Mellow AM, *et al.* A peptide enhancement strategy in Alzheimer's disease: pilot study with TRH-physostigmine infusions. *Biol Psychiatry* 1993; **34:** 271–3.
4. Tanaka C, *et al.* Successful treatment of progressive myoclonus epilepsy with TRH. *Pediatr Neurol* 1998; **18:** 442–4.
5. Chemaly R, *et al.* Myélinolyse extra-pontine: traitement par T.R.H. *Rev Neurol (Paris)* 1998; **154:** 163–5.

Preparations

Proprietary Preparations (details are given in Part 3)
Aust.: Antepan; Relefact TRH; **Belg.:** TRH; **Canad.:** Relefact TRH; **Denm.:** Thyrefact; **Fr.:** Stimu-TSH; **Ger.:** Antepan; Relefact TRH; Thyroliberin; TRH; **Israel:** Relefact TRH; TRH; **Ital.:** Irtonin; Xantium; **Jpn:** Hirtonin; **Neth.:** Relefact TRH; **Spain:** TRH Prem; **Swed.:** Thyrefact; **Switz.:** Relefact TRH; **UK:** TRH; **USA:** Thypinone; Thyrel-TRH.

Somatomedins (16990-k)

IGFs; Insulin-like Growth Factors; Sulphation Factors.

A group of polypeptide hormones related to insulin and usually known individually as insulin-like growth factors (IGFs), with molecular weights of about 7000 to 8000. They are synthesised in the liver, kidney, muscle, and other tissues.

Mecasermin (15906-x)

Mecasermin *(BAN, USAN, rINN)*.
CEP-151; IGF-I; Insulin-like growth factor I (human); rhIGF-1; Somatomedin C.
$C_{331}H_{512}N_{94}O_{101}S_7 = 7648.6$.
CAS — 68562-41-4; 67763-96-6.
ATC — H01AC03.

Units

150 000 units of insulin-like growth factor I are contained in one ampoule of the first International Standard (1994). For practical purposes 1 international unit can be assumed to be equivalent to 1 μg of insulin-like growth factor I.

Adverse Effects

Since the somatomedins are considered to be responsible for many of the actions of growth hormone similar adverse effects (see p.1286) might be expected.

◊ Syncope in the absence of hypoglycaemia has been reported in patients receiving mecasermin by intravenous bolus, accompanied in some cases by convulsions, asystole, bradycardia, hypotension, or dizziness.[1] Reports appear to have ceased since recommendations that mecasermin should not be given intravenously at rates greater than 24 μg per kg body-weight per hour. In addition, mid- and long-term effects of treatment have resulted in adverse effects similar to those associated with growth hormone therapy, including benign intracranial hypertension, gynaecomastia, and acromegalic changes of the features.[1] Arthralgia, nerve palsies, and hypophosphataemia and dyspnoea have been associated with high-dose intravenous bolus therapy.[2]
For a reference to benign intracranial hypertension associated with mecasermin therapy, see under Growth Hormone, p.1286. For concerns about an increased risk of retinopathy in diabetic patients receiving mecasermin, see under Diabetes Mellitus, below.

1. Malozowski S, Stadel B. Risks and benefits of insulin-like growth factor. *Ann Intern Med* 1994; **121:** 549.
2. Usala A-L. Risks and benefits of insulin-like growth factor. *Ann Intern Med* 1994; **121:** 550.

Uses and Administration

The somatomedins are a group of polypeptide hormones, some of which are involved in mediating the effects of growth hormone in the body. IGF-I (mecasermin) is believed to be responsible for many of the anabolic effects of growth hormone. It is secreted primarily by the liver, regulated principally by growth hormone and insulin secretion; IGF-I may also be secreted in other tissues, where it may exert local hormonal (paracrine) effects. In the circulation, IGF-I is almost completely protein bound; 6 binding proteins have been identified, production of some of which is also under the control of growth hormone. In addition to its anabolic effects IGF-I, which is structurally related to insulin, also has potent hypoglycaemic properties.

IGF-I is available as mecasermin, a product of recombinant DNA technology. It has been used in the treatment of children with Laron-type dwarfism, in whom an abnormality of the growth hormone receptor results in an inability to secrete endogenous IGF-I. Long-term administration (several months) with a dose of 150 μg per kg body-weight daily by subcutaneous injection has been reported to produce significant improvement in linear growth in children with this condition. It has also been given to children with growth-attenuating antibodies to growth hormone.

Mecasermin is also being investigated in the management of diabetes mellitus and insulin resistance and is being tried in various other disorders including motor neurone disease, osteoporosis, cachexia, and some peripheral neuropathies.

IGF-II is thought to play an important role in fetal growth, although its function in adults is uncertain. It is closely related in structure to IGF-I, but is not under the control of growth hormone.

◊ General reviews.
1. Laron Z. Somatomedin-1 (insulin-like growth factor-I) in clinical use: facts and potential. *Drugs* 1993; **45:** 1–8.
2. Bondy CA, *et al.* Clinical uses of insulin-like growth factor I. *Ann Intern Med* 1994; **124:** 593–601.
3. Le Roith D. Insulin-like growth factors. *N Engl J Med* 1997; **336:** 633–40.

Diabetes mellitus. There has been considerable interest in the therapeutic potential of mecasermin in diabetes mellitus;[1,2] in particular, several reports and small studies have suggested it can improve insulin sensitivity in patients with insulin resistance.[3-7] Randomised studies[8,9] have found that mecasermin 40 μg per kg body-weight daily by subcutaneous injection improves metabolic control in the short term when added to insulin therapy in patients with type 1 diabetes. Although there was no evidence of an increase in diabetic complications in these studies the known proliferative effects of mecasermin have raised concern about a possibly increased risk of diabetic retinopathy;[10] some studies have been halted because of this possibility.

For a general discussion of diabetes mellitus and its management, see p.315.

1. Kolaczynski JW, Caro JF. Insulin-like growth factor-1 therapy in diabetes: physiologic basis, clinical benefits, and risks. *Ann Intern Med* 1994; **120:** 47–55.
2. Dunger DB. Insulin and insulin-like growth factors in diabetes. *Arch Dis Child* 1995; **72:** 469–71.
3. Usala A-L, *et al.* Brief report: treatment of insulin-resistant diabetic ketoacidosis with insulin-like growth factor I in an adolescent with insulin-dependent diabetes. *N Engl J Med* 1992; **327:** 853–7.
4. Hussain MA, Froesch ER. Treatment of type A insulin resistance with insulin-like growth factor-I. *Lancet* 1993; **341:** 1536–7.
5. Ishihara H, *et al.* Long term follow up in type A insulin resistant syndrome treated with insulin-like growth factor I. *Arch Dis Child* 1994; **71:** 144–6.
6. Moses AC, *et al.* Insulin-like growth factor I (rhIGF-I) as a therapeutic agent for hyperinsulinemic insulin-resistant diabetes mellitus. *Diabetes Res Clin Pract* 1995; **28** (suppl): 185–94.
7. Hirano T, Adachi M. Insulin-like growth factor 1 therapy for type B insulin resistance. *Ann Intern Med* 1997; **127:** 245–6.
8. Acerini CL, *et al.* Randomised placebo-controlled trial of human recombinant insulin-like growth factor I plus intensive insulin therapy in adolescents with insulin-dependent diabetes. *Lancet* 1997; **350:** 1199–1204.
9. Thrailkill KM, *et al.* Cotherapy with recombinant human insulin-like growth factor I and insulin improves glycemic control in type 1 diabetes. *Diabetes Care* 1999; **22:** 585–92.
10. Møller N, Ørskov H. Does IGF-I therapy in insulin-dependent diabetes mellitus limit complications? *Lancet* 1997; **350:** 1188–9.

Growth retardation. References[1,2] to the use of mecasermin in patients with Laron-type dwarfism (growth hormone resistance). For a discussion of growth retardation and its management see p.1273.
1. Laron Z, *et al.* Effect of acute administration of insulin-like growth factor I in patients with Laron-type dwarfism. *Lancet* 1988; **ii:** 1170–72.
2. Laron Z, *et al.* Effects of insulin-like growth factor on linear growth, head circumference, and body fat in patients with Laron-type dwarfism. *Lancet* 1992; **339:** 1258–61.

Motor neurone disease. Mecasermin is under investigation for the management of amyotrophic lateral sclerosis,[1] a form of motor neurone disease (p.1658).
1. Lai EC, *et al.* Effect of recombinant human insulin-like growth factor-1 on progression of ALS: a placebo-controlled study. *Neurology* 1997; **49:** 1621–30.

Osteoporosis. Mecasermin has been investigated as a stimulant of bone formation in osteoporosis (p.745).
References.
1. Ebeling PR, *et al.* Short-term effects of recombinant human insulin-like growth factor I on bone turnover in normal women. *J Clin Endocrinol Metab* 1993; **77:** 1384–7.
2. Rubin CG, *et al.* Treating a patient with the Werner syndrome and osteoporosis using recombinant human insulin-like growth factor. *Ann Intern Med* 1994; **121:** 655–8.
3. Boonen S, *et al.* The prevention or treatment of age-related osteoporosis in the elderly by systemic recombinant growth factor therapy (rhIGF-I or rhTGF beta): a perspective. *J Intern Med* 1997; **242:** 285–90.

Somatorelin (3765-j)

Somatorelin (rINN).
GHRF; GHRH; GRF; GRF-44; Growth Hormone-releasing Factor (Human); Growth Hormone-releasing Hormone; Somatoliberin.
$C_{215}H_{358}N_{72}O_{66}S = 5039.7$.
CAS — 83930-13-6.
ATC — V04CD05.

Sermorelin Acetate (2499-b)

Sermorelin Acetate (BANM, USAN, rINNM).
GRF(1-29)NH₂; Growth hormone-releasing factor (human)-(1-29)-peptide amide. Tyr-Ala-Asp-Ala-Ile-Phe-Thr-Asn-Ser-Tyr-Arg-Lys-Val-Leu-Gly-Gln-Leu-Ser-Ala-Arg-Lys-Leu-Leu-Gln-Asp-Ile-Met-Ser-Arg-NH₂ acetate hydrate.
$C_{149}H_{246}N_{44}O_{42}S.xC_2H_4O_2.yH_2O = 3357.9$ (sermorelin).
CAS — 86168-78-7 (sermorelin); 114466-38-5 (sermorelin acetate).

The symbol † denotes a preparation no longer actively marketed

Adverse Effects and Precautions

Facial flushing and pain at the injection site may occur after injection of sermorelin acetate. Headache, nausea and vomiting, dysgeusia, and tightness in the chest have also been reported. Antibodies to somatorelin may develop on repeated administration.

Sermorelin should be used with care in patients with epilepsy or diabetes mellitus. Sermorelin should not be used to treat growth retardation in children in whom the growth hormone response to stimulation tests is inadequate. Treatment should cease once the epiphyses have closed. Uncontrolled hypothyroidism may impair response to sermorelin.

Uses and Administration

Somatorelin is a peptide secreted by the hypothalamus which promotes the release of growth hormone from the anterior pituitary. It exists in 44-, 40-, and 37-amino-acid peptides; the 44-amino acid form may possibly be converted to the smaller forms but all are reported to be active, the activity residing in the first 29 amino-acid residues. Sermorelin is a synthetic peptide corresponding to the 1–29 amino acid sequence of somatorelin.

Sermorelin is used in the form of the acetate for the diagnosis of growth hormone deficiency. The usual dose is the equivalent of sermorelin 1 μg per kg body-weight by intravenous injection in the morning following an overnight fast. A normal response to sermorelin indicates that the somatotrophs are functional, but does not exclude growth hormone deficiency due to hypothalamic dysfunction; to establish a diagnosis it must be used in conjunction with other tests.

Sermorelin is also used for the treatment of growth hormone deficiency in children; doses equivalent to 30 μg per kg, as the acetate, may be given once daily at bedtime by subcutaneous injection.

Sermorelin has also been tried as an adjunct to gonadotrophin therapy in the induction of ovulation and has been investigated in the treatment of HIV-associated wasting.

◊ Somatorelin (in its 40- or 44-amino-acid forms) has been used in the assessment of growth hormone deficiency.[1-3] It has usually been given as a single intravenous injection in doses of 1 μg per kg body-weight or total doses of up to 200 μg. Subsequent normal or exaggerated increases in serum-growth hormone concentrations have occurred in healthy subjects,[1,2] and in patients with hypothalamic tumours[3] or acromegaly,[2] but not in patients with hypopituitarism.[2] A synthetic 29-amino-acid sequence of somatorelin, sermorelin acetate is now available for the diagnosis of growth hormone deficiency. However, it has been suggested that the test is not useful for screening as it does not test the hypothalamic-pituitary axis, and that it should not be used in routine clinical practice.[4] The use of sermorelin in combination with the synthetic hexapeptide growth-hormone-releasing peptide-6 has also been reported.[5]

The 44- and 40-amino-acid forms of somatorelin, known as GRF(1-44) and GRF(1-40) (hpGRF-40), as well as sermorelin, have been investigated for the treatment of growth hormone deficiency.[6-9] Generally an increase in growth-hormone secretion occurred accompanied by an increase in growth rate. Various treatment regimens have been tried. Patients have received somatorelin or sermorelin subcutaneously. Somatorelin has been given in 3-hourly pulses day and night,[6] in 4 nocturnal pulses,[7] or once daily.[9] Sermorelin has been given twice daily.[7,8] For a discussion of growth retardation and its management, including mention of the use of growth hormone releasing hormone as an alternative to growth hormone treatment, see p.1273.

Sermorelin has also been investigated for intranasal administration.[10]

1. Thorner MO, *et al.* Human pancreatic growth-hormone-releasing factor selectively stimulates growth-hormone secretion in man. *Lancet* 1983; **i:** 24–8. Correction. *ibid.;* 256.
2. Wood SM, *et al.* Abnormalities of growth hormone release in response to human pancreatic growth hormone releasing factor (GRF (1-44)) in acromegaly and hypopituitarism. *BMJ* 1983; **286:** 1687–91.
3. Grossman A, *et al.* Growth-hormone-releasing factor in growth hormone deficiency: demonstration of a hypothalamic defect in growth hormone release. *Lancet* 1983; **ii:** 137–8.
4. Hindmarsh PC, Swift PGF. An assessment of growth hormone provocation tests. *Arch Dis Child* 1995; **72:** 362–8.
5. Popovic V, *et al.* GH-releasing hormone and GH-releasing peptide-6 for diagnostic testing in GH-deficient adults. *Lancet* 2000; **356:** 1137–42.
6. Thorner MO, *et al.* Acceleration of growth in two children treated with human growth hormone-releasing factor. *N Engl J Med* 1985; **312:** 4–9.

7. Smith PJ, Brook CGD. Growth hormone releasing hormone or growth hormone treatment in growth hormone insufficiency? *Arch Dis Child* 1988; **63:** 629–34.
8. Ross RJM, *et al.* Treatment of growth-hormone deficiency with growth-hormone-releasing hormone. *Lancet* 1987; **i:** 5–8.
9. Wit JM, *et al.* Short-term effect on growth of two doses of GRF 1-44 in children with growth hormone deficiency: comparison with growth induced by methionyl-GH administration. *Horm Res* 1987; **27:** 181–9.
10. Vance ML, *et al.* The effect of intravenous, subcutaneous, and intranasal GH-RH analog, [Nle²⁷]GHRH(1-29)-NH₂, on growth hormone secretion in normal men: dose-response relationships. *Clin Pharmacol Ther* 1986; **40:** 627–33.

Preparations

Proprietary Preparations (details are given in Part 3)
Aust.: Geref; **Belg.:** GHRH; **Canad.:** Geref†; **Denm.:** Somatrel; **Fin.:** Geref; **Hong Kong:** Geref; **Irl.:** Geref; **Israel:** Geref; **Ital.:** Geref; GHRH; **Mex.:** Geref; **Neth.:** GHRH; Somatobis†; **Norw.:** Geref; **Port.:** Geref; **S.Afr.:** Geref; **Spain:** Geref; **Swed.:** Geref†; **Switz.:** Geref; **Thai.:** Geref; **UK:** Geref; GHRH; **USA:** Geref.

Somatostatin (5946-I)

Somatostatin (BAN, rINN).
GH-RIF; GHRIH; Growth-hormone-release-inhibiting Hormone; Somatostatinum; Somatotrophin-release-inhibiting Factor. Ala-Gly-Cys-Lys-Asn-Phe-Phe-Trp-Lys-Thr-Phe-Thr-Ser-Cys cyclic (3→14) disulphide.
$C_{76}H_{104}N_{18}O_{19}S_2 = 1637.9$.
CAS — 38916-34-6.
ATC — H01CB01.
Pharmacopoeias. In Eur. (see p.vi).

Pharmacopoeial description

Ph. Eur.: A cyclic tetradecapeptide having the structure of the hypothalamic hormone that inhibits the release of human growth hormone. It is produced by chemical synthesis and contains not more than 15% w/w of acetic acid. A white amorphous powder. Freely soluble in water and in acetic acid; practically insoluble in dichloromethane. Store in airtight containers at a temperature of 2° to 8°. Protect from light and moisture.

Adverse Effects and Precautions

Abdominal discomfort, flushing, nausea, and bradycardia have been associated with too rapid administration. Because of the short half-life of somatostatin adverse effects are generally transitory on stopping or reducing the infusion. Concomitant parenteral nutrition has been suggested because of the inhibitory effects of somatostatin on intestinal absorption; blood sugar should be monitored since somatostatin may interfere with carbohydrate metabolism.

Effects on the kidneys. Somatostatin has been reported to have an inhibitory effect on renal function[1,2] and severe water retention and hyponatraemia have been reported.[3]
1. Walker BJ, *et al.* Somatostatin and water excretion. *Lancet* 1983; **i:** 1101–2.
2. Vora JP, *et al.* Effect of somatostatin on renal function. *BMJ* 1986; **292:** 1701–2.
3. Halma C, *et al.* Life-threatening water intoxication during somatostatin therapy. *Ann Intern Med* 1987; **107:** 518–20.

Uses and Administration

Somatostatin is a polypeptide obtained from the hypothalamus or by synthesis. The naturally occurring form has a cyclic structure. Although somatostatin derived from the hypothalamus is a 14-amino-acid peptide, a longer, 28-amino-acid form also exists in some tissues. It inhibits the release of growth hormone (p.1286) from the anterior pituitary. Somatostatin also inhibits the release of thyrotrophin (p.1298) and corticotropin (p.1280) from the pituitary, glucagon and insulin from the pancreas, and appears to have a role in the regulation of duodenal and gastric secretions. In the CNS it appears to play a role in the perception of pain.

It has been tried in a variety of disorders such as upper gastrointestinal haemorrhage including variceal haemorrhage (p.1637), insulin resistance, and the management of hormone-secreting tumours and other hypersecretory disorders. However, it has a very short duration of action and several analogues of somatostatin have been produced in an attempt to prolong its activity as well as making its inhibitory effects more specific. Octreotide (p.1291) and lanreotide (p.1289) are such analogues.

Somatostatin is usually given as the acetate. In the treatment of gastrointestinal haemorrhage, somatostatin acetate equivalent to somatostatin

3.5 µg per kg body-weight per hour has been given by intravenous infusion.

◊ Somatostatin given with melatonin, bromocriptine, and a solution of retinoids (the Di Bella regimen) was ineffective in the treatment of advanced malignancies (see Malignant Neoplasms, under Uses and Administration of Octreotide, p.1293).

Preparations

Proprietary Preparations (details are given in Part 3)
Aust.: Curastatin; Somatin; Somatolan; Stilamin; *Belg.:* Modustatine; *Braz.:* Stilamin; *Canad.:* Stilamin; *Fr.:* Modustatine; *Ger.:* Aminopan; *Hong Kong:* Stilamin; *Ital.:* Etaxene; Ikestatina; Modustatina; Nastoren; Resurmide; Stilamin; Zecnil; *Mex.:* Stilamin; *Neth.:* Somatofalk; *Port.:* Stilamin; *S.Afr.:* Stilamin; *Singapore:* Stilamin; *Spain:* Biostatine; Somiaton; Somonal; *Switz.:* Stilamin; *Thai.:* Somatosan; Stilamin.

Taltirelin (5668-g)

Taltirelin *(rINN)*.

TA-0910. (−)-N-{[(S)-Hexahydro-1-methyl-2,6-dioxo-4-pyrimidinyl]carbonyl}-L-histidyl-L-prolinamide.
$C_{17}H_{23}N_7O_5 = 405.4$.
CAS — 103300-74-9.

Profile
Taltirelin is an analogue of protirelin (p.1295) and is claimed to have beneficial effects on CNS function. It is used in the treatment of spinocerebellar degeneration, and is under investigation for dementia.

Terlipressin (12796-g)

Terlipressin *(BAN, rINN)*.

Triglycyl-lysine-vasopressin. N-[N-(N-Glycylglycyl)glycyl]lypressin; Gly-Gly-Gly-Cys-Tyr-Phe-Gln-Asn-Cys-Pro-Lys-Gly-NH$_2$ cyclic (4→9) disulphide.
$C_{52}H_{74}N_{16}O_{15}S_2 = 1227.4$.
CAS — 14636-12-5.
ATC — H01BA04.

Adverse Effects, Treatment, and Precautions
As for Vasopressin, p.1300.

The pressor and antidiuretic effects of terlipressin are reported to be less marked than those of vasopressin.

Effects on electrolytes. A report of hypokalaemia in a patient receiving terlipressin.[1]

1. Stéphan F, Paillard F. Terlipressin-exacerbated hypokalaemia. *Lancet* 1998; **351:** 1249–50.

Uses and Administration
Terlipressin is an inactive prodrug which is slowly converted in the body to lypressin, and has the general physiological actions of vasopressin (p.1300).

It is used to control bleeding oesophageal varices and is given by intravenous injection in doses of terlipressin acetate 2 mg, followed by 1 or 2 mg every 4 to 6 hours if necessary, until bleeding is controlled, for up to 72 hours.

Variceal haemorrhage. Meta-analysis has indicated[1] that terlipressin is effective in the management of acute oesophageal variceal haemorrhage (p.1637), and reduces the relative risk of mortality by about one-third. Differences in effectiveness from other therapies could not be conclusively demonstrated. Comparison of a regimen of terlipressin given by intravenous bolus injection, plus glyceryl trinitrate given sublingually, with balloon tamponade in variceal bleeding has suggested similar efficacy.[2] However, tamponade was successful in all patients that were previously unresponsive to terlipressin plus glyceryl trinitrate whereas this drug combination failed in all patients previously unresponsive to tamponade. A comparison of terlipressin and endoscopic injection sclerotherapy found them to be equally effective for the control of acute variceal bleeding.[3]

1. Ioannou G, *et al.* Terlipressin for acute esophageal variceal hemorrhage (updated 22 May 2001). Available in The Cochrane Library; Issue 3. Oxford: Update Software; 2001.
2. Fort E, *et al.* A randomized trial of terlipressin plus nitroglycerin vs balloon tamponade in the control of acute variceal hemorrhage. *Hepatology* 1990; **11:** 678–81.
3. Escorsell À, *et al.* Multicenter randomized controlled trial of terlipressin versus sclerotherapy in the treatment of acute variceal bleeding: the TEST study. *Hepatology* 2000; **32:** 471–6.

Preparations

Proprietary Preparations (details are given in Part 3)
Aust.: Glycylpressin; *Belg.:* Glypressin; *Denm.:* Glypressin; *Fin.:* Glypressin; *Fr.:* Glypressine; *Ger.:* Glycylpressin; Haemopressin; *Hong Kong:* Glypressin; *Irl.:* Glypressin; *Ital.:* Glipressina; *Neth.:* Glypressin; *Singapore:* Glypressin; *Spain:* Glypressin; *Switz.:* Glypressine; *Thai.:* Glypressin; *UK:* Glypressin.

Tetracosactide (1465-s)

Tetracosactide *(BAN, rINN)*.

α$^{1-24}$-Corticotrophin; β$^{1-24}$-Corticotrophin; Cosyntropin *(USAN)*; Tetracosactido; Tetracosactidum; Tetracosactrin. Corticotrophin-(1-24)-tetracosapeptide; Ser-Tyr-Ser-Met-Glu-His-Phe-Arg-Trp-Gly-Lys-Pro-Val-Gly-Lys-Lys-Arg-Arg-Pro-Val-Lys-Val-Tyr-Pro.
$C_{136}H_{210}N_{40}O_{31}S = 2933.4$.
CAS — 16960-16-0.
ATC — H01AA02.

Pharmacopoeias. In *Eur.* (see p.vi).

Pharmacopoeial description
Ph. Eur.: A synthetic tetracosapeptide in which the sequence of amino acids is the same as that of the first 24 residues of human corticotropin. It is available as an acetate and contains water. It increases the rate at which corticoid hormones are secreted by the adrenal gland. The potency is not less than 800 units per mg. A white or yellow, amorphous powder. Sparingly soluble in water. Store under nitrogen at a temperature of 2° to 8°. Protect from light.

Units
490 units of tetracosactide for bioassay are contained in approximately 490 µg of synthetic tetracosactide with mannitol 20 mg in one ampoule of the first International Reference Preparation (1981).

Adverse Effects
As for Corticotropin, p.1280.

Withdrawal
As for Corticotropin, p.1280.

Precautions
As for Corticosteroids, p.1042. Tetracosactide is contra-indicated in patients with a history of allergic disorders such as asthma.

Since hypersensitivity reactions may not occur for up to 1 hour after injection sufficient time should be allowed for recovery after administration at the hospital or surgery. Self-administration is not recommended.

Interactions
As for Corticosteroids, p.1043.

Pharmacokinetics
Following intravenous injection tetracosactide exhibits triphasic pharmacokinetics. It is rapidly eliminated from plasma, mostly by distribution to the adrenal glands and kidneys. It is metabolised by serum endopeptidases into inactive oligopeptides, and then by aminopeptidases into free amino acids. Most of a dose is excreted in urine within 24 hours. The terminal half-life of tetracosactide is about 3 hours.

Uses and Administration
Tetracosactide is a synthetic polypeptide with general properties similar to those of corticotropin (p.1280). Tetracosactide is used diagnostically to investigate adrenocortical insufficiency (p.1046).

Although tetracosactide, like corticotropin, has also been used therapeutically for most of the conditions in which systemic corticosteroid therapy is indicated, it is now rarely used for such indications.

Tetracosactide is usually employed in the form of the acetate although doses are often expressed in terms of tetracosactide itself.

For diagnostic purposes tetracosactide acetate is used intramuscularly or intravenously as a plain injection in the first instance then, if results are inconclusive, intramuscularly as a long-acting depot injection. The initial test using the plain injection is based on the measurement of plasma-cortisol concentrations immediately before and exactly 30 minutes after an intramuscular or intravenous injection equivalent to 250 µg of tetracosactide; adrenocortical function may be regarded as normal if there is a rise in the cortisol concentration of at least 200 nmol per litre (70 µg per litre). A suggested intravenous dose in children has been 250 µg per 1.73 m² body-surface.

If the results of this test are equivocal the long-acting depot preparation may be used, the adult dose being

1 mg of tetracosactide acetate given intramuscularly with adrenocortical function being regarded as normal if plasma-cortisol concentrations have steadily increased to 1000 to 1800 nmol per litre 5 hours after the injection. A three day test, for example with 1 mg of the depot preparation given each morning, is also used to differentiate between primary and secondary adrenocortical insufficiency; this is preceded on the first day and followed on the fourth day by the test using the plain injection. A marked improvement in the second assessment suggests secondary adrenocortical insufficiency.

For therapeutic purposes tetracosactide acetate has been given by intramuscular injection as the long-acting depot preparation. The usual initial adult dose of tetracosactide acetate has been 1 mg daily (or 1 mg every 12 hours in acute cases), reduced after the acute symptoms have been controlled to 0.5 to 1 mg every 2 or 3 days or 1 mg weekly. For children aged 3 to 5 years, a dose of 250 to 500 µg intramuscularly has been given daily initially, and then every 2 to 8 days for maintenance. A dose of 0.25 to 1 mg has been used similarly in children aged 5 to 12 years.

Preparations

BP 2001: Tetracosactide Injection; Tetracosactide Zinc Injection.

Proprietary Preparations (details are given in Part 3)
Aust.: Synacthen; *Austral.:* Synacthen; *Belg.:* Synacthen; *Braz.:* Cortrosina; *Canad.:* Cortrosyn; Synacthen Depot; *Denm.:* Synacthen; *Fr.:* Synacthene; *Ger.:* Synacthen; Synacthen Depot; *Hong Kong:* Cortrosyn; *Irl.:* Synacthen; *Israel:* Cortrosyn; Synacthen†; *Ital.:* Cortrosyn; Synacthen; *Neth.:* Synacthen; *Norw.:* Synacthen†; *NZ:* Synacthen; *Port.:* Synacthen; *S.Afr.:* Synacthen Depot; *Spain:* Nuvacthen Depot; *Swed.:* Synacthen; *Switz.:* Synacthen; Synacthen Retard; *UK:* Synacthen; Synacthen Depot; *USA:* Cortrosyn.

Thyrotrophin (5947-y)

Thyrotrophin *(BAN, rINN)*.

Thyroid-stimulating Hormone; Thyrotrophic Hormone; Thyrotropin; TSH.
CAS — 9002-71-5.
ATC — H01AB01; V04CJ01.

A glycoprotein from the anterior pituitary with a molecular weight in man of about 30 000.

Thyrotropin Alfa (20062-j)

Thyrotropin Alfa *(BAN, USAN, rINN)*.

rhTSH.
CAS — 194100-83-9.

Units
0.037 units of human pituitary thyrotrophin for immunoassay and bioassay are contained in approximately 7.5 µg of thyrotrophin, with albumin 1 mg and lactose 5 mg, in one ampoule of the second International Reference Preparation (1983).

Adverse Effects
Infrequent side-effects of thyrotrophin include nausea, vomiting, headache, a desire to micturate, and flushing. High doses may produce excessive thyroid stimulation, with angina, tachycardia or arrhythmias, dyspnoea, sweating, nervousness and irritability. Hypersensitivity reactions, including skin rash and urticaria, erythema and swelling at the injection site, and anaphylaxis have occurred, particularly on repeated administration.

Precautions
Thyrotrophin should not be given to patients with recent myocardial infarction or uncorrected adrenocortical insufficiency, including adrenocortical insufficiency secondary to hypopituitarism. Care is also required in patients with cardiovascular disease.

Uses and Administration
Thyrotrophin is a glycoprotein secreted by the anterior lobe of the pituitary and with an alpha subunit essentially the same as that of the gonadotrophins. Its main actions are to increase iodine uptake by the thyroid and the formation and secretion of the thyroid hormones. It may produce hyperplasia of thyroid tissue. Thyrotrophin secretion is controlled by a hypothalamic releasing hormone (Protirelin, p.1295) and by circulating thyroid hormones; somatostatin (p.1297) may inhibit the release of thyrotrophin.

Thyrotrophin has been used in conjunction with radio-iodine in the diagnosis of hypothyroidism (p.1520) and to differentiate between primary and secondary hypothyroidism, but direct radio-immunoassay of circulating endogenous thyroid-stimulating hormone may be preferred. Thyrotrophin increases the uptake of radio-iodine by the thyroid and has been used as a diagnostic tool and as an adjunct in the treatment of certain types of thyroid cancer.

The usual dose is 10 units daily by intramuscular or subcutaneous injection; depending upon the indication this dose may be given for between 1 and 8 days.

Thyrotropin alfa is a recombinant form of thyrotrophin used in the follow-up of patients with thyroid cancer. The usual dose is 900 μg intramuscularly, every 24 hours for two doses, or every 72 hours for three doses, given before serum-thyroglobulin testing with or without radio-iodine imaging.

Malignant neoplasms of the thyroid. Patients with well-differentiated thyroid carcinoma (p.500) undergo surgery, with or without iodine-131 treatment, and then receive thyroid hormone therapy. Monitoring for tumour recurrence by iodine-131 total body scanning in subsequent years requires interruption of thyroid hormone treatment for at least 2 weeks, with consequent hypothyroidism. Studies[1,2] have compared administration of thyrotropin alfa with withdrawal of thyroid hormones as a prelude to radio-iodine scanning. They found that thyrotropin alfa did stimulate radio-iodine uptake, although the sensitivity of scanning may depend on the technique used, and that thyrotropin alfa might be considered an alternative to thyroid hormone withdrawal.

1. Ladenson PW, *et al.* Comparison of administration of recombinant human thyrotropin with withdrawal of thyroid hormone for radioactive iodine scanning in patients with thyroid carcinoma. *N Engl J Med* 1997; **337:** 888–96.
2. Haugen BR, *et al.* A comparison of recombinant human thyrotropin and thyroid hormone withdrawal for the detection of thyroid remnant or cancer. *J Clin Endocrinol Metab* 1999; **84:** 3877–85.

Preparations

Proprietary Preparations (details are given in Part 3)
Israel: Thytropar; *USA:* Thyrogen; Thytropar†.

Triptorelin   (16834-v)

Triptorelin *(BAN, USAN, rINN).*

AY-25650; BIM-21003; BN-52014; CL-118532; Triptoreline; D-Trp⁶-LHRH; [6-D-Tryptophan] luteinising hormone-releasing factor. 5-Oxo-L-prolyl-L-histidyl-L-tryptophyl-L-seryl-L-tyrosyl-D-tryptophyl-L-leucyl-L-arginyl-L-prolylglycinamide.

$C_{64}H_{82}N_{18}O_{13}$ = 1311.4.
CAS — 57773-63-4 *(triptorelin); 124508-66-3 (triptorelin embonate).*
ATC — L02AE04.

Adverse Effects and Precautions

As for Gonadorelin, p.1284.

◊ For a report of disease flare in patients given triptorelin for prostatic cancer, see Effects on the Bones, under Adverse Effects of Buserelin Acetate, p.1278.

Local reactions. For reference to local reactions occurring following injection of gonadorelin analogues, including triptorelin, see Leuprorelin Acetate, p.1289.

Sepsis. A report of 2 patients in whom triptorelin therapy led to sepsis caused by expulsion of necrotic fibroids through the cervix.[1]

1. Ellenbogen A, *et al.* Complication of triptorelin treatment for uterine myomas. *Lancet* 1989; **ii:** 167–8.

Interactions

As for Gonadorelin, p.1284.

Pharmacokinetics

Triptorelin is rapidly absorbed following subcutaneous injection, with peak plasma concentrations achieved about 40 minutes after a dose. The biological half-life has been stated to be about 7.5 hours, although longer half-lives have been reported in patients with prostate cancer, and shorter half-lives in some groups of healthy subjects.

◊ References.
1. Müller FO, *et al.* Pharmacokinetics of triptorelin after intravenous bolus administration in healthy males and in males with renal or hepatic insufficiency. *Br J Clin Pharmacol* 1997; **44:** 335–41.

Uses and Administration

Triptorelin is an analogue of gonadorelin (p.1284) with similar properties. It is used for the suppression of gonadal sex hormone production in the treatment of malignant neoplasms of the prostate, in precocious puberty, and in the management of endometriosis, female infertility, and uterine fibroids. It is used either as the base or as the acetate or embonate; doses are given in terms of the base. It is given as a daily subcutaneous injection or monthly as an intramuscular depot preparation.

In the treatment of prostate cancer 3 or 3.75 mg of the depot preparation is given intramuscularly every 4

weeks; the first dose may be preceded by 0.1 mg daily for 7 days by subcutaneous injection. An anti-androgen such as cyproterone acetate may be given for several days before beginning therapy with triptorelin and continued for about 3 weeks to avoid the risk of a disease flare.

Similar doses of the depot preparation may be given for up to 6 months in the management of endometriosis or uterine fibroids, with treatment begun during the first 5 days of the menstrual cycle. In the management of female infertility doses of 0.1 mg subcutaneously daily, in conjunction with gonadotrophins, have been recommended from the second day of the menstrual cycle for about 10 to 12 days. In children with precocious puberty a dose of 50 μg of depot triptorelin per kg body-weight may be given intramuscularly every 4 weeks.

Delayed and precocious puberty. Gonadorelin analogues such as triptorelin[1,2] are used in the management of central precocious puberty (see p.1277). They may also be effective in delayed puberty (p.1273) although they are most likely to be helpful where this is due to hypogonadism. Triptorelin has been used to differentiate gonadotrophin deficiency from constitutional delayed puberty.[3]

1. Roger M, *et al.* Long term treatment of male and female precocious puberty by periodic administration of a long-acting preparation of D-trp⁶-luteinizing hormone-releasing hormone microcapsules. *J Clin Endocrinol Metab* 1986; **62:** 670–7.
2. Oostdijk W, *et al.* Final height in central precocious puberty after long term treatment with a slow release GnRH agonist. *Arch Dis Child* 1996; **75:** 292–7.
3. Zamboni G, *et al.* Use of the gonadotropin-releasing hormone agonist triptorelin in the diagnosis of delayed puberty in boys. *J Pediatr* 1995; **126:** 756–8.

Disturbed behaviour. Combined therapy with triptorelin, which suppressed testosterone secretion by inhibiting the pituitary-gonadal axis, and supportive psychotherapy, has been tried in the treatment of men with paraphilias (see p.650): a reduction in abnormal sexual thoughts and behaviours has been reported, although the study was uncontrolled.[1]

1. Rösler A, Witztum E. Treatment of men with paraphilia with a long-acting analogue of gonadotropin-releasing hormone. *N Engl J Med* 1998; **338:** 416–22.

Endometriosis. Gonadorelin analogues are effective in the management of endometriosis (see p.1469), but the need for long-term therapy to prevent recurrence limits their value because of the risk of osteoporosis; 'add-back' therapy, with concomitant hormone replacement, is being investigated.

References.
1. Lindsay PC, *et al.* The effect of add-back treatment with tibolone (Livial) on patients treated with the gonadotropin-releasing hormone agonist triptorelin (Decapeptyl). *Fertil Steril* 1996; **65:** 342–8.

Fibroids. Gonadorelin analogues have been used as an alternative to surgery in the treatment of uterine fibroids (see p.1285), despite some concern that this may complicate the diagnosis of malignancy.

References to the use of triptorelin.
1. Schneider D, *et al.* GnRH analogue-induced uterine shrinkage enabling a vaginal hysterectomy and repair in large leiomyomatous uteri. *Obstet Gynecol* 1991; **78:** 540–1.
2. van Leusden HA. Symptom-free interval after triptorelin treatment of uterine fibroids: long-term results. *Gynecol Endocrinol* 1992; **6:** 189–98.
3. Golan A, *et al.* Pre-operative gonadotrophin-releasing hormone agonist treatment in surgery for uterine leiomyomata. *Hum Reprod* 1993; **8:** 450–2.
4. Broekmans FJ, *et al.* Two-step gonadotropin-releasing hormone agonist treatment of uterine leiomyomas: standard-dose therapy followed by reduced-dose therapy. *Am J Obstet Gynecol* 1996; **175:** 1208–16.
5. Vercellini P, *et al.* Treatment with a gonadotrophin releasing hormone agonist before hysterectomy for leiomyomas: results of a multicentre, randomised controlled trial. *Br J Obstet Gynaecol* 1998; **105:** 1148–54.

Growth retardation. As discussed on p.1273 gonadorelin analogues have been given in combination with growth hormone to short girls without growth hormone deficiency, in an attempt to delay puberty and bone maturation and thus maximise the final height achieved. However, there is some doubt about the extent of benefit, and in any case the concept of such treatment in children who are not clinically deficient in growth hormone is controversial, and some authorities do not consider it appropriate.

References to the use of triptorelin.
1. Saggese G, *et al.* Combination treatment with growth hormone and gonadotropin-releasing hormone analogs in short normal girls. *J Pediatr* 1995; **126:** 468–73.

Infertility. Gonadorelin analogues are used in the management of infertility related to hypogonadotrophic hypogonadism in both men and women. For a discussion of infertility and its management, including the role of gonadorelin analogues, see p.1275.

Malignant neoplasms. Two multicentre studies[1,2] found slow-release triptorelin (in the form of microcapsules releasing 100 μg daily, given intramuscularly once a month) to be ef-

fective as orchidectomy in the initial treatment of advanced prostatic cancer (p.497).

1. Parmar H, *et al.* Randomised controlled study of orchidectomy vs long-acting D-TRP-6-LHRH microcapsules in advanced prostatic carcinoma. *Lancet* 1985; **ii:** 1201–5.
2. Boccardo F, *et al.* D-TRP-6-LH-RH treatment of advanced prostatic cancer. *Lancet* 1986; **i:** 621.

Preparations

Proprietary Preparations (details are given in Part 3)
Aust.: Decapeptyl; *Belg.:* Decapeptyl; *Braz.:* Neo Decapeptyl; *Denm.:* Decapeptyl; *Fin.:* Decapeptyl; *Fr.:* Decapeptyl; *Ger.:* Decapeptyl; *Hong Kong:* Decapeptyl; *Irl.:* Decapeptyl; *Israel:* Decapeptyl; *Ital.:* Decapeptyl; *Neth.:* Decapeptyl; *NZ:* Decapeptyl; *Port.:* Decapeptyl; *S.Afr.:* Decapeptyl; *Singapore:* Decapeptyl; *Spain:* Decapeptyl; *Swed.:* Decapeptyl; *Switz.:* Decapeptyl; *Thai.:* Decapeptyl; *UK:* Decapeptyl; *USA:* Trelstar.

Urofollitropin   (12013-v)

Urofollitropin *(BAN, USAN, rINN).*
Urofollitrophin; Urofollitropinum.
CAS — 97048-13-0.
ATC — G03GA04.
Pharmacopoeias. In Eur. (see p.vi).

Pharmacopoeial description

Ph. Eur.: A dry preparation containing menopausal gonadotrophin obtained from the urine of postmenopausal women. It has follicle-stimulating activity and no or virtually no luteinising activity. The potency is not less than 90 units of follicle-stimulating hormone per mg; the ratio of units of luteinising hormone to units of follicle-stimulating hormone is not more than 1:60. An almost white or slightly yellow powder. Soluble in water. Store in airtight containers at a temperature of 2° to 8°. Protect from light.

Units

121 units of urofollitropin (purified urinary follicle-stimulating hormone) are contained in one ampoule of the first International Standard (1995).

Uses and Administration

Urofollitropin is a gonadotrophin, obtained from the urine of postmenopausal women, possessing follicle-stimulating hormone (FSH) activity but virtually no luteinising activity. For details of the actions of FSH, see p.1283.

Urofollitropin is used similarly to human menopausal gonadotrophins (p.1288) in the treatment of female infertility with the exception that, being without luteinising hormone activity, it can be used in patients where any increase in luteinising hormone activity is not required, as in polycystic ovarian disease. Urofollitropin is given subcutaneously or intramuscularly in a dosage adjusted according to the patient's response. Usually a dose providing 75 to 150 units of FSH daily is given initially. When an adequate response is achieved, as determined by oestrogen monitoring or ultrasonic visualisation of follicles, treatment is stopped and chorionic gonadotrophin is administered to induce ovulation. Treatment with urofollitropin should be discontinued if there is no response after 4 weeks although treatment may be attempted again in future cycles.

Urofollitropin is also used in conjunction with other agents as part of *in-vitro* fertilisation procedures. It is typically given in a dose providing 150 to 225 units of FSH daily, usually beginning from day 2 or 3 of the menstrual cycle. Alternatively, therapy has been initiated with clomifene citrate and continued with urofollitropin, or urofollitropin may be given after suppression of gonadotrophin release with a gonadorelin analogue. Treatment is continued until an adequate response is obtained and the final injection of urofollitropin is followed 1 to 2 days later by 5000 to 10 000 units of chorionic gonadotrophin. Oocyte retrieval is performed 34 to 35 hours later.

Urofollitropin is also used in conjunction with chorionic gonadotrophin to stimulate spermatogenesis in the treatment of male infertility, although a preparation with combined luteinising activity, such as human menopausal gonadotrophins, may be preferred. The usual dose provides 75 units of FSH daily, or 75 to 150 units 2 to 3 times a week, together with a simultaneous dose of chorionic gonadotrophin 1000 to 2000 units. Treatment should be continued for at least 3 or 4 months. For a brief discussion of hypogonadism see p.1274.

Infertility. For reference to the use of preparations with follicle-stimulating hormone activity in infertility, see p.1275. The management of women with polycystic ovary syndrome is discussed in more detail on p.1276. Some further references are listed below.

1. Remorgida V, *et al.* Administration of pure follicle-stimulating hormone during gonadotropin-releasing hormone agonist therapy in patients with clomiphene-resistant polycystic ovarian disease: hormonal evaluations and clinical perspectives. *Am J Obstet Gynecol* 1989; **160:** 108–13.
2. Buvat J, *et al.* Purified follicle-stimulating hormone in polycystic ovary syndrome: slow administration is safer and more effective. *Fertil Steril* 1989; **52:** 553–9.
3. McFaul PB, *et al.* Treatment of clomiphene citrate-resistant polycystic ovarian syndrome with pure follicle-stimulating hormone or human menopausal gonadotropin. *Fertil Steril* 1990; **53:** 792–7.
4. European Metrodin HP Study Group. Efficacy and safety of highly purified urinary follicle-stimulating hormone with human chorionic gonadotropin for treating men with isolated hypogonadotropic hypogonadism. *Fertil Steril* 1998; **70:** 256–62.

Preparations

BP 2001: Urofollitropin Injection.

Proprietary Preparations (details are given in Part 3)
Aust.: Fertinorm†; *Austral.:* Metrodin; *Braz.:* Metrodin; *Canad.:* Fertinorm; Metrodin†; *Fr.:* Fertiline†; Metrodine†; *Ger.:* Fertinorm; *Hong Kong:* Metrodin; *Irl.:* Metrodin; *Israel:* Metrodin; *Ital.:* Fostimon; Metrodin; *Mex.:* Follitrin; *Neth.:* Follegon; Metrodin†; *NZ:* Metrodin; *Port.:* Metrodin; *S.Afr.:* Metrodin; *Singapore:* Metrodin; *Spain:* Neo Fertinorm; *Swed.:* Fertinorm†; *Switz.:* Fostimon; *Thai.:* Metrodin; *UK:* Metrodin; Orgafol†; *USA:* Fertinex; Metrodin.

Vapreotide (13864-w)

Vapreotide (BAN, USAN, rINN).

BMY-41606; RC-160. D-Phenylalanyl-L-cysteinyl-L-tyrosyl-D-tryptophyl-L-lysyl-L-valyl-L-cysteinyl-L-tryptophanamide cyclic (2→7)-disulfide.
$C_{57}H_{70}N_{12}O_9S_2 = 1131.4.$
CAS — 103222-11-3.

Profile

Vapreotide is a somatostatin analogue similar to octreotide (p.1291). It is under investigation in the management of various gastrointestinal and neoplastic disorders.

◊ References.
1. Stiefel F, Morant R. Vapreotide, a new somatostatin analogue in the palliative management of obstructive ileus in advanced cancer. *Support Care Cancer* 1993; **1:** 57–8.
2. Eriksson B, *et al.* The use of new somatostatin analogues, lanreotide and octastatin, in neuroendocrine gastro-intestinal tumours. *Digestion* 1996; **57** (suppl 1): 77–80.
3. Calès P, *et al.* Early administration of vapreotide for variceal bleeding in patients with cirrhosis. *N Engl J Med* 2001; **344:** 23–8.

Vasopressin (5948-j)

ADH; Antidiuretic Hormone; Beta-Hypophamine.
CAS — 11000-17-2 (vasopressin injection).
ATC — H01BA01.

NOTE. Vasopressin Injection is *rINN*.
Pharmacopoeias. In *US*, which includes both argipressin and lypressin in this title.
Vasopressin Injection is included in *Jpn*.

Pharmacopoeial description

USP 25: A polypeptide hormone having the properties of causing the contraction of vascular and other smooth muscles, and of antidiuresis. It is prepared by synthesis or obtained from the posterior lobe of the pituitary of healthy, domestic animals used for food by humans. Its vasopressor activity is not less than 300 USP units per mg. Store in airtight containers at 2° to 8°.

Argipressin (5949-z)

Argipressin (BAN, rINN).

[8-Arginine]vasopressin; AVP; CI-107 (argipressin tannate). Cys-Tyr-Phe-Gln-Asn-Cys-Pro-Arg-Gly-NH₂ cyclic (1→6) disulphide.
$C_{46}H_{65}N_{15}O_{12}S_2 = 1084.2.$
CAS — 113-79-1.
ATC — H01BA06.

NOTE. Argipressin Tannate is *USAN*.

Argipressin is a form of vasopressin obtained from most mammals including man but excluding pig. It is usually prepared synthetically. Lypressin (see below) is vasopressin from pig.

Units

8.2 units of argipressin for bioassay are contained in approximately 20 µg of synthetic peptide acetate (with human albumin 5 mg and citric acid) in one ampoule of the first International Standard (1978).

Lypressin (5934-p)

Lypressin (BAN, USAN, rINN).

L-8; Lipressina; LVP. [8-Lysine]vasopressin; Cys-Tyr-Phe-Gln-Asn-Cys-Pro-Lys-Gly-NH₂ cyclic (1→6) disulphide.
$C_{46}H_{65}N_{13}O_{12}S_2 = 1056.2.$
CAS — 50-57-7.
ATC — H01BA03.

Pharmacopoeias. Lypressin Injection is included in *Eur.* (see p.vi). US includes Lypressin Nasal Solution.

Lypressin is the form of vasopressin present in the posterior pituitary of pigs.

Pharmacopoeial description

Ph. Eur.: Lypressin Injection is a clear colourless liquid with a pH of 3.7 to 4.3. Store at a temperature of 2° to 15°.

Units

7.7 units of lypressin are contained in approximately 23.4 µg of synthetic peptide (with albumin 5 mg and citric acid) in one ampoule of the first International Standard (1978).

Vasopressin Tannate (5950-p)

The water-insoluble tannate of the pressor principle of the posterior lobe of the pituitary.

Adverse Effects

Large parenteral doses of vasopressin may give rise to marked pallor, pounding headache, sweating, tremor, nausea, vomiting, diarrhoea, eructation, cramp, and a desire to defaecate; some of these effects may also be noted following large intranasal doses of lypressin. In women, vasopressin may cause uterine cramps of a menstrual character. Hyponatraemia with water retention and signs of water intoxication can occur.

Hypersensitivity reactions have occurred and include urticaria and bronchial constriction. Anaphylactic shock and cardiac arrest have been reported.

Vasopressin may constrict coronary arteries. Chest pain, myocardial ischaemia, and infarction have occurred following injection, and fatalities have been reported. Other cardiovascular effects include occasional reports of arrhythmias and bradycardia, as well as hypertension. Peripheral vasoconstriction has resulted in gangrene, and thrombosis as well as local irritation at the injection site may occur.

Following intranasal use (usually as lypressin) nasal congestion, irritation, and ulceration have been reported occasionally; systemic effects at usual intranasal doses are mostly reported to be mild.

Effects on the heart. Arrhythmias, including ventricular tachycardia and fibrillation,[1] torsade de pointes,[2-4] and asystole[5] are among the adverse effects of vasopressin administration. Paradoxical bradycardia and hypotension has also been reported.[6]

1. Kelly KJ, *et al.* Vasopressin provocation of ventricular dysrhythmia. *Ann Intern Med* 1980; **92:** 205–6.
2. Eden E, *et al.* Ventricular arrhythmia induced by vasopressin: torsade de pointes related to vasopressin-induced bradycardia. *Mt Sinai J Med* 1983; **50:** 49–51.
3. Stein LB, *et al.* Fatal torsade de pointes occurring in a patient receiving intravenous vasopressin and nitroglycerin. *J Clin Gastroenterol* 1992; **15:** 171–4.
4. Faigel DO, *et al.* Torsade de pointes complicating the treatment of bleeding esophageal varices: association with neuroleptics, vasopressin, and electrolyte imbalance. *Am J Gastroenterol* 1995; **90:** 822–4.
5. Fitz JD. Vasopressin induction of ventricular ectopy. *Arch Intern Med* 1982; **142:** 644.
6. Kraft W, *et al.* Paradoxical hypotension and bradycardia after intravenous arginine vasopressin. *J Clin Pharmacol* 1998; **38:** 283–6.

Ischaemia. Reports of ischaemia and infarction associated with vasopressin.
1. Greenwald RA, *et al.* Local gangrene: a complication of peripheral Pitressin therapy for bleeding esophageal varices. *Gastroenterology* 1978; **74:** 744–6.
2. Colombani P. Upper extremity gangrene secondary to superior mesenteric artery infusion of vasopressin. *Dig Dis Sci* 1982; **27:** 367–9.
3. Lambert M, *et al.* Reversible ischemic colitis after intravenous vasopressin therapy. *JAMA* 1982; **247:** 666–7.
4. Anderson JR, Johnston GW. Development of cutaneous gangrene during continuous peripheral infusion of vasopressin. *BMJ* 1983; **287:** 1657–8.
5. Reddy KR, *et al.* Bilateral nipple necrosis after intravenous vasopressin therapy. *Arch Intern Med* 1984; **144:** 835–6.
6. Brearly S, *et al.* A lethal complication of peripheral vein vasopressin infusion. *Hepatogastroenterology* 1985; **32:** 224–5.
7. Sweren BS, Bohlman ME. Gastric and splenic infarction: a complication of intraarterial vasopressin infusion. *Cardiovasc Intervent Radiol* 1989; **12:** 207–9.
8. Maceyko RF, *et al.* Vasopressin-associated cutaneous infarcts, alopecia, and neuropathy. *J Am Acad Dermatol* 1994; **31:** 111–13.

Treatment of Adverse Effects

The antidiuretic effects on water retention and sodium imbalance may be treated by water restriction and a temporary withdrawal of vasopressin. Severe cases may require osmotic diuresis alone or with frusemide [furosemide].

◊ A report of the localised intravenous and intra-arterial administration of guanethidine in the treatment of a patient with extravasation of vasopressin.[1] The intra-arterial administration of guanethidine was considered to have helped to avoid necrotic changes.

1. Crocker MC. Intravascular guanethidine in the treatment of extravasated vasopressin. *N Engl J Med* 1981; **304:** 1430.

Precautions

Vasopressin should not be used in patients with chronic nephritis with nitrogen retention. It should be avoided or given only with extreme care, and in small doses, to patients with vascular disease, especially of the coronary arteries.

It should be given with care to patients with asthma, epilepsy, migraine, heart failure, or other conditions which might be aggravated by water retention. Fluid intake should be adjusted to avoid hyponatraemia and water intoxication. Care is also required in hypertension or other conditions that may be exacerbated by a rise in blood pressure. Nasal absorption of vasopressin may be impaired in patients with rhinitis.

Abuse. Vasopressin or its analogues have been abused as so-called 'smart drugs' for their supposed effect on memory recall and cognition.

Resistance. Antibodies to vasopressin were detected in 6 of 28 patients being treated for diabetes insipidus, all of whom experienced a decrease in antidiuretic effect with previously effective argipressin or lypressin therapy;[1] desmopressin and chlorpropamide remained effective in these patients. There have been reports of patients with diabetes insipidus of pregnancy unresponsive to argipressin but responsive to desmopressin.[2] This was probably due to excessive placental production of vasopressinase, an enzyme which degrades argipressin.

1. Vokes TJ, *et al.* Antibodies to vasopressin in patients with diabetes insipidus: implications for diagnosis and therapy. *Ann Intern Med* 1988; **108:** 190–5.
2. Shah SV, Thakur V. Vasopressinase and diabetes insipidus of pregnancy. *Ann Intern Med* 1988; **109:** 435–6.

Interactions

The antidiuretic effects of vasopressins might be expected to be enhanced in some patients receiving chlorpropamide, clofibrate, carbamazepine, fludrocortisone, urea, or tricyclic antidepressants; lithium, heparin, demeclocycline, noradrenaline [norepinephrine], and alcohol may decrease the antidiuretic effect. Ganglion-blocking drugs may increase sensitivity to the pressor effects of vasopressins.

Cimetidine. A report of severe bradycardia and heart block leading to asystole in a patient given combined vasopressin and cimetidine therapy.[1]
1. Nikolic G, Singh JB. Cimetidine, vasopressin and chronotropic incompetence. *Med J Aust* 1982; **2:** 435–6.

Uses and Administration

Vasopressin is secreted by the hypothalamus and stored in the posterior lobe of the pituitary gland. It may be prepared from the gland of mammals or by synthesis. Vasopressin has a direct antidiuretic action on the kidney, increasing tubular reabsorption of water. It also constricts peripheral blood vessels and causes contraction of the smooth muscle of the intestine, gallbladder, and urinary bladder. It has practically no oxytocic activity.

Vasopressin, which is usually administered parenterally or intranasally in the synthetic forms of argipressin or lypressin, is used in the treatment of cranial diabetes insipidus due to a deficiency in antidiuretic hormone. It is ineffective in nephrogenic diabetes insipidus. It should not be used to raise the blood pressure. Argipressin has also been used in the prevention and treatment of postoperative abdominal distension, and was formerly given to remove gas in abdominal visualisation procedures. Argipressin or lypressin are used in the treatment of bleeding oesophageal varices.

In the treatment of cranial diabetes insipidus to control polyuria, argipressin may be administered subcutaneously or intramuscularly; the dose in the UK is 5 to 20 units every 4 hours. In the USA, 5 to 10 units given 2 or 3 times daily or more has been used. Alternatively, lypressin may be given as a nasal spray, the usual dose for diabetes insipidus being 4 to 10 units 3 or 4 times daily; an extra dose may be given at bedtime to eliminate nocturia. Dosage should be adjusted as required; more frequent administration may be needed. Argipressin has also been given intranasally. A long-acting oily suspension of vasopressin tannate was formerly used by intramuscular injection in diabetes insipidus.

In the initial control of variceal bleeding argipressin is given in an initial dose of 20 units in 100 mL of glucose 5% infused over 15 minutes. Lypressin is also sometimes administered intravenously for bleeding oesophageal varices.

Administration. Results[1] suggesting that although intravenous administration of argipressin produced much higher plasma concentrations than intranasal administration, the latter evoked a greater CNS response.

1. Pietrowsky R, *et al.* Brain potential changes after intranasal vs intravenous administration of vasopressin: evidence for a direct nose-brain pathway for peptide effects in humans. *Biol Psychiatry* 1996; **39:** 332–40.

Administration in children. Vasopressin given by continuous intravenous infusion in an average dose of 9 milliunits per kg body-weight per hour was safe and effective in five children who had diabetes insipidus as a manifestation of severe brain injury.[1] It has also been used safely in two children aged 3 years and under with postoperative diabetes insipidus; the dose used was 1.5 to 3 milliunits per kg per hour.[2] Similar initial doses of argipressin were used in 3 comatose children with cranial diabetes insipidus,[3] while a published algorithm for the management of acute cranial diabetes insipidus has recommended an initial dose of vasopressin of 0.25 to 1 milliunits per kg per hour, subsequently titrated to achieve an appropriate output and specific gravity of urine, and a serum sodium value of between 140 and 145 mEq per litre.[4]

1. Ralston C, Butt W. Continuous vasopressin replacement in diabetes insipidus. *Arch Dis Child* 1990; **65:** 896–7.
2. McDonald JA, *et al.* Treatment of the young child with postoperative central diabetes insipidus. *Am J Dis Child* 1989; **143:** 201–4.
3. Lee Y-J, *et al.* Continuous infusion of vasopressin in comatose children with neurogenic diabetes insipidus. *J Pediatr Endocrinol Metab* 1995; **8:** 257–62.
4. Lugo N, *et al.* Diagnosis and management algorithm of acute onset of central diabetes insipidus in critically ill children. *J Pediatr Endocrinol Metab* 1997; **10:** 633–9.

Advanced cardiac life support. In a preliminary study argipressin 40 units by intravenous injection appeared to be of value in the treatment of cardiac arrest due to ventricular fibrillation.[1] Spontaneous circulation returned in 16 of 20 patients so treated; 14 were successfully resuscitated on arrival in hospital and 8 survived to be discharged. In comparison, of 20 patients treated with 1 mg of adrenaline [epinephrine] intravenously only 7 were resuscitated and 3 survived till discharge. In contrast, a larger study[2] of patients who experienced cardiac arrest while in hospital and were treated with either vasopressin 40 units or adrenaline [epinephrine] 1 mg, found no difference in survival to discharge from hospital. Vasopressin (as argipressin) may be used as an alternative to adrenaline [epinephrine] in cardiopulmonary resuscitation (see p.790) although further evidence of benefit is required before such use can be recommended.

1. Lindner KH, *et al.* Randomised comparison of epinephrine and vasopressin in patients with out-of-hospital ventricular fibrillation. *Lancet* 1997; **349:** 535–7.
2. Stiell IG, *et al.* Vasopressin versus epinephrine for inhospital cardiac arrest: a randomised controlled trial. *Lancet* 2001; **358:** 105–9.

Diabetes insipidus. For a discussion of diabetes insipidus and its management, including reference to the use of vasopressin analogues (particularly desmopressin), see p.1273.

Nocturnal enuresis. For references to the use of the vasopressin analogue, desmopressin, in nocturnal enuresis, see p.1282.

Variceal haemorrhage. Vasopressin has been widely used to control bleeding from oesophageal varices, as discussed on p.1637. However, terlipressin, and more recently octreotide, have been found to have some advantages over vasopressin including bolus administration and fewer side-effects, and octreotide is increasingly preferred for this purpose. Glyceryl trinitrate has been given with the aim of counteracting the adverse cardiac effects of vasopressin while potentiating its beneficial effects on portal pressure.[1-4]

References listed below also give information on the use of vasopressin in the management of some other haemorrhagic disorders, including massive haemorrhage in Crohn's disease, blood loss in abortion or caesarean section, and haemoptysis.[5-8]

1. Stump DL, Hardin TC. The use of vasopressin in the treatment of upper gastrointestinal haemorrhage. *Drugs* 1990; **39:** 38–53.
2. Williams SGJ, Westaby D. Management of variceal haemorrhage. *BMJ* 1994; **308:** 1213–17.
3. Sung JJY. Non-surgical treatment of variceal haemorrhage. *Br J Hosp Med* 1997; **57:** 162–6.
4. McCormack G, McCormack PA. A practical guide to the management of oesophageal varices. *Drugs* 1999; **57:** 327–35.
5. Mellor JA, *et al.* Massive gastrointestinal bleeding in Crohn's disease: successful control by intra-arterial vasopressin infusion. *Gut* 1982; **23:** 872–4.
6. Schulz KF, *et al.* Vasopressin reduces blood loss from second-trimester dilatation and evacuation abortion. *Lancet* 1985; **ii:** 353–6.
7. Noseworthy TW, Anderson BJ. Massive hemoptysis. *Can Med Assoc J* 1986; **135:** 1097–9.
8. Lurie S, *et al.* Subendometrial vasopressin to control intractable placental bleeding. *Lancet* 1997; **349:** 698.

Preparations

Ph. Eur.: Lypressin Injection;
USP 25: Lypressin Nasal Solution; Vasopressin Injection.

Proprietary Preparations (details are given in Part 3)
Austral.: Pitressin; **Canad.:** Pressyn; **Fr.:** Diapid†; **Ger.:** Pitressin; Vasopressin†; **Irl.:** Pitressin; Syntopressin; **Neth.:** Vasopressine†; **NZ:** Pitressin; **S.Afr.:** Vasopressin†; **Spain:** Vasopresina†; **Swed.:** Postacton†; **UK:** Pitressin; Syntopressin†; **USA:** Diapid†; Pitressin.

Used as an adjunct in: **Ger.:** Neo-Lidocaton†; **Thai.:** Neo-Lidocaton.

Local Anaesthetics

Local anaesthetics produce reversible loss of function or sensation by preventing or diminishing the conduction of nerve impulses near to the site of their application or injection. Because their mode of action is to decrease permeability of the nerve cell membrane to sodium ions, they also have a membrane stabilising effect.

Clinically useful local anaesthetics have the same general chemical configuration of an amine portion joined to an aromatic residue by an ester or amide link. The type of linkage is important in determining the properties of the drug.

For a classification of local anaesthetics, see Table 1, below.

Table 1. Classification of local anaesthetics.

Amide type	Ester type
Articaine	*Esters of benzoic acid*
Bupivacaine	Amylocaine
Cinchocaine	Cocaine
Ethyl parapiperidino-acetylaminobenzoate	Propanocaine
Etidocaine	*Esters of meta-aminobenzoic acid*
Levobupivacaine	Proxymetacaine
Lignocaine [lidocaine]	
Mepivacaine	*Esters of para-aminobenzoic acid*
Oxetacaine	
Prilocaine	Amethocaine [tetracaine]
Ropivacaine	Benzocaine
Tolycaine	Butacaine
Trimecaine	Butoxycaine
Miscellaneous	Butyl aminobenzoate
Diperodon	Chloroprocaine
Dyclonine	Oxybuprocaine
Ethyl chloride	Parethoxycaine
Ketocaine	Procaine
Myrtecaine	Propoxycaine
Octacaine	Tricaine
Pramocaine	
Propipocaine	
Quinisocaine	

Adverse Effects

Adverse effects apparent after local anaesthesia may be caused by the anaesthetic or errors in technique, or may be the result of blockade of the sympathetic nervous system. Local anaesthetics may produce systemic adverse effects as a result of raised plasma concentrations that occur when the rate of uptake into the circulation exceeds the rate of breakdown, for example, following

- accidental intravascular injection
- excessive dosage or rate of administration
- absorption of large amounts through mucous membranes or damaged skin
- absorption of large amounts from inflamed or highly vascular areas.

The systemic toxicity of local anaesthetics mainly involves the CNS and the cardiovascular system. Excitation of the CNS may be manifested by restlessness, excitement, nervousness, paraesthesias, dizziness, tinnitus, blurred vision, nausea and vomiting, muscle twitching and tremors, and convulsions. Numbness of the tongue and perioral region, and lightheadedness followed by sedation may appear as early signs of systemic toxicity. Excitation when it occurs may be transient and followed by depression with drowsiness, respiratory failure, and coma. There may be effects on the cardiovascular system with myocardial depression and peripheral vasodilatation resulting in hypotension and bradycardia; arrhythmias and cardiac arrest may occur. Hypotension often accompanies spinal and epidural anaesthesia; inappropriate positioning of the patient may be a contributory factor for women in labour.

Hypersensitivity reactions are rare and generally limited to local anaesthetics of the ester type. There ap-

pears to be no cross-sensitivity between ester- and amide-type local anaesthetics. Idiosyncrasy to local anaesthetics has been reported. Hypersensitivity reactions to preservatives in local anaesthetic preparations have also occurred.

Some local anaesthetics cause methaemoglobinaemia.

Fetal intoxication has occurred following the use of local anaesthetics in labour, either as a result of transplacental diffusion or after accidental injection of the fetus.

Prolonged use of topical anaesthetics in the eye causes corneal damage.

Adverse effects may also be caused by concomitantly administered vasoconstrictors.

◊ Reviews.
1. McCaughey W. Adverse effects of local anaesthetics. *Drug Safety* 1992; **7:** 178–189.
2. Berde CB. Toxicity of local anesthetics in infants and children. *J Pediatr* 1993; **122** (suppl): S14–S20.
3. Naguib M, *et al.* Adverse effects and drug interactions associated with local and regional anaesthesia. *Drug Safety* 1998; **18:** 221–50.
4. Dalens BJ, Mazoit J-X. Adverse effects of regional anaesthesia in children. *Drug Safety* 1998; **19:** 251–68.

Adverse effects of central block. Central nerve block (see Local Anaesthetic Techniques, below), comprising spinal or epidural block, is very widely used and certain adverse effects are particularly associated with the technique. Systemic effects (see Adverse Effects, above) are more likely with epidural than with spinal block, because of the larger doses used.

Total spinal anaesthesia from extreme spread of a block or accidental penetration of the dura during an epidural block produces unconsciousness, hypotension, and respiratory arrest. Less extensive spread to the cervical region is usually associated with nausea, agitation, and hypotension.

Hypotension (associated with venodilatation and decreased cardiac output secondary to sympathetic block) is the **cardiovascular** effect most often associated with the technique, and may be especially problematic in pregnancy. Other cardiovascular complications may include bradycardia or heart block; cardiac arrest has also been reported unexpectedly after spinal anaesthesia.

Post-dural puncture headache (see Treatment of Adverse Effects, below) is probably the most common **neurological complication** related to these procedures and may be accompanied by tinnitus or photophobia. Headache following spinal block may rarely be caused by meningitis. Backache is a frequent postoperative complication following epidural, spinal, or general anaesthesia. Cranial nerve lesions and reversible loss of hearing in the low frequency range, usually affecting both ears, have been reported rarely following spinal block. Neurological complications associated with these blocks may also rarely include paraplegia caused by arachnoiditis, or trauma or compression of the spinal cord following development of a haematoma or abscess. Transient radicular irritation involving the lower back, buttocks, and thighs may develop within 24 hours of spinal block; recovery is usually within 1 week. Cauda equina syndrome, the symptoms of which include urinary retention, loss of perineal sensation, loss of sexual function, and faecal incontinence, is also a rare complication which can present many months after spinal block.

Perioperative shivering has been associated with epidural block.

References.
1. Kalmanovitch DVA, Simmons P. Post-anaesthetic complications in the home. *Prescribers' J* 1988; **28:** 124–31.
2. Wildsmith JAW, Lee JA. Neurological sequelae of spinal anaesthesia. *Br J Anaesth* 1989; **63:** 505–7.
3. Parnass SM, Schmidt KJ. Adverse effects of spinal and epidural anaesthesia. *Drug Safety* 1990; **5:** 179–94.
4. Anonymous. Perioperative shivering. *Lancet* 1991; **338:** 547–8.
5. Broome IJ. Hearing loss and dural puncture. *Lancet* 1993; **341:** 667–8.
6. Russell R, *et al.* Assessing long term backache after childbirth. *BMJ* 1993; **306:** 1299–1303.
7. Harding SA, *et al.* Meningitis after combined spinal-extradural anaesthesia in obstetrics. *Br J Anaesth* 1994; **73:** 545–7.
8. Gielen M. Spinal anaesthesia: hearing loss, failure, transient radicular irritation. *Anaesthesia* 1998; **53** (suppl 2): 23–5.
9. Horlocker TT, Wedel DJ. Neurologic complications of spinal and epidural anesthesia. *Reg Anesth Pain Med* 2000; **25:** 88–98.

Effects on the ears. Symptoms such as vertigo, nausea, and nystagmus, which have been reported following the use of local anaesthetics in the external[1] or middle ear,[2] may result from penetration of the local anaesthetic into the inner ear. For reference to hearing loss associated with spinal block, see under Adverse Effects of Central Block, above.

1. Raine NMN, Whittet HB. Emla cream and induced vertigo. *Br J Hosp Med* 1994; **51:** 614–15.
2. Blair Simmons F, *et al.* Lidocaine in the middle ear: a unique cause of vertigo. *Arch Otolaryngol* 1973; **98:** 42–3.

Hypersensitivity. Local anaesthetics may provoke types I and IV hypersensitivity reactions. Type I reactions (e.g. anaphylaxis) to local anaesthetics are generally rare. They occur more frequently with the ester-type than with the amide-type drugs, probably because of the metabolism of the former to para-aminobenzoic acid (PABA). Nevertheless, severe or fatal reactions have been associated not only with ester-type local anaesthetics such as amethocaine [tetracaine][1] and procaine[2] but also with the amide-type local anaesthetics lignocaine [lidocaine][3-7] and prilocaine.[5] Intolerance may also have been the cause of death in a patient who received mepivacaine for paracervical anaesthesia.[8] Hypotension encountered during dental anaesthesia is usually a vasovagal response unrelated to the type of local anaesthetic used and may be prevented by the use of diazepam. Patients sensitised by topical application may subsequently develop anaphylactic reactions when treated systemically.[9] The use of drugs such as benzocaine or amethocaine [tetracaine] in lozenges or throat sprays may also sensitise patients.[10]

Some patients diagnosed as being hypersensitive to local anaesthetics may have reacted to preservatives in the preparations.[11] Cross-hypersensitivity reactions may also occur between some ester-type local anaesthetics and topical preparations, such as sunscreens, that contain PABA or related compounds.[12]

Skin testing may be of benefit in patients who will require future local anaesthesia and when a patient's history does not rule out a possible allergic reaction. However, testing itself can cause severe or anaphylactic reactions.[9,13]

Type IV reactions (i.e. delayed reactions) to local anaesthetics have also been reported, albeit rarely.[14-16]

For reports of the incidence of allergy to local anaesthetics determined by patch testing, see under individual monographs.

1. Moriwaki K, *et al.* A case report of anaphylactic shock induced by tetracaine used for spinal anesthesia. *Masui* 1986; **35:** 1279–84.
2. MacLachlan D, Forrest AL. Procaine and malignant hyperthermia. *Lancet* 1974; i: 355.
3. Fisher MM, Pennington JC. Allergy to local anaesthesia. *Br J Anaesth* 1982; **54:** 893–4.
4. Howard JJ, *et al.* Adult respiratory distress syndrome following administration of lidocaine. *Chest* 1982; **81:** 644–5.
5. Promisloff RA, DuPont DC. Death from ARDS and cardiovascular collapse following lidocaine administration. *Chest* 1983; **83:** 585.
6. Ruffles SP, Ayres JG. Fatal bronchospasm after topical lignocaine before bronchoscopy. *BMJ* 1994; **294:** 1658–9.
7. Ball IA. Allergic reactions to lignocaine. *Br Dent J* 1999; **186:** 224–6.
8. Grimes DA, Cates W. Deaths from paracervical anesthesia used for first-trimester abortion, 1972–1975. *N Engl J Med* 1976; **295:** 1397–9.
9. Mulvey PM. Allergy to local anaesthesia. *Med J Aust* 1980; **1:** 386.
10. Verbov J. Drug eruptions. *Practitioner* 1979; **222:** 400–9.
11. Wildsmith JAW, *et al.* Alleged allergy to local anaesthetic drugs. *Br Dent J* 1998; **184:** 507–10.
12. Parnass SM, Schmidt KJ. Adverse effects of spinal and epidural anesthesia. *Drug Safety* 1990; **5:** 179–94.
13. Brown DT, *et al.* Allergic reaction to an amide local anaesthetic. *Br J Anaesth* 1981; **53:** 435–7.
14. Klein CE, Gall H. Type IV allergy to amide-type local anesthetics. *Contact Dermatitis* 1991; **25:** 45–8.
15. Craft DV, Good RP. Delayed hypersensitivity reaction of the knee after injection of arthroscopy portals with bupivacaine (Marcaine). *Arthroscopy* 1994; **10:** 305–8.
16. Bircher AJ, *et al.* Delayed-type hypersensitivity to subcutaneous lidocaine with tolerance to articaine: confirmation by in vivo and in vitro tests. *Contact Dermatitis* 1996; **34:** 387–9.

Methaemoglobinaemia. Methaemoglobinaemia has been reported following the use of several local anaesthetics including amethocaine [tetracaine],[1] benzocaine,[1-3] and lignocaine [lidocaine][1] but is more commonly associated with the use of prilocaine.[4-6] It may occur following local injection or topical administration. It has been suggested that the effect is due to the presence of an aniline group in the structure or, in the case of lignocaine [lidocaine] and prilocaine, metabolism to an aniline-like structure. Methaemoglobinaemia may result from the use of usual doses as well as exposure to toxic concentrations of local anaesthetic;[1,6] with prilocaine doses of 8 mg per kg body-weight or more [above recommended maxima] usually produce symptoms.[7]

Methaemoglobinaemia has occurred following the topical application of a eutectic preparation of prilocaine and lignocaine [lidocaine].[5] Although increases in methaemoglobin concentrations are generally small following the use of this mixture in infants[8,9] and children,[10] some infants may be particularly susceptible to induced methaemoglobinaemia during the first 3 months of life probably due to their limited enzyme capacity.[8] In consequence the use of eutectic prilocaine/lignocaine [lidocaine] cream is not recommended in the UK below 1 year of age, although in some countries such preparations are licensed for limited use in neonates (see also Surface Anaesthesia, under Lignocaine p.1316).

Concomitant administration of other drugs such as sulfonamides[5] or antimalarials[7] may predispose to methaemoglobinaemia. Patients with haemoglobinopathies or glucose-6-

phosphate dehydrogenase deficiency may also be at greater risk.[1]

1. Olson ML, McEvoy GK. Methemoglobinemia induced by local anesthetics. *Am J Hosp Pharm* 1981; **38**: 89–93.
2. Rodriguez LF, *et al*. Benzocaine-induced methemoglobinemia: report of a severe reaction and review of the literature. *Ann Pharmacother* 1994; **28**: 643–9.
3. Tush GM, Kuhn RJ. Methemoglobinemia induced by an over-the-counter medication. *Ann Pharmacother* 1996; **30**: 1251–4.
4. Mandel S. Methemoglobinemia following neonatal circumcision. *JAMA* 1989; **261**: 702.
5. Jakobson B, Nilsson A. Methemoglobinemia associated with a prilocaine-lidocaine cream and trimetoprim-sulphamethoxazole: a case report. *Acta Anaesthesiol Scand* 1985; **29**: 453–5.
6. Knobeloch L, *et al*. Prilocaine-induced methemoglobinemia—Wisconsin, 1993. *JAMA* 1994; **272**: 1403–4.
7. Reynolds F. Adverse effects of local anaesthetics. *Br J Anaesth* 1987; **59**: 78–95.
8. Nilsson A, *et al*. Inverse relationship between age-dependent erythrocyte activity of methaemoglobin reductase and prilocaine-induced methaemoglobinaemia during infancy. *Br J Anaesth* 1990; **64**: 72–6.
9. Brisman M, *et al*. Methaemoglobin formation after the use of EMLA cream in term neonates. *Acta Paediatr* 1998; **87**: 1191–4.
10. Frayling IM, *et al*. Methaemoglobinaemia in children treated with prilocaine-lignocaine cream. *BMJ* 1990; **301**: 153–4.

Pregnancy. As mentioned under Adverse Effects of Central Block, above, hypotension may be particularly problematic for patients receiving epidural or spinal block for analgesia during labour. In addition it has been suggested that patients receiving epidural analgesia during labour may have an increased risk of pyrexia, which can lead to fetal compromise.[1] See also under Labour Pain on p.6.

For adverse effects on the fetus associated with paracervical block, see Peripheral Nerve Block under Local Anaesthetic Techniques, below.

1. Fusi L, *et al*. Maternal pyrexia associated with the use of epidural analgesia in labour. *Lancet* 1989; **i**: 1250–2.

Treatment of Adverse Effects

At the first signs of local anaesthetic toxicity due to parenteral administration, the injection should be stopped; in some cases it may also be possible to apply a tourniquet to limit further systemic absorption. Subsequent management, regardless of route of administration, is supportive. In the event of systemic reactions developing steps should be taken to maintain the circulation and respiration and to control convulsions. A patent airway must be established and oxygen given, together with assisted ventilation if necessary. The circulation should be maintained with infusions of intravenous fluids. Vasopressors have been suggested in the treatment of marked hypotension although their use is accompanied by a risk of CNS excitation. Ephedrine is preferred for the management of hypotension associated with spinal or epidural block, particularly in pregnancy. Vasopressors should not be given to patients receiving oxytocic drugs. Convulsions may be controlled by the intravenous administration of benzodiazepines such as diazepam although these drugs may also depress respiration and the circulation. Intravenous phenobarbital is used for persistent convulsions.

Methaemoglobinaemia may be treated by the intravenous administration of methylene blue [methylthioninium chloride].

Post-dural puncture headache. Headache following puncture of the dura mater (post-dural puncture headache) during procedures such as lumbar puncture or central nerve blocks is thought to be caused by subsequent leakage of CSF. The incidence of such headache is significantly reduced by the use of small, blunt needles which produce a smaller hole in the dura and separate its fibres rather than cutting them.

When treatment is necessary conservative therapy such as analgesics and hydration will relieve symptoms in the majority of patients with mild post-dural puncture headache within 1 to 2 days. Bed rest does not reduce the incidence but once headache develops the patient may feel some relief when recumbent. If the headache persists for a further 24 hours measures such as epidural saline or dextran or the use of intravenous caffeine and sodium benzoate may be effective; oral caffeine has also been shown to be of benefit. If such measures are unsuccessful then the epidural injection of autologous blood to form a blood patch over the dural puncture is extremely effective. There have been anecdotal reports of success using corticotropin or tetracosactide.

References.

1. Choi A, *et al*. Pharmacologic management of postdural puncture headache. *Ann Pharmacother* 1996; **30**: 831–9.
2. Broadley SA. Fuller GN. Lumbar puncture needn't be a headache. *BMJ* 1997; **315**: 1324–5.
3. Serpell MG, *et al*. Prevention of headache after lumbar puncture: questionnaire survey of neurologists and neurosurgeons in United Kingdom. *BMJ* 1998; **316**: 1709–10.

Precautions

As with any drug local anaesthetics are contra-indicated in patients with known hypersensitivity. However, it might be possible to avoid reactions by using a local anaesthetic of the alternative chemical type. Facilities for resuscitation should be available when local anaesthetics are administered parenterally.

Local anaesthetics should not be used in patients with complete heart block. They should be given cautiously to the elderly, to the debilitated, to children, and to patients with epilepsy, impaired cardiac conduction or respiratory function, shock, or hepatic impairment; patients with myasthenia gravis are particularly susceptible to the effects of local anaesthetics. Ester-type local anaesthetics are contra-indicated in patients with low plasma-cholinesterase concentrations. Techniques such as epidural or spinal block should not be employed in patients with cerebrospinal diseases, cardiogenic or hypovolaemic shock, or altered coagulation status. Because of the risk of transmitting infection into the CNS these techniques should not be employed where there is pyogenic infection of the skin at or adjacent to the injection site.

Because of the risk of systemic adverse effects when local anaesthetics are absorbed too rapidly, they should not be injected into or applied to inflamed or infected tissues or to damaged skin or mucosa. For similar reasons, the rate of injection should not be too rapid and great care must be taken to avoid inadvertent intravascular injection. The risk of adverse effects from the uptake of local anaesthetics into the circulation may be reduced by the inclusion of adrenaline [epinephrine] to produce vasoconstriction, but the lowest effective concentration of adrenaline [epinephrine] should be used. Solutions containing adrenaline [epinephrine] should not, however, be used for producing anaesthesia in appendages such as digits, because the profound ischaemia that follows may lead to gangrene. Mepivacaine and prilocaine tend to produce less vasodilatation at low concentrations than other local anaesthetics and may be useful where the addition of vasoconstrictors is contra-indicated (but see also under Action, below).

When used in the mouth or throat, local anaesthetics may impair swallowing and increase the risk of aspiration. Patients who have received local anaesthetics for procedures such as laryngoscopy or tracheoscopy should be cautioned not to eat or drink for at least 3 to 4 hours after the anaesthetic.

The cornea may be damaged by prolonged topical application of local anaesthetics, particularly cocaine. Patients should be warned not to rub or touch the eye while anaesthesia persists and the anaesthetised eye should be protected from dust and bacterial contamination.

Local anaesthetics may be ototoxic and should not be instilled into the middle ear.

The application of local anaesthetics to the skin for prolonged periods or to extensive areas should be avoided.

Precautions for central block. Epidural or spinal block may rarely result in paraplegia caused by an induced haematoma or abscess producing arachnoiditis, trauma, or compression of the spinal cord. These blocks have therefore in general been considered to be unsuitable for use in patients with pre-existing neurological disease, infection at the puncture site, or blood disorders or in those receiving aspirin or full-dose anticoagulant therapy. Such therapy may be discontinued at an appropriate time before surgery if central block is planned. It is necessary to balance the risk of withholding anticoagulation against the risk of bleeding in the individual patient. Epidural or spinal block in patients receiving low-dose anticoagulant therapy to prevent postoperative deep-vein thrombosis is still controversial. For further discussion and recommendations on concomitant use see p.903.

A study in the USA[1] involving 891 patients found that low-dose aspirin during pregnancy did not increase the risk of bleeding complications during epidural anaesthesia compared with placebo; it was considered that the recommendation to stop aspirin 7 to 10 days before delivery was unjustified.

1. Sibai BM, *et al*. Low-dose aspirin in correlation between bleeding time and maternal-neonatal bleeding complications. *Am J Obstet Gynecol* 1995; **172**: 1553–7.

Pregnancy. For discussions covering the precautions associated with the use of epidural or spinal blocks during labour, see under Labour Pain, p.6.

Tachyphylaxis. The effect of successive epidural injections of 2% solutions of lignocaine [lidocaine], mepivacaine, or prilocaine was reduced by 25 to 30% with each injection when the interval between the disappearance of analgesia and re-injection was more than 10 minutes but anaesthesia was augmented if this interval was less than 10 minutes.[1] Such tachyphylaxis, associated with the prolonged epidural administration of all local anaesthetics, has been reviewed more recently.[2]

1. Bromage PR, *et al*. Tachyphylaxis in epidural analgesia 1: augmentation and decay of local anesthesia. *J Clin Pharmacol* 1969; **9**: 30–8.
2. Mogensen T. Tachyphylaxis to epidural local anaesthetics. *Dan Med Bull* 1995; **42**: 141–6.

Test dose. A test dose is recommended in epidural block to check for accidental intravenous or intrathecal injection but negative results should be treated with caution.[1] Accidental intravenous placement of the needle is notoriously more difficult to detect than inadvertent subarachnoid placement. Adrenaline [epinephrine] has been added to the test solution to aid detection of intravenous injection but is considered by some to be of little value.[2,3]

1. Scott DB. Test doses in extradural block. *Br J Anaesth* 1988; **61**: 129–30.
2. Thornburn J. Limitations of adrenaline test doses in obstetric patients undergoing extradural anaesthesia. *Br J Anaesth* 1989; **62**: 578–81.
3. Narchi P, *et al*. Heart rate response to an iv test dose of adrenaline and lignocaine with and without atropine pretreatment. *Br J Anaesth* 1991; **66**: 583–6.

Interactions

The metabolism of ester-type local anaesthetics may be inhibited by anticholinesterases thus increasing the risk of systemic toxicity.

Ester derivatives such as amethocaine [tetracaine], benzocaine, or procaine that are hydrolysed to para-aminobenzoic acid may antagonise the activity of aminosalicylic acid or sulfonamides. Ester-type local anaesthetics such as procaine and cocaine that are hydrolysed by plasma cholinesterase may competitively enhance the neuromuscular blocking activity of suxamethonium; the amide local anaesthetic, lignocaine [lidocaine] may have a similar effect.

There is an increased risk of myocardial depression when amide-type local anaesthetics such as bupivacaine, lignocaine [lidocaine], or ropivacaine are administered concomitantly with antiarrhythmics.

If local anaesthetics containing adrenaline [epinephrine] are given for epidural or paracervical block during labour the use of an oxytocic drug post partum may lead to severe hypertension. Although there is no clinical evidence of dangerous interactions between adrenaline [epinephrine]-containing local anaesthetics and MAOIs or tricyclic antidepressants, great care should nevertheless be taken to avoid inadvertent intravenous administration of the local anaesthetic preparation.

For further details of interactions between local anaesthetics and other drugs, see under individual monographs.

Pharmacokinetics

Most local anaesthetics are readily absorbed through mucous membranes, and through damaged skin. Local anaesthetics are weak bases and at tissue pH can diffuse through connective tissue and cellular membranes to reach the nerve fibre where ionisation can occur.

Anaesthetics of the ester type are hydrolysed by esterases in the plasma and, to a lesser extent, in the liver. The effect of spinal anaesthetics lasts until the drug is taken up into the blood circulation since there is little esterase in the spinal fluid.

Amide-type anaesthetics are metabolised in the liver and, in some cases, the kidneys. While there is little protein binding with most ester-type anaesthetics, the amide types are considerably bound.

◊ References.

1. Tucker GT. Pharmacokinetics of local anaesthetics. *Br J Anaesth* 1986; **58**: 717–31.
2. Burm AGL. Clinical pharmacokinetics of epidural and spinal anaesthesia. *Clin Pharmacokinet* 1989; **16**: 283–311.
3. Smith C. Pharmacology of local anaesthetic agents. *Br J Hosp Med* 1994; **52**: 455–60.

Uses and Administration

Local anaesthetics act by preventing the generation and transmission of impulses along nerve fibres and at nerve endings; depolarisation and ion-exchange are inhibited. The effects are reversible. They are used for the local relief of painful conditions, and to prevent pain and discomfort of various medical and surgical procedure (see below). In general, loss of pain (analgesia) occurs before loss of sensory and autonomic function (anaesthesia) and loss of motor function (paralysis), but this may depend on the drug used and the site of administration.

Local anaesthetics vary in their potency and speed of onset and duration of action. The anaesthetic must penetrate the lipoprotein nerve sheath in its unionised form before it can act and therefore drugs with high lipid-solubility tend to have a greater potency and duration of action and a faster onset than drugs with low lipid-solubility. The most protein-bound drugs tend to have the longest duration of action.

The potency of local anaesthetics is traditionally compared against that of procaine, which is low; chloroprocaine, lignocaine [lidocaine], mepivacaine, and prilocaine are similar or somewhat more potent; etidocaine is of intermediate potency, bupivacaine and ropivacaine highly potent, and amethocaine [tetracaine] extremely potent.

Speed of onset and duration of action also depend on the technique employed (see below), the type of block, and the site of administration.

The speed of onset and duration of action of local anaesthetics may be increased by the addition of a vasoconstrictor, which has the effect of reducing the uptake of the local anaesthetic into the circulation from the injection site. Solutions containing adrenaline [epinephrine] 1 in 200 000 are generally advocated, although higher concentrations such as 1 in 80 000 may be used in dentistry where the total dose is small. The total amount of adrenaline [epinephrine] injected should not exceed 500 µg although the amount of adrenaline [epinephrine] absorbed varies considerably with the site of administration; some consider that the maximum dose should be 200 µg. Other vasoconstrictors including noradrenaline [norepinephrine] are also used, but authorities in the UK consider that noradrenaline [norepinephrine] should not be used since it presents no advantages and when administered at relatively high concentrations has occasionally been associated with severe hypertensive episodes. Vasoconstrictors should not be used when producing a nerve block in an appendage such as a digit, as gangrene may occur. Vasoconstrictors have been added to injections for spinal block, but their use is not recommended because of the danger of reducing the blood supply to the spinal cord.

Local anaesthetics are generally administered as acidic solutions of the water-soluble hydrochloride salts; alkalinisation of these solutions or formulation as a carbonated base may increase the speed of onset (see under Administration, below).

The dosage of individual local anaesthetics depends on the injection site and the procedure used. The smallest effective dose and the lowest effective concentration should be used. Smaller doses are usually needed in the elderly, in children, in debilitated patients, and in cardiac disease. Doses should also be reduced in the presence of hepatic disease. Meticulous attention to technique is essential particularly in nerve block and spinal procedures. Injections for central nerve blocks, such as epidural (including caudal block) and spinal block should not contain preservatives.

Action. The intrinsic vasoactivity of a local anaesthetic can influence its rate of removal from the site of action and therefore its duration of action. Ester-type local anaesthetics such as amethocaine [tetracaine] and procaine are more likely to produce vasodilatation than amide-type local anaesthetics such as cinchocaine, lignocaine [lidocaine], mepivacaine, and prilocaine following intradermal administration.[1] However, cocaine differs from other ester-type local anaesthetics in that it produces vasoconstriction. The amide-type local anaesthetics can pro-

duce vasoconstriction but, apart from prilocaine, their vasoconstrictor activity has generally been found to decline with increasing concentration,[1,2] and, in one study, lignocaine [lidocaine] and bupivacaine produced more vasodilatation than vasoconstriction at the higher concentrations tested.[2] Mepivacaine has produced greater and more consistent vasoconstriction than lignocaine [lidocaine], cinchocaine, or prilocaine following intradermal injection[1] but this greater vasoactivity is not always evident.[3]

1. Willatts DG, Reynolds F. Comparison of the vasoactivity of amide and ester local anaesthetics: an intradermal study. *Br J Anaesth* 1985; **57:** 1006–11.
2. Aps C, Reynolds F. The effect of concentration on vasoactivity of bupivacaine and lignocaine. *Br J Anaesth* 1976; **48:** 1171–4.
3. Goebel WM, *et al.* Comparative circulatory levels of 2 per cent mepivacaine and 2 per cent lignocaine. *Br Dent J* 1980; **148:** 261–4.

Administration. Systemic toxic effects of local anaesthetics are related to blood concentrations and, as absorption varies considerably according to the site of injection, it has been suggested[1,2] that recommendation of a single maximum dose without regard to the site of the procedure is meaningless. If a plasma-lignocaine [lidocaine] concentration of 5 µg per mL were required for toxicity then this would be achieved by injection of 300 mg in the intercostal area, 500 mg epidurally, 600 mg in the region of the brachial plexus, or 1000 mg subcutaneously. The reduction of peak concentrations obtained by the addition of adrenaline [epinephrine] was also dependent on the site of injection. Furthermore, most cases of severe toxicity did not result from overdosage but from inadvertent intravascular injection or too rapid injection.

1. Scott DB. "Maximum recommended doses" of local anaesthetic drugs. *Br J Anaesth* 1989; **63:** 373–4.
2. Scott DB. Safe use of lignocaine. *BMJ* 1989; **299:** 56.

CARBONATED SOLUTIONS. The use of carbonated solutions of local anaesthetics instead of the usual hydrochloride salts has been discussed in several reviews.[1-3] Although some early studies indicated that carbonated solutions of bupivacaine, lignocaine [lidocaine], or prilocaine produced earlier onset of anaesthesia and improved the quality of epidural or brachial plexus blocks not all subsequent studies have confirmed these results. A method for preparing carbonated solutions has been published[4] but proprietary preparations of such solutions of bupivacaine or lignocaine [lidocaine] may be available in some countries.

1. Covino BG. Pharmacology of local anaesthetic agents. *Br J Anaesth* 1986; **58:** 701–16.
2. Burm AGL. Clinical pharmacokinetics of epidural and spinal anaesthesia. *Clin Pharmacokinet* 1989; **16:** 283–311.
3. Carrie LES. Extradural, spinal or combined block for obstetric surgical anaesthesia. *Br J Anaesth* 1990; **65:** 225–33.
4. Bromage PR. Improved conduction blockade in surgery and obstetrics: carbonated local anaesthetics. *Can Med Assoc J* 1967; **97:** 1377–84.

PH OF SOLUTIONS. The pain associated with infiltration of local anaesthetics can be reduced by buffering the solution to physiological pH with sodium bicarbonate.[1,2] Although buffering itself does not appear to compromise the efficacy of anaesthesia,[2] alkalinisation of the solution may reduce the solubility of the local anaesthetic and cause precipitation.[2-4] To enhance stability local anaesthetic solutions are usually prepared to have an acidic pH and it is therefore recommended that if solutions are buffered they should be used immediately.[2] (Solutions containing adrenaline [epinephrine] require an acidic pH.)

Similar pH adjustments for solutions for intravenous regional anaesthesia have been reported to reduce the amount of local venous irritation and thrombophlebitis[5] and to increase the speed of onset and the duration of the block.[6] However, it has been noted that alkaline pH lignocaine [lidocaine] can lower surface tension, thereby altering drop size and potentially resulting in a decreased dose if such solutions are infused via a drop counting device rather than a volume pump.[7] Alkalinisation of a solution used for epidural block for caesarean section has been reported to result in a more rapid onset of action and denser block.[8]

Alkalinisation has also been used to hasten the onset of peripheral nerve block[9] by increasing the proportion of the lipid-soluble nonionised free base but the effect in epidural block has been inconsistent.[10,11]

1. McKay W, *et al.* Sodium bicarbonate attenuates pain on skin infiltration with lidocaine, with or without epinephrine. *Anesth Analg* 1987; **66:** 572–4.
2. Cristoph RA, *et al.* Pain reduction in local anesthetic administration through pH buffering. *Ann Emerg Med* 1988; **17:** 117–20.
3. Bourget P, *et al.* Factors influencing precipitation of pH-adjusted bupivacaine solutions. *J Clin Pharm Ther* 1990; **15:** 197–204.
4. Nakano NI. Temperature-dependent aqueous solubilities of lidocaine, mepivacaine, and bupivacaine. *J Pharm Sci* 1979; **68:** 667–8.
5. Yudenfreund SM, *et al.* pH-Buffered 2-chloroprocaine for intravenous regional anesthesia. *DICP Ann Pharmacother* 1989; **23:** 614–15.
6. Armstrong P, *et al.* Effect of alkalinization of prilocaine on IV regional anaesthesia. *Br J Anaesth* 1989; **63:** 625P–626P.
7. Leor R, *et al.* The influence of pH on the intravenous delivery of lidocaine solutions. *Eur J Clin Pharmacol* 1990; **39:** 521–3.
8. Fernando R, Jones HM. Comparison of plain and alkalinized local anaesthetic mixtures of lignocaine and bupivacaine for elective extradural caesarean section. *Br J Anaesth* 1991; **67:** 699–703.
9. Coventry DM, Todd JG. Alkalinization of bupivacaine for sciatic nerve blockade. *Br J Anaesth* 1989; **62:** 227P.

10. Burm AGL. Clinical pharmacokinetics of epidural and spinal anaesthesia. *Clin Pharmacokinet* 1989; **16:** 283–311.
11. Carrie LES. Extradural, spinal or combined block for obstetric surgical anaesthesia. *Br J Anaesth* 1990; **65:** 225–33.

Anorectal disorders. See under Surface Anaesthesia, below.

Cough. Drugs such as lignocaine [lidocaine] or bupivacaine have been given by inhalation in severe intractable cough (p.1082), including cough caused by malignant neoplasms.[1-4] Cough suppression is produced by an indirect peripheral action on sensory receptors, but as all protective pulmonary reflexes may be lost and bronchospasm may be induced, nebulised local anaesthetics should be used in controlled circumstances only; there may also be temporary loss of the swallowing reflex.

1. Howard P, *et al.* Lignocaine aerosol and persistent cough. *Br J Dis Chest* 1977; **71:** 19–24.
2. Stewart CJ, Coady TJ. Suppression of intractable cough. *BMJ* 1977; **i:** 1660–1.
3. Sanders RV, Kirkpatrick MB. Prolonged suppression of cough after inhalation of lidocaine in a patient with sarcoid. *JAMA* 1984; **252:** 2456–7.
4. Brown RC, Turton CWG. Cough and angiotensin converting enzyme inhibition. *BMJ* 1988; **296:** 1741.

Endoscopy. Local anaesthetics such as lignocaine [lidocaine] are sometimes used before endoscopy to improve patient comfort and facilitate passage of the endoscope. As mentioned in the discussion on drugs used in endoscopy (see p.652) some consider that the use of local anaesthetics for procedures such as gastrointestinal endoscopy should probably be reserved for those patients who prefer not to be sedated as their use in addition to premedication with opioids or benzodiazepines appears to serve little purpose.

References.
1. Chuah SY, *et al.* Topical anaesthesia in upper gastrointestinal endoscopy. *BMJ* 1991; **303:** 695.
2. Jameson JS, *et al.* Topical anaesthesia improves toleration for upper gastrointestinal endoscopy. *Gut* 1992; **33** (suppl): S51.
3. Randell T, *et al.* Topical anaesthesia of the nasal mucosa for fibreoptic airway endoscopy. *Br J Anaesth* 1992; **68:** 164–7.

Mouth ulceration. For the role of local anaesthetics in the management of mouth ulceration, see p.1206.

Pain. Pain and its general management are discussed on p.2. Local anaesthetics are used in a variety of situations for the management of pain. They are usually given by local injection or applied topically but are sometimes used intravenously in techniques such as intravenous regional anaesthesia, which involves the continuous infusion of local anaesthetics such as lignocaine [lidocaine] to produce general analgesia. However, the technique is potentially dangerous and seldom employed.

CANCER PAIN. For the role of local anaesthetics in the management of cancer pain, see p.5.

INTRAOPERATIVE AND POSTOPERATIVE PAIN. Local anaesthetic techniques can be used to prevent intraoperative pain and discomfort, see below. For details of the use of local anaesthetics in postoperative analgesia, see p.4 and also under Choice of Analgesics in Children, p.3.

LABOUR PAIN. For the role of epidural analgesia with local anaesthetics in the relief of labour pain, see p.6.

LOW BACK PAIN. For the role of local anaesthetics in the management of low back pain, see p.6.

Postherpetic neuralgia. For the role of local anaesthetics in the management of postherpetic neuralgia, see p.7.

Soft-tissue rheumatism. For the adjunctive use of local anaesthetics in the management of soft-tissue rheumatism, see p.10.

Spasticity. The management of spasticity (p.1322) involves physiotherapy together with the use of antispastic drugs. Other approaches to treatment include nerve blocks with local anaesthetics; these can improve spasticity but should generally only be used when further muscle relaxation would not increase disability.

Local Anaesthetic Techniques

Local anaesthetics are employed in several techniques. In order of increasing level of anaesthesia they are: surface or topical anaesthesia; infiltration anaesthesia; and regional nerve block, including peripheral nerve block, sympathetic nerve block, and central nerve block which includes epidural and spinal (intrathecal or subarachnoid) block. Local anaesthetics may also be given intravenously for regional anaesthesia in the extremities.

Surface anaesthesia

Surface or topical anaesthesia blocks the sensory nerve endings in the skin or mucous membranes. Many local anaesthetics are effective surface anaesthetics, a notable exception being procaine. Penetration of intact skin by most local anaesthetics is poor whereas absorption through mucous membranes may be rapid. However reliable percutaneous anaesthesia can be achieved by application of a eutectic mixture of lignocaine [lidocaine] and prilocaine to intact skin (see under Surface Anaesthesia in Lignocaine, p.1316). Eutectic mixtures may be of value in providing surface anaesthesia for a number of minor medical or surgical procedures. Amethocaine [tetracaine] also provides reliable percutaneous anaesthesia. Other methods of dermal delivery of local anaesthetics include a transdermal patch of lignocaine [lidocaine], and an iontophoretic drug delivery system incorporating lignocaine [lidocaine] and adrenaline [epinephrine]. Anaesthesia of the skin and subcutaneous tissues is also discussed under Infiltration Anaesthesia, below.

There are a number of special uses of topical anaesthesia including anaesthetising the cornea during ophthalmological procedures and the throat and larynx before intubation and bronchoscopy. Absorption from the respiratory tract is rapid and care is essential to avoid administering a toxic dose. Great care is also necessary when employing local anaesthetics to anaesthetise the urethra; if trauma has occurred, rapid absorption of the drug may occur and give rise to serious adverse effects.

Local anaesthetics have been included in topical preparations to relieve the pain of haemorrhoids (p.1205) but good evidence of their efficacy is lacking. Similar uses include pain relief in pruritus ani and anal fissure. Excessive application of local anaesthetics to the rectal mucosa should be avoided as absorption can occur; use for periods of no longer than a few days is recommended to prevent sensitisation of the anal skin. Local anaesthetics are sometimes included in topical preparations for the relief of pruritus (p.1106). However, they are only marginally effective and can very occasionally cause sensitisation. The use of local anaesthetics in rubefacient and topical analgesic preparations is discussed on p.4.

Infiltration anaesthesia

Infiltration anaesthesia is produced by injection of a local anaesthetic such as lignocaine [lidocaine] or bupivacaine directly into and around the field of operation without attempting to identify individual nerves. The drug used should not be absorbed too rapidly otherwise the anaesthesia will wear off too quickly for practical use; some local anaesthetics require the addition of a vasoconstrictor in low concentrations, which can increase the duration of infiltration anaesthesia and reduce peak plasma concentrations of the local anaesthetic. Infiltration anaesthesia is extensively used in dentistry.

Anaesthesia of small areas by infiltration techniques requires a relatively large amount of local anaesthetic, which is not a problem for minor surgery but would be for more extensive areas that required anaesthesia. The amount of local anaesthetic used can be reduced and the duration of anaesthesia increased by blocking specific nerves that innervate the area. This may be carried out at several levels. In *field block* anaesthesia subcutaneous injection of a local anaesthetic close to the nerves around the area to be anaesthetised blocks sensory nerve paths. This is a form of infiltration anaesthesia, but the technique requires less drug for a given area to be anaesthetised.

Regional nerve block

Regional nerve block anaesthesia involves specific blocks at the levels of major nerves or spinal roots, and may include peripheral nerve block, sympathetic nerve block, and central nerve block including epidural and spinal block. For a discussion of the use of nerve blocks in the management of pain, see p.3.

Peripheral nerve block. Peripheral nerve block anaesthesia involves injection into or around a peripheral nerve or plexus supplying the part to be anaesthetised; motor fibres may be blocked as well as sensory fibres. *Brachial plexus block* is widely used for procedures involving the arm; lower limb blocks are less simple although *sciatic* and *femoral blocks* may be combined to permit surgery below the knee. Other peripheral nerve blocks such as those for the head and neck, or *intercostal* or *paravertebral blocks* for local anaesthesia of the trunk, are mostly highly specialised techniques. Lignocaine [lidocaine], prilocaine, bupivacaine or ropivacaine have all been widely employed for peripheral nerve blocks. Adrenaline [epinephrine] is often added as a vasoconstrictor.

Pudendal block (usually with prilocaine) may be useful in obstetrics for forceps delivery, but as mentioned under Labour Pain on p.6, the technique of *paracervical local anaesthetic block* has largely fallen out of favour because of the high incidence of serious adverse effects on the fetus.

Sympathetic nerve block. Sympathetic nerve block such as *stellate ganglion blockade* and *lumbar sympathectomy* is used in the management of a range of painful conditions and vascular diseases (see under Sympathetic Pain Syndromes on p.8). Temporary block is obtained using local anaesthetics such as lignocaine [lidocaine] or bupivacaine but permanent block may be produced with use of neurolytic agents such as phenol (see Pain, p.1153) or alcohol (see Pain, p.1132).

Central nerve block. Central nerve block includes epidural and spinal block.

Epidural block (also referred to as *extradural* or *peridural block*) is widely used to provide analgesia or anaesthesia in surgical and obstetric procedures. It involves injecting a local anaesthetic such as lignocaine [lidocaine], bupivacaine, or ropivacaine, alone or with a small dose of an opioid analgesic into the epidural space in the lumbar, sacral (*caudal block*), thoracic, or cervical regions. Introduction of a cannula into the epidural space enables prolonged analgesia or anaesthesia (epidural anaesthesia) to be provided through the use of 'top-up' doses or continuous infusion of the drugs. A vasoconstrictor is sometimes added to reduce systemic exposure to the local an-

aesthetic. A test dose at the intended injection site is recommended before starting epidural anaesthesia to ensure that the main dose is not accidentally injected intravascularly or into the subarachnoid space.

Spinal block (also referred to as *subarachnoid* or *intrathecal block*) is produced by injecting a solution of a suitable drug such as bupivacaine within the spinal subarachnoid space, causing temporary paralysis of the nerves with which it comes into contact. It may be used, for example, to produce spinal anaesthesia in surgical procedures on the lower body. Vasoconstrictors have been added to prolong the duration of the block but the effect is not always clinically useful and there is a danger of restricting the blood supply to the spinal cord; therefore this practice is not recommended. The somatic level at which anaesthesia occurs depends on many factors including the specific gravity or baricity of the anaesthetic solution used and the positioning of the patient.

For the adverse effects of and precautions for central block, see above.

Intravenous regional anaesthesia

Intravenous regional anaesthesia (Bier's block) involves injection of a dilute solution of local anaesthetic into a suitable limb vein after exsanguination and application of a tourniquet, in order to produce anaesthesia distal to it. Arterial flow must remain occluded for at least 20 minutes after injection and adrenaline [epinephrine] should not be used. Intravenous regional anaesthesia may be used for short procedures where postoperative pain is not marked, such as manipulation of fractures and minor surgical procedures to the limbs. Although a safe procedure when performed correctly, complications have arisen; there have been fatalities associated with the use of bupivacaine and prilocaine is the drug of choice. Facilities for resuscitation should be available.

Amethocaine (7603-v)

Amethocaine (BAN).

Tetracaine (BAN, rINN). 2-Dimethylaminoethyl 4-butylaminobenzoate.

$C_{15}H_{24}N_2O_2$ = 264.4.

CAS — 94-24-6.

ATC — C05AD02; D04AB06; N01BA03; S01HA03.

Pharmacopoeias. In Chin. and US.

Pharmacopoeial description

USP 25: A white or light yellow waxy solid. M.p. 41° to 46°. Very slightly soluble in water; soluble 1 in 5 of alcohol and 1 in 2 of chloroform or of ether; soluble in benzene. Store in airtight containers. Protect from light.

Amethocaine Hydrochloride (7604-g)

Amethocaine Hydrochloride (BANM).

Tetracaine Hydrochloride (BANM, rINNM); Dicainum; Tetracaini Hydrochloridum; Tetracainii Chloridum.

$C_{15}H_{24}N_2O_2,HCl$ = 300.8.

CAS — 136-47-0.

NOTE. AME and TET are codes approved by the BP 2001 for use on single unit doses of eye drops containing amethocaine [tetracaine] hydrochloride where the individual container may be too small to bear all the appropriate labelling information.

Pharmacopoeias. In Chin., Eur. (see p.vi), Int., Jpn, Pol., and US.

Pharmacopoeial description

Ph. Eur.: A white, slightly hygroscopic, polymorphic, crystalline powder. Freely soluble in water; soluble in alcohol; practically insoluble in ether. A 1% solution in water has a pH of 4.5 to 6.5. Protect from light.

USP 25: A fine, white, odourless, hygroscopic, polymorphic, crystalline powder. Very soluble in water; soluble in alcohol; insoluble in ether and in benzene. Its solutions are neutral to litmus. Store in airtight containers. Protect from light.

Adverse Effects and Treatment

As for Local Anaesthetics in general, p.1302.

Amethocaine [tetracaine] has high systemic toxicity. Absorption of amethocaine [tetracaine] from mucous membranes is rapid and adverse reactions can occur abruptly without the appearance of prodromal signs or convulsions; fatalities have occurred.

A stinging sensation may occur when amethocaine [tetracaine] is used in the eye. Mild erythema at the site of application is frequently seen with topical administration; slight oedema or pruritus occur less commonly. Blistering of the skin may occur.

Urethral stricture. There has been a report[1] of a sudden increase in the incidence of urethral stricture following transurethral surgery, which may have been due to an increase in the concentration of amethocaine [tetracaine] hydrochloride in the lubricant gel from 0.1 to 3%.

1. Pansadoro V. Role of local anaesthetics in urethral strictures after transurethral surgery. *Lancet* 1990; **336:** 64.

Precautions

As for Local Anaesthetics in general, p.1303.

Amethocaine [tetracaine] should not be applied to inflamed, traumatised, or highly vascular surfaces. It should not be used to provide anaesthesia for bronchoscopy or cystoscopy, as lignocaine [lidocaine] is a safer alternative.

Interactions

For interactions associated with local anaesthetics, see p.1303.

Pharmacokinetics

See under Local Anaesthetics, p.1303. Amethocaine [tetracaine] is reported to be about 15% bioavailable following application of a 4% gel to intact skin, with a mean absorption and elimination half-life of about 75 minutes.

Uses and Administration

Amethocaine [tetracaine], a para-aminobenzoic acid ester, is a potent local anaesthetic with actions and uses similar to those described on p.1304. It is used for surface anaesthesia and spinal block; its use in other local anaesthetic techniques is restricted by its systemic toxicity.

Amethocaine [tetracaine] is generally used as the hydrochloride in solutions and creams, and as the base in gels or ointments.

For *anaesthesia of the eye*, solutions containing 0.5 to 1% amethocaine [tetracaine] hydrochloride and ointments containing 0.5% amethocaine [tetracaine] have been used. Instillation of a 0.5% solution produces anaesthesia within 25 seconds that lasts for 15 minutes or longer and is suitable for use before minor surgical procedures.

For *topical anaesthesia*, a 1% cream or a 0.5% ointment has been used. These preparations have been used for painful conditions of the *anus or rectum*. A 4% gel is used as a *percutaneous local anaesthetic* before *venepuncture or venous cannulation*. The gel is applied to the centre of the area to be anaesthetised and covered with an occlusive dressing. Gel and dressing are removed after 30 minutes for venepuncture and after 45 minutes for venous cannulation. A single application generally provides anaesthesia for 4 to 6 hours. This method is not suitable for premature infants or those less than 1 month of age.

Amethocaine [tetracaine] hydrochloride has also been used in the *mouth* in sprays and lozenges.

Amethocaine [tetracaine] hydrochloride has also been used for *spinal block* usually as a 0.5% solution.

Action. For a comparison of the vasoactivity of amethocaine [tetracaine] with some other local anaesthetics, see p.1304.

Spinal block. A study[1] in 40 patients indicated that for patients undergoing caesarean section with spinal anaesthesia (see Central Nerve Block, p.1305) doses of 12 or 14 mg of amethocaine [tetracaine] provided better intraoperative analgesia than doses of 8 or 10 mg without leading to excessive spread of the block.

1. Hirabayashi Y, *et al.* Visceral pain during Caesarean section: effect of varying dose of spinal amethocaine. *Br J Anaesth* 1995; **75:** 266–8.

Surface anaesthesia. A topical gel formulation of amethocaine [tetracaine] 4% appears to provide more rapid and prolonged surface anaesthesia (see p.1304) than a eutectic mixture of lignocaine [lidocaine] and prilocaine.[1,2] In a double-blind placebo-controlled study[3] the amethocaine [tetracaine] gel formulation was significantly better than the eutectic mixture in reducing pain caused by laser treatment of portwine stains. Similar findings were also seen in a comparative study in children requiring venous cannulation.[4] The same formulation appears to be equally effective when incorporated into a transdermal patch.[5]

There have been reports of seizures and death in children following the use of a mixture of amethocaine [tetracaine], adrenaline [epinephrine], and cocaine on mucosal surfaces;[6] application of preparations of amethocaine [tetracaine] to highly vascular surfaces is contra-indicated. A gel containing a mixture of lignocaine [lidocaine], adrenaline [epinephrine], and amethocaine [tetracaine] has been found to be an effective alternative to the cocaine-containing preparation.[7]

Amethocaine [tetracaine] has also been incorporated into a mucosa-adhesive polymer film to relieve the pain of oral lesions resulting from radiation and antineoplastic therapy.[8] Liposome-encapsulated amethocaine [tetracaine] has also been shown to provide adequate surface anaesthesia.[9]

1. McCafferty DF, et al. In vivo assessment of percutaneous local anaesthetic preparations. Br J Anaesth 1989; 62: 17–21.
2. Rømsing J, et al. Tetracaine gel vs EMLA cream for percutaneous anaesthesia in children. Br J Anaesth 1999; 82: 637–8.
3. McCafferty DF, et al. Effect of percutaneous local anaesthetics on pain reduction during pulse dye laser treatment of portwine stains. Br J Anaesth 1997; 78: 286–9.
4. Arrowsmith J, Campbell C. A comparison of local anaesthetics for venepuncture. Arch Dis Child 2000; 82: 309–10.
5. McCafferty DF, Woolfson AD. New patch delivery system for percutaneous local anaesthesia. Br J Anaesth 1993; 71: 370–4.
6. Wong S, Hart LL. Tetracaine/adrenaline/cocaine for local anesthesia. DICP Ann Pharmacother 1990; 24: 1181–3.
7. Ernst AA, et al. Lidocaine adrenaline tetracaine gel versus tetracaine adrenaline cocaine gel for topical anesthesia in linear scalp and facial lacerations in children aged 5 to 17 years. Pediatrics 1995; 95: 255–8.
8. Yotsuyanagi T, et al. Mucosa-adhesive film containing local analgesic. Lancet 1985; ii: 613.
9. Fisher R, et al. Topical anaesthesia of intact skin: liposome-encapsulated tetracaine vs EMLA. Br J Anaesth 1998; 81: 972–3.

Preparations

BP 2001: Tetracaine Eye Drops;
USP 25: Benzocaine, Butamben, and Tetracaine Hydrochloride Gel; Benzocaine, Butamben, and Tetracaine Hydrochloride Ointment; Benzocaine, Butamben, and Tetracaine Hydrochloride Topical Aerosol; Benzocaine, Butamben, and Tetracaine Hydrochloride Topical Solution; Cocaine and Tetracaine Hydrochlorides and Epinephrine Topical Solution; Procaine and Tetracaine Hydrochlorides and Levonordefrin Injection; Tetracaine and Menthol Ointment; Tetracaine Hydrochloride Cream; Tetracaine Hydrochloride for Injection; Tetracaine Hydrochloride in Dextrose Injection; Tetracaine Hydrochloride Injection; Tetracaine Hydrochloride Ophthalmic Solution; Tetracaine Hydrochloride Topical Solution; Tetracaine Ointment; Tetracaine Ophthalmic Ointment.

Proprietary Preparations (details are given in Part 3)
Braz.: Anestesico; **Canad.:** Ametop; Cepacol Viractin; Pontocaine; Supracaine†; **Ger.:** Oto-Flexiole N†; **Israel:** Pontocaine; **NZ:** Ametop; **Port.:** Anestesico; **S.Afr.:** Ametop; Anethaine; Covostet; **Spain:** Anest Compuesto†; Anestesia Topi Braun C/A; Anestesico; Hemonet; **UK:** Ametop; Anethaine; **USA:** Ak-T-Caine†; Cepacol Viractin Cold Sore Treatment; Pontocaine.

Multi-ingredient: Aust.: Dynexan; Herviros; Neocones; Tonexol†; **Belg.:** Anesthesique Double†; **Braz.:** Anesdente do Bebe; Anestesicol; Anevrase; Hexomedine; Osmogenol; Oto Betnovate; Oto-Biotic; UM Instante; **Canad.:** Endospray; Panocaine†; **Fr.:** Amygdospray†; Aphtoral; Broncorinol maux de gorge; Cantalene; Codetricine vitamine C; Drill; Eludril; Hexomedine; Lysofon; Oromedine; Oroseptol Lysozyme; Oroseptol†; Otylol; Solutricine Maux de Gorge; Solutricine Tetracaine; Tyrcine; **Ger.:** Acoin; Gingicain D; Herviros; Ophtocain; **Hong Kong:** Herviros; Norgotin; **Israel:** Anaesthetic Ear Drops; Otidin; **Ital.:** Corizzina; Donalg; Lasoproct†; Odongi; Recto-Reparil; Ruscoroid; **Port.:** Anucet; Davicaina†; Drill; Hemofissural; Xilonibsa; **S.Afr.:** Dynexan; **Spain:** Anesti Doble; Anestina Braun†; Blastoestimulina; Carbocaina; Dentikrisos; Neocones; Otogen Calmante; Resorborina; Topicaina; Vinciseptil Otico; **Switz.:** Adrectal†; Angidine; Dynexan; Eludril; Tonex; Tyrothricine + Gramicidine; **UK:** Eludril; **USA:** Cetacaine; Stypto-Caine.

Amylocaine Hydrochloride (7605-q)

Amylocaine Hydrochloride (BANM).
Amyleinii Chloridum; Amylocain. Hydrochlor.; Chlorhydrate d'Améléine. 1-(Dimethylaminomethyl)-1-methylpropyl benzoate hydrochloride.
$C_{14}H_{21}NO_2,HCl = 271.8$.
CAS — 532-59-2 (amylocaine hydrochloride); 644-26-8 (amylocaine hydrochloride).
Pharmacopoeias. In Belg.

Profile

Amylocaine, a benzoic acid ester, is a local anaesthetic (p.1302) used mainly as the hydrochloride in a range of preparations for application to the skin or mucous membranes. It has also been used in preparations for the relief of painful anorectal conditions and has been included in oral mixtures for the relief of coughs.

Preparations

Proprietary Preparations (details are given in Part 3)
Multi-ingredient: Belg.: Babygencal; Dentophar; Dequalinium†; Rectovasol; **Braz.:** Fonergin; **Canad.:** Pommade Midy; Rhino-Mex; **Fr.:** Amygdol; Artralgon†; Avenoc†; Bronchodermine; Campho-Pneumine; Collustan; Dolodent; Elenol; Frazoline; Glottyl; Parkipan; Pholcones†; Pulmoll; Sedaplaie; **Ital.:** Dentinale; Proctosedyl; **Spain:** Eucalyptospirine Lact†; Hemodren Compuesto†; **Thai.:** Lobacin; Mybacin.

Articaine Hydrochloride (7614-p)

Articaine Hydrochloride (BANM, USAN, rINNM).
40045; Articaini Hydrochloridum; Carticaine Hydrochloride; Hoe-045. Methyl 4-methyl-3-(2-propylaminopropionamido)thiophene-2-carboxylate hydrochloride.
$C_{13}H_{20}N_2O_3S,HCl = 320.8$.
CAS — 23964-58-1 (articaine); 23964-57-0 (articaine hydrochloride).
Pharmacopoeias. In Eur. (see p.vi).

Pharmacopoeial description

Ph. Eur.: A white or almost white crystalline powder. Freely soluble in water and in alcohol. A 1% solution in water has a pH of 4.2 to 5.2. Protect from light.

Profile

Articaine hydrochloride is an amide local anaesthetic (p.1302). It has been used as a 1 or 2% solution with or without adrenaline [epinephrine] for infiltration and regional anaesthesia. A 4% solution of articaine hydrochloride with adrenaline [epinephrine] is used similarly in dentistry. A 5% hyperbaric solution of articaine hydrochloride with glucose has been used for spinal block.

Porphyria. Articaine hydrochloride is considered to be unsafe in patients with porphyria because it has been shown to be porphyrinogenic in in-vitro systems.

Preparations

Proprietary Preparations (details are given in Part 3)
Aust.: Ubistesin; Ultracain Dental; **Canad.:** Astracaine; Ultracaine D-S; **Fin.:** Ultracain D-Suprarenin; **Fr.:** Alphacaine; Predesic; **Ger.:** Ubistesin; Ultracain; Ultracain D-S; Ultracain hyperbar; Ultracain-Suprarenin; **Ital.:** Cartidont; Citocartin; Septanest; Ubistesin; Ultracain D-S; **Neth.:** Ultracain D-S; Ultracain Hyperbaar; **Spain:** Ultracain; **Switz.:** Rudocaine; Septanest; Ubistesin; Ultracaine D-S; **UK:** Septanest; **USA:** Septocaine.

Benzocaine (7608-w)

Benzocaine (BAN, rINN).
Anaesthesinum; Anesthamine; Benzocainum; Ethoform; Éthoforme; Ethyl Aminobenzoate; Ethylis Aminobenzoas. Ethyl 4-aminobenzoate.
$C_9H_{11}NO_2 = 165.2$.
CAS — 94-09-7.
ATC — C05AD03; D04AB04; N01BA05; R02AD01.
Pharmacopoeias. In Chin., Eur. (see p.vi), Int., Jpn, Pol., and US.

Pharmacopoeial description

Ph. Eur.: Colourless crystals or a white crystalline powder. M.p. 89° to 92°. Very slightly soluble in water; freely soluble in alcohol and in ether. Protect from light.

USP 25: Small, white crystals or a white odourless crystalline powder. M.p. 88° to 92°. Soluble 1 in 2500 of water, 1 in 5 of alcohol, 1 in 2 of chloroform, 1 in 4 of ether, and 1 in 30 to 50 of almond oil or olive oil; dissolves in dilute acids.

Adverse Effects and Treatment

As for Local Anaesthetics in general, p.1302.

Hypersensitivity. The incidence of positive reactions in patients patch tested with benzocaine has ranged from 3.3 to 5.9%.[1,2] Patch testing with benzocaine has been recommended by The International Contact Dermatitis Research Group as an indicator of contact hypersensitivity to local anaesthetics. However, it was found that of 40 patients who had had positive reactions to benzocaine with amethocaine [tetracaine] and cinchocaine 21 were not allergic to benzocaine alone.[3]

1. Rudzki E, Kleniewska D. The epidemiology of contact dermatitis in Poland. Br J Dermatol 1970; 83: 543–5.
2. Bandmann H-J, et al. Dermatitis from applied medicaments. Arch Dermatol 1972; 106: 335–7.
3. Beck MH, Holden A. Benzocaine—an unsatisfactory indicator of topical local anaesthetic sensitization for the UK. Br J Dermatol 1988; 118: 91–4.

Precautions

As for Local Anaesthetics in general, p.1303.

Interactions

For interactions associated with local anaesthetics, see p.1303.

Pharmacokinetics

See under Local Anaesthetics, p.1303.

Uses and Administration

Benzocaine, a para-aminobenzoic acid ester, is a local anaesthetic used for surface anaesthesia (p.1304); it has low potency and systemic toxicity. It is used, often in combination with other drugs such as analgesics, antiseptics, antibacterials, antifungals, and antipruritics, for the temporary local relief of pain associated with dental conditions, oropharyngeal disorders, haemorrhoids, anal pruritus, and ear pain.

Lozenges containing benzocaine in usual doses of up to 10 mg are used for the relief of sore throat. Gels, pastes, solutions, and sprays containing benzocaine in concentrations of up to 20% have been used for surface anaesthesia of the mouth and throat.

Benzocaine is used in ear drops, creams, ointments, lotions, solutions, sprays, gels, and suppositories in concentrations up to 20% for topical analgesia and anaesthesia.

Benzocaine has also been used as the hydrochloride.

Obesity. It has been reported[1] that despite the inclusion of benzocaine in some over-the-counter appetite suppressants there is no good evidence of its value in obesity (p.1505).

1. Anonymous. A nasal decongestant and a local anesthetic for weight control? Med Lett Drugs Ther 1979; 21: 65–6.

Preparations

USP 25: Antipyrine and Benzocaine Otic Solution; Antipyrine, Benzocaine, and Phenylephrine Hydrochloride Otic Solution; Benzocaine and Menthol Topical Aerosol; Benzocaine Cream; Benzocaine Gel; Benzocaine Lozenges; Benzocaine Ointment; Benzocaine Otic Solution; Benzocaine Topical Aerosol; Benzo-

caine Topical Solution; Benzocaine, Butamben, and Tetracaine Hydrochloride Gel; Benzocaine, Butamben, and Tetracaine Hydrochloride Ointment; Benzocaine, Butamben, and Tetracaine Hydrochloride Topical Aerosol; Benzocaine, Butamben, and Tetracaine Hydrochloride Topical Solution.

Proprietary Preparations (details are given in Part 3)
Aust.: Anaestherit; **Austral.:** Applicaine; Topicaine†; **Canad.:** Anbesol Baby; Baby Orajel; Johnson & Johnson Burn Cream; Orajel; Outgro; Sirop Dentition; Topicaine†; Zilactin Baby; Zilactin-B; **Ger.:** Anaesthesin; Flavamed Halstabletten; Subcutin N; Zahnerol N; **Israel:** Anadent; Baby Gel; Lanacane; Maintain; **Ital.:** Gengivarium†; **Mex.:** Auralyt; **NZ:** Applicaine; **Port.:** Dentispray; **Spain:** Dentispray; Gartricin; Hurricaine; Lanacane; **Switz.:** Orajel†; **UK:** AAA; Burneze; Lanacane; Ultracare; Vicks Ultra Chloraseptic; **USA:** 3 in 1 Toothache Relief; Americaine; Americaine Anesthetic; Americaine Otic; Baby Anbesol; Baby Orajel; BanSmoke†; Benzodent; Chigger-Tox; Dent's Extra Strength Toothache Gum; Dent's Lotion-Jel; Dent's Maximum Strength Toothache Drops; Dermoplast; Detane; Diet Ayds†; Hurricaine; Lanacane; Mycinettes; Numzident; Orabase Baby; Orabase Gel; Orabase-B; Orajel; Otocain; Red Cross Canker Sore Medication†; SensoGARD; Slim Mint†; Spec-T; Trocaine; Vicks Children's Chloraseptic; Zilactin-B Medicated; ZilaDent†.

Multi-ingredient: numerous preparations are listed in Part 3.

Bupivacaine Hydrochloride (7609-e)

Bupivacaine Hydrochloride (BANM, USAN, rINNM).
AH-2250; Bupivacaini Hydrochloridum; LAC-43; Win-11318. (±)-(1-Butyl-2-piperidyl)formo-2',6'-xylidide hydrochloride monohydrate.
$C_{18}H_{28}N_2O,HCl,H_2O = 342.9$.
CAS — 2180-92-9 (bupivacaine); 18010-40-7 (anhydrous bupivacaine hydrochloride); 14252-80-3 (bupivacaine hydrochloride monohydrate).
Pharmacopoeias. In Chin., Eur. (see p.vi), Int., Pol., and US.

Pharmacopoeial description

Ph. Eur.: A white crystalline powder or colourless crystals. Soluble in water; freely soluble in alcohol. Protect from light.

USP 25: A white, odourless, crystalline powder. Freely soluble in water and in alcohol; slightly soluble in acetone and in chloroform. A 1% solution in water has a pH of 4.5 to 6.0.

Stability of solutions. For a discussion of the effect that pH has on the stability of local anaesthetic solutions and the pain associated with their injection, see p.1304.

For reference to the stability of admixtures of bupivacaine and fentanyl in solution, with or without adrenaline [epinephrine], see under Fentanyl, p.37.

Adverse Effects and Treatment

As for Local Anaesthetics in general, p.1302.

Bupivacaine appears to be more cardiotoxic than other local anaesthetics. Cardiac arrest due to bupivacaine can be resistant to electrical defibrillation and a successful outcome may require prolonged resuscitative efforts.

◊ For reference to the toxic threshold for bupivacaine plasma concentrations, see Absorption under Pharmacokinetics, below.

Effects on the cardiovascular system. Bupivacaine[1,2] and etidocaine[2] appear to be more cardiotoxic than most other commonly used local anaesthetics and marked cardiovascular depression may occur at plasma concentrations only slightly above those for CNS toxicity.[2] Fatalities have occurred. Simultaneous seizures and cardiovascular collapse may develop rapidly following inadvertent intravascular injection and even prompt oxygenation and blood pressure support might not prevent cardiac arrest.[2] Ventricular fibrillation which is very resistant to normal methods of defibrillation may develop. Since lignocaine [lidocaine] and the other local anaesthetics have additive effects on the CNS bretylium may be preferable to lignocaine [lidocaine] for the treatment of induced arrhythmias.[1] Fatal cardiotoxicity has occurred following the use of bupivacaine in intravenous regional anaesthesia, possibly due to leakage past the tourniquet, and the use of bupivacaine in this technique should be avoided.[1] Fatalities have also been associated with the use of 0.75% solutions for epidural anaesthesia in obstetric patients and this strength is no longer recommended for obstetric anaesthesia. See also Labour Pain under Uses and Administration, below.

1. Anonymous. Cardiotoxicity of local anaesthetic drugs. Lancet 1986; ii: 1192–4.
2. Albright GA. Cardiac arrest following regional anesthesia with etidocaine or bupivacaine. Anesthesiology 1979; 51: 285–7.

Effects on the eyes. Bilateral retinal haemorrhages developed in a 47-year-old woman[1] after receiving a caudal block with bupivacaine 0.5%. The haemorrhages cleared and her usual vision returned by 3 months.

1. Ling C, et al. Bilateral retinal haemorrhages following epidural injection. Br J Ophthalmol 1993; 77: 316–17.

Prolonged block. Reports of prolonged block following the use of bupivacaine in regional anaesthesia.[1,2]

1. Pathy GV, Rosen M. Prolonged block with recovery after extradural analgesia for labour. *Br J Anaesth* 1975; **47**: 520–2.
2. Brockway MS, *et al.* Prolonged brachial plexus block with 0.42% bupivacaine. *Br J Anaesth* 1989; **63**: 604–5.

Precautions

As for Local Anaesthetics in general, p.1303.

Bupivacaine is contra-indicated for use in intravenous regional anaesthesia (Bier's block) and for paracervical block in obstetrics. The 0.75% solution is contra-indicated for epidural block in obstetrics.

Renal impairment. Spinal block after the administration of 3 mL bupivacaine 0.75% was reported to be more rapid in onset and of shorter duration in patients with chronic renal failure when compared with control patients.[1]

1. Orko R, *et al.* Subarachnoid anaesthesia with 0.75% bupivacaine in patients with chronic renal failure. *Br J Anaesth* 1986; **58**: 605–9.

Interactions

For interactions associated with local anaesthetics, see p.1303.

Antiarrhythmics. There is an increased risk of myocardial depression when bupivacaine and antiarrhythmics are administered concomitantly.

Beta blockers. *Propranolol* reduced the clearance of bupivacaine by 35% in 6 healthy subjects.[1] There is therefore the risk of increased bupivacaine toxicity if these drugs are administered concomitantly.

1. Bowdle TA, *et al.* Propranolol reduces bupivacaine clearance. *Anesthesiology* 1987; **66**: 36–8.

Histamine H₂-antagonists. Studies of the effect of H₂-antagonists on the pharmacokinetics of bupivacaine have yielded variable results. While one group of workers[1] found that pretreatment with *cimetidine* decreased the clearance of bupivacaine, others have failed to find any significant pharmacokinetic effects.[2,3] Similarly, pretreatment with *ranitidine* has either increased plasma concentrations of bupivacaine[4] or had no significant effect.[3]

1. Noble DW, *et al.* Effects of H-2 antagonists on the elimination of bupivacaine. *Br J Anaesth* 1987; **59**: 735–7.
2. Pihlajamäki KK. Lack of effect of cimetidine on the pharmacokinetics of bupivacaine in healthy subjects. *Br J Clin Pharmacol* 1988; **26**: 403–6.
3. Flynn RJ, *et al.* Does pretreatment with cimetidine and ranitidine affect the disposition of bupivacaine? *Br J Anaesth* 1989; **62**: 87–91.
4. Wilson CM. Plasma bupivacaine concentrations associated with extradural anaesthesia for caesarean section: influence of pretreatment with ranitidine. *Br J Anaesth* 1986; **58**: 1330P–1331P.

Local anaesthetics. For reference to the effect of bupivacaine on the protein binding of lignocaine [lidocaine] and mepivacaine, see p.1314 and p.1317, respectively.

Pharmacokinetics

Bupivacaine is about 95% bound to plasma proteins. Reported half-lives are from 1.5 to 5.5 hours in adults and about 8 hours in neonates. It is metabolised in the liver and is excreted in the urine principally as metabolites with only 5 to 6% as unchanged drug.

Bupivacaine is distributed into breast milk in small quantities. It crosses the placenta but the ratio of fetal concentrations to maternal concentrations is relatively low. Bupivacaine also diffuses into the CSF.

See also under Local Anaesthetics, p.1303.

Absorption. The toxic threshold for bupivacaine plasma concentrations is considered by some[1] to lie in the range of 2 to 4 μg per mL and in the UK the maximum single recommended dose for anhydrous bupivacaine hydrochloride is 150 mg (equivalent to approximately 2 mg per kg body-weight). Administration of bupivacaine for regional anaesthesia of the head and neck in a mean total dose of 3.4 mg per kg body-weight has produced mean peak plasma concentrations of 3.56 and 4.95 μg per mL when administered with or without adrenaline [epinephrine] respectively, without producing toxicity.[2] Similarly, intrapleural administration of bupivacaine 0.5% in a dose of 2.5 mg per kg has produced mean peak plasma concentrations of 2.57 and 3.22 μg per mL when given with or without adrenaline [epinephrine] respectively, without producing toxicity.[3] A further study[4] in which a 72-hour interpleural infusion of bupivacaine hydrochloride with adrenaline [epinephrine] was administered to cholecystectomy patients showed appreciable interpatient variability in steady-state plasma drug concentrations (range 1.3 to 3.2 μg per mL; mean 2.1 μg per mL); no patient suffered any adverse effects. Bilateral intercostal nerve blocks using bupivacaine 2 mg per kg have also produced concentrations within the presumed toxic range without adverse effects but the use of adrenaline [epinephrine] with this block did not reliably reduce peak plasma-bupivacaine concentrations.[5]

The symbol † denotes a preparation no longer actively marketed

Stellate ganglion block with bupivacaine 0.25% has produced a mean peak plasma concentration of 0.34 and 0.47 μg per mL after doses of 10 or 20 mL respectively.[6] Administration of bupivacaine 0.5% in a dose of 3 mg per kg with or without adrenaline [epinephrine] for sciatic and femoral nerve block produced mean peak plasma concentrations below 0.8 μg per mL.[7]

Bupivacaine is rapidly absorbed from the synovial membrane of the knee during arthroscopy but plasma concentrations did not exceed 0.35 μg per mL after controlled pressure-irrigation with isotonic solutions containing up to 200 mg.[8] Although one group of workers found that maximum plasma concentrations of bupivacaine after intra-articular injection of 30 mL of a 0.5% solution for arthroscopy was 0.875 μg per mL they suggested that adrenaline [epinephrine] should probably be added to minimise absorption.[9]

1. Tucker GT. Pharmacokinetics of local anaesthetics. *Br J Anaesth* 1986; **58**: 717–31.
2. Neill RS, Watson R. Plasma bupivacaine concentrations during combined regional and general anaesthesia for resection and reconstruction of head and neck carcinomata. *Br J Anaesth* 1984; **56**: 485–92.
3. Gin T, *et al.* Effect of adrenaline on venous plasma concentrations of bupivacaine after interpleural administration. *Br J Anaesth* 1990; **64**: 662–6.
4. Kastrissios H, *et al.* The disposition of bupivacaine following a 72h interpleural infusion in cholecystectomy patients. *Br J Clin Pharmacol* 1991; **32**: 251–4.
5. Bodenham A, Park GR. Plasma concentrations of bupivacaine after intercostal nerve block in patients after orthotopic liver transplantation. *Br J Anaesth* 1990; **64**: 436–41.
6. Hardy PAJ, Williams NE. Plasma concentrations of bupivacaine after stellate ganglion block using two volumes of 0.25% bupivacaine plain solution. *Br J Anaesth* 1990; **65**: 243–4.
7. Misra U, *et al.* Plasma concentrations of bupivacaine following combined sciatic and femoral 3 in 1 nerve blocks in open knee surgery. *Br J Anaesth* 1991; **66**: 310–13.
8. Debruyne D, *et al.* Monitoring serum bupivacaine levels during arthroscopy. *Eur J Clin Pharmacol* 1985; **27**: 733–5.
9. Butterworth JF, *et al.* Effect of adrenaline on plasma concentrations of bupivacaine following intra-articular injection of bupivacaine for knee arthroscopy. *Br J Anaesth* 1990; **65**: 537–9.

SURFACE ANAESTHESIA. Studies of the absorption of bupivacaine following surface application.

1. McBurney A, *et al.* Absorption of lignocaine and bupivacaine from the respiratory tract during fibreoptic bronchoscopy. *Br J Clin Pharmacol* 1984; **17**: 61–6.

Pregnancy. Bupivacaine crosses the placenta to a lesser degree than lignocaine [lidocaine] or mepivacaine following maternal injection. Values of 0.2 to 0.4 have been reported[1,2] for the ratio of fetal to maternal concentrations for bupivacaine compared with values of 0.5 to 0.7 quoted[2,3] for lignocaine [lidocaine] and mepivacaine. The greater degree of protein-binding of bupivacaine compared with these other drugs not only limits the amount of bupivacaine available to cross the placenta but also reduces the relative amount of free drug in the fetal circulation[2] (see also under Protein Binding, below). Addition of adrenaline [epinephrine] to the injection does not appear to affect the placental transfer rate of bupivacaine.[4] Measurement of a beta-phase half-life of 25 hours in the neonate compared with 1.25 hours in mothers suggests that the neonate is less able to metabolise bupivacaine.[5]

1. Denson DD, *et al.* Serum bupivacaine concentrations in term parturients following continuous epidural analgesia for labor and delivery. *Ther Drug Monit* 1984; **6**: 393–8.
2. Blogg CE, Simpson BR. Obstetric analgesia and the newborn baby. *Lancet* 1974; **i**: 1283.
3. Poppers PJ. Evaluation of local anaesthetic agents for regional anaesthesia in obstetrics. *Br J Anaesth* 1975; **47**: 322–7.
4. Reynolds F, *et al.* Effect of time and adrenaline on the feto-maternal distribution of bupivacaine. *Br J Anaesth* 1989; **62**: 509–14.
5. Caldwell J, *et al.* Pharmacokinetics of bupivacaine administered epidurally during childbirth. *Br J Clin Pharmacol* 1976; **3**: 956P–957P.

Protein binding. The two major binding proteins for bupivacaine in the blood are α-1-acid glycoprotein, the influence of which is predominant at low concentrations, and albumin, which plays the major role at high concentrations. Reduction in pH from 7.4 to 7.0 decreases the affinity of the α₁-acid glycoprotein for bupivacaine but has no effect on albumin affinity.[1] Binding of bupivacaine is reduced during pregnancy but it is considered that the increase in free bupivacaine concentrations is unlikely to cause a clinically significant increase in the risk of CNS or cardiovascular toxicity.[2]

As fetal plasma contains little α₁-acid glycoprotein the binding capacity for bupivacaine is reduced and this may contribute to the difference between maternal and fetal plasma concentration at delivery[3] (see also under Pregnancy, above).

Ageing, uncomplicated by disease, does not affect the protein binding of bupivacaine.[4]

1. Denson D, *et al.* Alpha₁-acid glycoprotein and albumin in human serum bupivacaine binding. *Clin Pharmacol Ther* 1984; **35**: 409–15.
2. Denson DD, *et al.* Bupivacaine protein binding in the term parturient: effects of lactic acidosis. *Clin Pharmacol Ther* 1984; **35**: 702–9.
3. Petersen MC, *et al.* Relationship between the transplacental gradients of bupivacaine and α₁-acid glycoprotein. *Br J Clin Pharmacol* 1981; **12**: 859–62.
4. Veering BT, *et al.* Age does not influence the serum protein binding of bupivacaine. *Br J Clin Pharmacol* 1991; **32**: 501–3.

Uses and Administration

Bupivacaine hydrochloride is a local anaesthetic of the amide type with actions and uses similar to those described on p.1304. It has a slow onset and a long duration of action. The speed of onset and duration of action are increased by the addition of a vasoconstrictor, and absorption into the circulation from the site of injection is reduced. Slow accumulation occurs with repeated doses. It is used mainly for infiltration anaesthesia and regional nerve blocks, particularly epidural block, but is contra-indicated for obstetric paracervical block and for use in intravenous regional anaesthesia (Bier's block). The 0.75% solution is contra-indicated for epidural block in obstetrics. (Local anaesthetic techniques are discussed on p.1304.)

Bupivacaine is a racemic mixture but the S(−)-isomer levobupivacaine (see p.1312) is also used. The carbonated solution of bupivacaine is also available for injection in some countries (see p.1304).

In recommended doses bupivacaine produces complete sensory blockade but the concentration of bupivacaine solution used affects the extent of motor blockade achieved. A 0.25% solution generally produces incomplete motor block, a 0.5% solution will usually produce motor block and some muscle relaxation, and complete motor block and muscle relaxation can be achieved with a 0.75% solution.

The dosage of bupivacaine used depends on the site of injection and the procedure used, as well as the status of the patient. Doses of bupivacaine are expressed in terms of the anhydrous hydrochloride. In the UK the suggested general **maximum single dose** of bupivacaine hydrochloride is 150 mg with or without adrenaline [epinephrine] followed if necessary by doses of up to 50 mg every 2 hours. In the USA the recommended maximum single dose is 175 mg of the plain preparation or 225 mg when given with adrenaline [epinephrine]; doses may be repeated at intervals of not less than 3 hours but the total daily dose should not exceed 400 mg. The dose should be reduced in the elderly, in children, in debilitated patients, and in cardiac or hepatic disease.

A test dose of bupivacaine, preferably with adrenaline [epinephrine], should be given before commencing epidural block to detect inadvertent intravascular administration. Subsequent doses should be given in small increments.

Solutions with or without adrenaline [epinephrine] may be used for most **local anaesthetic techniques** and procedures apart from dental infiltration, when adrenaline [epinephrine] is added to the solution (see below).

For *infiltration anaesthesia* bupivacaine hydrochloride is typically used as a 0.25% solution in doses up to the recommended maximum (see above). When a longer duration of anaesthesia is required, as in dental or surgical procedures of the maxillary and mandibular area, a 0.5% solution with adrenaline [epinephrine] 1 in 200 000 has been used but a total dose of 90 mg (18 mL) should not be exceeded over a single dental sitting. For *peripheral nerve block* the usual dose is 12.5 mg (5 mL) as a 0.25% solution or 25 mg (5 mL) as a 0.5% solution, although doses up to the recommended maximum single dose (see above) may also be given. For *sympathetic nerve block* 50 to 125 mg (20 to 50 mL) as a 0.25% solution is recommended. A 0.75% solution has been used for *retrobulbar block* in ophthalmic surgery in a dose of 15 to 30 mg (2 to 4 mL).

For *lumbar epidural block* in surgery a 0.25% solution of bupivacaine hydrochloride may be used in a dose of 25 to 50 mg (10 to 20 mL) or as a 0.5% solution in a dose of 50 to 100 mg (10 to 20 mL). Lower doses of 15 to 30 mg (6 to 12 mL) as a 0.25% solution or 30 to 60 mg (6 to 12 mL) as the 0.5% solution have been recommended for analgesia during labour. A 0.75% solution is also used for induction of lumbar epidural block in non-obstetric surgery in a single dose of 75 to 150 mg (10 to 20 mL). For *caudal block* in surgery 37.5 to 75 mg (15 to 30 mL) as a 0.25%

solution or 75 to 150 mg (15 to 30 mL) as a 0.5% solution may be used. For analgesia during labour a dose of 25 to 50 mg (10 to 20 mL) as a 0.25% solution or 50 to 100 mg (10 to 20 mL) as a 0.5% solution has been recommended.

Hyperbaric solutions of bupivacaine hydrochloride without adrenaline [epinephrine] may be used for *spinal block*. Preparations containing 0.5% are available and are given in doses of 10 to 20 mg (2 to 4 mL).

Action. Addition of potassium chloride 0.2 mmol to 40 mL of bupivacaine 0.25% solution resulted in a more rapid onset of sensory loss than the same dose of plain bupivacaine in patients undergoing brachial plexus block for forearm or hand surgery.[1] Hyaluronidase did not increase the speed of onset of brachial plexus block produced by bupivacaine 0.5%, with or without adrenaline [epinephrine], but did reduce the duration of anaesthesia.[2]

Administration of bupivacaine encapsulated in liposomes can prolong postsurgical analgesic action without motor block.[3,4]

For a comparison of the vasoactivity of bupivacaine and some other local anaesthetics, see p.1304.

1. Parris MR, Chambers WA. Effects of the addition of potassium to prilocaine or bupivacaine: studies on brachial plexus blockade. *Br J Anaesth* 1986; **58:** 297–300.
2. Keeler JF, *et al.* Effect of addition of hyaluronidase to bupivacaine during axillary brachial plexus block. *Br J Anaesth* 1992; **68:** 68–71.
3. Boogaerts S, *et al.* Epidural administration of liposomal bupivacaine for the management of postsurgical pain. *Br J Anaesth* 1993; **70:** (suppl 1): 104.
4. Boogaerts JG, *et al.* Pharmacokinetic-pharmacodynamic specific behaviour of liposome-associated bupivacaine in humans. *Br J Anaesth* 1995; **74** (suppl 1): 74.

Administration in children. Bupivacaine 0.25% injected intra-operatively up to a maximum dose of 1.5 mg per kg bodyweight with adrenaline [epinephrine] has been used in infants for the control of postoperative pain due to pyloromyotomy and appears to attenuate some of the cardiac and respiratory effects associated with the use of general anaesthesia alone.[1] Doses of 2.5 mg of bupivacaine per year of age administered as a 0.5% solution has been used for ilio-inguinal nerve block in children undergoing herniotomy.[2] A study[3] in infants undergoing abdominal surgery found that an epidural infusion of bupivacaine produced comparable analgesia to an intravenous infusion of morphine. It was considered that bupivacaine might be preferable to morphine in neonates and young infants who are particularly prone to respiratory depression, but older children might require additional sedation or analgesia to prevent postoperative restlessness.

1. McNicol LR, *et al.* Peroperative bupivacaine for pyloromyotomy pain. *Lancet* 1990; **335:** 54–5.
2. Smith BAC, Jones SEF. Analgesia after herniotomy in a paediatric day unit. *BMJ* 1982; **285:** 1466.
3. Wolf AR, Hughes D. Pain relief for infants undergoing abdominal surgery: comparison of infusions of IV morphine and extradural bupivacaine. *Br J Anaesth* 1993; **70:** 10–16.

Labour pain. For a discussion of the management of labour pain, including mention of the use of local anaesthetics, see p.6. Early experience in nearly 1000 patients suggested that 8 mL of a 0.5% solution of bupivacaine with adrenaline [epinephrine] was the optimum dose for epidural block during labour;[1] pain relief lasted for about 2 hours. Decreasing the concentration of the final dose to 0.25% reduced the persistence of sensory and motor nerve block after delivery. Others[2] found that bupivacaine 0.375% was the most suitable concentration for epidural analgesia when using a regimen of regular 'top-up' doses of 0.5 mg per kg body-weight about every 90 minutes. However, the use of low doses of bupivacaine 0.25% for epidural analgesia in primiparous women was associated with a lower incidence of forceps delivery and oxytocin augmentation.[3] Although an even lower concentration of bupivacaine (0.0625%) used in combination with sufentanil[4] produced analgesia similar to that with 0.125% bupivacaine used alone, the duration of the second stage of labour and the incidence of instrumental and surgical delivery were not reduced. Similar results were obtained using bupivacaine 0.0625% with diamorphine 0.005%; in addition pruritus and drowsiness produced by diamorphine were considered to be troublesome in many patients.[5]

Intrathecal injections of bupivacaine with or without an opioid are sometimes used[6,7] with epidural injections to achieve a faster onset of analgesia and a reduced degree of motor block in the management of labour pain. Intrathecal injections containing bupivacaine have also been given alone[8,9] for the management of labour pain but the use of this route alone is usually associated with anaesthesia and management of postoperative pain in caesarean section. Bupivacaine has also been tried with lignocaine [lidocaine] for epidural anaesthesia in caesarean section in order to reduce the dose of bupivacaine and minimise cardiotoxicity.[10]

1. Crawford JS. Lumbar epidural block in labour: a clinical analysis. *Br J Anaesth* 1972; **44:** 66–74.
2. Purdy G, *et al.* Continuous extradural analgesia in labour: comparison between "on demand" and regular "top-up" injections. *Br J Anaesth* 1987; **59:** 319–24.
3. Turner MJ, *et al.* Primiparous women using epidural analgesia. *BMJ* 1990; **300:** 123.

---

4. Auroy Y, Benhamou D. Extradural analgesia for labour: 0.125% bupivacaine vs 0.0625% bupivacaine with 0.2 μg mL⁻¹ sufentanil. *Br J Anaesth* 1995; **74** (suppl 1): 105–6.
5. Bailey CR, *et al.* Diamorphine-bupivacaine mixture compared with plain bupivacaine for analgesia. *Br J Anaesth* 1994; **72:** 58–61.
6. Stacey RGW, *et al.* Single space combined spinal-extradural technique for analgesia in labour. *Br J Anaesth* 1993; **71:** 499–502.
7. Collis RE, *et al.* Randomised comparison of combined spinal-epidural and standard epidural analgesia in labour. *Lancet* 1995; **345:** 1413–16.
8. Kestin IG, *et al.* Analgesia for labour and delivery using incremental diamorphine and bupivacaine via a 32-gauge intrathecal catheter. *Br J Anaesth* 1992; **68:** 244–7.
9. McHale S, *et al.* Continuous subarachnoid infusion of 0.125% bupivacaine for analgesia during labour. *Br J Anaesth* 1992; **69:** 634–6.
10. Howell P, *et al.* Comparison of four local extradural anaesthetic solutions for elective Caesarean section. *Br J Anaesth* 1990; **65:** 648–53.

Preparations

BP 2001: Bupivacaine and Adrenaline Injection; Bupivacaine Injection;
USP 25: Bupivacaine Hydrochloride in Dextrose Injection; Bupivacaine Hydrochloride Injection.

Proprietary Preparations (details are given in Part 3)
Aust.: Bucain; Carboneural†; Carbostesin; **Austral.:** Marcain; **Belg.:** Marcaine; **Braz.:** Marcaina; Neocaina; **Canad.:** Marcaine; Sensorcaine; **Denm.:** Marcain; **Fin.:** Bicain; Marcain; **Fr.:** Marcaine; **Ger.:** Bucain; Carbostesin; Dolanaest; **Hong Kong:** Marcaine; **Irl.:** Marcain; **Israel:** Kamacaine; Marcaine; **Ital.:** Bupiforan; Bupyl; Marcaina; **Mex.:** Buvacaina; **Neth.:** Marcaine; **Norw.:** Marcain; **NZ:** Marcain; **Port.:** Marcaina†; **S.Afr.:** Macaine; Regibloc†; **Singapore:** Marcain; **Spain:** Svedocain Sin Vasoconstr; **Swed.:** Marcain; **Switz.:** Carbostesin; Duracain; **Thai.:** Marcaine; **UK:** Marcain; **USA:** Marcaine; Sensorcaine.

Multi-ingredient: Austral.: Marcain with Fentanyl; Marcain with Pethidine; **Fin.:** Solomet c bupivacain hydrochlorid; **NZ:** Marcain with Fentanyl; Marcain with Pethidine.

Butacaine Sulfate   (7610-b)

Butacaine Sulfate (rINNM).

Butacain. Sulph.; Butacaine Sulphate (BANM). 3-Dibutylaminopropyl 4-aminobenzoate sulphate.
(C₁₈H₃₀N₂O₂)₂,H₂SO₄ = 711.0.
CAS — 149-16-6 (butacaine); 149-15-5 (butacaine sulfate).

Profile
Butacaine, a para-aminobenzoic acid ester, is a local anaesthetic (p.1302) used for surface anaesthesia. It has been used topically, as the sulfate, in solutions for dental pain and in ear and nasal drops.

Preparations
Proprietary Preparations (details are given in Part 3)
Multi-ingredient: Fr.: Relaxoddi†; **Spain:** Topicaina.

Butoxycaine Hydrochloride   (11333-y)

Butoxycaini Hydrochloridum. 2-Diethylaminoethyl-(p-butoxybenzoate) hydrochloride.
C₁₇H₂₇NO₃,HCl = 329.9.
CAS — 3772-43-8 (butoxycaine); 2350-32-5 (butoxycaine hydrochloride).

Profile
Butoxycaine, a para-aminobenzoic acid ester, is a local anaesthetic (p.1302) that has been used as the base or hydrochloride for surface anaesthesia.

Preparations
Proprietary Preparations (details are given in Part 3)
Multi-ingredient: Braz.: Nene Dent; **Ger.:** Bismolan; Hamo-ratiopharm.

Butyl Aminobenzoate   (7613-q)

Butamben (USAN); Butoforme. Butyl 4-aminobenzoate.
C₁₁H₁₅NO₂ = 193.2.
CAS — 94-25-7.
Pharmacopoeias. In Fr. and US.

Pharmacopoeial description
USP 25: A white, odourless, crystalline powder. M.p. 57° to 59°. Soluble 1 in 7000 of water; soluble in alcohol, in ether, in chloroform, in fixed oils, and in dilute acids. It slowly hydrolyses when boiled with water.

Butyl Aminobenzoate Picrate   (9857-x)

Abbott-34842; Butamben Picrate (USAN).
(C₁₁H₁₅NO₂)₂,C₆H₃N₃O₇ = 615.6.
CAS — 577-48-0.

Profile
Butyl aminobenzoate, a para-aminobenzoic acid ester, is a local anaesthetic (p.1302) that has been used for surface anaesthesia of the skin and mucous membranes. It has also been used for relief of pain and pruritus associated with anorectal disor-

---

ders. A suspension of butyl aminobenzoate 5 or 10% has been given epidurally.

Butyl aminobenzoate picrate is applied to the skin as a 1% ointment.

◊ References.
1. Korsten HH, *et al.* Long-lasting epidural sensory blockade by n-butyl-p-aminobenzoate in the terminally ill intractable cancer pain patient. *Anesthesiology* 1991; **75:** 950–60.
2. Armstrong DG, Kanat IO. Analgesic efficacy of topical butamben picrate. *J Am Podiatr Med Assoc* 1995; **85:** 738–40.
3. Shulman M, *et al.* Nerve blocks with 5% butamben suspension for the treatment of chronic pain syndromes. *Reg Anesth Pain Med* 1998; **23:** 395–401.

Preparations
USP 25: Benzocaine, Butamben, and Tetracaine Hydrochloride Gel; Benzocaine, Butamben, and Tetracaine Hydrochloride Ointment; Benzocaine, Butamben, and Tetracaine Hydrochloride Topical Aerosol; Benzocaine, Butamben, and Tetracaine Hydrochloride Topical Solution; Erythromycin Ethylsuccinate Injection.

Proprietary Preparations (details are given in Part 3)
USA: Butesin Picrate.

Multi-ingredient: Austral.: Butesin Picrate; **Braz.:** Nestosyl; Predmicin; **Fr.:** Ginkor Procto†; Nestosyl; Preparation H; Tyrothricine Lafran†; **Spain:** Alvogil; Topicaina; **Switz.:** Alvogyl; **USA:** Cetacaine.

Chloroprocaine Hydrochloride   (7615-s)

Chloroprocaine Hydrochloride (rINNM).

2-Diethylaminoethyl 4-amino-2-chlorobenzoate hydrochloride.
C₁₃H₁₉ClN₂O₂,HCl = 307.2.
CAS — 133-16-4 (chloroprocaine); 3858-89-7 (chloroprocaine hydrochloride).
Pharmacopoeias. In US.

Pharmacopoeial description
USP 25: A white odourless crystalline powder. Soluble 1 in 20 of water and 1 in 100 of alcohol; very slightly soluble in chloroform; practically insoluble in ether. Solutions are acid to litmus.

pH of solutions. For a discussion of the effect that pH has on the stability of local anaesthetic solutions and the pain associated with their injection, see p.1304.

Adverse Effects, Treatment, and Precautions
As for Local Anaesthetics in general, p.1302. Chloroprocaine is said to be unsuitable for intravenous regional anaesthesia (Bier's block) because of a high incidence of thrombophlebitis associated with such use. It is also contra-indicated in spinal anaesthesia due to potential neurotoxicity.

Interactions
For interactions associated with local anaesthetics, see p.1303.

Pharmacokinetics
Chloroprocaine is hydrolysed rapidly in the circulation by plasma cholinesterase. It has a half-life of 19 to 26 seconds in adults. It is excreted in the urine mainly as metabolites.

See also under Local Anaesthetics, p.1303.

Uses and Administration
Chloroprocaine, a para-aminobenzoic acid ester, is a local anaesthetic with actions and uses similar to those described on p.1304. It has properties similar to those of procaine (p.1319). It has a rapid onset (6 to 12 minutes) and short duration (one hour) of action.

Chloroprocaine is used as the hydrochloride for infiltration, peripheral nerve block, and central nerve block including lumbar and caudal epidural blocks. It may be given, if necessary, with adrenaline [epinephrine] 1 in 200 000 to delay absorption and reduce toxicity. Chloroprocaine is not an effective surface anaesthetic. It should not be used for spinal anaesthesia. (Local anaesthetic techniques are discussed on p.1304.)

The dosage of chloroprocaine used depends on the site of injection and the procedure used. In adults the **maximum single dose** of chloroprocaine hydrochloride without adrenaline [epinephrine] should not exceed 800 mg; when given with adrenaline [epinephrine] 1 in 200 000 the maximum single dose should not exceed 1 g.

For *mandibular nerve block* a 2% solution is used in a dose of 40 to 60 mg (2 to 3 mL) and for *infra-orbital nerve block* a dose of 10 to 20 mg (0.5 to 1 mL) as a 2% solution is used. A 2% solution is also used for *brachial plexus block* in a dose of 600 to 800 mg (30 to 40 mL). For *digital nerve block* a 1% solution without adrenaline [epinephrine] is used in a dose of 30 to 40 mg (3 to 4 mL). In obstetrics a dose of 200 mg (10 mL) per side as a 2% solution is suggested for *pudendal block*, and for a *paracervical block* a 1% solution in a dose of 30 mg (3 mL) at each of 4 sites. For *lumbar epidural block* 40 to 50 mg (2 to 2.5 mL) as a 2% solution or 60 to 75 mg (2 to 2.5 mL) as a 3% solution is used for each segment to be anaesthetised, the usual total dose being 300 to 750 mg with smaller repeat doses being given at intervals of 40 to 50 minutes. For *caudal block* a dose of 300 to 500 mg (15 to 25 mL) as a 2% solution or 450 to 750 mg (15 to 25 mL) as a 3% solution may be given and repeated at intervals of 40 to 60 minutes.

Dosages should be reduced in children, elderly or debilitated patients, and those with cardiac or liver disease. For children concentrations of 0.5 to 1.0% are suggested for infiltration and 1.0 to 1.5% for nerve block procedures.

Preparations

USP 25: Chloroprocaine Hydrochloride Injection.

Proprietary Preparations (details are given in Part 3)
Canad.: Nesacaine; *Switz.:* Ivracain; Nesacain; *USA:* Nesacaine.

Cinchocaine (7616-w)

Cinchocaine *(BAN, rINN)*.

Cincainum; Dibucaine. 2-Butoxy-*N*-(2-diethylaminoethyl)cinchoninamide; 2-Butoxy-*N*-(2-diethylaminoethyl)quinoline-4-carboxamide.
$C_{20}H_{29}N_3O_2 = 343.5$.
CAS — 85-79-0.
ATC — C05AD04; D04AB02; N01BB06; S01HA06.
Pharmacopoeias. In US.

Pharmacopoeial description

USP 25: A white to off-white powder, with a slight characteristic odour. M.p. 62.5° to 66°. Soluble 1 in 4600 of water, 1 in 0.7 of alcohol, 1 in 0.5 of chloroform, and 1 in 1.4 of ether; soluble in 1N hydrochloric acid. It darkens on exposure to light. Store in airtight containers. Protect from light.

Cinchocaine Hydrochloride (7617-e)

Cinchocaine Hydrochloride *(BANM, rINNM)*.

Cincaini Chloridum; Cinchocaini Hydrochloridum; Dibucaine Hydrochloride; Dibucainium Chloride; Percainum; Sovcainum.
$C_{20}H_{29}N_3O_2,HCl = 379.9$.
CAS — 61-12-1.

NOTE. This compound was originally marketed under the name Percaine, but accidents occurred owing to the confusion of this name with procaine.

Pharmacopoeias. In Eur. (see p.vi), Jpn, and US.

Pharmacopoeial description

Ph. Eur.: A white or almost white, crystalline powder or colourless crystals; it is hygroscopic. It agglomerates very easily. Very soluble in water; freely soluble in alcohol, in acetone, and in dichloromethane. A 2% solution in water has a pH of 5.0 to 6.0. Store in airtight containers. Protect from light.

USP 25: Colourless or white to off-white crystals or white to off-white, crystalline powder. It is odourless, somewhat hygroscopic, and darkens on exposure to light. Freely soluble in water, in alcohol, in acetone, and in chloroform. Its solutions have a pH of about 5.5. Store in airtight containers. Protect from light.

Profile

Cinchocaine is an amide local anaesthetic (p.1302) that is now generally only used for surface anaesthesia. It is one of the most potent and toxic of the long-acting local anaesthetics and its parenteral use was restricted to spinal anaesthesia.

For surface anaesthesia cinchocaine has been used, as the base or hydrochloride, in creams and ointments containing up to 1% and in suppositories for the temporary relief of pain and itching associated with skin and anorectal conditions. Cinchocaine benzoate has also been used topically.

Action. For a comparison of the vasoactivity of cinchocaine and some other local anaesthetics, see p.1304.

Plasma cholinesterase deficiency. For mention of the use of cinchocaine in the determination of plasma cholinesterase activity, see under Precautions of Suxamethonium Chloride, p.1341.

Preparations

USP 25: Dibucaine Cream; Dibucaine Hydrochloride Injection; Dibucaine Ointment.

Proprietary Preparations (details are given in Part 3)
Austral.: Nupercaine Heavy; *Braz.:* Nupercainal; *Canad.:* Nupercainal; *Denm.:* Cincain; *Ger.:* DoloPosterine N; *Swed.:* Cincain; *Switz.:* Nupercainal†; *UK:* Nupercainal; *USA:* Nupercainal.

Multi-ingredient: *Aust.:* Ciloprin cum Anaesthetico; Scheriproct; Ultraproct; *Austral.:* Proctosedyl; Rectinol HC; Scheriproct; Ultraproct; *Belg.:* Hemosedan; Scheriproct; Trihistalex; Ultraproct; *Braz.:* Proctil; Senol; Ultraproct; *Canad.:* Nupercainal; Proctosedyl; Proctosone; *Denm.:* Proctosedyl; *Fin.:* Ciloprin cum Anaesthetico; Faktu; Proctosedyl; Scheriproct; *Fr.:* Anti-Hemorroidaires†; Deliproct; Ultraproct; *Ger.:* Anumedin; Faktu; Otobacid N; Procto-Kaban; Proctospre; Scheriproct; Ultraproct; *Hong Kong:* Borraginol-N; Decatylen; Faktu; Proctosedyl; Scheriproct; Protozone; Ultraproct; *Irl.:* Proctosedyl; Scheriproct; Ultraproct; *Israel:* Proctosedyl; *Ital.:* Ultraproct; *Mex.:* Proctoacid; Scheriproct; Ultraproct; *Neth.:* Proctosedyl; Ultraproct†; *Norw.:* Proctosedyl; Scheriproct; *NZ:* Proctosedyl; Ultraproct; Faktu; Scheriproct; *Port.:* Faktu; Scheriproct; *S.Afr.:* Cepacaine; Proctosedyl; Scheriproct; *Singapore:* Decatylen; Faktu; Proctosedyl; *Spain:* Anestesia Loc Braun S/A; Ruscus; Scheriproct; *Swed.:* Proctosedyl; Scheriproct N; *Switz.:* Ciloprine ca; Decatylene Neo; Faktu; Locaseptil-Neo; Proctospre; Scheriproct; Ultraproct†; *Thai.:* Faktu; Proctosedyl; Scheriproct; *UAE:* Supraproct-S; *UK:* Proctosedyl; Scheriproct; Ultraproct; Uniroid-HC; Uniroid†; *USA:* Corticaine.

Used as an adjunct in: *Aust.:* Butazolidin; Delta-Tomanol†; *Ger.:* Butazolidin; *Switz.:* Butazolidine†.

Coca (7618-I)

Coca Leaves; Hoja de Coca.

The dried leaves of *Erythroxylum coca* (Bolivian or Huanuco leaf) or of *E. truxillense* (Peruvian or Truxillo leaf) (Erythroxylaceae), indigenous to Bolivia and Peru and cultivated in Colombia and Indonesia.

Coca leaves contain about 0.7 to 1.5% of total alkaloids, of which cocaine, cinnamyl-cocaine, and α-truxilline are the most important.

Profile

Coca was formerly used for its stimulant action and for the relief of gastric pain, nausea, and vomiting, but it has no place in modern medicine. The practice of coca leaf chewing still continues in South America.

Cocaine (7619-y)

Cocaine *(BAN)*.

Cocaina; Methyl Benzoylecgonine. (1R,2R,3S,5S)-2-Methoxycarbonyltropan-3-yl benzoate.
$C_{17}H_{21}NO_4 = 303.4$.
CAS — 50-36-2.
ATC — N01BC01; R02AD03; S01HA01; S02DA02.

NOTE. The following names have also been used to describe various forms of cocaine: basuco, bazooka, bernice, blow, C, charlie, coke, crack, flake, freebase, girl, gold dust, her, lady, leaf, nose candy, pasta, rock, she, snow, space dust, toot, white girl, white lady.

Pharmacopoeias. In Br., It., and US.

Pharmacopoeial description

BP 2001: It may be obtained from the leaves of *Erythroxylum coca* and other spp. of *Erythroxylum*, or by synthesis. Colourless crystals or a white, crystalline powder. It is slightly volatile. M.p. 96° to 98°. Practically insoluble in water; freely soluble in alcohol and in ether; very soluble in chloroform; soluble in arachis oil; slightly soluble in liquid paraffin.

USP 25: Colourless to white crystals or white, crystalline powder. M.p. 96° to 98°. Soluble 1 in 600 of water, 1 in 7 of alcohol, 1 in 1 of chloroform, 1 in 3.5 of ether, 1 in 12 of olive oil, and 1 in 80 to 100 of liquid paraffin. A saturated solution in water is alkaline to litmus. Protect from light.

Cocaine Hydrochloride (7620-g)

Cocaine Hydrochloride *(BANM)*.

Chloridrato de Cocaína; Cocaine Hydrochlor.; Cocaini Hydrochloridum; Cocainium Chloratum.
$C_{17}H_{21}NO_4,HCl = 339.8$.
CAS — 53-21-4.

NOTE. CCN is a code approved by the BP 2001 for use on single unit doses of eye drops containing cocaine hydrochloride where the individual containers may be too small to bear all the appropriate labelling information.

Pharmacopoeias. In Chin., Eur. (see p.vi), Jpn, Pol., and US.

Cocaine hydrochloride 1.12 g is approximately equivalent to 1 g of cocaine. Solutions are adversely affected by alkalis.

Pharmacopoeial description

Ph. Eur.: Hygroscopic, colourless crystals or a white crystalline powder. M.p. about 197° with decomposition. Very soluble in water; freely soluble in alcohol; practically insoluble in ether. Protect from moisture and light.

USP 25: Colourless crystals or white, crystalline powder. Soluble 1 in 0.5 of water, 1 in 3.5 of alcohol, and 1 in 15 of chloroform; soluble in glycerol; insoluble in ether. Protect from light.

Stability of solutions. A stability study[1] was conducted in response to queries over conflicting data on the incompatibility of cocaine hydrochloride solutions and phenol. Some pharmacists had reported that cocaine hydrochloride eye drops preserved with phenol had shown no sign of physical incompatibility. The BPC 1973 states that cocaine hydrochloride is incompatible with phenol but suggests that cocaine hydrochloride solutions may be preserved with chlorocresol. The study found that there was no sign of physical incompatibility in aqueous solutions containing cocaine hydrochloride 5% and phenol 0.5% stored for a year at temperatures of 0° to 37° but there was a fall in pH, greatest at the higher temperatures, which was suggestive of chemical change. It was recommended that such solutions should be stored in a cool place.

1. *PSGB Lab Report P/75/14 1975.*

Adverse Effects

Because the therapeutic use of cocaine is now very restricted many reports of adverse effects occur in the context of abuse. However, both systemic and local effects have followed its use as a surface anaesthetic. Although some effects are similar to those of other local anaesthetics (p.1302), cocaine differs in that it acts as a potent indirect-acting sympathomimetic. It stimulates the CNS causing agitation, dilated pupils,

tachycardia, hypertension, hallucinations, hypertonia, and hyperreflexia. Convulsions, coma, and metabolic acidosis may develop. Symptoms of CNS stimulation and sympathetic overactivity are very marked in overdosage with cocaine. A single oral dose of 1.2 g or less may be fatal, but some persons have a cocaine idiosyncrasy and severe toxicity may occur after doses of only 10 mg intravenously. Systemic absorption of small doses may slow the heart, but with increasing doses tachycardia, hypertension, and ventricular fibrillation occur.

High concentrations of cocaine should not be used topically as, in addition to risks of systemic toxicity following absorption, lasting local damage may occur.

Topical application of cocaine to the cornea can cause corneal damage with clouding, pitting, sloughing, and occasionally ulceration. Topical application to the nose or mouth has been reported to cause loss of smell and taste respectively.

Prolonged use of cocaine by nasal inhalation may cause mucosal damage or perforation of the nasal septum.

Abuse. Cocaine abuse and its effects have been discussed in a number of reviews.[1-5]
Cocaine abuse was once only in the form of chewing of Coca leaves containing small amounts of cocaine but processing of the leaves has led to abuse with a variety of more dangerous preparations containing higher concentrations of cocaine.[6] Coca paste, produced by maceration of the leaves with petrol and sulfuric acid, contains about 40 to 90% of cocaine sulfate and is smoked with tobacco or cannabis. Treatment of coca paste with hydrochloric acid produces cocaine hydrochloride, which is abused by intravenous injection, either alone or with diamorphine, or by sniffing to achieve nasal absorption. Alkaloidal cocaine (cocaine base; 'freebase'), which is abused by smoking, is produced by treating cocaine hydrochloride with alkali, followed either by heating (to form 'crack' cocaine) or by extracting the base from ether or another organic solvent. The route of administration of cocaine determines the rate and extent of its absorption, although once absorbed, the pharmacokinetics are independent of route. The route of administration rather than the form of cocaine used is important in determining the abuse potential; intravenous cocaine hydrochloride and smoked cocaine base have a greater potential for abuse than intranasal cocaine hydrochloride because of their greater rapidity and intensity of effects.
The psychological effects of cocaine abuse may be described by a cycle of initial euphoria followed by dysphoria and finally schizophreniform psychosis.[6,7] Euphoria may be accompanied by other symptoms of stimulation such as sexual arousal, anorexia, insomnia, hyperexcitability, loquacity, and grandiosity, and users may appear manic. After a short time these feelings are replaced by symptoms of dysphoria including considerable anxiety, fear, depression, apathy, irritability, suspiciousness. Dysphoria may be ameliorated by repeated administration, so the user develops the need to take the drug continuously to feel relatively well, but repeated administration appears to diminish the intensity of the effects.[6] During euphoria and dysphoria users may experience a wide range of physical symptoms including palpitations, headache, dizziness, gastrointestinal effects, hyperhidrosis, tremors, tachycardia, hypertension, fever, and myoclonic jerks. Seizures can also occur following repeated use. In chronic abusers psychological deterioration may eventually occur, resulting in loss of mental function, compulsive disorders, suicidal ideation, psychopathic disorders, and ultimately a psychosis resembling acute paranoid schizophrenia similar to that seen with amfetamines.[6,7] Symptoms may include paranoia, stereotyped behaviour, delusions, loss of impulse control, violence, and visual, olfactory, auditory, gustatory, and tactile hallucinations. Overdosage can result in death due to status epilepticus, hyperthermia, ventricular tachycardia, and cardiac or respiratory arrest.[6]

For further details of the adverse effects of cocaine abuse, including effects due to use during pregnancy, see below.

1. Johanson C-E, Fischman MW. The pharmacology of cocaine related to its abuse. *Pharmacol Rev* 1989; **41:** 3–52.
2. Warner EA. Cocaine abuse. *Ann Intern Med* 1993; **119:** 226–35.
3. Strang J, *et al.* Cocaine in the UK—1991. *Br J Psychiatry* 1993; **162:** 1–13.
4. Das G. Cocaine abuse in North America: a milestone in history. *J Clin Pharmacol* 1993; **33:** 296–310.
5. Hatsukami DK, Fischman MW. Crack cocaine and cocaine hydrochloride: are the differences myth or reality? *JAMA* 1996; **276:** 1580–8.
6. Arif A, ed. *Adverse health consequences of cocaine abuse.* Geneva: WHO, 1987.
7. Leikin JB, *et al.* Clinical features and management of intoxication due to hallucinogenic drugs. *Med Toxicol Adverse Drug Exp* 1989; **4:** 324–50.

EFFECTS ON THE BLOOD. References.
1. Leissinger CA. Severe thrombocytopenia associated with cocaine use. *Ann Intern Med* 1990; **112:** 708–10.

The symbol † denotes a preparation no longer actively marketed

1310 Local Anaesthetics

EFFECTS ON THE CARDIOVASCULAR SYSTEM. There appears to be no relationship between underlying heart disease and the risk of cocaine-induced cardiac effects and cardiac events can occur regardless of the route of abuse.[1] Cardiovascular toxicity due to cocaine may be related to individual sensitivity and therefore may not be predictable or dose dependent.[2] Patients with plasma cholinesterase deficiency are particularly at risk for sudden death.[3] Other risk factors for cardiovascular disease, such as cigarette smoking, may exacerbate the cardiac toxicity of cocaine.[4,5] Cocaine blocks reuptake of catecholamines at adrenergic nerve endings and thus produces sympathetic stimulation of the cardiovascular system. Accumulation of catecholamines predisposes the myocardium to arrhythmias,[6] and sinus tachycardia, supraventricular or ventricular tachyarrhythmias, myocarditis, and sudden arrhythmic death may occur.[6-8] Severe hypertension can lead to cerebrovascular accidents and stroke has occurred even in young adults without other predisposing conditions.[9,10] Aortic dissection[11,12] and rupture of the aorta have also occurred.[3] Myocardial infarction and ischaemia have been associated with cocaine abuse[1,3,6] but self-limiting chest pain without signs of myocardial infarction also commonly occurs;[7] asymptomatic myocardial ischaemia manifesting as episodes of ST segment elevation has also been reported during withdrawal of cocaine.[13] The mechanism for these changes remains to be resolved but coronary vasospasm,[13] vasoconstriction,[14] coronary thrombosis,[15,16] and direct myocardiotoxicity[17] are among the suggested causes. Some workers[18] have found that the timing of the coronary vasoconstriction correlated with blood concentration of cocaine's active metabolites, benzoylecgonine and ethyl methyl ecgonine.

Vasoconstriction due to cocaine may also produce ischaemia in the fingers, toes, spinal cord,[7] kidneys,[19] spleen,[20] and intestines.[21] Other reported cardiovascular effects include dilated cardiomyopathy.[22]

1. VanDette JM, Cornish LA. Medical complications of illicit cocaine use. *Clin Pharm* 1989; **8:** 401–11.
2. Thadani PV. Cardiovascular toxicity of cocaine: underlying mechanisms. *J Appl Cardiol* 1990; **5:** 317–20.
3. Cregler LL, Mark H. Medical complications of cocaine abuse. *N Engl J Med* 1986; **315:** 1495–1500.
4. Moliterno DJ, et al. Coronary-artery vasoconstriction induced by cocaine, cigarette smoking, or both. *N Engl J Med* 1994; **330:** 454–9.
5. Higgins ST, et al. Influence of cocaine use on cigarette smoking. *JAMA* 1994; **272:** 1724.
6. Loper KA. Clinical toxicology of cocaine. *Med Toxicol Adverse Drug Exp* 1989; **4:** 174–85.
7. Anonymous. Acute reactions to drugs of abuse. *Med Lett Drugs Ther* 1990; **32:** 92–4.
8. Bauman JL, et al. Cocaine-related sudden cardiac death: a hypothesis correlating basic science and clinical observations. *J Clin Pharmacol* 1994; **34:** 902–11.
9. Kaku DA, Lowenstein DH. Emergence of recreational drug abuse as a major risk factor for stroke in young adults. *Ann Intern Med* 1990; **113:** 821–7.
10. Levine SR, et al. Cerebrovascular complications of the use of the "crack" form of alkaloidal cocaine. *N Engl J Med* 1990; **323:** 699–704.
11. Edwards J, Rubin RN. Aortic dissection and cocaine abuse. *Ann Intern Med* 1987; **107:** 779–80.
12. Jaffe BD, et al. Cocaine-induced coronary-artery dissection. *N Engl J Med* 1994; **330:** 510–11.
13. Nademanee K, et al. Myocardial ischemia during cocaine withdrawal. *Ann Intern Med* 1989; **111:** 876–80.
14. Lange RA, et al. Cocaine-induced coronary-artery vasoconstriction. *N Engl J Med* 1989; **321:** 1557–62.
15. Minor RL, et al. Cocaine-induced myocardial infarction in patients with normal coronary arteries. *Ann Intern Med* 1991; **115:** 797–806.
16. Kugelmass AD, Ware JA. Cocaine and coronary artery thrombosis. *Ann Intern Med* 1992; **116:** 776–7.
17. Peng S-K, et al. Direct cocaine cardiotoxicity demonstrated by endomyocardial biopsy. *Arch Pathol Lab Med* 1989; **113:** 842–5.
18. Brogan WC, et al. Recurrent coronary vasoconstriction caused by intranasal cocaine: possible role for metabolites. *Ann Intern Med* 1992; **116:** 556–61.
19. Sharff JA. Renal infarction associated with intravenous cocaine use. *Ann Emerg Med* 1984; **13:** 1145–7.
20. Novielli KD, Chambers CV. Splenic infarction after cocaine use. *Ann Intern Med* 1991; **114:** 251–2.
21. Freudenberger RS, et al. Intestinal infarction after intravenous cocaine administration. *Ann Intern Med* 1990; **113:** 715–16.
22. Chokshi SK, et al. Reversible cardiomyopathy associated with cocaine intoxication. *Ann Intern Med* 1989; **111:** 1039–40.

EFFECTS ON THE CNS. Severe CNS depression with deep coma has been seen in a few cocaine abusers after prolonged binges.[1]

1. Roberts JR, Greenberg MI. Cocaine washout syndrome. *Ann Intern Med* 2000; **132:** 679–80.

EFFECTS ON THE KIDNEYS. For reference to renal failure following rhabdomyolysis associated with cocaine abuse, see under Effects on the Muscles, below. There has been a report[1] of acute renal failure occurring in a 16-year-old girl secondary to cocaine abuse but without evidence of rhabdomyolysis.

For reference to renal ischaemia due to cocaine abuse, see under Effects on the Cardiovascular System, above.

1. Leblanc M, et al. Cocaine-induced acute renal failure without rhabdomyolysis. *Ann Intern Med* 1994; **121:** 721–2.

EFFECTS ON THE LUNGS. Smoking the free base has resulted in a range of pulmonary complications not previously encountered with other methods of abuse of cocaine. Associated adverse effects have included pulmonary oedema, hypersensitivity pneumonitis, pulmonary haemorrhage, obliterative bronchiolitis, abnormalities of pulmonary function, pneumomediasti-

num, and pneumothorax.[1] Severe or life-threatening exacerbations of asthma have also been reported.[2]

1. Ettinger NA, et al. A review of the respiratory effects of smoking cocaine. *Am J Med* 1989; **87:** 664–8.
2. Rubin RB, Neugarten J. Cocaine-associated asthma. *Am J Med* 1990; **88:** 438–9.

EFFECTS ON THE MOUTH. Gingival necrosis following the abuse of cocaine by local application to the gingivae has been reported.[1]

1. Parry J, et al. Mucosal lesions due to oral cocaine use. *Br Dent J* 1996; **180:** 462–4.

EFFECTS ON THE MUSCLES. Rhabdomyolysis, sometimes progressing to renal failure, has been associated with free-base smoking or injection of cocaine hydrochloride.[1-3]

1. Roth D, et al. Acute rhabdomyolysis associated with cocaine intoxication. *N Engl J Med* 1988; **319:** 673–7.
2. Herzlich BC, et al. Rhabdomyolysis related to cocaine abuse. *Ann Intern Med* 1988; **109:** 335–6.
3. Pogue VA, Nurse HM. Cocaine-associated acute myoglobinuric renal failure. *Am J Med* 1989; **86:** 183–6.

EFFECTS ON SEXUAL FUNCTION. While the initial euphoria of cocaine abuse may be accompanied by sexual arousal, sexual dysfunction can occur[1] and male infertility has been reported.[2] Priapism associated with cocaine abuse has also occurred.[3]

1. Cregler LL, Mark H. Medical complications of cocaine abuse. *N Engl J Med* 1986; **315:** 1495–1500.
2. Bracken MB, et al. Association of cocaine use with sperm concentration, motility, and morphology. *Fertil Steril* 1990; **53:** 315–22.
3. Altman AL, et al. Cocaine associated priapism. *J Urol* 1999; **161:** 1817–18.

EFFECTS ON THE SKIN. Urticarial vasculitis occurred in a young man following intranasal abuse of cocaine.[1]

1. Hofbauer GFL, et al. Uritcarial vasculitis following cocaine use. *Br J Dermatol* 1999; **141:** 600–601.

OVERDOSAGE. References to fatal overdosage from cocaine abuse.

1. Mittleman RE, Wetli CV. Death caused by recreational cocaine use. *JAMA* 1984; **252:** 1889–93.
2. Cowart V. National concern about drug abuse brings athletes under unusual scrutiny. *JAMA* 1986; **256:** 2457–65.
3. Greenland VC, et al. Vaginally administered cocaine overdose in a pregnant woman. *Obstet Gynecol* 1989; **74:** 476–7.
4. Peretti FJ, et al. Cocaine fatality: an unexplained blood concentration in a fatal overdose. *Forensic Sci Int* 1990; **48:** 135–8.
5. Karch SB, et al. Relating cocaine blood concentrations to toxicity–an autopsy study of 99 cases. *J Forensic Sci* 1998; **43:** 41–5.

PREGNANCY AND BREAST FEEDING. The effects of cocaine abuse during pregnancy have been reviewed.[1-3] Women who abuse cocaine during pregnancy appear to have an increased risk of spontaneous abortion,[4] abruptio placentae[5,6] and associated still-births,[7] premature labour,[8-10] and other birth complications.[8-10] These effects may be due to vasoconstriction by cocaine increasing maternal blood pressure and reducing placental blood flow.[11] Uterine rupture[12] during pregnancy and rupture of ectopic pregnancies[13] have also been associated with cocaine. Neonates born to mothers abusing cocaine have an increased risk of intra-uterine growth retardation and may have lower birth-weight, smaller head size, and shorter length.[5,7-9,14-16] Cocaine is possibly teratogenic and congenital abnormalities associated with abuse include cardiovascular abnormalities,[8,17,18] limb reduction defects,[19] intestinal atresia or infarction,[19] skull defects,[7] and genito-urinary tract anomalies.[20] Neurobehavioural impairment[21] and signs of transient CNS irritability[22] may also occur. Some workers[23,24] have found effects on cognition and motor delays while others have found effects on arousal and attention regulation rather than cognitive processes.[25] Cocaine can increase neonatal cerebral blood flow[26] and cerebral infarction and associated seizures have occurred in neonates whose mothers took cocaine near to the onset of labour.[27] Evidence on the risk of intraventricular haemorrhage is conflicting.[6,23]

Acute intoxication has been reported in a breast-fed child whose mother was using cocaine intranasally.[28]

1. Slutsker L. Risks associated with cocaine use during pregnancy. *Obstet Gynecol* 1992; **79:** 778–89.
2. Volpe JJ. Effects of cocaine use on the fetus. *N Engl J Med* 1992; **327:** 399–407. Correction. *ibid.*; 1039.
3. Wiggins RC. Pharmacokinetics of cocaine in pregnancy and effects on fetal maturation. *Clin Pharmacokinet* 1992; **22:** 85–93.
4. Chasnoff IJ, et al. Cocaine use in pregnancy. *N Engl J Med* 1985; **313:** 666–9.
5. Dombrowski MP, et al. Cocaine abuse is associated with abruptio placentae and decreased birth weight, but not shorter labor. *Obstet Gynecol* 1991; **77:** 139–41.
6. Dusick AM, et al. Risk of intracranial hemorrhage and other adverse outcomes after cocaine exposure in a cohort of 323 very low birth weight infants. *J Pediatr* 1993; **122:** 438–45.
7. Bingol N, et al. Teratogenicity of cocaine in humans. *J Pediatr* 1987; **110:** 93–6.
8. Little BB, et al. Cocaine abuse during pregnancy: maternal and fetal implications. *Obstet Gynecol* 1989; **73:** 157–60.
9. Mastrogiannis DS, et al. Perinatal outcome after recent cocaine usage. *Obstet Gynecol* 1990; **76:** 8–11.
10. Spence MR, et al. The relationship between recent cocaine use and pregnancy outcome. *Obstet Gynecol* 1991; **78:** 326–9.
11. Farrar HC, Kearns GL. Cocaine: clinical pharmacology and toxicology. *J Pediatr* 1989; **115:** 665–75.
12. Gonsoulin W, et al. Rupture of unscarred uterus in primigravid woman in association with cocaine abuse. *Am J Obstet Gynecol* 1990; **163:** 526–7.
13. Thatcher SS, et al. Cocaine use and acute rupture of ectopic pregnancies. *Obstet Gynecol* 1989; **74:** 478–9.
14. Zuckerman B, et al. Effects of maternal marijuana and cocaine use on fetal growth. *N Engl J Med* 1989; **320:** 762–8.

15. Chasnoff IJ, et al. Temporal patterns of cocaine use in pregnancy: perinatal outcome. *JAMA* 1989; **261:** 1741–4.
16. Little BB, Snell LM. Brain growth among fetuses exposed to cocaine in utero: asymmetrical growth retardation. *Obstet Gynecol* 1991; **77:** 361–4.
17. Lipshultz SE, et al. Cardiovascular abnormalities in infants prenatally exposed to cocaine. *J Pediatr* 1991; **118:** 44–51.
18. Shaw GM, et al. Maternal use of cocaine during pregnancy and congenital cardiac anomalies. *J Pediatr* 1991; **118:** 167–8.
19. Hoyme HE, et al. Prenatal cocaine exposure and fetal vascular disruption. *Pediatrics* 1990; **85:** 743–7.
20. Chávez GF, et al. Maternal cocaine use during early pregnancy as a risk factor for congenital urogenital anomalies. *JAMA* 1989; **262:** 795–8.
21. Singer LT, et al. Neurobehavioural sequelae of fetal cocaine exposure. *J Pediatr* 1991; **119:** 667–72.
22. Doberczak TM, et al. Neonatal neurologic and electroencephalographic effects of intrauterine cocaine exposure. *J Pediatr* 1988; **113:** 354–8.
23. Singer LT, et al. Increased incidence of intraventricular hemorrhage and developmental delay in cocaine-exposed, very low birth weight infants. *J Pediatr* 1994; **124:** 765–71.
24. Azuma SD, Chasnoff IJ. Outcome of children prenatally exposed to cocaine and other drugs: a path analysis of three-year data. *Pediatrics* 1993; **92:** 396–402.
25. Mayes LC, et al. Information processing and developmental assessments in 3-month-old infants exposed prenatally to cocaine. *Pediatrics* 1995; **95:** 539–45.
26. van der Bor M, et al. Increased cerebral blood flow velocity in infants of mothers who abuse cocaine. *Pediatrics* 1990; **85:** 733–6.
27. Chasnoff IJ, et al. Perinatal cerebral infarction and maternal cocaine use. *J Pediatr* 1986; **108:** 456–9.
28. Chasnoff IJ, et al. Cocaine intoxication in a breast-fed infant. *Pediatrics* 1987; **80:** 836–8.

Treatment of Adverse Effects
As for Local Anaesthetics in general, p.1303.

Cocaine overdosage. In the emergency management of overdosage with cocaine the general aims are to establish adequate ventilation and support the circulation. If oral ingestion of a large amount is suspected the stomach should be emptied and activated charcoal administered.[1] A tourniquet may be applied to limit absorption if the drug was injected. Patients who have swallowed packages containing cocaine for the purpose of smuggling, may be given laxatives but surgical intervention may be required if signs of toxicity appear.[2]

Sedation with intravenous diazepam may be sufficient to manage the symptoms of cocaine overdose. Sedation with benzodiazepines may also be appropriate initial therapy for hypertension or tachyarrhythmias since the excessive sympathetic tone is largely centrally mediated.[3] Severe life-threatening arrhythmias may require treatment with intravenous propranolol although, following a report of paradoxical hypertension presumably due to unopposed α-adrenergic stimulation, a beta blocker with both α- and β-adrenergic effects such as labetalol is preferred by some if hypertension is also present;[2,4] sodium nitroprusside[3,4] or phentolamine[3,5] may also be used. Although labetalol can reduce the hypertension it does not alleviate cocaine-induced coronary vasoconstriction;[6] it has therefore been suggested that glyceryl trinitrate would be preferable for patients with cocaine-induced chest pain.[5,6] Calcium-channel blockers such as verapamil may also be of use as an antagonist for coronary artery vasoconstriction induced by cocaine.[5] There is concern about the use of lignocaine [lidocaine] for the treatment of cocaine-induced arrhythmias as lignocaine [lidocaine] may enhance toxicity.[5] Diazepam should be used to manage seizures[1,4] but if they cannot be controlled phenytoin can be used as an adjunct.[1] Hyperthermia should be treated with physical cooling but the use of dantrolene may also be necessary.[1] Control of anxiety and agitation with benzodiazepines when combined with rapid cooling may also have the effect of decreasing heat production in hyperthermic patients.[3] Metabolic acidosis should be monitored and treated where necessary.[1,4] Short-acting barbiturates or benzodiazepines may be used for dysphoric agitation but drugs that lower the seizure threshold or aggravate hyperthermia such as phenothiazines or haloperidol should be avoided.[1]

1. Loper KA. Clinical toxicology of cocaine. *Med Toxicol Adverse Drug Exp* 1989; **4:** 174–85.
2. Ramrakha P, Barton I. Drug smuggler's delirium. *BMJ* 1993; **306:** 470–1.
3. Anonymous. Acute reactions to drugs of abuse. *Med Lett Drugs Ther* 1996; **38:** 43–6.
4. Farrar HC, Kearns GL. Cocaine: clinical pharmacology and toxicology. *J Pediatr* 1989; **115:** 665–75.
5. Hollander JE. The management of cocaine-associated myocardial ischemia. *N Engl J Med* 1995; **333:** 1267–72.
6. Boehrer JD, et al. Influence of labetalol on cocaine-induced coronary vasoconstriction in humans. *Am J Med* 1993; **94:** 608–10.

Withdrawal. Cocaine can produce psychological dependence but does not produce a major physical withdrawal syndrome. The management of cocaine abuse and dependence has been reviewed.[1-3] There is no advantage to gradual withdrawal and it is best for the patient to discontinue the drug abruptly.[1,4] The three major psychiatric complications associated with cocaine withdrawal are dysphoric agitation, severe depression, and psychotic symptoms.[1] Such complications are initially managed with psychosocial treatments. However patients with more severe dependence or those who fail to respond to psychosocial treatments should be considered for drug therapies. Dysphoric agitation is best treated with diazepam; propranolol may also be used in more persistent cases. Depressive symptoms during the acute post-cocaine phase are usually transient and require no treatment other than close observation. Desipramine has been used with equivocal results; it appears to be of most benefit in patients who have antecedent or consequent symptoms of severe depression.[3] Trazodone and imipramine have also been tried but had more adverse effects than desipramine.[3] Antipsychotics such as chlorpromazine, haloperidol, and promazine have been used successfully to manage patients with psychotic symptoms associated with cocaine dependence.[1]

Several drugs have been tried in the maintenance of abstinence from cocaine.[1] Lithium may be useful in patients with bipolar disorder or cyclothymic personality. Methylphenidate may be helpful in patients with attention deficit disorders but has potential for abuse itself. Phenothiazine derivatives have been tried in the control of impulsive behaviour and to decrease cocaine craving, although adverse effects may limit their acceptability. Carbamazepine has been reported to suppress the craving for cocaine although this has not been supported by subsequent trials.[3] Buprenorphine has been investigated to suppress cocaine and opioid use in patients dependent on both drugs.[3] Anxiolytics or antidepressants are considered unlikely to be of benefit in maintaining abstinence.[3] MAOIs such as phenelzine have been used in a manner analogous to the use of disulfiram in alcohol abuse to provoke unpleasant reactions if patients relapse.[5]

There is evidence to suggest that cocaine use affects the dopaminergic modulation of CNS function, and several drugs that interact with the dopamine system have been tried in the treatment of cocaine abuse and dependence, but with mixed results.[3]

1. Arif A, ed. *Adverse health consequences of cocaine abuse.* Geneva: WHO, 1987.
2. Kleber HD. Pharmacotherapy, current and potential, for the treatment of cocaine dependence. *Clin Neuropharmacol* 1995; **18** (suppl 1): S96–S109.
3. Mendelson JH, Mello NK. Management of cocaine abuse and dependence. *N Engl J Med* 1996; **334**: 965–72.
4. DoH. *Drug misuse and dependence: guidelines on clinical management.* London: HMSO, 1999.
5. Brewer C. Cocaine and crack. *BMJ* 1989; **299**: 792.

Precautions

As for Local Anaesthetics in general, p.1303.

Since some patients have a marked sensitivity to cocaine the administration of a test dose before use on mucous membranes has been suggested. Cocaine should not be applied to damaged mucosa because of the risk of systemic toxicity from enhanced absorption. Ophthalmic preparations of cocaine should not be applied to the eyes for prolonged periods as damage to the cornea may occur not only from the local action of cocaine, but also from loss of the protective eyelid reflexes. As with other mydriatics, there is also a risk of cocaine precipitating angle-closure glaucoma in patients predisposed to the condition. Patients receiving cocaine for surface anaesthesia should be monitored for possible cardiovascular effects. Cocaine should be used with great caution in patients with hypertension, cardiovascular disease, or thyrotoxicosis. It is not recommended for use during pregnancy or breast feeding.

Abuse. Cocaine is subject to abuse. See under Adverse Effects, above.

Gilles de la Tourette's syndrome. Gilles de la Tourette's syndrome, which had been well controlled for 10 years by haloperidol, was precipitated in a 27-year-old man following intranasal use of cocaine on one occasion.[1]

1. Mesulam M-M. Cocaine and Tourette's syndrome. *N Engl J Med* 1986; **315**: 398.

Myasthenia gravis. Report of a patient in whom cocaine abuse first unmasked and then exacerbated myasthenia gravis.[1]

1. Berciano J, *et al.* Myasthenia gravis unmasked by cocaine abuse. *N Engl J Med* 1991; **325**: 892.

Porphyria. Cocaine has been associated with acute attacks of porphyria and is considered unsafe in porphyric patients.

Interactions

For interactions associated with local anaesthetics, see p.1303.

Cocaine and adrenaline [epinephrine] enhance each other's sympathomimetic effects and should preferably not be used in association. Caution is needed if cocaine is used with other drugs that may also potentiate the action of catecholamines such as guanethidine or MAOIs.

Adrenaline [epinephrine]. In a report[1] of 3 cases of arrhythmias associated with the use of a paste containing cocaine 25% and adrenaline [epinephrine] 0.18% for local anaesthesia of the nasal mucosa, the amount of cocaine applied to the nasal mucosa ranged from about 2.5 to 4.5 mg per kg body-weight.

The symbol † denotes a preparation no longer actively marketed

The maximum recommended dose of cocaine alone in healthy adults is 1.5 mg per kg.

1. Nicholson KEA, Rogers JEG. Cocaine and adrenaline paste: a fatal combination? *BMJ* 1995; **311**: 250–1.

Alcohol. In the presence of alcohol, cocaine is metabolised to its ethyl homologue cocaethylene.[1] Cocaethylene appears to have the same stimulant effects as cocaine but it has a longer half-life and *animal* studies suggest that it is more toxic than the parent drug.

1. Randall T. Cocaine, alcohol mix in body to form even longer lasting, more lethal drug. *JAMA* 1992; **267**: 1043–4.

Beta blockers. *Propranolol* potentiated cocaine-induced coronary vasoconstriction following intranasal administration of cocaine in a placebo-controlled study.[1] Because of a possible risk of paradoxical hypertension associated with the use of propranolol to manage arrhythmias associated with cocaine overdosage some prefer the use of labetalol for this indication (see under Treatment of Adverse Effects, above).

1. Lange RA, *et al.* Potentiation of cocaine-induced coronary vasoconstriction by beta-adrenergic blockade. *Ann Intern Med* 1990; **112**: 897–903.

Haloperidol. For the effect of cocaine on haloperidol, see under Chlorpromazine, p.665.

Pharmacokinetics

Cocaine may be slowly absorbed from some sites because of the vasoconstriction it produces, but absorption occurs from all sites of application, including mucous membranes and the gastrointestinal tract, and may be enhanced when there is inflammation. Cocaine is rapidly absorbed when smoked.

Cocaine is rapidly metabolised by plasma esterases and hepatic esterases to ecgonine methyl ester. Benzoylecgonine, another major metabolite of cocaine, may be produced by spontaneous hydrolysis. Cocaine is also demethylated to the active metabolite norcocaine which is not excreted but undergoes further metabolism. There is considerable interindividual variation in the plasma half-life of cocaine possibly due to differences in esterase activity.

Cocaine and its metabolites are excreted in the urine, approximately 10% appearing as unchanged drug; they may be detectable in urine for several days or even weeks after administration. Cocaine crosses the blood-brain barrier and accumulates within the CNS. It does not appear to undergo rapid metabolism within the brain and concentrations in the CNS following acute intoxication may greatly exceed those in plasma.

Cocaine crosses the placenta and the presence of its metabolites in neonatal hair has been used to indicate intra-uterine exposure. Cocaine is distributed into breast milk.

See also under Local Anaesthetics, p.1303.

◊ References.
1. Busto U, *et al.* Clinical pharmacokinetics of non-opiate abused drugs. *Clin Pharmacokinet* 1989; **16**: 1–26.
2. Graham K, *et al.* Determination of gestational cocaine exposure by hair analysis. *JAMA* 1989; **262**: 3328–30.
3. Burke WM, Ravi NV. Urinary excretion of cocaine. *Ann Intern Med* 1990; **112**: 548–9.
4. Ravi NV, Burke WM. Cocaine and traffic accident fatalities in New York City. *JAMA* 1990; **263**: 2887.
5. Schenker S, *et al.* The transfer of cocaine and its metabolites across the term human placenta. *Clin Pharmacol Ther* 1993; **53**: 329–39.

Absorption. Cocaine is rapidly absorbed from the pulmonary vasculature when smoked and the speed of onset of its effects is similar to that obtained after intravenous injection.[1] Absorption from mucous membranes is delayed by vasoconstriction and peak plasma concentrations of up to 474 nanograms per mL have been obtained 15 to 120 minutes after application of doses of 1.5 to 2 mg per kg body-weight to the nasal mucosa as a 10% cocaine hydrochloride solution;[2,3] cocaine may still be detectable in the nose several hours later and this may result in prolonged systemic absorption.[2] In one study it was estimated that only 5% of the total dose of cocaine hydrochloride used prior to nasal surgery was absorbed from the nasal mucosa following application of 500 mg of cocaine hydrochloride as a 25% paste with adrenaline [epinephrine] or 200 mg as a 10% solution with adrenaline [epinephrine] (Moffett's solution) and blood concentrations were well below those associated with toxicity[4] (but see also Adrenaline [epinephrine], under Interactions, above). Peak serum concentrations of cocaine have been obtained after 50 to 90 minutes following oral administration and are similar to those obtained after nasal application.[3]

1. Farrar HC, Kearns GL. Cocaine: clinical pharmacology and toxicology. *J Pediatr* 1989; **115**: 665–75.
2. Van Dyke C, *et al.* Cocaine: plasma concentrations after intranasal application in man. *Science* 1976; **191**: 859–61.

3. Van Dyke C, *et al.* Oral cocaine: plasma concentrations and central effects. *Science* 1978; **200**: 211–13.
4. Quiney RE. Intranasal topical cocaine: Moffett's method or topical cocaine paste? *J Laryngol Otol* 1986; **100**: 279–83.

Uses and Administration

Cocaine, a benzoic acid ester, is a local anaesthetic with actions and uses similar to those described on p.1304. It is used as a surface anaesthetic but, because of systemic adverse effects and its abuse potential, its use is now almost entirely restricted to surgery of the ear, nose, and throat. It has been largely replaced by other drugs in ophthalmology because of its corneal toxicity, although it may still be useful in removal or debridement of the corneal epithelium. Cocaine also blocks the uptake of catecholamines at adrenergic nerve endings and potentiates the action of catecholamines. Its sympathomimetic actions cause tachycardia, peripheral vasoconstriction, a rise in blood pressure, and mydriasis. The use of cocaine in association with drugs such as adrenaline [epinephrine] increases the risk of cardiac arrhythmias. Despite this hazard some use this combination in otolaryngology to improve the operative field and reduce absorption.

When applied to mucous membranes, surface anaesthesia develops rapidly and persists for 30 minutes or longer depending on the concentration of cocaine used, the dose, and on the vascularity of the tissue.

Cocaine hydrochloride is used for the administration of cocaine in aqueous solutions. Solutions containing up to 4% have been used in ophthalmology (but see Precautions, above).

Solutions containing up to 10% of cocaine are applied to the nasal mucosa in otolaryngological procedures. Pastes containing up to 25% of cocaine have also been applied.

In order to avoid systemic effects, the usual maximum total dose recommended for application to the nasal mucosa in healthy adults is 1.5 mg per kg body-weight. It should be used only by those skilled in the precautions needed to minimise absorption and the consequent risk of arrhythmias.

Cocaine was used in conjunction with diamorphine or morphine for the relief of severe pain, especially in terminal illness, but this use is now obsolete.

Cocaine solutions should *never* be administered by injection; other local anaesthetics are equally effective and much safer.

◊ References.
1. Middleton RM, Kirkpatrick MB. Clinical use of cocaine: a review of the risks and benefits. *Drug Safety* 1993; **9**: 212–17.
2. Latorre F, Klimek L. Does cocaine still have a role in nasal surgery? *Drug Safety* 1999; **20**: 9–13.

Preparations

USP 25: Cocaine and Tetracaine Hydrochlorides and Epinephrine Topical Solution; Cocaine Hydrochloride Tablets for Topical Solution.

Diperodon Hydrochloride   (7624-w)

Diperodon Hydrochloride (BANM, rINNM).

Diperocaine Hydrochloride. 3-Piperidinopropylene bis(phenylcarbamate) hydrochloride.
$C_{22}H_{27}N_3O_4,HCl = 433.9.$
CAS — 101-08-6 (anhydrous diperodon); 51552-99-9 (diperodon monohydrate); 537-12-2 (diperodon hydrochloride).

Profile
Diperodon is a local anaesthetic (p.1302) that has been used as the base or the hydrochloride for surface anaesthesia.

Preparations
Proprietary Preparations (details are given in Part 3)
Multi-ingredient: *USA:* A-Caine†; Bactine First Aid Antibiotic Plus Anesthetic†.

Dyclonine Hydrochloride   (7625-e)

Dyclonine Hydrochloride (BANM, rINNM).

Dyclocaine Hydrochloride; Dyclocaini Chloridum. 4′-Butoxy-3-piperidinopropiophenone hydrochloride.
$C_{18}H_{27}NO_2,HCl = 325.9.$
CAS — 586-60-7 (dyclonine); 536-43-6 (dyclonine hydrochloride).
Pharmacopoeias. In US.

Pharmacopoeial description

USP 25: White crystals or white crystalline powder, with a slight odour. Soluble 1 in 60 of water, 1 in 24 of alcohol, and 1 in 2.3 of chloroform; soluble in acetone; practically insoluble in ether and in hexane. A 1% solution in water has a pH of 4.0 to 7.0. Store in airtight containers. Protect from light.

Profile

Dyclonine hydrochloride is a local anaesthetic (p.1302) used topically for surface anaesthesia of the skin and mucous membranes in concentrations of 0.5 or 1%. Single doses in excess of 200 mg should generally not be used. Lozenges containing up to 3 mg have been used for the temporary relief of pain associated with sore throats or mouth irritation. It may cause irritation at the site of application and should not be given by injection or used in the eyes.

Preparations

USP 25: Dyclonine Hydrochloride Gel; Dyclonine Hydrochloride Topical Solution.

Proprietary Preparations (details are given in Part 3)
Canad.: Sucrets; Sucrets for Kids; *Israel:* Childrens Cherry Sucrets; Sucrets Children's Formula; Sucrets Maximum Strength; *USA:* Dyclone; Sucrets.

Multi-ingredient: *Canad.:* Skin Shield†; Tanac; *USA:* Cepacol Maximum Strength Sore Throat; Skin Shield; Tanac.

Ethyl Chloride (3108-b)

Aethylium Chloratum; Chlorethyl; Cloruro de Etilo; Ethylis Chloridum; Hydrochloric Ether; Monochlorethane. Chloroethane.
$C_2H_5Cl = 64.51$.
CAS — 75-00-3.
ATC — N01BX01.
Pharmacopoeias. In Aust., Belg., Br., Pol., and US.

Pharmacopoeial description

BP 2001: Gaseous at ambient temperatures and pressures, but usually compressed to a colourless, mobile, flammable, and very volatile liquid, with an ethereal odour. If prepared from Industrial Methylated Spirit it may contain a small variable proportion of methyl chloride. Distillation range 12° to 12.5°. Slightly soluble in water; miscible with alcohol and with ether. The residual liquid from a solution in water after the ethyl chloride has evaporated is neutral to litmus. Store at a temperature not exceeding 20°. Protect from light.

USP 25: A colourless, mobile, very volatile liquid at low temperatures or under pressure, with a characteristic ethereal odour. B.p. 12° to 13°. Slightly soluble in water; freely soluble in alcohol and in ether. Store in airtight containers, preferably hermetically sealed.

◊ CAUTION. Ethyl chloride is highly flammable and mixtures of the gas with 5 to 15% of air are explosive.

Adverse Effects and Precautions

As for Chloroform, p.1257.
Cutaneous sensitisation can occur rarely. Thawing of frozen tissue following surgery may be painful and prolonged spraying onto the skin can cause chemical frostbite. Freezing may also distort the histological structure of biopsy specimens. Ethyl chloride should not be applied to broken skin or mucous membranes.

Uses and Administration

Owing to its low boiling-point and the intense cold produced by evaporation, ethyl chloride has been used as a local anaesthetic in minor surgery but such use is not generally recommended. It has also been used topically for the relief of pain. Ethyl chloride was formerly used as an inhalational anaesthetic but has no place in modern anaesthetic practice.

Preparations

Proprietary Preparations (details are given in Part 3)
Denm.: Kloraetyl; *Ger.:* Chloraethyl "Dr Henning"; Holsten aktiv†; WariActiv; *Hong Kong:* WariActiv; *Mex.:* Traumazol; *Spain:* Cloretilo Chemirosa; *Switz.:* Chlorethyl; *UK:* Cryogesic.

Multi-ingredient: *Ger.:* Olbas; *Spain:* Talgo Odontalgico†; *USA:* Fluro-Ethyl.

Ethyl p-Piperidinoacetylaminobenzoate

(8638-n)
EPAB; SA-7. 4-[(1-Piperidinylacetyl)amino]benzoic acid ethyl ester.
$C_{16}H_{22}N_2O_3 = 290.4$.
CAS — 41653-21-8.

Profile

Ethyl p-piperidinoacetylaminobenzoate is an amide local anaesthetic (p.1302) that has been given by mouth for the symptomatic relief of gastritis.

Preparations

Proprietary Preparations (details are given in Part 3)
Jpn: Sulcain.

Multi-ingredient: *Hong Kong:* Sulcain; *Singapore:* Sulcain; *Thai.:* Sulcain.

Etidocaine Hydrochloride (7626-l)

Etidocaine Hydrochloride (BANM, rINNM).
W-19053. (±)-2-(N-Ethylpropylamino)butyro-2',6'-xylidide hydrochloride.
$C_{17}H_{28}N_2O,HCl = 312.9$.
CAS — 36637-18-0 (etidocaine); 36637-19-1 (etidocaine hydrochloride).

NOTE. Etidocaine is *USAN*.

Adverse Effects, Treatment, and Precautions

As for Local Anaesthetics in general, p.1302.

Effects on the cardiovascular system. For a discussion of the cardiotoxicity of etidocaine, see under the Adverse Effects of Bupivacaine Hydrochloride, p.1306.

Porphyria. Etidocaine is considered to be unsafe in patients with porphyria because it has been shown to be porphyrinogenic in *animals*.

Interactions

For interactions associated with local anaesthetics, see p.1303.

Pharmacokinetics

Etidocaine is rapidly absorbed into the circulation after parenteral injection and is about 95% bound to plasma proteins. It crosses the placenta but the ratio of fetal to maternal concentrations is relatively low. It also diffuses across the blood-brain barrier. Etidocaine is metabolised in the liver and its numerous metabolites are excreted in the urine; less than 10% of the drug is excreted unchanged. The plasma elimination half-life of etidocaine is 2 to 3 hours in adults.
See also under Local Anaesthetics, p.1303.

Pregnancy. Following maternal injection etidocaine rapidly crosses the placenta[1] but the degree of transfer is less than for other local anaesthetics including bupivacaine.[2] The ratio of fetal to maternal concentrations of etidocaine varies but values up to about 0.35 are usual.[1,2] Some metabolites appear to be transferred to a greater degree than the parent compound[1]. Etidocaine is highly protein bound but the fraction of unbound drug in plasma increases in pregnant women during delivery.[1] Protein binding of etidocaine is also reduced in fetal plasma.[3] Although neonates are able to metabolise etidocaine it appears that they are less able to do so than adults; a mean elimination half-life of 6.42 hours has been reported in neonates.[3]

1. Morgan DJ, *et al.* Disposition and placental transfer of etidocaine in pregnancy. *Eur J Clin Pharmacol* 1977; **12:** 359–65.
2. Poppers PJ. Evaluation of local anaesthetic agents for regional anaesthesia in obstetrics. *Br J Anaesth* 1975; **47:** 322–7.
3. Morgan D, *et al.* Pharmacokinetics and metabolism of the anilide local anaesthetics in neonates: 11: etidocaine. *Eur J Clin Pharmacol* 1978; **13:** 365–71.

Uses and Administration

Etidocaine hydrochloride is a local anaesthetic of the amide type with actions and uses similar to those described on p.1304. It has a rapid onset and a long duration of action. Etidocaine is used for infiltration anaesthesia, peripheral nerve block, and epidural block, usually with adrenaline [epinephrine] 1 in 200 000. (Local anaesthetic techniques are discussed on p.1304.)

The dose of etidocaine hydrochloride varies with the site of injection and the **local anaesthetic technique** being used. The **maximum single dose** should not generally exceed 300 mg when given without adrenaline [epinephrine], or 400 mg when given with adrenaline [epinephrine]. Generally, additional incremental doses may be administered every 2 to 3 hours.

For *infiltration anaesthesia* a 0.5% solution of etidocaine hydrochloride may be used in a dose of 5 to 400 mg (1 to 80 mL). For dentistry a dose of 15 to 75 mg (1 to 5 mL) may be given as a 1.5% solution. For *peripheral nerve blocks* a 0.5% solution may be used in a dose of 25 to 400 mg (5 to 80 mL) or a 1% solution in a dose of 50 to 400 mg (5 to 40 mL). For *retrobulbar block* a 1% solution may be used in a dose of 20 to 40 mg (2 to 4 mL) or a 1.5% solution in a dose of 30 to 60 mg (2 to 4 mL).

When given by *epidural injection* etidocaine hydrochloride produces a profound degree of motor blockade and although the degree of abdominal muscle relaxation produced may be desirable in some obstetrical procedures it makes this drug unsuitable for use in vaginal deliveries. A dose of 100 to 300 mg (10 to 30 mL) may be injected as a 1% solution or 150 to 300 mg (10 to 20 mL) as a 1.5% solution for *lumbar epidural block* prior to surgery, including caesarean section. Lower doses of 50 to 150 mg (10 to 30 mL) as a 0.5% solution or 50 to 200 mg (5 to 20 mL) as a 1% solution are suggested for gynaecological procedures. For *caudal anaesthesia* 50 to 150 mg (10 to 30 mL) as a 0.5% solution or 100 to 300 mg (10 to 30 mL) as a 1% solution may be given.

Preparations

Proprietary Preparations (details are given in Part 3)
Aust.: Duranest†; *Fr.:* Duranest; *Ger.:* Duranest†; *USA:* Duranest.

Ketocaine Hydrochloride (12882-b)

Ketocaine Hydrochloride (rINNM).
Chetocaina Cloridrata. 2'-(2-Di-isopropylaminoethoxy)butyrophenone hydrochloride.
$C_{18}H_{29}NO_2,HCl = 327.9$.
CAS — 1092-46-2 (ketocaine); 1092-47-3 (ketocaine hydrochloride).

Profile

Ketocaine hydrochloride is a local anaesthetic (p.1302) that has been used as a surface anaesthetic in suppositories or ointments for anorectal disorders.

Preparations

Proprietary Preparations (details are given in Part 3)
Multi-ingredient: *Ital.:* Proctolyn.

Levobupivacaine (17525-d)

Levobupivacaine (BAN, rINN).
S(−)-Bupivacaine; Levobupivacaina; Lévobupivacaïne. (S)-1-Butyl-2-piperidylformo-2',6'-xylidide.
$C_{18}H_{28}N_2O = 288.4$.
CAS — 27262-47-1.
ATC — N01BB10.

Levobupivacaine Hydrochloride (675-e)

Levobupivacaine Hydrochloride (BANM, USAN, rINNM).
$C_{18}H_{28}N_2O,HCl = 324.9$.
CAS — 27262-48-2.

Adverse Effects, Treatment, and Precautions

As for Local Anaesthetics in general, p.1302.

Levobupivacaine is contra-indicated for use in intravenous regional anaesthesia (Bier's block) and for paracervical block in obstetrics. The 0.75% solution is contra-indicated for epidural block in obstetrics.

Effects on the cardiovascular system. It has been suggested[1] that levobupivacaine may have a lower risk of causing cardiotoxicity than bupivacaine (for the effects of bupivacaine on the cardiovascular system see p.1306).

1. Mather LE, Chang DH. Cardiotoxicity with modern local anaesthetics: is there a safer choice? *Drugs* 2001; **61:** 333–42.

Interactions

For interactions associated with local anaesthetics, see p.1303. Plasma concentrations of levobupivacaine may be reduced by enzyme-inducing drugs such as rifampicin. Levobupivacaine is metabolised by the cytochrome P450 isoenzymes CYP3A4 and CYP1A2 and there is a theoretical possibility that substrates for or inhibitors of these isoenzymes may adversely alter plasma concentrations of levobupivacaine.

Pharmacokinetics

The pharmacokinetics of levobupivacaine are similar to those of the racemic form, bupivacaine (p.1307). Levobupivacaine is at least 97% bound to plasma proteins. After intravenous administration the mean half-life is about 80 minutes. Levobupivacaine is extensively metabolised and excreted as its metabolites mainly in the urine, with smaller amounts appearing in the faeces. 3-Hydroxylevobupivacaine is a major metabolite and its formation is mediated by the cytochrome P450 isoenzyme CYP1A2; CYP3A4 is also involved in the metabolism of levobupivacaine.

Uses and Administration

Levobupivacaine is a local anaesthetic of the amide type with actions and uses similar to those described on p.1304. It is the S-enantiomer of bupivacaine (p.1306). Levobupivacaine is given as the hydrochloride for infiltration anaesthesia and regional nerve blocks including epidural block; however it is contraindicated for obstetric paracervical block and for use in intravenous regional anaesthesia (Bier's block). The 0.75% solution is contra-indicated for epidural blocks in obstetrics. (Local anaesthetic techniques are discussed on p.1304.)

Levobupivacaine hydrochloride is available in solutions containing the equivalent of 0.25 to 0.75% of levobupivacaine. The dosage depends on the site of injection and the procedure used as well as the status of the patient. The recommended **maximum single dose** is 150 mg. The total daily dose should not exceed 400 mg. A test dose of a suitable local anaesthetic, preferably with adrenaline [epinephrine], should be given before commencing epidural block with levobupivacaine to detect inadvertent intravascular administration. Subsequent doses of levobupivacaine should be given in small increments.

For **surgical anaesthesia** doses of levobupivacaine for *epidural block* are 50 to 100 mg (10 to 20 mL) as a 0.5% solution, or 75 to 150 mg (10 to 20 mL) as a 0.75% solution; for caesarean section, doses are 75 to 150 mg (15 to 30 mL) as a 0.5% solution. The dose for *spinal block* is 15 mg (3 mL) as a 0.5% solution. For *peripheral nerve blocks*, doses are 2.5 to 150 mg as a 0.25 or 0.5% solution; a volume of 40 mL should not be exceeded. Alternatively doses for peripheral block may be expressed on the basis of body-weight: 1 to 2 mg per kg body-weight (0.4 mL per kg) as a 0.25 or 0.5% solution. For *infiltration anaesthesia* up to 150 mg (60 mL) as a 0.25% solution may be used. For peribulbar block in *ophthalmic* procedures 37.5 to 112.5 mg (5 to 15 mL) as a 0.75% solution may be given. For ilioinguinal or iliohypogastric blocks in **children** under 12 years of age, doses of levobupivacaine are 1.25 to 2.5 mg per kg (0.25 to 0.5 mL per kg) as a 0.25 or 0.5% solution.

In the management of **acute pain** it may be given as an epidural bolus or by continuous infusion. For pain relief during *labour* 15 to 50 mg (6 to 20 mL) as a 0.25% solution is given as a bolus. Alternatively a 0.125% solution may be given as an infusion in a dose of 5 to 12.5 mg (4 to 10 mL) per hour. For *postoperative pain* 10 to 25 mg (4 to 10 mL) per hour as a 0.25% solution or 12.5 to 18.75 mg (10 to 15 mL) per hour as a 0.125% solution may be given as an epidural infusion. When necessary, dilutions should be made with sodium chloride 0.9%.

◊ Reviews
1. Foster RH, Markham A. Levobupivacaine: a review of its pharmacology and use as a local anaesthetic. *Drugs* 2000; **59**: 551–79.

Action. A comparison[1] of epidural bupivacaine with levobupivacaine in women in labour found that levobupivacaine had 98% of the potency of the racemate, a clinically insignificant difference. However it was pointed out that whereas the concentration of bupivacaine solutions was expressed in terms of the hydrochloride, solutions of levobupivacaine had their strength expressed in terms of the free base. When calculations were made in terms of molar equivalents levobupivacaine appeared to be 13% less potent then racemic bupivacaine. The difference in expression should be borne in mind when evaluating comparative studies.
1. Lyons G, *et al.* Epidural pain relief in labour: potencies of levobupivacaine and racemic bupivacaine. *Br J Anaesth* 1998; **81**: 899–901.

Preparations

Proprietary Preparations (details are given in Part 3)
Neth.: Chirocaine; **Swed.:** Chirocaine; **UK:** Chirocaine; **USA:** Chirocaine.

Lignocaine (7602-b)

Lignocaine (BAN).
Lidocaine (BAN, rINN); Lidocainum. 2-Diethylaminoaceto-2′,6′-xylidide.
$C_{14}H_{22}N_2O$ = 234.3.
CAS — 137-58-6.
ATC — C01BB01; C05AD01; D04AB01; N01BB02; R02AD02; S01HA07; S02DA01.
Pharmacopoeias. In *Eur.* (see p.vi), *Int., Jpn,* and *US.*

Lignocaine [lidocaine] forms a mixture with prilocaine that has a melting-point lower than that of either ingredient. This eutectic mixture is used in the preparation of topical dosage forms.

Pharmacopoeial description
Ph. Eur.: A white or almost white, crystalline powder. M.p. 66° to 70°. Practically insoluble in water; very soluble in alcohol and in dichloromethane; freely soluble in ether.

USP 25: A white to slightly yellow crystalline powder with a characteristic odour. M.p. 66° to 69°. Practically insoluble in water; very soluble in alcohol and in chloroform; freely soluble in ether and in benzene; dissolves in oils.

Lignocaine Hydrochloride (7601-m)

Lignocaine Hydrochloride (BANM).
Lidocaine Hydrochloride (BANM, rINNM); Lidocaini Hydrochloridum; Lignoc. Hydrochlor.
$C_{14}H_{22}N_2O,HCl,H_2O$ = 288.8.
CAS — 73-78-9 (anhydrous lignocaine [lidocaine] hydrochloride); 6108-05-0 (lignocaine [lidocaine] hydrochloride monohydrate).

NOTE. LIDFLN is a code approved by the BP 2001 for use on single unit doses of eye drops containing lignocaine [lidocaine] hydrochloride and fluorescein sodium where the individual container may be too small to bear all the appropriate labelling information.

Pharmacopoeias. In *Chin., Eur.* (see p.vi), *Int., Pol.,* and *US.*

Lignocaine [lidocaine] hydrochloride monohydrate 1.23 g or anhydrous lignocaine [lidocaine] hydrochloride 1.16 g is approximately equivalent to 1 g of lignocaine [lidocaine].

Pharmacopoeial description
Ph. Eur.: A white crystalline powder. M.p. 74° to 79°. Very soluble in water; freely soluble in alcohol; practically insoluble in ether. A 0.5% solution in water has a pH of 4.0 to 5.5. Protect from light.

USP 25: A white, odourless, crystalline powder. M.p. 74° to 79°. Very soluble in water and in alcohol; soluble in chloroform; insoluble in ether.

Incompatibility. Lignocaine [lidocaine] hydrochloride has been reported to be incompatible in solution with amphotericin B,[1] sulfadiazine sodium,[2] methohexital sodium,[2] cefazolin sodium,[3] or phenytoin sodium.[4]
Acid stable drugs such as adrenaline [epinephrine] hydrochloride, noradrenaline [norepinephrine] acid tartrate, or isoprenaline may begin to deteriorate within several hours of admixture with lignocaine [lidocaine] hydrochloride as lignocaine [lidocaine] solutions may raise the pH of the final solution above the maximum pH for their stability. Such extemporaneous mixtures should be used promptly after preparation.[5]
1. Whiting DA. Treatment of chromoblastomycosis with high local concentrations of amphotericin B. *Br J Dermatol* 1967; **79**: 345–51.
2. Riley BB. Incompatibilities in intravenous solutions. *J Hosp Pharm* 1970; **28**: 228–40.
3. Kleinberg ML, *et al.* Stability of antibiotics frozen and stored in disposable hypodermic syringes. *Am J Hosp Pharm* 1980; **37**: 1087–8.
4. Kirschenbaum HL, *et al.* Stability and compatibility of lidocaine hydrochloride with selected large-volume parenterals and drug additives. *Am J Hosp Pharm* 1982; **39**: 1013–15.
5. Parker EA. Xylocaine hydrochloride 2% injection. *Am J Hosp Pharm* 1971; **28**: 805.

pH of solutions. For the effect pH has on the surface tension and administration of lignocaine [lidocaine] solutions by infusion, see under Administration in Uses and Administration, p.1304. For its effect on the stability of local anaesthetic solutions and the pain associated with their injection, see p.1304.

Stability. Although there was no decrease in the lignocaine [lidocaine] content of lignocaine [lidocaine] hydrochloride and adrenaline [epinephrine] injection during transport and storage under tropical conditions, the content of adrenaline [epinephrine] fell to almost zero in some samples after several months; supply of the injection as a dry powder and separate solvent should be considered for the tropics.[1]
The lignocaine [lidocaine] content of buffered cardioplegic solutions has been reported[2] to decrease when stored in PVC containers at ambient temperature, but not when stored at 4°. This loss appeared to result from pH-dependent sorption of lignocaine [lidocaine] onto the plastic and did not occur when lignocaine [lidocaine] solutions were stored in glass bottles.
1. Abu-Reid IO, *et al.* Stability of drugs in the tropics: a study in Sudan. *Int Pharm J* 1990; **4**: 6–10.
2. Lackner TE, *et al.* Lidocaine stability in cardioplegic solution stored in glass bottles and polyvinyl chloride bags. *Am J Hosp Pharm* 1983; **40**: 97–101.

Adverse Effects and Treatment

As for Local Anaesthetics in general, p.1302.

Effects on the CNS. A report[1] of suspected psychotic reactions associated with the use of lignocaine [lidocaine] in 6 patients given intravenous lignocaine [lidocaine] for the treatment of cardiac disorders.
1. Turner WM. Lidocaine and psychotic reactions. *Ann Intern Med* 1982; **97**: 149–50.

Effects on the skin. Erythema and pigmentation of the upper lip in a child following local dental infiltration of lignocaine [lidocaine] was attributed to a type of fixed drug eruption.[1] Erythema may also occur after topical administration of some lignocaine [lidocaine] formulations, such as transdermal patches, while transient blanching of the skin is frequent after application of eutectic lignocaine [lidocaine]/prilocaine mixtures to the skin.[2]
True hypersensitivity reactions, including dermatitis, are rare (see also p.1302) but can occur.[3]
1. Curley RK, *et al.* An unusual cutaneous reaction to lignocaine. *Br Dent J* 1987; **162**: 113–14.
2. Villada G, *et al.* Local blanching after epicutaneous application of EMLA cream: a double-blind randomized study among 50 healthy volunteers. *Dermatologica* 1990; **181**: 38–40.
3. Bircher AJ, *et al.* Delayed-type hypersensitivity to subcutaneous lidocaine with tolerance to articaine: confirmation by in vivo and in vitro tests. *Contact Dermatitis* 1996; **34**: 387–9.

Overdosage. The most serious effects of lignocaine [lidocaine] intoxication are on the CNS and cardiovascular system and overdosage can result in severe hypotension, asystole, bradycardia, apnoea, seizures, coma, cardiac arrest, respiratory arrest, and death. Intoxication with lignocaine [lidocaine] is relatively common and can occur as a result of acute overdosage following poor control of intravenous maintenance infusions or after accidental injection of concentrated solutions. However, it more commonly results from inadvertent intravascular administration during regional anaesthesia, or from too rapid injection of antiarrhythmic doses, particularly in patients with circulatory insufficiency, or when clearance is reduced due to heart failure, liver disease, old age, or through interaction with other drugs.[1] Seizures have also been reported after excessive doses administered subcutaneously.[2] Although the bioavailability of lignocaine [lidocaine] is low it may be sufficient to result in significant toxicity when swallowed[1] and there have been reports of CNS toxicity, seizures, and death in children[3-7] and adults[8-10] following the ingestion of topical solutions and after the use of viscous preparations in the mouth. Death has also ensued after gargling with a 4% lignocaine [lidocaine] solution.[11] Lignocaine [lidocaine] is absorbed from mucous membranes and serious toxicity has been reported after urethral[12] or rectal[13] instillation of lignocaine [lidocaine] preparations.
1. Denaro CP, Benowitz NL. Poisoning due to class 1B antiarrhythmic drugs: lignocaine, mexiletine and tocainide. *Med Toxicol Adverse Drug Exp* 1989; **4**: 412–28.
2. Pelter MA, *et al.* Seizure-like reaction associated with subcutaneous lidocaine injection. *Clin Pharm* 1989; **8**: 767–8.
3. Sakai RI, Lattin JE. Lidocaine ingestion. *Am J Dis Child* 1980; **134**: 323.
4. Rothstein P, *et al.* Prolonged seizures associated with the use of viscous lidocaine. *J Pediatr* 1982; **101**: 461–3.
5. Mofenson HC, *et al.* Lidocaine toxicity from topical mucosal application. *Clin Pediatr (Phila)* 1983; **22**: 190–2.
6. Giard MJ, *et al.* Seizures induced by oral viscous lidocaine. *Clin Pharm* 1983; **2**: 110.
7. Amitai Y, *et al.* Death following accidental lidocaine overdose in a child. *N Engl J Med* 1986; **314**: 182–3.
8. Parish RC, *et al.* Seizures following oral lidocaine for esophageal anesthesia. *Drug Intell Clin Pharm* 1985; **19**: 199–201.
9. Fruncillo RJ, *et al.* CNS toxicity after ingestion of topical lidocaine. *N Engl J Med* 1982; **306**: 426–7.
10. Geraets DR, *et al.* Toxicity potential of oral lidocaine in a patient receiving mexiletine. *Ann Pharmacother* 1992; **26**: 1380–1.
11. Zuberi BF, *et al.* Lidocaine toxicity in a student undergoing upper gastrointestinal endoscopy. *Gut* 2000; **46**: 435.
12. Dix VW, Tresidder GC. Collapse after use of lignocaine jelly for urethral anaesthesia. *Lancet* 1963; **i**: 890.
13. Pottage A, Scott DB. Safety of "topical" lignocaine. *Lancet* 1988; **i**: 1003.

Pregnancy. The overall effect of maternal epidural anaesthesia appears to be beneficial for the fetus (see under Labour Pain, p.6) but lignocaine [lidocaine] may have transient effects on the neonatal auditory system.[1]
1. Bozynski MEA, *et al.* Effect of prenatal lignocaine on auditory brain stem evoked response. *Arch Dis Child* 1989; **64**: 934–8.

Precautions

As for Local Anaesthetics in general, p.1303.

In general lignocaine [lidocaine] should not be given to patients with hypovolaemia, heart block or other conduction disturbances, and should be used with caution in patients with congestive heart failure, bradycardia, or respiratory depression. Lignocaine [lidocaine] is metabolised in the liver and must be given with caution to patients with hepatic insufficiency. The plasma half-life of lignocaine [lidocaine] may be prolonged in conditions that reduce hepatic blood flow such as cardiac and circulatory failure.

The symbol † denotes a preparation no longer actively marketed

Metabolites of lignocaine [lidocaine] may accumulate in patients with renal impairment.

The intramuscular injection of lignocaine [lidocaine] may increase creatine phosphokinase concentrations that can interfere with the diagnosis of acute myocardial infarction.

Cerebrovascular disorders. Administration of lignocaine [lidocaine] 5 mg per kg body-weight by intravenous infusion over 30 minutes was associated with a 12% reduction in cerebral blood flow in healthy subjects although it returned to normal within 60 minutes.[1] Cerebral blood flow in patients with diabetes was lower than in healthy subjects, but was unaffected by lignocaine [lidocaine] infusion, indicating reduced cerebrovascular reactivity.

1. Kastrup J, et al. Intravenous lidocaine and cerebral blood flow: impaired microvascular reactivity in diabetic patients. *J Clin Pharmacol* 1990; **30:** 318–23.

Porphyria. Lignocaine [lidocaine] is considered to be unsafe in patients with porphyria because it has been shown to be porphyrinogenic in *animals*.

Renal impairment. The pharmacokinetics of lignocaine [lidocaine] and its metabolite monoethylglycinexylidide appear to be unaffected in patients with renal failure except that accumulation of the metabolite glycinexylidide may occur during infusions of 12 hours or more.[1] Data to predict the amount of lignocaine [lidocaine] and glycinexylidide removed during haemodialysis have been provided by several workers.[2,3] Lignocaine [lidocaine] does not appear to be removed during haemofiltration.[4]

1. Collinsworth KA, et al. Pharmacokinetics and metabolism of lidocaine in patients with renal failure. *Clin Pharmacol Ther* 1975; **18:** 59–64.
2. Gibson TP, Nelson HA. Drug kinetics and artificial kidneys. *Clin Pharmacokinet* 1977; **2:** 403–26.
3. Lee CC, Marbury TC. Drug therapy in patients undergoing haemodialysis: clinical pharmacokinetic considerations. *Clin Pharmacokinet* 1984; **9:** 42–66.
4. Saima S, et al. Negligible removal of lidocaine during arteriovenous hemofiltration. *Ther Drug Monit* 1990; **12:** 154–6.

Smoking. The effects of smoking on lignocaine [lidocaine] therapy are unclear. Studies in a limited number of patients have found reduced systemic bioavailability suggestive of induction of drug-metabolising activity[1] and an inconsistent effect on protein binding.[2,3]

1. Huet P-M, Lelorier J. Effects of smoking and chronic hepatitis B on lidocaine and indocyanine green kinetics. *Clin Pharmacol Ther* 1980; **28:** 208–15.
2. McNamara PJ, et al. Effect of smoking on binding of lidocaine to human serum proteins. *J Pharm Sci* 1980; **69:** 749–51.
3. Davis D, et al. The effects of age and smoking on the plasma protein binding of lignocaine and diazepam. *Br J Clin Pharmacol* 1985; **19:** 261–5.

Interactions

For interactions associated with local anaesthetics, see p.1303.

The clearance of lignocaine [lidocaine] may be reduced by propranolol and cimetidine (see below). The cardiac depressant effects of lignocaine [lidocaine] are additive with those of beta blockers and of other antiarrhythmics including intravenous phenytoin; long-term administration of enzyme-inducers such as phenytoin may increase dosage requirements of lignocaine [lidocaine] (see below). Hypokalaemia produced by acetazolamide, loop diuretics, and thiazides antagonises the effect of lignocaine [lidocaine].

Antiarrhythmics. Lignocaine [lidocaine] toxicity, arising from the use of an oral preparation containing lignocaine [lidocaine], has been reported[1] in a patient who was receiving *mexiletine*. There are isolated reports of seizures or heart failure and cardiac arrest in patients who received intravenous lignocaine [lidocaine] concomitantly with *ajmaline*,[2] *amiodarone*,[3,4] or *tocainide*.[5] Delirium has been reported in a patient who received lignocaine [lidocaine] together with *procainamide*.[6]

1. Geraets DR, et al. Toxicity potential of oral lidocaine in a patient receiving mexiletine. *Ann Pharmacother* 1992; **26:** 1380–1.
2. Bleifeld W. Side effects of antiarrhythmic drugs. *Naunyn Schmiedebergs Arch Pharmacol* 1971; **269:** 282–97.
3. Siegmund JB, et al. Amiodarone interaction with lidocaine. *J Cardiovasc Pharmacol* 1993; **21:** 513–15.
4. Keidar S, et al. Sinoatrial arrest due to lidocaine injection in sick sinus syndrome during amiodarone administration. *Am Heart J* 1982; **104:** 1384–5.
5. Forrence E, et al. A seizure induced by concurrent lidocaine-to-cainide therapy—is it just a case of additive toxicity? *Drug Intell Clin Pharm* 1986; **20:** 56–9.
6. Ilyas M, et al. Delirium induced by a combination of anti-arrhythmic drugs. *Lancet* 1969; **ii:** 1368–9.

Antiepileptics. Studies in healthy subjects and patients with epilepsy[1,2] suggest that long-term use of drugs such as *phenytoin* or *barbiturates* may increase dosage requirements for lignocaine [lidocaine] due to induction of drug-metabolising microsomal enzymes. Administration of phenytoin can also increase plasma concentrations of α_1-acid glycoprotein and

thereby reduce the free fraction of lignocaine [lidocaine] in plasma.[3]

The cardiac depressant effects of lignocaine [lidocaine] may be dangerously enhanced by intravenous phenytoin.[4]

1. Heinonen J, et al. Plasma lidocaine levels in patients treated with potential inducers of microsomal enzymes. *Acta Anaesthesiol Scand* 1970; **14:** 89–95.
2. Perucca E, Richens A. Reduction of oral bioavailability of lignocaine by induction of first pass metabolism in epileptic patients. *Br J Clin Pharmacol* 1979; **8:** 21–31.
3. Routledge PA, et al. Lignocaine disposition in blood in epilepsy. *Br J Clin Pharmacol* 1981; **12:** 663–6.
4. Wood RA. Sinoatrial arrest: an interaction between phenytoin and lignocaine. *BMJ* 1971; **1:** 645.

Beta blockers. Significant increases in plasma-lignocaine [lidocaine] concentrations have occurred during concomitant therapy with *propranolol*[1-4] owing to a reduction in the clearance of lignocaine [lidocaine] from plasma. A similar interaction has been observed with *nadolol*[3] and *metoprolol*,[2] although in another study[5] metoprolol did not alter the pharmacokinetics of lignocaine [lidocaine]. The hepatic metabolism of lignocaine [lidocaine] may be reduced as a result of a fall in hepatic blood flow associated with reduced cardiac output or it may be caused by direct inhibition of hepatic microsomal enzymes.[6] Significant impairment of lignocaine [lidocaine] clearance would therefore be most likely to occur with those drugs that lack intrinsic sympathomimetic activity and have a greater effect on cardiac output or the more lipid-soluble drugs that have greater effects on microsomal oxygenases. Results of one study[4] suggest that the reduction in clearance produced by propranolol is mainly by direct inhibition of metabolism rather than by lowering of hepatic blood flow.

1. Ochs HR, et al. Reduction in lidocaine clearance during continuous infusion and by coadministration of propranolol. *N Engl J Med* 1980; **303:** 373–7.
2. Conrad KA, et al. Lidocaine elimination: effects of metoprolol and of propranolol. *Clin Pharmacol Ther* 1983; **33:** 133–8.
3. Schneck DW, et al. Effects of nadolol and propranolol on plasma lidocaine clearance. *Clin Pharmacol Ther* 1984; **36:** 584–7.
4. Bax NDS, et al. The impairment of lignocaine clearance by propranolol—major contribution from enzyme inhibition. *Br J Clin Pharmacol* 1985; **19:** 597–603.
5. Miners JO, et al. Failure of 'therapeutic' doses of β-adrenoceptor antagonists to alter the disposition of tolbutamide and lignocaine. *Br J Clin Pharmacol* 1984; **18:** 853–60.
6. Tucker GT, et al. Effects of β-adrenoceptor antagonists on the pharmacokinetics of lignocaine. *Br J Clin Pharmacol* 1984; **17:** 21S–28S.

H_2-antagonists. There have been numerous studies[1-4] of the interaction between *cimetidine* and lignocaine [lidocaine] but differences between the studies makes interpretation of the overall clinical significance of the results difficult. Cimetidine appears to reduce the hepatic metabolism of lignocaine [lidocaine]; it may also reduce its clearance by decreasing hepatic blood flow. Significant increases in plasma-lignocaine [lidocaine] concentrations have been reported. Changes in protein binding are not generally important but patients with myocardial infarction who have increased levels of α_1-acid glycoprotein may be partially protected from increases in concentrations of free lignocaine [lidocaine].[5] Since it is not possible to identify those patients at risk all patients receiving these drugs concurrently should be closely monitored for signs of toxicity. The use of other H_2-antagonists may be preferable. In studies in healthy subjects *ranitidine* either had no effect on lignocaine [lidocaine] kinetics[6] or produced changes consistent with small reductions in hepatic blood flow.[7]

1. Feely J, et al. Increased toxicity and reduced clearance of lidocaine by cimetidine. *Ann Intern Med* 1982; **96:** 592–4.
2. Knapp AB, et al. The cimetidine-lidocaine interaction. *Ann Intern Med* 1983; **98:** 174–7.
3. Patterson JH, et al. Influence of a continuous cimetidine infusion on lidocaine plasma concentrations in patients. *J Clin Pharmacol* 1985; **25:** 607–9.
4. Bauer LA, et al. Cimetidine-induced decrease in lidocaine metabolism. *Am J Med* 1984; **108:** 413–15.
5. Berk SI, et al. The effect of oral cimetidine on total and unbound serum lidocaine concentrations in patients with suspected myocardial infarction. *Int J Cardiol* 1987; **14:** 91–4.
6. Feely J, Guy E. Lack of effect of ranitidine on the disposition of lignocaine. *Br J Clin Pharmacol* 1983; **15:** 378–9.
7. Robson RA, et al. The effect of ranitidine on the disposition of lignocaine. *Br J Clin Pharmacol* 1985; **20:** 170–3.

Local anaesthetics. Although a number of drugs were shown to reduce the amount of lignocaine [lidocaine] bound to α_1-acid glycoprotein only the displacement produced by *bupivacaine* was considered to be of possible clinical significance.[1]

There is concern about the use as lignocaine [lidocaine] to treat *cocaine*-induced arrhythmias as lignocaine [lidocaine] may enhance toxicity.[2]

1. Goolkasian DL, et al. Displacement of lidocaine from serum α_1-acid glycoprotein binding sites by basic drugs. *Eur J Clin Pharmacol* 1983; **25:** 413–17.
2. Hollander JE. The management of cocaine-associated myocardial ischemia. *N Engl J Med* 1995; **333:** 1267–72.

Neuromuscular blockers. The possible interaction between neuromuscular blockers and antiarrhythmics including lignocaine [lidocaine] is discussed under Atracurium, p.1334.

Oral contraceptives. For mention of the effect of oral contraceptives on the protein binding of lignocaine [lidocaine], see under Protein Binding in Pharmacokinetics, below.

Pharmacokinetics

Lignocaine [lidocaine] is readily absorbed from the gastrointestinal tract, from mucous membranes, and through damaged skin. Absorption through intact skin is poor. It is rapidly absorbed from injection sites including muscle.

After an intravenous dose lignocaine [lidocaine] is rapidly and widely distributed into highly perfused tissues followed by redistribution into skeletal muscle and adipose tissue. Lignocaine [lidocaine] is bound to plasma proteins, including α_1-acid glycoprotein (AAG). The extent of binding is variable but is approximately 66%. Plasma protein binding of lignocaine [lidocaine] depends in part on the concentrations of both lignocaine [lidocaine] and AAG. Any alteration in the concentration of AAG can greatly affect plasma concentrations of lignocaine [lidocaine] (see under Protein Binding, below).

Plasma concentrations decline rapidly after an intravenous dose with an initial half-life of less than 30 minutes; the elimination half-life is 1 to 2 hours but may be prolonged if infusions are given for longer than 24 hours or if hepatic blood flow is reduced.

Lignocaine [lidocaine] is largely metabolised in the liver and any alteration in liver function or hepatic blood flow can have a significant effect on its pharmacokinetics and dosage requirements. First-pass metabolism is extensive and bioavailability is about 35% after oral administration. Metabolism in the liver is rapid and approximately 90% of a given dose is dealkylated to form monoethylglycinexylidide and glycinexylidide. Both of these metabolites may contribute to the therapeutic and toxic effects of lignocaine [lidocaine] and since their half-lives are longer than that of lignocaine [lidocaine], accumulation, particularly of glycinexylidide, may occur during prolonged infusions. Further metabolism occurs and metabolites are excreted in the urine with less than 10% of unchanged lignocaine [lidocaine]. Reduced clearance of lignocaine [lidocaine] has been found in patients with heart failure, alcoholic liver disease, or chronic or viral hepatitis. Concomitant therapy with drugs that alter hepatic blood flow or induce drug-metabolising microsomal enzymes can also affect the clearance of lignocaine [lidocaine] (see under Interactions, above). Renal impairment does not affect the clearance of lignocaine [lidocaine] but accumulation of its active metabolites can occur.

Lignocaine [lidocaine] crosses the placenta and blood-brain barrier; it is distributed into breast milk.

See also under Local Anaesthetics, p.1303.

◊ References.

1. Nattel S, et al. The pharmacokinetics of lignocaine and β-adrenoceptor antagonists in patients with acute myocardial infarction. *Clin Pharmacokinet* 1987; **13:** 293–316.

Absorption. SURFACE APPLICATION. Serum-lignocaine [lidocaine] concentrations were usually so low as to be unmeasurable in patients who gargled and expectorated 15 mL (300 mg) of a 2% viscous solution before endoscopy[1] and mean peak serum concentrations of lignocaine [lidocaine] were below those associated with toxicity following endotracheal application of 100 mg of lignocaine [lidocaine] by spray.[2] The relative bioavailability of lignocaine [lidocaine] has been found to be higher when applied to the upper respiratory tract than after administration to the lower respiratory tract.[3] Acceptably low plasma-lignocaine [lidocaine] concentrations were noted with the following regimen used before bronchoscopy: a 4% lignocaine [lidocaine] solution gargled for 30 seconds, a 2% solution sprayed onto the oropharynx, a 2% jelly applied to the oropharynx and nasal passages, and a 1% solution injected through a bronchoscope.[4] However, a fatality has been reported following the use of lignocaine [lidocaine] as a gargle (see under Overdosage, above); the absorption of intranasal lignocaine [lidocaine] can also be highly variable.[5] For bronchoscopy, administration of lignocaine [lidocaine] by inhalation from a nebuliser rather than by direct spray may result in lower peak serum concentrations.[6]

Absorption of lignocaine [lidocaine] is generally poor through intact skin. However, there is some evidence that absorption may be greater following application to the skin of preterm infants.[7]

1. Fazio A, et al. Lidocaine serum concentrations following endoscopy. *Drug Intell Clin Pharm* 1987; **21:** 752–3.
2. Scott DB, et al. Plasma lignocaine concentrations following endotracheal spraying with an aerosol. *Br J Anaesth* 1976; **48:** 899–902.

3. McBurney A, *et al.* Absorption of lignocaine and bupivacaine from the respiratory tract during fibreoptic bronchoscopy. *Br J Clin Pharmacol* 1984; **17:** 61–6.
4. Ameer B, *et al.* Systemic absorption of topical lidocaine in elderly and young adults undergoing bronchoscopy. *Pharmacotherapy* 1989; **9:** 74–81.
5. Scavone JM, *et al.* The bioavailability of intranasal lignocaine. *Br J Clin Pharmacol* 1989; **28:** 722–4.
6. Labedzki L, *et al.* Reduced systemic absorption of intrabronchial lidocaine by high-frequency nebulization. *J Clin Pharmacol* 1990; **30:** 795–7.
7. Barrett DA, Rutter N. Percutaneous lignocaine absorption in newborn infants. *Arch Dis Child* 1994; **71:** F122–F124.

Protein binding. Lignocaine [lidocaine] is markedly bound to α_1-acid glycoprotein (AAG), a plasma protein which is increased after trauma, surgery, burns, myocardial infarction, in chronic inflammatory disorders such as Crohn's disease, and in cancer. Protein binding may therefore be greatly increased in these conditions and reduced in neonates, the nephrotic syndrome, and in liver disease when AAG concentrations are lower than normal. This can result in an eightfold variation in the free fraction of lignocaine [lidocaine] between these conditions.[1] Measurement of free drug concentrations may be a better guide to dosage requirements than measurement of total plasma concentrations.[2] AAG concentrations may also be reduced by oestrogens[3] leading to a higher free fraction of lignocaine [lidocaine] in women than in men and the free fraction is further increased during pregnancy and in women taking oral contraceptives.[3,4] Protein binding may also be affected by other concomitant drug therapy or smoking (for further details, see under Interactions, above and Precautions, Smoking, above).

1. Routledge PA. Pharmacological terms: protein binding. *Prescribers' J* 1988; **28:** 34–5.
3. Shand DG. α_1-Acid glycoprotein and plasma lidocaine binding. *Clin Pharmacokinet* 1984; **9** (suppl 1): 27–31.
3. Routledge PA, *et al.* Sex-related differences in the plasma protein binding of lignocaine and diazepam. *Br J Clin Pharmacol* 1981; **11:** 245–50.
4. Wood M, Wood AJJ. Changes in plasma drug binding and α_1-acid glycoprotein in mother and newborn infant. *Clin Pharmacol Ther* 1981; **29:** 522–6.

Uses and Administration

Lignocaine [lidocaine] is a local anaesthetic of the amide type with actions and uses similar to those described on p.1304. It is used for infiltration anaesthesia and regional nerve blocks. It has a rapid onset of action and anaesthesia is obtained within a few minutes depending on the site of administration; it has an intermediate duration of action. The speed of onset and duration of action of lignocaine [lidocaine] are increased by the addition of a vasoconstrictor and absorption into the circulation from the site of injection is reduced. It is generally given as the hydrochloride. The carbonated solution of lignocaine [lidocaine] is also available in some countries for injection (see p.1304). Lignocaine [lidocaine] is also a useful surface anaesthetic but it should be remembered that it may be rapidly and extensively absorbed following topical application to mucous membranes and systemic effects may occur. Hyaluronidase (p.1620) has been added to preparations of lignocaine [lidocaine] used for surface and infiltration anaesthesia but it may also enhance systemic absorption. (Local anaesthetic techniques are discussed on p.1304.)

Lignocaine [lidocaine] is included in some injections, such as depot corticosteroids, to prevent pain, itching, and other local irritation. Lignocaine [lidocaine] sodium has also been included in intramuscular injections of some antibacterials to reduce the pain on administration.

Lignocaine [lidocaine] is also a class Ib antiarrhythmic used in the treatment of ventricular arrhythmias, especially after myocardial infarction. It has been given by intravenous infusion in the treatment of refractory status epilepticus.

USE IN LOCAL ANAESTHESIA.

The dose of lignocaine [lidocaine] hydrochloride used for local anaesthesia depends on the site of injection and the procedure used. Specific licensed doses for individual procedures are not generally available in the UK, although US product information often includes them (see below). When given with adrenaline [epinephrine], the suggested general **maximum single dose** of lignocaine [lidocaine] hydrochloride is 500 mg; without adrenaline [epinephrine], the recommended maximum single dose in the UK is 200 mg and in the USA, 300 mg, except for spinal anaesthesia (see below). Lignocaine [lidocaine] hydrochloride solutions containing adrenaline [epinephrine] 1 in 200 000 are used for infiltration anaesthesia and nerve blocks; higher concentrations of adrenaline [epinephrine] are seldom necessary, except in dentistry, in which case, solutions of lignocaine [lidocaine] hydrochloride with adrenaline [epinephrine] 1 in 80 000 may be used. Doses should be reduced in children, the elderly, and in debilitated patients. A test dose, preferably with adrenaline [epinephrine], should be given before commencing epidural block to detect inadvertent intravascular or subarachnoid administration.

The following doses have been recommended for individual **local anaesthetic procedures** in the USA:

- For percutaneous *infiltration anaesthesia*, 5 to 300 mg (1 to 60 mL of a 0.5% solution, or 0.5 to 30 mL of a 1% solution).
- The dosage in *peripheral nerve block* depends on the route of administration. For brachial plexus block 225 to 300 mg (15 to 20 mL) as a 1.5% solution is used; for intercostal nerve block 30 mg (3 mL) is given as a 1% solution; for paracervical block a 1% solution is used in a dose of 100 mg (10 mL) on each side, repeated not more frequently than every 90 minutes; for paravertebral block a 1% solution may be used in doses of 30 to 50 mg (3 to 5 mL); a 1% solution is recommended for pudendal block in doses of 100 mg (10 mL) on each side; for retrobulbar block a 4% solution may be used in doses of 120 to 200 mg (3 to 5 mL).
- For *sympathetic nerve block* a 1% solution is recommended; doses are 50 mg (5 mL) for cervical block and 50 to 100 mg (5 to 10 mL) for lumbar block.
- For *epidural anaesthesia* 2 to 3 mL of solution is needed for each dermatome to be anaesthetised but usual total doses and recommended concentrations are: lumbar epidural 250 to 300 mg (25 to 30 mL) as a 1% solution for analgesia and 225 to 300 mg (15 to 20 mL) as a 1.5% solution or 200 to 300 mg (10 to 15 mL) as a 2% solution for anaesthesia, and for thoracic epidural a 1% solution may be used at doses of 200 to 300 mg (20 to 30 mL). In obstetric caudal analgesia 200 to 300 mg (20 to 30 mL) is used as a 1% solution and in surgical caudal anaesthesia a 1.5% solution may be used in doses of 225 to 300 mg (15 to 20 mL). For continuous epidural anaesthesia, the maximum doses should not be repeated more frequently than every 90 minutes.
- A hyperbaric solution of 1.5% or 5% lignocaine [lidocaine] hydrochloride in glucose 7.5% solution is available for *spinal anaesthesia*; adrenaline [epinephrine] should not be used. Doses of up to 50 mg (1 mL) as a 5% solution and 9 to 15 mg (0.6 to 1 mL) as a 1.5% solution have been used during labour for a normal vaginal delivery. Up to 75 mg (1.5 mL) as the 5% solution has been used for caesarean section and 75 to 100 mg (1.5 to 2 mL) for other surgical procedures.
- For *intravenous regional anaesthesia* a 0.5% solution without adrenaline [epinephrine] has been used in doses of 50 to 300 mg (10 to 60 mL); a maximum dose of 4 mg per kg body-weight has been recommended for adults.

Lignocaine [lidocaine] may be used in a variety of formulations for **surface anaesthesia**.

- Lignocaine [lidocaine] ointment is used for *anaesthesia of skin and mucous membranes* with a maximum recommended total dose of 20 g of 5% ointment (equivalent to 1 g of lignocaine [lidocaine] base) in 24 hours.
- Gels are used for *anaesthesia of the urinary tract* and the dose used varies in different countries. The manufacturers in the UK have suggested the following doses given as a 2% gel: in females 100 to 200 mg of lignocaine [lidocaine] hydrochloride inserted into the urethra several minutes before examination; in males 400 mg instilled in 2 portions, or 600 to 800 mg in 3 or 4 portions. The doses used in the USA are lower: in females 60 to 100 mg of lignocaine [lidocaine] hydrochloride inserted into the urethra several minutes before examination; in males 100 to 200 mg used before catheterisation and 600 mg before sounding or cystoscopy.
- A dose of 200 to 400 mg of a 2% gel is also recommended in the UK for *analgesia during endoscopy*. A quantity of the gel containing about 100 mg of lignocaine [lidocaine] hydrochloride is also used to lubricate tubing for *endotracheal insertion*.
- Topical solutions are used for *surface anaesthesia of mucous membranes of the mouth, throat, and upper gastrointestinal tract*. For painful conditions of the mouth and throat a 2% solution may be used: 300 mg (15 mL) may be rinsed and ejected or, for pharyngeal pain, the solution is gargled and swallowed if necessary; it should not be used more frequently than every 3 hours. The recommended maximum daily dose in the USA for topical oral solutions is 2.4 g. Doses of 40 to 300 mg as a 4% solution (1 to 7.5 mL) are used before bronchoscopy, bronchography, laryngoscopy, oesophagoscopy, endotracheal intubation, and biopsy in the mouth and throat. Lignocaine [lidocaine] in a strength of 10% has also been used as a spray for application to mucous membranes for the prevention of pain during various procedures including use in otorhinolaryngology, dentistry, introduction of instruments into the respiratory and gastrointestinal tracts, and in obstetrics. The dose depends on the extent of the site to be anaesthetised; 10 to 50 mg is generally sufficient for dentistry and otorhinolaryngology; for other procedures, the maximum dose in a 24-hour period is 200 mg. For laryngotracheal anaesthesia 160 mg of lignocaine [lidocaine] hydrochloride as a 4% spray is instilled as a single dose into the lumen of the larynx and trachea.
- Lignocaine [lidocaine] is used *rectally* as suppositories, ointments, and creams in the treatment of haemorrhoids and other painful perianal conditions.
- *Eye drops* containing lignocaine [lidocaine] hydrochloride 4% with fluorescein are used in tonometry.
- A *eutectic mixture* containing lignocaine [lidocaine] base 2.5% and prilocaine base 2.5% is applied as a cream under an occlusive dressing to produce *surface anaesthesia of the skin* before procedures requiring needle puncture, surgical treatment of localised lesions, and split skin grafting; it has been used similarly, but without an occlusive dressing, before removal of genital warts (see also under Surface Anaesthesia, below).
- Other methods of dermal delivery include a *transdermal patch* of lignocaine [lidocaine] 5% for the treatment of pain associated with postherpetic neuralgia, and an *iontophoretic drug delivery system* incorporating lignocaine [lidocaine] and adrenaline [epinephrine].

USE IN ARRHYTHMIAS.

For the treatment of **ventricular arrhythmias** lignocaine [lidocaine] is given *intravenously* as the hydrochloride. It may be used in advanced cardiac life support for cardiac arrest due to ventricular fibrillation and pulseless ventricular tachycardia when direct current shocks (together with adrenaline [epinephrine]) have failed to restore a normal rhythm. For adults, a dose of 1 to 1.5 mg per kg body-weight can be given and repeated after 3 to 5 minutes to a total dose of 3 mg per kg if necessary. The *endotracheal* route has been employed when intravenous access cannot be obtained, although doses should probably be larger than those employed intravenously; the precise endotracheal dose has not yet been established, however.

Lignocaine [lidocaine] is also used in other ventricular arrhythmias in which the patient is in a more stable condition. In these circumstances lignocaine [lidocaine] hydrochloride is usually given as a loading dose followed by an infusion. Usual doses are 50 to

100 mg or 1 to 1.5 mg per kg as a direct *intravenous injection* at a rate of 25 to 50 mg per minute. If no effect is seen within 5 to 10 minutes of this loading dose, it may be repeated once or twice to a maximum dose of 200 to 300 mg in 1 hour. A *continuous intravenous infusion* is usually commenced after loading, at a dose of 1 to 4 mg per minute. It is rarely necessary to continue this infusion for longer than 24 hours, but in the event that a longer infusion is required, the dose may need to be reduced to avoid potential toxicity resulting from an increase in the half-life. Dosage may need to be reduced in patients with heart failure or liver disorders.

In emergency situations, lignocaine [lidocaine] hydrochloride has also been given for arrhythmias by *intramuscular* injection into the deltoid muscle in a dose of 300 mg, repeated if necessary after 60 to 90 minutes.

Action. For a comparison of the vasoactivity of lignocaine [lidocaine] and some other local anaesthetics, see p.1304.

Burns. Lignocaine [lidocaine] given intravenously has been reported to have produced pain relief in a few patients with second-degree burns.[1]

1. Jönsson A, *et al.* Inhibition of burn pain by intravenous lignocaine infusion. *Lancet* 1991; **338**: 151–2.

Cardiac arrhythmias. Lignocaine [lidocaine] is classified as a class Ib antiarrhythmic drug (p.787) and may be used in the treatment of ventricular arrhythmias, including those associated with cardiac arrest and myocardial infarction. It is usually administered intravenously (see above). Some forms of ventricular tachycardia may be terminated by the use of lignocaine [lidocaine]; the overall treatment options are described under Cardiac Arrhythmias, p.794. Lignocaine [lidocaine] may also be used during advanced cardiac life support (p.790).

Lignocaine [lidocaine] has been considered for the *prophylaxis* of ventricular fibrillation in patients with proven or suspected myocardial infarction. However, while some studies have identified a protective effect,[1,2] in others this has not been shown to be accompanied by a reduction in mortality and might even have increased it.[3,4] Nevertheless, one review of the available evidence[5] concluded that lignocaine [lidocaine] prophylaxis was a reasonable policy for patients at highest risk of ventricular fibrillation such as those with acute transmural infarction, under 65 years of age, and within 6 hours of the onset of infarction symptoms.

It has been suggested that the increased mortality sometimes seen with lignocaine [lidocaine] might be associated with the duration of administration; one study[6] found that patients who received a bolus dose of lignocaine [lidocaine] followed by a 40-hour continuous infusion for prophylaxis of ventricular arrhythmias experienced more episodes of heart failure than patients who received the bolus dose followed by an 8-hour infusion.

1. Horwitz RI, Feinstein AR. Improved observational method for studying therapeutic efficacy: suggestive evidence that lidocaine prophylaxis prevents death in acute myocardial infarction. *JAMA* 1981; **246**: 2455–9.
2. Koster RW, Dunning AJ. Intramuscular lidocaine for prevention of lethal arrhythmias in the prehospitalization phase of acute myocardial infarction. *N Engl J Med* 1985; **313**: 1105–10.
3. MacMahon S, *et al.* Effects of prophylactic lidocaine in suspected acute myocardial infarction: an overview of results from the randomized, controlled trials. *JAMA* 1988; **260**: 1910–16.
4. Hine LK, *et al.* Meta-analytic evidence against prophylactic use of lidocaine in acute myocardial infarction. *Ann Intern Med* 1989; **149**: 2694–8.
5. Nattel S, Arenal A. Antiarrhythmic prophylaxis after acute myocardial infarction: is lidocaine still useful? *Drugs* 1993; **45**: 9–14.
6. Pharand C, *et al.* Lidocaine prophylaxis for fatal ventricular arrhythmias after acute myocardial infarction. *Clin Pharmacol Ther* 1995; **57**: 471–8.

Hiccup. A protocol for the management of intractable hiccups may be found under Chlorpromazine, p.667. Lignocaine [lidocaine] is one of a large number of drugs that has been tried in the treatment of hiccups without strong evidence of their efficacy. It has been given in the form of a 2% viscous solution taken by mouth. Nebulised lignocaine [lidocaine] has also been tried.[1]

1. Neeno TA, Rosenow EC. Intractable hiccups: consider nebulized lidocaine. *Chest* 1996; **110**: 1129–30.

Intubation. Lignocaine [lidocaine] has produced conflicting results when used to attenuate the pressor response and rise in intra-ocular pressure induced by procedures such as tracheal intubation.[1-5] For an overall discussion of this problem, see under Anaesthesia, p.1331.

1. Tam S, *et al.* Attenuation of circulatory responses to endotracheal intubation using intravenous lidocaine: a determination of the optimal time of injection. *Can Anaesth Soc J* 1985; **32**: S65.
2. Murphy DF, *et al.* Intravenous lignocaine pretreatment to prevent intraocular pressure rise following suxamethonium and tracheal intubation. *Br J Ophthalmol* 1986; **70**: 596–8.
3. Drenger B, Pe'er J. Attenuation of ocular and systemic responses to tracheal intubation by intravenous lignocaine. *Br J Ophthalmol* 1987; **71**: 546–8.

4. Miller CD, Warren SJ. IV lignocaine fails to attenuate the cardiovascular response to laryngoscopy and tracheal intubation. *Br J Anaesth* 1990; **65**: 216–19.
5. Mostafa SM, *et al.* Effects of nebulized lignocaine on the intraocular pressure responses to tracheal intubation. *Br J Anaesth* 1990; **64**: 515–17.

Migraine and cluster headache. Despite periodic renewed interest, lignocaine [lidocaine] has so far failed to find an accepted role in the management of migraine (p.449) or cluster headache (p.449). Lignocaine [lidocaine] has been tried for the emergency parenteral treatment of migraine, but in a comparative study with dihydroergotamine or chlorpromazine it was found to be less effective than either.[1] Intranasal instillation of lignocaine [lidocaine] has produced rapid relief of headache in some patients with acute migraine (though early relapse was common),[2] and has also been reported to be effective in aborting individual attacks of headache during cluster periods in patients with cluster headache.[3,4]

1. Bell R, *et al.* A comparative trial of three agents in the treatment of acute migraine headache. *Ann Emerg Med* 1990; **19**: 1070–82.
2. Maizels M, *et al.* Intranasal lidocaine for treatment of migraine: a randomized, double-blind, controlled trial. *JAMA* 1996; **276**: 319–21.
3. Kittrelle JP, *et al.* Cluster headache: local anesthetic abortive agents. *Arch Neurol* 1985; **42**: 496–8.
4. Robbins L. Intranasal lidocaine for cluster headache. *Headache* 1995; **35**: 83–4.

Neuropathic pain syndromes. Lignocaine [lidocaine] may be useful in the management of some types of neuropathic pain syndromes (p.7). The pain of *postherpetic neuralgia* has been significantly reduced by the application of lignocaine [lidocaine] 5% transdermal patches;[1,2] a eutectic mixture of lignocaine [lidocaine] and prilocaine has also been of benefit (see Surface Anaesthesia below). Syndromes where intravenous lignocaine [lidocaine] therapy has been tried include *diabetic neuropathy*[3] and *central neuropathic pain* associated with stroke or spinal cord injury.[4]

1. Rowbotham MC, *et al.* Lidocaine patch: double-blind controlled study of a new treatment method for post-herpetic neuralgia. *Pain* 1996; **65**: 39–44.
2. Comer AM, Lamb HM. Lidocaine patch 5%. *Drugs* 2000; **59**: 245–9.
3. Kastrup J, *et al.* Treatment of chronic painful diabetic neuropathy with intravenous lidocaine infusion. *BMJ* 1986; **292**: 173.
4. Attal N, *et al.* Intravenous lidocaine in central pain: a double-blind, placebo-controlled, psychophysical study. *Neurology* 2000; **54**: 564–74.

Pleurodesis. Lignocaine [lidocaine] has been instilled intrapleurally as a 1% solution in doses of up to 300 mg to relieve the severe chest pain associated with the use of tetracycline for pleurodesis.[1-3] While the larger doses were significantly more effective[2] toxic plasma concentrations were less likely to occur if a dose of 3 mg per kg body-weight or less was used.[3]

1. Harbecke RG. Intrapleurally given tetracycline with lidocaine. *JAMA* 1980; **244**: 1899–1900.
2. Sherman S, *et al.* Optimum anesthesia with intrapleural lidocaine during chemical pleurodesis with tetracycline. *Chest* 1988; **93**: 533–6.
3. Wooten SA, *et al.* Systemic absorption of tetracycline and lidocaine following intrapleural instillation. *Chest* 1988; **94**: 960–3.

Status epilepticus. Lignocaine [lidocaine] hydrochloride may be used to control status epilepticus (p.341) resistant to more conventional treatment. It has a rapid onset of action but its effect is short-lived and continuous infusion may be necessary.[1] It should also be noted that doses producing high plasma concentrations of lignocaine [lidocaine] can result in CNS toxicity including seizures.[1] Recurrence of seizures associated with the withdrawal of prolonged lignocaine [lidocaine] therapy may be due to its accumulated metabolites exerting an excitatory effect on the nervous system when the inhibitory effect of lignocaine [lidocaine] is being reduced.[2]

Lignocaine [lidocaine] was used instead of diazepam for 42 episodes of status epilepticus in 36 patients who either had limited pulmonary reserve or who had not responded to intravenous diazepam.[3] Lignocaine [lidocaine] 1.5 to 2 mg per kg body-weight (usually a dose of 100 mg) was administered as a single intravenous dose over 2 minutes. This dose was repeated once if there was no positive response to the first dose (11 episodes) or the seizures recurred (19 episodes). Subsequently a continuous infusion of lignocaine [lidocaine] at a rate of 3 to 4 mg per kg per hour was given in the 7 episodes that recurred after the second dose; 5 of these showed a positive response. The 11 episodes not responding to the first dose did not respond to the second dose or to a continuous infusion.

1. Bauer J, Elger CE. Management of status epilepticus in adults. *CNS Drugs* 1994; **1**: 26–44.
2. Wallin A, *et al.* Lidocaine treatment of neonatal convulsions, a therapeutic dilemma. *Eur J Clin Pharmacol* 1989; **36**: 583–6.
3. Pascual J, *et al.* Role of lidocaine in managing status epilepticus. *J Neurol Neurosurg Psychiatry* 1992; **55**: 49–51.

Surface anaesthesia. EUTECTIC MIXTURES. A cream, containing lignocaine [lidocaine] 2.5% and prilocaine 2.5% in a eutectic mixture, can produce local anaesthesia when applied topically to intact skin and appears to be of value in a number of minor medical or surgical procedures both in adults and in children.[1-3] Applications that have been tried include venepuncture for blood sampling, intravenous or arterial cannulation, retrobulbar injections, lumbar puncture, curettage of molluscum contagiosum lesions, genital wart removal, split skin grafting, laser treatment, extracorporeal shock wave therapy, separation of preputial adhesions, and circumcision. It has also been tried as

an anaesthetic for the ear drum in preparation for otological procedures such as myringotomy and grommet insertion but is potentially ototoxic and should not be used in the presence of a perforation. Postherpetic neuralgia (p.7) has also been treated with some success.[4,5]

The eutectic cream is usually applied to skin under an occlusive dressing for at least 60 minutes although it has been suggested that for children aged 1 to 5 years 30 minutes may be sufficient.[6] The manufacturers suggest a maximum application time of 5 hours. The onset and duration of the effect may be affected by the site of application.[2] When used for the removal of genital warts an occlusive dressing is not necessary and the application time recommended by the manufacturer is 5 to 10 minutes. The level of anaesthesia begins to decline after 10 to 15 minutes when applied to the genital mucosa and any procedure should be started immediately.

Systemic absorption of lignocaine [lidocaine] and prilocaine appears to be minimal when applied to intact skin[6] even after treating large areas or leaving the cream in place for many hours.[7] Nevertheless, the UK manufacturers recommend that it should not be used for children under 1 year of age as excessive absorption can lead to methaemoglobinaemia, owing to the presence of prilocaine (see under Methaemoglobinaemia, p.1302). However, eutectic mixtures of lignocaine [lidocaine] and prilocaine have been used to reduce the pain of puncture procedures[8] and for circumcision[9] in neonates, and appear to be safe and efficacious. Indeed, in some other countries including the USA, the cream is licensed for use in neonates provided that their gestational age is at least 37 weeks and that those aged 3 months or less are monitored for methaemoglobin levels; it should not be used in infants under the age of 1 year who are receiving treatment with methaemoglobin-inducing drugs.

The eutectic cream should not be used on wounds or mucous membranes (except for genital warts in adults) and should not be used for atopic dermatitis. It should not be applied to or near the eyes because it causes corneal irritation, and it should not be instilled in the middle ear. It should be used with caution in patients with anaemia or congenital or acquired methaemoglobinaemia. Transient paleness, redness, and oedema may occur following application.

Some studies suggest that a topical gel formulation of amethocaine [tetracaine] 4% can produce longer and more rapid anaesthesia than the above lignocaine [lidocaine] with prilocaine cream (see Surface Anaesthesia, under Uses and Administration of Amethocaine, p.1305). It has also been suggested[10] that topical amethocaine [tetracaine] may have practical advantages over the eutectic mixture of lignocaine [lidocaine] and prilocaine, which has to be applied for at least one hour, and causes vasoconstriction at the site of application which can make venepuncture difficult.

1. Lee JJ, Rubin AP. Emla cream and its current uses. *Br J Hosp Med* 1993; **50**: 463–6.
2. Buckley MM, Benfield P. Eutectic lidocaine/prilocaine cream: a review of the topical anaesthetic/analgesic efficacy of a eutectic mixture of local anaesthetics (EMLA). *Drugs* 1993; **46**: 126–51.
3. Koren G. Use of the eutectic mixture of local anesthetics in young children for procedure-related pain. *J Pediatr* 1993; **122** (suppl): S30–S35.
4. Litman SJ, *et al.* Use of EMLA cream in the treatment of postherpetic neuralgia. *J Clin Anesth* 1996; **8**: 54–7.
5. Kost RG, Straus SE. Postherpetic neuralgia—pathogenesis, treatment, and prevention. *N Engl J Med* 1996; **335**: 32–42.
6. Hanks GW, White I. Local anaesthetic creams. *BMJ* 1988; **297**: 1215–16.
7. Scott DB. Topical anaesthesia of intact skin. *Br J Parenter Ther* 1986; **7**: 134–5.
8. Gourrier E, *et al.* Use of EMLA® cream in a department of neonatology. *Pain* 1996; **68**: 431–4.
9. Taddio A, *et al.* Efficacy and safety of lidocaine-prilocaine cream for pain during circumcision. *N Engl J Med* 1997; **336**: 1197–1201.
10. Russell SCS, Doyle E. Paediatric anaesthesia. *BMJ* 1997; **314**: 201–3.

Tinnitus. Tinnitus is the perception of a noise that arises or appears to arise within the head.

Objective tinnitus may be audible to others and arises from lesions outside the auditory system. Subjective tinnitus (tinnitus aurium) originates from sites within the auditory system and is perceived only by the patient. A simple and remediable cause of tinnitus can be impacted ear wax. Tinnitus is often associated with head injury, vertigo, and hearing loss, including age-related and noise-induced hearing loss. It may also be a symptom of an underlying disorder such as Ménière's disease, may be associated with anxiety or depressive disorders, or may be a manifestation of drug toxicity (for example with aspirin or quinine). In such cases, treatment of the underlying disorder or removal of the offending drug can resolve the tinnitus.

Treatment of tinnitus is difficult although reassurance and counselling are often effective in helping patients to tolerate their condition. Maskers or, if the tinnitus is associated with hearing loss, hearing aids are also used; surgery is rarely indicated. Treatment with a wide variety of drugs has been tried. Intravenous lignocaine [lidocaine] has proven to be effective in reducing or eliminating tinnitus but the effect only lasts for a few hours and is, therefore, impractical for most patients. Efforts to find an effective oral analogue of lignocaine [lidocaine] have not, so far, been successful. Other drugs that have been tried include the antiepileptics carbamazepine and phenytoin, and the loop diuretic frusemide [furosemide], but unacceptable adverse effects limit their use.

References.
1. Luxon LM. Tinnitus: its causes, diagnosis, and treatment. *BMJ* 1993; **306:** 1490–1.
2. Robson AK, Birchall JP. Management of tinnitus. *Prescribers' J* 1994; **34:** 1–7.
3. Coles RRA. Drug treatment of tinnitus in Britain. In: Reich GE, Vernon JA, eds. *Proceedings of the fifth international tinnitus seminar.* Portland: American Tinnitus Association, 1995.
4. Vesterager V. Tinnitus—investigation and management. *BMJ* 1997; **314:** 728–31.
5. Simpson JJ, Davies WE. Recent advances in the pharmacological treatment of tinnitus. *Trends Pharmacol Sci* 1999; **20:** 12–18.

Preparations

BP 2001: Lidocaine and Adrenaline Injection; Lidocaine and Chlorhexidine Gel; Lidocaine Gel; Lidocaine Injection; Sterile Lidocaine Solution;
USP 25: Lidocaine Hydrochloride and Dextrose Injection; Lidocaine Hydrochloride and Epinephrine Injection; Lidocaine Hydrochloride Injection; Lidocaine Hydrochloride Jelly; Lidocaine Hydrochloride Oral Topical Solution; Lidocaine Hydrochloride Topical Solution; Lidocaine Ointment; Lidocaine Oral Topical Solution; Lidocaine Topical Aerosol; Neomycin and Polymyxin B Sulfates and Lidocaine Cream; Neomycin and Polymyxin B Sulfates, Bacitracin Zinc, and Lidocaine Ointment; Neomycin and Polymyxin B Sulfates, Bacitracin, and Lidocaine Ointment.

Proprietary Preparations (details are given in Part 3)
Aust.: Lidocorit; Neo-Xylestesin; Neo-Xylestesin forte and Neo-Xylestesin special; Neurolid†; Xylanaest; Xylocain; Xylocard; Xyloneural; **Austral.:** Fargo†; Lignospan; Nurocain; Nurocain with Sympathin; Seda-Gel; Stud 100; Xylocaine; Xylocaine Special Adhesive; Xylocard; **Belg.:** Linisol; Otoralgyl; Xylocaine; Xylocaine Visqueuse; Xylocard; **Braz.:** Hypocaina; Lidocord; Xylestesin; Xylocaina; **Canad.:** Afterburn; Family Medicated Sunburn Relief†; Lidodan; Solarcaine Lidocaine; Xylocaine; Xylocard; Zilactin-L; **Denm.:** Xylocain; **Fin.:** Lidocard; Xylocain; **Fr.:** Dynexan; Mesocaine; Otoralgyl†; Xylocaine; Xylocard; **Ger.:** Anaesthol†; Gelicain; Haemo-Exhirud Bufexamac Zäpfchen; Heweneural; Licain; Lidesthesin; Lidocaton†; Lidoject; LidoPosterine; Neo-Lidocaton†; Nor-Anaesthol†; Rowo-629; Sagittaproct; Xylestesin-A, Xylestesin centro; Xylestesin-S; Xylestesin, Xylestesin-F; Xylocain f.d. Kardiologie; Xylocitin; Xylocitin cor; Xyloneural; **Hong Kong:** Xylocaine; Xylocard; **Irl.:** Xylocaine; Xylocard; **Israel:** Esracain; LidoPen; Stud 100; Xylocaine; **Ital.:** Basicaina; Ecocain; Lident Adrenalina; Lident Andrenor; Lidosen; Lidrian; Luan; Odontalg; Ortodermina; Xilo-Mynol; Xylocaina; Xylonor; **Jpn:** Penles; **Mex.:** Pisacaina; Rucaina; Uvega; Xlyocaina; **Neth.:** Dentinox†; Otalgan; Xylocaine; Xylocard; **Norw.:** Xylocain; Xylocard†; **NZ:** Nurocain; Virasolve; Xylocaine; Xylocard; **Port.:** Lidonostrum; Lincaina; Xilonibsa; Xylocaina†; Xylocard†; **S.Afr.:** Lignospan Special; Peterkaien; Remicaine; Remicard; Xylocaine; Xylotox; **Singapore:** Xylocaine; Xylocard; **Spain:** Aeroderm; Curadent; Llorentecaina Noradrenal; Octocaine; Xilonibsa; Xylocaina; Xylonor 2% Sin Vasoconst; Xylonor Especial; **Swed.:** Xylocain; Xylocain lung; Xylocard; **Switz.:** Kenergon; Lidocaton†; Lignospan; Lubogliss†; Neurodol Tissugel; Sedagul; Sedagul; Solarcaine; Xylesine; Xylestesin-F; Xylestesin-S "special"; Xylocain; Xylocard; Xyloneural; Xylonor†; **Thai.:** Docaine; Lidocation; Lidocaton; Neo-Lidocaton; Xylocaine; Xylocard; **UAE:** Ecocain; **UK:** Laryng-O-Jet; Lignostab-A; Rinstead; Strepsils Pain Relief Spray; Vagisil; Xylocaine; Xylocaine 2% Plain; Xylocard†; Xylotox; **USA:** Anestacon; Dentipatch; Dermaflex†; Dilocaine; Dr Scholl's Cracked Heel Relief; Duo-Trach Kit; ELA-Max; Lidoderm; Lidoject; LidoPen; Nervocaine; Nulicaine†; Octocaine; Xylocaine; Zilactin-L.

Multi-ingredient: numerous preparations are listed in Part 3.

Mepivacaine Hydrochloride (7633-e)

Mepivacaine Hydrochloride (BANM, rINNM).

Mepivacaini Chloridum; Mepivacaini Hydrochloridum. (1-Methyl-2-piperidyl)formo-2′,6′-xylidide hydrochloride.
$C_{15}H_{22}N_2O,HCl = 282.8$.

CAS — 96-88-8 (mepivacaine); 22801-44-1 ((±)-mepivacaine); 1722-62-9 (mepivacaine hydrochloride).

Pharmacopoeias. In Eur. (see p.vi), Jpn, and US.

Pharmacopoeial description

Ph. Eur.: A white crystalline powder. Freely soluble in water and in alcohol; very slightly soluble in dichloromethane. A 2% solution in water has a pH of 4.0 to 5.0.

USP 25: A white, odourless, crystalline solid. Freely soluble in water and in methyl alcohol; very slightly soluble in chloroform; practically insoluble in ether. A 2% solution in water has a pH of about 4.5.

pH of solutions. For a discussion of the effect that pH has on the stability of local anaesthetic solutions and the pain associated with their injection, see p.1304.

Adverse Effects, Treatment, and Precautions

As for Local Anaesthetics in general, p.1302.

Porphyria. Mepivacaine is considered to be unsafe in patients with porphyria because it has been shown to be porphyrinogenic in *in-vitro* systems.

Interactions

For interactions associated with local anaesthetics, see p.1303.

◊ Studies *in vitro* showed that bupivacaine dramatically reduced the binding of mepivacaine to α-1-acid glycoprotein.[1]
1. Hartrick CT, *et al.* Influence of bupivacaine on mepivacaine protein binding. *Clin Pharmacol Ther* 1984; **36:** 546–50.

Pharmacokinetics

Mepivacaine is about 78% bound to plasma proteins. The plasma half-life has been reported to be about 2 to 3 hours in adults and about 9 hours in neonates. It is rapidly metabolised in the liver and less than 10% of a dose is reported to be excreted unchanged in the urine. Over 50% of a dose is excreted as metabolites into the bile but these probably undergo enterohepatic circulation as only small amounts appear in the faeces. Several metabolites are also excreted via the kidneys and include glucuronide conjugates of hydroxy compounds and an *N*-demethylated compound, 2′,6′-pipecoloxylidide. Mepivacaine crosses the placenta.

See also under Local Anaesthetics, p.1303.

Pregnancy. There is considerable transfer of mepivacaine across the placenta following maternal administration and the ratio of fetal to maternal concentrations[1] is about 0.7. Although neonates have a very limited capacity to metabolise mepivacaine it appears they are able to eliminate the drug.[2]
1. Lurie AO, Weiss JB. Blood concentration of mepivacaine and lidocaine in mother and baby after epidural anesthesia. *Am J Obstet Gynecol* 1970; **106:** 850–6.
2. Meffin P, *et al.* Clearance and metabolism of mepivacaine in the human neonate. *Clin Pharmacol Ther* 1973; **14:** 218–25.

Uses and Administration

Mepivacaine hydrochloride is a local anaesthetic of the amide type with actions and uses similar to those described on p.1304. It is mainly used for infiltration anaesthesia, peripheral nerve block, and epidural block. (Local anaesthetic techniques are discussed on p.1304.) Mepivacaine has a rapid onset and an intermediate duration of action. The speed of onset and duration of action are increased by the addition of a vasoconstrictor and absorption into the circulation from the site of injection is reduced.

The dosage of mepivacaine hydrochloride varies with the site of injection and the type of **local anaesthetic procedure**. In adults, the **maximum single dose** of mepivacaine hydrochloride should not generally exceed 400 mg and the total dose in 24 hours should not exceed 1 g. Doses should be reduced in the elderly, in debilitated patients, and in those with cardiac or hepatic impairment. A suggested maximum dose for children, especially for those less than 3 years of age, is 5 to 6 mg per kg body-weight. Concentrations of less than 2% should also be used for children less than 3 years of age.

For *infiltration anaesthesia* up to 400 mg as a 1% (40 mL) or 0.5% (80 mL) solution is used. For *dental infiltration and nerve block* a 2% solution with a vasoconstrictor or a 3% plain solution is used. For anaesthesia at a single site in the jaw a dose of 36 mg (1.8 mL) as the 2% solution or 54 mg (1.8 mL) as the 3% solution is used. For anaesthesia of the entire oral cavity 180 mg (9 mL) as the 2% solution or 270 mg (9 mL) as the 3% solution is used. Some recommend that no more than 400 mg should be administered at a single dental sitting.

For *peripheral nerve blocks*, namely *cervical, brachial plexus, intercostal,* and *pudendal blocks*, 1 or 2% solutions may be used in doses of 50 to 400 mg (5 to 40 mL) as a 1% solution, or 100 to 400 mg (5 to 20 mL) as a 2% solution. For pudendal block half of the dose is injected on each side. For *paracervical block* a dose of up to 100 mg (10 mL) as a 1% solution on each side has been suggested allowing an interval of 5 minutes between sides. This may be repeated at an interval of not less than 90 minutes, and for a combined paracervical and pudendal block up to 150 mg (15 mL) as a 1% solution is injected on each side. For therapeutic nerve block in the management of pain 10 to 50 mg (1 to 5 mL) as a 1% solution or 20 to 100 mg (1 to 5 mL) as a 2% solution may be given.

For *epidural block* usual doses are: 150 to 300 mg (15 to 30 mL) as a 1% solution, 150 to 375 mg (10 to 25 mL) as a 1.5% solution, or 200 to 400 mg (10 to 20 mL) as a 2% solution. Hyperbaric solutions of mepivacaine hydrochloride without adrenaline [epinephrine] have also been used for *spinal block*.

Mepivacaine has been included in the intramuscular injections of other drugs to minimise the pain produced at the injection site.

Mepivacaine has also been used as a surface anaesthetic but other local anaesthetics such as lignocaine [lidocaine] are more effective.

Action. For a comparison of the vasoactivity of mepivacaine and some other local anaesthetics, see p.1304.

Preparations

USP 25: Mepivacaine Hydrochloride and Levonordefrin Injection; Mepivacaine Hydrochloride Injection.

Proprietary Preparations (details are given in Part 3)
Aust.: Scandicain; Scandonest; **Austral.:** Carbocaine; Scandonest; **Belg.:** Scandicaine; **Canad.:** Carbocaine; Polocaine; **Denm.:** Carbocain; Scandonest; **Fr.:** Carbocaine; **Ger.:** Meaverin; Meaverin "A" mit Adrenalin†; Meaverin "N" mit Noradrenaline†; Meaverin hyperbar; Mecain; Mepicaton†; Mepihexal; Mepivastesin; Scandicain; **Israel:** Tevacaine; **Ital.:** Carbocaina; Mepi-Mynol; Mepicain; Mepident; Mepifloran; Mepyl; Optocain; Pericaina; Scandonest; **Neth.:** Scandicaine; **Norw.:** Carbocain; **Port.:** Scandinibsa; **S.Afr.:** Carbocaine; Scandonest; **Spain:** Isogaine; Scandinibsa; **Swed.:** Carbocain; **Switz.:** Mepicaton†; Scandicain; Scandonest; **Thai.:** Mepicaton; **USA:** Carbocaine; Carbocaine with Neo-Cobefrin; Isocaine; Polocaine.

Multi-ingredient: Ger.: Meaverin; Thesit.

Used as an adjunct in: **Aust.:** Estradurin; Triodurin†; **Belg.:** Estradurine; **Denm.:** Estradurin; **Fin.:** Estradurin; **Ger.:** Estradurin; **Hong Kong:** Nevramin; **Jpn:** Amasulin; Bestcall; Lilacillin; Pansporin; Takesulin; **Mex.:** Kedacillin; **Neth.:** Estradurin; **Norw.:** Estradurin; **Port.:** Linamin Plus; **Singapore:** Nevramin; **Swed.:** Estradurin; **Switz.:** Estradurin; **Thai.:** Nevramin; **UK:** Estradurin†.

Myrtecaine (12986-I)

Myrtecaine (rINN).

Nopoxamine. 2-[2-(10-Norpin-2-en-2-yl)ethoxy]triethylamine.
$C_{17}H_{31}NO = 265.4$.
CAS — 7712-50-7.

Profile

Myrtecaine is a local anaesthetic (p.1302) used topically as the base or laurilsulfate in rubefacient preparations for the treatment of muscle and joint pain. Myrtecaine laurilsulfate is also used in preparations with antacids for the symptomatic relief of gastrointestinal disorders.

Preparations

Proprietary Preparations (details are given in Part 3)
Multi-ingredient: Aust.: Acidrine; Algesal; Kalisyl†; Latesyl; Rheugesal; **Belg.:** Acidrine; **Fr.:** Acidrine; Algesal Suractive; **Ger.:** Acidrine; Algesal; Algesalona; **Ital.:** Acidrine; **Neth.:** Algesal Forte; **Port.:** Algesal; Latesil; **Spain:** Algesal; **Switz.:** Algesal; Algesalona.

Octacaine Hydrochloride (13036-x)

Octacaine Hydrochloride (pINNM).

3-Diethylaminobutyranilide hydrochloride.
$C_{14}H_{22}N_2O,HCl = 270.8$.
CAS — 13912-77-1 (octacaine); 59727-70-7 (octacaine hydrochloride).

Profile

Octacaine hydrochloride is a local anaesthetic (p.1302) that has been used for surface anaesthesia.

Preparations

Proprietary Preparations (details are given in Part 3)
Multi-ingredient: Ger.: Batrax; **Switz.:** Batramycine.

Oxetacaine (7638-c)

Oxetacaine (BAN, rINN).

Oxethazaine (USAN); Wy-806. 2,2′-(2-Hydroxyethylimino)bis[N-(αα-dimethylphenethyl)-N-methylacetamide].
$C_{28}H_{41}N_3O_3 = 467.6$.
CAS — 126-27-2 (oxetacaine); 13930-31-9 (oxetacaine hydrochloride).
ATC — C05AD06.
Pharmacopoeias. In Br. and Jpn.

Pharmacopoeial description

BP 2001: A white or almost white powder. Practically insoluble in water; freely soluble in methyl alcohol; very soluble in chloroform; soluble in ethyl acetate.

Profile

Oxetacaine is an amide anaesthetic (p.1302) that is stated to have a prolonged action. It is administered by mouth in conjunction with antacids for the symptomatic relief of gastro-

---

The symbol † denotes a preparation no longer actively marketed

oesophageal reflux disease (p.1204). It has also been used as the hydrochloride in ointments and suppositories for the relief of pain associated with haemorrhoids.

Preparations

Proprietary Preparations (details are given in Part 3)
Hong Kong: Strocain; *Ital.:* Emoren; *Jpn:* Strocain; *Singapore:* Strocain.

Multi-ingredient: *Aust.:* Tepilta; *Austral.:* Mucaine; *Belg.:* Muthesa†; *Braz.:* Droxaine; *Canad.:* Mucaine; *Fr.:* Mutesa; *Ger.:* Tepilta; *Hong Kong:* Mucaine; Oxema; *Irl.:* Mucaine; *Ital.:* Magnesia Bisurata Aromatic Plus; Mucoxin†; *NZ:* Mucaine; *Port.:* Betalgil; *S.Afr.:* Mucaine; *Singapore:* Mucaine; *Spain:* Natrocitral; Roberfarin; Tepilta†; *Switz.:* Muthesa; *Thai.:* Mucaine; Strocain; *UK:* Mucaine.

Oxybuprocaine Hydrochloride

(7639-k)

Oxybuprocaine Hydrochloride (BANM, rINNM).
Benoxinate Hydrochloride; Oxybuprocaini Hydrochloridum. 2-Diethylaminoethyl 4-amino-3-butoxybenzoate hydrochloride.
$C_{17}H_{28}N_2O_3,HCl = 344.9$.
CAS — 99-43-4 (oxybuprocaine); 5987-82-6 (oxybuprocaine hydrochloride).

NOTE. BNX is a code approved by the BP 2001 for use on single unit doses of eye drops containing oxybuprocaine hydrochloride where the individual container may be too small to bear all the appropriate labelling information.
Pharmacopoeias. In Eur. (see p.vi), *Jpn*, and US.

Pharmacopoeial description
Ph. Eur.: A white crystalline powder or colourless crystals. It exhibits polymorphism. Very soluble in water; freely soluble in alcohol. A 10% solution in water has a pH of 4.5 to 6.0. Protect from light.
USP 25: White or slightly off-white, crystals or crystalline powder, odourless or with a slight characteristic odour. Soluble 1 in 0.8 of water, 1 in 2.6 of alcohol, and 1 in 2.5 of chloroform; insoluble in ether. A 1% solution in water has a pH of 5.0 to 6.0.

Adverse Effects, Treatment, and Precautions

As for Local Anaesthetics in general, p.1302.

Effects on the eyes. Fibrinous iritis and moderate corneal swelling occurred in 2 patients following the use of a 0.4% or 1% solution of oxybuprocaine hydrochloride for topical anaesthesia of the eye for minor surgery.[1] The effects may have been due to inadvertent entry of the drug into the anterior chamber of the eye.
1. Haddad R. Fibrinous iritis due to oxybuprocaine. *Br J Ophthalmol* 1989; **73:** 76–7.

Interactions

For interactions associated with local anaesthetics, see p.1303.

Uses and Administration

Oxybuprocaine, a para-aminobenzoic acid ester, is a local anaesthetic with actions and uses similar to those described on p.1304. It is used for surface anaesthesia (p.1304) and is reported to be less irritant than amethocaine [tetracaine] when applied to the conjunctiva in therapeutic concentrations.

Oxybuprocaine is used as the hydrochloride in a 0.4% solution in short ophthalmological procedures. One drop instilled into the conjunctival sac anaesthetises the surface of the eye sufficiently to allow tonometry after 60 seconds and a further drop after 90 seconds provides adequate anaesthesia for the fitting of contact lenses. Three drops at 90-second intervals produces sufficient anaesthesia after 5 minutes for removal of a foreign body from the corneal epithelium, or for incision of a Meibomian cyst through the conjunctiva. The sensitivity of the cornea is normal again after about 1 hour.

A 1% solution of oxybuprocaine hydrochloride is used for surface anaesthesia of the ear nose, and throat.

Preparations

BP 2001: Oxybuprocaine Eye Drops;
USP 25: Benoxinate Hydrochloride Ophthalmic Solution; Fluorescein Sodium and Benoxinate Hydrochloride Ophthalmic Solution.

Proprietary Preparations (details are given in Part 3)
Aust.: Fortasept†; Novain; *Belg.:* Novesine†; Unicaine†; *Fin.:* Oftan Obucain; *Fr.:* Cebesine; Novesine SE; *Ger.:* Benoxinat SE; Conjuncain-EDO; Novesine; Oxbarukain; *Hong Kong:* Novesin; *Israel:* Localin; *Ital.:* Novesina; *Port.:* Anestocil; *S.Afr.:* Novesin;

Singapore: Novesin; *Spain:* Benoxinato†; Prescaina; *Switz.:* Novesin; *Thai.:* Novesin.
Multi-ingredient: *Aust.:* Flurekain; *Austral.:* Fluress; *Belg.:* Anesthesique Double†; *Canad.:* Fluress; *Fin.:* Oftan Flurekain; *Ger.:* Thilorbin; *Mex.:* Mentalgina; *NZ:* Fluress; *Port.:* Mebocaina; *Spain:* Anesti Doble; Fluotest†; *Swed.:* Fluress; *Switz.:* Collu-Blache; Mebucaine; *UAE:* B-Cool; *USA:* Flu-Oxinate; Fluorox; Flurate; Fluress; Flurox.

Parethoxycaine Hydrochloride (13082-m)

Parethoxycaine Hydrochloride (rINNM).
2-Diethylaminoethyl 4-ethoxybenzoate hydrochloride.
$C_{15}H_{23}NO_3,HCl = 301.8$.
CAS — 94-23-5 (parethoxycaine); 136-46-9 (parethoxycaine hydrochloride).

Profile
Parethoxycaine hydrochloride, a para-aminobenzoic acid ester, is a local anaesthetic (p.1302) that has been used in pastilles for painful conditions of the mouth and throat.

Preparations

Proprietary Preparations (details are given in Part 3)
Fr.: Maxicaine.

Pramocaine Hydrochloride (7642-l)

Pramocaine Hydrochloride (BANM, rINNM).
Pramoxine Hydrochloride; Pramoxinium Chloride. 4-[3-(4-Butoxyphenoxy)propyl]morpholine hydrochloride.
$C_{17}H_{27}NO_3,HCl = 329.9$.
CAS — 140-65-8 (pramocaine); 637-58-1 (pramocaine hydrochloride).
Pharmacopoeias. In US.

Pharmacopoeial description
USP 25: A white or almost white crystalline powder; it may have a faint aromatic odour. Freely soluble in water and in alcohol; soluble 1 in 35 of chloroform; very slightly soluble in ether. A 1% solution in water has a pH of about 4.5. Store in airtight containers.

Profile
Pramocaine hydrochloride is a local anaesthetic (p.1302) used for surface anaesthesia. It is used alone or with corticosteroids and other drugs, usually in a concentration of 1%, in a wide range of formulations for the relief of pain and itching associated with minor skin conditions and anorectal disorders. Initial burning or stinging may occur following topical application. It should not be used for the nose or eyes. The base has been used similarly .

Preparations

USP 25: Neomycin and Polymyxin B Sulfates and Pramoxine Hydrochloride Cream; Pramoxine Hydrochloride Cream; Pramoxine Hydrochloride Jelly.

Proprietary Preparations (details are given in Part 3)
Fr.: Tronothane; *Israel:* Anti Itch; *Ital.:* Tronotene; *S.Afr.:* Anugesic; *Spain:* Balsabit; Pramox; *USA:* Anti Itch†; Fleet Pain Relief; PramOtic; Prax; Proctofoam; Tronothane.

Multi-ingredient: *Belg.:* Nestosyl; *Canad.:* Anugesic-HC; Anusol Plus; Aveeno Anti-Itch; Hemorrhoid Ointment; Onguent Hemorrhoidal; PrameGel; Pramox HC; Proctodan-HC; Proctofoam-HC; Sarna-P; *Irl.:* Anugesic-HC; Proctofoam-HC; *Israel:* Epifoam; Proctofoam-HC; *Ital.:* Proctofoam-HC; *S.Afr.:* Anugesic; Proctofoam†; *UK:* Anugesic-HC; Proctocream HC†; Proctofoam-HC; *USA:* 1 + 1-F; Analpram-HC; Anusol; Aveeno Anti-Itch; Betadine Plus First Aid Antibiotics & Pain Reliever; Bite & Itch Lotion; Caladryl; Caladryl Clear; Cortane-B Otic; Cortic; Enzone; Epifoam; Hemorid For Women; Itch-X; Neosporin + Pain Relief; Oti-Med; Otomar-HC; Phicon; Phicon-F; PrameGel; Pramosone; Proctofoam-HC; Tri-Biozene; Tri-Otic; Tronolane; Zone-A; Zoto-HC.

Prilocaine Hydrochloride (7643-y)

Prilocaine Hydrochloride (BANM, USAN, rINNM).
Astra-1512; L-67; Prilocaine Hydrochloridum; Propitocaine Hydrochloride. 2-Propylaminopropiono-o-toluidide hydrochloride.
$C_{13}H_{20}N_2O,HCl = 256.8$.
CAS — 721-50-6 (prilocaine); 1786-81-8 (prilocaine hydrochloride).
Pharmacopoeias. In Eur. (see p.vi) *and* US. Eur. also includes Prilocaine.

Prilocaine forms a mixture with lignocaine [lidocaine] that has a melting-point lower than that of either ingredient. This eutectic mixture is used in the preparation of topical dosage forms.
Pharmacopoeial description
Ph. Eur.: A white crystalline powder or colourless crystals. M.p. 168° to 171°. Freely soluble in water and in alcohol; very slightly soluble in acetone.
USP 25: A white odourless crystalline powder. M.p. 166° to 169°. Soluble 1 in 3.5 of water, 1 in 4.2 of alcohol, and 1 in 175 of chloroform; very slightly soluble in acetone; practically insoluble in ether.

pH of solutions. For a discussion of the effect that pH has on the stability of local anaesthetic solutions and the pain associated with their injection, see p.1304.

Adverse Effects, Treatment, and Precautions

As for Local Anaesthetics in general, p.1302.

Prilocaine has relatively modest toxicity compared with most amide-type local anaesthetics. However, dose-related methaemoglobinaemia and cyanosis, attributed to the metabolite *o*-toluidine, appear to occur more frequently with prilocaine than with other local anaesthetics (see Methaemoglobinaemia, p.1302). Symptoms usually occur when doses of prilocaine hydrochloride exceed about 8 mg per kg body-weight but the very young may be more susceptible. Methaemoglobinaemia has been observed in neonates whose mothers received prilocaine shortly before delivery and it has also been reported following prolonged topical application of a prilocaine/lignocaine [lidocaine] eutectic mixture in children. (See under Surface Anaesthesia in Lignocaine, p.1316 for precautions to be observed with such a eutectic mixture.) Methaemoglobinaemia may be treated by administering oxygen followed, if necessary, by an injection of methylene blue [methylthioninium chloride].

Prilocaine should be avoided in patients with anaemia, congenital or acquired methaemoglobinaemia, cardiac or ventilatory failure, or hypoxia.

Effects on the CNS. For reference to the prilocaine serum concentrations associated with CNS toxicity, see under Absorption in Pharmacokinetics, below.

Porphyria. Prilocaine has been associated with acute attacks of porphyria and is considered unsafe in porphyric patients.

Interactions

For interactions associated with local anaesthetics, see p.1303.

Methaemoglobinaemia may occur at lower doses of prilocaine in patients receiving concomitant therapy with other drugs known to cause such conditions (e.g. sulfonamides such as sulfamethoxazole in co-trimoxazole).

Neuromuscular blockers. For a possible interaction between *mivacurium* and prilocaine, see under Atracurium, p.1335.

Pharmacokinetics

Prilocaine is reported to be 55% bound to plasma proteins. It is rapidly metabolised mainly in the liver and also in the kidneys and is excreted in the urine mainly as metabolites. One of the principal metabolites excreted in the urine is *o*-toluidine, which is believed to cause the methaemoglobinaemia observed after large doses. Prilocaine crosses the placenta and during prolonged epidural anaesthesia may produce methaemoglobinaemia in the fetus. It is distributed into breast milk.

See also under Local Anaesthetics, p.1303.

Absorption. Peak serum concentrations of prilocaine hydrochloride attained after the use of 8.5 mL of a 1% solution for retrobulbar and facial nerve block were well below the concentration of 20 µg per mL associated with CNS toxicity due to prilocaine.[1]
1. Goggin M, *et al.* Serum concentrations of prilocaine following retrobulbar block. *Br J Anaesth* 1990; **64:** 107–9.

Uses and Administration

Prilocaine is a local anaesthetic of the amide type with actions and uses similar to those described on p.1304. It has a similar anaesthetic potency to lignocaine [lidocaine]. However, it has a slower onset of action, less vasodilator activity, and a slightly longer duration of action; it is also less toxic. Prilocaine hydrochloride is used for infiltration anaesthesia and nerve blocks in solutions of 0.5%, 1%, and 2%; a 2% solution is used for epidural block and for analgesia, and for intravenous regional anaesthesia 0.5% solutions are used. A 3% solution with the vasoconstrictor felypressin (p.1283) or a 4% solution without are used for dental procedures. Carbonated solutions of prilocaine have also been tried in some countries in epidural and brachial plexus nerve blocks (see under Administration, p.1304). Prilocaine is used for surface anaesthesia in a eutectic mixture with lignocaine [lidocaine]. (Local anaesthetic techniques are discussed on p.1304.)

The dosage used in various **local anaesthetic procedures** varies with the site of injection and the procedure used. The recommended **maximum single dose** in adults for prilocaine hydrochloride is 400 mg if used alone, or 300 mg if used with felypressin. Doses should be reduced for elderly or debilitated patients. The dose for children over 6 months of age is up to 5 mg per kg body-weight. For *dental infiltration* or *dental nerve blocks*, the usual adult dose of prilocaine hydrochloride without felypressin is 40 to 80 mg (1 to 2 mL) as a 4% solution; children under 10 years of age generally require about 40 mg (1 mL). The usual adult dose of prilocaine hydrochloride with felypressin 0.03 units per mL is 30 to 150 mg (1 to 5 mL) as a 3% solution; children under 10 years of age generally require 30 to 60 mg (1 to 2 mL).

A eutectic mixture (see p.1316) of prilocaine base 2.5% and lignocaine [lidocaine] base 2.5% is applied as a cream under an occlusive dressing to produce *surface anaesthesia* of the skin before procedures requiring needle puncture, surgical treatment of localised lesions, and split skin grafting; it has been used similarly, but without an occlusive dressing, before removal of genital warts.

Action. For a comparison of the vasoactivity of prilocaine and some other local anaesthetics, see p.1304.

Infiltration anaesthesia. Addition of felypressin at a concentration of 0.03 units per mL to prilocaine 3% solution did not reduce plasma concentrations of prilocaine after infiltration of a 60-mg dose into the upper premolar region.[1]

1. Cannell H, Whelpton R. Systemic uptake of prilocaine after injection of various formulations of the drug. *Br Dent J* 1986; **160**: 47–9.

Preparations

BP 2001: Prilocaine Injection;
USP 25: Prilocaine and Epinephrine Injection; Prilocaine Hydrochloride Injection.

Proprietary Preparations (details are given in Part 3)
Austral.: Citanest; Citanest Dental; *Belg.:* Citanest; *Braz.:* Citanest; Citocaina; *Canad.:* Citanest; *Denm.:* Citanest Octapressin; *Fin.:* Citanest; Citanest Octapressin; *Ger.:* Xylonest; *Irl.:* Citanest; Citanest with Octapressin; *Ital.:* Citanest con Octapressin; *Mex.:* Citanest Octapresin; *Neth.:* Citanest; Citanest Octapressine; *Norw.:* Citanest Octapressin; *NZ:* Citanest; Citanest Octapressin; *Port.:* Citanest Octapressin†; *S.Afr.:* Citanest Octopressin†; *Spain:* Citanest; Citanest Octapressin; *Swed.:* Citanest; Citanest Octapressin; *Switz.:* Xylonest; Xylonest-Octapressin; *UK:* Citanest; Citanest with Octapressin; *USA:* Citanest.

Multi-ingredient: *Aust.:* Emla; *Austral.:* Emla; *Belg.:* Emla; *Braz.:* Emla; Medicaina; *Canad.:* Emla; *Denm.:* Emla; *Fin.:* Citanest; Emla; *Fr.:* Emla; Emlapatch; *Ger.:* Emla; *Hong Kong:* Emla; *Irl.:* Emla; *Israel:* Emla; *Ital.:* Emla; *Neth.:* Emla; *Norw.:* Citanest; Emla; *NZ:* Emla; *Port.:* Emla; *S.Afr.:* Emla; *Singapore:* Emla; *Spain:* Emla; *Swed.:* Emla; *Switz.:* Emla; *Thai.:* Emla; *UK:* Emla; *USA:* Emla.

Procaine Hydrochloride (7644-j)

Procaine Hydrochloride (BANM, rINNM).

Allocaine; Ethocaine Hydrochloride; Novocainum; Procaini Hydrochloridum; Procainii Chloridum; Procainium Chloride; Syncaine. 2-Diethylaminoethyl 4-aminobenzoate hydrochloride.
$C_{13}H_{20}N_2O_2,HCl = 272.8$.
CAS — 59-46-1 *(procaine);* 51-05-8 *(procaine hydrochloride).*
Pharmacopoeias. In *Chin., Eur.* (see p.vi), *Int., Jpn, Pol.,* and *US.*

Incompatibility has been reported with aminophylline, barbiturates, magnesium sulfate, phenytoin sodium, sodium bicarbonate, and amphotericin B.

Pharmacopoeial description

Ph. Eur.: A white crystalline powder or colourless crystals. Very soluble in water; soluble in alcohol; practically insoluble in ether. A 2% solution in water has a pH of 5.0 to 6.5. Protect from light.

USP 25: Odourless, small, white crystals or white, crystalline powder. Soluble 1 in 1 of water and 1 in 15 of alcohol; slightly soluble in chloroform; practically insoluble in ether.

Stability of solutions. Degradation of procaine in a cardioplegic solution containing magnesium, sodium, potassium, and calcium salts was found to be temperature dependent.[1] At a storage temperature of 6° the shelf-life of the solution was 5 weeks and this was increased to 9 weeks when the storage tem-

perature was −10°. Using carbon dioxide instead of nitrogen in the head space did not affect stability of procaine.

1. Synave R, *et al.* Stability of procaine hydrochloride in a cardioplegic solution containing bicarbonate. *J Clin Hosp Pharm* 1985; **10**: 385–8.

Adverse Effects, Treatment, and Precautions

As for Local Anaesthetics in general, p.1302.

Effects on the cardiovascular system. Severe hypotension leading to cardiac arrest and death developed in a patient following the infusion of 600 mg of procaine for malignant hyperthermia.[1]

1. MacLachlan D, Forrest AL. Procaine and malignant hyperthermia. *Lancet* 1974; **i**: 355.

Hypersensitivity. Of 600 persons with dermatitis or eczema submitted to patch testing with 2% aqueous solution of procaine hydrochloride, 4.8% gave a positive reaction.[1]

For reports of hypersensitivity including anaphylactic reactions associated with procaine and other local anaesthetics, see under Adverse Effects of Local Anaesthetics, p.1302.

1. Rudzki E, Kleniewska D. The epidemiology of contact dermatitis in Poland. *Br J Dermatol* 1970; **83**: 543–5.

Systemic lupus erythematosus. The limited theoretical risk from using procaine for local anaesthesia in patients who have had procainamide-induced systemic lupus erythematosus was aired some years ago.[1-3]

1. Dubois EL. Procaine anesthesia after procainamide-induced systemic erythematosus. *JAMA* 1977; **238**: 2201.
2. Alarcón-Segovia D. Procaine anesthesia after procainamide-induced systemic erythematosus. *JAMA* 1977; **238**: 2201.
3. Lee SL. Procaine anesthesia after procainamide-induced systemic erythematosus. *JAMA* 1977; **238**: 2201.

Interactions

For interactions associated with local anaesthetics, see p.1303.

Diuretics. Concomitant administration of *acetazolamide* extends the plasma half-life of procaine.[1]

1. Calvo R, *et al.* Effects of disease and acetazolamide on procaine hydrolysis by red blood cell enzymes. *Clin Pharmacol Ther* 1980; **27:** 179–83.

Pharmacokinetics

Procaine is poorly absorbed from mucous membranes but is readily absorbed following parenteral administration. It is rapidly hydrolysed by plasma cholinesterase to para-aminobenzoic acid and diethylaminoethanol; some may also be metabolised in the liver. Only about 6% is bound to plasma proteins. About 80% of the para-aminobenzoic acid is excreted unchanged or conjugated in the urine. About 30% of the diethylaminoethanol is excreted in the urine, the remainder being metabolised in the liver.

See also under Local Anaesthetics, p.1303.

Uses and Administration

Procaine hydrochloride, a para-aminobenzoic acid ester, is a local anaesthetic with actions and uses similar to those described on p.1304. Because of its poor penetration of intact mucous membranes, procaine is ineffective for surface application and has been chiefly used by injection, although in general it has been replaced by lignocaine [lidocaine] and other local anaesthetics. It has a slow onset of action and a short duration of action. It has vasodilator activity and therefore a vasoconstrictor may be added to delay absorption and increase the duration of action. Procaine has mainly been used for infiltration anaesthesia, peripheral nerve blocks, and spinal block. (Local anaesthetic techniques are discussed on p.1304.) It has also been used in cardioplegic solutions to protect the myocardium during cardiac surgery.

For *infiltration anaesthesia* 0.25 to 0.5% solutions of procaine hydrochloride have been used in doses of 350 to 600 mg.

For *peripheral nerve block* a usual dose of 500 mg of procaine hydrochloride has been given as a 0.5% (100 mL), 1% (50 mL), or 2% (25 mL) solution. Doses up to 1 g have been used. For infiltration and peripheral nerve block adrenaline [epinephrine] has been added to solutions, in general to give a final concentration of 1 in 200 000 to 1 in 100 000.

Procaine hydrochloride has been used with propoxycaine in dentistry.

Procaine forms poorly soluble salts or conjugates with some drugs, for example penicillin, and is used to prolong their action after injection. It may also reduce the pain of injection.

Procaine-*N*-glucoside hydrochloride has been included in a preparation for gastrointestinal disorders, and procaine ascorbate has been included in a multivitamin preparation.

Action. For a comparison of the vasoactivity of procaine and some other local anaesthetics, see p.1304.

Preparations

USP 25: Procaine and Tetracaine Hydrochlorides and Levonordefrin Injection; Procaine Hydrochloride and Epinephrine Injection; Procaine Hydrochloride Injection; Propoxycaine and Procaine Hydrochlorides and Levonordefrin Injection; Propoxycaine and Procaine Hydrochlorides and Norepinephrine Bitartrate Injection.

Proprietary Preparations (details are given in Part 3)
Aust.: Geroaslan H3; Gerovital H3; Novanaest; *Canad.:* Novocain; *Ger.:* Hewedolor Procain; Lophakomp-Procain N; Novocain; Pasconeural-Injektopas 1%†; Procaneural; *Hong Kong:*

Gerovital H3; *Ital.:* Lenident; *Spain:* Anestesia Loc Braun C/A; Venocaina†; *Switz.:* Syntocaine†; *USA:* Novocain.

Multi-ingredient: *Aust.:* Aslavital; Biolecit H3; Causat†; Gerontin; KH3; Regenerin; *Austral.:* Cardioplegia; *Belg.:* Otocalmine; Tympalgine; *Braz.:* Algidente; Auditol; Axol; Bismu-Jet; Claudemor; Colutoide; Dexa-Neuriberi; Dexador; Dexaneurin; Fonergin; Geri-Kan H3; KLGH 3; Malvosulfam; Otobel; Otoloide; Otonax; Oturga; Passaja; Pradente; Timpanol; Verlin; Visual; *Denm.:* Kardioplex; *Fr.:* Antiseptique-Calmante; Novitan†; Otylol; Rectophedrol†; X-Adene†; *Ger.:* Cardioplegin N; Causat B12 N; Causat N; Dodecatol N; Echtrovit-K†; Gero H3 Aslan; Hewedolor plus Coffein†; Impletol; KH3; NeyChondrin N (Revitorgan-Dilutionen N Nr 68); NeyPulpin N (Revitorgan-Dilutionen N Nr 10); Otalgan; Otodolor; Pasconeural-Injektopas; Revicain; Revicain comp; Revicain comp plus; Veno-Kattwiga N; *Hong Kong:* Cardioplegia; KH3; *Israel:* Bedodeka Antineuralgica; *Ital.:* Citroftalmina; Citroftalmina VC; Dentosedina; Ginvapast; Mios; Neo-Ustiol; Oftalzina; Otalgan; Otomidone; Otopax; Rinantipiol; Ustiosan; *NZ:* KH3; *Port.:* Claudemor; Gramixina; KH3†; Otalgan; Otocalma; *S.Afr.:* Universal Earache Drops; *Singapore:* Cardioplegia; *Spain:* Anestesia Loc Braun S/A; Anestina Braun†; Co Bucal; Coliriocilina Adren Astr; Dentol Topico; Eupnol; Hepadigest†; Higado Potenciado Medic†; Kanafosal; Kanafosal Predni; KH3 Powel; Neocolan; Nulacin Fermentos; Oftalmol Dexa†; Oftalmol Ocular; Otalgan; Otonasal; Otosedol; Tangenol; *Switz.:* Anaestalgin; Ginvapast; Nasello†; Otalgan; Otosan; *Thai.:* Cardioplegia; KH3; *UK:* KH3; *USA:* Ravocaine and Novocain†.

Used as an adjunct in: *Braz.:* Isacilin; *Ger.:* Eukalisan N; Redox-Injektopas†; *Ital.:* Neuroftal; *Singapore:* Alinamin B12; *Spain:* Sulmetin; Sulmetin Papaverina; *USA:* Hemocyte; Hytinic; Licoplex DS†.

Propanocaine Hydrochloride (7645-z)

Propanocaine Hydrochloride (rINNM).
467D₃. 3-Diethylamino-1-phenylpropyl benzoate hydrochloride.
$C_{20}H_{25}NO_2,HCl = 347.9$.
CAS — 493-76-5 *(propanocaine);* 1679-79-4 *(propanocaine hydrochloride).*

Profile
Propanocaine hydrochloride, a benzoic acid ester, is a local anaesthetic (p.1302) that has been used topically for surface anaesthesia.

Preparations

Proprietary Preparations (details are given in Part 3)
Multi-ingredient: *Fr.:* Lelong Irritations†; *Spain:* Detraine.

Propipocaine (19750-h)

Propipocaine (rINN).
Propoxypiperocaine. 3-Piperidino-4′-propoxypropiophenone.
$C_{17}H_{25}NO_2 = 275.4$.
CAS — 3670-68-6.

Profile
Propipocaine is a local anaesthetic (p.1302) that has been used for surface anaesthesia.

Preparations

Proprietary Preparations (details are given in Part 3)
Multi-ingredient: *Ger.:* Nifucin†.

Propoxycaine Hydrochloride (7646-c)

Propoxycaine Hydrochloride (rINNM).
Propoxycainium Chloride. 2-Diethylaminoethyl 4-amino-2-propoxybenzoate hydrochloride.
$C_{16}H_{26}N_2O_3,HCl = 330.9$.
CAS — 86-43-1 *(propoxycaine);* 550-83-4 *(propoxycaine hydrochloride).*
Pharmacopoeias. In *US.*

Pharmacopoeial description

USP 25: A white odourless crystalline solid. It discolours on prolonged exposure to light and air. Soluble 1 in 2 of water, 1 in 10 of alcohol, and 1 in 80 of ether; practically insoluble in acetone and in chloroform. A 2% solution in water has a pH of about 5.4. Protect from light.

Profile
Propoxycaine hydrochloride, a para-aminobenzoic acid ester, is a local anaesthetic (p.1302). It has been used in a concentration of 0.4% in combination with procaine hydrochloride 2% solution with a vasoconstrictor for infiltration anaesthesia and nerve block in dental procedures. Propoxycaine has a more rapid onset and a longer duration of action than that of procaine.

Preparations

USP 25: Propoxycaine and Procaine Hydrochlorides and Levonordefrin Injection; Propoxycaine and Procaine Hydrochlorides and Norepinephrine Bitartrate Injection.

Proprietary Preparations (details are given in Part 3)
Multi-ingredient: *USA:* Ravocaine and Novocain†.

The symbol † denotes a preparation no longer actively marketed

Proxymetacaine Hydrochloride

(7647-k)

Proxymetacaine Hydrochloride (BANM, rINNM).
Proparacaine Hydrochloride. 2-Diethylaminoethyl 3-amino-4-propoxybenzoate hydrochloride.
$C_{16}H_{26}N_2O_3,HCl = 330.9$.
CAS — 499-67-2 (proxymetacaine); 5875-06-9 (proxymetacaine hydrochloride).

NOTE. PROX is a code approved by the BP 2001 for use on single unit doses of eye drops containing proxymetacaine hydrochloride where the individual container may be too small to bear all the appropriate labelling information. PROXFLN is a similar code approved for eye drops containing proxymetacaine hydrochloride and fluorescein sodium.
Pharmacopoeias. In Br. and US.

Pharmacopoeial description

BP 2001: A white or almost white, odourless or almost odourless, crystalline powder. Soluble in water and in chloroform; very soluble in dehydrated alcohol; practically insoluble in ether. A 1% solution in water has a pH of 5.7 to 6.4. Protect from light.

USP 25: A white to off-white, or faintly buff-coloured, odourless, crystalline powder. Soluble in water, in warm alcohol, and in methyl alcohol; insoluble in ether and in benzene.

Adverse Effects, Treatment, and Precautions

As for Local Anaesthetics in general, p.1302.

A severe immediate-type corneal reaction to proxymetacaine may rarely occur. Allergic contact dermatitis has also been reported.

Effects on the skin. Exacerbation of Stevens-Johnson syndrome has been reported[1] in a woman after ophthalmic anaesthesia with proxymetacaine hydrochloride.

1. Ward B, et al. Dermatologic reaction in Stevens-Johnson syndrome after ophthalmic anaesthesia with proparacaine hydrochloride. *Am J Ophthalmol* 1978; **86**: 133–5.

Interactions

For interactions associated with local anaesthetics, see p.1303.

Pharmacokinetics

See under Local Anaesthetics, p.1303.

Uses and Administration

Proxymetacaine hydrochloride, a meta-aminobenzoic acid ester, is a local anaesthetic with actions and uses similar to those described on p.1304. It is used for surface anaesthesia (p.1304) in ophthalmology in a concentration of 0.5%. Proxymetacaine is of similar potency to amethocaine [tetracaine] in equal concentrations and induces anaesthesia within about 20 seconds. The duration of action may be 15 minutes or longer. Instillation of 1 or 2 drops permits tonometry after 30 seconds. For removal of foreign bodies or sutures from the cornea 1 or 2 drops are instilled every 5 to 10 minutes for up to three doses, or 1 or 2 drops are instilled 2 to 3 minutes before the procedure. For deeper anaesthesia such as needed for cataract extraction 1 drop is instilled every 5 to 10 minutes to a total of 5 to 7 applications.

Trigeminal neuralgia. There have been anecdotal reports that proxymetacaine eye drops relieved trigeminal neuralgia (p.8) refractory to carbamazepine.[1,2] However, a controlled study failed to demonstrate any benefit.[3]

1. Zavon MR, Fichte CM. Trigeminal neuralgia relieved by ophthalmic anesthetic. *JAMA* 1991; **265**: 2807.
2. Zavon MR, Fichte CM. Trigeminal neuralgia relieved by optical anesthesia. *JAMA* 1991; **266**: 1649.
3. Kondziolka D, et al. The effect of single-application topical ophthalmic anesthesia in patients with trigeminal neuralgia: a randomized double-blind placebo-controlled trial. *J Neurosurg* 1994; **80**: 993–7.

Preparations

BP 2001: Proxymetacaine Eye Drops;
USP 25: Fluorescein Sodium and Proparacaine Hydrochloride Ophthalmic Solution; Proparacaine Hydrochloride Ophthalmic Solution.

Proprietary Preparations (details are given in Part 3)
Austral.: Alcaine; Ophthetic; *Braz.:* Anestalcon; Visonest; *Canad.:* Ak-Taine; Alcaine; Diocaine; Ophthetic; *Ger.:* Chibro-Kerakain†; Proparakain-POS; *Hong Kong:* Alcaine; *Irl.:* Ophthaine†; *Mex.:* Alcaine; *Norw.:* Alcaine; *NZ:* Ophthetic; *S.Afr.:* Ophthetic†; *Singapore:* Alcaine; *Switz.:* Alcaine; *UK:* Ophthaine†; *USA:* Ak-Taine; Alcaine; Ocu-Caine; Ophthaine†; Ophthetic; Parcaine.

Multi-ingredient: *Canad.:* Fluoracaine; *USA:* Fluoracaine; Fluorescaine.

Quinisocaine Hydrochloride (7622-p)

Quinisocaine Hydrochloride (BANM, rINNM).
Chinisocainum Hydrochloride; Dimethisoquin Hydrochloride (USAN); Dimethisoquinium Chloride. 2-(3-Butyl-1-isoquinolyloxy)-NN-dimethylethylamine hydrochloride.
$C_{17}H_{24}N_2O,HCl = 308.8$.
CAS — 86-80-6 (quinisocaine); 2773-92-4 (quinisocaine hydrochloride).

Profile

Quinisocaine hydrochloride is a local anaesthetic (p.1302) available in some countries for use as a surface anaesthetic in the form of an ointment or cream in a concentration of 0.5% or as suppositories. It is used for the relief of pruritus, anogenital or anorectal irritation, and minor skin conditions.

Preparations

Proprietary Preparations (details are given in Part 3)
Fr.: Quotane; *Ger.:* Haenal†; Isochinol; *Switz.:* Isochinol.
Multi-ingredient: *Fr.:* Rectoquotane.

Ropivacaine Hydrochloride (7300-y)

Ropivacaine Hydrochloride (BANM, rINNM).
AL-281. (S)-2′,6′-Dimethyl-1-propylpiperidine-2-carboxanilide hydrochloride monohydrate.
$C_{17}H_{26}N_2O,HCl,H_2O = 328.9$.
CAS — 84057-95-4 (ropivacaine); 98717-15-8 (anhydrous ropivacaine hydrochloride); 132112-35-7 (ropivacaine hydrochloride monohydrate).

Adverse Effects, Treatment, and Precautions

As for Local Anaesthetics in general, p.1302.

Effects on the cardiovascular system. Ropivacaine is structurally related to bupivacaine, but data from extensive *animal* studies suggest that ropivacaine may be less cardiotoxic than bupivacaine.[1] Results from a study[2] in 12 healthy male volunteers support these data; at doses producing CNS symptoms cardiovascular changes, such as depression of conduction and diastolic function, were less pronounced with ropivacaine than with bupivacaine.

1. Cederholm I. Preliminary risk-benefit analysis of ropivacaine in labour and following surgery. *Drug Safety* 1997; **16**: 391–402.
2. Knudsen K, et al. Central nervous and cardiovascular effects of i.v. infusions of ropivacaine, bupivacaine and placebo in volunteers. *Br J Anaesth* 1997; **78**: 507–14.

Interactions

For interactions associated with local anaesthetics, see p.1303.

Concomitant administration of ropivacaine with general anaesthetics, opioid analgesics, or drugs structurally related to amide-type local anaesthetics (e.g. certain antiarrhythmics) may result in potentiation of adverse effects.

The metabolism of ropivacaine is mediated by the cytochrome P450 isoenzyme CYP1A2 and the potential exists for interactions between ropivacaine and other drugs which inhibit or act as a substrate for this isoenzyme. Prolonged administration of ropivacaine should be avoided in patients treated with potent CYP1A2 inhibitors, such as fluvoxamine and verapamil. Plasma concentrations of ropivacaine may be reduced by enzyme-inducing drugs such as rifampicin.

Pharmacokinetics

Ropivacaine is about 94% bound to plasma proteins. The terminal elimination half-life has been reported to be 1.8 hours. It is extensively metabolised in the liver, predominantly by aromatic hydroxylation which is mediated by the cytochrome P450 isoenzyme CYP1A2; CYP3A4 plays a minor role in the metabolism of ropivacaine. The metabolites are excreted mainly in the urine; about 1% of a dose is excreted as unchanged drug. Some metabolites also have a local anaesthetic effect but less than that of ropivacaine. Ropivacaine crosses the placenta.
See also under Local Anaesthetics, p.1303.

Uses and Administration

Ropivacaine hydrochloride is a local anaesthetic of the amide type with actions and uses similar to those described on p.1304. It is a long-acting local anaesthetic, although onset and duration of action are dependent upon the administration site; the presence of a vasoconstrictor such as adrenaline [epinephrine] has no effect. Ropivacaine is used for epidural block, peripheral nerve block, and infiltration anaesthesia and field block. (Local anaesthetic techniques are discussed on p.1304.) At high doses ropivacaine produces surgical anaesthesia, whereas at lower doses it is used for the management of acute pain such as labour pain (p.6) and in postoperative analgesia (p.4).

Like bupivacaine (p.1306), ropivacaine has a differential blocking effect on nerve fibres and, at the lowest concentration used, there is good differentiation between sensory and motor block. The onset and duration of sensory block produced by ropivacaine is generally similar to that obtained with bupivacaine but the motor block is often slower in onset, shorter in duration, and less intense.

Ropivacaine hydrochloride is administered in concentrations of 0.2 to 1%. The dosage depends on the site of injection and the procedure used, as well as the status of the patient. The dose of ropivacaine should be reduced in the elderly, and in acutely ill or debilitated patients. A test dose of lignocaine [lidocaine] with adrenaline [epinephrine] should be given before commencing epidural block with ropivacaine to detect inadvertent intravascular administration.

For **surgical anaesthesia**, doses of ropivacaine hydrochloride for *lumbar epidural block* are 75 to 150 mg (15 to 30 mL) as a 0.5% solution, or 112.5 to 187.5 mg (15 to 25 mL) as a 0.75% solution, or 150 to 200 mg (15 to 20 mL) as a 1% solution; for caesarean section, doses are 100 to 150 mg (20 to 30 mL) as a 0.5% solution or 112.5 to 150 mg (15 to 20 mL) as a 0.75% solution. Doses for *thoracic epidural block* to establish a block for postoperative pain relief are 25 to 75 mg (5 to 15 mL) as a 0.5% solution or 37.5 to 112.5 mg (5 to 15 mL) as a 0.75% solution; the actual dose used depends on the level of the injection. For *peripheral nerve block* of major nerves such as the brachial plexus, typical doses are 175 to 250 mg (35 to 50 mL) as a 0.5% solution; 225 to 300 mg (30 to 40 mL) as a 0.75% solution has also been recommended for brachial plexus block. For *infiltration anaesthesia* and *field block* up to 200 mg (40 mL) as a 0.5% solution or up to 225 mg (30 mL) as a 0.75% solution may be used.

In the management of **acute pain** ropivacaine hydrochloride is used as a 0.2% solution for epidural block (0.5% solutions may be used for infiltration). Doses for *lumbar epidural block* are 20 to 40 mg (10 to 20 mL) as an initial bolus followed by 20 to 30 mg (10 to 15 mL) at intervals of not less than 30 minutes. Alternatively, 12 to 20 mg (6 to 10 mL) per hour may be given as a continuous epidural infusion; if additional pain relief is required, doses of up to 28 mg (14 mL) per hour may be given. Doses for *thoracic epidural block* are 12 to 28 mg (6 to 14 mL) per hour as a continuous infusion. For *infiltration anaesthesia* doses are 2 to 200 mg (1 to 100 mL) as a 0.2% solution or 5 to 200 mg (1 to 40 mL) as a 0.5% solution.

In children aged 1 year and over, ropivacaine hydrochloride may be used for the management of pre- and postoperative pain. A 0.2% solution is given in doses of 2 mg per kg body-weight (1 mL per kg) to achieve a *caudal epidural block*.

◊ References.

1. Markham A, Faulds D. Ropivacaine: a review of its pharmacology and therapeutic use in regional anaesthesia. *Drugs* 1996; **52**: 429–49.
2. McClure JH. Ropivacaine. *Br J Anaesth* 1996; **76**: 300–307
3. Morton C. Ropivacaine. *Br J Hosp Med* 1997; **58**: 97–100.

Preparations

Proprietary Preparations (details are given in Part 3)
Aust.: Naropin; *Austral.:* Naropin; *Belg.:* Naropin; *Canad.:* Naropin; *Denm.:* Naropin; *Fin.:* Naropin; *Fr.:* Naropeine; *Ger.:* Naropin; *Hong Kong:* Naropin; *Irl.:* Naropin; *Israel:* Narop; *Ital.:* Naropina; *Mex.:* Naropin; *Neth.:* Naropin; *Norw.:* Naropin; *NZ:* Naropin; *Port.:* Naropeine; *S.Afr.:* Naropin; *Singapore:* Naropin; *Spain:* Naropin; *Swed.:* Narop; *Switz.:* Naropin; *UK:* Naropin; *USA:* Naropin.

Multi-ingredient: *Austral.:* Naropin with Fentanyl.

Tolycaine Hydrochloride (7649-t)

Tolycaine Hydrochloride (BANM, rINNM).

Methyl 2-(2-diethylaminoacetamido)-m-toluate hydrochloride.
$C_{15}H_{22}N_2O_3$,HCl = 314.8.
CAS — 3686-58-6 (tolycaine); 7210-92-6 (tolycaine hydrochloride).

Profile
Tolycaine hydrochloride is an amide local anaesthetic (p.1302) included in some preparations to reduce the pain of injection.

Preparations

Proprietary Preparations (details are given in Part 3)

Used as an adjunct in: **Ger.:** Tardocillin.

Tricaine Mesilate (11077-y)

Metacaine Mesylate; Tricaine Mesylate. Ethyl 3-aminobenzoate methanesulphonate.
$C_{10}H_{15}NO_5S$ = 261.3.
CAS — 886-86-2.

Profile
Tricaine mesilate is a derivative of an isomer of benzocaine (see p.1306) and although it has been used as a local anaesthetic in human medicine it is now mainly used as an anaesthetic and tranquilliser for fish and other cold-blooded animals.

Trimecaine Hydrochloride (7650-l)

Trimecaine Hydrochloride (rINNM).
Trimecainium Chloratum. 2-Diethylamino-2',4',6'-trimethylacetanilide hydrochloride.
$C_{15}H_{24}N_2O$,HCl = 284.8.
CAS — 616-68-2 (trimecaine); 1027-14-1 (trimecaine hydrochloride).

Profile
Trimecaine hydrochloride is an amide local anaesthetic (p.1302) included in some preparations to reduce the pain of injection.

Preparations

Proprietary Preparations (details are given in Part 3)

Used as an adjunct in: **Aust.:** Ketazon; **Ger.:** Ketazon.

Muscle Relaxants

The muscle relaxants included in this chapter are used in the management of musculoskeletal and neuromuscular disorders. There are 2 main types:

- **centrally acting relaxants**—these generally have a selective action on the CNS and are principally used for relieving painful muscle spasms or spasticity occurring in musculoskeletal and neuromuscular disorders. Their mechanism of action may be due to their CNS-depressant activity.

- **directly acting relaxants**—dantrolene is a drug which has a direct action on skeletal muscle and is used for the relief of spasticity associated with a variety of conditions.

Also included in this chapter are miscellaneous drugs, such as botulinum toxins A and B, which inhibit the release of acetylcholine at the motor nerve terminals.

Other drugs which block transmission at the neuromuscular junction and are used as adjuncts to general anaesthesia are discussed in the chapter on Neuromuscular Blockers, p.1331.

Drugs used to relax *smooth muscle* include antimuscarinics, which are described in a separate chapter (p.459), and some gastrointestinal drugs such as mebeverine (p.1233).

Muscle spasm

Spasm is a painful involuntary contraction of muscle which can cause involuntary movement, interfere with function, and cause distortion. It is a symptom of many muscular and other types of disorders and treatment should primarily be aimed at the underlying cause. Centrally acting muscle relaxants and benzodiazepines are used to treat muscle spasms such as *splinting* that occur in response to local trauma or musculoskeletal and joint disorders. Splinting is a reflex muscular spasm that produces muscular rigidity and acts as a protective mechanism to prevent movement and further damage of the affected part. Short courses of muscle relaxants may be considered in the management of acute low back pain (p.6).

Cramps are muscle spasms of abrupt onset that occur at rest and usually last for a few seconds or minutes. They are often precipitated by dehydration and hyponatraemia produced by vigorous exercise, excessive sweating, diarrhoea, and vomiting, or may be associated with drug therapy or haemodialysis. Pregnant women, the elderly, and those with peripheral vascular disease, appear to be particularly susceptible to *night cramps* of the feet or legs, the cause of which is not well understood.

The management of muscle cramps has been reviewed.[1] Quinine has traditionally been used for nocturnal cramps but there has been concern over its efficacy and potential for adverse effects, especially in the elderly. Meta-analyses[2,3] have indicated that although quinine was modestly effective in the treatment of nocturnal cramps in ambulatory patients the risk of serious adverse effects should be borne in mind; patients should be closely monitored over a period of at least 4 weeks while the efficacy of quinine was assessed. In the UK, it is recommended that treatment should be stopped every 3 months to see whether it is still needed.[4] In the USA, the FDA has ruled that quinine products should no longer be used for the management of nocturnal cramps.[5,6] A number of other drugs have been tried for nocturnal cramps but there is little convincing evidence to support their use.[1,5]

Haemodialysis-induced cramp (p.1184) is a common complication occurring during or after dialysis.[1,7] Its aetiology is not clear but response to blood volume expansion with hypertonic solutions such as glucose, mannitol, or saline suggests that hypovolaemia may be involved. Haemodialysis-induced cramp has also been reported to respond to quinine.

1. McGee SR. Muscle cramps. *Arch Intern Med* 1990; **150:** 511–18.
2. Man-Son-Hing M, Wells G. Meta-analysis of efficacy of quinine for treatment of nocturnal leg cramps in elderly people. *BMJ* 1995; **310:** 13–17.
3. Man-Son-Hing M, *et al.* Quinine for nocturnal leg cramps: a meta-analysis including unpublished data. *J Gen Intern Med* 1998; **13:** 600–606.
4. Anonymous. Quinine for nocturnal leg cramps? *Drug Ther Bull* 1996; **34:** 7–8.
5. FDA. Drug products for the treatment and/or prevention of nocturnal leg muscle cramps for over-the-counter human use. *Fed Regist* 1994; **59:** 43234–52.
6. Nightingale SL. Quinine for nocturnal leg cramps. *ACP J Club* 1995; **123:** 86.
7. Mujais SK. Muscle cramps during hemodialysis. *Int J Artif Organs* 1994; **17:** 570–2.

Spasticity

The term spasticity has been loosely applied to various disorders of motor control resulting from CNS disease and marked by effects such as increased muscle tone, exaggerated stretch reflexes, impaired voluntary movement, weakness, loss of dexterity, abnormal posture, and often disturbed gait. In some patients muscle spasm and pain may be more distressing than impaired movement. Other complications may include contractures, pressure sores, and infection. Spasticity is a feature of many neurological conditions, particularly spinal lesions, such as in multiple sclerosis, cerebral palsy, head injury, and stroke.

Spasticity is disabling and difficult to treat when severe, but mild or moderate forms may be effectively managed by conservative treatment. Some patients may even use spasticity to provide a means of posture control and care should be taken that treatment does not lead to increased disability.

Various discussions on the management of spasticity have been published.[1-5] The mainstay of management is physiotherapy together with antispastic drugs, although the evidence base for the latter is rather scanty.[6] Baclofen, dantrolene, and diazepam are the drugs most often used. These 3 drugs act via different mechanisms which are not fully understood.

Baclofen is thought to act at the spinal cord level but may also have supraspinal sites of action. It is a powerful neuronal depressant and may exert its inhibitory effects by acting as an agonist at GABA (gamma aminobutyric acid) receptors. *Diazepam* is also thought to act centrally by enhancing the response to GABA. In contrast, *dantrolene* acts directly on muscles, possibly by interfering with the release of calcium from muscular sarcoplasmic reticulum needed for contraction. All these are usually given by mouth but baclofen may also be given intrathecally in severe chronic spasticity.[7,8] Injection directly into the spinal subarachnoid space allows immediate delivery to the site of action in the spinal cord and hence allows considerably lower doses to be used than those given orally. It has been reported[9] that some patients receiving long-term intrathecal baclofen treatment have been able to stop their therapy without symptoms of spasticity re-appearing, and that others have been able to reduce the dosage required.

Tizanidine, a centrally acting relaxant and α-adrenergic agonist, may also be of value for spasticity. It can produce additive effects with baclofen thereby allowing a reduction in the dosage of both drugs; use with benzodiazepines is not recommended because of the potential for interactions.

Other drugs which may produce some benefit or are being studied in spasticity include *other benzodiazepines*, *clonidine*, and *memantine*.

Other approaches to treatment include nerve blocks using *local anaesthetics*; they should generally only be used when further muscle relaxation would not increase disability. *Chemical neurolysis* using alcohol or phenol is only considered when there is intractable continuous pain. Local injections of *botulinum A toxin* have produced some encouraging results in the management of limb spasticity in post-stroke patients and in children with cerebral palsy; its temporary effect may be an advantage over chemical neurolysis but the need for regular injections may limit acceptability to children.[10]

Nondrug treatments have included electrical stimulation techniques such as transcutaneous nerve stimulation and dorsal column stimulation; vibration applied to agonist spastic muscles to improve voluntary movement; cooling to decrease afferent inputs from peripheral receptors; and orthopaedic surgery or neurosurgery.

1. Young RR. Spasticity: a review. *Neurology* 1994; **44** (suppl 9): S12–S20.
2. Ko Ko C, Ward AB. Management of spasticity. *Br J Hosp Med* 1997; **58:** 400–5.
3. Kita M, Goodkin DE. Drugs used to treat spasticity. *Drugs* 2000; **59:** 487–95.
4. Anonymous. The management of spasticity. *Drug Ther Bull* 2000; **38:** 44–6.
5. Bhakta BB. Management of spasticity in stroke. *Br Med Bull* 2000; **56:** 476–85.
6. Taricco M, *et al.* Pharmacological interventions for spasticity following spinal cord injury (updated 26 September 2000). Available in The Cochrane Library; Issue 3. Oxford: Update Software; 2001.
7. McLean BN. Intrathecal baclofen in severe spasticity. *Br J Hosp Med* 1993; **49:** 262–7.
8. Anonymous. Intrathecal baclofen for spasticity. *Med Lett Drugs Ther* 1994; **36:** 21–2.
9. Dressnandt J, Conrad B. Lasting reduction of severe spasticity after ending chronic treatment with intrathecal baclofen. *J Neurol Neurosurg Psychiatry* 1996; **60:** 168–73.
10. Neville B. Botulinum toxin in the cerebral palsies. *BMJ* 1994; **309:** 1526–7.

Afloqualone (12331-t)

Afloqualone (*rINN*).

HQ-495. 6-Amino-2-fluoromethyl-3-*o*-tolylquinazolin-4(3*H*)-one.

$C_{16}H_{14}FN_3O = 283.3$.

CAS — 56287-74-2.

Profile

Afloqualone is a centrally acting skeletal muscle relaxant that has been given by mouth for the treatment of muscle spasm associated with musculoskeletal conditions. Photosensitivity reactions have been reported.

◊ References.

1. Ishikawa T, *et al.* Photoleukomelanodermatitis (Kobori) induced by afloqualone. *J Dermatol* 1994; **21:** 430–3.

Baclofen (5702-z)

Baclofen (*BAN, USAN, rINN*).

Aminomethyl Chlorohydrocinnamic Acid; Ba-34647; Baclofenum. β-Aminomethyl-*p*-chlorohydrocinnamic acid; (*RS*)-Amino-3-(4-chlorophenyl)butyric acid.

$C_{10}H_{12}CINO_2 = 213.7$.

CAS — 1134-47-0.

ATC — M03BX01.

Pharmacopoeias. In *Eur.* (see p.vi), *Jpn, Pol.*, and *US*.

Pharmacopoeial description

Ph. Eur.: A white or almost white powder. It exhibits polymorphism. Slightly soluble in water; very slightly soluble in alcohol; practically insoluble in acetone and in ether; dissolves in dilute mineral acids and in dilute solutions of alkali hydroxides.

USP 25: A white to off-white, odourless or practically odourless, crystalline powder. Slightly soluble in water; very slightly soluble in methyl alcohol; insoluble in chloroform. Store in airtight containers.

Adverse Effects

Adverse effects associated with baclofen are often transient and dose-related. They may be minimised by increasing doses gradually or controlled by a reduction in dosage.

The most common side-effects include drowsiness, nausea, dizziness, lightheadedness, confusion, fatigue, muscular pain and weakness, and hypotension. Other side-effects include euphoria, hallucinations, depression, headache, tinnitus, paraesthesias, slurred speech, dry mouth, taste alterations, vomiting, diarrhoea or constipation, ataxia, nystagmus, tremors, insomnia, visual disturbances, skin rashes, pruritus, increased sweating, urinary disturbances, respiratory or cardiovascular depression, blood sugar changes, alterations in liver function values, and a paradoxical increase in spasticity. Problems with erection and ejaculation have also been reported; these are usually reversible on withdrawal of therapy.

Overdosage may lead to muscular hypotonia, drowsiness, respiratory depression, coma, and convulsions (see also below).

Abrupt withdrawal of baclofen may result in a withdrawal syndrome (see under Precautions, below).

Effects on the nervous system. Epilepsy, progressing to status epilepticus, has been associated with the use of baclofen in a patient who had had no previous history of seizures.[1] Baclofen had been given in a dose of 80 mg daily and symptoms had resolved following gradual withdrawal and the use of antiepileptics.

1. Rush JM, Gibberd FB. Baclofen-induced epilepsy. *J R Soc Med* 1990; **83:** 115–16.

Treatment of Adverse Effects

Treatment of overdosage is symptomatic. Consideration should be given to gastric lavage or the use of activated charcoal in patients who have ingested more than 100 mg within an hour of presentation; activated charcoal is recommended in children who have taken more than 5 mg per kg body-weight or 100 mg within the last hour. Observation should continue for at least 6 hours after ingestion. For the use of physostigmine salicylate in the treatment of intrathecal baclofen overdosage, see below.

Overdosage. Atropine sulfate 600 µg intravenously[1] was used to treat a patient who had ingested 420 mg of baclofen and had failed to improve after gastric lavage and induced diuresis. Bradycardia, hypotension, hypothermia, and respiratory depression all improved and no further treatment was needed. The clinical course and management of acute intoxication in 8 adolescents, who ingested estimated amounts of baclofen ranging from 60 to more than 600 mg, has also been described.[2]

Accidental *intrathecal* overdosage has caused respiratory depression, decreased alertness, coma, muscle weakness, and vomiting.[3] Mild intrathecal bolus overdoses of baclofen in patients without cardiac compromise can be treated using physostigmine. Physostigmine salicylate is given intravenously in a dose of 1 to 2 mg over 5 minutes and may be repeated at intervals of 30 to 60 minutes.[3,4] Physostigmine was ineffective in a patient who accidentally received 10 mg of baclofen intrathecally;[5] in such severe overdosage, respiratory support and time to recover is needed.[4] A lumbar tap to remove about 30 to 50 mL of cerebrospinal fluid may help to reduce the intrathecal concentration of baclofen if implemented soon after the overdose.

1. Ferner RE. Atropine treatment for baclofen overdose. *Postgrad Med J* 1981; **57:** 580–1.
2. Perry HE, *et al.* Baclofen overdose: drug experimentation in a group of adolescents. *Pediatrics* 1998; **101:** 1045–8.
3. Müller-Schwefe G, Penn RD. Physostigmine in the treatment of intrathecal baclofen overdose. *J Neurosurg* 1989; **71:** 273–5.
4. Penn RD, Kroin JS. Failure of physostigmine in treatment of acute severe intrathecal baclofen intoxication. *N Engl J Med* 1990; **322:** 1533–4.
5. Saltuari L, *et al.* Failure of physostigmine in treatment of acute severe intrathecal baclofen intoxication. *N Engl J Med* 1990; **322:** 1533.

Precautions

Baclofen should be used with caution in patients with a history of peptic ulcer and avoided in those with active peptic ulcer disease. It should also be used with caution in patients with severe psychiatric disorders or epilepsy or convulsive disorders since these disorders may be exacerbated by baclofen. Liver function should be monitored in patients with liver disease; patients with renal impairment need a reduced dose. Baclofen should be used with caution in patients with respiratory impairment. Observations of increased blood sugar concentrations suggest caution in patients with diabetes mellitus. Care is also required in the elderly in whom adverse effects may be more common and in patients with cerebrovascular disease who tolerate baclofen poorly. It should be used with caution in patients who use their spasticity to maintain posture or to increase function. Urine retention may be exacerbated in patients with hypertonic bladder sphincters. Baclofen may cause drowsiness; patients affected should not drive or operate machinery.

Abrupt withdrawal of baclofen may result in a withdrawal syndrome and exacerbation of spasticity; dosage should be reduced gradually over at least 1 to 2 weeks, or longer if symptoms occur.

Anaesthesia. Acute bradycardia and hypotension occurred following rib retraction in 3 patients given baclofen 30 mg by mouth 90 minutes before thoracic surgery under general anaesthesia, but not in a further 3 patients given placebo.[1] Administration of atropine and ephedrine relieved bradycardia and hypotension in 2 patients, but a brief cardiac arrest occurred in 1. Baclofen may disturb autonomic control of the circulation during general anaesthesia and surgery.

1. Sill JC, *et al.* Bradycardia and hypotension associated with baclofen used during general anaesthesia. *Anesthesiology* 1986; **64:** 255–8.

Peptic ulcer. Results of a study of baclofen-stimulated gastric acid secretion in 10 healthy subjects given 600 µg per kg body-weight intravenously suggested that patients on baclofen might be at risk from baclofen-induced hyperacidity.[1]

1. Pugh S, *et al.* Clinical and experimental significance of the newly discovered activity of baclofen (PCP-GABA) as a stimulant of gastric acid secretion. *Gut* 1985; **26:** A545.

Porphyria. Baclofen is considered to be unsafe in patients with porphyria because it has been shown to be porphyrinogenic in *in-vitro* systems.

Renal impairment. Reports of baclofen toxicity in patients with severe renal impairment.[1] Most patients had received 15 mg or more of baclofen daily although one patient who had received the manufacturer's suggested dose of 5 mg daily still developed toxic symptoms after only 4 days of treatment.

1. Chen K-S, *et al.* Baclofen toxicity in patients with severely impaired renal function. *Ann Pharmacother* 1997; **31:** 1315–20.

Respiratory disorders. Baclofen might precipitate bronchoconstriction in susceptible individuals. A patient with asthma developed symptomatic bronchoconstriction after taking baclofen on two separate occasions.[1] Another patient who had a history of exercise-induced dyspnoea and wheezing was found to have bronchial hyperresponsiveness to methacholine only after taking baclofen.[1]

1. Dicpinigaitis PV, *et al.* Baclofen-induced bronchoconstriction. *Ann Pharmacother* 1993; **27:** 883–4.

Withdrawal. Psychiatric reactions including hallucinations, paranoia, delusions, psychosis, anxiety, confusion, and agitation have been reported[1-4] following abrupt withdrawal of baclofen; symptoms have generally resolved on restarting. Convulsions have also been reported.[5] Autonomic dysfunction including hyperthermia may also follow sudden withdrawal.[6,7] Except for serious adverse reactions, the dose of baclofen should be gradually reduced. In the UK the Committee on Safety of Medicines recommends reduction over at least 1 to 2 weeks or longer if symptoms occur.

1. Lees AJ, *et al.* Hallucinations after withdrawal of baclofen. *Lancet* 1977; **i:** 858.
2. Stein R. Hallucinations after sudden withdrawal of baclofen. *Lancet* 1977; **ii:** 44–5.
3. Harrison SA, Wood CA. Hallucinations after preoperative baclofen discontinuation in spinal cord injury patients. *Drug Intell Clin Pharm* 1985; **19:** 747–9.
4. Committee on Safety of Medicines/Medicines Control Agency. Severe withdrawal reactions with baclofen. *Current Problems* 1997; **23:** 3.
5. Barker I, Grant IS. Convulsions after abrupt withdrawal of baclofen. *Lancet* 1982; **ii:** 556–7.
6. Green LB, Nelson VS. Death after acute withdrawal of intrathecal baclofen: case report and literature review. *Arch Phys Med Rehabil* 1999; **80:** 1600–4.
7. Grenier B, *et al.* Hyperthermie grave liée à un sevrage brutal de baclofène administré de façon continue par voie intrathécale. *Ann Fr Anesth Reanim* 1996; **15:** 659–62.

Interactions

Alcohol and other CNS depressants may exacerbate the CNS effects of baclofen and should be avoided; severe aggravation of hyperkinetic symptoms may possibly occur in patients taking lithium. There may be increased weakness if baclofen is given to patients taking a tricyclic antidepressant and there may be an increased hypotensive effect if it is given to patients receiving antihypertensive therapy.

Dopaminergics. For reports of patients with Parkinson's disease taking levodopa who have experienced adverse effects when given baclofen, see under Levodopa, on p.1172.

NSAIDs. Report of an elderly patient who developed baclofen toxicity after concomitant ibuprofen therapy was started.[1] It appeared that acute renal insufficiency caused by ibuprofen had impaired baclofen excretion.

1. Dahlin PA, George J. Baclofen toxicity associated with declining renal clearance after ibuprofen. *Drug Intell Clin Pharm* 1984; **18:** 805–8.

Pharmacokinetics

Baclofen is rapidly and almost completely absorbed from the gastrointestinal tract following an oral dose. The peak plasma concentration occurs about 1 to 3 hours following ingestion, but the rate and extent of absorption vary between patients, and vary inversely with the dose. Following oral administration some baclofen crosses the blood-brain barrier with concentrations in CSF corresponding to about 12% of those in the plasma. Approximately 30% of baclofen is bound to plasma proteins. About 70 to 80% of a dose is excreted in the urine mainly as unchanged drug; about 15% is metabolised in the liver. The elimination half-life of baclofen is about 3 to 4 hours in plasma and about 5 hours in the CSF.

Absorption. A crossover study in 5 healthy subjects given baclofen 20 mg by mouth after an overnight fast or a standardised breakfast showed that baclofen was rapidly absorbed in both cases, and the rate and extent of absorption were not significantly altered by the presence of food.[1] There is no need to modify the current practice of giving baclofen with food to minimise gastrointestinal side-effects.

1. Peterson GM, *et al.* Food does not affect the bioavailability of baclofen. *Med J Aust* 1985; **142:** 689–90.

Uses and Administration

Baclofen, an analogue of gamma-aminobutyric acid (p.1613), is a centrally acting skeletal muscle relaxant. It interferes with the release of excitatory neurotransmitters and inhibits monosynaptic and polysynaptic transmission at the spinal cord level. It may also act at supraspinal sites producing CNS depression. Baclofen is one of the drugs commonly used for the symptomatic relief of severe chronic spasticity associated with a variety of conditions.

Baclofen is given by mouth in divided doses, preferably with or after food or milk. The initial dose of baclofen is 5 mg three times daily for 3 days, increased to 10 mg three times daily for 3 days, then in similar increments and intervals until either a dose of 20 mg three times daily is reached or until the desired therapeutic effect is obtained. Higher doses have been used. Doses of more than 80 to 100 mg daily are not generally recommended although doses of up to 150 mg daily have been given to carefully supervised patients.

In the UK a dosage range of 0.75 to 2 mg per kg body-weight daily has been used for children; in children over 10 years a maximum daily dosage of 2.5 mg per kg may be given. It is usual to start with a low dose of 2.5 mg given four times daily increased cautiously about every 3 days until the desired therapeutic effect is obtained. The recommended daily maintenance doses are: 12 months to 2 years of age, 10 to 20 mg; 2 to 6 years, 20 to 30 mg; 6 to 10 years, 30 to 60 mg.

Doses should be reduced in renal impairment; 5 mg daily has been suggested (but see also under Precautions, above). Elderly patients should also receive lower initial doses, although final maintenance doses may be in the same range as younger adults.

If no benefit is apparent within 6 weeks of achieving the maximum dosage, therapy should probably be gradually withdrawn.

Baclofen is also given by continuous intrathecal infusion in the treatment of spasticity in patients intolerant of or unresponsive to baclofen by mouth. Before beginning the intrathecal regimen any existing antispastic therapy should be gradually withdrawn to avoid overdosage or drug interactions. Intrathecal test doses are given initially to determine if there is going to be any benefit before implanting a controlled infusion pump. It is important that patients are monitored closely in experienced centres during screening and immediately following implantation of the infusion pump and that resuscitation equipment is available for immediate use. Test doses start at 25 or 50 µg given over at least 1 minute and are increased by 25 µg every 24 hours until a dose of 100 µg is reached or a positive response of about 4 to 8 hours is obtained. Patients who fail to respond to a test dose of up to 100 µg are considered to be unsuitable for intrathecal treatment. An initial test dose of 25 µg is recommended for patients under 18 years of age. However, the manufacturers do not recommend the use of intrathecal baclofen in patients in this age group with spasticity of spinal origin.

For patients showing a positive response lasting for longer than 8 to 12 hours, the test dose that was required to produce the response can then be given as a 24-hour infusion; if the response to the test dose lasted 8 to 12 hours or less, then a dose equivalent to twice the test dose is given. Daily dosage can then be adjusted as required. Maintenance doses range from about 10 to 2000 µg daily, depending on the cause of spasticity, with most patients being adequately maintained with 300 to 800 µg daily.

Dystonias. There have been isolated reports of improvement in patients with various forms of dystonia (p.1173) treated with baclofen[1-3] although there has also been a report[4] of a patient whose condition deteriorated during baclofen therapy.

1. Narayan RK, *et al.* Intrathecal baclofen for intractable axial dystonia. *Neurology* 1991; **41:** 1141–2.
2. Greene PE, Fahn S. Baclofen in the treatment of idiopathic dystonia in children. *Mov Disord* 1992; **7:** 48–52.

3. van Hilten BJ, *et al.* Intrathecal baclofen for the treatment of dystonia in patients with reflex sympathetic dystrophy. *N Engl J Med* 2000; **343**: 625–30.
4. Silbert PL, Stewart-Wynne EG. Increased dystonia after intrathecal baclofen. *Neurology* 1992; **42**: 1639–40.

Hiccup. Baclofen has been given by mouth in daily divided doses ranging from 10 to 80 mg for the management of intractable hiccup (p.667) poorly controlled by other drugs.
References.
1. Burke AM, *et al.* Baclofen for intractable hiccups. *N Engl J Med* 1988; **319**: 1354.
2. Lance JW, Bassil GT. Familial intractable hiccup relieved by baclofen. *Lancet* 1989; **ii**: 276–7.
3. Yaqoob M, *et al.* Baclofen for intractable hiccups. *Lancet* 1989; **ii**: 562–3.
4. Ramirez FC, Graham DY. Treatment of intractable hiccup with baclofen: results of a double-blind randomized, controlled, cross-over study. *Am J Gastroenterol* 1992; **87**: 1789–91.
5. Ramirez FC, Graham DY. Hiccups, compulsive water drinking, and hyponatremia. *Ann Intern Med* 1993; **118**: 649.

Pain. Like some other muscle relaxants baclofen is used in the management of painful conditions associated with muscle spasm or spasticity (see below). The use of muscle relaxants for conditions such as acute low back pain is referred to on p.6. Baclofen does not appear to possess conventional analgesic activity[1] but may potentiate the analgesia produced by opioid analgesics.[2] However, it appears to be of use in the management of trigeminal neuralgia (p.8) and is sometimes added to treatment when response to first-line drugs alone is inadequate.[3]
1. Terrence CF, *et al.* Is baclofen an analgesic? *Clin Neuropharmacol* 1983; **6**: 241–5.
2. Panerai AE, *et al.* Baclofen prolongs the analgesic effect of fentanyl in man. *Br J Anaesth* 1985; **57**: 954–5.
3. Fromm GH, *et al.* Baclofen in the treatment of trigeminal neuralgia: double-blind study and long-term follow-up. *Ann Neurol* 1984; **15**: 240–4.

Spasticity. Baclofen is one of the main drugs used in the management of spasticity (see p.1322). It is used in spasticity to reduce muscle spasm and pain especially in spinal cord lesions in conditions such as multiple sclerosis or paraplegia.
Patients with severe spasticity often require high doses of baclofen by mouth before a response occurs. Some may fail to respond because adverse effects limit increases in dosage. Intrathecal administration is therefore sometimes tried as this produces much higher concentrations in the CNS than oral administration.[1,2] Intrathecal administration may be by bolus injection or by continuous infusion; infusion is probably preferred[3] to minimise the risk of overdosage. There is a large interindividual variation in the dose required to produce improvement in spasticity; doses of 12 to 1500 μg per day by continuous infusion[2,4–9] have produced improvement in some adults and children with spinal cord injuries, multiple sclerosis, and cerebral spasticity. An increased dose of baclofen may be given at night to prevent spasms that interfere with sleep. Although reports of tolerance to the effect of intrathecal baclofen have raised doubt[10] over whether long-term benefit can be maintained, a number of workers have achieved long-term efficacy.[6,11] It has been reported[12] that some patients receiving long-term intrathecal baclofen treatment have been able to stop their therapy without symptoms of spasticity re-appearing and others have been able to reduce the dosage required.
1. McLean BN. Intrathecal baclofen in severe spasticity. *Br J Hosp Med* 1993; **49**: 262–7.
2. Anonymous. Intrathecal baclofen for spasticity. *Med Lett Drugs Ther* 1994; **36**: 21–2.
3. Penn RD, Kroin JS. Intrathecal baclofen. *N Engl J Med* 1989; **321**: 1414–15.
4. Penn RD, Kroin JS. Continuous intrathecal baclofen for severe spasticity. *Lancet* 1985; **ii**: 125–7.
5. Dralle D, *et al.* Intrathecal baclofen for spasticity. *Lancet* 1985; **ii**: 1003.
6. Penn RD, *et al.* Intrathecal baclofen for severe spinal spasticity. *N Engl J Med* 1989; **320**: 1517–21.
7. Dralle D, *et al.* Intrathecal baclofen for cerebral spasticity. *Lancet* 1989; **ii**: 916.
8. Albright AL, *et al.* Intrathecal baclofen for spasticity in cerebral palsy. *JAMA* 1991; **265**: 1418–22.
9. Albright AL, *et al.* Continuous intrathecal baclofen infusion for spasticity of cerebral origin. *JAMA* 1993; **270**: 2475–7.
10. Lewis KS, Mueller WM. Intrathecal baclofen for severe spasticity secondary to spinal cord injury. *Ann Pharmacother* 1993; **27**: 767–74.
11. Azouvi P, *et al.* Intrathecal baclofen administration for control of severe spinal spasticity: functional improvement and long-term follow-up. *Arch Phys Med Rehabil* 1996; **77**: 35–9.
12. Dressnandt J, Conrad B. Lasting reduction of severe spasticity after ending chronic treatment with intrathecal baclofen. *J Neurol Neurosurg Psychiatry* 1996; **60**: 168–73.

Stiff-man syndrome. There has been an anecdotal report[1] of benefit with intrathecal baclofen in a patient with stiff-man syndrome (p.681) inadequately controlled with other drugs or oral baclofen. However, in a double-blind placebo-controlled study[2] in 3 patients clinical improvement was evident in only one patient when receiving intrathecal baclofen.
1. Seitz RJ, *et al.* Stiff-person syndrome with anti-glutamic acid decarboxylase autoantibodies: complete remission of symptoms after intrathecal baclofen administration. *J Neurol* 1995; **242**: 618–22.
2. Silbert PL, *et al.* Intrathecal baclofen therapy in stiff-man syndrome: a double-blind, placebo-controlled trial. *Neurology* 1995; **45**: 1893–7.

Tardive dyskinesia. Baclofen is one of many drugs that have been tried in antipsychotic-induced tardive dyskinesia (see Extrapyramidal Disorders, p.662) but its efficacy is unclear. While

patients in some double-blind studies[1] have obtained improvement with baclofen other double-blind studies[2] suggest that it is unlikely to be more effective than placebo.
1. Ananth J, *et al.* Baclofen in the treatment of tardive dyskinesia. *Curr Ther Res* 1987; **42**: 111–14.
2. Glazer WM, *et al.* The treatment of tardive dyskinesia with baclofen. *Psychopharmacology (Berl)* 1985; **87**: 480–3.

Tetanus. The management of tetanus is described on p.1332 and p.142. There are case reports of beneficial responses with baclofen 1 or 2 mg daily by continuous intrathecal infusion.[1] However, the therapeutic range of intrathecal baclofen in severe tetanus may be very narrow and deep coma with loss of spontaneous respiration and reflexes has been reported[2] following an increase in dosage from 1.2 mg to 2 mg daily. This adverse effect could be fatal in the absence of ventilatory support. In an attempt to avoid the risk of secondary infection from an indwelling intraspinal catheter intermittent intrathecal administration of baclofen has also been employed.[3]
1. Müller H, *et al.* Intrathecal baclofen in tetanus. *Lancet* 1986; **i**: 317–18.
2. Romijn JA, *et al.* Reversible coma due to intrathecal baclofen. *Lancet* 1986; **ii**: 696.
3. Demaziere J, *et al.* Intermittent intrathecal baclofen for severe tetanus. *Lancet* 1991; **337**: 427.

Tourette's syndrome. Improvement was noted in children with Tourette's syndrome (see Tics, p.650) treated with baclofen compared with placebo in one small study.[1]
1. Singer HS, *et al.* Baclofen treatment in Tourette syndrome: a double-blind, placebo-controlled, crossover trial. *Neurology* 2001; **56**: 599–604.

Urinary incontinence. Baclofen has been used with some benefit in the management of urinary incontinence and retention (p.459) secondary to lesions of the spinal cord.
References.
1. Hachen HJ, Krucker V. Clinical and laboratory assessment of the efficacy of baclofen (Lioresal®) on urethral sphincter spasticity in patients with traumatic paraplegia. *Eur Urol* 1977; **3**: 237–40.
2. Leyson JFJ, *et al.* Baclofen in the treatment of detrusor-sphincter dyssynergia in spinal cord injury patients. *J Urol (Baltimore)* 1980; **124**: 82–4.
3. Kums JJM, Delhaas EM. Intrathecal baclofen infusion in patients with spasticity and neurogenic bladder disease. *World J Urol* 1991; **9**: 153–6.

Preparations

BP 2001: Baclofen Oral Solution; Baclofen Tablets;
USP 25: Baclofen Tablets.

Proprietary Preparations (details are given in Part 3)
Aust.: Lioresal; *Austral.:* Baclohexal; Clofen; Lioresal; *Belg.:* Lioresal; *Braz.:* Lioresal; *Canad.:* Lioresal; Liotec; Nu-Baclo; *Denm.:* Lioresal; *Fin.:* Baclon; Baclopar; Lioresal; *Fr.:* Lioresal; *Ger.:* Lebic; Lioresal; *Hong Kong:* Lioresal; *Irl.:* Lioresal; *Israel:* Baclosal; Lioresal; *Ital.:* Lioresal; *Neth.:* Lioresal; *Norw.:* Lioresal; *NZ:* Lioresal; Pacifen; *Port.:* Lioresal; *S.Afr.:* Clinispas†; Lioresal; *Singapore:* Lioresal; *Spain:* Lioresal; *Swed.:* Lioresal; *Switz.:* Lioresal; *Thai.:* Lioresal; *UK:* Baclospas; Balgifen; Lioresal; *USA:* Lioresal.

Botulinum Toxins (20959-s)

Botulinum A Toxin (18860-d)

Botulinum A toxin is a neurotoxin produced by *Clostridium botulinum.*
Residual botulinum A toxin or spillages should be inactivated by autoclaving or use of a dilute hypochlorite solution (0.5%).

Botulinum B Toxin (17169-t)

Botulinum B toxin is a neurotoxin produced by *Clostridium botulinum.* Like botulinum A toxin (above) residual or spilled toxin may be decontaminated by hypochlorite solution and autoclaving, or a strong caustic solution may be used.

Units

The dose of preparations containing botulinum toxins A or B is expressed in terms of units, but the available preparations are used at different doses for the same indications, and the units of one preparation cannot be considered to apply to another.

◊ It has been suggested that the difference between botulinum A toxin preparations may not only be confined to just a numerical dosage adjustment.[1] Reviews of the literature have suggested that there may also be a difference in the incidence of adverse effects. The reported frequency of dysphagia for Dysport (28% and 44%) in patients with spasmodic torticollis was greater than that for Botox (9.5 to 17%). This variation might relate to differences in bioactivity not recognised by the mouse lethality bioassay which is used to determine the potency of preparations.
1. Borodic G. Therapeutic botulinum toxin. *Lancet* 1994; **344**: 1370.

Adverse Effects

Injections of botulinum toxins have been associated with a transient burning sensation, bruising at the injection site, and local weakness. Deep or misplaced

injections may paralyse nearby muscle groups and excessive doses may paralyse distant muscles. Overdosage can produce a widespread paralysis.

There have been occasional reports of hypersensitivity reactions such as skin rashes and influenza-like symptoms.

The most common adverse effects following injection into muscles surrounding the eye, such as in the management of blepharospasm, hemifacial spasm, or strabismus are ptosis, lachrymation, photophobia, and ocular irritation. Some patients may be unable to close the eyelid completely. Other adverse effects that have been reported include ectropion and entropion, and diplopia. Patients experience a reduction in blinking and this can lead to dry eye, keratitis, and corneal damage. Angle-closure glaucoma has been reported. Vertical deviation has also occurred in patients treated for horizontal strabismus. Needle penetrations of the eye during treatment of strabismus have resulted in vitreous and retrobulbar haemorrhages.

Dysphagia is the most common adverse effect following injection into neck muscles in the treatment of spasmodic torticollis and there may be pooling of saliva with risk of aspiration in severely affected patients (*important*, see also under Precautions, below). Dry mouth, paralysis of the vocal cords, and weakness of the neck muscles may also occur. Generalised weakness, malaise, nausea, and visual disturbances have occasionally been reported. Other effects which have occurred rarely include drowsiness, numbness, stiffness, ptosis, and headache. Respiratory difficulties, associated with the use of large doses, have occurred on rare occasions.

Adverse effects most frequently associated with injection into the lower limb include falling, leg pain, and general weakness; lethargy and leg cramps have also been reported.

Angiosarcoma. It has been suggested[1] that botulinum A toxin injection might have acted as a triggering factor in the initiation of angiosarcoma in a 66-year-old patient being treated for blepharospasm.
1. Kárpáti S, *et al.* Human herpesvirus type 8-positive facial angiosarcoma developing at the site of botulinum toxin injection for blepharospasm. *Br J Dermatol* 2000; **143**: 660–2.

Antibody formation. Neutralising antibodies that reduce or abolish the beneficial effects of treatment have been found in a small proportion of patients who have received prolonged treatment with botulinum A toxin.[1] In a review[2] of the use of botulinum A toxin it was stated that there was growing concern over the development of antibodies after repeated injections, as many of the conditions for which botulinum toxin is indicated are chronic and require indefinite treatment. Antibody formation was reported to be more common with high-dose indications such as spasmodic torticollis than in low-dose indications such as blepharospasm. The occurrence of antibodies appeared to correlate with the dose per injection, the quantity of botulinum protein given per injection, the number of injections given, and the frequency of injections.

Antibodies have also developed following the use of botulinum B toxin. However, botulinum toxin B is antigenically distinct from botulinum A toxin, and may be of value in patients who develop resistance to treatment associated with antibody formation to type A toxin.[3] Botulinum F toxin is also antigenically distinct and is being studied in a similar way.
1. Hambleton P, *et al.* Antitoxins and botulinum toxin treatment. *BMJ* 1992; **304**: 959–60.
2. Borodic GE, Pearce LB. New concepts in botulinum toxin therapy. *Drug Safety* 1994; **11**: 145–52.
3. Brin MF, *et al.* Safety and efficacy of NeuroBloc (botulinum toxin type B) in type A-resistant cervical dystonia. *Neurology* 1999; **53**: 1431–8.

Biliary colic. A 43-year-old woman with no previous history of gallbladder disease experienced single episodes of biliary colic after each of 3 sessions of treatment with botulinum A toxin for blepharospasm.[1] Botulinum A toxin might have exerted a systemic effect to block acetylcholine release leading to gallbladder hypomotility with delayed emptying and stasis.
1. Schnider P, *et al.* Gallbladder dysfunction induced by botulinum A toxin. *Lancet* 1993; **342**: 811–12.

Dysphagia. By November 1993, the UK Committee on Safety of Medicines had received 4 reports of severe dysphagia with choking in patients who had received injections of botulinum A toxin into the neck muscles as a treatment for torticollis.[1] The dysphagia developed 5 to 7 days after the injection and in one patient it was persisting 6 weeks after the injection. The dysphagia led to aspiration of the stomach contents into the lungs and one patient with a history of poor lung function died from bronchopneumonia. Dysphagia is also reported to be a common adverse effect in patients with spasmodic torticollis being treated with Botulinum B toxin.[2]

See also under Units, above for further reference to dysphagia as an adverse effect.

1. Committee on Safety of Medicines/Medicines Control Agency. Reminder: botulinum type A toxin (Dysport)—severe dysphagia with unlicensed route of administration. *Current Problems* 1993; **19**: 11.
2. Lew MF, *et al.* The safety and efficacy of botulinum toxin type B in the treatment of patients with cervical dystonia: summary of three controlled clinical trials. *Neurology* 2000; **55** (suppl 5): S29–S35.

Effects on the eyes. Acute angle-closure glaucoma has been reported[1] in an 83-year-old woman after a series of injections of botulinum A toxin for the treatment of blepharospasm. Permanent extra-ocular muscle damage following botulinum toxin injection has been reported[2] in a 70-year-old man.

1. Corridan P, *et al.* Acute angle-closure glaucoma following botulinum toxin injection for blepharospasm. *Br J Ophthalmol* 1990; **74**: 309–10.
2. Mohan M, *et al.* Permanent extraocular muscle damage following botulinum toxin injection. *Br J Ophthalmol* 1999; **83**: 1309–10.

Treatment of Adverse Effects

The use of artificial tears may relieve keratitis and dry eye. In the event of overdosage general supportive care is required. The patient should be monitored for several days for signs of paralysis and artificial respiration may be necessary. It is doubtful that specific botulinum antitoxin (p.1534) will be of value although some consider that it might help if given within 30 minutes of overdosage.

Precautions

Botulinum toxin is contra-indicated in generalised disorders of muscle activity such as myasthenia gravis. Injections, especially those into the neck, should be made with great care to avoid unintended paralysis (see also below). It is also contra-indicated in pregnancy and breast feeding. As with other biological products, the potential for botulinum toxin to cause anaphylaxis should be considered. Deep or misplaced injections should be avoided; the relevant anatomy, and any alterations due to previous surgery, must be understood before injecting.

SPECIFIC CAUTIONS WHEN TREATING BLEPHAROSPASM, HEMIFACIAL SPASM, OR STRABISMUS. Reduced blinking can lead to corneal exposure, persistent epithelial defect, and corneal ulceration, especially in patients with seventh cranial nerve disorders; corneal sensation should be carefully tested in previously treated eyes, injection into the lower eyelid area avoided, and any resulting epithelial defect vigorously treated.

SPECIFIC CAUTIONS WHEN TREATING LOWER LIMB SPASTICITY IN CHILDREN WITH CEREBRAL PALSY OR SPASMODIC TORTICOLLIS. Botulinum toxin should only be used by specialists experienced in the diagnosis and management of these disorders and who have received training.

Interactions

Botulinum A toxin should not be given with (or before) aminoglycosides or spectinomycin. Interactions may also occur with other drugs that have neuromuscular blocking activity, including lincosamides, polymyxins, tetracyclines, and muscle relaxants. Likewise, administration of botulinum B toxin with aminoglycosides or neuromuscular blocking drugs should be undertaken with caution.

Uses and Administration

Botulinum toxins cause neuromuscular blockade by inhibiting the calcium-ion mediated release of acetylcholine at the motor nerve terminals, resulting in a diminished endplate potential and subsequent flaccid paralysis of the affected muscles. The paralysis persists until new nerve terminals form, usually within 2 to 4 months. Botulinum A toxin is given as a complex with haemagglutinin by local injection in the treatment of hemifacial spasm, blepharospasm, spasmodic torticollis, and lower limb spasticity in children with cerebral palsy. Botulinum A toxin is also used for the management of strabismus and hyperhidrosis, and is being investigated for use in the management of several other disorders. Botulinum B toxin is also used in the management of spasmodic torticollis and, being antigenically distinct, it has the potential for use

in patients who develop resistance to treatment due to the development of antibodies to type A toxin.

Doses of botulinum toxins A and B are expressed in terms of units, which have not been standardised between preparations (see Units, above). Doses are therefore specific to each individual preparation; details are given below.

Botulinum F toxin is under investigation for the treatment of similar neuromuscular disorders.

◊ Reviews.
1. Borodic GE, Pearce LB. New concepts in botulinum toxin therapy. *Drug Safety* 1994; **11**: 145–52.
2. Hughes AJ. Botulinum toxin in clinical practice. *Drugs* 1994; **48**: 888–93.

Achalasia. The treatment of choice for achalasia (see Oesophageal Motility Disorders, p.1208) is mechanical dilatation of the lower oesophageal sphincter, or if necessary surgery, but more recently injection of botulinum A toxin[1,2] has been found to be effective. However, one year after treatment only 7 of 22 (32%) patients who received botulinum A toxin were in symptomatic remission compared with 14 of 20 (70%) patients treated with mechanical dilatation.[3] It was recommended that its use would be better reserved for patients thought to be at risk from mechanical dilatation or surgery.[3,4] Another study[5] demonstrated that intrasphincteric injection of botulinum toxin A was safe and effective for the treatment of achalasia in the short and medium term, although only a weak correlation with dose emerged.

1. Pasricha PJ, *et al.* Intrasphincteric botulinum toxin for the treatment of achalasia. *N Engl J Med* 1995; **332**: 774–8. Correction. *ibid.*; **333**: 75.
2. Cuillière C, *et al.* Achalasia: outcome of patients treated with intrasphincteric injection of botulinum toxin. *Gut* 1997; **41**: 87–92.
3. Vaezi MF, *et al.* Botulinum toxin versus pneumatic dilatation in the treatment of achalasia: a randomised trial. *Gut* 1999; **44**: 231–9.
4. Spiess AE, Kahrilas PJ. Treating achalasia: from whalebone to laparoscope. *JAMA* 1998; **280**: 638–42.
5. Annesse V, *et al.* A multicentre randomised study of intrasphincteric botulinum toxin in patients with oesophageal achalasia. *Gut* 2000; **46**: 597–600.

Anal fissure. Anal fissure is a superficial tear in the mucosa of the distal anal canal characterised by pain on defaecation, rectal bleeding, and spasm of the anal sphincter. Healing, which is usually uneventful, may be helped by conservative management with bran and bulk laxatives and topical local anaesthetics for pain relief. Surgical treatment has been used for patients who develop a chronic condition but since this has been associated with high rates of long-term incontinence and recurrence, alternative treatments are being investigated. As hypertonicity of the internal anal sphincter may be involved in the pathophysiology of chronic anal fissure, local injections of botulinum A toxin have been used to produce paresis of this sphincter.[1,2] The duration of the effect appears to be long enough to allow complete healing of the fissure in most patients although some may relapse; temporary incontinence had been the only adverse effect reported. Although possibly less effective than botulinum toxin,[3] topical application of nitrates can relax the anal sphincter and a randomised controlled study[4] has produced encouraging results in the treatment of anal fissure using glyceryl trinitrate ointment. Follow-up[5] of patients treated with glyceryl trinitrate indicated that after 24 to 38 months most had not experienced further problems or had had occasional recurrences which in the majority of cases had responded to further topical treatment. Isosorbide dinitrate ointment has also been tried. Calcium antagonists may also be effective: nifedipine[6] and diltiazem[7] have both produced promising results in small studies.

1. Jost WH, Schimrigk K. Botulinum toxin in therapy of anal fissure. *Lancet* 1995; **345**: 188–9.
2. Maria G, *et al.* A comparison of botulinum toxin and saline for the treatment of chronic anal fissure. *N Engl J Med* 1998; **338**: 217–20.
3. Brisinda G, *et al.* A comparison of injections of botulinum toxin and topical nitroglycerin ointment for the treatment of chronic anal fissure. *N Engl J Med* 1999; **341**: 65–9. Correction. *ibid.*; 624.
4. Lund JN, Scholefield JH. A randomised, prospective, double-blind, placebo-controlled trial of glyceryl trinitrate ointment in treatment of anal fissure. *Lancet* 1997; **349**: 11–14. Correction. *ibid.*: 656.
5. Lund JN, Scholefield JH. Follow-up of patients with chronic anal fissure treated with topical glyceryl trinitrate. *Lancet* 1998; **352**: 1681.
6. Cook TA, *et al.* Oral nifedipine reduces resting anal pressure and heals chronic anal fissure. *Br J Surg* 1999; **86**: 1269–73.
7. Carapeti EA, *et al.* Topical diltiazem and bethanechol decrease anal sphincter pressure without side effects. *Gut* 1999; **45**: 719–22.

Anismus. Anismus is a condition in which inappropriate contraction of the anal sphincters occurs when bowel evacuation is attempted; it seems to be a form of dystonia.

Treatment with botulinum A toxin was investigated in 7 patients with intractable constipation due mainly to anismus.[1] The toxin was injected bilaterally into the puborectalis muscle using an electromyographically guided needle; patients were allowed to continue with their laxatives throughout the study if required. Symptoms improved in all but one of the patients, al-

though two patients could not be regarded as treatment successes because they developed faecal incontinence; four patients had an excellent clinical outcome.

1. Hallan RI, *et al.* Treatment of anismus in intractable constipation with botulinum A toxin. *Lancet* 1988; **ii**: 714–17.

Blepharospasm. Blepharospasm is a focal dystonia characterised by repeated involuntary blinking caused by spasms of the orbicularis oculi muscle of the eye, which may result in functional blindness. Blepharospasm is often associated with other dystonias of the head and neck, such as Meige syndrome in which patients also suffer from involuntary contractures of the muscles around the mouth. Oral drug treatment as used for dystonias in general (see p.1173) is usually ineffective, and surgery (facial nerve avulsion) is often followed by recurrent spasm.[1] Local injections of botulinum A toxin into the orbicularis oculi muscle mimic the effect of surgical denervation of the muscle and are reported[2-4] to have been effective in over 70% of patients, although there appear to be few controlled studies.[5] Symptomatic improvement has been reported to last from about 9 to 15 weeks; no increase in duration of effect is apparent following multiple injections. In one retrospective study in patients with blepharospasm and Meige syndrome, treatment with botulinum A toxin was still effective in most patients 11 years after the start of therapy.[4]

Doses of botulinum A toxin are expressed in terms of units, which have not been standardised between preparations. Doses are therefore *specific to each individual preparation*. For blepharospasm botulinum A toxin is injected into the orbicularis oculi of the upper and lower lids; injection into additional sites in the brow area and upper facial area may be indicated if the spasms interfere with vision. In the UK *the preparation Botox* is injected intramuscularly in an initial dose of 1.25 to 2.50 units at each site to a total of up to 25 units per eye. An effect is usually obtained within 3 days and reaches a peak after 1 to 2 weeks; each treatment lasts for about 3 months. If the response lasts less than 2 months the dose may be increased to 5 units at each site but the total dose administered in a 12-week period should not exceed 100 units. Administration more frequently than every 3 months confers no additional benefit. For *the preparation Dysport* the initial dose is a total of 120 units per eye given as subcutaneous injections of 20 or 40 units per site. Subsequently the total dose may need to be reduced to 60 to 80 units per eye. With this preparation the relief of symptoms may begin within 2 to 4 days with a maximum effect being obtained within 2 weeks. Injections of Dysport may need to be repeated every 8 weeks.

1. Kennedy RH, *et al.* Treatment of blepharospasm with botulinum toxin. *Mayo Clin Proc* 1989; **64**: 1085–90.
2. Grandas F. Blepharospasm: a review of 264 patients. *J Neurol Neurosurg Psychiatry* 1988; **51**: 767–72.
3. Elston JS. The management of blepharospasm and hemifacial spasm. *J Neurol* 1992; **239**: 5–8.
4. Mauriello JA, *et al.* Treatment selections of 239 patients with blepharospasm and Meige syndrome over 11 years. *Br J Ophthalmol* 1996; **80**: 1073–6.
5. Jankovic J, Orman J. Botulinum A toxin for cranial-cervical dystonia: a double blind, placebo-controlled study. *Neurology* 1987; **37**: 616–23.

Cosmetic use. Botulinum A toxin has been used for the cosmetic treatment of facial lines and wrinkles and age-related neck degeneration.[1-3]

1. Olver JM. Botulinum toxin A treatment of overactive corrugator supercilii in thyroid eye disease. *Br J Ophthalmol* 1998; **82**: 528–33.
2. Song KH. Botulinum toxin type A injection for the treatment of frown lines. *Ann Pharmacother* 1998 **32**: 1365–7.
3. Anonymous. Cosmetic use of botulinum toxin. *Med Lett Drugs Ther* 1999; **41**: 63–4.

Hand dystonia. Hand dystonia, or hand cramp, is a type of focal dystonia (p.1173). It is more commonly reported in people who perform repetitive movements with their hands, such as writers, keyboard operators, and musicians. Treatment has usually been with antimuscarinics, although with limited success. A double-blind study reported that 8 out of 10 patients had greater subjective improvement in focal hand dystonia, compared with placebo, after treatment with botulinum A toxin given by the intramuscular route; objective improvement in muscle strength was seen in 6 patients.[1] However, pain and severe weakness in the shoulder region resembling neuralgic amyotrophy has been reported[2] in 2 patients injected with botulinum A toxin for writer's cramp. It was considered that if unexplained pain occurred in the shoulder or upper arm after a first injection of botulinum A toxin further injections were contra-indicated.

1. Cole R, *et al.* Double-blind trial of botulinum toxin for treatment of focal hand dystonia. *Mov Disord* 1995; **10**: 466–71.
2. Sheean GL, *et al.* Pain and remote weakness in limbs injected with botulinum toxin A for writer's cramp. *Lancet* 1995; **346**: 154–6.

Headache. Pericranial injection of botulinum A toxin has shown promise[1] in the prophylactic treatment of migraine (p.449) although equivocal results[2,3] have been obtained in tension-type headache (p.450). Chronic cervical-associated headache following whiplash injury responded favourably to cervical injections.[4]

1. Silberstein S, *et al.* Botulinum toxin type A as a migraine preventive treatment. *Headache* 2000; **40**: 445–50.
2. Porta M. A comparative trial of botulinum toxin type A and methylprednisolone for the treatment of tension-type headache. *Curr Rev Pain* 2000; **4**: 31–5.

The symbol † denotes a preparation no longer actively marketed

3. Rollnik JD, *et al.* Treatment of tension-type headache with botulinum toxin type A: a double-blind, placebo-controlled study. *Headache* 2000; **40:** 300–305.
4. Freund B, Schwartz M. Treatment of chronic cervical-associated headache with botulinum toxin A: a pilot study. *Headache* 2000; **40:** 231–6.

Hemifacial spasm. Hemifacial spasm is characterised by involuntary unilateral synchronous contractions of muscles innervated by the facial nerve. The spasms usually begin with twitching of muscles around the eye or mouth but as the disease progresses their frequency increases and they spread to involve the rest of the facial muscles. Hemifacial spasm may be improved by surgery but there is a risk of irreversible paralysis. Few drugs are effective for hemifacial spasm but carbamazepine has been reported to have been of help on occasions. Reports suggest that injections of botulinum A toxin may be effective in relieving symptoms in about 75% of patients but there do not appear to be any studies comparing it against other treatments. Repeat injections are required by most patients every 3 to 4 months but long-term efficacy appears to be maintained. Dosage regimens of botulinum A toxin used in hemifacial spasm are similar to those used for blepharospasm (see above) although an electromyographically guided needle may be required to identify small muscles around the mouth.

References.
1. Elston JS. The management of blepharospasm and hemifacial spasm. *J Neurol* 1992; **239:** 5–8.
2. Chen R-S, *et al.* Botulinum toxin A injection in the treatment of hemifacial spasm. *Acta Neurol Scand* 1996; **94:** 207–11.

Hyperhidrosis. A number of drugs and surgical techniques have been used in the treatment of hyperhidrosis (p.1105). Botulinum A toxin is used in the management of focal hyperhidrosis because of its ability to block cholinergic transmission at nerve terminals innervating the sweat glands. Encouraging results have been obtained in patients with severe resistant focal hyperhidrosis using intradermal[1] or subcutaneous[2,3] injections and results from a larger multicentre study[4] confirm that intradermal injection of botulinum A is effective and well-tolerated for the treatment of axillary hyperhidrosis. In the UK, it is given for this purpose *as the preparation Botox*, by intradermal injection in doses of 50 units to each axilla, evenly distributed in multiple sites approximately 1 to 2 cm apart. Clinical improvement generally occurs within a week of injection, and may last for 4 to 7 months; repeat injections may be given once the effects of the previous injection have subsided. Some workers[5] prefer to use intradermal injections for palmar hyperhidrosis in order to minimise the risk of reversible weakness of the small muscles of the hand reported with subcutaneous injection.

1. Naumann M, *et al.* Focal hyperhidrosis: effective treatment with intracutaneous botulinum toxin. *Arch Dermatol* 1998; **134:** 301–4.
2. Schnider P, *et al.* Double-blind trial of botulinum A toxin for the treatment of focal hyperhidrosis of the palms. *Br J Dermatol* 1997; **136:** 548–52.
3. Schnider P, *et al.* Uses of botulinum toxin. *Lancet* 1997; **349:** 953.
4. Heckmann M, *et al.* Botulinum toxin A for axillary hyperhidrosis (excessive sweating). *N Engl J Med* 2001; **344:** 488–93.
5. Heckmann M, *et al.* Optimizing botulinum toxin therapy for hyperhidrosis. *Br J Dermatol* 1998; **138:** 553–4.

Laryngeal dystonias. Botulinum A toxin has been tried in the treatment of spasmodic dysphonia,[1,2] focal laryngeal dystonia,[3] and dysfunctional spasm following total laryngectomy.[4]

1. Ludlow CL. Treatment of speech and voice disorders with botulinum toxin. *JAMA* 1990; **264:** 2671–5.
2. Liu TC, *et al.* Prospective study of patients' subjective responses to botulinum toxin injection for spasmodic dysphonia. *J Otolaryngol* 1996; **25:** 66–74.
3. Marion M-H, *et al.* Stridor and focal laryngeal dystonia. *Lancet* 1992; **339:** 457–8.
4. Crary MA, *et al.* Using botulinum toxin A to improve speech and swallowing function following total laryngectomy. *Arch Otolaryngol Head Neck Surg* 1996; **122:** 760–3.

Nystagmus. Nystagmus is characterised by an involuntary, rapid, rhythmic movement of the eyeball. Various treatments including surgery, corrective spectacles, and drug therapy have been tried but none appears to be ideal. Retrobulbar injection of botulinum A toxin was associated with an improvement in visual acuity when tried in 6 patients with acquired nystagmus and debilitating symptoms such as oscillopsia (oscillating vision).[1] The amplitude of the nystagmus was reduced but the frequency was generally unchanged. However, the need for repeated injections and adverse effects such as diplopia limited patient acceptability.

1. Repka MX, *et al.* Treatment of acquired nystagmus with botulinum neurotoxin A. *Arch Ophthalmol* 1994; **112:** 1320–4.

Ocular surgery. Ptosis is a common adverse effect of botulinum A toxin (see Adverse Effects, above). Therapeutic ptosis induced with botulinum toxin may be a useful adjunct in the management of patients undergoing epikeratoplasty since it promotes stabilisation of the epithelium on the graft.[1]

1. Freegard T, *et al.* Therapeutic ptosis with botulinum toxin in epikeratoplasty. *Br J Ophthalmol* 1993; **77:** 820–2.

Pain. There have been anecdotal reports of the use of botulinum A toxin in the treatment of painful disorders such as post-cholecystectomy pain associated with sphincter of Oddi dysfunction,[1] and relief of orofacial pain associated with temporomandibular joint dysfunction[2] and facial arthromyalgia.[3] Promising results have been obtained from an open study[4]

investigating botulinum toxin as a treatment for chronic refractory tennis elbow in 14 patients. The general management of pain is discussed on p.2 with separate sections on biliary and renal colic (p.5), orofacial pain (p.7), postoperative analgesia (p.4), and soft-tissue rheumatism (p.10).

1. Pasricha PJ, *et al.* Intrasphincteric injection of botulinum toxin for suspected sphincter of Oddi dysfunction. *Gut* 1994; **35:** 1319–21.
2. Girdler NM. Use of botulinum toxin to alleviate facial pain. *Br J Hosp Med* 1994; **52:** 363.
3. Girdler NM. Uses of botulinum toxin. *Lancet* 1997; **349:** 953.
4. Morré HHE, *et al.* Treatment of chronic tennis elbow with botulinum toxin. *Lancet* 1997; **349:** 1746.

Spasmodic torticollis. Spasmodic torticollis (cervical dystonia) is a focal dystonia (p.1173) characterised by spasmodic rotation of the head as a result of dystonic spasm of the neck muscles. The head may turn to one side (torticollis), extend (retrocollis), or flex (antecollis). Spasms may be repetitive or sustained. Response of spasmodic torticollis to drug therapy is usually poor and surgery has been associated with potentially serious complications. Intramuscular injections of botulinum toxins have been shown to be effective but dysphagia, which can have severe consequences (see under Adverse Effects, above) occurs in a significant number of patients. Other side-effects have included lethargy, local weakness, vertigo, and dysphonia.

When injecting botulinum toxins localisation of the involved muscles with electromyographic guidance may be useful. Multiple injection sites allow more uniform contact with the innervation areas of the dystonic muscle and are especially useful in larger muscles. Bilateral injection of the sternocleidomastoid muscle is not recommended as there is an increased risk of adverse effects, especially dysphagia. Reduced doses may be required for patients with reduced muscle mass.

Doses of botulinum toxins, which are expressed in terms of units, have not been standardised between preparations. Doses are therefore *specific to each individual preparation.*

In the UK the usual initial dose of botulinum A toxin *as the preparation Dysport* is 500 units injected in divided doses into the two or three most active neck muscles.

- For *rotational torticollis*, 350 units is given initially into the splenius capitis muscle (ipsilateral to the direction of the chin/head rotation) and 150 units into the sternocleidomastoid muscle (contralateral to rotation).
- For *laterocollis*, 350 units is given initially into the ipsilateral splenius capitis muscle and 150 units into the ipsilateral sternocleidomastoid muscle; if associated with *shoulder elevation*, ipsilateral trapezoid or levator scapulae muscles may also require treatment; if 3 muscles need treatment, 300 units are injected into the splenius capitis muscle, 100 units into the sternocleidomastoid muscle, and 100 units into the third muscle.
- For *retrocollis*, 250 units is given into each of the splenius capitis muscles which may be followed after 6 weeks by bilateral trapezius injections in a dose of up to 250 units per muscle; bilateral splenii injections may increase the risk of neck muscle weakness.

Subsequent doses may range from 250 to 1000 units, although the higher doses may be accompanied by an increase in adverse effects such as dysphagia; doses above 1000 units are not recommended. An initial effect is usually observed within 1 week; injections usually need to be repeated every 8 to 12 weeks.

Recommended doses in the UK for botulinum A toxin *as the preparation Botox* are listed below but the manufacturer has stated that in practice the maximum total dose is not usually more than 200 units. No more than 50 units should be given at any one injection site; limiting the dose injected into the sternocleidomastoid muscle to less than 100 units may reduce the risk of dysphagia.

- *Type I* (head rotated toward side of shoulder elevation)—sternocleidomastoid muscle: total dosage of 50 to 100 units divided amongst at least 2 sites; levator scapulae: total of 50 units amongst 1 to 2 sites; scalene: total of 25 to 50 units amongst 1 to 2 sites; splenius capitis: total of 25 to 75 units amongst 1 to 3 sites; trapezius: total of 25 to 100 units amongst 1 to 8 sites.
- *Type II* (head rotation only)—sternocleidomastoid muscle: total dosage of 25 to 100 units divided amongst at least 2 sites if more than 25 units is given.
- *Type III* (head tilted toward side of shoulder elevation)—sternocleidomastoid muscle: total dosage of 25 to 100 units at posterior border divided amongst at least 2 sites if more than 25 units is given; levator scapulae: total of 25 to 100 units amongst at least 2 sites; scalene: total of 25 to 75 units amongst at least 2 sites; trapezius: total of 25 to 100 units amongst 1 to 8 sites.
- *Type IV* (bilateral posterior cervical muscle spasm with elevation of the face)—splenius capitis and splenius cervicis: a total dosage of 50 to 200 units divided amongst 2 to 8 sites and which include both sides of the neck.

In the UK the usual initial dose of botulinum B toxin *as the preparation NeuroBloc* is 5000 to 10 000 units given by intramuscular injection in divided doses into the two to four most affected muscles.

References.
1. Blackie JD, Lees AJ. Botulinum toxin treatment in spasmodic torticollis. *J Neurol Neurosurg Psychiatry* 1990; **53:** 640–3.

2. Greene P, *et al.* Double-blind, placebo-controlled trial of botulinum toxin injections for the treatment of spasmodic torticollis. *Neurology* 1990; **40:** 1213–18.
3. Anderson TJ, *et al.* Botulinum toxin treatment of spasmodic torticollis. *J R Soc Med* 1992; **85:** 524–9.
4. Brans JWM, *et al.* Botulinum toxin versus trihexyphenidyl in cervical dystonia: a prospective, randomized, double-blind controlled trial. *Neurology* 1996; **46:** 1066–72.
5. Brin MF, *et al.* Safety and efficacy of NeuroBloc (botulinum toxin type B) in type A-resistant cervical dystonia. *Neurology* 1999; **53:** 1431–8.
6. Brashear A, *et al.* Safety and efficacy of NeuroBloc (botulinum toxin B) in type A-resistant cervical dystonia. *Neurology* 1999; **53:** 1439–46.

Spasticity. The mainstay of management of spasticity, as discussed on p.1322, is physiotherapy together with antispastic drugs. Chemical neurolysis should only be considered when there is intractable continuous pain. Local injections of botulinum A toxin, as an alternative to chemical neurolysis, have been of benefit in the management of limb spasticity in poststroke patients[1-3] and children with cerebral palsy.[4-7]

In the UK, botulinum A toxin is used in the management of dynamic equinus foot deformity associated with spasticity in children with cerebral palsy. For children over 2 years of age the recommended total dose of botulinum A toxin *as the preparation Botox* is 4 units per kg body-weight injected into each of 2 sites in the medial and lateral heads of the gastrocnemius muscle. When both lower limbs are to be injected on the same occasion this total dose should be divided between the 2 limbs. Clinical improvement generally occurs within the first 2 weeks. Repeat doses should not be given more frequently than every 2 months. For children over 2 years of age the recommended total dose of botulinum A toxin *as the preparation Dysport* is 10 to 30 units per kg body-weight divided between both calf muscles, primarily targeted to the gastrocnemius muscle. The maximum dose administered should not exceed 1000 units per patient. Clinical improvement generally occurs within the first 2 weeks. Repeat doses should not be given more frequently than every 8 weeks.

1. Simpson DM, *et al.* Botulinum toxin type A in the treatment of upper extremity spasticity: a randomized, double-blind, placebo-controlled trial. *Neurology* 1996; **46:** 1306–10.
2. Bhakta BB, *et al.* Use of botulinum toxin in stroke patients with severe upper limb spasticity. *J Neurol Neurosurg Psychiatry* 1996; **61:** 30–5.
3. Burbaud P, *et al.* A randomised, double blind, placebo controlled trial of botulinum toxin in the treatment of spastic foot in hemiparetic patients. *J Neurol Neurosurg Psychiatry* 1996; **61:** 265–9.
4. Zelnik N, *et al.* The role of botulinum toxin in the treatment of lower limb spasticity in children with cerebral palsy—a pilot study. *Isr J Med Sci* 1997; **33:** 129–33.
5. Carr LJ, *et al.* Position paper on the use of botulinum toxin in cerebral palsy. *Arch Dis Child* 1998; **79:** 271–3.
6. Fehlings D, *et al.* An evaluation of botulinum-A toxin injections to improve upper extremity function in children with hemiplegic cerebral palsy. *J Pediatr* 2000; **137:** 331–7.
7. Ubhi T, *et al.* Randomised double blind placebo controlled trial of the effect of botulinum toxin on walking in cerebral palsy. *Arch Dis Child* 2000; **83:** 481–7.

Stiff-man syndrome. Report[1] of a patient with stiff-man syndrome (p.681) who had marked improvement of ambulation and cessation of pain following injection of botulinum A toxin into affected paraspinal muscles.

1. Davis D, Jabbari B. Significant improvement of stiff-person syndrome after paraspinal injection of botulinum toxin A. *Mov Disord* 1993; **8:** 371–3.

Strabismus. Botulinum A toxin has been used to weaken overactive extra-ocular muscles as an alternative or adjunct to surgery in the correction of strabismus (p.1414). Not all patients respond to botulinum A toxin and many patients who do respond require more than one injection to maintain improvement. Botulinum A toxin does not appear to offer a better degree of correction than traditional surgery, and it has been suggested that it should be reserved for use in patients unresponsive to, or unsuitable for, surgery. In the USA botulinum A toxin *as the preparation Botox* is indicated for the treatment of strabismus in patients 12 years of age or older. Depending on the direction and degree of deviation to be corrected the recommended initial dose of Botox to be injected into any one extra-ocular muscle ranges from 1.25 to 5.0 units. Paralysis is usually seen within the first 2 days and increases in intensity during the first week. The paralysis lasts for 2 to 6 weeks and gradually resolves over a further 2 to 6 weeks. It is recommended that patients are re-examined 7 to 14 days after injection to assess the effect of the dose given. If treatment is required for residual or recurrent strabismus, patients are either given treatment at the previous dosage if response is judged to have been adequate or up to twice the previous dose if paralysis had been incomplete. Repeat injections should not be administered until the effects of the previous dose have dissipated. No more than 25 units should be injected into any one muscle; the US manufacturer recommends that the cumulative dose in a 30-day period should not exceed 200 units. Injections should be diluted with 0.9% sodium chloride solution so that the volume administered is between 0.05 mL and 0.15 mL. Injections should also be made using an electromyographically guided needle to aid location of the target muscle.

References.
1. Biglan AW, *et al.* Management of strabismus with botulinum A toxin. *Ophthalmology* 1989; **96:** 935–43.
2. Carruthers JDA, *et al.* Botulinum vs adjustable suture surgery in the treatment of horizontal misalignment in adult patients lacking fusion. *Arch Ophthalmol* 1990; **108:** 1432–5.

3. Lyons CJ, *et al.* Botulinum toxin therapy in dysthyroid strabismus. *Eye* 1990; **4:** 538–42.
4. McNeer KW. An investigation of the clinical use of botulinum toxin A as a postoperative adjustment procedure in the therapy of strabismus. *J Pediatr Ophthalmol Strabismus* 1990; **27:** 3–9.
5. Scott AB, *et al.* Botulinum treatment of childhood strabismus. *Ophthalmology* 1990; **97:** 1434–8.
6. Petitto VB, Buckley EG. Use of botulinum toxin in strabismus after retinal detachment surgery. *Ophthalmology* 1991; **98:** 509–13.
7. Elston J. Is botulinum toxin helpful in squint management? *Br J Ophthalmol* 1998; **82:** 105.
8. Tejedor J, Rodríguez JM. Early retreatment of infantile esotropia: comparison of reoperation and botulinum toxin. *Br J Ophthalmol* 1999; **83:** 783–7.

Tourette's syndrome. Improvement in tics was noted in patients with Tourette's syndrome (see Tics, p.650) treated with botulinum A toxin.[1,2]

1. Kwak CH, *et al.* Botulinum toxin in the treatment of tics. *Arch Neurol* 2000; **57:** 1190–3.
2. Marras C, *et al.* Botulinum toxin for simple motor tics: a randomized, double-blind, controlled clinical trial. *Neurology* 2001; **56:** 605–10.

Tremor. Local injection of botulinum A toxin[1,2] has been tried in patients with essential tremor (p.848) that fails to respond to conventional treatment.

1. Henderson JM, *et al.* Botulinum toxin A in non-dystonic tremors. *Eur Neurol* 1996; **36:** 29–35.
2. Jankovic J, *et al.* A randomized, double-blind, placebo-controlled study to evaluate botulinum toxin type A in essential hand tremor. *Mov Disord* 1996; **11:** 250–6.

Urinary incontinence. Preliminary results[1] suggest that injection of botulinum A toxin into the detrusor muscle can increase functional bladder capacity and restore continence in patients with urinary incontinence (p.459) following spinal cord injury that is resistant to antimuscarinics.

1. Schurch B, *et al.* Botulinum-A toxin for treating detrusor hyperreflexia in spinal cord injured patients: a new alternative to anticholinergic drugs? Preliminary results. *J Urol (Baltimore)* 2000; **164:** 692–7.

Vaginismus. Report[1] of one patient who had relief of vaginismus (painful involuntary spasm of the vaginal or perianal muscles severe enough to prevent intercourse) for more than 24 months after injection of botulinum toxin into the vaginal wall muscles.

1. Brin MF, Vapnek JM. Treatment of vaginismus with botulinum toxin injections. *Lancet* 1997; **349:** 252–3.

Preparations

Proprietary Preparations (details are given in Part 3)
Aust.: Botox; Dysport; **Austral.:** Botox; Dysport; **Belg.:** Botox; Dysport; **Braz.:** Botox; **Canad.:** Botox; **Denm.:** Botox; Dysport; **Fin.:** Botox; Dysport; **Fr.:** Botox; Dysport; **Ger.:** Botox; Dysport; **Hong Kong:** Dysport; **Irl.:** Botox; Dysport; **Israel:** Botox; **Ital.:** Botox; Dysport; **Jpn:** Botox; **Mex.:** Botox; **Norw.:** Botox; **NZ:** Botox; Dysport; **S.Afr.:** Botox; **Singapore:** Botox; **Spain:** Botox; Dysport; **Swed.:** Botox; **Switz.:** Botox; **Thai.:** Botox; **UK:** Botox; Dysport; NeuroBloc; **USA:** Botox; Myobloc.

Carisoprodol (5704-k)

Carisoprodol (BAN, rINN).

Carisoprodolum; Isopropylmeprobamate. 2-Methyl-2-propyltrimethylene carbamate isopropylcarbamate.

$C_{12}H_{24}N_2O_4 = 260.3.$
$CAS — 78-44-4.$
$ATC — M03BA02.$

Pharmacopoeias. In *Eur.* (see p.vi) and *US*.

Pharmacopoeial description

Ph. Eur.: A white or almost white fine powder. M.p. 92° to 95°. Very slightly soluble in water; freely soluble in alcohol, in acetone, and in dichloromethane.

USP 25: A white crystalline powder having a mild characteristic odour. M.p. 91° to 94°. Soluble 1 in 2083 of water, 1 in 2.5 of alcohol and of acetone, and 1 in 2.3 of chloroform. Store in airtight containers.

Adverse Effects, Treatment, and Precautions

As for Meprobamate, p.691.

An idiosyncratic reaction may occur within minutes of a dose in patients who have not previously received carisoprodol. The symptoms, which include severe weakness and central disturbances, usually subside over several hours. There may be a short-lived quadriplegia. Cross reactivity can occur with its metabolite meprobamate.

Overdosage may result in stupor, coma, shock, respiratory depression, and rarely death.

It should be used with caution in patients with impaired hepatic or renal function. As carisoprodol is concentrated in breast milk, it is perhaps best avoided during breast feeding.

Carisoprodol may cause drowsiness, therefore patients affected should not drive or operate machinery.

Dependence. There has been a case report of carisoprodol dependence, probably due to its metabolism to meprobamate.[1] The patient experienced symptoms of meprobamate withdrawal which resolved with a dose-reducing schedule of meprobamate.

1. Luehr JG, *et al.* Mail-order (veterinary) drug dependence. *JAMA* 1990; **263:** 657.

Porphyria. Carisoprodol has been associated with acute attacks of porphyria and is considered unsafe in porphyric patients.

Interactions

The CNS effects of carisoprodol may be potentiated by alcohol or other CNS depressants.

Pharmacokinetics

Carisoprodol is absorbed from the gastrointestinal tract. It is metabolised in the liver and excreted in urine as metabolites, including meprobamate. It is distributed in substantial amounts into breast milk.

◊ References.

1. Olsen H, *et al.* Carisoprodol elimination in humans. *Ther Drug Monit* 1994; **16:** 337–40.

Uses and Administration

Carisoprodol is a centrally acting skeletal muscle relaxant whose mechanism of action is not completely understood but may be related to its sedative actions. Following administration by mouth its effects begin within about 30 minutes and last for 4 to 6 hours. It is used as an adjunct in the short-term symptomatic treatment of painful muscle spasm (p.1322) associated with musculoskeletal conditions. A usual dose is 350 mg given three to four times daily by mouth. Half the usual dose or less is recommended in elderly patients. It is also given with analgesics in compound preparations.

Headache. Carisoprodol is available in some countries in compound analgesic preparations for the treatment of tension-type headache (muscle-contraction headache), but results for muscle relaxants in general are disappointing and they appear to have little place in the management of tension-type headache (p.450).

Preparations

USP 25: Carisoprodol and Aspirin Tablets; Carisoprodol Tablets; Carisoprodol, Aspirin, and Codeine Phosphate Tablets.

Proprietary Preparations (details are given in Part 3)
Canad.: Soma; **Denm.:** Somadril; **Ger.:** Sanoma; **Mex.:** Dolaren; **Norw.:** Somadril; **Spain:** Mio Relax; Somalgit†; **Swed.:** Somadril; **Thai.:** Myolax; **UK:** Carisoma; **USA:** Soma.

Multi-ingredient: Braz.: Dorilax; Dorpinol; Dorserol; Mio-Citalgan; Mioflex; Mionevrix; Paceflex; Somaflex; Tandrilax; **Fin.:** Somadril Comp; **Ital.:** Flexidone†; Soma Complex; **Mex.:** Naxodol; Somalgesic; **Spain:** Flexagil; Relaxibys; **Swed.:** Somadril Comp; **Thai.:** Alaxan; Asialax; Cariso-Co; Carisoma Compound; Caritasone; Muscelax; Myophen; Polixan; **USA:** Sodol Compound; Soma Compound; Soma Compound with Codeine.

Chlorphenesin Carbamate (5705-a)

Chlorphenesin Carbamate (BANM, USAN, pINNM).

U-19646. 3-(4-Chlorophenoxy)propane-1,2-diol 1-carbamate.

$C_{10}H_{12}ClNO_4 = 245.7.$
$CAS — 104-29-0 (chlorphenesin); 886-74-8 (chlorphenesin carbamate).$

Pharmacopoeias. In *Jpn*.

Adverse Effects and Precautions

Chlorphenesin carbamate produces drowsiness and dizziness. There may also be nausea, headache, weakness, confusion, agitation, and insomnia. Hypersensitivity reactions have been reported. There are rare reports of blood disorders.

It should be used with caution in patients with hepatic impairment. Patients affected by drowsiness should not drive or operate machinery.

Interactions

The CNS effects of chlorphenesin carbamate may be potentiated by alcohol or other CNS depressants.

Pharmacokinetics

Chlorphenesin carbamate is readily and completely absorbed from the gastrointestinal tract and partly metabolised in the liver. It is excreted in the urine, mainly as the glucuronide.

Uses and Administration

Chlorphenesin carbamate is a centrally acting skeletal muscle relaxant related to mephenesin (p.1329). Its mode of action may be related to general depressant effects on the CNS. It is used as an adjunct in the symptomatic treatment of painful muscle spasm (p.1322) associated with musculoskeletal conditions. The usual initial dose is 800 mg three times daily given by mouth reduced to 400 mg four times daily or less once a response has been achieved. It has been recommended that chlorphenesin carbamate should not be administered for longer than 8 weeks.

Chlorphenesin base (p.381) is used as an antifungal.

Preparations

Proprietary Preparations (details are given in Part 3)
USA: Maolate.

Chlorzoxazone (5706-t)

Chlorzoxazone (BAN, rINN).

Chlorobenzoxazolinone. 5-Chlorobenzoxazol-2(3H)-one.
$C_7H_4ClNO_2 = 169.6.$
$CAS — 95-25-0.$
$ATC — M03BB03.$

Pharmacopoeias. In *US*.

Pharmacopoeial description

USP 25: A white or practically white, practically odourless, crystalline powder. Slightly soluble in water; sparingly soluble in alcohol, in isopropyl alcohol, and in methyl alcohol; soluble in solutions of alkali hydroxides and ammonia. Store in airtight containers.

Adverse Effects and Treatment

The most common side-effects of chlorzoxazone are drowsiness and dizziness. There may occasionally also be gastrointestinal irritation and gastrointestinal bleeding has been reported. Other effects that have occurred are headache, overstimulation, and rarely sensitivity reactions including skin rashes, petechiae, ecchymoses, urticaria and pruritus; very rarely, angioedema or anaphylactoid reactions may occur. Some patients taking chlorzoxazone have developed jaundice and liver damage suspected to be caused by the drug.

Following overdosage there may be gastrointestinal disturbances, drowsiness, dizziness, headache, malaise, and sluggishness followed by marked loss of muscle tone, hypotension, and respiratory depression. Treatment consists of emptying the stomach by lavage or emesis, followed by administration of activated charcoal and supportive therapy.

Effects on the liver. Hepatotoxicity, sometimes fatal, has been associated with chlorzoxazone treatment.[1]

1. Powers BJ, *et al.* Chlorzoxazone hepatotoxic reactions: an analysis of 21 identified or presumed cases. *Arch Intern Med* 1986; **146:** 1183–6.

Torticollis. There has been a report of a patient with a spasmodic torticollis-like syndrome, consisting of tonic deviation of the head to the right, clenching of the teeth, and dysarthria, which developed repeatedly within 2 hours of ingesting chlorzoxazone for low back pain.[1] Intravenous injection of benzatropine mesilate 1 mg gave rapid relief of symptoms.

1. Rosin MA. Chlorzoxazone-induced spasmodic torticollis. *JAMA* 1981; **246:** 2575.

Precautions

Chlorzoxazone should not be given to patients with impaired liver function and should be discontinued if signs of liver toxicity appear. Patients should be advised to report to their doctor any signs or symptoms of possible liver toxicity such as fever, rash, jaundice, dark urine, anorexia, nausea, vomiting, or right upper quadrant pain. Chlorzoxazone may cause drowsiness; patients affected should not drive or operate machinery.

The urine of patients taking chlorzoxazone may be coloured orange or reddish-purple by a phenolic metabolite.

Porphyria. Chlorzoxazone has been associated with acute attacks of porphyria and is considered unsafe in porphyric patients.

Interactions

The CNS effects of chlorzoxazone may be enhanced by alcohol and other CNS depressants.

Disulfiram. A study[1] of the efficacy of disulfiram as an inhibitor of the cytochrome P450 isoenzyme CYP2E1 (an enzyme involved in the metabolism of chlorzoxazone) found that a single 500-mg dose of disulfiram reduced plasma clearance of chlorzoxazone by 85%, resulting in a doubling of peak plasma concentrations and prolongation of chlorzoxazone's elimination half-life from a mean of 0.92 to 5.1 hours.

1. Kharasch ED, *et al.* Single-dose disulfiram inhibition of chlorzoxazone metabolism: a clinical probe for P450 2E1. *Clin Pharmacol Ther* 1993; **53:** 643–50.

Isoniazid. Isoniazid inhibited the clearance of chlorzoxazone by 56% when given to 10 slow acetylator subjects resulting in an increase in sedation, headache, and nausea.[1] Two days after discontinuation of isoniazid there had been a rebound increase in the clearance of chlorzoxazone by 56% over the pre-isoniazid clearance value. Similar but less pronounced effects have also been reported[2] in rapid acetylators with chlorzoxazone's pharmacokinetic parameters returning to baseline values in 2 days.

1. Zand R, *et al.* Inhibition and induction of cytochrome P4502E1-catalyzed oxidation by isoniazid in humans. *Clin Pharmacol Ther* 1993; **54:** 142–9.
2. O'Shea D, *et al.* Modulation of CYP2E1 activity by isoniazid in rapid and slow N-acetylators. *Br J Clin Pharmacol* 1997; **43:** 99–103.

Pharmacokinetics

Chlorzoxazone is reported to be completely absorbed after oral administration and peak plasma concentrations are achieved after 1 to 2 hours. It is rapidly metabolised in the liver, mainly to 6-hydroxychlorzoxazone, and excreted in the urine primarily as the glucuronide. The elimination half-life of chlorzoxazone is about 1 hour.

Uses and Administration

Chlorzoxazone is a centrally acting skeletal muscle relaxant with sedative properties. It is claimed to inhibit muscle spasm by exerting an effect primarily at the level of the spinal cord and subcortical areas of the brain. Following oral administration its effects begin within an hour and last for 3 to 4 hours.

It is used as an adjunct in the symptomatic treatment of painful muscle spasm (p.1322) associated with musculoskeletal conditions. The usual initial dose is 500 mg three or four times daily by mouth; the dose can often be reduced subsequently to 250 mg three or four times daily, although doses of up to 750 mg three or four times daily may be given if necessary. Chlorzoxazone is also given with analgesics in compound preparations.

Preparations

USP 25: Chlorzoxazone Tablets.

Proprietary Preparations (details are given in Part 3)
Denm.: Paraflex; **Hong Kong:** Solaxin; **S.Afr.:** Paraflex†; **Swed.:** Paraflex; **Thai.:** Chlorzox; **USA:** Paraflex; Parafon Forte DSC; Remular-S.
Multi-ingredient: Aust.: Parafon; **Canad.:** Acetazone Forte; Acetazone Forte C8; Back-Aid; Parafon Forte; Parafon Forte C8; Tylenol Aches & Strains; **Fin.:** Paraflex comp; **Hong Kong:** Relaxin-P; **Mex.:** Parafon Forte; Reumophan; **Swed.:** Paraflex comp; **Switz.:** Parafon†; Zafor†; **Thai.:** Cezox; Parafon; **USA:** Flexaphen.

Cyclobenzaprine Hydrochloride (5708-r)

Cyclobenzaprine Hydrochloride (USAN, rINNM).
MK-130 (cyclobenzaprine); Proheptatriene Hydrochloride; Ro-4-1557 (cyclobenzaprine); RP-9715 (cyclobenzaprine). 3-(5H-Dibenzo[a,d]cyclohepten-5-ylidene)-NN-dimethylpropylamine hydrochloride.
$C_{20}H_{21}N,HCl = 311.8$.
CAS — 303-53-7 (cyclobenzaprine); 6202-23-9 (cyclobenzaprine hydrochloride).
Pharmacopoeias. In US.

Pharmacopoeial description

USP 25: A white to off-white, odourless, crystalline powder. Freely soluble in water, in alcohol, and in methyl alcohol; sparingly soluble in isopropyl alcohol; slightly soluble in chloroform and in dichloromethane; insoluble in hydrocarbons.

Adverse Effects, Treatment, and Precautions

Cyclobenzaprine hydrochloride is structurally related to the tricyclic antidepressants and shares their adverse effects and precautions (see Amitriptyline, p.273).

It may cause drowsiness; patients affected should not drive or operate machinery.

Neuroleptic malignant syndrome. Report of a neuroleptic malignant-like syndrome associated with cyclobenzaprine in a 36-year-old man.[1] It was not clear whether the syndrome was due to an idiosyncratic reaction or to an overdose.

1. Theoharides TC, et al. Neuroleptic malignant-like syndrome due to cyclobenzaprine. J Clin Psychopharmacol 1995; **15:** 79–81.

Interactions

Cyclobenzaprine is structurally related to the tricyclic antidepressants and may be subject to similar interactions (see Amitriptyline, p.276). The CNS effects of cyclobenzaprine may be enhanced by alcohol or other CNS depressants.

◊ Report[1] of a patient with QT prolongation associated with concomitant use of cyclobenzaprine and *fluoxetine*. The patient developed torsade de pointes, progressing into ventricular fibrillation, when given *droperidol* as premedication prior to surgery. QT abnormalities resolved on discontinuation of cyclobenzaprine.

1. Michalets EL, et al. Torsade de pointes resulting from the addition of droperidol to an existing cytochrome P450 drug interaction. Ann Pharmacother 1998; **32:** 761–5.

Pharmacokinetics

Cyclobenzaprine hydrochloride is readily and almost completely absorbed from the gastrointestinal tract, although plasma concentrations vary considerably among individuals given the same dose. About 93% is bound to plasma proteins and has a reported elimination half-life of 1 to 3 days. It is extensively metabolised, principally to glucuronide conjugates, and excreted in the urine. Some unchanged drug appears in the bile and is excreted in the faeces.

Uses and Administration

Cyclobenzaprine hydrochloride is a centrally acting skeletal muscle relaxant, related to the tricyclic antidepressants. It acts mainly at the brain stem to decrease tonic somatic motor activity influencing both alpha and gamma motor systems. Additional activity at spinal cord sites may be involved. Following oral administration its effects begin within 1 hour; the effects of a single dose have been reported to last as long as 12 to 24 hours.

It is used as an adjunct in the symptomatic treatment of painful muscle spasm (p.1322) associated with musculoskeletal conditions. The usual dose is 10 mg three times daily given by mouth; the daily dose should not exceed 60 mg. Treatment for more than 2 or 3 weeks is not recommended.

◊ References.

1. Katz WA, Dube J. Cyclobenzaprine in the treatment of acute muscle spasm: review of a decade of clinical experience. Clin Ther 1988; **10:** 216–28.
2. Browning R, et al. Cyclobenzaprine and back pain: a meta-analysis. Arch Intern Med 2001; **161:** 1613–20.

Fibromyalgia. Studies of the efficacy of cyclobenzaprine in the management of fibromyalgia, a painful musculoskeletal disorder which usually responds poorly to analgesics, have produced conflicting results[1,2] but a small percentage of patients may obtain some relief.[2] In one study[2] involving 208 patients with fibromyalgia, improvement 1 month after starting treatment was shown in 21% of patients receiving amitriptyline, 12% of those receiving cyclobenzaprine, and in none of those given placebo. Although the percentage of patients with improvement had increased at the 3 and 6 month assessments, there was no longer a significant difference between the groups. Cyclobenzaprine had been given in an initial dosage of 10 mg at night and increased to 30 mg daily. An earlier study[3] found that 30 mg daily was not more effective than 10 mg at night but resulted in a higher incidence of adverse effects.

1. Reynolds WJ, et al. The effects of cyclobenzaprine on sleep physiology and symptoms in patients with fibromyalgia. J Rheumatol 1991; **18:** 452–4.
2. Carette S, et al. Comparison of amitriptyline, cyclobenzaprine, and placebo in the treatment of fibromyalgia: a randomized, double-blind clinical trial. Arthritis Rheum 1994; **37:** 32–40.
3. Santandrea S, et al. A double-blind crossover study of two cyclobenzaprine regimens in primary fibromyalgia syndrome. J Int Med Res 1993; **21:** 74–80.

Preparations

USP 25: Cyclobenzaprine Hydrochloride Tablets.

Proprietary Preparations (details are given in Part 3)
Canad.: Flexeril; Novo-Cycloprine; **Ital.:** Flexiban; **Port.:** Flexiban; **Spain:** Yurelax; **USA:** Flexeril.

Dantrolene Sodium (5709-f)

Dantrolene Sodium (BANM, USAN, rINNM).
F-440; F-368 (dantrolene). The hemiheptahydrate of the sodium salt of 1-[5-(4-nitrophenyl)furfurylideneamino]imidazolidine-2,4-dione.
$C_{14}H_9N_4NaO_5,3\frac{1}{2}H_2O = 399.3$.
CAS — 7261-97-4 (dantrolene); 14663-23-1 (anhydrous dantrolene sodium); 24868-20-0 (dantrolene sodium, hemiheptahydrate).
Pharmacopoeias. In Jpn.

Adverse Effects

Adverse effects associated with dantrolene sodium tend to occur at the start of treatment, but are often short lived and can be controlled by adjusting the dose. The most common side-effects are drowsiness, dizziness, fatigue, muscle weakness, and malaise. Diarrhoea may be severe enough to necessitate withdrawal. If diarrhoea recurs following reintroduction of dantrolene, then treatment should probably be stopped permanently. Other side-effects reported include nausea and vomiting, anorexia, constipation, abdominal cramps, gastrointestinal bleeding, tachycardia, unstable blood pressure, dyspnoea, rashes (often acneform), pruritus, chills and fever, headache, myalgia, nervousness, insomnia, confusion, visual disturbances, mental depression, dysphagia and speech disturbances, and seizures. Haematuria, crystalluria, urinary frequency and retention, and incontinence may occur. Rare but serious adverse effects include hepatotoxicity which may be fatal (see below) and pleural effusion with pericarditis.

Serious side-effects do not appear to be a problem with the short-term use of intravenous dantrolene sodium in the treatment of malignant hyperthermia.

Effects on the liver. Dantrolene has caused hepatotoxicity with raised liver enzyme values, jaundice, and hepatitis;[1-3] fatalities have been reported.[1,3] Not all patients experienced symptoms such as anorexia, nausea, or abdominal discomfort before the onset of disease and the severity of hepatic injury was unrelated to clinical presentation. In the first report[1] the 14 fatalities occurred with doses in excess of 200 mg daily; a later review[3] found the mean dose associated with 27 fatalities to be 582 mg daily, while reports of non-fatal liver toxicity (95 cases) were associated with a mean dose of 263 mg daily. The onset of hepatic injury was usually between 1 and 6 months after starting treatment and fatalities were not reported in the first 2 months. Only rarely did injury develop before 45 days of treatment. Females appeared to be at greater risk of serious liver injury and the severity of reaction appeared to be age-related with most fatalities occurring in patients over 30 years of age. The liver injury was usually hepatocellular and might include ascending cholangitis; there was little evidence of hypersensitivity.

1. Utili R, et al. Dantrolene-associated hepatic injury: incidence and character. Gastroenterology 1977; **72:** 610–16.
2. Wilkinson SP, et al. Hepatitis from dantrolene sodium. Gut 1979; **20:** 33–6.
3. Chan CH. Dantrolene sodium and hepatic injury. Neurology 1990; **40:** 1427–32.

Effects on the lungs. Pulmonary oedema associated with heart failure,[1] and pleural effusions with eosinophilia[2,3] have been reported rarely in patients receiving dantrolene. These reactions generally resolve on withdrawal of the drug but resolution may take several months; corticosteroid therapy may be of benefit in dantrolene-related eosinophilic pleural effusion.[3]

1. Robillart A, et al. Insuffisance cardiaque par surdosage en dantrolène. Ann Fr Anesth Reanim 1986; **5:** 617–19.
2. Mahoney JM, Bachtel MD. Pleural effusion associated with chronic dantrolene administration. Ann Pharmacother 1994; **28:** 587–9.
3. Felz MW, Haviland-Foley DJ. Eosinophilic pleural effusion due to dantrolene: resolution with steroid therapy. South Med J 2001; **94:** 502–4.

Lymphomas. Fatal lymphocytic lymphoma in one patient was associated with prolonged dantrolene therapy 600 mg daily for progressive spastic paraplegia.[1]

1. Wan HH, Tucker JS. Dantrolene and lymphocytic lymphoma. Postgrad Med J 1980; **56:** 261–2.

Precautions

It is recommended that dantrolene sodium should not be given to patients with active liver disease. Liver-function tests should be performed in all patients before and during treatment; if abnormal values are found, treatment should generally be discontinued. The risk of liver injury may be increased in patients over 30 years of age, in females (especially those taking oestrogens), and with doses above 400 mg per day (see under Effects on the Liver, above). Dantrolene sodium should be used with caution in patients with cardiac or pulmonary disorders. It should not be given to patients who use their spasticity to maintain posture or function or to patients with acute muscle spasm.

Dantrolene sodium may cause drowsiness; patients affected should not drive or operate machinery.

Interactions

The CNS effects of dantrolene sodium may be enhanced by alcohol or other CNS depressants. Concomitant administration with oestrogens may possibly increase the risk of liver damage.

Calcium-channel blockers. Severe hyperkalaemia and myocardial depression occurred following administration of dantrolene intravenously for prophylaxis of malignant hyperthermia in a patient also taking verapamil for angina.[1] The peak serum-potassium concentration was 7.1 mmol per litre 2.5 hours after the dantrolene infusion. Nifedipine was substituted for verapamil in a subsequent operation and only a small increase in serum potassium occurred following administration of dantrolene. Ventricular fibrillation and cardiovascular collapse associated with hyperkalaemia have been seen with this combination in *animal* studies, and the manufacturers recommend that calcium-channel blockers and intravenous dantrolene should not be used together.

1. Rubin AS, Zablocki AD. Hyperkalaemia, verapamil, and dantrolene. Anesthesiology 1987; **66:** 246–9.

Pharmacokinetics

Dantrolene sodium is slowly and incompletely absorbed from the gastrointestinal tract. It is metabolised in the liver mainly to the hydroxylated and acetamide metabolites, which have weak muscle relaxant activity. It is excreted in the urine, mainly as metabolites with a small amount of unchanged dantrolene; some is excreted in the bile. Dantrolene is bound extensively to plasma proteins. The elimination half-life following oral administration is about 9 hours.

Uses and Administration

Dantrolene sodium is a muscle relaxant with a direct action on skeletal muscle. It uncouples muscular contraction from excitation, probably by interfering with the release of calcium from the sarcoplasmic reticulum.

It has an important role when given by mouth, for the symptomatic relief of chronic, severe spasticity (p.1322) due to a variety of conditions. It is also given, usually by intravenous injection, for the treatment of malignant hyperthermia.

For **spasticity**, the initial dose is 25 mg daily by mouth increased gradually as necessary, at 7-day intervals, over about 7 weeks to a maximum dose of 100 mg four times daily. If no response is achieved within 45 days treatment should be discontinued. In the UK dantrolene is not recommended for use in children, but in the USA a suggested dose for children is 0.5 mg per kg body-weight once daily, increased gradually if necessary to 2 mg per kg three times daily; administration four times daily may be necessary for some children but a dose of 100 mg 4 times daily should not be exceeded.

In the treatment of **malignant hyperthermia**, dantrolene sodium is given, together with supportive measures, in an initial dose of 1 mg per kg body-weight by rapid intravenous injection, repeated, if necessary, to a total dose of 10 mg per kg. An average dose of 2.5 mg per kg is usually effective. If a relapse or recurrence occurs, dantrolene should be readministered at the last effective dose. In the USA, doses of 1 to 2 mg per kg by mouth 4 times daily have been recommended for up to 3 days after the crisis to prevent recurrence, and similar doses have been given for 1 to 2 days before surgery in individuals thought to be at risk of developing the syndrome. Prophylactic doses may also be given intravenously; 2.5 mg per kg has been recommended, infused over about 60 minutes, starting about 75 minutes before anticipated anaesthesia, with further administration during anaesthesia and surgery if signs of malignant hyperthermia develop.

Hyperthermia. Dantrolene is used in the treatment of hyperthermia associated with muscle rigidity and fulminant hypermetabolism of skeletal muscle which occurs in the neuroleptic malignant syndrome (see below and p.662) and in malignant hyperthermia (see below). There is also anecdotal evidence that dantrolene may produce beneficial effects for the treatment of similar symptoms resulting from poisoning with various agents such as carbon monoxide,[1] MAOIs,[2] and ethyltenamfetamine.[3] However, following suggestions that it may also be of use in cocaine intoxication, the manufacturers[4] warned physicians that they should not regard dantrolene as an effective treatment for all types of hyperthermia and rigidity accompanying poisoning.

Dantrolene may hasten cooling when used as part of treatment for heat stroke (see under Fever and Hyperthermia, p.8) but does not appear to affect outcome.[5]

1. Ten Holter JBM, Schellens RLLAM. Dantrolene sodium for treatment of carbon monoxide poisoning. *BMJ* 1988; **296:** 1772–3.
2. Kaplan RF, *et al.* Phenelzine overdose treatment with dantrolene sodium. *JAMA* 1986; **255:** 642–4.
3. Tehan B. Ecstasy and dantrolene. *BMJ* 1993; **306:** 146.
4. Fox AW. More on rhabdomyolysis associated with cocaine intoxication. *N Engl J Med* 1989; **321:** 1271.
5. Channa AB, *et al.* Is dantrolene effective in heat stroke patients? *Crit Care Med* 1990; **18:** 290–2.

MALIGNANT HYPERTHERMIA. Malignant hyperthermia (malignant hyperpyrexia) is a rare but potentially fatal syndrome associated with general anaesthesia. The aetiology is not completely understood but appears to be a disorder of muscle fibres in which a sudden increase in the concentration of calcium in muscle cytoplasm initiates a series of metabolic disturbances. The disorder appears to be genetically determined and is more common in males. In susceptible individuals a reaction may be induced by inhalation anaesthetics (mainly halogenated hydrocarbons), suxamethonium, prolonged anaesthesia, pre-operative exercise, muscle trauma, fever, or anxiety. However, many reactions occur in individuals who have had uneventful general anaesthesia previously. Early signs and symptoms of the syndrome include tachycardia, unstable blood pressure, hypercapnia, rising temperature, and hyperventilation followed by metabolic acidosis and hyperkalaemia. Muscle rigidity develops in many patients and later there may be evidence of muscle damage including raised serum concentrations of creatine phosphokinase and other enzymes, myoglobinaemia, and myoglobinuria. Hyperthermia develops relatively late. Other late complications may include renal failure, intravascular coagulopathy, and pulmonary oedema.

Treatment should be started as soon as possible after symptoms appear with dantrolene being given by rapid intravenous injection.[1,2] If symptoms reappear the regimen may be repeated. Supportive treatment must also be started including immediate withdrawal of anaesthesia, administration of oxygen, correction of acidosis with sodium bicarbonate, control of hyperkalaemia with insulin, and cooling procedures (see p.8). The incidence of reactions in susceptible individuals can be reduced by avoiding triggering agents. Prophylactic administration of dantrolene has also been used but one group of workers[3] who reported a high incidence of adverse effects in a small study of susceptible patients given dantrolene did not recommend its routine use. Susceptibility to malignant hyperthermia can be detected by histological examination of muscle fibres obtained by biopsy and study of their response to caffeine and/or halothane *in vitro*.

Dantrolene has been suggested[4] for use as a secondary drug in the treatment of a related and potentially fatal syndrome that

has developed in some children following induction of anaesthesia with halothane and suxamethonium (see also Children, under Precautions of Suxamethonium, p.1341).

1. Britt BA. Dantrolene. *Can Anaesth Soc J* 1984; **31:** 61–75.
2. Ward A, *et al.* Dantrolene: a review of its pharmacodynamic and pharmacokinetic properties and therapeutic use in malignant hyperthermia, the neuroleptic malignant syndrome and an update of its use in muscle spasticity. *Drugs* 1986; **32:** 130–68.
3. Wedel DJ, *et al.* Clinical effects of intravenously administered dantrolene. *Mayo Clin Proc* 1995; **70:** 241–6.
4. Rosenberg H, Gronert GA. Intractable cardiac arrest in children given succinylcholine. *Anesthesiology* 1992; **77:** 1054.

Neuroleptic malignant syndrome. Dantrolene has been used, usually alone or with bromocriptine, in the treatment of neuroleptic malignant syndrome (p.662), although some workers have not found it to be of use.[1] Doses reported for dantrolene have varied greatly.[2,3] For those patients unable to swallow and when rapid control of symptoms is required, doses of 1 mg or more per kg body-weight have been given initially by intravenous injection. Up to 600 mg has been given daily by mouth in divided doses.

1. Rosebush PI, *et al.* The treatment of neuroleptic malignant syndrome: are dantrolene and bromocriptine useful adjuncts to supportive care? *Br J Psychiatry* 1991; **159:** 709–12.
2. Ward A, *et al.* Dantrolene: a review of its pharmacodynamic and pharmacokinetic properties and therapeutic use in malignant hyperthermia, the neuroleptic malignant syndrome and an update of its use in muscle spasticity. *Drugs* 1986; **32:** 130–68.
3. Harpe C, Stoudemire A. Aetiology and treatment of neuroleptic malignant syndrome. *Med Toxicol* 1987; **2:** 166–76.

Preparations

Proprietary Preparations (details are given in Part 3)
Aust.: Dantamacrin; *Austral.:* Dantrium; *Belg.:* Dantrium; *Canad.:* Dantrium; *Denm.:* Dantrium; *Fr.:* Dantrium; *Ger.:* Dantamacrin; *Hong Kong:* Dantrium; *Irl.:* Dantrium; *Israel:* Dantrium; *Ital.:* Dantrium; *Neth.:* Dantrium; *NZ:* Dantrium; *Port.:* Dantrium; *S.Afr.:* Dantrium; *Switz.:* Dantamacrin; *UK:* Dantrium; *USA:* Dantrium.

Eperisone Hydrochloride   (16629-d)

Eperisone Hydrochloride (rINNM).
4'-Ethyl-2-methyl-3-piperidinopropiophenone hydrochloride.
$C_{17}H_{25}NO,HCl = 295.8$.
CAS — 64840-90-0 (eperisone).

Profile
Eperisone hydrochloride is a centrally acting skeletal muscle relaxant that has been given by mouth in the symptomatic treatment of muscle spasm (p.1322) and spasticity (p.1322). It may also have a vasodilator action.

Preparations

Proprietary Preparations (details are given in Part 3)
Jpn: Myonal; *Singapore:* Myonal; *Thai.:* Myonal.

Idrocilamide   (12842-t)

Idrocilamide (rINN).
LCB-29. N-(2-Hydroxyethyl)cinnamamide.
$C_{11}H_{13}NO_2 = 191.2$.
CAS — 6961-46-2.

Adverse Effects
When given by mouth idrocilamide was reported to produce abdominal pain, nausea, and drowsiness. Excitement, euphoria and hallucinations, and mental depression may occur.

Uses and Administration
Idrocilamide is a centrally acting muscle relaxant that has been given by mouth or intramuscular injection for the symptomatic treatment of painful muscle spasm associated with musculoskeletal conditions. It is reported to have local muscle relaxant and anti-inflammatory effects and is now mainly used topically.

Preparations

Proprietary Preparations (details are given in Part 3)
Belg.: Srilane; *Fr.:* Srilane; *Hong Kong:* Srilane; *Switz.:* Talval.

Mephenesin   (5722-t)

Mephenesin (BAN, rINN).
Cresoxydiol; Glykresin. 3-(o-Tolyloxy)propane-1,2-diol.
$C_{10}H_{14}O_3 = 182.2$.
CAS — 59-47-2.
ATC — M03BX06.
Pharmacopoeias. In It.

Adverse Effects
Given by mouth, mephenesin may produce lassitude, drowsiness, weakness, loss of appetite, nausea, and vomiting. Allergic reactions may rarely occur. Overdosage may produce visual disturbances, motor incoordination, hypotonia, a fall in blood pressure, and respiratory paralysis.

Precautions
Mephenesin may cause drowsiness; patients affected should not drive or operate machinery.

Porphyria. Mephenesin is considered to be unsafe in patients with porphyria because it has been shown to be porphyrinogenic in *in-vitro* systems.

Interactions
The CNS effects of mephenesin may be enhanced by alcohol or other CNS depressants.

Pharmacokinetics
Mephenesin is readily absorbed from the gastrointestinal tract and distributed throughout most tissues of the body. It is metabolised mainly in the liver and excreted in urine as metabolites and a small amount of unchanged drug.

Uses and Administration
Mephenesin is a centrally acting skeletal muscle relaxant used for the symptomatic treatment of painful muscle spasm (p.1322) associated with musculoskeletal conditions. Its clinical usefulness is considered to be limited by its brief duration of action. It is given by mouth in doses of 1.5 to 3 g daily in divided doses. It is also applied topically, usually with rubefacients.

Preparations

Proprietary Preparations (details are given in Part 3)
Fr.: Decontractyl; *Ger.:* DoloVisano M.

Multi-ingredient: *Belg.:* Algipan; Decontractyl†; *Canad.:* Decontractyl†; *Fr.:* Algipan; Decontractyl; Traumalgyl; *Ital.:* Relaxar; *S.Afr.:* Spasmend.

Metaxalone   (5724-r)

Metaxalone (BAN, USAN, rINN).
AHR-438. 5-(3,5-Xylyloxymethyl)oxazolidin-2-one.
$C_{12}H_{15}NO_3 = 221.3$.
CAS — 1665-48-1.

Adverse Effects, Treatment, and Precautions
As for Chlorzoxazone, p.1327.

Metaxalone may cause drowsiness; patients affected should not drive or operate machinery.

Patients taking metaxalone excrete in the urine a metabolite which gives a false positive reaction to copper sulfate-based tests for glycosuria.

Interactions
The CNS effects of metaxalone may be enhanced by alcohol and other CNS depressants.

Pharmacokinetics
Metaxalone is absorbed from the gastrointestinal tract, metabolised in the liver, and excreted in urine as metabolites. The plasma elimination half-life is about 2 to 3 hours.

Uses and Administration
Metaxalone is a centrally acting skeletal muscle relaxant. Its mode of action may be related to its sedative properties.

It is used as an adjunct in the symptomatic treatment of painful muscle spasm (p.1322) associated with musculoskeletal conditions. The usual dose is 800 mg three or four times daily by mouth.

Preparations

Proprietary Preparations (details are given in Part 3)
USA: Skelaxin.

Methocarbamol   (5725-f)

Methocarbamol (BAN, rINN).
Guaiphenesin Carbamate. 2-Hydroxy-3-(2-methoxyphenoxy)propyl carbamate.
$C_{11}H_{15}NO_5 = 241.2$.
CAS — 532-03-6.
ATC — M03BA03.
Pharmacopoeias. In US.

Pharmacopoeial description
USP 25: A white powder, odourless or having a slight characteristic odour. M.p. about 94° or, if previously ground to a fine powder, about 90°. Soluble 1 in 40 of water at 20°; sparingly soluble in chloroform; soluble in alcohol only with heating; insoluble in *n*-hexane and in benzene. Store in airtight containers.

Adverse Effects
Side-effects reported with methocarbamol include nausea, anorexia, lightheadedness, dizziness, lassitude, drowsiness, restlessness, anxiety, confusion, blurred vision, fever, headache, convulsions, and hypersensitivity reactions including rashes, pruritus, urticaria, angioedema, and conjunctivitis with nasal congestion.

After injection patients may experience flushing and a metallic taste; incoordination, diplopia, nystagmus, vertigo, syncope, hypotension, bradycardia, and anaphylaxis have been reported. There may be sloughing and thrombophlebitis at the site of injection.

Precautions
Methocarbamol is contra-indicated in coma or pre-coma states, brain damage, myasthenia gravis, or in patients with a history of epilepsy. Caution is advisable in renal or hepatic impairment. Methocarbamol may cause drowsiness; patients affected should not drive or operate machinery.

The symbol † denotes a preparation no longer actively marketed

Preparations for injection may contain, as a solvent, a macrogol which could increase existing acidosis and urea retention in patients with renal impairment; such preparations should not be used in patients with known or suspected renal disease.

◊ Methocarbamol has been reported to cause brown to black or green discoloration of the urine on standing.[1]

1. Baran RB, Rowles B. Factors affecting coloration of urine and feces. *J Am Pharm Assoc* 1973; **NS13:** 139–42.

Interactions
The CNS effects of methocarbamol may be potentiated by alcohol or other CNS depressants. Methocarbamol has also been reported to potentiate the effects of anorectics and antimuscarinics.

Pharmacokinetics
Methocarbamol is rapidly and almost completely absorbed from the gastrointestinal tract following oral administration. Its plasma half-life is reported to be about 1 to 2 hours. It is metabolised by dealkylation and hydroxylation and is excreted in urine primarily as the glucuronide and sulfate conjugates of its metabolites. A small amount is excreted in faeces.

Uses and Administration
Methocarbamol is a centrally acting skeletal muscle relaxant whose action may be due to general depressant effects on the CNS.

Methocarbamol is used as an adjunct in the short-term symptomatic treatment of painful muscle spasm (p.1322) associated with musculoskeletal conditions. It is sometimes given with analgesics in compound preparations for the treatment of musculoskeletal pain.

The usual initial dose by mouth for muscle spasm is 1.5 g four times daily, reduced to a maintenance dose of about 4 g daily after 2 to 3 days. A dose of 750 mg three times daily may be sufficient for a therapeutic effect. Half the maximum daily dose or less may be sufficient for elderly patients.

Methocarbamol has also been given intravenously at a rate of not more than 300 mg per minute, by slow injection or by infusion in sodium chloride or glucose injection. The parenteral route should not be used for more than 3 consecutive days and the dose should not exceed 3 g daily. The patient should remain lying down during, and for 10 to 15 minutes after, intravenous administration. The manufacturers state that the injection is hypertonic and extravasation should be avoided. However, it may also be given by intramuscular injection in a dose of up to 500 mg into each gluteal region at intervals of 8 hours.

Preparations
USP 25: Methocarbamol Injection; Methocarbamol Tablets.

Proprietary Preparations (details are given in Part 3)
Canad.: Robaxin; *Fin.:* Robaxin; *Fr.:* Lumirelax; *Ger.:* Ortoton; *Hong Kong:* Robaxin; *Mex.:* Labycarbol; Robaxin; *S.Afr.:* Robaxin; *Spain:* Robaxin; *Swed.:* Robaxin; *Thai.:* Laxan; Mebaxin; Muscan; Myocin; Myomethol; *UK:* Robaxin; *USA:* Robaxin.

Multi-ingredient: *Canad.:* Aspirin Backache; Methoxacet; Methoxacet-C; Methoxisal; Methoxisal-C; Muscle & Back Pain Relief; Robaxacet; Robaxacet-8; Robaxisal; Robaxisal-C; *Ger.:* Ortoton Plus; *Irl.:* Robaxisal†; *Mex.:* Carbager-Plus; Malival Compuesto; Robaxifen; Robaxisal; *S.Afr.:* Robaxisal; *Spain:* Robaxisal; Robaxisal Compuesto; *Swed.:* Robaxisal Forte; *Thai.:* Sancago; *UK:* Robaxisal Forte†; *USA:* Robaxisal.

Pridinol Mesilate (5729-m)

Pridinol Mesilate *(rINNM)*.

C-238 (pridinol); Pridinol Mesylate. 1,1-Diphenyl-3-piperidino-propan-1-ol methanesulphonate.

$C_{20}H_{25}NO,CH_3SO_3H = 391.5$.

CAS — 511-45-5 (pridinol); 968-58-1 (pridinol hydrochloride); 6856-31-1 (pridinol mesilate).

Profile
Pridinol mesilate is a centrally acting muscle relaxant used in the symptomatic treatment of muscle spasm (p.1322). The usual initial dose by mouth is 2 to 8 mg three times daily, reduced to 4 to 8 mg daily for maintenance treatment. It is also given by intramuscular injection or rectally, and has been applied in compound topical preparations.

Pridinol is used as the hydrochloride for its antimuscarinic properties in the management of parkinsonism (p.1160).

Preparations
Proprietary Preparations (details are given in Part 3)
Ger.: Lyseen†; Myoson; Parks; *Hong Kong:* Konlax; *Ital.:* Lyseen; *Thai.:* Konlax.
Multi-ingredient: *Ital.:* Algolisina.

Thiocolchicoside (13324-v)

Thiocolchicoside *(rINN)*.

3,10-Di(demethoxy)-3-glucopyranosyloxy-10-methylthiocolchicine.

$C_{27}H_{33}NO_{10}S = 563.6$.

CAS — 602-41-5.
ATC — M03BX05.

Pharmacopoeias. In Fr.

Profile
Thiocolchicoside is a muscle relaxant which has been claimed to possess GABA-mimetic and glycinergic actions. It is used in the symptomatic treatment of painful muscle spasm (p.1322). The usual initial dose is 16 mg daily by mouth. It has also been given intramuscularly, in doses up to 8 mg daily, or applied as cream or ointment. Photosensitivity reactions may occur.

Preparations
Proprietary Preparations (details are given in Part 3)
Braz.: Coltrax; *Fr.:* Coltramyl; Miorel; Myoplege; *Ital.:* Muscoril; *Port.:* Coltramyl; Relmus.

Multi-ingredient: *Ital.:* Tioscina†; *Mex.:* Neuroflax; *Port.:* Adalgur N; Relmus Compositum; *Spain:* Adalgur; Liviane Compuesto†.

Tizanidine Hydrochloride (13357-j)

Tizanidine Hydrochloride *(BANM, USAN, rINNM)*.
AN-021; DS-103-282; DS-103-282-ch. 5-Chloro-N-(2-imidazolin-2-yl)-2,1,3-benzothiadiazol-4-ylamine hydrochloride.

$C_9H_8CIN_5S,HCl = 290.2$.

CAS — 51322-75-9 (tizanidine); 64461-82-1 (tizanidine hydrochloride).

Tizanidine hydrochloride 1.14 mg is approximately equivalent to 1 mg of tizanidine.

Adverse Effects and Precautions
Tizanidine hydrochloride may cause drowsiness; patients affected should not drive or operate machinery. Other adverse effects include dry mouth, fatigue, dizziness or vertigo, muscle pain and weakness, insomnia, anxiety, headache, bradycardia, nausea, and gastrointestinal disturbances. Hallucinations have occurred on rare occasions. Many adverse effects have been found to be dose related and slow titration of doses appears to reduce the frequency of occurrence. Hypotension may occur. Increases in liver enzymes and rarely acute hepatitis have been associated with tizanidine and it is contra-indicated in patients with severe hepatic dysfunction. In the UK it is recommended that liver function should be monitored monthly in all patients for the first 4 months and in those who develop symptoms suggestive of hepatic dysfunction. Treatment should be discontinued if liver enzymes are persistently raised. Caution is required in the elderly and in patients with renal insufficiency.

Interactions
The CNS effects of tizanidine may be enhanced by alcohol or other CNS depressants. There may be an additive hypotensive effect when tizanidine is used in patients receiving antihypertensive therapy; bradycardia may also be enhanced if given with beta blockers or digoxin. Caution should be exercised when tizanidine is given with drugs known to increase the QT interval. The clearance of tizanidine has been reported to be lower in women receiving hormonal contraceptives.

Antiepileptics. For reference to an interaction between tizanidine and phenytoin, see p.361.

Pharmacokinetics
Tizanidine is absorbed from the gastrointestinal tract and peak plasma concentrations have occurred 1 to 2 hours after administration by mouth. Tizanidine undergoes extensive first-pass metabolism in the liver and is excreted mainly in the urine as inactive metabolites. Elimination half-lives of 2.1 to 4.2 hours have been reported.

Uses and Administration
Tizanidine hydrochloride is a centrally acting skeletal muscle relaxant. It is an α_2-adrenergic agonist structurally related to clonidine (p.860) and acts mainly at the level of the spinal cord. It is used for the symptomatic relief of spasticity associated with multiple sclerosis or with spinal cord injury or disease. It is also used in the symptomatic treatment of painful muscle spasm (p.1322) associated with musculoskeletal conditions.

Tizanidine hydrochloride is usually given in divided doses by mouth. The usual initial daily dose in the management of spasticity is the equivalent of 2 mg of the base given as a single dose. The daily dose may be increased thereafter according to response in steps of 2 mg at intervals of at least 3 to 4 days, usually up to 24 mg daily given in 3 to 4 divided doses. The maximum recommended dose is 36 mg daily. For patients with renal insufficiency, treatment is also started with 2 mg once daily, but thereafter it is advised to slowly increase the once-daily dose before increasing the frequency of administration. Maintenance doses have been given in some countries in the form of modified-release preparations.

In the treatment of painful muscle spasm tizanidine hydrochloride is given in doses of 2 to 4 mg three times daily.

◊ References.
1. Hutchinson DR. Modified release tizanidine: a review. *J Int Med Res* 1989; **17:** 565–73.

Headache. Although results from an open-label study[1] suggested that tizanidine might be of value in the prophylaxis of chronic daily headache, a controlled study[2] failed to demonstrate any significant advantage over placebo in the treatment of chronic tension-type headache.

1. Saper JR, *et al.* An open-label dose-titration study of the efficacy and tolerability of tizanidine hydrochloride tablets in the prophylaxis of chronic daily headache. *Headache* 2001; **41:** 357–68.
2. Murros K, *et al.* Modified-release formulation of tizanidine in chronic tension-type headache. *Headache* 2000; **40:** 633–7.

Premedication. The value of tizanidine as a premedicant is being studied.[1] A dose of tizanidine 12 mg appears to have sedative and sympatholytic effects comparable with clonidine 150 µg.

1. Meittinen TJ, *et al.* The sedative and sympatholytic effects of oral tizanidine in healthy volunteers. *Anesth Analg* 1996; **82:** 817–20.

Spasticity. The use of tizanidine in the management of spasticity (p.1322) associated with cerebral and spinal disorders has been discussed.[1,2] Its antispastic efficacy had been demonstrated in several placebo-controlled studies and in comparative studies it had produced similar improvements in muscle tone to baclofen or diazepam. Carefully titrated doses of tizanidine and baclofen used together may have additive beneficial effects[1,2] but use with benzodiazepines is not recommended because of potential interactions.[1] It was considered that tizanidine might have the advantage of being better tolerated than baclofen.

1. Wagstaff AJ, Bryson HM. Tizanidine: a review of its pharmacology, clinical efficacy and tolerability in the management of spasticity associated with cerebral and spinal disorders. *Drugs* 1997; **53:** 435–52.
2. Anonymous. Tizanidine for spasticity. *Med Lett Drugs Ther* 1997; **39:** 62–3.

Preparations
Proprietary Preparations (details are given in Part 3)
Aust.: Sirdalud; *Belg.:* Sirdalud; *Braz.:* Sirdalud; *Denm.:* Sirdalud; *Fin.:* Sirdalud; *Ger.:* Sirdalud; *Irl.:* Zanaflex; *Ital.:* Sirdalud; *Jpn:* Ternelin†; *Mex.:* Sirdalud; *Neth.:* Sirdalud; *Port.:* Sirdalud; *Spain:* Sirdalud; *Switz.:* Sirdalud; *Thai.:* Sirdalud; *UK:* Zanaflex; *USA:* Zanaflex.

Tolperisone Hydrochloride (5735-n)

Tolperisone Hydrochloride *(BANM, rINNM)*.
N-553. 2,4'-Dimethyl-3-piperidinopropiophenone hydrochloride.

$C_{16}H_{23}NO,HCl = 281.8$.

CAS — 728-88-1 (tolperisone); 3644-61-9 (tolperisone hydrochloride).

Pharmacopoeias. In Jpn.

Profile
Tolperisone hydrochloride is a centrally acting muscle relaxant that has been used for the symptomatic treatment of spasticity (p.1322) and muscle spasm (p.1322), in usual doses of 50 to 150 mg three times daily by mouth. It has also been given by intramuscular or slow intravenous injection.

Preparations
Proprietary Preparations (details are given in Part 3)
Aust.: Mydocalm†; *Ger.:* Mydocalm; *Hong Kong:* Mydocalm; *Switz.:* Mydocalm; *Thai.:* Biocalm; Mydocalm; Mydosone; Myolax; Myoxan; Risocalm; Soneriper; Tanderon.

Multi-ingredient: *Mex.:* Mydocalm-A.

Neuromuscular Blockers

Neuromuscular blockers (myoneuronal blockers) affect transmission at the neuromuscular junction and are used as adjuncts to general anaesthesia, particularly to enable adequate muscle relaxation to be achieved with light anaesthesia. There are 2 main types of neuromuscular blockers: competitive (non-depolarising neuromuscular blockers) and depolarising neuromuscular blockers (see Table 1, below).

Table 1. Classification of neuromuscular blockers.

Competitive		Depolarising
Aminosteroidal	*Benzylisoquinolinium*	Decamethonium
Pancuronium	Alcuronium	Suxamethonium
Pipecuronium	Atracurium	
Rapacuronium	Cisatracurium	
Rocuronium	Doxacurium	
Vecuronium	Gallamine	
	Metocurine	
	Mivacurium	
	Tubocurarine	

- **Competitive neuromuscular blockers** act by competing with acetylcholine for receptors on the motor end-plate. Their action can be opposed by increasing the local concentration of acetylcholine, for example by giving an anticholinesterase such as neostigmine (p.1419). Tubocurarine (p.1343) was formerly the standard reference drug of this type but its use has declined, therefore details of the actions and uses of competitive neuromuscular blockers are discussed under Atracurium, p.1333.

- **Depolarising neuromuscular blockers** act by depolarising the motor end-plate to prevent the normal response to acetylcholine; their action is not reversed by anticholinesterases. Suxamethonium (p.1340) is the standard reference drug of this type.

Other drugs with muscle relaxant properties which are used in the management of musculoskeletal and neuromuscular disorders are discussed in the chapter on Muscle Relaxants, p.1322.

◊ General references.

1. Agoston S, *et al.* Clinical pharmacokinetics of neuromuscular blocking drugs. *Clin Pharmacokinet* 1992; **22**: 94–115.
2. Book WJ, *et al.* Adverse effects of depolarising neuromuscular blocking agents: incidence, prevention and management. *Drug Safety* 1994; **10**: 331–49.
3. Abel M, *et al.* Adverse effects of nondepolarising neuromuscular blocking agents: incidence, prevention and management. *Drug Safety* 1994; **10**: 420–38.
4. Hunter JM. New neuromuscular blocking drugs. *N Engl J Med* 1995; **332**: 1691–9.
5. Naguib M, Magboul MMA. Adverse effects of neuromuscular blockers and their antagonists. *Drug Safety* 1998; **18**: 99–116.
6. Guay J, *et al.* Clinical pharmacokinetics of neuromuscular relaxants in pregnancy. *Clin Pharmacokinet* 1998; **34**: 483–96.
7. Atherton DPL, Hunter JM. Clinical pharmacokinetics of the newer neuromuscular blocking drugs. *Clin Pharmacokinet* 1999; **36**: 169–89.
8. Sparr HJ, *et al.* Newer neuromuscular blocking agents: how do they compare with established agents? *Drugs* 2001; **61**: 919–42.

Anaesthesia

Generally, *competitive neuromuscular blockers*, having a slower onset and a longer duration of action, are used in major operations, while the *depolarising neuromuscular blockers* (usually suxamethonium), with a much faster onset and shorter duration, are used for minor operations or manipulations and particularly for intubation. Following administration of suxamethonium to aid intubation, a longer-acting competitive drug may then be given to maintain muscle relaxation throughout the operation. Neuromuscular blockers can be classified by their onset and duration of action (see Table 2, below), but both onset and duration are dose-dependent and can therefore vary. Competitive neuromuscular blockers with a short to intermediate duration of action, such as atracurium and vecuronium, are more widely employed than those with a longer duration of action such as pancuronium. Because of the adverse effects such as myalgia associated with suxamethonium, alternative neuromuscular blockers have been investigated for intubation and some now

question the use of suxamethonium for elective procedures,[1] especially in day-case patients.[2] Some competitive blockers such as vecuronium have a relatively rapid onset of action but are considered to act too slowly to enable rapid intubation in an emergency[3] when suxamethonium remains the drug of choice. The newer competitive blocker rocuronium has an onset of action only slightly slower than that of suxamethonium and may be suitable for use in emergencies when suxamethonium is contra-indicated;[4] unfortunately it has a long duration of action. Competitive blockers with more rapid onset are being evaluated. One study found that it was necessary to use an opioid such as alfentanil as part of the induction regimen in order to obtain intubating conditions with rocuronium similar to those with suxamethonium alone.[5]

Combinations of competitive neuromuscular blockers have also been tried for rapid intubation.[6]

Competitive neuromuscular blockers have also been administered in divided doses in an attempt to shorten the onset to paralysis and thus provide an alternative to suxamethonium for intubation.[7] This so-called *priming principle* involves administration of a small initial dose, termed the priming dose, followed by a large paralysing dose. Priming may be with 2 doses of the same competitive relaxant or a combination of 2 different relaxants which may then exhibit synergism. However, some consider[7] that priming techniques are associated with an unacceptable incidence of adverse effects and that they have no role in clinical anaesthesia.

The use of anaesthetic regimens that avoid the need for a neuromuscular blocker during intubation has also been investigated. Although the general anaesthetic propofol has been tried alone,[8] some consider it to be inadequate[9,10] due to undesirable haemodynamic responses and intolerance of the tracheal tube. Propofol with alfentanil was considered to produce suitable conditions for intubation in studies in adults[11-13] and in children.[14,15] In one study[14] coughing and limb movements were more common with propofol and alfentanil than with propofol and suxamethonium, but it appears that the coughing may be reduced by concomitant administration of lignocaine [lidocaine].[13]

One group of workers[16] found that using a very low dose of suxamethonium after alfentanil and propofol produced good conditions for nasal intubation without the incidence of myalgia associated with full-dose suxamethonium. Low doses of rocuronium have also been found to improve conditions for tracheal intubation after induction with propofol and alfentanil.[17] Induction with propofol and alfentanil has enabled standard doses of vecuronium to produce conditions for rapid tracheal intubation comparable to those achieved with suxamethonium.[18]

Procedures such as intubation can cause an undesirable pressor response resulting in increased heart rate and arterial blood pressure. They can also cause an increase in intracranial pressure and intra-ocular pressure. Furthermore, the use of suxamethonium to facilitate intubation

Table 2. Relative speed of onset and duration of action of neuromuscular blockers.

Neuromuscular blocker	Onset*	Duration†
Alcuronium	Intermediate	Intermediate
Atracurium	Intermediate	Short/Intermediate
Cisatracurium	Intermediate	Short/Intermediate
Doxacurium	Slow	Long
Gallamine	Rapid	Intermediate
Mivacurium	Intermediate	Short
Pancuronium	Rapid	Long
Pipecuronium	Intermediate	Intermediate/Long
Rocuronium	Rapid	Intermediate
Suxamethonium	Ultra-rapid	Ultra-short
Tubocurarine	Intermediate/Slow	Intermediate
Vecuronium	Rapid	Intermediate

*Onset:
Ultra-rapid, less than 1 minute
Rapid, 1 to 2 minutes
Intermediate, 2 to 4 minutes
Slow, more than 4 minutes

†Duration:
Ultra-short, less than 8 minutes
Short, 8 to 20 minutes
Intermediate, 20 to 50 minutes
Long, more than 50 minutes

Onset and duration of action are dose-dependent

is itself associated with a transient increase in intra-ocular pressure. Small doses of a competitive neuromuscular blocker have been given before suxamethonium to prevent this rise in intra-ocular pressure, but such a measure is not considered to be effective.[19] Opioids such as alfentanil and fentanyl appear to be effective in attenuating both the pressor response[20-22] and the rise in intra-ocular pressure[23,24] associated with intubation, but the use of lignocaine [lidocaine] has produced conflicting results.[25-29] Many anaesthetics, with the exception of ketamine, reduce intra-ocular pressure to some extent and prior administration of thiopental may help to counteract the effect of suxamethonium.[30]

Other drugs that have been used or tried in the prevention of the haemodynamic response to intubation include magnesium sulfate[31] and propofol.[32,33]

1. Steyn M, Morton NS. Tracheal intubation without neuromuscular block. *Br J Anaesth* 1994; **73**: 862–7.
2. Cartwright DP. Suxamethonium in day-case anaesthesia. *Br J Anaesth* 1993; **71**: 918–19.
3. Williams A, *et al.* Clinical experience with Org NC45 (Norcuron) as the sole muscle relaxant. *Can Anaesth Soc J* 1982; **29**: 567–72.
4. Hunter JM. Rocuronium: the newest aminosteroid neuromuscular blocking drug. *Br J Anaesth* 1996; **76**: 481–3.
5. Sparr HJ, *et al.* Influence of induction technique on intubating conditions after rocuronium in adults: comparison with rapid-sequence induction using thiopentone and suxamethonium. *Br J Anaesth* 1996; **77**: 339–42.
6. Naguib M, *et al.* Comparison of suxamethonium and different combinations of rocuronium and mivacurium for rapid tracheal intubation in children. *Br J Anaesth* 1997; **79**: 450–5.
7. Jones RM. The priming principle: how does it work and should we be using it? *Br J Anaesth* 1989; **63**: 1–3.
8. Keaveny JP, Knell PJ. Intubation under induction doses of propofol. *Anaesthesia* 1988; **43S**: 80–1.
9. Saarnivaara L, Klemola U-M. Injection pain, intubating conditions and cardiovascular changes following induction of anaesthesia with propofol alone or in combination with alfentanil. *Acta Anaesthesiol Scand* 1991; **35**: 19–23.
10. Rodney GE, *et al.* Propofol or propofol/alfentanil compared to thiopentone/succinylcholine for intubation of healthy children. *Can J Anaesth* 1992; **39**: A129.
11. Alcock R, *et al.* Comparison of alfentanil with suxamethonium in facilitating nasotracheal intubation in day-case anaesthesia. *Br J Anaesth* 1993; **70**: 34–7.
12. Coghlan SFE, *et al.* Use of alfentanil with propofol for nasotracheal intubation without neuromuscular block. *Br J Anaesth* 1993; **70**: 89–91.
13. Davidson JAH, Gillespie JA. Tracheal intubation after induction of anaesthesia with propofol, alfentanil and i.v. lignocaine. *Br J Anaesth* 1993; **70**: 163–6.
14. Steyn MP, *et al.* Tracheal intubation without neuromuscular block in children. *Br J Anaesth* 1994; **72**: 403–6.
15. McConaghy P, Bunting HE. Assessment of intubating conditions in children after induction with propofol and varying doses of alfentanil. *Br J Anaesth* 1994; **73**: 596–9.
16. Nimmo SM, *et al.* Effectiveness and sequelae of very low-dose suxamethonium for nasal intubation. *Br J Anaesth* 1995; **74**: 31–4.
17. Barclay K, *et al.* Low-dose rocuronium improves conditions for tracheal intubation after induction of anaesthesia with propofol and alfentanil. *Br J Anaesth* 1997; **78**: 92–4.
18. Groener R, Moyes DG. Rapid tracheal intubation with propofol, alfentanil and a standard dose of vecuronium. *Br J Anaesth* 1997; **79**: 384–5.
19. Book WJ, *et al.* Adverse effects of depolarising neuromuscular blocking agents: incidence, prevention and management. *Drug Safety* 1994; **10**: 331–49.
20. Crawford DC, *et al.* Effects of alfentanil on the pressor and catecholamine responses to tracheal intubation. *Br J Anaesth* 1987; **59**: 707–12.
21. Scheinin B, *et al.* Alfentanil obtunds the cardiovascular and sympathoadrenal responses to suxamethonium-facilitated laryngoscopy and intubation. *Br J Anaesth* 1989; **62**: 385–92.
22. Chung F, Evans D. Low-dose fentanyl: haemodynamic response during induction and intubation in geriatric patients. *Can Anaesth Soc J* 1985; **32**: 622–8.
23. Mostafa SM, *et al.* Comparison of effects of fentanyl and alfentanil on intra-ocular pressure. *Anaesthesia* 1986; **41**: 493–8.
24. Sweeney J, *et al.* Modification by fentanyl and alfentanil of the intraocular pressure response to suxamethonium and tracheal intubation. *Br J Anaesth* 1989; **63**: 688–91.
25. Tam S, *et al.* Attenuation of circulatory responses to endotracheal intubation using intravenous lidocaine: a determination of the optimal time of injection. *Can Anaesth Soc J* 1985; **32**: S65.
26. Miller CD, Warren SJ. I.V. lignocaine fails to attenuate the cardiovascular response to laryngoscopy and tracheal intubation. *Br J Anaesth* 1990; **65**: 216–19.
27. Murphy DF, *et al.* Intravenous lignocaine pretreatment to prevent intraocular pressure rise following suxamethonium and tracheal intubation. *Br J Ophthalmol* 1986; **70**: 596–8.
28. Drenger B, Pe'er J. Attenuation of ocular and systemic responses to tracheal intubation by intravenous lignocaine. *Br J Ophthalmol* 1987; **71**: 546–8.
29. Mostafa SM, *et al.* Effects of nebulized lignocaine on the intraocular pressure responses to tracheal intubation. *Br J Anaesth* 1990; **64**: 515–17.
30. Holloway KB. Control of the eye during general anaesthesia for intraocular surgery. *Br J Anaesth* 1980; **52**: 671–9.
31. Ashton WB, *et al.* Attenuation of the pressor response to tracheal intubation by magnesium sulphate with and without alfentanil in hypertensive proteinuric patients undergoing caesarean section. *Br J Anaesth* 1991; **67**: 741–7.
32. Brossy MJ, *et al.* Haemodynamic and catecholamine changes after induction of anaesthesia with either thiopentone or propofol with suxamethonium. *Br J Anaesth* 1994; **72**: 596–8.
33. Gin T, *et al.* Plasma catecholamines and neonatal condition after induction of anaesthesia with propofol or thiopentone at caesarean section. *Br J Anaesth* 1993; **70**: 311–116.

The symbol † denotes a preparation no longer actively marke᠁

Intensive care

The use of neuromuscular blockers in patients requiring mechanical ventilation as part of intensive care has been discussed in a number of reviews.[1-3] Neuromuscular blockers are used to provide additional relaxation and facilitate ventilatory support in patients who fail to respond to sedation alone. It is important to ensure that such patients are adequately sedated before these drugs are used. Patients who are considered most likely to benefit are those with spontaneous respiration that is counterproductive to mechanical ventilation. Patients with little inherent respiratory muscle activity are less likely to obtain an improvement in oxygenation. Neuromuscular blockers may also improve control of intracranial pressure in patients with intracranial hypertension including prevention of rises in intracranial pressure associated with routine tracheobronchial suction.

Pancuronium has been widely used as a neuromuscular blocker in intensive care because of its tendency to increase arterial pressure but its long duration of action may be a problem in some circumstances, and it can also produce tachycardia. Vecuronium and atracurium have relatively few cardiovascular effects, but there has been some concern over the ability of the atracurium metabolite laudanosine to accumulate in the CNS (see under Pharmacokinetics, p.1336). Tachyphylaxis may occur and dosage requirements may be increased in patients with burns or in those receiving prolonged therapy. Dose modification may also be necessary in patients with renal or hepatic impairment.

When rapid reversal of paralysis is necessary an anticholinesterase such as neostigmine may be used, but relatively little is known about the efficacy of anticholinesterases in reversing prolonged paralysis.[4] Prolonged neuromuscular blockade may be related to dosage and, since the pharmacodynamics and pharmacokinetics of neuromuscular blockers may be altered in patients in intensive care, close monitoring of neuromuscular blockade is advised.[1-3] Other factors which may potentiate neuromuscular blockade include drug interactions, electrolyte imbalance, hypothermia, or changes in acid-base balance.[1,3] An acute myopathy has followed prolonged use, most commonly with aminosteroid neuromuscular blockers; there are case reports suggesting that concomitant use of corticosteroids might increase the risk.[5]

Neonatal intensive care. Neuromuscular blockers such as pancuronium bromide are used in neonatal intensive care to obtain muscle relaxation during mechanical ventilation in infants with severe pulmonary disease, especially in those whose respiratory efforts are out of phase with the ventilator.[6] They are only used in infants at high risk of complications such as *pneumothorax* or *intraventricular haemorrhage*.

Abolition of spontaneous respiration during mechanical ventilation has had variable effects on the incidence of *pneumothorax* in infants with respiratory distress syndrome. Although a reduced incidence was found in one study[7] involving infants of less than 33 weeks' gestation, in another study[8] the incidence was reduced only in infants with a gestational age of 27 to 32 weeks; no reduction was obtained in those below 26 weeks' gestation. Paralysis also failed to reduce the incidence of pneumothorax or interstitial emphysema in a study[9] of infants with hyaline membrane disease but did appear to speed recovery of lung function.

The aetiology of *intraventricular haemorrhage* remains obscure but there is a well recognised association with gestational age;[10] less mature neonates are more susceptible and the incidence decreases sharply after 30 weeks' gestation. There appears to be an association between fluctuating cerebral blood-flow velocity in the first day of life and subsequent development of intraventricular haemorrhage.[11] Respiratory paralysis from the first day of life until 72 hours of age has been reported[12] to stabilise both cerebral and arterial blood-flow velocity and to produce a decrease in the incidence and severity of intraventricular haemorrhage in infants with respiratory distress syndrome. However, respiratory paralysis has also been reported to have no effect on the development of intraventricular haemorrhage.[7,8]

The use of neuromuscular blockers in the newborn is not without complications. Multiple joint contractures, possibly potentiated by concomitant use of aminoglycosides or phenobarbital, have been reported[13,14] in infants given pancuronium, and regular passive limb movements should be performed during paralysis. Marked oedema, severe disturbances of fluid balance, and renal failure followed by death were reported in 2 neonates.[15] Hy-

poxaemia may develop following induction of paralysis unless a significant increase in ventilator support is made;[7,11,16] hypotension may also occur.[17] Drugs such as pancuronium which are metabolised in the liver and excreted in the urine have a prolonged action in premature infants.[6] As with adults (see above), continuous use of neuromuscular blockers in neonates has been associated with prolonged neuromuscular block on discontinuation.[18]

1. Coursin DB, *et al.* Muscle relaxants in critical care. *Curr Opin Anaesthesiol* 1993; **6:** 341–6.
2. Elliot JM, Bion JF. The use of neuromuscular blocking drugs in intensive care practice. *Acta Anaesthesiol Scand* 1995; **39** (suppl 106): 70–82.
3. Lewis KS, Rothenberg DM. Neuromuscular blockade in the intensive care unit. *Am J Health-Syst Pharm* 1999; **56:** 72–5.
4. Watling SM, Dasta JF. Prolonged paralysis in intensive care unit patients after the use of neuromuscular blocking agents: a review of the literature. *Crit Care Med* 1994; **22:** 884–93.
5. Fischer JR, Baer RK. Acute myopathy associated with combined use of corticosteroids and neuromuscular blocking agents. *Ann Pharmacother* 1996; **30:** 1437–45.
6. Levene MI, Quinn MW. Use of sedatives and muscle relaxants in newborn babies receiving mechanical ventilation. *Arch Dis Child* 1992; **67:** 870–3.
7. Greenough A, *et al.* Pancuronium prevents pneumothoraces in ventilated premature babies who actively expire against positive pressure inflation. *Lancet* 1984; **i:** 1–3.
8. Cooke RWI, Rennie JM. Pancuronium and pneumothorax. *Lancet* 1984; **i:** 286–7.
9. Pollitzer MJ, *et al.* Pancuronium during mechanical ventilation speeds recovery of lungs of infants with hyaline membrane disease. *Lancet* 1981; **i:** 346–8.
10. Miall-Allen VM, *et al.* Blood pressure fluctuation and intraventricular haemorrhage in the preterm infant of less than 31 weeks' gestation. *Pediatrics* 1989; **83:** 657–61.
11. Perlman JM, *et al.* Fluctuating cerebral blood-flow velocity in respiratory distress syndrome. *N Engl J Med* 1983; **309:** 204–9.
12. Perlman JM, *et al.* Reduction in intraventricular hemorrhage by elimination of fluctuating cerebral blood-flow velocity in preterm infants with respiratory distress syndrome. *N Engl J Med* 1985; **312:** 1353–7.
13. Sinha SK, Levene MI. Pancuronium bromide induced joint contractures in the newborn. *Arch Dis Child* 1984; **59:** 73–5.
14. Fanconi S, *et al.* Effects of paralysis with pancuronium bromide on joint mobility in premature infants. *J Pediatr* 1995; **127:** 134–6.
15. Reynolds EOR, *et al.* Muscle relaxation and periventricular hemorrhage. *N Engl J Med* 1985; **313:** 955–6.
16. Philips JB, *et al.* Hypoxaemia in ventilated neonates after pancuronium paralysis. *Lancet* 1979; **i:** 877.
17. McIntosh N. Hypotension associated with pancuronium use in the newborn. *Lancet* 1985; **ii:** 279.
18. Björklund LJ. Use of sedatives and muscle relaxants in newborn babies receiving mechanical ventilation. *Arch Dis Child* 1993; **69:** 544.

Tetanus

The clinical manifestations of tetanus following infection with *Clostridium tetani* are caused by the highly potent neurotoxin tetanospasmin produced by its germinating spores. For the antibacterial treatment and prevention of tetanus and neutralisation of tetanospasmin, see p.142.

The muscular symptoms of generalised tetanus include trismus (lockjaw), glottal spasm, generalised muscle spasm, opisthotonus (spasm of the back muscles resulting in backward arching of the body), respiratory spasm, and paralysis. Other complications include electrolyte disturbances and autonomic dysfunction leading to cardiovascular effects such as hypertension, tachycardia, and peripheral vasoconstriction. Patients may have a milder form in which the twitching and muscle spasms are limited to the area near the site of the injury, but such localised tetanus is rare and can progress to the generalised form.

Benzodiazepines such as diazepam are useful for controlling the neuromuscular manifestations and can also reduce patient anxiety and produce sedation. *Opioid analgesics* can be added to treatment to provide analgesia and additional sedation. *Chlorpromazine* is sometimes used with benzodiazepines to minimise rigidity and muscle spasms. Centrally acting muscle relaxants have also been used to control muscle spasms. *Baclofen* has been given by the intrathecal route, but its therapeutic range in severe tetanus may be very narrow and deep coma and loss of spontaneous respiration has been reported. When muscle spasms are severe or interfere with respiration, *competitive neuromuscular blockers* have been used in addition to benzodiazepine sedation, to control spasms and to induce therapeutic paralysis so mechanical ventilation can be initiated. Various drugs have been tried to control autonomic overactivity, including *beta blockers* and *morphine*. Electrolyte disturbance is corrected with calcium and magnesium salts.

References.

1. Attygalle D, Karalliedde L. Unforgettable tetanus. *Eur J Anaesthesiol* 1997; **14:** 122–33.
2. Ernst ME, *et al.* Tetanus: pathophysiology and management. *Ann Pharmacother* 1997; **31:** 1507–13.

Alcuronium Chloride (5701-j)

Alcuronium Chloride (BAN, USAN, rINN).

Alcuronii Chloridum; Allnortoxiferin Chloride; Diallylnortoxiferine Dichloride; Diallyltoxiferine Chloride; Ro-4-3816. NN′-Diallylbisnortoxiferinium dichloride.

$C_{44}H_{50}Cl_2N_4O_2 = 737.8.$

CAS — 23214-96-2 (alcuronium); 15180-03-7 (alcuronium chloride).

Pharmacopoeias. In Eur. (see p.vi).

Pharmacopoeial description

Ph. Eur.: A white or slightly greyish-white, crystalline powder. Freely soluble in water and in methyl alcohol; soluble in alcohol; practically insoluble in cyclohexane. Store under nitrogen in an airtight container. Protect from light.

Adverse Effects, Treatment, and Precautions

As for competitive neuromuscular blockers in general (see Atracurium, p.1333).

Alcuronium chloride can induce histamine release to some degree. Anaphylactoid reactions have been associated with the use of alcuronium. It has some vagolytic action and may produce tachycardia; hypotension may also occur.

Hypersensitivity. Reports of anaphylactoid reactions to alcuronium.

See also under Suxamethonium Chloride, p.1341.

1. Fisher M, Baldo B. Adverse reactions to alcuronium: an Australian disease? *Med J Aust* 1983; **1:** 630–2.
2. Fisher MM, Munro I. Life-threatening anaphylactoid reactions to muscle relaxants. *Anesth Analg* 1983; **62:** 559–64.

Porphyria. Alcuronium is considered to be unsafe in patients with porphyria because it has been shown to be porphyrinogenic in *animals*.

Pregnancy. Alcuronium crosses the placenta. No evidence of neuromuscular block was seen in any of the neonates born to 12 women who received alcuronium 15 to 30 mg by intravenous injection, 5.0 to 10.5 minutes before delivery[1] but caution was advised if alcuronium was given in obstetrics in high doses or for a prolonged period.

1. Ho PC, *et al.* Caesarean section and placental transfer of alcuronium. *Anaesth Intensive Care* 1981; **9:** 113–18.

Renal impairment. Alcuronium is excreted mainly by the kidneys and accumulation, with prolonged paralysis, may therefore be expected in patients with renal impairment given large or repeated doses. A prolonged elimination half-life has been reported in anuria.[1] However, doses of 160 μg per kg body-weight have been used without any problems in patients with chronic renal failure undergoing renal transplantation.[2] The average duration of action of this dose was 37 minutes and any residual neuromuscular blockade at the end of surgery was successfully reversed using atropine and neostigmine.

1. Raaflaub J, Frey P. Zur Pharmakokinetik von Diallyl-nor-toxiferin beim Menschen. *Arzneimittelforschung* 1972; **22:** 73–8.
2. Kaushik S, *et al.* Use of alcuronium in patients undergoing renal transplantation. *Br J Anaesth* 1984; **56:** 1229–33.

Interactions

For interactions associated with competitive neuromuscular blockers, see Atracurium, p.1334.

Pharmacokinetics

When given intravenously, alcuronium is widely distributed throughout the body tissues and crosses the placenta. It is excreted unchanged, mainly in urine. Small amounts are also excreted in bile. The elimination half-life is about 3 hours.

◊ References.

1. Raaflaub J, Frey P. Zur Pharmakokinetik von Diallyl-nor-toxiferin beim Menschen. *Arzneimittelforschung* 1972; **22:** 73–8.
2. Walker J, *et al.* Clinical pharmacokinetics of alcuronium chloride in man. *Eur J Clin Pharmacol* 1980; **17:** 449–57.

Uses and Administration

Alcuronium chloride is a benzylisoquinolinium competitive neuromuscular blocker (see Atracurium, p.1336) that is used for endotracheal intubation and to provide muscle relaxation in general anaesthesia for surgical procedures (see Anaesthesia, p.1331).

Doses of neuromuscular blockers need to be carefully titrated for individual patients according to response, and may vary with the procedure, the other drugs given, and the state of the patient; monitoring of the degree of block is recommended in order to reduce the risk of overdosage. An initial dose of 150 to 250 μg per kg body-weight has been given intravenously. Muscle relaxation occurs after about 2 minutes and the effect lasts for about 20 to 30 minutes. Supplementary doses of 30 μg per kg have been given to provide additional periods of muscle relaxation.

Preparations

Proprietary Preparations (details are given in Part 3)

Aust.: Alloferin; **Braz.:** Alloferine; **Ger.:** Alloferin; **Hong Kong:** Alloferin; **Israel:** Alloferin; **Neth.:** Alloferin†; **S.Afr.:** Alloferin; **Singapore:** Alloferin; **Thai.:** Alloferin.

Atracurium Besilate (12405-r)

Atracurium Besilate (BAN, rINN).

33A74; Atracurium Besylate (USAN); BW-33A. 2,2′-(3,11-Di-oxo-4,10-dioxatridecamethylene)bis(1,2,3,4-tetrahydro-6,7-dimethoxy-2-methyl-1-veratrylisoquinolinium) di(benzenesul-phonate).

$C_{53}H_{72}N_2O_{12},2C_6H_5O_3S = 1243.5$.
CAS — 64228-81-5.

Pharmacopoeias. In Br. and It.

The commercial preparation of atracurium is a mixture of 10 stereoisomers of which cisatracurium constitutes about 15%.

Pharmacopoeial description

BP 2001: A white to pale yellow hygroscopic powder or flaky crystals. It contains about 58% of the cis-cis isomer, about 36% of the cis-trans isomer, and about 6% of the trans-trans isomer. Soluble in water; very soluble in acetonitrile and in chloroform; practically insoluble in ether. A 1% solution in water has a pH of 3.5 to 5.0. Store in airtight containers at a temperature of 2° to 8°. Protect from light.

Cisatracurium Besilate (17507-r)

Cisatracurium Besilate (BAN, rINN).

Bésilate de Cisatracurium; BW-51W (cisatracurium); BW-51W89 (cisatracurium); Cisatracurium Besylate; 51W89 (cisatracurium). (1R,1′R,2R,2′R)-2,2′-(3,11-Dioxo-4,10-dioxatridecamethylene)bis(1,2,3,4-tetrahydro-6,7-dimethoxy-2-methyl-1-veratrylisoquinolinium) dibenzenesulfonate.

CAS — 96946-42-8.

Incompatibility. Neuromuscular blockers are generally incompatible with alkaline solutions, for example barbiturates such as thiopental sodium. It is good practice not to administer neuromuscular blockers in the same syringe, or simultaneously through the same needle, as other drugs.

Stability. In a stability study,[1] solutions of cisatracurium (as the besilate) in concentrations of 2 mg or 10 mg per mL were stable for at least 90 days when stored in the original vials at 4° either exposed to or protected from light; similar solutions stored at 23° were stable for at least 45 days. Solutions of 2 mg per mL stored in plastic syringes at 4° or 23° were stable for at least 30 days. Solutions of 0.1, 2, or 5 mg per mL in 5% glucose injection or 0.9% sodium chloride injection in PVC minibags were stable for at least 30 days stored at 4°; the 5 mg per mL solution was also stable for at least 30 days stored at 23°.

1. Xu QA, et al. Stability of cisatracurium besylate in vials, syringes, and infusion admixtures. Am J Health-Syst Pharm 1998; 55: 1037–41.

Adverse Effects

The adverse effects of competitive neuromuscular blockers are generally similar although they differ in their propensity to cause histamine release and cardiovascular effects. Histamine release and associated cardiovascular effects appear to be rare with the aminosteroidal blockers. Competitive neuromuscular blockers with vagolytic activity may produce tachycardia and a rise in blood pressure. The use of blockers which lack an effect on the vagus may result in bradycardia during anaesthesia due to the effects of other drugs employed or as a result of vagal stimulation. Reduction in blood pressure with compensatory tachycardia may occur with some competitive neuromuscular blockers due in part to sympathetic ganglion blockade or the release of histamine. Reduction in gastrointestinal motility and tone may occur as a result of ganglionic blockade.

Histamine release may also lead to wheal-and-flare effects at the site of injection, flushing, occasionally bronchospasm, and rarely anaphylactoid reactions.

Malignant hyperthermia has been associated rarely with competitive neuromuscular blockers.

In overdosage there is prolonged apnoea due to paralysis of the intercostal muscles and diaphragm, with cardiovascular collapse and the effects of histamine release.

Atracurium and its isomer cisatracurium have no significant vagal or ganglionic blocking activity at recommended doses. Unlike atracurium, cisatracurium does not induce histamine release and is therefore associated with greater cardiovascular stability.

For possible risks from their major metabolite laudanosine, see under Pharmacokinetics, below.

◊ In 3 large-scale surveillance studies involving a total of 6106 patients, 3346 of whom were given atracurium, the overall incidence of adverse events in the atracurium groups was 10%,[1] 13%,[2] and 29%.[3] This compared with an incidence of 18% in patients given alcuronium, 13% in patients given a neuromus-

cular blocker other than atracurium, and 40% in patients given vecuronium, respectively. Severe reactions with atracurium were infrequent. No patient experienced cardiac arrest or anaphylaxis and there were no reports of difficulty in antagonism of neuromuscular blockade. Adverse effects possibly related to histamine release in the atracurium groups were hypotension (in 3.4, 1.8, and 15% of patients), bronchospasm or wheezing (0.2, 1.5, and 0.4%), tachycardia (1.9, 0.1, and 0.4%), and rash (2.5, 0.3, and 1.0%). Other cardiovascular events reported included hypertension (1.1, 1.4, and 0.6%) and bradycardia (0.6, 0.8, and 12%). Hypotension and tachycardia occurred significantly less often in patients given atracurium compared with those given alcuronium but cutaneous reactions occurred more often. No other significant differences were observed in the incidence of adverse events in patients given atracurium compared with those receiving another neuromuscular blocker.

1. Beemer GH, et al. Adverse reactions to atracurium and alcuronium: a prospective surveillance study. Br J Anaesth 1988; 61: 680–4.
2. Jick H, et al. Atracurium—a post-marketing surveillance study: methods and US experience. Br J Anaesth 1989; 62: 590–5.
3. Lawson DH, et al. Atracurium—a post-marketing surveillance study: UK study and discussion. Br J Anaesth 1989; 62: 596–600.

Effects on body temperature. Malignant hyperthermia has been associated with competitive neuromuscular blockers on rare occasions. Two cases of mild malignant hyperthermia have been reported[1] where tubocurarine was probably the triggering drug. Each episode developed in a member of a known malignant hyperthermia family despite preventive measures such as prophylactic cooling, and avoidance of potent inhalation anaesthetics and depolarising neuromuscular blockers. Another case[2] was associated with the use of pancuronium.

1. Britt BA, et al. Malignant hyperthermia induced by curare. Can Anaesth Soc J 1974; 21: 371–5.
2. Waterman PM, et al. Malignant hyperthermia: a case report. Anesth Analg 1980; 59: 220–1.

Effects on the muscles. For reference to acute myopathy and prolonged muscle weakness after withdrawal of long-term continuous infusions of competitive neuromuscular blockers, see under Intensive Care, p.1332.

Hypersensitivity. Reports of severe anaphylactoid reactions following administration of atracurium[1,2] or cisatracurium.[3,4] For a discussion of hypersensitivity reactions associated with neuromuscular blockers, see under Suxamethonium Chloride, p.1341.

1. Stirton-Hopkins C. Life-threatening reaction to atracurium. Br J Anaesth 1988; 60: 597–8.
2. Oh TE, Horton JM. Adverse reactions to atracurium. Br J Anaesth 1989; 62: 467–8.
3. Briassoulis G, et al. Persistent anaphylactic reaction after induction with thiopentone and cisatracurium. Paediatr Anaesth 2000; 10: 429–34.
4. Legros CB, et al. Severe anaphylactic reaction to cisatracurium in a child. Anesth Analg 2001; 92: 648–9.

Treatment of Adverse Effects

It is essential to maintain assisted respiration in patients who have received a competitive neuromuscular blocker until spontaneous breathing is fully restored; in addition a cholinesterase inhibitor such as neostigmine is usually given intravenously, in association with atropine or glycopyrronium, to hasten reversal of the neuromuscular block. Patients need to be closely monitored after reversal of block to ensure that muscle relaxation does not return.

Severe hypotension may require intravenous fluid replacement and cautious administration of a pressor agent; the patient should be positioned to facilitate venous return from the muscles.

Administration of an antihistamine before induction of neuromuscular blockade may be of value in preventing histamine-induced adverse effects in patients with asthma or those susceptible to bronchospasm.

Reversal of neuromuscular blockade. For a discussion of the use of anticholinesterases for reversal of residual neuromuscular block produced by intermediate- or short-acting blockers after surgical or similar procedures, see under Neostigmine, p.1421.

Precautions

Patients who have received a neuromuscular blocker should always have their respiration assisted or controlled until the drug has been inactivated or antagonised.

Atracurium and other competitive neuromuscular blockers should be used with great care, if at all, in respiratory insufficiency or pulmonary disease and in the dehydrated or severely ill patient. The response to neuromuscular blockers is often unpredictable in patients with neuromuscular disorders and they should be used with great caution in these patients (see be-

low). Caution is also needed in patients with a history of conditions such as asthma where release of histamine would be a hazard. Care is also required in patients with a history of hypersensitivity to any neuromuscular blocker.

Resistance to the effects of competitive neuromuscular blockers may occur in patients with burns (see below). The effect of competitive neuromuscular blockers may vary in patients with hepatic impairment; resistance appears to occur to the actions of some blockers such as doxacurium, metocurine, pancuronium, and tubocurarine while for some other blockers, including mivacurium and rocuronium, a prolonged action in patients with hepatic impairment may necessitate a reduction in the usual dosage.

Competitive neuromuscular blockers excreted mainly in the urine should be used with caution in renal impairment; a reduction in dosage may be necessary. Doses may need to be reduced in infants and neonates due to increased sensitivity to competitive muscle relaxants. Doses in obese patients should usually be based upon the patient's ideal body-weight rather than actual body-weight.

The effects of competitive neuromuscular blockers are increased by metabolic or respiratory acidosis and hypokalaemia, hypermagnesaemia, hypocalcaemia, and hypophosphataemia. Competitive neuromuscular blockade may also be enhanced by raised body temperature and reduced in hypothermia.

In contrast to other competitive neuromuscular blockers, reduction in body temperature may necessitate a dosage reduction for atracurium and its isomer cisatracurium since cooling reduces the rate of inactivation of atracurium and cisatracurium, but physiological variations in body temperature and pH will not significantly affect their action.

Burns. The dose requirements of competitive neuromuscular blockers are increased in patients with burns,[1-3] the dose correlating with both the extent of the burn and time after injury. This resistance is usually not seen in patients with less than 10% body-surface burns but if more than 40% of the body-surface is affected the dose of competitive blocker may need to be up to five times higher than in patients without burns. Resistance peaks about 2 weeks after injury, persists for many months in patients with major burns, and decreases gradually with healing of the burn. The mechanism of resistance is multifactorial but may be partly explained by increased protein binding, increased volume of distribution, and increased numbers of acetylcholine receptors at the motor end-plate requiring more muscle relaxant to produce a given effect. Despite the high doses of competitive relaxants that are required, recovery from neuromuscular blockade is not seriously impaired and their effects can be reversed with usual doses of an anticholinesterase.

1. Martyn J, et al. Clinical pharmacology of muscle relaxants in patients with burns. J Clin Pharmacol 1986; 26: 680–5.
2. Anonymous. Neuromuscular blockers in patients with burns. Lancet 1988; ii: 1003–4.
3. Tschida SJ, et al. Resistance to nondepolarizing neuromuscular blocking agents. Pharmacotherapy 1996; 16: 409–18.

Cardiopulmonary bypass. The effect of cardiopulmonary bypass on the pharmacokinetics and pharmacodynamics of competitive neuromuscular blockers can be complex but generally their dosage may need to be reduced. Although the intensity of neuromuscular blockade of most competitive neuromuscular blockers is reduced by hypothermia[1] used during cardiopulmonary bypass, their administration during this procedure is associated with rises in plasma concentrations, reduced clearance, and prolongation of the elimination half-life.[2-5] Various mechanisms, including reduced distribution to highly perfused tissues such as the lungs, have been proposed to explain this.[2] For atracurium, it appears that it is a reduction in the temperature-dependent inactivation by Hofmann elimination during hypothermia which enables lower doses to be used.[6]

1. Buzello W, et al. Unequal effects of cardiopulmonary bypass-induced hypothermia on neuromuscular blockade from constant infusion of alcuronium, d-tubocurarine, pancuronium, and vecuronium. Anesthesiology 1987; 66: 842–6.
2. Walker JS, et al. Alcuronium kinetics in patients undergoing cardiopulmonary bypass surgery. Br J Clin Pharmacol 1983; 15: 237–44.
3. Walker JS, et al. Altered d-tubocurarine disposition during cardiopulmonary bypass surgery. Clin Pharmacol Ther 1984; 35: 686–94.
4. Wierda JMKH, Agoston S. Pharmacokinetics of vecuronium during hypothermic bypass. Br J Anaesth 1989; 63: 627P–628P.
5. Smeulers NJ, et al. Hypothermic cardiopulmonary bypass influences the concentration-response relationship and the biodisposition of rocuronium. Eur J Anaesthesiol 1995; 12 (suppl 11): 91–4.
6. Flynn PJ, et al. Use of atracurium in cardiac surgery involving cardiopulmonary bypass with induced hypothermia. Br J Anaesth 1984; 56: 967–72.

Hepatic impairment. The effect of competitive neuromuscular blockers may vary in patients with hepatic impairment (see Precautions, above) but alterations in the pharmacokinetics of atracurium and cisatracurium in patients with hepatic impairment (see under Pharmacokinetics, below) do not appear to be clinically significant and a reduction in dosage is not generally recommended.

Neuromuscular disorders. Caution is needed if competitive neuromuscular blockers are given to patients with neuromuscular disease since severe complications have been reported.[1] Increased response may be seen in patients with paraplegia or quadriplegia, but resistance has been reported in patients with hemiplegia. Increased response may also occur in patients with amyotrophic lateral sclerosis, neurofibromatosis, and poliomyelitis; this is of little concern unless the respiratory muscles are involved when prolonged apnoea may occur. Patients with myasthenia gravis usually show increased sensitivity to competitive relaxants although small doses have been given without complications. During remission of myasthenia gravis a normal response is usual but since remission is often incomplete, small intermittent doses are advised. A significantly greater exaggeration of response is seen in patients with the myasthenic syndrome. Both normal and increased responses have been reported in patients with myotonias or muscular dystrophies but exquisite sensitivity occurs in patients with ocular muscular dystrophy. A normal response to competitive relaxants may be expected in patients with multiple sclerosis, muscular denervation, Parkinson's disease, and tetanus.

1. Azar I. The response of patients with neuromuscular disorders to muscle relaxants: a review. *Anesthesiology* 1984; **61:** 173–87.

Pregnancy. Results of a controlled study[1] have indicated that the pharmacokinetics of atracurium are unaltered during pregnancy; it is concluded that atracurium could be given in usual doses during pregnancy or in the postpartum period. Atracurium 300 µg per kg body-weight given to 26 women undergoing caesarean section, with subsequent incremental doses of 100 or 200 µg per kg if necessary, produced good surgical relaxation in all patients without any complications.[2] Of the 26 neonates delivered, respiration was established within 90 seconds in 21, with an Apgar score of 10 at 5 minutes. The remaining 5 neonates were delivered by caesarean section because of fetal distress and were slower to start breathing.

1. Guay J, *et al.* Pharmacokinetics of atracurium in pregnant women. *Clin Drug Invest* 1996; **11:** 167–73.
2. Frank M, *et al.* Atracurium in obstetric anaesthesia: a preliminary report. *Br J Anaesth* 1983; **55:** 113S–114S.

Renal impairment. Although some differences in the pharmacokinetics of atracurium and cisatracurium have been reported in patients with renal impairment (see under Pharmacokinetics, below) duration of their neuromuscular blocking action is not significantly dependent on renal function and usual doses may be given to patients with renal impairment.[1,2] Atracurium has been given by infusion to patients with end-stage renal failure[3] when the initial dose required for induction of neuromuscular block was 37% higher than that required by patients without renal impairment. The increase could be explained by the larger extracellular fluid volume in patients with chronic renal failure.

Although the pharmacokinetics of atracurium and cisatracurium are not appreciably different in renal impairment, those of their metabolites may be (see under Pharmacokinetics, below) and therefore it has been suggested that neuromuscular function should be monitored during use of atracurium.[4]

1. Hunter JM, *et al.* Use of the muscle relaxant atracurium in anephric patients: preliminary communication. *J R Soc Med* 1982; **75:** 336–340.
2. Boyd AH, *et al.* Pharmacodynamics of the 1R cis-1′R cis isomer of atracurium (51W89) in health and chronic renal failure. *Br J Anaesth* 1995; **74:** 400–404.
3. Gramstad L. Atracurium, vecuronium and pancuronium in end-stage renal failure: dose-response properties and interactions with azathioprine. *Br J Anaesth* 1987; **59:** 995–1003.
4. Vandenbrom RHG, *et al.* Pharmacokinetics and neuromuscular blocking effects of atracurium besylate and two of its metabolites in patients with normal and impaired renal function. *Clin Pharmacokinet* 1990; **19:** 230–40.

Resistance. The aetiology of resistance to competitive blockers is not clear but might be due to pharmacodynamic or pharmacokinetic alterations associated with disease states such as burn injuries (see above) or hepatic impairment (see Precautions, above) or concomitant drug therapy (see Interactions, below). One review[1] noted that there had been numerous case reports of resistance to competitive neuromuscular blockers; most had been associated with single dose administration or short-term intermittent therapy, but more recent reports have documented resistance during continuous infusions in 9 patients of whom 7 had received atracurium and 2 rocuronium. Resistance to atracurium had followed 2 different patterns. Patients had required either usual or raised doses for initial control but both groups had subsequently required progressive increases. Most patients with resistance to atracurium were successfully managed by transfer to pancuronium or doxacurium.

1. Tschida SJ, *et al.* Resistance to nondepolarizing neuromuscular blocking agents. *Pharmacotherapy* 1996; **16:** 409–18.

Tourniquets. Atracurium might be unsuitable for neuromuscular blockade of a limb which has been isolated with a tourniquet in order to provide a bloodless field for surgery.[1] Atracu-

rium undergoes non-enzymatic degradation in plasma and would therefore continue to degrade locally leading to a loss of blockade in the limb, which could not be corrected by further doses unless the tourniquet was deflated.

1. Shannon PF. Neuromuscular block and tourniquets. *Br J Anaesth* 1994; **73:** 726.

Interactions

A number of drugs may influence neuromuscular transmission and thus interfere with the action of both competitive and depolarising neuromuscular blockers, resulting in potentiation or antagonism of neuromuscular block. Some interactions may be advantageous, such as the reversal of competitive neuromuscular block by anticholinesterases. In general, adverse interactions are potentially more serious in patients with impaired neuromuscular function (see Neuromuscular Disorders, above, and under Suxamethonium Chloride, p.1341).

Drug interactions affecting neuromuscular blockers of either type (competitive and depolarising) as well as those specific for competitive neuromuscular blockers are discussed below. For drug interactions specific to depolarising neuromuscular blockers see under Interactions in Suxamethonium Chloride, p.1342.

◊ Reviews.
1. Feldman S, Karalliedde L. Drug interactions with neuromuscular blockers. *Drug Safety* 1996; **15:** 261–73.

Antiarrhythmics. Lignocaine [lidocaine], procainamide, quinidine, and verapamil all have some neuromuscular blocking activity and may enhance the block produced by neuromuscular blockers. Large doses of *lignocaine [lidocaine]* may reduce the release of acetylcholine and act directly on the muscle membrane. *Quinidine* has a curare-like action at the neuromuscular junction and depresses the muscle action potential. If administered during recovery from neuromuscular block it can result in muscle weakness and apnoea and it should be avoided, if possible, in the immediate postoperative period. Calcium-channel blockers such as *verapamil* may interfere with the release of acetylcholine and prolonged administration may lead to a reduction in intracellular calcium concentration. Potentiation of neuromuscular blockade has been reported[1] and the block may be resistant to reversal with neostigmine; edrophonium may be required.

1. van Poorten JF, *et al.* Verapamil and reversal of vecuronium neuromuscular blockade. *Anesth Analg* 1984; **63:** 155–7.

Antibacterials. Some antibacterials in very high concentration can produce a muscle paralysis which may be additive to or synergistic with that produced by neuromuscular blockers. The neuromuscular block produced by antibacterials may be enhanced in patients with intracellular potassium deficiency, low plasma-calcium concentration, neuromuscular disease, or a tendency to a high plasma-antibacterial concentration, for example following large doses or in renal impairment. The interaction appears to be more important for competitive neuromuscular blockers. The antibacterials most commonly implicated are aminoglycosides, lincosamides, polymyxins, and, more rarely, tetracyclines.

The *aminoglycosides* diminish release of and sensitivity to acetylcholine and their effect can be reversed, at least in part, by calcium, fampridine, or an anticholinesterase. The interaction can occur with most routes of aminoglycoside administration. There are reports of potentiation of neuromuscular blockade occurring with many different aminoglycoside-neuromuscular blocker combinations[1-6] and all aminoglycosides should be used with extreme caution during surgery and in the postoperative period.

The *lincosamides* (*clindamycin* and *lincomycin*) can prolong the action of muscle relaxants producing a neuromuscular block that may be difficult to reverse with calcium or anticholinesterases.[7,8] Patients should be monitored for prolonged paralysis.

There have been reports of prolonged apnoea[2,5,8] following the use of *polymyxins* (*colistin, polymyxin B*) with a neuromuscular blocker. The block is difficult to reverse; calcium may be partially successful, but neostigmine may increase the block.

Tetracyclines have weak neuromuscular blocking properties; potentiation of neuromuscular block has been reported in patients with myasthenia gravis.[2] Reversal of the block may be partly achieved with calcium, but the value of anticholinesterases is questionable.

The *ureidopenicillins* (*azlocillin* and *mezlocillin*), and the closely related *piperacillin* and *apalcillin*, are reported to prolong the block produced by vecuronium.[9,10]

Vancomycin has been reported to increase neuromuscular blockade by vecuronium.[11] Prolonged paralysis and apnoea has occurred in a patient recovering from suxamethonium-induced blockade after being given vancomycin.[12]

1. Hall DR, *et al.* Gentamicin, tubocurarine, lignocaine and neuromuscular blockade. *Br J Anaesth* 1972; **44:** 1329–32.
2. Pittinger CB, *et al.* Antibiotic-induced paralysis. *Anesth Analg Curr Res* 1970; **49:** 487–501.

3. Waterman PM, Smith RB. Tobramycin-curare interaction. *Anesth Analg Curr Res* 1977; **56:** 587–8.
4. Regan AG, Perumbetti PPV. Pancuronium and gentamicin interaction in patients with renal failure. *Anesth Analg* 1980; **59:** 393.
5. Giala MM, Paradelis AG. Two cases of prolonged respiratory depression due to interaction of pancuronium with colistin and streptomycin. *J Antimicrob Chemother* 1979; **5:** 234–5.
6. Jedeikin R, *et al.* Prolongation of neuromuscular blocking effect of vecuronium by antibiotics. *Anaesthesia* 1987; **42:** 858–60.
7. Booij LHD, *et al.* Neostigmine and 4-aminopyridine antagonism of lincomycin-pancuronium neuromuscular blockade in man. *Anesth Analg* 1978; **57:** 316–21.
8. de Gouw NE, *et al.* Interaction of antibiotics on pipecuronium-induced neuromuscular blockade. *J Clin Anesth* 1993; **5:** 212–15.
9. Tryba M. Wirkungsverstäkung nicht-depolarisierender Muskelrelaxantien durch Acylaminopenicilline: Untersuchungen am Beispiel von Vecuronium. *Anaesthesist* 1985; **34:** 651–5.
10. Tryba M, Klemm D. Wechselwirkungen zwischen Acylaminopenicillinen und nicht depolarisierenden Muskelrelaxantien. *Fortschr Antimikrob Antineoplast Chemother* 1985; **4-7:** 1827–33.
11. Huang KC, *et al.* Vancomycin enhances the neuromuscular blockade of vecuronium. *Anesth Analg* 1990; **70:** 194–6.
12. Albrecht RF, Lanier WL. Potentiation of succinylcholine-induced phase II block by vancomycin. *Anesth Analg* 1993; **77:** 1300–2.

Anticholinesterases. Anticholinesterases, including *ecothiopate*, *edrophonium*, *neostigmine*, *pyridostigmine*, *rivastigmine*, and possibly *donepezil*, antagonise the effect of competitive neuromuscular blockers. Some anticholinesterases such as neostigmine inhibit both acetylcholinesterase and plasma cholinesterase, and are used clinically to antagonise competitive neuromuscular blockade. Conversely anticholinesterases enhance the action of depolarising muscle relaxants thus prolonging neuromuscular block, although suxamethonium-induced phase II block can be reversed with an anticholinesterase. See also Interactions in Suxamethonium Chloride, p.1342.

Antiepileptics. Resistance to competitive neuromuscular blockers has been reported in patients receiving chronic treatment with *carbamazepine*[1,2] or *phenytoin*[3] and rapid recovery from neuromuscular block may occur. However, atracurium[1] and mivacurium[4] appear to be unaffected by chronic carbamazepine therapy and the effect of chronic phenytoin treatment on atracurium has usually been minimal.[3] Although one study[5] did report that epileptic patients receiving one or more antiepileptics had significantly shorter times to recovery from atracurium, the authors pointed out that the patient populations were different from those in the previous studies.[1,3] A report of sensitivity to vecuronium[6] has suggested that acute administration of phenytoin may increase rather than decrease the effect of competitive neuromuscular blockers.

1. Ebrahim Z, *et al.* Carbamazepine therapy and neuromuscular blockade with atracurium and vecuronium. *Anesth Analg* 1988; **67:** S55.
2. Whalley DG, Ebrahim Z. Influence of carbamazepine on the dose-response relationship of vecuronium. *Br J Anaesth* 1994; **72:** 125–6.
3. Ornstein E, *et al.* The effect of phenytoin on the magnitude and duration of neuromuscular block following atracurium or vecuronium. *Anesthesiology* 1987; **67:** 191–6.
4. Spacek A, *et al.* Chronic carbamazepine therapy does not influence mivacurium-induced neuromuscular block. *Br J Anaesth* 1996; **77:** 500–502.
5. Tempelhoff R, *et al.* Resistance to atracurium-induced neuromuscular blockade in patients with intractable seizure disorders treated with anticonvulsants. *Anesth Analg* 1990; **71:** 665–9.
6. Baumgardner JE, Bagshaw R. Acute versus chronic phenytoin therapy and neuromuscular blockade. *Anaesthesia* 1990; **45:** 493–4.

Antineoplastics. It has been recommended that atracurium should be used with care in patients receiving anti-oestrogenic drugs,[1] following a case of prolonged neuromuscular blockade with atracurium in a patient receiving *tamoxifen*. See also under Interactions in Suxamethonium Chloride, p.1342.

1. Naguib M, Gyasi HK. Antiestrogenic drugs and atracurium—a possible interaction? *Can Anaesth Soc J* 1986; **33:** 682–3.

Aprotinin. Following reports of apnoea, caution has been advised when aprotinin and neuromuscular blockers are used concomitantly.[1,2]

1. Chasapakis G, Dimas C. Possible interaction between muscle relaxants and the kallikrein-trypsin inactivator "Trasylol". *Br J Anaesth* 1966; **38:** 838–9.
2. Marcello B, Porati U. Trasylol e blocco neuromuscolare: nota preventiva. *Minerva Anestesiol* 1967; **33:** 814–5.

Benzodiazepines. There are conflicting reports of the effect of *diazepam* on neuromuscular blockers; potentiation,[1] or antagonism[1] of neuromuscular block, and a lack of interaction[2-4] have all been reported.

1. Feldman SA, Crawley BE. Interaction of diazepam with the muscle-relaxant drugs. *BMJ* 1970; **2:** 336–8.
2. Driessen JJ, *et al.* Benzodiazepines and neuromuscular blocking drugs in patients. *Acta Anaesthesiol Scand* 1986; **30:** 642–6.
3. Bradshaw EG, Maddison S. Effect of diazepam at the neuromuscular junction. *Br J Anaesth* 1979; **51:** 955–60.
4. Asbury AJ, *et al.* Effect of diazepam on pancuronium-induced neuromuscular blockade maintained by a feedback system. *Br J Anaesth* 1981; **53:** 859–63.

Beta blockers. There is conflicting evidence for the effect of beta blockers on the activity of neuromuscular blockers. Lack of effect on depolarising neuromuscular block[1] and antagonism[2,3] or enhancement[4,5] of both competitive and depolarising block have been reported. The exact mechanism of interaction is not clear. There have also been reports of some neuromuscular blockers such as atracurium[6,7] and alcuronium[8] increasing the hypotension and bradycardia associated with the use of anaesthesia in patients receiving beta blockers; these include reports in patients using beta blockers in eye drops for glaucoma.

1. McCammon RL, *et al.* The effect of esmolol on the onset and duration of succinylcholine-induced neuromuscular blockade. *Anesthesiology* 1985; **63:** A317.
2. Varma YS, *et al.* Effect of propranolol hydrochloride on the neuromuscular blocking action of d-tubocurarine and succinylcholine in man. *Indian J Med Res* 1972; **60:** 266–72.
3. Varma YS, *et al.* Comparative effects of propranolol, oxprenolol and pindolol on neuromuscular blocking action of d-tubocurarine in man. *Indian J Med Res* 1973; **61:** 1382–6.
4. Rozen MS, Whan FM. Prolonged curarization associated with propranolol. *Med J Aust* 1972; **1:** 467–8.
5. Murthy VS, *et al.* Cardiovascular and neuromuscular effects of esmolol during induction of anesthesia. *J Clin Pharmacol* 1986; **26:** 351–7.
6. Glynne GL. Drug Interaction? *Anaesthesia* 1984; **39:** 293.
7. Rowlands DE. Drug Interaction? *Anaesthesia* 1984; **39:** 1252.
8. Yate B, Mostafa SM. Drug Interaction? *Anaesthesia* 1984; **39:** 728.

Botulinum A toxin. The neuromuscular block induced by botulinum toxins (p.1325) is enhanced by competitive neuromuscular blockers.

Calcium-channel blockers. Both *nifedipine* and *verapamil* enhance the effect of competitive neuromuscular blockers. See also under Antiarrhythmics, above.

Cardiac inotropes. Pancuronium or suxamethonium may interact with cardiac glycosides[1] resulting in an increased incidence of arrhythmias; the interaction is more likely with pancuronium.

1. Bartolone RS, Rao TLK. Dysrhythmias following muscle relaxant administration in patients receiving digitalis. *Anesthesiology* 1983; **58:** 567–9.

Corticosteroids. Antagonism of the neuromuscular blocking effects of pancuronium[1] and vecuronium[2] has been reported in patients taking corticosteroids. This interaction may occur only with long-term corticosteroid treatment and may be expected with all competitive neuromuscular blockers.

For reference to a suggestion that concomitant use of corticosteroids might increase the risk of acute myopathy associated with prolonged use of neuromuscular blockers, see under Intensive Care, p.1332.

1. Azar I, *et al.* Resistance to pancuronium in an asthmatic patient treated with aminophylline and steroids. *Can Anaesth Soc J* 1982; **29:** 280–2.
2. Parr SM, *et al.* Betamethasone-induced resistance to vecuronium: a potential problem in neurosurgery? *Anaesth Intensive Care* 1991; **19:** 103–5.

Diuretics. *Frusemide [furosemide]*, and possibly *mannitol*, have been reported to enhance tubocurarine neuromuscular block in patients with renal failure,[1] but antagonism of tubocurarine by frusemide [furosemide] has also occurred.[2] Small doses of frusemide [furosemide] (less than 100 µg per kg) may inhibit protein kinase, which inhibits muscle contraction and potentiates neuromuscular blockade, whereas high doses inhibit phosphodiesterase increasing cAMP activity and resulting in antagonism of neuromuscular blockade. The potassium-depleting effect of diuretics may enhance the effect of competitive neuromuscular blockers.

1. Miller RD, *et al.* Enhancement of d-tubocurarine neuromuscular blockade by diuretics in man. *Anesthesiology* 1976; **45:** 442–5.
2. Azar I, *et al.* Furosemide facilitates recovery of evoked twitch response after pancuronium. *Anesth Analg* 1980; **59:** 55–7.

Ganglion blockers. Prolonged neuromuscular blockade has been reported[1,2] in patients receiving neuromuscular blockers and *trimetaphan*. Trimetaphan may have direct neuromuscular blocking activity and some activity against plasma cholinesterase.

1. Wilson SL, *et al.* Prolonged neuromuscular blockade associated with trimethaphan: a case report. *Anesth Analg Curr Res* 1976; **55:** 353–6.
2. Poulton TH, *et al.* Prolonged apnea following trimethaphan and succinylcholine. *Anesthesiology* 1979; **50:** 54–6.

General anaesthetics. Neuromuscular blockers are potentiated in a dose-dependent manner by inhalation anaesthetics.[1-5] The dose of neuromuscular blocker may need to be reduced by up to 70%[1] depending on the anaesthetic used and its concentration, and on the choice of blocker; the interaction is of greater clinical importance with competitive blockers. *Isoflurane*, *enflurane*, *desflurane*, and *sevoflurane* produce the greater potentiation, followed by *halothane* and *cyclopropane*. Reversal of competitive block with an anticholinesterase has been reported to be reduced.[6,7] See also under Interactions in Suxamethonium Chloride, p.1342.

Potentiation of the neuromuscular blocking effects of tubocurarine[8] and atracurium[9] has been reported following the intravenous administration of *ketamine*. Results from studies *in vitro* suggest that ketamine decreases sensitivity to acetylcholine and it would therefore be expected to potentiate all neuromuscular blockers, but no interaction was reported for pancuronium.[8] Early data[10] suggesting that ketamine potentiates suxamethonium-induced blockade have not been confirmed by later studies.[8,11] For incompatibility between neuromuscular blockers and alkaline solutions such as thiopental sodium, see under Incompatibility, above.

1. Cannon JE, *et al.* Continuous infusion of vecuronium: the effect of anesthetic agents. *Anesthesiology* 1987; **67:** 503–6.

2. Swen J, *et al.* Interaction between nondepolarizing neuromuscular blocking agents and inhalation anesthetics. *Anesth Analg* 1989; **69:** 752–5.
3. Ghourin AF, White PF. Comparative effects of desflurane and isoflurane on vecuronium-induced neuromuscular blockade. *J Clin Anesth* 1992; **4:** 34–8.
4. Vanlinthout LEM, *et al.* Effect of isoflurane and sevoflurane on the magnitude and time course of neuromuscular block produced by vecuronium, pancuronium and atracurium. *Br J Anaesth* 1996; **76:** 389–95.
5. Wulf H, *et al.* Augmentation of the neuromuscular blocking effects of cisatracurium during desflurane, sevoflurane, isoflurane or total i.v. anaesthesia. *Br J Anaesth* 1998; **80:** 308–12.
6. Delisle S, Bevan DR. Impaired neostigmine antagonism of pancuronium during enflurane anaesthesia in man. *Br J Anaesth* 1982; **54:** 441–5.
7. Gill SS, *et al.* Edrophonium antagonism of atracurium during enflurane anaesthesia. *Br J Anaesth* 1990; **64:** 300–5.
8. Johnston RR, *et al.* The interaction of ketamine with d-tubocurarine, pancuronium, and succinylcholine in man. *Anesth Analg Curr Res* 1974; **53:** 496–501.
9. Toft P, Helbo-Hansen S. Interaction of ketamine with atracurium. *Br J Anaesth* 1989; **62:** 319–20.
10. Bovill JG, *et al.* Current status of ketamine anaesthesia. *Lancet* 1971; **i:** 1285–8.
11. Helbo-Hansen HS, *et al.* Ketamine does not affect suxamethonium-induced neuromuscular blockade in man. *Eur J Anaesthesiol* 1989; **6:** 419–23.

Histamine H2-antagonists. There are conflicting reports of the effects of histamine H2-antagonists on neuromuscular blockade. *Cimetidine* has been variously reported to prolong suxamethonium-induced paralysis[1] or to have no effect.[2] *Famotidine* and *ranitidine* have been reported[2] not to interact with suxamethonium. Cimetidine, but not ranitidine, has been reported[3] to delay recovery from vecuronium-induced neuromuscular block. Neither drug appeared to affect recovery after the use of atracurium.

1. Kambam JR, *et al.* Effect of cimetidine on duration of action of succinylcholine. *Anesth Analg* 1987; **66:** 191–2.
2. Turner DR, *et al.* Neuromuscular block by suxamethonium following treatment with histamine type 2 antagonists or metoclopramide. *Br J Anaesth* 1989; **63:** 348–50.
3. McCarthy G, *et al.* Effect of H2-receptor antagonist pretreatment on vecuronium- and atracurium-induced neuromuscular blockade. *Br J Anaesth* 1991; **66:** 713–15.

Immunosuppressants. Antagonism of the neuromuscular blocking effects of competitive neuromuscular blockers has been reported with *azathioprine*,[1] although the effect may not be clinically important. Azathioprine probably inhibits phosphodiesterase activity at the motor nerve terminal resulting in increased release of acetylcholine. There have been reports of prolonged neuromuscular blockade with atracurium, pancuronium, and vecuronium in some patients receiving *ciclosporin* intravenously.[2,3] This effect has been attributed to interaction with polyethoxylated castor oil used as the solvent for intravenous ciclosporin but a similar reaction has been reported in a patient receiving ciclosporin by mouth.[4]

1. Gramstad L. Atracurium, vecuronium and pancuronium in end-stage renal failure: dose-response properties and interaction with azathioprine. *Br J Anaesth* 1987; **59:** 995–1003.
2. Crosby E, Robblee JA. Cyclosporine-pancuronium interaction in a patient with a renal allograft. *Can J Anaesth* 1988; **35:** 300–2.
3. Sidi A, *et al.* Prolonged neuromuscular blockade and ventilatory failure after renal transplantation and cyclosporine. *Can J Anaesth* 1990; **37:** 543–8.
4. Ganjoo P, Tewari P. Oral cyclosporine-vecuronium interaction. *Can J Anaesth* 1994; **41:** 1017.

Lithium. There have been isolated reports of prolonged neuromuscular blockade following the use of neuromuscular blockers in patients receiving lithium.[1,2]

1. Borden H, *et al.* The use of pancuronium bromide in patients receiving lithium carbonate. *Can Anaesth Soc J* 1974; **21:** 79–82.
2. Hill GE, *et al.* Potentiation of succinylcholine neuromuscular blockade by lithium carbonate. *Anesthesiology* 1976; **44:** 439–42.

Local anaesthetics. Healthy subjects who had undergone regional anaesthesia of the forearm experienced symptoms suggestive of local anaesthetic toxicity on deflation of the tourniquet cuff when mivacurium and *prilocaine* had been used together for anaesthesia;[1] administration of prilocaine or mivacurium alone did not produce such an effect. It was considered unlikely that the effect was due entirely to prilocaine inhibition of metabolism of mivacurium by plasma cholinesterase.[2]

The interaction between neuromuscular blockers and *lignocaine [lidocaine]* is discussed under Antiarrhythmics above.

1. Torrance JM, *et al.* Low-dose mivacurium supplementation of prilocaine i.v. regional anaesthesia. *Br J Anaesth* 1997; **78:** 222–3.
2. Torrance JM, *et al.* Interactions between mivacurium and prilocaine. *Br J Anaesth* 1997; **78:** 262.

Magnesium salts. Parenteral magnesium salts may potentiate the effects of competitive and depolarising neuromuscular blockers;[1] the neuromuscular block is deepened and prolonged and a reduction in the dose of the blocker may be needed. Magnesium salts should be used with caution in the postoperative period since administration shortly after recovery from neuromuscular block can lead to recurarisation.[2] Magnesium salts reduce release of and sensitivity to acetylcholine, thus contributing to neuromuscular blockade.

1. Ghoneim MM, Long JP. The interaction between magnesium and other neuromuscular blocking agents. *Anesthesiology* 1970; **32:** 23–7.
2. Fuchs-Buder T, Tassonyi E. Magnesium sulphate enhances residual neuromuscular block induced by vecuronium. *Br J Anaesth* 1996; **76:** 565–6.

MAOIs. There appears to be a theoretical hazard with pancuronium in patients receiving MAOIs since it releases stored adrenaline;[1] alcuronium, atracurium, or vecuronium would appear to be suitable alternatives.

1. Stack CG, *et al.* Monoamine oxidase inhibitors and anaesthesia: a review. *Br J Anaesth* 1988; **60:** 222–7.

Neuromuscular blockers. A competitive neuromuscular blocker given shortly before a depolarising blocker antagonises the depolarising neuromuscular block. This interaction has been used clinically to reduce muscle fasciculations caused by suxamethonium (see Anaesthesia, p.1331 and Effects on the Muscles, p.1340) and tried for other adverse effects associated with suxamethonium (see Effects on Plasma-potassium Concentration, p.1340). To achieve this antagonism a small non-paralysing dose of a competitive blocker is given before suxamethonium. If a paralysing dose of a competitive blocker is followed some time later with a dose of suxamethonium, for example to facilitate abdominal closure, the resulting neuromuscular block is influenced by the competitive blocker used, the depth of residual block, the dose of suxamethonium, and whether an anticholinesterase is given; antagonism, enhancement, and a combination of the two have been observed.[1,2]

A competitive blocker is often given following the short-acting suxamethonium to maintain neuromuscular blockade during long procedures. The action of the competitive blocker has been reported to be considerably potentiated and prolonged in these circumstances,[3,4] and reduction in the dose of the competitive blocker may be appropriate.

Combination of competitive blockers may have additive or synergistic effects and the interaction may differ depending on which blocker is given first. Caution is needed if a small dose of a shorter-acting blocker is given near the end of an operation in which a long-acting blocker has been given previously, since the resulting block may be greater than expected and much longer than desired.[5-7]

1. Scott RPF, Norman J. Effect of suxamethonium given during recovery from atracurium. *Br J Anaesth* 1988; **61:** 292–6.
2. Black AMS. Effect of suxamethonium given during recovery from atracurium. *Br J Anaesth* 1989; **62:** 348–9.
3. d'Hollander AA, *et al.* Clinical and pharmacological actions of a bolus injection of suxamethonium: two phenomena of distinct duration. *Br J Anaesth* 1983; **55:** 131–4.
4. Ono K, *et al.* Influence of suxamethonium on the action of subsequently administered vecuronium or pancuronium. *Br J Anaesth* 1989; **62:** 324–6.
5. Rashkovsky OM, *et al.* Interaction between pancuronium bromide and vecuronium bromide. *Br J Anaesth* 1985; **57:** 1063–6.
6. Middleton CM, *et al.* Use of atracurium or vecuronium to prolong the action of tubocurarine. *Br J Anaesth* 1989; **62:** 659–63.
7. Kim KS, *et al.* Interactions between mivacurium and pancuronium. *Br J Anaesth* 1997; **79:** 19–23.

Sex hormones. Resistance to the neuromuscular blocking effects of suxamethonium and vecuronium in one patient was attributed to previous long-term therapy with *testosterone*,[1] although the exact mechanism could not be explained. See also under Interactions in Suxamethonium Chloride, p.1342.

1. Reddy P, *et al.* Resistance to muscle relaxants in patients receiving prolonged testosterone therapy. *Anesthesiology* 1989; **70:** 871–3.

Smoking. Preliminary work suggests that smoking might affect the dose requirements for neuromuscular blockers. One group of workers[1] found that smokers needed more vecuronium than non-smokers; it was considered that the effect might be explained at the receptor level, although possible increased metabolism of vecuronium could not be excluded. This was in contrast to an earlier study[2] in which the amount of atracurium required was reduced in smokers.

1. Teiriä H, *et al.* Effect of smoking on dose requirements for vecuronium. *Br J Anaesth* 1996; **76:** 154–5.
2. Kroeker KA, *et al.* Neuromuscular blockade in the setting of chronic nicotine exposure. *Anesthesiology* 1994; **81:** A1120.

Sympathomimetics. Intravenous *salbutamol* has been reported to enhance the blockade obtained with pancuronium and vecuronium.[1] See also under Interactions in Suxamethonium Chloride, p.1342.

1. Salib Y, Donati F. Potentiation of pancuronium and vecuronium neuromuscular blockade by intravenous salbutamol. *Can J Anaesth* 1993; **40:** 50–3.

Xanthines. Resistance to neuromuscular block with pancuronium, requiring an increase in dosage or transfer to vecuronium, has been reported in patients receiving *aminophylline* with[1] or without[2] corticosteroid therapy. It was suggested that this effect might be due to inhibition of phosphodiesterase by aminophylline resulting in increased release of acetylcholine at the nerve terminal.

1. Azar I, *et al.* Resistance to pancuronium in an asthmatic patient treated with aminophylline and steroids. *Can Anaesth Soc J* 1982; **29:** 280–2.
2. Daller JA, *et al.* Aminophylline antagonizes the neuromuscular blockade of pancuronium but not vecuronium. *Crit Care Med* 1991; **19:** 983–5.

Pharmacokinetics

Following intravenous injection both atracurium besilate and cisatracurium besilate undergo spontaneous degradation via Hofmann elimination (a non-enzymatic breakdown process occurring at physiological pH and temperature) to produce laudanosine and other metabolites. There is also ester hydrolysis by non-specific plasma esterases. The metabolites have no neuromuscular blocking activity.

About 80% of atracurium besilate is bound to plasma proteins. Atracurium besilate and its metabolites cross the placenta in clinically insignificant amounts. Excretion of atracurium and cisatracurium is in urine and bile, mostly as metabolites. The elimination half-life has been reported to be approximately 20 minutes for atracurium and 22 to 29 minutes for cisatracurium but laudanosine has an elimination half-life of about 3 hours.

◊ Reviews.
1. Kisor DF, Schmith VD. Clinical pharmacokinetics of cisatracurium besilate. *Clin Pharmacokinet* 1999; **36:** 27–40.

◊ Atracurium and cisatracurium are degraded by Hofmann elimination and metabolised by non-specific plasma esterases. Hofmann elimination is generally believed to be the main route of degradation but *in-vitro* work suggests ester hydrolysis is more important.[1] Both routes are independent of renal and hepatic function and no dosage reduction is recommended for elderly patients or those with impaired renal or hepatic function. However, the elimination half-life of atracurium has been found to be slightly longer in elderly patients[2] and in those with hepatic cirrhosis[3] compared with young and healthy patients, although others[4] have found no change in the pharmacokinetics of atracurium in the elderly. Renal and hepatic involvement in the metabolism of atracurium[2] may help to explain any tendency to reduced elimination but this does not appear to be clinically significant. Although clearance of cisatracurium has been reported to be reduced in patients with renal failure[5] this appears to have little significant effect on its pharmacodynamics.[6] Differences in the pharmacokinetics of cisatracurium in patients with hepatic impairment have been reported to be minor.[7] The major biotransformation product of atracurium and cisatracurium is *laudanosine*; it has no clinical neuromuscular blocking activity but has been associated with CNS stimulation in *animal* studies. It is more lipid soluble than atracurium and cisatracurium and has a half-life of around 3 hours compared with one of approximately 20 minutes for atracurium. Higher plasma-laudanosine concentrations have been reported in patients with renal failure[5,8,9] than in patients with normal renal function. The elimination half-life of laudanosine was found to be significantly greater in patients with hepatic cirrhosis[3] and in elderly patients[2] compared with healthy and young patients respectively. Laudanosine crosses the blood-brain barrier in man. The concentration of laudanosine in the CSF increases during an infusion of atracurium and the CSF-to-plasma ratio gradually increases. A ratio of 0.14 was found at 125 to 140 minutes[10] during an infusion of atracurium at a mean rate of 510 μg per kg per hour. No evidence of CNS stimulation has been reported in man although patients given atracurium[11] had a 20% higher mean arterial-thiopental concentration at awakening compared with patients given vecuronium, suggesting that laudanosine may have had a minor stimulatory effect on the CNS. The blood-brain barrier appears to be effective in preventing a very high concentration of laudanosine from reaching the CNS and it is considered unlikely[12] that concentrations great enough to provoke seizures will be reached. Cisatracurium may be associated with the production of less laudanosine than atracurium.[13]

1. Stiller RL, *et al.* In vitro degradation of atracurium in human plasma. *Br J Anaesth* 1985; **57:** 1085–8.
2. Kent AP, *et al.* Pharmacokinetics of atracurium and laudanosine in the elderly. *Br J Anaesth* 1989; **63:** 661–6.
3. Parker CJR, Hunter JM. Pharmacokinetics of atracurium and laudanosine in patients with hepatic cirrhosis. *Br J Anaesth* 1989; **62:** 177–83.
4. d'Hollander AA, *et al.* Clinical evaluation of atracurium besylate requirement for a stable muscle relaxation during surgery: lack of age-related effects. *Anesthesiology* 1983; **59:** 237–40.
5. Eastwood NB, *et al.* Pharmacokinetics of 1R-cis 1′R-cis atracurium besylate (51W89) and plasma laudanosine concentrations in health and chronic renal failure. *Br J Anaesth* 1995; **75:** 431–5
6. Boyd AH, *et al.* Pharmacodynamics of the 1R cis-1′R cis isomer of atracurium (51W89) in health and chronic renal failure. *Br J Anaesth* 1995; **74:** 400–404.
7. De Wolf AM, *et al.* Pharmacokinetics and pharmacodynamics of cisatracurium in patients with end-stage liver disease undergoing liver transplantation. *Br J Anaesth* 1996; **76:** 624–8.
8. Fahey MR, *et al.* Effect of renal failure on laudanosine excretion in man. *Br J Anaesth* 1985; **57:** 1049–51.
9. Vandenbrom RHG, *et al.* Pharmacokinetics and neuromuscular blocking effects of atracurium besylate and two of its metabolites in patients with normal and impaired renal function. *Clin Pharmacokinet* 1990; **19:** 230–40.
10. Eddleston JM, *et al.* Concentrations of atracurium and laudanosine in cerebrospinal fluid and plasma during intracranial surgery. *Br J Anaesth* 1989; **63:** 525–30.
11. Beemer GH, *et al.* Production of laudanosine following infusion of atracurium in man and its effects on awakening. *Br J Anaesth* 1989; **63:** 76–80.
12. Yate PM, *et al.* Clinical experience and plasma laudanosine concentrations during the infusion of atracurium in the intensive therapy unit. *Br J Anaesth* 1987; **59:** 211–17.
13. Boyd AH, *et al.* Comparison of the pharmacokinetics and pharmacodynamics of an infusion of cis-atracurium (51W89) or atracurium in critically ill patients undergoing mechanical ventilation in an intensive therapy unit. *Br J Anaesth* 1996; **76:** 382–8.

Uses and Administration

Competitive neuromuscular blockers act by competing with acetylcholine for receptors on the motor endplate of the neuromuscular junction to produce blockade. The muscles that produce fine rapid movements such as those of the face are the first to be affected followed by those of the limbs and torso; the last to be affected are those of the diaphragm. The paralysis is reversible with recovery occurring in reverse order. Restoration of normal neuromuscular function can be hastened by increasing the concentration of acetylcholine at the motor end-plate by giving an anticholinesterase such as neostigmine.

Atracurium besilate and cisatracurium besilate are competitive benzylisoquinolinium neuromuscular blockers. Cisatracurium besilate, the *R-cis,1′R-cis*-isomer of atracurium besilate, is about 3 times more potent than the mixture of isomers that constitute atracurium besilate. Following an intravenous dose of atracurium muscle relaxation begins in about 2 minutes and lasts for 15 to 35 minutes; onset may be slightly slower for cisatracurium.

Atracurium besilate and cisatracurium besilate are used for endotracheal intubation and to provide muscle relaxation in general anaesthesia for surgical procedures (see Anaesthesia, p.1331) and to aid controlled ventilation (see Intensive Care, p.1332).

Doses of neuromuscular blockers need to be carefully titrated for individual patients according to response, and may vary with the procedure, the other drugs given, and the state of the patient; monitoring of the degree of block is recommended in order to reduce the risk of overdosage.

For **atracurium besilate**, the usual initial dose for adults and children over 1 month of age is 300 to 600 μg per kg body-weight by intravenous injection. Subsequent doses of 100 to 200 μg per kg may be given as necessary, typically every 15 to 25 minutes. It is recommended that in patients with cardiovascular disease the initial dose should be administered over a period of 60 seconds.

Atracurium besilate may also be given by continuous intravenous infusion at a rate of 5 to 10 μg per kg per minute to maintain neuromuscular block during prolonged procedures. Somewhat higher infusion rates may be used in patients undergoing controlled ventilation in intensive care.

For **cisatracurium**, a usual initial dose for adults is the equivalent of 150 μg per kg body-weight, as the besilate. The neuromuscular block may be extended with a maintenance dose of 30 μg per kg about every 20 minutes.

The usual initial dose for children aged over 1 month is 150 μg per kg body-weight. The neuromuscular block may be extended in children between 2 and 12 years of age with a maintenance dose of 20 μg per kg about every 9 minutes.

Cisatracurium besilate may also be given by continuous intravenous infusion to adults and children over 2 years of age at an initial rate equivalent to 3 μg of cisatracurium per kg per minute followed by a rate of 1 to 2 μg per kg per minute after stabilisation.

◊ Reviews.
1. Hughes R. Atracurium—the first years. *Clin Anaesthesiol* 1985; **3:** 331–45.
2. Bryson HM, Faulds D. Cisatracurium besilate: a review of its pharmacology and clinical potential in anaesthetic practice. *Drugs* 1997; **53:** 848–66.

Administration in infants and children. Children generally require larger doses of competitive neuromuscular blockers on a weight basis than adolescents or adults to achieve similar degrees of neuromuscular blockade and may recover more quickly. However, neonates and infants under 1 year of age are more sensitive and usual doses may produce prolonged neuromuscular blockade.

Electroconvulsive therapy. Competitive neuromuscular blockers have been used to reduce the intensity of muscle contractions and minimise trauma in patients receiving electroconvulsive therapy, but suxamethonium (p.1340) is generally preferred because of its short duration of action.

Intravenous regional anaesthesia. Competitive neuromuscular blockers and/or opioid analgesics have been added to the local anaesthetic used in intravenous regional anaesthesia (p.1305) to improve the quality of anaesthesia. However atracurium (see Tourniquets under Precautions, above) and mivacurium (see Tourniquets, p.1337) might be unsuitable for such use.

Shivering. Various drugs have been tried in the treatment of postoperative shivering (p.1255). There are reports of neuromuscular blockers being used to treat shivering after cardiac surgery in order to reduce cardiovascular stress;[1] one study[2] has suggested that vecuronium might be preferable to pancuronium as it does not increase myocardial work and may be associated with fewer complications.

1. Cruise C, *et al.* Comparison of meperidine and pancuronium for the treatment of shivering after cardiac surgery. *Can J Anaesth* 1992; **39:** 563–8.
2. Dupuis J-Y, *et al.* Pancuronium or vecuronium for the treatment of shivering after cardiac surgery. *Anesth Analg* 1994; **79:** 472–81.

Tetanus. For a comment on the role of competitive neuromuscular blockers in the management of muscle spasms caused by tetanus, see p.1332.

Preparations

Proprietary Preparations (details are given in Part 3)
Aust.: Nimbex; Tracrium; **Austral.:** Nimbex; Tracrium; **Belg.:** Nimbex; Tracrium; **Braz.:** Tracrium; **Canad.:** Nimbex; Tracrium; **Denm.:** Nimbex; Tracrium; **Fin.:** Nimbex; Tracrium; **Fr.:** Nimbex; Tracrium; **Ger.:** Nimbex; Tracrium; **Hong Kong:** Nimbex; Tracrium; **Irl.:** Nimbex; Tracrium; **Israel:** Mycurium; Tracrium; **Ital.:** Nimbex; Tracrium; **Mex.:** Nimbex; Relatrac; Tracrium; **Neth.:** Nimbex; Tracrium; **Norw.:** Nimbex; Tracrium; **NZ:** Tracrium; **Port.:** Faulcurium; Nimbex; Tracrium; **S.Afr.:** Nimbex; Tracrium; **Singapore:** Nimbex; Tracrium; **Spain:** Nimbex; Tracrium; **Swed.:** Nimbex; Tracrium; **Switz.:** Nimbex; Tracrium; **Thai.:** Nimbex; Tracrium; **UK:** Nimbex; Tracrium; **USA:** Nimbex; Tracrium.

Decamethonium Iodide (5711-c)

Decamethonium Iodide (*BAN*).

Decamethonium Biiodatum; Decametonium Iodidum. *NN′*-Decamethylenebis(trimethylammonium) di-iodide.
$C_{16}H_{38}I_2N_2 = 512.3.$
CAS — 156-74-1 *(decamethonium); 541-22-0 (decamethonium bromide); 1420-40-2 (decamethonium iodide).*

NOTE. Decamethonium Bromide is *rINN*.

Profile

Decamethonium is a depolarising neuromuscular blocker with actions and uses similar to those of suxamethonium chloride (p.1340). The effect of a single intravenous injection lasts for 15 to 20 minutes, but onset of action is slower than with suxamethonium. It is excreted mainly in the urine as unchanged drug. It has been used mainly as the iodide salt, although the bromide was also formerly employed.

Doxacurium Chloride (4961-m)

Doxacurium Chloride (*BAN, USAN, rINN*).

BW-A938U. A mixture of the (1R,1′S,2S,2′R), (1R,1′R,2S,2′S), and (1S,1′S,2R,2′R) stereoisomers (a *meso* isomer and two enantiomers respectively) of 1,1′,2,2′,3,3′,4,4′-octahydro-6,6′,7,7′,8,8′-hexamethoxy-2,2′-dimethyl-1,1′-bis(3,4,5-trimethoxybenzyl)-2,2′-[butanedioylbis(oxytrimethylene)]di-isoquinolinium dichloride, all of which are in a *trans* configuration at the 1 and 2 positions of the isoquinolinium rings.
$C_{56}H_{78}Cl_2N_2O_{16} = 1106.1.$
CAS — 106819-53-8 (doxacurium chloride, meso isomer); 83348-52-1 (doxacurium chloride, total racemate).
ATC — M03AC07.

Adverse Effects, Treatment, and Precautions

As for competitive neuromuscular blockers in general (see Atracurium, p.1333). Doxacurium has little histamine-releasing activity and causes negligible vagal or sympathetic blockade so that significant cardiovascular side-effects are not a problem.

Renal impairment. Although the duration of neuromuscular block and speed of recovery following the use of doxacurium were found to be prolonged in patients with renal failure when compared with patients with normal renal function, the differences were considered not to be significant.[1]

1. Cashman JN, *et al.* Neuromuscular block with doxacurium (BW A938U) in patients with normal or absent renal function. *Br J Anaesth* 1990; **64:** 186–92.

Interactions

For interactions associated with competitive neuromuscular blockers, see Atracurium, p.1334.

Pharmacokinetics

Following intravenous administration, doxacurium chloride is excreted mainly unchanged in the urine and bile. The elimination half-life is reported to be about 2 hours.

Uses and Administration

Doxacurium chloride is a benzylisoquinolinium competitive neuromuscular blocker (see Atracurium, p.1336). It is used for endotracheal intubation and to provide muscle relaxation in general anaesthesia for surgical procedures (see Anaesthesia, p.1331) and to aid controlled ventilation (see below).

Doses of neuromuscular blockers need to be carefully titrated for individual patients according to response, and may vary with the procedure, the other drugs given, and the state of the patient; monitoring of the degree of block is recommended in order to reduce the risk of overdosage. Doses of doxacurium chloride are expressed in terms of the equivalent amount of doxacurium base. The usual initial dose is 50 µg per kg body-weight intravenously; maintenance doses of 5 to 10 µg per kg are employed. At the above dose muscle relaxation occurs within about 5 minutes and the effect lasts for about 100 minutes. For more prolonged procedures an initial dose of 80 µg per kg may be used, which produces muscle relaxation in about 4 minutes and the effects last for about 2½ hours.

◊ Reviews.
1. Mirakhur RK. Newer neuromuscular blocking drugs: an overview of their clinical pharmacology and therapeutic use. *Drugs* 1992; **44**: 182–99.

Administration in the elderly. Several studies have shown that the duration of action of doxacurium is prolonged in the elderly, although the precise mechanism for this prolongation is subject to debate.[1-3] Since both the onset of action and recovery are delayed, some consider[4] that doxacurium may not be suitable for use in the elderly for surgical procedures of less than one hour.
1. Levy G. Effect of advanced age on the pharmacodynamics of doxacurium. *Clin Pharmacol Ther* 1994; **55**: 359.
2. Varin F, *et al.* Effect of advanced age on the pharmacodynamics of doxacurium. *Clin Pharmacol Ther* 1994; **55**: 359–60.
3. Schmith VD, *et al.* Effect of advanced age on the pharmacodynamics of doxacurium. *Clin Pharmacol Ther* 1994; **55**: 360–2.
4. Martlew RA, Harper NJN. The clinical pharmacology of doxacurium in young adults and in elderly patients. *Anaesthesia* 1995; **50**: 779–82.

Administration in infants and children. As for some other neuromuscular blockers, children over 2 years of age have been found to require more doxacurium per kg body-weight than adults to achieve a similar degree of neuromuscular blockade,[1] and the dosage requirement may be almost twice as great as that for adults.[2] Children may also recover more quickly.[1] However, the sensitivity of infants under one year of age appears to be increased.[2]
1. Goudsouzian NG, *et al.* Neuromuscular and cardiovascular effects of doxacurium in children anaesthetized with halothane. *Br J Anaesth* 1989; **62**: 263–8.
2. Taivainen T, Meretoja OA. Doxacurium in infants, children and adolescents during balanced anaesthesia. *Br J Anaesth* 1995; **74** (suppl 1): 98–9.

Intensive care. Experience of the use of doxacurium to facilitate mechanical ventilation in patients in intensive care (see p.1332) is relatively limited. It appears to offer prolonged neuromuscular block without the tachycardia associated with pancuronium; recovery after prolonged administration may also be faster than with pancuronium.[1] There has been an anecdotal report of the successful management with doxacurium of 4 patients who had developed tachyphylaxis to long-term administration of atracurium.[2]
1. Murray MJ, *et al.* Double-blind, randomized multicenter study of doxacurium vs. pancuronium in intensive care unit patients who require neuromuscular-blocking agents. *Crit Care Med* 1995; **23**: 450–8.
2. Coursin DB, *et al.* Doxacurium infusion in critically ill patients with atracurium tachyphylaxis. *Am J Health-Syst Pharm* 1995; **52**: 635–9.

Preparations

Proprietary Preparations (details are given in Part 3)
Canad.: Nuromax; *USA:* Nuromax.

Gallamine Triethiodide (5720-k)

Gallamine Triethiodide (BANM, rINN).

Benzcurine Iodide; Gallamini Triethiodidum; Gallamone Triethiodide. 2,2′,2″-(Benzene-1,2,3-triyltrioxy)tris(tetraethylammonium) tri-iodide.

$C_{30}H_{60}I_3N_3O_3 = 891.5$.

CAS — 153-76-4 (gallamine); 65-29-2 (gallamine triethiodide).

Pharmacopoeias. In *Eur.* (see p.vi), *Int.*, and *US.*

Pharmacopoeial description

Ph. Eur.: A white, or almost white, hygroscopic powder. Very soluble in water; slightly soluble in alcohol; practically insoluble in dichloromethane and in ether. Store in airtight containers. Protect from light.

USP 25: A white, hygroscopic, odourless, amorphous powder. Very soluble in water; sparingly soluble in alcohol; very slightly soluble in chloroform. pH of a 2% solution in water is between 5.3 and 7.0. Store in airtight containers. Protect from light.

Adverse Effects, Treatment, and Precautions

As for competitive neuromuscular blockers in general (see Atracurium, p.1333). Tachycardia often develops due to the vagolytic action of gallamine triethiodide and blood pressure may be raised. It has a small histamine-releasing effect; occasional anaphylactoid reactions have been reported. It should be avoided in patients hypersensitive to iodine. Although competitive muscle relaxants have been given with great care to patients

with myasthenia gravis (see Neuromuscular Disorders, p.1334), the manufacturer of gallamine triethiodide recommends that it should not be used in such patients.

Cardiopulmonary bypass. Alterations in the pharmacokinetics of competitive neuromuscular blockers in patients undergoing surgery involving cardiopulmonary bypass usually necessitate the use of reduced doses (see p.1333). However, the pharmacokinetics of gallamine in patients undergoing cardiopulmonary bypass appear not to differ significantly from those in control patients.[1]
1. Shanks CA, *et al.* Gallamine disposition in open-heart surgery involving cardiopulmonary bypass. *Clin Pharmacol Ther* 1983; **33**: 792–9.

Renal impairment. Gallamine triethiodide is excreted unchanged in the urine and some consider that it should be avoided in severe renal impairment since prolonged paralysis may occur. Significantly prolonged elimination half-life and reduced clearance have been reported[1] in patients with chronic renal failure given gallamine triethiodide in initial doses of 2 mg per kg body-weight intravenously.
1. Ramzan MI, *et al.* Gallamine disposition in surgical patients with chronic renal failure. *Br J Clin Pharmacol* 1981; **12**: 141–7.

Interactions

For interactions associated with competitive neuromuscular blockers, see Atracurium, p.1334.

Pharmacokinetics

Following intravenous administration gallamine triethiodide is distributed throughout body tissues. It is not metabolised, and is excreted in the urine as unchanged drug.

Uses and Administration

Gallamine triethiodide is a benzylisoquinolinium competitive neuromuscular blocker (see Atracurium, p.1336). Muscle relaxation occurs within about 1 to 2 minutes following intravenous injection and lasts for about 20 to 30 minutes. It is used to provide muscle relaxation in general anaesthesia for surgical procedures (see Anaesthesia, p.1331) and to aid controlled ventilation (see Intensive Care, p.1332).

Doses of neuromuscular blockers need to be carefully titrated for individual patients according to response, and may vary with the procedure, the other drugs given, and the state of the patient; monitoring of the degree of block is recommended in order to reduce the risk of overdosage. An initial test dose of 20 mg may be given intravenously to the patient before anaesthesia to determine undue sensitivity. In the UK, initial doses of 80 to 120 mg by intravenous injection have been recommended, with further doses of 20 to 40 mg as required. In children, a dose of 1.5 mg per kg body-weight has been recommended, reduced to 600 µg per kg for neonates.

In the USA and some other countries lower doses have generally been employed; an initial dose of 1 mg per kg intravenously, up to a maximum of 80 mg, with additional doses of 0.5 to 1 mg per kg after about 50 to 60 minutes if required.

Gallamine triethiodide has also been given intramuscularly, with or without hyaluronidase.

Preparations

BP 2001: Gallamine Injection;
USP 25: Gallamine Triethiodide Injection.

Proprietary Preparations (details are given in Part 3)
Austral.: Flaxedil†; *Braz.:* Flaxedil; *Canad.:* Flaxedil†; *Denm.:* Relaxan†; *Neth.:* Flaxedil†; *Spain:* Miowas G; *UK:* Flaxedil.

Metocurine Iodide (5726-d)

Metocurine Iodide (USAN).

Dimethyl Tubocurarine Iodide; (+)-O,O′-Dimethylchondrocurarine Di-iodide; Dimethyltubocurarine Iodide; Trimethyltubocurarine Iodide. (+)-6,6′,7′,12′-Tetramethoxy-2,2,2′,2′-tetramethyltubocuraranium di-iodide.

$C_{40}H_{48}I_2N_2O_6 = 906.6$.

CAS — 5152-30-7 (metocurine); 7601-55-0 (metocurine iodide).

NOTE. The name dimethyltubocurarine iodide was based on the old empirical formula for tubocurarine (p.1343).

Profile

Metocurine iodide is a benzylisoquinolinium competitive neuromuscular blocker (see Atracurium, p.1336) that has been used for endotracheal intubation and to provide muscle relaxation in general anaesthesia for surgical and other procedures (see Anaesthesia, p.1331) and to aid controlled ventilation (see Intensive Care, p.1332).

Metocurine iodide has a moderate risk of inducing histamine release. Allergic reactions may occur in patients sensitive to iodine. Metocurine has some ganglion blocking activity and cardiovascular side-effects may occur.

Renal impairment. A study involving 5 patients with renal failure undergoing transplantation showed that the mean elimination half-life of metocurine was 11.4 hours, compared with 6.0 hours in 5 healthy subjects and plasma clearance was significantly reduced.[1] However, the serum concentration required to produce 90% blockade was significantly elevated in patients with renal failure. There was considerable variation in the duration of neuromuscular blockade in patients with renal failure, one remaining well relaxed for 6 hours while one was well re-

laxed for only 10 minutes. If patients with renal failure are given metocurine, monitoring is imperative to ensure adequate relaxation without overdosage.
1. Brotherton WP, Matteo RS. Pharmacokinetics and pharmacodynamics of metocurine in humans with and without renal failure. *Anesthesiology* 1981; **55**: 273–6.

Preparations

Proprietary Preparations (details are given in Part 3)
Canad.: Metubine†; *USA:* Metubine†.

Mivacurium Chloride (5500-v)

Mivacurium Chloride (BAN, USAN, rINN).

BW-B1090U. A mixture of the stereoisomers of (E)-1,1′,2,2′,3,3′,4,4′-octahydro-6,6′,7,7′-tetramethoxy-2,2′-dimethyl-1,1′-bis(3,4,5-trimethoxybenzyl)-2,2′-[oct-4-enedioyl-bis(oxytrimethylene)]di-isoquinolinium dichloride.

$C_{58}H_{80}Cl_2N_2O_{14} = 1100.2$.

CAS — 106861-44-3 (mivacurium chloride, total racemate).

ATC — M03AC10.

Adverse Effects, Treatment, and Precautions

As for competitive neuromuscular blockers in general (see Atracurium, p.1333). Mivacurium chloride has no significant vagal or ganglion blocking activity at recommended doses. It may induce histamine release especially when given in large doses rapidly.

Mivacurium should be used with caution, if at all, in patients with plasma cholinesterase deficiency, since its duration of action will be prolonged in such patients.

Burns. In common with other competitive muscle relaxants patients with burns may develop resistance to mivacurium and require increased doses (see under Atracurium, p.1333). However, as these patients may also have reduced plasma cholinesterase activity dosage requirements could also be reduced. The manufacturer recommends that such patients should be given a test dose of 15 to 20 µg per kg body-weight with subsequent dosage adjustments being guided by monitoring of the block.

Hepatic and renal impairment. The pharmacokinetics of mivacurium have been studied in patients with kidney[1-3] or liver impairment.[1,4,5] Compared with healthy subjects, the duration of relaxation produced by mivacurium was approximately 1.5 times greater than normal in patients with kidney disease and up to about 3 times greater than normal in patients with liver impairment. The reduced plasma-cholinesterase activity in the patients with liver impairment may have played an important part in this effect. Although an anticholinesterase such as neostigmine hastens recovery by only a few minutes in healthy subjects its use may be indicated in patients in whom recovery is delayed.[2]
1. Cook DR, *et al.* Pharmacokinetics of mivacurium in normal patients and in those with hepatic or renal failure. *Br J Anaesth* 1992; **69**: 580–5.
2. Phillips BJ, Hunter JM. Use of mivacurium chloride by constant infusion in the anephric patient. *Br J Anaesth* 1992; **68**: 492–8.
3. Head-Rapson AG, *et al.* Pharmacokinetics and pharmacodynamics of the three isomers of mivacurium in health, in end-stage renal failure and in patients with impaired renal function. *Br J Anaesth* 1995; **75**: 31–6.
4. Devlin JC, *et al.* Pharmacodynamics of mivacurium chloride in patients with hepatic cirrhosis. *Br J Anaesth* 1993; **71**: 227–31.
5. Head-Rapson AG, *et al.* Pharmacokinetics of the three isomers of mivacurium and pharmacodynamics of the chiral mixture in hepatic cirrhosis. *Br J Anaesth* 1994; **73**: 613–18.

Neuromuscular disorders. Neuromuscular blockade was successfully achieved with mivacurium in an obese elderly patient with myasthenia gravis requiring surgery.[1] Only about half the usual dose was required and even then recovery was delayed. See Atracurium, p.1334 for a discussion of the use of competitive neuromuscular blockers in patients with neuromuscular disorders.
1. Seigne RD, Scott RPF. Mivacurium chloride and myasthenia gravis. *Br J Anaesth* 1994; **72**: 468–9.

Plasma cholinesterase deficiency. There have been reports of prolonged neuromuscular block produced by mivacurium in patients with plasma cholinesterase deficiency.[1-4] Time to full recovery had varied; one patient required up to 8 hours.
1. Goudsouzian NG, *et al.* Prolonged neuromuscular block from mivacurium in two patients with cholinesterase deficiency. *Anesth Analg* 1993; **77**: 183–5.
2. Sockalingam I, Green DW. Mivacurium-induced prolonged neuromuscular block. *Br J Anaesth* 1995; **74**: 234–6.
3. Fox MH, Hunt PCW. Prolonged neuromuscular block associated with mivacurium. *Br J Anaesth* 1995; **74**: 237–8.
4. Zimmer S. Mivacurium and prolonged neuromuscular block. *Br J Anaesth* 1995; **75**: 823.

Tourniquets. It has been suggested that mivacurium might be unsuitable for neuromuscular blockade of a limb which has been isolated with a tourniquet in order to provide a bloodless field for surgery.[1] Mivacurium is largely inactivated by the enzymatic action of plasma cholinesterase and would therefore continue to degrade locally leading to a loss of blockade in the limb, which could not be corrected by further doses unless the tourniquet was deflated. However, Torrance et al.[2] found that, as for other competitive neuromuscular blockers, the use of mivacurium to supplement regional anaesthesia produced prolonged muscle weakness well beyond cuff deflation. This suggests that mivacurium is not broken down in the ischaemic limb and that recovery is not dependent on plasma concentrations of mivacurium.

See also Local Anaesthetics, under Interactions in Atracurium, p.1335, for a report of symptoms suggestive of local anaesthetic toxicity when prilocaine and mivacurium were used together.

1. Shannon PF. Neuromuscular block and tourniquets. Br J Anaesth 1994; 73: 726.
2. Torrance JM, et al. Low-dose mivacurium supplementation of prilocaine i.v. regional anaesthesia. Br J Anaesth 1997; 78: 222–3.

Interactions

For interactions associated with competitive neuromuscular blockers, see Atracurium, p.1334.

Metoclopramide. Metoclopramide, an inhibitor of plasma cholinesterase, was found to significantly prolong the duration of action of mivacurium in patients undergoing surgery, although in this study only marginal inhibition of plasma cholinesterase by metoclopramide could be demonstrated.

1. Skinner HJ, et al. Influence of metoclopramide on plasma cholinesterase and duration of action of mivacurium. Br J Anaesth 1999; 82: 542–5.

Pharmacokinetics

Mivacurium is administered as a mixture of 3 stereoisomers, 2 of which (cis-trans and trans-trans) are considered to account for most of the neuromuscular blocking effect. All 3 isomers are inactivated by plasma cholinesterase. Renal and hepatic mechanisms are involved in their elimination with excretion in urine and bile.

Uses and Administration

Mivacurium chloride is a benzylisoquinolinium competitive neuromuscular blocker (see Atracurium, p.1336).

Following intravenous injection muscle relaxation occurs within 2 to 2.5 minutes with a duration of action of about 10 to 20 minutes. It is used for endotracheal intubation and to provide muscle relaxation in general anaesthesia for surgical procedures (see Anaesthesia, p.1331) and to aid controlled ventilation (see Intensive Care, p.1332).

Doses of neuromuscular blockers need to be carefully titrated for individual patients according to response, and may vary with the procedure, the other drugs given, and the state of the patient; monitoring of the degree of block is recommended in order to reduce the risk of overdosage. Doses of mivacurium chloride are expressed in terms of mivacurium base. The initial dose by intravenous injection is 70 to 250 µg per kg body-weight. Doses up to 150 µg per kg may be administered over 5 to 15 seconds but higher doses should be given over 30 seconds. In patients with asthma or cardiovascular disease, or those who are sensitive to falls in arterial blood pressure, administration should be over 60 seconds. A suggested method for administration of a dose of 250 µg per kg for tracheal intubation is to give one injection of 150 µg per kg followed 30 seconds later by an injection of 100 µg per kg. Maintenance doses of 100 µg per kg may be given at intervals of 15 minutes. In children aged 2 to 6 months an initial dose of 150 µg per kg has been given; in children aged 7 months to 12 years, an initial dose of 200 µg per kg has been given. A maintenance dose of 100 µg per kg may be given every 6 to 9 minutes for children aged 2 months to 12 years. Reduced doses may be required in elderly patients. For obese patients weighing more than 30% over their ideal body-weight the manufacturer recommends that the initial dose should be based upon their ideal body-weight and not actual body-weight. Mivacurium chloride may also be administered by continuous intravenous infusion for maintenance of block. For adults the initial rate is 8 to 10 µg per kg per minute adjusted every 3 minutes if necessary by increments of 1 µg per kg per minute to a usual dose of 6 to 7 µg

per kg per minute; in children aged 2 months to 12 years the usual dose is 11 to 14 µg per kg per minute.

◊ Reviews.
1. Mirakhur RK. Newer neuromuscular blocking drugs: an overview of their clinical pharmacology and therapeutic use. Drugs 1992; 44: 182–99.
2. Frampton JE, McTavish D. Mivacurium: a review of its pharmacology and therapeutic potential in general anaesthesia. Drugs 1993; 45: 1066–89.
3. Feldman S. Mivacurium. Br J Hosp Med 1997; 57: 199–201.

Action. Mivacurium has a shorter duration of action than most other competitive neuromuscular blockers. Studies[1-3] suggest that it is a useful alternative to suxamethonium for the production of neuromuscular block of short duration and has the advantage that its block can be reversed with an anticholinesterase. For a discussion of the choice of anticholinesterase for reversal of neuromuscular block produced by short-acting blockers such as mivacurium, see under Neostigmine, p.1421. Although its onset of action may be accelerated by giving a priming dose,[4] mivacurium has a slower onset than suxamethonium and so may not be a suitable alternative[5] when rapid intubation is required. For a general review of neuromuscular blockers, see Anaesthesia, p.1331.

1. Brandom BW, et al. Comparison of mivacurium and suxamethonium administered by bolus and infusion. Br J Anaesth 1989; 62: 488–93.
2. Caldwell JE, et al. Comparison of the neuromuscular block induced by mivacurium, suxamethonium or atracurium during nitrous oxide-fentanyl anaesthesia. Br J Anaesth 1989; 63: 393–9.
3. Goldberg ME, et al. Comparison of tracheal intubating conditions and neuromuscular blocking profiles after intubating doses of mivacurium chloride or succinylcholine in surgical outpatients. Anesth Analg 1989; 69: 93–9.
4. Haxby EJ, et al. Mivacurium priming intervals. Br J Anaesth 1994; 72: 485P.
5. Anonymous. Mivacurium—a new neuromuscular blocker. Med Lett Drugs Ther 1992; 34: 82.

Administration in the elderly. In a study[1] comparing the effects of mivacurium in elderly and young adults the duration of neuromuscular effects was prolonged in elderly patients by about 30%. The mean infusion requirement in elderly patients was 3.67 µg per kg body-weight per minute compared with 5.5 µg per kg in young adults.

1. Maddineni VR, et al. Neuromuscular and haemodynamic effects of mivacurium in elderly and young adult patients. Br J Anaesth 1994; 73: 608–12.

Preparations

Proprietary Preparations (details are given in Part 3)
Aust.: Mivacron; *Austral.:* Mivacron; *Belg.:* Mivacron; *Canad.:* Mivacron; *Denm.:* Mivacron; *Fin.:* Mivacron; *Fr.:* Mivacron; *Ger.:* Mivacron; *Hong Kong:* Mivacron; *Irl.:* Mivacron; *Israel:* Mivacron; *Ital.:* Mivacron; *Mex.:* Mivacron; *Neth.:* Mivacron; *Norw.:* Mivacron; *NZ:* Mivacron; *Port.:* Mivacron; *S.Afr.:* Mivacron; *Singapore:* Mivacron; *Spain:* Mivacron; *Swed.:* Mivacron; *Switz.:* Mivacron; *Thai.:* Mivacron; *UK:* Mivacron; *USA:* Mivacron.

Pancuronium Bromide (5727-n)

Pancuronium Bromide (BAN, USAN, rINN).

NA-97; Org-NA-97; Pancuronii Bromidum. 1,1'-(3α,17β-Diacetoxy-5α-androstan-2β,16β-ylene)bis(1-methylpiperidinium) dibromide.

$C_{35}H_{60}Br_2N_2O_4 = 732.7$.

CAS — 15500-66-0.

Pharmacopoeias. In *Eur.* (see p.vi).

Pharmacopoeial description

Ph. Eur.: White or almost white, hygroscopic crystalline powder. Very soluble to freely soluble in water; freely soluble in alcohol; very soluble in dichloromethane. Store in airtight containers. Protect from light.

Adverse Effects, Treatment, and Precautions

As for competitive neuromuscular blockers in general (see Atracurium, p.1333).

Pancuronium has a vagolytic action but does not produce ganglionic blockade. It has little histamine-releasing effect. Hypersensitivity reactions are relatively rare but bradycardia, bronchospasm, hypotension, and cardiovascular collapse have been reported. Pancuronium has been associated with excessive salivation is some patients.

Pancuronium should be used with caution in patients with raised catecholamine concentrations, or who are receiving drugs with sympathomimetic effects, as cardiovascular side-effects are more likely in these patients.

Hepatic impairment. Prolonged neuromuscular blockade may occur in patients with liver disease given pancuronium bromide since increased elimination half-life with increased volume of distribution and reduced clearance has been reported.[1] However, the expanded distribution volume may necessi-

tate an increase in the dose of pancuronium in these patients[1,2] and may be interpreted as resistance to the neuromuscular blocking effects of pancuronium.

1. Duvaldestin P, et al. Pancuronium pharmacokinetics in patients with liver cirrhosis. Br J Anaesth 1978; 50: 1131–6.
2. Ward ME, et al. Althesin and pancuronium in chronic liver disease. Br J Anaesth 1975; 47: 1199–1204.

Hypersensitivity. Reports of anaphylactoid or anaphylactic reactions associated with pancuronium bromide.

1. Brauer FS, Ananthanarayan CR. Histamine release by pancuronium. Anesthesiology 1978; 49: 434–5.
2. Patriarca G, et al. Pancuronium allergy: a case report. Br J Anaesth 1989; 62: 210–12.
3. Moneret-Vautrin DA, et al. Simultaneous anaphylaxis to thiopentone and a neuromuscular blocker: a study of two cases. Br J Anaesth 1989; 64: 743–5.
4. Sanchez-Guerrero IM, et al. Anaphylactoid reaction induced by pancuronium during general anaesthesia. Eur J Anaesthesiol 1998; 15: 613–14.

Postoperative complications. Because of its prolonged duration of action, pancuronium may be more likely than other neuromuscular blockers to produce residual neuromuscular block; such residual block is associated with an increased incidence of postoperative respiratory complications.[1,2]

1. Berg H, et al. Residual neuromuscular block is a risk factor for postoperative pulmonary complications: a prospective, randomised, and blinded study of postoperative pulmonary complications after atracurium, vecuronium and pancuronium. Acta Anaesthesiol Scand 1997; 41: 1095–1103.
2. Bissinger U, et al. Postoperative residual paralysis and respiratory status: a comparative study of pancuronium and vecuronium. Physiol Res 2000; 49: 455–62.

Renal impairment. Prolonged neuromuscular blockade may occur following administration of pancuronium to patients with severe renal impairment. Pancuronium distributes rapidly into extracellular fluid following intravenous injection and the initial neuromuscular blockade produced will depend upon the peak drug concentration in this fluid. Since extracellular fluid volume is increased in chronic renal failure such patients may require a larger initial dose of pancuronium and a 45% increase in dose requirement has been reported[1] in patients with end-stage renal failure. Renal excretion is the main route of elimination and prolonged elimination half-life with reduced clearance may be expected in renal failure; total dose requirements may be reduced. The main infusion rate of pancuronium to maintain 90% blockade in patients with end-stage renal failure was reported to be 61.5% less than for patients with normal renal function.

1. Gramstad L. Atracurium, vecuronium and pancuronium in end-stage renal failure. Br J Anaesth 1987; 59: 995–1003.

Interactions

For interactions associated with competitive neuromuscular blockers, see Atracurium, p.1334.

Pharmacokinetics

Following intravenous injection pancuronium bromide is rapidly distributed into body tissues; about 80% may be bound to plasma proteins. A small proportion is metabolised in the liver to metabolites with weak neuromuscular blocking activity. It is largely excreted in urine as unchanged drug and metabolites; a small amount is excreted in bile. The plasma elimination half-life is about 2 hours.

Pregnancy. In 15 patients undergoing caesarean section[1] given pancuronium bromide 100 µg per kg body-weight intravenously with other agents, mean maternal arterial and umbilical venous serum concentrations of pancuronium bromide and metabolites were 520 and 120 nanograms per mL respectively at delivery (mean of 13 minutes after injection), giving a fetal to maternal ratio of 0.23.

1. Wingard LB, et al. Modified fluorometric quantitation of pancuronium bromide and metabolites in human maternal and umbilical serums. J Pharm Sci 1979; 68: 914–15.

Uses and Administration

Pancuronium bromide is an aminosteroidal competitive neuromuscular blocker (see Atracurium, p.1336). Muscle relaxation occurs within about 1.5 to 2 minutes of intravenous administration and lasts for about 45 to 60 minutes.

Pancuronium bromide is used for endotracheal intubation and to provide muscle relaxation in general anaesthesia for surgical procedures (see Anaesthesia, p.1331) and to aid controlled ventilation (see Intensive Care, p.1332).

Doses of neuromuscular blockers need to be carefully titrated for individual patients according to response, and may vary with the procedure, the other drugs given, and the state of the patient; monitoring of the degree of block is recommended in order to reduce the risk of overdosage. The initial dose for intubation is usually 50 to 100 µg per kg body-weight by intravenous injection, with maintenance doses of 10 to 20 μg per kg. Children may be given similar doses. The manufacturers recommend a reduction in the initial dose to 20 to 60 μg per kg when pancuronium is given following suxamethonium. Doses of 30 to 40 μg per kg initially have been suggested in neonates, with maintenance doses of 10 to 20 μg per kg as necessary; in the USA, dosage based on an initial test dose of 20 μg per kg has been advocated for the neonate. Adult patients under intensive care who require assisted ventilation for conditions such as intractable status asthmaticus or tetanus may be given 60 μg per kg intravenously every 1 to 1½ hours or less frequently.

Fetal paralysis. Pancuronium bromide 100 μg per kg estimated fetal-weight administered into the umbilical vein produced fetal paralysis for about 40 minutes during intravascular exchange transfusion.[1] A dose of 200 to 300 μg per kg produced fetal paralysis for about 1 to 8 hours for more complicated transfusion procedures.[2] No adverse effects were reported.

1. Copel JA, et al. The use of intravenous pancuronium bromide to produce fetal paralysis during intravascular transfusion. *Am J Obstet Gynecol* 1988; **158**: 170–1.
2. Moise KJ, et al. Intravenous pancuronium bromide for fetal neuromuscular blockade during intrauterine transfusion for red-cell alloimmunization. *Obstet Gynecol* 1989; **74**: 905–8.

Neuroleptic malignant syndrome. Pancuronium is one of several drugs for which there have been isolated reports[1] of success in the management of neuroleptic malignant syndrome (p.662).

1. Sangal R, Dimitrijevic R. Neuroleptic malignant syndrome: successful treatment with pancuronium. *JAMA* 1985; **254**: 2795–6.

Preparations

BP 2001: Pancuronium Injection.

Proprietary Preparations (details are given in Part 3)
Aust.: Pavulon; **Austral.:** Pavulon; **Braz.:** Pancuron; Pavulon; **Canad.:** Pavulon†; **Denm.:** Pavulon; **Fin.:** Pavulon; **Fr.:** Pavulon; **Hong Kong:** Pavulon; **Irl.:** Pavulon; **Israel:** Pavulon; **Ital.:** Pavulon; **Mex.:** Bromurex; Minopres; Panlem; Parulon; Pavulon; **Neth.:** Pavulon; **Norw.:** Pavulon; **Port.:** Pancurox; Pavulon; **S.Afr.:** Curon-B; Pavulon; **Singapore:** Pavulon; **Spain:** Pavulon; **Swed.:** Pavulon; **Switz.:** Pavulon; **Thai.:** Pavulon; **UK:** Pavulon; **USA:** Pavulon.

Pipecuronium Bromide (19664-b)

Pipecuronium Bromide (BAN, USAN, rINN).

Pipecurium Bromide; RGH-1106. 1,1,1′,1′-Tetramethyl-4,4′-(3α,17β-diacetoxy-5α-androstan-2β,16β-diyl)dipiperazinium dibromide.

$C_{35}H_{62}Br_2N_4O_4 = 762.7$.
CAS — 52212-02-9 (anhydrous pipecuronium bromide); 68399-57-5 (pipecuronium bromide dihydrate).
ATC — M03AC06.

Adverse Effects, Treatment, and Precautions

As for competitive neuromuscular blockers in general (see Atracurium, p.1333). Pipecuronium is reported to have no significant cardiovascular adverse effects or histamine-related effects.

Interactions

For interactions associated with competitive neuromuscular blockers, see Atracurium, p.1334.

Pharmacokinetics

Following intravenous administration, pipecuronium is excreted in the urine mainly unchanged and as the less active 3-desacetyl metabolite. Values of about 1.7 and 2.3 hours have been reported for the mean elimination half-life.

Uses and Administration

Pipecuronium bromide is an aminosteroidal competitive neuromuscular blocker (see Atracurium, p.1336). Following intravenous injection muscle relaxation occurs within 2.5 to 3 minutes with a duration of action of about 30 minutes to 2 hours, depending on the dose.

Pipecuronium bromide is used for endotracheal intubation and to provide muscle relaxation in general anaesthesia for surgical procedures (see Anaesthesia, p.1331) and to aid mechanical ventilation (see Intensive Care, p.1332).

Doses of neuromuscular blockers need to be carefully titrated for individual patients according to response, and may vary with the procedure, the other drugs given, and the state of the patient; monitoring of the degree of block is recommended in order to reduce the risk of overdosage. Doses of 70 to 85 μg per kg body-weight intravenously have been recommended with subsequent doses of 10 to 15 μg per kg. Doses may need to be reduced in the presence of renal impairment; a dose of 50 μg per kg has been recommended for patients with a creatinine clearance of less than 40 mL per minute. A similar reduction

The symbol † denotes a preparation no longer actively marketed

---

has been recommended for the initial dose when pipecuronium is given following suxamethonium.

◊ Reviews.
1. Mirakhur RK. Newer neuromuscular blocking drugs: an overview of their clinical pharmacology and therapeutic use. *Drugs* 1992; **44**: 182–99.

Preparations

Proprietary Preparations (details are given in Part 3)
Aust.: Arpilon; **Ital.:** Arduan†; **Neth.:** Arpilon†; **USA:** Arduan.

Rapacuronium Bromide (17374-n)

Rapacuronium Bromide (BAN, USAN, rINN).

Org-9487. 1-(3α-Acetoxy-2β-piperidino-17β-propionyloxy-5α-androstan-16β-yl)-1-allylpiperidinium bromide; 1-Allyl-1-(3α,17β-dihydroxy-2β-piperidino-5α-androstan-16β-yl)piperidinium bromide, 3-acetate 17-propionate.

$C_{37}H_{61}BrN_2O_4 = 677.8$.
CAS — 156137-99-4.

Profile

Rapacuronium bromide, an analogue of vecuronium (p.1343), is an aminosteroidal competitive neuromuscular blocker (see Atracurium, p.1336). It was used to provide muscle relaxation in general anaesthesia for surgical procedures and for endotracheal intubation, but was withdrawn from the market following reports of severe bronchospasm, including fatalities.

Preparations

Proprietary Preparations (details are given in Part 3)
USA: Raplon.

Rocuronium Bromide (13930-b)

Rocuronium Bromide (BAN, USAN, rINN).

Org-9426. 1-Allyl-1-(3α,17β-dihydroxy-2β-morpholino-5α-androstan-16β-yl)pyrrolidinium bromide 17-acetate; 1-(17β-Acetoxy-3α-hydroxy-2β-morpholino-5α-androstan-16β-yl)-1-allylpyrrolidinium bromide.

$C_{32}H_{53}BrN_2O_4 = 609.7$.
CAS — 119302-91-9.
ATC — M03AC09.

Adverse Effects, Treatment, and Precautions

As for competitive neuromuscular blockers in general (see Atracurium, p.1333). Rocuronium is reported to have minimal cardiovascular and histamine-releasing effects. High doses have mild vagolytic activity. It should be used with caution in patients with hepatic or renal impairment.

Hepatic impairment. There have been conflicting reports of the pharmacokinetics and pharmacodynamics of rocuronium in patients with hepatic impairment. In contrast to earlier studies,[1,2] one group of workers[3] found a significant reduction in the plasma clearance of rocuronium in patients with cirrhosis. The elimination half-life has been variously reported to be unchanged[1] or prolonged[2,3] with delayed recovery.[3] Some studies[2,3] found that the onset of action was not affected while one group of workers[1] reported a delay.

1. Khalil M, et al. Pharmacokinetics and pharmacodynamics of rocuronium in patients with cirrhosis. *Anesthesiology* 1994; **80**: 1241–7.
2. Magorian T, et al. The pharmacokinetics and neuromuscular effects of rocuronium bromide in patients with liver disease. *Anesth Analg* 1995; **80**: 754–9.
3. van Miert MM, et al. The pharmacokinetics and pharmacodynamics of rocuronium in patients with hepatic cirrhosis. *Br J Clin Pharmacol* 1997; **44**: 139–44.

Hypersensitivity. Although rocuronium is considered to have minimal histamine-releasing effects, histaminoid reactions have been reported[1] on induction of anaesthesia in 3 patients who had been given rocuronium.

1. Neal SM, et al. Histaminoid reactions associated with rocuronium. *Br J Anaesth* 2000; **84**: 108–11.

Pain on administration. Severe transient burning pain associated with injection of rocuronium was considered[1] to be responsible for the spontaneous movement sometimes seen in the arm or wrist into which rocuronium is administered. It is recommended that rocuronium should be administered only when a deep stage of unconsciousness has been achieved.

1. Borgeat A, Kwiatkowski D. Spontaneous movements associated with rocuronium: is pain on injection the cause? *Br J Anaesth* 1997; **79**: 382–3.

Renal impairment. In a study[1] of the pharmacokinetics and neuromuscular effects of rocuronium, the clearance of rocuronium was reduced in patients with renal failure when compared with healthy patients, but the accompanying increase in duration of clinical relaxation did not reach statistical significance. However, it was recommended that rocuronium should be used with caution in the presence of renal failure as there were large interpatient variations in both clinical response and pharma-

---

cokinetic parameters in patients with renal failure. It has been suggested[2] that chronic renal failure may have played a role in the prolongation of neuromuscular blockade in a 47-year-old woman following administration of rocuronium in a dose of 1 mg per kg body-weight. Although this dose is within the recommended adult dose range, it was criticised[3] as being excessive for a patient with renal impairment.

1. Cooper RA, et al. Time course of neuromuscular effects and pharmacokinetics of rocuronium bromide (ORG 9426) during isoflurane anaesthesia in patients with and without renal failure. *Br J Anaesth* 1993; **71**: 222–6.
2. Lewis KS, et al. Prolonged neuromuscular blockade associated with rocuronium. *Am J Health-Syst Pharm* 1999; **56**: 1114–18.
3. Cozanitis DA, Booij HD. Muscle relaxants and renal failure. *Am J Health-Syst Pharm* 2000; **57**: 1713–14.

Interactions

For interactions associated with competitive neuromuscular blockers, see Atracurium, p.1334.

Pharmacokinetics

Following intravenous administration plasma concentrations of rocuronium follow a three compartment open model. There is an initial distribution phase with a half-life of 1 to 2 minutes followed by a slower distribution phase with a half-life of 14 to 18 minutes. It is reported to be about 30% bound to plasma proteins. The elimination half-life is about 1.4 to 1.6 hours. Up to 40% of a dose may be excreted in the urine within 24 hours; rocuronium is also excreted in the bile. The main metabolite of rocuronium, 17-desacetylrocuronium, is reported to have a weak neuromuscular blocking effect.

◊ References.
1. Khuenl-Brady KS, Sparr H. Clinical pharmacokinetics of rocuronium bromide. *Clin Pharmacokinet* 1996; **31**: 174–83.
2. McCoy EP, et al. Pharmacokinetics of rocuronium after bolus and continuous infusion during halothane anaesthesia. *Br J Anaesth* 1996; **76**: 29–33.
3. Wierda JMKH, et al. Pharmacokinetics and pharmacokinetic-dynamic modelling of rocuronium in infants and children. *Br J Anaesth* 1997; **78**: 690–5.
4. Proost JH, et al. Urinary, biliary and faecal excretion of rocuronium in humans. *Br J Anaesth* 2000; **85**: 717–23.

Intensive care. The pharmacokinetics of rocuronium appear to differ between intensive care patients receiving prolonged administration and surgical patients.[1] The volume of distribution at steady state may be increased, the plasma clearance decreased, and the terminal half-life prolonged. Recovery time on discontinuation may also be longer.

1. Sparr HJ, et al. Pharmacodynamics and pharmacokinetics of rocuronium in intensive care patients. *Br J Anaesth* 1997; **78**: 267–73.

Pregnancy. The mean concentration of rocuronium in venous plasma of 32 patients given a dose of 600 μg per kg body-weight before undergoing caesarean section was 2412 nanograms per mL at delivery;[1] the ratio of mean concentrations of rocuronium in umbilical venous plasma to maternal venous plasma at this time was 0.16. In 12 of these patients the mean concentration of rocuronium in umbilical arterial plasma was 271 nanograms per mL giving a ratio of 0.62 for the mean concentration of rocuronium in arterial to venous umbilical plasma. The concentration of 17-desacetylrocuronium in maternal venous plasma was 178 nanograms per mL and was less than 25 nanograms per mL in umbilical plasma.

1. Abouleish E, et al. Rocuronium (Org 9426) for Caesarean section. *Br J Anaesth* 1994; **73**: 336–41.

Uses and Administration

Rocuronium bromide is an aminosteroidal competitive neuromuscular blocker (see Atracurium, p.1336). Following intravenous injection it produces muscle relaxation within 1 to 2 minutes with a duration of about 30 to 50 minutes. Rocuronium bromide is used for endotracheal intubation and to provide muscle relaxation in general anaesthesia for surgical procedures (see Anaesthesia, p.1331) and to aid controlled ventilation (see Intensive Care, p.1332).

Doses of neuromuscular blockers need to be carefully titrated for individual patients according to response, and may vary with the procedure, the other drugs given, and the state of the patient; monitoring of the degree of block is recommended in order to reduce the risk of overdosage. A usual initial dose is 600 μg per kg body-weight by intravenous injection with maintenance doses of 150 μg per kg by injection; maintenance may also be by infusion at a rate of 300 to 600 μg per kg per hour although higher rates have been used in the USA. Similar doses to those used in adults have been used in infants and children older than one month but maintenance doses may be required more frequently.

For obese patients weighing more than 30% over their ideal body-weight the UK manufacturer recommends that doses should be reduced by taking into account lean body-mass; in the USA the manufacturer recommends that dosage should be based on actual body-weight. The UK manufacturer also recommends reduced maintenance doses of 75 to 100 µg per kg in the elderly or patients with renal or hepatic impairment.

◊ Reviews and discussions.
1. Mirakhur RK. Newer neuromuscular blocking drugs: an overview of their clinical pharmacology and therapeutic use. *Drugs* 1992; **44:** 182–9.
2. Hunter JM. Rocuronium: the newest aminosteroid neuromuscular blocking drug. *Br J Anaesth* 1996; **76:** 481–3.

Administration in children. Conditions for intubation in a study involving 70 children were judged to be good to excellent within one minute of intravenous administration of rocuronium 600 or 900 µg per kg body-weight with a trend to better conditions with the higher dose.[1]
1. Fuchs-Buder T, Tassonyi E. Intubating conditions and time course of rocuronium-induced neuromuscular block in children. *Br J Anaesth* 1996; **77:** 335–8.

INTRAMUSCULAR ROUTE. Intramuscular injection of rocuronium 1 mg per kg body-weight into the deltoid muscle permitted tracheal intubation to be carried out in lightly anaesthetised infants after 2.5 minutes.[1] In children a dose of 1.8 mg per kg enabled tracheal intubation after 3 minutes. However, the mean time to initial recovery after these doses was 57 minutes in infants and 70 minutes in children.
1. Reynolds LM, *et al.* Intramuscular rocuronium in infants and children: dose-ranging and tracheal intubating conditions. *Anesthesiology* 1996; **85:** 231–9.

Preparations

Proprietary Preparations (details are given in Part 3)
Aust.: Esmeron; *Austral.:* Esmeron; *Belg.:* Esmeron; *Canad.:* Zemuron; *Denm.:* Esmeron; *Fin.:* Esmeron; *Fr.:* Esmeron; *Ger.:* Esmeron; *Hong Kong:* Esmeron; *Irl.:* Esmeron; *Israel:* Esmeron; *Ital.:* Esmeron; *Neth.:* Esmeron; *Norw.:* Esmeron; *NZ:* Esmeron; *Port.:* Esmeron; *S.Afr.:* Esmeron; *Singapore:* Esmeron; *Spain:* Esmeron; *Swed.:* Esmeron; *Switz.:* Esmeron; *Thai.:* Esmeron; *UK:* Esmeron; *USA:* Zemuron.

Suxamethonium Chloride (5732-r)

Suxamethonium Chloride (BAN, pINN).

Choline Chloride Succinate; Succicurarium Chloride; Succinylcholine Chloride; Suxamethonium Chloridum; Suxametonklorid. 2,2′-Succinyldioxybis(ethyltrimethylammonium) dichloride dihydrate.
$C_{14}H_{30}Cl_2N_2O_4,2H_2O = 397.3$.
CAS — 306-40-1 (suxamethonium); 55-94-7 (suxamethonium bromide); 71-27-2 (anhydrous suxamethonium chloride); 6101-15-1 (suxamethonium chloride dihydrate); 541-19-5 (suxamethonium iodide).

Pharmacopoeias. In *Chin., Eur.* (see p.vi), *Int., Jpn, Pol.,* and *US.*

Suxamethonium 1 mg is equivalent to 1.37 mg of suxamethonium chloride dihydrate and to 1.24 mg of anhydrous suxamethonium chloride.

Pharmacopoeial description

Ph. Eur.: A white or almost white, hygroscopic, crystalline powder. Freely soluble in water; slightly soluble in alcohol; practically insoluble in ether. A 0.5% solution in water has a pH of 4.0 to 5.0. Protect from light.

USP 25: A white, odourless, crystalline powder. The anhydrous form is hygroscopic. Soluble 1 in 1 of water and 1 in 350 of alcohol; slightly soluble in chloroform; practically insoluble in ether. Its solutions in water have a pH of about 4. Store in airtight containers.

Incompatibility. Incompatibilities of neuromuscular blockers are discussed under Atracurium, p.1333.

Stability. A study of the loss of potency of suxamethonium chloride 20 mg per mL in water indicated that decomposition occurred at a considerably higher rate at 40° than at 25° and that the pH range of maximum stability was 3.75 to 4.50 for unbuffered solutions.[1] Assuming usual conditions of manufacturing, transit, and storage the total loss of potency was estimated to be 7% and 9% respectively for injections kept at room temperature for 4 and 6 weeks. If unbuffered, suxamethonium chloride injection complying with USP pH limits (3.0 to 4.5) must be stored at room temperature; it should not be kept for longer than 4 weeks.
1. Boehm JJ, *et al.* Shelf life of unrefrigerated succinylcholine chloride injection. *Am J Hosp Pharm* 1984; **41:** 300–2.

Adverse Effects

The neuromuscular blocking action of suxamethonium chloride is terminated by the enzyme plasma cholinesterase and prolonged apnoea may occur in patients with an atypical enzyme or with low enzyme

activity. Apnoea may also occur following development of phase II block (see Uses and Administration, below) after high or repeated doses of suxamethonium chloride, although tachyphylaxis may also occur with repeated doses.

Administration of suxamethonium chloride results in transient fasciculations during the onset of depolarising block. Rhabdomyolysis, myoglobinaemia, and myoglobinuria have been reported and may be associated with muscle damage following fasciculations. Postoperative muscle pain occurs in some patients but is not directly related to the degree of fasciculation. A transient rise in intra-gastric pressure may occur secondary to fasciculation of abdominal muscles. A transient increase in intra-ocular pressure often occurs. Depolarisation of skeletal muscle produces an immediate increase in plasma-potassium concentration and this can have serious consequences in some patients (see below).

Stimulation of the vagus nerve and parasympathetic ganglia by suxamethonium chloride may be followed by bradycardia, other arrhythmias, and hypotension, and may be exacerbated by the raised plasma-potassium concentration; cardiac arrest has been reported. Tachycardia and an increase in blood pressure due to stimulation of sympathetic ganglia have also been reported.

Suxamethonium chloride may cause an increase in salivary, bronchial, and gastric secretion and other muscarinic effects. Salivary gland enlargement has occurred.

Direct release of histamine from mast cells occurs but this is not the main mechanism of hypersensitivity reactions (see Hypersensitivity, below). Flushing, skin rash, bronchospasm, and shock have been reported.

Other reported effects include prolonged respiratory depression and apnoea.

Administration of suxamethonium chloride is implicated in the development of malignant hyperthermia (p.1329) in those patients with a genetic predisposition to the syndrome.

◊ Reviews of the adverse effects of suxamethonium.
1. Book WJ, *et al.* Adverse effects of depolarising neuromuscular blocking agents: incidence, prevention and management. *Drug Safety* 1994; **10:** 331–49.

Effects on intra-ocular pressure. Administration of suxamethonium is often followed 20 to 30 seconds later by a transient increase in intra-ocular pressure, which may be due in part to contracture of extra-ocular muscles. If suxamethonium is administered during eye surgery after incision of the eyeball or to patients with a penetrating eye injury, there is a theoretical risk that any increase in intra-ocular pressure may result in extrusion of ocular contents and loss of sight. However, there appear to be few reports of vitreous extrusion associated with suxamethonium,[1] and a large retrospective study[2] has failed to find any evidence that suxamethonium caused additional eye damage in patients with penetrating eye injuries. Furthermore, the procedure of intubation is associated with a greater increase in intra-ocular pressure than that seen with suxamethonium. Nonetheless, opinion on the safety of suxamethonium in eye surgery varies. While some suggest that a rapid competitive neuromuscular blocker would be preferable to aid intubation in patients with penetrating eye injuries, after incision of the eyeball, and in glaucoma, others advocate that the risk of a transient rise of intra-ocular pressure in these situations should be weighed against the need for rapid intubation.[1,3] For a discussion on the use of various agents to counteract the rise in intra-ocular pressure associated with suxamethonium and intubation in general, see under Anaesthesia, p.1331.
1. Book WJ, *et al.* Adverse effects of depolarising neuromuscular blocking agents: incidence, prevention and management. *Drug Safety* 1994; **5:** 331–49.
2. Libonati MM, *et al.* The use of succinylcholine in open eye surgery. *Anesthesiology* 1985; **62:** 637–40.
3. Edmondson L. Intraocular pressure and suxamethonium. *Br J Anaesth* 1997; **79:** 146.

Effects on the muscles. Muscle fasciculations and postoperative muscle pain commonly follow administration of suxamethonium. Fasciculations (generalised and desynchronised contractions of skeletal muscle fibres) occur during the onset of depolarising block in almost all patients given suxamethonium and may cause muscle damage. They are seen especially in the 'fine' muscles of the hands and face, and can be useful as an indication that suxamethonium is working. Attempts have been made to prevent their development with the aim of reducing postoperative muscle pain. However, there appears to be no direct correlation between the extent of visible fasciculations and

muscle pain.[1,2] Slow infusion of suxamethonium[3] or administration in divided doses[4] reduces fasciculations but not muscle pain.

Postoperative muscle pain is one of the most common side-effects of suxamethonium and has been noted in about 50% of patients, although the reported incidence varies widely from around 1.5 to about 90%.[2] It usually occurs on the first postoperative day and lasts for 2 or 3 days, and most commonly affects muscles of the neck, shoulders, and upper abdomen.[2] The incidence and severity of muscle pain is increased in patients who are mobile soon after surgery and in females, but it occurs less often in children, the physically fit, pregnant women, and the elderly.[2]

The mechanism of suxamethonium-induced muscle pain is not fully understood; there have been many attempts to prevent it. Most commonly, pretreatment with a small dose of a competitive neuromuscular blocker has reduced both visible fasciculations and the incidence and severity of muscle pain,[1,2,5-8] but has the disadvantage that it may delay the onset and reduce the intensity of subsequent suxamethonium block[9] and impair conditions for intubation[1,9] (see Neuromuscular Blockers, under Interactions in Atracurium, p.1335). Pretreatment with a small dose (10 mg) of suxamethonium in a 'self-taming' technique appears to offer no protection against muscle pain.[1,2] The choice of anaesthetic induction agent has been suggested to be significant, as has the timing of administration, but despite claims for benefit with, for example, propofol, this remains questionable.[2] Pretreatment with benzodiazepines or NSAIDs has produced conflicting results.[2] Other drugs that have been tried include lignocaine [lidocaine], calcium gluconate, and vitamin C; there is some evidence that lignocaine [lidocaine] may be the most effective pretreatment.[2] Not all methods have concentrated on drug treatment. A simple regimen of stretching exercises before premedication has reduced the incidence of both fasciculations and postoperative muscle pain.[10]

Suxamethonium may also produce an increase in jaw tension (masseter spasm or trismus)[11] in both adults[12] and children[13,14] during the onset of neuromuscular blockade. Tracheal intubation is greatly hindered in affected patients. It is not possible to predict which patients will show this response and the mechanism is unknown, although in about 50% of patients it may indicate the onset of malignant hyperthermia. Pretreatment with a paralysing dose of a competitive neuromuscular blocker prevents the response[14] but it is not known whether this is clinically useful.
1. O'Sullivan EP, *et al.* Differential effects of neuromuscular blocking agents on suxamethonium-induced fasciculations and myalgia. *Br J Anaesth* 1988; **60:** 367–71.
2. Wong SF, Chung F. Succinylcholine-associated postoperative myalgia. *Anaesthesia* 2000; **55:** 144–52.
3. Feingold A, Velazquez JL. Suxamethonium infusion rate and observed fasciculations: a dose-response study. *Br J Anaesth* 1979; **51:** 241–5.
4. Wilson DB, Dundee JW. Failure of divided doses of succinylcholine to reduce the incidence of muscle pains. *Anesthesiology* 1980; **52:** 273–5.
5. Bennetts FE, Khalil KI. Reduction of post-suxamethonium pains by pretreatment with four non-depolarising agents. *Br J Anaesth* 1981; **53:** 531–6.
6. Erkola O, *et al.* Five non-depolarizing muscle relaxants in precurarization. *Acta Anaesthesiol Scand* 1983; **27:** 427–32.
7. Sosis M, *et al.* Comparison of atracurium and d-tubocurarine for prevention of succinylcholine myalgia. *Anesth Analg* 1987; **66:** 657–9.
8. Findlay GP, Spittal MJ. Rocuronium pretreatment reduces suxamethonium-induced myalgia: comparison with vecuronium. *Br J Anaesth* 1996; **76:** 526–9.
9. Pauca AL, *et al.* Inhibition of suxamethonium relaxation by tubocurarine and gallamine pretreatment during induction of anaesthesia in man. *Br J Anaesth* 1975; **47:** 1067–73.
10. Magee DA, Robinson RJS. Effect of stretch exercises on suxamethonium induced fasciculations and myalgia. *Br J Anaesth* 1987; **59:** 596–601.
11. Saddler JM. Jaw stiffness—an ill understood condition. *Br J Anaesth* 1991; **67:** 515–16.
12. Leary NP, Ellis FR. Masseteric muscle spasm as a normal response to suxamethonium. *Br J Anaesth* 1990; **64:** 488–92.
13. Van Der Spek AFL, *et al.* Changes in resistance to mouth opening induced by depolarizing and non-depolarizing muscle relaxants. *Br J Anaesth* 1990; **64:** 21–7.
14. Smith CE, *et al.* Pretreatment with non-depolarizing neuromuscular blocking agents and suxamethonium-induced increases in resting jaw tension in children. *Br J Anaesth* 1990; **64:** 577–81.

Effects on plasma-potassium concentration. Suxamethonium administration is followed by depolarisation of motor end-plates in skeletal muscle resulting in an immediate increase in plasma-potassium concentration. The rise is usually small, being about 0.5 mmol or less per litre, but suxamethonium is best avoided in patients whose plasma-potassium concentration is already high, such as those with renal impairment. An exaggerated response, with severe hyperkalaemia resulting in ventricular fibrillation and cardiac arrest, has been reported in patients with burns,[1,2] massive trauma, neuromuscular disease (see under Neuromuscular Disorders in Precautions, below), and severe long-lasting sepsis.[3] See also Children in Precautions, below for reference to fatal cardiac arrest associated with hyperkalaemia in children. With burns or trauma the period of greatest risk is from about 10 to 90 days after the injury, but may be further prolonged if there is delayed healing or persistent infection. These patients may still react abnormally to suxamethonium 2 years after the injury. In neuromuscular disease the greatest risk period is usually from 3 weeks to 6 months after onset, but severe hyperkalaemia may occur after 24 to 48 hours or later than 6 months. Patients with severe sepsis for more than a week should be considered at risk of hyperkalaemia and no suxamethonium should be given until the infection has cleared. The mechanism of this hyperkalaemic response appears to be a supersensitivity of acetylcholine receptors in which the entire muscle fibre membrane, rather than discrete motor end-plate sites, becomes directly excitable by depolarising drugs. Depolarisation by suxamethonium thus results in release of potassium over the entire muscle fibre membrane and hyperkalaemia results.

Various methods have been tried to attenuate the hyperkalaemia, including pretreatment with a small dose of a competitive neuromuscular blocker[3,4] or with suxamethonium itself.[5,6] No method is reliable enough to be used clinically.

Anaesthetics such as thiopental and halothane can increase the hyperkalaemic response.[4]

1. Martyn J, et al. Clinical pharmacology of muscle relaxants in patients with burns. *J Clin Pharmacol* 1986; **26:** 680–5.
2. Anonymous. Neuromuscular blockers in patients with burns. *Lancet* 1988; **ii:** 1003–4.
3. Kohlschütter B, et al. Suxamethonium-induced hyperkalaemia in patients with severe intra-abdominal infections. *Br J Anaesth* 1976; **48:** 557–62.
4. Dhanaraj VJ, et al. A study of the changes in serum potassium concentration with suxamethonium using different anaesthetic agents. *Br J Anaesth* 1975; **47:** 516–19.
5. Magee DA, Gallagher EG. "Self-taming" of suxamethonium and serum potassium concentration. *Br J Anaesth* 1984; **56:** 977–9.
6. Plötz J, Schreiber W. Side effects induced by suxamethonium on the skeletal muscle and their prevention. *Br J Anaesth* 1985; **57:** 1044–5.

Hypersensitivity. Hypersensitivity reactions to neuromuscular blockers occur more commonly in women than in men,[1,2] in atopic patients and those who have a history of asthma or allergy,[2] and in patients who have had a previous reaction to anaesthetic drugs.[2] Circulatory collapse, flushing, skin rash, urticaria, and bronchospasm have occurred in hypersensitivity reactions associated with suxamethonium;[1,3,4] deaths have been reported.[3,5] The exact mechanism by which neuromuscular blockers produce hypersensitivity reactions is still uncertain; they all have a direct effect on mast cells, releasing histamine without immunological involvement, and could cause anaphylactoid reactions. Histamine release associated with use of aminosteroidal blockers is rare compared with the benzylisoquinolinium blockers.[6] Tubocurarine is considered to be the most potent releaser of histamine, with pancuronium and vecuronium having only very weak activity. Suxamethonium is considered to have only 1% of the histamine-releasing activity of tubocurarine but is more likely to produce serious hypersensitivity reactions. A type I immediate hypersensitivity reaction involving IgE antibodies is considered to be the mechanism of most hypersensitivity reactions associated with neuromuscular blockers.[2,5,7,8] Antibodies reacting with neuromuscular blockers, including suxamethonium, have been demonstrated.[5,8] The antibodies appear to be directed against quaternary or tertiary ammonium-ion groups which are present in neuromuscular blockers; such groups are also found in other drugs, cosmetics, disinfectants, and foods. This may help explain the cross-reactivity reported between different neuromuscular blockers[1,2,5,8,9] and how sensitisation occurs without prior exposure to any neuromuscular blocker.[2,5] At least 50% of patients sensitive to one neuromuscular blocker will react to one or more others[10] with some patients sensitive to most.[1] Intradermal skin tests are used to investigate and predict sensitivity to neuromuscular blockers, but their interpretation is controversial and it cannot be concluded that all patients with positive skin tests will have clinical sensitivity.[1,10] Although radioallergosorbent tests can detect antibodies to suxamethonium, alcuronium, and thiopental[3,11] some consider that their routine use is not justified as reactions could be avoided by taking an adequate patient history.[12]

1. Youngmen PR, et al. Anaphylactoid reactions to neuromuscular blocking agents: a commonly undiagnosed condition? *Lancet* 1983; **i:** 597–9.
2. Fisher MM, Munro I. Life-threatening anaphylactoid reactions to muscle relaxants. *Anesth Analg* 1983; **62:** 559–64.
3. Brahams D. Fatal reaction to suxamethonium: case for screening by radioallergosorbent test? *Lancet* 1989; **i:** 1400–1.
4. Moneret-Vautrin DA, et al. Simultaneous anaphylaxis to thiopentone and a neuromuscular blocker: a study of two cases. *Br J Anaesth* 1990; **64:** 743–5.
5. Fisher M, Baldo B. Adverse reactions to alcuronium: an Australian disease? *Med J Aust* 1983; **1:** 630–2.
6. Naguib M, et al. Histamine-release haemodynamic changes produced by rocuronium, vecuronium, mivacurium, atracurium and tubocurarine. *Br J Anaesth* 1995; **75:** 588–92.
7. Vervloet D. Anaphylactoid reactions to suxamethonium. *Lancet* 1983; **ii:** 1197.
8. Harle DG, et al. Detection of IgE antibodies to suxamethonium after anaphylactoid reactions during anaesthesia. *Lancet* 1984; **I:** 930–2.
9. Harle DG, et al. Cross-reactivity of metocurine, atracurium, vecuronium and fazadinium with IgE antibodies from patients unexposed to these drugs but allergic to other myoneural blocking drugs. *Br J Anaesth* 1985; **57:** 1073–6.
10. Withington DE. Relevance of histamine to the anaesthetist. *Br J Hosp Med* 1988; **40:** 264–70.
11. Assem ESK. Anaphylactic anaesthetic reactions: the value of paper radioallergosorbent tests for IgE antibodies to muscle relaxants and thiopentone. *Anaesthesia* 1990; **45:** 1032–8.
12. Noble DW, Yap PL. Screening for antibodies to anaesthetics. *BMJ* 1989; **299:** 2.

Treatment of Adverse Effects

Following administration of suxamethonium chloride assisted respiration should be maintained until spontaneous respiration has been fully restored. Transfusion of fresh whole blood, frozen plasma, or other source of plasma cholinesterase will help the destruction of the suxamethonium when prolonged paralysis is a result of atypical or low serum concentrations of plasma cholinesterase. Anticholinesterases should not normally be used since they potentiate the usual phase I block (see under Uses and Administration, below). If the neuromuscular block ceases to be depolarising in type and acquires some features of a competitive block (phase II block) the cautious use of an anticholinesterase may be considered. A short-acting anticholinesterase such as edrophonium may be given intravenously and if an obvious improvement is maintained for several minutes, neostigmine may be given with atropine.

Severe hypersensitivity reactions should be treated promptly with supportive and symptomatic measures. If malignant hyperthermia develops, it may be treated as described on p.1329.

The muscarinic effects of suxamethonium chloride, such as bradycardia and excessive salivary secretion, may be reduced by giving an antimuscarinic such as atropine before suxamethonium. A small dose of a competitive neuromuscular blocker given before suxamethonium has been used to reduce some of the adverse effects of suxamethonium on the muscles (see Effects on the Muscles, above).

Precautions

Patients who have received a neuromuscular blocker should always have their respiration assisted or controlled until the drug has been inactivated or antagonised.

Suxamethonium chloride is contra-indicated in patients with atypical plasma cholinesterase and should be used with caution in patients with reduced plasma cholinesterase activity (see below), which may occur in certain disease states and following exposure to certain drugs. Plasma cholinesterase concentrations fall during pregnancy and the puerperium and therefore maternal paralysis may be mildly prolonged. Suxamethonium is contra-indicated in patients with burns, massive trauma, renal impairment with a raised plasma-potassium concentration, severe long-lasting sepsis, and severe hyperkalaemia, since suxamethonium-induced rises in plasma-potassium concentration can have serious consequences in such patients. It is contra-indicated in patients with a history of hypersensitivity to the drug and, because of the possibility of cross-sensitivity (see above), should be used with caution when hypersensitivity to any neuromuscular blocker has previously occurred. Suxamethonium should be avoided in patients with a penetrating eye injury, raised intra-ocular pressure or glaucoma, or those about to undergo incision of the eyeball in eye surgery, because of the risks from increased intra-ocular pressure. Suxamethonium chloride produces muscle contractions before relaxation and should therefore be used with caution in patients with bone fractures. It is contra-indicated in patients with a family history of malignant hyperthermia.

The response to suxamethonium chloride is often unpredictable in patients with neuromuscular disorders and it should be used with great caution in these patients (see below). Caution is also needed if it is given to a patient with cardiac or respiratory disease. Children may be at special risk from cardiac arrest associated with hyperkalaemia, see below.

Hypothermia may enhance the neuromuscular blocking effects of suxamethonium chloride and an increase in body temperature may reduce them.

Children. Reports of fatal cardiac arrests[1,2] in apparently healthy children and adolescents, who were subsequently found to have had undiagnosed myopathies, led to restrictions in the USA on the use of suxamethonium in this age group, contra-indicating it except for emergency tracheal intubation or where an immediate securing of an airway is essential. Many anaesthetists disagreed[2] with this contra-indication and an FDA Committee advised[3] that the contra-indication should be replaced by a warning about the possibility of cardiac arrest associated with hyperkalaemia with special attention being paid to male children who are considered to be at the highest risk. One British anaesthetist who questioned the rationale behind restricting the elective use of suxamethonium pointed out that alternatives to suxamethonium had not been demonstrated to be as safe or effective for airway management.[4] The rare occurrence of cardiac arrest in children might be further reduced by taking a careful family history to exclude undiagnosed myopathies and by using an intravenous as opposed to inhalation induction when suxamethonium is to be used. A survey had found that most cases of cardiac arrest in children in the UK associated with the use of suxamethonium had been caused by vagal overactivity in non-atropinised patients.[4]

1. Rosenberg H, Gronert GA. Intractable cardiac arrest in children given succinylcholine. *Anesthesiology* 1992; **77:** 1054.
2. Book WJ, et al. Adverse effects of depolarizing neuromuscular blocking agents: incidence, prevention and management. *Drug Safety* 1994; **10:** 331–49.
3. *FDC Reports Pink Sheet* 1994; June 13: 16.
4. Hopkins PM. Use of suxamethonium in children. *Br J Anaesth* 1995; **75:** 675–7.

Neuromuscular disorders. Caution is needed if suxamethonium is to be given to patients with neuromuscular disease, since severe complications have been reported.[1] Hyperkalaemia and cardiac arrhythmias or cardiac arrest have been reported following administration of suxamethonium to patients with hemiplegia, diffuse intracranial lesions (head injury, encephalitis, ruptured cerebral aneurysm), tetanus, paraplegia, acute anterior horn cell disease, and muscular dystrophies. An exaggerated response to suxamethonium has been reported in the myasthenic syndrome but resistance may occur in patients with neurofibromatosis. Resistance may also occur in patients with myasthenia gravis, but uneventful administration has also been reported, although early onset of phase II block is possible in these patients. Muscle contractures and hyperkalaemia may be expected in amyotrophic lateral sclerosis and muscular denervation. Suxamethonium should be avoided in patients with myotonias, as response is unpredictable. It is recommended that suxamethonium is also avoided in hemiplegia, paraplegia, muscular denervation, and muscular dystrophies.

1. Azar I. The response of patients with neuromuscular disorders to muscle relaxants: a review. *Anesthesiology* 1984; **61:** 173–87.

Plasma cholinesterase deficiency. Suxamethonium is normally rapidly hydrolysed by plasma cholinesterase and the clinical effects usually last for only several minutes. Activity of the enzyme varies between individuals and prolonged paralysis following suxamethonium is commonly due to a hereditary or acquired reduction in plasma cholinesterase activity. The genes involved in the control of plasma cholinesterase production are termed usual, atypical (dibucaine-resistant), fluoride-resistant, and silent. About 96% of the population are homozygous for the normal gene. The commonest variant in western populations is the atypical form with about 3 to 4% of the population being heterozygous for this variant. They exhibit a slightly prolonged response to suxamethonium. Homozygotes for the atypical variant have a frequency of about 0.04%. They exhibit markedly prolonged apnoea following a standard dose of suxamethonium but can be readily identified by biochemical tests. The fluoride-resistant and silent variants occur very rarely. A measure of plasma cholinesterase activity can be obtained from the percentage inhibition of the enzyme by the local anaesthetic cinchocaine (commonly known in this context by its American name, dibucaine) to give the dibucaine number. Most normal people have a dibucaine number of about 80.

Acquired plasma cholinesterase deficiency is clinically less important than genetically determined deficiency. The enzyme is synthesised in the liver and **severe liver impairment** or malnutrition may cause abnormally low enzyme levels with some prolongation of suxamethonium activity. Reduced enzyme activity may also be found in severe anaemia, burns, cancer, collagen diseases, severe dehydration, severe infections, malnutrition, myocardial infarction, myxoedema, and renal impairment; plasmapheresis or plasma exchange removes significant amounts of plasma cholinesterase.

During **pregnancy** there is a rapid fall in plasma cholinesterase concentration which persists throughout pregnancy and for up to several weeks into the puerperium. The concentration of atypical plasma cholinesterase is also reduced in pregnancy and the puerperium. A number of **drugs** reduce plasma cholinesterase synthesis or activity and may prolong suxamethonium paralysis as discussed under Interactions, below.

References.
1. Wood GJ, Hall GM. Plasmapheresis and plasma cholinesterase. *Br J Anaesth* 1978; **50:** 945–9.
2. Evans RT, Wroe JM. Plasma cholinesterase changes during pregnancy: their interpretation as a cause of suxamethonium-induced apnoea. *Anaesthesia* 1980; **35:** 651–4.
3. Lumley J. Prolongation of suxamethonium following plasma exchange. *Br J Anaesth* 1980; **52:** 1149–50.
4. Williams FM. Clinical significance of esterases in man. *Clin Pharmacokinet* 1985; **10:** 392–403.
5. Robson N, et al. Plasma cholinesterase changes during the puerperium. *Anaesthesia* 1986; **41:** 243–9.
6. Cherala SR, et al. Placental transfer of succinylcholine causing transient respiratory depression in the newborn. *Anaesth Intensive Care* 1989; **17:** 202–4.

The symbol † denotes a preparation no longer actively marketed

Renal impairment. Suxamethonium chloride may be given in usual doses to patients with renal failure[1] but should be avoided if hyperkalaemia is also present (see Effects on Plasma-potassium Concentration above).

1. Ryan DW. Preoperative serum cholinesterase concentration in chronic renal failure. *Br J Anaesth* 1977; **49**: 945–9.

Interactions

A number of drugs may interact with depolarising neuromuscular blockers such as suxamethonium. The mechanisms of interaction may include a direct effect on neuromuscular transmission or an alteration of enzyme activity and may result in potentiation or antagonism of neuromuscular block. In general, interactions with suxamethonium are potentially more serious in patients with impaired neuromuscular function (see Neuromuscular Disorders, above) and in patients with reduced activity of plasma cholinesterase enzyme (see above).

Interactions common to competitive and depolarising neuromuscular blockers are covered under Atracurium, p.1334 whereas those specific for depolarising blockers are discussed below.

Antiarrhythmics. See under Atracurium, p.1334.

Antibacterials. See under Atracurium, p.1334.

Anticholinesterases. The action of suxamethonium can be markedly prolonged in patients using eye drops containing *ecothiopate*, a long-acting anticholinesterase which inhibits both acetylcholinesterase and plasma cholinesterase. Following systemic absorption of ecothiopate, plasma cholinesterase activity may rapidly be reduced to 5% or less of normal and prolonged apnoea after use of suxamethonium has occurred. On discontinuing ecothiopate, enzyme activity remains depressed for 1 to 2 months. If a patient has used ecothiopate eye drops in the previous 2 months, suxamethonium should not be given unless normal plasma cholinesterase activity can be demonstrated; a competitive neuromuscular blocker is preferable. Exposure to *organophosphorus insecticides* may also reduce plasma cholinesterase activity resulting in prolonged paralysis after use of suxamethonium; enzyme activity may be totally abolished. Anticholinesterases including *edrophonium, neostigmine, pyridostigmine, rivastigmine, tacrine,* and possibly *donepezil* enhance the action of suxamethonium, although suxamethonium-induced phase II block can be reversed with an anticholinesterase. Care should be taken if there is a need to use suxamethonium for urgent short procedures after a competitive-neuromuscular-induced block has been antagonised with an anticholinesterase, as the resulting block may be greatly prolonged.[1]

1. Fleming NW, *et al.* Neuromuscular blocking action of suxamethonium after antagonism of vecuronium by edrophonium, pyridostigmine or neostigmine. *Br J Anaesth* 1996; **77**: 492–5.

Antiepileptics. The mean time to recovery from suxamethonium-induced neuromuscular block was 14.3 minutes in 9 patients receiving chronic treatment with phenytoin and/or carbamazepine compared with 10.0 minutes in 9 patients not receiving antiepileptics.[1]

1. Melton AT, *et al.* Prolonged duration of succinylcholine in patients receiving anticonvulsants: evidence for mild upregulation of acetylcholine receptors. *Can J Anaesth* 1993; **40**: 939–42.

Antineoplastics. *Cyclophosphamide* has been reported to prolong the neuromuscular block produced by suxamethonium through reduction of plasma cholinesterase activity, possibly by alkylation of the enzyme.[1] Since enzyme activity may be reduced by up to 70% for several days to several weeks, it was suggested[2] that suxamethonium should be avoided if possible in patients receiving cyclophosphamide. Other alkylating agents also reported to reduce plasma cholinesterase activity include *mustine [chlormethine], thiotepa,* and *tretamine.*[2]

1. Walker IR, *et al.* Cyclophosphamide, cholinesterase and anaesthesia. *Aust N Z J Med* 1972; **3**: 247–51.
2. Zsigmond EK, Robins G. The effect of a series of anti-cancer drugs on plasma cholinesterase activity. *Can Anaesth Soc J* 1972; **19**: 75–82.

Aprotinin. See under Atracurium, p.1334.

Benzodiazepines. See under Atracurium, p.1334.

Beta blockers. See under Atracurium, p.1334.

Cardiac inotropes. See under Atracurium, p.1335.

Ganglion blockers. See under Atracurium, p.1335.

General anaesthetics. Tachyphylaxis and phase II block (see below) develop earlier, and after smaller total doses of suxamethonium, when inhalation anaesthetics are used. Halothane may increase the incidence of arrhythmias associated with suxamethonium and may potentiate suxamethonium-induced muscle damage.[1] Suxamethonium should be used with caution with other drugs that might produce additive cardiovascular effects. Severe bradycardia and asystole have occurred when used in

anaesthetic regimens with propofol and opioids such as fentanyl.

See also under Interactions in Atracurium, p.1335.

1. Laurence AS, Henderson P. Serum myoglobin after suxamethonium administration to children: effect of pretreatment before iv and inhalation induction. *Br J Anaesth* 1986; **58**: 126P.

Histamine H$_2$ antagonists. See under Atracurium, p.1335.

Lithium. See under Atracurium, p.1335.

Local anaesthetics. *Procaine, cocaine,* and *chloroprocaine* are ester-type local anaesthetics which are hydrolysed by plasma cholinesterase and may competitively enhance the neuromuscular blocking activity of suxamethonium. See also Antiarrhythmics under Atracurium, p.1334.

Magnesium salts. See under Atracurium, p.1335.

MAOIs. Reduction of plasma cholinesterase activity by *phenelzine* has been reported[1] to cause significant prolongation of suxamethonium paralysis. Enzyme activity may be reduced to 10% of normal and recovery may take up to a month. The dosage of suxamethonium may need to be substantially reduced or a competitive neuromuscular blocker used.

1. Bodley PO, *et al.* Low serum pseudocholinesterase levels complicating treatment with phenelzine. *BMJ* 1969; **3**: 510–12.

Metoclopramide. Dose-dependent prolongation of suxamethonium-induced neuromuscular blockade has been reported in patients given metoclopramide.[1,2] The potent inhibitory effect of metoclopramide on plasma cholinesterase may account for this interaction.

1. Turner DR, *et al.* Neuromuscular block by suxamethonium following treatment with histamine type 2 antagonists or metoclopramide. *Br J Anaesth* 1989; **63**: 348–50.
2. Kao YJ, *et al.* Dose-dependent effect of metoclopramide on cholinesterases and suxamethonium metabolism. *Br J Anaesth* 1990; **65**: 220–4.

Neuromuscular blockers. See under Atracurium, p.1335.

Sex hormones. *Oestrogens* and oestrogen-containing *oral contraceptives* reduce plasma cholinesterase activity[1] possibly due to suppression of hepatic synthesis of the enzyme, but little prolongation of suxamethonium paralysis may be expected since activity is reduced by only about 20%. See also under Atracurium, p.1335.

1. Robertson GS, Aberd MB. Serum protein and cholinesterase changes in association with contraceptive pills. *Lancet* 1967; **i**: 232–5.

Sympathomimetics. *Bambuterol* can inhibit plasma cholinesterase activity and so prolong the activity of suxamethonium.[1] Phase II block has been reported in some patients with abnormal plasma cholinesterase.[2]

1. Staun P, *et al.* The influence of 10 mg and 20 mg bambuterol on the duration of succinylcholine-induced neuromuscular blockade. *Acta Anaesthesiol Scand* 1990; **34**: 498–500.
2. Bang U, *et al.* The effect of bambuterol on plasma cholinesterase activity and suxamethonium-induced neuromuscular blockade in subjects heterozygous for abnormal plasma cholinesterase. *Acta Anaesthesiol Scand* 1990; **34**: 600–4.

Pharmacokinetics

After injection, suxamethonium is rapidly hydrolysed by plasma cholinesterase in plasma. One molecule of choline is split off rapidly to form succinylmonocholine which is then slowly hydrolysed to succinic acid and choline. Only a small proportion of suxamethonium is excreted unchanged in the urine. Succinylmonocholine has weak muscle-relaxant properties mainly of a competitive nature.

The gene responsible for the expression of plasma cholinesterase exhibits polymorphism and enzyme activity varies between individuals (see under Precautions, above).

Small amounts of suxamethonium do cross the placenta but clinical experience indicates that the neonate is not adversely affected when it has been used for caesarean section.

Uses and Administration

Suxamethonium is a depolarising neuromuscular blocker used to produce muscle relaxation. It acts as an acetylcholine agonist at the neuromuscular junction, combining with cholinergic receptors of the motor end-plate to produce depolarisation which may produce transient fasciculations. Suxamethonium is resistant to breakdown by acetylcholinesterase, the depolarisation is prolonged, and the refractory period of the motor end-plate extended. This prevents repolarisation and subsequent depolarisation and a flaccid muscle paralysis occurs. This initial depolarisation block is commonly known as a **phase I block.** The muscles that produce fine rapid movements such as

those of the face are the first to be affected followed by those of the limbs, abdomen, and chest; the diaphragm is affected last. Recovery occurs in reverse order. When excessive amounts of suxamethonium accumulate at the neuromuscular junction, for example following high or prolonged dosage, the nature of the block may change to one with characteristics similar to competitive block. This is commonly termed **phase II block** or **dual block** and may be associated with prolonged neuromuscular blockade and apnoea.

Following intravenous injection suxamethonium chloride acts in about 30 to 60 seconds and has a duration of action of about 2 to 6 minutes. Following intramuscular injection it acts in 2 to 3 minutes and has a duration of action of about 10 to 30 minutes. It is used in surgical and other procedures in which a rapid onset and brief duration of muscle relaxation is needed (see Anaesthesia, p.1331), including intubation, endoscopies, and electroconvulsive therapy. It is normally given by intravenous injection, usually as the chloride (but the bromide and iodide have also been used). Suxamethonium has to be given after induction of general anaesthesia because paralysis is usually preceded by painful muscle fasciculations. A competitive neuromuscular blocker may sometimes be given before suxamethonium to try to reduce some of the adverse effects on the muscles (see under Effects on the Muscles, above). Premedication with an antimuscarinic may be of value in reducing bradycardia and excessive salivation. Assisted respiration is necessary.

An initial test dose of 0.1 mg per kg of suxamethonium chloride may be given intravenously if increased sensitivity is suspected. Doses of neuromuscular blockers need to be carefully titrated for individual patients according to response, and may vary with the procedure, the other drugs given, and the state of the patient; monitoring of the degree of block is recommended in order to reduce the risk of overdosage. The response to suxamethonium varies considerably and the usual single dose of suxamethonium chloride for an adult is 0.3 to 1.1 mg per kg body-weight by intravenous injection with a usual range of 20 mg to a maximum total of 100 mg. Supplementary doses of 50 to 100% of the initial dose may be administered at 5 to 10 minute intervals if required but the total dose given by repeated intravenous injection or continuous infusion (see below) should not exceed 500 mg per hour. Infants and children are more resistant to suxamethonium than adults. A recommended intravenous dose for infants under one year of age is 2 mg per kg; a dose of 1 mg per kg is recommended for children 1 to 12 years old.

When a suitable vein is inaccessible suxamethonium chloride has been given by intramuscular injection in a dose of 3 to 4 mg per kg body-weight to a maximum total of 150 mg. The intramuscular dose for infants is up to 4 to 5 mg per kg and for older children up to 4 mg per kg to a maximum total of 150 mg.

For prolonged procedures in adults sustained relaxation may be obtained by continuous intravenous infusion of a 0.1 to 0.2% solution. A rate of 2 to 5 mg per minute is usually adequate but may be adjusted as necessary. The total dose given by repeated intravenous injection (see above) or continuous infusion should not exceed 500 mg per hour.

Preparations

BP 2001: Suxamethonium Chloride Injection;
USP 25: Succinylcholine Chloride for Injection; Succinylcholine Chloride Injection.

Proprietary Preparations (details are given in Part 3)

Aust.: Lysthenon; *Austral.:* Scoline; *Belg.:* Myoplegine; *Braz.:* Quelicin; *Canad.:* Anectine; Quelicin; *Fin.:* Sukolin; *Fr.:* Celocurine; *Ger.:* Lysthenon; Pantolax; Succicuran; *Irl.:* Anectine; *Israel:* Succinyl; *Ital.:* Midarine; Myotenlis; *Mex.:* Anectine; Ectinex; Uxicolin; *Neth.:* Succinyl†; *Norw.:* Curacit; *NZ:* Ethicholine; *Port.:* Mioflex; *S.Afr.:* Scoline; *Singapore:* Ethicholine; *Spain:* Anectine; Mioflex; *Swed.:* Celocurin; *Switz.:* Lysthenon; Midarine; Succinolin; *Thai.:* Succinyl; *UK:* Anectine; Scoline†; *USA:* Anectine; Quelicin.

Tubocurarine Chloride   (5736-h)

Tubocurarine Chloride (BAN, rINN).

d-Tubocurarine Chloride; (+)-Tubocurarine Chloride Hydrochloride Pentahydrate; Tubocurarini Chloridum. (+)-7′,12′-Dihydroxy-6,6′-dimethoxy-2,2′,2′-trimethyltubocuraranium dichloride pentahydrate.

$C_{37}H_{42}Cl_2N_2O_6,5H_2O = 771.7$ (The empirical formula of tubocurarine chloride was formerly considered to be $C_{38}H_{44}Cl_2N_2O_6,5H_2O$).

CAS — 57-95-4 (tubocurarine); 57-94-3 (anhydrous tubocurarine chloride); 6989-98-6 (tubocurarine chloride, pentahydrate).

Pharmacopoeias. In Eur. (see p.vi), Int., Jpn, and US.

The chloride of (+)-tubocurarine. It may be obtained from extracts of the stems of Chondodendron tomentosum (Menispermaceae) and is one of the active principles of curare, by which name it is sometimes referred to in anaesthetic literature.

Pharmacopoeial description

Ph. Eur.: A white or slightly yellowish crystalline powder. Soluble in water and in alcohol; practically insoluble in acetone and in ether; dissolves in solutions of alkali hydroxides. A 1% solution in water has a pH of 4.0 to 6.0. Store in airtight containers.

USP 25: A white or yellowish-white to greyish-white, crystalline powder. Soluble 1 in 20 of water and 1 in 45 of alcohol. Store in airtight containers.

Adverse Effects, Treatment, and Precautions

As for competitive neuromuscular blockers in general (see Atracurium, p.1333). A transient fall in blood pressure commonly occurs, due in part to ganglionic blockade and the release of histamine; there may be an increase in heart rate. Tubocurarine has a greater propensity to cause histamine release than other competitive neuromuscular blockers in clinical use. Tubocurarine should be used with caution in patients with renal impairment. Resistance to the effect of tubocurarine may occur in patients with hepatic impairment.

Interactions

For interactions associated with competitive neuromuscular blockers, see Atracurium, p.1334.

Pharmacokinetics

Tubocurarine chloride is a quaternary ammonium compound and absorption from the gastrointestinal tract following oral administration is extremely poor. Absorption is slow and irregular when given intramuscularly. Following intravenous injection tubocurarine is widely distributed throughout body tissues; less than 50% is bound to plasma proteins. Following a single dose extensive redistribution to tissues is responsible for the termination of activity, but after a large single dose or repeated small doses tissue saturation occurs and renal excretion becomes the main determinant of duration. When given in usual doses it does not pass the blood-brain barrier, and does not appear to cross the placenta in significant amounts. Up to 75% of a dose is excreted unchanged in the urine in 24 hours, and up to 12% in bile. Biliary excretion is increased in renal impairment. A small proportion of a dose is metabolised in the liver.

Uses and Administration

Tubocurarine is a benzylisoquinolinium competitive neuromuscular blocker (see Atracurium, p.1336). Following intravenous injection of tubocurarine chloride neuromuscular block appears within one minute and lasts for about 30 minutes; the maximum effect is attained within 2 to 5 minutes. Tubocurarine chloride has been used similarly to other competitive neuromuscular blockers to produce muscle relaxation in various procedures but has largely been replaced by other drugs with fewer cardiovascular effects and a lower potential for histamine release.

Doses used have varied according to the degree of muscle relaxation required. Doses of neuromuscular blockers need to be carefully titrated for individual patients according to response, and may vary with the procedure, the other drugs given, and the state of the patient; monitoring of the degree of block is recommended in order to reduce the risk of overdosage. An initial dose of 6 to 9 mg intravenously has been suggested followed by 3 to 4.5 mg after 3 to 5 minutes if necessary; additional doses of 3 mg may be given as required for prolonged procedures. Higher doses have been given in some countries. Tubocurarine should be given with caution in reduced doses to patients with renal impairment; if large or repeated doses are given neuromuscular block may be prolonged. Tubocurarine chloride has also been used to control the muscle spasms of tetanus (p.1332).

Preparations

USP 25: Tubocurarine Chloride Injection.

Proprietary Preparations (details are given in Part 3)
Israel: Curarine; Tubarine; *Spain:* Curarina Miro†.

Vecuronium Bromide   (14012-x)

Vecuronium Bromide (BAN, USAN, rINN).

Org-NC-45.   1-(3α,17β-Diacetoxy-2β-piperidino-5α-androstan-16β-yl)-1-methylpiperidinium bromide.

$C_{34}H_{57}BrN_2O_4 = 637.7$.

CAS — 50700-72-6.

Incompatibility. A solution containing vecuronium bromide 1 mg per mL was found to be visually incompatible with frusemide [furosemide].[1] For incompatibilities of competitive neuromuscular blockers in general, see under Atracurium on p.1333.

1. Chiu MF, Schwartz ML. Visual compatibility of injectable drugs used in the intensive care unit. Am J Health-Syst Pharm 1997; 54: 64–5.

Adverse Effects, Treatment, and Precautions

As for competitive neuromuscular blockers in general (see Atracurium, p.1333).

Vecuronium bromide has little histamine-releasing activity although a local reaction at the site of injection has been reported; bronchospasm and anaphylactoid reactions have been rarely reported. Also it has little vagolytic or ganglion-blocking activity and produces no significant adverse cardiovascular effects at usual doses.

Caution may be needed in patients with hepatic or renal impairment (see below); dosage adjustments may be required in renal failure.

Elderly. It has been recommended that neuromuscular function should be monitored in elderly patients receiving vecuronium since there may be a risk of prolonged block.[1]

1. Slavov V, et al. Comparison of duration of neuromuscular blocking effect of atracurium and vecuronium in young and elderly patients. Br J Anaesth 1995; 74: 709–11.

Hepatic impairment. The duration of action of vecuronium is reported to be significantly prolonged in patients with cholestasis[1] or cirrhosis with oesophageal varices[2] given a dose of 200 μg per kg body-weight intravenously. Plasma clearance was significantly reduced and the elimination half-life significantly increased from a mean of 58 to 98 minutes.[1] A dose of 150 μg per kg was found to have a similar onset and duration of action in patients with hepatic impairment and healthy controls,[2] but a dose of 100 μg per kg had a slower onset and slightly shorter duration of action in those with liver disturbance.[3] Following a dose of vecuronium, rapid and extensive hepatic uptake occurs, which largely determines its short duration of action. However, as the dose increases this mechanism becomes saturated, and hepatic elimination becomes more important in terminating activity. This would help to explain the variation in results seen with the different doses. Caution is needed if large single doses or repeated doses are given to patients with hepatic impairment.

1. Lebrault C, et al. Pharmacokinetics and pharmacodynamics of vecuronium in patients with cholestasis. Br J Anaesth 1986; 58: 983–7.
2. Hunter JM, et al. The use of different doses of vecuronium in patients with liver dysfunction. Br J Anaesth 1985; 57: 758–64.
3. Bell CF, et al. Use of atracurium and vecuronium in patients with oesophageal varices. Br J Anaesth 1985; 57: 160–8.

Renal impairment. A small proportion of vecuronium bromide is excreted in urine and it may be given in usual doses to patients with renal failure.[1,2] No clinically significant difference in elimination half-life, clearance, or duration of action were reported[1] between patients with renal failure and those with normal renal function. The onset of neuromuscular block may be slightly slower in renal failure[2] and these patients may require an increase of around 20% in the initial dose of vecuronium.[3] However, the dosage requirement for maintenance of neuromuscular block may be reduced by about 20%[3] and slight prolongation of block may occur if dosage is not adjusted, but reversal of residual block with neostigmine is prompt and effective.[2]

Resistance to vecuronium has been reported[2] in 2 anephric patients. Total doses of 620 and 660 μg per kg body-weight produced maximum neuromuscular block of 77% and 36% but, despite the high doses used, there were no adverse effects or residual curarisation.

1. Fahey MR, et al. Pharmacokinetics of Org NC 45 (Norcuron) in patients with and without renal failure. Br J Anaesth 1981; 53: 1049–53.
2. Hunter JM, et al. Comparison of vecuronium, atracurium and tubocurarine in normal patients and in patients with no renal function. Br J Anaesth 1984; 56: 941–51.
3. Gramstad L. Atracurium, vecuronium and pancuronium in end-stage renal impairment: dose-response properties and interactions with azathioprine. Br J Anaesth 1987; 59: 995–1003.

Interactions

For interactions associated with competitive neuromuscular blockers, see Atracurium, p.1334.

Pharmacokinetics

Following intravenous administration vecuronium is rapidly distributed. It is taken up by the liver and partly metabolised; the metabolites have some neuromuscular blocking activity. It is excreted mainly in bile as unchanged drug and metabolites; some is also excreted in urine. The plasma elimination half-life is reported to range from about 30 to 80 minutes.

Pregnancy. The proportion of vecuronium crossing the placenta following doses of 60 to 80 μg per kg body-weight was considered clinically insignificant and its use during obstetric anaesthesia was considered safe for the newborn.[1]

1. Demetriou M, et al. Placental transfer of Org NC 45 in women undergoing caesarean section. Br J Anaesth 1982; 54: 643–5.

Uses and Administration

Vecuronium bromide is an aminosteroidal competitive neuromuscular blocker (see Atracurium, p.1336).

Following intravenous injection muscle relaxation occurs within about 1.5 to 2 minutes and lasts for about 20 to 30 minutes.

Vecuronium bromide is used for endotracheal intubation and to provide muscle relaxation in general anaesthesia for surgical procedures (see Anaesthesia, p.1331) and to aid controlled ventilation (see Intensive Care, p.1332).

Doses of neuromuscular blockers need to be carefully titrated for individual patients according to response, and may vary with the procedure, the other drugs given, and the state of the patient; monitoring of the degree of block is recommended in order to reduce the risk of overdosage. The usual initial dose for intubation is 80 to 100 μg per kg body-weight by intravenous injection, although reduced initial doses of 30 to 50 μg per kg are suggested following the use of suxamethonium. Higher initial doses ranging from 150 to 300 μg per kg have sometimes been used for other procedures. However, it is recommended that the dose should not exceed 100 μg per kg in caesarean section or neonatal surgery. Maintenance doses of 20 to 30 μg per kg may be given as required during prolonged procedures; in the USA a lower maintenance dose of 10 to 15 μg per kg is recommended. Neuromuscular blockade may also be maintained with an intravenous infusion given at a rate of 0.8 to 1.4 μg per kg per minute but should be preceeded by an initial bolus injection of 40 to 100 μg per kg. The manufacturers recommend that in obese patients the dosage of vecuronium should be reduced taking into account lean body-mass.

Children older than 5 months can be given adult doses but children up to 1 year may have a more rapid response and the high initial dose for intubation may not be necessary. Neonates and infants below 5 months of age may be more sensitive to vecuronium and it is recommended that they should be given an initial test dose of 10 to 20 μg per kg, followed by increments according to response. The duration of action and recovery is longer in neonates and infants than in children and adults and they may require smaller maintenance doses given less frequently.

◊ Reviews of vecuronium.

1. Miller RD, et al. Clinical pharmacology of vecuronium and atracurium. Anesthesiology 1984; 61: 444–53.
2. Reilly CS, Nimmo WS. New intravenous anaesthetics and neuromuscular blocking drugs: a review of their properties and clinical use. Drugs 1987; 34: 98–135.

Preparations

Proprietary Preparations (details are given in Part 3)
Aust.: Norcuron; *Austral.:* Norcuron; *Belg.:* Norcuron; *Braz.:* Norcuron; *Canad.:* Norcuron; *Denm.:* Norcuron†; *Fin.:* Norcuron; *Fr.:* Norcuron; *Ger.:* Norcuron; *Hong Kong:* Norcuron; *Irl.:* Norcuron; *Israel:* Norcuron; *Ital.:* Curlem; Norcuron; *Neth.:* Norcuron; *Norw.:* Norcuron; *NZ:* Norcuron; *Port.:* Norcuron; *S.Afr.:* Norcuron; *Singapore:* Norcuron; *Spain:* Norcuron; *Swed.:* Norcuron; *Switz.:* Norcuron; *Thai.:* Norcuron; *UK:* Norcuron; *USA:* Norcuron.

The symbol † denotes a preparation no longer actively marketed

Nonionic Surfactants

A surfactant is a compound that can reduce the interfacial tension between 2 immiscible phases. This is due to the molecule containing 2 localised regions, one being hydrophilic in nature and the other hydrophobic.

The properties of nonionic surfactants are largely dependent on the proportions of these 2 groups in the molecule. Hydrophilic groups include the oxyethylene group ($-O.CH_2.CH_2-$) and the hydroxyl group ($-OH$). By varying the number of these groups in a hydrophobic molecule, such as a fatty acid, substances are obtained which range from strongly hydrophobic and water-insoluble compounds, such as glyceryl monostearate, to strongly hydrophilic and water-soluble compounds, such as the macrogols. These 2 extreme types are not satisfactory as emulsifying agents, though they are useful stabilisers in the presence of efficient emulsifying agents. Between these extremes are the nonionic emulsifying agents in which the proportions of hydrophilic and hydrophobic groups are more evenly balanced; these include some of the macrogol esters and ethers and sorbitan derivatives. By virtue of the processes used in their manufacture, nonionic surfactants are usually mixtures of related compounds; the properties of a particular material may vary from one manufacturer to another and there may be variation in batches from an individual source.

Nonionic surfactants differ from anionic surfactants (p.1496) by the absence of charge on, or ionisation of, the molecule; they are generally less irritant than anionic or cationic surfactants.

In addition to their use as emulsifiers some nonionic surfactants are also used in pharmacy as solubilising and wetting agents. Nonionic surfactants have applications in the food, cosmetic, paint, pesticide, and textile industries as well as being used as oil slick dispersants. Some macrogol ethers such as nonoxinol 9 are used as spermicides.

Since nonionic surfactants do not ionise to any great extent in solution, they are generally compatible with both anionic and cationic substances, but they reduce the antimicrobial action of many preservatives.

Nonionic surfactants may be classified according to their hydrophilic-lipophilic balance (HLB). This is an arbitrary scale of values denoting the relative affinity of the surfactant for oil and water. Lipophilic surfactants have low HLB values (less than 10) and are generally used as antifoaming agents, water-in-oil emulsifying agents, and as wetting agents; hydrophilic surfactants have higher HLB values (greater than 10) and are generally used as oil-in-water emulsifying agents and solubilising agents.

The range of nonionic surfactants used in pharmaceutical practice is large and their classification can be varied and complex. The principal groups of nonionic surfactants are outlined below.

Glycol and glycerol esters are a group of nonionic surfactants consisting of fatty acid esters of glycols and glycerol. Hydrophobic properties predominate and these compounds are poor emulsifying agents if used alone, though they are useful stabilisers for both oil-in-water and water-in-oil emulsions. If a small amount of soap, sulfated fatty alcohol, or other surfactant is added to the esters, a 'self-emulsifying' product is formed which is capable of producing satisfactory oil-in-water emulsions. **Acetoglycerides** are mixed glyceryl esters in which the glycerol is esterified partly with a fatty acid and partly with acetic acid.

Macrogol esters are polyoxyethylene esters of fatty acids, mainly stearates. The hydrophilic properties of the oxyethylene group are weaker than those of the hydroxyl group but by introducing a sufficient number into a fatty acid molecule, substances are produced in which the hydrophilic and hydrophobic properties are sufficiently well balanced for the esters to act as efficient oil-in-water emulsifying agents. They may also be used as wetting and solubilising agents. Since the ester linkage is prone to hydrolysis, these compounds are less resistant to acids and alkalis than the macrogol ethers.

Macrogol ethers are condensation products prepared by reaction between fatty alcohols or alkylphenols and ethylene oxide. The ether linkage confers good stability to acids and alkalis. Macrogol ethers are widely used in the preparation of oil-in-water emulsions and as wetting and solubilising agents.

Sorbitan derivatives are derivatives of the cyclic mono- or di-anhydrides of sorbitol. They consist of *sorbitan esters* which are prepared by esterification of one or more of the hydroxyl groups in the anhydrides with a fatty acid such as stearic, palmitic, oleic, or lauric acid, and *polysorbates* which are polyoxyethylene derivatives of the sorbitan esters. Sorbitan esters are oil-soluble, water-dispersible, nonionic surfactants which are effective water-in-oil emulsifiers. Polysorbates are more hydrophilic, water-soluble compounds and are used as oil-in-water emulsifying agents. By varying the number of oxyethylene groups in the molecule, and the type of fatty acid in the sorbitan ester, surfactants with a wide range of properties may be obtained.

Poloxamers are copolymers of polyoxyethylene and polyoxypropylene. They are used as oil-in-water emulsifiers and as solubilising and wetting agents in a variety of pharmaceutical preparations intended for internal use.

Other nonionic compounds with surface activity such as the higher fatty alcohols are covered in the chapter on Paraffins and Similar Bases (p.1407).

Diacetylated Monoglycerides (486-g)

Pharmacopoeias. In *USNF*.

Pharmacopoeial description
USNF 20: Consists of glycerol esterified with edible fat-forming fatty acids and acetic acid. A clear liquid. Very soluble in alcohol 80%, in vegetable oils, and in mineral oils; sparingly soluble in alcohol 70%. Store in airtight containers. Protect from light.

Profile
Diacetylated monoglycerides have been used as plasticisers.

p-Di-isobutyl-phenoxypolyethoxyethanol
(9985-v)

Profile
p-Di-isobutyl-phenoxypolyethoxyethanol has been used as a spermicide.

Preparations
Proprietary Preparations (details are given in Part 3)
Canad.: Ortho-Gynol†; *Neth.:* Ortho-Gynol†; *NZ:* Ortho-Gynol.

Ethylene Glycol Monopalmitostearate
(433-c)

Ethylene Glycol Monostearate; Ethylene Glycol Stearate; Éthylène Glycol (Stéarate d'); Ethylenglycoli Monostearas; Ethylenglycoli Monostearas; Ethyleni Glycoli Stearas.
CAS — 111-60-4 *(ethylene glycol monostearate)*; 4219-49-2 *(ethylene glycol monopalmitate)*.
Pharmacopoeias. In *Eur.* (see p.vi).

Pharmacopoeial description
Ph. Eur.: A mixture of ethylene glycol mono- and di-esters of stearic and palmitic acids. It contains not less than 50% of monoesters produced from the condensation of ethylene glycol and stearic acid and not more than 5% of free ethylene glycol.

A white or almost white, waxy solid. Practically insoluble in water; soluble in hot alcohol and in acetone. M.p. 54° to 60°. Protect from light.

Profile
Ethylene glycol monopalmitostearate has the properties of, and is used for the same purposes as, glyceryl monostearate or self-emulsifying glyceryl monostearate (below). Ethylene glycol monolaurate and mono-oleate, and diethylene glycol monostearate, monolaurate, and mono-oleate, have also been used.

Glyceryl Behenate (3270-j)

Pharmacopoeias. In *USNF. Eur.* (see p.vi) includes Glycerol Dibehenate (Glyceroli Dibehenas).

Pharmacopoeial description
Ph. Eur.: Glycerol Dibehenate is a mixture of diacylglycerols, mainly dibehenoylglycerol, together with variable quantities of mono- and triacylglycerols. It contains 13 to 21% of monoacylglycerols, 40 to 60% of diacylglycerols, and 21 to 35% of triacylglycerols, obtained by esterification of glycerol and behenic acid. A hard, waxy mass or powder or white or almost white, unctuous flakes. Insoluble in water; partly soluble in hot alcohol; soluble in dichloromethane. M.p. 65° to 77°.
USNF 20: Glyceryl Behenate is a mixture of glycerides of fatty acids, mainly behenic acid. A fine powder with a faint odour. M.p. about 70°. Practically insoluble in water and in alcohol; soluble in chloroform. Store in airtight containers at a temperature not exceeding 35°.

Profile
Glyceryl behenate is used as a lubricant and binder in tablet-making.

Glyceryl Mono-oleate (434-k)

Monolein.
CAS — 25496-72-4.
Pharmacopoeias. Eur. (see p.vi) includes a monograph covering a range of compounds defined by their monoacylglycerol content.

Pharmacopoeial description
Ph. Eur.: Glycerol Mono-oleates are mixtures of monoacylglycerols, mainly mono-oleoylglycerol, together with variable quantities of di- and triacylglycerols. They are defined by the nominal content of monoacylglycerols and obtained by partial glycerolysis of vegetable oils mainly containing triacylglycerols of oleic acid, or by esterification of glycerol by oleic acid. A suitable antioxidant may be added.

Amber, oily liquids which may be partially solidified at room temperature. Practically insoluble in water; freely soluble in dichloromethane. Store in airtight containers. Protect from light.

Profile
Glyceryl mono-oleate has similar properties to glyceryl monostearate or self-emulsifying glyceryl monostearate (below).

Glyceryl Monostearate (435-a)

Glycérol (Monostéarate de); Glyceroli Monostearas; GMS; Monostearin.
CAS — 31566-31-1 *(glyceryl monostearate)*; 26657-96-5 *(glyceryl monopalmitate)*.
Pharmacopoeias. In *Eur.* (see p.vi), *Int.*, *Jpn*, and *Pol.* Also in *USNF*.

Pharmacopoeial description
Ph. Eur.: Glycerol Monostearate 40-55 is a mixture of monoacylglycerols, mainly monostearoylglycerol, together with variable quantities of di- and triacylglycerols. It contains 40 to 55% of monoacylglycerols, 30 to 45% of diacylglycerols, and 5 to 15% of triacylglycerols, obtained by partial glycerolysis of vegetable oils mainly containing triacylglycerols of palmitic and stearic acid, or by esterification of glycerol with stearic acid.

A white or almost white, hard, waxy mass or unctuous powder or flakes. Practically insoluble in water; soluble in alcohol at 60°. M.p. 54° to 64°.
USNF 20: Glyceryl Monostearate contains not less than 90% of monoglycerides of saturated fatty acids, chiefly glyceryl monostearate ($C_{21}H_{42}O_4 = 358.6$) and glyceryl monopalmitate ($C_{19}H_{38}O_4 = 330.5$). It may contain a suitable antioxidant.

A white wax-like solid, beads, or flakes with a slight, agreeable, fatty odour. M.p. not below 55°. Insoluble in water but may be dispersed in hot water with the aid of a small amount of soap or other suitable surfactant; soluble 1 in 10 of chloroform, 1 in 100 of ether and of methyl alcohol, 1 in 33 of isopropyl alcohol; dissolves in hot organic solvents such as alcohol, acetone, mineral or fixed oils, and benzene. Store in airtight containers. Protect from light.

Self-emulsifying Glyceryl Monostearate

(436-t)

Monostearin Emulsificans; Self-emulsifying Mono- and Diglycerides of Food Fatty Acids; Self-emulsifying Monostearin.

Pharmacopoeias. In Br.

Because of the presence of soap, it is incompatible with acids and high concentrations of ionisable salts, hard water, calcium compounds, zinc oxide, and oxides of heavy metals.

Pharmacopoeial description

BP 2001: A mixture consisting principally of mono-, di-, and triglycerides of stearic and palmitic acids, and of minor proportions of other fatty acids; it may also contain free fatty acids, free glycerol, and soap. It contains not less than 30% of monoglycerides, not more than 7% of free glycerol, and not more than 6% of soap, calculated as sodium oleate, all calculated with reference to the anhydrous substance.

A white to cream-coloured, hard, waxy solid with a faint fatty odour. Dispersible in hot water; soluble in hot dehydrated alcohol and in hot liquid paraffin; soluble in hot vegetable oils, but may give turbid solutions at concentrations below 20%.

Profile

Glyceryl monostearate is a poor water-in-oil emulsifying agent but it is a useful stabiliser of water-in-oil and oil-in-water emulsions in preparations for internal and external use. It has emollient properties. Glyceryl monostearate is also used in the food and cosmetic industries.

It is usual to add a small amount of soap, sulfated fatty alcohol, or other surfactant, to glyceryl monostearate, which has the effect of making the product self-emulsifying and capable of producing satisfactory oil-in-water emulsions. Self-emulsifying glyceryl monostearate is used as an emulsifying agent for oils, fats, solvents, and waxes in the preparation of bases of the non-emulsified, emulsified, and vanishing-cream types. It is not intended for inclusion in preparations for internal use.

Aqueous preparations containing self-emulsifying glyceryl monostearate should contain a preservative to prevent fungal or bacterial growth.

Macrogol Cetostearyl Ethers (10485-r)

Macrogoli Aetherum Cetostearylicum.

Pharmacopoeias. In Eur. (see p.vi), which gives standards for compounds containing from 2 to 33 units of ethylene oxide per molecule (nominal value).

Pharmacopoeial description

Ph. Eur.: Macrogol cetostearyl ether is a mixture of ethers of mixed macrogols with linear fatty alcohols, mainly cetostearyl alcohol. It may contain some free macrogols and it contains various amounts of free cetostearyl alcohol. The amount of ethylene oxide reacted with cetostearyl alcohol is from 2 to 33 units per molecule (nominal value). White or yellowish-white waxy, unctuous mass, pellets, microbeads, or flakes. Macrogol cetostearyl ether with low numbers of ethylene oxide units per molecule is practically insoluble in water; soluble in alcohol and in dichloromethane. Macrogol cetostearyl ether with higher numbers of ethylene oxide units per molecule is dispersible or soluble in water; soluble in alcohol and in dichloromethane. Macrogol cetostearyl ether solidifies at 32° to 52°. Store in airtight containers. The labelling states the amount of ethylene oxide reacted with cetostearyl alcohol (nominal value).

Cetomacrogol 1000 (445-x)

Cetomacrogol 1000 (BAN, rINN).
Polyethylene Glycol 1000 Monocetyl Ether; Polyoxyethylene Glycol 1000 Monocetyl Ether.
CAS — 9004-95-9; 68439-49-6.

Pharmacopoeias. In Int.

A macrogol ether containing 20 to 24 oxyethylene groups in the polyoxyethylene chain. It is represented by the formula $CH_3.[CH_2]_m.[O.CH_2.CH_2]_n.OH$, where m may be 15 or 17 and n may be 20 to 24.

It has been reported to be incompatible with phenols and to reduce the antibacterial activity of quaternary ammonium compounds. Cetomacrogol may separate from solutions in the presence of a high concentration of electrolytes.

Polyoxyl 20 Cetostearyl Ether (459-m)

Pharmacopoeias. In USNF.

Pharmacopoeial description

USNF 20: A mixture of the monocetostearyl (mixed hexadecyl and octadecyl) ethers of mixed macrogols, the average polymer length being equivalent to 17.2 to 25.0 oxyethylene units. A cream-coloured waxy unctuous mass melting, when heated, to a clear brownish-yellow liquid. Soluble in water, in alcohol, and in acetone; insoluble in petroleum spirit. A 10% solution in water has a pH of 4.5 to 7.5. Store at a temperature of 8° to 15° in airtight containers.

Profile

Macrogol cetostearyl ethers are used as surfactants and emulsifiers. Macrogol cetostearyl ether (22) is used with cetostearyl

The symbol † denotes a preparation no longer actively marketed

alcohol (for example, in the form of Cetomacrogol Emulsifying Wax BP 2001) as an emulsifying agent for making oil-in-water emulsions that are unaffected by moderate concentrations of electrolytes and that are stable over a wide pH range. It is also used to disperse volatile oils in water to form transparent sols.

Preparations

BP 2001: Cetomacrogol Emulsifying Wax.

Macrogol Lauril Ethers (13605-j)

α-Dodecyl-ω-hydroxypoly(oxyethylene); Laureth Compounds; Lauromacrogols; Macrogol Lauryl Ethers; Macrogoli Aetherum Laurilicum; Polyoxyl Lauryl Ethers.
CAS — 9002-92-0.

Pharmacopoeias. In Eur. (see p.vi), which gives standards for compounds containing from 3 to 23 units of ethylene oxide per molecule (nominal value). *Jpn.* also contains a general monograph.

Mixtures of ethers of mixed macrogols with linear fatty alcohols, mainly lauril alcohol, represented by the formula $C_{12}H_{25}(OCH_2CH_2)_nOH$.

Pharmacopoeial description

Ph. Eur.: Macrogol lauril ether is a mixture of ethers of mixed macrogols with linear fatty alcohols, mainly lauril alcohol. It may contain some free macrogols and it contains various amounts of free lauril alcohol. Macrogol lauril ether with 3 to 5 units of ethylene oxide per molecule is a colourless liquid. Practically insoluble in water and in petroleum spirit; soluble or dispersible in alcohol. Macrogol lauril ether with 9 to 23 units of ethylene oxide per molecule is a white, waxy mass. Soluble or dispersible in water; soluble in alcohol; practically insoluble in petroleum spirit. Macrogol lauril ether should be stored in airtight containers.

Laureth 4 (447-f)

Laureth 4 (USAN).
CAS — 9002-92-0.

A mixture of monolauril ethers of macrogols where the average value of n in the formula given above is 4.

Lauromacrogol 400 (448-d)

Lauromacrogol 400 (rINN).
Laureth 9 (USAN); Polidocanol.
CAS — 9002-92-0; 3055-99-0.
ATC — C05BB02.

NOTE. Lauromacrogol 400 has sometimes been erroneously described as containing 8, rather than 9, oxyethylene groups.

A mixture of monolauril ethers of macrogols where the average value of n in the formula given above is 9.

Adverse Effects

There have been occasional reports of allergic skin reactions following the topical application of preparations containing laureth compounds.

◊ A 63-year-old man developed pulmonary oedema, a dramatic fall in heart rate, transient left pyramidal syndrome and died following sclerotherapy with lauromacrogol 400 to control gastric variceal bleeding;[1] the fatality was attributed to the action of the drug that had passed into the systemic circulation. Another patient has been described[2] who suffered a reversible ischaemic neurological deficit after sclerotherapy with lauromacrogol 400 for varicose veins of the leg.

1. Paterlini A, *et al.* Heart failure and endoscopic sclerotherapy of variceal bleeding. *Lancet* 1984; **i:** 1241.
2. Van der Plas JPL, *et al.* Reversible ischaemic neurological deficit after sclerotherapy of varicose veins. *Lancet* 1994; **343:** 428.

Uses and Administration

Macrogol lauril ethers (laureth compounds) have been used as surfactants and spermicides. Lauromacrogol 400 is used as a sclerosant in the treatment of oesophageal and gastric varices (p.1637) and varicose veins (p.1637), and has been used as a local anaesthetic and antipruritic in combination topical preparations.

Preparations

Proprietary Preparations (details are given in Part 3)
Aust.: Aethoxysklerol; *Belg.:* Aethoxysklerol; *Denm.:* Aethoxysklerol; *Fin.:* Aethoxysklerol; *Fr.:* Aetoxisclerol; *Ger.:* Aethoxysklerol; Anaesthesulf; Hamo-Europuran N†; Recessan; *Ital.:* Atossisclerol Kreussler; *Mex.:* Farmaflebon; *Neth.:* Aethoxysklerol; *Spain:* Etoxisclerol; *Swed.:* Aethoxysklerol; *Switz.:* Aethoxysklerol; *Thai.:* Aethoxysklerol.

Multi-ingredient: *Aust.:* Balneum Plus; Dentinox; Optiderm; Paididont; Prurimix; Recessan†; Solcoseryl Dental; Vonum; *Austral.:* TAGG; *Belg.:* Neo-Alcos-Anal; *Ger.:* Acoin; Alcos-Anal; Balneum Plus; Brand- u. Wundgel-Medice N; Collomack; Corti-Dynexan; Dentinox N; Haemo-Exhirud; Hexamon; Inflam; Meaverin; Medigel; Optiderm; Rectosellan H†; Sagittaproct S; Solcoseryl Dental; Tamposit N; Thesit; Thesit P; Varitan N; Vaxicum N†; Vivisun†; *Hong Kong:* Collomack; Solcoseryl Dental; *Irl.:* Balneum Plus; *Israel:* Balneum Plus; Derma-Care; *Ital.:* Optiderm; Pruriden; *Norw.:* Alcos-Anal; *Port.:* Anacal; Optiderme†; *S.Afr.:* Tyrogel†; *Singapore:* Collomack; *Switz.:* Balneum Hermal Plus; Decasept N; Dentinox†; Optiderm; Oxydermine; Pruri-med;

Ralur; Remexal; Sclerovein; Solcoseryl Dental; Sportusal; Sportusal Spray sine heparino; Venucreme; Venugel; *Thai.:* Collomack; Solcoseryl Dental; *UK:* Anacal; Balneum Plus; E45 Itch Relief; *USA:* Lubrin.

Macrogol Monomethyl Ethers (15825-t)

Polyethylene Glycol Monomethyl Ethers. α-Methyl-ω-hydroxy-poly(oxyethylene).
CAS — 9004-74-4.

Pharmacopoeias. In USNF which gives standards for compounds having nominal average molecular weights in the range of 350 to 10 000.

Pharmacopoeial description

USNF 20: Addition polymers of ethylene oxide and methyl alcohol, represented by the formula $CH_3(OCH_2CH_2)_nOH$, where n represents the average number of oxyethylene groups. The name is usually designated by a number that corresponds approximately to its average molecular weight.

As the average molecular weight increases, the water solubility, vapour pressure, hygroscopicity, and solubility in organic solvents decrease while congealing temperature, specific gravity, flash-point, and viscosity increase. Liquid grades occur as clear to slightly hazy, colourless or practically colourless, slightly hygroscopic, viscous liquids with a slight characteristic odour. Solid grades occur as practically odourless, white, waxy, plastic material with a consistency similar to beeswax, or as creamy white flakes, beads, or powders. Liquid grades are miscible with water; solid grades are freely soluble in water; all grades are soluble in alcohol, in acetone, in chloroform, in ethyl acetate, in ethylene glycol monoethyl ether, and in toluene; all grades are insoluble in ether and in hexane. Store in airtight containers.

Profile

Macrogol monomethyl ethers may be used as ointment bases, solvents, and plasticisers.

Macrogol Oleyl Ethers (10492-x)

Macrogoli Aetherum Oleicum.

Pharmacopoeias. In Eur. (see p.vi), which gives standards for compounds containing from 2 to 20 units of ethylene oxide per molecule (nominal value).

Pharmacopoeial description

Ph. Eur.: Macrogol oleyl ether is a mixture of ethers of mixed macrogols with linear fatty alcohols, mainly oleyl alcohol. It may contain some free macrogols and it contains various amounts of free oleyl alcohol. Macrogol oleyl ether with 2 to 5 units of ethylene oxide per molecule is a yellow liquid. Practically insoluble in water and in petroleum spirit; soluble in alcohol. Macrogol oleyl ether with 10 to 20 units of ethylene oxide per molecule is a yellowish-white, waxy mass. Dispersible or soluble in water; soluble in alcohol; practically insoluble in petroleum spirit. Macrogol oleyl ethers should be stored in airtight containers. Protect from light.

Polyoxyl 10 Oleyl Ether (460-t)

Polyethylene Glycol Mono-oleyl Ether.
CAS — 9004-98-2.

Pharmacopoeias. In USNF.

Pharmacopoeial description

USNF 20: A mixture of the mono-oleyl ethers of mixed macrogols, the average polymer length being equivalent to 8.6 to 10.4 oxyethylene units. It may contain suitable stabilisers.

A soft white semisolid or pale yellow liquid with a bland odour. Soluble in water and in alcohol; dispersible in liquid paraffin and in propylene glycol with possible separation on standing. Store at a temperature of 8° to 15° in airtight containers.

Profile

Macrogol oleyl ethers such as polyoxyl 10 oleyl ether are used as surfactants.

Macrogol Stearates (13602-e)

Macrogoli Stearas; Polyoxyethylene Glycol Stearates; Polyoxyethylene Stearates; Polyoxyl Stearates.
CAS — 9004-99-3.

NOTE. There are two systems of nomenclature used for these compounds; these substances have the general formula $C_{17}H_{35}COO.[O.CH_2CH_2]_n.H$. In the systems used by BAN and USAN the numbers in the names refer to the approximate polymer length in oxyethylene units whereas in the system used by INN the number refers to the average molecular weight of the polymer chain. Thus, the names Macrogol Stearate 8 (BAN), Polyoxyl 8 Stearate (USAN), and Macrogol Stearate 400 (rINNM) all describe the same compound and similarly Macrogol 40 Stearate (BAN), Polyoxyl 40 Stearate (USAN), and Macrogol Stearate 2000 (rINNM) all refer to another.

Pharmacopoeias. In Eur. (see p.vi). *USNF* includes a monograph for Polyoxyl 40 Stearate.

Pharmacopoeial description

Ph. Eur.: Macrogol Stearate is a mixture of the mono- and di-esters of mainly stearic acid and/or palmitic acid and macrogols. It may be obtained by ethoxylation or by esterification of macrogols with stearic acid 50 (type I) or stearic acid 95 (type II). The average polymer length is equivalent to 6 to 100 ethylene oxide units per molecule (nominal value). It may contain free macrogols. White or slightly yellowish waxy mass. Soluble in alcohol and in isopropyl alcohol. Compounds containing 6 to 9 units of ethylene oxide per molecule are practically insoluble but freely dispersible in water; miscible with fatty oils and with waxes. Compounds containing 20 to 100 units of ethylene oxide per molecule are soluble in water; practically insoluble in fatty oils and in waxes. Store in airtight containers.

USNF 20: Polyoxyl 40 Stearate is a mixture of the mono- and di-esters of stearic acid and mixed macrogols, the average polymer length being about 40 oxyethylene units. It contains not less than 17% and not more than 27% of free macrogols. It is a waxy, white to light tan solid, odourless or with a faint fat-like odour. Congealing range 37° to 47°. Soluble in water, in alcohol, in acetone, and in ether; insoluble in liquid paraffin and in vegetable oils. Store in airtight containers.

Incompatibilities. Macrogol stearates have been reported to be generally stable with electrolytes and weak acids or bases although strong acids or bases may cause hydrolysis and saponification. Discoloration or precipitation may occur with phenolic substances and complexation with preservatives. Decrease in the antimicrobial activity of bacitracin, chloramphenicol, phenoxymethylpenicillin, and tetracycline has been stated to occur with concentrations of macrogol stearates exceeding 5%.

Profile
Macrogol stearates are macrogol esters which are used as emulsifying and solubilising agents.

Menfegol (748-l)

Menfegol (rINN).

Menphegol. α-[p-(p-Menthyl)phenyl]-ω-hydroxypoly(oxyethylene).

CAS — 57821-32-6.

Menthylphenyl ethers of macrogols represented by the formula $C_{16}H_{23}(OCH_2CH_2)_nOH$.

Profile
Menfegol is a nonionic surfactant used as a spermicide.

Preparations

Proprietary Preparations (details are given in Part 3)
Hong Kong: Neo Sampoon; **Singapore:** Neo Sampoon.

Mono- and Di-glycerides (487-q)

E471 (mono- and di-glycerides of fatty acids).

Pharmacopoeias. In USNF.

Pharmacopoeial description

USNF 20: A mixture of glycerol mono- and di-esters, with minor amounts of tri-esters, of fatty acids from edible oils. It contains not less than 40% of monoglycerides. It may contain suitable stabilisers. Store in airtight containers. Protect from light.

Profile
Mono- and di-glycerides is used as an emulsifying agent.

Nonoxinols (450-k)

Macrogol Nonylphenyl Ethers; Nonoxynols. α-(4-Nonylphenyl)-ω-hydroxypoly(oxyethylene).

CAS — 26027-38-3.

NOTE. Nonoxinol is *BAN* and *rINN*. The name may be followed by a figure indicating the approximate number of oxyethylene groups in the polyoxyethylene chain. *USAN* specifies Nonoxynol 4, Nonoxynol 9, Nonoxynol 15, and Nonoxynol 30.

A series of nonylphenyl ethers of macrogols of differing chain lengths, represented by the formula $C_{15}H_{23}.[O.CH_2.CH_2]_n.OH$.

Nonoxinol 9 (452-t)

Nonoxinol 9 (BAN, rINN).

Nonoxinolum 9; Nonoxynol 9 (USAN). α-(4-Nonylphenyl)-ω-hydroxynona(oxyethylene).

$C_{33}H_{60}O_{10}$ (nominal) = 616.8.

Pharmacopoeias. In Eur. (see p.vi) and US.

Pharmacopoeial description

Ph. Eur.: A liquid mixture consisting mainly of monononylphenyl ethers of macrogols corresponding to the formula: $C_{15}H_{23}.(O.CH_2.CH_2)_n.OH$ where the average value of n is

about 9 but can be between 4 and 16. A clear colourless to light yellow viscous liquid. Miscible with water, with alcohol, and with olive oil. Store in airtight containers.

USP 25: An anhydrous liquid mixture consisting chiefly of monononylphenyl ethers of macrogols corresponding to the formula $C_{15}H_{23}.[O.CH_2.CH_2]_n.OH$, in which the average value of n is about 9. A clear, colourless to light yellow, viscous liquid. Soluble in water, in alcohol, and in maize oil. Store in airtight containers.

Nonoxinol 10 (453-x)

Nonoxinol 10 (BAN, rINN).

Nonoxynol 10. α-(4-Nonylphenyl)-ω-hydroxydeca(oxyethylene).

$C_{35}H_{64}O_{11}$ (nominal) = 660.9.

Nonoxinol 11 (9983-m)

Nonoxinol 11 (BAN, rINN).

Nonoxynol 11. α-(4-Nonylphenyl)-ω-hydroxyundeca(oxyethylene).

$C_{37}H_{68}O_{12}$ (nominal) = 704.9.

Adverse Effects and Precautions
Nonoxinols used as vaginal spermicides may cause local irritation.

Pregnancy. Although maternal use of spermicidal contraceptives has been linked to an increased frequency of congenital abnormalities, including trisomy, such studies may be flawed by recall bias.[1] Meta-analysis of 9 studies also supported the view that peri- and postconceptual maternal use of spermicides was not associated with adverse fetal outcome.[2]

1. Mishell DR. Contraception. *N Engl J Med* 1989; **320:** 777–87.
2. Einarson TR, *et al.* Maternal spermicide use and adverse reproductive outcome: a meta-analysis. *Am J Obstet Gynecol* 1990; **162:** 655–60.

Toxic shock syndrome. Thirteen cases of toxic shock syndrome associated with the use of a vaginal contraceptive sponge impregnated with nonoxinol 9 were reviewed.[1] These had been reported in the USA up to November 1984. In 4 of the cases, there were other predisposing conditions: postpartum use, use during menstruation, and prolonged retention.

1. Faich G, *et al.* Toxic shock syndrome and the vaginal contraceptive sponge. *JAMA* 1986; **255:** 216–18.

Urinary-tract infection. Use of spermicidal foam or jelly containing nonoxinol 9 may disturb the normal vaginal flora and predispose to colonisation with *Escherichia coli* and the development of bacteriuria.[1] An increased risk of acute *E. coli* urinary-tract infection has been reported[2] associated with the use of condoms coated with nonoxinol 9.

1. Hooton TM, *et al.* Escherichia coli bacteriuria and contraceptive method. *JAMA* 1991; **265:** 64–9.
2. Fihn SD, *et al.* Association between use of spermicide-coated condoms and Escherichia coli urinary tract infection in young women. *Am J Epidemiol* 1996; **144:** 512–20.

Uses
Nonoxinols have surface active properties and may be used as solubilising agents. Nonoxinol 9 is used as a spermicide for contraception (p.1460).

Antimicrobial activity. Nonoxinol 9 has activity *in vitro* against a number of bacteria and viruses and it has been suggested that, when used as a spermicidal contraceptive, it may also provide some protection against sexually transmitted diseases, including chlamydial and gonococcal infections,[1,2] and human immunodeficiency virus (HIV) infection.[2] However, the results of *in vitro* testing may not apply to *in vivo* use and it is not clear whether it is of clinical benefit.[2] Indeed, a double-blind placebo-controlled study[3] involving 1292 HIV-negative female sex workers found that it did not reduce the rate of new HIV, gonorrhoea, or chlamydia infection. Furthermore, there has also been concern that the irritant action of nonoxinol 9 may increase the risk of infection by HIV,[2] a view re-iterated by the United Nations,[4] who advised against its use by women at high risk.

1. North BB. Vaginal contraceptives: effective protection from sexually transmitted diseases for women? *J Reprod Med* 1988; **33:** 307–311.
2. Anonymous. Multipurpose spermicides. *Lancet* 1992; **340:** 211–13.
3. Roddy RE, *et al.* A controlled trial of nonoxinol 9 film to reduce male-to-female transmission of sexually transmitted diseases. *N Engl J Med* 1998; **339:** 504–10.
4. Anonymous. UN warns against use of spermicide. *BMJ* 2000; **321:** 194.

Preparations

Proprietary Preparations (details are given in Part 3)
Aust.: Delfen; Patentex; **Austral.:** Delfen; Lubarol; Ortho-Creme; **Belg.:** Gynintim Film; Patentex; **Braz.:** Pessarios Profilaticos Rendel; **Canad.:** Advantage 24; Comfort; Delfen; Encare†; K-Y Personal Lubricant; Lifestyles; Ortho Shields; Ortho-Gynol II; Ramses; Sheik; Titan; Trojan; **Fr.:** Patentex; Semicid†; **Ger.:** Ortho-Gel†; Patentex; Patentex Oval N; **Hong Kong:** VCF; **Irl.:** Delfen; Gynol II; Ortho-Creme; Orthoforms; **Israel:** Delfen; **Ital.:** C-Film; Delfen; **NZ:** Lorophyn; Preforms; **NZ:** Rendells Plus; **Port.:** Delfen; Rendells; **S.Afr.:** Delfen; Emko†; Patentex†; **Spain:** Lineafarm†; Nacha; Nobliten†; Yadalan†; **Switz.:** C-Film; Delfen; Pat-

entex Oval N; Syn-A-Gen†; **UK:** C-Film; Delfen; Double Check; Duracreme; Duragel; Gynol II; Ortho-Creme; Orthoforms; Prelude; Today; **USA:** Advantage 24; Because; Delfen; Emko; Encare; Excita†; Gynol; Koromex; Ramses; Semicid; Sheik Elite; Shur-Seal; Today†; VCF.

Multi-ingredient: Canad.: Protectaid; **Ger.:** A-gen 53; **Hong Kong:** Protectaid; **Israel:** Glovan; **Ital.:** Agena†; Betaform Habitat; Florigien; Vironox; **Spain:** Lavolen; **UK:** Protectaid.

Octoxinols (456-d)

Macrogol Tetramethylbutylphenyl Ethers; Octoxynols; Octylphenoxy Polyethoxyethanol. α-[4-(1,1,3,3-Tetramethylbutyl)phenyl]-ω-hydroxypoly(oxyethylene).

CAS — 9002-93-1.

NOTE. Octoxinol is *BAN* and *rINN*. The name may be followed by a figure indicating the approximate number of oxyethylene groups in the polyoxyethylene chain.
USAN specifies Octoxynol 9.

A series of tetramethylbutylphenyl ethers of macrogols of differing chain lengths, represented by the formula $C_{14}H_{21}.[O.CH_2.CH_2]_n.OH$.

Octoxinol 9 (457-n)

Octoxinol 9 (BAN, rINN).

Octoxynol 9 (USAN).

$C_{32}H_{58}O_{10}$ (nominal) = 602.8.

Pharmacopoeias. In USNF.

Pharmacopoeial description

USNF 20: An anhydrous liquid mixture consisting chiefly of mono-octylphenyl ethers of macrogols, corresponding to the formula $C_{14}H_{21}.[O.CH_2.CH_2]_n.OH$, in which the average value of n is about 9. A clear, pale yellow, viscous liquid with a faint odour. Miscible with water, with alcohol, and with acetone; soluble in toluene and in benzene; practically insoluble in petroleum spirit. Store in airtight containers.

Profile
Octoxinols have surface active properties and may be used as solubilising agents. They are also used as spermicides.

Preparations

Proprietary Preparations (details are given in Part 3)
Austral.: Ortho-Gynol; Summers Eve Disposable†; **USA:** Koromex; Ortho-Gynol; Vagi-Gard Medicated Disposable Douche.

Multi-ingredient: Austral.: Summers Eve Feminine; **Canad.:** Aseptone Quat; **USA:** Feminique; Massengill; Massengill Disposable; Summers Eve Disposable.

Poloxamers (463-f)

Polyethylene-polypropylene glycol. α-Hydro-ω-hydroxypoly(oxyethylene)poly(oxypropylene)poly(oxyethylene) block copolymer.

CAS — 9003-11-6.

NOTE. Poloxamer is *BAN* and *rINN*. The name is followed by a figure, the first 2 digits of which, when multiplied by 100, correspond to the approximate average molecular weight of the polyoxypropylene portion and the third digit, when multiplied by 10, corresponds to the percentage by weight of the polyoxyethylene portion.
USAN specifies Poloxamer 182D, Poloxamer 182LF, Poloxamer 188, Poloxamer 188LF, and Poloxamer 331.
Poloxalene (BAN, USAN, rINN) is also a poloxamer.
Pharmacopoeias. In Eur. (see p.vi) under the title Poloxamers where specifications are given for Poloxamer 124, Poloxamer 188, Poloxamer 237, Poloxamer 338, and Poloxamer 407. Also in *USNF* under the title Poloxamer where specifications are given for Poloxamer 124, Poloxamer 188, Poloxamer 237, Poloxamer 338, and Poloxamer 407.

Poloxamers have been reported to be incompatible with phenols.

Pharmacopoeial description

Ph. Eur.: Poloxamer is a synthetic block copolymer of ethylene oxide and propylene oxide represented by the general formula: $HO(C_2H_4O)_a(C_3H_6O)_b(C_2H_4O)_aH$. It may contain a suitable antioxidant. Poloxamer 124 is a colourless or almost colourless liquid. Poloxamer 188, poloxamer 237, poloxamer 338, and poloxamer 407 are white or almost white, waxy powders, microbeads or flakes; m.p. about 50°. All poloxamers are very soluble in water and in alcohol; practically insoluble in petroleum spirit (50° to 70°). pH of a 10% solution in water is 5.0 to 7.5. Store in airtight containers.

USNF 20: Poloxamer is a synthetic block copolymer of ethylene oxide and propylene oxide with the general formula $HO(C_2H_4O)_a(C_3H_6O)_b(C_2H_4O)_aH$. It may contain a suitable antioxidant. Poloxamer 124 is a colourless liquid with a mild odour. Poloxamers 188, 237, 338, and 407 are white, prilled or cast solids, odourless or with a mild odour. All poloxamers are freely soluble in water and in alcohol. Poloxamers 124 and 407 are freely soluble in isopropyl alcohol and in propylene glycol; poloxamer 237 is sparingly soluble in isopropyl alcohol and in xylene; poloxamer 338 is sparingly soluble in propylene glycol; poloxamer 124 is freely soluble in xylene. A 2.5% solution in water has a pH of 5.0 to 7.5. Store in airtight containers.

Poloxalene (464-d)

Poloxalene (BAN, USAN, rINN).

SKF-18667.

Pharmacopoeias. In *US* for veterinary use only.

Pharmacopoeial description

USP 25: A synthetic block copolymer of ethylene oxide and propylene oxide. A colourless or pale yellow liquid. Soluble in water, in chloroform, and in ethylene dichloride. A 2.5% solution in water has a pH of 5.0 to 7.5. Store in airtight containers.

Poloxamer 188 (465-n)

Poloxamer 188 (BAN, USAN, rINN).

Poloxalkol.

NOTE. Compounded preparations of poloxamer 188 may be represented by the following names:

• Co-danthramer *x/y* (*BAN*)—where *x* and *y* are the strengths in milligrams of dantron and poloxamer respectively.

Pharmacopoeias. In *Eur.* (see p.vi) under the group title Poloxamers. Also in *USNF* under the group title Poloxamer.

Pharmacopoeial description

Ph. Eur.: Poloxamer 188 is a poloxamer in which *a* in the general formula given above is 75 to 85 and *b* is 25 to 30; it has an average molecular weight of 7680 to 9510. It is a white or almost white, waxy powder, microbeads, or flakes. M.p. about 50°. Very soluble in water and in alcohol: practically insoluble in petroleum spirit (50° to 70°). pH of a 10% solution is 5.0 to 7.5. Store in airtight containers.

USNF 20: A poloxamer in which *a* in the general formula averages 80 and *b* averages 27; it has an average molecular weight of 7680 to 9510. A white prilled or cast solid, odourless or with a very mild odour. M.p. about 52°. Freely soluble in water and in alcohol. Store in airtight containers.

Poloxamer 407 (9988-p)

Poloxamer 407 (BAN, rINN).

Pharmacopoeias. In *Eur.* (see p.vi) under the group title Poloxamers. Also in *USNF* under the group title Poloxamer.

Pharmacopoeial description

Ph. Eur.: Poloxamer 407 is a poloxamer in which *a* in the general formula given above is 95 to 105 and *b* is 54 to 60; it has an average molecular weight of 9840 to 14 600. It is a white or almost white, waxy powder, microbeads, or flakes. M.p. about 50°. Very soluble in water and in alcohol: practically insoluble in petroleum spirit (50° to 70°). pH of a 10% solution in water is 5.0 to 7.5. Store in airtight containers.

USNF 20: A poloxamer in which *a* in the general formula averages 101 and *b* averages 56; it has an average molecular weight of 9840 to 14 600. A white, prilled or cast solid, odourless or with a very mild odour. M.p. about 56°. Freely soluble in water, in alcohol, and in isopropyl alcohol. Store in airtight containers.

Precautions

Poloxamers may increase the absorption of liquid paraffin and other fat-soluble substances.

Uses and Administration

Poloxamers are used as emulsifying agents for intravenous fat emulsions, as solubilising agents to maintain clarity in elixirs and syrups, and as wetting agents for antibiotics. They may also be used in ointment or suppository bases and as tablet binders or coaters.

Poloxamer 188 is used as a wetting agent in the treatment of constipation. It is usually administered in combination with a laxative such as dantron. Poloxamer 188 has also been used as an emulsifying agent in fluorocarbon blood substitutes. Poloxamer 188 has been investigated for its ability to improve blood flow in sickle-cell crisis; it has also been tried in myocardial infarction. Other investigational uses include the treatment of burns.

Poloxamer 407 is used in solutions for contact lens care, as is poloxamer 338.

Poloxalene is used as a defoaming agent in the treatment of bloat in ruminants.

Preparations

Proprietary Preparations (details are given in Part 3)

Austral.: Clerz; Coloxyl; Pliagel; *Braz.:* Pliagel; *Canad.:* Clerz; *Fr.:* Alkenide; Idrocol; *NZ:* Coloxyl; Pliagel.

Multi-ingredient: *Aust.:* Actizyme; *Austral.:* Comfortcare GP Dual Action†; *Irl.:* Ailax; Codalax; Cotron; *NZ:* Codalax; *UK:* Ailax; Codalax; Danlax; *USA:* Baby Orajel Tooth and Gum Cleanser.

Polyoxyl Castor Oils (9982-h)

Macrogolglycerol Ricinoleate; Macrogolglyceroli Ricinoleas; Polyethoxylated Castor Oils; Polyoxyethylene Castor Oils.

Pharmacopoeias. In *Eur.* (see p.vi).

Pharmacopoeial description

Ph. Eur.: Polyoxyl castor oil contains mainly ricinoleyl glycerol ethoxylated with 30 to 50 molecules of ethylene oxide (nominal value), with small amounts of macrogol ricinoleate and of the corresponding free glycols. It results from the reaction of castor oil with ethylene oxide. A clear, yellow, viscous liquid or semi-solid. Relative density about 1.05; viscosity, at 25°, 500 to 800 mPa s. Freely soluble in water and in alcohol; very soluble in dichloromethane. Protect from light.

Polyoxyl 35 Castor Oil (18355-g)

Pharmacopoeias. In *USNF.*

Polyethoxylated castor oils are reported to affect polyvinyl chloride containers and apparatus adversely.

Pharmacopoeial description

USNF 20: A mixture of the triricinoleate ester of ethoxylated glycerol with smaller amounts of macrogol ricinoleate and the corresponding free glycols. It is produced by reacting 1 mole of glycerol ricinoleate with about 35 moles of ethylene oxide.

A yellow oily liquid with a faint characteristic odour. Sp. gr. 1.05 to 1.06; viscosity, at 25°, 650 to 850 mPa s. Very soluble in water, producing a practically odourless and colourless solution; soluble in alcohol and in ethyl acetate; insoluble in mineral oils. Store in airtight containers.

Adverse Effects

Polyoxyl castor oils (such as Cremophor EL), used as vehicles in various intravenous injections, have been associated with severe anaphylactoid reactions, hyperlipidaemias, alterations in blood viscosity, and erythrocyte aggregation.

◊ References.
1. Bagnarello AG, *et al.* Unusual serum lipoprotein abnormality induced by the vehicle of miconazole. *N Engl J Med* 1977; **296:** 497–9.
2. Forrest ARW, *et al.* Long-term Althesin infusion and hyperlipidaemia. *BMJ* 1977; **2:** 1357–8.
3. Dye D, Watkins J. Suspected anaphylactic reaction to Cremophor EL. *BMJ* 1980; **280:** 1353.
4. Howrie DL, *et al.* Anaphylactoid reactions associated with parenteral cyclosporine use: possible role of Cremophor EL. *Drug Intell Clin Pharm* 1985; **19:** 425–7.
5. Chapuis B, *et al.* Anaphylactic reaction to intravenous cyclosporine. *N Engl J Med* 1985; **312:** 1259.
6. Siddall SJ, *et al.* Anaphylactic reactions to teniposide. *Lancet* 1989; **i:** 394.

Uses

Polyoxyl castor oils are macrogol esters used as emulsifying and solubilising agents. Polyoxyl 35 castor oil has been used as a solvent in vehicles for various intravenous injections.

Polyoxyl Hydrogenated Castor Oils (19834-g)

Macrogolglycerol Hydroxystearate; Macrogolglyceroli Hydroxystearas.

Pharmacopoeias. In *Eur.* (see p.vi).

Pharmacopoeial description

Ph. Eur.: Polyoxyl hydrogenated castor oil contains mainly trihydroxystearyl glycerol ethoxylated with 7 to 60 molecules of ethylene oxide (nominal value), with small amounts of macrogol hydroxystearate and of the corresponding free glycols. It results from the reaction of hydrogenated castor oil with ethylene oxide. Polyoxyl hydrogenated castor oil with less than 10 units of ethylene oxide per molecule is a yellowish, turbid, viscous liquid. Practically insoluble in water; dispersible in alcohol; soluble in acetone. Polyoxyl hydrogenated castor oil with more than 20 units of ethylene oxide per molecule is a white or yellowish, semi-liquid or pasty mass. Freely soluble in water, in alcohol, and in acetone; practically insoluble in petroleum spirit.

Polyoxyl 40 Hydrogenated Castor Oil

(18356-q)

Pharmacopoeias. In *USNF.*

Pharmacopoeial description

USNF 20: A mixture of mainly the trihydroxystearate ester of ethoxylated glycerol, with smaller amounts of macrogol trihydroxystearate and the corresponding free glycols. It is produced by reacting 1 mole of glycerol trihydroxystearate with about 40 to 45 moles of ethylene oxide.

A white to yellowish paste or pasty liquid with a faint odour. Congealing range 20° to 30°. Very soluble in water, producing an odourless, colourless solution; soluble in alcohol and in ethyl acetate; insoluble in liquid paraffin. Store in airtight containers.

Profile

Polyoxyl hydrogenated castor oils are used as surfactants.

Polysorbates (13603-l)

A series of mixtures of fatty acid esters of sorbitol and its anhydrides copolymerised with approximately 20 moles of ethylene oxide for each mole of sorbitol and its anhydrides.

Incompatibilities. Polysorbates have been reported to be stable with electrolytes and weak acids and bases although saponification may occur in the presence of strong acids and bases. Discoloration or precipitation may occur with phenolic substances. The oleic acid esters are sensitive to oxidation. For reference to the possible incompatibility of polysorbate 80 with hydroxybenzoates, see p.1148.

Polysorbate 20 (472-d)

Polysorbate 20 (BAN, USAN, rINN).

E432; Polyoxyethylene 20 Sorbitan Monolaurate; Polysorbatum 20; Sorbimacrogol Laurate 300; Sorboxaethenum Laurinicum.

$C_{58}H_{114}O_{26}$ (approximate).

CAS — 9005-64-5.

Pharmacopoeias. In *Eur.* (see p.vi) and *Int.* Also in *USNF.*

Pharmacopoeial description

Ph. Eur.: A mixture of partial lauric esters of sorbitol and its anhydrides copolymerised with approximately 20 moles of ethylene oxide for each mole of sorbitol and its anhydrides. The lauric acid used for esterification may contain other fatty acids. A clear or slightly opalescent yellowish or brownish-yellow oily liquid. Relative density about 1.1. Miscible with water, with dehydrated alcohol, with methyl alcohol, and with ethyl acetate; practically insoluble in liquid paraffin and in fatty oils. Store in airtight containers. Protect from light.

USNF 20: A laurate ester of sorbitol and its anhydrides copolymerised with approximately 20 moles of ethylene oxide for each mole of sorbitol and its anhydrides. A lemon to amber liquid with a faint characteristic odour. Soluble in water, in alcohol, in dioxan, in ethyl acetate, and in methyl alcohol; insoluble in liquid paraffin. Store in airtight containers.

Polysorbate 40 (427-a)

Polysorbate 40 (BAN, USAN, rINN).

E434; Polyoxyethylene 20 Sorbitan Monopalmitate; Sorbimacrogol Palmitate 300.

$C_{62}H_{122}O_{26}$ (approximate).

CAS — 9005-66-7.

Pharmacopoeias. In *USNF.*

Pharmacopoeial description

USNF 20: A palmitate ester of sorbitol and its anhydrides copolymerised with approximately 20 moles of ethylene oxide for each mole of sorbitol and its anhydrides. A yellow liquid with a faint characteristic odour. Soluble in water and in alcohol; insoluble in liquid paraffin and in vegetable oils. Store in airtight containers.

Polysorbate 60 (474-h)

Polysorbate 60 (BAN, USAN, rINN).

E435; Polyoxyethylene 20 Sorbitan Monostearate; Polysorbatum 60; Sorbimacrogol Stearate 300; Sorboxaethenum Stearinicum.

$C_{64}H_{126}O_{26}$ (approximate).

CAS — 9005-67-8.

Pharmacopoeias. In *Eur.* (see p.vi), *Int.*, and *Pol.* Also in *USNF.*

Pharmacopoeial description

Ph. Eur.: A mixture of partial stearic esters of sorbitol and its anhydrides copolymerised with approximately 20 moles of ethylene oxide for each mole of sorbitol and its anhydrides. The stearic acid used for esterification may contain other fatty acids, especially palmitic acid. A yellowish-brown gelatinous mass which becomes a clear liquid at temperatures above 25°. Relative density about 1.1. Miscible with water, with dehydrated alcohol, with ethyl acetate, and with methyl alcohol; practically insoluble in liquid paraffin and in fatty oils. Store in airtight containers. Protect from light.

USNF 20: A mixture of stearate and palmitate esters of sorbitol and its anhydrides copolymerised with approximately 20 moles of ethylene oxide for each mole of sorbitol and its anhydrides. A lemon to orange-coloured oily liquid or semi-gel with a faint characteristic odour. Soluble in water, in ethyl acetate, and in toluene; insoluble in liquid paraffin and in vegetable oils. Store in airtight containers.

Polysorbate 80 (476-b)

Polysorbate 80 (BAN, USAN, rINN).

E433; Olethytan 20; Polyäthylenglykol-Sorbitanoleat; Polyoxyethylene 20 Sorbitan Mono-oleate; Polysorbatum 80; Polysorbitanum 80 Oleinatum; Sorbimacrogol Oleate 300; Sorboxaethenum Oleinicum; Sorethytan 20 Mono-oleate.

$C_{64}H_{124}O_{26}$ (approximate).

CAS — 9005-65-6.

Pharmacopoeias. In *Chin.*, *Eur.* (see p.vi), *Int.*, *Jpn*, and *Pol.* Also in *USNF.*

Pharmacopoeial description

Ph. Eur.: A mixture of partial oleic esters of sorbitol and its anhydrides copolymerised with approximately 20 moles of ethylene oxide for each mole of sorbitol and its anhydrides. A clear yellowish or brownish-yellow oily liquid. Relative density about 1.08; viscosity, at 25°, about 400 mPa s. Miscible with water, with dehydrated alcohol, with ethyl acetate, and with methyl alcohol; practically insoluble in liquid paraffin and in fatty oils. Store in airtight containers. Protect from light.

USNF 20: An oleate ester of sorbitol and its anhydrides copolymerised with approximately 20 moles of ethylene oxide for each mole of sorbitol and its anhydrides. A lemon to amber-coloured oily liquid with a faint characteristic odour. Sp. gr. between 1.06 and 1.09; viscosity, at 25°, between 300 and 500 mPa s. Very soluble in water, producing an odourless and practically colourless solution; soluble in alcohol and in ethyl acetate; insoluble in liquid paraffin. Store in airtight containers.

Polysorbate 85 (477-v)

Polysorbate 85 (BAN, USAN, rINN).
Polyoxyethylene 20 Sorbitan Trioleate; Sorbimacrogol Trioleate 300.
$C_{100}H_{188}O_{28}$ (approximate).
CAS — 9005-70-3.

A mixture of mainly trioleate esters of sorbitol and its anhydrides copolymerised with approximately 20 moles of ethylene oxide for each mole of sorbitol and its anhydrides.

Adverse Effects and Precautions

Polysorbates may increase the absorption of fat-soluble substances.

There have been occasional reports of hypersensitivity following topical application of preparations containing polysorbates. Fatalities in low birth-weight infants associated with the injection of a polysorbate-containing preparation are discussed below.

Effects in infants. Following the introduction in the USA of an intravenous preparation of vitamin E (E-Ferol) there were a number of reports of unusual liver and kidney disorders with 38 deaths being reported among treated low birth-weight infants. Affected infants had unexplained hypotension, thrombocytopenia, renal dysfunction, hepatomegaly, cholestasis, ascites, and metabolic acidosis;[1-3] the preparation was subsequently withdrawn from the market in April 1984 about 5 months after it was introduced. In-vitro evidence was produced demonstrating that E-Ferol suppressed the response of human lymphocytes to phytohaemagglutinin. However, it was the mixture of polysorbates, polysorbate 20 and in particular polysorbate 80, that was shown to be responsible for this suppression rather than the α-tocopherol acetate component. Despite this in-vitro data, overwhelming infection was not a feature in the affected infants.[2] Large doses of polysorbates were unavoidably injected when E-Ferol was used and it was suggested that polysorbates may accumulate as a result of an alteration in the metabolism by low birth-weight infants; polysorbate-induced alteration of membrane fluidity in cells of vessel walls may have led to changes in structure and function.[2]

1. Alade SL, et al. Polysorbate 80 and E-Ferol toxicity. Pediatrics 1986; **77:** 593–7.
2. Balistreri WF, et al. Lessons from the E-Ferol tragedy. Pediatrics 1986; **78:** 503–6.
3. Golightly LK, et al. Pharmaceutical excipients: adverse effects associated with inactive ingredients in drug products. Med Toxicol 1988; **3:** 128–65 and 209–240.

Hypersensitivity. Local inflammatory reactions following intramuscular injection of a vitamin A preparation were considered[1] to be due to a hypersensitivity reaction to polysorbate 80, included as an excipient.
1. Shelley WB, et al. Polysorbate 80 hypersensitivity. Lancet 1995; **345:** 1312–13.

Uses

Polysorbates are hydrophilic nonionic surfactants which are used as emulsifying agents for the preparation of stable oil-in-water emulsions in pharmaceutical products; they are frequently used with a sorbitan ester in varying proportions to produce products with a range of texture and consistency. Polysorbates have also been used in the formulation of insecticide and herbicide sprays, industrial detergents, and cosmetic products. They are also used as emulsifiers in the food industry.

Polysorbates are used as solubilising agents for a variety of substances including essential oils and oil-soluble vitamins such as vitamins A, D, and E, and as wetting agents in the formulation of oral and parenteral suspensions. However, see Adverse Effects and Precautions, above.

Polysorbates may also be used for their surfactant properties in preparations for the removal of ear wax, and for the management of dry eyes and upper respiratory-tract disorders.

Preparations

Proprietary Preparations (details are given in Part 3)
Belg.: Oleosorbate†; *Canad.:* Tears Encore; *Fr.:* Cerumenol; *USA:* Viva-Drops.

Multi-ingredient: *Aust.:* Expigen; Nasimild; *Fin.:* Expigen; *Fr.:* Fluisedal; Fluisedal sans promethazine; Prorhinel; *Ger.:* Prorhinel†; *Israel:* Lubrin; *Norw.:* Expigen; *S.Afr.:* Dilinct; Expigen; *Switz.:* Prorhinel; Rhinocure Simplex†; Rhinocure†.

Propylene Glycol Diacetate (18363-g)

Propanediol diacetate.
$C_7H_{12}O_4 = 160.2$.
CAS — 623-84-7 (1,2-isomer); 628-66-0 (1,3-isomer).

Profile

Propylene glycol diacetate is an emulsifying and/or solubilising agent, and a solvent. It is included in some external preparations for ear infection.

Preparations

Proprietary Preparations (details are given in Part 3)
Austral.: VoSoL.

Multi-ingredient: *Canad.:* VoSoL; VoSoL HC; *NZ:* VoSoL; *USA:* AA-HC Otic†; Acetasol; Acetasol HC; VoSoL; VoSoL HC.

Propylene Glycol Monopalmitostearate (437-x)

E477 (propylene glycol esters of fatty acids); Propylene Glycol Monostearate; Propylene Glycol Stearate; Propylèneglycol (Stéarate de); Propylenglycoli Monopalmitostearas; Propylenglycoli Monostearas; Prostearin.

CAS — 1323-39-3 (propylene glycol monostearate); 29013-28-3 (propylene glycol monopalmitate).
Pharmacopoeias. In Eur. (see p.vi). Also in USNF.

Propylene glycol monopalmitostearate is obtainable commercially in the pure, non-dispersible form, or in the self-emulsifying form containing a small proportion of soap or other primary emulsifying agent.

Pharmacopoeial description

Ph. Eur.: A mixture of the propylene glycol mono- and di-esters of stearic and palmitic acids. It contains a minimum of 50% of mono-esters produced from the condensation of propylene glycol and stearic acid 50. A white or almost white, waxy solid. M.p. 33° to 40°. Practically insoluble in water; soluble in hot alcohol and in acetone. Protect from light.

USNF 20: A mixture of the propylene glycol mono- and di-esters of stearic and palmitic acids. It contains not less than 90% of mono-esters of saturated fatty acids, chiefly propylene glycol monostearate and propylene glycol monopalmitate. A white, wax-like solid, beads, or flakes, with a slight agreeable fatty odour. Congealing temperature not less than 45°. Insoluble in water but it may be dispersed in hot water with the aid of a small amount of soap or other suitable surfactant; soluble in organic solvents such as alcohol, acetone, ether, benzene, and fixed or mineral oils.

Profile

Propylene glycol monopalmitostearate is used as a stabiliser or emulsifier similarly to glyceryl monostearate or self-emulsifying glyceryl monostearate (p.1345). Propylene glycol monolaurate and mono-oleate have also been used.

Quillaia (469-v)

E999 (quillaia extract); Panama Wood; Quillaia Bark; Quillaiae Cortex; Seifenrinde; Soap Bark.

CAS — 631-01-6 (quillaic acid).
Pharmacopoeias. In Aust., Br., Fr., and Swiss.

It contains 2 amorphous saponin glycosides, quillaic acid and quillaiasapotoxin.

Pharmacopoeial description

BP 2001: The dried inner part of the bark of *Quillaja saponaria* and other species of *Quillaja* containing not less than 22% of alcohol (45%)-soluble extractive. It is odourless or almost odourless, but the dust or powder is strongly sternutatory.

Adverse Effects

Quillaia taken by mouth has been reported to produce gastro-intestinal irritation. It has been suggested that the ingestion of large amounts may produce liver damage, respiratory failure, convulsions, and coma.

Uses

Quillaia is used as an emulsifying agent and frothing agent; it is often used with tragacanth mucilage or another thickening agent. Quillaia is also used for its surfactant properties in preparations for skin and respiratory-tract disorders.

Preparations

BP 2001: Quillaia Liquid Extract; Quillaia Tincture.

Proprietary Preparations (details are given in Part 3)
Multi-ingredient: *Braz.:* Bluderm; *Fin.:* Kvilla; *Fr.:* Coaltar Saponine le Beuf; *Hong Kong:* Pectoral; *Ital.:* Soluzione Composta Alcoolica Saponosa di Coaltar†; *Swed.:* Quilla simplex; *Switz.:* Expectoran Codein.

Sorbitan Esters (13604-y)

A series of mixtures of the partial esters of sorbitol and its mono- and di-anhydrides with fatty acids.

Sorbitan Laurate (478-g)

Sorbitan Laurate (BAN, rINN).
E493; Sorbitan Monolaurate (USAN); Sorbitani Lauras.
$C_{18}H_{34}O_6$ (approximate).
CAS — 1338-39-2.
Pharmacopoeias. In Eur. (see p.vi). Also in USNF.

Pharmacopoeial description

Ph. Eur.: A mixture of the partial esters of sorbitol and its mono- and di-anhydrides with lauric acid. A brownish-yellow viscous liquid. Relative density about 0.98. Practically insoluble but dispersible in water; miscible with alcohol; slightly soluble in cottonseed oil. Protect from light.

USNF 20: A partial ester of sorbitol and its mono- and di-anhydrides with lauric acid. A yellow to amber oily liquid with a bland characteristic odour. Insoluble in water; soluble in liquid paraffin; slightly soluble in cottonseed oil and in ethyl acetate. Store in airtight containers.

Sorbitan Oleate (479-q)

Sorbitan Oleate (BAN, rINN).
E494; NSC-406239; Sorbitan Monooleate (USAN); Sorbitan Mono-oleate; Sorbitani Oleas.
$C_{24}H_{44}O_6$ (approximate).
CAS — 1338-43-8.
Pharmacopoeias. In Eur. (see p.vi). Also in USNF.

Pharmacopoeial description

Ph. Eur.: A mixture usually obtained by esterification of 1 mole of sorbitol and its mono- and di-anhydrides per mole of oleic acid. A suitable antioxidant may be added. A brownish-yellow viscous liquid. Relative density about 0.99. Practically insoluble but dispersible in water; miscible with alcohol; soluble in fatty oils producing a hazy solution. Protect from light.

USNF 20: A partial oleate ester of sorbitol and its mono- and di-anhydrides. A yellow to amber-coloured, viscous, oily liquid with a bland characteristic odour. Insoluble in water and in propylene glycol; miscible with mineral and vegetable oils. Store in airtight containers.

Sorbitan Palmitate (480-d)

Sorbitan Palmitate (BAN, rINN).
E495; Sorbitan Monopalmitate (USAN); Sorbitani Palmitas.
$C_{22}H_{42}O_6$ (approximate).
CAS — 26266-57-9.
Pharmacopoeias. In Eur. (see p.vi). Also in USNF.

Pharmacopoeial description

Ph. Eur.: A mixture of the partial esters of sorbitol and its mono- and di-anhydrides with palmitic acid. A yellowish or yellow powder, waxy flakes, or hard masses. M.p. 44° to 51°. Practically insoluble in water; slightly soluble in alcohol; soluble in fatty oils. Protect from light.

USNF 20: A partial ester of sorbitol and its mono- and di-anhydrides with palmitic acid. A cream-coloured, waxy solid with a faint fatty odour. Insoluble in water; soluble in warm dehydrated alcohol; soluble with haze in warm liquid paraffin and in warm arachis oil.

Sorbitan Sesquioleate (482-h)

Sorbitan Sesquioleate (BAN, USAN, rINN).
Sorbitani Sesquioleas.
$C_{33}H_{60}O_{6.5}$ (approximate).
CAS — 8007-43-0.
Pharmacopoeias. In Eur. (see p.vi) and Jpn. Also in USNF.

Pharmacopoeial description

Ph. Eur.: A mixture usually obtained by esterification of 2 moles of sorbitol and its mono- and di-anhydrides per 3 moles of oleic acid. A suitable antioxidant may be added. A pale yellow or slightly brownish-yellow paste, which becomes a viscous oily, brownish-yellow liquid at about 25°. Dispersible in water; slightly soluble in dehydrated alcohol; soluble in fatty oils. Protect from light.

USNF 20: A partial oleate ester of sorbitol and its mono- and di-anhydrides. A yellow to amber-coloured, oily viscous liquid. Insoluble in water and in propylene glycol; soluble in alcohol, in isopropyl alcohol, in cottonseed oil, and in liquid paraffin. Store in airtight containers.

Sorbitan Stearate (481-n)

Sorbitan Stearate (BAN, rINN).
E491; Sorbitan Monostearate (USAN); Sorbitani Stearas.
$C_{24}H_{46}O_6$ (approximate).
CAS — 1338-41-6.
Pharmacopoeias. In Eur. (see p.vi). Also in USNF.

Pharmacopoeial description

Ph. Eur.: A mixture of the partial esters of sorbitol and its mono- and di-anhydrides with stearic acid. A pale yellow, waxy solid. M.p. 50° to 55°. Practically insoluble but dispersible in water; slightly soluble in alcohol. Protect from light.

USNF 20: A partial ester of sorbitol and its mono- and di-anhydrides with stearic acid. A cream-coloured to tan, hard, waxy solid with a bland odour. Insoluble in cold water and in acetone; dispersible in warm water; soluble, with haze, above 50° in ethyl acetate and in liquid paraffin.

Sorbitan Trioleate   (483-m)

Sorbitan Trioleate (BAN, USAN, rINN).

Sorbitani Trioleas.

$C_{60}H_{108}O_8$ (approximate).

CAS — 26266-58-0.

Pharmacopoeias. In Eur. (see p.vi). Also in USNF.

Pharmacopoeial description

Ph. Eur.: A mixture usually obtained by esterification of 1 mole of sorbitol and its mono- and di-anhydrides per 3 moles of oleic acid. A suitable antioxidant may be added. A pale yellow, light yellowish or brown solid which becomes a brownish-yellow, viscous, oily liquid at 25°. Practically insoluble but dispersible in water; slightly soluble in alcohol; soluble in fatty oils. Protect from light.

USNF 20: A tri-ester of sorbitol and its mono- and di-anhydrides with oleic acid. A yellow to amber-coloured, oily liquid. Insoluble in water, in ethylene glycol, and in propylene glycol; soluble in alcohol, in isopropyl alcohol, in methyl alcohol, in maize oil, in cottonseed oil, and in liquid paraffin. Store in airtight containers.

Sorbitan Tristearate   (484-b)

Sorbitan Tristearate (BAN, USAN, rINN).

E492.

$C_{60}H_{114}O_8$ (approximate).

CAS — 26658-19-5.

A mixture of the partial tri-esters of sorbitol and its mono- and di-anhydrides with stearic acid.

Adverse Effects

There have been occasional reports of hypersensitive skin reactions following the topical application of creams containing sorbitan esters.

◊ References.
1. Finn OA, Forsyth A. Contact dermatitis due to sorbitan monolaurate. *Contact Dermatitis* 1975; **1:** 318.
2. Hannuksela M, *et al.* Allergy to ingredients of vehicles. *Contact Dermatitis* 1976; **2:** 105–10.
3. Austad J. Allergic contact dermatitis to sorbitan monooleate (Span 80). *Contact Dermatitis* 1982; **8:** 426–7.
4. Boyle J, Kennedy CTC. Contact urticaria and dermatitis to Alphaderm. *Contact Dermatitis* 1984; **10:** 178.

Uses

Sorbitan esters are lipophilic nonionic surfactants which are used as emulsifying agents in the preparation of emulsions, creams, and ointments for pharmaceutical and cosmetic use. When used alone they produce stable water-in-oil emulsions but they are frequently used in combination with a polysorbate in varying proportions to produce water-in-oil or oil-in-water emulsions or creams with a variety of different textures and consistencies. Sorbitan esters are also used as emulsifiers and stabilisers in food.

Sucrose Esters   (485-v)

E473 (sucrose esters of fatty acids).

Esterification of 1 or more hydroxyl groups in sucrose with a fatty acid such as stearic or palmitic acid produces nonionic compounds which possess surface-active properties. Commercial sucrose esters are mixtures of the mono-, di-, and tri-esters of palmitic and stearic acids with sucrose; various grades are available.

Profile

The sucrose esters are used as dispersing and emulsifying agents in food and cosmetic preparations.

Tyloxapol   (461-x)

Tyloxapol (BAN, USAN, rINN).

Superinone.

CAS — 25301-02-4.

ATC — R05CA01.

Pharmacopoeias. In US.

Pharmacopoeial description

USP 25: A polymer of 4-(1,1,3,3-tetramethylbutyl)phenol with ethylene oxide and formaldehyde. A viscous amber liquid, sometimes slightly turbid, with a slight aromatic odour. Slowly but freely miscible with water; soluble in chloroform, in glacial acetic acid, in carbon disulfide, in carbon tetrachloride, in toluene, and in benzene. A 5% solution has a pH of 4.0 to 7.0. Tyloxapol should not be allowed to come into contact with metals. Store in airtight containers.

Adverse Effects

Slight inflammation of the eyelids has been reported after prolonged use of aqueous inhalations. It has been reported that occasional febrile reactions may occur.

Uses and Administration

Tyloxapol is a nonionic surfactant of the alkyl aryl polyether alcohol type. Solutions have been used as an aqueous inhalation as a mucolytic for tenacious bronchopulmonary secretions. It is also employed in solutions used to cleanse contact lenses. It has also been used as a vehicle for aerosol medication and for antibacterials administered in irrigation solutions for pyogenic bone or joint infections.

Preparations

Proprietary Preparations (details are given in Part 3)
Aust.: Tacholiquin; **Canad.:** Enuclene; **Fr.:** Translight†; **Ger.:** Enuclen N; Tacholiquin; **NZ:** Enuclene; **Spain:** Lacermucin; **USA:** Enuclene.

Multi-ingredient: **Ger.:** Complete†; **Israel:** Complete All-In-One.

The symbol † denotes a preparation no longer actively marketed

Nutritional Agents and Vitamins

The principal constituents of food are carbohydrates, fats, minerals, proteins, vitamins, indigestible fibre, and water. Energy is provided by the metabolism of carbohydrates, fats, surplus protein, and alcohol.

Carbohydrates found in foods may be classified according to their degree of polymerisation into three main groups, namely sugars, oligosaccharides, and polysaccharides; all of these are made up only of carbon, hydrogen, and oxygen. Sugars can be further subdivided into *monosaccharides* (single-molecule sugars), such as fructose and glucose, *disaccharides* (whose molecules consist of two monosaccharides joined together), such as lactose and sucrose, and *sugar alcohols* (polyols) such as sorbitol and mannitol. *Oligosaccharides* typically consist of 3 to 9 monosaccharides joined together, and include malto-oligosaccharides such as maltodextrins. *Polysaccharides* consist of many monosaccharides joined together and include starches and non-starch polysaccharides such as cellulose. Non-starch polysaccharides are the major fraction of dietary fibre, and many authorities now consider this term is preferable to dietary fibre.

Fats have the same elemental composition as carbohydrates, but with a lower proportion of oxygen. Dietary fat is usually in the form of triglycerides, esters of glycerol with three fatty acid molecules. Essential fatty acids are ones which cannot be made in the body and which must be supplied by the food.

Proteins are made up of carbon, hydrogen, oxygen, and nitrogen; most proteins also contain sulfur and some contain phosphorus. They are required for the regulation of body processes such as growth and tissue maintenance, and excess protein can be converted into carbohydrate and used to provide energy.

Proteins consist of chains of **amino acids** of which there are *essential* and *non-essential* types. Essential amino acids (indispensable amino acids) cannot be synthesised in sufficient amounts in the body and must therefore be present in food; non-essential amino acids can be synthesised in the body. There are eight essential amino acids: isoleucine, leucine, lysine, methionine, phenylalanine, threonine, tryptophan, and valine. Arginine and histidine are also essential for infant growth while synthesis of cysteine, taurine, and tyrosine may be inadequate in premature infants.

Several inorganic elements, or minerals, are essential dietary constituents; those which are required in relatively small amounts are known as **trace elements** (see below). Their main function is to act as essential cofactors in various enzyme systems.

Vitamins and their general role in health are described below.

Dietary Modification

Infants, children, elderly people, and pregnant or lactating women have particular nutritional requirements, but in most cases, provided that they are in good general health, adjustment to intake is all that is required rather than extensive modification or supplementation.

Dietary modification is important in the management of a variety of disorders. Calorie restriction is fundamental to the management of obesity, although it may be difficult to motivate patients to accept long-term changes to their eating habits, and some fashionable diets are at best of little value.

The role of diet in the aetiology of cardiovascular disorders (such as salt intake in hypertension and fat intake in ischaemic heart disease) is recognised to be of importance and has lead to public health campaigns for healthier eating patterns.

Dietary modification is also an accepted part of the management of diabetes mellitus, while protein restriction is important in the management of uraemia or hepatic encephalopathy.

There are also various metabolic disorders such as phenylketonuria, or forms of intolerance to dietary components, such as coeliac disease, in which the diet must be modified to exclude or drastically reduce certain food components.

Amino acid metabolic disorders. Various inborn errors of amino-acid metabolism are known. They are not common but their consequences are often serious or fatal. Although in some cases there is no effective treatment, early diagnosis is important as some conditions can be managed by dietary modification and/or the use of vitamins. Two of the better known syndromes, homocystinuria and phenylketonuria, are discussed briefly below. Cystinosis, another disorder of amino acid metabolism, is discussed on p.1633. Urea cycle disorders are discussed under Hyperammonaemia on p.1354.

Homocystinuria. Homocystinuria in its classical form is an autosomal recessive disorder due to a genetic deficiency of the enzyme cystathionine synthetase, resulting in accumulation of homocysteine (oxidised extracellularly to homocystine).[1] Manifestations may include mental retardation, atherosclerosis, thromboembolism, osteoporosis, and ocular symptoms including lens dislocation, glaucoma, cataract, and retinal detachment. Dietary restriction of methionine together with cystine supplements has been used for treatment; some patients may respond to treatment with B vitamins (pyridoxine, cobalamins, and folic acid),[1,2] or to betaine.[3-6]

Phenylketonuria. Phenylketonuria is an autosomal recessive disorder which is usually due to a defect in the enzyme phenylalanine hydroxylase. This results in raised blood concentrations of phenylalanine in the neonate, and if untreated produces a syndrome of skin rash, depigmentation, hypertonia, seizures, and severe mental retardation. The disease is controlled by use of a synthetic diet very low in phenylalanine,[7-11] and if started early this can permit relatively normal intellectual development. High-dose tyrosine does not appear to be an effective alternative to a diet low in phenylalanine.[12,13]

1. Isherwood DM. Homocystinuria. *BMJ* 1996; **313**: 1025–6.
2. Schuh S, *et al.* Homocystinuria and megaloblastic anemia responsive to vitamin B₁₂ therapy. *N Engl J Med* 1984; **310**: 686–90.
3. Smolin LA, *et al.* The use of betaine for the treatment of homocystinuria. *J Pediatr* 1981; **99**: 467–72.
4. Wilcken DEL, *et al.* Homocystinuria—the effects of betaine in the treatment of patients not responsive to pyridoxine. *N Engl J Med* 1983; **309**: 448–53.
5. Holme E, *et al.* Betaine for treatment of homocystinuria caused by methylenetetrahydrofolate reductase deficiency. *Arch Dis Child* 1989; **64**: 1061–4.
6. Anonymous. Betaine for homocystinuria. *Med Lett Drugs Ther* 1997; **39**: 12.
7. Rylance G. Outcome of early detected and early treated phenylketonuria patients. *Postgrad Med J* 1989; **65** (suppl 2): S7–9.
8. Link R. Phenylketonuria diet in adolescents— energy and nutrient intake—is it adequate? *Postgrad Med J* 1989; **65** (suppl 2): S21–4.
9. American Academy of Pediatrics Committee on Genetics. Maternal phenylketonuria. *Pediatrics* 1991; **88**: 1284–5.
10. Thompson GN, *et al.* Pregnancy in phenylketonuria: dietary treatment aimed at normalising maternal plasma phenylalanine concentration. *Arch Dis Child* 1991; **66**: 1346–9.
11. Medical Research Council. Report of the Medical Research Council Working Party on Phenylketonuria. Recommendations on the dietary management of phenylketonuria. *Arch Dis Child* 1993; **68**: 426–7.
12. Pietz J, *et al.* Effect of high-dose tyrosine supplementation on brain function in adults with phenylketonuria. *J Pediatr* 1995; **127**: 936–43.
13. Smith ML, *et al.* Randomised controlled trial of tyrosine supplementation on neuropsychological performance in phenylketonuria. *Arch Dis Child* 1998; **78**: 116–21.

Cardiovascular disease. Modification of the diet may be helpful in patients with, or at risk of, cardiovascular disease. In patients with hypertension (p.802), reduction in salt intake may be tried before commencing drug therapy or used as an adjunct to such therapy. Reduction in the total intake of dietary fat, and in particular of saturated fatty acids, is considered important for both the general population and those considered at high risk of ischaemic heart disease. An increased intake of long chain n-3 polyunsaturated fatty acids has been recommended and also a restriction on *trans* fatty acids. Dietary cholesterol should be restricted although it may make less of a contribution to plasma cholesterol levels than dietary saturates.[1] For a discussion on the control of blood lipid levels to modify the risk of ischaemic heart disease, see Cardiovascular Risk Reduction, p.797.

For discussion of the possibility that antioxidant vitamins may reduce the risk of ischaemic heart disease see under Vitamins, below. The link between folic acid, homocysteine, and ischaemic heart disease is discussed on p.1362.

1. DoH. Nutritional aspects of cardiovascular disease. *Report on health and social subjects 46.* London: HMSO, 1994. [COMA report.]

Coeliac disease. Coeliac disease (gluten-sensitive enteropathy) is an inflammatory disorder of the small intestine that results from an immunological reaction to the gliadin fraction of gluten (p.1616). The inflammation leads to mucosal atrophy with subsequent malabsorption, although the extent and severity of mucosal inflammation varies widely, and some patients are asymptomatic. In adults, anaemia and mild gastrointestinal symptoms that may be confused with irritable bowel syndrome are the usual symptoms. In infants and children there may be growth retardation or failure to thrive, and gastrointestinal symptoms may be more marked. Other nutritional deficiencies, including calcium malabsorption leading to osteopenia, may also occur, and mouth ulcers are also common.

Treatment of coeliac disease involves a strict, life-long, gluten-free diet. Nutritional supplements may be necessary at the start of treatment but can usually be stopped once mucosal recovery has occurred. Diagnosis is confirmed by normalisation of the mucosa on repeat biopsy after 3 to 4 months. Dermatitis herpetiformis (p.1104) is a non-gastrointestinal manifestation of coeliac disease. Patients may have no gastrointestinal symptoms, although mucosal abnormalities are generally apparent on biopsy. These patients also respond to a gluten-free diet.

Coeliac disease is associated with a number of auto-immune diseases, including type 1 diabetes, thyroid disease, and IgA deficiency. Patients with coeliac disease have an increased incidence of small-bowel lymphoma and a slight increase in the incidence of some other gastrointestinal cancers. There is some evidence that this incidence is reduced in patients maintaining a strict diet.

Reviews.
1. Duggan JM. Recent developments in our understanding of adult coeliac disease. *Med J Aust* 1997; **166**: 312–15.
2. Ferguson A. Coeliac disease. *Prescriber's J* 1997; **37**: 206–12.
3. Mäki M, Collin P. Coeliac disease. *Lancet* 1997; **349**: 1755–9.
4. Barr GD, Grehan MJ. Coeliac disease. *Med J Aust* 1998; **169**: 109–14.
5. Branski D, Troncone R. Celiac disease: a reappraisal. *J Pediatr* 1998; **133**: 181–7.
6. Feighery C. Coeliac disease. *BMJ* 1999; **319**: 236–9.

Diabetes mellitus. Dietary control is important in both type 1 and type 2 diabetes mellitus (p.315); in the latter condition such control, combined possibly with increased exercise, may be all that is required to correct the condition. In addition to reduction in the intake of sugar, and an increase in fibre intake (which may also lower blood sugar concentrations), the correction of obesity removes one of the factors associated with insulin resistance.

Fish odour syndrome. Fish odour syndrome (trimethylaminuria) is an inherited metabolic disorder in which there is impaired hepatic N-oxidation of trimethylamine. Trimethylamine is formed in the intestine by bacterial degradation of foods rich in choline and carnitine, and is readily absorbed from the gut. If not oxidised in the liver, it is excreted in the breath, urine, sweat, and vaginal secretions. It smells of rotting fish, and has a high olfactory potency. Treatment involves dietary modification to avoid choline-rich foods such as eggs, liver, peas, soya beans, and sea fish. Short-term treatments to reduce the intestinal flora, and thereby decrease the production of trimethylamine, are occasionally used; examples include metronidazole, neomycin, and lactulose.

References.
1. Pike MG, *et al.* Lactulose in trimethylaminuria, the fish-odour syndrome. *Helv Paediat Acta* 1988; **43**: 345–8.
2. Rehman HU. Fish odour syndrome. *Postgrad Med J* 1999; **75**: 451–2.

Hepatic encephalopathy. Restriction of dietary protein intake is a mainstay of the treatment of hepatic encephalopathy, but care is required to avoid malnutrition (see p.1205).

Inflammatory bowel disease. In inflammatory bowel diseases (p.1205) dietary modification or supplementation may often be necessary to maintain the nutritional status of the patient. Such supplementation may be oral, nasogastric, or parenteral.

Enteral feeding, particularly with elemental diets has been shown to be effective in the treatment of active Crohn's disease,[1] but is probably less effective than corticosteroids.[2-4] The terminology surrounding the use of these diets has been elucidated.[5] The term elemental diet was originally coined to describe diets containing free amino acids and glucose and was often prefixed by the phrase 'chemically defined'. However, it came to embrace diets whose nitrogen sources included peptides and were often also called predigested diets. It was suggested[5] that the term elemental diet could be used for either type but that for those with an amino acid nitrogen source the term chemically defined elemental diet should be used whereas for those with a peptide nitrogen source predigested elemental diet was suitable. The term polymeric diet should be used for those diets with a whole protein nitrogen source.

1. Teahon K, *et al.* Ten years' experience with an elemental diet in the management of Crohn's disease. *Gut* 1990; **31**: 1133–7.
2. Griffiths AM, *et al.* Meta-analysis of enteral nutrition as a primary treatment of active Crohn's disease. *Gastroenterology* 1995; **108**: 1056–67.
3. Messori A, *et al.* Defined-formula diets versus steroids in the treatment of active Crohn's disease: a meta-analysis. *Scand J Gastroenterol* 1996; **31**: 267–72.

4. Zachos M, *et al.* Enteral nutritional therapy for inducing remission of Crohn's disease (updated 25 May 2001). Available in The Cochrane Library; Issue 3. Oxford: Update Software; 2001.
5. Payne-James JJ, Silk DBA. Use of elemental diets in the treatment of Crohn's disease by gastroenterologists. *Gut* 1990; **31:** 1424.

Malignant neoplasms. For a discussion of the possible link between an increased intake of antioxidant vitamins and a reduced risk of developing malignancies, see under Vitamins, below.

Obesity. Obesity is relatively common in the developed world, and is accompanied by an increased risk of cardiovascular disease, diabetes, and other disorders. Methods such as dietary modification, behaviour therapy, and exercise with adjunctive drug therapy, where indicated (see p.1505) can produce weight loss, but the essence of treatment is a reduction in calorific intake, usually by about 300 to 500 kcal per day in patients with a body-mass index (BMI) of 27 to 35, and 500 to 1000 kcal in those with a BMI greater than 35. This would be expected to produce a weight loss of about 0.25 to 1 kg per week. Very low calorie diets (less than 600 to 800 kcal per day) should only be considered after the failure of determined attempts to lose weight by conventional calorie restriction. For weight loss to be achieved and sustained, eating behaviour must be permanently modified, which may pose difficulties. The proportion of calories from fat in particular, and also alcohol and sugars should be reduced and those from high carbohydrate foods increased. It is obviously important to maintain an adequate intake of essential nutrients.

Artificial sweeteners or other non-sucrose sweeteners are often used as part of weight-reducing diets.

Renal failure. A resurgence of interest in possible interventions that may be of value in preventing or slowing the progression of chronic renal failure (p.1185) has led again to evaluation of low-protein diets. Patients with renal failure who adopt a protein-restricted diet have fewer symptoms of uraemia than those on a normal diet.[1] Some results have also suggested that protein restriction can slow the progression of renal failure,[2] but the value of low-protein diets in delaying the onset of end-stage renal disease has been the subject of much controversy. Two large multicentre studies provided little evidence of a substantial benefit,[3,4] but meta-analyses have consistently provided support for dietary protein restriction.[5,6] It has been suggested that the benefit of other interventions such as the use of ACE inhibitors,[7] as well as the difficulties in obtaining patient compliance with such a restrictive diet,[8] may have limited the benefits to be obtained from protein restriction, but there is also evidence that response and outcome vary depending on the cause of renal failure.[4,9]

1. Klahr S. Chronic renal failure: management. *Lancet* 1991; **338:** 423–7.
2. Mallick NP. Dietary protein and progression of chronic renal disease. *BMJ* 1994; **309:** 1101–2.
3. Locatelli F, *et al.* Prospective, randomised, multicentre trial of effect of protein restriction on progression of chronic renal insufficiency. *Lancet* 1991; **337:** 1299–1304.
4. Klahr S, *et al.* The effects of dietary protein restriction and blood-pressure control on the progression of chronic renal disease. *N Engl J Med* 1994; **330:** 877–84.
5. Fouque D, *et al.* Controlled low protein diets in chronic renal insufficiency: meta-analysis. *BMJ* 1992; **304:** 216–20.
6. Pedrini MT, *et al.* The effect of dietary protein restriction on the progression of diabetic and nondiabetic renal diseases: a meta-analysis. *Ann Intern Med* 1996; **124:** 627–32.
7. Shiigai T, *et al.* Dietary protein restriction and blood-pressure control in chronic renal insufficiency. *N Engl J Med* 1994; **331:** 405.
8. Barsotti G, Giovannetti S. Low-protein diet and chronic renal failure. *Lancet* 1991; **338:** 442.
9. Locatelli F, *et al.* Low-protein diet and chronic renal failure. *Lancet* 1991; **338:** 442–3.

Enteral and Parenteral Nutrition

Malnutrition of varying degrees is not uncommon in hospitalised patients, and some form of nutritional support is important in patients who cannot eat an adequate normal diet. Such support should provide for the patient's requirements for energy, in the form of carbohydrate and fat, nitrogen as amino acids or protein, water and electrolytes; where appropriate, vitamins and trace elements should also be supplied. The decision to initiate nutritional support depends on the patient's clinical condition: indications may include unconsciousness, obstruction or inability to swallow, inflammatory bowel disease, fistula, short bowel syndrome, and weakness and malnutrition associated with trauma, surgery, or malignant disease. If possible, nutritional support should be by the enteral route; it is easier, more physiological, and less prone to complications than the parenteral route.

Enteral nutrition includes feeding by mouth, by nasogastric or nasoenteric tube, or directly into a gastrostomy or other enterostomy. It may be supplemental, if normal food intake is possible but inadequate, or total. Individual patients vary in their requirements according to age, size, and metabolic state, but a diet supplying 2000 to 3000 kcal of energy and 10 to 15 g of nitrogen (as 60 to 90 g of protein) in 2 to 3 litres of fluid is fairly typical; because absorption from the gastrointestinal tract is incomplete requirements are higher than by the parenteral route. Preparations containing whole protein (often derived from milk or soya) are generally preferred; elemental diets, in which nitrogen is supplied as amino acids or oligopeptides, are less well tolerated and less palatable, although they may have a role in impaired digestion or when a zero-residue diet is desired.

Although preferred to parenteral nutrition, enteral feeding is not without complications. Patients may be at risk of oesophagitis, aspiration, and regurgitation as a result of the tube insertion; other potential problems include diarrhoea, nausea and vomiting, gastric retention, hyperglycaemia, fluid and electrolyte disturbances, and microbial contamination of the feed regimen.

Parenteral nutrition is reserved for situations in which it is impossible to meet nutritional requirements by the enteral route. Like enteral nutrition it may be given supplementally or as the sole source of body requirements (total parenteral nutrition or TPN). The normal route of administration is via a dedicated central venous catheter. However, peripheral administration is increasingly used for short-term feeding. This reduces some complications and insertion is less complex, but because of the risk of thrombophlebitis feeds used should have low osmolality and neutral pH. Other measures to delay the development of peripheral thrombophlebitis are mentioned under Adverse Effects and Precautions, below.

The formulation of the nutritional solution must be adjusted according to the patient's requirements. The solution should supply sufficient energy to allow for the resting energy expenditure (around 25 kcal per kg body-weight in the average adult) but must also take into account any increased energy expenditure of illness. Conversely, starvation can reduce resting metabolism and energy requirements. Various formulae exist for the calculation of energy expenditure in patients. Energy is best supplied in the form of carbohydrate (at least 30%, and preferably 60% of energy requirements should be in this form) and fat. Glucose is the optimal carbohydrate energy source, while fat is supplied as a lipid emulsion, often of soya oil. Nitrogen is supplied as amino acids, but to ensure that these are used for protein synthesis rather than as sources of energy it is important to control the ratio of non-protein energy to nitrogen in the solution. A ratio of 150 to 200 kcal per g of nitrogen is usually considered optimal but in hypercatabolic patients (e.g. in sepsis) lower ratios of 120 kcal per g or less may be appropriate. All essential amino acids are supplied although there is some variation between solutions as to which non-essential amino acids are present.

Parenteral nutrition must also supply the patient's requirements for fluid, essential electrolytes such as sodium, potassium, magnesium, bicarbonate, and calcium (as well as phosphate, since glucose infusion may provoke hypophosphataemia), and, particularly if treatment is prolonged, vitamins and trace elements. If glucose loading produces signs of hyperglycaemia insulin may be added to correct it.

The major complication of parenteral nutrition is bacterial colonisation of the catheter, which can lead to septicaemia. Other problems may include venous thrombosis or air embolism, extravasation due to misplacement of the catheter tip, and metabolic disturbances. Adverse effects of overfeeding include respiratory and hepatic dysfunction. Complications of long-term total parenteral nutrition include gallbladder sludging, gallstones, cholestasis, and abnormal liver function tests.

Stability and compatibility. The complex nature of solutions for parenteral nutrition renders them susceptible to compatibility problems.[1-12] Stability is dependent upon several factors including pH and relative concentrations of the components. Amino acids exert a buffering effect on the overall pH of mixed solutions containing amino acids, glucose, and fat emulsions but amino acids with glucose undergo the Maillard reaction (browning) and the life of combined solutions is therefore limited. Solutions containing electrolytes, particularly divalent cations, are not stable, and aggregation will eventually occur. Additives should be added only if there is known compatibility, and any additions performed aseptically before the start of the infusion. In general mixed parenteral nutrition solutions should be used immediately after preparation and administered to the patient within 24 hours.

1. Allwood MC. Compatibility and stability of TPN mixtures in big bags. *J Clin Hosp Pharm* 1984; **9:** 181–98.
2. Niemiec PW, Vanderveen TW. Compatibility considerations in parenteral nutrient solutions. *Am J Hosp Pharm* 1984; **41:** 893–911.
3. Parry VA, *et al.* Effect of various nutrient ratios on the emulsion stability of total nutrient admixtures. *Am J Hosp Pharm* 1986; **43:** 3017–22.
4. Hardy G. Ten years of TPN with 3 litre bags. *Pharm J* 1987; **239:** HS26–HS28.
5. Johnson OL, *et al.* The destabilization of parenteral feeding emulsions by heparin. *Int J Pharmaceutics* 1989; **53:** 237–40.
6. Takagi J, *et al.* Sterility of total parenteral nutrient solutions stored at room temperature for seven days. *Am J Hosp Pharm* 1989; **46:** 973–7.
7. Tripp MG, *et al.* Stability of total nutrient admixtures in a dual-chamber flexible container. *Am J Hosp Pharm* 1990; **47:** 2496–503.
8. Vaughan LM, *et al.* Incompatibility of iron dextran and a total nutrient admixture. *Am J Hosp Pharm* 1990; **47:** 1745–6.
9. Washington C. The stability of intravenous fat emulsions in total parenteral nutrition mixtures. *Int J Pharmaceutics* 1990; **66:** 1–21.
10. Manning RJ, Washington C. Chemical stability of total parenteral nutrition mixtures. *Int J Pharmaceutics* 1992; **81:** 1–20.
11. Neuzil J, *et al.* Oxidation of parenteral lipid emulsion by ambient and phototherapy lights: potential toxicity of routine parenteral feeding. *J Pediatr* 1995; **126:** 785–90.
12. Trissel LA, *et al.* Compatibility of parenteral nutrient solutions with selected drugs during simulated Y-site administration. *Am J Health-Syst Pharm* 1997; **54:** 1295–1300.

Adverse effects and precautions. ENTERAL NUTRITION. Reviewing the complications of enteral nutrition it was noted[1] that many of the problems encountered could be avoided by using a fine bore tube, administering the feed by continuous infusion, and by careful monitoring of the patient for metabolic abnormalities.

Complexation of the nutrients with aluminium-containing antacids, also given via the tube, may occur and this deposition of solid masses may cause oesophageal obstruction.[2]

Diarrhoea in patients receiving enteral nutrition may not necessarily be caused by the tube feeding itself;[3,4] concomitant drug therapy can often be implicated. However, enteral feeding has been shown to be associated with increased colonic secretion, which can be reversed by infusion of short-chain fatty acids.[5]

1. Bastow MD. Complications of enteral nutrition. *Gut* 1986; **21** (suppl 1): 51–5.
2. Valli C, *et al.* Interaction of nutrients with antacids: a complication during enteral tube feeding. *Lancet* 1986; **i:** 747–8.
3. Edes TE, *et al.* Diarrhea in tube-fed patients: feeding formula not necessarily the cause. *Am J Med* 1990; **88:** 91–3.
4. Heimburger DC. Diarrhea with enteral feeding: will the real cause please stand up? *Am J Med* 1990; **88:** 89–90.
5. Bowling TE, *et al.* Reversal by short-chain fatty acids of colonic fluid secretion induced by enteral feeding. *Lancet* 1993; **342:** 1266–8.

PARENTERAL NUTRITION. A common complication of parenteral nutrition is infection of the intravenous feeding catheter site which can lead to septicaemia. Infection and colonisation of central venous catheters may be reduced if the catheter is tunnelled through subcutaneous tissue before emerging through the skin.[1] Strict aseptic techniques should be used for changing the dressing or bags containing the nutrient fluids.

Thrombophlebitis can occur following the use of either peripheral or central veins. Although it has been suggested that infusion of hyperosmolar solutions via a central line is less likely to produce thrombophlebitis, because the feed is immediately diluted by a large volume of blood, major thrombotic complications such as pulmonary embolism and right atrial thrombosis could be more common than hitherto recognised in children and adolescents receiving long term parenteral nutrition via central catheters.[2,3] The use of a fine-bore silicone catheter peripherally may avoid the need for central vein cannulation[4] and there is a lower incidence of thrombophlebitis when fine-bore silicone catheters rather than teflon ones are used for peripheral administration of parenteral nutrition.[5] The addition of heparin to the feed, and the use of local hydrocortisone and glyceryl trinitrate, has also been reported to prolong the survival of peripheral infusion sites.[6] Extravasation may also be a problem, particularly with hyperosmolar solutions, and has led to severe tissue damage; hyaluronidase or thiomucase may be used in the treatment of such extravasation.[7]

Parenteral nutrition may be associated with atrophic changes in the mucosal structure and enzymic activity of the intestine, leading to increased permeability with a possible increased risk of bacteraemia and endotoxaemia. These changes, which have been attributed to lack of glutamine (which is unstable in solution), can reportedly be prevented by addition of glutamine-releasing dipeptides to solutions for total parenteral nutrition—see p.1365.

1. de Cicco M, *et al.* Source and route of microbial colonisation of parenteral nutrition catheters. *Lancet* 1989; **ii:** 1258–61.

2. Dollery CM, et al. Thrombosis and embolism in long-term central venous access for parenteral nutrition. *Lancet* 1994; **344:** 1043–5.
3. Dollery CM. Pulmonary embolism in parenteral nutrition. *Arch Dis Child* 1996; **74:** 95–8.
4. Kohlhardt SR, Smith RC. Fine bore silicone catheters for peripheral intravenous nutrition in adults. *BMJ* 1989; **299:** 1380–1.
5. Madan M, et al. Influence of catheter type on occurrence of thrombophlebitis during peripheral intravenous nutrition. *Lancet* 1992; **339:** 101–103.
6. Moclair AE, et al. Total parenteral nutrition via a peripheral vein: a comparison of heparinised and non-heparinised regimens. *Int J Pharm Pract* 1991; **1:** 38–40.
7. Gil M-E, Mateu J. Treatment of extravasation from parenteral nutrition solution. *Ann Pharmacother* 1998; **32:** 51–5.

Uses. Parenteral and enteral nutrition now have an established place either for supplemental use or for providing total nutritional requirements in many conditions. General reviews as well as those pertaining to special groups of patients or disorders have been published.[1-11]

1. Driscoll DF, Blackburn GL. Total parenteral nutrition 1990: a review of its current status in hospitalised patients, and the need for patient-specific feeding. *Drugs* 1990; **40:** 346–63.
2. Pennington C. Parenteral nutrition at home. *Prescribers' J* 1990; **30:** 271–8.
3. The Veterans Affairs Total Parenteral Nutrition Cooperative Study Group. Perioperative total parenteral nutrition in surgical patients. *N Engl J Med* 1991; **325:** 525–32.
4. Matuchansky C, et al. Cyclical parenteral nutrition. *Lancet* 1992; **340:** 588–92.
5. ASPEN Board of Directors. Guidelines for the use of parenteral and enteral nutrition in adult and pediatric patients. *J Parenter Enteral Nutr* 1993; **17** (suppl): 1SA–52SA.
6. Elia M. Changing concepts of nutrient requirements in disease: implications for artificial nutritional support. *Lancet* 1995; **345:** 1279–84.
7. Mattox TW, et al. Recent advances: parenteral nutrition support. *Ann Pharmacother* 1995; **29:** 174–80.
8. American Gastroenterological Association. Guidelines for the use of enteral nutrition. *Gastroenterology* 1995; **108:** 1280.
9. Souba WW. Nutritional support. *N Engl J Med* 1997; **336:** 41–8.
10. Cerra FB, et al. Applied nutrition in ICU patients: a consensus statement of the American College of Chest Physicians. *Chest* 1997; **111:** 769–78.
11. Heyland DK, et al. Total parenteral nutrition in the critically ill patient: a meta-analysis. *JAMA* 1998; **280:** 2013–19.

Trace Elements

Trace elements are inorganic substances found in small amounts in the tissues and required for various metabolic processes; together with the vitamins (see below) they are sometimes referred to as micronutrients. The elements considered essential are chromium, copper, fluorine, iodine, iron, manganese, molybdenum, selenium, and zinc. Iron, in the form of haem, plays an essential role in oxygen transport while iodine is required by the thyroid for the formation of thyroid hormones; most of the other essential trace elements are cofactors for various enzymes. Boron, nickel, silicon, and vanadium may also be essential, and it has been suggested on the basis of *animal* studies that there might be a requirement for tin.

Well-defined deficiency syndromes exist for copper, iodine, iron, selenium, and zinc; although deficiency of other trace elements is possible, their deficiency syndromes are not well defined because of their ubiquity in the diet. Guidance concerning the intake of various trace elements has been published—see also Human Requirements under Vitamins, below.

◊ References.
1. WHO. *Trace elements in human nutrition and health.* Geneva: WHO, 1996.

Vitamins

Vitamins are organic substances required by the body in small amounts for various metabolic processes. Most are not synthesised in the body, or are synthesised in small or insufficient quantities. Vitamins are sometimes classified as fat soluble or water soluble. Substances in the vitamin A, D, E, and K groups are generally fat soluble, and biotin, folic acid, niacin, pantothenic acid, vitamins B_1, B_2, B_6, and B_{12}, and vitamin C substances are generally water soluble.

Vitamin deficiency may result from an inadequate diet, perhaps due to increased requirements such as during pregnancy, or may be induced by disease or drugs. Vitamins may be used clinically for the prevention and treatment of specific vitamin deficiency states and details of these uses are provided under the individual drug monographs.

Large doses of vitamins (megavitamin therapy) have been proposed for a variety of disorders, but adequate evidence of their value is lacking. Excessive intakes of most water-soluble vitamins have little effect due to their rapid excretion in urine, but excessive intakes of fat-soluble vitamins accumulate in the body and are potentially dangerous.

Stability. Water-soluble vitamins are liable to degrade in solution especially if exposed to light. Addition of vitamin mixtures to infusion solutions for parenteral nutrition should therefore be carried out as soon as possible before infusion. Solutions should be used within 24 hours of preparation and be protected from light.

Human requirements. Vitamins and trace elements are essential nutrients and in many countries guidance has been published concerning their intake.

In the UK various terms are used to define intake:[1]

- estimated average requirement (EAR) is used for the requirements of energy, proteins, vitamins, or minerals of a group of people and usually about half will need more and half less than the specified figure
- lower reference nutrient intake (LRNI) is applied to proteins, vitamins, or minerals and is that amount that is enough for only a few people who have low needs
- reference nutrient intake (RNI) is also applied to proteins, vitamins, or minerals and is an amount that is enough, or more than enough, for about 97% of people in a group
- a safe intake is used to indicate an intake or range of intakes where there is not enough information to estimate EAR, LRNI, or RNI, but where it is an amount enough for almost everyone but is not so large as to cause undesirable effects
- dietary reference value (DRV) is used to cover EAR, LRNI, RNI, and safe intake.

It is emphasised in the report that these intakes are not meant to be recommendations for any individual or group; they do not reflect either a recommendation that such an amount should be taken daily in the diet or as a supplement. They are intended rather as yardsticks for the assessment of dietary surveys and food supply statistics; to provide guidance on appropriate dietary composition and meal provision; or for food labelling purposes in which case it is envisaged that an EAR will be used.

In the USA the National Academy of Sciences has traditionally set recommended dietary allowances (RDAs),[2] defined as the levels of intake of essential nutrients that, on the basis of scientific knowledge, are judged to be adequate to meet the known nutrient needs of practically all healthy persons. The allowances are amounts that are intended to be consumed as part of a normal diet. However, new dietary reference intakes (DRIs) are being developed,[3] which will include 3 reference values in addition to the traditional RDA as follows:

- the estimated average requirement is the intake that meets the needs of half the individuals in a group
- the adequate intake is the mean intake level that appears to sustain a desired marker of health, and will be set when there is insufficient evidence to establish an RDA
- the tolerable upper intake level is the maximum intake that is not likely to adversely affect health.

Information pertaining to the requirements of specific vitamins and minerals is provided under the individual monographs.

1. DoH. Dietary reference values for food energy and nutrients for the United Kingdom: report of the panel on dietary reference values of the committee on medical aspects of food policy. *Report on health and social subjects 41.* London: HMSO, 1991.
2. Subcommittee on the tenth edition of the RDAs, Food and Nutrition Board, Commission on Life Sciences, National Research Council. *Recommended dietary allowances.* 10th ed. Washington, DC: National Academy Press, 1989.
3. Standing Committee on the Scientific Evaluation of Dietary Reference Intakes of the Food and Nutrition Board. *Dietary Reference Intakes: applications in dietary assessment.* Washington DC: National Academy Press, 2001.

Supplementation. An adequate dietary intake of vitamins is necessary for good health but whether vitamin supplementation in the absence of any demonstrable deficiency is beneficial or even worthwhile remains debatable.

It is generally considered that healthy persons eating a normal balanced diet should have no need for vitamin supplementation. A review of the topic[1] pointed out that the vitamins that people chose for self medication are often not the ones that are actually present in inadequate amounts in their diets and that the commercial preparations available often do not make it clear whether the amounts they contain are near the physiological requirements or many times greater. Supplementation should concentrate on groups of people at risk of deficiency such as neonates, who need vitamin K; pregnant and lactating women, who need calcium, folic acid, and iron; and certain groups who need vitamin D; vegans and their infants may require vitamin B_{12} supplements. A multivitamin supplement might be considered for some groups such as the elderly and those with reduced calorie intake. However, one might have difficulty in finding a good multivitamin preparation containing all 13 vitamins but no non-vitamins. Also with many of the multivitamin preparations the doses and ratios varied inexplicably.

A review[2] of supplementation specifically in children concluded that, provided schoolchildren and adolescents eat a wide variety of foods, there was no need for vitamin supplementation. However, it was recommended that supplementation with vitamins A, C, and D should be given to those between the ages of 6 months and 2 years and preferably up to the age of 5 years.

A subsequent study[3] supports the suggestion that supplementation may be of some benefit in the elderly. Supplementation with modest, physiological doses of vitamins and trace elements resulted in an improvement in immune response and a decreased frequency of infection in elderly subjects. It was suggested that dosage might be crucial and that excessive doses of micronutrients could impair rather than improve immune response.

1. Truswell S. Who should take vitamin supplements? *BMJ* 1990; **301:** 135–6. Correction. *ibid.*; 354.
2. Kendall HE. Vitamin and mineral supplements for children. *Pharm J* 1990; **245:** 460–2.
3. Chandra RK. Effect of vitamin and trace-element supplementation on immune responses and infection in elderly subjects. *Lancet* 1992; **340:** 1124–7.

MENTAL FUNCTION. Administration of vitamin and mineral supplements to children was reported in 1988 to increase non-verbal intelligence[1] and the topic has since remained highly controversial. In the following two years more studies were published but these failed to substantiate the earlier possible effect and concluded that vitamin supplementation did not improve mental functioning or reasoning in children.[2,3] Suggestions were made shortly after these publications that there might be a subset of children with poor nutritional status who would receive some benefit[4] but this again was disputed.[5] In 1991 another study was published,[6] this time coinciding with the launch of the proprietary product used in the study, with the publication of a book on the subject, and with the showing on British television of a documentary concerning the study. This study purported to demonstrate that supplementation with exactly the recommended dietary allowances of vitamins improved the IQ of children, a finding that was said not to occur significantly with other quantities of vitamin supplementation. This view attracted extremely harsh criticism[7-9] from physicians, nutritionists, psychologists, and epidemiologists.

1. Benton D, Roberts G. Effect of vitamin and mineral supplementation on intelligence of a sample of schoolchildren. *Lancet* 1988; **i:** 140–3.
2. Naismith DJ, et al. Can children's intelligence be increased by vitamin and mineral supplements? *Lancet* 1988; **ii:** 335.
3. Crombie IK, et al. Effect of vitamin and mineral supplementation on verbal and non-verbal reasoning of schoolchildren. *Lancet* 1990; **335:** 744–7.
4. Benton D, Buts J-P. Vitamin/mineral supplementation and intelligence. *Lancet* 1990; **335:** 1158–60.
5. Crombie IK, et al. Vitamin/mineral supplementation and intelligence. *Lancet* 1990; **336:** 175.
6. Schoenthaler SJ, et al. Controlled trial of vitamin-mineral supplementation: effects on intelligence and performance. *Personality Indiv Diff* 1991; **12:** 351–62.
7. Whitehead RG. Vitamins, minerals, schoolchildren, and IQ. *BMJ* 1991; **302:** 548.
8. Peto R. Vitamins and IQ. *BMJ* 1991; **302:** 906.
9. Anonymous. Brains and vitamins. *Lancet* 1991; **337:** 587–8.

PROPHYLAXIS OF ISCHAEMIC HEART DISEASE. Hypercholesterolaemia is a major risk factor for the development of atherosclerosis and consequently ischaemic heart disease. Since oxidation of lipids, particularly low-density-lipoprotein (LDL) cholesterol,[1] has been proposed as a factor in atherogenesis, the possibility of preventing atherosclerosis by the use of dietary antoxidants such as vitamins E and C and betacarotene has been investigated. Prospective epidemiological studies have revealed a reduced risk of ischaemic heart disease in individuals taking vitamin E supplements,[2,3] and those with a high carotene intake (particularly smokers).[2] In a further prospective cohort study,[4] dietary vitamin E consumption, but not vitamin E supplementation, was associated with decreased risk of death from ischaemic heart disease. Conversely, in these studies,[2-4] intake of vitamin C did not appear to be associated with a decreased risk of ischaemic heart disease. Data from some studies assessing serum or fat concentrations also provide evidence that high betacarotene concentrations are associated with decreased cardiovascular disease.[5-7]

However, despite these promising epidemiological data, results from randomised placebo-controlled trials have failed to find any benefit for betacarotene supplements in the primary or secondary prevention of ischaemic heart disease, and those for vitamin E supplements are inconclusive. In the Alpha Tocopherol, Beta Carotene Cancer Prevention (ATBC) study, which monitored cardiovascular disease as a secondary end-point, vitamin E was not associated with a decreased incidence of ischaemic heart disease, and betacarotene was associated with a small increased risk.[8] In further analyses, neither supplement appreciably altered the incidence of angina pectoris,[9] nor showed any beneficial effect on cardiovascular deaths in the subset of men with previous myocardial infarction.[10] It has been suggested that the lack of effect of vitamin E in this study may be due to an insufficiently high dose of tocopherol. Similarly, neither the Betacarotene and Retinol Efficacy Trial (CARET)[11] nor the Skin Cancer Prevention Study[7] found an effect for betacarotene supplementation on the risk of death from cardiovascular disease. In studies specifically on cardiovascular end-points, no benefit from betacarotene supplements was seen in a large, randomised, placebo-controlled study[12] in healthy men, and an initial study[13] of supplementation with high-dose vitamin E in patients with evidence of ischaemic heart disease failed to show any beneficial effect on cardiovascular deaths. However, there was a reduction in non-fatal myocardial infarction and major cardiovascular events. The Heart Outcomes Prevention Evaluation (HOPE) study also showed that vitamin E treatment for 4 to 6 years had no effect on cardiovascular events in high-risk patients.[14] Another large-scale study is underway; the Heart Protection Study is assessing the effect of a 'cocktail' of vitamin E, vitamin C, and betacarotene on the development of ischaemic heart disease in high risk subjects.[15] Until results from all studies are known, it has been recommended that the emphasis should be on consuming a balanced diet including antioxidant-rich fruits, vegetables, and whole grains rather than vitamin supplements.[16] For a discussion of the possibility that folic acid may reduce ischaemic heart disease through its homocysteine-lowering effect, see p.1362.

1. Jha P, et al. The antioxidant vitamins and cardiovascular disease: a critical review of epidemiologic and clinical trial data. Ann Intern Med 1995; 123: 860–72. Correction. ibid. 1996; 124: 934.
2. Rimm EB, et al. Vitamin E consumption and the risk of coronary heart disease in men. N Engl J Med 1993; 328: 1450–6.
3. Stampfer MJ, et al. Vitamin E consumption and the risk of coronary disease in women. N Engl J Med 1993; 328: 1444–9.
4. Kushi LH, et al. Dietary antioxidant vitamins and death from coronary heart disease in postmenopausal women. N Engl J Med 1996; 334: 1156–62.
5. Morris DL, et al. Serum carotenoids and coronary heart disease: the Lipid Research Clinics Coronary Primary Prevention Trial and Follow-up Study. JAMA 1994; 272: 1439–41.
6. Kardinaal AFM, et al. Antioxidants in adipose tissue and risk of myocardial infarction: the EURAMIC study. Lancet 1993; 342: 1379–84.
7. Greenberg ER, et al. Mortality associated with low plasma concentration of beta carotene and the effect of oral supplementation. JAMA 1996; 275: 699–703.
8. The Alpha-Tocopherol, Beta-Carotene Cancer Prevention Study Group. The effect of vitamin E and beta carotene on the incidence of lung cancer and other cancers in male smokers. N Engl J Med 1994; 330: 1029–35.
9. Rapola JM, et al. Effect of vitamin E and beta carotene on the incidence of angina pectoris. JAMA 1996; 275: 693–8. Correction. ibid. 1998; 279: 1528.
10. Rapola JM, et al. Randomised trial of α-tocopherol and β-carotene supplements on incidence of major coronary events in men with previous myocardial infarction. Lancet 1997; 349: 1715–20.
11. Omenn GS, et al. Effects of a combination of beta carotene and vitamin A on lung cancer and cardiovascular disease. N Engl J Med 1996; 334: 1150–5.
12. Hennekens CH, et al. Lack of effect of long-term supplementation with beta carotene on the incidence of malignant neoplasms and cardiovascular disease. N Engl J Med 1996; 334: 1145–9.
13. Stephens NG, et al. Randomised controlled trial of vitamin E in patients with coronary disease: Cambridge Heart Antioxidant Study (CHAOS). Lancet 1996; 347: 781–6.
14. Yusuf S, et al. Vitamin E supplementation and cardiovascular events in high-risk patients. The Heart Outcomes Prevention Evaluation Study Investigators. N Engl J Med 2000; 342: 154–60.
15. Lonn EM, Yusuf S. Is there a role for antioxidant vitamins in the prevention of cardiovascular diseases? An update of epidemiological and clinical trials data. Can J Cardiol 1997; 13: 957–65.
16. Tribble DL. Antioxidant consumption and risk of coronary heart disease: emphasis on vitamin C, vitamin E, and β-carotene: a statement for healthcare professionals from the American Heart Association. Circulation 1999; 99: 591–5.

PROPHYLAXIS OF MALIGNANT NEOPLASMS. There is evidence that a diet rich in fruit and vegetables is associated with a lower incidence of malignant disease, particularly of the respiratory and digestive tracts.[1] It has been hypothesised that some of the benefits of such a diet derive from the role of antioxidant vitamins such as the carotenoids and vitamins C and E in scavenging free radicals.[2,3] However, it is by no means certain that these are the only, or necessarily the most important, dietary components responsible for benefit, since components such as dietary fibre may also play a role. In addition, different antioxidants may vary in their properties and efficacy,[3,4] and the appropriate dosage remains largely conjectural, and perhaps as a result the evidence of benefit is often conflicting.

Several clinical trials of the use of **vitamin A** or **betacarotene** in the secondary or primary prevention of malignancy have been reported. Prolongation of disease-free interval in patients with various malignant neoplasms was reported in 1 study of betacarotene,[5] and another reported remission of oral leukoplakia in patients treated with betacarotene and vitamin A.[6] Vitamin A alone was reported to reduce the incidence of primary tobacco-related neoplasms in a study of patients treated surgically for lung cancer.[7] However, other results have largely failed to substantiate any benefit for secondary prevention. No reduction in the incidence of new skin cancers,[8] or in malignant transformation of cervical dysplasia,[9] or in new colorectal adenomas[10] was reported in 3 other studies. In a primary prevention study, a combination of betacarotene, vitamin E, and selenium was associated with a reduction in stomach and oesophageal cancers in a population at high risk of these cancers and with a diet low in micronutrients in China.[11] In contrast, other primary prevention studies have failed to show any benefit, and possibly some harm, from betacarotene supplements in well-nourished populations. A study in smokers[12,13] showed an increase in lung cancer and associated mortality in those receiving betacarotene (20 mg daily), but not those receiving vitamin E (50 mg daily). Similarly, an increased risk of lung cancer was noted in recipients of betacarotene (30 mg daily) with vitamin A (25 000 units daily) in another study in individuals at high risk of lung cancer, and this study was stopped early as a result.[14,15] A third study in healthy men found no benefit or harm for betacarotene supplements (50 mg on alternate days) in terms of incidence of malignant neoplasms, including those of the lung.[16]

Vitamin C has also been proposed for this purpose but there is no real evidence to justify it. It certainly appears to be ineffec-

tive as adjuvant therapy in the treatment of advanced malignancy,[17] and combination with betacarotene and vitamin E failed to show any effect in preventing colorectal adenoma.[10] At physiological concentrations vitamin C is an important antioxidant,[3] but supplementation is unlikely to be justified in anyone eating a balanced diet.[1]

Vitamin E substances are also known to play an important antioxidant role in the body. Animal studies have suggested that they should inhibit tumour production, and the Chinese study mentioned above found combined antioxidant therapy including vitamin E to be of benefit in the primary prevention of stomach and oesophageal cancers.[11] Other studies in western populations have generally been disappointing; vitamin E had no effect on lung cancer incidence in those at risk,[12,13] and did not prevent the development of new colorectal adenomas.[10] However, further analysis of the lung-cancer study[18] suggests that vitamin E may have protected against prostate cancer.

Results from the Nurses' Health Study have indicated that prolonged use of multivitamins was associated with reduced risk of developing cancer of the colon.[19] This effect was thought to be due to the **folate** component and could be demonstrated after 15 years of use, but not after shorter-term ingestion. Dietary folate was also associated with a modest reduction in risk for colon cancer.

At present, therefore, the only conclusion that appears uncontroversial is that a diet involving frequent consumption of fruit and vegetables is likely to be beneficial.[1] However, given the present difficulties in treating many malignancies once they develop interest in the topic seems likely to continue.

1. Austoker J. Diet and cancer. BMJ 1994; 308: 1610–14.
2. Hennekens CH. Antioxidant vitamins and cancer. Am J Med 1994; 97 (suppl 3A): 2S–4S.
3. Halliwell B. Free radicals, antioxidants, and human disease: curiosity, cause, or consequence? Lancet 1994; 344: 721–4.
4. Hankinson SE, Stampfer MJ. All that glitters is not beta carotene. JAMA 1994; 272: 1455–6.
5. Santamaria L, et al. First clinical report (1980-1988) of cancer chemoprevention with betacarotene plus canthaxanthin supplemented to patients after radical treatment. Boll Chim Farm 1988; 127: 57S–60S.
6. Stich HF, et al. Remission of oral leukoplakias and micronuclei in tobacco/betel quid chewers treated with beta-carotene and with beta-carotene plus vitamin A. Int J Cancer 1988; 42: 195–9.
7. Pastorino U, et al. Adjuvant treatment of stage I lung cancer with high-dose vitamin A. J Clin Oncol 1993; 11: 1216–22.
8. Greenberg ER, et al. A clinical trial of beta carotene to prevent basal-cell and squamous-cell cancers of the skin. N Engl J Med 1990 323: 789–95.
9. de Vet HCW, et al. The effect of beta-carotene on the regression and progression of cervical dysplasia: a clinical experiment. J Clin Epidemiol 1991; 44: 273–83.
10. Greenberg ER, et al. A clinical trial of antioxidant vitamins to prevent colorectal adenoma. N Engl J Med 1994; 331: 141–7.
11. Blot WJ, et al. Nutrition intervention trials in Linxian, China: supplementation with specific vitamin/mineral combinations, cancer incidence, and disease-specific mortality in the general population. J Natl Cancer Inst 1993; 85: 1483–92.
12. The Alpha-Tocopherol, Beta-Carotene Cancer Prevention Study Group. The effect of vitamin E and beta carotene on the incidence of lung cancer and other cancers in male smokers. N Engl J Med 1994; 330: 1029–35.
13. Albanes D, et al. α-Tocopherol and β-carotene supplements and lung cancer incidence in the alpha-tocopherol, beta-carotene cancer prevention study: effects of base-line characteristics and study compliance. J Natl Cancer Inst 1996; 88: 1560–70.
14. Omenn GS, et al. Effects of a combination of beta carotene and vitamin A on lung cancer and cardiovascular disease. N Engl J Med 1996; 334: 1150–5.
15. Omenn GS, et al. Risk factors for lung cancer and for intervention effects in CARET, the Beta-Carotene and Retinol Efficacy Trial. J Natl Cancer Inst 1996; 88: 1550–9.
16. Hennekens CH, et al. Lack of effect of long-term supplementation with beta carotene on the incidence of malignant neoplasms and cardiovascular disease. N Engl J Med 1996; 334: 1145–9.
17. Moertel CG, et al. High-dose vitamin C versus placebo in the treatment of patients with advanced cancer who have had no prior chemotherapy: a randomized double-blind comparison. N Engl J Med 1985; 312: 137–41.
18. Heinonen OP, et al. Prostate cancer and supplementation with α-tocopherol and β-carotene: incidence and mortality in a controlled trial. J Natl Cancer Inst 1998; 90: 440–6.
19. Giovannucci E, et al. Multivitamin use, folate, and colon cancer in women in the Nurses' Health Study. Ann Intern Med 1998; 129: 517–24.

Acesulfame Potassium (14035-b)

Acesulfame Potassium (BANM, rINNM).

Acesulfame K; Acesulfamum Kalicum; E950; H73-3293; Hoe-095K. 6-Methyl-1,2,3-oxathiazin-4(3H)-one 2,2-dioxide potassium.

$C_4H_4KNO_4S = 201.2$.

CAS — 55589-62-3.

Pharmacopoeias. In Eur. (see p.vi).

Pharmacopoeial description

Ph. Eur.: A white, crystalline powder or colourless crystals. Soluble in water; very slightly soluble in alcohol and in acetone.

Profile

Acesulfame potassium is an intense sweetener about 200 times as sweet as sucrose. It is used in foods and does not appear to be affected by cooking.

Alanine (572-b)

Alanine (USAN, rINN).

A; Ala; L-Alanine; Alaninum. L-2-Aminopropionic acid.

$C_3H_7NO_2 = 89.09$.

CAS — 56-41-7.

Pharmacopoeias. In Eur. (see p.vi) and US.

Pharmacopoeial description

Ph. Eur.: A white or almost white crystalline powder or colourless crystals. Freely soluble in water; very slightly soluble in alcohol; practically insoluble in ether. Protect from light.

USP 25: White, odourless, crystals or crystalline powder. Freely soluble in water; slightly soluble in 80% alcohol; insoluble in ether. pH of a 5% solution in water is between 5.5 and 7.0.

Profile

Alanine is an aliphatic amino acid. It is used as a dietary supplement. The dipeptide N(2)-L-alanyl-L-glutamine is used similarly.

Hypoglycaemia. References to the investigational use of alanine in the management of insulin-induced hypoglycaemia.[1-3]

1. Wiethop BV, Cryer PE. Glycemic actions of alanine and terbutaline in IDDM. Diabetes Care 1993; 16: 1124–30.
2. Wiethop BV, Cryer PE. Alanine and terbutaline in treatment of hypoglycemia in IDDM. Diabetes Care 1993; 16: 1131–6.
3. Saleh TY, Cryer PE. Alanine and terbutaline in the prevention of nocturnal hypoglycemia in IDDM. Diabetes Care 1997; 20: 1231–6.

Preparations

Proprietary Preparations (details are given in Part 3)
Aust.: Dipetiven; *Denm.:* Dipetiven; *Fin.:* Dipetiven; *Fr.:* Dipetiven; *Ger.:* Dipetamin; *Ital.:* Dipetiven; *Mex.:* Dipetiven; *Port.:* Dipetiven; *Spain:* Dipetiven; *Swed.:* Dipetiven; *UK:* Dipetiven.

Multi-ingredient: *Port.:* Tebetane Composto; *Spain:* Tebetane Compuesto; *UK:* Amino MS.

Arginine (573-v)

Arginine (rINN).

Arg; L-Arginine; Argininum; R. L-2-Amino-5-guanidinovaleric acid.

$C_6H_{14}N_4O_2 = 174.2$.

CAS — 74-79-3.

Pharmacopoeias. In Eur. (see p.vi) and US.

Pharmacopoeial description

Ph. Eur.: A white or almost white crystalline powder, or colourless crystals. Freely soluble in water; very slightly soluble in alcohol; practically insoluble in ether. Protect from light.

USP 25: White, practically odourless crystals. Freely soluble in water; sparingly soluble in alcohol; insoluble in ether.

Arginine Glutamate (574-g)

Arginine Glutamate (BAN, USAN, rINNM).

L-Arginine L-glutamate.

$C_6H_{14}N_4O_2,C_5H_9NO_4 = 321.3$.

CAS — 4320-30-3.

ATC — A05BA01.

Arginine Hydrochloride (575-q)

Arginine Hydrochloride (USAN, rINNM).

L-Arginine Monohydrochloride; Arginini Hydrochloridum.

$C_6H_{14}N_4O_2,HCl = 210.7$.

CAS — 1119-34-2.

ATC — B05XB01.

Pharmacopoeias. In Chin., Eur. (see p.vi), Jpn, and US.
Fr. also includes Arginine Aspartate.

Pharmacopoeial description

Ph. Eur.: A white or almost white crystalline powder, or colourless crystals. Freely soluble in water; very slightly soluble in alcohol; practically insoluble in ether.

USP 25: White, practically odourless, crystals or crystalline powder. Freely soluble in water.

Adverse Effects and Precautions

Nausea, vomiting, flushing, headache, numbness, and local venous irritation may occur if arginine solutions are infused too rapidly. Elevated plasma-potassium concentrations have been reported in uraemic patients and arginine should therefore be administered with caution to patients with renal disease or anuria. Arginine hydrochloride should be administered cautiously to patients with electrolyte disturbances as its high chloride content could lead to the development of hyperchloraemic acidosis.

Extravasation. A report[1] of necrosis following extravasation of a 10% solution of arginine hydrochloride. Both osmotic and local hyperkalaemic effects had been proposed as a mechanism for the injury.

1. Bowlby HA, Elanjian SI. Necrosis caused by extravasation of arginine hydrochloride. *Ann Pharmacother* 1992; **26:** 263–4.

Hyperkalaemia. Two alcoholic patients with severe liver disease and moderate renal insufficiency developed severe hyperkalaemia following administration of arginine hydrochloride and one died.[1] Both patients had received a total dose of 300 mg of spironolactone some time before arginine hydrochloride administration, but the contribution of spironolactone to the hyperkalaemia was not known.

1. Bushinsky DA, Gennari FJ. Life-threatening hyperkalemia induced by arginine. *Ann Intern Med* 1978; **89:** 632–4.

Hypersensitivity. A 10-year-old boy experienced an anaphylactic reaction 5 minutes after the start of an infusion of a 5% arginine hydrochloride solution in a test for growth-hormone output.[1] This was considered to be a very rare event and only one other apparent allergic reaction had been reported to the manufacturers.

1. Tiwary CM, *et al.* Anaphylactic reaction to arginine infusion. *N Engl J Med* 1973; **288:** 218.

Uses and Administration

Arginine is an aliphatic amino acid which is essential for infant growth. It is used as a dietary supplement.

Arginine stimulates the release of growth hormone by the pituitary gland and may be used instead of, or in addition to, other tests such as insulin-induced hypoglycaemia, for the evaluation of growth disorders; false-positive and false-negative results are relatively common and evaluation therefore should not be made on the basis of a single arginine test. It is used as a 10% solution of the hydrochloride in usual doses of 30 g by intravenous infusion given over 30 minutes; children should be given 500 mg per kg body-weight.

Arginine is used in certain conditions accompanied by hyperammonaemia; for further details see below.

Arginine hydrochloride has also been used as an acidifying agent. In severe metabolic alkalosis intravenous doses (in grams) have been calculated by multiplying the desired decrease in plasma-bicarbonate concentration (mEq or mmol per litre) by the patient's body-weight (in kg) and then dividing by 9.6. In forced acid diuresis to hasten drug elimination after overdose a suggested dose has been 10 g intravenously over 30 minutes.

Arginine may also be employed in the form of the acetylasparaginate, aspartate, citrate, glutamate, oxoglurate, tidiacicate (thiazolidine-2,4-dicarboxylate), and timonacicate (thiazolidine-4-carboxylate). Formulation as an arginine salt is used to improve the solubility of a number of drugs, notably analgesics and antibiotics.

Hyperammonaemia. Hyperammonaemia is a characteristic feature of inborn errors of the urea cycle and is particularly severe in ornithine carbamoyl transferase (OCT) deficiency and carbamoyl phosphate synthetase (CPS) deficiency. During the urea cycle, waste ammonia, in the form of the ammonium ion, is normally condensed with bicarbonate and ATP to form carbamoyl phosphate which undergoes several more reactions, including one leading to the synthesis of arginine, and ultimate transformation to urea for excretion. Thus, in defects of this cycle ammonia accumulates and arginine synthesis is deficient. Hyperammonaemia is often associated with respiratory alkalosis in patients with urea cycle disorders.

The basis of treatment is dietary protein restriction, to decrease the requirement for waste nitrogen synthesis, and the administration of drugs to stimulate alternative pathways of waste nitrogen excretion. These include arginine, citrulline, sodium benzoate, sodium phenylacetate, and sodium phenylbutyrate. In the initial management of severe hyperammonaemia, haemodialysis is required.[1]

Arginine supplements are given except in hyperargininaemia,[2] although citrulline may be used in some cases instead.[3] One review[2] quoted oral doses of arginine 0.5 to 2 g daily for long-term management of OCT and CPS deficiency, and up to 700 mg per kg daily for argininosuccinate synthetase (AS) or argininosuccinate lyase (AL) deficiencies. Intravenous doses quoted for the treatment of severe hyperammonaemia or encephalopathy were arginine 200 to 800 mg per kg body-weight given as a loading dose over 4 hours, followed by a constant infusion of 200 to 800 mg per kg daily, the dose range varying with the specific defect in the cycle.

Patients also receive concomitant treatment with sodium benzoate and sodium phenylacetate[3-6] or sodium phenylbutyrate[6-8] unless suffering from AL deficiency, which can usually be managed with protein restriction and arginine alone.[5] When so-

dium benzoate is conjugated with glycine and excreted as hippuric acid it provides an alternative pathway of nitrogen excretion, while sodium phenylacetate and sodium phenylbutyrate provide a second and even more effective pathway by conjugation with glutamine.

The usual initial doses of sodium benzoate and sodium phenylacetate in affected infants are 250 mg of each per kg body-weight daily by intravenous infusion, followed by 250 to 500 mg of each per kg daily by constant infusion.[5,6] Infusion is continued until the drugs can be taken orally; although earlier oral protocols were based on sodium benzoate, sodium phenylbutyrate is now preferred at a dosage of 450 to 600 mg per kg daily.[6-8] It has been suggested that carnitine supplementation should be added to minimise the adverse effects in patients treated with benzoate.[9]

Hyperammonaemia and hepatic encephalopathy (p.1205) can also arise from a variety of other causes and although arginine has been advocated many authorities do not consider such use beneficial.

1. Summar M. Current strategies for the management of neonatal urea cycle disorders. *J Pediatr* 2001; **138** (suppl): S30–S39.
2. Walter JH, Leonard JV. Inborn errors of the urea cycle. *Br J Hosp Med* 1987; **38:** 176–83.
3. Msall M, *et al.* Neurologic outcome in children with inborn errors of urea synthesis: outcome of urea-cycle enzymopathies. *N Engl J Med* 1984; **310:** 1500–5.
4. Brusilow SW, *et al.* New pathways of nitrogen excretion in inborn errors of urea synthesis. *Lancet* 1979; **ii:** 452–4.
5. Brusilow SW, *et al.* Treatment of episodic hyperammonemia in children with inborn errors of urea synthesis. *N Engl J Med* 1984; **310:** 1630–4.
6. Maestri NE, *et al.* Prospective treatment of urea cycle disorders. *J Pediatr* 1991; **119:** 923–8.
7. Maestri NE, *et al.* Long-term survival of patients with argininosuccinate synthetase deficiency. *J Pediatr* 1995; **127:** 929–35.
8. Maestri NE, *et al.* Long-term treatment of girls with ornithine transcarbamylase deficiency. *N Engl J Med* 1996; **335:** 855–9.
9. Sakuma T. Alteration of urinary carnitine profile induced by benzoate administration. *Arch Dis Child* 1991; **66:** 873–5.

Hypotensive action. Arginine is the physiological precursor of nitric oxide and this has been suggested as an explanation for the hypotensive effect that has been reported in healthy subjects[1-3] and hypertensive patients[1,4] given infusions of arginine, although effects of arginine unrelated to nitric oxide generation cannot be excluded.[4] Decrease in plasma-cholesterol concentrations has also been reported in 2 hypercholesterolaemic patients given arginine infusions.[5] It has even been suggested that arginine might be suitable for the short-term control of hypertension,[3] although in the absence of controlled studies of its effect this must be considered speculative. Some interest has surrounded its potential role in other cardiovascular diseases.[6]

1. Nakaki T, *et al.* L-arginine-induced hypotension. *Lancet* 1990; **336:** 696.
2. Hishikawa K, *et al.* L-arginine-induced hypotension. *Lancet* 1991; **337:** 683–4.
3. Petros AJ, *et al.* L-arginine-induced hypotension. *Lancet* 1991; **337:** 1044–5.
4. Pedrinelli R, *et al.* Pressor, renal and endocrine effects of L-arginine in essential hypertensives. *Eur J Clin Pharmacol* 1995; **48:** 195–201.
5. Korbut R, *et al.* Effect of L-arginine on plasminogen-activator inhibitor in hypertensive patients with hypercholesterolemia. *N Engl J Med* 1993; **328:** 287–8.
6. Cheng JWM, Balwin SN. L-arginine in the management of cardiovascular diseases. *Ann Pharmacother* 2001; **35:** 755–64.

Preparations

BP 2001: Arginine Hydrochloride Intravenous Infusion;
USP 25: Arginine Hydrochloride Injection.

Proprietary Preparations (details are given in Part 3)
Aust.: Sangenor; *Belg.:* Dynamisan†; *Braz.:* Desfatigan; Targifor; *Fr.:* Dynamisan; Energitum†; Eucol; Sargenor; Tiadilon; *Ger.:* Eubiol; *Ital.:* Bioarginina; Dynamisan; Sargenor; Sulfile; *Mex.:* Fertibion; *Port.:* Asparten; Bio-Energol Plus; Dynamisan; Sargenor; Sulfile; *Spain:* Hepacitol; Livercom; Potenciator; Sargenor; Sorbenor; *Switz.:* Dynamisan; *USA:* R-Gene.

Multi-ingredient: *Aust.:* Leberinfusion; Rocmaline; *Braz.:* Necroplex; Ornihepat; Ornitargin; Targifor C; *Fr.:* Arginotri-B; Arnilose†; Citrarginine; Epuram; Fastenyl; Hepagrome; Hepargitol; Rocmaline; Sargenor a la Vitamine C; *Ger.:* Glutarsin E; Infumal; Polilevo N; *Ital.:* Calciofix; Glutargin; Ipoazotal; Ipoazotal Complex; Isoram; Polilevo; Somatron; Tonoplus; Vitasprint Complex; *Spain:* Dynamogen; Sanieb; *Switz.:* Activital; Arginotri-B; Vitasprint Complex.

Arrowroot (12393-w)

Amylum Marantae; Araruta; Maranta.

The starch granules of the rhizomes of *Maranta arundinacea* (Marantaceae).

Profile
Arrowroot has the general properties of starch (p.1379). It has been used as a suspending agent in the preparation of barium meals and has sometimes been used in place of starch in tablet manufacture.

Aspartame (2374-j)

Aspartame (BAN, USAN, rINN).

APM; Aspartamum; E951; SC-18862. Methyl *N*-L-α-aspartyl-L-phenylalaninate; 3-Amino-*N*-(α-methoxycarbonylphenethyl)succinamic acid; *N*-L-α-aspartyl-L-phenylalanine, 1-methyl ester.
$C_{14}H_{18}N_2O_5 = 294.3.$
CAS — 22839-47-0.

Pharmacopoeias. In *Eur.* (see p.vi). Also in *USNF*.

In the presence of moisture it hydrolyses to form aspartylphenylalanine and a diketopiperazine derivative, with a resulting loss of sweetness.

Pharmacopoeial description

Ph. Eur.: A white, slightly hygroscopic, crystalline powder. Sparingly or slightly soluble in water and in alcohol; practically insoluble in dichloromethane and in *n*-hexane. Store in airtight containers.

USNF 20: White, odourless, crystalline powder having a sweet taste. Sparingly soluble in water; slightly soluble in alcohol. pH of a 0.8% solution in water is about 5.

Adverse Effects and Precautions
Excessive use of aspartame should be avoided by patients with phenylketonuria since one of its metabolic products is phenylalanine. Aspartame's sweetness is lost during prolonged cooking.

◊ The safety and side-effects of aspartame as a pharmaceutical excipient have been reviewed.[1,2]

Aspartame is hydrolysed in the gastrointestinal tract to its 3 primary constituents, methanol, aspartic acid, and phenylalanine. However, even with extraordinary consumption, methanol toxicity stemming from aspartame use is extremely unlikely. Aspartate concentrations in blood do not rise significantly following a very large dose (50 to 100 mg per kg body-weight) and therefore toxicity related to aspartate is also not expected to occur. Despite the similarity of aspartate to glutamate studies in glutamate-sensitive persons have shown that they are not affected by aspartame consumption. Plasma concentrations of phenylalanine are also unlikely to be markedly elevated following modest consumption of aspartame by healthy persons but persons with phenylketonuria should avoid or limit their use of aspartame.

A number of adverse effects have been reported[1,2] following the use of aspartame, either as spontaneously recorded complaints from consumers or as published case reports in the medical literature. Most frequently reported problems have been headache, neuropsychiatric or behavioural symptoms, seizures, gastrointestinal symptoms, and hypersensitivity or dermatological symptoms. Available data do not provide evidence for serious widespread health consequences attendant upon the use of aspartame but it would appear that certain individuals may have an unusual sensitivity to the product.

Studies have confirmed aspartame's lack of effect on children's behaviour or cognitive function.[3,4]

An increased incidence of brain cancer was postulated to be related to aspartame use in a recent report;[5] however, the USA Food and Drug Administration maintain that the available evidence does not support an association.[6]

1. Golightly LK, *et al.* Pharmaceutical excipients: adverse effects associated with 'inactive' ingredients in drug products (part II). *Med Toxicol* 1988; **3:** 209–40.
2. American Academy of Pediatrics. "Inactive" ingredients in pharmaceutical products: update. *Pediatrics* 1997; **99:** 268–78.
3. Shaywitz BA, *et al.* Aspartame, behavior, and cognitive function in children with attention deficit disorder. *Pediatrics* 1994; **93:** 70–5.
4. Wolraich ML, *et al.* Effects of diets high in sucrose or aspartame on the behavior and cognitive performance of children. *N Engl J Med* 1994; **330:** 301–7.
5. Olney JW, *et al.* Increasing brain tumor rates: is there a link to aspartame? *J Neuropathol Exp Neurol* 1996; **55:** 1115–23.
6. Anonymous. Aspartame: no apparent link with brain tumours. *WHO Drug Inf* 1997; **11:** 18–19.

Uses
Aspartame is an intense sweetening agent about 180 to 200 times as sweet as sucrose. It is used in foods, beverages, and pharmaceuticals. Each g provides approximately 17 kJ (4 kcal).

Sickle-cell disease. There is some preliminary evidence that aspartame may have beneficial effects in sickle-cell disease.[1]

1. Manion CV, *et al.* Aspartame effect in sickle cell anemia. *Clin Pharmacol Ther* 2001; **69:** 346–55.

Preparations

Proprietary Preparations (details are given in Part 3)
Braz.: Dietacil; Finn; Stetic; Sucret; *Fr.:* D Sucril†; *Ital.:* Aspartina; Miripel†; Futura; Suaviter; Sweet Touch; Vantaggio†; Weight Watchers Punto; *Mex.:* Canderel; *NZ:* Equal; *Port.:* Canderel†; Dolcevita; Neo Dulceril†; *Thai.:* Equal; Espar; Sweetabb.

Multi-ingredient: *Ital.:* Doldieta†; Weight Watchers Punto.

Aspartic Acid (576-p)

Aspartic Acid (USAN, rINN).

Acidum Asparticum; Asp; L-Aspartic Acid; D. L-Aminosuccinic acid.

$C_4H_7NO_4 = 133.1$.

CAS — 56-84-8.

Pharmacopoeias. In Eur. (see p.vi) and US.

Pharmacopoeial description

Ph. Eur.: A white or almost white crystalline powder, or colourless crystals. Slightly soluble in water; practically insoluble in alcohol and in ether. It dissolves in dilute solutions of alkali hydroxides and in dilute mineral acids. Protect from light.

USP 25: A white or almost white crystalline powder, or colourless crystals. Slightly soluble in water; practically insoluble in alcohol and in ether; soluble in dilute solutions of alkali hydroxides and in dilute mineral acids.

Profile

Aspartic acid is an aliphatic amino acid. It is used as a dietary supplement.

Betacarotene (7824-a)

Betacarotene (rINN).

all-trans-β-Carotene; Beta Carotene (USAN); Betacarotenum; E160(a); Provitamin A. β,β-Carotene; (all-E)-1,1'-(3,7,12,16-Tetramethyl-1,3,5,7,9,11,13,15,17-octadecanonaene-1,18-diyl)bis[2,6,6-trimethylcyclohexene].

$C_{40}H_{56} = 536.9$.

CAS — 7235-40-7.

ATC — D02BB01.

Pharmacopoeias. In Eur. (see p.vi) and US.

Carotene exists in 3 isomeric forms, all of which are converted to some extent into vitamin A in the livers of man and animals. Of the 3 isomers of carotene, the *beta* compound is more active than the *alpha*- or *gamma*-isomers. The vitamin A activity of plants is due to the presence of *alpha*-, *beta*-, and *gamma*-carotenes and to kryptoxanthine; that of animal tissues is due to both vitamin A and carotene, while fish-liver oils contain vitamin A but no carotene.

Pharmacopoeial description

Ph. Eur.: A brown-red or brownish-red crystalline powder. Practically insoluble in water and in dehydrated alcohol; slightly soluble in cyclohexane and in ether. It is sensitive to air, heat and light, especially in solution. Store in airtight containers at a temperature not exceeding 25°. Protect from light.

USP 25: Red or reddish-brown to violet-brown crystals or crystalline powder. Insoluble in water, in acids, and in alkalis; practically insoluble in alcohol and in methyl alcohol; soluble in carbon disulfide, in chloroform, and in benzene; sparingly soluble in ether, in petroleum spirit, and in vegetable oils. Store in airtight containers. Protect from light.

Units

Vitamin A activity in foods is expressed in terms of retinol equivalents: 6 µg of betacarotene represents 1 retinol equivalent (or 10 of the former International units for provitamin A—see p.1382).

Adverse Effects and Precautions

Loose stools may occasionally occur during treatment with betacarotene and the skin may assume a slightly yellow discoloration. Bruising and arthralgia have been reported rarely.

Excessive intake of betacarotene does not result in hypervitaminosis A (see Pharmacokinetics, below).

Carcinogenicity. For reference to the finding of an increased incidence of lung cancers in individuals receiving betacarotene supplements, compared with those receiving placebo, in studies investigating the ability of betacarotene to protect against malignancy, see under Prophylaxis of Malignant Neoplasms, p.1353.

Effects on the skin. Yellow pigmentation of the skin may result from an unusually high consumption of carrots or other source of carotene,[1] or from a defect in the enzyme that normally metabolises betacarotene to vitamin A.[2] Hypercarotenaemia can be distinguished from jaundice by the fact that the sclerae retain their normal white colour. Pigmentation occurs first on the palms and soles and may extend to the nasolabial folds. Although it has been stated that the condition is harmless as the body converts carotene to retinol only as required,[1] others consider that long-standing hypercarotenaemia can have clinical sequelae:[2] neutropenia[3] and amenorrhoea[4] have been reported to be associated with the condition.

1. Sharman IM. Hypercarotenaemia. *BMJ* 1985; **290:** 95.
2. Vaughan Jones SA, Black MM. Metabolic carotenaemia. *Br J Dermatol* 1994; **131:** 145.
3. Shoenfeld Y, et al. Neutropenia induced by hypercarotenaemia. *Lancet* 1982; **i:** 1245.
4. Kemmann E, et al. Amenorrhoea associated with carotenemia. *JAMA* 1983; **249:** 926–9.

Pharmacokinetics

Gastrointestinal absorption of betacarotene depends on the presence of bile and is increased by dietary fat. About 20 to 60% of betacarotene is metabolised to retinol in the intestinal wall, and a small amount is converted to vitamin A in the liver. The proportion of betacarotene converted to vitamin A decreases as the intake of betacarotene increases, and high doses of betacarotene do not lead to abnormally high serum concentrations of vitamin A. Unchanged betacarotene is distributed to various tissues including fat, the adrenal glands, and ovaries.

◊ References.
1. Wang X-D. Review: absorption and metabolism of β-carotene. *J Am Coll Nutr* 1994; **13:** 314–25.

Human Requirements

Carotenes, of which betacarotene has the highest activity, are major dietary sources of vitamin A—see p.1383.

Uses and Administration

Betacarotene is a carotenoid precursor of vitamin A (p.1382). It is used for the prevention of vitamin A deficiency at a dose of 6 to 15 mg daily. In the treatment of vitamin A deficiency, vitamin A is preferred to betacarotene.

Betacarotene may be given by mouth to reduce the severity of photosensitivity reactions in patients with erythropoietic protoporphyria (see also below). Doses are in the range of 30 to 300 mg daily for adults and 30 to 150 mg daily for children, depending upon severity; they may be taken as either single daily doses or divided doses but should preferably be taken with meals. The protection offered by betacarotene is not total and generally 2 to 6 weeks of treatment resulting in a yellow coloration of palms and soles is necessary before patients should attempt to increase their exposure to sunlight.

Betacarotene and other carotenoids (alphacarotene and gammacarotene) are used as colouring agents for foods.

Betacarotene has antioxidant activity and has been studied for its possible protective benefit in a number of disorders.

Age-related macular degeneration. A study in patients with age-related macular degeneration indicated that the risk of developing this disorder (a leading cause of irreversible blindness among elderly persons) was markedly decreased amongst those with the highest carotenoid intake;[1] in particular, lutein and zeaxanthin, or green leafy vegetables (which contain high concentrations of these carotenoids) were associated with a lower risk. Increasing the intake of these carotenoids may be of benefit in reducing the development of this disorder.

1. Seddon JM, et al. Dietary carotenoids, vitamins A, C, and E, and advanced age-related macular degeneration. *JAMA* 1994; **272:** 1413–20.

Deficiency states. A study in Senegalese children suffering from vitamin A deficiency as defined by abnormal results on eye cytology found that supplementation with betacarotene (in a single dose equivalent to 200 000 units of vitamin A) was as effective as a single 200 000 unit dose of vitamin A palmitate in reversing the ocular changes.[1] Since betacarotene is less toxic than vitamin A itself it would have some advantages for vitamin A supplementation, either as an oral supplement or by encouraging the consumption of carotenoid-rich fruit and vegetables. A study in Indonesian women found that a betacarotene supplement improved vitamin A status, whereas an additional daily portion of dark-green leafy vegetables containing a similar amount of betacarotene did not.[2] However, others contend that consumption of food sources of carotenoids are effective in improving vitamin A status in deficiency states,[3,4] and that it may not be appropriate to extrapolate these findings to vitamin A deficient children.[3,5] WHO policy is still to promote dietary adjustment wherever vitamin A deficiency is endemic.[5]

For further discussion of vitamin A deficiency and the value of supplementation in various disease states, see under Vitamin A Substances, p.1383.

1. Carlier C, et al. A randomised controlled trial to test equivalence between retinyl palmitate and β carotene for vitamin A deficiency. *BMJ* 1993; **307:** 1106–10.
2. de Pee S, et al. Lack of improvement in vitamin A status with increased consumption of dark-green leafy vegetables. *Lancet* 1995; **346:** 75–81.
3. Reddy V. Vitamin A status and dark green leafy vegetables. *Lancet* 1995; **346:** 1634–5.
4. Underwood BA. Vitamin A status and dark green leafy vegetables. *Lancet* 1995; **346:** 1635.
5. WHO. Vitamin A status: is dietary replacement practicable. *WHO Drug Inf* 1995; **9:** 141.

Ischaemic heart disease. There are results from epidemiological studies suggesting the potential benefits of dietary betacarotene in preventing ischaemic heart disease, particularly in smokers; however, randomised placebo-controlled studies of betacarotene supplements have returned negative results, as discussed on p.1352.

Malignant neoplasms. Some evidence from epidemiological studies suggested that higher dietary intakes of carotenoids and especially betacarotene had a protective effect against cancer. Consequently several randomised placebo-controlled trials examining the use of betacarotene supplements in the primary or secondary prevention of malignancy were instigated. However, the results of studies so far published have generally been disappointing. Moreover, some results suggest that supplementation with betacarotene may actually be harmful: an increase in lung cancer was seen in those at risk for this malignancy (see p.1353).

Porphyria. Betacarotene is the most widely used systemic drug for the management of erythropoietic protoporphyria,[1] a non-acute porphyria characterised by cutaneous photosensitivity (p.1011). It is often administered with canthaxanthin to reduce the skin discoloration caused by betacarotene alone.

1. Todd DJ. Erythropoietic protoporphyria. *Br J Dermatol* 1994; **131:** 751–66.

Preparations

USP 25: Beta Carotene Capsules.

Proprietary Preparations (details are given in Part 3)
Aust.: Carotaben; **Austral.:** B-Tene; **Ger.:** BellaCarotin mono; Carotaben; **Ital.:** Tannisol; **Neth.:** Carotaben; **Swed.:** Karotena ACO†; **Switz.:** Carotaben; **UK:** Arocin; Biocarotine; Pervita.

Multi-ingredient: Aust.: Oleovit A; Oleovit A + D; **Austral.:** Antioxidant Forte Tablets; Antioxidant Tablets; Beta A-C; Beta-Ace Tablets; Cold Sore Tablets; Eye Health Herbal Plus Formula 4; Ginkgo ACE†; Lifesystem Herbal Plus Formula 5 Eye Relief; Lifesystem Herbal Plus Formula 8 Echinacea†; Odourless Garlic; Sinus and Hayfever; **Braz.:** Purpuralin; **Fr.:** Difrarel; Phenoro; **Ger.:** Carotin; Sonnenbraun; **Hong Kong:** Purpuralin; **Ital.:** Aclon Lievit; Agedin Plus; Angstrom Viso/Labbra Alta Protezione; Ecamannan; Keratolip; Levudin; Mirtilene; Solecin; Tannidin Plus; **Mex.:** Unitone; **Spain:** Aceite Acalorico; Mirtilus; **Switz.:** Apotrin; Linola gras; Visaline; **USA:** Antiox.

Biotin (7859-g)

Biotin (rINN).

Biotinum; Coenzyme R; Vitamin H. cis-5-(Hexahydro-2-oxo-1H-thieno[3,4-d]imidazol-4-yl)valeric acid.

$C_{10}H_{16}N_2O_3S = 244.3$.

CAS — 58-85-5.

ATC — A11HA05.

Pharmacopoeias. In Eur. (see p.vi) and US.

Pharmacopoeial description

Ph. Eur.: A white crystalline powder or colourless crystals. Very slightly soluble in water and in alcohol; practically insoluble in acetone. It dissolves in dilute solutions of alkali hydroxides. Protect from light.

USP 25: A practically white crystalline powder. Very slightly soluble in water and in alcohol; insoluble in other common organic solvents. Store in airtight containers.

Profile

Biotin is traditionally considered to be a vitamin B substance. It is an essential coenzyme in fat metabolism and in other carboxylation reactions. Biotin deficiency may result in the urinary excretion of organic acids and changes in skin and hair. Deficiency of biotin is very unlikely in man because of its widespread distribution in food. Egg-yolk and offal are especially good sources. Biotin deficiency has been reported however during long-term parenteral nutrition and in patients with biotinidase deficiency, an inherited metabolic disorder.

Biotin combines with avidin, a glycoprotein present in raw eggwhite, to form an inactive compound.

Adverse effects. For reference to life-threatening pleuropericarditis in a patient receiving biotin and pantothenic acid see p.1374.

Deficiency states. References to the successful use of biotin to treat deficiency of biotinidase or holocarboxylase synthetase, enzymes responsible for the recycling and incorporation of biotin.

1. Wolf B, et al. Clinical findings in four children with biotinidase deficiency detected through a statewide neonatal screening program. *N Engl J Med* 1985; **313:** 16–19.
2. Hurvitz H, et al. Biotinidase deficiency associated with severe combined immunodeficiency. *Lancet* 1989; **ii:** 228–9.
3. McVoy JRS, et al. Partial biotinidase deficiency: clinical and biochemical features. *J Pediatr* 1990; **116:** 78–83.
4. Lara EB, et al. Biotinidase deficiency in black children. *J Pediatr* 1990; **116:** 750–2.
5. Baumgartner ER, Suormala T. Multiple carboxylase deficiency: inherited and acquired disorders of biotin metabolism. *Int J Vitam Nutr Res* 1997; **67:** 377–84.

Human requirements. In the UK neither a reference nutrient intake (RNI) nor an estimated average requirement (EAR—see p.1352) has been set for biotin although it was considered that an intake of between 10 and 200 µg daily was both safe and

The symbol † denotes a preparation no longer actively marketed

adequate.[1] Similarly in the USA an adequate intake of 30 μg daily has been set for adults.[2]

1. DoH. Dietary reference values for food energy and nutrients for the United Kingdom: report of the panel on dietary reference values of the committee on medical aspects of food policy. *Report on health and social subjects 41*. London: HMSO, 1991.
2. Standing Committee on the Scientific Evaluation of Dietary Reference Intakes of the Food and Nutrition Board. *Dietary Reference Intakes for thiamin, riboflavin, niacin, vitamin B6, folate, vitamin B12, pantothenic acid, biotin, and choline*. Washington, DC: National Academy Press, 2000.

Preparations

Proprietary Preparations (details are given in Part 3)
Aust.: Bio-H-Tin; Medobiotin; **Ger.:** Bio-H-Tin; Biokur; Biotin-Asmedic; Deacura; Gabunat; Medobiotin; Priorin Biotin†; Rombellin; **Ital.:** Biodermatin; Diathynil; **Switz.:** Bio-H-Tin; Rombellin.

Multi-ingredient: Fr.: Arbum; Forcapil; **Ger.:** Carotin; Sonnenbraun; **Ital.:** Herbavit; **Spain:** Doctodermis; Lacerdermol.

Calcium Fluoride (12507-b)

CaF₂ = 78.07.

CAS — 7789-75-5.

Pharmacopoeias. In Ger.

Profile

Calcium fluoride is used as a fluoride supplement (see Sodium Fluoride, p.1375) for the prevention of dental caries. Calcium fluoride is also used as a source of calcium.

Native calcium fluoride (Calcarea Fluorica; Calc. Fluor.) is used in homoeopathic medicine.

Preparations

Proprietary Preparations (details are given in Part 3)
Denm.: Bifluorid; **Fr.:** Calcifluor.

Multi-ingredient: Austral.: Cirflo†; **Fr.:** Fluopate; **Spain:** Calcio Faes DYC†; Calcio Geve D y C; **Swed.:** Bifluorid 12.

Carnitine (20298-e)

Carnitine *(rINN)*.

Vitamin B_T. (3-Carboxy-2-hydroxypropyl)trimethylammonium hydroxide, inner salt; 3-Hydroxy-4-trimethylammoniobutyrate.

C₇H₁₅NO₃ = 161.2.

CAS — 461-06-3.

Levocarnitine (12528-s)

Levocarnitine *(BAN, USAN, rINN)*.

L-Carnitine. (R)-(3-Carboxy-2-hydroxypropyl)trimethylammonium hydroxide, inner salt; (R)-3-Hydroxy-4-trimethylammoniobutyrate.

C₇H₁₅NO₃ = 161.2.

CAS — 541-15-1.

ATC — A16AA01.

Pharmacopoeias. In Eur. (see p.vi) and US.

Pharmacopoeial description

Ph. Eur.: A white, hygroscopic, crystalline powder or colourless crystals. Freely soluble in water; soluble in warm alcohol; practically insoluble in acetone. A 5% solution in water has a pH of 6.5 to 8.5. Store in airtight containers.

USP 25: White, hygroscopic, crystals or crystalline powder. Freely soluble in water and in hot alcohol; practically insoluble in acetone, in ether, and in benzene. pH of a 5% solution in water is between 5.5 and 9.5. Store in airtight containers.

Adverse Effects and Precautions

Gastrointestinal disturbances such as nausea, vomiting, diarrhoea, and abdominal cramps have been reported following the administration of levocarnitine. Body odour has also been noticed in some patients.

The US manufacturer advises that patients with severe renal impairment should not be given high doses of levocarnitine by mouth for long periods, because of the accumulation of the metabolites trimethylamine and trimethylamine N-oxide. This is said not to occur to the same extent after intravenous administration.

◊ Of 30 patients given DL-carnitine intravenously after dialysis sessions 3 developed myasthenia-like symptoms but when these 3 were given only levocarnitine the symptoms did not occur.[1] It was considered that in anuric uraemic patients the D-isomer was not excreted adequately and that accumulation had blocked neuromuscular transmission. It was therefore suggested that levocarnitine, rather than the DL-form, should be used. (High and prolonged oral doses of levocarnitine should, however, be avoided—see above.)

1. Bazzato G, *et al.* Myasthenia-like syndrome after D.L but not L-carnitine. *Lancet* 1981; i: 1209.

Uses and Administration

Carnitine is an amino acid derivative which is an essential cofactor of fatty acid metabolism.

Carnitine is used in the treatment of primary carnitine deficiency and in carnitine deficiency secondary to a variety of defects of intermediary metabolism or other conditions such as haemodialysis. Both the L- and the DL-isomers have been used, but it is believed that only levocarnitine is effective and in addition, that DL-carnitine supplementation can lead to carnitine deficiency.

In the UK, depending on the condition, up to 200 mg of levocarnitine per kg body-weight daily by mouth is given, administered in 2 to 4 divided doses. Rarely, higher doses of up to 400 mg per kg daily may be needed. In the USA, lower doses of about 1 to 3 g daily are recommended.

When administered intravenously, up to 100 mg per kg daily is given in 3 to 4 divided doses by slow intravenous injection over 2 to 3 minutes. Higher intravenous doses have been given, but are associated with an increased incidence of adverse effects.

In patients with carnitine deficiency secondary to haemodialysis, the recommended dose of levocarnitine is 10 to 20 mg per kg intravenously after each dialysis session, adjusted according to plasma-carnitine concentrations. A maintenance dose of 1 g daily by mouth may be considered (but see Adverse Effects and Precautions, above).

Levocarnitine is under investigation for the treatment of zidovudine-induced mitochondrial myopathy.

Carnitine hydrochloride, carnitine orotate, and bicarnitine chloride have also been used.

◊ Carnitine, which has been the subject of several reviews,[1-4] occurs as distinct L- and D-isomers although naturally-occurring carnitine is almost exclusively the L-isomer. In higher animals carnitine is an essential co-factor of fatty acid metabolism in the heart, liver, and skeletal muscle. It is normally synthesised in the liver, brain, and kidneys in sufficient quantities to meet human requirements but dietary sources such as meat and dairy products also provide carnitine. In plasma and tissues carnitine is present in the free form and as acylcarnitine esters of which acetylcarnitine (see p.1572) is the most abundant.

It has been pointed out that levocarnitine should be used in therapeutics in preference to DL-carnitine, which is the form often present in over-the-counter preparations and dietary supplements. This is because the biochemical and pharmacological profiles of the two isomers differ: levocarnitine acts as a substrate for carnitine acetyltransferase while D-carnitine acts as a competitive inhibitor; also, levocarnitine-induced stimulation of palmitate oxidation is competitively inhibited by D-palmitoylcarnitine. Such differences are believed to account for findings of benefit only with the L-isomer, or unwanted effects when D-carnitine or DL-carnitine was administered.[1,3]

Primary carnitine deficiency is a disorder of the membrane transport of carnitine and patients have presented with hypoglycaemia and encephalopathy, skeletal myopathy, and cardiomyopathy. Therapy with carnitine in these primary deficiency states is considered to have a rational basis.[1,2] Secondary carnitine deficiency occurs in many inherited metabolic disorders and especially in the organic acidurias and disorders of beta-oxidation. Some authors have said that the benefit of carnitine is limited in organic acidurias[2] and unproven or doubtful in disorders of beta-oxidation[2,5,6] while others have disagreed with this view believing treatment may be worthwhile.[7,8]

Carnitine deficiency may also arise during the long-term administration of drugs such as valproic acid,[1] pivampicillin,[9,10] or pivmecillinam,[9] which are conjugated with carnitine. Whether carnitine supplementation can prevent or reverse this type of carnitine deficiency is unclear: treatment with carnitine, although it raised plasma-carnitine concentrations, had no more effect than placebo on the well-being of children receiving valproic acid therapy in one study,[11] but others have found levocarnitine supplementation of value in attenuating valproate-induced hyperammonaemia after a protein-rich meal,[12] and some paediatric neurologists consider supplementation justified in selected children with epilepsy,[13] including those with, or at risk of, valproate-induced hepatotoxicity.

Since carnitine supplementation has been associated with a reduction[14] in the incidence of haemodialysis-induced cramps (p.1322) it has been suggested that these cramps might be due in part to carnitine deficiency.

There is also some evidence[1,15] that carnitine supplements may be of benefit to low birth-weight preterm infants, but a double-blind study[16] failed to confirm this effect. However, premature infants at particular risk of carnitine deficiency, such as those on long-term parenteral nutrition, may benefit.[4,17] Some workers consider that carnitine supplements may be advisable in full-term infants receiving formula feeds.[18]

Low concentrations of carnitine have also been reported to occur in a variety of other conditions and there is some evidence that carnitine supplementation may exert a cardioprotective role. Benefit in patients with cardiomyopathies,[1,19] reduction of infarct size and prevention of arrhythmias in patients with myocardial infarction,[1,2] increased exercise tolerance in patients with angina[1,2] or intermittent claudication,[2] and protection from the cardiotoxicity of the anthracycline antineoplastics[1] have all been described in patients given carnitine supplementation. However, the use of carnitine in healthy subjects in an attempt to improve athletic performance is controversial.[20]

One case report has described a dramatic response of longstanding leg ulcers to carnitine therapy in a patient with sickle-cell disease.[21]

1. Goa KL, Brogden RN. L-Carnitine: a preliminary review of its pharmacokinetics, and its therapeutic use in ischaemic cardiac disease and primary and secondary carnitine deficiencies in relationship to its role in fatty acid metabolism. *Drugs* 1987; **34:** 1–24.
2. Anonymous. Carnitine deficiency. *Lancet* 1990; **335:** 631–3.
3. Li Wan Po A. Carnitine: a scientifically exciting molecule. *Pharm J* 1990; **245:** 388–9.
4. Walter JH. L-Carnitine. *Arch Dis Child* 1996; **74:** 475–8.
5. Anonymous. Medium chain acyl CoA dehydrogenase deficiency. *Lancet* 1991; **338:** 544–5.
6. Rinaldo P, *et al.* Effect of treatment with glycine and L-carnitine in medium-chain acyl-coenzyme A dehydrogenase deficiency. *J Pediatr* 1993; **122:** 580–4.
7. Winter SC, *et al.* Carnitine deficiency. *Lancet* 1990; **335:** 981–2.
8. Chalmers RA, *et al.* Carnitine deficiency. *Lancet* 1990; **335:** 982.
9. Holme E, *et al.* Carnitine deficiency induced by pivampicillin and pivmecillinam therapy. *Lancet* 1989; ii: 469–73.
10. Melegh B. Carnitine supplementation in pivampicillin treatment. *Lancet* 1989; ii: 1096.
11. Freeman JM, *et al.* Does carnitine administration improve the symptoms attributed to anticonvulsant medications?: a double-blinded, crossover study. *Pediatrics* 1994; **93:** 893–5.
12. Gidal BE, *et al.* Diet- and valproate-induced transient hyperammonemia: effect of L-carnitine. *Pediatr Neurol* 1997; **16:** 301–5.
13. De Vivo DC, *et al.* L-carnitine supplementation in childhood epilepsy: current perspectives. *Epilepsia* 1998; **39:** 1216–25.
14. Ahmad S, *et al.* Multicenter trial of L-carnitine in maintenance hemodialysis patients II: clinical and biochemical effects. *Kidney Int* 1990; **38:** 912–8.
15. Shortland GJ, Walter JH. L-carnitine. *Lancet* 1990; **335:** 1215.
16. Shortland GJ, *et al.* Randomised controlled trial of L-carnitine as a nutritional supplement in preterm infants. *Arch Dis Child Fetal Neonatal Ed* 1998; **78:** F185–F188.
17. Sulkers EJ, *et al.* L-carnitine. *Lancet* 1990; **335:** 1215.
18. Giovannini M, *et al.* Is carnitine essential in children? *J Int Med Res* 1991; **19:** 88–102.
19. Helton E, *et al.* Metabolic aspects of myocardial disease and a role for L-carnitine in the treatment of childhood cardiomyopathy. *Pediatrics* 2000; **105:** 1260–70. Correction. *ibid.*; **106:** 623.
20. Tonda ME, Hart LL. N,N-dimethylglycine and L-carnitine as performance enhancers in athletes. *Ann Pharmacother* 1992; **26:** 935–7.
21. Harrell HL. L-Carnitine for leg ulcers. *Ann Intern Med* 1990; **113:** 412.

Preparations

USP 25: Levocarnitine Injection; Levocarnitine Oral Solution; Levocarnitine Tablets.

Proprietary Preparations (details are given in Part 3)
Canad.: Carnitor; **Fr.:** Levocarnil; **Ger.:** Biocarn; L-Carn; Nefrocarnit; **Hong Kong:** Carnitor; **Ital.:** Anetin; Briocar; Cardimet†; Cardiobil; Cardiogen; Carnicor; Carnitene; Carnitolo; Carnitop; Carnovis; Carnum; Carrier; Carvis†; Carvit; Elleci; Eucar; Eucarnil; Farnitin; Framil†; Karrer; Kernit; Lefcar; Levocarvit; Medocarnitin; Megavis; Metina; Miocardin; Miocor; Miotonal; Neo Cardiol; Transfert; **Mex.:** Cardispan; **Port.:** Discocor; **Spain:** Carnicor; Secabiol; **UK:** Carnitor; Elcarn; **USA:** Carnitor; VitaCarn.

Multi-ingredient: Braz.: Hepanisan; Nutrimaiz SM; Pepsivit; **Fr.:** Arkotonic†; **Ital.:** Biocarnil; Carpantin; Co-Carnetina B12; Memorandum; **Mex.:** Lipovitasi-Or; **Spain:** Hepadif; Malandil; Pranzo.

Choline Chloride (7875-g)

Choline Chloride *(rINN)*.

Cholinii Chloridum. 2-Hydroxyethyltrimethylammonium chloride.

C₅H₁₄ClNO = 139.6.

CAS — 62-49-7 (choline); 67-48-1 (choline chloride).

Pharmacopoeias. In Aust. and Fr.

Profile

Choline is an acetylcholine precursor. It is involved in lipid metabolism and acts as a methyl donor in various other metabolic processes. Choline has traditionally been considered to be a vitamin B substance although its functions do not justify its classification as a vitamin. Choline can be synthesised in the body. However, its absence in total parenteral nutrition causes hepatic steatosis, and it is also thought to be a requirement in the diet of neonates. Sources of choline, which occurs mostly as lecithin, include egg-yolk and vegetable and animal fat.

Choline is used as a dietary supplement and has been used to treat liver disorders such as fatty liver and cirrhosis. It has been tried in the management of Alzheimer's disease (see Dementia, p.1412) but without success. Choline is used as the bitartrate, dihydrogen citrate, and orotate salts as well as the chloride.

Human requirements. In the USA, an adequate intake (see p.1352) of 550 mg daily in men and 425 mg daily in women has been determined for choline.[1] The tolerable upper intake level for adults is 3.5 g daily.[1]

1. Standing Committee on the Scientific Evaluation of Dietary Reference Intakes of the Food and Nutrition Board. *Dietary Reference Intakes for thiamin, riboflavin, niacin, vitamin B6, folate, vitamin B12, pantothenic acid, biotin, and choline.* Washington, DC: National Academy Press, 2000.

Preparations

Proprietary Preparations (details are given in Part 3)
Ger.: neurotropan; *Hong Kong:* Athero.

Multi-ingredient: *Aust.:* Orocholin; *Austral.:* Gingo A; Ginkgo ACE†; Anekron; Betaliver; Biofigado; Boldobeba; Colagotil; Colinvintol; Cynatrop; Epacrosil; Epativan B6; Epocler; Ergohepat B12; Eviepar; Extrato Hepatico Composto; Figadobil; Hepalin; Hepasedan; Hepatocler; Hepatotris; Hepofilina; Hormo Hepatico; Lisotox; Litrison; Mesitol; Metiocolin B12; Metiocolin Composto; Metionina Composta; Necrohepat; Neofarmotox; Olocynan; Olohepat; Panvitrop; Scolybil; Vesibil; Xantina B12; Xantinon B12; Xantinon Complex; *Fr.:* Citrocholine; Cystichol; Desintex-Choline; Hepacholine Sorbitol; Hepagrume; Kalicitrine†; Phosphocholine; Romarinex-Choline†; *Ger.:* Hepalipon N†; Hepatofalk; Hepatofalk Neu; Lipovitan; *Hong Kong:* Bilsan; Hepatofalk; *Ital.:* Epa-Treis; *Port.:* Metionina; *S.Afr.:* Hepavite; Prohep; *Spain:* Antibiofilus; Hepato Fardi; *Thai.:* Liporon; Proheparum; *UK:* Fat-Solv; Lipotropic Factors; *USA:* Ak-Biocholine†; Ilopan-Choline.

Chondroitin Sulfate–Iron Complex (14169-a)

Chondroitin Sulphate–Iron Complex; Ferropolichondrum.
CAS — 54391-57-0.

Profile

Chondroitin sulfate-iron complex is employed as a source of iron (p.1366) for iron-deficiency anaemia (p.716). It is given by mouth in doses of up to 900 mg daily, equivalent to up to 90 mg of iron daily.

Preparations

Proprietary Preparations (details are given in Part 3)
Ital.: Condrofer; Ferrol†; Isairon; *Jpn:* Blutal†.

Chromium (18958-w)

Cr = 51.9961.

Chromium Picolinate (11769-a)

Chromium Tripicolinate.
$C_{18}H_{12}N_3O_6Cr$ = 418.3.
Pharmacopoeias. In USNF.

Pharmacopoeial description

USNF 20: Store in airtight containers.

Chromium Trichloride (12560-s)

Chromic Chloride.
$CrCl_3$ = 158.4.
CAS — 10025-73-7 (anhydrous chromium trichloride); 10060-12-5 (chromium trichloride hexahydrate).
Pharmacopoeias. US has a monograph for chromium trichloride hexahydrate.

Pharmacopoeial description

USP 25: Chromium trichloride hexahydrate occurs as dark green, odourless, slightly deliquescent crystals. Soluble in water and in alcohol; slightly soluble in acetone; practically insoluble in ether. Store in airtight containers.

Adverse Effects

Trivalent salts of chromium, such as chromium trichloride, are generally considered to produce few adverse effects. However, hexavalent forms of chromium are notably toxic (see under Chromium Trioxide, p.1594).

Effects on the kidneys. Two cases of renal failure were attributed to ingestion of excessive doses of chromium picolinate (a trivalent chromium salt) in women with no previous history of renal dysfunction.[1,2] For mention of decreases in glomerular filtration rate in children receiving chromium-supplemented total parenteral nutrition, see below.

1. Wasser WG, *et al.* Chronic renal failure after ingestion of over-the-counter chromium picolinate. *Ann Intern Med* 1997; **126:** 410.
2. Cerulli J, *et al.* Chromium picolinate toxicity. *Ann Pharmacother* 1998; **32:** 428–31.

Uses and Administration

Chromium is an essential trace element that potentiates insulin action thus influencing carbohydrate, lipid, and protein metabolism. Dietary sources rich in chromium include brewers' yeast, meat, whole grains, and nuts. Chromium trichloride has been given as a chromium supplement in total parenteral nutrition. Chromium picolinate is used as a chromium supplement, and is being investigated for improving glycaemic control in patients with diabetes mellitus.

Human requirements. In the UK neither a reference nutrient intake (RNI) nor an estimated average requirement (EAR—see p.1352) has been set for chromium although a safe and ad-

equate intake was believed to be above 25 µg daily for adults.[1] Similarly, in the USA a recommended dietary allowance has not been published but the adequate intake was estimated to be 35 µg daily for young men and 25 µg daily for young women.[2] WHO considers that the minimum population mean intake likely to meet normal needs for chromium might be approximately 33 µg daily, and that supplementation of this element should not exceed 250 µg daily until more is known.[3]

1. DoH. Dietary reference values for food energy and nutrients for the United Kingdom: report of the panel on dietary reference values of the committee on medical aspects of food policy. *Report on health and social subjects 41.* London: HMSO, 1991.
2. Standing Committee on the Scientific Evaluation of Dietary Reference Intakes of the Food and Nutrition Board. *Dietary Reference Intakes for vitamin A, vitamin K, arsenic, boron, chromium, copper, iodine, iron, manganese, molybdenum, nickel, silicon, vanadium, and zinc.* Washington DC: National Academy Press, 2001.
3. WHO. Chromium. In: *Trace elements in human nutrition and health.* Geneva: WHO, 1996: 155–60.

Supplementation. Although a daily chromium intake of 200 nanograms per kg body-weight has been suggested in children receiving total parenteral nutrition (TPN), a study in 15 children[1] receiving long-term parenteral nutrition found that supplementation at about this level was associated with serum-chromium concentrations 4 to 42 times higher than the mean value in 15 children not receiving TPN. Raised serum-chromium concentrations were associated with a decrease in glomerular filtration rate; one year after discontinuing chromium supplementation, which reduced intake to 50 nanograms per kg daily (as contaminants of water and TPN solutions), chromium concentrations, although lower, were still higher than controls and renal function had not altered. The authors subsequently discontinued chromium supplementation in both children and adults, since chromium contamination of TPN solutions appeared adequate to prevent deficiency, although it was acknowledged that signs of chromium deficiency might take some years to appear. Chromium contamination in various preparations used in paediatric parenteral nutrition has been studied.[2]

1. Moukarzel AA, *et al.* Excessive chromium intake in children receiving total parenteral nutrition. *Lancet* 1992; **339:** 385–8.
2. Hak EB, *et al.* Chromium and zinc contamination of parenteral nutrient solution components commonly used in infants and children. *Am J Health-Syst Pharm* 1998; **55:** 150–4.

Preparations

USP 25: Chromic Chloride Injection.

Proprietary Preparations (details are given in Part 3)
Austral.: Chrome; *Canad.:* Micro Cr†; *USA:* Chroma-Pak.

Multi-ingredient: *Austral.:* Bio-Chromium; Bioglan 3B Beer Belly Buster; Citri Slim+Trim; Digestaid; Pro-Shape; *Canad.:* Formula CI†; *Fr.:* Bio-Chrome†.

Citrulline (16582-n)

N^5-(Aminocarbonyl)-L-ornithine; N^6-Carbamylornithine. α-Amino-δ-ureidovaleric acid.
$C_6H_{13}N_3O_3$ = 175.2.
CAS — 372-75-8.

Profile

Citrulline is an amino acid which is involved in the urea cycle. Citrulline and citrulline malate are used as dietary supplements.

◊ Citrulline has been given as an alternative to arginine in the management of hyperammonaemia due to urea cycle disorders (p.1354).

Lysinuric protein intolerance is another condition associated with hyperammonaemia and similar neurological sequelae. In this condition there is no deficiency of urea-cycle enzymes but a deficiency of urea-cycle substrate, such as ornithine, which results in reduced synthesis of citrulline. Supplements of citrulline given with meals have been reported to have resulted in a substantial increase in protein tolerance, striking acceleration in linear growth, and an increase in bone mass in a child with this disorder who presented with osteoporosis.[1]

1. Carpenter TO, *et al.* Lysinuric protein intolerance presenting as childhood osteoporosis: clinical and skeletal response to citrulline therapy. *N Engl J Med* 1985; **312:** 290–4.

Preparations

Proprietary Preparations (details are given in Part 3)
Fr.: Stimol; *Port.:* Dynergum.

Multi-ingredient: *Braz.:* Necroplex; Ornihepat; Ornitargin; *Fr.:* Epuram; *Ger.:* Polilevo N; *Ital.:* Ideolider; Ipoazotal; Ipoazotal Complex; Polilevo.

Cod-liver Oil (7890-v)

Cod-liver Oil *(BAN)*.

Aceite de Hígado de Bacalao; Cod Liver Oil; Huile de Foie de Morue; Iecoris Aselli Oleum; Lebertran; Ol. Morrh.; Óleo de Bacalhau; Oleum Jecoris Aselli; Oleum Morrhuae; Olio di Fegato di Merluzzo.
CAS — 8001-69-2.
Pharmacopoeias. In Eur. (see p.vi), Jpn, Pol., and US.

Pharmacopoeial description

Ph. Eur.: The purified fatty oil obtained from the fresh livers of *Gadus morrhua* and other species of Gadidae, solid substances being removed by cooling and filtering. Cod-liver Oil (Type A) and Cod-liver Oil (Type B) both contain not less than 600 units (180 µg) and not more than 2500 units (750 µg) of vitamin A per g and not less than 100 units (1.5 µg) and not more than 250 units (6.25 µg) of vitamin D3 (colecalciferol) per g. Authorised antioxidants in concentrations not exceeding those prescribed by the competent authority may be added.

A clear yellowish viscous liquid. Practically insoluble in water; slightly soluble in alcohol; miscible with petroleum spirit. Store in well-filled airtight containers preferably under an inert gas. Protect from light.

USP 25: The partially destearinated fixed oil obtained from the fresh livers of *Gadus morrhua* and other species of Gadidae. It contains not less than 850 units (255 µg) of vitamin A and not less than 85 units (2.125 µg) of vitamin D per g, and permits up to 1% of a suitable flavour or flavours.

A thin, oily liquid, having a characteristic, slightly fishy but not rancid odour. Slightly soluble in alcohol; freely soluble in carbon disulfide, in chloroform, in ether, and in ethyl acetate. Store in airtight containers. It may be bottled or packaged in containers from which air has been expelled by the production of a vacuum or by an inert gas.

Uses and Administration

Cod-liver oil is a rich source of vitamin D (p.1391) and a good source of vitamin A (p.1382). It also contains several essential fatty acids.

Cod-liver oil dressings or ointment have been advocated to accelerate healing in burns, ulcers, pressure sores, and superficial wounds, but controlled observations have failed to substantiate claims of their value.

Preparations

Proprietary Preparations (details are given in Part 3)
Aust.: Adecaps; *Austral.:* Hypol; *Belg.:* Surmoruine†; *Ger.:* Unguentolan; *Ital.:* Dermovitamina; *Spain:* Aceite Geve Concentrado; *Switz.:* Morrhulan.

Multi-ingredient: *Aust.:* Dermilon; Dermowund; Desitin; Leukichtan; Linobion-Globuli; Mirfulan; Pudan-Lebertran-Zinksalbe; Vitapan; Vulpuran; *Austral.:* Hypol; *Belg.:* Mitosyl; Newderm; Polyseptol; Pyal†; Vitamorrhuine; *Braz.:* Blumen; Dermoglos; Hiposan; Preparado H; Topo Worth; Vitacolor; *Canad.:* Caldesene; Desitin; *Fr.:* Eryteal; Halivite; *Ger.:* Dermilon; Desitin; Leukona-Wundsalbe; Mirfulan; Mirfulan Spray N; Mitosyl; Zinksalbe; *Hong Kong:* Scott's Emulsion Orange; *Irl.:* Caldease; Morhulin; *Israel:* Desitin; Rekasitin; Zincod; *Ital.:* Fosfarsile Yunior; Idustatin†; Neo-Ustiol; Steril Zeta; Trofo 5; Viocidina; *Mex.:* Desitin; Glossderm; *Norw.:* Aselli; *Port.:* Pomaglos; *S.Afr.:* Achromide; Daromide; Ung Vernleigh; *Spain:* Avril; Recto Menaderm†; Siete Mares Higado Bacal†; *Switz.:* Keroderm; Perles d'huile de foie de morue du Dr Geistlich; Phlogidermil†; Vita-Hexin; *UK:* Clogar; M & M; Morhulin; Scott's Emulsion; Woodwards Nappy Rash Ointment†; *USA:* A and D Medicated; Caldesene; Clocream; Desitin; Diaper Rash; Dyprotex; Medicone Dressing†; Primaderm-B†.

Copper (5284-y)

Cu = 63.546.
CAS — 7440-50-8.

Calcium Copperedetate (12505-h)

Calcium [ethylenediaminetetra-acetato{4—}-N,N',O,O']copper (II) dihydrate.
$C_{10}H_{12}CaCuN_2O_8,2H_2O$ = 427.9.
CAS — 66317-91-7 (anhydrous calcium copperedetate).
Pharmacopoeias. In BP(Vet).

Pharmacopoeial description

BP(Vet) 2001: A blue, odourless or almost odourless, crystalline powder. It contains 9.1 to 9.7% of Ca and 14.4 to 15.3% of Cu. Freely soluble in water, the solution gradually precipitating the tetrahydrate; practically insoluble in alcohol.

Copper Chloride (5288-k)

Cupric Chloride.
$CuCl_2,2H_2O$ = 170.5.
CAS — 7447-39-4 (anhydrous copper chloride); 10125-13-0 (copper chloride dihydrate).
Pharmacopoeias. In US.

Pharmacopoeial description

USP 25: Bluish-green, deliquescent crystals. Freely soluble in water; soluble in alcohol; slightly soluble in ether. Store in airtight containers.

Copper Gluconate (18507-g)

Copper D-gluconate (1:2); Bis(D-gluconato-O^1,O^2) copper.
$C_{12}H_{22}CuO_{14}$ = 453.8.
CAS — 527-09-3.
Pharmacopoeias. In US.

The symbol † denotes a preparation no longer actively marketed

Copper Sulfate (5285-j)

Copper Sulph.; Copper Sulphate; Cuivre (Sulfate de); Cupri Sulfas; Cupri Sulphas; Cupric Sulfate; Kupfersulfat; Sulfato de Cobre. Copper (II) sulphate pentahydrate.

$CuSO_4,5H_2O = 249.7$.
CAS — 7758-98-7 (anhydrous copper sulfate); 7758-99-8 (copper sulfate pentahydrate).
ATC — V03AB20.

NOTE. Crude copper sulfate is sometimes known as 'blue copperas', 'blue stone', and 'blue vitriol'.
Pharmacopoeias. In Eur. (see p.vi) and US. Eur. also includes Anhydrous Copper Sulphate.

Pharmacopoeial description

Ph. Eur.: A blue crystalline powder or transparent blue crystals. Freely soluble in water; practically insoluble in alcohol; soluble in methyl alcohol.
Anhydrous Copper Sulphate is a greenish-grey, very hygroscopic, powder. Freely soluble in water; practically insoluble in alcohol; slightly soluble in methyl alcohol. Store in airtight containers.

USP 25: Deep blue, triclinic crystals, or blue, crystalline granules or powder. It effloresces slowly in dry air. Soluble 1 in 3 of water, 1 in 0.5 of boiling water, 1 in 500 of alcohol, and 1 in 3 of glycerol. Its solutions are acid to litmus. Store in airtight containers.

Adverse Effects and Treatment

Adverse effects from copper have tended to arise following absorption of the metal from cooking utensils and during dialysis. Ingestion of copper from cooking utensils is associated mainly with hepatotoxicity. Dialysis procedures may supply copper through the water supply or from parts of the equipment and when this happens patients may suffer haemolysis and other haematological reactions with kidney involvement as well as hepatotoxicity; the toxicity is generally a result of poor equipment maintenance.

Adverse effects attributed to copper have been reported in women with copper-containing intra-uterine devices. There have been isolated case reports of various effects such as allergy and endometrial changes. However, with these devices it is difficult to separate those adverse effects that are due to the device from those due solely to the copper.

The symptoms of Wilson's disease (hepatolenticular degeneration) (see p.1019) are due to an accumulation of copper in various parts of the body.

Copper salts if ingested can produce severe gastrointestinal effects and there may be systemic absorption of copper leading to the effects discussed above. The use of sprays of copper salts in agriculture has been associated with lung changes. Treatment of copper poisoning is symptomatic and may involve the use of a chelating agent to remove any absorbed metal. Dialysis has been tried.

Effects on the liver. A report of cirrhosis and acute liver failure attributable to chronic excessive copper supplement ingestion.[1]

1. O'Donohue J, *et al.* Micronodular cirrhosis and acute liver failure due to chronic copper self-intoxication. *Eur J Gastroenterol Hepatol* 1993; **5:** 561–2.

Interactions

Large doses of zinc supplements may inhibit the gastrointestinal absorption of copper.

Uses and Administration

Copper is an essential trace element although severe copper deficiency, which is associated with anaemia, neutropenia, and bone demineralisation, is rare in humans. Copper sulfate is added to parenteral feeds as a source of copper in the prophylaxis and treatment of deficiency states. Doses that have been employed for prophylaxis range from 0.5 to 1.5 mg (7.9 to 23.6 μmol) of copper daily although up to 3 mg daily has been suggested in established deficiency; infants have received 20 μg (0.3 μmol) of copper per kg body-weight daily. The dose should be governed by the serum-copper concentration which in healthy adults ranges between 0.7 and 1.6 μg per mL (0.01 to 0.025 μmol per mL).

Copper sulfate and other soluble salts of copper have an astringent action on mucous surfaces and in strong solutions they are corrosive.

Copper has a contraceptive effect when present in the uterus and is added to some intra-uterine contraceptive devices; for further details, see below. It is also reported to have an antimicrobial action.

Copper sulfate has been used to prevent the growth of algae in reservoirs, ponds, and swimming pools and as a molluscicide in the control of fresh-water snails that act as intermediate hosts in the life-cycle of the parasites causing schistosomiasis.

Reagents containing copper sulfate are used in tests for reducing sugars.

In veterinary medicine calcium copperedetate, copper methionate, and cuproxoline are used for the prevention and treatment of copper deficiency.

Copper bracelets are worn as a folk remedy for rheumatic disorders: there is no good evidence to justify such a practice.

Copper (Cuprum Metallicum; Cuprum Met.) is used in homoeopathic medicine.

Contraception. In a statement from the Medical Advisory Committee of the Family Planning Association and the National Association of Family Planning Doctors in Great Britain the following points were made.[1] Intra-uterine devices (IUDs) are believed to exert their contraceptive effect (p.1460) by interfering with the reproductive process before the ovum reaches the intra-uterine cavity and the copper released from copper-bearing IUDs probably potentiates this effect. Like all devices which are placed in the uterus, copper IUDs are subject to deposition of cellular debris and of calcium and magnesium salts. The calcium and magnesium salts were once thought to reduce the effectiveness of IUDs, but this is not so as the copper ions are still able to diffuse. Copper IUDs first became available in the 1970s and in the early models the thin copper wire wound around the stem of the device sometimes fragmented or disappeared completely. Subsequent development led to devices that are both more effective and have a longer life. This has been achieved by increasing the wire thickness, by the preparation of a silver-core copper wire, and by the use of solid copper collars or sleeves on the device. The modern copper IUDs in use today should be regarded as being clinically effective and safe for at least five years. Copper IUDs are the most effective available method for emergency contraception (p.1460). Traditional copper IUDs are T-shaped and rigid or semi-rigid. Newer forms include an implantable frameless device, which may be more suitable for nulliparous women.

1. Newton J, Tacchi D. Long-term use of copper intrauterine devices. *Lancet* 1990; **335:** 1322–3.

Deficiency states. Acquired copper deficiency is very rare and the small number of cases have usually involved patients on total parenteral nutrition or in one case[1] enteral nutrition.

Menkes' disease is an X-linked genetic disorder associated with a defect in copper transport, which almost invariably results in death due to progressive cerebral degeneration by the age of 3 years. Early initiation of treatment with copper-histidine complex may be of benefit in such children.[2]

1. Masugi J, *et al.* Copper deficiency anemia and prolonged enteral feeding. *Ann Intern Med* 1994; **121:** 386.
2. Sarkar B, *et al.* Copper-histidine therapy for Menkes' disease. *J Pediatr* 1993; **123:** 828–30.

Human requirements. In the UK dietary reference values (see p.1352) have been published for copper.[1] Although an estimated average requirement (EAR) could not be derived a reference nutrient intake (RNI) of 1.2 mg (19 μmol) daily was set for adults; RNIs of lower values were also specified for infants and children.[1]

In the USA the recommended dietary allowance (RDA) for copper is 900 μg daily in adults, and the tolerable upper intake level is 10 mg daily.[2]

WHO has estimated a minimum population mean intake of 1.2 mg daily for women and 1.3 mg daily for men, and safe upper limits of population mean intakes of 10 mg daily for women and 12 mg daily for men;[3] values are also estimated for infants and children.

1. DoH. Dietary reference values for food energy and nutrients for the United Kingdom: report of the panel on dietary reference values of the committee on medical aspects of food policy. *Report on health and social subjects 41.* London: HMSO, 1991.
2. Standing Committee on the Scientific Evaluation of Dietary Reference Intakes of the Food and Nutrition Board. *Dietary Reference Intakes for vitamin A, vitamin K, arsenic, boron, chromium, copper, iodine, iron, manganese, molybdenum, nickel, silicon, vanadium, and zinc.* Washington DC: National Academy Press, 2001.
3. WHO. Copper. In: *Trace elements in human nutrition and health.* Geneva: WHO, 1996: 123–43.

Schistosomiasis. Although most control programmes for schistosomiasis (p.94) use niclosamide as a molluscicide, and copper salts have largely been abandoned for snail control, copper sulfate was still used for this purpose in Egypt.[1]

1. WHO. The control of schistosomiasis: second report of the WHO expert committee. *WHO Tech Rep Ser 830* 1993.

Preparations

BPC 1973: Compound Ferrous Sulphate Tablets;
USP 25: Cupric Chloride Injection; Cupric Sulfate Injection.

Proprietary Preparations (details are given in Part 3)
Austral.: Multiload; *Braz.:* Multiload; *Canad.:* Gyne-T; Micro Cu†; *Denm.:* CuNova T; Gyne-T; Multiload†; *Fr.:* Gyne-T; Gynefix; Gynelle 375; Ionarthrol; Metacuprol; ML Cu 250†; ML Cu 375†; Multiload; Remoplexe†; *Ger.:* Gyne-T†; Multiload; *Hong Kong:* Gyne-T; Multiload; *Irl.:* Multiload; Ortho Gyne-T†; *Israel:* Anticon; Gyne-T; Mona-Lisa; Multiload; *Ital.:* Gravigard†; Mini-Gravigard†; Multiload; No-Gravid; Telo Cypro; *Mex.:* Multiload; Protec T; *Mon.:* Sertalia; *Neth.:* Gyne-T†; Multiload; *NZ:* Multiload; *Port.:* Multiload; *S.Afr.:* Cuprocept CCL; Dalcept; Multiload; Tricept; *Singapore:* Multiload; *Switz.:* Fincoid†; Multiload†; SOF-T†; *Thai.:* Multiload; *UK:* Gyne-T; Gynefix; Multiload; Novagard†; *USA:* Paragard T380A.

Multi-ingredient: *Austral.:* Alcusal; Alcusal Sport†; APR Cream; Ascoxal; *Braz.:* Belagin; *Canad.:* Nova-T; *Fin.:* Ascoxal; *Fr.:* Bioceanat; Dermalibour; Dermo-Sulfuryl; Dermocreme†; Dermocuivre; Eryase; Femiplexe†; Nova-T; Oligoderm; Ramet Dalibour; Ramet Pain; Ruboderm; Sanoformine†; Septalibour; *Ger.:* Nova-T; *Hong Kong:* Aderma Dermalibour; Nova-T; *Irl.:* Ferrotab; *Israel:* Nova-T; *Ital.:* Cuprosodio; Emmenoiasi; Nova-T; *Mex.:* Ascoxal; Dalidome; Nova-T; *Norw.:* Ascoxal; *NZ:* Nova-T; *Port.:* Cobalti; *S.Afr.:* Nova-T; *Singapore:* Ferromex; Neogobion; Nova-T; *Spain:* Acnosan; *Swed.:* Ascoxal;

Switz.: Nova-T; *Thai.:* Nova-T; *UK:* Foresight Iron Formula; Nova-T; *USA:* ORA5.

Cyclamic Acid (2389-r)

Cyclamic Acid *(BAN, USAN)*.

Cyclam. Acid; E952; Hexamic Acid. *N*-Cyclohexylsulphamic acid.
$C_6H_{13}NO_3S = 179.2$.
CAS — 100-88-9.

Calcium Cyclamate (2379-t)

Calc. Cyclam.; Calcium Cyclohexanesulfamate; Cyclamate Calcium; E952. Calcium *N*-cyclohexylsulphamate dihydrate.
$C_{12}H_{24}CaN_2O_6S_2,2H_2O = 432.6$.
CAS — 139-06-0 (anhydrous calcium cyclamate); 5897-16-5 (calcium cyclamate dihydrate).

Sodium Cyclamate (2409-s)

Sodium Cyclamate *(BAN, rINN)*.

Cyclamate Sodium; E952; Natrii cyclamas; Sod. Cyclam.; Sodium Cyclohexanesulphamate. Sodium *N*-cyclohexylsulphamate.
$C_6H_{12}NNaO_3S = 201.2$.
CAS — 139-05-9.

Pharmacopoeias. In Eur. (see p.vi).

Pharmacopoeial description

Ph. Eur.: A white crystalline powder or colourless crystals. Freely soluble in water; slightly soluble in alcohol. A 10% solution in water has a pH of 5.5 to 7.5.

Profile

Cyclamic acid and its calcium and sodium salts are intense sweetening agents. In dilute solutions (up to about 0.17%) sodium cyclamate is about 30 times as sweet as sucrose but this factor decreases at higher concentrations. When the concentration approaches 0.5%, a bitter taste becomes noticeable. It is stable to heat.

The use of cyclamates as artificial sweeteners in food, soft drinks, and artificial sweetening tablets was at one time prohibited in Great Britain and some other countries because of concern about the metabolite cyclohexylamine, but has since been reappraised to allow their use.

Preparations

Proprietary Preparations (details are given in Part 3)
Braz.: Sucaryl; *Canad.:* Sucaryl.

Multi-ingredient: *Austral.:* Sucaryl; *Braz.:* Adocante Docura; Adocyl C; Belpen; *Fr.:* Sucaryl; *Israel:* Sucrin; *Ital.:* Diet Sucaryl; *NZ:* Sucaryl; *Port.:* Dulceril.

Cysteine (16183-s)

Cysteine *(rINN)*.

C; Cys; L-Cysteine. L-2-Amino-3-mercaptopropionic acid.
$C_3H_7NO_2S = 121.2$.
CAS — 52-90-4.
Pharmacopoeias. In Ger.

Cysteine Hydrochloride (579-e)

Cysteine Hydrochloride *(rINNM)*.

920; Cys Hydrochloride; L-Cysteine Hydrochloride Monohydrate; Cysteini Hydrochloridum Monohydricum. L-2-Amino-3-mercaptopropionic acid hydrochloride monohydrate.
$C_3H_7NO_2S,HCl,H_2O = 175.6$.
CAS — 52-89-1 (anhydrous L-cysteine hydrochloride); 7048-04-6 (L-cysteine hydrochloride monohydrate).
Pharmacopoeias. In Eur. (see p.vi) and US.

Pharmacopoeial description

Ph. Eur.: A white crystalline powder or colourless crystals. Freely soluble in water; slightly soluble in alcohol; practically insoluble in ether. Protect from light.

USP 25: White crystals or crystalline powder. Soluble in water, in alcohol, and in acetone.

Profile

Cysteine is an aliphatic amino acid. Cysteine and cysteine hydrochloride are used as dietary supplements.

Cysteine and cysteine hydrochloride are included in preparations used in ophthalmology; eye drops have been used to prevent corneal ulceration after chemical burns.

Precautions. Cysteine, like other sulfhydryl-containing drugs, could produce a false-positive result in the nitroprusside test for ketone bodies used in diabetes and suspected hepatocellular injury.[1]

1. Csako G, Elin RJ. Unrecognized false-positive ketones from drugs containing free-sulfhydryl group(s). *JAMA* 1993; **269:** 1634.

Preparations

USP 25: Cysteine Hydrochloride Injection.

Proprietary Preparations (details are given in Part 3)
Multi-ingredient: *Austral.:* Ginkgo ACE†; *Fr.:* Lobamine-Cysteine; Phakan; Vita-Iodurol ATP†; Vita-Iodurol†; *Ger.:* Hepatofalk Neu; *Hong Kong:* Hepatofalk; *Port.:* Phakan; *S.Afr.:* Prohep; *Switz.:* Lobamine-Cysteine†; Phakolen; *Thai.:* Proheparum.

Cystine (580-b)

Cystine *(USAN, rINN).*

L-Cystine; Cystinum; Di(α-aminopropionic)-β-disulphide; β,β′-Dithiodialanine. L-3,3′-Dithiobis(2-aminopropionic acid).
$C_6H_{12}N_2O_4S_2 = 240.3.$
CAS — 56-89-3.
Pharmacopoeias. In *Eur.* (see p.vi).

Pharmacopoeial description

Ph. Eur.: A white crystalline powder. Practically insoluble in water and in alcohol. It dissolves in dilute solutions of alkali hydroxides. Protect from light.

Profile

Cystine is an aliphatic amino acid. It is used as a dietary supplement.

Low-methionine diets in conjunction with cystine supplementation have been used in the treatment of congenital homocystinuria (see Amino Acid Metabolic Disorders, p.1350).

Preparations

Proprietary Preparations (details are given in Part 3)
Fr.: Gelucystine; *Ital.:* Cistidil; Mavigen Sebo; *Spain:* Crecil.
Multi-ingredient: *Aust.:* Gelacet; *Canad.:* Amino-Cerv; *Fr.:* Cystichol; Cystine B$_6$; Forcapil; Solacy; *Ger.:* Gelacet N; Gerontamin; Pantovigar; *Switz.:* Gelacet; *USA:* Amino-Cerv.

Dectaflur (3487-p)

Dectaflur *(USAN, rINN).*
SKF-38094. 9-Octadecenylamine hydrofluoride.
$C_{18}H_{38}NF = 287.5.$
CAS — 36505-83-6 (nonstereospecific); 1838-19-3 (9-octadecenylamine).

Profile

Dectaflur is used as a source of fluoride (see Sodium Fluoride, p.1375) in the prevention of dental caries.

Preparations

Proprietary Preparations (details are given in Part 3)
Multi-ingredient: *Aust.:* Elmex; *Belg.:* Elmex; *Fin.:* Elmex; *Ger.:* Elmex; Multifluorid; *Israel:* Elmex; *Ital.:* Elmex; *Neth.:* Elmex; *S.Afr.:* Elmex; *Spain:* Elmex; *Switz.:* Elmex.

Dextrin (581-v)

Dextrin *(BAN).*
British Gum; Dextrinum; Dextrinum Album; Starch Gum.
$[C_6H_{10}O_5]_n.xH_2O.$
CAS — 9004-53-9.
Pharmacopoeias. In *Eur.* (see p.vi), *Chin.,* and *Jpn.* Also in *USNF.*

Pharmacopoeial description

Ph. Eur.: Maize starch or potato starch partially hydrolysed by heat with or without the presence of acids, alkalis, or pH control agents. A white or almost white, free-flowing powder. Very soluble in boiling water forming a mucilaginous solution; slowly soluble in cold water; practically insoluble in alcohol. A 5% dispersion in water has a pH of 2.0 to 8.0.

USNF 20: It is starch, or partially hydrolysed starch, modified by heating in a dry state, with or without acids, alkalis, or pH control agents. A white, yellow, or brown free-flowing powder. Its solubility in water varies; it is usually very soluble, but often contains an insoluble portion.

Icodextrin (17088-a)

Icodextrin *(BAN, rINN).*
$[C_6H_{10}O_5]_n.$
CAS — 9004-53-9.

(1→4)-α-D-Glucan with a weight-average molecular weight of about 20 000 and more than 85% of its molecules with molecular weights between 1640 and 45 000.

Profile

Dextrin, a glucose polymer, is a source of carbohydrate sometimes used in oral dietary supplements and tube feeding. Glucose is rapidly released in the gastrointestinal tract but because of the high average molecular weight of dextrin, solutions have a lower osmolarity than isocaloric solutions of glucose. Additionally, preparations based on dextrin and intended for dietary supplementation usually have a low electrolyte content and are free of lactose and sucrose. These properties make such preparations suitable for dietary supplementation in a variety of diseases including certain gastrointestinal disorders where malabsorption is a problem, in disaccharide intolerance (without isomaltose intolerance), and in acute and chronic hepatic and

renal diseases where protein, mineral, and fluid restriction are often necessary.

Dextrin is also used as a tablet and capsule diluent, and as a binding, suspending, and viscosity-increasing agent. It has also been used as an adhesive and stiffening agent for surgical dressings.

Dextrin sulfate is under investigation in the treatment of HIV infection and AIDS.

Icodextrin is used in dialysis fluids as an alternative to glucose-based solutions (see also below). Icodextrin-based fluids are used as vehicles for administration of drugs via the peritoneal cavity. They may also be instilled intraperitoneally to reduce adhesions after abdominal surgery.

Dialysis. Glucose-based solutions are commonly used in dialysis solutions for continuous ambulatory peritoneal dialysis (CAPD). However, there is rapid absorption of glucose across the peritoneal membrane, reducing the duration of ultrafiltration and leading to long-term metabolic complications such as hyperglycaemia, hyperinsulinaemia, hyperlipidaemia and obesity. Other osmotic agents have been investigated. One study reported results in 11 patients[1] receiving CAPD who had suffered repeated fluid overload from glucose-based dialysis solutions, and suggested that replacement of glucose with dextrin as the osmotic agent could reverse fluid overload and possibly reduce the frequency of exchange. However, others[2] considered that the proposed frequency of exchange would not provide adequate removal of urea, and that in addition to underdialysis there would be an accumulation of poorly-metabolisable glucose polymers in the blood.

Icodextrin is another alternative. It is a glucose polymer, given in iso-osmolar solution. Studies supported by the manufacturers have found that it can be used in ultrafiltration for up to 12 hours, with lower transperitoneal absorption and potential calorie load than glucose solutions.[3,4] It can also be metabolised by amylases in the blood stream, so is less likely to accumulate than other glucose polymers if absorbed.[4] In a study in CAPD patients, icodextrin was well-tolerated and produced at least equivalent ultrafiltration to glucose solutions.[3]

1. Stein A, *et al.* Glucose polymer for ultrafiltration failure in CAPD. *Lancet* 1993; **341:** 1159.
2. Martis L, *et al.* CAPD with dialysis solution containing glucose polymer. *Lancet* 1993; **342:** 176–7.
3. Mistry CD, *et al.* A randomized multicenter clinical trial comparing isosmolar icodextrin with hyperosmolar glucose solutions in CAPD. *Kidney Int* 1994; **46:** 496–503.
4. Peers E, Gokal R. Icodextrin provides long dwell peritoneal dialysis and maintenance of intraperitoneal volume. *Artif Organs* 1998; **22:** 8–12.

Hypersensitivity. Skin reactions, sometimes severe and generalised, have occurred in patients receiving icodextrin.[1-3] Reactions have sometimes been delayed up to about 2 weeks after administration.[3]

1. Fletcher S, *et al.* Icodextrin allergy in a peritoneal dialysis patient. *Nephrol Dial Transplant* 1998; **13:** 2656–8.
2. Goldsmith D, *et al.* Allergic reactions to the polymeric glucose-based peritoneal dialysis fluid icodextrin in patients with renal failure. *Lancet* 2000; **355:** 897.
3. Queffeulou G, *et al.* Allergy to icodextrin. *Lancet* 2000; **356:** 75.

Preparations

USNF 20: Liquid Glucose.

Proprietary Preparations (details are given in Part 3)
Austral.: Poly-Joule; *Fr.:* Caloreen; *Irl.:* Caloreen†; *S.Afr.:* Caloreen†; *Spain:* Icodial; *UK:* Adept; Caloreen; Dexmel.
Multi-ingredient: *Fr.:* Picot.

Ferric Ammonium Citrate (5034-a)

381; Ferricum Citricum Ammoniatum; Iron and Ammonium Citrate.
CAS — 1185-57-5.
ATC — V08CA07.
Pharmacopoeias. In *Chin.* and *US.*

A complex of ammonium ferric citrate.

Pharmacopoeial description

USP 25: It contains between 16.5% and 18.5% of iron. Store in airtight containers at a temperature of 8° to 15°. Protect from light.

Profile

Ferric ammonium citrate is given by mouth as a source of iron (see p.1366) for iron-deficiency anaemia (p.716). It is also used as a food additive to fortify bread.

Preparations

USP 25: Ferric Ammonium Citrate for Oral Solution.

Proprietary Preparations (details are given in Part 3)
Braz.: Vinho Ferruginoso; Vinho Tonificante; *Ital.:* Ferriseltz; Sciroppo Fenoglio; *Spain:* Ferriseltz.
Multi-ingredient: *Aust.:* Ferrovin-Chinaeisenwein; *Belg.:* Ferrifol B12; *Braz.:* Anemokol; Carneferrol; Cobalplex; Emotonico; Ferroben; Ferrotonico B12; Ferrotrat B12; Gladiaton; Hematiase B12; Hepavitose; Rubrobion; Tonico Prata; Tonosai; Veafer; *Canad.:* Geritol; Heparos; Maltlevol; *Ger.:* Praefeminon plus; *Hong Kong:* Nutroplex; *Ital.:* Emopon; *Port.:* Cobalti; *Singapore:* Nutroplex; *UK:* Ironorm; Lexpec with Iron; Lexpec with Iron-M; *USA:* Geritol; Geritonic.

Ferric Pyrophosphate (11422-j)

Iron Pyrophosphate.
$Fe_4(P_2O_7)_3 = 745.2.$
CAS — 10058-44-3.

Profile

Ferric pyrophosphate is given by mouth as a source of iron (see p.1366) for iron-deficiency anaemia (p.716).

Preparations

Proprietary Preparations (details are given in Part 3)
Multi-ingredient: *Austral.:* Incremin Iron; *Mex.:* Incremin Con Hierro; *USA:* Incremin with Iron†; Kovitonic; Vitafol; Vitalize.

Ferritin (3934-z)

Ferritin is the major iron storage protein of vertebrates found mainly in the liver, spleen, intestinal mucosa, and bone marrow and consisting of a soluble protein shell (apoferritin) with a core of crystalline ferric hydroxyphosphate complex.

Profile

Ferritin has been given by mouth as a source of iron (p.1366) in iron-deficiency anaemias (p.716).

Preparations

Proprietary Preparations (details are given in Part 3)
Ital.: Femit; Profer; *Mex.:* Ferroprotina; *Spain:* Ferroprotina; Hierco; Profer†; Tedec Profer.

Ferrocholinate (5042-a)

Ferrocholinate *(rINN).*
$C_{11}H_{20}FeNO_9,2H_2O = 402.2.$
CAS — 1336-80-7.

A chelate prepared by reacting equimolar quantities of freshly precipitated ferric hydroxide with choline dihydrogen tartrate.

Profile

Ferrocholinate is given by mouth as a source of iron (see p.1366) for iron-deficiency anaemia (p.716).

Preparations

Proprietary Preparations (details are given in Part 3)
Spain: Podertonic.

Ferrous Ascorbate (12749-f)

$C_{12}H_{14}FeO_{12} = 406.1.$
CAS — 24808-52-4.
ATC — B03AA10.

Profile

Ferrous ascorbate is used as a source of iron (see p.1366) for iron-deficiency anaemia (p.716). It is given by mouth as the anhydrous form in usual dose units of 245 mg and as a hydrated form in usual dose units of 275 mg; both forms provide about 33 mg of iron per dose unit; the total dose is usually up to the equivalent of 200 mg of iron daily.

Preparations

Proprietary Preparations (details are given in Part 3)
Canad.: Ascofer; *Fr.:* Ascofer; *Spain:* Ferro Semar.
Multi-ingredient: *Aust.:* China-Eisenwein.

Ferrous Aspartate (5044-x)

$C_8H_{12}FeN_2O_8,4H_2O = 392.1.$
ATC — B03AA09.

Profile

Ferrous aspartate is used as a source of iron (see p.1366) for iron-deficiency anaemia (p.716). It has been given by mouth in doses of up to 1.4 g daily (equivalent to about 200 mg of iron daily).

Preparations

Proprietary Preparations (details are given in Part 3)
Belg.: Spartocine; *Fin.:* Spartocine; *Ger.:* Spartocine N.

Ferrous Chloride (18204-j)

Iron (II) chloride tetrahydrate.
$FeCl_2,4H_2O = 198.8.$
CAS — 7758-94-3 (anhydrous ferrous chloride); 13478-10-9 (ferrous chloride tetrahydrate).
ATC — B03AA05.

Profile

Ferrous chloride is used as a source of iron (see p.1366) for iron-deficiency anaemia (p.716). It is given by mouth in usual doses of about 350 to 700 mg daily in divided doses (equivalent to about 100 to 200 mg of iron daily).

Preparations

Proprietary Preparations (details are given in Part 3)
Fr.: Fer UCB; *Ger.:* Ferro 66†; Vitaferro; *Switz.:* Ferrascorbin.
Multi-ingredient: *Switz.:* Ferrascorbin.

The symbol † denotes a preparation no longer actively marketed

Ferrous Fumarate (5054-f)

Ferrosi Fumaras.
$C_4H_2FeO_4 = 169.9$.
CAS — 141-01-5.
ATC — B03AA02; B03AD02.
Pharmacopoeias. In Chin., Eur. (see p.vi), Int., and US.

200 mg of ferrous fumarate contains about 65 mg of iron.

Pharmacopoeial description

Ph. Eur.: A fine, reddish-orange or reddish-brown powder. Slightly soluble in water; very slightly soluble in alcohol. Store in airtight containers. Protect from light.

USP 25: A reddish-orange to red-brown, odourless powder, which may contain soft lumps that produce a yellow streak when crushed. Slightly soluble in water; very slightly soluble in alcohol. Its solubility in dilute hydrochloric acid is limited by the separation of fumaric acid.

Profile

Ferrous fumarate is used as a source of iron (see p.1366) for iron-deficiency anaemia (p.716). It is given by mouth in usual doses of up to 600 mg daily (equivalent to about 200 mg of iron daily); doses of up to 1.2 g daily (equivalent to about 400 mg of iron daily) may be used if necessary.

Preparations

BP 2001: Ferrous Fumarate and Folic Acid Tablets; Ferrous Fumarate Capsules; Ferrous Fumarate Oral Suspension; Ferrous Fumarate Tablets;
USP 25: Ferrous Fumarate and Docusate Sodium Extended-release Tablets; Ferrous Fumarate Tablets.

Proprietary Preparations (details are given in Part 3)
Aust.: Ferretab; Ferrobet; *Belg.:* Ferrum Hausmann; Ferumat; *Braz.:* Ferrin; *Canad.:* Neo-Fer; Novo-Fumar; Palafer; *Fr.:* Fumafer; *Ger.:* Ferrokapsul; Ferrum Hausmann; *Hong Kong:* Ferosof; Triniscon; *Irl.:* Galfer; *Ital.:* Ferro-12; *Mex.:* Biofuroso; Croferron; Fernadin; Ferro-Terapina; Ferval; Gestaferron; Medifer; Regufer; Reufirron; *Neth.:* Ferumat†; *Norw.:* Neo-Fer; *Swed.:* Erco-Fer; *Switz.:* Ferretab; Ferrum Hausmann; *Thai.:* Ferdek; Fermasian; Fermate; *UK:* Fersaday; Fersamal; Galfer; *USA:* Femiron; Feostat; Ferancee†; Ferocyl†; Ferretts†; Ferro-Dok; Ferro-Sequels†; Ferromar†; Fumasorb†; Fumerin†; Hemaspan; Hemocyte; Hemocyte-F; Span-FF†; Vitron-C.
Multi-ingredient: *Aust.:* Ferretab comp; Trinsicon†; *Austral.:* Blackmores for Women Bio Iron; Children's Calcium With Minerals†; Extralife PMS-Care; Medinat PMT-Eze; *Belg.:* Gestiferrol; *Braz.:* Betozone; Iloban; Renutrin; Rubralong; *Canad.:* Appedrine; Caltrate + Iron & Vitamin D†; Dexatrim†; Fortiplex; Palafer CF; Prevencal & D & Fer†; *Fin.:* Matrifolin; *Ger.:* Blutquick Forte S; *Hong Kong:* Fortifier; *Irl.:* BC 500 with Iron; Ferrocap F; Folex; Galfer FA; Givitol; Israel: Folex; Foric; *Mex.:* Autrin; Ferrotemp; *S.Afr.:* Autrin; Pregamal; Trinsicon†; *Singapore:* Odiron-C; *Spain:* Foliferron; *Swed.:* Erco-Fer vitamin†; *Switz.:* Duofer; Duofer Fol; *Thai.:* Adnemic; Adnemic F; Biocalron; FBC; Ferplus-B; Hemarate; Hemolax; Intricon; Polycolvit; Polyvit; Trinsicon; *UK:* Folex; Galfer FA; Givitol; Iron Jelloids†; Meterfolic; Pregaday; *USA:* ABC to Z; Anemagen; Anemagen OB; Berocca Plus; Berplex†; Caltrate + Iron & Vitamin D; Certagen; Cevi-Fer; Chromagen; Chromagen FA; Chromagen Forte; Contrin; Estrostep Fe; Ferotrinsic; Fetrin; Formula B Plus; Fumatinic; Geriot; Gevral T; Hem Fe; Hemocyte Plus; Hemocyte-F; Livitrinsic-f; Loestrin Fe; Nephro-Fer Rx; Parvlex; Polytinic†; Pronemia Hematinic; Stuartinic†; Thera Hematinic; Theragenerix-H; Tolfrinic; TriHEMIC; Trinsicon; Vitafol; Yelets; Zodeac.

Ferrous Gluceptate (13440-s)

Ferrous Glucoheptonate.
$Fe(C_7H_{13}O_8)_2 = 506.2$.
CAS — 25126-38-9.

Profile

Ferrous gluceptate is given by mouth as a source of iron (see p.1366) for iron-deficiency anaemia (p.716).

Preparations

Proprietary Preparations (details are given in Part 3)
Multi-ingredient: *Spain:* Clamarvit; Normovite Antianemico; Normovite Antianemico Inyectable†.

Ferrous Gluconate (5058-m)

Eisen(II)-Gluconat; Ferrosi Gluconas. Iron (II) di(D-gluconate).
$C_{12}H_{22}FeO_{14},xH_2O$.
CAS — 299-29-6 (anhydrous ferrous gluconate); 12389-15-0 (ferrous gluconate dihydrate).
ATC — B03AA03.
Pharmacopoeias. In Eur. (see p.vi).
Pol. and US. specify the dihydrate.

600 mg of ferrous gluconate dihydrate contains about 70 mg of iron.

Pharmacopoeial description

Ph. Eur.: A greenish-yellow to grey powder or granules. It contains not less than 11.8% and not more than 12.5% of ferrous iron calculated with reference to the dried substance. Free-

ly but slowly soluble in water producing a greenish-brown solution, more readily soluble in hot water; practically insoluble in alcohol. A 10% solution in water has a pH of 4.0 to 5.5 three to four hours after preparation. Protect from light.

USP 25: A yellowish-grey or pale greenish-yellow, fine powder or granules having a slight odour resembling that of burnt sugar. Soluble 1 in 5 of water; practically insoluble in alcohol. A 5% solution in water is acid to litmus. Store in airtight containers.

Profile

Ferrous gluconate is used as a source of iron (see p.1366) for iron-deficiency anaemia (p.716). It is given by mouth in doses of up to 1.8 g daily (equivalent to up to 210 mg of iron daily).

A ferric iron compound, ferric sodium gluconate has been employed similarly. It may also be given by slow intravenous injection or infusion in the treatment of iron-deficiency anaemia in haemodialysis patients. The equivalent of 125 mg of iron is administered per dose; a cumulative dose of up to 1 g may be required. Hypersensitivity reactions have been reported.

Preparations

BP 2001: Ferrous Gluconate Tablets;
USP 25: Ferrous Gluconate Capsules; Ferrous Gluconate Elixir; Ferrous Gluconate Tablets.

Proprietary Preparations (details are given in Part 3)
Aust.: Ferro-Agepha; Losferron; *Austral.:* Fergon; *Belg.:* Fenrore; Losferron; *Braz.:* Ferrin; *Canad.:* Fertinic; Novo-Ferrogluc; *Fr.:* Losferron†; *Ger.:* Eisen-Sandoz; Ferrlecit; Ferrum Verla; Losan Fe†; Losferron; Rulofer G; Vitaferro; *Irl.:* Fergon; *Israel:* Ferrlecit; Ferri Nat; Actiferro; Cromatonferro; Emoferrina†; Epaplex 40; Extrafer; Ferlixit; Ferrematos†; Ferri-Emina; Ferritin Oti; Ferrosprint; Fevital Simplex; Fisiofer; Gibifer; Glucoferro; Hemocromo; Inferil; Ipocromo; Ironax†; Lisiofer; Losferron; Rossepar; Rubroferrina; Sanifer; Sustemial; *Neth.:* Losferron; *NZ:* Fergon; *Port.:* Anemital; Hemototal; Losferron; *Switz.:* Loesfer; *USA:* Fergon; Ferralet†; Ferrlecit; Simron†.

Multi-ingredient: *Aust.:* Losferron-Fol; *Braz.:* Apefer; *Fr.:* Tot'Hema; Triogene†; *Ger.:* Biovital Forte N; Blutquick Forte; Blutquick Forte S; Ferro-C-Calcium; Folsana†; *Ital.:* Ferritin Complex; *Port.:* Tot'Hema; *S.Afr.:* Kiddie Vite; *Singapore:* Neogobion; Sangobion; *Spain:* Clamarvit; *Switz.:* Duofer; Duofer Fol; Ferrascorbin; Loesfer + acide folique†; *Thai.:* Ferro-Be-Sian; Glufer-C; Sangobion; *UK:* Ferfolic SV; Foresight Iron Formula; *USA:* Compete; Ferralet Plus; Hemocyte; Hemocyte-V; Hytinic; Iromin-G; Licoplex DS†; Mission Surgical Supplement.

Ferrous Glycine Sulfate (5059-b)

Ferrous Aminoacetosulphate; Ferrous Glycine Sulphate.
CAS — 14729-84-1.

A chelate of ferrous sulfate and glycine.

Profile

Ferrous glycine sulfate is used as a source of iron (see p.1366) for iron-deficiency anaemia (p.716). It is given by mouth in doses containing the equivalent of up to 150 mg of iron daily.

Preparations

Proprietary Preparations (details are given in Part 3)
Denm.: Glycifer; *Fin.:* Obsidan; *Ger.:* Ferro sanol; Ferro sanol duodenal; *Irl.:* Plesmet; *Port.:* Ferrocutid†; *Spain:* Glutaferro; *Switz.:* Ferrosanol duodenal; *UK:* Ferrocontin Continus†; Plesmet.

Multi-ingredient: *Fin.:* Obsidan comp; *UK:* Ferrocontin Folic Continus†.

Ferrous Lactate (5060-x)

Iron Lactate.
$C_6H_{10}FeO_6,3H_2O = 288.0$.
CAS — 5905-52-2 (anhydrous ferrous lactate); 6047-24-1 (ferrous lactate trihydrate).

Profile

Ferrous lactate is used as a source of iron (see p.1366) for iron-deficiency anaemia (p.716).

Preparations

Proprietary Preparations (details are given in Part 3)
S.Afr.: Ferro Drops L; *Spain:* Cromatonbic Ferro.

Multi-ingredient: *Aust.:* Anthozym.

Ferrous Oxalate (5061-r)

Ferrum Oxalicum Oxydulatum; Iron Protoxalate.
$C_2FeO_4,2H_2O = 179.9$.
CAS — 516-03-0 (anhydrous ferrous oxalate); 6047-25-2 (ferrous oxalate dihydrate).
Pharmacopoeias. In Belg.

Profile

Ferrous oxalate has been used as a source of iron (see p.1366) for iron-deficiency anaemia (p.716).

Preparations

Proprietary Preparations (details are given in Part 3)
Multi-ingredient: *Fr.:* Disulone; Ducase†.

Ferrous Succinate (5062-f)

$C_4H_4FeO_4 = 171.9$.
CAS — 10030-90-7.
ATC — B03AA06.

Profile

Ferrous succinate is used as a source of iron (see p.1366) for iron-deficiency anaemia (p.716). It is given by mouth in doses of up to about 600 mg daily (equivalent to up to about 200 mg of iron daily).

Preparations

Proprietary Preparations (details are given in Part 3)
Canad.: Cerevon†; *Denm.:* Ferromyn†; *Fr.:* Inofer; *Ger.:* Ferrlecit 2; *Swed.:* Ferromyn S.

Multi-ingredient: *Belg.:* Ferrifol.

Ferrous Sulfate (5063-d)

Eisen(II)-Sulfat; Ferreux (Sulfate); Ferrosi Sulfas; Ferrous Sulphate; Ferrum Sulfuricum Oxydulatum; Iron (II) Sulphate Heptahydrate; Iron Sulphate.
$FeSO_4,7H_2O = 278.0$.
CAS — 7720-78-7 (anhydrous ferrous sulfate); 7782-63-0 (ferrous sulfate heptahydrate).
ATC — B03AA07; B03AD03.

NOTE. Crude ferrous sulfate is known as Green Vitriol or Green Copperas.
Pharmacopoeias. In Chin., Eur. (see p.vi), Int., Jpn, and US. Swiss also includes ferrous sulfate sesquihydrate.

Ferrous sulfate contains about 60 mg of iron in 300 mg.

Pharmacopoeial description

Ph. Eur.: A light green crystalline powder or bluish-green crystals, efflorescent in air. It is oxidised in moist air, becoming brown. Freely soluble in water; very soluble in boiling water; practically insoluble in alcohol. A 5% solution in water has a pH of 3.0 to 4.0.

USP 25: Pale bluish-green, odourless, crystals or granules. It is efflorescent in dry air and oxidises readily in moist air to form brownish-yellow basic ferric sulfate. Soluble 1 in 1.5 of water and 1 in 0.5 of boiling water; insoluble in alcohol. A 10% solution in water is acid to litmus, having a pH of about 3.7. Store in airtight containers.

Dried Ferrous Sulfate (5064-n)

Dried Ferrous Sulfate (USAN).
Dried Ferrous Sulphate; Exsiccated Ferrous Sulphate; Ferrosi Sulfas Exsiccatus.
CAS — 13463-43-9.
Pharmacopoeias. In Aust., Br., Int., and US.

Pharmacopoeial description

BP 2001: Ferrous sulfate deprived of part of its water of crystallisation by drying at 40°. It contains 86.0 to 90.0% of FeSO₄. A greyish white powder. It dissolves slowly, but almost completely, in freshly boiled and cooled water.

USP 25: A greyish-white to buff-coloured powder consisting primarily of ferrous sulfate monohydrate with varying amounts of ferrous sulfate tetrahydrate. It contains 86.0 to 89.0% of FeSO₄. Slowly soluble in water; insoluble in alcohol.

Profile

Ferrous sulfate is used as a source of iron (see p.1366) for iron-deficiency anaemia (p.716). It is given by mouth and the dried form is frequently used in solid dosage forms and the heptahydrate in liquid dosage forms. Usual doses of dried ferrous sulfate are up to 600 mg daily (equivalent to 180 to 195 mg of iron daily, this figure being somewhat variable depending on the purity and water content of the salt).

Ferrous sulfate oxidised with nitric and sulfuric acids yields ferric subsulfate solution, also known as Monsel's solution, which has been used as a haemostatic.

Preparations

BP 2001: Ferrous Sulphate Tablets; Paediatric Ferrous Sulphate Oral Solution; Prolonged-release Ferrous Sulphate Tablets;
BPC 1973: Compound Ferrous Sulphate Tablets;
USP 25: Ferric Subsulfate Solution; Ferrous Sulfate Oral Solution; Ferrous Sulfate Syrup; Ferrous Sulfate Tablets.

Proprietary Preparations (details are given in Part 3)
Aust.: Ferro-Gradumet; Ferrograd C; Infa-Tardyferon; Tardyferon; *Austral.:* Ferro-Gradumet; Ferrograd C; *Belg.:* Fero-Grad; Fero-Gradumet; Resoferon†; *Braz.:* Fer-In-Sol; Ferroklinge; *Canad.:* Fer-In-Sol; Fero-Grad; Ferodan; Novo-Ferrosulfate; Slow-Fe; *Denm.:* Ferro; *Fin.:* Duroferon; Retafer; *Fr.:* Fero-Grad vitamine C; *Ger.:* Aktiferrin N; Ceferro†; Dreisafer; Eisen-Diasporal;

Eisendragees-ratiopharm; Eryfer; Ferrogamma; FERROinfant N; Haemoprotect; Hamatopan; Kendural C; Plastufer; Tardyferon; Vitaferro; **Hong Kong:** Feospan; Fer-In-Sol; Sorbifer; **Irl.:** Feospan; Fer-In-Sol; Ferrograd; Ferrograd C; **Israel:** Ferro-Gradumet; Slow-Fe; **Ital.:** Fer-In-Sol; Ferrograd; Ferrograd C; **Mex.:** Elfer; Fer-In-Sol; Feriler; Forcil; Hemobion; Hemofer; Ifersol; Regucel; Sulfafer; Tardyferon; Valdefer; **Neth.:** Fero-Gradumet; Liquifer; **Norw.:** Duroferon; Ferro-Retard; Ferromax; **NZ:** Ferro-Gradumet; Ferrograd C; **Port.:** Ferro-Gradumet; Tardyferon; **S.Afr.:** Fero-Grad; Fesofor†; **Singapore:** Retafer; **Spain:** Ferro-Gradumet; Tardyferon; **Swed.:** Duroferon; Tardyferon; **Switz.:** Ferro-Gradumet; Resoferon; **Thai.:** Fer-In-Sol; **UAE:** Kdiron; **UK:** Feospan; Ferrograd; Ferrograd C; Ironorm; Slow-Fe; **USA:** Ed-in-Sol; Fe⁵⁰; Feosol; Fer-gen-sol; Fer-In-Sol; Fer-Iron; Feratab; Fero-Grad; Fero-Gradumet†; Ferospace†; Ferra-TD†; Ferralyn†; Irospan; Mol-Iron†; Slow-Fe.

Multi-ingredient: Aust.: Aktiferrin; Aktiferrin compositum; Ferrograd Fol; Ferrum-Quarz; Kephalodoron; Tardyferon-Fol; **Austral.:** Fefol; FGF Tabs; Irontona; **Braz.:** Anemofer; Betozone; Biotonico Fontoura; Combiron B 12; Coraben; Dobiron; Ferroben; Ferrocomplex; Ferrofran; Ferroplex; Ferrotrat; Iberin Folico; Iberol; Novofer; Rubrargil; Teutonico; Tonico No 1; Trifacta; **Canad.:** Iberet; Slow-Fe Folic; **Fr.:** Tardyferon; Tardyferon B₉; **Ger.:** Biovital N; Eryfer comp; Ferro sanol comp; Ferro sanol gyn; Ferro-Folgamma; Ferro-Folsan; Hamatopan F; Kendural-Fol-500; Kendural-Plus; Plastulen N; Tardyferon-Fol; **Hong Kong:** Iberet; Iberet-Folic; **Irl.:** Fefol; Ferrograd Folic; Ferrotab; Fesovit; **Israel:** Aktiferrin-F; Ferrograd Folic; Slow-Fe Folic; **Ital.:** Cura†; Ferrograd Folic; **Mex.:** Ferro Folico; Iberet; Iberol; Orafer Comp; **Norw.:** Ferrograd Folic; **NZ:** Ferrograd Folic; **Port.:** Ferro-Folsan; Ferrograd Folico; Folifer; Tardyferon-Fol; **S.Afr.:** Effee†; Fefol; Fefol-Vit†; Fero-Folic; Foliglobin; Iberet; Laxicaps†; **Singapore:** Fefol; Ferromex; Iberet; Iberet-Folic; **Spain:** Iberet†; Pildoras Ferrug Sanatori; Vitagama Fluor Complex†; **Switz.:** Actiferrine; Actiferrine-F Nouvelle formule; Fero-Folic; Gyno-Tardyferon; Kendural; Tardyferon; **Thai.:** Iberet; **UK:** Bidor; Dencyl†; Ditemic†; Fefol; Fefol Z†; Ferrograd Folic; Fesovit Z†; Fortespan†; Ironorm; Pregnavite Forte F; Slow-Fe Folic; **USA:** Aqua Ban Plus; Fero-Folic; Generet; Gerivites; Iberet; Iberet-Folic; Slow Fe with Folic Acid.

Ferrous Tartrate (5065-h)

Ferrosi Tartras.

$C_4H_4FeO_6,2\frac{1}{2}H_2O = 249.0$.

CAS — 2944-65-2 *(anhydrous ferrous tartrate).*

ATC — B03AA08.

Profile
Ferrous tartrate has been used as a source of iron (see p.1366) for iron-deficiency anaemia (p.716).

Folic Acid (7860-f)

Folic Acid *(BAN, rINN).*

Acidum Folicum; Folacin; Folinsyre; PGA; Pteroylglutamic Acid; Pteroylmonoglutamic Acid; Vitamin B₉; Vitamin B₁₁. *N*-[4-(2-Amino-4-hydroxypteridin-6-ylmethylamino)benzoyl]-L(+)-glutamic acid.

$C_{19}H_{19}N_7O_6 = 441.4$.

CAS — 59-30-3 *(folic acid);* 6484-89-5 *(sodium folate).*

ATC — B03BB01.

Pharmacopoeias. In *Chin., Eur.* (see p.vi), *Int., Jpn, Pol.,* and *US.*

Pharmacopoeial description
Ph. Eur.: A yellowish or orange crystalline powder. Practically insoluble in water and in most organic solvents. It dissolves in dilute acids and in alkaline solutions. Protect from light.

USP 25: A yellow, yellow-brownish, or yellowish-orange, odourless crystalline powder. Very slightly soluble in water; insoluble in alcohol, in acetone, in chloroform, and in ether. It readily dissolves in dilute solutions of alkali hydroxides and carbonates; soluble in hot, 3N hydrochloric acid and in hot, 2N sulfuric acid; soluble in hydrochloric acid and in sulfuric acid, yielding pale yellow solutions. Protect from light.

Adverse Effects
Folic acid is generally well tolerated. Gastrointestinal disturbances and hypersensitivity reactions have been reported rarely.

Precautions
Folic acid should never be given alone or in conjunction with inadequate amounts of vitamin B₁₂ for the treatment of undiagnosed megaloblastic anaemia, since folic acid may produce a haematopoietic response in patients with a megaloblastic anaemia due to vitamin B₁₂ deficiency without preventing aggravation of neurological symptoms. This masking of the true deficiency state can lead to serious neurological damage, such as subacute combined degeneration of the spinal cord (see also below).

Vitamin B₁₂ deficiency. The issue of fortification of food with folic acid to reduce the number of infants born with neural tube defects (see below) has created debate on the risks of masking vitamin B₁₂ deficiency, particularly in the elderly. As

mentioned in Precautions, above, it is accepted that folic acid should not be used in megaloblastic anaemia due to vitamin B₁₂ deficiency, because it will not prevent the neurological manifestations of this deficiency, and may delay the diagnosis. Masking of vitamin B₁₂ deficiency has been noted with daily doses of folic acid of 5 mg, and it is generally considered that very low doses do not have this effect. It has also been stated that folic acid may precipitate the neurological manifestations of vitamin B₁₂ deficiency; however, a review of the evidence suggests this is unlikely.[1]

Nevertheless, concerns regarding neurological effects of vitamin B₁₂ deficiency in the elderly have led to adoption of a level of folic acid fortification in the USA that is accepted will not provide optimum protection against neural tube defects, but that is hoped will minimise any risks.[2] It has been suggested that concomitant fortification with vitamin B₁₂ might also be a solution.

1. Dickinson CJ. Does folic acid harm people with vitamin B₁₂ deficiency? *Q J Med* 1995; **88:** 357–64.
2. Tucker KL, *et al.* Folic acid fortification of the food supply: potential benefits and risks for the elderly population. *JAMA* 1996; **276:** 1879–85. Correction. *ibid.* 1997; **277:** 714.

Interactions
Folate deficiency states may be produced by a number of drugs including antiepileptics, oral contraceptives, antituberculous drugs, alcohol, and folic acid antagonists such as aminopterin, methotrexate, pyrimethamine, trimethoprim, and sulfonamides. In some instances, such as during methotrexate or antiepileptic therapy, replacement therapy with folinic acid or folic acid may become necessary in order to prevent megaloblastic anaemia developing; folate supplementation has reportedly decreased serum-phenytoin concentrations in a few cases (see Interactions, Vitamins, p.362) and there is a possibility that such an effect could also occur with barbiturate antiepileptics.

Antiepileptic-associated folate deficiency is discussed further under Adverse Effects of Phenytoin, p.358.

◊ References.
1. Lambie DG, Johnson RH. Drugs and folate metabolism. *Drugs* 1985; **30:** 145–55.

Pharmacokinetics
Folic acid is rapidly absorbed from the gastrointestinal tract, mainly from the duodenum and jejunum. Dietary folates are stated to have about half the bioavailability of crystalline folic acid. The naturally occurring folate polyglutamates are largely deconjugated and reduced by dihydrofolate reductase in the intestines to form 5-methyltetrahydrofolate, which appears in the portal circulation, where it is extensively bound to plasma proteins. Folic acid administered therapeutically enters the portal circulation largely unchanged since it is a poor substrate for reduction by dihydrofolate reductase. It is converted to the metabolically active form 5-methyltetrahydrofolate in the plasma and liver.

The principal storage site of folate is the liver; it is also actively concentrated in the CSF.

Folate undergoes enterohepatic circulation. Folate metabolites are eliminated in the urine and folate in excess of body requirements is excreted unchanged in the urine. Folate is distributed into breast milk. Folic acid is removed by haemodialysis.

Human Requirements
Body stores of folate in healthy persons have been reported as being between 5 to 10 mg, but may be much higher. In the UK about 150 to 200 µg of folate daily is considered a suitable average intake for all healthy persons except women of child-bearing potential and pregnant women who require additional folic acid to protect against neural tube defects in their offspring (see below). In the US the recommended dietary allowance is 400 µg of dietary folate equivalents (see below) in both men and women. Folate is present, chiefly combined with several L(+)-glutamic acid moieties, in many foods, particularly liver, kidney, yeast, nuts, and leafy green vegetables. The vitamin is readily oxidised to unavailable forms and is easily destroyed during cooking.

◊ In the UK dietary reference values (see p.1352) have been published for folate.[1] In the USA recommended dietary allow-

ances (RDAs) had been set, and have recently been reviewed[2] under the programme to set Dietary Reference Intakes (see p.1352). Differing amounts are recommended for infants and children of varying ages, for adult males and females, and for pregnant and lactating women. In the UK the Reference Nutrient Intake (RNI) for adult males and females is 200 µg daily and the Estimated Average Requirement (EAR) is 150 µg daily. In the USA the RDA is expressed in terms of dietary folate equivalents (DFEs) where 1 µg DFE is equivalent to 1 µg folate from natural sources, 0.5 µg of a folic acid supplement taken on an empty stomach, or 0.6 µg of folic acid from fortified food or as a supplement taken with meals. An RDA of 400 µg DFE daily for adult men and women has been set; the EAR is 320 µg DFE daily and the tolerable upper intake level is 1 mg daily.

Folate requirements are increased during pregnancy; an RNI of 300 µg daily has been suggested for pregnant women in the UK and an RDA of 600 µg daily in the USA. In view of the value of folate in preventing neural tube defects, it is now recommended that women planning a pregnancy receive supplemental folic acid before conception and during the first trimester (see Neural Tube Defects, below). To increase the intake in women of child-bearing age, folic acid fortification of grain-based foods has been adopted in the USA, and advocated in other countries including the UK. However, there remains some debate over the appropriate level of fortification to optimise prevention of neural tube defects and to minimise the risks of masking underlying vitamin B₁₂ deficiency in the elderly.

1. DoH. Dietary reference values for food energy and nutrients for the United Kingdom: report of the panel on dietary reference values of the committee on medical aspects of food policy. *Report on health and social subjects 41.* London: HMSO, 1991.
2. Standing Committee on the Scientific Evaluation of Dietary Reference Intakes of the Food and Nutrition Board. *Dietary Reference Intakes for thiamin, riboflavin, niacin, vitamin B₆, folate, vitamin B₁₂, pantothenic acid, biotin, and choline.* Washington, DC: National Academy Press, 2000.

Uses and Administration
Folic acid is a member of the vitamin B group. Folic acid is reduced in the body to tetrahydrofolate, which is a coenzyme for various metabolic processes including the synthesis of purine and pyrimidine nucleotides, and hence in the synthesis of DNA; it is also involved in some amino-acid conversions, and in the formation and utilisation of formate. Deficiency, which can result in megaloblastic anaemia (p.717), develops when the dietary intake is inadequate (as in malnutrition), when there is malabsorption (as in sprue), increased utilisation (as in pregnancy or conditions such as haemolytic anaemia), increased loss (as in haemodialysis), or as a result of the administration of folate antagonists and other drugs that interfere with normal folate metabolism (see Interactions, above).

Folic acid is used in the treatment and prevention of the folate deficiency state. It does not correct folate deficiency due to dihydrofolate reductase inhibitors; calcium folinate (p.1363) is used for this purpose. Folic acid is also used in women of child-bearing potential and pregnant women to protect against neural tube defects in their offspring. This is discussed in more detail in Neural Tube Defects, below.

For the treatment of folate-deficient megaloblastic anaemia it is recommended in the UK that folic acid is given by mouth in doses of 5 mg daily for 4 months; up to 15 mg daily may be necessary in malabsorption states. Continued administration of folic acid 5 mg every 1 to 7 days by mouth may be necessary in chronic haemolytic states such as thalassaemia major or sickle-cell anaemia, depending on the diet and rate of haemolysis; similar doses may be necessary in some patients receiving renal dialysis in order to prevent deficiency.

In the USA the usual recommended therapeutic dose for folate deficiency is lower; folic acid 0.25 to 1 mg daily by mouth is suggested until a haematopoietic response has been obtained, although some patients require higher doses, especially in malabsorption states. The usual maintenance dose is 0.4 mg daily.

In the prophylaxis of megaloblastic anaemia of pregnancy, the usual dose is 0.2 to 0.5 mg daily in the UK, and up to 1 mg daily in the USA.

For women of child-bearing potential at high risk of having a pregnancy affected by neural tube defect, the dose of folic acid is 4 or 5 mg daily starting before pregnancy (in the USA the recommendation is 4 weeks before) and continued through the first trimester. For other women of child-bearing potential the dose in the UK is 0.4 mg daily.

Folic acid may also be given by intramuscular, intravenous, or subcutaneous injection as the sodium salt.

Deficiency states. Reviews of the use of folic acid in conditions associated with folate deficiency.

1. Davis RE. Clinical chemistry of folic acid. *Clin Chem* 1986; **25:** 233–94.
2. Crellin R, *et al.* Folates and psychiatric disorders: clinical potential. *Drugs* 1993; **45:** 623–36.
3. Wickramasinghe SN. Folate and vitamin B$_{12}$ deficiency and supplementation. *Prescribers' J* 1997; **37:** 88–95.

Ischaemic heart disease. Elevated blood-homocysteine concentrations appear to be an independent risk factor for atherosclerosis and ischaemic heart disease (p.793),[1] and there is evidence that they are inversely related to blood-folate concentrations.[2] Epidemiological studies[3,4] indicate that individuals with a high intake of folate or vitamin B$_6$ from vitamin supplements or food are at lower risk of ischaemic heart disease. Furthermore, meta-analyses suggest that administration of folic acid reduces blood-homocysteine levels,[2,5] and that vitamin B$_{12}$, but not B$_6$, may have an additional effect.[5] Thus, there is growing interest in conducting prospective randomised trials to assess the effect of folic acid in the primary or secondary prevention of ischaemic heart disease. The American Heart Association has stated that until the results of these trials become available routine testing of plasma-homocysteine concentrations cannot be justified.[6] However all patients should be encouraged to consume the recommended dietary allowance (RDA) of folate, vitamin B$_6$ and vitamin B$_{12}$.[6]

In a study[7] in renal transplant recipients with hyperhomocysteinaemia, vitamin B$_6$ was effective in reducing post-methionine-loading plasma homocysteine concentrations, and folic acid plus vitamin B$_{12}$ was effective in lowering fasting plasma-homocysteine concentrations. The authors concluded that all three of these B-group vitamins may have a role in reducing atherosclerotic outcomes in this patient group.[7]

1. Welch GN, Loscalzo J. Homocysteine and atherothrombosis. *N Engl J Med* 1998; **338:** 1042–50.
2. Boushey CJ, *et al.* A quantitative assessment of plasma homocysteine as a risk factor for vascular disease: probable benefits of increasing folic acid intakes. *JAMA* 1995; **274:** 1049–57.
3. Morrison HI, *et al.* Serum folate and risk of fatal coronary heart disease. *JAMA* 1996; **275:** 1893–6.
4. Rimm EB, *et al.* Folate and vitamin B$_6$ from diet and supplements in relation to risk of coronary heart disease among women. *JAMA* 1998; **279:** 359–64.
5. Homocysteine Lowering Trialists' Collaboration. Lowering blood homocysteine with folic acid based supplements: meta-analysis of randomised trials. *BMJ* 1998; **316:** 894–8.
6. Malinow MR, *et al.* Homocyst(e)ine, diet, and cardiovascular diseases: a statement for healthcare professionals from the Nutrition Committee, American Heart Association. *Circulation* 1999; **99:** 178–82.
7. Bostom AG, *et al.* Treatment of hyperhomocysteinemia in renal transplant recipients. *Ann Intern Med* 1997; **127:** 1089–92.

Neural tube defects. Failure of the fetal neural tube to fuse normally during the first 4 weeks of pregnancy may result in one of several congenital defects. These include anencephaly (absence of the brain and cranial vault) and spina bifida (failure of the vertebrae to fuse). The latter ranges from spina bifida occulta, where neurological abnormalities are rare, to meningocoele or meningomyelocoele, where the meninges, or meninges and spinal cord, herniate outwards through the vertebral defect and which may be associated with hydrocephalus and paralysis of the lower limbs and sphincters.

The reasons for this failure in normal development are not well understood and appear to include both environmental and genetic factors. The risk is increased in certain geographical areas, and in the offspring of parents with previous children who had neural tube defects, or of parents who themselves suffer from the condition.

A defect in the methylenetetrahydrofolate reductase gene has been identified, which is estimated to occur in about 5 to 15% of white populations, and appears to result in an increased requirement for folates, and an increased risk of recurrent early pregnancy loss and neural tube defects.[1,2] Since the 1960s there has been some evidence that the mother's folate status was significant, and in the early 1980s two groups published evidence for claims that the oral administration of folic acid, with or without other vitamins, in the period around conception, reduced the incidence of neural tube defect in the offspring of mothers who had previously borne children with the defect.[3,4]

Although criticised on several grounds, the conclusions of these studies were borne out by a large multicentre study initiated by the Medical Research Council (MRC) of the UK.[5] This study was terminated early because of overwhelming evidence that folic acid 4 mg daily taken from before conception until the twelfth week of gestation by women with a history of a previous pregnancy affected by a neural tube defect reduced the incidence of such defect by about two-thirds. Other studies and systematic reviews have since confirmed the benefits of supplementation.[6,7] Multivitamins alone (A, D, B$_1$, B$_2$, nicotinamide, B$_6$, and C) did not demonstrate a similar benefit.

Prevention of recurrence. In the light of the MRC study, it is recommended in the UK that in couples with spina bifida or a history of previous offspring with neural tube defect, all those women who may become pregnant should receive folic acid 5 mg daily (in the absence of a commercially-available 4 mg

dosage form) until the twelfth week of pregnancy.[8] In the USA, recommendations are 4 mg of folic acid daily from at least four weeks before conception through the first 3 months of pregnancy.[9] It must be borne in mind that only about 60 to 70% of neural tube defects appear to be folate-sensitive, and parents should be counselled appropriately.

The investigators in the MRC trial acknowledged that a 4 mg dose may not be optimal, and both early[3,4] and later[10] studies imply that much lower doses of folic acid may reduce the risk of recurrence, but this has yet to be clearly demonstrated. Furthermore, the optimum length of time that supplements should be given to these women before conception is unknown.

Prevention of occurrence. First occurrences of neural tube defects account for about 95% of cases, and there are obvious public health implications if the benefits of folate in mothers known to be at risk can be extended to the general population. A study in Hungary[11] indicated that folic acid 0.8 mg daily with multivitamins, taken for at least one month before conception and until the third month of gestation decreased the incidence of first occurrence of neural tube defects. A case control study in the USA[12] (where the normal incidence of neural tube defect is much lower than Hungary) suggested that a periconceptional folic acid intake of as little as 0.4 mg daily reduced the occurrence of the disorder by 60%.

With such results in mind the US Public Health Service has recommended that all women of child-bearing age who are capable of pregnancy should receive folic acid 0.4 mg daily although care should be taken to keep folate consumption below 1 mg daily except under medical supervision.[13] Such universal coverage would allow for the problem of unplanned pregnancies but would be difficult to achieve, other than by fortification of dietary staples with folate. Food fortification has therefore been adopted in the USA, at a level of 140 µg of folic acid per 100 g of cereal-grain product. While this amount will probably be insufficient to provide maximum reduction in the incidence of neural tube defects,[14,15] there is some evidence of benefit,[16] and it was chosen to minimise the risk of masking vitamin B$_{12}$ deficiency in the elderly.[17] Efforts to increase the use of folic acid supplements in women of child-bearing potential are still advocated.

In the UK, the current recommendation is that all women planning a pregnancy should take an extra 0.4 mg of folic acid daily before conception and during the first twelve weeks of pregnancy, bringing the average folate intake to about 0.6 mg daily.[8] In unplanned pregnancies, supplementation should begin as soon as pregnancy is suspected. As in the USA food fortification is being considered and some food is already fortified on a voluntary basis; however, the current emphasis is on education. Patients receiving antiepileptic drugs are at increased risk of neural tube defect and it has been suggested that folic acid supplementation for such patients should be at the level used for prevention of recurrence,[18] i.e. 4 or 5 mg daily.

The mechanism by which folic acid protects against neural tube defects is unknown, but various theories have been postulated including a positive effect in promoting neural tube closure,[19] or a selective abortifacient effect on affected fetuses (teratanasia),[20] although the latter has been disputed.[21] There is some evidence that low maternal vitamin B$_{12}$ concentrations are an independent risk factor for neural tube defects,[22,23] perhaps indicating a role for methionine synthase in their aetiology, and suggesting that additional supplementation with cobalamins may be warranted, or that methionine supplements could be investigated as an alternative to folic acid.[24] Interestingly, the results from the Hungarian programme[25,26] and from other studies[27,28] suggest that multivitamin supplements (including folic acid) may also reduce the occurrence of other congenital abnormalities.

1. Molloy AM, *et al.* Thermolabile variant of 5,10-methylenetetrahydrofolate reductase associated with low red-cell folates: implications for folate intake recommendations. *Lancet* 1997; **349:** 1591–3.
2. Nelen WLDM, *et al.* Recurrent early pregnancy loss and genetic-related disturbances in folate and homocysteine metabolism. *Br J Hosp Med* 1997; **58:** 511–13.
3. Smithells RW, *et al.* Apparent prevention of neural tube defects by periconceptional vitamin supplementation. *Arch Dis Child* 1981; **56:** 911–18.
4. Laurence KM, *et al.* Double-blind randomised controlled trial of folate treatment before conception to prevent recurrence of neural tube defects. *BMJ* 1981; **282:** 1509–11.
5. MRC Vitamin Study Research Group. Prevention of neural tube defects: results of the Medical Research Council vitamin study. *Lancet* 1991; **338:** 131–7.
6. Berry RJ, *et al.* Prevention of neural-tube defects with folic acid in China. *N Engl J Med* 1999; **341:** 1485–90. Correction. *ibid.*; 1864.
7. Lumley J, *et al.* Periconceptional supplementation with folate and/or multivitamins for preventing neural tube defects (updated 31 May 2001). Available in The Cochrane Library; Issue 3. Oxford: Update Software; 2001.
8. DoH. *Folic acid and the prevention of neural tube defects: report from an expert advisory group.* London: Department of Health, 1992.
9. Centers for Disease Control. Use of folic acid for prevention of spina bifida and other neural tube defects—1983-1991. *MMWR* 1991; **40:** 513–16.
10. Kirke PN, *et al.* A randomised trial of low dose folic acid to prevent neural tube defects. *Arch Dis Child* 1992; **67:** 1442–6.
11. Czeizel AE, Dudás I. Prevention of the first occurrence of neural-tube defects by periconceptional vitamin supplementation. *N Engl J Med* 1992; **327:** 1832–5.
12. Werler MM, *et al.* Periconceptional folic acid exposure and risk of occurrent neural tube defects. *JAMA* 1993; **269:** 1257–61.

13. Centers for Disease Control. Recommendations for use of folic acid to reduce number of spina bifida cases and other neural tube defects. *JAMA* 1993; **269:** 1233–8.
14. Daly S, *et al.* Minimum effective dose of folic acid for food fortification to prevent neural-tube defects. *Lancet* 1997; **350:** 1666–9.
15. Brown JE, *et al.* Predictors of red cell folate level in women attempting pregnancy. *JAMA* 1997; **277:** 548–52.
16. Honein M, *et al.* Impact of folic acid fortification of the US food supply on the occurrence of neural tube defects. *JAMA* 2001; **285:** 2981–6.
17. Tucker KL, *et al.* Folic acid fortification of the food supply: potential benefits and risks for the elderly population. *JAMA* 1996; **276:** 1879–85. Correction. *ibid.* 1997; **277:** 714.
18. Girling JC, Shennan AH. Epilepsy and pregnancy. *BMJ* 1993; **307:** 937.
19. Zhao Q, *et al.* Prenatal folic acid treatment suppresses acrania and meroanencephaly in mice mutant for the Cart1 homeobox gene. *Nat Genet* 1996; **13:** 275–83.
20. Hook EB, Czeizel AE. Can teratanasia explain the protective effect of folic-acid supplementation on birth defects? *Lancet* 1997; **350:** 513–15.
21. Burn J, Fisk NM. Teratanasia, folic acid, and birth defects. *Lancet* 1997; **350:** 1322–3.
22. Kirke PN, *et al.* Maternal plasma folate and vitamin B$_{12}$ are independent risk factors for neural tube defects. *Q J Med* 1993; **86:** 703–8.
23. Mills JL, *et al.* Homocysteine metabolism in pregnancies complicated by neural-tube defects. *Lancet* 1995; **345:** 149–51.
24. Klein NW. Folic acid and prevention of spina bifida. *JAMA* 1996; **275:** 1636.
25. Czeizel AE. Prevention of congenital abnormalities by periconceptional multivitamin supplementation. *BMJ* 1993; **306:** 1645–8.
26. Czeizel AE. Reduction of urinary tract and cardiovascular defects by periconceptional multivitamin supplementation. *Am J Med Genet* 1996; **62:** 179–83.
27. Shaw GM, *et al.* Risks of orofacial clefts in children born to women using multivitamins containing folic acid periconceptionally. *Lancet* 1995; **346:** 393–6.
28. Botto LD, *et al.* Periconceptional multivitamin use and the occurrent of conotruncal heart defects: results from a population-based, case-control study. *Pediatrics* 1996; **98:** 911–17.

Prophylaxis of malignant neoplasms. For reference to an epidemiological study suggesting that long-term use of folate-containing multivitamin supplements may be associated with a reduced risk of colon cancer, see p.1353.

Preparations

BP 2001: Ferrous Fumarate and Folic Acid Tablets; Folic Acid Tablets;
USP 25: Folic Acid Injection; Folic Acid Tablets.

Proprietary Preparations (details are given in Part 3)

Aust.: Folsan; *Austral.:* Megafol; *Belg.:* Folavit; *Braz.:* Acfol; Endofolin; Folacin; *Canad.:* Folvite†; Novo-Folacid†; *Fin.:* Folvite; *Fr.:* Speciafoldine; *Ger.:* Fol-Asmedic; Folarell; Folgamma Mono; Folsan; Folverlan; Lafol; RubieFol; *Hong Kong:* Foliamin; Triniscon; *Irl.:* Cardioguard; Clonfolic; *Ital.:* Folina; Folingrav; *Mex.:* AF; Ferranina Fol; Folitab; Precileucin; *Port.:* Folicil; *Spain:* Acfol; *Swed.:* Folacin; *Switz.:* Andreafol; Foli-Rivo; Folvite; *Thai.:* Foliamin; Folivit; Lafol; *Turk.:* Folatine; Folicare; Lexpec; Preconceive; *USA:* Fe-Tinic Forte; Folvite.

Multi-ingredient: *Aust.:* Aktiferrin compositum; Beneuran compositum; Ferretab comp; Ferrograd Fol; Losferron-Fol; Tardyferon-Fol; Trinicon†; *Austral.:* Antioxidant Forte Tablets; Children's Calcium With Minerals†; Fefol; FGF Tabs; Pre Natal; VitaPreg; *Belg.:* Ferrifol; Ferrifol B12; Gestiferrol; *Braz.:* Anemofer; Betozone; Cobalplex; Coraben; Ferroplex; Ferrotrat; Folacin; Iberin Folico; Iloban; Noripurum Folico; Vi-Ferrin; *Canad.:* Folacin 12; Palafer CF; Slow-Fe Folic; *Fin.:* Folina; Obsidan comp; *Fr.:* Tardyferon B$_9$; *Ger.:* B$_{12}$ Fol-Vicotrat; Eryfer comp; Ferro sanol comp; Ferro sanol gyn; Ferro-Folgamma; Ferro-Folsan; Folgamma; Folicombin; Folsana†; Hamatopan F; Hepagrisevit Forte-N; Kendural-Fol-500; Medivitan N; Medyn; MerSol; Plastulen N; Selectafer N; Tardyferon-Fol; *Hong Kong:* Epargriseovit; Hepatofalk; Iberet-Folic; *Irl.:* Fefol; Ferrocap F; Ferrograd Folic; Folex; Galfer FA; Givitol; *Israel:* Aktiferrin-F; Ferrifol-3; Ferrograd Folic; Folex; Foric; Slow-Fe Folic; *Ital.:* Efargen; Epargriseovit; Ferrograd Folic; Folepar B12; Oro B12; *Mex.:* Ferro Folico; Orafer Comp; *Norw.:* Pregnifer; *NZ:* Ferrograd Folic; *Port.:* Ferro-Folsan; Ferrograd Folico; Ferrum Fol; Folifer; Tardyferon-Fol; *S.Afr.:* Effee†; Fefol; Fefol-Vit†; Fero-Folic; Ferrimed; Foliglobin; Hepabionta; Pregamal; Trinicon†; *Singapore:* Fefol; Iberet-Folic; Neogobion; Sangobion; *Spain:* Foliferron; Hepa Factor†; Normovite Antianemico; Normovite Antianemico Inyectable†; *Switz.:* Actiferrine-F Nouvelle formule; Duofer Fol; Fero-Folic; Gyno-Tardyferon; Losferron-Fol; Maltofer Fol; *Thai.:* Ademic F; Cilfer-12-F; Sangobion; Triniscon; *UK:* Dencyl†; Fefol; Fefol Z†; Ferfolic SV; Ferrocontin Folic Continus†; Ferrograd Folic; Folex; Folic Plus; Fortespan†; Galfer FA; Givitol; Hematinic; Ironorm; Lexpec with Iron; Lexpec with Iron-M; Meterfolic; Pregaday; Pregnavite Forte F; Slow-Fe Folic; *USA:* ABC to Z; Berocca Plus; Berplex†; Bevitamel; Centurion A–Z; Certagen; Cevi-Fer; Chromagen FA; Chromagen Forte; Compete; Contrin; Feocyte; Fero-Folic; Ferotrinsic; Ferralet Plus; Ferrex Forte; FOLTX; Formula B Plus; Geriot; Geritol Complete; Gevral T; Hemocyte Plus; Hemocyte-F; Iberet-Folic; Iromin-G; Kovitonic; Livitrinsic-f; Nephro-Fer Rx; Niferex Forte; Nu-Iron Plus; Nu-Iron V; Parvlex; Poly-Iron Forte; Polytinic†; PremesisRx; Pronemia Hematinic; Slow Fe with Folic Acid; Thera Hematinic; Theragenerix-H; Theravee Hematinic; TriHEMIC; Triniscon; Vita-Feron†; Vitafol; Yelets; Zodeac.

Folinic Acid (7862-n)

Citrovorum Factor; Leucovorin. 5-Formyltetrahydropteroylglutamic acid; N-[4-(2-Amino-5-formyl-5,6,7,8-tetrahydro-4-hydroxypteridin-6-ylmethylamino)benzoyl]-L(+)-glutamic acid.

$C_{20}H_{23}N_7O_7 = 473.4$.
CAS — 58-05-9.

Calcium Folinate (7863-h)

Calcium Folinate (BAN, rINN).

Calcium Folinate-SF; Calcium Leucovorin; Leucovorin Calcium; NSC-3590. The calcium salt of folinic acid (1:1).

$C_{20}H_{21}CaN_7O_7 = 511.5$.
CAS — 1492-18-8 (anhydrous calcium folinate); 41927-89-3 (calcium folinate pentahydrate); 6035-45-6 (calcium folinate pentahydrate).
ATC — V03AF03.

Pharmacopoeias. In Eur. (see p.vi), Int., Jpn, and US.

Pharmacopoeial description

Ph. Eur.: A white or light yellow, amorphous or crystalline powder. Sparingly soluble in water; practically insoluble in alcohol and in acetone. A 2.5% solution in water has a pH of 6.8 to 8.0. Store in airtight containers. Protect from light.

USP 25: A yellowish-white or yellow, odourless, powder. Very soluble in water; practically insoluble in alcohol. Protect from light.

Incompatibility. Calcium folinate and fluorouracil, with or without 5% glucose, were incompatible when mixed in various ratios and stored in polyvinyl chloride containers at various temperatures.[1]

1. Trissel LA, *et al.* Incompatibility of fluorouracil with leucovorin calcium or levoleucovorin calcium. *Am J Health-Syst Pharm* 1995; **52:** 710–15.

Calcium Levofolinate (15422-d)

Calcium Levofolinate (BAN, rINN).

Calcii Levofolinas; Levofolinate; Levoleucovorin Calcium (USAN). The calcium salt of the isomer of S-folinic acid (1:1).

$C_{20}H_{21}CaN_7O_7 = 511.5$.
CAS — 80433-71-2.
ATC — V03AF04.

Pharmacopoeias. Eur. (see p.vi) includes the pentahydrate.

Pharmacopoeial description

Ph. Eur.: Calcium Levofolinate Pentahydrate is a white or light yellow, amorphous or crystalline, hygroscopic powder. Slightly soluble in water; practically insoluble in alcohol and in acetone. A 0.8% solution in water has a pH of 7.5 to 8.5. Store in airtight containers. Protect from light.

Adverse Effects

Occasional hypersensitivity reactions have been reported; pyrexia has occurred rarely after injections.

Precautions

As for Folic Acid, p.1361.

Interactions

As for Folic Acid, p.1361.

Folinic acid should not be administered simultaneously with a folic acid antagonist such as methotrexate as this may nullify the effect of the antagonist. Folinic acid enhances the toxicity, as well as the antineoplastic action, of fluorouracil, especially on the gastrointestinal tract.

Pharmacokinetics

Calcium folinate is well absorbed after oral and intramuscular administration and, unlike folic acid (p.1361), is rapidly converted to biologically active folates. Folate is concentrated in the liver and CSF although distribution occurs to all body tissues. Folates are mainly excreted in the urine, with small amounts in the faeces.

◊ References.

1. McGuire BW, *et al.* Pharmacokinetics of leucovorin calcium after intravenous, intramuscular, and oral administration. *Clin Pharm* 1988; **7:** 52–8.
2. Wolfrom C, *et al.* Pharmacokinetic study of methotrexate, folinic acid and their serum metabolites in children treated with high-dose methotrexate and leucovorin rescue. *Eur J Clin Pharmacol* 1990; **39:** 377–83.
3. Zittoun J, *et al.* Pharmacokinetic comparison of leucovorin and levoleucovorin. *Eur J Clin Pharmacol* 1993; **44:** 569–73.
4. Mader RM, *et al.* Pharmacokinetics of rac-leucovorin vs [S]-leucovorin in patients with advanced gastrointestinal cancer. *Br J Clin Pharmacol* 1994; **37:** 243–8.
5. Schmitz JC, *et al.* Disposition of folic acid and its metabolites: a comparison with leucovorin. *Clin Pharmacol Ther* 1994; **55:** 501–8.

The symbol † denotes a preparation no longer actively marketed

Uses and Administration

Folinic acid is the 5-formyl derivative of tetrahydrofolic acid, the active form of folic acid. Folinic acid is used principally as an antidote to folic acid antagonists, such as methotrexate (p.554), which block the conversion of folic acid to tetrahydrofolate by binding the enzyme dihydrofolate reductase. It does not block the antimicrobial action of folate antagonists such as trimethoprim or pyrimethamine, but may reduce their haematological toxicities.

Folinic acid is given as calcium folinate, although doses are stated in terms of folinic acid. It can be administered by mouth, by intramuscular injection, or by intravenous injection or infusion. Intravenous injections should be given over several minutes because of their calcium content; the maximum recommended rate is the equivalent of 160 mg of folinic acid per minute when used as an antidote to folic acid antagonists. It has been recommended that oral doses should not be greater than 50 mg, since absorption is saturable. Calcium levofolinate, the active laevo-isomer, which is used similarly to calcium folinate, is given in doses half those recommended for the racemic form.

In cases of inadvertent **overdosage of a folic acid antagonist**, folinic acid should be administered as soon as possible and preferably within the first hour. Doses equal to or greater than the dose of methotrexate have been recommended. Alternatively it has been stated that where large overdoses of methotrexate have been given, calcium folinate may be given by intravenous infusion in a dose equivalent to 75 mg of folinic acid within 12 hours, followed by 12 mg intramuscularly every 6 hours for 4 doses. Although vincristine is not a folic acid antagonist, folinic acid has also been proposed for some manifestations of vincristine toxicity overdosage—see p.579.

Folinic acid is used in conjunction with high-dose methotrexate antineoplastic therapy to reduce the toxicity of the methotrexate ('**folinic acid rescue**'; 'calcium leucovorin rescue'). Folinic acid is given after an appropriate interval, usually 24 hours, has elapsed for methotrexate to exert its antineoplastic effect and the objective is to maintain plasma concentrations of reduced folates at a level equivalent to or greater than the plasma-methotrexate concentration. Dosage must therefore be adapted according to the methotrexate regimen, and the patient's ability to clear the antineoplastic. In general, doses of up to 120 mg have been given over 12 to 24 hours, by intramuscular injection or intravenous injection or infusion, followed by 12 to 15 mg intramuscularly, or 15 mg by mouth, every 6 hours for the next 48 to 72 hours. With doses of methotrexate below 100 mg, folinic acid 15 mg by mouth every 6 hours for 48 to 72 hours may suffice.

Folinic acid is also used **with fluorouracil** to enhance the cytotoxic effect in advanced colorectal cancer (see Administration, under Fluorouracil, p.542). One suggested regimen is folinic acid 200 mg per m^2 body-surface by slow intravenous injection over at least 3 to 5 minutes followed by fluorouracil at an initial dose of 370 mg per m^2 intravenously; the treatment is given daily for 5 consecutive days and may be repeated at intervals of 21 to 28 days. Lower doses of folinic acid (20 mg per m^2 by intravenous injection followed by fluorouracil 425 mg per m^2) have also been used. Sodium folinate has been used similarly. It may also be given by intravenous infusion over 2 hours at a dose equivalent to 500 mg per m^2 folinic acid. An intravenous injection of 600 mg per m^2 fluorouracil is administered one hour after the start of the folinate infusion. Treatment is given weekly for 6 weeks, and may be repeated after 2 weeks.

Folinic acid, like folic acid, is effective in the treatment of folate-deficient **megaloblastic anaemia** (see p.717). Doses of 15 mg daily by mouth have been suggested. If given intramuscularly a dose of up to 1 mg daily has been recommended on the grounds that higher doses have not been proven to be any more effective. It is unsuitable for megaloblastic anaemia secondary to vitamin-B_{12} deficiencies.

Folinic acid has been used in the form of calcium mefolinate.

HIV infection and AIDS. Calcium folinate has been used to reduce the toxicity of pyrimethamine and trimethoprim in patients with HIV infection. However, adjunctive administration of oral calcium folinate to patients with AIDS receiving co-trimoxazole for the treatment of *Pneumocystis carinii* pneumonia (PCP) was associated with a higher rate of therapeutic failure and a decrease in survival and did not reduce the frequency of dose-limiting co-trimoxazole toxicity.[1] Calcium folinate did not reduce the toxicity of co-trimoxazole being used for the primary prophylaxis of PCP.[2]

1. Safrin S, *et al.* Adjunctive folinic acid with trimethoprim-sulfamethoxazole for Pneumocystis carinii pneumonia in AIDS patients is associated with an increased risk of therapeutic failure and death. *J Infect Dis* 1994; **170:** 912–17.
2. Bozzette SA, *et al.* The tolerance for zidovudine plus thrice weekly or daily trimethoprim-sulfamethoxazole with and without leucovorin for primary prophylaxis in advanced HIV disease. *Am J Med* 1995; **98:** 177–82.

Preparations

BP 2001: Calcium Folinate Injection; Calcium Folinate Tablets;
USP 25: Leucovorin Calcium Injection; Leucovorin Calcium Tablets.

Proprietary Preparations (details are given in Part 3)

Aust.: Cehafolin; Isovorin; Levorin; Ribofolin†; *Belg.:* Elvorine; Ledervorin; *Braz.:* Tecnovorin; *Denm.:* Isovorin; Rescuvolin; *Fin.:* Antrex; Isovorin; Rescuvolin; *Fr.:* Elvorine; Folinoral; Lederfoline; Osfolate; Perlolate; *Ger.:* FOLI-cell; Lederfolat; O-folin; Rescuvolin; Ribofolin; *Israel:* Rescuvolin; *Ital.:* Biofolic; Calcifolin; Calfolex; Calinat; Citofolin; Ecofol; Emovis; Folaren; Foliben; Folidar; Folinac; Folinvit; Foliplus; Folix†; Furoic; Lederfolin; Levofolene; Osfolato; Perfolin; Prefolic; Resfolin; Sanifolin; Tonofolin; *Mex.:* Dalisol; Flynoken A; Folcane; Lenovor; Medsavorina; Tecfoline; *Neth.:* Isovorin; Ledervorin; *Norw.:* Isovorin; Rescuvolin; *NZ:* Rescuvolin; *Port.:* Lederfoline; Medifolin; *S.Afr.:* Isovorin; Refolinon†; Rescuvolin; *Singapore:* Rescuvolin; *Spain:* Cromatonbic Folinico; Folaxin; Folidan; Isovorin; Lederfolin; *Swed.:* Citrec; Isovorin; Rescuvolin; *Switz.:* Isovorin†; Osfolate†; *Thai.:* Rescuvolin; *UK:* Isovorin; Lederfolin; Refolinon; Sodiofolin; *USA:* Wellcovorin.

Multi-ingredient: *Ital.:* Divical; Emazian B12; Emoantitossina; Emopon; Eparmefolin; Ferritin Complex; Ferrofolin; For Liver†; Hepa-Factor; Idropan B; Ipavit; Sulton.

Fructose (595-e)

D-Fructose; Fructosum; Fruit Sugar; Laevulose; Laevulosum; Levulose. D-(–)-Fructopyranose.

$C_6H_{12}O_6 = 180.2$.
CAS — 57-48-7.
ATC — V06DC02.

Pharmacopoeias. In Eur. (see p.vi), Jpn, and US.

Pharmacopoeial description

Ph. Eur.: A white crystalline powder with a very sweet taste. Very soluble in water; soluble in alcohol.

USP 25: Colourless crystals or a white crystalline powder. Is odourless and has a sweet taste. Freely soluble in water; soluble 1 in 15 of alcohol and 1 in 14 of methyl alcohol.

Adverse Effects

Large doses of fructose given by mouth may cause flatulence, abdominal pain, and diarrhoea. Lactic acidosis and hyperuricaemia may follow intravenous infusions; fatalities have occurred.

◊ Urticaria in a patient associated with the ingestion of certain foods was found to be caused by D-psicose, a minor constituent of high-fructose syrup, which is used as a sweetening agent.[1]

1. Nishioka K, *et al.* Urticaria induced by D-psicose. *Lancet* 1983; **ii:** 1417–18.

Precautions

Fructose should not be given to patients with hereditary fructose intolerance.

It should be given with caution to patients with impaired kidney function or severe liver damage.

Pharmacokinetics

Fructose is absorbed from the gastrointestinal tract but more slowly than glucose. It is metabolised more rapidly than glucose, mainly in the liver where it is phosphorylated and a part is converted to glucose; other metabolites include lactic acid and pyruvic acid. Although it has often been considered that the metabolism of fructose is not dependent on insulin and that insulin is not necessary for its conversion to glycogen, glucose is a metabolic product of fructose and requires the presence of insulin for its further metabolism.

Uses and Administration

Fructose is sweeter than sucrose or sorbitol. It is used as a sweetener in foods for diabetics; in the UK it has been advised that the intake of fructose be limited to 25 g daily in persons with diabetes mellitus.

Fructose has been employed as an alternative to glucose in parenteral nutrition but its use is not recommended because of the risk of lactic acidosis. Use by intravenous infusion in the treatment of severe alcohol poisoning is also no longer recommended.

Solutions of fructose with glucose have been used in the treatment of nausea and vomiting (p.1206) including vomiting of pregnancy.

◊ Reiterations of the view that the use of intravenous infusions containing fructose and sorbitol, which remained popular in some countries, should be abandoned,[1,2] Not only can they lead to life-threatening build-up of lactic acid, they have led to fatalities in patients with undiagnosed hereditary fructose intolerance.
1. Collins J. Time for fructose solutions to go. *Lancet* 1993; **341:** 600.
2. Committee on Safety of Medicines/Medicines Control Agency. Reminder: fructose and sorbitol containing parenteral solutions should not be used. *Current Problems* 2001; **27:** 13.

Preparations

BP 2001: Fructose Intravenous Infusion;
USP 25: Fructose and Sodium Chloride Injection; Fructose Injection.

Proprietary Preparations (details are given in Part 3)
Aust.: Laevoral; Laevosan; *Fr.:* Fruxucre†; *Ital.:* Fructal; Fructan; Fructofin; Fructopiran; Fructosil; Laevosan; *Spain:* Levulosado; Suero Levulosado Vitulia; *UK:* Levugen.

Multi-ingredient: *Austral.:* Emetrol; *Braz.:* Dramin B-6 DL; *Fr.:* Arnilose†; *Ger.:* Gallexier; *Ital.:* Eparema-Levul; Giflorex; Liozim; Vitalmix; Weight Watchers Punto; *Norw.:* Invertos†; *Spain:* Levulosalino Isot; Levupotasico†; Levusalino; *USA:* Emecheck†; Emetrol; Formula EM; Naus-A-Way†.

Gleptoferron (16821-d)

Gleptoferron *(BAN, USAN, rINN)*.
$C_7H_{14}O_8.(C_6H_{10}O_5)_n.FeOOH$.
CAS — 57680-55-4.

A macromolecular complex of ferric hydroxide and dextran-glucoheptonic acid.

Profile

Gleptoferron has been employed for iron-deficiency anaemia in veterinary medicine. It was given by intramuscular injection.

Glucose (17536-m)

ATC — B05CX01; V04CA02; V06DC01.

Anhydrous Glucose (582-g)

Anhydrous Dextrose; Anhydrous Glucose; Dextrosum Anhydricum; D-Glucose; Glucosum Anhydricum. D-(+)-Glucopyranose.
$C_6H_{12}O_6 = 180.2$.
CAS — 50-99-7.

Pharmacopoeias. In Eur. (see p.vi), Int., Jpn, Pol., and US.
Some pharmacopoeias include anhydrous glucose and/or glucose monohydrate as separate monographs whereas others permit the anhydrous and/or monohydrate under a single monograph.

Anhydrous glucose 0.9 g is approximately equivalent to glucose monohydrate 1 g. A 5.05% solution of anhydrous glucose in water is iso-osmotic with serum.

Both Glucose Intravenous Infusion (BP 2001) and Dextrose Injection (USP 25) may be prepared from either anhydrous glucose or glucose monohydrate. However, the potency of the BP 2001 preparation is expressed in terms of anhydrous glucose whereas that of the USP 25 is expressed in terms of glucose monohydrate.

Pharmacopoeial description

Ph. Eur.: Anhydrous glucose is a white crystalline powder with a sweet taste. Freely soluble in water; sparingly soluble in alcohol.

BP 2001 directs that when glucose is required as a diluent for official injections or intravenous infusions, Glucose Intravenous Infusion 5% should be used.

USP 25: Dextrose contains one molecule of water of hydration or is anhydrous. Colourless crystals or white, crystalline or granular powder. It is odourless and has a sweet taste. Soluble 1 in 1 of water and 1 in 100 of alcohol; very soluble in boiling water; soluble in boiling alcohol.

Glucose Monohydrate (584-p)

Dextrosum Monohydridicum; D-Glucose Monohydrate; Glucosum Monohydridicum; Glycosum; Grape Sugar. D-(+)-Glucopyranose monohydrate.
$C_6H_{12}O_6,H_2O = 198.2$.
CAS — 5996-10-1.

Pharmacopoeias. In Chin., Eur. (see p.vi), Int., and US.
Some pharmacopoeias include anhydrous glucose and/or glucose monohydrate as separate monographs whereas others permit the anhydrous and/or monohydrate under a single monograph.
Eur. includes Liquid Glucose and Spray-dried Liquid Glucose. *USNF* includes Dextrose Excipient and Liquid Glucose.

Glucose monohydrate 1.1 g is approximately equivalent to anhydrous glucose 1 g. A 5.51% solution of glucose monohydrate in water is iso-osmotic with serum.

Pharmacopoeial description

Ph. Eur.: Glucose Monohydrate is a white crystalline powder with a sweet taste. Freely soluble in water; sparingly soluble in alcohol.

Liquid Glucose is a clear, colourless, or brown viscous liquid containing a mixture of glucose, di- and polysaccharides obtained by hydrolysis of starch, in aqueous solution. It contains not less than 70.0% of dry matter. Miscible with water. It may partly or totally solidify at room temperature, liquefying again on heating to 50°. Spray-dried Liquid Glucose is a white or almost white, slightly hygroscopic powder or granules. Freely soluble in water.

USP 25: Dextrose contains one molecule of water of hydration or is anhydrous. Colourless crystals or white, crystalline or granular powder. It is odourless and has a sweet taste. Soluble 1 in 1 of water and 1 in 100 of alcohol; very soluble in boiling water; soluble in boiling alcohol.

Liquid Glucose (USNF 20) is obtained by incomplete hydrolysis of starch; it consists chiefly of glucose, dextrins, maltose, and water. It is a colourless or yellowish, thick, syrupy, odourless or nearly odourless liquid. Miscible with water; sparingly soluble in alcohol.

Adverse Effects and Precautions

Intravenous administration of glucose solutions (particularly hyperosmotic solutions, which also have a low pH) may cause local pain, vein irritation, and thrombophlebitis, and tissue necrosis if extravasation occurs. Some of these reactions may be due to degradation products present after autoclaving or to poor administration technique. Intravenous infusion can lead to the development of fluid and electrolyte disturbances including hypokalaemia, hypomagnesaemia, and hypophosphataemia. Prolonged administration or rapid infusion of large volumes of iso-osmotic solutions may cause oedema or water intoxication; conversely, prolonged or rapid administration of hyperosmotic solutions may result in dehydration as a consequence of the induced hyperglycaemia.

The use of hyperosmotic glucose solutions is contra-indicated in patients with anuria, intracranial or intraspinal haemorrhage, and in delirium tremens where there is dehydration.

It has been suggested that glucose solutions should not be used after acute ischaemic strokes as hyperglycaemia has been implicated in increasing cerebral ischaemic brain damage and in impairing recovery.

Glucose solutions should not be administered through the same infusion equipment as whole blood as haemolysis and clumping can occur.

Pregnancy. Glucose solutions are commonly employed as hydrating fluids and as vehicles for the administration of other drugs. It has been suggested that if used during labour the glucose load on the mother may lead to fetal hyperglycaemia, hyperinsulinaemia, and acidosis, with subsequent neonatal hypoglycaemia and jaundice.[1,2] Others[3] have found no evidence of such an effect, and note that the number of patients included in such reports is often small and the selection criteria not homogeneous.
1. Kenepp NB, *et al.* Fetal and neonatal hazards of maternal hydration with 5% dextrose before caesarean section. *Lancet* 1982; **i:** 1150–2.
2. Singhi S, *et al.* Hazards of maternal hydration with 5% dextrose. *Lancet* 1982; **ii:** 335–6.
3. Piquard F, *et al.* Does fetal acidosis develop with maternal glucose infusion during normal labor? *Obstet Gynecol* 1989; **74:** 909–14.

Stroke. Hyperglycaemia may be caused by physiological stress during ischaemic stroke, and this worsens cerebral ischaemic damage and impairs recovery. During cerebral ischaemia, cellular hypoxia causes a shift from aerobic to anaerobic metabolism of glucose leading to intracellular lactic acidosis, which is toxic to the cell. Hyperglycaemia provides more glucose for anaerobic metabolism, further worsening intracellular

acidosis. Blood-glucose concentrations should therefore be monitored and hyperglycaemia avoided or treated. Glucose infusions should not be used routinely after ischaemic stroke, unless specifically indicated. Hypoglycaemia must also be avoided and for patients who do require glucose, it should be administered by continuous infusion, avoiding large infusions or boluses that can cause hyperglycaemia.[1]
1. Wass CT, Lanier WL. Glucose modulation of ischemic brain injury: review and clinical recommendations. *Mayo Clin Proc* 1996; **71:** 801–12.

Pharmacokinetics

Glucose is rapidly absorbed from the gastrointestinal tract. Peak plasma concentrations of glucose occur about 40 minutes after oral administration of glucose to hypoglycaemic patients. It is metabolised via pyruvic or lactic acid to carbon dioxide and water with the release of energy. All body cells are capable of oxidising glucose and it forms the principal source of energy in cellular metabolism.

Uses and Administration

Glucose, a monosaccharide, is administered by mouth or by intravenous infusion in the treatment of carbohydrate and fluid depletion. It is the preferred source of carbohydrate in parenteral nutrition regimens (p.1351) and is used in oral rehydration solutions (p.1185) for the prevention and treatment of dehydration due to acute diarrhoeal diseases (p.1203).

Glucose is also used in the treatment of hypoglycaemia (see below) and is administered orally in the glucose tolerance test as a diagnostic aid for diabetes mellitus (see p.315).

The way in which the strengths of glucose solutions for intravenous use are expressed varies in different countries. Although the BP 2001 requires that the strength be expressed in terms of anhydrous glucose, the USP 25 states that strengths are expressed in terms of glucose monohydrate. Thus, the term glucose 5% may represent, depending on origin, either 50 g per litre of anhydrous glucose (equivalent to about 55 g per litre of glucose monohydrate) or 50 g per litre of glucose monohydrate (equivalent to about 45 g per litre of anhydrous glucose). As the manner in which such preparations are referred to in the medical literature is sometimes ambiguous, it has not always been possible to state clearly in *Martindale* whether the strengths of glucose solutions mentioned relate to the anhydrous or hydrated form; however, in *Martindale*, unless otherwise specified, glucose injection is a 5% solution to distinguish it from more concentrated forms. For many practical purposes it is probably less important to know the exact way in which the strength of a given concentration is expressed than to avoid confusion between completely different strengths such as 5, 10, and 50% as the more concentrated forms are associated with special side-effects and precautions.

Glucose solution 5% (5.05% anhydrous, 5.51% monohydrate) is iso-osmotic with blood and is the strength often employed for fluid depletion; it may be administered via a peripheral vein. Glucose solutions with a concentration greater than 5% are hyperosmotic and are generally used as a carbohydrate source; a 50% solution is often employed in the treatment of severe hypoglycaemia (but see also Hypoglycaemia, below). Hyperosmotic solutions should generally be administered via a central vein although the *American Hospital Formulary Service* suggests that concentrations up to 10% may be administered via a peripheral vein for short periods provided the site is alternated regularly. In the emergency treatment of hypoglycaemia it may be necessary to use a peripheral vein but the solution should be given slowly; a suggested rate for glucose 50% in such circumstances is 3 mL per minute.

The dose of glucose is variable and is dependent on individual patient requirements; serum-glucose concentrations may need to be carefully monitored. The maximum rate of glucose utilisation has been estimated to be about 500 to 800 mg per kg body-weight per hour.

Strongly hyperosmotic glucose solutions (25 to 50%) have also been used to reduce cerebrospinal pressure (p.811) and cerebral oedema caused by delirium tremens or acute alcohol intoxication (p.1131) although they do not appear to be widely employed. Glucose solution 50% has also been used as a sclerosing agent in the treatment of varicose veins (p.1637) and as an irritant to produce adhesive pleuritis.

Ectopic pregnancy. Ectopic pregnancy (implantation of the fertilised ovum outside the womb) is now recognised at earlier stages as a result of improved diagnostic techniques. Surgery remains the mainstay of treatment, but although conservative surgical techniques may be employed in an attempt to preserve fertility, nonsurgical methods have been increasingly investigated. The best established therapy is with methotrexate (p.556), but prostaglandins or hyperosmolar glucose solutions have also been employed.

The local instillation of 10 to 20 mL of glucose 50% into unruptured tubes has been found to be a safe and satisfactory alternative to combined therapy consisting of dinoprost injected into the gestational sac, sulprostone intramuscularly, and oestrogens to effect luteolysis.[1] No side-effects were reported by 16 women who received glucose in this manner whereas 9 of 15 who received the prostaglandins and oestrogens reported abdominal cramps which ceased only after discontinuation of sulprostone, 6 were subfebrile, and 2 had signs of imminent tubal rupture. It was believed that the action of hyperosmolar glucose in destroying the developing ectopic pregnancy was probably due to necrobiosis by dehydrating the cells.

Others subsequently queried whether methotrexate was likely to cause any more local damage to the fallopian tubes than glucose.[2] In reply the original authors[3] still believed that damage to the tubal wall with glucose was unlikely and additionally pointed out corrections to the urinary concentrations of chorionic gonadotrophin as published in the original article.

1. Lang PF, et al. Conservative treatment of ectopic pregnancy with local injection of hyperosmolar glucose solution or prostaglandin-F₂α: a prospective randomised study. *Lancet* 1990; **336:** 78–81.
2. Thompson GR. Hyperosmolar glucose solution or prostaglandin-F₂α for ectopic pregnancy. *Lancet* 1990; **336:** 685.
3. Lang PF, Hönigl W. Hyperosmolar glucose solution or prostaglandin-F₂α for ectopic pregnancy. *Lancet* 1990; **336:** 685.

Glycogen storage disease. Starch may be a more acceptable alternative to glucose in the control of the hypoglycaemia of type I glycogen storage disease, see p.1380.

Haemodialysis-induced cramp. Suggestions that haemodialysis-induced cramps (p.1184) are due to hypovolaemia (see p.1322) are supported by the efficacy of volume expansion with hypertonic solutions in the management of such cramps. Intravenous infusion of 50 mL of glucose 50% solution has been used as an effective alternative to infusion of sodium chloride or mannitol.[1,2]

1. Milutinovich J, et al. Effect of hypertonic glucose on the muscular cramps of hemodialysis. *Ann Intern Med* 1979; **90:** 926–8.
2. Canzanello VJ, et al. Comparison of 50% dextrose water, 25% mannitol, and 23.5% saline for the treatment of hemodialysis-associated muscle cramps. *Trans Am Soc Artif Intern Organs* 1991; **37:** 649–52.

Hyperkalaemia. Insulin, together with glucose to prevent hypoglycaemia, is given to stimulate the cellular uptake of potassium in the emergency treatment of moderate to severe hyperkalaemia (p.1182). Usually, 50 mL of glucose 50% is administered.

Hypoglycaemia. Glucose is used to correct insulin-induced hypoglycaemia, as discussed on p.325, either by mouth or by infusion of a hypertonic solution. For intravenous infusion up to 50 mL of a 50% solution is given. Glucose 10 or 20% may be used but larger volumes are required. Although 50% glucose solution has been generally used to correct hypoglycaemia in children, some workers consider that so concentrated a solution is associated with unacceptable morbidity and possible mortality, and that it should be replaced by the 10% solution for this purpose.[1] A 5 or 10% solution is used to prevent the hypoglycaemia associated with insulin infusion for the treatment of diabetic ketoacidosis, once blood-glucose concentrations have fallen below 10 mmol per litre (see p.318).

1. Winrow AP, et al. Paediatric resuscitation: don't use 50% dextrose. *BMJ* 1993; **306:** 1612.

Myocardial infarction. Some results in diabetic and nondiabetic patients have suggested that the value of a glucose, insulin, and potassium combination in patients with myocardial infarction should be further investigated (see p.331).

Pain. Oral glucose solution has been used similarly to sucrose solution (p.1381) to alleviate mild pain in neonates requiring heel-prick tests.[1]

1. Skogsdal Y, et al. Analgesia in newborns given oral glucose. *Acta Paediatr Scand* 1997; **86:** 217–20.

Preparations

BP 2001: Glucose Intravenous Infusion; Glucose Irrigation Solution; Potassium Chloride and Glucose Intravenous Infusion; Potassium Chloride, Sodium Chloride and Glucose Intravenous Infusion; Sodium Chloride and Glucose Intravenous Infusion;
Ph. Eur.: Anticoagulant Acid-Citrate-Glucose Solutions (ACD); Anticoagulant Citrate-Phosphate-Glucose Solution (CPD);

USNF 20: Dextrose Excipient; Liquid Glucose;
USP 25: Alcohol in Dextrose Injection; Anticoagulant Citrate Dextrose Solution; Anticoagulant Citrate Phosphate Dextrose Adenine Solution; Anticoagulant Citrate Phosphate Dextrose Solution; Dextrose and Sodium Chloride Injection; Dextrose Injection; Half-strength Lactated Ringer's and Dextrose Injection; Lactated Ringer's and Dextrose Injection; Multiple Electrolytes and Dextrose Injection Type 1; Multiple Electrolytes and Dextrose Injection Type 2; Multiple Electrolytes and Dextrose Injection Type 4; Potassium Chloride in Dextrose and Sodium Chloride Injection; Potassium Chloride in Dextrose Injection; Potassium Chloride in Lactated Ringer's and Dextrose Injection; Ringer's and Dextrose Injection; Sodium Chloride and Dextrose Tablets.

Proprietary Preparations (details are given in Part 3)
Aust.: Glucosan†; ***Austral.:*** Insta-Glucose; ***Braz.:*** Glicosado; ***Canad.:*** Glucodex; ***Fin.:*** Glucosteril; ***Ger.:*** Glucosteril; ***Irl.:*** Hycal; ***Ital.:*** Energen; ***Mex.:*** Dextralpha; ***Port.:*** Glucosada; Glucosado; Glucosteril; ***Spain:*** Apir Glucoibys†; Apir Glucosado; Apiroflex Glucosada; Glucosmon; Plast Apyr Glucosado; Suero Glucosado Vitulia; ***USA:*** Dex4 Glucose; Glutose; Insulin Reaction.

Multi-ingredient: numerous preparations are listed in Part 3.

Glutamic Acid (586-w)

Glutamic Acid (USAN, rINN).
Acidum Glutamicum; E; E620; Glu; L-Glutamic Acid; Glutaminic Acid. L-(+)-2-Aminoglutaric acid.
$C_5H_9NO_4 = 147.1$.
CAS — 56-86-0.
Pharmacopoeias. In Chin. and Eur. (see p.vi).

Pharmacopoeial description

Ph. Eur.: A white crystalline powder or colourless crystals. Freely soluble in boiling water; slightly soluble in cold water; practically insoluble in alcohol, in acetic acid, in acetone, and in ether. Protect from light.

Glutamic Acid Hydrochloride (587-e)

Glutamic Acid Hydrochloride (rINNM).
Aciglumin; Glu Hydrochloride. L-(+)-2-Aminoglutaric acid hydrochloride.
$C_5H_9NO_4,HCl = 183.6$.
CAS — 138-15-8.
ATC — A09AB01.
Pharmacopoeias. In Ger.

Levoglutamide (598-j)

Levoglutamide (pINN).
Gln; L-Glutamine; Q. L-Glutamic acid 5-amide; L-(+)-2-Aminoglutaramic acid.
$C_5H_{10}N_2O_3 = 146.1$.
CAS — 56-85-9.
ATC — A16AA03.
Pharmacopoeias. In Ger. and US.

Pharmacopoeial description

USP 25: Glutamine occurs as white crystals or crystalline powder. Soluble in water; practically insoluble in alcohol and in ether. Store at a mean temperature not exceeding 25°.

Profile

Glutamic acid is an aliphatic amino acid which is degraded readily in the body to form levoglutamide (glutamine). Glutamic acid and levoglutamide are used as dietary supplements. The dipeptide N(2)-L-alanyl-L-glutamine (Ala-Gln) is used similarly.

Glutamic acid hydrochloride, which releases hydrochloric acid in the stomach, has been used in the symptomatic treatment of achlorhydria or hypochlorhydria in usual doses by mouth of 0.5 to 1 g with meals.

Parenteral and enteral nutrition. Evidence that glutamine is involved in the regulation of muscle protein synthesis, maintenance of gut mucosal barrier function, and possibly enhanced immunological response has led to studies of supplementation with levoglutamide or more stable peptide derivatives in parenteral and enteral nutrition regimens for patients with injury and infection.[1]

Supplementation of parenteral nutrition regimens with levoglutamide has been shown to reduce clinical infection in patients who have undergone bone-marrow transplantation[2] or who have suffered multiple trauma.[3] Improved mortality has been reported among intensive-care patients given parenteral feeds supplemented with glutamine,[4] although a larger study found it difficult to demonstrate benefit.[5]

In patients undergoing major uncomplicated surgery on the lower gastrointestinal tract, a significantly better postoperative nitrogen balance was achieved in those whose total parenteral nutrition regimen had been supplemented with about 20 g daily of levoglutamide coupled with alanine (L-alanyl-L-glutamine) (equivalent to about 12 g daily of glutamine) when compared with a control group.[6] Others[7] have shown that supplementation of total parenteral nutrition solutions with a glutamine dipeptide (glycyl-L-glutamine), in quantities equivalent to 0.23 g of glutamine per kg body-weight daily, prevented the increased intestinal permeability and atrophic changes in the intestinal mucosa associated with unsupplemented solutions. Supplementation of total parenteral nutrition with α-ketoglutarate or a dipeptide, ornithine-α-ketoglutarate, reduced muscle

protein depletion in one study,[8] suggesting that this may be a more physiological way of providing glutamine.

1. Sacks GS. Glutamine supplementation in catabolic patients. *Ann Pharmacother* 1999; **33:** 348–54.
2. Ziegler TR, et al. Clinical and metabolic efficacy of glutamine-supplemented parenteral nutrition after bone marrow transplantation: a randomized, double-blind, controlled study. *Ann Intern Med* 1992; **116:** 821–8.
3. Houdijk APJ, et al. Randomised trial of glutamine-enriched enteral nutrition on infectious morbidity in patients with multiple trauma. *Lancet* 1998; **352:** 772–6.
4. Griffiths RD, et al. Six-month outcome of critically ill patients given glutamine-supplemented parenteral nutrition. *Nutrition* 1997; **13:** 295–302.
5. Powell-Tuck J, et al. A double blind, randomised, controlled trial of glutamine supplementation in parenteral nutrition. *Gut* 1999; **45:** 82–8.
6. Stehle P, et al. Effect of parenteral glutamine peptide supplements on muscle glutamine loss and nitrogen balance after major surgery. *Lancet* 1989; **i:** 231–3.
7. van der Hulst RRWJ, et al. Glutamine and the preservation of gut integrity. *Lancet* 1993; **334:** 1363–5.
8. Wernerman J, et al. α-Ketoglutarate and postoperative muscle catabolism. *Lancet* 1990; **335:** 701–3.

Vincristine neurotoxicity. Vincristine neurotoxicity has been reduced by the use of oral glutamic acid (see Administration Error, p.579).

Preparations

Proprietary Preparations (details are given in Part 3)
Aust.: Dipeptiven; Neuroglutamin; ***Denm.:*** Dipeptiven; ***Fin.:*** Dipeptiven; Hypochylin; ***Fr.:*** Dipeptiven; ***Ger.:*** Dipeptamin; Glutamin; Gluti-Agil mono; Pepsaletten N; ***Ital.:*** Dipeptiven; Glutacerebro; Glutaven; Memoril; ***Mex.:*** Dipeptiven; ***Norw.:*** Glutacid; ***Port.:*** Dipeptiven; ***Spain:*** Dipeptiven; ***Swed.:*** Dipeptiven; Hypochylin; ***UK:*** Dipeptiven.

Multi-ingredient: ***Aust.:*** Aslavital; Pansan; ***Austral.:*** Aspartatol; Bioglan Digestive Zyme; Liv-Detox; Prozyme; ***Braz.:*** Espasmo Novozyme; Taludon; ***Fr.:*** Phakan; Vita-Dermacide; YSE Glutamique; ***Ger.:*** Glutarsin E; Vitasprint B₁₂; ***Hong Kong:*** Esafosfina Glutammica; ***Ital.:*** Acutil Fosforo; Briogen; Deadyn†; Esaglut; Fosfo Plus; Glutamin Fosforo; Memoserina S; Memovit B12; Vitasprint; Vitasprint Complex; ***Port.:*** Espasmo Canulase; Phakan; Relavit Fosforo; Tebetane Composto; ***S.Afr.:*** Lentogesic; Spasmo-Canulase; ***Spain:*** Agudil; Espasmo Canulasa†; Gammamida Complex†; Gastro Gobens; Gastroglutal; Jorkil†; Mederebro Complex†; Nuclerserina; Tebetane Compuesto; ***Switz.:*** Phakolen; Spasmo-Canulase; Vitasprint Complex; ***UK:*** Amino MS; Fat-Solv.

Glycine (589-y)

Glycine (rINN).
Aminoacetic Acid; E640 (glycine or glycine sodium); G; Gly; Glycinum; Glycocoll; Sucre de Gélatine.
$C_2H_5NO_2 = 75.07$.
CAS — 56-40-6.
ATC — B05CX03.
Pharmacopoeias. In Eur. (see p.vi), Jpn, and US.

Pharmacopoeial description

Ph. Eur.: A white crystalline powder. Freely soluble in water; very slightly soluble in alcohol; practically insoluble in ether. A 5% solution in water has a pH of 5.9 to 6.4.

USP 25: A white, odourless crystalline powder. Soluble 1 in 4 of water at 25°, 1 in 2.6 at 50°, 1 in 1.9 at 75°, and 1 in 1.5 at 100°; soluble 1 in 1254 of alcohol; very slightly soluble in ether. Its solutions are acid to litmus.

Adverse Effects and Precautions

Systemic absorption of glycine irrigation solutions can lead to disturbances of fluid and electrolyte balance and cardiovascular and pulmonary disorders.

Glycine irrigation should be used cautiously in patients with hepatic impairment since any absorption and consequent metabolism may cause hyperammonaemia. The possible effects on fluid and electrolyte balance warrant cautious use in patients with cardiopulmonary or renal dysfunction; glycine irrigation is contra-indicated in anuric patients.

◊ Reports and discussions concerning adverse effects, including disturbances of fluid and electrolyte balance, after the use of glycine irrigation solutions and precautions to be observed.

1. Ovassapian A, et al. Visual disturbances: an unusual symptom of transurethral prostatic resection reaction. *Anesthesiology* 1982; **57:** 332–4.
2. Sinclair JF, et al. Absorption of 1.5% glycine after percutaneous ultrasonic lithotripsy for renal stone disease. *BMJ* 1985; **291:** 691–2.
3. Goble NM, et al. Absorption of 1.5% glycine after percutaneous ultrasonic lithotripsy for renal stone disease. *BMJ* 1985; **291:** 966–7.
4. Miller RA, Whitfield HN. Absorption of 1.5% glycine after percutaneous ultrasonic lithotripsy for renal stone disease. *BMJ* 1985; **291:** 967.
5. Hahn RG, Rundgren M. Vasopressin and amino acid concentrations in serum following absorption of irrigating fluid containing glycine and ethanol. *Br J Anaesth* 1989; **63:** 337–9.
6. Baumann R, et al. Absorption of glycine irrigating solution during transcervical resection of endometrium. *BMJ* 1990; **300:** 304–5.
7. Boto TCA, et al. Absorption of irrigating fluid during transcervical resection of endometrium. *BMJ* 1990; **300:** 748.
8. Rao PN. Absorption of irrigating fluid during transcervical resection of endometrium. *BMJ* 1990; **300:** 748–9.
9. Wiener J, Gregory L. Absorption of irrigating fluid during transcervical resection of endometrium. *BMJ* 1990; **300:** 749.

The symbol † denotes a preparation no longer actively marketed

10. Magos AL, *et al.* Absorption of irrigating fluid during transcervical resection of endometrium. *BMJ* 1990; **300:** 1079.
11. Istre O, *et al.* Postoperative cerebral oedema after transcervical endometrial resection and uterine irrigation with 1.5% glycine. *Lancet* 1994; **344:** 1187–9.
12. Beutler JJ, Koomans HA. Safety and transcervical endometrial resection. *Lancet* 1995; **345:** 55.
13. Hahn RG, Persson P-G. Acute myocardial infarction after prostatectomy. *Lancet* 1996; **347:** 355.

Uses and Administration

Glycine is the simplest of the amino acids. It is used as a dietary supplement.

Glycine is sometimes used in conjunction with antacids in the treatment of gastric hyperacidity. It is also used as an ingredient of some aspirin preparations with the object of reducing gastric irritation.

Sterile solutions of glycine 1.5% in water, which are hypotonic and non-conductive, are used as urogenital irrigation solutions during certain surgical procedures, particularly transurethral resection of the prostate.

Glycine hydrochloride has also been used.

Preparations

BP 2001: Glycine Irrigation Solution;
USP 25: Glycine Irrigation.

Proprietary Preparations (details are given in Part 3)
Fr.: Gyn-Hydralin; Uro 3000†; *Mex.:* Glisuret.

Multi-ingredient: *Aust.:* Centramin; *Austral.:* Cal Alkyline; Proacid†; *Fr.:* Cristopal; Phakan; *Ital.:* Detoxicon; Digestivo Antonetto; *Mex.:* Segel; *Mon.:* Magnesium Glycocolle Lafarge; *Port.:* Phakan; Tebetane Composto; *Spain:* Sanieb; Tebetane Compuesto; *Switz.:* Phakolen; Regla pH†; *USA:* Calglycine Antacid†.

Used as an adjunct in: *Austral.:* Disprin Direct; *Fr.:* Juvepirine†; Sargepirine†; *Ger.:* Godamed; Praecineural; *Hong Kong:* Cardiprin; *Israel:* Lysoprin; *Ital.:* Aspiglicina; Geyfritz; *Singapore:* Cardiprin; *Thai.:* Cardiprin; *UK:* Beechams Lemon Tablets.

Halibut-liver Oil (7825-t)

Aceite de Hígado de Hipogloso; Heilbuttleberöl; Ol. Hipogloss.; Oleum Hippoglossi; Oleum Jecoris Hippoglossi.
CAS — 8001-46-5.
Pharmacopoeias. In Aust. and Br.

Halibut-liver oil containing 30 000 units of vitamin A in 1 g contains approximately 4000 units in 0.15 mL.

Pharmacopoeial description

BP 2001: The fixed oil extracted from the fresh or suitably preserved liver of the halibut species belonging to the genus *Hippoglossus*. It contains not less than 30 000 units of vitamin A activity per g. Halibut-liver oil may contain up to about 3000 units of vitamin D activity per g. A pale to golden yellow liquid with a fishy, but not rancid, odour and taste. Practically insoluble in alcohol; miscible with chloroform, with ether and with petroleum spirit. Store in well-filled containers. Protect from light.

Profile

Halibut-liver oil is used as a means of administering vitamins A (p.1382) and D (p.1391); the proportion of vitamin A to vitamin D is usually greater in halibut-liver oil than in cod-liver oil (p.1357). It is usually given in capsules.

Preparations

BP 2001: Halibut-liver Oil Capsules.

Proprietary Preparations (details are given in Part 3)
Switz.: Halibut.

Multi-ingredient: *Aust.:* Vitawund; *Fr.:* Eryteal; Preparation H; *Port.:* Halibut; *Switz.:* A Vogel Capsules polyvitaminees; Perles d'huile de foie de morue du Dr Geistlich.

Histidine (591-q)

Histidine (USAN, rINN).
H; His; ʟ-Histidine; Histidinum. ʟ-2-Amino-3-(1*H*-imidazol-4-yl)propionic acid.
$C_6H_9N_3O_2 = 155.2.$
CAS — 71-00-1 (L-histidine); 645-35-2 (anhydrous L-histidine hydrochloride).
Pharmacopoeias. In Eur. (see p.vi) and US.
Eur. also includes Histidine Hydrochloride Monohydrate.

Pharmacopoeial description

Ph. Eur.: Colourless crystals or a white crystalline powder. Soluble in water; very slightly soluble in alcohol; practically insoluble in ether. Protect from light.

Histidine Hydrochloride Monohydrate is a white crystalline powder or colourless crystals. Freely soluble in water; slightly soluble in alcohol; practically insoluble in ether. A 5% solution in water has a pH of 3.0 to 5.0. Protect from light.

USP 25: White, odourless crystals. Soluble in water; very slightly soluble in alcohol; insoluble in ether. pH of a 2% solution in water is between 7.0 and 8.5.

Profile

Histidine is a heterocyclic amino acid which is essential for infant growth and which may be essential for some other groups, such as patients with uraemia. Histidine and histidine hydrochloride are used as dietary supplements.

Histidine, like glycine, is sometimes used in conjunction with antacids in the treatment of gastric hyperacidity.

Purified Honey (592-p)

Clarified Honey; Gereinigter Honig; Mel Depuratum; Mel Despumatum; Miel Blanc; Purified Honey; Strained Honey.
Pharmacopoeias. In Br., Chin., Fr., Ger., and Jpn.

Pharmacopoeial description

BP 2001: It is obtained by purification of the honey from the comb of the bee, *Apis mellifera* and other species of Apis. A thick, syrupy, translucent, pale yellow or yellowish-brown liquid with a pleasant, characteristic odour, and a sweet, characteristic taste which varies according to the floral origin.

Profile

Honey, which contains about 70 to 80% of glucose and fructose, is used as a demulcent and sweetening agent, especially in linctuses and cough mixtures (p.1082).

Precautions. Honey has been identified as a source of *Clostridium botulinum* spores and thus recommendations have been made that honey should not be given to infants because of the risk of causing infant botulism.[1]

1. Arnon SS, *et al.* Honey and other environmental risk factors for infant botulism. *J Pediatr* 1979; **94:** 331–6.

Wounds. Anecdotal reports and traditional usage dating back to Ancient Egypt suggest that honey may be of some value as a wound dressing (p.1108). Its antibacterial properties are attributed both to high osmolality and the liberation of hydrogen peroxide, but may vary with the source:[1,2] in Europe, some of the best activity has been seen with lime-flower honey.[2] A group from India[3] has reported that these properties offer a potentially simple and cheap means of preserving skin grafts in developing countries, with 100% uptake of reconstituted grafts stored for up to 6 weeks and 80% uptake of those stored for 7 to 12 weeks. However, concern has been expressed since honey may contain not only chemical contaminants but clostridial spores (see also above), and it has been suggested[2] that to be medically acceptable honey must be sterile, residue-free, and of measured antibacterial activity.

Sugar (p.1381) has been used similarly to honey in treating wounds.

1. Greenwood D. Honey for superficial wounds and ulcers. *Lancet* 1993; **341:** 90–1.
2. Postmes T, *et al.* Honey for wounds, ulcers, and skin graft preservation. *Lancet* 1993; **341:** 756–7.
3. Subrahmanyam M. Storage of skin grafts in honey. *Lancet* 1993; **341:** 63–4.

Preparations

Proprietary Preparations (details are given in Part 3)
Ital.: Oramil.

Multi-ingredient: *Aust.:* Anifer Fenchelhonig; Thierry; *Braz.:* Broncmel; Expectomel; Mel Jatahy; Melagriao; Melxi; *Canad.:* Herbal Cough Expectorant; Mielocol; *Ital.:* Apiserum con Telergon 1; Bebimix; Bioton; Biovigor†; Cocktail Reale; Fon Wan Eleuthero; Fon Wan Ginsenergy; Fon Wan Pocket Energy†; Fon Wan Pollen; Liozim; Miegel†; Nerex; Nutrigel; Vitalmix; *Neth.:* Melrosum; *Switz.:* Neo-Angin au miel et citron; *UK:* Adult Meltus for Chesty Coughs & Catarrh; Buttercup Syrup (Honey and Lemon flavour); Herb and Honey Cough Elixir; Honey & Molasses; Jackson's Lemon Linctus; Jackson's Troublesome Coughs; Lemsip Cough & Cold Dry Cough; Lockets; Lockets Medicated Linctus; M & M; Meltus Honey & Lemon; Potters Children's Cough Pastilles; Regina Royal Five; Sanderson's Throat Specific; Throaties Catarrh Pastilles†; Throaties Family Cough Linctus†; Venos Honey & Lemon; Zubes Honey & Lemon.

Invert Sugar (661-v)

CAS — 8013-17-0.
ATC — C05BB03.
Pharmacopoeias. Br. and US include preparations of invert sugar.

An equimolecular mixture of glucose and fructose which may be prepared by the hydrolysis of sucrose with a suitable mineral acid such as hydrochloric acid.

Profile

Invert sugar has similar actions and uses to those of glucose (p.1364) and fructose (p.1363). It has been used as a 5 or 10% solution as an alternative to glucose in parenteral nutrition but, as with fructose, such use cannot be recommended.

A syrup of invert sugar is used as a stabilising agent; when mixed with suitable proportions of sucrose-based syrup it will help to prevent crystallisation of the sucrose.

Preparations

BP 2001: Invert Syrup;
USP 25: Invert Sugar Injection; Multiple Electrolytes and Invert Sugar Injection Type 1; Multiple Electrolytes and Invert Sugar Injection Type 2; Multiple Electrolytes and Invert Sugar Injection Type 3.

Proprietary Preparations (details are given in Part 3)
Multi-ingredient: *Norw.:* Travert†; *S.Afr.:* Emex; *USA:* Travert.

Iron (5031-z)

Ferrum.
$Fe = 55.845.$
CAS — 7439-89-6.
Pharmacopoeias. Aust. and It. include a monograph for reduced iron.

Practically **insoluble** in water and alcohol; almost completely soluble in dilute mineral acids.

Adverse Effects

The astringent action of iron preparations sometimes produces gastrointestinal irritation and abdominal pain with nausea and vomiting when administered orally. These irritant side-effects are usually related to the amount of elemental iron taken rather than the type of preparation. Other gastrointestinal effects may include either diarrhoea or constipation. Side-effects may be reduced by administration with or after food (rather than on an empty stomach) or by beginning therapy with a small dose and increasing gradually. Modified-release products are claimed to produce fewer side-effects but this may only reflect the lower availability of iron from these preparations. Oral liquid preparations containing iron salts may blacken the teeth and should be drunk through a straw. The faeces of patients taking iron salts may be coloured black.

The adverse effects associated with iron given parenterally are described under iron dextran (see p.1368).

Since absorbed iron is conserved by the body, iron overload, with increased storage of iron in various tissues (haemosiderosis), may occur as a result of excessive oral or, in particular, parenteral therapy. Patients mistakenly given iron therapy when not suffering from iron-deficiency anaemia are also at risk as those with pre-existing iron storage or absorption diseases.

Acute iron overdosage can be divided into four stages. In the first phase, which occurs up to 6 hours after oral ingestion, gastrointestinal toxicity, notably vomiting and diarrhoea, predominates. Other effects may include cardiovascular disorders such as hypotension and tachycardia, metabolic changes including acidosis and hyperglycaemia, and CNS depression ranging from lethargy to coma. Patients with only mild to moderate poisoning do not generally progress past this first phase. The second phase may occur at 6 to 24 hours after ingestion and is characterised by a temporary remission or clinical stabilisation. In the third phase gastrointestinal toxicity recurs together with shock, metabolic acidosis, convulsions, coma, hepatic necrosis and jaundice, hypoglycaemia, coagulation disorders, oliguria or renal failure, and pulmonary oedema. The fourth phase may occur several weeks after ingestion and is characterised by gastrointestinal obstruction and possibly late hepatic damage.

Relatively small amounts of iron may produce symptoms of toxicity. It has been stated that more than the equivalent of 30 mg of iron per kg body-weight could lead to some symptoms of toxicity and that in a young child the equivalent of about 75 mg of iron per kg should be regarded as extremely dangerous. Estimates of acute lethal dosages have ranged from the equivalent of 180 mg of iron per kg upwards. Serum-iron concentrations have also been employed as an indication of the severity of overdosage: a peak concentration of 5 μg or more per mL is reportedly associated with moderate to severe poisoning in many patients.

Effects on the cardiovascular system. For a suggestion that iron overload may contribute to ischaemic heart disease, see under Precautions, below.

Effects on growth. Iron supplementation in iron-replete children has been reported to adversely affect their growth—see below, under Precautions.

Iron overload. Because the body lacks a mechanism for the excretion of excess iron, abnormally high absorption or repeated blood transfusion will result in iron overload, leading eventually to haemochromatosis. The consequences of haemochromatosis include pigment deposition in skin and other organs, mild liver dysfunction, endocrine dysfunction (failure of the adolescent growth spurt, hypogonadism, sometimes diabetes and hypothyroidism), and heart disease (pericarditis, heart failure, and arrhythmias). If unchecked, the iron build-up can lead to death, mainly through heart failure or arrhythmia. Where the increased iron intake cannot be avoided (as in patients receiving regular transfusions for β-thalassaemia—see p.718) treatment with the iron chelator desferrioxamine is used to retard accumulation.

Treatment of Adverse Effects

In treating acute iron poisoning, speed is essential to reduce absorption of iron from the gastrointestinal tract. Lavage should be considered and serum-iron concentrations may be an aid to estimating the severity of poisoning. Chelation therapy with desferrioxamine (p.1004) may be necessary.

Other measures include the symptomatic management and therapy of metabolic and cardiovascular disorders.

◊ General references.
1. Proudfoot AT, *et al.* Management of acute iron poisoning. *Med Toxicol* 1986; **i:** 83–100.
2. Mann KV, *et al.* Management of acute iron overdose. *Clin Pharm* 1989; **8:** 428–40.

Overdosage. References highlighting the specific problem of iron overdose in children.[1-3] Child-resistant packaging and warning labels may be helpful in reducing the problem.
1. Anonymous. Iron-containing drugs and supplements: accidental poisoning. *WHO Drug Inf* 1995; **9:** 159–60.
2. Fitzpatrick R, Murray V. Iron toxicity: dietary supplements. *Pharm J* 1996; **256:** 18.
3. Committee on Safety of Medicines/Medicines Control Agency. Oral iron supplements: accidental overdose may be fatal in children. *Current Problems* 2001; **27:** 14.

Pregnancy. Limited data on the treatment of iron overdose in pregnancy from the UK National Teratology Information Service, suggested that treatment with desferrioxamine should not be withheld if clinically indicated.[1-3] Most pregnancies had a normal outcome.
1. McElhatton PR, *et al.* The consequences of iron overdose and its treatment with desferrioxamine in pregnancy. *Hum Exp Toxicol* 1991; **10:** 251–9.
2. McElhatton PR, *et al.* Outcome of pregnancy following deliberate iron overdose by the mother. *Hum Exp Toxicol* 1993; **12:** 579.
3. McElhatton PR, *et al.* The outcome of pregnancy following iron overdose by the mother. *Br J Clin Pharmacol* 1998; **45:** 212P–213P.

Precautions

Iron compounds should not be given to patients receiving repeated blood transfusions or to patients with anaemias not produced by iron deficiency unless iron deficiency is also present. Oral iron therapy should not be administered concomitantly with parenteral iron. Care should be taken in patients with iron-storage or iron-absorption diseases such as haemochromatosis, haemoglobinopathies, or existing gastrointestinal diseases such as inflammatory bowel disease, intestinal strictures and diverticulae.

Liquid preparations containing iron salts should be well diluted with water and swallowed through a straw to prevent discoloration of the teeth.

◊ There has been concern, for a number of reasons, about the potential consequences of iron supplementation in individuals and groups who are not actually iron-deficient. Apart from the suggestion that certain populations may be at somewhat increased risk of microbial infection following supplementation (see Infections, below), there is some evidence that supplementation in non-iron-deficient children may retard their growth.[1] It has also been proposed that iron may be associated with ischaemic heart disease, by modifying low-density lipoprotein in ways which increase its atherogenic potential and by sensitising the myocardium to ischaemic injury.[2,3] Although the role of iron in the pathogenesis of coronary heart disease is at present undecided, the use of iron should, it has been suggested, be restricted to patients with proven iron deficiency or to pregnancy.[2]
1. Idjradinata P, *et al.* Adverse effect of iron supplementation on weight gain of iron-replete young children. *Lancet* 1994; **343:** 1252–4.
2. Burt MJ, *et al.* Iron and coronary heart disease. *BMJ* 1993; **307:** 575–6.
3. Sullivan JL. Iron and coronary heart disease: iron makes myocardium vulnerable to ischaemia. *BMJ* 1993; **307:** 1066–7.

Infections. Iron is not only an essential element for humans but is also essential for many micro-organisms. Thus, it has been suggested that persons with either adequate iron stores or iron overload may provide optimum conditions for microbial growth and therefore be susceptible to an increased incidence and severity of infection; conversely, iron-deficiency anaemia may offer some protection against infections. The topic has been reviewed[1] and although there is no evidence that small amounts of iron supplements or iron-fortified food in normal

people will render them more prone to infection[2] there is some evidence that in populations with a high prevalence of endemic infectious disease such as malaria, iron therapy may be followed by a higher incidence of infectious complications or by a flare-up of existing low-grade disease. Therefore, the routine use of iron supplements in such communities has been questioned;[3,4] however, an increasing number of studies have failed to demonstrate a detrimental effect.[5-8]
1. Hershko C, *et al.* Iron and infection. *BMJ* 1988; **296:** 660–4.
2. Bullen JJ, Ward CG. Iron and infection. *BMJ* 1988; **296:** 1539.
3. Oppenheimer SJ, *et al.* Iron supplementation increases prevalence and effects of malaria: report on clinical studies in Papua New Guinea. *Trans R Soc Trop Med Hyg* 1986; **80:** 603–12.
4. Smith AW. The effects on malaria of treatment of iron-deficiency anaemia with oral iron in Gambian children. *Ann Trop Paediatr* 1989; **9:** 17–23.
5. Harvey PWJ, *et al.* The effect of iron therapy on malarial infection in Papua New Guinean schoolchildren. *Am J Trop Med Hyg* 1989; **40:** 12–18.
6. Boele van Hensbroek M, *et al.* Iron, but not folic acid, combined with effective antimalarial therapy promotes haematological recovery in African children after acute falciparum malaria. *Trans R Soc Trop Med Hyg* 1995; **89:** 672–6.
7. van den Hombergh J, *et al.* Does iron therapy benefit children with severe malaria-associated anaemia? A clinical trial with 12 weeks supplementation of oral iron in young children from the Turiani Division, Tanzania. *J Trop Pediatr* 1996; **42:** 220–7.
8. Menendez C, *et al.* Randomised placebo-controlled trial of iron supplementation and malaria chemoprophylaxis for prevention of severe anaemia and malaria in Tanzanian infants. *Lancet* 1997; **350:** 844–50.

Interference with diagnostic tests. Although studies *in vitro* demonstrated that iron (ferrous sulfate) caused a false-positive result in the Hemoccult test for blood in faeces, this did not occur *in vivo* in persons receiving oral iron therapy.[1,2] An explanation for the difference in these findings was that hydrogen peroxide in the Hemoccult developer converted ferrous ions in solution to ferric ions, which caused oxidation in the test, whereas *in vivo* the iron was probably eliminated in the faeces in the form of non-reactive insoluble iron precipitates.[2]
1. Kulbaski MJ, *et al.* Oral iron and the Hemoccult test: a controversy on the teaching wards. *N Engl J Med* 1989; **320:** 1500.
2. McDonnell M, Elta G. More on oral iron and the Hemoccult test. *N Engl J Med* 1989; **321:** 1684.

Porphyria. Erythropoietic protoporphyria was exacerbated by oral iron therapy in four patients;[1] a further patient had a variable reaction to iron, being able to tolerate it on some occasions but suffering from exacerbation of porphyria on others.[2]
1. Milligan A, *et al.* Erythropoietic protoporphyria exacerbated by oral iron therapy. *Br J Dermatol* 1988; **119:** 63–6.
2. McClements BM, *et al.* Erythropoietic protoporphyria and iron therapy. *Br J Dermatol* 1990; **122:** 423–6.

Interactions

Iron salts are not well absorbed by mouth, and administration with food may further impair their absorption.

Compounds containing calcium and magnesium, including antacids and mineral supplements, and bicarbonates, carbonates, oxalates, or phosphates, may also impair the absorption of iron by the formation of insoluble complexes. Similarly the absorption of both iron salts and tetracyclines is diminished when they are taken concomitantly by mouth. If treatment with both drugs is required, a time interval of about 2 to 3 hours should be allowed between them. A suitable interval is also advised if an iron supplement is required in patients receiving trientine. Zinc salts may decrease the absorption of iron.

Some agents, such as ascorbic acid and citric acid, may actually increase the absorption of iron.

The response to iron may be delayed in patients receiving systemic chloramphenicol.

Iron salts can also decrease the absorption of other drugs and thus reduce their bioavailability and clinical effect. Drugs so affected include bisphosphonates, entacapone, fluoroquinolones, levodopa, methyldopa, penicillamine, and tetracycline. Iron salts may reduce the efficacy of thyroxine [levothyroxine] (p.1528).

Interactions with parenteral iron are mentioned under Iron Dextran, p.1369.

◊ Reviews.
1. Campbell NRC, Hasinoff BB. Iron supplements: a common cause of drug interactions. *Br J Clin Pharmacol* 1991; **31:** 251–5.

Pharmacokinetics

Iron is irregularly and incompletely absorbed from the gastrointestinal tract, the main sites of absorption being the duodenum and jejunum. Absorption is aided by the acid secretion of the stomach and by some dietary acids (such as ascorbic acid) and is more readily effected when the iron is in the ferrous state or is part of the haem complex (haem-iron). Absorption is also increased in conditions of iron deficiency or in the fasting state but is decreased if the body stores are overloaded. Only about 5 to 15% of the iron ingested in food is normally absorbed.

Following absorption the majority of iron is bound to transferrin and transported to the bone marrow where it is incorporated into haemoglobin; the remainder is contained within the storage forms, ferritin (p.1359) or haemosiderin, or as myoglobin, with smaller amounts occurring in haem-containing enzymes or in plasma bound to transferrin.

Only very small amounts of iron are excreted as the majority released after the destruction of the haemoglobin molecule is re-used. This conservation of body iron, and lack of an excretory mechanism for excess iron, is the reason for the development of iron overload with excessive iron therapy or repeated transfusions.

◊ General references.
1. Harju E. Clinical pharmacokinetics of iron preparations. *Clin Pharmacokinet* 1989; **17:** 69–89.

Human Requirements

The body contains about 4 g of iron most of which is present as haemoglobin.

Apart from haemorrhage, iron is mainly lost from the body in the faeces, urine, from skin, and sweat, but the total loss is very small. Iron is also lost in small amounts in breast milk and in menstrual blood. In healthy men and postmenopausal women the loss is replaced by the absorption of about 1 mg of iron daily; about 1.5 to 2 mg needs to be absorbed daily by premenopausal women. In childhood and adolescence, the need is proportionately greater because of growth. Iron absorption is variable but is usually between 5 and 15% and therefore a dietary allowance containing the equivalent of about 10 mg of iron daily is usually sufficient for men and postmenopausal women; up to 15 mg daily may be necessary for premenopausal women with normal menstrual blood losses; some authorities recommend higher amounts or supplements during pregnancy. For further details concerning dietary requirements, see below and for a discussion of prophylactic iron given during pregnancy, see Iron-deficiency Anaemia, under Uses and Administration, below.

Good dietary sources of haem-iron are animal products such as meat and fish; non-haem-iron is also found in animal products and in vegetable products such as legumes and some leafy vegetables, but some vegetable products with a high iron content also contain phosphates or phytates which inhibit absorption by the formation of unabsorbable complexes.

◊ In the United Kingdom, dietary reference values (DRV)[1] and in the USA, recommended dietary allowances (RDA)[2] have been published for iron.

In the UK the estimated average requirement (EAR) for adult males and postmenopausal females is 6.7 mg daily and the reference nutrient intake (RNI) is 8.7 mg daily; for premenopausal females, but without heavy menstrual blood losses, the EAR and RNI are 11.4 and 14.8 mg daily respectively. Amounts for infants, children, and adolescents, which are proportionately higher than those for adults, are also given. No increase is considered necessary during pregnancy or lactation.[1]

In the USA the RDA for adult males and postmenopausal females is 8 mg daily and that for premenopausal women is 18 mg daily. The tolerable upper intake level is 45 mg daily. Amounts for infants, children, and adolescents, again proportionately higher than for adults, are also provided. The RDA for pregnant women is 27 mg daily. An RDA of 9 mg for lactating adult women has been estimated from the EAR of non-menstruating women plus the average iron content of human milk.[2]

The Food and Agriculture Organization of the United Nations together with the World Health Organization has also published guidelines concerning iron requirements and these take into account many factors including bioavailability of iron in the diet.[3]

For the definitions of DRV, EAR, RNI, and RDA, see under Vitamins, p.1352.

1. DoH. Dietary reference values for food energy and nutrients for the United Kingdom: report of the panel on dietary reference values of the committee on medical aspects of food policy. *Report on health and social subjects 41.* London: HMSO, 1991.
2. Standing Committee on the Scientific Evaluation of Dietary Reference Intakes of the Food and Nutrition Board. *Dietary reference intakes for vitamin A, vitamin K, arsenic, boron, chromium, copper, iodine, iron, manganese, molybdenum, nickel, silicon, vanadium, and zinc.* Washington DC: National Academy Press, 2001.
3. FAO/WHO. *Requirements of vitamin A, iron, folate and vitamin B₁₂: report of a joint FAO/WHO expert consultation.* Rome: Food and Agriculture Organization of the United Nations, 1988.

Uses and Administration

Iron is an essential constituent of the body, being necessary for haemoglobin formation and for the oxidative processes of living tissues. Iron deficiency results in defective erythropoiesis and anaemia. Iron and iron salts should only be given for the treatment or prophylaxis of iron-deficiency anaemias (see below). They should not be given for the treatment of other types of anaemia except where iron deficiency is also present. Iron-deficiency anaemias respond readily to iron therapy but the underlying cause of the anaemia should be determined and treated.

The preferred route for the administration of iron is by mouth, usually as soluble ferrous salts, which are better absorbed than ferric salts. The usual adult dose for the treatment of iron-deficiency anaemia is 100 to 200 mg of iron daily in divided doses. The usual adult prophylactic dose is 60 to 120 mg of iron daily. There are various recommendations for children's doses and up to 2 mg of iron per kg body-weight three times daily for treatment and 1 mg per kg daily for prophylaxis of iron-deficiency anaemia has been employed. Therapy is generally continued until haemoglobin concentrations reach normal values, which may take some weeks, and then for a further 3 months or more to restore body-iron stores.

Further information concerning the dosage of iron salts and compounds used is provided in the individual monographs; this information, however, tends to reflect the amounts of iron contained in different salts or available commercial preparations and therefore, in some instances, may not be within the general range of iron dosages as quoted above.

The iron content of various iron salts is tabulated in Table 1, below.

Some oral preparations of iron are presented in modified-release dosage forms and these preparations are claimed to result in reduced gastrointestinal side-effects and have the advantage of once-daily dosing. The preparations are designed to release the iron gradually along the gut but in some instances the iron may not be released until the preparation reaches a part of the gut where absorption is poor thus resulting in sub-optimal dosing.

Iron can also be given parenterally in circumstances where oral therapy cannot be undertaken and such use is typified by iron dextran (see below).

Anoxic seizures. Findings[1] of a reduction in the frequency of breath-holding episodes in children treated with iron suggest that there might be a relationship between anoxic seizures (p.462) and iron deficiency.[2]

1. Daoud AS, *et al.* Effectiveness of iron therapy on breath-holding spells. *J Pediatr* 1997; **130:** 547–50.
2. Hannon DW. Breath-holding spells: waiting to inhale, waiting for systole, or waiting for iron therapy? *J Pediatr* 1997; **130:** 510–12.

Table 1. Approximate amounts of different iron salts that supply 60 mg of elemental iron.

Iron salt	Amount
Ferrous ascorbate (anhydrous)	437 mg
Ferrous aspartate (tetrahydrate)	422 mg
Ferrous chloride (tetrahydrate)	214 mg
Ferrous fumarate (anhydrous)	183 mg
Ferrous gluconate (dihydrate)	518 mg
Ferrous succinate (anhydrous)	185 mg
Ferrous sulfate (dried)	186 mg
Ferrous sulfate (heptahydrate)	300 mg

Iron-deficiency anaemia. Iron deficiency eventually results in anaemia (p.716), usually of a microcytic, hypochromic type, and because iron requirements are increased during infancy, puberty, pregnancy, and menstruation, such anaemias are most common in women and children.[1] Although any underlying cause for the iron deficiency should be sought and treated, most iron-deficiency anaemias respond well to treatment with oral iron.[2] The usual dose is sufficient of a ferrous salt to supply about 100 to 200 mg of elemental iron daily, with the aim of increasing haemoglobin concentrations by 0.1 to 0.2 g per 100 mL per day or 2 g per 100 mL over 3 to 4 weeks.[2] Treatment is continued for about 3 months once haemoglobin concentrations have returned to the normal range, in order to aid replenishment of iron stores. Parenteral iron therapy is rarely indicated. Prophylactic administration may be justifiable in certain groups, such as in pregnancy and in pre-school children, but there is some debate as to its value, and its use in the former has declined.[3-7] (For the possible problems associated with iron supplementation in those who are not deficient, see under Precautions, above.) Usual prophylactic doses provide about 60 to 120 mg of elemental iron daily. Intermittent iron supplementation is under study.[8]

1. De Maayer EM, *et al. Preventing and controlling iron deficiency anaemia through primary health care: a guide for health administrators and programme managers.* Geneva: WHO, 1989.
2. Smith AG. Prescribing iron. *Prescribers' J* 1997; **37:** 82–7.
3. Hibbard BM. Iron and folate supplements during pregnancy: supplementation is valuable only in selected patients. *BMJ* 1988; **297:** 1324 and 1326.
4. Horn E. Iron and folate supplements during pregnancy: supplementing everyone treats those at risk and is cost effective. *BMJ* 1988; **297:** 1325 and 1327.
5. US Preventive Services Task Force. Routine iron supplementation during pregnancy: policy statement. *JAMA* 1993; **270:** 2846–8.
6. US Preventive Services Task Force. Routine iron supplementation during pregnancy: review article. *JAMA* 1993; **270:** 2848–54.
7. Anonymous. Routine iron supplements in pregnancy are unnecessary. *Drug Ther Bull* 1994; **32:** 30–1.
8. Cook JD. Iron supplementation: is less better? *Lancet* 1995; **346:** 587.

Preparations

Proprietary Preparations (details are given in Part 3)
Thai.: Pediron; *USA:* Icar.

Multi-ingredient: *Austral.:* Clements Iron; *Braz.:* Ferrocitol; Fortonal; Hemofer; Nervoforcan; Norden; Olohepat; Sadol; *Denm.:* Ferroplex-frangula; *Thai.:* Cilfer-12-F; Hemo-Cyto-Serum; *UK:* Hematinic; *USA:* Centurion A–Z; Feocyte; Geritol Complete; I-L-X; Theravee Hematinic; Ultra-Natal; Vita-Feron†.

Iron Dextran (5066-m)

Iron-Dextran Complex.
CAS — 9004-66-4.

Pharmacopoeias. Br., Chin., and US include Iron Dextran Injection.

Pharmacopoeial description

BP 2001: Iron Dextran Injection is a sterile colloidal solution containing a complex of ferric hydroxide and dextrans of weight average molecular weight between 5000 and 7000. It contains 4.75 to 5.25% of iron and 17.0 to 23.0% of dextrans. pH 5.2 to 6.5.

USP 25: Iron Dextran Injection is a sterile colloidal solution of ferric hydroxide in complex with partially hydrolysed dextran of low molecular weight. It may contain not more than 0.5% of phenol as a preservative. pH 5.2 to 6.5.

Adverse Effects and Treatment

Severe anaphylactoid reactions may occur after administration of iron dextran and fatalities have been reported. It is therefore recommended that administration takes place where there are facilities for the emergency treatment of such reactions, that certain precautions be observed, and that test doses be employed (see Precautions, below).

Intravenous administration may be associated with peripheral vascular flushing, tachycardia, and hypotension and syncope; thrombophlebitis may also occur at the site of injection, although the incidence may be reduced by giving iron dextran in sodium chloride 0.9% rather than glucose 5%. Intramuscular injection is associated with local reactions, pain, and staining at the site of injection; leakage along the injection track may occur unless the proper administration technique is used (see Uses and Administration, below). Other immediate reactions with either route include nausea, vomiting, and taste disturbance.

Patients may also experience delayed reactions 1 to 2 days after administration of iron dextran, such as arthralgia, myalgia, regional lymphadenopathy, chills,

fever, paraesthesia, dizziness, malaise, headache, nausea, vomiting, and haematuria.

Overdose of parenteral iron is unlikely to be associated with any acute manifestations. Unwarranted parenteral iron therapy will result in iron overload and excess storage of iron (haemochromatosis) in the long term. The consequences of this include liver and endocrine dysfunction and heart disease (see Iron Overload, p.1366), and possibly an increased risk of infection (see Infections, under Precautions for Iron, p.1367). Iron overload may require chelation therapy with desferrioxamine (p.1004).

Intramuscular injection of iron complexes such as iron dextran has resulted in sarcomas at the injection site in *animals*. There is some evidence that this may occur in humans.

Effects on the blood. A 1-year-old girl with Down's syndrome and iron-deficiency anaemia was given three intramuscular injections of iron dextran over 6 days (to a total of 30 mg per kg body-weight). Pancytopenia developed subsequently, which reappeared when challenged with iron dextran. Tests indicated an allergic pathogenesis for the pancytopenia.[1]

For further discussion of hypersensitivity reactions to iron dextran, see under Hypersensitivity, below.

1. Hurvitz H, *et al.* Pancytopenia caused by iron-dextran. *Arch Dis Child* 1986; **61:** 194–6.

Hypersensitivity. The Boston Collaborative Drug Surveillance Program monitored consecutively 32 812 medical inpatients. Drug-induced anaphylaxis occurred in 1 of 169 patients given iron dextran; the route of administration was not stated in this report.[1]

An investigation of 481 persons who received a total of 2099 intravenous injections of iron dextran found 3 life-threatening immediate anaphylactoid reactions; 8 severe delayed reactions were also observed, and many reactions of a less serious nature.[2] In a more recent series,[3] 10 of 573 patients experienced anaphylactoid reactions after intravenous administration of iron dextran. Other serious reactions included 1 case of cardiac arrest, and 3 cases of dyspnoea, hypertension, or chest pain.

In a report of a lupus-like disorder associated with administration of iron dextran,[4] the illness resolved with appropriate treatment but recurred on rechallenge.

For discussion of pancytopenia believed to have an underlying allergic pathogenesis, see under Effects on the Blood, above.

1. Porter J, Jick H. Drug-induced anaphylaxis, convulsions, deafness, and extrapyramidal symptoms. *Lancet* 1977; **i:** 587–8.
2. Hamstra RD, *et al.* Intravenous iron dextran in clinical medicine. *JAMA* 1980; **243:** 1726–31.
3. Fishbane S, *et al.* The safety of intravenous iron dextran in hemodialysis patients. *Am J Kidney Dis* 1996; **28:** 529–34.
4. Oh VMS. Iron dextran and systemic lupus erythematosus. *BMJ* 1992; **305:** 1000.

Overdosage. A 29-year-old woman was given 32 mL iron dextran (Imferon) intravenously. Twenty-four hours later she developed muscle cramps, bilateral frontal headaches, with subsequent neck stiffness, and marked opisthotonia with photophobia.[1] The haemoglobin concentration did not rise following the infusion of iron which indicated there had been no iron deficiency. Thus, abnormally high concentrations of free iron had followed the iron therapy and this free iron was able to cross into the cerebrospinal fluid and was responsible for the meningitic symptoms.

1. Shuttleworth D, *et al.* Meningism due to intravenous iron dextran. *Lancet* 1983; **ii:** 453.

Precautions

Iron dextran is contra-indicated in patients with severe liver damage or acute kidney infection. It is also contra-indicated in persons with a history of hypersensitivity to the preparation. Teratogenicity has been demonstrated in non-anaemic *animals* given the equivalent of about three times the maximum human dose and its use should be avoided in pregnancy if possible.

Additionally, iron dextran should be employed with caution in patients with a history of allergic disorders or asthma and in these patients the intramuscular, and not the intravenous, route should be employed. Patients with rheumatoid arthritis may experience a worsening of symptoms when given iron dextran intravenously. Patients with other inflammatory disorders such as lupus erythematosus may be at increased risk of delayed reactions. Large doses of iron dextran by infusion may lead to serum discoloration; this should not be mistaken as evidence of haemolysis. Oral iron salts should be discontinued before administration of parenteral iron.

A test dose should be given before administration of a full therapeutic dose (see Uses and Administration, below) and emergency measures for the treatment of allergic reactions should be available (see Anaphylactic Shock, p.832). Patients should be kept under observation for at least 1 hour after administration of a test dose or following intravenous administration.

Iron dextran formulated with phenol as a preservative is intended for administration by the intramuscular route only.

Interactions

Enalapril. There is some evidence that enalapril may potentiate the adverse systemic reactions seen with intravenous iron therapy.[1]
1. Rolla G, et al. Systemic reactions to intravenous iron therapy in patients receiving angiotensin-converting enzyme inhibitor. *J Allergy Clin Immunol* 1994; **93:** 1074–5.

Pharmacokinetics

After intramuscular injection iron dextran is absorbed primarily through the lymphatic system: about 60% is absorbed after 3 days and up to 90% after 1 to 3 weeks. The reticuloendothelial cells gradually separate iron from the iron-dextran complex; the distribution and elimination of iron is described on p.1367. Absorption of drug inadvertently deposited in subcutaneous tissue may take months or even years.

◊ References.
1. Spruill WJ. Timing iron dextran doses when plasmapheresis is required. *Clin Pharm* 1990; **9:** 419–20.

Uses and Administration

Iron dextran should be used only in the treatment of proven iron-deficiency anaemia (p.716) where oral therapy, as described on p.1368, is ineffective or impracticable.

It is given by deep intramuscular injection into the upper outer quadrant of the buttock; to prevent leakage along the injection track, the subcutaneous tissue is drawn to one side before the needle is inserted. It may also be given intravenously at a rate not exceeding the equivalent of 50 mg iron (1 mL) per minute.

Prior to commencing therapy, all patients should receive a test dose of 0.5 mL administered via the intended route, and should be observed for adverse reactions (see Precautions, above).

For iron-deficiency anaemia, total dosage is calculated according to the haemoglobin concentration and body-weight of the patient; allowance is also made for additional iron to replenish iron stores. Iron dextran injection is usually supplied with a table from which the recommended dose can be obtained for patients of different weights and haemoglobin (Hb) status. There may be variations between countries in the doses obtained from such tables. Doses can also be calculated from various formulae. Typical formulae used for a preparation containing the equivalent of 50 mg of iron per mL are as follows:

$$\text{Dose in mL} =$$
$$\{0.0476 \times \text{body-weight (kg)} \times [14.8 - \text{Hb level (g/100 mL)}]\}$$
$$+$$
1 mL per 5 kg body-weight, to a maximum of 14 mL

$$\text{Dose in mL for children up to 15 kg} =$$
$$\{0.0476 \times \text{body-weight (kg)} \times [12 - \text{Hb level (g/100 mL)}]\}$$
$$+$$
1 mL per 5 kg body-weight.

Using these formulae a 70-kg man with a haemoglobin value of 5.9 g per 100 mL would be given a total of 2.2 g of iron (44 mL of the iron dextran preparation). An alternative formula is:

$$\text{Dose in mL} =$$
$$\{0.0442 \times \text{body-weight (kg)} \times$$
$$[\text{desired Hb level (g/100 mL)} - \text{measured Hb level}]\}$$
$$+$$
$$(0.26 \times \text{body-weight})$$

In adults, the calculated lean body-weight should normally be used in this formula rather than the actual

body-weight. Note that doses obtained from tables or the above formulae are for iron-deficiency anaemia, and are not suitable for iron replacement for simple blood loss.

The total dose requirement may be administered as a series of intramuscular injections daily or once or twice weekly in inactive patients. A suggested dosage per intramuscular injection for children is: less than 5 kg body-weight, up to 0.5 mL (25 mg); 5 to 9 kg, up to 1 mL (50 mg). Adults and larger children normally receive 2 mL (100 mg).

Iron dextran is also administered intravenously either by total-dose infusion (TDI) or as an undiluted injection. In total-dose infusion, the total dose calculated according to the haemoglobin concentration (as outlined above) is given by slow intravenous infusion in about 500 mL of sodium chloride 0.9% or glucose 5%; sodium chloride may be preferable due to the reduced incidence of thrombophlebitis. The initial rate for the 0.5 mL test dose should not exceed 5 drops per minute but provided that this is well tolerated the rate of infusion may be increased progressively to 45 to 60 drops per minute.

For undiluted administration the total dose is also calculated according to the haemoglobin concentration. A test dose of 0.5 mL of the iron dextran preparation should be given by slow intravenous injection. If, after an observation period of about 1 hour, this test dose has been well tolerated, the therapeutic dose may be given either as a single dose, or divided and given as a series of injections. Patients given iron dextran intravenously should be observed closely for at least one hour after administration.

Anaemia of chronic renal failure. US guidelines for the treatment of anaemia of chronic renal failure[1] recommend the regular use of small intravenous doses of iron dextran to prevent iron deficiency and promote improved erythropoiesis; oral iron is usually insufficient to maintain adequate iron stores in these patients, particularly when also treated with erythropoietin.
1. National Kidney Foundation. NKF-DOQI clinical practice guidelines for the treatment of anemia of chronic renal failure. *Am J Kidney Dis* 1997; **30** (suppl 3): S192–S240.

Preparations

BP 2001: Iron Dextran Injection;
USP 25: Iron Dextran Injection.

Proprietary Preparations (details are given in Part 3)
Belg.: Fercayl; **Canad.:** Dexiron; Infufer; **Mex.:** Driken; Ferrocel; Ferroin; Imferon; **Spain:** Imferon; **Switz.:** Ferrum Hausmann; **UK:** Cosmofer; **USA:** DexFerrum; INFeD.

Iron Polymaltose (12864-h)

Ferromaltose; Ferrum Polyisomaltose.

A complex of ferric hydroxide and isomaltose.

Profile

Iron polymaltose is used as a source of iron (p.1366) for iron-deficiency anaemia (p.716). It is given by mouth in usual doses containing the equivalent of up to 200 mg of iron daily. It is also given parenterally, the total dose being calculated and given by intravenous infusion or, preferably, as a series of intramuscular injections containing the equivalent of up to 200 mg of iron in a single day; injections are usually given only every few days. For further information relating to the parenteral use of iron, see Iron Dextran, p.1368.

Preparations

Proprietary Preparations (details are given in Part 3)
Aust.: Ferrum Hausmann; **Austral.:** Ferrum H; **Braz.:** Noripurum; **Fin.:** Colleofer; Maltofer; **Fr.:** Maltofer; **Ger.:** Ferrum Hausmann; **Hong Kong:** Ferrum Hausmann; **Irl.:** Ferrum H; **Israel:** Ferripel-3; **Ital.:** Intrafer; **Mex.:** Ferranina; Ferranina Fol; **NZ:** Ferrum H; **Port.:** Ferrum Hausmann; **S.Afr.:** Ferrimed; Ferrimed DS; **Singapore:** Ferrum Hausmann; **Switz.:** Maltofer.

Multi-ingredient: Braz.: Noripurum Folico; **Israel:** Ferrifol-3; **Port.:** Ferrum Fol; **S.Afr.:** Ferrimed; **Switz.:** Maltofer Fol.

Iron Sorbitol (5070-f)

Astra-1572; Iron Sorbitex (USAN); Iron-Sorbitol-Citric Acid Complex.
CAS — 1338-16-5.

Pharmacopoeias. Br. and *US* include injections of iron sorbitol.

A complex of ferric iron, sorbitol, and citric acid, stabilised with dextrin and sorbitol.

Adverse Effects, Treatment, and Precautions

As for Iron Dextran, p.1368.

There may be severe systemic reactions, and cardiac complications, such as complete atrioventricular block, ventricular tachycardia, or ventricular fibrillation, may be fatal. The urine of patients treated with iron sorbitol may become dark on standing.

Iron sorbitol should not be administered intravenously. It should preferably be avoided in patients with pre-existing cardiac abnormalities.

◊ A description of adverse events in three patients with the malabsorption syndrome treated with intramuscular injections of iron sorbitol.[1] Two patients died; in one, findings were consistent with anaphylaxis and in the other cardiac toxicity was considered to be due to a direct effect. In the third patient direct cardiac toxicity was also implicated.
1. Karhunen P, et al. Reaction to iron sorbitol injection in three cases of malabsorption. *BMJ* 1970; **2:** 521–2.

Interactions

As for Iron Dextran, p.1369.

Pharmacokinetics

About 66% of iron sorbitol is absorbed within 3 hours of intramuscular injection, most of it directly into the blood circulation, and some via the lymphatic system. Almost all is absorbed within about 10 days. Clearance of iron sorbitol from the plasma is rapid, and is mainly via the reticuloendothelial system, as described for Iron Dextran, p.1369.

Uses and Administration

Iron sorbitol should be used only in the treatment of proven iron-deficiency anaemia (p.716) where oral therapy, as described on p.1368, is ineffective or impracticable.

It is given by deep intramuscular injection into the upper outer quadrant of the buttock; to prevent leakage along the injection track, the subcutaneous tissue is drawn to one side before the needle is inserted.

Total dosage is calculated according to body-weight and the haemoglobin concentration of the blood, and tables are usually provided with iron sorbitol injections for this purpose. The recommended single dose is the equivalent of 1.5 mg of iron per kg body-weight up to a maximum of 100 mg per injection; these doses are then given daily until the total dosage has been achieved. Iron sorbitol is not recommended in children under 3 kg in body-weight.

Iron sorbitol should not be given intravenously.

Preparations

BP 2001: Iron Sorbitol Injection;
USP 25: Iron Sorbitex Injection.

Proprietary Preparations (details are given in Part 3)
Aust.: Jectofer; **Canad.:** Jectofer; **Denm.:** Jectofer; **Ger.:** Jectofer; **Irl.:** Jectofer; **Neth.:** Jectofer; **Norw.:** Jectofer; **Spain:** Yectofer; **Swed.:** Jectofer; **UK:** Jectofer.

Iron Succinyl-Protein Complex (19370-y)

Iron Proteinsuccinylate; ITF-282.
CAS — 93615-44-2.

Profile

Iron succinyl-protein complex is a source of iron (p.1366) used for iron-deficiency anaemia (p.716). It is given by mouth in doses of up to 1.6 g daily (equivalent to up to 80 mg of iron daily).

◊ References.
1. Köpcke W, Sauerland MC. Meta-analysis of efficacy and tolerability data on iron proteinsuccinylate in patients with iron deficiency anemia of different severity. *Arzneimittelforschung* 1995; **45:** 1211–16.

Preparations

Proprietary Preparations (details are given in Part 3)
Braz.: Fisiofer; **Ital.:** Ferlatum; Ferplex; Ferremon; Ferrofolin Simplex†; Folinemic Ferro; Legofer; Pernexin; Proteoferrina; Rekord Ferro; **Mex.:** Ferxal; **Port.:** Fetrival; Legofer; **Spain:** Ferplex; Ferrocur; Lactoferrina.

Multi-ingredient: Ital.: Ferrofolin.

Iron Sucrose (5067-b)

Iron Sucrose (BAN, USAN).
Eisenzucker; Ferric Hydroxide Sucrose; Ferric Oxide, Saccharated; Ferrum Oxydatum Saccharatum; Iron (III) hydroxide-sucrose complex; Oxyde de Fer Sucré; Saccharated Iron Oxide; XI-921.
CAS — 8047-67-4.
ATC — B03AB02; B03AC02.
Pharmacopoeias. In Aust. and Swiss.

A complex of iron(III) hydroxide with sucrose containing traces of sodium chloride and sodium hydroxide and having an approximate molecular weight of 43 200.

Adverse Effects, Treatment, and Precautions

For parenteral iron, see Iron Dextran, p.1368. Iron sucrose injection is strongly alkaline and must not be administered subcutaneously or intramuscularly. The injection should be used with caution in patients with a history of asthma, eczema, anaphylaxis, or other allergic disorders.

Pharmacokinetics

Iron sucrose is rapidly cleared from the plasma after intravenous injection with a terminal half-life of about 6 hours. A competitive exchange of iron takes place from the iron sucrose complex to the iron-binding protein transferrin. About 5% of a dose is eliminated via the kidneys in the first 4 hours after administration.

Uses and Administration

Iron sucrose is used as a source of iron (p.1366) for iron-deficiency anaemia (p.716). It is given when oral iron therapy is ineffective or impractical, by slow intravenous injection or intravenous infusion in sodium chloride 0.9%. The dose is calculated according to body-weight and iron deficit, a usual dose being the equivalent of 100 mg of iron administered not more than 3 times per week. The maximum single dose is 200 mg of iron. A small test dose should be administered initially. Iron sucrose has also been given by mouth.

Preparations

Proprietary Preparations (details are given in Part 3)
Aust.: Ferrivenin†; Fr.: Venofer; Ger.: FERROinfant Neu; Venofer; Hong Kong: Venofer; Israel: Venofer; Ital.: Ferroven†; Ferrum Hausmann; Unifer; Mex.: Venoferrum; Port.: Venofer; Switz.: Venofer; Thai.: Venofer; UK: Venofer; USA: Venofer.
Multi-ingredient: Aust.: Ferrovin-Eisenelixier; Ger.: Hicoton; Selectafer N.

Isoleucine (593-s)

Isoleucine (USAN, rINN).
I; Ile; L-Isoleucine; Isoleucinum. L-2-Amino-3-methylvaleric acid.
$C_6H_{13}NO_2 = 131.2$.
CAS — 73-32-5.
Pharmacopoeias. In Eur. (see p.vi), Jpn, and US.

Pharmacopoeial description

Ph. Eur.: A white or almost white, crystalline powder or flakes. Sparingly soluble in water; slightly soluble in alcohol; practically insoluble in ether. It dissolves in dilute mineral acids and in dilute solutions of alkali hydroxides. Protect from light.
USP 25: White, practically odourless crystals. Soluble in water; slightly soluble in hot alcohol; insoluble in ether. pH of a 1% solution in water is between 5.5 and 7.0.

Profile

Isoleucine is a branched-chain amino acid which is an essential constituent of the diet. It is used as a dietary supplement. It is also an ingredient of several preparations that have been promoted for disorders of the liver.

Preparations

Proprietary Preparations (details are given in Part 3)
Multi-ingredient: Ger.: Bramin-hepa; Falkamin; Ital.: Falkamin; Isobranch; Isoram.

Isomalt (14038-q)

Isomalt (BAN).
Bay-i-3930; E953; Isomaltitol; Isomaltum.
Pharmacopoeias. In Eur. (see p.vi).

Pharmacopoeial description

Ph. Eur.: A mixture of 6-O-α-D-glucopyranosyl-D-glucitol ($C_{12}H_{24}O_{11} = 344.3$) and 1-O-α-D-glucopyranosyl-D-mannitol dihydrate ($C_{12}H_{24}O_{11},2H_2O = 380.3$) and neither of the two components is less than 3%, calculated with reference to the anhydrous substance. A white or almost white powder or granules. Freely soluble in water; very slightly soluble in dehydrated alcohol.

Profile

Isomalt is a sugar alcohol (polyol) used as a bulk sweetener in foods. The ingestion of large quantities may produce flatulence and have a laxative effect.

◊ A WHO Expert Committee reported[1] that isomalt is partly metabolised in the small intestine to glucose, mannitol, and sorbitol and the remaining isomalt is completely metabolised by the flora of the large intestine. The Australian manufacturers

have commented that the hydrolysis and absorption is minimal and does not significantly affect blood-sugar or insulin concentrations; they consider isomalt to be suitable for use by diabetic patients.[2]

1. FAO/WHO. Evaluation of certain food additives and contaminants: twenty-ninth report of the joint FAO/WHO expert committee on food additives. WHO Tech Rep Ser 733 1986.
2. Barnes JA. Martindale and isomalt. Aust J Pharm 1994; 75: 183.

Lactose (594-w)

Lactosum; Lattosio; Milk Sugar; Saccharum Lactis.
CAS — 63-42-3 (anhydrous lactose); 5989-81-1 (lactose monohydrate); 10039-26-6 (lactose monohydrate, cyclic); 64044-51-5 (lactose monohydrate, open form).
Pharmacopoeias. In Chin., Eur. (see p.vi), Int., Jpn, and Pol. Also in USNF. Some pharmacopoeias include separate monographs for Anhydrous Lactose and Lactose Monohydrate.

A 9.75% solution in water is iso-osmotic with blood.
A disaccharide obtained from the whey of milk. Lactose may exist in a number of distinct forms depending upon the crystallisation and drying processes employed. The forms can vary in the contents of crystalline and amorphous lactose, the amounts of α-lactose (O-β-D-galactopyranosyl-(1→4)-α-D-glucopyranose) and β-lactose (O-β-D-galactopyranosyl-(1→4)-β-D-glucopyranose), and in their hydration states. The α-form of lactose exists in either the anhydrous ($C_{12}H_{22}O_{11} = 342.3$) or monohydrate ($C_{12}H_{22}O_{11},H_2O = 360.3$) state whereas the β-form exists only in the anhydrous state. Commercial lactose is mainly the α-monohydrate.

Pharmacopoeial description

Ph. Eur.: Anhydrous Lactose is β-lactose or a mixture of α-lactose and β-lactose. A white or almost white, crystalline powder. Freely but slowly soluble in water; practically insoluble in alcohol.
Lactose Monohydrate is the monohydrate of α-lactose. It may be modified as to its physical characteristics and may contain varying proportions of amorphous lactose. A white or almost white, crystalline powder. Freely but slowly soluble in water; practically insoluble in alcohol. Store in airtight containers.
USNF 20: Anhydrous Lactose is primarily β-lactose or a mixture of α- and β-lactose. It is a white or almost white powder. Freely soluble in water; practically insoluble in alcohol.
Lactose Monohydrate is a natural disaccharide, obtained from milk, which consists of one glucose and one galactose moiety. It may be modified as to its physical characteristics, and may contain varying proportions of amorphous lactose. It is a white, free-flowing powder. Freely, but slowly soluble in water; practically insoluble in alcohol. Store in airtight containers.

Adverse Effects and Precautions

Lactose intolerance occurs due to a deficiency of the intestinal enzyme lactase. Ingestion of lactose by patients with lactase deficiency leads to a clinical syndrome of abdominal pain, diarrhoea, distension, and flatulence; symptoms may also occur in persons without such a deficiency who have ingested excessive amounts of lactose.

Lactose is contra-indicated in patients with galactosaemia, the glucose-galactose malabsorption syndrome, or lactase deficiency.

Lactose intolerance. A review of lactose intolerance.[1] The capacity of the infant intestine to produce lactase, the enzyme responsible for digesting lactose, is retained into adulthood only by a minority of the world's population, mostly of north European descent; in Africa and Asia more than 90% of the population are lactase deficient. Because of the ubiquity of lactose in the diet and the consequent frequency of abdominal symptoms, attempts have been made to treat lactose intolerance by dietary exclusion (which need not be complete since lactase deficiency is rarely absolute). An alternative is enzyme replacement therapy with β-galactosidase from micro-organisms (see Tilactase, p.1673), but the role of such therapy has yet to be fully determined. The findings of one study[2] suggested that, in adults with lactose intolerance, the use of lactose-digestive aids is unnecessary if lactose intake is limited to the equivalent of 240 mL of milk or less daily.
For the use of soya in infants intolerant to cows' milk, see p.1379.

1. Anonymous. Lactose intolerance. Lancet 1991; 338: 663–4.
2. Suarez FL, et al. A comparison of symptoms after the consumption of milk or lactose-hydrolysed milk by people with self-reported severe lactose intolerance. N Engl J Med 1995; 333: 1–4.

Pharmacokinetics

Lactose is hydrolysed by lactase in the small intestine to glucose and galactose, which are then absorbed.

Uses and Administration

Lactose, the carbohydrate component of milk, is less sweet than sucrose.

Lactose is widely used in pharmaceutical manufacturing. In the production of capsules or tablets it may be employed as a diluent, bulking agent, filler, or excipient and in powders as a bulking agent. Lactose is also used as a carrier for drugs in dry powder inhalers. Characteristics such as particle size make different grades of lactose suitable for different applications.

Preparations

Proprietary Preparations (details are given in Part 3)
Aust.: Vitawund Baby; Canad.: Novo-Plus†.
Multi-ingredient: Aust.: Ichth-Oestren; Joghurt Milkitten†; Braz.: Lacto-Purga; Ger.: Eugalan Topfer forte; Eugalan Topfer forte LC.

Leucine (597-y)

Leucine (USAN, rINN).
α-Aminoisocaproic Acid; L; Leu; L-Leucine; Leucinum. L-2-Amino-4-methylvaleric acid.
$C_6H_{13}NO_2 = 131.2$.
CAS — 61-90-5.
Pharmacopoeias. In Eur. (see p.vi), Jpn, and US.

Pharmacopoeial description

Ph. Eur.: A white or almost white, crystalline powder or shiny flakes. Sparingly soluble in water; practically insoluble in alcohol and in ether. It dissolves in dilute mineral acids and in dilute solutions of alkali hydroxides. Protect from light.
USP 25: White, practically odourless crystals. Sparingly soluble in water; insoluble in ether. pH of a 1% solution in water is between 5.5 and 7.0.

Profile

Leucine is a branched-chain amino acid which is an essential constituent of the diet. It is used as a dietary supplement. It is also an ingredient of several preparations that have been promoted for disorders of the liver.

Preparations

Proprietary Preparations (details are given in Part 3)
Multi-ingredient: Fr.: Revitalose; Ger.: Bramin-hepa; Falkamin; Ital.: Falkamin; Isobranch; Isoram.

Lysine (12141-y)

Lysine (USAN, rINN).
K; Lys; L-Lysine. L-2,6-Diaminohexanoic acid.
$C_6H_{14}N_2O_2 = 146.2$.
CAS — 56-87-1.
ATC — B05XB03.
Pharmacopoeias. In Ger. as the monohydrate.

Lysine Acetate (669-y)

Lysine Acetate (rINNM).
Lys Acetate; L-Lysine Monoacetate. L-2,6-Diaminohexanoic acid acetate.
$C_6H_{14}N_2O_2,C_2H_4O_2 = 206.2$.
CAS — 57282-49-2.
Pharmacopoeias. In US.

Pharmacopoeial description

USP 25: White, odourless crystals or crystalline powder. Freely soluble in water.

Lysine Hydrochloride (599-z)

Lysine Hydrochloride (USAN, rINNM).
Lys Hydrochloride; L-Lysine Monohydrochloride; Lysini Hydrochloridum. L-2,6-Diaminohexanoic acid hydrochloride.
$C_6H_{14}N_2O_2,HCl = 182.6$.
CAS — 657-27-2.
Pharmacopoeias. In Eur. (see p.vi), Jpn, and US.

Pharmacopoeial description

Ph. Eur.: A white crystalline powder or colourless crystals. Freely soluble in water; slightly soluble in alcohol; practically insoluble in ether. Protect from light.
USP 25: A white, odourless powder. Freely soluble in water.

Profile

Lysine is an aliphatic amino acid which is an essential constituent of the diet. Lysine and lysine hydrochloride are used as dietary supplements.

Preparations

Proprietary Preparations (details are given in Part 3)
Port.: Incremin.
Multi-ingredient: Austral.: Cold Sore Relief; Cold Sore Tablets; Vitaline; Braz.: Lisin Sorb; Fr.: Acti 5†; Curasten; Revitalose; Ital.: Biocarnil; Calciofix; Mex.: Corpotasin CL; Spain: Acticinco; Calcioretard; Euzymina Lisina I; Euzymina Lisina II; Malandil; Pranzo; UK: Amino MS; USA: Klorvess.

Maize Oil (7361-m)

Corn Oil; Huile de Maïs; Ol. Mayd.; Oleum Maydis.

Pharmacopoeias. In *Eur* (see p.vi) and *Jpn*. Also in *USNF*.

Pharmacopoeial description

Ph. Eur.: The refined fatty oil obtained from the seeds of *Zea mays*. A clear, light yellow or yellow oil. Practically insoluble in water and in alcohol; miscible with dichloromethane and with petroleum spirit (b.p.: 40° to 60°). Store at a temperature not exceeding 25°. Protect from light.

USNF 20: The refined fixed oil obtained from the embryos of *Zea mays* (Gramineae). A clear, light yellow, oily liquid having a faint characteristic odour. Slightly soluble in alcohol; miscible with chloroform, with ether, with petroleum spirit, and with benzene. Store in airtight containers at a temperature not exceeding 40°. Protect from light.

Profile

Maize oil has a high content of unsaturated acids and has been used in patients with familial hypercholesterolaemia and as a high-calorie nutritional supplement. It is also used as an oily vehicle.

Preparations

Proprietary Preparations (details are given in Part 3)

Multi-ingredient: *USA:* Lipomul.

Malt Extract (601-c)

Extractum Bynes.

It contains 50% or more of maltose, together with dextrin, glucose, and small amounts of other carbohydrates, and protein. It is prepared from malted grain of barley (*Hordeum distichon* or *H. vulgare*) or a mixture of this with not more than 33% of malted grain of wheat (*Triticum aestivum* or *T. turgidum*).

Profile

Malt extract has nutritive properties. It is chiefly used as a vehicle in preparations containing cod-liver oil (p.1357) and halibut-liver oil (p.1366). It is a useful flavouring agent for masking bitter tastes.

A product known as malt soup extract, obtained from barley grains, and containing 73% maltose together with 12% other polymeric carbohydrates as well as small amounts of proteins, electrolytes, and vitamins, is sometimes used as a laxative.

Preparations

Proprietary Preparations (details are given in Part 3)
USA: Maltsupex.

Multi-ingredient: *Braz.:* Anemokol; Pinosil; *Fr.:* Elixir Contre La Toux Weleda†; Galactogil; *Switz.:* Optilax†; *USA:* Syllamalt†.

Maltitol (13690-b)

Maltitol (*BAN*).

E965; Hydrogenated Maltose; D-Maltitol; Maltitolum. α-D-Glucopyranosyl-1,4-D-glucitol.

$C_{12}H_{24}O_{11} = 344.3$.
CAS — 585-88-6.
Pharmacopoeias. In *Eur.* (see p.vi).

Pharmacopoeial description

Ph. Eur.: A white crystalline powder. Very soluble in water; practically insoluble in dehydrated alcohol.

Maltitol Syrup (10169-s)

E965; Hydrogenated Glucose Syrup; Hydrogenated High Maltose-glucose Syrup; Liquid Maltitol; Maltitol Solution; Maltitolum Liquidum.

Pharmacopoeias. In *Eur.* (see p.vi). Also in *USNF*.

Pharmacopoeial description

Ph. Eur.: An aqueous solution of a hydrogenated, part hydrolysed starch, containing not less than 68.0% w/w and not more than 85.0% w/w of anhydrous substance composed of a mixture of mainly D-maltitol with D-sorbitol and hydrogenated oligo- and polysaccharides. It contains not less than 50.0% w/w of D-maltitol and not more than 8.0% w/w of D-sorbitol, both calculated with reference to the anhydrous substance. A clear, colourless, syrupy liquid. Miscible with water and with glycerol.

USNF 20: Maltitol Solution is a water solution of a hydrogenated, partially hydrolysed starch. It contains, on an anhydrous basis, not less than 50.0% of D-maltitol (w/w) and not more than 16.0% of D-sorbitol (w/w). Store in airtight containers.

◊ Hydrogenated glucose syrup is a generic term encompassing products of widely varying composition and it was concluded that such products containing up to 90% of maltitol should more properly be called maltitol syrup.[1] This was subsequently amended to include products containing up to 98% maltitol.[2]

The symbol † denotes a preparation no longer actively marketed

---

Preparations containing a minimum of 98% of maltitol were designated the title maltitol.

1. FAO/WHO. Evaluation of certain food additives and contaminants: thirty-third report of the joint FAO/WHO expert committee on food additives. *WHO Tech Rep Ser 776* 1989.
2. FAO/WHO. Evaluation of certain food additives and contaminants: forty-first report of the joint FAO/WHO expert committee on food additives. *WHO Tech Rep Ser 837* 1993.

Profile

Maltitol and maltitol syrup are bulk sweeteners used in foods; they are considered to be less cariogenic than sucrose. The ingestion of large quantities may produce flatulence and diarrhoea.

Preparations

USNF 20: Maltitol Solution.

Maltodextrin (602-k)

Maltodextrinum.

Pharmacopoeias. In *Eur.* (see p.vi). Also in *USNF*.

Pharmacopoeial description

Ph. Eur.: A mixture of glucose, disaccharides, and polysaccharides, obtained by the partial hydrolysis of starch. The degree of hydrolysis, expressed as dextrose equivalent (DE) is not more than 20. A white or almost white, slightly hygroscopic powder or granules. Freely soluble in water.

USNF 20: A nonsweet, nutritive saccharide mixture of polymers that consists of D-glucose units with a Dextrose Equivalent of less than 20. It is prepared by the partial hydrolysis of food grade starch with suitable acids and/or enzymes. White, hygroscopic powder or granules. Freely soluble or readily dispersible in water; slightly soluble to insoluble in dehydrated alcohol. pH of a 20% solution in water is between 4.0 and 7.0. Store in airtight containers at a temperature not exceeding 30° and a relative humidity not exceeding 50%.

Profile

Maltodextrin, a malto-oligosaccharide, is a source of carbohydrate often used in oral dietary supplements and tube feeding. It rapidly releases glucose in the gastrointestinal tract but because of the high average molecular weight of maltodextrin, solutions have a lower osmolarity than isocaloric solutions of glucose. Additionally, preparations based on maltodextrin and intended for dietary supplementation usually have a low electrolyte content and are free of other sugars such as fructose, galactose, lactose, and sucrose. These properties make such preparations suitable for dietary supplementation in a variety of diseases including certain gastrointestinal disorders where malabsorption is a problem, in disaccharide intolerance (without isomaltose intolerance), and in acute and chronic hepatic and renal diseases where protein, mineral, and fluid restriction are often necessary.

Maltodextrin is also employed as a pharmaceutical excipient.

Preparations

Proprietary Preparations (details are given in Part 3)
Austral.: Maxijul; *Fin.:* Fantomalt; *Irl.:* Fibrosine†; *Israel:* Maxijul; *Ital.:* Energen; Fantomalt; Maltovis; Nidex; *NZ:* Moducal; *Port.:* Fantomalt; Fibrosine.

Multi-ingredient: *Austral.:* Moducal; *Fr.:* Gumilk; *Ital.:* Doldieta†; Giflorex.

Maltose (603-a)

4-O-α-D-Glucopyranosyl-β-D-glucopyranose.

$C_{12}H_{22}O_{11} = 342.3$.
CAS — 69-79-4 (anhydrous maltose); 6363-53-7 (maltose monohydrate).
Pharmacopoeias. In *Jpn*.

It is obtained from starch by hydrolysis with amylase. The hydration of maltose depends on the solvent from which it is crystallised.

Profile

Maltose, a disaccharide composed of two glucose molecules, is less sweet than sucrose. It is often present with other sugars in mixtures used as carbohydrate sources.

Adverse effects. Hyponatraemia developed in a patient with acute renal failure after liver transplantation following intravenous infusion of normal immunoglobulin in 10% maltose.[1] The effect which recurred on each of four successive infusions resembled that of hyperglycaemia and was thought to be due to accumulation of maltose and other osmotically active metabolites in the extracellular fluid.

1. Palevsky PM, *et al.* Maltose-induced hyponatremia. *Ann Intern Med* 1993; **118:** 526–8.

Preparations

USNF 20: Liquid Glucose.

Proprietary Preparations (details are given in Part 3)
Jpn: Martos-10†.

Multi-ingredient: *Fr.:* Picot.

Manganese (5303-d)

Mn = 54.938049.
CAS — 7439-96-5.

Manganese Chloride (18463-w)

$MnCl_2.4H_2O = 197.9$.
CAS — 7773-01-5 (anhydrous manganese chloride); 13446-34-9 (manganese chloride tetrahydrate).
Pharmacopoeias. In *US*.

Pharmacopoeial description

USP 25: Large, irregular, pink, odourless, translucent crystals. Soluble in water and in alcohol; insoluble in ether. Store in airtight containers. pH of a 5% solution in water is between 3.5 and 6.0.

Manganese Gluconate (18506-v)

Bis(D-gluconato-O^1,O^2)manganese; Manganese D-gluconate.
$C_{12}H_{22}MnO_{14} = 445.2$.
Pharmacopoeias. In *US* which allows either the anhydrous or dihydrate form.

Manganese Sulfate (5304-n)

Manganese Sulphate; Mangani Sulfas. Manganese (II) sulphate tetrahydrate.
$MnSO_4.4H_2O = 223.1$.
CAS — 7785-87-7 (anhydrous manganese sulfate); 10034-96-5 (manganese sulfate monohydrate); 10101-68-5 (manganese sulfate tetrahydrate).
Pharmacopoeias. In *Br.* and *Fr.*
Eur. (see p.vi) and *US* include the monohydrate.

Pharmacopoeial description

BP 2001: Manganese Sulphate (the tetrahydrate form) occurs as pale pink, odourless or almost odourless, crystals or crystalline powder. Freely soluble in water; practically insoluble in alcohol.

Ph. Eur.: Manganese Sulphate Monohydrate occurs as a pale pink, slightly hygroscopic, crystalline powder. Freely soluble in water; practically insoluble in alcohol.

USP 25: Manganese Sulfate (monohydrate) occurs as pale red, slightly efflorescent crystals, or as a purple, odourless powder. Soluble in water; insoluble in alcohol. Store in airtight containers.

Adverse Effects and Precautions

Acute poisoning due to ingestion of manganese or manganese salts is rare. The main symptoms of chronic poisoning, either from injection or usually inhalation of manganese dust or fumes in air, include extrapyramidal effects which may be followed by progressive deterioration in the CNS. Parenteral manganese should be used cautiously in patients with reduced biliary excretion, especially in cholestatic liver disease. When the duration of total parenteral nutrition is likely to exceed 1 month, serum-manganese concentration and liver function should be checked before commencing treatment and regularly during treatment; additives containing manganese should be discontinued if serum-manganese concentrations are raised or cholestasis develops.

◊ Cholestatic liver disease, and possibly changes in the basal ganglia have been reported to be associated with hypermanganesaemia in children receiving long-term parenteral nutrition;[1,2] manganese accumulation may be secondary to impaired biliary excretion.[3] Manganese supplementation in such patients requires re-appraisal and whole blood manganese concentrations should be monitored regularly. A low-dose regimen of not more than 1 μg (0.018 μmol) per kg body-weight daily has been suggested,[2,3] which is the dose recommended by the American Society of Clinical Nutrition.[4] Hypermanganesaemia and basal ganglia manganese deposition resolved over time in 2 children when the manganese dose in their parenteral nutrition was reduced.[5] Manganese accumulation in the basal ganglia has been observed in patients with liver cirrhosis.[6]

1. Reynolds AP, *et al.* Manganese in long term paediatric parenteral nutrition. *Arch Dis Child* 1994; **71:** 527–8.
2. Fell JME, *et al.* Manganese toxicity in children receiving long-term parenteral nutrition. *Lancet* 1996; **347:** 1218–21.
3. Beath SV, *et al.* Manganese toxicity and parenteral nutrition. *Lancet* 1996; **347:** 1773–4. Correction. *ibid.* **348:** 416.
4. Greene HL, *et al.* Guidelines for the use of vitamins, trace elements, calcium, magnesium, and phosphorus in infants and children receiving total parenteral nutrition: report of the Subcommittee on Pediatric Parenteral Nutrient Requirements from the Committee on Clinical Practice Issues of The American Society for Clinical Nutrition. *Am J Clin Nutr* 1988; **48:** 1324–42.
5. Kafritsa Y, *et al.* Long term outcome of brain manganese deposition in patients on home parenteral nutrition. *Arch Dis Child* 1998; **79:** 263–5.
6. Krieger D, *et al.* Manganese and chronic hepatic encephalopathy. *Lancet* 1995; **346:** 270–4.

Pharmacokinetics

Absorption of manganese from the gastrointestinal tract is variable, ranging from 3 to 50%. There is some evidence that the amount absorbed decreases as intake increases, suggesting a homoeostatic response. In the circulation, manganese is bound to transmanganin, a beta-1-globulin. Manganese is stored in the brain, kidneys, pancreas, and liver. It is excreted in bile, and undergoes enterohepatic circulation.

Uses and Administration

Manganese is an essential trace element and small amounts of a salt such as the chloride or sulfate are sometimes added to solutions for total parenteral nutrition. Suggested doses are 275 μg (5 μmol) elemental manganese daily for adults and children over 40 kg body-weight, and 1 μg (0.0182 μmol) per kg body-weight for infants and children to a maximum of 15 μg (see also under Adverse Effects, above).

Manganese compounds or salts that have been used in therapeutics in addition to those mentioned above include manganese amino acid chelate, manganese dioxide, manganese gluconate, and manganese hydrogen citrate.

Human requirements. In the UK neither a reference nutrient intake (RNI) nor an estimated average requirement (EAR) (see p.1352) has been set for manganese although a safe intake for adults was believed to lie above 1.4 mg (26 μmol) daily.[1] Similarly, in the USA a recommended dietary allowance has not been published, although an adequate intake has been estimated to be 2.3 mg daily for men and 1.8 mg daily for women.[2] A tolerable upper intake level of 11 mg has also been set.[2] WHO has not proposed a safe range of mean population intakes for manganese since neither intakes resulting in deficiency nor threshold toxicity levels have been established.[3] Diets high in unrefined cereals, nuts, leafy vegetables, and tea will be high in manganese.

1. DoH. Dietary reference values for food energy and nutrients for the United Kingdom: report of the panel on dietary reference values of the committee on medical aspects of food policy. *Report on health and social subjects 41.* London: HMSO, 1991.
2. Standing Committee on the Scientific Evaluation of Dietary Reference Intakes of the Food and Nutrition Board. *Dietary Reference Intakes for vitamin A, vitamin K, arsenic, boron, chromium, copper, iodine, iron, manganese, molybdenum, nickel, silicon, vanadium, and zinc.* Washington DC: National Academy Press, 2001.
3. WHO. Manganese. In: *Trace elements in human nutrition and health.* Geneva: WHO, 1996; 163–7.

Preparations

BPC 1973: Compound Ferrous Sulphate Tablets;
USP 25: Manganese Chloride Injection; Manganese Chloride for Oral Solution; Manganese Sulfate Injection.

Proprietary Preparations (details are given in Part 3)
Canad.: Micro Mn†; *Fr.:* Mangaplexe; *Mex.:* MN-Fusin.

Multi-ingredient: *Austral.:* Bio Magnesium; *Braz.:* Xantina B12; Xantinon B12; *Fr.:* Megasthenyl†; Oligoderm; *Hong Kong:* Eviprostat; *Irl.:* Ferrotab; *Port.:* Cobalti; *Singapore:* Eviprostat; Ferromex; Neogobion.

Medium-chain Triglycerides (7357-q)

Triglycerida Saturata Media.
Pharmacopoeias. In *Eur.* (see p.vi).

Pharmacopoeial description

Ph. Eur.: They are obtained from the oil extracted from the hard, dried fraction of the endosperm of *Cocos nucifera* or from the dried endosperm of *Elaeis guineensis.* They consist of a mixture of triglycerides of saturated fatty acids, mainly of octanoic acid (p.1643) and of capric acid ($C_{10}H_{20}O_2$). They contain not less than 95% of saturated fatty acids with 8 and 10 carbon atoms.

A colourless or slightly yellowish, oily liquid. Practically insoluble in water; miscible with alcohol, with dichloromethane, with petroleum spirit, and with fatty oils. Store in well-filled containers. Protect from light.

Profile

Medium-chain triglycerides are used for enteral and parenteral nutrition (p.1351) in conditions associated with malabsorption of fat, such as cystic fibrosis, enteritis, and steatorrhoea, and following intestinal resection. Medium-chain triglycerides are more readily hydrolysed than long-chain triglycerides and are not dependent upon biliary or pancreatic secretions for absorption from the gastrointestinal tract. They provide 35 kJ (8.3 kcal) per g. They do not provide essential fatty acids.

Medium-chain triglycerides have also been used as bases for pharmaceutical preparations.

Preparations

Proprietary Preparations (details are given in Part 3)
Austral.: Liquigen; MCT Oil; *Canad.:* MCT Oil; *Fin.:* Liquigen; MCT Oljymoduli; *Fr.:* Liquigen; *Israel:* MCT; *Ital.:* MCT; *NZ:* Liquigen; *Port.:* MCT Oil; *Singapore:* Liquigen; MCT; *Thai.:* MCT Oil; *UK:* Alembicol D; *USA:* MCT.

Multi-ingredient: *Aust.:* Lipofundin mit MCT; *Belg.:* Medialipide; *Fin.:* Nutriflex Lipid; Vasolipid; *Fr.:* Liprocil; Medialipide; *Ger.:* Gleitgelen; Lipofundin MCT; Lipovenos MCT; *Hong Kong:* Lipofundin MCT/LCT; *Irl.:* Caprilon; Liquigen; MCT Duocal; *Israel:* Lipofundin MCT/LCT; *Ital.:* Lipofundin MCT; *Norw.:* Vasolipid; *Port.:* Lipofundin MCT/LCT; Nutribraun; *S.Afr.:* Lipofundin MCT/LCT; *Singapore:* Lipofundin MCT/LCT; *Spain:* Lipofundina MCT/LCT; *Swed.:* Structolipid; Vasolipid; *Switz.:* Lipofundin MCT; *Thai.:* Lipofundin MCT/LCT; *UK:* Caprilon; Imuderm; Lipofundin MCT/LCT; Liquigen; MCT Oil; MCT Pepdite.

Molybdenum (16901-d)

Mo = 95.94.

Ammonium Molybdate (18365-p)

Hexaammonium molybdate tetrahydrate.
$(NH_4)_6Mo_7O_{24},4H_2O = 1235.9.$
CAS — 12054-85-2.
Pharmacopoeias. In *US.*

Pharmacopoeial description

USP 25: Colourless or slightly greenish or yellowish crystals. Soluble in water; practically insoluble in alcohol. Store in airtight containers.

Sodium Molybdate (18511-h)

Natrii Molybdas.
$Na_2MoO_4 = 205.9.$
Pharmacopoeias. In *Ger. Eur.* (see p.vi) includes a monograph for the dihydrate.

Pharmacopoeial description

Ph. Eur.: Sodium Molybdate Dihydrate occurs as a white powder or colourless crystals. Freely soluble in water.

Adverse Effects

Very high intakes of molybdenum, and associated increases in xanthine oxidase activity, may result in hyperuricaemia, and possibly gout. Molybdenum intoxication may impair the utilisation of copper.

Uses and Administration

Molybdenum is an essential trace element and small amounts, in the form of ammonium molybdate or sodium molybdate, are sometimes added to solutions for total parenteral nutrition. A suggested dose is about 20 to 120 μg (0.2 to 1.2 μmol) elemental molybdenum daily.

Ammonium molybdate is used in veterinary medicine to treat copper poisoning in sheep.

Human requirements. In the UK neither a reference nutrient intake (RNI) nor an estimated average requirement (EAR) (see p.1352) has been set for molybdenum although a safe intake was believed to be between 50 and 400 μg (0.5 and 4 μmol) daily for adults.[1] In the USA, the recommended dietary allowance is 45 μg daily for adults.[2] The tolerable upper intake level is 2 mg daily.[2] WHO make the suggestion that the adult basal requirement for molybdenum could be about 25 μg daily, corresponding to approximately 0.4 μg per kg body-weight.[3]

Foods contributing to dietary molybdenum include milk, beans, breads, and cereals; however, extreme regional variations occur in molybdenum contents of food crops due to soil differences.

1. DoH. Dietary reference values for food energy and nutrients for the United Kingdom: report of the panel on dietary reference values of the committee on medical aspects of food policy. *Report on health and social subjects 41.* London: HMSO, 1991.
2. Standing Committee on the Scientific Evaluation of Dietary Reference Intakes of the Food and Nutrition Board. *Dietary Reference Intakes for vitamin A, vitamin K, arsenic, boron, chromium, copper, iodine, iron, manganese, molybdenum, nickel, silicon, vanadium, and zinc.* Washington DC: National Academy Press, 2001.
3. WHO. Molybdenum. In: *Trace elements in human nutrition and health.* Geneva: WHO, 1996; 144–54.

Preparations

USP 25: Ammonium Molybdate Injection.

Proprietary Preparations (details are given in Part 3)
Fr.: Molybdene Injectable; *USA:* Molypen.

Monosodium Glutamate (617-n)

Chinese Seasoning; E621; MSG; Natrii Glutamas; Sodium Glutamate. Sodium hydrogen L-(+)-2-aminoglutarate monohydrate.
$C_5H_8NNaO_4,H_2O = 187.1.$
CAS — 142-47-2 (anhydrous monosodium glutamate).
Pharmacopoeias. In *USNF. Chin.* includes the injection.

Monosodium glutamate 32 g is approximately equivalent to anhydrous monosodium glutamate 29 g or glutamic acid 25 g.

Pharmacopoeial description

USNF 20: White, practically odourless, free-flowing crystals or crystalline powder. It may have either a slightly sweet or slightly salty taste. Freely soluble in water; sparingly soluble in alcohol. pH of a 5% solution in water is between 6.7 and 7.2. Store in airtight containers.

Profile

Monosodium glutamate is widely used as a flavour enhancer and imparts a meaty flavour.

In susceptible individuals, ingestion of foods containing monosodium glutamate may result in flushing, facial pressure, chest pain, headache, and nausea. The symptoms tend to occur within an hour of eating 3 g or more of monosodium glutamate on an empty stomach.

Preparations

Proprietary Preparations (details are given in Part 3)
Multi-ingredient: *Thai.:* Hemo-Cyto-Serum.

Nicotinic Acid (7865-b)

Nicotinic Acid (rINN).
375; Acidum Nicotinicum; Niacin; Nikotinsäure. Pyridine-3-carboxylic acid.
$C_6H_5NO_2 = 123.1.$
CAS — 59-67-6.
ATC — C04AC01; C10AD02.

NOTE. Some published sources use the term niacin as a generic term to include both nicotinic acid and nicotinamide; in the USP 25 the title niacin is applied specifically to nicotinic acid.
Pharmacopoeias. In *Chin., Eur.* (see p.vi), *Int., Jpn,* and *US.*

Pharmacopoeial description

Ph. Eur.: A white, crystalline powder. Sparingly soluble in water; soluble in boiling water and in boiling alcohol; practically insoluble in ether. It dissolves in dilute solutions of alkali hydroxides and carbonates. Protect from light.

USP 25: White crystals or crystalline powder, odourless or has a slight odour. Soluble 1 in 60 of water; freely soluble in boiling water, in boiling alcohol, and in solutions of alkali hydroxides and carbonates; practically insoluble in ether.

Nicotinamide (7864-m)

Nicotinamide (rINN).
Niacinamide; Nicotinamidum; Nicotinic Acid Amide; Nicotylamide; Vitamin B₃; Vitamin PP. Pyridine-3-carboxamide.
$C_6H_6N_2O = 122.1.$
CAS — 98-92-0.
ATC — A11HA01.
Pharmacopoeias. In *Chin., Eur.* (see p.vi), *Int., Jpn, Pol.,* and *US.*

Pharmacopoeial description

Ph. Eur.: A white crystalline powder or colourless crystals. Freely soluble in water and in dehydrated alcohol. A 5% solution in water has a pH of 6.0 to 7.5.

USP 25: A white crystalline powder, odourless or practically so. Soluble 1 in 1.5 of water, 1 in 10 of boiling water, and 1 in 5.5 of alcohol; soluble in glycerol. Its solutions are neutral to litmus. Store in airtight containers.

Adverse Effects and Treatment

Nicotinic acid has a vasodilator action and when given by mouth or by injection in therapeutic doses it may cause flushing, a sensation of heat, faintness, and a pounding in the head. These symptoms are transient and various strategies have been proposed to reduce them (see below). Nicotinamide does not have a vasodilator action.

Other adverse effects which have been reported, especially following high doses of nicotinic acid, include dryness of the skin, pruritus, hyperpigmentation, abdominal cramps, diarrhoea, nausea and vomiting, anorexia, activation of peptic ulcer, amblyopia, jaundice and impairment of liver function, decrease in glucose tolerance, hyperglycaemia, and hyperuricaemia. Most of these effects subside on withdrawal of the drug.

Topical nicotinamide may cause dryness of the skin and, less frequently, pruritus, erythema, burning sensation, and irritation. Frequency of application should be reduced if these effects occur.

◊ Nicotinic acid produces frequent adverse effects, but they are not usually serious, tend to decrease with time, and some can be minimised by following appropriate instructions for use.[1,2] Dermal and gastrointestinal reactions are most common. Truncal and facial flushing are reported in 90 to 100% of treated patients in large clinical trials; they appear to be prostaglandin-mediated and can be reduced with aspirin 75 mg or 325 mg given shortly before nicotinic acid administration, or simply by giving the nicotinic acid with food, and by starting therapy with a low dose and gradually increasing this. Flushing may be less common with modified-release formulations.[2] Significant elevations of liver enzymes are occasionally seen with nicotinic acid therapy. They are more common in patients given large dosage increases over short periods of time, and in patients treated with modified-release formulations. It has been suggested[3] that since effects on liver function may in some instances lead to hepatic failure and are more common with modified-release dosage forms the use of crystalline immediate-release preparations should be preferred, a view shared by other commentators.[4] However, although studies appear to confirm a more frequent association of hepatotoxicity with modified-release dosage forms[5-7] it should be borne in mind that these effects can also occur with the immediate-release preparations, especially at high doses. There is also a suggestion that not all modified-release preparations are alike in their effects.[8] (For further references to hepatotoxicity, see Effects on the Liver, below.)

Nicotinic acid can reduce glucose tolerance, and this may be problematic in patients with diabetes mellitus,[2,4] although nicotinamide has been investigated in the prevention of diabetes mellitus (see below). Nicotinic acid also decreases urinary excretion of uric acid, which may result in elevation of serum uric acid and exacerbation of pre-existing gout.[2]

1. Knodel LC, Talbert RL. Adverse effects of hypolipidaemic drugs. *Med Toxicol* 1987; **2**: 10–32.
2. American Society of Health-System Pharmacists. ASHP therapeutic position statement on the safe use of niacin in the management of dyslipidemias. *Am J Health-Syst Pharm* 1997; **54**: 2815–19.
3. Palumbo PJ. Rediscovery of crystalline niacin. *Mayo Clin Proc* 1991; **66**: 112–13.
4. Kreisberg RA. Niacin: a therapeutic dilemma—"one man's drink is another's poison". *Am J Med* 1994; **97**: 313–16.
5. McKenney JM, et al. A comparison of the efficacy and toxic effects of sustained- vs immediate-release niacin in hypercholesterolemic patients. *JAMA* 1994; **271**: 672–7.
6. Rader JI, et al. Hepatic toxicity of unmodified and time-release preparations of niacin. *Am J Med* 1992; **92**: 77–81.
7. Gray DR, et al. Efficacy and safety of controlled-release niacin in dyslipoproteinemic veterans. *Ann Intern Med* 1994; **121**: 252–8.
8. Lavie CJ, Milani RV. Safety and side-effects of sustained-release niacin. *JAMA* 1994; **272**: 513–14.

Effects on the eyes. Retrospective survey of hyperlipidaemic patients suggested that dry eyes (sicca syndromes), blurred vision, and swollen eyelids might be associated with nicotinic acid therapy in some patients.[1] The effects appeared to be dose-related and reversible. In 2 patients treatment was discontinued because of symptoms suggestive of cystoid macular oedema. Three other cases of nicotinic acid maculopathy have been reported.[2]

1. Fraunfelder FW, et al. Adverse ocular effects associated with niacin therapy. *Br J Ophthalmol* 1995; **79**: 54–6.
2. Callanan D, et al. Macular edema associated with nicotinic acid (niacin). *JAMA* 1998; **279**: 1702.

Effects on the liver. As mentioned above hepatotoxicity may occur with nicotinic acid, particularly at high doses or with modified-release dosage forms, but toxicity at low doses and with immediate-release preparations has also been seen. Further references.

1. Mullin GE, et al. Fulminant hepatic failure after ingestion of sustained-release nicotinic acid. *Ann Intern Med* 1989; **iii**: 253–5.
2. Knopp RH. Niacin and hepatic failure. *Ann Intern Med* 1989; **iii**: 769.
3. Henkin Y, et al. Rechallenge with crystalline niacin after drug-induced hepatitis from sustained-release niacin. *JAMA* 1990; **264**: 241–3.
4. Hodis HN. Acute hepatic failure associated with the use of low-dose sustained-release niacin. *JAMA* 1990; **264**: 181.
5. Etchason JA, et al. Niacin-induced hepatitis: a potential side effect with low-dose time-release niacin. *Mayo Clin Proc* 1991; **66**: 23–8.
6. Rader JI, et al. Hepatic toxicity of unmodified and time-release preparations of niacin. *Am J Med* 1992; **92**: 77–81.

Effects on the muscles. Myopathy has been noted with nicotinic acid.[1] Rhabdomyolysis has occurred when nicotinic acid was given with lovastatin (see p.923).

1. Litin SC, Anderson CF. Nicotinic-acid associated myopathy: a report of three cases. *Am J Med* 1989; **86**: 481–3.

Precautions

Nicotinic acid should be given cautiously to patients with a history of peptic ulcer disease, and to patients with diabetes mellitus, gout, or impaired liver function.

Interactions

There may be an increased risk of myopathy or rhabdomyolysis when nicotinic acid is used concurrently with statins (see Effects on Skeletal Muscle, p.923). Nicotinic acid may increase the requirements for insulin or oral hypoglycaemics.

Antiepileptics. For the effect of nicotinamide on *carbamazepine*, see p.345.

Nicotine. In a patient receiving nicotinic acid as part of her regular medication, addition of therapy with transdermal nicotine patches was followed by flushing and dizziness after usual doses of nicotinic acid.[1] The patient had experienced such reactions 3 years previously on commencing nicotinic acid therapy, but not subsequently, and it was suggested that on this occasion an interaction might have been responsible.

1. Rockwell KA. Potential interaction between niacin and transdermal nicotine. *Ann Pharmacother* 1993; **27**: 1283–4.

Pharmacokinetics

Nicotinic acid and nicotinamide are readily absorbed from the gastrointestinal tract following oral administration and widely distributed in the body tissues. Nicotinic acid appears in breast milk. The main route of metabolism is their conversion to *N*-methylnicotinamide and the 2-pyridone and 4-pyridone derivatives; nicotinuric acid is also formed. Small amounts of nicotinic acid and nicotinamide are excreted unchanged in urine following therapeutic doses; however the amount excreted unchanged is increased with larger doses.

The symbol † denotes a preparation no longer actively marketed

◊ References.

1. Gugler R. Clinical pharmacokinetics of hypolipidaemic drugs. *Clin Pharmacokinet* 1978; **3**: 425–39.
2. Weiner M. Clinical pharmacology and pharmacokinetics of nicotinic acid. *Drug Metab Rev* 1979; **9**: 99–106.

Human Requirements

The daily human requirement of nicotinic acid, though not definitely known, is probably about 15 to 20 mg. Yeast, meat, fish, potatoes, green vegetables, and wholemeal cereals are good sources of nicotinic acid and nicotinamide. However they may be present in a bound, unabsorbable form in cereals, especially maize. Nicotinic acid can also be obtained from the conversion of tryptophan in the body, 60 mg of dietary tryptophan being considered equivalent to 1 mg of dietary nicotinic acid, so requirements are influenced by dietary protein intake and if protein intake is adequate there is little need for any preformed vitamin in the diet. There is generally little loss of nicotinic acid from foods during cooking.

◊ In the UK dietary reference values (see p.1352) have been published for nicotinic acid[1] and in the USA recommended dietary allowances (RDAs) have been set.[2] In the UK the reference nutrient intake (RNI) is 6.6 mg niacin equivalent per 1000 kcal daily and the estimated average requirement (EAR) is 5.5 mg niacin equivalent per 1000 kcal daily for adult males and females. One niacin equivalent is equal to 1 mg of dietary nicotinic acid or 60 mg of dietary tryptophan. In the US the RDAs are also expressed in niacin equivalents and are 16 mg daily for adult males and 14 mg daily for adult females; the EAR is 12 mg daily in males and 11 mg daily in females. The tolerable upper intake level for adults is 35 mg daily.[2]

1. DoH. Dietary reference values for food energy and nutrients for the United Kingdom: report of the panel on dietary reference values of the committee on medical aspects of food policy. *Report on health and social subjects 41.* London: HMSO, 1991.
2. Standing Committee on the Scientific Evaluation of Dietary Reference Intakes of the Food and Nutrition Board. *Dietary Reference Intakes for thiamin, riboflavin, niacin, vitamin B₆, folate, vitamin B₁₂, pantothenic acid, biotin, and choline.* Washington, DC: National Academy Press, 2000.

Uses and Administration

Nicotinic acid and nicotinamide, the form which occurs naturally in the body, are water-soluble vitamin B substances which are converted to nicotinamide adenine dinucleotide (Nadide, p.1639) and nicotinamide adenine dinucleotide phosphate (NADP). These coenzymes are involved in electron transfer reactions in the respiratory chain.

Nicotinic acid deficiency develops when the dietary intake is inadequate. Deficiency leads to the development of a syndrome known as pellagra, characterised by skin lesions, especially on areas exposed to sunlight, with hyperpigmentation and hyperkeratinisation. Other symptoms include diarrhoea, abdominal pain, glossitis, stomatitis, loss of appetite, headache, lethargy, and mental and neurological disturbances. Nicotinic acid deficiency may occur in association with other vitamin B-complex deficiency states, for example in alcoholism.

Nicotinic acid and nicotinamide are used in the treatment and prevention of nicotinic acid deficiency. Nicotinamide is preferred as it does not cause vasodilatation. They are usually given by mouth, the preferred route, but may also be given by the intramuscular route or by slow intravenous administration. Doses of up to 500 mg daily (of either compound) in divided doses have been recommended.

Nicotinic acid has been employed for its vasodilator action in the treatment of a variety of disorders; its value is not considered to be established.

In high doses, nicotinic acid has beneficial effects on blood lipid profiles, and has been used, in conjunction with dietary modification and often in association with other lipid regulating drugs, in hyperlipidaemias (see below). For the immediate-release preparations, up to 600 mg daily by mouth in 3 divided doses has been given initially, gradually increased over 2 to 4 weeks to doses of up to 6 g daily; side-effects may be a limiting factor. Alternatively, initial doses of 500 mg at night have been given as a modified-release preparation and gradually increased according to response to a maintenance dose of 1 to 2 g at bedtime.

Topical nicotinamide is used in the treatment of mild to moderate inflammatory acne (see below), typically as a 4% gel applied twice daily.

Nicotinamide has been shown to inhibit the destruction of pancreatic beta cells *in vitro* and is therefore being investigated in the prevention and treatment of type 1 diabetes mellitus (see below).

Acne. Topical nicotinamide may be used in the treatment of inflammatory acne (p.1103); nicotinamide 4% was as effective as clindamycin 1% when applied topically twice daily for 8 weeks.[1]

1. Shalita AR, et al. Topical nicotinamide compared with clindamycin gel in the treatment of inflammatory acne vulgaris. *Int J Dermatol* 1995; **34**: 434–7.

Diabetes mellitus. Nicotinic acid can affect glucose tolerance and should be used with care in established diabetes (see under Adverse Effects and Treatment, above). However, the drug has been used successfully in patients with diabetes. Nicotinamide has been reported to induce remission in patients with newly diagnosed type 1 diabetes mellitus (p.315), and may delay the onset of disease.[1,2] Nicotinic acid can also raise high-density lipoprotein (HDL)-cholesterol concentrations (see below), and one study found that changes in glucose tolerance were mild enough for the drug to be used as an alternative to statins and fibrates in diabetic patients.[3]

1. Elliott RB, Chase HP. Prevention or delay of type 1 (insulin-dependent) diabetes mellitus in children using nicotinamide. *Diabetologia* 1991; **34**: 362–5.
2. Pozzilli P, et al. Meta-analysis of nicotinamide treatment in patients with recent-onset IDDM. *Diabetes Care* 1996; **19**: 1357–63.
3. Elam MB, et al. Effect of niacin on lipid and lipoprotein levels and glycemic control in patients with diabetes and peripheral arterial disease: the ADMIT study: a randomized trial. *JAMA* 2000; **284**: 1263–70.

Hyperlipidaemias. Nicotinic acid is reported to have a favourable effect on blood-lipid profiles, raising high-density lipoprotein (HDL)-cholesterol and lowering low-density lipoprotein (LDL)-cholesterol. Immediate-release preparations exhibit this effect to a greater degree than modified-release preparations (although modified-release preparations may be better at lowering LDL-cholesterol).[1] Nicotinic acid was less effective than lovastatin at reducing LDL-cholesterol in patients with primary hypercholesterolaemia, but more effective at increasing HDL-cholesterol; lovastatin was better tolerated.[2] The first-line treatment for hyperlipidaemias remains dietary and lifestyle modification; where this fails, drug therapy may be considered (p.800). Nicotinic acid is used particularly in familial hypertriglyceridaemia, or in familial combined hyperlipidaemia when both triglyceride and cholesterol concentrations are similarly elevated.

1. McKenney JM, et al. A comparison of the efficacy and toxic effects of sustained- vs immediate-release niacin in hypercholesterolemic patients. *JAMA* 1994; **271**: 672–7.
2. Illingworth DR, et al. Comparative effects of lovastatin and niacin in primary hypercholesterolemia: a prospective trial. *Arch Intern Med* 1994; **154**: 1586–95.

Pemphigus. Oral treatment with nicotinamide and a tetracycline[1,2] has controlled lesions in pemphigus and pemphigoid (p.1106).

1. Sawai T, et al. Pemphigus vegetans with oesophageal involvement: successful treatment with minocycline and nicotinamide. *Br J Dermatol* 1995; **132**: 668–70.
2. Kolbach DN, et al. Bullous pemphigoid successfully controlled by tetracycline and nicotinamide. *Br J Dermatol* 1995; **133**: 88–90.

Preparations

BP 2001: Nicotinamide Tablets; Nicotinic Acid Tablets; Vitamins B and C Injection;
BPC 1973: Compound Vitamin B Tablets; Strong Compound Vitamin B Tablets;
USP 25: Niacin Injection; Niacin Tablets; Niacinamide Injection; Niacinamide Tablets.

Proprietary Preparations (details are given in Part 3)
Aust.: Nicovitol; *Austral.:* Papulex†; Tri-B3†; *Belg.:* Ucemine PP; *Canad.:* Papulex†; *Fr.:* Nicobion; *Ger.:* Nicobion; *Hong Kong:* Papulex; *Irl.:* Papulex; *Mex.:* Hipocol; Nacro; Nicotinoid; Pepevit; *Swed.:* Nicangin; *Thai.:* Natinate; *UK:* Papulex; *USA:* Nia-Bid†; Niacels†; Niacor; Niaspan; Nico-400†; Nicobid Tempules†; Nicotinex†; Nicotinex; Slo-Niacin.

Multi-ingredient: *Aust.:* Beneuran Vit B-Komplex; Cosaldon; Diligan; Spasmocor; *Austral.:* Bio-Chromium; Bioglan Cirflo; Bioglan Fingers & Toes†; Chilblain Formula; Cirflo†; Gingo A; Prochol; Silybum Complex; *Belg.:* Trihistalex; Vitapantol; *Braz.:* Gaba; Hepato-Flux; Necrohepat; Nicopaverina; Nicopaverina B6; *Fin.:* Neurovitan; Vertipam; *Fr.:* Bio-Chrome†; Glutamag Vitamine; Paranico†; TTD-B₃-B₄; Vita-Dermacide; Vita-Iodurol ATP†; Vita-Iodurol†; Vitaphakol; Vitarutine; *Ger.:* Antisklerosin S; Eukalisan forte; Eukalisan N; Hepagrisevit Forte-N; MerSol; Peteha; Telbibur N; Vitreolent plus; *Hong Kong:* Epargriseovit; *Israel:* Babyzim; *Ital.:* Efargen; Emazian B12; Emoantitossina; Emopon; Epargriseovit; Flar; Folepar B12; For Liver†; Fosforilasi; Neuroftal; Solvobil; Vit-Porphyrin; *Port.:* Diligan†; Vitaphakol; *S.Afr.:* Cosaldon; *Spain:* Depurativo Richelet; Espasmo Digestomen; Euzymina Lisina I; Euzymina Lisina II; Vitaphakol; *Swed.:* Histilos; Theranyl; *Switz.:* Vitaphakol†; *UK:* Crampex; Epopa; Quiet Life; S.P.H.P.

Olaflur (2496-n)

Olaflur (BAN, USAN, rINN).

Amine Fluoride 297; GA-297; SKF-38095. 2,2'-(3-[N-(2-Hydroxyethyl)octadecylamino]propylimino)diethanol dihydrofluoride.

$C_{27}H_{60}F_2N_2O_3 = 498.8$.
CAS — 6818-37-7.
ATC — A01AA03.

Profile

Olaflur is used as a source of fluoride (see Sodium Fluoride, p.1375) in the prevention of dental caries.

Preparations

Proprietary Preparations (details are given in Part 3)
Fr.: Elmex; *Israel:* Elmex.

Multi-ingredient: *Aust.:* Elmex; *Belg.:* Elmex; *Fin.:* Elmex; *Fr.:* Elmex; Meridol; *Ger.:* Elmex; Multifluorid; *Israel:* Elmex; Meridol; *Ital.:* Elmex; *Neth.:* Elmex; *S.Afr.:* Elmex; *Spain:* Elmex; *Switz.:* Elmex.

Ornithine (608-d)

Ornithine (rINN).

α,δ-Diaminovaleric Acid; L-Ornithine. L-2,5-Diaminovaleric acid.

$C_5H_{12}N_2O_2 = 132.2$.
CAS — 70-26-8.
Pharmacopoeias. Ger. includes Ornithine Aspartate and Ornithine Hydrochloride.

Profile

Ornithine is an aliphatic amino acid. It is used as a dietary supplement.

The aspartate, hydrochloride, and oxoglurate have been used in the treatment of hyperammonaemia (p.1354) and hepatic encephalopathy (p.1205).

◊ References.
1. Kircheis G, *et al.* Therapeutic efficacy of L-ornithine-L-aspartate infusions in patients with cirrhosis and hepatic encephalopathy: results of a placebo-controlled, double-blind study. *Hepatology* 1997; **25:** 1351–60.
2. Stauch S, *et al.* Oral L-ornithine-L-aspartate therapy of chronic hepatic encephalopathy: results of a placebo-controlled double-blind study. *J Hepatol* 1998; **28:** 856–64.

Preparations

Proprietary Preparations (details are given in Part 3)
Aust.: Cere; Hepa; Ornicetil; *Fr.:* Cetornan; Ornicetil; *Ger.:* Hepa-Merz; Hepa-Merz KT; Hepa-Vibolex; *Hong Kong:* Hepa-Merz; *Ital.:* Ornicetil; Ornicetil S; Ornil; Ornil KG; *Spain:* Ornicetil; *Switz.:* Ornicetil.

Multi-ingredient: *Braz.:* Necroplex; Ornihepat; Ornitargin; *Fr.:* Arnilose†; Epuram; Ornitaine; *Ger.:* Polilevo N; *Ital.:* Ipoazotal; Ipoazotal Complex; Polilevo; Somatron.

Pantothenic Acid (7866-v)

Pantothenic Acid (BAN).

Vitamin B₅. (+)-(R)-3-(2,4-Dihydroxy-3,3-dimethylbutyramido)propionic acid.

$C_9H_{17}NO_5 = 219.2$.
CAS — 79-83-4 (D-pantothenic acid); 599-54-2 (DL-pantothenic acid).

Calcium Pantothenate (7867-g)

Calcium Pantothenate (BANM, rINN).

Calcii Pantothenas; Dextro Calcium Pantothenate.

$(C_9H_{16}NO_5)_2Ca = 476.5$.
CAS — 137-08-6 (calcium D-pantothenate); 6381-63-1 (calcium DL-pantothenate);.
ATC — A11HA31; D03AX04.

Pharmacopoeias. In Chin., Eur. (see p.vi), Jpn, Pol. and US.
US also has a monograph for Racemic Calcium Pantothenate.
Ger. also includes Sodium Pantothenate.

Pharmacopoeial description

Ph. Eur.: A white, slightly hygroscopic powder. Freely soluble in water; slightly soluble in alcohol; practically insoluble in ether. A 5% solution has a pH of 6.8 to 8.0. Store in airtight containers.

USP 25: Calcium Pantothenate is the calcium salt of the dextrorotatory isomer of pantothenic acid. A white, odourless, slightly hygroscopic powder. Soluble 1 in 3 of water; practically insoluble in alcohol, in chloroform, and in ether; soluble in glycerol. Store in airtight containers.

Racemic Calcium Pantothenate is a mixture of the calcium salts of the dextrorotatory and laevorotatory isomers of pantothenic acid. The physiological activity of Racemic Calcium Pantothenate is approximately one-half that of Calcium Pantothenate. A white, slightly hygroscopic powder, having a faint characteristic odour. Freely soluble in water; practically insoluble in alcohol, in chloroform, and in ether; soluble in glycerol. Its solutions are neutral or alkaline to litmus. Store in airtight containers.

Adverse Effects

Pantothenic acid is reported to be generally non-toxic.

◊ A report of life-threatening eosinophilic pleuropericarditis associated with the use of biotin and pantothenic acid.[1] Symptoms resolved on discontinuation of the vitamins.
1. Debourdeau PM, *et al.* Life-threatening eosinophilic pleuropericardial effusion related to vitamins B₅ and H. *Ann Pharmacother* 2001; **35:** 424–6.

Pharmacokinetics

Pantothenic acid is readily absorbed from the gastrointestinal tract following oral administration. It is widely distributed in the body tissues and appears in breast milk. About 70% of pantothenic acid is excreted unchanged in the urine and about 30% in the faeces.

Human Requirements

Pantothenic acid is widely distributed in foods. Meat, legumes, and whole grain cereals are particularly rich sources; other good sources include eggs, milk, vegetables, and fruits.

◊ In the UK neither a reference nutrient intake (RNI) nor an estimated average requirement (EAR) has been set (see p.1352) for pantothenic acid although an intake of 3 to 7 mg daily for adults was believed to be adequate.[1] Similarly, in the USA a recommended dietary allowance has not been published but an adequate intake for adults was believed to be 5 mg daily, increased to 6 mg in pregnancy and 7 mg during lactation.[2]
1. DoH. Dietary reference values for food energy and nutrients for the United Kingdom: report of the panel on dietary reference values of the committee on medical aspects of food policy. *Report on health and social subjects 41.* London: HMSO, 1991.
2. Standing Committee on the Scientific Evaluation of Dietary Reference Intakes of the Food and Nutrition Board. *Dietary Reference Intakes for thiamin, riboflavin, niacin, vitamin B₆, folate, vitamin B₁₂, pantothenic acid, biotin, and choline.* Washington, DC: National Academy Press, 2000.

Uses and Administration

Pantothenic acid is traditionally considered to be a vitamin B substance. It is a component of coenzyme A which is essential in the metabolism of carbohydrate, fat, and protein.

Deficiency of pantothenic acid is unlikely in man because of its widespread distribution in food.

Pantothenic acid has no accepted therapeutic uses in human medicine, though it has been administered by mouth as a nutritional supplement, often as the calcium salt and usually in conjunction with other vitamins of the B group.

Preparations

USP 25: Calcium Pantothenate Tablets.

Proprietary Preparations (details are given in Part 3)
Austral.: Pantonate; *Canad.:* Calpan†; *Ger.:* Kerato Biciron N; *Switz.:* Panthon; *UK:* Cantopal.

Multi-ingredient: *Aust.:* Lemuval; Salbei-Halspastillen; *Austral.:* Bioglan Zn-A-C; Hair and Skin Formula; *Belg.:* Sili-MetSan; Vitapantol; *Braz.:* Gaba; Luftgaz; Pantevit; *Fr.:* Dossifil†; Forcapil; Modane; Thiopon Pantothenique†; *Ger.:* Azupanthenol; Carotin; Pantovigar; Potsilo; Regepithel; Sonnenbraun; *Hong Kong:* Regepithel; *Ital.:* Esaglut; Lasonil H; Lasoproct†; Nuleron; Silisan; Vitecaf; *Mex.:* Espaven; Modaton; *Spain:* Calcio 20 Complex; Hubergrip; Lacerdermol; Lupidon; Pantenil; Pulmofasa; Pulmofasa Antihist; Tri Hachemina; *Switz.:* Cortifluid N; Decasept N; Osa†; Sili-Met-San; *Thai.:* Chinta.

Phenylalanine (610-k)

Phenylalanine (USAN, rINN).

α-Aminohydrocinnamic Acid; F; Phe; L-Phenylalanine; Phenylalaninum. L-2-Amino-3-phenylpropionic acid.

$C_9H_{11}NO_2 = 165.2$.
CAS — 63-91-2.
Pharmacopoeias. In Eur. (see p.vi), Jpn, and US.

Pharmacopoeial description

Ph. Eur.: A white or almost white, crystalline powder, or shiny, white flakes. Sparingly soluble in water; very slightly soluble in alcohol; practically insoluble in ether. It dissolves in dilute mineral acids and in dilute solutions of alkali hydroxides. Protect from light.

USP 25: White, odourless crystals. Sparingly soluble in water; very slightly soluble in alcohol, in methyl alcohol, and in dilute mineral acids. pH of a 1% solution in water is between 5.4 and 6.0.

Profile

Phenylalanine is an aromatic amino acid which is an essential constituent of the diet. It is used as a dietary supplement.

Phenylalanine intake should be restricted in patients with phenylketonuria (see Amino Acid Metabolic Disorders, p.1350).

Vitiligo. There is no totally effective treatment for vitiligo (localised hypopigmentation, p.1106). Oral or topical photochemotherapy with psoralens is generally considered to be the best available treatment, but experimental therapy includes UVA phototherapy with phenylalanine. Administration of phenylalanine in doses of up to 100 mg per kg body-weight by mouth in conjunction with UVA/sunlight led to beneficial results in more than 90% of 200 patients with vitiligo.[1] Optimal repigmentation of the vitiliginous macules was noted in early disease, but prolonged treatment still induced repigmentation in long-standing cases. Repigmentation occurred mainly in areas rich in follicles. Such treatment is contra-indicated in phenylketonuria and in pregnancy.

Similarly a further open study reported responses in 94 of 149 patients receiving 50 to 100 mg of phenylalanine per kg daily plus twice weekly UVA treatment.[2] However, only 22% of responders had repigmentation in more than 60% of the affected area. Higher doses did not seem to be more effective than 50 mg per kg daily. Another group reported on 6 years experience of treatment of vitiligo using 50 or 100 mg of phenylalanine per kg daily, together with application of 10% phenylalanine gel and daily sun exposure.[3] Although not ideal, they considered the treatment useful, especially for its ability to rapidly repigment the face.
1. Cormane RH, *et al.* Treatment of vitiligo with L-phenylalanine and light. *Br J Dermatol* 1986; **115:** 587.
2. Siddiqui AH, *et al.* L-Phenylalanine and UVA irradiation in the treatment of vitiligo. *Dermatology* 1994; **188:** 215–18.
3. Camacho F, Mazuecos J. Treatment of vitiligo with oral and topical phenylalanine: 6 years of experience. *Arch Dermatol* 1999; **135:** 216–17.

Preparations

Proprietary Preparations (details are given in Part 3)
USA: Endorphenyl†.

Multi-ingredient: *Fr.:* Revitalose.

Polysaccharide-Iron Complex (11509-r)

Profile

Polysaccharide-iron complex is used as a source of iron (p.1366) for iron-deficiency anaemia (p.716). It is given by mouth in doses containing the equivalent of up to 300 mg of iron daily.

Preparations

Proprietary Preparations (details are given in Part 3)
Belg.: Ferricure; *Canad.:* Niferex; *UK:* Niferex; *USA:* Fe-Tinic; Fe-Tinic Forte; Ferrex; Hytinic; Niferex; Niferex with Vitamin C†; Nu-Iron; Poly-Iron.

Multi-ingredient: *USA:* Ferrex Forte; Ferrex PC; Hemocyte-F; Niferex Forte; Nu-Iron Plus; Nu-Iron V; Poly-Iron Forte.

Proline (613-x)

Proline (USAN, rINN).

P; Pro; L-Proline; Prolinum. L-Pyrrolidine-2-carboxylic acid.

$C_5H_9NO_2 = 115.1$.
CAS — 147-85-3.
Pharmacopoeias. In Eur. (see p.vi) and US.

Pharmacopoeial description

Ph. Eur.: A white or almost white, crystalline powder or colourless crystals. Very soluble in water; freely soluble in alcohol; practically insoluble in ether. Protect from light.

USP 25: White, odourless crystals. Freely soluble in water and in dehydrated alcohol; insoluble in butyl alcohol, in ether, and in isopropyl alcohol.

Profile

Proline is a heterocyclic amino acid. It is used as a dietary supplement.

Preparations

Proprietary Preparations (details are given in Part 3)
Multi-ingredient: *Port.:* Creme Laser Hidrante.

Saccharin (2404-b)

Benzoic Acid Sulphimide; Benzoic Sulfimide; Benzosulphimide; E954; Gluside; Sacarina; Saccarina; Saccharinum; o-Sulfobenzimide; Zaharina. 1,2-Benzisothiazolin-3-one 1,1-dioxide.

$C_7H_5NO_3S = 183.2$.
CAS — 81-07-2.
Pharmacopoeias. In Eur. (see p.vi). Also in USNF.

Pharmacopoeial description

Ph. Eur.: A white, crystalline powder or colourless crystals. Slightly soluble in cold water and in ether; sparingly soluble in boiling water and in alcohol. It dissolves in dilute solutions of alkali hydroxides and carbonates. A saturated solution, prepared without heating, is acid to litmus.

USNF 20: White crystals or white, crystalline powder. Is odourless or has a faint, aromatic odour. In dilute solutions, it is intensely sweet. Soluble 1 in 290 of water, 1 in 25 of boiling water, and 1 in 31 of alcohol; slightly soluble in chloroform and in ether; is readily dissolved by dilute solutions of ammonia, by solutions of alkali hydroxides, and by solutions of alkali carbonates with the evolution of carbon dioxide. Its solutions are acid to litmus.

Saccharin Calcium (2405-v)

Calcium Benzosulphimide; Calcium Saccharin; E954.

$C_{14}H_8CaN_2O_6S_2,3\frac{1}{2}H_2O = 467.5$.
CAS — 6485-34-3 (anhydrous saccharin calcium); 6381-91-5 (hydrated saccharin calcium).
Pharmacopoeias. In US.

Pharmacopoeial description

USP 25: White crystals or white, crystalline powder. Is odourless, or has a faint, aromatic odour, and has an intensely sweet taste, even in dilute solutions. Its dilute solution is about 300 times as sweet as sucrose. Soluble 1 in 2.6 of water and 1 in 4.7 of alcohol.

Saccharin Sodium (2406-g)

E954; Saccharin Sod.; Saccharinnatrium; Saccharinum Natricum; Saccharoidum Natricum; Sodium Benzosulphimide; Sodium Saccharin; Soluble Gluside; Soluble Saccharin.
$C_7H_4NNaO_3S = 205.2$.
CAS — 128-44-9 (anhydrous saccharin sodium); 6155-57-3 (saccharin sodium dihydrate).
Pharmacopoeias. In Chin., Eur. (see p.vi), Int., Jpn, and US. Some pharmacopoeias specify the dihydrate but it may contain a variable quantity of water as a result of efflorescence.

Pharmacopoeial description

Ph. Eur.: A white crystalline powder or colourless crystals. It may contain a variable quantity of water. Efflorescent in dry air. Freely soluble in water; sparingly soluble in alcohol; practically insoluble in ether. Store in airtight containers.

USP 25: White crystals or white, crystalline powder. Is odourless, or has a faint, aromatic odour, and has an intensely sweet taste, even in dilute solutions. Its dilute solution is about 300 times as sweet as sucrose. When in powdered form, it usually contains about one-third the theoretical amount of water of hydration as a result of efflorescence. Soluble 1 in 1.5 of water and 1 in 50 of alcohol.

Adverse Effects

There have been rare reports of hypersensitivity and photosensitivity reactions with saccharin.

Saccharin-associated bladder tumours in *rats* given high doses have been the cause of much concern and investigation. However, it is now generally accepted that these are not applicable to saccharin use as a sweetener by man.

Effects on the liver. Elevated liver enzyme values in an elderly woman followed administration of two different medications sweetened with saccharin sodium.[1] Findings resolved on discontinuation of all preparations containing saccharin, and were subsequently found to recur on rechallenge with a small amount of saccharin sodium.
1. Negro F, et al. Hepatotoxicity of saccharin. N Engl J Med 1994; **331:** 134–5.

Pharmacokinetics

Saccharin is readily absorbed from the gastrointestinal tract. It is almost all excreted unchanged in the urine within 24 to 48 hours.

Uses and Administration

Saccharin and its salts are intense sweeteners, a dilute solution having about 300 times the sweetening power of sucrose. They are used in pharmaceuticals and in foods and beverages and are heat stable. They have no food value. The salts are more often used than saccharin itself as they are considered to be more palatable.

Preparations

USP 25: Saccharin Sodium Oral Solution; Saccharin Sodium Tablets.

Proprietary Preparations (details are given in Part 3)
Braz.: Sukir; *Fr.:* Sucredulcor; *NZ:* Sactabs; Sweetex.
Multi-ingredient: *Austral.:* Sucaryl; *Braz.:* Adocante Docura; Adocyl C; Belpen; *Fr.:* Sucaryl; *Israel:* Sucrin; *Ital.:* Diet Sucaryl; *NZ:* Sucaryl; *Port.:* Dulceril.

Safflower Oil (7367-s)

Pharmacopoeias. In US.
Jpn includes Safflower, the flower of Carthamus tinctorius.

The refined fixed oil obtained from the seeds of the safflower, or false (bastard) saffron, Carthamus tinctorius (Compositae). It contains about 75% of linoleic acid as well as various saturated fatty acids.

Pharmacopoeial description

USP 25: The refined fixed oil yielded from the seed of Carthamus tinctorius (Compositae). A light yellow oil. It thickens and becomes rancid on prolonged exposure to air. Insoluble in water; miscible with chloroform and with ether. Store in airtight containers. Protect from light.

Profile

Safflower oil has similar actions and uses to those of soya oil, p.1378. Emulsions containing a mixture of safflower oil 5% and soya oil 5%, or 10% and 10% respectively, are given as part of total parenteral nutrition regimens.

◊ For reference to the association of lipid emulsion administration, as part of a parenteral nutrition regimen, with the development of sinus bradycardia, see Effects on the Cardiovascular System, under Soya Oil, p.1378.

Preparations

Proprietary Preparations (details are given in Part 3)
Multi-ingredient: *Canad.:* GLA-130; *Denm.:* Liposyn; *Fin.:* Liposyn; Novamix; *Ger.:* Abbolipid; *Israel:* Liposyn; *Ital.:* Liposyn; *Mex.:* Liposyn; *Swed.:* Liposyn; Novamix; *Switz.:* A Vogel Capsules polyvitaminees; *UK:* Efamol Safflower & Linseed; Epopa; Exzem Oil; *USA:* Liposyn II; Microlipid.

Selenium (16982-k)

Se = 78.96.

Potassium Selenate (13159-p)

$K_2SeO_4 = 221.2$.
CAS — 7790-59-2.
Pharmacopoeias. In BP(Vet).

Pharmacopoeial description

BP(Vet) 2001: Colourless, odourless or almost odourless crystals or a white crystalline powder. Freely soluble in water.

Selenious Acid (3941-j)

Monohydrated selenium dioxide .
$H_2SeO_3 = 129.0$.
CAS — 7783-00-8.
Pharmacopoeias. In US.

Pharmacopoeial description

USP 25: Store in airtight containers.

Sodium Selenite (16987-f)

$Na_2SeO_3 = 172.9$.
CAS — 10102-18-8.
Pharmacopoeias. In BP(Vet).

Pharmacopoeial description

BP(Vet) 2001: White to slightly greyish pink granular powder. Freely soluble in water; practically insoluble in alcohol and in ether.

Adverse Effects

Overdosage of selenium has been associated with loss of hair, nail changes, diarrhoea, dermatitis, garlic odour of breath, fatigue, and peripheral neuropathy.

◊ References.
1. Clark RF, et al. Selenium poisoning from a nutritional supplement. JAMA 1996; **275:** 1087–8.

Pharmacokinetics

Selenium compounds are generally readily absorbed from the gastrointestinal tract. Selenium is stored in red blood cells, the liver, spleen, heart, and nails. It is converted in tissues to its metabolically active forms. Selenium is excreted in the urine, and to a lesser extent in the faeces.

Uses and Administration

Selenium is an essential trace element and is an integral part of the enzyme system glutathione peroxidase; this enzyme protects intracellular structures against oxidative damage. Deficiency of selenium has been associated with an endemic form of cardiomyopathy, Keshan disease, seen in certain areas of China. Selenium is present in foods mainly as the amino acids selenomethionine and selenocysteine and derivatives.

Selenious acid and its sodium salt, sodium selenite, are used as a source of selenium, especially for patients with deficiency states following prolonged parenteral nutrition. Suggested doses for addition to total parenteral nutrition are 31.5 μg elemental selenium daily for adults and children greater than 40 kg body-weight, and 2 μg per kg body-weight daily for infants and children to a maximum of 30 μg daily.

Selenate and selenite salts are used for selenium deficiency states in veterinary medicine.

Human requirements. In the UK dietary reference values (see p.1352)[1] and in the USA recommended dietary allowances (RDA)[2] have been published for selenium. In the UK the reference nutrient intake for adults is 75 and 60 μg daily respectively; values are also given for infants and children of varying ages and for lactating women. The UK report also noted that there was no convincing evidence that high intakes protected against cancer or cardiovascular disease; indeed, there was even some evidence that high intakes disturbed selenium homoeostasis and it was recommended that the maximum safe intake from all sources should be set at 450 μg daily for adult males. In the USA, the RDA for adult males and females is 55 μg daily, and again values are also given for infants and children as well as pregnant and lactating women. The tolerable upper intake level is 400 μg daily.[2] WHO have recommended a lower limit of the safe range of population mean intakes of dietary selenium of 40 μg daily for adult males and 30 μg daily for adult females.[3] A maximum daily safe dietary selenium intake of 400 μg was suggested for adults.
1. DoH. Dietary reference values for food energy and nutrients for the United Kingdom: report of the panel on dietary reference values of the committee on medical aspects of food policy. *Report on health and social subjects 41.* London: HMSO, 1991.
2. Standing Committee on the Scientific Evaluation of Dietary Reference Intakes of the Food and Nutrition Board. *Dietary Reference Intakes for vitamin C, vitamin E, selenium, and carotenoids.* Washington DC: National Academy Press, 2000.
3. WHO. Selenium. In: *Trace elements in human nutrition and health.* Geneva: WHO, 1996; 105–22.

Prophylaxis of malignant neoplasms. Selenium supplementation did not protect against the development of new basal or squamous cell carcinomas of the skin in a study of patients with a history of these cancers.[1] However, analysis of secondary end-points indicated a reduced incidence of various other cancers in this study group.[1] Subsequent study has suggested, in particular, an association between low selenium intake and the risk of prostate cancer; incidence was reduced by 63% in

patients receiving the supplement.[2] Another group has also reported an inverse correlation between surrogate measurements of long-term selenium intake and the risk of advanced prostate cancer.[3]
1. Clark LC, et al. Effects of selenium supplementation for cancer prevention in patients with carcinoma of the skin: a randomized controlled trial. JAMA 1996; **276:** 1957–63. Correction. ibid. 1997; **277:** 1520.
2. Clark LC, et al. Decreased incidence of prostate cancer with selenium supplementation: results of a double-blind cancer prevention trial. Br J Urol 1998; **81:** 730–4.
3. Yoshizawa K, et al. Study of prediagnostic selenium level in toenails and the risk of advanced prostate cancer. J Natl Cancer Inst 1998; **90:** 1219–24.

Preparations

USP 25: Selenious Acid Injection.

Proprietary Preparations (details are given in Part 3)
Aust.: Selen; *Canad.:* Micro Se†; *Fr.:* Celnium; Plexium; Selenion; *Ger.:* Cefasel; selenase; Selit; Seltrans; *Hong Kong:* Selepen; *Mex.:* Selefusin; *Swed.:* Selen†; *USA:* Sele-Pak; Selepen.
Multi-ingredient: *Austral.:* Vitaglow Selemite B; *Canad.:* Selenium Plus; Vita-E Plus Selenium; *Fr.:* Bio-Selenium; Selenium-ACE; *Ital.:* Fosfarsile Forte; Neomyrt Plus; Tannidin Plus; *Port.:* Selenium-ACE; *Swed.:* Selen + E†; *UK:* Se-Power; Selenium-ACE.

Serine (616-d)

Serine (USAN, rINN).
β-Hydroxyalanine; S; Ser; L-Serine; Serinum. L-2-Amino-3-hydroxypropionic acid.
$C_3H_7NO_3 = 105.1$.
CAS — 56-45-1.
Pharmacopoeias. In Eur. (see p.vi) and US.

Pharmacopoeial description

Ph. Eur.: White or almost white crystalline powder or colourless crystals. Freely soluble in water; practically insoluble in alcohol and in ether. Protect from light.
USP 25: White, odourless crystals. Soluble in water; practically insoluble in dehydrated alcohol and in ether.

Profile

Serine is an aliphatic amino acid. It is used as a dietary supplement.

Sodium Feredetate (5071-d)

Sodium Feredetate (BAN, rINN).
Sodium Ironedetate. The monohydrated iron chelate of the monosodium salt of ethylenediamine-NNN'N'-tetra-acetic acid; Iron (III) sodium ethylenediaminetetra-acetate monohydrate.
$C_{10}H_{12}FeN_2NaO_8,H_2O = 385.1$.
CAS — 15708-41-5 (anhydrous sodium feredetate).
ATC — B03AB03.
Pharmacopoeias. In Br.

Pharmacopoeial description

BP 2001: A yellow or yellowish brown, hygroscopic, crystalline powder. A 1% solution in water has a pH of 4.0 to 6.5. Store in airtight containers.

Profile

Sodium feredetate is used as a source of iron (p.1366) for iron-deficiency anaemia (p.716). It is given by mouth in doses of up to 1.42 g daily (equivalent to up to about 205 mg of iron daily).

Preparations

BP 2001: Sodium Feredetate Oral Solution.

Proprietary Preparations (details are given in Part 3)
Fr.: Ferrostrane; *Ital.:* Ferro Complex; *UK:* Sytron.

Sodium Fluoride (7733-z)

Natrii Fluoridum; Natrium Fluoratum.
NaF = 41.99.
CAS — 7681-49-4.
ATC — A01AA01; A12CD01.
Pharmacopoeias. In Eur. (see p.vi), Pol., and US.

Sodium fluoride 2.2 mg is approximately equivalent to 1 mg of fluoride. Each g provides approximately 23.8 mmol of sodium and fluoride.

Pharmacopoeial description

Ph. Eur.: A white powder or colourless crystals. Soluble in water; practically insoluble in alcohol.
USP 25: A white, odourless powder. Soluble 1 in 25 of water; insoluble in alcohol.

Adverse Effects and Treatment

In the controlled amounts recommended for fluoridation of drinking water and at the recommended doses employed in dentistry for caries prophylaxis, sodium fluoride has not been shown to have significant side-effects.

In acute poisoning, sodium fluoride taken by mouth is corrosive, forming hydrofluoric acid in the stomach. Effects include hypocalcaemia, hyperkalaemia, tremors, hyperreflexia, paraesthesia, tetany, convulsions, cardiac arrhythmias, shock, respiratory arrest, and cardiac failure. Death may occur within 2 to 4 hours. Although there is much interindividual variation, a single oral dose of 5 to 10 g of sodium fluoride would be considered lethal in an untreated adult by most authorities. However, dangerous poisoning has been reported after oral doses of less than 1 g, and the minimum dose that can cause possibly fatal toxicity has been suggested to be 5 mg per kg body-weight.

Treatment of acute poisoning involves gastric lavage with lime water or a weak solution of another calcium salt to precipitate fluoride, maintenance of high urine output, slow intravenous injections of calcium gluconate 10% for hypocalcaemia and tetany, and symptomatic and supportive measures. Magnesium sulfate, or aluminium hydroxide may also reduce fluoride absorption. Haemodialysis may be considered.

Chronic fluoride poisoning may result in skeletal fluorosis, manifestations of which include increased density and coarsened trabeculation of bone and calcification in ligaments, tendons, and muscle insertions. Clinical signs are bone pain, stiffness, limited movement, and in severe cases, crippling deformities. Prolonged excessive intake by children during the period of tooth development before eruption can result in dental fluorosis characterised by mottled enamel. At fluoride concentrations in drinking water of 1 to 2 ppm (1 to 2 mg per litre) dental fluorosis is mild with white opaque flecks on the teeth. At higher concentrations, enamel defects become more severe with brown to black staining and the teeth have a pitted corroded appearance.

The fluoridation of water has been a subject of considerable controversy. Suggestions that it increases the incidence of thyroid disorders, chromosome aberrations, and cancer have not been substantiated.

◊ Reviews of the toxic effects of fluoride salts.
1. Fluorine and Fluorides. *Environmental Health Criteria 36.* Geneva: WHO 1984.
2. Whitford GM. The physiological and toxicological characteristics of fluoride. *J Dent Res* 1990; **69** (Spec Iss): 539–49.

Carcinogenicity. Based on comparisons of cancer mortality rates for communities residing in fluoridated and non-fluoridated cities, Yiamouyiannis and Burk[1] alleged that artificial fluoridation of water might be associated with an increased risk of cancer. Re-examination of their data by others failed to confirm this relationship nor did further studies in a number of countries.[2] In Great Britain, the Working Party on Fluoridation of Water and Cancer[3] found nothing which could lead them to conclude that either fluoride occurring naturally in water, or fluoride added to water supplies, was capable of inducing cancer, or of increasing the mortality from cancer. In this respect, fluoridation of drinking water was considered safe. Further study in *animal* models by the USA National Toxicology Programme[4] found no evidence of carcinogenicity in female *rats* or in *mice* of either sex. A small number of osteosarcomas was found in male *rats* in the medium- and high-dose groups, although the association between sodium fluoride administration and the tumour was uncertain.
1. Yiamouyiannis J, Burk D. Fluoridation and cancer: age-dependence of cancer mortality related to artificial fluoridation. *Fluoride* 1977; **10**: 102–25S.
2. Clemmesen J. The alleged association between artificial fluoridation of water supplies and cancer: a review. *Bull WHO* 1983; **61**: 871–83.
3. DHSS. *Fluoridation of water and cancer: a review of the epidemiological evidence: report of the working party.* London: HMSO, 1985.
4. Public Health Service report on fluoride benefits and risks. *JAMA* 1991; **266**: 1061–2, 1066–7.

Effects on bone and joints. Exacerbation of rheumatoid arthritis in a 68-year-old woman was attributed to sodium fluoride given in a dose equivalent to 22 mg of fluorine daily for osteoporosis.[1] An increased risk of hip fracture in the elderly has been suggested as being associated with fluoridated water,[2] although another study[3] reported that this association was confined to fluoride concentrations of more than 0.11 mg per litre. Use of fluoride, particularly in doses of 40 mg or more daily, may be associated with a peripheral pain syndrome, usually manifested as bone pain in the distal lower limbs, but sometimes involving the upper limbs and axial skeleton. The cause is uncertain: both stress fractures and increased bone growth at the site of pain have been proposed.[4] For comment on the influence of therapeutic doses of fluoride on the incidence of frac-

tures, see below under Osteoporosis in Uses and Administration.
1. Duell PB, Chesnut CH. Exacerbation of rheumatoid arthritis by sodium fluoride treatment of osteoporosis. *Arch Intern Med* 1991; **151**: 783–4.
2. Danielson C, *et al.* Hip fractures and fluoridation in Utah's elderly population. *JAMA* 1992; **268**: 746–8
3. Jacqmin-Gadda H, *et al.* Fluorine concentration in drinking water and fractures in the elderly. *JAMA* 1995; **273**: 775–6.
4. Jones G, Sambrook PN. Drug-induced disorders of bone metabolism: incidence, management and avoidance. *Drug Safety* 1994; **10**: 480–9.

Effects on the kidneys. Nephrotoxicity has been associated with high plasma concentrations of fluoride during anaesthesia with fluorine-containing anaesthetics such as methoxyflurane (p.1264). Elevated fluoride ion concentrations have also been noted in the plasma of patients receiving enflurane or isoflurane, although no clinical effect on renal function was found (see p.1258 and p.1261).

Fluorosis. Discussions of chronic fluorosis.[1,2] In temperate climates, teeth seem not to be affected if fluoride concentrations in drinking water are not greatly above 1 ppm; fluorosis affecting bone has not been detected at concentrations of 4 to 8 ppm in temperate regions, although it can occur at concentrations of more than 6 ppm in tropical areas.[3] Swallowing of fluoridated toothpaste by infants may be related to fluorosis of permanent incisors.[4]
1. Anonymous. Chronic fluorosis. *BMJ* 1981; **282**: 253–4.
2. Mason JO. A message to health professionals about fluorosis. *JAMA* 1991; **265**: 2939.
3. WHO. *Fluorides and oral health: report of a WHO expert committee on oral health status and fluoride use. WHO Tech Rep Ser 846* 1994.
4. Rock WP, Sabieha AM. The relationship between reported toothpaste usage in infancy and fluorosis of permanent incisors. *Br Dent J* 1997; **183**: 165–70.

Hypersensitivity. Rash and other hypersensitivity reactions have been reported following use of oral sodium fluoride preparations including fluoride-containing toothpastes and drinking water.[1]
1. Mummery RV. Claimed fluoride allergy. *Br Dent J* 1984; **157**: 48.

Overdosage. References.
1. McIvor ME. Acute fluoride toxicity: pathophysiology and management. *Drug Safety* 1990; **5**: 79–85.
2. Gessner BD, *et al.* Acute fluoride poisoning from a public water system. *N Engl J Med* 1994; **330**: 95–9.
3. Arnow PM, *et al.* An outbreak of fatal fluoride intoxication in a long-term hemodialysis unit. *Ann Intern Med* 1994; **121**: 339–44.

Precautions
When considering fluoride supplementation, allowance should be made for fluorides ingested from other sources; fluoride supplements in children are not generally recommended when the fluoride content of drinking water is over 0.7 ppm (0.6 ppm in the USA) (see also Uses and Administration, below). Care should be taken to prevent children swallowing excessive fluoride after topical application to teeth.

Patients with impaired renal function may be particularly susceptible to fluorosis. Regular dialysis with fluoridated water may result in additional fluoride absorption; a maximum concentration of 0.2 ppm of fluoride in the dialysate has been recommended. Dialysis patients not using deionised water are at risk from changes in the fluoride content of the water supply.

Interactions
Aluminium, calcium, and magnesium salts may decrease the absorption of fluoride.

Pharmacokinetics
Sodium fluoride and other soluble fluorides are readily absorbed from the gastrointestinal tract. Inhaled fluorides (from industrial fumes and dusts) are absorbed through the lungs. Fluoride is deposited predominantly in the bones and teeth. It is principally excreted in the urine but small amounts may also be excreted in faeces and sweat. It readily crosses the placenta and is present in saliva, nails, and hair. There is some evidence of distribution into breast milk.

Uses and Administration
Sodium fluoride is used to prevent dental caries and may be used to increase bone density in osteoporosis (see below). Sodium fluoride is used as a source of fluoride in total parenteral nutrition.

For **dental caries prophylaxis**, sodium fluoride is used as an adjunct to diet and oral hygiene. It may render the enamel of teeth more resistant to acid, pro-

mote remineralisation, or reduce microbial acid production. Fluoride may be administered through fluoridation of the public water supply to achieve a usual fluoride concentration of 1 ppm in temperate regions. The concentration may vary from 0.6 to 1.2 ppm depending on the climatic temperature with the lower concentrations being used in hotter regions where more water is likely to be consumed. Fluoridation of salt at a minimum concentration of 200 mg fluoride per kg is an alternative.

Alternatively, sodium fluoride may be administered as an oral supplement to children considered to be at high risk of caries. The daily dosage should be adjusted for the fluoride content of the drinking water, for fluorides ingested from other sources such as the diet, and for the age of the child. Guidelines have recently been amended in the USA and the UK. In both countries it is suggested that, where the drinking water contains less than 0.3 ppm of fluoride, children aged 6 months to 3 years may be given sodium fluoride 0.55 mg (equivalent to 0.25 mg of fluoride) daily; those aged 3 to 6 years, 1.1 mg (equivalent to 0.5 mg of fluoride) daily; and those aged 6 years and over, 2.2 mg (equivalent to 1 mg of fluoride) daily. Supplements are not recommended for infants under 6 months of age. When drinking water contains 0.3 to 0.7 ppm (0.3 to 0.6 ppm in the USA) of fluoride lower doses should be considered. Specifically, it is recommended that no additional fluoride should be given to children less than 3 years of age and for older children the above doses should be halved. If the water contains more than 0.7 ppm (0.6 ppm in the USA) of fluoride, supplementation is not recommended. Tablets should be sucked or chewed before swallowing since the topical action of fluoride on enamel and plaque is considered to be more important than the systemic effect. The value of giving fluoride during pregnancy, to benefit the child, is not established. Dental benefits from the use of dietary fluoride supplements by adults are unsubstantiated.

After tooth eruption, local fluoride application is effective. Daily mouth-rinses of sodium fluoride 0.05% (about 225 ppm fluoride) or weekly to monthly mouth-rinses of sodium fluoride 0.2% (900 ppm) may be used, but are not recommended for children aged under 6 years because they are unable to effectively spit the rinse out after use. Fluoridated toothpastes are now widely available and are a convenient source of fluoride. In the UK, the maximum permitted fluoride level in toothpastes is sodium fluoride 0.32% (0.15% or 1500 ppm fluoride). Low-dose formulations for children under 7 years of age usually contain sodium fluoride 0.11% (500 ppm), and their use should be supervised to avoid excessive use or ingestion. Sodium fluoride has also been applied topically as a varnish or 2% (about 9090 ppm fluoride) solution under professional supervision. Alternatively, sodium fluoride solutions or gels acidified with phosphoric acid and commonly known as acidulated phosphate fluoride preparations may be used. These preparations are considered to increase the fluoride uptake by the enamel and protect the enamel from demineralisation. For maximum benefit, eating, drinking, or rinsing should be avoided for at least 30 minutes after topical fluoride application.

Other fluoride compounds used in oral hygiene products and toothpastes include aluminium fluoride, ammonium fluoride, calcium fluoride (p.1356), dectaflur (p.1359), olaflur (p.1374), potassium fluoride, sodium monofluorophosphate (p.1377), sodium silicofluoride (p.1377), and stannous fluoride (p.1379). Other fluorides used in the fluoridation of water supplies include sodium silicofluoride.

Sodium fluoride has also been used, like some other fluoride compounds, in rodenticides and insecticides.

Human requirements. In the USA dietary reference intakes have been set for fluoride. These propose an adequate intake (AI—see p.1352) for dental caries prevention to be 4 mg daily in adult men and 3 mg in women;[1] lower values are suggested in children and adolescents, depending on age. The tolerable upper intake level is 10 mg daily in adults.[1]

1. Standing Committee on the Scientific Evaluation of Dietary Reference Intakes of the Food and Nutrition Board. *Dietary Reference Intakes for calcium, phosphorus, magnesium, vitamin D, and fluoride.* Washington, DC: National Academy Press, 1999.

Dental caries prophylaxis. References.

1. WHO. Fluorides and oral health: report of a WHO expert committee on oral health status and fluoride use. *WHO Tech Rep Ser* 846 1994.
2. Lewis DW, *et al.* Periodic health examination, 1995 update: 2: prevention of dental caries. *Can Med Assoc J* 1995; **152:** 836–46.
3. American Academy of Pediatrics, Committee on Nutrition. Fluoride supplementation for children: interim policy recommendations. *Pediatrics* 1995; **95:** 777.
4. Holt RD, *et al.* British Society of Paediatric Dentistry: a policy document on fluoride dietary supplements and fluoride toothpastes for children. *Int J Paediatr Dent* 1996; **6:** 139–42.
5. Anonymous. Fluoride supplement dosage: a statement by the British Dental Association, the British Society of Paediatric Dentistry and the British Association for the Study of Community Dentistry. *Br Dent J* 1997; **182:** 6–7.

Osteoporosis. Fluoride has been used in the treatment of osteoporosis (p.745) to improve bone strength by inducing subclinical fluorosis. The predominant effect of fluoride on the skeleton is to stimulate osteoblasts and increase trabecular bone mass. Because antiresorptive drugs cannot restore lost bone mass, this is potentially valuable in the treatment of osteoporosis. However, too much fluoride can increase bone fragility, and the overall effect of sodium fluoride on the incidence of fracture has not been established.

A controlled study in patients with postmenopausal osteoporosis[1] found that sodium fluoride 75 mg daily with a calcium supplement increased trabecular bone mass of the spine but did not reduce the incidence of vertebral fractures. Patients given sodium fluoride also had a higher incidence of nonvertebral fractures. An extension and reanalysis of the study,[2] however, showed that gradual increases in bone mass observed in patients receiving lower doses of sodium fluoride (down to about 40 mg daily) were associated with a decrease in the incidence of fractures. A previous study[3] had reported a beneficial effect in vertebral fracture rate in patients with primary osteoporosis and at least one vertebral crush fracture. In this study sodium fluoride was given in a daily dose of 50 mg; calcium and vitamin D were also given. Interim analysis of a subsequent study using a slow-release formulation of sodium fluoride 50 mg daily taken intermittently with a regular calcium supplement showed a decrease in vertebral fractures of 50% at 2.5 years.[4] At 4 years the beneficial effect was sustained, the main effect being seen in a reduced incidence of new vertebral fractures;[5] no reduction was seen in the incidence of recurrent fractures but this study found no evidence of an increase in nonvertebral fractures. Some consider that low-dose fluoride can be of benefit in established postmenopausal osteoporosis, but the therapeutic window is narrow, and calcium and vitamin D must be given concomitantly to meet the calcium demand and avoid resorption of established bone.[6] A further double-blind study failed to demonstrate a reduction in vertebral fracture rates in women with osteoporosis treated with fluoride, and calcium and vitamin D compared with women who received only calcium and vitamin D.[7] This was despite a significant increase in bone mass density of the spine in the fluoride-treated groups. Fluoride regimens consisted of 50 mg enteric-coated sodium fluoride daily, or 150 or 200 mg sodium monofluorophosphate daily. In contrast, a further 4-year study found a decrease in vertebral fracture rates in women with moderate osteoporosis treated with sodium monofluorophosphate 156 mg daily plus calcium compared with those receiving calcium alone.[8]

A systematic review of 11 studies concluded that fluoride can increase bone mineral density at the lumbar spine, but this does not reduce the rate of vertebral fractures.[9] The authors of this review considered that fluoride should not be used in the first-line therapy of postmenopausal osteoporosis.

1. Riggs BL, *et al.* Effect of fluoride treatment on the fracture rate in postmenopausal women with osteoporosis. *N Engl J Med* 1990; **322:** 802–9.
2. Riggs BL, *et al.* Clinical trial of fluoride therapy in postmenopausal osteoporotic women: extended observations and additional analysis. *J Bone Miner Res* 1994; **9:** 265–75.
3. Mamelle N, *et al.* Risk-benefit ratio of sodium fluoride treatment in primary vertebral osteoporosis. *Lancet* 1988; **ii:** 361–5.
4. Pak CYC, *et al.* Slow-release sodium fluoride in the management of postmenopausal osteoporosis: a randomized controlled trial. *Ann Intern Med* 1994; **120:** 625–32.
5. Pak CYC, *et al.* Treatment of postmenopausal osteoporosis with slow-release sodium fluoride: final report of a randomized controlled trial. *Ann Intern Med* 1995; **123:** 401–8.
6. Anonymous. New drugs for osteoporosis. *Med Lett Drugs Ther* 1996; **38:** 1–3.
7. Meunier PJ, *et al.* Fluoride salts are no better at preventing new vertebral fractures than calcium-vitamin D in postmenopausal osteoporosis: the FAVOStudy. *Osteoporosis Int* 1998; **8:** 4–12.
8. Reginster JY, *et al.* The effect of sodium monofluorophosphate plus calcium on vertebral fracture rate in postmenopausal women with moderate osteoporosis: a randomized, controlled trial. *Ann Intern Med* 1998; **129:** 1–8.
9. Haguenauer D, *et al.* Fluoride for treating postmenopausal osteoporosis (updated 30 November 2000). Available in The Cochrane Library; Issue 2. Oxford: Update Software; 2001.

The symbol † denotes a preparation no longer actively marketed

Preparations

BP 2001: Sodium Fluoride Mouthwash; Sodium Fluoride Oral Drops; Sodium Fluoride Tablets;
USP 25: Sodium Fluoride and Acidulated Phosphate Topical Solution; Sodium Fluoride and Phosphoric Acid Gel; Sodium Fluoride and Phosphoric Acid Topical Solution; Sodium Fluoride Oral Solution; Sodium Fluoride Tablets.

Proprietary Preparations (details are given in Part 3)
Aust.: Duraphat; Fluodont; Osteofluor; Zymafluor; **Austral.:** Denta-Mint Topical Fluoride Solution†; Floran Effervescent†; Fluor; Flurets; Hi-Fluor†; Neutrafluor; Orofluor†; Phos-Flur†; **Belg.:** Procal; **Braz.:** Fluocaril; Fluodel; Fluornatrium; Novodentin; **Canad.:** Duraflor†; Fluor-A-Day; Fluoridrops; Fluorinse; Fluoritabs; Fluorosol; Fluotic; Karidium; Oral-B Anti-Cavity Dental Rinse; Oro-NaF; Pedi-Dent; Solu-Flur†; **Denm.:** Bifluorid; Duraphat; Fluorette; **Fin.:** Duraphat; Fludent; Fluorilette; **Fr.:** Fluodontyl; Fluogum; Fluoplexe; Fluor; Fluor Microsol; Fluorex; Osteofluor; Sanogyl; Zymafluor; **Ger.:** Duraphat; Fluoretten; Fluoros; Koreberon; NaFril; Ospur F; Ossin; Zymafluor; **Irl.:** Reach Junior Fluoride; **Israel:** Denticare; Duraphat; Fluden; Fluvium; Teeth Tough; Zymafluor; **Ital.:** Dentosan Extra Fluor; Fluodent†; Fluordent†; Fluorigard; Fluorvitin; Oral-B Collutorio Protezione Anti-Carie Fluorinse; Oralsan; Sensifluor†; Zymafluor; **Mex.:** Audifluor; **Neth.:** Dagra Fluor†; Davitamon Fluor†; Zymafluor; **Norw.:** Duraphat; Fluorette; Flux; **Port.:** Fluor-In; Fluorigard Ortho†; Medusit; Oratol F; Zymafluor; **S.Afr.:** Dentil Gum F†; Fluorogum†; Listerfluor; Zymafluor; **Spain:** Fluodontyl; Zymafluor; **Swed.:** Dentan; Duraphat; Fludent; Fluorette; Top dent fluor; **Switz.:** Fluortop; Ossin; Ossofluor; Zymafluor; **Thai.:** Zymafluor; **UK:** Duraphat; En-De-Kay; Fluor-A-Day; Fluorigard; **USA:** ACT; APF; Fluorigard; Fluorinse; Fluoritab; Flura; Karidium; Karigel; Karigel-N; Luride; Minute-Gel; MouthKote F/R†; Pediaflor; Pharmaflur; Phos-Flur; Point-Two; Prevident; SF Gel; Thera-Flur.

Multi-ingredient: **Aust.:** Elmex; Ossiplex; **Austral.:** Macleans Sensitive; Oral-B Sensitive; **Belg.:** Elmex; **Braz.:** Calcigenol Irradiado; Fluotrat; Malvatricin; Poly-Vi-Fluor; Tri-Vi-Fluor; **Canad.:** Cepacol with Fluoride; Oral Plan; Oral-B Anti-Bacterial with Fluoride; Poly-Vi-Flor; Sensodyne-F; Tri-Vi-Flor; Tri-Vi-Sol with Fluoride; **Fin.:** Elmex; Xerodent; **Fr.:** Elmex; Fluocaril Bi-Fluore; Fluogel; Fluopate; Fluoselgine; Fluosept†; Sanoformine†; Sanogyl; Sanogyl Fluo; Sanogyl Junior; Zymaduo; **Ger.:** D-Fluoretten; Elmex; Fluor-Vigantoletten; Multifluorid; Natabec F; Ossiplex; Zymafluor D; **Irl.:** Listermint with Fluoride†; **Israel:** Elmex; **Ital.:** Actifluor; Aqua Emoform; AZ Junior†; AZ Protezione Completa; AZ Protezione Gengive; Benodent; Broxo al Fluoro; Clorexident Ortodontico†; Dentosan Junior; Dentosan Placca & Carie; Dentosan Sensibile; Eburdent F; Elmex; Eudent con Glysan; Fluocaril Bi-Fluore; Fluorin; Lacalut; Merfluan Sali Dentali; Oral-B Collutorio per la Protezione di Denti e Gengive; Ossiplex; Otofluor; Plax; Pronto Emoform†; Ridiodent; Tetrafluor†; Valda F3†; **Neth.:** Davitamon AD Fluor†; Elmex; **NZ:** Luborant; **Port.:** Biofluor; Biofluor Sensitive; **S.Afr.:** Denti Gum CF†; Elmex; Ossiplex; **Spain:** Elmex; Vitagama Fluor; **Swed.:** Bifluorid 12; Xerodent; **Switz.:** Elmex; **Thai.:** Poly-Vi-Flor; **UK:** Dentyl pH; Listermint with Fluoride; Macleans Mouthguard; Saliva Orthana; Sensodyne-F; **USA:** Adeflor M; Apatate with Fluoride; Florical; Florvite; Mulvidren-F Softab; Poly-Vi-Flor; Polytabs-F; Sensitivity Protection Crest; Soluvite; Tri Vit with Fluoride; Tri-Flor-Vite with Fluoride†; Tri-Vi-Flor; Trivitamin Fluoride Drops; Vi-Daylin/F.

Sodium Monofluorophosphate   (7735-k)

MFP Sodium; Natrii Monofluorophosphas; Sodium Fluorophosphate. Disodium phosphorofluoridate.
$Na_2PO_3F = 143.9.$
CAS — 10163-15-2.
ATC — A01AA02; A12CD02.
Pharmacopoeias. In US.

Pharmacopoeial description

USP 25: A white to slightly grey, odourless powder. Freely soluble in water. pH of a 2% solution in water is between 6.5 and 8.0.

Profile

Sodium monofluorophosphate is used as a source of fluoride (see Sodium Fluoride, p.1375) in toothpastes for the prevention of dental caries. It may also be given by mouth in the management of osteoporosis.

In the UK, the maximum permitted fluoride level in toothpastes is 1.14% of sodium monofluorophosphate (0.15% or 1500 ppm of fluoride). Low-dose formulations for children under 7 years of age typically contain sodium monofluorophosphate 0.38% (500 ppm fluoride), and their use should be supervised to avoid excessive use or ingestion.

Other monofluorophosphate salts permitted for use in oral hygiene products and dentifrices include ammonium monofluorophosphate, calcium monofluorophosphate, and potassium monofluorophosphate.

Osteoporosis. For reference to the use of fluorides, including sodium monofluorophosphate, in the treatment of osteoporosis, see under Uses of Sodium Fluoride, p.1377.

Preparations

Proprietary Preparations (details are given in Part 3)
Austral.: Fluorocare; Nicodent†; **Ger.:** Mono-Tridin†; **Ital.:** Neo Fluostomygen; Neo-Emoform; Oralsan; Stomygen.

Multi-ingredient: **Aust.:** Fluocalcic; **Austral.:** Thermodent†; **Belg.:** Fluocalcic; **Canad.:** Sensodyne-F; Viadent; **Fr.:** Architex; Fluocalcic†; Fluocaril Bi-Fluore; Fluorocalciforte†; Sanogyl; Sanogyl Fluo; Sanogyl Junior; **Ger.:** Calcivit F; Fluoril; Tridin; **Ital.:** Aqua Emoform; Biogreen; Broxo al Fluoro; Cepacol†; Dentosan Carie & Alito; Dentosan Junior; Eudent con Glysan; Fluocaril Bi-

---

Fluore; Formedico; Neo-Stomygen; Orosanyl; Periogard; Pronto Emoform†; Sanogyl Bianco†; Tetrafluor†; **Port.:** Periogard†; Sensitive Care†; **Switz.:** Emoform-F au fluor; Fluo-calc; **USA:** Optimoist; Sensodyne-F.

Sodium Silicofluoride   (7736-a)

Sodium Fluorosilicate; Sodium Fluosilicate; Sodium Hexafluorosilicate.
$Na_2SiF_6 = 188.1.$
CAS — 16893-85-9.

Profile

Sodium silicofluoride is used as a source of fluoride (see Sodium Fluoride, p.1375) for the fluoridation of drinking water. It has also been considered for inclusion in oral hygiene products.

Other silicofluoride (fluorosilicate) salts permitted for use in oral hygiene products include ammonium silicofluoride, magnesium silicofluoride, and potassium silicofluoride.

Sodium silicofluoride has also been used in insecticides.

Sorbitol   (619-m)

E420; D-Sorbitol; Sorbitolum. D-Glucitol.
$C_6H_{14}O_6 = 182.2.$
CAS — 50-70-4.
ATC — A06AG07; B05CX02; V04CC01.

Pharmacopoeias. In Chin., Eur. (see p.vi), Jpn, and Pol. Also in USNF.
US includes only Sorbitol Solution.

A 5.48% solution of sorbitol hemihydrate is iso-osmotic with serum.

Pharmacopoeial description

Ph. Eur.: A white or almost white crystalline powder. It exhibits polymorphism. Very soluble in water; practically insoluble in alcohol.

USNF 20: White, hygroscopic powder, granules, or flakes having a sweet taste. Soluble 1 in 0.45 of water; slightly soluble in alcohol, in methyl alcohol, and in acetic acid. Store in airtight containers.

Incompatibility. For reference to the incompatibility of sorbitol with hydroxybenzoates, see p.1148.

Adverse Effects and Precautions

As for Fructose, p.1363.

Effects on electrolyte balance. Sorbitol is employed as a vehicle in some proprietary preparations of activated charcoal intended to reduce drug absorption after poisoning; the sorbitol increases the palatability of the preparation and also produces an osmotic diarrhoea that facilitates elimination of the activated charcoal and adsorbed drug. Repeated doses of such preparations are often advocated but a case report has described a patient with end-stage renal failure in whom profuse watery diarrhoea and subsequent hypernatraemia was induced by the sorbitol.[1] For debate about such multiple dose therapy see Poisoning under Activated Charcoal, p.1001.

1. Gazda-Smith E, Synhavsky A. Hypernatraemia following treatment of theophylline toxicity with activated charcoal and sorbitol. *Arch Intern Med* 1990; **150:** 689 and 692.

Effects on the gastrointestinal tract. Sorbitol is often used as a sweetener in sugar-free liquid preparations and the risk of sorbitol-induced diarrhoea associated with such products has been highlighted.[1-3] Chronic sorbitol-induced diarrhoea with associated pneumatosis intestinalis has been reported in a child receiving 21.7 g sorbitol daily in liquid medications.[4]

Colonic necrosis in a renal transplant recipient who received sodium polystyrene sulfonate suspension in sorbitol enemas for hyperkalaemia has been attributed to the sorbitol component.[5] It was subsequently pointed out that the manufacturers' instructions to give a cleansing enema both before and after the resin enema had not been followed and that this complication had never been reported when the product was administered properly.[6] It has also been suggested that sorbitol contributed to the morbidity in a patient who developed septicaemia as a complication of intestinal pseudo-obstruction, following the use of charcoal with sorbitol to treat self-poisoning with theophylline.[7] It was suggested that gaseous distension following bacterial metabolism of sorbitol had rendered the bowel wall ischaemic, facilitating passage of bacteria or of endotoxin into the systemic circulation.

1. Brown AM, Masson E. 'Hidden' sorbitol in proprietary medicines - a cause for concern? *Pharm J* 1990; **245:** 211.
2. Edes TE, *et al.* Diarrhea in tube-fed patients: feeding formula not necessarily the cause. *Am J Med* 1990; **88:** 91–3.
3. Johnston KR, *et al.* Gastrointestinal effects of sorbitol as an additive in liquid medications. *Am J Med* 1994; **97:** 185–91.
4. Duncan B, *et al.* Medication-induced pneumatosis intestinalis. *Pediatrics* 1997; **99:** 633–6.
5. Wootton FT, *et al.* Colonic necrosis with Kayexalate-Sorbitol enemas after renal transplantation. *Ann Intern Med* 1989; **111:** 947–9.

6. Shepard KV. Cleansing enemas after sodium polystyrene sulfonate enemas. *Ann Intern Med* 1990; **112:** 711.
7. Longdon P, Henderson A. Intestinal pseudo-obstruction following the use of enteral charcoal and sorbitol and mechanical ventilation with papaveretum sedation for theophylline poisoning. *Drug Safety* 1992; **7:** 74–7.

Pharmacokinetics

Sorbitol is poorly absorbed from the gastrointestinal tract following oral or rectal administration. It is metabolised mainly in the liver, to fructose (see p.1363), a reaction catalysed by the enzyme sorbitol dehydrogenase. Some sorbitol may be converted directly to glucose by the enzyme aldose reductase.

Uses and Administration

Sorbitol is a polyhydric sugar alcohol (polyol) with half the sweetening power of sucrose. It occurs naturally in many fruits and vegetables and is prepared commercially by the reduction of glucose.

It has been employed as a 30% solution as an alternative to glucose in parenteral nutrition (p.1351) but its use is not recommended because of the risk of lactic acidosis.

Sorbitol may be administered by mouth or rectally as an osmotic laxative in the management of constipation (p.1202); doses of 20 to 50 g have been suggested.

Solutions containing about 3% of sorbitol are used as irrigating fluids in transurethral surgical procedures.

Sorbitol was formerly given intravenously as a 50% solution as an osmotic diuretic.

Sorbitol also acts as a bulk sweetening agent. It is used in limited quantities as a sweetener in energy-reduced diabetic food products. It is also used as an alternative to sucrose in many sugar-free oral liquid preparations and in sugar-free foods as it is less likely to cause dental caries.

Sorbitol also has humectant and stabilising properties and is used in various pharmaceutical and cosmetic products including toothpaste.

Preparations

BP 2001: Sorbitol Intravenous Infusion;
Ph. Eur.: Sorbitol, Liquid (Crystallising); Sorbitol, Liquid (Noncrystallising);
USNF 20: Noncrystallizing Sorbitol Solution;
USP 25: Sorbitol Solution.

Proprietary Preparations (details are given in Part 3)
Austral.: Sorbilax; **Belg.:** Syn MD†; **Braz.:** Minilax; **Swed.:** Cystosol; Resulax; Sorbitur†; **Switz.:** Syn MD.

Multi-ingredient: Aust.: Glandosane; Lemazol; Microklist; Resectal; Tromgallol†; Yal; **Austral.:** Aquae; Carbosorb S; Fleet Micro-Enema; Medevac; Microlax; **Belg.:** Bilagol†; Microlax; **Braz.:** Anekron; Biliflux; Biofigado; Colachofra; Hepalin; Hormo Hepatico; Scolybil; **Canad.:** Charcodote; Microlax; Moi-Stir; Salivart; **Denm.:** Klyx; **Fin.:** Klyx; Microlax; Somanol + Ethanol; **Fr.:** Apilaxe; Arnilose†; Artisial; Hepacholine Sorbitol; Hepagrume; Hepargitol; Megabyt†; Microlax; Modulite†; Nivabetol; Norbiline; Ornitaine; Parapsyllium; Schoum; Spagulax au Sorbitol; Vitaphakol; **Ger.:** Artisial†; Dr. Hotz Vollbad†; Flacar; Freka-Drainjet Purisole; Glandosane; Klysma Sorbit; Microklist; Tutofusin S; Yal; **Hong Kong:** Aquae; Microlax; Salivart; **Irl.:** Luborant; **Israel:** Glandosane; **Ital.:** Citroepatina; Macrolax; Magisbile; Norbiline; Novilax; Si-Cliss†; Sorbiclis; Weight Watchers Punto; **Mex.:** Clyss-Go; **Neth.:** Microlax; **Norw.:** Klyx; Microlax; **NZ:** Carbosorb S; Medevac; Microlax; **Port.:** Clyss-Go; Glandosane; Purisole; Vitaphakol; **S.Afr.:** Agofell; Microlax; **Spain:** Hepadif; Levaliver; Polisilan Gel†; Primperan Complex†; Sualyn†; Sugarbil; Sugarceton†; Vitaphakol; **Swed.:** Klyx; Microlax; Somanol†; Vi-Siblin S; **Switz.:** Agarol Soft; Cital†; Glandosane; Microklist; Microlax; Purisole†; Pursana; Vitaphakol†; Yal; **Thai.:** Glandosane; **UK:** Glandosane; Luborant; Relaxit; SST; **USA:** Actidose with Sorbitol; Glandosane†; Moi-Stir; Salivart.

Soya Bean   (20958-p)

Soja Bean; Soyabean; Soybean.

Soya bean is the seed of the soya plant *Glycine max* (*G. hispida*) or *G. soja*. It is a source of soya oil and soya protein.

Soya Oil   (7369-e)

Soja Bean Oil; Sojae Oleum; Soyabean Oil; Soya-bean Oil; Soybean Oil.

Pharmacopoeias. In Chin., Jpn, and US.
Eur. (see p.vi) includes Hydrogenated Soya-bean Oil and Refined Soya-bean Oil. *Ger.* also includes Partially Hydrogenated Soya Oil.

Pharmacopoeial description
Ph. Eur.: Refined Soya-bean Oil is the fatty oil obtained from seeds of *Glycine soja* and *G. max* (*G. hispida*) by extraction and

---

subsequent refining. It may contain a suitable antioxidant and is a clear, pale yellow liquid. Practically insoluble in alcohol; miscible with petroleum spirit. Store in well-filled containers at a temperature not exceeding 25°. Protect from light.

Hydrogenated Soya-bean Oil is obtained by refining, bleaching, hydrogenation, and deodorisation of soya oil. It consists mainly of triglycerides of palmitic and stearic acids and is a white mass or powder which melts to a clear, pale yellow liquid when heated. Practically insoluble in alcohol; very slightly soluble in alcohol; freely soluble in dichloromethane, in petroleum spirit after heating, and in toluene. Protect from light.

USP 25: Soyabean Oil is the refined fixed oil obtained from the seeds of the soya plant *Glycine soja* (Leguminosae). A clear, pale yellow, oily liquid having a characteristic odour. Insoluble in water; miscible with chloroform and with ether. Store in airtight containers at a temperature not exceeding 40°. Protect from light.

Incompatibility. For mention of the compatibility and stability of solutions and emulsions for parenteral nutrition see under Enteral and Parenteral Nutrition, p.1351.

Adverse Effects

Hypersensitivity reactions including fever and chills have been reported following the infusion of soya oil emulsion although they are considered to be fairly rare. Other rare immediate reactions include dyspnoea, cyanosis, nausea, vomiting, headache, and chest and back pain.

Too rapid infusion of soya oil emulsion or prolonged infusion or its administration to patients with impaired fat metabolism has been associated with the 'overload syndrome'. This is manifested by blood disorders such as bone-marrow depression, anaemia, thrombocytopenia, and spontaneous bleeding, hepatosplenomegaly, raised liver enzyme values, hyperlipidaemia, seizures, and shock. Pigmentation of tissues after prolonged therapy with lipid emulsion infusions has also been reported.

Soya protein-based infant feeds can be antigenic and cause gastrointestinal adverse effects in sensitive individuals.

Bacteraemia. A strong association has been demonstrated between the administration of lipids through peripheral venous catheters made of Teflon and development of coagulase-negative staphylococcal bacteraemia in neonates.[1] It was suggested that investigation of catheters made of other materials, or other delivery systems, might reduce the opportunity for coagulase-negative staphylococci to adhere and come into contact with nutrient-rich growth media in the form of lipid emulsions. Others also took the view that this work should not lead to the abandonment of parenteral lipids in premature infants.[2]

1. Freeman J, *et al.* Association of intravenous lipid emulsion and coagulase-negative staphylococcal bacteremia in neonatal intensive care units. *N Engl J Med* 1990; **323:** 301–8.
2. Klein JO. From harmless commensal to invasive pathogen: coagulase-negative staphylococci. *N Engl J Med* 1990; **323:** 339–40.

Effects on the cardiovascular system. Development of sinus bradycardia has been reported in a patient receiving total parenteral nutrition that included soya oil-based emulsion via a central line.[1] The authors suggested that it might be wise to administer fat emulsion only through a peripheral vein. However, sinus bradycardia has been reported following the administration of a safflower oil-based emulsion via a peripheral vein as part of a TPN regimen.[2]

1. Sternberg A, *et al.* Intralipid-induced transient sinus bradycardia. *N Engl J Med* 1981; **304:** 422–3.
2. Traub SL, *et al.* Sinus bradycardia associated with peripheral lipids and total parenteral nutrition. *J Parenter Enteral Nutr* 1985; **9:** 358–60.

Effects on the endocrine system. Soya bean is a rich source of phyto-oestrogens including isoflavones, and it has recently been demonstrated that infants fed soya-based formulae have high serum concentrations of these substances.[1] It has been suggested that these may be sufficient to exert biological effects, bringing the safety of soya-based formulae into question. As yet, effects have not been observed clinically, but further studies are needed to assess the short- and long-term effects of soya-based products.[2]

1. Setchell KDR, *et al.* Exposure of infants to phyto-oestrogens from soy-based infant formula. *Lancet* 1997; **350:** 23–7.
2. Essex C. Phytoestrogens and soy based infant formula. *BMJ* 1996; **313:** 507–8.

Effects on the nervous system. CNS disorders in 2 patients receiving infusions of fractionated soya emulsion included convulsions, coma, and cortical blindness in one young woman.[1] A similar case was attributed to fat embolism,[2] but occurring after what the manufacturers pointed out was a faster than recommended infusion[3] may perhaps have represented a fat-overload syndrome.

1. Jellinek EH. Dangers of intravenous fat infusions. *Lancet* 1976; **ii:** 967.

---

2. Estebe JP, Malledant Y. Fat embolism after lipid emulsion infusion. *Lancet* 1991; **337:** 673.
3. McCracken M. Fat embolism after lipid emulsion infusion. *Lancet* 1991; **337:** 983.

Hypersensitivity. Urticaria has been reported in two patients following the administration intravenously of soya oil emulsions.[1,2] In one case the patient had previously received the emulsion for 19 days without ill-effect.[1]

Anaphylactic reactions have been documented after the ingestion of several foods or foodstuffs containing, or prepared from, soya beans, although the exact allergen remains unknown. In one patient who suffered anaphylactic attacks after eating such products a specific IgE-antibody response to the allergen Kunitz soybean trypsin inhibitor was demonstrated.[3] This was not, however, the only allergen present in soya beans as other patients who had a negative response to this allergen had positive responses in whole soya bean tests.

IgE antibodies to soya bean antigens have also been found in workers who suffered from asthma after handling soya beans[4,5] leading to the suggestion that an allergic mechanism had been responsible; the asthma was believed to have been due to the dust released during the handling of the beans.

1. Kamath KR, *et al.* Acute hypersensitivity reaction to Intralipid. *N Engl J Med* 1981; **304:** 360.
2. Hiyama DT, *et al.* Hypersensitivity following lipid emulsion infusion in an adult patient. *J Parenter Enteral Nutr* 1989; **13:** 318–20.
3. Moroz LA, Yang WH. Kunitz soybean trypsin inhibitor: a specific allergen in food anaphylaxis. *N Engl J Med* 1980; **302:** 1126–8.
4. Sunyer J, *et al.* Case-control study of serum immunoglobulin-E antibodies reactive with soybean in epidemic asthma. *Lancet* 1989; **i:** 179–82.
5. Hernando L, *et al.* Asthma epidemics and soybean in Cartagena (Spain). *Lancet* 1989; **i:** 502.

Pulmonary fat emboli. Pulmonary fat emboli or microemboli, sometimes fatal, have occurred in several infants who received infusions of fat emulsions based on soya oil.[1-3]

In one case[3] the patient's serum, which contained a high concentration of C-reactive protein, agglutinated the fat emulsion and this finding was considered to support the hypothesis that microemboli are formed by agglutination of fat emulsion in the blood stream by C-reactive protein. The authors of this report did not consider the precise pathogenesis to be clear, nor did they know whether the condition was preventable, but did suggest that it may be prudent either to ensure that the C-reactive protein concentration was normal (less than 10 mg per litre) or to perform a creaming test to determine which babies may embolise the infused fat emulsion. However, other studies,[4] while not excluding any role of C-reactive protein in agglutination, have failed to find any correlation between raised concentrations of this protein and the rate of agglutination.

1. Barson AJ, *et al.* Fat embolism in infancy after intravenous fat infusions. *Arch Dis Child* 1978; **53:** 218–23.
2. Levene MI, *et al.* Pulmonary fat accumulation after Intralipid infusion in the preterm infant. *Lancet* 1980; **ii:** 815–8.
3. Hulman G, Levene M. Intralipid microemboli. *Arch Dis Child* 1986; **61:** 702–3.
4. Zagara G, *et al.* C-reactive protein and serum agglutination in vivo of intravenous fat emulsions. *Lancet* 1989; **i:** 733.

Precautions

Intravenous soya oil emulsion should not be given to patients with severe liver disease, acute shock, or severe or pathological hyperlipidaemia, or when the ability to metabolise fat may otherwise be impaired. Caution has also been advised in patients with pulmonary disease, renal insufficiency, uncompensated diabetes mellitus, hyperthyroidism, sepsis, and some disorders of blood coagulation. However, if administration is considered in such patients, the elimination of fat should be monitored daily.

Intravenous soya oil emulsion may interfere with some laboratory tests if blood is taken before fat has adequately cleared; this may take 4 to 6 hours.

Egg-yolk phospholipids may be used as emulsifiers in some preparations and therefore such fat emulsions should not be given to patients with severe egg allergy.

Fat emulsions may extract phthalate plasticisers from administration bags and sets and therefore non-phthalate containing equipment should be used wherever possible. Soya-based infant feeds should be avoided in infants with documented cows' milk protein-induced enteropathy or enterocolitis, as these infants are frequently also sensitive to soya protein.

Neonatal hyperbilirubinaemia. In neonates with hyperbilirubinaemia, intravenous lipid emulsions should be used with caution because of the risk of displacing bilirubin from albumin. The risk appears to be higher in preterm infants,[1] at higher doses,[1] and with intermittent rather than continuous dosing.[2]

1. Spear ML, *et al.* The effect of 15-hour fat infusions of varying dosage on bilirubin binding to albumin. *J Parenter Enteral Nutr* 1985; **9:** 144–7.
2. Brans YW, *et al.* Influence of intravenous fat emulsion on serum bilirubin in very low birthweight neonates. *Arch Dis Child* 1987; **62:** 156–60.

Uses and Administration

Emulsions of fractionated soya oil containing 10, 20, or 30% are given by slow intravenous infusion as part of total parenteral nutrition regimens (p.1351), usually in conjunction with amino acid and carbohydrate solutions. The solutions and emulsions may be administered at separate sites, administered at the same site through a Y-connector, or combined in one admixture. Fat emulsions provide a high energy intake in a relatively small volume. They may also be used to prevent or correct essential fatty acid deficiency. When used as a calorie source the dose of the emulsion is determined by the energy requirements and clinical status of the patient; the amount, generally, should not comprise more than 60% of patients' total calorie intake. For the prevention and correction of fatty acid deficiency about 5 to 10% of total calorific intake should be as an intravenous fat emulsion.

The composition and dosage recommendations of commercial preparations do differ slightly but they should be started slowly. Suggested initial rates for the 10% and 20% products are 1 mL per minute and 0.5 mL per minute respectively for 15 to 30 minutes. The rate may then be increased and up to about 500 mL (or 10 mL per kg body-weight) of 10% or 250 mL (or 5 mL per kg) of 20% emulsion may be given on the first day. The total daily dosage may then be increased gradually on subsequent days; suggested daily dose ranges are 500 to 1500 mL of a 10% or 500 to 1000 mL of a 20% emulsion and suggested rates of administration are 500 mL of a 10% emulsion over a period of not less than 3 hours, and 500 mL of a 20% emulsion over not less than 5 hours. Where a 30% emulsion is used, a dose of 333 mL or about 4.75 mL per kg body-weight has been recommended, given over 5 hours or more; the first dose should not exceed 3 mL per kg.

Soya oil also has emollient properties and is used as a bath additive in the treatment of dry skin conditions.

Preparations made from whole soya beans, containing soya oil and soya protein, are used as the basis of lactose-free vegetable milks for infants and patients with lactose or similar disaccharide intolerance or with an allergy to cows' milk protein (see also below).

Administration. It has been suggested[1] that it is the concentration of phospholipid solubilisers, and particularly the excess present as free phospholipid liposomes, that determines the effect of lipid emulsions on plasma-lipid concentrations. In 20 premature infants requiring parenteral nutrition, infusion of up to 4 g of fat per kg body-weight daily as a 20% emulsion (twice the usual maximum dose) had less effect on plasma lipid concentrations than 2 g per kg daily as a 10% emulsion; the difference was thought to be due to the fact that the 20% emulsion was relatively liposome-poor, with a ratio of phospholipids to triglycerides of 0.06, whereas the liposome-rich 10% emulsion had a ratio of 0.12. The authors suggested that the 10% emulsion should not be used in preterm infants.

For mention of the risk of kernicterus if lipid infusions are given to hyperbilirubinaemic neonates, see under Precautions, above.

1. Haumont D, *et al.* Effect of liposomal content of lipid emulsions on plasma lipid concentrations in low birth weight infants receiving parenteral nutrition. *J Pediatr* 1992; **121:** 759–63.

Food intolerance. The American Academy of Pediatrics currently recommends[1] that soya-based infant feeds are appropriate for use in galactosaemia and hereditary lactase deficiency, and documented allergy to cows' milk protein. However, infants with documented cows' milk protein enteropathy or enterocolitis should receive hydrolysed protein formula, as they are likely to be sensitive to soya protein. They conclude that soya-based infant feeds have no proven role in the prevention of atopic disease or in the management of infantile colic.

The FDA has warned against the use of soya-based drinks intended for adults as the sole source for nutrition for infants.[2] It was stated that soya drinks can lead to severe protein and calorie malnutrition, multiple vitamin and mineral deficiency, and death in infants who receive no other source of nourishment, and should not be confused with soya-based infant formulas,

which are specially formulated to meet the nutritional needs of infants.

For reference to the use of soya-based foods themselves causing allergic reactions, see under Hypersensitivity, above.

1. American Academy of Pediatrics. Soy protein-based formulas: recommendations for use in infant feeding. *Pediatrics* 1998; **101:** 148–53.
2. Nightingale S. Warnings issued about practices, products: soy drink warning. *JAMA* 1985; **254:** 1428.

Hyperlipidaemias. Soya protein has been tried in the treatment of hyperlipidaemia (p.800). Soya isoflavones such as genistein and daidzein are able to mimic oestrogen and may therefore have a beneficial effect on blood lipids.[1,2] Other constituents of soya protein, including phytic acid and saponins may also contribute to this, and some authorities consider that intact soya protein will provide the maximum cholesterol-lowering effect.[2] A meta-analysis of controlled trials found that the substitution of soya protein for animal protein in the diet resulted in significant decreases in serum total cholesterol, low-density lipoprotein (LDL)-cholesterol, and triglyceride concentrations.[3] A subsequent systematic review of studies reached similar conclusions,[1] and the FDA considers that a low-fat diet including 25 g daily of soya protein may reduce the risk of ischaemic heart disease.[2] Soya protein does not appear to have a cholesterol-lowering effect in subjects with normal cholesterol concentrations,[2] although a small study found it to be beneficial in type 2 diabetes patients with near-normal lipid concentrations.[4]

1. Costa RL, Summa MA. Soy protein in the management of hyperlipidemia. *Ann Pharmacother* 2000; **34:** 931–5.
2. Erdman JW. Soy protein and cardiovascular disease: a statement for healthcare professionals from the Nutrition Committee of the AHA. *Circulation* 2000; **102:** 2555–9.
3. Anderson JW, *et al.* Meta-analysis of the effects of soy protein intake on serum lipids. *N Engl J Med* 1995; **333:** 276–82.
4. Hermansen K, *et al.* Beneficial effects of a soy-based dietary supplement on lipid levels and cardiovascular risk markers in type 2 diabetic subjects. *Diabetes Care* 2001; **24:** 228–33.

Menopausal disorders. Soya contains isoflavones, in particular genistein and daidzein, which have been investigated for their oestrogen-modulating effects in the treatment of menopausal symptoms (p.1464).[1] A small reduction in the incidence of hot flushes has been noted.[2] Isoflavones may have a beneficial effect on cholesterol and lipid concentrations (see above). Some epidemiological studies and *animal* data suggest that they may also provide protection against breast cancer.[1] A few small studies have shown that soya isoflavones can decrease bone turnover, leading to speculation that they could be used to prevent osteoporosis.[1] The effects of these isoflavones should be investigated in larger trials before they can be recommended as alternatives to conventional HRT.[3]

1. Vincent A, Fitzpatrick LA. Soy isoflavones: are they useful in menopause? *Mayo Clin Proc* 2000; **75:** 1174–84.
2. Upmalis DH, *et al.* Vasomotor symptom relief by soy isoflavone extract tablets in postmenopausal women: a multicenter, double-blind, randomized, placebo-controlled study. *Menopause* 2000; **7:** 236–42. Correction. *ibid.*; 422.
3. Anonymous. The role of isoflavones in menopausal health: consensus opinion of the North American Menopause Society. *Menopause* 2000; **7:** 215–29.

Preparations

Proprietary Preparations (details are given in Part 3)
Aust.: Balneum; Elolipid; Intralipid; Lipofundin; Lipovenos; Olbad Cordes; Solipid; *Austral.:* Intralipid; *Belg.:* Intralipid†; Ivelip; Lipovenoes†; *Braz.:* Lipofundin S; Lipovenos; *Canad.:* Intralipid; *Denm.:* Intralipid; Lipofundin†; Lipovenos; Vasolipid†; *Fin.:* Intralipid; *Fr.:* Endolipide; Intralipide; Ivelip; Lipoven; *Ger.:* Balneovit; Balneum; Deltalipid; Eucerin Omega Fettsauren Olbad; Hoecutin Olbad†; Intralipid; Kneipp Neurodermatitis-Bad†; Lipofundin N; Lipopharm N; Olbad Cordes; Penatoel; salvilipid; *Hong Kong:* Balneum Hermal; Intralipid; *Irl.:* Balneum; Intralipid; Lipofundin S†; *Israel:* Balneum; Intralipid; Ivelip; *Ital.:* Balneum Hermal; Elolipid; Intralipid; Ivelip; Lipofundin S; Lipovenos; *Jpn:* Intrafat; *Mex.:* Lipovenos; *Neth.:* Intralipid; Lipovenos; *Norw.:* Intralipid; Lipovenos; *NZ:* Intralipid; *Port.:* Balneum†; Banholeum†; Intralipid; Lipovenoes; *S.Afr.:* Intralipid; Lipovenos; *Singapore:* Intralipid; Intralipos; *Spain:* Ivelip; Lipovenos; Soyacal; *Swed.:* Emulsan†; Intralipid; Lipovenos; *Switz.:* Balneum Hermal; Intralipid; Lipidem; Lipovenos; *Thai.:* Intralipid; Lipofundin S; Lipovenos; *UK:* Balneum; Intralipid; Ivelip; Lipofundin; Lipovenos; Soyacal†; *USA:* Intralipid; Liposyn III.

Multi-ingredient: *Aust.:* Badeol; Balneum mit Teer; Balneum Plus; Clinomel; Gesamtnahrlosung; KabiMix; Lipofundin mit MCT; Olbad Cordes comp; Oleosint; PE-Mix; TriMix E; *Austral.:* Bioglan Mens Super Soy/Clover; Bioglan Soy Power Plus; Extralife Meno-Care; Hypol; Lifechange Menopause Formula; Phytolife; Soy Forte with Block Cohosh; *Belg.:* Clinoleic; Clinomel; Medialipide; *Denm.:* Clinoleic; Liposyn; Vitrimix; *Fin.:* Clinoleic; Complemen; KabiMix Basal; Kabiven; Liposyn; Novamix; Nutriflex Lipid; Structolipid; Vamin Glukos Combi; Vasolipid; *Fr.:* Clinoleic; Clinomel; Ivemix†; KabiMix; Medialipide; Piascledine; Structolipide; Trive; Vitrimix KV; *Ger.:* Abbolipid; Balneoconzen; Balneum Plus; Clinoleic; Clinomel; Complemen; Lipofundin MCT; Lipovenos; Lipovenos MCT; Nutriflex Lipid; Oleobal; Sulfo-Olbad Cordes; Windol Basisbad; *Hong Kong:* Lipofundin MCT/LCT; Vitrimix KV; *Irl.:* Balneum Plus; Balneum mit Tar; Vitrimix KV; *Israel:* Balneum Plus; Lipofundin MCT/LCT; Liposyn; Piascledine; *Ital.:* Clinoleic; KabiMix; Lipofundin MCT; Liposyn; Piascledine; *Mex.:* Liposyn; Soyaloid; Soydex; *Neth.:* KabiMix; Vitrimix KV; *Norw.:* Ivamix; KabiMix; Vasolipid; Vitrimix; *Port.:* Banholeum Composto†; Banholeum Gel†; Lipofundina MCT/LCT; Nutribraun; Structolipid; Vitrimix; *S.Afr.:* Lipofundin MCT/LCT; Lipovenoes; *Singapore:* Lipofundin MCT/LCT; Vitrimix KV; *Spain:* Clinoleic; Clinomel; KabiMix;

Lipofundina MCT/LCT; Nutriplasmal; Trive; *Swed.:* Complemen; KabiMix; Kabiven; Liposyn; Novamix; Nutriflex Lipid N; Structolipid; Vasolipid; Vitrimix; *Switz.:* Antidry; Balneum Hermal Plus; Demosvelte N†; Lipofundin MCT; Melisol†; Nutriflex 1680; Vitrimix; *Thai.:* Lipofundin MCT/LCT; Trive; Vitrimix KV; *UK:* Balneum Plus; Balneum with Tar†; Clinoleic; Clinomel; Complemen; KabiMix; Lipofundin MCT/LCT; Phytolife Plus; Vitrimix KV; *USA:* Anusol; Liposyn II.

Stannous Fluoride (7737-t)

Stannosi Fluoridum. Tin fluoride.
$SnF_2 = 156.7.$
CAS — 7783-47-3.
Pharmacopoeias. In US.

Aqueous solutions decompose within a few hours with the formation of a white precipitate; they slowly attack glass.

Pharmacopoeial description

USP 25: A white crystalline powder. Freely soluble in water; practically insoluble in alcohol, in chloroform, and in ether. pH of a freshly prepared 0.4% solution in water is between 2.8 and 3.5.

Profile

Stannous fluoride is used as a source of fluoride (see Sodium Fluoride, p.1375) for the prophylaxis of dental caries. Dental gels containing concentrations of stannous fluoride 0.4% are available for daily use. Higher concentrations have been applied under professional supervision. Stannous fluoride has also been used in dentifrices and mouth rinses.

Stannous fluoride has an unpleasant taste.

Preparations

USP 25: Stannous Fluoride Gel.

Proprietary Preparations (details are given in Part 3)
Port.: Gel Kam†; *UK:* Fluorigard Gel-Kam; Omnigel†; Stop; *USA:* Gel Kam; Gel-Tin; Stop.

Multi-ingredient: *Fr.:* Meridol; *Israel:* Meridol; *Ital.:* Actifluor; *Port.:* Meridol.

Stanol Esters (20343-d)

Profile

Stanol esters are formed by the esterification of plant stanols with unsaturated fatty acids. Sitostanol, the main plant stanol used, is produced by the saturation of sitosterol (p.970) derived from wood pulp. Stanol esters reduce plasma levels of total cholesterol and low-density lipoprotein (LDL)-cholesterol by inhibiting the intestinal absorption of cholesterol. They are incorporated into foods such as margarine, which are used as part of a cholesterol-lowering diet in the management of hyperlipidaemias (p.800).

◊ References.

1. Miettinen TA, *et al.* Reduction of serum cholesterol with sitostanol-ester margarine in a mildly hypercholesterolemic population. *N Engl J Med* 1995; **333:** 1308–12.
2. Gylling H, *et al.* Reduction of serum cholesterol in postmenopausal women with previous myocardial infarction and cholesterol malabsorption induced by dietary sitostanol ester margarine: women and dietary sitostanol. *Circulation* 1997; **96:** 4226–31.
3. Nguyen TT, *et al.* Cholesterol-lowering effect of stanol ester in a US population of mildly hypercholesterolemic men and women: a randomized controlled trial. *Mayo Clin Proc* 1999; **74:** 1198–1206.
4. Hallikainen MA, Uusitupa MIJ. Effects of 2 low-fat stanol ester-containing margarines on serum cholesterol concentrations as part of a low-fat diet in hypercholesterolemic subjects. *Am J Clin Nutr* 1999; **69:** 403–10.

Starch (1641-s)

Almidón; Amido; Amidon; Amilo; Amylum; Stärke.
CAS — 9005-25-8 (starch); 9005-82-7 (α-amylose); 9004-34-6 (β-amylose); 9037-22-3 (amylopectin).

NOTE. Starch (BP 2001) may be maize starch, rice starch, potato starch, wheat starch, or tapioca starch (cassava starch). Starch (USNF 20) is maize starch, wheat starch, tapioca starch, or potato starch.

Pharmacopoeias. Some or all of the starches described are included in *Chin., Eur.* (see p.vi), *Int., Jpn,* and *Pol.* Also in *USNF. Eur.* also includes Pregelatinised Starch, *USNF* also includes Pregelatinized Starch, and *US* includes Absorbable Dusting Powder and Topical Starch.

Polysaccharide granules obtained from the caryopsis of maize, *Zea mays,* rice, *Oryza sativa,* wheat, *Triticum aestivum* (T. vulgare), from the tubers of potato, *Solanum tuberosum* (T. tuberosum), from the rhizomes of cassava, *Manihot utilissima*. Maize starch is also known as corn starch. Starch contains amylose and amylopectin, both polysaccharides based on α-glucose.

Pharmacopoeial description

Ph. Eur.: Maize Starch is obtained from the caryopsis of *Zea mays*. It is a tasteless, matt, white to slightly yellowish, very fine powder which creaks when pressed between the fingers. The presence of granules with cracks or irregularities on the edge is exceptional. Practically insoluble in cold water and in alcohol. Store in airtight containers.

Potato Starch is obtained from the tuber of *Solanum tuberosum*. It is a very fine, white powder which creaks when pressed between the fingers. It does not contain starch grains of any other origin but may contain a minute quantity, if any, of fragments of the tissue of the original plant. Practically insoluble in cold water and in alcohol. The pH of a 20% mixture in water after 15 minutes is 5.0 to 8.0. Store in airtight containers.

Rice Starch is obtained from the caryopsis of *Oryza sativa*. It is a tasteless, very fine, white powder which creaks when pressed between the fingers. The presence of granules with cracks or irregularities on the edge is exceptional. Practically insoluble in cold water and in alcohol. Store in airtight containers.

Wheat Starch is obtained from the caryopsis of *Triticum aestivum* (*T. vulgare*). It is a very fine, white powder which creaks when pressed between the fingers. It does not contain starch grains of any other origin but may contain a minute quantity, if any, of fragments of the tissue of the original plant. Practically insoluble in cold water and in alcohol. The pH of a 20% mixture in water after 15 minutes is 5.0 to 8.0. Store in airtight containers.

BP 2001: Tapioca Starch is obtained from the rhizomes of *Manihot utilssima*. It is a very fine powder which creaks when pressed between the fingers. Practically insoluble in cold water and in alcohol. Store in airtight containers.

The BP directs that when starch is specified and the type is not indicated, Maize Starch, Potato Starch, Rice Starch, Wheat Starch, or in tropical countries where these are not available, Tapioca Starch may be supplied or used.

USNF 20: Granules separated from the mature grain of corn, *Zea mays* (Gramineae) or of wheat, *Triticum aestivum* (Gramineae), or from tubers of the potato, *Solanum tuberosum* (Solanaceae) or of tapioca, *Manihot utilissima* (Euphorbi Aceae). Irregular, angular, odourless, white masses or fine powder. Insoluble in cold water and in alcohol.

Adverse Effects

◊ The use of starch glove powders by surgeons has resulted in contamination of surgical wounds by starch and in the development of complications such as inflammation, adhesions, and granulomatous lesions. In addition, glove starch powder may be a risk factor in the development of latex allergy, and may act as a vector for bacterial pathogens. Because of these risks, it has been proposed that the use of powder in latex gloves be banned.[1,2]

1. Haglaund U, Junghanns K, eds. Glove powder—the hazards which demand a ban. *Eur J Surg* 1997; **163** (suppl 579): 1–55.
2. AAAAI and ACAAI joint statement concerning the use of powdered and non-powdered natural latex gloves. *Ann Allergy Asthma Immunol* 1997; **79**: 487.

Effects of cassava. In 1985 WHO added malnutrition-related diabetes (which included the type previously known as tropical diabetes) to its classification of diabetes mellitus.[1] Epidemiological evidence had suggested an association between fibrocalculous pancreatic diabetes (a subclass of malnutrition-related diabetes) and the consumption of cassava root (tapioca, manioc), which for many people living in tropical developing countries, where protein intake was low, was the main source of food energy. Cassava root contains several cyanogenic substances and although food preparation and processing could reduce the cyanide content, there was the possibility that in persons with an inadequate protein intake, particularly if deficient in sulfur-containing amino acids which are involved in detoxification pathways, accumulation of cyanides might occur. WHO, however, did consider that further research was necessary to firmly establish any relation between this type of diabetes and high levels of cassava consumption. In a review which appeared in the following year[2] the cassava/malnutrition hypothesis was thought to be attractive, but unproven; also there was strong evidence against it being the only cause.

WHO deleted malnutrition-related diabetes from its most recent report on the classification of diabetes.[3] Fibrocalculous pancreatic diabetes is now fibrocalculous pancreatopathy, a disease which may cause diabetes mellitus but is not considered a form of diabetes.

Neurotoxicity including spastic paraparesis[4] and optic neuropathy[5] caused by exposure to cyanide after ingestion of cassava root has been reported.

1. WHO. Diabetes mellitus: report of a WHO study group. *WHO Tech Rep Ser 727* 1985.
2. Abu-Bakare A, *et al.* Tropical or malnutrition-related diabetes: a real syndrome? *Lancet* 1986; **i:** 1135–8.
3. Alberti KGMM, Zimmet PZ. Definition, diagnosis, and classification of diabetes mellitus and its complications. Part I: diagnosis and classification of diabetes mellitus. Provisional report of a WHO consultation. *Diabetic Med* 1998; **15**: 539–53.
4. Cliff J, *et al.* Association of high cyanide and low sulphur intake in cassava-induced spastic paraparesis. *Lancet* 1985; **ii:** 1211–3.
5. Freeman AG. Optic neuropathy and chronic cyanide toxicity. *Lancet* 1986; **i:** 441–2.

Uses and Administration

Starch is absorbent and is widely used in dusting powders, either alone or mixed with zinc oxide or other similar substances. Starch is used as a surgical glove powder, but such use has been discouraged (see

above). It is incorporated in many tablets as a disintegrating agent.

A starch mucilage is given by mouth in the treatment of iodine poisoning.

Rice-based solutions may be used in the prevention and treatment of dehydration due to acute diarrhoeal diseases (p.1203) and may have advantages under certain circumstances over conventional oral rehydration solutions.

Glycogen storage diseases. Type I glycogen storage disease, in which hypoglycaemia is a predominant symptom, has been successfully managed by continuous nocturnal nasogastric infusion of glucose and frequent daytime feedings. However, such a regimen requires good patient compliance and monitoring of the night-time infusions. As an alternative, a more standard diet together with uncooked corn starch suspensions prepared with tap water at room temperature and taken every 6 hours in doses of 1.75 to 2.5 g per kg body-weight has been reported[1] to be very satisfactory in maintaining normoglycaemia. In one infant, in whom starch was not satisfactory, the lack of response was considered to be due to inadequate pancreatic amylase activity and although it was subsequently reported[2] that addition of a pancreatic enzyme concentrate had produced some improvement, the response was still inadequate to maintain normoglycaemia for more than 2 hours. It was considered that other amylase preparations should be identified for possible use in such patients.

Renal complications can also arise in type I glycogen storage disease as a consequence of a range of metabolic abnormalities. Corn starch therapy has been reported to have caused the amelioration of proximal renal tubular dysfunction in 3 patients who had previously only received frequent daytime feeding as therapy. In 16 other patients who had previously received treatment with corn starch or glucose infusions such renal dysfunction was not identified and it was considered that the rapid response to therapy may explain why renal tubular dysfunction is not found more frequently in these patients.[3]

1. Chen Y-T, *et al.* Cornstarch therapy in type 1 glycogen-storage disease. *N Engl J Med* 1984; **310:** 171–5.
2. Chen Y-T, Sidbury JB. Cornstarch therapy in type 1 glycogen-storage disease. *N Engl J Med* 1984; **311:** 128–9.
3. Chen Y-T, *et al.* Amelioration of proximal renal tubular dysfunction in type I glycogen storage disease with dietary therapy. *N Engl J Med* 1990; **323:** 590–3.

Preparations

BP 2001: Compound Zinc Paste; Dithranol Paste; Talc Dusting Powder;
Ph. Eur.: Pregelatinised Starch;
USNF 20: Pregelatinized Starch;
USP 25: Absorbable Dusting Powder; Topical Starch.

Proprietary Preparations (details are given in Part 3)
Fr.: Pyoralene; **Mex.:** Panaline; **NZ:** Karicare Food Thickener.

Multi-ingredient: Aust.: Myrtilen; **Austral.:** Karicare Food Thickener; Nucolox; ZSC; **Braz.:** Pantopept; **Fr.:** Magic Mix; **Israel:** Baby Paste; **Ital.:** Lenipasta; **Port.:** Cuidaderma; **UK:** Herbheal Ointment; Psoralsolv; Skin Clear; **USA:** Balmex Baby; Desitin with Zinc Oxide; Diaparene Corn Starch; Mexsana; Norforms; Yeast-X.

Stevioside (16994-r)

Eupatorin; Rebaudin; Stevin; Steviosin.
$C_{38}H_{60}O_{18} = 804.9$.
CAS — 57817-89-7.

A glycoside extracted from the leaves of yerba dulce, *Stevia rebaudiana* (Compositae).

Profile
Stevioside has about 300 times the sweetness of sucrose and has been used as a sweetening agent in foods. An extract of the leaves of *Stevia rebaudiana* which contains stevioside as well as other glycosides including rebaudioside A, has been used similarly.

◊ **References.**
1. Hanson JR, De Oliveira BH. Stevioside and related sweet diterpenoid glycosides. *Nat Prod Rep* 1993; **10:** 301–9.

Hypertension. The antihypertensive action of stevioside has been investigated in a randomised, double-blind trial.[1] A dose of 250 mg three times daily was found to lower blood pressure in patients with mild to moderate hypertension.

1. Chan P, *et al.* A double-blind placebo-controlled study of the effectiveness and tolerability of oral stevioside in human hypertension. *Br J Clin Pharmacol* 2000; **50:** 215–20.

Sucralose (5781-q)

Sucralose *(BAN)*.
TGS; Trichlorogalactosucrose. 1,6-Dichloro-1,6-dideoxy-β-D-fructofuranosyl 4-chloro-4-deoxy-α-D-galactopyranoside.
$C_{12}H_{19}Cl_3O_8 = 397.6$.
CAS — 56038-13-2.
Pharmacopoeias. In *USNF.*

Pharmacopoeial description
USNF 20: A white to off-white, crystalline powder. Freely soluble in water, in alcohol, and in methyl alcohol; slightly soluble in ethyl acetate. Store in a cool, dry place at a temperature not exceeding 21°.

Profile
Sucralose is used as a sweetening agent in foods and beverages. It has between about 300 and 1000 times the sweetening power of sucrose and is stable to heat. It has no food value.

◊ **References.**
1. Anonymous. Sucralose—a new artificial sweetener. *Med Lett Drugs Ther* 1998; **40:** 67–8.

Sucrose (660-b)

Azúcar; Cane Sugar; Refined Sugar; Sacarosa; Saccharose; Saccharum; Sucre; Sucrosum; Zucker. β-D-Fructofuranosyl-α-D-glucopyranoside.
$C_{12}H_{22}O_{11} = 342.3$.
CAS — 57-50-1.

Pharmacopoeias. In *Chin., Eur.* (see p.vi), *Jpn,* and *Pol.* Also in *USNF.*
USNF also includes Compressible Sugar, Confectioner's Sugar, and Sugar Spheres.

It is obtained from sugar-cane, *Saccharum officinarum* (Gramineae), sugar-beet, *Beta vulgaris* (Chenopodiaceae), and other sources.

A solution in water is neutral to litmus. Sucrose may be contaminated by traces of heavy metals or sulfites and this may lead to incompatibility with active ingredients when sucrose is used as a pharmaceutical excipient. Syrup preserved with hydroxybenzoates has been reported to be incompatible with a range of compounds.

Pharmacopoeial description
Ph. Eur.: A white, crystalline powder or lustrous, dry, colourless or white crystals. Very soluble in water; slightly soluble in alcohol; practically insoluble in dehydrated alcohol.

USNF 20: A sugar obtained from *Saccharum officinarum* (Gramineae), *Beta vulgaris* (Chenopodiaceae), and other sources. White, crystalline powder or lustrous, dry, colourless or white crystals. Soluble 1 in 0.5 of water, 1 in 0.2 of boiling water, and 1 in 170 of alcohol; practically insoluble in dehydrated alcohol.

Adverse Effects and Precautions
Sucrose consumption increases the incidence of dental caries.

Sucrose use should be avoided in patients with the glucose-galactose malabsorption syndrome, fructose intolerance, or sucrase-isomaltase deficiency. The intake of sucrose from dietary and other sources must be controlled in patients with diabetes mellitus.

◊ Conclusions and recommendations of the Panel on Dietary Sugars after reviewing the evidence relating to sugars in the diet and the health of the population in the UK.[1]

No evidence was found that the consumption of most sugars naturally incorporated into the cellular structure of foods (intrinsic sugars) represented a threat to health and consideration was therefore mainly directed towards the dietary use of sugars not so incorporated (extrinsic sugars), of which sucrose was the principal non-milk extrinsic sugar.

There was extensive evidence suggesting that sugars were the most important dietary factor in the cause of dental caries and it was recommended that consumption of non-milk extrinsic sugars should be decreased.

It was considered that dietary sugars may contribute to the development of obesity, a condition which plays an important part in the aetiology of a number of diseases. For the majority of the population, who had normal plasma lipids and normal glucose tolerance, the consumption of sugars within the present range carried no special metabolic risks but those persons consuming more than about 200 g daily should replace the excess with starch. It was, however, recommended that those with special medical problems such as diabetes or hypertriglyceridaemia should restrict non-milk extrinsic sugar to less than about 20 to 50 g daily unless otherwise instructed by their own physician or dietitian. It was also concluded that current consumption of sugars, particularly sucrose, played no direct causal role in the development of cardiovascular (atherosclerotic coronary, peripheral, or cerebral vascular) disease, essential hypertension, or diabetes mellitus, and also had no significant specific effects on behaviour or psychological function. Although links between sucrose intake and certain other diseases (such as colorectal cancer, renal and biliary calculi, and Crohn's disease) had been proposed it was not felt that the evidence was adequate to justify any general dietary recommendations.

The conclusions of a joint FAO/WHO consultation on carbohydrates in human nutrition[2] were broadly in agreement with the above. However, they note that the terms intrinsic and extrinsic sugars have not gained wide acceptance, either in the UK or other countries in the world, and they recommended against the use of these terms.

1. DoH. Dietary sugars and human disease: report of the panel on dietary sugars of the committee on medical aspects of food policy. *Report on health and social subjects 37.* London: HMSO, 1989.
2. FAO/WHO. *Carbohydrates in human nutrition: report of a joint FAO/WHO expert consultation. FAO Food and Nutrition 66.* Rome: Food and Agriculture Organization of the United Nations, 1998.

Effects on the kidneys. Acute renal failure with severe hyponatraemia has followed the use of granulated sugar to treat an infected pneumonectomy wound cavity.[1] It was noted that intravenous sucrose had long been known to be nephrotoxic in both animal models and man and that mild renal insufficiency before sucrose intoxication might have contributed to the nephrosis. Others, however, considered that the nephrotoxicity might have been caused by gentamicin, a solution of which had been used to irrigate the cavity prior to packing the wound.[2]

1. Debure A, *et al.* Acute renal failure after use of granulated sugar in deep infected wound. *Lancet* 1987; **i:** 1034–5.
2. Archer H, *et al.* Toxicity of topical sugar. *Lancet* 1987; **i:** 1485–6.

Pharmacokinetics

Sucrose is hydrolysed in the small intestine by the enzyme sucrase to glucose and fructose, which are then absorbed. Sucrose is excreted unchanged in the urine when given intravenously.

Uses and Administration

Sucrose, a disaccharide, is used as a sweetening agent. It is commonly used as household sugar. If the sweetness of sucrose is taken as 100, fructose has a value of about 173, glucose 74, maltose 32, galactose 32, and lactose 16.

Sucrose is used as a tablet excipient and lozenge basis, and as a suspending and viscosity-increasing agent. Syrups prepared from concentrated solutions of sucrose form the basis of many linctuses.

Cough. Sucrose syrups are used as demulcents in linctuses used for treating cough (p.1082).

Diagnostic test for gastrointestinal damage. Sucrose is not absorbed from the healthy gastrointestinal tract. It has been proposed[1] that the absorption of sucrose could be used as a diagnostic test of gastrointestinal damage.

1. Sutherland LR, *et al.* A simple non-invasive marker of gastric damage: sucrose permeability. *Lancet* 1994; **343:** 998–1000.

Gastrointestinal spasm. For mention of a beneficial effect of sucrose solution in infant colic, see p.1204.

Hiccup. Administration of a teaspoon of dry granulated sugar resulted in the immediate cessation of hiccup in 19 of 20 patients;[1] 12 of the patients had suffered from hiccup for less than 6 hours but in the remaining 8 persistent hiccup had been present for 24 hours to 6 weeks. The effect may be due to stimulation of the pharynx. A protocol for the treatment of intractable hiccup (p.667) suggests that swallowing dry granulated sugar is one of the first treatments that should be tried.

1. Engleman EG, *et al.* Granulated sugar as treatment for hiccups in conscious patients. *N Engl J Med* 1971; **285:** 1489.

Pain. A systematic review[1] concluded that sucrose solutions could reduce physiological and behavioural indicators of stress and pain in neonates undergoing painful procedures although there had been some doubt expressed[2] over whether this indicated effective analgesia. The review[1] was unable to determine an optimal dose, but 1 mL of a 25% solution or 2 mL of a 50% solution has been reported to reduce crying time in premature[3] and full-term[4] infants, respectively, when administered 2 minutes before heel prick sampling. Similarly, 2 mL of a 75% sucrose solution by mouth reduced crying time in infants receiving intramuscular vaccines.[5] The route of administration of the sucrose solution may also be important: a reduced pain response was only noted after intraoral administration; administration via a nasogastric tube was ineffective.[6] For choice of analgesic in children, see p.3.

1. Stevens B, *et al.* Sucrose for analgesia in newborn infants undergoing painful procedures (updated 28 August 2001). Available in The Cochrane Library; Issue 4. Oxford: Update Software; 2001.
2. Anonymous. Pacifiers, passive behaviour, and pain. *Lancet* 1992; **339:** 275–6.
3. Ramenghi LA, *et al.* Reduction of pain response in premature infants using intraoral sucrose. *Arch Dis Child* 1996; **74:** F126–F128.
4. Haouari N, *et al.* The analgesic effect of sucrose in full term infants: a randomised controlled trial. *BMJ* 1995; **310:** 1498–1500.
5. Lewindon PJ, *et al.* Randomised controlled trial of sucrose by mouth for the relief of infant crying after immunisation. *Arch Dis Child* 1998; **78:** 453–6.
6. Ramenghi LA, *et al.* "Sucrose analgesia": absorptive mechanism or taste perception. *Arch Dis Child Fetal Neonatal Ed* 1999; **80:** F146–F147.

Wound healing. Sugar, either in the form of granulated sugar[1,2] or pastes composed of caster sugar and icing sugar,[3,4] has been used successfully in the treatment of a variety of wounds (p.1108) including open mediastinitis after cardiac surgery,[1] large abscesses and bed sores,[3,4] and diabetic ulcers.[2] De-

---

bridement of the wound is believed to be due partly to the osmotic effect of sugar and partly to the mechanical cleansing action but it is not known how sugar stimulates granulation tissue to form.[3,4] Once granulation tissue is well established and the wound is shrinking, an alternative wound preparation, such as an alginate, hydrocolloid, or hydrogel, should be used as sugar pastes cause bleeding.[5] Sugar is also effective at deodorising malodorous wounds. The use of the combined caster and icing sugar pastes, of which details of the formulas used are provided in the original publications,[3,4] has been advocated as a way to overcome the problems of possible non-sterility and contamination of commercial granulated sugar.[3,4]

Honey (p.1366) has been used similarly.

1. Trouillet JL, *et al.* Use of granulated sugar in treatment of open mediastinitis after cardiac surgery. *Lancet* 1985; **ii:** 180–4.
2. Quatraro A, *et al.* Sugar and wound healing. *Lancet* 1985; **ii:** 664.
3. Gordon H, *et al.* Sugar and wound healing. *Lancet* 1985; **ii:** 663–4.
4. Middleton KR, Seal D. Sugar as an aid to wound healing. *Pharm J* 1985; **235:** 757–8.
5. Seal DV, Middleton K. Healing of cavity wounds with sugar. *Lancet* 1991; **338:** 571–2.

Preparations

BP 2001: Compressible Sugar; Syrup;
Ph. Eur.: Sugar Spheres;
USNF 20: Compressible Sugar; Confectioner's Sugar; Sugar Spheres; Syrup.

Proprietary Preparations (details are given in Part 3)
Fr.: Gelodiet.

Multi-ingredient: *S.Afr.:* Emetrol.

Sucrose Polyesters   (16716-f)
Profile
A sucrose polyester that is a mixture of hexa-, hepta-, and octa-fatty acid esters of sucrose is used as a nondigestible fat substitute by the food industry. Fat substitutes have been promoted as part of a strategy to reduce fat and calories in the diet to aid body-weight control.

Possible adverse effects of sucrose polyesters are flatulence, anal leakage, abdominal cramps, and loose bowel movements. They may also reduce the absorption of fat-soluble vitamins.

◊ References.
1. Cotton JR, *et al.* Replacement of dietary fat with sucrose polyester: effects on energy intake and appetite control in non-obese males. *Am J Clin Nutr* 1996; **63:** 891–6.
2. Goldman P. Olestra: assessing its potential to interact with drugs in the gastrointestinal tract. *Clin Pharmacol Ther* 1997; **61:** 613–18.
3. Cheskin LJ, *et al.* Gastrointestinal symptoms following consumption of olestra or regular triglyceride potato chips: a controlled comparison. *JAMA* 1998; **279:** 150–2.
4. Sandler RS, *et al.* Gastrointestinal symptoms in 3181 volunteers ingesting snack foods containing olestra or triglycerides. *Ann Intern Med* 1999; **130:** 253–61.

Sunflower Oil   (7370-b)
Helianthi Annui Oleum; Huile de Tournesol; Oleum Helianthi; Sunflowerseed Oil.

Pharmacopoeias. In Eur. (see p.vi).

Pharmacopoeial description
Ph. Eur.: The fatty oil obtained from the seeds of *Helianthus annuus* by mechanical expression or by extraction and then refined. A suitable antioxidant may be added. A clear, light yellow liquid. Practically insoluble in water and in alcohol; miscible with petroleum spirit (b.p.: 40° to 60°). Store in well-filled airtight containers. Protect from light.

Profile
Sunflower oil is used in pharmaceutical preparations. It is rich in linoleic acid (p.1613).

Multiple sclerosis. As discussed on p.633, the role of dietary lipids in multiple sclerosis remains to be proven,[1] although many patients modify their diets and take supplements of sunflower and other oils. Some studies have shown a reduction in severity and duration of relapse in patients taking linoleic acid supplements (as sunflower oil)[2] and another[3] has reported benefit in patients who limit their intake of dietary saturated fatty acids and supplement their diet with polyunsaturated fatty acids.

1. Anonymous. Lipids and multiple sclerosis. *Lancet* 1990; **336:** 25–6.
2. Millar JHD, *et al.* Double-blind trial of linoleate supplementation of the diet in multiple sclerosis. *BMJ* 1973; **1:** 765–8.
3. Swank RL, Dugan BB. Effect of low saturated fat diet in early and late cases of multiple sclerosis. *Lancet* 1990; **336:** 37–9.

Preparations
Proprietary Preparations (details are given in Part 3)
Port.: Oleoban.

Multi-ingredient: *Aust.:* Pelsana Med; Piniment; *Ger.:* dermalogues N; *Port.:* Oleoban Composto; Oleoban Gel; *Switz.:* Huile de millepertuis A. Vogel (huile de St. Jean); Pelsano; *UK:* Snor-Away; Snorenz.

Thaumatin   (12877-q)
Thaumatin *(BAN).*
E957; Katemfe.
CAS — 53850-34-3.

A mixture in the ratio of 2:1 of two polypeptides thaumatin I and thaumatin II, each consisting of 207 amino acid residues and having a molecular weight of about 22 000, derived from the fruit of *Thaumatococcus danielii* (Scitamineae).

An odourless, cream-coloured, proteinaceous powder with an intensely sweet taste.

Profile
Thaumatin is a protein whose amino-acid range excludes histidine. It produces an intense sweetness that builds up gradually but persists for up to an hour, and is considered to be by far the sweetest of such compounds in use. It is approved as a sweetener and flavour modifier in foods and drinks.

Threonine   (662-g)
Threonine *(USAN, rINN).*
β-Methylserine; T; Thr; L-Threonine; Threoninum. L-2-Amino-3-hydroxybutyric acid.
$C_4H_9NO_3 = 119.1.$
CAS — 72-19-5.
Pharmacopoeias. In Eur. (see p.vi), Jpn, and US.

Pharmacopoeial description
Ph. Eur.: A white, crystalline powder or colourless crystals. Soluble in water; practically insoluble in alcohol and in ether. A 2.5% solution in water has a pH of 5.0 to 6.5. Protect from light.

USP 25: White, odourless crystals. Freely soluble in water; insoluble in dehydrated alcohol, in chloroform, and in ether. pH of a 5% solution in water is between 5.0 and 6.5.

Profile
Threonine is an aliphatic amino acid which is an essential constituent of the diet. It is used as a dietary supplement.

Threonine has been investigated for the treatment of various spastic disorders.

Tyrosine   (665-s)
Tyrosine *(USAN, rINN).*
Tyr; L-Tyrosine; Tyrosinum; Y. L-2-Amino-3-(4-hydroxyphenyl)propionic acid.
$C_9H_{11}NO_3 = 181.2.$
CAS — 60-18-4.
Pharmacopoeias. In Eur. (see p.vi) and US.

Pharmacopoeial description
Ph. Eur.: A white crystalline powder or colourless crystals. Very slightly soluble in water; practically insoluble in alcohol. It dissolves in dilute mineral acids and in dilute solutions of alkali hydroxides. Protect from light.

USP 25: White, odourless crystals or crystalline powder. Very slightly soluble in water; insoluble in alcohol and in ether.

Profile
Tyrosine is an aromatic amino acid. It is used as a dietary supplement.

Phenylketonuria. Tyrosine was not an effective alternative to a diet low in phenylalanine in patients with phenylketonuria, see under Amino Acid Metabolic Disorders, p.1350.

Preparations
Proprietary Preparations (details are given in Part 3)
Multi-ingredient: *Austral.:* Aussie Tan Pre-Tan; Bioglan Zellulean with Escin; Tyroseng; *UK:* Amino MS; *USA:* Catemine†.

Valine   (666-w)
Valine *(USAN, rINN).*
α-Aminoisovaleric Acid; V; Val; L-Valine; Valinum. (S)-2-Amino-3-methylbutanoic acid.
$C_5H_{11}NO_2 = 117.1.$
CAS — 72-18-4.
Pharmacopoeias. In Eur. (see p.vi), Jpn, and US.

Pharmacopoeial description
Ph. Eur.: A white or almost white, crystalline powder or colourless crystals. Soluble in water; very slightly soluble in alcohol; practically insoluble in ether. Protect from light.

USP 25: White, odourless crystals. Soluble in water; practically insoluble in alcohol, in acetone, and in ether. pH of a 5% solution in water is between 5.5 and 7.0.

Profile
Valine is a branched-chain amino acid which is an essential constituent of the diet. It is used as a dietary supplement. It is also an ingredient of several preparations that have been promoted for disorders of the liver.

The symbol † denotes a preparation no longer actively marketed

Preparations

Proprietary Preparations (details are given in Part 3)
Multi-ingredient: *Fr.:* Revitalose; *Ger.:* Bramin-hepa; Falkamin; *Ital.:* Falkamin; Isobranch; Isoram.

Vitamin A (7823-k)

Vitamin A *(USAN)*.
Retinol *(BAN, rINN)*; Antixerophthalmic Vitamin; Axerophtholum; Oleovitamin A; Vitamin A Alcohol; Vitaminum A. 15-Apo-β-caroten-15-ol; 3,7-Dimethyl-9-(2,6,6-trimethylcyclohex-1-enyl)nona-2,4,6,8-tetraen-1-ol.
$C_{20}H_{30}O = 286.5$.
CAS — 68-26-8.
ATC — D10AD02; R01AX02; S01XA02.

Pharmacopoeias. In *Eur.* (see p.vi) and *US*, which permit retinol or its esters.

Chin. includes a monograph for the acetate. *Jpn* and *Pol.* include monographs for the acetate and the palmitate. *Br.* includes a monograph for Natural Vitamin A Ester Concentrate. *Eur.* also includes monographs for Synthetic Vitamin A Concentrate (Oily Form), Synthetic Vitamin A Concentrate (Powder Form), and Synthetic Vitamin A Concentrate (Solubilisate/Emulsion). *Br.* uses Retinol in the title of preparations containing synthetic Vitamin A, and Vitamin A in the title of preparations containing material of natural origin.

Vitamin A Acetate. Retinol Acetate; Retinyl Acetate; $C_{22}H_{32}O_2 = 328.5$; CAS — 127-47-9
Vitamin A Palmitate. Retinol Palmitate; Retinyl Palmitate; $C_{36}H_{60}O_2 = 524.9$; CAS — 79-81-2
Vitamin A Propionate. Retinol Propionate; Retinyl Propionate; $C_{23}H_{34}O_2 = 342.5$; CAS — 7069-42-3.

Pharmacopoeial description

Ph. Eur.: Under the name Vitamin A are included a number of substances of very similar structure (including (*Z*)-isomers) found in animal tissues and possessing similar activity. The principal and biologically most active substance is all-(*E*) retinol.

Vitamin A is generally used in the form of esters such as the acetate, propionate, and palmitate. Synthetic retinol ester refers to an ester of synthetic retinol (acetate, propionate, or palmitate) or a mixture of synthetic retinol esters.

Retinol acetate occurs as pale yellow crystals. M.p. about 60°; once melted it tends to yield a supercooled melt. Retinol propionate occurs as a reddish-brown oily liquid. Retinol palmitate occurs as a fat-like, light yellow solid, or as a yellow oily liquid, if melted. M.p. about 26°. All retinol esters are practically insoluble in water; soluble or partly soluble in dehydrated alcohol; miscible with organic solvents. Vitamin A and its esters are sensitive to the action of air, oxidising agents, acids, light, and heat. Store in well-filled airtight containers. Protect from light. Once the container has been opened, its contents should be used as soon as possible and any part of the contents not used should be protected by an atmosphere of inert gas.

Synthetic Vitamin A Concentrate (Oily Form) is prepared from synthetic retinol ester as is or by dilution with a suitable vegetable oil. It contains not less than 500 000 units of vitamin A per g. It is a yellow or brownish-yellow, oily liquid; practically insoluble in water; soluble or partly soluble in dehydrated alcohol; miscible with organic solvents. Partial crystallisation may occur in highly concentrated solutions. Store in well-filled airtight containers. Protect from light. Once the container has been opened, its contents should be used as soon as possible and any part of the contents not used at once should be protected by an atmosphere of inert gas.

Synthetic Vitamin A Concentrate (Powder Form) is obtained by dispersing a synthetic retinol ester in a matrix of gelatin or acacia or other suitable material. It contains not less than 250 000 units of vitamin A per g. It is a yellowish powder usually in the form of particles of almost uniform size. Practically insoluble in water or may swell or form an emulsion, depending on formulation. Store in well-filled airtight containers. Protect from light. Once the container has been opened, its contents should be used as soon as possible and any part of the contents not used at once should be protected by an atmosphere of inert gas.

Synthetic Vitamin A Concentrate (Solubilisate/Emulsion) is a liquid form (water is generally used as solvent) of synthetic retinol ester and a suitable solubiliser. It contains not less than 100 000 units of vitamin A per g. It is a yellow or yellowish liquid of variable opalescence and viscosity. Highly concentrated solutions may become cloudy at low temperatures or take the form of a gel. A mixture of 1 g with 10 mL of water previously warmed to 50° gives after cooling to 20°, a uniform, slightly opalescent and slightly yellow dispersion. Store in airtight containers. Protect from light. Once the container has been opened, its contents should be used as soon as possible and any part of the contents not used at once should be protected by an atmosphere of inert gas.

BP 2001: Natural Vitamin A Ester Concentrate consists of a natural ester or a mixture of natural esters of retinol or of a solution of the ester or mixture of esters in arachis oil or other suitable vegetable oil. It contains not less than 485 000 units of

vitamin A per g. It is a yellow oil or a mixture of oil and crystalline material, with a faint odour. Practically insoluble in water; soluble or partly soluble in alcohol; miscible with chloroform, with ether, and with petroleum spirit. Store in airtight containers at 8° to 15°. Protect from light.

USP 25: It may consist of retinol or its esters formed from edible fatty acids, principally acetic and palmitic acids. In liquid form, it is a light yellow to red oil that may solidify upon refrigeration. In solid form, has the appearance of any diluent that has been added. It may be practically odourless or may have a mild fishy odour but no rancid odour or taste. It is unstable in air and light. In liquid form, it is insoluble in water and in glycerol; soluble in dehydrated alcohol and in vegetable oils; very soluble in chloroform and in ether. In solid form, may be dispersible in water. Store in airtight containers, preferably under an atmosphere of inert gas. Protect from light.

Units

The International Standards for vitamin A and for provitamin A were discontinued in 1954 and 1956 respectively but the International units for these substances have continued to be widely used. In 1960–1, the WHO Expert Committee on Biological Standardization stated that the International unit for vitamin A is equivalent to the activity of 0.000344 mg of pure all-*trans* vitamin A acetate and the International unit for provitamin A is equivalent to the activity of 0.0006 mg of pure all-*trans* β-carotene.

The activity of one International unit is contained in 0.0003 mg of all-*trans* retinol, in 0.00055 mg of all-*trans* retinol palmitate, and in 0.000359 mg of all-*trans* retinol propionate.

USP 25 defines the USP unit as the specific biologic activity of 0.0003 mg of the all-*trans* isomer of retinol, and is equivalent to the International unit.

Vitamin A activity in foods is currently expressed in terms of retinol equivalents: 1 retinol equivalent is defined as 1 µg of all-*trans* retinol, 6 µg of all-*trans* beta carotene, or 12 µg of other provitamin A carotenoids.

Adverse Effects and Precautions

The administration of excessive amounts of vitamin A substances over long periods can lead to toxicity, known as hypervitaminosis A. This is characterised by fatigue, irritability, anorexia and loss of weight, vomiting and other gastrointestinal disturbances, low-grade fever, hepatosplenomegaly, skin changes (yellowing, dryness, sensitivity to sunlight), alopecia, dry hair, cracking and bleeding lips, anaemia, headache, hypercalcaemia, subcutaneous swelling, nocturia, and pains in bones and joints. Symptoms of chronic toxicity may also include raised intracranial pressure and papilloedema mimicking brain tumours, tinnitus, and visual disturbances which may be severe. Symptoms usually clear on withdrawal of vitamin A, but in children premature closure of the epiphyses of the long bones may result in arrested bone growth.

Acute vitamin A intoxication may occur with very high doses and is characterised by sedation, dizziness, nausea and vomiting, erythema, pruritus, desquamation, and increased intracranial pressure (resulting in bulging fontanelle in infants).

Hypervitaminosis A does not appear to be a problem with large doses of carotenoids (see Pharmacokinetics under Betacarotene, p.1355).

Enhanced susceptibility to the effects of vitamin A may be seen in children and in patients with liver disease.

Excessive doses of vitamin A should be avoided in pregnancy because of potential teratogenic effects; for further details see Pregnancy, below.

Gastrointestinal absorption of vitamin A may be impaired in cholestatic jaundice and fat-malabsorption conditions.

Benign intracranial hypertension. High doses of vitamin A cause increased intracranial pressure, and, in infants, this is manifested as bulging of the fontanelle. In one study,[1] 11.5% of infants receiving 3 doses of 50 000 units of vitamin A at monthly intervals had bulging fontanelle, compared with 1% of infants receiving placebo. The bulging lasted between 24 and 72 hours and subsided without treatment,[1] and did not appear to be associated with any physical or developmental abnormalities on long-term follow-up.[2] In another study in neonates, bulging fontanelle occurred in 4.6% of recipients of vitamin A

50 000 units and 2.7% of placebo recipients 24 hours after administration.[3] In contrast, less than 1% of infants given 3 doses of 25 000 units of vitamin A at monthly intervals had bulging fontanelle in a further study.[4]

1. de Francisco A, *et al.* Acute toxicity of vitamin A given with vaccines in infancy. *Lancet* 1993; **342:** 526–7.
2. van Dillen J, *et al.* Long-term effect of vitamin A with vaccines. *Lancet* 1996; **347:** 1705.
3. Agoestina T, *et al.* Safety of one 52 µmol (50 000 IU) oral dose of vitamin A administered to neonates. *Bull WHO* 1994; **72:** 859–68.
4. WHO/CHD Immunisation-Linked Vitamin A Supplementation Study Group. Randomised trial to assess benefits and safety of vitamin A supplementation linked to immunisation in early infancy. *Lancet* 1998; **352:** 1257–63. Correction. *ibid.* 1999; **353:** 154.

Carcinogenicity. For mention of the *increased* risk of lung cancer in high-risk individuals receiving betacarotene and vitamin A, when compared with placebo, in a study investigating vitamins in lung cancer prevention, see Prophylaxis of Malignant Neoplasms, p.1353.

Effects on the blood. Normochromic macrocytic anaemia developed in a patient who had been receiving vitamin A 150 000 IU daily by mouth for several months.[1] The patient's haemoglobin returned to normal when vitamin A was discontinued, and the accompanying symptoms of perioral dermatitis and glossitis also disappeared.

1. White JM. Vitamin-A-induced anaemia. *Lancet* 1984; **ii:** 573.

Effects on bone. Excessive dietary intake of vitamin A may be associated with osteoporosis. In an epidemiological study,[1] a dietary intake of retinol greater than 1500 µg per day (5000 units) doubled the risk of hip fracture compared with an intake of less than 500 µg per day (about 1670 units) in women (odds ratio, 2.1; 95% confidence interval 1.1 to 4.0).

1. Melhus H, *et al.* Excessive dietary intake of vitamin A is associated with reduced bone mineral density and increased risk for hip fracture. *Ann Intern Med* 1998; **129:** 770–8.

Effects on the immune system. Vitamin A deficiency is generally associated with impaired immunity, and treatment of deficiency results in reductions in morbidity and mortality from a number of infectious diseases (see Deficiency States, below). However, a few studies have shown increased prevalence of diarrhoea and/or respiratory-tract infections with high doses of vitamin A. There is a possibility that high single doses of vitamin A may temporarily attenuate the immune response in non-deficient children.[1] For mention that high-dose vitamin A supplements have been associated with a reduced response to measles vaccine in some studies, see p.1547.

1. Anonymous. Childhood morbidity, immunity and micronutrients. *WHO Drug Inf* 1996; **10:** 12–16.

Effects on the liver. Vitamin A is stored in the Dissë space of liver cells and excess administration can lead to fibrosis and obstruction of sinusoidal blood flow, causing non-cirrhotic portal hypertension and hepatocellular dysfunction.[1] Although hepatotoxicity has typically been reported with habitual ingestion of doses of vitamin A greater than 50 000 units daily, a case of severe hepatic fibrosis, with jaundice and hepatomegaly, has been reported in a patient who had been taking 25 000 units daily for at least 6 years in a multivitamin supplement.[2]

1. Sherlock S. The spectrum of hepatotoxicity due to drugs. *Lancet* 1986; **ii:** 440–4.
2. Kowalski TE, *et al.* Vitamin A hepatotoxicity: a cautionary note regarding 25,000 IU supplements. *Am J Med* 1994; **97:** 523–8.

Hypersensitivity. Local inflammatory reactions and severe anaphylactoid reactions have occurred in patients receiving vitamin A injections, and are usually attributed to solubilisers such as polyoxyl castor oils (p.1347), and, less commonly, polysorbates (p.1348).

A case of cutaneous hypersensitivity to retinol palmitate, and not other injection ingredients, has been described.[1]

1. Shelley WB, *et al.* Hypersensitivity to retinol palmitate injection. *BMJ* 1995; **311:** 232.

Pregnancy. The fact that synthetic vitamin A derivatives such as isotretinoin are teratogenic (p.1117) has prompted concern about the potential teratogenicity of high doses of vitamin A.

A prospective cohort study found that a total daily intake of vitamin A from all sources of greater than 15 000 units during early pregnancy was associated with a significantly increased risk of birth defects of structures arising from the cranial neural crest.[1] When vitamin A intake from supplements was analysed separately, an apparent vitamin A threshold dose for the development of birth defects of 10 000 units daily was suggested. However, this study has been criticised[2,3] and some suggest the data allows for a higher threshold dose.[3] A further study found no significant difference in birth defect rates between women consuming greater than 8000 or 10 000 units of vitamin A daily in the period around conception (as supplements and fortified cereals) and those consuming less than 5000 units daily.[4]

Following earlier case reports in the USA suggesting that large doses of vitamin A (equivalent to about ten times the daily recommended dietary allowance of 2250 units) taken in early pregnancy may cause birth defects, the UK Chief Medical Officer cautioned women against the use of vitamin A supplements except under medical supervision.[5] Additionally, advice was given that liver or liver products should not be eaten because high concentrations of vitamin A had been detected in some samples of animal liver. However, others thought that the avoidance of liver or liver products might result in inadequate nutrition in some and that a less alarmist view might have been to suggest a limitation on intake rather than total prohibition.[6,7]

The American College of Obstetricians and Gynecologists has recommended that women who are pregnant or planning pregnancy should ensure that any vitamin supplements they take contain a daily dose of vitamin A of no more than 5000 units.[8] The Australian Adverse Drug Reactions Advisory Committee has advised women in this category to avoid vitamin A supplements and to not exceed the recommended daily allowance of 2500 units from all sources.[9]

1. Rothman KJ, *et al.* Teratogenicity of high vitamin A intake. *N Engl J Med* 1995; **333:** 1369–73.
2. Werler MM, *et al.* Teratogenicity of high vitamin A intake. *N Engl J Med* 1996; **334:** 1195–6.
3. Watkins M, *et al.* Teratogenicity of high vitamin A intake. *N Engl J Med* 1996; **334:** 1196.
4. Mills JL, *et al.* Vitamin A and birth defects. *Am J Obstet Gynecol* 1997; **177:** 31–6.
5. Department of Health. *Women cautioned: watch your vitamin A intake.* London: Department of Health, 1990 (18 October).
6. Nelson M. Vitamin A, liver consumption, and risk of birth defects. *BMJ* 1990; **301:** 1176.
7. Sanders TAB. Vitamin A and pregnancy. *Lancet* 1990; **336:** 1375.
8. American College of Obstetricians and Gynecologists. Vitamin A supplementation during pregnancy. *Int J Gynecol Obstet* 1993; **40:** 175.
9. Adverse Drug Reactions Advisory Committee. Vitamin A and birth defects. *Aust Adverse Drug React Bull* 1996; **15:** 14–15.

Interactions

Absorption of vitamin A from the gastrointestinal tract may be reduced by the presence of neomycin, colestyramine, or liquid paraffin.

There is an increased risk of hypervitaminosis A if vitamin A is coadministered with synthetic retinoids such as acitretin, isotretinoin, and tretinoin.

There is conflicting evidence regarding the effect of vitamin A on the response to measles vaccine (see p.1547).

Pharmacokinetics

Vitamin A substances are readily absorbed from the gastrointestinal tract but absorption may be reduced in the presence of fat malabsorption, low protein intake, or impaired liver or pancreatic function. Vitamin A esters are hydrolysed by pancreatic enzymes to retinol, which is then absorbed and re-esterified. Some retinol is stored in the liver. It is released from the liver bound to a specific α_1-globulin (retinol-binding protein) in the blood. The retinol not stored in the liver undergoes glucuronide conjugation and subsequent oxidation to retinal and retinoic acid; these and other metabolites are excreted in urine and faeces. Vitamin A does not readily diffuse across the placenta (but see Pregnancy, above), but is present in breast milk.

◊ References.

1. Hartmann D, *et al.* Pharmacokinetic modelling of the plasma concentration-time profile of the vitamin retinyl palmitate following intramuscular administration. *Biopharm Drug Dispos* 1990; **11:** 689–700.

Human Requirements

Dietary vitamin A is derived from 2 sources, *preformed retinoids* from animal sources such as liver, kidney, dairy produce, and eggs (fish-liver oils are the most concentrated natural source), and *provitamin carotenoids* which can be obtained from many plants; the latter are converted to retinol in the body but are less effectively utilised. Carotenes (α, β, and γ) are major sources and of these, β-carotene (betacarotene—see p.1355) has the highest vitamin A activity and is the most plentiful in food. Variable amounts of β-carotenes are found in carrots and dark green or yellow vegetables. Red palm oil is a good source of α- and β-carotenes.

◊ In the UK dietary reference values (see p.1352) have been published[1] for vitamin A and similarly in the USA recommended dietary allowances (RDAs) have been set.[2] Differing amounts are recommended for infants and children of varying ages, for adult males and females, and for pregnant and lactating women (but see Pregnancy, above). In the UK the reference nutrient intake (RNI) for adult males and females is 700 and 600 µg retinol equivalents (approximately 2330 and 2000 units) daily, respectively and the estimated average requirement (EAR) is 500 and 400 µg retinol equivalents (approximately 1660 and 1330 units) daily, respectively. This UK report[1] also highlighted the toxicity associated with large doses of vitamin A and recommended that regular intakes should not

exceed 9000 µg (30 000 units) daily in adult men and 7500 µg (25 000 units) daily in adult women. Figures were also given for infants and children who were said to be more sensitive to the effects of vitamin A. These limits did not apply to therapeutic doses of vitamin A used under medical supervision.[1] In pregnancy the RNI is 700 µg retinol equivalents (2330 units) daily and in nursing mothers 950 µg (3160 units) daily. In the USA the RDA for adults is 900 µg daily for men and 700 µg daily for women.[2] The tolerable upper intake level is 3000 µg daily.

1. DoH. Dietary reference values for food energy and nutrients for the United Kingdom: report of the panel on dietary reference values of the committee on medical aspects of food policy. *Report on health and social subjects 41.* London: HMSO, 1991.
2. Standing Committee on the Scientific Evaluation of Dietary Reference Intakes of the Food and Nutrition Board. *Dietary Reference Intakes for vitamin A, vitamin K, arsenic, boron, chromium, copper, iodine, iron, manganese, molybdenum, nickel, silicon, vanadium, and zinc.* Washington DC: National Academy Press, 2001.

Uses and Administration

Vitamin A, a fat-soluble vitamin, is essential for growth, for the development and maintenance of epithelial tissue, and for vision, particularly in dim light. Vitamin A deficiency develops when the dietary intake is inadequate and is seen more frequently in young children than in adults. It is rare in developed countries but remains a major problem in many developing countries. Prolonged deficiency leads to xerophthalmia or "dry eye", the initial symptom of which is night blindness which may progress to severe eye lesions and blindness. Other symptoms include changes in the skin and mucous membranes.

Vitamin A is used in the treatment and prevention of vitamin A deficiency. It may be administered by mouth in an oil- or water-based form, the oil-based generally being the preferred type. It can also be administered by intramuscular injection of a water-miscible form; oil-miscible preparations of vitamin A are poorly absorbed from injection sites following intramuscular injection and are not usually used for administration by this route. For further details concerning vitamin A supplementation, including doses for the treatment and prophylaxis of xerophthalmia, see under Deficiency States, below.

Vitamin A supplements are often given to patients with primary biliary cirrhosis or chronic cholestatic liver disease as deficiencies are common in these disorders. An intramuscular dose of 100 000 units every 2 to 4 months has been suggested.

Vitamins A and D have been used together as cream or ointment in the treatment of minor skin disorders including abrasions. Vitamin A has also been used alone to treat various skin disorders including acne and psoriasis. It has been tried in patients with retinitis pigmentosa to retard the decline in retinal function.

Deficiency states. Vitamin A deficiency is relatively rare in developed countries and is usually only seen in certain medical conditions such as biliary cirrhosis or cholestatic jaundice. However, it is a continuing problem in many developing countries and children appear to be particularly vulnerable.

In the developing countries where dietary intake may often be less than desirable, infections such as measles, acute respiratory diseases, and diarrhoea can be major precipitating factors of vitamin A deficiency. Thus WHO have targeted elimination of vitamin A deficiency as an important strategy in child health,[1,2] and as part of the Expanded Programme on Immunization. They recommend the use of vitamin A supplements in the treatment of vitamin A deficiency (see Xerophthalmia, below) and to prevent vitamin A deficiency where the periodic administration of supplements is determined to be the most feasible and effective method of improving vitamin A status. In universal distribution programmes,[2] supplemental doses are given to all preschool-age children at a dose of 200 000 units every 4 to 6 months, with infants between the ages of 6 and 12 months receiving half this dose. Infants aged less than 6 months may receive 50 000 units if they are not breast fed or if they are breast fed and their mothers have not received supplemental vitamin A. Mothers in high-risk regions should receive 200 000 units within 8 weeks of delivery of a child. Targeted distribution programmes involve vitamin A supplementation to children and pregnant women in specific high-risk areas.[2] Doses used in children are similar to those used in universal programmes, but doses used in pregnant women should not exceed 10 000 units daily, or 25 000 units weekly.

A number of studies have indicated that general supplementation with vitamin A decreases both mortality rates and morbidity among children in developing countries with a high prevalence of vitamin A deficiency.[3-6] Although not all studies have

confirmed these findings,[7,8] two meta-analyses concur that the effect is likely to be genuine at least as regards measles infection,[9,10] and researchers and commentators have agreed that overall improvement of vitamin A status is worthwhile and necessary.[7,11] Supplementation with vitamin A 23 300 units per week, or the equivalent amount of betacarotene, in women of child-bearing age reduced pregnancy-related mortality.[12] Some studies have evaluated mortality specifically in infants less than 6 months of age. In one study there was no overall benefit on early infant mortality with a tendency for the relative risk of mortality to increase with improved nutritional status,[13] whereas another reported a decrease in mortality in the first year of life.[14] A further study found no sustained benefit of vitamin A supplements on vitamin A status or morbidity beyond the age of 6 months, in infants receiving supplements with immunisation at 6, 10, and 14 weeks.[15] A study in vitamin-A-deficient children has demonstrated abnormalities in T-cell subsets which are corrected by vitamin A supplementation,[16] and it has been proposed that the apparent effects of vitamin A on morbidity and mortality may be due to modulation of immune function (see also Effects on the Immune System, above).

In countries in which vitamin A deficiency is not widespread some form of supplementation may still be considered. In the UK, the Department of Health has recommended routine supplementation with 700 units of vitamin A daily, together with ascorbic acid and vitamin D, in children aged 1 to 5 years; some breast-fed infants from 1 or 6 months of age may also benefit. Preterm infants have low vitamin A status at birth, which may increase their risk of developing chronic lung disease.[17] A meta-analysis of trials in low birth-weight infants found that vitamin A supplementation was associated with a reduced requirement for oxygen at 36 weeks postmenstrual age.[17]

Anaemia. There has been a study among pregnant Indonesian women with nutritional anaemia that demonstrated a beneficial effect for vitamin A on haemoglobin when given with iron supplementation.[18]

Diarrhoea. Several of the large mortality trials already mentioned reported that vitamin A supplementation was associated with reduced mortality attributed to diarrhoea,[4-6] but one did not.[7] The effect on morbidity from diarrhoea is even less clear. A reduction in the severity, but not the incidence, of diarrhoea has been noted in two studies.[19,20] However, in one study in children with subclinical vitamin A deficiency, there was an increased prevalence of diarrhoea for 2 weeks after vitamin A supplementation,[21] and in another study, vitamin A increased the incidence of diarrhoea in children aged less than 30 months.[22]

Measles. Vitamin A supplementation has an important role in the prevention of complications from measles.[9,10] Two studies specifically addressing vitamin A status and measles have found that complications such as pneumonia and diarrhoea were less common in children who had received supplements at the time of diagnosis than in those given a placebo.[23,24] A meta-analysis of randomised trials concluded that a dose of 200 000 units of vitamin A given on two consecutive days reduced mortality in children with measles.[25] WHO has recommended treating children in populations where vitamin A deficiency is common with high-dose vitamin A supplements during episodes of measles.[2] A dose of 200 000 units should be given on two consecutive days to all children over 12 months of age. This should be followed by a further dose at least 2 weeks later. Infants less than 6 months of age should receive doses of 50 000 units and those between 6 and 12 months should be given 100 000 units. Studies in the USA have indicated that even among well-nourished children from a developed country, vitamin A deficiency in measles patients is not uncommon,[26,27] and vitamin A supplementation needs to be considered in children at risk.[28]

Respiratory-tract infections. The mortality trials mentioned did not show a consistent impact for vitamin A supplementation on death from non-measles-related respiratory infections.[4-6] Similarly, other studies have found no benefit of vitamin A on subsequent respiratory morbidity.[19,20,29] A meta-analysis of trials reporting pneumonia morbidity and mortality found no overall benefit or harm from vitamin A supplementation.[30] However, an increased prevalence of symptoms of respiratory infections associated with vitamin A supplementation has been noted in two studies,[21,22] particularly in children with adequate nutritional status.

Vitamin A was not effective for the treatment of childhood non-measles-related lower respiratory-tract infections[31] or pneumonia.[32] Similarly, there was no benefit from vitamin A in the treatment of respiratory syncytial virus infection in children in two studies.[33,34] In one of these studies there was a tendency for vitamin A to improve outcomes in the subgroup of severely ill children,[33] and in the other there was a slight increase in duration of hospitalisation in low-risk children receiving vitamin A.[34]

Shigellosis. A single high-dose vitamin A supplement reduced the severity of acute shigellosis in children in Bangladesh.[35]

Xerophthalmia. Vitamin A deficiency is responsible in many developing countries for visual problems which may culminate in xerophthalmia and blindness. Supplementation with vitamin A as recommended by WHO and discussed above will raise the vitamin A status of the individual and act prophylactically against the development of xerophthalmia. For the treatment of xerophthalmia (which includes night blindness, conjunctival xerosis with Bitot's spots, corneal xerosis, corneal ulceration, and keratomalacia) WHO have stated that oral doses of vitamin A, preferably in an oil-based preparation, are the treatment of choice and should be given immediately the disorder is recognised.[2] All patients over 1 year of age (with the exception of women of reproductive age, see below) should receive 200 000 units by mouth immediately on diagnosis; infants aged 6 to 12 months should receive 100 000 units, and those aged less than 6 months, 50 000 units. The dose should be repeated the next day, and again at least 2 weeks later. In women of reproductive age there is a need to balance the possible teratogenic effects of vitamin A should they be pregnant (see under Precautions, above) with the serious consequences of xerophthalmia. WHO recommend that when there are severe signs of active xerophthalmia (i.e. acute corneal lesions) high dose vitamin A treatment should be given as described above for those aged over 1 year. When only less severe signs are present (night blindness, Bitot's spots), women of reproductive age should receive a daily oral dose of 5000 to 10 000 units for at least 4 weeks. Alternatively, a weekly dose of not more than 25 000 units may be substituted.

Although xerophthalmia is far less common in developed countries, vitamin A deficiency should be considered in all patients with recurrent conjunctival or corneal disorders associated with gastrointestinal or liver disease.[36]

1. Potter AR. Reducing vitamin A deficiency. *BMJ* 1997; **314:** 317–18.
2. WHO/UNICEF/IVACG Task Force. *Vitamin A supplements: a guide to their use in the treatment and prevention of vitamin A deficiency and xerophthalmia.* 2nd ed. Geneva: WHO, 1997.
3. Rahmathullah L, *et al.* Reduced mortality among children in southern India receiving a small weekly dose of vitamin A. *N Engl J Med* 1990; **323:** 929–35.
4. West KP, *et al.* Efficacy of vitamin A in reducing preschool child mortality in Nepal. *Lancet* 1991; **338:** 67–71.
5. Daulaire NMP, *et al.* Childhood mortality after a high dose of vitamin A in a high risk population. *BMJ* 1992; **304:** 207–10.
6. Ghana VAST Study Team. Vitamin A supplementation in northern Ghana: effects on clinic attendances, hospital admissions, and child mortality. *Lancet* 1993; **342:** 7–12.
7. Vijayaraghavan K, *et al.* Effect of massive dose of vitamin A on morbidity and mortality in Indian children. *Lancet* 1990; **336:** 1342–5.
8. Herrera MG, *et al.* Vitamin A supplementation and child survival. *Lancet* 1992; **340:** 267–71.
9. Glasziou PP, Mackerras DEM. Vitamin A supplementation in infectious diseases: a meta-analysis. *BMJ* 1993; **306:** 366–70.
10. Fawzi WW, *et al.* Vitamin A supplementation and child mortality: a meta-analysis. *JAMA* 1993; **269:** 898–903.
11. Anonymous. Vitamin A and malnutrition/infection complex in developing countries. *Lancet* 1990; **336:** 1349–51.
12. West KP, *et al.* Double blind, cluster randomised trial of low dose supplementation with vitamin A or β carotene on mortality related to pregnancy in Nepal. *BMJ* 1999; **318:** 570–5. Correction. *ibid.*; 1386.
13. West KP, *et al.* Mortality of infants <6 mo of age supplemented with vitamin A: a randomized double-masked trial in Nepal. *Am J Clin Nutr* 1995; **62:** 143–8.
14. Humphrey JH, *et al.* Impact of neonatal vitamin A supplementation on infant morbidity and mortality. *J Pediatr* 1996; **128:** 489–96.
15. WHO/CHD Immunisation-Linked Vitamin A Supplementation Study Group. Randomised trial to assess benefits and safety of vitamin A supplementation linked to immunisation in early infancy. *Lancet* 1998; **352:** 1257–63. Correction. *ibid.* 1999; **353:** 154.
16. Semba RD, *et al.* Abnormal T-cell subset proportions in vitamin-A-deficient children. *Lancet* 1993; **341:** 5–8.
17. Darlow BA, Graham PJ. Vitamin A supplementation for preventing morbidity and mortality in very low birthweight infants (updated 23 February 2000). Available in The Cochrane Library; Issue 4. Oxford: Update Software; 2001.
18. Suharno D, *et al.* Supplementation with vitamin A and iron for nutritional anaemia in pregnant women in West Java, Indonesia. *Lancet* 1993; **342:** 1325–8.
19. Barreto ML, *et al.* Effect of vitamin A supplementation on diarrhoea and acute lower-respiratory-tract infections in young children in Brazil. *Lancet* 1994; **344:** 228–31.
20. Bhandari N, *et al.* Impact of massive dose of vitamin A given to preschool children with acute diarrhoea on subsequent respiratory and diarrhoeal morbidity. *BMJ* 1994; **309:** 1404–7.
21. Stansfield SK, *et al.* Vitamin A supplementation and increased prevalence of childhood diarrhoea and acute respiratory infections. *Lancet* 1993; **342:** 578–82.
22. Dibley MJ, *et al.* Vitamin A supplementation fails to reduce incidence of acute respiratory illness and diarrhea in preschool-age Indonesian children. *J Nutr* 1996; **126:** 434–42.
23. Barclay AJG, *et al.* Vitamin A supplements and mortality related to measles: a randomised clinical trial. *BMJ* 1987; **294:** 294–6.
24. Hussey GD, Klein M. A randomized, controlled trial of vitamin A in children with severe measles. *N Engl J Med* 1990; **323:** 160–4.
25. D'Souza RM, D'Souza R. Vitamin A for treating measles in children (updated 18 July 2001). Available in The Cochrane Library; Issue 4. Oxford: Update Software; 2001.
26. Arrieta AC, *et al.* Vitamin A levels in children with measles in Long Beach, California. *J Pediatr* 1992; **121:** 75–8.
27. Butler JC, *et al.* Measles severity and serum retinol (vitamin A) concentration among children in the United States. *Pediatrics* 1993; **91:** 1176–81.
28. Committee on Infectious Diseases of the American Academy of Pediatrics. Vitamin A treatment of measles. *Pediatrics* 1993; **91:** 1014–15.
29. Kartasasmita CB, *et al.* Plasma retinol level, vitamin A supplementation and acute respiratory infections in children of 1-5 years old in a developing country. *Tubercle Lung Dis* 1995; **76:** 563–9.
30. The Vitamin A and Pneumonia Working Group. Potential interventions for the prevention of childhood pneumonia in developing countries: a meta-analysis of data from field trials to assess the impact of vitamin A supplementation on pneumonia morbidity and mortality. *Bull WHO* 1995; **73:** 609–19.

31. Kjolhede CL, *et al.* Clinical trial of vitamin A as adjuvant treatment for lower respiratory tract infections. *J Pediatr* 1995; **126:** 807–12.
32. Nacul LC, *et al.* Randomised, double blind, placebo controlled clinical trial of efficacy of vitamin A treatment in non-measles childhood pneumonia. *BMJ* 1997; **315:** 505–10.
33. Dowell SF, *et al.* Treatment of respiratory syncytial virus infection with vitamin A: a randomised placebo-controlled trial in Santiago, Chile. *Pediatr Infect Dis J* 1996; **15:** 782–6.
34. Bresee JS, *et al.* Vitamin A therapy for children with respiratory syncytial virus infection: a multicenter trial in the United States. *Pediatr Infect Dis J* 1996; **15:** 777–82.
35. Hossain S, *et al.* Single dose vitamin A treatment in acute shigellosis in Bangladeshi children: randomised double blind controlled trial. *BMJ* 1998; **316:** 422–6.
36. Watson NJ, *et al.* Vitamin A deficiency and xerophthalmia in the United Kingdom. *BMJ* 1995; **310:** 1050–1. Correction. *ibid.*: 1320.

HIV infection and AIDS. A study in Malawi found that the rates of vertical transmission of HIV infection (birth of seropositive infants to seropositive mothers) were inversely related to maternal vitamin A status;[1] vitamin A deficiency during pregnancy was associated with a threefold to fourfold increased risk of mother-to-child transmission of HIV. This was not incompatible with the role of vitamin A in immunity and maintenance of mucosal surfaces, and since both HIV infection and pregnancy are risk factors for vitamin A deficiency, it was suggested that nutritional intervention to reduce vitamin A deficiency might help combat mother-to-child transmission. However, another study[2] in Tanzania, for which vertical transmission data were not available, found no evidence of an effect of vitamin A on birth outcomes in HIV-infected women and the authors pointed out that serum concentrations of vitamin A might be a marker for the stage of HIV disease rather than being causally related to outcome. The study did however find that multivitamin supplements reduced the risk of low-birth-weight and size for age, and of premature birth, in the offspring of these women.[2] Means of reducing the risk of HIV infection in neonates (see HIV Infection Prophylaxis, p.610) are of considerable interest.

1. Semba RD, *et al.* Maternal vitamin A deficiency and mother-to-child transmission of HIV-1. *Lancet* 1994; **343:** 1593–7.
2. Fawzi WW, *et al.* Randomised trial of effects of vitamin supplements on pregnancy outcomes and T-cell counts in HIV-1-infected women in Tanzania. *Lancet* 1998; **351:** 1477–82.

Malignant neoplasms. Epidemiological studies suggest that antioxidant vitamins such as the vitamin A substances may play a role in preventing the development of malignancy but there is currently little evidence from prospective studies to support this (see p.1353). Conversely, synthetic retinoids such as tretinoin (all-*trans*-retinoic acid) have an established role in treating some cancers (see p.1127).

Retinitis pigmentosa. Retinitis pigmentosa is the name applied to a group of slowly progressive hereditary degenerative diseases of the retina that often results in blindness in adulthood. The rod and cone photoreceptors in the retina are primarily affected and initial symptoms include night blindness and intolerance to light. Later signs include infiltration of pigment from the retinal pigmentary epithelium into the retinal layers. Various treatments have been tried but none appear to have any proven benefit. Results of one large double-blind study[1] suggest that whereas treatment with vitamin A might slow the decline in visual acuity treatment with vitamin E appears to have a deleterious effect on the rate of decline. In 3 patients with retinitis pigmentosa and a defect in α-tocopherol-transfer protein associated with vitamin E deficiency, vitamin E administration did appear to delay the rate of vision decline.[2] Transplantation of the retina is being investigated as a treatment for retinitis pigmentosa.[3]

1. Berson EL, *et al.* A randomized trial of vitamin A and vitamin E supplementation for retinitis pigmentosa. *Arch Ophthalmol* 1993; **111:** 761–2.
2. Yokota T, *et al.* Retinitis pigmentosa and ataxia caused by a mutation in the gene for the α-tocopherol-transfer protein. *N Engl J Med* 1996; **335:** 1770–1.
3. Anonymous. Transplantation as a therapy for retinitis pigmentosa? *Br J Ophthalmol* 1997; **81:** 430.

Preparations

BPC 1973: Vitamins A and D Capsules;
USP 25: Oleovitamin A and D; Oleovitamin A and D Capsules; Vitamin A Capsules.

Proprietary Preparations (details are given in Part 3)
Aust.: Arcavit A; Avitol; Oleovit A; *Austral.:* Dermalife†; *Belg.:* Dagravit A; *Braz.:* Arovit; Nalfan; *Canad.:* A-Mulsion; Arovit; *Denm.:* A-vitamin; *Fin.:* A-Vitamiini; *Fr.:* A 313; Arovit; Avibon; *Ger.:* A-Mulsin; A-Vicotrat; Augenkraft; Oculotect; Oculotect sine; Ophtol-A; Ophtosan; Solan-M; Vitadral; *Hong Kong:* Aquasol A; *Israel:* Avipur; *Ital.:* Akeral; Arovit; Euvitol; Repervit; Vit-A-N; *Mex.:* A Grin; A-Vitex; Acon; Avinal-Ex; Pertamin; *Neth.:* Dagravit A Forte; Dermalife; Ro-A-Vit; Ungvita; *Port.:* A-Vite; Vitaminoftalmina; *S.Afr.:* Arovit; *Spain:* Auxina Masiva; Biominol A; Dif Vitamin A Masivo; Ido A 50; Mulsal A Megadosis; Rinocusi Vitaminico; *Swed.:* Arovit; *Switz.:* Arovit; Oculotect; *UK:* Biovit-A; Ro-A-Vit; *USA:* Aquasol A; Del-Vi-A†; Palmitate-A; Pedi-Vit-A; Retinol-A.

Multi-ingredient: *Aust.:* A-E-Mulsin; Arcavit A/E; Coldistop; Gelacet; Gerogelat; Lemuval; Maagersan†; Oleovit; Oleovit A; Oleovit A + D; Regenerin; Rovigon; Ultren; Vasovitol; *Austral.:* Althaea Complex; Arthriforte; Bioglan Micelle A plus E; Bioglan Zn-A-C; Dermalife Plus; Garlic, Horseradish, A & C Capsules; Halivol†; Hydrastis Complex; John Plunketts Protective Day Cream; Macro Natural Vitamin E Cream; Natures Way Total Zinc; Proyeast; Sambucus Complex; Trifolium Complex; Ungvita; Ver-

bascum Complex; *Belg.:* Ad-Vitan†; Dagravit A-E; Neo-Cutigenol; Neo-Debiol AD3; Newderm; Rovigon; Vita-Mefren; Vitaminic A-D†; Vitamorrhuine; Vitapantol; *Braz.:* AD Til; ADE 2; Adrofix D3; Aderogil D3; Epitezan; Gaduol; Gotil-AD; Hipoderme; Hipodermon; Hipodex; Hipoglos; Hipoglos com Hidrocortisona; Hipoglos Oftalmico; Preparado H; *Canad.:* A & D Ointment; Antiseptic Skin Cream; Aquasol A†; Cirkan a la Prednacinolone; Dermocalm†; Pommade Lelong†; Rovigon; Solacy; *Ger.:* A + D + E-Vicotrat; A + D₃-Vicotrat†; A + E Thilo; A-E-Mulsin; Augentonikum; Coldastop; Corti-Fixcole†; Cosaldon A; duraultra; Gelacet N; Golden Star; Hewekzem novo; Kollateral A + E; Magopsor†; Oculotect; Regepithel; Remederm; Rovigon G; Salus Augenschutz-Kapseln N; Unguentacid; *Hong Kong:* Aderma Epitheliale; Regepithel; *Israel:* Aquitol; Aronal Forte; Oleovit A + D₃; Vita-Merfen NF; Vitamidyne A and D; *Ital.:* AD Pabyrn; Adiboran AD; Adisterolo; Aminotril; Babysteril; Derman-Oil; Dermana; Dicalcium; Evitex; Granoleina; Lasonil H; Lasoproct†; Midium; NeoCeuticals Spot Treatment; Provitamin A-E; Rinopanteina; Rovigon; Tocalfa; *Mex.:* Adekon; Adekon C; Adeloren; Adibal; Hipoglos Plus; Kamiloderm; *Neth.:* Dagravit A-E Forte; Davitamon AD Fluor†; Davitamon AD†; Dohyfral Vitamine AD3†; Halitran†; *NZ:* Dermalife Plus; Ungvita; *Port.:* Esclerobion; Rovigon; Zelderme†; *S.Afr.:* Corti-Fixcole†; Vandol; *Spain:* Adiod; Antihemorroidal; Auxina A + E; Biominol A D; Bronquimar Vit A†; Calcio 20 Complex; Cicatral; Dermo H Infantil; Dimayon†; Epitelizante; Evitex A E Fuerte; Gramoce A; Grietalgen; Grietalgen Hidrocort; Halibut; Halibut Hidrocortisona; Hubergrip; Lacerdermol; Lacerdermol Complex; Mastiol; Mitosyl; Noquema†; Poli ABE; Queratil; Ravigona†; Trivitan†; Vicomin A C; Vitaber A E; Wobenzimal; *Swed.:* AD-vitamin; *Switz.:* Alphastria; Antikeloides Creme; Carbamide Creme; Coldistop; Demosept; Gelacet; Kamillosan†; Malvedrin; Oravil; Riccomycine†; Riccovitan; Rovigon; Sanhelios Capsules a la vitamine A; Unatol; Vita-Hexin; Vita-Merfen; *Thai.:* Rovigon; *UK:* S.P.H.P.; Se-Power; *USA:* A and D Medicated; Aloe Grande; Clocream; Comfortine; Diaper Guard; Lazercreme; Lobana Derm-Aide; Lobana Peri-Garde; Phicon; Vitanumonyl†.

Vitamin B Substances (17537-b)

The B vitamin group includes the B₁ substances (thiamine and its derivatives), B₂ (riboflavin), B₆ (pyridoxine and derivatives), and B₁₂ (the cobalamins). In addition, nicotinic acid and its derivatives (p.1372) and folic acid (p.1361) are held to be part of the group, as is pantothenic acid (p.1374), but these latter substances are not generally referred to by their traditional B nomenclature.

Vitamin B₁ Substances (14738-l)

Acetiamine Hydrochloride (12309-r)

Acetiamine Hydrochloride (*rINNM*).

Acethiamine Hydrochloride; Diacethiamine Hydrochloride. *N*-(5-Acetoxy-3-acetylthiopent-2-en-2-yl)-*N*-(4-amino-2-methylpyrimidin-5-ylmethyl)formamide hydrochloride monohydrate.
$C_{16}H_{22}N_4O_4S,HCl,H_2O = 420.9$.
CAS — 299-89-8 (acetiamine).

Benfotiamine (7831-k)

Benfotiamine (*rINN*).

S-Benzoylthiamine O-Monophosphate. *N*-(4-Amino-2-methylpyrimidin-5-ylmethyl)-*N*-(2-benzoylthio-4-dihydrophosphinyloxy-1-methylbut-1-enyl)formamide.
$C_{19}H_{23}N_4O_6PS = 466.4$.
CAS — 22457-89-2.

Bisbentiamine (7832-a)

Bisbentiamine (*rINN*).

O-Benzoylthiamine Disulphide. NN'-{Dithiobis[2-(2-benzoyloxyethyl)-1-methylvinylene]}bis[*N*-(4-amino-2-methylpyrimidin-5-ylmethyl)formamide].
$C_{38}H_{42}N_8O_6S_2 = 770.9$.
CAS — 2667-89-2.

Cycotiamine (7837-d)

Cycotiamine (*rINN*).

CCT; Cyclocarbothiamine. *N*-(4-Amino-2-methylpyrimidin-5-ylmethyl)-*N*-[1-(2-oxo-1,3-oxathian-4-ylidene)ethyl]formamide.
$C_{13}H_{16}N_4O_3S = 308.4$.
CAS — 6092-18-8.

Fursultiamine (7838-n)

Fursultiamine (*rINN*).

Thiamine Tetrahydrofurfuryl Disulphide; TTFD. *N*-(4-Amino-2-methylpyrimidin-5-ylmethyl)-*N*-[4-hydroxy-1-methyl-2-(tetrahydrofurfuryldithio)but-1-enyl]formamide.
$C_{17}H_{26}N_4O_3S_2 = 398.5$.
CAS — 804-30-8.

Octotiamine (7839-h)

Octotiamine (rINN).

TATD; Thiocotthiamine. N-[2-(3-Acetylthio-7-methoxycarbo-nylheptyldithio)-4-hydroxy-1-methylbut-1-enyl]-N-(4-amino-2-methylpyrimidin-5-ylmethyl)formamide.

$C_{23}H_{36}N_4O_5S_3 = 544.8$.
CAS — 137-86-0.

Prosultiamine (13182-q)

Prosultiamine (rINN).

DTPT; Thiamine Propyl Disulphide. N-(4-Amino-2-methylpyri-midin-5-ylmethyl)-N-(4-hydroxy-1-methyl-2-propyldithiobut-1-enyl)formamide.

$C_{15}H_{24}N_4O_2S_2 = 356.5$.
CAS — 59-58-5.

Sulbutiamine (7834-x)

Sulbutiamine (rINN).

Bisibutiamine; O-Isobutyrylthiamine Disulphide. NN'-{Dithio-bis[2-(2-isobutyryloxyethyl)-1-methylvinylene]}bis[N-(4-ami-no-2-methylpyrimidin-5-ylmethyl)formamide].

$C_{32}H_{46}N_8O_6S_2 = 702.9$.
CAS — 3286-46-2.
ATC — A11DA02.

Thiamine Hydrochloride (7829-d)

Thiamine Hydrochloride (BANM, rINNM).

Aneurine Hydrochloride; Thiamin Hydrochloride; Thiamine Chloride; Thiamini Hydrochloridum; Thiaminii Chloridum; Vita-min B₁. 3-(4-Amino-2-methylpyrimidin-5-ylmethyl)-5-(2-hy-droxyethyl)-4-methylthiazolium chloride hydrochloride.

$C_{12}H_{17}ClN_4OS,HCl = 337.3$.
CAS — 59-43-8 (thiamine); 67-03-8 (thiamine hydrochlo-ride).

Pharmacopoeias. In Chin., Eur. (see p.vi), Int., Jpn, Pol., and US. Thiamine hydrobromide is included in Int.

Sterile solutions of pH 4 or less lose activity only very slowly but neutral or alkaline solutions deteriorate rapidly, especially in contact with air.

Pharmacopoeial description

Ph. Eur.: A white or almost white, crystalline powder or col-ourless crystals. Freely soluble in water; slightly soluble in al-cohol; practically insoluble in ether; soluble in glycerol. A 2.5% solution in water has a pH of 2.7 to 3.3. Store in nonme-tallic containers. Protect from light.

USP 25: White crystals or crystalline powder, usually having a slight, characteristic odour. When exposed to air, the anhydrous product rapidly absorbs about 4% of water. Soluble 1 in 1 of water and 1 in 170 of alcohol; insoluble in ether and in ben-zene; soluble in glycerol. pH of a 1% solution in water is be-tween 2.7 and 3.4. Store in airtight containers. Protect from light.

Thiamine Nitrate (7830-c)

Thiamine Nitrate (BANM, rINNM).

Aneurine Nitrate; Thiamine Mononitrate; Thiamini Nitras; Vitamin B₁ Mononitrate. 3-(4-Amino-2-methylpyrimidin-5-yl-methyl)-5-(2-hydroxyethyl)-4-methylthiazolium nitrate.

$C_{12}H_{17}N_5O_4S = 327.4$.
CAS — 532-43-4.

Pharmacopoeias. In Eur. (see p.vi), Int., Jpn, Pol., and US.

Pharmacopoeial description

Ph. Eur.: A white or almost white, crystalline powder or small, colourless crystals. Sparingly soluble in water; freely soluble in boiling water; slightly soluble in alcohol and in methyl alcohol. A 2% solution in water has a pH of 6.8 to 7.6. Store in nonme-tallic containers. Protect from light.

USP 25: White crystals or crystalline powder, usually having a slight characteristic odour. Soluble 1 in 44 of water; slightly soluble in alcohol; very slightly soluble in chloroform. pH of a 2% solution in water is between 6.0 and 7.5. Store in airtight containers. Protect from light.

Adverse Effects and Precautions

Adverse effects seldom occur following administration of thiamine, but hypersensitivity reactions have occurred, mainly after parenteral administration. These reactions have ranged in severity from very mild to, very rarely, fatal anaphylactic shock (see be-low).

Hypersensitivity. The UK Committee on Safety of Medi-cines had received, between 1970 and July 1988, 90 reports of adverse reactions associated with the use of an injection con-taining high doses of vitamins B and C. The most frequent re-actions were 41 cases of anaphylaxis, 13 cases of dyspnoea or bronchospasm, and 22 cases of rash or flushing; 78 of the reac-tions occurred during, or shortly after, intravenous injection and the other 12 after intramuscular injection.[1] They recom-mended that parenteral treatment be used only when essential, and that, when used, facilities for treating anaphylaxis should

be available. They also recommended that, when the intrave-nous route was used, the injection be administered slowly (over 10 minutes). Various authors[2,3] have noted that parenteral treat-ment is *essential* for the prophylaxis and treatment of Wer-nicke's encephalopathy (see below).

1. Committee on Safety of Medicines. Parentrovite & allergic reac-tions. *Current Problems* 24 1989.
2. Wrenn KD, Slovis CM. Is intravenous thiamine safe? *Am J Emerg Med* 1992; **10:** 165.
3. Thomson AD, Cook CCH. Parenteral thiamine and Wernicke's encephalopathy: the balance of risks and concerns. *Alcohol Alco-hol* 1997; **32:** 207–9.

Pharmacokinetics

Small amounts of thiamine are well absorbed from the gastrointestinal tract following oral administra-tion, but the absorption of doses larger than about 5 mg is limited. It is also rapidly absorbed following intramuscular administration. It is widely distributed to most body tissues, and appears in breast milk. Within the cell thiamine is mostly present as the di-phosphate. Thiamine is not stored to any appreciable extent in the body and amounts in excess of the body's requirements are excreted in the urine as unchanged thiamine or as metabolites.

◊ References.
1. Weber W, *et al.* Nonlinear kinetics of the thiamine cation in hu-mans: saturation of nonrenal clearance and tubular reabsorption. *J Pharmacokinet Biopharm* 1990; **18:** 501–23.
2. Tallaksen CME, *et al.* Kinetics of thiamin and thiamin phosphate esters in human blood, plasma and urine after 50 mg intrave-nously or orally. *Eur J Clin Pharmacol* 1993; **44:** 73–8.

Human Requirements

Thiamine requirements are directly related to the car-bohydrate intake and the metabolic rate. A daily die-tary intake of about 0.9 to 1.5 mg of thiamine is rec-ommended for healthy men and about 0.8 to 1.1 mg for healthy women. Cereals, nuts, peas, beans, and yeast are rich sources of thiamine. Pork and some oth-er meats especially liver, heart, or kidneys, and also fish, contain significant amounts. Flour and bakery products are often enriched with thiamine. Consider-able losses of thiamine may result from cooking proc-esses.

◊ In the UK dietary reference values (see p.1352) have been published for thiamine[1] and similarly in the USA recommend-ed dietary allowances (RDAs) have been set.[2] In the UK for adult males and females the reference nutrient intake (RNI) is 0.4 mg per 1000 kcal daily and the estimated average require-ment (EAR) is 0.3 mg per 1000 kcal daily. In the USA an RDA of 1.2 mg daily in adult males and 1.1 mg daily in females is recommended.
1. DoH. Dietary reference values for food energy and nutrients for the United Kingdom: report of the panel on dietary reference val-ues of the committee on medical aspects of food policy. *Report on health and social subjects 41*. London: HMSO, 1991.
2. Standing Committee on the Scientific Evaluation of Dietary Ref-erence Intakes of the Food and Nutrition Board. *Dietary Refer-ence Intakes for thiamin, riboflavin, niacin, vitamin B₆, folate, vitamin B₁₂, pantothenic acid, biotin, and choline*. Washington, DC: National Academy Press, 2000.

Uses and Administration

Thiamine is a water-soluble vitamin, although some of its derivatives have greater lipophilicity. It is an es-sential coenzyme for carbohydrate metabolism in the form of the diphosphate (thiamine pyrophosphate, cocarboxylase). Thiamine deficiency develops when the dietary intake is inadequate; severe deficiency leads to the development of a syndrome known as beri-beri. Chronic 'dry' beri-beri is characterised by peripheral neuropathy, muscle wasting and muscle weakness, and paralysis. Acute 'wet' beri-beri is characterised by cardiac failure and oedema. Wer-nicke-Korsakoff syndrome (demyelination of the CNS) may develop in severe cases of thiamine defi-ciency. Severe thiamine deficiency, characterised by lactic acidosis and neurological deterioration, has been reported within a relatively short time of the in-itiation of thiamine-free total parenteral nutrition; some deaths have occurred.

Thiamine is used in the treatment and prevention of thiamine deficiency. It is given by mouth, the pre-ferred route, or if necessary by the intramuscular or intravenous routes (but see Hypersensitivity, above); intravenous injections should be given slowly over 10 minutes. In the treatment of mild chronic thiamine de-ficiency usual doses of 10 to 25 mg daily by mouth, in

single or divided doses have been recommended. In severe thiamine deficiency doses of up to 300 mg daily are given, and even higher daily doses may be employed in Wernicke-Korsakoff syndrome by the intravenous route.

Thiamine is usually given as either the hydrochloride or nitrate salts although other salts such as the dicam-sylate, disulfide, monophosphate (monophosphothia-mine) or pyrophosphate may be employed.

Other compounds that possess vitamin B₁ activity and may be used as alternatives to thiamine include ben-fotiamine, cycotiamine, octotiamine, prosultiamine, and sulbutiamine. Acetiamine, bisbentiamine, and fursultiamine have also been used.

Wernicke-Korsakoff syndrome. The Wernicke-Korsakoff syndrome is a manifestation of thiamine deficiency seen partic-ularly in alcoholics, but which may accompany other condi-tions including starvation or prolonged fasting, or persistent vomiting. It was originally classified as two separate disorders, Wernicke's encephalopathy and Korsakoff's syndrome, but these are now thought to represent aspects of a single patholog-ical process.

Classical Wernicke's symptoms comprise confusion, ataxia, ophthalmoplegia, and nystagmus. Ophthalmoplegia and ataxia may precede the mental symptoms by some days. Hypothermia may be seen, and collapse and sudden death may occur in some patients. The manifestations of Korsakoff's syndrome are short-term memory loss, learning deficits, and confabulation. The conditions are associated with demyelination and glial pro-liferation, as well as haemorrhagic lesions, mainly in the periv-entricular regions of the brain; characteristic biochemical ab-normalities include raised serum-pyruvate concentration, which has been postulated as a cause of encephalopathy.[1]

Early recognition and treatment is important, both because of the risk of collapse and sudden death,[2] and to prevent irrevers-ible damage to the CNS. Korsakoff symptoms respond less well to treatment than those associated with Wernicke's en-cephalopathy,[3] and may indeed only become evident on treat-ment.

Treatment is with parenteral thiamine, preferably intravenous-ly, to ensure adequate absorption; any risks of parenteral treat-ment are considered justifiable.[4] Although as little as 2 or 3 mg may be enough to reverse the ocular symptoms, which general-ly begin to improve in 1 to 6 hours, doses of at least 100 mg should be given initially. (In practice a typical dose is 500 mg given intravenously with other vitamins every 8 hours, for 2 days if symptoms persist, and followed by 100 mg twice daily by mouth, or 250 mg daily intravenously until the patient can take oral thiamine.[4,5]) The ataxia and acute confusional state may also resolve dramatically although improvement may not be noted for days or months. The effects of the syndrome on memory are much harder to reverse. Some 25% of patients make a full, and 50% a partial, recovery.[3]

1. Petrie WM, Ban TA. Vitamins in psychiatry: do they have a role? *Drugs* 1985; **30:** 58–65.
2. Reuler JB, *et al.* Wernicke's encephalopathy. *N Engl J Med* 1985; **312:** 1035–9.
3. Anonymous. Korsakoff's syndrome. *Lancet* 1990; **336:** 912–13.
4. Cook CCH, Thomson AD. B-complex vitamins in the prophylax-is and treatment of Wernicke-Korsakoff syndrome. *Br J Hosp Med* 1997; **57:** 461–5.
5. Chataway J, Hardman E. Thiamine doses for alcohol withdrawal. *Br J Hosp Med* 1994; **51:** 615.

Preparations

BP 2001: Thiamine Injection; Thiamine Tablets; Vitamins B and C Injection;
BPC 1973: Compound Vitamin B Tablets; Strong Compound Vi-tamin B Tablets;
USP 25: Thiamine Hydrochloride Elixir; Thiamine Hydrochlo-ride Injection; Thiamine Hydrochloride Tablets; Thiamine Mononitrate Elixir.

Proprietary Preparations (details are given in Part 3)
Aust.: Beneuran; Bevitol; *Austral.:* Beta-Sol; Betamin; *Belg.:* Aneurol†; Benerva; Beneural; Betamine; *Braz.:* Arcalion; Be-caps; Benerva; Proton; *Canad.:* Betaxin; Bewon†; *Fin.:* Neu-ramin; Vita-B1; *Fr.:* Arcalion; Benerva; Bevitine; *Ger.:* Aneurin; B1-Asmedic; B₁ Vicotrat; Betabion; Imilgamma; Lophakomp-B1; *Hong Kong:* Arcalion; *Irl.:* Benerva; *Ital.:* Benerva; Betabion; Bivitasi; *Jpn:* Biotamin†; Cometamin†; Neuvita; *Mex.:* Benal-500; Benerva; Calsein; Carzilasa; TTC; X-2; *Port.:* Arcalion; Tri-fosfaneurina; *Singapore:* Arcalion; *Spain:* Arcalion; Benerva; Neurostop; Surmenalit; *Swed.:* Benerva; Betabion; *Switz.:* Arcal-ion; Benerva; *Thai.:* Arcalion; Menamin; *UAE:* Thiavit; *UK:* Ben-erva; *USA:* Thiamilate†.

Multi-ingredient: *Aust.:* Ambene N; Arca-Be; Beneuran com-positum; Beneuran Vit B-Komplex; Calcisan B + C; Cellobexon; Diclovit; Dilaescol; Dolo-Neurobion; Neurobion; Noxenur; Pronerv; *Austral.:* Berberis Complex; *Belg.:* Betapyr; Neurobion; Vioneurin; Vithathion†; *Braz.:* 6 Copena; Aminocid; Betinjectol; Bituelve; Boldobeba; Citoneurin; Dexa-Citoneurin; Dexa-Neurib-eri; Dexacobal; Dexador; Dexadoze; Dexagil; Dexaneurin; Doxal; Dozeneurin; Espasmocron; Fol Saag B12; Thiaminase; Trinalgen; Trinevral; Trirubin; Venofortan; Vibetrat; Vibetrat Dexa; Vipirim; Vitaneuron; *Canad.:* Penta-3B; Penta-3B + C; Penta-Thion; Pen-tathion-ATP; *Fin.:* Neurobion; Neurovitan; *Fr.:* Algo-Nevriton; Enuretine†; Hexaquine; Paranico†; Vita-Iodurol ATP†; Vita-Iodu-rol†; Vitathion; *Ger.:* B₁/₆ Effekton†; Bevit Forte; Discmigon; Hewedolor neuro; Medivitan N Neuro; milgamma; milgamma N;

milgamma-NA; Neuralysan S; Neuro; Neuro uno; Neuro-AS N; neuro-B forte; Neuro-Effekton B; Neuro-Lichtenstein; Neuro-Lichtenstein N; Neuro-ratiopharm; Neuro-ratiopharm N; Neuro-Vibolex; Neurobion; Neurobion N; Neurogrisevit N; Neurotrat; Neurotrat S; Novirell B; Pantovigar; Pleomix-B; Recatol N; Regepithel; Vitaject; Vitamin B duo; Vitobasan N†; *Hong Kong:* 3B; Childrens Coltalin with Vit B₁; Coltalin with Vit B₁; Magesto; Neuro B1-6-12; Neurobion; Neurorubine; Princi-B Fort; Regepithel; Tonterin; *Israel:* Betrivit; Calmanervin; Tribemin; *Ital.:* Adenobeta; Adenoplex Forte; Adenovit; Antiadiposo; Benexol B12; Emazian B12; Emoantitossina; Emopon; Esaglut; Fibronevrina; Firmavit; Folepar B12; For Liver†; Fosforilasi; Fosfoutipi Vitaminico; Menalgon B6; Mionevrasi; Neurobionta; Neuroftal; Nevril†; Novaneurina B12; Odontalgico Dr. Knapp con Vit. B1; OH B12 B1†; Punginot†; Rubjovit; Sinevrile†; Triferon; Trinevrina B6; *Jpn:* Neurovitan; *Mex.:* Benexol B12; Dexabion; Dolo-Neurobion; Dolo-Tiaminal; Ferrotemp; Lipovitasi-Or; Neurobion; Pangavit; Selectadoce; Tiaminal B₁₂; Tiaminal B₁₂ Trivalente; Tribedoxyl; *Neth.:* Princi B1 + B6; *Port.:* Linamin Plus; Neurobion; Tridocemine; *S.Afr.:* Kiddie Vite; Neurobion; *Singapore:* 3B; Alinamin B12; Alinamin-F; Neurobion; Neuroforte; Neurorubine; Nevramin; Princi-B Fort; *Spain:* Acetuber; Antineurina; Benexol B1 B6 B12; Bester Complex; Calmante Vitaminado P G; Calmante Vitaminado PG Efervescente; Calmante Vitaminado Rinver; Dalamon; Epixian†; Gammamida Complex†; Hidroxil B12 B6 B1; Inzitan; Mederebro; Mederebro Compuesto†; Meloka; Menalgil B6; Nervobion; Neuromade; Neurostop Complex; Pazbronquial; Quimpedor; Refulgin; Sugarcetón†; Teovit; Viadetres; *Swed.:* Neurobion; *Switz.:* Neurotrat; Tribeton; *Thai.:* 3B; Beromin; Cydoxmine-B; Cyriamine; Diasgest; Digestin; Douzabox; Endogest; Genavit; Hemolax; Neurobex; Neurobion; Nevramin; Nuvit; Princi-B; Tribesian; Trivit-B; Vioneurin; Vita-B; Vitamedin; Vitron; *UAE:* 3V; *UK:* Labiton; Quiet Life; *USA:* Nervidox 6†; Nervidox†; Neuro B-12†; Neurobion†; Tia Doce†.

Vitamin B₂ Substances (14733-q)

Riboflavin (7843-r)

Riboflavin (BAN, rINN).

E101; Lactoflavin; Riboflavine; Riboflavinum; Vitamin B₂; Vitamin G. 7,8-Dimethyl-10-(1′-D-ribityl)isoalloxazine; 3,10-Dihydro-7,8-dimethyl-10-(D-ribo-2,3,4,5-tetrahydroxypentyl)benzopteridine-2,4-dione.

$C_{17}H_{20}N_4O_6 = 376.4$.
CAS — 83-88-5.
ATC — A11HA04.
Pharmacopoeias. In Chin., Eur. (see p.vi), Int., Jpn, Pol., and US.

Pharmacopoeial description

Ph. Eur.: A yellow or orange-yellow crystalline powder. Very slightly soluble in water; more soluble in sodium chloride 0.9%; practically insoluble in alcohol and in ether. Store in airtight containers. Protect from light. Solutions deteriorate on exposure to light, especially in the presence of alkali.

USP 25: A yellow to orange-yellow crystalline powder, having a slight odour. When dry, it is not appreciably affected by diffused light, but in solution light induces quite rapid deterioration, especially in the presence of alkalis. Very slightly soluble in water, in alcohol, and in isotonic sodium chloride solution; insoluble in chloroform and in ether; soluble in dilute solutions of alkalis. Its saturated solution in water is neutral to litmus. Store in airtight containers. Protect from light.

Riboflavin Sodium Phosphate (7842-x)

Riboflavin Sodium Phosphate (BANM, rINNM).

Riboflavin 5′-Phosphate Sodium; Riboflavine Phosphate (Sodium Salt); Riboflavine Sodium Phosphate; Riboflavini Natrii Phosphas; Vitamin B₂ Phosphate. The sodium salt of riboflavine 5′-phosphate.

$C_{17}H_{20}N_4NaO_9P = 478.3$.
CAS — 130-40-5.
Pharmacopoeias. In Eur. (see p.vi) and Jpn.
US specifies the dihydrate salt.

Riboflavin sodium phosphate 1.27 g is approximately equivalent to 1 g of riboflavin.

Pharmacopoeial description

Ph. Eur.: A yellow or orange-yellow, hygroscopic, crystalline powder. Soluble in water; very slightly soluble in alcohol; practically insoluble in ether. A 1% solution in water has a pH of 5.0 to 6.5. Store in airtight containers. Protect from light.

USP 25: A fine, orange-yellow, hygroscopic, crystalline powder, having a slight odour. When dry, it is not affected by diffused light, but when in solution light induces rapid deterioration. Sparingly soluble in water. pH of a 1% solution in water is between 5.0 and 6.5. Store in airtight containers. Protect from light.

Adverse Effects and Precautions

Large doses of riboflavin result in a bright yellow discoloration of the urine which may interfere with certain laboratory tests.

Pharmacokinetics

Riboflavin is absorbed from the gastrointestinal tract. Although riboflavin is widely distributed to body tissues little is stored in the body.

Riboflavin is converted in the body to the coenzyme flavine mononucleotide (FMN; riboflavin 5′-phosphate) and then to another coenzyme flavine adenine dinucleotide (FAD). About 60% of FMN and FAD are bound to plasma proteins. Riboflavin is excreted in urine, partly as metabolites. As the dose increases, larger amounts are excreted unchanged. Riboflavin crosses the placenta and is distributed into breast milk.

Human Requirements

The riboflavin requirement is often related to the energy intake but it appears to be more closely related to resting metabolic requirements. A daily dietary intake of about 1.1 to 1.7 mg of riboflavin is recommended. Liver, kidney, fish, eggs, milk, cheese, yeast, and some green vegetables such as broccoli and spinach are the richest sources of riboflavin. In general, little loss of riboflavin occurs during cooking, but considerable losses may occur if foods, especially milk, are exposed to sunlight.

◊ In the UK dietary reference values (see p.1352) have been published for riboflavin[1] and similarly in the USA recommended dietary allowances (RDAs) have been set.[2] Differing amounts are recommended for infants and children of varying ages, for adult males and females of varying ages, and for pregnant and lactating women; the differences between age groups are intended to reflect the changes in caloric intakes at these ages. In the UK the reference nutrient intake (RNI) is 1.3 mg daily and 1.1 mg daily for adult males and females respectively; the estimated average requirement (EAR) is 1.0 mg daily and 0.9 mg daily respectively. In the USA the RDAs for adult males and females are 1.3 and 1.1 mg daily respectively.

1. DoH. Dietary reference values for food energy and nutrients for the United Kingdom: report of the panel on dietary reference values of the committee on medical aspects of food policy. *Report on health and social subjects 41.* London: HMSO, 1991.
2. Standing Committee on the Scientific Evaluation of Dietary Reference Intakes of the Food and Nutrition Board. *Dietary Reference Intakes for thiamin, riboflavin, niacin, vitamin B₆, folate, vitamin B₁₂, pantothenic acid, biotin, and choline.* Washington, DC: National Academy Press, 2000.

Uses and Administration

Riboflavin, a water-soluble vitamin, is essential for the utilisation of energy from food. The active, phosphorylated forms, flavine mononucleotide (FMN) and flavine adenine dinucleotide (FAD), are involved as coenzymes in oxidative/reductive metabolic reactions. Riboflavin is also necessary for the functioning of pyridoxine and nicotinic acid.

Riboflavin deficiency develops when the dietary intake is inadequate. Deficiency leads to the development of a well-defined syndrome known as ariboflavinosis, characterised by cheilosis, angular stomatitis, glossitis, keratitis, surface lesions of the genitalia, and seborrhoeic dermatitis. There may also be normocytic anaemia and ocular symptoms including itching and burning of the eyes, photophobia, and corneal vascularisation. Some of these symptoms may, in fact, be due to other vitamins such as pyridoxine or nicotinic acid which do not function correctly in the absence of riboflavin. Riboflavin deficiency may also occur in association with other vitamin B-complex deficiency states such as pellagra.

Riboflavin is used in the treatment and prevention of riboflavin deficiency. It is usually given in doses of 1 or 2 mg by mouth for prophylaxis, and doses of up to 30 mg daily in divided doses are used for treatment. Riboflavin is also a component of intramuscular or intravenous vitamins B and C injections.

Riboflavin tetrabutyrate has also been used.

Riboflavin is also used as a colouring agent for food.

Migraine. Results from an open pilot study[1] and a placebo-controlled trial[2] have suggested that riboflavin in high doses (400 mg daily) might be of some benefit in the prophylaxis of migraine attacks (p.449).

1. Schoenen J, et al. High-dose riboflavin as a prophylactic treatment of migraine: results of an open pilot study. *Cephalalgia* 1994; **14:** 328–9.
2. Schoenen J, et al. Effectiveness of high-dose riboflavin in migraine prophylaxis: a randomized controlled trial. *Neurology* 1998; **50:** 466–70.

Preparations

BP 2001: Vitamins B and C Injection;
BPC 1973: Compound Vitamin B Tablets; Strong Compound Vitamin B Tablets;
USP 25: Riboflavin Injection; Riboflavin Tablets.

Proprietary Preparations (details are given in Part 3)
Belg.: Berivine; Ribon; *Fin.:* Vita-B2; *Fr.:* Beflavine; *Ger.:* B2-Asmedic; *Hong Kong:* Hibon; *Thai.:* Boflavin.

Multi-ingredient: *Aust.:* Beneuran Vit B-Komplex; *Austral.:* Antioxidant Forte Tablets; Antioxidant Tablets; Extralife Eye-Care; Liv-Detox; *Fr.:* Glutamag Vitamine; *Ger.:* Golden Star; Salus Augenschutz-Kapseln N; *Hong Kong:* Alinamin-F; *Ital.:* Emazian B12; Emoantitossina; Facovit; For Liver†; Fosforilasi; Neuroftal; *Jpn:* Neurovitan; *Singapore:* Alinamin-F; *Spain:* Aftasone B C; Balneogel; *Thai.:* Alinamin-F; *UK:* Quiet Life; Se-Power.

Vitamin B₆ Substances (14734-p)

Vitamin B₆ is usually available as pyridoxine but the term is also used to refer to the related compounds, pyridoxal and pyridoxamine.

Pyridoxine Hydrochloride (7847-h)

Pyridoxine Hydrochloride (BANM, rINNM).

Adermine Hydrochloride; Piridossina Cloridrato; Pyridoxini Hydrochloridum; Pyridoxinii Chloridum; Pyridoxinium Chloride; Pyridoxol Hydrochloride; Vitamin B₆. 3-Hydroxy-4,5-bis(hydroxymethyl)-2-picoline hydrochloride.

$C_8H_{11}NO_3,HCl = 205.6$.
CAS — 65-23-6 (pyridoxine); 58-56-0 (pyridoxine hydrochloride).
Pharmacopoeias. In Chin., Eur. (see p.vi), Int., Jpn, Pol., and US.

Pharmacopoeial description

Ph. Eur.: A white or almost white, crystalline powder. Freely soluble in water; slightly soluble in alcohol; practically insoluble in ether. A 5% solution in water has a pH of 2.4 to 3.0. Protect from light.

USP 25: White or practically white crystals or crystalline powder. Soluble 1 in 5 of water and 1 in 115 of alcohol; insoluble in ether. Its solutions in water have a pH of about 3. Store in airtight containers. Protect from light.

Adverse Effects and Precautions

Long-term administration of large doses of pyridoxine is associated with the development of severe peripheral neuropathies; the dose below which these do not occur is controversial (see below).

Effects on the nervous system. Severe sensory neuropathy has been described in patients receiving large doses of pyridoxine (2 to 6 g daily) for periods of 2 to 40 months.[1] It has, however, been debated as to whether smaller doses may produce such effects. Some contend that amounts of pyridoxine below this level are unlikely to produce toxic effects[2,3] although there have been some case reports[4,5] with amounts up to about 500 mg daily. Following a review of the possible toxicity associated with lower doses of pyridoxine, proposals were put forward in the UK to limit the dose freely available in dietary supplements to 10 mg daily; products supplying up to 50 mg daily would continue to be available from pharmacies and higher doses would only be available on prescription.[6] These proposals have been heavily contested.[6,7] An upper limit of 100 mg daily has been suggested in the USA.[7]

1. Schaumburg H, et al. Sensory neuropathy from pyridoxine abuse: a new megavitamin syndrome. *N Engl J Med* 1983; **309:** 445–8.
2. Pauling L. Sensory neuropathy from pyridoxine abuse. *N Engl J Med* 1984; **310:** 197.
3. Baker H, Frank O. Sensory neuropathy from pyridoxine abuse. *N Engl J Med* 1984; **310:** 197.
4. Berger A, Schaumburg HH. More on neuropathy from pyridoxine abuse. *N Engl J Med* 1984; **311:** 986.
5. Waterston JA, Gilligan BS. Pyridoxine neuropathy. *Med J Aust* 1987; **146:** 640–2.
6. Collier J. Vitamin B-6: food or medicine? *BMJ* 1998; **317:** 92–3.
7. Anonymous. Still time for rational debate about vitamin B₆. *Lancet* 1998; **351:** 1523.

Interactions

Pyridoxine reduces the effects of levodopa (see p.1172), but this does not occur if a dopa decarboxylase inhibitor is also given. Pyridoxine reduces the activity of altretamine. It has also been reported to decrease serum concentrations of phenobarbital (p.356). Many drugs may increase the requirements for pyridoxine; such drugs include isoniazid, penicillamine, and oral contraceptives.

Pharmacokinetics

Pyridoxine, pyridoxal, and pyridoxamine are readily absorbed from the gastrointestinal tract following oral administration and are converted to the active forms pyridoxal phosphate and pyridoxamine phosphate. They are stored mainly in the liver where there is oxidation to 4-pyridoxic acid and other inactive metabolites which are excreted in the urine. As the dose increases, proportionally greater amounts are excreted unchanged in the urine. Pyridoxal crosses the placenta and is distributed into breast milk.

Human Requirements

For adults, the daily requirement of pyridoxine is probably about 1.5 to 2 mg and this amount is present in most normal diets. The requirement tends to increase as protein intake increases due to the role of the vitamin in amino acid metabolism. Meats, especially chicken, kidney, and liver, cereals, eggs, fish, and certain vegetables and fruits are good sources of pyridoxine.

◊ In the UK[1] dietary reference values (see p.1352) have been published for vitamin B₆ and similarly in the USA recommended dietary allowances (RDAs) have been set.[2] Differing amounts are recommended for infants and children of varying ages, for adult males and females, and during pregnancy and lactation. In the UK the reference nutrient intake (RNI) is 15 µg per g of protein daily for adult males and females and the estimated average requirement (EAR) is 13 µg per g of protein daily for the same group. In the USA the RDA for adult men ranges from 1.3 to 1.7 mg daily and that for adult women ranges from 1.3 to 1.5 mg daily.[2] The tolerable upper intake level is 100 mg daily.[2]

1. DoH. Dietary reference values for food energy and nutrients for the United Kingdom: report of the panel on dietary reference values of the committee on medical aspects of food policy. *Report on health and social subjects 41.* London: HMSO, 1991.
2. Standing Committee on the Scientific Evaluation of Dietary Reference Intakes of the Food and Nutrition Board. *Dietary Reference Intakes for thiamin, riboflavin, niacin, vitamin B₆, folate, vitamin B₁₂, pantothenic acid, biotin, and choline.* Washington, DC: National Academy Press, 2000.

Uses and Administration

Pyridoxine, a water-soluble vitamin, is involved principally in amino acid metabolism, but is also involved in carbohydrate and fat metabolism. It is also required for the formation of haemoglobin.

Deficiency of pyridoxine is rare in humans because of its widespread distribution in foods. Pyridoxine deficiency may however be drug-induced and can occur, for instance, during isoniazid therapy. Inadequate utilisation of pyridoxine may result from certain inborn errors of metabolism. Pyridoxine deficiency may lead to sideroblastic anaemia, dermatitis, cheilosis, and neurological symptoms such as peripheral neuritis, and convulsions.

Pyridoxine is used in the treatment and prevention of pyridoxine deficiency states. It is usually given by mouth, the preferred route, but may also be given by the subcutaneous, intramuscular, or intravenous routes. Doses of up to 150 mg daily are used in general deficiency states; higher doses of up to 400 mg daily are used in the treatment of sideroblastic anaemias (see below); and similar doses have been used to treat certain metabolic disorders such as homocystinuria (see Amino Acid Metabolic Disorders, below) or primary hyperoxaluria (below). Pyridoxine has also been used to treat seizures due to hereditary syndromes of pyridoxine deficiency or dependency in infants.

Pyridoxine has also been tried in a wide variety of other disorders, including the treatment of depression and other symptoms associated with the premenstrual syndrome (see below) and the use of oral contraceptives, although its efficacy has been questioned.

Pyridoxine is usually administered as the hydrochloride although other salts such as the citrate, oxoglutarate, phosphate, and phosphoserinate, have also been employed. The pidolate (metadoxine) has been investigated in alcoholism (see below).

For the use of pyridoxine in the prophylaxis of isoniazid-induced peripheral neuritis and for the treatment of acute isoniazid toxicity, see under Isoniazid, p.216.

Pyridoxal phosphate may be used to treat vitamin B₆ deficiency.

◊ Reviews.
1. Bender DA. Non-nutritional uses of vitamin B₆. *Br J Nutr* 1999; **81:** 7–20.

Alcoholism and alcohol poisoning. Pyridoxine and its pidolate, known as metadoxine, have been tried in the treatment of alcohol poisoning and alcoholism. One study showed pyridoxine to be ineffective in acute alcohol poisoning[1] but another[2] suggested that the pidolate might be of benefit as an adjunct in the management of alcohol withdrawal (p.1131).
1. Mardel S, *et al.* Intravenous pyridoxine in acute ethanol intoxication. *Hum Exp Toxicol* 1994; **13:** 321–3.
2. Rizzo A, *et al.* Uso terapeutico della metadoxina nell'alcolismo cronico: studio clinico in doppio cieco su pazienti ricoverati in un reparto di medicina generale. *Clin Ter* 1993; **142:** 243–50.

Amino acid metabolic disorders. Reports of the use of pyridoxine in various inborn errors of amino acid metabolism.[1,2] Some patients with homocystinuria respond to pyridoxine with or without cobalamins and folate. Dietary methionine restriction and betaine or choline may also be required (see p.1350). For the use of pyridoxine in primary hyperoxaluria, another inherited metabolic disorder, see below.
1. Boers GHJ, *et al.* Heterozygosity for homocystinuria in premature peripheral and cerebral occlusive arterial disease. *N Engl J Med* 1985; **313:** 709–15.
2. Hayasaka S, *et al.* Clinical trials of vitamin B₆ and proline supplementation for gyrate atrophy of the choroid and retina. *Br J Ophthalmol* 1985; **69:** 283–90.

Anaemias. Some patients with acquired or hereditary sideroblastic anaemia (p.717) that is severe enough to require treatment will respond to high doses (up to 400 mg daily) of pyridoxine, and a trial is considered worthwhile in all patients.

Carpal tunnel syndrome. Pyridoxine has been advocated by some[1] for patients with carpal tunnel syndrome (see Soft-tissue Rheumatism, p.10), but there is controversy surrounding its efficacy,[2] and a study found pyridoxine to be no more effective than placebo.[3]
1. Lewis PJ. Pyridoxine supplements may help patients with carpal tunnel syndrome. *BMJ* 1995; **310:** 1534.
2. Copeland DA, Stoukides CA. Pyridoxine in carpal tunnel syndrome. *Ann Pharmacother* 1994; **28:** 1042–4.
3. Spooner GR, *et al.* Using pyridoxine to treat carpal tunnel syndrome. *Can Fam Physician* 1993; **39:** 2122–7.

Epilepsy. Pyridoxine-dependent epilepsy is an autosomal recessive disorder associated with decreased central γ-aminobutyric acid (GABA) concentrations and elevated cerebral glutamate concentrations. Untreated patients suffer from progressive encephalopathy, mental retardation, and intractable epilepsy; lifelong supplementation with pyridoxine can control epileptic symptoms but mental retardation may still develop. Test doses of pyridoxine intravenously, repeated at intervals of 10 minutes up to a total of 500 mg if necessary, have been suggested in the diagnosis of pyridoxine-dependent epilepsy; if the patient responds then a daily oral dose of 5 mg per kg body-weight is suggested although there is no real consensus on the appropriate dosage.[1] A study in one patient[2] found that although pyridoxine 5 mg per kg body-weight reduced glutamate concentrations in cerebrospinal fluid from their untreated value of 200 times normal limits, it did so only to 10 times the normal value, despite remission of symptoms. Doses of 10 mg per kg daily were required to normalise CSF glutamate, and it was suggested that this was a more appropriate target for therapy.
1. Gospe SM. Current perspectives on pyridoxine-dependent seizures. *J Pediatr* 1998; **132:** 919–23.
2. Baumeister FAM, *et al.* Glutamate in pyridoxine-dependent epilepsy: neurotoxic glutamate concentration in the cerebrospinal fluid and its normalization by pyridoxine. *Pediatrics* 1994; **94:** 318–21.

Ischaemic heart disease. For mention of the possible link between vitamin B₆, hyperhomocysteinaemia, and atherosclerosis and ischaemic heart disease, see under Folic Acid, p.1362.

Premenstrual syndrome. Pyridoxine has been widely used in the premenstrual syndrome (p.1475) despite controversy over its effectiveness. Some consider that depressive symptoms may be provoked by pyridoxine deficiency because of its role as a coenzyme in the production of certain neurotransmitters, but it is difficult to attribute any of the other symptoms of the premenstrual syndrome to pyridoxine deficiency and doses of 50 mg are no more effective than a placebo.[1] A systematic review found that although treatment with pyridoxine was more effective than placebo, there was insufficient high-quality evidence to recommend its routine use in premenstrual syndrome.[2] If pyridoxine is used, the dosage should be restricted (see Effects on the Nervous System, above) because of concerns about neurotoxicity.[3]
1. West CP. The premenstrual syndrome. *Prescribers' J* 1987; **27** (2): 9–15.
2. Wyatt KM, *et al.* Efficacy of vitamin B-6 in the treatment of premenstrual syndrome: systematic review. *BMJ* 1999; **318:** 1375–81.
3. Severino SK, Moline ML. Premenstrual syndrome: identification and management. *Drugs* 1995; **49:** 71–82.

Primary hyperoxaluria. Primary hyperoxaluria (as distinct from the various forms secondary to other disorders) is a genetic disorder characterised by excessive synthesis and urinary excretion of oxalic acid. Two forms are known, type I (glycolic aciduria) and type II (L-glyceric aciduria), associated with different enzyme defects. They are marked by recurrent calcium oxalate kidney stones, or nephrocalcinosis, leading to renal failure, together with extrarenal deposition of calcium oxalate and frequently severe peripheral vascular insufficiency. Treatment with high doses of pyridoxine may help decrease oxalate excretion particularly in type I disease.[1-3] A few patients may respond to lower (physiological) doses.[4] Such treatment can be

combined with an oral orthophosphate supplement, which helps reduce renal deposition of calcium oxalate, and the combination appears to preserve renal function.[5] Therapy with magnesium salts, citrate, and thiazide diuretics has also been suggested. In patients in whom renal failure develops, the results of kidney transplantation have been disappointing, due to deposition of calcium oxalate in the new kidney, although concomitant liver transplantation can correct the enzyme defect.[3,6]
1. Alinei P, *et al.* Pyridoxine treatment of type 1 hyperoxaluria. *N Engl J Med* 1984; **311:** 798.
2. de Zegher F, *et al.* Successful treatment of infantile type I primary hyperoxaluria complicated by pyridoxine toxicity. *Lancet* 1985; **ii:** 392–3.
3. Cochat P, Basmaison O. Current approaches to the management of primary hyperoxaluria. *Arch Dis Child* 2000; **82:** 470–3.
4. Yendt ER, Cohanim M. Response to a physiologic dose of pyridoxine in type I primary hyperoxaluria. *N Engl J Med* 1985; **312:** 953–7.
5. Milliner DS, *et al.* Results of long-term treatment with orthophosphate and pyridoxine in patients with primary hyperoxaluria. *N Engl J Med* 1994; **331:** 1553–8.
6. Watts RWE, *et al.* Combined hepatic and renal transplantation in primary hyperoxaluria type I: clinical report of nine cases. *Am J Med* 1991; **90:** 179–88.

Preparations

BP 2001: Pyridoxine Tablets; Vitamins B and C Injection;
BPC 1973: Strong Compound Vitamin B Tablets;
USP 25: Pyridoxine Hydrochloride Injection; Pyridoxine Hydrochloride Tablets.

Proprietary Preparations (details are given in Part 3)

Aust.: Benadon; *Austral.:* Pyroxin; Vita B6; *Belg.:* Bedoxine; *Canad.:* Carthamex; *Fin.:* Heksavit; Vita-B6; *Fr.:* Becilan; Dermo 6; *Ger.:* B6-Asmedic; B₆ Vicotrat; Bonasanit; Hexobion; Lophakomp-B6; *Irl.:* Benadon; Complement Continus; *Israel:* Anacrodyne; B Six; *Ital.:* Benadon; Memosprint; Metadoxil; Xanturenasi; *Mex.:* Benadon; *Norw.:* AFI-B₆; *Port.:* Benadon; Metadoxil; *S.Afr.:* Beesix†; Lactosec; *Spain:* Beglunina†; Benadon; Conductasa; Godabion B6; Serfoxide; *Swed.:* Benadon; *Switz.:* Benadon; Complement Continus; *Thai.:* Metadoxil; *UK:* Benadon†; Complement Continus; Orovite Complement B₆; Woman Kind; *USA:* Aminoxin†; Vitelle Nestrex.

Multi-ingredient: *Aust.:* Arca-Be; Aslavital; Astronautal; Beneuran compositum; Beneuran Vit B-Komplex; Contravert B₆; Diclovit; Dolo-Neurobion; Echnatol B₆; Neurobion; Pronerv; Sigmalin B₆; Sigmalin B₆ forte; Sigmalin B₆ ohne Coffein; Vertirosan Vitamin B₆; *Austral.:* Bio Magnesium; Extralife Flow-Care; Extralife Fluid-Care; Extralife PMS-Care; Extralife Uri-Care; Formula Three Triple Strength†; Formula Three†; Liv-Detox; Mag-Oro; Medinat PMT-Eze; Natures Way Total Zinc; Zinc Zenith; *Belg.:* Betapyr; Neurobion; Postadoxine; R Calm + B6†; Vioneurin; *Braz.:* Alergo Filinal; Aminocid; Aminotox; Anekron; Betaliver; Benjectol; Biofigado; Bronquitos; Citoneurin; Colivintol; Dexa-Citoneurin; Dexa-Neuriberi; Dexacobal; Dexador; Dexadoze; Dexagil; Dexaneurin; Diagrin; Doxal; Dramavit; Dramin B-6; Dramin B-6 DL; Epacrosil; Epativan B6; Epocler; Estac; Eviepar; Extrato Hepatico Composto; Figadobil; Gabax; Hepalin; Hormo Hepatico; Lisomalen; Nicopaverina B6; Pantevit; Plagon; Plasonil; Trinalgen; Trineval; Trirubin; Vibetrat; Vibetrat Dexa; Vipirim; Vominil; Vomistop; Vopax; Xantinon Complex; *Canad.:* Diclectin; Formula Gyn; Penta-3B; Penta-3B + C; *Fin.:* Neurobion; Neurovitan; Wicnecarb; Wicnevit; *Fr.:* Acnestrol†; Alphanet†; Anebtor B₆†; Arbum; Catarstat; Cystelle Shampooing Cheveux Gras; Cysti-Z; Cystine B₆; Forcapil; Lyso-6; Magne-B₆; Osteogen†; Phakan; Uvimag B₆; *Ger.:* AntiFocal N; B₁/₆ Effekton†; Bevit Forte; Bramin-hepa; Hepagrisevit Forte-N; Hewedolor neuro; Medivitan N; Medivitan N Neuro; Medyn; milgamma; milgamma N; milgamma-NA; Neuralysan S; Neuro; Neuro uno; Neuro-AS N; neuro-B forte; Neuro-Effekton B; Neuro-Lichtenstein; Neuro-Lichtenstein N; Neuro-ratiopharm; Neuro-ratiopharm N; Neuro-Vibolex; Neurobion; Neurobion N; Neurogrisevit N; Neurotrat; Neurotrat S; Nifurantin B 6; Novirell B; Pleomix-B; Recatol N; Reisegold; Telbibur N; Vitaject; Vitamin B duo; Vitobasan N†; *Hong Kong:* 3B; Navidoxine; Neuro B1-6-12; Neurobion; Neurorubine; Nevramin; Princi-B Fort; *Irl.:* Optimax; *Israel:* Betrivit; Calmanervin; Tribemin; *Ital.:* Acutil Fosforo; Adenoplex Forte; Adenovit; Alcalosio; Antemesyl; Antimicotico; Benexol B12; Coxanturenasi; Detoxergon†; Efargen; Emoantitossina; Esaglut; Firmavit; For Liver†; Fosforil Calcium†; Fosforilasi; Furanvit; Lozione Same AS†; Menalgon B6; Miazide B6; Midium; Mionevrasi; Neo-Geynevral; Neuraben; Neurobionta; Triferon; Trinevrina B6; *Jpn:* Neurovitan; *Mex.:* Benexol B12; Bonadoxina; Dexabion; Dolo-Neurobion; Dolo-Tiaminal; Emediba; Liatriz; Meclifar; Neurobion; Pangavit; Selectadoxe; Tiaminal B₁₂ Trivalente; Tribedoxyl; *Neth.:* Emesafene; Princi B1 + B6; *Port.:* Esclerobion; Linamin Plus; Nausefe; Neurobion; Phakan; Tridocemine; *S.Afr.:* Asic; Neurobion; Nicene†; Vomifene; *Singapore:* 3B; Navidoxine; Neurobion; Neuroforte; Neurorubine; Nevramin; Princi-B Fort; *Spain:* Acetuber; Aftasone B C; Agudil; Antineurina; Benexol B1 B6 B12; Bester Complex; Biodramina Cafeina; Cariban; Cefabol; Dalamon; Duplicalcio 150; Epixian†; Gamalate B6; Gammamida Complex†; Hidroxil B12 B6 B1; Levaliver; Mederebro; Mederebro Compuesto†; Menalgil B6; Nervobion; Neuromade; Neurostop Complex; Nucleserina; Pazbronquial; Pleocortex B6; Poli ABE; Quimpedor; Redutona; Relaxedans†; Sirodina; Taurobetina; Teovit; Tepazepan; Trivitan†; Trofi Milina†; Vertigum†; *Swed.:* Neurobion; *Switz.:* Acne Gel; Antemin compositum; Catarstat; Demodenal compositum; Itinerol B₆; Linervidol; Magnesplus; Medramine retard†; Medramine-B₆ Rectocaps†; Neurotrat; Phakolen; Tribeton; *Thai.:* 3B; Beromin; Cydoxmine-B; Cyriamine; Douzabox; Genavit; Hemolax; Neurobex; Neurobion; Nevramin; Nuvit; Princi-B; Tribesian; Tricortin; Trivit-B; Vita-B; Vitamedin; Vitron; *UAE:* 3V; *UK:* Fat-Solv; HealthAid Boldo-Plus; Kelp Plus 3; Rapi-snooze; *USA:* Beelith; Catemine†; FOLTX; KLB6; Lurline PMS; Marlyn Formula 50; Nervidox 6†; Neurobion†; PremesisRx; Releaf for PMS.

Used as an adjunct in: *Ger.:* Isozid comp N; tebesium; *Ital.:* Etanicozid B6; *Spain:* Cemidon B6; Isoetam†.

The symbol † denotes a preparation no longer actively marketed

Vitamin B₁₂ Substances (14752-w)

Vitamin B_{12} is the name generally used for a group of related cobalt-containing compounds, also known as cobalamins, of which cyanocobalamin and hydroxocobalamin are the principal forms in clinical use.

Cyanocobalamin (7853-d)

Cyanocobalamin (BAN, rINN).

Cobamin; Cyanocobalaminum; Cycobemin. Coα-[α-(5,6-Dimethylbenzimidazolyl)]-Coβ-cyanocobamide.

$C_{63}H_{88}CoN_{14}O_{14}P = 1355.4$.

CAS — 68-19-9.

ATC — B03BA01.

Pharmacopoeias. In Chin., Eur. (see p.vi), Int., Jpn, Pol., and US.

Pharmacopoeial description

Ph. Eur.: A dark red, crystalline powder or dark red crystals. The anhydrous substance is very hygroscopic. Sparingly soluble in water and in alcohol; practically insoluble in acetone and in ether. Store in airtight containers. Protect from light.

USP 25: Dark red crystals or amorphous or crystalline red powder. In the anhydrous form it is very hygroscopic and when exposed to air it may absorb about 12% of water. Soluble 1 in 80 of water; soluble in alcohol; insoluble in acetone, in chloroform, and in ether. Store in airtight containers. Protect from light.

Hydroxocobalamin (7854-n)

Hydroxocobalamin (BAN, USAN, rINN).

Hydroxocobalaminum; Idrossocobalamina. Coα-[α-(5,6-Dimethylbenzimidazolyl)]-Coβ-hydroxocobamide.

$C_{62}H_{89}CoN_{13}O_{15}P = 1346.4$.

CAS — 13422-51-0.

ATC — B03BA03; V03AB33.

Pharmacopoeias. In Int., It., and US.

Int. also includes Hydroxocobalamin Chloride and Hydroxocobalamin Sulfate. Jpn has Hydroxocobalamin Acetate. Eur. (see p.vi) includes the acetate, chloride, and sulfate.

Hydroxocobalamin occurs either as the acetate ($C_{64}H_{93}CoN_{13}O_{17}P$), the chloride ($C_{62}H_{90}ClCoN_{13}O_{15}P$) or the sulfate ($C_{124}H_{180}Co_2N_{26}O_{34}P_2S$). The hydrated form of hydroxocobalamin has been referred to as aquocobalamin.

Pharmacopoeial description

Ph. Eur.: Hydroxocobalamin acetate is a dark red, very hygroscopic, crystalline powder or dark red crystals. Soluble in water. Some decomposition may occur on drying. Store at a temperature between 2° and 8° in airtight containers. Protect from light.

Hydroxocobalamin chloride is a dark red, very hygroscopic, crystalline powder or dark red crystals. Soluble in water. Some decomposition may occur on drying. Store at a temperature between 2° and 8° in airtight containers. Protect from light.

Hydroxocobalamin sulfate is a dark red, very hygroscopic, crystalline powder or dark red crystals. Soluble in water. Some decomposition may occur on drying. Store at a temperature between 2° and 8° in airtight containers. Protect from light.

USP 25: Dark red crystals or red crystalline powder. Is odourless or has not more than a slight acetone odour. The anhydrous form is very hygroscopic. Soluble 1 in 50 of water and 1 in 100 of alcohol; practically insoluble in acetone, in chloroform, in ether, and in benzene; sparingly soluble in methyl alcohol. pH of a 2% solution in water is between 8.0 and 10.0. Store in airtight containers at a temperature of 8° to 15°. Protect from light.

Adverse Effects and Precautions

Allergic hypersensitivity reactions have occurred rarely following the parenteral administration of the vitamin B_{12} compounds cyanocobalamin and hydroxocobalamin. Antibodies to hydroxocobalamin-transcobalamin II complex have developed during hydroxocobalamin therapy.

Arrhythmias secondary to hypokalaemia have occurred at the beginning of parenteral treatment with hydroxocobalamin.

Intranasal cyanocobalamin may cause rhinitis, nausea, and headache.

Cyanocobalamin or hydroxocobalamin should, if possible, not be given to patients with suspected vitamin B_{12} deficiency without first confirming the diagnosis. Regular monitoring of the blood is advisable. Administration of doses greater than 10 μg daily may produce a haematological response in patients with folate deficiency; indiscriminate use may mask the precise diagnosis. Conversely, folate may mask vitamin B_{12} deficiency (see p.1361).

Cyanocobalamin should not be used for Leber's disease or tobacco amblyopia since these optic neuropathies may degenerate further.

◊ Analysis, by the Boston Collaborative Drug Surveillance Program, of data on 15 438 patients hospitalised between 1975 and 1982 detected 3 allergic skin reactions attributed to cyanocobalamin among 168 recipients of the drug.[1] For the purposes of the study, reactions were defined as being generalised morbilliform exanthems, urticaria, or generalised pruritus only.

1. Bigby M, et al. Drug-induced cutaneous reactions: a report from the Boston Collaborative Drug Surveillance Program on 15 438 consecutive inpatients, 1975 to 1982. JAMA 1986; 256: 3358–63.

Interactions

Absorption of vitamin B_{12} from the gastrointestinal tract may be reduced by neomycin, aminosalicylic acid, histamine H_2-receptor antagonists, and colchicine. Serum concentrations may be decreased by concurrent administration of oral contraceptives. Many of these interactions are unlikely to be of clinical significance but should be taken into account when performing assays for blood concentrations. Parenteral chloramphenicol may attenuate the effect of vitamin B_{12} in anaemia.

Pharmacokinetics

Vitamin B_{12} substances bind to intrinsic factor, a glycoprotein secreted by the gastric mucosa, and are then actively absorbed from the gastrointestinal tract. Absorption is impaired in patients with an absence of intrinsic factor, with a malabsorption syndrome or with disease or abnormality of the gut, or after gastrectomy. Absorption from the gastrointestinal tract can also occur by passive diffusion; little of the vitamin present in food is absorbed in this manner although the process becomes increasingly important with larger amounts such as those used therapeutically. After intranasal administration, peak plasma concentrations of cyanocobalamin have been reached in 1 to 2 hours. The bioavailability of the intranasal preparation is about 7 to 11% of that by intramuscular injection.

Vitamin B_{12} is extensively bound to specific plasma proteins called transcobalamins; transcobalamin II appears to be involved in the rapid transport of the cobalamins to tissues. Vitamin B_{12} is stored in the liver, excreted in the bile, and undergoes extensive enterohepatic recycling; part of an administered dose is excreted in the urine, most of it in the first 8 hours; urinary excretion, however, accounts for only a small fraction in the reduction of total body stores acquired by dietary means. Vitamin B_{12} diffuses across the placenta and also appears in breast milk.

◊ After injection of cyanocobalamin a large proportion is excreted in the urine within 24 hours; the body retains only 55% of a 100-μg dose and 15% of a 1000-μg dose. Body stores of vitamin B_{12} amount to 2000 to 3000 μg which is believed to be enough for 3 to 4 years. If 1000 μg is injected monthly, the 150 μg retained lasts for about 1 month. Hydroxocobalamin is better retained than cyanocobalamin; 90% of a 100-μg dose and 30% of a 1000-μg dose are retained and that range is believed to be enough for 2 to 10 months.[1]

1. Anonymous. Time to drop cyanocobalamin? Drug Ther Bull 1984; 22: 43.

Human Requirements

For adults, the daily requirement of vitamin B_{12} is probably about 1 to 2 μg and this amount is present in most normal diets. Vitamin B_{12} occurs only in animal products; it does not occur in vegetables, therefore strict vegetarian (vegan) diets that exclude dairy products may provide an inadequate amount although it has been said that many years of vegetarianism are necessary before a deficiency is produced, if at all. Meats, especially liver and kidney, milk, eggs, and other dairy products, and fish are good sources of vitamin B_{12}.

◊ In the UK[1] dietary reference values (see p.1352) have been published for vitamin B_{12} and similarly in the USA recommended dietary allowances (RDAs) have been set.[2] Differing amounts are recommended for infants and children of varying ages, adults and pregnant and lactating women. In the UK the reference nutrient intake (RNI) is 1.5 μg daily for adult males

and females and the estimated average requirement (EAR) is 1.25 μg daily. In the USA the RDA for adults is 2.4 μg daily.

1. DoH. Dietary reference values for food energy and nutrients for the United Kingdom: report of the panel on dietary reference values of the committee on medical aspects of food policy. Report on health and social subjects 41. London: HMSO, 1991.
2. Standing Committee on the Scientific Evaluation of Dietary Reference Intakes of the Food and Nutrition Board. Dietary Reference Intakes for thiamin, riboflavin, niacin, vitamin B_6, folate, vitamin B_{12}, pantothenic acid, biotin, and choline. Washington, DC: National Academy Press, 2000.

Uses and Administration

Vitamin B_{12}, a water-soluble vitamin, occurs in the body mainly as methylcobalamin (mecobalamin) and as adenosylcobalamin (cobamamide) and hydroxocobalamin. Mecobalamin and cobamamide act as coenzymes in nucleic acid synthesis. Mecobalamin is also closely involved with folic acid in several important metabolic pathways.

Vitamin B_{12} deficiency can occur in strict vegetarians with an inadequate dietary intake, although it may take many years before a deficiency is produced. Deficiency is more likely in patients with malabsorption syndromes or metabolic disorders, nitrous oxide-induced megaloblastosis, or following gastrectomy or extensive ileal resection. Deficiency leads to the development of megaloblastic anaemias and demyelination and other neurological damage. A specific anaemia known as pernicious anaemia develops in patients with an absence of the intrinsic factor necessary for good absorption of the vitamin from dietary sources.

Vitamin B_{12} preparations are used in the treatment and prevention of vitamin B_{12} deficiency. It is essential to identify the exact cause of deficiency, preferably before commencing therapy. Hydroxocobalamin is generally preferred to cyanocobalamin; it binds more firmly to plasma proteins and is retained in the body longer (see under Pharmacokinetics, above). Cyanocobalamin and hydroxocobalamin are generally administered by the intramuscular route, although cyanocobalamin may be given by mouth or intranasally (see also under Administration, below). Oral cyanocobalamin may be used in treating or preventing vitamin B_{12} deficiency of dietary origin.

In the UK, recommended doses for pernicious anaemia and other macrocytic anaemias without neurological involvement are hydroxocobalamin (or cyanocobalamin) 250 to 1000 μg intramuscularly on alternate days for 1 to 2 weeks, then 250 μg weekly until the blood count returns to normal. Maintenance doses of 1000 μg of hydroxocobalamin are administered every 2 to 3 months (or monthly for cyanocobalamin). If there is neurological involvement, hydroxocobalamin or cyanocobalamin may be given in doses of 1000 μg on alternate days and continued for as long as improvement occurs. For the prophylaxis of anaemia associated with vitamin B_{12} deficiency resulting from gastrectomy or malabsorption syndromes hydroxocobalamin may be given in doses of 1000 μg intramuscularly every 2 or 3 months or cyanocobalamin in doses of 250 to 1000 μg intramuscularly each month. For vitamin B_{12} deficiency of dietary origin, cyanocobalamin 50 to 150 μg may be taken daily by mouth between meals.

Lower doses for the administration of both cyanocobalamin and hydroxocobalamin are recommended in the USA. For the treatment of pernicious anaemia, the usual intramuscular dose of cyanocobalamin is 100 μg daily for 7 days then on alternate days for 7 further doses then every 3 to 4 days for 2 to 3 weeks. For hydroxocobalamin the dose is 30 μg daily for 5 to 10 days. For maintenance, both cyanocobalamin and hydroxocobalamin are given at a dose of 100 to 200 μg monthly, based on haematological monitoring. An intranasal preparation of cyanocobalamin is also available for maintenance therapy, the recommended dose being 500 μg once weekly. Oral doses of up to 1000 μg of cyanocobalamin have also been used. In patients with normal gastrointestinal absorption, doses of 1 to 25 μg daily are considered sufficient as a dietary supplement.

Treatment usually results in rapid haematological improvement and a striking clinical response. However, neurological symptoms respond more slowly and in some cases remission may not be complete.

Hydroxocobalamin may also be given in the treatment of tobacco amblyopia and Leber's optic atrophy; initial doses are 1000 µg daily for 2 weeks intramuscularly followed by 1000 µg twice weekly for as long as improvement occurs. Thereafter, 1000 µg is administered every 1 to 3 months.

Cyanocobalamin and hydroxocobalamin are also used in the Schilling test to investigate vitamin B$_{12}$ absorption and deficiency states. They are administered in a non-radioactive form together with cyanocobalamin radioactively-labelled with cobalt-57 (p.1449) or cobalt-58 (p.1449) and the amount of radioactivity excreted in the urine can be used to assess absorption status. A differential Schilling test, in which the forms of cyanocobalamin are given under different conditions can provide information concerning the cause of the malabsorption. Cobamamide and mecobalamin may also be used for vitamin B$_{12}$ deficiency.

Administration. The small amounts of vitamin B$_{12}$ present in the diet are absorbed from the gastrointestinal tract by an active process which involves binding with intrinsic factor. As intrinsic factor is absent in patients who have developed pernicious anaemia it has often been assumed that oral treatment with vitamin B$_{12}$ preparations will therefore be ineffective. However, about 1% of an oral dose is absorbed by passive diffusion, and with large doses this amount may be sufficient for therapy. Thus attention has been given again to the use of oral cobalamins for the treatment of pernicious anaemia.[1-3] Oral cyanocobalamin 2000 µg daily was as effective as intramuscular therapy in patients with vitamin B$_{12}$ deficiency in a comparative study.[4] Some now consider that oral doses of 1000 µg daily are a suitable alternative to injections given at monthly or so intervals.[3] Cyanocobalamin is also effective when given intranasally,[5] with peak plasma concentrations greater than those achievable orally, and this may offer another alternative to injection. The intranasal absorption of hydroxocobalamin has also been studied.[6,7]

1. Lederle FA. Oral cobalamin for pernicious anemia: medicine's best kept secret? *JAMA* 1991; **265:** 94–5.
2. Hathcock JN, Troendle GJ. Oral cobalamin for treatment of pernicious anemia? *JAMA* 1991; **265:** 96–7.
3. Elia M. Oral or parenteral therapy for B12 deficiency. *Lancet* 1998; **352:** 1721–2.
4. Kuzminski AM, *et al.* Effective treatment of cobalamin deficiency with oral cobalamin. *Blood* 1998; **92:** 1191–8.
5. Romeo VD, *et al.* Intranasal cyanocobalamin. *JAMA* 1992; **268:** 1268–9.
6. van Asselt DZB, *et al.* Nasal absorption of hydroxocobalamin in healthy elderly adults. *Br J Clin Pharmacol* 1998; **45:** 83–6.
7. Slot WB, *et al.* Normalization of plasma vitamin B12 concentration by intranasal hydroxocobalamin in vitamin B12-deficient patients. *Gastroenterology* 1997; **113:** 430–3.

Amino acid metabolic disorders. References to the use of hydroxocobalamin in the treatment of inborn errors of vitamin B$_{12}$ metabolism.[1-6] Some patients with homocystinuria (p.1350) or methylmalonic aciduria have responded to cobalamins.

1. Schuh S, *et al.* Homocystinuria and megaloblastic anemia responsive to vitamin B$_{12}$ therapy. *N Engl J Med* 1984; **310:** 686–90.
2. Hoffbrand AV, *et al.* Hereditary abnormal transcobalamin II previously diagnosed as congenital dihydrofolate reductase deficiency. *N Engl J Med* 1984; **310:** 789–90.
3. Shinnar S, Singer HS. Cobalamin C mutation (methylmalonic aciduria and homocystinuria) in adolescence. *N Engl J Med* 1984; **311:** 451–4.
4. Bhatt HR, *et al.* Treatment of hydroxocobalamin-resistant methylmalonic acidaemia with adenosylcobalamin. *Lancet* 1986; **ii:** 465.
5. van der Meer SB, *et al.* Prenatal treatment of a patient with vitamin B$_{12}$-responsive methylmalonic acidemia. *J Pediatr* 1990; **117:** 923–6.
6. Andersson HC, Shapira E. Biochemical and clinical response to hydroxocobalamin versus cyanocobalamin treatment in patients with methylmalonic acidemia and homocystinuria (cblC). *J Pediatr* 1998; **132:** 121–4.

Cyanide toxicity. Hydroxocobalamin combines with cyanide to form cyanocobalamin, and thus may be used as an antidote to cyanide toxicity (p.1433). Hydroxocobalamin is reported to be effective in controlling cyanide toxicity due to nitroprusside infusion,[1] and after exposure to inhaled combustion products in residential fires.[2]

1. Zerbe NF, Wagner BKJ. Use of vitamin B12 in the treatment and prevention of nitroprusside-induced cyanide toxicity. *Crit Care Med* 1993; **21:** 465–7.
2. Houeto P, *et al.* Relation of blood cyanide to plasma cyanocobalamin concentration after a fixed dose of hydroxocobalamin in cyanide poisoning. *Lancet* 1995; **346:** 605–8.

Deficiency states. The emergence of new metabolic assays for homocysteine and methylmalonic acid has led to the identification of subtle vitamin B$_{12}$ deficiency[1,2] without the overt manifestations of megaloblastic anaemia (p.717) or neurologi-

cal disease; this condition appears to be particularly common in the elderly.[1] At present, there is no clear clinical rationale for treating subtle deficiency.[1] However, preliminary findings from a recent study suggest it may be linked to some immunological impairment, identified as impaired antibody responses to pneumococcal vaccine.[3] Moreover, raised homocysteine concentrations have been identified as a risk factor for atherosclerosis and ischaemic heart disease, and there is increasing interest in the potential of B vitamins, including B$_{12}$, to reduce homocysteine concentrations and therefore atherosclerotic outcomes (see Ischaemic Heart Disease, under Uses of Folic Acid, p.1362).

Dietary vitamin B$_{12}$ deficiency in infants may lead to developmental abnormalities.[4,5]

1. Carmel R. Subtle cobalamin deficiency. *Ann Intern Med* 1996; **124:** 338–40.
2. Green R. Screening for vitamin B$_{12}$ deficiency: caveat emptor. *Ann Intern Med* 1996; **124:** 509–11.
3. Fata FT, *et al.* Impaired antibody responses to pneumococcal polysaccharide in elderly patients with low serum vitamin B$_{12}$ levels. *Ann Intern Med* 1996; **124:** 299–304.
4. Emery ES, *et al.* Vitamin B12 deficiency: a cause of abnormal movements in infants. *Pediatrics* 1997; **99:** 255–6.
5. von Schenck U, *et al.* Persistence of neurological damage induced by dietary vitamin B-12 deficiency in infancy. *Arch Dis Child* 1997; **77:** 137–9.

Neural tube defects. It has been found that an abnormality in homocysteine metabolism is present in many women who give birth to children with neural tube defects (p.1362); the enzyme methionine synthase, which converts homocysteine to methionine, requires both folate and vitamin B$_{12}$ as cofactors, and low maternal vitamin B$_{12}$ concentrations may be an independent risk factor for neural tube defects.[1] If confirmed, this would suggest that additional supplementation with cobalamins may be warranted.

1. Mills JL, *et al.* Homocysteine metabolism in pregnancies complicated by neural-tube defects. *Lancet* 1995; **345:** 149–51.

Preparations

BP 2001: Cyanocobalamin Tablets; Hydroxocobalamin Injection;
USP 25: Cyanocobalamin Injection; Hydroxocobalamin Injection.

Proprietary Preparations (details are given in Part 3)

Aust.: Erycytol; Hepavit; **Austral.:** Cytamen; Neo-Cytamen; **Belg.:** Forta B; Hydroxo†; Novobedouze; **Braz.:** Bedozil; Cronobe; Enzicoba; Rubranova; Zinabol; **Canad.:** Bedoz; Rubion; Rubramin; **Denm.:** Behepan; Betolvex; Vibeden; **Fin.:** Betolvex; Cohemin; **Fr.:** Cobanzyme; Cyanokit; Dibencozan†; Dodecavit; Indusil T†; **Ger.:** Ambe 12; Aquo-Cytobion; B 12-L 90; B12 Depot-Rotexmedica; B12 Ehrl†; B12-Horfervit; B12-Rotexmedica; B12-Steigerwald; B$_{12}$ Ankermann; B$_{12}$ Depot-Hevert; B$_{12}$ Depot-Vicotrat; B$_{12}$ Vicotrat; B$_{12}$-AS; Cytobion; Hamo-Vibolex; Lophakomp-B 12; Lophakomp-B 12 Depot; Neurotrat B$_{12}$; Novidroxin; Vicapan N; Vita-Brachont†; **Hong Kong:** Methycobal; Triniscon; **Irl.:** Cytacon; Cytamen; Neo-Cytamen; **Israel:** Bedodeka; **Ital.:** Cobaforte; Dobetin; Eritrovit B12; Indusil; Neo-Cytamen; OH B12; Reticulogen†; **Jpn:** Calomide-S†; Methycobal; **Mex.:** Axofor; Biocobal; Biotrefon-L; Compensal; Doprit; Droxibit; Duradoce; Exorvit; Hidrowil; Lentorem; Leo-Doce; Maxibol; Nebal; Neurofor; Parol; Rubrina; Valamin 12; Vidavit; **Neth.:** Hydrocobamine; **Norw.:** Betolvex; **NZ:** Neo-Cytamen; **Port.:** Bedoze; Co-Vibedoze; Cobamet; Cobaxid; Jaba B$_{12}$; Made B12; OH B12; Permadoze; Tridocemine; **S.Afr.:** Betolvex†; Cobalatec; Norivite-12; **Singapore:** Methycobal; Neuromethyn; **Spain:** Ambritan†; Asimil B12; Cromatonbic B12; Isopto B 12; Lifaton B12; Megamilbedoce; Optovite B12; Reticulogen Fortificado; Zimadoce; **Swed.:** Behepan; Betolvex; **Switz.:** Betolvex; Vitarubin; **Thai.:** Ampavit; Hitocobamin; Methycobal; Neuromet; Redisol; Sicobal; **UAE:** Cynovit; **UK:** Cemac B12; Cobalin-H; Cytacon; Cytamen; Neo-Cytamen; **USA:** Crystamine; Crysti 1000; Cyanoject; Cyomin; Ener-B†; Fe-Tinic Forte; Hydro Cobex; Hydro-Crysti-12; LA-12; Nascobal; Rubramin PC†.

Multi-ingredient: Aust.: Aktiferrin compositum; Ambene; Ambene N; Arca-Be; Beneuran compositum; Clinit†; Delta-Tomanol†; Diclovit; Dolo-Neurobion; Neurobion; Pronerv; Rheumesser; Trinsicon†; **Austral.:** Medinat PMT-Eze; **Belg.:** Ferrifol B12; Neurobion; Vioneurin; **Braz.:** Aminocid; Anemofer; Betinjectol; Bituelve; Citoneurin; Cobactin; Cobaglobal; Coduract; Coraben; Dexa-Citoneurin; Dexa-Neuriberi; Dexacobal; Dexador; Dexadoze; Dexagil; Dexalgen; Dexaneurin; Dozeneurin; Ergohepat B12; Ferroplex; Ferrotrat; Fol Sang B12; Hematiase B12; Hepasedan; Hepatotris; Iloban; Lisotox; Metiocolin B12; Metiocolin Composto; Nucleo CMP; Trinalgen; Trineval; Trirubin; Vibetrat; Vibetrat Dexa; Vipirim; Vitaneuron; Xantinon B12; Xantinon Complex; Acti-B$_{12}$; Folacin 12; Fortiplex; Heparos; Penta-3B; Penta-3B + C; **Fin.:** Neurobion; Neurovitan; **Fr.:** Nuclevit B$_{12}$†; Vibalgan†; **Ger.:** Ambene Comp; AntiFocal N; B$_{12}$ Fol-Vicotrat; Causat B12 N; Dodecavit N; Eryfer comp; Eukalisan forte; Eukalisan N; Ferro sanol comp; Ferro-Folgamma; Folgamma; Hepagrisevit Forte-N; Hepatofalk; Medivitan N; Medyn; milgamma N; Neuro-Lichtenstein; Neuro-ratiopharm; Neuro-Vibolex; Neurobion; Neurotrat; NeyNormin N (Revitorgan-Dilutionen N Nr 65); NeyTumorin N (Revitorgan-Dilutionen N Nr 66); Novirell B; Pernaemyl†; Selectafer N; Telbibur N; Vitaject; Vitasprint B$_{12}$; **Hong Kong:** 3B; Epargriseovit; Hepatofalk; Neuro B1-6-12; Neurobion; Neurorubine; Nevramin; Princi-B Fort; Trabit; **Israel:** Betrivit; Tribemin; **Ital.:** Adenobeta; Adenoplex Forte; Adenovit; Benexol B12; Betascor B12†; Briogen; Calcio Dobetin; Co-Carnetina B12; Efargen; Emazian B12; Emoantitossina; Emopon; Epargriseovit; Eparmefolin; Fibronevrina; Firmavit; Folepar B12; For Liver†; Fosfo Plus; Fosfoutipi Vitaminico; Gluta Complex; Glutamin Fosforo; Hepa-Factor; Hepatos B12; Memoserina S; Memovissus; Memovit B12; Menalgon; Menalgon B6; Mionevrasi; Neo-Eparbiol; Neo-Geynevral; Neuraben; Neurobionta; Nevril†; Novaneurina B12†; OH B12 B1†; Oro B12; Porfirin 12; Sinevrile†; Tonogen; Tricortin; Triferon; Trinevrina B6; Vitasprint; Vitasprint Complex; **Jpn:** Neurovitan; **Mex.:** Benexol

B12; Ciprolisina; Dexabion; Dolo-Neurobion; Dolo-Tiaminal; Gonakor; Neurobion; Neuroflax; Orafer Comp; Pangavit; Selectadoce; Tiaminal B$_{12}$; Tiaminal B$_{17}$ Trivalente; Tribedoxyl; **Port.:** Linamin Plus; Neurobion; Tridocemine; **S.Afr.:** Foliglobin; Neurobion; Prohep; Revaton†; Trinsicon†; **Singapore:** 3B; Alinamin B12; Neogobion; Neurobion; Neuroforte; Neurorubine; Nevramin; Princi-B Fort; Sangobion; **Spain:** Antineurina; Bexeol B1 B6 B12; Bester Complex; Calcio 20 Complex; Covitasa B12; Dalamon; Duplicalcio B12; Enoton; Gammamida Complex†; Hepa Factor†; Hidroxil B12 B6 B1; Inzitan; Malandil; Mederebro; Mederebro Compuesto†; Menalgil B6; Meneparol; Metabolicum; Milbedoce Anabolico; Nervobion; Neuromade; Neurostop Complex; Prodessal; Refulgin; Rubrocortin; Sugarceton†; Taurobetina; Teovit; Tonico Juventus; Trofalgon; Trofi Milina†; Viadetres; Vitafardi C B12; **Swed.:** Neurotrat; Tribeton; Vitasprint Complex; **Thai.:** 3B; Alinamin B12; Beromin; Cilfer-12-F; Cydoxmine-B; Cyriamine; Douzabox; Genavit; Hemolax; Neurobex; Neurobion; Nevramin; Nuvit; Ostone-B12; Princi-B; Sangobion; Trabit; Tribesian; Tricortin; Trinsicon; Trivit-B; Vioneurin; Vita-B; Vitamedin; Vitron; **UAE:** 3V; **UK:** Dicopac; Hematinic; **USA:** Anemagen; Bevitamel; Chromagen; Chromagen FA; Chromagen Forte; Contrin; Ferotrinsic; Ferralet Plus; Ferrex Forte; Fetrin; FOLTX; Fumatinic; Hem Fe; Hemocyte-F; Livitrinsic-f; Nervidox 6†; Nervidox†; Neuro B-12†; Neurobion†; Niferex Forte; Nu-Iron Plus; Poly-Iron Forte; PremesisRx; Pronemia Hematinic; Tia Doce†; Tolfrinic; Tri-HEMIC; Trinsicon; Vita-Feron†.

Vitamin C Substances   (14732-g)

Several substances have vitamin C activity, notably ascorbic acid and its calcium and sodium salts. Natural products with a high vitamin C content are black currant and rose fruit.

Ascorbic Acid   (7881-b)

Ascorbic Acid (BAN, rINN).

Acidum Ascorbicum; L-Ascorbic Acid; Cevitamic Acid; E300; Vitamin C. The enolic form of 3-oxo-L-gulofuranolactone; 2,3-Didehydro-L-*threo*-hexono-1,4-lactone.

$C_6H_8O_6 = 176.1$.

CAS — 50-81-7.

ATC — A11GA01.

Pharmacopoeias. In Chin., Eur. (see p.vi), Int., Jpn, Pol., and US.

Pharmacopoeial description

Ph. Eur.: A white or almost white crystalline powder or colourless crystals becoming discoloured on exposure to air and moisture. Freely soluble in water; soluble in alcohol; practically insoluble in ether. A 5% solution in water has a pH of 2.1 to 2.6. Store in nonmetallic containers. Protect from light.

USP 25: White or slightly yellow crystals or powder. On exposure to light, it gradually darkens. In the dry state, is reasonably stable in air, but in solution rapidly oxidises. Soluble 1 in 3 of water and 1 in 40 of alcohol; insoluble in chloroform, in ether, and in benzene. Store in airtight containers. Protect from light.

Black Currant   (7882-v)

Cassis; Rib. Nig.; Ribes Nigrum.

Pharmacopoeias. In Br.

Pharmacopoeial description

BP 2001: The fresh ripe fruits of *Ribes nigrum* together with their pedicels and rachides. It has a strong, characteristic odour and a pleasantly acidic taste.

Calcium Ascorbate   (16560-a)

Calcium Ascorbate (BANM, rINNM).

Calcii Ascorbas; E302.

$(C_6H_7O_6)_2Ca,2H_2O = 426.3$.

CAS — 5743-27-1.

Pharmacopoeias. In Eur. (see p.vi) and US.

Pharmacopoeial description

Ph. Eur.: A white or slightly yellowish crystalline powder. Freely soluble in water; practically insoluble in alcohol. A 10% solution in water has a pH between 6.8 and 7.4. Store in non-metallic containers. Protect from light.

USP 25: A white to slightly yellow, practically odourless, powder. Freely soluble in water (about 1 in 2); slightly soluble in alcohol; insoluble in ether. pH of a 10% solution in water is between 6.8 and 7.4. Store in airtight containers. Protect from light.

Rose Fruit   (7883-g)

Brier Fruit; Cynosbati Fructus; Cynosbati Pseudofructus; Dog Rose Fruits; Églantier; Hips; Hypanthium Rosae; Rosae Fructus; Rosae Pseudo-fructus; Rose Hips.

Pharmacopoeias. In Eur. (see p.vi) and Jpn.

Pharmacopoeial description

Ph. Eur.: The rose hips made up by the receptacle and the remains of the dried sepals of *Rosa canina*, *R. pendulina*, and other *Rosa* spp. with the achenes removed. It contains not less than 0.3% of ascorbic acid, calculated with reference to the dried drug. Protect from light.

The symbol † denotes a preparation no longer actively marketed

Sodium Ascorbate (7880-m)

Sodium Ascorbate (BANM, rINN).

E301; Monosodium L-Ascorbate; Natrii Ascorbas. 3-Oxo-L-gulofuranolactone sodium enolate.

$C_6H_7NaO_6 = 198.1$.

CAS — 134-03-2.

Pharmacopoeias. In Eur. (see p.vi) and *US.*

Pharmacopoeial description

Ph. Eur.: A white or yellowish crystalline powder or crystals. Freely soluble in water; sparingly soluble in alcohol; practically insoluble in dichloromethane. A 10% solution in water has a pH of 7.0 to 8.0. Store in non-metallic containers. Protect from light.

USP 25: White or very faintly yellow, odourless or practically odourless, crystals or crystalline powder. On exposure to light it gradually darkens. Soluble 1 in 1.3 of water; very slightly soluble in alcohol; insoluble in chloroform and in ether. pH of a 10% solution in water is between 7.0 and 8.0. Store in airtight containers. Protect from light.

Adverse Effects and Precautions

Ascorbic acid is usually well tolerated. Large doses are reported to cause diarrhoea and other gastrointestinal disturbances. It has also been stated that large doses may result in hyperoxaluria and the formation of renal calcium oxalate calculi and ascorbic acid should therefore be given with care to patients with hyperoxaluria (see Effects on the Kidneys, below). Tolerance may be induced with prolonged use of large doses, resulting in symptoms of deficiency when intake is reduced to normal.

Large doses of ascorbic acid have resulted in haemolysis in patients with glucose-6-phosphate dehydrogenase (G6PD) deficiency (see Effects on the Blood, below).

Effects on the blood. There are reports of haemolysis in patients with glucose-6-phosphate dehydrogenase deficiency following large doses of ascorbic acid either intravenously[1,2] or in soft drinks.[3] There has also been a report[4] of a patient with paroxysmal nocturnal haemoglobinuria suffering haemolysis following the ingestion of large amounts of ascorbic acid in a soft drink. There is concern that the large quantities of vitamin C in feeds for premature neonates may have a pro-oxidant effect, and lead to haemolysis. However, a double-blind study found no increase in erythrocyte destruction or hyperbilirubinaemia in premature neonates receiving vitamin C.[5]

1. Campbell GD, *et al.* Ascorbic acid-induced hemolysis in G-6-PD deficiency. *Ann Intern Med* 1975; **82:** 810.
2. Rees DC, *et al.* Acute haemolysis induced by high dose ascorbic acid in glucose-6-phosphate dehydrogenase deficiency. *BMJ* 1993; **306:** 841–2.
3. Mehta JB, *et al.* Ascorbic-acid-induced hemolysis in G-6-PD deficiency. *Lancet* 1990; **336:** 944.
4. Iwamoto N, *et al.* Haemolysis induced by ascorbic acid in paroxysmal nocturnal haemoglobinuria. *Lancet* 1994; **343:** 357.
5. Doyle J, *et al.* Does vitamin C cause hemolysis in premature newborn infants? Results of a multicenter double-blind, randomized, controlled trial. *J Pediatr* 1997; **130:** 103–9.

Effects on the kidneys. Although renal impairment associated with excessive oxalate excretion has been reported following the administration of large doses of ascorbic acid[1-3] it has been considered that healthy persons can ingest large amounts of ascorbic acid with relatively small increases in oxalate excretion[4,5] and without an increased risk of oxalate stone formation.

1. Reznik VM, *et al.* Does high-dose ascorbic acid accelerate renal failure? *N Engl J Med* 1980; **302:** 1418–19.
2. Swartz RD, *et al.* Hyperoxaluria and renal insufficiency due to ascorbic acid administration during total parenteral nutrition. *Ann Intern Med* 1984; **100:** 530–1.
3. Balcke P, *et al.* Ascorbic acid aggravates secondary hyperoxalemia in patients on chronic hemodialysis. *Ann Intern Med* 1984; **101:** 344–5.
4. Tsao CS. Ascorbic acid administration and urinary oxalate. *Ann Intern Med* 1984; **101:** 405–6.
5. Wandzilak TR, *et al.* Effect of high dose vitamin C on urinary oxalate levels. *J Urol (Baltimore)* 1994; **151:** 834–7.

Effects on the teeth. A report of dental enamel erosion which was attributed to the daily ingestion of chewable ascorbic acid tablets over a period of 3 years.[1] The tablets lowered the pH of the saliva to a level at which calcium was lost from the tooth enamel.

1. Giunta JL. Dental erosion resulting from chewable vitamin C tablets. *J Am Dent Assoc* 1983; **107:** 253–6.

Interference with laboratory tests. Ascorbic acid, a strong reducing agent, interferes with laboratory tests involving oxidation and reduction reactions. Falsely-elevated or false-negative test results may be obtained from plasma, faeces, or urine samples depending on such factors as the dose of ascorbic acid and specific method employed.

Interactions

For the effect of ascorbic acid on various drugs see under desferrioxamine (p.1004), hormonal contra-

ceptives (p.1459), fluphenazine (p.665), and warfarin (p.997). Ascorbic acid may increase the absorption of iron in iron-deficiency states.

Pharmacokinetics

Ascorbic acid is readily absorbed from the gastrointestinal tract and is widely distributed in the body tissues. Plasma concentrations of ascorbic acid rise as the dose ingested is increased until a plateau is reached with doses of about 90 to 150 mg daily. Body stores of ascorbic acid in health are about 1.5 g although more may be stored at intakes above 200 mg daily. The concentration is higher in leucocytes and platelets than in erythrocytes and plasma. In deficiency states the concentration in leucocytes declines later and at a slower rate, and has been considered to be a better criterion for the evaluation of deficiency than the concentration in plasma.

Ascorbic acid is reversibly oxidised to dehydroascorbic acid; some is metabolised to ascorbate-2-sulfate, which is inactive, and oxalic acid which are excreted in the urine. Ascorbic acid in excess of the body's needs is also rapidly eliminated unchanged in the urine; this generally occurs with intakes exceeding 200 mg daily. Ascorbic acid crosses the placenta and is distributed into breast milk. It is removed by haemodialysis.

Human Requirements

A daily dietary intake of about 30 to 100 mg of vitamin C has been recommended for adults. There is, however, wide variation in individual requirements. Humans are unable to form their own ascorbic acid and so a dietary source is necessary. Most dietary ascorbic acid is obtained from fruit and vegetable sources; only small amounts are present in milk and animal tissues. Relatively rich sources include rose hips (rose fruit), black currant, citrus fruits, leafy vegetables, tomatoes, potatoes, and green and red peppers.

Ascorbic acid is readily destroyed during cooking processes. Considerable losses may also occur during storage.

◊ In the UK[1] dietary reference values (see p.1352) have been published for vitamin C and similarly in the USA recommended dietary allowances (RDAs) have been set.[2] Differing amounts are recommended for infants and children of varying ages, for adult males and females, and for pregnant and lactating women. In the UK the reference nutrient intake (RNI) is 40 mg daily for adult males and females and the estimated average requirement (EAR) is 30 mg daily. In general the amount recommended in the USA for all ages and groups is higher than that set in the UK; the RDA is 90 mg daily for men and 75 mg daily for women.[2] The RDA is increased in smokers by 35 mg daily. The tolerable upper intake level is 2 g daily.[2] The EAR is 75 mg daily for men and 60 mg daily for women.

1. DoH. Dietary reference values for food energy and nutrients for the United Kingdom: report of the panel on dietary reference values of the committee on medical aspects of food policy. *Report on health and social subjects 41.* London: HMSO, 1991.
2. Standing Committee on the Scientific Evaluation of Dietary Reference Intakes of the Food and Nutrition Board. *Dietary Reference Intakes for vitamin C, vitamin E, selenium, and carotenoids.* Washington DC: National Academy Press, 2000.

Uses and Administration

Vitamin C, a water-soluble vitamin, is essential for the synthesis of collagen and intercellular material. Vitamin C deficiency develops when the dietary intake is inadequate. It is rare in adults, but may occur in infants, alcoholics, or the elderly. Deficiency leads to the development of a well-defined syndrome known as scurvy. This is characterised by capillary fragility, bleeding (especially from small blood vessels and the gums), normocytic or macrocytic anaemia, cartilage and bone lesions, and slow healing of wounds.

Vitamin C is used in the treatment and prevention of deficiency. It completely reverses symptoms of deficiency. It is usually given by mouth, the preferred route, as ascorbic acid, and has been given to children in the form of a suitable fruit juice such as orange juice or as black currant or rose hip syrups. Ascorbic acid may be administered, as sodium ascorbate, by the intramuscular route, and also by the intravenous

or subcutaneous routes. Doses of 25 to 75 mg daily in the prevention of deficiency, and 250 mg or more daily in divided doses for the treatment of deficiency, have been recommended.

Ascorbic acid 100 to 200 mg daily may be given with desferrioxamine in the treatment of patients with thalassaemia, to improve the chelating action of desferrioxamine, thereby increasing the excretion of iron (see p.1004). In iron deficiency states ascorbic acid may increase gastrointestinal iron absorption and ascorbic acid or ascorbate salts are therefore included in some oral iron preparations. Ascorbic acid or sodium ascorbate have been used in treating methaemoglobinaemia. Ascorbic acid has been used to acidify urine. It has also been tried in the treatment of many other disorders, as discussed in the review below, but there is little evidence of beneficial effect.

Eye drops containing potassium ascorbate have been used for the treatment of chemical burns. Potassium ascorbate 10% is used alternately with sodium citrate 10%; it is believed that the ascorbate works by mopping up free oxygen radicals thus aiding in the prevention of corneal epithelial damage.

Ascorbic acid and calcium and sodium ascorbates are used as antioxidants in pharmaceutical manufacturing and in the food industry.

◊ A beneficial effect of 'megadose' ascorbic acid therapy has been claimed for an extraordinary number of conditions and the subject has been reviewed.[1] These conditions include the common cold, asthma, atherosclerosis, cancer, psychiatric disorders, increased susceptibility to infections due to abnormal leucocyte function, infertility, and osteogenesis imperfecta; it has also been tried in treatment of wound healing, pain in Paget's disease, and opioid withdrawal. The reviewer concluded that generally there were only few properly controlled studies which substantiate these claims, and confirmation by controlled studies was required. This is certainly true of the proposed use of vitamin C to prevent cancer. Data from the few studies that have been conducted have failed to show any benefit from vitamin C (see Prophylaxis of Malignant Neoplasms, p.1353).

As for the common cold (p.605), published findings suggest that ascorbic acid might produce a reduction in the severity of a cold but not in its incidence,[2,3] except perhaps in men with a low vitamin C intake.[4]

Another field in which it has been proposed that vitamin C might produce benefit is in the prevention of ischaemic heart disease, in which oxidation by free radicals is thought to play a role. However, in general, data from prospective epidemiological studies have not revealed a link between vitamin C intake and ischaemic heart disease (see p.1352). Ascorbic acid is also one of a number of agents for which reports of benefit exist in idiopathic thrombocytopenic purpura (see p.1052).

1. Ovesen L. Vitamin therapy in the absence of obvious deficiency: what is the evidence? *Drugs* 1984; **27:** 148–70.
2. Hemilä H. Does vitamin C alleviate the symptoms of the common cold?—a review of current evidence. *Scand J Infect Dis* 1994; **26:** 1–6.
3. Douglas RM, *et al.* Vitamin C for preventing and treating the common cold (updated 18 July 2001). Available in The Cochrane Library; Issue 4. Oxford: Update Software; 2001.
4. Hemilä H. Vitamin C intake and susceptibility to the common cold. *Br J Nutr* 1997; **77:** 59–72.

Preparations

BP 2001: Ascorbic Acid Injection; Ascorbic Acid Tablets; Black Currant Syrup; Vitamins B and C Injection;
USP 25: Ascorbic Acid Injection; Ascorbic Acid Oral Solution; Ascorbic Acid Tablets.

Proprietary Preparations (details are given in Part 3)

Aust.: Ascorbin; Bioagil; C-Vit; Calcascorbin; Ce-Limo; Cebion; Cetebe; Cevitol; Irocovit C†; Mel-C; Redoxon; Tetesept Vitamin C; Vicedent; *Austral.:* Bioglan Cal C; Cecon†; Potent C†; Pro-C; Redoxon; Sugarless C; Supa C; Vita C; *Belg.:* C-Dose; C-Will; Cenol†; Cetamine; Redoxon; Upsavit C; *Braz.:* Ascortil; Cebion; Ceklin; Cewin; Citrovit; Energil C; Lento C; Redoxon; Vi-Ce; Vitafran; Vitascorb; Vitax; *Canad.:* Action; Apo-C; Ascorbex; Balanced C Complex; C Forte†; C-1000; C-3000; Ester-C; Kamu Jay; Kyolic Formula 103; Nutrol C; Ortic C; Redoxon; Revitalose C; Super C; Timed Release C; Vita-C; *Fin.:* Ascorbin; Bio-C-Vitamin; C-Poretta; C-Tabs; C-vimin; Cevi-Tabs; Poremax-C; Puru-C; Vita-C; *Fr.:* Arkovital C†; Laroscorbine; Midy Vitamine C; Tempodia†; Vitascorbol; *Ger.:* Ascorell; Ascorvit; ASS OPT†; ASS-Kreuz; Cebion; Cebion N; Cetebe; Hermes Cevitt; Vagi-C; *Hong Kong:* C Rose Hips; C-1000; Cecap; Cegrovit; Celin; Cetrinets; Chewies; Delrosa; Flavettes; Redoxon; Vicemex; *Irl.:* Redoxon; Rubex; *Israel:* C500; Cereon; Redoxon; Vi-C; Vitascarbol; *Ital.:* Acidylina†; Agrumina; Ascomed†; Bio-Ci; C Monovit; C-Lisa; C-Tard; Cebion; Cecon; Duo-C; Dynaphos-C; Ergofit†; Idro-C†; Lemonvit; Redoxon; Vici; Vicitina†; Zig C; *Mex.:* Ascortil; Cebion; Cevalin; Infa-C-Vit; Redoxon; *Neth.:* C-Will; Dagravit C†; Redoxon; *Norw.:* AFI-C; *NZ:* Citravite; Redoxon; *Port.:* Anti-rugas C; C'Nergil; Cebiolon; Cebion; Cecrisina; Citavi†; Redoxon; Vivin C; *S.Afr.:* Redoxon; Scorbex; *Singapore:* Ascorbin; Cetrinets; Dumovit C; Flavettes; Redoxon; Vorange; *Spain:* Caramelos Vit C†; Cebion; Citrolider; Citrovit; Junce†; Ledovit C; Redoxon; Upsa C; *Swed.:* C-vimin; Ido-C; *Switz.:* C-Naryl; Cegrovit; Cetebe; Demovit C; Redoxon; Vicemex; Vita-Ce; **Thai.:** Bio-C; C Mon; C-Will; Hicee; Mymin C; Redoxon; Vitacimin; **UK:** Buffered C; Buffered C 500; Haliborange Halibonbons; Redoxon; **USA:** Alba CE†; Ascorbicap†; Ce-Vi-Sol†; Cebid†; Cecon; Cenolate; Cevalin†; Cevi-Bid; Dull-C; Flavorcee†; N'ice Vitamin C; Sunkist; Vita-C.

Multi-ingredient: numerous preparations are listed in Part 3.

Vitamin D Substances (7892-q)

The term vitamin D is used for a range of closely related sterol compounds including alfacalcidol, calcifediol, calcitriol, colecalciferol, dihydrotachysterol, and ergocalciferol. Newer vitamin D analogues include doxercalciferol, paricalcitol, and maxacalcitol.

Alfacalcidol (7885-p)

Alfacalcidol (BAN, rINN).

EB-644; 1α-Hydroxycholecalciferol; 1α-Hydroxyvitamin D$_3$; 1α-OHD$_3$.   (5Z,7E)-9,10-Secocholesta-5,7,10(19)-triene-1α,3β-diol.
$C_{27}H_{44}O_2 = 400.6$.
CAS — 41294-56-8.
ATC — A11CC03.
Pharmacopoeias. In Eur. (see p.vi).

Pharmacopoeial description
Ph. Eur.: White or almost white crystals which are sensitive to air, heat, and light. Practically insoluble in water; freely soluble in alcohol; soluble in fatty oils. Reversible isomerisation to pre-alfacalcidol takes place in solution, depending on temperature and time. Activity is due to both compounds. Store at 2° to 8° under an atmosphere of nitrogen in airtight containers. The contents of an opened container should be used immediately. Protect from light.

Calcifediol (7886-s)

Calcifediol (BAN, USAN, rINN).

Calcidiol; 25-Hydroxycholecalciferol; 25-Hydroxyvitamin D$_3$; 25-(OH)D$_3$; U-32070E. (5Z,7E)-9,10-Secocholesta-5,7,10(19)-triene-3β,25-diol monohydrate.
$C_{27}H_{44}O_2,H_2O = 418.7$.
CAS — 19356-17-3 (anhydrous calcifediol); 63283-36-3 (calcifediol monohydrate).
ATC — A11CC06.
Pharmacopoeias. In Eur. (see p.vi) and US.

Pharmacopoeial description
Ph. Eur.: White or almost white crystals which are sensitive to air, heat, and light. Practically insoluble in water; freely soluble in alcohol; soluble in fatty oils. Reversible isomerisation to pre-calcifediol takes place in solution, depending on temperature and time. The activity is due to both compounds. Store at 2° to 8° under an atmosphere of nitrogen in airtight containers. The contents of an opened container should be used immediately. Protect from light.
USP 25: Store in airtight containers. Protect from light.

Calcitriol (7887-w)

Calcitriol (BAN, USAN, rINN).

Calcitriolum; 1,25-Dihydroxycholecalciferol; 1α,25-Dihydroxycholecalciferol; 1α,25-Dihydroxyvitamin D$_3$; 1α,25(OH)$_2$D$_3$; Ro-21-5535.   (5Z,7E)-9,10-Secocholesta-5,7,10(19)-triene-1α,3β,25-triol.
$C_{27}H_{44}O_3 = 416.6$.
CAS — 32222-06-3.
ATC — A11CC04; D05AX03.
Pharmacopoeias. In Eur. (see p.vi).

Pharmacopoeial description
Ph. Eur.: White or almost white crystals. Practically insoluble in water; freely soluble in alcohol; soluble in fatty oils. It is sensitive to air, heat, and light. A reversible isomerisation to pre-calcitriol takes place in solution, depending on temperature and time. The activity is due to both compounds. Store at 2° to 8° under an atmosphere of nitrogen in airtight containers. The contents of an opened container should be used immediately. Protect from light.

Colecalciferol (7888-e)

Colecalciferol (BAN, rINN).

Activated 7-Dehydrocholesterol; Cholecalciferol; Cholecalciferolum; Vitamin D$_3$. (5Z,7E)-9,10-Secocholesta-5,7,10(19)-trien-3β-ol.
$C_{27}H_{44}O = 384.6$.
CAS — 67-97-0.
ATC — A11CC05.
Pharmacopoeias. In Chin., Eur. (see p.vi), Int., Jpn, Pol., and US. Eur. also includes monographs for Cholecalciferol Concentrate (Oily Form), Cholecalciferol Concentrate (Powder Form), and Cholecalciferol Concentrate (Water-dispersible Form). US also includes Cholecalciferol Solution.

The symbol † denotes a preparation no longer actively marketed

---

The naturally occurring form of vitamin D. It is produced from 7-dehydrocholesterol, a sterol present in mammalian skin, by ultraviolet irradiation.

Pharmacopoeial description
Ph. Eur.: White or almost white crystals which are sensitive to air, heat, and light. Practically insoluble in water; freely soluble in alcohol; soluble in fatty oils. Solutions in volatile solvents are unstable and should be used immediately. A reversible isomerisation to pre-colecalciferol takes place in solution, depending on temperature and time. The activity is due to both compounds. Store under nitrogen in airtight containers at a temperature of 2° to 8°. The contents of an opened container should be used immediately. Protect from light.
USP 25: White, odourless crystals. Insoluble in water; soluble in alcohol, in chloroform, and in fatty oils. M.p. about 85°. It is affected by air and light. Store under nitrogen in hermetically sealed containers at a temperature of 8° to 15°. Protect from light.

Dihydrotachysterol (7891-g)

Dihydrotachysterol (BAN, rINN).

Dichysterol.   (5E,7E,22E)-10α-9,10-Secoergosta-5,7,22-trien-3β-ol.
$C_{28}H_{46}O = 398.7$.
CAS — 67-96-9.
ATC — A11CC02.
Pharmacopoeias. In US.

Pharmacopoeial description
USP 25: Colourless or white, odourless crystals, or white, odourless, crystalline powder. Practically insoluble in water; soluble in alcohol; freely soluble in chloroform and in ether; sparingly soluble in vegetable oils. Store in hermetic glass containers from which the air has been displaced by an inert gas. Protect from light.

Doxercalciferol (15029-j)

Doxercalciferol (USAN, rINN).

1α-Hydroxyergocalciferol; 1α-Hydroxyvitamin D$_2$; 1α-OH-D$_2$. (5Z,7E,22E)-9,10-Secoergosta-5,7,10(19),22-tetraene-1α,3β-diol.
$C_{28}H_{44}O_2 = 412.6$.
CAS — 54573-75-0.

Ergocalciferol (7884-q)

Ergocalciferol (BAN, rINN).

Calciferol; Ergocalciferolum; Irradiated Ergosterol; Viosterol; Vitamin D$_2$. (5Z,7E,22E)-9,10-Secoergosta-5,7,10(19),22-tetraen-3β-ol.
$C_{28}H_{44}O = 396.6$.
CAS — 50-14-6.
ATC — A11CC01.
Pharmacopoeias. In Chin., Eur. (see p.vi), Int., Jpn, and US.

An antirachitic substance obtained from ergosterol, a sterol present in fungi and yeasts, by ultraviolet irradiation.

Pharmacopoeial description
Ph. Eur.: White or almost white, crystals or white or slightly yellowish crystalline powder. It is sensitive to air, heat, and light. Practically insoluble in water; freely soluble in alcohol; soluble in fatty oils. Solutions in volatile solvents are unstable and should be used immediately. A reversible isomerisation to pre-ergocalciferol takes place in solution, depending on temperature and time. The activity is due to both compounds. Store under nitrogen in airtight containers at a temperature of 2° to 8°. The contents of an opened container should be used immediately. Protect from light.
USP 25: White, odourless crystals. It is affected by air and light. Insoluble in water; soluble in alcohol, in chloroform, in ether, and in fatty oils. Store in hermetically sealed containers under nitrogen at a temperature of 8° to 15°. Protect from light.

Maxacalcitol (5594-b)

Maxacalcitol (USAN, rINN).

1α,25-Dihydroxy-22-oxavitamin D$_3$; OCT; 22-Oxacalcitriol; Sch-209579.   (+)-(5Z,7E,20S)-20-(3-Hydroxy-3-methylbutoxy)-9,10-secopregna-5,7,10(19)-triene-1α,3β-diol.
$C_{26}H_{42}O_4 = 418.6$.
CAS — 103909-75-7.

Paricalcitol (19956-c)

Paricalcitol (USAN, rINN).

Compound 49510. (7E,22E)-19-Nor-9,10-secoergosta-5,7,22-triene-1α,3β,25-triol.
$C_{27}H_{44}O_3 = 416.6$.
CAS — 131918-61-1.

Units
The Second International Standard Preparation (1949) of vitamin D consisted of bottles containing approximately 6 g of a solution of colecalciferol in vegetable oil (1000 units per g). This standard has now been discontinued.

NOTE. One unit of vitamin D is contained in 25 nanograms of colecalciferol or ergocalciferol (i.e. 1 mg of colecalciferol or ergocalciferol is equivalent to 40 000 units of vitamin D as determined by bioassay in *rats*).

Adverse Effects and Treatment
Excessive intake of vitamin D leads to the development of hypercalcaemia and its associated effects including hypercalciuria, ectopic calcification, and renal and cardiovascular damage (for a discussion of vitamin-D mediated hypercalcaemia and its treatment, see p.1181). Symptoms of overdosage include anorexia, lassitude, nausea and vomiting, diarrhoea, polyuria, sweating, headache, thirst, and vertigo. Interindividual tolerance to vitamin D varies considerably; infants and children are generally more susceptible to its toxic effects. The vitamin should be withdrawn if toxicity occurs. It has been stated that vitamin D dietary supplementation may be detrimental in persons already receiving an adequate intake through diet and exposure to sunlight, since the difference between therapeutic and toxic concentrations is relatively small.

The most potent forms of vitamin D, such as alfacalcidol and calcitriol, might reasonably be expected to pose a greater risk of toxicity; however, their effects are reversed rapidly on withdrawal.

Hypersensitivity reactions have occurred.

◊ Vitamin D is the most likely of all vitamins to cause overt toxicity. Doses of 60 000 units per day can cause hypercalcaemia, with muscle weakness, apathy, headache, anorexia, nausea and vomiting, bone pain, ectopic calcification, proteinuria, hypertension, and cardiac arrhythmias. Chronic hypercalcaemia can lead to generalised vascular calcification, nephrocalcinosis, and rapid deterioration of renal function.[1] A number of reports of accidental overdosage, leading to hypercalcaemia or nephrocalcinosis, occurred in the UK following introduction of a concentrated alfacalcidol oral solution that was 10 times stronger than the former presentation.[2]

Hypercalcaemia has been reported in one person following brief industrial exposure to colecalciferol.[3]

A study in children treated for renal osteodystrophy has provided some evidence that hypercalcaemia may occur more frequently with calcitriol than with ergocalciferol.[4] Another such study has suggested that vitamin D has nephrotoxic properties independent of the degree of induced hypercalcaemia, and that the decline in renal function may be more marked with calcitriol.[5]

Topical calcitriol may affect calcium homoeostasis, and hypercalcaemia has been reported in some studies.[6] For mention of the effect of other vitamin D analogues used in psoriasis on calcium homoeostasis, see p.1112.

1. Anonymous. *Med Lett Drugs Ther* 1984; **26:** 73.
2. Committee on Safety of Medicines/Medicines Control Agency. Accidental overdose with alfacalcidol (One-Alpha drops). *Current Problems* 2001; **27:** 3.
3. Jibani M, Hodges NH. Prolonged hypercalcaemia after industrial exposure to vitamin D$_3$. *BMJ* 1985; **290:** 748–9.
4. Hodson EM, *et al.* Treatment of childhood renal osteodystrophy with calcitriol or ergocalciferol. *Clin Nephrol* 1985; **24:** 192–200.
5. Chan JCM, *et al.* A prospective, double-blind study of growth failure in children with chronic renal insufficiency and the effectiveness of treatment with calcitriol versus dihydrotachysterol. *J Pediatr* 1994; **124:** 520–8.
6. Bourke JF, *et al.* Vitamin D analogues in psoriasis: effects on systemic calcium homeostasis. *Br J Dermatol* 1996; **135:** 347–54.

Precautions
Vitamin D should not be administered to patients with hypercalcaemia. It should be administered with caution to infants as they may have increased sensitivity to its effects and should be used with care in patients with renal impairment or calculi, or heart disease, who might be at increased risk of organ damage if hypercalcaemia occurred. Plasma phosphate concentrations should be controlled during vitamin D therapy to reduce the risk of ectopic calcification.

It is advised that patients receiving pharmacological doses of vitamin D should have their plasma-calcium concentration monitored at regular intervals, especially initially and if symptoms suggest toxicity (see above). Similar monitoring is recommended in infants if they are breast fed by mothers receiving pharmacological doses of vitamin D.

Pregnancy. Hypercalcaemia during pregnancy may produce congenital disorders in the offspring, and neonatal hypoparathyroidism. However, the risks to the fetus of untreated maternal hypoparathyroidism are considered greater than the risks of hypercalcaemia due to vitamin D therapy. Indeed, one report noted increased requirements for vitamin D preparations during pregnancy for the treatment of hypoparathyroidism;[1] the doses tended to need increasing during the second half of pregnancy. In one woman in whom the dose of calcitriol was kept at the increased level after delivery (in an attempt to allow for the calcium loss involved in breast feeding) hypercalcaemia developed; this did not occur in 2 women who did not breast feed and in whom the dose of the vitamin D preparations was reduced soon after delivery.[1]

1. Caplan RH, Beguin EA. Hypercalcemia in a calcitriol-treated hypoparathyroid woman during lactation. *Obstet Gynecol* 1990; **76:** 485–9.

Interactions
There is an increased risk of hypercalcaemia if vitamin D is coadministered with thiazide diuretics and calcium. Plasma-calcium concentrations should be monitored in patients receiving the drugs concurrently. Some antiepileptics may increase vitamin D requirements (e.g. carbamazepine, phenobarbital, phenytoin, and primidone).

Danazol. A report of hypercalcaemia associated with danazol in a patient maintained on alfacalcidol therapy for hypoparathyroidism.[1] Introduction of danazol appeared to reduce the maintenance requirement for alfacalcidol.

1. Hepburn NC, *et al.* Danazol-induced hypercalcaemia in alpha-calcidol-treated hypoparathyroidism. *Postgrad Med J* 1989; **65:** 849–50.

Thyroxine [levothyroxine]. Three patients receiving dihydrotachysterol and calcium for postoperative hypoparathyroidism, following thyroidectomy, developed hypercalcaemia when their concomitant thyroxine [levothyroxine] therapy was discontinued before a radio-iodine scan.[1] The dose of dihydrotachysterol should be reduced and serum-calcium concentrations should be monitored when thyroid treatment is interrupted, since elimination of dihydrotachysterol may be delayed in hypothyroidism.

1. Lamberg B-A, Tikkanen MJ. Hypercalcaemia due to dihydrotachysterol treatment in patients with hypothyroidism after thyroidectomy. *BMJ* 1981; **283:** 461–2.

Pharmacokinetics
Vitamin D substances are well absorbed from the gastrointestinal tract. The presence of bile is essential for adequate intestinal absorption; absorption may be decreased in patients with decreased fat absorption.

Vitamin D and its metabolites circulate in the blood bound to a specific α-globulin. Vitamin D can be stored in adipose and muscle tissue for long periods of time. It is slowly released from such storage sites and from the skin where it is formed in the presence of sunlight or ultraviolet light. Ergocalciferol and colecalciferol have a slow onset and a long duration of action; calcitriol and its analogue alfacalcidol, however, have a more rapid action and shorter half-lives.

Colecalciferol and ergocalciferol are hydroxylated in the liver by the enzyme vitamin D 25-hydroxylase to form 25-hydroxycholecalciferol (calcifediol) and 25-hydroxyergocalciferol respectively. These compounds undergo further hydroxylation in the kidneys by the enzyme vitamin D 1-hydroxylase to form the active metabolites 1,25-dihydroxycholecalciferol (calcitriol) and 1,25-dihydroxyergocalciferol respectively. Further metabolism also occurs in the kidneys, including the formation of the 1,24,25-trihydroxy derivatives. Of the synthetic analogues, alfacalcidol is converted rapidly in the liver to calcitriol, and dihydrotachysterol is hydroxylated, also in the liver, to its active form 25-hydroxydihydrotachysterol.

Vitamin D compounds and their metabolites are excreted mainly in the bile and faeces with only small amounts appearing in urine; there is some enterohepatic recycling but it is considered to have a negligible contribution to vitamin D status. Certain vitamin D substances may be distributed into breast milk.

Human Requirements
The daily requirements of vitamin D in adults are small and may be met mainly by exposure to sunlight and/or obtained from the diet. A daily dietary intake of about 200 to 400 units (5 to 10 µg of colecalciferol or ergocalciferol) of vitamin D is generally considered adequate for healthy adults. In comparison with

older adults (in the age range of 25 years upwards) the requirements per kg body-weight are greater in infants, children, and young adults and during pregnancy and lactation. Requirements may also be higher in people who are not exposed to adequate sunlight such as the elderly or housebound.

Vitamin D is present in few foods. Fish-liver oils, especially cod-liver oil, are good sources of vitamin D. Other sources, which contain much smaller amounts, include butter, eggs, and liver. Some foods are fortified with vitamin D, and milk and margarine may therefore also supply the vitamin. Cooking processes do not appear to affect the activity of vitamin D.

◊ In the UK dietary reference values (see p.1352) for vitamin D have only been published for selected groups of the population.[1] In the USA recommended dietary allowances had been set, and have recently been replaced by dietary reference intakes[2] (see p.1352). Differing amounts are recommended for infants and children of varying ages, for adults, and for pregnant and lactating women. In the UK a dietary intake was considered unnecessary for adults living a normal lifestyle who were being exposed to solar radiation; for those confined indoors a reference nutrient intake (RNI) of 10 µg [as colecalciferol or ergocalciferol] daily was set. This RNI of 10 µg daily was also considered to be applicable to all persons aged 65 years or more and to pregnant and lactating women. RNIs were set for children up to the age of 3 years; dietary intake was considered unnecessary for older children. Mention was made that in order to achieve the above reference nutrient intakes, supplementation of the diet may actually be required and supplementation was also recommended for Asian women and children in the UK. In the USA,[2] adequate intakes for vitamin D are: 5 µg daily (as colecalciferol) for all persons from birth through to age 50 years, including pregnant or lactating women; 10 µg daily for adults aged 51 to 70 years; and 15 µg daily for those aged greater than 70 years. The tolerable upper intake level is 50 µg daily.

1. DoH. Dietary reference values for food energy and nutrients for the United Kingdom: report of the panel on dietary reference values of the committee on medical aspects of food policy. *Report on health and social subjects 41.* London: HMSO, 1991.
2. Standing Committee on the Scientific Evaluation of Dietary Reference Intakes of the Food and Nutrition Board. *Dietary Reference Intakes for calcium, phosphorus, magnesium, vitamin D, and fluoride.* Washington, DC: National Academy Press, 1999.

Uses and Administration
Vitamin D compounds are fat-soluble sterols, sometimes considered to be hormones or hormone precursors, which are essential for the proper regulation of calcium and phosphate homoeostasis and bone mineralisation.

Vitamin D deficiency develops when there is inadequate exposure to sunlight or a lack of the vitamin in the diet. Deficiency generally takes a prolonged period of time to develop due to slow release of the vitamin from body stores. Deficiency may occur in some infants who are breast fed without supplemental vitamin D or exposure to sunlight, in the elderly whose mobility and thus exposure to light may be impaired, and in persons with fat malabsorption syndromes; certain disease states such as renal failure may also affect the metabolism of vitamin D substances to metabolically active forms and thus result in deficiency. Deficiency leads to the development of a syndrome characterised by hypocalcaemia, hypophosphataemia, undermineralisation or demineralisation of bone, bone pain, bone fractures, and muscle weakness, known in adults as osteomalacia (see below). In children, in whom there may be growth retardation and skeletal deformity, especially of the long bones, it is known as rickets.

Vitamin D compounds are used in the treatment and prevention of vitamin D deficiency states and hypocalcaemia associated with disorders such as hypoparathyroidism and secondary hyperparathyroidism as indicated by the cross-references given below.

A variety of forms and analogues of vitamin D are available, and the choice of agent depends on the cause of the condition to be treated and the relative properties of the available agents. Colecalciferol and ergocalciferol are equal in potency, and have a slow onset and relatively prolonged duration of action. Dihydrotachysterol has relatively weak antirachitic activity, but its actions are faster in onset and less persistent than those of the calciferols and it does not

require renal hydroxylation. Calcifediol, an intermediate metabolite, has some action of its own but is also converted to the more potent 1,25-dihydroxycholecalciferol (calcitriol); calcitriol and its analogue alfacalcidol are the most potent and rapidly acting of the vitamin D substances.

• For the treatment of simple nutritional deficiencies **colecalciferol** or **ergocalciferol** are generally preferred. They are usually given by mouth, but may also be administered by intramuscular injection. A dose of 10 µg (400 units) daily is generally sufficient in adults for the prevention of simple deficiency states; in the UK, 20 µg (800 units) daily is recommended in some ethnic groups consuming unleavened bread, and in the elderly living alone. Deficiency due to malabsorption states or liver disease often requires higher doses for treatment, of up to 1 mg (40 000 units) daily. Doses of up to 2.5 mg (100 000 units) daily may be used in the treatment of hypocalcaemia due to hypoparathyroidism.

• Where large doses are required it may be preferable to use one of the more potent derivatives. In particular, when renal function is impaired as in secondary hyperparathyroidism associated with chronic renal failure, with consequent reduction in the conversion of calciferols to their active metabolites, then alfacalcidol, calcitriol, or doxercalciferol, which do not require renal hydroxylation, should be given. Paricalcitol and maxacalcitol are newer vitamin D analogues used similarly. **Calcitriol** is given by mouth or by intravenous injection. Usual initial adult doses of 0.25 µg daily or on alternate days are given by mouth, increased if necessary, in steps of 0.25 µg at intervals of 2 to 4 weeks, to a usual dose of 0.5 to 1 µg daily. Initial doses intravenously are usually 0.5 µg three times a week increased if necessary in steps of 0.25 to 0.5 µg at intervals of 2 to 4 weeks, to a usual dose of 0.5 to 3 µg three times a week. Alternatively, **alfacalcidol** is given in initial doses of 1 µg daily by mouth, or 0.5 µg for elderly patients. Doses of 0.25 to 1 µg daily may be given for maintenance. Suggested doses for children under 20 kg are 0.05 µg (50 nanograms) per kg body-weight daily and for premature infants and neonates a dose of 0.05 to 0.1 µg (50 to 100 nanograms) per kg daily. Doses of alfacalcidol may also be given by intravenous injection over 30 seconds. **Doxercalciferol** is given by mouth or intravenous injection. The initial oral dose is 10 µg three times weekly at dialysis, increased by increments of 2.5 µg after 8 weeks if necessary. The maximum recommended dose by mouth is 20 µg three times weekly. The initial intravenous dose is 4 µg given three times weekly, and increased after 8 weeks in increments of 1 to 2 µg if required. **Paricalcitol** is administered intravenously at a dose of 0.04 to 0.1 µg (40 to 100 nanograms) per kg body-weight on alternate days or less frequently. The dose may be increased if necessary by 2 to 4 µg at intervals of 2 to 4 weeks.

• Of the other available forms, **calcifediol**, the 25-hydroxylated metabolite of colecalciferol, is given in usual adult doses of 50 to 100 µg daily or 100 to 200 µg on alternate days by mouth. For hypocalcaemic tetany due to hypoparathyroidism, **dihydrotachysterol** is given in initial adult doses of 250 to 2500 µg daily by mouth, depending on severity. Maintenance doses have ranged from 250 µg per week to 1000 µg daily.

When vitamin D substances are given in pharmacological doses, dosage must be individualised for each patient, and should be based on regular monitoring of plasma-calcium concentrations (initially weekly, and then every 2 to 4 weeks), to optimise clinical response and avoid hypercalcaemia.

Vitamin D, usually in the form of calcitriol, may be used in the treatment of osteoporosis (see below). In established postmenopausal osteoporosis, calcitriol 0.25 µg twice daily is recommended. Vitamin D and calcium supplements are often given as adjuncts to other therapies in osteoporosis.

Calcitriol has been used in the management of psoriasis (see below).

Calciferol derivatives are used as a rodenticide.

◊ General references.
1. Fraser DR. Vitamin D. *Lancet* 1995; **345:** 104–7.
2. van der Wielen RPJ, *et al.* Serum vitamin D concentrations among elderly people in Europe. *Lancet* 1995; **346:** 207–10.
3. Gloth FM, *et al.* Vitamin D deficiency in homebound elderly persons. *JAMA* 1995; **274:** 1683–6.
4. Nellen JFJB, *et al.* Hypovitaminosis D in immigrant women: slow to be diagnosed. *BMJ* 1996; **312:** 570–2.
5. Thomas MK, *et al.* Hypovitaminosis D in medical inpatients. *N Engl J Med* 1998; **338:** 777–83.
6. Compston JE. Vitamin D deficiency: time for action. *BMJ* 1998; **317:** 1466–7.

Hyperparathyroidism. Vitamin D has been employed for certain forms of hyperparathyroidism. The secondary hyperparathyroidism of renal osteodystrophy (p.746) may respond to oral or intravenous treatment with calcitriol, or its analogue alfacalcidol,[1-3] which do not require renal hydroxylation for activation. Newer analogues for this indication include paricalcitol,[4] doxercalciferol,[5] and falecalcitriol.[6] However, doses capable of suppressing parathyroid hormone secretion may lead to hypercalcaemia[3] and a decline in renal function[7] (see also under Adverse Effects, above).

1. Andress DL, *et al.* Intravenous calcitriol in the treatment of refractory osteitis fibrosa of chronic renal failure. *N Engl J Med* 1989; **321:** 274–9.
2. Argilés À, *et al.* High-dose alfacalcidol for anaemia in dialysis. *Lancet* 1993; **342:** 378–9.
3. Quarles LD, *et al.* Prospective trial of pulse oral versus intravenous calcitriol treatment of hyperparathyroidism in ESRD. *Kidney Int* 1994; **45:** 1710–21.
4. Martin KJ, *et al.* Therapy of secondary hyperparathyroidism with 19-nor-1α,25-dihydroxyvitamin D₂. *Am J Kidney Dis* 1998; **32** (suppl 2): S61–6.
5. Frazão JM, *et al.* Intermittent doxercalciferol (1α-hydroxyvitamin D₂) therapy for secondary hyperparathyroidism. *Am J Kidney Dis* 2000; **36:** 550–61.
6. Akiba T, *et al.* Controlled trial of falecalcitriol versus alfacalcidol in suppression of parathyroid hormone in hemodialysis patients with secondary hyperparathyroidism. *Am J Kidney Dis* 1998; **32:** 238–46.
7. Chan JCM, *et al.* A prospective, double-blind study of growth failure in children with chronic renal insufficiency and the effectiveness of treatment with calcitriol versus dihydrotachysterol. *J Pediatr* 1994; **124:** 520–8.

Hypoparathyroidism. Although parenteral calcium salts may be given acutely for hypocalcaemic tetany, long-term treatment of hypoparathyroidism (p.747) usually aims at correction of associated hypocalcaemia with oral vitamin D compounds, which increase the intestinal absorption of calcium. If dietary calcium is inadequate these may be combined with calcium supplementation.

Hypoparathyroidism in *pregnancy* poses severe risks of fetal hyperparathyroidism with neonatal hypocalcaemic rickets, which may be fatal. Treatment with calcium and either colecalciferol or ergocalciferol in doses of 1.25 to 2.5 mg daily, or dihydrotachysterol 0.25 to 1.0 mg daily is essential.[1]

1. Hague WM. Treatment of endocrine diseases. *BMJ* 1987; **294:** 297–300.

Malignant neoplasms. The active form of vitamin D, calcitriol (1,25-dihydroxycholecalciferol) has been found to promote tissue differentiation and to inhibit cellular proliferation *in vitro*. These findings have prompted workers to investigate the potential role and efficacy of vitamin D metabolites or analogues (sometimes referred to as deltanoids) in malignant neoplasms and in other disorders of cell growth such as psoriasis (see below).

Animal and *in vitro* studies with alfacalcidol have led to the suggestion that evaluation should be undertaken in malignant disease of the human breast.[1] A study in humans has been performed with the calcitriol derivative calcipotriol (p.1112); in this trial calcipotriol used topically in advanced or cutaneous metastatic breast cancer was considered to exert some positive effects and further investigation was considered warranted.[2] Regression of T-cell lymphoma of the skin (mycosis fungoides, p.489) has been reported following application of calcipotriol,[3] and following systemic treatment with calcitriol and a retinoid in a patient who failed to respond to topical calcipotriol.[4] However, 3 other patients with cutaneous T-cell lymphoma failed to respond to calcitriol and isotretinoin,[5] which may have been because of the phenotype or stage of the disease.[6]

1. Colston KW, *et al.* Possible role for 1,25-dihydroxyvitamin D in controlling breast cancer cell proliferation. *Lancet* 1989; **i:** 188–91.
2. Bower M, *et al.* Topical calcipotriol treatment in advanced breast cancer. *Lancet* 1991; **337:** 701–2. Correction. *ibid.*; 1618.
3. Scott-Mackie P, *et al.* Calcipotriol and regression in T-cell lymphoma of skin. *Lancet* 1993; **342:** 172.
4. French LE, *et al.* Remission of cutaneous T-cell lymphoma with combined calcitriol and acitretin. *Lancet* 1994; **344:** 686–7.
5. Thomsen K. Cutaneous T-cell lymphoma and calcitriol and isotretinoin treatment. *Lancet* 1995; **345:** 1583.
6. French LE, Saurat J-H. Treatment of cutaneous T-cell lymphoma by retinoids and calcitriol. *Lancet* 1995; **346:** 376–7.

Osteomalacia. Treatment of osteomalacia (p.744) primarily aims at correcting any underlying deficiency states, and vitamin D substances, calcium, or phosphate supplements may be given by mouth as necessary. Where rickets is due to impaired synthesis of calcitriol (type I pseudodeficiency) or receptor resistance (type II pseudodeficiency) replacement therapy with calcitriol may be indicated (in the latter case with very high dose calcium),[1] while X-linked hypophosphataemic rickets is generally treated with phosphate supplementation and calcitriol, although vitamin D alone is also effective.[2] The use of single large doses of a vitamin D substance (stosstherapie), for the prophylaxis of rickets, is highly controversial because of problems with toxicity, although it may be effective in patients with rickets due to proven vitamin D deficiency.[3]

1. Hochberg Z, *et al.* Calcium therapy for calcitriol-resistant rickets. *J Pediatr* 1992; **121:** 803–8.
2. Seikaly MG, *et al.* The effect of phosphate supplementation on linear growth in children with X-linked hypophosphatemia. *Pediatrics* 1994; **94:** 478–81.
3. Shah BR, Finberg L. Single-day therapy for nutritional vitamin D-deficiency rickets: a preferred method. *J Pediatr* 1994; **125:** 487–90.

The symbol † denotes a preparation no longer actively marketed

PREGNANCY AND THE NEONATE. Most infants receive adequate calcium and vitamin D during pregnancy and during breast feeding or bottle feeding to prevent the development of rickets. However, it is considered that there are certain groups of women whose infants may be at special risk of neonatal rickets and these include those suffering economic deprivation, those living at high latitudes, and Asian immigrants in northern Europe, especially in winter. It is therefore suggested that pregnant women in such circumstances should receive supplements as the diet and sunshine exposure may not be providing adequate calcium (1 to 1.2 g daily) or vitamin D (400 units daily).[1]

Rickets may be more problematical in the premature infant as vitamin D requirements may be increased. Although there is no evidence that routine administration is necessary or desirable, healing of illness as a result of rickets may be achieved rapidly by the use of alfacalcidol 100 to 200 nanograms per kg bodyweight daily.[2]

1. Misra R, Anderson DC. Providing the fetus with calcium. *BMJ* 1990; **300:** 1220–1.
2. Brooke OG. Supplementary vitamin D in infancy and childhood. *Arch Dis Child* 1983; **58:** 573–4.

Osteopetrosis. For mention of the use of high-dose calcitriol in the management of juvenile osteopetrosis, see under Corticosteroids, p.1053.

Osteoporosis. Studies using vitamin D in pharmacological[1-3] or supplemental[4-6] doses for the treatment of osteoporosis (p.745) have produced conflicting results.[1-7] However, in patients over 75 years of age, in whom dietary deficiencies are common, calcium and vitamin D supplements are recommended.

Vitamin D may be used in the prevention of corticosteroid-induced osteoporosis, see Effects on Bones and Joints, p.1040.

1. Ott SM, Chesnut CH. Calcitriol treatment is not effective in postmenopausal osteoporosis. *Ann Intern Med* 1989; **110:** 267–74.
2. Gallagher JC, Goldgar D. Treatment of postmenopausal osteoporosis with high doses of synthetic calcitriol: a randomized controlled study. *Ann Intern Med* 1990; **113:** 649–55.
3. Tilyard MW, *et al.* Treatment of postmenopausal osteoporosis with calcitriol or calcium. *N Engl J Med* 1992; **326:** 357–62.
4. Chapuy MC, *et al.* Effect of calcium and cholecalciferol treatment for three years on hip fractures in elderly women. *BMJ* 1994; **308:** 1081–2.
5. Lips P, *et al.* Vitamin D supplementation and fracture incidence in elderly persons. *Ann Intern Med* 1996; **124:** 400–6.
6. Dawson-Hughes B, *et al.* Effect of calcium and vitamin D supplementation on bone density in men and women 65 years of age or older. *N Engl J Med* 1997; **337:** 670–6.
7. Gillespie WJ, *et al.* Vitamin D and vitamin D analogues for preventing fractures associated with involutional and post-menopausal osteoporosis (updated 30 August 2001). Available in The Cochrane Library; Issue 4. Oxford: Update Software; 2001.

Psoriasis. A vitamin D analogue, calcipotriol (p.1112), is often used as an alternative to more traditional topical agents such as coal tar or dithranol in the initial management of mild to moderate psoriasis (p.1106). Another vitamin D analogue, tacalcitol (p.1124), is used similarly, and maxacalcitol[1] is being investigated. Calcitriol itself has been tried, both topically[2,3] and orally.[4]

1. Barker JNWN, *et al.* Topical maxacalcitol for the treatment of psoriasis vulgaris: a placebo-controlled, double-blind, dose-finding study with active comparator. *Br J Dermatol* 1999; **141:** 274–8.
2. Sips AJAM, *et al.* Topically applied low-dose calcitriol has no calciotropic effect in patients with stable plaque psoriasis. *J Am Acad Dermatol* 1994; **30:** 966–9.
3. Langner A, *et al.* A long-term multicentre assessment of the safety and tolerability of calcitriol ointment in the treatment of chronic plaque psoriasis. *Br J Dermatol* 1996; **135:** 385–9.
4. Perez A, *et al.* Safety and efficacy of oral calcitriol (1,25-dihydroxyvitamin D₃) for the treatment of psoriasis. *Br J Dermatol* 1996; **134:** 1070–8.

Renal osteodystrophy. See under Hyperparathyroidism, above.

Rickets. See Osteomalacia, above.

Preparations

BP 2001: Calcitriol Capsules; Calcium and Colecalciferol Tablets; Calcium and Ergocalciferol Tablets; Colecalciferol Injection; Colecalciferol Tablets; Ergocalciferol Injection; Ergocalciferol Tablets;
BPC 1973: Calcium with Vitamin D Tablets; Vitamins A and D Capsules;
USP 25: Calcifediol Capsules; Calcium with Vitamin D Tablets; Dihydrotachysterol Capsules; Dihydrotachysterol Oral Solution; Dihydrotachysterol Tablets; Ergocalciferol Capsules; Ergocalciferol Oral Solution; Ergocalciferol Tablets; Oleovitamin A and D; Oleovitamin A and D Capsules.

Proprietary Preparations (details are given in Part 3)
Aust.: AT 10; Calcijex; Etalpha; Laeovit D₃; Oleovit D₃; Rocaltrol; Vi-De₃; *Austral.:* AT 10†; Calcijex; Citrihexal; Ostelin; Rocaltrol; Sitriol; *Belg.:* 1-Alpha; AT 10; D-Cure; Dedrogyl; Dihydral†; Rocaltrol; Sterogyl†; *Braz.:* Rocaltrol; *Canad.:* Calcijex†; D-Tabs†; D-Vi-Sol; Drisdol; Hytakerol; One-Alpha; Ostoforte; Rocaltrol; *Denm.:* Dygratyl; Etalpha; Rocaltrol; *Fin.:* Calcijex; Deetipat; Devitol; Dygratyl; Etalpha; Jekovit; *Fr.:* Adrigyl; Dedrogyl; Densical vitamine D₃; Rocaltrol; Sterogyl; Un-Alfa; Uvedose; Uvesterol D; Zyma-D2; *Ger.:* AT 10; Bondiol; D-Mulsin; D-Tracetten; D₃ Vicotrat; Decostriol; Dedrei; Dedrogyl; Dekristol; Doss; EinsAlpha; Ospur D₃; Rocaltrol; Tachystin; Vigantol; Vigantoletten; Vigorsan; *Hong Kong:* Alfarol; Alpha D3; Calcijex; One-Alpha; Rocaltrol; *Irl.:* AT 10†; Calcijex; One-Alpha; Rocaltrol; *Israel:* Alpha D3; Calcijex; One-Alpha; Osteo D; *Ital.:* Alpha D3; Atiten; Dediol; Deril; Didrogyl; Difix; Diseon; Diserinal; Ostelin; Ostidil; Rocaltrol; Tridelta; *Jpn:* Alfarol; *Mex.:*

Alfad; Calcijex; Doferol; Genevis D2; Rocaltrol; Tirocal; Vita-D-Grin; *Neth.:* Devaron; Dihydral; Etalpha; Neo Dohyfral; Rocaltrol; *Norw.:* AFI-D₂; Calcijex; Etalpha; Rocaltrol; *NZ:* One-Alpha; Rocaltrol; *Port.:* Dedrogyl; Rocaltrol; Vigantol; *S.Afr.:* AT 10†; One-Alpha; Rocaltrol; *Singapore:* Alpha D3; Bongreen; Calcijex; One-Alpha; Rocaltrol; Roical; *Spain:* Alfadelta; Calcijex; Etalpha; Hidroferol; Rocaltrol; *Swed.:* Calcijex; Detrixin†; Devitre; Dygratyl; Etalpha; Rocaltrol; *Switz.:* AT 10; Calcijex; Rocaltrol; Vi-De₃; *Thai.:* Alpha D3; Bon-One; One-Alpha; Rocaltrol; *UK:* Alfad; AT 10; Calcijex; One-Alpha; Rocaltrol; *USA:* Calciferol; Calcijex; Calderol; Delta-D; DHT; Drisdol; Hectorol; Hytakerol; Rocaltrol; Zemplar.

Multi-ingredient: *Aust.:* Cal-De; Cal-De-Ce†; Calcipot D₃; Calcisan D; Maagersan†; Maxi-Kalz Vit D3; Oleovit A + D; Ruticalzon; Vitapan; *Austral.:* Bio Magnesium; Caltrate + Vitamin D; Caltrate Plus; Calvita Osti†; Children's Calcium With Minerals†; FAB Tri-Cal; Halivol†; Lifesystem Mineral Plus Formula 10 Osteoporosis†; Natures Way Total Calcium Plus; Osteoporosis Mineral Plus Formula 9†; Prosteo; Red Seal Liquid Calcium; Soy Forte with Block Cohosh; *Belg.:* Ad-Vitan†; Cacit Vitamine D₃; D-Vital; Neo-Debiol AD3; Newderm; Pyal†; Vitaminic A-D†; Vitamorrhuine; *Braz.:* AD Til; ADE 2; Aderofix D3; Aderogil D3; Gaduol; Gotil-AD; Hipoderme; Hipodermon; Hipodex; Hipoglos; Hipoglos com Hidrocortisona; Hipoglos Oftalmico; Hormoginase; Normagrin; *Canad.:* A & D Ointment; Antiseptic Skin Cream; Cal D; Calcite D; Caltrate + Iron & Vitamin D†; Caltrate + Vitamin D; Caltrate Plus; Neo Cal D; Nutrol A D; Os-Cal D; Prevencal & D & Fer†; Prevencal & D & Magnesium†; Prevencal & D†; *Denm.:* Calcichew D₃; CaviD; *Fin.:* Calcichew D₃; D-Calsor; Ideos; Kalcipos-D; Ostram-Vit D₃; *Fr.:* Auxergyl D₃; Cacit Vitamine D₃; Calcidose Vitamine D; Calciprat D₃; Calperos D₃; Caltrate Vitamine D; Dossifil†; Fixical Vitamine D; Frubiose Vitamine D; Ideos; Osseans D3; Ostram Vitamine D₃; Zymaduo; *Ger.:* A + D + E-Vicotrat; A + D₃-Vicotrat†; Calcigen D; Calcimagon D3; Calcimed D₃; Calcium Verla D; Calcium-D-Sandoz; Calcium-dura Vit D₃; Calcivit D; calcivitase; D-Fluoretten; Fluor-Vigantoletten; Frubiase Calcium forte 500; Ideos; Ossofortin; Ossofortin forte; Osspulvit S; Sandocal-D; Strafortin; Zymafluor D; *Hong Kong:* Bone Plus; Calcichew D₃; Calcioday-D; Calperos D₃; Caltrate + D; Caltrate Plus; Citracal + D; Mega-Cal with Vit D; Os-Cal + D; Osteocare; Tri-Cal; *Irl.:* Bio-Calcium + D₃; Bio-Calcium + D₃ + K; Calcichew D₃; Chocovite; Decal; Ideos; *Israel:* Aquitol; Caltrate + Vit D; Oleovit A + D₃; Vitamidyne A and D; *Ital.:* AD Pabyrn; Adiboran AD; Adisterolo; Cacit Vitamina D3; Calcidon; Calciovit Urto; Calisvit; Caltrate; Dialcium; Eurocal D; Fosforil Calcium†; Fruttocal; Granoleina; Ideos; Ostram-D₃; *Mex.:* Adekon; Adekon C; Adeloren; Adibal; Dical; *Mon.:* Orocal D₃; *Neth.:* Calcium-D†; Davitamon AD Fluor†; Davitamon AD†; Dohyfral Vitamine AD; Halitran†; Zwitsavit-D†; *Norw.:* Calcigran; Ideos; *NZ:* Oscal D; *Port.:* Calcium 600; Caltrate; Caltrate Plus; Decalcit; Frucalde; Ideos; Zelderme†; *S.Afr.:* Vandol; *Singapore:* Cal-D3; Calcioday-D; Caltrate + Vit D; Caltrate Plus; Dumocalcin; Os-Cal + D; Procal-D; *Spain:* Adiod; Biominol A D; Calcio 20 Complex; Calcio 20 Fuerte; Calcio Faes DYC†; Calcio Geve D y C; Calcio Vitam D3†; Calcium-Sandoz Forte D; Cicatral; Cimascal D; Creacal; Duplicalcio†; Grietalgen; Grietalgen Hidrocort; Ideos; Mencalisvit; Mitosyl; Natecal D; Noquema†; Osteomerck; Ostine; Osvical†; Queratil; Redoxon Calciovit; Veriscal D; *Swed.:* AD-vitamin; Cal-D-Vita; Calcichew D₃; Ideos; Kalcipos-D; Ostram-Vit D₃; *Switz.:* Cal-De; Calcimagon-D3; Calciplus; Calcium D Sauter; Calcivit; Calperos D₃; Decalcit; Demosept; Frubiose Calcium†; Linola gras; Malvedrin; Riccomycine†; Riccovitan; *Thai.:* Cal-D-Vita; Caltrate + D; Caltrate Plus; Ostone-B12; *UK:* Adcal-D₃; Cacit D3; Calceos; Calcichew D₃; Calcium and Ergocalciferol Tablets; Caltrate; Caltrate Plus; Chocovite; Crampex; Folic Plus; Haliborange Calcium Plus Vitamin D; Osteocare; Porosis D; S.P.H.P.; *USA:* A and D Medicated; Calcarb with Vitamin D; Calcet; Calcium 600; Calel-D; Caltrate + Iron & Vitamin D; Caltrate + Vitamin D; Caltrate Plus; Citracal + D; Clocream; Desert Pure Calcium; Diaper Guard; FemCal; Lobana Derm-Aide; Lobana Peri-Garde; Os-Cal + D; Posture-D; Vitanumonyl†.

Vitamin E Substances (7893-p)

NOTE. The food additive number E306 is used for tocopherols.

Vitamin E is a generic term applied to a large number of natural or synthetic compounds. The most important substances are the **tocopherols** of which **alpha tocopherols** are the most active and widely distributed in nature; other naturally occurring tocopherols include beta, gamma, and delta tocopherols, but these are not used in therapeutics. The other group of compounds with vitamin E activity are the tocotrienols.

Alpha tocopherols occur naturally in the *d* optical isomer form, which is more active than the synthetic racemic *dl* form; for further details concerning the comparative activities of the different forms and isomers of vitamin E compounds, see under Units, below.

d-Alpha Tocopherol (7894-s)

Natural Alpha Tocopherol; Natural α-Tocopherol; RRR-α-Tocopherol; d-α-Tocopherol; RRR-α-Tocopherolum. (+)-2,5,7,8-Tetramethyl-2-(4,8,12-trimethyltridecyl)chroman-6-ol.

$C_{29}H_{50}O_2 = 430.7$.

CAS — 59-02-9.

Pharmacopoeias. In *Eur.* (see p.vi). *US* allows it under the title Vitamin E.

Pharmacopoeial description

Ph. Eur.: A clear, colourless, or yellowish-brown viscous oily liquid. Practically insoluble in water; freely soluble in dehydrated alcohol, in acetone, in dichloromethane, and in fatty oils. Store under an inert gas in airtight containers. Protect from light.

USP 25: A clear, yellow, or greenish-yellow, practically odourless, viscous oil. It is unstable to air and light, particularly in alkaline media. Insoluble in water; soluble in alcohol; miscible with acetone, with chloroform, with ether, and with vegetable oils. Store under an inert gas in airtight containers. Protect from light.

dl-Alpha Tocopherol (7895-w)

Alpha Tocopherol; E307; Synthetic Alpha Tocopherol; Synthetic α-Tocopherol; α-Tocopherol; dl-α-Tocopherol; all-rac-α-Tocopherol; α-Tocopherolum. (±)-2,5,7,8-Tetramethyl-2-(4,8,12-trimethyltridecyl)chroman-6-ol.
$C_{29}H_{50}O_2 = 430.7$.
CAS — 10191-41-0.
Pharmacopoeias. In Eur. (see p.vi) and Jpn. US allows it under the title Vitamin E.

Pharmacopoeial description

Ph. Eur.: A clear, colourless or yellowish-brown viscous oily liquid. Practically insoluble in water; freely soluble in dehydrated alcohol, in acetone, in dichloromethane, in ether, and in fatty oils. Store under an inert gas in airtight containers. Protect from light.

USP 25: A clear, yellow, or greenish-yellow, practically odourless, viscous oil. It is unstable to air and light, particularly in alkaline media. Insoluble in water; soluble in alcohol; miscible with acetone, with chloroform, with ether, and with vegetable oils. Store under an inert gas in airtight containers. Protect from light.

d-Alpha Tocoferil Acetate (18520-m)

d-Alpha Tocopheryl Acetate; RRR-α-Tocopheroli Acetas; d-α-Tocopheryl Acetate; RRR-α-Tocopheryl Acetate. (+)-α-Tocopherol acetate.
$C_{31}H_{52}O_3 = 472.7$.
CAS — 58-95-7.
Pharmacopoeias. In Eur. (see p.vi). US allows it under the title Vitamin E.

Pharmacopoeial description

Ph. Eur.: A clear, pale greenish-yellow, viscous oily liquid. Practically insoluble in water; soluble in alcohol; freely soluble in dehydrated alcohol, in acetone, and in fatty oils. Protect from light.

USP 25: A clear, yellow, or greenish-yellow, practically odourless, viscous oil. It may solidify in the cold. It is stable to air and light, but unstable to alkali. Insoluble in water; soluble in alcohol; miscible with acetone, with chloroform, with ether, and with vegetable oils. Store under an inert gas in airtight containers. Protect from light.

dl-Alpha Tocoferil Acetate (7896-e)

Alpha Tocopheryl Acetate; dl-Alpha Tocopheryl Acetate; α-Tocopherol Acetate; α-Tocopheroli Acetas; dl-α-Tocopheryl Acetate; all-rac-α-Tocopheryl Acetate. (±)-α-Tocopherol acetate.
$C_{31}H_{52}O_3 = 472.7$.
CAS — 7695-91-2.
Pharmacopoeias. In Chin., Eur. (see p.vi), Jpn, and Pol. US allows it under the title Vitamin E.
Eur. also has a monograph for the concentrated powdered form.

Pharmacopoeial description

Ph. Eur.: A clear, slightly greenish-yellow, viscous, oily liquid. Practically insoluble in water; soluble in alcohol; freely soluble in dehydrated alcohol, in acetone, in ether, and in fatty oils. The concentrate (powder form) consists of almost white, yellowish, or light-brown small particles which, depending on their formulation, may be practically insoluble in water or may swell to form a dispersion. Store in airtight containers. Protect from light.

USP 25: A clear, yellow, or greenish-yellow, practically odourless, viscous oil. It is stable to air and light, but unstable to alkali. Insoluble in water; soluble in alcohol; miscible with acetone, with chloroform, with ether, and with vegetable oils. Store in airtight containers. Protect from light.

d-Alpha Tocoferil Acid Succinate (7897-l)

d-Alpha Tocopheryl Acid Succinate; RRR-α-Tocopheroli Hydrogenosuccinas; d-α-Tocopheryl Acid Succinate; RRR-α-Tocopheryl Hydrogen Succinate. (+)-α-Tocopherol hydrogen succinate.
$C_{33}H_{54}O_5 = 530.8$.
CAS — 4345-03-3.
Pharmacopoeias. In Eur. (see p.vi). US allows it under the title Vitamin E. USNF also includes Vitamin E Polyethylene Glycol Succinate, a mixture formed by the esterification of d-alpha tocoferil acid succinate with a macrogol.

Pharmacopoeial description

Ph. Eur.: A white or almost white crystalline powder. Practically insoluble in water; soluble in dehydrated alcohol, in acetone, and in ether; very soluble in dichloromethane. Protect from light.

USP 25: A white, practically odourless, powder. M.p. about 75°; it is unstable when held molten. It is stable to air and light, but unstable to alkali. Insoluble in water; soluble in alcohol, in acetone, in ether, and in vegetable oils; very soluble in chloroform; slightly soluble in alkaline solution. Store in airtight containers. Protect from light.

dl-Alpha Tocoferil Acid Succinate (11236-l)

dl-Alpha Tocopheryl Acid Succinate; Alpha Tocopheryl Hydrogen Succinate; DL-α-Tocopheryl Hydrogenosuccins; dl-α-Tocopheryl Acid Succinate; DL-α-Tocopheryl Hydrogen Succinate. (±)-α-Tocopherol hydrogen succinate.
$C_{33}H_{54}O_5 = 530.8$.
CAS — 17407-37-3.
Pharmacopoeias. In Eur. (see p.vi). US allows it under the title Vitamin E.

Pharmacopoeial description

Ph. Eur.: A white or almost white, crystalline powder. Practically insoluble in water; soluble in dehydrated alcohol, in acetone, and in ether; very soluble in dichloromethane. Protect from light.

USP 25: A white, practically odourless, powder. M.p. about 70°; it is unstable when held molten. It is stable to air and light, but unstable to alkali. Insoluble in water; soluble in alcohol, in acetone, in ether, and in vegetable oils; very soluble in chloroform; slightly soluble in alkaline solution. Store in airtight containers. Protect from light.

Units

Though the potency of preparations of vitamin E is still sometimes expressed in units, the International Standard for vitamin E was discontinued in 1956. The International Unit was the activity contained in 1 mg of a standard preparation of α-tocoferil acetate. Past editions of the USP have stated that in expressing vitamin E activity of tocopherol products, the following equivalents of 1 mg were to be employed:

- *dl*-alpha tocoferil acetate, 1 unit
- *dl*-alpha tocoferil acid succinate, 0.89 unit
- *dl*-alpha tocopherol, 1.1 units
- *d*-alpha tocoferil acetate, 1.36 units
- *d*-alpha tocopherol, 1.49 units
- *d*-alpha tocoferil acid succinate, 1.21 units.

For dietary purposes, vitamin-E activity may now be expressed in terms of alpha tocopherol equivalents (α-TEs). One α-TE is the activity contained in 1 mg of *d*-alpha tocopherol (natural alpha tocopherol; *RRR*-α-tocopherol), 1.4 mg *dl*-alpha tocopherol, 1.1 mg *d*-alpha tocoferil acetate, 1.5 mg *dl*-alpha tocoferil acetate, 1.2 mg *d*-alpha tocoferil acid succinate, or 1.7 mg *dl*-alpha tocoferil acid succinate.

Adverse Effects and Precautions

Vitamin E is usually well tolerated. Large doses may cause diarrhoea, abdominal pain, and other gastrointestinal disturbances, and have also been reported to cause fatigue and weakness. Contact dermatitis has occurred following topical application.

Large doses of vitamin E have been reported to increase bleeding tendency in vitamin-K deficient patients such as those taking oral anticoagulants. However, it has also been suggested that it may increase the risk of thrombosis in some patients, such as those taking oestrogens. The clinical significance of these effects is not known.

A higher incidence of necrotising enterocolitis has been noted in premature infants weighing less than 1.5 kg treated with vitamin E.

◊ For a review and discussion of liver and kidney toxicity in premature neonates associated with an intravenous preparation of vitamin E (E-Ferol) and attributed to the inclusion of polysorbates, see p.1348.

Interactions

Various drugs may interfere with the absorption of vitamin E including colestyramine, colestipol, and orlistat. High doses of vitamin E may increase the effects of oral anticoagulants.

Pharmacokinetics

Absorption of vitamin E from the gastrointestinal tract is dependent on the presence of bile and on normal pancreatic function. The amount of vitamin E absorbed varies widely between about 20% and 80% and appears to decrease as the dose is increased. It enters the blood via the chylomicrons in the lymph and is bound to beta lipoproteins. It is widely distributed to all tissues, and stored in adipose tissue. Some vitamin E is metabolised in the liver to glucuronides of tocopheronic acid and its γ-lactone. Some is excreted in the urine, but most of a dose is slowly excreted in the bile. Vitamin E appears in breast milk but is poorly transferred across the placenta.

Human Requirements

The daily requirement of vitamin E has not been clearly defined but is probably about 3 to 12 mg of *d*-alpha tocopherol or the equivalent of other vitamin E substances. Requirements increase with increased dietary amounts of polyunsaturated fatty acids. There appears to be no evidence that supplements are required in subjects on balanced diets.

Vitamin E is widely distributed in food. The richest sources are vegetable oils especially wheat-germ oil, sunflower oil, and cottonseed oil; cereals and eggs are also good sources. It does not appear to be destroyed by cooking processes.

◊ In the UK neither a reference nutrient intake (RNI—see p.1352) nor an estimated average requirement (EAR) has been set for vitamin E although daily intakes of 4 mg and 3 mg α-tocopherol equivalents (see under Units, above) were considered adequate for men and women, respectively.[1]

In the USA the recommended dietary allowance for adults is 15 mg daily of alpha tocopherol, and the tolerable upper intake level is 1000 mg daily.[2]

1. DoH. Dietary reference values for food energy and nutrients for the United Kingdom: report of the panel on dietary reference values of the committee on medical aspects of food policy. *Report on health and social subjects 41.* London: HMSO, 1991.
2. Standing Committee on the Scientific Evaluation of Dietary Reference Intakes of the Food and Nutrition Board. *Dietary Reference Intakes for vitamin C, vitamin E, selenium, and carotenoids.* Washington DC: National Academy Press, 2000.

Uses and Administration

Vitamin E, a fat-soluble vitamin, prevents the oxidation of polyunsaturated fatty acids. It reacts with free radicals, which are the cause of oxidative damage to cell membranes, without the formation of another free radical in the process.

Vitamin E deficiency is rare but develops when the dietary intake is inadequate. In children with cystic fibrosis or biliary atresia, malabsorption of fat may lead to a vitamin E deficiency; deficiency may also occur in children with abnormalities of lipid transport, as in abetalipoproteinaemia. Low vitamin E concentrations are also found in premature, very low birth-weight infants. In previously healthy adults malabsorption and low intake of vitamin E must continue for a number of years before signs of deficiency appear. The major signs of vitamin E deficiency are the development of myopathic and neurological disorders.

Vitamin E is used in the treatment and prevention of vitamin E deficiency. It is usually given by mouth, generally the preferred route, but may also be given by intramuscular or intravenous routes. It may be given as *d*- or *dl*-alpha tocopherol or as the respective acetates or acid succinates.

Recommended doses vary, in part because of differences in the activity of different preparations; however, a daily dose of several times the recommended dietary allowance (RDA), or around 40 to 50 mg of *d*-alpha tocopherol, has been suggested for deficiency syndromes; somewhat higher daily doses have been given in cystic fibrosis (100 to 200 mg of *dl*-alpha tocoferil acetate, or about 67 to 135 mg of *d*-alpha tocopherol) and much higher daily doses in abetalipoproteinaemia (50 to 100 mg of *dl*-alpha tocoferil acetate per kg body-weight, or about 33 to 67 mg d-alpha tocopherol per kg).

Vitamin E has also been tried in retinopathy of prematurity and intraventricular haemorrhage in neonates (see Perinatal Disorders, below), and in a wide variety of other disorders, for which the evidence of value is generally lacking (see Prophylaxis of Ischaemic Heart Disease, p.1352, and Prophylaxis of Malignant Neoplasms, p.1353).

Other substances with vitamin-E activity which have been used include dl-alpha tocoferil palmitate and tocofersolan (tocophersolan), a water-soluble substance which is d-alpha tocoferil acid succinate combined with a macrogol. Wheat-germ oil is also widely used as a source of vitamin E.

Vitamin E is also often used as an antioxidant in pharmaceutical manufacturing.

◊ General references.
1. Meydani M. Vitamin E. Lancet 1995; 345: 170–5.

Dementia. A hypothesis that free radicals may initiate and maintain mechanisms responsible for neurodegeneration in Alzheimer's disease (p.1412) has prompted the investigation of various drugs for antioxidant therapy. Preliminary studies[1] suggest that alpha tocopherol may possibly slow progression. A prospective cohort study found that self-administration of combined vitamin C and vitamin E was associated with a lower risk of vascular dementia in elderly men.[2] However, no significant protective effect was seen against Alzheimer's disease.
1. Sano M, et al. A controlled trial of selegiline, alpha-tocopherol, or both as treatment for Alzheimer's disease. N Engl J Med 1997; 336: 1216–22.
2. Masaki KH, et al. Association of vitamin E and C supplement use with cognitive function and dementia in elderly men. Neurology 2000; 54: 1265–72.

Muscle spasm. Vitamin E is one of a number of drugs that have been tried in the management of nocturnal cramps (p.1322) but there is little convincing evidence to support its use.[1,2] It has also been tried for haemodialysis-induced cramp.[3]
1. Connolly PS, et al. Treatment of nocturnal leg cramps: a crossover trial of quinine vs vitamin E. Arch Intern Med 1992; 152: 1877–80.
2. FDA. Drug products for the treatment and/or prevention of nocturnal leg muscle cramps for over-the-counter human use. Fed Regist 1994; 59: 43234–52.
3. Roca AO, et al. Dialysis leg cramps: efficacy of quinine versus vitamin E. ASAIO J 1992; 38: M481–M485.

Muscular dystrophies. Vitamin E substances have been used in some countries in the management of muscular dystrophies, but controlled studies[1] have failed to demonstrate any benefit.
1. Örndahl G, et al. Functional deterioration and selenium-vitamin E treatment in myotonic dystrophy: a placebo-controlled study. J Intern Med 1994; 235: 205–10.

Parkinsonism. Vitamin E has been tried (as dl-alpha tocoferol) in an attempt to slow neurodegeneration in patients with Parkinson's disease (p.1160) but has proved ineffective.[1]
1. The Parkinson Study Group. Effects of tocopherol and deprenyl on the progression of disability in early Parkinson's disease. N Engl J Med 1993; 328: 176–83.

Perinatal disorders. The primary biological action of vitamin E is known to be the protection of polyunsaturated fatty acids, and thus membranes, from oxidation. Two disorders which may particularly affect premature and very low birthweight infants are retinopathy of prematurity (below) and intraventricular haemorrhage (p.723) and as both may have some association with the occurrence of excess oxygen or oxidant stress, interest has been shown in the possible role vitamin E may have in their prevention.

Retinopathy of prematurity. Retinopathy of prematurity (retrolental fibroplasia) is a disease associated with immature vascularisation of the retina. Formation of retinal lesions may interfere with normal development, resulting in neovascularisation and fibrovascular proliferation. Some cases regress spontaneously but advanced cases can lead to tractional retinal detachment and loss of vision. The pathogenesis of retinopathy of prematurity is not clearly understood, but is likely to be multifactorial.[1]

Following the acknowledgement of a link between retinopathy of prematurity and oxygen therapy, the use of oxygen was reduced and the incidence of this disorder declined. The rising incidence since then probably reflects the larger numbers of extremely premature infants who are surviving due to improved neonatal care. A safe concentration of arterial oxygen has not been defined and antioxidants such as vitamin E have been used prophylactically for several decades. However, this use is controversial. Studies assessing the efficacy of vitamin E prophylaxis have not produced clear results. Some considered that vitamin E prophylaxis had a beneficial effect and recommended routine prophylaxis as soon as possible after birth for infants less than 1.5 kg body-weight.[2] However, others feel that there is no data to support prophylaxis with vitamin E[3,4] and that antioxidants cannot be recommended for routine use.[1] The various studies have been re-evaluated by meta-analysis, the results of which suggest that vitamin E may reduce the incidence

of stage 3+ retinopathy of prematurity.[5] The authors recommended that a well-controlled trial should be conducted.

Other agents suggested for prophylaxis include penicillamine and antenatal dexamethasone, with some suggestion of benefit.[6,7] Reduction in ambient-light exposure did not alter the incidence of retinopathy of prematurity.[8,9]
1. Holmström G. Retinopathy of prematurity. BMJ 1993; 307: 694–5.
2. Johnson L, et al. Effect of sustained pharmacologic vitamin E levels on incidence and severity of retinopathy of prematurity: a controlled clinical trial. J Pediatr 1989; 114: 827–38.
3. Law MR, et al. Is routine vitamin E administration justified in very low-birthweight infants? Dev Med Child Neurol 1990; 32: 442–50.
4. Ehrenkranz RA. Vitamin E and retinopathy of prematurity: still controversial. J Pediatr 1989; 114: 801–3.
5. Raju TNK, et al. Vitamin E prophylaxis to reduce retinopathy of prematurity: a reappraisal of published trials. J Pediatr 1997; 131: 844–50.
6. Higgins RD, et al. Antenatal dexamethasone and decreased severity of retinopathy of prematurity. Arch Ophthalmol 1998; 116: 601–5.
7. Phelps DL, et al. D-Penicillamine for preventing retinopathy of prematurity in preterm infants (updated 5 December 2000). Available in The Cochrane Library; Issue 4. Oxford: Update Software; 2001.
8. Reynolds JD, et al. Lack of efficacy of light reduction in preventing retinopathy of prematurity. N Engl J Med 1998; 338: 1572–6.
9. Phelps DL, Watts JL. Early light reduction for preventing retinopathy of prematurity in very low birth weight infants (updated 27 February 2001). Available in The Cochrane Library; Issue 4. Oxford: Update Software; 2001.

Tardive dyskinesia. Reviews[1,2] on the use of vitamin E in the management of antipsychotic-induced tardive dyskinesia (p.662) concluded that evidence of benefit has generally come from small studies with methodological problems. One review[1] concluded that whereas vitamin E may protect against deterioration of tardive dyskinesia there was no evidence that it produced symptomatic improvement. It was suggested[2] that vitamin E therapy may be most beneficial in those patients with tardive dyskinesia of less than 5-years duration. Further large-scale studies are required to establish its place in treatment.
1. Soares KVS, McGrath JJ. Vitamin E for neuroleptic-induced tardive dyskinesia (updated 20 August; 2001). Available in the Cochrane Library; Issue 4. Oxford: Update Software; 2001.
2. Boomershine KH, et al. Vitamin E in the treatment of tardive dyskinesia. Ann Pharmacother 1999; 33: 1195–1202.

Preparations

BP 2001: Alpha Tocopheryl Succinate Tablets;
USNF 20: Tocopherols Excipient;
USP 25: Vitamin E Capsules; Vitamin E Preparation.

Proprietary Preparations (details are given in Part 3)
Aust.: Avigilen; Ephynal; Etocoderm; Etocovit; Evit; Evitol; Tetefit Vitamin E; **Austral.:** Alpha Keri Silky Smooth†; Bio E; Bio Enhaced Natural E; Bioglan Micelle E; Bioglan Natural E; Bioglan Water Soluble E; Chew-E; Dal-E; Macro E; Mega E; Vita E; **Belg.:** Ephynal; **Braz.:** E Radicaps; Ephynal; Tesurene; Vita-E; Vitabase; **Canad.:** Aquasol E; Novo E; Nutrol E; Organex; Vita-E; **Fin.:** Bio-E-Vitamin; Equiday; Esol; Ido-E; Tokovitan; Vita-E; **Fr.:** Ephynal; Tocalfa†; Toco; Tocolion; Tocomine; Tocopa; **Ger.:** Antioxidans E; Biogenis One-a-Day; Biopto-E; Biosan E; Detulin; E-Mulsin; E-Vicotrat; Ecoro†; Embial; Ephynal; Eplonat; Equiday E†; Eusovit; Evion; Evit; Malton E; Mowivit; Optovit; Pexan E; Puncto E; Sanavitan S; Spondyvit; Tocorell; Tocovenos†; Tocovital; Togasan; Uno-Vit; Vibolex E; Vitagutt Vitamin E; Vitazell E; **Hong Kong:** Natopheryl; Topher-E; **Irl.:** Ephynal; **Israel:** Ephynal; Evitol; **Ital.:** E-Vitum; Ephynal; Evasen Crema; Evion; Evitina; Na-To-Caps; Sursum; Tocogen; **Mex.:** Ekanin; Elibet; Ephynal; Eugerminal; **Neth.:** Davitamon E†; **Norw.:** AFI-E; Bio-E-Vitamin; Ido-E; **NZ:** Micelle E; **Port.:** Ephynal; Oxivite Ve; **S.Afr.:** Ephynal; Ephynal; Evit; Opto Vit-E; **Thai.:** Bio-E; Chew-E; E-Drops; **UK:** Bio E; Ephynal; Prairie Gold; Vita-E; **USA:** Amino-Opti-E†; Aquasol E†; Aquavit-E; E-Gems; Nutr-E-Sol; VitaPlus E; Vitec.

Multi-ingredient: Aust.: A-E-Mulsin; Arcavit A/E; Colagain†; Coldistop; Dr Schmidgall Halsweh; Gerogelat; Lecivital; Magnesium Tonil Vitamine E; Mamellin; Pasuma-Dragees†; Regenerin; Rovigon; Ulcurilen; Vasovitol; **Austral.:** Althaea Complex; Antioxidant Forte Tablets; Antioxidant Tablets; Arthriforte; Beta A-C; Beta-Ace Tablets; Bioglan Bioage Peripheral; Bioglan E-Plus†; Bioglan Fingers & Toes†; Bioglan Maxepa; Bioglan Micelle A plus E; Bioglan Primrose-E; Blistex Aloe & Vitamin E†; Curash Baby Wipes; Curash Babycare; Echinacea & Antioxidants; Epo + Maxepa + Vitamin E-Herbal Plus Formula 8†; Eye Health Herbal Plus Formula 4; Ginkgo ACE†; Ginkgo Complex; Ginzing E; Hair and Skin Formula; Lifechange Circulation Aid; Lifesystem Herbal Plus Formula 5 Eye Relief; Lifesystem Herbal Plus Formula 8 Echinacea†; Lifesystem Herbal Plus Formula 9 Fatty Acids And Vitamin E†; Macro Natural Vitamin E Cream; ML 20; Sambucus Complex; Selenium E; Serenoa Complex; Trillium Complex; Viburnum Complex; **Belg.:** Dagravit A-E; Rovigon; **Braz.:** Gerosenil; Ioimbina Composta; Neurofitol; Sexormon; **Canad.:** Bionagre plus E; Bye Bye Burn†; Super Gamma Oil with Vitamin E; Vita-E Plus Selenium; **Fin.:** Aesol; **Fr.:** Arkotonic†; Bio-Selenium; Cicatryl; Circularine; Cirkan a la Prednacinolone; Difrarel E; Enuretine†; Ophtadil; Rovigon; Trisolvit†; **Ger.:** A + D + E-Vicotrat; A + E Thilo; A-E-Mulsin; Alsicur†; Alsiroyal†; anabolloges; Antimyopikum; Biogenis†; Buer Vitamin E + Magnesium; Coldastop; Dr. Hotz Vollbad†; Dynef; E-Vicotrat + Magnesium; Elex; Hewekzem novo; Kollateral A + E; Lasar; Lipidavit; Lipovitan; Magium E; Magnesium Tonil; Magnesium-Plus-Hevert; Magopsor†; Mapurit; NeyChondrin N (Revitorgan-Dilutionen N Nr 68); NeyNormin N (Revitorgan-Dilutionen N Nr 65); Ney-Pulpin N (Revitorgan-Dilutionen N Nr 10); NeyTumorin N (Revitorgan-Dilutionen N Nr 66); Protecor; Remederm; Rovigon G; RubieMag + E; Salus Herz-Schutz-Kapseln; Supplevit Magnum†;

Ulcurilen N; Unguentacid; Ureata S; Vaso-E-Bion; **Hong Kong:** Aderma Epitheliale; Difrarel E; Karoyan S; **Ital.:** Angstrom Viso/Labbra Alta Protezione; Babysteril; Derman-Oil; Dermana; Ecamannan; Efagel; Ener-E; Forticrin; Granoleina; Ictom 3; Midium; Mirtilene; Pasta Dicofarm; Provitamin A-E; Rovigon; Royal E; Rutisan CE; Tannidin Plus; Tocalfa; Ultravisin; Vit Eparin; **Mon.:** Tocogestan; **Neth.:** Dagravit A-E Forte; **Port.:** Antiestrias; Creme Laser Hidrante; Disoderme; Esclerobion; Nutrasidin; Rovigon; Synchrorose; **S.Afr.:** Haemonase P†; **Spain:** Auxina A + E; Difrarel E; Poli ABE; Ravigona†; Trivitan†; Vitaber A E; Wobenzimal; **Swed.:** Selen + E†; **Switz.:** Alphastria; Coldistop; Linola gras; Oravil; Rovigon; Visaline; **Thai.:** Men Hormone; Rovigon; **UK:** Efatime; Exzem Oil; Octacosanol; Se-Power; **USA:** Aloe Grande; Anusol; Comfortine; Diaper Guard; Lactinol-E; Lazercreme; Lobana Derm-Aide; Phicon; Stay Moist Lip Conditioner†; Yeast-Gard Advanced Sensitive Formula†; Ze Caps.

Vitamin K Substances (7902-c)

The term vitamin K is used for a range of naphthoquinone compounds which include acetomenaphthone, menadiol, menadione, and phytomenadione.

Acetomenaphthone (7904-a)

Acetomenaphthone (BAN).

Acetomenadione; Acetomenaph.; Menadiol Diacetate; Vitamin K$_4$ Diacetate. 2-Methyl-1,4-naphthylene diacetate.

$C_{15}H_{14}O_4 = 258.3$.
CAS — 573-20-6.

Menadiol Sodium Phosphate (7905-t)

Menadiol Sodium Phosphate (BANM).

Menadiol Sodium Diphosphate; Menadiolum Solubile; Vitamin K$_4$ Sodium Phosphate. 2-Methylnaphthalene-1,4-diyl bis(disodium phosphate) hexahydrate.

$C_{11}H_8Na_4O_8P_2,6H_2O = 530.2$.
CAS — 481-85-6 (menadiol); 131-13-5 (anhydrous menadiol sodium phosphate); 6700-42-1 (menadiol sodium phosphate hexahydrate); 84-98-0 (menadiol diphosphate).

NOTE. Menadiol Potassium Sulfate (Potassium Menaphthosulfate) is BAN and Menadiol Sodium Sulfate is rINN.

Pharmacopoeias. In Br. and US.

Pharmacopoeial description

BP 2001: A white to pink, hygroscopic, crystalline powder with a characteristic odour. Very soluble in water; practically insoluble in alcohol.

USP 25: A white to pink, hygroscopic, powder having a characteristic odour. Very soluble in water; insoluble in alcohol. Its solutions in water are neutral or slightly alkaline to litmus having a pH of about 8. Store in airtight containers at a temperature not exceeding 8°. Protect from light.

Menadione (7906-x)

Menadione (BAN).

Menadionum; Menaph.; Menaphthene; Menaphthone; Methylnaphthochinonum; Vitamin K$_3$. 2-Methyl-1,4-naphthoquinone.

$C_{11}H_8O_2 = 172.2$.
CAS — 58-27-5.
ATC — B02BA02.

Pharmacopoeias. In Eur. (see p.vi) and US.

Pharmacopoeial description

Ph. Eur.: A pale yellow crystalline powder. It is unstable in light. Practically insoluble in water; sparingly soluble in alcohol and in methyl alcohol; soluble in ether; freely soluble in toluene. Protect from light.

USP 25: A bright yellow, practically odourless, crystalline powder. It is affected by sunlight. Practically insoluble in water; soluble 1 in 60 of alcohol, 1 in 50 of vegetable oils, and 1 in 10 of benzene; sparingly soluble in chloroform. Protect from light.

◊ CAUTION. The powder is irritating to the respiratory tract and to the skin. The alcoholic solution has vesicant properties.

Menadione Sodium Bisulfite (7907-r)

Menadione Sodium Bisulfite (rINN).

Kavitanum; Menadione Sodium Bisulphite (BANM); Menaph. Sod. Bisulphite; Menaphthone Sodium Bisulphite; Methylnaphthochinonumnatrium Bisulfurosum; Vikasolum; Vitamin K$_3$ Sodium Bisulphite. Sodium 1,2,3,4-tetrahydro-2-methyl-1,4-dioxonaphthalene-2-sulphonate trihydrate.

$C_{11}H_8O_2NaHSO_3,3H_2O = 330.3$.
CAS — 130-37-0 (anhydrous menadione sodium bisulfite); 6147-37-1 (menadione sodium bisulfite trihydrate).
Pharmacopoeias. In Belg. and Pol.

Phytomenadione (7903-k)

Phytomenadione (BAN, rINN).

Methylphytylnaphthochinonum; Phylloquinone; Phytomenad.; Phytomenadionum; Phytonadione; Vitamin K_1. 2-Methyl-3-[3,7,11,15-tetramethylhexadec-2-enyl] naphthalene-1,4-dione.

$C_{31}H_{46}O_2 = 450.7$.
CAS — 84-80-0.
ATC — B02BA01.

Pharmacopoeias. In Chin., Eur. (see p.vi), Int., Jpn, and US.

Aqueous dispersions of phytomenadione for injection should not be allowed to freeze.

Pharmacopoeial description

Ph. Eur.: Phytomenadione is a mixture of the *trans* (*E*) and *cis* (*Z*) isomers. It contains not less than 75% of *trans*-phytomenadione, and also allows not more than 4% of *trans*-epoxyphytomenadione.

A clear, intense yellow, viscous, oily liquid, which decomposes on exposure to actinic light. Practically insoluble in water; sparingly soluble in alcohol; miscible with ether and with fatty oils. Protect from light.

USP 25: A mixture of the *E* and *Z* isomers. It contains not more than 21% of the *Z* isomer. A clear, yellow to amber, very viscous, odourless or practically odourless, liquid. It is stable in air, but decomposes on exposure to sunlight. Insoluble in water; slightly soluble in alcohol; soluble in dehydrated alcohol, in chloroform, in ether, in vegetable oils, and in benzene. Store in airtight containers. Protect from light.

Stability. A polyethoxylated castor oil formulation of phytomenadione was stable for at least 30 days at room temperature when repackaged in amber glass dropper bottles.[1] When refrigerated at 4° to 8°, it was stable in both plastic and amber glass bottles.

1. Wong VK, Ho PC. Stability of Konakion repacked in dropper bottles for oral administration. *Aust J Hosp Pharm* 1996; **26:** 641-4.

Adverse Effects and Precautions

Intravenous administration of *phytomenadione* has caused severe reactions resembling hypersensitivity or anaphylaxis. Symptoms have included facial flushing, sweating, chest constriction and chest pain, dyspnoea, cyanosis, and cardiovascular collapse; fatalities have been reported. Anaphylactic reactions have generally been associated with an overly rapid rate of infusion but have also been reported even when the solution was diluted and infused slowly. They are generally thought to be due to polyethoxylated castor oil which is present as a surfactant in some parenteral formulations; reports of such reactions with formulations that do not contain polyethoxylated castor oil are rare.

Pain, swelling, and phlebitis may occur at the injection site following administration of phytomenadione. Localised skin reactions including atrophy or necrosis have been reported following intramuscular or subcutaneous injection of phytomenadione.

Phytomenadione formulations solubilised with lecithin and a bile salt should be given with caution to patients with severely impaired liver function and to premature neonates weighing less than 2.5 kg, since the bile salt may displace bilirubin.

Administration of *menadione* and *menadiol sodium phosphate* to neonates, especially premature infants, or to the mother during late pregnancy has been associated with the development in the infant of haemolytic anaemia, hyperbilirubinaemia, and kernicterus, and such use is not recommended. Phytomenadione has a lower risk of haemolysis. Menadione and menadiol sodium phosphate have also been reported to cause haemolysis in patients with glucose-6-phosphate dehydrogenase deficiency or vitamin E deficiency.

Carcinogenicity. A case-control study from the UK[1] suggested an increased risk of cancer in children who had received vitamin K at birth for the prevention of haemorrhagic disease of the newborn (see below). A further study[2] by the same authors indicated that this risk was associated with intramuscular, but not oral, administration, and was strongest for childhood leukaemia. In response to these data, the British Paediatric Association recommended that the oral route of administration be preferred for prophylaxis,[3] whereas the American Academy of Pediatrics continued to advocate the intramuscular route.[4] Subsequent studies from the USA,[5] Sweden,[6] Denmark,[6,7] Germany,[8] and England[9] did not confirm an increased risk of childhood cancer, including leukaemias, after the use of intramuscular vitamin K. More recently, 4 further studies were published.[10-13] Two of the reports, a case-control study in

Scotland[10] and an ecological study in Britain,[11] showed no increased risk of any cancers with the use of intramuscular vitamin K. A third case-control study in England and Wales[12] found a borderline association between intramuscular vitamin K and cancers, particularly leukaemia. In the fourth study, a case-control study in northern England,[13] there was an increased risk (odds ratio 1.79) of acute lymphoblastic leukaemia developing 1 to 6 years after birth in children who had received intramuscular vitamin K. In 1998 an expert working group formed by the UK Medicines Control Agency and the Committee on Safety of Medicines reviewed all the available studies.[14] They concluded that there was no increased risk of solid tumours with vitamin K, and that, although an increased risk of leukaemia could not be excluded, observed results were compatible with chance. Moreover, they could not identify a plausible mechanism for a carcinogenic effect of vitamin K. The UK Department of Health[15] now advocates either oral or intramuscular prophylaxis, and recommends that the parents should be involved in the decision on which route of administration is used.

1. Golding J, *et al.* Factors associated with childhood cancer in a national cohort study. *Br J Cancer* 1990; **62:** 304-8.
2. Golding J, *et al.* Childhood cancer, intramuscular vitamin K, and pethidine given during labour. *BMJ* 1992; **305:** 341-6.
3. British Paediatric Association. *Vitamin K prophylaxis in infancy.* London, 1992: British Paediatric Association.
4. American Academy of Pediatrics Vitamin K Ad Hoc Task Force. Controversies concerning vitamin K and the newborn. *Pediatrics* 1993; **91:** 1001-3.
5. Klebanoff MA, *et al.* The risk of childhood cancer after neonatal exposure to vitamin K. *N Engl J Med* 1993; **329:** 905-8.
6. Ekelund H, *et al.* Administration of vitamin K to newborn infants and childhood cancer. *BMJ* 1993; **307:** 89-91.
7. Olsen JH, *et al.* Vitamin K regimens and incidence of childhood cancer in Denmark. *BMJ* 1994; **308:** 895-6.
8. von Kries R, *et al.* Vitamin K and childhood cancer: a population based case-control study in Lower Saxony, Germany. *BMJ* 1996; **313:** 199-203.
9. Ansell P, *et al.* Childhood leukaemia and intramuscular vitamin K: findings from a case-control study. *BMJ* 1996; **313:** 204-5.
10. McKinney PA, *et al.* Case-control study of childhood leukaemia and cancer in Scotland: findings for neonatal intramuscular vitamin K. *BMJ* 1998; **316:** 173-7.
11. Passmore SJ, *et al.* Ecological studies of relation between hospital policies on neonatal vitamin K administration and subsequent occurrence of childhood cancer. *BMJ* 1998; **316:** 184-9.
12. Passmore SJ, *et al.* Case-control studies of relation between childhood cancer and neonatal vitamin K administration. *BMJ* 1998; **316:** 178-184.
13. Parker L, *et al.* Neonatal vitamin K administration and childhood cancer in the north of England: retrospective case-control study. *BMJ* 1998; **316:** 189-93.
14. Committee on Safety of Medicines/Medicines Control Agency. Safety of intramuscular vitamin K (Konakion). *Current Problems* 1998; **24:** 3-4.
15. Department of Health. *Vitamin K for newborn babies.* London, 1998: Department of Health.

Effects on the blood. Cerebral arterial thrombosis developed in 2 patients with malabsorption syndromes due to coeliac disease during treatment with vitamin K for severe deficiency of vitamin-K-dependent coagulation factors. An increased tendency to thrombotic events had previously been reported to be present in patients with intestinal inflammatory disorders. It was suggested that if bleeding did occur in such patients treatment should be with plasma infusions or small doses of vitamin K but that vitamin K deficiency should not be specifically treated since a gluten-free diet or corticosteroids given for the gastrointestinal disorder will result in a gradual correction.[1]

1. Florholmen J, *et al.* Cerebral thrombosis in two patients with malabsorption syndrome treated with vitamin K. *BMJ* 1980; **281:** 541.

Interactions

Vitamin K decreases the effects of oral anticoagulants (see p.997), and is used to counteract excessive effects of these drugs, see below. Vitamin K may reduce the response to resumed therapy with anticoagulants for a week or more.

Pharmacokinetics

The fat-soluble vitamin K compounds phytomenadione and menadione require the presence of bile for their absorption from the gastrointestinal tract; the water-soluble derivatives of menadione can be absorbed in the absence of bile. Vitamin K accumulates mainly in the liver but is stored in the body only for short periods of time. Vitamin K does not appear to cross the placenta readily and it is poorly distributed into breast milk. Phytomenadione is rapidly metabolised to more polar metabolites and is excreted in bile and urine as glucuronide and sulfate conjugates.

Absorption. Absorption of phytomenadione from the colloidal (micellar) preparation was more irregular and unpredictable after intramuscular than intravenous administration in healthy adults;[1] when used as an antidote to anticoagulant drugs, this formulation should be given intravenously. In neonates, plasma phytomenadione concentrations were within or above the adult fasting plasma range 24 days after receiving a single dose of the

colloidal preparation either orally (3 mg) or intramuscularly (1.5 mg).[2]

1. Soedirman JR, *et al.* Pharmacokinetics and tolerance of intravenous and intramuscular phylloquinone (vitamin K_1) mixed micelles formulation. *Br J Clin Pharmacol* 1996; **41:** 517-23.
2. Schubiger G, *et al.* Vitamin K_1 concentration in breast-fed neonates after oral or intramuscular administration of a single dose of a new mixed-micellar preparation of phylloquinone. *J Pediatr Gastroenterol Nutr* 1993; **16:** 435-9.

Human Requirements

The minimum daily requirements of vitamin K are not clearly defined but an intake of about 1 μg per kg body-weight daily appears to be adequate. Vitamin K requirements in normal adults can be met from the average diet and from the synthesis of menaquinones (also known as vitamin K_2) by bacterial action in the intestine. Vitamin K occurs naturally as phytomenadione (vitamin K_1) which is present in many foods, especially leafy green vegetables such as cabbage and spinach, and is also present in liver, cows' milk, egg-yolk, and some cereals.

◊ In the UK neither a reference nutrient intake (RNI) nor an estimated average requirement (EAR—see p.1352) has been set for vitamin K although an intake of 1 μg per kg body-weight daily was considered to be both safe and adequate for adults; a higher intake of about 2 μg per kg body-weight daily (10 μg daily) was believed to be justified in infants because of the absence of hepatic menaquinones in early life and reliance on dietary vitamin K alone. It was stated that all babies should receive prophylactic vitamin K at birth[1] and for further details concerning neonatal use, see Haemorrhagic Disease of the Newborn below.

In the USA, adequate intake levels have been determined to be 120 μg daily for adult men and 90 μg daily for adult women.[2]

1. DoH. Dietary reference values for food energy and nutrients for the United Kingdom: report of the panel on dietary reference values of the committee on medical aspects of food policy. *Report on health and social subjects 41.* London: HMSO, 1991.
2. Standing Committee on the Scientific Evaluation of Dietary Reference Intakes of the Food and Nutrition Board. *Dietary Reference Intakes for vitamin A, vitamin K, arsenic, boron, chromium, copper, iodine, iron, manganese, molybdenum, nickel, silicon, vanadium, and zinc.* Washington DC: National Academy Press, 2001.

Uses and Administration

Vitamin K is an essential cofactor in the hepatic synthesis of prothrombin (factor II) and other blood clotting factors (factors VII, IX, and X, and proteins C and S) and in the function of proteins such as osteocalcin important for bone development.

Vitamin K deficiency may develop in neonates, and can lead to haemorrhagic disease of the newborn. Vitamin K deficiency is uncommon in adults, but may occur in patients with malabsorption syndromes, obstructive jaundice or hepatic disease. Deficiency leads to the development of hypoprothrombinaemia, in which the clotting time of the blood is prolonged and spontaneous bleeding can occur. Coumarin anticoagulants interfere with vitamin K metabolism, and their effects can be antagonised by giving vitamin K.

Vitamin K compounds are used in the treatment and prevention of haemorrhage associated with vitamin K deficiency. The dose of vitamin K should be carefully controlled by prothrombin-time estimations.

Phytomenadione is a naturally occurring vitamin K substance. It is the only vitamin K compound used to reverse hypoprothrombinaemia and haemorrhage caused by anticoagulant therapy. It is not effective as a heparin antidote. For over-anticoagulation, the dose depends on the international normalised ratio (INR) and the degree of haemorrhage. Typical doses of phytomenadione are 0.5 to 5 mg by slow intravenous injection or up to 5 mg orally (see also Over-anticoagulation, below). Depending on the solubilising agents used, some formulations of phytomenadione are more suitable for intravenous use than others, and administration details vary. Phytomenadione has also been used in hypoprothrombinaemia due to certain cephalosporins (see Cefamandole, Adverse Effects, p.163).

In the treatment of haemorrhagic disease of the newborn phytomenadione may be given in a dose of 1 mg intravenously or intramuscularly and, if necessary, further doses may be given 8-hourly. As a prophylactic measure, a single dose of 0.5 to 1 mg may be given intramuscularly to the newborn infant, or 2 mg orally followed by a second dose of 2 mg after 4 to 7 days; for further details see below.

Menadiol sodium phosphate is a water-soluble derivative of menadione, a synthetic lipid-soluble vitamin K analogue. It may be used for the prevention of vitamin K deficiency in patients with malabsorption syndromes in whom oral phytomenadione may be inefficiently absorbed. It is given in usual doses equivalent to 10 to 40 mg of menadiol phosphate daily by mouth.

Menadiol dibutyrate and menatetrenone have also been used and the latter has been investigated in the management of osteoporosis. Acetomenaphthone has been used in preparations promoted for the relief of chilblains.

Action. References to the action of vitamin K and the role of vitamin K-dependent coagulation proteins and carboxyglutamate-containing proteins such as osteocalcin.

1. Friedman PA. Vitamin K-dependent proteins. *N Engl J Med* 1984; **310:** 1458–60.
2. Rick ME. Protein C and protein S: vitamin K-dependent inhibitors of blood coagulation. *JAMA* 1990; **263:** 701–3.
3. Shearer MJ. Vitamin K. *Lancet* 1995; **345:** 229–34.

Haemorrhagic disease of the newborn. Haemorrhagic disease of the newborn (HDN; vitamin K deficiency bleeding; VKDB) of which 3 types have been recognised, is associated with a clotting defect due to vitamin K deficiency. In early HDN bleeding occurs at the time of delivery or during the first 24 hours of life and is typically seen in infants whose mothers have taken drugs that affect vitamin K metabolism such as warfarin, some antiepileptics, rifampicin, or isoniazid. Classic HDN, the most common type, usually occurs at 2 to 5 days of age and breast feeding is an important factor as human breast milk has a much lower content of vitamin K than either cow's milk or infant formulas. Late HDN presents frequently as intracranial haemorrhage in infants over one month of age. The vitamin-K deficiency in these cases can be either idiopathic (usually in breast-fed infants who did not receive vitamin K at birth) and/or can be a secondary manifestation of other disorders such as chronic diarrhoea, cystic fibrosis or other malabsorption syndromes, biliary atresia, or α_1-antitrypsin deficiency.[1]

Treatment of HDN involves use of parenteral phytomenadione, usually 1 mg initially with further doses depending on response. More immediate treatment, in the form of blood transfusion or blood clotting factors, may be needed to compensate for severe blood loss and delayed response to vitamin K. HDN, particularly the late type, carries a high risk of morbidity or death; therefore, the emphasis has been on prevention. It has long been known that administration of vitamin K to the neonate soon after birth can reduce the incidence of HDN. Menadiol sodium phosphate was formerly used, but reports in the 1950s of jaundice and kernicterus in infants given this vitamin K analogue caused concern, and led to the preferential use of phytomenadione either intramuscularly or orally. Administration of phytomenadione, usually as a single intramuscular injection, has been standard practice for neonates considered at high risk of HDN, such as those who had a complicated delivery, those born prematurely, and those whose mothers were receiving antiepileptic therapy. Since it is not possible to selectively identify all neonates that are at risk for HDN, the routine administration of phytomenadione to all neonates has been advocated. However, such practice has been controversial, particularly as regards the route of administration.[2,3] Some have considered that oral administration is less invasive and more acceptable to parents.[3] However, there has also been concern about the adequacy of absorption of orally administered phytomenadione, and the lack of a suitable oral formulation. In addition, there was some evidence[4-6] to suggest that a single intramuscular dose was more effective than a single oral dose in preventing late HDN, and that repeated oral doses might be required, which may be less convenient and carry the risk of poor compliance. More recently, a possible increased risk of childhood cancer in neonates treated with intramuscular, but not oral, phytomenadione has been reported (see Carcinogenicity, above). Although the association remains controversial, it led to recommendations for the preferential use of oral vitamin K in neonates at low-risk of HDN in some countries, including the UK[7] and Germany,[8] whereas other countries, including the USA,[9] still preferred the intramuscular route for all neonates. There is still no agreement on the most effective oral dose and its frequency of administration, and study of this has been complicated by the lack of a suitable oral preparation of phytomenadione.[10,11] Options currently available for oral administration include the polyethoxylated castor oil and polysorbate-80 containing preparations (unlicensed for oral use) and the colloidal, micelle formulation (licensed for oral use in some countries). These preparations are packaged in glass ampoules, therefore are unsuitable for parents to administer at home. The colloidal preparation may be absorbed more reliably (see under Pharmacokinetics, above).

The 1992 recommendations of the British Paediatric Society[7] for oral use of the polyethoxylated castor oil formulation suggested a single dose of 0.5 mg on the day of birth. For breast-fed babies, additional doses of 0.5 mg at 7 to 10 days and at 4

to 6 weeks, or 0.2 mg at weekly intervals for 26 weeks, or 0.05 mg daily for 26 weeks, were recommended. Current UK doses[12] for the colloidal preparation in healthy term neonates are 2 mg soon after birth, then 2 mg at 4 to 7 days. Exclusively breast-fed infants should be given a third oral dose of 2 mg one month after birth. Further monthly doses of 2 mg have been recommended while the infant remains exclusively breast-fed. A report[13] of the failure of prophylaxis in 3 breast-fed babies (2 of whom had unidentified cholestatic liver disease) who received 2 doses of this formulation, as recommended in Switzerland, emphasises the importance of the third, and possibly, other, follow-up doses. Plasma vitamin K concentrations in breast-fed infants receiving 3 oral doses of this formulation were at least equal to concentrations in those receiving a single intramuscular dose.[14] The most recent advice from the UK Department of Health[12] advocates that all newborn infants should receive vitamin K prophylaxis, both oral and intramuscular administration should be available, and that parents should be involved in the decision on which route of administration is used.

Various other oral regimens have been investigated or are in use. In the Netherlands a regimen of 1 mg orally or intramuscularly at birth, followed by 25 µg daily or 1 mg weekly by mouth from 1 week to 3 months of age has been found satisfactory.[15,16] In Germany[8,16] and Australia[16] the suggested oral regimen for the polyethoxylated castor oil formulation was 1 mg at birth, at 3 to 10 days and at weeks 3 to 6, although some failures have been reported in babies receiving this regimen,[8] and the Australian data confirm it is less effective than a single intramuscular dose.[16] One hospital in the USA has satisfactorily used, for many years, a single 2-mg dose administered via nasogastric tube to neonates after birth.[17] In Denmark, a 2-mg dose at birth followed by a weekly dose of 1 mg during the first 3 months of life has effectively prevented any late HDN in healthy breast-fed babies.[18]

Although phytomenadione crosses the placenta slowly and to a limited extent, it is nevertheless recommended that pregnant women receiving drugs that are vitamin K antagonists (particularly antiepileptics) should receive phytomenadione 10 to 20 mg daily from 36 weeks gestation.[19] This is in addition to the requirement that their neonates, who are at high risk of HDN, receive intramuscular phytomenadione soon after birth. Maternal phytomenadione administration has been investigated as a means of improving vitamin K status in breast-fed neonates. In 1 study,[20] 5 mg daily for 12 weeks was effective for this purpose.

1. Hathaway WE. Haemostatic disorders in the newborn. In: Bloom AL, Thomas DP, eds. *Haemostasis and thrombosis.* 2nd ed. Edinburgh: Churchill Livingstone, 1987: 554–69.
2. Tripp JH, McNinch AW. Haemorrhagic disease and vitamin K. *Arch Dis Child* 1987; **62:** 436–7.
3. Brown SG, *et al.* Should intramuscular vitamin K prophylaxis for haemorrhagic disease of the newborn be continued? A decision analysis. *N Z Med J* 1989; **102:** 3–5.
4. Clarkson PM, James AG. Parenteral vitamin K₁: the effective prophylaxis against haemorrhagic disease for all newborn infants. *N Z Med J* 1990; **103:** 95–6.
5. McNinch AW, Tripp JH. Haemorrhagic disease of the newborn in the British Isles: two year prospective study. *BMJ* 1991; **303:** 1105–9.
6. Von Kries R. Neonatal vitamin K. *BMJ* 1991; **303:** 1083–4.
7. British Paediatric Association. *Vitamin K prophylaxis in infancy.* London, 1992: British Paediatric Association.
8. von Kries R, *et al.* Repeated oral vitamin K prophylaxis in West Germany: acceptance and efficacy. *BMJ* 1995; **310:** 1097–8.
9. American Academy of Pediatrics Vitamin K Ad Hoc Task Force. Controversies concerning vitamin K and the newborn. *Pediatrics* 1993; **91:** 1001–3.
10. Barton JS, *et al.* Neonatal vitamin K prophylaxis in the British Isles: current practice and trends. *BMJ* 1995; **310:** 632–3.
11. Rennie JM, Kelsall AWR. Vitamin K prophylaxis in the newborn—again. *Arch Dis Child* 1994; **70:** 248–51.
12. Department of Health. *Vitamin K for newborn babies.* London, 1998: Department of Health.
13. Baenziger O, *et al.* Oral vitamin K prophylaxis for newborn infants: safe enough? *Lancet* 1996; **348:** 1456.
14. Greer FR, *et al.* A new mixed micellar preparation for oral vitamin K prophylaxis: randomised controlled comparison with an intramuscular formulation in breast fed infants. *Arch Dis Child* 1998; **79:** 300–5.
15. Cornelissen M, Hirasing R. Vitamin K for neonates. *BMJ* 1994; **309:** 1441–2.
16. Cornelissen M, *et al.* Prevention of vitamin K deficiency bleeding: efficacy of different multiple oral dose schedules of vitamin K. *Eur J Pediatr* 1997; **156:** 126–30.
17. Clark FI, James EJP. Twenty-seven years of experience with oral vitamin K₁ therapy in neonates. *J Pediatr* 1995; **127:** 301–4.
18. Nørgaard Hansen N, Ebbesen F. Neonatal vitamin K prophylaxis in Denmark: three years' experience with oral administration during the first three months of life compared with one oral administration at birth. *Acta Paediatr Scand* 1996; **85:** 1137–9.
19. Delgado-Escueta AV, Janz D. Consensus guidelines: preconception counseling, management, and care of the pregnant woman with epilepsy. *Neurology* 1992; **42** (suppl 5): 149–60.
20. Greer FR, *et al.* Improving the vitamin K status of breastfeeding infants with maternal vitamin K supplements. *Pediatrics* 1997; **99:** 88–92.

Neonatal intraventricular haemorrhage. Vitamin K crosses the placenta slowly and to a limited extent,[1,2] but sufficiently to warrant studies to assess whether antenatal administration of phytomenadione to the mother may reduce the incidence or severity of intraventricular haemorrhage (p.723) in the preterm neonate. Two studies found that antenatal administration had a beneficial outcome[3,4] but this finding was not confirmed by a subsequent study.[5] Moreover, a larger randomised controlled study failed to find any benefit from vitamin K prophylaxis.[6] A systematic review of trials concluded

that vitamin K did not significantly prevent periventricular haemorrhage, and could not be recommended for routine clinical use.[7]

1. Yang Y-M, *et al.* Maternal-fetal transport of vitamin K₁ and its effects on coagulation in premature infants. *J Pediatr* 1989; **115:** 1009–13.
2. Kazzi NJ, *et al.* Placental transfer of vitamin K₁ in preterm pregnancy. *Obstet Gynecol* 1990; **75:** 334–7.
3. Pomerance JJ, *et al.* Maternally administered antenatal vitamin K₁: effect on neonatal prothrombin activity, partial thromboplastin time, and intraventricular hemorrhage. *Obstet Gynecol* 1987; **70:** 235–41.
4. Morales WJ, *et al.* The use of antenatal vitamin K in the prevention of early neonatal intraventricular hemorrhage. *Am J Obstet Gynecol* 1988; **159:** 774–9.
5. Kazzi NJ, *et al.* Maternal administration of vitamin K does not improve the coagulation profile of preterm infants. *Pediatrics* 1989; **84:** 1045–50.
6. Thorp JA, *et al.* Antepartum vitamin K and phenobarbital for preventing intraventricular hemorrhage in the premature newborn: a randomized, double-blind, placebo-controlled trial. *Obstet Gynecol* 1994; **83:** 70–6.
7. Crowther CA, Henderson-Smart DJ. Vitamin K prior to preterm birth for preventing neonatal periventricular haemorrhage (updated 30 November 2000). Available in The Cochrane Library; Issue 4. Oxford: Update Software; 2001.

Over-anticoagulation. Doses of vitamin K for over-anticoagulation with warfarin have traditionally been large, and this continues to be reflected in manufacturers' literature for these products, where recommended parenteral doses range from 2.5 to 10 mg up to 25 mg initially, with a maximum dose of 40 to 50 mg. However, large doses of vitamin K may result in over-correction, and increase the delay before resumed anticoagulant therapy becomes effective. In addition, the time to onset of action is a minimum of 1 to 2 hours, irrespective of dose. There is increasing evidence that lower doses of vitamin K are effective in over-anticoagulation.[1,2] The British Society of Haematology currently recommends doses of phytomenadione of 5 mg by slow intravenous injection for patients with major bleeding, and 0.5 mg intravenously or 5 mg orally for those with risk factors for bleeding (see Treatment of Adverse Effects of Warfarin, p.993).

1. Weibert RT, *et al.* Correction of excessive anticoagulation with low-dose oral vitamin K₁. *Ann Intern Med* 1997; **125:** 959–62.
2. Fetrow CW, *et al.* Antagonism of warfarin-induced hypoprothrombinemia with use of low-dose subcutaneous vitamin K₁. *J Clin Pharmacol* 1997; **37:** 751–7.

Preparations

BP 2001: Menadiol Phosphate Injection; Menadiol Phosphate Tablets; Phytomenadione Injection; Phytomenadione Tablets;
USP 25: Menadiol Sodium Diphosphate Injection; Menadiol Sodium Diphosphate Tablets; Menadione Injection; Phytonadione Injection; Phytonadione Tablets.

Proprietary Preparations (details are given in Part 3)

Aust.: Kavitol; Konakion; Vikaman; *Austral.:* K Thrombin; Konakion; *Belg.:* Konakion; Vitamon K; *Braz.:* Kanakion; *Denm.:* Konakion; *Fin.:* Konakion; *Ger.:* Kanavit; Konakion; *Hong Kong:* Konakion; *Irl.:* Konakion; *Israel:* Konakion; *Ital.:* Konakion; *Jpn:* Glakay; Kaytwo; *Mex.:* K-50; Konakion; *Neth.:* Konakion; *Norw.:* Konakion Novum; *NZ:* K-Thrombin; Konakion; *Port.:* Kanakion; *S.Afr.:* Konakion; *Singapore:* Konakion; *Spain:* Kaergona Hidrosoluble; Konakion; *Swed.:* Konakion; *Switz.:* Konakion; *Thai.:* Konakion; KP; *UK:* Synkavit; *USA:* Aquamephyton†; Konakion†; Mephyton.

Multi-ingredient: *Austral.:* Chilblain Formula; *Braz.:* Enteromicina; Frenovex; *Fr.:* Bilkaby†; *Hong Kong:* Haemosol; *Irl.:* Bio-Calcium + D₃ + K; *Mex.:* Hemosin-K; *Spain:* Caprofides Hemostatico; Cromoxin K; Quercetol K†; Vitaendil C K P†; *Thai.:* Siduol.

Xylitol (667-e)

Xylitol *(BAN).*
E967; Xylit; *meso*-Xylitol.
$C_5H_{12}O_5 = 152.1.$
CAS — 87-99-0 *(xylitol);* 16277-71-7 *(D-xylitol).*
Pharmacopoeias. In Eur. (see p.vi) and Jpn. Also in USNF.

A polyhydric alcohol (polyol) related to the pentose sugar, xylose (p.1681).

Pharmacopoeial description

Ph. Eur.: White crystals or crystalline powder. M.p. is 92° to 96°. Very soluble in water; sparingly soluble in alcohol.

USNF 20: White crystals or crystalline powder. Crystalline xylitol has a melting range between 92° and 96°. It has a sweet taste and produces a cooling sensation in the mouth. Soluble 1 in about 0.65 of water; sparingly soluble in alcohol.

Adverse Effects

Large amounts taken by mouth may cause diarrhoea and flatulence. Ingestion of xylitol is not likely to lead to hyperoxaluria which can occur with intravenous infusion. Hyperuricaemia, changes in liver-function tests, and acidosis (including lactic acidosis) have occurred after intravenous infusion.

Uses and Administration

Xylitol is used as a bulk sweetener in foods. It is also used as a sweetening agent in sugar-free preparations as it is non-cariogenic and is less likely to cause dental caries than sucrose. It is under investigation for the prevention of dental caries and acute otitis media. It was formerly considered as a substitute for glucose in intravenous nutrition but such use has generally been abandoned due to adverse effects.

The symbol † denotes a preparation no longer actively marketed

Dental caries. Chewing-gum containing xylitol appears to have a useful role in the prevention of dental caries (p.130).[1,2]

1. Edgar WM. Sugar substitutes, chewing gum and dental caries—a review. *Br Dent J* 1998; **184:** 29–32.
2. Gales MA, Nguyen T-M. Sorbitol compared with xylitol in prevention of dental caries. *Ann Pharmacother* 2000; **34:** 98–100.

Otitis media. It has been suggested that xylitol chewing gum[1,2] and xylitol syrup[2] may have a preventative effect against acute otitis media (p.132).

1. Uhari M, *et al.* Xylitol chewing gum in prevention of acute otitis media: double blind randomised trial. *BMJ* 1996; **313:** 1180–4.
2. Uhari M, *et al.* A novel use of xylitol sugar in preventing acute otitis media. *Pediatrics* 1998; **102:** 879–84.

Preparations

Proprietary Preparations (details are given in Part 3)
Canad.: Trident; *Ger.:* Xylit; *Irl.:* Oralbalance†.

Multi-ingredient: *Austral.:* Saliva Orthana†; *Braz.:* Fluotrat; *Ger.:* Cardioplegin N; Duocal; Kalium-Magnesium-Asparaginat; Kaloplasmal†; salvi CAL GX; *Ital.:* Neo-Stomygen; *Swed.:* Salivin†; *UK:* Saliva Orthana; Salivace; *USA:* Optimoist.

Dried Yeast (7840-a)

Brewers' Yeast; Cerevisiae Fermentum Siccatum; Faex Siccata; Fermento de Cerveja; Levedura Sêca; Levure de Bière; Saccharomyces Siccum; Trockenhefe.

Pharmacopoeias. In Aust., Chin., and Jpn.

Unicellular fungi belonging to the family Saccharomycetaceae, dried by a process which avoids decomposition of the vitamins present. The chief species are *Saccharomyces cerevisiae*, *S. carlsbergensis*, and *S. monacensis*. Dried yeast contains thiamine, nicotinic acid, riboflavin, pyridoxine, pantothenic acid, biotin, folic acid, cyanocobalamin, aminobenzoic acid, inositol, and chromium.

Profile

Dried yeast is a rich source of vitamins of the B group. It has been used for the prevention and treatment of vitamin B deficiency in doses of 1 to 8 g daily by mouth. Yeast is an ingredient of some preparations for treating haemorrhoids, and some preparations intended to restore normal gastrointestinal flora. Yeast is widely used in brewing.

Preparations

Proprietary Preparations (details are given in Part 3)
Belg.: Preparation H Sperti†; *Fr.:* Microlev; *Ger.:* Faexojodan†; Furunkulosin; Levurinetten N†; *Ital.:* Lievitovit 300†; Nutrivit; Zimocel; *Mex.:* Cervekanin; Levadin; Levifusa; Leza; *Port.:* Lio-Levedura†; *Thai.:* Brewers Yeast; *UK:* Bio-Strath.

Multi-ingredient: *Aust.:* Levurinetten; Sperti Praparation H; *Austral.:* Bio-Chromium; ML 20; Plantiodine Plus; Preparation H; Vitaglow Selemite B; *Braz.:* Preparado H; Staphylase; *Canad.:* Preparation H; *Fr.:* Actisoufre; Calciforte; Carbolevure; Carbophagix; Fluorocalciforte†; Phytophanere; Preparation H; Solacy; Spasmag; *Ger.:* Haut-Vital N; Imbak; Pantovigar; Sperti Preparation H; *Irl.:* Preparation H; *Israel:* Preparation H; *Ital.:* Aclon Lievit; Alvear Complex†; Bifilact 6; Bio-Real†; Eurogel; Florelax; Lactisporin; Lactivis; Lactolife; Lactovit†; Levudin; Lievistar; Lievitosohn; Lievitovit; Preparazione H; Sillix; Vigogel†; *Neth.:* Sperti Preparation H; *Port.:* Bioregime Fort; Sperti Preparacao H; *S.Afr.:* Revaton†; *Singapore:* Preparation H; *Spain:* Preparacion H; *Switz.:* A Vogel Capsules polyvitaminees; Carbolevure; Sperti Preparation H; *UK:* B Complex; Bio-Strath Artichoke Formula; Bio-Strath Valerian Formula; Bio-Strath Willow Formula; Brewers Yeast; Brewers Yeast with Garlic; Phillips P.T.Y. Yeast Tablets; Preparation H; Yeast Vite; *USA:* Medicone; Preparation H; Rectagene Medicated Balm; Wyanoids Relief Factor.

Zinc (5327-p)

Zn = 65.39.
CAS — 7440-66-6.

Zinc Acetate (5328-s)

Zinci Acetas Dihydricus.
$(CH_3CO_2)_2Zn,2H_2O = 219.5$.
CAS — 557-34-6 (anhydrous zinc acetate); 5970-45-6 (zinc acetate dihydrate).

NOTE. Zinc Acetate, Basic is *rINN*.
Pharmacopoeias. In Eur. (see p.vi) and US.

Pharmacopoeial description

Ph. Eur.: A white crystalline powder or leaflets. Freely soluble in water; soluble in alcohol. A 5% solution in water has a pH of 5.8 to 7.0. Store in nonmetallic containers.

USP 25: White crystals or granules having a slight acetous odour. Is slightly efflorescent. Soluble 1 in 2.5 of water and 1 in 30 of alcohol; freely soluble in boiling alcohol. pH of a 5% solution in water is between 6.0 and 8.0. Store in airtight containers.

Zinc Chloride (5329-w)

Zinci Chloridum; Zincum Chloratum.
$ZnCl_2 = 136.3$.
CAS — 7646-85-7.
ATC — B05XA12.

Pharmacopoeias. In Eur. (see p.vi), Jpn, Pol., and US.

Zinc chloride almost always contains some oxychloride which produces a slightly turbid aqueous solution. Turbid solutions, except when intended for ophthalmic use, may be cleared by adding gradually a small amount of dilute hydrochloric acid. Solutions of zinc chloride should be filtered through asbestos or sintered glass, since they dissolve paper and cotton wool.

Pharmacopoeial description

Ph. Eur.: A white, deliquescent, crystalline powder or cast in white sticks. Very soluble in water; freely soluble in alcohol and in glycerol. An approximately 10% solution in water has a pH of 4.6 to 5.5. Store in nonmetallic containers.

USP 25: A white or practically white, odourless, crystalline powder, or white or practically white crystalline granules. May also be in porcelain-like masses or moulded into cylinders. It is very deliquescent. Soluble 1 in 0.5 of water, 1 in 1.5 of alcohol, and 1 in 2 of glycerol. Its solution in water or in alcohol is usually slightly turbid, but the turbidity disappears when a small quantity of hydrochloric acid is added. A 10% solution in water is acid to litmus. Store in airtight containers.

Zinc Gluconate (17035-v)

$C_{12}H_{22}O_{14}Zn = 455.7$.
CAS — 4468-02-4.
ATC — A12CB02.
Pharmacopoeias. In US.

Zinc gluconate 350 mg is approximately equivalent to 50 mg of zinc.

Pharmacopoeial description

USP 25: White or practically white powder or granules. Soluble in water; very slightly soluble in alcohol. pH of a 1% solution in water is between 5.5 and 7.5.

Zinc Sulfate (5330-m)

Zinc Sulphate; Zinci Sulfas; Zincum Sulfuricum.
$ZnSO_4,7H_2O = 287.6$.
CAS — 7733-02-0 (anhydrous zinc sulfate); 7446-20-0 (zinc sulfate heptahydrate).
ATC — A12CB01.

NOTE. 'White vitriol' or 'white copperas' is crude zinc sulfate. ZSU is a code approved by the BP 2001 for use on single unit doses of eye drops containing zinc sulfate where the individual container may be too small to bear all the appropriate labelling information.

Pharmacopoeias. In Chin., Eur. (see p.vi), Jpn, and Pol.
US includes the monohydrate and the heptahydrate.

Each g of zinc sulfate represents 3.5 mmol of zinc. Zinc sulfate 220 mg is approximately equivalent to 50 mg of zinc.

Pharmacopoeial description

Ph. Eur.: Colourless, transparent, crystals or a white crystalline powder; efflorescent. Very soluble in water; practically insoluble in alcohol. A 5% solution in water has a pH of 4.4 to 5.6. Store in nonmetallic containers.

USP 25: It contains one or seven molecules of water of hydration. Colourless, transparent, prisms, or small needles. May occur as a white, granular, crystalline powder. It is odourless and is efflorescent in dry air. Very soluble in water (heptahydrate); freely soluble in water (monohydrate); practically insoluble in alcohol (monohydrate); insoluble in alcohol (heptahydrate); freely soluble in glycerol (heptahydrate). Its solutions are acid to litmus. Store in airtight containers.

Adverse Effects, Treatment, and Precautions

The most frequent adverse effects of zinc salts (the gluconate and sulfate) administered by mouth are gastrointestinal and include abdominal pain, dyspepsia, nausea, vomiting, diarrhoea, gastric irritation, and gastritis. These are particularly common if zinc salts are taken on an empty stomach, and may be reduced by administration with meals.

In acute overdosage zinc salts are corrosive, due to the formation of zinc chloride by stomach acid; treatment consists of administration of milk or alkali carbonates and activated charcoal. The use of emetics or gastric lavage should be avoided.

Prolonged administration of high doses of zinc supplements by mouth or parenterally leads to copper deficiency with associated sideroblastic anaemia and neutropenia. Zinc toxicity has occurred after the use of contaminated water in haemodialysis solutions. High serum zinc concentrations may be reduced by using a chelating drug such as sodium calcium edetate (p.1022).

Metal fume fever is an occupational disease associated with inhalation of freshly-oxidised metal fumes, most commonly from zinc, iron or copper. It is characterised by fever, nausea, dyspnoea, and chest pain, and is generally self-limiting and does not appear to be associated with long-term sequelae.

Parenteral nutrition. Zinc was found to be a common contaminant of various components used for total parenteral nutrition (TPN), and rubber stoppers or glass may have been the source.[1] Levels of zinc found may exceed daily requirements even before the addition of supplementary zinc. The authors suggested it may be important to routinely monitor zinc status in patients receiving long-term TPN, particularly infants and children.

1. Hak EB, *et al.* Chromium and zinc contamination of parenteral nutrient solution components commonly used in infants and children. *Am J Health-Syst Pharm* 1998; **55:** 150–4.

Interactions

The absorption of zinc may be reduced by iron supplements, penicillamine, phosphorus-containing preparations, and tetracyclines. Zinc supplements reduce the absorption of copper, fluoroquinolones (see Antacids and Metal Ions, under Interactions of Ciprofloxacin, p.184), iron, penicillamine, and tetracyclines (p.259).

Pharmacokinetics

Zinc is incompletely absorbed from the gastrointestinal tract, and absorption is reduced in the presence of some dietary constituents such as phytates. Bioavailability of dietary zinc varies widely between different sources, but is approximately 20 to 30%. Zinc is distributed throughout the body with the highest concentrations found in muscle, bone, skin, and prostatic fluids. It is primarily excreted in the faeces, and regulation of faecal losses is important in zinc homoeostasis. Small amounts are lost in urine and perspiration.

Human Requirements

◊ In the UK dietary reference values (DRV)[1] and in the USA recommended dietary allowances (RDA)[2] have been published for zinc (see p.1352 for an explanation of these terms). In the UK the reference nutrient intake (RNI) for adult males and females is 9.5 and 7.0 mg daily respectively; values are also given for infants and children of varying ages and for lactating women. In the USA the RDA for adults is 11 mg daily for men and 8 mg daily for women.[2] The tolerable upper intake level is 40 mg daily. WHO recommend lower limits of the safe ranges of population mean intakes of dietary zinc for 3 categories of diets based on high, moderate, and low zinc bioavailability: values are 4.0, 6.5, and 13.1 mg dietary zinc daily for women, and 5.6, 9.4, and 18.7 mg dietary zinc daily for men, respectively.[3] They recommend an upper limit of the safe range of population mean intakes of zinc of 35 mg per day for women, and 45 mg per day for men.

1. DoH. Dietary reference values for food energy and nutrients for the United Kingdom: report of the panel on dietary reference values of the committee on medical aspects of food policy. *Report on health and social subjects 41.* London: HMSO, 1991.
2. Standing Committee on the Scientific Evaluation of Dietary Reference Intakes of the Food and Nutrition Board. *Dietary Reference Intakes for vitamin A, vitamin K, arsenic, boron, chromium, copper, iodine, iron, manganese, molybdenum, nickel, silicon, vanadium, and zinc.* Washington DC: National Academy Press, 2001.
3. WHO. Zinc. In: *Trace elements in human nutrition and health.* Geneva: WHO, 1996: 72–104.

Uses and Administration

Zinc is an essential element of nutrition and traces are present in a wide range of foods. It is a constituent of many enzyme systems and is present in all tissues. Features of zinc deficiency include growth retardation and defects of rapidly-dividing tissues such as the skin, the immune system, and the intestinal mucosa. Water-soluble zinc salts are used as supplements to correct zinc deficiency; for example, in malabsorption syndromes, during parenteral feeding, in conditions with increased body losses (trauma, burns, and protein-losing states), and in acrodermatitis enteropathica (a rare genetic disorder characterised by severe zinc deficiency). They have been tried in the treatment of a large number of conditions that may be related to zinc deficiency. In deficiency states, zinc is usually given by mouth as the sulfate, the sulfate monohydrate, or the gluconate, in doses of up to 50 mg of elemental zinc three times daily. When intravenous supplements are required, zinc chloride or zinc sulfate may be given; a suggested dose for parenteral nutrition is 6.5 mg of elemental zinc (100 μmol) daily.

Oral zinc salts, commonly the acetate, may be used as copper absorption inhibitors in Wilson's disease (p.1019).

Zinc sulfate is used topically in a variety of skin conditions mainly for its astringent properties. The insoluble zinc salts, commonly the oxide (p.1128), are used similarly. A 1.2% solution of zinc acetate is used topically in combination with erythromycin in the treatment of acne vulgaris (p.1103). Zinc sulfate is also used as an astringent in eye drops. Zinc chloride has been employed for its powerful caustic and astringent properties, usually in very dilute solution, in, for example, mouthwashes.

Common cold. Zinc salts, in the form of lozenges, have been tried in the treatment of the common cold (p.605) with variable results.[1-5] A systematic review of randomised trials found that there was no strong evidence to recommend their use.[6]

1. Al-Nakib W, *et al.* Prophylaxis and treatment of rhinovirus colds with zinc gluconate lozenges. *J Antimicrob Chemother* 1987; **20:** 893–901.
2. Douglas RM, *et al.* Failure of effervescent zinc acetate lozenges to alter the course of upper respiratory tract infections in Australian adults. *Antimicrob Agents Chemother* 1987; **31:** 1263–5.
3. Smith DS, *et al.* Failure of zinc gluconate in treatment of acute upper respiratory tract infections. *Antimicrob Agents Chemother* 1989; **33:** 646–8.
4. Mossad SB, *et al.* Zinc gluconate lozenges for treating the common cold: a randomized, double-blind, placebo-controlled study. *Ann Intern Med* 1996; **125:** 81–8.
5. Macknin ML, *et al.* Zinc gluconate lozenges for treating the common cold in children: a randomized controlled trial. *JAMA* 1998; **279:** 1962–7.
6. Marshall I. Zinc for the common cold (updated 29 August 2001). Available in The Cochrane Library; Issue 4. Oxford: Update Software; 2001.

Deficiency states. General references.

1. Bryce-Smith D. Zinc deficiency—the neglected factor. *Chem Br* 1989; **25:** 783–6.

DIARRHOEA. Chronic diarrhoea can be a sign of zinc deficiency, and diarrhoea can lead to excessive zinc losses and zinc deficiency when dietary zinc is inadequate. Zinc supplements have been shown to reduce the incidence, intensity, or duration of acute diarrhoea (p.1203) in children in developing countries.[1-4] A pooled analysis of 10 trials performed in developing countries found that zinc supplementation was associated with a 25% reduction in prevalence of diarrhoea.[5]

1. Sazawal S, *et al.* Zinc supplementation in young children with acute diarrhea in India. *N Engl J Med* 1995; **333:** 839–44.
2. Roy SK, *et al.* Randomised controlled trial of zinc supplementation in malnourished Bangladeshi children with acute diarrhoea. *Arch Dis Child* 1997; **77:** 196–200.
3. Ruel MT, *et al.* Impact of zinc supplementation on morbidity from diarrhea and respiratory infections among rural Guatemalan children. *Pediatrics* 1997; **99:** 808–13.
4. Penny ME, *et al.* Randomized, community-based trial of the effect of zinc supplementation, with and without other micronutrients on the duration of persistent childhood diarrhea in Lima, Peru. *J Pediatr* 1999; **135:** 208–17.
5. Bhutta ZA, *et al.* Prevention of diarrhea and pneumonia by zinc supplementation in children in developing countries: pooled analysis of randomized controlled trials. *J Pediatr* 1999; **135:** 689–97.

GROWTH RETARDATION. Growth retardation (p.1273) in a group of short Japanese children without endocrine abnormalities was found to be associated with mild to moderate zinc deficiency; supplementation with zinc sulfate 5 mg per kg body-weight daily by mouth over 6 months resulted in an improvement in growth velocity despite unchanged growth hormone production.[1]

1. Nakamura T, *et al.* Mild to moderate zinc deficiency in short children: effect of zinc supplementation on linear growth velocity. *J Pediatr* 1993; **123:** 65–9.

TASTE DISORDERS. Zinc appears to be effective for the treatment of taste disturbances (p.667) associated with zinc deficiency but there is insufficient evidence to determine its efficacy for taste dysfunction secondary to conditions that do not involve low serum zinc concentrations.[1]

1. Heyneman CA. Zinc deficiency and taste disorders. *Ann Pharmacother* 1996; **30:** 186–7.

Wilson's disease. References.

1. Anderson LA, *et al.* Zinc acetate treatment in Wilson's disease. *Ann Pharmacother* 1998; **32:** 78–87.

Preparations

BP 2001: Zinc Sulphate Eye Drops; Zinc Sulphate Lotion; **USP 25:** White Lotion; Zinc Chloride Injection; Zinc Sulfate Injection; Zinc Sulfate Ophthalmic Solution.

Proprietary Preparations (details are given in Part 3)

Aust.: Solvezink; *Austral.:* Bioglan Zinc Chelate; Zincaps; *Braz.:* Zincopan; *Canad.:* Anu-Aide; Anusol; Anuzinc; Egozinc; Micro Zn†; PMS-Egozinc†; Rivasol; *Denm.:* Solvezink; *Fin.:* Solvezink; *Fr.:* Rubozinc; Vitazinc†; Zymizinc; *Ger.:* Nefro-Zinc; Solvezink; Virudermin; Zink beta; Zink Verla; Zink-D Longoral; Zink-Sandoz; Zinkamin; Zinkbrause; Zinkit; Zinkorot; *Hong Kong:* Anuzinc; Egozinc; Zincaps; *Israel:* Avazinc; Zincol; *Ital.:* Pontefix; *Mex.:* Metazinc; *Norw.:* Solvezink; *NZ:* Zincaps; *S.Afr.:* ZN 220; *Swed.:* Solvezink; *Switz.:* Collazin; Virudermin; *Thai.:* Zincaps; Zinctab; *UK:* Cold-Gard; Solvazinc; Tartar Control Listerine; Z Span; Zincosol; *USA:* Eye-Sed; Halls Zinc Defense; Ivy Dry; Orazinc; Verazinc; Zinca-Pak; Zincate.

Multi-ingredient: *Aust.:* Ophtaguttal; *Austral.:* Antioxidant Forte Tablets; Antioxidant Tablets; APR Cream; Beta A-C; Beta-Ace Tablets; Bio-Chromium; Bioglan Joint Mobility; Bioglan The Blue One; Bioglan Zn-A-C; Caprilate; Children's Calcium With Minerals†; Cold and Flu Relief; Cold Sore Relief; Cold Sore Tablets; Echinacea & Antioxidants; Echinacea 4000; Echinacea ACE + Zinc; Echinacea ACE Plus Zinc; Echinacea Complex; Echinacea Herbal Plus Formula†; Extralife Eye-Care; Extralife Flow-Care; Formula Three Triple Strength†; Formula Three†; Galium Complex; Ginkgo ACE†; Goodnight Formula; Horse Radish and Garlic Tablets; In A Wink; Lifechange Mens Complex with Saw Palmetto; Lifesystem Herbal Plus Formula 8 Echinacea†; Macro C + Garlic with Zinc†; Natures Way Total Zinc; Odourless Garlic; Optazine A†; Prefrin Z; Proyeast; Serenoa Complex; Sinus and Hayfever; Strepsils Zinc Cold Relief; Trifolium Complex; Urapro; Visine Allergy; Vita-Minis Cold & Flu; Z-Acne; ZBM; Zinc +

C250; Zinc C Plus; Zinc Plus; Zinc Supplement; Zinc Zenith; Zincfrin; Zinvit; Zinvit C; Zinvit G; *Belg.:* Zincfrin; Zincfrin Antihistaminicum; Zineryt; *Braz.:* Belagin; Borato de Sodio; Colirio Blumen; Colirio Helios; Colirio Legrand; Colirio Moura Brasil; Colirio Vima; Dexa-Vastrictol; Fluo-Vaso; Kalloplast; Mirabel; Mirorroidin; Neo Vastrictol; Pomada Blumen; Vastrictol; Verlin; Visiplex; Visolon; Visual; Zincolok; *Canad.:* Anodan-HC; Anugesic-HC; Anusol Plus; Anusol-HC; Beminal Z†; Hemcort HC; Hemorrhoid Ointment; Lipactin; Onguent Hemorrhoidal; Orajel Mouth Aid; PMS-Egozinc-HC; Proctodan-HC; Rectogel; Rectogel HC; Rivasol HC; Visine Allergy; Zinc Plus; Zincfrin; Zincfrin-A; *Denm.:* Zincfrin; *Fin.:* Wicnelact; Zincfrin; Zincfrin-A; *Fr.:* Aftagel; Alphane†; Arbum; Cystelle Shampooing Cheveux Gras; Cysti-Z; Dermalibour; Dermo-Sulfuryl; Femiplexe†; Kelual Zinc; Keralac Plus; Keraliss 14; Ramet Dalibour; Ramet Pain; Ruboderm; Septalibour; Visiolyre; Vitasedine†; YSE; YSE Glutamique; *Ger.:* Baran-mild N; Efadermin; Gehwol Nagelpilz; Lipactin; Oculosan N; Zincfrin; Zineryt; *Hong Kong:* Aderma Dermalibour; Chelated Zinc; Hemcort HC; Oculosan; Osteocare; Irl.: Efalith; Zineryt; *Israel:* Hemo; Visine AC; *Ital.:* Acnesan; Bagno Oculare; Cuprosodio; Emmenoiasi; Formedico; Indaco; Lozione Same AS†; Meziv; Zinc-Imizol; Zincometil; Zineryt; *Mex.:* Afazol Z; Dalidome; Z Frin; *Neth.:* Zincfrin†; Zineryt; *NZ:* Clear Eyes ACR; Efalith; Prefrin Z; Zincfrin; *Port.:* Kemphor; Mentofenol; Oralbiotico; Oratol; Zineryt; *S.Afr.:* Nazene; Oculoforte; Oculosan; Zincfrin-A†; Zincfrin†; *Singapore:* New Daigaku; Redoxon Double Action; *Spain:* Acnosan; Buco Regis; Cilinavagin Neomicina; Clo Zinc†; Cloranfenic Zinc; Coliriocilina Adren Astr; Dexa Vasoc†; Fluo Vasoc; Mirantal†; Odamida; Odontocromil c Sulfamida; Regal†; Vasocon Ant; Vasoconstr; Zincfrin; Zineryt; *Swed.:* Mezinc; Zincfrin; *Switz.:* Acne Lotion; Bonactin†; Collypan; Efalith; Hima-Pasta nouvelle formule; Lipactin; Oculosan; Oculosan forte; Rocanal Permanent Gangrene†; Rocanal Permanent Vital†; Zincfrin†; *Thai.:* Oculosan; Opplin; Visotone; Zincfrin; *UK:* Brushtox; Ceezinc; Dencyl†; Ditemic†; Efalith; Fefol Z†; Fesovit Z†; Flavo-Zinc; Listermint; Lypsyl Cold Sore Gel; Osteocare; Redoxon Double Action; Se-Power; Strepsils Zinc Defence; Vicks Vital; Zineryt; *USA:* Amerigel; Astring-O-Sol†; Benadryl Itch; Caladryl Clear; Clear Eyes ACR; Clearly Calagel†; Dermasept Antifungal; Geneye AC Allergy†; Gets-It; Nasal-Ease; Orajel Mouth Aid; Sulpho-Lac; Super Ivy Dry; VasoClear A; Visine Allergy Relief; Ze Caps; Zincfrin.

The symbol † denotes a preparation no longer actively marketed

Organic Solvents

Most of the solvents described in this chapter have no specific therapeutic use. Additional solvents used in pharmacy and described in other chapters include alcohols, chlorinated hydrocarbons such as chloroform and trichloroethylene, fixed oils, glycols, paraffins, and water.

Organic solvents are widely used in industry and toxicity may follow acute or chronic exposure. Adverse effects may occur due to inhalation, ingestion, or absorption through the skin. Organic solvents are irritant to the skin and mucous membranes, and also commonly affect the CNS. They may sensitise the myocardium to catecholamines and cardiac arrhythmias may occur. Chronic exposure may lead to central and peripheral neurotoxicity, as well as to renal toxicity and hepatotoxicity.

◊ References.
1. White RF, Proctor SP. Solvents and neurotoxicity. *Lancet* 1997; **349:** 1239–43.

Abuse. Since they are volatile liquids and have CNS effects many organic solvents are implicated in volatile substance abuse. Clinical features of intoxication are similar to those of alcohol intoxication, with initial CNS stimulation followed by CNS depression, which may progress to delirium, convulsions, coma, and death. Sudden death due to cardiac arrhythmias has also been reported.
1. Proceedings of a meeting on substance abuse. *Hum Toxicol* 1989; **8:** 253–334.
2. Ashton CH. Solvent abuse. *BMJ* 1990; **300:** 135–6.

Acetone (6501-j)
Dimethyl Ketone; 2-Propanone.
$C_3H_6O = 58.08$.
CAS — 67-64-1.
Pharmacopoeias. In Eur. (see p.vi). *Also in USNF.*

Pharmacopoeial description
Ph. Eur.: A volatile, clear, colourless liquid; the vapour is flammable. Miscible with water, with alcohol, and with ether. Protect from light.

USNF 20: A transparent, colourless, mobile, volatile, very flammable liquid, having a characteristic odour. Sp. gr. not more than 0.789. Miscible with water, with alcohol, with chloroform, with ether, and with most volatile oils. A 50% solution in water is neutral to litmus. Store in airtight containers remote from fire.

Adverse Effects and Treatment
Inhalation of acetone vapour causes excitement followed by CNS depression with headache, restlessness, fatigue, and possibly convulsions, leading to coma and respiratory depression in severe cases. Vomiting and haematemesis may occur. There may be a latent period before the onset of symptoms of acetone poisoning. Similar symptoms may be observed after ingestion of acetone although hyperglycaemia has also been reported. The vapour is irritant to mucous membranes in high concentrations.

Acetone is commonly implicated in volatile substance abuse (p.1400).

Treatment of adverse effects consists of removal from exposure and general supportive and symptomatic measures; activated charcoal may be administered.

◊ For the possible effect of acetone on the metabolism of acetonitrile, see under Acetonitrile, below.

Pharmacokinetics
Acetone is absorbed through the lungs following inhalation. Some absorption occurs from the gastrointestinal tract. It is mostly excreted unchanged, predominantly through the lungs and also in the urine.

Uses
Acetone is widely used as an industrial, pharmaceutical, and domestic solvent; it is also used as an extraction solvent in food processing.

Preparations
Proprietary Preparations (details are given in Part 3)
Multi-ingredient: *Ital.:* Benzogen Ferri.

Acetonitrile (6502-z)
Ethanenitrile; Methyl Cyanide.
$C_2H_3N = 41.05$.
CAS — 75-05-8.

A colourless liquid with an aromatic odour. Wt per mL about 0.79 g. B.p. about 81°.

Acetonitrile emits highly toxic fumes of hydrogen cyanide when heated to decomposition or when reacted with acids or oxidising agents. Store in airtight containers.

Adverse Effects and Treatment
As for cyanides (see Hydrocyanic Acid, p.1433).

◊ There have been several reports, including a fatality, of cyanide poisoning in infants following ingestion of artificial nail removers containing acetonitrile.[1,2] As acetonitrile is slowly metabolised to cyanide, serious toxic effects may not occur until several hours after ingestion and there is the danger that these products may be confused with acetone-based nail polish removers which are less toxic. In a report of an adult who died after ingestion of acetonitrile, the onset of symptoms was delayed for 24 hours. It was considered that concomitant ingestion of acetone had slowed the metabolism of acetonitrile.[3]
1. Caravati EM, Litovitz TL. Pediatric cyanide intoxication and death from an acetonitrile-containing cosmetic. *JAMA* 1988; **260:** 3470–3.
2. Losek JD, *et al.* Cyanide poisoning from a cosmetic nail remover. *Pediatrics* 1991; **88:** 337–40.
3. Boggild MD, *et al.* Acetonitrile ingestion: delayed onset of cyanide poisoning due to concurrent ingestion of acetone. *Postgrad Med J* 1990; **66:** 40–1.

Pharmacokinetics
Acetonitrile undergoes metabolism to cyanide. Cyanide is responsible for the toxicity of acetonitrile.

Uses
Acetonitrile is used as an industrial solvent. It may also be present in artificial nail removers.

Amyl Acetate (6503-c)
$C_7H_{14}O_2 = 130.2$.
CAS — 123-92-2 (iso-amyl acetate); 53496-15-4 (sec-amyl acetate); 628-63-7 (n-amyl acetate).

A mixture of isomers, principally *iso-*, *sec-*, and *n*-amyl acetate. *iso*-Amyl acetate is a clear colourless liquid with a sharp, fruity odour. Wt per mL about 0.87 g. B.p. about 140°. Slightly soluble in water; miscible with alcohol and with ether. Store in airtight containers.

Adverse Effects
Prolonged exposure to amyl acetate may produce headache, fatigue, and depression of the CNS. Irritation of mucous membranes may also occur.

Effects on the heart. A 27-year-old man developed headache, nausea, and vomiting after using a paint containing amyl acetate as the solvent in an unventilated room.[1] Some days later chest pain and dyspnoea developed; he was admitted to hospital 2 weeks after exposure with heart failure which slowly responded to treatment.
1. Weissberg PL, Green ID. Methyl-cellulose paint possibly causing heart failure. *BMJ* 1979; **ii:** 1113–14.

Uses
Amyl acetate is used as a pharmaceutical and industrial solvent.

Amylene Hydrate (4004-b)
Aethyldimethylmethanolum; Dimethylethyl Carbinol; Tertiary Amyl Alcohol. 2-Methylbutan-2-ol.
$C_5H_{12}O = 88.15$.
CAS — 75-85-4.
Pharmacopoeias. In Aust. Also in USNF.

Pharmacopoeial description
USNF 20: A clear, colourless, liquid having a camphoraceous odour. Sp. gr. 0.803 to 0.807. Distilling range 97° to 103°. Freely soluble in water; miscible with alcohol, with chloroform, with ether, and with glycerol. Its solutions are neutral to litmus. Store in airtight containers.

Adverse Effects
Amylene hydrate is irritant and has a depressant effect on the CNS.

Uses
Amylene hydrate is used as a pharmaceutical solvent. It was formerly used as a hypnotic.

Aniline (6504-k)
Phenylamine.
$C_6H_7N = 93.13$.
CAS — 62-53-3.

A colourless or pale yellow oily liquid with a characteristic odour, readily darkening to brown on exposure to air and light. Wt per mL about 1.02 g. B.p. about 183°. Store in airtight containers. Protect from light.

◊ CAUTION. *Suitable precautions should be taken to avoid skin contact with aniline as it can penetrate skin and produce systemic toxicity.*

Adverse Effects and Treatment
Inhalation, ingestion, or cutaneous absorption of aniline results in methaemoglobinaemia, with cyanosis, headache, weakness, stupor, convulsions, and coma. Irritation, nausea and vomiting, and cardiac arrhythmias may occur. Haemolysis has been reported and may give rise to renal damage or jaundice. Death is usually a result of cardiovascular collapse.

Treatment may involve methylene blue [methylthioninium chloride] (p.1013), transfusions, or haemodialysis. Gastric lavage may be performed after ingestion; activated charcoal may be administered.

Bladder papillomas have been reported in workers previously exposed to aniline. Commercial aniline may be contaminated with β-naphthylamine, a potential carcinogen.

Uses
Aniline is a solvent with wide industrial applications.

Benzene (6505-a)
Phenyl Hydride.
$C_6H_6 = 78.11$.
CAS — 71-43-2.

NOTE. Benzene may be known as 'benzina', 'benzol', 'benzole', or 'benzolum'. However, 'benzol' is also used to describe a mixture of hydrocarbons and 'benzin' or 'benzine' is used as a name for a petroleum distillate (see also Petroleum Spirit, p.1405).
Pharmacopoeias. In Aust.

A clear colourless flammable liquid with a characteristic aromatic odour. Wt per mL about 0.88 g. B.p. about 80°. Store in airtight containers.

Adverse Effects, Treatment, and Precautions
Symptoms of acute poisoning following inhalation or ingestion of benzene include initial excitement or euphoria followed by CNS depression with headache, dizziness, blurred vision, and ataxia, which in severe cases may progress to coma (accompanied by hyperactive reflexes), convulsions, and death from respiratory failure. Other symptoms include nausea and irritation of the mucous membranes; ventricular arrhythmias may occur. Direct skin contact with liquid benzene may result in marked irritation, and dermatitis may develop on prolonged or repeated exposure.

Prolonged industrial exposure to benzene vapour has been associated with adverse effects on the gastrointestinal tract and the CNS but in particular with marked effects on the bone marrow and blood. Decreases in the numbers of red or white blood cells or of platelets may occur, producing symptoms of headache, fatigue, anorexia, pallor, and petechiae. In severe cases pancytopenia or aplastic anaemia may develop. Leukaemia, particularly acute myeloid leukaemia, has also developed, often many years after exposure to benzene has ceased. These effects have been reported in workers exposed to relatively high concentrations of the vapour (around 200 ppm or more) but reduced red blood cell counts and anaemia have also been reported at lower concentrations. Chromosome abnormalities have been observed after prolonged exposure to benzene, particularly at the higher concentrations associated with blood dyscrasias; however, the significance of these abnormalities in the development of leukaemia is unclear.

Treatment of poisoning consists of symptomatic and supportive measures. Gastric lavage may be performed for acute intoxication if the patient presents soon after ingestion but care must be taken to avoid aspiration. Activated charcoal may be administered. In chronic poisoning, repeated blood transfusions may be necessary. Adrenaline [epinephrine] and other sympathomimetics should be avoided because of the risk of precipitating cardiac arrhythmias.

◊ Reviews.
1. Health and Safety Executive. Benzene. *Toxicity Review 4.* London: HMSO, 1982.

Malignant neoplasms. Epidemiological data have supported an association between benzene exposure and acute myeloid leukaemia, but the risk following low levels of exposure (1 to 10 ppm) was not clear.[1] A large cohort study[2] has suggested that there is an increased risk of acute myeloid leukaemia and of non-Hodgkin's lymphoma with benzene exposure at levels below 10 ppm.
1. Austin H, *et al.* Benzene and leukemia: a review of the literature and a risk assessment. *Am J Epidemiol* 1988; **127:** 419–39.
2. Hayes RB, *et al.* Benzene and the dose-related incidence of hematologic neoplasms in China. *J Natl Cancer Inst* 1997; **89:** 1065–71.

Pregnancy. An evaluation of the USA National Natality and Fetal Mortality Survey noted that maternal or paternal occupational exposure to agents such as benzene was associated with an increased risk of still-birth and that paternal exposure to benzene increased the risk of low-birth-weight infants.[1]
1. Savitz DA, *et al.* Effect of parents' occupational exposures on risk of stillbirth, preterm delivery, and small-for-gestational-age infants. *Am J Epidemiol* 1989; **129:** 1201–18.

Pharmacokinetics

Benzene is absorbed by inhalation, and ingestion, but is not significantly absorbed through the skin. Some is excreted unchanged from the lungs. Oxidation to phenol and related quinol compounds occurs, the metabolites being excreted in the urine as conjugates of sulfuric or glucuronic acid.

Uses

Benzene was formerly applied as a pediculicide. Its use as an industrial solvent is decreasing.

Butyl Acetate (12482-e)

n-Butyl acetate.
$C_6H_{12}O_2 = 116.2$.
CAS — 123-86-4.

A clear, colourless flammable liquid with a strong fruity odour. Wt per mL about 0.88 g. B.p. 123° to 126°. Slightly soluble in water; miscible with alcohol. Store in airtight containers.

Adverse Effects

Butyl acetate is irritant. High concentrations may cause CNS depression.

Uses

Butyl acetate is used as an industrial solvent and as an extraction solvent in food processing.

Butyl Alcohol (16556-f)

n-Butanol; *n*-Butyl Alcohol. Butan-1-ol.
$C_4H_{10}O = 74.12$.
CAS — 71-36-3.
Pharmacopoeias. In USNF.

Pharmacopoeial description

USNF 20: A clear, colourless, mobile liquid having a characteristic, penetrating vinous odour. Sp. gr. 0.807 to 0.809. It distils within a range of 1.5°, including 117.7°. Soluble in water; miscible with alcohol, with ether, and with many other organic solvents. Store in airtight containers at a temperature not exceeding 40°.

◊ CAUTION. *Suitable precautions should be taken to avoid skin contact with butyl alcohol as it can penetrate skin and produce systemic toxicity.*

Adverse Effects

Butyl alcohol may be irritant and may cause mild CNS depression with headache, dizziness, and drowsiness.

◊ References to the toxicity of butyl alcohol.
1. Butanols—four isomers: 1-butanol, 2-butanol, tert-butanol, isobutanol. *Environmental Health Criteria 65.* Geneva: WHO, 1987.
2. 1-Butanol. *Health and Safety Guide.* Geneva: WHO, 1987.

Uses

Butyl alcohol is used as an industrial and pharmaceutical solvent and as an extraction solvent in food processing.

Butylamine (12484-y)

n-Butylamine.
$C_4H_{11}N = 73.14$.
CAS — 109-73-9.

A colourless to pale yellow flammable liquid with an ammoniacal odour. Wt per mL about 0.744 g. B.p. about 78°. Miscible with water, with alcohol, and with ether. Store in airtight containers.

◊ CAUTION. *Suitable precautions should be taken to avoid skin contact with butylamine as it can penetrate skin and produce systemic toxicity.*

Adverse Effects

Butylamine is irritant. Symptoms of CNS depression may be observed after exposure to high concentrations of the vapour.

Uses

Butylamine is used as a solvent.

Carbon Disulfide (6506-t)

Carbon Bisulphide; Carbon Disulphide; Carbonei Sulfidum; Carboneum Bisulfuratum; Carboneum Sulfuratum; Schwefelkohlenstoff.
$CS_2 = 76.14$.
CAS — 75-15-0.
Pharmacopoeias. In Aust.

A clear, colourless, volatile, flammable liquid with a chloroform-like odour. Commercial grades have an unpleasant odour described by some as being reminiscent of decaying radishes. Wt per mL about 1.26 g. B.p. about 46°. Store in airtight containers.

The vapour mixed with air in the proportions of 1 to 50% is highly explosive.

◊ CAUTION. *Suitable precautions should be taken to avoid skin contact with carbon disulfide as it can penetrate skin and produce systemic toxicity.*

Adverse Effects and Treatment

Carbon disulfide is irritant. Toxic effects may occur as a result of inhalation, ingestion, or absorption through the skin.

Acute poisoning may result in gastrointestinal disturbances and euphoria, followed by CNS depression. Symptoms include headache, dizziness, mood changes, and in severe cases, manic psychoses, delirium, hallucinations, coma, convulsions, and death due to respiratory failure.

Chronic poisoning has been associated with occupational exposure to carbon disulfide vapour for prolonged periods. It is characterised by peripheral neuropathies; CNS effects such as headache, fatigue, insomnia, tremor, emotional lability, extrapyramidal disorders, bipolar disorder, and encephalopathy; gastrointestinal effects including anorexia, dyspepsia, and ulcerative changes; and effects on the eye. Occupational exposure to carbon disulfide has been shown to be associated with an increased incidence of mortality from coronary heart disease. The action of carbon disulfide on endocrine function has resulted in menstrual irregularities, an increased incidence of spontaneous abortions and premature births, loss of libido, sperm abnormalities, and decreased serum-thyroxine concentrations; there is limited evidence of impaired glucose tolerance.

Treatment consists of removal from exposure and general supportive and symptomatic measures. Gastric lavage may be performed after ingestion; activated charcoal may be administered. Adrenaline [epinephrine] and other sympathomimetics should be avoided because of the risk of precipitating cardiac arrhythmias. Peripheral neuropathies may be only slowly reversible.

◊ Reviews of the toxicity of carbon disulfide.
1. Carbon Disulfide. *Environmental Health Criteria 10.* Geneva: WHO, 1979.
2. WHO. Recommended health-based limits in occupational exposure to selected organic solvents. *WHO Tech Rep Ser 664* 1981.
3. Health and Safety Executive. Carbon disulphide. *Toxicity Review 3.* London: HMSO, 1981.

Effects on endocrine function. A retrospective study of 265 female workers in the rayon industry exposed for at least one year to carbon disulfide, and 291 non-exposed female workers.[1] Levels of exposure to carbon disulfide varied over the study period from 0.7 to 30.6 mg per m^3. Women exposed to carbon disulfide had a higher risk of menstrual disturbances than non-exposed women. However, there was no difference between the 2 groups in incidence of toxaemia, emesis gravidarum, spontaneous abortion, premature or overdue delivery, or congenital malformation.

1. Zhou SY, *et al.* Effects of occupational exposure to low-level carbon disulfide (CS$_2$) on menstruation and pregnancy. *Ind Health* 1988; **26:** 203–14.

Effects on the heart. Studies demonstrating an increased incidence of mortality from cardiovascular disease in workers occupationally exposed to carbon disulfide.[1-3] The evidence suggests that the risk decreases after cessation of exposure.

1. Nurminen M, Hernberg S. Effects of intervention on the cardiovascular mortality of workers exposed to carbon disulphide: a 15 year follow up. *Br J Ind Med* 1985; **42:** 32–5.
2. Sweetnam PM, *et al.* Exposure to carbon disulphide and ischaemic heart disease in a viscose rayon factory. *Br J Ind Med* 1987; **44:** 220–7.
3. MacMahon B, Monson RR. Mortality in the US rayon industry. *J Occup Med* 1988; **30:** 698–705.

Pharmacokinetics

Carbon disulfide is rapidly absorbed after inhalation and ingestion, and is also absorbed through intact skin. It is excreted unchanged through the lungs and in the urine predominantly as metabolites.

Uses

Carbon disulfide is used as an industrial solvent and has been used, in the vapour form, as an insecticide.

Carbon Tetrachloride (767-z)

Tetrachloromethane.
$CCl_4 = 153.8$.
CAS — 56-23-5.
Pharmacopoeias. In Belg.

A clear, colourless, mobile, liquid with a chloroform-like odour. Sp. gr. 1.588 to 1.590. B.p. 76° to 78°. Practically insoluble in water; miscible with alcohol, chloroform, ether, petroleum spirit, and fixed and volatile oils. Store in airtight containers at a temperature not exceeding 30°. Protect from light.

◊ CAUTION. *Avoid contact with carbon tetrachloride; the vapour and liquid are poisonous. Care should be taken not to vaporise carbon tetrachloride in the presence of a flame because of the production of harmful gases, mainly phosgene.*

Adverse Effects

Individual response to carbon tetrachloride varies widely; a few mL of carbon tetrachloride inhaled or ingested have proved fatal and its toxicity appears to be increased by alcohol. Symptoms of poisoning follow inhalation, ingestion, or topical application but develop more rapidly after inhalation.

Carbon tetrachloride is irritant; repeated application of carbon tetrachloride to the skin may result in dermatitis. Aspiration may result in pulmonary oedema.

Adverse effects after acute exposure from any route include gastrointestinal disturbances such as nausea, vomiting, and abdominal pain, and CNS disturbances such as headache, dizziness, and drowsiness, with progression to convulsions, coma, and death from respiratory depression or circulatory collapse. Death may also occur as a result of ventricular arrhythmia. Hepatic and renal cellular necrosis can occur and are associated with free radical production; symptoms usually begin a few days or up to 2 weeks after acute exposure to carbon tetrachloride. Renal damage may present as oliguria, progressing to proteinuria, anuria, weight gain, and oedema. Symptoms of hepatic damage include anorexia, jaundice, and hepatomegaly. If hepatorenal necrosis is not fatal recovery is eventually complete.

Symptoms of chronic poisoning are similar to those of acute poisoning; in addition, paraesthesias, visual disturbances, anaemia, and aplastic anaemia have occurred. Carcinogenicity has been demonstrated in *animals.*

◊ References.
1. Melamed E, Lavy S. Parkinsonism associated with chronic inhalation of carbon tetrachloride. *Lancet* 1977; **i:** 1015.
2. Johnson BP, *et al.* Cerebellar dysfunction after acute carbon tetrachloride poisoning. *Lancet* 1983; **ii:** 968.
3. Perez AJ, *et al.* Acute renal failure after topical application of carbon tetrachloride. *Lancet* 1987; **i:** 515–6.
4. Health and Safety Executive. Carbon tetrachloride, chloroform. *Toxicity Review 23.* London: HMSO, 1992.
5. Manno M, Rezzadore M. Critical role of ethanol abuse in carbon tetrachloride poisoning. *Lancet* 1994; **343:** 232.

Treatment of Adverse Effects

If carbon tetrachloride vapour has been inhaled the patient should be removed to the fresh air. Clothing contaminated by liquid should be removed and the skin washed. If carbon tetrachloride has been recently ingested gastric lavage may be performed and activated charcoal may be administered.

The usual symptomatic and supportive measures should be instituted. Hepatic and renal function should be monitored closely. Haemodialysis or peritoneal dialysis may be needed if renal function is impaired. Adrenaline [epinephrine] or other sympathomimetics should be avoided because of the risk of precipitating cardiac arrhythmias.

Acetylcysteine (p.1084) may be administered to patients recently exposed to carbon tetrachloride in an attempt to prevent or modify hepatic and renal damage.

◊ Experimental studies and anecdotal reports suggest that hyperbaric oxygen therapy is of potential benefit in the treatment of carbon tetrachloride poisoning.[1]
1. Burkhart KK, *et al.* Hyperbaric oxygen treatment for carbon tetrachloride poisoning. *Drug Safety* 1991; **6:** 332–8.

Pharmacokinetics

Carbon tetrachloride is readily absorbed after inhalation and from the gastrointestinal tract. It is also absorbed through the skin. Metabolism to reactive free radicals is thought to account for the hepatorenal toxicity of carbon tetrachloride.

Carbon tetrachloride is slowly excreted from the body via the lungs and the urine.

Uses

Carbon tetrachloride is employed in industry as a solvent and degreaser. It was formerly used in certain types of fire extinguisher and as an industrial and domestic dry cleaner but has been largely replaced for this purpose by less toxic substances. Carbon tetrachloride has also been used for the fumigation of cereals.

Carbon tetrachloride was formerly given by mouth as an anthelmintic but it has been superseded by equally effective and less toxic drugs.

Cyclohexane (6507-x)

Hexahydrobenzene; Hexamethylene.
$C_6H_{12} = 84.16$.
CAS — 110-82-7.

A colourless, flammable liquid. Wt per mL about 0.78 g. B.p. about 81°. Store in airtight containers.

Adverse Effects

Cyclohexane is irritant, and may also have effects on the CNS.

◊ Reviews of the toxicity of cyclohexane.
1. Health and Safety Executive. Cyclohexane, cumene, para-dichlorobenzene (p-DCB), chlorodifluoromethane (CFC 22). *Toxicity Review 25.* London: HMSO, 1991.

Uses

Cyclohexane is used as an industrial solvent.

Dichloromethane (6521-a)

Methylene Chloride; Methyleni Chloridum.
$CH_2Cl_2 = 84.93$.
CAS — 75-09-2.
Pharmacopoeias. In Eur. (see p.vi). Also in USNF.

Its vapour is not explosive when mixed with air. Phosgene is produced on heating of dichloromethane.

Pharmacopoeial description

Ph. Eur.: A clear, colourless, volatile liquid. Relative density 1.320 to 1.332. It may contain not more than 2% of alcohol and/or not more than 0.03% of 2-methylbut-2-ene as stabiliser. Sparingly soluble in water; miscible with alcohol and with ether. Store in airtight containers. Protect from light.

USNF 20: A clear, colourless, mobile liquid having an odour resembling chloroform. Sp. gr. 1.318 to 1.322. Miscible with alcohol, with ether, and with fixed and volatile oils. Store in airtight containers.

Adverse Effects and Treatment

Acute exposure to dichloromethane vapour may depress the CNS; symptoms progress from headache and dizziness to coma and death in severe cases. Pulmonary oedema has been reported. Significant exposure may result in raised blood concentrations of carboxyhaemoglobin and symptoms of carbon monoxide poisoning. Cardiovascular effects have been attributed to hypoxia secondary to carboxyhaemoglobinaemia. There has been a report of haemolysis following acute ingestion of dichloromethane.

Chronic occupational exposure to dichloromethane vapour has produced gastrointestinal disturbances in addition to symptoms observed after acute poisoning. Dichloromethane is a common constituent of paint strippers and may be implicated in volatile substance abuse (p.1400).

The liquid is irritant and high concentrations of the vapour are irritant to the eyes.

Treatment of acute poisoning consists of removal from exposure and symptomatic and supportive measures. Carboxyhaemoglobinaemia should be managed as for carbon monoxide poisoning (p.1198) by administration of 100% oxygen; hyperbaric oxygen may be indicated. Activated charcoal may be administered following ingestion. Adrenaline [epinephrine] and other sympathomimetics should be avoided because of the risk of precipitating cardiac arrhythmias.

◊ References.
1. Methylene Chloride. *Environmental Health Criteria 32.* Geneva: WHO, 1984.
2. Health and Safety Executive. Dichloromethane (methylene chloride). *Toxicity Review 12.* London: HMSO, 1985.
3. Methylene chloride. *Health and Safety Guide 6.* Geneva: WHO, 1987.
4. Rioux JP, Myers RAM. Methylene chloride poisoning: a paradigmatic review. *J Emerg Med* 1988; **6:** 227–38.
5. Manno M, *et al.* Double fatal inhalation of dichloromethane. *Hum Exp Toxicol* 1992; **11:** 540–5.

Pharmacokinetics

Dichloromethane is rapidly absorbed following inhalation and is also absorbed after ingestion and slowly through intact skin. It appears to be partially metabolised to carbon dioxide and carbon monoxide which are exhaled, although significant blood-carboxyhaemoglobin concentrations may be attained. Some unchanged dichloromethane is exhaled and small amounts are excreted in the urine.

Uses

Dichloromethane is used as a pharmaceutical and industrial solvent. It is also employed as an extraction solvent in food processing.

Dichloromethane is widely used in paint strippers.

Dichloropropane (19073-b)

Propylene Dichloride. 1,2-Dichloropropane.
$C_3H_6Cl_2 = 113.0$.
CAS — 78-87-5.

A colourless, mobile, flammable liquid. Wt per mL about 1.16 g. B.p. about 96°. Store in airtight containers.

Adverse Effects

Dichloropropane is irritant; high concentrations may result in CNS depression.

◊ A report of acute renal failure, haemolytic anaemia, acute liver disease, and disseminated intravascular coagulation following intentional inhalation of a stain remover containing dichloropropane; the patient recovered following blood transfusions and haemodialysis.[1]
1. Locatelli F, Pozzi C. Relapsing haemolytic-uraemic syndrome after organic solvent sniffing. *Lancet* 1983; **ii:** 220.

Uses

Dichloropropane is used as an industrial solvent, dry cleaning agent, and agricultural defumigant.

Diethyl Phthalate (6508-r)

Diethylis Phthalas; Ethyl Phthalate. The diethyl ester of benzene-1,2-dicarboxylic acid .
$C_{12}H_{14}O_4 = 222.2$.
CAS — 84-66-2.
Pharmacopoeias. In Eur. (see p.vi). Also in USNF.

Pharmacopoeial description

Ph. Eur.: A clear, colourless or very slightly yellow, oily liquid. Relative density 1.117 to 1.121. Practically insoluble in water; miscible with alcohol and with ether. Store in airtight containers.

USNF 20: A colourless, practically odourless, oily liquid. Sp. gr. 1.118 to 1.122 at 20°. Insoluble in water; miscible with alcohol, with ether, and with other usual organic solvents. Store in airtight containers.

Adverse Effects

Diethyl phthalate is irritant and, in high concentrations, causes CNS depression.

◊ References.
1. Health and Safety Executive. Review of the toxicity of the esters of o-phthalic acid (phthalate esters). *Toxicity Review 14.* London: HMSO, 1986.
2. Kamrin MA, Mayor GH. Diethyl phthalate: a perspective. *J Clin Pharmacol* 1991; **31:** 484–9.

Uses

Diethyl phthalate is used as a denaturant of alcohol, for example in surgical spirit, and as a solvent and plasticiser.

Preparations

BP 2001: Surgical Spirit.

Dimethyl Sulfoxide (6509-f)

Dimethyl Sulphoxide; Dimethylis Sulfoxidum; DMSO; Methyl Sulphoxide; NSC-763; SQ-9453; Sulphinylbismethane.
$C_2H_6OS = 78.13$.
CAS — 67-68-5.
ATC — M02AX03.
Pharmacopoeias. In Eur. (see p.vi) and US.

Pharmacopoeial description

Ph. Eur.: A colourless hygroscopic liquid or crystals. F.p. not lower than 18.3°. Relative density 1.100 to 1.104. Miscible with water, with alcohol, and with ether. Store in airtight glass containers. Protect from light.

USP 25: A clear, colourless, odourless, hygroscopic liquid. M.p. about 18.4°. Sp. gr. 1.095 to 1.097. Soluble in water; practically insoluble in alcohol, in acetone, in chloroform, in ether, and in benzene. Store in airtight containers. Protect from light.

Adverse Effects and Treatment

High concentrations of dimethyl sulfoxide applied to the skin may cause burning discomfort, itching, erythema, vesiculation, and urticaria. Continued use may result in scaling.

Systemic effects may occur after administration by any route and include gastrointestinal disturbances, drowsiness, headache, and hypersensitivity reactions. A garlic-like odour on the breath and skin is attributed to the formation of dimethyl sulfide (see Pharmacokinetics, below). Intravascular haemolysis has been reported following intravenous administration. Local discomfort and spasm may occur when given by bladder instillation.

Treatment of adverse effects consists of symptomatic and supportive measures. Gastric lavage may be helpful after acute ingestion, although it should be remembered that absorption is rapid.

◊ Reviews.
1. Brobyn RD. The human toxicology of dimethyl sulfoxide. *Ann N Y Acad Sci* 1975; **243:** 497–506.
2. Willhite CC, Katz PI. Toxicology updates: dimethyl sulfoxide. *J Appl Toxicol* 1984; **4:** 155–60.

◊ Dimethyl sulfoxide given by intravenous infusion for spinal cord injury to 14 patients caused transient haemolysis and haemoglobinuria.[1] Infusion strengths greater than 10% were associated with grossly discoloured urine but there was no evidence of renal damage. In 2 patients, raised liver and muscle enzyme concentrations, mild jaundice, and evidence of haemolysis developed after receiving dimethyl sulfoxide intravenously for arthritis.[2] One also developed acute renal tubular necrosis, deterioration in level of consciousness, and evidence of cerebral infarction. Acute, reversible neurological deterioration in a patient has been associated with intravenous dimethyl sulfoxide.[3] Serum hyperosmolality[4] has been reported in a patient who had pre-existing diabetes insipidus after receiving haematopoietic stem cells cryopreserved in dimethyl sulfoxide following chemotherapy for a malignant germ-cell tumour; symptoms included severe headache, confusion, and abdominal pain.
1. Muther RS, Bennett WM. Effects of dimethyl sulfoxide on renal function in man. *JAMA* 1980; **244:** 2081–3.
2. Yellowlees P, *et al.* Dimethylsulphoxide-induced toxicity. *Lancet* 1980; **ii:** 1004–6.
3. Bond GR, *et al.* Dimethylsulphoxide-induced encephalopathy. *Lancet* 1989; **i:** 1134–5.
4. Thomé S, *et al.* Dimethylsulphoxide-induced serum hyperosmolality after cryopreserved stem-cell graft. *Lancet* 1994; **344:** 1431–2.

Precautions

When used as a penetrating basis for other drugs applied topically, dimethyl sulfoxide may enhance their toxic effects.

Since dimethyl sulfoxide has been associated with lens changes in *animals*, the manufacturers recommend assessment of ophthalmic function every 6 months during long-term treatment of cystitis with intravesical instillation of dimethyl sulfoxide. Hepatic and renal function should also be assessed at intervals of 6 months. Bladder instillation may be harmful in patients with urinary-tract malignancy because of vasodilatation.

Interactions

◊ For mention of an interaction between dimethyl sulfoxide and *sulindac,* see p.86.

Pharmacokinetics

Dimethyl sulfoxide is readily absorbed after administration by all routes. It is metabolised by oxidation to dimethyl sulfone and by reduction to dimethyl sulfide. Dimethyl sulfoxide and the sulfone metabolite are excreted in the urine and faeces. Dimethyl sulfide is excreted through the lungs and skin and is responsible for the characteristic odour from patients.

Uses and Administration

Dimethyl sulfoxide is a highly polar substance which has exceptional solvent properties for both organic and inorganic chemicals, and is widely used as an industrial solvent.

It has been reported to have a wide spectrum of pharmacological activity including membrane penetration, anti-inflammatory effects, local analgesia, weak bacteriostasis, diuresis, vasodilatation, dissolution of collagen, and free-radical scavenging.

The principal use of dimethyl sulfoxide is as a vehicle for drugs such as idoxuridine (p.625); it aids penetration of the drug into the skin, and so may enhance the drug's effect. It is also used as a 50% aqueous solution for bladder instillation for the symptomatic relief of interstitial cystitis; doses of 50 mL are instilled and allowed to remain for 15 minutes. Treatment is repeated every 2 weeks initially.

Dimethyl sulfoxide has been administered orally, intravenously, or topically for a wide range of indications including cutaneous and musculoskeletal disorders, but evidence of beneficial effects is limited.

Dimethyl sulfoxide is used as a cryoprotectant for various human tissues.

◊ Reviews.
1. Trice JM, Pinals RS. Dimethyl sulfoxide: a review of its use in the rheumatic disorders. *Semin Arthritis Rheum* 1985; **15:** 45–60.
2. Swanson BN. Medical use of dimethyl sulfoxide (DMSO). *Rev Clin Basic Pharm* 1985; **5:** 1–33.

Cryopreservation. Dimethyl sulfoxide is used as a cryoprotectant in various assisted conception techniques.[1] Adverse effects have been reported in patients receiving haematopoietic stem cells cryopreserved in dimethyl sulfoxide (see under Adverse Effects, above).
1. Trounson AO. Cryopreservation. *Br Med Bull* 1990; **46:** 695–708.

Extravasation of antineoplastics. Several reports have suggested a role for topical dimethyl sulfoxide in the treatment of anthracycline extravasation.[1-4] The problem of antineoplastic extravasation and its management is discussed further on p.480.
1. Lawrence HJ, Goodnight SH. Dimethyl sulfoxide and extravasation of anthracycline agents. *Ann Intern Med* 1983; **98:** 1025.
2. Olver IN, *et al.* A prospective study of topical dimethyl sulfoxide for treating anthracycline extravasation. *J Clin Oncol* 1988; **6:** 1732–5.
3. Rospond RM, Engel LM. Dimethyl sulfoxide for treating anthracycline extravasation. *Clin Pharm* 1993; **12:** 560–1.
4. Bertelli G, *et al.* Dimethylsulphoxide and cooling after extravasation of antitumour agents. *Lancet* 1993; **341:** 1098.

Gallstones. For mention of the use of dimethyl sulfoxide to dissolve gallstones, see Methyl *tert-*Butyl Ether, p.1404.

Interstitial cystitis. Interstitial cystitis is an inflammatory condition of the bladder of unknown aetiology. Symptoms include pain, urinary frequency, urinary urgency, and nocturia. Many treatments have been tried, including local and systemic drug therapy and surgery.

Bladder instillations of a 50% aqueous solution of dimethyl sulfoxide appear to alleviate symptoms.[1,2] The chief effect of dimethyl sulfoxide may be on sensory nerves since there appears to be no significant alteration in the endoscopic or morphological appearance of the bladder after treatment.[3] Treatment has successfully been repeated at relapse.[3]

Oral administration of pentosan polysulfate sodium may also provide some relief of symptoms.
1. Fowler JE. Prospective study of intravesical dimethyl sulfoxide in treatment of suspected early interstitial cystitis. *Urology* 1981; **18:** 21–6.
2. Perez-Marrero R, *et al.* A controlled study of dimethyl sulfoxide in interstitial cystitis. *J Urol (Baltimore)* 1988; **140:** 36–9.
3. Ryan PG, Wallace DMA. Are we making progress in the drug treatment of disorders of the bladder, prostate, and penis? *J Clin Pharm Ther* 1990; **15:** 1–12.

Raised intracranial pressure. Intravenous osmotic diuretics, particularly mannitol, are used to lower raised intracranial pressure (p.811). Small preliminary studies[1,2] indicate that intravenous administration of dimethyl sulfoxide can control raised intracranial pressure refractory to other treatments but some workers[1] have encountered problems with fluid overload and difficulties with administration.
1. Marshall LF, *et al.* Dimethyl sulfoxide for the treatment of intracranial hypertension: a preliminary trial. *Neurosurgery* 1984; **14:** 659–63.
2. Karaca M, *et al.* Dimethyl sulphoxide lowers ICP after closed head trauma. *Eur J Clin Pharmacol* 1991; **40:** 113–14.

Preparations

USP 25: Dimethyl Sulfoxide Irrigation.

Proprietary Preparations (details are given in Part 3)
Canad.: Kemsol; Rimso; *Ger.:* Rheumabene; *UK:* Rimso; *USA:* Rimso.

Multi-ingredient: *Aust.:* Dolobene; *Ger.:* Dolobene; Verrumal; *Hong Kong:* Dolobene; Verrumal; *Israel:* Verrumal; Verucid; *Singapore:* Verrumal; *Spain:* Artrodesmol Extra; *Switz.:* Dolo Demotherm; Dolobene; Histalgane; Histalgane mite; Remexal; Rollbene; Sportusal; Sportusal Spray sine heparino; Venucreme; Venugel; Verra-med; Verrumal; *Thai.:* Verrumal.

Dimethylacetamide   (6510-z)

Acetyldimethylamine; DMAC. *NN*-Dimethylacetamide.
$C_4H_9NO = 87.12$.
CAS — 127-19-5.

A clear, colourless liquid. Wt per mL about 0.94 g. B.p. about 165°. Miscible with water and most organic solvents.

◊ CAUTION. *Suitable precautions should be taken to avoid skin contact with dimethylacetamide as it can penetrate skin and produce systemic toxicity.*

Adverse Effects

As for Dimethylformamide (below), although a disulfiram-like reaction with alcohol has not been reported.

◊ A review[1] of the toxicology of dimethylacetamide with reference to its use as a vehicle for antineoplastic agents.

1. Kim S-N. Preclinical toxicology and pharmacology of dimethylacetamide, with clinical notes. *Drug Metab Rev* 1988; **19:** 345–68.

Uses

Dimethylacetamide is used as an industrial and pharmaceutical solvent.

Dimethylformamide   (6511-c)

DMF. *NN*-Dimethylformamide.
$C_3H_7NO = 73.09$.
CAS — 68-12-2.

A colourless liquid. Wt per mL about 0.95 g. B.p. about 153°.

◊ CAUTION. *Suitable precautions should be taken to avoid skin contact with dimethylformamide as it can penetrate skin and produce systemic toxicity.*

Adverse Effects and Precautions

Dimethylformamide is irritant. Gastrointestinal effects including nausea, vomiting, loss of appetite, and abdominal pain, CNS effects such as headache, dizziness, and weakness, exposed to the liquid or vapour. Some workers exposed to dimethylformamide have experienced a disulfiram-like effect after consumption of alcohol.

◊ Reviews of the adverse effects of dimethylformamide.

1. Dimethylformamide. *Environmental Health Criteria 114.* Geneva: WHO, 1991.

Effects on the liver. Exposure to the solvent, dimethylformamide, was considered to be the most likely cause of elevated liver enzyme values in 36 of 58 (62%) workers in a fabric coating factory.[1] Symptoms reported were generally mild and included anorexia, abdominal pain, nausea, headache, dizziness, and a disulfiram-type reaction to alcohol.

Hepatotoxicity has occurred following acute poisoning with a veterinary drug formulated in dimethylformamide. There were only minor increases in liver enzyme values in a patient who was treated early with acetylcysteine.[2]

1. Redlich CA, *et al.* Liver disease associated with occupational exposure to the solvent dimethylformamide. *Ann Intern Med* 1988; **108:** 680–6.
2. Buylaert W, *et al.* Hepatotoxicity of N,N-dimethylformamide (DMF) after acute poisoning with the veterinary euthanasia drug T-61. *Hum Exp Toxicol* 1996; **15:** 607–11.

Malignant neoplasms. There have been reports of testicular cancer in men occupationally exposed to dimethylformamide.[1] Such an association could not, however, be substantiated by epidemiological data[2] on 3859 male employees exposed to dimethylformamide between 1950 and 1970 and followed up to 1984. It has been suggested that although dimethylformamide may not itself be carcinogenic, it may increase absorption through the skin of heavy metal carcinogens, possibly including chromates.[3]

1. Levin SM, *et al.* Testicular cancer in leather tanners exposed to dimethylformamide. *Lancet* 1987; **ii:** 1153.
2. Chen JL, Kennedy GL. Dimethylformamide and testicular cancer. *Lancet* 1988; **i:** 55.
3. Ducatman AM. Dimethylformamide, metal dyes, and testicular cancer. *Lancet* 1989; **i:** 911.

Pharmacokinetics

Dimethylformamide is absorbed after inhalation and through intact skin. It is excreted mainly in the urine as metabolites.

Uses

Dimethylformamide is used as an industrial solvent.

Dioxan   (6512-k)

Diethylene Dioxide; Diethylene Ether; Dioxane. 1,4-Dioxane.
$C_4H_8O_2 = 88.11$.
CAS — 123-91-1.

NOTE. Do not confuse dioxan and dioxin (p.1604).

A colourless flammable liquid with an ethereal odour. Wt per mL about 1.03 g. B.p. about 101°. Store in airtight containers.

◊ CAUTION. *It is dangerous to distil or evaporate dioxan unless precautions have been taken to remove explosive peroxides. Suitable precautions should be taken to avoid skin contact with dioxan as it can penetrate skin and produce systemic toxicity.*

Adverse Effects and Treatment

Dioxan vapour is irritant to mucous membranes. High concentrations may cause nausea and vomiting, and CNS depression with headache, dizziness, drowsiness, and in severe cases unconsciousness. On repeated exposure, severe hepatic and renal damage, including necrotic changes, can occur and may be fatal. Direct contact with liquid dioxan can result in dermatitis. Dioxan has been shown to be carcinogenic in *animals.*

Treatment consists of removal from exposure and general supportive and symptomatic measures.

Pharmacokinetics

Dioxan is absorbed after inhalation and through the skin. It is metabolised by oxidation to β-hydroxyethoxy-acetic acid.

Uses

Dioxan is used as an industrial solvent.

Epichlorohydrin   (16293-z)

1-Chloro-2,3-epoxypropane.
$C_3H_5ClO = 92.52$.
CAS — 106-89-8.

A colourless, flammable liquid. Wt per mL about 1.18 g. B.p. 115° to 118°. The vapour forms explosive mixtures with air. Harmful gases including phosgene are liberated on heating of epichlorohydrin. Store in airtight containers.

◊ CAUTION. *Suitable precautions should be taken to avoid skin contact with epichlorohydrin as it can penetrate skin and produce systemic toxicity.*

Adverse Effects

Epichlorohydrin is irritant. It has been shown to be carcinogenic to *animals.*

◊ References to the toxicity of epichlorohydrin.

1. Epichlorohydrin. *Environmental Health Criteria 33.* Geneva: WHO, 1984.
2. Epichlorohydrin. *Health and Safety Guide 8.* Geneva: WHO, 1987.
3. Health and Safety Executive. Ammonia, 1-chloro-2,3-epoxypropane (epichlorohydrin), carcinogenicity of cadmium and its compounds. *Toxicity Review 24.* London: HMSO, 1991.

Uses

Epichlorohydrin is used as an industrial solvent.

Solvent Ether   (6513-a)

Aether; Aether Aethylicus; Aether Solvens; Diethyl Ether; Eter; Ether; Éther rectifié; Ethyl Ether; Ethyl Oxide.
$(C_2H_5)_2O = 74.12$.
CAS — 60-29-7.

NOTE. Solvent ether is not intended for anaesthesia; only ether of a suitable quality (see p.1259) should be so used.

Pharmacopoeias. In *Eur.* (see p.vi) and *Jpn, Pol.,* and *US.*

It volatilises very quickly and by so doing reduces temperature. Though ether is one of the lightest of liquids, its vapour is very heavy, being 2½ times heavier than air.

Pharmacopoeial description

Ph. Eur.: A colourless, clear, volatile, highly flammable liquid. It may contain a suitable non-volatile antioxidant at a suitable concentration. Relative density 0.714 to 0.716. Distillation range 34° to 35°. Soluble in water; miscible with alcohol, with dichloromethane, and with fatty oils. Store at 8° to 15° in airtight containers. Protect from light.

USP 25: A colourless, mobile, volatile, flammable liquid, having a characteristic sweet, pungent odour. It is slowly oxidised by the action of air and light, with the formation of peroxides. B.p. about 35°. Sp. gr. 0.713 to 0.716. Soluble 1 in 12 of water; miscible with alcohol, with chloroform, with dichloromethane, with petroleum spirit, with benzene, and with fixed and volatile oils; soluble in hydrochloric acid. Store in partly filled airtight containers at a temperature not exceeding 30° and remote from fire. Protect from light.

◊ CAUTION. *Ether is very volatile and flammable and mixtures of its vapour with oxygen, nitrous oxide, or air at certain concentrations are explosive. It should not be used in the presence of an open flame or any electrical apparatus liable to produce a spark; precautions should be taken against the production of static electrical discharge. Explosive peroxides are generated by the atmospheric oxidation of solvent ether and it is dangerous to distil a sample which contains peroxides.*

Adverse Effects

As for Anaesthetic Ether, p.1259. Ingestion of 30 to 60 mL may be fatal.

Uses

Solvent ether is widely used as a pharmaceutical and industrial solvent, and is used as an extraction solvent in food processing.

Preparations

Proprietary Preparations (details are given in Part 3)
Multi-ingredient: *S.Afr.:* Famstim.

Ethyl Acetate   (6514-t)

Acetic Ether; Aethylis Acetas; Aethylium Aceticum; Ethyl Ethanoate; Ethylis Acetas.
$C_4H_8O_2 = 88.11$.
CAS — 141-78-6.
Pharmacopoeias. In *Eur.* (see p.vi) and *Pol.* Also in *USNF.*

Pharmacopoeial description

Ph. Eur.: A colourless, clear, volatile liquid. Relative density 0.898 to 0.902. B.p. 76° to 78°. Soluble in water; miscible with alcohol, with acetone, and with dichloromethane. Store at a temperature not exceeding 30°. Protect from light.

USNF 20: A transparent, colourless, flammable liquid having a fragrant, refreshing, slightly acetous odour. Sp. gr. 0.894 to 0.898. Soluble in water; miscible with alcohol, with ether, and with fixed and volatile oils. Store in airtight containers at a temperature not exceeding 40°.

Adverse Effects

Ethyl acetate is irritant to mucous membranes. High concentrations may cause CNS depression. Ethyl acetate may be implicated in volatile substance abuse (p.1400).

◊ For discussion of neurotoxicity after occupational exposure to solvents and the absence of such an effect with ethyl acetate, see under Toluene, p.1406.

Uses

Ethyl acetate is used as a flavour and solvent in pharmaceutical preparations. It is also employed in industry as a solvent and is used as an extraction solvent in food processing.

Formamide   (6516-r)

Carbamaldehyde; Methanamide.
$CH_3NO = 45.04$.
CAS — 75-12-7.

A colourless, oily liquid. B.p. 210°. Wt per mL, about 1.13 g.

Profile

Formamide is used as an industrial solvent. It is reported to be irritant.

Glycofurol   (9935-a)

Glycofurol 75; Tetraglycol; Tetrahydrofurfuryl Alcohol Polyethylene Glycol Ether. α-(Tetrahydrofuranyl)-ω-hydroxypoly(oxyethylene).
CAS — 9004-76-6.

A clear, colourless, almost odourless liquid. Wt per mL about 1.08 g. B.p. 80° to 100°. Incompatible with oxidising agents. Store under nitrogen in airtight containers. Protect from light.

Profile

Glycofurol is used as a pharmaceutical solvent for injections.

Hexachloroethane   (780-l)

$C_2Cl_6 = 236.7$.
CAS — 67-72-1.
Pharmacopoeias. In *Aust.*

Profile

Hexachloroethane is a chlorinated hydrocarbon used in industry as a solvent. Eye irritation and photophobia have resulted from industrial exposure to the vapour. It was formerly used in veterinary medicine as an anthelmintic, but has been superseded by less toxic drugs.

n-Hexane   (9931-j)

$C_6H_{14} = 86.18$.
CAS — 110-54-3.

A colourless, flammable, volatile liquid with a faint odour. Wt per mL about 0.66 g. B.p. about 69°. Store in airtight containers.

Adverse Effects

n-Hexane is irritant. Acute exposure to the vapour may result in CNS depression with headache, drowsiness, dizziness, and in severe cases unconsciousness. Chronic occupational exposure and abuse of *n*-hexane have been associated with the development of peripheral neuropathies. *n*-Hexane is a constituent of some adhesives and may be implicated in volatile substance abuse (p.1400). Some adverse effects of petrol have been attributed to its content of *n*-hexane.

◊ References.
1. Health and Safety Executive. *n-Hexane. Toxicity Review 18.* London: HMSO, 1987.
2. *n-Hexane. Environmental Health Criteria 122.* Geneva: WHO, 1991.
3. *n-Hexane. Health and Safety Guide 59.* Geneva: WHO, 1991.

Effects on the nervous system. There have been many reports of peripheral neuropathy attributed to the abuse of, and occupational exposure to, *n*-hexane, although symptoms tend to be milder in the latter.[1] Tetraplegia has occurred in severe cases. There is typically a clinical deterioration several weeks after exposure followed by a slow recovery which, in severe cases, may not be complete. It has been suggested that methyl ethyl ketone potentiates the peripheral neuropathy induced by *n*-hexane. Occupational exposure to *n*-hexane has also been associated with cranial nerve neuropathy.

Parkinsonism in a leather worker, possibly associated with exposure to solvents, predominantly *n*-hexane, has been noted.[2]

For further discussion of neurotoxicity after occupational exposure to solvents including *n*-hexane, see under Toluene, p.1406.

1. Lolin Y. Chronic neurological toxicity associated with exposure to volatile substances. *Hum Toxicol* 1989; **8:** 293–300.
2. Pezzoli G, *et al.* Parkinsonism due to n-hexane exposure. *Lancet* 1989; **ii:** 874.

Pharmacokinetics
n-Hexane is absorbed by inhalation and to a limited extent through the skin. Oxidative metabolites, including 2,5-hexanedione are excreted in the urine largely as conjugates. Some unchanged *n*-hexane is excreted via the lungs.

Uses
n-Hexane is widely used as an industrial solvent, as a solvent in glues, and as an extraction solvent in food processing.

Preparations
Proprietary Preparations (details are given in Part 3)
Multi-ingredient: *Austral.:* Sacsol.

Isobutyl Alcohol (13804-r)
Isobutanol.
$C_4H_{10}O = 74.12$.
CAS — 78-83-1.

Profile
Isobutyl alcohol is used as an industrial solvent. It is also used as an anaesthetic in the American lobster, *Homarus americanus*, in which it is given by injection into the intra-abdominal sinus.

Kerosene (6517-f)
Kerosine; 'Paraffin'.
CAS — 8008-20-6.

Kerosene is a mixture of hydrocarbons, chiefly members of the alkane series, distilled from petroleum. It is a clear, colourless liquid with a characteristic odour. Sp. gr. about 0.8 g. B.p. 180° to 300°. An odourless grade is available. Store in airtight containers.

Adverse Effects
The chief danger from ingestion of kerosene is pneumonitis and attendant pulmonary complications resulting from aspiration. Spontaneous or induced vomiting increases the risk of aspiration. Ingestion of kerosene results in a burning sensation in the mouth and throat, gastrointestinal disturbances, and possibly cough, dyspnoea, and transient cyanosis. There may be excitation followed by CNS depression, with weakness, dizziness, drowsiness, confusion, incoordination, and restlessness progressing to convulsions, coma, and respiratory depression in severe cases. Cardiac arrhythmias have been reported.

The course of poisoning from inhalation is similar to that following ingestion although CNS and cardiac effects are more likely. Kerosene is irritant.

Abuse. A case of volatile substance abuse (p.1400) involving kerosene by inhalation and ingestion has been reported.[1]

1. Das PS, *et al.* Kerosene abuse by inhalation and ingestion. *Am J Psychiatry* 1992; **149:** 710.

Treatment of Adverse Effects
Treatment of kerosene poisoning is supportive and symptomatic. Every precaution should be taken to avoid aspiration of kerosene into the lungs. Most authorities agree that gastric lavage should generally be avoided unless a very large amount of kerosene or an additional toxin such as a pesticide has been ingested. Activated charcoal may be administered. Adrenaline [epinephrine] and other sympathomimetics should be avoided because of the risk of precipitating cardiac arrhythmias.

Uses
Kerosene is used as a degreaser and cleaner and as an illuminating and fuel oil in kerosene ('paraffin') lamps and stoves. The odourless grade has been used as a solvent in the preparation of some insecticide sprays.

2-Methoxyethanol (12943-n)
Ethylene Glycol Monomethyl Ether.
$C_3H_8O_2 = 76.09$.
CAS — 109-86-4.

A clear, colourless to slightly yellow liquid. Wt per mL about 0.96 g. B.p. about 125°. Miscible with water, with alcohol, with acetone, with dimethylformamide, with ether, and with glycerol. Store in airtight containers.

◊ CAUTION. *Suitable precautions should be taken to avoid skin contact with 2-methoxyethanol as it can penetrate skin and produce systemic toxicity.*

Adverse Effects
2-Methoxyethanol is irritant to mucous membranes. Ingestion may result in CNS depression with confusion, weakness, and in severe cases coma and death from respiratory depression. Nausea, metabolic acidosis, and renal damage may also occur. Prolonged industrial exposure to the vapour has been associated with severe effects on the CNS characterised by headache, dizziness, lethargy, weakness, ataxia, tremor, disorientation, mental changes, weight loss, and visual disturbances. Anaemia has also been reported.

◊ References to the toxicity of 2-methoxyethanol and other glycol ethers.

1. Health and Safety Executive. Glycol ethers. *Toxicity Review 10.* London: HMSO, 1985.
2. 2-Methoxyethanol, 2-ethoxyethanol, and their acetates. *Environmental Health Criteria 115.* Geneva: WHO, 1990.
3. Browning RG, Curry SC. Clinical toxicology of ethylene glycol monoalkyl ethers. *Hum Exp Toxicol* 1994; **13:** 325–35.

Uses
2-Methoxyethanol is used as an industrial solvent.

Methyl Alcohol (556-b)
Methanol.
$CH_3OH = 32.04$.
CAS — 67-56-1.
Pharmacopoeias. In Br. and Ger. Also in USNF.

Pharmacopoeial description
BP 2001: A colourless, clear, hygroscopic liquid. B.p. 65°. Relative density 0.791 to 0.793. Miscible with water, with dehydrated alcohol, and with ether. Store at a temperature not exceeding 25°. Protect from moisture.

USNF 20: A clear, colourless, flammable liquid having a characteristic odour. Miscible with water, with alcohol, with ether, with benzene, and with most other organic solvents. Store in airtight containers remote from heat, sparks, and open flames.

◊ CAUTION. *Suitable precautions should be taken to avoid skin contact with methyl alcohol as it can penetrate skin and produce systemic toxicity.*

Adverse Effects
Immediate signs of acute poisoning following ingestion of methyl alcohol resemble those of ethanol (alcohol; ethyl alcohol) intoxication (see p.1131), but are milder. Characteristic symptoms of methyl alcohol poisoning are caused by toxic metabolites and develop after a latent period of about 12 to 24 hours or longer with concomitant ethanol consumption. The outstanding features of poisoning are metabolic acidosis with rapid, shallow breathing, visual disturbances which often proceed to irreversible blindness, and severe abdominal pain. Other symptoms include headache, gastrointestinal disturbances, pain in the back and extremities, and coma which in severe cases may terminate in death due to respiratory failure or, rarely, to circulatory collapse. Mania and convulsions occasionally occur. Individual response to methyl alcohol varies widely. Ingestion of 30 mL is considered to be potentially fatal.

Absorption of methyl alcohol through the skin or inhalation of the vapour may also lead to toxic systemic effects.

◊ References to the adverse effects of methyl alcohol.

1. Jacobsen D, McMartin KE. Methanol and ethylene glycol poisonings: mechanism of toxicity, clinical course, diagnosis and treatment. *Med Toxicol* 1986; **1:** 309–34.
2. Anderson TJ, *et al.* Neurologic sequelae of methanol poisoning. *Can Med Assoc J* 1987; **136:** 1177–9.
3. Cavalli A, *et al.* Severe reversible cardiac failure associated with methanol intoxication. *Postgrad Med J* 1987; **63:** 867–8.
4. Shapiro L, *et al.* Unusual case of methanol poisoning. *Lancet* 1993; **341:** 112.

Treatment of Adverse Effects
Gastric lavage may be considered if the patient presents within 1 hour of ingesting methyl alcohol. Activated charcoal is probably of little use as it does not absorb significant amounts of methyl alcohol. Metabolic acidosis (p.1180) should be corrected immediately with intravenous sodium bicarbonate. Treatment with ethanol, which delays the oxidation of methyl alcohol to its toxic metabolites formaldehyde and formic acid, should also be initiated, the dosage being adjusted to achieve and maintain a blood-ethanol concentration of 1 to 1.5 mg per mL. An oral dose of about 50 g (equivalent to 150 mL of 40% v/v ethanol) for an adult of around 70 kg body-weight has been suggested; the ethanol should be well diluted before administration. If required, an ethanol infusion may then be given for which the following doses have been used: for an average adult, 110 mg per kg body-weight per hour (1.38 mL per kg per

hour of 10% ethanol, or 2.76 mL per kg per hour of 5% ethanol); for a non-drinker or child, 66 mg per kg per hour (0.825 mL per kg per hour of 10% ethanol, or 1.65 mL per kg per hour of 5% ethanol); for a chronic drinker, 153.78 mg per kg per hour (1.95 mL per kg per hour of 10% ethanol, or 3.9 mL per kg per hour of 5% ethanol).

Haemodialysis may be indicated to increase the removal of methyl alcohol and its toxic metabolites. Peritoneal dialysis has been used but is less efficient. Some authorities recommend initiation of haemodialysis if the amount of methyl alcohol ingested exceeds 30 mL (equivalent to about 24 g), if the blood-methyl alcohol concentration is greater than 500 μg per mL, or if severe metabolic acidosis or visual complications develop. If haemodialysis is used, a constant blood-ethanol concentration may be ensured either by increasing the ethanol infusion rate or by addition of ethanol to the dialysate fluid. Treatment should not be discontinued prematurely since oxidation and excretion of methyl alcohol may continue for several days; patients should, therefore, be closely observed and monitored. Suitable supportive treatment should be carried out as required.

Folinic acid and folic acid have been given in the treatment of methyl alcohol toxicity because they may enhance the metabolism of formic acid. Fomepizole (p.1009), an inhibitor of alcohol dehydrogenase, is also used; it inhibits the metabolism of methyl alcohol to its toxic metabolites.

Pharmacokinetics
Methyl alcohol is readily absorbed from the gastrointestinal tract and distributed throughout the body fluids. It may also be absorbed by inhalation or through large areas of skin. Oxidation by alcohol dehydrogenase with formation of formaldehyde and formic acid takes place mainly in the liver and also in the kidneys. These metabolites are thought to be largely responsible for the characteristic symptoms of methyl alcohol poisoning. Metabolism is much slower than for ethanol, which competitively inhibits the metabolism of methyl alcohol. Oxidation and excretion may continue for several days after ingestion. Elimination of unchanged methyl alcohol via the lungs and in the urine is a minor route of excretion.

Uses
Methyl alcohol is used as a pharmaceutical and industrial solvent. It is also used as 'wood naphtha' to denature ethanol in the preparation of industrial methylated spirits. Methyl alcohol is also used as an extraction solvent in food processing.

Preparations
Proprietary Preparations (details are given in Part 3)
Multi-ingredient: *Ger.:* Acarex.

Methyl tert-Butyl Ether (19482-r)
Methyl Terbutyl Ether; Methyl Tertiary Butyl Ether; MTBE. 2-Methoxy-2-methylpropane.
$C_5H_{12}O = 88.15$.
CAS — 1634-04-4.

A volatile, flammable liquid. Wt per mL about 0.74 g. B.p. about 55°. Store in airtight containers.

◊ CAUTION. *Explosive peroxides may be generated by the atmospheric oxidation of methyl tert-butyl ether, but the risk is lower than with solvent ether.*

Adverse Effects
Methyl *tert*-butyl ether is irritant and may cause CNS depression. Adverse effects that have been reported after use as a gallstone solvent are described under Uses and Administration, below.

Uses and Administration
Methyl *tert*-butyl ether is a solvent which is used for the rapid dissolution of cholesterol gallstones.

Gallstones. An alternative to bile acid therapy in patients with gallstones (p.1678) who are not considered suitable for surgery is direct instillation of a solvent into the gallbladder.

Methyl *tert*-butyl ether has been used to dissolve cholesterol gallstones; stones rich in calcium or pigments are not dissolved.[1] Unfortunately incomplete dissolution and residual debris can lead to recurrence of stone formation.[2] The solvent is most commonly instilled via a percutaneous transhepatic catheter,[1,3] although other routes have been used.[4] Gallbladder stones were treated in 75 patients with continuous infusion and aspiration of methyl *tert*-butyl ether 4 to 6 times per minute for an average of 5 hours daily for 1 to 3 days.[1] At least 95% of the stone mass was dissolved in 72 patients. Gallbladder stones recurred in 4 patients between 6 and 16 months after the procedure; 7 of 51 patients with residual stone fragments had an episode of biliary colic during 6 to 42 months of follow-up. Nausea, sometimes with emesis, occurred in about one-third of patients. Overflow of solvent from the gallbladder can result in absorption from the gastrointestinal tract; methyl *tert*-butyl ether is detected on the breath and sedation can occur. One patient in whom overflow occurred developed ulcerative duodenitis and intravascular haemolysis. Coma and acute renal failure have also complicated treatment and have been attributed to leakage alongside the catheter rather than overflow of solvent.[5] Other workers[6,7] have obtained similar results for the dissolution of gallstones. One group[6] found that nausea and vomiting could be reduced if the treatment time was kept short and the perfusion volume was kept as low as possible; they also managed to prevent bile leakage and haemorrhage using a tissue adhesive or subcutaneous administration of ceruletide to contract the gallbladder. Dissolution of gallbladder stones with methyl *tert*-butyl ether is likely to remain confined to specialist centres for use in patients unsuitable for surgical treatment.[1] A combination of litholytic modalities such as dissolution with solvents or bile acids, or lithotripsy may overcome some of the disadvantages of individual treatments.[8]

Methyl *tert*-butyl ether has been instilled via a nasobiliary catheter to dissolve stones in the common bile duct. Although effective in some cases,[9] further study has indicated disappointing overall results.[1,10]

Various combinations of drugs have been investigated to dissolve pigment-rich or mixed stones. For common bile-duct stones these include a cocktail of dimethyl sulfoxide 60%, methyl *tert*-butyl ether 20%, and sodium bicarbonate 20%, and a regimen of alternating infusions of pentyl ether and edetic acid-urea 10%.[11] A similar regimen of methyl hexyl ether and edetic acid-urea has been used successfully in 2 patients with calcified gallbladder stones.[12]

1. Bouchier IAD. Gall stones. *BMJ* 1990; **300:** 592–7.
2. Maudgal DP, Northfield TC. A practical guide to the nonsurgical treatment of gallstones. *Drugs* 1991; **41:** 185–92.
3. Thistle JL, *et al.* Dissolution of cholesterol gallbladder stones by methyl *tert*-butyl ether administered by percutaneous transhepatic catheter. *N Engl J Med* 1989; **320:** 633–9.
4. Foerster E-Ch, *et al.* Direct dissolution of gallbladder stones. *Lancet* 1989; **i:** 954.
5. Ponchon T, *et al.* Renal failure during dissolution of gallstones by methyl-*tert*-butyl ether. *Lancet* 1988; **ii:** 276–7.
6. Hellstern A, *et al.* Gall stone dissolution with methyl tert-butyl ether: how to avoid complications. *Gut* 1990; **31:** 922–5.
7. McNulty J, *et al.* Dissolution of cholesterol gall stones using methyltertbutyl ether: a safe effective treatment. *Gut* 1991; **32:** 1550–3.
8. Salen G, Tint GS. Nonsurgical treatment of gallstones. *N Engl J Med* 1989; **320:** 665–6.
9. Murray WR, *et al.* Choledocholithiasis—in vivo stone dissolution using methyl tertiary butyl ether (MTBE). *Gut* 1988; **29:** 143–5.
10. Neoptolemos JP, *et al.* How good is methyl tert-butyl (MTBE) for common bile duct (CBD) stone dissolution? *Gut* 1989; **30:** A736–7.
11. Anonymous. Gallstones, bile acids, and the liver. *Lancet* 1989; **ii:** 249–51.
12. Swobodnik W, *et al.* Dissolution of calcified gallbladder stones by treatment with methyl-hexyl ether and urea-EDTA. *Lancet* 1988; **ii:** 216.

Methyl Butyl Ketone   (10649-h)

2-Hexanone; Methyl *n*-Butyl Ketone. Hexan-2-one.
$C_6H_{12}O = 100.2$.
CAS — 591-78-6.

A colourless, volatile liquid. Wt per mL about 0.82 g. B.p. about 127°. Store in airtight containers.

◊ CAUTION. *Suitable precautions should be taken to avoid skin contact with methyl butyl ketone as it can penetrate skin and produce systemic toxicity.*

Methyl Isobutyl Ketone   (6520-k)

Hexone; Isopropylacetone; MIBK. 4-Methylpentan-2-one.
$C_6H_{12}O = 100.2$.
CAS — 108-10-1.
Pharmacopoeias. In *USNF.*

Pharmacopoeial description

USNF 20: A transparent, colourless, mobile, volatile liquid having a faint ketonic and camphoraceous odour. Sp. gr. not more than 0.799. Distilling range 114° to 117°. Slightly soluble in water; miscible with alcohol, with ether, and with benzene. Store in airtight containers.

◊ CAUTION. *Suitable precautions should be taken to avoid skin contact with methyl isobutyl ketone as it can penetrate skin and produce systemic toxicity.*

Adverse Effects

Methyl butyl ketone and methyl isobutyl ketone may depress the CNS in high concentrations. Their vapours are irritating to mucous membranes. Methyl isobutyl ketone may be implicated in volatile substance abuse (p.1400).

◊ References.
1. Methyl isobutyl ketone. *Environmental Health Criteria 117.* Geneva: WHO, 1990.
2. Methyl isobutyl ketone. *Health and Safety Guide 58.* Geneva: WHO, 1991.

Effects on the nervous system. Peripheral neuropathy[1] has occurred following occupational exposure to methyl butyl ketone, particularly an outbreak of neuropathy in a printing plant after the replacement of methyl isobutyl ketone by methyl butyl ketone in a solvent mixture with methyl ethyl ketone. Methyl ethyl ketone may have potentiated the neurotoxicity induced by methyl butyl ketone.

For further discussion of neurotoxicity after occupational exposure to solvents including methyl butyl ketone, see under Toluene, p.1406.
1. Lolin Y. Chronic neurological toxicity associated with exposure to volatile substances. *Hum Toxicol* 1989; **8:** 293–300.

Uses
Methyl isobutyl ketone is used as an industrial and pharmaceutical solvent and also as an alcohol denaturant. Methyl butyl ketone is used as an industrial solvent.

Methyl Chloride   (6519-n)

Monochloromethane. Chloromethane.
$CH_3Cl = 50.49$.
CAS — 74-87-3.

A colourless gas compressed to a colourless liquid with an ethereal odour. B.p. about −24°. Store in airtight containers.

Adverse Effects and Treatment

Symptoms of methyl chloride intoxication often appear after a latent period of several hours and are similar after acute or chronic exposure to the vapour. Symptoms include gastrointestinal disturbances such as nausea, vomiting, and abdominal pain, and signs of CNS depression including headache, weakness, drowsiness, confusion, visual disturbances, and incoordination progressing to convulsions, coma, and death from respiratory depression in severe cases. There have been a few reports of hepatic and renal damage.

Treatment consists of removal from exposure and supportive and symptomatic measures. Neurological effects may persist for many months.

◊ References to the toxicity of methyl chloride.
1. Repko JD, Lasley SM. Behavioral, neurological, and toxic effects of methyl chloride: a review of the literature. *CRC Crit Rev Toxicol* 1979; **6:** 283–302.

Uses
Methyl chloride is used as an industrial solvent. It has been used as an aerosol propellant and refrigerant and was formerly used as a local anaesthetic.

Methyl Ethyl Ketone   (16890-y)

Ethyl Methyl Ketone; MEK. Butan-2-one.
$C_4H_8O = 72.11$.
CAS — 78-93-3.

A colourless flammable liquid with an acetone-like odour. Wt per mL about 0.81 g. B.p. 79° to 81°. Soluble in water; miscible with alcohol and with ether. Store in airtight containers.

Adverse Effects

Methyl ethyl ketone is irritant. Inhalation may result in mild CNS effects including headache and dizziness; nausea and vomiting may also occur.

Methyl ethyl ketone may be implicated in volatile substance abuse (p.1400).

Effects on the nervous system. There are isolated reports of neurotoxicity produced by methyl ethyl ketone alone.[1] These include one of retrobulbar neuritis and one of peripheral neuropathy. It has been suggested, however, that methyl ethyl ketone potentiates the peripheral neuropathy induced by methyl butyl ketone and *n*-hexane.

For further discussion of neurotoxicity after occupational exposure to solvents including methyl ethyl ketone, see under Toluene, p.1406.
1. Lolin Y. Chronic neurological toxicity associated with exposure to volatile substances. *Hum Toxicol* 1989; **8:** 293–300.

Uses
Methyl ethyl ketone is used as an industrial solvent and as an extraction solvent in food processing.

Octyldodecanol   (6347-x)

Octyldodecanolum.
$C_{20}H_{42}O = 298.5$.
Pharmacopoeias. In *Eur.* (see p.vi). Also in *USNF.*

Pharmacopoeial description

Ph. Eur.: A condensation product of saturated liquid fatty alcohols. It contains not less than 90% of (*RS*)-2-octyldodecan-1-ol the remainder consisting mainly of related alcohols. A clear, colourless to yellowish, oily liquid. Relative density 0.830 to 0.850. Practically insoluble in water; miscible with alcohol. Protect from light.

USNF 20: It contains not less than 90% of 2-octyldodecanol, the remainder consisting chiefly of related alcohols. A clear, water-white, free-flowing liquid. Insoluble in water; soluble in alcohol and in ether. Store in airtight containers.

Profile
Octyldodecanol is used as a pharmaceutical solvent.

Petroleum Spirit   (6518-d)

Light Petroleum; Petroleum Benzin; Petroleum Ether; Solvent Hexane.

Pharmacopoeias. In *Aust., Ger., Jpn.,* and *Pol.* Various boiling ranges are specified.

Swiss describes Benzinum Medicinale, consisting mainly of hexane and heptane.

A purified distillate of petroleum, consisting of a mixture of the lower members of the paraffin series of hydrocarbons. It is a colourless, transparent, very volatile, highly flammable liquid with a characteristic odour. It is available in a variety of boiling ranges.

◊ NOTE. The motor fuel termed 'petrol' in the UK and 'gasoline' in the USA is a mixture of volatile hydrocarbons of variable composition containing paraffins (alkanes), olefins (alkenes), cycloparaffins, and aromatic compounds.

Adverse Effects and Treatment

As for Kerosene, p.1404. Petroleum spirit and petrol, being more volatile and of lower viscosity than kerosene, are more likely to be inhaled and to cause aspiration pneumonitis. The toxicity of petrol varies with its composition; some adverse effects have been attributed to lead additives or to the content of *n*-hexane or benzene. Petrol may be implicated in volatile solvent abuse (p.1400).

◊ References to the toxicity of petroleum spirit.[1-3]
For discussion of neurotoxicity after occupational exposure to solvents including petrol, see under Toluene, p.1406.
1. Selected petroleum products. *Environmental Health Criteria 20.* Geneva: WHO, 1982.
2. Daniels AM, Latcham RW. Petrol sniffing and schizophrenia in a Pacific island paradise. *Lancet* 1984; **i:** 389.
3. Eastwell HD. Elevated lead levels in petrol "sniffers". *Med J Aust* 1985; **143** (suppl): S63–4.

Uses
Petroleum spirit and other petroleum distillates are used as pharmaceutical solvents.

Propylene Carbonate   (5451-l)

4-Methyl-1,3-dioxolan-2-one.
$C_4H_6O_3 = 102.1$.
CAS — 108-32-7.
Pharmacopoeias. In *USNF.*

A clear colourless mobile liquid. Freely soluble in water; miscible with alcohol and with chloroform; practically insoluble in petroleum spirit.

Pharmacopoeial description

USNF 20: Sp. gr. 1.203 to 1.210 at 20°. Store in airtight containers.

Profile

Propylene carbonate is used as a solvent in oral and topical pharmaceuticals and for cellulose-based polymers and plasticisers. It has been used as a nonvolatile, stabilising liquid carrier in hard gelatin capsules.

Tetrachloroethane   (6522-t)

Acetylene Tetrachloride. 1,1,2,2-Tetrachloroethane.
$C_2H_2Cl_4 = 167.8$.
CAS — 79-34-5.

A colourless liquid with a chloroform-like odour. B.p. about 146°. Wt per mL about 1.59 g. Store in airtight containers.

◊ CAUTION. *Suitable precautions should be taken to avoid skin contact with tetrachloroethane as it can penetrate skin and produce systemic toxicity.*

Adverse Effects and Treatment

As for Carbon Tetrachloride, p.1401. Tetrachloroethane is probably the most toxic of the chlorinated hydrocarbons. Poisoning can occur through percutaneous absorption as well as ingestion or inhalation.

Uses
Tetrachloroethane is used as an industrial solvent.

Tetrachloroethylene   (813-v)

Perchloroethylene; Tetrachloroethene; Tetrachloroethylenum.
$C_2Cl_4 = 165.8$.
CAS — 127-18-4.

Adverse Effects and Treatment

As for Carbon Tetrachloride, p.1401. Symptoms, especially following administration by mouth, are less severe with tetrachloroethylene than with carbon tetrachloride.

The vapour or liquid may be irritating to skin or mucous membranes.

Tetrachloroethylene may be implicated in volatile substance abuse (p.1400). Dependence may follow habitual inhalation of small quantities of tetrachloroethylene vapour.

◊ References to adverse effects of tetrachloroethylene.
1. Bagnell PC, Ellenberger HA. Obstructive jaundice due to a chlorinated hydrocarbon in breast milk. *Can Med Assoc J* 1977; **117:** 1047–8.
2. Tetrachloroethylene. *Environmental Health Criteria 31.* Geneva: WHO, 1984.
3. Tetrachloroethylene. *Health and Safety Guide.* Geneva: WHO, 1987.
4. Health and Safety Executive. Tetrachloroethylene (tetrachloroethene, perchloroethylene). *Toxicity Review 17.* London: HMSO, 1987.
5. Mutti A, *et al.* Nephropathies and exposure to perchloroethylene in dry-cleaners. *Lancet* 1992; **340:** 189–93.

The symbol † denotes a preparation no longer actively marketed

Pharmacokinetics

Tetrachloroethylene is slightly absorbed from the gastrointestinal tract; absorption is increased in the presence of alcohol and fats or oils. It is absorbed following inhalation and after direct contact with the skin. It is excreted unchanged in expired air; initial elimination is rapid but a proportion may be retained and excreted slowly.

Metabolites of tetrachloroethylene, mainly trichloroacetic acid, have been found in the urine.

Uses and Administration

Tetrachloroethylene is a chlorinated hydrocarbon widely used as a solvent in industry. It was formerly given by mouth as an anthelmintic, but has been superseded by equally effective and less toxic drugs.

Toluene (6523-x)

Methylbenzene; Phenylmethane; Toluol; Toluole.

$C_7H_8 = 92.14$.

CAS — 108-88-3.

A colourless, volatile, flammable liquid with a characteristic odour. Wt per mL about 0.87 g. B.p. about 111°. Store in airtight containers.

◊ CAUTION. *Suitable precautions should be taken to avoid skin contact with toluene as it can penetrate skin and produce systemic toxicity.*

Adverse Effects, Treatment, and Precautions

Toluene has similar acute toxicity to benzene (p.1400) but is a less serious industrial hazard. Adverse effects are treated similarly to benzene. It is a common constituent of adhesives and is frequently implicated in volatile substance abuse (p.1400). Commercial toluene may contain benzene, and this may perhaps influence the pattern of adverse effects. In addition to acute toxic effects, toluene abuse has been associated with damage to the nervous system, kidneys, liver, heart, and lungs (see below). Chronic poisoning caused by occupational exposure to toluene has resulted mainly in nervous system disorders.

◊ Reviews.
1. WHO. Recommended health-based limits in occupational exposure to selected organic solvents. *WHO Tech Rep Ser 664* 1981.
2. Toluene. *Environmental Health Criteria 52*. Geneva: WHO, 1985.
3. Health and Safety Executive. Toluene. *Toxicity Review 20*. London: HMSO, 1989.

◊ The non-neurological toxicity following volatile substance abuse has been reviewed.[1] Chronic toluene abuse may result in damage to the *kidneys*; renal tubular acidosis and glomerulonephritis have been described, although evidence for the latter is only circumstantial. Renal tubular acidosis has been regarded as reversible; however, there are reports suggesting that damage to renal tubules is permanent.

The few reports linking chronic toluene abuse with *liver* damage cover hepatomegaly and hepatorenal failure. Effects on the *heart* are usually acute; sudden death has resulted from ventricular arrhythmias. Chronic myocarditis with fibrosis has been reported. Chronic toluene inhalation can cause damage to the *lungs*. Autopsies in a few patients have shown changes indicative of emphysema.

Nervous system toxicity has also been reviewed.[2] Cerebellar dysfunction has occurred after toluene abuse; an acute intoxication phase, which usually subsides within weeks of abstinence, is followed by a chronic phase which may be permanent. Diffuse CNS disease such as encephalopathy, dementia, and multifocal brain injury may also develop. An association between toluene abuse and peripheral neuropathy has not been confirmed; muscle weakness may be a result of electrolyte and fluid disturbances. The review cites individual reports of choreoathetosis, epilepsy, and optic atrophy with anosmia and deafness after toluene abuse. Some of these neurological effects, particularly cerebellar effects and diffuse CNS disease have also occurred after occupational exposure to toluene.

Some studies have noted an excess mortality from motor neurone diseases among leather workers,[3] although this has not been confirmed by others.[4] Occupational exposure to solvents has been postulated as the cause.[3] Of the many agents currently used in leather work, those with known or probable neurotoxic effects are *n*-hexane, methyl butyl ketone, toluene, and methyl ethyl ketone. Ethyl acetate is commonly used but has no recognised neurological side-effects.[3] A Swedish study of workers in a range of occupations has found some support for an increased risk of amyotrophic lateral sclerosis after occupational exposure to solvents, probably toluene and petrol.[5] Another Swedish study found an association between multiple sclerosis and occupational exposure to solvents, especially white spirit and petrol.[5]

1. Marjot R, McLeod AA. Chronic non-neurological toxicity from volatile substances. *Hum Toxicol* 1989; **8**: 301–6.
2. Lolin Y. Chronic neurological toxicity associated with exposure to volatile substances. *Hum Toxicol* 1989; **8**: 293–300.
3. Hawkes CH, *et al.* Motoneuron disease: a disorder secondary to solvent exposure? *Lancet* 1989; **i**: 73–6.

4. Martyn CN. Motoneuron disease and exposure to solvents. *Lancet* 1989; **i**: 394.
5. Gunnarsson L-G, Lindberg G. Amyotrophic lateral sclerosis in Sweden 1970-83 and solvent exposure. *Lancet* 1989; **i**: 958.

Pregnancy. Retrospective surveys of pregnancies in mothers with a history of solvent abuse suggested that toluene abuse during pregnancy can cause preterm delivery and perinatal death. It was suggested that toluene may be teratogenic as intrauterine exposure was associated with prenatal and postnatal growth retardation, microcephaly, impairment of mental development, and facial dysmorphia.[1-3] It is uncertain if these results can be extrapolated to cover occupational exposure. Although some studies of occupational exposure to solvents during pregnancy have suggested an association,[4,5] exposure is usually to a number of solvents[5] and there is little consistent evidence to link exposure to any particular one with spontaneous abortion, retarded fetal development, still-birth, or congenital malformation.[6]

1. Wilkins-Haug L, Gabow PA. Toluene abuse during pregnancy: obstetric complications and perinatal outcomes. *Obstet Gynecol* 1991; **77**: 504–9.
2. Pearson MA, *et al.* Toluene embryopathy: delineation of the phenotype and comparison with fetal alcohol syndrome. *Pediatrics* 1994; **93**: 211–15.
3. Arnold GL, *et al.* Toluene embryopathy: clinical delineation and developmental follow-up. *Pediatrics* 1994; **93**: 216–20.
4. McDonald JC, *et al.* Chemical exposures at work in early pregnancy and congenital defect: a case-referent study. *Br J Ind Med* 1987; **44**: 527–33.
5. Khattak S, *et al.* Pregnancy outcome following gestational exposure to organic solvents: a prospective controlled study. *JAMA* 1999; **281**: 1106–9.
6. Scott A. *BMJ* 1992; **304**: 369.

Pharmacokinetics

Toluene is absorbed by inhalation, ingestion, and to some extent through the skin. It is rapidly metabolised mainly by oxidation to benzoic acid which is excreted in the urine largely as the glycine conjugate hippuric acid; *o*-, *m*-, and *p*-cresol are minor urinary metabolites. Some unchanged toluene is excreted through the lungs.

Uses

Toluene is widely used as an industrial solvent.

Trichloroethane (6524-r)

Methylchloroform; α-Trichloroethane. 1,1,1-Trichloroethane.

$C_2H_3Cl_3 = 133.4$.

CAS — 71-55-6.

A colourless, slightly hygroscopic liquid. Sp. gr. about 1.31. B.p. about 74°. Practically insoluble in water; miscible with alcohol, with chloroform, and with ether. Non-flammable. Store in airtight containers.

Adverse Effects and Treatment

Acute intoxication with trichloroethane may result in initial excitement followed by CNS depression with dizziness, drowsiness, headache, lightheadedness, and ataxia, progressing to coma and death from respiratory depression in severe cases. Death may also occur from ventricular arrhythmias. Fatalities have occurred following accidental exposure to high concentrations of trichloroethane in confined spaces. Trichloroethane is commonly used in dry cleaning, typewriter correction fluids, and as a solvent for plaster removal and is frequently implicated in volatile substance abuse (p.1400).

Nausea, vomiting, and diarrhoea have been reported following ingestion. Trichloroethane is a mild irritant.

Treatment of adverse effects consists of removal from exposure and general supportive and symptomatic measures. Activated charcoal may be administered. Adrenaline [epinephrine] and other sympathomimetics should be avoided because of the risk of precipitating cardiac arrhythmias.

◊ Reviews.
1. Health and Safety Executive. 1,1,1-Trichloroethane. *Toxicity Review 9*. London: HMSO, 1984.

◊ According to a brief review of non-neurological toxicity from volatile substance abuse,[1] there were no reports of damage to the *liver* after the abuse of trichloroethane. There was a report of hepatotoxicity following acute occupational exposure, but this might have been a hypersensitivity reaction. There was another report[2] of fatty liver disease in 4 patients with a history of occupational exposure to trichloroethane although there has been some debate over the validity of the association for 2 of these cases.[3,4]

Effects on the *heart* were considered usually to be acute and sudden death from ventricular arrhythmias had occurred in abusers. There have, however, been a few cases of chronic cardiac toxicity after both abuse and occupational exposure.[1]

1. Marjot R, McLeod AA. Chronic non-neurological toxicity from volatile substance abuse. *Hum Toxicol* 1989; **8**: 301–6.
2. Hodgson MJ, *et al.* Liver disease associated with exposure to 1,1,1-trichloroethane. *Arch Intern Med* 1989; **149**: 1793–8.
3. Guzelian PS. 1,1,1-Trichloroethane and the liver. *Arch Intern Med* 1991; **151**: 2321–2.
4. Hodgson MJ, Vanthiel DH. 1,1,1-Trichloroethane and the liver. *Arch Intern Med* 1991; **151**: 2322 and 2325–6.

Effects on the skin. A report of scleroderma in 3 patients occupationally exposed to trichloroethylene and, in 2 cases, also to trichloroethane.[1]

1. Flindt-Hansen H, Isager H. Scleroderma after occupational exposure to trichlorethylene and trichlorethane. *Acta Derm Venereol* (Stockh) 1987; **67**: 263–4.

Pharmacokinetics

Trichloroethane is absorbed after inhalation, ingestion, and through intact skin. Small amounts are metabolised to trichloroethanol and trichloroacetic acid and excreted in the urine, but it is largely excreted unchanged through the lungs over a period of days.

Uses

Trichloroethane has wide applications as an industrial solvent. It is commonly used in dry cleaning, typewriter correction fluids, and as a solvent for plaster removal.

Preparations

Proprietary Preparations (details are given in Part 3)
UK: Zoff.
Multi-ingredient: *Austral.:* Sacsol NF.

White Spirit (6525-f)

A mixture of hydrocarbons available as a colourless liquid. Store in airtight containers.

Adverse Effects and Treatment

As for Kerosene, p.1404.

◊ References to the toxicity of white spirit.[1]

For discussion of neurotoxicity after occupational exposure to solvents including white spirit, see under Toluene, p.1406.

1. Selected petroleum products. *Environmental Health Criteria 20*. Geneva: WHO, 1982.

Uses

White spirit is used as an industrial solvent.

Xylene (6526-d)

Dimethylbenzene; Xylol; Xylole.

$C_8H_{10} = 106.2$.

CAS — 1330-20-7; 108-38-3 (m-xylene); 95-47-6 (o-xylene); 106-42-3 (p-xylene).

Pharmacopoeias. In Aust.

A mixture of the *o*-, *m*-, and *p*-isomers in which the *m*-isomer predominates.

A colourless, volatile, flammable liquid. Wt per mL about 0.86 g. B.p. about 138° to 142°. Store in airtight containers.

◊ CAUTION. *Suitable precautions should be taken to avoid skin contact with xylene as it can penetrate skin and produce systemic toxicity.*

Adverse Effects, Treatment, and Precautions

The acute toxicity of xylene is similar to that of benzene (p.1400) but is less marked. Adverse effects are treated similarly to benzene.

Xylene has been implicated in volatile substance abuse (p.1400). Commercial xylene may contain benzene, and this may perhaps influence the pattern of adverse effects.

Xylene should not be used to dissolve ear wax if the tympanic membrane is perforated.

◊ References.
1. WHO. Recommended health-based limits in occupational exposure to selected organic solvents. *WHO Tech Rep Ser 664* 1981.
2. Health and Safety Executive. Xylenes. *Toxicity Review 26*. London: HMSO, 1992.

Effects on the eyes. Eye injuries due to accidental contact with paints containing xylene have been reported.[1] The injuries resembled alkali burns and were treated in a similar manner.

1. Ansari EA. Ocular injury with xylene - a report of two cases. *Hum Exp Toxicol* 1997; **16**: 273–5.

Effects on the nervous system. References to the adverse effects of xylene on the nervous system.

1. Arthur LJH, Curnock DA. Xylene-induced epilepsy following innocent glue sniffing. *BMJ* 1982; **284**: 1787.
2. Roberts FP, *et al.* Near-pure xylene causing reversible neuropsychiatric disturbance. *Lancet* 1988; **ii**: 273.

Pharmacokinetics

Xylene is absorbed after inhalation, ingestion, and to some extent through the skin. It is rapidly metabolised by oxidation to the corresponding *o*-, *m*-, or *p*-methylbenzoic (toluic) acids and excreted in the urine largely as the glycine conjugate, methylhippuric acid (toluric acid). Xylenols are minor metabolites and are excreted in the urine as the glucuronide and sulfate conjugates. Some unchanged xylene is excreted through the lungs.

Uses

Xylene is used as an industrial and pharmaceutical solvent and in preparations to dissolve ear wax.

Preparations

Proprietary Preparations (details are given in Part 3)
Fr.: Cerulyse; *Ital.:* Cerulisina; *Switz.:* Novo-Cerusol.

Paraffins and Similar Bases

This chapter includes a number of substances used mainly as bases for the preparation of creams, ointments, other topical preparations, and suppositories. They are used either as inert carriers for drugs or for their various emulsifying and emollient properties. Some are also used to improve the texture, stability, or water repellent properties of the final preparation. The bases discussed include petroleum hydrocarbons, animal fats and waxes, vegetable oils, and silicones. Other substances used in the preparation of bases can be found in Soaps and other Anionic Surfactants (p.1496) and in Nonionic Surfactants (p.1344).

Hard Paraffin (6401-w)

905 (mineral hydrocarbons); Hartparaffin; Paraff. Dur.; Paraffin; Paraffin Wax; Paraffinum Durum; Paraffinum Solidum.

CAS — 8002-74-2.

Pharmacopoeias. In Chin., Eur. (see p.vi), Int., Jpn, and Pol. Also in USNF.
USNF includes additionally Synthetic Paraffin.

Pharmacopoeial description

Ph. Eur.: A purified mixture of solid saturated hydrocarbons, generally obtained from petroleum. M.p. 50° to 61°. It is a colourless or white mass. The melted substance is free from fluorescence in daylight. Practically insoluble in water and in alcohol; freely soluble in dichloromethane. Protect from light.

USNF 20: Paraffin is a purified mixture of solid hydrocarbons obtained from petroleum. It is a colourless or white, odourless, more or less translucent mass showing a crystalline structure, and is slightly greasy to the touch. It has a congealing range of 47° to 65°. Insoluble in water and in alcohol; slightly soluble in dehydrated alcohol; freely soluble in chloroform, in ether, in volatile oils, and in most warm fixed oils. An alcoholic extract is neutral to litmus. Store at a temperature not exceeding 40°.

Synthetic Paraffin is a very hard odourless white wax containing mostly long-chain, unbranched, saturated hydrocarbons, with a small amount of branched hydrocarbons. The average molecular weight may range from 400 to 1400. Insoluble in water; very slightly soluble in aliphatic, oxygenated, and halogenated hydrocarbon solvents; slightly soluble in aromatic and normal paraffinic solvents.

Profile

Hard paraffin is employed principally as a stiffening ingredient in ointment bases. It is also used in creams, and as a coating for capsules and tablets.

A variety of hard paraffin (m.p. 43° to 46°) is employed in physiotherapy in the form of paraffin-wax baths for the relief of pain in inflamed joints and sprains.

The injection of paraffins may produce granulomatous reactions.

Preparations

BP 2001: Paraffin Ointment; Simple Ointment; Wool Alcohols Ointment.

Proprietary Preparations (details are given in Part 3)
Multi-ingredient: *UK:* Melrose.

Liquid Paraffin (6402-e)

905 (mineral hydrocarbons); Dickflüssiges Paraffin; Heavy Liquid Petrolatum; Huile de Vaseline Épaisse; Liquid Petrolatum; Mineral Oil; Oleum Petrolei; Oleum Vaselini; Paraffinum Liquidum; Paraffinum Subliquidum; Vaselinöl; Vaselinum Liquidum; White Mineral Oil.

CAS — 8012-95-1.
ATC — A06AA01.

Pharmacopoeias. In Chin., Eur. (see p.vi), Jpn, Pol., and US.

Pharmacopoeial description

Ph. Eur.: A purified mixture of liquid saturated hydrocarbons obtained from petroleum. It is a transparent, colourless, oily liquid, free from fluorescence in daylight. Practically insoluble in water; slightly soluble in alcohol; miscible with hydrocarbons. Protect from light.

USP 25: A mixture of liquid hydrocarbons obtained from petroleum. It may contain a suitable stabiliser. It is a transparent, colourless, odourless or almost odourless, oily liquid, free, or practically free, from fluorescence. Insoluble in water and in alcohol; soluble in volatile oils; miscible with fixed oils (except castor oil). Store in airtight containers.

Light Liquid Paraffin (6403-l)

Dünnflüssiges Paraffin; Huile de Vaseline Fluide; Light Liquid Petrolatum; Light Mineral Oil; Light White Mineral Oil; Paraff. Liq. Lev.; Paraffinum Liquidum Leve; Paraffinum Liquidum Tenue; Paraffinum Perliquidum; Spray Paraffin; Vaselina Liquida.

Pharmacopoeias. In Eur. (see p.vi) and Jpn. Also in USNF. US also includes Topical Light Mineral Oil .

Pharmacopoeial description

Ph. Eur.: Light Liquid Paraffin is a purified mixture of liquid saturated hydrocarbons. It has similar characteristics to Liquid Paraffin, but a lower relative density and viscosity. Protect from light.

USNF 20: Light Mineral Oil is a mixture of liquid hydrocarbons obtained from petroleum. It may contain a suitable stabiliser. It has similar characteristics to Mineral Oil but a lower kinematic viscosity. Store in airtight containers.

Adverse Effects and Precautions

Excessive dosage by mouth, or rectum, may result in anal seepage and irritation. Liquid paraffin is absorbed to a slight extent and may give rise to foreign-body granulomatous reactions. Similar reactions have followed the injection of liquid paraffin and may be considerably delayed in onset. Injection may also cause vasospasm and prompt surgical removal may be required to prevent severe damage. Lipoid pneumonia has been reported following the aspiration of liquid paraffin.

Chronic ingestion of liquid paraffin may rarely be associated with impaired absorption of fat-soluble vitamins and possibly other compounds. It should not be used when abdominal pain, nausea, or vomiting is present. Prolonged use should be avoided. Also it should not be used in children under 3 years of age.

◊ Haematological changes and deposition of food grade liquid paraffins in the liver, spleen, and lymph nodes has occurred during feeding studies in *rats*.[1]

1. FAO/WHO. Evaluation of certain food additives and contaminants: forty-fourth report of the joint FAO/WHO expert committee on food additives. *WHO Tech Rep Ser* 859 1995.

Granuloma. References.
1. Bloem JJ, van der Waal I. Paraffinoma of the face: a diagnostic and therapeutic problem. *Oral Surg* 1974; **38**: 675–80.
2. Albers DD, *et al.* Oil granuloma of the ureter. *J Urol (Baltimore)* 1984; **132**: 114.

Lipoid pneumonia. References.
1. Varkey B, Kutty AVP. Lipoid pneumonia with lipoid granuloma in scalene node. *Ann Intern Med* 1976; **84**: 176–7.
2. Anonymous. Case records of the Massachusetts general hospital. *N Engl J Med* 1977; **296**: 1105–11.
3. Becton DL, *et al.* Lipoid pneumonia in an adolescent girl secondary to use of lip gloss. *J Pediatr* 1984; **105**: 421–3.
4. Beermann B, *et al.* Lipoid pneumonia: an occupational hazard of fire eaters. *BMJ* 1984; **289**: 1728–9.

Uses and Administration

Taken internally, liquid paraffin acts as a lubricant and, since it keeps the stools soft, it has been used in the symptomatic treatment of constipation (p.1202), although its use is generally not recommended. Up to 45 mL is given daily by mouth, usually in the evening although it should not be taken immediately before going to bed. Liquid paraffin is an ingredient of several preparations that contain other laxatives such as cascara, magnesium hydroxide, or phenolphthalein. It has also been given as an enema in a usual dose of 120 mL.

Externally, liquid paraffin may be used as an ingredient of ointment bases, as an emollient and cleanser in certain skin conditions, and as an ophthalmic lubricant in the management of dry eye (p.1498).

Light liquid paraffin has similar uses to liquid paraffin.

Preparations

BP 2001: Cetomacrogol Emulsifying Ointment; Cetrimide Emulsifying Ointment; Emulsifying Ointment; Light Liquid Paraffin Eye Drops; Liquid Paraffin and Magnesium Hydroxide Oral Emulsion; Liquid Paraffin Oral Emulsion; Simple Eye Ointment; Wool Alcohols Ointment;
USP 25: Bland Lubricating Ophthalmic Ointment; Mineral Oil Emulsion; Mineral Oil, Rectal; Topical Light Mineral Oil.
Proprietary Preparations (details are given in Part 3)
Austral.: Agarol; Hamilton Dry Skin; Oilatum Bar; Oilatum Shower Gel; **Belg.:** Lansoyl; **Braz.:** Purol; **Canad.:** Fleet Enema Mineral Oil; Lansoyl; Nujol; Skin Conditioner & Bath Oil†; Therapeutic Bath Oil; **Fr.:** Lansoyl; Laxamalt; Lubentyl; Nujol; Nutra Nutraderme†; Oleatum Bar; Oleatum Emollient; Oleatum Gel; Parlax; Restrical; **Ger.:** Agarol N; Obstinol M; Oleatum; **Hong Kong:** Agarol; Body Wash; Keri; Oilatum Bar; Oilatum Emollient; Oilatum Gel; **Irl.:** Alcoderm; Oilatum Gel; **Ital.:** Agarol CM; Duratirs; **NZ:** Oilatum; **Singapore:** Nutraderm; Oilatum Bar; Oilatum Emollient; Oilatum Gel; **Spain:** Emuliquen Simple; Hodernal; **Switz.:** Lansoyl; Laxamalt; **Thai.:** Nutraderm; Oilatum Bar; Oilatum Emollient; Oilatum Gel; **UK:** Cetraben Bath Oil; Keri; Oilatum Bath Formula; Oilatum Fragrance Free; Oilatum Gel; Oilatum Junior; Oilatum Skin Therapy†; Oilatum Soap; **USA:** Agoral Plain†; Kondremul; Liqui-Doss†; Milkinol†; Neo-Cultol†.
Multi-ingredient: **Aust.:** Balneum F; **Austral.:** Alpha Keri; Alpha Keri Tar; Body Lotion; Cleansing Lotion; DermaVeen Shower and Bath; Dermeze; Duratears; E45; Ego Prickly Heat Powder†; Egozite Baby Cream; Granugen; Hamilton Dry Skin; Lacri-Lube; Oilatum Emollient; Oilatum Plus; Parachoc; Riko-

---

derm; Soov Prickly Heat; **Belg.:** Agarol†; Duratears; Lacrytube; **Braz.:** Agarol; **Canad.:** Agarol Plain; Agarol†; Akwa Tears; Alpha Keri; Duolube; Duratears; Episec; Huile de Bain Therapeutique; Hypotears; Lacri-Lube; Laxarol†; Lubriderm; Magnolax; Oculube†; Optilube; Penederm; Puralube; Stancare†; Therapeutic Bath Oil; Therapeutic Skin Lotion; Ti-Lub; **Denm.:** Ojensalve Neutral; **Fr.:** Balmex; Balneum surgras†; Cerat Inalterable; Cold Cream Naturel; Dexeryl; Lubentyl a la Magnesie; Melaxose; Oilatum Cream; Parapsyllium†; Transitol; Transulose; **Ger.:** Balneum F; Befelka-Oel; Coliquifilm; Gleitgelen; Hoecutin Olbad F†; Obstinol†; Oleobal; Parfenac Basisbad; Windol Basisbad; **Hong Kong:** Alpha Keri; Duratears; Ego Skin Cream; Egozite Baby Cream; Hydromol; Oilatum Plus; Soov Prickly Heat; **Irl.:** Agarol†; Diprobath; Emulsiderm; Hydromol; Lacri-Lube; Milpar†; Oilatum Emollient; Oilatum Junior Flare-up; Oilatum Plus; Petrolagar No. 2†; Petrolagar with Phenolphthalein; Polytar Emollient; **Israel:** Balneum F; Duratears; Emulsiderm; Hypotears; Lacri-Lube; Lacrimol; **Ital.:** Agarol†; Balneum Hermal Forte; Lacrilube; **Neth.:** Agarol†; Duratears Z†; Siccatears†; **Norw.:** Simplex; **NZ:** Alpha Keri; BK; DP; Duratears; E45; Egozite Baby; Hydroderm; Karicare Baby Bath Oil; Karicare Breast Care; Karicare Mother and Baby; Lacrilube; Oilatum Plus; Pharmacycare Bath Oil; Pharmacycare Hand & Body; Polytar Emollient; **Port.:** Balmex; Banholeum Gel†; Oleoban Gel; **S.Afr.:** Agarol; Lacrilube; Millypar†; Oilatum Plus; **Singapore:** Alpha Keri; Duratears; Egozite; Lacrilube; Lubrifilm; Oilatum Plus; Soov Prickly Heat; **Spain:** Aceite Acalorico; Agarol†; Emuliquen Laxante; Lubrifilm; Vaselatum; **Switz.:** Agarol†; Antidry; Balmandol; Balneum Hermal F; Coliquifilm; Duratears†; Falqui†; Melisol†; Paragar; Paragol; **Thai.:** Agarol; Duratears; Emulax; Oilatum Plus; **UK:** 50:50; Agarol; Alpha Keri; Cetraben; Dermalo; Dermol; Diprobase; Diprobath; Doublebase; Emulsiderm; Epaderm; Hydromol; Imuderm; Infaderm; Lacri-Lube; Lubri-Tears; Mil-Par; Oilatum Cream; Oilatum Emollient; Oilatum Junior; Oilatum Junior Flare-up; Oilatum Plus; Polytar Emollient; Refresh Night Time†; **USA:** Agoral; Akwa Tears; Alpha Keri; Desitin Creamy; Dry Eyes; Duratears Naturale; Haley's M-O; Hemorid For Women; Hypotears; Kondremul with Phenolphthalein†; Lacri-Gel; Lacri-Lube; Lacticare; LubriTears; Puralube; Refresh PM; Tears Again; Tears Renewed; Throat Discs; Vagisil; ZBT.

White Soft Paraffin (6404-y)

905 (mineral hydrocarbons); Paraff. Moll. Alb.; Paraffinum Molle Album; Vaselina Branca; Vaseline Officinale; White Petrolatum; White Petroleum Jelly.

Pharmacopoeias. In Aust., Br., Chin., Fr., Ger., Int., It., Jpn, Pol., Port., Swiss, and US. Many pharmacopoeias use the title Vaselinum Album; in Great Britain the name 'Vaseline' is a trade-mark.

Pharmacopoeial description

BP 2001: A semi-solid mixture of hydrocarbons obtained from petroleum and bleached. A white, translucent, soft unctuous mass, not more than slightly fluorescent by daylight even when melted, and odourless when rubbed on the skin. It has a drop point of 42° to 60°. Practically insoluble in water and in alcohol; soluble in chloroform, in ether, and in petroleum spirit (boiling range, 40° to 60°), the solutions sometimes showing a slight opalescence. Protect from light.

USP 25: A purified mixture of semisolid hydrocarbons obtained from petroleum, and wholly or nearly decolorised. A white or faintly yellowish unctuous mass, transparent in thin layers even after cooling to 0°. Insoluble in water; slightly soluble in cold or hot alcohol and in cold dehydrated alcohol; freely soluble in chloroform, in benzene, and in carbon disulfide; soluble in ether, in petroleum spirit, and in most fixed and volatile oils.

Yellow Soft Paraffin (6405-j)

Paraff. Moll. Flav.; Paraffinum Molle Flavum; Petrolatum; Petroleum Jelly; Vaselina Amarela; Yellow Petrolatum; Yellow Petroleum Jelly.

CAS — 8009-03-8.

Pharmacopoeias. In Chin., Eur. (see p.vi), Jpn, Pol., and US. Many pharmacopoeias use the title Vaselinum Flavum; in Great Britain the name 'Vaseline' is a trade-mark.

Pharmacopoeial description

Ph. Eur.: A purified mixture of semi-solid hydrocarbons obtained from petroleum. A yellow, translucent, unctuous mass, slightly fluorescent in daylight when melted. It has a drop point of 40° to 60°. Practically insoluble in water, in alcohol, and in glycerol; soluble in dichloromethane. Protect from light.

USP 25: A purified mixture of semi-solid hydrocarbons obtained from petroleum. It may contain a suitable stabiliser. It is an unctuous yellowish to light amber mass, having not more than a slight fluorescence even after being melted. It is transparent in thin layers. It is free or practically free from odour. M.p. 38° to 60°. Insoluble in water; practically insoluble in cold or hot alcohol and in cold dehydrated alcohol; freely soluble in benzene, in carbon disulfide, in chloroform, and in turpentine oil; soluble in ether, in petroleum spirit, and in most fixed and volatile oils.

Adverse Effects

Adverse effects of white soft paraffin or yellow soft paraffin are rare when used in topical preparations, but sensitivity reactions and acne have been reported following topical use. Granulomatous reactions following absorption or injection and lipoid pneumonia following aspiration have occurred.

◊ A report of burns to the scalp, face, and hands in 5 patients who accidentally ignited their hair following the application of paraffin-based hair grease.[1] Four patients suffered inhalation injury, 2 of whom required intubation.

1. Bascom R, *et al.* Inhalation injury related to use of petrolatum-based hair grease. *J Burn Care Rehabil* 1984; **5:** 327–30.

Hypersensitivity. Studies on the allergenicity of white soft paraffin and yellow soft paraffin products.[1-3] Considering their widespread use there are very few reports of sensitivity; white soft paraffin is generally less sensitising than yellow soft paraffin, although allergenicity differs from product to product. The allergenic components are probably polycyclic aromatic hydrocarbons present as impurities and quantities found in a particular paraffin depend on the source and purification method. Only the purest forms should be used in pharmaceuticals, cosmetics, and for patch testing, and highly purified white soft paraffin is preferred to white soft paraffin.

1. Dooms-Goossens A, Degreef H. Contact allergy to petrolatums (I). Sensitising capacity of different brands of yellow and white petrolatums. *Contact Dermatitis* 1983; **9:** 175–85.
2. Dooms-Goossens A, Degreef H. Contact allergy to petrolatums (II). Attempts to identify the nature of the allergens. *Contact Dermatitis* 1983; **9:** 247–56.
3. Dooms-Goossens A, Dooms M. Contact allergy to petrolatums (III). Allergenicity prediction and pharmacopoeial requirements. *Contact Dermatitis* 1983; **9:** 352–9.

Uses and Administration

Soft paraffin is used as an ointment basis and as an emollient in the management of skin disorders. It is not readily absorbed by the skin. Sterile dressings containing soft paraffin are used for wound dressing and as a packing material. Soft paraffin is also included in ointments used as ophthalmic lubricants in the management of dry eye (p.1498). Application of soft paraffin has also been used for the eradication of pubic lice from the eyelashes (p.1427).

Preparations

BP 2001: Cetomacrogol Emulsifying Ointment; Cetrimide Emulsifying Ointment; Emulsifying Ointment; Paraffin Ointment; Simple Eye Ointment; Simple Ointment; Wool Alcohols Ointment;
USP 25: Bland Lubricating Ophthalmic Ointment; Hydrophilic Ointment; Hydrophilic Petrolatum; Petrolatum Gauze; White Ointment; Yellow Ointment.

Proprietary Preparations (details are given in Part 3)

Austral.: Jelonet; Uni Salve; Unitulle; *Canad.:* Aquaphor; Vaseline; *Fr.:* Jelonet; Unitulle†; *Ital.:* Jelonet; Lomatuell H; *Mex.:* Lubrilin; *S.Afr.:* Jelonet; *Spain:* Lacrilube; *UK:* Dermamist; Jelonet; Paratulle; Vaseline; *USA:* Ocu-Lube.

Multi-ingredient: *Aust.:* Tiroler Steinol; *Austral.:* Blistex Medicated Lip Conditioner†; DermaVeen Moisturising; Dermeze; E45; Lacri-Lube; Poly Visc; *Belg.:* Duratears; Lacrytube; *Canad.:* Akwa Tears; Chapstick Medicated Lip Balm; Diaper Guard†; Duolube; Duratears; Hydrophil; Hypotears; Lacri-Lube; Moisturel; Oculube†; Optilube; Prevex; Puralube; *Denm.:* Ojensalve Neutral; *Fr.:* Dexeryl; Oilatum Cream; Transitol; Transulose; *Ger.:* Coliquifilim; *Hong Kong:* Duratears; Dyprotex; *Irl.:* Lacri-Lube; *Israel:* Duratears; Hypotears; Kamil Blue; Lacri-Lube; Lacrimol; *Ital.:* Lacrilube; *Neth.:* Duratears Z†; Siccatears†; *Norw.:* Simplex; *NZ:* Duratears; Lacrilube; *S.Afr.:* Lacrilube; *Singapore:* Duratears; Lacrilube; Lubrifilm; *Spain:* Lubrifilm; Tears Lubricante; Vaselina Boricada; Vaselina Simple; *Switz.:* Coliquifilm; *Thai.:* Duratears; *UK:* 50:50; Cetraben; Diprobase; Epaderm; Hewletts; Imuderm; Lacri-Lube; Lubri-Tears; Melrose; Oilatum Cream; Oilatum Junior; Refresh Night Time†; *USA:* Akwa Tears; Bottom Better; Chapstick Medicated Lip Balm; Desitin Creamy; Diaper Guard; Dry Eyes; Duratears Naturale; Hemorid For Women; Hypotears; Lacri-Gel; Lacri-Lube; LubriTears; Puralube; Refresh PM; Tears Again; Tears Renewed; Triple Care Extra Protective Cream†.

Alkyl Benzoate (19787-z)

Alkyl (C12-15) Benzoate.
Pharmacopoeias. In USNF.

Pharmacopoeial description

USNF 20: Alkyl benzoate consists of esters of a mixture of C_{12} to C_{15} primary and branched alcohols and benzoic acid. It is a clear, practically colourless, oily liquid. Insoluble in water, in glycerol, and in propylene glycol; soluble in alcohol, in acetone, in ethyl acetate, in isopropyl alcohol, in isopropyl myristate, in isopropyl palmitate, in liquid paraffin, in vegetable oils, in volatile silicones, and in wool fat. Store in airtight containers. Protect from light.

Profile

Alkyl benzoate has emollient properties. It may be used as an oily vehicle.

White Beeswax (6407-c)

Cera Alba; Cera Blanca; Cêra Branca; Cire Blanche; E901; Gebleichtes Wachs; White Wax.
CAS — 8012-89-3.
Pharmacopoeias. In Eur. (see p.vi), Jpn, and Pol. Also in USNF.

Pharmacopoeial description

Ph. Eur.: Bleached yellow beeswax. It occurs as white or yellowish-white pieces or plates, translucent when thin, with an odour similar to that of yellow beeswax, though fainter and never rancid, and with a fine-grained, matt and non-crystalline fracture, becoming soft and malleable when warmed in the hand. Drop point 61° to 65°. Practically insoluble in water; partially soluble in hot alcohol; completely soluble in fatty and essential oils.

USNF 20: Bleached and purified yellow beeswax. A yellowish-white solid, somewhat translucent in thin layers. It has a faint characteristic odour and is free from rancidity. M.p. 62° to 65°. Insoluble in water; sparingly soluble in cold alcohol; boiling alcohol dissolves the cerotic acid and a portion of the myricin, that are constituents of the wax; completely soluble in chloroform, in ether, in fixed oils, and in volatile oils; partly soluble in cold benzene and in cold carbon disulfide; completely soluble in these liquids at about 30°.

Yellow Beeswax (6408-k)

Cêra Amarela; Cera Amarilla; Cera Flava; Cire Jaune; E901; Gelbes Wachs; Yellow Wax.
CAS — 8012-89-3.
Pharmacopoeias. In Chin., Eur. (see p.vi), and Jpn. Also in USNF.

Pharmacopoeial description

Ph. Eur.: The wax obtained by melting with hot water the walls of the honeycomb of the bee, *Apis mellifera*, and removing the foreign matter. It occurs as yellow or light brown pieces or plates with a faint and characteristic odour of honey, and with a fine-grained, matt and non-crystalline fracture, becoming soft and malleable when warmed in the hand. Drop point 61° to 65°. Practically insoluble in water; partially soluble in hot alcohol and in ether; completely soluble in fatty and essential oils.

USNF 20: The purified wax from the honeycomb of the bee, *Apis mellifera* (Apidae). It is a solid, varying in colour from yellow to greyish-brown with an agreeable honey-like odour, somewhat brittle when cold, pliable when warmed in the hand, and presenting a dull, granular, noncrystalline fracture when broken. M.p. 62° to 65°. Insoluble in water; sparingly soluble in cold alcohol; boiling alcohol dissolves the cerotic acid and a portion of the myricin, that are constituents of the wax; completely soluble in chloroform, in ether, in fixed oils, and in volatile oils; partly soluble in cold benzene and in cold carbon disulfide; completely soluble in these liquids at about 30°.

Profile

Yellow beeswax is used as a stiffening agent in ointments and creams, and enables water to be incorporated to produce water-in-oil emulsions. White beeswax is similarly employed; it is occasionally used to adjust the melting-point of suppositories.

A sterile preparation of white beeswax, hard paraffin, and isopropyl palmitate (Sterile Surgical Bone Wax) is used to control bleeding from damaged bone in orthopaedic surgery. It should not be confused with Aseptic Surgical Wax (BPC 1949), also known as Horsley's Wax, which contained yellow beeswax, olive oil, and phenol in a mercuric chloride solution and was used to control haemorrhage in bone or cranial surgery.

Hypersensitivity to beeswax has been reported.

Preparations

BP 2001: Paraffin Ointment;
USP 25: Rose Water Ointment; White Ointment; Yellow Ointment.

Proprietary Preparations (details are given in Part 3)

Multi-ingredient: *Aust.:* Tiroler Steinol; *Fr.:* Balmex; Cerat Inalterable; Cold Cream Naturel; *Port.:* Balmex.

Cetostearyl Alcohol (6410-e)

Alcohol Cetylicus et Stearylicus; Alcool Cetostearilico; Cetearyl Alcohol; Cetostearyl Alc.; Cetylstearylalkohol.
CAS — 8005-44-5; 67762-27-0.
Pharmacopoeias. In Eur. (see p.vi), Int., and Pol. Also in USNF.

Pharmacopoeial description

Ph. Eur.: A mixture of solid aliphatic alcohols. It contains not less than 90% of stearyl plus cetyl alcohols and not less than 40% of stearyl alcohol. A white or pale yellow wax-like mass, plates, flakes, or granules. M.p. 49° to 56°. Practically insoluble in water; soluble in alcohol and in petroleum spirit; freely soluble in ether. When melted, it is miscible with fatty oils, with liquid paraffin, and with melted wool fat.

Emulsifying Cetostearyl Alcohol (Type A) is a mixture containing not less than 80% cetostearyl alcohol and not less than 7% sodium cetostearyl sulfate, both calculated with reference to the anhydrous substance. A suitable buffer may be added. Emulsifying Cetostearyl Alcohol (Type B) is a mixture containing not less than 80% cetostearyl alcohol and not less than 7% sodium laurilsulfate, both calculated with reference to the

anhydrous substance. A suitable buffer may be added. Both types are a white or pale yellow, wax-like mass, plates, flakes, or granules. Soluble in hot water giving an opalescent solution; practically insoluble in cold water; slightly soluble in alcohol.

USNF 20: It contains not less than 40% of stearyl alcohol ($C_{18}H_{38}O$ = 270.5) and the sum of the stearyl alcohol content and the cetyl alcohol ($C_{16}H_{34}O$ = 242.4) content is not less than 90%. Unctuous, white flakes or granules, having a faint, characteristic odour. M.p. 48° to 55°. Insoluble in water; soluble in alcohol and in ether.

Profile

Cetostearyl alcohol is used in creams, ointments, and other topical preparations as a stiffening agent and emulsion stabiliser. In conjunction with suitable hydrophilic substances as in Emulsifying Wax, it produces oil-in-water emulsions which are stable over a wide pH range. It is also used to improve the emollient properties of paraffin ointments.

Cetostearyl alcohol can cause hypersensitivity.

Preparations

BP 2001: Cetomacrogol Emulsifying Wax; Cetrimide Emulsifying Ointment; Emulsifying Wax;
USNF 20: Emulsifying Wax.

Cetyl Alcohol (6411-l)

Alcohol Cetylicus; Álcool Cetílico; Cetanol; 1-Hexadecanol; Hexadecyl Alcohol.
CAS — 36653-82-4; 124-29-8.
Pharmacopoeias. In Eur. (see p.vi), Int., Jpn, and Pol. Also in USNF.

Pharmacopoeial description

Ph. Eur.: A mixture of solid alcohols consisting mainly of cetyl alcohol ($C_{16}H_{33}OH$ = 242.4). It occurs as a white unctuous mass, powder, flakes, or granules. M.p. 46° to 52°. Practically insoluble in water; freely to sparingly soluble in alcohol; freely soluble in ether; miscible when melted with animal and vegetable oils, with liquid paraffin, and with melted wool fat.

USNF 20: A mixture containing not less than 90% of cetyl alcohol ($C_{16}H_{34}O$ = 242.4), the remainder consisting chiefly of related alcohols. White unctuous flakes, cubes, granules, or castings, with a faint characteristic odour. M.p. 45° to 50°. Insoluble in water; soluble in alcohol and in ether, the solubility increasing with increasing temperature.

Profile

Cetyl alcohol is used in topical preparations for its emollient, water absorptive, stiffening, and weak emulsifying properties. It may be incorporated into suppositories to raise the melting-point and may be used in the coating of modified-release solid dose forms.

Cetyl alcohol can cause hypersensitivity.

Preparations

Proprietary Preparations (details are given in Part 3)
Multi-ingredient: *Hong Kong:* Ego Skin Cream.

Cetyl Esters Wax (6430-z)

Synthetic Spermaceti.
Pharmacopoeias. In Int. Also in USNF.

Pharmacopoeial description

USNF 20: A mixture consisting primarily of esters of saturated fatty alcohols (C_{14} to C_{18}) and saturated fatty acids (C_{14} to C_{18}). White to off-white somewhat translucent flakes with a crystalline structure and a pearly lustre when caked; it has a faint odour and is free from rancidity. M.p. 43° to 47°. Insoluble in water; practically insoluble in cold alcohol; soluble in boiling alcohol, in chloroform, in ether, and in fixed and volatile oils; slightly soluble in cold petroleum spirit. Store in a dry place at a temperature not exceeding 40°.

Profile

Cetyl esters wax is used as a stiffening agent and emollient in creams and ointments as a replacement for natural spermaceti obtained from the sperm whale and the bottle-nosed whale.

Preparations

USP 25: Rose Water Ointment.

Cholesterol (6412-y)

Cholesterin; Cholesterolum. Cholest-5-en-3β-ol.
$C_{27}H_{46}O$ = 386.7.
CAS — 57-88-5.
Pharmacopoeias. In Eur. (see p.vi), Jpn, and Pol. Also in USNF.

Pharmacopoeial description

Ph. Eur.: A white or almost white, crystalline powder. It is sensitive to light. M.p. 147° to 150°. Practically insoluble in water; sparingly soluble in alcohol and in acetone. Protect from light.
USNF 20: White or faintly yellow, practically odourless, pearly leaflets, needles, powder, or granules. It acquires a yellow to pale tan colour on prolonged exposure to light. M.p. 147° to 150°. Insoluble in water; slowly soluble 1 in 100 of alcohol; soluble 1 in 50 of dehydrated alcohol; soluble in ace-

tone, in chloroform, in dioxan, in ether, in ethyl acetate, in petroleum spirit, and in vegetable oils. Protect from light.

Profile
Cholesterol imparts water-absorbing power to ointments and is used as an emulsifying agent. It has emollient activity. Cholesteryl benzoate is used as an ingredient in dermatological preparations.

Coconut Oil (6413-j)

Aceite de Coco; Coconut Butter; Oleum Cocois; Oleum Cocos Raffinatum; Oleum Cocosis.
CAS — 8001-31-8.
Pharmacopoeias. In Eur. (see p.vi) and Jpn.

NOTE. Fractionated coconut oil (thin vegetable oil) is used as a source of medium-chain triglycerides (p.1372).

Pharmacopoeial description
Ph. Eur.: The refined fatty oil obtained from the dried, solid part of the endosperm of *Cocos nucifera*. A white or almost white, unctuous mass. M.p. 23° to 26°. Practically insoluble in water; very slightly soluble in alcohol; freely soluble in dichloromethane and in petroleum spirit (b.p. 65° to 70°). Store in well-filled containers. Protect from light.

Profile
Coconut oil forms a readily absorbable ointment basis. It is also used in food manufacturing.

Preparations
Proprietary Preparations (details are given in Part 3)
Ger.: Aesculo Gel L; *UK:* Nitlotion.
Multi-ingredient: *Fin.:* Structolipid; *Fr.:* Structolipide; *Port.:* Structolipid.

Emulsifying Wax (6021-r)

Anionic Emulsifying Wax; Cera Emulsificans; Cetylanum; Emulsif. Wax.
CAS — 8014-38-8.
Pharmacopoeias. In Br. Also in USNF.

Pharmacopoeial description
BP 2001: It is prepared from 9 parts of cetostearyl alcohol and 1 part of sodium laurilsulfate or sodium salts of similar sulfated higher primary aliphatic alcohols. An almost white or pale yellow, waxy solid or flakes, becoming plastic when warmed, with a faint characteristic odour. Practically insoluble in water, forming an emulsion; partly soluble in alcohol.
USNF 20: It is prepared from cetostearyl alcohol containing a polyoxyethylene derivative of a fatty acid ester of sorbitan. M.p. 50° to 54°. It is a creamy-white, wax-like solid, with a mild characteristic odour. Insoluble in water; soluble in alcohol; freely soluble in chloroform, in ether, in most hydrocarbon solvents, and in aerosol propellants.

Profile
Emulsifying wax added to fatty or paraffin bases facilitates the preparation of oil-in-water emulsions which are absorbed and are nongreasy when rubbed into the skin. It is a constituent of many hydrophilic ointment bases for so-called 'washable' ointments.

◊ Emulsifying ointment, which contains emulsifying wax with white soft paraffin and liquid paraffin, was found to have major sunscreen activity in clinically normal skin.[1] It should not be used before phototherapy or in phototesting procedures.
1. Cox NH, Sharpe G. Emollients, salicylic acid, and ultraviolet erythema. *Lancet* 1990; **335:** 53–4.

Preparations
BP 2001: Aqueous Cream; Emulsifying Ointment.
Proprietary Preparations (details are given in Part 3)
Multi-ingredient: *UK:* Epaderm.

Hard Fat (6415-c)

Adeps Neutralis; Adeps Solidus; Glycérides Semi-synthétiques Solides; Hartfett; Massa Estearínica; Neutralfett.
Pharmacopoeias. In Eur. (see p.vi), Int., and Pol. Also in USNF.

Pharmacopoeial description
Ph. Eur.: A mixture of triglycerides, diglycerides, and monoglycerides obtained either by esterification of fatty acids of natural origin with glycerol or by transesterification of natural fats.
A white or almost white, waxy, brittle mass. M.p. 30° to 45°; it does not differ by more than 2° from the nominal value. Practically insoluble in water; slightly soluble in dehydrated alcohol; freely soluble in ether. When heated to 50°, it melts giving a colourless or slightly yellowish liquid. Protect from light and heat.
USNF 20: A mixture of glycerides of saturated fatty acids. A white mass, almost odourless and free from rancid odour, and greasy to the touch. M.p. is between 27° and 44° and does not differ by more than 2° from the nominal value. The melted substance is colourless or slightly yellowish and forms a white

emulsion when shaken with an equal amount of hot water. Practically insoluble in water; slightly soluble in alcohol; freely soluble in ether. Store in airtight containers at a temperature 5° or more below the melting-point.

Profile
The name Hard Fat is applied to a range of bases with varying degrees of hardness and differing melting ranges used for the preparation of suppositories.

Isopropyl Myristate (6416-k)

Isopropylis Myristas. Tetradecanoic acid 1-methylethyl ester; Isopropyl tetradecanoate.
$C_{17}H_{34}O_2 = 270.5$.
CAS — 110-27-0.
Pharmacopoeias. In Eur. (see p.vi). Also in USNF.

Incompatible with hard paraffin.

Pharmacopoeial description
Ph. Eur.: A clear, colourless, oily liquid. Immiscible with water; miscible with alcohol, with dichloromethane, with ether, with fatty oils, and with liquid paraffin. Protect from light.
USNF 20: A clear practically colourless, almost odourless, oily liquid; congeals at about 5°. Insoluble in water, in glycerol and in propylene glycol; freely soluble in alcohol. Miscible with most organic solvents and with fixed oils. Store in airtight containers. Protect from light.

Profile
Isopropyl myristate is resistant to oxidation and hydrolysis and does not become rancid. It is absorbed fairly readily by the skin and is used as a basis for relatively nongreasy emollient ointments and creams. It is also used as a solvent for many substances applied externally.
Other isopropyl fatty acid esters, including di-isopropyl adipate, isopropyl laurate, isopropyl linoleate, and isopropyl palmitate (below) have similar properties and are used for similar purposes to those of isopropyl myristate.

Preparations
Proprietary Preparations (details are given in Part 3)
Spain: Nucoa.
Multi-ingredient: *Hong Kong:* Hydromol; *Irl.:* Diprobath; Emulsiderm; Hydromol; *Israel:* Emulsiderm; *UK:* Dermol; Diprobath; Doublebase; Emulsiderm; Hydromol.

Isopropyl Palmitate (6417-a)

Isopropylis Palmitas. Hexadecanoic acid 1-methylether ester; Isopropyl hexadecanoate.
$C_{19}H_{38}O_2 = 298.5$.
CAS — 142-91-6.
Pharmacopoeias. In Eur. (see p.vi). Also in USNF.

Pharmacopoeial description
Ph. Eur.: A clear, colourless, oily liquid. Immiscible with water; miscible with alcohol, with dichloromethane, with ether, with fatty oils, and with liquid paraffin. Protect from light.
USNF 20: A colourless, mobile, liquid with a very slight odour. Insoluble in water, in glycerol, and in propylene glycol; soluble in alcohol, in acetone, in castor oil, in chloroform, in cottonseed oil, in ethyl acetate, and in mineral oil. Store in airtight containers. Protect from light.

Profile
Isopropyl palmitate has properties and uses similar to those of isopropyl myristate (above).

Laurocapram (16870-s)

Laurocapram (USAN, rINN).
N-0252. 1-Dodecylazacycloheptan-2-one; 1-Dodecylhexahydro-2H-azepin-2-one.
$C_{18}H_{35}NO = 281.5$.
CAS — 59227-89-3.

Profile
Laurocapram (Azone®) has been investigated for enhancing the penetration of drugs through the skin.

Microcrystalline Wax (6422-z)

907 (refined microcrystalline wax).
Pharmacopoeias. In USNF.

Pharmacopoeial description
USNF 20: A mixture of straight-chain, branched-chain, and cyclic hydrocarbons, obtained by solvent fractionation of the still bottom fraction of petroleum by suitable dewaxing or de-oiling means. A white or cream-coloured odourless waxy solid. Melting range 54° to 102°. Insoluble in water; sparingly soluble in dehydrated alcohol; soluble in chloroform, in ether, in volatile oils, and in most warm fixed oils. Store in airtight containers.

Profile
Microcrystalline wax is used as a stiffening agent in creams and ointments and as a tablet and capsule coating agent.

Oleic Acid (1319-f)

Acidum Oleicum; Ölsäure.
CAS — 112-80-1 ($C_{18}H_{34}O_2$).
Pharmacopoeias. In Eur. (see p.vi). Also in USNF.

Pharmacopoeial description
Ph. Eur.: It contains 65% to 88% of (Z)-octadec-9-enoic acid [$C_{18}H_{34}O_2 = 282.5$] together with varying amounts of saturated and other unsaturated fatty acids. It may contain a suitable antioxidant. It is a clear, yellowish or brownish, oily liquid. Practically insoluble in water; miscible with alcohol and with dichloromethane. Store in well-filled airtight containers. Protect from light.
USNF 20: Oleic acid is manufactured from fats and oils derived from edible sources, and consists chiefly of (Z)-9-octadecenoic acid [$CH_3.(CH_2)_7.CH:CH.(CH_2)_7.COOH = 282.5$]. It is a colourless to pale yellow oily liquid when freshly prepared with a characteristic lard-like odour. On exposure to air it gradually absorbs oxygen and darkens in colour. When strongly heated in air, it is decomposed with the production of acid vapours. Congealing point not above 10°. Practically insoluble in water; miscible with alcohol, with chloroform, with ether, with benzene and with fixed and volatile oils. Store in airtight containers.

Profile
Oleic acid forms soaps with alkaline substances and is used as an emulsifying or solubilising agent. It occurs in edible fats and oils which are used as foods or food components and has been used as a choleretic.

Preparations
BP 2001: Chloroxylenol Solution; White Liniment.
Proprietary Preparations (details are given in Part 3)
Multi-ingredient: *Fr.:* Relaxoddi†.

Oleyl Alcohol (6423-c)

CAS — 143-28-2.
Pharmacopoeias. In USNF.

Pharmacopoeial description
USNF 20: A mixture of unsaturated and saturated high molecular weight fatty alcohols consisting chiefly of oleyl alcohol ($C_{18}H_{36}O = 268.5$). A clear colourless to light yellow oily liquid with a faint characteristic odour. Insoluble in water; soluble in alcohol, in ether, in isopropyl alcohol, and in light liquid paraffin. Store in well-filled airtight containers at a temperature not exceeding 25°.

Profile
Oleyl alcohol is used as an emollient and as an emulsifying and solubilising agent. The acetate has also been used.

Fractionated Palm Kernel Oil (6425-a)

Pharmacopoeias. In Br.

Pharmacopoeial description
BP 2001: It is obtained by expression of the natural oil from the kernels of *Elaeis guineensis* followed by selective solvent fractionation and hydrogenation. A white, odourless or almost odourless, solid, brittle fat. M.p. 31° to 36°. Practically insoluble in water and in alcohol; miscible with chloroform, with ether, and with petroleum spirit (boiling range, 40° to 60°). Store at a temperature not exceeding 25°.

Profile
Fractionated palm kernel oil is used as a basis for suppositories. It has also been used in food manufacturing. The unfractionated oil has been used as an emollient and as an ointment basis.

Shea Butter (13235-b)

A natural fat obtained from the kernel of the fruit of *Butyrospermum parkii* (Sapotaceae) indigenous to West Africa.

Profile
Shea butter is used as an ointment and cream basis.

Silicones (13600-s)

ATC — A03AX13.

Silicones are polymers with a structure consisting of alternate atoms of silicon and oxygen, with organic groups attached to the silicon atoms. As the degree of polymerisation increases, the products become more viscous and the various grades are distinguished by a number, approximately corresponding to the viscosity of the particular grade. Silicones may be fluids (or oils), greases, waxes, resins, or rubbers depending on the degree of polymerisation.

The symbol † denotes a preparation no longer actively marketed

Dimeticones (6428-r)

Dimethicone; Dimethicones; Dimethyl Silicone Fluid; Dimethylpolysiloxane; Dimethylsiloxane; Dimeticonum; E900; Huile de Silicone; Methyl Polysiloxane; Permethylpolysiloxane; Silicone Oil; Siliconum Liquidum; Poly(dimethylsiloxane).
$CH_3.[Si(CH_3)_2.O]_nSi(CH_3)_3$.
CAS — 9006-65-9.

NOTE. Dimeticone is *BAN* and *rINN*, and Dimethicone is *USAN*.
Pharmacopoeias. In *Chin.* and *Eur.* (see p.vi). Also in *USNF.*
USNF also includes Cyclomethicone, a fully methylated cyclic siloxane.

Dimeticones are fluid silicones in which the organic group is a methyl radical.
Simeticone (activated dimeticone), a mixture of liquid dimeticones with silicon dioxide, is described on p.1249.

Pharmacopoeial description

Ph. Eur.: Dimeticone is a poly(dimethylsiloxane). The degree of polymerisation is such that the kinematic viscosities are nominally between 20 and 1300 mm^2 per second; dimeticones with a nominal viscosity of 50 mm^2 per second or lower are intended for external use only. Dimeticones are clear, colourless, liquids of various viscosities. Practically insoluble in water; very slightly soluble to practically insoluble in dehydrated alcohol; miscible with ethyl acetate, with methyl ethyl ketone, and with toluene.

USNF 20: Dimethicone is a mixture of fully methylated linear siloxane polymers containing repeating units of the formula $[-(CH_3)_2SiO-]_n$, stabilised with trimethylsiloxy end-blocking units of the formula $[(CH_3)_3SiO-]$, wherein *n* has an average value such that the corresponding nominal viscosity is in a discrete range between 20 and 30 000 centistokes. It is a clear colourless, odourless liquid. Insoluble in water, in alcohol, in acetone, and in methyl alcohol; very slightly soluble in isopropyl alcohol; soluble in amyl acetate, in chlorinated hydrocarbons, in ether, in *n*-hexane, in petroleum spirit, in benzene, in toluene, and in xylene. Store in airtight containers.

Adverse Effects

Adverse effects from the clinical use of silicones appear to be rare. Foreign-body reactions have been reported following their use as joint implants. Other implants, notably breast implants, usually for reconstruction following mastectomy or for cosmetic purposes, carry the risk of migration of silicone with cyst formation and other complications; accidental intravascular injection has been fatal. Late adverse ocular effects can follow the intravitreal injection of liquid silicone in the management of retinal detachment (see below).

Connective-tissue disorders. Since the introduction of silicone breast implants in the early 1960s there have been numerous anecdotal reports of various connective-tissue disorders occurring in women who have undergone breast reconstruction or augmentation with these implants. Scleroderma has been the most frequently reported disorder; others have included systemic lupus erythematosus, rheumatoid arthritis, and inflammatory myopathies. A syndrome of vague musculoskeletal symptoms, fever, and fatigue has also been reported. These cases led the FDA to call for a moratorium in the US on the use of silicone breast implants in January 1992. However, with the exception of one study of self-reported symptoms which showed only a small increase in risk,[1] large epidemiological studies,[2-5] meta-analyses,[6] and a review by the Medical Devices Agency in the UK have so far failed to show any association between silicone breast implants and connective-tissue disorders.

1. Hennekens CH, *et al.* Self-reported breast implants and connective-tissue diseases in female health professionals: a retrospective cohort study. *JAMA* 1996; **275:** 616–21.
2. Gabriel SE, *et al.* Risk of connective-tissue diseases and other disorders after breast implantation. *N Engl J Med* 1994; **330:** 1697–1702.
3. Sánchez-Guerrero J, *et al.* Silicone breast implants and the risk of connective-tissue diseases and symptoms. *N Engl J Med* 1995; **332:** 1666–70.
4. Silverman BG, *et al.* Reported complications of silicone gel breast implants: an epidemiologic review. *Ann Intern Med* 1996; **124:** 744–56.
5. Nyrén O, *et al.* Risk of connective tissue disease and related disorders among women with breast implants: a nation-wide retrospective cohort study in Sweden. *BMJ* 1998; **316:** 417–22.
6. Janowsky EC, *et al.* Meta-analyses of the relation between silicone breast implants and the risk of connective-tissue diseases. *N Engl J Med* 2000; **342:** 781–90.

Uses and Administration

Dimeticones and other silicones are water-repellent and have a low surface tension. They are used in topical barrier preparations for protecting the skin against water-soluble irritants. Creams, lotions, and ointments containing a dimeticone are employed for the prevention of bedsores and napkin rash and to protect the skin against trauma due to incontinence or stoma discharge. Silicone preparations should not be applied where free drainage is necessary or to inflamed or abraded skin. Silicones, usually a dimeticone, are also used topically as wound dressings.

Silicones have also been used for arthroplasty in rheumatic disorders, by intravitreal injection for retinal detachment, and by subcutaneous injection or implantation in reconstructive or cosmetic surgery.

Dimeticones, in particular simeticone (activated dimeticone) (p.1249), are used in the treatment of flatulence.

Retinal detachment. Retinal detachment is separation of the retina from the underlying retinal pigmentary epithelium and usually requires surgical repair. Intravitreal injection of liquid silicone may be used for retinal tamponade following or in conjunction with surgery in complicated or persistent detachment of the retina.[1,2] Late complications following its use may include cataract, glaucoma, and keratopathy.

1. Chan C, Okun E. The question of ocular tolerance to intravitreal liquid silicone: a long-term analysis. *Ophthalmology* 1986; **93:** 651–60.
2. Gray RH, *et al.* Fluorescein angiographic findings in three patients with long-term intravitreal liquid silicone. *Br J Ophthalmol* 1989; **73:** 991–5.

Preparations

Proprietary Preparations (details are given in Part 3)
Austral.: Egozite Protective Baby Lotion; Instru-Safe; Rosken Skin Repair; Silic 15; **Canad.:** Barrier Cream; Barriere; Protecto-Derm†; **Fr.:** Cica-Care; Ophtasiloxane; **Ger.:** Jaikin N; Symadal M; **Hong Kong:** Silic 15; Skin Repair; **Israel:** Adato-Sil Ol; **Ital.:** Radioced†; **NZ:** Aquim; DP Barrier Cream; Egozite Protective Baby; Pharmacycare Barrier; **Singapore:** DP; Egozite; Silic 15; Skin Repair; **UK:** Cica-Care; Silgel.

Multi-ingredient: *Aust.:* Ceolat Compositum; Evalgan; Riker Silicone-Spray†; *Austral.:* Dermalife Plus; Dimethicream; Eczema Cream; Egoderm Ointment; Egozite Baby Cream; Formicare Skin Relief†; Hamilton Skin Repair; Nappy-Mate; Silcon; *Canad.:* Blistex Lip Balm; Blistex Lip Tone; Complex 15; Diaper Guard†; Moisturel; Soft Lips; Zilactin-Lip; *Denm.:* Silan; *Fr.:* Balmex; *Hong Kong:* Dyprotex; Egozite Baby Cream; Hamilton Skin Repair; *Irl.:* Conotrane; Siopel; Sprilon; Vasogen; *Israel:* Kamil Blue; *Ital.:* Angstrom Viso/Labbra Alta Protezione; Rikospray; *NZ:* Dermalife Plus; E45; Egoderm; Egozite Baby; Karicare Barrier Cream; Rosken Skin Repair; Silic; Ungvita; *Port.:* Balmex; *S.Afr.:* Arola Rosebalm; Siopel; Siopel; *Singapore:* Egozite; *Spain:* Dermo H Infantil; Proskin; Silidermil; Tegunal; *Swed.:* Silon; *UK:* Bioglan Effervescent Granules†; Cobadex; Conotrane; Cymex; Silastic; Siopel; Sprilon; Vasogen; *USA:* Blistex Lip Balm; Dermasil†; Diaper Guard; Dyprotex; Maxilube; Medacote†; Mentholatum Cherry Ice; Mentholatum Natural Ice; Mentholatum Softlips; Mentholatum Softlips Lipbalm; Mentholatum Softlips Lipbalm (UV).

Squalane (6431-c)

Cosbiol; Dodecahydrosqualene; Perhydrosqualène; Spinacane. 2,6,10,15,19,23-Hexamethyltetracosane.
$C_{30}H_{62} = 422.8$.
CAS — 111-01-3.
Pharmacopoeias. In *USNF.*

Pharmacopoeial description

USNF 20: A saturated hydrocarbon obtained by hydrogenation of squalene, an aliphatic triterpene occurring in some fish oils. It is a colourless, almost odourless, transparent oil. Insoluble in water; very slightly soluble in dehydrated alcohol; miscible with chloroform and with ether; slightly soluble in acetone. Store in airtight containers.

Profile

Squalane is a saturated derivative of squalene, a constituent of human sebum. It is miscible with human sebum and is included in topical preparations to increase skin permeability. It is also used as an emollient.

Preparations

Proprietary Preparations (details are given in Part 3)
Multi-ingredient: *Port.:* Creme Laser Hidrante; Lactonico.

Stearyl Alcohol (6432-k)

Alcohol Stearylicus; Alcool Stéarylique; 1-Octadecanol; Octadecyl Alcohol.
CAS — 112-92-5.
Pharmacopoeias. In *Eur.* (see p.vi), *Jpn*, and *Pol.* Also in *USNF.*

Pharmacopoeial description

Ph. Eur.: A mixture of solid alcohols; it contains not less than 95.0% of stearyl alcohol ($C_{18}H_{38}O = 270.5$). White, unctuous flakes, granules, or mass. M.p. 57° to 60°. Practically insoluble in water; soluble in alcohol; freely soluble in ether. When melted, it is miscible with fatty oils, with liquid paraffin, and with melted wool fat.

USNF 20: It contains not less than 90% of stearyl alcohol ($C_{18}H_{38}O = 270.5$), the remainder consisting chiefly of related alcohols. White unctuous flakes or granules with a faint characteristic odour. M.p. 55° to 60°. Insoluble in water; soluble in alcohol and in ether.

Profile

Stearyl alcohol is used to thicken ointments and creams and to increase their water-holding capacity; it has emollient and weak emulsifying properties. It is also used in modified-release solid dose formulations.

Stearyl alcohol can cause hypersensitivity.

Preparations

Proprietary Preparations (details are given in Part 3)
USA: SFC Lotion.

Theobroma Oil (6435-x)

Beurre de Cacao; Burro di Cacao; Butyrum Cacao; Cacao Butter; Cocoa Butter; Kakaobutter; Manteca de Cacao; Manteiga de Cacau; Ol. Theobrom.; Oleum Cacao; Oleum Theobromatis.
CAS — 8002-31-1.
Pharmacopoeias. In *Aust., Br., Fr., Ger., It., Jpn, Neth.,* and *Pol.* Also in *USNF.*

Pharmacopoeial description

BP 2001: The solid fat obtained from the roasted seeds of *Theobroma cacao.* A yellowish-white, somewhat brittle, solid fat, with a slight odour of cocoa. M.p. 31° to 34°. Slightly soluble in alcohol; freely soluble in chloroform, in ether, and in petroleum spirit (boiling range, 40° to 60°). Store at a temperature not exceeding 25°.

USNF 20: A fat obtained from the seeds of *Theobroma cacao* (Sterculiaceae). It is a yellowish-white, usually brittle solid with a faint agreeable odour. M.p. 31° to 35°. Slightly soluble in alcohol; soluble in boiling dehydrated alcohol; freely soluble in chloroform and in ether.

Profile

Theobroma oil is employed as a basis for suppositories. If it is heated to more than 36° during preparation the solidification point will be appreciably lowered due to the formation of metastable states, leading to subsequent difficulty in setting. It is a major ingredient of chocolate.

Wool Alcohols (6436-r)

Alcoholes Adipis Lanae; Alcoholia Lanae; Alcolanum; Lanalcolum; Lanolin Alcohols; Wollwachsalkohole; Wool Wax Alcohols.
CAS — 8027-33-6.
Pharmacopoeias. In *Eur.* (see p.vi). Also in *USNF.*

Incompatible with coal tar, ichthammol, resorcinol, and phenol.

Pharmacopoeial description

Ph. Eur.: A mixture of sterols and higher aliphatic alcohols obtained from wool fat and containing not less than 30.0% of cholesterol. It may contain not more than 200 ppm of butylated hydroxytoluene. A pale yellow to brownish-yellow, brittle mass becoming plastic when warm. M.p. not lower than 58°. Practically insoluble in water; slightly soluble in alcohol; soluble in boiling dehydrated alcohol, in dichloromethane, and in ether. Store in well-filled containers. Protect from light.

USNF 20: A mixture of sterols, aliphatic alcohols, and triterpenoid alcohols obtained by the hydrolysis of wool fat. It may contain not more than 0.1% of a suitable antioxidant. It is a hard, waxy amber solid with a characteristic odour. M.p. not below 56°. Insoluble in water; slightly soluble in alcohol; freely soluble in chloroform, in ether, and in petroleum spirit. Store at a temperature not exceeding 25°. Protect from light.

Profile

Wool alcohols is an emulsifying agent and emulsion stabiliser used in the preparation of water-in-oil creams and ointments. It increases the water absorbing capacity of hydrocarbon mixtures; the addition of 5% of wool alcohols permits a threefold increase in the amount of water which can be incorporated in soft paraffin and such emulsions are not 'cracked' by the addition of weak acids.

It has an emollient action on the skin and is used in preparations for dry skin and dry eyes.

Derivatives of wool alcohols with similar uses include acetylated wool alcohols and ethoxylated wool alcohols.

Wool alcohols may cause hypersensitivity.

Preparations

BP 2001: Wool Alcohols Ointment

Proprietary Preparations (details are given in Part 3)
Austral.: Eucerin.

Multi-ingredient: *Austral.:* Oilatum Emollient; *Canad.:* Lacri-Lube; *Ger.:* Coliquifilm; *Irl.:* Oilatum Emollient; *Israel:* Adinol; *Ital.:* Lacrilube; *NZ:* Lacrilube; *S.Afr.:* Lacrilube; *Switz.:* Coliquifilm; *UK:* Dermalo; Lacri-Lube; Oilatum Emollient; Refresh Night Time†; *USA:* Refresh PM.

Wool Fat (6437-f)

Adeps Lanae; Anhydrous Lanolin; Cera Lanae; Graisse de Suint Purifiée; Lanoléine; Lanolin; Lanolina; Purified Lanolin; Refined Wool Fat; Suarda; Wollfett; Wollwachs.
CAS — 8006-54-0.
Pharmacopoeias. In *Chin., Eur.* (see p.vi), *Int., Jpn, Pol.,* and *US.* Some pharmacopoeias include Hydrous Wool Fat which is prepared by the addition of water to wool fat.
US also includes under the title Modified Lanolin a grade that has been processed to reduce the contents of free lanolin alcohols and detergent and pesticide residues.

Pharmacopoeial description

Ph. Eur.: A purified, anhydrous, waxy material obtained from the wool of the sheep (*Ovis aries*). It may contain not more than 200 ppm of butylated hydroxytoluene. A pale yellow, unctuous substance. When melted, it is a clear or almost clear, yellow liquid. Drop point 38° to 44°. 10 g absorbs not less than 20 mL of water. Practically insoluble in water; slightly soluble in boiling dehydrated alcohol; soluble in ether; it forms an opalescent solution in petroleum spirit. Store at a temperature not exceeding 25°.

Hydrogenated Wool Fat is a mixture of higher aliphatic alcohols and sterols obtained from the direct, high-pressure, high-temperature hydrogenation of anhydrous wool fat during which the esters and acids present are reduced to corresponding alcohols. It may contain butylated hydroxytoluene. A white or pale yellow, unctuous substance. M.p. 45° to 55°. Practically insoluble in water; soluble in boiling alcohol and in petroleum spirit. Store in well-filled containers. Protect from light.

Hydrous Wool Fat is a mixture of 75% of wool fat and 25% of water. It may contain not more than 150 ppm of butylated hydroxytoluene. A pale yellow, unctuous substance. Drop point 38° to 44°. Store at a temperature not exceeding 25°.

USP 25: A purified wax-like substance obtained from the wool of the sheep, *Ovis aries* (Bovidae). It is a yellow tenacious unctuous mass with a slight characteristic odour. Melting range 38° to 44°. It may contain a suitable antioxidant. It contains not more than 0.25% of water. Insoluble in water, but mixes without separation with about twice its weight of water; sparingly soluble in cold alcohol; more soluble in hot alcohol; free-ly soluble in chloroform and in ether. Store at a temperature preferably between 15° and 30°.

Profile

Wool fat is used in the formulation of water-in-oil creams and ointments. When mixed with a suitable vegetable oil or with soft paraffin it gives emollient creams which penetrate the skin. It can absorb about 30% of water.

Derivatives and modifications of wool fat include poloxyl lanolin (ethoxylated lanolin), isopropyl lanolate, lanolin oil, and lanolin wax. Hydrogenated wool fat (hydrogenated lanolin) is a mixture of higher aliphatic alcohols and sterols obtained from the hydrogenation of wool fat.

Hydrous wool fat (hydrous lanolin) is an ointment basis prepared by the addition of water to wool fat. The Ph. Eur. specifies wool fat 75% and water 25%.

Wool fat can cause sensitivity reactions.

◊ General reviews.
1. Barnett G. Lanolin and derivatives. *Cosmet Toilet* 1986; **101** (Mar): 23–44.

◊ Reports of pesticide residues in wool fat and comments on risks.
1. Copeland CA, *et al.* Pesticide residue in lanolin. *JAMA* 1989; **261**: 242.
2. Cade PH. Pesticide in lanolin. *JAMA* 1989; **262**: 613.
3. Copeland CA, Wagner SL. Pesticide in lanolin. *JAMA* 1989; **262**: 613.

◊ Lanolin treated to remove both detergent and natural free fatty alcohols reduced the incidence of hypersensitivity in lanolin-sensitive patients to almost zero.[1]

1. Clark EW, *et al.* Lanolin with reduced sensitizing potential. *Contact Dermatitis* 1977; **3**: 69–74.

Preparations

BP 2001: Simple Eye Ointment; Simple Ointment;
USP 25: Modified Lanolin.

Proprietary Preparations (details are given in Part 3)
Austral.: Lansinoh; *Canad.:* Lanolelle†; *S.Afr.:* Duratears; *UK:* Medilan.

Multi-ingredient: *Aust.:* Tiroler Steinol; *Austral.:* Alpha Keri; Alpha Keri Tar; Duratears; E45; Lacri-Lube; Poly Visc; Rikoderm; Silcon; Soothe'n Heal; *Belg.:* Duratears; Lacrytube; *Canad.:* Akwa Tears; Alpha Keri; Duratears; Huile de Bain Therapeutique; Lubriderm; Optilube; Stancare†; Therapeutic Bath Oil; Therapeutic Skin Lotion; *Hong Kong:* Alpha Keri; Duratears; *Irl.:* Lacri-Lube; *Israel:* Duratears; Kamil Blue; Lacrimol; Pedisol; *Neth.:* Duratears Z†; *NZ:* Alpha Keri; BK; DP; Hydroderm; Karicare Baby Bath Oil; Karicare Mother and Baby; Oralife Peppermint; Pharmacycare Bath Oil; Pharmacycare Hand & Body; *Singapore:* Alpha Keri; Duratears; Lacrilube; Lubrifilm; *Spain:* Lubrifilm; Tears Lubricante; *Switz.:* Duratears†; *Thai.:* Duratears; *UK:* Alpha Keri; Hewletts; Lubri-Tears; Melrose; *USA:* Akwa Tears; Alpha Keri; Bottom Better; Dry Eyes; Duratears Naturale; Lacri-Gel; Lacri-Lube; LubriTears.

Parasympathomimetics

Parasympathomimetics may be classified into 2 distinct pharmacological groups:

- cholinergic agonists, such as bethanechol, carbachol, methacholine, and pilocarpine which act directly on effector cells to mimic the effects of acetylcholine. They are sometimes referred to as cholinomimetics or true parasympathomimetics; some such as bethanechol, carbachol, and methacholine are choline esters

- anticholinesterases (cholinesterase inhibitors) which inhibit the enzymic hydrolysis of acetylcholine by acetylcholinesterase and other cholinesterases, thereby prolonging and enhancing its actions in the body. They may be classified by the length of time taken to restore active enzyme following binding of enzyme to drug. The 'reversible' anticholinesterases such as ambenonium, neostigmine, physostigmine, and pyridostigmine generally produce enzyme inhibition for a few hours, whereas 'irreversible' anticholinesterases such as dyflos and ecothiopate produce extremely prolonged inhibition, and return of cholinesterase activity depends on synthesis of new enzyme. Centrally acting reversible anticholinesterases include donepezil, galantamine, rivastigmine, and tacrine.

Parasympathomimetics may be administered topically for their miotic action in the treatment of glaucoma and strabismus, given systemically to reverse the neuromuscular blockade of neuromuscular blockers or may be used in myasthenia gravis and for dementia of the Alzheimer's type. Other uses have included treatment of paralytic ileus or other disorders of decreased gastrointestinal motility (p.1202), and postoperative urinary retention (p.459).

A number of drugs, such as fampridine and guanidine, which enhance the release of acetylcholine from nerve terminals are also discussed in this chapter.

◊ References.
1. Goyal RK. Muscarinic receptor subtypes: physiology and clinical implications. *N Engl J Med* 1989; **321:** 1022–9.

Dementia

Dementia is a syndrome in which impairment of cortical or subcortical function leads to deterioration of cognitive processes or intellectual abilities including memory, judgement, language, communication, and abstract thinking. Unlike delirium there is no gross clouding of consciousness. There may be changes in personality and behaviour disturbances. Dementia is usually progressive, though not always irreversible, and loss of social and other skills often leads to complete dependence on others.

Although dementia is more prevalent in the elderly it is not an inevitable consequence of ageing. Dementia can result from many conditions including:

- *neurodegenerative diseases*: Alzheimer's disease, Pick's disease, Huntington's chorea, Parkinson's disease, Lewy-body disease, multiple sclerosis, progressive supranuclear palsy
- *vascular diseases*: multiple cerebral infarcts, occlusion of carotid artery, cranial arteritis
- *trauma*: subdural haematoma
- *neoplasms*
- *CNS infections*: encephalitis, syphilis, toxoplasmosis, AIDS, Creutzfeldt-Jakob disease
- *endocrine/metabolic disorders*: hypothyroidism, uraemia, hepatic failure, cardiac failure, respiratory failure, hypoxia
- *toxic insults*: alcohol, solvents, heavy metals, drug therapy
- *hydrocephalus*
- *nutritional deficiency*: vitamin B$_{12}$, folic acid, thiamine
- *depression*

Of the above, Alzheimer's disease is the most common cause of dementia and accounts for over half of all patients; about one-third of dementia cases are due to vascular disease.

Treatment of dementia can be broadly divided into that which controls disturbed behaviour (p.650) and that which tries to improve or preserve cognitive function (see below). Although many drugs have been tried in the management of cognitive impairment most have produced little or no benefit.

Alzheimer's disease is a progressive degenerative condition affecting mainly patients over 60 years of age. The rare early-onset form of Alzheimer's disease (familial Alzheimer's disease) is sometimes referred to as pre-senile dementia. Death usually occurs within 10 years of onset. Apart from age other risk factors include Down's syndrome and a family history of Alzheimer's disease. Presence of the ε4 allele of apolipoprotein E is another risk factor; it correlates with prevalence and age of onset in some forms of Alzheimer's disease but use for routine clinical or predictive testing is controversial. Dialysis dementia, an irreversible condition which has occurred in dialysis patients, has been associated with excess aluminium in the dialysing fluid but the role of aluminium in Alzheimer's disease, if any, is unclear.

Deficiencies in numerous neurotransmitters have been found in patients with Alzheimer's disease but reduced choline acetyltransferase activity leading to reduced synthesis of acetylcholine remains the most consistent defect correlating with the severity of the condition. A number of methods have been tried in an attempt to increase acetylcholine concentrations in the brain including administration of *acetylcholine precursors, cholinesterase inhibitors, enhancers of acetylcholine release,* and *cholinergic agonists*. However, none replace lost cholinergic neurones and therefore none affect overall progression of the disease.

Treatments using *precursors of acetylcholine* such as lecithin or choline alone are not considered to produce useful improvements.

Donepezil, galantamine, tacrine, and rivastigmine are the main *cholinesterase inhibitors* used. All have produced modest improvement in cognition and global clinical impression in patients with mild to moderately severe disease; but there is a lack of long-term studies and little evidence of their effectiveness in advanced disease. Tacrine is often poorly tolerated and may cause serious hepatotoxicity; donepezil, galantamine, and rivastigmine may be more acceptable to patients. Other cholinesterase inhibitors which have been tried or are under study for use in Alzheimer's disease include metrifonate and physostigmine.

Fampridine and linopirdine, which *enhance acetylcholine release from nerve terminals* have also been tried in Alzheimer's disease but there is little evidence of clinical benefit.

Limited improvement has been reported with some *cholinergic agonists* but pilocarpine may exacerbate the dementia. Muscarinic M$_1$ agonists such as cevimeline and xanomeline have been investigated on the basis that muscarinic M$_1$ receptors appear to be preserved throughout the course of Alzheimer's disease. However, these drugs have not been successful in improving symptoms of the disease. An alternative line of investigation is the *stimulation of nicotinic receptors* using nicotine.

A hypothesis that free radicals may initiate and maintain mechanisms responsible for neurodegeneration in Alzheimer's disease has prompted the investigation of drugs such as α-tocopherol and selegiline for *antioxidant* therapy but their value remains to be confirmed.

Neurotropic or nootropic drugs such as piracetam have also been tried in Alzheimer's disease and other dementias but there is little convincing evidence of clinical usefulness.

The *N-methyl-D-aspartate (NMDA) receptor antagonist* memantine has shown some benefit in various dementias including Alzheimer's disease; it is thought to act through modulation of the effects of the neurotransmitter glutamate.

Many drugs with *vasodilator activity* were originally tried in dementia when it was believed that the condition was due to 'cerebrovascular insufficiency' (p.798), and overall there is little convincing evidence of benefit. Ergot derivatives such as co-dergocrine mesilate and nicergoline have been the most commonly used; however, any effectiveness is now attributed to their action as metabolic enhancers or nootropic drugs and their place in therapy has still to be established.

The *calcium-channel blocker* nimodipine has been investigated in dementia of various aetiologies but so far results have been unclear.

Observations in women receiving HRT have suggested that *oestrogens* may reduce the risk and delay the onset of Alzheimer's disease in elderly women and a long-term study on the value of HRT for prevention of Alzheimer's disease is in progress. The effect of oestrogens on cognitive function in postmenopausal women who already have mild or moderate Alzheimer's disease is also being studied. Some retrospective studies also indicate an inverse association between the use of *anti-inflammatory drugs* such as NSAIDs and the risk of developing Alzheimer's disease. The possibility of an association between *statin* therapy and a reduced risk of developing dementia has also been mooted.

A vaccine for Alzheimer's disease is being investigated.

Vascular dementia is a syndrome produced by ischaemic, hypoxic, or haemorrhagic brain lesions. Vessel occlusion is the most common cause of vascular dementia and produces a variety of cognitive deficits depending on the site of ischaemia. Among the major forms of dementia recognised are those due to multiple infarcts, single strategic infarcts, and subcortical white matter ischaemia (Binswanger's disease). Vascular dementia has a more acute onset than dementia due to Alzheimer's disease and in contrast to the continuous progression of Alzheimer's disease often has a stepwise progression. Risk factors for vascular dementia parallel those for stroke (p.813) and similar methods for prevention and treatment may be of use.

Lewy-body dementia is distinguished from other types of dementia by a state of fluctuating cognitive impairment and confusion; hallucinations, paranoid delusions, a tendency to fall for no apparent reason, and transient clouding or loss of consciousness are also characteristic symptoms. In addition, mild extrapyramidal symptoms may be present and there is increased susceptibility to the extrapyramidal adverse effects of antipsychotics (see the Elderly, under Precautions of Chlorpromazine on p.663).

References.

1. Cummings JL. Dementia: the failing brain. *Lancet* 1995; **345:** 1481–4. Correction. *ibid.*; 1551.
2. Fleming KC, *et al.* Dementia: diagnosis and evaluation. *Mayo Clin Proc* 1995; **70:** 1093–1107.
3. Gooch MD, Stennett DJ. Molecular basis of Alzheimer's disease. *Am J Health-Syst Pharm* 1996; **53:** 1545–57.
4. Amar K, Wilcock G. Vascular dementia. *BMJ* 1996; **312:** 227–31.
5. Konno S, *et al.* Classification, diagnosis and treatment of vascular dementia. *Drugs Aging* 1997; **11:** 361–73.
6. Parnetti L, *et al.* Cognitive enhancement therapy for Alzheimer's disease: the way forward. *Drugs* 1997; **53:** 752–68.
7. American Psychiatric Association. Practice guideline for the treatment of patients with Alzheimer's disease and other dementias of late life. *Am J Psychiatry* 1997; **154** (suppl): 1–39.
8. Benzi G, Moretti A. Is there a rationale for the use of acetylcholinesterase inhibitors in the therapy of Alzheimer's disease? *Eur J Pharmacol* 1998; **346:** 1–13.
9. Small GW. Treatment of Alzheimer's disease: current approaches and promising developments. *Am J Med* 1998; **104** (suppl 4A): 32S–38S.
10. Eccles M, *et al.* North of England evidence based guidelines development project: guideline for the primary care management of dementia. *BMJ* 1998; **317:** 802–8.
11. Sachdev PS, *et al.* Vascular dementia: diagnosis, management and possible prevention. *Med J Aust* 1999; **170:** 81–5.
12. Flynn BL. Pharmacologic management of Alzheimer disease: Part I: hormonal and emerging investigational drug therapies. *Ann Pharmacother* 1999; **33:** 178–87.
13. Flynn BL, Ranno AE. Pharmacologic management of Alzheimer disease: Part II: antioxidants, antihypertensives, and ergoloid derivatives. *Ann Pharmacother* 1999; **33:** 188–97.
14. Flicker L. Acetylcholinesterase inhibitors for Alzheimer's disease. *BMJ* 1999; **318:** 615–6.
15. Krall WJ, *et al.* Cholinesterase inhibitors: a therapeutic strategy for Alzheimer disease. *Ann Pharmacother* 1999; **33:** 441–50.
16. Korczyn AD. Muscarinic M(1) agonists in the treatment of Alzheimer's disease. *Expert Opin Invest Drugs* 2000; **9:** 2259–67.
17. Grutzendler J, Morris JC. Cholinesterase inhibitors for Alzheimer's disease. *Drugs* 2001; **61:** 41–52.
18. Scott HD, Laake K. Statins for the prevention of Alzheimer's disease (updated 29 August 2001). Available in The Cochrane Library; Issue 4. Oxford: Update Software; 2001.
19. National Institute for Clinical Excellence. Guidance on the use of donepezil, rivastigmine and galantamine for the treatment of Alzheimer's disease (issued January 2001). Available at: http://www.nice.org.uk/pdf/ALZHEIMER_full_guidance.pdf (accessed 20/11/01).

Eaton-Lambert myasthenic syndrome

Eaton-Lambert myasthenic syndrome is a rare auto-immune disease of the neuromuscular junction. Unlike myasthenia gravis (below), in which auto-antibodies affect acetylcholine receptors, antibodies in Eaton-Lambert syndrome act presynaptically to reduce release of acetylcholine. Weakness mostly affects the proximal muscles, particularly those of the limbs; respiratory and ocular muscles are usually spared. Autonomic symptoms including dry mouth, constipation, and impotence are common. Over half of patients also develop small cell carcinoma of the lung. Response to treatment with anticholinesterases alone is poor; treatment with 3,4-diaminopyridine, which increases acetylcholine release, appears to be more effective. The use of similar drugs such as guanidine and fampridine is limited by severe adverse effects. Low-dose guanidine has been tried in combination with pyridostigmine where 3,4-diaminopyridine is not readily available. Although there has been some improvement with the combination, the incidence of side-effects, especially gastrointestinal reactions, is still high. Some patients may obtain additional benefit when anticholinesterases are used in addition to 3,4-diaminopyridine. Immunosuppressive treatment and plasma exchange are also used, and unlike myasthenia gravis, treatment with corticosteroids does not appear to induce an initial exacerbation of symptoms.

References.

1. Newsom-Davis J. Myasthenia gravis and the Lambert-Eaton myasthenic syndrome. *Prescribers' J* 1993; **33**: 205–12.
2. Oh SJ, *et al.* Low-dose guanidine and pyridostigmine: relatively safe and effective long-term symptomatic therapy in Lambert-Eaton myasthenic syndrome. *Muscle Nerve* 1997; **20**: 1146–52.

Glaucoma and ocular hypertension

Intra-ocular pressure rises when there is an imbalance between production and drainage of aqueous humour in the eye. Aqueous humour is secreted by the ciliary body and flows into the posterior chamber of the eye. It then passes through the pupil into the anterior chamber from where about 75% drains from the eye through the trabecular meshwork into Schlemm's canal and then into the episcleral veins. The remainder is removed by the uveoscleral route, passing through the ciliary muscle and finally into the episcleral tissues.

The term **ocular hypertension** is used to describe intra-ocular pressure above an upper normal value of 21 mmHg when there are no signs of optic nerve damage. The term **glaucoma** is used to describe a group of conditions characterised by cupping (excavation) of the optic disc and damage of the optic nerve leading to gradual visual loss. Although it is now recognised that glaucoma can occur and progress in patients with an intra-ocular pressure within the normal range, raised intra-ocular pressure is an important risk factor for glaucoma, and as it is the only one that can be altered, current therapy for glaucoma is directed at lowering it. The aim is not just to reduce intra-ocular pressure to a normal value but to a level at which damage to the optic nerve ceases.[1-4] Some patients may have raised intra-ocular pressure for many years without evidence of glaucoma. Whether these patients would receive long-term benefit from a reduction in intra-ocular pressure is under study but many ophthalmologists consider that therapy is indicated if the intra-ocular pressure is higher than 30 mmHg.

Raised intra-ocular pressure associated with glaucoma is usually due to reduced outflow of aqueous humour from the eye. Glaucoma is described as open-angle or angle-closure depending on the mechanism of the obstruction of drainage and may be acute or chronic. Glaucoma may also be referred to as primary or secondary. Primary glaucoma is usually associated with a direct disturbance of aqueous outflow whereas secondary glaucoma develops as a consequence of a number of diseases or of trauma.

The most common form of glaucoma is **chronic open-angle glaucoma** (simple glaucoma; wide-angle glaucoma) which is due to blockage in drainage through the trabecular meshwork. Intra-ocular pressure increases gradually, and the condition is usually asymptomatic until well advanced and severe damage has occurred. Usually, both eyes are affected. Risk factors include old age, diabetes, Afro-Caribbean race, a family history of glaucoma, and myopia. A 'steroid glaucoma' may be produced, after a few weeks of treatment with eye drops containing corticosteroids, in patients predisposed to open-angle glaucoma; the risk with systemic corticosteroids appears to be less.

In contrast, **angle-closure glaucoma** (closed-angle glaucoma; narrow-angle glaucoma) usually occurs as an acute emergency. Patients present with a painful red eye, sweating, and nausea and vomiting as a result of a rapid rise in intra-ocular pressure. This can result from blockage of the flow of aqueous humour into the anterior chamber. The resulting rise in intra-ocular pressure bows the iris against the trabecular meshwork restricting aqueous outflow and thereby further raising intra-ocular pres-

sure. It usually occurs in patients with hypermetropia who have a shallow anterior chamber and a narrow filtration angle. The use of mydriatics in such patients is contra-indicated as dilatation of the pupil can precipitate an acute attack of angle-closure glaucoma.

ANTIGLAUCOMA DRUGS. Although many drugs are effective in reducing intra-ocular pressure there is little data on their long-term effect on visual field changes in glaucoma.[3,5] Drugs used in the treatment of glaucoma lower intra-ocular pressure by a variety of mechanisms and their effects are often additive. Their use has been discussed in a number of reviews.[1,2,4,6,7]

* *Beta blockers* inhibit beta receptors in the ciliary epithelium and thereby reduce the secretion of aqueous humour. They are often the drugs of first choice for initial and maintenance treatment of open-angle and other chronic glaucomas and of ocular hypertension; other drugs are used with them when further reductions in intra-ocular pressure are required. They are better tolerated than miotics but can produce systemic effects, and their safety, particularly in the elderly, has been questioned.[8,9] Studies suggest that individual topical beta blockers are probably equally effective in reducing intra-ocular pressure but if a nonselective beta blocker is used an additional reduction in pressure may not be obtained with adrenaline [epinephrine] (see below).

* *Parasympathomimetic miotics* facilitate trabecular drainage by constricting the pupil and pulling open the trabecular meshwork. However, this can cause blurred vision and browache, especially in younger patients, and the small pupil may cause problems if central vision is already limited. Parasympathomimetic miotics also reduce uveoscleral outflow and this can cause a paradoxical increase in intra-ocular pressure in patients with a recessed anterior angle. They should not be used in the presence of inflammation as adhesions may form between the pupil and the lens (posterior synechiae). Pilocarpine is the miotic most frequently employed and is indicated in the treatment of open-angle glaucoma and other chronic glaucomas. It is often added to treatment with other drugs when further reductions in intra-ocular pressure are required. It requires frequent instillation and this may lead to problems with compliance. Carbachol is sometimes used when resistance or intolerance to pilocarpine develops. Physostigmine is more potent than pilocarpine but is poorly tolerated and is rarely used now; it was used with pilocarpine but rarely alone. Stronger or longer-acting anticholinesterase miotics such as demecarium and ecothiopate can cause pupillary block and induce angle-closure glaucoma. They are usually only used in patients refractory to other antiglaucoma treatment or in those in whom the lens of the eye has been removed (aphakic patients). Pilocarpine is also used in the emergency treatment of angle-closure glaucoma before surgery or laser therapy.

* *Sympathomimetics* such as adrenaline [epinephrine] or dipivefrine increase outflow of aqueous humour through the trabecular meshwork and the uveoscleral route and may also reduce its rate of production. They are used in open-angle glaucoma and other chronic glaucomas usually when further reductions in intra-ocular pressure are required in patients receiving beta blockers (but may not produce an additive effect if used with a nonselective beta blocker).[10] As they produce pupillary dilatation they can induce an acute attack if used in angle-closure glaucoma. Adrenaline [epinephrine] can cause eye irritation and produce systemic effects. Dipivefrine is converted into adrenaline [epinephrine] by corneal esterases and ocular adverse effects are usually less than with adrenaline [epinephrine] itself. Guanethidine, an adrenergic neurone blocker, reduces aqueous secretion and is used either alone or in combination to enhance and prolong the effect of adrenaline [epinephrine]; prolonged use can cause fibrosis and corneal changes. The alpha$_2$-adrenoceptor agonist clonidine has also been used in some countries, while more recent introductions include apraclonidine and brimonidine. Alpha$_2$-adrenoceptor agonists lower intra-ocular pressure by reducing production of aqueous humour. Apraclonidine is used alone or as an adjunct to other drugs in the control of intra-ocular pressure associated with ocular surgery or in the short-term to delay laser treatment or surgery for patients with glaucoma not adequately controlled with other drugs; tachyphylaxis and ocular irritation limit

its long-term use. Brimonidine is another alpha$_2$-adrenoceptor agonist used similarly.

* *Carbonic anhydrase inhibitors* such as acetazolamide, reduce production of aqueous humour by a mechanism independent of their diuretic action. They are used as part of the emergency treatment of angle-closure glaucoma to produce a rapid reduction in intra-ocular pressure before surgery or laser therapy. They are also added to treatment in open-angle glaucoma and other chronic glaucomas in patients refractory to treatment with beta blockers, sympathomimetics, and short-acting miotics, but many patients are unable to tolerate prolonged therapy when they are given systemically. More recently introduced topical carbonic anhydrase inhibitors, such as dorzolamide, have a lower potential to produce adverse effects. Dorzolamide is used similarly to other topical drugs either alone or as an adjunct in patients resistant to or intolerant of beta blockers.

* *Osmotic diuretics* reduce vitreous volume and can produce a marked reduction in intra-ocular pressure. They are used in the short-term management of glaucoma when a rapid reduction in intra-ocular pressure is required before surgery. Mannitol and urea are both given intravenously and have a faster onset than glycerol or isosorbide given orally.

* *Several other drugs* are used topically in glaucoma and ocular hypertension. Latanoprost is a prostaglandin $F_{2\alpha}$ analogue which is effective when used topically once a day and is currently indicated for use in patients intolerant of or not adequately controlled by other drugs. It lowers intra-ocular pressure by increasing uveoscleral outflow. It appears to be well-tolerated but may cause a potentially irreversible increase in brown pigmentation of the iris; the long-term significance of this effect is unknown. The alpha-adrenergic antagonist dapiprazole and the prostaglandin $F_{2\alpha}$ analogue unoprostone are also used in some countries.

DIAGNOSIS OF GLAUCOMA. *Open-angle glaucoma* is asymptomatic in its early stages and the use of screening methods for detecting early disease is of great importance. Measurement of intra-ocular pressure alone is a poor diagnostic tool and a combination of direct examination of the optic nerve together with visual field examination and intra-ocular pressure tonometry is considered to be more reliable.[4] Provocative tests such as placing the patient prone in a dark room are sometimes used to identify eyes suffering from or at risk of *angle-closure glaucoma*. Short-acting mydriatics have also been used but are not without risk. Long-term follow-up of patients whose treatment had been determined by the use of a provocative test using phenylephrine with pilocarpine has suggested that this test is neither sensitive nor specific.[11]

TREATMENT OF GLAUCOMA. *Open-angle glaucoma* is frequently treated first with a topical beta blocker. Adrenaline [epinephrine] and a miotic such as pilocarpine are then added as necessary to control intra-ocular pressure. Other drugs such as a topical carbonic anhydrase inhibitor may also be required. It has been suggested that each type of drug should be tried alone first before resorting to combination therapy. If further reduction of intra-ocular pressure is required a systemic carbonic anhydrase inhibitor may be used but long-term treatment is poorly tolerated. If this is unsuccessful, surgery (trabeculectomy) or laser treatment (trabeculoplasty) is usually indicated. Laser treatment appears to be as effective as topical drug therapy[12] although its effects may be short-lived.[13] It has been suggested that it might be of use in the initial treatment of older patients who cannot use eye drops or when surgery needs to be postponed or is contra-indicated.[4] However, the early use of surgery is now often advocated in Europe, especially for younger patients, although this is still a subject of debate in the USA. Some consider that there is an unnecessary risk of continuing visual loss while drug treatment is being evaluated, and they advocate surgery as the primary treatment.[14] The earlier use of surgical intervention is supported by evidence that long-term drug therapy[15] or laser treatment[4] may have a deleterious effect on the outcome of subsequent surgery and by evidence that surgery is more effective than drug or laser treatment in producing long-term intra-ocular pressure control.[13]

It is essential to start treatment for an *acute attack of angle-closure glaucoma* within 24 to 48 hours. If treatment is delayed adhesions may form between the iris and the cornea (peripheral anterior synechiae) and the trabecular meshwork may be damaged. *Chronic angle-closure glaucoma* may then develop with permanently raised intra-ocular pressure which ultimately leads to total loss of vision (absolute glaucoma). The initial treatment aims to produce a rapid reduction in intra-ocular pressure. A miotic such as pilocarpine is used topically to constrict the pupil while a carbonic anhydrase inhibitor such as acetazolamide is given by mouth or by intravenous injection. Osmotic diuretics such as mannitol or urea given intravenously or glycerol or isosorbide given orally may also be used. When intra-ocular pressure has been reduced sufficiently, laser therapy or surgery is performed on both eyes to increase drainage of aqueous humour. If further topical treatment is required after surgery, treatment is usually as for open-angle glaucoma. Beta blockers, with or without adrenaline [epinephrine], are preferred to pilocarpine as there is a risk of posterior synechiae forming when pilocarpine is used.

Glaucoma filtering surgery such as trabeculectomy can be highly effective in reducing intra-ocular pressure, but in some groups of patients, such as children, Afro-Caribbeans, or those who have had previous ocular surgery, there is a high failure rate, usually due to formation of scar tissue.[16] The scar formation is associated with proliferation of fibroblasts and the subconjunctival injection of antiproliferative drugs such as fluorouracil has been shown to reduce the failure rate of surgery but at a cost of increased epithelial toxicity and conjunctival wound leaks.[16] A study group[17] reporting on the long-term follow-up of patients treated with fluorouracil recommended that fluorouracil should still be used in the surgical management of glaucoma in patients with a history of ocular surgery, but in view of the increased incidence of late-onset conjunctival wound leaks, suggested caution in its use in eyes with good prognoses at the dosage they employed. The use of a single intraoperative topical application of mitomycin has been investigated as an alternative to the regimen of multiple injections required with fluorouracil. Rates of success comparable with those for fluorouracil have been achieved but a plea for caution has been made[18] over the risk of adverse effects that could affect vision and the need to determine long-term safety of antiproliferative drugs. Other drugs are also being studied as antiproliferative agents. Whether the use of antiproliferative drugs is of benefit to all patients undergoing glaucoma surgery is under study.[8]

Postoperative ocular hypertension may occur following surgery on the anterior chamber of the eye or procedures such as trabeculoplasty. Acetylcholine or carbachol instilled directly into the anterior chamber of the eye (intracameral instillation) are used intra-operatively to reduce early postoperative rises in intra-ocular pressure in procedures such as cataract extraction. The short action of acetylcholine can be an advantage as prolonged miosis is associated with severe postoperative pain. However, some consider carbachol to be the more effective drug;[19,20] standard antiglaucoma drugs including beta blockers, pilocarpine, apraclonidine, and carbonic anhydrase inhibitors have also been used for prophylaxis of postoperative ocular hypertension.

1. Hurvitz LM, *et al.* New developments in the drug treatment of glaucoma. *Drugs* 1991; **41**: 514–32.
2. Quigley HA. Open-angle glaucoma. *N Engl J Med* 1993; **328**: 1097–1106.
3. Liesegang TJ. Glaucoma: changing concepts and future directions. *Mayo Clin Proc* 1996; **71**: 689–94.
4. Anonymous. The management of primary open angle glaucoma. *Drug Ther Bull* 1997; **35**: 4–6.
5. Rossetti L, *et al.* Randomized clinical trials on medical treatment of glaucoma: are they appropriate to guide clinical practice? *Arch Ophthalmol* 1993; **111**: 96–103.
6. Taniguchi T, Kitazawa Y. A risk-benefit assessment of drugs used in the management of glaucoma. *Drug Safety* 1994; **11**: 68–74.
7. Alward WLM. Medical management of glaucoma. *N Engl J Med* 1998; **339**: 1298–1307.
8. Diggory P, Franks W. Medical treatment of glaucoma—a reappraisal of the risks. *Br J Ophthalmol* 1996; **80**: 85–9.
9. O'Donoghue E. β Blockers and the elderly with glaucoma: are we adding insult to injury? *Br J Ophthalmol* 1995; **79**: 794–6.
10. Sorensen SJ, Abel SR. Comparison of the ocular beta-blockers. *Ann Pharmacother* 1996; **30**: 43–54.
11. Wishart PK. Does the pilocarpine phenylephrine provocative test help in the management of acute and subacute angle closure glaucoma? *Br J Ophthalmol* 1991; **75**: 284–7.
12. Glaucoma Laser Trial Research Group. The glaucoma laser trial (GLT) and glaucoma laser trial follow-up study: 7. results. *Am J Ophthalmol* 1995; **120**: 718–31.
13. Migdal C, *et al.* Long-term functional outcome after early surgery compared with laser and medicine in open-angle glaucoma. *Ophthalmology* 1994; **101**: 1651–7.
14. Hitchings RA. Primary surgery for primary open angle glaucoma—justified or not? *Br J Ophthalmol* 1993; **77**: 445–8.
15. Broadway D, *et al.* Adverse effects of topical antiglaucomatous medications on the conjunctiva. *Br J Ophthalmol* 1993; **77**: 590–6.
16. Khaw PT, *et al.* 5-Fluorouracil and beyond. *Br J Ophthalmol* 1991; **75**: 577–8.
17. The Fluorouracil Filtering Surgery Study Group. Five-year follow-up of the Fluorouracil Filtering Surgery Study. *Am J Ophthalmol* 1996; **121**: 349–66.
18. Khaw PT. Antiproliferative agents and the prevention of scarring after surgery: friend or foe? *Br J Ophthalmol* 1995; **79**: 627.
19. Ruiz RS, *et al.* Effects of carbachol and acetylcholine on intraocular pressure after cataract extraction. *Am J Ophthalmol* 1989; **107**: 7–10.
20. Hollands RH, *et al.* Control of intraocular pressure after cataract extraction. *Can J Ophthalmol* 1990; **25**: 128–32.

Myasthenia gravis

Myasthenia gravis is a disorder characterised by defective neuromuscular transmission and consequent muscular weakness due to formation of auto-antibodies to acetylcholine receptors. The thymus appears to be involved in many patients and some have a thymoma. There appear to be several types of myasthenia and a number of classifications have been proposed. Classifications based on the distribution and severity of symptoms include ocular myasthenia, where the disease is clinically confined to the extra-ocular muscles and mild or moderate generalised myasthenia, also affecting muscles other than the extra-ocular muscles; acute fulminating myasthenia; and late severe myasthenia. Another classification, based on the age of onset and the presence, or absence of thymoma, divides patients into those with thymoma; those without thymoma and onset before age of 40; and those without thymoma and onset after 40 years of age. Other types of myasthenia include transient neonatal myasthenia, which may persist for 1 to 6 weeks in the infants of myasthenic mothers due to transplacental passage of receptor antibodies, penicillamine-induced myasthenia, and congenital myasthenia (see under 3,4-Diaminopyridine, p.1416).

DIAGNOSIS OF MYASTHENIA GRAVIS.

Although all patients have circulating antibodies to acetylcholine receptors they are undetectable by radio-immunoassay in about 15% of patients who are described as having seronegative myasthenia. Patients may often be tested first for their reaction to an anticholinesterase. Intravenous edrophonium preceded by atropine (Tensilon test) is the most commonly used anticholinesterase test because of its rapid onset and short duration of action. However severe adverse effects can occasionally occur so testing should only be undertaken when facilities for endotracheal intubation and controlled ventilation are immediately available. A positive result is considered to be a rapid but temporary increase in muscle strength. Repetitive nerve stimulation is also used as a diagnostic test but, like the anticholinesterase test, is not specific for myasthenia gravis.

TREATMENT OF MYASTHENIA GRAVIS.

• Symptomatic treatment is with an *anticholinesterase*; pyridostigmine and neostigmine are those most commonly used. Most patients prefer pyridostigmine as it produces less muscarinic adverse effects and has a longer duration of action, although the quicker onset of action of neostigmine may offer an advantage at the beginning of the day. The dose must be adjusted to give the optimum therapeutic response but muscle strength may not be restored to normal and some patients must live with a degree of disability. The effect may vary for different muscles and the dosage should be adjusted so that the bulbar and respiratory muscles receive optimum treatment. Overdosage may lead to a 'cholinergic crisis' (see Adverse Effects of Neostigmine, p.1420). Edrophonium may be employed to establish whether the patient is underdosed or overdosed.

• *Corticosteroids* are the main immunosuppressive drugs used and are indicated for patients who are seriously ill prior to thymectomy, for those unsuitable for thymectomy (see below), and for those who are insufficiently improved postoperatively. They are also useful in patients with ocular myasthenia, who as a group respond poorly to anticholinesterases and to thymectomy, provided that their disability is severe enough to warrant long-term corticosteroid treatment with its attendant side-effects. Various dosage regimens appear to be in use. Some start with low doses such as 5 to 20 mg of prednisolone daily (or on alternate days to reduce the risk of steroid-induced exacerbations of weakness) and increase the dose slowly thereafter according to response; an improvement is usually seen after a few weeks. Others use more aggressive regimens to obtain a more rapid response and start with large doses such as 60 to 100 mg of prednisolone daily. Whichever method is used, once clinical benefit has been obtained the regimen should be modified to administration on alternate days with the dose being slowly tapered when the patient is in remission. It should be remembered that patients receiving corticosteroids require less anticholinesterase therapy and, if the dosage of the anticholinesterase is not reduced, an initial deterioration in the myasthenia may occur in the first few weeks of treatment (see also under Interactions of Neostigmine, p.1420). In the majority of patients it is not usually possible to withdraw corticosteroids completely but some patients may be maintained satisfactorily on as little as 10 mg on alternate days. If remission cannot be maintained on low-dose prednisolone, addition of azathioprine at a dosage of 2 to 3 mg per kg body-weight daily may be considered.

• Addition of *azathioprine* to treatment may allow a reduction in the dose of both corticosteroids and anticholinesterases. Azathioprine may also be of use when corticosteroids are contra-indicated or when response to corticosteroids alone is insufficient, but since it has a much slower onset of action than corticosteroids it is not usually used alone. *Ciclosporin* has been effective in some patients unresponsive to anticholinesterases and corticosteroids but serious adverse effects including nephrotoxicity may limit its use; the time to response is similar to that with corticosteroids. Other drugs such as *cyclophosphamide* and *methotrexate* have also been tried.

• Plasma exchange provides a dramatic but short-lived improvement and is useful as a short-term measure in myasthenic crisis to improve ill patients while other therapies take effect, but there is no evidence that repeated plasma exchange combined with immunosuppression is superior to immunosuppression alone.

• Thymectomy may be offered to all patients sufficiently fit to undergo surgery unless they have minimal symptoms, purely ocular disease, or late onset or seronegative disease. Thymectomy is usually avoided in prepubertal children because of concern over the effect on growth and the development of the immune system and it has been suggested that symptomatic treatment with anticholinesterases should be continued until adolescence, when the disease often improves spontaneously. Following thymectomy, remission or improvement may be expected in about 80% of patients without thymomas, although this may take some years; the response is poorer in those with thymomas.

• Other forms of treatment, such as high-dose intravenous normal immunoglobulins are mostly non-specific and have generally been used only in patients refractory to all other treatment.

References.
1. Havard CWH, Fonseca V. New treatment approaches to myasthenia gravis. *Drugs* 1990; **39**: 66–73.
2. Keys PA, Blume RP. Therapeutic strategies for myasthenia gravis. *DICP Ann Pharmacother* 1991; **25**: 1101–8.
3. Newsom-Davis J. Myasthenia gravis and the Lambert-Eaton myasthenic syndrome. *Prescribers' J* 1993; **33**: 205–12.
4. Drachman DB. Myasthenia gravis. *N Engl J Med* 1994; **330**: 1797–1810.
5. Evoli A, *et al.* A practical guide to the recognition and management of myasthenia gravis. *Drugs* 1996; **52**: 662–70.
6. Yi Q, Lefvert AK. Current and future therapies for myasthenia gravis. *Drugs Aging* 1997; **11**: 132–9.

Reversal of mydriasis

Topical miotics (mydriolytics) are sometimes used to reverse the effects of mydriatics following surgery or ophthalmoscopic examination but do not appear to be in routine clinical use. Pilocarpine can counteract the mydriatic effect of topical sympathomimetics, such as phenylephrine and hydroxyamfetamine, but is ineffective against mydriasis produced by antimuscarinics, such as homatropine, and may impair vision further when used with tropicamide. Furthermore, there is also the risk that pilocarpine might precipitate angle-closure glaucoma in susceptible patents. Dapiprazole appears to be safer than pilocarpine when used to reverse sympathomimetic-induced mydriasis and is effective to some degree against tropicamide-induced mydriasis. It also appears to enhance recovery of accommodation after the use of cycloplegics.

The rate of reversal of mydriasis is generally slower in patients with dark irides than in those with lighter irides.

Strabismus

Strabismus, sometimes referred to as a squint or cast, is a lack of coordination of the visual axes of the eyes so that the eyes are usually either turned towards (convergent strabismus) or away (divergent strabismus) from each other. It can arise from a physical defect of the attachment of the extra-ocular muscles to the eye or from paralysis, spasms, or overactivity affecting the extra-ocular muscles of one of the eyes. In young children strabismus or other conditions which prevent a clear image being formed on the retina can result in visual impairment (amblyopia) in the affected eye if not treated.

Treatment for strabismus often consists of eye exercises, and methods to force preferential use of the affected eye by restricting vision through the healthy eye. This is accomplished either by using an eye patch or by penalisation with glasses or the cycloplegic drug atropine. However, as prolonged use of atropine eye drops may be required there is a risk of systemic toxicity. Surgery may sometimes be necessary. Extra-ocular injection of botulinum A toxin has been used to weaken an overactive extra-ocular eye muscle as an aid to eye realignment; repeated injections may be required. Long-acting parasympathomimetic miotics such as demecarium, dyflos, and ecothiopate have been used in the diagnosis and management of convergent strabismus (esotropia) due to excessive accommodation. With any form of treatment care has to be taken not to induce amblyopia in the healthy eye.

Aceclidine Hydrochloride (4503-d)

Aceclidine Hydrochloride (rINNM).

3-Acetoxyquinuclidine hydrochloride; 3-Quinuclidinyl acetate hydrochloride.

$C_9H_{15}NO_2,HCl = 205.7$.

CAS — 827-61-2 (aceclidine); 6109-70-2 (aceclidine hydrochloride).

NOTE. Aceclidine is *USAN*.

Adverse Effects, Treatment, and Precautions

As for Neostigmine, p.1420. For adverse effects and precautions of miotics, see also Pilocarpine, p.1422.

Uses and Administration

Aceclidine hydrochloride is a parasympathomimetic miotic which is a cholinergic agonist. It is used in eye drops to lower intra-ocular pressure in patients with glaucoma (p.1413).

Preparations

Proprietary Preparations (details are given in Part 3)
Belg.: Glaucocare†; **Fr.:** Glaucostat; **Ger.:** Glaucotat; **Ital.:** Glaunorm; **Neth.:** Glaucocare†; **Port.:** Glaucostat; **Spain:** Glaucostat; **Switz.:** Glaucostat.

Multi-ingredient: Belg.: Glaucofrin†; **Fr.:** Glaucadrine; **Neth.:** Glaucofrin†; **Switz.:** Glaucadrine†.

Acetylcholine Chloride (4506-m)

Acetylcholine Chloride (BAN, rINN).

Acetylcholini Chloridum. (2-Acetoxyethyl)trimethylammonium chloride.

$C_7H_{16}ClNO_2 = 181.7$.

CAS — 51-84-3 (acetylcholine); 60-31-1 (acetylcholine chloride).

Pharmacopoeias. In Eur. (see p.vi) and US.

Jpn includes Acetylcholine Chloride for Injection.

Pharmacopoeial description

Ph. Eur.: A very hygroscopic, white crystalline powder or colourless crystals. Very soluble in water; freely soluble in alcohol; slightly soluble in dichloromethane. Protect from light.

USP 25: White or off-white crystals or crystalline powder. Very soluble in water; freely soluble in alcohol; insoluble in ether. It is decomposed by hot water and by alkalis. Store in airtight containers.

Adverse Effects

Because it is rapidly hydrolysed in the body by cholinesterases the toxicity of acetylcholine is normally relatively low.

Adverse effects of the choline esters include nausea and vomiting, abdominal pain, flushing, sweating, salivation, lachrymation, rhinorrhoea, eructation, diarrhoea, urinary frequency, headache, difficulty in visual accommodation, bradycardia, peripheral vasodilatation leading to hypotension, and bronchoconstriction.

Treatment of Adverse Effects

Atropine sulfate may be given intravenously, intramuscularly, or subcutaneously to control the muscarinic effects of the choline esters. Supportive treatment may be required.

Precautions

Choline esters are contra-indicated in intestinal or urinary obstruction or where increased muscular activity of the urinary or gastrointestinal tract is liable to be harmful. They are also contra-indicated in asthma and obstructive airways disease, in cardiovascular disorders including bradycardia or heart block and recent myocardial infarction, and in hypotension, vagotonia, epilepsy, parkinsonism, hyperthyroidism, peptic ulceration, and pregnancy.

Interactions

As for Neostigmine, p.1420. Acetylcholine is hydrolysed in the body by cholinesterase and its effects are markedly prolonged and enhanced by prior administration of anticholinesterases.

The symbol † denotes a preparation no longer actively marketed

Beta blockers. A report[1] of severe bronchospasm with subsequent pulmonary oedema following intra-ocular injection of acetylcholine chloride in a patient also receiving *metoprolol* by mouth.

1. Rasch D, *et al.* Bronchospasm following intraocular injection of acetylcholine in a patient taking metoprolol. *Anesthesiology* 1983; **59:** 583–5.

NSAIDs. According to a manufacturer of acetylcholine chloride ophthalmic preparations there have been reports of acetylcholine and carbachol being ineffective when used in patients treated with topical (ophthalmic) NSAIDs.

Uses and Administration

Acetylcholine is an endogenous chemical transmitter with a very wide range of actions in the body; it is a powerful quaternary ammonium parasympathomimetic but its action is transient as it is rapidly destroyed by cholinesterase. It is released from postganglionic parasympathetic nerves and also from some postganglionic sympathetic nerves to produce peripheral actions which correspond to those of muscarine. It is accordingly a vasodilator and cardiac depressant, a stimulant of the vagus and the parasympathetic nervous system, and it has a tonic action on smooth muscle. It also increases lachrymal, salivary, and other secretions. All the muscarinic actions of acetylcholine are abolished by atropine.

Acetylcholine also has actions which correspond to those of nicotine and is accordingly a stimulant of skeletal muscle, the autonomic ganglia, and the adrenal medulla. The nicotinic actions of acetylcholine on skeletal muscle are blocked by competitive neuromuscular blockers; they are also inhibited by massive administration or discharge of acetylcholine itself which has clinical application in relation to the mode of action of suxamethonium (p.1342).

Acetylcholine chloride is used as a miotic to reduce postoperative rises in intra-ocular pressure associated with cataract surgery, penetrating keratoplasty, iridectomy, and other anterior segment surgery (p.1413) but is ineffective when applied topically as it is hydrolysed more rapidly than it can penetrate the cornea. Doses of 0.5 to 2 mL of a freshly prepared 1% solution of acetylcholine chloride are therefore instilled directly into the anterior chamber of the eye (intracameral instillation). Miosis occurs within seconds and lasts for about 20 minutes.

Diagnosis and testing. AUTONOMIC FAILURE. Acetylcholine has been used in a sweat-spot test for autonomic neuropathy in diabetic patients.[1] An area on the dorsum of the foot is painted with iodine and starch, followed by intradermal injection of acetylcholine into the centre of the area. Sweat produced in response to acetylcholine reacts with the iodine and starch to produce fine black dots corresponding to the pores of the sweat glands; a normal response is indicated by a uniform distribution of dark spots whereas in diabetic autonomic neuropathy this pattern is lost to a varying degree. A similar test has been carried out[2] to assess sympathetic nerve function and therefore predict the success of lumbar sympathectomy in patients with critical limb ischaemia.

1. Ryder REJ, *et al.* Acetylcholine sweatspot test for autonomic denervation. *Lancet* 1988; **i:** 1303–5.
2. Altomare DF. Acetylcholine sweat test: an effective way to select patients for lumbar sympathectomy. *Lancet* 1994; **344:** 976–8.

Preparations

USP 25: Acetylcholine Chloride for Ophthalmic Solution.

Proprietary Preparations (details are given in Part 3)
Austral.: Miochol; **Belg.:** Miochol†; **Canad.:** Miochol; **Fin.:** Miochol; **Fr.:** Miochole; **Ger.:** Miochol-E; **Hong Kong:** Miochol-E; **Israel:** Miochol; **Ital.:** Miochol-E; **Miovisin;** **NZ:** Miochol; **S.Afr.:** Covochol; Miochol; **Singapore:** Miochol-E; **Swed.:** Miochol†; **Switz.:** Miochol; **Thai.:** Miochol; **UK:** Miochol; **USA:** Miochol.

Ambenonium Chloride (4507-b)

Ambenonium Chloride (BAN, rINN).

Ambestigmini Chloridum; Win-8077. N,N'-Oxalylbis(N-2-aminoethyl-N-2-chlorobenzyldiethylammonium) dichloride.

$C_{28}H_{42}Cl_4N_4O_2 = 608.5$.

CAS — 7648-98-8 (ambenonium); 115-79-7 (anhydrous ambenonium chloride); 52022-31-8 (ambenonium chloride tetrahydrate).

Pharmacopoeias. In Jpn.

Adverse Effects, Treatment, and Precautions

As for Neostigmine, p.1420.

Ambenonium produces fewer muscarinic side-effects than neostigmine. As there is only slight warning of overdosage, routine administration of atropine with ambenonium is contra-indicated because the muscarinic symptoms of overdosage may be suppressed leaving only the more serious nicotinic effects (fasciculation and paralysis of voluntary muscle).

Pharmacokinetics

Ambenonium chloride is poorly absorbed from the gastrointestinal tract. It does not appear to be hydrolysed by cholinesterases.

Uses and Administration

Ambenonium is a quaternary ammonium compound which is a reversible inhibitor of cholinesterase activity with actions similar to those of neostigmine (p.1420), but of longer duration. Ambenonium chloride is given by mouth in the treatment of

myasthenia gravis (p.1414) and may be of value in patients who cannot tolerate neostigmine or pyridostigmine. It is administered 3 or 4 times daily, usually in doses of 5 to 25 mg, adjusted according to individual response.

Preparations

Proprietary Preparations (details are given in Part 3)
Fr.: Mytelase; **Swed.:** Mytelase; **USA:** Mytelase.

Bethanechol Chloride (4509-g)

Bethanechol Chloride (BAN).

Carbamylmethylcholine Chloride. (2-Carbamoyloxypropyl)trimethylammonium chloride.

$C_7H_{17}ClN_2O_2 = 196.7$.

CAS — 674-38-4 (bethanechol); 590-63-6 (bethanechol chloride).

Pharmacopoeias. In Jpn and US.

The manufacturers state that solutions of bethanechol chloride may be autoclaved at 120° for 20 minutes without discoloration or loss of potency.

Pharmacopoeial description

USP 25: Colourless or white crystals, or white crystalline powder, usually having a slight, amine-like odour. It is hygroscopic and exhibits polymorphism. Freely soluble in water and in alcohol; insoluble in chloroform and in ether. pH of a 1% solution in water is between 5.5 and 6.5. Store in airtight containers.

Stability. References to the stability of oral liquid preparations of bethanechol chloride prepared extemporaneously from tablets.

1. Schlatter JL, Saulnier J-L. Bethanechol chloride oral solutions: stability and use in infants. *Ann Pharmacother* 1997; **31:** 294–6.
2. Allen LV, Erickson MA. Stability of bethanechol chloride, pyrazinamide, quinidine sulfate, rifampin, and tetracycline hydrochloride in extemporaneously compounded oral liquids. *Am J Health-Syst Pharm* 1998; **55:** 1804–9.

Adverse Effects and Treatment

As described for choline esters under Acetylcholine Chloride, p.1415.

Precautions

As described for choline esters under Acetylcholine Chloride, p.1415.

Bethanechol should not be given by the intravenous or intramuscular routes as very severe muscarinic adverse effects are liable to occur, calling for emergency administration of atropine.

Autonomic neuropathy. Patients with autonomic neuropathy might be more susceptible to the adverse effects of bethanechol and they should be started on low-dosage regimens and observed closely for signs of toxicity.[1]

1. Caraco Y, *et al.* Bethanechol-induced cholinergic toxicity in diabetic neuropathy. *DICP Ann Pharmacother* 1990; **24:** 327–8.

Interactions

As for Neostigmine, p.1420.

Pharmacokinetics

Bethanechol chloride is poorly absorbed from the gastrointestinal tract. It is not hydrolysed by cholinesterases. At standard doses bethanechol does not cross the blood-brain barrier.

Uses and Administration

Bethanechol chloride, a choline ester, is a quaternary ammonium parasympathomimetic which has predominantly the muscarinic actions of acetylcholine (p.1415). It is not inactivated by cholinesterases so its actions are more prolonged than those of acetylcholine. Bethanechol chloride has little if any nicotinic activity and is used for its actions on the bladder and gastrointestinal tract. It has been used as an alternative to catheterisation in the treatment of urinary retention and has also been used for gastric atony and retention, abdominal distension following surgery, congenital megacolon, and gastro-oesophageal reflux disease.

It is given in usual doses of 5 mg subcutaneously or 10 to 50 mg by mouth, both up to 4 times daily, but dosage must be adjusted individually. Oral doses should be taken on an empty stomach. The effects usually occur within 5 to 15 minutes of a subcutaneous dose, or 30 to 90 minutes of an oral dose, and disappear within about 1 to 2 hours depending on the dose and route of administration used. For a warning to avoid intravenous or intramuscular administration, see under Precautions, above.

Decreased gastrointestinal motility. Parasympathomimetics such as bethanechol enhance gastric contractions and increase intestinal motility and form just one of many treatments that have been used in conditions associated with decreased gastrointestinal motility (p.1202).

Gastro-oesophageal reflux disease. Prokinetic drugs such as bethanechol have been tried in gastro-oesophageal reflux disease (p.1204) but their value is not clear.

References.

1. Thanick KD, *et al.* Reflux esophagitis: effect of oral bethanechol on symptoms and endoscopic findings. *Ann Intern Med* 1980; **93:** 805–8.
2. Saco LS, *et al.* Double-blind controlled trial of bethanechol and antacid versus placebo and antacid in the treatment of erosive esophagitis. *Gastroenterology* 1982; **82:** 1369–73.

3. Thanick K, *et al.* Bethanechol or cimetidine in the treatment of symptomatic reflux esophagitis: a double-blind control study. *Arch Intern Med* 1982; **142:** 1479–81.
4. Strickland AD, Chang JHT. Results of treatment of gastro-esophageal reflux with bethanechol. *J Pediatr* 1983; **103:** 311–15.

Stuttering. A double-blind placebo-controlled study[1] in 10 patients with stuttering (p.687) on the whole failed to confirm an earlier report[2] of benefit using bethanechol although 2 patients who did respond elected to continue treatment after the study.

1. Kampman K, Brady JP. Bethanechol in the treatment of stuttering. *J Clin Psychopharmacol* 1993; **13:** 284–5.
2. Hays P. Bethanechol chloride in treatment of stuttering. *Lancet* 1987; **i:** 271.

Urinary incontinence and retention. Bethanechol is one of the parasympathomimetics that have been given to increase detrusor activity in patients with overflow incontinence, but there have been doubts about the effectiveness of such treatment (see p.459). Bethanechol was also one of the parasympathomimetics used in the management of postoperative urinary retention but they have generally been superseded by catheterisation.

References.
1. Finkbeiner AE. Is bethanechol chloride clinically effective in promoting bladder emptying: a literature review. *J Urol (Baltimore)* 1985; **134:** 443–9.

Preparations

USP 25: Bethanechol Chloride Injection; Bethanechol Chloride Tablets.

Proprietary Preparations (details are given in Part 3)
Aust.: Myocholine; *Austral.:* Urecholine; Urocarb; *Belg.:* Muscaran; *Canad.:* Duvoid; Myotonachol; Urecholine; *Ger.:* Myocholine; *Israel:* Urecholine; *Ital.:* Urecholine†; *S.Afr.:* Urecholine; *Spain:* Myo Hermes; *Switz.:* Myocholine; *Thai.:* Urecholine; *UK:* Myotonine; *USA:* Duvoid; Myotonachol; Urecholine†.

Carbachol (4511-d)

Carbachol *(BAN, rINN)*.

Carbach.; Carbacholine; Carbacholum; Carbacholum Chloratum; Choline Chloride Carbamate. *O*-Carbamoylcholine chloride; (2-Carbamoyloxyethyl)trimethylammonium chloride.
$C_6H_{15}ClN_2O_2 = 182.6$.
CAS — 51-83-2.
ATC — N07AB01; S01EB02.

NOTE. CAR is a code approved by the BP 2001 for use on single unit doses of eye drops containing carbachol where the individual container may be too small to bear all the appropriate labelling information.

Pharmacopoeias. In *Eur.* (see p.vi), *Pol.*, and *US*.

Pharmacopoeial description
Ph. Eur.: A white, crystalline, hygroscopic powder. Very slightly soluble in water; sparingly soluble in alcohol; practically insoluble in acetone. Store in airtight containers. Protect from light.
USP 25: Store in airtight containers.

Incompatibility. Chlorocresol (0.025 to 0.1%) and chlorobutanol (0.5%) were both found to be incompatible with a solution of carbachol (0.8%) and sodium chloride (0.69%), very slight precipitates forming on heating and increasing on standing.[1]
1. *PSGB Lab Report No.911* 1962.

Adverse Effects and Treatment
As described for choline esters under Acetylcholine Chloride, p.1415. Carbachol has substantial nicotinic activity which may be unmasked by the use of atropine to counteract muscarinic effects. Carbachol also produces adverse effects similar to those of other miotics such as pilocarpine (p.1422) when used in the eye but may produce more ciliary spasm than pilocarpine.

Effects on the gastrointestinal tract. A report[1] of fatal oesophageal rupture following subcutaneous injection of carbachol to relieve urinary retention.
1. Cochrane P. Spontaneous oesophageal rupture after carbachol therapy. *BMJ* 1973; **1:** 463–4.

Overdosage. A report[1] of life-threatening attacks of profuse sweating, intestinal cramps, explosive defaecation, hypothermia, hypotension, and bradycardia in a 36-year-old man following deliberate poisoning with 30 to 40 mg of carbachol. The patient's 10-year-old son had died after poisoning with a similar dose of carbachol.
1. Sangster B, *et al.* Two cases of carbachol intoxication. *Neth J Med* 1979; **22:** 27–8.

Precautions
As described for choline esters under Acetylcholine Chloride, p.1415. For precautions when used as a miotic see under Pilocarpine, p.1422. Carbachol should not be given by the intravenous or intramuscular routes as very severe muscarinic adverse effects are liable to occur, calling for emergency treatment with atropine.

Interactions

NSAIDs. According to a manufacturer of acetylcholine chloride ophthalmic preparations there have been reports of acetyl-

choline and carbachol being ineffective when used in patients treated with topical (ophthalmic) NSAIDs.

Uses and Administration
Carbachol, a choline ester, is a quaternary ammonium parasympathomimetic with the muscarinic and nicotinic actions of acetylcholine (p.1415). It is not inactivated by cholinesterases so its actions are more prolonged than those of acetylcholine.
Carbachol has a miotic action and eye drops containing 0.75 to 3% are sometimes used up to four times daily to lower intra-ocular pressure in glaucoma usually in conjunction with other miotics. Miosis occurs within 10 to 20 minutes of instillation of carbachol eye drops and lasts for 4 to 8 hours; reduction in intra-ocular pressure lasts for 8 hours.
Carbachol is also administered intra-ocularly, up to 0.5 mL of a 0.01% solution being instilled into the anterior chamber of the eye (intracameral instillation), to produce miosis in ocular surgery, and reduce postoperative rises in intra-ocular pressure. The maximum degree of miosis is usually obtained within 2 to 5 minutes of intra-ocular instillation and miosis lasts for 24 to 48 hours.
Carbachol has been used for the treatment of urinary retention (p.459) in a dose of 2 mg given three times daily by mouth on a empty stomach, although catheterisation is generally preferred. For the acute symptoms of postoperative urinary retention doses of 250 µg have been given subcutaneously repeated twice if necessary at 30-minute intervals. For a warning to avoid intravenous or intramuscular administration, see under Precautions, above. Carbachol has also been used in some countries for the treatment of decreased gastrointestinal motility (p.1202).

Dry mouth. Carbachol has been used as an alternative to pilocarpine in the treatment of radiation-induced xerostomia.[1] The overall treatment of dry mouth is discussed on p.1498.
1. Joensuu H. Treatment for post-irradiation xerostomia. *N Engl J Med* 1994; **330:** 141–2.

Glaucoma and ocular hypertension. Carbachol is sometimes used as an alternative to pilocarpine in the management of glaucoma (p.1413) when resistance or intolerance to pilocarpine develops. It is also instilled into the anterior chamber of the eye (intracameral instillation) to minimise postoperative rises in intra-ocular pressure associated with ocular surgery, and is considered by some[1,2] to be more effective than acetylcholine.
1. Ruiz RS, *et al.* Effects of carbachol and acetylcholine on intramuscular pressure after cataract extraction. *Am J Ophthalmol* 1989; **107:** 7–10.
2. Hollands RH, *et al.* Control of intraocular pressure after cataract extraction. *Can J Ophthalmol* 1990; **25:** 128–32.

Preparations

USP 25: Carbachol Intraocular Solution; Carbachol Ophthalmic Solution.

Proprietary Preparations (details are given in Part 3)
Austral.: Miostat; *Belg.:* Miostat; *Canad.:* Carbastat; Miostat; *Fin.:* Doryl; *Ger.:* Carbamann; Doryl; Jestryl; *Hong Kong:* Miostat; *Israel:* Miostat; *Ital.:* Mioticol; *NZ:* Miostat; *Singapore:* Miostat; *Swed.:* Isopto Karbakolin; *Switz.:* Doryl; Miostat; Spersacarbachol; *Thai.:* Miostat; *USA:* Carbastat; Miostat.

Multi-ingredient: *Ital.:* Mios.

Cevimeline Hydrochloride (9712-m)

Cevimeline Hydrochloride *(USAN, rINNM)*.
AF-102; AF-102B; FKS-508; SND-5008; SNI-2011; SNK-508. (±)-*cis*-2-Methylspiro[1,3-oxathiolane-5,3′-quinuclidine] hydrochloride hemihydrate.
$C_{10}H_{17}NOS,HCl,\frac{1}{2}H_2O = 244.8$.
CAS — 107233-08-9 (cevimeline); 153504-70-2 (cevimeline hydrochloride).

Profile
Cevimeline hydrochloride is a selective muscarinic M_1 agonist used to improve the symptoms of dry mouth in patients with Sjögren's syndrome. It is given by mouth in doses of 30 mg three times daily.

Dementia. Muscarinic M_1 agonists such as cevimeline have proved unsuccessful in relieving the symptoms of Alzheimer's disease (see p.1412).

Preparations

Proprietary Preparations (details are given in Part 3)
USA: Evoxac.

Choline Alfoscerate (4848-h)

Choline Alfoscerate *(rINN)*.
Choline Glycerophosphate; L-α-Glycerylphosphorylcholine. Choline hydroxide, (*R*)-2,3-dihydroxypropyl hydrogen phosphate, inner salt.
$C_8H_{20}NO_6P = 257.2$.
CAS — 28319-77-9.
ATC — N07AX02.

Profile
Choline alfoscerate is reported to be a precursor of acetylcholine and has been tried in the treatment of Alzheimer's disease

and other dementias (p.1412), although this type of treatment is not considered to produce useful improvement.

◊ References.
1. Di Perri R, *et al.* A multicentre trial to evaluate the efficacy and tolerability of α-glycerylphosphorylcholine versus cytosine diphosphocholine in patients with vascular dementia. *J Int Med Res* 1991; **19:** 330–41.
2. Parnetti L *et al.* Multicentre study of l-α-glyceryl-phosphorylcholine vs ST200 among patients with probable senile dementia of Alzheimer's type. *Drugs Aging* 1993; **3:** 159–64.

Preparations

Proprietary Preparations (details are given in Part 3)
Ital.: Brezal; Delicit; Gliatilin.

Demecarium Bromide (4512-n)

Demecarium Bromide *(BAN, rINN)*.
BC-48. *N,N'*-Decamethylenebis(*N,N,N*-trimethyl-3-methylcarbamoyloxyanilinium) dibromide.
$C_{32}H_{52}Br_2N_4O_4 = 716.6$.
CAS — 56-94-0.
Pharmacopoeias. In *US*.

Pharmacopoeial description
USP 25: A white or slightly yellow, slightly hygroscopic, crystalline powder. Freely soluble in water and in alcohol; sparingly soluble in acetone; soluble in ether. pH of a 1% solution in water is between 5.0 and 7.0. Store in airtight containers. Protect from light.

Adverse Effects
As for Neostigmine, p.1420 and Ecothiopate Iodide, p.1418. For adverse effects of miotics, see also Pilocarpine, p.1422.

Treatment of Adverse Effects
As for Ecothiopate Iodide, p.1418.
Pralidoxime has been reported to be more active in counteracting the effects of dyflos and ecothiopate than of demecarium.

Precautions
As for Neostigmine, p.1420 and Ecothiopate Iodide, p.1418. For precautions of miotics, see also Pilocarpine, p.1422.

Interactions
As for Ecothiopate Iodide, p.1418.

Uses and Administration
Demecarium is a quaternary ammonium compound which is a reversible inhibitor of cholinesterase with a long duration of action similar to that of ecothiopate iodide (p.1418). Its miotic action begins within about 15 to 60 minutes of its application and may persist for a week or more. It causes a reduction in intra-ocular pressure that is maximal in 24 hours and may persist for 9 days or more.
Demecarium bromide has been used in the treatment of open-angle glaucoma (p.1413), particularly in aphakic patients and when other drugs have proved inadequate. The dosage varies, 1 or 2 drops of a 0.125% or 0.25% solution being instilled from twice weekly, preferably at bedtime, to twice daily. Demecarium bromide has also been used in the diagnosis and management of accommodative convergent strabismus (p.1414).

Preparations

USP 25: Demecarium Bromide Ophthalmic Solution.

Proprietary Preparations (details are given in Part 3)
USA: Humorsol.

3,4-Diaminopyridine (19064-m)

Profile
3,4-Diaminopyridine has similar actions and uses to fampridine (p.1419) but is reported to be more potent in enhancing the release of acetylcholine from nerve terminals. It is used in the Eaton-Lambert myasthenic syndrome and other myasthenic conditions. It has been tried in multiple sclerosis and in botulism. There have been isolated reports of seizures and 3,4-diaminopyridine is therefore contra-indicated in patients with epilepsy.

Congenital myasthenia. Congenital or hereditary myasthenia is a heterogeneous group of rare disorders associated with various defects in neuromuscular transmission including presynaptic impairment of acetylcholinesterase release, postsynaptic abnormality of acetylcholine receptors, or a deficiency of acetylcholinesterase.[1] Symptoms may be similar to those of myasthenia gravis (p.1414) but there are no immunological abnormalities. Although some forms may respond to anticholinesterases, therapy is usually unsatisfactory. Experience in 16 patients[2] has suggested that 3,4-diaminopyridine used alone or with anticholinesterases may be of benefit. Clinical improvement was seen in 5 of 11 patients with congenital myasthenia who were given 3,4-diaminopyridine as part of a placebo-controlled trial; 3 of the 11 responded to placebo.[3] There have also been reports of benefit from the use of quinidine sulfate in patients with the slow-channel congenital myasthenic syndrome.[4]
1. Engel AG. Congenital myasthenic syndromes. *Neurol Clin North Am* 1994; **12:** 401–37.
2. Palace J, *et al.* 3,4-Diaminopyridine in the treatment of congenital (hereditary) myasthenia. *J Neurol Neurosurg Psychiatry* 1991; **54:** 1069–72.

3. Anlar B, *et al.* 3,4-Diaminopyridine in childhood myasthenia: double-blind, placebo-controlled trial. *J Child Neurol* 1996; **11:** 458–61.
4. Harper CM, Engel AG. Quinidine sulfate therapy for the slow-channel congenital myasthenic syndrome. *Ann Neurol* 1998; **43:** 480–4.

Eaton-Lambert myasthenic syndrome. Administration of 3,4-diaminopyridine by mouth in daily doses of up to 100 mg has been found[1] to be effective in the treatment of both the motor and autonomic deficits of patients with Eaton-Lambert syndrome (p.1412). A usual starting dose of 10 mg given three or four times daily increasing if necessary to a maximum of 20 mg given five times daily has been used.[2] Adverse effects appear to be mainly mild and dose related,[1] although there is a report of cardiac arrest following toxicity.[3] Most patients experience some form of paraesthesia up to 60 minutes after administration.[1,2] 3,4-Diaminopyridine can produce mild excitatory effects and some patients may experience difficulty in sleeping.

1. McEvoy KM, *et al.* 3,4-Diaminopyridine in the treatment of Lambert-Eaton myasthenic syndrome. *N Engl J Med* 1989; **321:** 1567–71.
2. Newsom-Davis J. Myasthenia gravis and the Lambert-Eaton myasthenic syndrome. *Prescribers' J* 1993; **33:** 205–212.
3. Boerma CE, *et al.* Cardiac arrest following an iatrogenic 3,4-diaminopyridine intoxication in a patient with Lambert-Eaton myasthenic syndrome. *J Toxicol Clin Toxicol* 1995; **33:** 249–51.

Multiple sclerosis. 3,4-Diaminopyridine has been tried in the management of multiple sclerosis (p.633). In a crossover study[1] involving 36 patients with multiple sclerosis, 3,4-diaminopyridine given in a dosage of up to 100 mg daily improved symptoms of leg weakness to a greater extent than placebo but paraesthesia and abdominal pain which occurred in most patients were dose-limiting in some.

1. Bever CT, *et al.* Treatment with oral 3,4-diaminopyridine improves leg strength in multiple sclerosis patients: results of a randomized, double-blind, placebo-controlled, crossover trial. *Neurology* 1996; **47:** 1457–62.

Distigmine Bromide (4513-h)

Distigmine Bromide (*BAN, rINN*).

BC-51; Bispyridostigmine Bromide; Hexamarium Bromide. 3,3′-[*N,N*′-Hexamethylenebis(methylcarbamoyloxy)]bis(1-methylpyridinium bromide).
$C_{22}H_{32}Br_2N_4O_4 = 576.3$.
CAS — 15876-67-2.

Pharmacopoeias. In Jpn.

Adverse Effects, Treatment, and Precautions
As for Neostigmine, p.1420. The anticholinesterase action of distigmine, and hence its adverse effects, may be prolonged, and if treatment with atropine is required it should be maintained for at least 24 hours. Distigmine may stimulate uterine contractions and the UK manufacturer has advised that it should be avoided in pregnancy.

Interactions
As for Neostigmine, p.1420.

Pharmacokinetics
Distigmine is poorly absorbed from the gastrointestinal tract.

Uses and Administration
Distigmine is a quaternary ammonium compound which is a reversible inhibitor of cholinesterase activity with actions similar to those of neostigmine (p.1420) but more prolonged. Maximum inhibition of plasma cholinesterase occurs 9 hours after a single intramuscular dose, and persists for about 24 hours.

Distigmine bromide has been administered by intramuscular injection or by mouth on an empty stomach. It is one of several drugs that have been used in the prevention and treatment of postoperative gastrointestinal atony (p.1202). It has also been used in postoperative urinary retention (p.459), although it has been superseded by catheterisation. A dose of 500 μg of distigmine bromide was injected intramuscularly about 24 to 72 hours after surgery and repeated at intervals of 1 to 3 days until normal function was restored. Alternatively it has been given by mouth in a dose of 5 mg daily thirty minutes before breakfast. A similar dose by mouth, given daily or on alternate days, has been employed in the management of neurogenic bladder.

Distigmine bromide in conjunction with short-acting parasympathomimetics may also be given by mouth for the treatment of myasthenia gravis (p.1414), but patients being treated with parasympathomimetics tend to prefer pyridostigmine. The initial dose is 5 mg daily before breakfast, increased at intervals of 3 to 4 days if necessary to a maximum of 20 mg daily; children may be given up to 10 mg daily according to age.

Preparations

Donepezil Hydrochloride (3627-b)

Donepezil Hydrochloride (*BANM, USAN, rINNM*).

BNAG; E-2020; ER-4111 (donepezil). (±)-2-[(1-Benzyl-4-piperidyl)methyl]-5,6-dimethoxy-1-indanone hydrochloride.
$C_{24}H_{29}NO_3,HCl = 416.0$.
CAS — 120014-06-4 (donepezil); 142057-79-2 (donepezil); 120011-70-3 (donepezil hydrochloride); 142057-77-0 (donepezil hydrochloride).

Adverse Effects, Treatment, and Precautions
Generally as for Neostigmine, p.1420. Adverse effects of donepezil notably include nausea, vomiting, diarrhoea, fatigue, insomnia, and muscle cramps. Less frequent adverse effects reported include headache and dizziness; syncope, bradycardia, convulsions, and sinoatrial and atrioventricular block have occurred rarely. Individual cases of increased liver transaminases and, rarely, hepatitis have also been noted. Psychiatric disturbances, including hallucinations, agitation, and aggressive behaviour, have been reported. Minor increases in plasma-creatine kinase have occurred and there is potential for bladder outflow obstruction.

◊ Review[1] of the safety profile of donepezil.
1. Committee on Safety of Medicines/Medicines Control Agency. Donepezil (Aricept). *Current Problems* 1999; **25:** 7.

Effects on the skin. A report[1] of purpuric rash associated with donepezil.
1. Bryant CA, *et al.* Purpuric rash with donepezil treatment. *BMJ* 1998; **317:** 787.

Interactions
As for Neostigmine, p.1420. Hepatic metabolism of donepezil via the cytochrome P450 system has been demonstrated; plasma concentrations of donepezil may be raised by drugs that inhibit the isoenzyme CYP3A4 such as ketoconazole, itraconazole, and erythromycin and by those that inhibit the isoenzyme CYP2D6 such as fluoxetine and quinidine. Plasma concentrations may be reduced by enzyme inducers such as rifampicin, phenytoin, carbamazepine, and alcohol.

Pharmacokinetics
Donepezil hydrochloride is well absorbed from the gastrointestinal tract, maximum plasma concentrations being achieved within 3 to 4 hours. It is about 95% bound to plasma proteins. Donepezil undergoes partial metabolism via the cytochrome P450 system to 4 major metabolites. About 11% of a dose is present in plasma as 6-*O*-desmethyl donepezil, which has similar activity to the parent compound. Over 10 days, about 57% of a dose is recovered from the urine as unchanged drug and metabolites, and about 15% from the faeces; 28% remains unrecovered suggesting accumulation. The elimination half-life is about 70 hours. Steady-state concentrations are achieved within 3 weeks of the start of therapy.

◊ References.
1. Tiseo PJ, *et al.* Metabolism and elimination of ¹⁴C-donepezil in healthy volunteers: a single-dose study. *Br J Clin Pharmacol* 1998; **46** (suppl 1): 19–24.

Uses and Administration
Donepezil hydrochloride, a piperidine derivative, is a reversible and specific inhibitor of acetylcholinesterase with actions similar to those of neostigmine (p.1420). It is highly selective for the CNS and is used for the symptomatic treatment of mild to moderately severe dementia in Alzheimer's disease. Donepezil hydrochloride is given in an initial dose of 5 mg by mouth once daily in the evening and increased if necessary after 4 to 6 weeks to a maximum of 10 mg once daily. Clinical benefit should be reassessed on a regular basis.

Alzheimer's disease. Donepezil hydrochloride is used in the symptomatic treatment of mild to moderately severe dementia in Alzheimer's disease (p.1412). In individual trials, it appears to produce modest benefits in some patients.[1,2] These findings are also supported by the results of a meta-analysis[3] which concluded that, in the short-term, donepezil produces modest improvements in cognitive function and global clinical state. Although there are no comparative studies of donepezil and

tacrine it has been suggested[4-6] that donepezil may prove preferable as it appears to be better tolerated and hepatotoxicity has not been reported to be a problem (but see Adverse Effects, above). Longer-term randomised trials of donepezil were considered necessary to evaluate benefits and costs.[7] UK guidelines recommend that treatment with donepezil should be under specialist supervision, that benefit should be assessed 2 to 4 months after reaching maintenance dosage, and every 6 months thereafter, and treatment only continued if there is evidence of benefit.[8]

1. Rogers SL, Friedhoff LT. Donepezil Study Group. The efficacy and safety of donepezil in patients with Alzheimer's disease: results of a US multicentre, randomized, double-blind, placebo-controlled trial. *Dementia* 1996; **7:** 293–303.
2. Rogers SL, *et al.* A 24-week, double-blind, placebo-controlled trial of donepezil in patients with Alzheimer's disease. *Neurology* 1998; **50:** 136–45.
3. Birks JS, *et al.* Donepezil for mild and moderate Alzheimer's disease (updated 30 May 2001). Available in The Cochrane Library; Issue 4. Oxford: Update Software; 2001.
4. American Psychiatric Association. Practice guideline for the treatment of patients with Alzheimer's disease and other dementias of late life. *Am J Psychiatry* 1997; **154** (suppl): 1–39.
5. Shintani EY, Uchida KM. Donepezil: an anticholinesterase inhibitor for Alzheimer's disease. *Am J Health-Syst Pharm* 1997; **54:** 2805–10.
6. Barner EL, Gray SL. Donepezil use in Alzheimer disease. *Ann Pharmacother* 1998; **32:** 70–7.
7. Eccles M, *et al.* North of England evidence based guidelines development project: guideline for the primary care management of dementia. *BMJ* 1998; **317:** 802–8.
8. National Institute for Clinical Excellence. Guidance on the use of donepezil, rivastigmine, and galantamine for the treatment of Alzheimer's disease (issued January 2001). Available at: http://www.nice.org.uk/pdf/ALZHEIMER_full_guidance.pdf (accessed 20/11/01).

Preparations

Dyflos (4514-m)

Dyflos (*BAN*).

DFP; Difluorophate; Di-isopropyl Fluorophosphate; Di-isopropylfluorophosphonate; Fluostigmine; Isoflurophate. Di-isopropyl phosphorofluoridate.
$C_6H_{14}FO_3P = 184.1$.
CAS — 55-91-4.
ATC — S01EB07.
Pharmacopoeias. In US.

Pharmacopoeial description
USP 25: A clear, colourless, or faintly yellow liquid. Specific gravity about 1.05. Sparingly soluble in water; soluble in alcohol and in vegetable oils. It is decomposed by moisture with the evolution of hydrogen fluoride. Store at 8° to 15° in sealed containers.

◊ CAUTION. *The vapour of dyflos is very toxic. The eyes, nose, and mouth should be protected when handling dyflos, and contact with the skin should be avoided. Dyflos can be removed from the skin by washing with soap and water. Contaminated material should be immersed in a 2% aqueous solution of sodium hydroxide for several hours.*

Adverse Effects
As for Neostigmine, p.1420 and Ecothiopate Iodide, p.1418. For adverse effects of miotics, see also Pilocarpine, p.1422.
The anticholinesterase action of dyflos, and hence its adverse effects, may be prolonged. Its vapour is extremely irritating to the eye and mucous membranes.
Systemic toxicity also occurs after inhalation of the vapour. Prolonged use of dyflos in the eye may cause slowly reversible depigmentation of the lid margins in dark-skinned patients.

Treatment of Adverse Effects
As for Ecothiopate Iodide, p.1418.

Precautions
As for Neostigmine, p.1420 and Ecothiopate Iodide, p.1418. For precautions of miotics, see also Pilocarpine, p.1422.

Interactions
As for Ecothiopate Iodide, p.1418.

Pharmacokinetics
Dyflos is readily absorbed from the gastrointestinal tract, from skin and mucous membranes, and from the lungs. Dyflos interacts with cholinesterases producing stable phosphonylated and phosphorylated derivatives which are then hydrolysed and excreted mainly in the urine.

Uses and Administration
Dyflos is an irreversible inhibitor of cholinesterases with actions similar to those of ecothiopate iodide (p.1418). Dyflos has a powerful miotic action which begins within 5 to 10 minutes and persists for up to 4 weeks; it causes a reduction in intra-ocular pressure which is maximal in 24 hours and may persist for a week.

The symbol † denotes a preparation no longer actively marketed

Dyflos has been used mainly in the treatment of open-angle glaucoma (p.1413), particularly in aphakic patients and when other drugs have proved inadequate. It was also employed in the diagnosis and management of accommodative convergent strabismus (p.1414).

Dyflos is administered locally usually as a 0.025% ophthalmic ointment preferably at night before retiring.

Preparations

USP 25: Isoflurophate Ophthalmic Ointment.
Proprietary Preparations (details are given in Part 3)
USA: Floropryl†.

Ecothiopate Iodide (4515-b)

Ecothiopate Iodide (*BAN, rINN*).

Echothiophate Iodide; Ecostigmine Iodide; MI-217. (2-Diethoxyphosphinylthioethyl)trimethylammonium iodide.

$C_9H_{23}INO_3PS = 383.2$.

CAS — 6736-03-4 (ecothiopate); 513-10-0 (ecothiopate iodide).

Pharmacopoeias. In Jpn and US.

Pharmacopoeial description

USP 25: A white, crystalline, hygroscopic solid having a slight mercaptan-like odour. Soluble 1 in 1 of water, 1 in 25 of dehydrated alcohol, and 1 in 3 of methyl alcohol; practically insoluble in other organic solvents. Its solutions in water have a pH of about 4. Store in airtight containers preferably at a temperature below 0°. Protect from light.

Adverse Effects

As for Neostigmine, p.1420. For adverse effects of miotics, see also Pilocarpine, p.1422.

Ecothiopate is an irreversible cholinesterase inhibitor; its action, and hence its adverse effects, may be prolonged.

Plasma and erythrocyte cholinesterases may be diminished by treatment with eye drops of ecothiopate, or other long-acting anticholinesterases and systemic toxicity occurs more frequently than with shorter-acting miotics. Acute iritis, retinal detachment, or precipitation of acute glaucoma may occasionally follow treatment with ecothiopate and iris cysts (especially in children) or lens opacities may develop following prolonged treatment.

Treatment of Adverse Effects

In systemic poisoning, atropine sulfate may be given parenterally with pralidoxime chloride as for intoxication with organophosphorus insecticides (see p.1020); subconjunctival injection of pralidoxime has been employed to reverse severe ocular adverse effects. Supportive treatment, including assisted ventilation, should be given as necessary.

To prevent or reduce development of iris cysts in patients receiving ecothiopate eye drops, phenylephrine eye drops may be given simultaneously.

Precautions

As for Neostigmine, p.1420. For precautions of miotics, see also under Pilocarpine, p.1422. In general ecothiopate, in common with other long-acting anticholinesterases, should be used only where therapy with other drugs has proved ineffective. Ecothiopate iodide should not be used in patients with iodine hypersensitivity.

Interactions

As for Neostigmine, p.1420. The possibility of an interaction remains for a considerable time after discontinuation of long-acting anticholinesterases such as ecothiopate.

Uses and Administration

Ecothiopate is an irreversible inhibitor of cholinesterase with actions similar to those of neostigmine (p.1420), but much more prolonged. Its miotic action begins within 10 to 30 minutes of its application and may persist for 1 to 4 weeks; it causes a reduction in intra-ocular pressure which is maximal after 24 hours and may persist for days or weeks.

Ecothiopate iodide is used mainly in the treatment of open-angle glaucoma (p.1413), particularly in aphak-

ic patients and when other drugs have proved inadequate. It is administered as drops of a 0.03 to 0.25% solution. The manufacturers recommend twice daily administration to allow for diurnal variations in intra-ocular pressure, although a single dose has also been used once daily or on alternate days. It is advisable to give the single dose or one of the two daily doses at bedtime.

Ecothiopate iodide eye drops are also used in the diagnosis and management of accommodative convergent strabismus (p.1414).

Preparations

USP 25: Echothiophate Iodide for Ophthalmic Solution.
Proprietary Preparations (details are given in Part 3)
Austral.: Phospholine Iodide; *Belg.:* Phospholine Iodide†; *Canad.:* Phospholine Iodide; *Fr.:* Phospholine Iodide; *Israel:* Phospholine Iodide; *Neth.:* Phospholine Iodide†; *UK:* Phospholine Iodide; *USA:* Phospholine Iodide.

Edrophonium Chloride (4516-v)

Edrophonium Chloride (*BAN, rINN*).

Edrophonii Chloridum. Ethyl(3-hydroxyphenyl)dimethylammonium chloride.

$C_{10}H_{16}ClNO = 201.7$.

CAS — 312-48-1 (edrophonium); 116-38-1 (edrophonium chloride).

Pharmacopoeias. In Br., Int., Jpn, and US.

Pharmacopoeial description

BP 2001: A white crystalline powder. Very soluble in water; freely soluble in alcohol; practically insoluble in chloroform and in ether. Protect from light.

USP 25: A white odourless crystalline powder. Soluble 1 in 0.5 of water and 1 in 5 of alcohol; insoluble in chloroform and in ether. A 10% solution in water is practically colourless and the pH is between 4.0 and 5.0.

Adverse Effects, Treatment, and Precautions

As for Neostigmine, p.1420.

Interactions

As for Neostigmine, p.1420.

Uses and Administration

Edrophonium is a quaternary ammonium compound which is a reversible inhibitor of cholinesterase activity. It has actions similar to those of neostigmine (p.1420) but its effect on skeletal muscle is claimed to be particularly prominent. Its action is rapid in onset and of short duration. In patients with myasthenia gravis, there is immediate subjective improvement and muscle strength increases. This effect usually lasts only for about 5 to 15 minutes, after which time the typical signs and symptoms return; because of its brief action the drug is not suitable for the routine treatment of myasthenia gravis.

Edrophonium chloride is used in **myasthenia gravis** (p.1414) both diagnostically and to distinguish between under- or over-treatment with other anticholinesterases. The usual *diagnostic procedure* is to inject 2 mg intravenously and, if no adverse reaction occurs within 30 to 45 seconds, to continue with the injection of a further 8 mg. In the UK the recommended total dose for children is 100 µg per kg body-weight, one-fifth of the dose being given initially, followed 30 seconds later by the remainder if no adverse effect develops. In the USA the manufacturers recommend a total dose of 5 mg for children weighing less than 34 kg and 10 mg for heavier children with one-fifth of the dose being given initially followed by increments of 1 mg every 30 to 45 seconds; the recommended total dose for infants is 0.5 mg.

When intravenous injection is difficult edrophonium chloride may be given by intramuscular injection; the usual dose in adults is 10 mg while children below 34 kg in weight may be given 2 mg and heavier children 5 mg; a suggested dose for infants is 0.5 to 1 mg given intramuscularly or subcutaneously. Atropine should always be available when the test is carried out in order to treat any severe muscarinic reactions that may occur.

To *detect under- or over-treatment*, test doses of 1 to 2 mg of edrophonium chloride are given intravenously to distinguish severe symptoms of myasthenia gravis due to inadequate therapy from the effects of overdosage with anticholinesterase drugs. If treatment has been inadequate, edrophonium chloride will produce an immediate amelioration of symptoms, whereas in cholinergic crises due to over-treatment the symptoms will be temporarily aggravated. The manufacturers suggest administration one hour after the last dose of treatment but the *British National Formulary* recommends administration just before the next dose is due. Testing should only be undertaken when facilities for endotracheal intubation and controlled ventilation are immediately available.

Edrophonium chloride was originally introduced for the **reversal of neuromuscular blockade** in anaesthesia. In the UK, the recommended dose for the reversal of the effects of competitive neuromuscular blockers is 500 to 700 µg per kg body-weight, given by intravenous injection over several minutes either with or after atropine sulfate 0.6 mg; in the USA a dose of 10 mg of edrophonium chloride is given over 30 to 45 seconds and repeated as required up to a maximum of 40 mg. The brevity of its action limits its value. Where prolonged apnoea occurs in a patient treated with a depolarising neuromuscular blocker, such as suxamethonium, edrophonium 10 mg may be given intravenously with atropine to determine the presence of phase II block (see p.1342).

Edrophonium bromide has been used similarly to edrophonium chloride.

Reversal of neuromuscular blockade. For a discussion of whether edrophonium might be more suitable than neostigmine for reversal of residual block after the use of the shorter-acting competitive neuromuscular blockers, see under Uses and Administration of Neostigmine, p.1421.

Snake bite. For the use of anticholinesterases in the treatment of snake bite, see under Uses and Administration of Neostigmine, p.1421.

Tetrodotoxin poisoning. Management of poisoning due to tetrodotoxin, a heat stable neuromuscular blocking toxin found in various marine animals, such as puffer fish, is mainly symptomatic and supportive. Reports[1,2] on the effectiveness of intravenous anticholinesterases such as edrophonium or neostigmine in reversing muscle weakness in tetrodotoxin poisoning have been conflicting. Although it appears that anticholinesterases may only be effective during partial block produced by tetrodotoxin, some consider[3] that, as there is no specific antidote, any measure that brings about improvement may be tried.

1. Chew SK, *et al.* Anticholinesterase drugs in the treatment of tetrodotoxin poisoning. *Lancet* 1984; **ii:** 108.
2. Tibballs J. Severe tetrodotoxic fish poisoning. *Anaesth Intensive Care* 1988; **16:** 215–17.
3. Karalliedde L. Management of puffer fish poisoning. *Br J Anaesth* 1995; **75:** 500.

Preparations

BP 2001: Edrophonium Injection;
USP 25: Edrophonium Chloride Injection.

Proprietary Preparations (details are given in Part 3)
Canad.: Enlon; Tensilon†; *S.Afr.:* Tensilon†; *Spain:* Anticude; *UK:* Camsilon; *USA:* Enlon; Enlon-Plus; Reversol; Tensilon.

Eptastigmine (13786-l)

Eptastigmine (*rINN*).

N-Demethyl-N-heptylphysostigmine. (3aS,8aR)-1,2,3,3a,8,8a-Hexahydro-1,3a,8-trimethylpyrrolo[2,3-b]indol-5-yl heptylcarbamate.

$C_{21}H_{33}N_3O_2 = 359.5$.

CAS — 101246-68-8.

Profile

Eptastigmine is a long-acting inhibitor of cholinesterase activity; it is a lipophilic derivative of physostigmine (p.1421). It has been studied in the oral treatment of Alzheimer's disease (see Dementia, p.1412) but development was stopped after reports of aplastic anaemia.

◊ References.

1. Imbimbo BP, *et al.* Relationship between pharmacokinetics and pharmacodynamics of eptastigmine in young healthy volunteers. *J Clin Pharmacol* 1995; **35:** 285–90.
2. Canal N, Imbimbo BP. Eptastigmine Study Group. Relationship between pharmacodynamic activity and cognitive effects of eptastigmine in patients with Alzheimer's disease. *Clin Pharmacol Ther* 1996; **60:** 218–28.

3. Canal N, *et al.* Eptastigmine Study Group. A 25-week, double-blind, randomized, placebo-controlled, trial of eptastigmine in patients with diagnosis of probable Alzheimer's disease. *Eur J Neurol* 1996; **3** (suppl 5): 238.
4. Imbimbo BP, *et al.* Efficacy and safety of eptastigmine for the treatment of patients with Alzheimer's disease. *Neurology* 1999; **52**: 700–8.

Eseridine Salicylate (4522-m)

Eseridine Salicylate *(rINNM)*.

Eserine Aminoxide Salicylate; Eserine Oxide Salicylate; Physostigmine Aminoxide Salicylate; Physostigmine *N*-Oxide Salicylate. (4aS,9aS)-2,3,4,4a,9,9a-Hexahydro-2,4a,9-trimethyl-1,2-oxazino[6,5-*b*]indol-6-ylmethylcarbamate salicylate.

$C_{15}H_{21}N_3O_3,C_7H_6O_3 = 429.5$.

CAS — 25573-43-7 (eseridine); 5995-96-0 (eseridine salicylate).

Profile
Eseridine salicylate, a derivative of physostigmine, is an inhibitor of cholinesterase activity that has been given by mouth in preparations for dyspepsia and other gastric disorders.

Preparations
Proprietary Preparations (details are given in Part 3)
Fr.: Geneserine.

Fampridine (12364-v)

Fampridine *(USAN, rINN)*.

EL-970. 4-Aminopyridine; 4-Pyridinamine.

$C_5H_6N_2 = 94.11$.

CAS — 504-24-5.

Profile
Fampridine enhances the release of acetylcholine from nerve terminals and has been used intravenously to reverse the effects of competitive neuromuscular blockers. It has also been tried by mouth and intravenously in the management of a number of neurological disorders including Eaton-Lambert myasthenic syndrome (p.1412), multiple sclerosis (p.633), spinal cord injury, and Alzheimer's disease (see Dementia, p.1412), and for the reversal of neuromuscular blockade in patients with botulism (p.1534).

Fampridine has also been considered as a specific antidote in poisoning with calcium-channel blockers such as verapamil (p.990).

Adverse effects, especially seizures, may limit its use.

◊ References.
1. Ter Wee PM, *et al.* 4-Aminopyridine and haemodialysis in the treatment of verapamil intoxication. *Hum Toxicol* 1985; **4**: 327–9.
2. Davidson M, *et al.* 4-Aminopyridine in the treatment of Alzheimer's disease. *Biol Psychiatry* 1988; **23**: 485–90.
3. Hansebout RR, *et al.* 4-Aminopyridine in chronic spinal cord injury: a controlled, double-blind, crossover study in eight patients. *J Neurotrauma* 1993; **10**: 1–18.

Multiple sclerosis. Fampridine has potassium-channel blocking activity and has been tried in the treatment of multiple sclerosis to improve conduction in demyelinated fibres; improvements have been reported in walking, dexterity, and vision, but only small numbers of patients have been studied.

References.
1. Davis FA, *et al.* Orally administered 4-aminopyridine improves clinical signs in multiple sclerosis. *Ann Neurol* 1990; **27**: 186–92.
2. van Dieman HAM, *et al.* The effect of 4-aminopyridine on clinical signs in multiple sclerosis: a randomized, placebo-controlled, double-blind, cross-over study. *Ann Neurol* 1992; **32**: 123–30.
3. Van Diemen HAM, *et al.* 4-Aminopyridine in patients with multiple sclerosis: dosage and serum level related to efficacy and safety. *Clin Neuropharmacol* 1993; **16**: 195–204.
4. Bever CT, *et al.* The effects of 4-aminopyridine in multiple sclerosis patients: results of a randomized, placebo-controlled, double-blind, concentration-controlled, crossover trial. *Neurology* 1994; **44**: 1054–9.
5. Schwid SR, *et al.* Quantitative assessment of sustained-release 4-aminopyridine for symptomatic treatment of multiple sclerosis. *Neurology* 1997; **48**: 817–21.

Galantamine Hydrobromide (4517-g)

Galantamine Hydrobromide *(BANM, USAN, rINNM)*.

Galanthamine Hydrobromide; Galanthamini Hydrobromidum. (4aS,6R,8aS)-4a,5,9,10,11,12-Hexahydro-3-methoxy-11-methyl-6*H*-benzofuro[3a,3,2-*ef*][2]benzazepin-6-ol hydrobromide.

$C_{17}H_{21}NO_3,HBr = 368.3$.

CAS — 357-70-0 (galantamine); 1953-04-4 (galantamine hydrobromide).

Pharmacopoeias. In *Chin.*

The hydrobromide of galantamine, an alkaloid which has been obtained from the Caucasian snowdrop (Voronov's snowdrop), *Galanthus woronowii* (Amaryllidaceae), and related species.

The symbol † denotes a preparation no longer actively marketed

Adverse Effects, Treatment, and Precautions
As for Rivastigmine, p.1424. Galantamine is contra-indicated in patients with severe renal or severe hepatic impairment.

Uses and Administration
Galantamine hydrobromide is a reversible inhibitor of cholinesterase activity, with actions similar to those of neostigmine (p.1420). It is used in mild to moderately severe Alzheimer's disease (see Dementia, p.1412). An initial dose of 4 mg is given twice daily with food for four weeks, then increased to 8 mg twice daily. This dose should be maintained for at least four weeks; thereafter, according to individual patient response and tolerability, the dose may be further increased to 12 mg twice daily. The clinical benefit of galantamine should be reassessed on a regular basis. The initial dose in patients with moderate hepatic impairment should be 4 mg once daily for at least one week, preferably in the morning, increased thereafter as above to a maximum of 8 mg twice daily. Galantamine is contra-indicated in severe hepatic impairment.

Galantamine hydrobromide has also been used in various neuromuscular disorders, and to curtail the muscle relaxation produced by competitive neuromuscular blockers.

Dementia. Reviews[1,2] suggest that galantamine is of benefit in patients with mild to moderate symptoms of Alzheimer's disease; evidence in more severely impaired subjects is lacking. In the UK, guidelines recommend the use of galantamine in such patients under specialist supervision, with benefits assessed 2 to 4 months after achieving maintenance dosage, and every 6 months thereafter; treatment should only continue where there is evidence of benefit.[3]

1. Scott LJ, Goa KL. Galantamine: a review of its use in Alzheimer's disease. *Drugs* 2000; **60**: 1095–1122.
2. Olin J, Schneider L. Galantamine for Alzheimer's disease (updated 24 August 2001). Available in The Cochrane Library; Issue 4. Oxford: Update Software; 2001.
3. National Institute for Clinical Excellence. Guidance on the use of donepezil, rivastigmine and galantamine for the treatment of Alzheimer's disease (issued January 2001). Available at: http://www.nice.org.uk/pdf/ALZHEIMER_full_guidance.pdf (accessed 20/11/01).

Preparations
Proprietary Preparations (details are given in Part 3)
Aust.: Nivalin; *Fr.:* Reminyl; *Irl.:* Reminyl; *Swed.:* Reminyl; *UK:* Reminyl; *USA:* Reminyl.

Guanidine Hydrochloride (12807-c)

Carbamidine Hydrochloride; Iminourea Hydrochloride.

$CH_5N_3,HCl = 95.53$.

CAS — 113-00-8 (guanidine); 50-01-1 (guanidine hydrochloride).

Profile
Guanidine hydrochloride enhances the release of acetylcholine from nerve terminals. It has been given by mouth to reverse neuromuscular blockade in patients with botulism (p.1534), but its efficacy has not been established. Guanidine hydrochloride has also been tried in Eaton-Lambert myasthenic syndrome (p.1412) and other neurological disorders, but its use has been associated with bone-marrow suppression in some patients.

◊ References.
1. Kaplan JE, *et al.* Botulism, type A, and treatment with guanidine. *Ann Neurol* 1979; **6**: 69–71.
2. Critchley EMR, *et al.* Outbreak of botulism in North West England and Wales. *Lancet* 1989; **ii**: 849–53.
3. Neal KR, Dunbar EM. Improvement in bulbar weakness with guanoxan in type B botulism. *Lancet* 1990; **335**: 1286–7.
4. Oh SJ, *et al.* Low-dose guanidine and pyridostigmine: relatively safe and effective long-term symptomatic therapy in Lambert-Eaton myasthenic syndrome. *Muscle Nerve* 1997; **20**: 1146–52.

Linopirdine (10977-a)

Linopirdine *(USAN, rINN)*.

DuP-996. 1-Phenyl-3,3-bis(4-pyridylmethyl)-2-indolinone; 1,3-Dihydro-1-phenyl-3,3-bis(4-pyridinylmethyl)-2*H*-indol-2-one.

$C_{26}H_{21}N_3O = 391.5$.

CAS — 105431-72-9.

ATC — N06BX09.

Profile
Linopirdine is reported to enhance the release of acetylcholine, and possibly other neurotransmitters, from nerve terminals. It has been given by mouth in studies of the treatment of Alzheimer's disease (see Dementia, p.1412) but there is little evidence of clinical benefit.

◊ References.
1. Pieniaszek HJ, *et al.* Single-dose pharmacokinetics, safety, and tolerance of linopirdine (DUP 996) in healthy young adults and elderly volunteers. *J Clin Pharmacol* 1995; **35**: 22–30.
2. Rockwood K, *et al.* A randomized, controlled trial of linopirdine in the treatment of Alzheimer's disease. *Can J Neurol Sci* 1997; **24**: 140–5.

Methacholine Chloride (4520-n)

Methacholine Chloride *(BAN, rINN)*.

Acetyl-β-methylcholine Chloride; Amechol Chloride; Methacholinium Chloratum. (2-Acetoxypropyl)trimethylammonium chloride.

$C_8H_{18}ClNO_2 = 195.7$.

CAS — 55-92-5 (methacholine); 62-51-1 (methacholine chloride).

Pharmacopoeias. In *Fr., It., Swiss,* and *US.*

Pharmacopoeial description
USP 25: Colourless or white crystals, or a white crystalline powder. It is odourless or has a slight odour, and is very hygroscopic. Soluble 1 in 1.2 of water, 1 in 1.7 of alcohol, and 1 in 2.1 of chloroform. Its solutions are neutral to litmus. Store in airtight containers.

Adverse Effects and Treatment
As for Acetylcholine Chloride, p.1415. Severe adverse cholinergic effects have followed the oral and parenteral administration of methacholine and these routes are no longer used.

Precautions
As for Neostigmine, p.1420.
Methacholine has the potential to produce severe bronchoconstriction and it should not be used for inhalation challenge tests in patients with clinically apparent asthma, wheezing, or poor pulmonary function.
Methacholine should not be given orally or parenterally.

Interactions
As for Neostigmine, p.1420. Methacholine is slowly hydrolysed by acetylcholinesterase, and its effects are markedly enhanced by prior administration of anticholinesterases.

Uses and Administration
Methacholine is a quaternary ammonium parasympathomimetic with the muscarinic actions of acetylcholine (p.1415). It is hydrolysed by acetylcholinesterase at a considerably slower rate than acetylcholine and is more resistant to hydrolysis by non-specific cholinesterases so that its actions are more prolonged.
Inhalation of nebulised solutions of methacholine chloride are used to provoke bronchoconstriction in the diagnosis of bronchial airway hypersensitivity (but see Precautions, above).
Methacholine chloride has been used in eye drops as a miotic.

Preparations
Proprietary Preparations (details are given in Part 3)
Canad.: Provocholine; *USA:* Mecholyl; Provocholine.
Multi-ingredient: *Braz.:* Frixodon; Pomalgex; Rubi-Dex.

Milameline (3156-l)

Milameline *(rINN)*.

CI-979 (milameline hydrochloride); Milamelina; Milaméline; RU-35926 (milameline hydrochloride). 1,2,5,6-Tetrahydro-1-methylnicotinaldehyde (E)-O-methyloxime.

$C_8H_{14}N_2O = 154.2$.

CAS — 139886-32-1 (milameline); 139886-04-7 (milameline hydrochloride).

NOTE. Milameline Hydrochloride is *USAN*.

Profile
Milameline is reported to be a selective muscarinic M_1 agonist; it has been investigated for the management of Alzheimer's disease but drugs of this type have not generally produced benefit.

Neostigmine (15576-a)

Neostigmine *(BAN)*.

3-(Dimethylcarbamoyloxy)trimethylanilinium ion.

$C_{12}H_{19}N_2O_2 = 223.3$.

CAS — 59-99-4.

ATC — N07AA01; S01EB06.

Neostigmine Bromide (4501-r)

Neostigmine Bromide *(BANM, pINN)*.

Neostig. Brom.; Neostigmini Bromidum; Neostigminii Bromidum; Neostigminum Bromatum; Synstigminium Bromatum.

$C_{12}H_{19}BrN_2O_2 = 303.2$.

CAS — 114-80-7.

Pharmacopoeias. In *Chin., Eur.* (see p.vi), *Int.,* and *US.*

Pharmacopoeial description

Ph. Eur.: Hygroscopic, colourless crystals or a white crystal-line powder. Very soluble in water; freely soluble in alcohol. Protect from light.

USP 25: Store in airtight containers.

Stability. References.
1. Porst H, Kny L. Kinetics of the degradation of neostigmine bromide in aqueous solution. *Pharmazie* 1985; **40:** 713–17.

Neostigmine Metilsulfate (4502-f)

Neostig. Methylsulph.; Neostigmine Methylsulfate; Neostigmine Methylsulphate *(BANM)*; Neostigmini Metilsulfas; Proserinum.

$C_{13}H_{22}N_2O_6S = 334.4.$
CAS — 51-60-5.
Pharmacopoeias. In *Chin., Eur.* (see p.vi), *Int., Jpn, Pol.,* and *US.*

Pharmacopoeial description

Ph. Eur.: Hygroscopic, colourless crystals or a white crystal-line powder. Very soluble in water; freely soluble in alcohol; practically insoluble in ether. Store in airtight containers. Protect from light.

USP 25: Store in airtight containers.

Adverse Effects

The side-effects of neostigmine are chiefly due to excessive cholinergic stimulation and most commonly include increased salivation, nausea and vomiting, abdominal cramps, and diarrhoea. Allergic reactions have been reported; rashes have been associated with the use of the bromide salt. Neostigmine penetrates the blood-brain barrier poorly and CNS effects are usually only seen with high doses.

Overdosage may lead to a 'cholinergic crisis', characterised by both muscarinic and nicotinic effects. These effects may include excessive sweating, lachrymation, increased peristalsis, involuntary defaecation and urination or desire to urinate, miosis, ciliary spasm, nystagmus, bradycardia and other arrhythmias, hypotension, muscle cramps, fasciculations, weakness and paralysis, tight chest, wheezing, and increased bronchial secretion combined with bronchoconstriction. CNS effects include ataxia, convulsions, coma, slurred speech, restlessness, agitation, and fear. Death may result from respiratory failure, due to a combination of the muscarinic, nicotinic and central effects, or cardiac arrest.

It has been reported that a paradoxical increase in blood pressure and heart rate may result from nicotinic stimulation of sympathetic ganglia, especially where atropine has been given to reverse the muscarinic effects (see under Treatment of Adverse Effects, below).

In patients with myasthenia gravis, in whom other symptoms of overdosage may be mild or absent, the major symptom of cholinergic crisis is increased muscular weakness, which must be differentiated from the muscular weakness caused by an exacerbation of the disease itself (myasthenic crisis).

The adverse effects of parasympathomimetics applied topically for their miotic action are discussed under Pilocarpine on p.1422.

Treatment of Adverse Effects

If neostigmine has been taken by mouth the stomach should be emptied by lavage. When necessary maintenance of respiration should take priority. Atropine sulfate should be given in usual doses of 1 to 2 mg, preferably intravenously, or else intramuscularly and repeated as necessary to control the muscarinic effects; some authorities suggest doses of up to 4 mg. Nicotinic effects, including muscle weakness and paralysis, are not antagonised by atropine; the use of small doses of a competitive neuromuscular blocker has been suggested for the control of muscle twitching. Use of the cholinesterase reactivator pralidoxime as an adjunct to atropine has also been suggested (see p.1020). Further supportive treatment should be given as required.

Precautions

Neostigmine is contra-indicated in patients with mechanical intestinal or urinary-tract obstruction, or peritonitis. It should be used with extreme caution in patients who have undergone recent intestinal or bladder surgery and in patients with bronchial asthma. It should be used with caution in patients with cardiovascular disorders including arrhythmias, bradycardia, recent myocardial infarction, and hypotension, as well as in patients with vagotonia, epilepsy, hyperthyroidism, parkinsonism, renal impairment, or peptic ulcer disease. When neostigmine is given by injection, atropine should always be available to counteract any excessive muscarinic reactions; atropine may also be given before, or with, neostigmine to prevent or minimise muscarinic side-effects but this may mask the initial symptoms of overdosage and lead to cholinergic crisis.

The UK manufacturer has advised that as the severity of myasthenia gravis often fluctuates considerably during pregnancy, particular care is needed to avoid cholinergic crisis caused by overdosage; it has also been reported that neonatal myasthenia may follow administration of large doses during pregnancy. The amount of neostigmine distributed into breast milk is very small but breast-fed infants need to be monitored.

Large doses of neostigmine by mouth should be avoided in conditions where there may be increased absorption from the gastrointestinal tract. It should be avoided in patients known to be hypersensitive to neostigmine; the bromide ion from neostigmine bromide may contribute to the allergic reaction.

The precautions of parasympathomimetics applied topically for their miotic action are discussed under Pilocarpine on p.1422.

Neuromuscular disorders. Treatment of residual non-depolarising neuromuscular block by administration of neostigmine in association with atropine to a patient with dystrophia myotonica was only partly effective, and following a second dose of both drugs complete neuromuscular block developed.[1] In a second patient, with a history of progressive muscle dystrophy, the administration of neostigmine to reverse residual non-depolarising blockade gave rise to a tonic response in the indirectly stimulated muscle. The type and degree of the response to neostigmine, and probably other anticholinesterases, cannot be predicted in patients with neuromuscular disease.

A patient with sero-negative ocular myasthenia gravis had exaggerated responses to both vecuronium and neostigmine.[2] The dose of neuromuscular blockers and their antagonists used in patients with myasthenia gravis should be titrated carefully regardless of the severity of the condition.

1. Buzello W, *et al.* Hazards of neostigmine in patients with neuromuscular disorders: report of two cases. *Br J Anaesth* 1982; **54:** 529–34.
2. Kim J-M, Mangold J. Sensitivity to both vecuronium and neostigmine in a sero-negative myasthenic patient. *Br J Anaesth* 1989; **63:** 497–500.

Renal impairment. The dosage of neostigmine may need to be adjusted in patients with renal impairment. One group of workers found[1] that a mean serum elimination half-life of 79.8 minutes obtained in patients with normal renal function was prolonged to 181.1 minutes in anephric patients.

1. Cronnelly R, *et al.* Renal function and the pharmacokinetics of neostigmine in anesthetized man. *Anesthesiology* 1979; **51:** 222–6.

Interactions

Drugs that possess neuromuscular blocking activity, such as the aminoglycosides, clindamycin, colistin, cyclopropane, and the halogenated inhalational anaesthetics, may antagonise the effects of neostigmine. A number of drugs, including quinine, chloroquine, hydroxychloroquine, quinidine, procainamide, propafenone, lithium, and the beta blockers, that have the potential to aggravate myasthenia gravis may reduce the effectiveness of treatment with parasympathomimetics. Prolonged bradycardia has also occurred in patients receiving beta blockers following administration of neostigmine. Anticholinesterases, such as neostigmine, can inhibit the metabolism of suxamethonium and enhance and prolong its action.

Concomitant ophthalmic use of anticholinesterases, such as ecothiopate, should be undertaken with care in patients receiving neostigmine systemically for myasthenia gravis, because of possible additive toxicity.

Antimuscarinics such as atropine antagonise the muscarinic effects of neostigmine.

Beta blockers. There have been several reports of bradycardia and hypotension following administration of neostigmine or physostigmine to patients receiving beta blockers[1-4] but no significant changes in heart rate were noted in a study of pyridostigmine given to 8 patients taking beta blockers.[5] Beta blockers have the potential to aggravate the symptoms of myasthenia gravis and may therefore reduce the effectiveness of parasympathomimetic treatment.

1. Sprague DH. Severe bradycardia after neostigmine in a patient taking propranolol to control paroxysmal atrial tachycardia. *Anesthesiology* 1975; **42:** 208–10.
2. Seidl DC, Martin DE. Prolonged bradycardia after neostigmine administration in a patient taking nadolol. *Anesth Analg* 1984; **63:** 365–7.
3. Baraka A, Dajani A. Severe bradycardia following physostigmine in the presence of beta-adrenergic blockade: a case report. *Middle East J Anesthesiol* 1984; **7:** 291–3.
4. Eldor J, *et al.* Prolonged bradycardia and hypotension after neostigmine administration in a patient receiving atenolol. *Anaesthesia* 1987; **42:** 1294–7.
5. Arad M, *et al.* Safety of pyridostigmine in hypertensive patients receiving beta blockers. *Am J Cardiol* 1992; **69:** 518–22.

Calcium-channel blockers. Concomitant use of calcium-channel blockers such as verapamil and neuromuscular blockers may produce an enhanced muscle block which is resistant to reversal with neostigmine[1] but which may be reversed by edrophonium.[2]

1. van Poorten JF, *et al.* Verapamil and reversal of vecuronium neuromuscular blockade. *Anesth Analg* 1984; **63:** 155–7.
2. Jones RM, *et al.* Verapamil potentiation of neuromuscular blockade: failure of reversal with neostigmine but prompt reversal with edrophonium. *Anesth Analg* 1985; **64:** 1021–5.

Corticosteroids. Although use of glucocorticoids alone may improve strength in myasthenic patients, administration of methylprednisolone to patients receiving neostigmine or pyridostigmine has exacerbated symptoms and produced profound weakness often necessitating assisted ventilation.[1] Since the adverse effects of concomitant therapy usually occur before any expected benefits it has been suggested that the glucocorticoid should be given on alternate days in small doses which are increased gradually until the optimal effect is achieved.[2]

1. Brunner NG, *et al.* Corticosteroids in management of severe, generalized myasthenia gravis: effectiveness and comparison with corticotrophin therapy. *Neurology* 1972; **22:** 603–10.
2. Jubiz W, Meikle AW. Alterations of glucocorticoid actions by other drugs and disease states. *Drugs* 1979; **18:** 113–21.

Pharmacokinetics

Neostigmine is a quaternary ammonium compound and as the bromide is poorly absorbed from the gastrointestinal tract. Following parenteral administration as the metilsulfate, neostigmine is rapidly eliminated and is excreted in the urine both as unchanged drug and metabolites. Neostigmine undergoes hydrolysis by cholinesterases and is also metabolised in the liver. Protein binding to human serum albumin is reported to range from 15 to 25%. Penetration into the CNS is poor. Neostigmine crosses the placenta and very small amounts are distributed into breast milk.

◊ Neostigmine appears to be poorly and variably absorbed when administered by mouth. In 3 myasthenic patients peak plasma concentrations were obtained 1 to 2 hours after a single 30-mg dose by mouth and the mean plasma half-life was 0.87 hours; bioavailability was estimated to be 1 to 2%.[1] Mean plasma half-lives of 0.89 and 1.20 hours have been obtained following intravenous[1] and intramuscular[2] injections of neostigmine metilsulfate respectively, although again only a few patients were studied. Metabolism and biliary excretion may play significant roles in the elimination of neostigmine.[2] About 80% of a dose may be excreted in the urine within 24 hours: about 50% of a dose as unchanged drug and 15% as 3-hydroxyphenyltrimethylammonium.[2] Mean plasma elimination half-lives for neostigmine have been found to be shorter in infants (0.65 hours) and children (0.80 hours) compared with adults (1.12 hours) but this does not appear to be related to its duration of effect in antagonising neuromuscular blockade.[3] For the half-life in anephric patients, see Renal Impairment, above.

1. Aquilonius S-M, *et al.* A pharmacokinetic study of neostigmine in man using gas chromatography–mass spectrometry. *Eur J Clin Pharmacol* 1979; **15:** 367–71.
2. Somani SM, *et al.* Kinetics and metabolism of intramuscular neostigmine in myasthenia gravis. *Clin Pharmacol Ther* 1980; **28:** 64–8.
3. Fisher DM, *et al.* The neuromuscular pharmacology of neostigmine in infants and children. *Anesthesiology* 1983; **59:** 220–5.

Uses and Administration

Neostigmine is a quaternary ammonium compound which inhibits cholinesterase activity and thus prolongs and intensifies the physiological actions of acetylcholine (p.1415). It probably also has direct effects on skeletal muscle fibres. The anticholinesterase actions of neostigmine are reversible.

Neostigmine is used in the treatment of myasthenia gravis, and has been used as an alternative to edrophonium in the diagnosis of myasthenia gravis (p.1414). It is used in anaesthesia to reverse the neuromuscular blockade produced by competitive neuromuscular blockers (see below). It is also used in the management of paralytic ileus. Neostigmine has been used in the management of postoperative urinary retention (p.459) but has generally been superseded by catheterisation. It is sometimes used to lower intraocular pressure in the management of glaucoma (p.1413) and to reduce rises in intra-ocular pressure associated with ophthalmic surgery, although other parasympathomimetics are usually used when such miotics are required.

Neostigmine is given as the bromide and as the metilsulfate. Neostigmine bromide is given by mouth and has been used topically as eye drops; the metilsulfate is administered by intramuscular, intravenous, or subcutaneous injection.

The manufacturers state that 0.5 mg of neostigmine metilsulfate by intravenous injection is approximately equivalent in effect to 1 to 1.5 mg of neostigmine metilsulfate by intramuscular or subcutaneous injection, or 15 mg of neostigmine bromide by mouth.

In the treatment of **myasthenia gravis**, neostigmine is given by mouth as the bromide in a total daily dose usually between 75 and 300 mg, divided throughout the day, and if necessary the night, according to individual response; larger portions of the total dose may be given at times of greater fatigue. The maximum daily dose that most patients can tolerate is 180 mg. A usual total daily dose in children is 15 to 90 mg by mouth. In patients in whom oral therapy is impractical neostigmine metilsulfate may be given in doses of 0.5 to 2.5 mg by intramuscular or subcutaneous injection at intervals, giving a total daily dose usually in the range 5 to 20 mg. Single doses in children have ranged from 200 to 500 µg.

In the treatment of neonatal myasthenia gravis doses in the range 50 to 250 µg of the metilsulfate by intramuscular or subcutaneous injection, or 1 to 5 mg of the bromide by mouth, have been given usually every 4 hours; treatment is rarely needed beyond 8 weeks of age.

To **reverse neuromuscular blockade** produced by competitive neuromuscular blockers, the usual adult dose used in the UK is 50 to 70 µg per kg bodyweight given by intravenous injection over a period of 60 seconds; in the USA lower doses of 0.5 to 2 mg are used. Additional neostigmine may be given until the muscle power is normal but a total of 5 mg should not be exceeded. The patient should be well ventilated until complete recovery of normal respiration is assured. To counteract any muscarinic effects 0.6 to 1.2 mg of atropine sulfate is administered by intravenous injection with or before the dose of neostigmine; it has been suggested that in the presence of bradycardia atropine sulfate should be administered several minutes before neostigmine. Glycopyrronium bromide has been used as an alternative to atropine sulfate.

In the treatment of paralytic **ileus** and postoperative **urinary retention**, doses of 15 to 30 mg of the bromide by mouth, or more usually 0.5 mg of the metilsulfate by subcutaneous or intramuscular injection, have been used.

Decreased gastrointestinal motility. Parasympathomimetics enhance gastric contractions and increase intestinal motility and have been used in a variety of conditions associated with decreased gastrointestinal motility (p.1202). Some workers[1,2] have reported good results using intravenous neostigmine in the treatment of acute colonic pseudo-obstruction, a condition that appears to be due to parasympathomimetic dysfunction. These results have been confirmed in a randomised double-blind study.[3] It has therefore been suggested that parasympathomimetics should be tried before colonic decompression or surgery when conservative management has failed or a rapid resolution is required.[3] Neostigmine has also been used in the treatment of severe constipation due to disrupted intestinal motility.[4,5]

1. Hutchinson R, Griffiths C. Acute colonic pseudo-obstruction: a pharmacological approach. *Ann R Coll Surg Engl* 1992; **74:** 364–7.
2. Stephenson BM, *et al.* Parasympathomimetic decompression of acute colonic pseudo-obstruction. *Lancet* 1993; **342:** 1181–2.
3. Ponec RJ, *et al.* Neostigmine for the treatment of acute colonic pseudo-obstruction. *N Engl J Med* 1999; **341:** 137–41.
4. Miller LS. Neostigmine for severe constipation with spinal cord lesions. *Ann Intern Med* 1984; **101:** 279.
5. Thurtle OA, *et al.* Intractable constipation in malignant phaeochromocytoma: combined treatment with adrenergic blockade and cholinergic drugs. *J R Soc Med* 1984; **77:** 327–8.

Growth hormone deficiency. For reference to the potential value of intranasal administration of neostigmine with somatorelin in the treatment of short stature in children, see under Uses and Administration of Pyridostigmine, p.1424.

Reversal of neuromuscular blockade. Anticholinesterases have commonly been used after surgery to antagonise residual neuromuscular block induced by the long-acting competitive neuromuscular blockers. However, since the introduction of intermediate-acting blockers such as atracurium and vecuronium and shorter-acting blockers such as mivacurium there has been continuing debate[1,2] on whether anticholinesterases can be used in reduced doses or even omitted for these blockers. Decreasing the dosage of the anticholinesterase may reduce its adverse effects. Nausea and vomiting may be less common in patients not given neostigmine after the use of a competitive blocker,[3,4] and omission of neostigmine also avoids any adverse effects it may have on gut anastomoses. One commentator[1] considered that the wide variation in recovery time with aminosteroid blockers such as rocuronium was an indication for always using at least a small dose of anticholinesterase when these drugs were used. However, it was suggested that, if the block was being carefully monitored and recovery was established, a reduced dose of 1.25 mg of neostigmine might be preferable during use of a benzylisoquinolinium blocker such as atracurium or mivacurium. In children, smaller doses of an anticholinesterase could be used, even after an aminosteroid blocker, and after a blocker such as mivacurium, they might not be needed at all.

It has been suggested that because of its shorter duration of action edrophonium might be more suitable than neostigmine to antagonise residual block for neuromuscular blockers with shorter actions and in particular, that edrophonium might be more appropriate than neostigmine for use with mivacurium. Neostigmine inhibits plasma cholinesterase responsible for the metabolism of mivacurium and its use can in theory delay rather than speed recovery, although in practice there is considered to be little evidence for such an effect.[1] Edrophonium also has lesser effects on the vagus, a more rapid onset of action, and may be associated with a lower incidence of nausea and vomiting than neostigmine.[5] Neostigmine can cause clinically significant neuromuscular blockade if it is given to a patient who has already recovered a large degree of neuromuscular function[6,7] but edrophonium appears not to re-induce blockade on repeat administration.[8] However, the antagonism produced by edrophonium is not adequately and reliably sustained especially following profound block.[9,10]

1. Hunter JM. Is it always necessary to antagonize residual neuromuscular block? Do children differ from adults? *Br J Anaesth* 1996; **77:** 707–9.
2. Fawcett WJ. Neuromuscular block in children. *Br J Anaesth* 1997; **78:** 627.
3. King MJ, *et al.* Influence of neostigmine on postoperative vomiting. *Br J Anaesth* 1988; **61:** 403–6.
4. Ding Y, *et al.* Use of mivacurium during laparoscopic surgery: effect of reversal drugs on postoperative recovery. *Anesth Analg* 1994; **78:** 450–4.
5. Watcha MF, *et al.* Effect of antagonism of mivacurium-induced neuromuscular block on postoperative emesis in children. *Anesth Analg* 1995; **80:** 713–17.
6. Hughes R, *et al.* Neuromuscular blockade by neostigmine. *Br J Anaesth* 1979; **51:** 568P.
7. Payne JP, *et al.* Neuromuscular blockade by neostigmine in anaesthetized man. *Br J Anaesth* 1980; **52:** 69–75.
8. Astley BA, *et al.* Electrical and mechanical responses after neuromuscular blockade with vecuronium, and subsequent antagonism with neostigmine or edrophonium. *Br J Anaesth* 1987; **59:** 983–8.
9. Caldwell JE, *et al.* Antagonism of profound neuromuscular blockade induced by vecuronium or atracurium: comparison of neostigmine with edrophonium. *Br J Anaesth* 1986; **58:** 1285–9.
10. Mirakhur RK, *et al.* Antagonism of vecuronium-induced neuromuscular blockade with edrophonium or neostigmine. *Br J Anaesth* 1987; **59:** 473–7.

Snake bite. The general management of snake bites is discussed on p.1564. Numerous reports from India have claimed benefit for anticholinesterases in the treatment of neurotoxic envenoming from snake bites but failure to distinguish between cobra and krait bites, lack of controls, and inadequate information about other therapy vitiate the claims.[1] However, edrophonium has been shown in 2 double-blind studies to be more effective than placebo[2] and antivenom[3] in the treatment of snake bite due to the Philippine cobra (*Naja naja philippinensis*). Neostigmine has also been reported[4] to have been effective in reversing paralysis in 2 patients bitten by *Micrurus frontalis* (a coral snake). Anticholinesterases would be expected to be of little value for bites from snakes whose venom contains neurotoxins which act presynaptically, including the Asian krait, the Australian tiger snake, and the taipan[5] and, although beneficial results have been reported in individual patients,[6] overall results are considered to be inconsistent.[2,7] However, it is recommended that a test dose of edrophonium preceded by atropine should be given to patients with neurological signs following a snake bite by any species and if improvement occurs, a longer acting anticholinesterase such as neostigmine can be administered.[2,3]

1. Reid HA. Venoms and antivenoms. *Trop Dis Bull* 1983; **80:** 23.
2. Watt G, *et al.* Positive response to edrophonium in patients with neurotoxic envenoming by cobras (Naja naja philippinensis). *N Engl J Med* 1986; **315:** 1444–8.
3. Watt G, *et al.* Comparison of Tensilon® and antivenom for the treatment of cobra-bite paralysis. *Trans R Soc Trop Med Hyg* 1989; **83:** 570–3.
4. Vital Brazil O, Vieira RJ. Neostigmine in the treatment of snake accidents caused by Micrurus frontalis: report of two cases. *Rev Inst Med Trop S Paulo* 1996; **38:** 61–7.
5. Brophy T, Sutherland SK. Use of neostigmine after snake bite. *Br J Anaesth* 1979; **51:** 264–5.
6. Warrell DA, *et al.* Severe neurotoxic envenoming by the Malayan krait Bungarus candidus (Linnaeus): response to antivenom and anticholinesterase. *BMJ* 1983; **286:** 678–80.
7. Trevett AJ, *et al.* Failure of 3,4-diaminopyridine and edrophonium to produce significant clinical benefit in neurotoxicity following the bite of Papuan taipan (Oxyuranus scutellatus carini). *Trans R Soc Trop Med Hyg* 1995; **89:** 444–6.

Tetrodotoxin poisoning. For reference to the use of neostigmine in the treatment of tetrodotoxin poisoning caused by eating puffer fish, see under Uses and Administration of Edrophonium Chloride, p.1418.

Preparations

BP 2001: Neostigmine Injection; Neostigmine Tablets;
USP 25: Neostigmine Bromide Tablets; Neostigmine Methylsulfate Injection.

Proprietary Preparations (details are given in Part 3) *Aust.:* Normastigmin; Prostigmin; *Austral.:* Prostigmin; *Belg.:* Prostigmine; Robinul-Neostigmine; *Braz.:* Prostigmin; *Canad.:* Prostigmin; *Denm.:* Robinul-Neostigmin; *Fin.:* Glycostigmin; Robinul-Neostigmin; *Fr.:* Prostigmine; *Ger.:* Neostig-Reu; *Hong Kong:* Prostigmin; *Irl.:* Prostigmin†; Robinul-Neostigmine; *Israel:* Prostigmine; *Ital.:* Intrastigmina; Prostigmina; *Mex.:* Prostigmine; *Neth.:* Prostigmin†; *Norw.:* Prostigmin†; Robinul-Neostigmin; *Port.:* Prostigmine; *Spain:* Prostigmine; *Swed.:* Robinul-Neostigmin; *Switz.:* Prostigmine; Robinul-Neostigmine; *Thai.:* Prostigmin; *UK:* Robinul-Neostigmine; *USA:* Neostigmine Min-I-Mix; Prostigmin.

Multi-ingredient: *Aust.:* Normastigmin mit Pilocarpin; Pilostigmin Puroptal; *Ger.:* Syncarpin.

Paraoxon (14240-s)

E-600. Diethyl *p*-nitrophenyl phosphate.
$C_{10}H_{14}NO_6P = 275.2$.
CAS — 311-45-5.
ATC — S01EB10.

Profile
Paraoxon is a potent inhibitor of cholinesterase activity which has been used with other miotics in the treatment of glaucoma. It is the active metabolite of the organophosphorus insecticide parathion (p.1435) and therefore produces similar toxicity but with a faster onset.

Preparations
Proprietary Preparations (details are given in Part 3)
Multi-ingredient: *Ital.:* Mios.

Physostigmine (4521-h)

Physostigmine (BAN).
Eserine. (3aS,8aR)-1,2,3,3a,8,8a-Hexahydro-1,3a,8-trimethylpyrrolo[2,3-b]indol-5-yl methylcarbamate.
$C_{15}H_{21}N_3O_2 = 275.3$.
CAS — 57-47-6.
ATC — S01EB05; V03AB19.
Pharmacopoeias. In US.

An alkaloid obtained from the calabar bean (ordeal bean; chopnut), the seed of *Physostigma venenosum* (Leguminosae).

Pharmacopoeial description
USP 25: An alkaloid usually obtained from the dried ripe seed of *Physostigma venenosum* (Leguminosae). It is a white, odourless, microcrystalline powder which acquires a red tint on exposure to heat, light, air, or contact with traces of metals. M.p. not lower than 103°. Slightly soluble in water; freely soluble in alcohol; very soluble in chloroform and in dichloromethane; soluble in fixed oils and in benzene. Store in airtight containers. Protect from light.

Physostigmine Salicylate (4523-b)

Physostigmine Salicylate (BANM).
Eserine Salicylate; Eserini Salicylas; Physostig. Sal.; Physostigmine Monosalicylate; Physostigmini Salicylas.
$C_{15}H_{21}N_3O_2,C_7H_6O_3 = 413.5$.
CAS — 57-64-7.
Pharmacopoeias. In Eur. (see p.vi), Int., Pol., and US.

Solutions for injection should not be used if more than slightly discoloured.

Pharmacopoeial description
Ph. Eur.: Colourless or almost colourless crystals. It becomes red on exposure to air and light; the colour develops more quickly in the presence of moisture. Sparingly soluble in water; soluble in alcohol; very slightly soluble in ether. A 0.9% solution in water has a pH of 5.1 to 5.9. Store in airtight containers. Protect from light. Aqueous solutions are unstable.

USP 25: White, shining, odourless, crystals or white powder. It acquires a red tint on exposure to heat, light, air, or contact with traces of metals for long periods. Soluble 1 in 75 of water, 1 in 16 of alcohol, 1 in 6 of chloroform, and 1 in 250 of ether. Store in airtight containers. Protect from light.

Physostigmine Sulfate (4524-v)

Eserine Sulphate; Eserini Sulfas; Physostig. Sulph.; Physostigmine Sulphate (BANM); Physostigmini Sulfas.
$(C_{15}H_{21}N_3O_2)_2,H_2SO_4 = 648.8.$
CAS — 64-47-1.
Pharmacopoeias. In *Eur.* (see p.vi) and *US.*

Pharmacopoeial description

Ph. Eur.: A white or almost white, hygroscopic crystalline powder. It becomes red on exposure to air and light; the colour develops more quickly in the presence of moisture. Very soluble in water; freely soluble in alcohol; practically insoluble in ether. A 1% solution in water has a pH of 3.5 to 5.5. Store in well-filled airtight glass containers. Protect from light. Aqueous solutions are unstable.

USP 25: A white, odourless, microcrystalline powder. It is deliquescent in moist air, and acquires a red tint on exposure to heat, light, air, and on contact with traces of metals for long periods. Soluble 1 in 4 of water, 1 in 0.4 of alcohol, and 1 in 1200 of ether. Store in airtight containers. Protect from light.

Adverse Effects, Treatment, and Precautions

Systemic effects as for Neostigmine, p.1420. For adverse effects and precautions for topical miotics see also under Pilocarpine, p.1422.

Systemic toxic effects of physostigmine are usually more severe than those occurring with neostigmine. Physostigmine crosses the blood-brain barrier and may therefore produce CNS effects. Physostigmine is not well tolerated when used in the eyes for long periods and may produce follicles in the conjunctiva; hypersensitivity reactions are also common. Prolonged use of ophthalmic ointments containing physostigmine may cause depigmentation of the lid margins in dark-skinned patients.

Overdosage. The use of atropine in the management of a patient who had taken 1 g of physostigmine had to be abandoned after it produced tachycardia and multifocal ventricular ectopic beats.[1] However, in a similar case of severe poisoning a slow intravenous injection of propranolol 5 mg reduced the high pulse rate and controlled pulse irregularities despite frequent intravenous administration of atropine.[2]

1. Cumming G, *et al.* Treatment and recovery after massive overdosage of physostigmine. *Lancet* 1968; ii: 147–9.
2. Valero A. Treatment of severe physostigmine poisoning. *Lancet* 1968; ii: 459–60.

Interactions

As for Neostigmine, p.1420.

Pharmacokinetics

Physostigmine is readily absorbed from the gastrointestinal tract, subcutaneous tissues, and mucous membranes. It is largely destroyed in the body by hydrolysis of the ester linkage by cholinesterases; a 1-mg dose injected subcutaneously has been claimed to be destroyed in 2 hours. It crosses the blood-brain barrier. Little is excreted in the urine.

◊ From studies in 5 subjects there appear to be marked interindividual differences in the absorption and metabolism of physostigmine salicylate after administration of doses of up to 4 mg by mouth and it has been suggested that physostigmine may undergo a saturable presystemic metabolism.[1-3] Oral bioavailability has ranged from 5.2 to 11.7% in 3 of the subjects.[3]

In a study[4] of a single application of a physostigmine (base) transdermal system in 6 subjects, the mean absolute bioavailability was 36% (range 12.6 to 53.2%); the interindividual variability in absolute bioavailability was decreased by about 30% in comparison with administration of an oral solution of physostigmine salicylate. There was continued absorption of physostigmine following removal of the transdermal system, indicating a drug reservoir in the skin.

In a study[5] of 9 patients with Alzheimer's disease, a mean elimination half-life for physostigmine of 16.4 minutes was reported following intravenous administration of physostigmine salicylate. Cholinesterase inhibition was more prolonged than that suggested by its elimination half-life.

1. Gibson M, *et al.* Physostigmine concentrations after oral doses. *Lancet* 1985; i: 695–6.
2. Sharpless NS, Thal LJ. Plasma physostigmine concentrations after oral administration. *Lancet* 1985; i: 1397–8.
3. Whelpton R, Hurst P. Bioavailability of oral physostigmine. *N Engl J Med* 1985; 313: 1293–4.
4. Walker K, *et al.* Pharmacokinetics of physostigmine in man following a single application of a transdermal system. *Br J Clin Pharmacol* 1995; 39: 59–63.
5. Asthana S, *et al.* Clinical pharmacokinetics of physostigmine in patients with Alzheimer's disease. *Clin Pharmacol Ther* 1995; 58: 299–309.

Uses and Administration

Physostigmine is a reversible tertiary amine inhibitor of cholinesterase activity with actions similar to those of neostigmine (p.1420). Physostigmine has been used, alone or more usually in combination with other miotics such as pilocarpine, to decrease intra-ocular pressure in glaucoma (p.1413). It is a more potent miotic than pilocarpine but is rarely tolerated for prolonged periods. When it is used in glaucoma physostigmine has usually been administered as eye drops containing 0.25 or

0.5% of the salicylate or as an ophthalmic ointment containing 0.25% of the sulfate.

Physostigmine crosses the blood-brain barrier and has been used to reverse the central as well as the peripheral effects of agents with antimuscarinic actions following overdosage but such treatment is not usually recommended. Physostigmine is also under investigation in the management of Alzheimer's disease.

Alzheimer's disease. Physostigmine is being studied in the symptomatic management of Alzheimer's disease (see Dementia, p.1412). However, a systematic review concluded that the evidence of its effectiveness was limited and the benefits shown were not convincing.[1] Small early studies with oral physostigmine in Alzheimer's disease were inconclusive; a larger multicentre study[2] using controlled-release physostigmine found that it produced some improvement in cognitive and global function, but gastrointestinal adverse effects were common and led to a high drop-out rate. Transdermal patches[3] have also been studied to overcome the problems associated with physostigmine's short half-life.

1. Coelho Filho JM, Birks J. Physostigmine for Alzheimer's disease (updated 9 May 2001). Available in The Cochrane Library; Issue 4. Oxford: Update Software; 2001.
2. Thal LJ, *et al.* A 24-week randomized trial of controlled-release physostigmine in patients with Alzheimer's disease. *Neurology* 1999; 52: 1146–52.
3. Levy A, *et al.* Transdermal physostigmine in the treatment of Alzheimer's disease. *Alzheimer Dis Assoc Disord* 1994; 8: 15–21.

Antimuscarinic poisoning. As physostigmine penetrates the blood-brain barrier it has been used to reverse the central effects of poisoning with agents that have antimuscarinic actions including tricyclic antidepressants, antihistamines, some antiemetics, some antiparkinsonian drugs, and phenothiazines. However, reviewers agree that in general such a use is inappropriate and hazardous. Physostigmine does not appear to affect the mortality rate in tricyclic antidepressant poisoning[1] and its use can lead to severe cardiac[2,3] and respiratory effects[2,3] and to convulsions.[3,4] In uncomplicated cases of overdosage the safest treatment could be to await the spontaneous remission of toxicity.[2] If used at all, physostigmine should be reserved for treatment of life-threatening symptoms such as uncontrollable convulsions, coma with respiratory depression, or severe hypertension.[5] Physostigmine has a shorter duration of action than most antimuscarinics and a considerably shorter duration of action than most tricyclics, therefore reports of the successful use of physostigmine have highlighted the need for repeated doses or continuous administration over periods of hours or days.[6,7]

1. Aquilonius S-M, Hedstrand U. The use of physostigmine as an antidote in tricyclic anti-depressant intoxication. *Acta Anaesthesiol Scand* 1978; 22: 40–5.
2. Caine ED. Anticholinergic toxicity. *N Engl J Med* 1979; 300: 1278.
3. Newton RW. Physostigmine salicylate in the treatment of tricyclic antidepressant overdosage. *JAMA* 1975; 231: 941–3.
4. Knudsen K, Heath A. Effects of self poisoning with maprotiline. *BMJ* 1984; 288: 601–3.
5. Anonymous. Treatment of acute drug abuse reactions. *Med Lett Drugs Ther* 1987; 29: 83–5.
6. Pall H, *et al.* Experiences with physostigminesalicylate in tricyclic antidepressant poisoning. *Acta Pharmacol Toxicol* 1977; 41 (suppl 2): 117–8.
7. Brier RH. Physostigmine dose for tricyclic drug overdose. *Ann Intern Med* 1978; 89: 579.

Baclofen overdosage. For references to the use of physostigmine in the treatment of baclofen overdosage, see p.1323.

Cerebellar ataxias. Double-blind controlled studies indicate that physostigmine[1,2] can produce symptomatic improvement in some patients with cerebellar ataxia including those with hereditary forms of spinocerebellar degeneration such as Friedreich's ataxia.

1. Rodriguez-Budelli MM, *et al.* Action of physostigmine on inherited ataxias. *Adv Neurol* 1978; 21: 195–202.
2. Aschoff JC, *et al.* Physostigmin in der behandlung von kleinhirnataxien. *Nervenarzt* 1996; 67: 311–18.

Preparations

USP 25: Physostigmine Salicylate Injection; Physostigmine Salicylate Ophthalmic Solution; Physostigmine Sulfate Ophthalmic Ointment.

Proprietary Preparations (details are given in Part 3)
Aust.: Anticholium; *Ger.:* Anticholium; *USA:* Antilirium.

Multi-ingredient: *Belg.:* Miotic Double†; *Braz.:* Enterotonus; *Ger.:* Isopto Pilomin; Pilo-Eserin.

Pilocarpine (4525-g)

Pilocarpine (BAN).
(3S,4R)-3-Ethyldihydro-4-[(1-methyl-1H-imidazol-5-yl)methyl]furan-2(3H)-one.
$C_{11}H_{16}N_2O_2 = 208.3.$
CAS — 92-13-7.
ATC — N07AX01; S01EB01.
Pharmacopoeias. In *US.*

An alkaloid obtained from the leaves of jaborandi, *Pilocarpus microphyllus* (Rutaceae) and other species of *Pilocarpus*.

Pharmacopoeial description

USP 25: A viscous, exceedingly hygroscopic, oily liquid or crystals. M.p. about 34°. Soluble in water, in alcohol, and in chloroform; sparingly soluble in ether and in benzene; practically insoluble in petroleum spirit. Store in airtight containers at a temperature not exceeding 8°. Protect from light.

Pilocarpine Borate (16189-z)

$C_{11}H_{16}N_2O_2,xBH_3O_3.$
CAS — 16509-56-1.

Pilocarpine Hydrochloride (4526-q)

Pilocarpine Hydrochloride (BANM).
Pilocarp. Hydrochlor.; Pilocarpine Monohydrochloride; Pilocarpini Chloridum; Pilocarpini Hydrochloridum; Pilocarpinium Chloratum.
$C_{11}H_{16}N_2O_2,HCl = 244.7.$
CAS — 54-71-7.
NOTE. PIL is a code approved by the BP 2001 for use on single unit doses of eye drops containing pilocarpine hydrochloride where the individual container may be too small to bear all the appropriate labelling information.
Pharmacopoeias. In *Eur.* (see p.vi), *Int., Jpn, Pol.,* and *US.*

Pharmacopoeial description

Ph. Eur.: Hygroscopic, colourless crystals or white or almost white crystalline powder. Very soluble in water and in alcohol. A 5% solution in water has a pH of 3.5 to 4.5. Store in airtight containers. Protect from light.
USP 25: Colourless, translucent, odourless, hygroscopic crystals. Soluble 1 in 0.3 of water, 1 in 3 of alcohol, and 1 in 360 of chloroform; insoluble in ether. Its solutions are acid to litmus. Store in airtight containers. Protect from light.

Stability. Pilocarpine hydrochloride oral solution, prepared from powder or eye drops and buffered at pH 5.5, was found[1] to be stable for 60 days at 25° and for 90 days at 4°.
1. Fawcett JP, *et al.* Formulation and stability of pilocarpine oral solution. *Int J Pharm Pract* 1994; 3: 14–18.

Pilocarpine Nitrate (4527-p)

Pilocarpine Nitrate (BANM).
Pilocarp. Nit.; Pilocarpine Mononitrate; Pilocarpini Nitras; Pilocarpinii Nitras; Pilocarpinium Nitricum.
$C_{11}H_{16}N_2O_2,HNO_3 = 271.3.$
CAS — 148-72-1.
NOTE. PIL is a code approved by the BP 2001 for use on single unit doses of eye drops containing pilocarpine nitrate where the individual container may be too small to bear all the appropriate labelling information.
Pharmacopoeias. In *Chin., Eur.* (see p.vi), *Int.,* and *US.*

Pharmacopoeial description

Ph. Eur.: Colourless crystals, or white or almost white crystalline powder. Freely soluble in water; sparingly soluble in alcohol; practically insoluble in ether. A 5% solution in water has a pH of 3.5 to 4.5. Protect from light.
USP 25: Shining white crystals. Soluble 1 in 4 of water and 1 in 75 of alcohol; insoluble in chloroform and in ether. Its solutions are acid to litmus. Store in airtight containers. Protect from light.

Adverse Effects, Treatment, and Precautions

Systemic effects and cautions are as for Neostigmine, p.1420.

In relation to the *oral* use of pilocarpine as a sialogogue, sweating is noted as a common problem; caution is needed to avoid dehydration in patients who may sweat excessively and who cannot maintain an adequate fluid intake. Paradoxical hypertension and constipation, confusion, and increased urinary frequency are also specifically included among the adverse effects reported. Additionally, contra-indications include pregnancy. The manufacturer recommends that it should not be given when miosis is undesirable such as in patients with acute iritis or angle-closure glaucoma. An eye examination should be carried out before starting treatment. Blurred vision may affect the performance of skilled tasks. In addition pilocarpine should be given with care to those with cognitive or psychiatric disturbances, with renal calculi or renal impairment, or with biliary-tract disorders. Dosage should be reduced in patients with hepatic impairment.

Following *ocular* administration pilocarpine is usually better tolerated than the anticholinesterases, but in common with other miotics may produce ciliary spasm, ocular pain and irritation, blurred vision, lachrymation, myopia, and browache. Conjunctival vascular congestion, superficial keratitis, vitreous haemorrhage, and increased pupillary block have been reported. Lens opacities have occurred following prolonged use. Treatment with miotics should be stopped if symptoms of systemic toxicity develop.

Miotics are contra-indicated in conditions where pupillary constriction is undesirable such as acute iritis, acute uveitis, anterior uveitis, and some forms of secondary glaucoma. They should be avoided in acute inflammatory disease of the anterior segment of the eye. If possible, treatment with long-acting miotics should be discontinued before surgery on the eye as there is an increased risk of hyphaema. Miotics should be used with extreme caution in patients with a history of retinal detachment and in young patients with myopia. Care is also needed in patients with corneal or conjunctival damage. Miosis may cause blurred vision and difficulty with dark adaptation and caution is necessary with night driving or when hazardous tasks are undertaken in poor illumination. Miotics should not be used by patients wearing soft contact lenses.

◊ Systemic adverse effects after the ophthalmic use of pilocarpine are thought to be rare and reports of toxicity appear to involve elderly patients treated for acute angle-closure glaucoma prior to surgery and who received 2 to 5 times the usual daily dose of pilocarpine in a few hours.[1]

1. Everitt DE, Avorn J. Systemic effects of medications used to treat glaucoma. *Ann Intern Med* 1990; **112:** 120–5.

Alzheimer's disease. In patients with dementia of Alzheimer type, CNS symptoms may be induced or exacerbated by the use of pilocarpine eye drops.[1,2]

1. Reyes PF, *et al.* Mental status changes induced by eye drops in dementia of the Alzheimer type. *J Neurol Neurosurg Psychiatry* 1987; **50:** 113–15.
2. Fraunfelder FT, Morgan R. The aggravation of dementia by pilocarpine. *JAMA* 1994; **271:** 1742–3.

Asthma. A reminder that topical miotics can precipitate bronchospasm in susceptible patients.[1] However, the severity of bronchospasm induced by carbachol has been reported to be less than that produced by timolol. Bronchospastic complications are much less likely to occur with pilocarpine but have nevertheless been reported. As inhalations of methacholine are used to induce bronchospasm in the diagnosis of latent asthma, the risk of exacerbating asthma should be considered before methacholine is used in the eye.

1. Prakash UBS, *et al.* Pulmonary complications from ophthalmic preparations. *Mayo Clin Proc* 1990; **65:** 521–9.

Glaucoma. Miotics usually lower intra-ocular pressure by decreasing the resistance to outflow of aqueous humour from the anterior chamber through the trabecular network. However, they appear to reduce uveoscleral outflow and this may cause a paradoxical rise in intra-ocular pressure in patients with severely compromised trabecular outflow as was reported in a patient with post-traumatic angle-recession glaucoma.[1] It has been recommended that the use of pilocarpine should be avoided after drainage operations for glaucoma because its miotic effect can increase the occurrence of posterior pupillary synechiae; a topical beta blocker is usually adequate if control of intra-ocular pressure is required.[2] Pilocarpine-induced miosis was shown to cause a significant deterioration in visual field in patients with chronic open-angle glaucoma in one study.[3] It was suggested that this factor should be an important consideration when choosing therapy for glaucoma, particularly in cases where field loss approaches the permitted legal minimum for driving. Of 53 patients receiving long-term therapy with pilocarpine gel, 15 developed a corneal haze which persisted for at least 2 years in 13; although the patients remained asymptomatic the long-term effects were unknown.[4] Many patients using the gel also developed superficial punctate keratitis which usually cleared spontaneously during treatment.

1. Bleiman BS, Schwartz AL. Paradoxical intraocular pressure response to pilocarpine: a proposed mechanism and treatment. *Arch Ophthalmol* 1979; **97:** 1305–6.
2. Phillips CI, *et al.* Posterior synechiae after glaucoma operations: aggravation by shallow anterior chamber and pilocarpine. *Br J Ophthalmol* 1987; **71:** 428–32.
3. Webster AR, *et al.* The effect of pilocarpine on the glaucomatous visual field. *Br J Ophthalmol* 1993; **77:** 721–5.
4. Johnson DH, *et al.* Corneal changes during pilocarpine gel therapy. *Am J Ophthalmol* 1986; **101:** 13–15.

Hypersensitivity. Contact urticaria involving the eyelids has been reported[1] in a patient following treatment with pilocarpine eye drops for glaucoma.

1. O'Donnell BF, Foulds IS. Contact allergic dermatitis and contact urticaria due to topical ophthalmic preparations. *Br J Ophthalmol* 1993; **77:** 740–1.

Retinal detachment. The use of miotics has been implicated in numerous reports as a cause of retinal detachment but reviews of the subject have concluded that there is little factual evidence to support the association.[1,2] However, there is circumstantial evidence that retinal detachment is more likely to occur with strong miotics. Furthermore, patients with myopia

The symbol † denotes a preparation no longer actively marketed

or pre-existing retinal damage appear to be at greater risk and there is the possibility that even low concentrations of relatively mild miotics such as 1% pilocarpine might precipitate retinal detachment.

1. Alpar JJ. Miotics and retinal detachment: a survey and case report. *Ann Ophthalmol* 1979; **11:** 395–401.
2. Beasley H, Fraunfelder FT. Retinal detachments and topical ocular miotics. *Ophthalmology* 1979; **86:** 95–8.

Interactions
As for Neostigmine, p.1420.

Pharmacokinetics
Mean elimination half-lives for pilocarpine have been reported to be 0.76 and 1.35 hours following oral administration of 5 and 10 mg doses of the hydrochloride respectively. Inactivation of pilocarpine is thought to occur at neuronal synapses and probably in plasma. Pilocarpine and its inactive metabolites, including pilocarpic acid, are excreted in the urine.

Uses and Administration
Pilocarpine is a tertiary amine direct-acting parasympathomimetic with primarily the muscarinic effects of acetylcholine (p.1415). It is used mainly in the treatment of glaucoma and dry mouth, and has also been used as a diaphoretic in diagnostic tests for cystic fibrosis and leprosy. Topical application of pilocarpine to the eye produces miosis (pupil constriction) by contraction of the iris sphincter muscle; contraction of the ciliary muscle results in increased accommodation. Constriction of the pupil also pulls open the trabecular meshwork in the eye and this in turn facilitates drainage of aqueous humour and reduction of intra-ocular pressure. Following the use of eye drops, miosis occurs in about 10 to 30 minutes and lasts 4 to 8 hours while peak reduction in intra-ocular pressure occurs within 75 minutes and the reduction usually persists for 4 to 14 hours.

Pilocarpine is used in the treatment of open-angle **glaucoma** (p.1413 but see also Adverse Effects, above) and is commonly administered with topical beta blockers or sympathomimetic drugs. It is used as the hydrochloride or the nitrate, usually as 0.5 to 4% eye drops administered 4 times daily, the dose being adjusted individually. Solutions containing 0.25 to 10% of the hydrochloride are also available and the higher strengths may sometimes be required in patients with heavily pigmented irides. A modified-release system inserted into the conjunctival sac and releasing 20 or 40 µg of pilocarpine per hour for 7 days and a 4% ophthalmic gel have also been used. Pilocarpine may also be used as part of the emergency treatment of acute attacks of angle-closure glaucoma prior to surgery.

The miotic action of pilocarpine has been used to antagonise the effects of sympathomimetic mydriatics on the eye and in surgical procedures on the eye. Pilocarpine borate has been used similarly in ophthalmology to the hydrochloride and nitrate.

Pilocarpine hydrochloride is used in the treatment of **dry mouth** following radiotherapy for malignant neoplasms of the head and neck. It increases salivary flow only in patients with residual salivary gland function. The initial dose is 5 mg by mouth three times daily with or immediately after meals, increased gradually if necessary after 4 to 8 weeks until an adequate response is obtained, up to a maximum of 10 mg three times daily. Doses of 5 mg by mouth 4 times daily are used to treat dry mouth and eye in patients with Sjögren's syndrome; this dose may be increased to a maximum of 30 mg daily. Treatment should be discontinued if no improvement is obtained after 3 months of use.

Diagnosis and testing. CYSTIC FIBROSIS. The fact that individuals with cystic fibrosis have abnormally high concentrations of sodium and chloride in their sweat has been used in the diagnosis of this condition and pilocarpine iontophoresis has been used to promote sweating as part of that test.[1]

1. Gibson LE, Cooke RE. A test for concentration of electrolytes in sweat in cystic fibrosis of the pancreas utilizing pilocarpine by iontophoresis. *Pediatrics* 1959; **23:** 545–9.

LEPROSY. The induction of sweat secretion by intradermal injection of pilocarpine nitrate has been used to assess the functional status of dermal nerves in patients with leprotic skin lesions.[1]

1. Joshi PB. Pilocarpine test in assesment of therapeutic efficacy in maculoanaesthetic leprosy. *Lepr India* 1976; **48:** 55–60.

Dry mouth. Pilocarpine is used as a sialogogue in the treatment of dry mouth (p.1498) following radiotherapy for head and neck cancer. It is also used as a treatment for dry mouth in the auto-immune disease, Sjögren's syndrome.[1-3]

1. Wiseman LR, Faulds D. Oral pilocarpine: a review of its pharmacological properties and clinical potential in xerostomia. *Drugs* 1995; **49:** 143–55.
2. Nelson JD, *et al.* Oral pilocarpine for symptomatic relief of keratoconjunctivitis sicca in patients with Sjögren's syndrome. *Adv Exp Med Biol* 1998; **438:** 979–83.
3. Vivino FB, *et al.* Pilocarpine tablets for the treatment of dry mouth and dry eye symptoms in patients with Sjögrens syndrome: a randomized, placebo-controlled, fixed-dose, multicenter trial. *Arch Intern Med* 1999; **159:** 174–81.

Reversal of mydriasis. Pilocarpine has been used to reverse the effects of mydriatics following surgery or ophthalmoscopic examination but other miotics may be preferred (see p.1414). It counteracts the mydriatic effects of sympathomimetics, such as phenylephrine and hydroxyamfetamine,[1] but is ineffective against mydriasis produced by antimuscarinics, such as homatropine,[1] and may impair vision further when used with tropicamide.[2] Furthermore, there is also the risk of pilocarpine precipitating angle-closure glaucoma in susceptible patients (see under Glaucoma, above).

1. Anastasi LM, *et al.* Effect of pilocarpine in counteracting mydriasis. *Arch Ophthalmol* 1968; **79:** 710–15.
2. Nelson ME, Orton HP. Counteracting the effects of mydriatics: does it benefit the patient? *Arch Ophthalmol* 1987; **105:** 486–9.

Preparations
BP 2001: Pilocarpine Hydrochloride Eye Drops; Pilocarpine Nitrate Eye Drops;
USP 25: Pilocarpine Hydrochloride Ophthalmic Solution; Pilocarpine Nitrate Ophthalmic Solution; Pilocarpine Ocular System.

Proprietary Preparations (details are given in Part 3)
Aust.: Pilax; Piloftal; Pilogel; Salagen; **Austral.:** Isopto Carpine; Ocusert; Pilopt; PV Carpine; **Belg.:** Isopto Carpine; Pilo; **Braz.:** Isopto Carpine; **Canad.:** Diocarpine; Isopto Carpine; Miocarpine; Pilopine HS; Salagen; **Fin.:** Isopto Carpine; **Fr.:** Chibro-Pilocarpine; Pilo; **Ger.:** Asthenopin†; Borocarpin-S; Pilo-Stulln; Pilocarpol; Pilogel; Pilomann; Pilomann-Ol; Pilopos; Spersacarpin; Vistacarpin†; **Hong Kong:** Isopto Carpine; Spersacarpine; **Irl.:** Isopto Carpine; Pilogel; Salagen; **Israel:** Glaucocarpine; Isopto Carpine; Mi-Pilo; Pilogel; Salagen; **Ital.:** Dropilton; Liocarpina; Pilogel; Pilotonina; Salagen; **Mex.:** Pilo; Pilof Nicolich; **Neth.:** Isopto Carpine†; Pilogel†; Salagen; **Norw.:** Isopto Carpine; Pilo; **NZ:** Isopto Carpine; Ocusert; Pilopt; PV Carpine; **Port.:** Pilocarcil; Piloplex; **S.Afr.:** Isopto Carpine; Pilogel; PV Carpine†; **Singapore:** Pilogel; Spersacarpine; **Spain:** Isopto Carpina; **Swed.:** Licarpin†; Spersacarpine†; **Switz.:** Isopto Carpine†; Pilo; Pilogel HS†; Spersacarpine; **Thai.:** Isopto Carpine; Pilogel; Pilomann; **UK:** Isopto Carpine†; Ocusert†; Pilogel; Salagen; Sno Pilo†; **USA:** Adsorbocarpine; Akarpine; Isopto Carpine; Ocu-Carpine; Ocusert; Pilagan†; Pilocar; Pilopine HS; Piloptic; Pilopto-Carpine; Pilostat; Salagen; Storzine†.

Multi-ingredient: *Aust.:* Betacarpin; Normastigmin mit Pilocarpin; Pilostigmin Puroptal; Thiloadren; Timpilo; **Austral.:** Timpilo; **Belg.:** Carteopil; Miotic Double†; Normoglaucon; **Canad.:** E-Pilo†; Timpilo; **Denm.:** Fotil; Timpilo; **Fin.:** Fotil; Timpilo; **Fr.:** Carpilo; Montavon†; Timpilo; **Ger.:** Fotil; Glauko Biciron; Isopto Pilomin; Normoglaucon; Pilo-Eserin; Syncarpin; Thiloadren N; Timpilo; TP-Ophtal; **Hong Kong:** Timpilo; **Israel:** Timpilo; **Ital.:** Equiton; Mios; Pilobloc; Pilodren; Ripix; Timicon; **Mex.:** Timpilo; **Neth.:** Normoglaucon; Timpilo; **Norw.:** Fotil; Timpilo; **NZ:** Timpilo; **Port.:** Normoglaucon; Timoglau Plus; **Singapore:** Normoglaucon; Timpilo; **Swed.:** Fotil; Timpilo; **Switz.:** Fotil; Ripix; Timpilo; **Thai.:** Fotil; Normoglaucon; **USA:** E-Pilo; PE†.

Pyridostigmine Bromide (4528-s)
Pyridostigmine Bromide (BAN, rINN).
Pyridostig. Brom.; Pyridostigmini Bromidum. 3-Dimethylcarbamoyloxy-1-methylpyridinium bromide.
$C_9H_{13}BrN_2O_2 = 261.1$.
CAS — 155-97-5 (pyridostigmine); 101-26-8 (pyridostigmine bromide).
Pharmacopoeias. In *Chin.*, *Eur.* (see p.vi), *Int.*, *Jpn*, and *US*.

Pharmacopoeial description
Ph. Eur.: A white or almost white deliquescent crystalline powder. Very soluble in water and in alcohol; practically insoluble in ether. Store in airtight containers. Protect from light.
USP 25: A white or practically white, hygroscopic, crystalline powder, having an agreeable characteristic odour. Freely soluble in water, in alcohol, and in chloroform; practically insoluble in ether; slightly soluble in petroleum spirit. Store in airtight containers.

Adverse Effects, Treatment, and Precautions
As for Neostigmine, p.1420. It has been stated that muscarinic adverse effects occur less frequently with pyridostigmine treatment than with neostigmine.

Psychosis. Postoperative psychosis which developed in a patient with myasthenia gravis who received large doses of pyridostigmine bromide has been attributed to bromide intoxication[1] but this diagnosis has been challenged.[2]

1. Rothenberg DM, *et al.* Bromide intoxication secondary to pyridostigmine bromide therapy. *JAMA* 1990; **263:** 1121–2.
2. Senecal P-E, Osterloh J. Confusion from pyridostigmine bromide: was there bromide intoxication? *JAMA* 1990; **264:** 454–5.

Renal impairment. In patients receiving pyridostigmine for the reversal of non-depolarising muscular blockade following anaesthesia, pyridostigmine kinetics were not significantly different in 5 following renal transplantation from those in 5 with normal renal function. However, in 4 anephric patients the elimination half-life was significantly increased and the plasma clearance significantly decreased.[1] It appeared that approximately 75% of the plasma clearance of pyridostigmine depended on renal function.

1. Cronnelly R, *et al.* Pyridostigmine kinetics with and without renal function. *Clin Pharmacol Ther* 1980; **28:** 78–81.

Interactions
As for Neostigmine, p.1420.

Pharmacokinetics
Pyridostigmine bromide is poorly absorbed from the gastrointestinal tract. It undergoes hydrolysis by cholinesterases and is also metabolised in the liver. Pyridostigmine is excreted mainly in the urine as unchanged drug and metabolites. Pyridostigmine crosses the placenta and very small amounts are distributed into breast milk. Penetration into the CNS is poor.

◊ One group of workers[1] suggest that data from previous pharmacokinetic studies of pyridostigmine may be at variance due to the analytical methods used or inappropriate storage conditions of plasma samples and recommended that samples should be acidified and stored at −75°. They measured a mean terminal elimination half-life of 200 minutes in 11 healthy subjects given 60 mg of pyridostigmine by mouth; maximum plasma concentrations were obtained 1 to 5 hours after dosing. The mean terminal elimination half-life following a 4-mg intravenous infusion in 10 of these subjects was 97 minutes. Oral bioavailability was calculated to vary from 11.5 to 18.9%. In an earlier study administration of food did not appear to affect bioavailability but did delay the time taken to achieve peak plasma concentrations.[2] It appears that 75% of the plasma clearance of pyridostigmine depends on renal function.[3] 3-Hydroxy-*N*-methylpyridinium has been identified as one of the 3 metabolites isolated from the urine of patients taking pyridostigmine.[4]

1. Breyer-Pfaff U, *et al.* Pyridostigmine kinetics in healthy subjects and patients with myasthenia gravis. *Clin Pharmacol Ther* 1985; **37:** 495–501.
2. Aquilonius S-M, *et al.* Pharmacokinetics and oral bioavailability of pyridostigmine in man. *Eur J Clin Pharmacol* 1980; **18:** 423–8.
3. Cronnelly R, *et al.* Pyridostigmine kinetics with and without renal function. *Clin Pharmacol Ther* 1980; **28:** 78–81.
4. Somani SM, *et al.* Pyridostigmine in man. *Clin Pharmacol Ther* 1972; **13:** 393–9.

Distribution into breast milk. Pyridostigmine was present in breast milk from 2 nursing mothers receiving maintenance therapy for myasthenia gravis in a concentration between 36 and 113% of that in maternal plasma,[1] but in both cases the dose ingested per kg body-weight by the nursing infant was 0.1% or less of that ingested by the mother. Maternal medication with pyridostigmine should be no obstacle to breast feeding, at least with doses in the range of 180 to 300 mg daily.

1. Hardell L-I, *et al.* Pyridostigmine in human breast milk. *Br J Clin Pharmacol* 1982; **14:** 565–7.

Uses and Administration
Pyridostigmine is a quaternary ammonium compound which is a reversible inhibitor of cholinesterase activity with actions similar to those of neostigmine (p.1420), but is slower in onset and of longer duration. It is administered as the bromide.

Pyridostigmine is mainly used in the treatment of myasthenia gravis (p.1414). It has also been used in the treatment of paralytic ileus. Pyridostigmine is sometimes used to reverse the neuromuscular blockade produced by competitive neuromuscular blockers but is generally considered less satisfactory than neostigmine. Pyridostigmine has been used in the management of postoperative urinary retention (p.459) but has generally been superseded by catheterisation.

In **myasthenia gravis**, total daily doses may range from 0.3 to 1.2 g by mouth; some authorities advise that the daily dose should not exceed 720 mg. The dose should be divided throughout the day and, if necessary, the night according to the response of the patient; larger portions of the total daily dose may be given at times of greater fatigue. A suggested dose for children is 7 mg per kg body-weight daily in 5 or 6 divided doses. An alternative regimen is an initial

dose of 30 mg for children under 6 years or 60 mg for those aged 6 to 12 years. This is increased gradually by increments of 15 to 30 mg daily until a satisfactory response is obtained, which is usually within the dosage range of 30 to 360 mg daily. It has been given as modified-release tablets, usually once or twice daily but these offer less flexibility of dosage. If necessary it has also been given by intramuscular injection or in severe cases by very slow intravenous injection. However, administration by the intravenous route is hazardous and, if used, atropine must be available to counteract any severe muscarinic reactions.

In the treatment of neonatal myasthenia doses in the range 50 to 150 µg per kg by intramuscular injection or 5 to 10 mg by mouth have been given every 4 to 6 hours; however, neostigmine has generally been preferred. Treatment is rarely needed beyond 8 weeks of age.

To **reverse neuromuscular blockade** produced by competitive neuromuscular blockers, doses of 10 to 20 mg have been given intravenously, preceded by atropine sulfate 0.6 to 1.2 mg to counteract any muscarinic effects. Glycopyrronium bromide has been used as an alternative to atropine.

In the treatment of paralytic **ileus** and postoperative **urinary retention** pyridostigmine bromide has been given by mouth in doses of 60 to 240 mg.

Decreased gastrointestinal motility. Parasympathomimetics such as pyridostigmine enhance gastric contractions and increase intestinal motility and form one of many treatments that have been used in a variety of conditions associated with decreased gastrointestinal motility (p.1202).

Pyridostigmine, generally in doses of 60 mg up to 3 times daily, has been used to relieve severe constipation in patients with impaired intestinal motility due to Parkinson's disease.[1]

1. Sadjadpour K. Pyridostigmine bromide and constipation in Parkinson's disease. *JAMA* 1983; **249:** 1148.

Growth hormone deficiency. The hypothalamic cholinergic system plays an important role in mechanisms for releasing growth hormone.[1] Activation of muscarinic receptors induces growth hormone release probably through inhibition of somatostatin release. Pyridostigmine greatly potentiates rises in growth hormone induced by somatorelin but, unexpectedly, direct muscarinic agonists apparently fail to induce growth hormone release. Studies in children indicate that intravenous administration of somatorelin preceded by pyridostigmine given by mouth is the most powerful single test to differentiate growth hormone deficiency due to pituitary secretory inability from that due to a hypothalamic defect. However, pyridostigmine given alone or with somatorelin does not appear to be useful for the *treatment* of short stature in children, although intranasal administration of neostigmine and somatorelin may be.

The management of growth retardation is discussed on p.1273, and includes a comment that there is some dispute over whether stimulated growth hormone secretion tests are superior to measurements of circulating somatomedins in detecting growth hormone deficiency.

1. Müller EE, *et al.* Involvement of brain catecholamines and acetylcholine in growth hormone deficiency states: pathophysiological, diagnostic and therapeutic implications. *Drugs* 1991; **41:** 161–77.

Nerve gas poisoning. Pyridostigmine has been administered prophylactically to protect soldiers against attack with nerve gas agents (p.1640) which inhibit acetylcholinesterase.[1] Pyridostigmine binds reversibly to acetylcholinesterase and provides a protected store from which acetylcholinesterase is later released.[1,2] Prophylaxis with pyridostigmine greatly enhances the efficacy of treatment with atropine and pralidoxime against exposure to soman but it is not effective alone and may not be uniformly effective against other nerve agents.[1] Administration of 30 mg of pyridostigmine every 8 hours provides the optimum level of protection[2] and, although adverse effects are common at this dosage, the performance of military duties is not impaired.[3] However, neurological symptoms in veterans suffering the so-called Gulf War Syndrome appear to be more common in those who reported exposure to a range of potentially toxic substances which include pyridostigmine.[4] It has been suggested that these symptoms may be evidence of organophosphate-induced polyneuropathy resulting from exposure to a combination of organophosphorus compounds and other cholinesterase inhibitors such as pyridostigmine.[5] A study in *hens*[6] (a species susceptible to anticholinesterases) has also found symptoms of enhanced neurotoxicity when pyridostigmine, the insect repellent diethyltoluamide, and the pyrethroid insecticide permethrin were used together.

1. Dunn MA, Sidell FR. Progress in medical defense against nerve agents. *JAMA* 1989; **262:** 649–52.
2. Ministry of Defence. *Medical manual of defence against chemical agents.* London: HMSO, 1987. (JSP312).
3. Keeler JR, *et al.* Pyridostigmine used as a nerve agent pretreatment under wartime conditions. *JAMA* 1991; **266:** 693–5.

4. The Iowa Persian Gulf Study Group. Self-reported illness and health status among gulf war veterans: a population-based study. *JAMA* 1997; **277:** 238–45.
5. Haley RW, Kurt TL. Self-reported exposure to neurotoxic chemical combinations in the gulf war: a cross-sectional epidemiologic study. *JAMA* 1997; **277:** 231–7.
6. Abou-Donia MB, *et al.* Neurotoxicity resulting from coexposure to pyridostigmine bromide, DEET, and permethrin: implications of gulf war chemical exposure. *J Toxicol Environ Health* 1996; **48:** 35–56.

Post-poliomyelitis syndrome. Pyridostigmine has been reported to be of benefit in reducing fatigue associated with post-poliomyelitis syndrome.[1] A suggested[2] dose is 30 mg daily increased gradually to about 60 mg three times daily but side effects are common.

1. Trojan DA, Cashman NR. Anticholinesterases in post-poliomyelitis syndrome. *Ann N Y Acad Sci* 1995; **753:** 285–95.
2. Thorsteinsson G. Management of postpolio syndrome. *Mayo Clin Proc* 1997; **72:** 627–38.

Preparations
BP 2001: Pyridostigmine Tablets;
USP 25: Pyridostigmine Bromide Injection; Pyridostigmine Bromide Syrup; Pyridostigmine Bromide Tablets.
Proprietary Preparations (details are given in Part 3)
Aust.: Mestinon; **Austral.:** Mestinon; **Belg.:** Mestinon; **Braz.:** Mestinon; **Canad.:** Mestinon; Regonol†; **Denm.:** Mestinon; **Fin.:** Mestinon; **Fr.:** Mestinon; **Ger.:** Kalymin; Mestinon; **Hong Kong:** Mestinon; **Irl.:** Mestinon; **Israel:** Mestinon; **Ital.:** Mestinon; **Mex.:** Mestinon; **Neth.:** Mestinon†; **Norw.:** Mestinon; **NZ:** Mestinon; **Port.:** Mestinon; **S.Afr.:** Mestinon; **Singapore:** Mestinon; **Spain:** Mestinon; **Swed.:** Mestinon; **Switz.:** Mestinon; **Thai.:** Mestinon; **UK:** Mestinon; **USA:** Mestinon; Regonol.

Rivastigmine Hydrogen Tartrate
(20664-k)

Rivastigmine Hydrogen Tartrate (BANM, rINNM).
ENA-713 (rivastigmine or rivastigmine hydrogen tartrate); Rivastigmine Bitartrate; Rivastigmine Tartrate; SDZ-212-713 (rivastigmine); SDZ-ENA-713 (rivastigmine or rivastigmine hydrogen tartrate). (*S*)-*N*-Ethyl-*N*-methyl-3-[1-(dimethylamino)ethyl]-phenyl carbamate hydrogen-(2*R*,3*R*)-tartrate.
$C_{14}H_{22}N_2O_2.C_4H_6O_6 = 400.4$.
CAS — 123441-03-2 (*rivastigmine*).
ATC — N06DA03.
NOTE. Rivastigmine is *USAN*.

Adverse Effects, Treatment, and Precautions
Generally as for Neostigmine, p.1420. Adverse effects with rivastigmine notably include nausea, vomiting, anorexia, dizziness, somnolence, and asthenia. Other common adverse effects include abdominal pain, diarrhoea, dyspepsia, agitation, confusion, depression, headache, insomnia, sweating, tremor, malaise, and upper-respiratory-tract and urinary-tract infections. Rare cases of angina, atrioventricular block, gastrointestinal haemorrhage, and syncope have been observed. There is a potential for bladder outflow obstruction and seizures. Use of rivastigmine has been associated with weight loss and monitoring of patients' weight during treatment is recommended. Female patients have been found to be more susceptible to nausea, vomiting, anorexia, and weight loss.

Interactions
As for Neostigmine, p.1420.

Pharmacokinetics
Rivastigmine is readily absorbed from the gastrointestinal tract and peak plasma concentrations are reached in about one hour. Administration with food delays absorption by about 1.5 hours and reduces maximum plasma concentrations. Rivastigmine is about 40% bound to plasma proteins and readily crosses the blood-brain barrier. It is rapidly and extensively metabolised, primarily by cholinesterase-mediated hydrolysis to the weakly active decarbamylated metabolite. The plasma half-life of rivastigmine is reported to be about one hour and more than 90% of a dose is excreted in the urine within 24 hours. Less than 1% of a dose appears in the faeces.

Uses and Administration
Rivastigmine is a carbamate type reversible acetylcholinesterase inhibitor. It is selective for the CNS and is used for the symptomatic treatment of mild to

moderately severe dementia in Alzheimer's disease (p.1412). It is given as the hydrogen tartrate but doses are expressed in terms of the equivalent amount of base. An initial dose is 1.5 mg given twice daily with food. Thereafter, the dose may be increased according to response by increments of 1.5 mg twice daily at intervals of at least 2 weeks to a maximum dose of 6 mg twice daily. If treatment is interrupted for more than a few days, it should be re-initiated at 1.5 mg twice daily, and then increased, if required, as described above. Clinical benefit should be reassessed on a regular basis.

◊ Studies[1-3] and a systematic review[4] indicate that rivastigmine may be of benefit in the management of patients with mild to moderate Alzheimer's disease. UK guidelines[5] recommend its use in such patients under specialist supervision, with benefits assessed 2 to 4 months after achieving maintenance dosage and every 6 months thereafter; treatment should only continue where there is evidence of benefit.

1. Anand R, et al. Efficacy and safety results of the early phase studies with Excelon™ (ENA-713) in Alzheimer's disease: an overview. J Drug Dev Clin Pract 1996; 8: 109–116.
2. Agid Y, et al. Efficacy and tolerability of rivastigmine in patients with dementia of the Alzheimer type. Curr Ther Res 1998; 59: 837–45.
3. Rösler M, et al. Efficacy and safety of rivastigmine in patients with Alzheimer's disease: international randomised controlled trial. BMJ 1999; 318: 633–8.
4. Birks J, et al. Rivastigmine for Alzheimer's disease (updated 23 August 2001). Available in The Cochrane Library; Issue 4. Oxford: Update Software; 2001.
5. National Institute for Clinical Excellence. Guidance on the use of donepezil, rivastigmine and galantamine for the treatment of Alzheimer's disease (issued January 2001). Available at: http://www.nice.org.uk/pdf/ALZHEIMER_full_guidance.pdf (accessed 20/11/01).

Preparations

Proprietary Preparations (details are given in Part 3)
Aust.: Exelon; **Austral.:** Exelon; **Belg.:** Exelon; **Canad.:** Exelon; **Denm.:** Exelon; **Fin.:** Exelon; **Fr.:** Exelon; **Ger.:** Exelon; **Hong Kong:** Exelon; **Irl.:** Exelon; **Israel:** Exelon; **Ital.:** Exelon; **Mex.:** Exelon; **Neth.:** Exelon; **Norw.:** Exelon; **NZ:** Exelon; **Port.:** Exelon; Prometax; **S.Afr.:** Exelon; **Singapore:** Exelon; **Spain:** Exelon; Prometax; **Swed.:** Exelon; **Switz.:** Exelon; **Thai.:** Exelon; **UK:** Exelon; **USA:** Exelon.

Tacrine Hydrochloride (1447-q)

Tacrine Hydrochloride (BANM, USAN, rINNM).
CI-970; Tetrahydroaminoacridine Hydrochloride; THA. 1,2,3,4-Tetrahydroacridin-9-ylamine hydrochloride.
$C_{13}H_{14}N_2$,HCl = 234.7.
CAS — 321-64-2 (tacrine); 1684-40-8 (tacrine hydrochloride).

Adverse Effects and Treatment
As for Neostigmine, p.1420.

Hepatotoxicity is common, and may be severe.

Effects on the CNS. A report of tonic or tonic-clonic seizures in 6 of 78 patients given tacrine for mild or moderate dementia of the Alzheimer's type.[1]

1. Lebert F, et al. Convulsive effects of tacrine Lancet 1996; 347: 1339–40.

Effects on the liver. A major adverse effect of tacrine therapy is hepatotoxicity. Examination of data from 2446 patients aged at least 50 years who received tacrine for Alzheimer's disease suggested that raised serum-alanine aminotransferase (ALT) concentrations are likely to occur in about 50% of patients; most cases developed within the first 12 weeks of therapy.[1] The increase is usually asymptomatic and mild, and resolves upon dosage reduction or discontinuation of treatment. However, a small percentage of patients may develop life-threatening hepatotoxicity, which cannot be predicted before treatment starts. No significant correlation has been found between plasma-tacrine concentrations and hepatotoxicity,[2] although frequent monitoring of serum-ALT concentrations during the first 12 weeks of therapy can identify these highly susceptible individuals. However, hepatotoxicity may occur after this time and an asymptomatic increase in serum-ALT concentrations has been reported in a patient after more than 80 weeks of therapy.[3]

For guidelines on the monitoring of serum-alanine aminotransferase concentrations during tacrine therapy, see Precautions, below.

1. Watkins PB, et al. Hepatotoxic effects of tacrine administration in patients with Alzheimer's disease. JAMA 1994; 271: 992–8.
2. Ford JM, et al. Serum concentrations of tacrine hydrochloride predict its adverse effects in Alzheimer's disease. Clin Pharmacol Ther 1993; 53: 691–5.
3. Terrell PS, et al. Late-onset alanine aminotransferase increase with tacrine. Ann Pharmacother 1996; 30: 301.

The symbol † denotes a preparation no longer actively marketed

Precautions
As for Neostigmine, p.1420. Tacrine should be used with care in patients with impaired liver function or who have a history of such impairment.

Serum-alanine aminotransferase concentrations should be monitored in patients receiving continuous treatment with tacrine. Monitoring should be carried out every other week from at least week 4 to week 16 of therapy, and then every 3 months thereafter. Weekly monitoring is recommended in patients with elevated aminotransferase levels that are greater than twice the upper limit of the normal range.

If signs of liver involvement worsen, the dose should be reduced or the drug withdrawn. It has been recommended that a threefold to fivefold increase of alanine aminotransferase concentrations calls for a reduction in the dose by 40 mg daily. If increases are above that tacrine should be withdrawn. Treatment with tacrine may be reconsidered once signs of liver dysfunction return to normal; more frequent monitoring of liver enzyme values will be required. Withdrawal is also imperative should jaundice develop, confirmed by elevated total bilirubin levels. Patients who develop jaundice should not be treated again with tacrine.

Abrupt discontinuation of tacrine therapy or a large reduction in the dose may be associated with behavioural disturbances and a decline in cognitive function.

Interactions
As for Neostigmine, p.1420. Since tacrine is metabolised in the liver by the cytochrome P450 enzyme system (principally CYP1A2), drugs that either inhibit or induce the same isoenzymes may raise or lower plasma concentrations of tacrine.

◊ Cimetidine, a non-specific inhibitor of the cytochrome P450 enzyme system, has been shown to inhibit the metabolism of tacrine resulting in reduced oral clearance and an increase in plasma concentrations.[1,2] A similar effect has been reported[3] with fluvoxamine which inhibits the cytochrome P450 isoenzyme CYP1A2, but quinidine, an inhibitor of CYP2D6, appears to have no effect on tacrine metabolism.[1] Cigarette smoking has been reported to markedly reduce plasma-tacrine concentrations.[4] Tacrine may inhibit the metabolism of other drugs, such as theophylline (see p.782), which are metabolised by the same cytochrome P450 isoenzyme.

1. de Vries TM. Effect of cimetidine and low-dose quinidine on tacrine pharmacokinetics in humans. Pharm Res 1993; 10: S337.
2. Forgue ST, et al. Inhibition of tacrine oral clearance by cimetidine. Clin Pharmacol Ther 1996; 59: 444–9.
3. Becquemont L, et al. Influence of the CYP1A2 inhibitor fluvoxamine on tacrine pharmacokinetics in humans. Clin Pharmacol Ther 1997; 61: 619–27.
4. Welty D, et al. The effect of smoking on the pharmacokinetics and metabolism of Cognex® in healthy volunteers. Pharm Res 1993; 10: S334.

Pharmacokinetics
Tacrine is rapidly absorbed from the gastrointestinal tract but large interindividual variations in oral bioavailability and the time to achieve peak plasma concentrations have been reported. The presence of food in the stomach reduces the absorption of tacrine by about 30 to 40%. Tacrine is subject to an extensive first-pass effect in the liver, and is metabolised by the cytochrome P450 system (principally CYP1A2) to several metabolites, the main one of which is the 1-hydroxy metabolite velnacrine (p.1425). Tacrine is 55% bound to plasma proteins. Little unchanged drug is excreted in urine.

◊ In 3 studies in a total of 21 patients peak plasma concentrations of tacrine hydrochloride have been achieved 0.5 to 3 hours after oral administration of doses of 25 or 50 mg and oral bioavailability has ranged from less than 5% to up to 36%.[1-3] Mean elimination half-lives were 1.37 and 1.59 hours after the 25 mg dose and 2.14 and 3.2 hours after the 50 mg dose. Tacrine's elimination appears to be mainly by metabolism in the liver and less than 3% of a dose was recovered unchanged in the urine of one patient.[1] Plasma concentrations of tacrine's main metabolite 1-hydroxy-9-aminotetrahydroacridine (velnacrine) rapidly exceed those of the parent compound and elimination half-lives of 43 and 81 minutes were found for this metabolite in 2 patients studied.[2] Tacrine's pharmacokinetics have been reviewed.[4]

1. Forsyth DR, et al. Pharmacokinetics of tacrine hydrochloride in Alzheimer's disease. Clin Pharmacol Ther 1989; 46: 634–41.
2. Hartvig P, et al. Clinical pharmacokinetics of intravenous and oral 9-amino-1,2,3,4-tetrahydroacridine, tacrine. Eur J Clin Pharmacol 1990; 38: 259–63.
3. Sitar DS, et al. Bioavailability and pharmacokinetic disposition of tacrine HCl in elderly patients with Alzheimer's disease. Clin Pharmacol Ther 1995; 57: 198.
4. Madden S, et al. Clinical pharmacokinetics of tacrine. Clin Pharmacokinet 1995; 28: 449–57.

Uses and Administration
Tacrine hydrochloride is a centrally acting reversible cholinesterase inhibitor used in the treatment of mild to moderately severe dementia in Alzheimer's disease.

The initial dose of tacrine hydrochloride, expressed in terms of tacrine, is 10 mg four times a day for a minimum of 4 weeks. Dosage should not be increased during this period because the potential exists for a delay in onset of increased liver enzyme concentrations. Serum-alanine aminotransferase concentrations should be monitored regularly (see Precautions, above) and, if there is no significant increase, doses may be increased by 40 mg daily at four- to six-week intervals until a satisfactory response is obtained, up to a maximum of 160 mg daily in four divided doses. Tacrine should be taken on an empty stomach to improve absorption, although it can be taken with food by patients in whom gastrointestinal adverse effects may be a problem.

Tacrine has been used to antagonise competitive neuromuscular blockers and as a postoperative respiratory stimulant.

Alzheimer's disease. Tacrine is used in the symptomatic management of Alzheimer's disease (see Dementia, p.1412). It may delay cognitive decline in some patients with mild or moderate Alzheimer's disease but many cannot tolerate the dosage required and have to stop treatment because of gastrointestinal effects or signs of hepatotoxicity. There have been numerous studies of the use of tacrine in Alzheimer's disease and a meta-analysis[1] found tacrine to have a small beneficial effect on both cognition and global clinical impression, although it was considered that the clinical relevance of these findings was unclear and that there were no data from long-term controlled studies. Some have considered[2-6] that a cautious trial of tacrine may be warranted in patients with mild to moderately severe Alzheimer's disease (although alternative drugs are now available) and various guidelines on its use have been issued.[5,6]

1. Qizilbash N, et al. Cholinesterase inhibition for Alzheimer disease: a meta-analysis of the tacrine trials. JAMA 1998; 280: 1777–82.
2. Crimson ML. Tacrine: first drug approved for Alzheimer's disease. Ann Pharmacother 1994; 28: 744–51.
3. Davis KL, Powchik P. Tacrine. Lancet 1995; 345: 625–30.
4. Samuels SC, Davis KL. A risk-benefit assessment of tacrine in the treatment of Alzheimer's disease. Drug Safety 1997; 16: 66–77.
5. Lyketsos CG, et al. Guidelines for the use of tacrine in Alzheimer's disease: clinical application and effectiveness. J Neuropsychiatr Clin Neurosci 1996; 8: 67–73.
6. American Psychiatric Association. Practice guideline for the treatment of patients with Alzheimer's disease and other dementias of late life. Am J Psychiatry 1997; 154 (suppl): 1–39.

Preparations
Proprietary Preparations (details are given in Part 3)
Aust.: Cognex; **Austral.:** Cognex; THA; **Belg.:** Cognex†; **Braz.:** Cognex; Tacrinal; **Fr.:** Cognex; **Ger.:** Cognex; **Hong Kong:** Cognex; **Israel:** Cognex; **NZ:** Cognex; **Port.:** Cognex; **Spain:** Cognex; **Swed.:** Cognex†; **Switz.:** Cognex; **USA:** Cognex.

Velnacrine Maleate (5350-q)

Velnacrine Maleate (BANM, USAN, rINNM).
HP-029; P-83-6029A. (±)-9-Amino-1,2,3,4,-tetrahydro-1-acridinol maleate (1:1).
$C_{13}H_{14}N_2O$,$C_4H_4O_4$ = 330.3.
CAS — 104675-29-8 (velnacrine); 112964-98-4 (velnacrine); 118909-22-1 (velnacrine maleate); 112964-99-5 (velnacrine maleate).

Profile
Velnacrine inhibits cholinesterase activity and has actions similar to those of tacrine (above) of which it is a metabolite. Velnacrine maleate has been studied in the treatment of Alzheimer's disease but the manufacturer stopped development in 1994.

◊ References.

1. Clipp EC, Moore MJ. Caregiver time use: an outcome measure in clinical trial research of Alzheimer's disease. Clin Pharmacol Ther 1995; 58: 228–36.
2. Zemlan FP, et al. Velnacrine for the treatment of Alzheimer's disease: a double-blind, placebo-controlled trial. J Neural Transm 1996; 103: 1105–16.

Xanomeline (17456-m)

Xanomeline *(USAN, rINN)*.

LY-246708. 3-[4-(Hexyloxy)-1,2,5-thiadiazol-3-yl]-1,2,5,6-tetrahydro-1-methylpyridine.

$C_{14}H_{23}N_3OS = 281.4$.

CAS — 131986-45-3.

Profile

Xanomeline is a selective muscarinic M_1 agonist. The tartrate has been studied in the management of Alzheimer's disease but drugs of this type have not generally produced benefit.

◊ References.
1. Sramek JJ, *et al.* The safety and tolerance of xanomeline tartrate in patients with Alzheimer's disease. *J Clin Pharmacol* 1995; **35:** 800–806.
2. Bodick NC, *et al.* Effects of xanomeline, a selective muscarinic receptor agonist, on cognitive function and behavioral symptoms in Alzheimer disease. *Arch Neurol* 1997; **54:** 465–73.

Zifrosilone (17651-g)

Zifrosilone *(USAN, rINN)*.

MDL-73745. 2,2,2-Trifluoro-3'-(trimethylsilyl)acetophenone.

$C_{11}H_{13}F_3OSi = 246.3$.

CAS — 132236-18-1.

Profile

Zifrosilone is an inhibitor of cholinesterase activity that has been investigated for the management of Alzheimer's disease.

◊ References.
1. Cutler NR, *et al.* Acetylcholinesterase inhibition by zifrosilone: pharmacokinetics and pharmacodynamics. *Clin Pharmacol Ther* 1995; **58:** 54–61.

Pesticides and Repellents

This chapter describes compounds used as pesticides and as insect repellents. The term pesticide covers fungicides, herbicides, insecticides (including acaricides), molluscicides, and rodenticides, among others. Most of the pesticides included here are used in clinical or veterinary practice or in vector control against human or animal disease. Some are used primarily in an agricultural or horticultural setting and are included because of their potential toxicity.

Pesticides can be absorbed during application, by consumption of treated or contaminated products or by accidental contamination, and they may be stored or retained in the tissues. International regulations and controls operate to reduce the risk to both public and user. Values for acceptable daily intakes of pesticides are provided by the Food and Agriculture Organization of the United Nations and the World Health Organization (WHO) through the WHO Technical Report series of publications or, more recently, through *Pesticides Residues in Food: yearly evaluations*, FAO Plant Production and Protection Papers, Rome.

Classification of the main pesticides included in this chapter is given in Table 1, below.

The **fungicides** included in this chapter are some of those used in the management of plant disease.

Herbicides are used for weed control both in the domestic setting and professionally in agriculture and horticulture. Those here have been included primarily because they are toxic and have been associated with many cases of poisoning.

Many biting insects can cause unpleasant reactions and the use of **insect repellents** can help to overcome this. Perhaps more importantly, the correct use of insect repellents plays a major role in personal protection against a number of communicable diseases transmitted by insect vectors. Examples are babesiosis (ticks), Lyme disease (ticks), malaria (mosquitoes), relapsing fevers (lice and ticks), spotted fevers (ticks), and typhus fever (fleas, lice, and mites). Some compounds, such as diethyltoluamide and dimethyl phthalate, are effective as repellents while others, such as benzyl benzoate and some of the pyrethroids, are effective both as repellents and as insecticides.

Insecticides have numerous applications. They are used in the treatment of ectoparasitic infections such as pediculosis (lice infections) (below) and in the vector control (below) of a number of communicable diseases that are spread by insects. Acaricides are used to treat scabies (mite infections) (below) and are included within the broad classification of insecticides, although acari (mites) are not, technically, insects. Insecticides are also widely used in veterinary practice and in agriculture and horticulture.

The insecticides used in veterinary practice are often classified as topical or systemic ectoparasiticides. Topical ectoparasiticides, as the name implies, are applied topically to the host animal (such as dogs or cats) to kill its ectoparasites (such as fleas). In the case of systemic ectoparasiticides the term 'systemic' refers to the ingestion of the insecticide by the ectoparasite from the host's blood; the insecticide may be present in the host's blood either as a result of absorption through the skin after topical application or after systemic administration.

Molluscicides are used in agriculture or horticulture or in the domestic garden to control snail and slug pests. Additionally, molluscicides such as niclosamide (described in the Anthelmintics chapter on p.104)

are used against the freshwater snail vector *Bulinus* in the control of schistosomiasis.

Rodenticides may be used to exterminate rats and mice which may be vectors for diseases such as leptospirosis, plague, rat-bite fever, and some haemorrhagic fevers. Many rodenticides are anticoagulants. Warfarin is a commonly used rodenticide but is described elsewhere (p.992).

Clinical Uses of Pesticides and Repellents

Pediculosis

Two species of louse cause pediculosis in man; these are *Pediculus humanus* with its two varieties, *Pediculus humanus capitis* (the head louse) and *Pediculus humanus humanus* (the body louse), and *Pthirus pubis* (*Phthirus pubis*) (the pubic or crab louse). Unlike the head louse, the body louse is an important vector for a number of infections including epidemic typhus (p.146), trench fever (p.143), and relapsing fever (p.137).

Insecticides used in the treatment of pediculosis include malathion, and some pyrethroids such as bioallethrin, permethrin, phenothrin, and tetramethrin. Carbaryl is also effective, although there has been some concern over a theoretical risk of carcinogenicity. Lindane has been used for pubic lice, but many strains of head lice are resistant.

In the UK it has been common for the recommended drugs for the treatment of head lice to be rotated periodically to reduce the emergence of resistance, a problem observed with the newer pyrethroids as well as older insecticides such as lindane, although the value of such rotation policies is debatable. Lotions are preferred to shampoos for head lice since contact time with the insecticide is longer and treatment is thus more effective. Treatment is usually repeated after 7 days. Egg cases ('nits') can be removed by combing the wet hair with a fine tooth comb. A head louse repellent containing piperonal is available.

Malathion has also been suggested for treatment of infestation of the eye lashes and brows with pubic lice (pthiriasis or phthiriasis palpebrarum). Other treatments have included the application of a thick layer of yellow soft paraffin or application of yellow mercuric oxide 1% eye ointment twice daily for about 7 or 8 days or a single application of fluorescein eye drops.

Clothing and bed linen of persons with body lice should be washed in hot water or dry cleaned and ironed.

Topical or systemic antimicrobials should be given as necessary for secondary infections.

References.
1. Burgess IF. Human lice and their management. *Adv Parasitol* 1995; **36:** 271–342.
2. Dodd CS. Interventions for treating headlice (updated 13 March 2001). Available in The Cochrane Library; Issue 4. Oxford: Update Software; 2001.
3. Chosidow O. Scabies and pediculosis. *Lancet* 2000; **355:** 819–26.

Scabies

Scabies is a parasitic infection of the skin by the mite *Sarcoptes scabiei*. The predominant symptom is pruritus, which is caused by an allergic reaction to the parasite and may not occur until several weeks after infection for the first time. Subsequent infections usually result in pruritus after a few days. Pruritus may persist for some months after effective treatment with an acaricide, but is not necessarily an indication for further acaricidal treatment; rather, antipruritics should be used. A severe crusted form (Norwegian scabies) may occur rarely, particularly in immunocompromised or incapacitated patients.

Treatment is with the acaricides permethrin or malathion applied, preferably as aqueous lotions, to clean, cool, dry skin over the entire body and left on for 8 to 24 hours, depending upon the preparation. The preparation should be reapplied to the hands whenever they are washed during this period. In adults, it is not usually necessary to treat the face and scalp, but these areas should be treated in young children or patients with atypical or crusted scabies. A single treatment is usually effective, but treatment may be repeated after 7 to 10 days if necessary. Close family and personal contacts should be treated at the same time. Other drugs used topically in the treatment of scabies include benzyl benzoate, crotamiton, lindane,

Table 1. Classification of pesticides.

Fungicides	Benomyl, cicloheximide, hexachlorobenzene, pentachlorophenol
Herbicides	Dichlorophenoxyacetic acid, dinitro-*o*-cresol, dinitrophenol, diquat, glyphosate, paraquat, pentachlorophenol, trichlorophenoxyacetic acid
Insect repellents	Butopyronoxyl, dibutyl phthalate, diethyltoluamide, dimethyl phthalate, dioctyl adipate, ethohexadiol, piperonal
Insecticides	
Carbamate	Bendiocarb, carbaryl, carbosulfan, methomyl, propoxur
Chlorinated	Chlordane, clofenotane, dieldrin, endosulfan, endrin, heptachlor, lindane
Organophosphorus	Azamethiphos, bromophos, chlorpyrifos, clofenvinfos, coumafos, cythioate, dichlorvos, dimethoate, dimpylate, dioxation, ethion, famphur, fenitrothion, fenthion, heptenophos, iodofenphos, malathion, naled, parathion, phosmet, phoxim, pirimiphos-methyl, propetamphos, pyraclofos, temefos
Pyrethroid	Bioallethrin, cyfluthrin, cyhalothrin, cypermethrin, deltamethrin, esdepallethrine, fenvalerate, flumethrin, permethrin, phenothrin, pyrethrum flower, resmethrin, tetramethrin
Miscellaneous	Amitraz, benzyl benzoate, chloropicrin, copper oleate, cymiazole, cyromazine, diflubenzuron, emamectin, ethylene dibromide, ethylene dichloride, fipronil, fluazuron, fluvalinate, lufenuron, methoprene, methyl bromide, pyriproxyfen, rotenone, sulfiram, triflumuron
Molluscicides	Endod, metaldehyde, pentachlorophenol
Rodenticides	Aluminium phosphide, antu, brodifacoum, bromadiolone, chloralose, chlorophacinone, coumatetralyl, difenacoum, diphenadione, flocoumafen, fluoroacetamide, norbormide, red squill, sodium fluoroacetate

and sulfur; sulfiram is used in combination with benzyl benzoate. A single oral dose of ivermectin may be effective.

In addition to treatment with an acaricide, symptomatic treatment of the itching with crotamiton, calamine lotion, or systemic antihistamines or corticosteroids may be required.

References.
1. Elgart ML. A risk-benefit assessment of agents used in the treatment of scabies. *Drug Safety* 1996; **14:** 386–93.
2. Walker GJA, Johnstone PW. Interventions for treating scabies (updated 30 August 2001). Available in The Cochrane Library; Issue 4. Oxford: Update Software; 2001.
3. Chosidow O. Scabies and pediculosis. *Lancet* 2000; **355:** 819–26.

Vector control

Many pests are involved in the transmission of communicable diseases, and vector control[1,2] is an important part of the fight against such diseases. Insecticides are employed in the control of filariasis (p.94) (*Aedes, Anopheles, Culex,* and *Mansonia* mosquitoes);[3] leishmaniasis (p.584) (*Phlebotomus* or *Lutzomyia* sandflies);[4] malaria (p.428) (*Anopheles* mosquitoes);[5-8] onchocerciasis (p.94) (*Simulium* blackflies);[9] African trypanosomiasis (p.586) (*Glossina* tsetse flies);[10] and South American trypanosomiasis (p.587) (*Triatoma* bugs).[11] The insecticide temefos is useful in dracunculiasis (p.92) (crustacean host to the guinea worm larvae). In some cases, as in filariasis or onchocerciasis, the insecticides employed act primarily against the larval stage of the insect vector, whereas in other situations, as in malaria, activity is against the adult insect; in trypanosomiasis, activity is directed against both adult and immature stages. The majority of the experience gained in insecticidal vector control has probably been in malaria, and, for instance, a positive effect seen in the control of leishmaniasis has been considered to be mainly a byproduct of the concomitant malaria control programmes.

Insect repellents can provide personal protection against many insect vectors. For example, in malaria, insect repellents as well as the use of insecticides are important in preventing mosquito bites.

Molluscicides are employed in the control of schistosomiasis (p.94) (*Bulinus* snails).[12]

Rodenticides are also extremely valuable in the vector control of some diseases such as leptospirosis (p.127), plague (p.135), rat-bite fever (p.115), and some haemorrhagic fevers (p.605).

1. Chavasse DC, Yap HH, eds. *Chemical methods for the control of vectors and pests of public health importance.* Geneva: WHO, 1997.
2. Rozendaal JA. *Vector control: methods for use by individuals and communities.* Geneva: WHO, 1997.
3. WHO. *Lymphatic filariasis: the disease and its control. WHO Tech Rep Ser 821* 1992.
4. WHO. *Control of the leishmaniases. WHO Tech Rep Ser 793* 1990.
5. WHO. *Vector control for malaria and other mosquito-borne diseases. WHO Tech Rep Ser 857* 1995.
6. Lengeler C. Insecticide-treated bednets and curtains for preventing malaria (updated 29 May 2001). Available in The Cochrane Library; Issue 4. Oxford: Update Software; 2001.
7. WHO. *International travel and health: vaccination requirements and health advice.* Geneva: WHO, 2001.
8. WHO. *Malaria vector control: insecticides for indoor residual spraying.* Geneva: WHO, 2001.
9. WHO. Report of a WHO expert committee on onchocerciasis control. *WHO Tech Rep Ser 852* 1995.
10. WHO. Epidemiology and control of African trypanosomiasis: report of a WHO expert committee. *WHO Tech Rep Ser 739* 1986.
11. WHO. Control of Chagas disease: report of a WHO expert committee. *WHO Tech Rep Ser 811* 1991.
12. WHO. The control of schistosomiasis: second report of the WHO expert committee. *WHO Tech Rep Ser 830* 1993.

Aluminium Phosphide (16410-b)

Aluminum Phosphide.
AlP = 57.96.
CAS — 20859-73-8 (aluminium phosphide); 7803-51-2 (phosphine); 1314-84-7 (zinc phosphide).

Profile
Aluminium phosphide is used for the fumigation of grain and as a rodenticide. It releases phosphine (PH₃) in the presence of moisture and this accounts for its pesticidal activity. Phosphine gas has a garlic-like odour repulsive to man and domestic animals but apparently not to *rats*. Zinc phosphide is used similarly.

◊ References to poisoning associated with aluminium phosphide.
1. Wilson R, *et al.* Acute phosphine poisoning aboard a grain freighter. *JAMA* 1980; **244:** 148–50.
2. Singh S, *et al.* Aluminium phosphide ingestion. *BMJ* 1985; **290:** 1110–11.

3. Anger F, *et al.* Fatal aluminium phosphide poisoning. *J Anal Toxicol* 2000; **24:** 90–2.
4. Nocera A, *et al.* Dangerous bodies: a case of fatal aluminium phosphide poisoning. *Med J Aust* 2000; **173:** 133–5.

Amitraz (18372-q)

Amitraz (BAN, USAN, pINN).
U-36059. N,N′-[(Methylimino)dimethylidyne]di-2,4-xylidine.
C₁₉H₂₃N₃ = 293.4.
CAS — 33089-61-1.
Pharmacopoeias. In BP(Vet). Also in US for veterinary use only.

Pharmacopoeial description
BP(Vet) 2001: A white to buff powder. Practically insoluble in water; decomposes slowly in alcohol; freely soluble in acetone.

Profile
Amitraz is used as a topical ectoparasiticide in veterinary practice. It is effective against various lice, mites, and ticks.

◊ References to poisoning with amitraz.
1. Jorens PG, *et al.* An unusual poisoning with the unusual pesticide amitraz. *Hum Exp Toxicol* 1997; **16:** 600–1.
2. Aydin K, *et al.* Amitraz poisoning in children: clinical and laboratory findings of eight cases. *Hum Exp Toxicol* 1997; **16:** 680–2.
3. Leung VK, *et al.* Amitraz poisoning in humans. *J Toxicol Clin Toxicol* 1999; **37:** 513–14.
4. Yaramis A, *et al.* Amitraz poisoning in children. *Hum Exp Toxicol* 2000; **19:** 431–3.

Antu (16411-v)

1-(1-Naphthyl)-2-thiourea; α-Naphthylthiourea.
C₁₁H₁₀N₂S = 202.3.
CAS — 86-88-4.

Profile
Antu was formerly used as a rodenticide. The carcinogenic risk from naphthylamine impurities restricted its use.

Azamethiphos (15581-z)

Azamethiphos (BAN).
CGA-18809; OMS-1825. S-[(6-Chloro-2,3-dihydro-2-oxo-1,3-oxazolo[4,5-b]pyridin-3-yl)methyl] O,O-dimethyl phosphorothioate.
C₉H₁₀ClN₂O₅PS = 324.7.
CAS — 35575-96-3.

Profile
Azamethiphos is an organophosphorus insecticide (p.1435) used in veterinary practice for the control of sea-lice infestation in salmon and for the control of ectoparasites in the environment.

Bendiocarb (18020-g)

2,3-Isopropylidenedioxyphenyl methylcarbamate.
C₁₁H₁₃NO₄ = 223.2.
CAS — 22781-23-3.

Profile
Bendiocarb is a carbamate insecticide (p.1429) for agricultural and household use.

Benomyl (18837-n)

Methyl 1-(butylcarbamoyl)benzimidazol-2-ylcarbamate.
C₁₄H₁₈N₄O₃ = 290.3.
CAS — 17804-35-2.

Profile
Benomyl is a fungicide used for the treatment and control of fungal plant diseases.

Toxicity. Although experimental evidence in *animals* has suggested a possible link between benomyl and congenital eye defects (anophthalmia) the association could not be substantiated in humans.[1-4]
1. Gilbert R. "Clusters" of anophthalmia in Britain. *BMJ* 1993; **307:** 340–1.
2. Bianchi F, *et al.* Clusters of anophthalmia. *BMJ* 1994; **308:** 205.
3. Kristensen P, Irgens LM. Clusters of anophthalmia. *BMJ* 1994; **308:** 205–6.
4. Castilla EE. Clusters of anophthalmia. *BMJ* 1994; **308:** 206.

Benzyl Benzoate (3569-w)

Benzoato de Bencilo; Benzoato de Benzilo; Benzoesäurebenzylester; Benzyl Benz.; Benzylis Benzoas.
C₆H₅.CO.O.CH₂.C₆H₅ = 212.2.
CAS — 120-51-4.
ATC — P03AX01.
Pharmacopoeias. In Eur. (see p.vi), Int., Jpn, and US.

Pharmacopoeial description
Ph. Eur.: Colourless or almost colourless crystals, or a colourless or almost colourless oily liquid. F.p. is not below 17°. Practically insoluble in water; miscible with alcohol, with dichlo-

romethane, with ether, and with fatty and essential oils. Store in well-filled airtight containers. Protect from light.
USP 25: A clear, colourless, oily liquid with a slight aromatic odour. Practically insoluble in water and in glycerol; miscible with alcohol, with chloroform, and with ether. Store at a temperature not exceeding 40° in well-filled airtight containers. Protect from light.

Adverse Effects and Treatment
Benzyl benzoate is irritant to the eyes and mucous membranes and it may be irritant to the skin. Hypersensitivity reactions have been reported. If ingested, benzyl benzoate may cause stimulation of the CNS and convulsions. Systemic symptoms have been reported following excessive topical use. Treatment of poisoning involves gastric lavage if accidentally ingested, or washing of the skin following topical use; appropriate symptomatic measures should also be instituted.

Uses and Administration
Benzyl benzoate is an acaricide used in the treatment of scabies (p.1427) although other treatments are generally preferred. A 25% emulsion is applied to the whole body, usually from the neck down; if the application is thorough, one treatment may suffice, although the possibility of failure is lessened by a second application within 5 days. Alternatively, three applications at 12-hour intervals, without bathing, may be made, followed by bathing 12 hours after the last application. Another alternative regimen recommended by the *British National Formulary* is one application to the whole body, repeated, without bathing, on the next day, and washed off 24 hours later; a third application may sometimes be necessary. Benzyl benzoate is not generally recommended for infants and children, but if used the application should be diluted to minimise the risk of irritation, although this also reduces efficacy.

Benzyl benzoate has also been used as a pediculicide.

Benzyl benzoate is also used as a solubilising agent.

Preparations
BP 2001: Benzyl Benzoate Application;
USP 25: Benzyl Benzoate Lotion.

Proprietary Preparations (details are given in Part 3)
Austral.: Ascabiol; Benzemul; *Braz.:* Acarsan; Miticocan; Sarnigal; Sarnisan; Sarnodex; *Ger.:* Acaril; Acarosan; Antiscabiosum; *Irl.:* Ascabiol; *Israel:* Scabiex; *Ital.:* Mom Lozione Preventiva; *Mex.:* Ansar; Escacin; *Port.:* Acarilbial; Neo-Acarina; *S.Afr.:* Ascabiol; *UK:* Ascabiol.

Multi-ingredient: *Austral.:* Anusol; *Belg.:* Pulmex; Pulmex Baby; *Braz.:* Anusol-HC; Benzilol; *Fr.:* Allerbiocid S; Ascabiol; Sanytol; *Ger.:* Kontakto Derm Lotio; Labocane; *Hong Kong:* Anusol-HC; *Irl.:* Anugesic-HC; Anusol-HC; Sudocrem†; *Ital.:* Antiscabbia Candioli al DDT Terapeutico; Dekar 2; Mom Zanzara; *Mex.:* Scabisan Plus; *NZ:* Anusol; *S.Afr.:* Anugesic; Anusol-HC†; *Singapore:* Anusol; *Spain:* Tulgrasum Cicatrizante; Yacutin; *Swed.:* Tenutex; *Switz.:* Anusol†; *Thai.:* Anusol; *UK:* Anugesic-HC; Anusol-HC; Plus HC; Sudocrem; *USA:* Anumed; Anumed HC; Hemril; Rectagene II†.

Bioallethrin (16537-t)

Bioallethrin (BAN).
Allethrin I; Depallethrin. (RS)-3-Allyl-2-methyl-4-oxocyclopent-2-enyl (1R,3R)-2,2-dimethyl-3-(2-methylprop-1-enyl)cyclopropanecarboxylate.
C₁₉H₂₆O₃ = 302.4.
CAS — 584-79-2 (RS-bioallethrin); 28434-00-6 (S-bioallethrin).
ATC — P03AC02.

Profile
Bioallethrin is a pyrethroid insecticide (p.1436). It is used topically, in conjunction with the synergist piperonyl butoxide (p.1436), in the treatment of pediculosis (p.1427). It is also used in anti-mosquito devices and for the control of household insect pests.

Preparations
Proprietary Preparations (details are given in Part 3)
UK: Actomite.

Multi-ingredient: *Austral.:* Paralice; *Belg.:* Para; *Braz.:* Vapio; *Canad.:* Para; *Denm.:* Para; *Fr.:* Para Special Poux; *Ger.:* Jacutin N; Spregal; *Israel:* Monocide; *Neth.:* Para-Speciaal; *UK:* Fortefog.

Brodifacoum (16545-t)

WBA-8119. 3-[3-(4′-Bromobiphenyl-4-yl)-1,2,3,4-tetrahydro-1-naphthyl]-4-hydroxycoumarin.
C₃₁H₂₃BrO₃ = 523.4.
CAS — 56073-10-0.

Profile
Brodifacoum is an anticoagulant rodenticide. It is reported to be effective in warfarin-resistant strains of rodents.

Toxicity. Brodifacoum, a second-generation anticoagulant rodenticide, inhibits prothrombin synthesis to cause bleeding that may be occult.[1,2] It is absorbed from the gastrointestinal tract; dermal absorption is possible. Poisons containing 100 mg per kg of bait are not hazardous to man; more concentrated forms are particularly hazardous and their availability should be restricted. Baits, which should be prepared only by trained personnel, should contain a suitable marker-dye.

There have been reports of poisoning with brodifacoum.[3-8]

1. WHO. Safe use of pesticides: ninth report of the WHO expert committee on vector biology and control. *WHO Tech Rep Ser 720* 1985.
2. Anticoagulant rodenticides. *Environmental Health Criteria 175.* Geneva: WHO, 1995.
3. Watts RG, *et al.* Accidental poisoning with a superwarfarin compound (brodifacoum) in a child. *Pediatrics* 1990; **86:** 883–7.
4. Ross GS, *et al.* An acquired hemorrhagic disorder from long-acting rodenticide ingestion. *Arch Intern Med* 1992; **152:** 410–12.
5. Kruse JA, Carlson RW. Fatal rodenticide poisoning with brodifacoum. *Ann Emerg Med* 1992; **21:** 331–6.
6. Tecimer C, Yam LT. Surreptitious superwarfarin poisoning with brodifacoum. *South Med J* 1997; **90:** 1053–5.
7. Corke PJ. Superwarfarin (brodifacoum) poisoning. *Anaesth Intensive Care* 1997; **25:** 707–9.
8. La Rosa FG, *et al.* Brodifacoum intoxication with marijuana smoking. *Arch Pathol Lab Med* 1997; **121:** 67–9.

Bromadiolone   (3862-z)

3-[3-[4′-Bromobiphenyl-4-yl)-3-hydroxy-1-phenylpropyl]-4-hydroxycoumarin.
$C_{30}H_{23}BrO_4 = 527.4$.
CAS — 28772-56-7.

Profile
Bromadiolone is an anticoagulant rodenticide.

Toxicity. Bromadiolone, a second-generation anticoagulant rodenticide, inhibits prothrombin synthesis to cause bleeding that may be occult.[1,2] It is absorbed from the gastrointestinal tract; dermal absorption is possible. Poisons containing 100 mg per kg of bait are not hazardous to man; more concentrated forms are particularly hazardous and their availability should be restricted. Baits, which should be prepared only by trained personnel, should contain a suitable marker-dye.

There have been reports of poisoning with bromadiolone.[3]

1. WHO. Safe use of pesticides: ninth report of the WHO expert committee on vector biology and control. *WHO Tech Rep Ser 720* 1985.
2. Anticoagulant rodenticides. *Environmental Health Criteria 175.* Geneva: WHO, 1995.
3. Greeff MC, *et al.* "Superwarfarin" (bromodialone) poisoning in two children resulting in prolonged anticoagulation. *Lancet* 1987; **ii:** 1269.

Bromophos   (18104-w)

OMS-658. *O*-4-Bromo-2,5-dichlorophenyl *O,O*-dimethyl phosphorothioate.
$C_8H_8BrCl_2O_3PS = 366.0$.
CAS — 2104-96-3.

Profile
Bromophos is an organophosphorus insecticide (p.1435) used in veterinary practice for the control of ectoparasites in the environment. It has also been used as an agricultural insecticide.

Butopyronoxyl   (2551-z)

Indalone. Butyl 3,4-dihydro-2,2-dimethyl-4-oxo-2*H*-pyran-6-carboxylate.
$C_{12}H_{18}O_4 = 226.3$.
CAS — 532-34-3.

Profile
Butopyronoxyl has been used as an insect repellent.

Carbamate Insecticides   (3561-h)

The carbamate insecticides are *N*-substituted esters of carbamic acid.

◊ References.
1. WHO. Carbamate pesticides: a general introduction. *Environmental Health Criteria 64.* Geneva: WHO, 1986.

Adverse Effects
As for Organophosphorus Insecticides, p.1435.

The carbamates are cholinesterase inhibitors, differing from the organophosphorus insecticides in that the inhibition they produce is generally less intense and more rapidly reversible. In addition, they do not appear to enter the CNS as readily and severe central effects are therefore uncommon.

Treatment of Adverse Effects
If carbamate insecticides have been ingested the stomach should be emptied by lavage. Contaminated clothing should be removed and the skin washed with soap and water. Treatment is largely symptomatic and supportive and includes atropine, but this may not always be necessary due to the rapidly reversible nature of the cholinesterase inhibition produced. Pralidoxime has usually been contra-indicated as some *animal* studies have suggested that it may increase the toxicity of carbamates. However, the evidence is not conclusive and some authorities state that it may be given in severe cases unresponsive to atropine and supportive care.

The symbol † denotes a preparation no longer actively marketed

◊ References.
1. WHO. Safe use of pesticides: fourteenth report of the WHO expert committee on vector biology and control. *WHO Tech Rep Ser 813* 1991.
2. Proudfoot A, ed. *Pesticide poisoning: notes for the guidance of medical practitioners.* 2nd ed. London: DoH, The Stationery Office, 1996.

Carbaryl   (3570-m)

Carbaryl (*BAN*).
Carbaril (*pINN*); OMS-29. 1-Naphthyl methylcarbamate.
$C_{12}H_{11}NO_2 = 201.2$.
CAS — 63-25-2.
Pharmacopoeias. In Br.

Pharmacopoeial description
BP 2001: A white to off-white or light grey powder which darkens on exposure to light. Very slightly soluble in water; soluble in alcohol and in acetone. Store at a temperature not exceeding 25°. Protect from light.

Adverse Effects and Treatment
As for Carbamate Insecticides, above. Carbaryl may be absorbed following ingestion, inhalation, or skin contamination. Carbaryl has been reported to produce neoplasms in *mice* and *rats* and in late 1995 the UK Department of Health advised that it would be prudent to consider carbaryl as a potential human carcinogen; its medicinal use was limited to prescription only. However, the Department of Health emphasised that the risk was a theoretical one and that any risk from the intermittent use of head lice preparations was likely to be very small.

Uses and Administration
Carbaryl is a carbamate insecticide (above). It is used as a 0.5 or 1.0% lotion or shampoo in the treatment of head and pubic pediculosis (p.1427). Lotions are generally preferred to shampoos as the contact time is longer. Aqueous lotions are preferred to treat pubic lice because alcoholic lotions are irritant to excoriated skin and the genitalia; aqueous lotions may also be preferable in asthmatic subjects or children to avoid alcoholic fumes. Skin or hair treated with an alcohol-based preparation should be allowed to dry naturally.

Carbaryl is also used as a topical ectoparasiticide in veterinary practice and as an agricultural, horticultural, and household insecticide.

Preparations
BP 2001: Carbaryl Lotion.

Proprietary Preparations (details are given in Part 3)
Irl.: Carylderm; Derbac-C†; *Israel:* Carbacide; Hafif; *UK:* Carylderm; Clinicide†; Mitchell Expel Anti Lice Spray; Suleo-C†.
Multi-ingredient: *Fr.:* Acarcid perles.

Carbosulfan   (5368-k)

2,3-Dihydro-2,2-dimethylbenzofuran-7-yl (dibutylaminothio)methylcarbamate.
$C_{20}H_{32}N_2O_3S = 380.5$.

Profile
Carbosulfan is a carbamate insecticide (p.1429) used in agriculture and for the larvicidal treatment of rivers in the control of onchocerciasis (p.94).

Chloralose   (4022-g)

Chloralose (*rINN*).
Alphachloralose; Chloralosane; α-Chloralose; Glucochloral. (*R*)-1,2-*O*-(2,2,2-Trichloroethylidene)-α-D-glucofuranose.
$C_8H_{11}Cl_3O_6 = 309.5$.
CAS — 15879-93-3.

Profile
Chloralose has general properties similar to those of cloral hydrate (p.669), of which it is a derivative. It is used as a rodenticide. It was formerly used for its hypnotic properties.

Chlordane   (18055-k)

1,2,4,5,6,7,8,8-Octachloro-2,3,3a,4,7,7a-hexahydro-4,7-methanoindene.
$C_{10}H_6Cl_8 = 409.8$.
CAS — 57-74-9.

Profile
Chlordane is a chlorinated insecticide (p.1429). Its use is limited, or even prohibited, in some countries because of toxicity due to its persistent nature.

◊ References.
1. Chlordane. *Environmental Health Criteria 34.* Geneva: WHO, 1984.
2. Kutz FW, *et al.* A fatal chlordane poisoning. *J Toxicol Clin Toxicol* 1983; **20:** 167–74.
3. Olanoff LS, *et al.* Acute chlordane intoxication. *J Toxicol Clin Toxicol* 1983; **20:** 291–306.

Chlorinated Insecticides   (3562-m)

The chlorinated or organochlorine insecticides were widely used but, because of persistence in man, many have been banned or restricted.

◊ References.
1. WHO. Polychlorinated biphenyls and terphenyls. *Environmental Health Criteria 2.* Geneva: WHO, 1976.

Adverse Effects
Chlorinated or organochlorine insecticides form a very wide group and the toxicity of individual members varies considerably. In general these insecticides produce symptoms consistent with CNS stimulation. They may be absorbed through the respiratory and gastrointestinal tracts and through the skin.

Symptoms of acute poisoning include nausea and vomiting, paraesthesia, giddiness, tremors, convulsions, coma, and respiratory failure. Liver, kidney, and myocardial toxicity have been reported. Effects on the blood include agranulocytosis and aplastic anaemia. Symptoms may be complicated by the effects of the solvent.

Chlorinated insecticides have been reported to enhance microsomal hepatic enzyme activity. Skin reactions can occur after contact.

Polychlorinated biphenyl (PCB) and terphenyl compounds were formerly used as insecticides in many countries. They accumulate in body fat and are not readily excreted, although they are distributed into breast milk and possibly cross the placenta; because of this and because of accidental contamination they remain a cause for concern. The related polybrominated biphenyl compounds (PBB), which have no insecticidal uses, have also been absorbed by humans following accidental contamination of the food chain.

Some chlorinated insecticides have weak oestrogenic effects; it has been proposed that exposure may increase the risk of breast cancer.

Treatment of Adverse Effects
If chlorinated insecticides have been ingested the stomach should be emptied by lavage. Contaminated clothing should be removed and the skin washed with soap and water. Treatment is largely symptomatic and supportive with treatment of CNS stimulation such as hyperactivity and convulsions.

◊ References.
1. WHO. Safe use of pesticides: fourteenth report of the WHO expert committee on vector biology and control. *WHO Tech Rep Ser 813* 1991.
2. Proudfoot A, ed. Pesticide poisoning: notes for the guidance of medical practitioners. 2nd ed. London: DoH, The Stationery Office, 1996.

Chlorophacinone   (18199-w)

LM-91. 2-[2-(4-Chlorophenyl)-2-phenylacetyl]indane-1,3-dione.
$C_{23}H_{15}ClO_3 = 374.8$.
CAS — 3691-35-8.

Profile
Chlorophacinone is an indanedione derivative used as an anticoagulant rodenticide. It is also reported to uncouple oxidative phosphorylation with consequent stimulation of cellular metabolism which may contribute to its toxicity.

◊ References.
1. Burucoa C, *et al.* Chlorophacinone intoxication: biological and toxicological study. *J Toxicol Clin Toxicol* 1989; **27:** 79–89.
2. Anticoagulant rodenticides. *Environmental Health Criteria 175.* Geneva: WHO, 1995.

Chloropicrin   (12554-e)

Nitrochloroform. Trichloronitromethane.
$CCl_3NO_2 = 164.4$.
CAS — 76-06-2.

Profile
Chloropicrin is a lachrymatory agent with an intense odour. It is intensely irritating to the skin and mucous membranes. It is an insecticide and is used for fumigating stored grain and soil. Chloropicrin is also added to other fumigants as a warning gas.

Chlorpyrifos   (18112-w)

Chlorpyrifos (*BAN*).
O,O-Diethyl *O*-3,5,6-trichloro-2-pyridyl phosphorothioate.
$C_9H_{11}Cl_3NO_3PS = 350.6$.
CAS — 2921-88-2.

Profile
Chlorpyrifos is an organophosphorus insecticide (p.1435) used in agriculture.

Cicloheximide (12620-v)

Cicloheximide (rINN).

Cycloheximide (USAN); U-4527. 3-{(2R)-2-[(1S,3S,5S)-3,5-Dimethyl-2-oxocyclohexyl]-2-hydroxyethyl}glutarimide.
$C_{15}H_{23}NO_4 = 281.3$.
CAS — 66-81-9.

Profile

Cicloheximide is an antimicrobial substance produced by strains of *Streptomyces griseus*. It has antifungal properties and has been used for the treatment and control of certain mycotic plant diseases.

Clofenotane (3578-e)

Clofenotane (rINN).

Chlorofenotano; Chlorophenothane; Chlorphenothanum; DDT; Dichlorodiphenyltrichloroethane; Dichophanum; Dicophane. 1,1,1-Trichloro-2,2-bis(4-chlorophenyl)ethane.
$C_{14}H_9Cl_5 = 354.5$.
CAS — 50-29-3.
ATC — P03AB01.

Pharmacopoeias. In Aust. and It.

Adverse Effects and Treatment

As for Chlorinated Insecticides, p.1429.

◊ References.
1. DDT and its derivatives. *Environmental Health Criteria 9.* Geneva: WHO, 1979.
2. DDT and its derivatives—environmental aspects. *Environmental Health Criteria 83.* Geneva: WHO, 1989.

Carcinogenicity. Some small epidemiological studies have suggested that certain organochlorines, namely 1,1-dichloro-2,2-bis(*p*-chlorophenyl)ethylene (DDE), a metabolite of clofenotane, and polychlorinated biphenyls (PCBs), might increase the risk of breast cancer in women. However, re-analysis[1,2] of the available data indicated that an association with breast cancer was unlikely for clofenotane; there was no evidence for an association with the PCBs. Any link between exposure to clofenotane and the development of testicular cancer in men was also refuted[3] following long-term monitoring of populations in Scandinavia.
1. Key T, Reeves G. Organochlorines in the environment and breast cancer. *BMJ* 1994; **308:** 1520–1.
2. van't Veer P, *et al.* DDT (dicophane) and postmenopausal breast cancer in Europe: case-control study. *BMJ* 1997; **315:** 81–5.
3. Ekbom A, *et al.* DDT and testicular cancer. *Lancet* 1996; **347:** 553–4.

Effects on fertility. A metabolite of clofenotane, 1,1-dichloro-2,2-bis(*p*-chlorophenyl)ethylene (DDE), was reported[1] to have anti-androgenic properties in *rats* and exposure to clofenotane might account for a previously reported decline in male fertility and an increase in male reproductive abnormalities.
1. Keke WR, *et al.* Persistent DDT metabolite p,p'-DDE is a potent androgen receptor antagonist. *Nature* 1995; **375:** 581–5.

Pharmacokinetics

Clofenotane may be absorbed after ingestion or inhalation or through the skin. Clofenotane is stored in the body, particularly in body fat, and is very slowly eliminated. It crosses the placenta and appears in breast milk. It is metabolised in the body to the ethylene derivative, 1,1-dichloro-2,2-bis(*p*-chlorophenyl)ethylene (DDE); the acetic acid derivative (DDA) also appears in the urine.

Uses

Clofenotane is a chlorinated insecticide (p.1429). It is a stomach and contact poison and retains its activity for long periods under a variety of conditions. It is effective against disease vectors such as fleas, lice, and mosquitoes and has been applied topically for pediculosis (p.1427) and scabies (p.1427), although more suitable alternatives exist.

Because of the extreme persistence of clofenotane, concern over its effect in the environment, and the problem of resistance, the widespread use of clofenotane is now generally discouraged. It is no longer used in some countries while in others its use is limited.

◊ Despite reservations regarding the use of clofenotane for vector control, many endemic countries have relied on it for the control of both malaria and visceral leishmaniasis. A WHO study group[1] reviewed the current situation and concluded that clofenotane might be used, provided that all the following conditions were met: that it was used only for indoor spraying; that it was known to be effective; that it was manufactured to WHO's specifications; and that the necessary safety precautions were taken in its use and disposal. However, they recommended further investigation of the effects of clofenotane in breast milk and of suspected carcinogenicity, as well as clarification of the significance of the reduced density of muscarinic receptors caused by clofenotane.
1. WHO. Vector control for malaria and other mosquito-borne diseases. *WHO Tech Rep Ser 857* 1995.

Preparations

Proprietary Preparations (details are given in Part 3)
Multi-ingredient: *Ital.:* Antiscabbia Candioli al DDT Terapeutico.

Clofenvinfos (18108-j)

Clofenvinfos (BAN, rINN).

Chlorfenvinphos. 2-Chloro-1-(2,4-dichlorophenyl)vinyl diethyl phosphate.
$C_{12}H_{14}Cl_3O_4P = 359.6$.
CAS — 470-90-6.

Profile

Clofenvinfos is an organophosphorus insecticide (p.1435) used in agriculture.

Copper Oleate (12608-s)

$Cu(C_{18}H_{33}O_2)_2 = 626.5$.
CAS — 1120-44-1.

Profile

Copper oleate has been used topically as an insecticide for the treatment of pediculosis (p.1427).

Coumafos (18115-y)

Coumafos (BAN, rINN).

Bayer-21199; Coumaphos. O-3-Chloro-4-methyl-7-coumarinyl O,O-diethyl phosphorothioate.
$C_{14}H_{16}ClO_5PS = 362.8$.
CAS — 56-72-4.

Profile

Coumafos is an organophosphorus insecticide (p.1435) used as a topical ectoparasiticide in veterinary practice.

Coumatetralyl (16406-p)

4-Hydroxy-3-(1,2,3,4-tetrahydro-1-naphthyl)coumarin.
$C_{19}H_{16}O_3 = 292.3$.
CAS — 5836-29-3.

Profile

Coumatetralyl is an anticoagulant rodenticide.

◊ References.
1. Anticoagulant rodenticides. *Environmental Health Criteria 175.* Geneva: WHO, 1995.

Cyfluthrin (3855-c)

Cyfluthrin (BAN).

Bay-VI-1704; Cyfluthin. (RS)-α-Cyano-4-fluoro-3-phenoxybenzyl (1RS,3RS;1RS,3SR)-3-(2,2-dichlorovinyl)-2,2-dimethylcyclopropanecarboxylate.
$C_{22}H_{18}Cl_2FNO_3 = 434.3$.
CAS — 68359-37-5.
ATC — P03BA01.

Profile

Cyfluthrin is a pyrethroid insecticide (p.1436) used in agriculture.

Preparations

Proprietary Preparations (details are given in Part 3)
Ital.: Responsar; Solfac EW.

Cyhalothrin (15318-d)

Cyhalothrin (BAN).

PP-563. (RS)-α-Cyano-3-phenoxybenzyl (Z)-(1RS,3RS)-3-(2-chloro-3,3,3-trifluoropropenyl)-2,2-dimethylcyclopropanecarboxylate.
$C_{23}H_{19}ClF_3NO_3 = 449.9$.
CAS — 68085-85-8.

Profile

Cyhalothrin is a pyrethroid insecticide (p.1436) that is used, particularly as a mixture of the (Z)-(1R,3R) S ester and the (Z)-(1S,3S) R ester (known as lambda-cyhalothrin), for the control of insect pests in public health. It has also been used in agriculture.

◊ References.
1. Cyhalothrin. *Environmental Health Criteria 99.* Geneva: WHO, 1990.

Cymiazole (3886-d)

CGA-50439; CGA-192357 (cymiazole hydrochloride); Xymiazole. 2,4-Dimethyl-N-(3-methyl-2(3H)-thiazolylidene)benzenamine.
$C_{12}H_{14}N_2S = 218.3$.
CAS — 61676-87-7 (cymiazole); 121034-85-3 (cymiazole hydrochloride).

Profile

Cymiazole is a pesticide used in beekeeping.

Cypermethrin (19015-k)

Cypermethrin (BAN).

(RS)-α-Cyano-3-phenoxybenzyl (1RS,3RS)-(1RS,3RS)-3-(2,2-dichlorovinyl)-2,2-dimethylcyclopropanecarboxylate.
$C_{22}H_{19}Cl_2NO_3 = 416.3$.
CAS — 52315-07-8.
ATC — P03BA02.

Profile

Cypermethrin, an isomeric mixture containing alpha-cypermethrin, is a pyrethroid insecticide (p.1436) used in veterinary practice as a topical ectoparasiticide and to control sea-lice infestation in salmon. It is also used in agriculture. Zeta-cypermethrin is also used.

◊ References.
1. Cypermethrin. *Environmental Health Criteria 82.* Geneva: WHO, 1989.
2. Alpha-cypermethrin. *Environmental Health Criteria 142.* Geneva: WHO, 1992.

Preparations

Proprietary Preparations (details are given in Part 3)
Multi-ingredient: *UK:* Fortefog.

Cyromazine (4874-b)

Cyromazine (BAN, rINN).

CGA-72662. N-Cyclopropyl-1,3,5-triazine-2,4,6-triamine.
$C_6H_{10}N_6 = 166.2$.
CAS — 66215-27-8.

Profile

Cyromazine is used as a topical ectoparasiticide in veterinary practice.

Cythioate (3573-g)

Cythioate (BAN).

O,O-Dimethyl O-(4-sulphamoylphenyl) phosphorothioate.
$C_8H_{12}NO_5PS_2 = 297.3$.
CAS — 115-93-5.

Profile

Cythioate is an organophosphorus insecticide (p.1435) used as a systemic ectoparasiticide in veterinary practice; it is administered by mouth to the host animal.

Daminozide (10683-b)

N-Dimethylaminosuccinamic acid.
$C_6H_{12}N_2O_3 = 160.2$.
CAS — 1596-84-5.

Profile

Daminozide is a plant growth regulator that has been used in pesticides to improve fruit crops. There have been concerns about residues of the chemical in the fruit.

Deltamethrin (16614-c)

Deltamethrin (BAN).

Decamethrin; NRDC-161. (S)-α-Cyano-3-phenoxybenzyl (1R,3R)-3-(2,2-dibromovinyl)-2,2-dimethylcyclopropanecarboxylate.
$C_{22}H_{19}Br_2NO_3 = 505.2$.
CAS — 52918-63-5.
ATC — P03BA03.

Pharmacopoeias. In BP(Vet).

Pharmacopoeial description

BP(Vet) 2001: A white to buff-coloured crystalline powder. Insoluble in water; soluble in alcohol and in acetone.

Profile

Deltamethrin is a pyrethroid insecticide (p.1436) used in the vector control of malaria (p.428). It is also used as a topical ectoparasiticide in veterinary practice and as an agricultural and household insecticide.

◊ References.
1. Deltamethrin health and safety guide. *IPCS Health and Safety Guide 30.* Geneva: WHO, 1989.
2. Deltamethrin. *Environmental Health Criteria 97.* Geneva: WHO, 1990.

Preparations

Proprietary Preparations (details are given in Part 3)
Braz.: Deltacid; Hexafen; *Mex.:* Difexon.

Multi-ingredient: *Braz.:* Deltacid Plus; Nopucid Composto.

Dibromochloropropane (12642-e)

1,2-Dibromo-3-chloropropane.
$C_3H_5Br_2Cl = 236.3.$
CAS — 96-12-8.

Profile
Dibromochloropropane has been used as a pesticide. Low sperm counts and evidence of testicular damage have occurred in workers exposed to dibromochloropropane.

Dibutyl Phthalate (2553-k)

Butyl Phthalate; DBP. Dibutyl benzene-1,2-dicarboxylate.
$C_{16}H_{22}O_4 = 278.3.$
CAS — 84-74-2.
Pharmacopoeias. In Eur. (see p.vi).

Pharmacopoeial description
Ph. Eur.: A clear, oily, colourless or very slightly yellow liquid. Practically insoluble in water; miscible with alcohol and with ether. Store in airtight containers.

Adverse Effects and Precautions
Dibutyl phthalate has occasionally caused hypersensitivity reactions. As with other phthalates contact with plastics should be avoided.

Uses and Administration
Dibutyl phthalate has been used as an insect repellent although it is slightly less effective than dimethyl phthalate (p.1431). It is less volatile and less easily removed by washing than dimethyl phthalate, and its chief use therefore has been for the impregnation of clothing.

Dibutyl phthalate has also been employed as a plasticiser.

Preparations
Proprietary Preparations (details are given in Part 3)
Multi-ingredient: *S.Afr.:* Mylol†.

Dichlorophenoxyacetic Acid (3576-s)

2,4-D. 2,4-Dichlorophenoxyacetic acid.
$C_8H_6Cl_2O_3 = 221.0.$
CAS — 94-75-7.

Adverse Effects, Treatment, and Precautions
Most cases of poisoning with dichlorophenoxyacetic acid have involved its ingestion with other herbicides; the solvent may also play a part in any toxicity. There is little pattern to the range of adverse effects which may occur following ingestion, inhalation, or topical exposure.

Observed adverse effects have involved the central and peripheral nervous system, muscles, and the cardiovascular system. Gastrointestinal effects are common with poisoning. Hepatotoxicity, nephrotoxicity, and pulmonary disorders have been observed but it is not clear that dichlorophenoxyacetic acid contributed to the toxicity. The role of phenoxyacetic acids in cancer is discussed under trichlorophenoxyacetic acid (p.1437).

Ingested material should be removed by lavage. Contaminated clothing should be removed and the skin washed with soap and water. Forced alkaline diuresis or haemodialysis has been reported to be effective in removing dichlorophenoxyacetic acid. Further treatment is symptomatic.

◊ References.
1. 2,4-Dichlorophenoxyacetic acid (2,4-D). *Environmental Health Criteria 29.* Geneva: WHO, 1984.
2. 2,4-Dichlorophenoxyacetic acid (2,4-D)—environmental aspects. *Environmental Health Criteria 84.* Geneva: WHO, 1989.
3. Bradberry SM, *et al.* Mechanisms of toxicology, clinical features, and management of acute chlorophenoxy herbicide poisoning: a review. *J Toxicol Clin Toxicol* 2000; **38:** 111–22.

Uses
Dichlorophenoxyacetic acid is a herbicide widely used for weed control in cereals and other crops. It is usually used as its salts or esters in combination with other herbicides.

Dichlorvos (3577-w)

Dichlorvos *(BAN, USAN, rINN).*
DDVP; NSC-6738; OMS-14; SD-1750. 2,2-Dichlorovinyl dimethyl phosphate.
$C_4H_7Cl_2O_4P = 221.0.$
CAS — 62-73-7.
Pharmacopoeias. In Fr. for veterinary use.

Profile
Dichlorvos is an organophosphorus insecticide (p.1435) of short persistence, effective against a wide range of insects. It is sometimes used as a fumigant. It has been used for the extermi-

nation of insects in aircraft (disinsection). It is also used as a topical ectoparasiticide and as an anthelmintic in veterinary practice.

◊ References.
1. Dichlorvos health and safety guide. *IPCS Health and Safety Guide 18.* Geneva: WHO, 1988.
2. Dichlorvos. *Environmental Health Criteria 79.* Geneva: WHO, 1989.

Dieldrin (3579-l)

Dieldrin *(BAN, pINN).*
CAS — 60-57-1 (HEOD).

Dieldrin contains about 85% of (1R,4S,5S,8R)-1,2,3,4,10,10-hexachloro-6,7-epoxy-1,4,4a,5,6,7,8,8a-octahydro-1,4:5,8-dimethanonaphthalene (HEOD), $C_{12}H_8Cl_6O = 380.9.$ The remaining 15% is mainly chlorinated organic compounds related to HEOD.

Adverse Effects and Treatment
As for Chlorinated Insecticides, p.1429.

Dieldrin is more toxic than clofenotane (p.1430) and is readily absorbed through the skin.

◊ References.
1. Aldrin and dieldrin. *Environmental Health Criteria 91.* Geneva: WHO, 1989.
2. Aldrin and dieldrin health and safety guide. *IPCS Health and Safety Guide 21.* Geneva: WHO, 1989.
3. Høyer AP, *et al.* Organochlorine exposure and risk of breast cancer. *Lancet* 1998; **352:** 1816–20.

Uses
Dieldrin is a chlorinated insecticide (p.1429) formerly used as a sheepdip. Its use is now limited to a few specified purposes such as termite control.

Diethyltoluamide (2554-a)

Diethyltoluamide *(BAN, rINN).*
DEET. NN-Diethyl-m-toluamide.
$C_{12}H_{17}NO = 191.3.$
CAS — 134-62-3.
ATC — P03BX01.
Pharmacopoeias. In US.

Pharmacopoeial description
USP 25: A colourless liquid with a faint pleasant odour. Practically insoluble in water and in glycerol; miscible with alcohol, with carbon disulfide, with chloroform, with ether, and with isopropyl alcohol. Store in airtight containers.

Adverse Effects and Precautions
Occasional hypersensitivity to diethyltoluamide has been reported. Diethyltoluamide should not be applied near the eyes, to mucous membranes, to broken skin, or to areas of skin flexion as irritation or blistering may occur. Systemic toxicity has been reported following application of large topical doses, particularly in children.

◊ Hypersensitivity and anaphylaxis has been described in a patient after exposure to diethyltoluamide.[1] Toxic encephalopathy has been noted in children who received liberal applications of this compound;[2] seizures have also been reported,[3] and there have been cases of manic psychosis[4] and cardiovascular toxicity (sinus bradycardia and orthostatic hypotension)[5] associated with topical application. However, an assessment[6] of both published and unpublished data concluded that there had been remarkably few problems considering the widespread use of diethyltoluamide and that the encephalopathy in children had not been substantiated by detailed surveillance.

Toxic reactions, including death, have been reported following the ingestion of large amounts of diethyltoluamide-containing insect repellents.[7]

1. Miller JD. Anaphylaxis associated with insect repellent. *N Engl J Med* 1982; **307:** 1341–2.
2. Roland EH, *et al.* Toxic encephalopathy in a child after brief exposure to insect repellents. *Can Med Assoc J* 1985; **132:** 155–6.
3. Anonymous. Seizures temporally associated with use of DEET insect repellent—New York and Connecticut. *Arch Dermatol* 1989; **125:** 1619–20.
4. Snyder JW, *et al.* Acute manic psychosis following the dermal application of N,N-diethyl-m-toluamide (DEET) in an adult. *J Toxicol Clin Toxicol* 1986; **24:** 429–39.
5. Clem JR, *et al.* Insect repellent (N,N-diethyl-m-toluamide) cardiovascular toxicity in an adult. *Ann Pharmacother* 1993; **27:** 289–93.
6. Goodyer L, Behrens RH. Short report: the safety and toxicity of insect repellents. *Am J Trop Med Hyg* 1998; **59:** 323–4.
7. Tenenbein M. Severe toxic reactions and death following the ingestion of diethyltoluamide-containing insect repellents. *JAMA* 1987; **258:** 1509–11.

Uses
Diethyltoluamide is an insect repellent which is effective against mosquitoes as well as blackflies, harvest-bugs or chiggers, midges, ticks, and fleas. It is considered to be of value for personal protection against malaria (p.428). It has also been used as a repellent against leeches. It may be applied to skin and clothing.

Preparations
USP 25: Diethyltoluamide Topical Solution.

Proprietary Preparations (details are given in Part 3)
Fr.: Insect Ecran; Item Antipoux; Moskizol; *Ger.:* Autan†; *Ital.:* Zanzipik; *S.Afr.:* Mylol†; *UK:* Bens; Bug Guards; Dusk†; Jungle Formula Insect Repellent; Mijex; Ultrathon.

Multi-ingredient: *Canad.:* Muskol; *Fr.:* Tiq'Aouta; *Hong Kong:* Pellit; *Israel:* Yatushan Plus; *Ital.:* Cruzzy; Entom; *S.Afr.:* Mylol†; No-Bite; *Thai.:* Pellit; *UK:* Jungle Formula Insect Repellent Plus U.V. Sunscreens.

Difenacoum (3864-k)

3-(3-Biphenyl-4-yl-1,2,3,4-tetrahydro-1-naphthyl)-4-hydroxycoumarin.
$C_{31}H_{24}O_3 = 444.5.$
CAS — 56073-07-5.

Profile
Difenacoum is an anticoagulant rodenticide.

Toxicity. Difenacoum, a second-generation anticoagulant rodenticide inhibits prothrombin synthesis to cause bleeding that may be occult.[1,2] It is absorbed from the gastrointestinal tract; dermal absorption is possible. Poisons containing 100 mg per kg of bait are not hazardous to man; more concentrated forms are particularly hazardous and their availability should be restricted. Baits, which should be prepared only by trained personnel, should contain a suitable marker-dye.

There have been reports of poisoning with difenacoum.[3-5]
1. WHO. Safe use of pesticides: ninth report of the WHO expert committee on vector biology and control. *WHO Tech Rep Ser 720* 1985.
2. Anticoagulant rodenticides. *Environmental Health Criteria 175.* Geneva: WHO, 1995.
3. Barlow AM, *et al.* Difenacoum (Neosorexa) poisoning. *BMJ* 1982; **285:** 541.
4. Butcher GP, *et al.* Difenacoum poisoning as a cause of haematuria. *Hum Exp Toxicol* 1992; **11:** 553–4.
5. McCarthy PT, *et al.* Covert poisoning with difenacoum: clinical and toxicological observations. *Hum Exp Toxicol* 1997; **16:** 166–70.

Diflubenzuron (18066-x)

1-(4-Chlorophenyl)-3-(2,6-difluorobenzoyl)urea.
$C_{14}H_9ClF_2N_2O_2 = 310.7.$
CAS — 35367-38-5.

Profile
Diflubenzuron is an insecticide and larvicide that acts as a growth regulator by interfering with the formation of cuticle. It is used in agriculture and for the control of disease vectors.

Diflubenzuron possesses residual activity against mosquito larvae.

Dimethoate (11646-q)

Fosfamid. O,O-Dimethyl S-methylcarbamoylmethyl phosphorodithioate.
$C_5H_{12}NO_3PS_2 = 229.3.$
CAS — 60-51-5.

Profile
Dimethoate is an organophosphorus insecticide (p.1435) used in agriculture.

◊ References.
1. Dimethoate health and safety guide. *IPCS Health and Safety Guide 20.* Geneva: WHO, 1988.
2. Dimethoate. *Environmental Health Criteria 90.* Geneva: WHO, 1989.
3. Jovanović D, *et al.* A case of unusual suicidal poisoning by the organophosphorus insecticide dimethoate. *Hum Exp Toxicol* 1990; **9:** 49–51.

Dimethyl Phthalate (2555-t)

DMP; Methyl Phthalate. Dimethyl benzene-1,2-dicarboxylate.
$C_{10}H_{10}O_4 = 194.2.$
CAS — 131-11-3.
Pharmacopoeias. In Br. and Fr.

Pharmacopoeial description
BP 2001: A colourless or faintly coloured liquid, odourless or almost odourless. Slightly soluble in water; miscible with alcohol, with ether, and with most organic solvents.

Adverse Effects and Precautions
Dimethyl phthalate may cause temporary smarting and should not be applied near the eyes or to mucous membranes. As with other phthalates contact with plastics should be avoided.

Uses
Dimethyl phthalate is an insect repellent.

Preparations
Proprietary Preparations (details are given in Part 3)
Multi-ingredient: *Fr.:* Tiq'Aouta; *Hong Kong:* Pellit; *Israel:* Yatushan Plus; *S.Afr.:* Mylol†; *Thai.:* Pellit.

The symbol † denotes a preparation no longer actively marketed

Dimpylate (18132-j)

Dimpylate (BAN, rINN).

Diazinon. O,O-Diethyl O-(2-isopropyl-6-methylpyrimidin-4-yl) phosphorothioate.

$C_{12}H_{21}N_2O_3PS = 304.3$.

CAS — 333-41-5.

Pharmacopoeias. In BP(Vet).

Pharmacopoeial description

BP(Vet) 2001: A clear, yellowish-brown, slightly viscous liquid. Practically insoluble in water; miscible with alcohol, with ether, and with most organic solvents.

Profile

Dimpylate is an organophosphorus insecticide (p.1435) used as a systemic ectoparasiticide in veterinary practice; it is applied topically to the host animal. It is also employed as an insecticide in agriculture and horticulture.

◊ References.
1. Wagner SL, Orwick DL. Chronic organophosphate exposure associated with transient hypertonia in an infant. *Pediatrics* 1994; **94:** 94–7.

Dinitro-o-cresol (18085-d)

DNOC. 4,6-Dinitro-o-cresol.

$C_7H_6N_2O_5 = 198.1$.

CAS — 534-52-1.

Profile

Dinitro-o-cresol is a dinitrophenol formerly used as an insecticide and a herbicide. It increases metabolism by uncoupling oxidative phosphorylation and was also formerly used in obesity. Fatal poisoning has occurred.

Dinitrophenol (3580-v)

2,4-Dinitrophenol.

$C_6H_4N_2O_5 = 184.1$.

CAS — 51-28-5.

Profile

Dinitrophenol has been used as a herbicide. Since dinitrophenol increases metabolism by uncoupling oxidative phosphorylation it was formerly used in the treatment of obesity. Fatal poisoning has occurred.

Dioctyl Adipate (19235-g)

DEHA; Di-(2-ethylhexyl)adipate.

$C_{22}H_{42}O_4 = 370.6$.

Profile

Dioctyl adipate is used as an insect repellent. It is also used as a plasticiser by the plastics industry; concern about the migration of this and other plasticisers into foodstuffs from polythene films used to wrap them ('cling film') have led to its use at lower concentrations.

Preparations

Proprietary Preparations (details are given in Part 3)

UK: Protec.

Dioxation (3581-g)

Dioxation (BAN, rINN).

Dioxathion. It consists mainly of cis and trans isomers of S,S'-1,4-dioxan-2,3-diyl bis(O,O-diethyl phosphorodithioate).

$C_{12}H_{26}O_6P_2S_4 = 456.5$.

CAS — 78-34-2.

Profile

Dioxation is an organophosphorus insecticide (p.1435) that has been used in agriculture and as a topical ectoparasiticide in veterinary practice.

Diphenadione (4812-y)

Diphenadione (BAN, pINN).

Diphacinone. 2-(Diphenylacetyl)indan-1,3-dione.

$C_{23}H_{16}O_3 = 340.4$.

CAS — 82-66-6.

ATC — B01AA10.

Profile

Diphenadione is used as an anticoagulant rodenticide.

Diquat Dibromide (3584-s)

9,10-Dihydro-8a,10a-diazoniaphenanthrene dibromide; 1,1'-Ethylene-2,2'-bipyridyldiylium dibromide.

$C_{12}H_{12}Br_2N_2 = 344.0$.

CAS — 2764-72-9 (diquat); 85-00-7 (diquat dibromide).

Profile

Diquat dibromide is a contact herbicide used in agriculture and horticulture. It has similar adverse effects to those of paraquat (p.1435).

◊ References.
1. Paraquat and diquat. *Environmental Health Criteria 39.* Geneva: WHO, 1984.
2. Proudfoot A, ed. Pesticide poisoning: notes for the guidance of medical practitioners. 2nd ed. London: DoH, The Stationery Office, 1996.
3. Jones GM, Vale JA. Mechanisms of toxicity, clinical features, and management of diquat poisoning: a review. *J Toxicol Clin Toxicol* 2000; **38:** 123–8.

Emamectin (20772-r)

A mixture of (4″-R)-5-O-Demethyl-4″-deoxy-4″-(methylamino)avermectin A_{1a} and (4″-R)-5-O-Demethyl-25-de(1-methylpropyl)-4″-deoxy-4″-(methylamino)-25-(1-methylethyl)avermectin A_{1a} in the ratio of 9:1.

CAS — 121124-29-6 (major component); 121424-52-0 (minor component); 137335-79-6.

Profile

Emamectin is an avermectin insecticide used for the control of sea-lice infestation in salmon.

Endod (19131-r)

Profile

Endod is obtained from the dried fruits of *Phytolacca dodecandra* (Phytolaccaceae) and has molluscicidal properties. It has been investigated for the control of the snail vector of schistosomiasis.

◊ References.
1. Goldsmith MF. Out of Africa comes the fruit of long research: possible self-reliant control of schistosomiasis. *JAMA* 1991; **265:** 2650–1.

Endosulfan (18067-r)

1,4,5,6,7,7-Hexachloro-8,9,10-trinorborn-5-en-2,3-ylenebismethylene sulphite.

$C_9H_6Cl_6O_3S = 406.9$.

CAS — 115-29-7.

Profile

Endosulfan is a chlorinated insecticide (p.1429) used in agriculture.

◊ References.
1. Endosulfan. *Environmental Health Criteria 40.* Geneva: WHO, 1984.
2. Endosulfan health and safety guide. *IPCS Health and Safety Guide 17.* Geneva: WHO, 1988.
3. Blanco-Coronado JL, et al. Acute intoxication by endosulfan. *J Toxicol Clin Toxicol* 1992; **30:** 575–83.
4. Boereboom FT, et al. Nonaccidental endosulfan intoxication: a case report with toxicokinetic calculations and tissue concentrations. *J Toxicol Clin Toxicol* 1998; **36:** 345–52.
5. Chugh SN, et al. Endosulfan poisoning in Northern India: a report of 18 cases. *Int J Clin Pharmacol Ther* 1998; **36:** 474–7.

Endrin (18068-f)

(1R,4S,4aS,5S,6S,7R,8R,8aR)-1,2,3,4,10,10-Hexachloro-1,4,4a,5,6,7,8,8a-octahydro-6,7-epoxy-1,4:5,8-dimethanonaphthalene.

$C_{12}H_8Cl_6O = 380.9$.

CAS — 72-20-8.

Profile

Endrin is a chlorinated insecticide (p.1429), but its use was prohibited, at least in some countries, because of toxicity and persistence in the environment.

◊ General references to endrin,[1-4] including reports of poisoning.[2,3]
1. Anonymous. Acute convulsions associated with endrin poisoning—Pakistan. *JAMA* 1985; **253:** 334–5.
2. Runhaar EA, et al. A case of fatal endrin poisoning. *Hum Toxicol* 1985; **4:** 241–7.
3. Endrin health and safety guide. *IPCS Health and Safety Guide 60.* Geneva: WHO, 1991.
4. Endrin. *Environmental Health Criteria 130.* Geneva: WHO, 1992.

Esdepallethrine (13425-w)

(S)-3-Allyl-2-methyl-4-oxocyclopent-2-enyl (1R,3R)-2,2-dimethyl-3-(2-methylprop-1-enyl)-cyclopropanecarboxylate.

$C_{19}H_{26}O_3 = 302.4$.

CAS — 28434-00-6.

Profile

Esdepallethrine is a pyrethroid insecticide (p.1436). It is employed as an acaricide in combination with piperonyl butoxide (p.1436) in the topical treatment of scabies (p.1427).

Esdepallethrine is also used in devices and sprays to control insects, including mosquitoes.

Preparations

Proprietary Preparations (details are given in Part 3)

Multi-ingredient: Canad.: Scabene; **Fr.:** A-Par; Acardust; Spregal; **Israel:** Acardust; **Ital.:** Acardust; **S.Afr.:** Spregal; **Switz.:** Acardust†.

Ethion (18138-x)

Diethion. O,O,O',O'-Tetraethyl S,S'-methylenediphosphorodithioate.

$C_9H_{22}O_4P_2S_4 = 384.5$.

CAS — 563-12-2.

Profile

Ethion is an organophosphorus insecticide used as a topical ectoparasiticide in veterinary practice.

Ethohexadiol (2556-x)

Ethylhexanediol. 2-Ethylhexane-1,3-diol.

$C_8H_{18}O_2 = 146.2$.

CAS — 94-96-2.

Profile

Ethohexadiol is an insect repellent. It may be applied topically to the skin and to clothing. It has been used in conjunction with dimethyl phthalate.

Preparations

Proprietary Preparations (details are given in Part 3)

Fr.: Insect Ecran.

Ethylene Dibromide (12710-q)

EDB. 1,2-Dibromoethane.

$C_2H_4Br_2 = 187.9$.

CAS — 106-93-4.

Profile

Ethylene dibromide is an insecticidal fumigant and a lead scavenger used in the petroleum industry. Its use has been restricted in certain areas because of carcinogenicity in *animals* and because of evidence of persistence in fruit and cereals that have undergone fumigation.

Ethylene dibromide is more toxic than carbon tetrachloride or ethylene dichloride. It is irritant to the eyes, skin, and mucous membranes. Inhalation leads to drowsiness, CNS depression, and possibly pulmonary oedema. Contact with the skin causes blistering and it is readily absorbed. Kidney and liver damage may occur.

◊ Reports of poisoning due to ethylene dibromide.
1. Letz GA, et al. Two fatalities after acute occupational exposure to ethylene dibromide. *JAMA* 1984; **252:** 2428–31.
2. Singh S, et al. Non-fatal ethylene dibromide ingestion. *Hum Exp Toxicol* 2000; **19:** 152–3.

Ethylene Dichloride (12711-p)

Brocide; Dutch Liquid. 1,2-Dichloroethane.

$C_2H_4Cl_2 = 98.96$.

CAS — 107-06-2.

Profile

Ethylene dichloride is an insecticidal fumigant. It is also used in the petroleum industry and as an industrial solvent. Exposure to the vapour may cause lachrymation and corneal clouding, nasal irritation, and vertigo due to the depressant effect on the CNS. Contact with the skin may cause dermatitis. Kidney and liver damage, hypotension and cardiac impairment, gastrointestinal disturbances, haemorrhage, coma, and pulmonary oedema may follow absorption after inhalation, topical application, or ingestion.

Ethylene dichloride has been reported to be carcinogenic in *animals*.

◊ References.
1. 1,2 Dichloroethane. *Environmental Health Criteria 62.* Geneva: WHO, 1987.
2. 1,2-Dichloroethane health and safety guide. *IPCS Health and Safety Guide 55.* Geneva: WHO, 1991.
3. Proudfoot A, ed. Pesticide poisoning: notes for the guidance of medical practitioners. 2nd ed. London: DoH, The Stationery Office, 1996.

Famphur (20580-y)

Famophos.

$C_{10}H_{16}NO_5PS_2 = 325.3$.

CAS — 52-85-7.

Profile

Famphur is an organophosphorus insecticide (p.1435) used as a systemic ectoparasiticide in veterinary practice; it is applied topically to the host animal.

Fenitrothion (18142-c)

Fenitrothion *(BAN)*.

O,O-Dimethyl *O*-4-nitro-*m*-tolyl phosphorothioate.

$C_9H_{12}NO_5PS = 277.2$.

CAS — 122-14-5.

Profile
Fenitrothion is an organophosphorus insecticide (p.1435) used as a topical ectoparasiticide in veterinary practice. It is also used as an agricultural insecticide.

◊ References.
1. Fenitrothion. *Environmental Health Criteria 133.* Geneva: WHO, 1992.
2. Bouma MJ, Nesbit R. Fenitrothion intoxication during spraying operations in the malaria programme for Afghan refugees in North West Frontier Province of Pakistan. *Trop Geogr Med* 1995; **47:** 12–14.

Fenthion (3586-e)

Fenthion *(BAN)*.

Bayer-29493; S-752. *O,O*-Dimethyl *O*-4-methylthio-*m*-tolyl phosphorothioate.

$C_{10}H_{15}O_3PS_2 = 278.3$.

CAS — 55-38-9.

Pharmacopoeias. In BP(Vet).

Pharmacopoeial description
BP(Vet) 2001: A yellowish-brown oily substance. Immiscible with water; miscible with alcohol and with chloroform.

Profile
Fenthion is an organophosphorus insecticide (p.1435) used as a systemic ectoparasiticide in veterinary practice; it is applied topically to the host animal. Fenthion has also been used in agriculture.

Toxicity. Macular changes have been detected in the eyes of workers regularly exposed to fenthion.[1] It was considered that there was a need for long-term studies on subjects exposed to different organophosphorus compounds to assess their role in producing macular changes.
1. Misra UK, *et al.* Some observations on the macula of pesticide workers. *Hum Toxicol* 1985; **4:** 135–45.

Fenvalerate (11799-n)

Fenvalerate *(BAN)*.

(RS)-α-Cyano-3-phenoxybenzyl *(RS)*-2-(4-chlorophenyl)-3-methylbutyrate.

$C_{25}H_{22}ClNO_3 = 419.9$.

CAS — 51630-58-1.

Profile
Fenvalerate is a pyrethroid insecticide (p.1436) used as a topical ectoparasiticide in veterinary practice. It has also been used as an insecticide in agriculture and horticulture.

Esfenvalerate, one of the stereoisomers of fenvalerate, is also used as an agricultural insecticide.

Fipronil (672-p)

Fipronil *(BAN)*.

MB-46030; RM-1601. *(RS)*-5-Amino-1-(2,6-dichloro-4-trifluoromethylphenyl)-4-(trifluoromethylsulfinyl)pyrazole-3-carbonitrile.

$C_{12}H_4Cl_2F_6N_4OS = 437.1$.

CAS — 120068-37-3.

Profile
Fipronil is used as a topical ectoparasiticide in veterinary practice.

Flocoumafen (3073-s)

Flocoumafene; OMS-3047. 4-Hydroxy-3-[1,2,3,4-tetrahydro-3-[4-(4-trifluoromethylbenzyloxy)phenyl]-1-naphthyl]coumarin.

$C_{33}H_{25}F_3O_4 = 542.5$.

CAS — 90035-08-8.

Profile
Flocoumafen is a coumarin derivative used as an anticoagulant rodenticide. It is said to be effective in rodents resistant to other anticoagulant rodenticides.

◊ References.
1. Anticoagulant rodenticides. *Environmental Health Criteria 175.* Geneva: WHO, 1995.

Fluazuron (15426-b)

Fluazuron *(rINN)*.

CGA-157419. 1-(4-Chloro-3-{[3-chloro-5-(trifluoromethyl)-2-pyridyl]oxy}phenyl)-3-(2,6-difluorobenzoyl)urea.

$C_{20}H_{10}Cl_2F_5N_3O_3 = 506.2$.

CAS — 86811-58-7.

The symbol † denotes a preparation no longer actively marketed

Profile
Fluazuron is used as a topical ectoparasiticide in veterinary practice.

Flumethrin (15321-a)

Flumethrin *(BAN)*.

α-Cyano-4-fluoro-3-phenoxybenzyl 3-(β,4-dichlorostyryl)-2,2-dimethylcyclopropanecarboxylate.

$C_{28}H_{22}Cl_2FNO_3 = 510.4$.

CAS — 69770-45-2.

Profile
Flumethrin is a pyrethroid insecticide (p.1436) used as a topical ectoparasiticide in veterinary practice.

◊ Reports of poisoning with flumethrin.
1. Box SA, Lee MR. A systemic reaction following exposure to a pyrethroid insecticide. *Hum Exp Toxicol* 1996; **15:** 389–90.

Fluoroacetamide (7731-y)

Compound 1081.

$FCH_2.CONH_2 = 77.06$.

CAS — 640-19-7.

Profile
Fluoroacetamide is a rodenticide and produces adverse effects similar to those of sodium fluoroacetate (p.1437).

Fluvalinate (3885-f)

ZR-3210. Cyano(3-phenoxyphenyl)methyl ester of *N*-[2-chloro-4-(trifluoromethyl)phenyl]-DL-valine.

$C_{26}H_{22}ClF_3N_2O_3 = 502.9$.

CAS — 69409-94-5.

Profile
Fluvalinate is a pesticide used in beekeeping.

Glyphosate (11805-g)

N-(Phosphonomethyl)glycine.

$C_3H_8NO_5P = 169.1$.

CAS — 1071-83-6.

Profile
Glyphosate is used as a herbicide.

Toxicity. Reports of poisoning with glyphosate products[1-3] and guidelines for treatment[4] have been published. The toxicity has been believed to be largely due to the inclusion of a surfactant, polyoxyethyleneamine, in the herbicide (Roundup) formulation.
1. Sawada Y, *et al.* Probable toxicity of surface-active agent in commercial herbicide containing glyphosate. *Lancet* 1988; **i:** 299.
2. Talbot AR, *et al.* Acute poisoning with a glyphosate-surfactant herbicide ('Roundup'): a review of 93 cases. *Hum Exp Toxicol* 1991; **10:** 1–8.
3. Menkes DB, *et al.* Intentional self-poisoning with glyphosate-containing herbicides. *Hum Exp Toxicol* 1991; **10:** 103–7.
4. Proudfoot A, ed. *Pesticide poisoning: notes for the guidance of medical practitioners.* 2nd ed. London: DoH, The Stationery Office, 1996.

Heptachlor (18074-x)

1,4,5,6,7,8,8-Heptachloro-3a,4,7,7a-tetrahydro-4,7-methanoindene.

$C_{10}H_5Cl_7 = 373.3$.

CAS — 76-44-8.

Profile
Heptachlor is a chlorinated insecticide (p.1429), but its use was prohibited, at least in some countries, because of its persistent nature.

◊ References.
1. Heptachlor. *Environmental Health Criteria 38.* Geneva: WHO, 1984.
2. Heptachlor health and safety guide. *IPCS Health and Safety Guide 14.* Geneva: WHO, 1988.

Heptenophos (18147-r)

Hoe-02982. 7-Chlorobicyclo[3.2.0]hepta-2,6-dien-6-yl dimethyl phosphate.

$C_9H_{12}ClO_4P = 250.6$.

CAS — 23560-59-0.

Profile
Heptenophos is an organophosphorus insecticide (p.1435) that has been used in veterinary practice for the control of ectoparasites. It is also used in agriculture.

Hexachlorobenzene (12823-c)

HCB.

$C_6Cl_6 = 284.8$.

CAS — 118-74-1.

NOTE. Hexachlorobenzene should not be confused with gamma benzene hexachloride (lindane).

Profile
Hexachlorobenzene has been used as an agricultural fungicide. It is not biodegradable to any significant extent and hexachlorobenzene residues in food have arisen as a result of its occurrence in industrial wastes as well as its use as a fungicide; its use is banned in some countries.

Hexachlorobenzene is reported to be distributed into breast milk.

Toxicity. Porphyria cutanea tarda[1] and parkinsonism[2] have both been reported in subjects who had ingested seed crops treated with hexachlorobenzene. In a further report the symptoms of porphyria in some patients have been said to persist for many years.[3]
1. Cam C, Nigogosyan G. Acquired toxic porphyria cutanea tarda due to hexachlorobenzene. *JAMA* 1963; **183:** 88–91.
2. Chapman LJ, *et al.* Parkinsonism and industrial chemicals. *Lancet* 1987; **i:** 332–3.
3. Cripps DJ, *et al.* Porphyria turcica due to hexachlorobenzene: a 20 to 30 year follow-up study on 204 patients. *Br J Dermatol* 1984; **111:** 413–22.

Hydrocyanic Acid (7751-k)

Prussic Acid.

CAS — 74-90-8.

An aqueous solution containing hydrogen cyanide, $HCN = 27.03$. A colourless liquid with a characteristic almond odour.

◊ CAUTION. *Hydrocyanic acid and its vapour are intensely poisonous.*

Adverse Effects and Precautions
Cyanides interfere with the oxygen uptake of cells by inhibition of cytochrome oxidase, an enzyme necessary for cellular oxygen transport.

Poisoning by cyanides may occur from inhalation of the vapour, ingestion, or absorption through the skin. Poisoning may arise from cyanide pesticides, industrial accidental exposure, or the inhalation of fumes from some burning plastics. Poisoning may also occur from cyanide-containing plants or fruits.

When large doses of hydrocyanic acid are taken, unconsciousness occurs within a few seconds and death within a few minutes. With smaller toxic doses the symptoms, which occur within a few minutes, may include constriction of the throat, nausea, vomiting, giddiness, headache, palpitation, hyperpnoea then dyspnoea, bradycardia (although initially there may be tachycardia), unconsciousness, and violent convulsions, followed by death. The characteristic smell of bitter almonds may not be obvious and not all individuals can detect it. Cyanosis is not prominent. Similar but usually slower effects occur with cyanide salts.

The fatal dose of hydrocyanic acid (HCN) for man is considered to be about 50 mg and of the cyanides about 250 mg.

Treatment of Adverse Effects
Treatment must be given rapidly but should not involve the use of antidotes unless it is certain that cyanide has been absorbed and poisoning is severe.

Cyanide is absorbed very rapidly on inhalation and the poisoned patient should be removed from the area and given oxygen. Steps should be taken to ensure that the airway is adequate. Contaminated clothing should be removed and skin washed. If the patient is conscious, amyl nitrite may be inhaled for up to 30 seconds in every minute but the value of this practice is questionable. Should the patient be unconscious or nearly so, then in the UK and some other countries it is the practice to give dicobalt edetate (p.1006) by injection since it forms a stable complex with the cyanide ion. However, cyanide poisoning should be confirmed, as absence of cyanide puts the patient at risk from the adverse effects of dicobalt edetate. The recommended dose of dicobalt edetate is 300 mg given intravenously over about 1 to 5 minutes, depending on the severity of the poisoning, and repeated once or twice depending on the response. It is customary to give 50 mL of glucose 50% intravenously after each injection, although the value of this has been questioned. An alternative treatment is to inject, as soon as possible, 10 mL of sodium nitrite injection (3%) intravenously over 3 to 5 minutes, then, using the same needle and vein, to continue with an injection of 12.5 g of sodium thiosulfate (50 mL of a 25% solution or 25 mL of a 50% solution) administered over a period of about 10 minutes. Sodium nitrite converts haemoglobin to methaemoglobin which competes with cytochrome oxidase for cyanide, with the formation of cyanmethaemoglobin; sodium thiosulfate aids the conversion or inactivation of cyanide from cyanmethaemoglobin to thiocyanate. If toxic symptoms recur, the injections of nitrite and thiosulfate may be repeated at half the initial doses. Appropriate measures should be instituted to correct hypotension and acidosis. Hydroxocobalamin has also been investigated in the management of cyanide toxicity.

If cyanide has been ingested, one of the above procedures should be instituted and the stomach then rapidly emptied by lavage.

◊ Some references concerning the management of cyanide poisoning.[1-3] The use of solutions A and B (15.8% ferrous sulfate in 0.3% citric acid, and 6% sodium carbonate respectively) as so-called oral antidotes in persons exposed to cyanide has been condemned as ineffective and lacking scientific evidence.[2]

1. Langford RM, Armstrong RF. Algorithm for managing injury from smoke inhalation. *BMJ* 1989; **299:** 902–5.
2. Koizumi A. Fighting myths. *Lancet* 1994; **344:** 559–60.
3. Proudfoot A, ed. *Pesticide poisoning: notes for the guidance of medical practitioners.* 2nd ed. London: DoH, The Stationery Office, 1996.

Uses
Cyanides have various industrial applications. Hydrocyanic acid and cyanide salts produce hydrogen cyanide which has been used as a gas for the eradication of rabbits, rodents, and some other pests. Cyanide salts that might be encountered include calcium cyanide, mercuric cyanide, potassium cyanide, potassium ferricyanide, potassium sodium cyanide, and sodium cyanide.

Preparations
Proprietary Preparations (details are given in Part 3)
Multi-ingredient: *Spain:* Oftalmol Dexa†; Oftalmol Ocular.

Imidacloprid   (8311-n)
Bay-NTN-33893.   1-[(6-Chloro-3-pyridinyl)methyl]-4,5-dihydro-N-nitro-1H-imidazol-2-amine.
$C_9H_{10}ClN_5O_2 = 255.7.$
CAS — 105827-78-9; 138261-41-3.

Profile
Imidacloprid is used as a topical ectoparasiticide in veterinary practice. It is also used as an insecticide in agriculture.

Iodofenphos   (3863-c)
Iodofenphos *(BAN)*.
Jodfenphos. *O*-2,5-Dichloro-4-iodophenyl *O,O*-dimethyl phosphorothioate.
$C_8H_8Cl_2IO_3PS = 413.0.$
CAS — 18181-70-9.

Profile
Iodofenphos is an organophosphorus insecticide (p.1435) used in veterinary practice for the control of ectoparasites in the environment. It has also been used as an agricultural insecticide. It is an effective mosquito larvicide.

Lindane   (3587-l)
Lindane *(BAN, USAN, rINN)*.
666; Benhexachlor; Gamma Benzene Hexachloride; Gamma-BHC; Gamma-HCH; HCH; Hexicide. 1α,2α,3β,4α,5α,6β-Hexachlorocyclohexane.
$C_6H_6Cl_6 = 290.8.$
CAS — 58-89-9.
ATC — P03AB02.
Pharmacopoeias. In Eur. (see p.vi), *Int.*, and *US.*

Pharmacopoeial description
Ph. Eur.: A white or almost white crystalline powder. Practically insoluble in water; soluble in dehydrated alcohol; freely soluble in acetone and in ether. Protect from light.

USP 25: A white, crystalline powder with a slight musty odour. Practically insoluble in water; soluble in dehydrated alcohol; freely soluble in chloroform; sparingly soluble in ether; slightly soluble in ethylene glycol.

Adverse Effects, Treatment, and Precautions
As for Chlorinated Insecticides, p.1429.

There has been some concern over the application of higher than normal concentrations of lindane to the skin in the treatment of scabies and pediculosis; children are considered to be particularly at risk. Resistance has limited its use in pediculosis, so children with that infection tend not to be exposed to it anyway. However, use has continued in scabies and here treatment should be avoided in young children and in women who are breast feeding or are pregnant. Lindane should also be avoided in patients who have a low body-weight or a history of epilepsy.

◊ Seizures have been reported following the topical use of lindane.[1] In reply, one of the manufacturers stated that up to the end of 1983 they were aware of 21 cases of convulsive disorders apparently associated with the use of their product; it had been used by over 40 million people. Of the 21 cases, the seizures were definitely or probably caused by the product in 11, but in 9 cases the seizures were associated with ingestion or excessive use.[2]

Isolated reports of adverse effects associated with lindane include disseminated intravascular coagulation and subsequent

death after oral ingestion[3] and aplastic anaemia after prolonged topical exposure (twice daily application for three weeks).[4]

1. Etherington JD. Major epileptic seizures and topical gammabenzene hexachloride. *BMJ* 1984; **289:** 228.
2. Kelly VT. Major epileptic seizures and topical gammabenzene hexachloride. *BMJ* 1984; **289:** 837.
3. Rao CVSR, *et al.* Disseminated intravascular coagulation in a case of fatal lindane poisoning. *Vet Hum Toxicol* 1988; **30:** 132–4.
4. Rauch AE, *et al.* Lindane (Kwell)-induced aplastic anemia. *Arch Intern Med* 1990; **150:** 2393–5.

Uses and Administration
Lindane is a chlorinated insecticide (p.1429). It has been used topically in a concentration of 1% for scabies (p.1427) in selected patients and has also been used in pediculosis (p.1427), but use for head lice is restricted by resistance.

Lindane has been used for the control of disease vectors including mosquitoes, lice, and fleas, but resistance has developed. It has also been used as an agricultural and a horticultural insecticide, but its use is prohibited or restricted in many countries.

Preparations
USP 25: Lindane Cream; Lindane Lotion; Lindane Shampoo.

Proprietary Preparations (details are given in Part 3)
Aust.: Jacutin; *Belg.:* Quellada†; *Braz.:* Escabin; Lendianon; Lindanoxil; Pediletan; Pilensar; Piodrex; Pioletal; Pionax; Plurisan; Pruritrat; Sarnapin; Sarpiol; *Canad.:* Hexit; Kwellada†; *Fr.:* Aphtiria†; Elentol; Scabecid; *Ger.:* Delitex N; Jacutin; Quellada H; *Irl.:* Quellada; *Israel:* Bicide; *Mex.:* Escarbicida; Herklin; Scabene; Scabisan; War Lin; *NZ:* Benhex; *Port.:* Musside†; Sarcoderma; *S.Afr.:* Gambex; Quellada; *Switz.:* Jacutin; *Thai.:* Jacutin; *USA:* G-well.

Multi-ingredient: *Braz.:* Lindanoxil; *Fr.:* Elenol; *Mex.:* Herklin; Scabisan Plus; *Spain:* Sudosin; Yacutin.

Lufenuron   (15417-m)
Lufenuron *(BAN, rINN)*.
CGA-184699.   1-[2,5-Dichloro-4-(1,1,2,3,3,3-hexafluoropropoxy)phenyl]-3-(2,6-difluorobenzoyl)urea; *(RS)*-N-[2,5-Dichloro-4-(1,1,2,3,3,3-hexafluoropropoxy)phenylcarbamoyl]-2,6-difluorobenzamide.
$C_{17}H_8Cl_2F_8N_2O_3 = 511.2.$
CAS — 103055-07-8.

Profile
Lufenuron is used as a systemic ectoparasiticide in veterinary practice; it is given by mouth or injection to the host animal.

Malathion   (3590-q)
Malathion *(BAN)*.
Carbofos; Compound 4047; OMS-1. Diethyl 2-(dimethoxyphosphinothioylthio)succinate.
$C_{10}H_{19}O_6PS_2 = 330.4.$
CAS — 121-75-5.
ATC — P03AX03.
Pharmacopoeias. In Eur. (see p.vi) and *US.*

Pharmacopoeial description
Ph. Eur.: A clear, colourless or slightly yellowish liquid. It freezes at about 3°. Slightly soluble in water; miscible with alcohol, with acetone, with cyclohexane, and with vegetable oils. Store in airtight containers. Protect from light.

USP 25: A yellow to deep brown liquid with a characteristic odour. Congeals at about 2.9°. Slightly soluble in water; miscible with alcohols, with ethers, with esters, with ketones, with aromatic and alkylated aromatic hydrocarbons, and with vegetable oils. Store in airtight containers. Protect from light.

Stability. The manufacturers have reported that malathion is sensitive to heat and is degraded at temperatures above 30°.

Adverse Effects and Treatment
As for Organophosphorus Insecticides, p.1435.

Malathion is one of the safer organophosphorus insecticides but its toxicity may be increased by the presence of impurities.

◊ Acute renal insufficiency has been described in a patient associated with excessive exposure to a malathion spray.[1] The condition resolved without specific treatment. Renal toxicity had not previously been associated with organophosphorus pesticides. In a second case of acute poisoning,[2] due to ingestion of malathion, mild transient renal insufficiency and proteinuria, together with several other late complications including cardiac arrhythmias, pulmonary oedema and diffuse interstitial fibrosis, and muscle weakness due to peripheral neuropathy, were seen subsequent to recovery from the initial cholinergic toxicity.

1. Albright RK, *et al.* Malathion exposure associated with acute renal failure. *JAMA* 1983; **250:** 2469.
2. Dive A, *et al.* Unusual manifestations after malathion poisoning. *Hum Exp Toxicol* 1994; **13:** 271–4.

Uses and Administration
Malathion is an organophosphorus insecticide (p.1435). It is used in the treatment of head and pubic pediculosis (p.1427) and in scabies (p.1427); lotions of 0.5% and shampoos of 1% are commonly available. Lotions are generally preferred to shampoos as the contact time is longer. Aqueous lotions are preferred to treat pubic lice and scabies because alcoholic

lotions are irritant to excoriated skin and the genitalia; aqueous lotions may also be preferable in asthmatic subjects or children to avoid alcoholic fumes. Skin or hair treated with an alcohol-based preparation should be allowed to dry naturally.

Malathion is also used in veterinary practice, agriculture, and horticulture. It is widely used for adult and larval mosquito control although resistance occurs.

Preparations
USP 25: Malathion Lotion.

Proprietary Preparations (details are given in Part 3)
Austral.: Cleensheen; Lice Rid; *Belg.:* Prioderm; Radikal; *Denm.:* Prioderm; *Fin.:* Prioderm; *Fr.:* Prioderm; *Irl.:* Derbac-M; Prioderm; *Israel:* Prioderm; *Ital.:* Aftir Gel; *Neth.:* Noury Hoofdlotion†; Prioderm; *Norw.:* Prioderm; *NZ:* Derbac-M; Prioderm; *Port.:* Olicide†; *Singapore:* A-Lices; *Swed.:* Prioderm; *Switz.:* Lusap; Prioderm; *UK:* Derbac-M; Prioderm; Quellada-M; Suleo-M; *USA:* Ovide.

Multi-ingredient: *Belg.:* Para Plus; *Fr.:* Para Plus; *Israel:* Para Plus; *NZ:* Para Plus.

Metaldehyde   (3591-p)
$(C_2H_4O)_x.$
CAS — 9002-91-9.

A cyclic polymer of acetaldehyde.

Adverse Effects and Treatment
Symptoms of poisoning by metaldehyde may be delayed and include vomiting and diarrhoea, fever, drowsiness, convulsions, and coma. Death from respiratory failure may occur within 48 hours. Kidney and liver damage may occur.

Treatment is symptomatic, although lavage may be considered if ingestion was within the preceding hour.

◊ References.
1. Longstreth WT, Pierson DJ. Metaldehyde poisoning from slug bait ingestion. *West J Med* 1982; **137:** 134–7.
2. Proudfoot A, ed. *Pesticide poisoning: notes for the guidance of medical practitioners.* 2nd ed. London: DoH, The Stationery Office, 1996.

Uses
Metaldehyde is a molluscicide used in pellets against slugs and snails. It is an ingredient of some firelighters.

'Meta' is compressed metaldehyde which has been used as a solid fuel burning with a non-luminous carbon-free flame.

Methomyl   (18035-y)
S-Methyl N-(methylcarbamoyloxy)thioacetimidate.
$C_5H_{10}N_2O_2S = 162.2.$
CAS — 16752-77-5.

Profile
Methomyl is a carbamate insecticide (p.1429) that has been used in agriculture.

◊ Reports of poisoning with methomyl and its management.
1. Martinez-Chuecos J, *et al.* Management of methomyl poisoning. *Hum Exp Toxicol* 1990; **9:** 251–4.

Methoprene   (3592-s)
Methoprene *(rINN)*.
ZR-515.   Isopropyl   11-methoxy-3,7,11-trimethyldodeca-2(E),4(E)-dienoate.
$C_{19}H_{34}O_3 = 310.5.$
CAS — 40596-69-8.

Profile
Methoprene is an insect growth regulator which mimics the action of insect juvenile hormones and, if it is applied at the appropriate period of sensitivity, it causes death by preventing the transformation of larva to pupa. It is used against a variety of insects including fleas and mosquitoes. It is used in veterinary practice for the control of ectoparasites in the environment, rather than being applied to the animals themselves. It is also used in agriculture.

Preparations
Proprietary Preparations (details are given in Part 3)
Multi-ingredient: *Fr.:* Acarcid perles.

Methyl Bromide   (2257-s)
Bromomethane; Monobromomethane.
$CH_3Br = 94.94.$
CAS — 74-83-9.

Adverse Effects, Treatment, and Precautions
Methyl bromide is a vesicant. Toxic effects after inhalation or percutaneous absorption are mainly due to neurotoxicity and include dizziness, headache, nausea, blurred vision, weakness, ataxia, confusion, mania, hallucinations, mental depression, convulsions, pulmonary oedema, and coma. Renal and hepatic toxicity may also occur and death may be due to circulatory collapse or respiratory failure. Onset of symptoms may be preceded by a latent period. Concentrations of 1% or more

are irritant to the eyes. Treatment is symptomatic although dimercaprol or acetylcysteine therapy has been tried.

Rubber absorbs and retains methyl bromide and should not therefore be used in protective clothing.

◊ References to toxicity of methyl bromide including reports of poisoning.
1. Chavez CT, *et al.* Methyl bromide optic atrophy. *Am J Ophthalmol* 1985; **99**: 715–19.
2. Langard S, *et al.* Fatal accident resulting from methyl bromide poisoning after fumigation of a neighbouring house: leakage through sewage pipes. *J Appl Toxicol* 1996; **16**: 445–8.
3. De Haro L, *et al.* Central and peripheral neurotoxic effects of chronic methyl bromide intoxication. *J Toxicol Clin Toxicol* 1997; **35**: 29–34.
4. Michalodimitrakis MN, *et al.* Death following intentional methyl bromide poisoning: toxicological data and literature review. *Vet Hum Toxicol* 1997; **39**: 30–4.
5. Horowitz BZ, *et al.* An unusual exposure to methyl bromide leading to fatality. *J Toxicol Clin Toxicol* 1998; **36**: 353–7.

Uses
Methyl bromide has been used as an insecticidal fumigant for soil and some foodstuffs.

When supplied for fumigation it usually contains chloropicrin as a lachrymatory warning agent.

Methyl bromide has been used as a gaseous disinfectant; it has low antimicrobial activity but good penetrating power.

Methyl bromide was formerly used with carbon tetrachloride in some fire extinguishers. It has also been used as a refrigerant.

◊ General references.
1. Methyl bromide. *Environmental Health Criteria 166*. Geneva: WHO, 1995.

Naled (18164-f)
Bromchlophos. Dimethyl 1,2-dibromo-2,2-dichloroethyl phosphate.
$C_4H_7Br_2Cl_2O_4P = 380.8$.
CAS — 300-76-5.

Profile
Naled is an organophosphorus insecticide used as a topical ectoparasiticide in veterinary practice.

Naphthalene (3596-y)
Naphthalin.
$C_{10}H_8 = 128.2$.
CAS — 91-20-3.

Adverse Effects, Treatment, and Precautions
Ingestion of naphthalene can produce headache, nausea and vomiting, diarrhoea, profuse perspiration, dysuria, coma, and convulsions. Doses as low as 2 g have proved fatal to the small child. Treatment is symptomatic and includes emptying the stomach by lavage. The vapour is irritating to the eyes; chronic exposure has led to cataract formation. Haemolytic anaemia and haematuria leading to acute renal failure may occur particularly in persons with glucose-6-phosphate dehydrogenase deficiency. Blood transfusions may be required.

Pregnancy. Haemolytic anaemia in a neonate has been attributed to inhalation of naphthalene by the mother during the twenty-eighth week of gestation.[1]
1. Athanasion M, *et al.* Hemolytic anemia in a female newborn infant whose mother inhaled naphthalene before delivery. *J Pediatr* 1997; **130**: 680–1.

Uses
Naphthalene has been used in lavatory deodorant discs and in mothballs. It has also been used as a soil fumigant.

Norbormide (3597-j)
McN-1025. 5-[α-Hydroxy-α-(2-pyridyl)benzyl]-7-[α-(2-pyridyl)benzylidene]-8,9,10-trinorborn-5-ene-2,3-dicarboximide.
$C_{33}H_{25}N_3O_3 = 511.6$.
CAS — 991-42-4.

Profile
Norbormide is a selective rodenticide effective against most species of rats, in which it produces extreme irreversible peripheral vasoconstriction. It is not very toxic to other rodents.

Organophosphorus Insecticides (3564-v)
The organophosphorus or organophosphate insecticides may be esters, amides, or thiol derivatives of phosphoric, phosphonic, phosphorothioic, or phosphonothioic acids.

◊ References.
1. WHO. Organophosphorus insecticides: a general introduction. *Environmental Health Criteria 63*. Geneva: WHO, 1986.

Adverse Effects
Organophosphorus insecticides are potent cholinesterase inhibitors and can be very toxic. This inhibition results in both muscarinic and nicotinic effects with some central involvement.

Toxic effects may include abdominal cramps, nausea, vomiting, diarrhoea, pancreatitis, urinary incontinence, miosis or mydriasis, weakness, respiratory disturbances, lachrymation, increased salivation and sweating, bradycardia or tachycardia, hypotension or hypertension, cyanosis, muscular twitching, and convulsions. Some organophosphorus compounds cause delayed neuropathy. CNS symptoms include restlessness, anxiety, dizziness, confusion, coma, and depression of the respiratory or cardiovascular system. Patients may experience mental disturbances. Inhalation or external contact can cause local as well as systemic effects.

Repeated exposure may have a cumulative effect though the organophosphorus insecticides are, in contrast to the chlorinated insecticides, rapidly metabolised and excreted and are not appreciably stored in body tissues.

◊ References to the adverse effects and poisoning encountered with organophosphorus compounds such as insecticides (including sheepdips).
1. WHO. Safe use of pesticides: fourteenth report of the WHO expert committee on vector biology and control. *WHO Tech Rep Ser 813* 1991.
2. Proudfoot A, ed. *Pesticide poisoning: notes for the guidance of medical practitioners*. 2nd ed. London: DoH, The Stationery Office, 1996.
3. Minton NA, Murray VSG. A review of organophosphate poisoning. *Med Toxicol* 1988; **3**: 350–75.
4. Dunn MA, Sidell FR. Progress in medical defense against nerve agents. *JAMA* 1989; **262**: 649–52.
5. Karalliedde L, Senanayake N. Organophosphorus insecticide poisoning. *Br J Anaesth* 1989; **63**: 736–50.
6. Öztürk MA, *et al.* Anticholinesterase poisoning in Turkey—clinical, laboratory and radiologic evaluation of 269 cases. *Hum Exp Toxicol* 1990; **9**: 273–9.
7. Murray VSG, Volans GN. Management of injuries due to chemical weapons. *BMJ* 1991; **302**: 129–30.
8. Lotti M. Treatment of acute organophosphate poisoning. *Med J Aust* 1991; **154**: 51–5.
9. Casey P, Vale JA. Deaths from pesticide poisoning in England and Wales: 1945–1989. *Hum Exp Toxicol* 1994; **13**: 95–101.
10. Eyer P. Neuropsychopathological changes by organophosphorus compounds—a review. *Hum Exp Toxicol* 1995; **14**: 857–64.
11. Steenland K. Chronic neurological effects of organophosphate pesticides. *BMJ* 1996; **312**: 1312–13.
12. Brown AA, Brix KA. Review of health consequences from high-, intermediate-, and low-level exposure to organophosphorus nerve agents. *J Appl Toxicol* 1998; **18**: 393–408.

Treatment of Adverse Effects
Rapid treatment is essential. If organophosphorus insecticides have been ingested the stomach should be emptied by lavage. Contaminated clothing should be removed and the skin, including any areas contaminated by vomiting or hypersecretion, should receive copious and prolonged washing with soap and water. Contamination of the eye is treated by washing of the conjunctiva. The patient should be treated with atropine (see Poisoning, p.462) and either pralidoxime (p.1020) or obidoxime (p.1016) and symptomatic treatment should be instituted. Diazepam is sometimes given; it may be necessary to give it parenterally in moderate to severe poisoning to control muscle fasciculations and convulsions; oral administration in mild poisoning may be helpful in relieving anxiety. The patient should be observed for signs of deterioration due to delayed absorption.

Paraquat (3600-c)
1,1′-Dimethyl-4,4′-bipyridyldiylium ion.
$C_{12}H_{14}N_2 = 186.3$.
CAS — 4685-14-7.

Paraquat Dichloride (3601-k)
$C_{12}H_{14}Cl_2N_2 = 257.2$.
CAS — 1910-42-5.

Adverse Effects
Concentrated solutions of paraquat may cause irritation, inflammation, and possibly blistering of the skin, cracking and shedding of the nails, and delayed healing of cuts and wounds. It is not significantly absorbed from undamaged skin. A few fatalities have occurred following skin contact, but these appear to have been associated with prolonged contact and concentrated solutions.

Splashes in the eye cause severe inflammation, which may be delayed for 12 to 24 hours, corneal oedema, reduced visual acuity, and extensive superficial stripping of the corneal and conjunctival epithelium, which usually slowly heals. Inhalation of dust or spray may cause nasal bleeding.

Paraquat weedkillers available for use in domestic gardens contain 2.5% w/v paraquat, sometimes in association with other herbicides such as diquat. While this strength of paraquat can cause nausea and vomiting as well as some respiratory changes when ingested, it is not considered to be a lethal form.

Most of the cases of severe poisoning follow the ingestion or sometimes injection of the concentrated forms of paraquat herbicide (20% w/v), the distribution of which is restricted to agriculturalists and horticulturalists. In many cases this ingestion is intentional. It is considered that patients who ingest 20 to 40 mg per kg body-weight suffer moderate to severe poisoning; most, but not all, die up to about 2 or 3 weeks after ingestion. Severe acute poisoning occurs with ingestion of higher doses. The irritant effects of paraquat are reflected in oesophageal ulceration and gastrointestinal effects. There is widespread organ

damage, most notably involving the kidneys and lungs. In such poisoning death is virtually certain and occurs rapidly.

Preparations of paraquat may contain an emetic or a laxative and some contain a malodorous agent to deter ingestion.

◊ General references concerning paraquat toxicity and its treatment.
1. Paraquat and diquat. *Environmental Health Criteria 39*. Geneva: WHO, 1984.
2. Bismuth C, *et al.* Paraquat poisoning. *Drug Safety* 1990; **5**: 243–51.
3. Pond SM. Manifestations and management of paraquat poisoning. *Med J Aust* 1990; **152**: 256–9.
4. Paraquat Health and Safety Guide. *Health and Safety Guide 51*. Geneva: WHO, 1991.
5. WHO. Safe use of pesticides: fourteenth report of the WHO expert committee on vector biology and control. *WHO Tech Rep Ser 813* 1991.
6. Proudfoot A, ed. *Pesticide poisoning: notes for the guidance of medical practitioners*. 2nd ed. London: DoH, The Stationery Office, 1996.

Treatment of Adverse Effects
Following contact with paraquat, contaminated clothing should be removed and the skin washed with soap and water. The eyes, if splashed, should be irrigated; later topical therapy may involve the symptomatic use of antibacterials or corticosteroids.

There is no specific treatment for paraquat poisoning and the immediate aim is to remove or inactivate the paraquat. Initial management involves the oral administration of an adsorbent, preferably activated charcoal given in a dose of 100 g, together with a laxative, and followed by 50 g of charcoal every 4 hours until the charcoal is seen in the stool. Gastric lavage is considered to be of doubtful value. Fuller's earth and bentonite are alternative oral adsorbents. When none of these adsorbents is available, a suspension of clay or of uncontaminated soil should be considered if medical attention is likely to be delayed. A 30% suspension of Fuller's earth has been used in a dose of 200 to 500 mL every 2 hours for three doses. Alternatively a suspension of 7% bentonite may be employed. Magnesium sulfate or mannitol are used with Fuller's earth or bentonite in order to hasten bowel evacuation and prevent obstruction due to the adsorbent. Patients may require intensive supportive therapy, but oxygen should not be given initially as it appears to enhance the pulmonary toxicity of paraquat; however, it may be needed in later stages as part of palliative care.

Methods aimed at hastening elimination such as forced diuresis, peritoneal dialysis, haemodialysis, and haemoperfusion have been tried but the former two appear to be ineffective and results with the latter two methods have varied; no method is of proven value.

◊ For some general references concerning the treatment of paraquat toxicity, see under Adverse Effects, above.

Once paraquat has been absorbed, moderate to severe poisoning may result in acute renal failure, hepatitis, and pulmonary fibrosis; death may occur after 2 to 3 weeks. Pulse therapy with cyclophosphamide and methylprednisolone might be of benefit in such patients.[1]
1. Lin J-L, *et al.* Pulse therapy with cyclophosphamide and methylprednisolone in patients with moderate to severe paraquat poisoning: a preliminary report. *Thorax* 1996; **51**: 661–3.

Uses
Paraquat is a contact herbicide widely used as the dichloride in agriculture and horticulture. Liquid concentrates are supplied in the UK only to approved users.

Parathion (18168-m)
O,O-Diethyl O-4-nitrophenyl phosphorothioate.
$C_{10}H_{14}NO_5PS = 291.3$.
CAS — 56-38-2.

Profile
Parathion is an organophosphorus insecticide (p.1435) that has been used in agriculture and horticulture. Its metabolite diethyl nitrophenyl phosphate (paraoxon, p.1421) contributes to its toxicity.

◊ Reports of poisoning with parathion.
1. Anastassiades CJ, Ioannides M. Organophosphate poisoning and auricular fibrillation. *BMJ* 1984; **289**: 290.
2. Golsousidis H, Kokkas V. Use of 19 590 mg of atropine during 24 days of treatment, after a case of unusually severe parathion poisoning. *Hum Toxicol* 1985; **4**: 339–40.
3. Clifford NJ, Nies AS. Organophosphate poisoning from wearing a laundered uniform previously contaminated with parathion. *JAMA* 1989; **262**: 3035–6.
4. Wang M-H, *et al.* Q-T interval prolongation and pleomorphic ventricular tachyarrhythmia ('Torsade de pointes') in organophosphate poisoning: report of a case. *Hum Exp Toxicol* 1998; **17**: 587–90.

Pentachlorophenol (6655-s)
PCP; Penta.
$C_6HCl_5O = 266.3$.
CAS — 87-86-5.
NOTE. The name PCP has also been used as a synonym for phencyclidine hydrochloride.

The symbol † denotes a preparation no longer actively marketed

Adverse Effects, Treatment, and Precautions

Pentachlorophenol may be absorbed in toxic amounts through the skin or by inhalation, as well as by ingestion. Pentachlorophenol and its aqueous solutions are irritant to the eyes, mucous membranes, and to the skin, and may produce caustic burns. The systemic effects are due to uncoupling of oxidative phosphorylation with consequent stimulation of cellular metabolism. Acute poisoning with pentachlorophenol increases metabolic rate, leading to raised temperature with copious sweating and thirst, restlessness, fatigue, increased rate and depth of respiration, and tachycardia. There may be abdominal pain and nausea, and death has occurred from respiratory failure. Symptoms of subacute or chronic poisoning include hyperpyrexia and CNS, haematological, renal, reproductive, respiratory, and skin disorders.

Treatment is symptomatic; it has been suggested that forced alkaline diuresis may be useful. The use of antipyretics is not recommended since they can increase toxicity.

◊ Reviews of the toxicity of pentachlorophenol.
1. Health and Safety Executive. Pentachlorophenol. *Toxicity Review 5.* London: HMSO, 1982.
2. Pentachlorophenol. *Environmental Health Criteria 71.* Geneva: WHO, 1987.
3. Pentachlorophenol health and safety guide. *Health and Safety Guide 19.* Geneva: WHO, 1989.
4. Jorens PG, Schepens PJC. Human pentachlorophenol poisoning. *Hum Exp Toxicol* 1993; **12:** 479–95.

◊ There have been reports of malignant neoplasms,[1,2] aplastic anaemia,[3] pancreatitis,[4] intravascular haemolysis,[5] and urticaria[6] associated with exposure to pentachlorophenol.
1. Greene MH, *et al.* Familial and sporadic Hodgkin's disease associated with occupational wood exposure. *Lancet* 1978; **ii:** 626–7.
2. Hardell L. Malignant lymphoma of histiocytic type and exposure to phenoxyacetic acids or chlorophenols. *Lancet* 1979; **i:** 55–6.
3. Roberts HJ. Aplastic anemia due to pentachlorophenol. *N Engl J Med* 1981; **305:** 1650–1.
4. Cooper RG, Macaulay MB. Pentachlorophenol pancreatitis. *Lancet* 1982; **i:** 517.
5. Hassan AB, *et al.* Intravascular haemolysis induced by pentachlorophenol. *BMJ* 1985; **291:** 21–2.
6. Kentor PM. Urticaria from contact with pentachlorophenate. *JAMA* 1986; **256:** 3350.

Pharmacokinetics

Pentachlorophenol may be absorbed after ingestion or inhalation or through the skin. Following ingestion, the majority of a dose is eliminated in the urine as unchanged pentachlorophenol and its glucuronide, with small amounts appearing in the faeces.

Uses

Pentachlorophenol has been used mainly as the sodium salt ($C_6Cl_5NaO = 288.3$), as a preservative for a wide range of industrial and agricultural products, including wood and other building materials, textiles, glues, and starch. It has also been used for the control of slime and algae, and as a molluscicide, fungicide, and herbicide.

Permethrin (13097-w)

Permethrin *(BAN, USAN, rINN).*

3-Phenoxybenzyl (1RS,3RS)-(1RS,3SR)-3-(2,2-dichlorovinyl)-2,2-dimethylcyclopropanecarboxylate.
$C_{21}H_{20}Cl_2O_3 = 391.3$.
CAS — 52645-53-1.
ATC — P03AC04.

Profile

Permethrin is a pyrethroid insecticide (p.1436). It is used in the treatment of head pediculosis (p.1427) as a 1% application; there have been signs of resistance. It is also employed as an acaricide in the treatment of scabies (p.1427) as a 5% cream.

Permethrin is also used as a topical ectoparasiticide in veterinary practice and as an agricultural, horticultural, and household insecticide.

Permethrin is active against mosquitoes and is widely used for the impregnation of bednets and curtains in the control of malaria (p.428). It is also active against blackflies in the adult and larval stages and is used for the larvicidal treatment of rivers in the control of onchocerciasis (p.94). It is also active against tsetse flies.

Permethrin is suitable for aircraft disinsection.

◊ References.
1. Permethrin. *Environmental Health Criteria 94.* Geneva: WHO, 1990.

Preparations

Proprietary Preparations (details are given in Part 3)
Austral.: Lyclear; Nix†; Pyrifoam; Quellada; *Belg.:* Nix; Zalvor; *Canad.:* Kwellada-P; Nix; *Denm.:* Nix; *Fin.:* Nix; *Fr.:* Insect Ecran; Moskizol; Nix; *Ger.:* Delixi; InfectoPedicul; *Irl.:* Lyclear; *Israel:* Lyclear; Mite-X; Nok; Zehu-Ze; *Ital.:* Nix; *Mex.:* Novo-Herklin 2000; *Neth.:* Loxazol; *Norw.:* Nix; *NZ:* Lyclear; Lyderm; Quellada P; *Port.:* Desintan P; Nix; *S.Afr.:* Lyclear; *Swed.:* Nix; *Switz.:* Loxazol; UK: Bug Proof; Lyclear; Residex P55; *USA:* Acticin; Elimite; Nix.

Multi-ingredient: *Belg.:* Para Plus; Shampoux†; *Fr.:* Acarcid perles; Anti-Ac; Charlieu Anti-Poux; Para Plus; Pyreflor; Sanytol; *Israel:* Para Plus; *NZ:* Para Plus.

Phenothrin (3602-a)

Phenothrin *(BAN, rINN).*

3-Phenoxybenzyl (1RS,3RS)-(1RS,3SR)-2,2-dimethyl-3-(2-methylprop-1-enyl)cyclopropanecarboxylate.
$C_{23}H_{26}O_3 = 350.5$.
CAS — 26002-80-2.
ATC — P03AC03.

Profile

Phenothrin is a pyrethroid insecticide (p.1436). It is used for the treatment of head and pubic pediculosis (p.1427) as a 0.2% alcoholic or 0.5% aqueous lotion, or as a 0.5% alcoholic foam; as with permethrin there have been signs of resistance.

Phenothrin is also used in veterinary practice as a topical ectoparasiticide, as a household insecticide, and for the disinsection of public areas and aircraft.

◊ General references.
1. d-Phenothrin. *Environmental Health Criteria 96.* Geneva: WHO, 1990.
2. d-Phenothrin health and safety guide. *IPCS Health and Safety Guide 32.* Geneva: WHO, 1989.

◊ References to the use of phenothrin for aircraft disinsection.
1. Russell RC, Paton R. In-flight disinsection as an efficacious procedure for preventing international transport of insects of public health importance. *Bull WHO* 1989; **67:** 543–7.

Preparations

Proprietary Preparations (details are given in Part 3)
Fr.: Itax Antipoux; Item Antipoux; Parasidose; *Irl.:* Headmaster; *Ital.:* Cruzzy; Mediker; Mom Gel; Mom Shampoo Schiuma; Ottocid; *Mon.:* Hegor Antipoux; *NZ:* Parasidose; *UK:* Full Marks; *USA:* Pronto.

Multi-ingredient: *Fr.:* Itax Antipoux†; Sanytol; *Ital.:* Mom Shampoo Antiparassitario; Neo Mom.

Phosmet (18175-h)

Phosmet *(BAN).*

O,O-Dimethyl phthalimidomethyl phosphorodithioate.
$C_{11}H_{12}NO_4PS_2 = 317.3$.
CAS — 732-11-6.

Profile

Phosmet is an organophosphorus insecticide (p.1435) used as a systemic ectoparasiticide in veterinary practice; it is applied topically to the host animal. It has also been used in agriculture and horticulture.

Phoxim (18178-v)

Phoxim *(BAN).*

Bayer-9053. 2-(Diethoxyphosphinothioyloxyimino)-2-phenylacetonitrile.
$C_{12}H_{15}N_2O_3PS = 298.3$.
CAS — 14816-18-3.

Profile

Phoxim is an organophosphorus insecticide (p.1435) used as a topical ectoparasiticide in veterinary practice. It is also used for the larvicidal treatment of rivers in the control of onchocerciasis (p.94).

Preparations

Proprietary Preparations (details are given in Part 3)
Ital.: Baython EC.

Piperonal (17600-a)

Heliotropin; Piperonylaldehyde. 1,3-Benzodioxole-5-carboxaldehyde.
$C_8H_6O_3 = 150.1$.
CAS — 120-57-0.

Profile

Piperonal is used as an insect repellent against head lice (p.1427).

Preparations

Proprietary Preparations (details are given in Part 3)
Fr.: Para Repulsif; *UK:* Rappell.

Piperonyl Butoxide (3603-t)

Piperonyl Butoxide *(BAN).*

5-[2-(2-Butoxyethoxy)ethoxymethyl]-6-propyl-1,3-benzodioxole.
$C_{19}H_{30}O_5 = 338.4$.
CAS — 51-03-6.

Pharmacopoeias. In BP(Vet).

Pharmacopoeial description

BP(Vet) 2001: A yellow or pale brown oily liquid with a faint characteristic odour. Very slightly soluble in water; miscible with alcohol, with chloroform, with ether, and with petroleum oils.

Profile

Piperonyl butoxide is used as a synergist for pyrethrin and pyrethroid insecticides. Mixtures of piperonyl butoxide and pyrethrins or pyrethroids are used in the treatment of pediculosis (p.1427).

Piperonyl butoxide is considered to cause a variety of gastrointestinal effects as well as mild CNS depression.

Preparations

Proprietary Preparations (details are given in Part 3)
Multi-ingredient: *Austral.:* Banlice; Lyban†; Paralice; Sundown with Insect Repellent; *Belg.:* Para; Para Plus; Pyriderm†; Shampoux†; *Braz.:* Deltacid Plus; Nopucid Composto; Vapio; *Canad.:* Para; Pronto; R & C; Scabene; *Denm.:* Para; *Fr.:* A-Par; Acarcid perles; Acardust; Anti-Ac; Charlieu Anti-Poux; Itax Antipoux†; Para Plus; Para Special Poux; Pyreflor; Spray-Pax; Spregal; *Ger.:* Goldgeist; Jacutin N; Quellada P; Spregal; *Israel:* A-200; Acardust; Kin Soff; Para Plus; *Ital.:* Acardust; Baygon N; Cruzzy; Cruzzy Antiparassitario; Entom; Mafu; Mom Piretro Emulsione; *Neth.:* Crinopex-N†; Para-Speciaal; *Norw.:* Rinsoderm†; *NZ:* Para Plus; *Port.:* Para-Pio; Quitoso; *S.Afr.:* Quell P†; Spregal; *Swed.:* Crinopex†; *Switz.:* A-Par†; Acardust†; *UK:* Buzpel; Fortefog; Patriot; Prevent; *USA:* A-200†; Barc; Blue; Clear Total Lice Elimination System; End Lice; InnoGel Plus; Licide; Pronto; Pyrinex; Pyrinyl II; Pyrinyl Plus; R & C; RID; Tegrin-LT; Tisit; Triple X.

Pirimiphos-Methyl (18181-d)

O-2-Diethylamino-6-methylpyrimidin-4-yl O,O-dimethyl phosphorothioate.
$C_{11}H_{20}N_3O_3PS = 305.3$.
CAS — 29232-93-7.

Profile

Pirimiphos-methyl is an organophosphorus insecticide (p.1435). It is used in agriculture and domestically.

Propetamphos (18182-n)

Propetamphos *(BAN).*

Isopropyl (E)-3-[(ethylamino)(methoxy)phosphinothiooxy]but-2-enoate.
$C_{10}H_{20}NO_4PS = 281.3$.
CAS — 31218-83-4.

Profile

Propetamphos is an organophosphorus insecticide (p.1435) used as a topical ectoparasiticide in veterinary practice.

Propoxur (18039-k)

Propoxur *(BAN).*

2-Isopropoxyphenyl methylcarbamate.
$C_{11}H_{15}NO_3 = 209.2$.
CAS — 114-26-1.

Profile

Propoxur is a carbamate insecticide (p.1429) used as a topical ectoparasiticide in veterinary practice. It is also used as a fumigant in agriculture.

Preparations

Proprietary Preparations (details are given in Part 3)
Ital.: Pulvis-3†.

Multi-ingredient: *Ital.:* Baygon N.

Pyraclofos (5372-y)

(RS)-[O-1-(4-Chlorophenyl)pyrazol-4-yl O-ethyl S-propyl phosphorothioate].
$C_{14}H_{18}ClN_2O_3PS = 360.8$.
CAS — 77458-01-6.

Profile

Pyraclofos is an organophosphorus insecticide (p.1435) used for the larvicidal treatment of rivers in the control of onchocerciasis (p.94).

Pyrethrum Flower (3604-x)

Chrysanthème Insecticide; Dalmatian Insect Flowers; Insect Flowers; Insektenblüten; Piretro; Pyrethri Flos.
CAS — 8003-34-7 (pyrethrum); 121-21-1 (pyrethrin I); 121-29-9 (pyrethrin II); 25402-06-6 (cinerin I); 121-20-0 (cinerin II).
ATC — P03AC01.

Pharmacopoeias. In Aust. Also in BP(Vet). US includes Pyrethrum Extract.

Pharmacopoeial description

BP(Vet) 2001: The dried flowerheads of *Chrysanthemum cinerariaefolium* containing not less than 1% of pyrethrins of which not less than one-half consists of pyrethrin I. It has a faint but characteristic odour.

USP 25: Pyrethrum Extract is a mixture of three naturally occurring, closely related insecticidal esters of chrysanthemic acid (pyrethrins I: pyrethrin 1, cinerin 1, and jasmolin 1) and three closely related esters of pyrethric acid (pyrethrins II: pyrethrin 2, cinerin 2, and jasmolin 2). It contains not less than 19% and not more than 21% of the sum of pyrethrins I and II in a mixture consisting of approximately 20 to 25% of light isoparaffins. The ratio of pyrethrins I to pyrethrins II is not less than 0.8 and not more than 2.8. It may also contain 3 to 5% of butylated hydroxytoluene as an antioxidant and 23 to 25% of phytochemical extracts containing triglyceride oils, terpenoids, and carotenoid plant colours. It contains no other added substances. It is a pale yellow liquid having a bland, flowery odour. Insoluble in water; soluble in liquid paraffin and in most organic solvents. Store in airtight containers. Protect from light.

Adverse Effects and Precautions
Pyrethrum is irritant to the eyes and mucosa. Hypersensitivity reactions have been reported.

Uses
Pyrethrum flower is mainly used for the preparation of pyrethrum extracts containing a mixture of chrysanthemic acid and pyrethric acid esters (pyrethrins I and II).

Pyrethrins in the form of pyrethrum extract have a long history of use as insecticides. Pyrethrum is rapidly toxic to many insects. It has a much quicker knock-down effect than clofenotane or lindane, but it is less persistent and less stable. Its action can be enhanced by certain substances such as piperonyl butoxide (p.1436), and pyrethrins with piperonyl butoxide are used clinically in the treatment of pediculosis (p.1427).

Pyrethroid insecticides (synthetic analogues of pyrethrins), such as permethrin and phenothrin, are also used clinically; deltamethrin and permethrin are among those used for the vector control of malaria.

Pyrethrum, pyrethrins, and pyrethroids are also used as topical ectoparasiticides in veterinary practice and as agricultural, horticultural, and household insecticides.

Preparations
Proprietary Preparations (details are given in Part 3)
Multi-ingredient: *Belg.*: Pyriderm†; ***Fr.*:** Spray-Pax; ***Ger.*:** Goldgeist; Quellada P; ***Israel:*** Kin Soff; ***Ital.*:** Cruzzy; Cruzzy Antiparassitario; Entom; ***Neth.*:** Crinopex-N†; ***Norw.*:** Rinsoderm†; ***Swed.*:** Crinopex†; ***Switz.*:** A-Par†; ***UK:*** Savlon Natural First Aid for Insect Bites & Stings; ***USA:*** Clear Total Lice Elimination System; Licide.

Pyriproxyfen (15068-r)
S-9318; S-31183. 2-[1-Methyl-2-(4-phenoxyphenoxy)ethoxy]pyridine.
$C_{20}H_{19}NO_3 = 321.4$.
CAS — 95737-68-1.

Profile
Pyriproxyfen is used as a topical ectoparasiticide in veterinary practice.

Red Squill (2028-t)
CAS — 507-60-8 (scilliroside).

A red variety of *Urginea maritima*, which contains, in addition to cardiac glycosides, an active principle, scilliroside.

Profile
Red squill is very toxic to *rats* and has been incorporated in rat poisons; it has neurotoxic and cardiotoxic properties.

Resmethrin (11863-c)
5-Benzyl-3-furylmethyl (1RS,3RS)-(1RS,3SR)-2,2-dimethyl-3-(2-methylprop-1-enyl)cyclopropanecarboxylate.
$C_{22}H_{26}O_3 = 338.4$.
CAS — 10453-86-8.

Profile
Resmethrin is a pyrethroid insecticide (p.1436) used in veterinary practice for the control of ectoparasites in the environment. Resmethrin is also used as an agricultural, horticultural, and household insecticide, but is not synergised by pyrethrum synergists such as piperonyl butoxide (p.1436).

Rotenone (3606-f)
Rotenonum. (2R,6aS,12aS)-1,2,6,6a,12,12a-Hexahydro-2-isopropenyl-8,9-dimethoxychromeno[3,4-b]furo[2,3-h]chromen-6-one.
$C_{23}H_{22}O_6 = 394.4$.
CAS — 83-79-4.

Profile
Rotenone is a non-systemic insecticide used in agriculture and in horticulture.

Rotenone is the active ingredient of derris (the dried rhizome and roots of *Derris elliptica*; also known as tuba root or aker-

tuba) and of lonchocarpus (the dried root of *Lonchocarpus utilis*; also known as cube root, timbo, or barbusco). Powdered forms of derris and of lonchocarpus have been used as insecticides and fish poisons.

Sodium Fluoroacetate (7734-c)
Compound 1080; Sodium Monofluoroacetate.
$FCH_2.CO_2Na = 100.0$.
CAS — 62-74-8.

Adverse Effects, Treatment, and Precautions
Sodium fluoroacetate is highly toxic, the lethal dose if ingested being about 2 to 10 mg per kg body-weight. Toxic effects may be delayed for several hours after absorption by mouth or inhalation, and include nausea and vomiting, apprehension, muscle twitching, cardiac irregularities, convulsions, respiratory failure, coma, and death usually due to ventricular fibrillation.

Treatment is generally supportive and symptomatic.

◊ References to sodium fluoroacetate toxicity.
1. Chi CH, *et al.* Clinical presentation and prognostic factors in sodium monofluoroacetate intoxication. *J Toxicol Clin Toxicol* 1996; **34:** 707–12.
2. Chi CH, *et al.* Hemodynamic abnormalities in sodium monofluoroacetate intoxication. *Hum Exp Toxicol* 1999; **18:** 351–3.

Uses
Sodium fluoroacetate is a highly effective rodenticide but must be used with great caution because of its toxicity to other animals and to man.

Sulfiram (3595-l)
Sulfiram (BAN, rINN).

Monosulfiram; Sulfiramum. Tetraethylthiuram monosulphide.
$C_{10}H_{20}N_2S_3 = 264.5$.
CAS — 95-05-6.

Pharmacopoeias. In Aust. .

Adverse Effects and Precautions
An erythematous rash has occasionally been reported. Sulfiram produces effects similar to those of disulfiram (p.1605) if ingested with alcohol. As there may be a risk of absorption following the application of sulfiram to the whole body, patients are advised to abstain from alcohol for at least 48 hours.

◊ The reactions to alcohol occasionally reported in patients who have applied sulfiram solution[1,2] resemble those seen with disulfiram. Analysis has shown that sulfiram solutions exposed to room light undergo photochemical conversion to disulfiram, and that the concentration of disulfiram, and the ability of the solution to inhibit aldehyde dehydrogenase and hence the metabolism of alcohol, increases with the duration of such storage.[3,4] Whether patients who have applied sulfiram solution should avoid direct light immediately afterwards remains to be elucidated.[4]
1. Blanc D, Deprez P. Unusual adverse reaction to an acaricide. *Lancet* 1990; **335:** 1291–2.
2. Burgess I. Adverse reactions to monosulfiram. *Lancet* 1990; **336:** 873.
3. Mays DC, *et al.* Photolysis of monosulfiram: a mechanism for its disulfiram-like reaction. *Clin Pharmacol Ther* 1994; **55:** 191.
4. Lipsky JJ, *et al.* Monosulfiram, disulfiram, and light. *Lancet* 1994; **343:** 304.

Uses and Administration
Sulfiram is a pesticide that has been used as an acaricide, either alone or in conjunction with benzyl benzoate, in the treatment of scabies (p.1427), although other treatments are now preferred.

Sulfiram has also been used as a pesticide in veterinary practice.

Preparations
Proprietary Preparations (details are given in Part 3)
Braz.*:** Tetmosol; Tiosol; ***Mex.*:** Tetmosol; ***Port.*:** Thiosan; ***S.Afr.*:** Tetmosol; ***Singapore: Tetmosol.

Multi-ingredient: *Fr.*: Ascabiol.

Temefos (3609-h)
Temefos (USAN, rINN).

27165; Temephos. *O,O'*-(Thiodi-*p*-phenylene) *O,O,O',O'*-tetramethyl bis(phosphorothioate).
$C_{16}H_{20}O_6P_2S_3 = 466.5$.
CAS — 3383-96-8.

Profile
Temefos is an organophosphorus insecticide (p.1435). It is effective against the larvae of mosquitoes, blackflies, and other insects, and is used for the larvicidal treatment of rivers in the control of onchocerciasis (p.94). It is also effective against the crustacean host to the larvae of the guinea worm and is used in

the control of dracunculiasis (p.92); treatment of drinking water is both effective and acceptable.

Tetrachlorvinphos (18193-b)
ENT-25841; SD-8447. 2-Chloro-1-(2,4,5-trichlorophenyl)vinyl dimethyl phosphate.
$C_{10}H_9Cl_4O_4P = 366.0$.
CAS — 961-11-5; 22248-79-9 (Z-tetrachlorvinphos); 22350-76-1 (E-tetrachlorvinphos).

Profile
Tetrachlorvinphos is an organophosphorus insecticide (p.1435) used as an ectoparasiticide in veterinary practice.

Tetramethrin (3610-a)
Tetramethrin (rINN).

Cyclohex-1-ene-1,2-dicarboximidomethyl (1RS,3RS)-(1RS,3SR)-2,2-dimethyl-3-(2-methylprop-1-enyl)cyclopropanecarboxylate.
$C_{19}H_{25}NO_4 = 331.4$.
CAS — 7696-12-0.
ATC — P03BA04.

Profile
Tetramethrin is a pyrethroid insecticide (p.1436) used in the treatment of pediculosis (p.1427). It is also used in veterinary practice for the control of ectoparasites in the environment and as a household insecticide.

Preparations
Proprietary Preparations (details are given in Part 3)
Multi-ingredient: *Fr.*: Itax Antipoux†; ***Ital.*:** Baygon N; Mafu; Mom Piretro Emulsione; Mom Shampoo Antiparassitario; Neo Mom.

Trichlorophenoxyacetic Acid (3611-t)
2,4,5-T. 2,4,5-Trichlorophenoxyacetic acid.
$C_8H_5Cl_3O_3 = 255.5$.
CAS — 35915-18-5.

Profile
Trichlorophenoxyacetic acid is a selective herbicide with similar actions to dichlorophenoxyacetic acid (p.1431). It is usually used in ester formulations. It was used as a defoliating agent in the Vietnam war in conjunction with dichlorophenoxyacetic acid.

Toxicity. Swedish studies initially indicated that there was an increased incidence of soft tissue sarcoma, Hodgkin's disease, and non-Hodgkin's lymphoma with phenoxy herbicides. Other studies have failed to demonstrate such a connection with the exception of non-Hodgkin's lymphoma.[1-4]

These herbicides were used for defoliation in Vietnam as Agent Orange, which consisted of a mixture of dichlorophenoxyacetic acid, trichlorophenoxyacetic acid, and the impurity TCDD (dioxin), and concern has been expressed that they may have contributed to an increased incidence of cancer among exposed subjects as well as an adverse effect on the offspring of those subjects. This has been a matter of considerable debate,[5] prompting a series of biennial reassessments of the health effects of Agent Orange by the US National Academy of Sciences' Institute of Medicine.[6]
1. Anonymous. Phenoxy herbicides, trichlorophenols, and soft-tissue sarcomas. *Lancet* 1982; **i:** 1051–2.
2. Coggon D, Acheson ED. Do phenoxy herbicides cause cancer in man? *Lancet* 1982; **i:** 1057–9.
3. Hoar SK, *et al.* Agricultural herbicide use and risk of lymphoma and soft-tissue sarcoma. *JAMA* 1986; **256:** 1141–7.
4. The Selected Cancers Cooperative Study Group. The association of selected cancers with service in the US military in Vietnam. *Arch Intern Med* 1990; **150:** 2473–83, 2485–92, and 2495–2505.
5. McCarthy M. Agent Orange. *Lancet* 1993; **342:** 362.
6. Stephenson J. New IOM report links Agent Orange exposure to risk of birth defect in Vietnam vets' children. *JAMA* 1996; **275:** 1066–7.

Triflumuron (15690-x)
Trifluron. 2-Chloro-*N*-([{4-(trifluoromethoxy)phenyl}amino]carbonyl)benzamide.
$C_{15}H_{10}ClF_3N_2O_3 = 358.7$.
CAS — 64628-44-0.

Profile
Triflumuron is an insecticide used in agriculture and as a topical ectoparasiticide in veterinary practice.

Preparations
Proprietary Preparations (details are given in Part 3)
***Ital.*:** Baycidal.

The symbol † denotes a preparation no longer actively marketed

Prostaglandins

The prostaglandins, along with thromboxanes and leukotrienes, are all derived from 20-carbon poly-unsaturated fatty acids and are collectively termed *eicosanoids*. In man, the most common precursor is arachidonic acid (eicosatetraenoic acid) whereas eicosapentaenoic acid is a predominant precursor in fish and marine animals.

Arachidonic acid is released from cell-membrane phospholipids by the enzyme phospholipase A_2 and is then rapidly metabolised by several enzymes, the major ones being cyclo-oxygenase (prostaglandin synthetase) and lipoxygenase. The prostaglandins, thromboxanes, and prostacyclin (sometimes collectively termed *prostanoids*) all contain ring structures and are products of arachidonic acid oxidation by cyclo-oxygenase, an enzyme with 2 isoforms widely distributed in cell membranes. The leukotrienes are products of the lipoxygenase pathway. The initial step in the cyclo-oxygenase pathway is the formation of cyclic endoperoxide prostaglandin G_2 (PGG_2) which is then reduced to the endoperoxide prostaglandin H_2 (PGH_2). Prostaglandin H_2 is then converted to the primary prostaglandins prostaglandin D_2, prostaglandin E_2, and prostaglandin $F_{2\alpha}$, to thromboxane A_2 (TXA_2) via the enzyme thromboxane synthetase, or to prostacyclin (PGI_2) via the enzyme prostacyclin synthetase. These products are further metabolised and rapidly inactivated in the body. The secondary prostaglandins, prostaglandin A_2 (PGA_2), prostaglandin B_2 (PGB_2), and prostaglandin C_2 (PGC_2) are derived from prostaglandin E_2, but are formed during extraction and probably do not occur biologically.

The prostaglandins are all derivatives of the carbon skeleton 7-(2-octilcyclopentyl)heptanoic acid (also known as prostanoic acid). All natural prostaglandins have a double bond at position 1,2 and a hydroxyl group at position 3 of the octil side-chain. Depending on the substitutions on the cyclopentane ring, the main series of prostaglandins are distinguished by the letters A, B, C, D, E, and F; the members of each series are further subdivided by subscript numbers which indicate the degree of unsaturation in the side-chains—hence, those derived from eicosatrienoic acid (dihomo-γ-linolenic acid) have the subscript 1, those derived from arachidonic acid have the subscript 2, and those derived from eicosapentaenoic acid have the subscript 3. In man, only prostaglandins of the '2' series appear to be of physiological importance. Thromboxane A_2 has an oxane rather than a cyclopentane ring; it is chemically unstable and breaks down to thromboxane B_2. Prostacyclin has a double-ring structure and breaks down to 6-keto-prostaglandin $F_{1\alpha}$.

Endogenous prostaglandins are autacoids; they can be formed by virtually all tissues and cells in response to a variety of stimuli, have a wide range of **actions**, and are involved in the regulation of virtually all biological functions. Prostaglandins appear to act through various receptor-mediated mechanisms. Some of their effects are mediated within cells by activation or inhibition of adenylate cyclase and the regulation of cyclic adenosine monophosphate production. At one time prostaglandin E_2 and prostaglandin $F_{2\alpha}$ were thought to be of paramount importance, but with the discovery of thromboxane A_2, prostacyclin, and the leukotrienes it was realised that these primary prostaglandins belong to a large family of physiologically active eicosanoids. Thromboxane A_2 induces platelet aggregation and constricts arterial smooth muscle whereas prostacyclin causes vasodilatation and prevents platelet aggregation; the balance between these opposing actions has an important role in the regulation of intravascular platelet aggregation and thrombus formation. The leukotrienes are important mediators of inflammation.

The pharmacological properties of prostaglandins are wide-ranging and include contraction or relaxation of smooth muscle in the blood vessels, bronchi, uterus, and gastrointestinal tract; inhibition of gastric acid secretion; and effects on platelet aggregation, the endocrine system, and metabolic processes.

Individual prostaglandins vary greatly in their activities and potencies; their actions also depend on the animal species, on the tissues in which they are acting, and on the concentration present, and entirely opposite actions may be elicited with very small structural changes in the molecule.

The diverse **clinical applications** of prostaglandins reflect their wide-ranging physiological and pharmacological properties. Synthetic analogues have been developed with the aim of obtaining compounds which are more stable, have a longer duration of action, and a more specific effect. Applications include:

- softening and dilating the cervix and for uterine stimulation, e.g. dinoprost (prostaglandin $F_{2\alpha}$) (p.1441) and its analogue carboprost (p.1441); dinoprostone (prostaglandin E_2) (p.1441) and its analogue sulprostone (p.1447); and gemeprost (p.1445) and misoprostol (p.1446), analogues of prostaglandin E_1
- vasodilators and inhibitors of platelet aggregation, e.g. alprostadil (prostaglandin E_1) (p.1439) and its analogue limaprost (p.1446); and epoprostenol (prostacyclin) (p.1443) and its analogue iloprost (p.1445)
- inhibition of gastric acid secretion and protection of the gastrointestinal mucosa, e.g. misoprostol (p.1446)
- glaucoma treatment, e.g. bimatoprost (p.1440), latanoprost (p.1445), travoprost (p.1447), and unoprostone (p.1447)
- as luteolytics (causing regression of the corpus luteum in the ovary) in veterinary medicine, e.g. synthetic analogues of prostaglandin F_1 and $F_{2\alpha}$.

◊ References.

1. Moncada S, Vane JR. Arachidonic acid metabolites and the interactions between platelets and blood-vessel walls. *N Engl J Med* 1979; **300:** 1142–7.
2. Higgs GA, Vane JR. Inhibition of cyclo-oxygenase and lipoxygenase. *Br Med Bull* 1983; **39:** 265–70.
3. Halushka PV, *et al.* Thromboxane, prostaglandin and leukotriene receptors. *Annu Rev Pharmacol Toxicol* 1989; **29:** 213–39.
4. Smith WL, *et al.* Prostaglandin and thromboxane biosynthesis. *Pharmacol Ther* 1991; **49:** 153–79.
5. O'Neill C. The biochemistry of prostaglandins: a primer. *Aust N Z J Obstet Gynaecol* 1994; **34:** 332–7.
6. Wu KK. Molecular regulation and augmentation of prostacyclin biosynthesis. *Agents Actions Suppl* 1995; **45:** 11–17.

Labour induction and augmentation

The uterus is normally spontaneously contractile but during pregnancy various physiological mechanisms maintain it in a quiescent state; retention of the fetus is also aided by a firm and contracted cervix. During the final 4 to 5 weeks of pregnancy the cervix normally undergoes a 'ripening' process in which it becomes softened and dilated, so that at parturition it is not a barrier to delivery of the fetus. Endogenous prostaglandins play an important role in this process, and also sensitise the uterus in preparation for labour. Labour usually begins spontaneously but in some cases it may be necessary to induce labour, for example in pregnancies that go beyond term, or where premature rupture of the membranes occurs or there are other maternal or fetal indications for early delivery.[1] Once labour has commenced, augmentation of uterine activity may be necessary if contractions fail to progress satisfactorily. A process of active management of labour, where augmentation is initiated at an early stage, has been advocated; however, a study[2] in nulliparous women found no reduction in the rate of caesarean section when active management was used.

Various techniques are available for induction of labour. Before pharmacological methods are used, women may be offered sweeping of the membranes.[3] This can avoid the use of drugs in some cases, but it is associated with increased maternal discomfort, irregular contractions, and bleeding.[4] When formal induction of labour is required, prostaglandins are preferred to oxytocin in all women with intact membranes, but either may be used in women who have ruptured membranes,[3] as neither method then offers any particular advantage.[5]

Dinoprostone (prostaglandin E_2) is the most widely used prostaglandin and has been given by various routes. It is usually given intravaginally as gel, vaginal tablets, or pessaries; although some have found the gel to be more effective,[6] a systematic review[7] considered the clinical benefits equivalent, and UK guidelines favour use of vaginal tablets.[3] Dinoprostone given this way produces similar results to oxytocin infusions[8] with the advantage of lower rates of neonatal jaundice and postpartum haemorrhage. It is also less invasive and, as its effects are more akin to spontaneous labour, it is more popular with the mother than oxytocin. The intravenous and oral routes have been associated with frequent adverse, particularly gastrointestinal, effects[9,10] and intravaginal administration is now preferred. Intracervical administration has also been used but it is no more effective than the intravaginal route, and is no longer recommended.[3]

Oxytocin should not be started for 6 hours after use of vaginal prostaglandins.[3] Whenever possible, amniotomy (deliberate rupture of the fetal membranes) should be performed before oxytocin administration in women with intact membranes.[3] Oxytocin is given by slow intravenous infusion. UK guidelines favour a starting dose of 1 to 2 milliunits per minute, increased at intervals of 30 minutes, and titrated against contractions.[3] However, there have been conflicting findings about the dose. Some have used low doses effectively[11-13] (e.g. starting at 0.5 or 0.7 milliunits per minute) and found them to be as effective as higher doses and to cause less uterine hyperstimulation.[12] In contrast, a double-blind study[14] reported that high doses of oxytocin (starting at 4.5 milliunits per minute) were associated with a shorter duration of labour without a demonstrable increase in adverse fetal or neonatal effects. Others also found that the failure of induction was less frequent with higher doses (starting at 6 milliunits per minute), although there was a higher rate of caesarean section for fetal distress.[15]

Misoprostol has also been investigated. Most studies have used the intravaginal route and have suggested it may be more effective than standard methods of labour induction.[16] Oral administration may also be effective, although less so than intravaginal.[17] However, the risk of uterine hyperstimulation may be increased with misoprostol and there is as yet insufficient evidence of its safety to recommend routine use.

The antiprogestogen mifepristone also produces cervical dilatation and stimulates uterine contraction and has been tried for cervical ripening and for induction of labour. A systematic review of trials found that it may be effective, but its place in therapy has yet to be established.[18]

In pregnancies at term, premature rupture of the fetal membranes (i.e. before labour begins) might increase the risk of both maternal and fetal infection.[19] The usual practice in such situations has often been to induce labour immediately, either with oxytocin intravenously or dinoprostone vaginally. Some have suggested expectant management as an alternative to immediate induction,[20] but this has been criticised.[19]

Oxytocin or a prostaglandin may also be used for **labour augmentation**. Doses of oxytocin are similar to those used for induction. Low-dose regimens, starting at 1 milliunit per minute intravenously, have proved successful[21,22] and are increasingly used, although higher doses starting at 6 milliunits per minute[23] have been given. Comparison of the two approaches[15] found that high doses led to shorter labour, fewer forceps deliveries, and a lower incidence of caesarean section for dystocia, but more commonly resulted in uterine hyperstimulation.

Dinoprostone is the prostaglandin most often used for augmentation of labour. As with its use for induction, dinoprostone results in lower incidences of neonatal jaundice and of postpartum haemorrhage, and is more popular with mothers than oxytocin. It is usually given intravaginally as a gel or pessaries. A gel may be given intracervically, but this is a more invasive route. Oral dinoprostone tablets have been used despite their gastrointestinal side-effects, and are considered to be more useful for augmentation than for induction.

Once delivery has successfully been initiated, management of the third stage of labour may be considered to reduce the risks of postpartum haemorrhage. Ergometrine or oxytocin or both are usually employed for this purpose, as discussed on p.1607. Misoprostol has also been tried, although it is not as effective as oxytocin.[24]

1. Chamberlain G, Zander L. ABC of labour care: induction. *BMJ* 1999; **318:** 995–8. Correction. *ibid.*; 1584.
2. Frigoletto FD, *et al.* A clinical trial of active management of labor. *N Engl J Med* 1995; **333:** 745–50.
3. Royal College of Obstetricians and Gynaecologists. Induction of labour: evidence-based clinical guideline number 9 (issued June 2001). Available at: http://www.nice.org.uk/pdf/inductionoflabourrcogrep.pdf (accessed 12/09/01).
4. Boulvain M, *et al.* Membrane sweeping for induction of labour (updated 14 February 2001). Available in The Cochrane Library; Issue 4. Oxford: Update Software; 2001.
5. Tan BP, Hannah ME. Prostaglandins versus oxytocin for prelabour rupture of membranes at or near term (updated 1 November 1999). Available in The Cochrane Library; Issue 4. Oxford: Update Software; 2001.
6. Mahmood TA. A prospective comparative study on the use of prostaglandin E₂ gel (2 mg) and prostaglandin E₂ tablet (3 mg) for the induction of labour in primigravid women with unfavourable cervices. *Eur J Obstet Gynecol Reprod Biol* 1989; **33:** 169–75.
7. Kelly AJ, *et al.* Vaginal prostaglandin (PGE2 and PGF2a) for induction of labour at term (updated 12 March 2001). Available in The Cochrane Library; Issue 4. Oxford: Update Software; 2001.
8. Silva-Cruz A, *et al.* Prostaglandin E₂ gel compared to oxytocin for medically-indicated labour induction at term: a controlled clinical trial. *Pharmatherapeutica* 1988; **5:** 228–32.
9. Luckas M, Bricker L. Intravenous prostaglandin for induction of labour (updated 30 August 2000). Available in The Cochrane Library; Issue 4. Oxford: Update Software; 2001.
10. French L. Oral prostaglandin E2 for induction of labour (updated 3 April 2001). Available in The Cochrane Library; Issue 4. Oxford: Update Software; 2001.
11. Blakemore KJ, *et al.* A prospective comparison of hourly and quarter-hourly prostaglandin E₂ dose increase intervals for the induction of labor at term. *Obstet Gynecol* 1990; **75:** 757–61.
12. Mercer B, *et al.* Labor induction with continuous low-dose oxytocin infusion: a randomized trial. *Obstet Gynecol* 1991; **77:** 659–63.
13. Wein P. Efficacy of different starting doses of oxytocin for induction of labor. *Obstet Gynecol* 1989; **74:** 863–8.
14. Merrill DC, Zlatnik FJ. Randomized, double-masked comparison of oxytocin dosage in induction and augmentation of labor. *Obstet Gynecol* 1999; **94:** 455–63.
15. Satin AJ, *et al.* High- versus low-dose oxytocin for labor stimulation. *Obstet Gynecol* 1992; **80:** 111–16.
16. Hofmeyr GJ, Gulmezoglu AM. Vaginal misoprostol for cervical ripening and induction of labour (updated 26 August 2001). Available in The Cochrane Library; Issue 4. Oxford: Update Software; 2001.
17. Alfirevic Z. Oral misoprostol for induction of labour (updated 22 February 2001). Available in The Cochrane Library; Issue 4. Oxford: Update Software; 2001.
18. Neilson JP. Mifepristone for induction of labour (updated 22 May 2001). Available in The Cochrane Library; Issue 4. Oxford: Update Software; 2001.
19. Duff P. Premature rupture of the membranes at term. *N Engl J Med* 1996; **334:** 1053–4.
20. Hannah ME, *et al.* Induction of labor compared with expectant management for prelabor rupture of the membranes at term. *N Engl J Med* 1996; **334:** 1005–10.
21. Seitchik J, Castillo M. Oxytocin augmentation of dysfunctional labor I: clinical data. *Am J Obstet Gynecol* 1982; **144:** 899–905.
22. Seitchik J, Castillo M. Oxytocin augmentation of dysfunctional labor III: multiparous patients. *Am J Obstet Gynecol* 1983; **145:** 777–80.
23. Akoury HA, *et al.* Oxytocin augmentation of labor and perinatal outcome in nulliparas. *Obstet Gynecol* 1991; **78:** 227–30.
24. Gülmezoglu AM, *et al.* WHO multicentre randomised trial of misoprostol in the management of the third stage of labour. *Lancet* 2001; **358:** 689–95.

Termination of pregnancy

Termination of pregnancy can be achieved medically or surgically. One of the main factors influencing the choice of method is the stage of gestation.[1,2]

• EARLY PREGNANCY

Surgical methods are commonly used in early pregnancy.[2] Menstrual extraction (menstrual regulation), which usually involves aspiration of the uterine cavity and induction of uterine bleeding is sometimes used when menstruation is no more than **14 days** overdue. Dilatation and vacuum aspiration has been widely used at up to **63 days** of amenorrhoea although other methods may be preferred before 49 days since most failures occur during this period. Cervical preparation is sometimes performed, commonly with prostaglandins; isosorbide mononitrate has also been tried.[3]

Medical methods of termination are also effective at this stage[4] and usually involve administration of the oral antiprogestogenic drug mifepristone followed by a prostaglandin. Mifepristone blocks the effects of progesterone on the uterus, leading to uterine contractions; it may also increase the myometrial sensitivity to prostaglandins. Prostaglandins soften and dilate the cervix and stimulate uterine contractions. Although both mifepristone and prostaglandins have been used alone, mifepristone is probably not sufficiently effective as a single agent,[4] while the doses of prostaglandins required are associated with adverse effects. Mifepristone is given orally, followed 36 to 48 hours later by a low dose of prostaglandin. Gemeprost, administered intravaginally, is commonly used; misoprostol, given orally or vaginally is a widely used and effective alternative.[2] Sulprostone has been used but has to be given by intravenous infusion.

The antimetabolite methotrexate has a role in the management of ectopic pregnancy and has also been investigated for termination of pregnancy. Intramuscular methotrexate followed 3 days later by intravaginal misoprostol was more effective than misoprostol alone for termination at 56 days or less;[5] the combination was reported to be less successful after 57 to 63 days' gestation.[6] Later studies[7,8] however found the combination to be safe and effective in terminating pregnancies up to 63 days' gestation; misoprostol was administered up to 7 days after the methotrexate. Oral administration is also effective.[4] A disadvantage of methotrexate is that its effect may be delayed by several weeks.

The combination of tamoxifen with misoprostol[9-11] has also been studied for the early termination of pregnancy but it is unclear whether it has any advantage over the prostaglandin alone.

• LATER PREGNANCY

Termination at later stages of pregnancy is generally associated with higher morbidity and mortality.

Standard methods at **9 to 14 weeks** of gestation are surgical (dilatation and vacuum aspiration). There has been very little clinical study of medical methods although preparation of the cervix with intravaginal prostaglandins is common. Preliminary evidence suggests that mifepristone with a prostaglandin may be effective.[12]

At **more than 14 weeks** cervical preparation is essential. Medical induction of labour is then usually performed with mifepristone followed by a prostaglandin, although surgical termination by dilatation and evacuation may be used. Gemeprost or misoprostol have been given intravaginally, but usually in repeated doses. Parenteral administration can involve carboprost intramuscularly or sulprostone intravenously. Intra-amniotic dinoprost or extra-amniotic dinoprostone have been used when none of the above prostaglandins were available but such methods of administration carry additional risks. The frequency of side-effects with prostaglandins is reported to be generally higher with intra-amniotic than with extra-amniotic administration. Other methods have included the intra-amniotic administration of hypertonic sodium chloride and the intra-amniotic administration of hyperosmolar urea augmented with dinoprost.

1. WHO. Medical methods for termination of pregnancy: report of a WHO scientific group. *WHO Tech Rep Ser 871* 1997.
2. Royal College of Obstetricians and Gynaecologists. The care of women requesting induced abortion. Available at: http://www.rcog.org.uk/guidelines/induced_abortion.html (accessed 26/09/00).
3. Thomson AJ, *et al.* Randomised trial of nitric oxide donor versus prostaglandin for cervical ripening before first-trimester termination of pregnancy. *Lancet* 1998; **352:** 1093–6.
4. Christin-Maitre S, *et al.* Medical termination of pregnancy. *N Engl J Med* 2000; **342:** 946–56.
5. Creinin MD, Vittinghoff E. Methotrexate and misoprostol vs misoprostol alone for early abortion: a randomized controlled trial. *JAMA* 1994; **272:** 1190–5.
6. Creinin MD. Methotrexate and misoprostol for abortion at 57-63 days gestation. *Contraception* 1994; **50:** 511–15.
7. Hausknecht RU. Methotrexate and misoprostol to terminate early pregnancy. *N Engl J Med* 1995; **333:** 537–40.
8. Creinin MD. A randomized trial comparing misoprostol three and seven days after methotrexate for early abortion. *Am J Obstet Gynecol* 1995; **173:** 1578–84.
9. Mishell DR, *et al.* A medical method of early pregnancy termination using tamoxifen and misoprostol. *Contraception* 1998; **58:** 1–6.
10. Wiebe ER. Tamoxifen compared to methotrexate when used with misoprostol for abortion. *Contraception* 1999; **59:** 265–70.
11. Jain JK, *et al.* A comparison of tamoxifen and misoprostol to misoprostol alone for early pregnancy termination. *Contraception* 1999; **60:** 353–6.
12. Ashok PW, *et al.* Termination of pregnancy at 9-13 weeks' amenorrhoea with mifepristone and misoprostol. *Lancet* 1998; **352:** 542–3.

Alfaprostol (18611-g)

Alfaprostol *(BAN, USAN, rINN).*

K-11941; Ro-22-9000. Methyl (Z)-7-{(1R,2S,3R,5S)-2-[(3S)-5-cyclohexyl-3-hydroxypent-1-ynyl]-3,5-dihydroxycyclopentyl}hept-5-enoate.

$C_{24}H_{38}O_5 = 406.6.$

CAS — 74176-31-1.

Profile

Alfaprostol is a synthetic analogue of dinoprost (prostaglandin F₂α). It is used as a luteolytic in veterinary medicine.

Alprostadil (8071-n)

Alprostadil *(BAN, USAN, rINN).*

Alprostadilum; PGE₁; Prostaglandin E₁; U-10136. (E)-(8R,11R,12R,15S)-11,15-Dihydroxy-9-oxoprost-13-enoic acid; 7-{(1R,2R,3R)-3-Hydroxy-2-[(E)-(3S)-3-hydroxyoct-1-enyl]-5-oxocyclopentyl}heptanoic acid.

$C_{20}H_{34}O_5 = 354.5.$

CAS — 745-65-3.

ATC — C01EA01; G04BE01.

NOTE. In *Martindale* the term alprostadil is used for the exogenous substance and prostaglandin E₁ for the endogenous substance.

Pharmacopoeias. In *Eur.* (see p.vi) and *US.*

Jpn includes Alprostadil Alfadex.

Pharmacopoeial description

Ph. Eur.: A white or slightly yellowish crystalline powder. Practically insoluble in water; freely soluble in alcohol; soluble in acetone; slightly soluble in ethyl acetate.

USP 25: A white to off-white crystalline powder. M.p. about 110°. Soluble in water; freely soluble in alcohol; soluble in acetone; very slightly soluble in chloroform and in ether; slightly soluble in ethyl acetate. Store between 2° and 8° in airtight containers.

Adverse Effects, Treatment, and Precautions

The adverse effects reported most commonly in infants with congenital heart disease treated with alprostadil are apnoea, fever, flushing, hypotension, bradycardia, tachycardia, diarrhoea, and convulsions. Other adverse effects reported include oedema, cardiac arrest, hypokalaemia, disseminated intravascular coagulation, and cortical proliferation of the long bones. Weakening of the wall of the ductus arteriosus and pulmonary artery may occur following prolonged infusion. Alprostadil should be avoided in neonates with respiratory distress syndrome and should be used with caution in those with bleeding tendencies; blood pressure and respiratory status should be monitored during infusion.

Adverse effects reported in adults given alprostadil have included headache, flushing, hypotension, diarrhoea, and pain and inflammation at the infusion site.

Following intracavernosal or intra-urethral administration of alprostadil for the treatment of erectile dysfunction, the most frequently reported adverse effect is pain during erection. Local reactions including penile fibrosis, fibrotic nodules, and Peyronie's disease have been reported. Priapism may occur (see below). Systemic effects are less common but hypotension and other adverse effects have been reported. Intracavernosal or intra-urethral administration of alprostadil should be avoided in patients with complicating penile deformities or with sickle-cell disease, myeloma, leukaemias, or other conditions predisposing to prolonged erection.

◊ A review[1] of adverse effects associated with alprostadil administration in infants with congenital heart disease.

1. Lewis AB, *et al.* Side effects of therapy with prostaglandin E₁ in infants with critical congenital heart disease. *Circulation* 1981; **64:** 893–8.

Effects on the bones. Periosteal or cortical hyperostosis has been reported in infants following therapy with alprostadil for cyanotic congenital heart disease.[1-4] A retrospective review of 30 infants[2] treated with alprostadil revealed radiographic signs of periosteal reactions in 5. Changes could be detected after even short courses of therapy; 3 developed relatively mild periosteal changes in the ribs after infusions ranging from 9 to 205 hours and one had involvement of the left femur after infusion for 71 hours. Resolution of lesions had occurred in most bones 6 to 12 months later. In a further study,[5] radiological evidence of cortical hyperostosis was found in 53 of 86 infant heart transplant recipients who had received alprostadil infusion pre-operatively. Of 53 of the infants who had received alprostadil for less than 30 days, 21 were affected (2 severely). Correspondingly, of those treated for 30 to 60 days, 18 of 22 were affected (13 severely). All 14 infants treated for more than 60 days were affected (7 severely). Since the associated bone changes may persist for months after discontinuation of alprostadil, caution should be exercised to avoid misdiagnosis.

1. Ueda K, *et al.* Cortical hyperostosis following long-term administration of prostaglandin E₁ in infants with cyanotic congenital heart disease. *J Pediatr* 1980; **97:** 834–6.
2. Ringel RE, *et al.* Periosteal changes secondary to prostaglandin administration. *J Pediatr* 1983; **103:** 251–3.
3. Williams JL. Periosteal hyperostosis resulting from prostaglandin therapy. *Eur J Radiol* 1986; **6:** 231–2.

4. Kalloghlian AK, *et al.* Cortical hyperostosis simulating osteomyelitis after short-term prostaglandin E₁ infusion. *Eur J Pediatr* 1996; **155:** 173–4.
5. Woo K, *et al.* Cortical hyperostosis: a complication of prolonged prostaglandin infusion in infants awaiting cardiac transplantation. *Pediatrics* 1994; **93:** 417–20.

Effects on the gastrointestinal tract. Hyperplasia of the gastric mucosa, resulting in gastric outlet obstruction, has been reported in several neonates receiving alprostadil infusion.[1-3] It was suggested that this effect was dose-dependent.[1] Regression of the obstruction usually occurred after cessation of therapy.

1. Peled N, *et al.* Gastric-outlet obstruction induced by prostaglandin therapy in neonates. *N Engl J Med* 1992; **327:** 505–10.
2. Merkus PJFM, *et al.* Prostaglandin E1 and gastric outlet obstruction in infants. *Lancet* 1993; **342:** 747.
3. Kobayashi N, *et al.* Acute gastric outlet obstruction following the administration of prostaglandin: an additional case. *Pediatr Radiol* 1997; **27:** 57–9.

Effects on the metabolism. Severe hyperglycaemia with apparent ketoacidosis occurred during postoperative infusion of alprostadil in the infant of a diabetic mother.[1] The manufacturers had received reports of hyperglycaemia associated with alprostadil in 5 infants, one of whom had a diabetic mother. Hypoglycaemia has also been reported in a few infants.[2]

1. Cohen MH, Nihill MR. Postoperative ketotic hyperglycaemia during prostaglandin E₁ infusion in infancy. *Pediatrics* 1983; **71:** 842–4.
2. Lewis AB, *et al.* Side effects of therapy with prostaglandin E₁ in infants with critical congenital heart disease. *Circulation* 1981; **64:** 893–8.

Effects on the skin. A 63-year-old man with Peyronie's disease[1] developed toxic pustuloderma (acute generalised exanthematous pustulosis) 6 days after receiving a single intracavernosal injection of alprostadil to define the penile morphology. He was treated with antihistamines and topical corticosteroids and the condition resolved completely within a week.

1. Gallego I, *et al.* Toxic pustuloderma induced by intracavernous prostaglandin E₁. *Br J Dermatol* 1997; **136:** 975–6.

Priapism. If priapism occurs following the use of alprostadil for erectile dysfunction, its treatment should not be delayed more than 6 hours. Initial therapy is by penile aspiration. If aspiration is unsuccessful a sympathomimetic with action on alpha-adrenergic receptors is given by cautious intracavernosal injection, with continuous monitoring of blood pressure and pulse. Extreme caution is necessary in patients with coronary heart disease, hypertension, cerebral ischaemia, or if taking an antidepressant. Low doses and dilute solutions are recommended as follows:

• intracavernosal injection of phenylephrine 100 to 200 µg (0.5 to 1 mL of a 200 µg per mL solution) every 5 to 10 minutes; maximum total dose 1 mg

alternatively

• intracavernosal injection of adrenaline [epinephrine] 10 to 20 µg (0.5 to 1 mL of a 20 µg per mL solution) every 5 to 10 minutes; maximum total dose 100 µg

alternatively

• intracavernosal injection of metaraminol may be used, but it should be noted that fatal hypertensive crises have been reported; metaraminol 100 µg (5 mL of a 20 µg per mL solution) may be given by careful slow injection every 15 minutes; a maximum total dose of up to 1 mg has been suggested.

If necessary the sympathomimetic injections can be followed by further penile aspiration. If sympathomimetics are unsuccessful, urgent surgical referral is required.

Pharmacokinetics

Following infusion alprostadil is rapidly metabolised by oxidation during passage through the pulmonary circulation. It is excreted in the urine as metabolites within about 24 hours. Systemic absorption of alprostadil occurs following intracavernosal injection.

◊ References.
1. Cox JW, *et al.* Pulmonary extraction and pharmacokinetics of prostaglandin E₁ during continuous intravenous infusion in patients with adult respiratory distress syndrome. *Am Rev Respir Dis* 1988; **137:** 5–12.
2. Cawello W, *et al.* Dose proportional pharmacokinetics of alprostadil (prostaglandin E₁) in healthy volunteers following intravenous infusion. *Br J Clin Pharmacol* 1995; **40:** 273–6.
3. Lea AP, *et al.* Intracavernosal alprostadil: a review of its pharmacodynamic and pharmacokinetic properties and therapeutic potential in erectile dysfunction. *Drugs Aging* 1996; **8:** 56–74.

Uses and Administration

Alprostadil is a prostaglandin which causes vasodilatation and prevents platelet aggregation. The endogenous substance is termed prostaglandin E₁. Alprostadil is used mainly in congenital heart disease and in erectile dysfunction (p.1663).

Alprostadil is given to maintain the patency of the ductus arteriosus in neonates with **congenital heart disease** until surgery is possible. It is administered by continuous intravenous infusion beginning with doses of 50 to 100 nanograms per kg body-weight per minute; doses should be reduced as soon as possible to the lowest dosage necessary to maintain response. Some workers recommend a lower starting dose. It may also be given by continuous infusion through an umbilical artery catheter placed at the ductal opening.

In the management of **erectile dysfunction**, alprostadil is given by intracavernosal injection; preparations may contain alprostadil or alprostadil alfadex (a combination of alprostadil with α-cyclodextrin), but the dose is expressed in terms of the base. Alprostadil may also be given as an intra-urethral application.

By *intracavernosal injection*, the initial dose is 2.5 µg, increased incrementally until a suitable dose is established. The usual dose range is 5 to 20 µg and the maximum recommended dose is 60 µg. Normally, the second dose should be 5 µg if some response to the first dose is observed, or 7.5 µg if there is no response; subsequent increments should be of 5 to 10 µg until an effective dose is reached. In cases of erectile dysfunction of neurogenic origin secondary to spinal cord injury the initial dose is 1.25 µg, with a second dose of 2.5 µg, and third dose and subsequent increments of 2.5 to 5 µg. While finding a suitable dose, the interval between doses should be at least 1 day if there has been a partial response. If there is no response however, the next, higher dose may be given within one hour. Once established, the optimal dose should be administered not more than once daily and not more than three times per week.

Alprostadil may also be injected intracavernosally in the diagnosis of erectile dysfunction in doses ranging from 5 to 20 µg.

By *intra-urethral (transurethral) application*, the initial dose is 250 µg. The dose may be increased incrementally to 500 or 1000 µg or decreased to 125 µg according to response. The optimal dose should be given not more than twice daily or seven times per week. A dose of 500 µg may be used diagnostically.

Alprostadil is also available as a *topical* formulation for the treatment of erectile dysfunction in some countries.

Ergotamine poisoning. Alprostadil[1,2] is one of many drugs that have been used to treat the circulatory disturbances in ergotamine poisoning (p.452).
1. Levy JM, *et al.* Prostaglandin E₁ for alleviating symptoms of ergot intoxication: a case report. *Cardiovasc Intervent Radiol* 1984; **7:** 28–30.
2. Horstmann R, *et al.* Kritische extremitätenischämie durch ergotismus. *Dtsch Med Wochenschr* 1993; **118:** 1067–71.

Haemorrhagic cystitis. Bladder irrigation with alprostadil produced resolution of severe haemorrhagic cystitis in 5 of 6 children who had undergone bone-marrow transplantation.[1] Alprostadil was administered via a catheter and retained for 1 hour each day for at least 7 consecutive days.
1. Trigg ME, *et al.* Prostaglandin E₁ bladder instillations to control severe hemorrhagic cystitis. *J Urol (Baltimore)* 1990; **143:** 92–4.

Hepatic disorders. Benefit has been reported in patients with *viral hepatitis* (p.605) following intravenous administration of alprostadil alone or followed by oral dinoprostone or misoprostol.[1,2] Prostaglandins were studied because they had previously been shown to have a cytoprotective effect in experimentally induced hepatitis or in isolated hepatocytes, but the mechanism by which they exerted a beneficial effect was uncertain.

Combined intravenous therapy with glucagon, insulin, and alprostadil formulated in lipid microspheres has also been found effective in preventing *acute fulminant hepatic failure* after hepatic arterial infusion of antineoplastic chemotherapy.[3]
1. Sinclair SB, *et al.* Biochemical and clinical response of fulminant viral hepatitis to administration of prostaglandin E: a preliminary report. *J Clin Invest* 1989; **84:** 1063–9.
2. Flowers M, *et al.* Prostaglandin E in the treatment of recurrent hepatitis B infection after orthotopic liver transplantation. *Transplantation* 1994; **58:** 183–92.
3. Ikegami T, *et al.* Randomized control trial of lipo-prostaglandin E₁ in patients with acute liver injury induced by Lipiodol-targeted chemotherapy. *Clin Pharmacol Ther* 1995; **57:** 582–9.

Peripheral vascular disease. Various prostaglandins including alprostadil[1-9] have been used in the treatment of peripheral vascular disease (p.809), particularly in severe Raynaud's syndrome, but do not constitute mainline therapy.
1. Clifford PC, *et al.* Treatment of vasospastic disease with prostaglandin E₁. *BMJ* 1980; **281:** 1031–4.
2. Martin MFR, Tooke JE. Effects of prostaglandin E₁ on microvascular haemodynamics in progressive systemic sclerosis. *BMJ* 1982; **285:** 1688–90.
3. Anonymous. Prostaglandins and peripheral vascular disease. *Lancet* 1983; **i:** 1199.
4. Kyle V, Hazleman B. Prostaglandin E₁ and peripheral vascular disease. *Lancet* 1983; **ii:** 282.
5. Telles GS, *et al.* Prostaglandin E₁ in severe lower limb ischaemia: a double-blind controlled trial. *Br J Surg* 1984; **71:** 506–8.
6. Mohrland JS, *et al.* A multiclinic, placebo-controlled, double-blind study of prostaglandin E₁ in Raynaud's syndrome. *Ann Rheum Dis* 1985; **44:** 754–60.
7. Sethi GK, *et al.* Intravenous infusion of prostaglandin E₁ (PGE₁) in management of limb ischemia. *Am Surg* 1986; **52:** 474–8.
8. Langevitz P, *et al.* Treatment of refractory ischemic skin ulcers in patients with Raynaud's phenomenon with PGE₁ infusions. *J Rheumatol* 1989; **16:** 1433–5.
9. The ICAI Study Group. Prostanoids for chronic critical leg ischemia: a randomized, controlled, open-label trial with prostaglandin E₁. *Ann Intern Med* 1999; **130:** 412–21.

Preparations

USP 25: Alprostadil Injection.

Proprietary Preparations (details are given in Part 3)
Aust.: Caverject; Minprog; Muse; Prostavasin; *Austral.:* Caverject; Muse; Prostin VR; *Belg.:* Caverject; Prostin VR; *Canad.:* Caverject; Muse; Prostin VR; *Denm.:* Caverject; Muse; Prostivas; Rigidur; Viridal; *Fin.:* Caverject; Muse; Prostivas; Rigidur; *Fr.:* Caverject; Edex; Prostine VR; *Ger.:* Caverject; Minprog; Muse; Prostavasin; Viridal; *Hong Kong:* Caverject; Muse; Prostavasin; Prostin VR; *Irl.:* Caverject; Muse; Viridal; *Israel:* Caverject; Muse; Prostin VR; *Ital.:* Alprostar; Caverject; Prostavasin; Prostin VR; Viridal; *Jpn:* Liple; Prostandin; *Mex.:* Caverject; Muse; *Neth.:* Caverject; Prostin VR; *Norw.:* Bondil; Caverject; Prostivas; *NZ:* Caverject; Muse; Prostin VR; *Port.:* Caverject; Muse; Prostin VR; *S.Afr.:* Caverject; Muse; Prostin VR; *Singapore:* Caverject; Muse; Spain: Caverject; Muse; Sugiran; *Swed.:* Bondil; Caverject; Prostivas; Rigidur Duo; *Switz.:* Caverject; Muse; Prostin VR; *Thai.:* Caverject; Muse; Prostin VR; *UK:* Caverject; Muse; Prostin VR; Viridal; *USA:* Caverject; Edex; Muse; Prostin VR.

Beraprost Sodium (20711-p)

Beraprost Sodium (USAN, rINNM).

ML-1129; ML-1229 (beraprost); TRK-100. Sodium (±)-(1R,2R,3aS,8bS)-2,3,3a,8b-tetrahydro-2-hydroxy-1-[(E)-(3S,4RS)-3-hydroxy-4-methyl-1-octen-6-ynyl]-1H-cyclopenta[b]benzofuran-5-butyrate.

$C_{24}H_{29}NaO_5 = 420.5$.
CAS — 88430-50-6 (beraprost); 88475-69-8 (beraprost sodium).

Profile

Beraprost is a synthetic analogue of epoprostenol (prostacyclin) which causes vasodilatation and prevents platelet aggregation. It is given by mouth as the sodium salt in the management of peripheral vascular disease in a dose of 120 µg daily in three divided doses. It is also being studied in pulmonary hypertension and thrombotic thrombocytopenic purpura.

◊ References.
1. Nagaya N, *et al.* Effect of orally active prostacyclin analogue on survival of outpatients with primary pulmonary hypertension. *J Am Coll Cardiol* 1999; **34:** 1188–92.
2. Lievre M, *et al.* Oral beraprost sodium, a prostaglandin I₂ analogue, for intermittent claudication: a double-blind, randomized, multicenter controlled trial. *Circulation* 2000; **102:** 426–31.

Preparations

Proprietary Preparations (details are given in Part 3)
Jpn: Dorner.

Bimatoprost (8003-l)

Agn-192024. (Z)-7-{(1R,2R,3R,5S)-3,5-Dihydroxy-2-[(1E,3S)-3-hydroxy-5-phenyl-1-pentenyl]cyclopentyl}-N-ethyl-5-heptenamide.

$C_{25}H_{37}NO_4 = 415.6$.
CAS — 155206-00-1.

Adverse Effects and Precautions

As for Latanoprost, p.1445.

Pharmacokinetics

Following ophthalmic administration, small amounts of bimatoprost are absorbed, with peak blood concentrations seen within 10 minutes of dosing. Bimatoprost is metabolised by oxidation, de-ethylation and glucuronidation and is excreted in the urine and faeces. The elimination half-life is 45 minutes.

Uses and Administration

Bimatoprost is a synthetic prostaglandin analogue. It is used to reduce intra-ocular pressure in the treatment of open-angle glaucoma and ocular hypertension (p.1413), in patients who are resistant to other forms of treatment. It is administered once daily as a 0.03% ophthalmic solution.

◊ References.
1. Sherwood M, *et al.* Six-month comparison of bimatoprost once-daily and twice-daily with timolol twice-daily in patients with elevated intraocular pressure. *Surv Ophthalmol* 2001; **45** (suppl 4): S361–S368.
2. Brandt JD, *et al.* Comparison of once- or twice-daily bimatoprost with twice-daily timolol in patients with elevated IOP: a 3-month clinical trial. *Ophthalmology* 2001; **108:** 1023–31.

Preparations

Proprietary Preparations (details are given in Part 3)
USA: Lumigan.

Carboprost (8074-b)

Carboprost *(BAN, USAN, rINN)*.

15-Me-PGF$_{2\alpha}$; Methyldinoprost; (15S)-15-Methylprostaglandin F$_{2\alpha}$; U-32921. (5Z,13E)-(8R,9S,11R,12R,15S)-9,11,15-Trihydroxy-15-methylprosta-5,13-dienoic acid; (Z)-7-{(1R,2R,3R,5S)-3,5-Dihydroxy-2-[(E)-(3S)-3-hydroxy-3-methyloct-1-enyl]cyclopentyl}hept-5-enoic acid.

C$_{21}$H$_{36}$O$_5$ = 368.5.
CAS — 35700-23-3.
ATC — G02AD04.

Carboprost Methyl (8075-v)

Carboprost Methyl *(BANM, USAN, rINNM)*.
U-36384. The methyl ester of carboprost.
C$_{22}$H$_{38}$O$_5$ = 382.5.
CAS — 35700-21-1.

Carboprost Trometamol (8076-g)

Carboprost Trometamol *(BANM, rINNM)*.
Carboprost Tromethamine *(USAN)*; U-32921E.
C$_{21}$H$_{36}$O$_5$,C$_4$H$_{11}$NO$_3$ = 489.6.
CAS — 58551-69-2.

A compound of carboprost with trometamol in a ratio of 1:1. Carboprost trometamol 1.3 µg is approximately equivalent to 1 µg of carboprost.

Adverse Effects and Precautions

As for Dinoprostone, p.1441.

Carboprost may cause bronchospasm and, less frequently, dyspnoea and pulmonary oedema. Patients with cardiopulmonary disorders should be monitored for reductions in arterial-oxygen content.

Once a prostaglandin has been given to terminate pregnancy it is essential that termination take place; if the prostaglandin is unsuccessful other measures should be used.

Uses and Administration

Carboprost is a synthetic 15-methyl analogue of dinoprost (prostaglandin F$_{2\alpha}$). It is a uterine stimulant with a more prolonged action than dinoprost; the presence of the methyl group delays inactivation by enzymic dehydrogenation.

Carboprost is used for the termination of pregnancy (p.1439) and for the treatment of refractory postpartum haemorrhage due to uterine atony (p.1607). It is usually administered intramuscularly as the trometamol salt.

For the termination of second trimester pregnancy (between the 13th and 20th weeks of gestation) the equivalent of 250 µg of carboprost is given by deep intramuscular injection and repeated every 1½ to 3½ hours depending on the uterine response; if necessary the dose may be increased to 500 µg, but the total dose given should not exceed 12 mg. If preferred, a test dose of 100 µg may be given initially. Alternatively carboprost trometamol has been administered intra-amniotically in a dose equivalent to 2.5 mg of carboprost over five minutes; this dose may be repeated after 24 hours if termination has not occurred and the membranes are intact.

Carboprost methyl given as vaginal pessaries has been tried for termination of pregnancy in the second trimester.

For the treatment of postpartum haemorrhage the equivalent of 250 µg of carboprost is given by deep intramuscular injection as the trometamol salt at intervals of about 90 minutes; the interval may be reduced if necessary, but should not be less than 15 minutes. A total dose of 2 mg should not be exceeded.

Haemorrhagic cystitis. Carboprost trometamol instilled into the bladder successfully controlled cyclophosphamide-induced haemorrhagic cystitis (p.528) in 15 of 24 bone-marrow transplant patients.[1] The dose consisted of 50 mL of solutions containing 2 to 10 µg per mL instilled four times daily for 7 days.

1. Ippoliti C, *et al.* Intravesicular carboprost for the treatment of hemorrhagic cystitis after marrow transplantation. *Urology* 1995; **46:** 811–15.

The symbol † denotes a preparation no longer actively marketed

Preparations

Proprietary Preparations (details are given in Part 3)
Belg.: Prostin/15M; *Denm.:* Prostinfenem; *Hong Kong:* Hemabate; *Neth.:* Prostin/15M; *NZ:* Prostin 15M; *Swed.:* Prostinfenem; *UK:* Hemabate; *USA:* Hemabate.

Cicaprost (2842-m)

Cicaprost *(rINN)*.

ZK-96480. {2-[(2E,3aS,4S,5R,6aS)-Hexahydro-5-hydroxy-4-[(3S,4S)-3-hydroxy-4-methyl-1,6-nonadiynyl]-2-(1H)-pentalenylidene]ethoxy}acetic acid.

C$_{22}$H$_{30}$O$_5$ = 374.5.
CAS — 95722-07-9.

Profile

Cicaprost is a synthetic analogue of epoprostenol (prostacyclin) that has been studied for the oral treatment of peripheral vascular disease. It has also been given as cicaprost betadex.

◊ References.
1. Lau CS, *et al.* A randomised, double-blind study of cicaprost, an oral prostacyclin analogue, in the treatment of Raynaud's phenomenon secondary to systemic sclerosis. *Clin Exp Rheumatol* 1993; **11:** 35–40.

Cloprostenol Sodium (8077-q)

Cloprostenol Sodium *(BANM, USAN, rINNM)*.

ICI-80996. Sodium (±)-(Z)-7-{(1R,2R,3R,5S)-2-[(E)-(3R)-4-(3-chlorophenoxy)-3-hydroxybut-1-enyl]-3,5-dihydroxycyclopentyl}hept-5-enoate.

C$_{22}$H$_{28}$ClNaO$_6$ = 446.9.
CAS — 40665-92-7 (cloprostenol); 55028-72-3 (cloprostenol sodium).
Pharmacopoeias. In *BP(Vet)*.

Pharmacopoeial description

BP(Vet) 2001: A white or almost white amorphous hygroscopic powder. Freely soluble in water, in alcohol, and in methyl alcohol; practically insoluble in acetone. Protect from light and moisture.

Profile

Cloprostenol is a synthetic analogue of dinoprost (prostaglandin F$_{2\alpha}$). The sodium salt is used as a luteolytic in veterinary medicine.

Dinoprost (2931-b)

Dinoprost *(BAN, USAN, rINN)*.

PGF$_{2\alpha}$; Prostaglandin F$_{2\alpha}$; U-14583. (5Z,13E)-(8R,9S,11R,12R,15S)-9,11,15-Trihydroxyprosta-5,13-dienoic acid; (Z)-7-{(1R,2R,3R,5S)-3,5-Dihydroxy-2-[(E)-(3S)-3-hydroxyoct-1-enyl]cyclopentyl}hept-5-enoic acid.

C$_{20}$H$_{34}$O$_5$ = 354.5.
CAS — 551-11-1.
ATC — G02AD01.

NOTE. In *Martindale* the term dinoprost is used for the exogenous substance and prostaglandin F$_{2\alpha}$ for the endogenous substance.
Pharmacopoeias. In *Jpn.*

Dinoprost Trometamol (8081-m)

Dinoprost Trometamol *(BANM, rINNM)*.

Dinoprost Tromethamine *(USAN)*; Dinoprostum Trometamoli; PGF$_{2\alpha}$ THAM; Prostaglandin F$_{2\alpha}$ Trometamol; U-14583E.

C$_{20}$H$_{34}$O$_5$,C$_4$H$_{11}$NO$_3$ = 475.6.
CAS — 38562-01-5.
Pharmacopoeias. In *Eur.* (see p.vi).

Dinoprost trometamol 1.3 µg is approximately equivalent to 1 µg of dinoprost.

Pharmacopoeial description

Ph. Eur.: A white or almost white powder. Very soluble in water; freely soluble in alcohol; practically insoluble in acetonitrile.

Adverse Effects and Precautions

As for Dinoprostone, p.1441.

Dinoprost can cause bronchoconstriction, and bronchospasm with wheezing and dyspnoea has occurred, especially in asthmatic patients.

Once a prostaglandin has been given to terminate pregnancy it is essential that termination take place; if the prostaglandin is unsuccessful other measures should be used.

Uses and Administration

Dinoprost is a prostaglandin of the F series (p.1438) with actions on smooth muscle; the endogenous substance is termed prostaglandin F$_{2\alpha}$ and is rapidly metabolised in the body. It induces contraction of uterine muscle at any stage of pregnancy and is reported to act predominantly as a vasoconstrictor on blood vessels and as a bronchoconstrictor on bronchial muscle.

Dinoprost is used principally for the termination of pregnancy (p.1439). It may also be used for missed abortion, hydatidiform mole, and fetal death *in utero*. Dinoprost has also been given

for the induction of labour but, because it has a higher incidence of adverse effects than dinoprostone, is no longer recommended for routine use; more appropriate treatment is discussed on p.1438.

Dinoprost is usually administered intra-amniotically for termination of pregnancy. It has been given intravenously, but this route has been associated with a high incidence of adverse effects. The extra-amniotic route has also been used. Dinoprost is given as the trometamol salt, doses being expressed in terms of the equivalent amount of dinoprost. It should not be administered continuously for more than two days.

For the termination of pregnancy during the second trimester 40 mg of dinoprost is administered intra-amniotically by slowly injecting 8 mL of a solution containing 5 mg per mL into the amniotic sac. A further dose of 10 to 40 mg after 24 hours may be given if the membranes are still intact.

Ileus. Ileus induced by administration of vinca alkaloids to 3 patients with carcinoma of the lung was successfully relieved by the intravenous infusion of dinoprost 0.3 to 0.5 µg per kg body-weight per minute for 2 hours twice daily.[1]

1. Saito H, *et al.* Prostaglandin F$_{2\alpha}$ in the treatment of vinca alkaloid-induced ileus. *Am J Med* 1993; **95:** 549–51.

Preparations

BP 2001: Dinoprost Injection.

Proprietary Preparations (details are given in Part 3)
Austral.: Prostin F2 Alpha; *Fr.:* Prostine F$_2$ Alpha†; *Ger.:* Minprostin F$_{2\alpha}$; *Hong Kong:* Prostin F2 Alpha; *Irl.:* Prostin F2; *Israel:* Prostin F2 Alpha; *S.Afr.:* Prostin F2 Alpha; *UK:* Prostin F2 Alpha†.

Dinoprostone (8082-b)

Dinoprostone *(BAN, USAN, rINN)*.

Dinoprostonum; PGE$_2$; Prostaglandin E$_2$; U-12062. (5Z,13E)-(8R,11R,12R,15S)-11,15-Dihydroxy-9-oxoprosta-5,13-dienoic acid; (Z)-7-{(1R,2R,3R)-3-Hydroxy-2-[(E)-(3S)-3-hydroxyoct-1-enyl]-5-oxocyclopentyl}hept-5-enoic acid.

C$_{20}$H$_{32}$O$_5$ = 352.5.
CAS — 363-24-6.
ATC — G02AD02.

NOTE. In *Martindale* the term dinoprostone is used for the exogenous substance and prostaglandin E$_2$ for the endogenous substance.
Pharmacopoeias. In *Eur.* (see p.vi).

Pharmacopoeial description

Ph. Eur.: A white or almost white, crystalline powder or colourless crystals. Practically insoluble in water; freely soluble in alcohol; very soluble in methyl alcohol. Store at a temperature not exceeding −15°.

Adverse Effects

The incidence and severity of adverse reactions to dinoprostone are dose-related and also depend to some extent on the route of administration; the intravenous route has been associated with a high incidence of adverse effects. Nausea, vomiting, diarrhoea, and abdominal pain are common. Transient cardiovascular symptoms have included flushing, shivering, headache, dizziness, and hypotension; there have been rare reports of sudden cardiovascular collapse. Hypertension has also been reported. Convulsions and EEG changes have occurred rarely. Local tissue irritation and erythema, as well as pyrexia and raised white cell count, may follow intravenous administration but generally revert to normal after termination of the infusion. Local infection may follow intra- and extra-amniotic therapy. Excessive uterine activity may occur and there have been occasional reports of uterine rupture following the use of prostaglandins to terminate pregnancy or induce labour; fetal distress and, rarely, fetal death have occurred during the induction of labour.

Dinoprostone, although generally acting as a bronchodilator, may cause bronchoconstriction in some individuals. Hypersensitivity reactions have occurred.

◊ Side-effects were evaluated in 626 patients[1] undergoing abortion (usually in the second trimester), using extra-amniotic or intra-amniotic dinoprost or dinoprostone, often with oxytocin. Vomiting occurred in 291, diarrhoea in 28, pyrexia in 34, transient hypotension (fall in systolic blood pressure of at least 20 mmHg) in 25, transient bronchospasm in 2 patients given extra-amniotic dinoprost, and blood loss exceeding 250 mL in 68 (38 lost more than 500 mL). No patients had convulsions even though 8 were epileptics receiving antiepileptics. Three patients sustained lacerations to the cervix. Five patients complained of breast soreness or lactation; these symptoms may have been under-reported. Overall 14 patients were re-admitted; 13 because of excessive vaginal bleeding and 1 because of pelvic infection.

A later report describes the cumulative experience in 3313 pregnancies[2] in which dinoprostone gel was used for induction of term labour or cervical ripening. Adverse effects were rare. Vomiting, fever, and diarrhoea occurred in approximately 0.2% of mothers and were difficult to distinguish from the effects of concurrent drug therapy. Detectable myometrial activity was dose-related and more common after intravaginal than after intracervical administration. Myometrial activity was reported in 0.6 to 6% of patients following intravaginal application and hyperstimulation was virtually non-existent at an intracervical dose of 500 µg. Fetal effects were negligible in the absence of uterine hyperstimulation.

1. MacKenzie IZ, *et al.* Prostaglandin-induced abortion: assessment of operative complications and early morbidity. *BMJ* 1974; **4:** 683–6.
2. Rayburn WF. Prostaglandin E₂ gel for cervical ripening and induction of labor: a critical analysis. *Am J Obstet Gynecol* 1989; **160:** 529–34.

Effects on the bones. Reversible periosteal reactions of the long bones and bone thickening have occurred in infants receiving long-term therapy with prostaglandins of the E series (see p.1439). In addition, reversible widening of cranial sutures was reported[1] in 2 neonates given dinoprostone intravenously for 95 and 97 days respectively.

1. Hoevels-Guerich H, *et al.* Widening of cranial sutures after long-term prostaglandin E₂ therapy in two newborn infants. *J Pediatr* 1984; **105:** 72–4.

Effects on the cardiovascular system. Cardiovascular adverse effects are most common following intravenous administration of dinoprostone but may also occur with other routes. Severe cardiovascular disorders reported with the intra-amniotic or intravaginal administration of dinoprost or dinoprostone have included: cardiac arrhythmias in 3 patients,[1,2] fatal in 2 of them;[2] hypotension, tachypnoea, and tachycardia in 3 patients[3,4] with associated pyrexias in 2 patients;[3] and fatal myocardial infarction in a patient who had several high-risk factors for ischaemic heart disease.[5]

Severe hypertension occurred in a patient[6] who received dinoprostone by direct myometrial injection and by intravenous infusion concomitantly for postpartum haemorrhage.

1. Burt RL, *et al.* Hypokalemia and cardiac arrhythmia associated with prostaglandin-induced abortion. *Obstet Gynecol* 1977; **50:** 45S–46S.
2. Cates W, Jordaan HVF. Sudden collapse and death of women obtaining abortions induced with prostaglandin F₂α. *Am J Obstet Gynecol* 1979; **133:** 398–400.
3. Phelan JP, *et al.* Dramatic pyrexic and cardiovascular response to intravaginal prostaglandin E₂. *Am J Obstet Gynecol* 1978; **132:** 28–32.
4. Cameron IT, Baird DT. Sudden collapse after intra-amniotic prostaglandin E₂ injection. *Lancet* 1984; **ii:** 1046.
5. Patterson SP, *et al.* A maternal death associated with prostaglandin E₂. *Obstet Gynecol* 1979; **54:** 123–4.
6. Veber B, *et al.* Severe hypertension during postpartum haemorrhage after i.v. administration of prostaglandin E2. *Br J Anaesth* 1992; **68:** 623–4.

Effects on the fetus. A woman who failed to abort despite receiving carboprost intravaginally 7 weeks after conception gave birth at 34 weeks' gestation to an infant with hydrocephalus and abnormal digits.[1]

For reports of adverse effects on the fetus due to hyperstimulation of the uterus during labour, see under Effects on the Uterus, below.

1. Collins FS, Mahoney MJ. Hydrocephalus and abnormal digits after failed first-trimester prostaglandin abortion attempt. *J Pediatr* 1983; **102:** 620–1.

Effects on the gastrointestinal system. Hypotension and apnoea induced by dinoprostone infusions have been suggested by some[1] as a cause of necrotising enterocolitis in infants with symptomatic congenital heart disease although others[2] did not support this view.

1. Leung MP, *et al.* Necrotizing enterocolitis in neonates with symptomatic congenital heart disease. *J Pediatr* 1988; **113:** 1044–6.
2. Miller MJS, Clark DA. Congenital heart disease and necrotizing enterocolitis. *J Pediatr* 1989; **115:** 335–6.

Effects on the neonate. Aspiration of the undissolved remnants of a dinoprostone vaginal tablet caused neonatal respiratory distress due to mechanical obstruction of the airways: there was no evidence to suggest absorption of dinoprostone from the tablet matrix.[1]

1. Andersson S, *et al.* Neonatal respiratory distress caused by aspiration of a vaginal tablet containing prostaglandin. *BMJ* 1987; **295:** 25–6.

Effects on the nervous system. Convulsions and EEG changes have been occasionally reported during the administration of prostaglandins for termination of pregnancy. Convulsions occurred[1] in 5 of 320 women following intra-amniotic dinoprost administration, but in other large series[2-4] of patients given dinoprost or dinoprostone by various routes no problems were encountered despite the inclusion of patients with a history of epilepsy. However, convulsions were reported[5] in 3 of 4 epileptic patients following intramuscular administration of sulprostone.

1. Lyneham RC, *et al.* Convulsions and electroencephalogram abnormalities after intra-amniotic prostaglandin F₂α. *Lancet* 1973; **ii:** 1003–5.

2. MacKenzie IZ, *et al.* Convulsions and prostaglandin-induced abortion. *Lancet* 1973; **ii:** 1323.
3. Thiery M, *et al.* Prostaglandins and convulsions. *Lancet* 1974; **i:** 218.
4. Fraser IS, Gray C. Electroencephalogram changes after prostaglandin. *Lancet* 1974; **i:** 360.
5. Brandenburg H, *et al.* Convulsions in epileptic women after administration of prostaglandin E₂ derivative. *Lancet* 1990; **336:** 1138.

Effects on the uterus. Fatal amniotic fluid embolism occurred following induction of labour with dinoprostone pessaries in a 37-year-old woman.[1] Although administration of dinoprostone was not considered to be solely responsible, the high pressure gradient produced in the uterus could have been a predisposing factor. Amniotic fluid embolism was also found post mortem in a patient who died of intracerebral haemorrhage[2] following a precipitate labour induced by a dinoprostone pessary. The infant also died from intracranial haemorrhage following the spontaneous vaginal delivery. Again, hyperstimulation of the uterus could have been implicated.

Hypertonic uterine contractions also followed application of dinoprostone as a gel.[3] The intensity of the contractions was eventually decreased with terbutaline.

Uterine hyperstimulation may also lead to fetal distress. Intra-uterine fetal death occurred in 2 high-risk pregnancies[4] following insertion into the extra-amniotic space of a dinoprost gel. Placental abruption and neonatal death following the administration of a dinoprostone vaginal pessary was also reported in a woman with a retained IUD but an otherwise uncomplicated pregnancy.[5]

Uterine or cervical rupture has been reported following the termination of pregnancy with dinoprost given intra-amniotically;[6] dinoprostone given intra-amniotically,[7,8] intravenously,[9] or extra-amniotically;[10] and carboprost given intramuscularly.[11] It was noted[11] that uterine rupture was not always suspected, but should be considered if established uterine contractions disappear or there is vaginal blood loss without concomitant progressive dilatation. Rupture has also followed the use of dinoprostone pessaries for the induction of labour;[12,13] rupture of a uterine scar occurred in 2 patients.[14] Complications have also been reported[15] following the use of dinoprostone to induce labour in grand multiparae; one patient given dinoprostone by mouth developed severe postpartum haemorrhage due to uterine rupture and died and another given dinoprostone vaginally was found to have a ruptured uterus following delivery of a stillborn infant. The authors suggested that induction of labour with dinoprostone was not safer than carefully controlled oxytocin infusion with amniotomy and that the vaginal dose of dinoprostone should be restricted in grand multiparae to 3 mg if the cervix is unripe, and to 2 mg if the cervix is ripe, and should not be repeated for at least 24 hours.

1. Less A, *et al.* Vaginal prostaglandin E₂ and fatal amniotic fluid embolus. *JAMA* 1990; **263:** 3259–60.
2. Stronge J, *et al.* A neonatal and maternal death following the administration of intravaginal prostaglandin. *J Obstet Gynaecol* 1987; **7:** 271–2.
3. Chamberlin RO, *et al.* Uterine hyperstimulation resulting from intravaginal prostaglandin E₂: a case report. *J Reprod Med* 1987; **32:** 233–5.
4. Quinn MA, Murphy AJ. Fetal death following extra-amniotic prostaglandin gel: report of two cases. *Br J Obstet Gynaecol* 1981; **88:** 650–1.
5. Simmons K, Savage W. Neonatal death associated with induction of labour with intravaginal prostaglandin E₂: case report. *Br J Obstet Gynaecol* 1984; **91:** 598–9.
6. Karim SMM, Ratnam SS. Mid-trimester termination. *BMJ* 1974; **4:** 161–2.
7. Fraser IS. Complications of prostaglandin-induced abortion. *BMJ* 1974; **4:** 404.
8. Emery S, *et al.* Uterine rupture after intra-amniotic injection of prostaglandin E₂. *BMJ* 1979; **2:** 51.
9. Smith AM. Rupture of uterus during prostaglandin-induced abortion. *BMJ* 1975; **i:** 205.
10. Traub AI, Ritchie JWK. Rupture of the uterus during prostaglandin-induced abortion. *BMJ* 1979; **2:** 496.
11. Vergote I, *et al.* Uterine rupture due to 15-methyl prostaglandin F₂α. *Lancet* 1982; **ii:** 1402.
12. Claman P, *et al.* Uterine rupture with the use of vaginal prostaglandin E₂ for induction of labor. *Am J Obstet Gynecol* 1984; **150:** 889–90.
13. Keller F, Joyce TH. Uterine rupture associated with the use of vaginal prostaglandin E₂ suppositories. *Can Anaesth Soc J* 1984; **31:** 80–2.
14. Bromham DR, Anderson RS. Uterine scar rupture in labour induced with vaginal prostaglandin E₂. *Lancet* 1980; **ii:** 485–6.
15. Larsen JV, *et al.* Uterine hyperstimulation and rupture after induction of labour with prostaglandin E₂. *S Afr Med J* 1984; **65:** 615–16.

Overdosage. Severe adverse effects associated with intra-amniotic prostaglandins have been attributed to absorption into the systemic circulation of doses higher than would normally be given systemically. Rigors, vomiting, severe abdominal pain, and an intense desire to urinate and defaecate occurred[1] in 3 patients given dinoprostone intra-amniotically for mid-trimester abortion; one patient had peripheral vasoconstriction and a rapid low-volume pulse, with hypotension, and another had peripheral cyanosis. It was suggested[2] that this might have been due to displacement of the needle or cannula outside the amniotic sac, or that prior administration of urea, as in 2 of the patients, increased the rate of absorption of prostaglandins from the amniotic cavity. In a further report[3] flushing, severe headache, and nausea immediately after a test dose of dinoprost 2.5 mg was also thought to be due to incorrect positioning of the needle in the amniotic cavity with consequent injection into

the systemic circulation; at least part of the dose might have been injected into the peritoneal cavity.[4]

Severe reactions have also been reported with prostaglandins given to abort hydatidiform moles. A 20-year-old woman given 20 mg of dinoprostone by injection into the uterine cavity developed profound hypotension, bradycardia, and rigors, followed by nausea, vomiting, suprapubic pain, an increased pulse rate, pyrexia, and generalised flushing.[5] Since there are no fetal membranes in a molar pregnancy, intra-uterine administration is similar to extra-amniotic administration and the dose used was 100 times higher than the usual extra-amniotic dose.[4] However, in a similar patient[6] 'extra-amniotic' instillation of dinoprostone 200 µg was followed immediately by nausea, retching, severe abdominal pain, dizziness, difficulty in breathing and the production of frothy blood-stained sputum, an imperceptible pulse, and hypotension; the dinoprostone had probably been injected directly into the maternal circulation.

1. Ross AH, Whitehouse WL. Adverse reactions to intra-amniotic urea and prostaglandin. *BMJ* 1974; **1:** 642.
2. Craft I, Bowen-Simpkins P. Adverse reactions to intra-amniotic urea and prostaglandin. *BMJ* 1974; **2:** 446.
3. Brown R. Adverse reactions to intra-amniotic prostaglandin. *BMJ* 1974; **2:** 382.
4. Karim SMM. Adverse reactions to intra-amniotic prostaglandin. *BMJ* 1974; **3:** 347.
5. Smith AM. Adverse reactions to intra-amniotic prostaglandin. *BMJ* 1974; **2:** 382–3.
6. McNicol E, Gray H. Adverse reaction to extra-amniotic prostaglandin E₂. *Br J Obstet Gynaecol* 1977; **84:** 229–30.

Precautions

Dinoprostone should not be given to patients in whom oxytocin drugs are generally contra-indicated (see Oxytocin, p.1294), or in those with a history of pelvic inflammatory disease. Since prostaglandins enhance the effects of oxytocin use of the 2 drugs together or in sequence should be carefully monitored.

Dinoprostone is contra-indicated in active cardiac, pulmonary, renal, or hepatic disease. It should be used with caution in patients with glaucoma or raised intra-ocular pressure, asthma or a history of asthma, epilepsy or a history of epilepsy, hepatic or renal dysfunction, or cardiovascular disease.

In the induction of labour cephalopelvic relationships should be carefully evaluated before use. During use uterine activity, fetal status, and the progress of cervical dilatation should be carefully monitored to detect adverse responses, such as hypertonus, sustained uterine contractions, or fetal distress. In patients with a history of hypertonic uterine contractility or tetanic uterine contractions, uterine activity and the state of the fetus should be continuously monitored throughout labour. Where high-tone myometrial contractions are sustained the possibility of uterine rupture should be considered.

Dinoprostone should not be administered by the myometrial route, since there is a possible association with cardiac arrest in severely ill patients. The extra-amniotic route should not be used in patients with cervicitis or vaginal infections. Vaginal preparations of dinoprostone should not be used in the induction of labour once the membranes are ruptured. In some countries, intravenous prostaglandins are considered to be contra-indicated in women who smoke.

In the therapeutic termination of pregnancy, fetal damage has been observed in cases of incomplete termination and the appropriate treatment for complete evacuation of the uterus should therefore be instituted whenever termination is unsuccessful or incomplete. Dinoprostone should not be used for termination in patients with pelvic infection, unless adequate treatment has already been started.

Administration. For the hazards of unintentional systemic absorption of prostaglandins following their intra-uterine administration for the termination of pregnancy and abortion of hydatidiform moles, see Overdosage in Adverse Effects, above.

Interactions

Dinoprostone enhances the effects of oxytocin on the uterus.

◊ Marked hypertension, vomiting, and severe dyspnoea occurred following the sequential administration of oxytocin, methylergometrine, and dinoprost within the space of 10 minutes to a woman with postpartum haemorrhage.[1]

1. Cohen S, *et al.* Severe systemic reactions following administration of different ureotonic [uterotonic] drugs. *N Y State J Med* 1983; **83:** 1060–1.

Uses and Administration

Dinoprostone is a prostaglandin of the E series (p.1438) with actions on smooth muscle; the endogenous substance is termed prostaglandin E_2 and is rapidly metabolised in the body. It induces contraction of uterine muscle at any stage of pregnancy and is reported to act predominantly as a vasodilator on blood vessels and as a bronchodilator on bronchial muscle. In the UK, dinoprostone is used principally in the induction of labour (p.1438); it may also be used for the termination of pregnancy (p.1439), missed abortion, hydatidiform mole, and fetal death *in utero*.

Dinoprostone is usually administered vaginally. It may also be given intravenously, extra-amniotically, or by mouth, but the intravenous route has been associated with a high incidence of adverse effects and is generally only used for missed abortion or hydatidiform mole; continuous administration for more than two days is not recommended.

For the **induction of labour** dinoprostone is used to ripen (soften and dilate) the cervix before the membranes are ruptured and to induce labour at term. The cervical gel used for the former purpose contains 500 µg in 2.5 mL, whereas the vaginal gel used for induction of labour contains 1 or 2 mg per 2.5 mL; the vaginal gel should not be administered into the cervical canal. Pessaries containing 3 mg are also available for labour induction. These are not bioequivalent to the vaginal gel and their dosage is different.

To soften and dilate the cervix before induction of labour dinoprostone 500 µg is administered as *cervical gel*. For induction of labour the dose as *vaginal gel* is 1 mg (or 2 mg in primigravid patients with unfavourable induction features) followed, if necessary, by a further 1 or 2 mg after 6 hours; a total dose of 3 mg (or 4 mg in unfavourable primigravid patients) should not be exceeded. Alternatively a *vaginal pessary* containing 3 mg may be used and this may be followed, if necessary, by a further 3 mg after 6 to 8 hours; a total dose of 6 mg should not be exceeded.

A *modified-release pessary* delivering 5 mg over 12 hours can be employed for cervical ripening and subsequent labour induction. If it does not produce satisfactory cervical ripening within 8 to 12 hours then it should be removed and a second and final modified-release pessary administered to be retained for not more than 12 hours.

Dinoprostone may be given *by mouth* for the induction of labour in an initial dose of 500 µg, repeated hourly, and increased if necessary to 1 mg hourly until an adequate response is achieved; single doses of 1.5 mg should not be exceeded. Oral administration has, however, generally been replaced by intravaginal administration since the latter is associated with fewer gastrointestinal side-effects.

Dinoprostone has been given *intravenously* for the induction of labour but is no longer recommended for routine use by most authorities. A suggested intravenous dosage regimen has been 250 nanograms of dinoprostone per minute infused as a solution containing 1.5 µg per mL for 30 minutes, the dose being subsequently maintained or increased according to the patient's response; in fetal death *in utero* higher doses may be required and an initial rate of 500 nanograms per minute has been used with increases at intervals of not less than 1 hour.

For the **termination of pregnancy** in the second trimester 1 mL of a solution containing 100 µg of dinoprostone per mL may be instilled *extra-amniotically* through a suitable Foley catheter, with subsequent doses of 1 or 2 mL given at intervals usually of 2 hours, according to response. Dinoprostone has also been given *intravenously* for the termination of pregnancy and for missed abortion or hydatidiform mole. A solution containing 5 µg per mL may be infused at a rate of 2.5 µg per minute for 30 minutes, then maintained or increased to 5 µg per minute; this rate should be maintained for at least 4 hours before making further increases.

The symbol † denotes a preparation no longer actively marketed

In the USA dinoprostone pessaries are used for the termination of second trimester pregnancy, a dose of 20 mg being administered *intravaginally* and repeated every 3 to 5 hours according to response for up to 2 days; a total dose of 240 mg should not be exceeded. Pessaries are also used in the USA in missed abortion, fetal death *in utero*, and benign hydatidiform mole.

Dinoprostone is used in some centres to maintain the patency of the ductus arteriosus (see below).

Haemorrhagic cystitis. Dinoprostone instilled into the bladder for 4 hours and repeated for 4 days successfully improved severe cyclophosphamide-induced haemorrhagic cystitis (p.528) in a bone marrow transplant recipient.[1] Similar results were obtained in another series of 10 patients.[2]

1. Mohiuddin J, *et al.* Treatment of cyclophosphamide-induced cystitis with prostaglandin E_2. *Ann Intern Med* 1984; **101**: 142.
2. Laszlo D, *et al.* Prostaglandin E2 bladder instillation for the treatment of hemorrhagic cystitis after allogeneic bone marrow transplantation. *Haematologica* 1995; **80**: 421–5.

Hepatic disorders. See under Alprostadil, p.1440, for reference to the use of prostaglandins, including dinoprostone, in the treatment of viral hepatitis.

Patent ductus arteriosus. Prostaglandins, particularly alprostadil (p.1440), may be used to maintain the patency of the ductus arteriosus in infants with congenital heart disease until surgery can be performed to correct the malformation. Treatment for a longer period, especially with oral dinoprostone, may facilitate later surgery by allowing growth of the infants and their pulmonary arteries.

Beneficial responses to long-term use of dinoprostone have been reported.[1,2] Dinoprostone has been given orally in an initial dose of 20 to 25 µg per kg body-weight hourly, decreasing the frequency of doses after the first week; it was suggested that treatment should be continued for up to 4 weeks initially and a decision then made whether to proceed with surgery or to plan a longer course of treatment to encourage further growth. Intravenous administration may be an alternative when gastrointestinal absorption is expected to be poor or when oral treatment is ineffective. Dinoprostone has been given by intravenous infusion, beginning with a dose of 3 nanograms per kg per minute, adjusted according to response. Doses as high as 10 to 20 nanograms per kg per minute have been used but are reported to be exceptional, and severe adverse effects were encountered[2] in 4 of 11 infants given dinoprostone by intravenous infusion at an initial dose of 50 nanograms per kg per minute.

1. Silove ED, *et al.* Evaluation of oral and low dose intravenous prostaglandin E_2 in management of ductus dependent congenital heart disease. *Arch Dis Child* 1985; **60**: 1025–30.
2. Thanopoulos BD, *et al.* Prostaglandin E_2 administration in infants with ductus-dependent cyanotic congenital heart disease. *Eur J Pediatr* 1987; **146**: 279–82.

Pemphigus. Erosive oral lesions in 3 patients[1] with pemphigus vulgaris (p.1106) that had previously been refractory to standard corticosteroid therapy resolved on sucking oral dinoprostone tablets 1.5 to 3 mg daily. Symptoms recurred within weeks of ceasing dinoprostone therapy but could be controlled by courses of 0.5 to 1 mg daily for 1 to 2 weeks, when required.

1. Morita H, *et al.* Clinical trial of prostaglandin E_2 on the oral lesions of pemphigus vulgaris. *Br J Dermatol* 1995; **132**: 165–6.

Peripheral vascular disease. Various prostaglandins have been used in the treatment of peripheral vascular disease (p.809), particularly in severe Raynaud's syndrome, but do not constitute mainline therapy.

Postpartum haemorrhage. Dinoprostone and other prostaglandins have been used to control severe postpartum haemorrhage (p.1607) unresponsive to ergometrine and oxytocin. Beneficial response to continuous intra-uterine irrigation with dinoprostone solution 1.5 µg per mL was seen in 22 patients with postpartum haemorrhage unresponsive to other treatment.[1] Postpartum haemorrhage was controlled in another patient using a dinoprostone 3-mg vaginal suppository held against the uterine wall.[2]

1. Peyser MR, Kupfermine MJ. Management of severe postpartum hemorrhage by intrauterine irrigation with prostaglandin E_2. *Am J Obstet Gynecol* 1990; **162**: 694–6.
2. Markos AR. Prostaglandin E_2 intrauterine suppositories in the treatment of secondary postpartum hemorrhage. *J R Soc Med* 1989; **82**: 504–5.

Preparations

Proprietary Preparations (details are given in Part 3)
Aust.: Cerviprost†; Prepidil; Propess; Prostin E2; *Austral.:* Prostin E2; *Belg.:* Prepidil; Prostin E2; *Canad.:* Cervidil; Prepidil; Prostin E2; *Denm.:* Minprostin; Propess†; *Fin.:* Minprostin; Propess; *Fr.:* Prepidil; Propess; Prostine E_2; *Ger.:* Cerviprost†; Minprostin E_2; Prepidil; *Hong Kong:* Prepidil; Propess; Prostin E2; *Irl.:* Prostin E2; *Israel:* Prepidil; Propess; Prostin E2; *Ital.:* Prepidil; Prostin E2; *Mex.:* Prepidil; Prostin E2; *Neth.:* Cerviprost†; Prepidil; Propess; Prostin E2; *Norw.:* Minprostin; Prostin E2; *NZ:* Prepidil; Prostin E2; *Port.:* Propess; Prostin E2; *S.Afr.:* Prostin E2; *Singapore:* Prostin; *Spain:* Gravidex†; Prepidil; Propess; *Swed.:* Cerviprost†; Minprostin; Propess; *Switz.:* Cerviprost†; Prepidil; Propess; Prostin E2; *Thai.:* Prostin E2; *UK:* Prepidil†; Propess; Prostin E2; *USA:* Cervidil; Prepidil; Prostin E2.

Enisoprost (16621-z)

Enisoprost (*USAN, rINN*).

SC-34301. (±)-Methyl (Z)-7-{(1R,2R,3R)-3-hydroxy-2-[(E)-(4RS)-4-hydroxy-4-methyl-1-octenyl]-5-oxocyclopentyl}-4-heptenoate.

$C_{22}H_{36}O_5 = 380.5$.
CAS — 81026-63-3.

Profile

Enisoprost is a synthetic analogue of alprostadil (prostaglandin E_1) that has been investigated as an adjunct to ciclosporin therapy in organ transplant recipients to reduce acute transplant rejection and to diminish the nephrotoxic effects of ciclosporin; however, results have generally been disappointing.

◊ References.

1. Adams MB and The Enisoprost Renal Transplant Study Group. Enisoprost in renal transplantation. *Transplantation* 1992; **53**: 338–45.
2. Pollak R, *et al.* A trial of the prostaglandin E1 analogue, enisoprost, to reverse chronic cyclosporine-associated renal dysfunction. *Am J Kidney Dis* 1992; **20**: 336–41.
3. Ismail T, *et al.* Enisoprost in liver transplantation. *Transplantation* 1995; **59**: 1298–1301.

Enprostil (16628-f)

Enprostil (*BAN, USAN, rINN*).

RS-84135. Methyl (E)-(11R,15R)-11,15-dihydroxy-9-oxo-16-phenoxy-17,18,19,20-tetranorprosta-4,5,13-trienoate; Methyl 7-{(E)-(3R*)-3-hydroxy-2-[(1R*,2R*,3R*)-3-hydroxy-4-phenoxy-but-1-enyl]-5-oxocyclopentyl}hepta-4,5-dienoate.

$C_{23}H_{28}O_6 = 400.5$.
CAS — 73121-56-9.
ATC — A02BB02.

Profile

Enprostil, a synthetic analogue of dinoprostone (prostaglandin E_2), inhibits gastric acid secretion. It has been given by mouth in the treatment of peptic ulcer disease.

◊ References.

1. Goa KL, Monk JP. Enprostil: a preliminary review of its pharmacodynamic and pharmacokinetic properties, and therapeutic efficacy in the treatment of peptic ulcer disease. *Drugs* 1987; **34**: 539–59.
2. Sontag SJ, *et al.* Healing of NSAID-induced gastric ulcers with a synthetic prostaglandin analog (enprostil). *Am J Gastroenterol* 1994; **89**: 1014–20.
3. Ching CK, Lam SK. A comparison of two prostaglandin analogues (enprostil vs misoprostol) in the treatment of acute duodenal ulcer disease. *J Gastroenterol* 1995; **30**: 607–14.

Epoprostenol (8084-g)

Epoprostenol (*USAN, rINN*).

PGI₂; PGX; Prostacyclin; Prostaglandin I₂; Prostaglandin X; U-53217. (5Z,13E)-(8R,9S,11R,12R,15S)-6,9-Epoxy-11,15-dihydroxyprosta-5,13-dienoic acid; (Z)-5-{(3aR,4R,5R,6aS)-5-Hydroxy-4-[(E)-(3S)-3-hydroxyoct-1-enyl]perhydrocyclopenta[b]furan-2-ylidene}valeric acid.

$C_{20}H_{32}O_5 = 352.5$.
CAS — 35121-78-9.
ATC — B01AC09.

NOTE. In *Martindale* the term epoprostenol is used for the exogenous substance and prostacyclin for the endogenous substance.

Epoprostenol Sodium (8085-q)

Epoprostenol Sodium (*BAN, USAN, rINNM*).

U-53217A.
$C_{20}H_{31}NaO_5 = 374.4$.
CAS — 61849-14-7.

Stability in solution. Epoprostenol is unstable at physiological pH and solutions for infusion are prepared in an alkaline glycine buffer at pH 10.5. The half-life in aqueous solution of pH 7.4 has been reported[1] to be less than 3 minutes at 37°, but increased stability has been reported in plasma, albumin, or whole blood.[1,2]

1. El Tahir KEH, *et al.* Stability of prostacyclin in human plasma. *Clin Sci* 1980; **59**: 28P–29P.
2. Mikhailidis DP, *et al.* Infusion of prostacyclin (epoprostenol). *Lancet* 1982; **ii**: 767.

Adverse Effects and Precautions

The incidence of adverse reactions to epoprostenol is dose-related. Side-effects during intravenous infusion commonly include hypotension, increased heart rate, flushing, and headache. Dosage should be reduced or the epoprostenol infusion stopped if excessive hypotension occurs. Bradycardia together with pallor, sweating, nausea, and abdominal discomfort may occur. Erythema over the intravenous infusion site has been noted. Other side-effects reported have included nausea and vomiting, diarrhoea, jaw pain or non-specific musculoskeletal pain, anxiety, nervousness, tremor, flu-like symptoms, hyperglycaemia, drowsiness, and chest pain.

Coagulation of blood in the dialysis circuit has been reported rarely in patients given epoprostenol but no conventional anticoagulant. Haematological and cardiovascular monitoring is required in patients receiving epoprostenol infusions. Care should be taken to avoid extravasation.

◊ A study in 24 healthy subjects investigated the incidence of adverse effects with intravenous infusions of epoprostenol of up to 10 nanograms per kg body-weight per minute for up to 100 minutes.[1] Subjects varied in their susceptibility to epoprostenol but the same sequence of events was usually present. A change in pre-ejection period and facial flushing was often apparent at an infusion rate of 2 to 2.5 nanograms per kg per minute. A rise in heart rate and change in other cardiovascular variables was present when the infusion rate had increased to 4 to 5 nanograms per kg per minute; headache, generally the dose-limiting factor, was usually present at this dose and increased as the dose was raised, as did the other effects. Erythema over the vein and 'vagal reflex' only appeared after at least 1 hour of infusion; 'vagal reflex' took only a few seconds to develop.

Early studies showing that high doses were well tolerated had been conducted using a form of epoprostenol probably only half as potent as the commercially available product. It was proposed that 4 nanograms per kg per minute should in general be the maximum infusion rate for prolonged infusions, although higher rates could be tolerated in anaesthetised patients. Careful attention to infusion technique is necessary and monitoring of the heart rate is advisable in view of the suddenness with which the 'vagal reflex' can occur. Most of the adverse effects reported here have responded to a reduction in dosage.

1. Pickles H, O'Grady J. Side effects occurring during administration of epoprostenol (prostacyclin, PGI₂), in man. *Br J Clin Pharmacol* 1982; **14**: 177–85.

Effects on the blood. Reports of rebound platelet activation during continuous epoprostenol infusion.[1,2]

1. Yardumian DA, Machin SJ. Altered platelet function in patients on continuous infusion of epoprostenol. *Lancet* 1984; **i**: 1357.
2. Sinzinger H, et al. Rebound platelet activation after continuous epoprostenol infusion. *Lancet* 1984; **ii**: 759.

Effects on the cardiovascular system. Evidence that epoprostenol and its analogue iloprost can induce myocardial ischaemia in patients with coronary artery disease.[1]

1. Bugiardini R, et al. Myocardial ischemia induced by prostacyclin and iloprost. *Clin Pharmacol Ther* 1985; **38**: 101–8.

Effects on mental state. Symptoms of depression were associated with intravenous epoprostenol therapy in 4 patients.[1]

1. Ansell D, et al. Depression and prostacyclin infusion. *Lancet* 1986; **ii**: 509.

Interactions

Since epoprostenol is a potent vasodilator and inhibitor of platelet aggregation, care should be taken in patients receiving other vasodilators or anticoagulants. The hypotensive effects of epoprostenol may be exacerbated by using acetate in dialysis fluids.

Pharmacokinetics

Endogenous prostacyclin is a product of arachidonic acid metabolism with a very short half-life. Following intravenous infusion epoprostenol is hydrolysed rapidly to the more stable but much less active 6-keto-prostaglandin $F_{1\alpha}$ (6-oxo-prostaglandin $F_{1\alpha}$). Unlike many other prostaglandins, epoprostenol is not inactivated in the pulmonary circulation.

Uses and Administration

Epoprostenol is a prostaglandin (p.1438) which causes vasodilatation and prevents platelet aggregation. The endogenous substance is termed prostacyclin. It is used mainly in extracorporeal procedures and in pulmonary hypertension.

Epoprostenol is given as the sodium salt and doses are expressed in terms of the base. It is unstable in solution at physiological pH and also has a very short duration of action because of its rapid hydrolysis *in vivo*. It must therefore be administered by continuous infusion. Great care must be taken in preparing a suitably diluted solution for infusion and only diluent as supplied by the manufacturer should be used to reconstitute epoprostenol.

Epoprostenol is used to **prevent platelet aggregation** when blood is brought into contact with nonbiological surfaces such as in extracorporeal circulation, es-

pecially in renal dialysis patients. It is indicated for use when heparin carries a high risk of causing or exacerbating bleeding, or is otherwise contra-indicated. Epoprostenol is administered by continuous intravenous infusion or into the blood supplying the extracorporeal circulation. The usual dose for renal dialysis is 4 or 5 nanograms per kg body-weight per minute intravenously before dialysis, then 4 or 5 nanograms per kg per minute into the arterial inlet of the dialyser during dialysis.

In the long-term treatment of primary **pulmonary hypertension** a dose-ranging procedure is performed first in order to establish the maximum infusion rate that can be tolerated. Epoprostenol is then given by continuous infusion through a central venous catheter, the initial rate being 4 nanograms per kg body-weight per minute *less than* the maximum-tolerated infusion rate; if the maximum-tolerated infusion rate is less than 5 nanograms per kg per minute, then the initial rate should be one-half of this maximum rate. The maintenance dose is subsequently adjusted according to the patient's response. If symptoms recur or if adverse effects occur the dosage may be increased or decreased by steps of 1 to 2 nanograms per kg per minute at intervals of at least 15 minutes until a new maintenance dose is established.

◊ The discovery, properties, and clinical applications of prostacyclin have been reviewed.[1] Prostacyclin is the main product of arachidonic acid in vascular tissues, endothelial cells from vessel walls being the most active producers. It is a strong hypotensive agent through vasodilatation of vascular beds, including the pulmonary and cerebral circulations, and is also a potent endogenous inhibitor of platelet aggregation. Inhibition of aggregation is achieved by stimulation of adenylate cyclase, leading to an increase in cyclic adenosine monophosphate (cAMP) levels in the platelets. By inhibiting several steps in the activation of the arachidonic acid metabolic cascade, prostacyclin exerts an overall control of platelet aggregability.

Endogenous prostacyclin and thromboxane A_2 may be of more physiological and pathological importance[2] than the more classical prostanoids prostaglandin E_2 and prostaglandin $F_{2\alpha}$. They have directly opposing pharmacological actions in many systems, such as on platelet function, vascular smooth muscle, bronchopulmonary function, and gastrointestinal integrity. Thus prostanoid-mediated control of cellular and tissue function may reflect an interactive modulation between prostacyclin and thromboxane A_2 with imbalance resulting in dysfunction, for example in platelet and vascular disorders. Thromboxane A_2 has both bronchoconstrictor and pulmonary irritant actions and has brought about marked changes in respiratory function in experimental models; prostacyclin may oppose these effects on both the pulmonary vasculature and bronchial smooth muscle. Thromboxane A_2 has induced marked renal vasoconstriction *in vitro* whereas renal vasodilatation and stimulation of the release of renin has followed the administration of epoprostenol [exogenous prostacyclin] in *animals*. In contrast to the pro-ulcerogenic actions of thromboxane A_2, epoprostenol and its analogues, like other prostaglandins, have potent gastrointestinal anti-ulcer properties which can be disassociated from their gastric antisecretory properties. The term 'cytoprotection' has been used to describe this ability of exogenous prostaglandins to prevent gastrointestinal damage; endogenous prostaglandins might have a similar protective role. Epoprostenol also has a cytoprotective effect against experimental damage in the gastric mucosa, myocardium, and liver whereas thromboxane A_2 has a cytolytic effect.

1. Vane JR, Botting RM. Pharmacodynamic profile of prostacyclin. *Am J Cardiol* 1995; **75**: 3A–10A.
2. Whittle BJR, Moncada S. Pharmacological interactions between prostacyclin and thromboxanes. *Br Med Bull* 1983; **39**: 232–8.

Acute respiratory distress syndrome. Encouraging results[1,2] have been seen with inhaled epoprostenol in the treatment of acute respiratory distress syndrome (p.1046).

1. Walmrath D, et al. Aerosolised prostacyclin in adult respiratory distress syndrome. *Lancet* 1993; **342**: 961–2.
2. Walmrath D, et al. Direct comparison of inhaled nitric oxide and aerosolized prostacyclin in acute respiratory distress syndrome. *Am J Respir Crit Care Med* 1996; **153**: 991–6.

Heart failure. Epoprostenol has been investigated for the treatment of heart failure but development was abandoned due to an increase in mortality associated with long-term use of the drug.[1,2]

1. Phillips BB, Gandhi AJ. Epoprostenol in the treatment of congestive heart failure. *Am J Health-Syst Pharm* 1997; **54**: 2613–15.
2. Califf RM, et al. A randomized controlled trial of epoprostenol therapy for severe congestive heart failure: the Flolan International Randomized Survival Trial (FIRST). *Am Heart J* 1997; **134**: 44–54.

Peripheral vascular disease. Various prostaglandins including epoprostenol have been used for their vasodilating effect in the treatment of peripheral vascular disease (p.809), par-

ticularly in severe Raynaud's syndrome, but do not constitute mainline therapy.

References.
1. Szczeklik A, et al. Successful therapy of advanced arteriosclerosis obliterans with prostacyclin. *Lancet* 1979; **i**: 1111–14.
2. Belch JJF, et al. Intermittent epoprostenol (prostacyclin) infusion in patients with Raynaud's syndrome: a double-blind controlled trial. *Lancet* 1983; **i**: 313–15.
3. Belch JJF, et al. Epoprostenol (prostacyclin) and severe arterial disease: a double-blind trial. *Lancet* 1983; **i**: 315–17.
4. De San Lazaro C, et al. Prostacyclin in severe peripheral vascular disease. *Arch Dis Child* 1985; **60**: 370–84.
5. Leaker B, et al. Treatment of acute renal failure, symmetrical peripheral gangrene, and septicaemia with plasma exchange and epoprostenol. *Lancet* 1987; **i**: 156.
6. Negus D, et al. Intra-arterial prostacyclin compared to Praxilene in the management of severe lower limb ischaemia: a double-blind trial. *J Cardiovasc Surg* 1987; **28**: 196–9.
7. Isenberg DA, Black C. Raynaud's phenomenon, scleroderma, and overlap syndromes. In: Snaith ML, ed. *ABC of Rheumatology*. 2nd ed. London: BMJ Publishing Group, 1999: 65–8.

Pulmonary hypertension. Epoprostenol was originally introduced into the management of primary pulmonary hypertension (p.810) to sustain patients long enough for them to have heart-lung transplantation. However, long-term therapy may also have a role as an alternative to transplantation; sustained clinical improvement and improved survival have been reported in some patients given long-term[1-6] intravenous therapy using portable infusion pumps. Epoprostenol infusion may also have a role in patients with secondary pulmonary hypertension.[7,8]

Inhaled epoprostenol, a method of administration that may overcome some of the adverse effects associated with the parenteral route, has been used with some success in adults[9,10] with primary or secondary pulmonary hypertension and in neonates[11] with persistent pulmonary hypertension of the newborn.

1. Barst RJ, et al. Survival in primary pulmonary hypertension with long-term continuous intravenous prostacyclin. *Ann Intern Med* 1994; **121**: 409–15. Correction. *ibid.* 1995; **122**: 238.
2. Barst RJ, et al. A comparison of continuous intravenous epoprostenol (prostacyclin) with conventional therapy for primary pulmonary hypertension. *N Engl J Med* 1996; **334**: 296–301.
3. Shapiro SM, et al. Primary pulmonary hypertension: improved long-term effects and survival with continuous intravenous epoprostenol infusion. *J Am Coll Cardiol* 1997; **30**: 343–9.
4. McLaughlin VV, et al. Reduction in pulmonary vascular resistance with long-term epoprostenol (prostacyclin) therapy in primary pulmonary hypertension. *N Engl J Med* 1998; **338**: 273–7.
5. Higenbottam T, et al. Long term intravenous prostaglandin (epoprostenol or iloprost) for treatment of severe pulmonary hypertension. *Heart* 1998; **80**: 151–5.
6. Herner SJ, Mauro LS. Epoprostenol in primary pulmonary hypertension. *Ann Pharmacother* 1999; **33**: 340–7.
7. McLaughlin VV, et al. Compassionate use of continuous prostacyclin in the management of secondary pulmonary hypertension: a case series. *Ann Intern Med* 1999; **130**: 740–3.
8. Badesch DB, et al. Continuous intravenous epoprostenol for pulmonary hypertension due to the scleroderma spectrum of disease: a randomized, controlled trial. *Ann Intern Med* 2000; **132**: 425–34.
9. Olschewski H, et al. Aerosolized prostacyclin and iloprost in severe pulmonary hypertension. *Ann Intern Med* 1996; **124**: 820–4.
10. Mikhail G, et al. An evaluation of nebulized prostacyclin in patients with primary and secondary pulmonary hypertension. *Eur Heart J* 1997; **18**: 1499–1504.
11. Bindl L, et al. Aerosolised prostacyclin for pulmonary hypertension in neonates. *Arch Dis Child* 1994; **71**: F214–F216.

Stroke. Results with epoprostenol in patients with acute stroke have been inconclusive and a systematic review of randomised studies concluded that too few patients had been studied for the effect of epoprostenol on survival to be determined.[1]

1. Bath PMW, Bath FJ. Prostacyclin and analogues for acute ischaemic stroke (updated 21 October 1999). Available in The Cochrane Library; Issue 4. Oxford: Update Software; 2001.

Thrombotic microangiopathies. Platelet aggregation has a major role in the pathogenesis of thrombotic thrombocytopenic purpura and the related disorder, haemolytic-uraemic syndrome (p.740). Prostacyclin deficiency has been demonstrated in both conditions, but case reports of epoprostenol treatment have indicated variable results.[1-7]

1. Webster J, et al. Prostacyclin deficiency in haemolytic-uraemic syndrome. *BMJ* 1980; **281**: 271.
2. Beattie TJ, et al. Prostacyclin infusion in haemolytic-uraemic syndrome of children. *BMJ* 1981; **283**: 470.
3. Johnson JE, et al. Ineffective epoprostenol therapy for thrombotic thrombocytopenic purpura. *JAMA* 1983; **250**: 3089–91.
4. Payton CD, et al. Successful treatment of thrombotic thrombocytopenic purpura by epoprostenol infusion. *Lancet* 1985; **i**: 927–8.
5. Tardy B, et al. Intravenous prostacyclin in thrombotic thrombocytopenic purpura: case report and review of the literature. *J Intern Med* 1991; **230**: 279–82.
6. Bobbio-Pallavicini E, et al. Intravenous prostacyclin (as epoprostenol) infusion in thrombotic thrombocytopenic purpura: four case reports and review of the literature. *Haematologica* 1994; **79**: 429–37.
7. Series C, et al. Interet de la prostacycline dans le traitement du syndrome hémolytique et urémique: à propos d'un cas. *Rev Med Interne* 1996; **17**: 76–8.

Preparations

Proprietary Preparations (details are given in Part 3)
Aust.: Flolan; *Belg.*: Flolan; *Canad.*: Flolan; *Denm.*: Flolan; *Fr.*: Flolan; *Irl.*: Flolan; *Ital.*: Flolan; *Neth.*: Flolan; *Spain*: Flolan; *UK*: Flolan; *USA*: Flolan.

Etiproston Trometamol (10706-a)

Etiproston Trometamol (rINNM).

Etiproston Tromethamine. Trometamol salt of (Z)-7-[(1R, 2R,3R,5S)-3,5-dihydroxy-2-[(E)-2-[2-(phenoxymethyl)-1,3-dioxolan-2-yl]vinyl]cyclopentyl]-5-heptenoic acid.
$C_{24}H_{32}O_7,C_4H_{11}NO_3 = 553.6$.
CAS — 59619-81-7 (etiproston).

Profile
Etiproston trometamol is a synthetic analogue of dinoprost (prostaglandin $F_{2\alpha}$). It is used as a luteolytic in veterinary medicine.

Gemeprost (8088-w)

Gemeprost (BAN, USAN, rINN).

16,16-Dimethyl-trans-Δ^2-prostaglandin E_1 methyl ester; ONO-802; SC-37681. Methyl (2E,13E)-(8R,11R,12R,15R)-11,15-dihydroxy-16,16-dimethyl-9-oxoprosta-2,13-dienoate; Methyl (E)-7-{(1R,2R,3R)-3-hydroxy-2-[(E)-(3R)-3-hydroxy-4,4-dimethyl-oct-1-enyl]-5-oxocyclopentyl}hept-2-enoate.
$C_{23}H_{38}O_5 = 394.5$.
CAS — 64318-79-2.
ATC — G02AD03.

Adverse Effects and Precautions
Gemeprost is given vaginally as pessaries and systemic adverse effects such as nausea, vomiting, and diarrhoea are relatively mild. Other-reported side-effects have included headache, muscle weakness, dizziness, flushing, chills, backache, dyspnoea, chest pain, palpitations, and mild pyrexia. Vaginal bleeding and mild uterine pain may occur.

Uterine rupture has been reported rarely, most commonly in multiparous women and in those with a history of uterine surgery. There have also been rare reports of severe hypotension and coronary spasm with subsequent myocardial infarction.

The effects of gemeprost on the fetus are not known. Once a prostaglandin has been given to terminate pregnancy it is essential that termination take place; if the prostaglandin is unsuccessful other measures should be used.

Gemeprost should be used with caution in patients with obstructive airways disease, cardiovascular disease, raised intra-ocular pressure, cervicitis, or vaginitis. Blood pressure and pulse rate should be monitored following administration; when given in combination with mifepristone monitoring for 6 hours is recommended.

◊ The incidence of vomiting (19 or 35%) and diarrhoea (12 or 19%) in 2 studies of patients treated with gemeprost pessaries was similar to that seen with other prostaglandins, but gemeprost was reported to cause less uterine pain.[1,2]
1. Cameron IT, Baird DT. The use of 16,16-dimethyl-trans-Δ^2 prostaglandin E_1 methyl ester (gemeprost) vaginal pessaries for the termination of pregnancy in the early second trimester: a comparison with extra-amniotic prostaglandin E_2. Br J Obstet Gynaecol 1984; 91: 1136–40.
2. Andersen LF, et al. Termination of second trimester pregnancy with gemeprost vaginal pessaries and intra-amniotic $PGF_{2\alpha}$: a comparative study. Eur J Obstet Gynecol Reprod Biol 1989; 31: 1–7.

Effects on the cardiovascular system. Periods of ventricular standstill of up to 6 seconds were observed in a patient during treatment with gemeprost vaginal pessaries.[1] The patient required temporary cardiac pacing, but no persistent cardiac rhythm disturbances were detected on follow-up. Severe cardiogenic shock due to vasospasm, and subsequent stroke, has been reported in a patient who had received gemeprost pessaries some hours earlier; myocardial infarction ensuing from coronary spasm was reported in a second patient.[2]
1. Kalra PA, et al. Cardiac standstill induced by prostaglandin pessaries. Lancet 1989; i: 1460–1.
2. Lauer M, Berentelg J. Schwere kardiovaskuläre Komplikationen im Zusammenhang mit Gemeprost. Zentralbl Gynakol 2000; 122: 324–7.

Uses and Administration
Gemeprost is a synthetic analogue of alprostadil (prostaglandin E_1). It is used to soften and dilate the cervix and as a uterine stimulant in the termination of pregnancy (p.1439). In the first trimester, a pessary containing gemeprost 1 mg is inserted into the vagina 3 hours before surgery to ripen the cervix. Gemeprost may also be used for termination of pregnancy in the second trimester when a 1-mg pessary is inserted every 3 hours to a maximum of 5 pessaries. Should this

course be ineffective one further course may be given after an interval of 24 hours. In the case of intra-uterine fetal death only one course of five pessaries should be given. Vaginal gemeprost is also used following the administration of oral mifepristone (p.1483) in the termination of pregnancy.

Preparations
Proprietary Preparations (details are given in Part 3)
Austral.: Cervagem; Denm.: Cervagem; Fin.: Cervagem; Fr.: Cervageme; Ger.: Cergem; Hong Kong: Cervagem; Ital.: Cervidil; Jpn: Preglandin; Norw.: Cervagem; NZ: Cervagem; Singapore: Cervagem; Swed.: Cervagem.

Iloprost (16847-w)

Iloprost (BAN, rINN).

Ciloprost; ZK-36374. (E)-(3aS,4R,5R,6aS)-Hexahydro-5-hydroxy-4-[(E)-(3S,4RS)-3-hydroxy-4-methyl-1-octen-6-ynyl]-$\Delta^{2(1H),\delta}$-pentalenevaleric acid.
$C_{22}H_{32}O_4 = 360.5$.
CAS — 73873-87-7.
ATC — B01AC11.

Iloprost Trometamol (17902-s)

Iloprost Trometamol (BANM, rINNM).

Ciloprost Tromethamine; Iloprost Tromethamine.

Adverse Effects and Precautions
As for Epoprostenol, p.1443.

Effects on the cardiovascular system. Hypotension was observed[1] in 2 of 6 patients during administration of iloprost. Both patients recovered rapidly when iloprost was discontinued, although one required intravenous atropine to correct sinus bradycardia. Evidence of myocardial ischaemia was reported in 4 of 33 patients with coronary artery disease during iloprost infusion.[2] The same authors[3] noted a similar effect in 4 of 28 patients with stable angina in a subsequent study. According to one study,[4] there might be an increased risk of thromboembolism in some patients given iloprost, due to platelet activation and enhanced coagulation.
1. Upward JW, et al. Hypotension in response to iloprost, a prostacyclin analogue. Br J Clin Pharmacol 1986; 21: 241–3.
2. Bugiardini R, et al. Myocardial ischemia induced by prostacyclin and iloprost. Clin Pharmacol Ther 1985; 38: 101–8.
3. Bugiardini R, et al. Effects of iloprost, a stable prostacyclin analog, on exercise capacity and platelet aggregation in stable angina pectoris. Am J Cardiol 1986; 58: 453–9.
4. Kovacs IB, et al. Infusion of a stable prostacyclin analogue, iloprost, to patients with peripheral vascular disease: lack of antiplatelet effect but risk of thromboembolism. Am J Med 1991; 90: 41–6.

Uses and Administration
Iloprost, a vasodilator and platelet aggregation inhibitor, is a stable analogue of the prostaglandin epoprostenol (prostacyclin). It is given by intravenous infusion as the trometamol salt in the treatment of peripheral vascular disease. The usual dose is the equivalent of 0.5 to 2 nanograms of iloprost per kg bodyweight per minute for 6 hours each day.

Administration of iloprost by mouth is under investigation.

◊ Reviews.
1. Grant SM, Goa KL. Iloprost: a review of its pharmacodynamic and pharmacokinetic properties, and therapeutic potential in peripheral vascular disease, myocardial ischaemia and extracorporeal circulation procedures. Drugs 1992; 43: 889–924.

Peripheral vascular disease. Various prostaglandins including iloprost[1-9] have been used in the treatment of peripheral vascular disease (p.809), particularly in severe Raynaud's syndrome, but do not constitute mainline therapy. Systematic review[9] suggests that iloprost when given intravenously produces prolonged benefit in Raynaud's phenomenon secondary to scleroderma. The benefits of oral iloprost are less clear. It is also unclear whether iloprost infusion is of benefit in occlusive peripheral arterial disease due to atherosclerosis: although a meta-analysis of (conflicting) controlled trials did suggest an effect,[6] firm conclusions are difficult.
1. Waller PC, et al. Placebo controlled trial of iloprost in patients with stable intermittent claudication. Br J Clin Pharmacol 1986; 21: 562P–563P.
2. Rademaker M, et al. Comparison of intravenous infusions of iloprost and oral nifedipine in treatment of Raynaud's phenomenon in patients with systemic sclerosis: a double blind randomised study. BMJ 1989; 298: 561–4.
3. Fiessinger JN, Schäfer M. Trial of iloprost versus aspirin treatment for critical limb ischaemia of thromboangiitis obliterans. Lancet 1990; 335: 555–7.
4. Zahavi J, et al. Ischaemic necrotic toes associated with antiphospholipid syndrome and treated with iloprost. Lancet 1993; 342: 862.
5. Tait IS, et al. Management of intra-arterial injection injury with iloprost. Lancet 1994; 343: 419.
6. Loosemore TM, et al. A meta-analysis of randomized placebo control trials in Fontaine stages III and IV peripheral occlusive arterial disease. Int Angiol 1994; 13: 133–42.
7. Wigley FM, et al. Oral iloprost treatment in patients with Raynaud's phenomenon secondary to systemic sclerosis: a multi-center, placebo-controlled, double-blind study. Arthritis Rheum 1998; 41: 670–7.

8. Black CM, et al. Oral iloprost in Raynaud's phenomenon secondary to systemic sclerosis: a multicentre, placebo-controlled, dose-comparison study. Br J Rheumatol 1998; 37: 952–60.
9. Pope J, et al. Iloprost and cisaprost for Raynauds phenomenon in progressive systemic sclerosis (updated 29 August 2001). Available in The Cochrane Library: Issue 4. Oxford: Update Software; 2001.

Pulmonary hypertension. Epoprostenol is an accepted part of the management of pulmonary hypertension (p.810) and the use of iloprost, a stable analogue, has been studied. Both aerosolised[1-3] administration and continuous intravenous infusion[4] have been tried with beneficial results.
1. Olschewski H, et al. Aerosolized prostacyclin and iloprost in severe pulmonary hypertension. Ann Intern Med 1996; 124: 820–4.
2. Olschewski H, et al. Inhaled iloprost to treat severe pulmonary hypertension: an uncontrolled trial. Ann Intern Med 2000; 132: 435–43.
3. Hoeper MM, et al. Long-term treatment of primary pulmonary hypertension with aerosolized iloprost, a prostacyclin analogue. N Engl J Med 2000; 342: 1866–70.
4. Higenbottam TW, et al. Treatment of pulmonary hypertension with the continuous infusion of a prostacyclin analogue, iloprost. Heart 1998; 79: 175–9.

Preparations
Proprietary Preparations (details are given in Part 3)
Aust.: Ilomedin; Denm.: Ilomedin; Fin.: Ilomedin; Fr.: Ilomedine; Ger.: Ilomedin; Israel: Ilomedin; Ital.: Endoprost; Ilomedin†; Neth.: Ilomedine; Norw.: Ilomedin; NZ: Ilomedin; Port.: Ilomedin; Spain: Ilocit; Ilomedin; Swed.: Ilomedin; Switz.: Ilomedin.

Latanoprost (16780-q)

Latanoprost (BAN, USAN, rINN).

PhXA-41; XA-41. Isopropyl (Z)-7-{(1R,2R,3R,5S)-3,5-dihydroxy-2-[(3R)-3-hydroxy-5-phenylpentyl]cyclopentyl}-5-heptenoate.
$C_{26}H_{40}O_5 = 432.6$.
CAS — 130209-82-4.
ATC — S01EX03.

Adverse Effects and Precautions
Latanoprost eye drops may produce a gradual increase in the amount of brown pigment in the iris, due to increased melanin content of melanocytes. This change in eye colour is most evident in patients with mixed colour irises. Darkening, thickening, and lengthening of eye lashes may occur and darkening of the palpebral skin has been reported rarely. Ocular irritation and conjunctival hyperaemia may occur; there have also been rare reports of iritis and/or uveitis, and macular oedema.

◊ The use of latanoprost eye drops has been associated with systemic adverse reactions. In a case report[1] of 2 patients with latanoprost-associated hypertension the authors mentioned that other events including peripheral and facial oedema, dyspnoea, exacerbation of asthma, tachycardia, and chest pain or angina pectoris had been reported. Another case report[2] also referred to exacerbation of angina.
1. Peak AS, Sutton BM. Systemic adverse effects associated with topically applied latanoprost. Ann Pharmacother 1998; 32: 504–5.
2. Mitra M, et al. Exacerbation of angina associated with latanoprost. BMJ 2001; 323: 783.

Effects on the eyes. Latanoprost has been associated with various adverse effects on the eyes, including case reports of cystoid macular oedema[1] and bilateral optic disc oedema.[2] The manufacturers have stated that reports of macular oedema have mainly occurred in aphakic patients, in pseudophakic patients with torn posterior lens capsule or anterior chamber lenses, or in patients with risk factors for cystoid macular oedema such as those with diabetic retinopathy or retinal vein occlusion.
1. Wardrop DRA, Wishart PK. Latanoprost and cystoid macular oedema in a pseudophake. Br J Ophthalmol 1998; 82: 843–4.
2. Stewart O, et al. Bilateral optic disc oedema associated with latanoprost. Br J Ophthalmol 1999; 83: 1092–3.

Uses and Administration
Latanoprost is a synthetic analogue of dinoprost (prostaglandin $F_{2\alpha}$) that is used topically to reduce intra-ocular pressure in patients with open-angle glaucoma and ocular hypertension (p.1413). One drop of a 0.005% solution is instilled once daily in the evening.

◊ References.
1. Patel SS, Spencer CM. Latanoprost: a review of its pharmacological properties, clinical efficacy and tolerability in the management of primary open-angle glaucoma and ocular hypertension. Drugs Aging 1996; 9: 363–78.
2. Eisenberg DL, Camras CB. A preliminary risk-benefit assessment of latanoprost and unoprostone in open-angle glaucoma and ocular hypertension. Drug Safety 1999; 20: 505–14.

The symbol † denotes a preparation no longer actively marketed

3. Einarson TR, *et al.* Meta-analysis of the effect of latanoprost and brimonidine on intraocular pressure in the treatment of glaucoma. *Clin Ther* 2000; **22:** 1502–15.
4. Zhang WY, *et al.* Meta-analysis of randomised controlled trials comparing latanoprost with timolol in the treatment of patients with open angle glaucoma or ocular hypertension. *Br J Ophthalmol* 2001; **85:** 983–90.

Preparations

Proprietary Preparations (details are given in Part 3)
Aust.: Xalatan; *Austral.:* Xalatan; *Belg.:* Xalatan; *Canad.:* Xalatan; *Denm.:* Xalatan; *Fin.:* Xalatan; *Fr.:* Xalatan; *Ger.:* Xalatan; *Hong Kong:* Xalatan; *Irl.:* Xalatan; *Israel:* Xalatan; *Ital.:* Xalatan; *Mex.:* Xalatan; *Neth.:* Xalatan; *Norw.:* Xalatan; *NZ:* Xalatan; *Port.:* Xalatan; *S.Afr.:* Xalatan; *Singapore:* Xalatan; *Spain:* Xalatan; *Swed.:* Xalatan; *Switz.:* Xalatan; *Thai.:* Xalatan; *UK:* Xalatan; *USA:* Xalatan.

Multi-ingredient: *UK:* Xalacom.

Limaprost (2957-j)

Limaprost (*rINN*).

ONO-1206; OP-1206. (*E*)-7-{(1*R*,2*R*,3*R*)-3-Hydroxy-2-[(*E*)-(3*S*,5*S*)-3-hydroxy-5-methyl-1-nonenyl]-5-oxocyclopentyl}-2-heptenoic acid.

$C_{22}H_{36}O_5 = 380.5$.
CAS — 74397-12-9 (*limaprost*); 88852-12-4 (*limaprost alfadex*).

Profile
Limaprost is a synthetic analogue of alprostadil (prostaglandin E_1) used in the management of peripheral vascular disease (p.809). It is given by mouth as limaprost alfadex, in a dose equivalent to limaprost 30 µg daily in three divided doses.

◊ References.
1. Shono T, Ikeda K. Rapid effect of oral limaprost in Raynaud's disease in childhood. *Lancet* 1989; **i:** 908.
2. Murai Y, *et al.* Oral limaprost for Raynaud's phenomenon. *Lancet* 1989; **ii:** 1218.

Preparations

Proprietary Preparations (details are given in Part 3)
Jpn: Opalmon.

Luprostiol (8089-e)

Luprostiol (*BAN, rINN*).

(±)-(*Z*)-7-{(1*S*,2*R*,3*R*,5*S*)-2-[(2*S*)-3-(3-Chlorophenoxy)-2-hydroxypropylthio]-3,5-dihydroxycyclopentyl}hept-5-enoic acid.
$C_{21}H_{29}ClO_6S = 445.0$.
CAS — 67110-79-6.

Profile
Luprostiol is a synthetic analogue of dinoprost (prostaglandin $F_{2\alpha}$). It is used as a luteolytic in veterinary medicine.

Meteneprost (8090-b)

Meteneprost (*USAN, rINN*).

9-Deoxo-16,16-dimethyl-9-methylene-prostaglandin E_2; U-46785. (5*Z*,13*E*)-(8*R*,11*R*,12*R*,15*R*)-11,15-Dihydroxy-16,16-dimethyl-9-methyleneprosta-5,13-dienoic acid; (*Z*)-7-{(1*R*,2*R*,3*R*)-3-Hydroxy-2-[(*E*)-(3*R*)-3-hydroxy-4,4-dimethyloct-1-enyl]-5-methylenecyclopentyl}hept-5-enoic acid.
$C_{23}H_{38}O_4 = 378.5$.
CAS — 61263-35-2.

Profile
Meteneprost is a synthetic derivative of dinoprostone (prostaglandin E_2). It is a uterine stimulant and has been studied for the termination of pregnancy.

Misoprostol (16898-r)

Misoprostol (*BAN, USAN, rINN*).

SC-29333. (±)-Methyl 7-{(1*R*,2*R*,3*R*)-3-hydroxy-2-[(*E*)-(4*RS*)-4-hydroxy-4-methyloct-1-enyl]-5-oxocyclopentyl}heptanoate; (±)-Methyl (13*E*)-11,16-dihydroxy-16-methyl-9-oxoprost-13-enoate.
$C_{22}H_{38}O_5 = 382.5$.
CAS — 59122-46-2.
ATC — A02BB01.

Adverse Effects
The commonest side-effect occurring with misoprostol is diarrhoea. Other gastrointestinal effects include abdominal pain, dyspepsia, flatulence, and nausea and vomiting. Increased uterine contractility and abnormal vaginal bleeding (including menorrhagia and intermenstrual bleeding) have been reported with misoprostol. Other adverse effects include skin rashes, headache, and dizziness. Hypotension is rarely seen at recommended doses.

◊ A summary of data on misoprostol presented to the FDA.[1] During controlled studies the most common adverse effect was diarrhoea (8.2% compared with 3.1% for placebo); it was dose-related but usually mild, only 8 of 2003 subjects receiving misoprostol having withdrawn because of incapacitating diarrhoea. Headaches and abdominal discomfort were also reported. The effects of misoprostol on the uterus and the potential risks of uterine bleeding or abortion in pregnant women were of more concern. In nonpregnant women taking part in the controlled studies there were menstrual complaints in 15 of 410 (3.7%) receiving misoprostol compared with 2 of 115 (1.7%) given placebo. In a study in pregnant women who had elected to undergo first trimester abortion, all 6 who had a spontaneous expulsion of the uterine contents had received 1 or 2 doses of misoprostol 400 µg the previous evening, while none of those given placebo aborted spontaneously; overall 25 of the 56 women receiving misoprostol experienced uterine bleeding compared with only 2 of 55 on placebo.
1. Lewis JH. Summary of the 29th meeting of the Gastrointestinal Drugs Advisory Committee, Food and Drug Administration—June 10, 1985. *Am J Gastroenterol* 1985; **80:** 743–5.

Effects on the fetus. For reports of congenital malformations possibly associated with the misuse of misoprostol, see under Termination of Pregnancy in Uses and Administration, below.

Precautions
Misoprostol should not be given to patients who are pregnant or who may become pregnant because it can cause uterine contraction. It should be used with caution in patients in whom hypotension might cause severe complications.

Inflammatory bowel disease. Life-threatening diarrhoea was reported in a patient with unrecognised Crohn's disease following six doses of misoprostol.[1]
1. Kornbluth A, *et al.* Life-threatening diarrhea after short-term misoprostol use in a patient with Crohn ileocolitis. *Ann Intern Med* 1990; **113:** 474–5.

Pharmacokinetics
Misoprostol is reported to be rapidly absorbed and metabolised to its active form (misoprostol acid, SC-30695) following administration by mouth; peak plasma concentrations of misoprostol acid occur after about 30 minutes. Administration with food reduces the rate but not the extent of absorption. Misoprostol acid is further metabolised by oxidation in a number of body organs and is excreted mainly in the urine. The plasma elimination half-life is reported to be between 20 and 40 minutes.

◊ References.
1. Schoenhard G, *et al.* Metabolism and pharmacokinetic studies of misoprostol. *Dig Dis Sci* 1985; **30** (suppl): 126S–128S.
2. Karim A, *et al.* Effects of food and antacid on oral absorption of misoprostol, a synthetic prostaglandin E_1 analog. *J Clin Pharmacol* 1989; **29:** 439–43.
3. Foote EF, *et al.* Disposition of misoprostol and its active metabolite in patients with normal and impaired renal function. *J Clin Pharmacol* 1995; **35:** 384–9.
4. Zieman M, *et al.* Absorption kinetics of misoprostol with oral or vaginal administration. *Obstet Gynecol* 1997; **90:** 88–92.

Uses and Administration
Misoprostol is a synthetic analogue of alprostadil (prostaglandin E_1).

It is used in the treatment of benign gastric and duodenal ulceration including that associated with NSAIDs. The usual dose by mouth is 800 µg daily in two to four divided doses with food.

Misoprostol is also used in conjunction with NSAIDs to prevent NSAID-induced ulcers. The usual prophylactic dose is 200 µg two to four times daily. A dose of 100 µg four times daily may be used in patients not tolerating the higher dose. Some preparations of NSAIDs contain misoprostol in an attempt to limit their adverse effects on the gastrointestinal mucosa.

Misoprostol has been used for termination of pregnancy, for induction of labour, and in the management of postpartum haemorrhage (see below).

◊ General reviews.
1. Walley TJ. Misoprostol. *Prescribers' J* 1993; **33:** 78–82.
2. Goldberg AB, *et al.* Misoprostol and pregnancy. *N Engl J Med* 2000; **344:** 38–47.

Labour induction and augmentation. Prostaglandins are well established for the induction of labour (p.1438) and several studies have investigated the use of misoprostol. Given vaginally misoprostol was as effective as intravenous oxytocin[1] and more effective than intracervical dinoprostone gel.[2-5] Using misoprostol tablets, doses employed have been 50 µg vaginally increased every 2 hours[1] or every 4 hours[2,4,5] or 25 µg vaginally increased every 2 hours[3] according to the patient's

response. Misoprostol has also been given orally in doses of 50 µg every 4 hours;[6] other dosage regimens have been used.[7] Oral administration appears to be less effective than vaginal administration, but may have fewer adverse effects.[8] However, the risk of uterine hyperstimulation may be increased with misoprostol by either route and there is as yet insufficient evidence of its safety to recommend routine use.[7,9]

Misoprostol has also been tried for active management of the third stage of labour (see Postpartum Haemorrhage, below).
1. Margulies M, *et al.* Misoprostol to induce labour. *Lancet* 1992; **339:** 64.
2. Chuck FJ, Huffacker BJ. Labor induction with intravaginal misoprostol versus intracervical prostaglandin E_2 gel (Prepidil gel): randomized comparison. *Am J Obstet Gynecol* 1995; **173:** 1137–42.
3. Varaklis K, *et al.* Randomized controlled trial of vaginal misoprostol and intracervical prostaglandin E_2 gel for induction of labor at term. *Obstet Gynecol* 1995; **86:** 541–4.
4. Mundle WR, Young DC. Vaginal misoprostol for induction of labor: a randomized controlled trial. *Obstet Gynecol* 1996; **88:** 521–5.
5. Buser D, *et al.* A randomized comparison between misoprostol and dinoprostone for cervical ripening and labor induction in patients with unfavorable cervices. *Obstet Gynecol* 1997; **89:** 581–5.
6. Windrim R, *et al.* Oral administration of misoprostol for labor induction: a randomized controlled trial. *Obstet Gynecol* 1997; **89:** 392–7.
7. Alfirevic Z. Oral misoprostol for induction of labour (updated 22 February 2001). Available in The Cochrane Library; Issue 4. Oxford: Update Software; 2001.
8. Bennett KA, *et al.* A masked randomized comparison of oral and vaginal administration of misoprostol for labor induction. *Obstet Gynecol* 1998; **92:** 481–6.
9. Hofmeyr GJ, Gulmezoglu AM. Vaginal misoprostol for cervical ripening and induction of labour (updated 26 August 2001). Available in The Cochrane Library; Issue 4. Oxford: Update Software; 2001.

Organ and tissue transplantation. Misoprostol 200 µg four times daily improved renal function in ciclosporin-treated recipients of renal transplants.[1] The number of patients who had acute graft rejection was lower in the misoprostol group than in the placebo group. However, another study[2] did not indicate any difference in the incidence of rejection episodes or in renal function when misoprostol was added to immunosuppressant regimens for kidney transplantation, and misoprostol does not appear to have gained a role in the usual management of renal transplantation (p.503).
1. Moran M, *et al.* Prevention of acute graft rejection by the prostaglandin E_1 analogue misoprostol in renal-transplant recipients treated with cyclosporine and prednisone. *N Engl J Med* 1990; **322:** 1183–8.
2. Pouteil-Noble C, *et al.* Misoprostol in renal transplant recipients: a prospective, randomized, controlled study on the prevention of acute rejection episodes and cyclosporin A nephrotoxicity. *Nephrol Dial Transplant* 1994; **9:** 552–5.

Peptic ulcer disease. Misoprostol is used in the prophylaxis and treatment of peptic ulceration in patients taking NSAIDs (p.1208). There is good evidence that misoprostol can reduce the risk of gastric and duodenal ulcer formation in patients on long-term NSAID treatment,[1-4] and it appears more effective in this respect than histamine H_2-antagonists,[1] for which evidence of benefit against gastric injury is less persuasive. However, misoprostol's abdominal adverse effects, particularly diarrhoea and abdominal cramps, may limit its usefulness and patient acceptability. Omeprazole, which is equally effective in preventing NSAID-induced ulceration, is better tolerated.[3] Improved formulations, in which the active isomer of misoprostol is bound to a polymer, may reduce adverse effects.[5]
1. Koch M, *et al.* Prevention of nonsteroidal anti-inflammatory drug-induced gastrointestinal mucosal injury: a meta-analysis of randomized controlled clinical trials. *Arch Intern Med* 1996; **156:** 2321–32.
2. Champion GD, *et al.* NSAID-induced gastrointestinal damage: epidemiology, risk and prevention, with an evaluation of the role of misoprostol: an Asia-Pacific perspective and consensus. *Drugs* 1997; **53:** 6–19.
3. Hawkey CJ, *et al.* Omeprazole compared with misoprostol for ulcers associated with nonsteroidal antiinflammatory drugs. *N Engl J Med* 1998; **338:** 727–34.
4. Rostom A, *et al.* Prevention of NSAID-induced gastroduodenal ulcers (updated 16 February 2001). Available in The Cochrane Library; Issue 4. Oxford: Update Software; 2001.
5. Perkins WE, *et al.* Polymer delivery of the active isomer of misoprostol: a solution to the intestinal side effect problem. *J Pharmacol Exp Ther* 1994; **269:** 151–6.

Postpartum haemorrhage. Prostaglandins, usually administered parenterally, have an accepted role in the management of established postpartum haemorrhage (p.1607), and there has been a report[1] of the successful use of rectal misoprostol in 14 women to control refractory postpartum haemorrhage.

Misoprostol has also been tried in the active management of third-stage labour. An open study[2] of misoprostol, administered orally in a dose of 600 µg immediately after delivery, indicated that it was effective in preventing bleeding. In a later, randomised study[3] using a 400-µg dose, misoprostol was no more effective than placebo in reducing the number of women with blood loss greater than 1000 mL but the need for additional oxytocics was significantly reduced. No serious adverse effects were associated with misoprostol, although the incidence of shivering was significantly increased.
1. O'Brien P, *et al.* Rectally administered misoprostol for the treatment of postpartum hemorrhage unresponsive to oxytocin and ergometrine: a descriptive study. *Obstet Gynecol* 1998; **92:** 212–4.

2. El-Refaey H, *et al.* Use of oral misoprostol in the prevention of postpartum haemorrhage. *Br J Obstet Gynaecol* 1997; **104:** 336–9.

3. Hofmeyr GJ, *et al.* A randomised placebo controlled trial of oral misoprostol in the third stage of labour. *Br J Obstet Gynaecol* 1998; **105:** 971–5.

Termination of pregnancy. Prostaglandins are widely employed for the termination of pregnancy (p.1439) and misoprostol has been studied both for cervical preparation and for inducing uterine contractions.

Vaginal administration of misoprostol is effective for cervical ripening prior to surgical termination in the first trimester.[1] Oral administration of misoprostol following the administration of mifepristone orally is effective in terminating early pregnancy of up to 63 days and especially so at up to 49 days.[2,3] Misoprostol can also be given vaginally.[4,5] In addition, vaginal misoprostol has been studied in combination with intramuscular[6-8] or oral[9-11] methotrexate.

Misoprostol on its own is only a weak abortifacient and is often ineffective when used alone for the termination of pregnancy, although it has been widely misused for this purpose in some countries, notably Brazil.[12-14] Anecdotal reports[14-16] and one small controlled study[17] have associated such misuse during the first trimester of pregnancy with congenital malformations, particularly of the skull, though the manufacturers had found no evidence of teratogenicity in *animals*.[18]

Intravaginal misoprostol has been reported to be as effective as dinoprostone for termination of pregnancy during the second trimester.[19]

1. El-Refaey H, *et al.* Cervical priming with prostaglandin E1 analogues, misoprostol and gemeprost. *Lancet* 1994; **343:** 1207–9. Correction. *ibid.*; 1650.

2. Peyron R, *et al.* Early termination of pregnancy with mifepristone (RU 486) and the orally active prostaglandin misoprostol. *N Engl J Med* 1993; **328:** 1509–13.

3. Spitz IM, *et al.* Early pregnancy termination with mifepristone and misoprostol in the United States. *N Engl J Med* 1998; **338:** 1241–7.

4. El-Refaey H, *et al.* Induction of abortion with mifepristone (RU 486) and oral or vaginal misoprostol. *N Engl J Med* 1995; **332:** 983–7.

5. Ashok PW, *et al.* Termination of pregnancy at 9-13 weeks' amenorrhoea with mifepristone and misoprostol. *Lancet* 1998; **52:** 542–3.

6. Creinin MD, Vittinghoff E. Methotrexate and misoprostol vs misoprostol alone for early abortion: a randomized controlled trial. *JAMA* 1994; **272:** 1190–5.

7. Hausknecht RU. Methotrexate and misoprostol to terminate early pregnancy. *N Engl J Med* 1995; **333:** 537–40.

8. Creinin MD, *et al.* A randomized trial comparing misoprostol three and seven days after methotrexate for early abortion. *Am J Obstet Gynecol* 1995; **173:** 1578–84.

9. Creinin MD. Oral methotrexate and vaginal misoprostol for early abortion. *Contraception* 1996; **54:** 15–18.

10. Creinin MD, *et al.* Medical abortion with oral methotrexate and vaginal misoprostol. *Obstet Gynecol* 1997; **90:** 611–16.

11. Carbonell JLL, *et al.* Oral methotrexate and vaginal misoprostol for early abortion. *Contraception* 1998; **57:** 83–8.

12. Costa SH, Vessey MP. Misoprostol and illegal abortion in Rio de Janeiro, Brazil. *Lancet* 1993; **341:** 1258–61.

13. Coêlho HLL, *et al.* Misoprostol and illegal abortion in Fortaleza, Brazil. *Lancet* 1993; **341:** 1261–3. Correction. *ibid.*; 1486.

14. Fonseca W, *et al.* Misoprostol and congenital malformations. *Lancet* 1991; **338:** 56.

15. Shepard TH. Möbius syndrome after misoprostol: a possible teratogenic mechanism. *Lancet* 1995; **346:** 780.

16. Gonzalez CH, *et al.* Congenital abnormalities in Brazilian children associated with misoprostol misuse in the first trimester of pregnancy. *Lancet* 1998; **351:** 1624–7.

17. Pastuszak AL, *et al.* Use of misoprostol during pregnancy and Möbius' syndrome in infants. *N Engl J Med* 1998; **338:** 1881–5.

18. Downie WW. Misuse of misoprostol. *Lancet* 1991; **338:** 247.

19. Jain JK, Mishell DR. A comparison of intravaginal misoprostol with prostaglandin E2 for termination of second-trimester pregnancy. *N Engl J Med* 1994; **331:** 290–3.

Preparations

Proprietary Preparations (details are given in Part 3)
Aust.: Cyprostol; *Austral.:* Cytotec; *Belg.:* Cytotec; *Braz.:* Cytotec; *Canad.:* Cytotec; *Denm.:* Cytotec; *Fin.:* Cytotec; *Fr.:* Cytotec; *Ger.:* Cytotec; *Hong Kong:* Cytotec; *Irl.:* Cytotec; *Israel:* Cytotec; *Ital.:* Misodex; *Mex.:* Cytotec; *Neth.:* Cytotec; *Norw.:* Cytotec; *NZ:* Cytotec; *Port.:* Cytotec; *S.Afr.:* Cytotec; *Singapore:* Cytotec; *Spain:* Corrigast; Cytotec; Menpros†; *Swed.:* Cytotec; *Switz.:* Cytotec; *Thai.:* Cytotec; *UK:* Cytotec; *USA:* Cytotec.

Used as an adjunct in: Aust.: Arthrotec; *Austral.:* Arthrotec; *Canad.:* Arthrotec; *Denm.:* Arthrotec; *Fin.:* Arthrotec; *Fr.:* Arthrotec; *Ger.:* Arthrotec; *Hong Kong:* Arthrotec; *Irl.:* Arthrotec; *Israel:* Arthrotec; *Ital.:* Arthrotec; Misofenac; *Mex.:* Artrenac Pro; Arthrotec; *Neth.:* Arthrotec; *Norw.:* Arthrotec; *Port.:* Arthrotec; Diclotec;

S.Afr.: Arthrotec; *Singapore:* Arthrotec; *Spain:* Arthrotec; *Swed.:* Arthrotec; *Switz.:* Arthrotec; *Thai.:* Arthrotec; *UK:* Arthrotec; Condrotec†; Napratec; *USA:* Arthrotec.

Nocloprost   (3146-w)

Nocloprost *(rINN)*.

(Z)-7-[(1R,2R,3R,5R)-5-Chloro-3-hydroxy-2-[(E)-(3R)-3-hydroxy-4,4-dimethyl-1-octenyl]cyclopentyl]-5-heptenoic acid.

$C_{22}H_{37}ClO_4 = 401.0$.

CAS — 79360-43-3.

Profile
Nocloprost is a synthetic analogue of dinoprostone (prostaglandin E2) that has been investigated in the treatment of peptic ulcer disease.

◊ References.
1. Täuber U, *et al.* Pharmacokinetics of nocloprost in human volunteers and its relation to dose. *Eur J Clin Pharmacol* 1993; **44:** 497–500.

Ornoprostil   (2971-l)

Ornoprostil *(rINN)*.

OU-1308. Methyl (−)-(1R,2R,3R)-3-hydroxy-2-[(E)-(3S,5S)-3-hydroxy-5-methyl-1-nonenyl]-ε,5-dioxocyclopentaneheptanoate.

$C_{23}H_{38}O_6 = 410.5$.

CAS — 70667-26-4.

Profile
Ornoprostil is a synthetic prostaglandin analogue that has been used in the treatment of peptic ulcer disease.

Sulprostone   (8096-w)

Sulprostone *(USAN, rINN)*.

CP-34089; 16-Phenoxy-ω-17,18,19,20-tetranor-prostaglandin E2-methylsulfonylamide; SHB-286; ZK-57671. (Z)-7-{(1R,2R,3R)-3-Hydroxy-2-[(E)-(3R)-3-hydroxy-4-phenoxybut-1-enyl]-5-oxocyclopentyl}-N-(methylsulphonyl)hept-5-enamide.

$C_{23}H_{31}NO_7S = 465.6$.

CAS — 60325-46-4.

ATC — G02AD05.

Adverse Effects and Precautions
As for Dinoprostone, p.1441. Use of sulprostone is contra-indicated in smokers or those who have smoked in the last 2 years.

Once a prostaglandin has been given to terminate pregnancy it is essential that termination take place; if the prostaglandin is unsuccessful other measures should be used.

Effects on the cardiovascular system. A 31-year-old woman died from cardiovascular shock during an abortion induced by mifepristone followed by sulprostone. She had 12 children, one previous abortion, and was a heavy cigarette smoker.[1] Four other deaths with sulprostone had not been associated with abortion.

1. Anonymous. A death associated with mifepristone/sulprostone. *Lancet* 1991; **337:** 969–70.

Effects on the nervous system. Convulsions occurred in 3 of 4 epileptic patients following administration of sulprostone.[1]

1. Brandenburg H, *et al.* Convulsions in epileptic women after administration of prostaglandin E2 derivative. *Lancet* 1990; **336:** 1138.

Uses and Administration
Sulprostone is a synthetic derivative of dinoprostone (prostaglandin E2). It is a uterine stimulant and is used for dilatation of the cervix prior to surgical termination of pregnancy in the first trimester and for the termination of pregnancy in the second trimester (p.1439). It is also used to control postpartum haemorrhage (p.1607). Sulprostone is administered by intravenous infusion. A dose of 500 µg over 3 to 6 hours is used for cervical dilatation in the first trimester and a similar dose over about 2 hours is given for postpartum haemorrhage. For termination of pregnancy in the second trimester sulprostone is infused at a rate of 100 µg per hour for up to 10 hours; if necessary the in-

fusion rate may be increased to up to 500 µg per hour, to a maximum total dose of 1.5 mg. If unsuccessful the course may be repeated once 12 to 24 hours later. Sulprostone has also been administered extra-amniotically and locally into the cervix. It has also been administered by the intramuscular route, but this is no longer recommended.

Preparations
Proprietary Preparations (details are given in Part 3)
Aust.: Nalador; *Fin.:* Nalador; *Fr.:* Nalador; *Ger.:* Nalador; *Hong Kong:* Nalador; *Ital.:* Nalador; *Neth.:* Nalador; *Singapore:* Nalador; *Switz.:* Nalador; *Thai.:* Nalador.

Tiaprost Trometamol   (8097-e)

Tiaprost Trometamol *(BANM, rINN)*.

Trometamol salt of (±)-(Z)-7-{(1R,2R,3R,5S)-3,5-dihydroxy-2-[(E)-(3RS)-3-hydroxy-4-(3-thienyloxy)but-1-enyl]cyclopentyl}hept-5-enoic acid.

$C_{20}H_{28}O_6S,C_4H_{11}NO_3 = 517.6$.

CAS — 71116-82-0 (tiaprost).

Profile
Tiaprost trometamol is a synthetic analogue of dinoprost (prostaglandin F2α). It is used as a luteolytic in veterinary medicine.

Travoprost   (20240-c)

Travoprost *(BAN, USAN, rINN)*.

AL-6221. Isopropyl (Z)-7-((1R,2R,3R,5S)-3,5-dihydroxy-2-{(1E,3R)-3-hydroxy-4-[α,α,α-trifluoro-m-tolyl)oxy]-1-butenyl}cyclopentyl)-5-heptenoate.

$C_{26}H_{35}F_3O_6 = 500.5$.

CAS — 157283-68-6.

Adverse Effects and Precautions
As for Latanoprost, p.1445.

Uses and Administration
Travoprost is a synthetic analogue of dinoprost (prostaglandin F2α). It is used topically in the treatment of open-angle glaucoma and ocular hypertension (p.1413), in patients who are refractory to other therapies. It is administered as a 0.004% ophthalmic solution once daily in the evening.

Preparations
Proprietary Preparations (details are given in Part 3)
UK: Travatan; *USA:* Travatan.

Unoprostone Isopropyl   (5693-q)

Unoprostone Isopropyl *(rINNM)*.

Isopropyl Lunoprostone; Isopropyl Unoprostone; UF-021. Isopropyl (+)-(Z)-7-((1R,2R,3R,5S)-3,5-Dihydroxy-2-(3-oxodecyl)cyclopentyl)-5-heptenoate.

$C_{25}H_{44}O_5 = 424.6$.

CAS — 120373-36-6 (unoprostone); 120373-24-2 (unoprostone isopropyl).

Adverse Effects and Precautions
As for Latanoprost, p.1445.

Uses and Administration
Unoprostone is a synthetic analogue of dinoprost (prostaglandin F2α) that is used topically as the isopropyl ester for the treatment of glaucoma and ocular hypertension (p.1413). One drop of a solution containing unoprostone isopropyl 0.12 or 0.15% is instilled twice daily.

◊ References.
1. Yamamoto T, *et al.* Clinical evaluation of UF-021 (Rescula; isopropyl unoprostone). *Surv Ophthalmol* 1997; **41** (suppl 2): S99–S103.

2. Eisenberg DL, Camras CB. A preliminary risk-benefit assessment of latanoprost and unoprostone in open-angle glaucoma and ocular hypertension. *Drug Safety* 1999; **20:** 505–14.

Preparations
Proprietary Preparations (details are given in Part 3)
Jpn: Rescula; *Mex.:* Rescula; *Singapore:* Rescula; *Thai.:* Rescula; *USA:* Rescula.

Radiopharmaceuticals

Radioactive compounds are used in medicine as sources of radiation for radiotherapy and for diagnostic purposes. They have numerous uses in research and industry.

Sealed radioactive sources are bonded or encapsulated to prevent the escape of the radioactive material and are used as supplied. Unsealed sources, on the other hand, are radioactive materials usually in liquid, particulate, or gaseous form that are removed from their containers for application. Radiopharmaceuticals come within this category.

The aim of this chapter is to provide background information on the radionuclides that are used as radiopharmaceuticals. Care is required in the preparation, handling, use, and disposal of these compounds; they are thus best dealt with by those with suitable experience and training.

Atomic Structure

An atom is composed of a central positively charged nucleus around which negatively charged electrons revolve in orbits. The electrons are arranged round the atomic nucleus in a series of 'shells' in each of which is a limited number of orbits.

The nucleus consists of 2 main kinds of particles known as protons, each of unit positive charge, and neutrons, which are uncharged; the total number of these particles in the nucleus is known as the *mass number*.

Each electron carries a negative charge which is of the same size as the positive charge of the proton, so that in the neutral atom the number of electrons is equal to the number of protons in the nucleus.

The number of protons in the nucleus is known as the *atomic number*, which determines the number of electrons in the extranuclear structure. Thus all the atoms of a particular chemical element have the same atomic number. But while the number of protons (atomic number) in a given element is constant, the number of neutrons in the atoms, and thus their masses (mass numbers), may vary. These different forms of the same element are known as isotopes of the element and these isotopes differ in some of their physical properties.

Some isotopes may be stable, the differences between them arising solely from their difference in mass; others may be radioactive (*radioisotopes*), their nuclei changing spontaneously and emitting particles or electromagnetic waves, or both.

Most of the naturally occurring isotopes are stable, though there are a number which are unstable and therefore radioactive, for example, uranium-235. In addition, artificial radionuclides are prepared by converting stable nuclei into unstable forms and even naturally occurring radionuclides may be prepared by artificial means.

The symbol used for a nuclide is a development of the chemical symbol for the atom, with the mass number as a superscript and the atomic number as a subscript; thus the symbols for the three hydrogen isotopes—common hydrogen, deuterium, and tritium—are $^{1}_{1}H$, $^{2}_{1}H$, and $^{3}_{1}H$, and the symbols for the three naturally occurring uranium isotopes are $^{234}_{92}U$, $^{235}_{92}U$, and $^{238}_{92}U$; as the atomic number can be inferred from the chemical symbol it is the usual practice to omit the subscript. It is also common practice to write out the full name of the element followed by the mass number, e.g. chromium-51 for ^{51}Cr.

Emissions from Radioisotopes

The 3 main types of emission from radioactive substances are *alpha particles, beta particles,* and *gamma-rays.* Most sources emit more than one type of radiation.

Alpha particles are positively charged particles (helium nuclei), each consisting of 2 protons and 2 neutrons.

Beta particles (β^- or β^+) are identical with electrons or positrons but arise from the nucleus. They are emitted with great velocity and their energies are spread over a spectrum. Positrons are similar to electrons, having a similar mass but a positive charge.

Gamma-rays are electromagnetic radiations or *photons* with a wavelength much shorter than those of light.

In certain cases, e.g. chromium-51, *electron capture* (EC) occurs, an electron from an inner shell being absorbed by the nucleus with the production of an *X-ray* characteristic of the daughter atom or emission of an *Auger electron*.

The type of emission from a radionuclide largely determines its usefulness in medicine. Those emitting alpha particles are very little used partly because detection and measurement are difficult. Positron-emitters, such as carbon-11, fluorine-18, nitrogen-13, and oxygen-15, have become more popular in recent years and are used in positron-emission tomography where the radiation is measured from within the body as opposed to computed tomography where the energy is supplied from an external source. Single photon emission tomography is another technique like positron-emission tomography that provides views of slices through the body and this technique employs gamma-ray emitting radionuclides which are the most accessible and the most common radiation source in radiopharmaceuticals.

Decay of Radionuclides

A radionuclide will consist of unstable atoms which will at some time undergo an energy change with the emission of ionising radiation, those which are actually undergoing this change, and those which have undergone the change. In quantitative terms this transition occurs at a rate which is characteristic of the radionuclide and it is expressed as its half-life—the time required for the activity to fall by one-half. Many radionuclides have complex decay characteristics with several possible energies of emitted particles and radiation. Some radionuclides may be in an excited or metastable state denoted by the suffix m attached to the mass number (e.g. technetium-99m) and undergo *isomeric transition* (IT) with the release of gamma-rays.

The activity of radionuclides is measured in terms of the rate of transformation or disintegration. The unit is the becquerel (Bq) = 1 transformation per second; the curie (Ci) was formerly used as the unit of activity; 1 Ci = 3.7×10^{10} Bq.

Supply, Preparation, and Control

A wide range of radionuclides and specially formulated radiopharmaceuticals is available from specialised manufacturers. However, there are national controls on the use, transport, storage, and disposal of such compounds. Authority and guidance should be sought from the relevant bodies and authorities before using such compounds.

Generators are special features in the supply of radionuclides. They are receptacles containing a parent and daughter nuclide in equilibrium and from which the daughter nuclide, which usually has a short half-life, may be eluted. Generators are available for the production of indium-113m, krypton-81m, and technetium-99m. Generators are also available for some positron-emitters.

Storage conditions for radiopharmaceuticals should be such as to prevent the inadvertent emission of radioactivity as well as to meet the storage requirements for the pharmaceutical that has been labelled. Thus due account still has to be paid, for instance, to the effects of temperature and light. Radiopharmaceuticals are liable to decomposition by self-irradiation effects which may cause degradation of solvent, preservative, or other compounds. There can also be a

continuous formation of oxidising and reducing chemical species arising from the effect of the radioactivity on any chemical substances present in the radiopharmaceutical, even in minute amounts.

Adverse Effects

The internal irradiation of tissues following the administration of radionuclides carries similar dangers to exposure to ionising radiation from an external source, and local high irradiation doses may arise if these nuclides are specifically localised in a tissue. The most serious danger is genetic damage prior to and during the reproductive period. Tissues whose cells are in a continuous state of multiplication are particularly sensitive to the effects of radiation.

Untoward effects of exposure to the larger doses of irradiation include leucopenia, anaemia, inflammation of the skin, radiation sickness, and neoplasms.

In considering the effect of a given radionuclide it is usual to calculate the dose to the organ most critically affected, and also the dose to the whole body.

In considering the adverse effects of radiopharmaceuticals one should not forget the effects that might arise from the carrier or from contaminants.

General Uses

Radiopharmaceuticals are used widely in many branches of medicine and surgery, mainly for the diagnosis and sometimes for the treatment of disease. They can provide information not available using other diagnostic techniques such as contrast media, ultrasound, and computed tomography or other external irradiation. Interesting developments have followed the tagging of monoclonal antibodies with radionuclides.

Many investigations involve the oral or parenteral administration of radionuclides or labelled compounds followed usually by an imaging procedure. Some investigations involve the measurement of radioactive concentrations in organs, tissues, blood, urine, or faeces. The quantities used are always the smallest which will give the desired accuracy of image or of measurement.

◊ Reviews.
1. Schwaiger M, Melin J. Cardiological applications of nuclear medicine. *Lancet* 1999; **354:** 661–6.
2. Corstens FHM, van der Meer JWM. Nuclear medicine's role in infection and inflammation. *Lancet* 1999; **354:** 765–70.
3. Eary JF. Nuclear medicine in cancer diagnosis. *Lancet* 1999; **354:** 853–7.
4. Chatal J-F, Hoefnagel CA. Radionuclide therapy. *Lancet* 1999; **354:** 931–5.
5. Krag D, Moffat F. Nuclear medicine and the surgeon. *Lancet* 1999; **354:** 1019–22.
6. Costa DC, *et al.* Nuclear medicine in neurology and psychiatry. *Lancet* 1999; **354:** 1107–1111.

Radiological Terms

- Alpha particles–nuclei of helium atoms emitted by radioactive atomic nuclei
- annihilation–the interaction and disappearance of a positive and a negative electron with the conversion of their energy into electromagnetic radiation
- atomic number (Z)–the number of protons in the atomic nucleus
- Auger effect–the emission of an electron from an atom due to the filling of a vacancy in an inner electron shell
- becquerel (Bq)–the SI unit of activity, defined as 1 transformation per second. The curie was formerly used as the unit of activity. 1 Bq = 2.7×10^{-11} Ci
- beta particles–electrons or positrons emitted by radioactive atomic nuclei
- carrier-free–a preparation in which substantially all the atoms of the activated element present are radioactive. Material of high specific activity is often loosely referred to as 'carrier-free'
- curie (Ci)–now superseded as a unit of activity by the becquerel. A curie (Ci) represented 3.7×10^{10} transformations per second. 1 Ci = 3.7×10^{10} Bq
- daughter–of a given nuclide, any nuclide that originates from it by radioactive decay
- electron capture (EC)–a mode of radioactivity decay involving the capture of an orbital electron by its nucleus

- gamma-radiation–electromagnetic radiation emitted in the process of a change in configuration of a nucleus or particle annihilation and having wavelengths shorter than those of X-rays
- gray (Gy)–the SI unit of absorbed dose, defined as 1 J per kg. The rad was formerly used as the unit of absorbed dose. 1 Gy = 100 rads
- isomeric transition (IT)–the decay of one isomer to another having a lower energy state. The transition is accompanied by the emission of gamma-radiation
- isomers–nuclides with the same mass number and atomic number but with nuclei having different energy states
- isotopes–nuclides with the same atomic number but different mass numbers
- nuclide–a species of atom having a specific mass number, atomic number, and nuclear energy state
- photon–a quantum of electromagnetic radiation
- positron–a positive beta particle
- rad (radiation absorbed dose)–now superseded as a unit of absorbed dose by the gray. A rad is equal to 10^{-2} J per kg. The röntgen and the rad in soft tissue are approximately equivalent in magnitude for moderate energies. 1 rad = 10^{-2} Gy
- radioactive decay–the spontaneous change of a nucleus resulting in the emission of a particle or a photon
- radioactivity–the property of certain nuclides of spontaneously emitting particles or photons or of undergoing spontaneous fission
- radioisotope–an isotope that is radioactive
- radionuclide–a nuclide that is radioactive
- rem (röntgen-equivalent-man)–now superseded as a unit of dose equivalent by the sievert (Sv). A rem is numerically equal to the absorbed dose in rads multiplied by the appropriate quality factor defining the biological effect and by any other modifying factors. The sievert is the joule per kg (J kg^{-1}) equal to 100 rem
- röntgen (R)–a unit of exposure of X- or gamma-radiation, equal to 2.58×10^{-4} coulombs per kg in air superseded by the SI unit of exposure, the coulomb per kg (C kg^{-1}). 1 C kg^{-1} = 3.876×10^{3} R
- sievert (Sv)–the SI unit of dose equivalent numerically equal to the absorbed dose in grays multiplied by the appropriate quality factor defining the biological effect and by any other modifying factors expressed in J per kg body-weight
- specific activity–the activity per unit mass of a material containing a radioactive substance
- X-rays–electromagnetic radiation other than annihilation radiation originating in the extranuclear part of the atom and having wavelengths much shorter than those of visible light

Carbon-11   (9907-j)

CAS — 14333-33-6.

HALF-LIFE. 20.4 minutes.

Profile
Carbon-11 is a positron-emitter which is used in positron-emission tomography (see Emissions from Radioisotopes, p.1448). Compounds which have been labelled with carbon-11 include L-methionine for the detection of malignant neoplasms, acetic acid and palmitic acids for the study of myocardial metabolism, and raclopride for the study of CNS dopaminergic D_2 receptors. Labelled carbon monoxide may be used to assess blood volume.

Preparations
Ph. Eur.: L-Methionine ((^{11}C)Methyl) Injection;
USP 25: Carbon Monoxide C 11; Flumazenil C 11 Injection; Mespiperone C 11 Injection; Methionine C 11 Injection; Raclopride C 11 Injection; Sodium Acetate C 11 Injection.

Carbon-14   (5853-q)

CAS — 14762-75-5.

HALF-LIFE. 5730 years.

Profile
Carbon-14 has been used to label many organic compounds that may be employed in breath tests.
Urea (p.1127) labelled with carbon-14 is used in a breath test to detect *Helicobacter pylori* as an aid in the diagnosis of peptic ulcer disease (p.1208).

Preparations
USP 25: Urea C 14 Capsules.
Proprietary Preparations (details are given in Part 3)
USA: Pytest.

Chromium-51   (5854-p)

CAS — 14392-02-0.

HALF-LIFE. 27.7 days.

Profile
Chromium-51, as sodium chromate (^{51}Cr), is used to label red blood cells so that red cell survival and red cell volume can be measured. Chromium-51 activity in the faeces can be used to estimate gastrointestinal blood losses. Red blood cells labelled with chromium-51 and damaged by heat before re-injection have been used for spleen scanning.
As chromium edetate (^{51}Cr) given intravenously, chromium-51 is used in the determination of the glomerular filtration rate.
As chromic chloride (^{51}Cr), chromium-51 has been administered intravenously for the determination of loss of serum protein into the gastrointestinal tract.

Preparations
Ph. Eur.: Chromium(^{51}Cr) Edetate Injection; Sodium Chromate(^{51}Cr) Sterile Solution;
USP 25: Chromium Cr 51 Edetate Injection; Sodium Chromate Cr 51 Injection.

Proprietary Preparations (details are given in Part 3)
USA: Chromitope†.

Cobalt-57   (5855-s)

CAS — 13981-50-5.

HALF-LIFE. 271 days.

Profile
Cobalt-57, in the form of an aqueous solution or capsules of cyanocobalamin (^{57}Co), is given by mouth for the measurement of absorption of vitamin B_{12} in the diagnosis of pernicious anaemia and other malabsorption syndromes. It is also used with cyanocobalamin (^{58}Co), see below.

Preparations
Ph. Eur.: Cyanocobalamin(^{57}Co) Capsules; Cyanocobalamin(^{57}Co) Solution;
USP 25: Cyanocobalamin Co 57 Capsules; Cyanocobalamin Co 57 Oral Solution.

Proprietary Preparations (details are given in Part 3)
USA: Cobratope†.

Multi-ingredient: *UK:* Dicopac.

Cobalt-58   (5856-w)

CAS — 13981-38-9.

HALF-LIFE. 70.8 days.

Profile
Cobalt-58, in the form of an aqueous solution or capsules of cyanocobalamin (^{58}Co), is given by mouth for the measurement of absorption of vitamin B_{12} in the diagnosis of pernicious anaemia and other malabsorption syndromes.
The different energies of cobalt-57 and cobalt-58 facilitate separation of the isotopes in a mixture. Advantage is taken of this to differentiate between failure of absorption due to lack of intrinsic factor (pernicious anaemia) and that due to ileal malabsorption by the simultaneous administration of free cyanocobalamin (^{58}Co) and cyanocobalamin (^{57}Co) bound to intrinsic factor. A dual isotope kit has been used for this purpose.

Preparations
Ph. Eur.: Cyanocobalamin(^{58}Co) Capsules; Cyanocobalamin(^{58}Co) Solution.

Proprietary Preparations (details are given in Part 3)
USA: Rubratope†.

Multi-ingredient: *UK:* Dicopac.

Fluorine-18   (19185-l)

CAS — 13981-56-1.
ATC — V09AX02 *(fludeoxyglucose (^{18}F))*.

HALF-LIFE. 110 minutes.

Profile
Fluorine-18 is a positron-emitting radionuclide which is used in positron-emission tomography (see Emissions from Radioisotopes, p.1448).
Fludeoxyglucose (^{18}F) (2-deoxy-2-fluoro-^{18}F-α-D-glucopyranose; ^{18}F-fluorodeoxyglucose) is given by intravenous injection for the assessment of cerebral and myocardial glucose metabolism in various physiological or pathological states including stroke and myocardial ischaemia. It is also employed for the detection of malignant tumours including those of the brain, liver, lung, and thyroid gland. Fluorodopa (^{18}F) is also used in cerebral imaging.

Preparations
Ph. Eur.: Fludeoxyglucose (^{18}F) Injection;
USP 25: Fludeoxyglucose F 18 Injection; Fluorodopa F 18 Injection; Sodium Fluoride F 18 Injection.

Gallium-67   (5858-l)

CAS — 14119-09-6.

HALF-LIFE. 3.26 days.

Profile
Gallium-67 is used in the form of an intravenous injection of gallium citrate (^{67}Ga).
Gallium citrate (^{67}Ga) is concentrated in some malignant tumours of the lymphatic system, as well as in some other tissues, and is used for tumour visualisation. Concentration also occurs in inflammatory lesions and the injection is therefore employed for the localisation of focal inflammatory sites, such as may occur in abscesses, osteomyelitis, or sarcoidosis. Gallium scans have proved useful for the detection of the various infections and malignancies that may be encountered in patients with AIDS.

Preparations
Ph. Eur.: Gallium(^{67}Ga) Citrate Injection;
USP 25: Gallium Citrate Ga 67 Injection.

Gold-198   (5859-y)

CAS — 10043-49-9.

HALF-LIFE. 65 hours (2.7 days).

Profile
Gold-198, as colloidal gold (^{198}Au) with most of the activity associated with particles of diameter 5 to 20 nm, has been used by intrapleural or intraperitoneal injection in the treatment of malignant ascites and malignant pleural effusion, and by intravenous injection for the measurement of liver blood flow, in liver scanning, and for general investigations of the reticuloendothelial system. Since the gamma-ray energies are not particularly good for scanning and the radiation dose to the patient is relatively high, it has generally been superseded by more suitable agents such as technetium-99m-labelled compounds.

Indium-111   (5860-g)

CAS — 15750-15-9.

HALF-LIFE. 67 hours (2.8 days).

Profile
Indium-111 as indium (^{111}In) complexed with pentetic acid (pentetate) is used diagnostically in CSF studies.
Leucocytes labelled with indium (^{111}In) hydroxyquinoline are used for the location of inflammatory lesions; applications have been the detection or localisation of abscesses, infections including those occurring in patients with AIDS, inflammatory bowel diseases such as Crohn's disease or ulcerative colitis, and transplant rejection. Platelets have been similarly labelled and used for the detection of thrombi and for the investigation of thrombocytopenia. Labelled erythrocytes have been used to investigate gastrointestinal haemorrhage.
Colloids have been prepared using indium chloride (^{111}In) and have been used for investigation of the lymphatic system. Indium (^{111}In) bleomycin has been given by intravenous injection for the detection of tumours. Indium (^{111}In) pentetreotide is used for the detection and localisation of tumours originating from neuroendocrine cells.
Several different monoclonal antibodies, such as altumomab pentetate, capromab pendetide, imciromab pentetate, and satumomab pendetide, have been labelled with indium-111. Applications include the detection, diagnosis, and evaluation of malignant neoplasms of the colon, rectum, prostate, and ovaries as well as the detection and localisation of myocardial infarction.

Preparations
Ph. Eur.: Indium(^{111}In) Chloride Solution; Indium(^{111}In) Oxine Solution; Indium(^{111}In) Pentetate Injection;
USP 25: Indium In 111 Capromab Pentetide Injection; Indium In 111 Chloride Solution; Indium In 111 Oxyquinoline Solution; Indium In 111 Pentetate Injection; Indium In 111 Pentetreotide Injection; Indium In 111 Satumomab Pendetide Injection.

Proprietary Preparations (details are given in Part 3)
Ital.: Myoscint†; Octreoscan; OncoScint CR 103; *Spain:* OncoScint CR 103; *USA:* OncoScint CR/OV.

Indium-113m   (5861-q)

CAS — 14885-78-0 (indium-113).

HALF-LIFE. 99.5 minutes.

Profile
Indium-113m is a daughter of tin-113 (^{113}Sn, half-life 115 days) and because of its short half-life is normally prepared just before use by elution from a sterile generator consisting of tin-113 adsorbed on an ion-exchange material contained in a column.
Indium-113m may be used for labelling a variety of materials with differing physical properties including particles and colloids suited to scanning procedures for various organs and tissues. Chelates with pentetic acid have also been used. The short

half-life of indium-113m and its lack of beta-emission have allowed large doses to be given with a small radiation dose to the patient. High count rates for scanning are therefore achieved.

Iodine-123   (5862-p)

CAS — 15715-08-9.
ATC — V09IX01 (iobenguane (^{123}I)); V09CX01 (sodium iodohippurate (^{123}I)); V09FX02 (sodium iodide (^{123}I)).

HALF-LIFE. 13.2 hours.

Profile

Iodine-123 has similar adverse effects and precautions to those of iodine-131 (see below).

Its principal use is in thyroid uptake tests and thyroid imaging when it is given by mouth or intravenous injection as sodium iodide (^{123}I).

Sodium iodohippurate (^{123}I) is employed intravenously in tests of renal function and in renal imaging.

Iobenguane (^{123}I) (m-iodobenzylguanidine (^{123}I)) is given intravenously for the localisation of certain tumours, for example phaeochromocytomas, and for the evaluation of neuroblastoma. It is also used for functional studies of the adrenal medulla and myocardium.

Ioflupane (^{123}I) is given intravenously to detect loss of functioning dopaminergic neurones in the differential diagnosis of tremor and parkinsonism.

Various monoclonal antibodies have been labelled with iodine-123; potential applications include the detection of malignant neoplasms.

Preparations

USP 25: Iobenguane I 123 Injection; Iodohippurate Sodium I 123 Injection; Sodium Iodide I 123 Capsules; Sodium Iodide I 123 Solution.

Proprietary Preparations (details are given in Part 3)
UK: DaTSCAN.

Iodine-125   (5863-s)

CAS — 14158-31-7.
ATC — V09CX03 (sodium iotalamate (^{125}I)).

HALF-LIFE. 60.1 days.

Profile

Iodine-125 has similar adverse effects and precautions to those of iodine-131 (see below).

Iodine-125 is not very suitable for the external counting of radioactivity in the thyroid gland because its gamma-energy is weak and tissue absorption is high. However, it is very suitable for radio-immunoassays *in vitro* and because it has a long half-life it is preferred as a label for many compounds to detect and estimate drugs and hormones in body fluids.

Iodine-125 may be used orally as sodium iodide (^{125}I) in the diagnosis of thyroid disorders.

Sodium iotalamate (^{125}I) has been used intravenously in the determination of glomerular filtration rate and sodium iodohippurate (^{125}I) intravenously for the measurement of effective renal plasma flow.

Iodine-125, as iodinated (^{125}I) human fibrinogen, has been used intravenously to demonstrate and locate deep-vein thrombosis of the leg. Iodinated (^{125}I) fibrinogen has also been used in the measurement of fibrinogen metabolism in certain disturbances of blood coagulation.

Human albumin iodinated with iodine-125 has been used for the determination of blood or plasma volume.

Iodine-125 implants have been used for the local treatment of cancers. Titanium capsules containing iodine-125 adsorbed onto a silver rod have been used in the treatment of cancers of the head and neck, lung, pancreas, and prostate. Brain tumours have been treated with titanium capsules containing iodine-125 adsorbed onto anion exchange resin spheres.

Preparations

BP 2001: Iodinated(^{125}I) Albumin Injection;
Ph. Eur.: Human Iodinated(^{125}I) Fibrinogen; Sodium Iodide(^{125}I) Solution;
USP 25: Iodinated I 125 Albumin Injection; Iothalamate Sodium I 125 Injection.

Proprietary Preparations (details are given in Part 3)
USA: Glofil.

Iodine-131   (5864-w)

CAS — 10043-66-0.
ATC — V09IX02 (iobenguane (^{131}I)); V09CX02 (sodium iodohippurate (^{131}I)); V09FX03 (sodium iodide (^{131}I)); V10XA02 (iobenguane (^{131}I)); V10XA01 (sodium iodide (^{131}I)).

HALF-LIFE. 8.04 days.

Adverse Effects

A small percentage of patients treated with iodine-131 for hyperthyroidism become hypothyroid each year and eventually most patients will require thyroid replacement therapy. Hypoparathyroidism has also been reported. Radiation thyroiditis

with soreness may develop shortly after treatment. There may be severe and potentially dangerous swelling of the thyroid especially in patients with large goitres and this has on rare occasions produced asphyxiation. Leukaemia and carcinoma of the thyroid have occasionally been reported, particularly in young patients. Retrospective studies have shown an increased incidence of thyroid cancer in adults after iodine-131 treatment for hyperthyroidism. However, the absolute risk of thyroid cancer is small and the underlying thyroid disease may play a role.

In the treatment of thyroid carcinoma, the larger doses of radioactive iodine sometimes cause nausea and vomiting a few days after ingestion, which may be due to gastritis as iodine-131 is also concentrated in gastric mucosa. Large doses depress the bone marrow.

◊ References.
1. Ron E, *et al.* Cancer mortality following treatment for adult hyperthyroidism. *JAMA* 1998; **280:** 347–55.
2. Franklyn JA, *et al.* Cancer incidence and mortality after radioiodine treatment for hyperthyroidism: a population-based cohort study. *Lancet* 1999; **353:** 2111–15.

Precautions

The use of sodium iodide (^{131}I) is contra-indicated, even in diagnostic doses, during pregnancy and lactation. Sodium iodide (^{131}I) should not be given to patients with large toxic nodular goitres or to patients with severe thyrotoxic heart disease. There is some controversy as to whether radio-iodine therapy exacerbates Graves' ophthalmopathy (see Hyperthyroidism, p.1519).

Many drugs have been reported to interfere with thyroid- or other organ-function studies and checks should be made on any treatment the patient might be receiving before any estimations are carried out.

Uses and Administration

Iodine radioisotopes are mainly used in studies of thyroid function and in the treatment of hyperthyroidism (p.1519) and some forms of thyroid carcinoma (p.500).

Iodine radioisotopes can be incorporated into many compounds including liothyronine and thyroxine [levothyroxine], triglycerides and fatty acids, such as triolein and oleic acid, and proteins, such as iodinated human albumin, with varying degrees of stability and with little or no change in the biological activity of the labelled molecule. It is common practice to saturate the thyroid with non-radioactive iodine when uptake of radiation by the gland is not desired (see Radiation Protection, p.1524).

Sodium iodide (^{131}I) is given by mouth and by intravenous injection in studies of thyroid function, particularly in measurements of the uptake of iodine by the thyroid, and in thyroid scanning. It is also used in the treatment of hyperthyroidism and in the treatment of malignant neoplasms of the thyroid.

Injections containing iobenguane (^{131}I) (m-iodobenzylguanidine (^{131}I)) may be employed for the localisation and treatment of phaeochromocytoma (p.810) and neuroblastoma (p.500).

Human albumin iodinated with iodine-131 is employed in the determination of the blood or plasma volume.

Sodium iodohippurate (^{131}I) is used intravenously for renal-function tests and for renal imaging.

Rose bengal sodium (^{131}I) has been given intravenously in tests of liver function.

Iodinated (^{131}I) norcholesterol (6β-iodomethyl-19-norcholest-5(10)-en-3β-ol (^{131}I)) has been used for adrenal scintigraphy by slow intravenous injection.

Various monoclonal antibodies labelled with iodine-131 are used for the detection of malignant neoplasms and some are being investigated for therapeutic purposes, such as iodine (^{131}I) tositumomab for non-Hodgkin's lymphoma.

Preparations

Ph. Eur.: Iobenguane(^{131}I) Injection for Diagnostic Use; Iobenguane(^{131}I) Injection for Therapeutic Use; Iodinated(^{131}I) Norcholesterol Injection; Sodium Iodide(^{131}I) Capsules for Diagnostic Use; Sodium Iodide(^{131}I) Solution; Sodium Iodohippurate(^{131}I) Injection;
USP 25: Iobenguane I 131 Injection; Iodinated I 131 Albumin Aggregated Injection; Iodinated I 131 Albumin Injection; Iodohippurate Sodium I 131 Injection; Rose Bengal Sodium I 131 Injection; Sodium Iodide I 131 Capsules; Sodium Iodide I 131 Solution.

Proprietary Preparations (details are given in Part 3)
UK: Theracap; USA: Hipputope†; Iodotope.

Iron-59   (5866-l)

CAS — 14596-12-4.
ATC — V09XX04 (ferric citrate (^{59}Fe)).

HALF-LIFE. 44.6 days.

Profile

Iron-59, in the form of ferrous citrate (^{59}Fe) or ferric citrate (^{59}Fe), has been used by intravenous injection in the measurement of iron absorption and utilisation. Ferric chloride (^{59}Fe) has been given for the same purpose.

Krypton-81m   (18354-v)

CAS — 15678-91-8.

HALF-LIFE. 13.1 seconds.

Profile

Krypton-81m is a daughter of rubidium-81 (^{81}Rb, half-life 4.58 hours), and is prepared immediately before use by elution from a generator containing rubidium-81 adsorbed on a suitable ion-exchange column using air or oxygen as the eluent. Krypton-81m is used as a gas in lung ventilation studies. Such ventilation studies can be combined with lung perfusion studies to diagnose pulmonary embolism.

Preparations

Ph. Eur.: Krypton(^{81m}Kr) Inhalation Gas;
USP 25: Krypton Kr 81m.

Nitrogen-13   (16918-s)

CAS — 13981-22-1.

HALF-LIFE. 9.96 minutes.

Profile

Nitrogen-13 is a positron-emitting radionuclide which is used in positron-emission tomography (see Emissions from Radioisotopes, p.1448). In the form of ammonia (^{13}N) it is given intravenously for imaging blood flow in organs such as the heart, brain, and liver. Nitrogen gas (^{13}N) may be used for pulmonary ventilation studies.

Preparations

Ph. Eur.: Ammonia(^{13}N) Injection;
USP 25: Ammonia N 13 Injection.

Oxygen-15   (17602-x)

CAS — 13982-43-9.

HALF-LIFE. 2 minutes.

Profile

Oxygen-15 is a positron-emitting radionuclide used in positron-emission tomography (see Emissions from Radioisotopes, p.1448). It is employed in the form of water (^{15}O) and is given intravenously to study cerebral and myocardial perfusion.

Oxygen gas, carbon dioxide, and carbon monoxide have also been labelled with oxygen-15.

Preparations

Ph. Eur.: Carbon Monoxide(^{15}O); Oxygen(^{15}O); Water(^{15}O) Injection;
USP 25: Water O 15 Injection.

Phosphorus-32   (5869-z)

CAS — 14596-37-3.
ATC — V10XX01 (sodium phosphate (^{32}P)).

HALF-LIFE. 14.3 days.

Profile

Phosphorus-32, given as sodium phosphate (^{32}P), is used intravenously in the treatment of polycythaemia vera (p.486). Phosphorus-32 is taken up by the rapidly proliferating haematopoietic cells sufficiently to reduce their reproduction. Sodium phosphate (^{32}P) has also been employed intravenously in the treatment of chronic myeloid (p.486) and chronic lymphocytic leukaemia (p.485) and in the palliative treatment of bone metastases.

Chromic phosphate (^{32}P) is administered intraperitoneally or intrapleurally in the treatment of malignant effusions (p.489); it may also be given by interstitial injection for the treatment of ovarian (p.496) or prostatic carcinoma (p.497).

Preparations

Ph. Eur.: Sodium Phosphate(^{32}P) Injection;
USP 25: Chromic Phosphate P 32 Suspension; Sodium Phosphate P 32 Solution.

Proprietary Preparations (details are given in Part 3)
USA: Phosphocol.

Rhenium-186   (3879-n)

CAS — 14998-63-1.

HALF-LIFE. 90.6 hours.

Profile

Rhenium-186 has been used in colloidal form for the treatment of arthritic joint conditions. Rhenium (^{186}Re) etidronate has been investigated for the treatment of painful bone metastases. Monoclonal antibodies labelled with rhenium-186 have been investigated for the treatment of various malignant neoplasms.

Rubidium-82 (11869-f)

CAS — 14391-63-0.

HALF-LIFE. 75 seconds.

Profile
Rubidium-82 is a positron-emitting radionuclide which is used in positron-emission tomography (see Emissions from Radioisotopes, p.1448). Rubidium chloride (^{82}Rb) is administered intravenously for cardiac imaging.

Preparations
USP 25: Rubidium Chloride Rb 82 Injection.
Proprietary Preparations (details are given in Part 3)
USA: CardioGen 82†.

Samarium-153 (12226-a)

CAS — 15766-00-4.
ATC — V10BX02 (samarium (^{153}Sm) lexidronam).

HALF-LIFE. 47 hours.

Profile
Samarium-153, in the form of samarium (^{153}Sm) lexidronam (samarium (^{153}Sm) EDTMP) is used for the palliative treatment of painful bone metastases (p.490). It is given by intravenous injection.

Preparations
USP 25: Samarium Sm 153 Lexidronam Injection.
Proprietary Preparations (details are given in Part 3)
Austral.: Quadramet; **Fr.:** Quadramet; **Ital.:** Quadramet; **USA:** Quadramet.

Selenium-75 (5872-w)

CAS — 14265-71-5.

HALF-LIFE. 118.5 days.

Profile
Selenium-75 in the form of 6β-[(methyl[^{75}Se]seleno)methyl]-19-norcholest-5(10)-en-3β-ol (selenonorcholestenol (^{75}Se)) is used intravenously in adrenal scintigraphy.
Selenium-75 in the form of tauroselcholic acid (^{75}Se) (^{75}SeHCAT) is used orally in the measurement of bile acid absorption for the assessment of ileal function.

Preparations
Proprietary Preparations (details are given in Part 3)
UK: Scintadren.

Strontium-89 (3881-a)

CAS — 14158-27-1.
ATC — V10BX01 (strontium chloride (^{89}Sr)).

HALF-LIFE. 50.5 days.

Profile
Strontium-89, in the form of strontium chloride (^{89}Sr), is used for the palliation of pain in patients with bone metastases (p.490); it is given intravenously.

◊ References.
1. Robinson RG, *et al.* Strontium 89 therapy for the palliation of pain due to osseous metastases. *JAMA* 1995; **274:** 420–4.

Preparations
Ph. Eur.: Strontium(^{89}Sr) Chloride Injection;
USP 25: Strontium Chloride Sr 89 Injection.
Proprietary Preparations (details are given in Part 3)
Austral.: Metastron; **Canad.:** Metastron†; **Fr.:** Metastron; **Ital.:** Metastron; **Spain:** Metastron; **UK:** Metastron; **USA:** Metastron.

Technetium-99m (5878-c)

CAS — 14133-76-7 (technetium-99).

HALF-LIFE. 6.02 hours.

Adverse Effects
Hypersensitivity reactions have been reported with technetium-99m preparations.

Uses and Administration
Technetium-99m is a daughter of molybdenum-99 (^{99}Mo, half-life 66.2 hours) and because of its short half-life is normally prepared just before use by elution from a sterile generator consisting of molybdenum-99 adsorbed onto alumina in a glass column. Technetium-99m as pertechnetate (^{99m}TcO$_4^-$) is obtained by elution with a sterile solution of sodium chloride 0.9%. Radiopharmaceuticals of technetium-99m are prepared shortly after elution to reduce loss by decay.

Because it has a short half-life and can be administered in relatively large doses, and because the energy of its gamma-emission is readily detected, technetium-99m is very widely used, either as the pertechnetate or in the form of various labelled compounds, particles, and colloids for scanning bone and organs such as the brain, heart, kidney, liver, lung, spleen, and thyroid.

Sodium pertechnetate (^{99m}Tc) is used intravenously for angiography and for imaging blood pools, brain, salivary glands, and thyroid gland; the oral route may also be employed for brain and thyroid imaging. Topical application to the eye is used for studying nasolachrymal drainage and the intraurethral route for imaging the urinary tract. Potassium perchlorate may be given before administration of the pertechnetate to prevent uptake in the thyroid or choroid plexus and thus enhance visualisation in other organs.

Macroaggregates of human albumin labelled with technetium-99m [macrosalb (^{99m}Tc)] are used in lung scanning for the detection of abnormal lung perfusion patterns; following the intravenous injection of a suspension of suitable particle size, usually 10 to 100 μm, the particles become trapped in the lung capillaries enabling ischaemic areas to be defined. Labelled albumin microspheres of particle size 10 to 50 μm are used similarly. Labelled macroaggregates of albumin have also been used in venography for the detection of deep-vein thrombosis of the legs. Technetium (^{99m}Tc) apcitide is a labelled peptide that binds to the glycoprotein IIb/IIIa receptor of activated platelets, and is also used for imaging of deep-vein thrombosis.

When technetium-99m bound to human serum albumin is administered intravenously it becomes evenly distributed in the circulation and highly vascular organs or pools of blood may be readily located. Such a preparation is used in the examination of the heart.

Technetium-99m in the form of a colloid, such as albumin, sulfur, antimony sulfide, or tin, is used intravenously for the examination of the liver, spleen, and bone marrow. Sulfur colloid (^{99m}Tc) may be given orally for oesophageal and gastrointestinal imaging. Albumin colloid (^{99m}Tc) may be given subcutaneously for scanning of the lymphatic system.

Technetium-99m complexes of iminodiacetic acid derivatives, such as disofenin, etifenin, lidofenin, and mebrofenin are employed intravenously in the investigation of hepatic function and in the imaging of the hepatobiliary system.

Agents used intravenously in both brain and renal imaging are technetium-99m-labelled gluconate, gluceptate, and pentetate. Other technetium-99m-labelled compounds are used in brain and kidney scanning; for instance, labelled bicisate and exametazime have been employed in brain imaging and mertiatide and succimer have been used in kidney studies. The pentetate is also given by inhalation for lung ventilation imaging, and orally for studies of gastro-oesophageal reflux and gastric emptying.

For bone scanning various labelled phosphate compounds may be used and include medronate, oxidronate, and pyrophosphate, all given intravenously. Technetium-99m as the pyrophosphate is also used in cardiac scintigraphy. Technetium-99m as the medronate and pyrophosphate are also used to label red blood cells for use in blood pool scintigraphy, cardiac scintigraphy, detection of gastrointestinal bleeding, and testicular scintigraphy.

Compounds employed intravenously in cardiac imaging include technetium-99m-labelled sestamibi, teboroxime, and tetrofosmin. Technetium (^{99m}Tc) sestamibi is also used for breast imaging.

Technetium-99m-labelled leucocytes (prepared using exametazime) are employed for localisation of sites of inflammation or infection.

Monoclonal antibodies, such as arcitumomab, labelled with technetium-99m are used for the detection and localisation of malignant neoplasms. Technetium (^{99m}Tc) depreotide is a labelled peptide used intravenously for imaging of pulmonary malignancy.

Many other technetium-99m-labelled compounds have been prepared and used in different clinical studies for the examination of different organs or systems. Use with other radionuclides includes subtraction scanning with thallium-201 to detect parathyroid tumours.

Preparations
Ph. Eur.: Sodium Pertechnetate(^{99m}Tc) Injection (Fission); Sodium Pertechnetate(^{99m}Tc) Injection (Non-fission); Technetium(^{99m}Tc) Colloidal Rhenium Sulphide Injection; Technetium(^{99m}Tc) Colloidal Sulphur Injection; Technetium(^{99m}Tc) Colloidal Tin Injection; Technetium(^{99m}Tc) Etifenin Injection; Technetium(^{99m}Tc) Gluconate Injection; Technetium(^{99m}Tc) Human Albumin Injection; Technetium(^{99m}Tc) Macrosalb Injection; Technetium(^{99m}Tc) Medronate Injection; Technetium(^{99m}Tc) Mertiatide Injection; Technetium(^{99m}Tc) Microspheres Injection; Technetium(^{99m}Tc) Pentetate Injection; Technetium(^{99m}Tc) Succimer Injection; Technetium(^{99m}Tc) Tin Pyrophosphate Injection;
USP 25: Sodium Pertechnetate Tc 99m Injection; Technetium Tc 99m (Pyro- and trimeta-) Phosphates Injection; Technetium Tc 99m Albumin Aggregated Injection; Technetium Tc 99m Albumin Colloid Injection; Technetium Tc 99m Albumin Injection; Technetium Tc 99m Apcitide Injection; Technetium Tc 99m Arcitumomab Injection; Technetium Tc 99m Bicisate Injection; Technetium Tc 99m Disofenin Injection; Technetium Tc 99m Etidronate Injection; Technetium Tc 99m Exametazime Injection; Technetium Tc 99m Gluceptate Injection; Technetium Tc 99m Lidofenin Injection; Technetium Tc 99m Mebrofenin Injection; Technetium Tc 99m Medronate Injection; Technetium Tc 99m Mertiatide Injection; Technetium Tc 99m Nofetumomab Merpentan Injection; Technetium Tc 99m Oxidronate Injection; Technetium Tc 99m Pentetate Injection; Technetium Tc 99m Pyrophosphate Injection; Technetium Tc 99m Red Blood Cells Injection; Technetium Tc 99m Sestamibi Injection; Technetium Tc 99m Succimer Injection; Technetium Tc 99m Sulfur Colloid Injection; Technetium Tc 99m Tetrofosmin Injection.
Proprietary Preparations (details are given in Part 3)
Aust.: Cardiolite; **Austral.:** Ceretec; Myoview; **Belg.:** Cardiolite; Neurolite; **Canad.:** Choletec†; **Fr.:** Cardiolite; Ceretec†; Myo-

view; Neurolite; **Ital.:** CEA-Scan; Ceretec; LeukoScan; Myoview; TechneScan MAG3; **Spain:** Cardiolite; CEA-Scan; Ceretec; Myoview; Neurolite; TechneScan HDP; TechneScan Mag3; **UK:** Amerscan DMSA; Amerscan Hepatate; Amerscan Medronate; Amerscan Pentetate; Amerscan Pulmonate; Amerscan Stannous; Amertec; Cardiolite; CEA-Scan; Ceretec; Myoview; Nanocoll; **USA:** AcuTect; Cardiolite; CardioTec†; CEA-Scan; Choletec†; Macrotec†; MDP-Squibb†; Miraluma; NeoTect; Phosphotec†; Techneplex†; TechneScan HDP; Tesuloid†.

Thallium-201 (5879-k)

CAS — 15064-65-0.

HALF-LIFE. 73.1 hours.

Profile
Thallium-201, in the form of thallous chloride (^{201}Tl), is administered by intravenous injection for scanning the myocardium in the investigation of acute myocardial infarction. It is also used for myocardial perfusion imaging in cardiac stress testing of patients with ischaemic heart disease. Adenosine (p.829), dipyridamole (p.878), or dobutamine (p.881) may be used to induce pharmacological stress in those patients unable to tolerate exercise.

Other uses include muscle perfusion scintigraphy in peripheral vascular disorders, visualisation of brain and thyroid tumours and metastases, and the localisation of parathyroid adenomas and hyperplasia by thallium-201 and technetium-99m subtraction scanning.

Preparations
Ph. Eur.: Thallous(^{201}Tl) Chloride Injection;
USP 25: Thallous Chloride Tl 201 Injection.

Tritium (5881-e)

Hydrogen-3.
CAS — 10028-17-8.

HALF-LIFE. 12.3 years.

Profile
Tritium, in the form of tritiated water, has been used to determine the total body water by a dilution technique.

Preparations
Ph. Eur.: Tritiated(^{3}H) Water Injection.

Xenon-127 (9910-s)

CAS — 13994-19-9.

HALF-LIFE. 36.41 days.

Profile
Xenon-127 has similar physical properties to those of xenon-133 (see below) and is also used by inhalation for pulmonary function studies and lung imaging.

Preparations
USP 25: Xenon Xe 127.

Xenon-133 (5882-l)

CAS — 14932-42-4.

HALF-LIFE. 5.25 days.

Profile
Xenon-133 is an inert gas with relatively low solubility in plasma. In the gaseous form, it is mixed with air or oxygen in a bag or in a closed or open circuit spirometer. When the administration of gas is stopped, xenon-133 is excreted promptly and completely through the lungs. It is used by inhalation in pulmonary function studies and lung imaging as well as in cerebral blood flow studies. It has also been employed for these purposes in the form of an injection in sodium chloride 0.9%.

Preparations
Ph. Eur.: Xenon(^{133}Xe) Injection;
USP 25: Xenon Xe 133; Xenon Xe 133 Injection.

Yttrium-90 (5883-y)

CAS — 10098-91-6.

HALF-LIFE. 64.1 hours.

Profile
Yttrium-90, in the form of a colloidal suspension of yttrium silicate (^{90}Y) is suitable for instillation into pleural or peritoneal cavities in the treatment of malignant pleural effusion (p.489) or malignant ascites.

Yttrium-90, as either yttrium citrate (^{90}Y) or yttrium silicate (^{90}Y), is also used in the treatment of arthritic conditions of joints.

Yttrium-90 conjugated to various monoclonal antibodies is being investigated for the treatment of malignant neoplasms.

The symbol † denotes a preparation no longer actively marketed

Sex Hormones

The male and female sex organs, the adrenal cortex, and the placenta produce steroidal hormones which influence the development and maintenance of structures directly and indirectly associated with reproduction. The secretion of these sex hormones is controlled by gonadotrophic hormones of the anterior lobe of the pituitary gland; the secretion of these gonadotrophic hormones is in turn influenced by the hypothalamus and also by the concentration of circulating sex hormones. There are 3 groups of endogenous sex hormones, androgens, oestrogens, and progestogens, all of which are derived from the same steroidal precursors. The progestogenic hormone, progesterone is formed from pregnenolone, and both of these compounds may be converted to androgen precursors such as androstenedione. Androstenedione is converted to the androgenic hormone testosterone by hydroxysteroid dehydrogenases. Oestrogenic hormones are synthesised from androstenedione (and also from testosterone) by the action of aromatase.

Testosterone is the main androgenic hormone formed in the interstitial (Leydig) cells of the testes. A small proportion of circulating testosterone is also derived from the metabolism of less potent androgens secreted by the adrenal cortex and ovaries. In many target tissues testosterone is then converted to the more active dihydrotestosterone by 5α-reductase. Some testosterone also undergoes peripheral conversion to oestradiol.

Testosterone controls the development and maintenance of the male sex organs and the male secondary sex characteristics. It also produces systemic anabolic effects, such as increased retention of nitrogen, calcium, sodium, potassium, chloride, and phosphate. This leads to an increase in water retention and bone growth. The skin becomes more vascular and less fatty and erythropoiesis is increased.

Numerous derivatives of testosterone have been developed. Alkylation at the 17α position results in derivatives that are orally active (e.g. methyltestosterone, stanozolol) and esterification of the 17β-hydroxyl group increases lipid solubility and is used to prepare long-acting intramuscular preparations (e.g. testosterone enantate). Removal of the 19-methyl group is reported to improve the anabolic to androgenic ratio (e.g. nandrolone). The derivatives also vary in their plasma protein binding affinity, and degree of conversion to dihydrotestosterone and aromatic conversion to oestrogen. Numerous other structural modifications have been made.

Oestradiol is the most active of the naturally occurring oestrogens formed from androgen precursors in the ovarian follicles of premenopausal women. In men and postmenopausal women (and to an insignificant extent in premenopausal women) oestrogens are also formed in adipose tissue from adrenal androgens.

Oestrogens control the development and maintenance of the female sex organs, secondary sex characteristics, and mammary glands as well as certain functions of the uterus and its accessory organs (particularly the proliferation of the endometrium, the development of the decidua, and the cyclic changes in the cervix and vagina). Large amounts of oestradiol are also formed in the placenta; in late pregnancy, this increases the spontaneous activity of the uterine muscle and its response to oxytocic drugs. The additional activity of progesterone is essential for the complete biological function of the female sex organs.

A number of oestrogens are used therapeutically. Ethinyl substitution at the C17 position has led to the development of synthetic oestrogens such as ethinylestradiol and mestranol, which have greatly improved potency and oral activity. Oral activity of natural oestrogens is improved by esterification (e.g. estradiol valerate) or by conjugation (e.g. estrone sulfate). Es-

terification also increases solubility in lipid vehicles and is used to prepare long-acting intramuscular preparations.

A number of nonsteroidal oestrogens, including broparestrol, chlorotrianisene, dienestrol, hexestrol, and diethylstilbestrol, have also been used.

Progesterone is the main hormone secreted by the corpus luteum. It acts on the endometrium by converting the proliferative phase induced by oestrogen to a secretory phase thereby preparing the uterus to receive the fertilised ovum. Progesterone has a catabolic action and causes a slight rise in basal body temperature during the secretory phase of menstruation. Large quantities of progesterone are also produced by the placenta during pregnancy. During pregnancy it suppresses uterine motility and is responsible for the further development of the breasts.

Progestogens (gestagens, progestagens, progestins) are synthetic compounds with actions similar to those of progesterone. They are either progesterone derivatives or 19-nortestosterone analogues. The 19-nortestosterone analogues (such as norethisterone and norgestrel) possess some androgenic activity, but some newer norgestrel derivatives (desogestrel, gestodene, and norgestimate) have little androgenic activity. The progesterone derivatives dydrogesterone, hydroxyprogesterone, and medroxyprogesterone are less androgenic than the 19-nortestosterone analogues. The progesterone derivatives chlormadinone, and particularly cyproterone, have anti-androgenic activity.

The principal natural and synthetic sex hormones covered in this chapter are thus:

- **androgens and anabolic steroids**, typified by testosterone (p.1492)
- **oestrogens**, typified by estradiol (p.1473)
- **progestogens**, typified by progesterone (p.1488).

Other related substances also described in this chapter are:

- drugs with predominantly **weak androgenic** properties such as danazol (p.1468) and gestrinone (p.1479)
- drugs that combine **oestrogenic and progestogenic** properties such as tibolone (p.1495)
- drugs with predominantly **anti-androgenic** properties. These include the progesterone derivative cyproterone acetate, the nonsteroidal 5α-reductase inhibitor finasteride, and the plant extract saw palmetto. Those anti-androgens used principally in the hormonal treatment of prostate cancer are covered in the Antineoplastics chapter; they include the nonsteroidal drugs bicalutamide (p.511), flutamide (p.542), and nilutamide (p.562).
- drugs with predominantly **anti-oestrogenic** properties. These include the nonsteroidal anti-oestrogens clomifene, cyclofenil, and the more selective nonsteroidal anti-oestrogens ormeloxifene and raloxifene. Those anti-oestrogens used principally in the hormonal treatment of breast cancer are covered in the Antineoplastics chapter; they include the oestrogen receptor antagonists tamoxifen (p.571) and toremifene (p.576), and various nonsteroidal aromatase inhibitors such as formestane (p.543) and anastrozole (p.508)
- drugs with predominantly **antiprogestogenic** properties such as the progesterone derivative mifepristone.

The activity of endogenous sex hormones can be modulated by gonadotrophins, and gonadorelin and its analogues, and these are discussed in Hypothalamic and Pituitary Hormones, beginning on p.1271.

The therapeutic applications of sex hormones and related substances are broad and cover many circumstances where hormonal manipulation is desirable. Major applications are the use of oestrogens and progestogens for **contraception** (p.1460) and for the al-

leviation of **menopausal symptoms** (p.1464). A physiological application is the use of an androgen or an oestrogen in the management of **delayed puberty** and **hypogonadism**, (see Testosterone, p.1493 or Estradiol, p.1474). Other clinical applications include the management of **benign prostatic hyperplasia** (p.1477), **endometriosis** (p.1469), **gynaecomastia** (p.1470), **hirsutism** (p.1468), **infertility** (p.1275), **mastalgia** (p.1470), **menorrhagia** (p.1490), and **premenstrual syndrome** (p.1475). Hormonal manipulation also has an important role in the treatment of **malignant neoplasms** of the breast (p.491), prostate (p.497), and endometrium (p.493).

Hormonal Contraceptives (9021-f)

Hormonal contraceptives are currently only available for women although preparations for men are being evaluated. Oral hormonal contraceptives for women are divided into 2 main types: 'combined' (containing an oestrogen and a progestogen) and 'progestogen-only'. Parenteral progestogen-only preparations have also been developed and include subcutaneous implants and depot intramuscular injections. Progestogen-releasing intra-uterine devices are also available.

Progestogens inhibit ovulation by suppressing the necessary mid-cycle surge of luteinising hormone. However, the low doses in progestogen-only oral contraceptives do not suppress it reliably in all cycles. Contraceptive efficacy is instead achieved by thickening the cervical mucus so that it is not readily penetrated by sperm, and by preventing proliferation of the endometrium so that it remains unfavourable for implantation of any fertilised ova. Intra-uterine progestogen-only devices act similarly; the physical presence of the system in the uterus may also contribute to overall contraceptive efficacy. Parenteral progestogen-only contraceptives on the other hand provide reliable suppression of ovulation.

Oestrogens inhibit ovulation by suppressing the mid-cycle release of follicle-stimulating hormone. They act synergistically with progestogens in combined oral contraceptives to provide regular and consistent suppression of ovulation.

Oral preparations are also available for *emergency contraception* after unprotected coitus; they prevent implantation of any fertilised ova.

Adverse Effects

Many reports have been published of adverse effects associated with the use of **combined oral contraceptives**. The data has mostly been gained retrospectively and often involves older preparations containing higher doses of oestrogen and progestogen than are used currently.

There may be gastrointestinal side-effects such as nausea or vomiting, chloasma (melasma) and other skin or hair changes, headache, water retention, weight gain, breast tenderness, and changes in libido.

Menstrual irregularities such as spotting, breakthrough bleeding, or amenorrhoea can occur during treatment. These effects may result from the relative balance of oestrogenic and progestogenic effects of particular products and their incidence may be reduced by changing to a different product. For example, early or mid-cycle spotting or absence of withdrawal bleeding may require a preparation with a greater oestrogen to progestogen ratio, or less progestogen as in multiphasic preparations, or temporary supplementation with an oestrogen.

Intolerance to contact lenses has been reported and vision may deteriorate in myopic patients. Some patients may experience depression and other mental changes. Preparations containing a progestogen with androgenic properties such as levonorgestrel and norgestrel may be associated with increased oiliness of the skin and acne. Conversely, acne may be improved with progestogens such as norgestimate or desogestrel.

There is an increased risk of cardiovascular disease and associated mortality related, at least in part, to the oestrogen content of combined oral contraceptives. The incidence of cardiovascular side-effects is probably less with the newer lower-dose preparations than with the older higher-dose preparations. Increased mortality from myocardial infarction is much greater with increased age and in cigarette smokers, although some evidence suggests that healthy women aged over 35 years who do not smoke are not at increased risk. Other risk factors include a family history of arterial disease, diabetes mellitus, hypertension, obesity, and migraine. Thrombosis may be more common when factor V Leiden is present or in patients with blood groups A, B, or AB. Specific risk factors for venous thromboembolism include a family history of venous thromboembolism, varicose veins and, again, obesity. Recent evidence has also indicated that the risk of venous thromboembolism varies according to the progestogen component of combined oral contraceptives; a higher incidence has been associated with desogestrel and gestodene than with levonorgestrel, norethisterone, and etynodiol. For further discussion see Venous Thromboembolism, below.

Combined oral contraceptives may cause hypertension and there may be reduced glucose tolerance and changes in lipid metabolism. Liver function can be impaired, although jaundice is rare. There appears to be a marked increase (though the incidence is still very low) in the relative risk of benign liver tumours. Malignant liver tumours have also been reported.

Combined oral contraceptives are reported to slightly increase the risk of cervical cancer (although other factors may be involved) and breast cancer, but to protect against ovarian cancer and endometrial cancer. For further discussion, see Carcinogenicity, below.

As with combined oral contraceptives, **progestogen-only contraceptives** may cause nausea, vomiting, headache, breast discomfort, depression, skin disorders, and weight gain. Menstrual irregularities such as amenorrhoea, breakthrough bleeding, spotting, and menorrhagia are more common with progestogen-only contraceptives, and are particularly common with parenteral preparations. Available progestogen-only contraceptives carry less risk of thromboembolic and cardiovascular disease than combined oral contraceptives.

Carcinogenicity. Concern has often been expressed as to whether the use of hormonal contraceptives by normally healthy women may either cause or increase the risk of developing malignant neoplasms. To investigate any possible link between such use and cancer, two main types of study have been employed by epidemiologists, namely the prospective study and the case-control study. Many factors have made direct comparison of results difficult and such factors include the type and composition of oral contraceptive used (which has changed over the years), the age of the patient, the age at which use first began, and the sexual and obstetric history of the patient. Overall the evidence indicates that combined oral contraceptives in fact exert a protective effect against the development of endometrial and ovarian carcinoma. However, there is a small increase in risk of breast cancer during use and for 10 years after discontinuation. In addition, there does appear to be a slight risk of cervical cancer with the prolonged use of combined oral contraceptives and a negligible risk of liver cancer. For further details concerning the effects on individual organs, see the following sections. It should be noted that even where the relative risk has been shown to be substantially increased this will not translate into many new cases of a rare cancer, and this contributes to the difficulties of assessing clinical relevance. It is also worthy of note that two large prospective cohort studies (the Nurses' Health Study and the Royal College of General Practitioners' study) found no evidence of a difference in overall mortality between women who had used oral contraceptives and those who had not.[1,2] Some general reviews on hormonal contraceptives and cancer are cited below.[3,4]

1. Colditz GA, et al. Oral contraceptive use and mortality during 12 years of follow-up: the Nurses' Health Study. Ann Intern Med 1994; 120: 821–6.
2. Beral V, et al. Mortality associated with oral contraceptive use: 25 year follow up of cohort of 46 000 women from Royal College of General Practitioners' oral contraception study. BMJ 1999; 318: 96–100.
3. WHO. Oral contraceptives and neoplasia: report of a WHO scientific group. WHO Tech Rep Ser 817 1992.
4. La Vecchia C, et al. Oral contraceptives and cancer: a review of the evidence. Drug Safety 1996; 14: 260–72.

BREAST. Numerous epidemiological studies have been published on the potential link between hormonal contraceptives and breast cancer. Most of these data relate to **combined oral contraceptives**, which are the most widely used form. The breast cancer risk from use of these contraceptives will require monitoring for some time to come as the first users of oral contraceptives continue to age, and because of the changing patterns of use.

Early studies from the 1980s variously failed to show any significant increase in risk of breast cancer in women who had ever used hormonal contraceptives compared with those who had never done so,[1-4] or showed an increase in risk,[5] or identified a risk in specific sub-groups of users.[6-12] Potential identified risk factors, for which much of the evidence was conflicting, included current use,[10] duration of use,[7,11] age at first use,[6] duration of use before a first full-term pregnancy,[7,8] nulliparity,[9] high-dose preparations,[11] and family history of breast cancer.[12] It was also reported that use of oral contraceptives might lead to an accelerated presentation of breast cancer,[13] or an increased risk of invasive cancer.[4]

In response to these studies, the UK Committee on Safety of Medicines,[14] the FDA in the USA,[15] and the International Committee for Research in Reproduction[16] issued advice that the available evidence did not require a change in prescribing practice. This advice has not been subsequently changed, although patients should be informed of the possible small increase in risk of breast cancer, which has to be weighed against established benefits of therapy.[17]

From 1990 to 1995, over 20 major studies had been published on the oral contraceptive-breast cancer issue. A review[18] indicated that, in general, these studies showed some excess breast cancer risk in current or recent users of oral contraceptives, but no excess risk for use more than 5 years previously. In contrast to some earlier studies, duration of use tended not to affect risk, neither did any of the major recognised risk factors for breast cancer.

More recently, a Collaborative Group on Hormonal Factors in Breast Cancer was set up to re-analyse all the worldwide epidemiological evidence on breast cancer risk and hormonal contraceptives. The group identified individual data on 53 297 women with breast cancer, and 100 239 controls (women without breast cancer) from 54 studies, and have published a summary of their findings,[19] and a further detailed review.[20] They reported that women currently using oral contraceptives have a slight increase in the relative risk of breast cancer (1.24; 95% confidence intervals 1.15 to 1.33), and that this risk decreases after stopping use, and is no longer significant after 10 or more years. There was a weak trend towards an increase in risk with increasing duration of use. Thus, it appears that the risk of breast cancer increases soon after first exposure, does not increase with duration of exposure, and returns to normal 10 years after cessation of exposure.[19]

Cancers diagnosed in those who had ever used hormonal contraceptives were clinically less advanced than in those who had never done so.[19] Further information is required on whether this is related to earlier diagnosis or a biological effect of the hormones. In addition, data on breast cancer mortality are required.

When analysed by age at first use, the risk was largest in those women who started use as teenagers. Because of the trend towards earlier use, further review of long-term data is required.[19] The most important risk factor is, however, the age at which women discontinue the contraceptive; the greater the age at stopping, the more breast cancers are diagnosed.[17]

There was no difference in risk between nulliparous women, parous women who began use of oral contraceptives before their first child, and parous women who began use of oral contraceptives after the birth of their first child.[19]

Low-dose oral contraceptives were not associated with a decreased risk of breast cancer.[19] When preparations were grouped according to oestrogen dose (<50 µg, 50 µg, and >50 µg), there was, if anything, a decrease in breast cancer risk with increasing dose among women who had stopped use 10 or more years before, largely due to a reduction in breast cancer risk in those who had used the highest dose preparations.

The Collaborative Group's analysis did not note any difference in risk according to family history.[19] However, a subsequent cohort study found an increased risk of breast cancer among women with a strong family history of the disease who used earlier formulations of oral contraceptives.[21] It is not known whether this risk applies to newer lower-dosage formulations, or whether it is correlated with mutations in the BRCA1 or BRCA2 genes. These findings are of concern because women with BRCA1 or BRCA2 mutations are often encouraged to take oral contraceptives to reduce their risk of ovarian cancer.

There are far fewer data on risk of breast cancer with **progestogen-only contraceptives**, which are less frequently used than combined preparations.

A WHO study published in 1991 indicated that, overall, depot medroxyprogesterone acetate did not increase the risk of breast cancer (relative risk compared with never users 1.21; 95% confidence intervals 0.96 to 1.53) and that risk did not increase with duration of use.[22] However, there appeared to be a slight increase in risk within the first 4 years of use, especially in women under 35 years of age. These findings agreed with those of a smaller study[23] in which women who had used depot medroxyprogesterone acetate for 2 years or longer before the age of 25 had a relative risk of 4.6. Pooled analysis of these 2 studies indicated that current or recent use was the key factor.[24] The relative risk of breast cancer in women who had used medroxyprogesterone acetate in the last 5 years was 2.0, and there was no increased risk in women who had ceased use more than 5 years previously, regardless of their duration of use.

The Collaborative Group on Hormonal Factors in Breast Cancer reported that there was some evidence of an increased risk of breast cancer for use of oral or injectable progestogens in the previous 5 years (relative risk 1.17), and no risk 10 or more years after stopping use.[19] These findings were broadly similar to those for combined preparations. As for combined preparations, the most important factor is the age at discontinuation. For women who stop by age 30 after 5 years use of a progestogen-only preparation there would be an estimated increase from 44 to 46 or 47 cases per 10 000 compared with those who have never used a hormonal contraceptive. For 5 years use stopping by age 40 there would be an estimated increase from 160 to 170 cases diagnosed in the following 10 years.[17]

1. Ellery C, et al. A case-control study of breast cancer in relation to the use of steroid contraceptive agents. Med J Aust 1986; 144: 173–6.
2. Paul C, et al. Oral contraceptives and breast cancer: a national study. BMJ 1986; 293: 723–6.
3. The Cancer and Steroid Hormone Study of the Centers for Disease Control and the National Institute of Child Health and Human Development. Oral-contraceptive use and the risk of breast cancer. N Engl J Med 1986; 315: 405–11.
4. Stanford JL, et al. Oral contraceptives and breast cancer: results from an expanded case-control study. Br J Cancer 1989; 60: 375–81.
5. Miller DR, et al. Breast cancer before age 45 and oral contraceptive use: new findings. Am J Epidemiol 1989; 129: 269–80.
6. Pike MC, et al. Breast cancer in young women and use of oral contraceptives: possible modifying effect of formulation and age at use. Lancet 1983; ii: 926–30.
7. Meirik O, et al. Oral contraceptive use and breast cancer in young women: a joint national case-control study in Sweden and Norway. Lancet 1986; ii: 650–4.
8. McPherson K, et al. Early oral contraceptive use and breast cancer: results of another case-control study. Br J Cancer 1987; 56: 653–60.
9. Meirik O, et al. Breast cancer and oral contraceptives: patterns of risk among parous and nulliparous women—further analysis of the Swedish-Norwegian material. Contraception 1989; 39: 471–5.
10. Romieu I, et al. Prospective study of oral contraceptive use and risk of breast cancer in women. J Natl Cancer Inst 1989; 81: 1313–21.
11. UK National Case-Control Study Group. Oral contraceptive use and breast cancer risk in young women. Lancet 1989; i: 973–82.
12. UK National Case-Control Study Group. Oral contraceptive use and breast cancer risk in young women: subgroup analyses. Lancet 1990; 335: 1507–9.
13. Kay CR, Hannaford PC. Breast cancer and the pill—a further report from the Royal College of General Practitioners' contraception study. Br J Cancer 1988; 58: 675–80.
14. Committee on Safety of Medicines. Oral contraceptives and carcinoma of the breast. Current Problems 26 1989.
15. Anonymous. Cancer risks of oral contraception. Lancet 1989; i: 84.
16. International Committee for Research in Reproduction. Oral contraceptives and breast cancer. JAMA 1989; 262: 206–7.
17. Committee on Safety of Medicines/Medicines Control Agency. Oral contraceptives and breast cancer. Current Problems 1998; 24: 2–3.
18. La Vecchia C, et al. Oral contraceptives and cancer: a review of the evidence. Drug Safety 1996; 14: 260–72.
19. Collaborative Group on Hormonal Factors in Breast Cancer. Breast cancer and hormonal contraceptives: collaborative reanalysis of individual data on 53 297 women with breast cancer and 100 239 women without breast cancer from 54 epidemiological studies. Lancet 1996; 347: 1713–27.
20. Collaborative Group on Hormonal Factors in Breast Cancer. Breast cancer and hormonal contraceptives: further results. Contraception 1996; 54 (suppl): 1S–106S.
21. Grabrick DM, et al. Risk of breast cancer with oral contraceptive use in women with a family history of breast cancer. JAMA 2000; 284: 1791–8.
22. WHO Collaborative Study of Neoplasia and Steroid Contraceptives. Breast cancer and depot-medroxyprogesterone acetate: a multinational study. Lancet 1991; 338: 833–8.
23. Paul C, et al. Depot medroxyprogesterone (Depo-Provera) and risk of breast cancer. BMJ 1989; 299: 759–62.
24. Skegg DCG, et al. Depot medroxyprogesterone acetate and breast cancer: a pooled analysis of the World Health Organization and New Zealand studies. JAMA 1995; 273: 799–804.

CERVIX. It is often considered difficult to carry out satisfactory epidemiological studies on the relationship between hormonal contraceptives and cervical cancer because of the many known variables and factors which may influence the development of this type of neoplasm. For example, sexual activity per se, and multiple sexual partners (both of the woman and her partner) increase the risk, while the use of other non-hormonal barrier methods of contraception may offer some protection against cervical neoplasia. Nevertheless, there have been some suggestions that the use of oral contraceptives may be associated with an increased risk.

Two UK cohort studies from the 1980s revealed an increased risk of cervical cancer in women receiving oral contraceptives that was shown to increase with increasing duration of use.[1,2]

In 1992, WHO reviewed[3] these cohort data, and data from 18 case-controlled studies carried out up to 1990. They concluded that use of oral contraceptives for more than 5 years was associated with a modest increase in the relative risk of cervical squamous cell carcinoma (in the order of 1.3 to 1.8). Additional potential risk factors included recent or current use and high oestrogen dose. Of known risk factors for cervical cancer, women with multiple sexual partners, genital infection, or high parity had enhanced risks associated with oral contraceptives.[3]

Most cervical cancers are squamous cell carcinomas, but it has been proposed that oral contraceptive use might be a particular risk factor for the rarer adenocarcinoma of the cervix, the incidence of which has risen in younger women. Reviewing studies up to 1990, WHO concluded that data were insufficient to draw firm conclusions on links between oral contraceptives and the risk of cervical adenocarcinoma.[3] A case-controlled study from 1994 found an increased risk of adenocarcinoma of the cervix in users of oral contraceptives.[4] Any use of oral contraceptives was associated with an approximate doubling of risk, and use for more than 12 years was associated with a relative risk 4.4 times greater than that in women who never used an oral contraceptive. More recently, a WHO study reported that the strength of the observed relationship for cervical adenocarcinomas and adenosquamous carcinomas and oral contraceptives was about the same as that for invasive squamous cell cervical carcinomas.[5]

Human papilloma virus (HPV) has a role in the aetiology of cervical cancer and women who are HPV positive and using oral contraceptives may be at increased risk of cervical neoplasm.[6]

Data on the risk of cervical cancer with **progestogen-only contraceptives** are limited. WHO have investigated any possible link between the use of medroxyprogesterone acetate as a longacting injectable contraceptive and cervical neoplasia. Analysis showed a small non-significant elevated risk (1.11; 95% confidence interval 0.9 to 1.29), and no clear association with duration of use.[7]

1. Vessey MP, et al. Neoplasia of the cervix uteri and contraception: a possible adverse effect of the pill. *Lancet* 1983; **ii**: 930–4.
2. Beral V, et al. Oral contraceptive use, and malignancies of the genital tract: results from the Royal College of General Practitioners' oral contraception study. *Lancet* 1988; **ii**: 1331–5.
3. WHO. Oral contraceptives and neoplasia: report of a WHO scientific group. *WHO Tech Rep Ser 817* 1992.
4. Ursin G, et al. Oral contraceptive use and adenocarcinoma of cervix. *Lancet* 1994; **344**: 1390–4.
5. Thomas DB, Ray RM. Oral contraceptives and invasive adenocarcinomas and adenosquamous carcinomas of the uterine cervix. *Am J Epidemiol* 1996; **144**: 281–9.
6. La Vecchia C, et al. Oral contraceptives and cancer: a review of the evidence. *Drug Safety* 1996; **14**: 260–72.
7. WHO Collaborative Study of Neoplasia and Steroid Contraceptives. Depot-medroxyprogesterone acetate (DMPA) and risk of invasive squamous cell cervical cancer. *Contraception* 1992; **45**: 299–312.

ENDOMETRIUM. It has been reliably demonstrated that **combined oral contraceptives** decrease the risk of endometrial cancer. WHO analysed data from case-control and cohort studies published up to 1990,[1] including data from the large Cancer and Steroid Hormone Study (CASH) in the USA,[2] and reported that there was a highly significant trend of decreasing risk of endometrial cancer with increasing duration of use of combined oral contraceptives. The reduction in risk was estimated to be 20% after 1 year and 50% after 4 years' use.[1] The protective effect was observed for endometrial cancer with and without squamous elements,[1,2] and was found to persist for at least 15 years after cessation of use.[2] A more recent study with longer term follow-up indicated that the protection persists for at least 20 years.[3] Further follow-up is required to determine the true duration of protection.

The results of the WHO Collaborative Study on Neoplasia and Steroid Contraceptives suggested that protection may be greater with preparations containing high-dose progestogen.[4] However, a more recent study found that risk of endometrial cancer was unrelated to progestogen potency of the oral contraceptive, although this study also reported no protective effect for less than 5 years' use.[5]

Unopposed menopausal oestrogen replacement therapy is known to increase the risk of endometrial cancer (see p.1461), and there is some evidence[3,5] that it reduces the protective effect of previous oral contraception.

There are limited data on the effect of **progestogen-only contraceptives** on the risk of endometrial cancer, although they would be expected to be protective. Results from the WHO Collaborative Study[6] suggest that depot medroxyprogesterone acetate reduced the risk of endometrial cancer; the estimated relative risk in users was 0.21. However, many of the women in this study received supplemental oestrogen to control menstrual irregularity, and were therefore technically taking a form of combined therapy.[7] There was some evidence that the protective effect of medroxyprogesterone acetate was greater in women who had not received oestrogen,[7] and this requires further study.

1. WHO. Oral contraceptives and neoplasia: report of a WHO scientific group. *WHO Tech Rep Ser 817* 1992.

2. The Cancer and Steroid Hormone Study of the Centers for Disease Control and the National Institute of Child Health and Human Development. Combination oral contraceptive use and the risk of endometrial cancer. *JAMA* 1987; **257**: 796–800.
3. Stanford JL, et al. Oral contraceptives and endometrial cancer: do other risk factors modify the association? *Int J Cancer* 1993; **54**: 243–8.
4. Rosenblatt KA, et al. Hormonal content of combined oral contraceptives in relation to the reduced risk of endometrial carcinoma. *Int J Cancer* 1991; **49**: 870–4.
5. Voigt LF, et al. Recency, duration, and progestin content of oral contraceptives in relation to the incidence of endometrial cancer. *Cancer Causes Control* 1994; **5**: 227–33.
6. WHO Collaborative Study of Neoplasia and Steroid Contraceptives. Depot-medroxyprogesterone acetate (DMPA) and risk of endometrial cancer. *Int J Cancer* 1991; **49**: 186–90.
7. Szarewski A, Guillebaud J. Safety of DMPA. *Lancet* 1991; **338**: 1157–8.

GASTROINTESTINAL TRACT. A link between female sex hormones and the risk of colorectal cancer has been postulated. Epidemiological studies have variously shown a possible increased risk of rectal cancer,[1] a possible decreased risk of colorectal cancer[2] in women ever having used oral contraceptives, and no association between past oral contraceptive use and colorectal cancer[3] (see also under Hormone Replacement Therapy, p.1462.)

1. Kune GA, et al. Oral contraceptive use does not protect against large bowel cancer. *Contraception* 1990; **41**: 19–25.
2. Fernandez E, et al. Oral contraceptives, hormone replacement therapy and the risk of colorectal cancer. *Br J Cancer* 1996; **73**: 1431–5.
3. Troisi R, et al. Reproductive factors, oral contraceptive use, and risk of colorectal cancer. *Epidemiology* 1997; **8**: 75–9.

LIVER. The use of **combined oral contraceptives** has been rarely associated with liver tumours, both benign (hepatic adenomas and focal nodular hyperplasia)[1] and malignant (hepatocellular carcinoma).[1,2]

Hepatocellular carcinomas are associated with hepatitis B, and are relatively common in countries where this is endemic but rare elsewhere. Case-control studies in populations at high risk for hepatocellular carcinoma suggest that the use of oral contraceptives does not significantly affect the risk, although long-term data are scanty.[3,4] In contrast, case-control studies in countries where the prevalence of hepatitis B is low have shown an increased risk of hepatocellular carcinoma among users of oral contraceptives, particularly after long-term use (reviewed by WHO[1] and La Vecchia[2]). However, because the malignancy is so rare, this increased risk may be negligible.[2] For example, there has been no increase in mortality from liver cancer in young women in the UK since the introduction and use of oral contraceptives.[5] Similar findings have been reported for the USA and Sweden.[6]

There are limited data specifically on **progestogen-only contraceptives**. Results from a WHO study[7] provided no evidence that use of medroxyprogesterone acetate as a long-acting injectable contraceptive altered the risk of developing liver cancer but the power of the study to detect small alterations in risk was low.

1. WHO. Oral contraceptives and neoplasia: report of a WHO scientific group. *WHO Tech Rep Ser 817* 1992.
2. La Vecchia C, et al. Oral contraceptives and cancer: a review of the evidence. *Drug Safety* 1996; **14**: 260–72.
3. The WHO Collaborative Study of Neoplasia and Steroid Contraceptives. Combined oral contraceptives and liver cancer. *Int J Cancer* 1989; **43**: 254–9.
4. Kew MC, et al. Contraceptive steroids as a risk factor for hepatocellular carcinoma: a case/control study in South African black women. *Hepatology* 1990; **11**: 298–302.
5. Mant JWF, Vessey MP. Trends in mortality from primary liver cancer in England and Wales 1975-1992: influence of oral contraceptives. *Br J Cancer* 1995; **72**: 800–3.
6. Waetjen LE, Grimes DA. Oral contraceptives and primary liver cancer: temporal trends in three countries. *Obstet Gynecol* 1996; **88**: 945–9.
7. Anonymous. Depot-medroxyprogesterone acetate (DMPA) and cancer: memorandum from a WHO meeting. *Bull WHO* 1986; **64**: 375–82.

OVARY. There is convincing evidence that **combined oral contraceptives** reduce the risk of ovarian cancer,[1,2] possibly as a function of their inhibition of ovulation. Relative risks for ovarian cancer have variously been reported as 0.4 to 0.8 in those who have ever used oral contraceptives, and decrease with increasing duration of use. There is evidence that there may be a delay of several years before the protective effect becomes apparent, but that it persists for as long as 20 years after cessation of use.[3] The protective effect has been noted for both malignant and borderline malignant tumours, and for each of the major histological subtypes of epithelial ovarian cancer.[3]

It has been suggested that newer lower-dose oestrogen preparations may be slightly less protective than higher-dose preparations.[4] The relative risk for use of high-dose preparations was 0.68, and for low-dose preparations was 0.81.

The protective effect against ovarian cancer may have significant implications for public health. For example, it was estimated that oral contraceptive use may have prevented nearly one-quarter of deaths expected to occur due to ovarian cancer in 1986 in women aged 54 years or less in England and Wales.[5]

There are few data on the effects of **progestogen-only contraceptives** on the risk of ovarian cancer. WHO have investigated the effect of depot medroxyprogesterone acetate on ovarian cancer, and found that it was not associated with either a decrease or increase in risk (relative risk 1.07; 95% confidence

interval 0.6 to 1.8).[6] This is perhaps surprising since the preparation, like combined oral contraceptives, inhibits ovulation.

1. Franceschi S, et al. Pooled analysis of 3 European case-control studies of epithelial ovarian cancer III: oral contraceptive use. *Int J Cancer* 1991; **49**: 61–5.
2. Whittemore AS, et al. Characteristics relating to ovarian cancer risk: collaborative analysis of 12 US case-control studies II: invasive epithelial ovarian cancers in white women. *Am J Epidemiol* 1992; **136**: 1184–1203.
3. Rosenberg L, et al. A case-control study of oral contraceptive use and invasive epithelial ovarian cancer. *Am J Epidemiol* 1994; **139**: 654–61.
4. Rosenblatt KA, et al. High-dose and low-dose combined oral contraceptives: protection against epithelial ovarian cancer and the length of the protective effect. *Eur J Cancer* 1992; **28A**: 1872–6.
5. Villard-Mackintosh L, et al. The effects of oral contraceptives and parity on ovarian cancer trends in women under 55 years of age. *Br J Obstet Gynaecol* 1989; **96**: 783–8.
6. WHO Collaborative Study of Neoplasia and Steroid Contraceptives. Depot-medroxyprogesterone acetate (DMPA) and risk of epithelial ovarian cancer. *Int J Cancer* 1991; **49**: 191–5.

SKIN. Although there have been some suggestions of a possible association between the use of oral contraceptives and the development of malignant melanoma[1-3] most studies, including recent analyses of relatively large numbers of women suffering from malignant melanoma, found no such association with either current or prior use of oral contraceptive preparations.[4-9] A meta-analysis of 18 case-control studies confirmed the lack of association.[10]

1. Beral V, et al. Malignant melanoma and oral contraceptive use among women in California. *Br J Cancer* 1977; **36**: 804–9.
2. Lerner AB, et al. Effects of oral contraceptives and pregnancy on melanomas. *N Engl J Med* 1979; **301**: 47.
3. Beral V, et al. Oral contraceptive use and malignant melanoma in Australia. *Br J Cancer* 1984; **50**: 681–5.
4. Bain C, et al. Oral contraceptive use and malignant melanoma. *J Natl Cancer Inst* 1982; **68**: 537–9.
5. Helmrich SP, et al. Lack of an elevated risk of malignant melanoma in relation to oral contraceptive use. *J Natl Cancer Inst* 1984; **72**: 617–20.
6. Green A, Bain C. Hormonal factors and melanoma in women. *Med J Aust* 1985; **142**: 446–8.
7. Østerlind A, et al. The Danish case-control study of cutaneous malignant melanoma III: hormonal and reproductive factors in women. *Int J Cancer* 1988; **42**: 821–4.
8. Palmer JR, et al. Oral contraceptive use and risk of cutaneous malignant melanoma. *Cancer Causes Control* 1992; **3**: 547–54.
9. Holly EA. Cutaneous melanoma in women III: reproductive factors and oral contraceptive use. *Am J Epidemiol* 1995; **141**: 943–50.
10. Gefeller O, et al. Cutaneous malignant melanoma in women and the role of oral contraceptives. *Br J Dermatol* 1998; **138**: 122–4.

Ectopic pregnancy. Pregnancies in users of oral (but not parenteral) **progestogen-only contraceptives** are more likely to be ectopic than are pregnancies occurring in the general population. Oral progestogen-only contraceptives do not reliably inhibit ovulation and therefore offer less protection against ectopic pregnancy than against intra-uterine pregnancy. Early references to this effect are cited below.[1-5] Since parenteral progestogen-only contraceptives provide reliable suppression of ovulation, like combined oral contraceptives, they protect against both ectopic pregnancies and functional ovarian cysts. In the case of the levonorgestrel-releasing progestogen-only implant the risk of ectopic pregnancy is believed to be reduced overall, but the proportion of ectopic to intra-uterine pregnancies is increased among the very few pregnancies that do occur.

1. Bonnar J. Progestagen-only contraception and tubal pregnancies. *Lancet* 1974; **i**: 170–1.
2. Bonnar J. Progestagen-only contraception and tubal pregnancies. *BMJ* 1974; **1**: 287.
3. Huntington KM. Progestagen-only contraception and tubal pregnancies. *Lancet* 1974; **i**: 360.
4. Liukko P, Erkkola R. Low-dose progestogens and ectopic pregnancy. *BMJ* 1976; **2**: 1257.
5. Corcoran R, Howard R. Low-dose progestagens and ectopic pregnancy. *Lancet* 1977; **i**: 98–9.

Effects on carbohydrate metabolism. The potential effects of oral contraceptives on glucose tolerance are of particular concern because of the risk that impaired glucose tolerance will exacerbate their cardiovascular effects.[1] Early studies suggested that the prevalence of abnormal glucose tolerance in oral contraceptive users was increased from about 4 to 35% but subsequent studies produced conflicting results. Possible reasons for these discrepancies include failure to discriminate between differing doses of oestrogen and between the differing types and doses of progestogen used in the preparation. It has been shown that the decrease in glucose tolerance is related not only to oestrogen doses greater than 75 µg daily but also to the type of progestogen. As most oral contraceptives used currently contain lower doses of oestrogen the important question is whether such low-dose preparations have deleterious effects. Levonorgestrel has been reported to be the most potent progestogen in decreasing glucose tolerance[2] whereas preliminary results of another study has suggested that a combined oral contraceptive containing norethisterone does not result in a deterioration of glucose tolerance.[3] It was therefore considered[1] that preparations containing high doses of levonorgestrel should be prescribed for long-term use only after the most careful consideration, especially in patients with a past history of gestational diabetes or with impaired glucose tolerance.

However, a subsequent study has suggested that glucose tolerance testing may not be the best way of assessing the effects of oral contraceptives on carbohydrate metabolism.[4] In this study, in which insulin and C-peptide production was also measured, it was found that although levonorgestrel-containing combined preparations had a greater effect on glucose tolerance, desogestrel- or norethindrone-containing preparations produced a similar degree of insulin resistance, suggesting that this depends on the oestrogenic component, and is modified by the progestogen.

Despite these effects, data from the Nurses' Health Study indicate that oral contraceptives do not appear to increase the risk of developing type 2 diabetes mellitus.[5,6] However a study in the USA, in breast-feeding women of Hispanic origin who had experienced recent gestational diabetes, suggested that the use of progestogen-only, but not combined, contraceptives was associated with an increased risk of developing type 2 diabetes mellitus in this group.[7]

1. Taylor R. Drugs and glucose tolerance. *Adverse Drug React Bull* 1986; (Dec.): 452–5.
2. Perlman JA, *et al.* Oral glucose tolerance and the potency of contraceptive progestins. *J Chron Dis* 1985; **38:** 857–64.
3. Wynn V. Effect of duration of low-dose oral contraceptive administration on carbohydrate metabolism. *Am J Obstet Gynecol* 1982; **142:** 739–46.
4. Godsland IF, *et al.* Insulin resistance, secretion, and metabolism in users of oral contraceptives. *J Clin Endocrinol Metab* 1992; **74:** 64–70.
5. Rimm EB, *et al.* Oral contraceptive use and the risk of type 2 (non-insulin-dependent) diabetes mellitus in a large prospective study of women. *Diabetologia* 1992; **35:** 967–72.
6. Chasan-Taber L, *et al.* A prospective study of oral contraceptives and NIDDM among US women. *Diabetes Care* 1997; **20:** 330–5.
7. Kjos SL, *et al.* Contraception and the risk of type 2 diabetes mellitus in Latina women with prior gestational diabetes mellitus. *JAMA* 1998; **280:** 533–8.

Effects on the cardiovascular system. Soon after their introduction in the 1960s it became apparent that **combined oral contraceptives** were associated with an increased risk of cardiovascular effects including *hypertension, venous thromboembolism, myocardial infarction,* and *stroke*. Consequently, there are a number of contra-indications and precautions relating to their use in women with risk factors for cardiovascular disease (see under Precautions, below).

Changing patterns of use, and a progressive reduction in doses, have meant a continued need to evaluate the risks associated with oral contraceptives.

Current use of lower-dose combined oral contraceptives (less than 50 μg oestrogen) increases blood pressure in many women, and also results in a small but significant increased risk of venous thromboembolism. Any increased risk of myocardial infarction and stroke is low in women aged less than 35 years who do not smoke and who do not have pre-existing hypertension. Further details of these adverse effects are covered in the following sections.

The effect of progestogens on the cardiovascular risk profile of oral contraceptives has not been established. Some of the newer progestogens have been reported to have more favourable effects on plasma lipids (see Effects on Lipids, below) and there is some suggestion that they may have a lower risk of myocardial infarction, but there are insufficient data to confirm or refute this. Recently, however, it has been reported that desogestrel and gestodene are associated with 1.5 to 2 times the risk of venous thromboembolism than older progestogens.

The Nurses' Health Study found no association between ever having used oral contraceptives and death from cardiovascular disease.[1] The Royal College of General Practitioners' study reported an increase in death from cerebrovascular disease with current or recent (within 10 years) use of oral contraceptives, but not for past use (greater than 10 years).[2]

Some general reviews are cited below.[3-5]

1. Colditz GA, *et al.* Oral contraceptive use and mortality during 12 years of follow-up: the Nurses' Health Study. *Ann Intern Med* 1994; **120:** 821–6.
2. Beral V, *et al.* Mortality associated with oral contraceptive use: 25 year follow up of cohort of 46 000 women from Royal College of General Practitioners' oral contraception study. *BMJ* 1999; **318:** 96–100.
3. WHO. WHO Scientific Group Meeting on Cardiovascular Disease and Steroid Hormone Contraceptive: summary of conclusions. *Wkly Epidem Rec* 1997; **72:** 361–3.
4. Chasan-Taber L, Stampfer MJ. Epidemiology of oral contraceptives and cardiovascular disease. *Ann Intern Med* 1998; **128:** 467–77.
5. WHO. Cardiovascular disease and steroid hormone contraception. *WHO Tech Rep Ser 877* 1998.

HYPERTENSION. In a one-year prospective multicentre study[1] involving 704 women under the age of 35 using a combined oral contraceptive containing levonorgestrel 250 μg and ethinylestradiol 50 μg and 703 women using a non-hormonal intrauterine contraceptive device, those using the oral contraceptive developed higher systolic and diastolic blood pressures (systolic pressures were 3.6 to 5.0 mmHg higher, diastolic pressures were 1.9 to 2.7 mmHg higher). Only 4 women receiving oral contraceptives developed hypertension. A similar increase in blood pressure was noted in a study[2] involving 222 users of combined oral contraceptives containing 30 μg ethinylestradiol. There was a greater increase in blood pressure for those preparations containing 250 μg levonorgestrel than those containing 150 μg levonorgestrel.

More recently, data from the Nurses' Health Study[3] showed an increased risk (relative risk 1.8) for the development of hypertension in women taking lower-dose combined oral contraceptives. Increasing doses of progestogen were positively associated with hypertension, and the lowest risk occurred in women

receiving triphasic preparations, which have the lowest total dose of progestogen. A UK study[4] found a small increase in blood pressure of 2.3/1.6 mmHg associated with the use of combined oral contraceptives. In this study, progestogen-only oral contraceptives were not associated with an increase in blood pressure.

1. WHO Task Force on Oral Contraceptives. The WHO multicentre trial of the vasopressor effects of combined oral contraceptives 1: comparisons with IUD. *Contraception* 1989; **40:** 129–45.
2. Khaw K-T, Peart WS. Blood pressure and contraceptive use. *BMJ* 1982; **285:** 403–7.
3. Chasan-Taber L, *et al.* Prospective study of oral contraceptives and hypertension among women in the United States. *Circulation* 1996; **94:** 483–9.
4. Dong W, *et al.* Blood pressure in women using oral contraceptives: results from the Health Survey for England 1994. *J Hypertens* 1997; **15:** 1063–8.

MYOCARDIAL INFARCTION. Case-control studies from the 1970s and early 1980s revealed an increased risk of acute myocardial infarction in users of oral contraceptives (generally of the high-dose type) relative to those never having used them.[1,2] Several large cohort studies have provided similar findings.[3-6] Among current users the reported[1-3,5,6] relative risk of myocardial infarction has varied between about 1.8 and 6.4, whereas in women having used oral contraceptives in the past the reported[2-5] relative risk has varied between about 0.8 and 2.5. Women who smoke while using oral contraceptives are at a greatly increased risk,[1,5,7] those smoking more than 15 to 25 cigarettes per day having at least a twentyfold increased risk of myocardial infarction compared with non-smoking non-oral contraceptive users.[1,5]

More recently, data on combined oral contraceptives that have lower oestrogen doses have revealed at most small and non-significant increases in risk of acute myocardial infarction associated with oral contraceptive use,[8,9] although one case-control study has suggested that again, there may be a greatly increased risk in women who smoke more than 25 cigarettes per day.[10]

These studies have principally been from the USA or the UK. Most recently, the WHO Collaborative Study of Cardiovascular Disease and Steroid Hormone Contraception have reported the findings of an international multicentre case-control study.[11] The overall odds ratio for acute myocardial infarction in current users of combined oral contraceptives was 5.01 in Europe and 4.78 in Africa, Asia, and Latin America. This increase in risk reflected use in women who had coexistent risk factors such as smoking, and who had not had their blood pressure checked before use. Thus, when the background incidence of acute myocardial infarction is taken into account, use of combined oral contraceptives in non-smoking women aged less than 35 years is associated with an excess of 3 per million women-years, and this is likely to be lower in those women who have their blood pressure screened before and during use. However, in older women who smoke, the excess risk associated with the use of combined oral contraceptives is substantial (400 per million women-years). There was no increase in risk associated with past use of oral contraceptives irrespective of duration of use.

There has been interest in the effect of different progestogen components on the risk of myocardial infarction. Limited data from the WHO study[11] and from the USA[12] suggest no difference in risk between desogestrel or gestodene compared with levonorgestrel. Analysis of European data[13] suggests a reduction in risk with gestodene- and desogestrel-containing products compared with other progestogens (0.28; 95% confidence intervals 0.09 to 0.86). A WHO Scientific Group meeting concluded that available data did not allow the conclusion that risk of myocardial infarction is related to progestogen type.[14] Moreover, there is probably a small increased risk of venous thromboembolism associated with desogestrel or gestodene (see below).

1. Shapiro S, *et al.* Oral-contraceptive use in relation to myocardial infarction. *Lancet* 1979; **i:** 743–7.
2. Slone D, *et al.* Risk of myocardial infarction in relation to current and discontinued use of oral contraceptives. *N Engl J Med* 1981; **305:** 420–4.
3. Royal College of General Practitioners' Oral Contraception Study. Further analyses of mortality in oral contraceptive users. *Lancet* 1981; **i:** 541–6.
4. Stampfer MJ, *et al.* A prospective study of past use of oral contraceptive agents and risk of cardiovascular diseases. *N Engl J Med* 1988; **319:** 1313–17.
5. Croft P, Hannaford PC. Risk factors for acute myocardial infarction in women: evidence from the Royal College of General Practitioners' oral contraception study. *BMJ* 1989; **298:** 165–8.
6. Vessey MP, *et al.* Mortality among oral contraceptive users: 20 year follow up of women in a cohort study. *BMJ* 1989; **299:** 1487–91.
7. Goldbaum GM, *et al.* The relative impact of smoking and oral contraceptive use on women in the United States. *JAMA* 1987; **258:** 1339–42.
8. Thorogood M, *et al.* Is oral contraceptive use still associated with an increased risk of fatal myocardial infarction? Report of a case-control study. *Br J Obstet Gynaecol* 1991; **98:** 1245–53.
9. Sidney S, *et al.* Myocardial infarction and use of low-dose oral contraceptives: a pooled analysis of 2 US studies. *Circulation* 1998; **98:** 1058–63.
10. Rosenberg L, *et al.* Low-dose oral contraceptive use and the risk of myocardial infarction. *Arch Intern Med* 2001; **161:** 1065–70.
11. WHO Collaborative Study of Cardiovascular Disease and Steroid Hormone Contraception. Acute myocardial infarction and combined oral contraceptives: results of an international multicentre case-control study. *Lancet* 1997; **349:** 1202–9.
12. Jick H, *et al.* Risk of acute myocardial infarction and low-dose combined oral contraceptives. *Lancet* 1996; **347:** 627–8.

13. Lewis MA, *et al.* The use of oral contraceptives and the occurrence of acute myocardial infarction in young women: results from the transnational study on oral contraceptives and the health of young women. *Contraception* 1997; **56:** 129–40.
14. WHO. WHO Scientific Group Meeting on Cardiovascular Disease and Steroid Hormone Contraceptives: summary of conclusions. *Wkly Epidem Rec* 1997; **72:** 361–3.

STROKE. Current use of **combined oral contraceptives** has been associated with an increased risk of stroke, with most data relating to older high-dose oestrogen preparations. In general this association has been strongest for ischaemic stroke, and relatively weak for haemorrhagic stroke.[1] A Danish study found that low-dose oral contraceptives (30 to 40 μg of oestrogen) were associated with a lower risk of cerebral thromboembolism than preparations containing 50 μg oestrogen.[2]

Data on 2198 cases of stroke (haemorrhagic, ischaemic, and unclassified) and 6086 controls have been reported from the WHO Collaborative Study of Cardiovascular Disease and Steroid Hormone Contraception.[3,4] For all strokes combined, odds ratios for the current use of lower-dose (less than 50 μg oestrogen) and higher dose preparations were 1.41 (95% confidence intervals 0.90 to 2.20) and 2.71 (1.70 to 4.32), respectively, in Europe, and 1.86 (1.49 to 2.33) and 1.92 (1.48 to 2.50), respectively, in Africa, Asia, and Latin America. In Europe, it was estimated that the incidence rate of stroke in women aged 20 to 44 years was 4.8 per 100 000 women-years, and that this was increased to 6.7 per 100 000 in users of lower-dose preparations and 12.9 per 100 000 in users of higher-dose preparations.[3]

The risk of haemorrhagic stroke was significant only in women aged greater than 35 years, those who had a history of hypertension, and those who were current smokers.[3]

The overall odds ratio for ischaemic stroke was 2.99 (1.65 to 5.40) in Europe and 2.93 (2.15 to 4.00) in Africa, Asia, and Latin America.[4] Odds ratios were lower in women aged less than 35 years, those who did not smoke, those with no history of hypertension, and those who reported that their blood pressure had been checked before use. Duration of current use and past use were unrelated to risk.[4] Similar findings to those of the WHO study have also been published from the USA.[5] Low-dose preparations (less than 50 μg oestrogen) were associated with a nonsignificant increase in ischaemic stroke; the odds ratio was 1.18 (0.54 to 2.59).

As regards the effect of the type of progestogen on risk of stroke, one case-control study[6] reported that there was no significant difference in risk of ischaemic stroke between low-dose oral contraceptives containing second generation progestogens and those containing desogestrel, gestodene, or norgestimate. However, another study found that levonorgestrel- or norgestimate-containing preparations were associated with a higher risk of cerebral thrombosis than preparations containing desogestrel or gestodene.[7] A reanalysis of the WHO data led to the cautious conclusion that the risk for stroke between second and third generation progestogens was similar,[8] and this was also supported by analysis of the General Practice Research Database.[9]

Data for **progestogen-only contraceptives** are limited. The Danish study reported no increase in cerebral thromboembolic attacks in users of oral progestogen-only contraceptives; the odds ratio was 0.9 (0.4 to 2.4).[2]

1. Vessey MP, *et al.* Oral contraceptives and stroke: findings in a large prospective study. *BMJ* 1984; **289:** 530–1.
2. Lidegaard Ø. Oral contraception and risk of a cerebral thromboembolic attack: results of a case-control study. *BMJ* 1993; **306:** 956–63.
3. WHO Collaborative Study of Cardiovascular Disease and Steroid Hormone Contraception. Haemorrhagic stroke, overall stroke risk, and combined oral contraceptives: results of an international, multicentre, case-control study. *Lancet* 1996; **348:** 505–10.
4. WHO Collaborative Study of Cardiovascular Disease and Steroid Hormone Contraception. Ischaemic stroke and combined oral contraceptives: results of an international, multicentre, case-control study. *Lancet* 1996; **348:** 498–505.
5. Petitti DB, *et al.* Stroke in users of low-dose oral contraceptives. *N Engl J Med* 1996; **335:** 8–15.
6. Heinemann LAJ, *et al.* Case-control study of oral contraceptives and risk of thromboembolic stroke: results from international study on oral contraceptives and health of young women. *BMJ* 1997; **315:** 1502–4.
7. Lidegaard Ø, Kreiner S. Cerebral thrombosis and oral contraceptives: a case-control study. *Contraception* 1998; **57:** 303–14.
8. Poulter NR, *et al.* Effect on stroke of different progestagens in low oestrogen dose oral contraceptives. *Lancet* 1999; **354:** 301–2.
9. Jick SS, *et al.* Risk of idiopathic cerebral haemorrhage in women on oral contraceptives with differing progestagen components. *Lancet* 1999; **354:** 302–3.

VENOUS THROMBOEMBOLISM. Use of **combined oral contraceptives** has long been known to be associated with an increased risk of venous thromboembolic events, particularly deep-vein thrombosis and pulmonary embolism. This increased risk applies both to idiopathic events and events associated with surgery or trauma, is limited to current users and is probably highest in the first year of use. Most early data relate to high-dose combined preparations, and it has been suggested by some studies,[1] but not others,[2,3] that preparations containing lower doses of oestrogen may be associated with a decreased risk. More recently, reports have identified an increased risk of cerebral-vein thrombosis with oral contraceptives.[4,5]

The WHO Collaborative Study of Cardiovascular Disease and Steroid Hormone Contraception reported data from over 10 times more cases than any previous study.[6] The increased risk of idiopathic deep-vein thrombosis and/or pulmonary embolism associated with current use of combined oral contraceptives was 4.15 (95% confidence intervals 3.09 to 5.57) in Europe and 3.25 (2.59 to 4.08) in Africa, Asia, and Latin America. The increased risk was apparent within 4 months of starting use, was unaffected by duration of use, and had disappeared within 3 months of stopping use. Risk was unaffected by age, hypertension, or smoking (in contrast to myocardial infarction, see above), but was increased in those with a body mass index greater than 25 kg per m^2 and in those with a history of hypertension of pregnancy. Of preparations containing progestogens of the norethisterone or norgestrel type, risk was nonsignificantly less with lower-dose oestrogen than with high-dose oestrogen.

The progestogen component has generally been considered to be unrelated to thromboembolic events; therefore, it came as a surprise when WHO found a higher risk in combined oral contraceptives containing *desogestrel* or *gestodene* than in those containing older progestogens.[6] These risk data were the subject of a separate report,[7] and were subsequently confirmed by 3 further case-control studies.[8-10] The increased risk varied from 4.8 to 9.1 compared with non-users, and was found to be 1.5 to 2.6 times higher than for preparations containing levonorgestrel or other progestogens. The incidence of venous thromboembolic disease has been estimated to be 25 per 100 000 users per year for desogestrel- and gestodene-containing products and 15 per 100 000 users per year for products containing low-dose oestrogen with other progestogens, compared with 5 per 100 000 per year for non-users. The risk was especially high in women with the factor V Leiden mutation,[9] who are at increased risk of thrombosis, but screening to exclude these women from using oral contraceptives was not considered necessary.[11,12] Despite much debate about possible bias and confounding in these results,[13,14] and the ambiguous or contradictory results of subsequent studies,[15-17] many sources seem now to agree with the 1997 conclusion of a WHO scientific group meeting[18] that there is a modestly increased risk of venous thromboembolism associated with the use of products containing desogestrel or gestodene, compared with levonorgestrel.

Regulatory agencies have reacted in different ways to these data. The UK Committee on Safety of Medicines has advised caution in prescribing of these products (see Cardiovascular Disease under Precautions, below), as have some other European authorities.

The mechanism behind differences in thrombotic potential is not known, but there is evidence that oral contraceptives may increase concentrations of prothrombin and factor VIII, and induce a resistance to the blood's natural anticoagulation system.[12] These effects may be greater with products containing desogestrel and gestodene compared with older progestogens.[12,19]

1. Vessey M, et al. Oral contraceptives and venous thromboembolism: findings in a large prospective study. BMJ 1986; 292: 526.
2. Kierkegaard A. Deep vein thrombosis and the oestrogen content in oral contraceptives—an epidemiological analysis. Contraception 1985; 31: 29–41.
3. Helmrich SP, et al. Venous thromboembolism in relation to oral contraceptive use. Obstet Gynecol 1987; 69: 91–5.
4. de Bruijn SFTM, et al. Case-control study of risk of cerebral sinus thrombosis in oral contraceptive users and in carriers of hereditary prothrombotic conditions. BMJ 1998; 316: 589–92. Correction. ibid.: 822.
5. Martinelli I, et al. High risk of cerebral-vein thrombosis in carriers of a prothrombin-gene mutation and in users of oral contraceptives. N Engl J Med 1998; 338: 1793–7.
6. WHO Collaborative Study Group. Venous thromboembolic disease and combined oral contraceptives: results of international multicentre case-control study. Lancet 1995; 346: 1575–82.
7. WHO Collaborative Study Group. Effect of different progestagens in low oestrogen oral contraceptives on venous thromboembolic disease. Lancet 1995; 346: 1582–8.
8. Jick H, et al. Risk of idiopathic cardiovascular death and nonfatal venous thromboembolism in women using oral contraceptives with differing progestagen components. Lancet 1995; 346: 1589–93.
9. Bloemenkamp KWM, et al. Enhancement by factor V Leiden mutation of risk of deep-vein thrombosis associated with oral contraceptives containing a third-generation progestagen. Lancet 1995; 346: 1593–6.
10. Spitzer WO, et al. Third generation oral contraceptives and risk of venous thromboembolic disorders: an international case-control study. BMJ 1996; 312: 83–8.
11. Vandenbroucke JP, et al. Factor V Leiden: should we screen oral contraceptive users and pregnant women? BMJ 1996; 313: 1127–30.
12. Vandenbroucke JP, et al. Oral contraceptives and the risk of venous thromboembolism. N Engl J Med 2001; 344: 1527–35.
13. Lewis MA, et al. The increased risk of venous thromboembolism and the use of third generation progestagens: role of bias in observational research. Contraception 1996; 54: 5–13.
14. Farley TMM, et al. Oral contraceptives and thrombotic diseases: impact of new epidemiological studies. Contraception 1996; 54: 193–5.
15. Farmer RDT, et al. Population-based study of risk of venous thromboembolism associated with various oral contraceptives. Lancet 1997; 349: 83–8.
16. Farmer RDT, et al. Effect of 1995 pill scare on rates of venous thromboembolism among women taking combined oral contraceptives: analysis of General Practice Research Database. BMJ 2000; 321: 477–9.
17. Jick H, et al. Risk of venous thromboembolism among users of third generation oral contraceptives compared with users of oral contraceptives with levonorgestrel before and after 1995: cohort and case-control analysis. BMJ 2000; 321: 1190–5. Correction. ibid. 2001; 322: 28.
18. WHO. WHO Scientific Group Meeting on Cardiovascular Disease and Steroid Hormone Contraceptives: summary of conclusions. Wkly Epidem Rec 1997; 72: 361–3.
19. Rosing J, et al. Oral contraceptives and venous thrombosis: different sensitivities to activated protein C in women using second- and third-generation oral contraceptives. Br J Haematol 1997; 97: 233–8.

Effects on the ears. In the Royal College of General Practitioners' study of oral contraception in the UK,[1] by 1981 there had been 13 cases of newly occurring otosclerosis in each of the groups of oral contraceptive users (101 985 woman-years) and controls (146 534 woman-years); this showed a non-significant relative risk of 1.29. Although, by analogy with pregnancy, it may be prudent to suppose that oral contraceptives could exacerbate pre-existing otosclerosis, the data do not support the view that the condition is associated with their use.

1. Kay CR, Wingrave SJ. Oral contraceptives and otosclerosis. BMJ 1984; 288: 1164.

Effects on the eyes. Analysis of data from 2 large UK cohort studies suggested that oral contraceptive use does not increase the risk of eye disease, with the possible exception of retinal vascular lesions.[1]

1. Vessey MP, et al. Oral contraception and eye disease: findings in two large cohort studies. Br J Ophthalmol 1998; 82: 538–42.

Effects on fertility. Following the discontinuation of hormonal contraceptives some patients may experience amenorrhoea, anovulation, and infertility. This infertility, however, has been shown by most studies to be only temporary.

Data from the Oxford Family Planning Association study[1] have indicated that impairment of fertility after oral contraceptives was only very slight and short-lived in women who had previously had a baby. In nulliparous women aged 25 to 29 years impairment of fertility was more severe but the effect had almost entirely disappeared after 48 months. In the older, aged 30 to 34 years, nulliparous women there was even more impairment of fertility but this was not permanent as by 72 months after stopping oral contraceptive use the numbers of women who had not conceived were similar to a group who had previously used non-hormonal methods of contraception.

After injectable progestogen-only contraceptives, smaller studies have again indicated that there are no long-lasting effects on fertility;[2] but it has also been suggested that a return to ovulation occurs significantly earlier in prior norethisterone enantate users than in medroxyprogesterone users.[3]

Infertility may also be related to the presence of pelvic inflammatory disease; for further details concerning the role of oral contraceptives in this disorder, see Pelvic Inflammatory Disease, below.

1. Anonymous. "Pill" use appears to impair fertility in a certain group of women. Pharm J 1986; 236: 227.
2. Fotherby K, et al. Return of ovulation and fertility in women using norethisterone enanthate. Contraception 1984; 29: 447–55.
3. Garza-Flores J, et al. Return to ovulation following the use of long-acting injectable contraceptives: a comparative study. Contraception 1985; 31: 361–6.

Effects on the gallbladder. Data from the Royal College of General Practitioners' (RCGP) oral contraception study accumulated up to December 1979 revealed no overall increased risk of gallbladder disease in the long-term, despite the indications of earlier data and other studies relating to short-term use.[1] Further studies[2,3] have identified an increased risk of gallbladder disease in oral contraceptive users under the age of 30 or 20 respectively.[2] The latest data from the RCGP study show an increase in risk of mild hepatitis during the first 4 years of oral contraceptive use, possibly reflecting gallstone-associated cholestasis.[4] This risk then decreased to less than that seen in women who had never used oral contraceptives.

1. Wingrave SJ, Kay CR. Oral contraceptives and gallbladder disease: Royal College of General Practitioners' oral contraception study. Lancet 1982; ii: 957–9.
2. Scragg RKR, et al. Oral contraceptives, pregnancy, and endogenous oestrogen in gall stone disease—a case-control study. BMJ 1984; 288: 1795–9.
3. Strom BL, et al. Oral contraceptives and other risk factors for gallbladder disease. Clin Pharmacol Ther 1986; 39: 335–41.
4. Hannaford PC, et al. Combined oral contraceptives and liver disease. Contraception 1997; 55: 145–51.

Effects on the gastrointestinal tract. Several case-control and cohort studies,[1-5] and a meta-analysis,[6] have shown a weak association between oral contraceptive use and Crohn's disease or ulcerative colitis. However, the suggestion that oral contraceptives have an aetiological role in chronic inflammatory bowel disease cannot be regarded as established.

1. Rhodes JM, et al. Colonic Crohn's disease and use of oral contraception. BMJ 1984; 288: 595–6.
2. Vessey M, et al. Chronic inflammatory bowel disease, cigarette smoking, and use of oral contraceptives: findings in a large cohort study of women of childbearing age. BMJ 1986; 292: 1101–3.
3. Entrican JH, Sircus W. Chronic inflammatory bowel disease, cigarette smoking, and use of oral contraceptives. BMJ 1986; 292: 1464.
4. Logan RFA, Kay CR. Oral contraception, smoking and inflammatory bowel disease—findings in the Royal College of General Practitioners Oral Contraception Study. Int J Epidemiol 1989; 18: 105–7.
5. Timmer A, et al. Oral contraceptive use and smoking are risk factors for relapse in Crohn's disease. Gastroenterology 1998; 114: 1143–50.
6. Godet PG, et al. Meta-analysis of the role of oral contraceptive agents in inflammatory bowel disease. Gut 1995; 37: 668–73.

Effects on lipids. Combined oral contraceptives have been reported to be associated with an excess risk of various adverse cardiovascular events (see above). Because other epidemiological evidence suggests that the composition of blood lipids may be one of several factors involved in the aetiology of some of these disorders, many workers have investigated the biochemical profiles of women taking various formulations of oral contraceptives. Results have often been conflicting as the net effect is the result of opposing actions of the oestrogen and the progestogen components, and depends on the ratio between these. In general, the oestrogen component increases triglycerides, but decreases low-density lipoproteins, whereas the progestogen component tends to decrease high-density lipoproteins and increase low-density lipoproteins, particularly if it is androgenic (19-nortestosterone-derived progestogens). Newer non-androgenic progestogens such as desogestrel and gestodene appear to have a less detrimental effect on serum lipids. However, the contribution of these lipid changes to the incidence of cardiovascular disease in oral contraceptive users is uncertain. In particular, contrary to expectations, desogestrel and gestodene appear to be associated with a higher risk of venous thromboembolism than older progestogens (see above).

Some references to the effects of various oral contraceptives on serum lipid profiles are given below.[1-10]

For further details concerning the proposed role of the various serum lipids and subfractions in the aetiology of cardiovascular disease, see Cardiovascular Risk Reduction, p.797.

1. Smith RP, Sizto R. Metabolic effects of two triphasic formulations containing ethinyl estradiol and dl-norgestrel. Contraception 1983; 28: 189–99.
2. Wahl P, et al. Effect of estrogen/progestin potency on lipid/lipoprotein cholesterol. N Engl J Med 1983; 308: 862–7.
3. Deslypere JP, et al. Effect of long term hormonal contraception on plasma lipids. Contraception 1985; 31: 633–42.
4. WHO Task Force on Oral Contraceptives. A randomized double-blind study of the effects of two low-dose combined oral contraceptives on biochemical aspects: report from a seven-centred study. Contraception 1985; 32: 223–6.
5. Luoma PV, et al. One year study of effects of an oestrogen-dominant oral contraceptive on serum high-density lipoprotein cholesterol, apolipoproteins A-I and A-II and hepatic microsomal function. Eur J Clin Pharmacol 1987; 31: 563–8.
6. Bertolini S, et al. Effects of three low-dose oral contraceptive formulations on lipid metabolism. Acta Obstet Gynecol Scand 1987; 66: 327–32.
7. Burkman RT, et al. Lipid and lipoprotein changes associated with oral contraceptive use: a randomized clinical trial. Obstet Gynecol 1988; 71: 33–8.
8. Notelovitz M, et al. Lipid and lipoprotein changes in women taking low-dose, triphasic oral contraceptives: a controlled, comparative, 12-month clinical trial. Am J Obstet Gynecol 1989; 160: 1269–80.
9. Patsch W, et al. The effect of triphasic oral contraceptives on plasma lipids and lipoproteins. Am J Obstet Gynecol 1989; 161: 1396–1401.
10. Crook D, Godsland I. Safety evaluation of modern oral contraceptives: effects on lipoprotein and carbohydrate metabolism. Contraception 1998; 57: 189–201. Correction. ibid.: 420.

Effects on mental state. A review of drug-induced mental depression concluded that since mood disturbance is common during the menstrual cycle and particularly in the premenstrual phase it is difficult to evaluate the possible association of depression with oral contraceptives.[1] The evidence, however, suggests that the incidence is a little greater than with control subjects but it is still only 4 to 6%. A later review[2] came to a similar conclusion that in a number of surveys in which oral contraceptives have been compared with either placebo or an intra-uterine device no increase in depression or other nervous symptoms has been found.

1. Tyrer PJ. Drug-induced depression. Prescribers' J 1981; 21: 237–42.
2. King DJ. Drug-induced psychiatric syndromes. Prescribers' J 1986; 26: 50–8.

Effects on the musculoskeletal system. BONE DENSITY. Combined oral contraceptives do not have a detrimental effect on bone mineral density, and may exert a positive effect although data are scanty.[1] Postmenopausal women who had previously used combined oral contraceptives appeared to have improved bone mineral density compared with those who had not in a cross-sectional study.[2] In a case-control study, oral contraceptive use late in reproductive life appeared to reduce the risk of hip fracture.[3]

In contrast, users of the progestogen-only contraceptive medroxyprogesterone acetate may have reductions in bone mineral density, although these appear to be reversible on discontinuation of the drug.[4] A small study has prospectively analysed the effect of combined oral contraceptives and parenteral progestogen-only contraceptives on bone mass in adolescents.[5] After 1 year of use, bone mineral density decreased by 1.5% in users of depot medroxyprogesterone acetate, but increased in users of combined oral contraceptives or levonorgestrel implants, and in control subjects. A later study in women who had used depot medroxyprogesterone acetate for between 1 and 16 years found that, although there was a slight reduction in bone density compared with age-specific population means, this was not sufficient to be of clinical importance.[6]

1. Cromer BA. Effects of hormonal contraceptives on bone mineral density. Drug Safety 1999; 20: 213–22.
2. Kritz-Silverstein D, Barrett-Connor E. Bone mineral density in postmenopausal women as determined by prior oral contraceptive use. Am J Public Health 1993; 83: 100–2.
3. Michaëlsson K, et al. Oral-contraceptive use and risk of hip fracture: a case-control study. Lancet 1999; 353: 1481–4.

4. Cundy T, *et al.* Recovering of bone density in women who stop using medroxyprogesterone acetate. *BMJ* 1994; **308:** 247–8.
5. Cromer BA, *et al.* A prospective comparison of bone density in adolescent girls receiving depot medroxyprogesterone acetate (Depo-Provera), levonorgestrel (Norplant), or oral contraceptives. *J Pediatr* 1996; **129:** 671–6.
6. Gbolade B, *et al.* Bone density in long term users of depot medroxyprogesterone acetate. *Br J Obstet Gynaecol* 1998; **105:** 790–4.

RHEUMATOID ARTHRITIS. While reviews[1] have commented on the rare reports of arthritis or arthropathies attributed to oral contraceptives some large studies have investigated the incidence of rheumatoid arthritis in oral contraceptive users. A negative association between the use of oral contraceptives and the development of rheumatoid arthritis has been reported in four studies[2-5] thus giving rise to the suggestion that oral contraceptive use may, in fact, have some sort of protective role. These findings were not, however, substantiated by other workers[6-8] who found no association, either beneficial or detrimental, between the use of oral contraceptives and the later development of rheumatoid arthritis. A meta-analysis found no conclusive evidence of a protective effect of oral contraceptives on rheumatoid arthritis risk.[9]

1. Hart FD. Drug-induced arthritis and arthralgia. *Drugs* 1984; **28:** 347–54.
2. Wingrave SJ, Kay CR. Reduction in incidence of rheumatoid arthritis associated with oral contraceptives: Royal College of General Practitioners' oral contraception study. *Lancet* 1978; **i:** 569–71.
3. Vandenbroucke JP, *et al.* Oral contraceptives and rheumatoid arthritis: further evidence for a preventive effect. *Lancet* 1982; **ii:** 839–42.
4. Hazes JMW, *et al.* Reduction of the risk of rheumatoid arthritis among women who take oral contraceptives. *Arthritis Rheum* 1990; **33:** 173–9.
5. Spector TD, *et al.* The pill, parity, and rheumatoid arthritis. *Arthritis Rheum* 1990; **33:** 782–9.
6. Linos A, *et al.* Case-control study of rheumatoid arthritis and prior use of oral contraceptives. *Lancet* 1983; **i:** 1299–1300.
7. del Junco DJ, *et al.* Do oral contraceptives prevent rheumatoid arthritis? *JAMA* 1985; **254:** 1938–41.
8. Hannaford PC, *et al.* Oral contraceptives and rheumatoid arthritis: new data from the Royal College of General Practitioners' oral contraception study. *Ann Rheum Dis* 1990; **49:** 744–6.
9. Pladevall-Vila M, *et al.* Controversy of oral contraceptives and risk of rheumatoid arthritis: meta-analysis of conflicting studies and review of conflicting meta-analyses with special emphasis on analysis of heterogeneity. *Am J Epidemiol* 1996; **144:** 1–14.

Effects on the nervous system. Chorea has been reported following use of 2 oral contraceptives;[1,2] the choreic movements stopped within 2 to 8 weeks of discontinuing therapy.

1. Lane RJM, Routledge PA. Drug-induced neurological disorders. *Drugs* 1983; **26:** 124–47.
2. Wadlington WB, *et al.* Chorea associated with the use of oral contraceptives: report of a case and review of the literature. *Clin Pediatr (Phila)* 1981; **20:** 804–6.

Effects on the pancreas. Reports of pancreatitis secondary to hyperlipidaemia associated with the use of combined oral contraceptives.[1,2]

1. Parker WA. Estrogen-induced pancreatitis. *Clin Pharm* 1983; **2:** 75–9.
2. Stuyt PMJ, *et al.* Pancreatitis induced by oestrogen in a patient with type I hyperlipoproteinaemia. *BMJ* 1986; **293:** 734.

Effects on the skin. Oral contraceptives may cause chloasma, and those containing androgenic progestogens may cause or aggravate acne and hirsutism. More rarely, oral contraceptives have been implicated in photosensitivity associated with drug-induced lupus erythematosus.[1] A survey of people using UV-A sunbeds at commercial premises in the UK revealed that the prevalence of pruritus, nausea, and skin rashes as side-effects of the sunbeds was higher in women taking oral contraceptives than in women receiving no medication.[2] There has been a report of hidradenitis suppurativa, a condition resulting in the recurrence of boils at the axillary apocrine sweat glands, anogenital region, and breasts, occurring in 7 women using oral contraceptives.[3]

For mention of the refuted association between oral contraceptives and malignant melanoma, see Skin under Carcinogenicity above.

1. Smith AG. Drug-induced photosensitivity. *Adverse Drug React Bull* 1989; (Jun.): 508–11.
2. Diffey BL. Use of UV-A sunbeds for cosmetic tanning. *Br J Dermatol* 1989; **115:** 67–76.
3. Stellon AJ, Wakeling M. Hidradenitis suppurativa associated with use of oral contraceptives. *BMJ* 1989; **298:** 28–9.

Effects on the uterus. The Oxford Family Planning Association study found that the risk of developing uterine leiomyomas (uterine fibroids) was reduced by the use of oral contraceptives.[1] The observed reduction in risk was approximately 17% with each five years of oral contraceptive use, and was not thought to be due to selective prescribing.[2,3] The authors hypothesised that unopposed oestrogen may be a risk factor for uterine fibroids, and that the reduced risk with oral contraceptives might be analogous to the reduction in endometrial carcinoma seen with these drugs (see above).[1] However, another case-control study involving 390 women with leiomyomas failed to find a protective (or detrimental) effect with oral contraceptive use.[4]

1. Ross RK, *et al.* Risk factors for uterine fibroids: reduced risk associated with oral contraceptives. *BMJ* 1986; **293:** 359–62.
2. Ratner H. Risk factors for uterine fibroids: reduced risk associated with oral contraceptives. *BMJ* 1986; **293:** 1027.
3. Ross RK, *et al.* Risk factors for uterine fibroids: reduced risk associated with oral contraceptives. *BMJ* 1986; **293:** 1027.
4. Parazzini F, *et al.* Oral contraceptive use and risk of uterine fibroids. *Obstet Gynecol* 1992; **79:** 430–3.

Pelvic inflammatory disease. Although it is generally held that oral contraceptives protect against pelvic inflammatory disease, there was some debate during the 1980s about whether this was always the case, especially in view of an apparent association between oral contraceptive use and increased infection with *Chlamydia trachomatis*, the leading cause of non-gonococcal pelvic inflammatory disease.[1-3] Some have also suggested a link between use of oral contraceptives and gonococcal infection.[4] Interestingly, these authors found that rates of gonococcal infection appeared higher for preparations containing more androgenic progestogens. A case-control study involving 141 women with pelvic inflammatory disease and 739 controls suggested that oral contraceptive use protected against symptomatic pelvic inflammatory disease in women already infected with *C. trachomatis*, but not in those infected with *N. gonorrhoeae*.[5] There is also evidence that users of older oral contraceptives containing more than 50 μg of oestrogen may have been at increased risk of tubal infertility, particularly if first used before 20 years of age.[6] No increased risk, or an active decrease in risk (depending on age at first use) was reported for formulations containing 50 μg or less of oestrogen, which are now favoured.

1. Washington AE, *et al.* Oral contraceptives, Chlamydia trachomatis infection, and pelvic inflammatory disease: a word of caution about protection. *JAMA* 1985; **253:** 2246–50.
2. Gall SA. Oral contraceptives and Chlamydia infections. *JAMA* 1986; **255:** 38.
3. Washington AE, *et al.* Oral contraceptives and Chlamydia infections. *JAMA* 1986; **255:** 38–9.
4. Louv WC, *et al.* Oral contraceptive use and the risk of chlamydial and gonococcal infections. *Am J Obstet Gynecol* 1989; **160:** 396–402.
5. Wølner-Hanssen P, *et al.* Decreased risk of symptomatic chlamydial pelvic inflammatory disease associated with oral contraceptive use. *JAMA* 1990; **263:** 54–9.
6. Cramer DW, *et al.* The relationship of tubal infertility to barrier method and oral contraceptive use. *JAMA* 1987; **257:** 2446–50.

Precautions

Before hormonal contraceptives are given the woman should undergo an appropriate medical examination and her medical history should be carefully evaluated. Regular examination is recommended during use. The contraceptive effectiveness of combined and progestogen-only preparations may be reduced during episodes of vomiting or diarrhoea and extra contraceptive measures may be necessary during and for 7 days after recovery. For precautions to be observed if a 'pill' is missed, see under Uses and Administration, below.

Combined oral contraceptives are *contra-indicated* in women with markedly impaired liver function or cholestasis, the Dubin-Johnson or Rotor syndromes, hepatic adenoma, oestrogen-dependent neoplasms such as breast or endometrial cancer, cardiovascular disease (see also below) including previous or current thromboembolic disorders, or high risk of them, and arterial disease or multiple risk factors for it, disorders of lipid metabolism, undiagnosed vaginal bleeding, possible pregnancy, or a history during pregnancy of pruritus or cholestatic jaundice, chorea, herpes, pemphigoid gestationis, or deteriorating otosclerosis. They are also contra-indicated in severe or focal migraine (or where there are other risk factors for cardiovascular disease) and should be used with caution in other forms of migraine (for further details, see below). They should be *given with caution* to women with a history of clinical depression, gallbladder disease, sickle-cell disease, or conditions influenced by fluid retention. They should also be used with caution in those with varicose veins (and should be avoided where the restrictions outlined under Venous Thromboembolism apply, see Cardiovascular Disease, below). Where not actually contra-indicated, they should also be used with caution in those with a risk factor for cardiovascular disease such as diabetes mellitus, smoking, obesity, hypertension, or a family history of cardiovascular disorders (see also below). Current opinion is that low-dose combined oral contraceptives may be used in women over the age of 35 years provided they do not smoke and have no other risk factors for cardiovascular disease, but that they should be avoided over the age of 50 years. Use by those undergoing surgery or prolonged bed rest may increase the risk of thromboembolic episodes and it is generally recommended that combined oral contraceptives should be discontinued 4 to 6 weeks before major elective surgery (see also below). Combined oral contraceptives should not be used after recent evacuation of a hydatidiform mole until urine and plasma gonadotrophin concentrations have returned to normal. They should be avoided in nursing mothers as lactation may be reduced (see also below). Contact lenses may irritate. The use of combined oral contraceptives may influence the results of certain laboratory tests including liver, thyroid, adrenal, and renal function tests, plasma concentrations of binding proteins and lipid/lipoprotein fractions, and fibrinolysis and coagulation parameters.

Combined oral contraceptives should be stopped immediately, and appropriate investigations and treatment carried out, if any of the following occur:

- sudden severe chest pain, sudden breathlessness, or severe pain/swelling in calf of one leg (possibly indicative of thromboembolic complications)

- unusual, severe, prolonged headache, sudden disturbances of vision or hearing or other perceptual disorders, collapse, marked numbness or weakness affecting one side of the body, or other signs or symptoms suggestive of cerebrovascular accident

- hepatitis, jaundice, generalised itching, liver enlargement, severe upper abdominal pain

- onset of severe depression

- significant rise in blood pressure (above 160 mmHg systolic or 100 mmHg diastolic)

- clear exacerbation of other conditions known to be capable of deteriorating during oral contraception or pregnancy.

Progestogen-only contraceptives, whether oral or injectable, may be used when oestrogen-containing preparations are contra-indicated but certain contra-indications and precautions must still be observed. They are contra-indicated in women with undiagnosed vaginal bleeding, possible pregnancy, severe arterial disease, hormone-dependent neoplasms, and severe liver disease such as hepatic adenoma.

Like combined oral contraceptives they should not be used after recent evacuation of a hydatidiform mole. Progestogen-only contraceptives should be used with care in women with heart disease, malabsorption syndromes, liver dysfunction including recurrent cholestatic jaundice, or a history of jaundice in pregnancy. Oral progestogen-only contraceptives should also be used with care in past ectopic pregnancy (see above) or functional ovarian cysts. Despite unsatisfactory evidence of hazard, other suggested cautions for progestogen-only contraceptives include diabetes mellitus, hypertension, migraine, and thromboembolic disorders.

Cardiovascular disease. Combined oral contraceptives are associated with a number of arterial and venous risks. Progestogen-only contraceptives are associated with fewer risks, although they will need to be avoided when arterial disease is severe.

ARTERIAL DISEASE. In the UK the *British National Formulary* has recommended that combined oral contraceptives may be used with **caution** if any **one** of the following factors are present, but should be **avoided** if **two or more** factors are present: *family history of arterial disease* in first-degree relative aged under 45 years (avoid if there is also an atherogenic lipid profile); *diabetes mellitus* (avoid if diabetic complications are present); *hypertension* (avoid if blood pressure is above 160/100 mmHg); *smoking* (avoid if 40 or more cigarettes are smoked daily); *age over 35 years* (avoid if over 50 years); *obesity* (avoid if body-mass index exceeds 39 kg per m²); *migraine,* see under Migraine, below.

VENOUS THROMBOEMBOLISM. Combined oral contraceptives increase the risk of venous thromboembolism and should not be used in women with a personal history of venous or arterial thrombosis. In addition they should be used with caution if any of the following risk factors are present: *family history of venous thromboembolism* in a first-degree relative aged under 45 years (avoid if there is a known thrombotic coagulation abnormality such as antiphospholipid antibodies, which may occur in patients with systemic lupus erythematosus, or factor V Leiden); *long-term immobilisation* such as wheelchair use (avoid if confined to bed or with a leg in plaster); *varicose veins* (avoid during sclerosing treatment); and (as for arterial disease) *obesity* (avoid if body-mass index greater than 39 kg per m²).

In the light of evidence indicating an increased risk of venous thromboembolism with combined oral contraceptives containing *desogestrel* or *gestodene* (see Venous Thromboembolism, under Effects on the Cardiovascular System, above), the UK Committee on Safety of Medicines (CSM) advised additional precautions for these products. As well as the usual precautions, it was initially advised they should not be used by obese women (body-mass index greater than 30 kg per m²), those with varicose veins, or those with a history of thrombosis of any cause. Moreover, it was also recommended that they should be used only by women who were intolerant of other combined oral contraceptives and who were prepared to accept an increased risk of venous thromboembolism. Subsequently the CSM[1] has modified its advice as follows: they recommend that these products should be avoided in women with known risk factors for venous thromboembolism. However, in women without contra-indications, the type of combined contraceptive is considered a matter of clinical judgement and personal choice, as long as the woman is fully informed of the small excess risk associated with desogestrel- and gestodene-containing products.

1. Committee on Safety of Medicines/Medicines Control Agency. Combined oral contraceptives containing desogestrel or gestodene and the risk of venous thromboembolism. *Current Problems* 1999; **25**: 12.

Lupus erythematosus. A short comment that despite there being occasional reports of lupus being exacerbated by oral contraceptives, the vast majority of patients with systemic lupus erythematosus (SLE) experience no adverse effects, especially from low oestrogen preparations.[1] However, it is generally advised that combined oral contraceptives should be avoided in women with antiphospholipid antibodies (which includes about a third of all patients with SLE) because they are at increased risk of venous thromboembolism.

1. Hughes GRV. The management of systemic lupus erythematosus. *Prescribers' J* 1987; **27**: 1.

Migraine. In the UK the *British National Formulary* has recommended that combined oral contraceptives are **contra-indicated** in: migraine with typical focal aura; severe migraine regularly lasting longer than 72 hours despite treatment; and migraine treated with an ergot derivative. It also recommended **caution** in migraine without focal aura and migraine controlled with a serotonin (5-HT₁) agonist. A woman receiving a combined oral contraceptive should report any increase in headache frequency or the onset of focal symptoms. If focal neurological symptoms not typical of aura persist for longer than one hour the combined oral contraceptive should be discontinued and the woman referred urgently to a neurologist.

Porphyria. Oral contraceptives have been associated with acute attacks of porphyria and are considered unsafe in porphyric patients. The progestogen content is considered more hazardous than the oestrogen content. A progestogen-only contraceptive may be used with extreme caution if non-hormonal contraception is inappropriate and potential benefit outweighs the risk. The risk of an acute attack is greatest in women who have had a previous attack or are under 30 years of age. Long-acting progestogen preparations should never be used in those at risk.

Pregnancy and breast feeding. In contrast to the numerous cases of congenital malformations reported after the use of high doses of sex hormones for hormonal pregnancy tests, there have been only a few suggestions that continued administration of oral contraceptives during early pregnancy may result in congenital limb reduction deformities,[1-3] and one case of neonatal choreoathetosis following prenatal exposure to oral contraceptives.[4]

Many studies, conversely, have shown no evidence that the use of oral contraceptives is associated with congenital malformations or teratogenic effects, whether past use (discontinued before conception), use after the last menstrual period, or known use in early pregnancy.[5-10] A meta-analysis[11] of some of these, plus other studies, confirmed this. The relative risk for all malformations with use of oral contraceptives was estimated to be 0.99 (95% confidence intervals 0.83 to 1.19). The use of oral contraceptives in early pregnancy also appears unlikely to increase the risk of hypospadia in male fetuses (see also under Precautions of Estradiol, p.1473).[12] For a discussion of the ectopic pregnancy risk in users of hormonal contraceptives, see above.

1. Janerich DT, *et al.* Oral contraceptives and congenital limb reduction defects. *N Engl J Med* 1974; **291**: 697–700.
2. McCredie J, *et al.* Congenital limb defects and the pill. *Lancet* 1983; **ii**: 623.
3. Kricker A, *et al.* Congenital limb reduction deformities and use of oral contraceptives. *Am J Obstet Gynecol* 1986; **155**: 1072–8.
4. Profumo R, *et al.* Neonatal choreoathetosis following prenatal exposure to oral contraceptives. *Pediatrics* 1990; **86**: 648–9.
5. Robinson SC. Pregnancy outcome following oral contraceptives. *Am J Obstet Gynecol* 1971; **109**: 354–8.
6. Royal College of General Practitioners' Oral Contraception Study. The outcome of pregnancy in former oral contraceptive users. *Br J Obstet Gynaecol* 1976; **83**: 608–16.
7. Rothman KJ, Louik C. Oral contraceptives and birth defects. *N Engl J Med* 1978; **299**: 522–4.
8. Vessey M, *et al.* Outcome of pregnancy in women using different methods of contraception. *Br J Obstet Gynaecol* 1979; **86**: 548–56.
9. Linn S, *et al.* Lack of association between contraceptive usage and congenital malformations in offspring. *Am J Obstet Gynecol* 1983; **147**: 923–8.

10. Källén B. Maternal use of oral contraceptives and Down syndrome. *Contraception* 1989; **39**: 503–6.
11. Bracken MB. Oral contraception and congenital malformations in offspring: a review and meta-analysis of the prospective studies. *Obstet Gynecol* 1990; **76**: 552–7.
12. Raman-Wilms L, *et al.* Fetal genital effects of first trimester sex hormone exposure: a meta-analysis. *Obstet Gynecol* 1995; **85**: 141–9.

BREAST FEEDING. Combined oral contraceptives may diminish the volume of breast milk and should be avoided until weaning (or for at least 6 months after birth). Progestogen-only oral contraceptives do not affect lactation, but should not be given until 3 weeks after birth to avoid an increased risk of breakthrough bleeding. Similarly, progestogen-only parenteral contraceptives should not be given until 5 or 6 weeks after birth if a woman is breast feeding; they may be started within 5 days if she is not breast feeding, provided she is warned that heavy or prolonged bleeding may occur. Very small amounts of both oestrogens and progestogens are distributed into the breast milk.

Sickle-cell disease. In *sickle-cell disease* there is an increased risk of thrombosis; oral contraceptive use also carries an increased risk of thrombosis but it is by no means certain that the two risks are additive. Some manufacturers have specifically warned against the use of combined oral contraceptives in sickle-cell disease but it has also been considered that there is no contra-indication to the use of low-dose combined preparations[1,2] or that a progestogen-only pill[3] or depot injection of medroxyprogesterone acetate,[4] be used.

For *sickle-cell trait* there is no increased risk of thrombosis and no contra-indication to the use of a combined preparation, as well as none to the use of a progestogen-only preparation. Many women with sickle-cell trait have, unnecessarily, been denied the use of oral contraceptives in the mistaken belief that advice for sickle-cell disease applies to the trait.[3]

1. Freie HMP. Sickle cell diseases and hormonal contraception. *Acta Obstet Gynecol Scand* 1983; **62**: 211–17.
2. Howard RJ, *et al.* Contraceptives, counselling, and pregnancy in women with sickle cell disease. *BMJ* 1993; **306**: 1735–7.
3. Evans DIK. Should patients who say that they have "sickle cells" be prescribed the contraceptive pill? *BMJ* 1989; **289**: 425.
4. Guillebaud J. Sickle cell disease and contraception. *BMJ* 1993; **307**: 506–7.

Surgery. Case reports and epidemiological studies showing an increased risk of idiopathic deep-vein thrombosis and pulmonary embolism in young women taking **combined oral contraceptives** (see above) led to the widespread belief that oral contraceptives may predispose to deep-vein thrombosis postoperatively. In consequence, the advice commonly given in the UK has been that, if possible, combined oral contraceptives should be discontinued 4 weeks before major elective surgery and all surgery of the legs, and that prophylactic heparin should be considered where this was not possible.[1] They can normally be recommenced at the first menses occurring at least 2 weeks after full mobilisation. However, estimates of the size of the risk are variable;[2-5] one report[2] found that the incidence of deep-vein thrombosis postoperatively in young women taking combined oral contraceptives was about twice that of women not taking contraceptives but the difference was not statistically significant. Some have considered[6] that the risk to young women of becoming pregnant from discontinuing oral contraceptives or of developing side-effects from prophylaxis may be greater than the risk of developing postoperative deep-vein thrombosis. This is in line with the views of the Thromboembolic Risk Factors (THRIFT) Consensus Group.[7] They suggested that unless there were other risk factors there was insufficient evidence to support a policy of routinely stopping combined oral contraceptives before major surgery. Additionally, there was insufficient evidence to support routine specific thromboembolic prophylaxis in women without additional risk factors. A review[8] has subsequently recommended that women for whom major elective surgery was planned should continue taking the combined oral contraceptive but should receive thromboprophylaxis in the perioperative period. It has also been pointed out[9,10] that for patients awaiting surgery who require contraception, a progestogen-only oral contraceptive or an injection of medroxyprogesterone acetate may be suitable since neither preparation increases the risk of thrombosis.

1. Guillebaud J. Surgery and the pill. *BMJ* 1985; **291**: 498–9.
2. Vessey M, *et al.* Oral contraceptives and venous thromboembolism: findings in a large prospective study. *BMJ* 1986; **292**: 526.
3. Tso SC, *et al.* Deep vein thrombosis and changes in coagulation and fibrinolysis after gynaecological operations in Chinese: the effect of oral contraceptives and malignant disease. *Br J Haematol* 1980; **46**: 603–12.
4. Gallus AS, *et al.* Oral contraceptives and surgery: reduced antithrombin and antifactor XA levels without postoperative venous thrombosis in low-risk patients. *Thromb Res* 1984; **35**: 513–26.
5. Sagar S, *et al.* Oral contraceptives, antithrombin III activity, and postoperative deep-vein thrombosis. *Lancet* 1976; **i**: 509–11.
6. Sue-Ling H, Hughes LE. Should the pill be stopped preoperatively? *BMJ* 1988; **296**: 447–8.
7. Thromboembolic Risk Factors (THRIFT) Consensus Group. Risk of and prophylaxis for venous thromboembolism in hospital patients. *BMJ* 1992; **305**: 567–74.
8. Anonymous. Drugs in the peri-operative period: hormonal contraceptives and hormone replacement therapy. *Drug Ther Bull* 1999; **37**: 78–80.
9. Guillebaud J. Should the pill be stopped preoperatively? *BMJ* 1988; **296**: 1522.
10. Guillebaud J, Robinson GE. Stopping the pill. *BMJ* 1991; **302**: 789.

Interactions

Enzyme-inducing drugs may cause failure of combined oral contraceptives by increasing their metabolism and clearance. This effect is well established for a number of *antiepileptics, griseofulvin,* and *rifamycin antibacterials,* and has also been suggested for some *antivirals* and for *modafinil.* Although less well documented, these interactions would also be expected to apply to progestogen-only contraceptives. Orally administered *retinoids* may cause failure of low-dose progestogen-only contraceptives. Rarely, *broad-spectrum antibacterials* have been associated with combined oral contraceptive failure, possibly by reducing enterohepatic recycling of the oestrogen component. As the doses of oestrogen and progestogen in oral contraceptives have decreased, reports of menstrual irregularities and unintended pregnancies attributed to these drug interactions have increased. Further details of drugs affecting hormonal contraceptives are given below under specific headings.

Oral contraceptives may, as well as being affected themselves by drug interactions, *affect other drugs.* Compounds undergoing oxidative metabolism may have their plasma concentration raised by oral contraceptives through an inhibitory action. Conversely, oral contraceptives appear to induce glucuronidation of some drugs thus reducing their plasma concentration. Oral contraceptives may also antagonise the actions of a number of drugs. Drugs affected include the following:

- some analgesics (increased clearance of paracetamol and morphine)
- anticoagulants (increased and decreased effects reported; see p.997)
- some antidepressants (reduced effectiveness, but also increased toxicity; see p.277)
- antidiabetics (antagonism of effect)
- antihypertensives (antagonism of effect)
- benzodiazepines (increased or decreased clearance; see p.679)
- ciclosporin (increased toxicity; see p.522)
- clofibrate (increased clearance and antagonism of effect)
- corticosteroids (reduced clearance and enhanced effect; see p.1043)
- lignocaine [lidocaine] (increased free fraction due to altered protein binding; see Protein Binding, under Pharmacokinetics, p.1315)
- selegiline (decreased clearance; see p.1178)
- thyroxine [levothyroxine] (reduced free fraction due to increased binding globulin concentration; see p.1528)
- xanthines (decreased clearance; see p.782).

◊ Reviews.

1. Brodie MJ. Oral contraceptives. *Prescribers' J* 1983; **23**: 140–3.
2. D'Arcy PF. Drug interactions with oral contraceptives. *Drug Intell Clin Pharm* 1986; **20**: 353–62.
3. Back DJ, Orme ML'E. Pharmacokinetic drug interactions with oral contraceptives. *Clin Pharmacokinet* 1990; **18**: 472–84.
4. Shenfield GM. Oral contraceptives: are drug interactions of clinical significance? *Drug Safety* 1993; **9**: 21–37.

Antibacterials. An interaction between the *rifamycins (rifampicin* and *rifabutin)* and oral contraceptives is well established (see Rifamycins, below) and alternative contraceptive measures are necessary. A variety of *broad-spectrum antibacterials* have been reported to decrease oral contraceptive efficacy. Some studies have pointed to interference with intestinal flora involved in enterohepatic circulation of oestrogens as being a likely mechanism for this interaction. Although up until 1985 there had been 32 reports[1] of unintended pregnancies in women receiving *penicillins* (25 of them with *ampicillin*) the ability of antibacterials to inhibit oral contraceptive efficacy remains unproven. The data are consistent, however, with the supposition that efficacy is occasionally impaired. Several cases of unintended pregnancies have been reported following the use of *tetracyclines.* It is recommended that additional contraceptive precautions should be used while taking, and for 7 days after stopping, a short course of any broad-spectrum antibacterial. If the course of antibacterial exceeds 2 weeks resistance to impairment of intestinal flora develops and additional precautions become unnecessary.

With regard to other antibacterials, in theory any one with significant effects on intestinal flora could reduce contraceptive efficacy. Isolated cases of pregnancy have been reported following the use of *cephalosporins, chloramphenicol, dapsone, isoniazid, nitrofurantoin, sulfonamides,* and *co-trimoxazole* but it is impossible to determine which, if any, of these interactions is real.

1. Back DJ, *et al.* Evaluation of Committee on Safety of Medicines yellow card reports on oral contraceptive-drug interactions with anticonvulsants and antibiotics. *Br J Clin Pharmacol* 1988; **25:** 527–32.

RIFAMYCINS. *Rifampicin* regularly results in menstrual irregularities and occasionally in unintended pregnancies in women receiving oral contraceptives. It is a potent enzyme inducer and considerably enhances the metabolism of oral contraceptives. Because of its potent effect, a non-hormonal method of contraception such as an intra-uterine device is recommended during, and for 4 to 8 weeks after stopping, rifampicin therapy. Similarly, other forms of contraception are recommended during *rifabutin* therapy.

TROLEANDOMYCIN. Severe pruritus and jaundice may occur if oral contraceptives and troleandomycin are administered concurrently.[1] It has been suggested that their hepatic effects may be additive or synergistic, and that concurrent use should be avoided.

1. Miguet J-P, *et al.* Jaundice from troleandomycin and oral contraceptives. *Ann Intern Med* 1980; **92:** 434.

Antidiabetics. *Troglitazone* is an enzyme inducer and increases the clearance of oestrogens and progestogens. A high-dose oral contraceptive, or an alternative method of contraception should be considered in women receiving troglitazone and requiring contraception.[1]

1. Loi C-M, *et al.* Effect of troglitazone on the pharmacokinetics of an oral contraceptive agent. *J Clin Pharmacol* 1999; **39:** 410–17.

Antiepileptics. Oral contraceptive failure and breakthrough bleeding have been reported in numerous cases during periods of concurrent antiepileptic therapy.[1-4] *Phenytoin,* barbiturates such as *phenobarbital* and *primidone*, and *carbamazepine* have been most frequently implicated, and *oxcarbazepine, ethosuximide,* and *topiramate* may interact similarly. These drugs increase clearance of oral contraceptives by enzyme induction, so diminishing their effect. In women receiving such antiepileptics use of non-hormonal contraceptives such as the intra-uterine device should be considered. If these are unsuitable, an oral contraceptive with an increased oestrogen content of 50 to 100 µg is generally adequate. Alternatively, a standard monophasic preparation may be given for 3 cycles without a break followed by a tablet-free interval of 4 days (tricycling). Switching to a non-interacting antiepileptic such as valproate could be considered.

1. Kenyon IE. Unplanned pregnancy in an epileptic. *BMJ* 1972; **1:** 686–7.
2. Hempel E, Klinger W. Drug stimulated biotransformation of hormonal steroid contraceptives: clinical implications. *Drugs* 1976; **12:** 442–8.
3. Mattson RH, Cramer JA. Epilepsy, sex hormones, and antiepileptic drugs. *Epilepsia* 1985; **26** (suppl 1): S40–S51.
4. Back DJ, *et al.* Evaluation of Committee on Safety of Medicines yellow card reports on oral contraceptive-drug interactions with anticonvulsants and antibiotics. *Br J Clin Pharmacol* 1988; **25:** 527–32.

Antifungals. Menstrual irregularities and pregnancies have been reported in women receiving oral contraceptives and *griseofulvin* concurrently[1,2] and more studies are needed to confirm the existence of the interaction and the mechanism of action involved. Additional contraceptive measures should be considered in women using the two drugs concurrently (and for at least 7 days after stopping griseofulvin). There have also been anecdotal reports[3,4] of menstrual irregularities and contraceptive failure with *fluconazole, itraconazole,* and *ketoconazole,* and similar advice applies to these if pregnancy is to be avoided with certainty.

1. van Dijke CPH, Weber JCP. Interaction between oral contraceptives and griseofulvin. *BMJ* 1984; **288:** 1125–6.
2. Back DJ, *et al.* Evaluation of Committee on Safety of Medicines yellow card reports on oral contraceptive-drug interactions with anticonvulsants and antibiotics. *Br J Clin Pharmacol* 1988; **25:** 527–32.
3. Pillans PI, Sparrow MJ. Pregnancy associated with a combined oral contraceptive and itraconazole. *N Z Med J* 1993; **106:** 436.
4. Meyboom RHB, *et al.* Disturbance of withdrawal bleeding during concomitant use of itraconazole and oral contraceptives. *N Z Med J* 1997; **110:** 300.

Antivirals. A number of antivirals are likely to accelerate the metabolism of oestrogens and progestogens; theoretically therefore, they may decrease the efficacy of hormonal contraceptives. This has been suggested for *HIV-protease inhibitors* such as *nelfinavir* and *ritonavir,*[1] and for *nevirapine*. An alternative form of contraception should be considered.

Conversely, the area under the plasma-concentration-time curve for ethinylestradiol is reported to be increased by *efavirenz* although the clinical implications are unknown.

1. Ouellet D, *et al.* Effect of ritonavir on the pharmacokinetics of ethinyl oestradiol in healthy female volunteers. *Br J Clin Pharmacol* 1998; **46:** 111–16.

Hypericum. Hypericum may decrease blood concentrations of oral contraceptives. There have been reports of intermenstrual bleeding and altered menstrual bleeding in women on long-term oral contraceptives who started taking hypericum.[1]

1. Yue Q-Y, *et al.* Safety of St. John's wort (Hypericum perforatum). *Lancet* 2000; **355:** 576–7.

Retinoids. One woman taking an oral progestogen-only contraceptive (levonorgestrel 30 µg daily) showed a significant increase in plasma-progestogen while receiving *acitretin,* which

indicated ovulation had occurred.[1] However, progestogen-only contraceptives do not suppress ovulation in all cycles, and this is not thought to be their primary mechanism of contraceptive efficacy (see p.1452). Nevertheless, because it is imperative that women receiving retinoids do not conceive, some have concluded that oral progestogen-only contraceptives are not suitable for use with retinoids.[2]

The anti-ovulatory efficacy of combined oral contraceptives was not affected by acitretin in 8 women in the study above,[1] or by *etretinate* in a study[3] in 12 women, and plasma concentrations of ethinylestradiol and levonorgestrel were not significantly changed by *isotretinoin* in another study in 9 women.[4] Lehucher Ceyrac *et al.*[2] concluded that, unless otherwise contra-indicated, oral combined contraceptives are the contraceptive method of choice for women undergoing retinoid treatment.

Both isotretinoin and combined oral contraceptives can have adverse effects on plasma lipids;[5] it has therefore been recommended that plasma lipids should be monitored during concurrent retinoid and oral contraceptive therapy, and that an oral contraceptive containing a non-androgenic progestogen is preferred,[2] since these have less detrimental effects on lipids (p.1456).

1. Berbis P, *et al.* Acitretin (RO10-1670) and oral contraceptives: interaction study. *Arch Dermatol Res* 1988; **280:** 388–9.
2. Lehucher Ceyrac D, *et al.* Retinoids and contraception. *Dermatology* 1992; **184:** 161–70.
3. Berbis P, *et al.* Study on the influence of etretinate on biologic activity of oral contraceptives. *J Am Acad Dermatol* 1987; **17:** 302–3.
4. Orme M, *et al.* Isotretinoin and contraception. *Lancet* 1984; **ii:** 752–3.
5. Chen Y, *et al.* Elevation of serum triglyceride and cholesterol levels from isotretinoin therapy with concomitant oral contraceptives. *Pharmacoepidemiol Drug Safety* 1995; **4:** 91–6.

Stimulants. *Modafinil* induces hepatic enzymes and may reduce the efficacy of oral contraceptives. The UK manufacturer of modafinil has suggested that when oral contraceptives are used concurrently, a preparation containing at least 50 µg of ethinylestradiol should be used.

Vitamins. Large supplements of *vitamin C* have been reported to increase serum ethinylestradiol concentrations in women taking oral contraceptives,[1] but a further study showed no effect.[2]

1. Back DJ, *et al.* Interaction of ethinyloestradiol with ascorbic acid in man. *BMJ* 1981; **282:** 1516.
2. Zamag NM, *et al.* Absence of an effect of high vitamin C dosage on the systemic availability of ethinyl estradiol in women using a combination oral contraceptive. *Contraception* 1993; **48:** 377–91.

Pharmacokinetics

For a discussion of the pharmacokinetics of oestrogens and progestogens, see Estradiol, p.1474 and Progesterone, p.1489, respectively. The extent of binding of progestogens to serum sex-hormone binding globulin may be altered when they are administered with an oestrogen. Oestrogens increase serum concentrations of sex-hormone binding globulin, and progestogens differ in their ability to suppress this effect.

◊ Reference to the effects of hormonal contraceptives on binding proteins.[1]

1. Fotherby K. Interactions of contraceptive steroids with binding proteins and the clinical implications. *Ann N Y Acad Sci* 1988; **538:** 313–20.

Uses and Administration

The main use of hormonal contraceptives is for contraception, but combined oral contraceptives are also commonly used in menstrual disorders such as dysmenorrhoea (p.6), premenstrual syndrome (p.1475), and menorrhagia (p.1490), particularly where contraception is also required. Combined oral contraceptives are also used in polycystic ovary syndrome (p.1276) and Turner's syndrome (p.1276), and may be used in endometriosis (p.1469); those containing non-androgenic progestogens may be used in acne (p.1103) and hirsutism (p.1468).

Combined oral contraceptives containing both an oestrogen and a progestogen are the most effective type of oral contraceptive for general use. The synthetic ethinyl derivatives ethinylestradiol and mestranol are the oestrogens typically used in such preparations. The progestogenic component is usually a 19-nortestosterone derivative such as desogestrel, etynodiol diacetate, gestodene, levonorgestrel, lynestrenol, norethisterone, norethisterone acetate, norgestimate, or norgestrel. Preparations may be *monophasic* (containing a fixed dose of oestrogen and progestogen), or *biphasic* or *triphasic* (when the dose of progestogen, or both the progestogen and oestrogen, are varied

through the cycle). Phased preparations are designed to mimic more closely the pattern of endogenous hormone secretion and may provide better cycle control than monophasic preparations. More rarely, *sequential* preparations are used, which contain an oestrogen alone for part of the cycle. Combined oral contraceptives are taken for 21 days (or occasionally 22 days) followed by an interval of 7 days (or 6 days) when menstrual bleeding will occur. Some preparations include 21 (or 22) active tablets plus 7 (or 6) inert tablets to remove the need for counting days ('every day' preparations). The oestrogen content of most preparations is currently in the range of 20 to 50 µg daily although higher doses were often formerly used. A formulation containing the lowest dose of oestrogen compatible with good cycle control should be chosen, considering the following:

- *low-strength* preparations (ethinylestradiol 20 µg) are most appropriate for obese or older women, provided a combined oral contraceptive is considered otherwise suitable
- *standard strength* preparations (ethinylestradiol 30 or 35 µg if monophasic, or 30 to 40 µg if phased) are appropriate for most other women
- *high-strength* preparations (ethinylestradiol 50 µg or mestranol 50 µg) are generally used only in circumstances where bioavailability of the oestrogen is reduced, such as concomitant use of some enzyme-inducing drugs (see Interactions, above).

When first **starting** combined oral contraceptives, if the first tablet is taken on the first day of the menstrual cycle (the first day of bleeding) additional contraceptive precautions are unnecessary. If the first tablet is taken on the fourth day of the cycle or later, additional contraceptive precautions should be undertaken for 7 days (or 14 days for 'every day' preparations in case the inert tablets are inadvertently taken first). If amenorrhoea is present and pregnancy has been excluded, combined oral contraceptives may be started on any day, but additional precautions should be used for the first 7 days. Combined oral contraceptives should be started on the same day after abortion or miscarriage. In women not breast feeding, they may be started 3 weeks postpartum; progestogen-only contraceptives are preferred in breast-feeding women (see under Precautions, above). When **changing** to a combined preparation containing a different progestogen, the new preparation should be started on the day following the last active tablet of the old preparation. If a tablet-free interval is taken then extra contraceptive precautions are necessary for the first 7 days of the new preparation. In the case of 'every day' preparations, to allow for the fact that the inert tablets may inadvertently be taken first, extra contraceptive precautions are necessary during the first 14 days. Meticulous regularity of dosage is essential and contraceptive protection may be lost if a dose is not taken at the proper time or is missed, especially if the missed dose is at the beginning or end of a cycle. If a tablet is **missed** it should be taken as soon as possible (if more than one is missed, just the most recent dose should be taken and the others omitted); the remainder of the course should be taken as normal. If the gap in dosage is more than 12 hours, then extra contraceptive measures are required for the next 7 days. If these 7 days run into the last 7 days of the cycle, then the tablet-free interval (or the 7 inert tablets) should be omitted and the next cycle of tablets started immediately. Similarly, extra contraceptive measures are advised during, and for 7 days after recovery from, vomiting and diarrhoea.

Progestogen-only oral contraceptives are suitable for women when an oestrogen component is contra-indicated. They are taken continuously, usually **starting** on day one of the menstrual cycle, with no interval during menstrual bleeding. They may be associated with a higher failure rate than the combined preparations. Regularity in taking the doses is even more important with this type of preparation; contraceptive efficacy is reduced if a dose is delayed by more than 3 hours. Commonly used progestogens include the 19-nortestosterone derivatives etynodiol diacetate, levonorgestrel or norgestrel, and norethisterone. When **changing** from a combined oral contraceptive preparation to an oral progestogen-only contraceptive, the new tablets should be started immediately with no tablet-free interval (or, in the case of 'every day' preparations, omitting the inert tablets). If there is a gap in administration of active ingredients, then extra contraceptive precautions are required for 7 days. If a **missed tablet** is delayed by more than 3 hours, it should be taken as soon as possible and the next tablet taken at the correct time. Additional contraceptive methods should be used for the next 7 days. Additional contraceptive methods are also required during, and for 7 days after recovery from, vomiting and diarrhoea.

Progestogens are also used alone as **parenteral contraceptives** and provide a very high level of contraceptive efficacy. They are usually given within the first 5 days of the menstrual cycle. Medroxyprogesterone acetate is given by intramuscular injection as a long-acting depot preparation in a dose of 150 mg to provide contraception for up to 3 months. Norethisterone enantate is used similarly in a dose of 200 mg to provide protection for up to 2 months. Injectable contraceptives are usually used to provide short-term protection or are used in women unable to use other methods. Levonorgestrel is used in the form of a subcutaneous implant providing contraception for 5 years. A contraceptive implant containing etonogestrel, effective for 3 years, is also available. A combined parenteral contraceptive containing the oestrogen estradiol cipionate with medroxyprogesterone acetate, and given monthly by intramuscular injection, has been developed.

Progestogen-releasing intra-uterine devices are also available. One such device releases 20 μg of levonorgestrel every 24 hours and provides contraception for 5 years. It is usually inserted within 7 days of the onset of menstruation.

Postcoital hormonal contraceptives (emergency contraception) have to be taken within 72 hours after unprotected intercourse to be effective. A preparation available for such use consists of tablets each containing ethinylestradiol 50 μg and norgestrel 500 μg or levonorgestrel 250 μg. Two tablets should be taken within 72 hours and a further 2 tablets exactly 12 hours later. If vomiting occurs within 2 hours of taking the tablets the dose can be repeated together with an antiemetic (but preferably not metoclopramide because of the risk of extrapyramidal effects). An alternative to this combined regimen is levonorgestrel 750 μg given alone and repeated after 12 hours (for details see below).

Contraception. Contraception is used for fertility control, and some methods have additional non-contraceptive health benefits. There are a wide variety of regular methods including periodic abstinence (natural family planning), male and female barrier methods, intra-uterine devices (IUDs), female hormonal contraceptives, and female or male sterilisation. In addition, female hormonal contraceptives and copper IUDs are available for emergency (postcoital) contraception. The methods employed for contraceptive purposes can be grouped into three categories: those that prevent ovulation, those that prevent fertilisation of the ovum, and those that prevent implantation of the fertilised ovum. None of the available contraceptive methods are effective once implantation of a fertilised ovum has occurred, i.e. they are not abortifacients.

A large number of factors will influence the choice of contraceptive method. Those relating to the woman include age (and therefore likely fertility), parity, medical disorders, risk of sexually transmitted diseases, smoking status, breast feeding, and cultural and religious considerations. Those relating to the method include its failure rate, reversibility, ease of use, mechanism of action, adverse effects, and non-contraceptive benefits.

The most reliable reversible methods for contraception are those for which there can be no 'user' failure such as *progestogen injections* and *implants*, and progestogen or copper *intra-uterine devices* (IUDs). These methods have reported failure rates of between 0.09 and 2% during the first year of use. The duration of action of the various progestogen injections is up to 2 or 3 months, whereas progestogen implants and progestogen IUDs are effective for up to 5 years. These long-acting progestogen preparations thicken cervical mucus, so preventing sperm penetration, and suppress the endometrium, so preventing implantation. In addition, they suppress ovulation; the degree of suppression is complete for injectable preparations, about 50% for implants, and low for the progestogen IUDs. Copper IUDs were traditionally thought to act by preventing implantation, but it is now thought that the biochemical changes which they produce in the uterus also prevent fertilisation. They are effective and have a prolonged action (up to 5 or 10 years), but they have been associated with an increased rate of pelvic inflammatory disease and ectopic pregnancy. IUDs are generally unsuitable for nulliparous women and those at increased risk of sexually transmitted diseases.

Of methods subject to 'user' failure, *combined oral contraceptives* are the most effective. They have a reported failure rate during the first year of 0.1% if used perfectly, but 3% in typical practice. Their principal mechanism of action is to prevent ovulation, and they also decrease the chances of fertilisation and implantation. Combined oral contraceptives offer the non-contraceptive advantages of avoidance of dysmenorrhoea, premenstrual tension, and iron-deficiency anaemia, and in the long-term they protect against endometrial and ovarian cancer. However, they do not protect against sexually transmitted diseases, they are unsuitable for older women who smoke, and long-term use carries a slight increased risk of breast cancer.

Progestogen-only oral contraceptives have a 0.5% failure rate during the first year of use if taken correctly, which is slightly higher than that for combined preparations; in practice, failure rates of from 1 to 10% have been reported. Regularity in taking them is essential; a dose should not be delayed for more than 3 hours. They act primarily to decrease the chance of fertilisation and implantation since they prevent ovulation in only 14 to 40% of cycles. They are useful for women who are breast feeding, for those who smoke and are more than 35 years of age, and if medical conditions contra-indicate the use of oestrogens.

Barrier methods, including both male and female condoms, vaginal sponges containing spermicide, and diaphragms and cervical caps used in conjunction with spermicide, act as a mechanical barrier to prevent fertilisation, and inactivate sperm. Barrier methods decrease the risk of sexually transmitted diseases and a shift towards their use has occurred since the emergence of HIV infection in particular. However, barrier methods are not as effective in preventing conception as hormonal contraception and copper IUDs. Even when used correctly, failure rates in the first year of use vary from 3% for the male condom to 11.5% with the cervical cap plus spermicide. Spermicides, such as nonoxinol 9, may be used alone as foam or as dissolvable vaginal tablets or pessaries, or as a spermicide-containing polyvinyl alcohol film placed over the cervix. However, they are generally considered relatively ineffective when used as the sole method of contraception, and such use is not recommended.

Natural family planning methods such as periodic abstinence using the calendar, temperature, cervical mucus ('Billings') or sympto-thermal methods require high motivation to learn and practice effectively. However, they may be the only acceptable method to some people. More recently, daily measurement of urine hormone concentrations has been used as a predictor of the timing of ovulation and hence the risk of becoming pregnant; on 'unsafe' days abstinence or barrier methods are required. Traditional methods such as withdrawal (coitus interruptus) are widely used in some areas, but are considered relatively ineffective.

Various other methods of contraception are under investigation including injectable, transdermal, and vaginal forms of combined hormonal contraceptives, and the use of gonadorelin analogues or selective sex-hormone receptor modulators. Contraceptive vaccines are also being investigated. Although there has been some investigation of **male contraception**, and weekly intramuscular injection of high-dose testosterone or nandrolone to produce azoospermia has been investigated with some success, development of an oral contraceptive dosage form for males has been slow. Use of a progestogen pill, with 'add-back' testosterone, is being studied, as is the use of implants of synthetic androgens such as trestolone (7-α-methyl-19-nortestosterone; MENT).

The available irreversible methods of contraception are surgical male or female *sterilisation*. The use of mepacrine for non-surgical sterilisation has been attempted but has proved extremely controversial.

References.
1. WHO. Facts about once-a-month injectable contraceptives: memorandum from a WHO meeting. *Bull WHO* 1993; **71:** 677–89.
2. Matlin SA. Prospects for pharmacological male contraception. *Drugs* 1994; **48:** 851–63.
3. Baird DT, Glasier AF. Hormonal contraception. *N Engl J Med* 1993; **328:** 1543–9.
4. Flemming CF. Oral contraception. *Prescribers' J* 1994; **34:** 227–34.
5. Weisberg E. Prescribing oral contraceptives. *Drugs* 1995; **49:** 224–31.
6. Anonymous. Long-acting progestogen-only contraception. *Drug Ther Bull* 1996; **34:** 93–6.
7. Anonymous. Choice of contraceptives. *Med Lett Drugs Ther* 1995; **37:** 9–12. Additional note. *ibid.*: 36.
8. WHO. *Contraceptive Method Mix: guidelines for policy and service delivery.* Geneva: World Health Organization, 1994.
9. Belfield T, ed. *FPA Contraceptive Handbook: a guide for family planning and other health professionals.* 2nd ed. London: Family Planning Association, 1997.
10. Rowlands S. Contraception beyond the millennium. *Pharm J* 1998; **261:** 666–8.
11. Baird DT, Glasier AF. Contraception. *BMJ* 1999; **319:** 969–72.
12. Baird DT. Overview of advances in contraception. *Br Med Bull* 2000; **56:** 704–16.
13. Anderson RA. Hormonal contraception in the male. *Br Med Bull* 2000; **56:** 717–28.
14. Lähteenmäki P, Jukarainen H. Novel delivery systems in contraception. *Br Med Bull* 2000; **56:** 739–48.
15. Kubba A, *et al.* Contraception. *Lancet* 2000; **356:** 1913–19.

EMERGENCY CONTRACEPTION. Emergency contraception[1-4] can be used after unprotected intercourse but before a fertilised ovum has been implanted. Methods that act after implantation are considered abortifacients. The two most commonly used emergency contraceptives are *oral contraceptives* and *copper IUDs*.

The oral contraceptive used has typically been a preparation containing high-dose oestrogen together with a progestogen, taken within 72 hours of intercourse, and repeated 12 hours later (the Yuzpe regimen or so-called 'morning after pill'). This preparation is thought to act by a variety of mechanisms, which may depend on when in the menstrual cycle it is used. It may prevent implantation, prevent or delay ovulation, disrupt ovum transport, and alter corpus luteum function. Reported efficacy rates vary between 75 and 80%. Levonorgestrel alone (without an oestrogen) is also used as an emergency contraceptive. A large WHO multicentre study found that levonorgestrel 750 μg alone within 72 hours of intercourse and repeated after 12 hours was more effective than the Yuzpe regimen and better tolerated.[5] Both regimens were most effective when given within 24 hours of intercourse.[5,6]

Copper, but not progestogen, IUDs can be inserted up to 120 hours after unprotected intercourse for postcoital contraception. They have a failure rate of less than 1% when used for emergency contraception. Thus, when efficacy is a priority the IUD is the emergency contraceptive method of choice.

Drugs under investigation for use as emergency contraceptives include *mifepristone*. When taken as a single 600-mg dose within 72 hours of unprotected intercourse this has been reported to be 100% effective.[7] More recently, a very low dose of 10 mg was shown to be similar in efficacy to the 600-mg dose.[8] Although mifepristone is also effective after implantation (5 to 7 days after fertilisation), its action as an emergency contraceptive appears to depend on inhibiting ovulation or, if ovulation has occurred, preventing implantation.

1. Anonymous. Hormonal emergency contraception. *Drug Ther Bull* 1993; **31:** 27–8.
2. Glasier A. Emergency postcoital contraception. *N Engl J Med* 1997; **337:** 1058–64.
3. Kubba A, Wilkinson C. Emergency contraception update. *Br J Fam Plann* 1998; **23:** 135–7.
4. Cheng L, *et al.* Interventions for emergency contraception (updated 10 May 2001). Available in The Cochrane Library; Issue 3. Oxford: Update Software; 2001.
5. Task Force on Postovulatory Methods of Fertility Regulation. Randomised controlled trial of levonorgestrel versus the Yuzpe regimen of combined oral contraceptives for emergency contraception. *Lancet* 1998; **352:** 428–33.
6. Piaggio G, *et al.* Timing of emergency contraception with levonorgestrel or the Yuzpe regimen. *Lancet* 1999; **353:** 721.
7. Glasier A, *et al.* Mifepristone (RU 486) compared with high-dose estrogen and progestogen for emergency postcoital contraception. *N Engl J Med* 1992; **327:** 1041–4.
8. Task Force on Postovulatory Methods of Fertility Regulation. Comparison of three single doses of mifepristone as emergency contraception: a randomised trial. *Lancet* 1999; **353:** 697–702.

Hormone Replacement Therapy

(19996-n)

The menopause is defined as the permanent cessation of cyclical menstruation due to loss of ovarian follicular activity. It is therefore determined in retrospect, conventionally after a period of 1 year without menstruation. In the few years prior to the menopause (the menopausal transition), ovarian oestradiol secretion declines, sometimes in a fluctuating manner, and there is a resultant increase in pituitary follicle-stimulating hormone (FSH) secretion. The menopausal transition may be characterised by irregular menstrual cycles and dysfunctional uterine bleeding, and fertility is much reduced compared with the early reproductive years. The term perimenopause is used to cover the menopausal transition and the first year after the menopause, and may last 3 to 5 years. It has sometimes been referred to as the climacteric. Oestrogen concentrations reach their minimum and FSH concentrations their maximum about 4 years after the menopause. After the menopause the ovaries may continue to produce some androgens, which together with adrenal androgens are converted to oestrogens (predominantly oestrone) in the periphery, but oestrogen concentrations are much lower than in premenopausal women. The median age for the natural menopause is about 51 years. If the menopause occurs in women aged 40 years or less, it is considered premature. The menopause may be induced by surgical removal of both ovaries, or sometimes by antineoplastic drugs or radiotherapy.

The decline in oestrogen concentrations during the perimenopause may be associated with both acute and long-term effects. However, some of these may be difficult to differentiate from the effects of ageing, and the incidence varies geographically. Established *acute symptoms* can include vasomotor instability, manifesting as hot flushes and night sweats, and vaginal atrophy and dyspareunia. Non-specific symptoms include palpitations, headache, backache, and psychological symptoms such as tiredness, lack of concentration, loss of libido, irritability, insomnia, and depression. Insomnia may occur secondary to night sweats. There is little evidence that depressive illness is disproportionately increased at the menopause. Urinary problems are common in ageing women, and may occur in the perimenopause, but the extent that these are due to lack of oestrogens has not been determined. An established *long-term consequence* of the decline in oestrogen concentrations is an increased risk of bone fractures resulting from an increase in the rate of bone resorption. In addition, decline in oestrogen concentrations is associated with adverse effects on blood lipoproteins, and this may be a risk factor for cardiovascular disease.

Acute and longer term effects of the menopause may be managed by using hormone replacement therapy (HRT) with oestrogens, with or without progestogens.

Adverse Effects

When oestrogens are used for menopausal HRT, adverse effects include nausea and vomiting, abdominal cramps and bloating, weight changes, breast enlargement and tenderness, premenstrual-like syndrome, sodium and fluid retention, altered blood lipids, changes in liver function, cholestatic jaundice, rashes and chloasma (melasma), changes in libido, migraine, dizziness, depression, headache, leg cramps, and decreased tolerance of contact lenses. Transdermal delivery systems may cause contact sensitisation (possibly severe hypersensitivity reactions on continued exposure), and headache has been reported on vigorous exercise. Use of oestrogen without a progestogen results in endometrial hyperplasia and an increased risk of endometrial carcinoma (see below). The addition of a progestogen for 10 to 14 days of a 28-day cycle reduces this risk but results in regular withdrawal bleeding towards the end of the progestogen. Use of continuous progestogen and oestrogen avoids withdrawal bleeding, but may result in irregular breakthrough bleeding, particularly in the early stages of therapy, or if used within 12 months of the last menstrual period. Current use of menopausal HRT is associated with an increased risk of venous thromboembolism (see below). Long-term use of menopausal HRT may be associated with an increased risk of breast cancer (see below).

◊ Reviews.
1. Winship KA. Unopposed oestrogens. *Adverse Drug React Acute Poisoning Rev* 1987; **1**: 37–66.
2. Evans MP, *et al.* Hormone replacement therapy: management of common problems. *Mayo Clin Proc* 1995; **70**: 800–5.

Carcinogenicity. Use of unopposed oestrogen as menopausal HRT in women with a uterus increases the risk of endometrial cancer, irrespective of the route of administration. This risk is reduced, although possibly not eliminated completely, by the concomitant use of a progestogen. Although less well established, there is mounting evidence that long-term use of oestrogens as HRT is associated with an increased risk of breast cancer, and that the addition of a progestogen does not decrease or increase this risk. The exact extent of the risk and its implications for prescribing practice remain controversial.

Because of continuing modifications in regimens for HRT there is a continuing need to monitor the incidence of various cancers in users of this therapy.

BREAST. Early age at menarche and late age at menopause increase the risk of breast cancer, and surgical oophorectomy at an early age decreases the risk of breast cancer. In addition, higher concentrations of unbound endogenous oestrogens in postmenopausal women appear to increase the risk of developing breast cancer.[1] Such risk factors have prompted concerns that menopausal HRT might be associated with an increased risk of breast cancer.

Reviews and analyses[2-4] of studies published during the 1970s and/or 1980s on the use of unopposed oestrogen replacement therapy in postmenopausal women have generally shown that there is an associated moderate increase in the risk of breast cancer; figures for overall relative risk compared with non-oestrogen users ranged from under 1 to up to 2. One of these,[3] a meta-analysis of studies from 1976 to 1989, further showed that although the relative risk of breast cancer rose to 1.3 after 15 years of oestrogen use, it did not appear to rise at all until after 5 years' use. A similar meta-analysis[4] differentiated between low-dose oestrogens and high-dose oestrogens; those taking 0.625 mg daily of conjugated oestrogens had a risk of breast cancer 1.08 times higher than non-oestrogen users, whereas the relative risk in those taking 1.25 mg daily or more was up to 2. A subsequent meta-analysis[5] differentiated between current use of HRT, duration of use, and use at any time. The highest relative risk of breast cancer was associated with current use (1.4); use for 10 years or more was associated with a relative risk of about 1.2, and having ever used HRT was not associated with an increased risk. The most robust data to date have been provided by the Collaborative Group on Hormonal Factors in Breast Cancer, who reanalysed about 90% of the worldwide evidence on breast cancer and the use of HRT.[6] They reported that the relative risk of having breast cancer diagnosed was increased by a factor of 1.023 for each year of use, being 1.35 for 5 or more years of use. However, this effect was reduced on cessation of use, and had largely disappeared after about 5 years. In women who started therapy at age 50, the cumulative excess number of breast cancers diagnosed per 1000 women between age 50 and 70 were estimated to be 2, 6, and 12 for 5, 10, and 15 years use, respectively, from a baseline of 45 per 1000 in never-users.[6]

Most data relate to the use of unopposed oestrogen. There has been speculation both that the concomitant use of progestogen in HRT could reduce the risk of breast cancer and that it may increase it. An early indication from the study by Bergkvist *et al.*[7] suggested an increased relative risk of 4.4 in the small subgroup using long-term combined therapy, but because of the large confidence intervals they considered these results were inconclusive. Analysis of the Nurses' Health Study cohort has provided evidence that current use of oestrogen and progestogen is associated with a similar increased relative risk of breast cancer to that of unopposed oestrogen (1.4 versus 1.3).[8] The Collaborative Group on Hormonal Factors in Breast Cancer[6] found no evidence of marked differences between preparations containing oestrogens alone and those containing oestrogens and progestogens. However, in a randomised trial, oestrogen plus progestogen was associated with greater increases in radiographic breast density than unopposed oestrogen.[9] The results of a further cohort study[10] also suggested an increased risk of breast cancer associated with HRT use, but also that the risk may be higher for current or recent use of combined HRT compared with oestrogen alone.

The public health perspective of any increased risk of breast cancer will depend on the background risk. This is high in western countries, so a small increased relative risk would equate to a large absolute increase in number of cases.[11]

If menopausal oestrogen therapy increases the risk of breast cancer, there is a need to ascertain whether these cancers can be detected early, how aggressive they are, and what the mortality rate from them is. Currently, there are limited data on these points. There is evidence[12,13] that the use of HRT decreases the sensitivity and specificity of screening mammography (resulting in more false positives and more false negatives), apparently because it increases radiographic breast density,[14] so decreasing the ability to interpret the mammogram. This is of concern for the success of screening programmes, and has been suggested as a factor in the increased detection of interval cancers (those detected between screening appointments).[15] In addition, HRT-associated increases in radiographic breast density could actually be a marker for risk of breast cancer.[9] However, there are also data suggesting that breast cancers in women on HRT may be of better prognostic grade.[16,17] The Collaborative Group on Hormonal Factors in Breast Cancer reported that breast cancers were more likely to be localised in current or recent users of HRT, but that there was evidence of an increased risk of metastasis with increasing duration of use.[6] Follow-up of most studies is currently insufficient to give a clear indication of mortality risk with long-term use. Early data from a UK cohort study[18] suggested a decreased risk of breast cancer mortality, but after further follow-up the risk was no longer reduced.[19] Similarly, a study in 2614 women with breast cancer followed up for up to 22 years found that the use of HRT at the time of diagnosis was associated with a reduction in mortality, but the effect waned over time.[20] In contrast, data[8] from the Nurses' Health Study cohort suggest an increase in risk of death from breast cancer in the subset of women currently using HRT with 5 years or more of use (1.45). Similarly, although mortality was lower overall, a trend towards an increased risk of death from breast cancer (1.9; 95% confidence interval 0.4 to 8.4) was seen in a study of long-term use (mean of 17 years).[21]

The risk of breast cancer may be increased further by the use of HRT in women who are already at an increased risk. Although a recent study found a modest increase in risk in these women, it was not significantly higher, and there was a reduced total mortality rate.[22] It is unclear whether use of HRT in breast cancer survivors increases the risk of subsequent recurrence and associated mortality (see also under Precautions, below).

1. Toniolo PG, *et al.* A prospective study of endogenous oestrogens and breast cancer in postmenopausal women. *J Natl Cancer Inst* 1995; **87**: 190–7.
2. Henderson BE. The cancer question: an overview of recent epidemiologic and retrospective data. *Am J Obstet Gynecol* 1989; **161**: 1859–64.
3. Steinberg KK, *et al.* A meta-analysis of the effect of estrogen replacement therapy on the risk of breast cancer. *JAMA* 1991; **265**: 1985–90.
4. Dupont WD, Page DL. Menopausal estrogen replacement therapy and breast cancer. *Arch Intern Med* 1991; **151**: 67–72.
5. Colditz GA, *et al.* Hormone replacement therapy and risk of breast cancer: results from epidemiologic studies. *Am J Obstet Gynecol* 1993; **168**: 1473–80.
6. Collaborative Group on Hormonal Factors in Breast Cancer. Breast cancer and hormone replacement therapy: collaborative reanalysis of data from 51 epidemiological studies of 52 705 women with breast cancer and 108 411 women without breast cancer. *Lancet* 1997; **350**: 1047–59. Correction. *ibid.*; 1484.
7. Bergkvist L, *et al.* The risk of breast cancer after estrogen and estrogen—progestin replacement. *N Engl J Med* 1989; **321**: 293–7.
8. Colditz GA, *et al.* The use of estrogens and progestins and the risk of breast cancer in postmenopausal women. *N Engl J Med* 1995; **332**: 1589–93.
9. Greendale GA, *et al.* Effects of estrogen and estrogen-progestin on mammographic parenchymal density. *Ann Intern Med* 1999; **130**: 262–9.
10. Schairer C, *et al.* Menopausal estrogen and estrogen-progestin replacement therapy and breast cancer risk. *JAMA* 2000; **283**: 485–91
11. WHO. Research on the menopause in the 1990s: report of a WHO scientific group. *WHO Tech Rep Ser 866* 1996.
12. Laya MB, *et al.* Effect of estrogen replacement therapy on the specificity and sensitivity of screening mammography. *J Natl Cancer Inst* 1996; **88**: 643–9.
13. Kavanagh AM, *et al.* Hormone replacement therapy and accuracy of mammographic screening. *Lancet* 2000; **355**: 270–4.
14. Rutter CM, *et al.* Changes in breast density associated with initiation, discontinuation, and continuing use of hormone replacement therapy. *JAMA* 2001; **285**: 171–6.
15. Cohen EL. Effect of hormone replacement therapy on cancer detection by mammography. *Lancet* 1997; **349**: 1624.
16. Harding C, *et al.* Hormone replacement therapy and tumour grade in breast cancer: prospective study in screening unit. *BMJ* 1996; **312**: 1646–7. Correction. *ibid.*; **313**: 198.
17. Gapstur SM, *et al.* Hormone replacement therapy and risk of breast cancer with a favorable histology: results of the Iowa Women's Health Study. *JAMA* 1999; **281**: 2091–7.
18. Hunt K, *et al.* Long-term surveillance of mortality and cancer incidence in women receiving hormone replacement therapy. *Br J Obstet Gynaecol* 1987; **94**: 620–35.
19. Hunt K, *et al.* Mortality in a cohort of long-term users of hormone replacement therapy: an updated analysis. *Br J Obstet Gynaecol* 1990; **97**: 1080–6.
20. Schairer C, *et al.* Estrogen replacement therapy and breast cancer survival in a large screening study. *J Natl Cancer Inst* 1999; **91**: 264–70.
21. Ettinger B, *et al.* Reduced mortality associated with long-term postmenopausal estrogen therapy. *Obstet Gynecol* 1996; **87**: 6–12.
22. Sellers TA, *et al.* The role of hormone replacement therapy in the risk for breast cancer and total mortality in women with a family history of breast cancer. *Ann Intern Med* 1997; **127**: 973–80.

CERVIX. Studies of the effect of HRT on cervical cancer risk are likely to be subject to the potential confounding of other risk factors such as sexual activity. There are few data on this risk, but one recent study suggests oestrogens do not increase, and may decrease, the risk of cervical cancer.[1]

1. Parazzini, F, *et al.* Case-control study of oestrogen replacement therapy and risk of cervical cancer. *BMJ* 1997; **315**: 85–8.

ENDOMETRIUM. The increased incidence of endometrial hyperplasia and risk of cancer in women receiving unopposed oestrogen replacement therapy is well established. An analysis of case control studies published during the 1970s and 1980s revealed a relative risk of developing endometrial cancer of 1.4 to 7.6 in women who had ever used oestrogen, and a relative risk of 3.1 to 15 in long-term users, compared with nonusers.[1] Risk was also increased with higher doses of oestrogens. In general, endometrial cancer in oestrogen users was of a better prognostic stage, and survival rates were better, than in nonusers.[1] An elevated risk of endometrial cancer persists for a number of years after discontinuation of unopposed oestrogen therapy.[2]

Addition of a progestogen to oestrogen replacement therapy reduces the incidence of endometrial hyperplasia[3] and cancer. However, the extent to which the addition of a progestogen alters the risks and benefits of oestrogen replacement therapy, and the optimum progestogen type, and dose and duration, have not been fully elucidated.

As regards endometrial cancer, preliminary data from a cohort study revealed that the addition of cyclical progestogen to oestrogen therapy reduced this risk compared with oestrogen therapy alone.[4] A further case-control study confirmed that progestogens decreased the relative risk, and that the reduction in risk was greater when progestogens were used for 10 or more days per month than when they were used for less than 10 days per month.[5] Two much larger case-control studies have confirmed these findings.[6,7] However, 1 of these studies[6] reported that in long-term users the addition of a progestogen did not reduce the risk of endometrial cancer to that seen in nonusers— after 5 years of use, the relative risk of endometrial cancer with

HRT containing 10 or more days of progestogen per month was 2.5 (95% confidence intervals 1.1 to 5.5). This finding remains to be confirmed.

Use of progestogens for 10 days of an 84-day cycle (long cycle) has been suggested to improve acceptability of combined HRT. However one study of a long-cycle regimen was discontinued because of an increased risk of endometrial hyperplasia and atypia compared with a conventional monthly cycle regimen.[8]

Some newer regimens of HRT employ continuous low-doses of progestogen with oestrogen, which avoid withdrawal bleeding. Data on the incidence of endometrial hyperplasia from randomised trials of these regimens have been reassuring.[3,9,10] Continuous norethisterone plus ethinylestradiol,[9] and continuous medroxyprogesterone plus conjugated oestrogens,[10] protected the endometrium against the hyperplasia seen with the oestrogen alone. Continuous therapy was as effective as cyclical therapy containing 12 days' progestogen,[10] and there is a suggestion from meta-analysis[3] that continuous therapy may even be more effective than sequential when given over a prolonged period, although this remains to be confirmed. The first data on endometrial cancer risk from continuous combined HRT suggests that it is as protective as sequential therapy with the progestogen administered for 10 or more days per month (odds ratio 1.07 per 5 years of use for both regimens).[7]

1. Henderson BE. The cancer question: an overview of recent epidemiologic and retrospective data. Am J Obstet Gynecol 1989; 161: 1859–64.
2. Rubin GL, et al. Estrogen replacement therapy and the risk of endometrial cancer: remaining controversies. Am J Obstet Gynecol 1990; 162: 148–54.
3. Lethaby A, et al. Hormone replacement therapy in postmenopausal women: endometrial hyperplasia and irregular bleeding (updated 27 October 1999). Available in The Cochrane Library; Issue 3. Oxford: Update Software; 2001.
4. Persson I, et al. Risk of endometrial cancer after treatment with oestrogens alone or in conjunction with progestogens: results of a prospective study. BMJ 1989; 298: 147–51.
5. Voigt LF, et al. Progestagen supplementation of exogenous oestrogens and risk of endometrial cancer. Lancet 1991; 338: 274–7.
6. Beresford S, et al. Risk of endometrial cancer in relation to use of oestrogen combined with cyclic progestagen therapy in postmenopausal women. Lancet 1997; 349: 458–61.
7. Pike MC, et al. Estrogen-progestin replacement therapy and endometrial cancer. J Natl Cancer Inst 1997; 89: 1110–16.
8. Cerin A, et al. Adverse endometrial effects of long-cycle estrogen and progestagen replacement therapy. N Engl J Med 1996; 334: 668–9.
9. Speroff L, et al. The comparative effect on bone density, endometrium, and lipids of continuous hormones as replacement therapy (CHART Study). JAMA 1996; 276: 1397–1403.
10. The Writing Group for the PEPI trial. Effects of hormone replacement therapy on endometrial histology in postmenopausal women. JAMA 1996; 275: 370–5.

GASTROINTESTINAL TRACT. Evidence of an effect of oestrogen replacement therapy on colorectal cancer is ambiguous, since studies have reported both an increased and a decreased incidence; a meta-analysis in 1995 suggested no overall effect.[1] However, subsequent cohort studies did suggest a lower incidence of colon cancer in those who had received oestrogens.[2,3] This was most pronounced in current users in whom the relative risk was about one-third to one-half of that for women who had never taken oestrogen. Similarly, a large case-control study also reported a significant reduction in colon cancer, but not rectal cancer.[4] A later meta-analysis[5] concluded that the risk of colon cancer might be decreased among women who have recently used HRT, and that the risk of death from colon cancer might also be reduced.

1. MacLennan SC, et al. Colorectal cancer and oestrogen replacement therapy: a meta-analysis of epidemiological studies. Med J Aust 1995; 162: 491–3.
2. Calle EE, et al. Estrogen replacement therapy and risk of fatal colon cancer in a prospective cohort of postmenopausal women. J Natl Cancer Inst 1995; 87: 517–23.
3. Grodstein F, et al. Postmenopausal hormone use and risk for colorectal cancer and adenoma. Ann Intern Med 1998; 128: 705–12.
4. Newcomb PA, Storer BE. Postmenopausal hormone use and risk of large-bowel cancer. J Natl Cancer Inst 1995; 87: 1067–71.
5. Nanda K, et al. Hormone replacement therapy and the risk of colorectal cancer: a meta-analysis. Obstet Gynecol 1999; 93: 880–8.

OVARY. There was no clear evidence that the use of oestrogen replacement therapy altered the risk of invasive ovarian cancer in various case-control studies reviewed by the Collaborative Ovarian Cancer Group.[1] However, more recent study of a large cohort has suggested that long-term oestrogen replacement therapy may increase the risk of fatal ovarian cancer.[2,3] Similarly, a meta-analysis indicated an increased risk for invasive epithelial ovarian cancer, especially after long-term use of HRT.[4]

1. Whittemore AS, et al. Characteristics relating to ovarian cancer risk: collaborative analysis of 12 US case-control studies. Am J Epidemiol 1992; 136: 1184–1203.
2. Rodriguez C, et al. Estrogen replacement therapy and fatal ovarian cancer. Am J Epidemiol 1995; 141: 828–35.
3. Rodriguez C, et al. Estrogen replacement therapy and ovarian cancer mortality in a large prospective study of US women. JAMA 2001; 285: 1460–5.
4. Garg PP, et al. Hormone replacement therapy and the risk of epithelial ovarian carcinoma: a meta-analysis. Obstet Gynecol 1998; 92: 472–9.

Effects on the cardiovascular system. Various facts support the theory that oestrogens may be cardioprotective. For example, mortality rates for cardiovascular disease in women are lower than those in men at all ages. In addition, women who

have a surgically induced menopause at a young age are at increased risk of ischaemic heart disease compared with women who have a natural menopause.

Conversely, use of high doses of oestrogens for malignant disease is associated with an increased risk of cardiovascular events. Similarly, use of oestrogens in combined oral contraceptives carries a small increased risk of cardiovascular disease (see p.1455). Moreover, an early study in men surviving a myocardial infarction found that high doses of conjugated oestrogens (5 mg daily) were associated with a higher incidence of subsequent coronary events than placebo (see Effects on the Cardiovascular System, in Conjugated Oestrogens, p.1467).

However, the majority of large observational studies have revealed a decreased risk of ischaemic heart disease and mortality in women receiving menopausal HRT compared with those who have never received this therapy (see below). Although progestogens may reduce the beneficial effects of oestrogens on some lipids, available data suggest that use of combined HRT is still cardioprotective. The reduction in risk has been estimated as 30 to 50%, although biases such as the healthy user effect are likely to play a part in this estimate and some results from controlled studies have cast doubt on the extent of any reduction in risk. Whether HRT reduces the risk of stroke is even less clear (see below) and it appears to be associated with an increased risk of venous thromboembolism (see below).

The mechanisms by which oestrogen exerts its cardiovascular effects are not fully understood.[1] Oestrogen has beneficial effects on lipoproteins, but adverse effects on triglycerides (see below). Similarly, it has beneficial effects on some, and adverse effects on other, mediators of thrombosis. Oestrogen may also have a direct beneficial effect on the coronary vasculature.

1. Mendelsohn ME, Karas RH. The protective effects of estrogen on the cardiovascular system. N Engl J Med 1999; 340: 1801–11.

HYPERTENSION. Although high doses of oestrogens have been associated with increased blood pressure, in normotensive women, use of menopausal HRT has little effect on blood pressure or may be associated with a small decrease. Similarly, there is some evidence that HRT does not alter blood pressure in hypertensive women.[1]

1. Lip GYH, et al. Hormone replacement therapy and blood pressure in hypertensive women. J Hum Hypertens 1994; 8: 491–4.

ISCHAEMIC HEART DISEASE. In 1991, Stampfer and Colditz reviewed 31 case-control and cohort studies on the risk of ischaemic heart disease in women using menopausal HRT.[1] Four studies showed an adverse trend, 2 showed no effect on risk, and 25 showed a trend to reduction in risk or a significant reduction in risk. The summary relative risk was 0.56, with estimated 95% confidence intervals of 0.50 to 0.61. Other reviews have reported similar reductions in risk.[2,3] Much of the data relate to the use of unopposed oestrogen, which is no longer recommended in women with a uterus because of the risk of endometrial cancer (see above).

There has been concern that the addition of progestogen might negate or reduce the cardiovascular benefits of oestrogens by reducing the oestrogen-induced rise in serum high-density-lipoprotein cholesterol concentrations. It has been postulated that this may be particularly true for progestogens derived from nortestosterone rather than progesterone. Results from the Postmenopausal Estrogen/Progestin Interventions Trial (PEPI) indicated that the beneficial effects on blood lipoproteins and fibrinogen, although greatest with unopposed oestrogen, were still present when combined with medroxyprogesterone or micronised progesterone (micronised progesterone was preferable to medroxyprogesterone).[4] Moreover, the UK Medical Research Council Study reported a fairly even balance between possibly beneficial and adverse effects on lipid concentrations and coagulability when conjugated oestrogens alone were compared with conjugated oestrogens plus norgestrel (a nortestosterone derivative).[5] Similar results were reported in the CHART study for ethinylestradiol with or without norethisterone.[6] Although reassuring, these 3 studies provide information only on surrogate end-points.

Data from the Nurses' Health Study cohort[7] showed a greater reduction in the risk of major ischaemic heart disease among women receiving an oestrogen plus a progestogen (relative risk 0.4) than those receiving an oestrogen alone (0.6), as compared with the risk in women not using hormones. In-vitro data suggest that progestogens may actually protect against atherosclerosis via inhibition of smooth muscle cell proliferation.[8]

As regards duration of HRT use, it appears that current use is the most important factor for cardiovascular risk reduction. Users with coronary risk factors appear to derive greater benefit from HRT than those at low risk of coronary artery disease.[9] Of concern, the Nurses' Health Study reported that the apparent benefit from HRT decreased with increasing duration of use beyond 10 years because of an increase in mortality from breast cancer.[9]

In contrast to previous findings, a retrospective case-control study[10] did not find a decreased risk of myocardial infarction in women currently using combined HRT or oestrogens alone. The authors of this study suggested that the benefit of HRT may not be as large as has been estimated in some qualitative overviews, and emphasised the need for data from randomised trials.[10] This has been confirmed by results[11] of the Heart and Estrogen/progestin Replacement Study, a randomised placebo-controlled trial in women with established ischaemic heart dis-

ease. Combined HRT with conjugated oestrogens plus medroxyprogesterone produced no overall reduction in the occurrence of myocardial infarction or death due to ischaemic heart disease in these women. This overall lack of effect was due to an initial increase in cardiac events during the first year, with a later beneficial effect. Another study, the Estrogen Replacement and Atherosclerosis trial, found that a similar HRT regimen did not affect the progression of existing coronary atherosclerosis as measured by angiography.[12]

These worrying results have suggested that HRT should not be used for secondary prevention in women with heart disease, in contrast to some earlier suggestions (see also under Uses and Administration, below), but the extent to which they can be extrapolated to women without pre-existing heart disease is unclear. Observational data from the Nurses' Health Study[13] showed a reduced risk of major coronary events in women without previous heart disease who were users of HRT, compared with never-users. It is hoped that the results of other ongoing randomised studies such as the Women's Health Initiative will provide a more definitive answer. There is also some evidence that the risks and benefits of HRT may vary according to the presence or absence of particular prothrombotic mutations.[14]

1. Stampfer MJ, Colditz GA. Estrogen replacement therapy and coronary heart disease: a quantitative assessment of the epidemiologic evidence. Prev Med 1991; 20: 47–63.
2. Grady D, et al. Hormone therapy to prevent disease and prolong life in postmenopausal women. Ann Intern Med 1992; 117: 1016–37.
3. Barrett-Connor E, Bush TL. Estrogen and coronary heart disease in women. JAMA 1991; 265: 1861–7.
4. The Writing Group for the PEPI Trial. Effects of estrogen or estrogen/progestin regimens on heart disease risk factors in postmenopausal women: the Postmenopausal Estrogen/Progestin Interventions (PEPI) Trial. JAMA 1995; 273: 199–208. Correction. ibid.; 274: 1676.
5. Medical Research Council's General Practice Research Framework. Randomised comparison of oestrogen versus oestrogen plus progestogen hormone replacement therapy in women with hysterectomy. BMJ 1996; 312: 473–8.
6. Speroff L, et al. The comparative effect on bone density, endometrium, and lipids of continuous hormones as replacement therapy (CHART Study): a randomized controlled trial. JAMA 1996; 276: 1397–1403.
7. Grodstein F, et al. Postmenopausal estrogen and progestin use and the risk of cardiovascular disease. N Engl J Med 1996; 335: 453–61. Correction. ibid.; 1046.
8. Lee W-S, et al. Progesterone inhibits arterial smooth muscle cell proliferation. Nature Med 1997; 3: 1005–1008.
9. Grodstein F, et al. Postmenopausal hormone therapy and mortality. N Engl J Med 1997; 336: 1769–75.
10. Sidney S, et al. Myocardial infarction and the use of estrogen and estrogen-progestogen in postmenopausal women. Ann Intern Med 1997; 127: 501–8.
11. Hulley S, et al. Randomized trial of estrogen plus progestin for secondary prevention of coronary heart disease in postmenopausal women. JAMA 1998; 280: 605–13.
12. Herrington DM, et al. Effects of estrogen replacement on the progression of coronary-artery atherosclerosis. N Engl J Med 2000; 343: 522–9.
13. Grodstein F, et al. A prospective, observational study of postmenopausal hormone therapy and primary prevention of cardiovascular disease. Ann Intern Med 2000; 133: 933–41.
14. Psaty BM, et al. Hormone replacement therapy, prothrombotic mutations, and the risk of incident nonfatal myocardial infarction in postmenopausal women. JAMA 2001; 285: 906–13.

STROKE. The Framingham Study suggested a more than twofold increased risk of stroke in women using menopausal HRT.[1] However, subsequent studies reporting risk of stroke separately from other cardiovascular events have shown either no effect on risk[2] or a decreased risk in the order of 30 to 50%.[3,4]

Data from the Nurses' Health Study cohort[5] revealed little association between the risk of stroke of any type and current use of unopposed oestrogens or oestrogen plus progestogen. However, they reported a trend towards an increased risk of stroke in current users of high-dose oestrogen therapy (1.25 mg or higher). Similarly, a large Danish case-control study found that unopposed oestrogens or oestrogen plus progestogen had no effect on the risk of non-fatal haemorrhagic or thromboembolic stroke,[6] and data from the Heart and Estrogen/Progestin Replacement Study indicated that combined HRT in women with pre-existing ischaemic heart disease had no effect on risk of stroke.[7]

1. Wilson PWF, et al. Postmenopausal estrogen use, cigarette smoking, and cardiovascular morbidity in women over 50: the Framingham study. N Engl J Med 1985; 313: 1038–43.
2. Stampfer MJ, et al. Postmenopausal estrogen therapy and cardiovascular disease: ten-year follow-up from the Nurses' Health Study. N Engl J Med 1991; 325: 756–62.
3. Paganini-Hill A, et al. Postmenopausal oestrogen treatment and stroke: a prospective study. BMJ 1988; 297: 519–22.
4. Finucane FF, et al. Decreased risk of stroke among postmenopausal hormone users: results from a national cohort. Arch Intern Med 1993; 153: 73–9.
5. Grodstein F, et al. Postmenopausal estrogen and progestin use and the risk of cardiovascular disease. N Engl J Med 1996; 335: 453–61. Correction. ibid.; 1406.
6. Tønnes Pedersen A, et al. Hormone replacement therapy and risk of non-fatal stroke. Lancet 1997; 350: 1277–83.
7. Simon JA, et al. Postmenopausal hormone therapy and risk of stroke: the Heart and Estrogen-progestin Replacement Study (HERS). Circulation 2001; 103: 638–42.

VENOUS THROMBOEMBOLISM. Traditionally it has been assumed that, unlike combined oral contraceptives, menopausal HRT is not associated with an increased risk of venous thromboembolism.

However, 4 recent observational studies have provided substantial evidence that there is an increased risk of deep-vein thrombosis and/or pulmonary embolism in women receiving HRT.[1-4] The relative risk of venous thromboembolism was found to be 2.1 to 3.6 in current users compared with past-users or those who had never received HRT. This equates to an excess of 16 to 23 cases per 100 000 women per year. One study found that the increase in risk was restricted to the first year of use.[4] Another reported an increased risk with increasing oestrogen dose.[2]

The UK Committee on Safety of Medicines considers that these data do not affect the risk-benefit ratio of therapy in women without predisposing factors for venous thromboembolism.[5] However, in some women with predisposing factors, such as a personal or family history of venous thromboembolism, severe varicose veins, obesity, surgery, trauma or prolonged bed-rest, the risk of venous thromboembolism may be increased. Evidence from a randomised placebo-controlled trial[6,7] supports the findings of the observational studies above.

1. Daly E, et al. Risk of venous thromboembolism in users of hormone replacement therapy. Lancet 1996; 348: 977–80.
2. Jick H, et al. Risk of hospital admission for idiopathic venous thromboembolism among users of postmenopausal oestrogens. Lancet 1996; 348: 981–83.
3. Grodstein F, et al. Prospective study of exogenous hormones and risk of pulmonary embolism in women. Lancet 1996; 348: 983–7.
4. Pérez Gutthann S, et al. Hormone replacement therapy and risk of venous thromboembolism: population based case-control study. BMJ 1997; 314: 796–800.
5. Committee on Safety of Medicines/Medicines Control Agency. Risk of venous thromboembolism with hormone replacement therapy. Current Problems 1997; 22: 9–10.
6. Grady D, Furberg C. Venous thromboembolic events associated with hormone replacement therapy. JAMA 1997; 278: 477.
7. Grady D, et al. Postmenopausal hormone therapy increases risk for venous thromboembolic disease: the Heart and Estrogen/progestin Replacement Study. Ann Intern Med 2000; 132: 689–96. Correction. ibid. 2001; 134: 81.

Effects on lipids. Oestrogens increase serum high-density-lipoprotein cholesterol and decrease low-density-lipoprotein cholesterol concentrations, effects that are considered favourable and may be a mechanism behind their apparent reduction in ischaemic heart disease in postmenopausal women (see Effects on the Cardiovascular System, above). However, they may also increase serum triglyceride concentrations, which is undesirable. Severe hypertriglyceridaemia and pancreatitis have occurred in women with hypertriglyceridaemia treated with oestrogens.[1,2] Use of concomitant progestogen reduces oestrogen-induced hypertriglyceridaemia.[2]

1. Glueck CJ, et al. Severe hypertriglyceridemia and pancreatitis when estrogen replacement therapy is given to hypertriglyceridemic women. J Lab Clin Med 1994; 123: 59–64.
2. Isley WL, Oki J. Estrogen-induced pancreatitis after discontinuation of concomitant medroxyprogesterone therapy. Am J Med 1997; 102: 416–17.

Pancreatitis. Unopposed oestrogen has been associated with pancreatitis in women with hypertriglyceridaemia (see Effects on Lipids, above).

Precautions

Before menopausal HRT is given the woman should undergo an appropriate medical examination and her medical history should be carefully evaluated. Regular examination is recommended during use.

HRT should be avoided in women with active thrombophlebitis or thromboembolic disease or undiagnosed abnormal vaginal bleeding, and abnormal vaginal bleeding during therapy should be investigated (see below). HRT is also contra-indicated in women with oestrogen-dependent neoplasms such as those of the breast or endometrium, and is usually considered contra-indicated in women with a history of these conditions although this has been debated (see below). Active liver disease, Dubin-Johnson or Rotor syndromes, severe cardiac disease, and severe diabetes with vascular changes are also generally considered to be contra-indications.

Prolonged exposure to unopposed oestrogens increases the risk of endometrial cancer whatever the route of administration (see above). HRT should be used with caution in women with antiphospholipid antibodies or predisposing factors to thromboembolism (see also Venous Thromboembolism, above), and in migraine, a history of breast nodules or fibrocystic disease, uterine fibroids, or a history of endometriosis. Consideration should be given to temporarily stopping HRT 4 to 6 weeks prior to elective surgery (but see also below).

HRT should be stopped immediately, and appropriate investigations and treatment carried out, if any of the following occur:

- sudden severe chest pain, sudden breathlessness, or severe pain/swelling in calf of one leg (possibly indicative of thromboembolic complications)

- unusual, severe, prolonged headache, sudden disturbances of vision or hearing or other perceptual disorders, collapse, marked numbness or weakness affecting one side of the body, or other signs or symptoms suggestive of cerebrovascular accident
- hepatitis, jaundice, generalised itching, liver enlargement, severe upper abdominal pain
- onset of severe depression
- significant rise in blood pressure (above 160 mmHg systolic or 100 mmHg diastolic)
- clear exacerbation of other conditions known to be capable of deteriorating during HRT or pregnancy.

Although evidence is in many cases less well established, HRT should perhaps also be used with caution in diseases which may be exacerbated during pregnancy or oestrogen therapy including diabetes, asthma, epilepsy, hypertension, cardiac or renal disease, sickle-cell disease, melanoma, otosclerosis, multiple sclerosis, systemic lupus erythematosus, and chorea. Doses of oestrogen in HRT are insufficient to provide contraception. HRT is contra-indicated in known or suspected pregnancy, and in women who are breast feeding.

Endometriosis. Endometriosis may be reactivated by unopposed oestrogen use in postmenopausal women. This has occurred, even in women who have previously undergone hysterectomy and bilateral oophorectomy for endometriosis.[1,2] Reactivation of endometriosis can result in ureteric obstruction and consequent renal damage.[1,2] Use of combined HRT rather than unopposed oestrogen has been advocated for women who have had radical surgery for endometriosis.[1]

1. Manyonda IT, et al. Obstructive uropathy from endometriosis after hysterectomy and oophorectomy: two case reports. Eur J Obstet Gynecol Reprod Biol 1989; 31: 195–8.
2. Brough RJ, O'Flynn K. Recurrent pelvic endometriosis and bilateral ureteric obstruction associated with hormone replacement therapy. BMJ 1996; 312: 1221–2.

Malignant neoplasms. HRT is usually avoided in women who have been treated for breast cancer because of the concern that oestrogen will stimulate cancer recurrence, although there is a lack of clinical evidence to substantiate this concern.[1] A recent retrospective case-control study among women diagnosed with breast cancer did not find any evidence of an adverse effect in those who began HRT after diagnosis.[2] A systematic review[3] of studies of HRT in breast cancer survivors reached a similar conclusion, but also noted that these studies were small, not randomised, and many were uncontrolled. It has been suggested that such therapy should not necessarily be withheld from these patients provided that the possible risks are understood.[1] Short-term continuous combined HRT in selected women with severe menopausal symptoms has been suggested.[4] Others suggest that HRT should be combined with tamoxifen in such patients.[5,6] For osteoporosis management and coronary heart disease prevention, alternatives to HRT are likely to be preferred.[7]

1. Cobleigh MA, et al. Estrogen replacement therapy in breast cancer survivors: a time for change. JAMA 1994; 272: 540–5.
2. O'Meara ES, et al. Hormone replacement therapy after a diagnosis of breast cancer in relation to recurrence and mortality. J Natl Cancer Inst 2001; 93: 754–62.
3. Col NF, et al. Hormone replacement therapy after breast cancer: a systematic review and quantitative assessment of risk. J Clin Oncol 2001; 19: 2357–63.
4. Eden JA. Estrogen replacement therapy in survivors of breast cancer: a risk-benefit assessment. Drugs Aging 1996; 8: 127–33.
5. Powles TJ, et al. Hormone replacement after breast cancer. Lancet 1993; 342: 60–1.
6. Powles TJ, Hickish T. Breast cancer response to hormone replacement therapy withdrawal. Lancet 1995; 345: 1442.
7. Chlebowski RT, McTiernan A. Elements of informed consent for hormone replacement therapy in patients with diagnosed breast cancer. J Clin Oncol 1999; 17: 130–42.

Porphyria. HRT should be used with caution in patients with porphyria.

Surgery. A review[1] recommended that women receiving HRT and due to have major elective surgery or leg surgery should continue taking the HRT and should routinely receive thromboprophylaxis (e.g. subcutaneous low-molecular-weight heparins and the use of graduated elastic compression stockings) in the perioperative period. Similar management was proposed when undergoing emergency surgery but prophylaxis was considered unnecessary with minor surgery. These conclusions were based on the advice of specialist groups but it was noted that there was some conflict with the manufacturers' recommendations and those of the British National Formulary. The British National Formulary states that it may be prudent to stop HRT a month before surgery; failing that, prophylaxis as above is recommended.

1. Anonymous. Drugs in the peri-operative period: hormonal contraceptives and hormone replacement therapy. Drug Ther Bull 1999; 37: 78–80.

Vaginal bleeding. Menopausal HRT is contra-indicated in patients with undiagnosed abnormal vaginal bleeding, which may be a symptom of endometrial carcinoma. The causes of

abnormal vaginal bleeding in women receiving HRT and guidelines on their investigation and treatment have been reviewed.[1,2]

1. Good AE. Diagnostic options for assessment of postmenopausal bleeding. Mayo Clin Proc 1997; 72: 345–9.
2. Spencer CP, et al. Management of abnormal bleeding in women receiving hormone replacement therapy. BMJ 1997; 315: 37–42.

Interactions

Drugs that increase the hepatic metabolism of oestrogens and progestogens have been associated with failure of the combined oral contraceptive (see p.1458). Important examples include rifamycins, some antiepileptics, and griseofulvin. It is not unreasonable to assume that these drugs would also be associated with decreased effectiveness of HRT, but there appears to be little information on this (for one report, see Antiepileptics, below).

Although oral contraceptives may antagonise or reduce the effects of a number of drugs (see p.1458), the lower doses of oestrogens used in HRT are considered less likely to induce interactions, although the possibility remains.

Alcohol. Acute ingestion of an alcoholic beverage led to a threefold increase in circulating estradiol in women on menopausal HRT.[1] The authors suggest that drinking habits may need to be considered when deciding on an appropriate dose of HRT.

1. Ginsburg ES, et al. Effects of alcohol ingestion on estrogens in postmenopausal women. JAMA 1996; 276: 1747–51.

Antiepileptics. A report of phenytoin diminishing the effect of conjugated oestrogens in a menopausal woman.[1]

1. Notelovitz M, et al. Interaction between estrogen and Dilantin in a menopausal woman. N Engl J Med 1981; 304: 788–9.

Thyroxine [levothyroxine]. For comment on the potential need for increased doses of thyroxine [levothyroxine] in hypothyroid women who receive oestrogens for postmenopausal HRT see p.1528.

Pharmacokinetics

For a discussion of the pharmacokinetics of oestrogens and progestogens, see Estradiol, p.1474 and Progesterone, p.1489, respectively. The extent of binding of progestogens to serum sex-hormone binding globulin may be altered when they are administered with an oestrogen. Oestrogens increase serum concentrations of sex-hormone binding globulin, and progestogens differ in their ability to suppress this effect.

Uses and Administration

The most commonly used oestrogens in menopausal HRT are natural oestrogens such as estradiol, and conjugated oestrogens. Dosages of oestrogens used in HRT are generally lower than those used in combined oral contraceptives, and do not therefore provide contraception.

Various dosage forms of the different oestrogenic compounds used for HRT are available, including oral tablets, intranasal sprays, subcutaneous implants, topical applications for vulvovaginal use, intravaginal rings, and transdermal skin patches and gels. Generally, if prolonged therapy (for more than 2 to 4 weeks) with an oestrogen by any route is envisaged in a woman with an intact uterus, a progestogen is required to prevent endometrial proliferation. This may be administered by mouth cyclically for 10 to 14 days per cycle or continuously; transdermal preparations are now also available. Both progesterone derivatives such as medroxyprogesterone and dydrogesterone, and 19-nortestosterone analogues such as norethisterone and norgestrel are used. Doses of progestogens for HRT are similar to those used in combined oral contraceptives.

Administration. In a discussion of the relative merits of oral and transdermal oestrogen therapy[1] it was suggested that there was circumstantial and theoretical evidence to suppose that transdermal therapy might be preferable in women who smoke, who suffer from migraine, hepatobiliary disease, or hypertriglyceridaemia, or who have a history of thromboembolism. In contrast, oral medication might be preferable in patients with hypercholesterolaemia. However, studies to examine these suppositions were needed. Various alternatives to oral oestrogen therapy have been reviewed.[2,3] For reviews of estradiol administration as implants or given transdermally, see p.1474.

1. Lufkin EG, Ory SJ. Relative value of transdermal and oral estrogen therapy in various clinical situations. Mayo Clin Proc 1994; 69: 131–5.

2. Baker VL. Alternatives to oral estrogen replacement: transdermal patches, percutaneous gels, vaginal creams and rings, implants, and other methods of delivery. *Obstet Gynecol Clin North Am* 1994; **21:** 271–97.
3. Jewelewicz R. New developments in topical estrogen therapy. *Fertil Steril* 1997; **67:** 1–12.

Cardiovascular disorders. Observational studies have shown a decreased risk of ischaemic heart disease and consequent mortality in women receiving menopausal HRT (see Ischaemic Heart Disease, under Adverse Effects, above) and oestrogens are known to have some beneficial effects on the plasma lipid profile (see Effects on Lipids, above). Data from a randomised crossover study[1] showed that both simvastatin and continuous conjugated oestrogens plus medroxyprogesterone had beneficial effects on plasma lipoprotein concentrations, although simvastatin was more effective. (In addition, the hormones increased, whereas simvastatin decreased, triglyceride concentrations.) However, results from a randomised study[2] in women with established ischaemic heart disease have shown an initial increase in adverse cardiac events when HRT was given, and although some benefit was seen after 4 or 5 years there was no overall decrease in myocardial infarction or cardiac death. These results suggest that HRT should not be initiated for the secondary prevention of ischaemic heart disease, but it may be appropriate for women already receiving treatment to continue.[3] Cardiovascular risk reduction, including management of blood lipids, is discussed on p.797.

Some observational studies have reported that women receiving HRT have better survival rates after revascularisation procedures (p.812) than women not receiving this therapy.[4,5]

1. Darling GM, *et al.* Estrogen and progestin compared with simvastatin for hypercholesterolemia in postmenopausal women. *N Engl J Med* 1997; **337:** 595–601.
2. Hulley S, *et al.* Randomized trial of estrogen plus progestin for secondary prevention of coronary heart disease in postmenopausal women. *JAMA* 1998; **280:** 605–13.
3. Mosca L, *et al.* Guide to preventive cardiology for women. *J Am Coll Cardiol* 1999; **33:** 1751–5.
4. O'Keefe JH, *et al.* Estrogen replacement therapy after coronary angioplasty in women. *J Am Coll Cardiol* 1997; **29:** 1–5.
5. Sullivan JM, *et al.* Effect on survival of estrogen replacement therapy after coronary artery bypass grafting. *Am J Cardiol* 1997; **79:** 847–50.

Dementia. Several observational studies[1-3] in women receiving HRT have suggested that oestrogens can reduce the risk and delay the onset of Alzheimer's disease (p.1412) in postmenopausal women. However, subsequent meta-analyses[4,5] concluded that studies conducted so far had substantial methodological problems and that results were conflicting. A long-term study of the value of HRT in Alzheimer's disease (Women's Health Initiative Clinical Trial) is in progress. Preliminary reports[6,7] suggest that treatment with oestrogens may also be of benefit in women who already have Alzheimer's disease; results of further studies are awaited.

1. Tang M-X, *et al.* Effect of oestrogen during menopause on risk and age at onset of Alzheimer's disease. *Lancet* 1996; **348:** 429–32.
2. Paganini-Hill A, Henderson VW. Estrogen replacement therapy and risk of Alzheimer disease. *Arch Intern Med* 1996; **156:** 2213–17.
3. Kawas C, *et al.* A prospective study of estrogen replacement therapy and the risk of developing Alzheimer's disease: the Baltimore Longitudinal Study of Aging. *Neurology* 1997; **48:** 1517–21.
4. Yaffe K, *et al.* Estrogen therapy in postmenopausal women: effects on cognitive function and dementia. *JAMA* 1998; **279:** 688–95.
5. LeBlanc ES, *et al.* Hormone replacement therapy and cognition: systematic review and meta-analysis. *JAMA* 2001; **285:** 1489–99.
6. Ohkura T, *et al.* Long-term estrogen replacement therapy in female patients with dementia of the Alzheimer type: 7 case reports. *Dementia* 1995; **6:** 99–107.
7. Schneider LS, *et al.* Potential role for estrogen replacement in the treatment of Alzheimer's dementia. *Am J Med* 1997; **103** (suppl 3A): 46S–50S.

Hyperparathyroidism. Oestrogens may ameliorate some consequences of hyperparathyroidism in postmenopausal women as well as mitigate osteoporosis,[1-4] but any long-term benefits are, as mentioned on p.746, uncertain.

1. Anonymous. Medical management of primary hyperparathyroidism. *Lancet* 1984; **ii:** 727–8.
2. Marcus R, *et al.* Conjugated estrogens in the treatment of postmenopausal women with hyperparathyroidism. *Ann Intern Med* 1984; **100:** 633–40.
3. Selby PL, Peacock M. Ethinyl estradiol and norethindrone in the treatment of primary hyperparathyroidism in postmenopausal women. *N Engl J Med* 1986; **314:** 1481–5.
4. Coe FL, *et al.* Is estrogen preferable to surgery for postmenopausal women with primary hyperparathyroidism? *N Engl J Med* 1986; **314:** 1508–9.

Menopausal disorders. ACUTE MENOPAUSAL SYMPTOMS. Where symptoms are severe enough to warrant treatment, HRT with oestrogens is the mainstay of treatment for *vasomotor symptoms and atrophic vaginitis.* Commentators[1-3] have suggested that there are few absolute contra-indications to the treatment of women with acute symptoms, although undiagnosed vaginal bleeding, before or during therapy, should always be investigated, as it can be a sign of endometrial cancer. In addition, women with active thrombophlebitis or thromboembolic disorders should not receive HRT, and the risk-benefit should be considered carefully in women with predisposing risk factors for venous thromboembolism. HRT should also not be used in women with oestrogen-dependent cancer, although

some have suggested that short-term HRT need not necessarily be withheld in women who have survived breast cancer if menopausal symptoms are severe and unresponsive to other measures (see also Malignant Neoplasms under Precautions, above).

If the woman is in the perimenopause she is potentially fertile, and HRT does not provide contraception. It is now considered that, in women under 50 years of age and free of all risk factors for venous and arterial disease, a low-oestrogen dose combined oral contraceptive (p.1459) can be used to provide both relief of menopausal symptoms and contraception.[4] If HRT is used in perimenopausal women, then non-hormonal contraceptive measures should be used if required (see p.1460).

Perimenopausal women with a uterus should also receive a cyclical progestogen, which will cause regular withdrawal bleeding. An alternative is the levonorgestrel intra-uterine device with concomitant oral or transdermal oestrogen.[5] In women with a uterus who are postmenopausal (greater than 12 months) continuous combined HRT may be used, which induces an atrophic endometrium. An alternative is the hormonal agent tibolone, which does not require concomitant progestogen. Women without a uterus, and who have not had endometriosis, may receive continuous oestrogen alone. For a discussion of the risks of endometrial cancer with HRT, see under Adverse Effects, above.

- In women experiencing solely *vaginal symptoms,* HRT administered just for a few weeks may be sufficient. This may be administered vaginally.
- In women experiencing *vasomotor symptoms,* oral or transdermal HRT is required. Most women do not require exogenous oestrogens to control hot flushes for more than 3 to 5 years; the lowest dose that controls symptoms is given, and therapy is tapered over a few years and withdrawn if prophylactic use of long-term effects is not required.[6] Nonpharmacological measures that may benefit some women with vasomotor symptoms include regular physical activity and stress management. Alternative medical therapies that may be tried include the progestogens megestrol and medroxyprogesterone, clonidine, or veralipride.[7,8] However, evidence for the efficacy of these alternative therapies is less conclusive than that for HRT. Evening primrose oil is not effective.[9] Women in cultures with diets high in plant oestrogens have low incidences of menopausal vasomotor symptoms suggesting a potential benefit from such diets.[10]
- *Non-specific symptoms* may also improve in women administered HRT. For example, oestrogens have reduced the incidence of urinary-tract infections,[11] and dysuria and incontinence (see below), although good evidence is somewhat scanty. Similarly, many women report improved mood and well-being when given oestrogens, although it is unclear to what extent this is due to relief of other symptoms. True depression does not respond to HRT, and needs to be identified and treated appropriately.[1] Moreover, the addition of progestogens carries some risk of adverse effects on mood such as depression, anxiety, and irritability. Androgens such as testosterone are sometimes used as adjuncts to HRT to improve psychological well-being and libido.[1,2]

LONG-TERM EFFECTS. Reliable estimates of the true benefits and risks for long-term HRT in postmenopausal women are not available, and hence for many women the balance of these risks remains controversial.[12-14] There are extensive data[10] from observational studies on the beneficial effects on fracture rates and cardiovascular disease, on the risks for development of breast cancer and endometrial cancer, and on the possible effects on overall mortality. However, the women receiving HRT in these studies may differ from women not receiving HRT, and the extent of any bias resulting from this is unclear. Randomised prospective studies are underway, but the first results will not be reported for a number of years. In the meantime, various authors have used the available data to suggest clinical guidelines.[1-3,5,6,15,16]

- It is generally agreed that all women who have had a *premature natural or induced menopause* should receive HRT until the age of 50 years, unless there are specific contra-indications to therapy (mentioned in the discussion of acute symptoms above). Considerations as to how long they need to continue HRT after the usual age for the menopause are probably the same as for other women.
- Women who have, or who are at risk of developing, *osteoporosis* should generally receive long-term HRT (but see also below). Risk factors for osteoporosis include familial predisposition, sedentary lifestyle, cigarette smoking, low body-weight, corticosteroid therapy, and a subnormal peak bone mass, for example, due to a calcium-deficient diet in childhood and adolescence. Where possible, treatment should be combined with adequate dietary calcium, weight-bearing exercise, and cessation of smoking.
- Women who have, or are at risk of developing, *ischaemic heart disease* have also been considered likely to benefit from HRT but recent studies cast some doubt on this (see above).
- Women who are at high risk of *breast cancer* should probably not receive long-term HRT (see also Malignant Neoplasms under Precautions, above). Those with a family history of breast cancer may be at particular risk.

Most authors agree that a woman should make an informed choice regarding HRT based on how she values each potential

effect. In general, studies that have modelled the various risks have estimated that the overall benefits of long-term HRT starting at about age 50 are likely to outweigh the risks except in women who are at high risk of breast cancer.[16,17] An important consideration in these analyses is that the data on incidence of each of the diseases are specific to the USA. Incidence rates of hip fracture, cardiovascular disease, and breast cancer vary widely between countries,[10] which may affect the choice. For example, a preliminary analysis using data from Italy suggested that use of HRT for 10 years was likely to result in an overall reduction in life expectancy in Italian women, who are at a low risk of ischaemic heart disease.[18]

The appropriate duration of HRT is also debated. For optimal benefits on bone and vasculature it is anticipated that HRT should be continued for 10 to 20 years or more.[15] However, the breast cancer risk increases with increasing duration of use. Moreover, the incidence of breast cancer may exceed that of cardiovascular disease in women aged less than 60 years. Therefore, some have suggested[19] that the best age to start HRT in asymptomatic women for prevention of osteoporosis and heart disease may be at age 65.

Long-term HRT for the treatment and prevention of osteoporosis is administered orally or transdermally. As mentioned above, oestrogens alone are suitable for women without a uterus who have not had endometriosis. In other women, a progestogen is also required to reduce the risk of endometrial hyperplasia and carcinoma (see also Carcinogenicity under Adverse Effects, above) or recurrence of endometriosis. This may be administered cyclically in perimenopausal women, but continuous administration is likely to be preferred in women who have been postmenopausal for more than 1 year since it avoids withdrawal bleeding. Tibolone is an alternative in women who have been postmenopausal for more than 1 year. Nonhormonal options for osteoporosis prophylaxis or treatment include bisphosphonates, as discussed on p.745. The selective oestrogen-receptor modulator raloxifene is also available.

1. Greendale GA, *et al.* The menopause. *Lancet* 1999; **353:** 571–80.
2. McKinney KA, Thompson W. A practical guide to prescribing hormone replacement therapy. *Drugs* 1998; **56:** 49–57.
3. McNagny SE. Prescribing hormone replacement therapy for menopausal symptoms. *Ann Intern Med* 1999; **131:** 605–16.
4. The North American Menopause Society. Clinical challenges of perimenopause: consensus opinion of the North American Menopause Society. *Menopause* 2000; **7:** 5–13.
5. Anonymous. Hormone replacement therapy. *Drug Ther Bull* 1996; **34:** 81–4.
6. The North American Menopause Society. A decision tree for the use of estrogen replacement therapy or hormone replacement therapy in postmenopausal women: consensus opinion of the North American Menopause Society. *Menopause* 2000; **7:** 76–86.
7. Young RL, *et al.* Management of menopause when estrogen cannot be used. *Drugs* 1990; **40:** 220–30.
8. Luchero MA, McCloskey WW. Alternatives to estrogen for the treatment of hot flushes. *Ann Pharmacother* 1997; **31:** 915–17.
9. Chenoy R, *et al.* Effect of oral gamolenic acid from evening primrose oil on menopausal flushing. *BMJ* 1994; **308:** 501–3.
10. WHO. Research on the menopause in the 1990s. *WHO Tech Rep Ser* 866 1996.
11. Raz R, Stamm WE. A controlled trial of intravaginal estriol in postmenopausal women with recurrent urinary tract infections. *N Engl J Med* 1993; **329:** 753–6.
12. Toozs-Hobson P, Cardoz L. Hormone replacement therapy for all? Universal prescription is desirable. *BMJ* 1996; **313:** 350–1.
13. Jacobs HS. Hormone replacement therapy for all? Not for everybody. *BMJ* 1996; **313:** 351–2.
14. Clinical Synthesis Panel on HRT. Hormone replacement therapy. *Lancet* 1999; **354:** 152–5. Correction. *ibid.;* 870.
15. American College of Physicians. Guidelines for counselling postmenopausal women about preventive hormone therapy. *Ann Intern Med* 1992; **117:** 1038–41.
16. Grady D, *et al.* Hormone therapy to prevent disease and prolong life in postmenopausal women. *Ann Intern Med* 1992; **117:** 1016–37.
17. Col NF, *et al.* Patient-specific decisions about hormone replacement therapy in postmenopausal women. *JAMA* 1997; **277:** 1140–7.
18. Panico S, *et al.* Hormone replacement therapy may not always be right choice to prevent cardiovascular disease. *BMJ* 1996; **313:** 687.
19. Prince RL, Geelhoed EA. When should postmenopausal women start taking oestrogen replacement therapy? *Med J Aust* 1995; **162:** 173–4.

Osteoporosis. Oestrogens are currently the preferred method of treating and preventing postmenopausal osteoporosis, as discussed on p.745. They have a direct antiresorptive effect on bone, and will increase bone mass density (BMD). Suggested minimum daily doses are 0.625 mg of conjugated oestrogens by mouth, 2 mg of estradiol by mouth or 50 μg transdermally, and 15 μg of ethinylestradiol by mouth.[1] Addition of a progestogen (required to prevent endometrial hyperplasia in women with a uterus) does not impair the beneficial effect of oestrogens on BMD, whether administered cyclically or continuously,[2,3] and may provide a further reduction in risk of fractures.[4] Unresolved issues are the duration of therapy required to prevent fractures in old age,[4,5] and the ideal age to start therapy to obtain the maximum benefits to the bone with the minimum risk of breast cancer.[6] Worryingly, recent data from the Heart and Estrogen/Progestin Replacement Study, which has forced a re-evaluation of the potential cardiovascular benefits of HRT, also call into question the benefit of HRT in reducing the incidence of fractures.[6] A meta-analysis[7] including these data, most of which were from women without osteoporosis, consequently found only nonsignificant reduction in fracture risk in older women although overall the risk of fracture was reduced by between 20 and 30%.

Oestrogens are also used in women to reduce the risk of corticosteroid-induced osteoporosis (see Effects on Bones and Joints, p.1040).

1. Jacobs HS, Loeffler FE. Postmenopausal hormone replacement therapy. *BMJ* 1992; **305:** 1403–8.
2. The Writing Group for the PEPI trial. Effects of hormone therapy on bone mineral density: results from the Postmenopausal Estrogen/Progestin Interventions (PEPI) trial. *JAMA* 1996; **276:** 1389–96.
3. Speroff L, *et al.* The comparative effect on bone density, endometrium, and lipids of continuous hormones as replacement therapy (CHART Study): a randomized controlled trial. *JAMA* 1996; **276:** 1397–1403.
4. Michaëlsson K, *et al.* Hormone replacement therapy and risk of hip fracture: population based case-control study. *BMJ* 1998; **316:** 1858–63.
5. Schneider DL, *et al.* Timing of postmenopausal estrogen for optimal bone mineral density: the Rancho Bernardo study. *JAMA* 1997; **277:** 543–7.
6. Cauley JA, *et al.* Effects of hormone replacement therapy on clinical fractures and height loss: the Heart and Estrogen/Progestin Replacement Study (HERS). *Am J Med* 2001; **110:** 442–50.
7. Torgerson DJ, Bell-Syer SEM. Hormone replacement therapy and prevention of nonvertebral fractures: a meta-analysis of randomized trials. *JAMA* 2001; **285:** 2891–7.

Urinary incontinence. Urinary incontinence (p.459) may be one of a number of acute symptoms associated with a decline in oestrogen levels at the menopause (see Menopausal Disorders, above). Studies[1,2] suggest that oestrogens used with alpha-adrenoceptor agonists are effective in the management of female stress incontinence and this combination has been advocated for use in postmenopausal patients with mild symptoms. Unfortunately addition of a progestogen to treatment to reduce the risk of endometrial carcinoma in women with an intact uterus might exacerbate the incontinence.[3] The value of oestrogens used without an alpha-adrenoceptor agonist in urinary incontinence is less clear. Some workers[4] consider that oestrogens may be of use for symptoms of urgency, frequency, and nocturia in postmenopausal patients with urge incontinence; it has been suggested that hypoestrogenism may reduce the sensory threshold of the bladder.[5] A meta-analysis of 23 studies concluded that oestrogen therapy subjectively improved urinary incontinence in postmenopausal women but many of the studies examined were considered to be deficient in some respect.[6] A later well-designed study[7] found that HRT did not improve measures of incontinence in such patients although there was the possibility that concomitant progestogen therapy might have affected efficacy.

1. Walter S, *et al.* Stress urinary incontinence in postmenopausal women treated with oral estrogen (estriol) and an alpha-adrenoceptor-stimulating agent (phenylpropanolamine): a randomized double-blind placebo-controlled study. *Int Urogynecol J* 1990; **1:** 74–9.
2. Hilton P, *et al.* Oral and intravaginal estrogens alone and in combination with alpha-adrenergic stimulation in genuine stress incontinence. *Int Urogynecol J* 1990; **1:** 80–6.
3. Benness C, *et al.* Do progestogens exacerbate urinary incontinence in women on HRT? *Neurourol Urodyn* 1991; **10:** 316–17.
4. Cardozo L. Role of estrogens in the treatment of female urinary incontinence. *J Am Geriatr Soc* 1990; **38:** 326–8.
5. Fantl JA, *et al.* Postmenopausal urinary incontinence: comparison between non-estrogen-supplemented and estrogen-supplemented women. *Obstet Gynecol* 1988; **71:** 823–8.
6. Fantl JA *et al.* Estrogen therapy in the management of urinary incontinence in postmenopausal women: a meta-analysis: first report of the hormones and urogenital therapy committee. *Obstet Gynecol* 1994; **83:** 12–18.
7. Fantl JA, *et al.* Efficacy of estrogen supplementation in the treatment of urinary incontinence. *Obstet Gynecol* 1996; **88:** 745–9.

Algestone Acetophenide (9022-d)

Algestone Acetophenide *(USAN, rINNM)*.

Alphasone Acetophenide; Dihydroxyprogesterone Acetophenide; SQ-15101. 16α,17α-(1-Phenylethylidenedioxy)pregn-4-ene-3,20-dione; 16α,17α-Isopropylidenedioxypregn-4-ene-3,20-dione.
$C_{29}H_{36}O_4 = 448.6$.
CAS — 595-77-7 (algestone); 24356-94-3 (algestone acetophenide).

Profile
Algestone acetophenide is a progestogen (see Progesterone, p.1488) that is given by intramuscular injection in monthly doses of 150 mg in conjunction with estradiol enantate as a hormonal contraceptive (see p.1452). It has also been applied topically in the treatment of acne.

◊ References.
1. Martínez GH, *et al.* Vaginal bleeding patterns in users of Perlutal®, a once-a-month injectable contraceptive consisting of 10 mg estradiol enantate combined with 150 mg dihydroxyprogesterone acetophenide: a trial of 5462 woman-months. *Contraception* 1998; **58:** 21–7.

Preparations
Proprietary Preparations (details are given in Part 3)
Multi-ingredient: *Braz.:* Ciclovular; Evitas; Perlutan; Uno-Ciclo; *Hong Kong:* Progestrol†; *Mex.:* Anafertin; Patector; Perlutal; Yectames; *Port.:* Cicnor; *Spain:* Topasel.

Allylestrenol (9023-n)

Allylestrenol *(BAN, rINN)*.
Allyloestrenol. 17α-Allylestr-4-en-17β-ol.
$C_{21}H_{32}O = 300.5$.
CAS — 432-60-0.
ATC — G03DC01.

Profile
Allylestrenol is a progestogen (see Progesterone, p.1488) structurally related to progesterone that has been given in threatened and recurrent miscarriage, and to prevent premature labour. However, with the exception of proven progesterone deficiency, such use is no longer recommended. In threatened miscarriage in progesterone-deficient women a suggested dose is 5 mg three times daily by mouth for 5 to 7 days.

◊ A case-control study of allylestrenol use in pregnancy during 1980 to 1984 in Hungary indicated that it was not teratogenic.[1]

1. Czeizel A, Huiskes N. A case-control study to evaluate the risk of congenital anomalies as a result of allylestrenol therapy during pregnancy. *Clin Ther* 1988; **10:** 725–39.

Preparations
Proprietary Preparations (details are given in Part 3)
Aust.: Gestanon†; ***Braz.:*** Orageston; ***Hong Kong:*** Turinal; ***Mex.:*** Crestanon; Gestanon; ***Singapore:*** Turinal.

Altrenogest (12346-m)

Altrenogest *(BAN, USAN, rINN)*.
A-35957; A-41300; RH-2267; RU-2267. 17α-Allyl-17β-hydroxy-19-norandrosta-4,9,11-trien-3-one; 17β-Hydroxy-19,21,24-trinorchola-4,9,11,22-tetraen-3-one.
$C_{21}H_{26}O_2 = 310.4$.
CAS — 850-52-2.

Profile
Altrenogest is a progestogen (see Progesterone, p.1488) used in veterinary medicine.

Androstanolone (9103-n)

Androstanolone *(BAN, rINN)*.
Dihydrotestosterone; Stanolone. 17β-Hydroxy-5α-androstan-3-one.
$C_{19}H_{30}O_2 = 290.4$.
CAS — 521-18-6.
ATC — A14AA01; G03BB02.

Profile
Androstanolone (dihydrotestosterone) is formed naturally in the body from testosterone (p.1492) by the action of 5α-reductase, and is more active than the parent compound. It has anabolic and androgenic properties and is applied topically in the form of a 2.5% gel for male hypogonadism, gynaecomastia, and for lichen sclerosus in both men and women.

Lichen sclerosus. For references to the use of androgens such as androstanolone in lichen sclerosus, see under Testosterone, p.1494.

Preparations
Proprietary Preparations (details are given in Part 3)
Belg.: Andractim; ***Fr.:*** Andractim; ***Spain:*** Gelovit†; ***Thai.:*** Andractim.

Androstenedione (20324-x)

Androst-4-ene-3,17-dione.
$C_{19}H_{26}O_2 = 286.4$.
CAS — 63-05-8.

Profile
Androstenedione is a naturally occurring adrenal androgen which is a precursor of androgens and oestrogens (see p.1452). It has been employed in an attempt to enhance athletic performance and as hormone replacement for men.

◊ In young men with normal testosterone concentrations, androstenedione 300 mg daily did not increase serum testosterone but did increase serum oestrogen concentrations.[1] However another study in healthy male subjects found that a similar dose of androstenedione increased both serum testosterone and serum estradiol concentrations, although the change in the latter was more marked and there was considerable interindividual variation in response.[2] Androstenedione did not enhance the effects of resistance training.[1]

1. King DS, *et al.* Effect of oral androstenedione on serum testosterone and adaptations to resistance training in young men: a randomized controlled trial. *JAMA* 1999; **281:** 2020–8.
2. Leder BZ, *et al.* Oral androstenedione administration and serum testosterone concentrations in young men. *JAMA* 2000; **283:** 779–82.

Preparations
Proprietary Preparations (details are given in Part 3)
Multi-ingredient: *Thai.:* Metharmon-F.

Broparestrol (12456-s)

Broparestrol *(rINN)*.
α-Bromo-β-(4-ethylphenyl)stilbene.
$C_{22}H_{19}Br = 363.3$.
CAS — 479-68-5.

Profile
Broparestrol is a synthetic nonsteroidal oestrogen (see Diethylstilbestrol, p.1471) that has been used as an ingredient of preparations promoted for topical use in acne and similar skin disorders. It has been given in neoplastic disease.

Preparations
Proprietary Preparations (details are given in Part 3)
Multi-ingredient: *Fr.:* Acnestrol†.

Chlormadinone Acetate (9027-v)

Chlormadinone Acetate *(BANM, USAN, rINNM)*.
NSC-92338. 6-Chloro-17-hydroxypregna-4,6-diene-3,20-dione acetate.
$C_{23}H_{29}ClO_4 = 404.9$.
CAS — 1961-77-9 (chlormadinone); 302-22-7 (chlormadinone acetate).
Pharmacopoeias. In Fr., Jpn., and Pol.

Adverse Effects and Precautions
As for progestogens in general (see Progesterone, p.1488).

Effects on the skin. A report of auto-immune dermatitis in one patient associated with chlormadinone acetate.[1]
1. Katayama I, Nishioka K. Autoimmune progesterone dermatitis with persistent amenorrhoea. *Br J Dermatol* 1985; **112:** 487–91.

Interactions
As for progestogens in general (see Progesterone, p.1489).

Uses and Administration
Chlormadinone acetate is a progestogen structurally related to progesterone (p.1489) that may have some anti-androgenic activity. It is given by mouth either alone or in combination with an oestrogen in the treatment of menstrual disorders such as menorrhagia (p.1490) and endometriosis (p.1469) at doses of 2 to 10 mg daily either cyclically or continuously. It may also be used as the progestogen component of combined oral contraceptives (see p.1459) at a dose of 1 to 2 mg daily, particularly in women with androgen-dependent conditions such as acne and hirsutism. Chlormadinone acetate has been used in some countries in the management of prostate cancer.

Preparations
Proprietary Preparations (details are given in Part 3)
Fr.: Luteran; *Ger.:* Gestafortin; *Jpn:* Prostal; *Mex.:* Lutoral; Nidal.

Multi-ingredient: *Fr.:* Lutestral†; *Ger.:* Belara; Gestamestrol N; Neo-Eunomin; Ovosiston; *Mex.:* Lutoral E; Secuentex-21; *Switz.:* Neo-Eunomine.

Chlorotrianisene (9029-q)

Chlorotrianisene *(BAN, rINN)*.
NSC-10108; Tri-p-anisylchloroethylene. Chlorotris(4-methoxyphenyl)ethylene.
$C_{23}H_{21}ClO_3 = 380.9$.
CAS — 569-57-3.
ATC — G03CA06.
Pharmacopoeias. In Chin.

Profile
Chlorotrianisene is a synthetic nonsteroidal oestrogen structurally related to diethylstilbestrol (p.1471). It has a prolonged action, and has been given by mouth for the treatment of menopausal symptoms, female hypogonadism, and prostatic carcinoma.

Preparations
Proprietary Preparations (details are given in Part 3)
Mex.: Estregur; *Spain:* Tace†; *USA:* Tace†.

Clomifene Citrate (9031-n)

Clomifene Citrate *(BANM, rINNM)*.
Chloramiphene Citrate; Clomifeni Citras; Clomiphene Citrate *(USAN)*; MER-41; MRL-41; NSC-35770. A mixture of the *E* and *Z* isomers of 2-[4-(2-chloro-1,2-diphenylvinyl)phenoxy]triethylamine dihydrogen citrate.
$C_{26}H_{28}ClNO, C_6H_8O_7 = 598.1$.
CAS — 911-45-5 (clomifene); 15690-57-0 ((E)-clomifene); 15690-55-8 ((Z)-clomifene); 50-41-9 (clomifene citrate); 7599-79-3 ((E)-clomifene citrate); 7619-53-6 ((Z)-clomifene citrate).

NOTE. Clomifene may be separated into its *Z* and *E* isomers, zuclomifene and enclomifene.

Pharmacopoeias. In Chin., Eur. (see p.vi), Int., Jpn, and US.

Pharmacopoeial description

Ph. Eur.: A white or pale yellow, crystalline powder. It contains 30 to 50% of the *Z* isomer. Slightly soluble in water; sparingly soluble in alcohol; practically insoluble in ether. Protect from light.

USP 25: A white to pale yellow, essentially odourless powder. It contains 30 to 50% of the *Z* isomer. Slightly soluble in water and in chloroform; sparingly soluble in alcohol; insoluble in ether; freely soluble in methyl alcohol.

Adverse Effects

The incidence and severity of adverse effects of clomifene citrate tend to be related to the dose employed. The most commonly reported adverse effects are reversible ovarian enlargement and cyst formation, vasomotor flushes resembling menopausal symptoms, and abdominal or pelvic discomfort or pain, sometimes with nausea or vomiting. Ovarian hyperstimulation syndrome has occurred. Breast tenderness, abnormal uterine bleeding, weight gain, headache, and endometriosis have also been reported. Transient visual disturbances such as after-images and blurring of vision may occur, and there have been rare reports of cataracts. Skin reactions such as allergic rashes and urticaria have occasionally been reported and reversible hair loss has been reported rarely. CNS disturbances have included convulsions, dizziness, lightheadedness, nervous tension, fatigue, vertigo, insomnia, and depression. Abnormalities in liver function tests and jaundice have sometimes been reported.

Following therapy with clomifene citrate there is an increased risk of multiple births, but rarely more than twins. There is also an increased risk of ectopic pregnancy. Although there have been reports of congenital disorders such as neural tube defects or Down's syndrome in infants born to women treated with clomifene the role of the drug in the causation of these defects has not been established and the incidence is reported to be similar to that in women with other types of infertility problems.

Carcinogenicity. There have been a number of reports suggesting an association between drug therapy to treat infertility by stimulating ovulation and the subsequent development of ovarian cancer.[1-5] Concern has focussed in particular on the use of clomifene citrate and gonadotrophins, and a study has reported an increased risk of ovarian cancer in women who had prolonged clomifene therapy (for one year or more) although not in those who received the drug for a shorter period.[6] No association between gonadotrophin therapy and ovarian cancer was noted in this study. The conclusions of this study are only tentative, since the numbers who developed ovarian cancer were small, and it has been pointed out that a successfully achieved pregnancy may reduce the risk of some other cancers, and that the risks and benefits of the procedure are not easy to balance.[7] However, as a matter of prudence the UK Committee on Safety of Medicines has recommended that clomifene should not normally be used for more than 6 cycles.[8]

1. Fishel S, Jackson P. Follicular stimulation for high tech pregnancies: are we playing it safe? *BMJ* 1989; **299:** 309–11.
2. Kulkarni R, McGarry JM. Follicular stimulation and ovarian cancer. *BMJ* 1989; **299:** 740.
3. Dietl J. Ovulation and ovarian cancer. *Lancet* 1991; **338:** 445.
4. Willemsen W, *et al.* Ovarian stimulation and granulosa-cell tumour. *Lancet* 1993; **341:** 986–8.
5. Tewari K, *et al.* Fertility drugs and malignant germ-cell tumour of ovary in pregnancy. *Lancet* 1997; **351:** 957–8.
6. Rossing MA, *et al.* Ovarian tumors in a cohort of infertile women. *N Engl J Med* 1994; **331:** 77–6.
7. Whittemore AS. The risk of ovarian cancer after treatment for infertility. *N Engl J Med* 1994; **331:** 805–6.
8. Committee on Safety of Medicines/Medicines Control Agency. Clomiphene (Clomid, Serophene): possible association with ovarian cancer. *Current Problems* 1995; **21:** 7.

Effects on the CNS. A report of convulsions following administration of clomifene citrate to an infertile woman;[1] only five other cases had been reported since 1963.

1. Rimmington MR, *et al.* Convulsions after clomiphene citrate. *BMJ* 1994; **309:** 512.

Effects on the eyes. As mentioned above, clomifene may cause visual disturbances, which resolve on cessation of treatment. However, visual symptoms have persisted in a few cases.[1]

1. Purvin VA. Visual disturbance secondary to clomiphene citrate. *Arch Ophthalmol* 1995; **113:** 482–4.

Effects on the fetus. Discussions and individual reports of congenital disorders after treatment of the mother with clomifene,[1-10] plus evidence that the incidence of fetal disorders is not increased following infertility treatment.[11-13]

1. Dyson JL, Kohler HG. Anencephaly and ovulation stimulation. *Lancet* 1973; **i:** 1256–7.

2. Field B, Kerr C. Ovulation stimulation and defects of neural-tube closure. *Lancet* 1974; **ii:** 1511.
3. Singh M, Singhi S. Possible relationship between clomiphene and neural tube defects. *J Pediatr* 1978; **93:** 152.
4. Halal F, *et al.* Méga-urètre, hypospadias et anus imperforé chez un nouveau-né: rôle possible du clomiphène pris par la mère. *Can Med Assoc J* 1980; **122:** 1159–60.
5. Cornel MC, *et al.* Ovulation induction and neural tube defects. *Lancet* 1989; **i:** 1386.
6. Czeizel A. Ovulation induction and neural tube defects. *Lancet* 1989; **ii:** 167.
7. Cuckle H, Wald N. Ovulation induction and neural tube defects. *Lancet* 1989; **ii:** 1281.
8. Cornel MC, *et al.* Ovulation induction, in-vitro fertilisation, and neural tube defects. *Lancet* 1989; **ii:** 1530.
9. Vollset SE. Ovulation induction and neural tube defects. *Lancet* 1990; **337:** 178.
10. White L, *et al.* Neuroectodermal tumours in children born after assisted conception. *Lancet* 1990; **336:** 1577.
11. Mills JL, *et al.* Risk of neural tube defects in relation to maternal fertility and fertility drug use. *Lancet* 1990; **336:** 103–4.
12. Rosa F. Ovulation induction and neural tube defects. *Lancet* 1990; **336:** 1327.
13. Werler MM, *et al.* Ovulation induction and risk of neural tube defects. *Lancet* 1994; **344:** 445–6.

Precautions

Clomifene is contra-indicated in patients with liver disease and the potential for toxicity should be considered in patients with a history of liver dysfunction. It should not be used in pregnancy, or in patients with undiagnosed abnormal uterine bleeding; some sources suggest it should also be avoided in patients with hormone-dependent tumours, and in those with pre-existing mental depression or thrombophlebitis because of the risk of exacerbation. The cause of infertility should be investigated. The patient should be warned of the possibility of multiple births, particularly if higher doses are used.

Patients undergoing therapy with clomifene, particularly those with polycystic ovaries, should receive the lowest doses possible to minimise ovarian enlargement or cyst formation. The patient should be instructed to report any abdominal or pelvic pain as this may indicate the presence or enlargement of ovarian cysts. They should also be evaluated for the presence of ovarian cysts before each cycle of treatment. If abnormal enlargement occurs, clomifene should not be given until the ovaries have returned to pre-treatment size, and subsequent doses should be reduced. Clomifene should be used with caution in patients with uterine fibroids, due to the potential for enlargement of the fibroids.

Treatment should be discontinued if visual disturbances develop and the patient warned that this might affect his or her ability to drive or operate machinery. Long-term cyclic therapy is not recommended, because of the uncertainty regarding increased risk of ovarian cancer (see above): in the UK a maximum of 6 cycles of treatment is advised.

Pharmacokinetics

Clomifene citrate is absorbed from the gastrointestinal tract. It is metabolised in the liver and slowly excreted via the bile. Unchanged drug and metabolites are excreted in the faeces. The biological half-life is reported to be 5 days although traces are found in the faeces for up to 6 weeks. Enterohepatic recirculation takes place. The *E*-isomer is reported to be less well absorbed and more rapidly eliminated than the *Z*-isomer.

◊ References.

1. Szutu M, *et al.* Pharmacokinetics of intravenous clomiphene isomers. *Br J Clin Pharmacol* 1989; **27:** 639–40.

Uses and Administration

Clomifene is chemically related to chlorotrianisene (p.1465) and has both oestrogenic and anti-oestrogenic properties, the latter residing principally in the *E*-isomer. Its action in stimulating ovulation is believed to be related to its anti-oestrogenic properties. It stimulates the secretion of pituitary gonadotrophic hormones, probably by blocking the negative feedback effect of oestrogens at receptor sites in the hypothalamus and pituitary.

Clomifene is the most widely used drug in the treatment of anovulatory infertility (p.1275). Therapy with clomifene will not be successful unless the woman, though anovulatory, is capable of ovulation

and her partner is fertile. It is ineffective in primary pituitary or primary ovarian failure. The usual dose by mouth is 50 mg of the citrate daily for 5 days, starting on or about the 5th day of the menstrual cycle or at any time if there is amenorrhoea. If ovulation does not occur, a course of 100 mg daily for 5 days may be given starting as early as 30 days after the previous one. Women should be examined for pregnancy and ovarian enlargement or cysts between treatment cycles. In general, 3 courses of therapy are adequate to assess whether ovulation is obtainable. If ovulation has not occurred, the diagnosis should be re-evaluated. Once ovulation is established, each treatment cycle of clomifene should be started on or about the 5th day of the menstrual cycle. If pregnancy has not occurred after a total of about 6 treatment cycles, further clomifene therapy is not recommended (see Precautions, above).

Clomifene has also been used in conjunction with gonadotrophins and in *in-vitro* fertilisation programmes.

Clomifene has also been used in the treatment of male infertility due to oligospermia to stimulate gonadotrophin release and enhance spermatogenesis.

Infertility. Systematic reviews have indicated that clomifene therapy was effective in the management of unexplained subfertility[1] or oligo-amenorrhoea[2] in women, although the absolute treatment effect was small in the former case, and concerns about the adverse effects remained. Evidence of improved fertility following clomifene treatment in men with idiopathic oligospermia or asthenospermia was lacking,[3] although treatment appeared to have a beneficial effect on some endocrine outcomes.

1. Hughes E, *et al.* Clomiphene citrate for unexplained subfertility in women (updated 29 May 2001). Available in The Cochrane Library; Issue 3. Oxford: Update Software; 2001.
2. Hughes E, *et al.* Clomiphene citrate for ovulation induction in women with oligo-amenorrhoea (updated 29 May 2001). Available in The Cochrane Library; Issue 3. Oxford: Update Software; 2001.
3. Vandekerckhove P, *et al.* Clomiphene or tamoxifen for idiopathic oligo/asthenospermia (updated 28 May 2001). Available in The Cochrane Library; Issue 3. Oxford: Update Software; 2001.

Preparations

BP 2001: Clomifene Tablets;
USP 25: Clomiphene Citrate Tablets.

Proprietary Preparations (details are given in Part 3)

Aust.: Clomid; Serophene; **Austral.:** Clomhexal; Clomid; Serophene; **Belg.:** Clomid; **Braz.:** Clomid; Serofene; **Canad.:** Clomid; Serophene; **Denm.:** Clomivid; Pergotime; **Fin.:** Clomifen; **Fr.:** Clomid; Pergotime; **Ger.:** Clomhexal; Clostilbegyt†; Dyneric; Pergotime†; **Hong Kong:** Arcafen; Clomid; Clostilbegyt; Duinum; Fertilan; Ova-Mit; Serophene; **Irl.:** Clomid; Serophene; **Israel:** Ikaclomin; **Ital.:** Clomid; Prolifen; Serofene; **Mex.:** Omifin; Serofene; **Neth.:** Clomid; Serophene; **Norw.:** Clomid; Serophene; Pergotime; **NZ:** Clomid; Phenate; Serophene; **Port.:** Dufine; **S.Afr.:** Clomid; Fertomid; Serophene; **Singapore:** Clomid; Clostilbegyt; Duinum; Ova-Mit; Phenate; Serophene; **Spain:** Clomifeno; Omifin†; **Swed.:** Clomivid; Pergotime; **Switz.:** Clomid; Serophene; **Thai.:** Clomid; Duinum; Omicite; Ova-Mit; Ovinum; Serophene; **UK:** Clomid; Serophene†; **USA:** Clomid; Milophene†; Serophene.

Clostebol Acetate (9032-h)

Clostebol Acetate (BAN, rINNM).

4-Chlorotestosterone Acetate; Chlortestosterone Acetate. 4-Chloro-3-oxoandrost-4-en-17β-yl acetate; 4-Chloro-17β-hydroxyandrost-4-en-3-one acetate.

$C_{21}H_{29}ClO_3 = 364.9$.

CAS — 1093-58-9 (clostebol); 855-19-6 (clostebol acetate).

Profile

Clostebol acetate has anabolic properties (see Testosterone, p.1492) and is given in doses of 30 mg weekly by intramuscular injection, or 15 mg 2 or 3 times daily by mouth, for 3 weeks followed by a 3-week pause. It has also been applied topically to wounds and ulcers, and has been used as an ophthalmological preparation.

Preparations

Proprietary Preparations (details are given in Part 3)
Ger.: Megagrisevit; **Mex.:** Trofodermin-S.

Multi-ingredient: Braz.: Trofodermin; **Ital.:** Trofodermin; **Thai.:** Trofodermin.

Conjugated Oestrogens (9091-y)

Conjugated Estrogens; Estrogeni Coniuncti.
ATC — G03CA57.
Pharmacopoeias. In *Eur.* (see p.vi) and *US.*

Pharmacopoeial description
Ph. Eur.: A mixture of various conjugated forms of oestrogens obtained from the urine of pregnant mares or by synthesis, dispersed in a suitable powdered diluent. It contains two principal components, 52.5 to 61.5% of sodium estrone sulfate and 22.5 to 30.5% of sodium equilin sulfate; the total of the combined two is 79.5 to 88.0%. It also contains 2.5 to 9.5% of sodium 17α-estradiol sulfate, 13.5 to 19.5% of sodium 17α-dihydroequilin sulfate, and 0.5 to 4.0% of sodium 17β-dihydroequilin sulfate. All percentages are related to the labelled content. An almost white brownish amorphous powder. Do not freeze.
USP 25: A mixture of sodium estrone sulfate and sodium equilin sulfate, derived wholly or in part from equine urine or synthetically from estrone and equilin. It contains other conjugated oestrogenic substances of the type excreted by pregnant mares. It contains 52.5 to 61.5% of sodium estrone sulfate and 22.5 to 30.5% of sodium equilin sulfate; the total of the two combined should comprise 79.5 to 88.0% of the labelled content of conjugated oestrogens. It should contain, as sulfate conjugates, 13.5 to 19.5% of 17α-dihydroequilin, 2.5 to 9.5% of 17α-estradiol, and 0.5 to 4.0% of 17β-dihydroequilin, relative to the labelled content of conjugated oestrogens.
If it is obtained from natural sources it is a buff-coloured amorphous powder which is odourless or has a slight characteristic odour; the synthetic form is a white to light buff-coloured crystalline or amorphous powder, odourless or with a slight odour.

Adverse Effects and Precautions
As for oestrogens in general (see Estradiol, p.1473). See also under Hormone Replacement Therapy, p.1461.

Effects on the cardiovascular system. Treatment of men with a previous myocardial infarction with conjugated oestrogens 5 mg daily in the USA Coronary Drug Project was discontinued because of a higher incidence of subsequent coronary events.[1] Moreover, treatment with the lower 2.5 mg dose was later also discontinued because of suggestions of adverse trends including a greater incidence of venous thromboembolism.[2] In postmenopausal women, there was an increase in adverse cardiac events in the first year of use of hormone replacement therapy containing 0.625 mg conjugated oestrogens[3] (see also p.1462).

1. Coronary Drug Project Research Group. The Coronary Drug Project: initial findings leading to modifications of its research protocol. *JAMA* 1970; **214:** 1303–13.
2. Coronary Drug Project Research Group. The Coronary Drug Project: findings leading to discontinuation of the 2.5-mg/day estrogen group. *JAMA* 1973; **226:** 652–7.
3. Hulley S, *et al.* Randomized trial of estrogen plus progestin for secondary prevention of coronary heart disease in postmenopausal women. *JAMA* 1998; **280:** 605–13.

Effects on the gallbladder. Analysis of data obtained during the Coronary Drug Project indicated a significant increase in the development of gallbladder disease among men treated with conjugated oestrogens 2.5 and 5 mg daily, compared with those treated with placebo.[1]

1. The Coronary Drug Project Research Group. Gallbladder disease as a side effect of drugs influencing lipid metabolism: experience in the Coronary Drug Project. *N Engl J Med* 1977; **296:** 1185–90.

Effects on the nervous system. Reversible chorea developed in a 57-year-old woman receiving conjugated oestrogens and norgestrel;[1] the woman had a history of migraine and Sydenham's chorea.

1. Steiger MJ, Quinn NP. Hormone replacement therapy induced chorea. *BMJ* 1991; **302:** 762.

Hypersensitivity. A report of an anaphylactic reaction following the intravenous administration of conjugated oestrogens.[1]

1. Searcy CJ, *et al.* Anaphylactic reaction to intravenous conjugated estrogens. *Clin Pharm* 1987; **6:** 74–6.

Interactions
See under Hormone Replacement Therapy, p.1463.

Pharmacokinetics
Orally administered conjugated oestrogens are hydrolysed by enzymes present in the intestine that remove the sulfate group and allow absorption of the unconjugated oestrogen. Metabolism occurs primarily in the liver; there is some enterohepatic recycling (see also under Estradiol, p.1474).

Uses and Administration
Conjugated oestrogens have actions and uses similar to those described for estradiol (see p.1474).

When used as menopausal HRT (p.1463) doses of 0.3 to 1.25 mg daily are given by mouth either cyclically or continuously, in conjunction with a progestogen ei-

ther cyclically or continuously in women with a uterus. Topical vaginal therapy may be used specifically for menopausal atrophic vaginitis; 0.5 to 2 g of a 0.0625% cream may be employed daily for 3 weeks of a 4-week cycle. If used long-term in a woman with a uterus, cyclical progestogen is required.

Doses of 1.25 mg daily by mouth are used as replacement therapy for primary ovarian failure and doses of 0.3 to 0.625 mg daily administered on a cyclical basis are used for female hypogonadism, although higher doses were formerly used.

For the palliative treatment of prostatic carcinoma (p.497), a dose of 1.25 to 2.5 mg three times daily by mouth has been used. A dose of 10 mg three times daily for at least 3 months has been used for palliative treatment of breast carcinoma in men and postmenopausal women (p.491).

Abnormal uterine bleeding has been treated acutely by giving 25 mg of conjugated oestrogens by slow intravenous injection, repeated if required after 6 to 12 hours; the intramuscular route has also been used.

Synthetic conjugated oestrogens, A, contains a mixture of nine derivatives of estrone, equilin, estradiol, and equilenin. It is derived from plant material, and is not a generic equivalent of conjugated oestrogens described in USP 25 (see above). It is used in doses of 0.625 to 1.25 mg daily by mouth for the relief of vasomotor symptoms associated with the menopause.

Haemorrhagic disorders. Some references to the use of high-dose intravenous or oral conjugated oestrogens in the management of haemorrhagic disorders associated with renal failure.[1-6]

1. Liu YK, *et al.* Treatment of uraemic bleeding with conjugated oestrogen. *Lancet* 1984; **ii:** 887–90.
2. Livio M, *et al.* Conjugated estrogens for the management of bleeding associated with renal failure. *N Engl J Med* 1986; **315:** 731–5.
3. Bronner MH, *et al.* Estrogen-progesterone therapy for bleeding gastrointestinal telangiectasias in chronic renal failure: an uncontrolled trial. *Ann Intern Med* 1986; **105:** 371–4.
4. Seth S, Geier TM. Use of conjugated estrogens to control gastrointestinal tract bleeding in two patients with chronic renal failure. *Clin Pharm* 1988; **7:** 906–9.
5. Shemin D, *et al.* Oral estrogens decrease bleeding time and improve clinical bleeding in patients with renal failure. *Am J Med* 1990; **89:** 436–40.
6. Heunisch C, *et al.* Conjugated estrogens for the management of gastrointestinal bleeding secondary to uremia of acute renal failure. *Pharmacotherapy* 1998; **18:** 210–7.

Preparations
USP 25: Conjugated Estrogens Tablets.

Proprietary Preparations (details are given in Part 3)
Aust.: Conjugen; Oestro-Feminal; Premarin; *Austral.:* Premarin; *Belg.:* Premarin; *Braz.:* Menosedan; *Canad.:* CES; Congest; Premarin; *Denm.:* Premarin; *Fin.:* Premarin; *Fr.:* Premarin; *Ger.:* Climarest; Conjugen; Femavit; Oestrofeminal; Transannon; *Hong Kong:* Equin; Premarin; *Irl.:* Premarin; *Israel:* Premaril; Prevagin-Premaril; *Ital.:* Emopremarin; Premarin; *Mex.:* Premarin; *Neth.:* Dagynil; Premarin; *NZ:* Premarin; *S.Afr.:* Premarin; *Singapore:* Premarin; *Spain:* Carentil; Equin; Premarin; *Swed.:* Premarina; *Switz.:* Conjugen; Premarin; Transannon; *Thai.:* Premarin; *UK:* Premarin; *USA:* Cenestin; Premarin.
Multi-ingredient: *Aust.:* Cyclo-Premarin-MPA; Cyclo-Premella†; Perennia; Premarin compositum; Premarin Plus; Premarin-MPA; Premella†; Sequennia; *Austral.:* Menoprem; Premia 5; Premia Continuous; Provelle; *Belg.:* Premelle; Premplus; *Braz.:* Ero Test; Menostress; Menotensil; *Ger.:* Climopax; Climopax Cyclo; Premarin compositum; *Hong Kong:* Premelle; Premelle Cycle; *Irl.:* Premique; Premique Cycle; Prempak-C; *Israel:* Premaril MP; Premaril Plus MP; *Ital.:* Premelle C; Premelle S; Prempak; *Mex.:* Premarin Pak; Premelle; *Neth.:* Premarin Plus; Premelle; Premelle Cycle; Prempak-C; *NZ:* Menoprem; Premia; Premia Continuous; Prempak-C; Provette Continuous; Provette Sequential; *Port.:* Premarin Plus; Premelle; Premelle Cycle; *S.Afr.:* Premelle; Prempak N; *Singapore:* Premelle; Premelle Cycle; Prempak-C; *Spain:* Premelle; Premelle Ciclico; *Swed.:* Premelle; Premelle Sekvens; *Switz.:* Cyclo-Premella ST; Cyclo-Premella†; Premarin Plus; Premella; *Thai.:* Prempak; *UK:* Premique; Premique Cycle; Prempak-C; *USA:* PMB†; Premarin with Methyltestosterone†; Premphase; Prempro.

Cyclofenil (9033-m)

Cyclofenil (BAN, rINN).
F-6066; H-3452; ICI-48213. 4,4′-(Cyclohexylidenemethylene)bis(phenyl acetate).
$C_{23}H_{24}O_4 = 364.4$.
CAS — 2624-43-3.
ATC — G03GB01.

Profile
Cyclofenil is a nonsteroidal anti-oestrogen that has been used in the treatment of menstrual disturbances and anovulatory infertility due to hypothalamic-pituitary dysfunction.

It has been given by mouth in doses of 200 mg three times daily for 5 days, in a cyclical regimen for 3 to 4 cycles. It has also been given for menopausal symptoms.

Preparations
Proprietary Preparations (details are given in Part 3)
Braz.: Fertodur; Menopax; *Ital.:* Neoclym; *Mex.:* Fertodur.

Cyproterone Acetate (9034-b)

Cyproterone Acetate (BANM, USAN, rINNM).
Cyproteroni Acetas; NSC-81430; SH-714; SH-881 (cyproterone). 6-Chloro-1β,2β-dihydro-17α-hydroxy-3′H-cyclopropa[1,2]pregna-1,4,6-triene-3,20-dione acetate.
$C_{24}H_{29}ClO_4 = 416.9$.
CAS — 2098-66-0 (cyproterone); 427-51-0 (cyproterone acetate).
Pharmacopoeias. In *Eur.* (see p.vi).

Pharmacopoeial description
Ph. Eur.: A white or almost white, crystalline powder. Practically insoluble in water; sparingly soluble in dehydrated alcohol; freely soluble in acetone; very soluble in dichloromethane; soluble in methyl alcohol. Protect from light.

Adverse Effects
When given to men cyproterone inhibits spermatogenesis, reduces the volume of ejaculate, and causes infertility; these effects are slowly reversible. Abnormal spermatozoa may be produced. Gynaecomastia is common and permanent enlargement of the mammary glands may occur; galactorrhoea and benign nodules have been reported rarely. There may be initial sedation and depressive mood changes. Patients may experience alterations in hair pattern, skin reactions and rarely rashes or hypersensitivity, weight changes, and anaemia. Osteoporosis may occur rarely. Altered liver function and breathlessness may occur. There have also been reports of hepatitis, jaundice, and hepatic failure, sometimes fatal, developing usually after several months of high-dose cyproterone therapy, but its association with liver cancer is uncertain.

When low-dose cyproterone is given with ethinylestradiol to women, adverse effects associated with combined oral contraceptives (see p.1452) may occur.

Carcinogenicity. See Effects on the Liver, below.

Effects on the cardiovascular system. Combined oral contraceptives are associated with a small increased risk of cardiovascular disease (see p.1455). Deep-vein thrombosis associated with antibodies to cyproterone acetate in women using oral contraceptives containing cyproterone acetate and ethinylestradiol has been reported.[1,2]

1. Leroy O, *et al.* Deep venous thrombosis and antibodies to cyproterone acetate. *Lancet* 1990; **336:** 509.
2. Beaumont V, Beaumont J-L. Thrombosis and antibodies to cyproterone acetate. *Lancet* 1991; **337:** 113.

Effects on the eyes. Bilateral optic atrophy in one elderly male patient was thought to be associated with cyproterone.[1] No other cases were known either from the published literature or from the manufacturers' records.

1. Markus H, Polkey M. Visual loss and optic atrophy associated with cyproterone acetate. *BMJ* 1992; **305:** 159.

Effects on the liver. There have been numerous reports of hepatic reactions associated with cyproterone acetate. In February 1995, the UK Committee on Safety of Medicines noted that it had received 96 reports of reactions including hepatitis, cholestatic jaundice, and hepatic failure, following cyproterone treatment;[1] 33 cases had led to fatalities. Nearly all cases (91 of 96) were in elderly men typically receiving high doses (300 mg) for prostatic cancer, and toxicity usually developed after several months of treatment. In view of this it was recommended that the use of cyproterone acetate in prostatic cancer be restricted to short courses for the testosterone flare associated with the commencement of gonadorelin analogue therapy, or for hot flushes after surgical or chemical castration, or for patients unresponsive to, or intolerant of, other treatments.

Although there is little doubt of the risk of hepatotoxicity, suggestions of an association between cyproterone therapy and the development of liver cancer remain contentious. There are individual reports of hepatocellular carcinoma developing in patients receiving cyproterone,[2,3] and some evidence *in vitro* of the formation of DNA adducts in exposed hepatocytes,[4] but there does not seem to be clinical evidence to support any association between use of cyproterone acetate and the development of liver tumours.[4,5]

1. Committee on Safety of Medicines/Medicines Control Agency. Hepatic reactions with cyproterone acetate (Cyprostat, Androcur). *Current Problems* 1995; **21:** 1.

The symbol † denotes a preparation no longer actively marketed

2. Watanabe S, *et al.* Three cases of hepatocellular carcinoma among cyproterone users. *Lancet* 1994; **344:** 1567–8.
3. Rüdiger T, *et al.* Hepatocellular carcinoma after treatment with cyproterone acetate combined with ethinyloestradiol. *Lancet* 1995; **345:** 452–3.
4. Lewis S. Warning on cyproterone. *Lancet* 1995; **345:** 247.
5. Rabe T, *et al.* Liver tumours in women on oral contraceptives. *Lancet* 1994; **344:** 1568–9.

Precautions

When used for hypersexuality, cyproterone is contra-indicated in men with liver diseases or malignant or wasting diseases. In addition, it should not be given to men with severe chronic depression, severe diabetes with vascular changes, sickle-cell anaemia, or to those with a history of thromboembolic disorders. It may delay bone maturation and testicular development and so should not be given to immature youths. When used for prostate cancer, there are no absolute contra-indications to the use of cyproterone, but the above conditions should prompt cautious consideration of the risks and benefits.

In men treated with cyproterone, liver function should be monitored before treatment, and whenever any symptoms or signs suggestive of hepatotoxicity occur. If cyproterone-induced hepatotoxicity occurs, treatment should be withdrawn. In men with prostate cancer, it may be advisable to limit the duration of treatment (see Effects on the Liver, above). Men with diabetes require careful monitoring of diabetic control. Since anaemia has been observed, regular blood counts are recommended during treatment. Adrenocortical suppression has been reported and function should be monitored regularly during treatment. Patients should be advised that the initial sedative effects may interfere with driving and the operation of machinery.

When cyproterone is given in conjunction with ethinylestradiol to women the precautions for combined oral contraceptives (see p.1457) should be observed.

Pregnancy. Administration of cyproterone during pregnancy might carry a risk of feminisation of a male fetus. However, there are a few case reports of healthy male infants born to mothers who had inadvertently taken a combination of cyproterone acetate and ethinylestradiol during the early stages of pregnancy,[1,2] and of a male fetus that was found to have no malformations after abortion was induced.[3] For further information on oral contraceptive use in pregnancy, see p.1458.

1. Statham BN, *et al.* Conception during 'Diane' therapy—a successful outcome. *Br J Dermatol* 1985; **113:** 374.
2. Bye P. Comments on 'conception during "Diane" therapy—a successful outcome'. *Br J Dermatol* 1986; **114:** 516.
3. Bergh T, Bakos O. Exposure to antiandrogen during pregnancy: case report. *BMJ* 1987; **294:** 677–8.

Interactions

The manufacturers state that alcohol may reduce the effectiveness of cyproterone acetate as it is ineffective in chronic alcoholics.

When given in conjunction with ethinylestradiol to women, interactions similar to those for combined oral contraceptives (see p.1458) might be anticipated.

Pharmacokinetics

Cyproterone acetate is slowly absorbed from the gastrointestinal tract with peak plasma concentrations being achieved in 3 to 4 hours. It is about 96% bound to plasma proteins. The terminal elimination half-life is about 38 hours. Cyproterone is metabolised in the liver; about 35% of a dose is excreted in urine as free and conjugated metabolites, the remainder being excreted in the bile. The principal metabolite, 15β-hydroxycyproterone, has anti-androgenic activity.

Uses and Administration

Cyproterone acetate is a progestogen with anti-androgenic properties.

It is used for the control of libido in severe hypersexuality or sexual deviation in adult males (see Disturbed Behaviour, p.650). The usual dose by mouth is 50 mg twice daily after meals.

It is also used in males for the palliative treatment of prostatic carcinoma (p.497) where other drugs are ineffective or not tolerated, to control disease flare or hot flushes associated with gonadorelin analogue therapy, and to control hot flushes associated with or-

chidectomy. The usual initial dose for disease flare or palliation is 300 mg daily in 2 or 3 divided doses after meals and maintenance treatment is continued with doses of 200 to 300 mg daily, but there is a risk of hepatotoxicity with long-term therapy. For the treatment of hot flushes, doses of 50 to 150 mg daily in 1 to 3 divided doses are given.

Cyproterone acetate may be used in conjunction with ethinylestradiol in females for the control of acne (see below) and hirsutism (see below), and also provides contraception in these women. The usual doses are 2 mg of cyproterone acetate with 35 µg of ethinylestradiol given daily for 21 days of each menstrual cycle; the first treatment course is started on the first day of the menstrual cycle and each subsequent course is started after 7 tablet-free days have followed the preceding course.

Cyproterone acetate has also been given by depot intramuscular injection.

Acne. Comparisons of cyproterone acetate 2 mg with either 35 or 50 µg of ethinylestradiol in the treatment of refractory acne (p.1103) in women[1-3] have shown that, in general, both combinations were effective but that the lower dose of oestrogen was considered more acceptable for long-term therapy.

1. Colver GB, *et al.* Cyproterone acetate and two doses of oestrogen in female acne; a double-blind comparison. *Br J Dermatol* 1988; **118:** 95–9.
2. Fugère P, *et al.* Cyproterone acetate/ethinyl estradiol in the treatment of acne: a comparative dose-response study of the estrogen component. *Contraception* 1990; **42:** 225–34.
3. Anonymous. Dianette for women with acne. *Drug Ther Bull* 1990; **28:** 15–16.

Hidradenitis suppurativa. Some reports[1-3] of a beneficial response to cyproterone acetate with ethinylestradiol in women with hidradenitis suppurativa, an androgen-dependent disorder of the skin and hair in the pubic and axillary regions.

1. Mortimer PS, *et al.* A double-blind controlled cross-over trial of cyproterone acetate in females with hidradenitis suppurativa. *Br J Dermatol* 1986; **115:** 263–8.
2. Sawers RS, *et al.* Control of hidradenitis suppurativa in women using combined antiandrogen (cyproterone acetate) and oestrogen therapy. *Br J Dermatol* 1986; **115:** 269–74.
3. Mortimer PS, *et al.* Mediation of hidradenitis suppurativa by androgens. *BMJ* 1986; **292:** 961.

Hirsutism. Hirsutism is an abnormal growth in females of coarse pigmented terminal hair in an adult male pattern, and is one of the clinical expressions of hyperandrogenism. Most women with hirsutism have increased concentrations of circulating androgens from the ovaries associated with polycystic ovary syndrome (p.1276).[1] In rare cases, the adrenal gland is the primary source of increased androgens, for example, in congenital adrenal hyperplasia (p.1049). In a few cases, severe hirsutism is associated with frank virilisation due to massively increased circulating androgen concentrations from an androgen-secreting tumour.[2] Hirsutism is an adverse effect of androgenic progestogens, such as norgestrel, used in hormonal contraceptives and HRT. Androgens and anabolic steroids may also cause hirsutism in females.

Treatment for hirsutism employs topical cosmetic treatments such as bleaching, shaving, plucking, and electrolysis, and in the mildest cases this may be all that is required. However, such mechanical means of treatment are more usually combined with drug therapy to prevent further conversion of vellus to terminal hair, and to slow the regrowth of terminal hair, which may become lighter and softer. Because the growth cycle of hair is long, a response to therapy may not be seen for 6 to 12 months.

The mainstay of drug therapy for hirsutism is an anti-androgen, the most commonly used being the steroidal anti-androgens *cyproterone acetate* and *spironolactone*. To increase efficacy (by suppressing ovarian androgen production) and minimise the chance of conception (because of the risk of feminisation of a male fetus), cyclical *ethinylestradiol* is commonly used with cyproterone acetate, while combined (nonandrogenic) *hormonal contraceptives* are commonly used with spironolactone, which has no progestogenic activity. Cyproterone acetate may be used in a low-dose combined preparation containing cyproterone acetate 2 mg with ethinylestradiol 35 µg.[1,2] In more severe hirsutism, the two drugs may be prescribed separately in a 'reversed sequential regimen', with cyproterone acetate 50 to 150 mg given on days 5 to 15 of the menstrual cycle and ethinylestradiol 30 to 50 µg on days 5 to 26.[1-3] When a satisfactory response has been achieved, the cyproterone dosage is gradually reduced, and eventually the low-dose combination preparation may be sufficient.

In some countries spironolactone is the drug of choice for the treatment of hirsutism, particularly if there is associated obesity and hypertension; doses of up to 300 mg daily have been given initially, with the aim of reducing the dose when hair growth has been controlled.[3] Despite its wide use, however, evidence of benefit is considered scanty.[4] *Flutamide, finasteride,* and *leuprorelin* have also been shown to be effective, although some consider finasteride to be less active.[5] The condition has also been reported to respond to *ketoconazole. Eflornithine* is

used topically for the reduction of facial hair. It is thought to slow hair growth by the inhibition of ornithine decarboxylase in hair follicles.

Although non-androgenic oral contraceptives have a role in reducing hyperandrogenism in polycystic ovary syndrome and corticosteroids have a role in congenital adrenal hyperplasia, neither is generally considered sufficient to reduce the hirsutism associated with these diseases, and an anti-androgen is usually added to the therapy.[2,5] Combination with a corticosteroid may however produce more prolonged response in appropriate patients (see also p.1068).

1. Conway GS, Jacobs HS. Hirsutism. *BMJ* 1990; **301:** 619–20.
2. Rittmaster RS. Hirsutism. *Lancet* 1997; **349:** 191–5.
3. Delahunt JW. Hirsutism: practical therapeutic guidelines. *Drugs* 1993; **45:** 223–31.
4. Lee O, *et al.* Spironolactone versus placebo or in combination with steroids for hirsutism and/or acne (updated 28 May 2001). Available in The Cochrane Library; Issue 3. Oxford: Update Software; 2001.
5. Carmina E. A risk-benefit assessment of pharmacological therapies for hirsutism. *Drug Safety* 2001; **24:** 267–76.

Preparations

BP 2001: Cyproterone Tablets.

Proprietary Preparations (details are given in Part 3)

Aust.: Andro-Diane; Androcur; *Austral.:* Androcur; Cyprone; Procur; *Belg.:* Androcur; *Braz.:* Androcur; *Canad.:* Alti-CPA; Androcur; *Denm.:* Androcur; *Fin.:* Androcur; *Fr.:* Androcur; *Ger.:* Androcur; Virilit; *Hong Kong:* Androcur; *Irl.:* Androcur; *Israel:* Androcur; Armocur; Cypron; *Ital.:* Androcur; *Mex.:* Androcur; *Neth.:* Androcur; *Norw.:* Androcur; *NZ:* Androcur; *Port.:* Androcur; *S.Afr.:* Androcur; *Singapore:* Androcur; *Spain:* Androcur; *Swed.:* Androcur; *Switz.:* Androcur; *Thai.:* Androcur; *UK:* Androcur; Cyprostat.

Multi-ingredient: *Aust.:* Climen; Diane; *Austral.:* Brenda-35 ED; Climen; Diane ED; *Belg.:* Climen; Diane; *Braz.:* Climene; Diane; *Canad.:* Diane; *Denm.:* Climen; Diane; *Fin.:* Diane; Femilar; *Fr.:* Climene; Diane; *Ger.:* Climen; Diane; *Hong Kong:* Climen; Diane; *Irl.:* Dianette; *Israel:* Diane; *Ital.:* Climen; Diane; Pausal; *Mex.:* Climene; Diane; *Neth.:* Climene; Diane; *Norw.:* Climen; Diane; *NZ:* Diane; *Port.:* Climen; Diane; *S.Afr.:* Diane; Diane; *Singapore:* Climen; Diane; *Spain:* Climen; Clisin; Diane; *Switz.:* Climen; Diane; *Thai.:* Climen; Diane; Lady-35; Preme; Tina; *UK:* Dianette.

Danazol (9035-v)

Danazol (BAN, USAN, pINN).

Win-17757. 17α-Pregna-2,4-dien-20-yno[2,3-*d*]isoxazol-17β-ol.

$C_{22}H_{27}NO_2 = 337.5.$

CAS — 17230-88-5.

ATC — G03XA01.

Pharmacopoeias. In *Chin.* and *US.*

Pharmacopoeial description

USP 25: A white to pale yellow crystalline powder. Practically insoluble or insoluble in water and in petroleum spirit; sparingly soluble in alcohol and in benzene; soluble in acetone; freely soluble in chloroform; slightly soluble in ether. Store in airtight containers. Protect from light.

Adverse Effects

Side-effects of danazol that reflect inhibition of the pituitary-ovarian axis include amenorrhoea (occasionally persistent), hot flushes, sweating, reduction in breast size, changes in libido, vaginitis, emotional lability, and nervousness.

Side-effects attributable to androgenic activity include acne, oily skin or hair, mild hirsutism, oedema, gain in weight, deepening of the voice, androgenic alopecia, and rarely clitoral hypertrophy. Testicular atrophy and a reduction in spermatogenesis may occur.

Other side-effects include gastrointestinal disturbances, increased or decreased blood cell counts, thrombotic events, headache, backache, dizziness, tremor, depression, fatigue, sleep disorders, muscle spasm or cramp, skin rash, hyperglucagonaemia, abnormal glucose tolerance, decreased serum high-density-lipoprotein cholesterol, increased serum low-density-lipoprotein cholesterol, and elevation of liver-function test values and rarely cholestatic jaundice. Some patients may experience tachycardia and hypertension. Benign intracranial hypertension and visual disturbances have occurred.

Effects on carbohydrate metabolism. Diabetes mellitus developed in a patient receiving danazol 400 mg twice daily for endometriosis.[1] The diabetes developed 8 weeks after initiation of danazol therapy and resolved completely after the drug was discontinued.

1. Seifer DB, *et al.* Insulin-dependent diabetes mellitus associated with danazol. *Am J Obstet Gynecol* 1990; **162:** 474–5.

Effects on the liver. As with other 17α-alkylated steroids (see p.1492), cholestatis, peliosis hepatis, and hepatic adenomas have been associated with danazol.

References.
1. Ohsawa T, Iwashita S. Hepatitis associated with danazol. *Drug Intell Clin Pharm* 1986; **20**: 889.
2. Boue F, *et al.* Danazol and cholestatic hepatitis. *Ann Intern Med* 1986; **105**: 139–40.
3. Fermand JP, *et al.* Danazol-induced hepatocellular adenoma. *Am J Med* 1990; **88**: 529–30.
4. Bray GP. *et al.* Resolution of danazol-induced cholestatis with S-adenosylmethionine. *Postgrad Med J* 1993; **69**: 237–9.
5. Makdisi WJ, *et al.* Fatal peliosis of the liver and spleen in a patient with agnogenic myeloid metaplasia treated with danazol. *Am J Gastroenterol* 1995; **90**: 317–8.
6. Bork K, *et al.* Hepatocellular adenomas in patients taking danazol for hereditary angio-oedema. *Lancet* 1999; **353**: 1066–7.

Effects on the skin. Erythema multiforme developed in two patients receiving danazol for profuse bleeding.[1]
1. Gately LE, Andes WA. Danazol and erythema multiforme. *Ann Intern Med* 1988; **109**: 85.

Pancreatitis. Reports of pancreatitis in patients receiving danazol.
1. Chevalier X, *et al.* Danazol induced pancreatitis and hepatitis. *Clin Rheumatol* 1990; **9**: 239–41.
2. Balasch J, *et al.* Acute pancreatitis associated with danazol treatment for endometriosis. *Hum Reprod* 1994; **9**: 1163–5.

Precautions

Danazol should be used with caution in conditions which may be adversely affected by fluid retention, such as in cardiovascular, hepatic, and renal disorders, migraine, and epilepsy. It should also be used with care in patients with diabetes mellitus, polycythaemia or a history of thrombosis, and should not be used in patients with a thromboembolic disorder. Also, it should not be given to patients with marked hepatic, cardiac or kidney dysfunction, undiagnosed genital bleeding, or androgen-dependent tumours. As with other 17α-alkylated compounds, there is an increased risk of liver disorders and liver function should be monitored during therapy.

Danazol should not be given during pregnancy because of a possible androgenic effect on the female fetus (see below), and non-hormonal contraception is recommended during treatment. Danazol should also not be given to breast-feeding mothers. Caution is required in children and adolescents since precocious sexual development may occur in boys and virilisation in girls, and premature epiphyseal closure may occur in both sexes.

In the event of androgenic effects, danazol should be withdrawn, as they may prove irreversible on continued use.

Porphyria. Danazol has been associated with acute attacks of porphyria and is considered unsafe in porphyric patients.

Pregnancy. Reports of masculinisation of female infants born to mothers who had received danazol during pregnancy.[1-3]
1. Shaw RW, Farquhar JW. Female pseudohermaphroditism associated with danazol exposure in utero: case report. *Br J Obstet Gynaecol* 1984; **91**: 386–9.
2. Kingsbury AC. Danazol and fetal masculinization: a warning. *Med J Aust* 1985; **143**: 410–11.
3. Brunskill PJ. The effects of fetal exposure to danazol. *Br J Obstet Gynaecol* 1992; **99**: 212–15.

Interactions

Therapy with danazol may inhibit the hepatic metabolism of a number of drugs including carbamazepine (see p.345), ciclosporin (see p.522), warfarin (see p.997), and possibly tacrolimus (see p.570). Introduction of danazol appeared to reduce the maintenance requirement for alfacalcidol (see p.1392).

Pharmacokinetics

Danazol is absorbed from the gastrointestinal tract and metabolised in the liver; absorption is said to be markedly increased if it is taken with food. A half-life of about 4.5 hours has been reported. 2-Hydroxymethylethisterone is said to be the major metabolite.

Uses and Administration

Danazol suppresses the pituitary-ovarian axis by inhibiting pituitary output of gonadotrophins. It has weak androgenic activity.

Danazol has been given by mouth in the treatment of a variety of conditions including endometriosis, some benign breast disorders such as mastalgia and fibro-

The symbol † denotes a preparation no longer actively marketed

cystic breast disease, gynaecomastia, menorrhagia associated with dysfunctional uterine bleeding, and prevention of hereditary angioedema. It may also be employed for the pre-operative thinning of the endometrium prior to hysteroscopic endometrial ablation, and has been tried in a variety of other conditions including pubertal or pre-pubertal breast hypertrophy and various blood disorders.

When given to women, treatment with danazol should be started on day 1 of the menstrual cycle or after pregnancy has been otherwise excluded.

In **endometriosis** the usual dose is 200 to 800 mg daily in 2 to 4 divided doses, adjusted according to the response. Therapy is given for 3 to 6 months or continued for up to 9 months if necessary.

In the treatment of **benign breast disorders** the usual initial dose is 100 to 400 mg daily in 2 divided doses, subsequently adjusted according to response, and continued for 3 to 6 months. For **gynaecomastia** 200 mg daily has been given to male adolescents, increased after 2 months to 400 mg daily if no response occurs; adult men may be given 400 mg daily initially. Therapy is usually tried for 6 months.

In dysfunctional uterine bleeding manifesting as **menorrhagia** doses of 200 mg daily have been employed and treatment is reviewed after 3 months.

In the management of **hereditary angioedema** initial doses of 200 mg two or three times daily are given, and then reduced according to the patient's response.

For **pre-operative thinning** of the endometrium the usual dose is 400 to 800 mg daily for 3 to 6 weeks.

Blood disorders. While danazol may produce thrombocytopenia and leucopenia it may also have a beneficial effect in some blood disorders. It has been reported that danazol increases plasma concentrations of factor VIII and factor IX and may therefore be beneficial in the treatment of the haemorrhagic disorders (p.721) **haemophilia A** or **haemophilia B** (Christmas disease).[1,2] However, other workers have failed to substantiate these results and indeed have sometimes suggested that danazol may even increase the frequency of bleeding in such patients.[3-6]

In one report, danazol was found to increase plasma concentrations of protein C and protein S (inhibitors of blood coagulation) in a patient with end-stage renal disease.[7] This led to the suggestion that it and stanozolol may be useful in end-stage renal disease with hypercoagulability after dialysis.

Treatment with danazol has been reported to be beneficial in the treatment of **idiopathic thrombocytopenic purpura** (p.1052) resulting in increased platelet counts,[8-12] although in one study[10] 7 of 10 patients derived no benefit. A study investigating the possible mode of action in this disorder[13] indicated that danazol may mediate an effect by influencing the number of available binding sites for monomeric immunoglobulin G (Fc receptors) on monocytes. Another study[14] showed that sex, age (in women only), and the status of the spleen influenced the response of auto-immune thrombocytopenia to danazol. Thrombocytopenia associated with systemic lupus erythematosus[15] and the antiphospholipid antibody syndrome,[16] as well as rheumatoid arthritis[17] has also been reported to respond to treatment with danazol. For mention of the use of danazol in Henoch-Schönlein purpura see Hypersensitivity Vasculitis, p.1052.

Additionally there have been reports of response to danazol therapy in patients with auto-immune haemolytic anaemia,[18,19] myelodysplastic syndromes,[20,21] paroxysmal cold haemoglobinuria,[22] hereditary haemorrhagic telangiectasia,[23] and Evan's syndrome due to systemic lupus erythematosus.[24]

1. Gralnick HR, Rick ME. Danazol increases factor VIII and factor IX in classic hemophilia and Christmas disease. *N Engl J Med* 1983; **308**: 1393–5.
2. Gralnick HR, *et al.* Benefits of danazol treatment in patients with hemophilia A (classic hemophilia). *JAMA* 1985; **253**: 1151–3.
3. Garewal HS, *et al.* Effect of danazol on coagulation parameters and bleeding in hemophilia. *JAMA* 1985; **253**: 1154–6.
4. Ambriz R, *et al.* Danazol and hemophilia. *JAMA* 1985; **254**: 754.
5. Kasper CK, Boylen AL. Poor response to danazol in hemophilia. *Blood* 1985; **65**: 211–13.
6. Heaton DC, *et al.* Danazol therapy in haemophilia. *N Z Med J* 1986; **99**: 185–7.
7. Henke WJ. Protein C and S response to Danacrine in end-stage renal disease. *Ann Intern Med* 1988; **108**: 910.
8. Ahn YS, *et al.* Danazol for the treatment of idiopathic thrombocytopenic purpura. *N Engl J Med* 1983; **308**: 1396–9.
9. Buelli M, *et al.* Danazol for the treatment of idiopathic thrombocytopenic purpura. *Acta Haematol (Basel)* 1985; **74**: 97–8.
10. McVerry BA, *et al.* The use of danazol in the management of chronic immune thrombocytopenic purpura. *Br J Haematol* 1985; **61**: 145–8.
11. Mylvaganam R, *et al.* Very low dose danazol in idiopathic thrombocytopenic purpura and its role as an immune modulator. *Am J Med Sci* 1989; **298**: 215–20.
12. Edelmann DZ, *et al.* Danazol in non-splenectomised patients with refractory idiopathic thrombocytopenic purpura. *Postgrad Med J* 1990; **66**: 827–30.

13. Schreiber AD, *et al.* Effect of danazol in immune thrombocytopenic purpura. *N Engl J Med* 1987; **316**: 503–8.
14. Ahn YS, *et al.* Long-term danazol therapy in autoimmune thrombocytopenia: unmaintained remission and age-dependent response in women. *Ann Intern Med* 1989; **111**: 723–9.
15. West SG, Johnson SC. Danazol for the treatment of refractory autoimmune thrombocytopenia in systemic lupus erythematosus. *Ann Intern Med* 1988; **108**: 703–6.
16. Kavanaugh A. Danazol therapy in thrombocytopenia associated with the antiphospholipid antibody syndrome. *Ann Intern Med* 1994; **121**: 767–8.
17. Dasgupta B, Grahame R. Treatment with danazol for refractory thrombocytopenia in rheumatoid arthritis. *Br J Rheumatol* 1989; **28**: 550–1.
18. Ahn YS, *et al.* Danazol therapy for autoimmune hemolytic anemia. *Ann Intern Med* 1985; **102**: 298–301.
19. Tan AM, *et al.* Danazol for treatment of refractory autoimmune hemolytic anaemia. *Ann Acad Med Singapore* 1989; **18**: 707–9.
20. Cines DB, *et al.* Danazol therapy in myelodysplasia. *Ann Intern Med* 1985; **103**: 58–60.
21. Kornberg A, *et al.* Danazol and myelodysplastic syndromes. *Ann Intern Med* 1986; **104**: 445–6.
22. Gertz MA. Possible response of paroxysmal cold hemoglobinuria to danazol. *Ann Intern Med* 1987; **106**: 635.
23. Haq AU, *et al.* Hereditary hemorrhagic telangiectasia and danazol. *Ann Intern Med* 1988; **109**: 171.
24. Aranegui P, *et al.* Danazol for Evan's syndrome due to SLE. *DICP Ann Pharmacother* 1990; **24**: 641–2.

Endometriosis. Endometriosis is a condition affecting women in their reproductive years,[1] in which clusters of oestrogen-dependent cells, histologically indistinguishable from endometrium, develop outside their usual location in the uterine cavity. They occur most commonly in the pelvis, less commonly in the peritoneal cavity,[2] and occasionally elsewhere such as the thoracic cavity.[1,3] The aetiology is uncertain, although an immunological defect which permits endometrial cells carried in menstrual blood to implant and grow following reflux of menstrual blood has been suggested. The advent of laparoscopy has indicated that the condition is more common than was previously thought, and not all women with endometriosis are symptomatic.[4]

The most common symptom is pain, usually manifesting as secondary dysmenorrhoea, dyspareunia, or cyclical back or pelvic pain. Associated adenomyosis may cause menorrhagia; fibrosis and adhesions may develop. Endometriosis is also strongly associated with infertility, although whether it causes infertility is unclear. Management will depend in part on whether the presenting complaint leading to evaluation and diagnosis of endometriosis was pelvic pain or infertility, or whether the condition was discovered secondary to laparoscopy for other purposes.[2,5-9] Minimal asymptomatic disease may resolve spontaneously, and there is little evidence that conservative surgery or medical therapy[10] improves fertility. In women wishing to conceive, infertility treatments may be used as appropriate (see p.1275). For more extensive disease, the most commonly used initial treatment is conservative surgery followed by drugs to suppress the endometriosis if pain was the principal complaint or if removal of endometriotic deposits was incomplete. Because available drugs also tend to suppress ovulation they are potentially contraceptive, and their use will defer opportunities for conception in women wishing to conceive.[10] Commonly used drugs include danazol, progestogens such as medroxyprogesterone acetate, combined oral contraceptives, and gonadorelin analogues.

One of the most widely used treatments is *danazol*, which has been shown to produce subjective improvement in symptoms of pain and reduction of some pelvic abnormalities and tissue implants.[11] Its androgenic effects can be a problem and there is concern about its effect on blood lipids, therefore therapy is restricted to 6 months, or rarely up to 9 months. *Gestrinone* has been shown to be equally effective and may be a useful alternative.[12] *Progestogens* such as medroxyprogesterone acetate or norethisterone acetate are also commonly used. They appear to be as effective as danazol in relieving pain symptoms[12] but there is a suggestion that they are less effective in eliminating endometriotic deposits.[5] Despite this, some consider them to be the drugs of first choice for endometriosis.[2,6]

Combined oral contraceptives have been used in a continuous fashion, but such use is associated with a high incidence of breakthrough bleeding. However, it is now apparent that the usual cyclical use of combined oral contraceptives is associated with a decreased incidence of endometriosis,[13] and cyclical use is being investigated as a treatment although evidence of benefit remains scanty.[14]

The other major group of drugs that are used in endometriosis are *gonadorelin* and its analogues such as buserelin, goserelin, leuprorelin, nafarelin, and triptorelin. They are as effective as danazol[15] and their adverse effects, which resemble menopausal symptoms, may be better tolerated than the androgenic effects of danazol.[5,16] Long-term use is limited by the risk of osteoporosis, but the use of concomitant low-dose oestrogen and progestogen HRT[7,9,15] or tibolone[17] ('add-back' therapy) to prevent this is under investigation. Parathyroid hormone[18] may also be effective for 'add-back' therapy. It has been suggested that the gonadorelin analogues should be reserved for patients unable to tolerate conventional treatments,[16] or where rapid initial control is desired, or to facilitate laparoscopic procedures.[8]

Investigational drugs include the *antiprogestogens* such as mifepristone.[7]

There is a relatively high recurrence rate of endometriosis after conservative surgery and drug therapy. In women who can accept loss of child-bearing potential, definitive therapy is surgical oophorectomy and hysterectomy with complete excision or ablation of endometrial deposits. Oestrogen replacement therapy is given, but carries a risk of recurrence of the disease; some have suggested that combined HRT may be preferable (see p.1463).

1. Rock JA, Markham SM. Pathogenesis of endometriosis. *Lancet* 1992; **340:** 1264–7.
2. Wardle PG. Management of endometriosis. *Prescribers' J* 1994; **34:** 221–6.
3. Joseph J, Sahn SA. Thoracic endometriosis syndrome: new observations from an analysis of 110 cases. *Am J Med* 1996; **100:** 164–70.
4. Anonymous. Endometriosis: time for re-appraisal. *Lancet* 1992; **340:** 1073.
5. Shaw RW. Treatment of endometriosis. *Lancet* 1992; **340:** 1267–71.
6. Lu PY, Ory SJ. Endometriosis: current management. *Mayo Clin Proc* 1995; **70:** 453–63.
7. Kettel LM, Hummel WP. Modern medical management of endometriosis. *Obstet Gynecol Clin North Am* 1997; **24:** 361–73.
8. Adamson GD, Nelson HP. Surgical treatment of endometriosis. *Obstet Gynecol Clin North Am* 1997; **24:** 375–409.
9. Anonymous. Managing endometriosis. *Drug Ther Bull* 1999; **37:** 25–9.
10. Hughes E, *et al.* Ovulation suppression for endometriosis (updated 29 May 2001). Available in The Cochrane Library; Issue 3. Oxford: Update Software; 2001.
11. Selak V, *et al.* Danazol for pelvic pain associated with endometriosis (updated 28 May 2001). Available in The Cochrane Library; Issue 3. Oxford: Update Software; 2001.
12. Prentice A, *et al.* Progestagens and anti-progestagens for pain associated with endometriosis (updated 27 November 2000). Available in The Cochrane Library; Issue 3. Oxford: Update Software; 2001.
13. Vessey MP, *et al.* Epidemiology of endometriosis in women attending family planning clinics. *BMJ* 1993; **306:** 182–4.
14. Moore J, *et al.* Modern combined oral contraceptives for pain associated with endometriosis (updated 29 May 2001). Available in The Cochrane Library; Issue 3. Oxford: Update Software; 2001.
15. Prentice A, *et al.* Gonadotrophin-releasing hormone analogues for pain associated with endometriosis (updated 29 May 2001). Available in The Cochrane Library; Issue 3. Oxford: Update Software; 2001.
16. Anonymous. Gonadotropin releasing hormone analogues for endometriosis. *Drug Ther Bull* 1993; **31:** 21–2.
17. Lindsay PC, *et al.* The effect of add-back treatment with tibolone (Livial) on patients treated with gonadotrophin-releasing hormone agonist triptorelin (Decapetyl). *Fertil Steril* 1996; **65:** 342–8.
18. Finkelstein JS, *et al.* Parathyroid hormone for the prevention of bone loss induced by estrogen deficiency. *N Engl J Med* 1994; **331:** 1618–23.

Gynaecomastia. Gynaecomastia is a benign glandular enlargement of the male breast, caused either by increased oestrogenic activity or decreased androgenic activity. Examples of gynaecomastia caused by increased oestrogenic activity include oestrogen-secreting malignancies, increased aromatisation of androgens into oestrogens (associated with an increase in adipose tissue), and exposure to drugs with oestrogenic activity such as digitoxin. Neonatal and pubertal gynaecomastia (the former due to exposure to maternal oestrogens, the latter because oestrogen levels increase before androgens do) come into this category. Examples of gynaecomastia caused by decreased androgenic activity include the various forms of hypogonadism, increased metabolism of androgens (for example in alcoholism), and exposure to drugs with anti-androgenic properties such as spironolactone, cimetidine, ketoconazole, cyproterone acetate, or flutamide. Some systemic disorders may also be associated with gynaecomastia, including cirrhosis of the liver, hyperthyroidism, and renal failure; it may also occur on refeeding after starvation.

Gynaecomastia has a high rate of spontaneous regression, and specific therapy (other than the removal of any cause) need only be considered if the enlarged breast tissue causes sufficient pain, embarrassment, or emotional discomfort to interfere with the patient's daily life.[1] Drug therapy is only likely to be of benefit while tissue is still proliferating; once glandular tissue has become inactive and fibrotic (usually after more than 12 months) a complete response is unlikely.

Testosterone itself is unlikely to be of benefit (and may be aromatised to estradiol, exacerbating the situation), but a non-aromatisable androgen such as *androstanolone* (dihydrotestosterone) may produce some benefit.[1] *Danazol* has produced marked responses in some patients.[2] Quite good responses have also been reported with *tamoxifen*,[3-5] and this has been recommended as a drug of choice.[1] *Clomifene*[6,7] and *testolactone*,[8] have also been tried. Where drug therapy is unsuccessful, or the breast enlargement is long-standing, surgical removal of breast tissue is advocated.[1]

1. Braunstein GD. Gynecomastia. *N Engl J Med* 1993; **328:** 490–5.
2. Buckle R. Danazol therapy in gynaecomastia: recent experience and indications for therapy. *Postgrad Med J* 1979; **55** (suppl 5): 71–8.
3. Jefferys DB. Painful gynaecomastia treated with tamoxifen. *BMJ* 1979; **1:** 1119–20.
4. Hooper PD. Puberty gynaecomastia. *J R Coll Gen Pract* 1985; **35:** 142.
5. McDermott MT, *et al.* Tamoxifen therapy for painful idiopathic gynecomastia. *South Med J* 1990; **83:** 1283–5.
6. LeRoith D, *et al.* The effect of clomiphene citrate on pubertal gynaecomastia. *Acta Endocrinol (Copenh)* 1980; **95;** 177–80.
7. Plourde PV, *et al.* Clomiphene in the treatment of adolescent gynecomastia: clinical and endocrine studies. *Am J Dis Child* 1983; **137:** 1080–2.
8. Zachmann M, *et al.* Treatment of pubertal gynaecomastia with testolactone. *Acta Endocrinol (Copenh)* 1986; **279** (suppl): 218–24.

Hereditary angioedema. Danazol has been used successfully to prevent attacks of hereditary angioedema (p.743). Patients with lupus-erythematosus-like syndromes associated with hereditary angioedema have also benefited from danazol therapy.[1-3]

1. Masse R, *et al.* Reversal of lupus-erythematosus-like disease with danazol. *Lancet* 1980; **ii:** 651.
2. Donaldson VH, Hess EV. Effect of danazol on lupus-erythematosus-like disease in hereditary angioneurotic oedema. *Lancet* 1980; **ii:** 1145.
3. Duhra P, *et al.* Discoid lupus erythematosus associated with hereditary angioneurotic oedema. *Br J Dermatol* 1990; **123:** 241–4.

Mastalgia. Mastalgia is often associated with nodularity or other fibrocystic changes in the female breast, and is sometimes divided into cyclical mastalgia, which accounts for about two-thirds of all cases, non-cyclical mastalgia, and chest-wall or costochondral pain (Tietze's syndrome). Cyclical mastalgia is most common in the third decade of life, following a chronic relapsing course thereafter, and usually resolving at the menopause. Non-cyclical mastalgia tends to present later in life and the duration of symptoms is usually shorter, with spontaneous resolution occurring in 50% of cases; it tends to be more refractory to drug treatment.

Once clear pathological causes of pain have been excluded most patients can be managed by simple reassurance.[1-5] Drug treatment should rarely be considered unless pain has been present for about 6 months.[2] Patients who are receiving an oral contraceptive or HRT may find that symptoms improve on stopping treatment.[1,2,4] It has been suggested that reducing the intake of saturated fat in the diet may be worthwhile, and there is evidence that a low-fat diet reduces symptoms of tenderness and swelling.[6]

Danazol is probably the most effective drug for mastalgia,[3] and produces the most rapid response;[2,5] open studies suggest that it is of benefit in about 70% or more of patients with cyclical mastalgia[1-4] and somewhat fewer with the non-cyclical form.[1,3,4] However, adverse effects may require dosage reduction. *Gestrinone* has also been reported to be effective in cyclical mastalgia.[5]

Other drugs for cyclical mastalgia are *bromocriptine* or *gamolenic acid* (as evening primrose oil in most cases). Both are reported to produce a response in about 50% of cases, and appear to be equally effective.[1-3] However, gamolenic acid produces fewer adverse effects.[1,2,4,5] Again these drugs are less effective in non-cyclical mastalgia.[1,3]

A good response to danazol or bromocriptine would be expected within 2 months; gamolenic acid may take 3 to 4 months to show an effect.[1,4,5] When a response is achieved, therapy is withdrawn after 6 months to see if continued treatment is needed; even if pain recurs it may be less severe and therapy may be unnecessary.[1,2,5]

In refractory cyclical or non-cyclical mastalgia *tamoxifen*[7,8] has been shown to be effective; however, the concept of using tamoxifen in otherwise healthy premenopausal women has produced some concern.[9-11] *Goserelin* has also been shown to be effective.[12]

Other drugs that have been used for cyclical mastalgia include antibiotics, diuretics, pyridoxine, and the progestogens, but there is no evidence that they are any better than placebo.[1,2,5]

1. Gateley CA, Mansel RE. Management of the painful and nodular breast. *Br Med J* 1991; **47:** 284–9.
2. Anonymous. Cyclical breast pain—what works and what doesn't. *Drug Ther Bull* 1992; **30:** 1–3.
3. Gateley CA, *et al.* Drug treatments for mastalgia: 17 years experience in the Cardiff mastalgia clinic. *J R Soc Med* 1992; **85:** 12–15.
4. Mansel RE. Breast pain. *BMJ* 1994; **309:** 866–8.
5. Holland PA, Gateley CA. Drug therapy of mastalgia: what are the options. *Drugs* 1994; **48:** 709–16.
6. Boyd NF, *et al.* Effect of a low fat high-carbohydrate diet on symptoms of cyclical mastopathy. *Lancet* 1988; **ii:** 128–32.
7. Fentiman IS, *et al.* Double-blind controlled trial of tamoxifen therapy for mastalgia. *Lancet* 1986; **i:** 287–8.
8. Fentiman IS, *et al.* Studies of tamoxifen in women with mastalgia. *Br J Clin Pract* 1989; **43** (suppl 68): 34–6.
9. Anonymous. Tamoxifen for benign breast disease. *Lancet* 1986; **i:** 305.
10. Smallwood JA, Taylor I. Tamoxifen for mastalgia. *Lancet* 1986; **i:** 680–1.
11. Fentiman IS, *et al.* Tamoxifen for mastalgia. *Lancet* 1986; **i:** 681.
12. Hamed H, *et al.* LHRH analogue for treatment of recurrent and refractory mastalgia. *Ann R Coll Surg Engl* 1990; **72:** 221–4.

Menorrhagia. Danazol is effective in the treatment of menorrhagia (p.1490)[1-3] but it is only used short term because of its adverse effects.

1. Chimbira TH, *et al.* Reduction of menstrual blood loss by danazol in unexplained menorrhagia: lack of effect of placebo. *Br J Obstet Gynaecol* 1980; **87:** 1152–8.
2. Dockeray CJ, *et al.* Comparison between mefenamic acid and danazol in the treatment of established menorrhagia. *Br J Obstet Gynaecol* 1989; **96:** 840–4.
3. Bonduelle M, *et al.* A comparative study of danazol and norethisterone in dysfunctional uterine bleeding presenting as menorrhagia. *Postgrad Med J* 1991; **67:** 833–6.

Premenstrual syndrome. Danazol may be useful[1,2] in the management of the premenstrual syndrome (p.1475), but adverse effects limit its long-term use.

1. Halbreich U, *et al.* Elimination of ovulation and menstrual cyclicity (with danazol) improves dysphoric premenstrual syndromes. *Fertil Steril* 1991; **56:** 1066–9.
2. Deeny M, *et al.* Low dose danazol in the treatment of the premenstrual syndrome. *Postgrad Med J* 1991; **67:** 450–4.

Skin disorders. A patient with a skin condition involving cholinergic pruritus, erythema, and urticaria that was unresponsive to treatment with antihistamines and anti-inflammatory drugs was successfully treated with danazol 600 mg daily.[1] This dose of danazol also resolved a case of chronic actinic dermatitis.[2] In both of these patients, the skin disorder had been associated with low plasma concentrations of antiprotease.

1. Berth-Jones J, Graham-Brown RAC. Cholinergic pruritus, erythema and urticaria: a disease spectrum responding to danazol. *Br J Dermatol* 1989; **121:** 235–7.
2. Humbert P, *et al.* Chronic actinic dermatitis responding to danazol. *Br J Dermatol* 1991; **124:** 195–7.

Preparations

USP 25: Danazol Capsules.

Proprietary Preparations (details are given in Part 3)
Aust.: Danokrin; *Austral.:* Azol; Danocrine; *Belg.:* Danatrol; *Braz.:* Ladogal; *Canad.:* Cyclomen; *Denm.:* Danocrine; *Fin.:* Danocrine; *Fr.:* Danatrol; *Ger.:* Winobanin; *Hong Kong:* Anargil; Danazant; Danocrine; *Irl.:* Danazant; Danol; *Israel:* Danocrine; *Ital.:* Danatrol; *Mex.:* Danalem; Kendazol; Ladogal; Lisigon; Norciden; Zoldan-A; *Neth.:* Danatrol; Norw.: Danocrine; *NZ:* D-Zol; Danocrine; *Port.:* Danatrol; Mastodanatrol; *S.Afr.:* Ladazol; *Singapore:* Azol; Ladogal; *Spain:* Danatrol; *Swed.:* Danocrine; *Switz.:* Danatrol; *Thai.:* Anargil; Ectopal; Ladogal; Vabon; *UK:* Danol; *USA:* Danocrine.

Delmadinone Acetate (12628-y)

Delmadinone Acetate *(BANM, USAN, rINNM).*
RS-1301. 6-Chloro-17α-hydroxypregna-1,4,6-triene-3,20-dione acetate.
$C_{23}H_{27}ClO_4 = 402.9.$
CAS — 15262-77-8 (delmadinone); 13698-49-2 (delmadinone acetate).

Profile
Delmadinone acetate is a progestogen with anti-androgenic and anti-oestrogenic activity. It is used as an anti-androgen in veterinary practice.

Demegestone (12629-j)

Demegestone *(rINN).*
R-2453. 17α-Methyl-19-norpregna-4,9-diene-3,20-dione.
$C_{21}H_{28}O_2 = 312.4.$
CAS — 10116-22-0.
ATC — G03DB05.

Profile
Demegestone is a progestogen structurally related to progesterone (p.1488). It has been given cyclically or continuously, for its progestogenic effects, in doses of 1 to 2 mg daily by mouth.

Preparations
Proprietary Preparations (details are given in Part 3)
Fr.: Lutionex†.

Desogestrel (12633-w)

Desogestrel *(BAN, USAN, rINN).*
Org-2969. 13β-Ethyl-11-methylene-18,19-dinor-17α-pregn-4-en-20-yn-17β-ol.
$C_{22}H_{30}O = 310.5.$
CAS — 54024-22-5.
ATC — G03AC09.

Pharmacopoeias. In Br.

Pharmacopoeial description

BP 2001: A white, crystalline powder. Practically insoluble in water; slightly soluble in alcohol and in ethyl acetate; sparingly soluble in *n*-hexane.

Adverse Effects and Precautions
As for progestogens in general (see Progesterone, p.1488). See also under Hormonal Contraceptives, p.1452. Desogestrel is reported to have few androgenic effects, and to have less adverse effect on the serum lipid profile than older 19-nortestosterone derivatives. However, there is some evidence that desogestrel-containing combined oral contraceptives are associated with a small increased risk of venous thromboembolism (see p.1455, and for precautions, see p.1457).

Interactions
As for progestogens in general (see Progesterone, p.1489). See also under Hormonal Contraceptives, p.1458.

Pharmacokinetics
After oral administration, desogestrel undergoes oxidative transformation to its active metabolite 3-keto-desogestrel (see also Etonogestrel, p.1477) in the in-

testinal mucosa and liver. In the blood, about 32% of 3-keto-desogestrel is bound to sex hormone binding globulin, and 66% to albumin.

◊ References.
1. Madden S, *et al.* Metabolism of the contraceptive steroid desogestrel by the intestinal mucosa. *Br J Clin Pharmacol* 1989; **27:** 295–9.
2. Madden S, *et al.* Metabolism of the contraceptive steroid desogestrel by human liver in vitro. *J Steroid Biochem* 1990; **35:** 281–8.
3. Kuhnz W, *et al.* Protein binding of the contraceptive steroids gestodene, 3-keto-desogestrel and ethinyloestradiol in human serum. *J Steroid Biochem* 1990; **35:** 313–18.

Uses and Administration

Desogestrel is a progestogen (see Progesterone, p.1489) structurally related to levonorgestrel that is used as a hormonal contraceptive (see p.1459). A typical daily dose of 150 µg is used as the progestogenic component of combined oral contraceptive preparations. A dose of 75 µg daily by mouth is used as a progestogen-only contraceptive; unlike traditional progestogen-only contraceptives, desogestrel is said to reliably inhibit ovulation.

◊ Reviews.
1. Anonymous. Marvelon—an OC with a new progestagen. *Drug Ther Bull* 1984; **22:** 69–70.
2. Anonymous. Mercilon—a new low-dose combined oral contraceptive. *Drug Ther Bull* 1989; **27:** 51–2.
3. Anonymous. Desogestrel—a new progestin for oral contraception. *Med Lett Drugs Ther* 1993; **35:** 73–4.

Contraception. The effects of a progestogen-only contraceptive containing desogestrel have been reported.[1,2] Desogestrel has also been investigated as a male contraceptive in combination with low-dose testosterone.[3]

1. Collaborative study group on the desogestrel-containing progestogen-only pill. A double-blind study comparing the contraceptive efficacy, acceptability and safety of two progestogen-only pills containing desogestrel 75 micrograms/day or levonorgestrel 30 micrograms/day. *Eur J Contracept Reprod Health Care* 1998; **3:** 169–78.
2. Rice CF, *et al.* A comparison of the inhibition of ovulation achieved by desogestrel 75 µg and levonorgestrel 30 µg daily. *Hum Reprod* 1999; **14:** 982–5.
3. Wu FCW, *et al.* Oral progestogen combined with testosterone as a potential male contraceptive: additive effects between desogestrel and testosterone enanthate in suppression of spermatogenesis, pituitary-testicular axis, and lipid metabolism. *J Clin Endocrinol Metab* 1999; **84:** 112–22.

Preparations

Proprietary Preparations (details are given in Part 3)
Belg.: Cerazette; **Fr.:** Cerazette; **Ger.:** Cerazette; **Neth.:** Cerazette; **NZ:** Cerazette; **Swed.:** Cerazette.

Multi-ingredient: Aust.: Gracial; Marvelon; Mercilon; **Austral.:** Marvelon; **Belg.:** Gracial; Marvelon; Mercilon; Ovidol; **Braz.:** Mercilon; Microdiol; **Canad.:** Marvelon; Ortho-Cept; **Denm.:** Desorelle; Gracial; Marvelon; Mercilon; Novynette; **Fin.:** Gracial; Marvelon; Mercilon; **Fr.:** Cycleane; Mercilon; Varnoline; **Ger.:** Biviol; Cyclosa; Desmin; Lovelle; Lovina; Marvelon; Oviol; **Hong Kong:** Gracial; Marvelon; Mercilon; **Irl.:** Marviol; Mercilon; **Israel:** Mercilon; Microdiol; **Ital.:** Dueva; Gracial; Mercilon; Planum; Practil; Securgin; **Mex.:** Marvelon; Mercilon; **Neth.:** Gracial; Marvelon; Mercilon; Ovidol; **Norw.:** Marvelon; **NZ:** Marvelon; Mercilon; **Port.:** Gracial; Marvelon; Mercilon; **S.Afr.:** Marvelon; Mercilon; **Singapore:** Marvelon; Mercilon; **Spain:** Microdiol; Suavuret; **Swed.:** Desolett; Mercilon; Trimiron; **Switz.:** Gracial; Marvelon; Mercilon; Ovidol; **Thai.:** Marvelon; Mercilon; **UK:** Marvelon; Mercilon; **USA:** Apri; Desogen; Mircette; Ortho-Cept.

Dienestrol (9037-q)

Dienestrol (*BAN, rINN*).
Dehydrostilbestrol; Dienestrolum; Dienoestrol; Dienoestrolum; Oestrodienolum. (*E,E*)-4,4'-[Di(ethylidene)ethylene]diphenol; 4,4'-(1,2-Diethylidene-1,2-ethanediyl)bisphenol.
$C_{18}H_{18}O_2 = 266.3$.
$CAS — 84-17-3$ (dienestrol); $13029-44-2$ ((*E,E*)-dienestrol).
$ATC — G03CB01; G03CC02$.
Pharmacopoeias. In *Eur.* (see p.vi) and US.
Aust. also includes dienestrol diacetate, $C_{22}H_{22}O_4 = 350.4$.

Pharmacopoeial description

Ph. Eur.: A white or almost white, crystalline powder. Practically insoluble in water; freely soluble in alcohol and in acetone; soluble in ether; dissolves in dilute solutions of alkali hydroxides. Protect from light.

USP 25: Colourless, white, or practically white needle-like crystals, or white or practically white crystalline powder. It is odourless. Practically insoluble in water; soluble in alcohol, in acetone, in ether, in methyl alcohol, in propylene glycol, and in solutions of alkali hydroxides; slightly soluble in chloroform and in fatty oils.

Profile

Dienestrol is a synthetic nonsteroidal oestrogen structurally related to diethylstilbestrol (p.1471). It is used as a 0.01% cream in the treatment of menopausal atrophic vaginitis. If used on a

long-term basis in women with a uterus a progestogen is required.

Dienestrol diacetate has been used as an ingredient of topical preparations for skin disorders.

Porphyria. Dienestrol is considered to be unsafe in patients with porphyria because it has been shown to be porphyrinogenic in *animals* or *in-vitro* systems.

Preparations

USP 25: Dienoestrol Cream.

Proprietary Preparations (details are given in Part 3)
Belg.: Ortho-Dienoestrol; **Denm.:** Sexadien; **Irl.:** Ortho; **Israel:** Ortho-Dienoestrol; **UK:** Ortho-Dienoestrol†; **USA:** DV†; Ortho-Dienestrol.

Dienogest (1999-c)

Dienogest (*rINN*).
STS-557. 17-Hydroxy-3-oxo-19-nor-17α-pregna-4,9-diene-21-nitrite.
$C_{20}H_{25}NO_2 = 311.4$.
$CAS — 65928-58-7$.

Profile

Dienogest is a nonethinylated progestogen (see Progesterone, p.1488) structurally related to nortestosterone. It is reported to have anti-androgenic properties. Dienogest is used as the progestogen component of some combined oral contraceptives (see p.1452); a typical daily dose is 2 mg.

◊ Reviews.
1. Foster RH, Wilde MI. Dienogest. *Drugs* 1998; **56:** 825–33.

Preparations

Proprietary Preparations (details are given in Part 3)
Multi-ingredient: Ger.: Valette.

Diethylstilbestrol (9106-b)

Diethylstilbestrol (*BAN, rINN*).
DES; Diethylstilbestrolum; Diethylstilboestrol; NSC-3070; Stilbestrol; Stilboestrol. (*E*)-αβ-Diethylstilbene-4-4'-diol.
$C_{18}H_{20}O_2 = 268.4$.
$CAS — 56-53-1$.
$ATC — G03CB02; G03CC05; L02AA01$.
Pharmacopoeias. In *Chin., Eur.* (see p.vi), and US.

Pharmacopoeial description

Ph. Eur.: A white or almost white crystalline powder. Practically insoluble in water; freely soluble in alcohol and in ether; dissolves in solutions of alkali hydroxides. Protect from light.

USP 25: A white, odourless, crystalline powder. Practically insoluble in water; soluble in alcohol, in chloroform, in ether, in fatty oils, and in dilute alkali solutions. Store in airtight containers. Protect from light.

Diethylstilbestrol Dipropionate (9105-m)

Diethylstilbestrol Dipropionate (*BANM, rINNM*).
Stilboestrol Dipropionate. (*E*)-αβ-Diethylstilbene-4,4'-diol dipropionate.
$C_{24}H_{28}O_4 = 380.5$.
$CAS — 130-80-3$.
Pharmacopoeias. In *Aust.*

Adverse Effects and Precautions

Dose-related adverse effects of diethylstilbestrol include nausea, fluid retention, and arterial and venous thrombosis, and these effects are common at the doses used for palliation of cancer. Impotence and gynaecomastia occur in men, and withdrawal bleeding may occur in women, as may hypercalcaemia and bone pain in women treated for breast cancer. Diethylstilbestrol should be used with caution in those with cardiovascular disease or hepatic impairment. Use of diethylstilbestrol is contra-indicated if pregnancy is suspected.

Adverse effects and precautions of oestrogens in general (steroidal compounds) are covered under Estradiol, on p.1473.

Historically, high doses of diethylstilbestrol and related substances were used for 'hormonal support' in pregnant women to try to prevent miscarriages and preterm births, most commonly in the USA. This practice was later shown to be ineffective. Adverse effects on the genito-urinary tract of offspring of these women have been noted. In particular, an increased incidence of changes in the cervix and vagina including adenosis and rarely clear-cell adenocarcinoma has been seen in postpubertal daughters of

women who received diethylstilbestrol or related substances during pregnancy (see below). A possible increased incidence of abnormalities of the genital tract and of abnormal spermatozoa has been reported in male offspring similarly exposed (see below). The recipients themselves appear to be at a small increased risk of breast cancer (see below).

Carcinogenicity. BREAST. No statistically significant difference in the incidence of breast cancer was found among a group of 693 women who had received diethylstilbestrol during pregnancy 25 years earlier compared with a control group of 668 who had not.[1] This finding was, however, criticised[2] on the basis that the study lacked the statistical power to reject the null hypothesis. In another study[3] the incidence of breast cancer in 3033 women who had taken diethylstilbestrol in pregnancy during the period 1940 to 1960 was compared with the incidence in a comparable group of unexposed women. This study involved over 85 000 women-years of follow-up in each group and it was found that the incidence of breast cancer per 100 000 women-years was 134 in the exposed group and 93 in the unexposed group (a relative risk of 1.4). The authors concluded that in those women given diethylstilbestrol there was a moderately increased incidence of breast cancer but that some unrecognised concomitant of exposure could not be excluded as a possibility for the increase. Although this study suggested that the risk increased over time, subsequent follow-up,[4] while confirming a modest increase in risk overall, did not confirm a higher risk in these women as time went on. Two recent cases of breast cancer[5] in premenopausal women exposed to diethylstilbestrol *in utero* have raised the possibility that the risk of breast cancer may be increased in these women, in addition to the known genito-urinary risk (see below under Pregnancy, Effects on Female Offspring). However, a cohort study[6] involving 4536 women exposed *in utero* found no increased risk of other cancers overall, and did not show an increased risk of breast cancer (relative risk 1.18; 95% confidence intervals 0.56 to 2.49). Nonetheless, since these women were relatively young, continued follow-up was considered necessary.

1. Bibbo M, *et al.* A twenty-five-year follow up study of women exposed to diethylstilbestrol during pregnancy. *N Engl J Med* 1978; **298:** 763–7.
2. Clark LC, Portier KM. Diethylstilbestrol and the risk of cancer. *N Engl J Med* 1979; **300:** 263–4.
3. Greenberg ER, *et al.* Breast cancer in mothers given diethylstilbestrol in pregnancy. *N Engl J Med* 1984; **311:** 1393–8.
4. Colton T, *et al.* Breast cancer in mothers prescribed diethylstilbestrol in pregnancy. *JAMA* 1993; **269:** 2096–2100.
5. Huckell C, *et al.* Premenopausal breast cancer after in-utero exposure to stilboestrol. *Lancet* 1996; **348:** 331.
6. Hatch EE, *et al.* Cancer risk in women exposed to diethylstilbestrol in utero. *JAMA* 1998; **280:** 630–4.

GENITO-URINARY TRACT. See below under Pregnancy, Effects on Female Offspring.

KIDNEY. Renal carcinoma associated with the long-term use of diethylstilbestrol for prostate cancer in 2 men.[1]

1. Nissenkorn I, *et al.* Oestrogen-induced renal carcinoma. *Br J Urol* 1979; **51:** 6–8.

LIVER. Hepatic angiosarcoma developed in a 76-year-old man who had received diethylstilbestrol 3 mg daily for 12 years.[1] Hepatoma developed in another elderly man who had received a similar dose for 4.5 years.[2]

1. Hoch-Ligeti C. Angiosarcoma of the liver associated with diethylstilbestrol. *JAMA* 1978; **240:** 1510–11.
2. Brooks JJ. Hepatoma associated with diethylstilbestrol therapy for prostate carcinoma. *J Urol (Baltimore)* 1982; **128:** 1044–5.

Effects on the blood. Adverse haematological effects reported with diethylstilbestrol include severe bone-marrow changes in a 71-year-old man given diethylstilbestrol in a massive dose of 150 mg daily for 7 years[1] and fatal immune haemolytic anaemia in a 69-year-old man given weekly infusions of diethylstilbestrol 1 g for 9 weeks.[2] The latter reaction was due to an IgG antibody specific for diethylstilbestrol.

1. Anderson AL, Lynch EC. Myelodysplastic syndrome associated with diethylstilbestrol therapy. *Arch Intern Med* 1980; **140:** 976–7.
2. Rosenfeld CS, *et al.* Diethylstilbestrol-associated hemolytic anemia with a positive direct antiglobulin test result. *Am J Med* 1989; **86:** 617–18.

Pregnancy. EFFECTS ON FEMALE OFFSPRING. The DESAD (Diethylstilbestrol and Adenosis) Project carried out by the National Cancer Institute in the USA led to several reports linking exposure to diethylstilbestrol *in utero* to adverse genital-tract effects.[1-3] It was reported that of nearly 300 young females with clear-cell adenocarcinoma of the genital tract, more than 80% had been exposed *in utero* to diethylstilbestrol-type hormones.[1] Patients had been aged 7 to 28 years at the time of diagnosis. Doses and duration of treatment varied widely; 1.5 mg of diethylstilbestrol daily throughout pregnancy or varying amounts for a week or more during the first trimester had shown an association. Vaginal adenosis, in unexposed young women, was present in about a third of those exposed in the first 4 months of pregnancy, and cervical ectropion in more than two-thirds. Vaginal epithelial changes were most closely associated with early exposure to diethylstilbestrol, with the total dose, and with the duration of exposure; their incidence decreased with age. The risk of cancer in the first 25 years after exposure was small.[2] Fertility did not appear to be impaired in

The symbol † denotes a preparation no longer actively marketed

women who had been exposed *in utero* to diethylstilbestrol but the relative risk of an unfavourable outcome of pregnancy in such a group was 1.69. However, of the women who became pregnant, 81% of those exposed to diethylstilbestrol and 95% of control subjects had at least one full-term live birth.[3] In a review of vaginal adenosis and its association with maternal diethylstilbestrol ingestion during pregnancy[4] it was noted that the link between diethylstilbestrol and particularly the benign changes in the vagina and cervix (adenosis) seemed well established. The association between this drug and the development of genital malignancies was less clear, and the very low incidence in the prospective studies in the USA supported this concept. The size of the problem in the UK was small, but clinicians should be aware that it exists. Cases of vaginal adenosis in young women should be investigated and screened appropriately, and preferably referred to centres where colposcopic expertise is available. Treatment of simple vaginal adenosis should be avoided.

More recent reviews[5,6] have highlighted the fact that adverse effects are still emerging in women who had been exposed to diethylstilbestrol *in utero* several decades ago. The need for thorough medical screening of such women was emphasised; genital-tract examination was particularly important. It was pointed out[6] that many women exposed to diethylstilbestrol *in utero* were now in the reproductive stage of their lives and warranted special observation since a diethylstilbestrol-damaged genital tract posed a potential problem during pregnancy.[5,6] It has also been suggested, for example, that such women are at increased risk of developing pre-eclampsia.[7]

Further information on the adverse effects of diethylstilbestrol in females exposed to the drug *in utero* can be obtained from the references listed below.[8-18] For mention of the possible increased risk of breast cancer in these women, see Carcinogenicity, above.

1. Professional and Public Relations Committee of the DESAD (Diethylstilbestrol and Adenosis) Project of the Division of Cancer Control and Rehabilitation. Exposure in utero to diethylstilbestrol and related synthetic hormones: association with vaginal and cervical cancers and other abnormalities. *JAMA* 1976; **236**: 1107–9.
2. O'Brien PC, *et al.* Vaginal epithelial changes in young women enrolled in the National Cooperative Diethylstilbestrol Adenosis (DESAD) Project. *Obstet Gynecol* 1979; **53**: 300–8.
3. Barnes AB, *et al.* Fertility and outcome of pregnancy in women exposed in utero to diethylstilbestrol. *N Engl J Med* 1980; **302**: 609–13.
4. Emens M. Vaginal adenosis and diethylstilbestrol. *Br J Hosp Med* 1984; **31**: 42–8.
5. Anonymous. Diethylstilboestrol—effects of exposure in utero. *Drug Ther Bull* 1991; **29**: 49–50.
6. Wingfield M. The daughters of stilboestrol. *BMJ* 1991; **302**: 1414–15.
7. Mittendorf R, Williams MA. Stilboestrol exposure in utero and risk of pre-eclampsia. *Lancet* 1995; **345**: 265–6.
8. Herbst AL, *et al.* Prenatal exposure to stilbestrol: a prospective comparison of exposed female offspring with unexposed controls. *N Engl J Med* 1975; **292**: 334–9.
9. Herbst AL, *et al.* Age-incidence and risk of diethylstilbestrol-related clear cell adenocarcinoma of the vagina and cervix. *Am J Obstet Gynecol* 1977; **128**: 43–50.
10. Kaufman RH, *et al.* Upper genital tract changes associated with in-utero exposure to diethylstilbestrol. *Am J Obstet Gynecol* 1977; **128**: 51.
11. Fowler WC, Edelman DA. In utero exposure to DES: evaluation and followup of 199 women. *Obstet Gynecol* 1978; **51**: 459–63.
12. Anderson B, *et al.* Development of DES-associated clear-cell carcinoma: the importance of regular screening. *Obstet Gynecol* 1979; **53**: 293–9.
13. Noller KL, *et al.* Maturation of vaginal and cervical epithelium in women exposed in utero to diethylstilbestrol (DESAD project). *Am J Obstet Gynecol* 1983; **146**: 279–85.
14. Robboy SJ, *et al.* Increased incidence of cervical and vaginal dysplasia in 3980 diethylstilbestrol-exposed young women: experience of the National Collaborative Diethylstilbestrol Adenosis Project. *JAMA* 1984; **252**: 2979–83.
15. Kaufman RH, *et al.* Upper genital tract changes and infertility in diethylstilbestrol-exposed women. *Am J Obstet Gynecol* 1986; **154**: 1312–18.
16. Melnick S, *et al.* Rates and risks of diethylstilbestrol-related clear-cell adenocarcinoma of the vagina and cervix—an update. *N Engl J Med* 1987; **316**: 514–16.
17. Helmerhorst TJM, *et al.* Colposcopic findings and intraepithelial neoplasia in diethylstilbestrol-exposed offspring: the Dutch experience. *Am J Obstet Gynecol* 1989; **161**: 1191–4.
18. Giusti RM, *et al.* Diethylstilbestrol revisited: a review of the long-term health effects. *Ann Intern Med* 1995; **122**: 778–88.

EFFECTS ON MALE OFFSPRING. The effects of exposure to diethylstilbestrol *in utero* have been studied in male offspring.[1-4] Problems in passing urine and abnormalities of the penile urethra were found to be more common in young males exposed to diethylstilbestrol *in utero* than in controls in one study.[1] In another,[2] genital tract abnormalities such as epididymal cysts, capsular induration, and defective testicles occurred in 41 of 163 diethylstilbestrol-exposed men compared with 11 of 168 controls; sperm counts and motility were also reduced in exposed males. In contrast, comparison of 828 men exposed to diethylstilbestrol *in utero* with 676 unexposed men suggested that, overall, diethylstilbestrol exposure did not result in an increased risk of genito-urinary abnormalities, infertility, or testicular cancer.[3] It was suggested that previously reported increased frequencies of such abnormalities may have resulted from a selection bias and/or from a difference in diethylstilbestrol usage. Another study[4] in 253 exposed men found that although there was an increased incidence of congenital malformations of the genitalia (18 cases compared with 5 of 241 controls), this was not associated with any decrease in fertility or impairment of sexual function.

Isolated reports of adverse effects occurring in young men who were exposed to diethylstilbestrol *in utero* have included seminoma and epididymal cysts in one man.[5]

1. Henderson BE, *et al.* Urogenital tract abnormalities in sons of women treated with diethylstilbestrol. *Pediatrics* 1976; **58**: 505–7.
2. Anonymous. Offspring of women given DES remains under study. *JAMA* 1977; **238**: 932.
3. Leary FJ, *et al.* Males exposed in utero to diethylstilbestrol. *JAMA* 1984; **252**: 2984–9.
4. Wilcox AJ, *et al.* Fertility in men exposed prenatally to diethylstilbestrol. *N Engl J Med* 1995; **332**: 1411–16.
5. Conley GR, *et al.* Seminoma and epididymal cysts in a young man with known diethylstilbestrol exposure in utero. *JAMA* 1983; **249**: 1325–6.

Veterinary use. In the European Union, the use of diethylstilbestrol or other stilbenes in veterinary medicine is banned unless prior steps are taken to ensure the treated animal and its products are not available for human or animal consumption.

Pharmacokinetics

Diethylstilbestrol is readily absorbed from the gastrointestinal tract. It is slowly inactivated in the liver and excreted in the urine and faeces, mainly as the glucuronide.

Uses and Administration

Diethylstilbestrol is a synthetic nonsteroidal oestrogen that has been used in the palliation of breast and prostate cancer.

Daily doses of 10 to 20 mg are occasionally used by mouth in the palliative treatment of malignant neoplasms of the breast in postmenopausal women (p.491). The usual dose in carcinoma of the prostate (p.497) is 1 to 3 mg daily by mouth; higher doses were formerly given. Diethylstilbestrol has also been used in the treatment of prostatic carcinoma in the form of its diphosphate salts (see Fosfestrol, p.1478).

Diethylstilbestrol has been used as pessaries in the short-term management of menopausal atrophic vaginitis at a dose of 1 mg daily.

Preparations

BP 2001: Diethylstilbestrol Pessaries; Diethylstilbestrol Tablets;
USP 25: Diethylstilbestrol Injection; Diethylstilbestrol Tablets.

Proprietary Preparations (details are given in Part 3)
Fr.: Distilbene; *UK:* Apstil†.

Multi-ingredient: *Braz.:* Calmovarin; *S.Afr.:* Oestro-Gynedron†; Poly-Gynedron†; *Spain:* Cilinavagin Neomicina; *UK:* Tampovagan.

Drospirenone (14636-g)

Drospirenone (USAN, rINN).

Dihydrospirenone; ZK-30595. (6R,7R,8R,9S,10R,13S,14S,15S,16S,17S)-1,3′,4′,6,6a,7,8,9,10,11,12,13,14,15,15a,16-Hexadecahydro-10,13-dimethylspiro-[17H-dicyclopropa[6,7:15,16]cyclopenta[a]phenanthrene-17,2′(5′H)-furan]-3,5′(2H)-dione.
$C_{24}H_{30}O_3 = 366.5$.
CAS — 67392-87-4.

Adverse Effects and Precautions

As for progestogens in general (see Progesterone, p.1488). See also under Hormonal Contraceptives, p.1452. Drospirenone has antimineralocorticoid activity and therefore should not be used in patients at risk of hyperkalaemia, such as those with renal or hepatic impairment or adrenal insufficiency.

Interactions

As for progestogens in general (see Progesterone, p.1489). See also under Hormonal Contraceptives, p.1458.

Pharmacokinetics

After oral administration, drospirenone is about 97% bound to plasma proteins, though it does not bind to sex hormone binding globulin or corticosteroid binding globulin. It is extensively metabolised with a terminal half-life of about 30 hours. The metabolites are excreted in the urine and faeces.

Uses and Administration

Drospirenone is a progestogen (see Progesterone, p.1489) with antimineralocorticoid and anti-androgenic activity, that is used as the progestogenic component of a combined oral contraceptive (see p.1459) in doses of 3 mg daily.

◊ References.

1. Huber J, *et al.* Efficacy and tolerability of a monophasic oral contraceptive containing ethinylestradiol and drospirenone. *Eur J Contracept Reprod Health Care* 2000; **5**: 25–34.
2. Foidart JM. The contraceptive profile of a new oral contraceptive with antimineralocorticoid and antiandrogenic effects. *Eur J Contracept Reprod Health Care* 2000; **5** (suppl 3): 25–33.
3. Oelkers W, *et al.* Effect of an oral contraceptive containing drospirenone on the renin-angiotensin-aldosterone system in healthy female volunteers. *Gynecol Endocrinol* 2000; **14**: 204–13.
4. Krattenmacher R. Drospirenone: pharmacology and pharmacokinetics of a unique progestogen. *Contraception* 2000; **62**: 29–38.

Preparations

Proprietary Preparations (details are given in Part 3)
Multi-ingredient: *USA:* Yasmin.

Dutasteride (20134-j)

Dutasteride (BAN, USAN, rINN).

GG-745; GI-198745; GI-198745X. α,α,α,α′,α′,α′-Hexafluoro-3-oxo-4-aza-5α-androst-1-ene-17β-carboxy-2′,5′-xylidide; 3-Oxo-2′,5′-bis(trifluoromethyl)-4-aza-5α-androst-1-ene-17β-carboxanilide.
$C_{27}H_{30}F_6N_2O_2 = 528.5$.
CAS — 164656-23-9.

Profile

Dutasteride is a 5α-reductase inhibitor (see Finasteride, p.1477) under investigation for benign prostatic hyperplasia and in alopecia.

◊ References.

1. Gisleskog PO, *et al.* The pharmacokinetic modelling of GI198745 (dutasteride), a compound with parallel linear and nonlinear elimination. *Br J Clin Pharmacol* 1999; **47**: 53–8.

Dydrogesterone (9040-h)

Dydrogesterone (BAN, USAN, rINN).

Dehydroprogesterone; 6-Dehydro-*retro*-progesterone; 6-Dehydro-9β,10α-progesterone; Didrogesteron; Isopregnenone; NSC-92336. 9β,10α-Pregna-4,6-diene-3,20-dione.
$C_{21}H_{28}O_2 = 312.4$.
CAS — 152-62-5.
ATC — G03DB01.
Pharmacopoeias. In *Br., Jpn,* and *US.*

Pharmacopoeial description

BP 2001: A white or almost white crystalline powder; odourless or almost odourless. Practically insoluble in water; sparingly soluble in alcohol and in methyl alcohol; soluble in acetone; freely soluble in chloroform; slightly soluble in ether and in fixed oils. Protect from light.

USP 25: A white to pale yellow crystalline powder. Practically insoluble in water; soluble 1 in 40 of alcohol, 1 in 2 of chloroform, and 1 in 200 of ether.

Adverse Effects and Precautions

As for progestogens in general (see Progesterone, p.1488).

Porphyria. Dydrogesterone has been associated with acute attacks of porphyria and is considered unsafe in porphyric patients.

Pregnancy. Anomalies (non-virilising) of the genito-urinary tract were found in a 4-month-old baby whose mother had taken dydrogesterone 20 mg daily from the eighth to twentieth week of pregnancy and 10 mg daily from then until term.[1] She had also been given hydroxyprogesterone caproate 250 mg by intramuscular injection weekly from the eighth to twentieth week.

1. Roberts IF, West RJ. Teratogenesis and maternal progesterone. *Lancet* 1977; **ii**: 982.

Interactions

As for progestogens in general (see Progesterone, p.1489).

Uses and Administration

Dydrogesterone is a progestogen structurally related to progesterone (p.1489). It does not have oestrogenic or androgenic properties.

Dydrogesterone is given by mouth in the treatment of menstrual disorders such as menorrhagia (p.1490), usually in a dose of 10 mg twice daily in a cyclical regimen, and for the treatment of endometriosis (p.1469) in a dose of 10 mg two or three times daily cyclically or continuously. It is also given cyclically in doses of 10 mg once or twice daily, or continuously in doses of 5 mg daily, for endometrial protection during menopausal HRT (p.1460).

In threatened miscarriage suggested doses have been 40 mg initially followed by 10 mg or more every 8 hours, continued for a week after symptoms cease. In recurrent miscarriage suggested doses have been 10 mg twice daily. However, such use is not recommended unless there is proven progesterone deficiency. Cyclical dydrogesterone has also been used in infertility (p.1275) in doses of 10 mg twice daily.

Preparations

BP 2001: Dydrogesterone Tablets;
USP 25: Dydrogesterone Tablets.

Proprietary Preparations (details are given in Part 3)
Aust.: Duphaston; *Austral.:* Duphaston; *Belg.:* Duphaston; *Fin.:* Terolut; *Fr.:* Duphaston; *Ger.:* Duphaston; *Hong Kong:* Duphaston; *Irl.:* Duphaston; *Israel:* Biphaston; *Ital.:* Dufaston; *Neth.:* Duphaston; *NZ:* Duphaston; *Port.:* Duphaston; *S.Afr.:* Duphaston; *Singapore:* Duphaston; *Spain:* Duphaston; *Swed.:* Duphaston; *Switz.:* Duphaston; *Thai.:* Duphaston; *UK:* Duphaston.

Multi-ingredient: *Aust.:* Femoston; *Austral.:* Femoston; *Belg.:* Femoston; *Fin.:* Femoston; *Fr.:* Climaston; *Ger.:* Femoston; *Hong Kong:* Femoston; *Irl.:* Femoston; *Neth.:* Femoston; Zumeston†; *Port.:* Femoston; *Singa-*

pore: Femoston; *Switz.:* Femoston; Femoston Conti; *UK:* Fema-pak; Femoston; Femoston Conti.

Equilin (18357-p)

3-Hydroxyestra-1,3,5(10),7-tetraen-17-one.
$C_{18}H_{20}O_2 = 268.4$.
CAS — 474-86-2.
Pharmacopoeias. In US.

Pharmacopoeial description

USP 25: Store in airtight containers. Protect from light.

Profile

Equilin is a natural oestrogenic hormone found in horses. Sodium equilin sulfate is one of the components of both conjugated oestrogens (p.1467) and esterified oestrogens (see below) used for menopausal HRT.

Esterified Oestrogens (10069-v)

Esterified Estrogens.
Pharmacopoeias. In US.

Pharmacopoeial description

USP 25: A mixture of the sodium salts of the sulfate esters of the oestrogenic substances, principally estrone. It contains 75 to 85% of sodium estrone sulfate and 6 to 15% of sodium equilin sulfate, in such a proportion that the total of these two components is not less than 90%, of the labelled amount of esterified oestrogens. A white or buff-coloured amorphous powder; odourless or having a slight characteristic odour. Store in airtight containers.

Profile

Esterified oestrogens have actions and uses similar to those described for estradiol (see below). They are used for the same purposes (principally menopausal HRT), and in a similar dosage by mouth, as conjugated oestrogens (see p.1467), although higher cyclical doses of 2.5 to 7.5 mg daily are still licensed for use in female hypogonadism.

Preparations

USP 25: Esterified Estrogens Tablets.

Proprietary Preparations (details are given in Part 3)
Switz.: Oestro-Feminal; *USA:* Estratab; Menest.

Multi-ingredient: *USA:* Estratest; Menogen†; Menrium†.

Estradiol (9083-y)

Estradiol (*BAN, rINN*).
Beta-oestradiol; Dihydrofolliculin; Dihydrotheelin; Dihydroxyoestrin; Estradiolum; NSC-9895; NSC-20293 (alpha-estradiol); Oestradiol. Estra-1,3,5(10)-triene-3,17β-diol.
$C_{18}H_{24}O_2 = 272.4$.
CAS — 50-28-2 (anhydrous estradiol).
ATC — G03CA03.

NOTE. In *Martindale* the term oestradiol is used for the endogenous substance.
Pharmacopoeias. In Aust., Fr., and US.
Eur. (see p.vi) includes the hemihydrate.
Estradiol hemihydrate 1.03 g is approximately equivalent to 1 g of the anhydrous substance.

Pharmacopoeial description

Ph. Eur.: Estradiol hemihydrate is a white or almost white crystalline powder or colourless crystals. Practically insoluble in water; sparingly soluble in alcohol; soluble in acetone; slightly soluble in dichloromethane and in ether. Protect from light.

USP 25: White or creamy-white, odourless, hygroscopic small crystals or crystalline powder. Practically insoluble in water; soluble 1 in 28 of alcohol, 1 in 435 of chloroform, and 1 in 150 of ether; soluble in acetone, in dioxan, and in solutions of fixed alkali hydroxides; sparingly soluble in vegetable oils. Store in airtight containers. Protect from light.

Estradiol Benzoate (9084-j)

Estradiol Benzoate (*BAN, rINN*).
Beta-oestradiol Benzoate; Dihydroxyoestrin Monobenzoate; Estradioli Benzoas; NSC-9566; Oestradiol Benzoate. Estra-1,3,5(10)-triene-3,17β-diol 3-benzoate.
$C_{25}H_{28}O_3 = 376.5$.
CAS — 50-50-0.
Pharmacopoeias. In Chin., Eur. (see p.vi), *Jpn,* and *Pol.*

Pharmacopoeial description

Ph. Eur.: An almost white crystalline powder or colourless crystals. Practically insoluble in water; slightly soluble in alcohol and in fatty oils; sparingly soluble in acetone. Protect from light.

Estradiol Cipionate (9085-z)

Estradiol Cipionate (*BANM, rINNM*).
Estradiol Cypionate; Oestradiol Cyclopentylpropionate; Oestradiol Cypionate. Estra-1,3,5(10)-triene-3,17β-diol 17-(3-cyclopentylpropionate).
$C_{26}H_{36}O_3 = 396.6$.
CAS — 313-06-4.
Pharmacopoeias. In US.

Pharmacopoeial description

USP 25: A white to practically white crystalline powder, odourless or has a slight odour. Insoluble in water; soluble 1 in 40 of alcohol, 1 in 7 of chloroform, and 1 in 2800 of ether; soluble in acetone and in dioxan; sparingly soluble in vegetable oils. Store in airtight containers. Protect from light.

Estradiol Dipropionate (9086-c)

Estradiol Dipropionate (*BANM, rINNM*).
Dihydroxyoestrin Dipropionate; Oestradiol Dipropionate. Estra-1,3,5(10)-triene-3,17β-diol dipropionate.
$C_{24}H_{32}O_4 = 384.5$.
CAS — 113-38-2.
Pharmacopoeias. In Aust. and Swiss.

Estradiol Enantate (9087-k)

Estradiol Enantate (*BANM, rINNM*).
Estradiol Enanthate (*USAN*); Oestradiol Enanthate; Oestradiol 17-Heptanoate; SQ-16150. Estra-1,3,5(10)-triene-3,17β-diol 17-heptanoate.
$C_{25}H_{36}O_3 = 384.6$.
CAS — 4956-37-0.

Estradiol Hexahydrobenzoate (13039-d)

Estradiol Hexahydrobenzoate (*BANM, rINNM*).
Oestradiol Hexahydrobenzoate. Estra-1,3,5(10)-triene-3,17β-diol 17-cyclohexanecarboxylate.
$C_{25}H_{34}O_3 = 382.5$.
CAS — 15140-27-9.

Estradiol Phenylpropionate (10064-d)

Estradiol Phenylpropionate (*BANM, rINNM*).
Oestradiol Phenylpropionate. Estra-1,3,5(10)-triene-3,17β-diol 17-(3-phenylpropionate).
$C_{27}H_{32}O_3 = 404.5$.

Estradiol Undecylate (9088-a)

Estradiol Undecylate (*BANM, USAN, rINN*).
Oestradiol Undecanoate; SQ-9993. Estra-1,3,5(10)-triene-3,17β-diol 17-undecanoate.
$C_{29}H_{44}O_3 = 440.7$.
CAS — 3571-53-7; 33613-02-4.

Estradiol Valerate (9089-t)

Estradiol Valerate (*BANM, rINN*).
Estradioli Valeras; NSC-17590; Oestradiol Valerate. Estra-1,3,5(10)-triene-3,17β-diol 17-valerate.
$C_{23}H_{32}O_3 = 356.5$.
CAS — 979-32-8.
Pharmacopoeias. In Chin., Eur. (see p.vi), and *US.*

Pharmacopoeial description

Ph. Eur.: A white or almost white, crystalline powder or colourless crystals. Practically insoluble in water; soluble in alcohol. Protect from light.

USP 25: A white crystalline powder which is usually odourless or may have a faint fatty odour. Practically insoluble in water; soluble in benzyl benzoate, in dioxan, in methyl alcohol, and in castor oil; sparingly soluble in arachis oil and in sesame oil. Store in airtight containers. Protect from light.

Adverse Effects

The adverse effects of estradiol and other oestrogens are related, in part, to dose and duration of therapy, and to the gender and age of the recipient. In addition, adverse effects may be modified by concomitant administration of a progestogen in menopausal HRT or combined oral contraceptives. Whether adverse effects of natural and synthetic oestrogens differ, and whether the route of administration has an effect, is less clear.

The adverse effects of oestrogens used in HRT are considered in detail starting on p.1461. Those of oestrogens used in hormonal contraceptives are considered in detail starting on p.1452.

The use of oestrogens in girls may cause premature closure of the epiphyses resulting in decreased final adult height.

Large doses of oestrogens used in palliation of cancers have additionally been associated with nausea, fluid retention, venous and arterial thrombosis, and hepatic impairment. In men, they cause impotence and feminising effects such as gynaecomastia. In women, they may cause withdrawal bleeding, and, when used for breast cancer, they have caused hypercalcaemia and bone pain.

Effects on the skin. There is some evidence[1] that transdermal patches in which estradiol is dissolved in the adhesive matrix cause fewer skin reactions than those employing release of estradiol from an alcoholic reservoir.

1. Ross D. Randomised crossover comparison of skin irritation with two transdermal oestradiol patches. *BMJ* 1997; **315:** 288.

Precautions

The precautions for the use of estradiol and other oestrogens used as menopausal HRT are considered in detail starting on p.1463. Those for oestrogens used in hormonal contraceptives are considered in detail starting on p.1457.

High doses of oestrogen used in treating malignant disease should be used cautiously in patients with cerebrovascular disorders, coronary artery disease, or venous thromboembolism. They may exacerbate hypercalcaemia of malignancy.

Oestrogens should be used with caution in children because premature closure of the epiphyses may occur resulting in inhibited linear growth and small stature.

Oestrogens have been reported to interfere with some diagnostic tests such as those for thyroid function and glucose tolerance.

Cosmetic use. Use of cosmetic products containing oestrogens has led to adverse effects such as precocious puberty in children and gynaecomastia or postmenopausal bleeding in adults.[1]

1. Anonymous. Estrogens in cosmetics. *Med Lett Drugs Ther* 1985; **27:** 54–5.

Porphyria. Oestrogens are considered to be unsafe in patients with porphyria although there is conflicting experimental evidence of porphyrinogenicity.

Pregnancy. Although gross abnormalities of the genito-urinary tract have been reported in the male offspring of women who took diethylstilbestrol during pregnancy there is conflicting evidence as to whether the oestrogen produced an increased risk of abnormalities, infertility, or testicular cancer in such offspring (see p.1472). The male fetus is normally protected from the feminising effects of the natural oestrogens in the uterine environment by the early development of the testes and the secretion of male hormones.[1] However, there has been considerable concern about a rising incidence of disorders of the male reproductive tract, and a reduction in sperm counts, which has been noted in the last 20 to 30 years. It has been hypothesised that overexposure of male fetuses to environmental oestrogens derived from pollutants such as pesticides and plastics may be responsible for this decline,[2,3] although some dispute this.[4]

For discussion of the lack of effects of hormonal contraceptives on the fetus, including evidence that they are unlikely to increase the risk of hypospadia in the male fetus, see Pregnancy and Breast Feeding, under Precautions of Hormonal Contraceptives, p.1458.

1. Mittwoch U, *et al.* Male sexual development in "a sea of oestrogen". *Lancet* 1993; **342:** 123–4.
2. Sharpe RM, Skakkebaek NE. Are oestrogens involved in falling sperm counts and disorders of the male reproductive tract? *Lancet* 1993; **341:** 1392–5.
3. de Kretser DM. Declining sperm counts. *BMJ* 1996; **312:** 457–8.
4. Thomas JA. Falling sperm counts. *Lancet* 1995; **346:** 635.

Veterinary use. An FAO/WHO expert committee considered it unnecessary to establish an acceptable daily intake or acceptable residual level in food for endogenous hormones such as estradiol.[1] Residues resulting from the use of estradiol as a growth promotor in accordance with good animal husbandry practice were thought unlikely to pose a hazard to human health. However, it should be noted that, in the European Union the use of steroidal hormones such as oestrogens in veterinary practice is restricted, and their use as growth promotors is banned.

There is concern about the effect of environmental oestrogens on male fertility and development, see Pregnancy, above.

1. FAO/WHO. Evaluation of certain veterinary drug residues in food: thirty-second report of the joint FAO/WHO expert committee on food additives. *WHO Tech Rep Ser 763* 1988.

Interactions

Interactions involving estradiol and other oestrogens used in menopausal HRT are covered on p.1463. Interactions for oestrogens used in hormonal contraceptives are covered on p.1458.

The symbol † denotes a preparation no longer actively marketed

Pharmacokinetics

In general, estradiol and other oestrogens are readily absorbed from the gastrointestinal tract and through the skin or mucous membranes. However, the natural unconjugated oestrogens such as estradiol undergo extensive first-pass metabolism in the gastrointestinal tract and liver following oral administration. They are, therefore, generally not orally active, although a micronised preparation of estradiol has sufficient bioavailability (3 to 5%) to be orally active. Estradiol is metabolised in part to less active oestrogens such as estriol and estrone. Synthetic oestrogens produced by alkylation of the C17 position, such as ethinylestradiol, are more slowly metabolised and are therefore orally active. Conjugated oestrogens, which are essentially oestrogen metabolites, are also orally active because they are hydrolysed by enzymes in the lower gastrointestinal tract allowing absorption of the active oestrogen. Vaginal, transdermal, intranasal, or parenteral administration of oestrogens also avoids first-pass hepatic metabolism. Plasma-estradiol concentrations are reported to reach a peak 1.5 to 2 hours after oral administration, and again at about 8 hours due to enterohepatic recycling. Estradiol esters are rapidly hydrolysed to free estradiol when administered by mouth. Following intramuscular administration of the esters, absorption is prolonged.

Oestrogens are extensively bound to plasma proteins. Naturally occurring oestrogens such as estradiol are principally bound to sex-hormone binding globulin. Conversely, ethinylestradiol is mostly bound to albumin.

Oestrogens are metabolised in the liver. A variety of sulfate and glucuronide conjugates are formed, and these are excreted in the urine and the bile. Those excreted in the bile undergo enterohepatic recycling or are excreted in the faeces.

◊ References to the pharmacokinetics of estradiol[1-4] and other oestrogens.[5,6]

1. Kuhnz W, et al. Pharmacokinetics of estradiol, free and total estrone, in young women following single intravenous and oral administration of 17β-estradiol. Arzneimittelforschung 1993; 43: 966–73.
2. Schubert W, et al. Pharmacokinetic evaluation of oral 17β-oestradiol and two different fat soluble analogues in ovariectomized women. Eur J Clin Pharmacol 1993; 44: 563–8.
3. Baker VL. Alternatives to oral estrogen replacement: transdermal patches, percutaneous gels, vaginal creams and rings, implants, other methods of delivery. Obstet Gynecol Clin North Am 1994; 21: 271–9.
4. Price TM, et al. Single-dose pharmacokinetics of sublingual versus oral administration of micronized 17β-estradiol. Obstet Gynecol 1997; 89: 340–5.
5. Stumpf PG. Pharmacokinetics of estrogen. Obstet Gynecol 1990; 75 (suppl): 9S–14S.
6. O'Connell MB. Pharmacokinetic and pharmacologic variation between different estrogen products. J Clin Pharmacol 1995; 35 (suppl): 18S–24S.

Uses and Administration

Estradiol is the most active of the naturally occurring oestrogens (for further details, see p.1452). Estradiol and its semisynthetic esters and other natural oestrogens are primarily used as menopausal HRT (see p.1463) whereas synthetic derivatives such as ethinylestradiol and mestranol have a major role as components of combined oral contraceptives (see Hormonal Contraceptives, p.1459). Estradiol may also be used as replacement therapy for female hypogonadism or primary ovarian failure (p.1276). Replacement therapy ('add-back' therapy) may also be given to women in whom the pituitary-ovarian axis is suppressed by therapy with gonadorelin or its analogues.

For menopausal **HRT** orally administered preparations of estradiol are commonly used, as are transdermal patches. Transdermal gels, subcutaneous implants, and a nasal spray are also available. Intramuscular injections were also formerly used. In women with a uterus, associated administration of a progestogen is required, given cyclically or continuously and usually administered by mouth although some transdermal preparations are available. Local vaginal estradiol preparations are used specifically for the treatment of menopausal atrophic vaginitis; these are generally recommended for short-term use

only, if given without a progestogen in women with a uterus, although specific recommendations vary between products.

For administration by mouth estradiol or estradiol valerate are normally used; doses of 1 to 2 mg daily are given cyclically or more often continuously.

Estradiol may be used topically as transdermal skin patches to provide a systemic effect; a variety of patches are available which release between 25 and 100 μg of estradiol every 24 hours. Depending on the preparation, patches are replaced once or twice weekly. Each new patch is applied to a different area of skin in rotation, usually below the waistline; patches should not be applied on or near the breasts. Topical gel preparations are also applied for systemic effect: the usual dose is 0.5 to 1.5 mg of estradiol daily. The gel should not be applied on or near the breasts or on the vulval region. A nasal spray is also available, delivering 150 μg of estradiol hemihydrate per spray. The usual initial dose is 300 μg daily; maintenance doses are 150 to 600 μg daily.

In order to prolong the duration of action subcutaneous implants of estradiol may be employed. The dose of estradiol is generally 25 to 100 mg with a new implant being administered after about 4 to 8 months according to oestrogen concentrations.

Estradiol may be applied locally either as 25-μg vaginal tablets, at an initial dose of one tablet daily for 2 weeks followed by a maintenance dose of two tablets weekly, or as a 0.01% vaginal cream, in initial amounts of up to 4 g of cream daily followed by a maintenance dose of 1 g up to 3 times weekly. Another local delivery system employs a 3-month vaginal ring containing 2 mg of estradiol hemihydrate, which delivers about 7.5 μg of estradiol per 24 hours.

Intramuscular injections of estradiol benzoate or valerate esters have been used as oily solutions to provide a depot, usually administered once every 3 to 4 weeks. The cipionate, dipropionate, enantate, hexahydrobenzoate, phenylpropionate, and undecylate esters have been used similarly. The enantate and cipionate esters are used as the oestrogen component of combined injectable **contraceptives**.

Estradiol and other oestrogens have sometimes been used in higher doses for palliative treatment in **prostate cancer** (p.497) and **breast cancer** in men and postmenopausal women (p.491).

Administration. IMPLANTS. There may be a striking interpatient variation in blood-estradiol concentrations in women receiving estradiol implants,[1] and symptoms of oestrogen deficiency have re-appeared in some patients even though serum-estradiol concentrations were within or above the physiological range.[2] This has led to debate on the appropriateness of using serum concentrations of estradiol as a guide to implant administration, rather than symptoms.[3-7] Some felt that withholding an implant while a patient suffered symptoms of oestrogen deficiency was unacceptable[3,4] and that other oestrogens or routes of administration may be more suitable.[3,5] Although some suggest[2] that high estradiol concentrations are probably not harmful, others[6,7] have pointed out that there was evidence to the contrary, lending weight to the suggestion that estradiol concentration should be monitored during therapy with implants and this is now recommended by the manufacturers.

Cyclical progestogen may be required for a prolonged period after discontinuation of estradiol implants in women with a uterus.[7]

1. Guirgis RR. Oestradiol implants: what dose, how often? Lancet 1987; ii: 856.
2. Gangar K, et al. Symptoms of oestrogen deficiency associated with supraphysiological plasma oestradiol concentrations in women with oestradiol implants. BMJ 1989; 299: 601–2.
3. Ginsburg J, Hardiman P. Oestrogen deficiency and oestradiol implants. BMJ 1989; 299: 1031.
4. Studd J, et al. Symptoms of oestrogen deficiency in women with oestradiol implants. BMJ 1989; 299: 1400–1.
5. Swyer GIM. Symptoms of oestrogen deficiency in women with oestradiol implants. BMJ 1989; 299: 854.
6. Tobias JH, Chambers TJ. Symptoms of oestrogen deficiency in women with oestradiol implants. BMJ 1989; 299: 854.
7. Wardle P, Fox R. Symptoms of oestrogen deficiency in women with oestradiol implants. BMJ 1989; 299: 1102.

INTRANASAL ADMINISTRATION. The intranasal administration of estradiol for HRT has been studied,[1] and appears to be comparable in efficacy to transdermal administration.[2] As with

transdermal administration, the intranasal route avoids intestinal and hepatic first-pass metabolism.

1. Studd J, et al. Efficacy and acceptability of intranasal 17β-oestradiol for menopausal symptoms: randomised dose-response study. Lancet 1999; 353: 1574–8. Correction. ibid.; 354: 780.
2. Lopes P, et al. Randomized comparison of intranasal and transdermal estradiol. Obstet Gynecol 2000; 96: 906–12.

TRANSDERMAL ADMINISTRATION. The transdermal administration of estradiol via patches applied to the skin has been reviewed.[1-7] This method of delivery has certain advantages over oral administration in that gastrointestinal and hepatic first-pass metabolism is avoided, liver enzymes are not stimulated (although this may also mean that beneficial effects on serum lipids are absent), and the prolonged drug release from the patch means less frequent application is necessary and hence patient compliance may be improved. For oestrogen replacement in menopausal and postmenopausal women estradiol patches are administered continuously or in a cyclical manner, with added progestogen for part of the cycle in those women with an intact uterus. This does not lead to drug accumulation and produces blood-estradiol concentrations and estradiol to estrone ratios similar to those normally observed in premenopausal women. Administration of estradiol via a skin patch is well tolerated with skin irritation being the main problem. The patches are as effective as orally administered oestrogens in treating menopausal and postmenopausal symptoms such as flushing and vaginal atrophy and in preventing osteoporosis.

1. Anonymous. Transdermal estrogen. Med Lett Drugs Ther 1986; 28: 119–20.
2. Ridout G, et al. Pharmacokinetic considerations in the use of newer transdermal formulations. Clin Pharmacokinet 1988; 15: 114–31.
3. Utian WH. Transdermal oestradiol: a recent advance in oestrogen therapy. Drugs 1988; 36: 383–6.
4. Bauwens SF. Transdermal versus oral estrogen for postmenopausal replacement therapy. Clin Pharm 1989; 8: 364–6.
5. Balfour JA, Heel RC. Transdermal estradiol: a review of its pharmacodynamic and pharmacokinetic properties, and therapeutic efficacy in the treatment of menopausal complaints. Drugs 1990; 40: 561–82.
6. Cheang A, et al. A risk-benefit appraisal of transdermal estradiol therapy. Drug Safety 1993; 9: 365–79.
7. Jewelewicz R. New developments in topical estrogen therapy. Fertil Steril 1997; 67: 1–12.

Depression. The use of oestrogen therapy in the treatment of postnatal depression has been shown to be effective.[1] However, a meta-analysis[2] considered that although such therapy could be a useful adjunct after failure of conventional treatment (see Depression, p.271), the risk of serious adverse effects including thrombosis is likely to limit its value.

1. Gregoire AJP, et al. Transdermal oestrogen for treatment of severe postnatal depression. Lancet 1996; 347: 930–3.
2. Lawrie TA, et al. Oestrogens and progestogens for preventing and treating postnatal depression (updated 27 September 1999). Available in the Cochrane Library; Issue 2. Oxford: Update Software; 2000.

Gender reassignment. Oestrogens such as ethinylestradiol and conjugated oestrogens are used in male-to-female transsexuals to develop and maintain secondary sexual characteristics. There is some evidence that this use improves vascular function.[1]

1. New G, et al. Long-term estrogen therapy improves vascular function in male to female transsexuals. J Am Coll Cardiol 1997; 29: 1437–44.

Growth disorders. Early researchers found that supraphysiological doses of oestrogens inhibited somatic growth and from this experience oestrogens, such as ethinylestradiol in oral doses of over 200 μg daily, came to be used for the treatment of acromegaly and for the arrest of growth in tall girls.[1] One study has reported that treatment with conjugated oestrogens 7.5 to 11.25 mg daily resulted in an average decrease of about 5 cm from final predicted height.[2] However, treatment with physiological doses causes growth stimulation, not inhibition, and such physiological doses have been used to promote growth in girls with conditions such as female hypogonadism and Turner's syndrome (see p.1276). Oestrogen therapy has occasionally been used in girls with delayed puberty (see p.1273).

1. Rosenfield RL. Toward optimal estrogen-replacement therapy. N Engl J Med 1983; 309: 1120–1.
2. Weimann E, et al. Oestrogen treatment of constitutional tall stature: a risk-benefit ratio. Arch Dis Child 1998; 78: 148–51.

Haemorrhagic disorders. Limited evidence supports the use of oestrogens in various bleeding disorders such as hereditary haemorrhagic telangiectasia, and those associated with chronic renal failure and gastrointestinal vascular malformations.

References.

1. Vase P. Estrogen treatment of hereditary hemorrhagic telangiectasia. Acta Med Scand 1981; 209: 393–6.
2. Livio M, et al. Conjugated estrogens for the management of bleeding associated with renal failure. N Engl J Med 1986; 315: 731–5.
3. van Cutsem E, et al. Treatment of bleeding gastrointestinal vascular malformations with oestrogen-progesterone. Lancet 1990; 335: 953–5.

Lactation inhibition. Synthetic oestrogens (e.g. quinestrol) and nonsteroidal oestrogens (e.g. diethylstilbestrol) were historically employed to suppress lactation (p.1276). However, such use is now considered inappropriate because of an increased risk of puerperal thromboembolism.

Premenstrual syndrome. Premenstrual syndrome (PMS) presents as a variable combination of psychological and somatic symptoms occurring during the luteal phase of the menstrual cycle, which resolve during, and immediately following, menstruation.[1,2] Another term, premenstrual dysphoric disorder, has been proposed to cover severe cyclical mood disorder that is functionally incapacitating.[2,3] Whereas about 20 to 30% of women have complaints that may be classified as PMS, only 3 to 5% meet criteria for premenstrual dysphoric disorder.[3] The term premenstrual tension (PMT) has sometimes been applied to the psychological symptoms. Many symptoms of PMS are the same as normal premenstrual symptoms, but are more severe. Premenstrual syndrome is not fully understood although it is thought to be due to the effects of the normal luteal phase release of progesterone on CNS neurotransmitter function; the syndrome is abolished by surgical or medical suppression of ovarian function. A recent study has shown that oestrogens, as well as progestogens, can induce symptoms.[4] Findings from another study demonstrated that women with PMS may metabolise progesterone differently to those without PMS.[5]

Initial management includes non-medical interventions such as education and support, counselling, stress management, relaxation techniques, and exercise; caffeine and salt restriction are of unproven benefit. The herbal remedy agnus castus has been found to be of benefit.[6] For patients with moderate to severe symptoms, a number of drugs have been tried with varying degrees of success; objective assessment of efficacy has been hampered by varying diagnostic criteria, a marked placebo response, and difficulties in obtaining reproducible responses. Treatment may be aimed at modifying the menstrual cycle or treating specific symptoms.[2]

In women with predominantly psychological symptoms, *SSRIs* can be helpful.[7-10] Fluoxetine and sertraline have been shown in controlled trials to alleviate both the psychological and somatic symptoms in women with premenstrual syndrome. *Clomipramine*, a nonselective serotonin reuptake inhibitor, has also been tried with some success. The anxiolytic *alprazolam* has also been used, but use of this and other benzodiazepines should be restricted to the luteal phase of the cycle in selected patients to minimise the risk of dependence and tolerance.[2,7]

Abdominal bloating and swelling associated with PMS has traditionally been thought to be due to sodium and water retention. However, in most women with these symptoms there is no evidence of an increase in body-weight or in body sodium or total water, and use of *diuretics* is therefore not justified.[1] Nevertheless, in women with appreciable weight gain in the luteal phase diuretics may be useful.[1,7] Another symptom of PMS, cyclical mastalgia, is discussed on p.1470.

Pyridoxine has been tried on the basis that it is a cofactor in neurotransmitter (specifically serotonin) synthesis, and has been found to relieve depression induced by oral contraceptives in selected patients. However, its efficacy in premenstrual syndrome is equivocal, and high daily doses have been associated with neurotoxicity.[2,7,8,11] *Calcium* supplementation may relieve symptoms of PMS.[12]

Treatments that modify the menstrual cycle have often been used in women with PMS. In general, drugs with proven efficacy such as danazol, oestrogen implants, and gonadorelin analogues are reserved for women with severe PMS unresponsive to other treatments, because of their adverse effects. *Progestogen* therapy was once popular, but beneficial responses have not been universally achieved and the theory that progesterone was necessary to correct a hormone imbalance is now losing ground. Combined oral contraceptives have met with limited success[1,2,7,9] and in some women, PMS is caused or exacerbated by them. Young women with severe symptoms and women approaching the menopause may benefit from *oestrogen* delivered either as implants or transdermal patches. In women with a uterus, administration with a cyclical progestogen is required to avoid endometrial hyperplasia which unfortunately, may be associated with the return of symptoms, although they may be milder.[1,2] *Danazol* can be useful, but there is concern over its adverse effects during long-term use and over the risk of masculinisation of a female fetus should pregnancy occur. For patients with severe symptoms not amenable to other treatments, gonadorelin analogues such as *goserelin* can be used to eliminate ovarian function, 'add-back' treatment with oestrogen plus progestogen being given to protect against the side-effects of oestrogen deficiency including osteoporosis. This treatment is very effective for both physical and psychological symptoms. Short-term use (3 months) of a gonadorelin analogue alone has been used to confirm the diagnosis of PMS, or to predict the response to bilateral oophorectomy.[1,2] Immunological control using an analogue of *luteinising hormone-releasing hormone* (LHRH) to raise antibodies against natural LHRH and thus suppress ovarian function has also been proposed.

1. O'Brien PMS. Helping women with premenstrual syndrome. *BMJ* 1993; 307: 1471–5.
2. Severino SK, Moline ML. Premenstrual syndrome: identification and management. *Drugs* 1995; 49: 71–82.
3. Gold JH. Premenstrual dysphoric disorder. *JAMA* 1997; 278: 1024–5.
4. Schmidt PJ, et al. Differential behavioral effects of gonadal steroids in women with and those without premenstrual syndrome. *N Engl J Med* 1998; 338: 209–16.
5. Rapkin AJ, et al. Progesterone metabolite allopregnanolone in women with premenstrual syndrome. *Obstet Gynecol* 1997; 90: 709–14.

6. Schellenberg R. Treatment for the premenstrual syndrome with agnus castus fruit extract: prospective, randomised, placebo controlled study. *BMJ* 2001; 322: 134–7.
7. Mortola JF. A risk-benefit appraisal of drugs used in the management of premenstrual syndrome. *Drug Safety* 1994; 10: 160–9.
8. Barnhart KT, et al. A clinician's guide to the premenstrual syndrome. *Med Clin North Am* 1995; 79: 1457–72.
9. Steiner M. Premenstrual syndromes. *Annu Rev Med* 1997; 48: 447–55.
10. Dimmock PW, et al. Efficacy of selective serotonin-reuptake inhibitors in premenstrual syndrome: a systematic review. *Lancet* 2000; 356: 1131–6.
11. Wyatt KM, et al. Efficacy of vitamin B-6 in the treatment of premenstrual syndrome: systematic review. *BMJ* 1999; 318: 1375–81.
12. Thys-Jacobs S, et al. Calcium carbonate and the premenstrual syndrome: effects on premenstrual and menstrual symptoms. *Am J Obstet Gynecol* 1998; 179: 444–52.

Preparations

BP 2001: Estradiol Injection;
USP 25: Estradiol Cypionate Injection; Estradiol Injectable Suspension; Estradiol Pellets; Estradiol Tablets; Estradiol Vaginal Cream; Estradiol Valerate Injection.

Proprietary Preparations (details are given in Part 3)
Aust.: Climara; Estraderm; Estramon; Estring†; Estrofem; Estrogel; FemSeven; Klimapur; Linoladiol; Menorest; Progynon; Progynova; Substitol†; Systen; Vagifem; Zumenon; *Austral.:* Climara; Dermestril; Estraderm; Estring; Estrofem; Femtran; Menorest; Primogyn Depot; Progynova; Sandrena; Vagifem; Zumenon; *Belg.:* Climara; Dermestril; Estraderm; Estrofem; Feminova; Meno-Implant; Oestrogel; Progynova; Systen; Vagifem; Zumenon; *Braz.:* Benzo-Ginoestril; Climaderm; Estraderm; Ginedisc; Reglovar; *Canad.:* Climara; Delestrogen; Estrace; Estraderm; Estring; Estrogel; Femogex†; Oesclim; Vivelle; *Denm.:* Climara; Divigel; Estraderm; Estring; Estrofem; Estrogel; Evorel; Femanest; FemSeven; Menorest†; Progynon; Sandrena; Vagifem; *Fin.:* Climara; Dermestril; Divigel; Estraderm; Estring; Estrofem; Estrogel; Evorel; FemSeven; Menorest; Merimono; Progynova; Vagifem; Zumenon; *Fr.:* Benzo-Gynoestryl†; Climara; Delidose; Dermestril; Estraderm; Estrofem; Femsept; Menorest; Oesclim; Oestrodose; Oestrogel; Oromone; Progynova; Provames; Systen; Thais; *Ger.:* Cerella; Cutanum; Dermestril; Ell-Cranell alpha; Estrabeta; Estraderm; Estramon; Estrifam; Estring; Estronorm; Evorel; Fem 7; Femoston mono; Gynokadin; GynPolar; Linoladiol N; Menorest; Merimono; Pantostin; Progynon Depot 10; Progynova; Sandrena; Sisare mono; Tradelia; Vagifem; *Hong Kong:* Bisteron; Dermestril; Estraderm; Estreva; Estrofem; Oestrogel; Progynova; *Irl.:* Climara; Divigel; Epiestrol; Estraderm; Estramon; Estrofem; Evorel; Fematab; Fematrix; Menorest; Oestrogel; Vagifem; *Israel:* Climara; Dermestril; Estraderm; Estrofem; Evorel; Meno-Patch; Oestrogel; Progynova; Vagifem; *Ital.:* Armonil; Benztrone; Climara; Dermestril; Epiestrol; Estraderm; Estroclim; Estrofem; FemSeven; Gelestra; Menorest; Progynon Depot; Progynova; Sandrena; Systen; Vagifem; *Mex.:* Benzo-Ginestryl; Climaderm; Estraderm; Fem 7; Ginedisc; Primogyn; Systen; *Mon.:* Estreva; *Neth.:* Climara; Dermestril; Estraderm; Estring; Estrofem; Menorest; Progynon Depot 10; Progynova; Sandrena; Systen; Vagifem; Zumenon; *Norw.:* Climara; Estraderm; Estring; Evorel; Menorest; Progynova; *NZ:* Climara; Estraderm; Estring; Estrofem; Femtran; Progynova; Sandrena; Vagifem; *Port.:* Climara; Dermestril; Estraderm; Estrofem; Estronar; Menorest; Vagifem; Zumenon; *S.Afr.:* Climara; Estraderm; Estring; Estro-Pause; Estrofem; Evorel; Femigel; Menorest†; Primogyn Depot; Progynova; Vagifem; *Singapore:* Estraderm; Estrofem; Fem 7; Oestrogel; Progynova; Vagifem; *Spain:* Absorlent; Alcis; Cliogan; Dermestril; Esotran; Estraderm; Evopad; Menorest; Meriestra; Oestraclin; Progynon Depot; Progynova; Vagifem; *Swed.:* Climara; Divigel; Estraderm; Evorel; Femanest; FemSeven; Menorest; Oesclim; Oestring; Progynon; Vagifem; *Switz.:* Cerina; Climara; Dermestril; Divigel; Epiestrol; Estraderm; Estramon; Estring; Estrofem N; FemSeven; Menorest; Oestrogel; Progynon Depot 10; Progynova; Sandrena; Systen; Vagifem; Zumenon; *Thai.:* Climara; Estrofem; Oestrogel; Progynon; Progynova; Vagifem; *UK:* Adgyn Estro; Aerodiol; Climaval; Dermestril; Elleste-Solo; Estraderm; Estring; Evorel; Fematrix; FemSeven; Menorest; Oestrogel; Progynova; Sandrena; Vagifem; Zumenon; *USA:* Alora; Climara; Delestrogen; depGynogen; Depogen; Dioval†; Esclim; Estra-L†; Estrace; Estraderm; Estring; Estro-Cyp†; FemPatch; Gynodiol; Vagifem; Valergen; Vivelle.

Multi-ingredient: *Aust.:* Activelle; Climen; Cyclacur; Estandron†; Estracomb; Estragest; Femoston; Filena; Gravibinon; Gynodian Depot; Ichth-Oestren; Kliogest; Mericomb; Merigest; Ostrolut†; Perikliman; Primodian Depot†; Tri-Filena; Trisequens; *Austral.:* Climen; Divina; Estalis Continuous; Estalis Sequi; Estracombi; Estrapak; Femoston; Kliogest; Kliovance; Primodian Depot†; Trisequens; *Belg.:* Activelle; Climen; Cyclocur; Dimenformon; Diviplus; Diviva; Estracomb; Femoston; Kliogest; Trisequens; Trivina; *Braz.:* Cicloprimogyna; Ciclovular; Climene; Dilena; Estandron P; Estracomb; Evitas; Gestadinona; Ginecoside; Hormoginase; Mesigyna; Normomensil; Perlutan; Postoval; Progest; Trinestril; Uno-Ciclo; *Canad.:* Climacterion; Estracomb; *Denm.:* Activelle; Climen; Cyclo-Progynon; Divina; Divina Plus; Estracomb; Evo-Conti; Evo-Sequi; Femanest; Femasekvens; Klimalet; Klimaxil; Kliogest; Nuvelle; Ostranorm; Trevina; Trinorm; Trisekvens; *Fin.:* Activelle; Climara Duo; Cyclabil; Divina; Divitren; Estalis; Estalis Sekvens; Estracomb; Evorel Conti; Evorel Sequi; Femilar; Femoston; Kliogest; Mericomb; Merigest; Senikolp; Trisekvens; *Fr.:* Climaston; Climene; Divina; Kliogest; Trisequens; *Ger.:* Activelle; Aknefug-Emulsion; Alpicort F neu; Androfemon; Climen; Crinohermal fem neu; Cyclo-Menorette; Cyclo-Progynova; CycloOstrogynal; CycloPolar; Ell-Cranell; Estracomb; Estrafemol; Estragest; Femoston; Gravibinon; Gynamon; Gynodian Depot; Jephagynon; Klimonorm; Kliogest N; Linoladiol-H N; Mericomb; Merigest; NeoOstrognal; NeyNormin N (Revitorgan-Dilutionen Nr 65); Osmil; Ostronara†; Procyclo; Sisare; Syngynon; Trisequens; *Hong Kong:* Climen; Dilena; Estracomb; Femoston; Hormonin; Klimonorm; Kliogest; Progestrol†; Trisequens; *Irl.:* Activelle; Estracombi; Estrapak; Evorel Conti; Femoston; Femoston Conti; Femplan-MA; Kliogest; Nuv-

elle; Tridestra; Trisequens; *Israel:* Kliogest; Meno-MPA; Meno-Net; Progyluton; Trisequens; *Ital.:* Activelle; Biormon; Climen; Duo-Ormogyn†; Estracomb; Femoston; Filena; Gravibinan; Gynodian Depot; Kliogest; Menovis; Nuvelle; Nuvelle TS; Pausal; Tesor-C; Trisequens; *Mex.:* Anafertin; Binodian; Cliane; Climene; Cyclofemina; Despamen; Dilena; Estracomb; Estrapak; Gravidinona; Lutoginestryl F; Mesigyna; Metrigen Fuerte; Patector; Perlutal; Primosiston; Progediol; Proger-F; Progyluton; Yectames; *Neth.:* Activelle; Climene; Cyclocur; Divina; Estracomb; Femoston; Kliogest; Trisequens; Zumeston†; *Norw.:* Activelle; Climen; Cyclabil; Estracomb; Kliogest; Trisekvens; *NZ:* Estrapak; Kliogest; Kliovance; Nuvelle; Trisequens; *Port.:* Cicnor; Climara Duo; Climen; Dilena; Emmenovis; Estalis Sequi; Estracomb; Femoston; Kliogest; Nuvelle; Progyluton; Trisequens; *S.Afr.:* Climen; Divina; Estracombi; Evorel Conti; Kliogest; Mixogen; Postoval; Primodian Depot; Trisequens; Trivina; *Singapore:* Activelle; Climen; Estracomb; Femoston; Kliogest; Progyluton; Trisequens; *Spain:* Absorlent Plus; Activelle; Auroclim; Climen; Clisin; Estracomb; Gynodian Depot; Merigest; Merigest Combi; Nuvelle; Perifem; Progyluton; Topasel; Trisequens; *Swed.:* Activelle; Cyclabil; Divina; Divina Plus; Estalis; Estalis Sekvens; Estracomb; Evorel Micronor; Femanor; Femasekvens; Kliogest; Trisekvens; Trivina; *Switz.:* Activelle; Alpicort F; Climen; Cyclacur; Estracomb; Estragest; Femoston; Femoston Conti; Gynodian Depot; Kliogest N; Linoladiol; Mericomb; Merigest; Primosiston; Systen Conti; Systen Sequi; Triaval; Trisequens; *Thai.:* Climen; Cyclo-Progynova; Duoton; Klimonorm; Kliogest; Primodian Depot; Trisequens; *UK:* Adgyn Combi; Climagest; Climesse; Cyclo-Progynova 1 mg; Cyclo-Progynova 2 mg; Elleste Duet Conti; Elleste-Duet; Estracombi; Estrapak; Evorel Conti; Evorel Pak; Evorel Sequi; Femapak; Femoston; Femoston Conti; Hormonin; Indivina; Kliofem; Kliovance; Nuvelle; Nuvelle Continuous; Nuvelle TS; Tridestra; Trisequens; *USA:* Activella; CombiPatch; depAndrogyn†; Depo-Testadiol; Depotestogen; Duo-Cyp; Duratestrin†; Lunelle; Ortho-Prefest; Test-Estro†; Valertest.

Estrapronicate   (13426-e)

Estrapronicate (rINN).

Oestradiol 17-nicotinate 3-propionate.
$C_{27}H_{31}NO_4 = 433.5$.
$CAS — 4140-20-9$.

Profile
Estrapronicate is a derivative of estradiol (p.1473) with nicotinic acid. It has been used as an ingredient of a combined preparation with an anabolic steroid and a progestogen for osteoporosis.

Preparations

Proprietary Preparations (details are given in Part 3)
Multi-ingredient: *Mon.:* Trophobolene†.

Estriol   (9090-l)

Estriol (BAN).

Follicular Hormone Hydrate; Oestriol; Theelol. Estra-1,3,5(10)-triene-3,16α,17β-triol.
$C_{18}H_{24}O_3 = 288.4$.
$CAS — 50-27-1$.
$ATC — G03CA04$.

Pharmacopoeias. In *Eur.* (see p.vi), *Jpn*, and *US*.

Pharmacopoeial description

Ph. Eur.: A white or almost white crystalline powder. Practically insoluble in water; sparingly soluble in alcohol.

USP 25: A white or practically white, odourless, crystalline powder. Insoluble in water; sparingly soluble in alcohol; soluble in acetone, in chloroform, in dioxan, in ether, and in vegetable oils. Store in airtight containers.

Estriol Sodium Succinate   (10345-s)

Estriol Sodium Succinate (BAN, rINNM).

Oestriol Sodium Succinate. Disodium 3-hydroxyestra-1,3,5(10)-triene-16α,17β-diyl disuccinate.
$C_{26}H_{30}Na_2O_9 = 532.5$.
$CAS — 113-22-4$.

Estriol Succinate   (10068-b)

Estriol Succinate (BAN, rINN).

Oestriol Succinate. 3-Hydroxyestra-1,3,5(10)-triene-16α,17β-diyl di(hydrogen succinate).
$C_{26}H_{32}O_9 = 488.5$.
$CAS — 514-68-1$.

Profile
Estriol is a naturally occurring oestrogen with actions and uses similar to those described for estradiol (p.1473). It is claimed to have only a mild proliferative effect on the endometrium.

It is used for menopausal HRT (p.1460). When oestrogens are administered to women with a uterus, a progestogen is required, particularly if used long-term. For short-term treatment, doses of estriol by mouth have been 500 µg to 3 mg daily given for one month followed by 500 µg to 1 mg daily. Estriol has also been given in combination with other natural oestrogens such as estradiol and estrone (p.1476); usual doses of estriol have ranged from about 250 µg to 2 mg daily. It is also administered intravaginally for the short-term treatment of menopausal atrophic vaginitis as a 0.01% or 0.1% cream or as pessaries containing 500 µg.

Estriol succinate has also been given by mouth in the treatment of menopausal disorders. The sodium succinate salt has been administered parenterally in the treatment of haemorrhage and thrombocytopenia.

Preparations

Proprietary Preparations (details are given in Part 3)
Aust.: Ortho-Gynest; Ovestin; Styptanon; **Austral.:** Ovestin; **Belg.:** Aacifemine; Ortho-Gynest; **Braz.:** Ovestrion; Styptanon; **Denm.:** Ovestin; **Fin.:** Ovestin; Pausanol; **Fr.:** Gydrelle; Physiogine; Trophicreme; **Ger.:** Cordes Estriol; Gynasan; OeKolp; Oestro-Gynaedron M; Ortho-Gynest; Ovestin; Ovo-Vinces; Synapause E; Xapro; **Hong Kong:** Ovestin; **Irl.:** Ortho-Gynest; Ovestin; **Israel:** Ortho-Gynest; Ovestin; **Ital.:** Colpogyn; Ortho Gynest Depot; Ovestin; **Mex.:** Ortho-Gynest; Sinapause; **Neth.:** Ortho-Gynest†; Ovestin†; Synapause-E₃; **Norw.:** Oevesterin; **NZ:** Ovestin; **Port.:** Ovestin; Pausigin; Synapausa; **S.Afr.:** Synapause; **Singapore:** Ovestin; **Spain:** Ovestinon; Synapause; **Swed.:** Ovesterin; **Switz.:** Oestro-Gynaedron Nouveau; Ortho-Gynest; Ovestin; **Thai.:** Ovestin; **UK:** Ortho-Gynest; Ovestin.

Multi-ingredient: Aust.: Gynoflor; **Belg.:** Gynoflor; **Fr.:** Florgynal; Trophigil; **Ger.:** Cyclo-Menorette; CycloOstrogynal; Gynoflor; NeoOstrogynal; Oestrugol N; **Hong Kong:** Gyno-Flor E; Hormonin, **Switz.:** Gynoflor; **UK:** Hormonin.

Estrone (9092-j)

Estrone (BAN, rINN).
Follicular Hormone; Folliculin; Ketohydroxyoestrin; Oestrone.
3-Hydroxyestra-1,3,5(10)-trien-17-one.
$C_{18}H_{22}O_2 = 270.4$.
CAS — 53-16-7.
ATC — G03CA07; G03CC04.
Pharmacopoeias. In Aust., It., and US.

Pharmacopoeial description

USP 25: Odourless, small white crystals or white to creamy-white crystalline powder. Practically insoluble in water; soluble 1 in 250 of alcohol and 1 in 110 of chloroform at 15°; soluble 1 in 50 of boiling alcohol, 1 in 33 of boiling acetone, 1 in 145 of boiling benzene, and 1 in 80 of boiling chloroform; soluble 1 in 50 of acetone at 50°; soluble in dioxan and in vegetable oils; slightly soluble in solutions of fixed alkali hydroxides. Store in airtight containers. Protect from light.

Profile

Estrone is a naturally occurring oestrogen with actions and uses similar to those described for estradiol (see p.1473).

For menopausal HRT (see p.1460) estrone has been given by mouth at a dose of 1.4 to 2.8 mg daily in a cyclical or continuous regimen, as a combination product with estradiol and estriol. Estrone has also been administered by intramuscular injection in oily solutions and aqueous suspensions. When used specifically for menopausal atrophic vaginitis, estrone has been administered vaginally. If used in women with a uterus, estrone by any route should be given with a progestogen.

Preparations

USP 25: Estrone Injectable Suspension; Estrone Injection.
Proprietary Preparations (details are given in Part 3)
Canad.: Oestrilin; **USA:** Aquest†; Kestrone.
Multi-ingredient: Braz.: Gineburno; **Fr.:** Synergon; **Hong Kong:** Hormonin; **Spain:** Cicatral; Grietalgen; Grietalgen Hidrocort; **Thai.:** Metharmon-F; **UK:** Hormonin.

Estropipate (9042-b)

Estropipate (BAN).
Piperazine Estrone Sulfate; Piperazine Oestrone Sulphate. Piperazine 17-oxoestra-1,3,5-(10)-trien-3-yl hydrogen sulphate.
$C_{18}H_{22}O_5S,C_4H_{10}N_2 = 436.6$.
CAS — 7280-37-7.
Pharmacopoeias. In Br. and US.

Pharmacopoeial description

BP 2001: A white or almost white crystalline powder. Very slightly soluble in water, in alcohol, in chloroform, and in ether.
USP 25: A white to yellowish-white fine crystalline powder, odourless or may have a slight odour. Very slightly soluble in water, in alcohol, in chloroform, and in ether; soluble 1 in 500 of warm alcohol; soluble in warm water. Store in airtight containers.

Adverse Effects and Precautions

As for oestrogens in general (see Estradiol, p.1473). See also under Hormone Replacement Therapy, p.1461.

Interactions

See under Hormone Replacement Therapy, p.1463.

Uses and Administration

Estropipate is a semisynthetic conjugate of estrone with piperazine that is used for menopausal HRT (see p.1460). Its action is due to estrone (p.1476) to which it is hydrolysed in the body.

Estropipate is given by mouth for the short-term treatment of menopausal symptoms; suggested doses have ranged from 0.75 to 6 mg daily, given cyclically or continuously. When used longer term for the prevention of postmenopausal osteoporosis a daily dose of 0.75 or 1.5 mg is given cyclically or continuous-

ly. In women with a uterus estropipate should be used in conjunction with a progestogen. Estropipate has also been used short term for menopausal atrophic vaginitis as a vaginal cream containing 0.15%; 2 to 4 g of cream is applied daily. It is also given by mouth in the treatment of female hypogonadism, castration, and primary ovarian failure in doses of 1.5 to 9 mg daily, in a cyclical regimen.

Preparations

BP 2001: Estropipate Tablets;
USP 25: Estropipate Tablets; Estropipate Vaginal Cream.
Proprietary Preparations (details are given in Part 3)
Austral.: Genoral; Ogen; **Canad.:** Ogen; **Irl.:** Harmogen; **Mex.:** Ogen; **S.Afr.:** Ortho-Est; **UK:** Harmogen; **USA:** Ogen; Ortho-Est.
Multi-ingredient: UK: Improvera.

Ethinylestradiol (9043-v)

Ethinylestradiol (BAN, rINN).
Aethinyloestradiolum; Ethinyl Estradiol; Ethinyloestradiol; Etinilestradiol; NSC-10973. 17α-Ethynylestra-1,3,5(10)-triene-3,17β-diol; 19-Nor-17α-pregna-1,3,5(10)-trien-20-yne-3,17β-diol.
$C_{20}H_{24}O_2 = 296.4$.
CAS — 57-63-6.
ATC — G03CA01; L02AA03.
Pharmacopoeias. In Chin., Eur. (see p.vi), Int., Jpn, and US.

Pharmacopoeial description

Ph. Eur.: A white to slightly yellowish-white, crystalline powder. Practically insoluble in water; freely soluble in alcohol; dissolves in dilute alkaline solutions. Protect from light.

USP 25: A white to creamy white, odourless, crystalline powder. Insoluble in water; soluble in alcohol, in chloroform, in ether, in vegetable oils, and in solutions of fixed alkali hydroxides. Store in non-metallic airtight containers. Protect from light.

Adverse Effects and Precautions

As for oestrogens in general (see Estradiol, p.1473). See also under Hormonal Contraceptives, p.1452.

Effects on calcium homoeostasis. Two patients with metastatic breast cancer given ethinylestradiol developed rapidly progressive irreversible and fatal hypercalcaemia, considered to be due to stimulation of osteolysis by the oestrogen.[1]

1. Cornbleet M, et al. Fatal irreversible hypercalcaemia in breast cancer. BMJ 1977; **1:** 145.

Effects on the liver. Cholestasis and pruritus developed in a liver transplant recipient receiving ethinylestradiol at a dose of 50 µg daily for the treatment of menorrhagia.[1] Symptoms subsided on withdrawal of ethinylestradiol but returned on its reintroduction.

1. Fedorkow DM, et al. Cholestasis induced by oestrogen after liver transplantation. BMJ 1989; **299:** 1080–1.

Interactions

See under Hormonal Contraceptives, p.1458.

Pharmacokinetics

Ethinylestradiol is rapidly and well absorbed from the gastrointestinal tract. The presence of an ethinyl group at the 17-position greatly reduces hepatic first-pass metabolism compared with estradiol, enabling the compound to be much more active by mouth, but there is some initial conjugation by the gut wall, and the systemic bioavailability is only about 40%. Ethinylestradiol is highly protein bound, but unlike naturally occurring oestrogens, which are mainly bound to sex-hormone binding globulin, it is principally bound to albumin. It is metabolised in the liver, and excreted in urine and faeces. Metabolites undergo enterohepatic recycling.

◊ References.

1. Back DJ, et al. The gut wall metabolism of ethinyloestradiol and its contribution to the pre-systemic metabolism of ethinyloestradiol in humans. Br J Clin Pharmacol 1982; **13:** 325–30.

Uses and Administration

Ethinylestradiol is a synthetic oestrogen with actions similar to those of estradiol (see p.1474).

It is frequently used as the oestrogenic component of combined oral contraceptive preparations; a typical daily dose is 20 to 50 µg (for guidance on appropriate dose, see p.1459). Ethinylestradiol is also used as an emergency contraceptive (p.1460) combined with levonorgestrel or norgestrel. A combined preparation of ethinylestradiol with the anti-androgen cyproterone (p.1467) is used for the hormonal treatment of

acne (p.1103), particularly when contraception is also required.

Ethinylestradiol has also been used for menopausal HRT (p.1460); doses of 10 to 20 µg daily were given (in conjunction with a progestogen in women with a uterus), but natural oestrogens are usually preferred.

For the treatment of female hypogonadism, 50 µg has been given up to three times daily for 14 consecutive days in every 4 weeks, followed by a progestogen for the next 14 days.

For the palliative treatment of malignant neoplasms of the prostate (p.497) doses of 150 µg to 3 mg have been given daily. For palliation of malignant neoplasms of the breast (p.491) in postmenopausal women doses of 100 µg to 1 mg three times daily have been used.

Preparations

BP 2001: Ethinylestradiol Tablets; Levonorgestrel and Ethinylestradiol Tablets;
USP 25: Ethinyl Estradiol Tablets; Ethynodiol Diacetate and Ethinyl Estradiol Tablets; Levonorgestrel and Ethinyl Estradiol Tablets; Norethindrone Acetate and Ethinyl Estradiol Tablets; Norethindrone and Ethinyl Estradiol Tablets; Norgestrel and Ethinyl Estradiol Tablets.

Proprietary Preparations (details are given in Part 3)
Aust.: Progynon C; **Austral.:** Estigyn†; **Canad.:** Estinyl†; **Ger.:** Progynon C; Turisteron; **Israel:** Progynon C; **Neth.:** Lynoral; **Norw.:** Etifollin; **S.Afr.:** Estinyl; **USA:** Estinyl.

Multi-ingredient: Aust.: Cileste; Diane; Etalontin†; Gracial; Gynovin; Harmonette; Levlen; Liogynon; Lyndiol; Marvelon; Meliane; Mercilon; Microgynon; Minulet; Monogestin; Myvlar; Neo-Stediril; Neogynon; Neorlest†; Orlest†; Ovanon; Ovranette; Ovysmen; Perikursal; Primosiston; Restovar†; Sequilar; Stediril D; Tri-Minulet; TriCilest; Trigynon; Trinordiol; Trinovum; Triodena; Triogestena; Triogestin; Vivelle; Yermonil; **Austral.:** Biphasil; Brenda-35 ED; Brevinor; Diane ED; Femoden ED; Improvil; Levlen ED; Loette; Logynon ED; Marvelon; Microgynon; Minulet; Monofeme; Nordette; Nordiol; Norimin; Ovulen†; Sequilar ED; Synphasic; Tri-Minulet; Trifeme; Trioden ED; Triphasil; Triquilar; **Belg.:** Binordiol; Cilest; Conova; Diane; Femodene; Fysioquens†; Gracial; Harmonet; Lyndiol†; Marvelon; Meliane; Mercilon; Microgynon; Minestril; Ministat†; Minulet; Neo-Stediril; Neogynon; Ovidol; Ovostat†; Ovulen†; Ovysmen; Stediril 30; Stediril D; Stediril†; Tri-Minulet; Trigynon; Trinordiol; Trinovum; Triodene; **Braz.:** Anacyclin; Anfertil; Ciclo; Ciclomestril; Ciclovulon; Diane; Evanor; Gestinol; Gynera; Karin; Levordiol; Mercilon; Microdiol; Microvlar; Minulet; Neovlar; Nordette; Normamor; Normex; Primosiston; Primovlar; Progest; Trinordiol; Trinovum; Triquilar; Unidose; **Canad.:** Alesse; Brevicon; Cyclen; Demulen; Diane; Loestrin 1.5/30; Marvelon; Min-Ovral; Minestrin; Ortho 0.5/35; Ortho 1/35; Ortho 10/11; Ortho 7/7/7; Ortho-Cept; Ovral; Select 1/35; Synphasic; Tri-Cyclen; Triphasil; Triquilar; **Denm.:** Cilest; Conova†; Desorelle; Diane; Dystrol†; Econ; Fironetta; Gracial; Gynatrol; Gynera; Harmonet; Lyndiol†; Marvelon; Meloden; Mercilon; Microgyn; Milvane; Minulet; Neogentrol; Neogynon; Novynette; Tetragynon; Tri-Minulet; Trinordiol; Trinovum; Triquilar; **Fin.:** Cilest; Diane; Femoden; Gracial; Harmonet; Marvelon; Meliane; Mercilon; Microgynon; Minulet; Neo-Primovlar; Tri-Femoden; Tri-Minulet; Trikvilar; Trinordiol; **Fr.:** Adepal; Cilest; Cycleane; Diane; Effiprev; Harmonet; Lutestral†; Meliane; Melodia; Mercilon; Milli Anovlar†; Minesse; Minidril; Miniphase; Minulet; Moneva; Ortho-Novum 1/35; Ovanon; Phaeva; Physiostat; Planor; Stediril; Tetragynon; Tri-Minulet; Triella; Trinordiol; Varnoline; **Ger.:** Anacyclin†; Belara; Biviol; Cilest; Conceplan M; Cyclosa; Desmin; Diane; Eve; Femigoa; Femovan; Femranette mikro; Gravistat; Leios; Lovelle; Lovina; Lyn-ratiopharm; Lyn-ratiopharm-Sequenz; Lyndiol†; Marvelon; Microgynon; Minisiston; Minulet; Miranova; MonoStep; Neo-Eunomin; Neo-Stediril; Neogynon; Neorlest; Non-Ovlon; Nora-ratiopharm; NovaStep; Nuriphasic; Ostro-Primolut†; Ovanon; Oviol; Ovoresta M; Ovoresta†; Ovysmen; Perikursal; Pramino; Pregnon L; Primosiston; Prosiston; Sequilar; Sequostat; Sinovula; Stediril; Stediril 30; Stediril D; Synphasec; Tetragynon; Triette; Trigoa; Trinordiol; Trinovum; Triquilar; Trisiston; TriStep; Valette; Yermonil; **Hong Kong:** Brevinor; Diane; Duoluton; Eugynon; Gerivit; Gracial; Gynera; Harmonet; Lyndiol; Marvelon; Mercilon; Microgynon; Minulet; Neogynon; Nordette; Nordiol; Norimin; Ovral; Rigevidon; Synphase; Tri-Regol; Trinordiol; Trinovum; Triquilar; **Irl.:** Binovum; Brevinor; Cilest; Dianette; Femodene; Logynon; Marviol; Mercilon; Microgynon 30; Microlite; Minesse; Minulet; Normin†; Ovran; Ovran 30; Ovranette; Ovysmen; Tri-Minulet; Trinordiol; Trinovum; Triodene; **Israel:** Diane; Gynera; Harmonet; Logynon; Meliane; Mercilon; Microdiol; Microgynon; Minulet; Neogynon; Nordette; Ortho Cyclen; Trinordiol; **Ital.:** Diane; Dueva; Egogyn 30; Eugynon; Evanor-D; Fedra; Ginoden; Gracial; Harmonet; Loette; Mercilon; Microgynon; Milvane; Minulet; Novogyn; Ovranet; Planum; Practil; Securgin; Tri-Minulet; Trigynon; Trinordiol; Trinovum†; **Mex.:** Cilest; Diane; Gynovin; Marvelon; Mercilon; Microgynon; Minulet; Neogynon; Nordet; Nordiol; Ortho-Novum 1/35; Ovral; Trinordiol; Triquilar; **Neth.:** Binordiol; Cilest; Diane; Femodeen; Fysioquens; Gracial; Harmonet; Marvelon; Meliane; Mercilon; Microgynon; Mini Pregnon; Ministat; Minulet; Modicon; Neo-Stediril; Neocon; Neogynon; Ovanon; Ovidol; Ovostat; Ovulen†; Stediril; Tri-Minulet; Trigynon; Tri-nordiol; Trinovum; Triodeen; **Norw.:** Diane; Eugynon; Follimin; Marvelon; Microgynon; Synfase; Tetragynon; Trinordiol; Trionetta; **NZ:** Biphasil; Brevinor; Diane; Femodene; Levlen ED; Loette; Marvelon; Melodene; Mercilon; Microgynon; Minulet; Monofeme; Nordette; Nordiol; Norimin; Ovral; Synphasic; Trifeme; Triphasil; Triquilar; **Port.:** Diane; Gracial; Gynera; Harmonet; Marvelon; Mercilon; Microginon; Minigeste; Minulet; Neomonovar; Tetragynon; Tri-Gynera; Tri-Minulet; Trinordiol;

Triquilar; **S.Afr.:** Biphasil; Brevinor†; Demulen†; Diane; Femodene ED; Logynon ED; Marvelon; Melodene; Menoflush; Menoflush + ¼†; Mercilon; Minulette; Mixogen†; Nordette; Nordiol; Normovlar ED†; Ovostat†; Ovral; Tri-Minulet; TriCilest; Trinovum; Triodene; Triphasil; **Singapore:** Diane; Gynera; Marvelon; Meliane; Mercilon; Microgynon; Minulet; Nordette; Trinordiol; Triquilar; **Spain:** Diane; Eugynon†; Gynovin; Harmonet; Meliane; Microdiol; Microgynon; Minulet; Neo Lyndiol; Neogynona; Ovoplex; Primosiston; Suavuret; Tri-Minulet; Triagynon; Triciclor; Trinovum; **Swed.:** Cilest; Follimin; Follinett; Lyndiol†; Lyndiolett; Mercilon; Neovletta; Orthonett Novum; Regunon; Restovar; Sequilarum†; Synfase; Tetragynon†; Trimiron; Trinordiol; Trinovum; Trionetta; **Switz.:** Binordiol; Cilest; Diane; Gracial; Gynera; Harmonet; Marvelon; Meloden; Microgynon; Milvane; Minulet; Neo-Eunomine; Neo-Stediril†; Neogynon; Normophasic; Ologyn; Ovanon; Ovidol; Ovostat†; Ovulen†; Oysmen; Primosiston; Sequilar†; Stediril 30; Stediril D; Tetragynon; Tri-Minulet; Trinordiol; Trinovum; Triquilar; Yermonil†; **Thai.:** Anna; Diane; Eugynon 250; FMP; Gynera; Hormone Multicap; Horon; Lady-35; Lyndiol; Marvelon; Meliane; Mercilon; Microgest; Microgynon; Minulet; Nordette; Nordiol; Ovral; Preme; R-Den; Riget; Rigevidon; Tina; Trinordiol; Triquilar; **UK:** Binovum; Brevinor; Cilest; Dianette; Eugynon 30; Femodene; Femodette; Loestrin; Logynon; Marvelon; Mercilon; Microgynon 30; Minulet; Norimin; Ovran; Ovran 30; Ovranette; Ovysmen; Schering PC4†; Synphase; Tri-Minulet; Triadene; Trinordiol; Trinovum; **USA:** Alesse; Apri; Aviane; Brevicon; Demulen; Desogen; Enpresse; Estrostep; Estrostep Fe; femhrt; GenCept 0.5/35 and 1/35†; GenCept 10/11†; Genora 0.5/35 and 1/35†; Jenest; Levlen; Levlite; Levora; Lo/Ovral; Loestrin; Loestrin Fe; Mircette; Modicon; Necon 10/11; Necon 0.5/35, 1/35; NEE 1/35; Nelova 0.5/35E and 1/35E†; Nelova 10/11†; Nordette; Norethin 1/35E†; Norinyl 1 + 35; Ortho Cyclen; Ortho Tri-Cyclen; Ortho-Cept; Ortho-Novum 1/35; Ortho-Novum 10/11; Ortho-Novum 7/7/7; Ovcon 35; Ovcon 50; Ovral; Preven; Tri-Levlen; Tri-Norinyl; Triphasil; Trivora; Yasmin; Zovia.

Ethylestrenol (9045-q)

Ethylestrenol (BAN, USAN, rINN).

Ethyloestrenol. 17α-Ethylestr-4-en-17β-ol; 19-Nor-17α-pregn-4-en-17β-ol.

$C_{20}H_{32}O = 288.5$.
CAS — 965-90-2.
ATC — A14AB02.

Profile

Ethylestrenol is a 17α-alkylated anabolic steroid (see Testosterone, p.1492) with little androgenic effect and slight progestational activity. It has been used for the promotion of growth in boys with short stature or delayed bone growth. It is used in veterinary medicine.

Preparations

Proprietary Preparations (details are given in Part 3)
S.Afr.: Orabolin†.

Etonogestrel (15428-g)

Etonogestrel (BAN, USAN, rINN).

3-keto-Desogestrel; Org-3236. 13-Ethyl-17-hydroxy-11-methylene-18,19-dinor-17α-pregn-4-en-20-yn-3-one; 17β-Hydroxy-11-methylene-18-homo-19-nor-17α-pregn-4-en-20-yn-3-one.

$C_{22}H_{28}O_2 = 324.5$.
CAS — 54048-10-1.
ATC — G03AC08.

Profile

Etonogestrel, the active metabolite of desogestrel (p.1470), is available as a parenteral progestogen-only contraceptive administered as an implant containing 68 mg of etonogestrel, which is effective for 3 years. It is under investigation as the progestogen component of a combined contraceptive delivered via a vaginal ring device. It is also under investigation as a male contraceptive, taken orally daily, in combination with testosterone implants or injections.

◊ References.
1. Edwards JE, Moore A. Implanon: a review of clinical studies. *Br J Fam Plann* 1999; **24:** 3–16.
2. Le J, Tsourounis C. Implanon: a critical review. *Ann Pharmacother* 2001; **35:** 329–36.

Preparations

Proprietary Preparations (details are given in Part 3)
Austral.: Implanon; **Denm.:** Implanon; **Fin.:** Implanon; **Fr.:** Implanon; **Ger.:** Implanon; **Neth.:** Implanon; **Swed.:** Implanon; **UK:** Implanon.

Etynodiol Diacetate (9046-p)

Etynodiol Diacetate (BANM, pINNM).

Aethynodiolum Diaceticum; Ethynodiol Diacetate (USAN); SC-11800. 19-Nor-17α-pregn-4-en-20-yne-3β,17β-diol diacetate.

$C_{24}H_{32}O_4 = 384.5$.
CAS — 1231-93-2 (etynodiol); 297-76-7 (etynodiol diacetate).

Pharmacopoeias. In Br., Pol., and US.

Pharmacopoeial description

BP 2001: A white or almost white, odourless or almost odourless, crystalline powder. Very slightly soluble in water; soluble

The symbol † denotes a preparation no longer actively marketed

---

in alcohol; freely soluble in chloroform and in ether. Protect from light.

USP 25: A white, odourless, crystalline powder. Insoluble in water; soluble in alcohol; very soluble in chloroform; freely soluble in ether; sparingly soluble in fixed oils. Protect from light.

Adverse Effects and Precautions

As for progestogens in general (see Progesterone, p.1488). See also under Hormonal Contraceptives, p.1452.

Pregnancy. Fetal adrenal cytomegaly in a 17-week-old fetus was associated with the maternal ingestion of an oral contraceptive containing etynodiol diacetate 2 mg and mestranol 100 µg from the sixth to the fourteenth week of pregnancy.[1]
1. Gau SS, Bennett MJ. Fetal adrenal cytomegaly. *J Clin Pathol* 1979; **32:** 305–6.

Interactions

As for progestogens in general (see Progesterone, p.1489). See also under Hormonal Contraceptives, p.1458.

Pharmacokinetics

Etynodiol diacetate is readily absorbed from the gastrointestinal tract and rapidly metabolised, largely to norethisterone (p.1485). Following administration of a radiolabelled dose of etynodiol diacetate about 60% of the radioactivity is stated to be excreted in urine and about 30% in faeces; the half-life in plasma is about 25 hours.

Uses and Administration

Etynodiol diacetate is a progestogen (see Progesterone, p.1489) that is used as the progestogenic component of combined oral contraceptives and also alone as an oral progestogen-only contraceptive (see p.1459); typical daily doses are 1 to 2 mg in combination products and 500 µg for progestogen-only contraceptives.

Preparations

USP 25: Ethynodiol Diacetate and Ethinyl Estradiol Tablets; Ethynodiol Diacetate and Mestranol Tablets.

Proprietary Preparations (details are given in Part 3)
Fr.: Lutometrodiol†; **Israel:** Femulen; **NZ:** Femulen; **S.Afr.:** Femulen†; **UK:** Femulen.

Multi-ingredient: Austral.: Ovulen†; **Belg.:** Conova; Ovulen†; **Braz.:** Normex; Unidose; **Canad.:** Demulen; **Denm.:** Conova†; **Neth.:** Ovulen†; **S.Afr.:** Demulen†; **Switz.:** Ovulen†; **USA:** Demulen; Zovia.

Finasteride (5502-q)

Finasteride (BAN, USAN, rINN).

Finasteridum; MK-0906; MK-906. N-tert-Butyl-3-oxo-4-aza-5α-androst-1-ene-17β-carboxamide.

$C_{23}H_{36}N_2O_2 = 372.5$.
CAS — 98319-26-7.
ATC — D11AX10; G04CB01.

Pharmacopoeias. In Eur. (see p.vi) and US.

Pharmacopoeial description

Ph. Eur.: A white or almost white crystalline powder. It exhibits polymorphism. Practically insoluble in water; freely soluble in dehydrated alcohol and in dichloromethane. Protect from light.

USP 25: A white to off-white crystalline solid. Very slightly soluble in water; freely soluble in alcohol and in chloroform.

Adverse Effects

The most commonly reported adverse effects of finasteride are decreased libido, impotence, ejaculation disorders, and reduced volume of ejaculate.

Breast tenderness and enlargement (gynaecomastia) may occur, and there have been reports of hypersensitivity reactions such as swelling of the lips and face, pruritus, urticaria, and rashes. Testicular pain has also been reported.

◊ In a study using prescription event monitoring data,[1] the most commonly reported adverse effects of finasteride in 14 772 patients were impotence or ejaculatory failure (2.1% of patients), reduced libido (1%), and breast disorders such as gynaecomastia (0.4%). Adverse effects reported in a single patient each, and verified on recballenge, were exfoliative dermatitis, perioral numbness, and swollen glands. Finasteride appeared to be associated with ataxia in 1 patient and wheeziness in another.
1. Wilton L, et al. The safety of finasteride used in benign prostatic hypertrophy: a non-interventional observational cohort study in 14 772 patients. *Br J Urol* 1996; **78:** 379–84.

Effects on the breast. Gynaecomastia was the adverse effect of finasteride most frequently reported to the FDA between June 1992 and February 1995 (a total of 214 reports).[1] The onset after therapy ranged from 14 days to 2.5 years, and the condition could be unilateral or bilateral. Mastectomy was performed in 12 men. Of the 86 men for whom information after discontinuation was available, partial or complete remission of gynaecomastia occurred in 80%, and no change occurred in 20%. In 2 of the cases, primary intraductal breast carcinoma was subsequently found, although 1 probably had breast cancer

---

before finasteride therapy. Continued surveillance of the relationship between finasteride and breast cancer is required.
1. Green L, et al. Gynecomastia and breast cancer during finasteride therapy. *N Engl J Med* 1996; **335:** 823.

Precautions

Finasteride should be used with caution in men with hepatic impairment. When used for benign prostatic hyperplasia, finasteride should be used with caution in men at risk of obstructive uropathy. Patients should be evaluated for prostatic carcinoma before and during therapy. Use of finasteride decreases concentrations of serum markers of prostate cancer such as prostate specific antigen (PSA) by up to 50% even when cancer is present, and reference values should be adjusted accordingly; the ratio of free to total PSA (percent free PSA) remains constant.

Studies in *animals* suggest finasteride could produce feminisation (hypospadia) of a male fetus if used in pregnant women; therefore, its use is contra-indicated in women who are or may become pregnant. In addition, it is recommended that women in this category should not handle crushed or broken finasteride tablets. Finasteride has been detected in semen, therefore use of a condom is recommended if the patient's sexual partner is, or may become, pregnant.

Pharmacokinetics

Finasteride is absorbed following oral administration, and peak plasma concentrations are achieved in 1 to 2 hours. The mean bioavailability has variously been reported as 63% and 80%. It is about 90% bound to plasma protein. Finasteride is metabolised in the liver and excreted in urine and faeces as metabolites. The mean terminal half-life is about 6 hours in patients under 60 years of age but may be prolonged to about 8 hours in those 70 years of age or older.

◊ References.
1. Steiner JF. Clinical pharmacokinetics and pharmacodynamics of finasteride. *Clin Pharmacokinet* 1996; **30:** 16–27.

Uses and Administration

Finasteride is an azasteroid that inhibits 5α-reductase, the enzyme responsible for conversion of testosterone to the more active dihydrotestosterone, and therefore has anti-androgenic properties. It is given by mouth in a dose of 5 mg daily in the management of benign prostatic hyperplasia to cause regression of the enlarged prostate and to improve symptoms; it may reduce the incidence of acute urinary retention and the need for surgery. Response may be delayed and treatment for 6 months or more may be required to assess whether benefit has been achieved.

In the treatment of male-pattern baldness (alopecia androgenetica) in men, finasteride is given by mouth in a dose of 1 mg daily. In general, use for 3 months or more is required before benefit is seen, and effects are reversed within 12 months of ceasing therapy.

Alopecia. In men with male-pattern baldness (alopecia—see p.1104), treatment with finasteride for 12 months resulted in an 11% increase in vertex hair count, which was maintained in those who continued therapy.[1] The use of oral finasteride for this purpose has been reviewed.[2,3] Topical finasteride has also been investigated, and some efficacy demonstrated.[4]
1. Kaufman KD, et al. Finasteride in the treatment of men with androgenetic alopecia. *J Am Acad Dermatol* 1998; **39:** 578–89.
2. Anonymous. Propecia and Rogaine Extra Strength for alopecia. *Med Lett Drugs Ther* 1998; **40:** 25–7.
3. McClellan KJ, Markham A. Finasteride: a review of its use in male pattern hair loss. *Drugs* 1999; **57:** 111–26.
4. Mazzerella F, et al. Topical finasteride in the treatment of androgenic alopecia. *J Dermatol Treat* 1997; **8:** 189–92.

Benign prostatic hyperplasia. Benign enlargement of the prostate gland is common in men with increasing age: as many as 50% of men aged over 50 years have histological evidence of hyperplasia.[1] Men with an enlarged prostate may exhibit overt symptoms of obstruction, such as acute or chronic urinary retention, or irritative symptoms such as frequency, urgency, nocturia, or occasionally urge incontinence, resulting from secondary bladder instability.[1-3] Symptoms can fluctuate, and do not necessarily deteriorate with time; furthermore, they do not seem to relate directly to prostatic volume.

In men with mild or moderate symptoms no treatment may be required, although symptoms need to be monitored ('watchful waiting').[1-3] In those with more severe symptoms or complications the mainstay of treatment is *transurethral resection of the prostate* (TURP).[1,2,4,5] This is the most effective treatment, but is associated with the greatest risk of complications and morbidity, including potential impotence. In consequence drug therapy may be tried first in men with moderate symptoms but no definite indications for surgery.[1-6]

Therapy with an *alpha$_1$-adrenoceptor blocker* (such as alfuzosin, doxazosin, prazosin, tamsulosin, or terazosin) can produce rapid symptomatic relief, apparently by an action on smooth muscle in the hyperplastic tissue and in the bladder.[3-6] However, adverse effects include orthostatic hypotension.

In recent years the *5α-reductase inhibitor* finasteride has offered an alternative approach.[3-12] Finasteride produces moderate reductions in prostate volume, although this takes a number of months and is not always associated with much symptomatic improvement. Like the alpha blockers, therapy must be continued indefinitely for benefit to be maintained. A comparative 12-month study[13] found that the alpha blocker terazosin to be more effective than finasteride in relieving symptoms and improving peak urine flow rates; the combination of finasteride plus terazosin was no more effective than terazosin alone. Moreover, although finasteride reduced prostatic volume, it was no more effective than placebo, a finding that is at odds with previous placebo-controlled studies. It has been suggested that the smaller median prostate size in this study may explain the negative findings,[14] and that men with larger prostates do benefit from finasteride. However, others consider that the findings indicate that decreasing muscle tone may be more important than reducing prostate size, and that alpha blockers remain the drugs of first choice for the medical management of benign prostatic hyperplasia although finasteride may be useful in gross enlargement.[15] More recently, a 4-year study found that finasteride reduced the probability of surgery and acute urinary retention in men with symptomatic benign prostate hyperplasia with prostatic enlargement.[16] Although the need for prostatectomy was reduced by 55% it was pointed out[17] that only 6% extra patients would benefit from treatment with finasteride. For every 100 men treated, 7 finasteride and 13 placebo recipients required surgery.

Other drug therapies exist but are largely unproven or unsuitable for general use. Gonadorelin analogues such as leuprorelin or nafarelin can produce a reduction in prostate size, but adverse effects make these drugs unsuitable for indefinite therapy. More recently, gonadorelin antagonists such as cetrorelix have been tried. The antifungal mepartricin has been reported to produce symptomatic improvement, possibly by binding to oestrogen in the intestinal lumen and lowering plasma-oestrogen concentrations. A number of plant extracts such as saw palmetto and *Pygeum africanum* are also in use,[18-21] and the phytosterol sitosterol, which is a constituent of these, is reported to be effective.[22] However, the aromatase inhibitor atamestane, which can inhibit the rise in oestrogen biosynthesis, appears not to be of benefit.[23]

Various *surgical alternatives to TURP* are under investigation: these include transurethral microwave thermotherapy, laser prostatectomy, and the insertion of stents to hold the urethra open.[3,5]

1. Bullock N. Benign prostatic hyperplasia. *Prescribers' J* 1999; **39:** 9–15.
2. Cockett AT, *et al.* Recommendations of the International Consensus Committee In: Cockett AT, *et al*, eds. *The 2nd international consultation on benign prostatic hyperplasia (BPH).* Jersey: Scientific Communication International, 1993: 553–64.
3. Lee M, Sharifi R. Benign prostatic hyperplasia: diagnosis and treatment guideline. *Ann Pharmacother* 1997; **31:** 481–6.
4. Monda JM, Oesterling JE. Medical treatment of benign prostatic hyperplasia: 5α-reductase inhibitors and α-adrenergic antagonists. *Mayo Clin Proc* 1993; **68:** 670–9.
5. Oesterling JE. Benign prostatic hyperplasia: medical and minimally invasive treatment options. *N Engl J Med* 1995; **332:** 99–109.
6. Lieber MM. Pharmacologic therapy for prostatism. *Mayo Clin Proc* 1998; **73:** 590–6.
7. Peters DH, Sorkin EM. Finasteride: a review of its potential in the treatment of benign prostatic hyperplasia. *Drugs* 1993; **46:** 177–208.
8. Rittmaster RS. Finasteride. *N Engl J Med* 1994; **330:** 120–5.
9. Gormley GJ, *et al.* The effect of finasteride in men with benign prostatic hyperplasia. *N Engl J Med* 1992; **327:** 1185–91.
10. Finasteride Study Group. Finasteride (MK-906) in the treatment of benign prostatic hyperplasia. *Prostate* 1993; **22:** 291–9.
11. Nickel JC, *et al.* Efficacy and safety of finasteride therapy for benign prostatic hyperplasia: results of a 2-year randomized controlled trial (the PROSPECT study). *Can Med Assoc J* 1996; **155:** 1251–9.
12. Wilde MI, Goa KL. Finasteride: an update of its use in the management of symptomatic benign prostatic hyperplasia. *Drugs* 1999; **57:** 557–81.
13. Lepor H, *et al.* The efficacy of terazosin, finasteride, or both in benign prostatic hyperplasia. *N Engl J Med* 1996; **335:** 533–9.
14. Walsh PC. Treatment of benign prostatic hyperplasia. *N Engl J Med* 1996; **335:** 586–7.
15. Farmer A, Noble J. Drug treatment for benign prostatic hyperplasia. *BMJ* 1997; **314:** 1215–16.
16. McConnell JD, *et al.* The effect of finasteride on the risk of acute urinary retention and the need for surgical treatment among men with benign prostate hyperplasia. *N Engl J Med* 1998; **338:** 557–63.
17. Wasson JH. Finasteride to prevent morbidity from benign prostatic hyperplasia. *N Engl J Med* 1998; **338:** 612–13.
18. Lowe FC, Ku JC. Phytotherapy in treatment of benign prostatic hyperplasia: a critical review. *Urology* 1996; **48:** 12–20.
19. Buck AC. Phytotherapy for the prostate. *Br J Urol* 1996; **78:** 325–36.
20. Wilt TJ, *et al.* Saw palmetto extracts for treatment of benign prostatic hyperplasia: a systematic review. *JAMA* 1998; **280:** 1604–9. Correction. *ibid.* 1999; **281:** 515.
21. Lowe FC, Fagelman E. Phytotherapy in the treatment of benign prostatic hyperplasia: an update. *Urology* 1999; **53:** 671–8.
22. Wilt TJ, *et al.* β-Sitosterol for the treatment of benign prostatic hyperplasia: a systematic review. *BJU Int* 1999; **83:** 976–83.
23. Gingell JC, *et al.* Placebo controlled double-blind study to test the efficacy of the aromatase inhibitor atamestane in patients with benign prostatic hyperplasia not requiring operation. *J Urol (Baltimore)* 1995; **154:** 399–401.

Hirsutism. Finasteride is under investigation for the treatment of hirsutism (p.1468) in women.[1,2] It should be noted that finasteride should not be used in women who are or may become pregnant (see Precautions, above).

1. Wong IL, *et al.* A prospective randomized trial comparing finasteride to spironolactone in the treatment of hirsute women. *J Clin Endocrinol Metab* 1995; **80:** 233–8.
2. Falsetti L, *et al.* Comparison of finasteride versus flutamide in the treatment of hirsutism. *Eur J Endocrinol* 1999; **141:** 361–7.

Malignant neoplasms of the prostate. Finasteride appears to have little effect in men with established prostate cancer,[1,2] but is under investigation for the prevention of prostate cancer (see also p.497). The results of 1 small study[3] of its effects on the prostate found little evidence to support its use for prevention of malignancy in patients at high risk.

1. Presti JC, *et al.* Multicenter, randomized, double-blind placebo controlled study to investigate the effect of finasteride (MK-906) on stage D prostate cancer. *J Urol (Baltimore)* 1992; **148:** 1201–4.
2. Rittmaster RS. Finasteride. *N Engl J Med* 1994; **330:** 120–5.
3. Cote RJ, *et al.* The effect of finasteride on the prostate gland in men with elevated serum prostate-specific antigen levels. *Br J Cancer* 1998; **78:** 413–18.

Preparations

USP 25: Finasteride Tablets.

Proprietary Preparations (details are given in Part 3)
Aust.: Proscar; *Austral.:* Propecia; Proscar; *Belg.:* Proscar; *Braz.:* Proscar; Prostide; *Canad.:* Propecia; Proscar; *Denm.:* Propecia; Proscar; *Fin.:* Propecia; Proscar; *Fr.:* Chibro-Proscar; Propecia; *Ger.:* Propecia; Proscar; *Hong Kong:* Proscar; *Irl.:* Proscar; *Israel:* Pro-Cure; *Ital.:* Finastid; Genaprost; Propecia; Proscar; Prostide; *Mex.:* Propeshia; Proscar; *Neth.:* Proscar; *Norw.:* Proscar; NZ: Proscar; *Port.:* Propecia; Proscar; *S.Afr.:* Propecia; Proscar; *Singapore:* Propecia; Proscar; *Spain:* Eucoprost; Folitabs; Propecia; Proscar; Urprosan†; *Swed.:* Propecia; Proscar; *Switz.:* Propecia; Proscar; *Thai.:* Proscar; *UK:* Propecia; Proscar; *USA:* Propecia; Proscar.

Flugestone Acetate (9047-s)

Flugestone Acetate (BANM).

Flurogestone Acetate (USAN); NSC-65411; SC-9880; 9α-Fluoro-11β,17α-dihydroxypregn-4-ene-3,20-dione 17-acetate.
$C_{23}H_{31}FO_5 = 406.5$.
CAS — 337-03-1 (flugestone); 2529-45-5 (flugestone acetate).

Profile
Flugestone acetate is a progestogen (see Progesterone, p.1488) used in veterinary medicine.

Fluoxymesterone (9049-e)

Fluoxymesterone (BAN, rINN).

NSC-12165. 9α-Fluoro-11β,17β-dihydroxy-17α-methylandrost-4-en-3-one.
$C_{20}H_{29}FO_3 = 336.4$.
CAS — 76-43-7.
ATC — G03BA01.
Pharmacopoeias. In Jpn and US.

Pharmacopoeial description
USP 25: A white or practically white, odourless, crystalline powder. Practically insoluble in water; sparingly soluble in alcohol; slightly soluble in chloroform. Protect from light.

Adverse Effects and Precautions
As for androgens and anabolic steroids in general (see Testosterone, p.1492).

As with other 17α-alkylated compounds fluoxymesterone may cause hepatotoxicity, and is probably best avoided in patients with hepatic impairment, and certainly if this is severe. Hepatic function should be monitored during therapy.

Uses and Administration
Fluoxymesterone has androgenic properties (see Testosterone, p.1493). It is effective when given by mouth and is more potent than methyltestosterone.

In the treatment of male hypogonadism, fluoxymesterone has been given in a dosage of 5 to 20 mg daily. In the treatment of delayed puberty in the male it has been given in usual daily doses of 2.5 to 10 mg, adjusted according to response; care was necessary because of the risk of epiphyseal closure and treatment was generally only given for 4 to 6 months. In the palliation of inoperable neoplasms of the breast in postmenopausal women, it has been given in daily doses of up to 40 mg. Fluoxymesterone has also been used in the treatment of aplastic anaemia.

Growth retardation. Fluoxymesterone has been used to try to increase final adult height in boys with constitutional delay of growth associated with delayed puberty (see p.1273).

Preparations

USP 25: Fluoxymesterone Tablets.

Proprietary Preparations (details are given in Part 3)
Austral.: Halotestin; *Canad.:* Halotestin; *Fr.:* Halotestin†; *Hong Kong:* Halotestin; *Israel:* Halotestin; *Ital.:* Halotestin; *Mex.:* Stenox; *Neth.:* Halotestin; *Norw.:* Halotestin†; *S.Afr.:* Halotestin; *Singapore:* Halotestin; *Swed.:* Halotestin†; *Thai.:* Halotestin; *USA:* Halotestin.

Formebolone (9051-v)

Formebolone (BAN, rINN).

Formyldienolone. 11α,17β-Dihydroxy-17β-methyl-3-oxoandrosta-1,4-diene-2-carbaldehyde.
$C_{21}H_{28}O_4 = 344.4$.
CAS — 2454-11-7.

Profile
Formebolone has anabolic properties (see Testosterone, p.1492) and has been given by mouth or by intramuscular injection.

Fosfestrol (9052-g)

Fosfestrol (BAN, rINN).

Diethylstilbestrol Diphosphate; Phosphoestrolum; Stilboestrol Diphosphate. (E)-αα′-Diethylstilbene-4,4′-diol bis(dihydrogen phosphate); (E)-4,4′-(1,2-Diethylvinylene)bis(phenyl dihydrogen orthophosphate).
$C_{18}H_{22}O_8P_2 = 428.3$.
CAS — 522-40-7.
ATC — L02AA04.
Pharmacopoeias. In Jpn and US.

Pharmacopoeial description
USP 25: An off-white, odourless, crystalline powder. Sparingly soluble in water; soluble in alcohol and in dilute alkali. Store in airtight containers at a temperature not exceeding 21°.

Fosfestrol Sodium (9053-q)

Fosfestrol Sodium (BANM, rINNM).
$C_{18}H_{18}Na_4O_8P_2 = 516.2$.
CAS — 23519-26-8 (fosfestrol tetrasodium xH$_2$O); 4719-75-9 (anhydrous fosfestrol tetrasodium).
Pharmacopoeias. In Br., which specifies xH$_2$O.

Anhydrous fosfestrol sodium 100 mg is approximately equivalent to 83 mg of fosfestrol.

Pharmacopoeial description
BP 2001: A white or almost white powder. Freely soluble in water; practically insoluble in dehydrated alcohol and in ether. A 5% solution in water has a pH of 7.0 to 9.0. Protect from light.

Adverse Effects and Precautions
As for Diethylstilbestrol, see p.1471.

Following intravenous injection of fosfestrol sodium there may be a temporary burning sensation in the perineal region and pain at the site of bony metastases. Slow infusion is not recommended as cytotoxic concentrations of the drug may not be achieved.

Uses and Administration
Fosfestrol is a synthetic nonsteroidal oestrogen that requires dephosphorylation to diethylstilbestrol (p.1471) before it is active. It is used in the treatment of malignant neoplasms of the prostate (p.497).

Expressed in terms of fosfestrol sodium, initial therapy for at least the first 5 days may range from 600 to 1200 mg daily by slow intravenous injection. In terms of fosfestrol, these doses are equivalent to 500 to 1000 mg. Injections should be given preferably with the patient lying down. Maintenance intravenous therapy may be with 300 mg fosfestrol sodium one to four times a week or 300 to 600 mg fosfestrol sodium (250 to 500 mg fosfestrol) once or twice a week. Fosfestrol sodium may also be given by mouth, in a dose of up to 240 mg (200 mg of fosfestrol) three times daily for 7 days then reducing over 14 days to 120 to 360 mg (100 to 300 mg of fosfestrol) daily in divided doses.

Fosfestrol disodium has also been used.

Preparations

BP 2001: Fosfestrol Injection; Fosfestrol Tablets;
USP 25: Diethylstilbestrol Diphosphate Injection.

Proprietary Preparations (details are given in Part 3)
Aust.: Honvan; *Austral.:* Honvan; *Belg.:* Honvan; *Braz.:* Honvan; Ronvan; *Canad.:* Honvol; *Fr.:* ST-52; *Ger.:* Honvan; *Hong Kong:* Honvan; *Mex.:* Honvan; *Neth.:* Honvan; *Norw.:* Honvan†; *NZ:* Honvan; *Port.:* Honvan; *S.Afr.:* Honvan†; *Singapore:* Honvan; *Spain:* Honvan; *Swed.:* Honvan†; *Switz.:* Honvan; *UK:* Honvan; *USA:* Stilphostrol†.

Gestodene (18649-x)

Gestodene (BAN, USAN, rINN).

SH-B-331. 13β-Ethyl-17β-hydroxy-18,19-dinor-17α-pregna-4,15-dien-20-yn-3-one.

$C_{21}H_{26}O_2 = 310.4$.

CAS — 60282-87-3.

Adverse Effects and Precautions

As for progestogens in general (see Progesterone, p.1488). See also under Hormonal Contraceptives, p.1452. Gestodene is reported to have few androgenic effects, and to have less adverse effect on the serum lipid profile than older 19-nortestosterone derivatives. However, there is some evidence that gestodene-containing combined oral contraceptives are associated with a small increased risk of venous thromboembolism (see p.1455, and for precautions, see p.1457).

Interactions

As for progestogens in general (see Progesterone, p.1489). See also under Hormonal Contraceptives, p.1458.

Antiepileptics. Felbamate treatment significantly increased gestodene clearance from a low-dose combined oral contraceptive, and might decrease contraceptive efficacy.[1] See also p.1459.

1. Saano V, et al. Effects of felbamate on the pharmacokinetics of a low-dose combination oral contraceptive. Clin Pharmacol Ther 1995; 58: 523–31.

Pharmacokinetics

Gestodene is well absorbed with a high bioavailability when administered by mouth. It is extensively bound to plasma proteins (75 to 87% to sex hormone binding globulin, and 13 to 24% to albumin). Gestodene is metabolised in the liver, less than 1% of a dose being excreted in the urine unchanged.

Uses and Administration

Gestodene is a progestogen (see Progesterone, p.1488) structurally related to levonorgestrel. It is used as the progestogenic component of combined oral contraceptives (see p.1459); a typical daily dose is 75 µg in monophasic preparations, and 50 to 100 µg in triphasic preparations.

◊ Reviews.

1. Anonymous. Femodene/Minulet—how different is gestodene? Drug Ther Bull 1990; 28: 41–2.
2. Wilde MI, Balfour JA. Gestodene: a review of its pharmacology, efficacy and tolerability in combined contraceptive preparations. Drugs 1995; 50: 364–95.

Preparations

Proprietary Preparations (details are given in Part 3)

Multi-ingredient: Aust.: Gynovin; Harmonette; Meliane; Minulet; Monogestin; Myvlar; Tri-Minulet; Triodena; Triogestena; Triogestin; **Austral.:** Femoden ED; Minulet; Tri-Minulet; Trioden ED; **Belg.:** Femodene; Harmonet; Meliane; Minulet; Tri-Minulet; Triodene; **Braz.:** Gestinol; Gynera; Minulet; Denm.: Gynera; Harmonet; Meloden; Milvane; Minulet; Tri-Minulet; **Fin.:** Femoden; Harmonet; Meliane; Minulet; Tri-Femoden; Tri-Minulet; **Fr.:** Harmonet; Meliane; Melodia; Minesse; Minulet; Moneva; Phaeva; Tri-Minulet; **Ger.:** Femovan; Minulet; **Hong Kong:** Gynera; Harmonet; Minulet; **Irl.:** Femodene; Minesse; Minulet; Tri-Minulet; Triodene; **Israel:** Gynera; Harmonet; Meliane; Minulet; **Ital.:** Fedra; Ginoden; Harmonet; Milvane; Minulet; Tri-Minulet; **Mex.:** Gynovin; Minulet; **Neth.:** Femodeen; Harmonet; Meliane; Minulet; Tri-Minulet; Triodeen; **NZ:** Femodene; Melodene; Minulet; **Port.:** Gynera; Harmonet; Minigeste; Minulet; Tri-Minulet; **S.Afr.:** Femodene ED; Melodene; Minulette; Tri-Minulet; Triodene; **Singapore:** Gynera; Meliane; Minulet; **Spain:** Gynovin; Harmonet; Meliane; Minulet; Tri-Minulet; Trigynovin; **Switz.:** Gynera; Harmonet; Meloden; Milvane; Minulet; Tri-Minulet; **Thai.:** Gynera; Meliane; Minulet; **UK:** Femodene; Femodette; Minulet; Tri-Minulet; Triadene.

Gestonorone Caproate (9055-s)

Gestonorone Caproate (BANM, USAN, rINN).

Gestronol Hexanoate; NSC-84054; SH-582. 17α-Hydroxy-19-norpregn-4-ene-3,20-dione hexanoate.

$C_{26}H_{38}O_4 = 414.6$.

CAS — 1253-28-7.

Adverse Effects and Precautions

As for progestogens in general (see Progesterone, p.1488).

Local reactions have occurred at the site of injection. Rarely, coughing, dyspnoea, and circulatory disturbances may develop during or immediately after injection but can be avoided by injecting gestonorone very slowly. In males, spermatogenesis is temporarily inhibited.

The symbol † denotes a preparation no longer actively marketed

Interactions

As for progestogens in general (see Progesterone, p.1489).

Uses and Administration

Gestonorone caproate is a long-acting potent progestogen structurally related to progesterone (p.1489). It is given in an oily solution by intramuscular injection in doses of 200 to 400 mg every 5 to 7 days for the adjunctive treatment of endometrial carcinoma (p.493). It has also been used in the management of benign prostatic hyperplasia (p.1477) in doses of 200 mg weekly, increased to 300 to 400 mg weekly if necessary.

Preparations

Proprietary Preparations (details are given in Part 3)

Aust.: Depostat†; **Ger.:** Depostat; **Ital.:** Depostat; **Mex.:** Primostat; **Spain:** Depostat; **Switz.:** Depostat; **UK:** Depostat.

Gestrinone (12782-d)

Gestrinone (BAN, USAN, rINN).

A-46745; Ethylnorgestrienone; R-2323; RU-2323. 13β-Ethyl-17β-hydroxy-18,19-dinor-17α-pregna-4,9,11-trien-20-yn-3-one.

$C_{21}H_{24}O_2 = 308.4$.

CAS — 16320-04-0; 40542-65-2.

ATC — G03XA02.

Adverse Effects

As for Danazol, p.1468. Gestrinone may inhibit ovulation, and menstrual irregularities such as breakthrough bleeding may occur during treatment. Androgenic side-effects include acne, oily skin, fluid retention, weight gain, hirsutism, and voice change. Headache, gastrointestinal disturbances, increased liver enzyme values, altered libido, hot flushes, decreased breast size, nervousness, change in appetite, muscle cramp, and depression may also occur.

Precautions

As for Danazol, p.1469.

Interactions

Antiepileptic drugs and rifampicin may accelerate the metabolism of gestrinone.

Pharmacokinetics

Gestrinone is well absorbed after oral administration with negligible first-pass hepatic metabolism. Peak plasma concentrations occur about 3 hours after administration. The plasma half-life is about 24 hours. Gestrinone is metabolised in the liver with the formation of conjugated metabolites.

Uses and Administration

Gestrinone is a synthetic steroidal hormone reported to have androgenic, anti-oestrogenic, and antiprogestogenic properties. It is used in the treatment of endometriosis (p.1469) in doses of 2.5 mg twice weekly by mouth; the first dose is taken on the first day of the menstrual cycle with the second dose taken three days later; thereafter the doses should be taken on the same two days of each week, usually for a period of 6 months. If a dose is missed it should be given as soon as possible and the original dose sequence maintained thereafter; if 2 or more doses are missed gestrinone should be discontinued and restarted on the first day of a new cycle after a negative pregnancy test.

◊ References.

1. Thomas EJ, Cooke ID. Impact of gestrinone on the course of asymptomatic endometriosis. BMJ 1987; 294: 272–4.
2. Brosens IA, et al. The morphologic effect of short-term medical therapy of endometriosis. Am J Obstet Gynecol 1987; 157: 1215–21.
3. Coutinho EM, Azadian-Boulanger G. Treatment of endometriosis by vaginal administration of gestrinone. Fertil Steril 1988; 49: 418–22.
4. Coutinho EM, Gonçalves MT. Long-term treatment of leiomyomas with gestrinone. Fertil Steril 1989; 51: 939–46.
5. Hornstein MD, et al. A randomized double-blind prospective trial of two doses of gestrinone in the treatment of endometriosis. Fertil Steril 1990; 53: 237–41.
6. Peters F. Multicentre study of gestrinone in cyclical breast pain. Lancet 1992; 339: 205–8.

7. Worthington M, et al. A randomized comparative study of the metabolic effects of two regimens of gestrinone in the treatment of endometriosis. Fertil Steril 1993; 59: 522–6.
8. Gestrinone Italian Study Group. Gestrinone versus a gonadotropin-releasing hormone agonist for the treatment of pelvic pain associated with endometriosis: a multicenter, randomized, double-blind study. Fertil Steril 1996; 66: 911–19.

Preparations

Proprietary Preparations (details are given in Part 3)

Austral.: Dimetriose; **Belg.:** Dimetrose†; **Braz.:** Dimetrose; **Ital.:** Dimetriose; **Mex.:** Nemestran; **Neth.:** Nemestran; **NZ:** Dimetriose; **Port.:** Dimetriose; **S.Afr.:** Tridomose; **Singapore:** Dimetriose; **Spain:** Nemestran; **Switz.:** Nemestran; **Thai.:** Dimetriose; **UK:** Dimetriose.

Hydroxyestrone Diacetate (12833-a)

16α-Hydroxyoestrone Diacetate. 3,16α-Dihydroxyestra-1,3,5(10)-trien-17-one diacetate.

$C_{22}H_{26}O_5 = 370.4$.

CAS — 566-76-7 (hydroxyestrone); 1247-71-8 (hydroxyestrone diacetate).

Profile

Hydroxyestrone diacetate is an oestrogen (see Estradiol, p.1473). It has been given by mouth in vulvo-vaginal disorders and for female infertility.

Preparations

Proprietary Preparations (details are given in Part 3)

Braz.: Hormocervix; **Fr.:** Colpormon†.

Hydroxyprogesterone Caproate (9057-e)

Hydroxyprogesterone Caproate (BANM, rINN).

17-AHPC; Hydroxyprogesterone Hexanoate; NSC-17592. 3,20-Dioxopregn-4-en-17α-yl hexanoate; 17α-Hydroxypregn-4-ene-3,20-dione hexanoate.

$C_{27}H_{40}O_4 = 428.6$.

CAS — 68-96-2 (hydroxyprogesterone); 630-56-8 (hydroxyprogesterone caproate).

Pharmacopoeias. In Br., Chin., and US.

Pharmacopoeial description

BP 2001: A white or almost white, odourless or almost odourless, crystalline powder. Practically insoluble in water; freely soluble in alcohol and in ether; very soluble in chloroform; dissolves in fixed oils and esters. Protect from light.

USP 25: A white or creamy-white, crystalline powder. Odourless or having a slight odour. Insoluble in water; soluble in ether; slightly soluble in benzene. Protect from light.

Adverse Effects and Precautions

As for progestogens in general (see Progesterone, p.1488).

There may be local reactions at the site of injection. Rarely, coughing, dyspnoea, and circulatory disturbances may occur during or immediately after injection of hydroxyprogesterone caproate but can be avoided by injecting the drug very slowly.

Pregnancy. Abnormalities reported in infants born to mothers who had received hydroxyprogesterone during pregnancy have included tetralogy of Fallot in one infant,[1] genito-urinary abnormalities in 2 infants,[2] and adrenocortical carcinoma in one infant.[3]

1. Heinonen OP, et al. Cardiovascular birth defects and antenatal exposure to female sex hormones. N Engl J Med 1977; 296: 67–70.
2. Evans ANW, et al. The ingestion by pregnant women of substances toxic to the foetus. Practitioner 1980; 224: 315–19.
3. Mann JR, et al. Transplacental carcinogenesis (adrenocortical carcinoma) associated with hydroxyprogesterone hexanoate. Lancet 1983; ii: 580.

Interactions

As for progestogens in general (see Progesterone, p.1489).

Uses and Administration

Hydroxyprogesterone caproate is a progestogen structurally related to progesterone (p.1489) that has been used for recurrent miscarriage and various menstrual disorders. In recurrent miscarriage associated with proven progesterone deficiency, suggested doses have been 250 to 500 mg weekly by intramuscular injection during the first half of pregnancy.

Hydroxyprogesterone enantate has also been used.

Preparations

BP 2001: Hydroxyprogesterone Injection;
USP 25: Hydroxyprogesterone Caproate Injection.

Proprietary Preparations (details are given in Part 3)

Aust.: Proluton; **Austral.:** Proluton; **Fr.:** Progesterone-retard Pharlon; **Ger.:** Progesteron-Depot; Proluton Depot; **Hong Kong:** Proluton Depot; **Israel:** Depolut; Proluton Depot; **Ital.:** Lentogest; Proluton Depot; **Mex.:** Caposten; Primolut Depot; **Neth.:** Proluton Depot; **S.Afr.:** Primolut Depot†; **Singapore:** Proluton Depot; **Spain:** Proluton Depot†; **Switz.:** Proluton Depot; **Thai.:** Proluton Depot; **UK:** Proluton Depot; **USA:** Hylutin; Hyprogest†.

Multi-ingredient: Aust.: Gravibinon; Ostrolut†; **Braz.:** Gestadinona; Progest; Trinestril; **Ger.:** Gravibinon; Syngynon; **Ital.:** Gravibinon; **Mex.:** Gravidinova; Primosiston; **Mon.:** Tocogestan; Trophobolene†; **Switz.:** Primosiston.

Lynestrenol (9059-y)

Lynestrenol (BAN, USAN, rINN).

Ethinylestrenol; Linestrenol; Lynenol; Lynestrenolum; Lynoestrenol; NSC-37725. 19-Nor-17α-pregn-4-en-20-yn-17β-ol.

$C_{20}H_{28}O = 284.4$.
CAS — 52-76-6.
ATC — G03AC02; G03DC03.
Pharmacopoeias. In Eur. (see p.vi).

Pharmacopoeial description

Ph. Eur.: A white or almost white crystalline powder. Practically insoluble in water; soluble in alcohol, in acetone, and in ether. Protect from light.

Profile

Lynestrenol is a progestogen (see Progesterone, p.1488) structurally related to norethisterone that is used alone or as the progestogenic component of some oral contraceptives (see p.1452). Typical oral daily doses for contraception are 0.5 mg when used as a progestogen-only preparation, and 0.75 to 2.5 mg when combined with an oestrogen. When used alone for menstrual disorders, doses of 5 to 10 mg per day are used, often as cyclical regimens.

Porphyria. Lynestrenol has been associated with acute attacks of porphyria and is considered unsafe in porphyric patients.

Preparations

Proprietary Preparations (details are given in Part 3)
Aust.: Orgametril; *Belg.:* Exluton†; Orgametril; *Denm.:* Exlutona; Orgametril; *Fin.:* Exluton; Orgametril; *Fr.:* Exluton; Orgametril; *Ger.:* Exlutona; Orgametril; *Mex.:* Exluton; *Neth.:* Exluton†; Orgametril; *Norw.:* Exlutona; *Port.:* Exluton; Orgametril; *S.Afr.:* Exluton†; *Spain:* Orgametril; *Swed.:* Exlutena; Orgametril; *Switz.:* Exlutona; Orgametril†; *Thai.:* Exluton.

Multi-ingredient: *Aust.:* Lyndiol; Ovanon; Restovar†; Yermonil; *Belg.:* Fysioquens†; Lyndiol†; Ministat†; Ovanon; Ovostat†; *Braz.:* Anacyclin; *Denm.:* Lyndiol†; *Fr.:* Ovanon; Physiostat; *Ger.:* Anacyclin†; Lyn-ratiopharm; Lyn-ratiopharm-Sequenz; Lyndiol†; Nuriphasic; Ovanon; Ovoresta M; Ovoresta†; Pregnon L; Yermonil; *Hong Kong:* Lyndiol; *Neth.:* Fysioquens; Mini Pregnon; Ministat; Ovanon; Ovostat; *S.Afr.:* Ovostat; *Spain:* Neo Lyndiol; *Swed.:* Lyndiol†; Lyndiolett; Restovar; *Switz.:* Normophasic; Ovanon; Ovostat†; Yermonil†; *Thai.:* Lyndiol.

Medrogestone (9061-q)

Medrogestone (BAN, USAN, rINN).

AY-62022; Metrogestone; NSC-123018; R-13-615. 6,17α-Dimethylpregna-4,6-diene-3,20-dione.
$C_{23}H_{32}O_2 = 340.5$.
CAS — 977-79-7.
ATC — G03DB03.

Profile

Medrogestone is a progestogen structurally related to progesterone (p.1488) that is used in the treatment of menstrual disorders, and as the progestogen in menopausal HRT (see p.1460). It is usually administered in daily doses of 5 to 10 mg by mouth, generally in a cyclical regimen. Higher doses were used in the treatment of endometrial carcinoma, prostatic hyperplasia, and breast disorders including carcinoma. It has also been used for threatened or recurrent miscarriage, but such use is not recommended unless there is proven progesterone deficiency.

Preparations

Proprietary Preparations (details are given in Part 3)
Aust.: Colpron; *Belg.:* Colpro; *Canad.:* Colprone; *Fr.:* Colprone; *Ger.:* Prothil; *Hong Kong:* Colprone; *Ital.:* Colprone; *Neth.:* Colpro; *S.Afr.:* Colpro; *Spain:* Colpro; *Switz.:* Colpro; *Thai.:* Colprone.

Multi-ingredient: *Aust.:* Premarin compositum; Premarin Plus; *Belg.:* Premplus; *Ger.:* Presomen compositum; *Hong Kong:* Prempak; *Ital.:* Prempak; *Mex.:* Premarin Pak; *Neth.:* Premarin Plus; *Port.:* Premarin Plus; *S.Afr.:* Prempak N; *Switz.:* Premarin Plus; *Thai.:* Prempak.

Medroxyprogesterone Acetate

(9062-p)

Medroxyprogesterone Acetate (BANM, rINNM).

Medroxyprogesteroni Acetas; Methylacetoxyprogesterone; Metipregnone; NSC-26386. 6α-Methyl-3,20-dioxopregn-4-en-17α-yl acetate; 17α-Hydroxy-6α-methylpregn-4-ene-3,20-dione acetate.
$C_{24}H_{34}O_4 = 386.5$.
CAS — 520-85-4 (medroxyprogesterone); 71-58-9 (medroxyprogesterone acetate).
Pharmacopoeias. In Eur. (see p.vi), Int., and US.

Pharmacopoeial description

Ph. Eur.: A white or almost white crystalline powder. Practically insoluble in water; sparingly soluble in alcohol; soluble in acetone and in dioxan; freely soluble in dichloromethane. Protect from light.

USP 25: A white to off-white, odourless, crystalline powder. Insoluble in water; sparingly soluble in alcohol and in methyl alcohol; soluble in acetone and in dioxan; freely soluble in chloroform; slightly soluble in ether. Store in airtight containers. Protect from light.

Adverse Effects and Precautions

As for progestogens in general (see Progesterone, p.1488). See also under Hormonal Contraceptives, p.1452. Medroxyprogesterone acetate may have glucocorticoid effects when administered long term at high doses.

Carcinogenicity. The risk of various cancers associated with the use of depot medroxyprogesterone acetate as a contraceptive has been evaluated by WHO.[1] Overall, there was no increase in risk of breast cancer, although there is some evidence that current or recent use may be associated with a slight increase in risk (see also p.1453). There was no increased risk of cervical cancer (see also p.1453), and a protective effect against endometrial cancer (see p.1454). In contrast to combined oral contraceptives, there was no evidence of a protective effect against ovarian cancer (p.1454).

1. Anonymous. Depot-medroxyprogesterone acetate (DMPA) and cancer: memorandum from a WHO meeting. *Bull WHO* 1993; **71:** 669–76.

Effects on bone density. Use of medroxyprogesterone acetate as a parenteral progestogen-only contraceptive has been associated with reductions in bone density (see under Effects on the Musculoskeletal System, p.1456). This effect has also been reported after oral administration for menstrual disorders,[1] and is thought to be due to medroxyprogesterone-induced oestrogen deficiency.

1. Cundy T, *et al.* Short-term effects of high dose oral medroxyprogesterone acetate on bone density in premenopausal women. *J Clin Endocrinol Metab* 1996; **81:** 1014–17.

Glucocorticoid effects. There have been reports of Cushing's syndrome induced by medroxyprogesterone acetate in patients receiving long-term therapy with high doses for the treatment of malignant neoplasms.[1-5] Cushingoid symptoms regressed when treatment was stopped. Medroxyprogesterone possesses glucocorticoid activity and there is a risk of adrenal insufficiency during periods of stress or after sudden withdrawal of treatment. Some[4] consider that patients should be monitored for glucose intolerance and adrenal insufficiency during treatment.

1. Siminoski K, *et al.* The Cushing syndrome induced by medroxyprogesterone acetate. *Ann Intern Med* 1989; **111:** 758–60.
2. Donckier JE, *et al.* Cushing syndrome and medroxyprogesterone acetate. *Lancet* 1990; **335:** 1094.
3. Grenfell A, *et al.* Cushing's syndrome and medroxyprogesterone acetate. *Lancet* 1990; **336:** 256.
4. Merrin PK, Alexander WD. Cushing's syndrome induced by medroxyprogesterone. *BMJ* 1990; **301:** 345.
5. Shotlift K, Nussey SS. Medroxyprogesterone acetate induced Cushing's syndrome. *Br J Clin Pharmacol* 1997; **44:** 304.

Porphyria. Medroxyprogesterone has been associated with acute attacks of porphyria and is considered unsafe in porphyric patients. However, for a reference to the use of medroxyprogesterone acetate with buserelin acetate in the prevention of premenstrual exacerbations of porphyria in 2 women, see p.1279.

Interactions

As for progestogens in general (see Progesterone, p.1489). Enzyme-inducing drugs may reduce the contraceptive efficacy of parenteral medroxyprogesterone; some recommend a reduction in the interval between injections of medroxyprogesterone from 12 to 10 weeks when such drugs are used concomitantly. It should be noted that aminoglutethimide markedly reduces plasma concentrations of medroxyprogesterone so that an increase in medroxyprogesterone dosage is likely to be required.

Pharmacokinetics

Medroxyprogesterone is absorbed from the gastrointestinal tract. In the blood, it is highly protein bound, principally to albumin. It is metabolised in the liver and excreted mainly as glucuronide conjugates in the urine and faeces. It has a half-life of 24 to 30 hours after oral administration; the half-life may be as long as 50 days after intramuscular injection. Medroxyprogesterone is reported to be distributed into breast milk.

Uses and Administration

Medroxyprogesterone acetate is a progestogen structurally related to progesterone, with actions and uses similar to those of the progestogens in general (see Progesterone, p.1489). It is administered by mouth or, for prolonged action, by intramuscular injection as an aqueous suspension.

It is used for the treatment of **menorrhagia** (p.1490) and **secondary amenorrhoea** in doses of 2.5 to 10 mg daily by mouth for 5 to 10 days starting on the assumed or calculated 16th to 21st day of the menstrual cycle, although some sources suggest that treatment may begin on any day in secondary amenorrhoea.

In the treatment of mild to moderate **endometriosis** (p.1469) usual doses are 10 mg three times daily by mouth, or 50 mg weekly or 100 mg every 2 weeks by intramuscular injection. In the UK it is recommended that treatment continue for 90 consecutive days; US sources recommend treatment for at least 6 months.

Medroxyprogesterone acetate is also given by intramuscular injection as a **contraceptive** (see under Hormonal Contraceptives, p.1459). As a progestogen-only contraceptive a dose of 150 mg is given every 12 weeks. A combined contraceptive injection containing medroxyprogesterone acetate 25 mg with estradiol cipionate 5 mg is given monthly.

When used as the progestogen component of **menopausal HRT** (see p.1463), medroxyprogesterone acetate is administered orally in a variety of regimens including 2.5 or 5 mg daily continuously, 5 or 10 mg daily for 12 to 14 days of a 28-day cycle, and 20 mg daily for 14 days of a 91-day cycle.

Medroxyprogesterone acetate may also be used in the palliative treatment of some hormone-dependent malignant neoplasms. In **breast carcinoma** (see below) doses have ranged from 0.4 to 1.5 g daily by mouth and from 0.5 g twice weekly to 1 g daily by intramuscular injection. In **endometrial** and **renal carcinoma** (p.493 and p.495, respectively) doses have ranged from 100 to 500 mg daily by mouth and from 0.25 to 1 g weekly by intramuscular injection. Alternative regimens using intramuscular injections have started with twice-weekly or alternate-day dosing before reducing to the weekly dosage interval or have started treatment with weekly doses and reduced to a maintenance schedule of as little as 400 mg monthly. In **prostatic carcinoma** (p.497) doses have been 100 to 500 mg daily by mouth and 0.5 g weekly or twice weekly by intramuscular injection.

Cachexia. Medroxyprogesterone may improve appetite and prevent loss of body-weight in cachexia (p.1481) associated with severe chronic disorders.[1]

1. Simons JPFHA, *et al.* Effects of medroxyprogesterone acetate on appetite, weight, and quality of life in advanced-stage non-hormone-sensitive cancer: a placebo-controlled multicenter study. *J Clin Oncol* 1996; **14:** 1077–84.

Contraception. Medroxyprogesterone acetate has established use as a parenteral progestogen-only contraceptive (p.1460). It has also been developed as the progestogenic component of a combined injectable contraceptive.
References.
1. Garza-Flores J, *et al.* Introduction of Cyclofem® once-a-month injectable contraceptive in Mexico. *Contraception* 1998; **58:** 7–12.

Epilepsy. Preliminary findings[1] suggested that medroxyprogesterone acetate might be of value in the management of catamenial epilepsy (p.338). In a more recent review[2] it was suggested that hormonal manipulation with drugs such as medroxyprogesterone should be reserved for highly selected groups under close supervision.

1. Mattson RH, *et al.* Treatment of seizures with medroxyprogesterone acetate: preliminary report. *Neurology* 1984; **34:** 1255–8.
2. Herkes GK. Drug treatment of catamenial epilepsy. *CNS Drugs* 1995; **3:** 260–6.

Male hypersexuality. The anti-androgenic action of medroxyprogesterone has been used for suppression of libido in the control of men with deviant or disinhibited sexual behaviour[1-3] (see Disturbed Behaviour, p.650).

1. Kiersch TA. Treatment of sex offenders with Depo-Provera. *Bull Am Acad Psychiatry Law* 1990; **18:** 179–87.
2. Weiner MF, *et al.* Intramuscular medroxyprogesterone acetate for sexual aggression in elderly men. *Lancet* 1992; **339:** 1121–2.
3. Kravitz HM, *et al.* Medroxyprogesterone treatment for paraphiliacs. *Bull Am Acad Psychiatry Law* 1995; **23:** 19–33.

Malignant neoplasms. BREAST. Progestogens are used as second- or third-choice drugs in the hormonal therapy of advanced breast cancer (p.491). Some references to the use of medroxyprogesterone acetate in advanced breast cancer are cited below.[1-6] Comparative studies have shown that patients respond equally well to medroxyprogesterone and either mepitiostane,[4] aminoglutethimide,[5] or oophorectomy.[6]

1. Pannuti F, *et al.* A possible new approach to the treatment of metastatic breast cancer: massive doses of medroxyprogesterone acetate. *Cancer Treat Rep* 1978; **62:** 499–504.

2. Guarnieri A, et al. Oral route administration of medroxyprogesterone acetate (MAP) at high doses in the treatment of advanced breast cancer: clinical results. *Chemioterapia* 1984; **3**: 320–3.

3. Hedley D, et al. Advanced breast cancer: response to high dose oral medroxyprogesterone acetate. *Aust N Z J Med* 1984; **14**: 251–4.

4. Izuo M, et al. A phase III trial of oral high-dose medroxyprogesterone acetate (MPA) versus mepitiostane in advanced postmenopausal breast cancer. *Cancer* 1985; **56**: 2576–9.

5. Canney PA, et al. Randomized trial comparing aminoglutethimide with high-dose medroxyprogesterone acetate in therapy for advanced breast carcinoma. *J Natl Cancer Inst* 1988; **80**: 1147–51.

6. Martoni A, et al. High-dose medroxyprogesterone acetate versus oophorectomy as first-line therapy of advanced breast cancer in premenopausal patients. *Oncology* 1991; **48**: 1–6.

ENDOMETRIUM. Progestogens are used in the treatment of advanced endometrial carcinoma (p.493) but there are doubts about their value in the earlier stages of disease.[1] Medroxyprogesterone acetate was effective in a rare case of low-grade endometrial stromal sarcoma.[2]

1. Martin-Hirsch PL, et al. Progestagens for endometrial cancer (updated 24 May 2001). Available in The Cochrane Library: Issue 3. Oxford: Update Software; 2001.

2. Rand RJ, Lowe JW. Low-grade endometrial stromal sarcoma treated with a progestogen. *Br J Hosp Med* 1990; **43**: 154–6.

Respiratory disorders. Reviews of the use of medroxyprogesterone acetate in obstructive sleep apnoea have concluded that it has a limited role.[1,2]

Medroxyprogesterone is commonly used in the treatment of pulmonary lymphangioleiomyomatosis, a rare disease affecting only women.[3] Anecdotal evidence suggests some patients improve or stabilise on treatment, possibly those with chylous effusions or chylous ascites.[4]

Medroxyprogesterone acetate was reported to be effective in treating congenital central hypoventilation syndrome in 2 children.[5]

1. Millman RP. Medroxyprogesterone and obstructive sleep apnea. *Chest* 1989; **96**: 225–6.

2. Terra SG, Gherky KC. Medroxyprogesterone acetate in the treatment of obstructive sleep apnea. *Ann Pharmacother* 1997; **31**: 776–8.

3. Johnson S. Lymphangioleiomyomatosis: clinical features, management and basic mechanisms. *Thorax* 1999; **54**: 254–64.

4. Taylor JR, et al. Lymphangioleiomyomatosis: clinical course in 32 patients. *N Engl J Med* 1990; **323**: 1254–60.

5. Milerad J, et al. Alveolar hypoventilation treated with medroxyprogesterone. *Arch Dis Child* 1985; **60**: 150–5.

Sickle-cell disease. Intramuscular medroxyprogesterone reduced the frequency of painful crises in patients with homozygous sickle-cell disease (p.717),[1] and is considered a suitable contraceptive in women with the condition[2,3] in whom combined oral contraceptives should probably be avoided (see also p.1458).

1. de Ceulaer K, et al. Medroxyprogesterone acetate and homozygous sickle-cell disease. *Lancet* 1982; **ii**: 229–31.

2. Guillebaud J. Sickle cell disease and contraception. *BMJ* 1993; **307**: 506–7.

3. Kirkman REJ, Elstein M. Management of sickle cell disease: contraception with medroxyprogesterone may be beneficial. *BMJ* 1998; **316**: 935.

Preparations

USP 25: Medroxyprogesterone Acetate Injectable Suspension; Medroxyprogesterone Acetate Tablets.

Proprietary Preparations (details are given in Part 3)
Aust.: Depo-Provera; Depocon; Farlutal; Prodafem; Provera; **Austral.:** Depo-Provera; Depo-Ralovera; Farlutal†; Provera; Ralovera; **Belg.:** Depo-Provera; Farlutal; Provera; **Braz.:** Cycrin; Depo-Provera; Farlutal; Provera; **Canad.:** Alti-MPA; Depo-Provera; Gen-Medroxy; Proclim; Provera; **Denm.:** Depo-Provera; Perlutex; Provera; **Fin.:** Cykrina; Depo-Provera; Farlutal; Gestapuran; Lutopolar; Mepastat; Provera; **Fr.:** Depo-Prodasone; Depo-Provera; Farlutal; Gestoral; Prodasone; **Ger.:** Clinofem; Clinovir; Depo-Clinovir; Farlutal; G-Farlutal; GestaPolar; MPA; MPA Gyn; MPA-beta; MPA-Noury; **Hong Kong:** Depo-Provera; Farlutal; Provera; **Irl.:** Depo-Provera; Farlutal; Provera; **Israel:** Aragest; Depo-Provera; Provera; **Ital.:** Depo-Provera; Farlutal; Lutoral†; Provera; **Mex.:** Ciclotal; Cycrin; Depo-Provera; Farlutal; Provera; **Neth.:** Depo-Provera; Farlutal; Provera; **Norw.:** Depo-Provera; Farlutal; Perlutex; Provera; **NZ:** Depo-Provera; Farlutal; Provera; **Port.:** Depo-Provera; Provera; **S.Afr.:** Depo-Provera; Farlutal; Petogen; Provera; **Singapore:** Depo-Provera; Farlutal; Provera; **Spain:** Depo-Progevera; Farlutal; Progevera; Progevera 250; **Swed.:** Depo-Provera; Farlutal; Gestapuran; Provera; **Switz.:** Depo-Provera; Farlutal; Prodafem; Provera†; **Thai.:** Contracep; Depo-Gestin; Depo-Progesta; Depo-Provera; Farlutal; Medeton; Provera; **UK:** Adgyn Medro; Depo-Provera; Farlutal; Provera; **USA:** Amen; Cycrin; Depo-Provera; Provera.

Multi-ingredient: **Aust.:** Cyclo-Premarin-MPA; Cyclo-Premella†; Filena; Perennia; Premarin-MPA; Premella†; Sequennia; Tri-Filena; **Austral.:** Divina; Estrapak; Menoprem; Premia 5; Premia Continuous; Provelle; **Belg.:** Diviplus; Diviva; Premelle; Trivina; **Braz.:** Dilena; **Denm.:** Divina; Divina Plus; Klimalet; Klimaxil; Trevina; **Fin.:** Divina; Divitren; **Fr.:** Precyclan; **Ger.:** Climopax; Climopax Cyclo; CycloPolar; Estrafemol; Osmil; Procyclo; Sisare; **Hong Kong:** Dilena; Premelle; Premelle Cycle; **Irl.:** Femplan-MA; Premique; Premique Cycle; Tridestra; **Israel:** Meno-MPA; Premaril MP; Premaril Plus MP; **Ital.:** Filena; Premelle C; Premelle S; **Mex.:** Cyclofemina; Dilena; Premelle; **Neth.:** Divina; Premelle; Premelle Cycle; **NZ:** Menoprem; Premia; Premia Continuous; Provette Continuous; Provette Sequential; **Port.:** Dilena; Medrivas Antibiotico; Medrivas†; Premelle; Premelle Cycle; **S.Afr.:** Divina; Premelle; Trivina; **Singapore:** Premelle; Premelle Cycle; **Spain:** Medricol; Medrivas; Medrivas Antib; Perifem; Premelle; Premelle Ciclico; **Swed.:** Di-

vina; Divina Plus; Premelle; Premelle Sekvens; Trivina; **Switz.:** Cyclo-Premella ST; Cyclo-Premella†; Premella; Triaval; **UK:** Improvera; Indivina; Premique; Premique Cycle; Tridestra; **USA:** Lunelle; Premphase; Prempro.

Megestrol Acetate (9063-s)

Megestrol Acetate (BANM, USAN, rINNM).
BDH-1298; Compound 5071; Megestroli Acetas; NSC-71423; SC-10363. 6-Methyl-3,20-dioxopregna-4,6-dien-17α-yl acetate; 17α-Hydroxy-6-methylpregna-4,6-diene-3,20-dione acetate.
$C_{24}H_{32}O_4 = 384.5$.
CAS — 3562-63-8 (megestrol); 595-33-5 (megestrol acetate).

Pharmacopoeias. In *Eur.* (see p.vi) and *US*.

Pharmacopoeial description

Ph. Eur.: A white or almost white crystalline powder. Practically insoluble in water; sparingly soluble in alcohol; soluble in acetone. Protect from light.

USP 25: A white to creamy-white, essentially odourless, crystalline powder. Insoluble in water; sparingly soluble in alcohol; soluble in acetone; very soluble in chloroform; slightly soluble in ether and in fixed oils. Protect from light.

Adverse Effects and Precautions

As for progestogens in general (see Progesterone, p.1488). The weight gain that may be observed with megestrol acetate appears to be associated with an increased appetite and food intake rather than with fluid retention. Megestrol acetate may have glucocorticoid effects when administered long term.

◊ Severe pain of the hands reminiscent of carpal tunnel syndrome occurred in 4 women while taking megestrol acetate and melphalan;[1] megestrol appeared to be responsible.

1. DiSaia PJ, Morrow CP. Unusual side effect of megestrol acetate. *Am J Obstet Gynecol* 1977; **129**: 460–1.

Effects on carbohydrate metabolism. Megestrol therapy has been associated with hyperglycaemia[1,2] or diabetes mellitus[3] in AIDS patients being treated for cachexia. It has been suggested that megestrol produces peripheral insulin resistance due to a glucocorticoid action.[4]

1. Panwalker AP. Hyperglycemia induced by megestrol acetate. *Ann Intern Med* 1992; **116**: 878.

2. Bornemann M, Johnson AC. Endocrine effects of HIV infection. *N Engl J Med* 1993; **328**: 894.

3. Henry K, et al. Diabetes mellitus induced by megestrol acetate in a patient with AIDS and cachexia. *Ann Intern Med* 1992; **116**: 53–4.

4. Leinung MC, et al. Induction of adrenal suppression by megestrol acetate in patients with AIDS. *Ann Intern Med* 1995; **122**: 843–5.

Effects on the respiratory system. Two cases of hyperpnoea in patients receiving megestrol acetate 80 mg three times daily.[1]

1. Fessel WJ. Megestrol acetate and hyperpnea. *Ann Intern Med* 1989; **110**: 1034–5.

Glucocorticoid effects. Megestrol has glucocorticoid-like properties which can result in adrenocortical insufficiency severe enough to require replacement therapy with hydrocortisone.[1-5]

1. Leinung MC, et al. Induction of adrenal suppression by megestrol acetate in patients with AIDS. *Ann Intern Med* 1995; **122**: 843–5.

2. Maurer M. Megestrol for AIDS-related anorexia. *Ann Intern Med* 1995; **122**: 880.

3. Stoffer SS, Krakauer JC. Induction of adrenal suppression by megestrol acetate. *Ann Intern Med* 1996; **124**: 613–14.

4. Mann M, et al. Glucocorticoidlike activity of megestrol: a summary of Food and Drug Administration experience and a review of the literature. *Arch Intern Med* 1997; **157**: 1651–6.

5. Stockheim JA, et al. Adrenal suppression in children with the human immunodeficiency virus treated with megestrol acetate. *J Pediatr* 1999; **134**: 368–70.

Porphyria. Megestrol is considered to be unsafe in patients with porphyria because it has been shown to be porphyrinogenic in *animals*.

Interactions

As for progestogens in general (see Progesterone, p.1489).

Pharmacokinetics

Absorption of megestrol acetate from the gastrointestinal tract is variable following oral administration; peak drug concentrations in plasma occur 1 to 3 hours after a dose by mouth. Megestrol acetate is highly protein bound in plasma. It undergoes hepatic metabolism, with 57 to 78% of a dose being excreted in the urine and 8 to 30% in the faeces.

Uses and Administration

Megestrol acetate is a progestogen structurally related to progesterone (p.1489) that is used for the palliative treatment of various cancers.

It is given by mouth in endometrial carcinoma in doses of 40 to 320 mg daily in divided doses, and in doses of 40 mg four times daily or 160 mg once daily in breast cancer.

Megestrol acetate is also used in the treatment of anorexia and cachexia in patients with cancer or AIDS. The usual dose is 800 mg daily, as oral suspension, for one month, followed by a maintenance dose of 400 to 800 mg daily.

Cachexia. In some patients with severe chronic disorders or malignant neoplasms, anorexia (loss of appetite) forms part of a syndrome of metabolic abnormalities and progressive physical wasting known as cachexia. Improved nutrition and dietary counselling are usually insufficient to reverse cachexia, and therefore drug therapy has been tried to stimulate appetite and promote weight gain.

In **cancer-related cachexia**, corticosteroids are frequently used for appetite stimulation in patients with advanced malignancies. They appear to be effective in stimulating appetite, although do not appear to promote weight gain.[1-4] High-dose megestrol has produced weight gain in some randomised controlled trials,[5,6] and has been recommended,[2] particularly in slowly progressive disease accompanied by anorexia.[3] Similar properties have been reported with medroxyprogesterone.[4] Anabolic steroids have also been tried, but further evaluation is necessary:[1-3] a comparison of megestrol or dexamethasone with fluoxymesterone found the latter to be less effective than the progestogen or the corticosteroid.[7] Prokinetic drugs such as metoclopramide may be useful in patients whose symptoms are secondary to decreased gastrointestinal motility.[3] Other drugs studied but with little, if any, benefit include cannabinoids, cyproheptadine and hydralazine.[1-4] Megestrol has also been given in combination with ibuprofen.[8]

High-dose megestrol is also effective in adults and children with **HIV-related cachexia**,[9-11] a topic which is discussed further on p.610.

1. Loprinzi CL, et al. Cancer-associated anorexia and cachexia: implications for drug therapy. *Drugs* 1992; **43**: 499–506.

2. Loprinzi CL. Management of cancer anorexia/cachexia. *Support Care Cancer* 1995; **3**: 120–2.

3. Bruera E. Anorexia, cachexia, and nutrition. *BMJ* 1997; **315**: 1219–22.

4. Mantovani G, et al. Managing cancer-related anorexia/cachexia. *Drugs* 2001; **61**: 499–514.

5. Loprinzi CL, et al. Controlled trial of megestrol acetate for the treatment of cancer anorexia and cachexia. *J Natl Cancer Inst* 1990; **82**: 1127–32.

6. Tchekmedyian NS, et al. Megestrol acetate in cancer anorexia and weight loss. *Cancer* 1992; **69**: 1268–74.

7. Loprinzi CL, et al. Randomized comparison of megestrol acetate versus dexamethasone versus fluoxymesterone for the treatment of cancer anorexia/cachexia. *J Clin Oncol* 1999; **17**: 3299–3306.

8. McMillan DC, et al. A prospective randomized study of megestrol acetate and ibuprofen in gastrointestinal cancer patients with weight loss. *Br J Cancer* 1999; **79**: 495–500.

9. Von Roenn JH, et al. Megestrol acetate in patients with AIDS-related cachexia. *Ann Intern Med* 1994; **121**: 393–9.

10. Oster MH, et al. Megestrol acetate in patients with AIDS and cachexia. *Ann Intern Med* 1994; **121**: 400–8.

11. Clarick RH, et al. Megestrol acetate treatment of growth failure in children infected with human immunodeficiency virus. *Pediatrics* 1997; **99**: 354–7.

Hot flushes. Megestrol has been used in female patients with breast cancer who were experiencing hot flushes (to avoid the potentially tumour-stimulating effects of an oestrogen—see Malignant Neoplasms, under Precautions of HRT, p.1463), as well as in men with hot flushes after orchidectomy or anti-androgen therapy for prostate cancer.[1] Therapy, which involved low doses of 20 mg twice daily, was associated with a decrease in frequency of flushes of 50% or more in about three-quarters of all patients.

1. Loprinzi CL, et al. Megestrol acetate for the prevention of hot flashes. *N Engl J Med* 1994; **331**: 347–52.

Malignant neoplasms. Like some other progestogens megestrol acetate is used in endometrial cancer (p.493), and it has been reported to have similar efficacy to anastrozole[1] and tamoxifen[2] in postmenopausal women with advanced breast cancer (p.491). There was no advantage in terms of response or survival in escalating the standard dose of megestrol (160 mg daily) to 800 or 1600 mg daily in a randomised study in women with breast cancer.[3]

1. Buzdar A, et al. Anastrozole, a potent and selective aromatase inhibitor, versus megestrol acetate in postmenopausal women with advanced breast cancer: results of overview analysis of two phase III trials. *J Clin Oncol* 1996; **14**: 2000–11.

2. Stuart NSA, et al. A randomised phase III cross-over study of tamoxifen versus megestrol acetate in advanced and recurrent breast cancer. *Eur J Cancer* 1996; **32A**: 1888–92.

3. Abrams J, et al. Dose-response trial of megestrol acetate in advanced breast cancer: cancer and Leukemia Group B phase III study 8741. *J Clin Oncol* 1999; **17**: 64–73.

Preparations

BP 2001: Megestrol Tablets;
USP 25: Megestrol Acetate Tablets.

Proprietary Preparations (details are given in Part 3)
Aust.: Megace; Nia; **Austral.:** Megace; Megostat; **Belg.:** Megace; **Braz.:** Megestat; **Canad.:** Megace; **Denm.:** Megace; Megestin; **Fin.:** Megace; Megestin; **Fr.:** Megace; **Ger.:** Megestat; **Hong Kong:** Megace; **Irl.:** Megace; **Israel:** Megace; **Ital.:** Megace; Megestil; **Mex.:** Megace; Mestrel; Prazoken; **Neth.:** Megace; **Norw.:** Megace; **NZ:** Megace; Megostat; **Port.:** Acestrol; **Singapore:** Megace; **Spain:** Borea; Maygace; Megefren; Megostat; **Swed.:** Megace; **Switz.:** Megestat; **Thai.:** Megace; **UK:** Megace; **USA:** Megace.

Mepitiostane (12930-t)

Mepitiostane (rINN).

S-10364. 17β-(1-Methoxycyclopentyloxy)-2α,3α-epithio-5α-androstane; Cyclopentanone 2α,3α-epithio-5α-androstan-17β-yl methyl acetal.
$C_{25}H_{40}O_2S = 404.6$.
CAS — 21362-69-6.

Pharmacopoeias. In Jpn.

Profile

Mepitiostane has androgenic and anabolic properties (see Testosterone, p.1492) and is given by mouth in usual doses of 10 mg twice daily for the management of neoplasms of the breast and anaemia associated with renal failure.

Preparations

Proprietary Preparations (details are given in Part 3)
Jpn: Thioderon.

Mesterolone (9064-w)

Mesterolone (BAN, USAN, rINN).

Mesterolonum; NSC-75054; SH-723. 17β-Hydroxy-1α-methyl-5α-androstan-3-one.
$C_{20}H_{32}O_2 = 304.5$.
CAS — 1424-00-6.
ATC — G03BB01.

Pharmacopoeias. In Eur. (see p.vi).

Pharmacopoeial description

Ph. Eur.: A white or yellowish crystalline powder. Practically insoluble in water; sparingly soluble in acetone, in ethyl acetate, and in methyl alcohol.

Adverse Effects and Precautions

As for androgens in general (see Testosterone, p.1492).
Mesterolone is reported not to inhibit gonadotrophin secretion or spermatogenesis.

Uses and Administration

Mesterolone has androgenic properties (see Testosterone, p.1493) but is reported to have less inhibitory effect on intrinsic testicular function than testosterone.

Mesterolone is given by mouth in the treatment of androgen deficiency or male infertility associated with hypogonadism (p.1274) in initial doses of 75 to 100 mg daily followed by doses of 50 to 75 mg daily for maintenance.

Preparations

Proprietary Preparations (details are given in Part 3)
Aust.: Proviron; **Austral.:** Proviron; **Belg.:** Proviron; **Braz.:** Proviron; **Denm.:** Mestoranum; **Fin.:** Proviron; **Fr.:** Proviron†; **Ger.:** Proviron; Vistimon; **Hong Kong:** Proviron; **Israel:** Proviron; **Ital.:** Proviron; **Mex.:** Proviron; **Neth.:** Proviron; **Norw.:** Mestoranum†; **Port.:** Proviron; **S.Afr.:** Proviron; **Singapore:** Provironum; **Spain:** Proviron; **Swed.:** Mestoranum; **Switz.:** Proviron; **Thai.:** Provironum; **UK:** Proviron.

Mestranol (9065-e)

Mestranol (BAN, USAN, rINN).

Compound 33355; EE3ME; EE₃ME; Ethinyloestradiol-3-methyl Ether; Mestranolum. 3-Methoxy-19-nor-17α-pregna-1,3,5(10)-trien-20-yn-17β-ol.
$C_{21}H_{26}O_2 = 310.4$.
CAS — 72-33-3.

Pharmacopoeias. In Eur. (see p.vi), Jpn, Pol., and US.

Pharmacopoeial description

Ph. Eur.: A white or almost white crystalline powder. Practically insoluble in water; sparingly soluble in alcohol; soluble in ether. Protect from light.

USP 25: A white to creamy-white, odourless, crystalline powder. Insoluble in water; sparingly soluble in dehydrated alcohol; freely soluble in chloroform; soluble in dioxan; slightly soluble in methyl alcohol. Protect from light.

Adverse Effects and Precautions

As for oestrogens in general (see Estradiol, p.1473).
See also under Hormonal Contraceptives, p.1452.

Porphyria. Mestranol is considered to be unsafe in patients with porphyria because it has been shown to be porphyrinogenic in *animals* or *in-vitro* systems.

Interactions

See under Hormonal Contraceptives, p.1458.

Pharmacokinetics

Mestranol is readily absorbed from the gastrointestinal tract. It is metabolised in the liver to ethinylestradiol and its glucuronide. Excretion is via the kidneys and bile; metabolites undergo enterohepatic recycling. Compared with many other oestrogens, its metabolism is slow. The biological half-life is about 50 hours.

Uses and Administration

Mestranol is a synthetic oestrogen with actions similar to those of estradiol (see p.1474). It is a component of high-strength combined oral contraceptive preparations (dose 50 µg daily—see under Hormonal Contraceptives, p.1459). The progestogen component is often norethisterone. Mestranol has also been used as the oestrogen component of some preparations for menopausal HRT (see p.1460), although natural oestrogens are often preferred. Administration has usually been in a sequential regimen with doses ranging from 12.5 to 50 µg daily, in combination with a cyclical progestogen.

Preparations

USP 25: Ethynodiol Diacetate and Mestranol Tablets; Norethindrone and Mestranol Tablets.

Proprietary Preparations (details are given in Part 3)
Multi-ingredient: Aust.: Ortho-Novum; **Austral.:** Norinyl-1; **Belg.:** Ortho-Novum 1/50†; **Braz.:** Biofim; Megestran; **Canad.:** Norinyl 1/50; Ortho-Novum 1/50; **Ger.:** Gestamestrol N; Ortho-Novum 1/50†; Ovosiston; **Hong Kong:** Norinyl-1; **Irl.:** Menophase†; Norinyl-1†; Ortho-Novin; **Mex.:** Lutoral E; Norinyl; Secuentex-21; **Neth.:** Ortho-Novum 1/50†; **NZ:** Norinyl-1; **S.Afr.:** Norinyl-1/28; **Switz.:** Ortho-Novum 1/50†; **Thai.:** Anamai; **UK:** Menophase†; Norinyl-1; Ortho-Novin 1/50†; **USA:** Enovid†; Genora 1/50†; Necon 1/50; Nelova 1/50M†; Norethin 1/50M†; Norinyl 1 + 50; Ortho-Novum 1/50.

Metenolone Acetate (9069-z)

Metenolone Acetate (BANM, rINNM).

Methenolone Acetate (USAN); NSC-74226; SH-567; SQ-16496. 17β-Hydroxy-1-methyl-5α-androst-1-en-3-one acetate.
$C_{22}H_{32}O_3 = 344.5$.
CAS — 153-00-4 (metenolone); 434-05-9 (metenolone acetate).

Pharmacopoeias. In Jpn.

Metenolone Enantate (9070-p)

Metenolone Enantate (BANM, rINNM).

Methenolone Enanthate (USAN); Methenolone Oenanthate; NSC-64967; SH-601; SQ-16374. 17β-Hydroxy-1-methyl-5α-androst-1-en-3-one heptanoate.
$C_{27}H_{42}O_3 = 414.6$.
CAS — 303-42-4.

Pharmacopoeias. In Jpn.

Profile

Metenolone is an anabolic steroid (see Testosterone, p.1492) that has been used in treating aplastic anaemia, breast cancer, and postmenopausal osteoporosis. It has been given by mouth as the acetate in usual doses of 10 to 20 mg daily (although higher doses have been given), and intramuscularly as the enantate in doses of 100 mg every 2 to 4 weeks.

Preparations

Proprietary Preparations (details are given in Part 3)
Aust.: Primobolan; **Austral.:** Primobolan; **Ger.:** Primobolan; **Ital.:** Primobolan Depot†; **Mex.:** Primobolan; **Neth.:** Primobolan; **Norw.:** Primobolan†; **S.Afr.:** Primobolan; **Spain:** Primobolan Depot.

Multi-ingredient: Ger.: AntiFocal N; NeyChondrin N (Revitorgan-Dilutionen N Nr 68); NeyGeront N (Revitorgan-Dilutionen N Nr 64); NeyPulpin N (Revitorgan-Dilutionen N Nr 10); NeyTumorin N (Revitorgan-Dilutionen N Nr 66).

Methandienone (9067-y)

Methandienone (BAN).

Metandienone (pINN); Methandrostenolone; NSC-42722. 17β-Hydroxy-17α-methylandrosta-1,4-dien-3-one.
$C_{20}H_{28}O_2 = 300.4$.
CAS — 72-63-9.
ATC — A14AA03; D11AE01.

Pharmacopoeias. In Pol.

Adverse Effects and Precautions

As for androgens and anabolic steroids in general (see Testosterone, p.1492).

As with other 17α-alkylated compounds, methandienone is associated with hepatotoxicity and hepatic function should be monitored during therapy. It should probably be avoided in patients with hepatic impairment, and certainly if this is severe.

Effects on the liver. References to carcinoma of the liver in one patient[1] given methandienone and benign liver-cell adenoma in another.[2]

1. Johnson FL, *et al.* Association of androgenic-anabolic steroid therapy with development of hepatocellular carcinoma. *Lancet* 1972; **ii:** 1273–6.
2. Hernandez-Nieto L, *et al.* Benign liver-cell adenoma associated with long-term administration of an androgenic-anabolic steroid (methandienone). *Cancer* 1977; **40:** 1761–4.

Uses and Administration

Methandienone has anabolic and some androgenic properties (see Testosterone, p.1493). It has little progestogenic activity. Methandienone has been given by mouth as an anabolic drug.

Preparations

Proprietary Preparations (details are given in Part 3)
Thai.: Anabol; Melic.

Methyltestosterone (9071-s)

Methyltestosterone (BAN, rINN).

Methyltestosteronum; NSC-9701. 17β-Hydroxy-17α-methyl-androst-4-en-3-one.
$C_{20}H_{30}O_2 = 302.5$.
CAS — 58-18-4.
ATC — G03BA02; G03EK01.

Pharmacopoeias. In Chin., Eur. (see p.vi), Int., Jpn, Pol., and US.

Pharmacopoeial description

Ph. Eur.: A white or slightly yellowish-white, crystalline powder. Practically insoluble in water; freely soluble in alcohol; slightly soluble in ether. Protect from light.

USP 25: White or creamy-white, odourless, slightly hygroscopic, crystals or crystalline powder. Practically insoluble in water; soluble in alcohol, in ether, in methyl alcohol, and in other organic solvents; sparingly soluble in vegetable oils. Protect from light.

Adverse Effects and Precautions

As for androgens and anabolic steroids in general (see Testosterone, p.1492).

As with other 17α-alkylated compounds, methyltestosterone can produce a cholestatic hepatitis with jaundice, and has caused peliosis hepatis and hepatic neoplasms (see below). Methyltestosterone should be used with caution in patients with liver impairment, and is probably best avoided if this is severe. Liver function should be monitored during therapy.

Effects on the liver. Reports of peliosis hepatis[1] and liver damage[2-4] associated with methyltestosterone.

See also under Malignant Neoplasms, below.

1. Bagheri SA, *et al.* Peliosis hepatis associated with androgenic-anabolic steroid therapy: a severe form of hepatic injury. *Ann Intern Med* 1974; **81:** 610–18.
2. Westaby D, *et al.* Liver damage from long-term methyltestosterone. *Lancet* 1977; **ii:** 261–3.
3. Lowdell CP, Murray-Lyon IM. Reversal of liver damage due to long term methyltestosterone and safety of non-17 α-alkylated androgens. *BMJ* 1985; **291:** 637.
4. Borhan-Manesh F, Farnum JB. Methyltestosterone-induced cholestasis: the importance of disproportionately low serum alkaline phosphatase level. *Arch Intern Med* 1989; **124:** 2127–9.

MALIGNANT NEOPLASMS. Reports of hepatocellular carcinoma[1-6] and hepatic adenoma[5,7] associated with methyltestosterone.

1. Johnson FL, *et al.* Association of androgenic-anabolic steroid therapy with development of hepatocellular carcinoma. *Lancet* 1972; **ii:** 1273–6.
2. Henderson JT, *et al.* Androgenic-anabolic steroid therapy and hepatocellular carcinoma. *Lancet* 1973; **i:** 934.
3. Farrell GC, *et al.* Androgen-induced hepatoma. *Lancet* 1975; **i:** 430–2.
4. Goodman MA, Laden AMJ. Hepatocellular carcinoma in association with androgen therapy. *Med J Aust* 1977; **1:** 220–1.
5. Boyd PR, Mark GJ. Multiple hepatic adenomas and a hepatocellular carcinoma in a man on oral methyl testosterone for eleven years. *Cancer* 1977; **40:** 1765–70.
6. Gleeson D, *et al.* Androgen associated hepatocellular carcinoma with an aggressive course. *Gut* 1991; **32:** 1084–6.
7. Coombes GB, *et al.* An androgen-associated hepatic adenoma in a trans-sexual. *Br J Surg* 1978; **65:** 869–70.

Pregnancy. For reference to virilisation of a female fetus whose mother received methyltestosterone during pregnancy, see p.1493.

Interactions

As for androgens and anabolic steroids in general (see Testosterone, p.1493).

Pharmacokinetics

Methyltestosterone is absorbed from the gastrointestinal tract and from the oral mucosa. It undergoes less extensive first-pass hepatic metabolism than testosterone following oral administration, and has a longer half-life.

Uses and Administration

As for androgens and anabolic steroids in general (see Testosterone, p.1493).

Methyltestosterone is effective when given by mouth; its effect is increased about twofold when given buccally, as this avoids first-pass hepatic metabolism.

Suggested doses of methyltestosterone for androgen replacement therapy in male hypogonadism (p.1274) have been 10 to 50 mg daily by mouth or 5 to 25 mg daily buccally. Doses of 50 to 200 mg daily by mouth or 25 to 100 mg daily buccally have been given for metastatic breast carcinoma (p.491) in postmenopausal women. Doses of 1.25 to 2.5 mg daily by mouth have been given with oestrogens for the short-term treatment of menopausal vasomotor symptoms unresponsive to oestrogens alone.

Preparations

USP 25: Methyltestosterone Capsules; Methyltestosterone Tablets.

Proprietary Preparations (details are given in Part 3)
Canad.: Metandren†; *Israel:* Testotic B; *Ital.:* Testovis; *USA:* Android; Oreton Methyl†; Testred; Virilon.
Multi-ingredient: *Aust.:* Pasuma-Dragees†; *Braz.:* Ero Test; Gabormon; Gerosenil; Ioimbina Composta; Neurofitol; Sexormom; Testonus; *Fin.:* Potentol; *Hong Kong:* Gerivit; Wari-Procomil; *S.Afr.:* Mixogen†; *Thai.:* Hormone Multicap; Horon; Men Hormone; Wari-Procomil; *UK:* Prowess; *USA:* Estratest; Menogen†; Premarin with Methyltestosterone†.

Mibolerone (12957-q)

Mibolerone *(BAN, USAN, rINN)*.
NSC-72260; U-10997. 17β-Hydroxy-7α,17-dimethylestr-4-en-3-one.
$C_{20}H_{30}O_2 = 302.5$.
CAS — 3704-09-4.
Pharmacopoeias. In *US* for veterinary use only.

Pharmacopoeial description

USP 25: A white to off-white powder. Practically insoluble in water; slightly soluble in chloroform, in dioxan, and in dichloromethane.

Profile

Mibolerone is an androgen that is used in veterinary practice as a contraceptive for female dogs. It also has anabolic properties.

Mifepristone (19516-z)

Mifepristone *(BAN, USAN, rINN)*.
RU-486; RU-38486. 11β-(4-Dimethylaminophenyl)-17β-hydroxy-17α-prop-1-ynylestra-4,9-dien-3-one.
$C_{29}H_{35}NO_2 = 429.6$.
CAS — 84371-65-3.
ATC — G03XB01.

Adverse Effects

In a small proportion of patients given mifepristone uterine bleeding may be severe enough to warrant transfusion and curettage. Few patients have experienced pain after use of mifepristone although uterine pain is often experienced after subsequent prostaglandin administration. Malaise, faintness, headache, nausea, vomiting, and skin rashes have been reported. Uterine and urinary-tract infections have occurred in a small number of patients.

Effects on the cardiovascular system. A 31-year-old woman died from cardiovascular shock during an abortion induced by mifepristone followed by sulprostone.[1] She was a heavy cigarette smoker.

1. Anonymous. A death associated with mifepristone/sulprostone. *Lancet* 1991; **337:** 969–70.

Precautions

Mifepristone should not be given to women with a suspected ectopic pregnancy, to those with chronic adrenal failure or haemorrhagic disorders, or to those receiving anticoagulants or long-term corticosteroid therapy. Use in those with renal or hepatic impair-

The symbol † denotes a preparation no longer actively marketed

---

ment is also not recommended. Women over 35 years of age who are smokers should not receive mifepristone in combination with a prostaglandin for pregnancy termination, and smoking and alcohol should be avoided in all patients on the day of prostaglandin administration and for 2 days beforehand. Mifepristone should be given with care to patients with asthma or chronic obstructive airways diseases and to patients with cardiovascular disease or associated risk factors. Patients with prosthetic heart valves or those with a history of infective endocarditis should be given chemoprophylaxis when undergoing pregnancy termination. As with other means of terminating pregnancy, rhesus-negative women who have not been rhesus immunised will require protection with anti-D immunoglobulin.

Porphyria. Mifepristone is considered to be unsafe in patients with porphyria although there is conflicting experimental evidence of porphyrinogenicity.

Pregnancy. Studies in *rabbits,* but not *rats* or *mice,* suggest mifepristone causes fetal malformation. There have been reports of normal fetal development following the use of mifepristone alone in mothers who subsequently decided to continue their pregnancy.[1,2] However, in one woman, use of mifepristone was possibly related to malformations of the fetus including sirenomelia.[2]

1. Lim BH, *et al.* Normal development after exposure to mifepristone in early pregnancy. *Lancet* 1990; **336:** 257–8.
2. Pons J-C, *et al.* Development after exposure to mifepristone in early pregnancy. *Lancet* 1991; **338:** 763.

Interactions

Aspirin and NSAIDs should be avoided until complete termination of pregnancy has been confirmed, because of a theoretical risk that prostaglandin synthetase inhibitors may alter the efficacy of mifepristone.

Pharmacokinetics

Following administration by mouth peak plasma concentrations of mifepristone are reported to be obtained after 1.3 hours; bioavailability is about 70%. Elimination is biphasic; an initial slow phase is followed by a more rapid terminal phase, with an elimination half-life of about 18 hours. Mifepristone undergoes hepatic metabolism, and metabolites are excreted in the bile and eliminated in the faeces. Only a small fraction is detected in the urine. Mifepristone is about 98% bound to plasma proteins, predominantly α_1-acid glycoprotein.

Uses and Administration

Mifepristone is a steroid derived from norethisterone that has potent antiprogestogenic activity, and is used for the medical termination of pregnancy (p.1439) and for the induction of labour following fetal death *in utero.* In the UK the licensed regimen for the termination of pregnancies of up to 63 days' duration, is to give a single oral dose of 600 mg of mifepristone followed by the prostaglandin gemeprost 1 mg vaginally 36 to 48 hours later, unless abortion has already been completed. Lower doses of mifepristone have been employed effectively in some studies as have different prostaglandins. In the USA mifepristone is given in combination with misoprostol by mouth for pregnancies up to 49 days' duration. See also Termination of Pregnancy, below. For the termination of pregnancy between 13 and 24 weeks' gestation the licensed dose in the UK is a single oral dose of mifepristone 600 mg; this is given 36 to 48 hours prior to scheduled prostaglandin termination of pregnancy, thus shortening the duration of the procedure and reducing the dose of prostaglandin required. Mifepristone may also be used for softening and dilatation of the cervix prior to surgical termination of pregnancy; a single 600-mg dose is given 36 to 48 hours before the procedure.

For labour induction following intra-uterine fetal death, mifepristone 600 mg is given daily for 2 consecutive days; if labour has not started within 72 hours of the first dose, other methods of induction should be used.

Mifepristone has been used as a postcoital contraceptive. It has also been investigated for use in endometriosis and uterine fibroids (leiomyomas), and for progestogen-dependent neoplasms such as meningiomas. Mifepristone also has anti-glucocorticoid activity and has been used in the treatment of Cushing's syndrome.

◊ General references.

1. Brogden RN, *et al.* Mifepristone: a review of its pharmacodynamic and pharmacokinetic properties, and therapeutic potential. *Drugs* 1993; **45:** 384–409.
2. Glasier A. Mifepristone. *Prescribers' J* 1993; **33:** 156–60.
3. Spitz IM, Bardin CW. Mifepristone (RU 486)—a modulator of progestin and glucocorticoid action. *N Engl J Med* 1993; **329:** 404–12.
4. Heikinheimo O. Clinical pharmacokinetics of mifepristone. *Clin Pharmacokinet* 1997; **33:** 7–17.

Contraception. A single 600-mg dose of mifepristone has been established as an effective emergency contraceptive (p.1460) when given within 72 hours postcoitally (pre-implantation).[1,2] More recently, mifepristone has also been shown to be effective within 120 hours of unprotected coitus; a very low dose of 10 mg appeared to be similar in efficacy to the 600-mg dose and caused less disturbance of the menstrual cycle.[3] Mifepristone has also been used 2 to 3 weeks postcoitally (post-implantation).[4] The development of a mifepristone-based standard contraceptive (p.1460) has been less successful,[5-7] as yet, because mifepristone alters the length of the menstrual cycle.[4,6]

1. Glasier A, *et al.* Mifepristone (RU 486) compared with high-dose estrogen and progestogen for emergency postcoital contraception. *N Engl J Med* 1992; **327:** 1041–4.
2. Webb AMC, *et al.* Comparison of Yuzpe regimen, danazol, and mifepristone (RU 486) in oral postcoital contraception. *BMJ* 1992; **305:** 927–31.
3. Task Force on Postovulatory Methods of Fertility Regulation. Comparison of three single doses of mifepristone as emergency contraception: a randomised trial. *Lancet* 1999; **353:** 697–702.
4. Lähteenmäki P, *et al.* Late postcoital treatment against pregnancy with antiprogesterone RU 486. *Fertil Steril* 1988; **50:** 36–8.
5. Luukkainen T, *et al.* Inhibition of folliculogenesis and ovulation by the antiprogesterone RU 486. *Fertil Steril* 1988; **49:** 961–3.
6. Swahn ML, *et al.* Contraception with mifepristone. *Lancet* 1991; **338:** 942–3.
7. Marions L, *et al.* Contraceptive efficacy of low doses of mifepristone. *Fertil Steril* 1998; **70:** 813–16.

Cushing's syndrome. Mifepristone may be useful in Cushing's syndrome (p.1272) because of its glucocorticoid antagonist effects.

References.

1. Nieman LK, *et al.* Successful treatment of Cushing's syndrome with the glucocorticoid antagonist RU 486. *J Clin Endocrinol Metab* 1985; **61:** 536–40.
2. van der Lely A-J, *et al.* Rapid reversal of acute psychosis in the Cushing syndrome with the cortisol-receptor antagonist mifepristone (RU 486). *Ann Intern Med* 1991; **114:** 143–4.
3. Sartor O, Cutler GB. Mifepristone: treatment of Cushing's syndrome. *Clin Obstet Gynecol* 1996; **39:** 506–10.

Ectopic pregnancy. Methotrexate in combination with mifepristone may be more effective than methotrexate alone for the medical treatment of ectopic pregnancy (p.556).

References.

1. Gazvani MR, *et al.* Mifepristone in combination with methotrexate for the medical treatment of tubal pregnancy: a randomized, controlled trial. *Hum Reprod* 1998; **13:** 1987–90.

Endometriosis. Preliminary results[1,2] have suggested that mifepristone, which is capable of suppressing ovarian function, may be of benefit in patients with endometriosis (p.1469).

1. Kettel LM, *et al.* Endocrine responses to long-term administration of the antiprogesterone RU486 in patients with pelvic endometriosis. *Fertil Steril* 1991; **56:** 402–7.
2. Kettel LM, *et al.* Preliminary report on the treatment of endometriosis with low-dose mifepristone (RU 486). *Am J Obstet Gynecol* 1998; **178:** 1151–6.

Fibroids. Mifepristone has been reported to produce significant decreases in tumour volume when given to patients with uterine leiomyomas,[1,2] and produced comparable results to a gonadorelin analogue (p.1285) as an adjunct to surgery.

1. Murphy AA, *et al.* Regression of uterine leiomyomata in response to the antiprogesterone RU 486. *J Clin Endocrinol Metab* 1993; **76:** 513–17.
2. Murphy AA, *et al.* Regression of uterine leiomyomata to the antiprogesterone RU486: dose-response effect. *Fertil Steril* 1995; **64:** 187–90.

Induction of labour. Some references to the use of mifepristone for cervical ripening and labour induction where intrauterine fetal death has occurred,[1] or at term.[2-5] See also p.1438.

1. Cabrol D, *et al.* Induction of labor with mifepristone (RU 486) in intrauterine fetal death. *Am J Obstet Gynecol* 1990; **163:** 540–2.
2. Frydman R, *et al.* Labor induction in women at term with mifepristone (RU486): a double-blind, randomized, placebo-controlled study. *Obstet Gynecol* 1992; **80:** 972–5.
3. Giacalone PL, *et al.* Cervical ripening with mifepristone before labor induction: a randomized study. *Obstet Gynecol* 1998; **92:** 487–92.
4. Elliott CL, *et al.* The effects of mifepristone on cervical ripening and labor induction in primigravidae. *Obstet Gynecol* 1998; **92:** 804–9.
5. Stenlund PM, *et al.* Induction of labor with mifepristone—a randomized, double-blind study versus placebo. *Acta Obstet Gynecol Scand* 1999; **78:** 793–8.

Malignant neoplasms. Mifepristone has been used successfully in the treatment of inoperable meningioma,[1-3] a brain tumour that may be progestogen-receptor positive. Preliminary data on mifepristone in patients with breast cancer (p.491) were encouraging,[4] but in a later study response rates were low.[5]

1. Haak HR, *et al.* Successful mifepristone treatment of recurrent, inoperable meningioma. *Lancet* 1990; **336:** 124–5.
2. Grunberg SM, *et al.* Treatment of unresectable meningiomas with the antiprogesterone agent mifepristone. *J Neurosurg* 1991; **74:** 861–6.
3. Lamberts SWJ, *et al.* Mifepristone (RU 486) treatment of meningiomas. *J Neurol Neurosurg Psychiatry* 1992; **55:** 486–90.
4. Bakker G, *et al.* Treatment of breast cancer with different antiprogestins: preclinical and clinical studies. *J Steroid Biochem Mol Biol* 1990; **37:** 789–94.
5. Perrault D, *et al.* Phase II study of the progesterone antagonist mifepristone in patients with untreated metastatic breast carcinoma: a National Cancer Institute of Canada Clinical Trials Group study. *J Clin Oncol* 1996; **14:** 2709–12.

Termination of pregnancy. For the termination of early pregnancy (prior to 9 weeks' gestation), mifepristone combined with a prostaglandin is an effective alternative to surgical methods.[1,2] Termination success rates are highest prior to 7 weeks; after this the success rate for mifepristone with oral misoprostol tends to decrease compared with other regimens.[1,2] Mifepristone has been used alone, but it is not sufficiently effective as a single agent.[2] The usual dose of mifepristone is 600 mg, although lower doses of 200 and 400 mg have been studied in various regimens with prostaglandins and found to be as effective. However, the manufacturers have commented that there was no evidence that a lower dose was better tolerated, and that early studies using mifepristone without a prostaglandin had indicated a significantly higher risk of ongoing pregnancy with lower doses.[3] Mifepristone is also used to ripen the cervix prior to surgical termination of pregnancy,[4-8] and in combination with a prostaglandin for second trimester termination (13 to 20 weeks' gestation).[9-13] Similarly to early termination, a study found mifepristone 200 mg to be as effective as 600 mg when combined with misoprostol for second trimester termination.[13] Preliminary evidence indicated that mifepristone plus a prostaglandin is also effective for medical termination of pregnancy at 9 to 13 weeks' gestation.[14]

In the UK the Royal College of Obstetricians and Gynaecologists' guidelines[15] for both early and mid-trimester terminations include the following regimens:

• For gestation up to 7 weeks (and as an option for gestation of 7 to 9 weeks), mifepristone 200 mg by mouth followed 36 hours later by gemeprost 500 μg vaginally.

• For mid-trimester termination (over 15 weeks), mifepristone 200 mg by mouth followed 36 hours later by gemeprost 1 mg every 6 hours vaginally.

For a discussion of the termination of pregnancy, see p.1439.

1. Kahn JG, *et al.* The efficacy of medical abortion: a meta-analysis. *Contraception* 2000; **61:** 29–40.
2. Christin-Maitre S, *et al.* Medical termination of pregnancy. *N Engl J Med* 2000; **342:** 946–56.
3. Ulmann A, Barnard J. Termination of pregnancy with mifepristone. *BMJ* 1993; **307:** 684.
4. Rådestad A, *et al.* Induced cervical ripening with mifepristone in first trimester abortion: a double-blind randomized biomechanical study. *Contraception* 1988; **38:** 301–12.
5. Gupta JK, Johnson N. Effect of mifepristone on dilatation of the pregnant and non-pregnant cervix. *Lancet* 1990; **335:** 1238–40.
6. Lefebvre Y, *et al.* The effects of RU48486 on cervical ripening. *Am J Obstet Gynecol* 1990; **162:** 61–5.
7. WHO. The use of mifepristone (RU 486) for cervical preparation in first trimester pregnancy termination by vacuum aspiration. *Br J Obstet Gynaecol* 1990; **97:** 260–6.
8. Henshaw RC, Templeton AA. Pre-operative cervical preparation before first trimester vacuum aspiration: a randomized controlled comparison between gemeprost and mifepristone (RU 486). *Br J Obstet Gynaecol* 1991; **98:** 1025–30.
9. Gottlieb C, Bygdeman M. The use of antiprogestin (RU 486) for termination of second trimester pregnancy. *Acta Obstet Gynecol Scand* 1991; **70:** 199–203.
10. Urquhart DR, Templeton AA. The use of mifepristone prior to prostaglandin-induced mid-trimester abortion. *Hum Reprod* 1990; **5:** 883–6.
11. Rodger M, Baird D. Pretreatment with mifepristone (RU486) reduces interval between prostaglandin administration and expulsion in second trimester abortion. *Br J Obstet Gynaecol* 1990; **97:** 41–5.
12. Thong KJ, Baird DT. Induction of second trimester abortion with mifepristone and gemeprost. *Br J Obstet Gynaecol* 1993; **100:** 758–61.
13. Webster D, *et al.* A comparison of 600 and 200 mg mifepristone prior to second trimester abortion with the prostaglandin misoprostol. *Br J Obstet Gynaecol* 1996; **103:** 706–9.
14. Ashok PW, *et al.* Termination of pregnancy at 9-13 weeks' amenorrhoea with mifepristone and misoprostol. *Lancet* 1998; **352:** 542–3.
15. Royal College of Obstetricians and Gynaecologists. The care of women requesting induced abortion. Available at: http://www.rcog.org.uk/guidelines/induced_abortion.html (accessed 26/09/00).

Preparations

Proprietary Preparations (details are given in Part 3)
Denm.: Mifegyne; *Fr.:* Mifegyne; *Swed.:* Mifegyne; *Switz.:* Mifegyne; *UK:* Mifegyne; *USA:* Mifeprex.

Nandrolone (13507-I)

Nandrolone (BAN, rINN).

19-Nortestosterone. 17β-Hydroxyestr-4-en-3-one; 3-Oxoestr-4-en-17β-yl.
$C_{18}H_{26}O_2 = 274.4.$
CAS — 434-22-0.
ATC — A14AB01; S01XA11.

Nandrolone Cyclohexylpropionate (9072-w)

Nandrolone Cyclohexylpropionate (BANM, rINNM).

Nandrolone Cyclohexanepropionate; Nortestosterone Cyclohexylpropionate. 3-Oxoestr-4-en-17β-yl 3-cyclohexylpropionate; 17β-Hydroxyestr-4-en-3-one cyclohexylpropionate.
$C_{27}H_{40}O_3 = 412.6.$
CAS — 912-57-2.

Nandrolone Decanoate (9073-e)

Nandrolone Decanoate (BANM, USAN, rINNM).

Nortestosterone Decanoate; Nortestosterone Decylate. 3-Oxoestr-4-en-17β-yl decanoate; 17β-Hydroxyestr-4-en-3-one decanoate.
$C_{28}H_{44}O_3 = 428.6.$
CAS — 360-70-3.
Pharmacopoeias. In *Br.* and *US.*

Pharmacopoeial description

BP 2001: A white to creamy-white crystalline powder with a faint characteristic odour. Practically insoluble in water; freely soluble in alcohol, in chloroform, in ether, in fixed oils, and in esters. Store under nitrogen at 2° to 8°. Protect from light.

USP 25: A white to creamy-white fine crystalline powder, odourless or may have a slight odour. Practically insoluble in water; soluble in alcohol, in acetone, in chloroform, and in vegetable oils. Store at 2° to 8° in airtight containers. Protect from light.

Nandrolone Laurate (12998-c)

Nandrolone Laurate (BANM, rINNM).

Nandrolone Dodecanoate; Nortestosterone Laurate. 3-Oxoestr-4-en-17β-yl dodecanoate; 17β-Hydroxyestr-4-en-3-one dodecanoate.
$C_{30}H_{48}O_3 = 456.7.$
CAS — 26490-31-3.
Pharmacopoeias. In *BP(Vet).*

Pharmacopoeial description

BP(Vet) 2001: A white to creamy-white crystalline powder with a faint characteristic odour. Practically insoluble in water; freely soluble in alcohol, in chloroform, in ether, in fixed oils, and in esters of fatty acids. Store at 2° to 8°. Protect from light.

Nandrolone Phenylpropionate (9074-I)

Nandrolone Phenylpropionate (BANM, rINNM).

Nandrolone Hydrocinnamate; Nandrolone Phenpropionate; 19-Norandrostenolone Phenylpropionate; Nortestosterone Phenylpropionate; NSC-23162. 3-Oxoestr-4-en-17β-yl 3-phenylpropionate; 17β-Hydroxyestr-4-en-3-one 3-phenylpropionate.
$C_{27}H_{34}O_3 = 406.6.$
CAS — 62-90-8.
Pharmacopoeias. In *Br., Chin., Pol.,* and *US.*

Pharmacopoeial description

BP 2001: A white to creamy-white crystalline powder with a characteristic odour. Practically insoluble in water; soluble in alcohol. Protect from light.

USP 25: Store in airtight containers. Protect from light.

Nandrolone Sodium Sulfate (16489-b)

Nandrolone Sodium Sulfate (rINNM).

Nandrolone Sodium Sulphate (BANM); Nortestosterone Sodium Sulphate. 3-Oxoestr-4-en-17β-yl sodium sulphate; 17β-Hydroxyestr-4-en-3-one sodium sulphate.
$C_{18}H_{25}O_5SNa = 376.4.$
CAS — 60672-82-4.

Nandrolone Undecylate (10062-r)

Nandrolone Undecylate (rINNM).

Nandrolone Undecanoate (BANM); Nortestosterone Undecanoate. 3-Oxoestr-4-en-17β-yl undecanoate; 17β-Hydroxyestr-4-en-3-one undecanoate.
$C_{29}H_{46}O_3 = 442.7.$
CAS — 862-89-5.

Adverse Effects and Precautions

As for androgens and anabolic steroids in general (see Testosterone, p.1492).

Abuse. Nandrolone, like other anabolic compounds, has been abused by athletes and bodybuilders. However controversy has arisen over the methods used to detect abuse in the former group, and there is some evidence that metabolites of nandrolone may be produced endogenously (see under Precautions of Testosterone, p.1493).

Effects on the liver. Intrahepatic cholestasis occurred in a patient receiving nandrolone cyclohexylpropionate.[1]

1. Gil VG, *et al.* A non-C17-alkylated steroid and long-term cholestasis. *Ann Intern Med* 1986; **104:** 135–6.

Porphyria. Nandrolone has been associated with acute attacks of porphyria and is considered unsafe in porphyric patients.

Interactions

As for androgens and anabolic steroids in general (see Testosterone, p.1493).

Uses and Administration

Nandrolone is an anabolic steroid with anabolic and some androgenic properties (see Testosterone, p.1493). It is usually administered as the decanoate ester in the form of oily intramuscular injections. The hexyloxyphenylpropionate, propionate, phenylpropionate, and undecylate esters have also been used.

Doses of nandrolone decanoate 25 to 100 mg once every 3 to 4 weeks have been used as an anabolic after debilitating illness, for postmenopausal osteoporosis, and for postmenopausal metastatic breast carcinoma. Doses of between 50 and 200 mg weekly have been suggested for the treatment of aplastic anaemia and anaemia of chronic renal failure.

Nandrolone sodium sulfate has been used topically in the treatment of corneal damage.

Nandrolone cyclohexylpropionate, laurate, and phenylpropionate are used in veterinary medicine.

Cachexia. Nandrolone increased body-weight in patients with HIV-associated wasting[1] (p.610) and in patients with end-stage renal failure undergoing dialysis.[2]

1. Gold J, *et al.* Safety and efficacy of nandrolone decanoate for treatment of wasting in patients with HIV infection. *AIDS* 1996 **10:** 745–52.
2. Johansen KL, *et al.* Anabolic effects of nandrolone decanoate in patients receiving dialysis: a randomized controlled trial. *JAMA* 1999; **281:** 1275–81.

Male contraception. Preliminary findings showed that nandrolone suppressed spermatogenesis,[1-3] suggesting it may have potential as a male contraceptive (p.1460).

1. Schürmeyer T, *et al.* Reversible azoospermia induced by the anabolic steroid 19-nortestosterone. *Lancet* 1984; **i:** 417–20.
2. Knuth UA, *et al.* Combination of 19-nortestosterone-hexyloxyphenyl-propionate (Anadur) and depot-medroxyprogesterone-acetate (Clinovir) for male contraception. *Fertil Steril* 1989; **51:** 1011–18.
3. WHO Task Force on Methods for the Regulation of Male Fertility. Comparison of two androgens plus depot-medroxyprogesterone acetate for suppression to azoospermia in Indonesian men. *Fertil Steril* 1993; **60:** 1062–8.

Preparations

BP 2001: Nandrolone Decanoate Injection; Nandrolone Phenylpropionate Injection;
USP 25: Nandrolone Decanoate Injection; Nandrolone Phenpropionate Injection.

Proprietary Preparations (details are given in Part 3)
Aust.: Anadur†; *Austral.:* Deca-Durabolin; *Belg.:* Deca-Durabolin; *Braz.:* Deca-Durabolin; *Canad.:* Deca-Durabolin; *Fin.:* Deca-Durabolin; *Fr.:* Keratyl; *Ger.:* Deca-Durabolin; Keratyl; *Hong Kong:* Deca-Durabolin; *Irl.:* Deca-Durabolin; *Israel:* Deca-Durabolin; Deca-Noralone; Durabolin; Noralone; *Ital.:* Deca-Durabolin; Dynabolon; *Mex.:* Deca-Durabolin; *Mon.:* Dynabolon†; *Neth.:* Deca-Durabolin; *Norw.:* Deca-Durabolin; *NZ:* Deca-Durabolin; *Port.:* Deca-Durabolin; Nandain†; *S.Afr.:* Deca-Durabolin; *Singapore:* Deca-Durabolin; *Spain:* Deca-Durabolin; Nandrol; *Swed.:* Deca-Durabol; *Switz.:* Deca-Durabolin; Keratyl; *Thai.:* Deca-Durabolin; Keratyl; *UK:* Deca-Durabolin; *USA:* Androlone-D; Deca-Durabolin; Durabolin; Hybolin; Neo-Durabolic.

Multi-ingredient: *Braz.:* Topidexa; *Fin.:* Dexatopic; *Mon.:* Trophobolene†; *Neth.:* Dexatopic†.

Nomegestrol Acetate (3147-e)

Nomegestrol Acetate (BANM, rINNM).

Nomegestroli Acetas. 17-Hydroxy-6-methyl-19-norpregna-4,6-diene-3,20-dione acetate.
$C_{23}H_{30}O_4 = 370.5.$
CAS — 58691-88-6 (nomegestrol); 58652-20-3 (nomegestrol acetate).
Pharmacopoeias. In *Eur.* (see p.vi).

Pharmacopoeial description

Ph. Eur.: A white or almost white crystalline powder. Practically insoluble in water; soluble in alcohol; freely soluble in acetone. Protect from light.

Profile

Nomegestrol acetate is a progestogen structurally related to progesterone (p.1488) that has been used in the treatment of menstrual disorders and as the progestogen component of menopausal HRT (p.1463). Typical doses are 5 mg daily by mouth for 10 to 14 days of a 28-day cycle. A subdermal implant is under investigation as a long-acting progestogen-only contraceptive.

◊ References.

1. Coutinho EM, *et al.* Multicenter clinical trial on the efficacy and acceptability of a single contraceptive implant of nomegestrol acetate, Uniplant. *Contraception* 1996; **53:** 121–5.
2. Devoto L, *et al.* Hormonal profile, endometrial histology and ovarian ultrasound assessment during 1 year of nomegestrol acetate implant (Uniplant). *Hum Reprod* 1997; **12:** 708–13.

Preparations

Proprietary Preparations (details are given in Part 3)
Braz.: Lutenil; *Hong Kong:* Lutenyl; *Ital.:* Lutenyl; *Mon.:* Lutenyl; *Port.:* Lutenyl.

Norethandrolone (9075-y)

Norethandrolone *(BAN, rINN).*

17α-Ethyl-17β-hydroxyestr-4-en-3-one; 17β-Hydroxy-19-nor-17α-pregn-4-en-3-one.
$C_{20}H_{30}O_2 = 302.5.$
$CAS — 52-78-8.$
$ATC — A14AA09.$
Pharmacopoeias. In It.

Adverse Effects and Precautions

As for androgens and anabolic steroids in general (see Testosterone, p.1492). As with other 17α-alkylated compounds, norethandrolone may produce hepatotoxicity and liver function should be monitored. It should probably be avoided in patients with impaired liver function, and certainly if this is severe.

Uses and Administration

Norethandrolone is an anabolic steroid (see Testosterone, p.1493). It is given by mouth in the treatment of aplastic anaemia in a dose of 0.25 to 2 mg per kg body-weight daily.

Preparations

Proprietary Preparations (details are given in Part 3)
Fr.: Nilevar.

Norethisterone (9078-c)

Norethisterone *(BAN, pINN).*

Ethinylnortestosterone; Norethindrone; Norethisteronum; Noretisterona; Noretisterone; Norpregneninolone; NSC-9564. 17β-Hydroxy-19-nor-17α-pregn-4-en-20-yn-3-one.
$C_{20}H_{26}O_2 = 298.4.$
$CAS — 68-22-4.$
$ATC — G03AC01; G03DC02.$
Pharmacopoeias. In Chin., Eur. (see p.vi), Int., Jpn, and US.

Pharmacopoeial description

Ph. Eur.: A white or yellowish-white crystalline powder. Practically insoluble in water; slightly soluble in alcohol. Protect from light.

USP 25: A white to creamy-white odourless crystalline powder. Practically insoluble in water; sparingly soluble in alcohol; soluble in chloroform and in dioxan; slightly soluble in ether.

Norethisterone Acetate (9077-z)

Norethisterone Acetate *(BANM, pINNM).*

Norethindrone Acetate; Norethisteroni Acetas. 17β-Hydroxy-19-nor-17α-pregn-4-en-20-yn-3-one acetate; 3-Oxo-19-nor-17α-pregn-4-en-20-yn-17β-yl acetate.
$C_{22}H_{28}O_3 = 340.5.$
$CAS — 51-98-9.$
Pharmacopoeias. In Eur. (see p.vi), Int., and US.

Pharmacopoeial description

Ph. Eur.: A white or yellowish-white crystalline powder. Practically insoluble in water; soluble in alcohol and in ether. Protect from light.

USP 25: A white to creamy-white odourless crystalline powder. Practically insoluble in water; soluble 1 in 10 of alcohol, 1 in less than 1 of chloroform, 1 in 2 of dioxan, and 1 in 18 of ether.

Norethisterone Enantate (9076-j)

Norethisterone Enantate *(BANM, pINNM).*

Norethindrone Enanthate; Norethisterone Enanthate; Norethisterone Heptanoate. 17β-Hydroxy-19-nor-17α-pregn-4-en-20-yn-3-one heptanoate.
$C_{27}H_{38}O_3 = 410.6.$
$CAS — 3836-23-5.$
Pharmacopoeias. In Int.

Adverse Effects and Precautions

As for progestogens in general (see Progesterone, p.1488). See also under Hormonal Contraceptives, p.1452.

Effects on the liver. There were 6 cases of jaundice among 107 patients with breast cancer treated with high-dose norethisterone acetate;[1] the jaundice was reversible and of an obstructive type.

1. Langlands AO, Martin WMC. Jaundice associated with norethisterone-acetate treatment of breast cancer. *Lancet* 1975; **i:** 584–5.

Porphyria. Norethisterone has been associated with acute attacks of porphyria and is considered unsafe in porphyric patients.

Pregnancy. Abnormalities seen in the offspring of women who had received norethisterone during pregnancy (either alone or in combination with ethinylestradiol) included hypospadias,[1] masculinisation of female infants,[2] meningomyelocele or hydrocephalus,[3] and neonatal choreoathetosis associated with oral contraceptive use.[4] For reference to the fact that oral contraceptives have not generally been associated with teratogenicity, even when used inadvertently in pregnancy, see p.1458.

1. Aarskog D. Clinical and cytogenetic studies in hypospadias. *Acta Paediatr Scand* 1970; (suppl 203): 1–62.
2. Wilkins L. Masculinisation of female fetus due to use of orally given progestins. *JAMA* 1960; **172:** 1028–32.
3. Gal I, *et al.* Hormonal pregnancy tests and congenital malformation. *Nature* 1967; **216:** 83.
4. Profumo R, *et al.* Neonatal choreoathetosis following prenatal exposure to oral contraceptives. *Pediatrics* 1990; **86:** 648–9.

Venous thromboembolism. For mention that combined oral contraceptives containing older progestogens such as norethisterone appear to be associated with a lower incidence of venous thromboembolism than desogestrel- or gestodene-containing preparations, see p.1455.

Interactions

As for progestogens in general (see Progesterone, p.1489). See also under Hormonal Contraceptives, p.1458.

Pharmacokinetics

Norethisterone is absorbed from the gastrointestinal tract, undergoing first-pass hepatic metabolism, with peak plasma concentrations occurring 1 to 2 hours after a dose by mouth. It exhibits biphasic pharmacokinetics; an initial distribution phase is followed by a prolonged elimination phase with a half-life of about 8 hours or more. Norethisterone is highly protein bound; about 60% to albumin and 35% to sex hormone binding globulin. Administration with an oestrogen increases the proportion bound to sex hormone binding globulin. It is metabolised in the liver with 50 to 80% of a dose being excreted in the urine and up to 40% in the faeces.

Norethisterone acetate is reported to show a more prolonged elimination than norethisterone following oral administration. It is hydrolysed to norethisterone, principally by intestinal tissue.

Following intramuscular injection of norethisterone enantate peak concentrations of norethisterone in plasma are not attained for several days.

Uses and Administration

Norethisterone and its acetate and enantate esters are progestogens (see Progesterone, p.1489) derived from nortestosterone that have weak oestrogenic and androgenic properties. They are commonly used as **hormonal contraceptives** (see p.1459). Norethisterone and norethisterone acetate are both administered by mouth. Typical daily doses are 0.35 mg for norethisterone and 0.6 mg for norethisterone acetate when used alone, or 0.5 to 1 mg for norethisterone and 1 to 1.5 mg for norethisterone acetate when combined with an oestrogen. Norethisterone enantate is administered by intramuscular injection; a dose of 200 mg provides contraception for 8 weeks.

Norethisterone and norethisterone acetate are used as the progestogen component of **menopausal HRT** (p.1463) to oppose the effects of oestrogens on the endometrium. Typical regimens have included either continuous daily doses of norethisterone 0.7 mg or norethisterone acetate 0.5 to 1 mg, or cyclical regimens of norethisterone or norethisterone acetate 1 mg daily for 10 to 12 days of a 28-day cycle. Norethisterone acetate is also available as transdermal patches supplying 170 or 250 µg per 24 hours that are applied twice weekly for 2 weeks of a 4-week cycle; the lower strength may also be applied twice weekly on a continuous basis.

Norethisterone and norethisterone acetate may be given by mouth for the treatment of conditions such as **menorrhagia** (p.1490) and **endometriosis** (p.1469). In menorrhagia (dysfunctional uterine bleeding), norethisterone is given in usual doses of 10 to 15 mg daily and norethisterone acetate in doses of 2.5 to 10 mg daily, in a cyclical regimen. In endometriosis the dosage of norethisterone is 10 to 25 mg daily and of norethisterone acetate 5 to 15 mg daily.

Treatment of endometriosis is usually continuous for 4 to 9 months.

Norethisterone has been used in daily doses of up to 15 mg by mouth in a cyclical regimen in the treatment of **premenstrual syndrome** (p.1475).

In **breast cancer** (p.491) doses of up to 60 mg daily by mouth of norethisterone have been used.

Menorrhagia. Although cyclical norethisterone has been widely used for menorrhagia (p.1490), it is of limited efficacy during ovulatory cycles being most effective for anovulatory bleeding, which occurs in a minority of women with menorrhagia.

References.

1. Cameron IT, *et al.* The effects of mefenamic acid and norethisterone on measured menstrual blood loss. *Obstet Gynecol* 1990; **76:** 85–8.
2. Preston JT, *et al.* Comparative study of tranexamic acid and norethisterone in the treatment of ovulatory menorrhagia. *Br J Obstet Gynaecol* 1995; **102:** 401–6.

Preparations

BP 2001: Norethisterone Tablets;
USP 25: Norethindrone Acetate and Ethinyl Estradiol Tablets; Norethindrone Acetate Tablets; Norethindrone and Ethinyl Estradiol Tablets; Norethindrone and Mestranol Tablets; Norethindrone Tablets.

Proprietary Preparations (details are given in Part 3)

Aust.: Micronovum; Primolut-Nor; *Austral.:* Locilan; Micronor; Noriday; Primolut N; *Belg.:* Primolut-Nor; *Braz.:* Micronor; Primolut-Nor; *Canad.:* Micronor; Norlutate; *Denm.:* Mini-Pe; *Fin.:* Mini-Pill; Primolut N; Primolut-Nor; *Fr.:* Milligynon; Noristerat; Norluten†; Primolut-Nor; *Ger.:* Gestakadin; Micronovum†; Noristerat; Primolut-Nor; Sovel; *Hong Kong:* Noristerat; Primolut N; *Irl.:* Micronor; Noriday; Primolut N; *Israel:* Primolut-Nor; *Ital.:* Primolut-Nor; *Mex.:* Noristerat; Primolut-Nor; *Neth.:* Primolut N; *Norw.:* Conludag; Primolut-Nor; *NZ:* Noriday; Primolut N; *Port.:* Primolut-Nor; *S.Afr.:* Micronovum; Nur-Isterate; Primolut N; Singapore: Norcolut; Noristerat; Primolut N; *Spain:* Primolut-Nor; *Swed.:* Mini-Pe; Primolut-Nor; *Switz.:* Micronovum; Primolut N; Primolut-Nor; *Thai.:* Noristerat; Primolut N; Steron; *UK:* Menzol†; Micronor; Micronor HRT; Noriday; Noristerat; Primolut N; Utovlan; *USA:* Aygestin; Micronor; Nor-QD.

Multi-ingredient: *Aust.:* Activelle; Estracomb; Estragest; Etalontin†; Kliogest; Mericomb; Merigest; Neorlest†; Orlest†; Ortho-Novum; Ovysmen; Perikliman; Primosiston; Trinovum; Trisequens; *Austral.:* Brevinor; Estalis Continuous; Estalis Sequi; Estracombi; Improvil; Kliogest; Kliovance; Norimin; Norinyl-1; Synphasic; Trisequens; *Belg.:* Activelle; Estracombi; Kliogest; Minestril; Ortho-Novum 1/50†; Ovysmen; Trinovum; Trisequens; *Braz.:* Biofim; Ciclovulon; Estracomb; Megestran; Mesigyna; Primosiston; Trinovum; *Canad.:* Brevicon; Estracomb; Loestrin 1.5/30; Minestrin; Norinyl 1/50; Ortho 0.5/35; Ortho 1/35; Ortho 10/11; Ortho 7/7/7; Ortho-Novum 1/50; Select 1/35; Synphasic; *Denm.:* Activelle; Econ; Estracomb; Evo-Conti; Evo-Sequi; Femanor; Femasekvens; Kliogest; Ostranorm; Trinorm; Trinovum; Trisekvens; *Fin.:* Activelle; Estalis; Estalis Sekvens; Estracomb; Evorel Conti; Evorel Sequi; Kliogest; Mericomb; Merigest; Trisekvens; *Fr.:* Kliogest; Milli Anovlar†; Miniphase; Ortho-Novum 1/35; Triella; Trisequens; *Ger.:* Activelle; Conceplan M; Estracomb; Estragest; Eve; Gynamon; Kliogest N; Mericomb; Merigest; Neorlest; Non-Ovlon; Nora-ratiopharm; Ortho-Novum 1/50†; Ortho-Primolut†; Ovysmen; Primosiston; Prosiston; Sequostat; Sinovula; Synphasec; Trinovum; Trisequens; *Hong Kong:* Brevinor; Estracombi; Kliogest; Norimin; Norinyl-1; Synphase; Trinovum; Trisequens; *Irl.:* Activelle; Binovum; Brevinor; Estracombi; Estrapak; Evorel Conti; Kliogest; Menophase†; Norinyl-1†; Normin†; Ortho-Novin; Ovysmen; Trinovum; Trisequens; *Israel:* Kliogest; Meno-Net; Trisequens; *Ital.:* Activelle; Estracomb; Kliogest; Tesor-C; Trinovum†; Trisequens; *Mex.:* Cliane; Estracomb; Estrapak; Mesigyna; Norinyl; Ortho-Novum 1/35; *Neth.:* Activelle; Estracomb; Kliogest; Modicon; Neocon; Ortho-Novum 1/50†; Trinovum; Trisequens; *Norw.:* Activelle; Estracomb; Kliogest; Synfase; Trisekvens; *NZ:* Brevinor; Estrapak; Kliogest; Kliovance; Norimin; Norinyl-1; Synphasic; Trisequens; *Port.:* Estalis Sequi; Estracomb; Kliogest; Trisequens; *S.Afr.:* Brevinor†; Estracombi; Evorel Conti; Kliogest; Norinyl-1/28; Trinovum; Trisequens; *Singapore:* Activelle; Estracomb; Kliogest; Trisequens; *Spain:* Absorbent Plus; Activelle; Estracomb; Merigest; Merigest Combi; Primosiston; Trisequens; *Swed.:* Activelle; Estalis; Estalis Sekvens; Estracomb; Evorel Micronor; Femanor; Femasekvens; Kliogest; Orthonett Novum; Synfase; Trinovum; Trisekvens; *Switz.:* Activelle; Estracomb; Estragest; Kliogest N; Mericomb; Merigest; Ortho-Novum 1/50†; Ovysmen; Primosiston; Systen Conti; Systen Sequi; Trinovum; Trisequens; *Thai.:* Anamai; Kliogest; Trisequens; *UK:* Adgyn Combi; Binovum; Brevinor; Climagest; Climesse; Elleste Duet Conti; Elleste-Duet; Estracombi; Estrapak; Evorel Conti; Evorel Pak; Evorel Sequi; Kliofem; Kliovance; Loestrin; Menophase†; Norimin; Norinyl-1; Nuvelle Continuous; Ortho-Novin 1/50†; Ovysmen; Synphase; Trinovum; Trisequens; *USA:* Activella; Brevicon; CombiPatch; Estrostep; Estrostep Fe; femhrt; GenCept 0.5/35 and 1/35†; Gen-Cept 10/11†; Genora 0.5/35 and 1/35†; Genora 1/50†; Jenest; Loestrin; Loestrin Fe; Modicon; Necon 1/50; Necon 10/11; Necon 0.5/35, 1/35; NEE 1/35; Nelova 0.5/35E and 1/35E†; Nelova 1/50M†; Nelova 10/11†; Norethin 1/35E†; Norethin 1/50M†; Norinyl 1 + 35; Norinyl 1 + 50; Ortho-Novum 1/35; Ortho-Novum 1/50; Ortho-Novum 10/11; Ortho-Novum 7/7/7; Ovcon 35; Ovcon 50; Tri-Norinyl.

The symbol † denotes a preparation no longer actively marketed

Noretynodrel (9079-k)

Noretynodrel (BAN, rINN).

Norethynodrel (USAN); NSC-15432; SC-4642. 17β-Hydroxy-19-nor-17α-pregn-5(10)-en-20-yn-3-one.
$C_{20}H_{26}O_2 = 298.4$.
CAS — 68-23-5.

Pharmacopoeias. In It. and US.

Pharmacopoeial description
USP 25: A white or practically white, odourless, crystalline powder. Very slightly soluble in water and in petroleum spirit; sparingly soluble in alcohol; soluble in acetone; freely soluble in chloroform.

Profile
Noretynodrel is a progestogen (see Progesterone, p.1488) structurally related to norethisterone that has been given by mouth in conjunction with an oestrogen such as mestranol for the treatment of various menstrual disorders and endometriosis.

Porphyria. Noretynodrel is considered to be unsafe in patients with porphyria because it has been shown to be porphyrinogenic in animals or in-vitro systems.

Pregnancy. A woman who had received noretynodrel during pregnancy to prevent threatened miscarriage gave birth to a female infant showing evidence of masculinisation.[1]

1. Wilkins L. Masculinization of female fetus due to use of orally given progestins. JAMA 1960; 172: 1028–32.

Preparations
Proprietary Preparations (details are given in Part 3)
Multi-ingredient: USA: Enovid†.

Norgestimate (13031-z)

Norgestimate (BAN, USAN, rINN).

D-138; Dexnorgestrel Acetime; ORF-10131; RWJ-10131. 13β-Ethyl-3-hydroxyimino-18,19-dinor-17α-pregn-4-en-20-yn-17β-yl acetate.
$C_{23}H_{31}NO_3 = 369.5$.
CAS — 35189-28-7.

Profile
Norgestimate is a progestogen (see Progesterone, p.1488) structurally related to levonorgestrel (to which it is partly metabolised) that is used as the progestogenic component of combined oral contraceptives (see p.1452). A typical daily dose is 250 µg in monophasic preparations, and 180 to 250 µg in triphasic preparations.

Preparations
Proprietary Preparations (details are given in Part 3)
Multi-ingredient: Aust.: Cileste; TriCilest; Vivelle; Belg.: Cilest; Canad.: Cyclen; Tri-Cyclen; Denm.: Cilest; Fin.: Cilest; Fr.: Cilest; Effiprev; Ger.: Cilest; Pramino; Irl.: Cilest; Israel: Ortho Cyclen; Mex.: Cilest; Neth.: Cilest; S.Afr.: TriCilest; Swed.: Cilest; Switz.: Cilest; UK: Cilest; USA: Ortho Cyclen; Ortho Tri-Cyclen; Ortho-Prefest.

Norgestomet (6340-y)

Norgestomet (BAN, USAN, rINN).

SC-21009. 11β-Methyl-3,20-dioxo-19-norpregn-4-en-17α-yl acetate.
$C_{23}H_{32}O_4 = 372.5$.
CAS — 25092-41-5.

Profile
Norgestomet is a progestogen (see Progesterone, p.1488) used in veterinary medicine in combination with estradiol.

Norgestrel (9080-w)

Norgestrel (BAN, USAN, rINN).

dl-Norgestrel; DL-Norgestrel; Norgestrelum; Wy-3707. (±)-13-Ethyl-17β-hydroxy-18,19-dinor-17α-pregn-4-en-20-yn-3-one.
$C_{21}H_{28}O_2 = 312.4$.
CAS — 6533-00-2.

Pharmacopoeias. In Chin., Eur. (see p.vi), Jpn, and US.

Pharmacopoeial description
Ph. Eur.: A white or almost white crystalline powder. Practically insoluble in water; slightly soluble in alcohol; sparingly soluble in dichloromethane. Protect from light.

USP 25: A white or practically white, practically odourless crystalline powder. Insoluble in water; sparingly soluble in alcohol; freely soluble in chloroform.

Levonorgestrel (9081-e)

Levonorgestrel (BAN, USAN, rINN).

Levonorgestrelum; D-Norgestrel; Wy-5104. (–)-13β-Ethyl-17β-hydroxy-18,19-dinor-17α-pregn-4-en-20-yn-3-one.
CAS — 797-63-7.
ATC — G03AC03.

NOTE. The name Dexnorgestrel has also been used.

Pharmacopoeias. In Eur. (see p.vi), Int., and US.

The (–)-isomer of norgestrel.

Pharmacopoeial description
Ph. Eur.: A white or almost white crystalline powder. Practically insoluble in water; slightly soluble in alcohol; sparingly soluble in dichloromethane. Protect from light.

USP 25: A white or practically white, odourless powder. Practically insoluble in water; slightly soluble in alcohol; soluble in chloroform. Protect from light.

Adverse Effects and Precautions
As for progestogens in general (see Progesterone, p.1488). See also under Hormonal Contraceptives, p.1452.

◊ Following the introduction of levonorgestrel in a subdermal implant formulation in February 1991, the US FDA had received about 5800 reports of adverse effects as of December 1993 (out of an estimated 891 000 implants distributed).[1] Serious adverse effects associated with the implant included 24 cases of infection related to insertion of the implant, 15 cases of stroke and 39 of benign intracranial hypertension, 3 cases of thrombocytopenic purpura and 6 of thrombocytopenia (1 fatal). None of the reporting rates for these disorders exceeded the expected rate in this population.

1. Wysowski DK, Green L. Serious adverse events in Norplant users reported to the Food and Drug Administration's MedWatch Spontaneous Reporting System. Obstet Gynecol 1995; 85: 538–42.

Benign intracranial hypertension. Intracranial hypertension, presenting as headaches, vomiting, and visual obscuration associated with florid bilateral papilloedema developed in 2 patients four to five months after subdermal implantation of levonorgestrel.[1] Despite a further 56 cases reported to various drug monitoring centres, and 70 cases known to the manufacturers,[2] it remained unclear whether the drug actually caused intracranial hypertension, but removal of implants in patients in whom intracranial pressure increases is recommended.

1. Alder JB, et al. Levonorgestrel implants and intracranial hypertension. N Engl J Med 1995; 332: 1720–1.
2. Weber ME, et al. Levonorgestrel implants and intracranial hypertension. N Engl J Med 1995; 332: 1721.

Effects on the blood. A long-term study of the use of levonorgestrel subdermal implants (Norplant) in 100 Singaporean women indicated that during 12 months of use patients possibly had an increased tendency for thrombosis and an increased potential for hypercoagulation.[1] It was felt, however, that further investigation was required since some of the haematological changes observed after 1 year persisted throughout the second year of the study whereas others returned to normal.[2]

1. Viegas OAC, et al. The effects of Norplant on clinical chemistry in Singaporean acceptors after 1 year of use I: haemostatic changes. Contraception 1988; 38: 313–23.
2. Singh K, et al. Two-year follow-up of changes in clinical chemistry in Singaporean Norplant-2 rod acceptors: haemostatic changes. Contraception 1989; 39: 155–64.

Effects on carbohydrate metabolism. For a mention that levonorgestrel has been reported to be the most potent progestogen in decreasing glucose tolerance when used as a combined oral contraceptive, see p.1454.

Glucocorticoid effects. Reference to the minimal suppressive effect of subdermal levonorgestrel on adrenal function.[1]

1. Toppozada MK, et al. Effect of Norplant implants on the pituitary-adrenal axis function and reserve capacity. Contraception 1997; 55: 7–10.

Myasthenia gravis. Myasthenia gravis occurring after insertion of a levonorgestrel implant improved on removal of the implant.[1]

1. Brittain J, Lange LS. Myasthenia gravis and levonorgestrel implant. Lancet 1995; 346: 1556.

Porphyria. Levonorgestrel has been associated with acute attacks of porphyria and is considered unsafe in porphyric patients.

Pregnancy. Adverse effects in infants whose mothers had received oral contraceptives containing norgestrel during early pregnancy have included tracheo-oesophageal fistula in one infant[1] and inoperable hepatoblastoma in another.[2] However, many epidemiological studies have failed to show any association between fetal malformations and oral contraceptives, even when used inadvertently during pregnancy, see p.1458.

1. Frost O. Tracheo-oesophageal fistula associated with hormonal contraception during pregnancy. BMJ 1976; 2: 978.
2. Otten J, et al. Hepatoblastoma in an infant after contraceptive intake during pregnancy. N Engl J Med 1977; 297: 222.

Venous thromboembolism. For mention that levonorgestrel-containing combined oral contraceptives appeared to be associated with a lower incidence of venous thromboembolism than desogestrel- or gestodene-containing preparations, see p.1455. See also Effects on the Blood, above.

Interactions
As for progestogens in general (see Progesterone, p.1489). See also under Hormonal Contraceptives, p.1458.

Pharmacokinetics
Levonorgestrel is rapidly and almost completely absorbed after administration by mouth, and undergoes little first-pass hepatic metabolism. It is highly bound to plasma proteins; 42 to 68% to sex hormone binding globulin and 30 to 56% to albumin. The proportion bound to sex hormone binding globulin is higher when it is given with an oestrogen. Levonorgestrel and norgestrel are metabolised in the liver to sulfate and glucuronide conjugates, which are excreted in the urine and to a lesser extent in the faeces.

◊ References.
1. Fotherby K. Levonorgestrel: clinical pharmacokinetics. Clin Pharmacokinet 1995; 28: 203–15.

Uses and Administration
Norgestrel and its active isomer levonorgestrel are progestogens (see Progesterone, p.1489) derived from nortestosterone. They are more potent inhibitors of ovulation than norethisterone and have androgenic activity. Levonorgestrel is more commonly used than norgestrel and is twice as potent. For example, levonorgestrel 37.5 µg is equivalent to norgestrel 75 µg.

They are both used as hormonal contraceptives (see p.1459). The typical daily dose when used as an oral progestogen-only contraceptive is the equivalent of 30 or 37.5 µg of levonorgestrel, and when used as a combined oral contraceptive, is the equivalent of 150 to 250 µg of levonorgestrel in monophasic preparations, and 50 to 125 µg of levonorgestrel in triphasic preparations. Levonorgestrel is also used as a long-acting progestogen-only contraceptive administered by subcutaneous implantation; 6 implants each containing 36 mg of levonorgestrel are inserted under the skin on the first day of the menstrual cycle and are replaced at intervals of up to 5 years. Insertion and removal must be carried out by personnel fully trained in the technique. A 2-implant preparation providing 3 years of contraception has been investigated. Uterine, cervical, and vaginal devices containing levonorgestrel have also been investigated. An intra-uterine device is available for contraception or menorrhagia, containing a total of 52 mg of levonorgestrel which is released at an initial rate of 20 µg per 24 hours. The device is effective for 5 years.

For emergency contraception (p.1460), the equivalent of levonorgestrel 500 µg plus ethinylestradiol 100 µg is given within 72 hours of coitus and repeated after 12 hours. Alternatively, levonorgestrel may be given alone by mouth in a dose of 750 µg within 72 hours of coitus (and preferably as soon as possible), repeated after 12 hours.

Both levonorgestrel and norgestrel are used as the progestogenic component of menopausal HRT (see p.1463). Typical regimens are the equivalent of 75 to 250 µg of levonorgestrel by mouth for 10 to 12 days of a 28-day cycle. Levonorgestrel may also be given via a combined transdermal patch, releasing 20 µg per 24 hours together with an oestrogen, which is applied twice weekly for 2 weeks of a 4-week cycle. The intra-uterine levonorgestrel device is under investigation for use in combination with oestrogen for this indication.

Administration. IMPLANTS. Some references to the use of levonorgestrel by subcutaneous implant for hormonal contraception.[1-4]

1. Shoupe D, Mishell DR. Norplant: subdermal implant system for long-term contraception. Am J Obstet Gynecol 1989; 160: 1286–92.
2. Polaneczky M, et al. The use of levonorgestrel implants (Norplant) for contraception in adolescent mothers. N Engl J Med 1994; 331: 1201–6.
3. Anonymous. Long-acting progestogen-only contraception. Drug Ther Bull 1996; 34: 93–6.
4. Coukell AJ, Balfour JA. Levonorgestrel subdermal implants: a review of contraceptive efficacy and acceptability. Drugs 1998; 55: 861–87.

INTRA-UTERINE DEVICES. Some references to the use of levonorg-estrel-releasing intra-uterine contraceptive devices.[1,2]

1. Sturridge F, Guillebaud J. A risk-benefit assessment of the levonorgestrel-releasing intrauterine system. *Drug Safety* 1996; **15**: 430–40.
2. Backman T, et al. Length of use and symptoms associated with premature removal of the levonorgestrel intrauterine system: a nation-wide study of 17,360 users. *Br J Obstet Gynaecol* 2000; **107**: 335–9.

Menorrhagia. Although oral cyclical progestogens have limited efficacy in the treatment of menorrhagia (p.1490), the levonorgestrel-containing intra-uterine device appears to be particularly useful in reducing menstrual blood loss. References[1-4] and a systematic review[5] of the use of levonorgestrel are given below.

1. Andersson JK, Rybo G. Levonorgestrel-releasing intrauterine device in the treatment of menorrhagia. *Br J Obstet Gynaecol* 1990; **97**: 690–4.
2. Milsom I, et al. A comparison of flurbiprofen, tranexamic acid, and a levonorgestrel-releasing intrauterine contraceptive device in the treatment of idiopathic menorrhagia. *Am J Obstet Gynecol* 1991; **164**: 879–83.
3. Crosignani PC, et al. Levonorgestrel releasing intrauterine device versus hysteroscopic endometrial resection in the treatment of dysfunctional uterine bleeding. *Obstet Gynecol* 1997; **90**: 257–63.
4. Lähteenmäki P, et al. Open randomised study of use of levonorgestrel releasing intrauterine system as alternative to hysterectomy. *BMJ* 1998; **316**: 1122–6.
5. Lethaby AE, et al. Progesterone/progestogen releasing intrauterine systems versus either placebo or any other medication for heavy menstrual bleeding (updated 28 May 2001). Available in The Cochrane Library; Issue 3. Oxford: Update Software; 2001.

Preparations

BP 2001: Levonorgestrel and Ethinylestradiol Tablets;
USP 25: Levonorgestrel and Ethinyl Estradiol Tablets; Norgestrel and Ethinyl Estradiol Tablets; Norgestrel Tablets.

Proprietary Preparations (details are given in Part 3)
Aust.: Mirena; ***Austral.:*** Microlut; Microval; ***Belg.:*** Microlut; Microval; Mirena; ***Braz.:*** Nortrel; ***Canad.:*** Norplant; ***Denm.:*** Levonova; Microluton; Microval; ***Fin.:*** Jadelle; Levonova; Microluton; ***Fr.:*** Microval; Mirena; Norlevo; ***Ger.:*** 28 mini; Microlut; Mikro-30; Mirena; ***Hong Kong:*** Mirena; ***Irl.:*** Mirena; ***Israel:*** Mirena; Norplant; ***Ital.:*** Microlut; Mirena; ***Mex.:*** Microlut; Norplant; ***Neth.:*** Mirena; ***Norw.:*** Levonova; Microluton; ***NZ:*** Microlut; Microval; Mirena; Postinor-2; ***Port.:*** Mirena; ***S.Afr.:*** Microval; Mirena; ***Singapore:*** Mirena; Norplant; Postinor; ***Swed.:*** Follistrel; Levonova; Norplant; Postinor; ***Switz.:*** Microlut; Mirena; ***Thai.:*** Madonna; Norplant; Postinor; ***UK:*** Levonelle; Microval; Mirena; Neogest; Norgeston; Norplant†; Postinor-2; ***USA:*** Mirena; Norplant; Ovrette; Plan B.

Multi-ingredient: ***Aust.:*** Cyclacur; Levlen; Liogynon; Microgynon; Neo-Stediril; Neogynon; Ovranette; Perikursal; Sequilar; Stediril D; Trigynon; Trinordiol; ***Austral.:*** Biphasil; Levlen ED; Loette; Logynon ED; Microgynon; Monofeme; Nordette; Nordiol; Sequilar ED; Trifeme; Triphasil; Triquilar; ***Belg.:*** Binordiol; Cyclocur; Microgynon; Neo-Stediril; Neogynon; Stediril D; Stediril†; Trigynon; Trinordiol; ***Braz.:*** Anfertil; Ciclomestril; Cicloprimogyna; Evanor; Karin; Levordiol; Microvlar; Neovlar; Nordette; Postoval; Primovlar; Trinordiol; Triquilar; ***Canad.:*** Alesse; Min-Ovral; Ovral; Triphasil; Triquilar; ***Denm.:*** Cyclo-Progynon; Dystrol†; Fironetta; Gynatrol; Microgyn; Neogentrol; Neogynon; Nuvelle; Tetragynon; Trinordiol; Triquilar; ***Fin.:*** Climara Duo; Cyclabil; Microgynon; Neo-Primovlar; Trikvilar; Trinordiol; ***Fr.:*** Adepal; Minidril; Stediril; Tetragynon; Trinordiol; ***Ger.:*** Cyclo-Menorette; Cyclo-Progynova; CycloOstrogynal; Femigoa; Femranette mikro; Gravistat; Klimonorm; Leios; Microgynon; Minisiston; Miranova; MonoStep; Neo-Stediril; Neogynon; NovaStep; Ostronara†; Perikursal; Sequilar; Stediril; Stediril 30; Stediril D; Tetragynon; Triette; Trigoa; Trinordiol; Triquilar; Trisiston; TriStep; ***Hong Kong:*** Duoluton; Eugynon; Klimonorm; Microgynon; Neogynon; Nordette; Nordiol; Ovral; Rigevidon; Tri-Regol; Trinordiol; Triquilar; ***Irl.:*** Logynon; Microgynon 30; Microlite; Nuvelle; Ovran; Ovran 30; Ovranette; Prempak-C; Trinordiol; ***Israel:*** Logynon; Microgynon; Neogynon; Nordette; Progyluton; Trinordiol; ***Ital.:*** Egogyn 30; Eugynon; Evanor-D; Loette; Microgynon; Novogyn; Nuvelle; Nuvelle TS; Ovranet; Trigynon; Trinordiol; ***Mex.:*** Microgynon; Neogynon; Nordet; Nordiol; Ovral; Progyluton; Trinordiol; Triquilar; ***Neth.:*** Binordiol; Cyclocur; Microgynon; Neo-Stediril; Neogynon; Prempak-C; Stediril; Trigynon; Trinordiol; ***Norw.:*** Cyclabil; Eugynon; Follimin; Microgynon; Tetragynon; Trinordiol; Trionetta; ***NZ:*** Biphasil; Levlen ED; Loette; Microgynon; Monofeme; Nordette; Nordiol; Nuvelle; Ovral; Prempak-C; Trifeme; Triphasil; Triquilar; ***Port.:*** Climara Duo; Microgynon; Neomonovar; Nuvelle; Progyluton; Tetragynon; Trinordiol; Triquilar; ***S.Afr.:*** Biphasil; Logynon ED; Nordette; Nordiol; Normovlar ED†; Ovral; Postoval; Triphasil; ***Singapore:*** Microgynon; Nordette; Prempak-C; Progyluton; Trinordiol; Triquilar; ***Spain:*** Aurolim; Eugynon†; Microgynon; Neogynona; Nuvelle; Ovoplex; Progyluton; Triagynon; Triciclor; ***Swed.:*** Cyclabil; Follimin; Follinett; Neovletta; Regunon; Sequilarum†; Tetragynon†; Trionetta; ***Switz.:*** Binordiol; Cyclacur; Microgynon; Neo-Stediril†; Neogynon; Ologyn; Sequilar†; Stediril 30; Stediril D; Tetragynon; Trinordiol; Triquilar; ***Thai.:*** Anna; Cyclo-Progynova; Eugynon 250; FMP; Klimonorm; Microgest; Microgynon; Nordette; Nordiol; Ovral; R-Den; Riget; Rigevidon; Trinordiol; Triquilar; ***UK:*** Cyclo-Progynova 1 mg; Cyclo-Progynova 2 mg; Eugynon 30; Logynon; Microgynon 30; Nuvelle; Nuvelle TS; Ovran; Ovran 30; Ovranette; Prempak-C; Schering PC4†; Trinordiol; ***USA:*** Alesse; Aviane; Enpresse; Levlen; Levlite; Levora; Lo/Ovral; Nordette; Ovral; Preven; Tri-Levlen; Triphasil; Trivora.

Norgestrienone (13032-c)

Norgestrienone (*rINN*).
17β-Hydroxy-19-nor-17α-pregna-4,9,11-trien-20-yn-3-one.
$C_{20}H_{22}O_2 = 294.4$.
CAS — 848-21-5.
ATC — G03AC07.

Profile
Norgestrienone is a progestogen (see Progesterone, p.1488) structurally related to norethisterone that is used as an oral contraceptive (see p.1452). Typical doses are 2 mg daily when combined with an oestrogen, and 350 µg daily when used alone.

Preparations

Proprietary Preparations (details are given in Part 3)
Fr.: Ogyline.
Multi-ingredient: ***Fr.:*** Planor.

Ormeloxifene (18929-v)

Ormeloxifene (*rINN*).
Centchroman.   *trans*-1-{2-[4-(3,4-Dihydro-7-methoxy-2,2-dimethyl-3-phenyl-2H-1-benzopyran-4-yl)phenoxy]ethyl}pyrrolidine.
$C_{30}H_{35}NO_3 = 457.6$.
CAS — 31477-60-8.

Profile
Ormeloxifene is a nonsteroidal benzopyran derivative with anti-oestrogenic and antiprogestogenic actions that has been administered weekly as an oral contraceptive. Ormeloxifene has also been investigated in the management of osteoporosis. The *l*-isomer, levormeloxifene, has also been investigated.

◊ References.
1. Kamboj VP, et al. New products: centchroman. *Drugs Today* 1992; **28**: 227–32.
2. Gupta RC, et al. Centchroman: a new non-steroidal oral contraceptive in human milk. *Contraception* 1995; **52**: 301–5.
3. Lal J, et al. Pharmacokinetics of centchroman in healthy female subjects after oral administration. *Contraception* 1995; **52**: 297–300.
4. Lal J, et al. Optimization of contraceptive dosage regimen of centchroman. *Contraception* 2001; **63**: 47–51.

Ovary Extracts (11486-q)

Ovarian Extracts.

Profile
Ovary extracts of animal origin (usually porcine or bovine) have been used for a variety of disorders including gynaecological and menopausal disorders. They are often used in preparations containing other mammalian tissue extracts.

Preparations

Proprietary Preparations (details are given in Part 3)
Aust.: Ovibion†.
Multi-ingredient: ***Ger.:*** Intradermi N.

Oxabolone Cipionate (13050-a)

Oxabolone Cipionate (*rINN*).
FI-5852; Oxabolone Cypionate. 4,17β-Dihydroxyestr-4-en-3-one 17-(β-cyclopentylpropionate).
$C_{26}H_{38}O_4 = 414.6$.
CAS — 1254-35-9.
ATC — A14AB03.

Profile
Oxabolone cipionate has anabolic properties.

Preparations

Proprietary Preparations (details are given in Part 3)
Ital.: Steranabol Ritardo†.

Oxandrolone (9093-z)

Oxandrolone (*BAN, USAN, rINN*).
NSC-67068; SC-11585. 17β-Hydroxy-17α-methyl-2-oxa-5α-androstan-3-one.
$C_{19}H_{30}O_3 = 306.4$.
CAS — 53-39-4.
ATC — A14AA08.
Pharmacopoeias. In US.

Pharmacopoeial description
USP 25: A white odourless crystalline powder. Soluble 1 in 5200 of water, 1 in 57 of alcohol, 1 in 69 of acetone, 1 in less than 5 of chloroform, and 1 in 860 of ether. Protect from light.

Adverse Effects and Precautions
As for androgens and anabolic steroids in general (see Testosterone, p.1492). As with most of the 17α-alkylated compounds, oxandrolone may cause hepatotoxicity, and liver function should be monitored. It should be avoided if hepatic impairment is severe.

Pharmacokinetics
Oxandrolone is rapidly absorbed from the gastrointestinal tract. It is excreted mainly in the urine as metabolites and unchanged oxandrolone. A small amount is excreted in the faeces.

Uses and Administration
Oxandrolone has anabolic and androgenic properties (see Testosterone, p.1493) and is given in doses of 2.5 to 20 mg daily by mouth; the usual dose is 5 to 10 mg daily in divided doses for 2 to 4 weeks. In the promotion of growth in constitutional delayed growth and puberty in boys, daily doses of up to 0.1 mg per kg body-weight have been given (see also below). Courses of treatment should generally be short to avoid the risk of epiphyseal closure.

Cachexia. Oxandrolone has been used for its protein anabolic effect in a number of conditions associated with cachexia (p.1481) or wasting, including alcoholic hepatitis,[1] burn injury,[2] HIV-infection,[3,4] and muscular dystrophy.[5]

1. Mendenhall CL, et al. A study of oral nutritional support with oxandrolone in malnourished patients with alcoholic hepatitis: results of a Department of Veterans Affairs Cooperative Study. *Hepatology* 1993; **17**: 564–76.
2. Demling RH. Comparison of the anabolic effects and complications of human growth hormone and the testosterone analog, oxandrolone, after severe burn injury. *Burns* 1999; **25**: 215–21.
3. Berger JR, et al. Oxandrolone in AIDS-wasting myopathy. *AIDS* 1996; **10**: 1657–62.
4. Strawford A, et al. Resistance exercise and supraphysiological androgen therapy in eugonadal men with HIV-related weight loss. *JAMA* 1999; **281**: 1282–90.
5. Fenichel G, et al. A beneficial effect of oxandrolone in the treatment of Duchenne muscular dystrophy: a pilot study. *Neurology* 1997; **48**: 1225–6.

Growth retardation. A beneficial effect of oxandrolone on growth rate in *boys* with constitutional delay of growth and puberty (p.1273) has been shown in various studies,[1-5] two of which[2,5] were placebo-controlled. Doses used have included 1.25 or 2.5 mg daily[1-3] and 0.05 or 0.1 mg per kg body-weight daily,[4,5] generally for 3 to 12 months. Although a slight advance in bone age has been noted,[1,4,5] final predicted height[5] and actual adult height[3] was not compromised by oxandrolone therapy. Oxandrolone did not affect the rate of pubertal progression and as the aim of such therapy is primarily to relieve psychosocial difficulties associated with short stature and sexual immaturity, it is not clear that it achieves this.[5]

Oxandrolone is also under investigation for the promotion of growth in *girls* with Turner's syndrome (p.1276) in daily doses of 0.05 to 0.125 mg per kg.

1. Stanhope R, Brook CGD. Oxandrolone in low dose for constitutional delay of growth and puberty in boys. *Arch Dis Child* 1985; **60**: 379–81.
2. Stanhope R, et al. Double blind placebo controlled trial of low dose oxandrolone in the treatment of boys with constitutional delay of growth and puberty. *Arch Dis Child* 1988; **63**: 501–5.
3. Tse W-Y, et al. Long-term outcome of oxandrolone treatment in boys with constitutional delay of growth and puberty. *J Pediatr* 1990; **117**: 588–91.
4. Papadimitriou A, et al. Treatment of constitutional growth delay in prepubertal boys with a prolonged course of low dose oxandrolone. *Arch Dis Child* 1991; **66**: 841–3.
5. Wilson DM, et al. Oxandrolone therapy in constitutionally delayed growth and puberty. *Pediatrics* 1995; **96**: 1095–1100.

Preparations

USP 25: Oxandrolone Tablets.

Proprietary Preparations (details are given in Part 3)
Austral.: Lonavar; ***USA:*** Oxandrin.

Oxymetholone (9095-k)

Oxymetholone (*BAN, USAN, rINN*).
CI-406; HMD. 17β-Hydroxy-2-hydroxymethylene-17α-methyl-5α-androstan-3-one.
$C_{21}H_{32}O_3 = 332.5$.
CAS — 434-07-1.
ATC — A14AA05.
Pharmacopoeias. In Br., Jpn, and US.

Pharmacopoeial description
BP 2001: A white to creamy-white, odourless or almost odourless, crystalline powder. It exhibits polymorphism. Practically insoluble in water; soluble in alcohol; freely soluble in chloroform; slightly soluble in ether. Protect from light. Avoid contact with ferrous metals.

USP 25: A white to creamy-white, odourless crystalline powder. Practically insoluble in water; soluble 1 in 40 of alcohol, 1 in 5 of chloroform, 1 in 82 of ether, and 1 in 14 of dioxan.

Adverse Effects and Precautions
As for androgens and anabolic steroids in general (see Testosterone, p.1492).

Liver disturbances and jaundice are common with normal doses and hepatic neoplasms have also been reported (see below). Liver function should be monitored during therapy. As with other 17α-alkylated compounds, oxymetholone should probably be avoided in patients with liver impairment, and certainly if this is severe.

Effects on the blood. Leukaemia developed in 4 patients given oxymetholone for aplastic anaemia.[1] Although a causal relationship had not been established,[1] other cases have been

---

cited.[2] It has also been pointed out that of patients who present with aplastic anaemia, 1 to 5% actually have leukaemia.[3]

1. Delamore IW, Geary CG. Aplastic anaemia, acute myeloblastic leukaemia, and oxymetholone. *BMJ* 1971; **2:** 743–5.
2. Ginsburg AD. Oxymetholone and hematologic disease. *Ann Intern Med* 1973; **79:** 914.
3. Camitta BM, *et al.* Aplastic anemia (first of two parts): pathogenesis, diagnosis, treatment, and prognosis. *N Engl J Med* 1982; **306:** 645–52.

Effects on carbohydrate metabolism. Pronounced hyperglucagonaemia developed in 6 patients receiving oxymetholone.[1]

1. Williams G, *et al.* Severe hyperglucagonaemia during treatment with oxymetholone. *BMJ* 1986; **292:** 1637–8.

Effects on the liver. Reports of peliosis hepatis[1-4] and various liver tumours[1,5-11] associated with oxymetholone.

1. Bernstein MS, *et al.* Hepatoma and peliosis hepatis developing in a patient with Fanconi's anemia. *N Engl J Med* 1971; **284:** 1135–6.
2. Bagheri SA, Boyer JL. Peliosis hepatis associated with androgenic-anabolic steroid therapy: a severe form of hepatic injury. *Ann Intern Med* 1974; **81:** 610–18.
3. Groos G, *et al.* Peliosis hepatis after long-term administration of oxymetholone. *Lancet* 1974; **i:** 874.
4. McDonald EC, Speicher CE. Peliosis hepatis associated with administration of oxymetholone. *JAMA* 1978; **240:** 243–4.
5. Johnson FL, *et al.* Association of androgenic-anabolic steroid therapy with development of hepatocellular carcinoma. *Lancet* 1972; **ii:** 1273–6.
6. Henderson JT, *et al.* Androgenic-anabolic steroid therapy and hepatocellular carcinoma. *Lancet* 1973; **i:** 934.
7. Farrell GC, *et al.* Androgen-induced hepatoma. *Lancet* 1975; **i:** 430–2.
8. Anthony PP. Hepatoma associated with androgenic steroids. *Lancet* 1975; **i:** 685–6.
9. Bruguera M. Hepatoma associated with androgenic steroids. *Lancet* 1975; **i:** 1295.
10. Lesna M, *et al.* Liver nodules and androgens. *Lancet* 1976; **i:** 1124.
11. Mokrohisky ST, *et al.* Fulminant hepatic neoplasia after androgen therapy. *N Engl J Med* 1977; **296:** 1411–12.

Effects on the nervous system. Toxic confusional state and choreiform movements developed in an elderly man given oxymetholone 200 to 300 mg daily.[1]

1. Tilzey A, *et al.* Toxic confusional state and choreiform movements after treatment with anabolic steroids. *BMJ* 1981; **283:** 349–50.

Uses and Administration
Oxymetholone has anabolic and androgenic properties (see Testosterone, p.1493). It has been used mainly in the treatment of anaemias such as aplastic anaemia at a usual dosage by mouth of 1 to 5 mg per kg body-weight daily. Treatment for 3 to 6 months has been suggested, with the drug either withdrawn gradually on remission or reduced to an appropriate maintenance dose.

Aplastic anaemia. There have been mixed results[1-5] with oxymetholone in the treatment of aplastic anaemia (p.715); generally, the response and survival rates have been disappointing.

1. Davis S, Rubin AD. Treatment and prognosis in aplastic anaemia. *Lancet* 1972; **i:** 871–3.
2. Mir MA, Delamore IW. Oxymetholone in aplastic anaemia. *Postgrad Med J* 1974; **50:** 166–71.
3. Camitta BM, *et al.* A prospective study of androgens and bone marrow transplantation for treatment of severe aplastic anemia. *Blood* 1979; **53:** 504–14.
4. Mir MA, Geary CG. Aplastic anaemia: an analysis of 174 patients. *Postgrad Med J* 1980; **56:** 322–9.
5. Webb DKH, *et al.* Acquired aplastic anaemia: still a serious disease. *Arch Dis Child* 1991; **66:** 858–61.

Preparations
BP 2001: Oxymetholone Tablets;
USP 25: Oxymetholone Tablets.

Proprietary Preparations (details are given in Part 3)
Braz.: Hemogenin; **S.Afr.:** Anapolon†; **UK:** Anapolon†; **USA:** Anadrol.

Polyestradiol Phosphate (9097-t)
Polyestradiol Phosphate (*BAN, rINN*).
Leo-114; Polyoestradiol Phosphate. A water-soluble polymeric ester of estradiol and phosphoric acid with a molecular weight of about 26 000.
CAS — 28014-46-2.
ATC — L02AA02.

Adverse Effects and Precautions
As for oestrogens in general (see Estradiol, p.1473). Pain may occur at the site of injection, and mepivacaine is included in some preparations to minimise this.

Pharmacokinetics
Following intramuscular injection polyestradiol phosphate is released slowly into the blood stream where it is slowly metabolised to estradiol.

Uses and Administration
Polyestradiol phosphate is a polymer of estradiol (see p.1473) which has a prolonged duration of action, and is used in the treatment of prostatic carcinoma (p.497). It has been given by deep intramuscular injection in initial doses of 80 to 160 mg every 4 weeks for 2 to 3 months, reduced to 40 to 80 mg every 4 weeks for maintenance.

Preparations
Proprietary Preparations (details are given in Part 3)
Aust.: Estradurin; **Belg.:** Estradurine; **Denm.:** Estradurin; **Fin.:** Estradurin; **Ger.:** Estradurin; **Neth.:** Estradurin; **Norw.:** Estradurin; **Spain:** Estradurin†; **Swed.:** Estradurin; **Switz.:** Estradurin; **UK:** Estradurin†.

Polyestriol Phosphate (10067-m)
Polyoestriol Phosphate.
CAS — 37452-43-0.

Profile
Polyestriol phosphate is a polymer of estriol (see p.1475) and phosphoric acid and has the properties of oestrogens in general (see Estradiol, p.1473). It has been given by intramuscular injection in the treatment of menopausal disorders in doses of 80 mg every 4 to 8 weeks.

Preparations
Proprietary Preparations (details are given in Part 3)
Aust.: Triodurin†.

Prasterone (9036-g)
Prasterone (*rINN*).
Dehydroandrosterone; Dehydroepiandrosterone; Dehydroisoandrosterone; DHEA. 3β-Hydroxyandrost-5-en-17-one.
$C_{19}H_{28}O_2 = 288.4.$
CAS — 53-43-0.
ATC — A14AA07.

Prasterone Enantate (11513-k)
Prasterone Enantate (*rINNM*).
Dehydroepiandrosterone Enanthate; EDHEA; Prasterone Enanthate. 3β-Hydroxyandrost-5-en-17-one heptanoate.
$C_{26}H_{40}O_3 = 400.6.$
CAS — 23983-43-9.

Prasterone Sodium Sulfate (14252-y)
Prasterone Sodium Sulfate (*rINNM*).
Dehydroepiandrosterone Sulphate Sodium; DHA-S; DHEAS; Prasterone Sodium Sulphate. 3β-Hydroxyandrost-5-en-17-one hydrogen sulphate sodium.
$C_{19}H_{27}NaO_5S = 390.5.$
CAS — 651-48-9 (prasterone sulfate); 1099-87-2 (prasterone sodium sulfate).
Pharmacopoeias. In Jpn.

Profile
Prasterone is a naturally occurring adrenal androgen that is a precursor of androgens and oestrogens. Prasterone enantate is given by intramuscular depot injection as menopausal HRT (p.1463) in association with estradiol valerate. Prasterone is also being investigated in systemic lupus erythematosus, and the sodium sulfate is under investigation for the treatment of burns.

◊ General reviews.
1. Kroboth PD, *et al.* DHEA and DHEA-S: a review. *J Clin Pharmacol* 1999; **39:** 327–48.
2. Pepping J. DHEA: dehydroepiandrosterone. *Am J Health-Syst Pharm* 2000; **57:** 2048–56.

HIV infection and AIDS. Plasma concentrations of prasterone are reported to be abnormally low in patients with AIDS, and it has been suggested that use of prasterone might be of benefit; however controlled studies are lacking.[1]

1. Centurelli MA, *et al.* The role of dehydroepiandrosterone in AIDS. *Ann Pharmacother* 1997; **31:** 639–42.

Replacement therapy. There has been much speculation about the physiological role and importance of prasterone, which is the most abundant steroid hormone in the circulation. It is produced by the adrenal gland and is a precursor of androgens and oestrogens.[1] Serum concentrations of the sulfate conjugate peak at about 20 years then gradually decline with age. Epidemiological studies suggest that certain age-related diseases are linked to this decline, including an increased risk of cardiovascular disease in men, and breast cancer in premenopausal women.[1] It has been suggested, therefore, that replacement therapy with prasterone might alleviate some of the problems of ageing. However, there is insufficient evidence of safety and efficacy to recommend such use. A systematic review[2] of studies in healthy adults taking prasterone supplementation found that although there was limited support for improvement in a sense of well-being in a longer-term study, there was no support for an improvement in memory or cognitive function. A later study of healthy adults who took prasterone or placebo for one year reported improved bone turnover and skin condition, particularly in women over 70 years old.[3] A review[4] of the use of prasterone as a 'food supplement' noted that although it was being taken in the belief that it could reverse some of the effects of ageing there was no good evidence of this. Various androgenic effects, including hirsutism and voice changes, have been reported in women taking prasterone and there is a theoretical possibility that it might promote growth of hormone-sensitive tumours in both sexes.[1,4]

Prasterone has also been studied as replacement therapy for patients with adrenal insufficiency, who have subnormal levels of prasterone. Such therapy has been reported to raise serum levels of prasterone to normal, and improve measures of well-being, mood, and fatigue.[5,6]

1. Weksler ME. Hormone replacement for men. *BMJ* 1996; **312:** 859–60.
2. Huppert FA, *et al.* Dehydroepiandrosterone (DHEA) supplementation for cognition and well-being (updated 23 November 2000). Available in The Cochrane Library; Issue 1. Oxford: Update Software; 2001.
3. Baulieu E-E, *et al.* Dehydroepiandrosterone (DHEA), DHEA sulfate, and aging: contribution of the DHEAge study to a socio-biomedical issue. *Proc Natl Acad Sci U S A* 2000; **97:** 4279–84.
4. Anonymous. Dehydroepiandrosterone (DHEA). *Med Lett Drugs Ther* 1996; **38:** 91–2.
5. Arlt W, *et al.* Dehydroepiandrosterone replacement in women with adrenal insufficiency. *N Engl J Med* 1999; **341:** 1013–20.
6. Hunt PJ, *et al.* Improvement in mood and fatigue after dehydroepiandrosterone replacement in Addison's disease in a randomized, double blind trial. *J Clin Endocrinol Metab* 2000; **85:** 4650–6.

Systemic lupus erythematosus. Symptomatic improvement was seen in 8 of 10 women with systemic lupus erythematosus (p.1059) who received prasterone 200 mg daily by mouth for several months.[1] Improvement permitted a reduction in the dosage of concomitant corticosteroids. Similar findings have been reported by one group in a number of small studies,[2-5] but although these workers consider that there is clear evidence of benefit,[6] two larger, and thus far unpublished, studies have produced more statistically ambiguous results; as a result, as of July 2001 the FDA had not approved licensing of prasterone for this indication.

1. van Vollenhoven RF, *et al.* An open study of dehydroepiandrosterone in systemic lupus erythematosus. *Arthritis Rheum* 1994; **37:** 1305–10.
2. van Vollenhoven RF, *et al.* Dehydroepiandrosterone in systemic lupus erythematosus. *Arthritis Rheum* 1995; **38:** 1826–31.
3. van Vollenhoven RF, *et al.* Treatment of systemic lupus erythematosus with dehydroepiandrosterone: 50 patients treated up to 12 months. *J Rheumatol* 1998; **25:** 285–9.
4. Barry NN, *et al.* Dehydroepiandrosterone in systemic lupus erythematosus: relationship between dosage, serum levels, and clinical response. *J Rheumatol* 1998; **25:** 2352–6.
5. van Vollenhoven RF, *et al.* A double-blind, placebo-controlled, clinical trial of dehydroepiandrosterone in severe systemic lupus erythematosus. *Lupus* 1999; **8:** 181–7.
6. van Vollenhoven RF. Dehydroepiandrosterone in systemic lupus erythematosus. *Rheum Dis Clin North Am* 2000; **26:** 349–62.

Preparations
Proprietary Preparations (details are given in Part 3)
Port.: Dinistenile.

Multi-ingredient: Aust.: Gynodian Depot; **Ger.:** Gynodian Depot; **Ital.:** Gynodian Depot; Sinsurrene†; **Mex.:** Binodian; Sten; **Spain:** Gynodian Depot; **Switz.:** Gynodian Depot.

Progesterone (9098-x)
Progesterone (*BAN, rINN*).
Corpus Luteum Hormone; Luteal Hormone; Luteine; Luteohormone; NSC-9704; Pregnenedione; Progesteronum. Pregn-4-ene-3,20-dione.
$C_{21}H_{30}O_2 = 314.5.$
CAS — 57-83-0.
ATC — G03DA04.

Pharmacopoeias. In Chin., Eur. (see p.vi), Int., Jpn, Pol., and US.

Pharmacopoeial description
Ph. Eur.: A white or almost white crystalline powder or colourless crystals. It exhibits polymorphism. Practically insoluble in water; freely soluble in dehydrated alcohol; sparingly soluble in acetone and in fatty oils. Protect from light.

USP 25: A white or creamy-white, odourless, crystalline powder. Practically insoluble in water; soluble in alcohol, in acetone, and in dioxan; sparingly soluble in vegetable oils. Store in airtight containers. Protect from light.

Adverse Effects
Progesterone and the progestogens may cause gastrointestinal disturbances, changes in appetite or weight, fluid retention, oedema, acne, chloasma (melasma), allergic skin rashes, urticaria, mental depression, breast changes including discomfort or occasionally gynaecomastia, changes in libido, hair loss, hirsutism, fatigue, drowsiness or insomnia, fever, headache, premenstrual syndrome-like symptoms, and altered menstrual cycles or irregular menstrual bleeding. Anaphylaxis or anaphylactoid reactions may occur rarely. Alterations in the serum lipid profile may occur, and rarely alterations in liver-function tests and jaundice. Pain, diarrhoea, and flatulence have followed rectal administration. Injection-site reactions have followed parenteral use.

Adverse effects vary depending on the dose and type of progestogen. For example, androgenic effects such as acne and hirsutism are more likely to occur with nortestosterone derivatives such as norethisterone and norgestrel. These derivatives may also be more likely to adversely affect serum lipids. Conversely, adverse effects on serum lipids appear less likely with gestodene and desogestrel, but these 2 drugs have been associated with a higher incidence of thromboembolism than norethisterone and norgestrel when used in combined oral contraceptives (see p.1455). High doses of progestogens such as those used in treating cancer have also been associated with thromboembolism. For a discussion of the effect of progestogens on the cardiovascular risk profile of menopausal HRT see p.1462. Breakthrough uterine bleeding is more common with oral progestogen-only contraceptives than when progestogens are used for menstrual irregularities or as part of menopausal HRT.

Some progestogens when given during pregnancy have been reported to cause virilisation of a female fetus. This appears to have been associated with those progestogens with more pronounced androgenic activity such as norethisterone; the natural progestogenic hormone progesterone and its derivatives such as dydrogesterone and medroxyprogesterone do not appear to have been associated with such effects.

For the adverse effects of progestogens when administered either alone or with oestrogens as contraceptives, see p.1452. For those of menopausal HRT, see p.1461.

Effects on the skin. A case report and discussion of progesterone-induced urticaria.[1]

1. Wilkinson SM, et al. Progesterone-induced urticaria—need it be autoimmune? *Br J Dermatol* 1995; **133:** 792–4.

Precautions

Progesterone and the progestogens should be used with caution in patients with cardiovascular or renal impairment, diabetes mellitus, asthma, epilepsy, and migraine, or other conditions which may be aggravated by fluid retention. They should also be used with care in persons with a history of depression.

Progesterone and the progestogens should not be given to patients with undiagnosed vaginal bleeding, nor to those with a history or current high risk of arterial disease and should generally be avoided in hepatic impairment, especially if severe. Unless progestogens are being used as part of the management of breast or genital-tract carcinoma they should not be given to patients with these conditions.

Although progestogens have been given as hormonal support during early pregnancy such use is not now generally advised and many authorities now recommend that progestogens should not be used at all in early pregnancy. Some, however, allow the use of a progesterone-type progestogen for women who are progesterone-deficient. Such use may prevent spontaneous evacuation of a dead fetus, therefore careful monitoring of pregnancy is required. Progestogens should not be used diagnostically for pregnancy testing and should not be given in missed or incomplete abortion.

For precautions to be observed when progestogens are used as contraceptives, see p.1457. For those to be observed when progestogens are used in preparations for menopausal HRT, see p.1463.

Abuse. A case report of abuse of and dependency on progesterone.[1]

1. Keefe DL, Sarrel P. Dependency on progesterone in woman with self-diagnosed premenstrual syndrome. *Lancet* 1996; **347:** 1182.

Porphyria. Progesterone and progestogens have been associated with acute attacks of porphyria and are considered unsafe in patients with porphyria (but medroxyprogesterone has been used with buserelin to suppress premenstrual exacerbations of porphyria, see p.1279). Progestogens should generally be avoided by all women with porphyria; however, where non-hormonal contraception is inappropriate progestogens may be used with extreme caution if the potential benefit outweighs the risk. The risk of an acute attack is greatest in women who have had a previous attack or are under 30 years of age. Long-acting progestogen preparations should never be used in those at risk.

Pregnancy. In Hungary where 30% of all pregnant women were given hormonal support therapy with progestogens during the early 1980s, a case-control study suggested that there was a causal relationship between such treatment and hypospadias in their offspring.[1] Reports of abnormalities in infants following exposure *in utero* to progestogens have included hypospadias[2] with norethisterone and hydroxyprogesterone; other genitourinary anomalies with dydrogesterone[3] and hydroxyprogesterone;[4] tetralogy of Fallot[5] and adrenocortical carcinoma[6] with hydroxyprogesterone; fetal masculinisation[7] with norethisterone, noretynodrel, and ethisterone; and meningomyelocele or hydrocephalus[8] with norethisterone and ethisterone. For further details see under Pregnancy in the individual monographs. For the effects on the fetus when progestogens are used as contraceptives, see p.1458. For the risk of ectopic pregnancy with progestogen-only contraceptives, see p.1454.

1. Czeizel A. Increasing trends in congenital malformations of male external genitalia. *Lancet* 1985; **i:** 462–3.
2. Aarskog D. Clinical and cytogenetic studies in hypospadias. *Acta Paediatr Scand* 1970; (suppl 203): 1–62.
3. Roberts IF, West RJ. Teratogenesis and maternal progesterone. *Lancet* 1977; **ii:** 982.
4. Evans ANW, et al. The ingestion by pregnant women of substances toxic to the foetus. *Practitioner* 1980; **224:** 315–19.
5. Heinonen OP, et al. Cardiovascular birth defects and antenatal exposure to female sex hormones. *N Engl J Med* 1977; **296:** 67–70.
6. Mann JR, et al. Transplacental carcinogenesis (adrenocortical carcinoma) associated with hydroxyprogesterone hexanoate. *Lancet* 1983; **ii:** 580.
7. Wilkins L. Masculinization of female fetus due to use of orally given progestins. *JAMA* 1960; **172:** 1028–32.
8. Gal I, et al. Hormonal pregnancy tests and congenital malformation. *Nature* 1967; **216:** 83.

Veterinary use. An expert committee of the FAO and WHO considered it unnecessary to establish an acceptable daily intake or acceptable residue level in food for endogenous hormones such as progesterone.[1] Residues resulting from the use of progesterone as a growth promotor in accordance with good animal husbandry practice are unlikely to pose a hazard to human health. However, it should be noted that in the European Union the use of steroidal hormones such as progestogens in veterinary practice is restricted, and their use as growth promotors is banned.

1. FAO/WHO. Evaluation of certain veterinary drug residues in food: thirty-second report of the joint FAO/WHO expert committee on food additives. *WHO Tech Rep Ser 763* 1988.

Interactions

Enzyme-inducing drugs such as carbamazepine, griseofulvin, phenobarbital, phenytoin, and rifampicin may enhance the clearance of progesterone and the progestogens. These interactions are likely to reduce the efficacy of progestogen-only contraceptives (see p.1458), and additional or alternative contraceptive measures are recommended.

Aminoglutethimide markedly reduces the plasma concentrations of medroxyprogesterone acetate and megestrol, possibly through a hepatic enzyme-inducing effect; an increase in progestogen dose is likely to be required.

Since progesterone and other progestogens can influence diabetic control an adjustment in antidiabetic dosage could be required. Progestogens may inhibit ciclosporin metabolism leading to increased plasma-ciclosporin concentrations and a risk of toxicity (see p.522).

Pharmacokinetics

Progesterone has a short elimination half-life and undergoes extensive first-pass hepatic metabolism when given by mouth; oral bioavailability is very low although it may be increased somewhat by administration in an oily vehicle and by micronisation. Progesterone is absorbed when administered buccally, rectally, or vaginally, and rapidly absorbed from the site of an oily intramuscular injection.

Various derivatives have been produced to extend the duration of action and to improve oral activity. Esters of progesterone derivatives such as hydroxyprogesterone caproate are used intramuscularly, and megestrol acetate is orally active. The ester medroxyprogesterone acetate is used orally and parenterally. 19-Nortestosterone progestogens have good oral activity because the 17-ethinyl substituent slows hepatic metabolism.

Progesterone and the progestogens are highly protein bound; progesterone is bound to albumin and corticosteroid binding globulin; esters such as medroxyprogesterone acetate are principally bound to albumin; and 19-nortestosterone analogues are bound to

sex-steroid binding globulin and albumin. Progesterone is metabolised in the liver to various metabolites including pregnanediol, which are excreted in the urine as sulfate and glucuronide conjugates. Similarly, progestogens undergo hepatic metabolism to various conjugates, which are excreted in the urine.

◊ Reviews.
1. Kuhl H. Comparative pharmacology of newer progestogens. *Drugs* 1996; **51:** 188–215.
2. Stanczyk FZ. Structure-function relationships, metabolism, pharmacokinetics and potency of progestins. *Drugs Today* 1996; **32** (suppl H): 1–14.

Uses and Administration

Progesterone is a natural hormone whereas progestogens are synthetic compounds, derived from progesterone or 19-nortestosterone, with actions similar to those of progesterone (for further details, see p.1452).

Progestogens derived from 19-nortestosterone are used as **hormonal contraceptives** (see p.1459), either alone or combined with an oestrogen. The progesterone derivative medroxyprogesterone acetate is also used, and progesterone itself has been used.

Progestogens, and sometimes progesterone, are used in combination with oestrogens for **menopausal HRT** (p.1463) to reduce the increased risk of endometrial hyperplasia and carcinoma which occurs when unopposed long-term oestrogen therapy is employed.

Similarly, drugs with progestogenic actions may be used in **menstrual disorders** such as dysmenorrhoea (p.6) and menorrhagia associated with dysfunctional uterine bleeding (below). Progestogens may also be used in the management of endometriosis (p.1469). Although progestogens and progesterone have been used for the management of the premenstrual syndrome, such a practice is of debatable value (p.1475).

Progestogens may be valuable in advanced **endometrial cancer** (p.493) and have been tried in some other malignancies. The progestogens typically used for malignant disease include medroxyprogesterone acetate, megestrol, and norethisterone. Some progestogens such as megestrol and medroxyprogesterone are used for the **cachexia** or wasting associated with severe illness including cancer and AIDS (p.1481).

Progestogens have been widely advocated for either the prevention of **recurrent miscarriage** or the treatment of threatened miscarriage. However, many authorities now consider that there is little evidence of any benefit from such a practice and recommend against the use of progestogens in early pregnancy, with the exception of the use of progesterone or a progesterone derivative in women who are progesterone deficient (see also under Precautions, above).

USES AND ADMINISTRATION OF PROGESTERONE. Progesterone is usually administered as an oily intramuscular injection, a vaginal gel or pessaries, or as suppositories. An oral micronised preparation of progesterone is also available.

In dysfunctional uterine bleeding or amenorrhoea 5 to 10 mg daily of progesterone may be given by intramuscular injection for about 5 to 10 days until 2 days before the anticipated onset of menstruation. Alternatively, progesterone may be administered as a vaginal gel at a usual dose of 45 mg on alternate days from day 15 to 25 of the cycle, or orally at a dose of 400 mg daily for 10 days.

In women with a history of recurrent miscarriage and proven progesterone deficiency, twice weekly intramuscular injection (increased to daily if necessary) of 25 to 100 mg of progesterone from approximately day 15 of the pregnancy until 8 to 16 weeks has been used. A similar schedule has been used in *in vitro* fertilisation or gamete intra-fallopian transfer techniques with treatment beginning on the day of transfer of embryo or gametes. The dose may be increased to 200 mg daily if necessary. Alternatively, progesterone may be administered as a vaginal gel at a dose of 90 mg daily continued for 30 days after laboratory evidence of pregnancy; 90 mg twice daily has been used in women with ovarian failure.

Progesterone may be given vaginally or rectally in doses of 200 mg daily to 400 mg twice daily for the management of the premenstrual syndrome. Treatment usually starts on day 12 to 14 of the menstrual cycle and continues until the onset of menstruation. Similar vaginal or rectal doses have also been used in the treatment of puerperal (post-natal) depression.

Progesterone gel may be administered intravaginally at a dose of 45 mg on alternate days for 12 days of a 28-day cycle as the progestogen component of menopausal HRT.

A progesterone-releasing intra-uterine device has also been used as a hormonal contraceptive; the device contains 38 mg of progesterone and is effective for up to 12 months.

Menorrhagia. Menorrhagia, or excessive menstrual bleeding, is usually defined as a blood loss exceeding 80 mL per menstrual period,[1,2] compared with a normal loss of about 30 mL. However, many women consider losses below 80 mL to be excessive particularly if 'flooding' occurs. Although not life-threatening, menorrhagia can lead to iron deficiency anaemia as well as considerably impairing quality of life. Menorrhagia may be associated with pelvic disorders such as fibroids or endometriosis, or the use of copper intra-uterine devices, or some systemic disorders.[1,2] However, most commonly it is associated with dysfunctional uterine bleeding; a term used to denote frequent, prolonged or heavy uterine bleeding for which no specific cause is found (essential, idiopathic, or primary menorrhagia). Both ovulatory (regular) and anovulatory cycles may give rise to dysfunctional uterine bleeding.[2] If the patient has regular ovulatory cycles and does not require contraception or wish to take a hormonal treatment, then an NSAID or tranexamic acid is usually the preferred treatment.[1-3] These have the advantage that they are only taken during menstruation, which increases compliance.[2] Therapy is generally tried for 3 months, and continued if the response is good and there are no adverse effects; nonresponders may be switched to the alternative therapy while awaiting referral to a specialist.[3]

UK summary guidelines for the initial management of menorrhagia recommend the use of mefenamic acid as the *NSAID* of choice[3] but other NSAIDs such as ibuprofen or naproxen have been employed and there does not seem to be evidence to suggest that one NSAID is more effective than another. They reduce menstrual blood loss by about 30%,[2,4] and relieve dysmenorrhoea (p.6). Systematic review suggests that NSAIDs are less effective than tranexamic acid or danazol in reducing bleeding,[5] but they may have fewer adverse effects.

Administered during menstruation *tranexamic acid* reduces menstrual blood loss by about half;[2,4] the benefits of tranexamic therapy have been confirmed by systematic review.[6] However, gastrointestinal adverse effects are common and it is contraindicated in women with thromboembolic disorders. *Etamsylate* has been reported to have similar efficacy to an NSAID in 1 study,[7] but to be ineffective in another.[8] An analysis, which included these and 2 earlier studies, concluded that etamsylate reduced menstrual blood loss by about 10 to 15%.[4]

In women who require contraception, a *combined oral contraceptive* appears to be effective,[1,2] although good evidence of this is actually lacking.[9] UK summary guidelines recommend combination with mefenamic acid in those women in whom an oral contraceptive alone is inadequate.[3] Traditional therapy with *progestogens* such as norethisterone or medroxyprogesterone given during the luteal phase appears to be ineffective in women with normal ovulatory cycles,[2,10] although cyclical therapy may be of benefit in anovulatory patients as it imposes a cycle.[2] Progestogen therapy for 21 days of the cycle results in a significant reduction in menstrual blood loss,[10] but is associated with adverse effects that may limit its acceptability.

More recently, a *levonorgestrel-containing intra-uterine device* has been shown to be very effective in reducing menstrual blood loss,[11,12] and to be an alternative to hysterectomy in menorrhagia.[13,14] It has been suggested that this may become the preferred long-term medical treatment for menorrhagia,[1] although comparative data are scanty.[15]

Danazol is also effective, producing about a 50% reduction in menstrual blood loss,[4] but has significant adverse effects and treatment is usually limited to 3 to 6 months. *Gonadorelin analogues* are effective for menorrhagia associated with fibroids (p.1285), but can only be used short term because of the resultant ovarian suppression.[1] When used pre-operatively for endometrial thinning, gonadorelin analogues produce more consistent results than danazol.[16]

In patients who fail to respond to drug treatment, or in whom such therapy is inappropriate, various *surgical options* exist. Conservative surgical techniques, where the endometrium is ablated or resected, are increasingly being used, and appear to be an effective alternative to hysterectomy.[17] Hysterectomy is

the ultimate therapy, but is associated with significant morbidity.

1. Wood CE. Menorrhagia: a clinical update. *Med J Aust* 1996; **165:** 510–14.
2. Prentice A. Medical management of menorrhagia. *BMJ* 1999; **319:** 1343–5.
3. Royal College of Obstetricians and Gynaecologists. The initial management of menorrhagia. Available at: http://www.rcog.org.uk/guidelines/menorrhagia.html (accessed 31/07/01).
4. Coulter A, *et al.* Treating menorrhagia in primary care: an overview of drug trials and a survey of prescribing practice. *Int J Technol Assess Health Care* 1995; **11:** 456–71.
5. Lethaby A, *et al.* Nonsteroidal anti-inflammatory drugs for heavy menstrual bleeding (updated 27 October 1999). Available in The Cochrane Library; Issue 3. Oxford: Update Software; 2001.
6. Lethaby A, *et al.* Antifibrinolytics for heavy menstrual bleeding (updated 27 November 2000). Available in The Cochrane Library; Issue 3. Oxford: Update Software; 2001.
7. Chamberlain G, *et al.* A comparative study of ethamsylate and mefenamic acid in dysfunctional uterine bleeding. *Br J Obstet Gynaecol* 1991; **98:** 707–11.
8. Bonnar J, Sheppard BL. Treatment of menorrhagia during menstruation: randomised controlled trial of ethamsylate, mefenamic acid, and tranexamic acid. *BMJ* 1996; **313:** 579–82.
9. Iyer V, *et al.* Oral contraceptive pills for heavy menstrual bleeding (updated 28 May 2001). Available in The Cochrane Library; Issue 3. Oxford: Update Software; 2001.
10. Lethaby A, *et al.* Cyclical progestogens for heavy menstrual bleeding (updated 27 November 2000). Available in The Cochrane Library; Issue 3. Oxford: Update Software; 2001.
11. Andersson JK, Rybo G. Levonorgestrel-releasing intrauterine device in the treatment of menorrhagia. *Br J Obstet Gynaecol* 1990; **97:** 690–4.
12. Milsom I, *et al.* A comparison of flurbiprofen, tranexamic acid, and a levonorgestrel-releasing intrauterine contraceptive device in the treatment of idiopathic menorrhagia. *Am J Obstet Gynecol* 1991; **164:** 879–83.
13. Lähteenmäki P, *et al.* Open randomised study of use of levonorgestrel releasing intrauterine system as alternative to hysterectomy. *BMJ* 1998; **316:** 1122–6.
14. Hurskainen R, *et al.* Quality of life and cost-effectiveness of levonorgestrel-releasing intrauterine system versus hysterectomy for treatment of menorrhagia: a randomised trial. *Lancet* 2001; **357:** 273–77.
15. Lethaby A, *et al.* Progesterone/progestogen releasing intrauterine systems versus either placebo or any other medication for heavy menstrual bleeding (updated 28 May 2001). Available in The Cochrane Library; Issue 3. Oxford: Update Software; 2001.
16. Sowter MC, *et al.* Pre-operative endometrial thinning agents before hysteroscopic surgery for heavy menstrual bleeding (updated 28 May 2001). Available in The Cochrane Library; Issue 3. Oxford: Update Software; 2001.
17. Lethaby A, *et al.* Endometrial resection and ablation versus hysterectomy for heavy menstrual bleeding (updated 27 November 2000). Available in The Cochrane Library; Issue 3. Oxford: Update Software; 2001.

Premenstrual syndrome. Progestogen therapy was once popular for premenstrual syndrome, but beneficial responses have not been universally achieved and the theory that progesterone was necessary to correct a hormone imbalance is now losing ground (see p.1475). A double-blind, placebo-controlled crossover study[1] involving 168 women showed that progesterone 0.4 or 0.8 g daily by the vaginal route did not significantly improve symptoms of the premenstrual syndrome. However, the view has been expressed[2] that since absorption of progesterone from the vagina or rectum may vary between patients, the dose and frequency of administration needs to be individualised and that if the response to treatment is inadequate the intramuscular route should be tried. A more recent study found oral micronised progesterone, in an initial dose of 1.2 g daily in divided doses, increased as required to 3.6 g daily, to be no better than placebo in the management of severe premenstrual syndrome.[3]

1. Freeman E, *et al.* Ineffectiveness of progesterone suppository treatment for premenstrual syndrome. *JAMA* 1990; **264:** 349–53.
2. Dalton K. Treating the premenstrual syndrome. *BMJ* 1988; **297:** 490.
3. Freeman EW, *et al.* A double-blind trial of oral progesterone, alprazolam, and placebo in treatment of severe premenstrual syndrome. *JAMA* 1995; **274:** 51–7.

Preparations

BP 2001: Progesterone Injection;
USP 25: Progesterone Injectable Suspension; Progesterone Injection; Progesterone Intrauterine Contraceptive System; Progesterone Vaginal Suppositories.

Proprietary Preparations (details are given in Part 3)

Aust.: Utrogestan; *Austral.:* Proluton; *Belg.:* Progestogel; Utrogestan; *Canad.:* Gesterol†; Prometrium; *Fin.:* Lugesteron; *Fr.:* Estima; Progestasert†; Progestogel; Progestosol; Utrogestan; *Ger.:* Crinone; Progestogel; Utrogest; *Hong Kong:* Cyclogest; Utrogestan; *Irl.:* Crinone; Utrogestan; *Israel:* Gestone; Utrogestan; *Ital.:* Crinone; Esolut; Progestogel; Progestil; Prontogest; *Mex.:* Crinone; Cuerpo Amarillo Fuerte; Prolidon; *Neth.:* Progestan; *NZ:* Gestone; *Port.:* Progenar; Progestogel; Utrogestan; *S.Afr.:* Cyclogest; Utrogestan; *Singapore:* Crinone; Utrogestan; *Spain:* Cutifitol; Progeffik; Progestogel; Utrogestan; *Switz.:* Progestogel; Utrogestan; *Thai.:* Cyclogest; Gestone; Progestogel; Proluton; Utrogestan; *UK:* Crinone; Cyclogest; Gestone; *USA:* Crinone; Prochieve; Prometrium.

Multi-ingredient: *Braz.:* Ginecoside; Hormoginase; Normomensil; Progest; *Fr.:* Florgynal; Synergon; Trophigil; *Ger.:* Jephagynon; *Ital.:* Biormon; Duo-Ormogyn†; Menovis; *Mex.:* Lutoginestryl F; Metrigen Fuerte; Progediol; Proger-F; *Mon.:* Tocogestan; *Port.:* Emmenovis; *Thai.:* Duoton.

Proligestone (8219-v)

Proligestone *(BAN, rINN)*.

14α,17α-Propylidene dioxypregn-4-ene-3,20-dione.

$C_{24}H_{34}O_4 = 386.5.$

CAS — 23873-85-0.

Profile

Proligestone is a progestogen used in veterinary medicine.

Promegestone (3871-c)

Promegestone *(rINN)*.

R-5020. 17α-Methyl-17-propionylestra-4,9-dien-3-one.

$C_{22}H_{30}O_2 = 326.5.$

CAS — 34184-77-5.

ATC — G03DB07.

Profile

Promegestone is a progestogen structurally related to progesterone (p.1488). It has been given by mouth on a cyclical basis, in doses of 125 to 500 μg daily, in the treatment of menstrual disorders and mastalgia, and as the progestogen component of menopausal HRT.

Preparations

Proprietary Preparations (details are given in Part 3)
Fr.: Surgestone; *Port.:* Surgestone.

Promestriene (13176-s)

Promestriene *(rINN)*.

17β-Methoxy-3-propoxyestra-1,3,5(10)-triene.

$C_{22}H_{32}O_2 = 328.5.$

CAS — 39219-28-8.

ATC — G03CA09.

Profile

Promestriene is a derivative of estradiol (see p.1473) that has been used topically in menopausal atrophic vaginitis, and in seborrhoea.

Preparations

Proprietary Preparations (details are given in Part 3)
Braz.: Colpotrofine; *Hong Kong:* Colpotrophine; *Ital.:* Colpotrophine; *Mon.:* Colpotrophine; Deliporderm†; *Port.:* Colpotrophine; *Singapore:* Colpotrophine; *Spain:* Colpotrofin; Deliporderm; *Switz.:* Colpotrophine.

Multi-ingredient: *Hong Kong:* Colposeptine; *Mon.:* Colposeptine; *Port.:* Trophoseptine.

Pygeum Africanum (13542-z)

African Prune.

ATC — G04CX01.

Profile

An extract of the bark of the African prune tree, *Pygeum africanum* (Rosaceae), is used in the treatment of benign prostatic hyperplasia (p.1477). Like some other phytotherapies for this disorder, it appears to contain various sitosterols. A usual dosage is 100 mg daily by mouth.

◊ Pygeum africanum appears to produce a modest benefit on urological symptoms and measures of urinary flow.

References.
1. Andro M-C, Riffaud J-P. Pygeum africanum extract for the treatment of patients with benign prostatic hyperplasia: a review of 25 years of published experience. *Curr Ther Res* 1995; **56:** 796–817.
2. Buck AC. Phytotherapy for the prostate. *Br J Urol* 1996; **78:** 325–36.
3. Ishani A, *et al.* Pygeum africanum for the treatment of patients with benign prostatic hyperplasia: a systematic review and quantitative meta-analysis. *Am J Med* 2000; **109:** 654–64.

Preparations

Proprietary Preparations (details are given in Part 3)
Aust.: Tadenan; *Braz.:* Prolitrol; Prostem; *Fr.:* Tadenan; *Hong Kong:* Tadenan; *Ital.:* Pigenil; Tadenan; *Port.:* Tadenan; *Spain:* Acubiron; Bidrolar; Pronitol; Prostamal; Tuzanil; *Switz.:* Tadenan; *Thai.:* Tadenan.

Multi-ingredient: *Aust.:* Prostatonin; *Braz.:* Prostem Plus; *Port.:* Neo Urgenin†; *Spain:* Neo Urgenin; Prosurol; Tebetane Compuesto; *Switz.:* Prostatonin.

Quinestradol (9100-r)

Quinestradol *(BAN, rINN)*.

Oestriol 3-Cyclopentyl Ether; Quinestradiol. 3-Cyclopentyloxyestra-1,3,5(10)-triene-16α,17β-diol.

$C_{23}H_{32}O_3 = 356.5.$

CAS — 1169-79-1.

Profile

Quinestradol is a synthetic oestrogen that has been given by mouth for the treatment of menopausal vaginal symptoms in a dosage of 1 to 2 mg daily.

Preparations

Proprietary Preparations (details are given in Part 3)
Ital.: Colpovis.

Quinestrol (9101-f)

Quinestrol *(BAN, USAN, rINN)*.

17α-Ethinyloestradiol 3-cyclopentyl Ether; W-3566. 3-Cyclopentyloxy-19-nor-17α-pregna-1,3,5(10)-trien-20-yn-17β-ol.

$C_{25}H_{32}O_2 = 364.5$.

$CAS — 152-43-2$.

Profile
Quinestrol is a synthetic oestrogen that has a prolonged duration of action and is metabolised to ethinylestradiol (p.1476). Quinestrol has been given by mouth for the treatment of menopausal symptoms and other conditions arising from oestrogen deficiency.

Raloxifene Hydrochloride (19377-x)

Raloxifene Hydrochloride *(BANM, USAN, rINNM)*.

Keoxifene Hydrochloride; LY-156758; LY-139481 (raloxifene). 6-Hydroxy-2-(*p*-hydroxyphenyl)benzo[*b*]thien-3-yl-*p*-(2-piperidinoethoxy)phenyl ketone hydrochloride.

$C_{28}H_{27}NO_4S,HCl = 510.0$.

$CAS — 84449-90-1$ (raloxifene); $82640-04-8$ (raloxifene hydrochloride).

Adverse Effects
The most common adverse effects of raloxifene are hot flushes and leg cramps. Raloxifene is associated with an increased risk of venous thromboembolic events, particularly during the first 4 months of treatment. Peripheral oedema has also been reported. Rashes and gastrointestinal disturbances have occurred rarely.

Effects on the liver. Hepatitis, probably associated with the drug, occurred in a woman a month after starting raloxifene.[1]

1. Vilches AR, *et al.* Raloxifene-associated hepatitis. *Lancet* 1998; **352:** 1524–5.

Precautions
Raloxifene should be avoided in women with active venous thromboembolism, or a history of thromboembolic disorders. It should be discontinued at least 72 hours prior to periods of prolonged immobilisation, such as post-surgical recovery. Raloxifene should be used with caution in women with risk factors for venous thromboembolism including congestive heart failure or active malignancy. It should be avoided in hepatic and severe renal impairment.

Raloxifene had adverse effects in *animal* teratogenicity studies and should not be used in women who are or may become pregnant. It should not be given to women with undiagnosed vaginal bleeding.

Interactions
Colestyramine reduces the absorption and enterohepatic recycling of raloxifene, and should not be given concomitantly. Raloxifene may decrease the efficacy of warfarin.

Pharmacokinetics
Raloxifene is absorbed from the gastrointestinal tract and undergoes extensive first-pass hepatic metabolism to the glucuronide conjugates. It is highly bound to plasma proteins, principally albumin and α_1-acid glycoprotein. Raloxifene undergoes enterohepatic recycling, and has a half-life of about 27 hours. It is excreted almost entirely in the faeces.

Uses and Administration
Raloxifene hydrochloride is a benzothiophene nonsteroidal anti-oestrogen related to clomifene and tamoxifen. It is used, in doses of 60 mg daily by mouth, for the prevention and treatment of postmenopausal osteoporosis (p.745).

It is also under investigation for the prophylaxis of breast cancer (p.492).

◊ References.

1. Delmas PD, *et al.* Effects of raloxifene on bone mineral density, serum cholesterol concentrations, and uterine endometrium in postmenopausal women. *N Engl J Med* 1997; **337:** 1641–7.

2. Walsh BW, *et al.* Effects of raloxifene on serum lipids and coagulation factors in healthy postmenopausal women. *JAMA* 1998; **279:** 1445–51.
3. Balfour JA, Goa KL. Raloxifene. *Drugs Aging* 1998; **12:** 335–41.
4. Lufkin EG, *et al.* Treatment of established postmenopausal osteoporosis with raloxifene: a randomized trial. *J Bone Miner Res* 1998; **13:** 1747–54.
5. Khovidhunkit W, Shoback DM. Clinical effects of raloxifene hydrochloride in women. *Ann Intern Med* 1999; **130:** 431–9.
6. Ettinger B, *et al.* Reduction of vertebral fracture risk in postmenopausal women with osteoporosis treated with raloxifene: results from a 3-year randomized clinical trial. *JAMA* 1999; **282:** 637–45.
7. Clemett D, Spencer CM. Raloxifene: a review of its use in postmenopausal osteoporosis. *Drugs* 2000; **60:** 379–411.

Malignant neoplasms of the breast. References.

1. Cummings SR, *et al.* The effect of raloxifene on risk of breast cancer in postmenopausal women: results from the MORE randomized trial. *JAMA* 1999; **281:** 2189–97.
2. Chlebowski RT, *et al.* American Society of Clinical Oncology technology assessment on breast cancer risk reduction strategies: tamoxifen and raloxifene. *J Clin Oncol* 1999; **17:** 1939–55.

Preparations

Proprietary Preparations (details are given in Part 3)
Aust.: Evista; *Austral.:* Evista; *Belg.:* Evista; *Canad.:* Evista; *Denm.:* Evista; *Fin.:* Evista; *Fr.:* Evista; *Ger.:* Evista; *Irl.:* Evista; *Israel:* Evista; *Ital.:* Evista; Optruma; *Mex.:* Evista; *Neth.:* Evista; *Norw.:* Evista; *NZ:* Evista; *Port.:* Evista; Optruma; *S.Afr.:* Evista; *Singapore:* Evista; *Spain:* Evista; Optruma; *Swed.:* Evista; *Thai.:* Celvista; *UK:* Evista; *USA:* Evista.

Saw Palmetto (921-s)

American Dwarf Palm; *Brahea serrulata*; PA-109; *Sabal serrulata*; *Serenoa repens*; *Serenoa serrulatum*.

$ATC — G04CX02$.

Pharmacopoeias. In USNF.

The dried fruit of the American dwarf palm, *Serenoa repens* (Arecaceae).

Pharmacopoeial description
USNF 20: The partially dried, ripe fruit of *Serenoa repens* (Arecaceae). Store in airtight containers. Protect from light.

Profile
Saw palmetto contains various steroidal compounds with antiandrogenic and oestrogenic activities, one of which is sitosterol (p.970). Saw palmetto is used for the treatment of benign prostatic hyperplasia. Preparations of alcoholic or lipophilic extracts have typically been administered in doses of 160 mg twice daily, or 320 mg once daily, by mouth.

Adverse effects. EFFECTS ON THE LIVER. Cholestatic hepatitis occurred in a man who took a herbal preparation containing saw palmetto for 2 weeks to treat nocturia and hesitancy.[1]

1. Hamid S, *et al.* Protracted cholestatic hepatitis after the use of Prostata. *Ann Intern Med* 1997; **127:** 169–70.

Uses. BENIGN PROSTATIC HYPERPLASIA. A lipid hexane extract of saw palmetto has been shown to be generally superior to placebo,[1,2] and of similar efficacy to finasteride[3] in the treatment of benign prostatic hyperplasia (p.1477). A meta-analysis of randomised studies of various saw palmetto extracts concluded that they improve urological symptoms and flow measures.[4]

1. Champault G, *et al.* A double-blind trial of an extract of the plant Serenoa repens in benign prostatic hyperplasia. *Br J Clin Pharmacol* 1984; **18:** 461.
2. Plosker GL, Brogden RN. Serenoa repens (Permixon): a review of its pharmacology and therapeutic efficacy in benign prostatic hyperplasia. *Drugs Aging* 1996; **9:** 379–95.
3. Carraro J-C, *et al.* Comparison of phytotherapy (Permixon) with finasteride in the treatment of benign prostate hyperplasia: a randomized international study of 1,098 patients. *Prostate* 1996; **29:** 231–40.
4. Wilt T, *et al.* Serenoa repens for benign prostatic hyperplasia (updated 24 May 2001). Available in The Cochrane Library; Issue 3. Oxford: Update Software; 2001.

Preparations

Proprietary Preparations (details are given in Part 3)
Aust.: Permixon; Talso†; *Austral.:* Bioglan Pro-Guard; Prosta; *Belg.:* Prosta-Urgenin; Prostaserene; *Fr.:* Capistan†; *Ger.:* Eviprostat-S; Prosta Urgenin Uno; Prostess; Remiprostan uno; Sabacur uno; Sabal; Sabal uno; Sabalvit; Sita; Steiprostat; Strogen; SX Sabal; Talso; Valverde Sabal; *Ital.:* Permixon; Proser; Prosteren; Rilaprost; Saba; Sere-Mit; Serpens; *Mex.:* Permixon; Prostex; Urogutt; *Port.:* Permixon; *Singapore:* Permixon; *Spain:* Permixon; Sereprostat; *Switz.:* Permixon Novum; Prosta-Urgenine; Prostasan; *Thai.:* Permixon; Urogutt; *UK:* Sabalin.

Multi-ingredient: *Aust.:* Prostagutt; Spasmo-Urgenin; Urgenin; *Austral.:* Bioglan Mens Super Soy/Clover; Extralife Flow-Care; Lifechange Mens Complex with Saw Palmetto; Serenoa Complex; Urapro; Urgenin; Urinase; *Belg.:* Urgenin; *Fr.:* Sabal; Salucur; *Ger.:* Cefasabal; Nephroselect M; Prosta Fink N; *Hong Kong:* Urgenin; *Israel:* Urgenin; *Ital.:* Biothymus M Urto; *Port.:* Neo Urgenin†; Spasmo-Urgenin; *S.Afr.:* Spasmo-Urgenin; *Spain:* Neo Urgenin; Spasmo-Urgenin; *Switz.:* Phytomed Prosta; Prosta-Caps Chassot N; Prosta-Caps Fink; Prostagutt-F; Urgenine†; *Thai.:* Spasmo-Urgenin; *UK:* Antiglan; Daily Fatigue Relief; Damiana and Kola Tablets; Elixir Damiana and Saw Palmetto; Regina Royal Concorde; Serenoa-C; Strength.

Stanozolol (9104-h)

Stanozolol *(BAN, USAN, rINN)*.

Androstanazole; Methylstanazole; NSC-43193; Stanozololum; Win-14833. 17α-Methyl-2′H-5α-androst-2-eno[3,2-c]pyrazol-17β-ol.

$C_{21}H_{32}N_2O = 328.5$.

$CAS — 10418-03-8$.

$ATC — A14AA02$.

Pharmacopoeias. In Eur. (see p.vi) and US.

Pharmacopoeial description
Ph. Eur.: A white or almost white, hygroscopic crystalline powder. It exhibits polymorphism. Practically insoluble in water; slightly soluble in alcohol; very slightly soluble in dichloromethane; soluble in dimethylformamide. Store in airtight containers. Protect from light.

USP 25: An odourless crystalline powder occurring in 2 forms; needles melt at about 155° and prisms at about 235°. Insoluble in water; soluble 1 in 41 of alcohol, 1 in 74 of chloroform, and 1 in 370 of ether; slightly soluble in acetone and in ethyl acetate; soluble in dimethylformamide; very slightly soluble in benzene. Store in airtight containers. Protect from light.

Adverse Effects and Precautions
As for androgens and anabolic steroids in general (see Testosterone, p.1492). As with other 17α-alkylated compounds stanozolol may produce hepatotoxicity, and liver function should be monitored. It is probably best avoided in patients with hepatic impairment, and certainly if this is severe. Haematocrit and haemoglobin concentrations should also be monitored.

Because of its androgenic effects some recommend that stanozolol should not be used to treat hereditary angioedema in premenopausal women except in life-threatening situations.

Effects on the liver. Some reports of jaundice associated with stanozolol.[1,2]

1. Slater SD, *et al.* Jaundice induced by stanozolol hypersensitivity. *Postgrad Med J* 1976; **52:** 229–32.
2. Evely RS, *et al.* Severe cholestasis associated with stanozolol. *BMJ* 1987; **294:** 612–13.

Effects on the nervous system. Benign intracranial hypertension developed in an elderly woman receiving stanozolol; CSF pressure returned to normal after stanozolol was discontinued.[1]

1. Tully MP, *et al.* Intracranial hypertension associated with stanozolol. *DICP Ann Pharmacother* 1990; **24:** 1234.

Porphyria. Stanozolol is considered to be unsafe in patients with porphyria because it has been shown to be porphyrinogenic in *animals*.

Interactions
As mentioned under Testosterone, p.1493, anabolic steroids may enhance the activity of a number of drugs. For the effect of stanozolol on some anticoagulants, see p.997.

Uses and Administration
Stanozolol has anabolic and androgenic properties (see Testosterone, p.1493). It is used in the treatment of vascular manifestations of Behçet's syndrome in usual doses of 10 mg daily by mouth.

In the management of hereditary angioedema, an initial dose of 2.5 to 10 mg daily by mouth is given to prevent attacks. The dosage may then be reduced, according to the patient's response; maintenance doses of 2 mg daily or on alternate days, or 2.5 mg three times weekly have been used successfully. In the UK the initial daily dose by mouth for children is 2.5 mg for those aged 1 to 6 years and 2.5 to 5 mg for those aged 6 to 12 years. However, in the USA doses of 1 mg daily for children under 6 years and up to 2 mg in those aged 6 to 12 years have been suggested.

As with other anabolic steroids, stanozolol has been used for breast cancer in postmenopausal women, and for anaemias, osteoporosis, and catabolic disorders. Stanozolol has also been given by intramuscular injection in doses of 50 mg every 2 or 3 weeks.

Hereditary angioedema. Stanozolol has been used successfully to prevent attacks of hereditary angioedema (p.743).
References.

1. Sheffer AL, *et al.* Hereditary angioedema: a decade of management with stanozolol. *J Allergy Clin Immunol* 1987; **80:** 855–60.

Vascular disorders. Stanozolol is used in the treatment of vascular manifestations of Behçet's syndrome (p.1047). It has also been reported to promote fibrinolysis in vascular disorders, including long-standing liposclerosis of the leg,[1-3] necrobiosis lipoidica,[4] Raynaud's syndrome,[5,6] systemic sclerosis,[6] idiopathic recurrent superficial thrombophlebitis,[7] leg ulcers due to cryofibrinogenaemia,[8] and venous ulceration.[9-11] Most of these studies were noncomparative and in small numbers of patients, and results have been variable.

1. Browse NL, *et al.* Treatment of liposclerosis of the leg by fibrinolytic enhancement: a preliminary report. *BMJ* 1977; **2:** 434–5.
2. Burnand K, *et al.* Venous lipodermatosclerosis: treatment by fibrinolytic enhancement and elastic compression. *BMJ* 1980; **280:** 7–11.
3. Muston HL. Treatment of liposclerosis. *BMJ* 1980; **280:** 254–5 [criticism].
4. Rhodes EL. Fibrinolytic agents in the treatment of necrobiosis lipoidica. *Br J Dermatol* 1976; **95:** 673–4.
5. Jarrett PEM, *et al.* Treatment of Raynaud's phenomenon by fibrinolytic enhancement. *BMJ* 1978; **2:** 523–5.
6. Jayson MIV, *et al.* A controlled study of stanozolol in primary Raynaud's phenomenon and systemic sclerosis. *Ann Rheum Dis* 1991; **50:** 41–7.
7. Jarrett PEM, *et al.* Idiopathic recurrent superficial thrombophlebitis: treatment with fibrinolytic enhancement. *BMJ* 1977; **1:** 933–4.
8. Falanga V, *et al.* Stanozolol in treatment of leg ulcers due to cryofibrinogenaemia. *Lancet* 1991; **338:** 347–8.
9. Anonymous. Does stanozolol prevent venous ulceration? *Drug Ther Bull* 1985; **23:** 91–2.
10. Browse NL, Burnand KG. Getting the balance right. *BMJ* 1986; **292:** 825 [criticism].
11. Herxheimer A. Getting the balance right. *BMJ* 1986; **292:** 1014 [reply].

Preparations

BP 2001: Stanozolol Tablets;
USP 25: Stanozolol Tablets.

Proprietary Preparations (details are given in Part 3)
Belg.: Stromba; Strombaject; *Irl.:* Stromba; *Neth.:* Stromba; *Spain:* Winstrol; *UK:* Stromba; *USA:* Winstrol.

Multi-ingredient: *Thai.:* Cetabon.

Testis Extracts   (11567-p)

Testicular Extracts.

Profile

Testis extracts are usually of bovine origin and have been used in a variety of disorders. They have been given parenterally to elderly men as androgenic supplements. They have also been used topically, often in preparations containing other mammalian tissue extracts, in the treatment of peripheral circulatory or musculoskeletal disorders.

Preparations

Proprietary Preparations (details are given in Part 3)
Aust.: Testiculi; *Ger.:* Orchibion.

Multi-ingredient: *Canad.:* Heracline; Revitonus C; *Ger.:* Intradermi N; poliomyelan; tactu-nerval; *Hong Kong:* Wari-Procomil; *Thai.:* Wari-Procomil.

Testosterone   (9108-g)

Testosterone (BAN, rINN).
17β-Hydroxyandrost-4-en-3-one.
$C_{19}H_{28}O_2 = 288.4$.
CAS — 58-22-0.
ATC — G03BA03.
Pharmacopoeias. In *Eur.* (see p.vi) and *US.*

Pharmacopoeial description

Ph. Eur.: A white crystalline powder, or colourless or yellowish-white crystals. Practically insoluble in water and in fatty oils; freely soluble in alcohol and in dichloromethane. Protect from light.
USP 25: White or slightly creamy-white, odourless, crystals or crystalline powder. Practically insoluble in water; soluble 1 in 6 of dehydrated alcohol, 1 in 2 of chloroform, and 1 in 100 of ether; soluble in dioxan and in vegetable oils.

Testosterone Cipionate   (9110-d)

Testosterone Cipionate (BANM, rINNM).
Testosterone Cyclopentylpropionate; Testosterone Cypionate. 3-Oxoandrost-4-en-17β-yl 3-cyclopentylpropionate; 17β-Hydroxyandrost-4-en-3-one cyclopentanepropionate; 17β-(3-Cyclopentyl-1-oxopropoxy)androst-4-en-3-one.
$C_{27}H_{40}O_3 = 412.6$.
CAS — 58-20-8.
Pharmacopoeias. In *US.*

Pharmacopoeial description

USP 25: A white or creamy-white powder, odourless or has a slight odour. Insoluble in water; freely soluble in alcohol, in chloroform, in dioxan, and in ether; soluble in vegetable oils. Protect from light.

Testosterone Decanoate   (9111-n)

Testosterone Decanoate (BANM, rINNM).
3-Oxoandrost-4-en-17β-yl decanoate; 17β-Hydroxyandrost-4-en-3-one decanoate.
$C_{29}H_{46}O_3 = 442.7$.
CAS — 5721-91-5.
Pharmacopoeias. In *Br.*

Pharmacopoeial description

BP 2001: White to creamy-white crystals or crystalline powder. Practically insoluble in water; very soluble in alcohol and in chloroform. Store at a temperature not exceeding 15°. Protect from light.

Testosterone Enantate   (9112-h)

Testosterone Enantate (BANM, rINNM).
NSC-17591; Testosterone Enanthate; Testosterone Heptanoate; Testosteroni Enantas. 3-Oxoandrost-4-en-17β-yl heptanoate; 17β-Hydroxyandrost-4-en-3-one heptanoate.
$C_{26}H_{40}O_3 = 400.6$.
CAS — 315-37-7.
Pharmacopoeias. In *Eur.* (see p.vi), *Int., Jpn, Pol.,* and *US.*

Pharmacopoeial description

Ph. Eur.: A white or yellowish-white crystalline powder. Practically insoluble in water; very soluble in dehydrated alcohol and in ether; freely soluble in fatty oils. Store at a temperature of 2° to 8°. Protect from light.
USP 25: A white or creamy-white crystalline powder. It is odourless or has a faint odour characteristic of heptanoic acid. Insoluble in water; very soluble in ether; soluble in vegetable oils. Store in a cool place.

Testosterone Isocaproate   (9113-m)

Testosterone Isocaproate (BANM, rINNM).
Testosterone Isohexanoate. 3-Oxoandrost-4-en-17β-yl 4-methylpentanoate; 17β-Hydroxyandrost-4-en-3-one 4-methylpentanoate.
$C_{25}H_{38}O_3 = 386.6$.
CAS — 15262-86-9.
Pharmacopoeias. In *Br.*

Pharmacopoeial description

BP 2001: White to creamy-white crystals or crystalline powder. Practically insoluble in water; very soluble in alcohol and in chloroform. Store at a temperature not exceeding 15°. Protect from light.

Testosterone Phenylpropionate   (9114-b)

Testosterone Phenylpropionate (BANM, rINNM).
3-Oxoandrost-4-en-17β-yl 3-phenylpropionate; 17β-Hydroxyandrost-4-en-3-one 3-phenylpropionate.
$C_{28}H_{36}O_3 = 420.6$.
CAS — 1255-49-8.
Pharmacopoeias. In *BP(Vet).*

Pharmacopoeial description

BP(Vet) 2001: A white to almost white crystalline powder with a characteristic odour. Practically insoluble in water; sparingly soluble in alcohol. Protect from light.

Testosterone Propionate   (9115-v)

Testosterone Propionate (BANM, rINNM).
NSC-9166; Testosteroni Propionas. 3-Oxoandrost-4-en-17β-yl propionate; 17β-Hydroxyandrost-4-en-3-one propionate.
$C_{22}H_{32}O_3 = 344.5$.
CAS — 57-85-2.
Pharmacopoeias. In *Chin., Eur.* (see p.vi), *Int., Jpn, Pol.,* and *US.*

Pharmacopoeial description

Ph. Eur.: A white or almost white powder or colourless crystals. Practically insoluble in water; freely soluble in alcohol, in acetone, and in methyl alcohol; soluble in fatty oils. Protect from light.
USP 25: White or creamy-white, odourless, crystals or crystalline powder. Insoluble in water; freely soluble in alcohol, in dioxan, in ether, and in other organic solvents; soluble in vegetable oils. Protect from light.

Testosterone Undecylate   (9116-g)

Testosterone Undecylate (rINNM).
Testosterone Undecanoate (BANM). 3-Oxoandrost-4-en-17β-yl undecanoate; 17β-Hydroxyandrost-4-en-3-one undecanoate.
$C_{30}H_{48}O_3 = 456.7$.
CAS — 5949-44-0.

Adverse Effects

Testosterone and other **androgens** may give rise to side-effects which can be related to their androgenic or anabolic activities. They include increased retention of nitrogen, sodium, and water, oedema, increased vascularity of the skin, hypercalcaemia, im-

paired glucose tolerance, and increased bone growth and skeletal weight. Other effects include increased low-density-lipoprotein cholesterol, decreased high-density-lipoprotein cholesterol, increased haematocrit, and increased fibrinolytic activity. Androgens may cause headache, depression, and gastrointestinal bleeding. It has been suggested that androgens may induce sleep apnoea in susceptible patients.

Abnormal liver function tests may occur and there have been reports of liver toxicity including jaundice and cholestatic hepatitis. There have also been reports of peliosis hepatis and hepatic tumours in patients who have received high doses over prolonged periods. These adverse hepatic effects have occurred primarily with the 17α-alkylated derivatives (e.g. methyltestosterone, stanozolol).

In men, large doses suppress spermatogenesis and cause degenerative changes in the seminiferous tubules. Priapism is a sign of excessive dosage and may occur especially in elderly males. Gynaecomastia may occur. Androgens may cause prostatic hyperplasia and accelerate the growth of malignant neoplasms of the prostate.

In women, the inhibitory action of androgens on the activity of the anterior pituitary results in the suppression of ovarian activity and menstruation. Continued use produces symptoms of virilism, such as hirsutism or male-pattern baldness, deepening of the voice, atrophy of the breasts and endometrial tissue, oily skin, acne, and hypertrophy of the clitoris; libido is increased and lactation suppressed. Virilisation may not be reversible, even after stopping therapy.

Large and repeated doses in early puberty may cause closure of the epiphyses and stop linear growth. Children may experience symptoms of virilisation: in boys there may be precocious sexual development with phallic enlargement and increased frequency of erection, and in girls, clitoral enlargement. Gynaecomastia may also occur in boys.

Masculinisation of the external genitalia of the female fetus may occur if androgens are given during pregnancy.

Following transdermal application of testosterone, skin reactions may include irritation, erythema, allergic contact dermatitis, and sometimes burn-like lesions. Skin reactions are more common with patches that contain permeation enhancers.

The **anabolic steroids**, because they generally retain some androgenic activity, share the adverse effects of the androgens described above, but their virilising effects, especially in women, are usually less. There have been reports of adverse psychiatric effects in athletes taking large doses to try and improve performance. For adverse effects following the misuse of anabolic steroids, see Abuse under Precautions, below.

Carcinogenicity. Reports of malignant neoplasms associated with testosterone therapy have included prostatic cancer (with testosterone cipionate therapy),[1] and renal cell carcinoma (testosterone ester unspecified).[2] Concern has been expressed[3] about the possibility that long-term use of testosterone esters for male contraception may lead to an increase in the number of cases of prostatic cancer or benign prostatic hyperplasia. For reference to hepatic malignancies associated with androgens and anabolic steroids, see Effects on the Liver, below.

1. Jackson JA, *et al.* Prostatic complications of testosterone replacement therapy. *Arch Intern Med* 1989; **149:** 2365–6.
2. Rosner F, Khan MT. Renal cell carcinoma following prolonged testosterone therapy. *Arch Intern Med* 1992; **152:** 426, 429.
3. Schally AV, Comaru-Schally AM. Male contraception involving testosterone supplementation: possible increased risks of prostate cancer? *Lancet* 1987; **i:** 448–9.

Effects on the cardiovascular system. A cerebrovascular accident has been reported in a young man following the overzealous self-administration of testosterone enantate intramuscularly for hypogonadism.[1] It was noted that thromboembolic complications are not generally recognised as side-effects of androgen therapy although there is some experimental evidence that testosterone stimulates thrombus formation.

1. Nagelberg SB, *et al.* Cerebrovascular accident associated with testosterone therapy in a 21-year-old hypogonadal man. *N Engl J Med* 1986; **314:** 649–50.

Effects on the liver. As mentioned above, hepatotoxicity including elevations in liver enzymes, hepatic cholestasis and jaundice, and rarely peliosis hepatis and hepatic tumours has occurred on administration of androgens and anabolic steroids, particularly the 17α-alkylated derivatives. Prolonged treatment and high doses may be significant contributory factors. Tumours have included hepatocellular carcinomas, benign adenomas, and less commonly angiosarcomas and cholangiocarcinomas. Tumours and peliosis may regress on discontinuation of therapy, but they can also progress to liver failure and death. Some reviews of the hepatic effects of androgens and anabolic steroids are cited below.[1-4] There has been a specific report of benign hepatic adenoma in a patient treated with testosterone enantate for 11 years,[5] and of hepatocellular carcinoma in a patient receiving testosterone enantate and methyltestosterone.[6] Further specific references may be found under individual drug monographs.

1. Bagheri SA, Boyer JL. Peliosis hepatis associated with androgenic-anabolic steroid therapy. *Ann Intern Med* 1974; **81:** 610–18.
2. Ishak KG, Zimmerman HJ. Hepatotoxic effects of the anabolic/androgenic steroids. *Semin Liver Dis* 1987; **7:** 230–6.
3. Sooe KL, *et al.* Liver pathology associated with the use of anabolic-androgenic steroids. *Liver* 1992; **12:** 73–9.
4. Touraine RL, *et al.* Hepatic tumours during androgen therapy in Fanconi anaemia. *Eur J Pediatr* 1993; **152:** 691–3.
5. Carrasco D, *et al.* Hepatic adenomata and androgen treatment. *Ann Intern Med* 1984; **100:** 316.
6. Johnson FL. *et al.* Association of androgenic-anabolic steroid therapy with development of hepatocellular carcinoma. *Lancet* 1972; **ii:** 1273–6.

Effects on sexual function. Reports of severe priapism following the administration of testosterone for the management of delayed puberty.[1,2]

1. Zelissen PMJ, Stricker BHC. Severe priapism as a complication of testosterone substitution therapy. *Am J Med* 1988; **85:** 273–4.
2. Ruch W, Jenny P. Priapism following testosterone administration for delayed male puberty. *Am J Med* 1989; **86:** 256.

Precautions

Testosterone and other androgens and anabolic steroids should be used cautiously in patients with cardiovascular disorders, renal or hepatic impairment, epilepsy, migraine, diabetes mellitus or other conditions which may be aggravated by the possible fluid retention or oedema caused. They should not be given to patients with hypercalcaemia or hypercalciuria, and should be used cautiously in conditions in which there is a risk of these developing such as skeletal metastases. The use of the 17α-alkylated derivatives, which are associated with an increased risk of hepatotoxicity, is probably best avoided in patients with hepatic impairment, and certainly if this is severe. Hepatic function should be monitored during therapy.

In men, androgens and anabolic steroids should not be given to those with carcinoma of the breast or prostate (although in women they have been used in the treatment of certain breast carcinomas). The prostate should be examined regularly during treatment.

Androgens and anabolic steroids should not be given during pregnancy because of the risk of virilisation of the female fetus. They should be avoided in women who are breast feeding.

Androgens and anabolic steroids should be used with extreme care in children because of the masculinising effects and also because premature closure of the epiphyses may occur resulting in inhibited linear growth and small stature. Skeletal maturation should be monitored during therapy.

Androgens and anabolic steroids may interfere with a number of clinical laboratory tests such as those for glucose tolerance and thyroid function.

Abuse. The adverse effects arising from the illicit use of androgens and anabolic steroids by athletes, often taken together at doses well in excess of those used therapeutically, have been discussed.[1-4] Effects have included abnormal liver function and hepatic neoplasms (see also Effects on the Liver, above), an atherogenic blood lipid profile[5] and increased risk of cardiovascular disease,[6] and reduced glucose tolerance. Hypogonadal states are commonly induced (azoospermia or oligospermia and testicular atrophy in men, and amenorrhoea or oligomenorrhoea in women). Gynaecomastia is relatively common in men, and virilisation in women. Psychiatric disturbances such as mania, hypomania, depression, aggression, and emotional lability, have been described.[7,8] There is also some evidence that dependence associated with an acute withdrawal syndrome can occur.[9,10] Rare reports include alterations in immune response,[11,12] bleeding oesophageal varices,[13] tendon damage,[14] renal cell carcinoma,[15] and peliosis hepatis.[16]

There has been some dispute about the methods used to detect abuse of certain anabolic steroids in athletes; a study in healthy subjects has apparently confirmed endogenous production of small amounts of nandrolone metabolites.[17]

1. American Medical Association Council on Scientific Affairs. Drug abuse in athletes: anabolic steroids and human growth hormone. *JAMA* 1988; **259:** 1703–5.
2. Hallagan JB, *et al.* Anabolic-androgenic steroid use by athletes. *N Engl J Med* 1989; **321:** 1042–5.
3. Graham S, Kennedy M. Recent developments in the toxicology of anabolic steroids. *Drug Safety* 1990; **5:** 458–76.
4. Kennedy M. Drugs and athletes—an update. *Adverse Drug React Bull* 1994; (Dec): 639–42.
5. Glazer G. Atherogenic effects of anabolic steroids on serum lipid levels. *Arch Intern Med* 1991; **151:** 1925–33.
6. Madea G, Grellner W. Long-term cardiovascular effects of anabolic steroids. *Lancet* 1998; **352:** 33.
7. Su T-P, *et al.* Neuropsychiatric effects of anabolic steroids in male normal volunteers. *JAMA* 1993; **269:** 2760–4.
8. Pope HG, Katz DL. Psychiatric and medical effects of anabolic-androgenic steroid use: a controlled study of 160 athletes. *Arch Gen Psychiatry* 1994; **51:** 375–82.
9. Kashkin KB, Kleber HD. Hooked on hormones: an anabolic steroid addiction hypothesis. *JAMA* 1989; **262:** 3166–70.
10. Brower KJ, *et al.* Evidence for physical and psychological dependence on anabolic androgenic steroids in eight weight lifters. *Am J Psychiatry* 1990; **147:** 510–12.
11. Widder RA, *et al.* Candida albicans endophthalmitis after anabolic steroid abuse. *Lancet* 1995; **345:** 330–1.
12. Johnson AS, *et al.* Severe chickenpox in an anabolic steroid user. *Lancet* 1995; **345:** 1447–8.
13. Winwood PJ, *et al.* Bleeding oesophageal varices associated with anabolic steroid use in an athlete. *Postgrad Med J* 1990; **66:** 864–5.
14. Laseter JT, Russell JA. Anabolic steroid-induced tendon pathology: a review of the literature. *Med Sci Sports Exerc* 1991; **23:** 1–3.
15. Bryden AAG, *et al.* Anabolic steroid abuse and renal-cell carcinoma. *Lancet* 1995; **346:** 1306–7.
16. Cabasso A. Peliosis hepatis in a young adult bodybuilder. *Med Sci Sports Exerc* 1994; **26:** 2–4.
17. Reznik Y, *et al.* Urinary nandrolone metabolites of endogenous origin in man: a confirmation by output regulation under human chorionic gonadotropin stimulation. *J Clin Endocrinol Metab* 2001; **86:** 146–50.

Porphyria. Androgens are considered to be unsafe in patients with porphyria although there is conflicting experimental evidence of porphyrinogenicity.

A female patient with acute intermittent porphyria (p.1011) who suffered from severe attacks pre-menstrually was successfully managed with subcutaneous implants of testosterone when suppression of the menstrual cycle with buserelin met with limited success.[1]

1. Savage MW, *et al.* Acute intermittent porphyria treated by testosterone implant. *Postgrad Med J* 1992; **68:** 479–81.

Pregnancy. Reports of female fetal virilisation following maternal use of testosterone[1] or methyltestosterone[2] during pregnancy.

1. Reschini E, *et al.* Female pseudohermaphroditism due to maternal androgen administration: 25-year follow-up. *Lancet* 1985; **i:** 1226.
2. Dewhurst J, Gordon RR. Fertility following change of sex. *Lancet* 1984; **ii:** 1461.

Veterinary use. It was considered unnecessary to establish an acceptable daily intake or acceptable residual level in food for endogenous hormones such as testosterone. Residues resulting from the use of testosterone as a growth promotor in accordance with good animal husbandry practice are unlikely to pose a hazard to human health.[1] However, it should be noted that, in the European Union the use of androgens in veterinary practice is restricted and their use as growth promotors is banned. In addition, the use of anabolic steroids is banned in animals intended for human consumption.

1. FAO/WHO. Evaluation of certain veterinary drug residues in food: thirty-second report of the joint FAO/WHO expert committee on food additives. *WHO Tech Rep Ser 763* 1988.

Interactions

Testosterone and other androgens and anabolic steroids have been reported to enhance the activity of a number of drugs, with resulting increases in toxicity. Drugs affected include ciclosporin (see p.522), antidiabetics, thyroxine [levothyroxine] (see p.1528), and anticoagulants such as warfarin (see p.997). Resistance to the effects of neuromuscular blockers (p.1335) has also been reported.

Pharmacokinetics

Testosterone is absorbed from the gastrointestinal tract, the skin, and the oral mucosa. However, testosterone undergoes extensive first-pass hepatic metabolism when administered by mouth and is therefore usually administered intramuscularly, subcutaneously, or transdermally. In addition, the basic molecule of testosterone has been modified to produce orally active compounds and to extend the duration of action. Alkylation of the 17α position produces compounds that are more slowly metabolised by the liver, and hence may be administered orally. Esterification of the 17β hydroxyl group increases lipid solubility and results in slower systemic absorption following intramuscular administration. The rate of absorption of the esters is related to the size of the ester group. The undecylate ester undergoes less complete inactivation after oral administration due to distribution into the lymphatic system. Testosterone esters are hydrolysed to testosterone following absorption.

Testosterone is about 80% bound to sex-hormone binding globulin. Derivatives of 19-nortestosterone and 17-α-methylated compounds have reduced binding to this globulin. The plasma half-life of testosterone is reported to range from about 10 to 100 minutes. It is largely metabolised in the liver via oxidation at the 17-OH group with the formation of androstenedione, which is further metabolised to the weakly androgenic androsterone and inactive etiocholanolone which are excreted in the urine mainly as glucuronides and sulfates. About 6% is excreted unchanged in the faeces after undergoing enterohepatic recirculation. Testosterone is converted to the more active dihydrotestosterone in some target organs by 5α-reductase. 19-Nortestosterone derivatives appear to be less susceptible to this enzyme. Small amounts of testosterone are aromatised to form oestrogenic derivatives in the body. Compounds with a saturated A-ring, such as mesterolone, appear to be less likely to be aromatised to oestrogen.

◊ References to the pharmacokinetics of subcutaneous testosterone pellets,[1] scrotal[2,3] and non-scrotal[4,5] transdermal patches, and gel[6] are given below.

1. Handelsman DJ, *et al.* Pharmacokinetics and pharmacodynamics of testosterone pellets in man. *J Clin Endocrinol Metab* 1990; **71:** 216–22.
2. Findlay JC, *et al.* Transdermal delivery of testosterone. *J Clin Endocrinol Metab* 1987; **64:** 266–8.
3. Cunningham GR, *et al.* Testosterone replacement with transdermal therapeutic systems: physiological serum testosterone and elevated dihydrotestosterone levels. *JAMA* 1989; **261:** 2525–30.
4. Meikle AW, *et al.* Pharmacokinetics and metabolism of a permeation-enhanced testosterone transdermal system in hypogonadal men: influence of application site. *J Clin Endocrinol Metab* 1996; **81:** 1832–40.
5. Yu Z, *et al.* Transdermal testosterone administration in hypogonadal men: comparison of pharmacokinetics at different sites of application and at the first and fifth days of application. *J Clin Pharmacol* 1997; **37:** 1129–38.
6. Swerdloff RS, *et al.* Long-term pharmacokinetics of transdermal testosterone gel in hypogonadal men. *J Clin Endocrinol Metab* 2000; **85:** 4500–10.

Uses and Administration

The natural hormone testosterone and its derivatives have anabolic and androgenic properties (for further details, see p.1452).

The primary indication for androgens, such as testosterone or its esters, is as replacement therapy in **male hypogonadal disorders** (p.1274) caused by either pituitary or testicular disorders or in hypogonadism following orchidectomy. Testosterone may be used as a subcutaneous implant in a dose of 100 to 600 mg; plasma concentrations of testosterone are usually maintained within the physiological range for 4 to 5 months with a dose of 600 mg. It may also be administered by transdermal delivery systems. The scrotal patch contains 10 or 15 mg of testosterone and supplies approximately 4 or 6 mg of testosterone in 24 hours. Non-scrotal patches are applied to the back, abdomen, thighs or upper arms to supply 2.5 to 10 mg daily. A hydroalcoholic gel containing 1% testosterone, which is applied daily to the shoulders and upper arms and/or abdomen, is also available. Approximately 10% of the applied dose is absorbed across the skin to provide a systemic dose of testosterone 5 to 10 mg (see also Hypogonadism, below). Testosterone has also been given by intramuscular injection in a dose of up to 50 mg two or three times weekly, but testosterone esters are generally preferred by this route.

The testosterone esters are usually formulated as oily solutions for intramuscular use to give a prolonged duration of action. Suggested doses for the various esters are: 50 to 400 mg every 2 to 4 weeks for the cipionate; 50 to 400 mg every 2 to 4 weeks for the enantate (or an initial dose of 250 mg every 2 to 3 weeks followed by maintenance dosing every 3 to 6 weeks may be employed); and up to 50 mg two or three times weekly for the propionate. The isocaproate, phenylpropionate, and propionate esters may be given as a combined intramuscular preparation, sometimes also containing testosterone decanoate. Testosterone hexahydrobenzoate and testosterone hexahydrobenzylcarbonate have also been used. The undecylate ester is given by mouth in an initial dose of 120 to 160 mg daily for 2 to 3 weeks, followed by a maintenance dose of 40 to 120 mg daily.

Androgens and anabolic steroids have also been used in adolescent males with constitutionally delayed puberty or growth, and anabolic steroids have been used in the treatment of short stature in girls with Turner's syndrome. However, great care is necessary when using androgens for such conditions as bone growth may be inhibited by the early fusion of the epiphyses. This effect has been utilised by the administration of supraphysiological doses of androgens to reduce final height in boys with constitutionally tall stature.

In postmenopausal women androgens, and sometimes anabolic steroids are occasionally used in the hormonal therapy of disseminated breast carcinoma but care should be taken to choose a compound with a lower masculinising effect; the short-acting synthetic compounds are usually preferred for such purposes. Androgens and anabolic steroids have also sometimes been used in conjunction with oestrogens in the management of certain menopausal disorders, but the use of androgens and anabolic steroids in women with osteoporosis is no longer advocated because their adverse effects essentially outweigh any benefit they may produce.

Anabolic steroids, and sometimes androgens, have been used in the treatment of refractory anaemias characterised by deficient red cell production, such as aplastic anaemia. Anabolic steroids and synthetic androgens with an attenuated action (sometimes known as 'attenuated androgens') such as danazol are also used in the management of hereditary angioedema.

Topical androgens may be used in the treatment of lichen sclerosus. Anabolic steroids may be useful to relieve the itching associated with obstructive jaundice.

Androgens and anabolic steroids have been used for their anabolic properties in various catabolic states.

Some testosterone esters are being investigated as male contraceptives.

Testosterone hemisuccinate is an ingredient of preparations promoted for the management of cataracts.

◊ General reviews of androgens and anabolic steroids.
1. Hickson RC, et al. Adverse effects of anabolic steroids. Med Toxicol Adverse Drug Exp 1989; 4: 254–71.
2. Bagatell CJ, Bremner WJ. Androgens in men—uses and abuses. N Engl J Med 1996; 334: 707–14.
3. Conway AJ, et al. Use, misuse and abuse of androgens: the Endocrine Society of Australia consensus guidelines for androgen prescribing. Med J Aust 2000; 172: 220–4.

Anabolic effects. The androgens generally possess anabolic activity and were formerly used to increase weight in patients suffering from emaciation or debilitating diseases but effectiveness was doubtful. The anabolic steroids were developed in order to enhance the ability to build proteins and diminish the virilising and masculinising effects of the natural androgens, but all anabolics retain some androgenic activity. The anabolic steroids have again, like the androgens, been used in an attempt to produce weight gain in cachexia and wasting diseases (p.1481).

The anabolic steroids and androgens have been the subject of much misuse and abuse by athletes, sports persons, and body builders (see under Precautions, above) in an attempt to increase muscle mass and body-weight but such use cannot be justified.

References to the anabolic effects of testosterone.
1. Bhasin S, et al. The effects of supraphysiologic doses of testosterone on muscle size and strength in normal men. N Engl J Med 1996; 335: 1–7.
2. Grinspoon S, et al. Effects of androgen administration in men with the AIDS wasting syndrome: a randomized, double-blind, placebo-controlled trial. Ann Intern Med 1998; 129: 18–26.

Antineoplastic-induced infertility. For reference to the use of testosterone to preserve gonadal function during cyclophosphamide therapy, see Effects on Reproductive Potential, p.528.

Constitutionally delayed puberty. Testosterone enantate given by intramuscular injection every one to two months for periods ranging from 3 months to several years, produced beneficial effects in boys with constitutionally delayed puberty and growth;[1,2] growth rate increased, sexual and skeletal maturation were stimulated, and full height potential did not appear to be compromised. However it has been pointed out that repeated intramuscular injections are painful and are disliked by adolescents;[3] oral testosterone undecylate or oxandrolone have been shown to be effective in the treatment of delayed puberty and growth in boys.[4,5] and may be preferred.[3] It should be noted that giving androgens to boys with constitutional delay of growth and puberty is controversial (see p.1273). For reference to the use of testosterone in boys with delayed puberty due to hypogonadism see below.
1. Donaldson MDC, Savage DCL. Testosterone therapy in boys with delayed puberty. Arch Dis Child 1987; 62: 647–8.

2. Richman RA, Kirsch LR. Testosterone treatment in adolescent boys with constitutional delay in growth and development. N Engl J Med 1988; 319: 1563–7.
3. Kelnar CJH. Treatment of the short, sexually immature adolescent boy. Arch Dis Child 1994; 71: 285–7.
4. Albanese A, et al. Oral treatment for constitutional delay of growth and puberty in boys: a randomised trial of an anabolic steroid or testosterone undecanoate. Arch Dis Child 1994; 71: 315–17.
5. Brown DC, et al. A double blind, placebo controlled study of the effects of low dose testosterone undecanoate on the growth of small for age, prepubertal boys. Arch Dis Child 1995; 73: 131–5.

Constitutionally tall stature. Supraphysiological doses of androgens have been used to *reduce* final height in tall adolescent boys. Testosterone esters in monthly doses of up to 1000 mg have been used. Preliminary evidence after a mean of 10 years follow-up suggests that there was no long-term effect on reproductive function.[1] For reference to the use of testosterone to *increase* growth rate, see Constitutionally Delayed Puberty, above.
1. de Waal WJ, et al. Long term sequelae of sex steroid treatment in the management of constitutionally tall stature. Arch Dis Child 1995; 73: 311–15.

Gender reassignment. Testosterone is used in female-to-male transsexuals to develop and maintain secondary sexual characteristics. Suggested doses of the cipionate and enantate esters are 200 mg intramuscularly every 2 weeks.

Hypogonadism. Replacement therapy with testosterone or a testosterone ester is the standard treatment for primary hypogonadism in men (see p.1274). The androgen is often given as an intramuscular depot injection of one of the esters, although subcutaneous implants and oral formulations are also employed, and, more recently, transdermal systems and a topical gel have been developed (for doses see above).[1-7] A sublingual testosterone tablet is under investigation. Testosterone is also used to promote masculinisation in hypogonadal adolescent boys,[8,9] and is of value in the treatment of osteoporosis in hypogonadal men.[10] Testosterone has a negative feedback effect on gonadotrophin secretion, therefore any remaining spermatogenesis is generally suppressed; androgens are thus rarely useful in reversing male infertility (p.1275).

Transdermal testosterone may possibly be of benefit as an adjunct to oestrogen replacement in women who have undergone hysterectomy and oophorectomy.[11]
1. Bals-Pratch M, et al. Transdermal testosterone substitution therapy for male hypogonadism. Lancet 1986; ii: 943–6.
2. Korenman SG, et al. Androgen therapy of hypogonadal men with transscrotal testosterone systems. Am J Med 1987; 83: 471–8.
3. Findlay JC, et al. Treatment of primary hypogonadism in men by the transdermal administration of testosterone. J Clin Endocrinol Metab 1989; 68: 369–73.
4. Anonymous. Testosterone patches for hypogonadism. Med Lett Drugs Ther 1996; 38: 49–50.
5. Arver S, et al. Improvement of sexual function in testosterone deficient men treated for 1 year with a permeation enhanced testosterone transdermal system. J Urol (Baltimore) 1996; 155: 1604–8.
6. Anonymous. Replacing testosterone in men. Drug Ther Bull 1999; 37: 3–5.
7. Wang C, et al. Transdermal testosterone gel improves sexual function, mood, muscle strength, and body composition parameters in hypogonadal men. J Clin Endocrinol Metab 2000; 85: 2839–53.
8. Moorthy B, et al. Depot testosterone in boys with anorchia or gonadotrophin deficiency: effect on growth rate and adult height. Arch Dis Child 1991; 66: 197–9.
9. Zacharin MR, Warne GL. Treatment of hypogonadal adolescent boys with long acting subcutaneous testosterone pellets. Arch Dis Child 1997; 76: 495–9.
10. Finkelstein JS, et al. Increases in bone density during treatment of men with idiopathic hypogonadotropic hypogonadism. J Clin Endocrinol Metab 1989; 69: 776–83.
11. Shifren JL, et al. Transdermal testosterone treatment in women with impaired sexual function after oophorectomy. N Engl J Med 2000; 343: 682–8.

Lichen sclerosus. Topical androgens such as androstanolone and testosterone have been used to treat pruritus associated with vulvar lichen sclerosus in postmenopausal women.[1-4] However, a topical corticosteroid is likely to be preferred[5] (p.1054).
1. Friedrich EG, Kalra PS. Serum levels of sex hormones in vulvar lichen sclerosus, and the effect of topical testosterone. N Engl J Med 1984; 310: 488–91.
2. Paslin D. Treatment of lichen sclerosus with topical dihydrotestosterone. Obstet Gynecol 1991; 78: 1046–9.
3. Paslin D. Androgens in the topical treatment of lichen sclerosus. Int J Dermatol 1996; 35: 298–301.
4. Bracco GL, et al. Clinical and histologic effects of topical treatments of vulval lichen sclerosus: a critical evaluation. J Reprod Med 1993; 38: 37–40.
5. Powell JJ, Wojnarowska F. Lichen sclerosus. Lancet 1999; 353: 1777–83.

Male contraception. In male contraceptive trials it was found that high-dose testosterone severely reduced sperm production.[1] In those in whom azoospermia was not induced there was oligozoospermia with remaining sperm having a markedly diminished fertilising capacity. In a multicentre study carried out by the WHO[2] involving 271 healthy fertile men, weekly intramuscular injection of testosterone enantate 200 mg produced azoospermia in 157 men within 6 months. In a subsequent 12-month study of these azoospermic men, during which time testosterone enantate was the only contraceptive measure used, there was only 1 pregnancy. Spermatogenesis was re-established on withdrawal of testosterone. These findings have been confirmed in a larger trial of the same regimen, which ad-

ditionally assessed contraceptive efficacy in men who achieved oligozoospermia (less than 3×10^6 per mL).[3] No pregnancies occurred in couples where the man was azoospermic. However, the pregnancy rate was 8.1 per 100-person-years in the subgroup of couples where the man was oligozoospermic. This rate is sixfold higher than is generally seen with hormonal contraceptives in women.[4] Both studies found that consistent azoospermia was achieved in a higher percentage of Asian men (95%) than Western men (70%).[4]

An alternative approach being investigated is the suppression of spermatogenesis with a progestogen such as desogestrel combined with low-dose testosterone.

For a general discussion on choice of contraceptive method, including mention of male contraception, see p.1460.
1. Matsumoto AM. Is high dosage testosterone an effective male contraceptive agent? Fertil Steril 1988; 50: 324–8.
2. WHO Task Force on Methods for the Regulation of Male Fertility. Contraceptive efficacy of testosterone-induced azoospermia in normal men. Lancet 1990; 336: 955–9.
3. WHO Task Force on Methods for the Regulation of Male Fertility. Contraceptive efficacy of testosterone-induced azoospermia and oligozoospermia in normal men. Fertil Steril 1996; 65: 821–9.
4. Anonymous. An androgen contraceptive for men: preliminary findings. WHO Drug Inf 1996; 10: 50–3.

Menopausal hormone replacement therapy. In the UK menopausal women are sometimes given implants of testosterone (in a dose of 50 to 100 mg every 4 to 8 months) as an adjunct to menopausal HRT (p.1460). In the USA, preparations containing an androgen and an oestrogen are available for the treatment of menopausal vasomotor symptoms, but there is conflicting opinion as to their usefulness, and further data are needed.[1] For mention of the use of transdermal testosterone in women who have undergone oophorectomy see under Hypogonadism, above.
1. Abraham D, Carpenter PC. Issues concerning androgen replacement therapy in postmenopausal women. Mayo Clin Proc 1997; 72: 1051–5.

Rheumatoid arthritis. A hypogonadic condition characterised by low serum-testosterone concentrations appears to be associated with at least the active stages of rheumatoid arthritis (p.9) in men.[1] Clinical improvement and reductions in IgM rheumatoid factor concentration, tender joint count, and the daily dosage of NSAIDs required, were observed in men with rheumatoid arthritis given oral testosterone undecylate 40 mg three times daily for 6 months. Improvements in rheumatoid arthritis were also seen in 12 of 36 postmenopausal women treated with intramuscular testosterone 50 mg plus progesterone 2.5 mg once every 2 weeks compared with 2 of 32 women receiving placebo.[2]
1. Cutolo M, et al. Androgen replacement therapy in male patients with rheumatoid arthritis. Arthritis Rheum 1991; 34: 1–5.
2. Booij A, et al. Androgens as adjuvant treatment in postmenopausal female patients with rheumatoid arthritis. Ann Rheum Dis 1996; 55: 811–15.

Preparations

BP 2001: Testosterone Implants; Testosterone Propionate Injection;
USP 25: Testosterone Cypionate Injection; Testosterone Enanthate Injection; Testosterone Injectable Suspension; Testosterone Propionate Injection.

Proprietary Preparations (details are given in Part 3)

Aust.: Andriol; Testoderm; Testotop†; Testoviron 250; *Austral.:* Andriol; Androderm; Primoteston Depot; Sustanon 100; Sustanon 250; *Belg.:* Sustanon; Testoderm; Testoviron; Undestor; *Braz.:* Androxon; Deposteron; Testiormina; Tesurene; *Canad.:* Andriol; Delatestryl; Malogen Aqueous†; Malogen in Oil†; Malogex†; Scheinpharm Testone-Cyp†; *Denm.:* Atmos; Restandol; Testoviron Depot 135; Testoviron Depot 250; *Fin.:* Atmos; Pantestone; Sustanon 250; *Fr.:* Androtardyl; Pantestone; *Ger.:* Andriol; Androderm; Testoderm; Testoviron Depot 250; *Hong Kong:* Andriol; Sustanon; Testoviron Depot; *Irl.:* Andropatch; Restandol; Sustanon 100; Sustanon 250; Testoviron Depot†; *Israel:* Androxon; Sustanon 250; Testoviron Depot; *Ital.:* Andriol; Androderm; Sustanon; Testo-Enant; Testovis; *Mex.:* Andriol; Primoteston Depot; Sostenon; Testozzard; *Neth.:* Andriol; Sustanon 100; Sustanon 250; Testoderm; Testoviron Depot; *Norw.:* Androxon; Atmos; *NZ:* Pantestone; Primoteston Depot; Sustanon; *Port.:* Andriol; Testoviron Depot; *S.Afr.:* Androxon; Depotrone; Sustanon 250; *Singapore:* Andriol; Sustanon 250; Testoviron Depot; *Spain:* Testex; Testoviron Depot 250; *Swed.:* Atmos; Testoviron Depot; Undestor; *Switz.:* Andriol; Androderm; Testoviron Depot; *Thai.:* Andriol; Testoviron 100; Testoviron 250; Viromone; *UK:* Andropatch; Primoteston Depot; Restandol; Sustanon 100; Sustanon 250; Testoderm†; Testosterone Implants; Virormone†; *USA:* Androt; Androderm; AndroGel; Andropository†; Delatestryl; depAndro†; Depotest†; Duratest†; Durathate†; Everone†; Histerone†; Tesamone†; Testandro†; Testoderm; Testopel; Virilon.

Multi-ingredient: *Aust.:* Estandron†; Primodian Depot†; Testoviron 100; *Austral.:* Primodian Depot†; *Braz.:* Durateston; Estandron P; Trinestril; *Ger.:* Andromefon; Tachynerg N; Testoviron Depot 100; Testoviron Depot 50; *Ital.:* Facovit; Rubidiosin Composto; Testoviron Depot; *Mex.:* Despamen; Sten; *Norw.:* Primoteston Depot; *Port.:* Sustenon 250; *S.Afr.:* Mixogen; Primodian Depot; *Spain:* Testoviron Depot 100; *Thai.:* Metharmon-F; Primodian Depot; *USA:* depAndrogyn†; Depo-Testadiol; Depotestogen; Duo-Cyp; Duratestrin†; Test-Estro†; Valertest.

Tibolone (13342-q)

Tibolone *(BAN, USAN, rINN)*.

7α-Methylnorethynodrel; Org-OD-14. 17β-Hydroxy-7α-methyl-19-nor-17α-pregn-5(10)-en-20-yn-3-one.
$C_{21}H_{28}O_2 = 312.4$.
CAS — 5630-53-5.
ATC — G03DC05.

Adverse Effects

Irregular vaginal bleeding or spotting may occur with tibolone, mainly during the first few months of treatment, and particularly in women undergoing a natural menopause who use tibolone within 12 months of their last menstrual period. Unlike cyclical, but similar to continuous, combination HRT (p.1461), tibolone does not produce regular withdrawal bleeding. Other adverse effects have included changes in body-weight, ankle oedema, dizziness, skin reactions, headache, migraine, visual disturbances, gastrointestinal disturbances, increased growth of facial hair, altered liver function, depression, and arthralgia or myalgia.

◊ The UK Committee on Safety of Medicines had received reports of 2796 suspected adverse reactions with tibolone over 3 years, out of about 666 000 prescriptions.[1] The commonest reported effects were headache, dizziness, nausea, rash, itching, and weight gain. Vaginal bleeding appeared to occur in about 8 to 9% of recipients. There had also been 52 reports of migraine, 4 of exacerbation of migraine, and 49 reports of visual disturbances, some suggestive of migraine.

1. Committee on Safety of Medicines/Medicines Control Agency. Tibolone (Livial). *Current Problems* 1994; **20:** 14.

Effects on the endometrium. Endometrial hyperplasia and endometrial carcinoma have been rarely reported after investigation of uterine bleeding in women receiving tibolone therapy,[1,2] as has exacerbation of adenomyosis.[3] Some of these women had previously received oestrogens. The authors of 1 report concluded that it was unclear whether tibolone was an aetiological agent or a cofactor in these cases,[1] and they emphasised that, although tibolone has progestogenic properties, it cannot be expected to reverse pre-existing endometrial hyperplasia or to protect against the development of endometrial malignancy.[1]

1. von Dadelszen P, *et al.* Endometrial hyperplasia and adenocarcinoma during tibolone (Livial) therapy. *Br J Obstet Gynaecol* 1994; **101:** 158–61.
2. Ginsburg J, Prelevic GM. Cause of vaginal bleeding in postmenopausal women taking tibolone. *Maturitas* 1996; **24:** 107–10.
3. Prys Davies A, Oram D. Exacerbation of adenomyosis in a postmenopausal woman taking tibolone associated with an elevation in serum CA 125. *Br J Obstet Gynaecol* 1994; **101:** 632–3.

Precautions

Tibolone is contra-indicated in women with hormone-dependent tumours, cardiovascular or cerebrovascular disorders including thrombophlebitis, thromboembolic processes, or a history of these conditions, undiagnosed vaginal bleeding, and severe liver disorders. It should not be given to pregnant or lactating women and should not be used prior to the menopause because menstrual regularity may be disturbed. Use of tibolone within 12 months of a natural menopause is also not recommended because irregular vaginal bleeding is likely. In postmenopausal women, vaginal bleeding starting after 3 months or more of treatment, or recurrent or persistent bleeding should be investigated. Care should be taken when administering tibolone to patients with liver disease or disorders that may be exacerbated by fluid retention such as kidney dysfunction, epilepsy, or migraine, or with a history of these conditions. It should also be given with caution to patients with hypercho-

lesterolaemia and impaired glucose tolerance. Tibolone should be discontinued if there are signs of thromboembolism or if abnormal liver function tests or cholestatic jaundice occur. Consideration should be given to stopping tibolone 4 weeks before elective surgery when prolonged immobilisation after surgery is likely.

In women transferring from another form of HRT to tibolone it is suggested that a withdrawal bleed be induced with a progestogen prior to starting tibolone treatment since the endometrium may already be stimulated.

Interactions

On theoretical grounds, it is anticipated that compounds that induce liver enzymes such as phenytoin, carbamazepine, and rifampicin may enhance the metabolism of tibolone and thus reduce its activity.

Pharmacokinetics

After oral administration, peak-plasma concentrations are attained in 1 to 4 hours. Tibolone is rapidly metabolised into 3 active metabolites, 2 of which have predominantly oestrogenic activity while the third, like the parent compound, has predominantly progestogenic activity. Metabolites are excreted in the bile and eliminated in the faeces. A small amount is excreted in the urine.

Uses and Administration

Tibolone is a steroid derived from noretynodrel that has oestrogenic, progestogenic, and weak androgenic properties. It is used as menopausal hormone replacement therapy (see p.1463) in the treatment of menopausal vasomotor symptoms and the prevention of postmenopausal osteoporosis. The usual dose is 2.5 mg daily by mouth.

'Add-back' therapy. Tibolone reduces vasomotor symptoms associated with the use of gonadorelin analogues for endometriosis (p.1469) or fibroids.[1]

1. Lindsay PC, *et al.* The effect of add-back treatment with tibolone (Livial) on patients treated with the gonadotropin-releasing hormone agonist triptorelin (Decapetyl). *Fertil Steril* 1996; **65:** 342–8.

Menopausal disorders. References to the use of tibolone for menopausal symptoms[1-3] and prevention[4,5] or treatment[6] of postmenopausal bone loss.

1. Anonymous. Tibolone (Livial) – a new steroid for the menopause. *Drug Ther Bull* 1991; **29:** 77–8.
2. Egarter C, *et al.* Tibolone versus conjugated estrogens and sequential progestogen in the treatment of climacteric complaints. *Maturitas* 1996; **23:** 55–62.
3. Hammar M, *et al.* A double-blind, randomised trial comparing the effects of tibolone and continuous combined hormone replacement therapy in postmenopausal women with menopausal symptoms. *Br J Obstet Gynaecol* 1998; **105:** 904–11.
4. Berning B, *et al.* Effects of two doses of tibolone on trabecular and cortical bone loss in early postmenopausal women: a two-year randomized, placebo-controlled study. *Bone* 1996; **19:** 395–9.
5. Lippuner K, *et al.* Prevention of postmenopausal bone loss using tibolone or conventional peroral or transdermal hormone replacement therapy with 17β-estradiol and dydrogesterone. *J Bone Miner Res* 1997; **12:** 806–12.
6. Studd J, *et al.* A randomized study of tibolone on bone mineral density in osteoporotic postmenopausal women with previous fractures. *Obstet Gynecol* 1998; **92:** 574–9.

Preparations

Proprietary Preparations (details are given in Part 3)
Aust.: Liviel; *Austral.:* Livial; *Belg.:* Livial; *Braz.:* Livial; *Denm.:* Livial; *Fin.:* Livial; *Ger.:* Liviella; *Hong Kong:* Livial; *Irl.:* Livial; *Ital.:* Livial; *Mex.:* Livial; *Neth.:* Livial; *Norw.:* Livial; *NZ:* Livial; *Port.:* Livial; *S.Afr.:* Livifem; *Singapore:* Livial; *Spain:* Boltin; *Swed.:* Livial; *Switz.:* Livial; *Thai.:* Livial; *UK:* Livial.

Trenbolone Acetate (9117-q)

Trenbolone Acetate *(BANM, USAN, rINNM)*.

RU-1697; Trienbolone Acetate. 17β-Hydroxyestra-4,9,11-trien-3-one acetate.
$C_{20}H_{24}O_3 = 312.4$.
CAS — 10161-33-8 (trenbolone); 10161-34-9 (trenbolone acetate).
Pharmacopoeias. In US, for veterinary use only.

Pharmacopoeial description

USP 25: Store in airtight containers at a temperature of 2° to 8°.

Profile

Trenbolone acetate has been used as an anabolic agent in veterinary practice. The hexahydrobenzylcarbonate has also been used for its anabolic properties.

◊ WHO specifies an acceptable daily intake of trenbolone acetate as a residue in foods, and recommends maximum residue limits in various animal tissues.[1] However, it should be noted that, in the European Union the use of trenbolone acetate and other anabolic steroids is restricted to certain therapeutic indications in non-food producing animals and their use as growth promotors is banned.

1. FAO/WHO. Evaluation of certain veterinary drug residues in food: thirty-fourth report of the joint FAO/WHO expert committee on food additives. *WHO Tech Rep Ser 788* 1989.

Preparations

Proprietary Preparations (details are given in Part 3)
Fr.: Parabolan†.

Trimegestone (15930-x)

Trimegestone *(BAN, USAN, rINN)*.

RU-27987. 17β-(S)-Lactoyl-17-methylestra-4,9-dien-3-one; 17β-[(S)-2-Hydroxypropionyl]-17α-methylestra-4,9-dien-3-one.
$C_{22}H_{30}O_3 = 342.5$.
CAS — 74513-62-5.

Profile

Trimegestone is a progestogen (see Progesterone, p.1488) under investigation in combination with oestrogens for menopausal HRT and as a combined oral contraceptive.

◊ References.

1. Ross D. Endometrial effects of three doses of trimegestone, a new orally active progestogen, on the postmenopausal endometrium. *Maturitas* 1997; **28:** 83–8.
2. Al-Azzawi F, *et al.* Acceptability and patterns of uterine bleeding in sequential trimegestone-based hormone replacement therapy: a dose-ranging study. *Hum Reprod* 1999; **14:** 636–41.

Zeranol (14027-b)

Zeranol *(BAN, USAN, rINN)*.

MK-188; P-1496; THFES (HM); Zearalanol. (3S,7R)-3,4,5,6,7,8,9,10,11,12-Decahydro-7,14,16-trihydroxy-3-methyl-1H-2-benzoxacyclotetradecin-1-one.
$C_{18}H_{26}O_5 = 322.4$.
CAS — 26538-44-3.

Profile

Zeranol is a nonsteroidal oestrogen that has been used for the management of menopausal and menstrual disorders. It has also been used as a growth promotor in veterinary practice.

◊ WHO specifies an acceptable daily intake of zeranol as a residue in foods and recommends maximum residue limits in various animal tissues.[1] However, it should be noted that, in the European Union the use of zeranol in veterinary medicine is prohibited. Certain other steroidal hormones are permitted for restricted use but their use as growth promotors is banned.

1. FAO/WHO. Evaluation of certain veterinary drug residues in food: thirty-second report of the joint FAO/WHO expert committee on food additives. *WHO Tech Rep Ser 763* 1988.

Soaps and Other Anionic Surfactants

Soaps and other anionic surfactants dissociate in aqueous solution to form an anion, which is responsible for the surface activity, and a cation which is devoid of surface-active properties. They are widely used for their emulsifying and cleansing properties. The term detergent is used to describe a surface-active agent that concentrates at oil-water interfaces and possesses emulsifying and cleansing properties. The principal groups of anionic surfactants used in pharmaceutical preparations include:

Alkali-metal and **ammonium soaps** (monovalent alkyl carboxylates) which are the sodium, potassium, and ammonium salts of the higher fatty acids.

Metallic soaps (polyvalent alkyl carboxylates) are the calcium, zinc, magnesium, and aluminium salts of the higher fatty acids and produce water-in-oil emulsions; the soaps are often made by chemical reaction during the preparation of the emulsion.

Amine soaps are salts of amines with fatty acids.

Alkyl sulfates or **sulfated fatty alcohols** are salts of the sulfuric acid esters of the higher fatty alcohols.

Alkyl ether sulfates or **ethoxylated alkyl sulfates** are formed by sulfating ethoxylated alcohols.

Sulfated oils are prepared by treating fixed oils with sulfuric acid and neutralising with sodium hydroxide solution.

Many **sulfonated compounds** have been produced which possess surface-active properties and are used as detergents; they include alkyl sulfonates, alkyl aryl sulfonates, and amide sulfonates. Docusate sodium (p.1223), a sulfonated dibasic acid ester, is used in medicine and pharmacy.

Ampholytic (or amphoteric) surfactants possess at least one anionic group and at least one cationic group in the molecule and can therefore have anionic, nonionic, or cationic properties depending on the pH. When the strength of the cationic portion of the molecule is equivalent to that of the anionic portion the isoelectric point occurs at pH 7 and the molecule is said to be balanced. Ampholytic surfactants have the detergent properties of anionic surfactants and the disinfectant properties of cationic surfactants. Their activity depends on the pH of the media in which they are used. Compounds used include aminocarboxylic acids, aminopropionic acid derivatives, imidazoline derivatives, dodicin, and pendecamaine. Long-chain betaines are sometimes classed as ampholytic surfactants.

Balanced ampholytic surfactants are reputed to be non-irritant to the eyes and skin and have therefore been used in baby shampoos.

Soft Soap (6014-f)

Green Soap; Jabon Blando; Medicinal Soft Soap; Potassium Soap; Sabão Mole; Sapo Mollis; Soft soap.
Pharmacopoeias. In *Br., Chin.,* and *US.*

Pharmacopoeial description
BP 2001: Soft Soap is made by the interaction of potassium hydroxide or sodium hydroxide with a suitable vegetable oil or oils or their fatty acids. It may be coloured with chlorophyll or not more than 0.015% of a suitable green soap dye. A yellowish-white to green or brown, unctuous substance. Soluble in water and in alcohol.

USP 25: Green Soap is made by the saponification of suitable vegetable oils, excluding coconut oil and palm kernel oil, without the removal of glycerol. The method given in the USP 25 involves mixing the oil with oleic acid and to the heated mixture adding potassium hydroxide dissolved in glycerol and water. The homogeneous emulsion is then adjusted to weight with hot water. A yellowish-white to brownish- or greenish-yellow, transparent to translucent, soft unctuous mass with a slight, characteristic odour.

Adverse Effects and Treatment
Soaps and anionic detergents, in general, may be irritant to the skin by removing natural oils and may produce redness, soreness, cracking and scaling, and papular dermatitis. There may be some irritation of the eyes and mucous membranes and this limits the use of soap enemas. Ingestion of anionic detergents

may cause gastrointestinal irritation with nausea, diarrhoea, intestinal distension, and occasionally vomiting. Treatment is symptomatic.

Uses
Soft soap is used to remove incrustations in chronic scaly skin diseases such as psoriasis (p.1106) and to cleanse the scalp before the application of lotions. A solution in industrial methylated spirit, with the addition of solvent ether, has been used to cleanse the skin. A solution of soft soap in warm water has been used as an enema to soften impacted faeces but should be avoided as it may inflame the colonic mucosa; other measures are now employed to soften impacted faeces (see Constipation, p.1202). Soft soap is an ingredient of Soap Spirit (BP 2001) and Green Soap Tincture (USP 25).

Potash soap (linseed oil soap) has been used in the preparation of liquid soaps. Hard soap (castile soap) and curd soap were formerly used as pill excipients and hard soap was also formerly used in the preparation of plasters.

Preparations
BP 2001: Soap Spirit;
USP 25: Green Soap; Green Soap Tincture.
Proprietary Preparations (details are given in Part 3)
USA: Fleet Bagenema.
Multi-ingredient: *Aust.:* Abfuhrdragees; Abfuhrdragees mild; *Spain:* Linimento Naion; *USA:* Therevac Plus; Therevac SB.

Aluminium Monostearate (6015-d)

Aluminii Monostearas; Aluminum Monostearate. Dihydroxy(octadecanoato-O-)aluminium; Dihydroxy(stearato)aluminium.
CAS — 7047-84-9.
Pharmacopoeias. In *Jpn* and *Pol.* Also in *USNF.*

Pharmacopoeial description
USNF 20: A compound of aluminium with a mixture of solid organic acids obtained from fats and consisting mainly of variable proportions of aluminium monostearate and aluminium monopalmitate. A fine, white to yellowish-white, bulky powder with a faint characteristic odour. Insoluble in water, in alcohol, and in ether.

Profile
Aluminium monostearate forms gels with fixed or mineral oils when heated to about 60°; such gels are used to suspend medicaments in oily injections.

Calcium Stearate (6016-n)

Calcii Stearas. Octadecanoic Acid, Calcium Salt.
CAS — 542-42-7 (calcium palmitate); 1592-23-0 (calcium stearate).
Pharmacopoeias. In *Eur.* (see p.vi), *Int.,* and *Jpn.* Also in *USNF.*

Pharmacopoeial description
Ph. Eur.: A mixture of calcium salts of different fatty acids consisting mainly of stearic acid ($C_{36}H_{70}CaO_4 = 607.0$) and palmitic acid ($C_{32}H_{62}CaO_4 = 550.9$) with minor proportions of other fatty acids. The fatty acid fraction contains not less than 40.0% of stearic acid and the sum of stearic acid and palmitic acids is not less than 90.0%. A fine, white or almost white, crystalline powder. Practically insoluble in water, in alcohol, and in ether.

USNF 20: A compound of calcium with a mixture of solid organic acids obtained from fats, consisting mainly of variable proportions of calcium stearate ($C_{36}H_{70}CaO_4 = 607.0$) and calcium palmitate ($C_{32}H_{62}CaO_4 = 550.9$). A fine, white to yellowish-white bulky, unctuous powder, free from grittiness with a slight characteristic odour. Insoluble in water, in alcohol, and in ether.

Profile
Calcium stearate is added to granules as a lubricant in the manufacture of tablets and capsules.

Sulfated Castor Oil (6017-h)

Ol. Ricin. Sulphat.; Oleum Ricini Sulphatum; Sulfonated Castor Oil; Sulphated Castor Oil.
CAS — 8002-33-3.

Profile
Sulfated castor oil is a detergent and wetting agent that has been used as a skin cleanser and emulsifying agent.

Sulfated hydrogenated castor oil (hydroxystearin sulfate) has been used in the manufacture of hydrophilic ointment bases and other emulsions.

Sodium ricinoleate has been used for its surfactant properties.

Magnesium Stearate (6022-f)

572; Estearato de Magnésio; Magnesii Stearas.
CAS — 1555-53-9 (magnesium oleate); 2601-98-1 (magnesium palmitate); 557-04-0 (magnesium stearate).
Pharmacopoeias. In *Chin., Eur.* (see p.vi), *Int., Jpn,* and *Pol.* Also in *USNF.*

Pharmacopoeial description
Ph. Eur.: A mixture of the magnesium salts of different fatty acids consisting mainly of stearic acid ($C_{36}H_{70}MgO_4 = 591.2$) and palmitic acid ($C_{32}H_{62}MgO_4 = 535.1$) and in minor proportions other fatty acids. The fatty acid fraction contains not less than 40.0% of stearic acid and the sum of stearic acid and palmitic acid is not less than 90.0%. A white, very fine, light powder, greasy to the touch. Practically insoluble in water and in dehydrated alcohol.

USNF 20: A compound of magnesium with a mixture of solid organic acids, and consisting mainly of variable proportions of magnesium stearate ($C_{36}H_{70}MgO_4 = 591.2$) and magnesium palmitate ($C_{32}H_{62}MgO_4 = 535.1$). It is a very fine, light, white powder, slippery to touch. Insoluble in water, in alcohol, and in ether.

Profile
Magnesium stearate is added as a lubricant to the granules in tablet-making and has been used as a dusting powder and in barrier creams.

Sodium Cetostearyl Sulfate (6023-d)

Cetylstearylschwefelsaures Natrium; Natrii Cetylo- et Stearylosulfas; Natrium Cetylosulphuricum; Natrium Cetylstearylosulphuricum; Sodium Cetostearyl Sulphate.
CAS — 1120-01-0 (sodium cetyl sulfate); 1120-04-3 (sodium stearyl sulfate).
Pharmacopoeias. In *Eur.* (see p.vi) and *Pol.*

Pharmacopoeial description
Ph. Eur.: A mixture of sodium cetyl sulfate ($C_{16}H_{33}NaO_4S = 344.5$) and sodium stearyl sulfate ($C_{18}H_{37}NaO_4S = 372.5$). A white or pale yellow, amorphous or crystalline powder. Soluble in hot water giving an opalescent solution; practically insoluble in cold water; partly soluble in alcohol.

Profile
Sodium cetostearyl sulfate is used for similar purposes to sodium laurilsulfate (see below).

Sodium Laurilsulfate (6024-n)

Sodium Laurilsulfate (pINNM).
Laurilsulfato de Sódio; Natrii Laurilsulfas; Natrium Lauryl Sulphuricum; Sodium Dodecyl Sulphate; Sodium Lauryl Sulfate; Sodium Lauryl Sulphate.
CAS — 151-21-3.
Pharmacopoeias. In *Eur.* (see p.vi), *Jpn,* and *Pol.* Also in *USNF.*

Pharmacopoeial description
Ph. Eur.: A mixture of sodium alkyl sulfates, consisting mainly of sodium dodecyl sulfate ($C_{12}H_{25}NaO_4S = 288.4$). It contains not less than 85% of sodium alkyl sulfates and not more than a total of 8% of sodium chloride and sodium sulfate. A white or pale yellow powder or crystals. Freely soluble in water giving an opalescent solution; partly soluble in alcohol.

USNF 20: A mixture of sodium alkyl sulfates, consisting mainly of sodium laurilsulfate ($C_{12}H_{25}NaO_4S = 288.4$). The combined content of sodium chloride and sodium sulfate is not more than 8%. Small, white or light yellow crystals with a slight, characteristic odour. Soluble 1 in 10 of water giving an opalescent solution.

Incompatibilities.
Sodium laurilsulfate interacts with cationic surfactants such as cetrimide, resulting in a loss of activity. It is also incompatible with salts of polyvalent metal ions (e.g. aluminium, lead, tin, or zinc) and with acids of pH below 2.5. It is not affected by hard water on account of the solubility of the corresponding calcium and magnesium salts.

Profile
Sodium laurilsulfate is an anionic emulsifying agent. It is a detergent and wetting agent, effective in both acid and alkaline solution and in hard water. It is used in medicated shampoos and as a skin cleanser and in toothpastes. It is used in the preparation of Emulsifying Wax (p.1409).

Other salts of laurilsulfate have been used for their surfactant properties. These include monoethanolamine laurilsulfate, diolamine laurilsulfate, and trolamine laurilsulfate, and magnesium and ammonium laurilsulfates. Similar surfactants include sodium lauril ether sulfate and sodium alkyl sulfoacetates such as sodium lauril sulfoacetate.

Sodium laurilsulfate and related surfactants are also included in some combination preparations used rectally for the management of constipation.

Preparations

BP 2001: Emulsifying Wax.

Proprietary Preparations (details are given in Part 3)
Braz.: Endocris; *Canad.:* Pro-Sope; *Fr.:* Gyalme; *Hong Kong:* Lowila Cake; *Mex.:* Aquanil; *Spain:* Anticerumen; *UK:* Empicols.

Multi-ingredient: *Aust.:* Microklist; *Austral.:* Fleet Micro-Enema; Microlax; *Belg.:* Microlax; Neo-Sabenyl; *Canad.:* Aseptone 2; Microlax; Plax; *Denm.:* Microlax; Fin.:* Microlax; *Fr.:* Bactident; Microlax; Ysol 206†; *Ger.:* Dermofug; Microklist; *Hong Kong:* Fleet Micro-Enema; Microlax; *Irl.:* Micolette; Microlax; *Israel:* Microlet; *Ital.:* Florigien; Novilax; Si-Cliss†; *Mex.:* Microlax; *Neth.:* Microlax; *Norw.:* Microlax; *NZ:* Fleet Micro-Enema; Microlax; *Port.:* Microlax; *S.Afr.:* Medigel; Microlax; *Singapore:* Dentinox Cradle Cap; Microlax; *Spain:* Micralax; Microcasen; *Swed.:* Fleet Micro; Microlax; *Switz.:* Microklist; Microlax; Stellisept; *UK:* Dentinox Cradle Cap; Fleet Micro-Enema†; Micolette; Micralax; Relaxit; *USA:* Maxilube; Summers Eve Post-Menstrual; Trichotine; Trimo-San.

Sodium Oleate (6025-h)

CAS — 143-19-1.

Profile
Sodium oleate is an anionic surfactant used as an ingredient in preparations for the symptomatic relief of haemorrhoids and pruritus ani.

Zinc oleate and potassium oleate have also been used in skin preparations, while the sodium, potassium, and calcium salts have applications as food additives.

Preparations

Proprietary Preparations (details are given in Part 3)
Multi-ingredient: *Belg.:* Neo-Alcos-Anal; *Fr.:* Bilifluine†; *Ger.:* Alcos-Anal; *Neth.:* Epianal; *Norw.:* Alcos-Anal; *Swed.:* Alcos-Anal.

Sodium Stearate (6027-b)

Estearato de Sodio.
CAS — 408-35-5 (sodium palmitate); 822-16-2 (sodium stearate).
Pharmacopoeias. In It., Pol., Port., and Swiss. Also in USNF.

Pharmacopoeial description
USNF 20: A mixture containing not less than 90% of sodium stearate ($C_{18}H_{35}NaO_2$ = 306.5) and sodium palmitate ($C_{16}H_{31}NaO_2$ = 278.4); the content of sodium stearate is not less than 40% of the total. It contains small amounts of the sodium salts of other fatty acids. A fine, white powder, soapy to the touch, usually with a slight tallow-like odour. Slowly soluble in cold water and in cold alcohol; readily soluble in hot water and in hot alcohol. Protect from light.

Profile
Sodium stearate is an emulsifying and stiffening agent used in a variety of topical preparations. It is an ingredient of Glycerin Suppositories (USP 25).

Sodium Stearyl Fumarate (18350-n)

Natrii Stearylis Fumaras.
$C_{22}H_{39}NaO_4$ = 390.5.
Pharmacopoeias. In Eur. (see p.vi). Also in USNF.

Pharmacopoeial description
Ph. Eur.: A fine, white or almost white powder with agglomerates of flat, circular shaped particles. Practically insoluble in water, in alcohol, and in acetone; slightly soluble in methyl alcohol.

USNF 20: A fine white powder. Practically insoluble in water; slightly soluble in methyl alcohol.

Profile
Sodium stearyl fumarate is used as a lubricant in the manufacture of tablets and capsules.

Sodium Tetradecyl Sulfate (6028-v)

Sodium Tetradecyl Sulfate *(rINN)*.
Sodium Tetradecyl Sulphate. Sodium 4-ethyl-1-isobutyloctyl sulphate.
$C_{14}H_{29}NaO_4S$ = 316.4.
CAS — 139-88-8.
ATC — C05BB04.
Pharmacopoeias. Br. has a monograph for Sodium Tetradecyl Sulphate Concentrate.

Pharmacopoeial description
BP 2001: Sodium Tetradecyl Sulphate Concentrate is a clear, colourless gel. Store at a temperature not exceeding 25°. Protect from light.

Adverse Effects and Precautions
The complications of injection sclerotherapy with sclerosants such as sodium tetradecyl sulfate are discussed under Monoethanolamine Oleate, p.1636.

Uses and Administration
Sodium tetradecyl sulfate is an anionic surfactant. It has sclerosing properties and is used in the treatment of varicose veins (p.1637). It has also been given in the management of bleeding oesophageal varices (p.1637).

Sclerotherapy for varicose veins is a specialised technique. A solution of sodium tetradecyl sulfate is injected slowly into the lumen of an isolated segment of an emptied superficial vein, followed by compression. Solutions are available in a variety of strengths (0.2 to 3%); doses depend on the site and condition being treated. A test dose is advisable in patients with a history of allergy. Facilities for treating anaphylaxis should be available.

Preparations

BP 2001: Sodium Tetradecyl Sulphate Injection.

Proprietary Preparations (details are given in Part 3)
Austral.: Fibro-Vein; STD†; *Canad.:* Trombovar; *Fr.:* Trombovar; *Irl.:* Fibro-Vein; *Ital.:* Fibro-Vein; Trombovar; *NZ:* Fibro-Vein; *S.Afr.:* Fibrovein; STD†; *UK:* Fibro-Vein; *USA:* Sotradecol.

Zinc Stearate (6030-f)

Zinci Stearas.
CAS — 4991-47-3 (zinc palmitate); 557-05-1 (zinc stearate).
Pharmacopoeias. In Eur. (see p.vi), Pol., and US.

Pharmacopoeial description
Ph. Eur.: Zinc stearate [$(C_{17}H_{35}CO_2)_2Zn$ = 632.3] may contain varying proportions of zinc palmitate [$(C_{15}H_{31}CO_2)_2Zn$ = 576.2] and zinc oleate [$(C_{17}H_{33}CO_2)2Zn$ = 628.3]. A light, white, amorphous powder, free from gritty particles. Practically insoluble in water, in dehydrated alcohol, and in ether.

USP 25: A compound of zinc with a mixture of solid organic acids obtained from fats and consisting mainly of variable proportions of zinc stearate [$(C_{17}H_{35}CO_2)_2Zn$ = 632.3] and zinc palmitate [$(C_{15}H_{31}CO_2)_2Zn$ = 576.2]. A fine, white, bulky powder, free from grittiness, with a faint characteristic odour. Insoluble in water, in alcohol, and in ether.

Adverse Effects
Zinc stearate inhalation has caused fatal pneumonitis, particularly in infants.

Uses
Zinc stearate is used as a soothing and protective application in the treatment of skin inflammation. It is used either alone or with other powders or in the form of a cream.

Zinc stearate is also added as a lubricant to the granules in tablet-making.

Preparations

USP 25: Compound Clioquinol Topical Powder.

Proprietary Preparations (details are given in Part 3)
Multi-ingredient: *Aust.:* Mykozem†; *Belg.:* Baseler Haussalbe†; Pelsano†; *Ital.:* Neo Zeta-Foot†; Steril Zeta; *Switz.:* Adrectal†; Hydrocortisone comp; Rocanal Permanent Gangrene†; Rocanal Permanent Vital†; *Thai.:* Banocin; *UK:* Simpsons.

The symbol † denotes a preparation no longer actively marketed

Stabilising and Suspending Agents

The stabilising and suspending agents described in this chapter have the property of increasing the viscosity of water when dissolved or dispersed. The rheological properties of the dispersions can vary widely from thin liquids to thick gels.

These agents have wide applications both in pharmaceutical manufacturing and in the food industry. As well as being used as thickening and suspending agents many are used in emulsions as stabilisers and in some cases as emulsifying agents; some are also used in the manufacture of tablets as disintegrants, binding and granulating agents, and for film or enteric coating.

Some of the agents in this chapter are used in artificial tear and artificial saliva preparations which are employed in the management of dry eye and dry mouth respectively. The agents most commonly used are carbomers; cellulose ethers such as carmellose and hypromellose; polyvinyl alcohol; and povidone. Some agents, such as the alginates and methylcellulose, are also used in gastrointestinal disorders.

Dry eye

Dry eye is a chronic condition caused by instability of the tear film covering the eye; the tear film breaks up into dry spots rather than being maintained between blinks. Tears consist of a slightly alkaline fluid that is spread across the eye by blinking and is lost via the lachrymal ducts or by evaporation. Mucus secreted by the conjunctiva is also required to maintain tear film stability and dry eye can result from reduced production of either tears or conjunctival mucus. Reduced tear secretion is common in the elderly, but also occurs in some systemic disorders or as an adverse effect of drugs such as those, like tricyclic antidepressants, that have antimuscarinic effects. Tear film instability may also result from increased tear evaporation, for example due to corneal exposure in thyroid disease, or from lid, corneal, or other eye disorders.

The main symptoms of dry eye are discomfort, typically with a chronic gritty sensation, visual disturbances, and sometimes photophobia. If left untreated corneal ulceration and eventual loss of sight may occur. Keratoconjunctivitis sicca (corneal inflammation) may result from severe dry eye in Sjögren's syndrome (see below).

Treatment of dry eye is primarily symptomatic using 'artificial tears' preparations; eye drops containing hypromellose or other cellulose ethers (carmellose, hyetellose, methylcellulose); polyvinyl alcohol; or povidone are used. Carbomer, in liquid gel formulations, and ointments containing soft or liquid paraffins are also employed. Ointments have a longer duration of action than drops, but tend to blur the vision and are most suitable for use at night. Drops should be used as frequently as required, up to hourly or more often if necessary. Frequent use of eye drops may cause sensitivity to the preservative, in which case preservative-free preparations should be considered. An alternative in patients requiring very frequent instillation of drops is a slow-release ophthalmic insert of hyprolose. Punctal occlusion with gelatin rods or collagen implants is used diagnostically to block tear outflow and treatment by permanent occlusion may be considered. Mucus build-up due to reduced tear production may respond to mucolytics such as acetylcysteine or bromhexine applied topically.

Sjögren's syndrome is an auto-immune inflammatory disease primarily affecting the lachrymal and salivary glands, and manifests as dry eye and dry mouth. It is often secondary to an auto-immune disorder such as rheumatoid arthritis. Treatment is mainly symptomatic[1] using artificial tears and topical mucolytics for dry eye; dry mouth is treated with artificial saliva as outlined below. Systemic treatment with the mucolytic bromhexine has produced conflicting results.[2-4]

1. Oxholm P, et al. Rational drug therapy: recommendations for the treatment of patients with Sjögren's syndrome. Drugs 1998; 56: 345–53.

2. Frost-Larsen K, et al. Sjögren's syndrome treated with bromhexine: a randomised clinical study. BMJ 1978; i: 1579–81.

3. Tapper-Jones LM, et al. Sjögren's syndrome treated with bromhexine: a reassessment. BMJ 1980; 280: 1356.

4. Prause JU, et al. Lacrimal and salivary secretion in Sjögren's syndrome: the effect of systemic treatment with bromhexine. Acta Ophthalmol (Copenh) 1984; 62: 489–97.

Dry mouth

Dryness of the mouth (xerostomia) resulting from decreased salivary secretion is often an adverse effect of therapy with drugs such as antimuscarinics, antihistamines, tricyclic antidepressants, and diuretics. Other causes include dehydration, anxiety, Sjögren's syndrome (see Dry Eye, above), and radiotherapy of the head and neck. Dry mouth can cause eating difficulties and lead to oral disease such as candidiasis, dental caries, and bacterial infections.[1] Where possible any underlying disorder should be treated first.

Frequent sips of fluids help to relieve dry mouth. Artificial saliva products are also important in the symptomatic treatment of dry mouth. They aim to mimic normal saliva and generally contain the viscosity-increasing agents mucins or cellulose derivatives such as carmellose[2,3] as well as electrolytes, including fluoride; they seldom relieve symptoms for more than one or two hours. It may be possible to stimulate saliva production with sialogogues such as sugarless chewing gum or citrus products but the low pH of the latter can damage the teeth. Malic acid has also been used as a sialogogue.

A number of systemic therapies have also been tried. Pilocarpine is an effective sialogogue, increasing salivary production where some function remains,[4] and is used in dry mouth following radiotherapy; it may also be effective in Sjögren's syndrome or other causes of dry mouth. Adverse effects, particularly increased sweating, may, however, limit its use. Carbachol has been suggested as an alternative to pilocarpine with one study[5] reporting comparable efficacy but less sweating. Anethole trithione and cevimeline have been used similarly. Amifostine is used for dry mouth associated with radiotherapy.

1. Fox PC. Management of dry mouth. Dent Clin North Am 1997; 41: 863–75.

2. Vissink A, et al. A clinical comparison between commercially available mucin- and CMC-containing saliva substitutes. Int J Oral Surg 1983; 12: 232–8.

3. Duxbury AJ, et al. A double-blind cross-over trial of a mucin-containing artificial saliva. Br Dent J 1989; 166: 115–20.

4. Wiseman LR, Faulds D. Oral pilocarpine: a review of its pharmacological properties and clinical potential in xerostomia. Drugs 1995; 49: 143–55.

5. Joensuu H. Treatment for post-irradiation xerostomia. N Engl J Med 1994; 330: 141–2.

Acacia   (5402-m)

Acac.; Acaciae Gummi; E414; Gomme Arabique; Gomme de Sénégal; Gum Acacia; Gum Arabic; Gummi Africanum; Gummi Arabicum; Gummi Mimosae.

CAS — 9000-01-5.

Pharmacopoeias. In Eur. (see p.vi), Int., Jpn, and Pol. Also in USNF.

Incompatibilities have been reported with a number of substances including alcohol, aminophenazone, apomorphine, cresol, ferric salts, morphine, phenol, physostigmine, tannins, thymol, and vanillin. Acacia contains an oxidising enzyme which may affect preparations containing easily oxidised substances; the enzyme may be inactivated by heating at 100° for a short time.

Pharmacopoeial description

Ph. Eur.: The air-hardened gummy exudate from the trunk and branches of *Acacia senegal* and other species of *Acacia* of African origin. Yellowish-white, yellow, or pale amber tears, sometimes with a pinkish tint. It is friable, opaque, frequently with a cracked surface, easily broken into irregular, whitish or slightly yellowish angular fragments with conchoidal fracture and a glassy and transparent appearance. A spray-dried form is available. Very slowly but almost completely soluble in twice its mass of water leaving only a very small residue of vegetable particles; the liquid obtained is colourless or yellowish, dense, viscous, adhesive, translucent and weakly acid to blue litmus paper. Practically insoluble in alcohol. Protect from light.

USNF 20: The dried gummy exudate from the stems and branches of *Acacia senegal* (Leguminosae) or of other related African species of *Acacia*. Spheroidal tears or angular fragments of white to yellowish-white colour. It is translucent or somewhat opaque from the presence of numerous minute fissures. It is very brittle, the fractured surface is glassy and occasionally iridescent. It is also available as flakes, powder, granules, or as a spray-dried form. It is practically odourless. Insoluble in alcohol. Store in airtight containers.

Adverse Effects

Hypersensitivity reactions have occurred rarely after inhalation or ingestion of acacia.

Uses

Acacia is used in pharmaceutical manufacturing as a suspending and emulsifying agent, as a tablet binder, and in pastilles. It is often used with tragacanth.

It is used as an emulsifier and stabiliser in the food industry.

Agar   (5403-b)

Agar-agar; Colle du Japon; E406; Gelosa; Gélose; Japanese Isinglass; Layor Carang.

CAS — 9002-18-0.

Pharmacopoeias. In Chin., Eur. (see p.vi), and Jpn. Also in USNF.

Pharmacopoeial description

Ph. Eur.: Polysaccharides extracted from various species of Rhodophyceae algae, mainly those belonging to the genus *Gelidium*. It is prepared by treating the algae with boiling water; the extract is filtered while hot, concentrated, and dried. Colourless to pale yellow translucent strips, flakes, or powder; tough when damp but becoming more brittle on drying.

USNF 20: The dried, hydrophilic, colloidal substance extracted from *Gelidium cartilagineum* (Gelidiaceae), *Gracilaria confervoides* (Sphaerococcaceae), and related red algae (Class Rhodophyceae). It consists of thin, membranous, agglutinated strips, or in cut, flaked, or granulated forms. May be weak yellowish-orange, yellowish-grey to pale yellow, or colourless. It is tough when damp, brittle when dry. Odourless or has a slight odour. Insoluble in cold water; soluble in boiling water.

Uses and Administration

Agar is used as a suspending or thickening agent in pharmaceutical manufacturing and as an emulsifying and stabilising agent in the food industry.

It was formerly used similarly to methylcellulose (p.1502) as a bulk laxative. Preparations containing agar together with liquid paraffin and phenolphthalein are available to treat constipation, but the relatively small amount of agar in these probably acts solely as an emulsion stabiliser.

Preparations

Proprietary Preparations (details are given in Part 3)

Multi-ingredient: *Austral.:* Lexat; *Belg.:* Agarol†; *Braz.:* Agarol; *Canad.:* Agarol†; *Fr.:* Gelogastrine†; Pseudophage; *Irl.:* Agarol†; *Ital.:* Agarbil†; Agarol†; *Neth.:* Agarol†; *Port.:* Byl; *S.Afr.:* Agarol; *Switz.:* Agarol†; Demosvelte N†; Falquit†; Paragar†; *UK:* Agarol; *USA:* Agoral.

Alginic Acid   (12341-r)

Acidum Alginicum; E400; Polymannuronic Acid.

CAS — 9005-32-7.

ATC — A02BX13.

Pharmacopoeias. In Eur. (see p.vi) and Int. Also in USNF.

Pharmacopoeial description

Ph. Eur.: A mixture of polyuronic acids composed of residues of D-mannuronic and L-guluronic acids extracted from algae belonging to the Phaeophyceae. A white or pale yellowish-brown, crystalline or amorphous powder. It swells in water. Very slightly soluble or practically insoluble in alcohol; practically insoluble in organic solvents; dissolves in solutions of alkali hydroxides.

USNF 20: A hydrophilic colloidal carbohydrate extracted with dilute alkali from various species of brown seaweeds (Phaeophyceae). A white to yellowish-white, odourless or practically odourless, fibrous powder. Insoluble in water and in organic solvents; soluble in alkaline solutions. pH of a 3% dispersion in water is between 1.5 and 3.5.

Propylene Glycol Alginate   (10233-n)

E405. Propane-1,2-diol Alginate.

Pharmacopoeias. In USNF.

Pharmacopoeial description

USNF 20: A white to yellowish, practically odourless, fibrous or granular powder. Soluble in water, in solutions of dilute organic acids, and, depending on the degree of esterification, in hydroalcoholic mixture containing up to 60% by weight of alcohol to form stable, viscous colloidal solutions at a pH of 3.

Sodium Alginate   (5459-x)

Algin; E401; Natrii Alginas; Sodium Polymannuronate.

CAS — 9005-38-3.

Pharmacopoeias. In Eur. (see p.vi). Also in USNF.

Incompatibilities have been observed with acridine derivatives, methylrosanilinium chloride, phenylmercuric acetate and nitrate, calcium salts, alcohol in concentrations greater than 5%, and heavy metals. High concentrations of electrolytes cause an increase in viscosity until salting-out of sodium alginate occurs; salting-out occurs if more than 4% of sodium chloride is present.

Pharmacopoeial description

Ph. Eur.: It consists chiefly of the sodium salt of alginic acid. A white or pale yellowish-brown powder. Slowly soluble in water, forming a viscous, colloidal solution; practically insoluble in alcohol and in ether.

USNF 20: A yellowish-white, practically odourless, coarse or fine powder. Soluble in water, forming a viscous, colloidal solution; insoluble in alcohol, in chloroform, and in ether, in hydroalcoholic solutions in which the alcohol content is greater than 30% by weight, and in acids when the pH of the resulting solution becomes lower than about 3. Store in airtight containers.

Uses and Administration

Alginic acid and alginates such as propylene glycol alginate and sodium alginate are used in pharmaceutical manufacturing as suspending and thickening agents. They may be used as stabilisers for oil-in-water emulsions and as binding and disintegrating agents in tablets. Various grades are usually available commercially for different applications and yield solutions of varying viscosity. A reduction in viscosity has been said to occur following sterilisation by autoclaving of sodium alginate solutions.

Alginic acid and alginates (ammonium alginate, calcium alginate (p.728), potassium alginate, propylene glycol alginate, and sodium alginate) are also employed as emulsifiers and stabilisers in the food industry.

Alginic acid or the alginates, magnesium alginate and sodium alginate, are used with an antacid or a histamine H₂-antagonist such as cimetidine in the management of gastro-oesophageal reflux disease (p.1204). Alginic acid or the alginate reacts with gastric acid to form a viscous gel (often termed a raft) which floats on top of the gastric contents. This raft then acts as a mechanical barrier to reduce reflux.

Sodium alginate is used in the form of a mixed calcium-sodium salt of alginic acid as a haemostatic and wound dressing; it is employed in the form of a fibre made into a dressing or packing material.

Preparations

Proprietary Preparations (details are given in Part 3)
Fr.: Nu-Gel; **Irl.:** Kaltostat; **Israel:** Nu-Gel; **Ital.:** Kaltostat; **NZ:** Gaviscon; **S.Afr.:** Gaviscon; Kaltostat; **UK:** Comfeel Seasorb; Heartburn & Indigestion Liquid.

Multi-ingredient: **Aust.:** Cimetalgin†; Sodinon†; **Austral.:** Algicon†; Gaviscon; Meracote; Mylanta Heartburn Relief; **Belg.:** Gaviscon; **Braz.:** Algicote; **Canad.:** Gastrifom; Gastrocote†; Gaviscon; Gaviscon Heartburn Relief; Heartburn Relief; Maalox HRF; Rafton; **Denm.:** Gaviscon; **Fin.:** Gaviscon; Refluxin; **Fr.:** Comfeel Seasorb; Gaviscon; Hyalogran; Pseudophage; Rennie Refluxine; Topaal; **Ger.:** Gaviscon; Nu-Gel; Recatol Algin; **Hong Kong:** Gaviscon; **Irl.:** Acidex; Algicon; Gaviscon; Gaviscon Advance; Gaviscon Infant; Pyrogastrone; **Israel:** Gaviscon; Kaltocarb; Kaltostat; **Ital.:** Digerall; Gaviscon; **Mex.:** Algicon; **Neth.:** Aciflux; Algicon; Gaviscon; **Norw.:** Algicon†; Gaviscon; **NZ:** Gaviscon; Mylanta Heartburn Relief; **Port.:** Carboflex; Gaviscon†; Kaltostat; **S.Afr.:** Gastrocote†; Gaviscon; Infant Gaviscon; **Singapore:** Gaviscon; **Spain:** Dolcopin; Gaviscon; **Swed.:** Gaviscon; **Switz.:** Demosvelte N†; Gaviscon; Refluxine; **UK:** Acidex; Algicon; Algitec†; Asilone Heartburn; Bisodol Heartburn Relief; Gastrocote; Gaviscon; Gaviscon Advance; Gaviscon Infant; Peptac; Pyrogastrone; Rennie Duo; Setlers Heartburn & Indigestion Liquid; Tagamet Dual Action†; Topal; **USA:** Foamicon; Gaviscon; Genaton; Pretts Diet Aid.

Aluminium Magnesium Silicate (5405-g)

Aluminii Magnesic Silicas; Magnesium Aluminium Silicate; Magnesium Aluminum Silicate; Saponite.
CAS — 1327-43-1; 12511-31-8.
Pharmacopoeias. In Eur. (see p.vi) and Int. Also in USNF.

Pharmacopoeial description

Ph. Eur.: A mixture of particles with colloidal particle size of montmorillonite and saponite, free from grit and nonswellable ore. Almost white powder, granules, or plates. Practically insoluble in water and in organic solvents; swells in water to form a colloidal dispersion. A 5% dispersion in water has a pH of 9.0 to 10.0.

USNF 20: A blend of colloidal montmorillonite and saponite that has been processed to remove grit and nonswellable ore components. There are several types, differing in viscosity and in ratio of aluminium content to magnesium content. It is an odourless, fine (micronised) powder, small cream to tan granules, or small flakes that are creamy when viewed on their flat surfaces and tan to brown when viewed on their edges. Insoluble in water and in alcohol; swells when added to water or glycerol. Store in airtight containers. pH of a 5% suspension in water is between 9.0 and 10.0.

Uses

Aluminium magnesium silicate has a variety of pharmaceutical uses, including use as a suspending and thickening agent, as an emulsion stabiliser, and as a binder and disintegrating agent in tablets.

Other forms of aluminium magnesium silicate include an artificial hydrate known as almasilate (p.1210), which is used as an antacid, and attapulgite (p.1212), a purified native hydrated magnesium aluminium silicate that is highly adsorbent and is used in a wide range of products including fertilisers and pesti-

cides. Activated attapulgite, which is attapulgite that has been carefully heated to increase its adsorptive capacity, is used in combination preparations for diarrhoea.

Preparations

Proprietary Preparations (details are given in Part 3)
Multi-ingredient: **Braz.:** Hipoglos; Hipoglos com Hidrocortisona; **Denm.:** Alkasid; **Fr.:** Mucal†; **Ger.:** Mucal†; **Hong Kong:** GI; **Switz.:** TRI-OM; **Thai.:** Almaxane; Diasgest; **UAE:** Alkasid.

Bentonite (5407-p)

558; Bentonitum; Mineral Soap; Soap Clay; Wilkinite.
CAS — 1302-78-9.
Pharmacopoeias. In Eur. (see p.vi), Int., Jpn, and Pol. Also in USNF which includes additionally Purified Bentonite.

A native colloidal hydrated aluminium silicate consisting mainly of montmorillonite, Al₂O₃,4SiO₂,H₂O; it may also contain calcium, magnesium, and iron.

Pharmacopoeial description

Ph. Eur.: A natural clay containing a high proportion of montmorillonite, a native hydrated aluminium silicate in which some aluminium and silicon atoms may be replaced by other atoms such as iron and magnesium. A very fine, homogeneous, greyish-white powder with a more or less yellowish or pinkish tint. Practically insoluble in water and in aqueous solutions, but swells with a little water forming a malleable mass.

USNF 20: A native, colloidal, hydrated aluminium silicate. A very fine, odourless, hygroscopic, pale buff or cream-coloured to greyish powder, free from grit. Insoluble in water, but swells to approximately 12 times its volume when added to water; insoluble in, and does not swell in, organic solvents. pH of a 2% suspension in water, mixed vigorously to facilitate wetting, is between 9.5 and 10.5. Store in airtight containers.

Uses

Bentonite absorbs water readily to form sols or gels, depending on its concentration. It is used in pharmaceutical manufacturing as a suspending and stabilising agent and as an adsorbent or clarifying agent. It is also used as an anticaking agent in the food industry.

Bentonite may be used as an oral adsorbent in paraquat poisoning (p.1435).

Preparations

USNF 20: Bentonite Magma.
Proprietary Preparations (details are given in Part 3)
Multi-ingredient: **Braz.:** Cravo-Espin.

Carbomers (5409-w)

Acrylic Acid Polymers; Carbopols; Carboxypolymethylene; Carboxyvinyl Polymers; Polyacrylic Acid.
CAS — 9003-01-4; 54182-57-5.
NOTE. Carbomer is BAN, USAN, and rINN.
Pharmacopoeias. In Eur. (see p.vi), and Int. USNF has separate monographs for Carbomer 910, Carbomer 934, Carbomer 934P, Carbomer 940, Carbomer 941, and Carbomer 1342.

Pharmacopoeial description

Ph. Eur.: High molecular weight polymers of acrylic acid cross-linked with polyalkenyl ethers of sugars or polyalcohols. They are produced in several grades characterised by the viscosity of a defined solution. White, fluffy, hygroscopic powders. They swell in water and in other polar solvents after dispersion and neutralisation with sodium hydroxide solution. Store in airtight containers.

USNF 20: High molecular weight polymers of acrylic acid cross-linked with polyalkenyl ethers of sugars or polyalcohols. They are produced in several grades, Carbomer 910, Carbomer 934, Carbomer 934P, Carbomer 940, Carbomer 941, and Carbomer 1342, characterised by the viscosity of a defined solution.

White, fluffy, hygroscopic powders having a slight characteristic odour. pH of a 1% dispersion in water is about 3. When neutralised with alkali hydroxides or with amines, they dissolve in water, in alcohol, and in glycerol. Store in airtight containers.

Uses and Administration

Carbomers are used in pharmaceutical manufacturing as suspending agents, gel bases, emulsifiers, and binding agents in tablets.

Carbomers, in liquid gel formulations containing typically 0.2 or 0.3%, are used topically as tear substitutes in the management of dry eye (p.1498).

Preparations

Proprietary Preparations (details are given in Part 3)
Aust.: Lacrisic†; Vidisic; **Austral.:** Geltears; Poly Gel; Viscotears; **Belg.:** Alcon Eye Gel; Ocugel; Thilo Tears†; Vidisic; **Canad.:** Lacrinorm; Tear-Gel; **Denm.:** Viscotears; **Fin.:** Oftagel; Viscotears; **Fr.:** Aqualarm; Civigel; Gel-Larmes; Lacrinorm; Lacryvisc; Siccafluid; **Ger.:** Liposic; Siccapos; Thilo-Tears; Vidisic; Visc-Ophtal; **Hong Kong:** Lacryvisc; Viscotears; **Irl.:** Geltears; Vidisic; **Israel:** Viscotears; **Ital.:** Dacriogel; Dropgel; Lacrinorm; Siccafluid; Viscotirs; **Mex.:** Lubrigel; **Mon.:** Lacrifluid; Lacrigel;

Neth.: Dry Eye Gel†; Thilo-Tears†; Vidisic; **Norw.:** Viscotears; **NZ:** Viscotears; **Port.:** Lacryvisc; Vidisic; **S.Afr.:** Teargel; **Singapore:** Lacryvisc; Vidisic; **Spain:** Lacryvisc; Revic; Siccafluid; Viscotears; **Swed.:** Lacryvisc; Oftagel; Viscotears; **Switz.:** Lacrinorm; Lacryvisc; Thilo-Tears†; Viscotears; **Thai.:** Lacryvisc; Vidisic; **UK:** Geltears; Viscotears.

Multi-ingredient: **Ital.:** Dropyal; **Port.:** Hidratante; **USA:** Maxilube.

Carmellose (14163-l)

Carmellose (rINN).
Carboxymethylcellulose; CMC; E466.
Pharmacopoeias. In Jpn.

Carmellose Calcium (5410-m)

Calcium Carmellose (rINNM).
Calcium Carboxymethylcellulose; Carboxymethylcellulose Calcium; Carmellosum Calcicum.
CAS — 9050-04-8.
Pharmacopoeias. In Eur. (see p.vi) and Jpn. Also in USNF.

Pharmacopoeial description

Ph. Eur.: A white or yellowish-white hygroscopic powder. It swells in water to form a suspension; practically insoluble in alcohol, in acetone, and in toluene.

USNF 20: A white to yellowish-white, hygroscopic, powder. It swells in water to form a suspension; practically insoluble in alcohol, in acetone, in chloroform, in ether, and in benzene. pH of a 1% suspension in water is between 4.5 and 6.0. Store in airtight containers.

Carmellose Sodium (5411-b)

Carmellose Sodium (BAN, rINNM).
Carboxymethylcellulose Sodium; Carboxymethylcellulosum Natricum; Carmellosum Natricum; Cellulose Gum; E466; SCMC; Sodium Carboxymethylcellulose; Sodium Cellulose Glycollate.
CAS — 9004-32-4.
Pharmacopoeias. In Eur. (see p.vi), Int., Jpn, Pol., and US.
USNF also includes Carboxymethylcellulose Sodium 12.

Incompatibilities have been reported with strongly acidic solutions, with soluble salts of iron and some other metals, and with xanthan gum.

Pharmacopoeial description

Ph. Eur.: Carmellose Sodium is a white or almost white, hygroscopic granular powder. It has a sodium content of 6.5 to 10.8% calculated on the dry substance. Ph. Eur. also has standards for Low-substituted Carmellose Sodium which has a sodium content of 2.0 to 4.5%.

Easily dispersed in water forming colloidal solutions; practically insoluble in dehydrated alcohol, in acetone, in ether, and in toluene. A 1% colloidal solution in water has a pH of 6.0 to 8.0.

USP 25: Carboxymethylcellulose Sodium is a white to cream-coloured, hygroscopic, powder or granules. It contains not less than 6.5% and not more than 9.5% of sodium, calculated on the dried basis. Easily dispersed in water to form colloidal solutions; insoluble in alcohol, in ether, and in most other organic solvents. pH of a 1% solution in water is between 6.5 and 8.5. Store in airtight containers.

USNF 20: Carboxymethylcellulose Sodium 12 has a sodium content of 10.4 to 12.0%, calculated on the dry substance.

Croscarmellose Sodium (10208-d)

Croscarmellose Sodium (USAN).
Carmellosum Natricum Conexum; Crosslinked Carboxymethylcellulose Sodium; Modified Cellulose Gum.
Pharmacopoeias. In Eur. (see p.vi). Also in USNF.

Pharmacopoeial description

Ph. Eur.: A cross-linked polymer of carmellose sodium. A white or greyish-white powder. Practically insoluble in dehydrated alcohol, in acetone, and in toluene. A 1% suspension in water has a pH of 5.0 to 7.0.

USNF 20: A cross-linked polymer of carmellose sodium. A white, free flowing, powder. Partially soluble in water; insoluble in alcohol, in ether, and in other organic solvents. pH of a dispersion containing 1 g mixed with 99 mL of water for 1 hour is between 5.0 and 7.0. Store in airtight containers.

Uses and Administration

Carmellose calcium and carmellose sodium have a variety of pharmaceutical uses, including use as suspending, thickening, and emulsifying agents, and as disintegrants, binders, and coating agents in tablets. Carmellose sodium is also used as an emulsifier or stabiliser in the food industry. Croscarmellose sodium is employed as a tablet disintegrant.

Carmellose sodium is used topically as an ingredient of protective preparations for stoma care, in the management of wounds, and for the mechanical protection of oral and perioral lesions, such as mouth ulceration (p.1206). It is also used, in concentrations of up to 1%, in artificial saliva preparations for the treatment of dry mouth (p.1498), and in eye drops for the management of dry eye (p.1498).

The symbol † denotes a preparation no longer actively marketed

Carmellose sodium given orally absorbs water and acts as a bulk-forming agent; the volume of faeces is increased and peristalsis promoted. It is used in the treatment of constipation (p.1202). Carmellose sodium has been included in preparations to control appetite in the management of obesity (p.1505) but there is little evidence of efficacy. For precautions to be observed with bulk-forming agents, see under Methylcellulose, p.1502.

Preparations

USP 25: Carboxymethylcellulose Sodium Paste; Carboxymethylcellulose Sodium Tablets.

Proprietary Preparations (details are given in Part 3)
Austral.: Cellufresh; Celluvisc; **Canad.:** Cellufresh; Celluvisc; **Denm.:** Celluvisc; **Fin.:** Celluvisc; **Fr.:** Aquacel; Askina Biofilm; Celluvisc; Comfeel; Hydrocoll; Urgomed; **Ger.:** Celluvisc; **Hong Kong:** Celluvisc; **Ital.:** Celluvisc; **NZ:** Cellufresh; Celluvisc; **Port.:** Aquacel; Celluvisc; **S.Afr.:** Cellufresh; Celluvisc; **Singapore:** Cellufresh; Celluvisc; **Spain:** Cellufresh; Celluvisc; Optrelam; **Swed.:** Celluvisc; **Switz.:** Celluvisc; Comfeel†; **Thai.:** Cellufresh; **UK:** Celluvisc; Comfeel; Intrasite; Revive; **USA:** Cellufresh†; Celluvisc; Refresh Plus; Refresh Tears.

Multi-ingredient: Aust.: Glandosane; Sialin; **Austral.:** Aquae; Orabase; Orahesive; SoloSite; Stomahesive; United Soft Guard†; **Braz.:** Chofranina; **Canad.:** Appedrine; Dexatrim†; Moi-Stir; Orabase; Orahesive; Salivart; **Fr.:** Artisial; Comfeel Seasorb; Intrasite; Melgisorb; Sureskin; Tegasorb; **Ger.:** Artisial†; Glandosane; Nu-Gel; Recatol Algin; **Hong Kong:** Aquae; Salivart†; **Irl.:** Luborant; Orabase; **Israel:** Glandosane; Orabase; **Ital.:** Agena†; Idrum; **NZ:** Stomahesive; **Port.:** Carboflex; Combiderm; Glandosane; Varihesive; **S.Afr.:** Granugel; Stomahesive; **Spain:** Laxvital; **Switz.:** Glandosane; Varihesive Hydroactive†; **Thai.:** Bisolax; Emulax; Glandosane; **UK:** Comfeel Plus; Glandosane; Luborant; Orabase; Orahesive; Salivace; Seprafilm; Stomahesive; Varihesive†; **USA:** Dieutrim†; Disolan Forte†; Disoplex†; Entertainer's Secret; Glandosane†; Moi-Stir; Pretts Diet Aid; Salivart; Surgel; Tears Night & Day.

Carrageenan (5412-v)

Carrageenin; Carraghénates; Chondrus Extract; E407; Irish Moss Extract.
CAS — 9000-07-1 (carrageenan); 11114-20-8 (κ-carrageenan); 9064-57-7 (λ-carrageenan).
Pharmacopoeias. In Fr. Also in USNF.

Pharmacopoeial description

USNF 20: The hydrocolloid obtained by extraction with water or aqueous alkali from some members of the class Rhodophyceae (red seaweeds). It consists chiefly of a mixture of the ammonium, calcium, magnesium, potassium, and sodium sulfate esters of galactose and 3,6-anhydrogalactose copolymers. The prevalent copolymers in the hydrocolloids are κ-carrageenan, ι-carrageenan, and λ-carrageenan.

A yellowish or tan to white, coarse to fine, practically odourless, powder. Soluble in water at 80° forming a viscous, clear or slightly opalescent solution that flows readily. It disperses more readily in water if first moistened with alcohol, with glycerol, or with a saturated solution of glucose in water. Store in airtight containers at a temperature of 8° to 15°.

Uses and Administration

Carrageenan is used in pharmaceutical manufacturing and the food industry as a suspending and gelling agent.

It is included for its effect as a bulk-forming laxative in several preparations used to treat constipation (p.1202). For precautions to be observed with bulk-forming laxatives, see under Methylcellulose, p.1502. Carrageenan is also included in topical preparations for the symptomatic relief of anorectal disorders.

A degraded form of carrageenan also used to be given in gastrointestinal disorders but it was associated with lesions in *animals* and is no longer used.

◊ An acceptable daily intake (ADI) of 'not specified' was allocated to refined non-degraded carrageenan as a food additive since the total daily intake of this form of carrageenan (arising from its use at the levels necessary to achieve the desired effect and from its acceptable background in food) was not considered to represent a hazard to health. The toxic effects associated with degraded carrageenan and of the use of 'semi-refined' carrageenan as a food in some countries were considered and the ADI of 'not specified' was not applied to these forms of carrageenan. The ADI did, however, apply to furcellaran [a similar extract from Rhodophyceae] which is included in the specifications for food-grade carrageenan.[1]

In the UK the Food Advisory Committee has recommended that carrageenan should not be permitted as an additive for infant formulas because of the possibility of immunological consequences following absorption from the immature gut.[2] Carrageenans were known to affect the immune system of experimental *animals* after parenteral administration and immune effects have been noted in *rats* after oral administration of undegraded carrageenan. Small amounts of food-grade carrageenan cross the intestinal epithelium in *rats* and are taken up by gut-associated lymphoid tissue.[3]

1. FAO/WHO. Evaluation of certain food additives and contaminants: twenty-eighth report of the joint FAO/WHO expert committee on food additives. *WHO Tech Rep Ser 710* 1984.

2. MAFF. Food Advisory Committee: report on the review of the use of additives in foods specially prepared for infants and young children. FdAC/REP/12. London: HMSO, 1992.

3. MAFF. Food Advisory Committee: report on the review of the emulsifiers and stabilisers in food regulations. FdAC/REP/11. London: HMSO, 1992.

Preparations

Proprietary Preparations (details are given in Part 3)
Aust.: Coreine.

Multi-ingredient: Aust.: Anoreine; Anoreine mit Lidocain; **Austral.:** Bonningtons Irish Moss; **Belg.:** Tisane Pectorale; **Fr.:** Anoreine; Titanoreine; **Ital.:** Resource Gelificata; **NZ:** Bonningtons Irish Moss; **Spain:** Laxante Bescansa; Titanorein; **Switz.:** Flogecyl; Titanoreine; **UK:** Biobalm; Fam-Lax Senna; Liminate.

Cellacefate (5413-g)

Cellacefate (BAN, rINN).
CAP; Cellacephate; Cellulose Acetate Phthalate; Cellulosi Acetas Phthalas; Cellulosum Acetylphthalicum; Celophthalum.
CAS — 9004-38-0.
Pharmacopoeias. In Eur. (see p.vi), Int., Jpn, and Pol. Also in USNF.

Pharmacopoeial description

Ph. Eur.: Cellulose in which some of the hydroxyl groups are acetylated (21.5 to 26.0%) and some are phthalylated (30.0 to 36.0%), both calculated with reference to the anhydrous, acid-free substance.

A hygroscopic, white, free-flowing powder or colourless flakes. Practically insoluble in water, in dehydrated alcohol, and in dichloromethane; freely soluble in acetone; soluble in diethylene glycol; it dissolves in dilute solutions of alkalis. Store in airtight containers.

USNF 20: A reaction product of phthalic anhydride and a partial acetate ester of cellulose. It contains not less than 21.5% and not more than 26.0% of acetyl groups, and not less than 30.0% and not more than 36.0% of phthalyl(o-carboxy-benzoyl) groups, calculated on the anhydrous, acid-free basis. A white, free-flowing powder that may have a slight odour of acetic acid. Insoluble in water and in alcohol; soluble in acetone and in dioxan. Store in airtight containers.

Uses

Cellacefate is unaffected by immersion in acid media in the stomach but softens and swells in intestinal fluid. It is used in pharmaceutical manufacturing as an enteric-coating material for tablets and capsules, usually with a plasticiser. Films of cellacefate are reported to be permeable to some ionic substances such as ammonium chloride and potassium iodide, and such substances require a sealing coat.

Cellulose (15824-a)

An unbranched polysaccharide polymer consisting of 1,4-β-linked glucopyranose units. It is the chief constituent of fibrous plant material.

Dispersible Cellulose (5415-p)

Dispersible Cellulose (BAN).
Microcrystalline Cellulose and Carboxymethylcellulose Sodium.
Pharmacopoeias. In Br. Also in USNF.

Pharmacopoeial description

BP 2001: An odourless or almost odourless, white or off-white, coarse or fine powder consisting of a colloid-forming attrited mixture of microcrystalline cellulose and carmellose sodium. Disperses in water to produce a white, opaque dispersion or gel; practically insoluble in organic solvents and in dilute acids. Store at a temperature between 8° and 15°.

USNF 20: A colloid-forming, attrited mixture of microcrystalline cellulose and carmellose sodium. A white to off-white, odourless, coarse to fine, powder. It swells in water, producing, when dispersed, a white, opaque dispersion or gel; insoluble in organic solvents and in dilute acids. Store in airtight containers in a dry place, and at a temperature not exceeding 40°.

Microcrystalline Cellulose (5414-q)

Cellulosa Microgranulare; Cellulose Gel; Cellulosum Microcrystallinum; Crystalline Cellulose; E460.
CAS — 9004-34-6.
Pharmacopoeias. In Eur. (see p.vi), Int., Jpn, and Pol. Also in USNF.

Pharmacopoeial description

Ph. Eur.: A purified, partly depolymerised cellulose, prepared by treating alpha-cellulose, obtained as a pulp from fibrous plant materials, with mineral acids. It is a white or almost white, fine or granular powder. Practically insoluble in water, in dehydrated alcohol, in acetone, in toluene, in dilute acids, and in sodium hydroxide solution (1 in 20). The pH of the supernatant liquid obtained from a 12.5% mixture in water after 20 minutes of shaking is 5.0 to 7.5.

USNF 20: A purified, partially depolymerised cellulose, prepared by treating alpha-cellulose, obtained as a pulp from fibrous plant material, with mineral acids. It is a fine, white or almost white powder consisting of free-flowing, nonfibrous particles. Insoluble in water, in dilute acids, and in most organic solvents; practically insoluble in sodium hydroxide solution (1 in 20). The pH of the supernatant liquid obtained from a 12.5% mixture in water after 20 minutes of shaking is between 5.0 and 7.0. Store in airtight containers.

Powdered Cellulose (5416-s)

Cellulose Powder; Cellulosi Pulvis; E460.
Pharmacopoeias. In Eur. (see p.vi) and Jpn. Also in USNF.

Pharmacopoeial description

Ph. Eur.: A purified mechanically disintegrated cellulose prepared from alpha-cellulose obtained as a pulp from fibrous plant materials. It is a white or almost white, fine or granular powder. Practically insoluble in water, in dehydrated alcohol, in acetone, in toluene, in most organic solvents, and in dilute acids; slightly soluble in sodium hydroxide solution (1 in 20). The pH of the supernatant liquid of a 11.1% mixture in water is between 5.0 and 7.5 one hour after preparation.

USNF 20: A purified, mechanically disintegrated cellulose prepared by processing alpha-cellulose obtained as a pulp from fibrous plant materials. It is a white or almost white powder. Exhibits degrees of fineness ranging from a free-flowing, dense powder to a coarse, fluffy, nonflowing material. Insoluble in water, in nearly all organic solvents, and in dilute acids; slightly soluble in sodium hydroxide solution (1 in 20). The pH of the supernatant liquid of a 11.1% mixture in water is between 5.0 and 7.5 one hour after preparation. Store in airtight containers.

Uses and Administration

Powdered cellulose and microcrystalline cellulose are used in pharmaceutical manufacturing as tablet binders and disintegrants and as capsule and tablet diluents. These two forms of cellulose are also used in the food industry. Dispersible cellulose (which also contains some carmellose sodium) forms a thixotropic gel with water and is used pharmaceutically as a suspending and thickening agent.

Various forms of cellulose have been included in preparations employed in the management of constipation and obesity. Cellulose is also used in adsorbent powder preparations used for skin disorders including hyperhidrosis.

Preparations

Proprietary Preparations (details are given in Part 3)
Ital.: Fibrasan; **UK:** Nasaleze; Sterigel; **USA:** Unifiber.

Multi-ingredient: Austral.: ZeaSorb; **Canad.:** ZeaSorb; **Fr.:** Gelopectose; ZeaSorb; **Ger.:** ZeaSorb; **Irl.:** ZeaSorb; **Israel:** Celluspan; **Port.:** Fermetone Composto; **Thai.:** ZeaSorb.

Ceratonia (5417-w)

Carob Bean Gum; Carob Gum; Cerat.; Ceratonia Gum; E410; Gomme de Caroube; Locust Bean Gum.
CAS — 9000-40-2.
ATC — A07XA02.

The endosperms separated from the seeds of the locust bean tree, *Ceratonia siliqua* (Leguminosae).

Uses and Administration

Ceratonia is used as a thickening agent and stabiliser in the food industry.

Preparations

Proprietary Preparations (details are given in Part 3)
Aust.: Arobon; **Austral.:** Carobel†; **Irl.:** Carobel; **Ital.:** Arobon; **Norw.:** Arobon; **Switz.:** Nestargel; **UK:** Arobon†; Carobel; Nestargel.

Multi-ingredient: Aust.: China-Eisenwein; **Belg.:** Kestomatine Baby; **Braz.:** Enteroftal; Licor de Tayuya; **Fr.:** Gumilk; Polysilane Joullie; **Switz.:** Gastricure; Kestomatine Bebe.

Dextrates (5420-v)

Dextrates (USAN).
CAS — 39404-33-6.
Pharmacopoeias. In USNF.

Pharmacopoeial description

USNF 20: A purified, anhydrous or hydrated, mixture of saccharides obtained by the controlled enzymatic hydrolysis of starch. Free-flowing, porous, white, odourless, spherical granules consisting of aggregates of microcrystals. Freely soluble in water (heating increases its solubility in water); soluble in dilute acids and alkalis and in basic organic solvents such as pyridine; insoluble in the common organic solvents. pH of a 20% solution in water is between 3.8 and 5.8. Store in a dry place at a temperature of 8° to 15°.

Uses

Dextrates is used as a capsule and tablet diluent and as a tablet binding agent.

Ethylcellulose (5421-g)

Ethylcellulose (rINN).

Cellulose Ethyl Ether; E462; Ethylcellulosum.

CAS — 9004-57-3.

Pharmacopoeias. In Eur. (see p.vi) and Int. Also in USNF.

Pharmacopoeial description

Ph. Eur.: A partly O-ethylated cellulose. It contains 44 to 51% of ethoxy (–OC₂H₅) groups, calculated on the dried basis. A white to yellowish-white, odourless or almost odourless, powder or granular powder. Solutions of ethylcellulose may show a slight opalescence. Practically insoluble in water, in glycerol (85%), and in propylene glycol; soluble in dichloromethane and in a mixture of 20 parts alcohol and 80 parts toluene (w/w); slightly soluble in ethyl acetate and methyl alcohol.

USNF 20: The ethyl ether of cellulose. When dried at 105° for 2 hours, it contains not less than 44.0% and not more than 51.0% of ethoxy groups. A free-flowing white to light tan powder. Its aqueous suspensions are neutral to litmus. Insoluble in water, in glycerol, and in propylene glycol. Ethylcellulose containing less than 46.5% of ethoxy groups is freely soluble in chloroform, in methyl acetate, in tetrahydrofuran, and in mixtures of aromatic hydrocarbons with alcohol; ethylcellulose containing not less than 46.5% of ethoxy groups is freely soluble in alcohol, in chloroform, in ethyl acetate, in methyl alcohol, and in toluene.

Uses

Ethylcellulose is used as a binder in tablets and as a coating material for tablets, granules, and microcapsules. It is also used as a thickening agent.

Preparations

USNF 20: Ethylcellulose Aqueous Dispersion.

Gastric Mucin (2492-x)

Gastric Mucin (BAN).

Gastric mucin is a high molecular weight glycoprotein precipitated by alcohol (60%) after digestion of hogs' stomach linings by pepsin and hydrochloric acid.

Uses and Administration

Gastric mucin is used in artificial saliva formulations for dry mouth (p.1498). An aerosol spray containing 3.5% is employed; lozenges are also available.

Preparations

Proprietary Preparations (details are given in Part 3)
Ger.: Saliva medac.

Multi-ingredient: Austral.: Saliva Orthana†; UK: Saliva Orthana.

of medicated eye drops and, either alone or in combination with other viscosity-increasing agents, in artificial tears preparations for the management of dry eye (p.1498); solutions containing 0.3 to 1% of hypromellose are commonly used. Solutions for contact lens care (p.1129) and for lubricating artificial eyes contain similar concentrations. Hypromellose is also administered intra-ocularly, usually as a 2% solution, as an adjunct in ophthalmic surgery (below) and concentrations of up to 2.5% may be used topically to protect the cornea during gonioscopy procedures.

Hypromellose has been included in artificial saliva preparations used in the management of dry mouth (p.1498), but other drugs are usually preferred.

Ophthalmic surgery. Intra-ocular hypromellose may be used as a visco-elastic agent to protect the eye during surgery. In cataract extraction it is employed to maintain the anterior chamber and to coat the intra-ocular lens to facilitate its implantation. Although intra-ocular hypromellose is generally considered to be well tolerated, some workers[1] reported an increased incidence of pupil abnormalities (non-reactive semi-dilated pupils) following such use; others[2] did not confirm this. There has also been a report[3] of corneal opacities in a number of patients following the use of intra-ocular hypromellose.

1. Tan AKK, Humphry RC. The fixed dilated pupil after cataract surgery—is it related to intraocular use of hypromellose? *Br J Ophthalmol* 1993; **77**: 639–41.
2. Eason J, Seward HC. Pupil size and reactivity following hydroxypropyl methylcellulose and sodium hyaluronate. *Br J Ophthalmol* 1995; **79**: 541–3.
3. Newton JN, *et al.* Corneal opacities after cataract surgery with hypromellose. *Lancet* 2000; **355**: 290.

Preparations

BP 2001: Hypromellose Eye Drops;
USP 25: Hydroxypropyl Methylcellulose Ophthalmic Solution.

Proprietary Preparations (details are given in Part 3)
Aust.: Artelac; Okuzell; Prosicca; Puroptal†; *Austral.:* Genteal; Isopto Tears; Methopt; *Belg.:* Artelac; Isopto Tears; Ocucoat; *Braz.:* Filmcel; *Canad.:* Eyelube; Genteal; Isopto Tears; Lacril; Visine Contact Lens; *Fin.:* Artelac; Isopto Alkaline; Isopto Plain; *Fr.:* Contactol†; *Ger.:* Artelac; Celoftal; Hymecel†; Isopto Fluid; Methocel; Methocel Dispersa†; Sic-Ophtal; Sicca-Stulln; *Hong Kong:* Isopto Tears; Methocel; *Irl.:* Artelac; Isopto Alkaline; Isopto Plain; *Israel:* Adato-Cel; Ocucoat; *Ital.:* Gel 4000; Genteal; Lacrimill; Lacrisifi; Lacrisol; Methocel; *Mex.:* Cellusec; Meticel; Oftalmet; *NZ:* Genteal; Isopto Tears; Methocel; *Port.:* Hidrocil; *S.Afr.:* Methocel; Spersatear; Viscotraan; *Singapore:* Celoftal; Eye Mo Moist; Isopto Tears; Lacrisifi; Methocel; *Spain:* Acuolens; *Swed.:* Artelac; Isopto Plain; Ocucoat†; *Switz.:* Isopto Tears; Ultra Tears†; *Thai.:* Isopto Tears; Lac-Oph; Opsil Tears; Simoph Tears; *UK:* Artelac; Isopto Alkaline; Isopto Plain; Moisture Eyes; Ocucoat; Tears Naturale; *USA:* Artificial Tears; Genteal; Gonak; Goniosoft; Goniosol; Isopto Alkaline†; Isopto Plain; Isopto Tears; Lacril; Ocucoat; Tearisol; Tears Again MC; Ultra Tears.

Multi-ingredient: *Austral.:* Bausch & Lomb Sensitive Eyes Lens Lubricant†; Bion Tears; Murine Contact; Poly-Tears; Tears Naturale; *Belg.:* Alcon Adequad; Lacrystat; Tears Naturale; *Braz.:* Lacrima; Lacrima Plus; Opti-Tears; *Canad.:* Bion Tears; Moisture Drops; Ocutears†; Tears Naturale; *Denm.:* Dacriosol; *Ger.:* Isopto Naturale; Lacrisic; Oculotect†; *Irl.:* Ilube; Tears Naturale; *Israel:* Tears Naturale; V-Crima; *Ital.:* Dacriosol; Hamamilla; Tirs; *Neth.:* Duratears†; *NZ:* Poly-Tears; Tears Naturale; *Port.:* Tears Naturale; *S.Afr.:* Tears Naturale; *Singapore:* Bion Tears; Dacrolux; Tears Naturale; *Spain:* Dacrolux; Tears Humectante; *Swed.:* Bion Tears; Tears Naturale; *Switz.:* Tears Naturale; *Thai.:* Bion Tears; Tears Naturale; *UK:* Ilube; Tears Naturale; *USA:* Bion Tears; Clear Eyes CLR; Estivin†; Lacri-Tears; LubriTears; Maximum Strength Allergy Drops; Moisture Drops; Muro's Opcon†; Nature's Tears; Ocucoat; Tears Naturale; Tears Renewed.

Magnesium Silicate (5443-l)

E553(a).
CAS — 1343-88-0.
ATC — A02AA05.

NOTE. The code E553(a) has also been applied to magnesium trisilicate.

Pharmacopoeias. In Jpn. Also in USNF.

Pharmacopoeial description

USNF 20: A compound of magnesium oxide and silicon dioxide. It contains not less than 15.0% of magnesium oxide and not less than 67.0% of silicon dioxide, calculated on the ignited basis. It is a fine, white, odourless powder, free from grittiness. Insoluble in water and in alcohol. It is readily decomposed by mineral acids. pH of a well-mixed 10% suspension in water is between 7.0 and 10.8.

Uses

Magnesium silicate is used in the food industry and in pharmaceutical manufacturing as an anticaking agent.

Preparations

Proprietary Preparations (details are given in Part 3)

Multi-ingredient: *Belg.:* Mucal†; *Braz.:* Cutisanol; *Fr.:* Zea-Sorb; *Ital.:* Babigoz Crema Protettiva; *Port.:* Mucal; *Switz.:* Bigasan†.

Methylcellulose (5401-h)

Methylcellulose (*rINN*).

E461; Methylcellulosum; Metilcelulosa.
CAS — 9004-67-5.
ATC — A06AC06.

Pharmacopoeias. In Eur. (see p.vi), Int., Jpn, Pol., and US.

Incompatibilities have been reported with a number of compounds including chlorocresol, hydroxybenzoates, and phenol. Large amounts of electrolytes increase the viscosity of methylcellulose mucilages owing to salting-out of the methylcellulose; in very high concentrations of electrolytes, the methylcellulose may be completely precipitated.

Pharmacopoeial description

Ph. Eur.: A cellulose having some of the hydroxyl groups in the form of the methyl ether. Various grades of methylcellulose are available and are distinguished by appending a number indicating the apparent viscosity in millipascal seconds of a 2% w/w solution at 20°. It is a white, yellowish-white, or greyish-white powder or granules; hygroscopic after drying. Practically insoluble in hot water, in dehydrated alcohol, in acetone, in ether, and in toluene; dissolves in cold water, forming a colloidal solution. A 1% w/w solution in water has a pH of 5.5 to 8.0.

USP 25: A methyl ether of cellulose. When dried at 105° for 2 hours, it contains not less than 27.5% and not more than 31.5% of methoxy groups. It is a white, fibrous powder or granules. It swells in water and produces a clear to opalescent, viscous, colloidal suspension; insoluble in alcohol, in chloroform, and in ether; soluble in glacial acetic acid and in a mixture of equal volumes of alcohol and chloroform. Its aqueous suspension are neutral to litmus.

Adverse Effects

Large quantities of methylcellulose may temporarily increase flatulence and distension and there is a risk of intestinal obstruction. Oesophageal obstruction may occur if compounds like methylcellulose are swallowed dry.

Precautions

Methylcellulose and other bulk-forming agents should not be given to patients with intestinal obstruction or conditions likely to lead to intestinal obstruction. They should be taken with sufficient fluid to prevent faecal impaction or oesophageal obstruction, and should not be taken immediately before going to bed. Methylcellulose should not be used in infective bowel disease.

Interactions

Bulk laxatives such as methylcellulose lower the transit time through the gut and could affect the absorption of other drugs. Incompatibilities that have been reported *in vitro* with methylcellulose are listed above.

Uses and Administration

The various grades of methylcellulose are widely used in pharmaceutical manufacturing as emulsifying, suspending, and thickening agents and as binding, disintegrating, and coating agents in tablet manufacturing. Low-viscosity grades are preferred for use as emulsifying agents as the surface tension produced is lower than with the higher-viscosity grades. Low-viscosity grades may also be used as suspending or thickening agents for liquid oral dosage forms and solutions of methylcellulose may be used as replacements for sugar-based syrups or other suspension bases. For thickening topically applied products such as gels and creams a high-viscosity grade is usually employed. In tablet technology low- or medium-viscosity grades are used as binding agents while high-viscosity grades act as tablet disintegrants by swelling on contact with the disintegration medium. For tablet coating, highly substituted low-viscosity grades are usually used. Methylcellulose may also be included in modified-release tablet formulations.

Methylcellulose is also employed as an emulsifier and stabiliser in the food industry.

Methylcellulose is also used clinically as a bulk-forming agent. Medium- or high-viscosity grades are used as bulk laxatives in the treatment of constipation (p.1202); by taking up moisture they increase the volume of the faeces and promote peristalsis. Methylcellulose is usually given in a dosage of up to 6 g daily in divided doses, taken with plenty of fluid. It is also given in similar doses but with a minimum amount of water for the control of diarrhoea (p.1203) and for the control of faecal consistency in ostomies. It is also used in the management of diverticular disease (p.1203). Methylcellulose has also been used as an aid to appetite control in the management of obesity (p.1505) but there is little evidence of efficacy.

A 0.5 to 1% solution of a high-viscosity grade of methylcellulose has been used as a vehicle for eye drops, as artificial tears, and in contact lens care, but hypromellose (p.1501) is now generally preferred for this purpose.

Preparations

BP 2001: Methylcellulose Granules; Methylcellulose Tablets;
USP 25: Methylcellulose Ophthalmic Solution; Methylcellulose Oral Solution; Methylcellulose Tablets.

Proprietary Preparations (details are given in Part 3)
Aust.: Bulk; *Austral.:* Cellulone; *Canad.:* Murocel; *Fr.:* Dacryolarmes; *Irl.:* Celevac; *Ital.:* Lacrimart; *Port.:* Davilose; *Spain:* Muciplasma; *UK:* Celevac; *USA:* Citrucel; Murocel.

Multi-ingredient: *Aust.:* Cellobexon; *Austral.:* Bioglan 3B Beer Belly Buster; Citri Slim+Trim; Le Trim-BM; Neo-Trim Fibre; Parachoc; Pro-Shape; *Braz.:* Kolantyl; Kolantyl DMP; *Canad.:* Slim Mint; *Ital.:* Conta-Lens Wetting; *S.Afr.:* Kolantyl; Medigel; Merasyn; *Spain:* Humectante.

Pectin (5447-c)

E440 (amidated pectin or pectin).
CAS — 9000-69-5.
ATC — A07BC01.
Pharmacopoeias. In Aust. and US.

Pharmacopoeial description

USP 25: A purified carbohydrate product obtained from the dilute acid extract of the inner portion of the rind of citrus fruits or from apple pomace; it consists mainly of partially methoxylated polygalacturonic acids. A yellowish-white, almost odourless, coarse or fine powder. Almost completely soluble in 1 in 20 of water, forming a viscous, opalescent, colloidal solution which flows readily and is acid to litmus; practically insoluble in alcohol or in diluted alcohol and in other organic solvents. It dissolves more readily in water if first moistened with alcohol, glycerol, or simple syrup, or if mixed with 3 or more parts of sucrose. Store in airtight containers.

Interactions

Bulk-forming agents such as dietary fibre lower the transit time through the gut and may affect the absorption of other drugs.

Lipid regulating drugs. Pectin, employed as a source of fibre, together with a lipid-lowering diet and *lovastatin* has resulted in a paradoxical increase in low-density lipoprotein (LDL)-cholesterol in patients with hypercholesterolaemia. It was believed the pectin reduced the absorption of lovastatin from the gut.[1]

1. Richter WO, *et al.* Interaction between fibre and lovastatin. *Lancet* 1991; **338**: 706.

Uses and Administration

Pectins are used as emulsifiers and stabilisers in the food industry. They are non-starch polysaccharide constituents of dietary fibre (see Bran, p.1214).

Pectin is an adsorbent and bulk-forming agent and is present in multi-ingredient preparations for the management of diarrhoea, constipation, and obesity. Pectin has also been tried for reducing or slowing carbohydrate absorption in the dumping syndrome (p.1203).

Preparations

Proprietary Preparations (details are given in Part 3)
Fr.: Arhemapectine Antihemorragique; Hydrocoll.

Multi-ingredient: *Aust.:* Diarrhoesan; *Austral.:* Betaine Digestive Aid; Bioglan 3B Beer Belly Buster; Bioglan Psylli-Mucil Plus; Bioglan Zellulean with Escin; Citri Slim+Trim; Diarcalm; Diareze; Donnagel; Enterocare; Kaomagma with Pectin; Kaopectate; Natures Own Acidophilus Plus; Orabase; Orahesive; PC Regulax; Pro-Shape; Stomahesive; United Soft Guard†; *Belg.:* Kaopectate; Tanalone; *Braz.:* Atacoly; Atalin; Atapec; Colestase; Diapool; Enterobion; Enterocler; Enterodina; Enteropen; Fluocal com Pectina; Furazolin; Kal Sept; Kaomagma; Kaopectate; Kaopectin; Linadin; Magnostase; Parenterin; Pectalin; Pectimax; Plasmocolit; Plexo Enterin; Tratocoli; *Canad.:* Diarex; Diban; Donnagel-PG; Orabase; Orahesive; *Fr.:* Gastropax; Sureskin; *Ger.:* Diarrhoesan; Kaoprompt-H; *Hong Kong:* Uni-Kaotin; *Irl.:* Kaopectate; Orabase; *Israel:* Kaopectin; Kapectin Forte; Orabase; *Ital.:* Cruscasohn; Streptomagma; *Mex.:* Colfur; Coralzul; Dibapec Compuesto; Farpectol; Fuzotyl; Kaomycin; Kaopectate; Tapzol; Tapzol Con Neomicina; Treda; *NZ:* Stomahesive; *Port.:* Cloranpectina; Combidern; Varihesive; *S.Afr.:* Betapect; Bipectinol; Biskapect; Chloropect; Collodyne†; Diastat†; Enterolyte; Gastropect; Granugel; Kantrexil; Kao; Kaoneo†; Kaopectin; Kaostatex; Neopect†; Pectikon; Pectin-K; Pectolin†; Pectrolyte; *Spain:* Bio Hubber Fuerte†; Bio Hubber†; Dextricea; Estreptoenterol; *Switz.:* Demosvelte N†; HEC; Kaopectate; Varihesive Hydroactive†; *Thai.:* Biodan; Carbonpectate; Di-Su-Frone; Difuran; Diolin; Disento PF; Furasian; Furopectin; Kaopectal; Kaopectalin-N; Kaopectate; Med-Kafuzone; *UAE:* Kaptin; *UK:* Entrotabs; Goodypops; Kaopectate†; KLN; Orabase; Orahesive; Stomahesive; Varihesive†; *USA:* K-C; Kao-Paverin; Kao-Spen; Kaodene Non-Narcotic.

Polyethylene Oxide (3271-z)

Pharmacopoeias. In USNF.

Pharmacopoeial description

USNF 20: A nonionic homopolymer of ethylene oxide, represented by the formula $(OCH_2CH_2)_n$, in which n represents the average number of oxyethylene groups (about 2000 to over 100 000). It is obtainable in several grades, varying in viscosity profile in an aqueous isopropyl alcohol solution. It may contain not more than 3% of silicon dioxide. A white to off-white powder. Miscible with water; freely soluble in acetonitrile, in dichloromethane, in ethylene dichloride, and in trichloroethylene; insoluble in aliphatic hydrocarbons, in ethylene glycol, in diethylene glycol, and in glycerol. Store in airtight containers. Protect from light.

Uses

Polyethylene oxide is used as a tablet binder and as a suspending and thickening agent in pharmaceutical preparations. Polyethylene oxide is also used in a hydrogel wound dressing.

Preparations

Proprietary Preparations (details are given in Part 3)
UK: Vigilon.

Polyvinyl Acetate Phthalate (18369-l)

Pharmacopoeias. In USNF.

Pharmacopoeial description

USNF 20: Polyvinyl acetate phthalate is a reaction product of phthalic anhydride and a partially hydrolysed polyvinyl acetate. It contains not less than 55.0% and not more than 62.0% of phthalyl groups, calculated on an anhydrous acid-free basis. It is a free-flowing white powder that may have a slight odour of acetic acid. Insoluble in water, in chloroform, and in dichloromethane; soluble in alcohol and in methyl alcohol. Store in airtight containers.

Uses

Polyvinyl acetate phthalate is a viscosity-modifying agent that is used in the manufacture of enteric coating for tablets.

Polyvinyl Alcohol (468-b)

Poly(Alcohol Vinylicus); Poly(Vinyl Alcohol).
CAS — 9002-89-5.
Pharmacopoeias. In Eur. (see p.vi), Pol., and US.

Pharmacopoeial description

Ph. Eur.: It is obtained by polymerisation of vinyl acetate followed by partial or complete hydrolysis of polyvinyl acetate in the presence of catalytic amounts of alkali or mineral acids. Various grades are available and they differ in their degree of polymerisation and their degree of hydrolysis, which determine the physical properties of the different grades. They are characterised by the viscosity and the ester value of the substance. The mean relative molecular mass lies between 20 000 and 150 000. The viscosity is 3 to 70 millipascal seconds. The ester value, which characterises the degree of hydrolysis, is not greater than 280.
Polyvinyl alcohol occurs as a yellowish-white powder or translucent granules. Soluble in water; slightly soluble in dehydrated alcohol; practically insoluble in acetone. A 4% solution in water has a pH of 4.5 to 6.5.
USP 25: A synthetic resin represented by the formula $(CH_2CHOH)_n$, where the average value of n is 500 to 5000. It is prepared by 85 to 89% hydrolysis of polyvinyl acetate. White to cream-coloured, odourless, granules or powder. Freely soluble in water at room temperature; solution may be effected more rapidly at somewhat higher temperatures. pH of a 4% solution in water is between 5.0 and 8.0.

Uses and Administration

Polyvinyl alcohol is a nonionic surfactant that is used in pharmaceutical manufacturing as a stabilising agent and as a viscosity-increasing agent and lubricant.

Polyvinyl alcohol has also been used in the preparation of jellies which dry rapidly when applied to the skin to form a soluble plastic film.

Polyvinyl alcohols of various grades are used for a wide variety of industrial applications.

Polyvinyl alcohol has been used to increase the viscosity of ophthalmic preparations thus prolonging contact of the active ingredient with the eye. It is included in artificial tears preparations used for dry eye (p.1498) and in contact lens solutions (p.1129). For dry eye it is often used in a concentration of 1.4% with or without povidone.

Preparations

Proprietary Preparations (details are given in Part 3)
Aust.: Liquifilm; *Austral.:* Barnes-Hind Wetting Solution†; Liquifilm; *Belg.:* Liquifilm; *Braz.:* Duracare; Lacril; Totalens; *Canad.:* Artificial Tears; Cooper Tears†; Duracare; Hypotears; Liquifilm; Optilube PVA; PMS-Artificial Tears; Revitaleyes†; RO-Dry Eyes†; Scheinpharm Artificial Tears; Total; *Denm.:* Lacril; *Fin.:* Liquifilm; Oftan; *Fr.:* Liquifilm†; *Ger.:* Alltotal†; Contafilm†; Lacrimal; Liquifilm; Vistofilm†; *Hong Kong:* Liquifilm; PMS-Artificial Tears; *Irl.:* Liquifilm; Sno Tears; *Israel:* Liquifilm; Liquifilm Tears; *Ital.:* Lacrilux; *Mex.:* Lubrik; *Neth.:* Liquifilm†; *Norw.:* Ocufri; *NZ:* Liquifilm; *Port.:* Liquifilm; *S.Afr.:* Liquifilm Tears; *Singapore:* Hypotears; Liquifilm Tears; PMS-Artificial Tears; *Spain:* Hypo Tears; Liquifilm Lagrimas; *Swed.:* Sincon; *Switz.:* Liquifilm; *Thai.:* Liquifilm Tears; *UK:* Liquifilm Tears; Sno Tears; *USA:* Akwa Tears; Dry Eyes; Liquifilm; Nu-Tears; Ocu-Tears; Puralube; Tear Drop†; Tears Again.

Multi-ingredient: *Aust.:* Siccaprotect; *Austral.:* Murine Revital Eyes; Murine Sore Eyes; Murine Tears for Eyes; Refresh; Teardrops; Tears Plus; *Braz.:* Polipred; *Canad.:* Murine; PMS-Artificial Tears Plus; Refresh; Scheinpharm Artificial Tears Plus; Teardrops; Tears Plus; *Fr.:* Refresh; *Ger.:* Dispatenol; Duracare†; Lacrimal OK; Siccaprotect; *Hong Kong:* Hypotears; *Israel:* Hypotears PF; Refresh; *Ital.:* Collyria; Hypotears; *Mex.:* Lagrifilm

The symbol † denotes a preparation no longer actively marketed

---

Plus; *Neth.:* Tears Plus†; *NZ:* Refresh; Teardrops; Tears Plus; *S.Afr.:* Refresh; Tears Plus; *Singapore:* Refresh; *Spain:* Liquifresh; *Switz.:* Collylarm; Hypotears; Tears Plus; *Thai.:* Refresh; *UK:* Hypotears; Refresh; *USA:* Hypotears; Murine; Murine Plus; Nu-Tears II; Refresh; Tears Plus; VasoClear.

Povidone (5450-e)

Povidone (*BAN, USAN, rINN*).
E1201; Polyvidone; Polyvidonum; Polyvinylpyrrolidone; Povidonum; PVP; Vinylpyrrolidinone Polymer. Poly (2-oxopyrrolidin-1-ylethylene).
$(C_6H_9NO)_n$.
CAS — 9003-39-8.
Pharmacopoeias. In Eur. (see p.vi), Int., Jpn, Pol., and US.

Pharmacopoeial description

Ph. Eur.: A mixture of essentially linear synthetic polymers of 1-vinylpyrrolidin-2-one. A white or yellowish-white, hygroscopic powder or flakes. Freely soluble in water, in alcohol, and in methyl alcohol; slightly soluble in acetone; practically insoluble in ether. A 5% solution in water has a pH of 3.0 to 7.0. Protect from moisture
USP 25: A synthetic polymer consisting essentially of linear 1-vinyl-2-pyrrolidinone groups, the degree of polymerisation of which results in polymers of various molecular weights. A white to slightly creamy-white, hygroscopic, powder. Freely soluble in water, in alcohol, and in methyl alcohol; slightly soluble in acetone; practically insoluble in ether. pH of a 5% solution in water is between 3.0 and 7.0. Store in airtight containers.

Copovidone (17698-r)

Copolyvidone; Copolyvidonum; Copovidonum.
Pharmacopoeias. In Eur. (see p.vi).

Pharmacopoeial description

Ph. Eur.: A copolymer of 1-vinylpyrrolidin-2-one and vinyl acetate in the mass proportion 3:2. A white or yellowish-white, hygroscopic powder or flakes. Freely soluble in water, in alcohol, and in dichloromethane; practically insoluble in ether. Protect from moisture.

Crospovidone (10229-v)

Crospovidone (*rINN*).
Crospovidonum; Polyplasdone XL.
CAS — 9003-39-8.
ATC — A07BC03.
Pharmacopoeias. In Eur. (see p.vi). Also in USNF.

Pharmacopoeial description

Ph. Eur.: A cross-linked homopolymer of 1-vinylpyrrolidin-2-one. A white or yellowish-white, hygroscopic powder or flakes. Practically insoluble in water, in alcohol, and in dichloromethane. Protect from moisture.
USNF 20: A synthetic cross-linked homopolymer of *N*-vinyl-2-pyrrolidinone. A white to creamy-white, hygroscopic powder having a faint odour. Insoluble in water and in ordinary organic solvents. pH of a 1% suspension in water is between 5.0 and 8.0. Store in airtight containers.

Adverse Effects

Some products intended for parenteral administration contain povidone as an excipient and injection has led to deposition of povidone in various tissues with consequent lesions and pain. There have been occasional reports of liver involvement.

◊ Reviews of adverse effects associated with pharmaceutical excipients including povidone.
1. Golightly LK, *et al.* Pharmaceutical excipients: adverse effects associated with 'inactive ingredients' in drug products (part II). *Med Toxicol* 1988; **3:** 209–40.

Uses and Administration

Povidone is used in pharmaceutical manufacturing as a suspending and dispersing agent and as a tablet binding, granulating, and coating agent. It is used as a carrier for iodine (see Povidone-Iodine, p.1155). An insoluble cross-linked form of povidone known as crospovidone is used as a tablet disintegrant. Copovidone, a copolymer with vinyl acetate, is used as a tablet binding and coating agent.

Povidone is included in artificial tears preparations used in the management of dry eye (p.1498) and in solutions for contact lens care (p.1129). For dry eye it is often used in a concentration of 0.6% together with other viscosity-increasing agents (such as polyvinyl alcohol); it may also be used alone in solutions containing 1.5 to 5%.

Povidone has also been used as an adsorbent in gastrointestinal disorders.

Povidone was formerly used as a plasma expander but other compounds are now preferred.

Preparations

Proprietary Preparations (details are given in Part 3)
Aust.: Oculotect; Protagent; *Austral.:* Clerz Moisturising Drops; In A Wink Moisturing; *Belg.:* Protagent†; Siccagent†; *Denm.:* Oculac; *Fin.:* Oculac; *Fr.:* Bolinan; Dulcilarmes; Nu-Gel; *Ger.:* Arufil; Lacophtal; Lacri-Stulln; Oculotect Fluid; Protagent; Vidirakt S; Vidisept; Vidisept EDO; *Hong Kong:* Hypotears Plus; *Israel:* Lacrimol; *Ital.:* Clarover; Protagent; *Neth.:* Duratears Free†; Oculotect; Protagens†; *Norw.:* Oculac; *NZ:* In A

Wink; *Port.:* Oculotect; *S.Afr.:* Hypotears; *Singapore:* Oculotect; Vidisept N; *Spain:* Oculotect; *Swed.:* Oculac; *Switz.:* Oculac; Protagent; *Thai.:* Hypotears Plus; *UK:* Oculotect.

Multi-ingredient: *Austral.:* Bausch & Lomb Sensitive Eyes Lens Lubricant†; Murine Revital Eyes; Murine Sore Eyes; Murine Tears for Eyes; Refresh; Teardrops; Tears Plus; Visine Advanced Relief; *Canad.:* Moisture Drops; Murine; PMS-Artificial Tears Plus; Refresh; Scheinpharm Artificial Tears Plus; Teardrops; Tears Plus; *Fr.:* Poly-Karaya; Refresh; *Ger.:* Lacrimal OK; Lacrisic; *Israel:* Refresh; V-Crima; *Mex.:* Lagrifilm Plus; Soyaloid; Soydex; *Neth.:* Tears Plus†; *NZ:* Refresh; Teardrops; Tears Plus; *S.Afr.:* Refresh; Tears Plus; *Singapore:* Refresh; *Spain:* Liquifresh; *Switz.:* Collylarm; Poly-Karaya; Tears Plus; *Thai.:* Refresh; *UK:* Gelclair; Refresh; *USA:* Adsorbotear†; Advanced Relief Visine; Murine; Murine Plus; Refresh; Tears Night & Day; Tears Plus.

Silica (4000-d)

Silica or silicon dioxide is available in various forms.

Purified Siliceous Earth (5456-k)

Diatomaceous Earth; Diatomite; Purified Infusorial Earth; Purified Kieselguhr; Terra Silicea Purificada.
CAS — 7631-86-9.
Pharmacopoeias. In USNF.

Pharmacopoeial description

USNF 20: A form of silicon dioxide consisting of frustules and fragments of diatoms purified by calcining. A very fine, white, light grey, or pale buff mixture of amorphous powder and lesser amounts of crystalline polymorphs, including quartz and cristobalite. It is gritty and readily absorbs moisture, and retains about four times its weight of water before becoming fluid. Insoluble in water, in acids, and in dilute solutions of alkali hydroxides.

Silicon Dioxide (5455-c)

Colloidal Hydrated Silica; E551; Precipitated Silica; Silica Colloidalis Hydrica; Silica Gel.
$SiO_2, xH_2O = 60.08$ (anhydrous).
CAS — 63231-67-4; 7631-86-9.
Pharmacopoeias. In Eur. (see p.vi). Also in USNF.

Pharmacopoeial description

Ph. Eur.: A light, fine, white or almost white, amorphous powder. Practically insoluble in water, and in mineral acids except hydrofluoric acid; dissolves in hot solutions of alkali hydroxides.
Dental-Type Silica is an amorphous silica (precipitated, gel, or obtained by flame hydrolysis). A white or almost white, light, fine amorphous powder. Practically insoluble in water and in mineral acids; dissolves in hydrofluoric acid and in hot solutions of alkali hydroxides.
USNF 20: It is obtained by insolubilising the dissolved silica in sodium silicate solution. Where obtained by the addition of sodium silicate to a mineral acid, the product is termed silica gel; where obtained by the destabilisation of a solution of sodium silicate in such a manner as to yield very fine particles, the product is termed precipitated silica. A fine, white, odourless, hygroscopic, amorphous powder in which the diameter of the average particles ranges from 2 to 10 μm. Insoluble in water, in alcohol, and in other organic solvents; soluble in hot solutions of alkali hydroxides. pH of 5% slurry in water is between 4.0 and 8.0. Store in airtight containers. Protect from moisture.
Dental-Type Silica is obtained from sodium silicate solution by destabilising with acid in such a way as to yield very fine particles. A fine, white, odourless, hygroscopic, amorphous powder in which the diameter of the average particles ranges from 0.5 to 40 μm. Insoluble in water, in alcohol, and in acid (except hydrofluoric acid); soluble in hot solutions of alkali hydroxides. pH of 5% slurry in water is between 4.0 and 8.5. Store in airtight containers.

Colloidal Silicon Dioxide (5457-a)

Acidum Silicicum Colloidale; Colloidal Anhydrous Silica; Colloidal Silica; Hochdisperses Silicumdioxid; Silica Colloidalis Anhydrica.
$SiO_2 = 60.08$.
CAS — 7631-86-9.
Pharmacopoeias. In Eur. (see p.vi). Also in USNF.

Pharmacopoeial description

Ph. Eur.: A light, fine, white, amorphous powder. It has a particle size of about 15 nm. Practically insoluble in water and in mineral acids except hydrofluoric acid; dissolves in hot solutions of alkali hydroxides. A 3.3% suspension in water has a pH of 3.5 to 5.5.
USNF 20: A submicroscopic fumed silicon dioxide, prepared by the vapour-phase hydrolysis of a silicon compound. A light, white, non-gritty powder of extremely fine particle size (about 15 nm). Insoluble in water and in acid (except hydrofluoric acid); soluble in hot solutions of alkali hydroxides. pH of a 4% dispersion in water is between 3.5 and 5.5.

Adverse Effects

Prolonged inhalation of some forms of silica dust may be associated with the development of fibrosis of the lung (silicosis). The forms of silica described here and used as pharmaceutical excipients may cause irritation of the respiratory tract if inhaled but do not appear to be associated with silicosis.

Uses

The different forms of silica have various pharmaceutical uses. Purified siliceous earth is used as a filtering medium and adsorbent. Silicon dioxide is used as a suspending and thickening agent and, as silica gel, as a desiccant. Colloidal silicon dioxide is used as a suspending agent and thickener, as a stabiliser in emulsions, and as an anticaking agent and desiccant. Silicon dioxide is also used as an anticaking agent in the food industry. Silicon dioxide (Silicea) is used in homoeopathic medicine.

Preparations

Proprietary Preparations (details are given in Part 3)
Austral.: Celloids S 79; *Ger.:* Aktiv-Puder; Entero-Teknosal; Sklerosol; *Mon.:* Dissolvurol.

Multi-ingredient: *Aust.:* CO$_2$ Granulat; Kephalodoron; *Austral.:* Bio-Disc; Duo Celloids SCF; Duo Celloids SPS; Duo Celloids SSS; Silicic Complex; *Fin.:* Wicne; *Fr.:* Gelopectose; Topaal; *Ger.:* Aplona; CO$_2$ Granulat; Equisil; Rowarolan†; *Hong Kong:* Biscasil; Disflatyl; *Israel:* Adinol; *Ital.:* Gastrovison†; Lacalut; *Singapore:* Disflatyl; *Switz.:* Acne Creme; Cicafissan; Fissan; *UK:* Bidor; New Era Hymosa†; New Era Zief†; WCS Dusting Powder.

Sodium Starch Glycolate (5460-y)

Carboxymethylamylum Natricum; Sodium Carboxymethyl Starch; Sodium Starch Glycollate; Starch Sodium Glycolate.
CAS — 9063-38-1.
Pharmacopoeias. In *Chin.* Also in *USNF.*
Eur. (see p.vi) includes Sodium Starch Glycolate (Type A), Sodium Starch Glycolate (Type B), and Sodium Starch Glycolate (Type C).

Pharmacopoeial description

Ph. Eur.: The sodium salt of a carboxymethyl ether of starch. Sodium Starch Glycolate (Type A) contains 2.8 to 4.2% of sodium, Sodium Starch Glycolate (Type B) contains 2.0 to 3.4% of sodium, and Sodium Starch Glycolate (Type C) contains 2.8 to 5.0% of sodium, each calculated with reference to the substance washed with alcohol (80%) and dried. A fine, white or almost white, very hygroscopic, free-flowing powder. Practically insoluble in dichloromethane. Type A and Type B form a translucent suspension in water; pH of the supernatant of a 4% suspension is 5.5 to 7.5 (Type A) and 3.0 to 5.0 (Type B). Type C forms a translucent gel-like product in water; a 4% gel has a pH of 5.5 to 7.5.

Store in airtight containers. Protect from light.

USNF 20: The sodium salt of a carboxymethyl ether of starch. It contains not less than 2.8% and not more than 4.2% of sodi-

um on the dried, alcohol-washed basis. A white, odourless, relatively free-flowing powder available in several different viscosity grades. A 2% dispersion in cold water settles, on standing, in the form of a highly hydrated layer. Protect from variations in temperature and humidity which may cause caking. pH of a 1 g in 30 mL suspension in water is either between 3.0 and 5.0 or between 5.5 and 7.5.

Uses

Sodium starch glycolate is used as a disintegrating agent in tablet manufacture.

Tragacanth (5463-c)

E413; Goma Alcatira; Gomme Adragante; Gum Dragon; Gum Tragacanth; Trag.; Tragacantha; Tragacanto; Tragant.
CAS — 9000-65-1.
Pharmacopoeias. In *Eur.* (see p.vi), *Jpn,* and *Pol.* Also in *USNF.*

Pharmacopoeial description

Ph. Eur.: The air-hardened gummy exudation flowing naturally or obtained by incision from the trunk and branches of *Astragalus gummifer* and some other species of *Astragalus* (Leguminosae) from western Asia. It occurs as thin, flattened, ribbon-like, white or pale yellow, translucent, horny strips. When reduced to a powder it forms a mucilaginous gel with about ten times its weight of water. Protect from light.

USNF 20: The dried gummy exudation from *Astragalus gummifer* or other Asiatic species of *Astragalus* (Leguminosae). It occurs as odourless, flattened, lamellated, frequently curved fragments or straight or spirally twisted linear pieces. It is white to weak yellow, translucent, and horny in texture. Powdered tragacanth is white to yellowish-white.

Adverse Effects

Hypersensitivity reactions, sometimes severe, have occurred rarely after the ingestion of products containing tragacanth. Contact dermatitis has been reported following the external use of tragacanth.

Uses

Tragacanth forms viscous solutions or gels with water, depending on the concentration. It is used in pharmaceutical manufacturing as a suspending agent and as an emulsifying agent. In dispensing aqueous preparations of tragacanth, the powdered tragacanth is first dispersed in a wetting agent, such as alcohol, to prevent agglomeration on the addition of water.

Tragacanth is also used for similar purposes in the food industry.

Xanthan Gum (5465-a)

Corn Sugar Gum; E415; Polysaccharide B 1459; Xantham Gum; Xanthani Gummi.
CAS — 11138-66-2.
Pharmacopoeias. In *Eur.* (see p.vi). Also in *USNF.*

Pharmacopoeial description

Ph. Eur.: A gum produced by fermentation of a carbohydrate with *Xanthomonas campestris* and purified. It is the sodium, potassium, or calcium salt of a high molecular weight polysaccharide containing D-glucose, mannose, and glucuronic acid. It also contains not less than 1.5% of pyruvic acid, calculated with reference to the dried substance. A white or yellowish-white, free-flowing powder. Soluble in water giving a highly viscous solution; practically insoluble in organic solvents. A 1% solution in water has a pH of 6.0 to 8.0.

USNF 20: A high molecular weight polysaccharide gum produced by a pure-culture fermentation of a carbohydrate with *Xanthomonas campestris* and purified. It contains D-glucose, D-mannose, and D-glucuronic acid. It is prepared as the sodium, potassium, or calcium salt. A cream-coloured powder. Soluble in hot or cold water. Its solutions are neutral to litmus.

Uses

Xanthan gum is used in pharmaceutical manufacturing as a suspending, stabilising, thickening, and emulsifying agent. It is also used similarly in the food industry.

◊ Suspensions of crushed tablets or insoluble powders made with xanthan gum were reported to be preferable to those made with tragacanth.[1]

The stability was generally good and only a small number of drugs had been found to be incompatible (amitriptyline, tamoxifen, and verapamil).[1] For extemporaneous dispensing, a 1% solution of xanthan gum with hydroxybenzoate, prepared in advance, was diluted to 0.5% with water when preparing the suspension.

Xanthan gum was found to be a suitable suspending vehicle for delivering antispasmodics topically along the length of the oesophagus in patients with oesophageal spasm.[2] Coagulation of the gum had been observed when it was used for suspensions of certain film-coated tablets.

1. Anonymous. "Extremely useful" new suspending agent. *Pharm J* 1986; **237:** 665.
2. Evans BK, Fenton-May V. Keltrol. *Pharm J* 1986; **237:** 736–7.

Preparations

USNF 20: Xanthan Gum Solution.

Proprietary Preparations (details are given in Part 3)
Switz.: TenderWet; *UK:* Keltrol.

Multi-ingredient: *Ital.:* Resource Gelificata.

Stimulants and Anorectics

This chapter includes compounds used, generally under specialist supervision, for their central stimulant or their anorectic effects. Many are sympathomimetics and are subject to extensive abuse, which has led to strict limitations on their availability.

Hyperactivity

Attention deficit hyperactivity disorder (ADHD) is a heterogeneous behaviour disorder which first becomes evident during childhood and consists of developmentally inappropriate and socially disruptive behaviour characterised by varying degrees of hyperactivity, inattention, and impulsiveness. Children with this disorder are easily distracted and have difficulty in completing tasks. Associated features may include low frustration tolerance, mood lability, and defiance. Some children continue to have symptoms throughout adolescence and into adulthood. The terms hyperkinesis, hyperkinetic syndrome, minimal brain dysfunction, attention deficit disorder, and attention deficit disorder with hyperactivity have sometimes been used synonymously for ADHD, but patients described as having these disorders do not necessarily satisfy the diagnostic criteria for ADHD.

Treatment depends on the severity of the disorder. In the USA drug treatment for ADHD is quite common even in mild forms, and in the hands of specialists appears superior to behavioural therapy, but in the UK it is generally only used under specialist supervision for the more severely affected child who fails to respond to counselling and behaviour therapy. Drug therapy is useful for the management of symptoms but is not curative. Dexamfetamine and methylphenidate are usually the drugs of first choice but there is no consensus on which is the most effective. Pemoline has been used but is associated with hepatotoxicity. Prolonged administration of such central stimulants can retard growth and some recommend occasional drug holidays to allow catch-up growth and determine whether continued therapy is necessary; many authorities consider that young children should not receive stimulants. However, clinical experience suggests that most children who benefit from drug therapy will require several years of therapy. Stimulants appear to be of use when the disorder persists into adulthood.

Tricyclic antidepressants such as imipramine and desipramine are also used for ADHD in both children and adults and their effect in this condition appears to be independent of their antidepressant action. However, they tend to be reserved for patients who fail to respond to, or are intolerant of, central stimulants. Tricyclic antidepressants may be a useful alternative in patients with Tourette's syndrome (which co-exists in some patients with ADHD) or in those with a family history of the disorder as stimulants are believed to precipitate or exacerbate associated tics (p.650). Tricyclic antidepressants might also be preferred in patients with co-existing anxiety, depression, or enuresis, or in those with a history of drug abuse. Combined therapy with tricyclic antidepressants and central stimulants has been studied but careful monitoring is advised. MAOIs have been used successfully but problems with dietary restriction and potential drug interactions have limited their use. For further information concerning potential interactions between stimulants and tricyclic antidepressants or MAOIs, see under Dexamfetamine, p.1508. The SSRIs such as fluoxetine have produced beneficial results as an adjunct to central stimulants in a small number of patients with associated depression or obsessive-compulsive disorder, but there is insufficient evidence to assess their efficacy in ADHD without these co-existing disorders. Bupropion has shown promising results in controlled studies in children; however, it has been reported to exacerbate tics and may increase the risk of seizures in predisposed patients. Venlafaxine has been effective in open trials in a small number of adult patients.

There is some evidence that carbamazepine may be an effective alternative to central stimulants. Clonidine has been used successfully as adjunctive therapy to stimulants in children with an inadequate response to the latter. However, there have been reports of adverse cardiac events associated with such combinations. Antipsychotics can produce severe adverse effects and are probably rarely indicated in ADHD. Their use might be warranted as adjunctive therapy to central stimulants in severe cases or when there is also extremely violent or destructive behaviour. Dopaminergic agonists such as levodopa or pergolide have been tried with beneficial results for the treatment of restless legs syndrome and periodic limb movements in sleep associated with ADHD; some improvements in ADHD symptoms were also noted following resolution of the parasomnias (see under Levodopa, p.1173).

Much controversy has surrounded the hypothesis that certain synthetic food additives including preservatives and artificial flavours and colours are aetiological agents in ADHD. Controlled studies have not proved the efficacy of dietary manipulation.

References.

1. Fox AM, Rieder MJ. Risks and benefits of drugs used in the management of the hyperactive child. *Drug Safety* 1993; **9:** 38–50.
2. Barbaresi WJ. Primary-care approach to the diagnosis and management of attention-deficit hyperactivity disorder. *Mayo Clin Proc* 1996; **71:** 463–71.
3. Committee on Children With Disabilities and Committee on Drugs. Medication for children with attention disorders. *Pediatrics* 1996; **98:** 301–4.
4. Cyr M, Brown CS. Current drug therapy recommendations for the treatment of attention deficit hyperactivity disorder. *Drugs* 1998; **56:** 215–23.
5. Goldman LS, *et al.* Diagnosis and treatment of attention-deficit/hyperactivity disorder in children and adolescents. *JAMA* 1998; **279:** 1100–1107.
6. Wender PH. Pharmacotherapy of attention-deficit/hyperactivity disorder in adults. *J Clin Psychiatry* 1998; **59** (suppl 7): 76–9.
7. Swanson JM, *et al.* Attention-deficit hyperactivity disorder and hyperkinetic disorder. *Lancet* 1998; **351:** 429–33.
8. Zametkin AJ, Ernst M. Problems in the management of attention-deficit-hyperactivity disorder. *N Engl J Med* 1999; **340:** 40–6.
9. Elia J, *et al.* Treatment of attention-deficit-hyperactivity disorder. *N Engl J Med* 1999; **340:** 780–8.
10. The MTA Cooperative Group. A 14-month randomized clinical trial of treatment strategies for attention-deficit/hyperactivity disorder. *Arch Gen Psychiatry* 1999; **56:** 1073–86.
11. Overmeyer S, Taylor E. Annotation: principles of treatment for hyperkinetic disorder: practice approaches for the UK. *J Child Psychol Psychiatry* 1999; **40:** 1147–57.
12. Trollor JN. Attention deficit hyperactivity disorder in adults: conceptual and clinical issues. *Med J Aust* 1999; **171:** 421–5.
13. Jadad AR, *et al. Treatment of attention-deficit/hyperactivity disorder.* Rockville, MD: Agency for Healthcare Research and Quality; 1999. Available at: http://www.ahcpr.gov/clinic/adhdsum.htm (accessed 17/10/01).
14. Spencer T, *et al.* Pharmacotherapy of attention deficit hyperactivity disorder. *Child Adolesc Psychiatr Clin North Am* 2000; **9:** 77–97.
15. Anonymous. Stimulant drugs for severe hyperactivity in childhood. *Drug Ther Bull* 2001; **39:** 52–4.
16. Scottish Intercollegiate Guidelines Network. Attention deficit and hyperkinetic disorders in children and young people: a national clinical guideline (issued June 2001). Available at: http://www.sign.ac.uk/pdf/sign52.pdf (accessed 17/10/01).
17. National Institute for Clinical Excellence. Guidance on the use of methylphenidate (Ritalin, Equasym) for attention deficit/hyperactivity disorder (ADHD) in childhood (issued October 2000). Available at: http://www.nice.org.uk/pdf/Methylph-guidance13.pdf (accessed 13/11/01).

Narcoleptic syndrome

Narcolepsy is characterised by excessive daytime sleepiness and irresistible sleep attacks that last from a few minutes to hours. The narcoleptic syndrome may include other symptoms such as cataplexy, sleep paralysis, hypnagogic hallucinations, or disturbed sleep. Most patients with narcolepsy experience **cataplexy**, a sudden short-lived loss of muscle tone and paralysis of voluntary muscles induced by strong emotions. The severity of the attack can vary and some patients may experience complete collapse but there is no loss of consciousness. **Sleep paralysis** consists of transient episodes of complete paralysis that occur while falling asleep or during waking; respiration is unaffected. Some patients may complain of vivid auditory or visual hallucinations while falling asleep (**hypnagogic hallucinations**).

In the treatment of narcoleptic syndrome the patient is initially encouraged to take planned regular short periods of sleep during the day and to avoid stressful events that may provoke attacks. If drug treatment is required then central stimulants are the main drugs used for the sleep attacks of narcolepsy. However, most are ineffective against cataplexy. The selection, dose, and timing of administration of these drugs needs to be titrated for each patient and drug holidays have been suggested to reduce the risk of developing tolerance. Amfetamines were the first drugs used. However, methylphenidate is often preferred to dexamfetamine as it has a rapid action and is considered to have fewer adverse effects. Alternative non-amfetamine stimulants used in the treatment of narcolepsy include mazindol, which also appears to be effective in cataplexy, and modafinil. Selegiline has been reported to improve excessive daytime sleepiness and cataplexy. There is a wide range of other drugs for which there is anecdotal or other limited evidence of efficacy in narcolepsy but there appears to be no evidence that they are superior to the central stimulants.

Tricyclic antidepressants are the primary treatment for cataplexy and sleep paralysis. Imipramine appears to be one of the most widely used and has been reported to act more rapidly and to require a lower dose for cataplexy than when used as an antidepressant. The daily dose should be titrated to provide maximal protection for the time of day when symptoms usually occur. Clomipramine and protriptyline are also commonly used.

The use of sodium oxybate at night with stimulants during the day has been reported to improve the symptoms of patients with narcoleptic syndrome.

Patients requiring treatment for both narcolepsy and cataplexy may be given central stimulants and tricyclic antidepressants but require careful monitoring as the combination may produce serious adverse effects such as cardiac arrhythmias or hypertension; see also Interactions, under Dexamfetamine, p.1508.

References.

1. Richardson JW, *et al.* Narcolepsy update. *Mayo Clin Proc* 1990; **65:** 991–8.
2. Aldrich MS. Narcolepsy. *N Engl J Med* 1990; **323:** 389–94.
3. Parkes JD. Daytime sleepiness. *BMJ* 1993; **306:** 772–5.
4. Eisen J, *et al.* Psychotropic drugs and sleep. *BMJ* 1993; **306:** 1331–4.
5. Wise MS. Childhood narcolepsy. *Neurology* 1998; **50** (suppl 1): S37–S42.
6. Nishino S, Mignot E. Drug treatment of patients with insomnia and excessive daytime sleepiness. *Clin Pharmacokinet* 1999; **37:** 305–30.
7. Krahn LE, *et al.* Narcolepsy: new understanding of irresistible sleep. *Mayo Clin Proc* 2001; **76:** 185–94.

Obesity

Obesity results from an imbalance between energy intake and energy expenditure and increases the risk of cardiovascular disease, diabetes mellitus, gallstones, respiratory disease, osteoarthritis, and some forms of cancer. It may be defined in terms of the body mass index (BMI), which is the weight (kg) divided by the square of the height (m^2). Patients with a BMI of 25.0 to 29.9 are considered to be overweight, and a BMI of 30.0 or more represents obesity; a value of 30.0 to 34.9 represents a moderate, 35.0 to 39.9 a severe, and 40.0 or more a very severe, risk of co-morbidity. Weight loss appears to improve control of diabetes mellitus and hypertension, and to reduce cardiovascular risk factors but long-term benefits are difficult to assess as weight is often regained.

Initial management involves dietary modification and includes calorie restriction and changes in the dietary proportions of fat, protein, and carbohydrates. Physical activity should also be increased and excess alcohol avoided. These measures should be followed for at least 3 months. If there has been less than 10% reduction in weight and the BMI is still above 30, drug treatment may be considered. For patients with associated risk factors such as diabetes mellitus, ischaemic heart disease, hyperlipidaemias, hypertension, or sleep apnoea, drugs may be considered when the BMI is 27 or 28. Combination drug therapy is not recommended. Drugs should be given initially for 12 weeks. If weight loss is less than 5% then they should be considered a failure and discontinued. If weight loss is more than 5% they may be continued and the patient monitored at monthly intervals. Treatment should be stopped once the BMI falls below 30 (or 27/28 as appropriate, see above), or if weight is regained, or there is any suspicion of toxicity.

Many drugs are capable of reducing appetite and have been used as such in the treatment of obesity. However, toxicity has been a major problem and very few are still in current use.

Appetite suppressants (anorectics) can be divided into two main groups: central stimulants that act on central catecholamine pathways and drugs acting on central serotonin pathways. Stimulants such as the amfetamines and phenmetrazine are no longer recommended because of their addictive potential. Other stimulants that have been used include diethylpropion, phentermine, mazindol, and phenylpropanolamine but they are also no longer recommended. The serotonergic drugs dexfenfluramine and fenfluramine were formerly used in long-term therapy (up to 1 year) but have both been associated with valvular heart defects and have now been withdrawn worldwide. There have also been reports of valvular heart defects in patients receiving combinations of anorectics. Regulatory authorities in the European Union have called for the withdrawal of all anorectics from the market.

More recent introductions for use in obesity include orlistat (a gastric lipase inhibitor) and sibutramine (a serotonin and noradrenaline reuptake inhibitor).

Other drugs that have been investigated include fluoxetine, which has been tried with some success, and ephedrine with caffeine. Bulk-forming drugs such as methylcellulose and sterculia have been used in an attempt to control appetite by the local effect they might exert when they swell in the gastrointestinal tract, but there is little evidence of efficacy. A sucrose polyester is used as a nondigestible fat substitute by the food industry, and promoted as part of a strategy to reduce fat and calories in the diet to aid body-weight control.

The control of appetite and the mechanisms of obesity are under investigation. A gene, called the ob-gene, and its protein product, leptin, have been identified and appear to be involved in regulation of food intake.

References.
1. Rosenbaum M, et al. Obesity. N Engl J Med 1997; **337:** 396–407.
2. Björntorp P. Obesity. Lancet 1997; **350:** 423–6.
3. Wilding J. Obesity treatment. BMJ 1997; **315:** 997–1000.
4. Epstein LH, et al. Treatment of pediatric obesity. Pediatrics 1998; **101:** 554–70.
5. National Institutes of Health. Clinical guidelines on the identification, evaluation, and treatment of overweight and obesity in adults: the evidence report. Bethesda: National Heart, Lung, and Blood Institute, 1998.
6. Royal College of Physicians of London. Clinical management of overweight and obese patients with particular reference to the use of drugs. London: Royal College of Physicians of London, 1998.
7. Kolanowski J. A risk-benefit assessment of anti-obesity drugs. Drug Safety 1999; **20:** 119–31.
8. Carek PJ, Dickerson LM. Current concepts in the pharmacological management of obesity. Drugs 1999; **57:** 883–904.
9. Collazo-Clavell ML. Safe and effective management of the obese patient. Mayo Clin Proc 1999; **74:** 1255–60.
10. Egger G, et al. The effectiveness of popular, non-prescription weight loss supplements. Med J Aust 1999; **171:** 604–8.
11. WHO. Obesity: preventing and managing the global epidemic. WHO Tech Rep Ser 894 2000.
12. National Heart, Lung, and Blood Institute. The practical guide: identification, evaluation, and treatment of overweight and obesity in adults. Available at: http://www.nhlbi.nih.gov/guidelines/obesity/practgde.htm (accessed 17/10/01).
13. Glazer G. Long-term pharmacotherapy of obesity 2000: a review of efficacy and safety. Ann Intern Med 2001; **161:** 1814–24. Also available at: http://archinte.ama-assn.org/issues/v161n15/rfull/ira00112.html (accessed 04/09/01).

Prader-Willi syndrome

Compulsive eating and a voracious appetite are two of the many clinical features of Prader-Willi syndrome, a congenital disorder characterised by infantile hypotonia, hypogonadism, and facial dysmorphism, with subsequent development of abnormalities of behaviour and intellect.[1,2] Supervision and restricted access to food are the mainstay in preventing obesity, but are commonly not sufficient. Fluoxetine may decrease food intake in some patients. It has also been tried for self-mutilatory behaviour (skin picking) with variable results.[3,4] Growth hormone may be of benefit in increasing associated short stature and decreasing percentage body fat,[5,6] although close surveillance of glucose homoeostasis is advisable. Anorectics have been ineffective.[2]

1. Donaldson MDC, et al. The Prader-Willi syndrome. Arch Dis Child 1994; **70:** 58–63.
2. Couper RTL, Couper JJ. Prader-Willi syndrome. Lancet 2000; **356:** 673–5.
3. Warnock JK, Kestenbaum T. Pharmacologic treatment of severe skin-picking behaviors in Prader-Willi syndrome. Arch Dermatol 1992; **128:** 1623–5.
4. Schepis C, et al. Failure of fluoxetine to modify the skin-picking behaviour of Prader-Willi syndrome. Australas J Dermatol 1998; **39:** 57–60.
5. Lindgren AC, et al. Five years of growth hormone treatment in children with Prader-Willi syndrome. Acta Paediatr Suppl 1999; **433:** 109–11.
6. Myers SE, et al. Physical effects of growth hormone treatment in children with Prader-Willi syndrome. Acta Paediatr Suppl 1999; **433:** 112–14.

Adrafinil (3018-h)

Adrafinil (rINN).

CRL-40048. 2-[(Diphenylmethyl)sulfinyl]acetohydroxamic acid.

$C_{15}H_{15}NO_3S = 289.3$.
CAS — 63547-13-7.
ATC — N06BX17.

Profile

Adrafinil is a central stimulant and alpha$_1$-adrenergic agonist chemically related to modafinil (p.1512). It is given by mouth for mental function impairment in the elderly in doses of 600 mg to 1.2 g daily.

Preparations

Proprietary Preparations (details are given in Part 3)
Fr.: Olmifon.

Almitrine Dimesilate (12342-f)

Almitrine Dimesilate (BANM, rINNM).

Almistrine Mesylate (USAN); Almitrine Bismesylate; Almitrine Dimesylate; S-2620 (almitrine or almitrine dimesilate). NN′-Diallyl-6-[4-(4,4′-difluorobenzhydryl)piperazin-1-yl]-1,3,5-triazine-2,4-dyldiamine bis(methanesulphonate).

$C_{26}H_{29}F_2N_7, 2CH_4SO_3 = 669.8$.
CAS — 27469-53-0 (almitrine); 29608-49-9 (almitrine dimesilate).

Profile

Almitrine dimesilate has been used as a respiratory stimulant in acute respiratory failure associated with conditions such as chronic obstructive pulmonary disease. Usual oral doses range from 50 to 100 mg daily and treatment may be intermittent. Up to 3 mg per kg body-weight has been given daily by intravenous infusion in 2 or 3 divided doses, each dose being infused over 2 hours. It is also available in a compound preparation with raubasine for mental function impairment in the elderly.

Mental impairment. References.
1. Poitrenaud J, et al. Almitrine-raubasine and cognitive impairment in the elderly: results of a 6-month controlled multicenter study. Clin Neuropharmacol 1990; **13** (suppl 3): S100–S108.
2. Poitrenaud J, et al. Time course of age-associated memory impairment in 8037 patients treated with Duxil for 6 months. Rev Geriatr 1994; **19:** 531–8.
3. Poitrenaud J, et al. Memory disorders in 8037 elderly patients with age-associated memory impairment: multicenter trial with a 6-month follow-up under almitrine-raubasine. Eur Neurol 1995; **35** (suppl 1): 43–6.
4. Allain P, Bentue-Ferrer D. Clinical efficacy of almitrine-raubasine: an overview. Eur Neurol 1998; **39:** (suppl 1) 39–44.

Respiratory system disorders. Respiratory stimulants (such as almitrine) have a limited and short-term role in acute respiratory failure in chronic obstructive pulmonary disease (p.759). Almitrine has been reported[1-6] to improve ventilation and blood oxygenation, and to decrease the number of episodes of dyspnoea and hospital admissions. There are also reports[7,8] of beneficial effects when used with inhaled nitric oxide in patients with severe hypoxaemic acute respiratory distress syndrome (p.1046) as well as in patients with hypoxia caused by focal lung lesions.[9] However, these modest benefits may be outweighed by the adverse effects, which have included peripheral paraesthesia and weight loss,[4] and headache, urticaria, breathlessness, diarrhoea, chest pain, nausea, and vomiting.[6] The peripheral neuropathy which sometimes occurs during long-term use of almitrine[10,11] may be due to an underlying feature of the pulmonary disease being treated,[12-14] although some disagree with this.[15]

1. Huchon G. Advances in treatment of chronic obstructive lung disease with almitrine bis-mesylate. Postgrad Med J 1983; **59** (suppl 3): 66–7.
2. Bell RC, et al. The effect of almitrine bismesylate on hypoxemia in chronic obstructive pulmonary disease. Ann Intern Med 1986; **105:** 342–6.
3. Chung KF, Barnes PJ. Respiratory and allergic disease II: chronic obstructive airways disease and respiratory infections. BMJ 1988; **296:** 111–5.
4. Watanabe S, et al. Long-term effect of almitrine bismesylate in patients with hypoxaemic chronic obstructive pulmonary disease. Am Rev Respir Dis 1989; **140:** 1269–73.
5. Daskalopoulou E, et al. Comparison of almitrine bismesylate and medroxyprogesterone acetate on oxygenation during wakefulness and sleep in patients with chronic obstructive lung disease. Thorax 1990; **45:** 666–9.
6. Bakran I, et al. Double-blind placebo controlled clinical trial of almitrine bismesylate in patients with chronic respiratory insufficiency. Eur J Clin Pharmacol 1990; **38:** 249–53.
7. Jolliet P, et al. Additive beneficial effects of the prone position, nitric oxide, and almitrine bismesylate on gas exchange and oxygen transport in acute respiratory distress syndrome. Crit Care Med 1997; **25:** 786–94.
8. Gallart L, et al. The NO Almitrine Study Group. Intravenous almitrine combined with inhaled nitric oxide for acute respiratory distress syndrome. Am J Respir Crit Care Med 1998; **158:** 1770–7.
9. Payen D, et al. Inhaled nitric oxide, almitrine infusion, or their coadministration as a treatment of severe hypoxemic focal lung lesions. Anesthesiology 1998; **89:** 1157–65.
10. Chedru F, et al. Peripheral neuropathy during treatment with almitrine. BMJ 1985; **290:** 896.
11. Gherardi R, et al. Peripheral neuropathy in patients treated with almitrine dimesylate. Lancet 1985; **i:** 1247–50.
12. Suggett AJ, et al. Almitrine and peripheral neuropathy. Lancet 1985; **ii:** 830–1.

13. Alani SM, et al. Almitrine and peripheral neuropathy. Lancet 1985; **ii:** 1251.
14. Moore N, et al. Peripheral neuropathy in chronic obstructive lung disease. Lancet 1985; **ii:** 1311.
15. Louarn F, Gherardi R. Almitrine and peripheral neuropathy. Lancet 1985; **ii:** 1068.

Preparations

Proprietary Preparations (details are given in Part 3)
Belg.: Vectarion; **Braz.:** Vectarion; **Denm.:** Vectarion; **Fr.:** Vectarion; **Ger.:** Vectarion; **Irl.:** Vectarion; **Port.:** Vectarion; **Spain:** Sovarel†; Vectarion.

Multi-ingredient: Fr.: Duxil; **Hong Kong:** Duxaril; **Port.:** Duxil; Transoxyl; **Singapore:** Duxaril; **Spain:** Duxor; Salvalion; **Thai.:** Duxaril.

Amfetamine (1412-t)

Amfetamine (BAN, rINN).

Amphetamine; Anfetamina; Racemic Desoxynorephedrine. (R,S)-α-Methylphenethylamine.

$C_9H_{13}N = 135.2$.
CAS — 300-62-9 (amfetamine); 139-10-6 (amfetamine phosphate).
ATC — N06BA01.

Amfetamine Sulfate (1414-r)

Amfetamine Sulfate (rINNM).

Amphetamine Sulphate (BANM); Amphetamine Sulfate; Amphetamini Sulphas; Amphetamini Sulfas; Phenaminum; Phenylaminopropanum Racemicum Sulfuricum. (R,S)-α-Methylphenethylamine sulphate.

$(C_9H_{13}N)_2, H_2SO_4 = 368.5$.
CAS — 60-13-9.
Pharmacopoeias. In Eur. (see p.vi) and US.

Incompatible with alkalis and calcium salts.

Pharmacopoeial description

Ph. Eur.: A white powder. Freely soluble in water; slightly soluble in alcohol; practically insoluble in ether. Protect from light.

USP 25: A white odourless crystalline powder. Freely soluble in water; slightly soluble in alcohol; practically insoluble in ether. Its solutions are acid to litmus, having a pH of 5 to 6.

Profile

Amfetamine is an indirect-acting sympathomimetic with actions and uses similar to those of its isomer dexamfetamine (below). Amfetamine, amfetamine sulfate, and amfetamine aspartate are given by mouth in doses similar to those of dexamfetamine sulfate. The laevo-isomer, levamfetamine was formerly used in a similar manner. Amfetamine, being volatile, was formerly employed by inhalation.

Preparations

USP 25: Amphetamine Sulfate Tablets.

Proprietary Preparations (details are given in Part 3)
Spain: Centramina†.

Multi-ingredient: Belg.: Epipropane; **Fr.:** Ortenal†; **USA:** Adderall.

Amfetaminil (1415-f)

Amfetaminil (rINN).

Amphetaminil. α-(α-Methylphenethylamino)-α-phenylacetonitrile.

$C_{17}H_{18}N_2 = 250.3$.
CAS — 17590-01-1.

Profile

Amfetaminil is a central stimulant that has been given by mouth in doses of 10 to 30 mg daily in the treatment of narcolepsy.

Preparations

Proprietary Preparations (details are given in Part 3)
Ger.: AN 1.

Amiphenazole Hydrochloride (1411-a)

Amiphenazole Hydrochloride (BANM, rINNM).

Amiphenazole Chloride. 5-Phenylthiazole-2,4-diamine hydrochloride.

$C_9H_9N_3S, HCl = 227.7$.
CAS — 490-55-1 (amiphenazole); 942-31-4 (amiphenazole hydrochloride).

Profile

Amiphenazole hydrochloride has properties similar to those of doxapram hydrochloride (p.1509) and has been used intramuscularly or intravenously as a respiratory stimulant.

Lichenoid reactions have been reported in addition to those reactions expected from its central activity.

Ammonium Camphocarbonate (14455-n)

$C_{11}H_{19}NO_3 = 213.3$.
$CAS — 5972-75-8$.

Profile
Ammonium camphocarbonate has been used in preparations for the treatment of respiratory-tract disorders.

Preparations
Proprietary Preparations (details are given in Part 3)
Multi-ingredient: *Spain:* Pulmofasa; Pulmofasa Antihist.

Bemegride (1416-d)

Bemegride (BAN, rINN).
Bemegridum. 3-Ethyl-3-methylglutarimide; 4-Ethyl-4-methyl-piperidine-2,6-dione.
$C_8H_{13}NO_2 = 155.2$.
$CAS — 64-65-3$.
$ATC — R07AB05$.

Profile
Bemegride has properties similar to those of doxapram (p.1509). It has been given intravenously as a respiratory stimulant.

Porphyria. Bemegride has been associated with acute attacks of porphyria and is considered unsafe in porphyric patients.

Benzfetamine Hydrochloride (1471-q)

Benzfetamine Hydrochloride (BANM, rINNM).
Benzphetamine Hydrochloride. (+)-N-Benzyl-N,α-dimethyl-phenethylamine hydrochloride.
$C_{17}H_{21}N,HCl = 275.8$.
$CAS — 156-08-1$ (benzfetamine); $5411-22-3$ (benzfetamine hydrochloride).

Profile
Benzfetamine hydrochloride is a central stimulant and sympathomimetic with properties similar to those of dexamfetamine (below). It has been used as an anorectic given by mouth in the treatment of obesity (p.1505), although amfetamines are no longer recommended for this indication. The usual initial dose is 25 to 50 mg once daily, subsequently adjusted, according to requirements, to a dose of 25 to 50 mg up to three times daily.

Preparations
Proprietary Preparations (details are given in Part 3)
USA: Didrex.

Catha (12537-w)

Abyssinian, African, or Arabian Tea; Kat; Kath; Khat; Miraa; Qat.

The leaves of *Catha edulis* (Celastraceae), containing cathine, cathinone, celastrin, choline, tannins, and inorganic salts.

Cathine (12538-e)

Cathine (pINN).
(+)-Norpseudoephedrine. *threo*-2-Amino-1-phenylpropan-1-ol.
$C_9H_{13}NO = 151.2$.
$CAS — 492-39-7; 36393-56-3$.
$ATC — A08AA07$.

Cathinone (10136-d)

Cathinone (pINN).
(S)-2-Aminopropiophenone.
$C_9H_{11}NO = 149.2$.
$CAS — 71031-15-7$.

Profile
Catha is used for its stimulant properties among some cultures of Africa and the Middle East, usually by chewing the leaves. Its effects are reported to resemble those of the amfetamines (see Dexamfetamine Sulfate, below), and are thought to be largely due to the content of cathinone. Dependence and psychotic reactions have been reported. Cathine, another constituent, is used as the hydrochloride as an anorectic.

◊ References to the pharmacology and pharmacokinetics of catha and its constituents[1-7] and reports of adverse effects.[8-12]

1. Brenneisen R, *et al.* Metabolism of cathinone to (–)-norephedrine and (–)-norpseudoephedrine. *J Pharm Pharmacol* 1986; **38:** 298–300.
2. Brenneisen R, *et al.* Amphetamine-like effects in humans of the khat alkaloid cathinone. *Br J Clin Pharmacol* 1990; **30:** 825–8.
3. Kalix P. Pharmacological properties of the stimulant khat. *Pharmacol Ther* 1990; **48:** 397–416.
4. Kalix P. Chewing khat, an old drug habit that is new in Europe. *Int J Risk Safety Med* 1992; **3:** 143–56.
5. Kalix P. Cathinone, a natural amphetamine. *Pharmacol Toxicol* 1992; **70:** 77–86.
6. Widler P, *et al.* Pharmacodynamics and pharmacokinetics of khat: a controlled study. *Clin Pharmacol Ther* 1994; **55:** 556–62.

7. Kalix P. Catha edulis, a plant that has amphetamine effects. *Pharm World Sci* 1996; **18:** 69–73.
8. Rumpf KW, *et al.* Rhabdomyolysis after ingestion of an appetite suppressant. *JAMA* 1983; **250:** 2112.
9. Gough SP, Cookson IB. Khat-induced schizophreniform psychosis in UK. *Lancet* 1984; **i:** 455.
10. Roper JP. The presumed neurotoxic effects of Catha edulis—an exotic plant now available in the United Kingdom. *Br J Ophthalmol* 1986; **70:** 779–81.
11. Zureikat N, *et al.* Chewing khat slows the orocaecal transit time. *Gut* 1992; **33** (suppl): S23.
12. Yousef G, *et al.* Khat chewing as a cause of psychosis. *Br J Hosp Med* 1995; **54:** 322–6.

Preparations
Proprietary Preparations (details are given in Part 3)
Ger.: Antiadipositum X-112 S; Mirapront N; Vita-Schlanktropfen†; *Hong Kong:* Mirapront N; *Mex.:* Insacial; *S.Afr.:* Appetrol; Dietene; Eetless; Laser Slim 'n Trim†; Leanor; Nobese No. 1; Slim 'n Trim; Thinz; *Singapore:* Mirapront N; *Switz.:* Adistop; Antiadipositum X-112; Belloform nouvelle formule; Limit-X; Miniscap; *Thai.:* Mirapront N.

Chlorphentermine Hydrochloride (1472-p)

Chlorphentermine Hydrochloride (BANM, USAN, rINNM).
NSC-76098; S-62; W-2426. 4-Chloro-α,α-dimethylphenethylamine hydrochloride.
$C_{10}H_{14}ClN,HCl = 220.1$.
$CAS — 461-78-9$ (chlorphentermine); $151-06-4$ (chlorphentermine hydrochloride).
Pharmacopoeias. In Fr.

Profile
Chlorphentermine hydrochloride is a sympathomimetic with properties similar to those of dexamfetamine (below). It was formerly used as an anorectic but has been implicated in lipid storage disorders and pulmonary hypertension.

Clobenzorex Hydrochloride (1473-s)

Clobenzorex Hydrochloride (rINNM).
SD-271-12. (+)-N-(2-Chlorobenzyl)-α-methylphenethylamine hydrochloride.
$C_{16}H_{18}ClN,HCl = 296.2$.
$CAS — 13364-32-4$ (clobenzorex); $5843-53-8$ (clobenzorex hydrochloride).

Profile
Clobenzorex hydrochloride is a central stimulant and sympathomimetic with properties similar to those of dexamfetamine (below). It has been used as an anorectic in the treatment of obesity (p.1505) but regulatory authorities in the European Union have called for the withdrawal of all anorectics from the market.

Preparations
Proprietary Preparations (details are given in Part 3)
Fr.: Dinintel†; *Mex.:* Asenlix; *Port.:* Dinintel†; *Singapore:* Dinintel; *Spain:* Finedal.

Deanol (12624-s)

Deanol (BAN).
Démanol. 2-Dimethylaminoethanol.
$C_4H_{11}NO = 89.14$.
$CAS — 108-01-0$ (deanol); $3342-61-8$ (deanol aceglumate); $968-46-7$ (deanol benzilate); $71-79-4$ (deanol benzilate hydrochloride).
$ATC — N06BX04$.

NOTE. Deanol Aceglumate is *pINN*.

Profile
Deanol, a precursor of choline, may enhance central acetylcholine formation. It has been employed as a central stimulant in the treatment of hyperactivity in children but its efficacy has not been substantiated. It is included in preparations used as tonics and for the management of impaired mental function.

It has been used as a variety of salts and esters including deanol aceglumate, deanol acetamidobenzoate, deanol bisorcate, deanol cyclohexylpropionate (cyprodenate; cyprodemanol), deanol hemisuccinate, deanol pidolate, and deanol tartrate. Deanol benzilate (deanol diphenylglycolate; benzacine) has been used as the hydrochloride in antispasmodic preparations.

Preparations
Proprietary Preparations (details are given in Part 3)
Belg.: Actebral; *Fr.:* Actebral†; Astyl; Cleregil; Tonibral Adulte; *Ger.:* Medacaps N†; Risatarun†; *Ital.:* Rischiaril; *Port.:* Tonibral.

Multi-ingredient: *Aust.:* Prospervital†; *Fr.:* Debrumyl; *Ger.:* Rowachol comp; *Port.:* Actilam†; Debrumyl; Forticol; Projuvex; Tonice; *Spain:* Acticinco; Anti Anorex Triple; Denubil; *Switz.:* Vigoran.

Dexamfetamine Sulfate (1419-m)

Dexamfetamine Sulfate (pINNM).
Dexamfetamine Sulphate (BANM); Dexamphetamine Sulphate; Dexamphetamini Sulfas; Dextro Amphetamine Sulphate; Dextroamphetamine Sulfate; NSC-73713 (dexamfetamine). (S)-α-Methylphenethylammonium sulphate; (+)-α-Methylphenethylamine sulphate.
$(C_9H_{13}N)_2,H_2SO_4 = 368.5$.
$CAS — 51-64-9$ (dexamfetamine); $7528-00-9$ (dexamfetamine phosphate); $51-63-8$ (dexamfetamine sulfate).
Pharmacopoeias. In Br., Swiss, and US.

Pharmacopoeial description
BP 2001: A white or almost white, odourless or almost odourless, crystalline powder. Freely soluble in water; slightly soluble in alcohol; practically insoluble in ether.
USP 25: A white, odourless, crystalline powder. Soluble 1 in 10 of water and 1 in 800 of alcohol; insoluble in ether. pH of a 5% solution in water is between 5.0 and 6.0.

Adverse Effects
The adverse effects of dexamfetamine are commonly symptoms of overstimulation of the CNS and include insomnia, night terrors, nervousness, restlessness, irritability, and euphoria that may be followed by fatigue and depression. There may be dryness of the mouth, anorexia, abdominal cramps and other gastrointestinal disturbances, headache, dizziness, tremor, sweating, tachycardia, palpitations, increased or sometimes decreased blood pressure, altered libido, and impotence. Psychotic reactions have occurred, as has muscle damage with associated rhabdomyolysis and renal complications. Rarely, cardiomyopathy has occurred with chronic use. In children, growth retardation may occur during prolonged treatment.

In *acute overdosage*, the adverse effects are accentuated and may be accompanied by hyperpyrexia, mydriasis, hyperreflexia, chest pain, cardiac arrhythmias, confusion, panic states, aggressive behaviour, hallucinations, delirium, convulsions, respiratory depression, coma, circulatory collapse, and death. Individual patient response may vary widely and toxic manifestations may occur at relatively low overdoses.

Tolerance can develop to some of dexamfetamine's central effects leading to increased doses and habituation. Abrupt cessation after prolonged treatment or abuse of amfetamines has been associated with extreme fatigue, hyperphagia, and depression. However, it is generally accepted that the amfetamines, although widely abused, are not associated with substantial physical dependence.

Abuse of amfetamines for their euphoriant effects has resulted in personality changes, compulsive and stereotyped behaviour, and may induce a toxic psychosis with auditory and visual hallucinations and paranoid delusions.

Abuse. Abuse of amfetamines can lead to toxicity affecting many organs or body systems. There have been reports of *intracerebral haemorrhage*[1-3] and of *cardiomyopathy*.[4-6] *Acute myocardial infarction* has also occurred.[7]

A syndrome characterised by *circulatory collapse, fever, leukaemoid reaction, disseminated intravascular coagulation*, and *rhabdomyolysis* with *diffuse myalgias* and *muscle tenderness* has been described[8] in 5 drug abusers who had administered amfetamines or phenmetrazine intravenously. In an earlier study,[9] *necrotising angiitis* was associated with intravenous metamfetamine abuse. A 30-year-old man who had ingested 50 amfetamine sulfate tablets developed *rhabdomyolysis* and *myoglobinuric renal failure*, possibly secondary to a crush syndrome, but in the absence of prolonged coma or other major myotoxic factors.[10] However, *acute interstitial nephritis* and *acute renal failure* have followed oral amfetamine abuse without the associated factors of rhabdomyolysis, hyperpyrexia, or necrotising angiitis.[11]

Chronic use may result in adverse effects such as *hallucinations*, a *delusional disorder* resembling *paranoid schizrenia, stereotyped behaviour*, and *movement disorders*.[12] Although chronic intoxication is the most common precondition for psychosis, individual sensitivities are an important aspect of the drug reaction.

Increased serum concentrations of *thyroxine [levothyroxine]* have been associated with heavy amfetamine abuse in 4 psychiatric patients.[13]

Abrupt cessation after prolonged treatment or abuse of amfetamines may cause *extreme fatigue, hyperphagia*, and *depression. Depressive stupor* has been reported in 3 long-term abusers of amfetamine after sudden withdrawal.[14]

1. Delaney P, Estes M. Intracranial hemorrhage with amphetamine abuse. *Neurology* 1980; **30:** 1125–8.
2. Harrington H, *et al.* Intracerebral hemorrhage and oral amphetamine. *Arch Neurol* 1983; **40:** 503–7.
3. Salanova V, Taubner R. Intracerebral haemorrhage and vasculitis secondary to amphetamine use. *Postgrad Med J* 1984; **60:** 429–30.
4. Smith HJ, *et al.* Cardiomyopathy associated with amphetamine administration. *Am Heart J* 1976; **91:** 792–7.
5. Call TD, *et al.* Acute cardiomyopathy secondary to intravenous amphetamine abuse. *Ann Intern Med* 1982; **97:** 559–60.
6. Hong R, *et al.* Cardiomyopathy associated with the smoking of crystal methamphetamine. *JAMA* 1991; **265:** 1152–4.
7. Waksman J, *et al.* Acute myocardial infarction associated with amphetamine use. *Mayo Clin Proc* 2001; **76:** 323–6.
8. Kendrick WC, *et al.* Rhabdomyolysis and shock after intravenous amphetamine administration. *Ann Intern Med* 1977; **86:** 381–7.

9. Citron BP, *et al.* Necrotizing angiitis associated with drug abuse. *N Engl J Med* 1970; **283**: 1003–11.
10. Scandling J, Spital A. Amphetamine-associated myoglobinuric renal failure. *South Med J* 1982; **75**: 237–40.
11. Foley RJ, *et al.* Amphetamine-induced acute renal failure. *South Med J* 1984; **77**: 258–60.
12. Ellinwood EH, Kilbey MM. Fundamental mechanisms underlying altered behavior following chronic administration of psychomotor stimulants. *Biol Psychiatry* 1980; **15**: 749–57.
13. Morley JE, *et al.* Amphetamine-induced hyperthyroxinemia. *Ann Intern Med* 1980; **93**: 707–9.
14. Tuma TA. Depressive stupor following amphetamine withdrawal. *Br J Hosp Med* 1993; **49**: 361–3.

Effects on growth. The Pediatric Subcommittee of the FDA Psychopharmacologic Drugs Advisory Committee reviewed the growth-suppressing effects of stimulant medication in hyperkinetic children.[1] There was reasonable evidence that stimulant drugs, particularly in higher doses, moderately suppressed growth in weight and might have a minor suppressing effect on growth in stature. There were indications that some growth caught up during drug holidays, and that early growth suppression was not evident in adulthood. Careful monitoring during treatment was recommended.

See also under Methylphenidate Hydrochloride, p.1512.

1. Roche AF, *et al.* The effects of stimulant medication on the growth of hyperkinetic children. *Pediatrics* 1979; **63**: 847–50.

Treatment of Adverse Effects
Activated charcoal may be given to delay absorption; gastric lavage may be considered in recent ingestions, but emesis should not be induced because of the risk of seizures. In general the management of overdosage with amfetamines involves supportive and symptomatic therapy. Sedation is usually sufficient. Forced acid diuresis has been advocated to increase amfetamine excretion but is seldom necessary and should only be considered in severely poisoned patients; it requires close supervision and monitoring.

Precautions
Dexamfetamine is contra-indicated in patients with cardiovascular disease including moderate to severe hypertension, and in patients with hyperthyroidism, glaucoma, hyperexcitability, or agitated states. It should not be given to patients with a history of drug or alcohol abuse and it should be avoided in pregnant women or breast-feeding mothers. It should be given with caution to patients with mild hypertension, impaired kidney function, or unstable personality.

Height and weight in children should be monitored as growth retardation may occur. Behavioural disturbances and thought disorders may be exacerbated in psychotic children.

Prolonged high doses may need gradual withdrawal as abrupt cessation may produce fatigue and mental depression.

Care may be needed in certain patients predisposed to tics or Tourette's syndrome as symptoms may be provoked. Dexamfetamine is likely to reduce the convulsive threshold; caution is therefore advised in patients with epilepsy. However, it appears that in some countries amfetamines have been included in antiepileptic preparations containing phenytoin or phenobarbital in an attempt to increase their antiepileptic action. Amfetamines may impair patients' ability to drive or to operate machinery.

Diabetic control should be monitored when central stimulants are used for the control of obesity.

Abuse. Dexamfetamine is subject to extensive abuse and for this reason its availability is severely curtailed. For adverse effects associated with abuse, see above.

Porphyria. Amfetamines are considered to be unsafe in patients with porphyria although there is conflicting experimental evidence of porphyrinogenicity. Metamfetamine has been associated with acute attacks of porphyria.

Pregnancy. No difference was found in the incidence of severe congenital anomalies between 1824 children of mothers prescribed amfetamines or phenmetrazine during pregnancy and 8989 children of mothers who had not received these drugs.[1] Though an excess of oral clefts was noted in the offspring of mothers prescribed amfetamines, there was no excess of congenital heart disease.[1] This was contrary to a previous suggestion[2] in which congenital heart disease in 184 infants had been studied and a link to maternal dexamfetamine exposure postulated. There has been a report of a bradycardia followed by death in a fetus due to maternal intravenous self-administration of 500 mg of amfetamine.[3]

1. Milkovich L, van den Berg BJ. Effects of antenatal exposure to anorectic drugs. *Am J Obstet Gynecol* 1977; **129**: 637–42.
2. Nora JJ, *et al.* Dexamphetamine: a possible environmental trigger in cardiovascular malformations. *Lancet* 1970; **i**: 1290–1.
3. Dearlove JC, Betteridge TJ. Stillbirth due to intravenous amphetamine. *BMJ* 1992; **304**: 548.

Tourette's syndrome. A review[1] of clinical reports concluded that there was virtually no evidence that central stimulants caused or provoked Tourette's syndrome and weak or inadequate evidence that clinically appropriate doses of central stimulants caused tics in previously asymptomatic patients or exacerbated pre-existing symptoms. However, the authors suggested that there was evidence that high or toxic doses might exacerbate or provoke tics in predisposed patients. Long-term methylphenidate therapy did not appear to exacerbate motor or vocal tics in a study[2] of 34 children with ADHD and chronic multiple tic disorder who were followed up for 2 years.

However, the authors did point out that careful clinical monitoring is essential to eliminate the possibility of drug-induced exacerbation in individual patients. In contrast, a report[3] on 15 children who developed Tourette's syndrome while receiving stimulant medication for hyperactivity considered that such therapy was contra-indicated in children with motor tics or diagnosed Tourette's syndrome and should be used with caution in children with a family history of these symptoms. In addition, it suggested that the development of motor tic symptoms in any child receiving stimulants should be a clear indication for immediate discontinuation to minimise the possibility of eliciting a full-blown Tourette's syndrome.

1. Shapiro AK, Shapiro E. Do stimulants provoke, cause, or exacerbate tics and Tourette syndrome? *Compr Psychiatry* 1981; **22**: 265–73.
2. Gadow KD, *et al.* Long-term methylphenidate therapy in children with comorbid attention-deficit hyperactivity disorder and chronic multiple tic disorder. *Arch Gen Psychiatry* 1999; **56**: 330–6.
3. Lowe TL, *et al.* Stimulant medications precipitate Tourette's syndrome. *JAMA* 1982; **247**: 1729–31.

Interactions
Dexamfetamine is an indirect-acting sympathomimetic and may interact with a number of other drugs. To avoid precipitating a hypertensive crisis, it should not be given to patients being treated with an MAOI or within 14 days of stopping such treatment. Concurrent use of beta blockers and amfetamines may produce severe hypertension. Dexamfetamine may also diminish the effects of other antihypertensives, including guanethidine and similar drugs, and concurrent use should be avoided. Patients receiving amfetamines and tricyclic antidepressants require careful monitoring as the risk of cardiovascular effects including arrhythmias may be increased. The urinary excretion of amfetamines is reduced by urinary alkalinisers which may enhance or prolong their effects; excretion is increased by urinary acidifiers.

Amfetamines may delay the absorption of ethosuximide, phenobarbital, and phenytoin. The stimulant effects of amfetamines are inhibited by chlorpromazine, haloperidol, and lithium. Disulfiram may inhibit the metabolism and excretion of amfetamines.

Concurrent use of sympathomimetics with volatile liquid anaesthetics such as halothane is associated with an increased risk of cardiac arrhythmias.

Pharmacokinetics
Amfetamines are readily absorbed from the gastrointestinal tract and are distributed into most body tissues with high concentrations in the brain and CSF. They are partially metabolised in the liver but a considerable fraction may be excreted in the urine unchanged. Urinary elimination is pH-dependent and enhanced in acid urine. Amfetamines are distributed into breast milk.

◊ References.
1. Steiner E, *et al.* Amphetamine secretion in breast milk. *Eur J Clin Pharmacol* 1984; **27**: 123–4.

Uses and Administration
Dexamfetamine, the dextrorotatory isomer of amfetamine, is an indirect-acting sympathomimetic with alpha- and beta-adrenergic agonist activity. It has a marked stimulant effect on the CNS, particularly the cerebral cortex.

Dexamfetamine is used in the treatment of narcolepsy (p.1505) and as an adjunct in the management of refractory hyperactivity disorders in children (p.1505). Dexamfetamine has been given in the treatment of obesity (p.1505), although amfetamines are no longer recommended for this indication. Amfetamines have also been used to overcome fatigue but, again, such use is considered undesirable.

Dexamfetamine is used as the sulfate and is given by mouth.

In the treatment of **narcolepsy**, the usual starting dose is 5 to 10 mg in divided doses, increased if necessary by 5 to 10 mg at weekly intervals to a maximum of 60 mg daily. The lower initial dose of 5 mg daily is recommended for the elderly and any weekly increments should also be restricted to 5 mg in such patients.

In children with **hyperactivity** individualisation of treatment is especially important. In the UK, children aged 6 years and over usually start with a dose of 5 mg once or twice daily; the daily dose may be increased if necessary by 5 mg at weekly intervals to an upper limit of 20 mg daily, although older children might require up to 40 mg daily. Although dexamfetamine is licensed for the treatment of children younger than 6 years of age in some countries, including the UK, WHO has recommended against the use of stimulants in children under 5 years of age and the *British National Formulary* considers such use inappropriate below 6 years of age.

Dexamfetamine has also been given as the saccharate.

Preparations
BP 2001: Dexamfetamine Tablets;
USP 25: Dextroamphetamine Sulfate Capsules; Dextroamphetamine Sulfate Elixir; Dextroamphetamine Sulfate Tablets.

Proprietary Preparations (details are given in Part 3)
Canad.: Dexedrine; *Switz.:* Dexamin; *UK:* Dexedrine; *USA:* Dexedrine; Dextrostat; Oxydess II†; Spancap No. 1†.

Multi-ingredient: *USA:* Adderall.

Dexfenfluramine Hydrochloride (18628-z)
Dexfenfluramine Hydrochloride (*BANM, USAN, rINNM*).
S-5614 (dexfenfluramine). (S)-N-Ethyl-α-methyl-3-trifluoromethylphenethylamine hydrochloride.
$C_{12}H_{16}F_3N,HCl = 267.7$.
CAS — 3239-44-9 (dexfenfluramine); 3239-45-0 (dexfenfluramine hydrochloride).
Pharmacopoeias. In Fr.

Profile
Dexfenfluramine is the *S*-isomer of fenfluramine (p.1510). It stimulates the release of serotonin and selectively inhibits its reuptake, but differs from fenfluramine in not possessing any catecholamine agonist activity.

Dexfenfluramine was formerly given by mouth as the hydrochloride in the treatment of obesity but, like fenfluramine, was withdrawn worldwide following reports of valvular heart defects.

Porphyria. Dexfenfluramine is considered to be unsafe in patients with porphyria because it has been shown to be porphyrinogenic in *in-vitro* systems.

Preparations
Proprietary Preparations (details are given in Part 3)
Ital.: Glypolix†; Isomeride†; *Neth.:* Isomeride†.

Diethylaminoethanol (12648-k)
2-Diethylaminoethanol.
$C_6H_{15}NO = 117.2$.
CAS — 100-37-8.

Profile
Diethylaminoethanol is an analogue of deanol (p.1507) and has been used similarly as the malate. The hydrochloride has also been used.

Preparations
Proprietary Preparations (details are given in Part 3)
Fr.: Cerebrol.

Multi-ingredient: *Aust.:* Barokaton.

Diethylpropion Hydrochloride (1475-e)
Diethylpropion Hydrochloride (*BANM*).
Amfepramone Hydrochloride (*pINNM*). N-(1-Benzoylethyl)-NN-diethylammonium chloride; 2-Diethylaminopropiophenone hydrochloride; (RS)-α-Diethylaminopropiophenone hydrochloride.
$C_{13}H_{19}NO,HCl = 241.8$.
CAS — 90-84-6 (diethylpropion); 134-80-5 (diethylpropion hydrochloride).
Pharmacopoeias. In US.

Pharmacopoeial description
USP 25: A white to off-white, fine crystalline powder. Is odourless or has a slight characteristic odour. It may contain tartaric acid as a stabilising agent. Soluble 1 in 0.5 of water, 1 in 3 of alcohol, and 1 in 3 of chloroform; practically insoluble in ether. Protect from light.

Adverse Effects, Treatment, and Precautions
As for Dexamfetamine Sulfate, p.1507. In addition gynaecomastia has been reported rarely. The incidence of central adverse effects may be lower with diethylpropion than with dexamfetamine. Diethylpropion should not be given to patients with emotional instability or a history of psychiatric illness. It should be avoided in children and the elderly and it should be given with caution to patients with peptic ulceration or prostatic hyperplasia. Diethylpropion hydrochloride is subject to abuse.

Porphyria. Diethylpropion is considered to be unsafe in patients with porphyria because it has been shown to be porphyrinogenic in *animals*.

Interactions
Diethylpropion is an indirect-acting sympathomimetic and, similarly to dexamfetamine (p.1508), may interact with a number of other drugs.

Pharmacokinetics
Diethylpropion is readily absorbed from the gastrointestinal tract. It is extensively metabolised in the liver and possibly the gastrointestinal tract and is excreted in the urine. Diethylpropion crosses the blood-brain barrier and the placenta. Diethylpropion and its metabolites are distributed into breast milk.

Uses and Administration
Diethylpropion hydrochloride is a central stimulant and indirect-acting sympathomimetic with the actions of dexamfetamine (p.1508). It has been used as an anorectic administered by mouth in the treatment of obesity (p.1505), although stimulants are not generally recommended for this indication.

Doses of 25 mg three times daily 1 hour before meals or 75 mg once daily in mid-morning as a modified-release preparation, have been given. Diethylpropion is not recommended for long-term treatment (over 3 months) and, to reduce the risk of dependence, it is preferably given intermittently for a few weeks at a time followed by a drug-free period.

Regulatory authorities in the European Union have withdrawn diethylpropion from the market.

Preparations

USP 25: Diethylpropion Hydrochloride Tablets.

Proprietary Preparations (details are given in Part 3)
Aust.: Regenon†; *Austral.:* Tenuate; *Belg.:* Atractil†; Menutil†; Prefamone†; Regenon†; Tenuate Dospan†; *Braz.:* Dualid S; Hipofagin S; Inibex S; *Canad.:* Tenuate; *Denm.:* Dobesin†; Regenon†; *Fr.:* Moderatan†; Prefamone Chronules†; Tenuate Dospan†; *Ger.:* Regenon†; Tenuate Retard†; *Ital.:* Linea†; Tenuate Dospan†; *Mex.:* Ifa Norex; Neobes; Tenuate Dospan; *NZ:* Tenuate Dospan; *S.Afr.:* Tenuate Dospan; *Spain:* Delgamer†; *Switz.:* Prefamone Chronules; Regenon; Tenuate Retard; *Thai.:* Atractil; Prefamone; *USA:* Tenuate.

Multi-ingredient: *Braz.:* Fastium.

Dimefline Hydrochloride (1420-t)

Dimefline Hydrochloride (BANM, USAN, rINNM).
DW-62; NSC-114650; Rec-7/0267. 8-Dimethylaminomethyl-7-methoxy-3-methyl-2-phenylchromen-4-one hydrochloride.
$C_{20}H_{21}NO_3,HCl = 359.8$.
CAS — 1165-48-6 (dimefline); 2740-04-7 (dimefline hydrochloride).

Profile

Dimefline has actions similar to those of doxapram (below) and has been used by mouth and parenterally as the hydrochloride as a respiratory stimulant.

Preparations

Proprietary Preparations (details are given in Part 3)
Ital.: Remeflin.

Doxapram Hydrochloride (1421-x)

Doxapram Hydrochloride (BANM, USAN, rINNM).
AHR-619; Doxaprami Hydrochloridum. 1-Ethyl-4-(2-morpholinoethyl)-3,3-diphenyl-2-pyrrolidinone hydrochloride monohydrate.
$C_{24}H_{30}N_2O_2,HCl,H_2O = 433.0$.
CAS — 309-29-5 (doxapram); 113-07-5 (anhydrous doxapram hydrochloride); 7081-53-0 (doxapram hydrochloride monohydrate).
Pharmacopoeias. In Eur. (see p.vi), Jpn, and US.

Pharmacopoeial description

Ph. Eur.: A white or almost white crystalline powder. Sparingly soluble in water, in alcohol and in dichloromethane. A 1% solution in water has a pH of 3.5 to 5.0.

USP 25: A white to off-white, odourless, crystalline powder. Soluble 1 in 50 of water; soluble in chloroform; sparingly soluble in alcohol; practically insoluble in ether. pH of a 1% solution in water is between 3.5 and 5.0. Store in airtight containers.

Incompatibility. The commercial injection is reported to be incompatible with alkaline solutions such as aminophylline, frusemide [furosemide], or thiopental sodium.

Adverse Effects

As with other respiratory stimulants, there is a risk that doxapram will produce adverse effects due to general stimulation of the CNS.

Doxapram may produce dyspnoea and other respiratory problems such as coughing, bronchospasm, laryngospasm, hiccup, hyperventilation, and rebound hypoventilation. Muscle involvement may range from fasciculations to spasticity. Convulsions may occur. Headache, dizziness, hyperactivity, and confusion can occur as can sweating, flushing, fever or a sensation of warmth, particularly in the genital or perineal regions. Hallucinations may occur rarely. There may be nausea, vomiting, diarrhoea, and problems with urination. Cardiovascular effects include hypertension and various arrhythmias although sudden hypotension may also occur.

Thrombophlebitis may follow extravasation of doxapram during injection.

Effects on the heart. Second-degree atrioventricular block caused by prolongation of the QT interval has been associated with doxapram administration in 3 neonates.[1] Although the preparation in question contained benzyl alcohol this was not considered to play a role in the adverse effect.

1. De Villiers GS, et al. Second-degree atrioventricular heart block after doxapram administration. *J Pediatr* 1998; **133:** 149–50.

Effects on the liver. Acute hepatic necrosis in a patient was attributed to a 24-hour infusion of doxapram.[1] Liver function tests returned to normal over 3 weeks.

1. Fancourt GJ, et al. Hepatic necrosis with doxapram hydrochloride. *Postgrad Med J* 1985; **61:** 833–5.

Precautions

Doxapram should not be administered to patients with epilepsy or other convulsive disorders, cerebral oedema, cerebrovascular accident, head injury, acute severe asthma, physical obstruction of the airway, severe hypertension, ischaemic heart disease, hyperthyroidism, or phaeochromocytoma. Caution is also advisable if doxapram is used in patients with less severe de-

The symbol † denotes a preparation no longer actively marketed

---

grees of hypertension or impaired cardiac reserve. It should be given with care to patients with liver dysfunction.

Patients should be carefully supervised during administration of doxapram; special attention should be paid to changes in blood gas measurements. Doxapram should be given with oxygen in severe irreversible airways obstruction or severely decreased lung compliance because of the increased work of breathing. A beta$_2$ agonist should be given concomitantly in patients with bronchoconstriction.

Interactions

Additive pressor effects may occur when doxapram is administered concurrently with sympathomimetics or MAOIs. Cardiac arrhythmias may occur when doxapram is given with anaesthetics known to sensitise the myocardium, such as halothane, enflurane, and isoflurane; it has been recommended that doxapram should not be given for at least 10 minutes after discontinuation of these anaesthetics. Doxapram may temporarily mask the residual effects of neuromuscular blockers. The manufacturers have reported that there may be an interaction between doxapram and aminophylline manifested by agitation and increased skeletal muscle activity.

Pharmacokinetics

Doxapram is extensively metabolised in the liver after intravenous injection. Metabolites and a small amount of unchanged drug are excreted in the urine. Some absorption has been demonstrated when doxapram is given by mouth.

◊ References.
1. Robson RH, Prescott LF. A pharmacokinetic study of doxapram in patients and volunteers. *Br J Clin Pharmacol* 1978; **7:** 81–7.
2. Baker JR, et al. Normal pharmacokinetics of doxapram in a patient with renal failure and hypothyroidism. *Br J Clin Pharmacol* 1981; **11:** 305–6.

Uses and Administration

Doxapram hydrochloride is a central and respiratory stimulant with a brief duration of action. It acts by stimulation of peripheral chemoreceptors and central respiratory centres; at higher doses, it stimulates other parts of the brain and spinal cord. Doxapram has a pressor action and may also increase catecholamine release.

Doxapram has limited uses in the treatment of acute respiratory failure (for example where this is superimposed on chronic obstructive pulmonary disease), and of postoperative respiratory depression (see Respiratory Failure, p.1200).

Doxapram hydrochloride may be infused at a rate of 1.5 to 4.0 mg per minute in the treatment of acute respiratory failure.

For postoperative respiratory depression it has been given in a dose of 0.5 to 1.5 mg per kg body-weight by intravenous injection over a period of at least 30 seconds. This dose may be repeated at hourly intervals. It may also be given by intravenous infusion, initially administered at a rate of 2 to 5 mg per minute and then reduced, according to the patient's response, to 1 to 3 mg per minute; a recommended maximum total dosage is 4 mg per kg.

Doxapram hydrochloride has also been used to treat respiratory and CNS depression following drug overdose but its use for this indication is no longer recommended.

Chronic obstructive pulmonary disease. Respiratory stimulants such as doxapram have a limited and short-term role in hypercapnic respiratory failure in patients with chronic obstructive pulmonary disease (p.759). Benefit has been reported in such patients in whom doxapram was used as an alternative to intubation.[1,2] However, a systematic review suggested that despite short-term improvements in blood-gas exchange with doxapram, techniques such as non-invasive ventilation might be more effective.[3]

1. Hirshberg AJ, et al. Use of doxapram hydrochloride injection as an alternative to intubation to treat chronic obstructive pulmonary disease patients with hypercapnia. *Ann Emerg Med* 1994; **24:** 701–3.
2. Kerr HD. Doxapram in hypercapnic chronic obstructive pulmonary disease with respiratory failure. *J Emerg Med* 1997; **15:** 513–15.
3. Greenstone M. Doxapram for ventilatory failure due to exacerbations of chronic obstructive pulmonary disease (updated 30 July 2001). Available in The Cochrane Library; Issue 4. Oxford: Update Software; 2001.

Neonatal apnoea. Doxapram is effective in neonatal apnoea (p.784) and may be considered as an alternative, or in addition, to xanthines in infants with apnoea that does not respond to xanthine therapy alone. However, it is less convenient to use as it must be administered by continuous intravenous infusion and blood pressure must be monitored. Additionally, some preparations may contain benzyl alcohol as a preservative making them unsuitable for use in neonates. It has been used in doses of 2.5 mg per kg body-weight per hour.[1-3] Adverse CNS effects have been reported.[3] Lower doses of 0.25 or 1.5 mg per kg per hour have been shown to be effective.[4,5] However, use of low doses of 0.5 mg per kg per hour in very low birth-weight premature infants produced higher than expected plasma-doxapram concentrations and a greater increase in systolic blood pressure compared with controls.[6]

1. Sagi E, et al. Idiopathic apnoea of prematurity treated with doxapram and aminophylline. *Arch Dis Child* 1984; **59:** 281–3.
2. Eyal F, et al. Aminophylline versus doxapram in idiopathic apnea of prematurity: a double-blind controlled study. *Pediatrics* 1985; **75:** 709–13.
3. Dear PRF, Wheeler D. Doxapram and neonatal apnoea. *Arch Dis Child* 1984; **59:** 903–4.

---

4. Bairam A, Vert P. Low-dose doxapram for apnoea of prematurity. *Lancet* 1986; **i:** 793–4.
5. Peliowski A, Finer NN. A blinded, randomized, placebo-controlled trial to compare theophylline and doxapram for the treatment of apnea of prematurity. *J Pediatr* 1990; **116:** 648–53.
6. Huon C, et al. Low-dose doxapram for treatment of apnoea following early weaning in very low birthweight infants: a randomized, double-blind study. *Acta Paediatr* 1998; **87:** 1180–4.

Respiratory depression. References to the use of doxapram in postoperative respiratory depression.

1. Jansen JE, et al. Effect of doxapram on postoperative pulmonary complications after upper abdominal surgery in high-risk patients. *Lancet* 1990; **335:** 936–8.
2. Thangathurai D, et al. Doxapram for respiratory depression after epidural morphine. *Anaesthesia* 1990; **45:** 64–5.
3. Sajjad T. Comparison of the effects of doxapram or carbon dioxide on ventilatory frequency and tidal volume during induction of anaesthesia with propofol. *Br J Anaesth* 1994; **73:** 266P.
4. Alexander-Williams M, et al. Doxapram and the prevention of postoperative hypoxaemia. *Br J Anaesth* 1995; **75:** 233P.

Shivering. For references to the use of doxapram in postoperative shivering, see p.1255.

Preparations

BP 2001: Doxapram Injection;
USP 25: Doxapram Hydrochloride Injection.

Proprietary Preparations (details are given in Part 3)
Aust.: Dopram; *Austral.:* Dopram; *Belg.:* Dopram; *Canad.:* Dopram; *Denm.:* Dopram; *Fin.:* Dopram; *Hong Kong:* Dopram; *Irl.:* Dopram; *Neth.:* Dopram; *Norw.:* Dopram; *NZ:* Dopram; *S.Afr.:* Dopram; *Spain:* Docatone; *Switz.:* Dopram; *UK:* Dopram; *USA:* Dopram.

Etamivan (1422-r)

Etamivan (BAN, rINN).
Ethamivan (USAN); NSC-406087; Vanillic Acid Diethylamide; Vanillic Diethylamide. N,N-Diethylvanillamide.
$C_{12}H_{17}NO_3 = 223.3$.
CAS — 304-84-7.
ATC — R07AB04.

Profile

Etamivan has actions similar to those of doxapram (above). It was formerly used as a respiratory stimulant, but the risk of toxicity associated with effective doses is now considered to be unacceptable.

Etamivan is available in compound preparations for administration by mouth in cerebrovascular and circulatory disorders and hypotension, but such use is not recommended.

Preparations

Proprietary Preparations (details are given in Part 3)
Multi-ingredient: *Aust.:* Cinnarplus; Instenon; *Ger.:* Normotin-R; *Hong Kong:* Instenon; *Spain:* Vasperdil†; *Thai.:* Instenon.

Fencamfamin Hydrochloride (1423-f)

Fencamfamin Hydrochloride (BANM, rINNM).
H-610. N-Ethyl-3-phenylbicyclo[2.2.1]hept-2-ylamine hydrochloride.
$C_{15}H_{21}N,HCl = 251.8$.
CAS — 1209-98-9 (fencamfamin); 2240-14-4 (fencamfamin hydrochloride).

Profile

Fencamfamin hydrochloride has been given by mouth as a central stimulant.

Preparations

Proprietary Preparations (details are given in Part 3)
Multi-ingredient: *S.Afr.:* Reactivan.

Fenetylline Hydrochloride (12738-t)

Fenetylline Hydrochloride (BANM, rINNM).
Amfetyline Hydrochloride; 7-Ethyltheophylline Amphetamine Hydrochloride; Fenethylline Hydrochloride (USAN); H-814; R-720-11. 7-[2-(α-Methylphenethylamino)ethyl]theophylline hydrochloride.
$C_{18}H_{23}N_5O_2,HCl = 377.9$.
CAS — 3736-08-1 (fenetylline); 1892-80-4 (fenetylline hydrochloride).

Profile

Fenetylline is a theophylline derivative of amfetamine with properties similar to those of dexamfetamine (p.1507). It has been given by mouth in the management of hyperactivity disorders in children. Fenetylline is subject to abuse.

Preparations

Proprietary Preparations (details are given in Part 3)
Belg.: Captagon; *Ger.:* Captagon; *Israel:* Fitton.

Fenfluramine Hydrochloride (1478-j)

Fenfluramine Hydrochloride (BANM, USAN, rINNM).
AHR-3002;   S-768.   N-Ethyl-α-methyl-3-trifluoromethyl-phenethylamine hydrochloride.
$C_{12}H_{16}F_3N,HCl = 267.7$.
CAS — 458-24-2 (fenfluramine); 404-82-0 (fenfluramine hydrochloride).
Pharmacopoeias. In Fr.

Adverse Effects and Precautions

As for Dexamfetamine, p.1507, but fenfluramine usually depressed rather than stimulated the CNS. Fenfluramine has been associated with serious cardiovascular toxicity. Pulmonary hypertension led to certain precautions being imposed upon its use and subsequent reports of valvular heart defects led to its withdrawal worldwide.

Effects on the cardiovascular system. The association of primary *pulmonary hypertension* with the use of anorectics including fenfluramine, dexfenfluramine, and phentermine is well recognised.[1-3] Both reversible and irreversible cases have been reported and in some cases it has proved fatal.[1,4-9] The condition appears to be linked to prolonged or repeated therapy.[1,10] In 1992 the UK Committee on Safety of Medicines (CSM) advised that treatment should not exceed 3 months[1] but later in 1997 it revised its recommendations for fenfluramine and dexfenfluramine allowing treatment for up to 12 months under certain conditions.[2] The CSM stated that treatment could be continued beyond 3 months only if there had been a satisfactory response (more than 10% weight loss) and that this loss was maintained. Patients should also be monitored for symptoms of pulmonary hypertension. For other anorectics such as phentermine the maximum duration of treatment remained 3 months.

However, shortly after this, a report was published[11] that outlined an association between the use of a fenfluramine-phentermine combination and the development of *valvular heart disease* in 24 patients. Initially, the response by the CSM was to advise against the use of combinations of anorectics[12] although subsequently fenfluramine, along with dexfenfluramine, was withdrawn from the world market after more cases became known.[13,14] By September 1997 the FDA in the USA[14] had received 144 reports of valvulopathy, including the original 24, associated with fenfluramine or dexfenfluramine, with or without phentermine; none were associated with phentermine treatment alone. As a consequence the US authorities made recommendations[14] for the screening of all patients who had previously received fenfluramine or dexfenfluramine in order to detect heart valve lesions and to provide optimal care. Further studies[15-20] have supported the association with valvular abnormalities, and suggested that prolonged exposure or exposure to high doses of dexfenfluramine or fenfluramine increased the risk; clinically important changes would probably not develop in most patients with only short-term exposure.[21] Regulatory authorities in the European Union have called for the withdrawal of all anorectics from the market.

1. Committee on Safety of Medicines. Fenfluramine (Ponderax Pacaps), dexfenfluramine (Adifax) and pulmonary hypertension. *Current Problems 34* 1992.
2. Committee on Safety of Medicines/Medicines Control Agency. Anorectic agents: risks and benefits. *Current Problems* 1997; **23:** 1–2.
3. Abenhaim L, *et al.* Appetite-suppressant drugs and the risk of primary pulmonary hypertension. *N Engl J Med* 1996; **335:** 609–16.
4. Douglas JG, *et al.* Pulmonary hypertension and fenfluramine. *BMJ* 1981; **283:** 881–3.
5. McMurray J, *et al.* Irreversible pulmonary hypertension after treatment with fenfluramine. *BMJ* 1986; **292:** 239–40.
6. Fotiadis I, *et al.* Fenfluramine-induced irreversible pulmonary hypertension. *Postgrad Med J* 1991; **67:** 776–7.
7. Atanassoff PG, *et al.* Pulmonary hypertension and dexfenfluramine. *Lancet* 1992; **339:** 436.
8. Cacoub P, *et al.* Pulmonary hypertension and dexfenfluramine. *Eur J Clin Pharmacol* 1995; **48:** 81–3.
9. Roche N, *et al.* Pulmonary hypertension and dexfenfluramine. *Lancet* 1992; **339:** 436–7.
10. Thomas SHL, *et al.* Appetite suppressants and primary pulmonary hypertension in the United Kingdom. *Br Heart J* 1995; **74:** 600–63.
11. Connolly HM, *et al.* Valvular heart disease associated with fenfluramine-phentermine. *N Engl J Med* 1997; **337:** 581–8. Correction. *ibid.;* 1783.
12. Committee on Safety of Medicines/Medicines Control Agency. Anorectic agents and valvular heart disease. *Current Problems* 1997; **23:** 12.
13. Committee on Safety of Medicines/Medicines Control Agency. Fenfluramine and dexfenfluramine withdrawn. *Current Problems* 1997; **23:** 13–14.
14. Anonymous. Cardiac valvulopathy associated with exposure to fenfluramine or dexfenfluramine: US Department of Health and Human Services interim public health recommendations, November 1997. *MMWR* 1997; **46:** 1061–6.
15. Khan MA, *et al.* The prevalence of cardiac valvular insufficiency assessed by transthoracic echocardiography in obese patients treated with appetite-suppressant drugs. *N Engl J Med* 1998; **339:** 713–18.
16. Jick H, *et al.* A population-based study of appetite-suppressant drugs and the risk of cardiac-valve regurgitation. *N Engl J Med* 1998; **339:** 719–24.
17. Weissman NJ, *et al.* An assessment of heart-valve abnormalities in obese patients taking dexfenfluramine, sustained-release dexfenfluramine, or placebo. *N Engl J Med* 1998; **339:** 725–32.
18. Gardin JM, *et al.* Valvular abnormalities and cardiovascular status following exposure to dexfenfluramine or phentermine/fenfluramine. *JAMA* 2000; **283:** 1703–9.

19. Lepor NE, *et al.* Dose and duration of fenfluramine-phentermine therapy impacts the risk of significant valvular heart disease. *Am J Cardiol* 2000; **86:** 107–10.
20. Jollis JG, *et al.* Fenfluramine and phentermine and cardiovascular findings: effect of treatment duration on prevalence of valve abnormalities. *Circulation* 2000; **101:** 2071–7.
21. Devereux RB. Appetite suppressants and valvular heart disease. *N Engl J Med* 1998; **339:** 765–6.

Porphyria. Fenfluramine is considered to be unsafe in patients with porphyria because it has been shown to be porphyrinogenic in *animals*.

Uses and Administration

Fenfluramine is an indirect-acting sympathomimetic related to amfetamine, but at standard doses it usually depresses rather than stimulates the CNS. It appears to stimulate the release of serotonin and selectively inhibits its reuptake resulting in increased CNS serotonin concentrations. It may also increase glucose utilisation and lower blood-glucose concentrations.

Fenfluramine was formerly given by mouth as the hydrochloride in the treatment of obesity (p.1505) but was withdrawn worldwide following reports of valvular heart defects.

Preparations

Proprietary Preparations (details are given in Part 3)
Ital.: Dima-Fen†; Pesos†; Ponderal†; *Neth.:* Ponderal†; *S.Afr.:* Ponderax†; *USA:* Pondimin†.

Fenozolone (12741-j)

Fenozolone (rINN).
LD-3394;   Phenozolone.   2-Ethylamino-5-phenyl-2-oxazolin-4-one.
$C_{11}H_{12}N_2O_2 = 204.2$.
CAS — 15302-16-6.
ATC — N06BA08.

Profile

Fenozolone is a central stimulant and indirect-acting sympathomimetic with actions similar to those of dexamfetamine (p.1507). It has been given by mouth in the treatment of symptoms of mental function impairment.

Preparations

Proprietary Preparations (details are given in Part 3)
Fr.: Ordinator†.

Fenproporex Hydrochloride (1479-z)

Fenproporex Hydrochloride (rINNM).
N-2-Cyanoethylamphetamine Hydrochloride. (±)-3-(α-Methylphenethylamino)propionitrile hydrochloride.
$C_{12}H_{16}N_2,HCl = 224.7$.
CAS — 15686-61-0 (fenproporex); 18305-29-8 (fenproporex hydrochloride).

Profile

Fenproporex is a central stimulant and indirect-acting sympathomimetic with actions similar to those of dexamfetamine (p.1507). Following administration by mouth it is reported to be metabolised to amfetamine. Fenproporex has been given as the hydrochloride, the diphenylacetate, and as a resinate.

Fenproporex hydrochloride has been used as an anorectic in the treatment of obesity (p.1505) although the use of stimulants in this way is no longer recommended. Regulatory authorities in the European Union have called for the withdrawal of all anorectics from the market.

Preparations

Proprietary Preparations (details are given in Part 3)
Braz.: Desobesi-M; Inobesin; Lipomax; Nobese; *Mex.:* Delgafen; Fenisec; Ifa Dex; Ifa Diety; Obisin; *Port.:* Drenur†; Pesex-R†; Tegisec†; *Spain:* Antiobes; Dicel†; Grasmin†; Tegisec.

Multi-ingredient: *Mex.:* Esbelcaps.

Lobelia (1426-h)

Indian Tobacco.
Pharmacopoeias. In Aust.

The dried aerial parts of *Lobelia inflata* (Lobeliaceae). Lobeline is the main alkaloidal constituent.

Lobeline Hydrochloride (1427-m)

Lobeline Hydrochloride (BANM, rINNM).
Alpha-lobeline Hydrochloride; Lobelini Hydrochloridum. 2-[6-(β-Hydroxyphenethyl)-1-methyl-2-piperidyl]acetophenone hydrochloride.
$C_{22}H_{27}NO_2,HCl = 373.9$.
CAS — 90-69-7 (lobeline); 134-63-4 (lobeline hydrochloride).
Pharmacopoeias. In Eur. (see p.vi).

Pharmacopoeial description

Ph. Eur.: A white microcrystalline powder. Sparingly soluble in water; freely soluble in dichloromethane. A 1% solution in water has a pH of 4.6 to 6.4. Protect from light.

Lobeline Sulfate (1428-b)

Lobeline Sulfate (rINNM).
Lobeline Sulphate (BANM).
$(C_{22}H_{27}NO_2)_2,H_2SO_4 = 773.0$.
CAS — 134-64-5.

Adverse Effects

Side-effects of lobelia and lobeline include nausea and vomiting, coughing, tremor, and dizziness. Symptoms of overdosage include profuse diaphoresis, paresis, tachycardia, hypothermia, hypotension, and coma; fatalities have occurred.

Uses and Administration

Lobeline, which chiefly accounts for the activity of lobelia, has peripheral and central effects similar to those of nicotine (p.1640).

Lobelia has been used mainly in preparations aimed at relieving respiratory-tract disorders. Lobeline has been given by mouth as the hydrochloride or sulfate as a smoking deterrent (see Smoking Cessation, p.1642). Lobelia has been used similarly given either by mouth or incorporated into herbal cigarettes.

◊ Reviews of anti-smoking therapy generally consider lobeline to have little benefit compared with placebo.[1-3]
1. Nunn-Thompson CL, Simon PA. Pharmacotherapy for smoking cessation. *Clin Pharm* 1989; **8:** 710–20.
2. Gourlay SG, McNeil JJ. Antismoking products. *Med J Aust* 1990; **153:** 699–707.
3. Stead LF, Hughes JR. Lobeline for smoking cessation (updated 30 August 2000). Available in The Cochrane Library; Issue 4. Oxford: Update Software; 2001.

Preparations

Proprietary Preparations (details are given in Part 3)
Austral.: Cig-Ridettes; *Canad.:* Butt-Out; *Spain:* Nofum†; Smokeless; *UK:* Anti-Smoking Tablets; *USA:* Bantron†.

Multi-ingredient: *Austral.:* Potassium Iodide and Stramonium Compound; *Belg.:* Kamfeine; Sirop Toux du Larynx†; *Braz.:* Broncofenil; Broncotussan; Bronquidex; Efedronal; Expectolu; Lobelia Composta; MM Expectorante; Pinosil; Pulmoformil; Sedatux; Subitan; Tosseina; Xarope de Iodeto de Potassio Composto; Xarope de Lobelia Composto; *Fr.:* Broncorinol toux seches; *Port.:* Lactucol; *Spain:* Pazbronquial; *UK:* Antibron; Asthma & Catarrh Relief; Balm of Gilead; Chest Mixture; Herbelix; Horehound and Aniseed Cough Mixture; Lobelia Compound; Modern Herbals Cold & Congestion; Vegetable Cough Remover.

Mazindol (1482-w)

Mazindol (BAN, USAN, rINN).
42-548; AN-448; SaH-42548. 5-(4-Chlorophenyl)-2,5-dihydro-3H-imidazo[2,1-a]isoindol-5-ol.
$C_{16}H_{13}CIN_2O = 284.7$.
CAS — 22232-71-9.
ATC — A08AA05.
Pharmacopoeias. In US.

Pharmacopoeial description

USP 25: A white to off-white crystalline powder, having not more than a faint odour. Insoluble in water; slightly soluble in chloroform and in methyl alcohol. Store in airtight containers.

Adverse Effects, Treatment, and Precautions

As for Dexamfetamine Sulfate, p.1507.

Effects on the testes. A report of 8 men who developed testicular pain after taking mazindol.[1]
1. McEwen J, Meyboom RHB. Testicular pain caused by mazindol. *BMJ* 1983; **287:** 1763–4.

Interactions

As for Dexamfetamine Sulfate, p.1508.

Lithium. For a report of mazindol interacting with lithium to cause lithium toxicity, see p.295.

Pharmacokinetics

Mazindol is readily absorbed from the gastrointestinal tract and is excreted in the urine, partly unchanged and partly as metabolites.

Uses and Administration

Mazindol is a central stimulant with actions similar to those of dexamfetamine (p.1508), although structurally the two compounds are unrelated. It appears to inhibit reuptake of dopamine and noradrenaline. It has been used as an anorectic, given by mouth in the treatment of obesity (p.1505) although stimulants are no longer recommended for this indication.

Mazindol has been investigated in the treatment of Duchenne muscular dystrophy.

Narcolepsy. Mazindol has been reported[1-4] to be beneficial in patients with narcolepsy and associated cataplexy (p.1505). A wide range of doses has been employed: 3 to 8 mg daily in one study,[1] 1 mg weekly to 16 mg daily in another;[3] children have been given 1 to 2 mg daily.[4]
1. Parkes JD, Schachter M. Mazindol in the treatment of narcolepsy. *Acta Neurol Scand* 1979; **60:** 250–4.
2. Shindler J, *et al.* Amfetamine, mazindol, and fencamfamin in narcolepsy. *BMJ* 1985; **290:** 1167–70.
3. Alvarez B, *et al.* Mazindol in long-term treatment of narcolepsy. *Lancet* 1991; **337:** 1293–4.
4. Allsopp MR, Zaiwalla Z. Narcolepsy. *Arch Dis Child* 1992; **67:** 302–6.

Preparations

USP 25: Mazindol Tablets.

Proprietary Preparations (details are given in Part 3)
Braz.: Absten S; Dasten; Fagolipo; Magrinex; *Canad.:* Sanorex; *Israel:* Teronac; *Jpn:* Sanorex†; *Mex.:* Diestet; Liofindol; Sanorex; Solucaps; *Neth.:* Teronac†; *Singapore:* Teronac; *Switz.:* Teronac; *USA:* Mazanor†; Sanorex†.

Multi-ingredient: *Braz.:* Dobesix; Moderine; Nofagus.

Mefenorex Hydrochloride (1483-e)

Mefenorex Hydrochloride (USAN, pINNM).
Ro-4-5282. N-(3-Chloropropyl)-α-methylphenethylamine hydrochloride.
$C_{12}H_{18}ClN,HCl = 248.2$.
CAS — 17243-57-1 (mefenorex); 5586-87-8 (mefenorex hydrochloride).

Profile

Mefenorex hydrochloride is a central stimulant and indirect-acting sympathomimetic with actions similar to those of dexamfetamine (p.1507). It has been used as an anorectic in the treatment of obesity although stimulants are no longer recommended for this indication. Regulatory authorities in the European Union have called for the withdrawal of all anorectics from the market.

Preparations

Proprietary Preparations (details are given in Part 3)
Ger.: Rondimen.

Mepixanox (12931-x)

Mepixanox (rINN).
Mepixantone. 3-Methoxy-4-piperidinomethyl-9H-xanthen-9-one.
$C_{20}H_{21}NO_3 = 323.4$.
CAS — 17854-59-0.
ATC — R07AB09.

Profile

Mepixanox has been used as a respiratory stimulant given by mouth or by intravenous or intramuscular injection.

Preparations

Proprietary Preparations (details are given in Part 3)
Ital.: Pimexone†.

Metamfetamine Hydrochloride (1431-f)

Metamfetamine Hydrochloride (rINNM).
d-Deoxyephedrine Hydrochloride; d-Desoxyephedrine Hydrochloride; Methamphetamine Hydrochloride; Methamphetamini Hydrochloridum; Methylamphetamine Hydrochloride; Phenylmethylaminopropane Hydrochloride. (+)-N,α-Dimethylphenethylamine hydrochloride.
$C_{10}H_{15}N,HCl = 185.7$.
CAS — 537-46-2 (metamfetamine); 51-57-0 (metamfetamine hydrochloride).

NOTE. Metamfetamine in a smokeable form has been known as Crank, Crystal, Crystal Meth, Ice, Meth, and Speed.
Pharmacopoeias. In *Aust., Jpn, Swiss,* and *US.*

Pharmacopoeial description

USP 25: White, odourless or practically odourless, crystals or crystalline powder. Freely soluble in water, in alcohol, and in chloroform; very slightly soluble in ether. Its solutions in water have a pH of about 6. Store in airtight containers. Protect from light.

Adverse Effects, Treatment, and Precautions

As for Dexamfetamine Sulfate, p.1507.
Metamfetamine has been subject to extensive abuse, in particular by injection.

Abuse. Pulmonary oedema,[1,2] cardiomyopathy,[2] and choreoathetosis and rhabdomyolysis[3] have occurred following smoking of metamfetamine crystals. It is also abused by mouth and intravenously, and has been associated with fatalities.[4]

1. Nestor TA, *et al.* Acute pulmonary oedema caused by crystalline methamphetamine. *Lancet* 1989; **ii:** 1277–8.
2. Hong R, *et al.* Cardiomyopathy associated with the smoking of crystal methamphetamine. *JAMA* 1991; **265:** 1152–4.
3. Sperling LS, Horowitz JL. Methamphetamine-induced choreoathetosis and rhabdomyolysis. *Ann Intern Med* 1994; **121:** 986.
4. Albertson TE, *et al.* Methamphetamine and the expanding complications of amphetamines. *West J Med* 1999; **170:** 214–19.

Porphyria. Metamfetamine has been associated with acute attacks of porphyria and is considered unsafe in porphyric patients.

Interactions

As for Dexamfetamine Sulfate, p.1508.

Pharmacokinetics

Like most amfetamines (see Dexamfetamine Sulfate, p.1508) metamfetamine is readily absorbed from the gastrointestinal tract and is distributed into most body tissues. It is partially metabolised in the liver and excreted in the urine.

The symbol † denotes a preparation no longer actively marketed

---

◊ References.
1. Shappell SA, *et al.* Chronopharmacokinetics and chronopharmacodynamics of dextromethamphetamine in man. *J Clin Pharmacol* 1996; **36:** 1051–63.

Uses and Administration

Metamfetamine hydrochloride is a central stimulant and indirect-acting sympathomimetic with actions and uses similar to those of dexamfetamine (p.1508).

It has been given by mouth in the treatment of hyperactivity disorders in children aged 6 years and over, although dexamfetamine and methylphenidate are the main stimulants used (p.1505). Initial doses are 5 mg once or twice daily, increased if necessary by 5 mg at weekly intervals to the optimum effective dose, usually 20 to 25 mg daily. The maintenance dose may be given once daily if a modified-release preparation is used.

Metamfetamine hydrochloride has also been used as an anorectic in the management of obesity (p.1505), although amfetamines are no longer recommended for this indication. A dose of 5 mg before each meal has been given by mouth; alternatively 10 or 15 mg has been given once daily in the morning as a modified-release preparation. Treatment should be for no longer than a few weeks.

Metamfetamine hydrochloride has also been used parenterally as a pressor agent.

The laevorotatory form, levmetamfetamine (p.1094) is used as a nasal decongestant.

Preparations

USP 25: Methamphetamine Hydrochloride Tablets.
Proprietary Preparations (details are given in Part 3)
USA: Desoxyn.

Methylenedioxymethamfetamine (19493-n)

MDMA; Methylenedioxymethamfetamine; 3,4-Methylenedioxymethamphetamine. N,α-Dimethyl-1,3-benzodioxole-5-ethanamine.
$C_{11}H_{15}NO_2 = 193.2$.
CAS — 42542-10-9.

NOTE. Methylenedioxymethamfetamine has also been known as Adam, E, Ecstasy, M&M, MDM, and XTC.

Profile

Methylenedioxymethamfetamine is a phenylethylamine compound structurally related to amfetamine and mescaline and is an analogue of tenamfetamine (p.1515). It is subject to abuse. Its toxicity is similar to that of dexamfetamine (see below and p.1507) and may be treated similarly.

Abuse. The toxicity associated with abuse of methylenedioxymethamfetamine has been the subject of a number of discussions.[1-6] Acute effects can be severe and symptoms have included cardiac arrhythmias, fulminant hyperthermia, convulsions, disseminated intravascular coagulation, rhabdomyolysis, and acute renal failure; fatalities may occur. Repeated use may cause hepatic damage. Psychiatric effects reported include psychosis[7-9] and depression.[8-10] Damage to central serotonergic nerves has been implicated[7-11] and hence there is some concern regarding the long-term effects of methylenedioxymethamfetamine abuse.[12,13] Hyponatraemia, inappropriate antidiuretic hormone secretion, and cerebral oedema have also been reported;[14-19] the severity may be increased by excessive fluid intake that is frequently advocated to prevent dehydration and hyperthermia.[17-21] Urinary retention has also been reported.[22]

Concern has been expressed regarding abuse during pregnancy. Twelve congenital malformations, including two cases of congenital heart disease, have been noted among 78 liveborn infants whose mothers had taken methylenedioxymethamfetamine, often with other drugs of abuse, during their pregnancies.[23]

For reviews of the properties of other phenylethylamine compounds, see under Tenamfetamine, p.1515.

1. Henry JA. Ecstasy and the dance of death. *BMJ* 1992; **305:** 5–6.
2. Henry JA, *et al.* Toxicity and deaths from 3,4-methylenedioxymethamphetamine ("ecstasy"). *Lancet* 1992; **340:** 384–7.
3. O'Connor B. Hazards associated with the recreational drug 'ecstasy'. *Br J Hosp Med* 1994; **52:** 507–14.
4. McCann UD, *et al.* Adverse reactions with 3,4-methylenedioxymethamphetamine (MDMA; 'Ecstasy'). *Drug Safety* 1996; **15:** 107–115.
5. Hall AP. Ecstasy and the anaesthetist. *Br J Anaesth* 1997; **79:** 697–8.
6. Schwartz RH, Miller NS. MDMA (ecstasy) and the rave: a review. *Pediatrics* 1997; **100:** 705–8.
7. McGuire P, Fahy T. Chronic paranoid psychosis after misuse of MDMA ("ecstasy"). *BMJ* 1991; **302:** 697.
8. Winstock AR. Chronic paranoid psychosis after misuse of MDMA. *BMJ* 1991; **302:** 1150–1.
9. Schifano F. Chronic atypical psychosis associated with MDMA ("ecstasy") abuse. *Lancet* 1991; **338:** 1335.
10. Benazzi F, Mazzoli M. Psychiatric illness associated with "ecstasy". *Lancet* 1991; **338:** 1520.
11. McCann UD, *et al.* Positron emission tomographic evidence of toxic effect of MDMA ("Ecstasy") on brain serotonin neurons in human beings. *Lancet* 1998; **352:** 1433–7.
12. Green AR, Goodwin GM. Ecstasy and neurodegeneration. *BMJ* 1996; **312:** 1493–4.
13. Bolla KI, *et al.* Memory impairment in abstinent MDMA ("Ecstasy") users. *Neurology* 1998; **51:** 1532–7.
14. Maxwell DL, *et al.* Hyponatraemia and catatonic stupor after taking "ecstasy". *BMJ* 1993; **307:** 1399.

---

15. Kessel B. Hyponatraemia after ingestion of "ecstasy". *BMJ* 1994; **308:** 414.
16. Satchell SC, Connaughton M. Inappropriate antidiuretic hormone secretion and extreme rises in serum creatinine kinase following MDMA ingestion. *Br J Hosp Med* 1994; **51:** 495.
17. Holden R, Jackson MA. Near-fatal hyponatraemic coma due to vasopressin over-secretion after ecstasy (3,4-MDMA). *Lancet* 1996; **347:** 1052.
18. Matthai SM, *et al.* Cerebral oedema after ingestion of MDMA (ecstasy) and unrestricted intake of water. *BMJ* 1996; **312:** 1359.
19. Parr MJA, *et al.* Hyponatraemia and death after ecstasy ingestion. *Med J Aust* 1997; **166:** 136–7.
20. Cook TM. Cerebral oedema after MDMA ('ecstasy') and unrestricted water intake. *BMJ* 1996; **313:** 689.
21. Henry JA, *et al.* Low-dose MDMA ("ecstasy") induces vasopressin secretion. *Lancet* 1998; **351:** 1784.
22. Bryden AA, *et al.* Urinary retention with misuse of 'ecstasy'. *BMJ* 1995; **310:** 504.
23. McElhatton PR, *et al.* Congenital anomalies after prenatal ecstasy exposure. *Lancet* 1999; **354:** 1441–2.

Interactions. A psychotic reaction has been reported in a patient who took methylenedioxymethamfetamine while receiving therapy with *citalopram*.[1]

A patient receiving *phenelzine* and lithium therapy experienced a serotonin syndrome (p.304) after ingesting methylenedioxymethamfetamine.[2] Symptoms included markedly increased muscle tension, tremulousness, abnormal posturing, limited pain response, tachycardia, hypertension, hyperthermia, increased white blood cell count, increased creatine phosphokinase concentration, respiratory acidosis, metabolic acidosis, delirium, and agitation. Within 15 minutes of methylenedioxymethamfetamine ingestion the patient was comatose; within 5 hours the patient was alert with a normal muscle tone. An interaction between phenelzine and methylenedioxymethamfetamine was suggested as the cause of the serotonin syndrome.

A fatal serotonergic reaction to methylenedioxymethamfetamine possibly due to an interaction with *ritonavir* has been described.[3] A prolonged and exaggerated effect from a small dose of methylenedioxymethamfetamine has been reported[4] in another patient also receiving ritonavir. Although this patient was also receiving saquinavir, the authors postulated that the mechanism may be ritonavir-induced inhibition of the cytochrome P450 isoenzyme CYP2D6.

1. Lauerma H, *et al.* Interaction of serotonin reuptake inhibitor and 3,4-methylenedioxymethamphetamine? *Biol Psychiatry* 1998; **43:** 923–8.
2. Kaskey GB. Possible interaction between an MAOI and "ecstasy". *Am J Psychiatry* 1992; **149:** 411–12.
3. Henry JA, Hill IR. Fatal interaction between ritonavir and MDMA. *Lancet* 1998; **352:** 1751–2.
4. Harrington RD, *et al.* Life-threatening interactions between HIV-1 protease inhibitors and the illicit drugs MDMA and γ-hydroxybutyrate. *Arch Intern Med* 1999; **159:** 2221–4.

Methylphenidate Hydrochloride (1433-n)

Methylphenidate Hydrochloride (BANM, rINNM).
Methyl Phenidate Hydrochloride. Methyl α-phenyl-2-piperidylacetate hydrochloride.
$C_{14}H_{19}NO_2,HCl = 269.8$.
CAS — 113-45-1 (methylphenidate); 298-59-9 (methylphenidate hydrochloride).
Pharmacopoeias. In *Chin., Swiss,* and *US.*

Pharmacopoeial description

USP 25: A white, odourless, fine crystalline powder. Freely soluble in water and in methyl alcohol; soluble in alcohol; slightly soluble in acetone and in chloroform. Solutions are acid to litmus.

Adverse Effects, Treatment, and Precautions

As for Dexamfetamine Sulfate, p.1507. Hypersensitivity reactions have been reported. Skin reactions have included exfoliative dermatitis and erythema multiforme. Purpura, thrombocytopenia, and leucopenia have occurred. Blood counts should be monitored periodically during prolonged therapy.

◊ References.
1. Ahmann PA, *et al.* Placebo-controlled evaluation of Ritalin side effects. *Pediatrics* 1993; **91:** 1101–6.
2. Efron D, *et al.* Side effects of methylphenidate and dexamphetamine in children with attention deficit hyperactivity disorder: a double-blind, crossover trial. *Pediatrics* 1997; **100:** 662–6.
3. Rappley MD. Safety issues in the use of methylphenidate: an American perspective. *Drug Safety* 1997; **17:** 143–8.

Abuse. Reports of adverse effects following the abuse of methylphenidate by injecting solutions of crushed tablets.[1-3] Intravenous abuse of methylphenidate in combination with pentazocine has also been reported.[4,5] In addition, there are also reports of intranasal methylphenidate abuse,[6-8] including fatalities.[8]

See also under Effects on the Liver, below.

1. Wolf J, *et al.* Eosinophilic syndrome with methylphenidate abuse. *Ann Intern Med* 1978; **89:** 224–5.
2. Gunby P. Methylphenidate abuse produces retinopathy. *JAMA* 1979; **241:** 546.
3. Parran TV, Jasinski DR. Intravenous methylphenidate abuse: prototype for prescription drug abuse. *Arch Intern Med* 1991; **151:** 781–3.
4. Debooy VD, *et al.* Intravenous pentazocine and methylphenidate abuse during pregnancy: maternal lifestyle and infant outcome. *Am J Dis Child* 1993; **147:** 1062–5.
5. Carter HS, Watson WA. IV pentazocine/methylphenidate abuse—the clinical toxicity of another Ts and blues combination. *J Toxicol Clin Toxicol* 1994; **32:** 541–7.

6. Jaffe SL. Intranasal abuse of prescribed methylphenidate by an alcohol and drug abusing adolescent with ADHD. *J Am Acad Child Adolesc Psychiatry* 1991; **30:** 773–5.
7. Garland EJ. Intranasal abuse of prescribed methylphenidate. *J Am Acad Child Adolesc Psychiatry* 1998; **37:** 573–4.
8. Massello W, Carpenter DA. A fatality due to the intranasal abuse of methylphenidate (Ritalin®). *J Forensic Sci* 1999; **44:** 220–1.

Effects on growth. Concern has been expressed about the effects of central stimulants such as methylphenidate on growth rate when used to treat hyperactivity in children. One study showed that methylphenidate treatment resulted in decreases in weight percentiles after one year of treatment and progressive decrement in height percentiles that became significant after 2 years of treatment.[1] However, another suggested that moderate doses might have a lower risk for long-term height suppression than dexamfetamine.[2] There has also been a study which showed that, even when methylphenidate had an adverse effect on growth rate during active treatment, final height was not compromised and that a compensatory rebound of growth appeared to occur following discontinuation of the stimulant treatment.[3]

See also under Dexamfetamine Sulfate, p.1508.

1. Mattes JA, Gittelman R. Growth of hyperactive children on maintenance regimen of methylphenidate. *Arch Gen Psychiatry* 1983; **40:** 317–21.
2. Greenhill LL, *et al.* Prolactin, growth hormone and growth responses in boys with attention deficit disorder and hyperactivity treated with methylphenidate. *J Am Acad Child Adolesc Psychiatry* 1984; **23:** 58–67.
3. Klein RG, Mannuzza S. Hyperactive boys almost grown up III: methylphenidate effects on ultimate height. *Arch Gen Psychiatry* 1988; **45:** 1131–4.

Effects on the liver. Hepatotoxicity with raised liver enzyme values in a 67-year-old woman was associated with the administration of methylphenidate hydrochloride 30 mg daily by mouth.[1] Methylphenidate-induced hepatocellular injury was reported in a 19-year-old woman who developed jaundice, fever, and malaise after intravenous abuse of methylphenidate hydrochloride tablets.[2]

1. Goodman CR. Hepatotoxicity due to methylphenidate hydrochloride. *N Y State J Med* 1972; **72:** 2339–40.
2. Mehta H, *et al.* Hepatic dysfunction due to intravenous abuse of methylphenidate hydrochloride. *J Clin Gastroenterol* 1984; **6:** 149–51.

Effects on the skin. A fixed drug eruption of the scrotum has been reported in 2 children treated with methylphenidate for attention deficit disorder.[1]

1. Cohen HA, *et al.* Fixed drug eruption of the scrotum due to methylphenidate. *Ann Pharmacother* 1992; **26:** 1378–9.

Tourette's syndrome. For a discussion on whether central stimulants provoke Tourette's syndrome, see Dexamfetamine Sulfate, p.1508.

Interactions

As for Dexamfetamine Sulfate, p.1508.

Anticoagulants. For the effect of methylphenidate on ethyl biscoumacetate, see under Warfarin, p.996.

Antidepressants. For the effect of methylphenidate on tricyclic antidepressants, see under Amitriptyline, p.276.

Antiepileptics. Methylphenidate blood concentrations decreased, and symptoms of attention deficit hyperactivity disorder worsened, in a 13-year-old girl after starting therapy with *carbamazepine.*[1]

1. Schaller JL, *et al.* Carbamazepine and methylphenidate in ADHD. *J Am Acad Child Adolesc Psychiatry* 1999; **38:** 112–13.

NSAIDs. For the effect of methylphenidate on phenylbutazone, see p.78.

Pharmacokinetics

Methylphenidate is readily absorbed from the gastrointestinal tract. The presence of food in the stomach accelerates the rate of absorption but not the total amount absorbed. Peak plasma concentrations are reached about 2 hours after oral administration; methylphenidate undergoes extensive first-pass metabolism. Protein binding is low. It is excreted as metabolites mainly in the urine with small amounts appearing in the faeces; less than 1% appears in the urine as unchanged methylphenidate. The major metabolite is ritalinic acid (2-phenyl-2-piperidyl acetic acid). The plasma elimination half-life is about 2 hours.

◊ References.
1. Aoyama T, *et al.* Nonlinear kinetics of threo-methylphenidate enantiomers in a patient with narcolepsy and in healthy volunteers. *Eur J Clin Pharmacol* 1993; **44:** 79–84.
2. Aoyama T, *et al.* Pharmacokinetics and pharmacodynamics of (+)-threo-methylphenidate enantiomer in patients with hypersomnia. *Clin Pharmacol Ther* 1994; **55:** 270–6.
3. Shader RI, *et al.* Population pharmacokinetics of methylphenidate in children with attention-deficit hyperactivity disorder. *J Clin Pharmacol* 1999; **39:** 775–785.
4. Kimko HC, *et al.* Pharmacokinetics and clinical effectiveness of methylphenidate. *Clin Pharmacokinet* 1999; **37:** 457–70.
5. Modi NB, *et al.* Single- and multiple-dose pharmacokinetics of an oral once-a-day osmotic controlled-release OROS® (methylphenidate HCl) formulation. *J Clin Pharmacol* 2000; **40:** 379–88.

Uses and Administration

Methylphenidate hydrochloride is a central stimulant and indirect-acting sympathomimetic with actions and uses similar to those of dexamfetamine (p.1508). It is used in the treatment of narcolepsy (p.1505) and as an adjunct to psychological, educa-

tional, and social measures in the treatment of hyperactivity disorders in children.

In the treatment of **narcolepsy** the usual dose is 20 to 30 mg daily by mouth in divided doses, normally 30 to 45 minutes before meals, but the effective dose may range from 10 to 60 mg daily.

In **hyperactivity disorders** in children aged 6 years and over, the usual initial dose is 5 mg once or twice daily by mouth, increased if necessary by 5 to 10 mg at weekly intervals to a maximum of 60 mg daily in divided doses. Methylphenidate may be given before breakfast and lunch. A bedtime dose may be considered if the effect wears off in the evening causing rebound hyperactivity. The dosage of methylphenidate in the treatment of hyperactivity in children has sometimes been expressed in terms of body-weight; usual doses are 0.25 mg per kg daily, doubled each week, if necessary, to 2 mg per kg. Methylphenidate should be discontinued if there is no improvement in symptoms after appropriate adjustments in dosage over one month. It also needs to be discontinued from time to time in those who do respond to assess the patient's condition. Treatment is not usually continued beyond puberty, however, in some patients drug therapy may be required into adulthood. In such cases doses are similar to those used in the treatment of narcolepsy.

Methylphenidate hydrochloride is also administered as a modified-release preparation.

A single isomer form of methylphenidate, *d-threo*-methylphenidate (dexmethylphenidate; D-2785; d-MPH), is also used for hyperactivity disorders.

◊ References.
1. Challman TD, Lipsky JJ. Methylphenidate: its pharmacology and uses. *Mayo Clin Proc* 2000; **75:** 711–21.

Depression. Stimulants are no longer recommended as sole treatment for depression (p.271), although they have been tried in augmenting the effect of standard antidepressants such as the SSRIs[1] in patients with refractory depressive disorders.

1. Stoll AL, *et al.* Methylphenidate augmentation of serotonin selective reuptake inhibitors: a case series. *J Clin Psychiatry* 1996; **57:** 72–6.

Disturbed behaviour. Disturbed behaviour can have a number of causes and is usually treated with an antipsychotic or benzodiazepine (see p.650). However, a study of methylphenidate in patients who had sustained serious brain injury found that methylphenidate 30 mg daily reduced anger and temper outbursts and improved memory and general measure of psychopathological outcome.[1]

1. Mooney GF, Haas LJ. Effect of methylphenidate on brain injury-related anger. *Arch Phys Med Rehabil* 1993; **74:** 153–60.

Hyperactivity. Methylphenidate is one of the main drugs used in hyperactivity, including attention deficit hyperactivity disorder (ADHD) (p.1505).

Small studies have indicated that different aspects of attention deficit disorders in children might respond to different doses of methylphenidate.[1-4] In addition to the morning and noon doses commonly used in hyperactivity disorders, studies[5,6] have shown improved clinical outcome with little adverse effect on sleep patterns if a third late afternoon dose is given. Although modified-release preparations with a slow onset of action have been developed to overcome the short duration of action of methylphenidate they are considered to be less effective than immediate-release preparations. A study,[7] using a regimen to simulate the prolonged steady plasma concentration profile obtained with the slow-onset, modified-release preparations, has suggested that unlike twice daily treatment acute tolerance might develop with the use of modified-release preparations. However, a newer modified-release preparation has been reported to be as effective as an immediate release preparation in short-term studies.[8,9]

UK guidelines for the use of methylphenidate in children and adolescents with ADHD are available.[10]

1. Sprague RL, Sleator EK. Methylphenidate in hyperkinetic children: differences in dose effects on learning and social behavior. *Science* 1977; **198:** 1274–6.
2. Tannock R, *et al.* Dose-response effects of methylphenidate on academic performance and overt behavior in hyperactive children. *Pediatrics* 1989; **84:** 648–57.
3. Sebrechts MM, *et al.* Components of attention, methylphenidate dosage, and blood levels in children with attention deficit disorder. *Pediatrics* 1986; **77:** 222–8.
4. Barkley RA, *et al.* Attention deficit disorder with and without hyperactivity: clinical response to three dose levels of methylphenidate. *Pediatrics* 1991; **87:** 519–31.
5. Kent JD, *et al.* Effects of late-afternoon methylphenidate administration on behavior and sleep in attention-deficit hyperactivity disorders. *Pediatrics* 1995; **96:** 320–5.
6. Stein MA, *et al.* Methylphenidate dosing: twice daily versus three times daily. *Pediatrics* 1996; **98:** 748–56.
7. Swanson J, *et al.* Acute tolerance to methylphenidate in the treatment of attention deficit hyperactivity disorder in children. *Clin Pharmacol Ther* 1999; **66:** 295–305.
8. Pelham WE, *et al.* Once-a-day Concerta methylphenidate versus three-times-daily methylphenidate in laboratory and natural settings. *Pediatrics* 2001; **107:** 1417. Full version available at: http://www.pediatrics.org/cgi/content/full/107/6/e105
9. Wolraich ML, *et al.* Randomized, controlled trial of OROS methylphenidate once a day in children with attention-deficit/hyperactivity disorder. *Pediatrics* 2001; **108:** 883–92.
10. National Institute for Clinical Excellence. Guidance on the use of methylphenidate (Ritalin, Equasym) for attention deficit/hyperactivity disorder (ADHD) in childhood (issued October 2000). Available at: http://www.nice.org.uk/pdf/Methylph-guidance13.pdf (accessed 13/11/01)

Preparations

USP 25: Methylphenidate Hydrochloride Extended-release Tablets; Methylphenidate Hydrochloride Tablets.

Proprietary Preparations (details are given in Part 3)
Aust.: Ritalin; *Austral.:* Attenta; Ritalin; *Belg.:* Ritalin; *Braz.:* Ritalina; *Canad.:* Riphenidate; Ritalin; *Denm.:* Ritalin; *Fr.:* Ritaline; *Ger.:* Ritalin; *Hong Kong:* Ritalin; *Israel:* Ritalin; *Mex.:* Ritalin; *Neth.:* Ritalin; *Norw.:* Ritalin; *NZ:* Ritalin; *Singapore:* Ritalin; Rubifen; *Spain:* Rubifen; *Switz.:* Ritaline; *UK:* Equasym; Ritalin; *USA:* Concerta; Focalin; Metadate; Methylin; Ritalin.

Modafinil (2963-I)

Modafinil *(BAN, USAN, rINN).*
CEP-1538; CRL-40476. 2-[(Diphenylmethyl)sulfinyl]acetamide.
$C_{15}H_{15}NO_2S = 273.4.$
CAS — 68693-11-8.
ATC — N06BA07.

Adverse Effects, Treatment, and Precautions

Adverse effects of modafinil may be a result of CNS stimulation and effects such as nervousness, insomnia, excitation, aggressive tendencies, personality disorder, tremor, and euphoria have been noted. There may also be gastrointestinal disturbances, including nausea and abdominal pain, dry mouth, headache, anorexia, and cardiovascular effects such as hypertension, palpitations, and tachycardia. Pruritic skin rashes, dose-related increases in alkaline phosphatase and, very rarely, bucco-facial dyskinesia have been observed.

Modafinil is contra-indicated in patients with moderate to severe hypertension or cardiac arrhythmias. It is not recommended in patients with a history of left ventricular hypertrophy or ischaemic ECG changes, chest pain, or other signs of mitral valve prolapse.

As with other stimulants, there is the possibility of dependence with long-term use.

Interactions

Modafinil has enzyme-inducing activity and may impair the effectiveness of drugs such as oral contraceptives and antiepileptics when given concomitantly.

Pharmacokinetics

Modafinil is well absorbed from the gastrointestinal tract following oral administration with peak plasma concentrations occurring after 2 to 3 hours. Plasma protein binding is 62%. Modafinil is metabolised in the liver, the major metabolite being acid modafinil, which is inactive. Excretion is mainly through the kidneys with less than 10% of the dose being eliminated unchanged. The elimination half-life is 10 to 12 hours.

◊ References.
1. Wong YN, *et al.* A double-blind, placebo-controlled, ascending-dose evaluation of the pharmacokinetics and tolerability of modafinil tablets in healthy male volunteers. *J Clin Pharmacol* 1999; **39:** 30–40.
2. Wong YN, *et al.* Open-label, single-dose pharmacokinetic study of modafinil tablets: influence of age and gender in normal subjects. *J Clin Pharmacol* 1999; **39:** 281–8.

Uses and Administration

Modafinil is a central stimulant chemically related to adrafinil (p.1506). It is used in the treatment of the narcoleptic syndrome (p.1505). Modafinil is given by mouth in a dose of 200 to 400 mg daily, administered in two divided doses, in the morning and at midday, or as a single dose in the morning. An initial dose of 100 mg daily should be used in the elderly and adjusted as necessary. The total dose should be reduced to 100 to 200 mg daily in any patient with severe hepatic or renal impairment.

Modafinil has also been investigated for the treatment of fatigue associated with multiple sclerosis and excessive daytime sleepiness associated with sleep apnoea or circadian rhythm alterations.

◊ References.
1. Broughton RJ, *et al.* Randomized, double-blind, placebo-controlled crossover trial of modafinil in the treatment of excessive daytime sleepiness in narcolepsy. *Neurology* 1997; **49:** 444–51.
2. US Modafinil in Narcolepsy Multicenter Study Group. Randomized trial of modafinil for the treatment of pathological somnolence in narcolepsy. *Ann Neurol* 1998; **43:** 88–97.
3. McClellan KJ, Spencer CM. Modafinil: a review of its pharmacology and clinical efficacy in the management of narcolepsy. *CNS Drugs* 1998; **9:** 311–24.
4. Fry JM. Treatment modalities for narcolepsy. *Neurology* 1998; **50:** S43–S48.
5. Anonymous. Modafinil for narcolepsy. *Med Lett Drugs Ther* 1999; **41:** 30–1.
6. US Modafinil in Narcolepsy Multicenter Study Group. Randomized trial of modafinil as a treatment for the excessive daytime somnolence of narcolepsy. *Neurology* 2000; **54:** 1166–75.
7. Kingshott RN, *et al.* Randomized, double-blind, placebo-controlled crossover trial of modafinil in the treatment of residual excessive daytime sleepiness in the sleep apnea/hypopnea syndrome. *Am J Respir Crit Care Med* 2001; **163:** 918–23.

Preparations

Proprietary Preparations (details are given in Part 3)
Aust.: Modasomil; *Canad.:* Alertec; *Denm.:* Modiodal; *Fr.:* Modiodal; *Ger.:* Vigil; *Irl.:* Provigil; *Neth.:* Modiodal; *Port.:* Modiodal; *Spain:* Modiodal; *UK:* Provigil; *USA:* Provigil.

Nikethamide (1434-h)

Nikethamide (BAN, rINN).

Nicethamidum; Nicotinic Acid Diethylamide; Nicotinoyldiaethylamidum; Nikethylamide. N,N-Diethylnicotinamide; N,N-Diethylpyridine-3-carboxamide.

$C_{10}H_{14}N_2O = 178.2$.

CAS — 59-26-7.

ATC — R07AB02.

Pharmacopoeias. In Chin., Eur. (see p.vi), and Pol.

Pharmacopoeial description

Ph. Eur.: A colourless or slightly yellow oily liquid or crystalline mass. Miscible with water, with alcohol, and with ether. A 25% solution in water has a pH of 6.0 to 7.8.

Profile

Nikethamide has actions similar to those of doxapram (p.1509). It was formerly given parenterally or by mouth as a respiratory stimulant but its use for this indication has largely been abandoned as the risk of toxicity associated with effective doses is now considered to be unacceptable.

Nikethamide and its calcium thiocyanate salt have been given by mouth in some countries as central stimulants and in preparations for hypotensive disorders.

Porphyria. Nikethamide has been associated with acute attacks of porphyria and is considered unsafe in porphyric patients.

Preparations

BP 2001: Nikethamide Injection.

Proprietary Preparations (details are given in Part 3)
Braz.: Cinclamina.

Multi-ingredient: *Braz.:* Cardioregis; *Fr.:* Coramine Glucose; *Ger.:* Felsol Neo; Zellaforte N Plus; *Switz.:* Gly-Coramin.

Pemoline (1436-b)

Pemoline (BAN, USAN, rINN).

LA-956; NSC-25159; Phenoxazole; Phenylisohydantoin; Phenylpseudohydantoin. 2-Imino-5-phenyl-4-oxazolidinone.

$C_9H_8N_2O_2 = 176.2$.

CAS — 2152-34-3 (pemoline); 68942-31-4 (pemoline hydrochloride); 18968-99-5 (magnesium pemoline).

ATC — N06BA05.

Adverse Effects, Treatment, and Precautions

As for Dexamfetamine Sulfate, p.1507; however, the effects of over-stimulation and sympathomimetic activity are considered to be less with pemoline. Reports of liver toxicity in patients taking pemoline (see Effects on the Liver, below) have limited its use; it is contra-indicated in patients with liver disorders and there are stringent precautions to be observed with its use. Treatment should be initiated only in patients with normal baseline liver function tests and liver function should be monitored every 2 weeks. Pemoline should be discontinued if serum alanine aminotransferase is increased to a clinically significant level or there is any increase greater than or equal to twice the upper limit of normal, or if any clinical signs or symptoms suggestive of liver failure develop. Pemoline should also be withdrawn from patients who have failed to show a substantial clinical response within three weeks of completing dose titration. There have also been rare or isolated reports of chorea, tics, mania, and neutropenia.

Abuse. Paranoid psychosis was observed in a 38-year-old man taking pemoline 75 to 225 mg daily.[1] The patient's compulsive use of the drug, development of tolerance, depressive withdrawal syndrome, and inability to abstain indicated dependence and it was evident that the patient was addicted to pemoline.

Choreoathetosis and rhabdomyolysis developed in a patient following a marked increase in intake of pemoline.[2] Abnormal movements responded to diazepam.

1. Polchert SE, Morse RM. Pemoline abuse. *JAMA* 1985; **254:** 946–7.
2. Briscoe JG, *et al.* Pemoline-induced choreoathetosis and rhabdomyolysis. *Med Toxicol* 1988; **3:** 72–6.

Effects on growth. Results of a study in 24 hyperkinetic children suggested that growth suppression was a potential side-effect of prolonged treatment with clinically effective doses of pemoline and that this effect might be dose-related.[1]

See also under Dexamfetamine Sulfate, p.1508.

1. Dickinson LC, *et al.* Impaired growth in hyperkinetic children receiving pemoline. *J Pediatr* 1979; **94:** 538–41.

Effects on the liver. Pemoline has been associated with hepatotoxicity.

Elevated concentrations of serum aspartate aminotransferase and serum alanine aminotransferase have been noted in 2% of children taking pemoline for hyperactivity; the effect was stated to be transient and reversible.[1]

However, more serious reactions have also occurred. Acute hepatitis was associated with pemoline in a 10-year-old boy[2] and the drug was believed to be the cause of fatal fulminant liver failure in a 14-year-old boy and in 2 previously published cases.[3] The UK Committee on Safety of Medicines[4] subsequently became aware of 33 reports of serious hepatic reactions

in the USA, including a total of 6 fatalities and the need for liver transplantation in 2 cases. This prompted the withdrawal of pemoline for the treatment of hyperactivity in the UK.

1. Anonymous. 'Hyperkinesis' can have many causes, symptoms. *JAMA* 1975; **232:** 1204–16.
2. Patterson JF. Hepatitis associated with pemoline. *South Med J* 1984; **77:** 938.
3. Berkovitch M, *et al.* Pemoline-associated fulminant liver failure: testing the evidence for causation. *Clin Pharmacol Ther* 1995; **57:** 696–8.
4. Committee on Safety of Medicines/Medicines Control Agency. Volital (pemoline) has been withdrawn. *Current Problems* 1997; **23:** 10.

Effects on the prostate. Experience in one patient suggested that pemoline might adversely affect the prostate gland or interfere with tests for prostatic acid phosphatase used in the diagnosis of prostatic carcinoma.[1]

1. Lindau W, de Girolami E. Pemoline and the prostate. *Lancet* 1986; **i:** 738.

Interactions

A possibility of hypertensive crisis when pemoline is administered with MAOIs has been suggested. Reduced seizure threshold has been reported in epileptic patients receiving pemoline and antiepileptics.

Pharmacokinetics

Pemoline is readily absorbed from the gastrointestinal tract. About 50% is bound to plasma protein. It is metabolised in the liver and excreted in the urine as unchanged pemoline and metabolites.

◊ References.

1. Vermeulen NPE, *et al.* Pharmacokinetics of pemoline in plasma, saliva and urine following oral administration. *Br J Clin Pharmacol* 1979; **8:** 459–63.
2. Sallee F, *et al.* Oral pemoline kinetics in hyperactive children. *Clin Pharmacol Ther* 1985; **37:** 606–9.
3. Collier CP, *et al.* Pemoline pharmacokinetics and long term therapy in children with attention deficit disorder and hyperactivity. *Clin Pharmacokinet* 1985; **10:** 269–78.

Uses and Administration

Pemoline is a central stimulant with actions similar to those of dexamfetamine (p.1508).

It has been used in the management of hyperactivity disorders in children (p.1505). In the USA 37.5 mg is given by mouth each morning initially, increased gradually at weekly intervals by 18.75 mg; the usual range is 56.25 to 75 mg daily and the maximum recommended daily dose is 112.5 mg. In the UK, pemoline was withdrawn from use for hyperactivity in children after reports of serious hepatotoxicity in the USA.

Pemoline has been included in preparations also containing yohimbine hydrochloride and methyltestosterone that are claimed to combat failure of sexual desire and functioning in males and females; such preparations are not recommended.

Pemoline has been given with magnesium hydroxide (magnesium pemoline) in an attempt to increase its absorption.

Preparations

Proprietary Preparations (details are given in Part 3)
Belg.: Stimul; *Canad.:* Cylert†; *Ger.:* Hyperilex; Senior†; Tradon; *Israel:* Cylert; Nitan; *S.Afr.:* Dynalert; *Switz.:* Stimul†; *UK:* Volital†; *USA:* Cylert; PemADD.

Multi-ingredient: *Ital.:* Deadyn†; *S.Afr.:* Lentogesic; *UK:* Prowess.

Pentetrazol (1437-v)

Pentetrazol (BAN, rINN).

Corazol; Leptazol; Pentamethazol; 1,5-Pentamethylenetetrazole; Pentazol; Pentetrazolum; Pentylenetetrazol. 6,7,8,9-Tetrahydro-5H-tetrazoloazepine.

$C_6H_{10}N_4 = 138.2$.

CAS — 54-95-5.

ATC — R07AB03.

Pharmacopoeias. In Aust. and It.

Profile

Pentetrazol is a central and respiratory stimulant similar to doxapram (p.1509). It has been used in respiratory depression and in multi-ingredient preparations intended for the treatment of respiratory-tract disorders including cough, cardiovascular disorders including hypotension, and for the treatment of pruritus. Administration has been by mouth and by injection.

Porphyria. Pentetrazol has been associated with acute attacks of porphyria and is considered unsafe in porphyric patients.

Preparations

Proprietary Preparations (details are given in Part 3)

Multi-ingredient: *Aust.:* Prospervital†; *Braz.:* Belacodid; Piritosse; Revulsan; Suprasten; *Ital.:* Cardiazol-Paracodina; *Port.:* Broncodiazina.

Phendimetrazine Tartrate (1486-j)

Phendimetrazine Tartrate (BANM, rINNM).

Phendimetrazine Acid Tartrate; Phendimetrazine Bitartrate. (+)-3,4-Dimethyl-2-phenylmorpholine hydrogen tartrate.

$C_{12}H_{17}NO,C_4H_6O_6 = 341.4$.

CAS — 634-03-7 (phendimetrazine); 7635-51-0 (phendimetrazine hydrochloride); 50-58-8 (phendimetrazine tartrate).

Pharmacopoeias. In US.

Pharmacopoeial description

USP 25: A white odourless crystalline powder. Freely soluble in water; sparingly soluble in warm alcohol; insoluble in acetone, in chloroform, in ether, and in benzene. pH of a 2.5% solution in water is between 3.0 and 4.0. Store in airtight containers.

Adverse Effects, Treatment, and Precautions

As for Dexamfetamine Sulfate, p.1507.

Pulmonary hypertension and valvular heart defects have been reported in patients receiving phendimetrazine in combination with other anorectics; these adverse effects, together with the relevant precautions to be observed, are discussed under Fenfluramine Hydrochloride, p.1510. Phendimetrazine should not be used with other anorectics nor within a year of their use.

Interactions

Phendimetrazine is an indirect-acting sympathomimetic and, similarly to dexamfetamine (p.1508), may interact with a number of other drugs.

Pharmacokinetics

Phendimetrazine tartrate is readily absorbed from the gastrointestinal tract and is excreted in the urine, partly unchanged and partly as metabolites, including phenmetrazine.

Uses and Administration

Phendimetrazine tartrate is a central stimulant and indirect-acting sympathomimetic with actions similar to those of dexamfetamine (p.1508). It has been used as an anorectic in the short-term treatment of obesity (p.1505), although stimulants are no longer recommended for this indication. The usual dose is 35 mg two or three times daily by mouth before food. An alternative dose is 105 mg once daily in the morning as a modified-release preparation.

Phendimetrazine hydrochloride has been used similarly.

Regulatory authorities in the European Union have called for the withdrawal of all anorectics from the market.

Preparations

USP 25: Phendimetrazine Tartrate Capsules; Phendimetrazine Tartrate Tablets.

Proprietary Preparations (details are given in Part 3)

Belg.: Anoran; *Ital.:* Plegine†; *S.Afr.:* Obesan-X; Obex-LA; *USA:* Adipost†; Anorex†; Bontril; Dyrexan-OD†; Melfiat; Obalan†; Plegine†; Prelu-2; Rexigen Forte†; Trimstat†; Weh-less†; Weightrol†; X-trozine†.

Phenmetrazine Hydrochloride (1487-z)

Phenmetrazine Hydrochloride (BANM, rINNM).

Oxazimédrine. (±)-trans-3-Methyl-2-phenylmorpholine hydrochloride.

$C_{11}H_{15}NO,HCl = 213.7$.

CAS — 134-49-6 (phenmetrazine); 1707-14-8 (phenmetrazine hydrochloride); 13931-75-4 (phenmetrazine teoclate).

Pharmacopoeias. In US.

Pharmacopoeial description

USP 25: A white to off-white crystalline powder. Soluble 1 in 0.4 of water, 1 in 2 of alcohol, and 1 in 2 of chloroform. pH of a 2.5% solution in water is between 4.5 and 5.5. Store in airtight containers.

Profile

Phenmetrazine hydrochloride is a central stimulant and indirect-acting sympathomimetic with actions similar to those of dexamfetamine (p.1507). It has been used as an anorectic in the treatment of obesity. It has been subject to extensive abuse.

Abuse. For reference to a serious syndrome involving rhabdomyolysis following intravenous abuse of phenmetrazine, see Dexamfetamine Sulfate, p.1507.

Preparations

USP 25: Phenmetrazine Hydrochloride Tablets.

The symbol † denotes a preparation no longer actively marketed

Phentermine (1490-w)

Phentermine (BAN, USAN, rINN).

α,α-Dimethylphenethylamine.

$C_{10}H_{15}N = 149.2$.

CAS — 122-09-8.

ATC — A08AA01.

Phentermine Hydrochloride (1489-k)

Phentermine Hydrochloride (BANM, rINNM).

$C_{10}H_{15}N,HCl = 185.7$.

CAS — 1197-21-3.

Pharmacopoeias. In US.

Phentermine hydrochloride 1.24 mg is approximately equivalent to 1 mg of phentermine.

Pharmacopoeial description

USP 25: A white, odourless, hygroscopic, crystalline powder. Soluble in water and in the lower alcohols; slightly soluble in chloroform; insoluble in ether. pH of a 2% solution in water is between 5.0 and 6.0. Store in airtight containers.

Adverse Effects, Treatment, and Precautions

As for Dexamfetamine Sulfate, p.1507. Urticaria may occur with use of phentermine.

Pulmonary hypertension has been reported in patients receiving phentermine and valvular heart defects in patients receiving the drug in combination with other anorectics such as fenfluramine or dexfenfluramine; these adverse effects, together with the relevant precautions to be observed, are discussed under Fenfluramine Hydrochloride, p.1510.

Interactions

Phentermine is an indirect-acting sympathomimetic and, similarly to dexamfetamine (p.1508), may interact with a number of other drugs.

Pharmacokinetics

Phentermine is readily absorbed from the gastrointestinal tract and is excreted in the urine, partly unchanged and partly as metabolites.

Uses and Administration

Phentermine is a central stimulant and indirect-acting sympathomimetic with actions similar to those of dexamfetamine (p.1508). It has been given by mouth as the base or hydrochloride as an anorectic in the short-term treatment of moderate to severe obesity (p.1505), although stimulants are no longer recommended for this indication.

The usual dose of phentermine is 15 or 30 mg once daily before breakfast given as an ion-exchange resin complex that provides modified release. A suggested dose for phentermine hydrochloride is 8 mg three times daily before meals or 15 to 37.5 mg once daily in the morning. It should not be given for longer than a few weeks.

Regulatory authorities in the European Union have withdrawn phentermine from the market.

Preparations

USP 25: Phentermine Hydrochloride Capsules; Phentermine Hydrochloride Tablets.

Proprietary Preparations (details are given in Part 3)
Aust.: Adipex†; Mirapront†; Austral.: Duromine; Belg.: Ionamin†; Panbesy†; Canad.: Fastin†; Ionamin; Hong Kong: Duromine; Panbesy; Redusa; Irl.: Ionamin†; Israel: Novirasin; Mex.: Diminex; Ifa Reduccing S; Ionamin; Reducap; NZ: Duromine; Umine; S.Afr.: Duromine; Minobese; Singapore: Duromine; Ionamin; Panbesy; Umine; Switz.: Adipex; Ionamine; Normaform; Thai.: Duromine; Panbesy; UK: Duromine†; Ionamin†; USA: Adipex-P; Fastin†; Ionamin; Obe-Nix†; Obephen†; Oby-Cap†; Oby-Trim 30†; Zantryl†.

Pipradrol Hydrochloride (1440-d)

Pipradrol Hydrochloride (BANM, rINNM).

α-2-Piperidylbenzhydrol hydrochloride; α,α-Diphenyl-2-piperidinemethanol hydrochloride.

$C_{18}H_{21}NO,HCl = 303.8$.

CAS — 467-60-7 (pipradrol); 71-78-3 (pipradrol hydrochloride).

Profile

Pipradrol hydrochloride has been given by mouth in tonic preparations as a CNS stimulant.

Preparations

Proprietary Preparations (details are given in Part 3)
Multi-ingredient: Austral.: Alertonic; Canad.: Alertonic; S.Afr.: Alertonic.

Prethcamide (1443-m)

G-5668. N,N-Dimethyl-2-(N-propylcrotonamido)butyramide (cropropamide, $C_{13}H_{24}N_2O_2 = 240.3$); 2-(N-Ethylcrotonamido)-N,N-dimethylbutyramide (crotetamide, $C_{12}H_{22}N_2O_2 = 226.3$).

CAS — 8015-51-8 (prethcamide); 633-47-6 (cropropamide); 6168-76-9 (crotetamide).

ATC — R07AB06.

NOTE. Cropropamide is pINN, Crotetamide (crotethamide) is BAN and rINN.

A mixture of equal parts by weight of cropropamide and crotetamide.

Profile

Prethcamide has actions similar to those of doxapram (p.1509) and has been used as a respiratory stimulant. Doses of 100 mg have been given three times daily by mouth.

Preparations

Proprietary Preparations (details are given in Part 3)
Ital.: Micoren.

Prolintane Hydrochloride (1444-b)

Prolintane Hydrochloride (BANM, USAN, rINNM).

SP-732. 1-(α-Propylphenethyl)pyrrolidine hydrochloride.

$C_{15}H_{23}N,HCl = 253.8$.

CAS — 493-92-5 (prolintane); 1211-28-5 (prolintane hydrochloride).

Profile

Prolintane hydrochloride is a mild central stimulant and has properties similar to those of dexamfetamine (p.1507). It has been available mainly in tonic preparations that also contained vitamin supplements. It has also been used in narcolepsy (p.1505) in doses of up to 40 mg daily.

Preparations

Proprietary Preparations (details are given in Part 3)
Belg.: Catorid; S.Afr.: Catovit N.
Multi-ingredient: Austral.: Catovit†; S.Afr.: Catovit†; Spain: Katovit.

Propylhexedrine (1445-v)

Propylhexedrine (BAN, rINN).

Hexahydrodesoxyephedrine; Propylhexed. 2-Cyclohexyl-1-methylethyl-(methyl)amine; (±)-N-α-Dimethylcyclo-hexaneethylamine.

$C_{10}H_{21}N = 155.3$.

CAS — 101-40-6; 3595-11-7 ((±)-propylhexedrine).

Pharmacopoeias. In US.

Pharmacopoeial description

USP 25: A clear colourless liquid having a characteristic amine-like odour. It slowly volatilises at room temperature and absorbs carbon dioxide from the air. Very slightly soluble in water; soluble 1 in 0.4 of alcohol, 1 in 0.2 of chloroform, and 1 in 0.1 of ether. Its solutions are alkaline to litmus. Store in airtight containers.

Propylhexedrine Hydrochloride (1446-g)

Propylhexedrine Hydrochloride (BANM, rINNM).

$C_{10}H_{21}N,HCl = 191.7$.

CAS — 1007-33-6; 6192-95-6 ((±)-propylhexedrine hydrochloride).

Adverse Effects, Treatment and Precautions

As for Dexamfetamine Sulfate, p.1507.

Nasal inhalation may cause transient burning, stinging, mucosal dryness, and sneezing. Prolonged use can cause rebound congestion, redness, swelling, and rhinitis. Systemic effects such as headache, hypertension, nervousness, and increased heart rate may occur.

Propylhexedrine is subject to abuse; fatalities following oral and intravenous use have been reported due to myocardial infarction, heart failure, or pulmonary hypertension. Psychosis may occur.

Abuse. References.
1. White L, DiMaio VJM. Intravenous propylhexedrine and sudden death. N Engl J Med 1977; 297: 1071.
2. Anderson RJ, et al. Intravenous propylhexedrine (Benzedrex®) abuse and sudden death. Am J Med 1979; 67: 15–20.
3. Cameron J, et al. Possible association of pulmonary hypertension with an anorectic drug. Med J Aust 1984; 140: 595–7.

Uses and Administration

Propylhexedrine is a central stimulant and indirect-acting sympathomimetic with actions similar to those of dexamfetamine (p.1508). It has been used as an inhalant for nasal decongestion (p.1082).

Propylhexedrine hydrochloride has been given by mouth as an anorectic in the treatment of obesity (p.1505) but stimulants are no longer recommended for this indication. The (−)-isomer, levopropylhexedrine hydrochloride, has been used similarly.

Preparations

USP 25: Propylhexedrine Inhalant.

Proprietary Preparations (details are given in Part 3)
Mex.: Colloidine; USA: Benzedrex.
Multi-ingredient: S.Afr.: Reducealin.

Sibutramine Hydrochloride (20428-v)

Sibutramine Hydrochloride (BANM, USAN, rINNM).

BTS-54524. (±)-1-(p-Chlorophenyl)-α-isobutyl-N,N-dimethyl-cyclobutanemethylamine hydrochloride monohydrate.

$C_{17}H_{26}ClN,HCl,H_2O = 334.3$.

CAS — 106650-56-0 (sibutramine); 84485-00-7 (anhydrous sibutramine hydrochloride); 125494-59-9 (sibutramine hydrochloride monohydrate).

Adverse Effects

Commonly reported side-effects of sibutramine are dry mouth, headache, insomnia, and constipation. Diarrhoea, back pain, increased appetite, dizziness, influenza-like symptoms, and rhinitis have also occurred. Less frequently reported side-effects include dyspepsia, nausea, dysmenorrhoea, increased sweating and thirst, oedema, paraesthesia, skin rashes, taste perversion, palpitations, vasodilatation, anxiety, nervousness, drowsiness, and depression. Abnormal bleeding including Henoch-Schönlein purpura and thrombocytopenia, acute interstitial nephritis, glomerulonephritis, emotional lability, seizures, and blurred vision have been reported rarely. Clinically significant increases in heart rate and blood pressure may occur. Sibutramine may decrease salivary flow and therefore increase the risk of dental caries, periodontal disease, or other oral disorders. It may also produce mydriasis. Reversible increases in liver enzymes have been reported.

Precautions

Sibutramine should be avoided in patients with a history of eating disorders such as anorexia nervosa and bulimia nervosa. It is also contra-indicated in patients with uncontrolled or poorly controlled hypertension and should be used with caution in patients with a history of, or with, well-controlled hypertension. Blood pressure and heart rate should be monitored (see below for details). In the event of sustained elevations, the dose should be reduced or treatment discontinued.

Sibutramine should not be used in patients with a history of cerebrovascular disease or cardiovascular disorders such as cardiac arrhythmias, heart failure, peripheral arterial occlusive disease, and coronary artery disease; it should be avoided in patients with severe hepatic or renal impairment. Sibutramine should also not be used in patients with bipolar disorder, Tourette's syndrome, hyperthyroidism, phaeochromocytoma, benign prostatic hyperplasia, or a history of drug or alcohol abuse. It should be used with caution, if at all, in patients with glaucoma. Sibutramine should also be used with caution in patients with a history of seizures or gallstones (which may be precipitated or exacerbated by weight loss), or a family history of motor or verbal tics.

Ability to perform tasks requiring judgement or motor or cognitive skills may be impaired by sibutramine, and patients, if affected, should not drive or operate machinery.

Cardiovascular monitoring. Sibutramine may cause clinically significant increases in blood pressure and heart rate and monitoring is recommended in all patients during treatment. In the first 3 months, blood pressure and heart rate should be checked every 2 weeks; this may be reduced to every month for the next 3 months, and at least every 3 months thereafter. Treatment should be discontinued in patients who develop an increase in resting heart rate of 10 beats per minute or an increase in blood pressure of 10 mmHg at two consecutive visits. In patients with previously well-controlled hypertension, treatment should be discontinued if their blood pressure exceeds 145/90 mmHg at two consecutive visits.

Interactions

Sibutramine should not be given concurrently with, or within at least two weeks of stopping an MAOI; at least two weeks should elapse between discontinuation of sibutramine and starting therapy with a MAOI. There is a risk of the serotonin syndrome (p.304) developing if sibutramine is administered together with other serotonergic drugs such as SSRIs, sumatriptan, lithium, pethidine, fentanyl, dextromethorphan, and pentazocine. Caution is advised when sibutramine is given with other drugs that may increase heart rate or blood pressure such as ephedrine, phenylpropanolamine, and pseudoephedrine (which may be ingredients of some cough and cold remedies). It should not be used together with other centrally acting anorectics. Alcohol should be avoided.

Inhibitors of the cytochrome P450 isoenzyme CYP3A4, such as ketoconazole and erythromycin, may increase plasma concentrations of sibutramine. Conversely, inducers of this isoenzyme, such as rifampicin, phenytoin, carbamazepine, and phenobarbital, may reduce plasma concentrations of sibutramine.

Antibacterials. A study in 12 obese subjects indicated that addition of erythromycin to sibutramine therapy resulted in little significant alteration in sibutramine pharmacokinetics beyond a modest increase in maximum plasma concentration of one of the active metabolites.[1] A small increase in the QT interval was not considered clinically meaningful.

1. Hinson JL, *et al.* Steady-state interaction study of sibutramine (Meridia™) and erythromycin in uncomplicated obese subjects. *Pharm Res* 1996; **13** (suppl): S116.

Antifungals. A study in 12 obese subjects given sibutramine found that *ketoconazole* moderately increased steady-state plasma concentrations of sibutramine and its active metabolites.[1] There was a significant increase in heart rate but no clinically meaningful change in the QT interval.

1. Hinson JL, *et al.* Steady-state interaction study of sibutramine (Meridia™) and ketoconazole in uncomplicated obese subjects. *Pharm Res* 1996; **13** (suppl): S116.

Pharmacokinetics
Sibutramine is well-absorbed from the gastrointestinal tract; peak plasma concentrations appear after 1.2 hours (parent drug) and 3 to 4 hours (metabolites). It undergoes extensive first-pass hepatic metabolism, principally by the cytochrome P450 isoenzyme CYP3A4. Demethylation produces mono- and di-desmethylsibutramine (both of which are pharmacologically active) and is followed by hydroxylation and conjugation to inactive metabolites. Protein binding is 97%. Plasma-elimination half-life is 14 to 16 hours. Elimination is mainly in the urine as inactive metabolites, and partly in the faeces.

◊ References.
1. Hind ID, *et al.* Sibutramine pharmacokinetics in young and elderly healthy subjects. *Eur J Clin Pharmacol* 1999; **54:** 847–9.

Uses and Administration
Sibutramine, which is structurally related to amfetamine (p.1506), is a serotonin and noradrenaline reuptake inhibitor; it also inhibits dopamine reuptake but to a lesser extent. Sibutramine is used in the management of obesity. It may also be used in overweight patients (body mass index of 27 kg per m^2 or more) if other risk factors such as hypertension (but see Precautions, above), diabetes mellitus, or hyperlipidaemias are present.

Sibutramine hydrochloride is given by mouth in an initial daily dose of 10 mg, usually taken in the morning. Patients who cannot tolerate 10 mg daily may benefit from a dose of 5 mg daily. Treatment with sibutramine should be re-evaluated if weight loss is less than 2 kg in the first 4 weeks of therapy. At this stage, the dose may be increased to a maximum of 15 mg daily, taking into consideration effects on heart rate and blood pressure, or treatment may need to be discontinued. It should be reassessed again after a further 4 weeks at maximum dose, and discontinued if weight loss is less than 2 kg. Treatment should also be stopped if:

* weight loss stabilises at less than 5% of the initial body-weight
* weight loss after 3 months is less than 5% of the initial body-weight
* weight gain of 3 kg or more occurs after previous weight loss.

Treatment should not be given for longer than 1 year.

In patients with other risk factors (see above), it is recommended that sibutramine is continued only if weight loss is associated with other clinical benefits.

◊ References.
1. McNeely W, Goa KL. Sibutramine: a review of its contribution to the management of obesity. *Drugs* 1998; **56:** 1093–1124.
2. Luque CA, Rey JA. Sibutramine: a serotonin-norepinephrine reuptake-inhibitor for the treatment of obesity. *Ann Pharmacother* 1999; **33:** 968–78.
3. James WPT, *et al.* Effect of sibutramine on weight maintenance after weight loss: a randomised trial. *Lancet* 2000; **356:** 2119–25.
4. McMahon FG, *et al.* Efficacy and safety of sibutramine in obese white and African American patients with hypertension: a 1-year, double-blind, placebo-controlled, multicenter trial. *Arch Intern Med* 2000; **160:** 2185–91.

Preparations
Proprietary Preparations (details are given in Part 3)
Ger.: Reductil; *Mex.:* Raductil; *S.Afr.:* Reductil; *Switz.:* Reductil; *UK:* Reductil; *USA:* Meridia.

Tenamfetamine (1432-d)
Tenamfetamine *(rINN).*
MDA; Methylenedioxyamphetamine; 3,4-Methylenedioxyamphetamine; SKF-5. α-Methyl-3,4-methylenedioxyphenethylamine.
$C_{10}H_{13}NO_2 = 179.2$.
CAS — 4764-17-4; 51497-09-7.
NOTE. Tenamfetamine has also been known as Love Drug, Love Pill, and Mellow Drug of America.

Profile
Tenamfetamine is a phenylethylamine compound, structurally related to amfetamine and mescaline, with hallucinogenic effects. It has been subject to abuse and dependence. A number of similar compounds are known because of their abuse and include:

* brolamfetamine (4-bromo-2,5-dimethoxyamfetamine; bromo-DMA; bromo-DOM; 2,5-dimethoxy-4-bromoamfetamine; DOB);
* 4-bromo-2,5-methoxyphenylethylamine (afterburner; 2-CB; MFT);
* 2,5-dimethoxy-4-metamfetamine (DOM; methyl-2,5-dimethoxyamfetamine; Serenity, Tranquillity and Peace; STP);
* *N*-ethyltenamfetamine (Eve; MDE; MDEA; 3,4-methylenedioxyethamfetamine);
* *N*-hydroxytenamfetamine (*N*-hydroxy MDA; 3,4-methylenedioxy-*N*-hydroxyamfetamine);
* methoxyamfetamine (4-methoxyamfetamine; *p*-methoxyamfetamine; PMA);
* methylenedioxymethamfetamine (Ecstasy) (see p.1511);
* 2,4,5-trimethoxyamfetamine (TMA; TMA-2).

In large doses the side-effects of tenamfetamine and related compounds are similar to those of dexamfetamine and may be treated similarly (see p.1507). Fatalities have been associated with the abuse of some of these compounds.

◊ Reviews of the properties of some designer drugs, including phenylethylamine compounds.
1. Buchanan JF, Brown CR. 'Designer drugs': a problem in clinical toxicology. *Med Toxicol* 1988; **3:** 1–17.
2. Chesher G. Designer drugs—the "whats" and the "whys". *Med J Aust* 1990; **153:** 157–61.

Sunscreens

In normal healthy individuals **exposure to sunlight** causes an increase in pigmentation (tanning). However, excessive exposure to strong sunlight causes erythema and sunburn. Immediate tanning may occur resulting from the oxidation of melanin precursors in the uppermost layers of the skin. There may also be a delayed and indirect pigmentation due to the formation of new melanin. The ability of an individual to form a tan is genetically predetermined. Melanin provides some protection against further exposure, but the main protection is provided by thickening of the corneous layer.

Excessive and prolonged exposure to intense sunlight may lead to degenerative changes in the skin (premature ageing of the skin or photoageing), actinic (solar) keratoses (which are risk factors or precursors of skin cancers), and some skin cancers such as basal cell or squamous cell carcinomas and malignant melanomas (see Malignant Neoplasms of the Skin, p.498).

Ultraviolet (UV) light has different properties according to its wavelength.

- UVA (wavelengths 320 to 400 nm) produces immediate direct tanning of the skin with little erythema although it does contribute to the long-term harmful effects of photoageing and cancers.
- UVB (wavelengths 290 to 320 nm) is about 1000 times stronger than UVA in producing erythema and is that part of the sun's spectrum that is responsible for producing sunburn and it too contributes to long-term effects. UVB also produces tanning by indirect pigmentation.
- UVC (wavelengths 200 to 290 nm) produces erythema without tanning. The earth's surface is usually screened by the ozone layer from UVC radiation although UVC may be emitted by artificial sources such as bactericidal lamps and industrial welding arcs.

Reflected ultraviolet light from snow, white sand, or water adds to direct irradiation.

In some persons brief exposure to sunlight can induce a variety of skin complaints. *Polymorphic light eruption* is characterised by pruritic erythematous lesions which develop some hours after exposure to sunlight. *Chronic actinic dermatitis* is manifested by a persistent eczematous eruption which usually only affects the exposed areas although in a small number of patients the whole skin can be affected. Photosensitivity can also be produced by drugs administered either systemically or applied topically (see Drug-induced Skin Reactions, p.1104). Such photosensitivity can be either phototoxic or photoallergic in nature. In *phototoxicity*, tissues are damaged when the drug is energised by absorbing radiation. In *photoallergy*, a hypersensitivity reaction is produced when the drug is chemically altered after exposure to light. Other conditions that can be exacerbated by sunlight include the *cutaneous porphyrias, lupus erythematosus, solar urticaria, xeroderma pigmentosum*, and sometimes *herpes labialis*. In many of these cases the photosensitivity is particularly associated with the longer UVA wavelengths.

Protection against sunlight is therefore beneficial, both in healthy people to prevent skin damage, and in patients with the disorders mentioned above. Protection may also be necessary in patients with *hypopigmentation disorders* such as vitiligo or albinism and medical personnel exposed to ultraviolet bactericidal lamps may need protection against the whole of the UV spectrum.

Sunscreens are used topically and are of 2 types: *chemical* agents that because of their chromophore groups absorb a particular range of wavelengths within the UV spectrum and *physical* agents that are opaque and reflect most UV radiation. A classification of the chemical sunscreens included in this chapter is given in Table 1, below. Trolamine salicylate (p.90) is a chemical sunscreen that is also used as a topical analgesic. Physical sunscreens include titanium dioxide (p.1126) and zinc oxide (p.1128). Many of the available products combine sunscreens from the different groups in order to widen the protection afforded. Other agents used as physical sunscreens include calcium carbonate, kaolin, magnesium oxide, red veterinary petroleum, and talc. Powders may be dusted onto the skin or applied in an aqueous or oily basis but these types of sunscreens are usually cosmetically unappealing.

The efficacy of a particular sunscreen preparation is often expressed as its **sun protection factor (SPF)**. This is a ratio of the time required for irradiation to produce minimal perceptible erythema (minimal erythemal dose; MED) with the skin protected with the sunscreen compared with the MED without protection. Thus the SPF is predominantly an indication of efficacy against UVB light. Various systems have been suggested for classifying the relative efficacies of sunscreens against UVA light but none appears, as yet, to be universally accepted. The efficacy of a sunscreen is also highly dependent upon its correct application.

Adverse effects such as photosensitisation may occur with chemical agents, and skin irritation has also been reported. Sunscreens in highly alcoholic vehicles should not be used on patients with inflamed skin.

Several other agents including betacarotene (p.1355) and psoralens (see Methoxsalen, p.1118), which are neither chemical nor physical sunscreens, have been used to increase tolerance to sunlight in various diseases characterised by photosensitivity, although psoralens are themselves photosensitisers. Dihydroxyacetone (p.1113) and lawsone (p.1627) when employed together appear to provide some protection against UV light although neither is effective when used alone.

◊ General references to sunscreens.

1. Council on Scientific Affairs, American Medical Association. Harmful effects of ultraviolet radiation. *JAMA* 1989; **262:** 380–4.

2. Anonymous. Measuring sunscreen protection against UVA. *Lancet* 1990; **336:** 472.

3. Taylor CR, *et al.* Photoaging/photodamage and photoprotection. *J Am Acad Dermatol* 1990; **22:** 1–15.

4. Ratnavel RC, Norris PG. Sunscreens and their medical uses. *Prescribers' J* 1993; **33:** 63–71.

5. McGregor JM, Young AR. Sunscreens, suntans, and skin cancer. *BMJ* 1996; **312:** 1621–2.

6. Anonymous. Do sunscreens prevent skin cancer? *Drug Ther Bull* 1998; **36:** 49–51.

7. Anonymous. Sunscreens: are they safe and effective? *Med Lett Drugs Ther* 1999; **41:** 43–4.

Table 1. Chemical sunscreens.

UVA absorbers	UVB absorbers
Anthranilates	*Aminobenzoates*
Meradimate	Aminobenzoic acid
Dibenzoylmethanes	Lisadimate
Avobenzone	Padimate
Dibenzoylmethane	Padimate O
Isopropyldibenzoyl-	Roxadimate
methane	*Camphor derivatives*
UVA and UVB absorbers	Enzacamene
	Cinnamates
Benzophenones	Amiloxate
Benzophenone-6	Cinoxate
Dioxybenzone	Octinoxate
Mexenone	Octocrilene
Oxybenzone	*Salicylates*
Sulisobenzone	Homosalate
	Octisalate

Amiloxate (20540-v)

Amiloxate (USAN, rINN).

E-1000; Isoamyl p-Methoxycinnamate. Isopentyl p-methoxycinnamate.

$C_{15}H_{20}O_3 = 248.3$.

CAS — 71617-10-2.

Pharmacopoeias. In US.

Pharmacopoeial description

USP 25: Store in airtight containers.

Profile

Amiloxate, a substituted cinnamate, is a sunscreen with actions similar to those of octinoxate (below).

Preparations

Proprietary Preparations
Some preparations are listed in Part 3.

Aminobenzoic Acid (7871-h)

Amben; PAB; PABA; Pabacidum; Para-aminobenzoic Acid; Vitamin H'. 4-Aminobenzoic acid.

$C_7H_7NO_2 = 137.1$.

CAS — 150-13-0.

ATC — D02BA01.

Pharmacopoeias. In Aust., Br., Swiss, and US.

Pharmacopoeial description

BP 2001: White or slightly yellow odourless or almost odourless crystals or crystalline powder. It gradually darkens on exposure to air and light. Slightly soluble in water; freely soluble in alcohol; it dissolves in solutions of alkali hydroxides or carbonates. Protect from light.

USP 25: White or slightly yellow, odourless crystals or crystalline powder. It discolours on exposure to air or light. Slightly soluble in water and in chloroform; freely soluble in alcohol and in solutions of alkali hydroxides or carbonates; sparingly soluble in ether. Store in airtight containers. Protect from light.

Adverse Effects

Contact and photocontact allergic dermatitis has been reported following the topical administration of aminobenzoate sunscreens.

◊ Adverse skin reactions have been reported following the topical use[1-6] of aminobenzoic acid or its esters. Skin reactions (vitiligo) have also been reported following the oral administration of aminobenzoic acid[7] and the adverse effects associated with the former use of high oral doses for various conditions have been highlighted.[8]

1. Parrish JA, *et al.* Facial irritation due to sunscreen products. *Arch Dermatol* 1975; **111:** 525.

2. Mathias CGT, *et al.* Allergic contact photodermatitis to para-aminobenzoic acid. *Arch Dermatol* 1978; **114:** 1665–6.

3. Horio T, Higuchi T. Photocontact dermatitis from p-aminobenzoic acid. *Dermatologica* 1978; **156:** 124–8.

4. Marmelzat J, Rapaport MJ. Photodermatitis with PABA. *Contact Dermatitis* 1980; **6:** 230–1.

5. Thune P. Contact and photocontact allergy to sunscreens. *Photodermatology* 1984; **1:** 5–9.

6. English JSC, *et al.* Sensitivity to sunscreens. *Contact Dermatitis* 1987; **17:** 159–62.

7. Hughes CG. Oral PABA and vitiligo. *J Am Acad Dermatol* 1983; **9:** 770.

8. Worobec S, LaChine A. Dangers of orally administered para-aminobenzoic acid. *JAMA* 1984; **251:** 2348.

Precautions

Aminobenzoate sunscreens should not be used by those with a history of photosensitivity or hypersensitivity reactions to chemically related drugs such as sulfonamides, thiazide diuretics, and certain local anaesthetics, particularly benzocaine.

Aminobenzoic acid may stain clothing.

Pharmacokinetics

If administered by mouth, aminobenzoic acid is absorbed from the gastrointestinal tract. It is metabolised in the liver and excreted in the urine as unchanged drug and metabolites.

Uses and Administration

Aminobenzoic acid is used by topical application as a sunscreen. Aminobenzoic acid and its derivatives effectively absorb light throughout the UVB range but absorb little or no UVA light (for definitions, see above). Aminobenzoate sunscreens may therefore be used to prevent sunburn, but are unlikely to prevent drug-related or other photosensitivity reactions associated with UVA light; combination with a benzophenone may give some added protection against such photosensitivity.

Aminobenzoic acid has sometimes been included as a member of the vitamin-B group, but deficiency of aminobenzoic acid in man or animals has not been demonstrated.

Aminobenzoic acid has been used in conjunction with bentiromide (p.1584) in the PABA or BTPABA test of pancreatic function.

Preparations

USP 25: Aminobenzoic Acid Gel; Aminobenzoic Acid Topical Solution.

Proprietary Preparations
Some preparations are listed in Part 3.

Avobenzone (10926-q)

Avobenzone (*USAN, rINN*).
Butylmethoxydibenzoylmethane; 4-*tert*-Butyl-4′-methoxydibenzoylmethane; Parsol 1789. 1-(p-*tert*-Butylphenyl)-3-(p-methoxyphenyl)-1,3-propanedione; 1-[4-(1,1-dimethylethyl)phenyl]-3-(4-methoxyphenyl)-1,3-propanedione.
$C_{20}H_{22}O_3 = 310.4$.
CAS — 70356-09-1.
Pharmacopoeias. In US.

Pharmacopoeial description
USP 25: M.p. 81° to 86°. Store in airtight containers. Protect from light.

Profile
Avobenzone is a substituted dibenzoylmethane used by topical application as a sunscreen. Dibenzoylmethanes absorb light in the UVA range (for definitions, see above) and may therefore be used in conjunction with other sunscreens that absorb UVB light to prevent sunburn; they will also provide some protection against drug-related or other photosensitivity reactions associated with UVA light.
Contact and photocontact allergic dermatitis has occasionally been reported following the topical use of dibenzoylmethane sunscreens.

Preparations

Proprietary Preparations
Numerous preparations are listed in Part 3.

Benzophenone-6 (9318-c)

2,2′-Dihydroxy-4,4′-dimethoxybenzophenone.
$C_{15}H_{14}O_5 = 274.3$.
CAS — 131-54-4.

Profile
Benzophenone-6 is a sunscreen with actions similar to those of oxybenzone (p.1518). It is effective against UVB and some UVA light (for definitions, see above).

Preparations

Proprietary Preparations
Some preparations are listed in Part 3.

Cinoxate (9302-p)

Cinoxate (*USAN, rINN*).
2-Ethoxyethyl p-methoxycinnamate.
$C_{14}H_{18}O_4 = 250.3$.
CAS — 104-28-9.
Pharmacopoeias. In US.

Pharmacopoeial description
USP 25: A slightly yellow, practically odourless, viscous liquid. Very slightly soluble in water; slightly soluble in glycerol; soluble in propylene glycol; miscible with alcohol and with vegetable oils. Store in airtight containers. Protect from light.

Profile
Cinoxate, a substituted cinnamate, is a sunscreen with actions similar to those of octinoxate (below). It is effective against UVB light (for definitions, see above).

Preparations

USP 25: Cinoxate Lotion.
Proprietary Preparations
Some preparations are listed in Part 3.

Dibenzoylmethane (13410-m)

1,3-Diphenyl-1,3-propanedione.
$C_{15}H_{12}O_2 = 224.3$.
CAS — 120-46-7.

Profile
Dibenzoylmethane is a sunscreen with actions similar to those of avobenzone (p.1517). It absorbs UVA light (for definitions, see p.1516).

Preparations

Proprietary Preparations
Some preparations are listed in Part 3.

Dioxybenzone (9303-s)

Dioxybenzone (*USAN, rINN*).
Benzophenone-8; NSC-56769. 2,2′-Dihydroxy-4-methoxybenzophenone.
$C_{14}H_{12}O_4 = 244.2$.
CAS — 131-53-3.
Pharmacopoeias. In US.

Pharmacopoeial description
USP 25: A yellow powder. Practically insoluble in water; freely soluble in alcohol and in toluene. Store in airtight containers. Protect from light.

Profile
Dioxybenzone, a substituted benzophenone, is a sunscreen with actions similar to those of oxybenzone (below). It is effective against UVB and some UVA light (for definitions, see p.1516).

Preparations

USP 25: Dioxybenzone and Oxybenzone Cream.
Proprietary Preparations
Some preparations are listed in Part 3.

Ensulizole (9329-t)

Ensulizole (*rINN*).
Phenylbenzimidazole Sulphonic Acid. 2-Phenyl-1H-benzimidazole-5-sulphonic acid.
$C_{13}H_{10}N_2O_3S = 274.3$.
CAS — 27503-81-7.
Pharmacopoeias. In US.

Pharmacopoeial description
USP 25: A white to ivory-coloured, odourless powder. Practically insoluble in water and in oily solvents; soluble in alcohol; its salts are freely soluble in water. Store in airtight containers at a temperature of 8° to 15°.

Profile
Ensulizole is used topically as a sunscreen.

Preparations

Proprietary Preparations
Some preparations are listed in Part 3.

Enzacamene (9327-k)

Enzacamene (*USAN, rINN*).
Methyl Benzylidene Camphor; 3-(4-Methylbenzylidene)bornan-2-one; 3-(4-Methylbenzylidene)camphor. 1,7,7-Trimethyl-3-[(4-methylphenyl)methylene]bicyclo[2.2.1]heptan-2-one.
$C_{18}H_{22}O = 254.4$.
CAS — 36861-47-9 (D,L-form); 38102-62-4 (form unspecified).
Pharmacopoeias. In US.

Pharmacopoeial description
USP 25: A white, fine crystalline powder. M.p. between 66° and 68°. Practically insoluble in water; freely soluble in alcohol; very soluble in chloroform. Store in airtight containers.

Profile
Enzacamene is a camphor derivative used as a sunscreen. It is effective against UVB light (for definitions, see p.1516).

◊ A case report of allergic contact dermatitis from enzacamene.[1]
1. Hunloh W, Goerz G. Contact dermatitis from Eusolex® 6300. *Contact Dermatitis* 1983; **9:** 333–4.

Preparations

Proprietary Preparations
Some preparations are listed in Part 3.

Homosalate (9306-l)

Homosalate (*USAN, rINN*).
Homomenthyl Salicylate. 3,3,5-Trimethylcyclohexyl salicylate.
$C_{16}H_{22}O_3 = 262.3$.
CAS — 118-56-9.
Pharmacopoeias. In US.

Pharmacopoeial description
USP 25: Store in airtight containers.

Profile
Homosalate, a substituted salicylate, is a sunscreen with actions similar to those of octisalate (below). It is effective against UVB light (for definitions, see p.1516).

Preparations

Proprietary Preparations
Some preparations are listed in Part 3.

Isopropyldibenzoylmethane (15708-j)

1-[4-(1-Methylethyl)phenyl]-3-phenyl-1,3-propanedione.
$C_{18}H_{18}O_2 = 266.3$.
CAS — 63250-25-9.

Profile
Isopropyldibenzoylmethane, a substituted dibenzoylmethane, is a sunscreen with actions similar to those of avobenzone (p.1517). It absorbs UVA light (for definitions, see p.1516).

Preparations

Proprietary Preparations
Some preparations are listed in Part 3.

Lisadimate (9305-e)

Lisadimate (*USAN, rINN*).
Glyceryl Aminobenzoate; Glyceryl PABA. Glyceryl 1-(4-aminobenzoate).
$C_{10}H_{13}NO_4 = 211.2$.
CAS — 136-44-7.

Profile
Lisadimate is a sunscreen with actions similar to those of aminobenzoic acid (p.1516). It is effective against UVB light (for definitions, see p.1516).

Preparations

Proprietary Preparations
Some preparations are listed in Part 3.

Meradimate (19515-j)

Meradimate (*USAN, rINN*).
Menthyl O-Aminobenzoate; Menthyl Anthranilate. 5-Methyl-2-(1-methylethyl)-cyclohexyl 2-aminobenzoate.
$C_{17}H_{25}NO_2 = 275.4$.
CAS — 134-09-8.
Pharmacopoeias. In US.

Pharmacopoeial description
USP 25: Store in airtight containers.

Profile
Meradimate is used as a sunscreen. It is effective against UVA light (for definitions, see p.1516).

Preparations

Proprietary Preparations
Some preparations are listed in Part 3.

Mexenone (9310-p)

Mexenone (*BAN, pINN*).
Benzophenone-10. 2-Hydroxy-4-methoxy-4′-methylbenzophenone.
$C_{15}H_{14}O_3 = 242.3$.
CAS — 1641-17-4.
Pharmacopoeias. In Br.

Pharmacopoeial description
BP 2001: A pale yellow odourless or almost odourless crystalline powder. Practically insoluble in water; sparingly soluble in alcohol; freely soluble in acetone.

Profile
Mexenone, a substituted benzophenone, is a sunscreen with actions similar to those of oxybenzone (below). It is effective against UVB and some UVA light (for definitions, see p.1516)

Preparations

BP 2001: Mexenone Cream.
Proprietary Preparations
Some preparations are listed in Part 3.

Octinoxate (9324-j)

Octinoxate (*USAN, rINN*).
Octyl methoxycinnamate; Parsol MCX. 2-Ethylhexyl-p-methoxycinnamate.
$C_{18}H_{26}O_3 = 290.4$.
CAS — 5466-77-3.
ATC — D02BA02.
Pharmacopoeias. In US.

Pharmacopoeial description
USP 25: Pale yellow oil. Insoluble in water. Store in airtight containers at a temperature of 8° to 15°.

Profile
Octinoxate, a substituted cinnamate, is used by topical application as a sunscreen. Cinnamate sunscreens effectively absorb light throughout the UVB range but absorb little or no UVA light (for definitions, see p.1516). Cinnamate sunscreens may therefore be used to prevent sunburn but are unlikely to prevent drug-related or other photosensitivity reactions associated with UVA light; combination with a benzophenone may give some added protection against such photosensitivity. Cinnamates may occasionally produce photosensitivity reactions.

Preparations

Proprietary Preparations
Numerous preparations are listed in Part 3.

Octisalate (18470-s)

Octisalate (USAN, rINN).
Octyl Salicylate. 2-Ethylhexyl salicylate.
$C_{15}H_{22}O_3 = 250.3$.
CAS — 118-60-5.
Pharmacopoeias. In US.

Pharmacopoeial description
USP 25: Store in airtight containers.

Profile
Octisalate is a substituted salicylate used by topical application as a sunscreen. Salicylates effectively absorb light throughout the UVB range but absorb little or no UVA light (for definitions, see p.1516). Salicylate sunscreens may therefore be used to prevent sunburn, but are unlikely to prevent drug-related or other photosensitivity reactions associated with UVA light; combination with a benzophenone may give some added protection.
Salicylates may occasionally produce photosensitivity reactions.

Preparations

Proprietary Preparations
Numerous preparations are listed in Part 3.

Octocrilene (9328-a)

Octocrilene (rINN).
2-Ethylhexyl α-cyano-β-phenylcinnamate; Octocrylene (USAN). 2-Ethylhexyl 2-cyano-3,3-diphenylacrylate.
$C_{24}H_{27}NO_2 = 361.5$.
CAS — 6197-30-4.
Pharmacopoeias. In US.

Pharmacopoeial description
USP 25: Store in airtight containers.

Profile
Octocrilene, a substituted cinnamate, is a sunscreen with actions similar to those of octinoxate (above). It is effective against UVB light (for definitions, see p.1516).

Preparations

Proprietary Preparations
Some preparations are listed in Part 3.

Oxybenzone (9312-w)

Oxybenzone (USAN, rINN).
Benzophenone-3. 2-Hydroxy-4-methoxybenzophenone.
$C_{14}H_{12}O_3 = 228.2$.
CAS — 131-57-7.
Pharmacopoeias. In US.

Pharmacopoeial description
USP 25: A pale yellow powder. Practically insoluble in water; freely soluble in alcohol and in toluene. Store in airtight containers. Protect from light.

Profile
Oxybenzone is a substituted benzophenone used by topical application as a sunscreen. Benzophenones effectively absorb light throughout the UVB range (wavelengths 290 to 320 nm) and also absorb some UVA light with wavelengths of 320 to about 360 nm and some UVC light with wavelengths of about 250 to 290 nm (for definitions, see p.1516). Benzophenones may therefore be used to prevent sunburn and may also provide some protection against drug-related or other photosensitivity reactions associated with UVA light; in practice they are usually combined with a sunscreen from another group.
Contact and photocontact allergic dermatitis has occasionally been reported following the topical administration of benzophenone sunscreens.

◊ References to allergic and photoallergic reactions in a few patients using oxybenzone sunscreens.[1-4]

1. Thompson G, et al. Allergic contact dermatitis from sunscreen preparations complicating photodermatitis. Arch Dermatol 1977; **113**: 1252–3.
2. Thune P. Contact and photocontact allergy to sunscreens. Photodermatology 1984; **1**: 5–9.
3. Knoler E, et al. Photoallergy to benzophenone. Arch Dermatol 1989; **125**: 801–4.
4. Collins P, Ferguson J. Photoallergic contact dermatitis to oxybenzone. Br J Dermatol 1994; **131**: 124–9.

Preparations

USP 25: Dioxybenzone and Oxybenzone Cream.

Proprietary Preparations
Numerous preparations are listed in Part 3.

Padimate (9313-e)

Padimate (BAN, rINN).
Amyl Dimethylaminobenzoate; Isoamyl Dimethylaminobenzoate; Padimate A (USAN). A mixture of pentyl, isopentyl, and 2-methylbutyl 4-dimethylaminobenzoates .
$C_{14}H_{21}NO_2 = 235.3$.
CAS — 14779-78-3 (pentyl 4-dimethylaminobenzoate); 21245-01-2 (isopentyl 4-dimethylaminobenzoate).

Profile
Padimate, a substituted aminobenzoate, is a sunscreen with actions similar to those of aminobenzoic acid (p.1516). It is effective against UVB light (for definitions, see p.1516).

Preparations

Proprietary Preparations
Some preparations are listed in Part 3.

Padimate O (9314-l)

Padimate O (BANM, USAN).
Octyl Dimethyl PABA. 2-Ethylhexyl 4-(dimethylamino)benzoate.
$C_{17}H_{27}NO_2 = 277.4$.
CAS — 21245-02-3.
Pharmacopoeias. In US.

Pharmacopoeial description
USP 25: A light yellow, mobile liquid with a faint aromatic odour. Practically insoluble in water, in glycerol, and in propylene glycol; soluble in alcohol, in isopropyl alcohol, and in liquid paraffin. Store in airtight containers. Protect from light.

Profile
Padimate O, a substituted aminobenzoate, is a sunscreen with actions similar to those of aminobenzoic acid (p.1516). It is effective against UVB light (for definitions, see p.1516).

◊ References to contact or photocontact allergy to padimate O.

1. Weller P, Freeman S. Photocontact allergy to octyldimethyl PABA. Australas J Dermatol 1984; **25**: 73–6.
2. Thune P. Contact and photocontact allergy to sunscreens. Photodermatology 1984; **1**: 5–9.
3. English JSC, et al. Sensitivity to sunscreens. Contact Dermatitis 1987; **17**: 159–62.

Preparations

USP 25: Padimate O Lotion.

Proprietary Preparations
Some preparations are listed in Part 3.

Roxadimate (9322-l)

Roxadimate (USAN, rINN).
Ethyl Dihydroxypropyl PABA. Ethyl (±)-4-[bis(2-hydroxypropyl)amino]benzoate.
$C_{15}H_{23}NO_4 = 281.3$.
CAS — 58882-17-0.

Profile
Roxadimate, a substituted aminobenzoate, is a sunscreen with actions similar to those of aminobenzoic acid (p.1516). It is effective against UVB light (for definitions, see p.1516).

Preparations

Proprietary Preparations
Some preparations are listed in Part 3.

Sodium 3,4-Dimethoxyphenylglyoxylate (9330-l)

$C_{10}H_9NaO_5 = 232.2$.
CAS — 37891-88-6.

Profile
Sodium 3,4-dimethoxyphenylglyoxylate has been used topically as a sunscreen.

Sulisobenzone (9316-j)

Sulisobenzone (USAN, rINN).
Benzophenone-4; NSC-60584. 5-Benzoyl-4-hydroxy-2-methoxybenzenesulphonic acid.
$C_{14}H_{12}O_6S = 308.3$.
CAS — 4065-45-6.
Pharmacopoeias. In US.

Pharmacopoeial description
USP 25: Light tan powder. M.p. about 145°. Freely soluble in water, in alcohol, and in methyl alcohol; sparingly soluble in ethyl acetate. Store in airtight containers. Protect from light.

Profile
Sulisobenzone, a substituted benzophenone, is a sunscreen with actions similar to those of oxybenzone (above). It is effective against UVB and some UVA light (for definitions, see p.1516).

Preparations

Proprietary Preparations
Some preparations are listed in Part 3.

Thyroid and Antithyroid Drugs

The principal role of the thyroid gland is to regulate tissue metabolism through production of the **thyroid hormones** 3,5,3',5'-tetra-iodo-L-thyronine (L-thyroxine; T_4) and, in smaller amounts, 3,5,3'-tri-iodo-L-thyronine (liothyronine, or triiodothyronine; T_3). In infants and children thyroid hormones are also necessary for the development of the CNS and for normal growth and bone maturation.

The production of hormones by the thyroid gland is dependent on an adequate supply of dietary iodine. Iodine is reduced to iodide in the gastrointestinal tract and is readily absorbed. Iodide is actively transported into the gland and undergoes oxidation. Oxidised iodide is incorporated into the tyrosyl residues of the glycoprotein thyroglobulin to form L-mono-iodotyrosine (MIT) and L-di-iodotyrosine (DIT), which are inactive. A coupling reaction yields the hormonally active iodothyronines, T_3 and T_4, joined by a peptide bond to thyroglobulin for storage in the follicular colloid. The secretion of thyroid hormones is mediated by the release of proteolytic enzymes from lysosomes to degrade the thyroglobulin into its constituent amino acids releasing T_3 and T_4 into the circulation; iodide resulting from this reaction is recycled.

Thyroid hormones are extensively protein bound in plasma, principally to thyroxine-binding globulin (TBG) but also to a lesser extent to thyroxine-binding pre-albumin (TBPA) or to albumin.

Whereas T_4 enters the circulation only by direct glandular secretion, very little T_3 is secreted by a normal thyroid gland and most of the extra-thyroid T_3 is produced by the mono-deiodination of T_4 in the peripheral tissues. About 35% of secreted T_4 is converted to T_3 and about 40% is converted to inactive reverse triiodothyronine (reverse T_3; rT_3). The metabolic activity of T_3 is about 3 to 5 times that of T_4 and it has been suggested that T_3 is the active thyroid hormone with T_4 acting primarily as a prohormone.

Thyroid hormone homoeostasis is maintained by autoregulatory mechanisms within the gland, and by the hypothalamic-pituitary-thyroid axis. In response to falling plasma concentrations of unbound T_3 and T_4, the hypothalamus secretes thyrotropin releasing hormone (protirelin; TRH—see p.1295), which in turn stimulates the synthesis and release of thyroid stimulating hormone (thyrotropin; TSH—see p.1298) by the anterior pituitary gland. TSH acts on its receptor in the thyroid gland to increase production of T_3 and T_4, and also to release hormone stored in the gland. As thyroid hormone concentrations in blood increase the secretion of TSH and possibly TRH will be suppressed. The term euthyroidism is used when the thyroid gland is functioning normally and there are normal amounts of thyroid hormone in the blood.

Goitre and thyroid nodules

Goitre is the enlargement of the thyroid gland. The swelling may be focal (caused by a solitary thyroid nodule, adenoma, or cyst) or generalised, in which case it is usually diffuse at first, later becoming multinodular. Non-toxic goitres may be associated with hypothyroidism (below) or euthyroidism. The management of toxic goitres is discussed under Hyperthyroidism, below.

Non-toxic goitres are generally attributed to intrinsic defects in hormone production or extrinsic factors such as dietary-iodine deficiency in endemic goitre (see Iodine Deficiency Disorders, p.1523). Decreased secretion of thyroid hormone results in an excessive output of thyroid-stimulating hormone (TSH) from the pituitary. This stimulates thyroid-hormone production but also leads to hypertrophy and hyperplasia of the thyroid gland. If the response to TSH overcomes the deficiency in thyroid-hormone synthesis then the patient is goitrous and euthyroid but if the compensatory response to TSH is inadequate then goitre with hypothyroidism is observed. Other factors such as autoantibodies might stimulate thyroid growth and thyroid autonomy, where the gland functions independently of TSH control, can also occur.

The general aims in the management of thyroid masses are:

- the detection and treatment of malignancy
- the reduction of goitre or prevention of further enlargement, and the relief of obstructive symptoms
- the maintenance of a euthyroid state.

Ultrasound or radionuclide imaging may be employed to determine the number and size of any nodules present but cannot distinguish a benign from a malignant nodule. Cytological analysis is the most reliable means of diagnosing malignancy.[1-3] Thyroxine [levothyroxine] has been given short-term in an attempt to distinguish benign from malignant nodules, with failure of the nodule to shrink being regarded as an indication of malignancy, but it is much less reliable.[2]

In established **malignancy**, surgery, followed by thyroxine [levothyroxine] replacement therapy, is the usual course (for further discussion of the treatment of thyroid cancer, see p.500).

The treatment of **benign solitary** non-toxic nodules is a matter of dispute. Many workers prefer simply to observe patients with benign solitary nodules.[1,2] Suppressive therapy with doses of thyroxine [levothyroxine] (or, less often, liothyronine) sufficient to suppress TSH production and reduce the size of the nodule has been widely practised, but results conflict as to whether such therapy is effective;[2-4] meta-analysis of 7 studies[5] suggested that although thyroxine [levothyroxine] treatment produced some benefit, the number of patients who responded was quite small. There has been some concern about the possible risk of osteoporosis[1,2,6] (see Effects on the Bones, p.1526). An alternative to thyroxine [levothyroxine] is treatment with potassium iodide, although it is somewhat less effective,[7] and has adverse effects of its own.[6] Sclerotherapy by alcohol injection has been investigated.[8,9]

Thyroxine [levothyroxine] suppression therapy is effective in patients with **diffuse** non-toxic goitre, and may be of benefit in some patients with **multinodular** disease.[3] However, many patients with large multinodular goitres have autonomous thyroid hormone production, and in such patients thyroxine [levothyroxine] is of no benefit and may cause overt hyperthyroidism. Radio-iodine (^{131}I) treatment of multinodular non-toxic goitre has been a useful alternative to surgery in selected cases.[3,10]

1. Mazzaferri EL. Management of a solitary thyroid nodule. *N Engl J Med* 1993; **328:** 553–9.
2. Giuffrida D, Gharib H. Controversies in the management of cold, hot, and occult thyroid nodules. *Am J Med* 1995; **99:** 642–50.
3. Hermus AR, Huysmans DA. Treatment of benign nodular thyroid disease. *N Engl J Med* 1998; **338:** 1438–47.
4. Gharib H, Mazzaferri EL. Thyroxine suppressive therapy in patients with nodular thyroid disease. *Ann Intern Med* 1998; **128:** 386–94.
5. Zelmanovitz F, *et al.* Suppressive therapy with levothyroxine for solitary thyroid nodules: a double-blind controlled clinical study and cumulative meta-analyses. *J Clin Endocrinol Metab* 1998; **83:** 3881–5.
6. Blum M. Why do clinicians continue to debate the use of levothyroxine in the diagnosis and management of thyroid nodules? *Ann Intern Med* 1995; **122:** 63–4.
7. La Rosa GL, *et al.* Levothyroxine and potassium iodide are both effective in treating benign solitary cold nodules of the thyroid. *Ann Intern Med* 1995; **122:** 1–8.
8. Bennedbaek FN *et al..* Effect of percutaneous ethanol injection therapy versus suppressive doses of L-thyroxine on benign solitary cold thyroid nodules: a randomized trial. *J Clin Endocrinol Metab* 1998; **83:** 830–5.
9. Bennedbaek FN, Hegedüs L. Percutaneous ethanol injection therapy in benign solitary solid cold thyroid nodules: a randomized trial comparing one injection with three injections. *Thyroid* 1999; **9:** 225–33.
10. Nygaard B, *et al.* Radio iodine treatment of multinodular non-toxic goitre. *BMJ* 1993; **307:** 828–32.

Hyperthyroidism

Hyperthyroidism is overactivity of the thyroid gland with consequent excess secretion of hormones. The terms thyrotoxicosis and hyperthyroidism are used interchangeably, although some apply 'thyrotoxicosis' to the *effects* of excessive thyroid hormone. The most common causes of hyperthyroidism are Graves' disease and hyperactivity arising from single or multiple thyroid nodules (toxic nodular goitre). Graves' disease (or Basedow's disease) is an auto-immune condition in which thyroid-stimulating antibodies in the plasma are directed against the thyroid-stimulating hormone (TSH) receptor or a closely associated protein on the thyroid cell. Graves' disease, which is more prevalent in females, frequently occurs in association with other auto-immune diseases such as rheumatoid arthritis and there may be a genetic predisposition. Iodine and its salts, or iodine-containing drugs

such as amiodarone, can also be a cause of both hyperthyroidism and hypothyroidism.

Subclinical hyperthyroidism is characterised by normal thyroid hormone concentrations, decreased TSH concentrations, but no clinical symptoms. It has been reported to occur less frequently than subclinical hypothyroidism. Some clinicians recommend treatment for these patients, but consensus is lacking.[1-3]

The major symptoms associated with clinical hyperthyroidism include goitre, nervousness, agitation, tremor, tachycardia or atrial fibrillation, weight loss (often despite increased appetite), emotional lability, muscle weakness, fatigue, heat intolerance and excessive perspiration, and increased bowel frequency. Exaggerated growth may occur in children. Females may occasionally experience amenorrhoea or oligomenorrhoea and males may develop gynaecomastia. Occasionally there is subcutaneous deposition of mucopolysaccharides around the ankles and/or feet.

In Graves' ophthalmopathy, oedematous swelling of the muscles around the eyes produces exophthalmos or proptosis and diplopia. On rare occasions patients may develop papilloedema and loss of vision.

A **diagnosis** of hyperthyroidism may be confirmed by demonstration of a high concentration of free T_4 or T_3 in the circulation. Determination of thyroid-stimulating hormone (TSH) concentration, which is low in hyperthyroidism due to negative feedback, allows differential diagnosis of hyperthyroidism from pituitary tumour and is the test of choice in the elderly as physiological changes and non-thyroidal illness present problems with interpretation of T_4 and T_3 concentrations.

There are three forms of **treatment**: drug therapy, use of radio-iodine, or surgery.

Drug therapy. Initially, many patients are given an antithyroid drug. The main **antithyroid drugs** are the thiourea derivatives (thiocarbamides, thionamides, or thioureylenes); this group comprises the imidazole derivatives (carbimazole and methimazole [thiamazole]) and the thiouracils (benzylthiouracil, methylthiouracil, and propylthiouracil). The thiourea compounds block the production of thyroid hormones through inhibition of thyroid peroxidase. The place of immunosuppression in the antithyroid activity of these drugs is subject to debate. Antithyroid drugs do not block the release of stored thyroid hormones and it is only when the preformed hormones are depleted and concentrations of circulating hormones decline that clinical effects become apparent. An additional action of propylthiouracil is inhibition of the peripheral deiodination of thyroxine to tri-iodothyronine.

Carbimazole (in the UK) or methimazole [thiamazole] (in the USA), or propylthiouracil, are the mainstays of treatment. Patients receive high doses initially until they become euthyroid, generally within 1 to 2 months. Once a response to the antithyroid drug has been obtained, patients with more severe or recurrent disease may require ablative treatment with either radio-iodine or surgery (see below), while those with mild to moderate disease may be best managed with lower maintenance doses of antithyroid drug therapy, either indefinitely, or more usually for at least a year, and often for 18 months, followed by observation to see if remission is maintained in the absence of therapy.[1,4-6] Relapse at some stage following cessation of therapy is fairly common but unpredictable. Addition of thyroxine [levothyroxine] to the maintenance dose of methimazole [thiamazole] has been reported to reduce the rate of relapse in patients with Graves' disease when therapy is subsequently withdrawn,[7] but later studies have not shown benefit.[8-11] An alternative maintenance regimen is to add the thyroid hormone while maintaining the high initial doses of antithyroid drug. This 'blocking-replacement therapy' has been suggested to help to prevent hypothyroidism which may be induced when antithyroid drugs are used alone. Because of the high doses of thioureas required the blocking-replacement regimen should not be used in pregnancy.

More rapid relief of the symptoms of hyperthyroidism can be achieved with beta blockers or iodide.[4,6] Beta blockers usually achieve a response within 48 hours, and are given as short-term adjuncts to antithyroid drugs to control severe sympathetic overactivity in patients such as those with thyroid storm (see below), but their use in heart failure associated with thyrotoxicosis is controversial because of the risk of cardiac deterioration.[12] The use of beta blockers in patients with mild to moderate hyperthyroidism is usually unnecessary.

Iodine and iodides are given in conjunction with antithyroid drugs for 7 to 14 days as pre-operative preparation for patients who are to undergo thyroidectomy (but see also under Surgical Therapy, below); a combination of iodide and a beta blocker has also been used. Iodide has been used with antithyroid drugs, for control of thyroid storm. It is suggested that the antithyroid drugs should always be given first to prevent incorporation of iodide into new hormone stores.[4]

Other drugs tried in hyperthyroidism have included lithium, though its practical value is a matter of debate.[4] Potassium and sodium perchlorate have been used and by increasing responsiveness to conventional antithyroid drugs they may be useful in patients with iodine-induced hyperthyroidism.[13]

In those patients in whom drug therapy fails to achieve long-term remission, ablative therapy may be considered in the form of radio-iodine therapy or surgery.

Radio-iodine therapy with ^{131}I as oral ^{131}I-sodium iodide cures hyperthyroidism by destroying the functioning cells of the thyroid gland. It is increasingly used as initial therapy.[4,14] It is also useful for patients who have not responded to antithyroid drug therapy or who have relapsed following it.[1,5]

Pretreatment of patients with an antithyroid drug for 2 to 8 weeks before radio-iodine therapy has been advocated, to avoid the risk of precipitating thyroid storm. However, many no longer consider this to be necessary for all patients,[4,14] although it is generally agreed that the elderly or those with severe disease or increased risk of cardiac symptoms should receive some form of pretreatment. In younger patients, a study has suggested that antithyroid pretreatment may exacerbate the risks when the drugs are withdrawn.[15] Such withdrawal, 2 to 4 days before radio-iodine is given, is standard practice to maximise the latter's effect, although some consider it unnecessary.[4] There is also some evidence that pretreated patients respond less well, and an increased dose of radio-iodine has been advocated in such patients.[14] Pretreatment or ancillary treatment with a beta blocker is a possible alternative to antithyroid drugs in patients receiving radio-iodine.[4,6,14]

The dose of radio-iodine required to achieve euthyroidism is difficult to predict and there is little agreement on the most appropriate dosage schedule.[1,6,14] Radio-iodine therapy may take up to 10 weeks to achieve a clinical response, and cover with an antithyroid drug may be required during this period. Radio-iodine is not generally considered to increase the risk of malignancy,[4,14,16] but it is contra-indicated in pregnancy. The commonest unwanted effect of radio-iodine therapy is hypothyroidism and all patients require long-term follow-up and possible thyroxine [levothyroxine] replacement therapy. Iodide may be given after radio-iodine therapy to help the return of normal thyroid function.[4] Controversy exists as to whether radio-iodine therapy exacerbates Graves' ophthalmopathy.[4,17,18]

Surgical treatment is usually reserved for patients with severe hyperthyroidism or for those with extreme thyroid enlargement or a single nodule. Euthyroidism is first established using antithyroid drugs and then iodide is given for 7 to 14 days before surgery to reduce the vasculature of the gland. Alternatively, a beta blocker and iodide may be used together for the pre-operative preparation. However, a consensus view[2] suggested that pre-operative iodine probably has no beneficial effect. Thyroxine [levothyroxine] replacement therapy may be required following surgical treatment.

Failure to control symptoms of hyperthyroidism with antithyroid drugs during **pregnancy** may indicate the need for surgery which is often delayed where possible until after the first trimester.[19] Iodide and radio-iodine should not be used during pregnancy.[6,19] **Neonatal hyperthyroidism** may occur rarely due to transfer of thyroid-stimulating immunoglobulins across the placenta, and should be treated with antithyroid drugs, iodide, and appropriate therapy for cardiovascular complications.

Thyroid storm (also known as thyroid crisis or thyrotoxic crisis) is an extreme accentuation of the hyperthyroid state and should be treated as a medical emergency. It is usually abrupt in onset and is often related to some precipitating factor such as inadequate preparation for thyroidectomy or radio-iodine therapy, or infection in previously unrecognised hyperthyroid subjects. The most common symptoms are hyperpyrexia and extreme tachycardia; others may include arrhythmia, heart failure, shock, agitation, tremor, mania, delirium, stupor, coma, abdominal pain, diarrhoea, vomiting, jaundice, and hepatomegaly. Treatment consists of high-dose antithyroid drugs, gradually reduced as the condition improves, along with a beta blocker and iodide to control cardiovascular symptoms and prevent thyroid hormone release from the thyroid gland. Additional symptomatic treatment may also be required.

The symptoms of **Graves' ophthalmopathy** may not occur in conjunction with signs of systemic hyperthyroidism, and it has been characterised as an independent manifestation of the immunological abnormality in Graves' disease.[20] The treatment of Graves' ophthalmopathy is generally unsatisfactory and signs of disease may persist indefinitely.[21] Opinions differ as to whether controlling associated hyperthyroidism improves ocular symptoms.[20] Reports that radio-iodine therapy may exacerbate Graves' ophthalmopathy are disputed,[4,14,17,18] but some workers prefer to avoid its use in active ocular disease.[1] Most patients with mild ocular involvement in hyperthyroidism require no specific therapy; dry eye should be managed appropriately (see p.1498). Patients with moderate to severe ophthalmopathy may be treated with high-dose systemic corticosteroids such as oral prednisone or prednisolone or intravenous methylprednisolone, or with orbital radiotherapy, which appears to be equally effective.[22] Other immunosuppressants, particularly ciclosporin, have also been used and have produced equivocal results.[20] Surgical decompression may be required if patients do not respond to such therapy or cannot tolerate its adverse effects, or if vision is threatened by severe optic nerve compression.

1. Gittoes NJL, Franklyn JA. Hyperthyroidism: current treatment guidelines. *Drugs* 1998; **55:** 543–53.
2. Vanderpump MPJ, *et al.* Consensus statement for good practice and audit measures in the management of hypothyroidism and hyperthyroidism *BMJ* 1996; **33:** 539–44.
3. Helfand M, Redfern CC. Screening for thyroid disease: an update. *Ann Intern Med* 1998; **129:** 144–58. Correction. *ibid.*; **130:** 246.
4. Klein I, *et al.* Treatment of hyperthyroid disease. *Ann Intern Med* 1994; **121:** 281–8.
5. Cheetham TD, *et al.* Treatment of hyperthyroidism in young people. *Arch Dis Child* 1998; **78:** 207–9.
6. Franklyn J. Thyrotoxicosis. *Prescribers' J* 1999; **39:** 1–8.
7. Hashizume K, *et al.* Administration of thyroxine in treated Graves' disease: effects on the level of antibodies to thyroid-stimulating hormone receptors and on the risk of recurrence of hyperthyroidism. *N Engl J Med* 1991; **324:** 947–53.
8. Tamai H, *et al.* Lack of effect of thyroxine administration on elevated thyroid stimulating hormone receptor antibody levels in treated Graves' disease patients. *J Clin Endocrinol Metab* 1995; **80:** 1481–4.
9. Hershman JM. Does thyroxine therapy prevent recurrence of Graves' hyperthyroidism? *J Clin Endocrinol Metab* 1995; **80:** 1479–80.
10. McIver B, *et al.* Lack of effect of thyroxine in patients with Graves' hyperthyroidism who are treated with an antithyroid drug. *N Engl J Med* 1996; **334:** 220–4.
11. Rittmaster RS, *et al.* Effect of methimazole, with or without L-thyroxine, on remission rates in Graves' disease. *J Clin Endocrinol Metab* 1998; **83:** 814–18.
12. Ko GTC, *et al.* Should β-blocking agents be used in thyrotoxic heart disease? *Med J Aust* 1995; **162:** 426–7.
13. Wolff J. Perchlorate and the thyroid gland. *Pharmacol Rev* 1998; **50:** 89–105.
14. Kaplan MM, *et al.* Treatment of hyperthyroidism with radioactive iodine. *Endocrinol Metab Clin North Am* 1998; **27:** 205–23.
15. Burch HB, *et al.* Discontinuing antithyroid drug therapy before ablation with radioiodine in Graves disease. *Ann Intern Med* 1994; **121:** 553–9.
16. Ron E, *et al.* Cancer mortality following treatment for adult hyperthyroidism. *JAMA* 1998; **280:** 347–55.
17. Tallstedt L, *et al.* Occurrence of ophthalmopathy after treatment for Graves' hyperthyroidism. *N Engl J Med* 1992; **326:** 1733–8.
18. Bartalena L, *et al.* Relation between therapy for hyperthyroidism and the course of Graves' ophthalmopathy. *N Engl J Med* 1998; **338:** 73–8.
19. Masiukiewicz US, Burrow GN. Hyperthyroidism in pregnancy: diagnosis and treatment. *Thyroid* 1999; **9:** 647–52.
20. Char DH. Thyroid eye disease. *Br J Ophthalmol* 1996; **80:** 922–6.
21. Fleck BW, Toft AD. Graves' ophthalmopathy. *BMJ* 1990; **300:** 1352–3.
22. Prummel MF, *et al.* Randomised double-blind trial of prednisone versus radiotherapy in Graves' ophthalmopathy. *Lancet* 1993; **342:** 949–54.

Hypothyroidism

Hypothyroidism is the clinical syndrome resulting from deficiency of thyroid hormones. It predominantly affects women and is more prevalent in the middle-aged and elderly. The symptoms of hypothyroidism may be due to general deceleration of metabolism or to accumulation of mucopolysaccharide in the subcutaneous tissues and vocal cords. Common symptoms include weakness, fatigue, lethargy, physical and mental slowness, and weight gain; puffy, nonpitted swelling of subcutaneous tissue often develops, particularly around the eyes. Menstrual disorders, hyperlipidaemia, and constipation can occur and goitre may develop despite associated cell destruction.

The term **myxoedema** is often reserved for severe or advanced hypothyroidism. In the most severely affected patients, progressive somnolence and torpor combine with cold intolerance and bradycardia to induce a state of coma often known as 'hypothyroid' or 'myxoedema coma' (see below).

In children, untreated hypothyroidism results in retardation of growth and mental development. Endemic cretinism is a result of maternal, and hence fetal, iodine deficiency and consequent lack of thyroid hormone production (see Iodine Deficiency Disorders, p.1523). **Subclinical hypothyroidism** is a condition in which there are normal concentrations of thyroid hormones, raised concentrations of thyroid-stimulating hormone (TSH), but no clinical symptoms.

Hypothyroidism is usually primary, resulting from malfunction of the thyroid gland. In areas where iodine intake is sufficient the commonest cause of hypothyroidism is auto-immune lymphocytic thyroiditis of which there are two major variants. In **Hashimoto's thyroiditis** there is also goitre whereas in **idiopathic** or **primary myxoedema (atrophic thyroiditis)** there is no thyroid enlargement. Hypothyroidism can also be caused by either an excess or a deficiency of iodine. An excess may result from intake of iodine or its salts or iodine-containing drugs such as amiodarone. Drugs that decrease thyroid hormone synthesis such as lithium can also be a cause of hypothyroidism. In some patients hypothyroidism may be secondary to disorders of the hypothalamus or pituitary gland.

The **diagnosis** of hypothyroidism is essentially clinical but, given the non-specific nature of many of the symptoms, biochemical tests are performed for confirmation.[1,2] Protirelin and thyrotrophin have also been used for the differential diagnosis of hypothyroidism. Patients with subclinical hypothyroidism are at a greater risk of developing clinical hypothyroidism if they also have thyroid antibodies against thyroid peroxidase/microsomal antigen although the best strategy for identifying those at risk is not yet known.[2]

Hypothyroidism is readily **treated** by lifelong replacement therapy with thyroxine [levothyroxine].[1-4] Although the thyroid gland produces both T_3 (liothyronine) and T_4 (thyroxine), T_3 is mainly produced by peripheral monodeiodination of circulating T_4 and it is therefore sufficient to administer thyroxine [levothyroxine] alone. There is no rationale for the use of combined preparations containing liothyronine and thyroxine [levothyroxine], or of dried thyroid hormone extracts, which may lead to elevated serum concentrations of T_3 and thyrotoxic symptoms. Liothyronine may, however, be used initially for its rapid onset of action in severe hypothyroid states such as myxoedema coma (see below). There is a need to check that thyroid replacement treatment is just restoring deficiencies in thyroid hormone and not providing an excess. While most workers accept that this is best done by monitoring hormone concentrations, there has been considerable debate as to whether T_3, T_4, TSH, or a combination of these should be measured, and whether the free or the total hormone concentrations should be used. Extremely sensitive assays for TSH have been developed and the goal of replacement therapy has been advocated as a normal TSH value, which is generally associated with a normal or slightly elevated T_4 value.[2,4]

In subclinical hypothyroidism, treatment with thyroxine [levothyroxine] is recommended[2,3] if thyroid peroxidase antibodies are present or if TSH levels are above 10 milliunits per litre.

Although titres of antithyroid antibodies may fall during **pregnancy**, some patients may require progressive increases in thyroxine [levothyroxine] dosage,[5] and therefore serum TSH concentrations should be measured in each trimester.[1-3]

The diagnosis of **congenital hypothyroidism** (neonatal hypothyroidism) is now most commonly made on the basis of screening programmes.[6] Early treatment with adequate doses of thyroxine [levothyroxine] is required to minimise the effects of hypothyroidism on mental and physical development. Administration should be started as soon as possible after birth and should be reviewed regularly.[6] However, it is generally accepted that in those with more severe hypothyroidism at diagnosis some small degree of deficit and incoordination remains, although they should be mild enough to permit a normal life.[7]

Hypothyroid (myxoedema) coma is a medical emergency requiring prompt treatment usually with liothyronine given by intravenous injection because of its rapid action, although some centres use intravenous thyroxine [levothyroxine]. Alternatively, the nasogastric route may be employed. In some patients, liothyronine given intravenously is followed by oral thyroxine [levothyroxine]. Other treatment includes intravenous hydrocortisone (because of the likelihood of adrenocortical insufficiency) and intravenous fluids (to maintain plasma-glucose and electrolyte concentrations). Respiratory function should be supported by assisted ventilation and oxygen administration.

1. Singer PA, et al. Treatment guidelines for patients with hyperthyroidism and hypothyroidism. JAMA 1995; 273: 808–12.
2. Lindsay RS, Toft AD. Hypothyroidism. Lancet 1997; 349: 413–17. Correction. ibid.; 1023.
3. Vanderpump MPJ, et al. Consensus statement for good practice and audit measures in the management of hypothyroidism and hyperthyroidism. BMJ 1996; 313: 539–44.
4. Toft AD. Thyroxine therapy. N Engl J Med 1994; 331: 174–80.
5. Drake WM, Wood DF. Thyroid disease in pregnancy. Postgrad Med J 1998; 74: 583–6.
6. LaFranchi S. Congenital hypothyroidism: etiologies, diagnosis, and management. Thyroid 1999; 9: 735–40.
7. Rovet JF. Congenital hypothyroidism: long term outcome. Thyroid 1999; 9: 741–8.

Benzylthiouracil (832-p)

6-Benzyl-2,3-dihydro-2-thioxopyrimidin-4(1H)-one; 6-Benzyl-2-mercaptopyrimidin-4-ol; 6-Benzyl-2-thiouracil.
$C_{11}H_{10}N_2OS = 218.3.$
CAS — 33086-27-0; 6336-50-1.
ATC — H03BA03.

Profile
Benzylthiouracil is a thiourea antithyroid drug. It is given by mouth in the treatment of hyperthyroidism (p.1519) in an initial dose of 150 to 200 mg daily, reducing to a maintenance dose of 100 mg daily after several weeks.

Porphyria. Benzylthiouracil is considered to be unsafe in patients with porphyria although there is conflicting experimental evidence of porphyrinogenicity.

Preparations
Proprietary Preparations (details are given in Part 3)
Fr.: Basdene.

Carbimazole (831-q)

Carbimazole (BAN, rINN).
Carbimazolum. Ethyl 3-methyl-2-thioxo-4-imidazoline-1-carboxylate.
$C_7H_{10}N_2O_2S = 186.2.$
CAS — 22232-54-8.
ATC — H03BB01.
Pharmacopoeias. In Chin. and Eur. (see p.vi).

Pharmacopoeial description
Ph. Eur.: A white or yellowish-white crystalline powder. Slightly soluble in water; soluble in alcohol and in acetone.

Adverse Effects and Precautions
Adverse effects from carbimazole and other thiourea antithyroid drugs occur most frequently during the first 8 weeks of treatment. The most common minor adverse effects are nausea and vomiting, gastric discomfort, headache, arthralgia, skin rashes, and pruritus. Hair loss has also been reported.

Bone-marrow depression may occur and mild leucopenia is common. Rarely, agranulocytosis can develop and this is the most serious adverse reaction associated with this class of drugs. Patients or their carers should be told how to recognise such toxicity and should be advised to seek immediate medical attention if mouth ulcers or sore throat, fever, bruising, malaise, or non-specific illness develop. Full blood counts should be performed, and treatment should be discontinued immediately if there is any clinical or laboratory evidence of neutropenia. Aplastic anaemia or isolated thrombocytopenia have been reported rarely, as has hypoprothrombinaemia.

There have been several reports of liver damage, most commonly jaundice, in patients taking thiourea antithyroid drugs; the drug should be withdrawn if hepatic effects occur.

Other adverse effects sometimes observed with the thiourea antithyroid compounds include fever, a lupus-like syndrome, myopathy, vasculitis and nephritis, and taste disturbances. Creatine phosphokinase values should be measured if patients experience myalgia.

Excessive doses of antithyroid drugs may cause hypothyroidism and goitre. High doses in pregnancy may result in fetal hypothyroidism and goitre (see Pregnancy and Breast Feeding, below).

An immune mechanism has been implicated in many of these reactions and cross-sensitivity between the thiourea antithyroid drugs may occur.

Effects on the blood. While leucopenia is considered to be a common adverse effect of the thiourea antithyroid drugs, occurring in up to a quarter of patients, it is usually mild and improves as treatment continues.[1]
Agranulocytosis, a more serious hazard, is usually reported to affect 0.03% of patients in Europe,[2] who are mostly treated with carbimazole. However the incidence has been reported to be higher (0.4%) in areas where methimazole [thiamazole] is used.[3,4] Fatalities have been reported.[1,2,4,5] Although a direct toxic effect had been suggested, the agranulocytosis associated with the thiourea drugs is now generally considered to be immunologically mediated.[1,6] The onset of agranulocytosis is usually rapid and monitoring of the blood count is not always of predictive value;[3] routine monitoring is not indicated.[2] Agranulocytosis has occurred in patients receiving propylthiouracil for a second time who had no such complications in their first course of therapy.[7] There is limited evidence that agranulocytosis is more common at higher doses, and in older patients. However this has not been proved conclusively.[1]
There have been some case reports of aplastic anaemia being produced by antithyroid drugs, but the excess risk associated with their use is considered to be very low[6,8] and complete recovery has been reported following withdrawal of the antithyroid drug. An immune mechanism has been implicated.
Carbimazole has produced haemolytic anaemia.[9] In this case the immune reaction was specific to carbimazole and could not be demonstrated with methimazole [thiamazole].
On very rare occasions patients taking propylthiouracil have experienced a reduction in prothrombin values and bleeding.[10-12] In one patient bleeding was linked to propylthiouracil-induced thrombocytopenia.[13]

1. Bartalena L et al. Adverse effects of thyroid hormone preparations and antithyroid drugs. Drug Safety 1996; 15: 53–63.
2. Committee on Safety of Medicines/Medicines Control Agency. Reminder: agranulocytosis with antithyroid drugs. Current Problems 1999; 25: 3.
3. Tajiri J, et al. Antithyroid drug-induced agranulocytosis: the usefulness of routine white blood cell count monitoring. Arch Intern Med 1990; 150: 621–4.
4. Anonymous. Elaboration: drug-induced agranulocytosis–monitoring antithyroid treatment. Drug Ther Bull 1997; 35: 88.
5. Anonymous. Drug-induced agranulocytosis. Drug Ther Bull 1997; 35: 49–52.
6. International Agranulocytosis and Aplastic Anaemia Study. Risk of agranulocytosis and aplastic anaemia in relation to use of antithyroid drugs. BMJ 1988; 297: 262–5.
7. Shiran A, et al. Propylthiouracil-induced agranulocytosis in four patients previously treated with the drug. JAMA 1991; 266: 3129–30.
8. Bishara J. Methimazole-induced aplastic anemia. Ann Pharmacother 1996; 30: 684.
9. Salama A, et al. Carbimazole-induced immune haemolytic anaemia: role of drug-red blood cell complexes for immunization. Br J Haematol 1988; 68: 479–82.
10. D'Angelo G, Le Gresley LP. Severe hypoprothrombinaemia after propylthiouracil therapy. Can Med Assoc J 1959; 81: 479–81.
11. Naeye RL, Terrien CM. Hemorrhagic state after therapy with propylthiouracil. Am J Clin Pathol 1960; 34: 254–7.
12. Gotta AW, et al. Prolonged intraoperative bleeding caused by propylthiouracil-induced hypoprothrombinemia. Anesthesiology 1972; 37: 562–3.
13. Ikeda S, Schweiss JF. Excessive blood loss during operation in the patient treated with propylthiouracil. Can Anaesth Soc J 1982; 29: 477–80.

Effects on the ears. Earache, high-frequency hearing loss, and tinnitus in a patient with Graves' disease were considered to be associated with hypersensitivity to carbimazole therapy;[1] hearing loss, but not the tinnitus, resolved when carbimazole was replaced with propylthiouracil.

1. Hill D, et al. Hearing loss and tinnitus with carbimazole BMJ 1994; 309: 929.

Effects on the kidneys. There have been reports of glomerulonephritis associated with the development of antineutrophil cytoplasmic antibodies in patients receiving thiourea antithyroid drugs.[1-5]

1. Vogt BA, et al. Antineutrophil cytoplasmic autoantibody-positive crescentic glomerulonephritis as a complication of treatment with propylthiouracil in children. J Pediatr 1994; 124: 986–8.
2. D'Cruz D, et al. Antineutrophil cytoplasmic antibody-positive crescentic glomerulonephritis associated with anti-thyroid drug treatment. Br J Rheumatol 1995; 34: 1090–1.
3. Yuasa S, et al. Antineutrophil cytoplasmic antibodies (ANCA)-associated crescentic glomerulonephritis and propylthiouracil therapy. Nephron 1996; 73: 701–3.
4. Kudoh Y, et al. Propylthiouracil-induced rapidly progressive glomerulonephritis associated with antineutrophil cytoplasmic autoantibodies. Clin Nephrol 1997; 48: 41–3.
5. Prasad GVR, et al. Propylthiouracil-induced diffuse proliferative lupus nephritis: review of immunological complications. J Am Soc Nephrol 1997; 8: 1205–10.

Effects on the liver. Jaundice, usually cholestatic, has been reported with methimazole [thiamazole] and carbimazole.[1-5] An immune-mediated mechanism rather than a toxic reaction has been proposed. Hepatitis (sometimes progressing to cirrhosis[6]) and hepatic necrosis have been associated with pro-

pylthiouracil,[6-9] sometimes with fatal consequences.[7,8] However, in one study[10] almost 30% of patients being treated with propylthiouracil developed asymptomatic liver changes (increased alanine aminotransferase values) that were mostly reversible as treatment continued at a reduced dose.
Despite reports of liver damage, propylthiouracil has been investigated in the treatment of patients with alcoholic liver disease (see p.1526).

1. Becker CE, et al. Hepatitis from methimazole during adrenal steroid therapy for malignant exophthalmos. JAMA 1968; 206: 1787–9.
2. Fischer MG, et al. Methimazole-induced jaundice. JAMA 1973; 223: 1028–9.
3. Blom H, et al. A case of carbimazole-induced intrahepatic cholestasis. Arch Intern Med 1985; 145: 1513–15.
4. Schmidt G, et al. Methimazole-associated cholestatic liver injury: case report and brief literature review. Hepatogastroenterology 1986; 33: 244–6.
5. Arab DM, et al. Severe cholestatic jaundice in uncomplicated hyperthyroidism treated with methimazole. J Clin Endocrinol Metab 1995; 80: 1083–5.
6. Özenírler S, et al. Propylthiouracil-induced hepatic damage. Ann Pharmacother 1996; 30: 960–3.
7. Hanson JS. Propylthiouracil and hepatitis. Two cases and a review of the literature. Arch Intern Med 1984; 144: 994–6.
8. Limaye A, Ruffolo PR. Propylthiouracil-induced fatal hepatic necrosis. Am J Gastroenterol 1987; 82: 152–4.
9. Ichiki Y, et al. Propylthiouracil-induced severe hepatitis: a case report and review of the literature. J Gastroenterol 1998; 33: 747–50.
10. Liaw Y-F, et al. Hepatic injury during propylthiouracil therapy in patients with hyperthyroidism. Ann Intern Med 1993; 118: 424–8.

Effects on the lungs. A report of a diffuse interstitial pneumonitis in 2 patients who had received propylthiouracil.[1] A hypersensitivity reaction to propylthiouracil was suggested. Propylthiouracil was also implicated in two cases of alveolar haemorrhage, associated with antineutrophil cytoplasmic antibody.[2,3]

1. Miyazono K, et al. Propylthiouracil-induced diffuse interstitial pneumonitis. Arch Intern Med 1984; 144: 1764–5.
2. Ohtsuka M, et al. Propylthiouracil-induced alveolar haemorrhage associated with antineutrophil cytoplasmic antibody. Eur Respir J 1997; 10: 1405–7.
3. Dhillon SS, et al. Diffuse alveolar hemorrhage and pulmonary capillaritis due to propylthiouracil. Chest 1999; 116: 1485–8.

Effects on the muscles. Myositis with pain, weakness, and increased creatine kinase concentrations has been reported with carbimazole.[1,2] This effect might be explained by 'tissue hypothyroidism', and might respond to dosage reduction.[3]

1. Page SR, Nussey SS. Myositis in association with carbimazole therapy. Lancet 1989; i: 964.
2. Pasquier E, et al. Biopsy-proven myositis with microvasculitis in association with carbimazole. Lancet 1991; 338: 1082–3.
3. O'Malley B. Carbimazole-induced cramps. Lancet 1989; i: 1456.

Hypersensitivity. Many of the adverse effects associated with the thiourea antithyroid drugs, including those involving the blood, kidneys, and liver appear to have an immune basis. These effects may be associated with polyarthritis[1] or hypersensitivity vasculitis.[2-6] The latter is sometimes severe and multisystemic, and fatalities have occurred. Hypersensitivity reactions may also be associated with the development of antineutrophil cytoplasmic antibodies (ANCA), or sometimes with a lupus-like syndrome with or without the presence of antinuclear antibodies.[2,5] Serum sickness with arthralgias and raised immunoglobulin M (IgM) concentrations has been reported with methimazole [thiamazole][7] and the production of antibodies to insulin resulting in episodes of hypoglycaemia has been associated with methimazole [thiamazole][8] and carbimazole.[9]

The thiourea antithyroid drugs all contain a thioamide group and cross-sensitivity between them might be expected; in particular, complete cross-reactivity may be expected between methimazole [thiamazole] and carbimazole since the latter is converted in-vivo to methimazole [thiamazole]. Cross-sensitivity between propylthiouracil and carbimazole[10] or methimazole [thiamazole][11] has been reported but the incidence and clinical importance is not clear. Although it has been suggested that carbimazole or methimazole [thiamazole] may be substituted for propylthiouracil in hypersensitive patients, it is safer to discontinue antithyroid drugs in such patients.[10]

1. Bajaj S, et al. Antithyroid arthritis syndrome. J Rheumatol 1998; 25: 1235–9.
2. Kawachi Y, et al. ANCA-associated vasculitis and lupus-like syndrome caused by methimazole. Clin Exp Dermatol 1995; 20: 345–7.
3. Chastain MA, et al. Propylthiouracil hypersensitivity: report of two patients with vasculitis and review of the literature. J Am Acad Dermatol 1999; 41: 757–64.
4. Gunton JE, et al. Clinical case seminar: antithyroid drugs and antineutrophil cytoplasmic antibody positive vasculitis. A case report and review of the literature. J Clin Endocrinol Metab 1999; 84: 13–16.
5. Mathieu E, et al. Systemic adverse effect of antithyroid drugs. Clin Rheumatol 1999; 18: 66–8.
6. Dolman KM, et al. Vasculitis and antineutrophil cytoplasmic autoantibodies associated with propylthiouracil therapy. Lancet 1993; 342: 651–2.
7. Van Kuyk M, et al. Methimazole-induced serum sickness. Acta Clin Belg 1983; 38: 68–9.
8. Hakamata M, et al. Insulin autoimmune syndrome after the third therapy with methimazole. Intern Med 1995; 34: 410–12.
9. Burden AC, Rosenthal FD. Methimazole and insulin autoimmune syndrome. Lancet 1983; ii: 1311.

The symbol † denotes a preparation no longer actively marketed

10. Smith A, *et al*. Cross sensitivity to antithyroid drugs. *BMJ* 1989; **298:** 1253.
11. De Weweire A, *et al*. Failure to control hyperthyroidism with a thionamide after potassium perchlorate withdrawal in a patient with amiodarone associated thyrotoxicosis. *J Endocrinol Invest* 1987; **10:** 529.

Pregnancy and breast feeding. Thiourea antithyroid drugs have been used successfully in pregnancy (see Hyperthyroidism, p.1519).

Methimazole [thiamazole] (the metabolite of carbimazole) has been the antithyroid drug most frequently involved in the few reports of **congenital defects** following maternal use of such compounds. Several infants exposed to methimazole [thiamazole] *in utero* have been born with scalp defects (aplasia cutis congenita—a localised absence of skin at birth)[1,2] although hyperthyroidism itself may give rise to such defects.[3] Individual case reports of other congenital defects associated with methimazole [thiamazole] have included choanal atresia (an upper respiratory-tract defect), oesophageal atresia, and tracheo-oesophageal fistula[3] but the incidence of congenital abnormalities is not increased compared with the general population.[4] There have been some reports of neonates exposed to thiourea antithyroid drugs *in utero* displaying signs of **hypothyroidism** including goitre.[5,6]

The safety of **breast feeding** during maternal treatment depends partly on how much drug is distributed into the breast milk. Thiourea antithyroid drugs may be used with care in breast-feeding mothers; neonatal development and thyroid function of the infant should be closely monitored and the lowest effective dose used. Propylthiouracil has been preferred to carbimazole or methimazole [thiamazole] since it enters breast milk less readily.[7,8] The infant's intake of methimazole [thiamazole] following administration of carbimazole [or methimazole [thiamazole]] might be greatly reduced by discarding the breast milk produced 2 to 4 hours after a dose,[9] since the highest concentration was found at this time. One study found no adverse effects on thyroid function or thyroid hormone levels in breast-fed infants during up to 6 months of maternal treatment with methimazole [thiamazole].[10]

1. Milham S. Scalp defects in infants of mothers treated for hyperthyroidism with methimazole or carbimazole during pregnancy. *Teratology* 1985; **32:** 321.
2. Vogt T, *et al*. Aplasia cutis congenita after exposure to methimazole: a causal relationship? *Br J Dermatol* 1995; **133:** 994–6.
3. Johnsson E, *et al*. Severe malformations in infant born to hyperthyroid woman on methimazole. *Lancet* 1997; **350:** 1520.
4. Wing DA, *et al*. A comparison of propylthiouracil versus methimazole in the treatment of hyperthyroidism in pregnancy. *Am J Obstet Gynecol* 1994; **170:** 90–5.
5. O'Doherty MJ, *et al*. Treating thyrotoxicosis in pregnant or potentially pregnant women. *BMJ* 1999; **318:** 5–6.
6. Masiukiewicz US, Barrow GN. Hyperthyroidism in pregnancy: diagnosis and treatment. *Thyroid* 1999; **9:** 647–52.
7. Kampmann JP, *et al*. Propylthiouracil in human milk: revision of a dogma. *Lancet* 1980; **i:** 736–8.
8. Johansen K, *et al*. Excretion of methimazole in human milk. *Eur J Clin Pharmacol* 1982; **23:** 339–41.
9. Rylance GW, *et al*. Carbimazole and breastfeeding. *Lancet* 1987; **i:** 928.
10. Azizi F. Effect of methimazole treatment of maternal thyrotoxicosis on thyroid function in breast-feeding infants. *J Pediatr* 1996; **128:** 855–8.

Pharmacokinetics

The pharmacokinetics of carbimazole and methimazole [thiamazole] can be considered together since carbimazole is rapidly and completely metabolised to methimazole [thiamazole] in the body. The antithyroid activity of carbimazole is dependent upon this conversion to methimazole [thiamazole].

Carbimazole and other thiourea antithyroid drugs are rapidly absorbed from the gastrointestinal tract with peak plasma concentrations occurring about 1 to 2 hours following administration by mouth.

They are concentrated in the thyroid gland and, since their duration of action is more closely related to the intrathyroidal drug concentration than their plasma half-life, this results in a prolongation of antithyroid activity such that single daily doses are possible. Methimazole [thiamazole] is not bound to plasma proteins.

Methimazole [thiamazole] has an elimination half-life from plasma of about 3 to 6 hours and is metabolised, probably by the liver, and excreted in the urine. Less than 12% of a dose of methimazole [thiamazole] may be excreted as unchanged drug. 3-Methyl-2-thiohydantoin has been identified as a metabolite of methimazole [thiamazole]. The elimination half-life may be increased in hepatic and renal impairment.

Methimazole [thiamazole] crosses the placenta and is distributed into breast milk.

◊ References to the pharmacokinetics of carbimazole and methimazole [thiamazole].

1. Skellern GG, *et al*. The pharmacokinetics of methimazole after oral administration of carbimazole and methimazole, in hyperthyroid patients. *Br J Clin Pharmacol* 1980; **9:** 137–43.

2. Kampmann JP, Hansen JM. Clinical pharmacokinetics of antithyroid drugs. *Clin Pharmacokinet* 1981; **6:** 401–28.
3. Jansson R, *et al*. Intrathyroidal concentrations of methimazole in patients with Graves' disease. *J Clin Endocrinol Metab* 1983; **57:** 129–32.
4. Cooper DS, *et al*. Methimazole pharmacology in man: studies using a newly developed radioimmunoassay for methimazole. *J Clin Endocrinol Metab* 1984; **58:** 473–9.
5. Jansson R, *et al*. Pharmacokinetic properties and bioavailability of methimazole. *Clin Pharmacokinet* 1985; **10:** 443–50.

Uses and Administration

Carbimazole is a thiourea antithyroid drug that acts by blocking the production of thyroid hormones (see p.1519). It is used in the management of hyperthyroidism (p.1519), including the treatment of Graves' disease, the preparation of hyperthyroid patients for thyroidectomy, use as an adjunct to radio-iodine therapy, and the treatment of thyroid storm.

Carbimazole is completely metabolised to methimazole [thiamazole] and it is this metabolite that is responsible for the clinical antithyroid activity of carbimazole.

Carbimazole is given by mouth typically in an initial dosage of 15 to 40 mg daily. It has often been given in divided daily doses but once daily administration is also possible. Improvement is usually seen in 1 to 3 weeks and control of symptoms is achieved in 1 to 2 months. When the patient is euthyroid the dose is gradually reduced to the smallest amount that will maintain the euthyroid state. Typical maintenance doses are 5 to 15 mg daily. Alternatively, the dose may be continued at the initial level in combination with supplemental thyroxine (levothyroxine) as a blocking-replacement regimen. Either form of maintenance treatment is usually continued for at least a year, and often for 18 months. Children may be given an initial dose of 250 μg per kg body-weight three times daily, adjusted according to response; treatment in children should be undertaken by a specialist.

Action. There is evidence to suggest that thiourea antithyroid drugs suppress the immune response. However, it is not clear whether this immunosuppressive effect contributes to their antithyroid action or has any clinical significance in the treatment of auto-immune thyroid disorders.[1-5] Increasing the daily dose of methimazole [thiamazole] with the aim of immunosuppression was of no benefit in a large study of patients with Graves' disease.[6]

A number of the adverse effects of the thiourea drugs are considered to have an immune basis (see under Hypersensitivity, above).

1. Kendall-Taylor P. Are antithyroid drugs immunosuppressive? *BMJ* 1984; **288:** 509–11.
2. Ludgate ME, *et al*. Analysis of T cell subsets in Graves' disease: alterations associated with carbimazole. *BMJ* 1984; **288:** 526–30.
3. Jansson R, *et al*. Thyroxine, methimazole, and thyroid microsomal autoantibody titres in hypothyroid Hashimoto's thyroiditis. *BMJ* 1985; **290:** 11–12.
4. Tötterman TH, *et al*. Induction of circulating activated suppressor-like T cells by methimazole therapy for Graves' disease. *N Engl J Med* 1987; **316:** 15–22.
5. Volpé R. Immunoregulation in autoimmune thyroid disease. *N Engl J Med* 1987; **316:** 44–6.
6. Reinwein D, *et al*. A prospective randomised trial of antithyroid drug dose in Graves' disease therapy. *J Clin Endocrinol Metab* 1993; **76:** 1516–21.

Preparations

BP 2001: Carbimazole Tablets.

Proprietary Preparations (details are given in Part 3)
Aust.: Carbistad; *Austral.:* Neo-Mercazole; *Denm.:* Neo-Mercazole; *Fin.:* Tyrazol; *Fr.:* Neo-Mercazole; *Ger.:* Neo-Thyreostat; *Hong Kong:* Cazole; Neo-Mercazole; *Irl.:* Neo-Mercazole; *Norw.:* Neo-Mercazole; *NZ:* Neo-Mercazole; *S.Afr.:* Neo-Mercazole; *Singapore:* Camazole; Cazole; Neo-Mercazole; *Spain:* Neo Tomizol; *Switz.:* Neo-Mercazole; *UK:* Neo-Mercazole.

Dibromotyrosine (12643-l)

3,5-Dibromo-L-tyrosine.
$C_9H_9Br_2NO_3 = 339.0$.
CAS — 300-38-9.
ATC — H03BX02.

Profile
Dibromotyrosine is an antithyroid drug used in the treatment of hyperthyroidism (p.1519) in doses of 300 to 900 mg daily by mouth.

Preparations
Proprietary Preparations (details are given in Part 3)
Ital.: Bromotiren.

Multi-ingredient: *Ital.:* Bromazolo.

Diiodotyrosine (9005-f)

Diotyrosine; Iodogorgoic Acid. 3,5-Di-iodo-L-tyrosine dihydrate.
$C_9H_9I_2NO_3,2H_2O = 469.0$.
CAS — 66-02-4 (anhydrous diiodotyrosine); 300-39-0 (anhydrous L-diiodotyrosine).
ATC — H03BX01.
Pharmacopoeias. In Aust.

Profile
Diiodotyrosine is an antithyroid drug. It is given by mouth in usual doses of 177.5 to 355 μg daily for the treatment of hyperthyroidism and iodine deficiency disorders.

Preparations
Proprietary Preparations (details are given in Part 3)
Ger.: Strumedical 400.

Fluorotyrosine (19714-r)

Fluorotyrosinum; Fluortyrosine. 3-Fluorotyrosine.
$C_9H_{10}FNO_3 = 199.2$.
CAS — 139-26-4.

Profile
Fluorotyrosine is an antithyroid drug used in the treatment of hyperthyroidism.

Preparations
Proprietary Preparations (details are given in Part 3)
Aust.: Fluorthyrin.

Iodine (4571-l)

Iode; Iodum; Jodum; Yodo.
$I_2 = 253.80894$.
CAS — 7553-56-2.
ATC — D08AG03.
Pharmacopoeias. In Chin., Eur. (see p.vi), Int., Jpn, Pol., and US.

With acetone iodine forms a pungent irritating compound.

Pharmacopoeial description
Ph. Eur.: Greyish-violet, brittle plates or fine crystals, with a metallic sheen. It is slowly volatile at room temperature. Very slightly soluble in water; soluble in alcohol; slightly soluble in glycerol; very soluble in concentrated solutions of iodides.
USP 25: Heavy, greyish-black plates or granules with a metallic sheen and a characteristic odour. Soluble 1 in 3000 of water, 1 in 13 of alcohol, 1 in 4 of carbon disulfide, and 1 in 80 of glycerol; freely soluble in chloroform, in ether, and in carbon tetrachloride; soluble in solutions of iodides. Store in airtight containers.

Potassium Iodide (4579-x)

Iodeto de Potássio; Kalii Iodetum; Kalii Iodidum; Kalii Jodidum; Kalium Iodatum; Kalium Jodatum; Pot. Iod.; Potassii Iodidum; Potassium (Iodure de).
$KI = 166.0$.
CAS — 7681-11-0.
ATC — R05CA02; S01XA04; V03AB21.
Pharmacopoeias. In Chin., Eur. (see p.vi), Int., Jpn, Pol., and US.

Each g represents 6 mmol of potassium and of iodide.

Pharmacopoeial description
Ph. Eur.: A white powder or colourless crystals. Very soluble in water; soluble in alcohol; freely soluble in glycerol. Protect from light.
USP 25: Hexahedral crystals, either transparent and colourless or somewhat opaque and white, or a white, granular powder. It is slightly hygroscopic. Soluble 1 in 0.7 of water and 1 in 0.5 of boiling water, 1 in 22 of alcohol, and 1 in 2 of glycerol. Its solutions are neutral or alkaline to litmus.

Sodium Iodide (4581-j)

Iodeto de Sódio; Natrii Iodetum; Natrii Iodidum; Natrii Jodidum; Natrium Iodatum; Sod. Iod.; Sodii Iodidum; Sodium (Iodure de).
$NaI = 149.9$.
CAS — 7681-82-5.
Pharmacopoeias. In Chin., Eur. (see p.vi), Jpn, Pol., and US.

Pharmacopoeial description
Ph. Eur.: Colourless crystals or white crystalline powder. It is hygroscopic. Very soluble in water; freely soluble in alcohol. Protect from light.
USP 25: Colourless, odourless crystals, or white crystalline powder. It is deliquescent in moist air and develops a brown tint upon decomposition. Soluble 1 in 0.6 of water, 1 in 2 of alcohol, and 1 in 1 of glycerol. Store in airtight containers.

Adverse Effects and Treatment

Iodine and iodides, whether applied topically or administered systemically, can give rise to hypersensitivity reactions which may include urticaria, angioedema, cutaneous haemorrhage or purpuras, fever, arthralgia, lymphadenopathy, and eosinophilia.

Inhalation of iodine vapour is very irritating to mucous membranes.

Iodine and iodides have variable effects on the thyroid (see below) and can produce goitre and hypothyroidism as well as hyperthyroidism (the Iod-Basedow or Jod-Basedow phenomenon). Goitre and hypothyroidism have also occurred in infants born to mothers who had taken iodides during pregnancy.

Prolonged administration may lead to a range of adverse effects, often called 'iodism' although some of the effects could be considered to be due to hypersensitivity. These include adverse effects on the mouth such as metallic taste, increased salivation, burning or pain; there may be acute rhinitis and swelling and inflammation of the throat. Eyes may be irritated and swollen and there may be increased lachrymation. Pulmonary oedema and bronchitis may develop. Skin reactions include acneform or, more rarely, severe eruptions (ioderma). Other reported effects include depression, insomnia, impotence, headache, and gastrointestinal disturbances, notably diarrhoea (which may be bloody).

The symptoms of acute poisoning from ingestion of iodine are mainly due to its corrosive effects on the gastrointestinal tract; a disagreeable metallic taste, vomiting, abdominal pain, and diarrhoea occur. Thirst and headache have been reported. Systemic toxicity may lead to shock, tachycardia, fever, metabolic acidosis and renal impairment. Death may be due to circulatory failure, oedema of the epiglottis resulting in asphyxia, aspiration pneumonia, or pulmonary oedema. Oesophageal stricture may occur if the patient survives the acute stage.

Victims of acute poisoning have been given copious draughts of milk or starch mucilage; lavage should probably not be attempted, and certainly not unless iodine has been ingested in sufficiently dilute form not to produce gastrointestinal corrosion. Other treatments include activated charcoal and sodium thiosulfate solution 1% or 5% to reduce iodine to the less toxic iodides.

Effects on the thyroid. Iodide may be isolated by the body from a variety of sources, including an iodine-rich diet, or some disinfectants and drugs containing iodine (see also under Amiodarone, p.837). Although iodine is required for the production of thyroid hormones, excessive quantities can cause hyperthyroidism, or even goitre and hypothyroidism (which are seen more often in iodine deficiency).

The normal daily requirement ranges from 100 to 300 μg.[1,2] Quantities of 500 μg to 1 mg daily probably have no untoward effects on thyroid function in most cases.[2] When progressively larger doses are given there is an initial rise in thyroid hormone production, but at still higher doses, production decreases (the Wolff-Chaikoff effect). This effect is usually seen with doses of more than about 2 mg daily, but is normally transient, adaptation occurring on repeated administration. In certain individuals a lack of adaptation produces a chronic inhibition of thyroid hormone synthesis leading to goitre and **hypothyroidism**.[1,2]

Excess iodine may also induce **hyperthyroidism** (the Iod-Basedow or Jod-Basedow phenomenon). Iodine-induced hyperthyroidism has been associated with iodine prophylaxis programmes in developing countries.[3] The highest incidence of hyperthyroidism has been reported to occur 1 to 3 years after supplementation commences, with the incidence returning to normal within 3 to 10 years despite continued iodine exposure.[4] Elderly subjects and those with nodular goitres have been found to be at greatest risk.

To overcome any adverse effects on thyroid function as a result of iodine prophylaxis during **pregnancy**, WHO has issued guidelines on the safe use of iodised oil during gestation.[5,6] There is some evidence that the use of iodine-containing antiseptics on pregnant women and neonates may cause disturbances in thyroid function.[7,8]

1. Arthur JR, Beckett GJ. Thyroid function. *Br Med Bull* 1999; **55:** 658–68.
2. WHO. Iodine. In *Trace elements in human nutrition and health.* Geneva: WHO, 1996: 49–71.
3. Delange F, *et al.* Risks of iodine-induced hyperthyroidism after correction of iodine deficiency by iodized salt. *Thyroid* 1999; **9:** 545–56.
4. Fradkin JE, Wolff J. Iodide-induced thyrotoxicosis. *Medicine (Baltimore)* 1983; **62:** 1–20.
5. WHO. Safe use of iodized oil to prevent iodine deficiency in pregnant women. *Bull WHO* 1996; **74:** 1–3.
6. Delange F. Administration of iodized oil during pregnancy: a summary of the published evidence. *Bull WHO* 1996; **74:** 101–8.

The symbol † denotes a preparation no longer actively marketed

7. Linder N *et al.* Topical iodine-containing antiseptics and subclinical hypothyroidism in preterm infants. *J Pediatr* 1997; **131:** 434–9.
8. Weber G *et al.* Neonatal transient hypothyroidism: aetiological study. *Arch Dis Child Fetal Neonatal Ed* 1998; **79:** F70–2.

Precautions

Caution is necessary if preparations containing iodine or iodides are taken for prolonged periods, and such preparations should not be taken regularly during pregnancy except when iodine supplementation is required. Iodine or iodides are contra-indicated during breast feeding. Caution is also required when giving iodine or iodides to children. Patients over the age of 45 years or with nodular goitres are especially susceptible to hyperthyroidism when given iodine supplementation. Reduced doses should therefore be employed and supplementation with iodised oil may not be appropriate.

Solutions of iodine applied to the skin should not be covered with occlusive dressings. The disinfectant activity of iodine is reduced by alkalis as well as by protein.

As iodine and iodides can affect the thyroid gland the administration of such preparations may interfere with tests of thyroid function.

Interactions

The effects of iodine and iodides on the thyroid may be altered by other compounds including amiodarone and lithium.

Pharmacokinetics

Iodine is slightly absorbed when applied to the skin. When taken by mouth iodine preparations (which are converted to iodide) and iodides are trapped by the thyroid gland (see p.1519). Iodides not taken up by the thyroid are excreted mainly in the urine, with smaller amounts appearing in the faeces, saliva, and sweat. They cross the placenta and are distributed into breast milk.

Uses and Administration

Iodine is an essential trace element in the human diet, necessary for the formation of thyroid hormones (see p.1519), and consequently it is used in iodine deficiency and thyroid disorders. It also has antimicrobial activity.

For the prophylaxis and treatment of **iodine deficiency disorders** (below) it may be administered as potassium or sodium iodide, as iodised oil, or as potassium iodate.

In the pre-operative management of **hyperthyroidism** (p.1519) iodine and iodides are used in conjunction with antithyroid drugs such as carbimazole, methimazole [thiamazole], or propylthiouracil. Iodine may be given as a solution with potassium iodide (Aqueous Iodine Oral Solution BP 2001: Lugol's Solution or Strong Iodine Solution USP 25) which contains in each mL 130 mg of free and combined iodine; a dose of 0.1 to 0.3 mL in milk or water three times daily for 10 to 14 days renders the thyroid firm and avoids the increased vascularity and friability with increased risk of haemorrhage that may result from the use of an antithyroid agent alone. Alternatively, potassium iodide has been given in doses of up to 250 mg three times daily with food. Solutions of potassium iodide intended for oral administration should be given well diluted to avoid gastric irritation. Potassium iodide may also be given as part of the management of thyroid storm one hour after administration of an antithyroid drug; doses of 50 to 100 mg have been given twice daily; higher doses have sometimes been employed. Sodium iodide has been given by intravenous injection as part of the management of thyroid storm.

Potassium iodide has been tried in the treatment of benign **thyroid nodules** (p.1519).

Potassium iodide or potassium iodate are taken by mouth for **radiation protection** (below) to saturate the thyroid when uptake of radio-iodine by the gland is not desired.

Iodine has a powerful bactericidal action. It is also active against fungi, viruses, protozoa, cysts, and spores. Iodine is used as an **antiseptic** and **disinfectant** generally as a 2.0% or 2.5% solution. Its activity is reduced in the presence of organic matter, though not to the same extent as with the other halogen disinfectants. If industrial methylated spirit is used for the solution, it should be free from acetone with which iodine forms an irritant and lachrymatory compound. Iodine solutions may be applied to small wounds or abrasions as well as to unbroken skin, but an iodophore such as povidone-iodine (p.1155) may be preferred.

Iodine may also be used to sterilise drinking water; 5 drops of a 2% alcoholic solution added to about one litre (one US quart) of water is reported to kill amoebae and bacteria within 15 minutes. Water contaminated with *Giardia* requires 12 drops of a 2% alcoholic solution for each litre which may take one hour to achieve its effect.

When iodine combines chemically it is decolorised and so-called colourless iodine preparations do not have the disinfectant properties of iodine.

Iodine stains the skin a deep reddish-brown; the stain can be readily removed by dilute solutions of alkalis or sodium thiosulfate. A dilute solution of iodine (Schiller's Iodine) has been used as a **diagnostic** stain in colposcopy.

There have been numerous other uses of iodine and iodides. Potassium iodide has been used in the treatment of fungal infections such as sporotrichosis (below). Iodides have long been used as ingredients of expectorant mixtures (see Cough, p.1082) but there is little evidence of their effectiveness. A diatomic iodine formulation is under investigation for the treatment of fibrocystic breast disease. Iodinated organic compounds including iodised oil are used as X-ray contrast media (p.1030). Iodine radionuclides are often administered as preparations of sodium iodide.

Fungal infections. Potassium iodide is used in the treatment of cutaneous sporotrichosis (p.376), although how it acts is unclear since antifungal activity was not demonstrated *in vitro* against *Sporothrix schenkii*.[1] It is usually given by mouth in a gradually increasing dosage up to the limit of tolerance. The recommended initial dose is 5 drops of a saturated solution of potassium iodide (1 g per mL) given three times daily; treatment should be continued for at least 1 month after the disappearance or stabilisation of the lesions.

Potassium iodide has also been found to be effective in the treatment of phycomycosis caused by *Basidiobolus haptosporus*;[2,3] once again the mode of action is unclear.

Potassium iodide and sodium iodide have been tried by local intracavitary instillation for the treatment of life-threatening haemoptysis from pulmonary aspergillomas.[5] Mechanical factors may have accounted for a beneficial effect rather than any antifungal action. Aspergillomas are usually managed conservatively or, in more severe disease, with antifungals or surgery (see p.372).

1. WHO. *WHO model prescribing information: drugs used in skin diseases.* Geneva: WHO, 1997.
2. Kelly S, *et al.* Subcutaneous phycomycosis in Sierra Leone. *Trans R Soc Trop Med Hyg* 1980; **74:** 396–7.
3. Kamalam A, Thambiah AS. Muscle invasion by Basidiobolus haptosporus. *Sabouraudia* 1984; **22:** 273–7.
4. Yangco BG, *et al.* In vitro susceptibilities of human and wild-type isolates of Basidiobolus and Conidiobolus species. *Antimicrob Agents Chemother* 1984; **25:** 413–16.
5. Rumbak M, *et al.* Topical treatment of life threatening haemoptysis from aspergillomas. *Thorax* 1996; **51:** 253–5.

Iodine deficiency disorders. Iodine is an essential trace element required for thyroid hormone production. Daily adult requirements are about 100 to 300 μg. In the UK the reference nutrient intake (RNI) for adults is 140 μg (1.1 μmol) of iodine daily[1] and in the USA the recommended dietary allowance (RDA) is 150 μg daily.[2] A full explanation of the terms RNI and RDA can be found under Human Requirements of Vitamins, p.1352.

When iodine requirements are not met, a range of disorders can develop. These iodine deficiency disorders include endemic goitre (enlargement of the thyroid), endemic cretinism (a syndrome characterised by deaf-mutism, intellectual deficit, spasticity, and sometimes hypothyroidism), impaired mental function in children and adults, and an increased incidence of still-births as well as perinatal and infant mortality.[3]

Iodine deficiency disorders can be prevented by iodine supplementation. The incidence of endemic goitre and endemic cretinism can be reduced and some of the effects of established iodine deficiency ameliorated.

Although various methods of iodine supplementation, including iodination of water and bread as well as the administration of potassium iodide, have been investigated, the two methods generally used are iodination of culinary salt and the administration of iodised oil.[3] Salt may be iodinated by the addition of potassium iodide. However, in countries where impurities or environmental factors such as moisture and temperature are likely to cause a reduction in the iodine content of the salt, potassium iodate is the preferred compound since it is more stable than iodide under varying climatic conditions.[4] The concentration used in different countries varies over a wide range from 10 to 80 ppm of elemental iodine.[4]

The chief alternative to supplementation with iodinated salt is iodised oil, usually by intramuscular injection; it is useful where salt consumption is unreliable or inadequate or where immediate action is necessary to correct severe iodine deficiency.[3] A commonly used type of iodised oil has been a poppyseed oil containing about 38% w/w of iodine (see Iodised Oil, p.1034). The Pan American Health Organization has proposed[5] that children in the first year of life receive a dose of 0.5 mL with 1 mL being given to all other subjects. Single intramuscular doses of 1 mL can provide adequate protection from iodine deficiency for at least 3 years while a dose of 2 mL provides adequate coverage for 3½ to 5 years.

Subjects over the age of 45 years and those with nodular goitre are susceptible to hyperthyroidism when given iodine, and iodised oil may not be a suitable means of supplementation. If it is used then doses of 0.2 mL should be employed.[5]

Iodised oil has been tried by mouth. A single dose of 1 mL is reported to provide protection for 1 year and 2 mL for 2 years[5] although there is some evidence that much smaller doses of 0.1 or 0.25 mL can provide protection for about 1 year.[6]

Indirect iodine supplementation, by addition of potassium iodate to the water used to irrigate crops, has been tried in areas of iodine deficiency where other methods had proved difficult to implement.[7]

Iodine or iodides may suppress neonatal thyroid function and it is generally recommended that iodine compounds should be avoided during **pregnancy**. However, where it is essential to prevent neonatal goitre and cretinism, iodine supplementation should not be withheld from pregnant women.[8,9] Iodine supplementation has been found to be effective in preventing brain-damage in the fetus provided it is given to the mother in the first or second trimester;[8] treatment later in pregnancy was not effective in improving neurological status, although some developmental improvement was seen and hypothyroidism will be corrected. WHO has stated that in areas where iodine deficiency disorders are moderate to severe, iodised oil given either before or at any stage of gestation is beneficial.[9] A dose of 480 mg iodine intramuscularly each year or 300 to 480 mg iodine by mouth each year or 100 to 300 mg iodine by mouth every 6 months is recommended for pregnant women and for at least one year postpartum. Similar intramuscular doses are recommended for non-pregnant fertile women with oral doses being 400 to 960 mg iodine every year or 200 to 480 mg every 6 months.

1. DoH. Dietary reference values for food energy and nutrients for the United Kingdom: report of the panel on dietary reference values of the Committee on Medical Aspects of Food Policy. *Report on health and social subjects 41.* London: HMSO, 1991.
2. Standing Committee on the Scientific Evaluation of Dietary Reference Intakes of the Food and Nutrition Board. *Dietary Reference Intakes for Vitamin A, Vitamin K, Arsenic, Boron, Chromium, Copper, Iodine, Iron, Manganese, Molybdenum, Nickel, Silicon, Vanadium, and Zinc.* Washington DC: National Academy Press, 2001.
3. WHO. Iodine. In *Trace elements in human nutrition and health.* Geneva: WHO, 1996: 49–71.
4. Mannar MGV. Control of iodine deficiency disorders by iodination of salt: strategy for developing countries. In: Hetzel BS, *et al.,* eds. *The prevention and control of iodine deficiency disorders.* Amsterdam: Elsevier, 1987: 111–25.
5. Dunn JT. Iodized oil in the treatment and prophylaxis of IDD. In: Hetzel BS, *et al.,* eds. *The prevention and control of iodine deficiency disorders.* Amsterdam: Elsevier, 1987: 127–34.
6. Tonglet R, *et al.* Efficacy of low oral doses of iodized oil in the control of iodine deficiency in Zaire. *N Engl J Med* 1992; **326:** 236–41.
7. Cao X-Y, *et al.* Iodination of irrigation water as a method of supplying iodine to a severely iodine-deficient population in Xinjiang, China. *Lancet* 1994; **344:** 107–10.
8. Delange F. Administration of iodized oil during pregnancy: a summary of the published evidence. *Bull WHO* 1996; **74:** 101–8.
9. WHO. Safe use of iodized oil to prevent iodine deficiency in pregnant women. *Bull WHO* 1996; **74:** 1–3.

Radiation protection. The administration of a radiologically stable form of iodine to saturate the thyroid gland confers thyroid protection from iodine radionuclides.[1,2] When thyroid protection from a *medical procedure* involving radio-iodine is needed, a dose of 100 to 150 mg of potassium iodide may be given 24 hours before the procedure and daily for up to 10 days following it.

In the USA a dose of 130 mg of potassium iodide given daily for 10 days has been recommended in the event of a *nuclear accident.*[1,3] In the UK the Department of Health[4] recommends a single dose of 100 mg of stable iodine (as 170 mg of potassium iodate) for adults (including pregnant women and women who are breast feeding) as soon as possible after exposure and before evacuation. Dosages for children are: 3 to 12 years, 50 mg of stable iodine (85 mg of potassium iodate); 1 month to 3 years, 25 mg of stable iodine (42.5 mg of potassium iodate);

and for neonates, 12.5 mg of stable iodine (21.25 mg of potassium iodate) given as a single dose. When evacuation is delayed, repeated daily administration is recommended.

1. Halperin JA. Potassium iodide as a thyroid blocker— Three Mile Island today. *Drug Intell Clin Pharm* 1989; **23:** 422–7.
2. Nauman J, Wolff J. Iodide prophylaxis in Poland after the Chernobyl reactor accident: benefits and risks. *Am J Med* 1993; **94:** 524–32.
3. Schleien B, *et al.* Recommendations on the use of potassium iodide as a thyroid-blocking agent in radiation accidents: an FDA update. *Bull N Y Acad Med* 1983; **59:** 1009–19.
4. DoH. Nuclear accident countermeasures: iodine prophylaxis: report of the United Kingdom working group on iodine prophylaxis following nuclear accidents. *Report on health and social subjects 39.* London: HMSO, 1991.

Preparations

BP 2001: Alcoholic Iodine Solution; Aqueous Iodine Oral Solution; Sodium Iodide Injection;

BPC 1968: Compound Iodine Paint;

USP 25: Iodine Tincture; Iodine Topical Solution; Potassium Iodide Delayed-release Tablets; Potassium Iodide Oral Solution; Potassium Iodide Tablets; Strong Iodine Solution; Strong Iodine Tincture.

Proprietary Preparations (details are given in Part 3)

Aust.: Jodonorm; Leukona-Jod-Bad; **Belg.:** Iodex†; **Canad.:** Micro I†; Thyro-Block; **Fin.:** Jodix; **Fr.:** Axyol†; **Ger.:** Jodetten; Jodid; jodminerase†; Kaliklora Jod med†; Leukona-Jod-Bad; Mono-Jod; Strumex; **Ital.:** Goccemed; Iodosan Collutorio; Sol-Jod; **Mex.:** Yodolactina; **Norw.:** Jodosan; **Port.:** Iodisis; **USA:** Iodopen; Pima; SSKI; Thyro-Block.

Multi-ingredient: Aust.: Jodthyrox; Jopinol†; **Austral.:** Asa Tones; Ayrton's Iodised†; Potassium Iodide and Stramonium Compound; **Belg.:** Aperop; ITC†; **Braz.:** Antiphlogistine; Atatosse Balsamico; Axol; Becantosse; Boralina; Broncofisin; Bronquidex; CAM; Dermicon; Dermofytol; Dermycose; Elixir de Marinheiro; Eterciclina; Expec; Expectolu; Formitonicum; Frenotossil; Fungol; Glicodin; Glycon; Hebrin; Iodepol; Iodermol; Iodesin; Iodetal; Iodeto de Potassio Composto; Iodeto de Potassium Composto; Iodobec; KI-Expectorante; Locao Mancha Branca; Micocid; Micofim; Micotiazol; Micotissim; MM Expectorante; Pulmonix; Salutina; Sanoclorofila; Sedatux; Subitan; Tetrabronco; Teutoss; Thiodeol; Tolusil; Tussin-Pinho; Tuzo; Xarope de Iodeto de Potassio Composto; **Canad.:** Diodine; IDM Solution†; Iode; Mathieu Cough Syrup; Theo-Bronc; Vito Bronches; **Fr.:** Marinol; Nitrol; Vita-Iodurol ATP†; Vita-Iodurol†; **Ger.:** Adelheid-Jodquelle, Tolzer; Jodthyrox; Krophan N; Thyreocomb N; Thyronajod; Varigloban; **Hong Kong:** Colircusi Iodine-Thio-Calcic; Vitreolent; **Israel:** Iodax; **Ital.:** Antiadiposo; Esoform Jod 20 and 50; Facovit; Fertomcidina-U; Jodo-Calcio-Vitaminico; Polijodurato; Rubidiosin Composto; Rubistenol†; Rubjovit; **Port.:** Fluidin Adulto; Fluidin Antiasmatico; Prelus†; **S.Afr.:** Efcospect†; **Singapore:** Vitreolent; **Spain:** Adiod; Audione; Callicida Rojo; Depurativo Richelet; Encialina; Lasa Antiasmatico†; Nitroina; Yodo Tio Calci; **Switz.:** Dental-Phenjoca†; Perpector; Variglobin; Vitreolent; **UK:** Nasciodine; TCP; **USA:** Elixophyllin-KI; Iodex with Methyl Salicylate; KIE; Mudrane; ORA5; Pediacof; Pedituss Cough; Phylorinol; Quadrinal.

Liothyronine Sodium   (9006-d)

Liothyronine Sodium *(BANM, rINNM)*.

Liothyroninum Natricum; Sodium Liothyronine; L-Tri-iodothyronine Sodium; 3,5,3′-Tri-iodo-L-thyronine Sodium. Sodium 4-O-(4-hydroxy-3-iodophenyl)-3,5-di-iodo-L-tyrosine.

$C_{15}H_{11}I_3NNaO_4 = 673.0$.

CAS — 6893-02-3 (liothyronine); 55-06-1 (liothyronine sodium); 8065-29-0 (liotrix).

ATC — H03AA02.

NOTE. The abbreviation T_3 is often used for endogenous tri-iodothyronine in medical and biochemical reports. Liotrix is the *USAN* name for a mixture of liothyronine sodium with thyroxine [levothyroxine] sodium.

Pharmacopoeias. In Eur. (see p.vi), Jpn, and US.

Liothyronine sodium 10.3 μg is approximately equivalent to 10 μg of liothyronine.

Pharmacopoeial description

Ph. Eur.: A white or slightly coloured powder. Practically insoluble in water; slightly soluble in alcohol; practically insoluble in ether. It dissolves in dilute solutions of alkali hydroxides. Store at 2° to 8° in airtight containers. Protect from light.

USP 25: A light tan, odourless, crystalline powder. Very slightly soluble in water; slightly soluble in alcohol; practically insoluble in most other organic solvents. Store in airtight containers.

Adverse Effects, Treatment, and Precautions

As for Thyroxine Sodium, p.1526.

Interactions

As for Thyroxine Sodium, p.1527.

Pharmacokinetics

Liothyronine is readily and almost completely absorbed from the gastrointestinal tract following oral administration. Once in the circulation, liothyronine binds principally to thyroxine-binding globulin (TBG), although less strongly than thyroxine [levothyroxine]; some is also bound to thyroxine-binding pre-albumin (TBPA) or to albumin. Liothyronine has a plasma half-life in euthyroidism of about 1 to 2 days; the half-life is prolonged in hypothyroidism and reduced in hyperthyroidism.

Liothyronine is metabolised by deiodination to inactive di-iodothyronine and mono-iodothyronine. Iodine released by deiodination is largely reused within the thyroid cells. Further metabolites result from deamination and decarboxylation to tiratricol (triac).

Uses and Administration

Liothyronine is a thyroid hormone (see p.1519). It is used in the treatment of hypothyroidism (p.1520), and is believed to be more active than thyroxine [levothyroxine] (p.1528). The onset of action of liothyronine is rapid, developing within a few hours of administration, and therefore it tends to be used in circumstances where this, and its short duration of action, are useful, particularly in hypothyroid (myxoedema) coma.

With regular dosing the peak therapeutic effect is usually achieved by 3 days; on withdrawal its effects may persist for 1 to 3 days.

The dose of liothyronine should be individualised on the basis of clinical response and biochemical tests and should be monitored regularly. Although liothyronine is administered as the sodium salt, doses can be expressed in terms of liothyronine sodium or liothyronine; the doses below are in terms of liothyronine sodium. Liothyronine sodium 20 to 25 μg is generally considered to be approximately equivalent in activity to thyroxine [levothyroxine] sodium 100 μg.

In hypothyroidism a usual initial adult dose is 5 to 25 μg daily by mouth increased gradually to a maintenance dose of 60 to 75 μg daily in 2 to 3 divided doses, although up to 100 μg daily may be required in some patients. In elderly patients, in those with cardiovascular disorders, or in those with severe long-standing hypothyroidism, treatment should be introduced with doses at the low end of the range, with smaller increments, and longer intervals between increases, as necessary.

In myxoedema coma liothyronine sodium may be given intravenously in a dose of 5 to 20 μg by slow intravenous injection, repeated as necessary, usually at intervals of 12 hours; the minimum interval between doses is 4 hours. Some authorities have advocated an initial dose of 50 μg intravenously followed by further injections of 25 μg every 8 hours until improvement occurs; the dosage may then be reduced to 25 μg intravenously twice daily.

Liothyronine has also been given in the diagnosis of hyperthyroidism in adults. Failure to suppress the take up of radio-iodine after several days of receiving liothyronine sodium suggests a diagnosis of hyperthyroidism.

Liothyronine hydrochloride has also been used.

Preparations

BP 2001: Liothyronine Tablets;
USP 25: Liothyronine Sodium Tablets; Liotrix Tablets.

Proprietary Preparations (details are given in Part 3)

Austral.: Tertroxin; **Belg.:** Cytomel†; **Braz.:** Cynomel; **Canad.:** Cytomel†; **Fr.:** Cynomel; **Ger.:** Thybon; Thyrotardin N; **Ital.:** Dispon; Ti-Tre; **Mex.:** Cynomel; Triyodisan; Triyotex; **Neth.:** Cytomel; **NZ:** Tertroxin; **Port.:** Neo-Tiroimade; **S.Afr.:** Tertroxin; **Thai.:** Tertroxin; **UK:** Tertroxin; Triiodothyronine Injection; **USA:** Cytomel; Triostat.

Multi-ingredient: Aust.: Combithyrex; Novothyral; Prothyrid; **Belg.:** Novothyral; **Braz.:** Levotiroxina; Tyroplus; **Fr.:** Euthyral; **Ger.:** AntiFocal N; NeyNormin N (Revitorgan-Dilutionen N Nr 65); NeyTumorin N (Revitorgan-Dilutionen N Nr 66); Novothyral; Prothyrid; Threeotom†; **Ital.:** Tiroide Amsa; **Mex.:** Novotiral; Proloid S; **S.Afr.:** Diotroxin; **Switz.:** Novothyral; **USA:** Thyrolar.

Methimazole (835-e)

Thiamazole *(BAN, rINN)*; Mercazolylum; Methylmercaptoimidazole; Tiamazol. 1-Methylimidazole-2-thiol.
$C_4H_6N_2S = 114.2$.
CAS — 60-56-0.
ATC — H03BB02.
Pharmacopoeias. In Chin., It., Jpn, Pol., and US.

Pharmacopoeial description

USP 25: A white to pale buff crystalline powder having a faint characteristic odour. Soluble 1 in 5 of water, 1 in 5 of alcohol, 1 in 4.5 of chloroform, and 1 in 125 of ether. Its solutions are practically neutral to litmus. Protect from light.

Adverse Effects and Precautions

As for Carbimazole, p.1521.

Pharmacokinetics

The pharmacokinetics of methimazole [thiamazole] can be considered together with those of carbimazole (p.1522) since the latter is rapidly and completely metabolised to methimazole [thiamazole] in the body.

Uses and Administration

Methimazole [thiamazole] is a thiourea antithyroid drug that acts by blocking the production of thyroid hormones (see p.1519). It is used in the management of hyperthyroidism (p.1519), including the treatment of Graves' disease, the preparation of hyperthyroid patients for thyroidectomy, use as an adjunct to radio-iodine therapy, and the treatment of thyroid storm.

Methimazole [thiamazole] is given by mouth usually in an initial dosage of 15 to 60 mg daily. It has often been given in divided doses but once daily administration is also possible. Improvement is usually seen in 1 to 3 weeks and control of symptoms in 1 to 2 months. When the patient is euthyroid the dose is gradually reduced to a maintenance dose, usually 5 to 15 mg daily. Alternatively, the dose may be continued at the initial level in combination with supplemental thyroxine [levothyroxine] as a blocking-replacement regimen. Either form of maintenance treatment is usually continued for at least a year, and often for 18 months. A recommended initial dose for children is 400 μg per kg body-weight daily; for maintenance this dose may be halved.

Action. For reference to the possible immunosuppressant effects of thiourea antithyroid drugs, see under Uses and Administration of Carbimazole, p.1522.

Preparations

USP 25: Methimazole Tablets.

Proprietary Preparations (details are given in Part 3)
Aust.: Favistan; *Belg.:* Strumazol; *Braz.:* Tapazol; *Canad.:* Tapazole; *Denm.:* Thycapzol; *Ger.:* Favistan; Thyrozol; *Hong Kong:* Tapazole; *Israel:* Mercaptizol; Tapazole; *Ital.:* Tapazole; *Mex.:* Tapazol; *Neth.:* Strumazol; *Port.:* Metibasol; *S.Afr.:* Tapazole†; *Singapore:* Thyrozol; *Spain:* Tirodril; *Swed.:* Thacapzol; *Switz.:* Tapazole; *Thai.:* Tapazole; *USA:* Tapazole.
Multi-ingredient: *Ital.:* Bromazolo.

Methylthiouracil (836-l)

Methylthiouracil *(rINN)*.
2,3-Dihydro-2-thioxo-6-methylpyrimidin-4(1*H*)-one; 2-Mercapto-6-methylpyrimidin-4-ol; 6-Methyl-2-thiouracil.
$C_5H_6N_2OS = 142.2$.
CAS — 56-04-2.
ATC — H03BA01.
Pharmacopoeias. In Aust., It., and Pol.

Profile

Methylthiouracil is a thiourea antithyroid drug that has been used in the treatment of hyperthyroidism.

Potassium Iodate (13154-m)

$KIO_3 = 214.0$.
CAS — 7758-05-6.
Pharmacopoeias. In Br. and It.

Pharmacopoeial description

BP 2001: A white crystalline powder with a slight odour. Slowly soluble in water; insoluble in alcohol. A 5% solution in water has a pH of 5.0 to 8.0.

Profile

Potassium iodate has the actions of iodine (p.1522) and the io-

dides. It is used for the prophylaxis and treatment of iodine deficiency disorders (p.1523).

It may be used similarly to potassium iodide as an adjunct to antithyroid drugs in the pre-operative management of hyperthyroidism (p.1519) and for radiation protection to prevent the uptake of radio-iodine by the thyroid (see p.1524 for doses).

Preparations

BP 2001: Potassium Iodate Tablets.

Proprietary Preparations (details are given in Part 3)
UK: Bioiodine.

Potassium Perchlorate (837-y)

Kalii Perchloras.
$KClO_4 = 138.5$.
CAS — 7778-74-7.
ATC — H03BC01.
Pharmacopoeias. In Eur. (see p.vi) and US.

Pharmacopoeial description

Ph. Eur.: A white crystalline powder or colourless crystals. Sparingly soluble in water; practically insoluble in alcohol.
USP 25: pH of a 0.1M solution in water is between 5.0 and 6.5.

◊ WARNING. *Potassium perchlorate has been used for the illicit preparation of explosives or fireworks; care is required with its supply. Great caution should be taken in handling potassium perchlorate in solution or in the dry state as explosions may occur if it is brought into contact with organic or other readily oxidisable substances.*

Adverse Effects

Fever and rashes have been observed following administration of potassium perchlorate. Some patients may experience nausea and vomiting. Potassium perchlorate seldom produces adverse effects when given as a single dose for diagnostic purposes. Prolonged administration of potassium perchlorate as an antithyroid drug has been associated with serious dose-related adverse effects. Aplastic anaemia (with some fatalities), agranulocytosis, leucopenia, pancytopenia, and the nephrotic syndrome have been reported. Excessive doses may cause hypothyroidism and goitre.

Effects on the blood. Reports of fatal aplastic anaemia[1,2] and of leucopenia and agranulocytosis[1] associated with the use of potassium perchlorate for the treatment of hyperthyroidism. A review[3] in 1998 noted that despite an increase in perchlorate use in recent years there did not appear to have been any further cases of aplastic anaemia since the 1960s.

1. Anonymous. Potassium perchlorate and aplastic anaemia. *BMJ* 1961; **i:** 1520–1.
2. Krevans JR, *et al.* Fatal aplastic anemia following use of potassium perchlorate in thyrotoxicosis. *JAMA* 1962; **181:** 182–4.
3. Wolff J. Perchlorate and the thyroid gland. *Pharmacol Rev* 1998; **50:** 89–105.

Uses and Administration

Potassium perchlorate reduces the uptake and concentration of iodide, pertechnetate, and other anions by the thyroid, choroid plexus, gastric mucosa, and salivary glands probably by competitive inhibition of active transport mechanisms.

It is used diagnostically as an adjunct to pertechnetate (^{99m}Tc) to enhance visualisation of the brain, Meckel's diverticulum, or the placenta by reducing unwanted images of other organs. The usual adult dose is 200 to 400 mg by mouth given 30 to 60 minutes before the administration of pertechnetate (^{99m}Tc). For children aged 2 to 12 years, a dose of 200 mg by mouth has been recommended; for children younger than 2 years of age, 100 mg may be given by mouth.

Potassium perchlorate is also used in conjunction with sodium iodide (^{131}I) in the perchlorate discharge test of thyroid function. The release of radio-iodine from the gland following an oral dose of potassium perchlorate indicates a defect in the binding of iodide by the thyroid and thus a defect in thyroid hormone synthesis. The test has also been used to investigate the action of antithyroid drugs.

Potassium perchlorate has been used in the treatment of hyperthyroidism (p.1519), but because of its toxicity it has been largely replaced by alternative treatments. However, it may be useful in patients with iodine-induced hyperthyroidism such as that associated with amiodarone therapy, by increasing respon-

siveness to conventional antithyroid drugs. An adult dose of 600 mg to 1 g daily by mouth in 3 or 4 divided doses is used as initial therapy with maintenance doses of 200 to 500 mg daily in divided doses. The total daily dose should not exceed 1 g.

◊ References.
1. Wolff J. Perchlorate and the thyroid gland. *Pharmacol Rev* 1998; **50:** 89–105.

Preparations

USP 25: Potassium Perchlorate Capsules.
Proprietary Preparations (details are given in Part 3)
Ital.: Pertiroid; *USA:* Perchloracap.

Prolonium Iodide (13175-p)

Prolonium Iodide *(rINN)*.
NN-(2-Hydroxytrimethylene)bis(trimethylammonium) di-iodide.
$C_9H_{24}I_2N_2O = 430.1$.
CAS — 123-47-7.
Pharmacopoeias. In Chin.

Profile

Prolonium iodide has been given by injection as a source of iodine (p.1522) as part of the treatment of thyroid storm and for the pre-operative management of hyperthyroidism.

Propylthiouracil (838-j)

Propylthiouracilum. 2,3-Dihydro-6-propyl-2-thioxopyrimidin-4(1*H*)-one; 2-Mercapto-6-propylpyrimidin-4-ol; 6-Propyl-2-thiouracil.
$C_7H_{10}N_2OS = 170.2$.
CAS — 51-52-5.
ATC — H03BA02.
Pharmacopoeias. In Chin., Eur. (see p.vi), Int., Jpn, and US.

Pharmacopoeial description

Ph. Eur.: White or almost white crystals or crystalline powder. Very slightly soluble in water and in ether; sparingly soluble in alcohol; dissolves in solutions of alkali hydroxides. Protect from light.
USP 25: A white, powdery, crystalline substance. It is starch-like in appearance and to the touch. Slightly soluble in water, in chloroform, and in ether; sparingly soluble in alcohol; soluble in ammonium hydroxide and in alkali hydroxides. Protect from light.

Adverse Effects and Precautions

As for Carbimazole, p.1521.

Propylthiouracil has been associated with greater hepatotoxicity than other thiourea antithyroid drugs (such as carbimazole or methimazole [thiamazole]). Rarely hepatitis, hepatic necrosis, encephalopathy, and death have occurred; asymptomatic liver damage is more common (see Effects on the Liver, p.1521).

Propylthiouracil should be given with care, and in reduced doses, to patients with renal impairment.

Pharmacokinetics

Propylthiouracil is rapidly absorbed from the gastrointestinal tract with peak plasma concentrations occurring about 1 to 2 hours following administration by mouth. It is concentrated in the thyroid gland and, since its duration of action is more closely related to the intrathyroidal drug concentration than its plasma half-life, this results in a prolongation of antithyroid activity such that single daily doses are possible. Propylthiouracil is 75 to 80% bound to plasma proteins.

Propylthiouracil has an elimination half-life of about 1 to 2 hours and is metabolised, probably by the liver, and excreted in the urine as unchanged drug (less than 2% of a dose) and metabolites; more than 50% of a dose is excreted as the glucuronic acid conjugate. The elimination half-life may be increased in renal and hepatic impairment.

Propylthiouracil crosses the placenta and is distributed into breast milk.

◊ References.
1. Kampmann JP, Hansen JM. Clinical pharmacokinetics of antithyroid drugs. *Clin Pharmacokinet* 1981; **6:** 401–28.
2. Giles HG, *et al.* Disposition of intravenous propylthiouracil. *J Clin Pharmacol* 1981; **21:** 466–71.
3. Kampmann JP, Hansen JEM. Serum protein binding of propylthiouracil. *Br J Clin Pharmacol* 1983; **16:** 549–52.

The symbol † denotes a preparation no longer actively marketed

Uses and Administration

Propylthiouracil is a thiourea antithyroid drug that acts by blocking the production of thyroid hormones (see p.1519); it also inhibits the peripheral deiodination of thyroxine to tri-iodothyronine. It is used in the management of hyperthyroidism (p.1519), including the treatment of Graves' disease, preparation of hyperthyroid patients for thyroidectomy, use as an adjunct to radio-iodine therapy, and the treatment of thyroid storm.

Propylthiouracil is given by mouth typically in an initial dosage of 200 to 400 mg daily. It has often been given in divided daily doses but once daily administration is also possible. Improvement is usually seen in 1 to 3 weeks and control of symptoms is achieved in 1 to 2 months. When the patient is euthyroid the dose is gradually reduced to a maintenance dose, usually 50 to 150 mg daily. Treatment is usually continued for at least a year, and often for 18 months. A suggested initial dose for children aged 6 to 10 years is 50 to 150 mg daily, and for children over 10 years 150 to 300 mg daily.

Doses should be reduced by 25% in mild to moderate renal impairment and by 50% in severe renal impairment. Doses may also need to be reduced in hepatic impairment.

Alcoholic liver disease. Propylthiouracil has been said to reduce hyperoxic liver injury in hypermetabolic *animals* and despite reports of hepatotoxicity, including some fatalities, associated with propylthiouracil (see Effects on the Liver, p.1521), it has been investigated in the treatment of patients with alcoholic liver disease. In a 2-year double-blind study[1] the 13% mortality rate in patients receiving propylthiouracil 300 mg daily was significantly lower than the 25% mortality rate in patients receiving placebo. The main effect of propylthiouracil appeared to be on acute alcoholic hepatitis as the difference in mortality rate was greatest during the first 12 weeks. However, Sherlock commented[2] that propylthiouracil had never gained general acceptance for the treatment of alcoholic liver disease.

1. Orrego H, *et al.* Long-term treatment of alcoholic liver disease with propylthiouracil. *N Engl J Med* 1987; **317:** 1421–7.
2. Sherlock S. Alcoholic liver disease. *Lancet* 1995; **345:** 227–9.

Psoriasis. Propylthiouracil has been tried orally[1] and topically[2] in a few patients with psoriasis (p.1106). The beneficial effects may be due to its immunomodulatory properties.

1. Elias AN, *et al.* Propylthiouracil in psoriasis: results of an open trial. *J Am Acad Dermatol* 1993; **29:** 78–81.
2. Elias AN, *et al.* A controlled trial of topical propylthiouracil in the treatment of patients with psoriasis. *J Am Acad Dermatol* 1994; **31:** 455–8.

Preparations

BP 2001: Propylthiouracil Tablets;
USP 25: Propylthiouracil Tablets.

Proprietary Preparations (details are given in Part 3)
Aust.: Prothiucil; **Canad.:** Propyl-Thyracil; **Ger.:** Propycil; Thyreostat II; **Israel:** Propylthiocil; **Port.:** Propycil; **Swed.:** Tiotil; **Thai.:** Propacil; Propyl; Uracil.

Sodium Perchlorate (13255-p)

NaClO$_4$ = 122.4.
CAS — 7601-89-0 (anhydrous sodium perchlorate); 7791-07-3 (sodium perchlorate, monohydrate).

◊ WARNING. *Sodium perchlorate has been used for the illicit preparation of explosives or fireworks; care is required with its supply.*

Profile

Sodium perchlorate has actions and uses similar to those of potassium perchlorate (p.1525). A dose of 200 to 400 mg by mouth has been given 30 to 60 minutes before radionuclide brain scanning.

It has been used to treat hyperthyroidism (p.1519) in an initial dose of 800 mg to 1 g daily by mouth in divided doses, reduced as required to a maintenance dose of 400 mg daily. Because of their toxicity the perchlorates have largely been replaced by other antithyroid drugs.

Preparations

Proprietary Preparations (details are given in Part 3)
Aust.: Irenat; **Ger.:** Irenat.

Thyroglobulin (9007-n)

Thyroglobulin (USAN, rINN).
CAS — 9010-34-8.

Profile

Thyroglobulin is an extract obtained by the fractionation of porcine thyroid glands, which yields thyroxine [levothyroxine] and liothyronine on hydrolysis. It has been used in the treatment of hypothyroidism, but such treatment with mixtures of thyroid hormones and preparations of animal extracts is not recommended.

Preparations

Proprietary Preparations (details are given in Part 3)
S.Afr.: Proloid†.

Thyroid (9001-a)

Dry Thyroid; Getrocknete Schilddrüse; NSC-26492; Thyreoidin; Thyroid Extract; Thyroid Gland; Thyroidea; Thyroideum Siccum; Tiroide Secca.
Pharmacopoeias. In Aust., Chin., Fr., Jpn, and US.

Pharmacopoeial description

USP 25: Thyroid is the cleaned, dried, and powdered thyroid gland, previously deprived of connective tissue and fat, obtained from domesticated animals used for food by humans. On hydrolysis it yields not less than 90% and not more than 110% each of the labelled amounts of thyroxine [levothyroxine] and liothyronine calculated on the dried basis. It is free from iodine in inorganic or any form of combination other than that peculiar to the thyroid gland. It may contain a suitable diluent such as glucose, lactose, sodium chloride, starch, or sucrose. A yellowish to buff-coloured amorphous powder, having a slight, characteristic, meat-like odour. Store in airtight containers.

Profile

Thyroid has been used in the treatment of hypothyroidism, but such treatment with mixtures of thyroid hormones and preparations of animal extracts is not recommended.

Preparations

USP 25: Thyroid Tablets.
Proprietary Preparations (details are given in Part 3)
Ital.: Cinetic; **USA:** S-P-T†; Thyrar†.
Multi-ingredient: **Braz.:** Emagrex; Esbelt; Esbeltrat; Macroten; Magroton; Normagrin; Obesidex; Obesifran; **Ger.:** AntiFocal; **Thai.:** Metharmon-F.

Thyroxine Sodium (9008-h)

Thyroxine Sodium (BANM).
Levothyroxine Sodium (BANM, rINN); Levothyroxinnatrium; Levothyroxinum Natricum; 3,5,3',5'-Tetra-iodo-L-thyronine Sodium; L-Thyroxine Sodium; Thyroxinum Natricum; Tirossina; Tiroxina Sodica. Sodium 4-O-(4-hydroxy-3,5-di-iodophenyl)-3,5-di-iodo-L-tyrosine hydrate.
C$_{15}$H$_{10}$I$_4$NNaO$_4$,xH$_2$O = 798.9 (anhydrous).
CAS — 51-48-9 (L-thyroxine [levothyroxine]); 55-03-8 (anhydrous thyroxine [levothyroxine] sodium); 25416-65-3 (thyroxine [levothyroxine] sodium; hydrate); 8065-29-0 (liotrix).
ATC — H03AA01.

NOTE. The abbreviation T$_4$ is often used for endogenous thyroxine in medical and biochemical reports. Liotrix is the *USAN* name for a mixture of liothyronine sodium with thyroxine [levothyroxine] sodium.
Pharmacopoeias. In Eur. (see p.vi), Int., Jpn, and US.
Int. includes the anhydrous. Aust. also includes a monograph on DL-thyroxine.

Pharmacopoeial description

Ph. Eur.: An almost white or slightly brownish-yellow powder or a fine, crystalline powder. Very slightly soluble in water; slightly soluble in alcohol; practically insoluble in ether. It dissolves in dilute solutions of alkali hydroxides. Store at 2° to 8° in airtight containers. Protect from light.

USP 25: The sodium salt of the laevo-isomer of thyroxine [levothyroxine], obtained from the thyroid gland of domesticated animals used for food by man or prepared synthetically. A light yellow to buff-coloured, odourless, hygroscopic, powder. It may assume a slight pink colour on exposure to light. Soluble 1 in 700 of water and 1 in 300 of alcohol; insoluble in acetone, in chloroform, and in ether; soluble in solutions of alkali hydroxides and in hot solutions of alkali carbonates. pH of a saturated solution in water is about 8.9. Store in airtight containers. Protect from light.

Adverse Effects and Treatment

The adverse effects of thyroxine [levothyroxine] are generally associated with excessive dosage and correspond to symptoms of hyperthyroidism. They may include tachycardia, palpitations, cardiac arrhythmias, anginal pain, headache, nervousness, excitability, insomnia, tremors, muscle weakness and cramps, heat intolerance, sweating, flushing, fever, weight loss, menstrual irregularities, diarrhoea, and vomiting. These adverse reactions usually disappear after dosage reduction or temporary withdrawal of treatment. Thyroid storm has occasionally been reported following massive or chronic intoxication and convulsions,

cardiac arrhythmias, heart failure, coma, and death have occurred.

In acute overdosage, gastrointestinal absorption may be reduced by activated charcoal. Treatment is usually symptomatic and supportive; propranolol may be useful in controlling the symptoms of sympathetic overactivity. Thyroxine [levothyroxine] overdosage requires an extended follow-up period as symptoms may be delayed for up to 6 days due to the gradual peripheral conversion of thyroxine [levothyroxine] to tri-iodothyronine.

Carcinogenicity. An association between the use of thyroid hormones and an increased risk of breast cancer in women has been proposed,[1] but a further analysis of the data did not confirm such an association,[2] and nor did later studies.[3-5]

1. Kapdi CC, Wolfe JN. Breast cancer. Relationship to thyroid supplements for hypothyroidism. *JAMA* 1976; **236:** 1124–7.
2. Mustacchi P, Greenspan F. Thyroid supplementation for hypothyroidism. An iatrogenic cause of breast cancer? *JAMA* 1977; **237:** 1446–7.
3. Wallace RB, *et al.* Thyroid hormone use in patients with breast cancer. Absence of an association. *JAMA* 1978; **239:** 958.
4. Shapiro S, *et al.* Use of thyroid supplements in relation to the risk of breast cancer. *JAMA* 1980; **244:** 1685–7.
5. Hoffman DA, *et al.* Breast cancer in hypothyroid women using thyroid supplements. *JAMA* 1984; **251:** 616–19.

Effects on the bones. Hyperthyroidism is a known risk factor for osteoporosis and some studies have indicated that women receiving long-term thyroxine [levothyroxine] therapy may have decreased bone density or accelerated bone mineralisation and thus be at greater risk of developing osteoporosis.[1-5] The bone changes were greatest in those who had some degree of overtreatment resulting in subclinical hyperthyroidism (usually indicated by low TSH concentrations) and therefore strict attention to monitoring of therapy by using sensitive TSH assays, and possibly the use of bone studies, has been advised.[1-6] A meta-analysis of the effects of thyroid hormones on bone density also suggested that prolonged therapy (some 10 years) reduced bone density.[7] Conversely, other studies have not found thyroxine [levothyroxine] treatment to affect bone density,[8,9] and even in postmenopausal women receiving relatively high doses of thyroxine [levothyroxine] there is evidence that any deleterious effect on the bones may be prevented by oestrogen replacement therapy.[10]

1. Paul TL, *et al.* Long-term L-thyroxine therapy is associated with decreased hip bone density in premenopausal women. *JAMA* 1988; **259:** 3137–41.
2. Stall GM, *et al.* Accelerated bone loss in hypothyroid patients overtreated with L-thyroxine. *Ann Intern Med* 1990; **113:** 265–9.
3. Adlin EV, *et al.* Bone mineral density in postmenopausal women treated with L-thyroxine. *Am J Med* 1991; **90:** 360–6.
4. Kung AWC, Pun KK. Bone mineral density in premenopausal women receiving long-term physiological doses of levothyroxine. *JAMA* 1991; **265:** 2688–91.
5. Greenspan SL, *et al.* Skeletal integrity in premenopausal and postmenopausal women receiving long-term L-thyroxine therapy. *Am J Med* 1991; **91:** 5–14.
6. Greenspan SL, Greenspan FS. The effect of thyroid hormone on skeletal integrity. *Ann Intern Med* 1999; **130:** 750–8.
7. Uzzan B, *et al.* Effects on bone mass of long-term treatment with thyroid hormones: a meta-analysis. *J Clin Endocrinol Metab* 1996; **81:** 4278–89.
8. Franklyn JA, *et al.* Long-term thyroxine treatment and bone mineral density. *Lancet* 1992; **340:** 9–13.
9. Ross DS. Bone density is not reduced during the short-term administration of levothyroxine to postmenopausal women with subclinical hypothyroidism: a randomized prospective study. *Am J Med* 1993; **95:** 385–8.
10. Schneider DL, *et al.* Thyroid hormone use and bone mineral density in elderly women: effects of estrogen. *JAMA* 1994; **271:** 1245–9.

Effects on the nervous system. Two children aged 8 and 11 years developed pseudotumour cerebri (benign intracranial hypertension) shortly after the initiation of thyroxine [levothyroxine] therapy for hypothyroidism.[1] There have been further reports on individual children[2,3] and infants.[4]

Partial complex status epilepticus, with confusion, agitation, and continuous myoclonic jerks in the left side of the face and left hand, was seen in a hypothyroid patient with Turner's syndrome who was receiving treatment with thyroxine [levothyroxine] for myxoedema coma.[5] The condition responded to anticonvulsant therapy; the patient subsequently remained seizure-free on a reduced dose of thyroxine [levothyroxine] and concomitant phenytoin.

1. Van Dop C, *et al.* Pseudotumor cerebri associated with initiation of levothyroxine therapy for juvenile hypothyroidism. *N Engl J Med* 1983; **308:** 1076–80.
2. McVie R. Pseudotumor cerebri and thyroid-replacement therapy. *N Engl J Med* 1983; **309:** 731.
3. Hymes LC, *et al.* Pseudotumor cerebri and thyroid-replacement therapy. *N Engl J Med* 1983; **309:** 732.
4. Raghavan S, *et al.* Pseudotumor cerebri in an infant after L-thyroxine therapy for transient neonatal hypothyroidism. *J Pediatr* 1997; **130:** 478–80.
5. Duarte J, *et al.* Thyroxine-induced partial complex status epilepticus. *Ann Pharmacother* 1993; **27:** 1139.

Hypersensitivity. A hypersensitivity reaction to synthetic thyroid hormones was reported in a 63-year-old hypothyroid woman with Hashimoto's thyroiditis.[1] Fever, eosinophilia, and liver dysfunction developed after replacement treatment with liothyronine or thyroxine [levothyroxine], but disappeared when therapy was discontinued. After an interval of 4 months liothyronine was gradually reintroduced without adverse effect.

Urticaria and angioedema has been described in a patient who received thyroid and thyroxine [levothyroxine].[2] In a further case similar reactions were attributed to the presence of sunset yellow as colouring agent in the proprietary thyroxine [levothyroxine] preparation.[3]

1. Shibata H, *et al.* Hypersensitivity caused by synthetic thyroid hormones in a hypothyroid patient with Hashimoto's thyroiditis. *Arch Intern Med* 1986; **146:** 1624–5.
2. Pandya AG, *et al.* Chronic urticaria associated with exogenous thyroid use. *Arch Dermatol* 1990; **126:** 1238–9.
3. Lévesque H, *et al.* Reporting adverse drug reactions by proprietary name. *Lancet* 1991; **338:** 393.

Overdosage. The clinical features and management of overdosage with thyroid drugs have been reviewed.[1] Although aggressive therapy is not normally justified in asymptomatic patients, various regimens have been tried.

Massive overdoses of thyroxine [levothyroxine] ranging from 70 to 1200 mg over 2 to 12 days have been described in 6 patients.[2] All the patients developed symptoms of thyrotoxicosis within 3 days of taking the first dose. Treatment was tried using propranolol 120 to 140 mg daily, with hydrocortisone 400 mg daily, and in 3 patients, propylthiouracil 400 to 1200 mg daily, but the benefits of such therapy were considered doubtful. Seven to 10 days after the first dose of thyroxine [levothyroxine], all 6 patients developed neurological complications and 5 went into coma. Cardiac disturbances were also noted; 2 had left ventricular failure and 3 developed severe arrhythmias. Plasmapheresis and charcoal haemoperfusion were both found to increase the elimination of L-thyroxine [levothyroxine] from serum. Plasmapheresis appeared to be the more effective procedure, though the magnitude of the extraction of L-thyroxine [levothyroxine] depended on the serum concentration of L-thyroxine [levothyroxine]. One patient died of septic shock and acute renal failure; the other 5 recovered after troubled courses.

In another report,[3] fever, confusion, agitation, and tachycardia developed 5 days after ingestion of approximately 720 mg of thyroxine [levothyroxine], despite treatment with activated charcoal and a cathartic at the time of ingestion (at which point the patient was asymptomatic). Despite treatment with diazepam 380 mg and phenobarbital 1 g intravenously complete sedation could not be achieved; the patient remained tachycardic and febrile for a further 7 days, during which propranolol 10 mg was given intravenously about every 6 hours, along with further diazepam as required. Symptoms subsequently resolved over about 2 weeks.

In a further study[4] of 41 children aged 1 to 5 years who had accidentally ingested estimated amounts of thyroxine [levothyroxine] sodium ranging from 0.05 to 13 mg, symptoms of hyperthyroidism occurred in only 11 between 12 hours and 11 days after ingestion. Treatment was limited to initial measures to decrease absorption; no adverse effect was considered severe enough to warrant specific symptomatic treatment and all symptoms fully resolved within 14 days. These findings appeared to be consistent with previous reports, although there has been a report[5] of a 2-year-old boy who developed clinical signs of hyperthyroidism and suffered 2 episodes of tonic-clonic seizures 7 days after the ingestion of up to 18 mg of thyroxine [levothyroxine] sodium. However, since serious complications appeared to be uncommon and most symptoms remitted without treatment, a conservative approach to the management of acute thyroxine [levothyroxine] overdosage in children was recommended.[4]

1. Lin T-H, *et al.* Clinical features and management of overdosage with thyroid drugs. *Med Toxicol* 1988; **3:** 264–72.
2. Binimelis J, *et al.* Massive thyroxine intoxication: evaluation of plasma extraction. *Intensive Care Med* 1987; **13:** 33–8.
3. Hack JB, *et al.* Severe symptoms following a massive intentional L-thyroxine ingestion. *Vet Hum Toxicol* 1999; **41:** 323–6.
4. Golightly LK, *et al.* Clinical effects of accidental levothyroxine ingestion in children. *Am J Dis Child* 1987; **141:** 1025–7.
5. Kulig K, *et al.* Levothyroxine overdosage associated with seizures in a young child. *JAMA* 1985; **254:** 2109–10.

Precautions

Thyroxine [levothyroxine] is contra-indicated in untreated hyperthyroidism. It should be used with extreme caution in patients with cardiovascular disorders including angina, heart failure, myocardial infarction, and hypertension; lower initial doses, smaller increments, and longer intervals between increases should be used as necessary. An ECG performed before starting treatment with thyroxine [levothyroxine] may help to distinguish underlying myocardial ischaemia from changes induced by hypothyroidism. Thyroxine [levothyroxine] should also be introduced very gradually in elderly patients and those with long-standing hypothyroidism to avoid any sudden increase in metabolic demands. It should not be given to patients with adrenal insufficiency without adequate corticosteroid cover otherwise the thyroid replacement therapy might precipitate an acute adrenal crisis. Care is also required when

thyroxine [levothyroxine] is given to patients with diabetes mellitus or diabetes insipidus.

Tests of thyroid function are subject to alteration by a number of nonthyroidal clinical conditions and by a wide variety of drugs, some of which are mentioned under Interactions, below.

Abuse. For mention of abuse of thyroxine [levothyroxine] by athletes for weight loss see Obesity, under Uses and Administration, below.

Adrenocortical insufficiency. Thyroid-hormone replacement without concomitant treatment with corticosteroids may precipitate acute adrenocortical insufficiency in patients with impaired adrenocortical function, including those with subclinical or unrecognised adrenocortical disease.[1] Prompt diagnosis and replacement of corticosteroids can prevent the development of a potentially fatal crisis. It has been pointed out that a raised concentration of thyroid-stimulating-hormone alone may not necessarily imply hypothyroidism in patients with chronic adrenocortical insufficiency.[2] Even confirmed hypothyroidism in these patients may not be permanent.

1. Fonseca V, *et al.* Acute adrenal crisis precipitated by thyroxine. *BMJ* 1986; **292:** 1185–6.
2. Davis J, Sheppard M. Acute adrenal crisis precipitated by thyroxine. *BMJ* 1986; **292:** 1595.

Cardiovascular disorders. There is a complex relationship between the heart and thyroid.[1] Cardiovascular abnormalities may be associated with hypothyroidism as well as with thyroxine [levothyroxine] replacement therapy, hence the need for caution.

1. Gammage M, Franklyn J. Hypothyroidism, thyroid treatment, and the heart. *Heart* 1997; **77:** 189–90.

Myasthenia. Thyroid hormones may occasionally precipitate or exacerbate a pre-existing myasthenic syndrome.[1,2]

1. Mastaglia FL. Adverse effects of drugs on muscle. *Drugs* 1982; **24:** 304–21.
2. Lane RJM, Routledge PA. Drug-induced neurological disorders. *Drugs* 1983; **26:** 124–47.

Pregnancy and breast feeding. Most authorities consider that thyroid hormones do not readily cross the placenta. Placental transfer has been reported,[1] but in amounts so limited that a mother with physiological concentrations of thyroxine and tri-iodothyronine would not provide normal thyroid hormone concentrations to a fetus with congenital hypothyroidism.[2-4]

Minimal amounts of thyroid hormones are distributed into breast milk.[5] There is insufficient thyroid hormone to meet the biological needs of a suckling infant with a nonfunctioning thyroid gland but it has been suggested that thyroxine [levothyroxine] in breast milk might mask any hypothyroidism in the suckling newborn.[6]

1. Vulsma T, *et al.* Maternal-fetal transfer of thyroxine in congenital hypothyroidism due to a total organification defect or thyroid agenesis. *N Engl J Med* 1989; **321:** 13–16.
2. Sack J, *et al.* Maternal-fetal transfer of thyroxine. *N Engl J Med* 1989; **321:** 1549–50.
3. Bachrach LK, Burrow GN. Maternal-fetal transfer of thyroxine. *N Engl J Med* 1989; **321:** 1549.
4. Vulsma T, *et al.* Maternal-fetal transfer of thyroxine. *N Engl J Med* 1989; **321:** 1550.
5. Bennett PN, ed. *Drugs and human lactation.* Amsterdam: Elsevier, 1988.
6. Anonymous. Can a woman on thyroxine safely breast-feed her baby? *BMJ* 1977; **2:** 1589.

Interactions

Antiarrhythmics. *Amiodarone*[1] may inhibit the de-iodination of thyroxine to tri-iodothyronine resulting in a decreased concentration of tri-iodothyronine with a concomitant rise in the concentration of inactive reverse tri-iodothyronine.

1. Hershman JM, *et al.* Thyroxine and triiodothyronine kinetics in cardiac patients taking amiodarone. *Acta Endocrinol (Copenh)* 1986; **111:** 193–9.

Antibacterials. Enzyme induction by *rifampicin*[1] enhances thyroid hormone metabolism resulting in reduced serum concentrations of thyroid hormones.

1. Ohnhaus EE, Studer H. A link between liver microsomal enzyme activity and thyroid hormone metabolism in man. *Br J Clin Pharmacol* 1983; **15:** 71–6.

Anticoagulants. Thyroid hormones enhance the effects of *oral anticoagulants.* Patients on anticoagulant therapy therefore require careful monitoring when treatment with thyroid drugs is initiated or altered as the oral anticoagulant dose may need to be adjusted (see under the interactions of Warfarin, p.997).

Antidepressants. Some drugs such as *lithium* act directly on the thyroid gland and inhibit the release of thyroid hormones leading to clinical hypothyroidism.[1]

The effects of thyroxine [levothyroxine] in hypothyroid patients may be decreased by concomitant administration of *sertraline*, and the dose of thyroxine [levothyroxine] may need to be increased.[2]

For the effects of thyroid hormones on *tricyclic antidepressants* see under Amitriptyline, p.278.

1. Ramsay I. Drugs and non-thyroid induced changes in thyroid function tests. *Postgrad Med J* 1985; **61:** 375–7.

2. McCowen KC, *et al.* Elevated serum thyrotropin in thyroxine-treated patients with hypothyroidism given sertraline. *N Engl J Med* 1997; **337:** 1010–11.

Antidiabetics. As thyroid status influences metabolic activity and most body systems, correction of hypothyroidism with thyroid drugs may affect other disease states and their treatment. In hypothyroid diabetics for instance, the initiation of thyroid replacement therapy may increase their *insulin* or *oral hypoglycaemic* requirements.[1]

1. Refetoff S. Thyroid hormone therapy. *Med Clin North Am* 1975; **59:** 1147–62.

Antiepileptics. Enzyme induction by drugs such as *carbamazepine*,[1,2] *phenytoin*,[2,3] or *barbiturates*[4] enhances thyroid hormone metabolism resulting in reduced serum concentrations of thyroid hormones. Therefore, patients on thyroid replacement therapy may require an increase in their dose of thyroid hormone if these drugs are given concurrently[5] and a decrease if the enzyme-inducing drug is withdrawn.[6] *Phenytoin*,[3] and *carbamazepine* may reduce protein binding by displacing the thyroid hormones from their plasma-binding sites. As thyroid hormones are highly protein bound, changes in binding might be expected to influence requirements in thyroid replacement therapy, but in practice there is little clinical evidence of any problems except with thyroid-function testing.

1. Connell JMC, *et al.* Changes in circulating thyroid hormones during short-term hepatic enzyme induction with carbamazepine. *Eur J Clin Pharmacol* 1984; **26:** 453–6.
2. Larkin JG, *et al.* Thyroid hormone concentrations in epileptic patients. *Eur J Clin Pharmacol* 1989; **36:** 213–6.
3. Franklyn JA, *et al.* Measurement of free thyroid hormones in patients on long-term phenytoin therapy. *Eur J Clin Pharmacol* 1984; **26:** 633–4.
4. Ohnhaus EE, Studer H. A link between liver microsomal enzyme activity and thyroid hormone metabolism in man. *Br J Clin Pharmacol* 1983; **15:** 71–6.
5. Blackshear JL, *et al.* Thyroxine replacement requirements in hypothyroid patients receiving phenytoin. *Ann Intern Med* 1983; **99:** 341–2.
6. Hoffbrand BI. Barbiturate/thyroid-hormone interaction. *Lancet* 1979; **ii:** 903–4.

Antimalarials. Increased thyroid-stimulating hormone concentration has been noted following the use of combined *chloroquine* and *proguanil* chemoprophylaxis for malaria in a patient stabilised on thyroxine [levothyroxine].[1] Induction of liver enzymes by chloroquine resulting in increased metabolism of thyroxine [levothyroxine] was suggested as the mechanism.

1. Munera Y, *et al.* Interaction of thyroxine sodium with antimalarial drugs. *BMJ* 1997; **314:** 1593.

Antivirals. There has been an isolated report of an interaction between *ritonavir* and thyroxine [levothyroxine], resulting in an increased requirement for thyroxine [levothyroxine] supplementation.[1]

1. Tseng A, Fletcher D. Interaction between ritonavir and levothyroxine. *AIDS* 1998; **12:** 2235–6.

Beta blockers. Studies have indicated that plasma concentrations of *propranolol* are reduced in hyperthyroidism compared with the euthyroid state, probably due to increased clearance[1-4] and hypothyroid patients receiving chronic propranolol therapy have had a reduction in plasma-propranolol concentrations when given thyroxine [levothyroxine] treatment.[2]

Propranolol[5,6] may inhibit the de-iodination of thyroxine to tri-iodothyronine resulting in a decreased concentration of tri-iodothyronine with a concomitant rise in the concentration of inactive reverse tri-iodothyronine.

1. Feely J, *et al.* Increased clearance of propranolol in thyrotoxicosis. *Ann Intern Med* 1981; **94:** 472–4.
2. Feely J, *et al.* Plasma propranolol steady state concentrations in thyroid disorders. *Eur J Clin Pharmacol* 1981; **19:** 329–33.
3. Aro A, *et al.* Pharmacokinetics of propranolol and sotalol in hyperthyroidism. *Eur J Clin Pharmacol* 1982; **21:** 373–7.
4. Hallengren B, *et al.* Influence of hyperthyroidism on the kinetics of methimazole, propranolol, metoprolol, and atenolol. *Eur J Clin Pharmacol* 1982; **21:** 379–84.
5. Chambers JB, *et al.* The effects of propranolol on thyroxine metabolism and triiodothyronines production in man. *J Clin Pharmacol* 1982; **22:** 110–16.
6. Wilkins MR, *et al.* Effect of propranolol on thyroid homeostasis of healthy volunteers. *Postgrad Med J* 1985; **61:** 391–4.

Cardiac glycosides. Serum-digoxin concentrations appear to be lower in hyperthyroidism and higher in hypothyroidism[1] which may contribute in part to the observed insensitivity of hyperthyroid patients to *digoxin* therapy[2] although other mechanisms have been proposed.[3]

1. Croxson MS, Ibbertson HK. Serum digoxin in patients with thyroid disease. *BMJ* 1975; **3:** 566–8.
2. Huffman DH, *et al.* Digoxin in hyperthyroidism. *Clin Pharmacol Ther* 1977; **22:** 533–8.
3. Lawrence JR, *et al.* Digoxin kinetics in patients with thyroid dysfunction. *Clin Pharmacol Ther* 1977; **22:** 7–13.

Gastrointestinal drugs. *Sucralfate* reduces absorption of thyroxine [levothyroxine] from the gastrointestinal tract[1,2] as does *aluminium hydroxide*,[3] and *calcium carbonate*.[4]

1. Sherman SI, *et al.* Sucralfate causes malabsorption of L-thyroxine. *Am J Med* 1994; **96:** 531–5.
2. Campbell JA, *et al.* Sucralfate and the absorption of L-thyroxine. *Ann Intern Med* 1994; **121:** 152.
3. Liel Y, *et al.* Nonspecific intestinal adsorption of levothyroxine by aluminium hydroxide. *Am J Med* 1994; **97:** 363–5.
4. Schneyer CR. Calcium carbonate and reduction of levothyroxine efficacy. *JAMA* 1998; **279:** 750.

General anaesthetics. Severe hypertension and tachycardia have been reported[1] when *ketamine* was used in patients taking thyroxine [levothyroxine].

1. Kaplan JA, Cooperman LH. Alarming reactions to ketamine in patients taking thyroid medication-treatment with propranolol. *Anesthesiology* 1971; **35**: 229–30.

Ion-exchange resins. *Colestyramine* significantly reduces the absorption of ingested thyroxine [levothyroxine] by binding with thyroid hormones in the gastrointestinal tract. The malabsorption of thyroxine [levothyroxine] is minimised by allowing an interval of 4 to 5 hours to elapse between the ingestion of the two drugs.[1] A similar effect has been observed with *sodium polystyrene sulfonate*.[2]

1. Northcutt RC, *et al.* The influence of cholestyramine on thyroxine absorption. *JAMA* 1969; **208**: 1857–61.
2. McLean M, *et al.* Cation-exchange resin and inhibition of intestinal absorption of thyroxine. *Lancet* 1993; **341**: 1286.

Iron salts. *Ferrous sulfate* reduces absorption of thyroxine [levothyroxine] from the gastrointestinal tract.[1]

1. Campbell NRC, *et al.* Ferrous sulfate reduces thyroxine efficacy in patients with hypothyroidism. *Ann Intern Med* 1992; **117**: 1010–13.

Lipid regulating drugs. Both decreased efficacy[1] and increased efficacy[2] of thyroxine [levothyroxine] have been reported in individual patients given *lovastatin*.

1. Demke DM. Drug interaction between thyroxine and lovastatin. *N Engl J Med* 1989; **321**: 1341–2.
2. Gormley GJ, Tobert JA. Drug interaction between thyroxine and lovastatin. *N Engl J Med* 1989; **321**: 1342.

NSAIDs. Falsely low total plasma concentrations of thyroxine [levothyroxine] have reportedly been observed during concurrent treatment with some anti-inflammatory drugs.

Sex hormones. *Oestrogen* therapy increases serum concentrations of thyroxine-binding globulin, thus increasing the amount of bound thyroxine. Normal thyroid function stimulates thyroxine synthesis to compensate for this effect and maintain normal free-thyroxine serum concentrations. In hypothyroidism, however, patients treated with exogenous thyroxine [levothyroxine] who receive oestrogens, as in oral contraceptives or hormone replacement therapy,[3] may require an increase in thyroxine [levothyroxine] dose. In contrast, *androgens* reduce the concentration of the binding globulin, which has resulted in clinical hyperthyroidism when given to postmenopausal women maintained on thyroxine [levothyroxine] replacement therapy.[2]

2. Arafah BM. Decreased levothyroxine requirement in women with hypothyroidism during androgen therapy for breast cancer. *Ann Intern Med* 1994; **121**: 247–51.
3. Arafah BM. Increased need for thyroxine in women with hypothyroidism during estrogen therapy. *N Engl J Med* 2001; **344**: 1743–9.

Sympathomimetics. Thyroid drugs increase metabolic demands and should therefore be used with caution with other drugs known to influence cardiac function, such as the *sympathomimetics*, as they may enhance this effect. In addition, thyroid hormones may increase receptor sensitivity to catecholamines.

Pharmacokinetics

Thyroxine [levothyroxine] is variably but adequately absorbed from the gastrointestinal tract following oral administration. Fasting increases absorption. Once in the circulation, thyroxine [levothyroxine] is extensively protein bound, principally to thyroxine-binding globulin (TBG) but also to a lesser extent to thyroxine-binding pre-albumin (TBPA) or to albumin. Thyroxine [levothyroxine] has a plasma half-life in euthyroidism of about 6 to 7 days; the half-life is prolonged in hypothyroidism and reduced in hyperthyroidism.

Thyroxine [levothyroxine] is primarily metabolised in the liver and kidney to tri-iodothyronine (liothyronine) and, about 40%, to inactive reverse triiodothyronine (reverse T_3) both of which undergo further deiodination to inactive metabolites. Further metabolites result from the deamination and decarboxylation of thyroxine [levothyroxine] to tetrac.

Thyroxine [levothyroxine] is reported to undergo enterohepatic recycling and excretion in the faeces.

The distribution of thyroid hormones across the placenta and into breast milk is discussed under Pregnancy and Breast Feeding (above).

Uses and Administration

Thyroxine [levothyroxine] is a thyroid hormone (see p.1519 for a description of the endogenous hormones) used as replacement therapy in the treatment of hypothyroidism (p.1520). It is given in conditions such as diffuse non-toxic goitre (see Goitre and Thyroid Nodules, p.1519) and Hashimoto's thyroiditis (see Hypothyroidism, p.1520) to suppress the secretion of thyroid-stimulating hormone (TSH) and hence prevent or reverse enlargement of the thyroid gland. Thyroxine [levothyroxine] is also used to suppress TSH production in the treatment of thyroid carcinoma (p.500) and as a diagnostic agent for the differential diagnosis of hyperthyroidism. It is given with antithyroid drugs in the management of hyperthyroidism (p.1519).

The peak therapeutic effect of regular oral administration of thyroxine [levothyroxine] may not be achieved until after several weeks and there is a slow response to changes in dosage. Similarly, effects may persist for several weeks after withdrawal. Thyroxine [levothyroxine] is given as the sodium salt in a single daily dose. Its absorption can be irregular and it is probably best taken on an empty stomach, usually before breakfast.

The dose of thyroxine [levothyroxine] sodium for the treatment of any thyroid disorder should be individualised on the basis of clinical response and biochemical tests and should be monitored regularly.

In **hypothyroidism** an initial adult dose of 50 to 100 µg of thyroxine [levothyroxine] sodium daily by mouth may be increased by 25 to 50 µg at intervals of about 4 weeks until the thyroid deficiency is corrected and a maintenance dose is established. The adult maintenance dose is usually between 100 and 200 µg daily. In elderly patients, in those with cardiovascular disorders, or in those with severe hypothyroidism of long standing, treatment should be introduced more gradually: an initial dose of 12.5 to 50 µg daily increased by increments of 12.5 to 25 µg at intervals of 4 weeks may be appropriate.

In children, individualisation of dosage and monitoring of treatment is especially important. One recommended regimen for the treatment of congenital hypothyroidism is 10 to 15 µg per kg body-weight daily, adjusted as necessary. Another regimen suggests an initial dose of 5 to 10 µg per kg daily in children up to 1 month of age (or 5 µg per kg in children over 1 month), adjusted in steps of 25 µg every 2 to 4 weeks until mild toxic symptoms appear, at which time the dosage is slightly reduced. For juvenile myxoedema, children over 1 year of age may be given 2.5 to 5 µg per kg body-weight daily initially.

Thyroxine [levothyroxine] sodium may also be given by the nasogastric route or by intravenous injection. It has also been given intramuscularly. In myxoedema (hypothyroid) coma doses of 200 to 500 µg by intravenous injection may be given initially, followed by daily supplements of 75 to 100 µg until the patient is euthyroid and can tolerate administration by mouth.

◊ General references.

1. Mandel SJ, *et al.* Levothyroxine therapy in patients with thyroid disease. *Ann Intern Med* 1993; **119**: 492–502.
2. Toft AD. Thyroxine therapy. *N Engl J Med* 1994; **331**: 174–80. Correction. *ibid.*; 1035.

Administration. There has been controversy over the bioequivalence or otherwise of different brands of thyroxine [levothyroxine]. Most studies and reports have come from the USA and results may have depended to some extent on the particular brands compared. Formulations may also have changed which makes comparison of results difficult. A recently published study[1] concluded that 2 generic thyroxine [levothyroxine] products were bioequivalent and interchangeable with 2 branded products.

1. Dong BJ, *et al.* Bioequivalence of generic and brand-name levothyroxine products in the treatment of hypothyroidism. *JAMA* 1997; **277**: 1205–13.

Cardiomyopathies. Management of dilated cardiomyopathy (p.796) usually involves conventional therapy for symptoms of heart failure, but a small study has reported benefit from short-term administration of thyroxine.[1] Thyroxine administration was well tolerated but thyroid-stimulating hormone levels were reduced and this might limit long-term therapy with thyroxine.

1. Moruzzi P, *et al.* Medium-term effectiveness of L-thyroxine treatment in idiopathic dilated cardiomyopathy. *Am J Med* 1996; **101**: 461–7.

Depression. While thyroid hormones may increase the activity of tricyclic antidepressants (see Thyroid Hormones, under Interactions of Amitriptyline, p.278), the benefits in the augmentation treatment of refractory depression (p.271) are debatable. A meta-analysis[1] of 8 studies involving 292 patients treated with liothyronine in addition to tricyclic antidepressants indicated that such therapy was effective in a subgroup of cases but that the small number of patients studied made additional placebo-controlled data desirable. It was also noted that current trends in the treatment of depression favoured drugs other than tricyclics, so that future trials with liothyronine may need to investigate combination treatment with selective serotonin reuptake inhibitors.

1. Aronson R, *et al.* Triiodothyronine augmentation in the treatment of refractory depression: a meta-analysis. *Arch Gen Psychiatry* 1996; **53**: 842–8.

Obesity. Thyroid drugs have been tried in the treatment of obesity (p.1505) in euthyroid patients, but they produce only temporary weight loss, mainly of lean body-mass, and can produce serious adverse effects, especially cardiac complications.[1] Hypothyroidism has also been reported[2] when these drugs were withdrawn from previously euthyroid patients being treated for simple obesity. It has also been noted that thyroxine [levothyroxine] is probably being abused by some athletes to promote weight loss.[3]

1. Rivlin RS. Therapy of obesity with hormones. *N Engl J Med* 1975; **292**: 26–9.
2. Dornhorst A, *et al.* Possible iatrogenic hypothyroidism. *Lancet* 1981; **i**: 52.
3. MacAuley D. Drugs in sport. *BMJ* 1996; **313**: 211–15.

Urticaria. There is some suggestion that chronic urticaria (p.1107) may be associated with thyroid autoimmunity and that treatment with thyroid hormones may result in clinical remission.[1] In one study, a nine-year-old boy was successfully treated for chronic urticaria with thyroxine [levothyroxine] therapy at doses of 50 to 100 µg daily.[2] The workers advised screening for thyroid function and anti-thyroid microsomal antibodies in cases of chronic urticaria as these patients may benefit from thyroid hormone therapy.

1. Rumbyrt JS, *et al.* Resolution of chronic urticaria in patients with thyroid autoimmunity. *J Allergy Clin Immunol* 1995; **96**: 901–5.
2. Dreyfus DH, *et al.* Steroid-resistant chronic urticaria associated with anti-thyroid microsomal antibodies in a nine-year-old boy. *J Pediatr* 1996; **128**: 576–8.

Preparations

BP 2001: Levothyroxine Tablets;
USP 25: Levothyroxine Sodium Tablets; Liotrix Tablets.

Proprietary Preparations (details are given in Part 3)

Aust.: Euthyrox; Thyrex; **Austral.:** Oroxine; **Belg.:** Elthyrone; Euthyrox; Thyrax; **Braz.:** Puran T4; Tetroid; **Canad.:** Elthroxin; Levo-T†; Levotec; Synthroid; **Denm.:** Eltroxin; **Fr.:** Levothyrox; **Ger.:** Berlthyrox; Eferox; Euthyrox; Thevier; **Hong Kong:** Eltroxin; **Irl.:** Eltroxin; **Israel:** Eltroxin; **Ital.:** Eutirox; Tiracrin; Tirosint; **Jpn.:** Thyradin-S; **Mex.:** Daltroid; Eutirox; Tiroidine; **Neth.:** Eltroxin; Euthyrox; Thyrax; **NZ:** Eltroxin; **Port.:** Letequatro; Letter; Thyrax; **S.Afr.:** Eltroxin; **Singapore:** Eltroxin; Euthyrox; Oroxine; **Spain:** Dexnon; Levothroid; Thyrax; **Swed.:** Levaxin; **Switz.:** Eltroxin; **Thai.:** Eltroxin; Thyrosit; **UK:** Eltroxin; **USA:** Eltroxin; Levo-T; Levothroid; Levoxyl; Synthroid; Unithroid.

Multi-ingredient: Aust.: Combithyrex; Jodthyrox; Novothyral; Prothyrid; **Belg.:** Novothyral; **Braz.:** Levotiroxina; Tyroplus; **Fr.:** Euthyral; **Ger.:** Jodthyrox; Novothyral; Prothyrid; Thyreocomb N; Thyreotom; Thyronajod; **Ital.:** Dermocinetic; Somatoline; Tiroide Amsa; **Mex.:** Novotiral; Proloid S; **S.Afr.:** Diotroxin; **Switz.:** Novothyral; **USA:** Thyrolar.

Tiratricol (9009-m)

Tiratricol *(rINN)*.

Triac; Triiodothyroacetic Acid. [4-(4-Hydroxy-3-iodophenoxy)-3,5-di-iodophenyl]acetic acid.

$C_{14}H_9I_3O_4 = 621.9.$
$CAS — 51-24-1.$
$ATC — D11AX08; H03AA04.$

NOTE. Tri-ac has also been used as a name for proprietary preparations containing other drugs.

Profile

Tiratricol, a metabolite of tri-iodothyronine, is reported to be less active than the thyroid hormones but is given by mouth to suppress the secretion of thyroid-stimulating hormone.

Obesity. Abnormal thyroid function tests, severe diarrhoea, fatigue, lethargy, and profound weight loss have occurred in patients taking dietary supplements containing tiratricol.[1] The FDA has warned that tiratricol may cause heart attacks and strokes, and has advised consumers not to take these products.[1]

1. Anonymous. Triax®: a harmful product sold on the internet. *WHO Drug Inf* 2000; **14**: 30.

Preparations

Proprietary Preparations (details are given in Part 3)

Braz.: Dimagress; Obelin; Triac; Trimag; **Fr.:** Teatrois; Triacana.

Vaccines Immunoglobulins and Antisera

Described in this section are immunological agents used for both active immunisation and passive immunisation.

Active immunisation is a process of increasing resistance to infection whereby micro-organisms or products of their activity act as antigens and stimulate certain body cells to produce antibodies with a specific protective capacity. It may be a natural process following recovery from an infection, or an artificial process following the administration of *vaccines*. It is inevitably a slow process dependent upon the rate at which the antibody formation can be developed. Although the terms vaccination and immunisation are often used synonymously and interchangeably, *vaccination* simply refers to the administration of a vaccine whereas *immunisation* implies the development of protective levels of antibodies confirmed usually by serological testing.

Passive immunisation, which results in immediate protection of short duration, may be achieved by the administration of the antibodies themselves usually in the form of *antisera* (of animal origin) or *immunoglobulins*.

Antisera (7931-r)

Antisera (immunosera) are sterile preparations containing immunoglobulins obtained from the serum of immunised animals by purification. The term antisera includes antitoxins, which are antibodies that combine with and neutralise specific toxins, and antivenins (antivenoms), which are antitoxins directed against the toxic principle of the venoms of poisonous animals such as certain snakes and arthropods.

Antisera are obtained from healthy animals immunised by injections of the appropriate toxins or toxoids, venins, or suspensions of micro-organisms or other antigens. The specific immunoglobulins may be obtained from the serum by fractional precipitation and enzyme treatment or by other chemical or physical means. A suitable antimicrobial preservative may be added, and is invariably added if the product is issued in multidose containers. The Ph. Eur. directs that when antisera contain phenol, the concentration is not more than 0.25%. The antiserum is distributed aseptically into sterile containers which are sealed so as to exclude micro-organisms. Alternatively they may be supplied as freeze-dried preparations for reconstitution immediately before use.

Adverse Effects and Precautions
Reactions are liable to occur after the injection of any serum of animal origin. Anaphylaxis (type I hypersensitivity reaction, p.404) may occur, with hypotension, dyspnoea, urticaria, and shock which requires management as a medical emergency (see p.832).

Serum sickness (type III hypersensitivity reaction, p.404) may occur, frequently 7 to 10 days after the injection of serum of animal origin.

Before injecting serum, information should be obtained whenever possible as to whether previous injections of serum have been received and whether the patient is subject to hypersensitivity disorders. Sensitivity testing should be performed before the administration of antisera. The patient must be kept under observation after the administration of full doses of antisera. Adrenaline [epinephrine] injection and resuscitation facilities should be available.

Uses and Administration
Antisera have the specific power of neutralising venins or bacterial toxins, or combining with the bacterium, virus, or other antigen used for their preparation. Most antisera in current use are antitoxins or antivenins. The use of antisera to induce passive immunity has declined; immunoglobulins are preferred. Although antisera are defined as being of animal origin (see above), the term antisera has been used in some countries to describe antitoxins of human origin (immunoglobulins).

Immunoglobulins (3893-f)

Immunoglobulins are produced by B lymphocytes as part of the humoral response to foreign antigens. Immunoglobulins used in clinical practice are preparations containing antibodies, usually prepared from human plasma or serum, and mainly comprise IgG. Normal immunoglobulin, prepared from material from blood donors, contains several antibodies against infectious diseases prevalent in the general population, whereas specific immunoglobulins contain minimum specified levels of one antibody. Antibodies may also be prepared by genetic engineering techniques.

Adverse Effects
Local reactions with pain and tenderness at the site of intramuscular injection may follow the administration of immunoglobulins. Hypersensitivity reactions, including, rarely, anaphylactic reactions, have also been reported; such reactions, though, are far less frequent than following the use of antisera of animal origin.

Some immunoglobulins are available as intravenous preparations. Systemic reactions with fever, chills, facial flushing, headache, and nausea may occur following their administration, particularly at high rates of infusion.

Precautions
Strenuous efforts are made to screen human donor material used in the preparation of immunoglobulins; the transmission of infections (including hepatitis B and HIV) which has been associated with the use of certain blood products (see p.726) does not appear to be a problem with the immunoglobulins currently in use.

IgA, present in some immunoglobulin preparations, may give rise to the production of anti-IgA antibodies in patients with IgA deficiencies with the consequent risk of anaphylactic reactions. For precautions in such patients see Hypersensitivity under Adverse Effects and Precautions in Normal Immunoglobulins, p.1552.

Interactions
Immunoglobulins may interfere with the ability of live vaccines to induce an immune response and a suitable interval should separate administration of the two (see Vaccines, Interactions, p.1530).

◊ Reviews of possible interactions between immunoglobulins and other drugs.
1. Grabenstein JD. Drug interactions involving immunologic agents. Part I. Vaccine-vaccine, vaccine-immunoglobulin, and vaccine-drug interactions. *DICP Ann Pharmacother* 1990; **24:** 67–81.
2. Grabenstein JD. Drug interactions involving immunologic agents. Part II. Immunodiagnostic and other immunologic drug interactions. *DICP Ann Pharmacother* 1990; **24:** 186–93.

Uses and Administration
Immunoglobulins are used for passive immunisation, thus conferring immediate protection against some infectious diseases. They are preferred to antisera of animal origin as the incidence of adverse reactions is less.

It is generally important to follow the conferment of passive immunity, which is largely an emergency procedure, by the injection of suitable antigens to produce active immunity.

Vaccines (7930-x)

Vaccines are traditionally preparations of antigenic materials which are administered with the object of inducing in the recipient active immunity to specific infecting agents or toxins or antigens produced by them. They may contain living or killed micro-organisms, bacterial toxoids, or antigenic material from particular parts of the infecting organism which may be derived from the organism or produced by recombinant DNA technology. Vaccines may be single-component vaccines or mixed combined vaccines. Vaccines against non-infective diseases are being developed.

Storage. Advice concerning the effects of temperature on vaccines.
1. Miller LG, Loomis JH. Advice of manufacturers about effects of temperature on biologicals. *Am J Hosp Pharm* 1985; **42:** 843–8.
2. Longland PW, Rowbotham PC. Stability at room temperature of medicines normally recommended for cold storage. *Pharm J* 1987; **238:** 147–51. Correction. *ibid.*; 220.
3. Anonymous. Stability of vaccines. *Bull WHO* 1990; **68:** 118–20.
4. Casto DT, Brunell PA. Safe handling of vaccines. *Pediatrics* 1991; **87:** 108–12.
5. André FE. Stability of vaccines. *BMJ* 1993; **307:** 939.

Adverse Effects
Administration of a vaccine by injection may be followed by a local reaction, possibly with inflammation and lymphangitis. An induration or sterile abscess may develop at the site of injected vaccine. Administration may be followed by fever, headache, and malaise starting a few hours after injection and lasting for 1 or 2 days. Hypersensitivity reactions may occur and anaphylaxis has been reported rarely.

Further details, if appropriate, of adverse effects of vaccines may be found in the respective individual monographs.

◊ The introduction of routine childhood vaccination has been accompanied by concerns over the safety and possible long term sequelae of some commonly used vaccines. Difficulties have arisen in distinguishing temporal and causal associations and in some cases the perceived dangers of vaccination have impeded uptake. Among the disorders that have been temporally associated with childhood vaccination are neurological disorders, sudden infant death syndrome, type 1 diabetes mellitus, and demyelinating disorders. Information on adverse effects associated with specific vaccines can be found under individual monographs.

References.
1. Stratton KR, *et al.* Adverse events associated with childhood vaccines other than pertussis and rubella: summary of a report from the Institute of Medicine. *JAMA* 1994; **271:** 1602–5.
2. Mitchell EA, *et al.* Immunisation and the sudden infant death syndrome. *Arch Dis Child* 1995; **73:** 498–501.
3. Freed GL, *et al.* Safety of vaccinations: Miss America, the media, and public health. *JAMA* 1996; **276:** 1869–72.
4. Centers for Disease Control. Update: vaccine side effects, adverse reactions, contraindications, and precautions: recommendations of the Advisory Committee on Immunization Practices (ACIP). *MMWR* 1996; **45** (RR-12): 1–45.
5. Braun MM, Ellenberg SS. Descriptive epidemiology of adverse events after immunization: reports to the vaccine adverse event reporting system (VAERS), 1991–1994. *J Pediatr* 1997; **131:** 529–35.
6. Jefferson T. Vaccination and its adverse effects: real or perceived. *BMJ* 1998; **317:** 159–60.
7. Ball LK, *et al.* Risky business: challenges in vaccine risk communication. *Pediatrics* 1998; **101:** 453–8.
8. Hiltunen M, *et al.* Immunisation and type 1 diabetes mellitus: is there a link? *Drug Safety* 1999; **20:** 207–12.
9. Institute for Vaccine Safety Diabetes Workshop Panel. Childhood immunizations and type 1 diabetes: summary of an Institute for Vaccine Safety workshop. *Pediatr Infect Dis J* 1999; **18:** 217–22.

Effects on the nervous system. GUILLAIN-BARRÉ SYNDROME. Guillain-Barré syndrome (see p.1554) has occasionally been associated with vaccination, although causal relationships have been difficult to evaluate. Vaccines implicated include a swine influenza vaccine, diphtheria and tetanus vaccines, some rabies vaccines, and oral poliomyelitis vaccines.[1] A report by the Institute of Medicine in the USA, summarised by Stratton and colleagues,[2] concluded that there was evidence favouring a causal relation with tetanus or diphtheria and tetanus vaccines (mainly in immunocompromised patients), and with oral poliomyelitis vaccines, but that the evidence was inadequate for measles vaccines, inactivated poliomyelitis vaccines, hepatitis

B vaccines, or haemophilus influenzae vaccines. See individual monographs for further details.

1. Awong IE, *et al.* Drug-associated Guillain-Barré syndrome: a literature review. *Ann Pharmacother* 1996; **30:** 173–80.
2. Stratton KR, *et al.* Adverse events associated with childhood vaccines other than pertussis and rubella: summary of a report from the Institute of Medicine. *JAMA* 1994; **271:** 1602–5.

Effects on the skin. Granuloma was reported in 3 patients at the injection site of adsorbed vaccines.[1] Biopsy and microscopy suggested that the granuloma was due to aluminium used as the adsorbant in the vaccines.

1. Fawcett HA, Smith NP. Injection-site granuloma due to aluminum. *Arch Dermatol* 1984; **120:** 1318–22.

Precautions

Vaccination should be postponed in patients suffering from any acute illness although minor infections without fever or systemic upset are not regarded as contra-indications.

Enquiry regarding previous hypersensitivity, either local or generalised, should precede the administration of a vaccine and measures to treat hypersensitivity reactions up to and including anaphylactic shock (p.832) should be immediately available. Immunisation should not be carried out in individuals who have previously had a severe local or generalised reaction to the vaccine. Reactions which should be regarded as severe include extensive redness and swelling with induration involving large areas of the vaccinated limb, fever of 39.5° or more within 48 hours of vaccination, anaphylaxis, bronchospasm, laryngeal oedema, generalised collapse, prolonged unresponsiveness, prolonged inconsolable or high-pitched screaming (more than 4 hours), convulsions, or encephalopathy within 72 hours. Some vaccines contain small amounts of antibacterials and should not be given to patients with a history of anaphylaxis to the agent used. Caution should be observed in patients with less severe manifestations of antibacterial hypersensitivity. Additionally some vaccines are prepared using hens' eggs and a history of anaphylaxis to the ingestion of eggs is a contra-indication to the use of such vaccines. Similarly, caution should be observed in patients with less severe manifestations of egg hypersensitivity. Asthma, eczema, hay fever, or a history of other allergies, should not be regarded as contra-indications to vaccination.

Before injection of a vaccine any alcohol or disinfectant used for cleansing the skin should be allowed to evaporate otherwise inactivation of live vaccines may occur.

It is recommended that immunisation of infants should not be postponed because of prematurity and that the normal schedules and timings based on the actual birth date should be adhered to.

Certain precautions and contra-indications apply specifically to vaccines containing live attenuated microorganisms.

Live vaccines should not be given to patients receiving immunosuppressive therapy (see under Interactions, below); to patients suffering from certain malignant conditions such as lymphoma, leukaemia, Hodgkin's disease, or other tumours of the reticuloendothelial system; to patients who have received bone-marrow transplants within the previous 6 months (after which time they should have their immune status checked and be immunised appropriately); or to patients with other types of impaired immunological responses, such as hypogammaglobulinaemia.

It should be remembered that the immune response to all vaccines (live or inactivated) may be diminished in immunocompromised patients.

Live vaccines should not be administered during pregnancy because of a theoretical risk to the fetus, unless it is considered there is a significant risk of exposure to infection.

HIV-infected patients. A review[1] of experience of the safety and efficacy of vaccines in patients infected with HIV found that the theoretical risk of accelerating HIV infection by immunisation is not supported by the limited clinical information available and the risks may be trivial compared with other nat-

ural sources of antigenic stimulation especially in areas of the world with high levels of endemic infectious diseases.

Recommendations for immunisation of HIV-positive individuals vary, particularly with regard to the use of live vaccines[2] (see Immunisation of Immunocompromised Patients, below for UK recommendations). Where an alternative is available an inactivated vaccine may be preferred to a live one (for example, poliomyelitis vaccines), but in general, vaccines recommended for routine immunisation in childhood may be given to HIV-positive individuals. For HIV-positive persons, WHO and UNICEF[3] recommend that routine immunisation should be carried out according to their usual EPI schedule (see below) in asymptomatic individuals. In addition, an extra dose of measles vaccine should be given at 6 months of age with the standard dose given as soon after 9 months of age as possible. BCG vaccines and yellow fever vaccines (pending further studies) should not be given to those with symptomatic disease. See individual monographs for further information.

1. von Reyn CF, *et al.* Human immunodeficiency virus infection and routine childhood immunisation. *Lancet* 1987; **ii:** 669–72.
2. Centers for Disease Control. Recommendations of the Advisory Committee on Immunization Practices (ACIP): use of vaccines and immune globulins for persons with altered immunocompetence. *Clin Pharm* 1993; **12:** 675–84.
3. WHO. *EPI vaccines in HIV-infected individuals: 5 October 2001.* Available at: http://www.who.int/vaccines-diseases/diseases/HIV.shtml (accessed 7/12/2001).

Premature infants. References.

1. Anonymous. Routine immunisation of preterm infants. *Lancet* 1990; **335:** 23–4.
2. Khalak R, *et al.* Three-year follow-up of vaccine response in extremely preterm infants. *Pediatrics* 1998; **101:** 597–603.

Interactions

The ability of vaccines to induce an immune response can be influenced by the recent administration of other vaccines or immunoglobulins. Live vaccines should either be given simultaneously (but at different sites) or an interval of at least 3 weeks allowed between administration. Live vaccines should normally be given at least 2 to 3 weeks before or at least 3 months after the administration of immunoglobulin. However, travellers should receive appropriate vaccines regardless of these limitations if time is short.

Patients receiving immunosuppressant therapy, including antineoplastics or therapeutic doses of corticosteroids, may also display a reduced response to vaccines, and there is a possibility of generalised infections with live viral vaccines. In the UK, the Department of Health suggests that immunosuppression may be expected in children receiving the equivalent of 2 mg prednisolone per kg body-weight daily for at least 1 week or 1 mg per kg daily for 1 month, and in adults receiving the equivalent of 40 mg prednisolone daily for more than 1 week. Vaccination should also be postponed for at least 6 months after the end of antineoplastic chemotherapy and for at least 3 months after high-dose systemic corticosteroid therapy.

Any agent that is active against the bacterial or viral strain present in the vaccine may interfere with development of a protective immune response but treatment with antibacterials should not be considered to be a contra-indication to immunisation.

◊ References.

1. Grabenstein JD. Drug interactions involving immunologic agents. Part I. Vaccine-vaccine, vaccine-immunoglobulin, and vaccine-drug interactions. *DICP Ann Pharmacother* 1990; **24:** 67–81.
2. Grabenstein JD. Drug interactions involving immunologic agents. Part II. Immunodiagnostic and other immunologic drug interactions. *DICP Ann Pharmacother* 1990; **24:** 186–93.

Uses and Administration

Vaccines are used for active immunisation as a prophylactic measure against some infectious diseases. They provide partial or complete protection for months or years. For inactivated vaccines a slight and rather slow antibody response of primarily immunoglobulin M (IgM) (the primary response) is produced after the first or second dose but, when a further dose is given after a suitable interval, a prompt antibody response follows and high concentrations of IgG occur in the blood (the secondary response). Though the antibody concentration may later fall, a further dose of vaccine promptly restores it. For most live vaccines only one dose is required although 3 doses of live (oral) poliomyelitis vaccines are needed to achieve

complete immunisation. Some inactivated vaccines contain an adjuvant such as aluminium hydroxide or aluminium phosphate to enhance the immune response.

Protection against several infectious diseases may be provided in early life by active immunisation and national schedules for childhood immunisation are regularly reviewed and updated. Schedules for routine immunisation of infants and children are generally designed to fit in with routine health checks and landmark events such as school starting and leaving ages. National immunisation schedules should be consulted for full details of local recommendations.

In the **UK** the following schedule of vaccination and immunisation is recommended:

- at 2, 3, and 4 months of age, doses of an adsorbed diphtheria, tetanus, and pertussis vaccine (p.1537) together with a *Haemophilus influenzae* vaccine (p.1540), a live (oral) poliomyelitis vaccine (p.1558), and a meningococcal C conjugate vaccine (p.1550). If pertussis vaccine is contra-indicated an adsorbed diphtheria and tetanus vaccine (p.1537) should be given

- at 12 to 15 months, measles, mumps, and rubella vaccine (p.1549)

- at 3 to 5 years, reinforcing doses of an adsorbed diphtheria, tetanus, and pertussis vaccine and a live (oral) poliomyelitis vaccine and a second dose of measles, mumps, and rubella vaccine

- between 10 and 14 years, BCG vaccine (p.1533) may be given to tuberculin-negative children if it has not been given in infancy

- before leaving school (age 13 to 18 years), reinforcing doses of an adsorbed tetanus with low-dose diphtheria vaccine (p.1565) and a live (oral) poliomyelitis vaccine

- a further reinforcing dose of tetanus vaccine may be given after 10 years. Adults who have received 5 doses of tetanus should not require further routine boosters.

The following schedule is recommended in the **USA**:

- at birth or up to 2 months of age, the first dose of hepatitis B vaccine (p.1542)

- at age 1 to 4 months, a second dose of hepatitis B vaccine, not less than 1 month after the first

- at 2 months and 4 months, diphtheria, tetanus, and pertussis vaccine, together with a *Haemophilus influenzae* vaccine, a pneumococcal conjugate vaccine (p.1557), and a poliomyelitis vaccine

- at 6 months, the third dose of *Haemophilus influenzae* vaccine if necessary (depending on the type of vaccine used), a third dose of diphtheria, tetanus, and pertussis vaccine, and a third dose of pneumococcal conjugate vaccine

- at 6 to 18 months, the third doses of hepatitis B and poliomyelitis vaccines

- at 12 to 15 months, a reinforcing dose of *Haemophilus influenzae* vaccine, the first dose of measles, mumps, and rubella vaccine, and the fourth dose of pneumococcal conjugate vaccine

- at 12 to 18 months (or at age 11 to 12 years), a varicella-zoster vaccine (p.1568)

- at 15 to 18 months, the fourth dose of diphtheria, tetanus, and pertussis vaccine

- at 2 to 18 years, hepatitis A vaccine in selected geographical areas and for certain high-risk groups

- at 4 to 6 years, the fifth dose of diphtheria, tetanus, and pertussis vaccine and the fourth dose of poliomyelitis vaccine; the second dose of measles, mumps, and rubella vaccine may be given at this age (or at age 11 to 12 years)

- at 11 to 12 years, varicella-zoster vaccine (if not previously given), the second dose of measles, mumps, and rubella vaccine (if not previously given), and a 3-dose course of hepatitis B vaccine (if not previously given)

- at age 11 to 16 years, tetanus and low-dose diphtheria toxoids. Susceptible children 13 years of age and older should receive 2 doses of varicella vaccine, at least 1 month apart
- subsequently routine booster doses of tetanus and low-dose diphtheria toxoids are recommended every 10 years.

Immunisation schedules for older children and adults are also produced, along with recommendations for vaccination of high risk groups, including the immunocompromised and the elderly, and of travellers.

In addition to vaccines directed against bacteria and viruses, advances are being made in producing vaccines against fungi, protozoa, and helminths, and for non-infective diseases including cancer and auto-immune disorders.

Development of novel vaccine formulations and delivery methods is continuing, including transdermal and transmucosal systems. Genetic manipulations of foodstuffs is being investigated with the aim of producing edible vaccines.

◊ Some general references to vaccines and immunisation including vaccine development and research.

1. Moxon ER. The scope of immunisation. *Lancet* 1990; **335:** 448–51.
2. Ada GL. The immunological principles of vaccination. *Lancet* 1990; **335:** 523–6.
3. Anderson RM, May RM. Immunisation and herd immunity. *Lancet* 1990; **335:** 641–5.
4. Gilligan CA, Li Wan Po A. Oral vaccines: design and delivery. *Int J Pharmaceutics* 1991; **75:** 1–24.
5. O'Hagan DT. Oral delivery of vaccines: formulation and clinical pharmacokinetic considerations. *Clin Pharmacokinet* 1992; **22:** 1–10.
6. McDonnell WM, Askari FK. Molecular medicine: DNA vaccines. *N Engl J Med* 1996; **334:** 42–5.
7. McCarthy M. DNA vaccination: a direct line to the immune system. *Lancet* 1996; **348:** 1232.
8. Various. Vaccine series. *Lancet* 1997; **350.**
9. McDonnell WM, Askari FK. Immunization. *JAMA* 1997; **278:** 2000–2007.
10. Lambert P-H, Siegrist C-A. Vaccines and vaccination. *BMJ* 1997; **315:** 1595–8.
11. Eskola J. Childhood immunisation today. *Drugs* 1998; **55:** 759–66.
12. Seder RA, Gurunathan S. DNA vaccines—designer vaccines for the 21st century. *N Engl J Med* 1999; **341:** 277–8.
13. Ellis RW. New technologies for making vaccines. *Vaccine* 1999; **17:** 1596–1604.
14. Lewis PJ, Babiuk LA. DNA vaccines: a review. *Adv Virus Res* 1999; **54:** 129–88.
15. Leitner WW, *et al.* DNA and RNA-based vaccines: principles, progress and prospects. *Vaccine* 2000; **18:** 765–77.
16. Restifo NP, *et al.* The promise of nucleic acid vaccines. *Gene Ther* 2000; **7:** 89–92.

Eradication of infections. Eradication of infectious diseases has proved more difficult than was hoped, and smallpox is the only disease to have been recognised officially as having been eradicated so far. Eradication is defined as the extinction of the pathogen that causes the infectious disease in question whereas in elimination the disease disappears but the causative agent remains. Of the 6 target diseases of WHO's Expanded Programme on Immunization, many of the factors necessary for elimination are present for each of the diseases, but some are not.[1] *Measles* is so highly communicable a disease that a vaccine efficacy rate of about 95% is probably not high enough even to eliminate, much less eradicate the disease.[1] However, immunisation campaigns have produced substantial reductions of infection rate in some countries although repeated vaccination may be necessary.[2] *Pertussis* is also highly infectious and the vaccine is almost certainly not effective enough. *Tetanus* is not eradicable as the causative organism is ubiquitous. However, elimination of neonatal tetanus may be possible although it depends on protection of more than 80% of infants at birth. This depends not only on maternal vaccination but also on delivery practices.[2] For *poliomyelitis*, countries that are efficient at giving vaccines have proved remarkably successful not only in practically eliminating the disease but also in virtually eradicating the organism. *Tuberculosis* is clearly not eradicable at present and *diphtheria* has many features that suggest it cannot be easily eradicated. Prospects for eradicating *congenital rubella syndrome* are more encouraging and the prospects for elimination or eradication of *mumps* are probably similar to those of rubella.

Other factors which may contribute to the failure of vaccination policies in eradicating disease include: concern, often unfounded, over the safety of vaccines and the perpetuation of invalid contra-indications, the use of inappropriate indicators for the effectiveness of vaccines, the suitability of different types of vaccine and of vaccination schedules, difficulties in vaccine supply, and social and behavioural pressures which reduce compliance with vaccination schedules.[2,3]

1. Noah ND, Begg NT. Smallpox ten years gone: what next? *BMJ* 1987; **295:** 1013–14.
2. Stanwell-Smith R. Immunization: celebrating the past and injecting the future. *J R Soc Med* 1996; **89:** 509–13.
3. Preston NW. Smallpox could be but one of many diseases that vaccination confines to the history of medicine. *Trop Dis Bull* 1994; **91:** R151–R165.

Immunisation schedules. Recommendations and discussions of routine immunisation schedules in the UK,[1,2] the USA[3-10] and the developed world in general.[11] See below for discussion of the Expanded Programme on Immunization.

1. Mayon-White RT. Vaccination for the elderly. *Br J Hosp Med* 1994; **51:** 265–7.
2. Salisbury DM, Begg NT (eds), Joint Committee on Vaccination and Immunisation. *Immunisation against infectious disease.* London: HMSO, 1996.
3. Fedson DS, National Vaccine Advisory Committee. Adult immunization: summary of the National Vaccine Advisory Committee report. *JAMA* 1994; **272:** 1133–7.
4. Halsey NA, Hall CB. Workshop on conflicting guidelines for the use of vaccines. *Pediatrics* 1995; **95:** 938–41.
5. Somani J, *et al.* Reimmunization after allogeneic bone marrow transplantation. *Am J Med* 1995; **98:** 389–98.
6. Gardner P, *et al.* Adult immunizations. *Ann Intern Med* 1996; **124:** 35–40.
7. American Academy of Pediatrics Committee on Infectious Diseases. Immunization of adolescents: recommendations of the Advisory Committee on Immunization Practices, the American Academy of Pediatrics, the American Academy of Family Physicians, and the American Medical Association. *Pediatrics* 1997; **99:** 479–88.
8. Reid KC, *et al.* Adult immunizations: recommendations for practice. *Mayo Clin Proc* 1999; **74:** 377–84.
9. American Academy of Pediatrics. Combination vaccines for childhood immunization: recommendations of the Advisory Committee on Immunization Practices (ACIP), the American Academy of Pediatrics (AAP), and the American Academy of Family Physicians (AAFP). *Pediatrics* 1999; **103:** 1064–77.
10. American Academy of Pediatrics Committee on Infectious Diseases. Recommended childhood immunization schedule—United States, January-December 2001. *Pediatrics* 2001; **107:** 202–4.
11. Hinman AR, Orenstein WA. Immunisation practice in developed countries. *Lancet* 1990; **335:** 707–10.

EXPANDED PROGRAMME ON IMMUNIZATION. In 1974 the World Health Assembly adopted a resolution creating the Expanded Programme on Immunization, the aim of which was to provide immunisation against six target diseases (diphtheria, measles, pertussis, poliomyelitis, tetanus, and tuberculosis) for all children throughout the world by 1990. Although the attention of WHO had been focussed primarily on the developing countries, it was emphasised that the programme was not created exclusively for these countries. Besides WHO, many other organisations, including UNICEF, were involved.

Vaccine uptake was around 70% in 1990 compared with less than 5% in 1974. Although many cases of the target diseases and many deaths have been prevented, vaccine coverage, especially for measles and neonatal tetanus is still low. It is particularly important to immunise children as early in life as possible and not to withhold vaccines from those suffering with minor illness or malnutrition.

A schedule designed to provide protection at the earliest possible age consists of: trivalent oral poliomyelitis vaccine together with BCG vaccine at birth; trivalent oral poliomyelitis vaccine together with diphtheria, tetanus, and pertussis vaccine at 6, 10, and 14 weeks of age; and measles vaccine at 9 months of age. Tetanus vaccine is also administered to all women of childbearing age. Other vaccines included in the programme are: yellow fever vaccine in parts of Africa and Japanese encephalitis vaccine in parts of the Far East. Further expansion to include vaccination against other diseases, particularly hepatitis B, (see Administration, p.1543) is under continued consideration.

Some references to the Expanded Programme on Immunization.

1. Hayden GF, *et al.* Progress in worldwide control and elimination of disease through immunization. *J Pediatr* 1989; **114:** 520–7.
2. Hall AJ, *et al.* Practice in developing countries. *Lancet* 1990; **335:** 774–7.

Immunisation of immunocompromised patients. Immunocompromised and asplenic patients and recipients of bone marrow transplants may require immunisation against opportunistic infections. As discussed under Precautions, above, immune response to vaccination may be impaired, and there is a risk of disseminated infection with live vaccines.

In the UK, the Department of Health recommends that HIV-positive individuals (whether symptomatic or asymptomatic) may receive, where appropriate, live vaccines against measles, mumps, poliomyelitis, and rubella and inactivated vaccines against cholera, diphtheria, *Haemophilus influenzae* type b infections, hepatitis B, pertussis, poliomyelitis, tetanus, and typhoid. Hepatitis A, meningococcal, pneumococcal, and rabies vaccines may also be given. In the UK it is recommended that BCG vaccine should not be given to HIV-positive individuals; WHO have, however, advised immunisation of asymptomatic infants when the risk of tuberculosis is high. There is as yet insufficient data on the safety of yellow fever vaccine in HIV-positive individuals. In the UK administration of yellow fever vaccine to all HIV-positive individuals, whether asymptomatic or not, is not recommended. WHO advise that the vaccine may be administered to asymptomatic persons, but that, pending further studies, it should not be given to those with symptomatic infection.

As with other causes of immunosuppression, the efficacy of vaccines may be reduced in HIV-positive individuals. Administration of normal immunoglobulins is suggested for HIV-positive individuals exposed to measles.

Further references.

1. Ljungman P, Hammarström V. Immunisation of transplant recipients. *Clin Immunother* 1995; **3:** 330–7.

2. Henning KJ, *et al.* A national survey of immunization practices following allogeneic bone marrow transplantation. *JAMA* 1997; **277:** 1148–51.
3. Loutan L. Vaccination of the immunocompromised patient. *Biologicals* 1997; **25:** 231–6.
4. Pirofski L-A, Casadevall A. Use of licensed vaccines for active immunization of the immunocompromised host. *Clin Microbiol Rev* 1998; **11:** 1–26.
5. Centers for Disease Control. 1999 USPHS/IDSA guidelines for the prevention of opportunistic infections in persons infected with human immunodeficiency virus. *MMWR* 1999; **48** (RR-10): 1–66.
6. WHO. *EPI vaccines in HIV-infected individuals: 5 October 2001.* Available at: http://www.who.int/vaccines-diseases/diseases/HIV.shtml (accessed 7/12/01).

Immunisation for travellers. A booklet entitled *International Travel and Health: Vaccination Requirements and Health Advice* is published annually by WHO. In the 2001 edition the following information regarding certification of vaccination was given.

A *yellow fever* vaccination certificate is now the only one that should be required in international travel, and then only for a limited number of travellers. The vaccine used must be approved by WHO and administered at a designated vaccinating centre. Vaccination is strongly recommended for travel outside the urban areas of countries in the yellow fever endemic zone even if these countries have not officially reported the disease and do not require evidence of vaccination on entry. Many countries require a certificate from travellers arriving from infected areas or from countries with infected areas, or who have been in transit through those areas. Some countries require a certificate from all entering travellers including those in transit; although there is no epidemiological justification for this requirement, and it is clearly in excess of the International Health Regulations (WHO recommendations for prevention of the international spread of diseases), travellers may find that it is strictly enforced, particularly for persons going to Asia from Africa or South America. The validity period of international certificates of vaccination against yellow fever is 10 years, beginning 10 days after vaccination.

No country or territory any longer requires a certificate of *cholera* immunisation as the introduction of cholera into any country cannot be prevented by cholera vaccination.

Now that *smallpox* has been eradicated, smallpox vaccination is no longer required by any country.

Apart from vaccinations required by countries for entry to their territory, other vaccinations are either recommended by WHO for general protection against certain diseases or advised in certain circumstances. A vaccination plan should be established, taking into account the traveller's destination, overall state of health and current immune status, the duration and type of travel, and the time available.

Further information for international travellers is also often provided by national authorities. In the UK the Department of Health issues *Health Advice for Travellers* for the public and *Health Information for Overseas Travel* for the medical profession. In the USA guidelines are produced by the Centers for Disease Control.

AIDS Immunoglobulins   (11739-l)

HIV Immunoglobulins.

Profile

AIDS immunoglobulin preparations containing HIV-neutralising antibodies have been prepared from the plasma of asymptomatic HIV-positive subjects. They are being tried for passive immunisation in patients with AIDS or AIDS-related complex.

◊ References.

1. Lambert JS, *et al.* Pediatric AIDS Clinical Trials Group Protocol 185 Pharmacokinetic Study Group. Safety and pharmacokinetics of hyperimmune anti-human immunodeficiency virus (HIV) immunoglobulin administered to HIV-infected pregnant women and their newborns. *J Infect Dis* 1997; **175:** 283–91.
2. Stiehm ER, *et al.* Efficacy of zidovudine and human immunodeficiency virus (HIV) hyperimmune immunoglobulin for reducing perinatal HIV transmission from HIV-infected women with advanced disease: results of Pediatric AIDS Clinical Trials Group protocol 185. *J Infect Dis* 1999; **179:** 567–75.
3. Stiehm ER, *et al.* Use of human immunodeficiency virus (HIV) human hyperimmune immunoglobulin in HIV type 1-infected children (Pediatric AIDS Clinical Trials Group protocol 273). *J Infect Dis* 2000; **181:** 548–54.

AIDS Vaccines   (18734-k)

HIV Vaccines.

Profile

Many prototype vaccines against the acquired immunodeficiency syndrome have been or are being developed but the results of clinical studies have generally been disappointing.

◊ Research into AIDS vaccines has continued into both therapeutic vaccines, aimed at reducing the rate of disease progression in HIV-infected individuals, and prophylactic vaccines, aimed at preventing primary infection. It is now appreciated that both humoral and cell-mediated immune mechanisms play a vital role in controlling HIV infection. Among a number of possible approaches, subunit recombinant viral envelope proteins (gp120 or gp160) have been candidates for both therapeutic and prophylactic vaccines, either as monovalent or polyvalent formulations. They mainly produce a humoral (antibody) response although cell-mediated responses, possibly to other components of the vaccine, have been detected. Clinical studies have not demonstrated a delay in disease progression. Attenuated live viral vaccines are potentially useful for prophylaxis but were initially dismissed because the risk of reversion to virulent strains was felt to be too great. However, they are now being re-examined since they are capable of producing both cell-mediated and humoral immune responses, although the problem of safety remains to be resolved. Another recent development is investigation of nucleic acid vaccines. Free DNA encoding for viral antigens injected into the muscle results in expression of the encoded antigens promoting a humoral and cell-mediated response. Although these vaccines are still at an early stage of development, they may represent a safer alternative to live viral vaccines.

Reviews.

1. Graham BS, Wright PF. Candidate AIDS vaccines. *N Engl J Med* 1995; **333:** 1331–9.
2. Anonymous. Update on AIDS: vaccines and genetic manipulation. *WHO Drug Inf* 1995; **9:** 201–9.
3. Esparaza J, *et al.* HIV prospective vaccines: progress to date. *Drugs* 1991; **50:** 792–804.
4. Stott EJ, Schild GC. Strategies for AIDS vaccines. *J Antimicrob Chemother* 1996; **37** (suppl B): 185–98.
5. Haynes BF. HIV vaccines: where we are and where we are going. *Lancet* 1996; **348:** 933–7.
6. Bangham CRM, Phillips RE. What is required of an HIV vaccine? *Lancet* 1997; **350:** 1617–21.
7. Frey SE. HIV vaccines. *Infect Dis Clin North Am* 1999; **13:** 95–112.
8. Rousseau MC, *et al.* Vaccination and HIV: a review of the literature. *Vaccine* 1999; **18:** 825–31.

Anthrax Vaccines (7933-d)

ATC — J07AC01.

Adverse Effects and Precautions
As for vaccines in general, p.1529.

Interactions
As for vaccines in general, p.1530.

Uses and Administration
In the UK an anthrax vaccine which is an alum precipitate of the antigen found in the sterile filtrate of suitable cultures of the Sterne strain of *Bacillus anthracis* is available for human use. It is used for active immunisation against anthrax and is recommended for persons working with potentially infected animals or animal products. It is given in 4 doses, each of 0.5 mL, administered by intramuscular injection. The first 3 doses are separated by intervals of 3 weeks and the fourth dose follows after an interval of 6 months. In the USA, where an anthrax vaccine is also available, 6 doses, each of 0.5 mL, are given subcutaneously, the first 3 at intervals of 2 weeks and the last 3 at intervals of 6 months. Reinforcing doses of 0.5 mL are required each year.

◊ References.

1. Hambleton P, *et al.* Anthrax: the disease in relation to vaccines. *Vaccine* 1984; **2:** 125–32.
2. Turnbull PCB. Thoroughly modern anthrax. *Abstr Hyg* 1986; **61:** R1–R13.
3. Turnbull PCB. Anthrax vaccines: past, present and future. *Vaccine* 1991; **9:** 533–9.
4. Farrar WE. Anthrax: virulence and vaccines. *Ann Intern Med* 1994; **121:** 379–80.
5. Centers for Disease Control. Use of anthrax vaccine in the United States: recommendations of the Advisory Committee on Immunization Practices (ACIP). *MMWR* 2000; **49** (RR-15): 1–20.

Anti-D Immunoglobulins (1234-k)

ATC — J06BB01.

Human Anti-D Immunoglobulin (Ph. Eur.) (Anti-D (Rho) Immunoglobulin (BP 2001); Immunoglobulinum Humanum Anti-D) is a liquid or freeze-dried preparation containing immunoglobulins, mainly immunoglobulin G (IgG). It is obtained from plasma from D-negative donors who have been immunised against the D-antigen. It contains specific antibodies against the erythrocyte D-antigen and may also contain small quantities of other blood group antibodies, such as anti-C, anti-E, anti-A, and anti-B. Normal immunoglobulin may be added. The liquid and freeze-dried preparations should be stored, protected from light, in a colourless, glass container. The freeze-dried preparation should be stored under vacuum or under an inert gas.

Rho (D) Immune Globulin (USP 25) is a sterile solution of globulins derived from human plasma containing antibody to the erythrocyte factor Rho (D). It contains 10 to 18% of protein, of which not less than 90% is gamma globulin. It contains glycine as a stabilising agent, and a suitable preservative. It should be stored at 2° to 8°.

Adverse Effects and Precautions
As for immunoglobulins in general, p.1529.

Anti-D immunoglobulin should be administered with caution to rhesus-positive persons for the treatment of blood disorders; the resultant haemolysis may exacerbate pre-existing anaemia.

Interactions
As for immunoglobulins in general, p.1529.

Uses and Administration
Anti-D immunoglobulin is used to prevent a rhesus-negative mother actively forming antibodies to fetal rhesus-positive red blood cells that may pass into the maternal circulation during childbirth, abortion, or certain other sensitising events. In subsequent rhesus-positive pregnancies these antibodies could produce haemolytic disease of the newborn (erythroblastosis foetalis). The injection of anti-D immunoglobulin is not effective once the mother has formed anti-D antibodies. Anti-D immunoglobulin is also used in the management of some blood disorders, primarily idiopathic thrombocytopenic purpura.

Anti-D immunoglobulin should always be given to rhesus-negative mothers with no anti-D antibodies in their serum and who have just delivered rhesus-positive infants. It should be given as soon as possible after delivery but may give some protection even if administration is delayed beyond 72 hours. In the UK, the Blood Transfusion Services recommend a dose of 500 units (100 µg) by intramuscular injection and this will clear up to 4 mL of fetal red cells. An additional dose may be required depending on the amount of transplacental bleeding as assessed by the Kleihauer test; for bleeds exceeding 4 mL an additional 125 units for each mL of red cells will be required.

For routine antenatal prophylaxis 500 units of anti-D immunoglobulin may be given at 28 and 34 weeks' gestation. Alternatively a single dose, usually of 1500 units, may be given at 28 weeks. Postnatal prophylaxis is still necessary.

There is also a risk of sensitisation during pregnancy from spontaneous, induced, or threatened abortion, amniocentesis, or external version. Any rhesus-negative woman at risk of transplacental haemorrhage during pregnancy and not known to be sensitised should be given 250 units at up to 20 weeks' gestation and 500 units of anti-D immunoglobulin after 20 weeks' gestation.

Anti-D immunoglobulin is also given to rhesus-negative women of child-bearing potential after the inadvertent transfusion of Rh-incompatible blood, or after receiving blood components containing rhesus-positive red cells or organ donations from rhesus-positive donors. The dose is based on the amount of red blood cells transfused; up to 125 units per mL of transfused cells may be used.

In Europe and the USA doses of anti-D immunoglobulins have traditionally been higher than in the UK; WHO and the European Commissions Committee for Proprietary Medicinal Products have recommended a standard dose of 200 to 300 µg (1000 to 1500 units) but do not include a requirement for Kleihauer screening. A dose of approximately 250 µg (1250 units) will suppress the immune response to up to 10 mL of red blood cells. In the USA the dosage recommendations are based on a standard dose which is capable of suppressing the immune response to 15 mL of incompatible red blood cells. One sixth of this dose may be used up to 12 weeks of gestation for sensitising episodes.

For idiopathic thrombocytopenic purpura, an initial dose of 250 units (50 µg) per kg body-weight of anti-D immunoglobulin by intravenous injection is given. Maintenance doses will depend on the clinical response.

Haemolytic disease of the newborn. Rhesus (Rh) incompatibility, in particular Rh(D) incompatibility, is a major cause of potentially severe haemolytic disease of the newborn, although other blood group antibodies may also cause the disease.[1] The use of anti-D immunoglobulin to suppress the production of anti-D antibodies in a Rh(D)-negative mother in response to leakage of red blood cells across the placenta from a Rh(D)-positive fetus has produced a major reduction in the incidence of this disorder.[1]

Postnatal prophylaxis of Rh(D)-negative mothers following the birth of a Rh(D)-positive infant is well established. In 1971 WHO[2] suggested a standard dose of 200 to 300 µg but stated that a 100-µg dose was likely to have a success rate only slightly inferior to that of a 200-µg dose, thus allowing optimum use to be made of a limited resource. Clinical experience in the UK has confirmed the efficacy of the 100-µg (500 units) dose and this is the amount officially recommended in the UK in such situations.[3]

Despite the success of anti-D prophylaxis, sensitisations have continued to occur.[4] There are several possible reasons for this. Failures may occur when an inadequate dose has been administered or when anti-D prophylaxis is omitted following a sensitising event.[5,6] Postpartum doses may be omitted due to oversight or loss to follow-up. Sensitisation may occur spontaneously during the first pregnancy without any identifiable event causing feto-maternal haemorrhage. Inadequate dosing can be avoided by application of the Kleihauer test to estimate the size of any transplacental haemorrhage.[1]

Significant feto-maternal transfusion may also occur following still-birth, abortion (both therapeutic and spontaneous), threatened abortion, external fetal version, abdominal injury, or amniocentesis.

The efficacy of postpartum prophylaxis is not in question but opinions differ on the need for prophylaxis during pregnancy. It is generally agreed that prophylaxis is necessary following therapeutic terminations at any stage of pregnancy,[7,8] including medical termination utilising mifepristone,[9] but there is no generally accepted policy for other possibly sensitising events. A study of 655 Rh(D)-negative women in Denmark,[10] where antepartum prophylaxis is not common practice, suggested that the sensitisation rate following amniocentesis was no higher than the spontaneous sensitisation rate. Surveys of general medical practitioners and consultant obstetricians and haematologists in the UK[11,12] have suggested that many do not recommend routine prophylaxis following early complete or threatened miscarriages; 74% of general practitioners in one survey[12] never gave anti-D after threatened miscarriages. Spontaneous miscarriages during early pregnancy might not cause sensitisation so long as there is no surgical intervention.[7,8,13] Nonetheless the Royal College of Obstetricians and Gynaecologists and other authorities in the UK urge routine antenatal prophylaxis for all Rh(D)-negative women. Others[14,15] represent the alternative opinion that, with the shortage of anti-D, indiscriminate use of anti-D should be avoided[14] and attention should be focussed upon administration of adequate doses following term deliveries and terminations of pregnancy in Rh(D)-negative women.[5,15]

Further debate arises over the significance of spontaneous sensitisation during the first pregnancy. In one study,[16] administration of anti-D to 2069 Rh(D)-negative primigravidas at 28 and 34 weeks as well as standard postpartum administration was more effective at preventing immunisation than standard postpartum prophylaxis in 2000 primigravidas. In a subsequent analysis of women from this study[17] following further pregnancies, comparison with a group of Rh(D)-positive mothers showed no detrimental effects to mothers or infants. In addition antenatal prophylaxis may not need to be given beyond the first pregnancy. Nevertheless, concerns have been expressed[18] over the consequent unnecessary administration of anti-D to women who are carrying Rh(D)-negative fetuses and the possible long-term effects, although anti-D has had a good safety record.[19] Both factions agree[18,20] on the desirability of identifying high-risk women to reduce the indiscriminate use of anti-D. A remaining major stumbling block, in the UK at least, is the continuing expense and scarcity of anti-D immunoglobulin. Supplies are derived from plasma collected from Rh-negative donors who have to undergo potentially hazardous sensitisation with Rh-positive red blood cells. The development of genetically-engineered anti-D should help to improve availability. The UK[3] and WHO[2] guidelines may represent a counsel of perfection, but until difficulties with supply are overcome, prophylaxis during the first pregnancy for Rh(D)-negative women, thus ensuring the possibility of two unaffected infants, would seem a reasonable priority.

Treatment. In mild cases, the resultant hyperbilirubinaemia can be managed with phototherapy. In severe cases, exchange transfusions may be necessary and intra-uterine transfusions may be considered in pregnancies of less than about 34 weeks' gestation; beyond this, premature delivery is often preferable.[21] Some clinicians[22] have reported treatment failures with intra-uterine transfusions but have found the intravenous administration of normal immunoglobulin 400 mg per kg body-weight daily for 5 days every 2 to 3 weeks to the mother to be effective. There are several case reports[23,24] of beneficial responses using similar doses, but no benefit was seen in 4 patients receiving 1000 mg per kg once a week.[25] This dose, however, appeared to reduce the severity of the disease in a patient with Kell sensitisation.[25] Reductions in bilirubin concentrations have been reported following intravenous administration of normal immunoglobulin 500 mg per kg as a single dose to newborn infants.[26] Preliminary studies in small numbers of infants[27,28] suggest that epoetins may be of value in controlling anaemia which develops 2 to 8 weeks after birth.

1. Tovey LAD. Haemolytic disease of the newborn and its prevention. *BMJ* 1990; **300:** 313–16.
2. WHO. Prevention of Rh sensitization: report of a WHO scientific group. *WHO Tech Rep Ser 468* 1971.

3. McClelland DBL, ed. *Handbook of transfusion medicine: Blood Transfusion Services of the United Kingdom.* 3rd ed. London: The Stationery Office, 2001.
4. Robson SC, *et al.* Anti-D immunoglobulin in RhD prophylaxis. *Br J Obstet Gynaecol* 1998; **105:** 129–34.
5. James D. Anti-D prophylaxis in 1997: the Edinburgh consensus statement. *Arch Dis Child* 1998; **78:** F161–F165.
6. Howard HL, *et al.* Preventing rhesus D haemolytic disease of the newborn by giving anti-D immunoglobulin: are the guidelines being adequately followed? *Br J Obstet Gynaecol* 1997; **104:** 37–41.
7. Contreras M. Is anti-D immunoglobulin unnecessary in the domiciliary treatment of miscarriages? *BMJ* 1988; **297:** 733.
8. Tovey LAD. Anti-D and miscarriages. *BMJ* 1988; **297:** 977–8.
9. Lee D. Recommendations for the use of anti-D immunoglobulin. *Prescribers' J* 1991; **31:** 262–3.
10. Tabor A, *et al.* Incidence of rhesus immunisation after genetic amniocentesis. *BMJ* 1986; **293:** 533–6.
11. Contreras M, *et al.* Why women are not receiving anti-Rh prophylaxis. *BMJ* 1986; **293:** 1373.
12. Everett C, *et al.* Reported management of threatened miscarriage by general practitioners in Wessex. *BMJ* 1987; **295:** 583–6.
13. Everett CB. Is anti-D immunoglobulin unnecessary in the domiciliary treatment of miscarriages? *BMJ* 1988; **297:** 732.
14. Everett CB. Anti-D immunoglobulin for bleeding in early pregnancy. *BMJ* 1990; **301:** 1329.
15. Hussey RM. Why women are not receiving anti-Rh prophylaxis. *BMJ* 1987; **294:** 119.
16. Tovey LAD, *et al.* The Yorkshire antenatal anti-D immunoglobulin trial in primigravidae. *Lancet* 1983; **ii:** 244–6.
17. Thornton JG, *et al.* Efficacy and long term effects of antenatal prophylaxis with anti-D immunoglobulin. *BMJ* 1989; **298:** 1671–3.
18. Hussey R. Antenatal prophylaxis with anti-D immunoglobulin. *BMJ* 1989; **299:** 568.
19. Lee D. Antenatal prophylaxis with anti-D immunoglobulin. *BMJ* 1989; **299:** 920.
20. Thornton JG, Tovey LAD. Antenatal prophylaxis with anti-D immunoglobulin. *BMJ* 1989; **299:** 919–20.
21. Whittle MJ. Rhesus haemolytic disease. *Arch Dis Child* 1992; **67:** 65–8.
22. Margulies M, Voto LS. High-dose intravenous gamma globulin: does it have a role in the treatment of severe erythroblastosis fetalis? *Obstet Gynecol* 1991; **77:** 804–5.
23. Berlin G, *et al.* Rhesus haemolytic disease treated with high-dose intravenous immunoglobulin. *Lancet* 1985; **i:** 1153.
24. de la Cámara C, *et al.* High-dose intravenous immunoglobulin as the sole prenatal treatment for severe Rh immunization. *N Engl J Med* 1988; **318:** 519–20.
25. Chitkara U, *et al.* High-dose intravenous gamma globulin: does it have a role in the treatment of severe erythroblastosis fetalis? *Obstet Gynecol* 1990; **76:** 703–8.
26. Rübo J, *et al.* High-dose intravenous immune globulin therapy for hyperbilirubinemia caused by Rh hemolytic disease. *J Pediatr* 1992; **121:** 93–7.
27. Ohls RK, *et al.* Recombinant erythropoietin as treatment for the late hyporegenerative anemia of Rh hemolytic disease. *Pediatrics* 1992; **90:** 678–80.
28. Scaradavou A, *et al.* Suppression of erythropoiesis by intrauterine transfusions in hemolytic disease of the newborn: use of erythropoietin to treat the late anemia. *J Pediatr* 1993; **123:** 279–84.

Idiopathic thrombocytopenic purpura. Normal immunoglobulin is used for chronic idiopathic thrombocytopenic purpura (p.1052), and anti-D immunoglobulin has been found to have similar properties.[1] Treatment of an Rh(D)-positive patient with a long history of severe immune thrombocytopenic purpura with a single dose of 500 units (100 µg) of anti-D immunoglobulin intravenously was reported to result in a steady rise in platelet count and rapid resolution of a cephalic haematoma.[2] Responses to anti-D immunoglobulin were reported in 23 of 25 children with chronic idiopathic thrombocytopenia[3] following treatment with 25 µg per kg body-weight on each of two consecutive days. It has been stated[4] that children with *acute* disease usually recover regardless of therapy but the small risk of intracranial haemorrhage leads many to recommend treatment. In one study[4] involving children with acute disease, a similar dose of anti-D immunoglobulin was less effective in restoring platelet count and produced a greater fall in haemoglobin than either normal immunoglobulin or corticosteroids.

Beneficial results in both rhesus-positive and rhesus-negative patients with HIV-related thrombocytopenia were reported[5-8] with doses in the order of 1 to 3 mg daily, given intravenously.

1. Anonymous. Rho(D) immunoglobulin iv for prevention of Rh isoimmunization and for treatment of ITP. *Med Lett Drugs Ther* 1996; **38:** 6–8.
2. Baglin TP, *et al.* Rapid and complete response of immune thrombocytopenic purpura to a single injection of rhesus anti-D immunoglobulin. *Lancet* 1986; **i:** 1329–30.
3. Andrew M, *et al.* A multicenter study of the treatment of childhood chronic idiopathic thrombocytopenic purpura with anti-D. *J Pediatr* 1992; **120:** 522–7.
4. Blanchette V, *et al.* Randomised trial of intravenous immunoglobulin G, intravenous anti-D, and oral prednisone in childhood acute immune thrombocytopenic purpura. *Lancet* 1994; **344:** 703–7.
5. Durand JM, *et al.* Anti-Rh(D) immunoglobulin for immune thrombocytopenic purpura. *Lancet* 1986; **ii:** 49–50.
6. Biniek R, *et al.* Anti-Rh(D) immunoglobulin for AIDS-related thrombocytopenia. *Lancet* 1986; **ii:** 627.
7. Bierling P, *et al.* Anti-rhesus antibodies, immune thrombocytopenia, and human immunodeficiency virus infection. *Ann Intern Med* 1987; **106:** 773–4.
8. Landonio G, *et al.* HIV-related severe thrombocytopenia in intravenous drug users: prevalence, response to therapy in a medium-term follow-up, and pathogenetic evaluation. *AIDS* 1990; **4:** 29–34.

Preparations

Ph. Eur.: Human Anti-D Immunoglobulin; Human Anti-D Immunoglobulin for Intravenous Administration;
USP 25: Rh₀ (D) Immune Globulin.

Proprietary Preparations (details are given in Part 3)
Aust.: Partobulin; Rhesogam; *Belg.:* Rhesuman†; *Braz.:* Matergam; Partogamma; Rhesonativ; *Canad.:* HypRho-D†; WinRho; *Fr.:* Natead; *Ger.:* Partobulin; Rhesogamma; *Hong Kong:* BayRho-D; Partobulin; Rhesuman†; RhoGAM; *Israel:* BayRho-D; IgRho; KamRho-D; WinRho; *Ital.:* Gamma-Men†; Haima-D; Immunorho; Parto-Gamma; Partobulin; Rhesuman†; Venogamma Anti-Rho (D)†; *Mex.:* BayRho-D; Probi-Rho D; Rhesogamma; *Norw.:* Rhesogamma; Rhesonativ; *NZ:* WinRho; *Port.:* Rhesuman†; *S.Afr.:* Rhesugam; *Spain:* Beriglobina Anti D-P†; Gamma Anti D; Gamma Glob Anti Rh†; Gammaglob Anti D; Globulina Lloren Anti RH; Rhesogamma; Rhesuman†; *Swed.:* Rhesogamma; Rhesonativ; *Switz.:* Rhesuman†; Rhophylac; *Thai.:* Rhesuman†; *UK:* Partobulin; WinRho; *USA:* BayRho-D; Gamulin Rh†; MICRhoGAM; Mini-Gamulin Rh†; RhoGAM; WinRho.

Argentine Haemorrhagic Fever Vaccines

(14682-l)

Junin Haemorrhagic Fever Vaccines.

Profile

A live attenuated vaccine has been investigated for active immunisation against Argentine haemorrhagic fever.

◊ References.

1. Maiztegui JI, *et al.* Protective efficacy of a live attenuated vaccine against Argentine hemorrhagic fever. *J Infect Dis* 1998; **177:** 277–83.

BCG Vaccines (7936-m)

Bacillus Calmette-Guérin Vaccines.
ATC — J07AN01; L03AX03.

Freeze-dried BCG Vaccine (Ph. Eur.) (Bacillus Calmette-Guérin Vaccine (BP 2001); BCG Vaccine; Dried Tub/Vac/BCG; Vaccinum Tuberculosis (BCG) Cryodesiccatum) is a freeze-dried preparation containing live bacteria obtained from a strain derived from the bacillus of Calmette and Guérin (*Mycobacterium bovis* BCG) and known to protect man against tuberculosis. It may contain a stabiliser. The dried vaccine should be stored at 2° to 8° and be protected from sunlight.

BCG Vaccine (USP 25) is a dried living culture of the bacillus Calmette-Guérin strain of *Mycobacterium tuberculosis* var. *bovis*; it is grown from a strain that has been maintained to preserve its capacity for conferring immunity. It contains an amount of viable bacteria such that inoculation, in the recommended dose, of tuberculin-negative persons results in an acceptable tuberculin conversion rate. It contains a suitable stabiliser and no antimicrobial agent. The dried vaccine should be stored at 2° to 8°. The reconstituted vaccine should be used immediately after preparation and any portion not used within 2 hours should be discarded.

Percutaneous Bacillus Calmette-Guérin Vaccine (BP 2001) (Percut. BCG Vaccine) is a suspension of living cells of an authentic strain of the bacillus of Calmette and Guérin with a higher viable bacterial count than Bacillus Calmette-Guérin Vaccine. It is supplied as a dried vaccine (Tub/Vac/BCG(Perc)) and is reconstituted immediately before use by the addition of a suitable sterile liquid. The dried vaccine should be stored at a temperature below −20° and be protected from light.

Adverse Effects

As for vaccines in general, p.1529.

Side-effects occur rarely with BCG vaccines. They include ulceration of the inoculation site, lymphadenitis, and keloid formation. Serious local reactions are usually due to faulty injection techniques. Very rarely, a lupoid type of reaction has occurred. Generalised, possibly hypersensitivity, reactions with a few fatalities have been reported. Disseminated BCG infection may occur. Osteitis has been reported with some BCG vaccines.

◊ Reviews and studies of the adverse effects of BCG vaccines.[1-3] An increased incidence of local effects has followed intradermal injection of high doses of BCG vaccines.[4,5]

1. Lotte A, *et al.* Second IUATLD study on complications induced by intradermal BCG-vaccination. *Bull Int Union Tuberc Lung Dis* 1988; **63:** 47–59.
2. Milstien JB, Gibson JJ. Quality control of BCG vaccine by WHO: a review of factors that may influence vaccine effectiveness and safety. *Bull WHO* 1990; **68:** 93–108.
3. Grange JM. Complications of bacille Calmette-Guérin (BCG) vaccination and immunotherapy and their management. *Commun Dis Public Health* 1998; **1:** 84–8.
4. Miles MM, Shaw RJ. Effect of inadvertent intradermal administration of high dose percutaneous BCG vaccine. *BMJ* 1996; **312:** 1014.
5. Puliyel JM, *et al.* Adverse local reactions from accidental BCG overdose in infants. *BMJ* 1996; **313:** 528–9.

Effects on the bones and joints. The risk of osteitis following BCG vaccination varies from country to country and appears to be linked to the strain of bacillus used.[1]

Osteitis or arthritis has also been reported following intravesicular administration of BCG (see below).

1. Milstien JB, Gibson JJ. Quality control of BCG vaccine by WHO: a review of factors that may influence vaccine effectiveness and safety. *Bull WHO* 1990; **68:** 93–108.

Effects on the eyes. Follicular conjunctivitis occurred following accidental contamination of the eye with BCG vaccine.[1] The conjunctivitis responded to topical corticosteroid therapy, but a course of isoniazid was given as a precautionary measure.

1. Pollard AJ, George RH. Ocular contamination with BCG vaccine. *Arch Dis Child* 1994; **70:** 71.

Effects on the lymphatic system. Increases in the incidence and severity of lymphadenitis have been reported following changes in BCG vaccine to one containing more virulent strains or with different dosage recommendations.[1,2]

1. Hengster P, *et al.* Occurrence of suppurative lymphadenitis after a change of BCG vaccine. *Arch Dis Child* 1992; **67:** 952–5.
2. Kabra SK, *et al.* BCG-associated adenitis. *Lancet* 1993; **341:** 970.

Intravesicular administration. Intravesicular instillation of BCG can give rise to both localised and systemic adverse effects.[1] Local effects include bladder irritation and urinary-tract infections. A case of local infection with vaccine-derived *Mycobacterium bovis* has been reported.[2] Symptoms of hypersensitivity reactions include malaise, fever, and chills. The most serious reactions are severe sepsis with cardiorespiratory manifestations and a disseminated mycobacterial infection with lung granulomas and impaired liver function; both require prompt treatment with antimycobacterials.[1] There have been case reports of systemic granulomatous disease[3] and of arthritis and osteitis[4-6] following intravesicular administration of BCG.

1. Lamm DL, *et al.* Incidence and treatment of complications of bacillus Calmette-Guérin intravesical therapy in superficial bladder cancer. *J Urol (Baltimore)* 1992; **147:** 596–600.
2. Ribera M, *et al.* Mycobacterium bovis-BCG infection of the glans penis: a complication of intravesical administration of bacillus Calmette-Guérin. *Br J Dermatol* 1995; **132:** 309–10.
3. Mooren FC, *et al.* Systemic granulomatous disease after intravesical BCG instillation. *BMJ* 2000; **320:** 219.
4. Puett DW, Fuchs HA. Arthritis after bacillus Calmette-Guérin therapy. *Ann Intern Med* 1992; **117:** 537.
5. Devlin M, *et al.* Arthritis as a complication of intravesical BCG vaccine. *BMJ* 1994; **308:** 1638.
6. Morgan MB, Iseman MD. Mycobacterium bovis vertebral osteomyelitis as a complication of intravesical administration of Bacille Calmette-Guérin. *Am J Med* 1996; **100:** 372–3.

Precautions

As for vaccines in general, p.1530. BCG vaccines may be given concomitantly with other live vaccines, but if they are not given at the same time it is preferable to allow an interval of 3 weeks between administration although the period may be reduced to 10 days if absolutely necessary. However, routine immunisation with live poliomyelitis vaccine need not be delayed. No further vaccination should be given in the arm used for BCG vaccination for at least 3 months because of the risk of lymphadenitis. Because of the possible risk of disseminated infections, it is recommended in the UK that BCG vaccines should not be given to HIV-positive persons or those with impaired immune systems from other causes. WHO has, however, advised immunisation of asymptomatic HIV-positive children when the risk of tuberculosis is high. In patients with eczema, BCG vaccines should be given at a site free from lesions. They should not be given to patients receiving antimycobacterial therapy.

Immunocompromised patients. Like other live vaccines, BCG vaccine should not be given to immunocompromised patients including those with symptomatic HIV infections and AIDS. However, the risk of possible adverse effects in patients with asymptomatic HIV infections may be outweighed by the possible advantages of vaccination (see Tuberculosis, HIV-infected Patients, below). Disseminated BCG infections have been reported in children with HIV infections,[1] but large studies have shown that infants born to HIV-positive mothers had only a slightly increased risk of adverse reactions, and many of these were generally mild.[2,3]

1. Ryder RW, *et al.* Safety and immunogenicity of bacille Calmette-Guérin, diphtheria-tetanus-pertussis, and oral polio vaccines in newborn children in Zaire infected with human immunodeficiency virus type 1. *J Pediatr* 1993; **122:** 697–702.
2. Besnard M, *et al.* Bacillus Calmette-Guérin infection after vaccination of human immunodeficiency virus-infected children. *Pediatr Infect Dis J* 1993; **12:** 993–7.
3. O'Brien KL, *et al.* Bacillus Calmette-Guérin complications in children born to HIV-1-infected women with a review of the literature. *Pediatrics* 1995; **95:** 414–18.

The symbol † denotes a preparation no longer actively marketed

Interactions

As for vaccines in general, p.1530.

Theophylline. For a report of increased theophylline half-life and serum concentrations after BCG vaccination, see under Theophylline Hydrate, p.782.

Uses and Administration

BCG vaccines are used for active immunisation against tuberculosis, principally for the vaccination of selected groups of the population and of persons likely to be exposed to infection. In some countries it is administered only to persons who give a negative tuberculin reaction, but in countries with a high prevalence of tuberculosis, routine vaccination in infancy is recommended (see below under Tuberculosis for further details). It is also used locally in the treatment of bladder cancers (see below under Malignant Neoplasms, Bladder for further details).

In the UK vaccination is recommended in the following groups of persons, if there is *no evidence of previous immunisation* and they are found to be *tuberculin-negative* (see under Tuberculins, p.1675):

- children aged 10 to 14 years (as part of the standard schedule for immunisation—see p.1530)
- contacts of persons suffering from active respiratory tuberculosis
- immigrants in whose communities there is known to be a high incidence of tuberculosis and all their children wherever born
- health service staff at high risk of infection
- veterinary and other staff who handle animals known to be susceptible to tuberculosis
- staff in any institution where the incidence of tuberculosis is high
- persons intending to stay in Asia, Africa, or Central or South America for more than a month
- any other individual upon request.

Sensitivity testing to tuberculin need not be performed for infants less than 3 months old.

The BCG vaccine is given intradermally (intracutaneously) at the insertion of the deltoid muscle in a dose of 0.1 mL; infants under 3 months of age are given 0.05 mL. For cosmetic reasons, the injection may be given into the upper and lateral surface of the thigh.

A BCG vaccine approximately 10 times the strength of the intradermal vaccine may be given percutaneously using a multiple-puncture device, but such administration is only recommended in infants and young children (up to 5 years of age).

Contacts of patients with active pulmonary tuberculosis may require chemoprophylaxis despite previous vaccination (see under Tuberculosis, p.143). Neonates and children under 2 years of age should be given chemoprophylaxis and immunised, if appropriate, once the course is completed. An isoniazid-resistant form of the vaccine has been produced for use in patients who have received isoniazid, but its use is not recommended.

◊ General references and reviews.
1. Lugosi L. Theoretical and methodological aspects of BCG vaccine from the discovery of Calmette and Guérin to molecular biology: a review. *Tubercle Lung Dis* 1992; **73:** 252–61.

Leishmaniasis. For reference to the use of BCG vaccines in leishmaniasis, see Leishmaniasis Vaccines, p.1546.

Leprosy. BCG vaccination has been shown to protect recipients against leprosy[1] and is considered to be one of the factors responsible for the decrease in the incidence of leprosy. As in tuberculosis considerable variation has been noted in the efficacy of BCG in leprosy, and it appears to be more effective in Africa[2-4] and South America than in Asia.[5,6] Protection appears to be afforded against both multibacillary and paucibacillary leprosy[7,8] and a second dose may provide additional protection.[9] Adding killed *Mycobacterium leprae* did not improve the response further.[9] BCG is considered to be an important addition to multidrug treatment in long-term eradication programmes.[1] Specific vaccines against leprosy are under development (see p.1546).
1. Lienhardt C, Fine PEM. Controlling leprosy. *BMJ* 1992; **305:** 206–7.
2. Stanley SJ, *et al.* BCG vaccination of children against leprosy in Uganda: final results. *J Hyg (Camb)* 1981; **87:** 233–48.
3. Fine PEM, *et al.* Protective efficacy of BCG against leprosy in northern Malawi. *Lancet* 1986; **ii:** 499–502.
4. Baker DM, Nguyen-Van-Tam JS. BCG vaccine and leprosy. *Lancet* 1992; **339:** 1236.

5. Lwin KW, *et al.* BCG vaccination of children against leprosy: fourteen-year findings of the trial in Burma. *Bull WHO* 1985; **63:** 1069–78.
6. Tripathy SP. The case for BCG. *Ann Natl Med Sci (India)* 1983; **19:** 11–21.
7. Pönnighaus JM, *et al.* Efficacy of BCG vaccine against leprosy and tuberculosis in northern Malawi. *Lancet* 1992; **339:** 636–9.
8. Muliyil J, *et al.* Effect of BCG on the risk of leprosy in an endemic area: case control study. *Int J Lepr* 1991; **59:** 229–36.
9. Karonga Prevention Trial Group. Randomised controlled trial of single BCG, repeated BCG, or combined BCG and killed mycobacterium leprae vaccine for prevention of leprosy and tuberculosis in Malawi. *Lancet* 1996; **348:** 17–24.

Malignant neoplasms. Immunotherapy with BCG vaccines has been tried in various malignant disorders and is most successful when administered locally. The possibility that BCG vaccination might protect children against malignancies has been discussed.[1]
1. Grange JM, Stanford JL. BCG vaccination and cancer. *Tubercle* 1990; **71:** 61–4.

BLADDER. Immunotherapy with adjuvant intravesicular BCG is used in the management of bladder cancers and is the treatment of choice for carcinoma *in situ* (p.490). Local and systemic adverse effects, although rarely severe, are relatively common. Treatment is not started until 7 to 14 days after bladder biopsy or transurethral resection. A number of regimens have been tried, but the UK manufacturers recommend that BCG is instilled into the bladder once weekly for 6 weeks, followed after a 6-week pause by further instillations once weekly for 1 to 3 weeks. Maintenance therapy is recommended and consists of instillations every 1 to 3 weeks at 6 months after initiation of treatment and then every 6 months thereafter until 36 months. Urine voided for 6 hours after instillation of BCG vaccines should be disinfected with sodium hypochlorite solution. Reviews.
1. Moss JT, Kadmon D. BCG and the treatment of superficial bladder cancer. *DICP Ann Pharmacother* 1991; **25:** 1355–67.
2. Alexandroff AB, *et al.* BCG immunotherapy of bladder cancer: 20 years on. *Lancet* 1999; **353:** 1689–94.

SKIN. Several studies have reported that BCG vaccine injected into intradermal metastases of melanoma can result in regression of the injected, and sometimes also the uninjected nodules. BCG therapy has been disappointing for visceral metastases. Many anecdotal reports and nonrandomised studies have shown benefit from BCG vaccine as adjuvant therapy, but these results have not been confirmed in large randomised, controlled studies.[1] More specific immunological interventions such as therapeutic vaccines are now being investigated in the treatment of melanomas (p.499).
1. Ho VC, Sober AJ. Therapy for cutaneous melanoma: an update. *J Am Acad Dermatol* 1990; **22:** 159–76.

Tuberculosis. Studies from many parts of the world have evaluated the efficacy of BCG vaccine to protect against tuberculosis. Levels of protection have varied from 0 to over 80%.[1] Many explanations for such variability have been proposed: interaction with the immune response to other mycobacterial infections; antigenic, microbiological, or formulation differences between BCG vaccines; differences in the natural history of infection and disease; variations in host genetics or nutrition; methodological differences between studies.[1,2] It has been noted that in general the efficacy of BCG vaccine in any region is proportional to its distance from the equator and this possibly reflects differences in exposure to environmental mycobacteria.[3] This could be the strongest influence on efficacy,[3] with the implication that BCG may be least effective in areas of the world where the risk of tuberculosis is greatest. BCG also appears to be more effective against systemic (miliary and meningitic tuberculosis) than against pulmonary tuberculosis. It is likely that BCG cannot produce complete protection against infection, and the development of new vaccines is underway.[4] National policies of BCG vaccination vary widely. In the USA vaccination is recommended only for tuberculin-negative infants and children at high risk of tuberculosis.[5] Most other countries recommend routine vaccination (the UK recommendations are described above).[1] Schedules vary from single vaccination at birth (as recommended by WHO),[6] to single vaccination at age 10 to 14 (as in the UK), to repeated vaccination every few years (particularly in eastern Europe). These policy differences appear to be related as much to differences of opinion about the mechanism of action and effectiveness of vaccines as to local differences in the epidemiology of tuberculosis.[1] WHO considers BCG vaccination to be an adjunct to case detection and treatment in the control of tuberculosis,[6] and recommends that neither tuberculin skin testing nor repeat vaccination should be used.
1. Fine PEM, Rodrigues LC. Modern vaccines: mycobacterial diseases. *Lancet* 1990; **335:** 1016–20.
2. Fine PEM. BCG vaccination against tuberculosis and leprosy. *Br Med Bull* 1988; **44:** 691–703.
3. Fine PEM. Variation in protection by BCG: implications of and for heterologous immunity. *Lancet* 1995; **346:** 1339–45. Correction. *ibid.*; **347:** 340.
4. Malin AS, Young DB. Designing a vaccine for tuberculosis. *BMJ* 1996; **312:** 1495.
5. Centers for Disease Control. The role of BCG vaccine in the prevention and control of tuberculosis in the United States: a joint statement by the Advisory Council for the Elimination of Tuberculosis and the Advisory Committee on Immunization Practices. *MMWR* 1996; **45** (RR-4): 1–18.
6. Anonymous. WHO statement on BCG revaccination for the prevention of tuberculosis. *Bull WHO* 1995; **73:** 805–6.

HIV-INFECTED PATIENTS. Like other live vaccines, BCG vaccine should not be given to immunocompromised patients including patients with symptomatic HIV infection or AIDS. Doubts about the safety (see under Precautions, above) and efficacy of BCG vaccines in patients with asymptomatic HIV infection have resulted in differing national policies. WHO recommends that the national policy should depend on the local prevalence of tuberculosis.[1] In countries where prevalence is high, the possible benefits of immunisation outweigh the possible disadvantages, and routine BCG vaccination should be given to all children except those with symptomatic HIV infection or AIDS. In countries with low tuberculosis prevalence, BCG vaccination should not be given to children with HIV infections. In the UK[2] and USA,[3] BCG vaccination is not recommended for HIV-positive patients. Similar policies apply to infants born to HIV-positive mothers, although it is not necessary to screen mothers for HIV infection before giving routine BCG vaccination.[2]
1. WHO. *TB/HIV: a clinical manual.* Geneva: WHO, 1996.
2. Salisbury DM, Begg NT, (eds), Joint Committee on Vaccination and Immunisation. *Immunisation against infectious disease.* London: HMSO, 1996.
3. Centers for Disease Control. The role of BCG vaccine in the prevention and control of tuberculosis in the United States: a joint statement by the Advisory Council for the Elimination of Tuberculosis and the Advisory Committee on Immunization Practices. *MMWR* 1996; **45** (RR-4) 1–18.

Preparations

BP 2001: Percutaneous Bacillus Calmette-Guérin Vaccine;
Ph. Eur.: Freeze-dried BCG Vaccine;
USP 25: BCG Vaccine.

Proprietary Preparations (details are given in Part 3)
Aust.: ImmuCyst, OncoTICE; *Austral.:* ImmuCyst; OncoTICE; *Belg.:* ImmuCyst; Pastimmun†; *Canad.:* ImmuCyst; OncoTICE; Pacis; *Denm.:* OncoTICE; *Fin.:* OncoTICE; *Fr.:* ImmuCyst; Monovax; *Ger.:* ImmuCyst†; OncoTICE; *Hong Kong:* ImmuCyst; OncoTICE; *Israel:* ImmuCyst; OncoTICE; *Ital.:* ImmuCyst; Imovax BCG; OncoTICE; *Mex.:* Cultivo BCG; *Neth.:* OncoTICE; *Norw.:* OncoTICE; *NZ:* ImmuCyst; OncoTICE; *Port.:* ImmuCyst; *Singapore:* ImmuCyst; *Spain:* ImmuCyst; OncoTICE; *Swed.:* OncoTICE; *Switz.:* ImmuCyst; OncoTICE; *Thai.:* ImmuCyst; *UK:* ImmuCyst; OncoTICE; *USA:* Pacis; TheraCys; Tice.

Botulism Antitoxins (7939-g)

ATC — J06AA04.

Botulinum Antitoxin (Ph. Eur.) (Bot/Ser; Immunoserum Botulinicum) is a sterile preparation containing the specific antitoxic globulins that have the power of neutralising the toxins formed by type A, type B, type E, or any mixture of types A, B, and E, of *Clostridium botulinum*. It contains not less than 500 international units of each of type A and type B and not less than 50 units of type E per mL. It should be stored at 2° to 8°, and not be allowed to freeze. The BP 2001 states that when Mixed Botulinum Antitoxin or Botulinum Antitoxin is prescribed or demanded and the types to be present are not stated, Botulinum Antitoxin prepared from types A, B, and E shall be dispensed or supplied. It should be noted, however, that some antitoxins available in the UK have not conformed to the requirements of the BP 2001 and Ph. Eur. (having a higher phenol content than the pharmacopoeias allow), and thus have been referred to as botulism antitoxin rather than botulinum antitoxin.

Botulism Antitoxin (USP 25) is a sterile solution of the refined and concentrated antitoxic antibodies, chiefly globulins, obtained from the blood of healthy horses that have been immunised against the toxins produced by type A and type B and/or E strains of *Clostridium botulinum*. It contains a suitable antimicrobial agent. It should be stored at 2° to 8° in single-use containers.

Adverse Effects and Precautions

As for antisera in general, p.1529.

Uses and Administration

Botulism antitoxins are used in the postexposure prophylaxis and treatment of botulism. Treatment should be given as early as possible in the course of the disease. Botulism antitoxins are generally not effective for infant botulism.

Since the type of botulism toxin is seldom known the polyvalent antitoxin is usually given. Sensitivity testing should always be performed before administration of the antitoxin.

In the UK a trivalent antitoxin containing not less than 500 units per mL of each of antitoxins types A, B, and E is employed. For the treatment of botulism, 20 mL of this antitoxin should be diluted to 100 mL with sodium chloride 0.9% and given by slow intravenous infusion over at least 30 minutes; another 10 mL may be given 2 to 4 hours later if necessary, and further doses at 12- to 24-hour intervals if indicated. Persons who have been exposed to the toxin and in whom symptoms have not developed should be given 20 mL intramuscularly as a prophylactic measure.

In some countries the mixed antitoxin contains differing amounts of type A, B, and E antitoxin.

Botulism. Botulism is caused by the exotoxin of *Clostridium botulinum*, a spore-forming, Gram-positive anaerobe which occurs in soil and mud. The disease usually follows ingestion of contaminated preserved foodstuffs, but may develop from infected wounds or following gastrointestinal colonisation in infants. The toxin is heat labile, but the spores can survive temperatures of up to 120°. Eight types of *C. botulinum* can be distinguished, each producing a different exotoxin; human disease is usually caused by types A, B and E.

Symptoms arise from inhibition of acetylcholine-mediated neurotransmission and include descending weakness or paralysis, gastrointestinal symptoms, postural hypotension, dry mouth, and dilated pupils. Death is usually from respiratory arrest.

Treatment of botulism is with antitoxins and intensive respiratory and supportive therapy. Antitoxins should be given as early as possible but may still be beneficial if treatment is delayed.

Drug therapy aimed at reversing the neuromuscular blockade has included fampridine, guanidine, and guanoxan, and some patients may benefit from this treatment.

Oral penicillins have been tried to eliminate any organisms remaining in the gastrointestinal tract.

Infant botulism is of increasing importance, especially in the USA where it is reported to be the most commonly occurring form of botulism, with honey (see p.1366) reputed to be the most frequent source of infection. Treatment is with intensive supportive care; antitoxins are not considered to be effective.

Reviews.

1. Shapiro RL, et al. Botulism in the United States: a clinical and epidemiologic review. *Ann Intern Med* 1998; **129:** 221–8.

Preparations

Ph. Eur.: Botulinum Antitoxin;
USP 25: Botulism Antitoxin.

Proprietary Preparations (details are given in Part 3)
Ital.: Liosiero.

Bovine Colostrum (3802-m)

Profile

Bovine colostrum has been used similarly to antisera and human immunoglobulin preparations to provide passive immunity against infectious diseases. Hyperimmune bovine colostra have been prepared from cows previously immunised with specific antigens. In particular, these specific hyperimmune bovine colostra have been tried in cryptosporidiosis and in the prevention of rotavirus diarrhoea in infants.

Preparations

Proprietary Preparations (details are given in Part 3)
Austral.: Gastrogard-R.

Brucellosis Vaccines (5171-b)

ATC — J07AD01.

Profile

A brucellosis vaccine prepared from an antigenic extract of *Brucella abortus* has been used for active immunisation against brucellosis in persons at high risk of contracting the disease.

Preparations

Proprietary Preparations (details are given in Part 3)
Braz.: Bruvac.

Campylobacter Jejuni Vaccines (12181-r)

Profile

An oral vaccine is under development to provide active immunisation against *Campylobacter jejuni* infection.

Cancer Vaccines (3041-n)

Profile

Vaccines are under investigation for a variety of neoplastic diseases including breast, cervical, colorectal, lung, ovarian, pancreatic, prostate, and renal cancers, lymphomas and melanoma. BCG vaccine (p.1534) is used locally in the treatment of bladder cancer and has been tried in other neoplastic diseases. Human papilloma virus vaccines (p.1544) are under investigation for the treatment of some cancers.

◊ General review of cancer vaccines under development.

1. Herlyn D, Birebent B. Advances in cancer vaccine development. *Ann Med* 1999; **31:** 66–78.
2. Minev BR, et al. Cancer vaccines: novel approaches and new promise. *Pharmacol Ther* 1999; **81:** 121–39.
3. Greten TF, Jaffee EM. Cancer vaccines. *J Clin Oncol* 1999; **17:** 1047–60.
4. Chamberlain RS. Prospects for the therapeutic use of anticancer vaccines. *Drugs* 1999; **57:** 309–25.
5. Jaffee EM. Immunotherapy of cancer. *Ann N Y Acad Sci* 1999; **886:** 67–72.
6. Sinkovics JF, Horvath JC. Vaccination against human cancers (review). *Int J Oncol* 2000; **16:** 81–96.

Melanoma. Reviews.

1. Bonn D. Getting under the skin with melanoma vaccines. *Lancet* 1996; **348:** 396.

The symbol † denotes a preparation no longer actively marketed

2. Haigh PI, et al. Vaccine therapy for patients with melanoma. *Oncology (Huntingt)* 1999; **13:** 1561–74.
3. Brinckerhoff LH, et al. Melanoma vaccines. *Curr Opin Oncol* 2000; **12:** 163–73.

Cholera Vaccines (7941-d)

ATC — J07AE01; J07AE02.

Cholera Vaccine (Ph. Eur.) (Cho/Vac; Vaccinum Cholerae) is a sterile homogeneous suspension of a suitable killed strain or strains of *Vibrio cholerae*. It consists of a mixture of equal parts of vaccines prepared from smooth strains of 2 main serological types, Inaba and Ogawa of the classical biotype with or without the El Tor biotype. A single strain or several strains of each type may be included. All strains must contain, in addition to their type O antigens, the heat-stable O antigen common to the Inaba and Ogawa types. If more than one strain each of Inaba and Ogawa are used they may be selected to contain other O antigens. It contains not less than 8000 million *V. cholerae* per dose, which does not exceed 1 mL. It contains not more than 0.5% of phenol. It should be stored at 2° to 8° and protected from light. It may also be supplied as a dried vaccine (Dried Cho/Vac; Freeze-dried Cholera Vaccine (Ph. Eur.); Vaccinum Cholerae Cryodesiccatum) which is reconstituted immediately before use by the addition of a suitable sterile liquid. Phenol may not be used in the preparation of the dried vaccine. It should be stored at 2° to 8° and be protected from light.

Cholera Vaccine (USP 25) is a sterile suspension, in sodium chloride injection or other suitable diluent, of killed *Vibrio cholerae* selected for high antigenic efficiency. It is prepared from equal parts of suspensions of cholera vibrios of the Inaba and Ogawa strains. It has a labelled potency of 8 units per serotype per mL. It contains a suitable antimicrobial agent. It should be stored at 2° to 8° and not be allowed to freeze.

Adverse Effects and Precautions

As for vaccines in general, p.1529.

Slight swelling, erythema, and tenderness occasionally occur at the injection site. Fever and malaise have been reported and general reactions, including anaphylaxis and hypersensitivity reactions, have occurred. Neurological and psychiatric reactions have occasionally occurred.

Interactions

As for vaccines in general, p.1530.

◊ For reference to the effect of cholera vaccination on the response to *yellow fever vaccines*, see under Yellow Fever Vaccines, p.1568.

Uses and Administration

Injectable inactivated whole-cell cholera vaccines have been used for active immunisation against cholera but are not considered to be very effective and the immunity conferred is short-lived. They have no role in the management of contacts of cases or in controlling the spread of infection. The WHO International Health Regulations do not require cholera vaccination for travellers as the introduction of cholera into any country cannot be prevented by cholera vaccination. However, travellers may still be asked for evidence of immunisation at some borders.

In the UK, a vaccine containing not less than 8000 million *V. cholerae* per mL has been used and a primary prophylactic course of 2 injections at an interval of at least a week and preferably 4 weeks has been given. Further doses should be given at intervals of 6 months.

Oral vaccines containing either live attenuated or inactivated strains are available in some countries and appear to be more effective than parenteral vaccines (see below).

Oral cholera vaccines. Since parenteral cholera vaccines are not considered to be very effective, providing at best 50% protection and confer immunity lasting only 3 to 6 months, attention has turned towards oral vaccines which stimulate intestinal immunity. Both killed and living oral vaccines have been developed, and both types have been shown to be non-toxic and immunogenic.

Killed vaccines contain inactivated whole *V. cholerae* O1 either alone or with B subunit component of cholera toxin.[1-6] These vaccines produce a protective efficacy of about 60 to 70%[1,2,6] and both modify established infections and prevent new ones. Although the vaccines are effective in areas where the El Tor biotype predominates,[5,6] they are more effective against classical strains.[1] Immunity particularly against El Tor may be less

sustained in children under 5 years of age than in older children and adults.[1,2,7] The main drawback is the need to administer two or more doses at 1- to 2-week intervals to achieve a protective effect.[4,5,8] The protective effect is rapidly established[5] but wanes over time[1,7] and booster doses after 1 year may be necessary to maintain a high level of immunity.[9]

The most widely investigated live attenuated vaccine is CVD 103-HgR in which the genes encoding the toxic A subunit are deleted by recombinant techniques.[10-14] This vaccine is effective 8 days after a single dose but less so against El Tor than against classical strains. Live oral vaccines effective against El Tor are now being developed,[15,16] and promising responses have also been reported with a live attenuated O139 vaccine.[17]

The efficacy and cost-effectiveness of oral vaccines to control cholera outbreaks in refugee populations remains uncertain.[18,19]

1. Clemens JD, et al. Field trial of oral cholera vaccines in Bangladesh: results from three-year follow-up. *Lancet* 1990; **335:** 270–3.
2. Clemens JD, et al. Evidence that inactivated oral cholera vaccines both prevent and mitigate Vibrio cholerae O1 infections in a cholera-endemic area. *J Infect Dis* 1992; **166:** 1029–34.
3. Jertborn M, et al. Evaluation of different immunization schedules for oral cholera B subunit-whole cell vaccine in Swedish volunteers. *Vaccine* 1993; **11:** 1007–12.
4. Sanchez JL, et al. Safety and immunogenicity of the oral, whole cell/recombinant B subunit cholera vaccine in North American volunteers. *J Infect Dis* 1993; **167:** 1446–9.
5. Sanchez JL, et al. Protective efficacy of oral whole-cell/recombinant-B-subunit cholera vaccine in Peruvian military recruits. *Lancet* 1994; **344:** 1273–6.
6. Trach DD, et al. Field trial of a locally produced, killed, oral cholera vaccine in Vietnam. *Lancet* 1997; **349:** 231–5.
7. van Loon FPL, et al. Field trial of inactivated oral cholera vaccines in Bangladesh: results from 5 years of follow-up. *Vaccine* 1996; **14:** 162–6.
8. Sanchez JL, et al. Immunological response to Vibrio cholerae O1 infection and an oral cholera vaccine among Peruvians. *Trans R Soc Trop Med Hyg* 1995; **89:** 542–5.
9. Begue RE, et al. Immunogenicity in Peruvian volunteers of a booster dose of oral cholera vaccine consisting of whole cells plus recombinant B subunit. *Infect Immun* 1995; **63:** 3726–8.
10. Levine MM, et al. Safety, immunogenicity, and efficacy of recombinant live oral cholera vaccines, CVD 103 and CVD 103-HgR. *Lancet* 1988; **ii:** 467–70.
11. Suharyono, et al. Safety and immunogenicity of single-dose live oral cholera vaccine CVD 103-HgR in 5-9-year-old Indonesian children. *Lancet* 1992; **340:** 689–94.
12. Su-Arehawaratana P, et al. Safety and immunogenicity of different immunization regimens of CVD 103-HgR live oral cholera vaccine in soldiers and civilians in Thailand. *J Infect Dis* 1992; **165:** 1042–8.
13. Barrett P, et al. Oral cholera vaccine well tolerated. *BMJ* 1993; **307:** 1425.
14. Tacket CO, et al. Onset and duration of protective immunity in challenged volunteers after vaccination with live oral cholera vaccine CVD 103-HgR. *J Infect Dis* 1992; **166:** 837–41.
15. Tacket CO, et al. Volunteer studies investigating the safety and efficacy of live El Tor Vibrio cholerae O1 vaccine strain CVD 111. *Am J Trop Med Hyg* 1997; **56:** 533–7.
16. Sack DA, et al. Evaluation of Peru-15, a new live oral vaccine for cholera, in volunteers. *J Infect Dis* 1997; **176:** 201–5.
17. Coster TS, et al. Safety, immunogenicity, and efficacy of live attenuated Vibrio cholerae O139 vaccine prototype. *Lancet* 1995; **345:** 949–52.
18. Naficy A, et al. Treatment and vaccination strategies to control cholera in sub-Saharan refugee settings: a cost-effectiveness analysis. *JAMA* 1998; **279:** 521–5.
19. Waldman RJ. Cholera vaccination in refugee settings. *JAMA* 1998; **279:** 552–3.

Preparations

Ph. Eur.: Cholera Vaccine; Freeze-dried Cholera Vaccine;
USP 25: Cholera Vaccine.

Proprietary Preparations (details are given in Part 3)
Austral.: Orochol; *Canad.:* Mutacol; *Denm.:* Dukoral; *Ital.:* Imovax Colera†; *Norw.:* Dukoral; *NZ:* Orochol; *Swed.:* Dukoral; *Switz.:* Orochol.

Contraceptive Vaccines (3865-a)

Profile

Various approaches to development of a contraceptive vaccine are under investigation. A synthetic contraceptive vaccine which stimulates the production of an antibody against human chorionic gonadotrophin has been studied in human trials.

◊ References.

1. Jones WR, et al. Phase I clinical trial of a World Health Organisation birth control vaccine. *Lancet* 1988; **i:** 1295–8.
2. Talwar GP, et al. A vaccine that prevents pregnancy in women. *Proc Natl Acad Sci U S A* 1994; **91:** 8532–6.

Crimean-Congo Haemorrhagic Fever Immunoglobulins (14731-v)

Profile

Preparations containing antibodies against Crimean-Congo haemorrhagic fever are available in some countries for passive immunisation against the disease.

◊ References.

1. Vassilenko SM, et al. Specific intravenous immunoglobulin for Crimean-Congo haemorrhagic fever. *Lancet* 1990; **335:** 791–2.

Cytomegalovirus Immunoglobulins (3896-h)

ATC — J06BB09.

Cytomegalovirus immunoglobulins containing high levels of specific antibody against cytomegalovirus have been prepared from human plasma.

Adverse Effects and Precautions
As for immunoglobulins in general, p.1529.

Interactions
As for immunoglobulins in general, p.1529.

Uses and Administration
Cytomegalovirus immunoglobulins are used for passive immunisation against cytomegalovirus infection. They may be used prophylactically, especially in patients undergoing certain transplant procedures, or therapeutically for the treatment of established cytomegalovirus infections. For therapeutic and some prophylactic uses, they are commonly given with ganciclovir.

In the USA a cytomegalovirus immunoglobulin G is available for use in recipients of heart, kidney, liver, lung, and pancreas transplants from cytomegalovirus seropositive donors. The dosage schedule for kidney transplant recipients is 150 mg per kg body-weight by intravenous infusion within 72 hours of transplantation, then 100 mg per kg once every 2 weeks for 4 doses, then 50 mg per kg every 4 weeks for 2 doses. The rate of infusion should start at 15 mg per kg per hour increasing to a maximum rate of 60 mg per kg per hour. For recipients of transplants other than kidney, the recommended dosage schedule is 150 mg per kg within 72 hours of transplantation and then once every 2 weeks for 4 further doses, then 100 mg per kg every 4 weeks for 2 doses. Ganciclovir should be given concomitantly. The name sevirumab is applied to a χ-chain human monoclonal cytomegalovirus immunoglobulin G1.

Preparations

Proprietary Preparations (details are given in Part 3)
Aust.: Cytotect; *Austral.:* CMV Immunoglobulin; *Canad.:* CMV Iveegam†; *Fin.:* Megalotect; *Ger.:* Cytoglobin; Cytotect; *Irl.:* Megalotect; *Israel:* Megalotect; *Ital.:* Cytotect; Haimacig; Immunoendocig; Uman-Cig; *Port.:* Megalotect; *S.Afr.:* Megalotect; *Swed.:* Megalotect; *Switz.:* Cytotect; Globuman iv CMV; *Thai.:* Megalotect; *USA:* CytoGam.

Cytomegalovirus Vaccines (16597-p)

Profile
A live attenuated cytomegalovirus vaccine containing human cytomegalovirus Towne strain has been investigated in humans since the late 1970s, particularly for the prevention of cytomegalovirus infection in renal transplant recipients. However, there are doubts over its safety. Vaccines produced by recombinant technology are also being studied.

◊ In a placebo-controlled study involving 237 renal transplant patients[1] no effect of the cytomegalovirus vaccine (Towne strain) (administered subcutaneously) could be demonstrated on the overall incidence of cytomegalovirus infection or disease, but there was less severe disease in seronegative recipients who received kidneys from seropositive donors. The vaccine also appeared to prolong graft survival in this subset of patients. However, the Towne vaccine failed to prevent infection in immunocompetent women exposed to infectious young children.[2]

Studies of subunit vaccines have produced some promising results.[3-5]

1. Plotkin SA, *et al.* Effect of Towne live virus vaccine on cytomegalovirus disease after renal transplant. *Ann Intern Med* 1991; **114:** 525–31.
2. Adler SP, *et al.* Immunity induced by primary human cytomegalovirus infection protects against secondary infection among women of childbearing age. *J Infect Dis* 1995; **171:** 26–32.
3. Britt WJ. Vaccines against human cytomegalovirus: time to test. *Trends Microbiol* 1996; **4:** 34–8.
4. Pass RF, *et al.* A subunit cytomegalovirus vaccine based on recombinant envelope glycoprotein B and a new adjuvant. *J Infect Dis* 1999; **180:** 970–5.
5. Frey SE, *et al.* Effects of antigen dose and immunization regimens on antibody responses to a cytomegalovirus glycoprotein B subunit vaccine. *J Infect Dis* 1999; **180:** 1700–3.

Dengue Fever Vaccines (16601-e)

Profile
Live attenuated vaccines under study for active immunisation against dengue fever contain dengue virus types 1, 2, 3, and 4 alone or in various combinations. The ultimate aim is to produce a vaccine active against all types of dengue virus. Recombinant vaccines are also under investigation.

◊ References.
1. Bhamarapravati N, *et al.* Immunization with a live attenuated dengue 2 virus candidate vaccine (16681-PDK 53): clinical, immunological and biological responses in adult volunteers. *Bull WHO* 1987; **65:** 189–95.
2. Bhamarapravati N, Yoksan S. Study of bivalent dengue vaccine in volunteers. *Lancet* 1989; **i:** 1077.
3. Brandt WE (WHO). Development of dengue and Japanese encephalitis vaccines. *J Infect Dis* 1990; **162:** 577–83.
4. Barrett ADT. Japanese encephalitis and dengue vaccines. *Biologicals* 1997; **25:** 27–34.

5. Cardosa MJ. Dengue vaccine design: issues and challenges. *Br Med Bull* 1998; **54:** 395–405.
6. Velzing J, *et al.* Induction of protective immunity against dengue virus type 2: comparison of candidate live attenuated and recombinant vaccines. *Vaccine* 1999; **17:** 1312–30.

Dental Caries Vaccines (1883-b)

Profile
Dental caries vaccines consisting of purified proteins from *Streptococcus mutans* are under investigation. Monoclonal antibodies are also being studied for local passive immunisation.

◊ References.
1. Russell MW. Immunization against dental caries. *Curr Opin Dent* 1992; **2:** 72–80.
2. Hajishengallis G, Michalek SM. Current status of a mucosal vaccine against dental caries. *Oral Microbiol Immunol* 1999; **14:** 1–20.
3. Ma JK-C. The caries vaccine: a growing prospect. *Dent Update* 1999; **26:** 374–80.

Diphtheria Antitoxins (7951-h)

ATC — J06AA01.

Diphtheria Antitoxin (Ph. Eur.) (Dip/Ser; Immunoserum Diphthericum) is a sterile preparation containing the specific antitoxic globulins that have the power of neutralising the toxin formed by *Corynebacterium diphtheriae.* It has a potency of not less than 1000 international units per mL when obtained from horse serum and not less than 500 international units per mL when obtained from other mammals. It should be stored at 2° to 8°, and not be allowed to freeze.

Diphtheria Antitoxin (USP 25) is a sterile solution of the refined and concentrated proteins, chiefly globulins, containing antitoxic antibodies obtained from the serum or plasma of healthy horses that have been immunised against diphtheria toxin or toxoid. It contains not less than 500 units per mL. It should be stored at 2° to 8°.

Adverse Effects and Precautions
As for antisera in general, p.1529.

Uses and Administration
Diphtheria antitoxins neutralise the toxin produced by *Corynebacterium diphtheriae* locally at the site of infection and in the circulation.

Diphtheria antitoxin is used for passive immunisation in suspected cases of diphtheria and should be given without waiting for bacteriological confirmation of the infection. An antibacterial is usually given concomitantly (see p.118). Diphtheria antitoxin is generally not used for the prophylaxis of diphtheria because of the risk of provoking a hypersensitivity reaction. Contacts of a diphtheria case should be promptly investigated, given antibacterial prophylaxis and active immunisation with a suitable diphtheria-containing vaccine as appropriate (see p.1536), and kept under observation.

A test dose of diphtheria antitoxin should always be given to exclude hypersensitivity. For the treatment of diphtheria of mild or moderate severity doses of 10 000 to 30 000 units of diphtheria antitoxin may be given intramuscularly; doses of 40 000 to 100 000 units may be given in severe cases. Higher doses have been used in some countries. For doses of more than 40 000 units a portion of the dose is given intramuscularly followed by the bulk of the dose intravenously after about 0.5 to 2 hours.

Preparations

Ph. Eur.: Diphtheria Antitoxin;
USP 25: Diphtheria Antitoxin.

Diphtheria Immunoglobulins (3894-d)

ATC — J06BB10.

Profile
A diphtheria immunoglobulin containing high levels of specific antibody to the toxin of *Corynebacterium diphtheriae* has been prepared from human plasma. It has been used similarly to diphtheria antitoxins (above) in suspected cases of diphtheria in conjunction with a suitable antibacterial. It has also been suggested for prophylaxis in subjects exposed to diphtheria.

Preparations

Proprietary Preparations (details are given in Part 3)
Switz.: Diphuman†.

Diphtheria Vaccines (7961-b)

ATC — J07AF01.

Diphtheria Vaccine (Adsorbed) (Ph. Eur.) (Adsorbed Diphtheria Vaccine (BP 2001); Adsorbed Diphtheria Prophylactic; Dip/Vac/Ads(Child); Vaccinum Diphtheriae Adsorbatum) is a preparation of diphtheria formol toxoid adsorbed on a mineral carrier. The formol toxoid is prepared from the toxin produced by the growth of *Corynebacterium diphtheriae.* The mineral carrier may be hydrated aluminium hydroxide, aluminium

phosphate, or calcium phosphate and the resulting mixture is approximately isotonic with blood. The antigenic properties are adversely affected by certain antimicrobial preservatives, particularly those of the phenolic type. It contains not less than 30 international units per dose. It should be stored at 2° to 8°, not be allowed to freeze, and be protected from light.

Diphtheria Vaccine (Adsorbed) for Adults and Adolescents (Ph. Eur.) (Dip/Vac/Ads(Adults); Adsorbed Diphtheria Vaccine for Adults and Adolescents (BP 2001); Vaccinum Diphtheriae Adulti et Adulescentis Adsorbatum); is adsorbed diphtheria vaccine containing not less than 2 international units per dose. For use in the UK, it contains not more than 2 Limes flocculationis per dose.

Diphtheria Toxoid (USP 25) is a sterile solution of the formaldehyde-treated products of growth of *Corynebacterium diphtheriae.* It contains a non-phenolic preservative. It should be stored at 2° to 8° and not be allowed to freeze.

Diphtheria Toxoid Adsorbed (USP 25) is a sterile preparation of plain diphtheria toxoid that has been precipitated or adsorbed by alum, aluminium hydroxide, or aluminium phosphate adjuvants. It should be stored at 2° to 8° and not be allowed to freeze.

Units
0.5 mL of the injection of absorbed diphtheria vaccine available in the UK for use in children is equivalent to 30 international units; 0.5 mL of the diluted vaccine for use in adults and older children is equivalent to 2 international units. The toxoid content is represented by flocculation equivalents or Limes flocculationis (Lf). There is no simple correlation between international units and Lf equivalents.

Adverse Effects and Precautions
As for vaccines in general, p.1529.

Local reactions may occur but are generally not severe in young children; the frequency and severity of reactions is reported to be less in children under 2 years of age than in older children and adults.

If diphtheria vaccines or vaccines containing a diphtheria component need to be given to children over the age of 10 years or to adults, vaccines with a reduced content of diphtheria toxoid and intended for adults and adolescents should be used. For further details see under Uses and Administration, below.

Uses and Administration
Diphtheria vaccines are used for active immunisation against diphtheria. The non-adsorbed vaccine has poor immunogenic properties and its effects are enhanced by administration as an adsorbed preparation. For primary immunisation combined diphtheria, tetanus, and pertussis vaccines (p.1537) or combined diphtheria and tetanus vaccines (p.1537) are usually used. For discussion of immunisation schedules see under Vaccines, p.1530.

A single-component diphtheria vaccine may sometimes be used for example in the event of contact with an infected patient or a carrier. In the UK a single-component adsorbed vaccine suitable for infants and children and one containing a low dose of toxoid suitable for children over 10 years of age and adults are available and are given by deep subcutaneous or by intramuscular injection in usual doses of 0.5 mL. For primary immunisation three doses are given at intervals of one month. For children who receive primary immunisation during infancy reinforcing doses should be given at school entry (preferably at least 3 years after primary immunisation) and again on leaving school, in the latter case using the low-dose preparation.

Individuals coming into contact with a case of diphtheria or carriers of a toxigenic strain, or those travelling to an endemic or epidemic area should receive a complete primary course or a reinforcing dose according to age and immunisation history; those not previously immunised should receive a 3-dose primary course using the appropriate vaccine as outlined above, those previously immunised should receive a single 0.5 mL dose. Unimmunised contacts of a case of diphtheria should in addition receive a prophylactic course of a suitable antibacterial (see p.118). Individuals at repeated risk of exposure to infection may be offered booster doses every 10 years.

If the low-dose vaccine for adults is not available, then 0.1 mL of the standard paediatric vaccine may be given as an alternative for both primary and reinforcing doses.

Schick testing (p.1661) to ascertain immune status is no longer considered necessary before administering diphtheria vaccine to adults provided that a low dose is given; antibody testing is used to check immunity in those regularly exposed to diphtheria.

In some countries, booster doses of diphtheria in combination with tetanus vaccine are recommended every 10 years (see under Diphtheria and Tetanus Vaccines, p.1537).

Conjugation to diphtheria toxoid has been used to increase the immunogenicity of other vaccines (see Haemophilus Influenzae Vaccines, p.1540).

Preparations
Ph. Eur.: Diphtheria Vaccine (Adsorbed); Diphtheria Vaccine (Adsorbed) for Adults and Adolescents;
USP 25: Diphtheria Toxoid; Diphtheria Toxoid Adsorbed.

Proprietary Preparations (details are given in Part 3)
Ital.: H-Adiftal; **NZ:** Di Anatoxal; **Switz.:** Anatoxal Di.

Diphtheria and Tetanus Vaccines

(7949-p)

ATC — J07AM51.

Diphtheria and Tetanus Vaccine (Adsorbed) (Ph. Eur.) (Adsorbed Diphtheria-Tetanus Prophylactic; DT/Vac/Ads(Child); Adsorbed Diphtheria and Tetanus Vaccine (BP 2001); Vaccinum Diphtheriae et Tetani Adsorbatum) is a preparation of diphtheria formol toxoid and tetanus formol toxoid adsorbed on a mineral carrier. The mineral carrier may be hydrated aluminium hydroxide, aluminium phosphate, or calcium phosphate and the resulting mixture is approximately isotonic with blood. The antigenic properties are adversely affected by certain antimicrobial preservatives particularly those of the phenolic type. It contains not less than 30 international units of diphtheria toxoid and not less than 40 international units of tetanus toxoid per dose. It should be stored at 2° to 8°, not be allowed to freeze, and be protected from light.

Diphtheria and Tetanus Vaccine (Adsorbed) for Adults and Adolescents (Ph. Eur.) (DT/Vac/Ads(Adult); Adsorbed Diphtheria and Tetanus Vaccine for Adults and Adolescents (BP 2001); Vaccinum Diphtheriae et Tetani Adulti et Adulescentis Adsorbatum) is adsorbed diphtheria and tetanus vaccine containing not less than 2 units of diphtheria toxoid and not less than 20 units of tetanus toxoid per dose. For use in the UK, it contains not more than 2 Limes flocculationis (Lf) per dose.

Diphtheria and Tetanus Toxoids (USP 25) is a sterile solution prepared by mixing suitable quantities of fluid diphtheria toxoid and fluid tetanus toxoid. The antigenicity or potency and the proportions of the toxoids are such as to provide an immunising dose of each toxoid in the labelled dose. It should be stored at 2° to 8° and be allowed to freeze.

Diphtheria and Tetanus Toxoids Adsorbed (USP 25) is a sterile suspension prepared by mixing suitable quantities of plain or adsorbed diphtheria toxoid and plain or adsorbed tetanus toxoid and, if plain toxoids are used, an aluminium adsorbing agent. The antigenicity or potency and the proportions of the toxoids are such as to provide an immunising dose of each toxoid in the labelled dose. It should be stored at 2° to 8° and not be allowed to freeze.

Tetanus and Diphtheria Toxoids Adsorbed for Adult Use (USP 25) is a sterile suspension prepared by mixing suitable quantities of adsorbed diphtheria toxoid and adsorbed tetanus toxoid using the same precipitating or adsorbing agent for both toxoids. The antigenicity or potency and the proportions of the toxoids are such as to provide, in the labelled dose, an immunising dose of adsorbed tetanus toxoid and one-tenth of the immunising dose of adsorbed diphtheria toxoid specified for children and not more than 2 Lf of diphtheria toxoid. It should be stored at 2° to 8° and not be allowed to freeze.

Units
0.5 mL of the injection of adsorbed diphtheria and tetanus vaccine available in the UK for use in children is equivalent to not less than 30 international units of diphtheria toxoid and not less than 40 international units of tetanus toxoid. The BP 2001 and Ph. Eur. injections for adults and adolescents contain the equivalent of not less than 2 international units of diphtheria toxoid and not less than 20 international units of tetanus toxoid per dose. However, the available UK preparation for adults and children over 10 years of age contains in each 0.5-mL dose not less than 4 in-

ternational units of diphtheria toxoid and not less than 40 international units of tetanus toxoid.

Adverse Effects and Precautions
As for vaccines in general, p.1529. See also under Diphtheria Vaccines, p.1536, and Tetanus Vaccines, p.1565. Diphtheria and tetanus vaccines are reported to produce fewer adverse effects than diphtheria, tetanus, and pertussis vaccines (see under Adverse Effects, p.1538).

Dose-related effects. A high incidence of adverse effects was reported in teenagers inadvertently given a high-dose diphtheria and tetanus vaccine intended for use in infants.[1] Most reactions were classified as mild or moderately severe, but severe local or systemic reactions occurred in a third of those reporting reactions.

1. Sidebotham PD, Lenton SW. Incidence of adverse reactions after administration of high dose diphtheria with tetanus vaccine to school leavers: retrospective questionnaire study. *BMJ* 1996; **313:** 533–4.

Effects on the nervous system. Encephalopathy more commonly follows vaccination with diphtheria, tetanus, and pertussis vaccine than with diphtheria and tetanus vaccine (p.1538). However, several cases of encephalopathy occurred in a small region in Italy in children following immunisation against diphtheria and tetanus,[1] although it was not possible to infer a causal relationship. A case of polyradiculoneuritis has been reported in a patient following the use of a diphtheria-tetanus vaccine and was considered most likely to have been due to the tetanus component.[2]

1. Greco D. Case-control study on encephalopathy associated with diphtheria-tetanus immunization in Campania, Italy. *Bull WHO* 1985; **63:** 919–25.
2. Holliday PL, Bauer RB. Polyradiculoneuritis secondary to immunization with tetanus and diphtheria toxoids. *Arch Neurol* 1983; **40:** 56–7.

GUILLAIN-BARRÉ SYNDROME. Evidence mainly from case reports and uncontrolled studies favoured a causal relationship between vaccination with diphtheria and tetanus vaccines or single-antigen tetanus vaccines and Guillain-Barré syndrome. The data came primarily from immunocompromised patients.[1]

1. Stratton KR, et al. Adverse events associated with childhood vaccines other than pertussis and rubella: summary of a report from the Institute of Medicine. *JAMA* 1994; **271:** 1602–5.

Uses and Administration
Combined adsorbed diphtheria and tetanus vaccines are used for active immunisation against diphtheria and tetanus; they are used in the UK for reinforcing doses following primary immunisation with diphtheria, tetanus, and pertussis vaccine, and also for primary immunisation. For discussion of immunisation schedules see under Vaccines, p.1530.

In the UK a combined adsorbed diphtheria and tetanus vaccine suitable for use in infants and young children and one with a lower dose of diphtheria toxoid suitable for use in children over 10 years of age and adults are each given in usual doses of 0.5 mL by deep subcutaneous or intramuscular injection. For primary immunisation 3 injections of 0.5 mL of the appropriate vaccine are given at intervals of 4 weeks. For children who receive primary immunisation during infancy reinforcing doses are given at school entry (preferably at least 3 years after primary immunisation) and again on leaving school, in the latter case using the low-dose preparation. For adults a reinforcing dose may be given after 10 years.

The non-adsorbed combined diphtheria and tetanus vaccines have weaker immunogenic properties than adsorbed vaccines and are no longer recommended.

◊ In some countries booster doses of combined diphtheria and tetanus vaccines are recommended every 10 years, and studies have been conducted to assess whether this is necessary. Since the incidence of clinical diphtheria in many countries in western Europe and North America approaches zero it had been considered that there was no need for booster doses in adults despite low antibody titres, so long as the policy of immunisation during infancy was maintained.[1,2] However, following a report[3] of an outbreak of clinical diphtheria in Sweden after a period of many years when no indigenous cases of diphtheria had occurred and the disease was regarded as being eliminated from the country, the question of immunity in adults and the need for revaccination again arose. In the USA it was considered[4] that re-immunisation every 10 years with a diphtheria and tetanus combined vaccine was mandatory and that this combined vaccine should be used whenever, as in treating emergency wounds, a tetanus vaccine was indicated. Outbreaks of diphtheria in Russia and neighbouring countries[5] have prompted recommendations for booster doses in travellers to these countries and, in the UK, for an additional dose to be

added to the routine immunisation schedule at school-leaving age.[6]
A study has shown that an intranasal formulation could produce an adequate booster response and may be advantageous in some patients.[7]

1. Mathias RG, Schechter MT. Booster immunisation for diphtheria and tetanus: no evidence of need in adults. *Lancet* 1985; **i:** 1089–91.
2. Anonymous. Diphtheria and tetanus boosters. *Lancet* 1985; **i:** 1081–2.
3. Rappuoli R, et al. Molecular epidemiology of the 1984–1986 outbreak of diphtheria in Sweden. *N Engl J Med* 1988; **318:** 12–14.
4. Karzon DT, Edwards KM. Diphtheria outbreaks in immunized populations. *N Engl J Med* 1988; **318:** 41–3.
5. Anonymous. Diphtheria immunisation—advice from the Chief Medical Officer. *Commun Dis Rep* 1993; **3:** 27.
6. Chief Medical Officer, Department of Health. Immunisation update. *CMO's Update 2* 1994.
7. Aggerbeck H, et al. Intranasal booster vaccination against diphtheria and tetanus in man. *Vaccine* 1997; **15:** 307–16.

Preparations
Ph. Eur.: Diphtheria and Tetanus Vaccine (Adsorbed); Diphtheria and Tetanus Vaccine (Adsorbed) for Adults and Adolescents;
USP 25: Diphtheria and Tetanus Toxoids; Diphtheria and Tetanus Toxoids Adsorbed; Tetanus and Diphtheria Toxoids Adsorbed for Adult Use.

Proprietary Preparations (details are given in Part 3)
Aust.: Anatoxal Di Te; Ditanrix; DT-reduct; Td-pur; **Austral.:** ADT Vaccine; CDT; **Belg.:** Anatoxal Di Te†; Ditemer; Tedivax; **Braz.:** Vacina Dupla DT; **Fr.:** Diftavax†; DT Bis†; DT Vax†; **Ger.:** DT-Impfstoff; DT-Rix†; DT-Vaccinol†; Td-Impfstoff; Td-pur; Td-Rix; Td-Vaccinol; **Hong Kong:** Adsorbed DT Vax; DiTe Anatoxal; **Irl.:** Diftavax; **Ital.:** Anatoxal Di Te; Dif-Tet-All; Ditanrix; H-Adiftetal; Imovax DT; Vaccino Difto Tetano; **NZ:** ADT; CDT; DiTe Anatoxal; **Port.:** Anatoxal Di Te; **S.Afr.:** DT Vax; **Singapore:** Di Te Anatoxal; **Spain:** Anatoxal Di Te; Anatoxal Te Di; Diftavax; Ditanrix; Divacuna DT; **Swed.:** Duplex†; **Switz.:** Anatoxal Di Te; Ditanrix; **Thai.:** Di Te Anatoxal; Dif-Tet-All; DT Vax; **UK:** Diftavax.

Diphtheria, Tetanus, and Haemophilus Influenzae Vaccines (17901-p)

Profile
Combined adsorbed diphtheria, tetanus, and *Haemophilus influenzae* type b vaccines have been used in some countries for active immunisation of infants. For discussion of immunisation schedules see under Vaccines, p.1530. For concern over the antigenicity of *Haemophilus influenzae* type b vaccine in combined vaccines, see under Haemophilus Influenzae Vaccines, Interactions, p.1540.

Preparations
Proprietary Preparations (details are given in Part 3)
Ger.: HIB-DT; **Swed.:** DT-HIB†.

Diphtheria, Tetanus, and Pertussis Vaccines (7955-g)

Diphtheria, Tetanus and Pertussis Vaccine (Adsorbed) (Ph. Eur.) (Adsorbed Diphtheria–Tetanus–Whooping-cough Prophylactic; DTPer/Vac/Ads; Adsorbed Diphtheria, Tetanus and Pertussis Vaccine (BP 2001); Vaccinum Diphtheriae, Tetani et Pertussis Adsorbatum) is a preparation of diphtheria formol toxoid and tetanus formol toxoid on a mineral carrier to which a suspension of killed *Bordetella pertussis* has been added. The mineral carrier may be hydrated aluminium hydroxide, aluminium phosphate, or calcium phosphate and the resulting mixture is approximately isotonic with blood. The antigenic properties are adversely affected by certain antimicrobial preservatives particularly those of the phenolic type. It contains not less than 30 international units of diphtheria toxoid, not less than 40 international units if the test is performed in *guinea-pigs*, or 60 international units if the test is performed in *mice*, of tetanus toxoid, and not less than 4 international units of the pertussis component per dose. It should be stored at 2° to 8°, not be allowed to freeze, and be protected from light.

Diphtheria, Tetanus and Pertussis (Acellular, Component) Vaccine (Adsorbed) (Ph. Eur.) (Vaccinum Diphtheriae, Tetani et Pertussis Sine Cellulis ex Elementis Praeparatum Adsorbatum) is a combined vaccine composed of diphtheria formol toxoid, tetanus formol toxoid, individually purified antigenic components of *Bordetella pertussis*, and a mineral carrier such as aluminium hydroxide or hydrated aluminium phosphate. It should be stored at 2° to 8°, not be allowed to freeze, and be protected from light.

Diphtheria and Tetanus Toxoids and Pertussis Vaccine (USP 25) is a sterile suspension prepared by mixing suitable quantities of pertussis vaccine component of killed *Bordetella pertussis*, or a fraction of this organism, fluid diphtheria toxoid, and fluid tetanus toxoid. The antigenicity or potency and the proportions of the components are such that the labelled dose provides an immunising dose of each component. It should be stored at 2° to 8° and not be allowed to freeze.

Diphtheria and Tetanus Toxoids and Pertussis Vaccine Adsorbed (USP 25) is a sterile suspension prepared by mixing suitable quantities of plain or adsorbed diphtheria toxoid, plain or adsorbed tetanus toxoid, plain or adsorbed pertussis vaccine, and, if plain antigen components are used, an aluminium adsorbing agent. The antigenicity or potency and the proportions of the components are such that the labelled dose provides an immunising dose of each component. It should be stored at 2° to 8° and not be allowed to freeze.

Units

0.5 mL of the injection of adsorbed diphtheria, tetanus, and pertussis (whole-cell) vaccine available in the UK is equivalent to not less than 30 international units of diphtheria toxoid, not less than 40 international units (or 60 international units if the *mouse* assay is employed) of tetanus toxoid, and not less than 4 international units of the *Bordetella pertussis* component. 0.5 mL of the injection of adsorbed diphtheria, tetanus, and pertussis (acellular) vaccine available in the UK is equivalent to the same amounts of diphtheria and tetanus toxoids, with 25 µg of pertussis toxoid, 25 µg of filamentous haemagglutinin, and 8 µg of pertactin.

Adverse Effects and Precautions

As for vaccines in general, p.1529. See also under Diphtheria Vaccines, p.1536, Pertussis Vaccines, p.1555, and Tetanus Vaccines, p.1565.

The incidence of local reactions and fever is reported to be lower with the accelerated immunisation schedule currently used in the UK than schedules spreading primary immunisation over 6 months. Local reactions and pyrexia occur less commonly after acellular pertussis vaccines, especially in children older than 6 months.

In infants with a personal or close family history of seizures, precautions should be taken to avoid pyrexia. See under Pertussis Vaccines for further details of precautions and contra-indications in individuals with a history of neurological problems.

As with other vaccines, immunisation should not be carried out in individuals with a definite history of severe reactions. However, in individuals with a history of a less severe general reaction to a preceding dose, immunisation should be completed using diphtheria and tetanus vaccine; acellular pertussis vaccine can be used if the previous reaction was a local one.

◊ Local and systemic reactions are more common following diphtheria, tetanus, and pertussis (DTP) vaccines than diphtheria and tetanus (DT) vaccines. However, they are generally mild and self-limiting.[1] Infrequently, high fever, persistent or inconsolable crying (possibly as a reaction to pain), hypotonic-hyporesponsive collapse, or short-lived convulsions (frequently febrile convulsions) may occur, and have been reported after both DT and DTP vaccines.[2] These reactions do not appear to have any long-term consequences.[1] Rare but serious acute neurological complications including encephalopathy and prolonged seizures have been reported after DTP and have been attributed to the whole-cell pertussis component (see p.1556) but the association could be coincidental. Epidemiological studies have shown that such events are exceedingly rare and only occasionally followed by long-term neurological damage. Analysis of these studies has been difficult but the National Vaccine Advisory Committee and the Advisory Committee on Immunization Practices[1] concluded that the evidence was insufficient for a link, and this was also the view of the Joint Committee on Vaccination and Immunisation in the UK.[2]

The risk of febrile convulsions following DTP vaccination is reported not to be increased in children immunised before 6 months of age,[2] but there appears to be an increased risk beyond this. Children with a personal or close family history of epilepsy may also be at increased risk of seizures after DTP vaccination. Current recommendations are that immunisation should be given to children with stable neurological conditions, using precautions (such as paracetamol administration and tepid sponging) to prevent pyrexia.

Children experiencing a seizure during the course of immunisation should be carefully assessed before deciding whether to continue immunisation with DTP or DT vaccine. A causal relationship between DTP vaccination and sudden infant death syndrome (SIDS) has not been established and any temporal relationship is likely to be due to chance.[3,4] There is evidence that the risk of SIDS is lower in infants who have been vaccinated.[5]

Immediate anaphylactic reactions have been reported and are regarded as a contra-indication to further use of DTP vaccine. However, the appearance of a rash is not generally regarded as a contra-indication to further doses.

1. Centers for Disease Control. Update: vaccine side effects, adverse reactions, contraindications, and precautions: recommendations of the Advisory Committee on Immunization Practices (ACIP). *MMWR* 1996; **45** (RR-12): 1–45.
2. Salisbury DM, Begg NT (eds), Joint Committee on Vaccination and Immunisation. *Immunisation against infectious disease.* London: HMSO, 1996.
3. Hoffman HJ, *et al.* Diphtheria-tetanus-pertussis immunization and sudden infant death: results of the National Institute of Child Health and Human Development Cooperative Epidemiological Study of Sudden Infant Death Syndrome Risk Factors. *Pediatrics* 1987; **79**: 598–611.
4. Griffin MR, *et al.* Risk of sudden infant death syndrome after immunization with the diphtheria-tetanus-pertussis vaccine. *N Engl J Med* 1988; **319**: 618–23.
5. Mitchell EA, *et al.* Immunisation and the sudden infant death syndrome. *Arch Dis Child* 1995; **73**: 498–501.

Interactions

As for vaccines in general, p.1530.

For a report of a diminished immune response to the pertussis component of diphtheria, tetanus, and pertussis vaccine when mixed with inactivated poliomyelitis vaccine, see Pertussis Vaccines, p.1556.

For a report of a diminished immune response to *Haemophilus influenzae* conjugated vaccine when mixed with diphtheria, tetanus, and acellular pertussis vaccine, see Haemophilus Influenzae Vaccines, p.1540.

Uses and Administration

Combined diphtheria, tetanus, and pertussis vaccines are used for active immunisation of children against diphtheria, tetanus, and pertussis (whooping cough). For discussion of immunisation schedules see below.

In the UK a combined adsorbed vaccine is given by deep subcutaneous or intramuscular injection (vaccines with acellular pertussis components are for intramuscular injection only) in usual doses of 0.5 mL. For primary immunisation of infants over 2 months of age and children under 10 years (or under 7 years with acellular pertussis component vaccines) three doses are given at intervals of one month. The acellular pertussis component vaccine may also be given as a booster in children who have previously received primary immunisation. The combined vaccine is not suitable for older children or adults. In the USA, three doses are given at intervals of 2 months, a fourth dose at least 6 months after the third, and a fifth dose at school entry.

For a discussion of vaccines containing an acellular pertussis component rather than the standard whole-cell component, which are now preferred in some countries, see under Uses and Administration of Pertussis Vaccines, p.1556. The non-adsorbed type of combined diphtheria, tetanus, and pertussis vaccines have weaker immunogenic properties than adsorbed vaccines and are no longer recommended.

Immunisation schedules. In 1990 the schedule for primary immunisation of infants for diphtheria, tetanus, pertussis, and polio in the UK changed[1] from three injections at 3, 4½ to 5, and 8½ to 11 months to 2, 3, and 4 months, with no further doses recommended until the child was 4 years of age (see also under Vaccines, p.1530). The aim was to improve compliance and to provide protection against pertussis at a younger age. An improvement of vaccine coverage has been achieved[2] and fewer adverse effects are associated with this accelerated schedule.[3] However, the accelerated schedule has been shown to be less immunogenic for diphtheria and tetanus than the old schedule at a month after completion of the vaccination course.[4] This could be due partly to the immaturity of the immune system at 2 months of age and an inhibitory effect of maternal tetanus toxoid antibodies. Nevertheless, differences in antibody concentrations produced by the two schedules were less marked at 12 months[5] and it was considered that adequate immunity would be maintained until the booster dose when the child is 4 years of age.

1. Department of Health. *Immunisation against infectious disease.* London: HMSO, 1990.
2. White JM, *et al.* Vaccine coverage: recent trends and future prospects. *BMJ* 1992; **304**: 682–4.
3. Ramsay MEB, *et al.* Symptoms after accelerated immunisation. *BMJ* 1992; **304**: 1534–6.
4. Booy R, *et al.* Immunogenicity of combined diphtheria, tetanus, and pertussis vaccine given at 2, 3, and 4 months versus 3, 5, and 9 months of age. *Lancet* 1992; **339**: 507–10.
5. Ramsay MEB *et al.* Antibody response to accelerated immunisation with diphtheria, tetanus, and pertussis vaccine. *Lancet* 1993; **342**: 203–5.

Preparations

Ph. Eur.: Diphtheria, Tetanus and Pertussis (Acellular, Component) Vaccine (Adsorbed); Diphtheria, Tetanus and Pertussis Vaccine (Adsorbed);

USP 25: Diphtheria and Tetanus Toxoids and Pertussis Vaccine; Diphtheria and Tetanus Toxoids and Pertussis Vaccine Adsorbed.

Proprietary Preparations (details are given in Part 3)
Aust.: Anatoxal Di Te Per; Infanrix; Tritanrix-DTPw†; *Austral.:* Boostrix; Infanrix; Tripacel; Triple Antigen; *Belg.:* Anatoxal Di Te Per†; Combivax; Infanrix; Triamer; *Braz.:* DTCOQ/DTP; Vacina Triplice DPT; *Canad.:* Tri-Immunol†; Tripacel†; *Fin.:* Di-Te-Kik; Infanrix; *Fr.:* DT Coq; *Ger.:* Boostrix; DPT Merieux; DPT-Impfstoff†; DPT-Vaccinol†; DTP-Rix†; Infanrix; *Hong Kong:* Adsorbed DT Coq; Di Te Per Anatoxal†; Tripacel; Triple Antigen; *Irl.:* Infanrix; Trivax-AD†; Trivax†; *Israel:* DT Coq DTP; Infanrix; *Ital.:* Adifteper†; Anatoxal Di Te Per†; Dif-Per-Tet-All; Imovax DTP†; Infanrix†; Triacelluvax; Tritanrix†; Vaccino DPT; *Mex.:* Infanrix; *Norw.:* Infanrix; *NZ:* DiTePer Anatoxal; Infanrix; Tripacel; *Port.:* Anatoxal Di Te Per†; Infanrix; *S.Afr.:* DTP-Merieux; *Singapore:* Di Te Per Anatoxal†; Infanrix; Tripacel; *Spain:* Anatoxal Di Te Per†; DTP-Merieux; Infanrix; Trivacuna; *Swed.:* Di-Te-Kik; Infanrix; *Switz.:* Acel-Imune; Anatoxal Di Te Per†; Infanrix DTPa; *Thai.:* Acelluvax DTP; Di Te Per Anatoxal†; Dif-Per-Tet-All; DTCOQ/DTP; Infanrix; Tripacel; *UK:* Infanrix; Trivax-AD; *USA:* Acel-Imune†; Certiva; Infanrix; Tri-Immunol†; Tripedia.

Diphtheria, Tetanus, Pertussis, and Haemophilus Influenzae Vaccines (17266-x)

Diphtheria, Tetanus, Pertussis (Acellular, Component) and Haemophilus type b Conjugate Vaccine (Adsorbed) (Ph. Eur.) (Vaccinum Diphtheriae, Tetani, Pertussis Sine Cellulis ex Elementis Praeparatum et Haemophili Stirpe b Conjugatum Adsorbatum) is a combined vaccine composed of diphtheria formol toxoid, tetanus formol toxoid, individually purified antigenic components of *Bordetella pertussis*, polyribosylribitol phosphate derived from a suitable strain of *Haemophilus influenzae* type b and covalently bound to a carrier protein, and a mineral carrier such as aluminium hydroxide or hydrated aluminium phosphate. The product may be presented with the Haemophilus type b component in a separate container, the contents of which are mixed with the other components immediately before use. It should be stored at 2° to 8°, not be allowed to freeze, and be protected from light.

Adverse Effects and Precautions
As for vaccines in general, p.1529.

Interactions
As for vaccines in general, p.1530.

Uses and Administration
Combined adsorbed diphtheria, tetanus, whole-cell or acellular pertussis, and *Haemophilus influenzae* type b vaccines are used for active immunisation of infants. For discussion of immunisation schedules, see under Vaccines, p.1530.

In the UK, primary immunisation should begin at 2 months of age, with three doses given by deep subcutaneous or intramuscular injection at intervals of at least one month. In the USA, three doses are given at two-month intervals, with a fourth dose given at 15 months of age. Some combined vaccines are not licensed for use in primary immunisation regimens because of concerns over the response to the *Haemophilus influenzae* type b component (see under Interactions of Haemophilus Influenzae Vaccines, p.1540).

◊ References.
1. Centers for Disease Control, Advisory Committee on Immunization Practices. Recommendations for use of Haemophilus b conjugate vaccines and a combined diphtheria, tetanus, pertussis, and haemophilus b vaccine. *MMWR* 1993; **42** (RR-13): 1–15.

Preparations
Ph. Eur.: Diphtheria, Tetanus, Pertussis (Acellular, Component) and Haemophilus Type b Conjugate Vaccine (Adsorbed).

Proprietary Preparations (details are given in Part 3)
Aust.: Act-HIB plus DPT; Infanrix+Hib; *Austral.:* Infanrix-Hib; *Belg.:* Infanrix + Hib; Tetract-HIB; *Canad.:* Tetramune†; *Ger.:* HIB-DPT; Infanrix + Hib; *Hong Kong:* Tetramune; *Israel:* Tetract-HIB; *Ital.:* Tetract-HIB†; *Mex.:* Tetramune; *NZ:* Tetramune; *S.Afr.:* Combact-HIB; TetraTITER; *Singapore:* Tetract-HIB; Tetramune; *Spain:* Infanrix Hib; Tetract-HIB; *Switz.:* Infanrix DTPa-Hib; ProHIBiT-DPT†; Tetramune; *Thai.:* Tetract-HIB; *UK:* Act-HIB DTP; Infanrix-Hib; Trivax-Hib†; *USA:* Tetramune†; Tri-HIBit.

Diphtheria, Tetanus, Pertussis, and Hepatitis B Vaccines (10051-a)
ATC — J07CA05.

Diphtheria, Tetanus, Pertussis (Acellular, Component) and Hepatitis B (rDNA) Vaccine (Adsorbed) (Ph. Eur.) (Vaccinum Diphtheriae, Tetani, Pertussis Sine Cellulis ex Elementis Praeparatum et Hepatitidis B (ADNr) Adsorbatum) is a combined vaccine composed of diphtheria formol toxoid, tetanus formol toxoid, individually purified antigenic components of *Bordetella pertussis*, hepatitis B surface antigen, and a mineral carrier such as aluminium hydroxide or hydrated aluminium phosphate. It should be stored at 2° to 8°, not be allowed to freeze, and be protected from light.

Profile
Diphtheria, tetanus, pertussis, and hepatitis B vaccines are available in some countries for active immunisation against diphtheria, tetanus, pertussis, and hepatitis B.

Preparations

Ph. Eur.: Diphtheria, Tetanus, Pertussis (Acellular, Component) and Hepatitis B (rDNA) Vaccine (Adsorbed).

Proprietary Preparations (details are given in Part 3)
Austral.: Infanrix HepB; **Fin.:** Infanrix HepB; **Ital.:** Infanrix HepB; **NZ:** Infanrix HepB; **Spain:** Infanrix HepB; Tritanrix HB; **Swed.:** Infanrix HepB; **Switz.:** Infanrix DTPa-HepB; **Thai.:** Tritanrix HB.

Diphtheria, Tetanus, Pertussis, and Poliomyelitis Vaccines (7957-p)

ATC — J07CA02.

Diphtheria, Tetanus, Pertussis (Acellular, Component) and Poliomyelitis (Inactivated) Vaccine (Adsorbed) (Ph. Eur.) (Vaccinum Diphtheriae, Tetani, Pertussis Sine Cellulis ex Elementis Praeparatum et Poliomyelitidis Inactivatum Adsorbatum) is a combined vaccine containing diphtheria formol toxoid, tetanus formol toxoid, individually purified antigenic components of *Bordetella pertussis*, suitable strains of human polioviruses type 1, 2, and 3 grown in suitable cell cultures and inactivated by a validated method, and a mineral carrier such as aluminium hydroxide or hydrated aluminium phosphate. It should be stored at 2° to 8°, not be allowed to freeze, and be protected from light.

Profile

Diphtheria, tetanus, pertussis, and poliomyelitis vaccines are available in some countries for active immunisation of infants against diphtheria, tetanus, pertussis, and poliomyelitis. Preparations containing acellular pertussis vaccine are also available.

For discussion of immunisation schedules, see under Vaccines, p.1530.

Preparations

Ph. Eur.: Diphtheria, Tetanus, Pertussis (Acellular, Component) and Poliomyelitis (Inactivated) Vaccine (Adsorbed).

Proprietary Preparations (details are given in Part 3)
Belg.: Tetracoq; Tetravac; **Braz.:** Tetracoq; **Canad.:** Quadracel; **Denm.:** Di-Te-Ki-Pol; **Fin.:** Di-Te-Ki-Pol; **Fr.:** Infanrix Polio; Tetracoq; Tetravac; Vaccin DTCP; **Ger.:** Quatro-Virelon; Tetravac; **Hong Kong:** Tetracoq; **Israel:** Tetracoq; **Swed.:** Di-Te-Ki-Pol; DTap-IPV; **Switz.:** DiTePerPol Vaccin†; **Thai.:** Tetracoq.

Diphtheria, Tetanus, Pertussis, Poliomyelitis, and Haemophilus Influenzae Vaccines (10050-k)

ATC — J07CA06.

Profile

Combined diphtheria, tetanus, pertussis, poliomyelitis, and Haemophilus influenzae vaccines are available in some countries for active immunisation.

Preparations

Proprietary Preparations (details are given in Part 3)
Aust.: Infanrix-IPV+Hib; **Belg.:** Infanrix IPV + Hib; **Canad.:** Pentacel; **Fin.:** Infanrix Polio+Hib; **Fr.:** Infanrix Polio-Hib; Pentacoq; Pentavac; **Ger.:** Infanrix-IPV+Hib; Pentavac; **Hong Kong:** Pentact-HIB; **Israel:** Infanrix Polio-Hib; Pentact-HIB; **Ital.:** Cinquerix; Pentavac; **Singapore:** Infanrix-IPV+Hib; **Spain:** Pentavac; **Swed.:** Infanrix-Polio+Hib; Pentavac; **Switz.:** Infanrix DTPa-IPV+Hib; **Thai.:** Pentact-HIB.

Multi-ingredient: **Fr.:** Pent-HIBest.

Diphtheria, Tetanus, and Poliomyelitis Vaccines (7956-q)

ATC — J07CA01.

Profile

An adsorbed diphtheria, tetanus, and poliomyelitis vaccine may be used for both primary immunisation against diphtheria, tetanus, and poliomyelitis and to reinforce the immunity of those who have previously been immunised. For discussion of immunisation schedules see under Vaccines, p.1530.

In some countries a preparation with a low dose of diphtheria vaccine is available for use in older children and adults.

Preparations

Proprietary Preparations (details are given in Part 3)
Canad.: Td-Polio; **Denm.:** Di-Te-Pol†; **Fr.:** DT Polio; Revaxis; Vaccin DTP; **Ger.:** Revaxis.

Diphtheria, Tetanus, and Rubella Vaccines (13415-p)

ATC — J07CA03.

Profile

Diphtheria, tetanus, and rubella vaccines have been used in some countries for active immunisation against diphtheria, tetanus, and rubella.

Japanese Encephalitis Vaccines (16619-r)

ATC — J07BA02.

Adverse Effects and Precautions

As for vaccines in general, p.1529.

Hypersensitivity reactions including urticaria, angioedema, hypotension, and dyspnoea have been reported mainly in travellers from non-endemic areas.

◊ References.
1. Andersen MM, Rønne T. Side-effects with Japanese encephalitis vaccine. *Lancet* 1991; **337:** 1044.
2. Ruff TA, *et al.* Adverse reactions to Japanese encephalitis vaccine. *Lancet* 1991; **338:** 881–2.
3. Plesner A-M, *et al.* Neurological complications and Japanese encephalitis vaccination. *Lancet* 1996; **348:** 202–3.
4. Nothdurft HD, *et al.* Adverse reactions to Japanese encephalitis vaccine in travellers. *J Infect* 1996; **32:** 119–22.
5. Jelinek T, Nothdurft HD. Japanese encephalitis vaccine in travellers: is wider use prudent? *Drug Safety* 1997; **16:** 153–6.
6. Berg SW, *et al.* Systemic reactions in US Marine Corps personnel who received Japanese encephalitis vaccine. *Clin Infect Dis* 1997; **24:** 265–6.
7. Liu ZL, *et al.* Short-term safety of live attenuated Japanese encephalitis vaccine (SA14-14-2): results of a randomized trial with 26,239 subjects. *J Infect Dis* 1997; **176:** 1366–9.
8. Plesner A, *et al.* Case-control study of allergic reactions to Japanese encephalitis vaccine. *Vaccine* 2000; **18:** 1830–6.

Interactions

As for vaccines in general, p.1530.

Uses and Administration

Two types of inactivated Japanese encephalitis vaccine are used for active immunisation against encephalitis due to Japanese encephalitis virus, an infection against which there is currently no specific treatment. One type of vaccine is derived from mouse brain and the other from hamster kidney cells. The vaccines are widely used in Japan and other parts of Asia and may form part of the WHO Expanded Programme on Immunization.

Vaccination is recommended for visitors to rural areas of South East Asia and the Far East where infection is endemic and where the visit is to be for more than one month; it is also recommended for shorter visits in individuals likely to be at exceptional risk. Adults are usually given 3 doses each of 1 mL of the inactivated vaccine subcutaneously at 0, 7 to 14, and 28 to 30 days; full immunity will take up to one month to develop. A two-dose schedule with doses given 7 to 14 days apart is suggested to provide short-term immunity but is effective in only 80% of recipients; in the USA an abbreviated dosage schedule with administration at 0, 7, and 14 days is suggested if time is not available for the standard schedule. Children under 3 years of age may be given a dose of 0.5 mL; in the USA the vaccine is not recommended for children under 1 year. A reinforcing dose may be given after 2 years.

Live attenuated Japanese encephalitis vaccines are used in some countries.

◊ Inactivated Japanese encephalitis vaccines have been widely used in Asia for some years. In Japan the incidence of the disease has decreased since the introduction of nationwide vaccination in the mid-1960s.[1] A study in Thailand in 1984–5 compared a monovalent Nakayama strain vaccine (21 628 subjects), a bivalent Nakayama-Beijing 1 strain vaccine (22 080 subjects), and a tetanus toxoid placebo (21 516 subjects) in children aged 1 to 14 years.[2] Two subcutaneous 1-mL doses (0.5 mL for children under 3 years of age) were given seven days apart. The attack rate for encephalitis caused by Japanese encephalitis virus was 51 per 100 000 in the placebo group and 5 per 100 000 in both vaccine groups. Vaccine efficacy in both groups combined was calculated to be 91%. Results suggested that Japanese encephalitis vaccine does not prevent virus infection but protects against symptomatic Japanese encephalitis. Immunisation had no significant effect on the incidence of dengue haemorrhagic fever although the severity of episodes may be decreased. The vaccines were associated with minimal short-term side-effects. Findings suggested that postvaccine encephalomyelitis does not occur or is very rare with these vaccines.

A case-control study of a live attenuated vaccine (SA14-14-2) indicated that 2 doses given a year apart were 97% effective in an endemic region of rural China.[3] Similar results were obtained when the interval between doses was reduced to 1 to 3 months.[4]

Other vaccines are at early stages of development.[5]
1. Denning DW, Kaneko Y. Should travellers to Asia be vaccinated against Japanese encephalitis? *Lancet* 1987; **i:** 853–4.
2. Hoke CH, *et al.* Protection against Japanese encephalitis by inactivated vaccines. *N Engl J Med* 1988; **319:** 608–14.
3. Hennessy S, *et al.* Effectiveness of live-attenuated Japanese encephalitis vaccine (SA14-14-2): a case-control study. *Lancet* 1996; **347:** 1583–6.
4. Tsai TF, *et al.* Immunogenicity of live attenuated SA14-14-2 Japanese encephalitis vaccine—a comparison of 1- and 3-month immunization schedules. *J Infect Dis* 1998; **177:** 221–3.
5. Barrett ADT. Japanese encephalitis and dengue vaccines. *Biologicals* 1997; **25:** 27–34.

Preparations

Proprietary Preparations (details are given in Part 3)
Austral.: JE-Vax; **Canad.:** JE-Vax; **Thai.:** JE-Vaccine; **USA:** JE-Vax.

Tick-borne Encephalitis Immunoglobulins (11616-n)

ATC — J06BB12.

Profile

Preparations containing antibodies against tick-borne encephalitis are available in some countries for passive immunisation against the disease.

Preparations

Proprietary Preparations (details are given in Part 3)
Aust.: FSME-Bulin; **Ger.:** Encegam†; FSME-Bulin; **Switz.:** FSME-Bulin.

Tick-borne Encephalitis Vaccines (3869-f)

ATC — J07BA01.

Tick-borne Encephalitis Vaccine (Inactivated) (Ph. Eur.) (Vaccinum Encephalitidis Ixodibus Advectae Inactivatum) is a liquid preparation of a suitable strain of tick-borne encephalitis virus grown in cultures of chick-embryo cells or other suitable cell cultures and inactivated by a suitable method. It should be stored at 2° to 8°, not be allowed to freeze, and be protected from light.

Adverse Effects and Precautions

As for vaccines in general, p.1529.

Effects on the nervous system. Severe progressive sensorimotor spastic paralysis occurred in a 54-year-old man after a second booster dose of tick-borne encephalitis vaccine.[1] Partial recovery was noted after about 6 months.
1. Bohus M, *et al.* Myelitis after immunisation against tick-borne encephalitis. *Lancet* 1993; **342:** 239–40.

Interactions

As for vaccines in general, p.1530.

Uses and Administration

A vaccine is available for active immunisation against tick-borne viral encephalitis.

In the UK, vaccination against tick-borne encephalitis is recommended for those who anticipate prolonged exposure to the infective agent, for example persons visiting or working in the warm forested parts of Europe and Scandinavia. The vaccine is given by intramuscular injection in a dose of 0.5 mL. A two-dose regimen with an interval of 4 to 12 weeks will provide protection for 1 year. A third dose 9 to 12 months after the second will give protection for up to 3 years. A further reinforcing dose may be given up to six years later if required. Reinforcing doses every 3 years are recommended for those at continued risk of exposure.

Preparations

Ph. Eur.: Tick-borne Encephalitis Vaccine (Inactivated).

Proprietary Preparations (details are given in Part 3)
Aust.: Encepur; FSME-Immun; **Belg.:** FSME-Immun†; **Fin.:** Encepur; **Fr.:** Ticovac; **Ger.:** Encepur; FSME-Immun; **Swed.:** Encepur; **Switz.:** FSME-Immun.

Endotoxin Antibodies (19133-d)

Profile

Antibodies against the endotoxin of Gram-negative bacteria have been tried as adjunctive therapy for the treatment and prevention of Gram-negative bacteraemia and shock.

Early preparations consisted of antisera prepared from the sera of donors immunised with *Escherichia coli* J5; these were superseded by human and murine IgM monoclonal antibodies. Nebacumab (HA-1A) is a human monoclonal IgM antibody that binds specifically to the lipid A domain of endotoxin. Lipid A in the circulation releases tumour necrosis factor and other cytokines from macrophages and endothelial cells which may ultimately culminate in physiological effects such as multiple organ failure. Despite early promising results of clinical studies the safety of nebacumab in patients without Gram-negative septicaemia was questioned and the product was withdrawn.

A murine monoclonal IgM antibody (edobacomab; E5) has also undergone clinical trials.

◊ Initial promising results in patients with Gram-negative infections given antibodies against the endotoxin core glycolipid of Gram-negative bacteria[1,2] prompted further investigations using monoclonal antibodies to these endotoxins in the management of septicaemia (p.138).

Studies concentrated on preparations of either human or murine IgM monoclonal antibodies to the endotoxin of Gram-negative organisms. A study[3] of nebacumab in 543 patients with sepsis showed a reduction in mortality from 49 to 30% in patients with Gram-negative bacteraemia. However, the study was severely criticised on the grounds that this group of patients could only be identified retrospectively, and overall nebacumab had no effect on mortality. A subsequent study involving 2199 patients with septic shock[4] was stopped when the mortality rate in patients without Gram-negative bacteraemia was found to be higher in those receiving nebacumab than in those receiving the placebo. The mortality rate was unchanged in patients with Gram-negative bacteraemia. Doubts about the safety and clinical efficacy of nebacumab were sufficient to lead to its withdrawal.[5] In the meantime, doubts over the role of endotoxins in the development of the sepsis syndrome have been raised[6] although there has been a report[7] of the development of full clinical manifestations of septic shock in a man following self-administration of a single large dose of endotoxin in an attempt to treat a tumour.

An initial study of the murine monoclonal antibody edobacomab showed some benefit in patients with Gram-negative infections but not in shock, although there was no overall improvement in survival at 30 days.[8] A subsequent study of patients with similar characteristics to those who had responded in the first study also failed to show an improvement in survival at 30 days[9] although some beneficial responses were seen in patients with organ failure. More recently, a multicentre, randomised controlled trial[10] also found that edobacomab did not improve short-term survival in adults with severe sepsis due to Gram-negative infection.

1. Ziegler EJ, et al. Treatment of Gram-negative bacteremia and shock with human antiserum to a mutant Escherichia coli. N Engl J Med 1982; 307: 1225–30.
2. Baumgartner J-D, et al. Prevention of Gram-negative shock and death in surgical patients by antibody to endotoxin core glycolipid. Lancet 1985; ii: 59–63.
3. Ziegler EJ, et al. Treatment of Gram-negative bacteremia and septic shock with HA-1A human monoclonal antibody against endotoxin. N Engl J Med 1991; 324: 429–36.
4. McCloskey RV, et al. Treatment of septic shock with human monoclonal antibody HA-1A: a randomized, double-blind, placebo-controlled trial. Ann Intern Med 1994; 121: 1–5.
5. Horton R. Voluntary suspension of Centoxin. Lancet 1993; 341: 298.
6. Hurley JC. Reappraisal of the role of endotoxin in the sepsis syndrome. Lancet 1993; 341: 1133–5.
7. da Silva AMT, et al. Brief report: shock and multiple-organ dysfunction after self-administration of salmonella endotoxin. N Engl J Med 1993; 328: 1457–60.
8. Greenman RL, et al. A controlled clinical trial of E5 murine monoclonal IgM antibody to endotoxin in the treatment of Gram-negative sepsis. JAMA 1991; 266: 1097–1102.
9. Bone RC, et al. A second large controlled clinical study of E5, a monoclonal antibody to endotoxin: results of a prospective, multicenter, randomized controlled trial. Crit Care Med 1995; 23: 994–1005.
10. Angus DC, et al. E5 murine monoclonal antiendotoxin antibody in Gram-negative sepsis: a randomized controlled trial. JAMA 2000; 283: 1723–30.

Epstein-Barr Virus Vaccines (1742-j)

Profile
Several Epstein-Barr virus vaccines are under investigation for active immunisation against infectious mononucleosis and post-transplant lymphoproliferative disorders.

◊ References.
1. Moss DJ, et al. Candidate vaccines for Epstein-Barr virus. BMJ 1998; 317: 423–4.

Escherichia Coli Vaccines (3067-e)

Profile
Vaccines against enterotoxigenic strains of Escherichia coli are under investigation. Vaccine candidates include toxoids, inactivated whole bacteria, purified surface antigens, and live oral vaccines.

◊ References.
1. Levine MM. Modern vaccines: enteric infections. Lancet 1990; 335: 958–61.
2. Cross A, et al. Safety and immunogenicity of a polyvalent Escherichia coli vaccine in human volunteers. J Infect Dis 1994; 170: 834–40.
3. Tacket CO, et al. Enteral immunization and challenge of volunteers given enterotoxigenic E. coli CFA/II encapsulated in biodegradable microspheres. Vaccine 1994; 12: 1270–4.
4. Konadu EY, et al. Investigational vaccine for Escherichia coli O157: phase 1 study of O157 O-specific polysaccharide-Pseudomonas aeruginosa recombinant exoprotein A conjugates in adults. J Infect Dis 1998; 177: 383–7.
5. Savarino SJ, et al. Safety and immunogenicity of an oral, killed enterotoxigenic Escherichia coli-cholera toxin B subunit vaccine in Egyptian adults. J Infect Dis 1998; 177: 796–9.
6. Jertbron M, et al. Safety and immunogenicity of an oral inactivated enterotoxigenic Escherichia coli vaccine. Vaccine 1998; 16: 255–60.

Gas-gangrene Antitoxins (8039-n)
ATC — J06AA05.

Gas-gangrene Antitoxin (Novyi) (Ph. Eur.) (Gas-gangrene Antitoxin (Oedematiens); Immunoserum Gangraenicum (Clostridium Novyi); Nov/Ser) is a sterile preparation containing the specific antitoxic globulins that have the power of neutralising the alpha toxin formed by Clostridium novyi. It has a potency of not less than 3750 international units (iu) per mL.

Gas-gangrene Antitoxin (Perfringens) (Ph. Eur.) (Immunoserum Gangraenicum (Clostridium Perfringens); Perf/Ser) is a sterile preparation containing the specific antitoxic globulins that have the power of neutralising the alpha toxin formed by Clostridium perfringens. It has a potency of not less than 1500 iu per mL.

Gas-gangrene Antitoxin (Septicum) (Ph. Eur.) (Immunoserum Gangraenicum (Clostridium Septicum); Sep/Ser) is a sterile preparation containing the specific antitoxic globulins that

have the power of neutralising the alpha toxin formed by Clostridium septicum. It has a potency of not less than 1500 iu per mL.

Mixed Gas-gangrene Antitoxin (Ph. Eur.) (Immunoserum Gangraenicum Mixtum; Gas/Ser) is prepared by mixing Gas-gangrene Antitoxin (Novyi), Gas-gangrene Antitoxin (Perfringens), and Gas-gangrene Antitoxin (Septicum) in appropriate quantities. It has a potency of not less than 1000 iu of Gas-gangrene Antitoxin (Novyi), not less than 1000 iu of Gas-gangrene Antitoxin (Perfringens), and not less than 500 iu of Gas-gangrene Antitoxin (Septicum) per mL.

The above antitoxins should be stored at 2° to 8°, and not be allowed to freeze.

Profile
Gas-gangrene antitoxins have been used for the treatment of gas gangrene and for prophylaxis in patients at risk following injury. They are now seldom used and have been superseded by antibacterials.

Suggested doses for a mixed gas-gangrene antitoxin were 25 000 units intravenously or intramuscularly for prophylaxis and 75 000 units intravenously for treatment; these doses might have been repeated or larger doses given initially. Monovalent gas-gangrene antitoxins have been little used in practice owing to the difficulty of rapidly identifying the infecting organism.

Preparations
Ph. Eur.: Gas-gangrene Antitoxin (Novyi); Gas-gangrene Antitoxin (Perfringens); Gas-gangrene Antitoxin (Septicum); Mixed Gas-gangrene Antitoxin.

Proprietary Preparations (details are given in Part 3)
Ger.: Gasbrand-Antitoxin.

Gonococcal Vaccines (19267-j)
Gonorrhoea Vaccines.

Profile
Several experimental gonococcal vaccines, produced usually from the surface antigens of Neisseria gonorrhoeae, are under investigation.

Haemophilus Influenzae Vaccines
(16828-q)

ATC — J07AG01 (B, purified antig. conjugate).

Haemophilus Type B Conjugate Vaccine (Ph. Eur.) (Vaccinum Haemophili Stirpe B Conjugatum) is a liquid or freeze-dried preparation of a polysaccharide, polyribosylribitol phosphate (PRP), derived from a suitable strain of Haemophilus influenzae type b, covalently bound to a carrier protein. It should be stored at 2° to 8° and protected from light.

Haemophilus Influenzae Conjugate Vaccine (Diphtheria Toxoid Conjugate) (PRP-D) consists of the purified capsular polysaccharide of Haemophilus influenzae type b covalently linked to diphtheria toxoid.

Haemophilus Influenzae Conjugate Vaccine (Diphtheria CRM₁₉₇ Protein Conjugate) (HbOC) consists of oligosaccharides derived from the purified capsular polysaccharide of Haemophilus influenzae type b covalently linked to a non-toxic variant of diphtheria toxin isolated from Corynebacterium diphtheriae.

Haemophilus Influenzae Conjugate Vaccine (Meningococcal Protein Conjugate) (PRP-OMP or PRP-OMPC) consists of the purified capsular polysaccharide of Haemophilus influenzae type b covalently linked to an outer membrane protein complex of Neisseria meningitidis group B.

Haemophilus Influenzae Conjugate Vaccine (Tetanus Toxoid Conjugate) (PRP-T) consists of the purified capsular polysaccharide of Haemophilus influenzae type b covalently linked to tetanus toxoid.

Adverse Effects and Precautions
As for vaccines in general, p.1529.

Erythema multiforme, convulsions, and transient cyanosis of the lower limbs have been reported rarely in children receiving haemophilus influenzae vaccines.

Effects on the nervous system. Guillain-Barré syndrome has been reported[1] in 3 infants, with onset of symptoms within 1 week of vaccination with a haemophilus influenzae conjugate vaccine (diphtheria toxoid conjugate).

1. D'Cruz OF, et al. Acute inflammatory demyelinating polyradiculoneuropathy (Guillain-Barré syndrome) after immunization with Haemophilus influenzae type b conjugate vaccine. J Pediatr 1989; 115: 743–6.

Interactions
As for vaccines in general, p.1530.

Antineoplastics. Haemophilus influenzae infection occurred in a child who had received antineoplastic therapy despite having completed a primary course of immunisation before the neoplasia was diagnosed.[1] A subsequent booster dose produced

an adequate antibody response. Antineoplastic therapy may have impaired the T-cell response to infection.

1. Jenkins DR, et al. Childhood neoplasia and Haemophilus influenzae type b vaccine failure. Lancet 1996; 348: 131.

Diphtheria, tetanus, and pertussis vaccines. Some haemophilus influenzae conjugated vaccines may be mixed with diphtheria, tetanus, and pertussis vaccines before administration without adversely affecting the immunogenicity of the components.[1,2] However the immunogenicity of a haemophilus influenzae conjugated vaccine was reduced when mixed with a diphtheria, tetanus, and acellular pertussis vaccine.[3]

1. Miller MA, et al. Safety and immunogenicity of PRP-T combined with DTP: excretion of capsular polysaccharide and antibody response in the immediate post-vaccination period. Pediatrics 1995; 95: 522–7.
2. Mulholland EK, et al. The use of Haemophilus influenzae type b-tetanus toxoid conjugate vaccine mixed with diphtheria-tetanus-pertussis vaccine in Gambian infants. Vaccine 1996; 14: 905–9.
3. Eskola J, et al. Randomised trial of the effect of co-administration with acellular pertussis DTP vaccine on immunogenicity of Haemophilus influenzae type b conjugated vaccine. Lancet 1996; 348: 1688–92.

Uses and Administration
Haemophilus influenzae (Hib) vaccines are used for active immunisation against Haemophilus influenzae type b infections. Vaccines are prepared from the capsular polysaccharide of H. influenzae type b and immunogenicity, especially in young children, is improved by linking the polysaccharide to a protein carrier to form a conjugate vaccine (see above for description of different conjugate vaccines). For discussion of immunisation schedules see below.

Different proprietary vaccines may be conjugated to differing proteins (see above) but are generally regarded as interchangeable.

In the UK a conjugate vaccine is given by deep subcutaneous or intramuscular injection in doses of 0.5 mL. For primary immunisation of infants from 2 months of age, three doses are given at intervals of one month. The vaccine may be administered at the same time as combined diphtheria, tetanus, and pertussis vaccines of the primary immunisation schedule. Children aged under 13 months who have already commenced or completed the rest of their primary immunisation schedule should receive three doses of Hib vaccine at intervals of one month. Children aged 13 to 48 months should be given a single dose as they are at lower risk and the vaccine is effective after a single dose in this age group. Routine use in older children or adults is not recommended in the UK. Unimmunised household contacts of a case of invasive disease who are under 4 years of age, and asplenic children and adults, should receive a single dose of Hib vaccine, or three doses for children under 1 year of age.

In the USA, primary immunisation is also carried out in conjunction with diphtheria, tetanus, and pertussis vaccination. If a meningococcal protein conjugate vaccine is used, only 2 doses are given for the primary course. A reinforcing dose using any of the available vaccines is given at 12 to 15 months of age.

Where compatibility has been demonstrated, Hib vaccines may be administered as mixtures with diphtheria, tetanus, and pertussis vaccines (but see Interactions, above).

Immunisation schedules. Various regimens for vaccination against Haemophilus influenzae type b infection (Hib) have been tried. In the USA a reinforcing dose is given at 12 to 15 months of age to children who have received a primary course and studies in other countries have shown that a booster dose substantially reduces the risk of infection.[1] In the UK this is considered unnecessary[2,3] and a reinforcing dose is not included in the routine schedule (see under Vaccines, p.1530). Follow-up of children vaccinated using this schedule have shown that satisfactory serum-antibody concentrations persist at 4.5 years of age.[4] This difference in recommendations may reflect the high vaccine uptake, the use of a three-dose primary schedule, and the use of a highly immunogenic vaccine in the UK.[1] Studies have shown that two-dose schedules[5,6] or giving one-half or one-third of the full dose at 2, 4, and 6 months of age[7] can produce an adequate immune response although the usual three-dose schedule produces higher antibody concentrations.[6]

Differing immunogenicity of conjugate vaccines led to concern over the interchangeability of vaccines during primary immunisation.[8] In general, studies have shown that, despite some differences in antibody concentrations when different vaccines are used for doses during the primary course, the immune response was usually adequate.[9-12]

Response to some Hib vaccines may be diminished in premature infants,[13,14] although adequate responses even in very premature infants have been reported.[15] Raised antibody titres have been reported in infants following maternal immunisation during the third trimester of pregnancy.[16]

1. Böhm O, von Kries R. Are Hib booster vaccinations redundant? *Lancet* 1997; **350:** 68.
2. Booy R, *et al.* Vaccine failures after primary immunisation with Haemophilus influenzae type-b conjugate vaccine without booster. *Lancet* 1997; **349:** 1197–1202.
3. Goldblatt D, *et al.* Immunological response to conjugate vaccines in infants: follow up study. *BMJ* 1998; **316:** 1570–1.
4. Heath PT, *et al.* Antibody persistence and Haemophilus influenzae type b carriage after infant immunisation with PRP-T. *Arch Dis Child* 1997; **77:** 488–92.
5. Kurikka S, *et al.* Immunologic priming by one dose of Haemophilus influenzae type b conjugate vaccine in infancy. *J Infect Dis* 1995; **172:** 1268–72.
6. Kurikka S, *et al.* Comparison of five different vaccination schedules with Haemophilus influenzae type b-tetanus toxoid conjugate vaccine. *J Pediatr* 1996; **128:** 524–30.
7. Lagos R, *et al.* Economisation of vaccination against Haemophilus influenzae type b: a randomised trial of immunogenicity of fractional-dose and two-dose regimens. *Lancet* 1998; **351:** 1472–6.
8. Granoff DM, *et al.* Differences in the immunogenicity of three Haemophilus influenzae type b vaccines in infants. *J Pediatr* 1992; **121:** 187–94.
9. Anderson EL, *et al.* Interchangeability of conjugated Haemophilus influenzae type b vaccines in infants. *JAMA* 1995; **273:** 849–53.
10. Greenberg DP, *et al.* Enhanced antibody responses in infants given different sequences of Haemophilus influenzae type b conjugate vaccines. *J Pediatr* 1995; **126:** 206–11.
11. Goldblatt D, *et al.* Interchangeability of conjugated Haemophilus influenzae type b vaccines during primary immunisation of infants. *BMJ* 1996; **312:** 817–18.
12. Bewley KM, *et al.* Interchangeability of Haemophilus influenzae type b vaccines in the primary series: evaluation of a two-dose mixed regimen. *Pediatrics* 1996; **98:** 898–904.
13. Munoz A, *et al.* Antibody response of low birth weight infants to Haemophilus influenzae type b polyribosylribitol phosphate-outer membrane protein conjugate vaccine. *Pediatrics* 1995; **96:** 216–19.
14. Kristensen K, *et al.* Antibody response to Haemophilus influenzae type b capsular polysaccharide conjugated to tetanus toxoid in preterm infants. *Pediatr Infect Dis J* 1996; **15:** 525–9.
15. D'Angio CT, *et al.* Immunologic response of extremely premature infants to tetanus, Haemophilus influenzae, and polio immunizations. *Pediatrics* 1995; **96:** 18–22.
16. Englund JA, *et al.* Haemophilus influenzae type b-specific antibody in infants after maternal immunization. *Pediatr Infect Dis J* 1997; **16:** 1122–30.

Preparations

Ph. Eur.: Haemophilus Type b Conjugate Vaccine.

Proprietary Preparations (details are given in Part 3)
Aust.: Act-HIB; HibTITER; ProHIBiT; ***Austral.:*** Hiberix; HibTITER; PedvaxHIB; ***Belg.:*** Act-HIB; Hiberix; HibTITER; ***Braz.:*** Act-HIB; HibTITER; ***Canad.:*** Act-HIB; HibTITER†; Pedvax-HIB; ***Denm.:*** Act-HIB; HibTITER; ***Fin.:*** Hiberix; HibTITER; ***Fr.:*** Act-HIB; HIBest; ***Ger.:*** Act-HIB; HIB Merieux; HIB-Vaccinol†; HibTITER; PedvaxHIB; ***Hong Kong:*** Act-HIB; Pedvax-HIB; ***Irl.:*** Act-HIB; Hiberix; HibTITER; ***Israel:*** Act-HIB; HibTITER; PedvaxHIB; ***Ital.:*** Act-HIB; Hiberix; HibTITER; Vaxem Hib; ***Mex.:*** HibTITER; PedvaxHIB; ***Neth.:*** Act-HIB; PedvaxHIB†; ***Norw.:*** Act-HIB; ***NZ:*** HibTITER; ***Port.:*** HibTITER; ***S.Afr.:*** Act-HIB; HibTITER; ***Singapore:*** Act-HIB; Hiberix; Hib-TITER; PedvaxHIB; ***Spain:*** Act-HIB; Hiberix; HibTITER; ***Swed.:*** Act-HIB; HibTITER; PedvaxHIB†; ProHIBiT†; ***Switz.:*** Act-HIB; Hiberix; HibTITER; ProHIBiT†; ***Thai.:*** Act-HIB; Hiberix; PedvaxHIB; ***UK:*** Act-HIB; HibTITER; ***USA:*** Act-HIB; HibTITER; OmniHIB; PedvaxHIB; ProHIBiT.

Multi-ingredient: ***Fr.:*** Pent-HIBest.

Haemophilus Influenzae and Hepatitis B Vaccines (9796-d)

Adverse Effects and Precautions
As for vaccines in general, p.1529.

Interactions
As for vaccines in general, p.1530.

Uses and Administration
Haemophilus influenzae type b (Hib) conjugate and hepatitis B vaccines are available in some countries for active immunisation as part of the primary immunisation of infants. In the USA, an Haemophilus influenzae type b conjugate (meningococcal protein conjugate) and hepatitis B (recombinant) vaccine is used. It is given in a schedule of 3 doses, 0.5 mL being administered intramuscularly at 2 months, 4 months, and 12 to 15 months of age. Administration to infants less than 6 weeks old is not recommended.

Preparations

Proprietary Preparations (details are given in Part 3)
Austral.: Comvax; ***Ger.:*** Procomvax; ***USA:*** Comvax.

Haemorrhagic Fever with Renal Syndrome Vaccines (9466-v)

HFRS Vaccine; Vaccinum Haemorrhagiae Febris cum Renis Sindronum.

A fluid or freeze-dried preparation of a suitable hantavirus grown in the neural tissue of suckling rodents or in cell cultures and inactivated. The fluid vaccine should be stored at 2° to 8° and not allowed to freeze. The freeze-dried form should be stored below 10°.

Profile
Inactivated viral vaccines against haemorrhagic fever with renal syndrome are being developed in several countries.

◊ References.
1. Lee HW, *et al.* Field trial of an inactivated vaccine against hemorrhagic fever with renal syndrome in humans. *Arch Virol* 1990; (suppl 1): 35–47.
2. Song G, *et al.* Preliminary trials of inactivated vaccine against haemorrhagic fever with renal syndrome. *Lancet* 1991; **337:** 801.
3. Zhu Z-Y, *et al.* Investigation on inactivated epidemic hemorrhagic fever tissue culture vaccine in humans. *Chin Med J* 1994; **107:** 167–70.

Helicobacter Pylori Vaccines (10802-a)
Profile
Vaccines against *Helicobacter pylori* are being developed for prophylaxis of peptic ulcer disease and gastric cancer.

◊ References.
1. Kreiss C, *et al.* Safety of oral immunisation with recombinant urease in patients with Helicobacter pylori infection. *Lancet* 1996; **347:** 1630–1.
2. Telford JL, Ghiara P. Prospects for the development of a vaccine against Helicobacter pylori. *Drugs* 1996; **52:** 799–804.
3. Haas R, Meyer TF. Vaccine development against Helicobacter pylori infections. *Biologicals* 1997; **25:** 175–7.
4. Kleanthous H, *et al.* Vaccine development against infection with Helicobacter pylori. *Br Med Bull* 1998; **54:** 229–41.
5. Blanchard TG, *et al.* Host response and vaccine development to Helicobacter pylori infection. *Curr Top Microbiol Immunol* 1999; **241:** 181–213.
6. Vyas SP, Sihorkar V. Exploring novel vaccines against Helicobacter pylori: protective and therapeutic immunization. *J Clin Pharm Ther* 1999; **24:** 259–72.

Hepatitis A Immunoglobulins (15378-l)
ATC — J06BB11.

Human Hepatitis A Immunoglobulin (Ph. Eur.) (Hepatitis A Immunoglobulin (BP 2001); Immunoglobulinum Humanum Hepatitidis A) is a liquid or freeze-dried preparation containing human immunoglobulins, mainly immunoglobulin G (IgG). It is obtained from plasma from selected donors having specific antibodies against the hepatitis A virus. Normal immunoglobulin may be added. It contains not less than 600 international units per mL. The liquid preparation should be stored, protected from light, in a sealed, colourless, glass container. The freeze-dried preparation should be stored, protected from light, in a colourless, glass container under vacuum or under an inert gas.

Profile
Immunoglobulins containing high levels of specific antibodies against hepatitis A are available in some countries for passive immunisation against hepatitis A infection; in the UK, normal immunoglobulin is usually given.

Preparations

Ph. Eur.: Human Hepatitis A Immunoglobulin.

Proprietary Preparations (details are given in Part 3)
Aust.: Globuman†; ***Belg.:*** Globuman Hepatite A†; ***Ger.:*** Gammabulin A†; ***Hong Kong:*** Globuman Hepatite A†; ***Port.:*** Globuman Hepatite A†; ***S.Afr.:*** Globuman Hepatite A; ***Switz.:*** Globuman Hepatite A†; ***Thai.:*** Globuman Hepatite A†.

Hepatitis A Vaccines (19290-y)

ATC — J07BC02.

Hepatitis A Vaccine (Inactivated, Adsorbed) (Ph. Eur.) (Inactivated Hepatitis A Vaccine (BP 2001); Hep A/Vac; Vaccinum Hepatitidis A Inactivatum Adsorbatum) is a liquid preparation of a suitable strain of hepatitis A virus grown in cell cultures, inactivated by a validated method, and adsorbed on a mineral carrier. It should be stored at 2° to 8°, not be allowed to freeze, and be protected from light.

Adverse Effects and Precautions
As for vaccines in general, p.1529.

◊ General references.
1. Niu MT, *et al.* Two-year review of hepatitis A vaccine safety: data from the Vaccine Adverse Event Reporting System (VAERS). *Clin Infect Dis* 1998; **26:** 1475–6.

Effects on the blood. WHO has received reports of 5 cases of thrombocytopenia, 3 with purpura, associated with hepatitis A vaccine.[1]
1. Meyboom RHB, *et al.* Thrombocytopenia reported in association with hepatitis B and A vaccines. *Lancet* 1995; **345:** 1638.

Effects on the nervous system. Neurological symptoms resembling encephalitis have followed a third dose of hepatitis A vaccine.[1] Other serious neurological reactions reported in patients receiving inactivated hepatitis A vaccine include transverse myelitis, Guillain-Barré syndrome, and neuralgic amyotrophy.[2] Such reactions appear to be very rare, and, since other vaccines have often been given simultaneously, may not be directly attributable to hepatitis A vaccine.
1. Hughes PJ, *et al.* Probable post-hepatitis A vaccination encephalopathy. *Lancet* 1993; **342:** 302.
2. Committee on Safety of Medicines/Medicines Control Agency. Hepatitis A vaccination (Havrix). *Current Problems* 1994; **20:** 16.

Interactions
As for vaccines in general, p.1530.

Uses and Administration
Hepatitis A vaccines are used for active immunisation against hepatitis A infections.

In the UK the use of an inactivated vaccine is recommended as an alternative to normal immunoglobulin for frequent travellers to areas of high or moderate hepatitis A endemicity or for those staying for more than 3 months in such areas; in some countries a hepatitis A immunoglobulin (p.1541) is available for those making shorter or less frequent journeys. Immunisation is also recommended in haemophiliacs and in those at risk of exposure to hepatitis A by virtue of their occupation, and should be considered in persons whose lifestyle is likely to place them at risk. The vaccine is given intramuscularly in the deltoid region, except in haemophiliacs in whom it should be given subcutaneously. In the UK vaccines containing 1440 ELISA units per mL (derived from the HM175 strain of virus), or 320 antigen units per mL (GBM strain) may be used: adult doses are 1 mL of the former, or 0.5 mL of the latter. The dose is repeated 6 to 12 months later. Alternatively a formulation containing 50 antigen units per 1-mL dose may be given, and repeated 6 to 12 months later. Children under the age of 15 years may be given a dose of 0.5 mL containing 720 ELISA units with a booster dose of 0.5 mL 6 to 12 months later. Alternatively 0.5 mL of a preparation containing 50 antigen units per mL may be given to adolescents or children over 2 years of age, and repeated after 6 to 18 months.

Immunity is provided for up to 10 years following these doses.

◊ Commercially available hepatitis A vaccines are usually produced from inactivated hepatitis A virus strains propagated in cell culture, commonly of human diploid fibroblast cells. Live attenuated hepatitis A vaccines have also been developed, although an oral live vaccine does not appear to have yet been produced. 'Virosome' hepatitis A vaccines consisting of inactivated hepatitis A virus epitopes formulated into liposomes are under investigation.
References.
1. Mao JS, *et al.* Primary study of attenuated live hepatitis A vaccine (H2 strain) in humans. *J Infect Dis* 1989; **159:** 621–4.
2. Loutan L, *et al.* Inactivated virosome hepatitis A vaccine. *Lancet* 1994; **343:** 322–4.
3. Strader DB, Seeff LB. New hepatitis A vaccines and their role in prevention. *Drugs* 1996; **51:** 359–66.
4. Committee on Infectious Diseases of the American Academy of Pediatrics. Prevention of hepatitis A infections: guidelines for use of hepatitis A vaccines and immune globulin. *Pediatrics* 1996; **98:** 1207–15.
5. Holzer BR, *et al.* Immunogenicity and adverse effects of inactivated virosome versus alum-adsorbed hepatitis A vaccine: a randomized controlled trial. *Vaccine* 1996; **14:** 982–6.
6. Lemon SM, Thomas DL. Vaccines to prevent viral hepatitis. *N Engl J Med* 1997; **336:** 196–204.

Preparations

Ph. Eur.: Hepatitis A Vaccine (Inactivated, Adsorbed).

Proprietary Preparations (details are given in Part 3)
Aust.: Avaxim; Havrix; ***Austral.:*** Avaxim; Havrix; VAQTA; ***Belg.:*** Epaxal; Havrix; VAQTA; ***Canad.:*** Epaxal; Havrix; VAQTA; ***Denm.:*** Avaxim†; Epaxal; Havrix; ***Fin.:*** Epaxal; Havrix; ***Fr.:*** Avaxim; Havrix; VAQTA; ***Ger.:*** Epaxal; Havrix; VAQTA; ***Hong Kong:*** Avaxim; Epaxal; Havrix; VAQTA; ***Irl.:*** Havrix; Vaqta; ***Israel:*** Avaxim; Epaxal; Havrix; Nothav; VAQTA; ***Mex.:*** Havrix; VAQTA; ***Neth.:*** Havrix; ***Norw.:*** Epaxal; Havrix; ***NZ:*** Epaxal; Havrix; VAQTA; ***Port.:*** Havrix; ***S.Afr.:*** Avaxim; Havrix; ***Singapore:*** Avaxim; VAQTA; ***Spain:*** Avaxim; Havrix; VAQTA; ***Swed.:*** Avaxim†; Epaxal; Ha-

vrix; VAQTA; *Switz.:* Epaxal; Havrix; VAQTA; *Thai.:* Havrix; VAQTA; *UK:* Avaxim; Havrix; VAQTA; *USA:* Havrix; VAQTA.

Hepatitis B Immunoglobulins (1235-a)

ATC — J06BB04.

Human Hepatitis B Immunoglobulin (Ph. Eur.) (Hepatitis B Immunoglobulin (BP 2001); Immunoglobulinum Humanum Hepatitidis B) is a liquid or freeze-dried preparation containing immunoglobulins, mainly immunoglobulin G (IgG). It is obtained from plasma from selected and/or immunised donors having specific antibodies against hepatitis B surface antigen. Normal immunoglobulin may be added. It contains not less than 100 international units per mL. The liquid preparation should be stored, protected from light, in a sealed, colourless, glass container. The freeze-dried preparation should be stored, protected from light, in a colourless, glass container, under vacuum or under an inert gas.

Human Hepatitis B Immunoglobulin for Intravenous Use (Ph. Eur.) (Human Hepatitis B Immunoglobulin for Intravenous Use (BP 2001); Immunoglobulinum Humanum Hepatitidis B ad Usum Intravenosum) is a liquid or freeze-dried preparation containing immunoglobulins, mainly immunoglobulin G (IgG). It is obtained from plasma from selected and/or immunised donors having antibodies against hepatitis B surface antigen. Normal immunoglobulin for intravenous use may be added. It contains not less than 50 international units per mL. Storage requirements are similar to those for Hepatitis B Immunoglobulin, except that the freeze-dried preparation is stored at a temperature not exceeding 25°.

Hepatitis B Immune Globulin (USP 25) is a sterile solution consisting of globulins derived from the plasma of human donors who have high titres of antibodies against hepatitis B surface antigen. It contains 10 to 18% of protein, of which not less than 80% is monomeric immunoglobulin G. It contains glycine as a stabilising agent, and a suitable preservative. It should be stored at 2° to 8°.

Adverse Effects and Precautions

As for immunoglobulins in general, p.1529.

◊ For a warning concerning possible lack of equivalence between different preparations of hepatitis B immunoglobulins, see under Uses and Administration, below.

Uses and Administration

Hepatitis B immunoglobulins are used for passive immunisation of persons exposed or possibly exposed to hepatitis B virus, including by sexual contact. They are not appropriate for treatment. Active immunisation with hepatitis B vaccine should always be commenced in conjunction with administration of hepatitis B immunoglobulins in patients exposed to hepatitis B virus.

In the UK a hepatitis B immunoglobulin containing 100 international units per mL is available for intramuscular use. The dose in adults and children over 10 years of age is a single dose of 500 international units by intramuscular injection given preferably within 48 hours of exposure and not more than 1 week after exposure. Children aged 5 to 9 years may be given 300 international units, and children under 5 years 200 international units. Hepatitis B immunoglobulin should also be given to newborn infants at risk whose mothers are persistent carriers of hepatitis B surface antigen or whose mothers are HBsAg-positive as a result of recent infection. The dose is 200 international units by intramuscular injection preferably at birth, and certainly within 48 hours of birth.

There is now a UK and European standard for a preparation for intravenous use containing not less than 50 international units per mL.

In the USA a hepatitis B immunoglobulin containing 15 to 18% of protein is available for intramuscular use. The dose for adults is 0.06 mL per kg bodyweight. A dose of 0.5 mL is given to infants perinatally exposed to hepatitis B; this appears to be a significantly lower dose than that employed in the UK.

◊ The US Immunization Practices Advisory Committee has issued recommendations on the use of hepatitis B vaccines and hepatitis B immunoglobulins.[1]

The content of hepatitis B immunoglobulin may vary between countries and between manufacturers. Care should be taken in interpreting dosage recommendations which are not given in terms of international units.[2] Products available in the USA have their strength expressed with reference to an FDA stand- ard but are considered to contain[3] the equivalent of at least 200 international units per mL.

1. Immunization Practices Advisory Committee. Hepatitis B virus: a comprehensive strategy for eliminating transmission in the United States through universal childhood vaccination. *MMWR* 1991; **40** (RR-13).
2. Vegnente A, *et al.* Universal hepatitis B immunization: the dose of HBIg that should be administered at birth. *Pediatrics* 1994; **94:** 242.
3. Halsey NA, Hall CB. Universal hepatitis B immunization: the dose of HBIg that should be administered at birth. *Pediatrics* 1994; **94:** 242–3.

Monoclonal antibodies. The name tuvirumab is applied to a human hepatitis B monoclonal antibody. A murine monoclonal antibody has been tried in a few patients with primary antibody deficiency.[1]

1. Lever AML, *et al.* Monoclonal antibody to HBsAg for chronic hepatitis B virus infection with hypogammaglobulinaemia. *Lancet* 1990; **335:** 1529.

Organ transplantation. Studies[1-5] in patients positive for hepatitis B surface antigen undergoing liver transplantation suggest that long-term passive immunisation with hepatitis B immunoglobulin could reduce hepatitis B re-infection and improve survival in these patients.

1. Samuel D, *et al.* Passive immunoprophylaxis after liver transplantation in HBsAg-positive patients. *Lancet* 1991; **337:** 813–15.
2. Nymann T, *et al.* Prevention of hepatitis B recurrence with indefinite hepatitis B immune globulin (HBIG) prophylaxis after liver transplantation. *Clin Transplant* 1996; **10:** 663–7.
3. McGory RW, *et al.* Improved outcome of orthotopic liver transplantation for chronic hepatitis B cirrhosis with aggressive passive immunization. *Transplantation* 1996; **61:** 1358–64.
4. Terrault NA, *et al.* Prophylaxis in liver transplant recipients using a fixed dosing schedule of hepatitis B immunoglobulin. *Hepatology* 1996; **24:** 1327–33.
5. Sanchez-Fueyo A, *et al.* Hepatitis B immunoglobulin discontinuation followed by hepatitis B virus vaccination: a new strategy in the prophylaxis of hepatitis B virus recurrence after liver transplantation. *Hepatology* 2000; **31:** 496–501.

Postexposure prophylaxis. For discussion of the use of hepatitis B immunoglobulins in patients exposed to hepatitis B virus, see Postexposure Prophylaxis under Uses and Administration of Hepatitis B Vaccines, below.

Preparations

Ph. Eur.: Human Hepatitis B Immunoglobulin; Human Hepatitis B Immunoglobulin for Intravenous Administration; *USP 25:* Hepatitis B Immune Globulin.

Proprietary Preparations (details are given in Part 3)
Aust.: Aunativ; Hepatect; *Belg.:* Hepuman†; *Canad.:* BayHep B; HyperHep†; *Denm.:* Aunativ; *Ger.:* Aunativ†; Hepatect; *Hong Kong:* BayHep B; Hepatect; Hepuman; *Irl.:* Hepatect; *Israel:* BayHep; Hepatect; Hepuman; *Ital.:* Haimabig; Hepatect; Hepuman B; ImmunoHBs; Uman-Big; Venbig; *Norw.:* Aunativ; *Port.:* Hepatect; *S.Afr.:* Hebagam IM; *Spain:* Gamma Antihep B; Gamma Glob Antihepa B†; Gammaglobin Antihep B P CE; Glogama Antihepatitis B†; Hepuman; *Swed.:* Aunativ; *Switz.:* Hepatect; Hepuman; *Thai.:* Hepuman; *USA:* BayHep B; H-BIG†; Nabi-HB.

Hepatitis B Vaccines (12818-t)

ATC — J07BC01.

Hepatitis B Vaccine (rDNA) (Ph. Eur.) (Hep B/Vac); (Vaccinum Hepatitidis B (ADNr)) is a preparation of hepatitis B surface antigen, that is obtained by recombinant DNA technology. It should be stored at a temperature of 2° to 8°, not be allowed to freeze, and be protected from light. Under these storage conditions it may be expected to retain its potency for 24 months.

Hepatitis B Virus Vaccine Inactivated (USP 25) is a sterile preparation consisting of a suspension of particles of hepatitis B surface antigen (HBsAg) isolated from the plasma of HBsAg carriers; it is treated so as to inactivate any hepatitis B virus and other viruses. It is adsorbed onto aluminium hydroxide and contains thiomersal as a preservative. It should be stored at 2° to 8° and not be allowed to freeze.

Adverse Effects

As for vaccines in general, p.1529.

In addition, hepatitis B vaccines have been reported to cause abdominal pain and gastrointestinal disturbance, and musculoskeletal and joint pain and inflammation. There may also be dizziness and sleep disturbance. Cardiovascular effects include occasional hypotension and, rarely, tachycardia. Other rare adverse effects include dysuria, visual disturbances, and earache.

◊ General references.

1. McMahon BJ, *et al.* Frequency of adverse reactions to hepatitis B vaccine in 43,618 persons. *Am J Med* 1992; **92:** 254–6.
2. Anonymous. Adverse events after hepatitis B vaccination. *Can Med Assoc J* 1992; **147:** 1023–6.

Effects on the blood. Rare cases of thrombocytopenia associated with hepatitis B vaccination have been reported.[1-3]

1. Poullin P, Gabriel B. Thrombocytopenic purpura after recombinant hepatitis B vaccine. *Lancet* 1994; **344:** 1293.

2. Meyboom RHB, *et al.* Thrombocytopenia reported in association with hepatitis B and A vaccines. *Lancet* 1995; **345:** 1638.
3. Ronchi F, *et al.* Thrombocytopenic purpura as adverse reaction to recombinant hepatitis B vaccine. *Arch Dis Child* 1998; **78:** 273–4.

Effects on bones and joints. Reactive arthritis[1,2] and Reiter's syndrome[2] have been reported after hepatitis B vaccination. A number of reports of arthralgia have been received by the UK Committee on Safety of Medicines and by the manufacturers of Engerix B, SmithKline Beecham.[2]

1. Rogerson SJ, Nye FJ. Hepatitis B vaccine associated with erythema nodosum and polyarthritis. *BMJ* 1990; **301:** 345.
2. Hassan W, Oldham R. Reiter's syndrome and reactive arthritis in health care workers after vaccination. *BMJ* 1994; **309:** 94–5.

Effects on the eyes. There have been isolated case reports of acute posterior uveitis,[1] visual loss associated with eosinophilia,[2] acute posterior multifocal placoid pigment epitheliopathy,[3] and central retinal vein occlusion[4] following vaccination against hepatitis B.

For mention of optic neuritis in patients receiving hepatitis B vaccine, see under Effects on the Nervous System, below.

1. Fried M, *et al.* Uveitis after hepatitis B vaccination. *Lancet* 1987; **ii:** 631–2.
2. Brézin AP, *et al.* Visual loss and eosinophilia after recombinant hepatitis B vaccine. *Lancet* 1993; **342:** 563–4.
3. Brézin AP, *et al.* Acute posterior multifocal placoid pigment epitheliopathy after hepatitis B vaccine. *Arch Ophthalmol* 1995; **113:** 297–300.
4. Devin F, *et al.* Occlusion of central retinal vein after hepatitis B vaccination. *Lancet* 1996; **347:** 1626.

Effects on the kidneys. Acute glomerulonephritis was reported in a patient following the third injection of hepatitis B vaccine.[1]

1. Carmeli Y, Oren R. Hepatitis B vaccine side-effect. *Lancet* 1993; **341:** 250–1.

Effects on the liver. There have been occasional reports of transient abnormalities in liver function associated with hepatitis B vaccine.[1-3] The appearance of autoantibodies has been reported in a patient,[2] and severe cytolysis consistent with an allergic mechanism in another.[3]

1. Rajendran V, Brooks AP. Symptomatic reaction to hepatitis B vaccine with abnormal liver function values. *BMJ* 1985; **290:** 1476.
2. Lilic D, Ghosh SK. Liver Dysfunction and DNA antibodies after hepatitis B vaccination. *Lancet* 1994; **344:** 1292–3.
3. Germanaud J, *et al.* A case of severe cytolysis after hepatitis B vaccination. *Am J Med* 1995; **98:** 595.

Effects on the nervous system. In the 3 years 1982 to 1985 the Centers for Disease Control, the FDA, and the manufacturer of plasma-derived hepatitis B vaccine received 41 reports of adverse neurological effects.[1] It was estimated that about 850 000 persons had received the vaccine in this time. Neurological events were convulsions (5 cases), Bell's palsy (10), Guillain-Barré syndrome (9), lumbar radiculopathy (5), brachial plexus neuropathy (3), optic neuritis (5), and transverse myelitis (4). In some analyses Guillain-Barré syndrome was reported significantly more often than expected. However, no conclusive epidemiological association could be made between any neurological adverse effect and the vaccine.

In France, spontaneous reports of multiple sclerosis and central demyelinating disease in patients who had received hepatitis B vaccine led to the suspension by the French authorities of hepatitis B vaccination in schools in 1998. This decision has been widely condemned by many authorities including WHO, the US National Multiple Sclerosis Society, and the Viral Hepatitis Prevention Board, and there is a fear that reduced confidence in the vaccine could have a profound effect on uptake. Arguments[2] against a link between hepatitis B vaccine and multiple sclerosis include the lack of correlation between the incidence of hepatitis B infection and demyelinating diseases, data from clinical studies including extensive postmarketing surveillance, and analysis of the French cases which concluded that the incidence of multiple sclerosis amongst vaccine recipients was not higher than would be expected in the population as a whole. A consultative group concluded[3] that, in the light of the evidence, the benefits of hepatitis B vaccination supported current WHO recommendations that all countries should have universal infant and/or adolescent hepatitis B immunisation programmes and that adults at increased risk of infection should also be immunised.

1. Shaw FE, *et al.* Postmarketing surveillance for neurologic adverse events reported after hepatitis B vaccination: experience of the first three years. *Am J Epidemiol* 1988; **127:** 337–52.
2. Anonymous. Expanded Programme on Immunization (EPI): lack of evidence that hepatitis B vaccine causes multiple sclerosis. *Wkly Epidem Rec* 1997; **72:** 149–52.
3. Halsey NA, *et al.* Hepatitis B vaccine and central nervous system demyelinating diseases. *Pediatr Infect Dis J* 1999; **18:** 23–4.

Effects on the skin. Skin reactions which have been reported in a few individuals after hepatitis B vaccination include erythema multiforme,[1,2] erythema nodosum,[3-5] lichen planus,[6,7] and vasculitis.[8,9]

1. Feldshon SD, Sampliner RE. Reaction to hepatitis B virus vaccine. *Ann Intern Med* 1984; **100:** 156–7.
2. Wakeel RA, White MI. Erythema multiforme associated with hepatitis B vaccine. *Br J Dermatol* 1992; **126:** 94–5.
3. Di Giusto CA, Bernhard JD. Erythema nodosum provoked by hepatitis B vaccine. *Lancet* 1986; **ii:** 1042.
4. Goolsby PL. Erythema nodosum after Recombivax HB vaccine. *N Engl J Med* 1989; **321:** 1198–9.

5. Rogerson SJ, Nye FJ. Hepatitis B vaccine associated with erythema nodosum and polyarthritis. *BMJ* 1990; **301:** 345.
6. Ciaccio M, Rebora A. Lichen planus following HBV vaccination: a coincidence? *Br J Dermatol* 1990; **122:** 424.
7. Ferrnado MF, *et al.* Lichen planus following hepatitis B vaccination. *Br J Dermatol* 1998; **139:** 350.
8. Cockwell P, *et al.* Vasculitis related to hepatitis B vaccine. *BMJ* 1990; **301:** 1281.
9. Le Helto C, *et al.* Suspected hepatitis B vaccination related vasculitis. *J Rheumatol* 1999; **26:** 191–4.

Hypersensitivity. Acute exacerbation of eczema[1] in a patient on the day after vaccination against hepatitis B; the pruritus experienced and the exacerbation of the eczema was probably due to the formaldehyde contained in the vaccine. Hypersensitivity to thiomersal included in recombinant hepatitis B vaccine has also been reported.[2]

There has also been a report of a hypersensitivity reaction after administration of a yeast-derived recombinant DNA hepatitis B vaccine to a patient with a history of reactions to mouldy foods.[3] The clinical history and skin-prick testing suggested a type I hypersensitivity reaction to small quantities of *Saccharomyces cerevisiae* remaining in the vaccine.

1. Ring J. Exacerbation of eczema by formalin-containing hepatitis B vaccine in formaldehyde-allergic patient. *Lancet* 1986; **ii:** 522–3.
2. Noel I, *et al.* Hypersensitivity to thiomersal in hepatitis B vaccine. *Lancet* 1991; **338:** 705.
3. Brightman CAJ, *et al.* Yeast-derived hepatitis B vaccine and yeast sensitivity. *Lancet* 1989; **i:** 903.

Precautions

As for vaccines in general, p.1530.

Reduced immune response. The immune response to hepatitis B vaccine is dependent on both host- and immunisation-related factors.[1] Host-related factors that appear to diminish the response include increasing age, increasing body-weight, smoking,[1,2] and male sex;[3] particular HLA haplotypes may also be associated with poor response.[4] Failure of hepatitis B immunisation in infants could be related to high perinatal maternal viraemia[5] rather than to inherent resistance to the vaccine.

Some studies have observed a defective response in chronic alcoholics[6,7] whereas others have not;[8] the degree of liver impairment may be a significant factor. It has been suggested that an increased dose of hepatitis B vaccine may be appropriate in those with a history of alcoholism.[9] Active infection with *Schistosoma mansoni* also appears to decrease the response to hepatitis B vaccination.[10] A diminished response occurs in HIV-positive patients[11-13] and in patients on haemodialysis;[1] an increased dose of hepatitis B vaccine is recommended in these patients. In patients with haemophilia who are not HIV-positive[14] immunity is reported to wane rapidly after vaccination and frequent booster doses may be required. Biological response modifiers such as thymopentin[15] and interferon,[16] have been used successfully in some patients on haemodialysis to overcome the immune deficit. Administration of interleukin-2 has met with variable success (see Vaccine Immunoadjuvant, in Uses and Administration of Aldesleukin, p.549).

The immune response to hepatitis B vaccine is affected by the site of intramuscular injection. The deltoid region is recommended for adults and the anterolateral thigh for infants. A diminished response has been associated with administration in the gluteal region (buttock).[1]

A related problem is posed by subjects who become infected with hepatitis B despite mounting an adequate response to immunisation. Evidence of viral replication was detected in 44 of 1590 hepatitis B vaccinees despite development of protective titres of antibody.[17] Acute hepatitis occurred in one patient. Although the infection may have been incubating at the time of vaccination, the virus isolated from the child with acute disease was an escape mutant with a different DNA sequence from that isolated from the mother.

1. Hollinger FB. Factors influencing the immune response to hepatitis b vaccine, booster dose guidelines, and vaccine protocol recommendations. *Am J Med* 1989; **87** (suppl 3A): 36S–40S.
2. Horowitz MM, *et al.* Duration of immunity after hepatitis B vaccination: efficacy of low-dose booster vaccine. *Ann Intern Med* 1988; **108:** 185–9.
3. Morris CA, *et al.* Intradermal hepatitis B immunization with yeast-derived vaccine: serological response by sex and age. *Epidemiol Infect* 1989; **103:** 387–94.
4. Alper CA, *et al.* Genetic prediction of nonresponse to hepatitis B vaccine. *N Engl J Med* 1989; **321:** 708–12.
5. del Canho R, *et al.* Failure of neonatal hepatitis B vaccination: the role of HBV-DNA levels in hepatitis B carrier mothers and HLA antigens in neonates. *J Hepatol* 1994; **20:** 483–6.
6. Degos F, *et al.* Hepatitis B vaccination and alcoholic cirrhosis. *Lancet* 1983; **ii:** 1498.
7. Mendenhall C, *et al.* Hepatitis B vaccination: response of alcoholic with and without liver injury. *Dig Dis Sci* 1988; **33:** 263–9.
8. McMahon BJ, *et al.* Response to hepatitis B vaccine in Alaska Natives with chronic alcoholism compared with non-alcoholic control subjects. *Am J Med* 1990; **88:** 460–4.
9. Rosman AS, *et al.* Efficacy of a high and accelerated dose of hepatitis B vaccine in alcoholic patients: a randomized clinical trial. *Am J Med* 1997; **103:** 217–22.
10. Ghaffar YA, *et al.* Response to hepatitis B vaccine in infants born to mothers with schistosomiasis. *Lancet* 1989; **i:** 272.
11. Carne CA, *et al.* Impaired responsiveness of homosexual men with HIV antibodies to plasma derived hepatitis B vaccine. *BMJ* 1987; **294:** 866–8.
12. Collier AC, *et al.* Antibody to human immunodeficiency virus (HIV) and suboptimal response to hepatitis B vaccination. *Ann Intern Med* 1988; **109:** 101–5.

13. Chan W, *et al.* Response to hepatitis B immunization in children with hemophilia: relationship to infection with human immunodeficiency virus type 1. *J Pediatr* 1990; **117:** 427–30.
14. Maris JM, *et al.* Loss of detectable antibody to hepatitis B surface antigen in immunized patients with hemophilia but without human immunodeficiency virus infection. *J Pediatr* 1995; **126:** 269–71.
15. Donati D, Gastaldi L. Controlled trial of thymopentin in hemodialysis patients who fail to respond to hepatitis B vaccination. *Nephron* 1988; **50:** 133–6.
16. Quiroga JA, Carreño V. Interferon and hepatitis B vaccine in haemodialysis patients. *Lancet* 1989; **i:** 1264.
17. Carman WF, *et al.* Vaccine-induced escape mutant of hepatitis B virus. *Lancet* 1990; **336:** 325–9.

Uses and Administration

Hepatitis B vaccines are used for active immunisation against hepatitis B infections. Two types of vaccine have been available each containing hepatitis B surface antigen (HBsAg) adsorbed onto aluminium hydroxide. In one type of vaccine the surface antigen is produced in yeast cells using recombinant DNA techniques. This type of vaccine is now widely used and there has been considerable interest in further developments to improve immunogenicity. The second type of vaccine, in which the surface antigen is obtained from plasma after purification and inactivation processes is now not generally available.

WHO had recommended that national immunisation policies should include routine hepatitis B immunisation for the whole population by 1997 and this has been implemented in some countries including the USA (see below). The current recommendations in the UK are for immunisation of persons at high risk of contracting hepatitis B. High-risk groups include: health care personnel, laboratory workers, or any other personnel who have direct contact with patients or their body fluids; staff and residents of accommodation for the mentally handicapped; patients with chronic renal failure including those requiring haemodialysis; haemophiliacs and those receiving regular blood transfusions or blood products; close family contacts or sexual partners of cases or carriers of hepatitis B; families adopting children from countries with a high prevalence of hepatitis B; individuals who frequently change sexual partners; parenteral drug abusers; inmates of custodial institutions; and some travellers to areas where hepatitis B is endemic. Immunisation should also be performed in infants born to women who are persistent carriers of hepatitis B surface antigen or infants born to women who are HBsAg-positive as a result of recent infection. Hepatitis C carriers who are not immunised against hepatitis B should also receive immunisation.

The basic immunisation schedule consists of 3 doses of a hepatitis B vaccine, with the second and third doses 1 and 6 months, respectively, after the first. In the USA, some products may be given in an alternative 2-dose regimen to adolescents with doses given 4 to 6 months apart. Doses should be given intramuscularly, with the deltoid region being the preferred site in adults and the anterolateral thigh the preferred site in infants; the gluteal region (buttock) should not be used as efficacy may be reduced. The dose of the recombinant vaccine depends on the product used. Typical doses for adults are 10 or 20 µg and for children 5 or 10 µg. Products containing 40 µg are available for patients on haemodialysis who have a reduced immune response to the vaccine. However, *the dose of one recombinant preparation should not be seen as equivalent to the dose of another.*

The recombinant vaccine has also been used where more rapid immunisation, for instance with travellers, is required. This schedule has involved the administration of the third dose 2 months after the initial dose with a further booster at 1 year. In exceptional circumstances in adults travelling to an endemic area who commence their vaccination course within a month of departure, an even more rapid schedule involving injections at 0, 7, and 21 days has been used; when this schedule is used, a booster dose is recommended after 1 year.

For newborn infants at risk combined active and passive immunisation against hepatitis B is recommended. The first dose of vaccine should preferably be giv-

en at birth, and certainly within 48 hours of birth. A single dose of hepatitis B immunoglobulin (200 international units) should be administered at the same time into a different site. Additionally, in any patient in whom immediate protection is required, combined active and passive immunisation may be considered with a single dose of 500 international units of hepatitis B immunoglobulin being the dose for adults. See under Hepatitis B Immunoglobulins, p.1542, for children's doses.

The subcutaneous route should be used in patients with haemophilia. Some authorities have suggested that intradermal administration, in a dose of about 2 µg, may be considered for haemophiliacs, but the likelihood of effective antibody response is reduced and the risk of local adverse effects may be increased.

◊ General references.
1. Buynak EB, *et al.* Vaccine against human hepatitis B. *JAMA* 1976; **235:** 2832–4.
2. Douglas RG. The heritage of hepatitis B vaccine. *JAMA* 1996; **276:** 1796–8.
3. Lemon SM, Thomas DL. Vaccines to prevent viral hepatitis. *N Engl J Med* 1997; **336:** 196–204.

Administration. The major public health burden of hepatitis B infection in the developing world is due to the consequences of chronic carriage of hepatitis B virus (hepatocellular carcinoma and chronic cirrhosis) rather than acute infection. WHO[1] considered that the most important means of controlling hepatitis B on a global scale and of reducing mortality from its sequelae was mass immunisation of infants. It stated that hepatitis B vaccine should be incorporated into the Expanded Programme on Immunization (EPI) and many countries have since done so. WHO later reiterated this aim[2] stating that hepatitis B vaccine should be integrated into national immunisation programmes in all countries with a hepatitis B carrier prevalence (HBsAg) of 8% or greater by 1995 and in all countries by 1997. WHO's aim was to reduce the incidence of new child carriers of hepatitis B by 80% by 2001. Results from Taiwan, where mass immunisation of infants has been in place since the mid-1980s have shown a marked decline in the number of child carriers under 10 years of age.[3,4] The incidence of hepatocellular carcinoma in children has also been reduced.[5,6]

Opinion remains divided in the UK regarding implementation of universal hepatitis B immunisation,[7-9] with some advising increased emphasis on alternative strategies already in place such as antenatal screening.[7,8]

The optimum vaccination strategy depends on the pattern of hepatitis B viral transmission in a particular country. In hyperendemic regions where most infections are acquired early in life, the vaccine should be administered shortly after birth and hepatitis B immunisation integrated into the EPI. Immunisation of all infants should be considered for population groups with chronic hepatitis B virus carrier rates greater than 2% and should be a public health priority where carrier rates are greater than 10%. Countries with a lower carrier rate might opt to immunise all adolescents as an alternative to infant immunisation. Immunisation of individuals at high risk of infection should be continued in addition to routine vaccination schedules[2] and, if hepatitis B is not integrated into infant vaccination schedules, screening pregnant women for HBsAg and immunising the infants of HBsAg-positive mothers should continue.[1]

If use of hepatitis B vaccine is integrated into the EPI, three doses should be given intramuscularly, the first dose being given as soon as possible after birth concomitantly with the first EPI immunisation. The exact timing of these doses will depend on the EPI schedule in operation. In the USA, these recommendations have been implemented by immunisation of all infants and of adolescents aged 11 to 12 years who have not previously received three doses of vaccine. The recommended schedule[10] is: infants of HBsAg-negative mothers, the initial dose is given at birth or at up to 2 months of age, a second dose at 1 to 4 months of age but at least 1 month after the first dose and the third dose at 6 to 18 months of age; infants of HBsAg-positive mothers, hepatitis B vaccine plus immunoglobulin at birth, then additional doses of vaccine at age 1 to 2 months and at 6 months; infants of mothers who HBsAg status is unknown, hepatitis B vaccine at birth, with maternal blood checked at delivery and, if positive for HBsAg, hepatitis B immunoglobulin as soon as possible (no later than 1 week of age). Adolescents aged 11 to 12 years who have not received immunisation as an infant should be given three doses with the second dose given at least one month after the first and third given at least 4 months after the first and 2 months after the second. Alternatively, some products may be administered in a two-dose regimen, with doses given 4 to 6 months apart. For further details, see p.1530. For premature infants of HBsAg-negative mothers, it has been suggested that the initial dose of vaccine could be delayed until the infant weighs at least 2000 g or until about 2 months of age.[11]

1. WHO. Progress in the control of viral hepatitis: memorandum from a WHO meeting. *Bull WHO* 1988; **66:** 443–55.
2. Anonymous. Hepatitis B vaccine. *WHO Drug Inf* 1993; **7:** 130–1.
3. Chen H-L, *et al.* Seroepidemiology of hepatitis B virus infection in children: ten years of mass vaccination in Taiwan. *JAMA* 1996; **276:** 906–8.

4. Hsu H-M, *et al.* Seroepidemiologic survey for hepatitis B virus infection in Taiwan: the effect of hepatitis B mass immunization. *J Infect Dis* 1999; **179:** 367–70.
5. Lee C-L, Ko Y-C. Hepatitis B vaccination and hepatocellular carcinoma in Taiwan. *Pediatrics* 1997; **99:** 351–3.
6. Chang M-H, *et al.* Universal hepatitis B vaccination in Taiwan and the incidence of hepatocellular carcinoma in children. *N Engl J Med* 1997; **336:** 1855–9.
7. Mortimer PP, Miller E. Commentary: antenatal screening and targeting should be sufficient in some countries. *BMJ* 1997; **314:** 1036–7.
8. Dunn J, *et al.* Integration of hepatitis B vaccination into national immunisation programmes: alternative strategies must be considered before universal vaccination is adopted. *BMJ* 1997; **315:** 121–2.
9. Goldberg D, McMenamin J. The United Kingdom's hepatitis B immunisation strategy—where now? *Commun Dis Public Health* 1998; **1:** 79–83.
10. American Academy of Pediatrics Committee on Infectious Diseases. Recommended childhood immunization schedule—United States, January-December 2001. *Pediatrics* 2001; **107:** 202–4.
11. Committee on Infectious Diseases. Update on timing of hepatitis B vaccination for premature infants and for children with lapsed immunization. *Pediatrics* 1994; **94:** 403–4.

BOOSTER DOSES. There has been considerable interest in the duration of immunity conferred by hepatitis B vaccination and the possible need for booster doses. However there are no official guidelines yet on administering booster doses after the recommended schedules, apart from recommendations that health care workers who have already been successfully vaccinated should be given a booster dose of vaccine after contamination of skin or eyes with blood from a HBsAg-positive person, unless they are known to have protective concentrations of antibody. A booster dose is also recommended for adults who receive a rapid immunisation schedule.

References.

1. Hollinger FB. Factors influencing the immune response to hepatitis B vaccine, booster dose guidelines, and vaccine protocol recommendations. *Am J Med* 1989; **87** (suppl 3A): 36S–40S.
2. Hadler SC. Are booster doses of hepatitis B vaccine necessary? *Ann Intern Med* 1988; **108:** 457–8.
3. Nommensen FE, *et al.* Half-life of HBs antibody after hepatitis B vaccination: an aid to timing of booster vaccination. *Lancet* 1989; **ii:** 847–9.
4. Gilks WR, *et al.* Timing of booster doses of hepatitis B vaccine. *Lancet* 1989; **ii:** 1273–4.
5. Coursaget P, *et al.* Scheduling of revaccination against hepatitis B virus. *Lancet* 1991; **337:** 1180–3.
6. Prince AM. Revaccination against hepatitis B. *Lancet* 1991; **338:** 61.
7. Hall AJ. Hepatitis B vaccination: protection for how long and against what? *BMJ* 1993; **307:** 276–7.
8. Tilzey AJ. Hepatitis B vaccine boosting: the debate continues. *Lancet* 1995; **345:** 1000–1.
9. Simó Miñana J, *et al.* Hepatitis B vaccine immunoresponsiveness in adolescents: a revaccination proposal after primary vaccination. *Vaccine* 1996; **14:** 103–6.
10. Edmunds WJ, *et al.* Vaccination against hepatitis B virus in highly endemic areas: waning vaccine-induced immunity and the need for booster doses. *Trans R Soc Trop Med Hyg* 1996; **90:** 436–40.
11. European Consensus Group on Hepatitis B Immunity. Are booster immunisations needed for lifelong hepatitis B immunity? *Lancet* 2000; **355:** 561–5.

Postexposure prophylaxis. A combination of passive immunisation with a hepatitis B immunoglobulin and active immunisation with a hepatitis B vaccine is generally recommended for postexposure prophylaxis against hepatitis B.

One group of patients who should be considered for postexposure prophylaxis are infants born to mothers who are persistent carriers of hepatitis B surface antigen (HBsAg). The risk is particularly high if the mother has detectable hepatitis B e antigen (HBeAg) or hepatitis B virus DNA or absence of detectable antibody to hepatitis e antigen (anti-HBe). Postexposure prophylaxis is also recommended in the UK for persons accidentally inoculated, or who contaminate the eye or mouth or breaks to the skin with blood from a known HBsAg-positive person, as well as in sexual contacts (and sometimes close family contacts) of sufferers from acute hepatitis B and who also seen with-in a week of the onset of jaundice in the contact.

In the UK, the recommended schedule for postexposure prophylaxis is the first dose of vaccine given preferably within 48 hours of exposure and no later than one week after exposure, or, for babies exposed to hepatitis B at birth, no later than 48 hours after birth, in conjunction with a single dose of hepatitis B immunoglobulin given at a separate site. The second and third doses of vaccine are given one and two months after the first dose, with a booster dose at 12 months. Health care workers who have been successfully immunised should be given a booster dose following subsequent contamination with blood from an infected person, unless they are known to have adequate antibody concentration.

Some references to postexposure prophylaxis against hepatitis B, including variations in the combined regimens used, the use of vaccine alone, and the use of accelerated regimens, are given below.

1. Polakoff S, Vandervelde EM. Immunisation of neonates at high risk of hepatitis B in England and Wales: national surveillance. *BMJ* 1988; **297:** 249–53.
2. WHO. Progress in the control of viral hepatitis: memorandum from a WHO meeting. *Bull WHO* 1988; **66:** 443–55.
3. Iwarson S. Post-exposure prophylaxis for hepatitis B: active or passive? *Lancet* 1989; **ii:** 146–8.
4. Vodopija I, *et al.* Post-exposure prophylaxis for hepatitis B. *Lancet* 1989; **ii:** 1161–2.

5. Ip HMH, *et al.* Prevention of hepatitis B virus carrier state in infants according to maternal serum levels of HBV DNA. *Lancet* 1989; **i:** 406–10.
6. Poovorawan Y, *et al.* Protective efficacy of a recombinant DNA hepatitis B vaccine in neonates of HBe antigen-positive mothers. *JAMA* 1989; **261:** 3278–81.
7. Polakoff S. Public Health Laboratory Service surveillance of prophylaxis by specific hepatitis B immunoglobulin in England and Wales during the period 1975-1987. *J Infect* 1990; **21:** 213–20.
8. O'Grady JG, Williams R. Liver transplantation for viral hepatitis. *Br Med Bull* 1990; **46:** 481–91.

Preparations

Ph. Eur.: Hepatitis B Vaccine (rDNA);
USP 25: Hepatitis B Virus Vaccine Inactivated.

Proprietary Preparations (details are given in Part 3)
Aust.: Engerix-B; Gen H-B-Vax; Hevac B†; *Austral.:* Engerix-B; H-B-Vax II; *Belg.:* Engerix-B; H-B-Vax II; *Braz.:* Engerix-B; Hevac B; *Canad.:* Engerix-B; Recombivax HB; *Denm.:* Engerix-B; H-B-Vax; *Fin.:* Engerix-B; *Fr.:* Engerix-B; GenHevac B; HB-Vax-DNA; *Ger.:* Engerix-B; Gen H-B-Vax; *Hong Kong:* Engerix-B; H-B-Vax II; *Irl.:* Engerix-B; H-B-Vax II; *Israel:* Engerix-B; Recombinant H-B Vax II; *Ital.:* Engerix-B; Recombivax HB; *Mex.:* Engerix-B; H-B-Vax II; Heberbiovac HB; *Neth.:* Engerix-B; HB-Vax-DNA; *Norw.:* Engerix-B; *NZ:* Engerix-B; H-B-Vax II; *Port.:* Engerix-B; Recombivax HB; *S.Afr.:* Engerix-B; H-B-Vax II; Hepaccine-B; *Singapore:* Engerix-B; H-B-Vax II; *Spain:* Engerix-B; Recombivax HB; *Swed.:* Engerix-B; H-B-Vax; *Switz.:* Engerix-B; Gen H-B-Vax; Heprecomb; *Thai.:* Engerix-B; Euvax-B; H-B-Vax II; Hepavax-Gene; *UK:* Engerix-B; H-B-Vax II; HBvaxPRO; *USA:* Engerix-B; Recombivax HB.

Hepatitis A and B Vaccines (6339-x)

Hepatitis A (Inactivated) and Hepatitis B (rDNA) Vaccine (Adsorbed) (Ph. Eur.) (Vaccinum Hepatitidis A Inactivatum et Hepatitidis B (ADNr)) is a suspension consisting of a suitable strain of hepatitis A virus, grown in cell cultures and inactivated by a validated method, and of hepatitis B surface antigen obtained by recombinant DNA technology; the antigens are adsorbed on a mineral carrier, such as aluminium hydroxide or hydrated aluminium phosphate. It should be stored at 2° to 8°, not be allowed to freeze, and be protected from light.

Adverse Effects and Precautions

As for vaccines in general, p.1529.

See also under Hepatitis A Vaccines, p.1541, and Hepatitis B Vaccines, p.1542.

Uses and Administration

Combined hepatitis A and B vaccines are used for active immunisation against hepatitis A and hepatitis B.

In the UK, a hepatitis A and B vaccine is available containing not less than 720 ELISA units of inactivated hepatitis A virus and not less than 20 µg of recombinant hepatitis B surface antigen (HBsAg) protein in 1 mL. For primary immunisation, three doses of 1 mL are given by intramuscular injection, with the second and third doses 1 and 6 months after the first. For children up to the age of 16 years a 0.5-mL dose is given.

Booster doses may be given as appropriate with the monovalent component vaccines since protection against hepatitis A and B declines at different rates, or a booster dose of the combined vaccine may be given after 5 years.

◊ References.

1. Leroux-Roels G, *et al.* Safety and immunogenicity of a combined hepatitis A and hepatitis B vaccine in young healthy adults. *Scand J Gastroenterol* 1996; **31:** 1027–31.
2. Bruguera M, *et al.* Immunogenicity and reactogenicity of a combined hepatitis A and B vaccine in young adults. *Vaccine* 1996; **14:** 1407–11.
3. Frey S, *et al.* Interference of antibody production to hepatitis B surface antigen in a combination hepatitis A/hepatitis B vaccine. *J Infect Dis* 1999; **180:** 2018–22.

Preparations

Ph. Eur.: Hepatitis A (Inactivated) and Hepatitis B (rDNA) Vaccine (Adsorbed).

Proprietary Preparations (details are given in Part 3)
Aust.: Twinrix; *Austral.:* Twinrix; *Belg.:* Twinrix; *Canad.:* Twinrix; *Denm.:* Twinrix; *Fin.:* Twinrix; *Fr.:* Twinrix; *Ger.:* Twinrix; *Irl.:* Twinrix; *Israel:* Twinrix; *Ital.:* Twinrix; *Mex.:* Twinrix; *Neth.:* Twinrix; *Norw.:* Twinrix; *NZ:* Twinrix; *Port.:* Twinrix; *Singapore:* Twinrix; *Spain:* Twinrix; *Swed.:* Twinrix; *Switz.:* Twinrix; *UK:* Twinrix; *USA:* Twinrix.

Hepatitis A and Typhoid Vaccines (20350-f)

Adverse Effects and Precautions

As for vaccines in general, p.1529.

Uses and Administration

A combined hepatitis A and typhoid vaccine is used for active immunisation. It consists of inactivated HM175 hepatitis A virus strain together with the Vi capsular polysaccharide from

Salmonella typhi Ty 2 strain. It is given to adults and adolescents over 15 years of age by intramuscular injection in a dose of 1 mL, containing not less than 1440 ELISA units of inactivated hepatitis A antigen and 25 µg of Vi polysaccharide antigen, at least 2 weeks prior to risk of exposure to typhoid and preferably one month before risk of exposure to hepatitis A. A booster dose may be given after 6 to 12 months to provide long-term protection.

Preparations

Proprietary Preparations (details are given in Part 3)
UK: Hepatyrix; ViATIM.

Herpes Simplex Vaccines (16841-b)

Profile

Several types of vaccines against herpes simplex virus types 1 and 2 have been developed. They have been tried in patients with both oral and genital herpes infections. They are also being studied for the prevention of infection in sexual partners of patients with genital herpes.

◊ References.

1. Stanberry LR, *et al.* Prospects for control of herpes simplex virus disease through immunization. *Clin Infect Dis* 2000; **30:** 549–66.

Preparations

Proprietary Preparations (details are given in Part 3)
Hong Kong: Lupidon G; *Ital.:* Lupidon G; Lupidon H; *Switz.:* Lupidon H+G.

Human Papilloma Virus Vaccines (14379-v)

Profile

Vaccines against human papilloma virus are under investigation for the treatment of genital warts and several malignant neoplasms including cervical and laryngeal cancers.

Influenza Vaccines (7967-w)

ATC — J07BB01; J07BB02.

Influenza Vaccine (Whole Virion, Inactivated) (Ph. Eur.); (Vaccinum Influenzae Inactivatum ex Viris Integris Praeparatum; Inactivated Influenza Vaccine (Whole Virion) (BP 2001); Flu/Vac) is a sterile aqueous suspension of a suitable strain or strains of influenza virus types A and B, either individually or mixed, grown individually in embryonated hen eggs and inactivated so that they retain their antigenic properties. The stated amount of haemagglutinin antigen for each strain present is usually 15 µg per dose. Suitable strains of influenza virus are those recommended by WHO. An antimicrobial preservative may be added. The vaccine should be stored at 2° to 8°, not be allowed to freeze, and be protected from light. Under these conditions it may be expected to be suitable for use for 1 year, provided that the strains of virus continue to be appropriate.

Influenza Vaccine (Split Virion, Inactivated) (Ph. Eur.) (Flu/Vac/Split; Inactivated Influenza Vaccine (Split Virion) (BP 2001); Vaccinum Influenzae Inactivatum ex Virorum Fragmentis Praeparatum) is a sterile aqueous suspension of a suitable strain or strains of influenza virus types A and B, either individually or mixed, grown individually in embryonated hen eggs and inactivated so that the integrity of the virus particles has been disrupted without diminishing their antigenic properties. The stated amount of haemagglutinin antigen for each strain present is usually 15 µg per dose. Suitable strains of influenza virus are those recommended by WHO. An antimicrobial preservative may be added. The vaccine should be stored at 2° to 8°, not be allowed to freeze, and be protected from light. Under these conditions it may be expected to be suitable for use for 1 year, provided that the strains of virus continue to be appropriate.

Influenza Vaccine (Surface Antigen, Inactivated) (Ph. Eur.) (Flu/Vac/SA; Inactivated Influenza Vaccine (Surface Antigen) (BP 2001); Vaccinum Influenzae Inactivatum ex Corticis Antigeniis Praeparatum) is a sterile aqueous suspension consisting predominantly of haemagglutinin and neuraminidase antigens of a suitable strain or strains of influenza virus types A and B either individually or mixed, grown individually in embryonated hen eggs and inactivated so that they retain their antigenic properties. The stated amount of haemagglutinin antigen for each strain is usually 15 µg per dose. Suitable strains of influenza virus are those recommended by WHO. An antimicrobial preservative may be added. The vaccine should be stored at 2° to 8°, not be allowed to freeze, and be protected from light. Under these conditions it may be expected to be suitable for use for 1 year, provided that the strains of virus continue to be appropriate.

The BP 2001 directs that when Inactivated Influenza Vaccine or Influenza Vaccine is prescribed or demanded and the form is not stated, Inactivated Influenza Vaccine (Whole Virion), (Split Virion), or (Surface Antigen) may be dispensed or supplied.

Influenza Virus Vaccine (USP 25) is a sterile aqueous suspension of suitably inactivated influenza virus types A and B, either individually or combined, or virus subunits prepared from the extra-embryonic fluid of virus-infected chick embryos.

Suitable strains of influenza virus are those designated by the US Government's Expert Committee on Influenza and recommended by the Surgeon General of the US Public Health Service. It may contain a suitable antimicrobial agent. It should be stored at 2° to 8° and not be allowed to freeze.

Nomenclature of strains. The strain designation for influenza virus types A, B, and C contains: a description of the antigenic specificity of the nucleoprotein antigen (types A, B, or C) (an internal antigen, the matrix antigen, has also been described); the host of origin (if not man, including, if appropriate, the inanimate source); the geographical origin; the strain number; and the year of isolation; e.g. A/lake water/Wisconsin/1/79. For type A viruses the antigenic description follows (in parenthesis) including the antigenic character of the haemagglutinin (e.g. H1) and the antigenic character of the neuraminidase (e.g. N1). There is no provision for describing subtypes of B and C viruses. Recombination between viruses within a type is readily accomplished; the letter R should be added after the strain description to indicate the recombinant nature of the virus, e.g. A/Hong Kong/1/68(H3N2)R. In addition the strain of origin of the H and N antigens of antigenic hybrid recombinant A and B viruses should be given, e.g. A/BEL/42(H1)—Singapore/1/57(N2)R.[1]

1. Assaad FA, et al. Revision of the system of nomenclature for influenza viruses: a WHO Memorandum. Bull WHO 1980; **58**: 585–91.

Adverse Effects
As for vaccines in general, p.1529.

Local and systemic reactions may occur but are usually mild. Fever and malaise sometimes occur and severe febrile reactions have been reported particularly after administration of whole-virion vaccine to children.

Various neurological syndromes have been temporally associated with administration of influenza vaccine, the most notable report being of the Guillain-Barré syndrome occurring after vaccination with inactivated swine influenza vaccine in 1976 (see below).

Effects on the nervous system. FACIAL PARALYSIS. For mention of temporary facial paralysis possibly associated with the intranasal administration of influenza vaccines, see under Uses and Administration, below.

GUILLAIN-BARRÉ SYNDROME. In 1976 a limited outbreak of influenza in the USA caused by a virus closely resembling the swine influenza virus led to the use of a killed swine influenza virus vaccine.[1] After about 45 million doses of the vaccine had been administered the vaccination programme ceased because there was some evidence of a temporal association between vaccination and the onset of a paralytic polyneuropathy of the Guillain-Barré type. An epidemiologic and clinical evaluation of these cases suggested a definite link between vaccination and the onset of the syndrome with extensive paralysis but no association with the onset of limited motor lesions. Influenza virus vaccines which lack a swine influenza virus component seem not to raise the risk of paralysis above background levels.

An increased number of reports of Guillain-Barré syndrome following vaccination with the 1993-94 influenza vaccine in the USA was not found to be associated with an increased risk from the vaccine itself, but was considered to be probably due to increases in vaccine coverage and in the baseline incidence of the syndrome.[2]

1. Anonymous. Influenza and the Guillain-Barré syndrome. Lancet 1984; **ii**: 850–1.
2. Lasky T, et al. The Guillain-Barré syndrome and the 1992-1993 and 1993-1994 influenza vaccines. N Engl J Med 1998; **339**: 1797–1802.

MULTIPLE SCLEROSIS. Analysis[1] indicating there was no association between the use in the USA during 1976 of influenza vaccines containing a swine virus component and the development of multiple sclerosis.

1. Kurland LT, et al. Swine flu vaccine and multiple sclerosis. JAMA 1984; **251**: 2672–5.

Henoch-Schönlein purpura. Influenza vaccination has been associated with both development[1] and exacerbation[2] of Henoch-Schönlein purpura.

1. Patel U, et al. Henoch-Schönlein purpura after influenza vaccination. BMJ 1988; **296**: 1800.
2. Damjanov I, Amato JA. Progression of renal disease in Henoch-Schönlein purpura after influenza vaccination. JAMA 1979; **242**: 2555–6.

Precautions
As for vaccines in general, p.1530.

Whole-virion influenza vaccine is not recommended for use in children because of the increased risk of febrile reactions.

Influenza vaccines should not be given to individuals with a known hypersensitivity to egg products.

Vaccination should be postponed in patients with active infection or acute febrile illness.

The symbol † denotes a preparation no longer actively marketed

Asthma. There have been reports of exacerbations of asthma following influenza vaccination[1,2] but reviews[3,4] have concluded that evidence of a causal relationship is lacking and that any risk of exacerbation which might exist is outweighed by the risk of influenza itself. Chronic respiratory disease, including asthma, is an indication for influenza vaccination in both the UK and USA. However, systematic reviews, while supporting the use of inactivated vaccines for patients with chronic obstructive pulmonary disease[5] have concluded that there is not enough evidence to assess the risks and benefits for people with asthma.[6]

1. Hassan WU, et al. Influenza vaccination in asthma. Lancet 1992; **339**: 194.
2. Nicholson KG, et al. Randomised placebo-controlled crossover trial on effect of inactivated influenza vaccine on pulmonary function in asthma. Lancet 1998; **351**: 326–31.
3. Watson JM, et al. Does influenza immunisation cause exacerbations of chronic airflow obstruction or asthma? Thorax 1997; **52**: 190–4.
4. Park CL, Frank A. Does influenza vaccination exacerbate asthma? Drug Safety 1998; **19**: 83–8.
5. Poole PJ, et al. Influenza vaccine for patients with chronic obstructive pulmonary disease (updated 30 July 2001). Available in The Cochrane Library; Issue 4. Oxford: Update Software; 2001.
6. Cates CJ, et al. Vaccines for preventing influenza in people with asthma (updated 21 August 2000). Available in The Cochrane Library; Issue 4. Oxford: Update Software; 2001.

Diagnostic tests. False-positive screening enzyme-linked immunosorbent assays (ELISAs) for antibodies to HIV-1, HTLV-1 and hepatitis C virus were reported in blood donors who had recently received influenza vaccine.[1] The reaction was attributed to cross-reactivity of the test kit in use at the time with non-specific IgM.

1. Anonymous. False-positive serologic tests for human T-cell lymphotropic virus type 1 among blood donors following influenza vaccination, 1992. JAMA 1993; **269**: 2076 and 2078.

Interactions
◊ For the effect of influenza vaccination on some other drugs see under Phenobarbital Sodium, p.356, Phenytoin Sodium, p.361, Theophylline Hydrate, p.782, and Warfarin Sodium, p.997.

Uses and Administration
Influenza vaccines are used for active immunisation against influenza.

Three types of the influenza virus occur, namely types A, B, and C, and the formulation and composition of influenza vaccines is constantly reviewed with changes made to accommodate the antigenic shifts and drifts of the influenza virus. Recommendations concerning the antigenic nature of influenza vaccines are made annually by WHO. Currently, influenza vaccines are of the inactivated type and may be available in three forms, as a whole-virion vaccine, as a split-virion vaccine, or as a surface-antigen vaccine.

Influenza vaccination is recommended for persons considered to be at special risk, particularly the elderly, those with chronic cardiac disease, chronic pulmonary disease including asthma (see above), chronic renal disease, diabetes or other endocrine disorders, and patients who are immunosuppressed. Vaccination should also be considered for residents, particularly elderly persons and children, in closed institutions. Medical personnel and other persons at risk from infection through contact with infected patients should also receive vaccination. Vaccination usually produces immunity after about 14 days, lasting for about 6 months to 1 year. Injections are therefore scheduled annually so that the period of maximum immunity coincides with the usual period of influenza infection. In the UK and USA they are generally given in October or November.

Influenza vaccines are administered in the UK by deep subcutaneous injection or intramuscular injection. The preferred site for injection is the deltoid muscle in adults and older children and, in infants and young children, the anterolateral aspect of the thigh. The recommended dose is 0.5 mL for adults and children aged over 3 years. In children aged 6 months to 3 years doses of 0.25 or 0.5 mL have been used. Children under 13 years of age should be given a second dose 4 to 6 weeks after the first if receiving the vaccine for the first time.

◊ Reviews.
1. Palache AM. Influenza vaccines: a reappraisal of their use. Drugs 1997; **54**: 841–56.
2. Demicheli V, et al. Vaccines for preventing influenza in healthy adults (updated 28 August 2001). Available in The Cochrane Library; Issue 4. Oxford: Update Software; 2001.

◊ Haemagglutinin on the surface of the influenza virus allows the virus to attach to the host cells, and antibody against it is the main form of immunity to influenza. Antibody to neuraminidase on the virus surface and cell-mediated immunity may be important as well. Adults with previous exposure to the relevant subtype usually get a fourfold or greater increase in haemagglutinin antibody after vaccination with 20 to 30 μg of haemagglutinin [approximately equivalent to one 0.5-mL dose], but in some cases most of the new antibody is against the original strain rather than the variant in the vaccine. Children and unprimed adults need two injections of a much larger dose of haemagglutinin (60 μg or more) for an adequate antibody response. The level of antibody falls by about 75% over 8 months after split-virus vaccine and by 50% over 6 months after whole-virus vaccine. Because of this decrease in antibody level, and antigenic drift, immunisation against influenza is required each year. After one or two doses of killed vaccine, clinical infection rates are reduced by 60 to 80% in children and young adults. Vaccination reduces clinical infection by only about 30% in elderly patients in institutions, but serious illness and death are probably cut by about 70%. The effectiveness of vaccination has varied widely in different studies, probably because of differences in previous exposure to the influenza subtype, vaccine dose, interval between vaccination and challenge, and matching of vaccine and challenge antigens.[1]

Various live influenza vaccines, all administered by the **intranasal** route, have been investigated,[1-10] and one such product was recently available in Switzerland but was withdrawn following reports of a possible link between its use and temporary facial paralysis. Cold-adapted and avian attenuated virus strains are considered to be potentially useful.[2,3,6-8,10] The intranasal route has also produced promising results with an inactivated split virion vaccine.[11] Preliminary *animal* studies are also under way[12] using microencapsulated inactivated influenza virus for **oral** administration.

A vaccine produced by inserting influenza haemagglutinin into **liposomes** produced higher concentrations of antibodies than conventional vaccines in a study in 126 elderly nursing-home residents,[13] an age group traditionally considered to respond poorly to the vaccine.

1. Shann F. Modern vaccines: pneumococcus and influenza. Lancet 1990; **335**: 898–901.
2. Clements ML, et al. Evaluation of the infectivity, immunogenicity, and efficacy of live cold-adapted influenza B/Ann Arbor/1/86 reassortant virus vaccine in adult volunteers. J Infect Dis 1990; **161**: 869–77.
3. Steinhoff MC, et al. Comparison of live attenuated cold-adapted and avian-human influenza A/Bethesda/85 (H3N2) reassortant virus vaccines in infants and children. J Infect Dis 1990; **162**: 394–401.
4. Clover RD, et al. Comparison of heterotypic protection against influenza A/Taiwan/86 (H1N1) by attenuated and inactivated vaccines to A/Chile/83-like viruses. J Infect Dis 1991; **163**: 300–4.
5. Gruber WC, et al. Evaluation of bivalent live attenuated influenza A vaccines in children 2 months to 3 years of age: safety, immunogenicity and dose-response. Vaccine 1997; **15**: 1379–84.
6. Belshe RB, et al. The efficacy of live attenuated, cold-adapted, trivalent, intranasal influenzavirus vaccine in children. N Engl J Med 1998; **338**: 1405–12.
7. King JC, et al. Safety and immunogenicity of low and high doses of trivalent live cold-adapted influenza vaccine administered intranasally as drops or spray to healthy children. J Infect Dis 1998; **177**: 1394–7.
8. Rudenko LG, et al. Clinical and epidemiological evaluation of a live, cold-adapted influenza vaccine for 3–14-year-olds. Bull WHO 1996; **74**: 77–84.
9. Nichol KL, et al. Effectiveness of live, attenuated intranasal influenza virus vaccine in healthy, working adults: a randomized controlled trial. JAMA 1999; **282**: 137–44.
10. Belshe RB, et al. Efficacy of vaccination with live attenuated, cold-adapted, trivalent, intranasal influenza virus vaccine against a variant (A/Sydney) not contained in the vaccine. J Pediatr 2000; **136**: 168–75.
11. Oh Y, et al. Local and systemic influenza haemagglutinin-specific antibody responses following aerosol and subcutaneous administration of inactivated split influenza vaccine. Vaccine 1992; **10**: 506–11.
12. Moldoveanu Z, et al. Oral immunization with influenza virus in biodegradable microspheres. J Infect Dis 1993; **167**: 84–90.
13. Glück R, et al. Immunogenicity of new virosome influenza vaccine in elderly people. Lancet 1994; **344**: 160–3.

Preparations
Ph. Eur.: Inactivated Influenza Vaccine (Split Virion); Inactivated Influenza Vaccine (Surface Antigen); Inactivated Influenza Vaccine (Whole Virion);
USP 25: Influenza Virus Vaccine.

Proprietary Preparations (details are given in Part 3)
Aust.: Begrivac; Fluarix; Inflexal; Influvac; Sandovac; Vaxigrip; *Austral.:* Fluarix; Fluvax; Fluvirin; Vaxigrip; Xflu; *Belg.:* α-Rix; Fluvirin; Influvac; Mutagrip; Vaxigrip; *Braz.:* Vaxigrip; *Canad.:* Fluviral; Fluzone; Vaxigrip; *Denm.:* Begrivac†; Fluarix; Influvac; Vaxigrip; *Fin.:* Begrivac; Fluarix; Flupar; Fluvirin; Influvac; Vaxigrip; *Fr.:* Fluarix; Fluvirine; Immugrip; Influvac; Mutagrip; Previgrip; Vaxigrip; *Ger.:* Begrivac; Fluarix; Inflexal; Influvac; Mutagrip; *Hong Kong:* Fluarix; Inflexal†; Vaxigrip; *Irl.:* Fluarix; Fluvirin; Fluzone; Influvac; Vaxigrip; *Israel:* Fluvirin; Influvac; Vaxigrip; *Ital.:* Adiugrip; Agrippal; Begrivac; Biaflu; Biaflu-Zonale SU; Fluad; Fluarix; Fluvirin†; Inflexal; Influpozzi; Influsplit; Influvac S; Influvirus; Isiflu Zonale; Mutagrip; Vaxigrip; *Mex.:* Fluarix; Flushield; *Neth.:* Fluarix; Influvac; Mutagrip†; Vaxigrip; *Norw.:* Begrivac; Fluarix; Fluvirin; Vaxigrip; *NZ:* Fluarix; Fluvax; Vaxigrip; *Port.:* Fluarix†; Fluvirin; Inflexal†; Influvac; Istivac; Vaxigrip; *S.Afr.:* Agrippal; Fluvirin; Inflexal; Influvac; Vaxigrip; Xflu; *Singapore:* Inflexal; Vaxigrip; *Spain:* Evagrip; Fluarix; Gripavac; Imuvac; Inflexal; Mutagrip; Vac Anti-

grip Frac; Vacuna Antigripal; ***Swed.:*** Begrivac; Fluarix; Fluvaccin†; Fluvirin; Fluzone†; Influvac; Vaxigrip; ***Switz.:*** Fluarix; Inflexal; Influvac; Mutagrip; Nasalflu; ***Thai.:*** Agrippal; Vaxigrip; ***UK:*** Agrippal; Begrivac; Fluarix; Fluvirin; Fluzone; Influvac; MFV-Ject; ***USA:*** Flu-Imune†; Fluogen†; Flushield; Fluvirin; Fluzone.

Jellyfish Venom Antisera (10837-g)

Jellyfish Antivenins; Jellyfish Antivenoms.

Adverse Effects and Precautions

As for antisera in general, p.1529.

Uses and Administration

An antiserum for use in the management of severe stings by the box jellyfish or sea wasp (*Chironex fleckeri*) is available in Australia. The preparation contains the specific antitoxic globulins that have the power of neutralising the venom of *Chironex fleckeri*. The globulins are obtained from the serum of sheep that have been immunised with the venom of the box jellyfish.

Box jellyfish antivenom is usually given by the intravenous route in a dose of 20 000 units. Alternatively, 60 000 units may be injected intramuscularly.

Box jellyfish sting. The sting of the box jellyfish (*Chironex fleckeri*) can be rapidly fatal so immediate first aid is vital. Fragments of tentacle adhering to the skin should be inactivated by the application of vinegar or 3 to 10% acetic acid solution. Artificial respiration and external cardiac massage may be necessary. The antiserum can be effective if administered quickly and in adequate dosage.[1-3] Studies in *rodents*[4] suggest that verapamil may be useful for treatment of the cardiotoxic effects of the venom and allow more time for the antiserum to exert its action. Some have suggested that the box jellyfish antiserum may be effective for severe envenomation by related species.[5]

1. Lumley J, *et al.* Fatal envenomation by Chironex fleckeri, the north Australian box jellyfish: the continuing search for lethal mechanisms. *Med J Aust* 1988; **148:** 527–34.
2. Horne TW. Box-jellyfish envenomation. *Med J Aust* 1988; **148:** 540.
3. Fenner PJ, *et al.* Successful use of chironex antivenom by members of the Queensland Ambulance Transport Brigade. *Med J Aust* 1989; **151:** 708–10.
4. Burnett JW. The use of verapamil to treat box-jellyfish stings. *Med J Aust* 1990; **153:** 363.
5. Fenner PJ, Williamson JA. Worldwide deaths and severe envenomation from jellyfish stings. *Med J Aust* 1996; **165:** 658–61.

Leishmaniasis Vaccines (16872-e)

Profile

Vaccines containing *Leishmania* spp. are under investigation in an attempt to prevent cutaneous leishmaniasis.

◊ The inoculation of an infective strain of a *Leishmania* sp. into the skin, a technique known as leishmanisation, has been used to protect against cutaneous leishmaniasis.[1] Although the technique has been standardised it is not generally recommended since large, slow-healing lesions have occurred in some patients.

Vaccines containing strains of killed leishmanial promastigotes have been developed and have conferred some protection against cutaneous leishmaniasis[1,2] although this has waned relatively quickly in some cases.[1] The safety and efficacy of killed *Leishmania* vaccines is under clinical investigation.[3] Killed vaccines combined with BCG as an adjuvant have also been tried.[4,5] Also under development are live vaccines containing stable mutants of *Leishmania* or recombinant subunit and synthetic vaccines.

Immunotherapy with a mixture of heat-killed promastigotes of *Leishmania mexicana amazonensis* and live BCG has compared favourably with meglumine antimoniate treatment in patients with cutaneous leishmaniasis.[6] Immunotherapy resulted in fewer side-effects than chemotherapy. For a discussion of the difficulties in treating cutaneous leishmaniasis, see p.584.

1. Playfair JHL, *et al.* Modern vaccines: parasitic diseases. *Lancet* 1990; **335:** 1263–6.
2. Nascimento E, *et al.* Vaccination of humans against cutaneous leishmaniasis: cellular and humoral immune responses. *Infect Immun* 1990; **58:** 2198–2203.
3. Modabber F. Vaccines against leishmaniasis. *Ann Trop Med Parasitol* 1995; **89:** 83–8.
4. Armijos RX, *et al.* Field trial of a vaccine against New World cutaneous leishmaniasis in an at-risk child population: safety, immunogenicity, and efficacy during the first 12 months of follow-up. *J Infect Dis* 1998; **177:** 1352–7.
5. Momeni AZ, *et al.* A randomised, double-blind, controlled trial of a killed L. major vaccine plus BCG against zoonotic cutaneous leishmaniasis in Iran. *Vaccine* 1999; **17:** 466–72.
6. Convit J, *et al.* Immunotherapy of localized, intermediate, and diffuse forms of American cutaneous leishmaniasis. *J Infect Dis* 1989; **160:** 104–15.

Leprosy Vaccines (16874-y)

Profile

Vaccines against leprosy including those using *Mycobacterium leprae* as well as other mycobacteria are under investigation. A killed vaccine has been developed in India for use as an adjunct to standard multidrug therapy in the treatment of leprosy. Although studies of new vaccines are continuing, BCG vaccine (p.1534) also appears to be effective.

◊ Attempts to develop a vaccine against leprosy are based on the assumption that induction of a cell-mediated immune response to *Mycobacterium leprae* will lead to protection against the bacillus.[1-4] Considerable protection against leprosy is afforded by BCG vaccination (see p.1534), and a study in Malawi showed that repeated vaccination provided additional protection.[5] However, the addition of killed *M. leprae* did not produce any further improvement, confirming preliminary results of a study in Venezuela.[6] The fortuitous finding that BCG vaccine, which is inexpensive and widely available, is effective against leprosy has important implications for leprosy control programmes.[7] Vaccines from non-pathogenic species of mycobacteria, *Mycobacterium w*, have been developed in India.

Leprosy vaccines are being studied both to prevent infection with *M. leprae* (immunoprophylaxis) and to prevent disease in infected individuals (immunotherapeutic). Beneficial responses have been reported[8-12] from the immunotherapeutic use of *Mycobacterium w* vaccine in combination with standard multidrug therapy (p.126) although a small increase in Type 1 lepra reactions has been observed.[13] A similar, and possibly identical, vaccine based on the ICRC bacillus is also being evaluated.[14,15] Immunotherapy with BCG and heat killed *M.leprae* has produced beneficial responses when given as an adjunct to chemotherapy.[16] WHO has suggested that the immunotherapeutic use of vaccines may ultimately prove to be more clinically relevant than the immunoprophylactic use,[14] and high compliance with immunotherapy appears to be attainable.[17]

1. Anonymous. Vaccines against leprosy. *Lancet* 1987; **i:** 1183–4.
2. WHO. WHO expert committee on leprosy: sixth report. *WHO Tech Rep Ser* 768 1988.
3. Fine PEM, Ponnighaus JM. Leprosy in Malawi 2: background, design and prospects of the Karonga Prevention Trial, a leprosy vaccine trial in northern Malawi. *Trans R Soc Trop Med Hyg* 1988; **82:** 810–17.
4. Anonymous. Bettering BCG. *Lancet* 1992; **339:** 462–3.
5. Karonga Prevention Trial Group. Randomised controlled trial of single BCG, repeated BCG, or combined BCG and killed Mycobacterium leprae vaccine for prevention of leprosy and tuberculosis in Malawi. *Lancet* 1996; **348:** 17–24.
6. Convit J, *et al.* Immunoprophylactic trial with combined Mycobacterium leprae/BCG vaccine against leprosy: preliminary results. *Lancet* 1992; **339:** 446–50.
7. Fine PEM, Smith PG. Vaccination against leprosy—the view from 1996. *Int Rev Immunol* 1996; **15:** 417–45.
8. Zaheer SA, *et al.* Combined multidrug and Mycobacterium w vaccine therapy in patients with multibacillary leprosy. *J Infect Dis* 1993; **167:** 401–10.
9. Zaheer SA, *et al.* Immunotherapy with Mycobacterium w vaccine decreases the incidence and severity of type 2 (ENL) reactions. *Lepr Rev* 1993; **64:** 7–14.
10. Zaheer SA, *et al.* Addition of immunotherapy with Mycobacterium w vaccine to multi-drug therapy benefits multibacillary leprosy patients. *Vaccine* 1995; **13:** 1102–10.
11. Katoch K, *et al.* Treatment of bacilliferous BL/LL cases with combined chemotherapy and immunotherapy. *Int J Lepr* 1995; **63:** 202–12.
12. Talwar GP. An immunotherapeutic vaccine for multibacillary leprosy. *Int Rev Immunol* 1999; **18:** 229–49.
13. Kar HK, *et al.* Reversal reaction in multibacillary leprosy patients following MDT with and without immunotherapy with a candidate for an antileprosy vaccine, Mycobacterium w. *Lepr Rev* 1993; **64:** 219–26.
14. Mangla B. Leprosy vaccine debate in India re-ignited. *Lancet* 1993; **342:** 233.
15. Jayaraman KS. Charges fly over rival leprosy vaccines. *Nature* 1994; **367:** 403.
16. Rada E, *et al.* A follow-up study of multibacillary Hansen's disease patients treated with multidrug therapy (MDT) or MDT + immunotherapy (IMT). *Int J Lepr* 1997; **65:** 320–7.
17. Walia R, *et al.* Field trials on the use of Mycobacterium w vaccine in conjunction with multidrug therapy in leprosy patients for immunotherapeutic and immunoprophylactic purposes. *Lepr Rev* 1993; **64:** 302–11.

Leptospirosis Vaccines (7688-m)

Leptospira Vaccines.

Profile

Leptospirosis vaccines prepared from killed *Leptospira interrogans* are available in some countries. They are used for active immunisation against leptospirosis icterohaemorrhagica (spirochaetal jaundice; Weil's disease) in persons at high risk of contracting the disease.

Preparations

Proprietary Preparations (details are given in Part 3)
Fr.: Spirolept.

Lyme Disease Vaccines (14348-r)

Adverse Effects and Precautions

As for antisera in general, p.1529.

Lyme arthritis refractory to treatment with antibacterials has occurred rarely as an immune reaction to vaccine-derived outer surface proteins of *Borrelia burgdorferi*.

Uses and Administration

Vaccines based on recombinant outer surface proteins of *Borrelia burgdorferi* have been developed and are available in some countries for active immunisation against Lyme disease. One such vaccine available in the USA consists of recombinant Osp A adsorbed onto aluminium hydroxide. It is given to individuals between the ages of 15 and 70 years who are at risk of contracting the disease; in most cases subjects are at risk because of their place of residence or occupation, or because they plan to travel to, or pursue recreational activities in, areas of risk. It is given in a dose of 0.5 mL, containing 30 μg of lipoprotein Osp A, repeated after one month and again after one year.

◊ References.

1. Centers for Disease Control. Recommendations for the use of lyme disease vaccine: recommendations of the Advisory Committee on Immunization Practices (ACIP). *MMWR* 1999; **48** (RR-7): 1–17. Correction. *ibid.:* 833.
2. Onrust SV, Goa KL. Adjuvanted Lyme disease vaccine: a review of its use in the management of Lyme disease. *Drugs* 2000; **59:** 281–99.

Preparations

Proprietary Preparations (details are given in Part 3)
Canad.: LYMErix; *USA:* LYMErix.

Malaria Vaccines (16882-y)

Profile

Malaria vaccines acting against the sporozoite, asexual, and sexual stages of the *Plasmodium falciparum* life cycle are under investigation, as well as multicomponent vaccines consisting of combined antigens from various stages.

◊ Chemoprophylaxis of malaria is becoming increasingly problematical (see p.428), resulting in the increased desirability of effective malaria vaccines, several of which have been, or are being, studied clinically.[1,2] Malaria vaccine development have been reviewed.[1,2] Malaria vaccines can be categorised into 3 main groups:

• vaccines against pre-erythrocytic forms of the parasite or specifically sporozoites would prevent development of clinical disease and interrupt transmission by insect vectors. However, infection acquired by blood transfusion would not be prevented. RTS/S, a recombinant circumsporozoite protein fused with the more immunogenic adjuvant hepatis B surface antigen, produced encouraging results in a preliminary study[3] although results in a follow-up study[4] were disappointing and it was considered that further development of vaccine composition was needed.

• vaccines against asexual stages of the parasite would inhibit development of clinical disease but would not interrupt transmission. Infection of the liver would not be impeded.

• vaccines against the sexual stages of the life cycle (so called 'altruistic' vaccines) would interrupt malaria transmission but would not prevent infection with sporozoites or development of asexual forms in the blood or liver.

A further approach that has been studied involves the development of vaccines to induce production of cytotoxic T-lymphocytes which confer immunity from malaria via destruction of parasite-infected hepatocytes.[5]

WHO envisages that different types of vaccine could be used in combination. Various malarial antigens have been identified and studied in the hope of developing a multicomponent vaccine. One such vaccine, SPf66, was developed in Colombia where it was shown to be effective in semi-immune populations in endemic areas.[6,7] The vaccine consists of a synthetic preparation of three antigens from the asexual phase of the parasite in the blood linked by a sporozoite antigen. Subsequent studies in Ecuador[8] and Venezuela[9] demonstrated efficacy of 67 and 55% respectively. However, the reproducibility of the results and the efficacy of this vaccine in highly endemic regions was the cause of considerable controversy[10-12] which, it was hoped, had been resolved by the results of a clinical study from Tanzania[13,14] where vaccine efficacy was reported to be 31%. Although low, it was thought that this degree of efficacy could substantially reduce mortality.[15] Unfortunately, however, SPf66 did not protect against clinical falciparum malaria in studies from The Gambia[16] and Thailand.[17]

Another multicomponent vaccine, NYVAC-Pf7, utilising a recombinant vaccinia viral vector that expresses 7 proteins from different stages of malarial infection, has also been studied,[18] but results have been disappointing. A further multicomponent vaccine, CDC/NIIMALVAC-1 has provided encouraging preliminary results in *animals* and *in vitro*.[19]

DNA vaccines against malaria are also under investigation.

1. Riley E. Malaria vaccines: current status and future prospects. *J Pharm Pharmacol* 1997; **49:** (suppl 2): 21–7.
2. Kwiatkowski D, Marsh K. Development of a malaria vaccine. *Lancet* 1997; **350:** 1696–1701.
3. Stoute JA, *et al.* A preliminary evaluation of a recombinant circumsporozoite protein vaccine against Plasmodium falciparum malaria. *N Engl J Med* 1997; **336:** 86–91.
4. Stoute JA, *et al.* Long-term efficacy and immune responses following immunization with the RTS, S malaria vaccine. *J Infect Dis* 1998; **178:** 1139–44.
5. Aidoo M, *et al.* Identification of conserved antigenic components for a cytotoxic T lymphocyte-inducing vaccine against malaria. *Lancet* 1995; **345:** 1003–7.
6. Valero MV, *et al.* Vaccination with SPf66, a chemically synthesised vaccine, against Plasmodium falciparum malaria in Colombia. *Lancet* 1993; **341:** 705–10.
7. Amador R, *et al.* The first field trials of the chemically synthesized malaria vaccine Spf66: safety, immunogenicity and protectivity. *Vaccine* 1992; **10:** 179–84.

8. Sempertergui F, *et al.* Safety, immunogenicity and protective effect of the SPf66 malaria synthetic vaccine against *Plasmodium falciparum* infection in a randomised double-blind placebo-controlled field trial in an endemic area of Ecuador. *Vaccine* 1994; **12:** 337–42.
9. Noya O, *et al.* A population based clinical trial with the SPf66 synthetic malaria vaccine in Venezuela. *J Infect Dis* 1994; **170:** 396–402.
10. Anonymous. Towards a malarial vaccine. *Lancet* 1992; **339:** 586–7.
11. Marsh K. Patarroyo's vaccine. *Lancet* 1993; **341:** 729–30.
12. Anonymous. Malaria: a first stride towards effective vaccination? *WHO Drug Inf* 1993; **7:** 45–7.
13. Teuscher T, *et al.* SPf66, a chemically synthesized subunit malaria vaccine, is safe and immunogenic in Tanzanians exposed to intense malaria transmission. *Vaccine* 1994; **12:** 328–36.
14. Alonso PL, *et al.* Randomised trial of efficacy of SPf66 vaccine against *Plasmodium falciparum* malaria in children in southern Tanzania. *Lancet* 1994; **344:** 1175–81.
15. White NJ. Tough test for malaria vaccine. *Lancet* 1994; **344:** 1172–3.
16. D'Alessandro U, *et al.* Efficacy trial of malaria vaccine SPf66 in Gambian infants. *Lancet* 1995; **346:** 462–7.
17. Nosten F, *et al.* Randomised double-blind placebo-controlled trial of SPf66 malaria vaccine in children in northwestern Thailand. *Lancet* 1996; **348:** 701–7.
18. Ockenhouse CF, *et al.* Phase I/IIa safety, immunogenicity, and efficacy trial of NYVAC-Pf7, a pox-vectored, multiantigen, multistage vaccine candidate for Plasmodium falciparum malaria. *J Infect Dis* 1998; **177:** 1664–73.
19. Shi YP, *et al.* Immunogenicity and in vitro protective efficacy of a recombinant multistage Plasmodium falciparum candidate vaccine. *Proc Natl Acad Sci U S A* 1999; **96:** 1615–20.

Measles Immunoglobulins (1236-t)

ATC — J06BB14.

Human Measles Immunoglobulin (Ph. Eur.) (Immunoglobulinum Humanum Morbillicum; Measles Immunoglobulin (BP 2001)) is a liquid or freeze-dried preparation containing immunoglobulins, mainly immunoglobulin G (IgG). It is obtained from plasma containing specific antibodies against the measles virus. Normal immunoglobulin may be added. It contains not less than 50 international units per mL. Both the liquid and freeze-dried preparations should be stored, protected from light, in a colourless, glass container. The freeze-dried preparation should be stored under vacuum or under an inert gas.

Adverse Effects and Precautions
As for immunoglobulins in general, p.1529.

Interactions
As for immunoglobulins in general, p.1529.

Uses and Administration
Measles immunoglobulins may be used for passive immunisation against measles. They have been used to prevent or modify measles in susceptible persons who have been exposed to infection; in the UK, normal immunoglobulin is usually given.

Preparations
Ph. Eur.: Human Measles Immunoglobulin.

Proprietary Preparations (details are given in Part 3)
Ital.: Immunomorb; Morbil; Moruman†; *S.Afr.:* Measlegam†; *Switz.:* Moruman†.

Measles Vaccines (7976-e)

ATC — J07BD01.

Measles Vaccine (Live) (Ph. Eur.) (Meas/Vac (Live); Measles Vaccine, Live (BP 2001); Vaccinum Morbillorum Vivum) is a freeze-dried preparation of a suitable live attenuated strain of measles virus grown in cultures of chick-embryo cells or human diploid cells. It is prepared immediately before use by reconstitution from the dried vaccine. The virus titre is not less than 1×10^3 CCID$_{50}$ per dose. The dried vaccine should be stored at $2°$ to $8°$ and be protected from light.

Measles Virus Vaccine Live (USP 25) is a bacterially sterile preparation of a suitable live strain of measles virus grown in cultures of chick-embryo cells. It contains not less than the equivalent of 1×10^3 TCID$_{50}$ in each immunising dose, and may contain suitable antimicrobial agents. It should be stored at $2°$ to $8°$ and be protected from light.

Adverse Effects
As for vaccines in general, p.1529.

Fever and skin rashes may occur following the administration of measles vaccines. The fever generally starts 5 to 10 days after the injection, lasts for about 1 or 2 days, and has sometimes been accompanied by convulsions. More serious effects reported rarely include encephalitis and thrombocytopenia.

◊ Reviews.
1. Duclos P, Ward BJ. Measles vaccines: a review of adverse events. *Drug Safety* 1998; **19:** 435–54.

◊ Some brief comments made by the Advisory Committee on Immunization in the USA on adverse effects of standard measles vaccines.[1] An excellent safety record of measles vaccines has been indicated by the experience gained through the use of more than 160 million doses up to 1986. Fever with a temper-

ature of $39.4°$ or more may develop in 5 to 15% of vaccinees beginning about the fifth day after vaccination and usually lasts several days. Transient rashes have been reported in about 5% of vaccinees. CNS disorders, including encephalitis and encephalopathy, have been reported with a frequency of less than one case per million doses administered. The incidence of encephalitis or encephalopathy following vaccination is lower than the incidence rate of encephalitis of unknown origin suggesting that such events following vaccination may be only temporally related to, rather than due to, vaccination.
1. Immunization Practices Advisory Committee. Measles prevention. *JAMA* 1987; **258:** 890–5.

Atypical measles. The atypical-measles syndrome has occurred in persons vaccinated against measles and later exposed to the natural infection. The syndrome has been characterised by high fever and atypical rash; abdominal pain has been common and pneumonia almost universal.[1] Although atypical measles has occurred particularly in patients given the no-longer used killed vaccine[1] it has been reported in recipients of live measles vaccines.[2-4]

Measles occurring in patients previously vaccinated with live measles vaccines may be mild and go unrecognised. However, secondary vaccine failure does not appear to be a major problem (see Immunisation Schedules under Uses, below).
1. Anonymous. The atypical-measles syndrome. *Lancet* 1979; **i:** 962–3.
2. Chatterji M, Mankad V. Failure of attenuated viral vaccine in prevention of atypical measles. *JAMA* 1977; **238:** 2635.
3. Henderson JAM, Hammond DI. Delayed diagnosis in atypical measles syndrome. *Can Med Assoc J* 1985; **133:** 211–13.
4. Hirose M, *et al.* Five cases of measles secondary vaccine failure with confirmed seroconversion after live measles vaccination. *Scand J Infect Dis* 1997; **29:** 187–90.

Effects on hearing. There have been individual case reports of sensorineural hearing loss after measles vaccination.[1,2] Similar reports have been made after vaccination with measles and rubella vaccines (p.1549), and measles, mumps, and rubella vaccines (p.1549).
1. Watson JG. Bilateral hearing loss in a 3-year-old girl following measles immunisation at the age of 15 months. *Int J Pediatr Otorhinolaryngol* 1990; **19:** 189–90.
2. Jayarajan V, Sedler PA. Hearing loss following measles vaccination. *J Infect* 1995; **30:** 184–5.

Effects on the nervous system. Subacute sclerosing panencephalitis (SSPE) is a rare complication of measles infection (p.611) and has been reported in children who have received measles vaccine but have no history of clinical disease. Nevertheless mass measles vaccination has been effective in reducing the incidence of SSPE in both developing and industrialised countries,[1] and the risks of remaining unimmunised are considered to be greater than those arising from immunisation.
1. Anonymous. SSPE in the developing world. *Lancet* 1990; **336:** 600.

GUILLAIN-BARRÉ SYNDROME. No association was found between measles vaccination and Guillain-Barré syndrome in an analysis of 2296 cases.[1]
1. da Silveira CM, *et al.* Measles vaccination and Guillain-Barré syndrome. *Lancet* 1997; **349:** 14–16.

OPTIC NEURITIS. For a report of optic neuritis in 2 children following administration of measles and rubella vaccine, see under Adverse Effects of Measles and Rubella Vaccines, p.1549.

Effects on the skin. Stevens-Johnson syndrome was associated with measles vaccination in a 10-month-old infant.[1]
1. Hazir T, *et al.* Stevens-Johnson syndrome following measles vaccination. *J Pakistan Med Assoc* 1997; **47:** 264–5.

High-titre vaccines and mortality. Following reports of excess mortality in children, especially among girls, who received the Edmonston-Zagreb (EZ) measles vaccine,[1] WHO reversed its recommendation for the use of this vaccine in its Expanded Programme on Immunization in developing countries.[2,3] Subsequent study[4] of children who had received high-titre EZ vaccine showed adverse effects on the nutritional status in either sex, confirming a generally deleterious effect of the vaccine. Others, however, have argued that the problems associated with the use of EZ vaccine have been exaggerated.[5]
1. Knudsen KM, *et al.* Child mortality following standard, medium or high titre measles immunization in West Africa. *Int J Epidemiol* 1996; **25:** 665–73.
2. Anonymous. High-titre measles vaccines dropped. *Lancet* 1992; **340:** 232.
3. WHO. Expanded Programme on Immunization; safety of high-titre measles vaccines. *Wkly Epidem Rec* 1992; **67:** 357–61.
4. Garenne M. Effect of Edmonston-Zagreb high-titre vaccine on nutritional status. *Lancet* 1994; **344:** 261–2.
5. Bennett JV, *et al.* Edmonston-Zagreb measles vaccine: a good vaccine with an image problem. *Pediatrics* 1999; **104:** 1123–4.

Precautions
As for vaccines in general, p.1530.

In the UK it was formerly recommended that children with a personal history of convulsions or those whose parents or siblings have a history of idiopathic epilepsy should receive measles vaccine but simultaneously with a specially diluted human normal immunoglobulin; it is now, however, recommended that such children be vaccinated with combined measles, mumps, and rubella vaccine in the same manner as normal

healthy children. The parents should understand that a febrile reaction is possible and that suitable prophylactic treatment against febrile convulsions be undertaken (see Fever and Hyperthermia, p.8, for comments on the prevention of fever following immunisation). Immunoglobulin should not be given with the combined vaccine.

Measles vaccines are not generally recommended for children below the age of 1 year in whom maternal antibodies might prevent a response, but they have been administered to younger infants when the risk of measles is particularly high (see Immunisation Schedules, under Uses, below, for further discussion).

Hypersensitivity. For discussion of precautions to be taken on administration of measles vaccines to children allergic to egg, see Measles, Mumps, and Rubella Vaccines, p.1549.

Immunocompromised patients. For a discussion of the use of live vaccines in immunocompromised patients including those with HIV infections, see under Uses on p.1531.

As with other live vaccines, measles vaccine is generally not recommended for use in patients with impaired immunity, although combined measles, mumps, and rubella vaccine may be given to HIV-positive individuals in the absence of other contra-indications. The WHO and UNICEF[1] recommend that children with suspected or confirmed HIV infection should receive a dose of measles vaccine at 6 months of age in addition to the scheduled dose at 9 months. The immunogenicity of measles vaccine in children with HIV infections has been shown to be low[2,3] although immunisation at 6 months of age was more effective than at 12 months of age.[3] Immunocompromised patients who come into contact with measles should be given normal immunoglobulin. Specific measles immunoglobulins are available in some countries. Although measles vaccines have been given to immunocompromised patients without causing adverse effects[2] there have been some reports of severe reactions; disseminated measles infection was reported in a child with severe congenital immunodeficiency,[4] and fatal giant-cell pneumonitis was reported in an adult with AIDS.[5] As a consequence of reports of adverse effects in severely immunocompromised individuals, the Advisory Committee on Immunization Practices in the USA is re-evaluating its recommendations for immunising patients with advanced HIV infection.[6] The American Academy of Pediatrics has recommended[7] that *severely* immunosuppressed HIV-infected children and young adults should not receive any measles-containing vaccines, whereas those with HIV infection but without evidence of severe immunosuppression should receive measles, mumps, and rubella vaccine. They also recommend that if HIV-infected children or adolescents are exposed to wild type measles, they should receive normal immunoglobulin regardless of their degree of immunosuppression or measles immunisation status.[7]
1. WHO. *EPI vaccines in HIV-infected individuals: 5 October 2001.* Available at: http://www.who.int/vaccines-diseases/diseases/HIV.shtml (accessed 7/12/01).
2. Krasinski K, Borkowsky W. Measles and measles immunity in children infected with human immunodeficiency virus. *JAMA* 1989; **261:** 2512–16.
3. Rudy BJ, *et al.* Responses to measles immunization in children infected with human immunodeficiency virus. *J Pediatr* 1994; **125:** 72–4.
4. Monafo WJ, *et al.* Disseminated measles infection after vaccination in a child with a congenital immunodeficiency. *J Pediatr* 1994; **124:** 273–6.
5. Angel JB, *et al.* Vaccine-associated measles pneumonitis in an adult with AIDS. *Ann Intern Med* 1998; **129:** 104–6.
6. Centers for Disease Control. Update: vaccine side effects, adverse reactions, contraindications, and precautions: recommendations of the Advisory Committee on Immunization Practices (ACIP). *MMWR* 1996; **45:** (RR-12): 1–35.
7. American Academy of Pediatrics Committee on Infectious Diseases and Committee on Pediatric AIDS. Measles immunization in HIV-infected children. *Pediatrics* 1999; **103:** 1057–60.

Inflammatory bowel disease. Measles vaccination has been suggested as a possible factor in the development of inflammatory bowel disease.[1] However a case-control study involving 140 patients with inflammatory bowel disease provided no support for this hypothesis,[2] and measles virus has not been detected in biopsy specimens from patients with inflammatory bowel disease.[3] A suggested link between measles vaccine-associated inflammatory bowel disease and autism has proved controversial (see p.1549).
1. Thompson NP, *et al.* Is measles vaccination a risk factor for inflammatory bowel disease? *Lancet* 1995; **345:** 1071–4.
2. Feeney M, *et al.* A case-control study of measles vaccination and inflammatory bowel disease. *Lancet* 2000; **350:** 764–6.
3. Afzal MA, *et al.* Absence of measles-virus genome in inflammatory bowel disease. *Lancet* 1998; **351:** 646–7.

Interactions
As for vaccines in general, p.1530

Vitamin A. Supplementation with vitamin A (p.1383) is now included as part of WHO's Expanded Programme on Immunization. There is conflicting evidence of the effects of such supplementation on the response to measles vaccination. One study[1] reported a reduced response if vaccination occurs at 6 months while another[2] found the response to be unaffected in children vaccinated at 9 months. This difference, if confirmed, could be due to the influence of maternal antibodies, which would still be present at 6 months but not at 9 months of age.[3]

1. Semba RD, et al. Reduced seroconversion to measles in infants given vitamin A with measles vaccination. Lancet 1995; 345: 1330–2.
2. Benn CS, et al. Randomised trial of effect of vitamin A supplementation on antibody response to measles vaccine in Guinea-Bissau, West Africa. Lancet 1997; 350: 101–5.
3. Semba RD. Vitamin A supplementation. Lancet 1997; 350: 1031–2.

Uses and Administration

Measles vaccines are used for active immunisation against measles.

For primary immunisation a combined measles, mumps, and rubella vaccine (p.1549) is usually used. For discussion of immunisation schedules, see below.

In the UK single-antigen measles vaccine prepared from the Schwarz strain of the measles virus was formerly used. It was given in a dose of 0.5 mL by deep subcutaneous or intramuscular injection.

Measles vaccines are not generally recommended for children below the age of 1 year in whom maternal antibodies might prevent a response. However, they have been administered to infants at 6 to 9 months in developing countries and in the USA in certain circumstances (see also below). A high-potency measles vaccine prepared from the Edmonston-Zagreb strain of measles virus was formerly used but was discontinued following evidence of increased mortality (see High-titre Vaccines and Mortality, under Adverse Effects, above).

Single-antigen measles vaccines have also been used for prophylaxis after exposure to measles provided they are given within 72 hours of contact.

Administration. Several alternative routes of administration of measles vaccines have been investigated in an attempt to overcome some of the disadvantages of subcutaneous or intramuscular injection.[1] Intradermal injection is effective if a needle is to be used but carries the same risk of secondary infection as subcutaneous administration; the use of a jet injector has produced less reliable immunisation. The conjunctival and oral routes are not sufficiently effective, and the intranasal route produced variable responses and could be influenced by concurrent upper respiratory-tract infections. A review of clinical studies[1] has shown that aerosol administration has produced good responses in children over 9 months of age, although this route was not so effective in younger children. The Edmonston-Zagreb strain generally produced higher rates of seroconversion than the Schwarz strain. Aerosol administration could be potentially useful for mass immunisation campaigns and this suggestion has been confirmed in a recent randomised study.[2]

1. Cutts FT, et al. Alternative routes of measles immunization: a review. Biologicals 1997; 25: 323–38.
2. Dilraj A, et al. Response to different measles vaccine strains given by aerosol and subcutaneous routes to schoolchildren: a randomised trial. Lancet 2000; 355: 798–803.

Immunisation schedules. In the developed world measles vaccine (usually as measles, mumps, and rubella vaccine) is usually given in the second year of life.[1] As a result of concern that measles vaccine would not elicit an appropriate immune response in young infants due to the persistence of maternal antibodies in circulation, vaccination has generally not been attempted in children under 12 months old. Studies have shown that seroconversion rates are similar following vaccination at 12, 13, 14, and 15 to 18 months.[2] However, infants born to vaccinated mothers tend to have lower levels of maternal antibodies and are susceptible to measles infection at under 12 months of age; vaccination has been shown to be effective at 6 to 9 months of age in such children,[3-5] although antibody titres were lower in infants vaccinated at 6 months of age than in those vaccinated later.[3,6]

In the UK and USA[7] routine vaccination is given at 12 to 15 months, with a second dose given at 3 to 6 years or 11 to 12 years of age (see the immunisation schedules summarised under Vaccines, p.1530). Similar schedules are used in other countries. There is evidence that these 2-dose strategies will produce high levels of immunity in the community.[8] During an outbreak of measles, vaccination may be given as early as 6 months of age;[9] revaccination is recommended in any child who is vaccinated before their first birthday. Vaccine may be given to non-immune persons of any age considered to be at risk of infection even if their immune status is uncertain.

Immunisation strategies involving a single dose of measles vaccine have not been successful in eradicating or eliminating the disease in developed countries.[10,11] Immunisation has changed the epidemiology of measles and several isolated outbreaks have occurred among both unvaccinated and vaccinated persons.[10] Primary vaccine failure (approximately 2 to 10% of vaccinees fail to seroconvert after measles vaccination) has played a substantial role in transmission of measles.[10] Furthermore, waning of immunity in the vaccinated cohort coupled with a reduction in the prevalence of the natural infection has

resulted in increasing numbers of young adults with low concentrations of antibodies.[12,13] As these young adults reach child-bearing age, their children in turn have lower, faster-waning immunity and are susceptible to infection before the usual age of immunisation.[14] Immunisation schedules which include a second dose of measles vaccine in adolescence would boost immunity in young adults and hence in their offspring, but there is evidence that revaccination is ineffective in a proportion of recipients.[15,16] The alternative is to give the first dose of vaccine earlier, for example at 6 months of age, and a second dose in early childhood. However this too would not overcome the problem of secondary vaccine failures in young adults. This dilemma over the most appropriate schedule is most pressing in developing countries where transmission rates are usually high. For discussion of immunisation schedules in the developing world, see under Expanded Programme on Immunization, below.

1. Isaacs D, Menser M. Modern vaccines: measles, mumps, rubella, and varicella. Lancet 1990; 335: 1384–7.
2. Kakakios AM, et al. Optimal age for measles and mumps vaccination in Australia. Med J Aust 1990; 152: 472–4.
3. Johnson CE, et al. Measles vaccine immunogenicity in 6- versus 15-month-old infants born to mothers in the measles vaccine era. Pediatrics 1994; 93: 939–44.
4. Carson MM, et al. Measles vaccination of infants in a well-vaccinated population. Pediatr Infect Dis J 1995; 14: 17–22.
5. Markowitz LE, et al. Changing levels of measles antibody titers in women and children in the United States: impact on response to vaccination. Pediatrics 1996; 97: 53–8.
6. Gans HA, et al. Deficiency of the humoral immune response to measles vaccine in infants immunized at age 6 months. JAMA 1998; 280: 527–32.
7. American Academy of Pediatrics Committee on Infectious Diseases. Recommended childhood immunization schedule—United States, January-December 2001. Pediatrics 2001; 107: 202–4.
8. Poland GA, et al. Measles reimmunization in children seronegative after initial immunization. JAMA 1997; 277: 1156–8.
9. De Serres G, et al. Effectiveness of vaccination at 6 to 11 months of age during an outbreak of measles. Pediatrics 1996; 97: 232–5.
10. Immunization Practices Advisory Committee. Measles prevention: supplementary statement. JAMA 1989; 261: 827 and 831.
11. Levy MH, Bridges-Webb C. "Just one shot" is not enough — measles control and eradication. Med J Aust 1990; 152: 489–91.
12. Mulholland K. Measles and pertussis in developing countries with good vaccine coverage. Lancet 1995; 345: 305–7.
13. McLean AR. After the honeymoon in measles control. Lancet 1995; 345: 272.
14. Maldonado YA, et al. Early loss of passive measles antibody in infants of mothers with vaccine-induced immunity. Pediatrics 1995; 96: 447–50.
15. Markowitz LE, et al. Persistence of measles antibody after revaccination. J Infect Dis 1992; 166: 205–8.
16. Cohn ML, et al. Measles vaccine failures: lack of sustained measles-specific immunoglobulin G responses in revaccinated adolescents and young adults. Pediatr Infect Dis J 1994; 13: 34–8.

EXPANDED PROGRAMME ON IMMUNIZATION. In the developed world measles vaccine (usually as measles, mumps, and rubella vaccine) is usually given in the second year of life. If given earlier, passively-acquired maternal antibodies against measles may interfere with development of protective immunity although this situation is changing as vaccinated women reach child-bearing age (see above). In the developing world, protection given by maternal antibodies is often rapidly lost.[1] Thus in hyperendemic areas, such as urban and peri-urban areas, clinical measles may occur in children as young as 5 to 6 months of age. Immunisation against measles is part of WHO's Expanded Programme on Immunization.[2] It is given as a single-antigen vaccine generally at 9 months of age. However control of measles in children less than 9 months of age is a major concern in some countries, in particular in areas of high population density.[3] WHO no longer recommends the use of high-titre Edmonston-Zagreb measles vaccine. Unlike conventional vaccines, this vaccine was shown to be effective at 6 months of age but, despite the resulting increase in immunity, increased mortality has been observed (see High-titre Vaccines and Mortality, under Adverse Effects, above). For comments on the possibility of a resurgence of measles infection in young adults and infants in countries with good vaccine coverage, see under Immunisation Schedules, above. WHO recognises that vaccination strategies will need to be formulated to cope with local disease patterns and available resources.[3]

In some situations high coverage with a single dose of vaccine can produce a high degree of immunity[3] and standard titre vaccines have been shown to be as effective as high-titre vaccines.[4,5] Mass immunisation campaigns can also be very effective[6] but can be expensive when a large proportion of the community is already immune.[7,8]

Early 2-dose schedules[3] may be more applicable in areas with high transmission rates among young infants. The first dose is typically given at 9 months of age and the second dose 3 to 6 months later. In very high-risk situations, such as refugee camps and following disasters, the first dose may be given at 6 months of age and the second dose as soon as possible after the child reaches 9 months of age.

Late 2-dose schedules[3] may be more appropriate in industrialised countries in which measles transmission among young infants is limited. The schedule is aimed at preventing infection in older children following primary or secondary vaccine failure. The first dose is typically given at 9 to 12 months of age, and the second dose at school entry.

Several studies have examined the effect of measles immunisation on mortality and morbidity in developing countries.[9] Data

suggest that the reduction in mortality following immunisation is greater than that expected simply from a reduction in death from acute measles. Measles immunisation may protect children dying not only from an acute measles attack but also from late causes which may be attributable to measles. It is also possible that measles vaccine has an immunostimulant effect.

For discussion of the link between vitamin A status and measles see Deficiency States, under Uses and Administration of Vitamin A Substances, p.1383.

1. Toole MJ, et al. Measles prevention and control in emergency settings. Bull WHO 1989; 67: 381–8.
2. Hall AJ, et al. Modern vaccines: practice in developing countries. Lancet 1990; 335: 774–7.
3. Rosenthal SR, Clements CJ. Two-dose measles vaccination schedules. Bull WHO 1993; 71: 421–8.
4. Garenne M, et al. Efficacy of measles vaccines after controlling for exposure. Am J Epidemiol 1993; 138: 182–95.
5. Diaz-Ortega J-L, et al. The relationship between dose and response of standard measles vaccines. Biologicals 1994; 22: 35–44.
6. de Quadros CA, et al. Measles elimination in the Americas: evolving strategies. JAMA 1996; 275: 224–9.
7. Cutts FT. Measles control in young infants: where do we go from here? Lancet 1993; 341: 290–1.
8. Global Programme for Vaccines of the World Health Organization. Role of mass campaigns in global measles control. Lancet 1994; 344: 174–5.
9. Aaby P, Clements CJ. Measles immunization research: a review. Bull WHO 1989; 67: 443–8.

Immunisation for travellers. The Immunization Practices Advisory Committee in the USA has recommended that administration of measles vaccine be considered for all persons travelling abroad who were born after 1956, regardless of their vaccination status.[1] Travellers who have had measles or were born before 1957 are considered immune secondary to natural infection.[2] Single-antigen measles vaccine or measles, mumps, and rubella vaccine may be used.[1] Children aged 6 to 11 months should receive a dose of single-antigen vaccine if travelling to areas where measles is endemic or epidemic.[1] A dose of measles, mumps, and rubella vaccine is given at 15 months, or 12 months if the child remains in a high-risk area.

1. Immunization Practices Advisory Committee. Measles prevention. JAMA 1987; 258: 890–5.
2. Hill DR, Pearson RD. Measles prophylaxis for international travel. Ann Intern Med 1989; 111: 699–701.

Preparations

Ph. Eur.: Measles Vaccine (Live);
USP 25: Measles Virus Vaccine Live.

Proprietary Preparations (details are given in Part 3)
Aust.: Attenuvax†; Rimevax†; **Austral.:** Rimevax; **Belg.:** Rimevax; **Braz.:** Attenuvax; Rouvax; **Denm.:** Attenuvax; **Fr.:** Rouvax; **Ger.:** Masern-Impfstoff Merieux; Masern-Lebend-Impfstoff†; Masern-Vaccinol†; Masern-Virus-Impfstoff†; **Hong Kong:** Moraten; Rouvax; **Israel:** Mevilin-L; Rimevax; Rouvax; **Ital.:** Attenuvax†; Lio-Morbillo; Moraten; Morbilvax; Rimevax†; Rouvax; **Mex.:** Rimevax; **Neth.:** Attenuvax†; **NZ:** Moraten; Rimevax; **Port.:** Moraten; **S.Afr.:** Diplovax; Moraten; Morbilvax; Rouvax; **Singapore:** Moraten; **Spain:** Amunovax†; Rimevax; **Switz.:** Attenuvax; Moraten; Rimevax; **Thai.:** Moraten; Morbilvax; Rimevax; Rouvax; **UK:** Mevilin-L†; **USA:** Attenuvax.

Measles and Mumps Vaccines (7971-g)
ATC — J07BD51.

Measles and Mumps Virus Vaccine Live (USP 25) is a bacterially sterile preparation of a suitable live strain of measles virus and a suitable live strain of mumps virus. It may contain suitable antimicrobial agents. Each labelled dose provides an immunising dose of each component. It should be stored at 2° to 8° and be protected from light.

Adverse Effects and Precautions
As for vaccines in general, p.1529.
See also under Measles Vaccines, p.1547, and Mumps Vaccines, p.1551.

Effects on the bones and joints. For a reference to arthritis occurring after administration of measles and mumps vaccine, see under Adverse Effects and Precautions of Measles, Mumps, and Rubella Vaccines, p.1549.

Interactions
As for vaccines in general, p.1530.
See also under Measles Vaccines, p.1547.

Uses and Administration
Measles and mumps vaccines may be used for active immunisation against measles and mumps. Vaccination against measles and mumps is normally performed using a combined measles, mumps, and rubella vaccine (p.1549) but the bivalent measles and mumps vaccine may be employed when vaccination against rubella is not indicated. For discussion of immunisation schedules, see under Vaccines, p.1530.

Two types of vaccine have been used. That usually available now is prepared from a more attenuated line of measles virus derived from Enders' attenuated Edmonston strain and the Jeryl Lynn (B level) strain of mumps virus. The second type of vaccine is prepared from the attenuated Schwarz strain of measles virus and the attenuated Urabe Am 9 strain of mumps virus. For both types, a 0.5-mL dose is given by intramuscular or subcutaneous injection.

Measles and mumps vaccines may also be used for prophylaxis after exposure to measles provided it is given within 72 hours of contact.

Preparations
USP 25: Measles and Mumps Virus Vaccine Live.

Proprietary Preparations (details are given in Part 3)
Aust.: M-M Vax†; *Belg.:* Duovax†; *Ger.:* M-M Vax; MM Diplovax; *S.Afr.:* Biviraten; *Switz.:* Biviraten†; M-M Vax.

Measles and Rubella Vaccines (7972-q)
ATC — J07BD53.

Measles and Rubella Virus Vaccine Live (USP 25) is a bacterially sterile preparation of suitable live strains of measles virus and live rubella virus. It may contain suitable antimicrobial agents. Each labelled dose provides an immunising dose of each component. It should be stored at 2° to 8° and be protected from light.

Adverse Effects and Precautions
As for vaccines in general, p.1529.

See also under Measles Vaccines, p.1547, and Rubella Vaccines, p.1562.

◊ Eight million children aged between 5 and 16 years were immunised with a measles and rubella vaccine in 1994 in the UK. By October 1995 the UK Committee on Safety of Medicines had received reports on 2735 suspected adverse reactions most of which were minor and self-limiting.[1] Serious suspected reactions were rare and generally the number of reported cases was consistent with the background frequency of the particular disorder.

1. Committee on Safety of Medicines/Medicines Control Agency. Adverse reactions to measles rubella vaccine. *Current Problems* 1995; **21:** 9–10.

Effects on hearing. Profound, irreversible sensorineural deafness was reported in a 27-year-old woman following administration of a measles and rubella vaccine.[1] Sensorineural deafness has also been reported following administration of measles, mumps, and rubella vaccine (p.1549), and monovalent measles vaccine (p.1547).

1. Hulbert TV, *et al.* Bilateral hearing loss after measles and rubella vaccination in an adult. *N Engl J Med* 1991; **325:** 134.

Effects on the nervous system. Optic neuritis was reported in two children who had received measles and rubella vaccine two to three weeks previously.[1]

1. Stevenson VL, *et al.* Optic neuritis following measles/rubella vaccination in two 13-year-old children. *Br J Ophthalmol* 1996; **80:** 1110–11.

Interactions
As for vaccines in general, p.1530.
See also under Measles Vaccines, p.1547.

Uses and Administration
Measles and rubella vaccines may be used for active immunisation against measles and rubella. For primary immunisation a combined measles, mumps, and rubella vaccine (p.1549) is usually used but the bivalent measles and rubella vaccine may be employed when vaccination against mumps is not indicated. For discussion of immunisation schedules, see under Vaccines, p.1530.

Vaccines have been prepared from either a more attenuated line of measles virus derived from Enders' attenuated Edmonston strain or attenuated Schwarz strain, and the Wistar RA 27/3 strain of rubella virus. The vaccine is generally given in a dose of 0.5 mL by subcutaneous or intramuscular injection to infants or to other susceptible children or adults considered to be at risk.

◊ Measles and rubella vaccine was successfully used in a mass immunisation campaign in children aged 5 to 16 years in the UK in order to avert an anticipated measles epidemic.[1,2]

1. Cutts FT. Revaccination against measles and rubella. *BMJ* 1996; **312:** 589–90.
2. Anonymous. Measles/rubella vaccine: a favourable balance of risk and benefit. *WHO Drug Inf* 1996; **10:** 43.

Preparations
USP 25: Measles and Rubella Virus Vaccine Live.

Proprietary Preparations (details are given in Part 3)
Canad.: MoRu-Viraten†; *Fr.:* Rudi-Rouvax†; *Ital.:* Morubel; *Switz.:* MoRu-Viraten†; *Thai.:* Rudi-Rouvax; *USA:* M-R-Vax II.

Measles, Mumps, and Rubella Vaccines (7973-p)
ATC — J07BD52.

Measles, Mumps and Rubella Vaccine (Live) (Ph. Eur.) (MMR/Vac (Live); Measles, Mumps and Rubella Vaccine, Live (BP 2001); Vaccinum Morbillorum, Parotitidis et Rubellae Vivum) is a freeze-dried preparation containing suitable live attenuated strains of measles virus, mumps virus (*Paramyxovirus parotitidis*), and rubella virus. The vaccine is prepared immediately before use by reconstitution from the dried vaccine. It contains in each dose not less than 1×10^3 CCID$_{50}$

The symbol † denotes a preparation no longer actively marketed

---

of infective measles virus, not less than 5×10^3 CCID$_{50}$ of infective mumps virus, and not less than 1×10^3 CCID$_{50}$ of infective rubella virus. The dried vaccine should be stored at 2° to 8° and be protected from light.

Measles, Mumps, and Rubella Virus Vaccine Live (USP 25) is a bacterially sterile preparation of suitable live strains of measles virus, mumps virus, and rubella virus. It may contain suitable antimicrobial agents. Each labelled dose provides an immunising dose of each component. It should be stored at 2° to 8° and be protected from light.

Adverse Effects and Precautions
As for vaccines in general, p.1529.

See also under Measles Vaccines, p.1547, Mumps Vaccines, p.1551, and Rubella Vaccines, p.1562.

Adverse effects tend to be less frequent after the second dose of vaccine than after the first dose.

Measles, mumps, and rubella vaccines should not be given to individuals hypersensitive to any antibacterial such as neomycin or kanamycin, that may be used in the manufacturing process.

Recommendations on vaccination in persons with egg allergy have been modified (see Hypersensitivity, below). A history of mild reactions to egg is not regarded as a contra-indication.

Children with a history of convulsions should receive measles, mumps, and rubella vaccination, but advice should be given on controlling fever.

◊ A double-blind placebo-controlled crossover study[1] in 581 pairs of twins showed that the true frequency of side-effects was between 0.5 and 4.0%, indicating that adverse reactions are much less common than was previously thought.

A study in the USA[2] showed that children receiving the vaccine at age 4 to 6 years had fewer adverse effects than those receiving it at 10 to 12 years.

A study[3] that assessed the effect of almost 3 million doses of vaccines in 1.8 million individuals revealed that 173 potentially serious reactions were claimed to have been caused by vaccination. There were 77 neurologic, 73 allergic, and 22 miscellaneous reactions recorded, and 1 death reported. However, 45% of the reactions were probably caused by some other factor. It was therefore concluded that serious events caused by measles, mumps, and rubella vaccine are rare and are greatly outweighed by the risks of the natural diseases.

1. Peltola H, Heinonen OP. Frequency of true adverse reactions to measles-mumps-rubella vaccine: a double-blind placebo-controlled trial in twins. *Lancet* 1986; **i:** 939–42.
2. Davis RL, *et al.* MMR2 immunization at 4 to 5 years and 10 to 12 years of age: a comparison of adverse clinical events after immunization in the vaccine safety datalink project. *Pediatrics* 1997; **100:** 767–71.
3. Patja A, *et al.* Serious adverse events after measles-mumps-rubella vaccination during a fourteen-year prospective follow-up. *Pediatr Infect Dis J* 2000; **19:** 1127–34.

Effects on the blood. Thrombocytopenia occurs rarely in children receiving measles, mumps, and rubella vaccine and usually resolves spontaneously. An increased incidence of thrombocytopenia following the second dose of the vaccine has been reported in children who developed thrombocytopenia after the first dose.[1]

1. Vlacha V, *et al.* Recurrent thrombocytopenic purpura after repeated measles-mumps-rubella vaccination. *Pediatrics* 1996; **97:** 738–9.

Effects on the bones and joints. Arthralgia and arthritis occurring in patients receiving mumps, measles, and rubella vaccines have generally been attributed to the rubella component.[1] However, arthritis has been reported in an infant following vaccination with measles and mumps vaccine.[2]

1. Benjamin CM, *et al.* Joint and limb symptoms in children after immunisation with measles, mumps, and rubella vaccine. *BMJ* 1992; **304:** 1075–8.
2. Nussinovitch M, *et al.* Arthritis after mumps and measles vaccination. *Arch Dis Child* 1995; **72:** 348–9.

Effects on hearing. Nine cases of sensorineural hearing loss following measles, mumps, and rubella (MMR) vaccine administration were reported to the UK Committee on Safety of Medicines between 1988 and 1993.[1] Of these, 3 cases were judged not to have been associated with MMR vaccine. In the remaining 6, the mumps virus component was considered to be the most likely cause of deafness if the vaccine was to blame, but the risk was considered to be small compared with the risks of natural infection. However, sensorineural deafness has also been reported following administration of measles and rubella vaccine (see p.1549), and monovalent measles vaccine (see p.1547).

1. Stewart BJA, Prabhu PU. Reports of sensorineural deafness after measles, mumps, and rubella immunisation. *Arch Dis Child* 1993; **69:** 153–4.

Effects on the nervous system. Although there have been case reports[1] linking Guillain-Barré syndrome with measles, mumps, and rubella vaccine (MMR) a retrospective study[2] that involved 189 patients with the syndrome and about 630 000 recipients of MMR could not find a causal association.

Prolonged tonic-clonic seizures were associated with prolonged hemiparesis in a 16-month-old girl six days after measles, mumps, and rubella vaccination.[3] There was evidence of transient encephalopathy. However, a causal relationship between measles-containing vaccines and encephalitis is generally considered to be unlikely. Other reported neurological effects following vaccination include gait disturbances[4] and transverse myelitis.[5]

For discussion of meningitis and encephalitis occurring after measles, mumps, and rubella vaccination, see under Adverse Effects of Mumps Vaccines, p.1551.

1. Morris K, Rylance G. Guillain-Barré syndrome after measles, mumps, and rubella vaccine. *Lancet* 1994; **343:** 60.
2. Patja A, *et al.* Risk of Guillain-Barré syndrome after measlesmumps-rubella vaccination. *J Pediatr* 2001; **138:** 250–4.
3. Sackey AH, Broadhead RL. Hemiplegia after measles, mumps, and rubella vaccination. *BMJ* 1993; **306:** 1169.
4. Plesner A-M. Gait disturbances after measles, mumps, and rubella vaccine. *Lancet* 1995; **345:** 316.
5. Joyce KA, Rees JE. Transverse myelitis after measles, mumps, and rubella vaccine. *BMJ* 1995; **311:** 422.

Hypersensitivity. Since the measles and mumps components of measles, mumps, and rubella vaccines are grown in cell cultures of chick embryos the vaccine has in the past been contraindicated in individuals with a history of anaphylactic reactions to egg. It is generally agreed that the vaccine can be given safely to children with less severe reactions to eggs. In both the UK and USA, even serious reactions to egg including anaphylaxis are no longer regarded as absolute contra-indications to vaccination,[1-4] and skin testing and desensitisation are considered to be of questionable value.[3,4] Nevertheless, a history of severe hypersensitivity to gelatin, kanamycin, or neomycin is regarded as a contra-indication to measles, mumps and rubella vaccines.[1,4]

1. Centers for Disease Control. Update: vaccine side effects, adverse reactions, contraindications, and precautions: recommendations of the Advisory Committee on Immunization Practices (ACIP). *MMWR* 1996; **45:** (RR-12): 1–45.
2. Salisbury DM, Begg NT (eds), Joint Committee on Vaccination and Immunisation. *Immunisation against infectious disease.* London: HMSO, 1996.
3. Khakoo GA, Lack G. Recommendations for using MMR vaccine in children allergic to eggs. *BMJ* 2000; **320:** 929–32.
4. Centers for Disease Control. Measles, mumps, and rubella—vaccine use and strategies for elimination of measles, rubella, and congenital rubella syndrome and control of mumps: recommendations of the Advisory Committee on Immunization Practices (ACIP). *MMWR* 1998; **47** (RR-8): 1–57.

Inflammatory bowel disease and autism. A controversial report[1] in 1998 by Wakefield and coworkers linking measles, mumps, and rubella (MMR) vaccination with the development of inflammatory bowel disease and behavioural abnormalities including autism was not supported by epidemiological evidence[2-4] and prompted the UK Committee on Safety of Medicines (CSM) to issue in 1999 a statement to this effect.[5] However, Wakefield, with another co-author,[6] in 2000 again raised issues concerning the safety of vaccination and alleged that the licensing procedures had not been properly carried out. The response by the UK Medicines Control Agency and Department of Health, reflecting additionally the view of the CSM and the Joint Committee on Vaccination and Immunisation,[7] was that the evidence did not support an association between MMR vaccine and inflammation of the bowel and autism. Moreover, it was re-iterated that this view was based not on a lack of evidence but, rather, that it was based on evidence that did not show an association. Other retrospective analyses[8-10] followed assessing the possible relationship of autism to MMR but again failed to document any association. Other suggestions of links between measles vaccines and inflammatory bowel disease have not been substantiated (see under Precautions for Measles Vaccines, p.1547).

1. Wakefield AJ, *et al.* Ileal-lymphoid-nodular hyperplasia, non-specific colitis, and pervasive developmental disorder in children. *Lancet* 1998; **351:** 637–41.
2. Peltola H, *et al.* No evidence for measles, mumps, and rubella vaccine-associated inflammatory bowel disease or autism in a 14-year prospective study. *Lancet* 1998; **351:** 1327–8.
3. Roberts R. There is no causal link between MMR vaccine and autism. *BMJ* 1998; **316:** 1824.
4. Taylor B, *et al.* Autism and measles, mumps, and rubella vaccine: no epidemiological evidence for a causal association. *Lancet* 1999; **353:** 2026–9.
5. Committee on Safety of Medicines. The safety of MMR Vaccine. *Current Problems* 1999; **25:** 9–10.
6. Wakefield AJ, Montgomery SM. Measles, mumps, rubella vaccine: through a glass, darkly. *Adverse Drug React Toxicol Rev* 2000; **19:** 265–83.
7. DoH. Measles, mumps and rubella vaccine (MMR). http://www.doh.gov.uk/mmrresponse.htm (accessed 14/02/01).
8. Kaye JA, *et al.* Mumps, measles, and rubella vaccine and the incidence of autism recorded by general practitioners: a time trend analysis. *BMJ* 2001; **322:** 460–3. Correction. *ibid.;* 720.
9. Dales L, *et al.* Time trends in autism and in MMR immunization coverage in California. *JAMA* 2001; **285:** 1183–5.
10. Halsey NA, *et al.* Measles-mumps-rubella vaccine and autistic spectrum disorder: report from the new challenges in childhood immunizations conference convened at Oak Brook, Illinois, June 12-13, 2000. Abstract: *Pediatrics* 2001; **107:** 1174. Full version: http://www.pediatrics.org/cgi/content/full/107/5/e84

Interactions
As for vaccines in general, p.1530.

See also under Measles Vaccines, p.1547.

Uses and Administration

Measles, mumps, and rubella vaccines are used for active immunisation against measles, mumps, and rubella. They are used for primary immunisation in children 12 months of age or older and to protect susceptible contacts during an outbreak of measles. For discussion of immunisation schedules, see under Vaccines, p.1530.

In the UK and USA the vaccine is prepared from an attenuated line of measles virus derived from Enders' attenuated Edmonston strain, the Jeryl Lynn (B level) strain of mumps virus, and the Wistar RA 27/3 strain of rubella virus. Another type, no longer used in several countries because of an increased risk of meningoencephalitis (see under Adverse Effects of Mumps Vaccines, p.1551), has been prepared from the Schwarz strain of measles virus, the Urabe Am 9 strain of mumps virus, and the Wistar RA 27/3 strain of rubella virus.

In the UK it is recommended that all children receive two doses of 0.5 mL of a measles, mumps, and rubella vaccine by deep subcutaneous or intramuscular injection. These are usually given shortly after the first birthday and before school entry, but may be given at any age if routine administration has been omitted, allowing 3 months between doses. The combined vaccine may also be used for prophylaxis after exposure to measles provided it is given within 72 hours of contact. However, it is not considered to be effective for postexposure prophylaxis against either mumps or rubella. If the vaccine is given before 12 months of age, re-immunisation will be necessary starting at between 12 and 15 months with a further dose according to national schedules.

In the USA, the second dose is recommended at age 4 to 6 years. Children who have not previously received the second dose should complete the vaccination schedule by age 11 to 12 years.

Preparations

Ph. Eur.: Measles, Mumps, and Rubella Vaccine (Live);
USP 25: Measles, Mumps, and Rubella Virus Vaccine Live.

Proprietary Preparations (details are given in Part 3)
Aust.: MMR Vax; ***Austral.:*** MMR II; Priorix; ***Belg.:*** MMR Vax; Priorix; ***Braz.:*** MMR II; Trimovax; ***Canad.:*** MMR II; Priorix; ***Denm.:*** MMR; Virivac†; ***Fin.:*** Priorix; ***Fr.:*** Priorix; R.O.R.; ***Ger.:*** MMR Triplovax; MMR Vax; Priorix; ***Hong Kong:*** MMR II; Trimovax; ***Irl.:*** MMR II; Priorix; ***Israel:*** MMR II; Priorix; ***Ital.:*** MMR II; Morupar; Priorix; Trimovax†; Triviraten; ***Mex.:*** MMR II; Priorix; ***NZ:*** Triviraten; ***Port.:*** Priorix; Triviraten; ***S.Afr.:*** MMR II†; Trimovax; Triviraten; ***Singapore:*** MMR II; Priorix; ***Spain:*** Priorix; Triviraten; Vac Triple MSD; ***Swed.:*** MMR II; Priorix; Virivac†; ***Switz.:*** MMR II; Priorix; Triviraten; ***Thai.:*** MMR II; Trimovax; Triviraten; ***UK:*** MMR II; Priorix; ***USA:*** MMR II.

Multi-ingredient: ***NZ:*** MMR II.

Meningococcal Vaccines (7979-j)

ATC — J07AH01; J07AH02; J07AH03; J07AH04; J07AH05; J07AH06.

Meningococcal Polysaccharide Vaccine (Ph. Eur.) (Neimen/Vac; Vaccinum Meningitidis Cerebrospinalis) consists of one or more purified capsular polysaccharides obtained from one or more suitable strains of *Neisseria meningitidis* group A, group C, group Y, and group W135; it may contain a single type of polysaccharide or any mixture of the types. It is prepared immediately before use by reconstitution from the stabilised freeze-dried vaccine with a suitable sterile liquid. The freeze-dried vaccine should be stored at 2° to 8° and be protected from light.

Meningococcal Polysaccharide Vaccine Group A (USP 25) is a sterile preparation of the group-specific polysaccharide antigen from *Neisseria meningitidis* group A.

Meningococcal Polysaccharide Vaccine Group C (USP 25) is a sterile preparation of the group-specific polysaccharide antigen from *Neisseria meningitidis* group C.

Meningococcal Polysaccharide Vaccine Groups A and C Combined (USP 25) is a sterile preparation of meningococcal polysaccharide group A and C specific antigens. All three USP 25 vaccines are supplied as dried vaccines containing lactose as a stabiliser which are reconstituted before use with bacteriostatic sodium chloride injection containing thiomersal. The dried vaccines should be stored at 2° to 8° and the reconstituted vaccines should be used immediately after preparation, or within 8 hours if stored at 2° to 8°.

Adverse Effects and Precautions

As for vaccines in general, p.1529.

Immunity to some meningococcal vaccines may be insufficient to confer adequate protection against infection in infants under about 2 years of age (for further discussion see under Uses, below).

Pregnancy and the neonate. A mixed meningococcal vaccine (A and C) was evaluated in pregnant women and infants during an epidemic of meningitis in Brazil.[1] Antibodies were detected in the women and there was some placental transfer of antibody although this was irregular. Vaccination of children in the first 6 months of life was unsuccessful.

These results were supported by a subsequent study in the Gambia.[2] Maternal antibodies were high in all women at the time of delivery, but only a proportion of the antibody crossed the placenta. There was considerable individual variation in the cord blood:maternal blood antibody ratios. Antibody concentrations declined rapidly in the infants and had effectively disappeared by 3 to 4 months of age.

1. Carvalho A de A, *et al.* Maternal and infant antibody response to meningococcal vaccination in pregnancy. *Lancet* 1977; **ii:** 809–11.
2. O'Dempsey TJD, *et al.* Meningococcal antibody titres in infants of women immunised with meningococcal polysaccharide vaccine during pregnancy. *Arch Dis Child* 1996; **74:** F43–6.

Interactions

As for vaccines in general, p.1530.

Uses and Administration

Meningococcal vaccines are used for active immunisation against *Neisseria meningitidis* infections which include meningitis and septicaemia. They are preparations of purified polysaccharide antigens from *N. meningitidis* and may be monovalent, containing the antigen of only one serotype of *N. meningitidis* or polyvalent, containing antigens of two or more serotypes. Vaccines available in the UK are a bivalent vaccine from groups A and C, a tetravalent vaccine from groups A, C, Y, and W135, and a meningococcal group C conjugate vaccine (diphtheria CRM$_{197}$ protein conjugate). In the USA, a tetravalent vaccine from groups A, C, Y, and W135 is used. Both the bivalent and the tetravalent vaccines are given in a dose of 0.5 mL; the bivalent vaccine is given by deep subcutaneous or intramuscular injection and the tetravalent vaccine by deep subcutaneous injection. The meningococcal C conjugate vaccine in the UK is given by intramuscular injection. Infants aged 2 to 4 months are given 3 doses of 0.5 mL at monthly intervals for primary immunisation. Children aged 5 to 12 months who have not received their primary immunisation should be given 2 doses of 0.5 mL one month apart. A single dose of 0.5 mL is given to adults and children over 1 year of age. For discussion of immunisation schedules see under Vaccines, p.1530.

Meningococcal vaccines are indicated in persons at risk, in epidemic or endemic areas, of meningococcal disease caused by the specific serotypes contained in the vaccines. They are given as an adjunct to chemoprophylaxis in close contacts of persons with the disease. Persons travelling to countries where the risk of infection is high should receive meningococcal polysaccharide A and C vaccine rather than the group C conjugate vaccine, and should be immunised even if they have already received the latter. The polysaccharide A and C vaccine is indicated particularly for visits of 1 month or more and for those backpacking or living or working with local residents. Asplenic persons or those who have terminal complement component deficiencies are at higher than normal risk of acquiring meningococcal infection. The polyvalent vaccine may also be considered in college students living in dormitories or halls of residence.

The minimum recommended age for administration of meningococcal vaccines has varied from 2 months to 2 years because of reports of poor immune response to the unconjugated polysaccharide vaccines in younger infants although the immunogenicity of the conjugate group C vaccine in these patients appears to be greater (see below).

◊ Reviews.
1. Peltola H. Meningococcal vaccines: current status and future possibilities. *Drugs* 1998; **55:** 347–66.

Immunisation. *Neisseria meningitidis* is an important cause of meningitis. About 60% of meningococcal infections (p.129) in the UK and the USA are caused by *Neisseria meningitidis* of

---

group B serotype. However, there is no available vaccine against these organisms because the purified group B polysaccharide is only poorly immunogenic, even after conjugation with proteins.[1] A number of avenues of research are being followed in the development of an effective vaccine against the group B serotype.[2-4] A number of candidate vaccines based on class 1 outer membrane proteins have been field-tested but efficacy has been variable. Favourable results with a fairly crude vaccine in Cuba were not confirmed by a study in Brazil using the same vaccine,[5] and the response in young children was especially disappointing. Similarly, a vaccine produced in Norway gave a protection rate of about 60%, judged to be too low for use in a general immunisation programme.[6] A direct comparison of the two vaccines[7] found that the Norwegian vaccine produced greater immunity in adolescents than the Cuban vaccine. A subsequent study,[8] however, has reiterated that neither vaccine would confer adequate protection during an epidemic with non-vaccine type strains of meningococcus. Other strategies have included vaccines based on other outer membrane proteins and lipopolysaccharide derivatives.[2-4]

Outbreaks of meningococcal infections are more commonly caused by group A or C meningococci. Epidemics of group A infection occur particularly in the meningitis belt of Africa in the dry season.

Polysaccharide vaccines of meningococci of groups A, C, W135, and Y have been successful in producing short-term immunity (up to about 5 years) and controlling epidemics and outbreaks, although vaccination does not influence nasopharyngeal carriage of the organism.[1,9] Antibody response to group A polysaccharide vaccine is reduced in infants under 2 years of age, but it is still sufficient to confer protection from infection in infants over 3 months.[10] Response can be improved in infants and young children by giving a second dose after 3 months. Infants and children do, however, show a poor immune response in areas where malaria is holoendemic.[11] Immunity to unconjugated group C meningococcal vaccine is low in infants below the age of 2 years and has been stated to be unlikely to persist for more than 1 to 2 years. However, a partial response has been demonstrated in children as young at 6 months of age following a mass vaccination campaign during an epidemic.[12] Therefore, the minimum age for administration recommended by manufacturers of polyvalent polysaccharide meningococcal vaccines varies from 2 months to 2 years. Attempts to enhance passive protection of infants by immunising their mothers during pregnancy has not been successful (see under Adverse Effects, above).

Conjugate vaccines against group A and C meningococci have been developed in an attempt to improve the immunogenicity[3,4] and are now in use. The results of clinical studies are encouraging[13] with greater immunogenicity in children under 2 years of age being produced than with polysaccharide vaccines and immunologic memory appears to be induced.[14,15]

1. Anonymous. Preventing meningococcal infection. *Drug Ther Bull* 1990; **28:** 34–6.
2. Zollinger WD, Moran E. Meningococcal vaccines—present and future. *Trans R Soc Trop Med Hyg* 1991; **85** (suppl 1): 37–43.
3. Herbert MA, *et al.* Meningococcal vaccines for the United Kingdom. *Commun Dis Rep* 1995; **5** (review 9): R130–5.
4. Ala'Aldeen DAA, Cartwright KAV. Neisseria meningitidis: vaccines and vaccine candidates. *J Infect* 1996; **33:** 153–7.
5. de Morales JC, *et al.* Protective efficacy of a serogroup B meningococcal vaccine in Sao Paulo, Brazil. *Lancet* 1992; **340:** 1074–8.
6. Bjune G, *et al.* Effect of outer membrane vesicle vaccine against group B meningococcal disease in Norway. *Lancet* 1991; **338:** 1093–6.
7. Perkins BA, *et al.* Immunogenicity of two efficacious outer membrane protein-based serogroup B meningococcal vaccines among young adults in Iceland. *J Infect Dis* 1998; **177:** 683–91.
8. Tappero JW, *et al.* Immunogenicity of 2 serogroup B outer-membrane protein meningococcal vaccines: a randomized controlled trial in Chile. *JAMA* 1999; **281:** 1520–7.
9. Anonymous. Meningococcal meningitis. *Lancet* 1989; **i:** 647–8. Correction. *ibid.*; 742.
10. Peltola H, *et al.* Clinical efficacy of meningococcus group A capsular polysaccharide vaccine in children three months to five years of age. *N Engl J Med* 1977; **297:** 686–91.
11. Moxon ER, Rappuoli R. Modern vaccines: Haemophilus influenzae infections and whooping cough. *Lancet* 1990; **335:** 1324–9.
12. King WJ, *et al.* Total and functional antibody response to a quadrivalent meningococcal polysaccharide vaccine among children. *J Pediatr* 1996; **128:** 196–202.
13. Lieberman JM, *et al.* Safety and immunogenicity of a serogroups A/C Neisseria meningitidis oligosaccharide-protein conjugate vaccine in young children: a randomized controlled trial. *JAMA* 1996; **275:** 1499–1503.
14. MacDonald NE, *et al.* Induction of immunologic memory by conjugated vs plain meningococcal C polysaccharide vaccine in toddlers: a randomized controlled trial. *JAMA* 1998; **280:** 1685–9.
15. Richmond P, *et al.* Meningococcal serogroup C conjugate vaccine is immunogenic in infancy and primes for memory. *J Infect Dis* 1999; **179:** 1569–72.

Preparations

Ph. Eur.: Meningococcal Polysaccharide Vaccine;
USP 25: Meningococcal Polysaccharide Vaccine Group A; Meningococcal Polysaccharide Vaccine Group C; Meningococcal Polysaccharide Vaccine Groups A and C Combined.

Proprietary Preparations (details are given in Part 3)
Aust.: Mencevax ACWY; ***Austral.:*** Mencevax ACWY; Menomune; ***Belg.:*** Mencevax ACWY; Meningovax A+C; ***Braz.:*** Meningo A+C; ***Denm.:*** Meningovax A+C; ***Fin.:*** Meningovax A+C; ***Ger.:*** Mencevax ACWY; Meningokokken-Impfstoff A + C; ***Hong Kong:*** Meningococcal A+C; ***Irl.:*** Mengivac (A+C); Meningitec;

Menjugate; *Israel:* Mencevax AC; *Ital.:* Mencevax ACWY; Menomune; Menpovax 4; Menpovax A+C; *Neth.:* Meningovax A+C; *Norw.:* Mencevax AC; Meningovax A+C; *NZ:* Mencevax ACWY; Menomune; *S.Afr.:* Imovax Meningo A & C; *Singapore:* Mencevax AC; Menomune; *Spain:* Mencevax AC; Vac Antimeningococic A+C; *Swed.:* Meningovax A+C; *Thai.:* Meningococcal A+C; Menpovax 4; Menpovax A+C; *UK:* AC Vax; ACWY Vax; Mengivac (A+C); Meningitec; Menjugate; Neisvac-C; *USA:* Menomune.

Multiple Sclerosis Vaccines (18390-s)

Profile
Vaccines based on T cells have been investigated for the management of multiple sclerosis.

◊ References.
1. Medaer R, *et al.* Depletion of myelin-basic-protein autoreactive T cells by T-cell vaccination: pilot trial in multiple sclerosis. *Lancet* 1995; **346:** 807–8.
2. Vandenbark AA, *et al.* Treatment of multiple sclerosis with T-cell receptor peptides: results of a double-blind pilot trial. *Nat Med* 1996; **2:** 1109–15. Correction. *ibid.* 1997; **3:** 240.
3. Goodkin DE, *et al.* A phase I trial of solubilized DR2:MBP84-102 (AG284) in multiple sclerosis. *Neurology* 2000; **54:** 1414–20.

Mumps Immunoglobulins (14232-s)
ATC — J06BB15.

Profile
Preparations containing antibodies against mumps virus are available in some countries for passive immunisation against mumps.

Preparations
Proprietary Preparations (details are given in Part 3)
Ital.: Haima-Parot; Immunoparot; Par-Gamma; Paruman†; *Switz.:* Paruman†.

Mumps Vaccines (7982-s)
ATC — J07BE01.

Mumps Vaccine (Live) (Ph. Eur.) (Mump/Vac (Live); Mumps Vaccine, Live (BP 2001); Vaccinum Parotitidis Vivum) is a freeze-dried preparation containing a suitable live attenuated strain of mumps virus (*Paramyxovirus parotitidis*) grown in cultures of human diploid cells or chick-embryo cells or the amniotic cavity of chick embryos. It is prepared immediately before use by reconstitution from the dried vaccine. The cell-culture medium may contain the lowest effective concentration of a suitable antibacterial. The virus titre is not less than 5×10^3 CCID$_{50}$ per dose. The dried vaccine should be stored at 2° to 8° and be protected from light.

Mumps Virus Vaccine Live (USP 25) is a bacterially sterile preparation of a suitable strain of mumps virus grown in cultures of chick-embryo cells. It contains not less than the equivalent of 5×10^3 TCID$_{50}$ in each immunising dose. It may contain suitable antimicrobial agents. It should be stored at 2° to 8° and be protected from light.

Adverse Effects and Precautions
As for vaccines in general, p.1529.

Parotid swelling may occur. Unilateral nerve deafness, meningitis, and encephalitis have occurred rarely (see below for further discussion).

Mumps vaccines are not generally recommended for children below the age of 1 year in whom maternal antibodies might prevent a response.

Effects on hearing. For a report of sensorineural hearing loss following measles, mumps, and rubella vaccination, see p.1549.

Effects on the nervous system. There have been a few reports of neurological reactions including meningitis and encephalitis after vaccination with measles, mumps, and rubella vaccines. These reactions have been attributed to the mumps component. However, it has not been possible to isolate the virus from the CSF in every case and identify it as either the vaccine strain or a wild-type strain. Meningitis develops up to 35 days after immunisation, is mild, and sequelae are rare.[1,2] One study[3] found the incidence of virus-positive post-immunisation meningitis from the Urabe strain of mumps vaccine to be approximately 1 in 11 000 immunised children with the incidence following Jeryl Lynn mumps vaccine being much lower. This result was supported by the incidence of 1 in about 4000 in another study,[4] making it less likely that this was a chance result, and much higher than the estimates of up to 1 in 1 million reported previously.[5] Subsequent research[6] identified the Urabe vaccine strain in CSF samples from all of 20 children with post-vaccination meningitis in the UK, and no isolates of the Jeryl Lynn strain in patients with meningitis among 80 samples tested. Thus, vaccines containing the Urabe strain, including combined measles, mumps, and rubella vaccines are no longer used in the UK and some other countries.[7] A relatively high incidence of about 1 in 1000 has also been observed after use of a measles and mumps vaccine prepared from the Leningrad-3 strain of mumps virus.[8,9]

Encephalitis has been associated with mumps vaccination less frequently than meningitis, but may be more serious.[1] The Immunization Practices Advisory Committee in the USA has reported that the incidence of encephalitis within 30 days of receiving a mumps-containing vaccine is 0.4 per one million doses.[10] This is no higher than the observed background incidence for CNS dysfunction in the general population.

In considering the above data it should be remembered that mumps is the most common cause of meningoencephalitis in children under 15 years of age in the UK and an important cause of permanent sensorineural deafness in childhood.[1] Meningitis after natural mumps infection is estimated to occur in 1 in 400 cases, an incidence that is very considerably above any reported with vaccination.

1. Anonymous. Mumps meningitis and MMR vaccination. *Lancet* 1989; **ii:** 1015–16.
2. Maguire HC, *et al.* Meningoencephalitis associated with MMR vaccine. *Commun Dis Rep* 1991; **1** (review 6): R60–R61.
3. Miller E, *et al.* Risk of aseptic meningitis after measles, mumps, and rubella vaccine in UK children. *Lancet* 1993; **341:** 979–82.
4. Colville A, Pugh S. Mumps meningitis and measles, mumps, and rubella vaccine. *Lancet* 1992; **340:** 786. Correction. *ibid.*: 986.
5. McDonald JC, *et al.* Clinical and epidemiologic features of mumps meningoencephalitis and possible vaccine-related disease. *Pediatr Infect Dis J* 1989; **8:** 751–5.
6. Forsey T, *et al.* Mumps vaccine and meningitis. *Lancet* 1992; **340:** 980.
7. Anonymous. Two MMR vaccines withdrawn. *Lancet* 1992; **340:** 722.
8. Čižman M, *et al.* Aseptic meningitis after vaccination against measles and mumps. *Pediatr Infect Dis J* 1989; **8:** 302–8.
9. Tešović G, *et al.* Aseptic meningitis after measles, mumps, and rubella vaccine. *Lancet* 1993; **341:** 1541.
10. Immunization Practices Advisory Committee. Mumps prevention. *MMWR* 1989; **38:** 388–400.

Interactions
As for vaccines in general, p.1530.

Uses and Administration
Mumps vaccines are used for active immunisation against mumps.

For primary immunisation a combined measles, mumps, and rubella vaccine (p.1549) is usually used. For discussion of immunisation schedules see under Vaccines, p.1530.

In the UK a vaccine prepared from the Jeryl Lynn (B level) strain of mumps virus was formerly available. The vaccine is, however, available in the USA, and may be given in a dose of 0.5 mL by subcutaneous injection.

Preparations
Ph. Eur.: Mumps Vaccine (Live);
USP 25: Mumps Vaccine Live.
Proprietary Preparations (details are given in Part 3)
Aust.: Mumpsvax†; *Braz.:* Imovax; Mumpsvax; *Canad.:* Mumpsvax; *Denm.:* Mumpsvax; *Fr.:* Imovax†; *Ger.:* Mumpsvax; *Hong Kong:* Imovax Mumps; Mumaten†; *Irl.:* Mumpsvax; *Ital.:* Mumaten†; Mumpsvax†; Vaxipar; *S.Afr.:* Mumaten; *Spain:* Vac Antiparotiditis†; *Switz.:* Mumaten†; Mumpsvax; *Thai.:* Mumaten†; *UK:* Mumpsvax; *USA:* Mumpsvax.

Mycobacterium Vaccae Vaccines (446-r)

Profile
Vaccines containing *Mycobacterium vaccae* are under investigation for the prevention and immunotherapy of tuberculosis and other mycobacterial infections. They are also being studied for therapeutic use in psoriasis and some neoplastic diseases.

Malignant neoplasms. References.
1. O'Brien ME, *et al.* A randomized phase II study of SRL172 (Mycobacterium vaccae) combined with chemotherapy in patients with advanced inoperable non-small-cell lung cancer and mesothelioma. *Br J Cancer* 2000; **83:** 853–7.

Psoriasis. References.
1. Balagon MV, *et al.* Improvement in psoriasis after intradermal administration of heat-killed Mycobacterium vaccae. *Int J Dermatol* 2000; **39:** 51–8.

Tuberculosis. IMMUNISATION. References.
1. von Reyn CF, *et al.* Cellular immune responses to mycobacteria in healthy and human immunodeficiency virus-positive subjects in the United States after a five-dose schedule of Mycobacterium vaccae vaccine. *Clin Infect Dis* 1998; **27:** 1517–20.
2. Waddell RD, *et al.* Safety and immunogenicity of a five-dose series of inactivated Mycobacterium vaccae vaccination for the prevention of HIV-associated tuberculosis. *Clin Infect Dis* 2000; **30** (suppl 3): S309–S315.

IMMUNOTHERAPY. A systematic review[1] found that immunotherapy with *Mycobacterium vaccae* produced no beneficial effects in patients with tuberculosis.
1. de Bruyn G, Garner P. Mycobacterium vaccae immunotherapy for treating tuberculosis (updated 29 November 2000). Available in The Cochrane Library; Issue 4. Oxford: Update Software; 2001.

Normal Immunoglobulins (1232-z)
ATC — J06BA01; J06BA02.

Human Normal Immunoglobulin (Ph. Eur.) (Normal Immunoglobulin Injection; Normal Immunoglobulin (BP 2001); Immunoglobulinum Humanum Normale) is a liquid or freeze-dried preparation containing immunoglobulins, mainly immunoglobulin G (IgG) antibodies, of normal subjects. Other proteins may be present; it contains not less than 10% and not more than 18% of total protein. It is intended for intramuscular injection. It is obtained from the pooled plasma collected from at least 1000 donors who must be healthy, must not have been treated with substances of human pituitary origin, and as far as can be ascertained be free from detectable agents of infection transmissible by transfusion of blood or blood components. No antibacterial is added to the plasma used. It is prepared as a stabilised solution and passed through a bacteria-retentive filter. Multidose, but not single dose, preparations contain an antimicrobial preservative. The pH of a solution in sodium chloride 0.9% containing 1% of protein is 6.4 to 7.2. The liquid preparation should be stored, protected from light, in a sealed, colourless, glass container. The freeze-dried preparation should be stored, protected from light, under vacuum or under an inert gas.

Human Normal Immunoglobulin for Intravenous Administration (Ph. Eur.) (Normal Immunoglobulin for Intravenous Use (BP 2001); Immunoglobulinum Humanum Normale ad Usum Intravenosum) is a liquid or freeze-dried preparation containing immunoglobulins, mainly immunoglobulin G (IgG); other proteins may be present and the total protein content is not less than 3%. It contains IgG antibodies of normal subjects; the standard does not apply to products intentionally prepared to contain fragments or chemically modified IgG. It is prepared as a stabilised solution and passed through a bacteria-retentive filter. It does not contain an antimicrobial preservative. The pH of a solution in sodium chloride 0.9% containing 1% of protein is 4.0 to 7.4. Storage requirements are similar to those for Human Normal Immunoglobulin, except that the freeze-dried preparation is stored at a temperature not exceeding 25°.

Immune Globulin (USP 25) is a sterile solution of globulins that contains many antibodies normally present in human adult blood. It is prepared from pooled material (approximately equal quantities of blood, plasma, serum, or placentas) from not fewer than 1000 donors. It contains 15 to 18% of protein, of which not less than 90% is gamma globulin. It is intended for intramuscular injection. It contains glycine as a stabiliser, and a suitable preservative. It contains antibodies against diphtheria, measles, and poliomyelitis. It should be stored at 2° to 8°.

Adverse Effects and Precautions
As for immunoglobulins in general, p.1529. Intravenous immunoglobulin preparations should be administered with caution to patients with renal insufficiency. Immunoglobulin products containing sucrose may be associated with an increased risk of inducing acute renal failure (see Effects on the Kidneys, below).

Antibody titres for some common pathogens can vary widely not only between products from different manufacturers, but also from lot to lot. Formulations of intravenous immunoglobulins should therefore not be regarded as equivalent.

◊ Reviews.
1. Nydegger UE, Sturzenegger M. Adverse effects of intravenous immunoglobulin therapy. *Drug Safety* 1999; **21:** 171–85.

Effects on the blood. Adverse effects on the blood have occasionally been reported following intravenous administration of normal immunoglobulin to increase the platelet count in patients with idiopathic thrombocytopenic purpura. Reduced platelet adhesiveness with multiple subcutaneous haematomas occurred in one patient.[1] Thrombotic events have occurred following intravenous immunoglobulin administration,[2,3] particularly in elderly subjects (sometimes fatal) suggesting that a rising platelet count during normal immunoglobulin treatment may represent a risk in patients with severe atherosclerotic disease.[2] A review in Scotland of 34 patients over 60 years of age treated with normal immunoglobulin could not, however, confirm the association.[4]

Passive transfer of anti-A, anti-B, or anti-D antibodies or active immunisation by blood group substances from normal immunoglobulin preparations has been implicated in the production of haemolytic reactions including a case of haemolytic disease of the newborn.[5,6] It has been suggested[6] that blood phenotyping be carried out before treatment with normal immunoglobulin is commenced.

Transient neutropenia has been observed after administration of normal immunoglobulin to patients with thrombocytopenic purpura, but the clinical significance of this effect has been disputed.[7-9]
1. Ljung R, Nilsson IM. High-dose intravenous gammaglobulin: a cautionary note. *Lancet* 1985; **i:** 467.

2. Woodruff RK, et al. Fatal thrombotic events during treatment of autoimmune thrombocytopenia with intravenous immunoglobulin in elderly patients. Lancet 1986; ii: 217–18.
3. Go RS, Call TG. Deep venous thrombosis of the arm after intravenous immunoglobulin infusion: case report and literature review of intravenous immunoglobulin-related thrombotic complications. Mayo Clin Proc 2000; 75: 83–5.
4. Frame WD, Crawford RJ. Thrombotic events after intravenous immunoglobulin. Lancet 1986; ii: 468.
5. Potter M, et al. ABO alloimmunisation after intravenous immunoglobulin infusion. Lancet 1988; i: 932–3.
6. Nicholls MD, et al. Haemolysis induced by intravenously-administered immunoglobulin. Med J Aust 1989; 150: 404–6.
7. Majer RV, Green PJ. Thrombocytopenia caused by intravenous immunoglobulin. BMJ 1988; 296: 1262.
8. Veys PA, et al. Neutropenia following intravenous immunoglobulin. BMJ 1988; 296: 1800.
9. Ben-Chetrit E, Putterman C. Transient neutropenia induced by intravenous immune globulin. N Engl J Med 1992; 326: 270–1.

Effects on the kidneys. Acute renal failure was reported after intravenous administration of normal immunoglobulin to a patient who had demonstrable serum rheumatoid factor associated with lymphoma.[1] A symptomless, transient rise in plasma-creatinine concentrations was also noted in 6 patients with nephrotic syndrome after administration of intravenous normal immunoglobulin.[2] A similar rise in plasma creatinine was observed in two other patients with pre-existing renal impairment but no nephrotic syndrome. An elderly patient with lymphoproliferative disorder and idiopathic thrombocytopenic purpura received normal immunoglobulin and developed acute renal failure within 48 hours, with subsequently fatal heart failure and pulmonary oedema.[3] The incidence of renal failure appears to be greatest with immunoglobulin products containing sucrose. As a consequence of such reports, the FDA in the USA has issued a warning alerting physicians to the potential risks of acute renal failure associated with intravenous administration of normal immunoglobulin products, particularly those containing sucrose.

1. Barton JC, et al. Acute cryoglobulinemic renal failure after intravenous infusion of gamma globulin. Am J Med 1987; 82: 624–9.
2. Schifferli J, et al. High-dose intravenous IgG treatment and renal function. Lancet 1991; 337: 457–8.
3. Winward DB, Brophy MT. Acute renal failure after administration of intravenous immunoglobulin: review of the literature and case report. Pharmacotherapy 1995; 15: 765–72.

Effects on the nervous system. Aseptic meningitis has been reported after intravenous administration of normal immunoglobulin.[1-5]

Migraine was associated with intravenous immunoglobulin therapy in a patient on two occasions.[6] Migraine did not recur after prophylaxis with propranolol was instituted.

Hemiplegia has been reported in a 4-year-old child receiving intravenous immunoglobulin for immune thrombocytopenic purpura.[7]

1. Kato E, et al. Administration of immune globulin associated with aseptic meningitis. JAMA 1988; 259: 3269–71.
2. Casteels-Van Daele M, et al. Intravenous immune globulin and acute aseptic meningitis. N Engl J Med 1990; 323: 614–15.
3. Sekul EA, et al. Aseptic meningitis associated with high-dose intravenous immunoglobulin therapy: frequency and risk factors. Ann Intern Med 1994; 121: 259–62.
4. Picton P, Chisholm M. Aseptic meningitis associated with high dose immunoglobulin: case report. BMJ 1997; 315: 1203–4.
5. Boyce TG, Spearman P. Acute aseptic meningitis secondary to intravenous immunoglobulin in a patient with Kawasaki syndrome. Pediatr Infect Dis J 1998; 17: 1054–6.
6. Constantinescu CS, et al. Recurrent migraine and intravenous immune globulin therapy. N Engl J Med 1993; 329: 583–4.
7. Tsiouris J, Tsiouris N. Hemiplegia as a complication of treatment of childhood immune thrombocytopenic purpura with intravenously administered immunoglobulin. J Pediatr 1998; 133: 717.

Effects on the skin. Diffuse alopecia has been reported[1] in 3 women within 1 to 4 weeks of treatment with intravenous normal immunoglobulin. There have been reports[2,3] of severe and extensive eczema in elderly patients up to 3 weeks after receiving normal immunoglobulin intravenously. There has also been a report of cutaneous vasculitic rash on the face of a woman receiving intravenous normal immunoglobulin.[4]

For mention of a patient with AIDS who developed erythema characteristic of fifth disease following intravenous normal immunoglobulin, see Infection, below.

1. Chan-Lam D, et al. Alopecia after immunoglobulin infusion. Lancet 1987; i: 1436.
2. Barucha C, McMillan JC. Eczema after intravenous infusion of immunoglobulin. BMJ 1987; 295: 1141.
3. Whittam LR, et al. Eczematous reactions to human immune globulin. Br J Dermatol 1997; 137: 481–2.
4. Howse M, et al. Facial vasculitic rash associated with intravenous immunoglobulin. BMJ 1998; 317: 1291.

Hypersensitivity. Hypersensitivity reactions may occasionally occur after intramuscular or intravenous administration of normal immunoglobulins particularly in hypogammaglobulinaemic or agammaglobulinaemic patients. Both immediate and late[1] reactions have occurred.

The IgA content of normal immunoglobulins can result in the development of IgE and IgG anti-IgA antibodies in immunodeficient patients with IgA deficiency. It has been suggested by some[2] that the IgE anti-IgA antibodies are responsible for anaphylaxis although others have disagreed.[3] Two patients who had reactions to conventional normal immunoglobulin preparations tolerated preparations with a low content of IgA.[2] Some manufacturers of normal immunoglobulin preparations recom-

mend that they should not be used in patients with selective IgA deficiencies who have known antibody against IgA.

The IgE content of some preparations has also been suggested as a cause of hypersensitivity reactions[4] although this has been disputed.[5] Complement-activating IgG aggregates may also be involved although the anticomplementary activity of the products does not appear to be related to the incidence of side-effects.[5]

1. Hachimi-Idrissi S, et al. Type III allergic reaction after infusion of immunoglobulins. Lancet 1990; 336: 55.
2. Burks AW, et al. Anaphylactic reactions after gamma globulin administration in patients with hypogammaglobulinemia. N Engl J Med 1986; 314: 560–4.
3. Hammarström L, Smith CIE. Anaphylaxis after administration of gamma globulin for hypogammaglobulinemia. N Engl J Med 1986; 315: 519.
4. Tovo P-A, et al. IgE content of commercial intravenous IgG preparations. Lancet 1984; i: 458.
5. Newland AC, et al. IgE in intravenous IgG. Lancet 1984; i: 1406–7.

Infection. An association between administration of certain intravenous immunoglobulin preparations and hepatitis C infections has led to changes in manufacturing procedures and withdrawal of the affected products from the market.[1-3]

In addition, there has been a report[4] of a patient with AIDS who developed fifth disease (erythema infectiosum) following intravenous normal immunoglobulin treatment for infection with parvovirus.

1. Quinti I, et al. Intravenous gammaglobulin may still infect patients. BMJ 1994; 308: 856.
2. Bader J-M. HCV and Gammagard in France. Lancet 1994; 343: 1628. Corrections. ibid.; 344: 201 and 206.
3. Anonymous. Outbreak of hepatitis C associated with intravenous immunoglobulin administration—United States, October 1993–June 1994. JAMA 1994; 272: 424–5.
4. French AL, et al. Fifth disease after immunoglobulin administration in an AIDS patient with parvovirus-induced red cell aplasia. Am J Med 1996; 101: 108–9.

Interactions

Administration of normal immunoglobulin may interfere with the immune response to live viral vaccines. Such vaccines should therefore be given at least 3 weeks before, or 3 months after, normal immunoglobulins. This does not apply to yellow fever vaccine for immunoglobulins prepared in the UK, nor for booster doses of oral poliomyelitis vaccines. Where such an interval is impractical for immunisation preceding foreign travel it may have to be ignored.

◊ For a study indicating that normal immunoglobulin has no effect on the antibody response to oral poliomyelitis vaccine, see p.1559.

Uses and Administration

Normal immunoglobulin is available as two distinct preparations and formulations. One type of injection generally containing 16% of protein is used for passive immunisation, and sometimes also for primary antibody deficiencies, and should only be given intramuscularly; Human Normal Immunoglobulin (Ph. Eur.) and Immune Globulin (USP 25) are intended for intramuscular use only. The second type of preparation is formulated for intravenous administration (Human Normal Immunoglobulin for Intravenous Administration (Ph. Eur.)) and is used in disorders such as primary antibody deficiencies and idiopathic thrombocytopenic purpura; solutions generally contain about 3 to 6% of protein, although some may contain up to 12%. Doses of normal immunoglobulin often appear confusing, being expressed variously in terms of weight (protein or immunoglobulin G content) or in terms of volume to be administered; the two do not always appear to correspond. It should be remembered that there may be differences between intravenous preparations of normal immunoglobulin including differing IgA content and IgG subclass distribution.

Normal immunoglobulin, being derived from the pooled plasma of blood donors, contains antibodies to bacteria and viruses currently prevalent in the general population; in the UK, and also in some other countries, typical antibodies present include those against hepatitis A, measles, mumps, rubella, and varicella. Normal immunoglobulin, therefore, may be used to provide passive immunisation against such diseases.

For the pre-exposure prophylaxis against **hepatitis A** in travellers going to endemic areas doses recommended in the UK for intramuscular injection are: for short-term exposure of up to 2 months, 125 mg for

children under 10 years of age and 250 mg for older children and adults; for longer-term exposure, 250 mg for children under 10 years of age and 500 mg for older children and adults. Alternative doses, expressed in terms of volume administered, have been 0.02 to 0.04 mL per kg body-weight for short-term exposure in both adults and children and 0.06 to 0.12 mL per kg for longer-term exposure. Hepatitis A vaccine (p.1541) may be preferred in adults visiting endemic countries frequently or staying for over 3 months or hepatitis A immunoglobulin (p.1541) for shorter or less frequent journeys. Normal immunoglobulin may also be used to control outbreaks of hepatitis A, the recommended dose for close contacts being 250 mg in those under 10 years of age and 500 mg in older children and adults.

Normal immunoglobulin may be used to prevent or possibly modify an attack of **measles** in children and adults at special risk (such as those who are immunocompromised) but should be given as soon as possible after contact with measles. In the UK recommended doses, administered intramuscularly, for the prevention of an attack are 250 mg for those under 1 year of age, 500 mg for those aged 1 to 2 years, and 750 mg for those aged 3 years and over; to modify an attack, recommended doses are 100 mg for those under 1 year of age and 250 mg for older children. Alternatively, doses (expressed in terms of volume) of 0.2 mL per kg body-weight have been suggested to prevent an attack and 0.04 mL per kg to modify an attack. The dose should be repeated after 3 weeks in the case of continued exposure to measles.

Normal immunoglobulin does not prevent **rubella** infection but may reduce the likelihood of clinical symptoms in pregnant women exposed to rubella thereby lessening the risk to the fetus; it should be given as soon as possible after exposure. The recommended dose is 750 mg by intramuscular injection. A dose of 20 mL has also been suggested.

Normal immunoglobulin may be used in the management of patients with **primary antibody deficiencies** such as congenital agammaglobulinaemia, hypogammaglobulinaemia, or **immunocompromised patients** including those with immunodeficiency syndromes; the immunoglobulin is given to provide protection against infectious diseases that such patients may suffer. The intramuscular preparation may be used but the intravenous route is usually preferred since administration is less painful for the doses required. For intravenous infusion, the dose, expressed in terms of weight (protein or immunoglobulin G content), is usually 400 to 800 mg per kg body-weight initially, then 200 mg per kg every 3 weeks adjusted as necessary according to trough-immunoglobulin concentrations; the maintenance dose is usually 200 to 800 mg per kg per month. In patients with secondary immunodeficiency syndromes doses of 200 to 400 mg per kg every 3 to 4 weeks have been recommended. Other dosage regimens have been used. When infused intravenously, normal immunoglobulin should always be given very carefully and slowly with gradual increases in the rate of administration. For the intramuscular type of preparation the usual initial dose, expressed in terms of volume, is 1.3 to 1.8 mL per kg in divided doses over 48 hours; the maximum recommended total initial dose is 60 mL. For maintenance, doses of 0.6 to 0.65 mL per kg (maximum 30 mL) may be given every 3 to 4 weeks.

For prophylaxis of infection after **bone marrow transplantation**, normal immunoglobulin is given intravenously in a dose of 500 mg per kg weekly, adjusted according to response.

Intravenous infusion of normal immunoglobulin is also employed to raise the platelet count in patients with **idiopathic thrombocytopenic purpura**. Doses of 400 mg per kg are given daily for 2 to 5 consecutive days. Alternatively doses of 800 to 1000 mg per kg may be given on day 1 and repeated on day 3 if necessary. Further doses may be given as necessary.

For **Kawasaki disease**, normal immunoglobulin (in conjunction with aspirin) is given intravenously in a dose of 1.6 to 2 g per kg in divided doses over 2 to 5 days, or 2 g per kg given as a single dose. Similar doses of intravenous normal immunoglobulin have been tried in a range of disorders believed to have an autoimmune origin. The precise mode of action of normal immunoglobulin in such disorders is unknown.

For the treatment of **Guillain-Barré syndrome**, normal immunoglobulin is given intravenously in a dose of 400 mg per kg for 5 consecutive days, repeated every 4 weeks if required.

Normal immunoglobulin is also given intramuscularly as an adjunct to plasma and blood in the treatment of burns; during the first week following the burns a total of about 50 g should be given from the third up to the tenth day, 2.5 to 5 g per day is administered.

◊ Reviews and discussions of the actions and uses of intravenous normal immunoglobulins.
1. National Institutes of Health Consensus Conference. Intravenous immunoglobulin: prevention and treatment of disease. *JAMA* 1990; **264:** 3189–93.
2. Anonymous. Consensus on IVIG. *Lancet* 1990; **336:** 470–2.
3. ASHP Commission on Therapeutics. ASHP therapeutic guidelines for intravenous immune globulin. *Clin Pharm* 1992; **11:** 117–36.
4. Dwyer JM. Manipulating the immune system with immune globulin. *N Engl J Med* 1992; **326:** 107–16.
5. Pirofsky B, Kinzey DM. Intravenous immune globulins: a review of their uses in selected immunodeficiency and autoimmune diseases. *Drugs* 1992; **43:** 6–14.
6. Keller T, et al. Indications for the use of intravenous immunoglobulin: recommendations of the Australasian Society of Blood Transfusion consensus symposium. *Med J Aust* 1993; **159:** 204–6.
7. Ratko TA, et al. Recommendations for off-label use of intravenously administered immunoglobulin preparations. *JAMA* 1995; **273:** 1865–70.
8. Stiehm ER. Appropriate therapeutic use of immunoglobulin. *Transfus Med Rev* 1996; **10:** 203–21.

Administration. In order to overcome some of the problems associated with ensuring regular venous access necessary for long term intravenous immunoglobulin therapy, administration by rapid subcutaneous infusion has been evaluated. Subcutaneous infusion of approximately 16% preservative-free solutions or solutions not containing a mercurial preservative were administered to adults[1] through 2 pumps at a rate of 17 to 20 mL per hour at each pump and to children[2,3] at a rate of 10 to 20 mL per hour. Adequate immunoglobulin concentrations were achieved and this route of administration was generally well tolerated. A subsequent review[4] of subcutaneous infusion therapy in 165 patients receiving doses of between 80 and 800 mg per kg body-weight per month in divided doses supported these results.

Oral administration of normal immunoglobulins has been proposed to reduce the incidence and severity of gastrointestinal infections,[5,6] particularly in patients with defective immune systems including neonates. Although the predominant immunoglobulin secreted into the gastrointestinal tract in subjects with a normal immune system is IgA, a species not present in large quantities in commercial normal immunoglobulins, beneficial responses, especially in viral infections,[7] have been reported following oral administration. Preparations of immunoglobulin A are available in some countries and have been tried, mainly in bacterial gastrointestinal infections.[8,9]
1. Gardulf A, et al. Home treatment of hypogammaglobulinaemia with subcutaneous gammaglobulin by rapid infusion. *Lancet* 1991; **338:** 162–6.
2. Thomas MJ, et al. Rapid subcutaneous immunoglobulin infusions in children. *Lancet* 1993; **342:** 1432–3.
3. Gaspar J, et al. Immunoglobulin replacement treatment by rapid subcutaneous infusion. *Arch Dis Child* 1998; **79:** 48–51.
4. Gardulf A, et al. Subcutaneous immunoglobulin replacement in patients with primary antibody deficiencies: safety and costs. *Lancet* 1995; **345:** 365–9.
5. Dattani SJ, Connelly JF. Oral immunoglobulins for gastroenteritis. *Ann Pharmacother* 1996; **30:** 1323–4.
6. Reilly RM, et al. Oral delivery of antibodies: future pharmacokinetic trends. *Clin Pharmacokinet* 1997; **32:** 313–23.
7. Guarino A, et al. Oral immunoglobulins for treatment of acute rotaviral gastroenteritis. *Pediatrics* 1994; **93:** 12–16.
8. Tjellström B, et al. Oral immunoglobulin A supplement in treatment of Clostridium difficile enteritis. *Lancet* 1993; **341:** 701–2.
9. Hammarström V, et al. Oral immunoglobulin treatment in Campylobacter jejuni enteritis. *Lancet* 1993; **341:** 1036.

Blood disorders. Intravenous normal immunoglobulins are used in the treatment of symptomatic severe acute and chronic idiopathic thrombocytopenic purpura (p.1052). Other blood disorders in which normal immunoglobulins have been tried include agranulocytosis[1] and haemolytic disease of the newborn (p.1532), aplastic and haemolytic anaemias (p.715), red cell aplasia caused by parvovirus B19 infections (see under Passive Immunisation, below), thrombotic thrombocytopenic purpura and haemolytic-uraemic syndrome (see Thrombotic Microangiopathies p.740), and thrombocytopenia with a variety of causes.[2-10]
1. Fasth A. Immunoglobulin for neonatal agranulocytosis. *Arch Dis Child* 1986; **61:** 86–7.

2. Hoffman DM, et al. Human immunodeficiency virus-associated thrombocytopenia. *DICP Ann Pharmacother* 1989; **23:** 157–160.
3. Frame JN, et al. Correction of severe heparin-associated thrombocytopenia with intravenous immunoglobulin. *Ann Intern Med* 1989; **111:** 946–7.
4. Howrie DL, et al. Use of iv immune globulin for treatment of phenytoin-induced thrombocytopenia. *Clin Pharm* 1989; **8:** 734–7.
5. Landonio G, et al. HIV-related severe thrombocytopenia in intravenous drug users: prevalence, response to therapy in a medium-term follow-up, and pathogenic evaluation. *AIDS* 1990; **4:** 29–34.
6. Goulder P, et al. Intravenous immunoglobulin in virus associated haemophagocytic syndrome. *Arch Dis Child* 1990; **65:** 1275–7.
7. Larner AJ, et al. Life threatening thrombocytopenia in sarcoidosis: response to vincristine, human immunoglobulin, and corticosteroids. *BMJ* 1990; **300:** 317–19.
8. Ray JB, et al. Intravenous immune globulin for treatment of presumed quinidine-induced thrombocytopenia. *DICP Ann Pharmacother* 1990; **24:** 693–5.
9. Salzman MB, Smith EM. Phenytoin-induced thrombocytopenia treated with intravenous immune globulin. *J Pediatr Hematol Oncol* 1998; **20:** 152–3.
10. Majluf-Cruz A, et al. Usefulness of a low-dose intravenous immunoglobulin regimen for the treatment of thrombocytopenia associated with AIDS. *Am J Hematol* 1998; **59:** 127–32.

Epilepsy. Normal immunoglobulins have sometimes been of benefit[1-3] in the treatment of children with intractable epilepsy, including Lennox-Gastaut syndrome or West's syndrome, but a review of the literature found that few well controlled studies had been conducted.[4] Although a positive trend in favour of intravenous immunoglobulin therapy for refractory epilepsy was noted in one double-blind controlled study[5] involving 61 patients, the results were not considered to be statistically significant.
1. Ariizumi M, et al. High dose gammaglobulin for intractable childhood epilepsy. *Lancet* 1983; **ii:** 162–3.
2. Sandstedt P, et al. Intravenous gammaglobulin for post-encephalitic epilepsy. *Lancet* 1984; **ii:** 1154–5.
3. van Engelen BGH, et al. High-dose intravenous immunoglobulin treatment in cryptogenic West and Lennox-Gastaut syndrome: an add-on study. *Eur J Pediatr* 1994; **153:** 762–9.
4. Duse M, et al. Intravenous immune globulin in the treatment of intractable childhood epilepsy. *Clin Exp Immunol* 1996; **104** (suppl 1): 71–6.
5. van Rijckevorsel-Harmant K, et al. Treatment of refractory epilepsy with intravenous immunoglobulins: results of the first double-blind/dose finding clinical study. *Int J Clin Lab Res* 1994; **24:** 162–6.

Hypogammaglobulinaemia. See under Primary Antibody Deficiency, below.

Immunocompromised patients. Immunodeficiency states may arise from primary disorders of the immune system, or, more commonly, they are secondary to immunosuppressive therapy, HIV infection, or haematological malignancies. Premature neonates may have deficits in their immune systems due to their immaturity; placental transfer of maternal antibodies usually occurs after about 32 weeks of gestation. Such immunodeficient patients and neonates may be deficient in gammaglobulins which increases their susceptibility to infections, and they could potentially benefit from the administration of normal immunoglobulins. For information on the use of immunoglobulins in specific conditions, see the following sections and under Neonatal Sepsis, below.

BONE-MARROW TRANSPLANTATION. In patients undergoing allogeneic bone-marrow transplantation (p.502), intravenous normal immunoglobulin has decreased the incidence of both bacterial infections[1] and of symptomatic cytomegalovirus infection, particularly interstitial pneumonia.[1,2] Overall survival[1] or overall incidence of cytomegalovirus infection[1,2] was not decreased. A combination of normal immunoglobulin and ganciclovir appears to improve the outcome of cytomegalovirus pneumonia subsequent to bone-marrow transplantation.[3] No patients treated with normal immunoglobulin alone survived. Cytomegalovirus immunoglobulins (p.1536) may be more appropriate for the specific prophylaxis and treatment of cytomegalovirus infections.

Intravenous immunoglobulin therapy has been found to be ineffective in preventing infections in patients receiving autologous bone-marrow transplants[4] and may have contributed to an increased incidence of fatal hepatic veno-occlusive disease.

Normal immunoglobulin administration has been associated with a reduced frequency of acute graft-versus-host disease, possibly as a result of a direct immunomodulatory effect.
1. Sullivan KM, et al. Immunomodulatory and antimicrobial efficacy of intravenous immunoglobulin in bone marrow transplantation. *N Engl J Med* 1990; **323:** 705–12.
2. Winston DJ, et al. Intravenous immune globulin for prevention of cytomegalovirus infection and interstitial pneumonia after bone marrow transplantation. *Ann Intern Med* 1987; **106:** 12–18.
3. Emanuel D, et al. Cytomegalovirus pneumonia after bone marrow transplantation successfully treated with the combination of ganciclovir and high-dose intravenous immune globulin. *Ann Intern Med* 1988; **109:** 777–82.
4. Wolff SN, et al. High-dose weekly intravenous immunoglobulin to prevent infections in patients undergoing autologous bone marrow transplantation or severe myelosuppressive therapy: a study of the American Bone Marrow Transplant Group. *Ann Intern Med* 1993; **118:** 937–42.

HIV INFECTION AND AIDS. Immunoglobulin levels are typically raised in patients with AIDS, but hypogammaglobulinaemia has been observed and, even in the presence of hypergammaglobulinaemia, patients exhibit signs of being hypogamma-

globulinaemic. Normal immunoglobulin has therefore been administered to some symptomatic HIV-positive children. A significant improvement was noted[1] in 8 children given intravenous normal immunoglobulin, in terms of weight gain, number of infectious episodes, and diarrhoea. HIV core antigen was detected in 4 children before treatment. All became core-antigen negative after treatment was commenced although the effect was only maintained in 3. The validity of these results was questioned.[2] Larger studies have reported improvements in the rate of decline of the CD4+ T lymphocyte count[3] and the incidence of serious bacterial infections[4,5] but could not demonstrate improved survival. However, a further controlled study[6] in adult patients with AIDS given intravenous normal immunoglobulin demonstrated both an increase in the time free from bacterial or viral infection and also an improvement in survival rate after 31 weeks, and a small study in 24 patients[7] has reported improved survival at up to 12 months in patients who received normal immunoglobulin.
1. Hague RA, et al. Intravenous immunoglobulin in HIV infection: evidence for the efficacy of treatment. *Arch Dis Child* 1989; **64:** 1146–50.
2. Gibb D, Levin M. Intravenous immunoglobulin in HIV infection. *Arch Dis Child* 1990; **65:** 247–8.
3. Mofenson LM, et al. Effect of intravenous immunoglobulin (IVIG) on CD4+ lymphocyte decline in HIV-infected children in a clinical trial of IVIG infection prophylaxis. *J Acquir Immune Defic Syndr* 1993; **6:** 1103–13.
4. The National Institute of Child Health and Human Development Intravenous Immunoglobulin Study Group. Intravenous immune globulin for the prevention of bacterial infections in children with symptomatic human immunodeficiency virus infection. *N Engl J Med* 1991; **325:** 73–80.
5. Spector SA, et al. A controlled trial of intravenous immune globulin for the prevention of serious bacterial infections in children receiving zidovudine for advanced human immunodeficiency virus infection. *N Engl J Med* 1994; **331:** 1181–7.
6. Kiehl MG, et al. A controlled trial of intravenous immune globulin for the prevention of serious infections in adults with advanced human immunodeficiency virus infection. *Arch Intern Med* 1996; **156:** 2545–50.
7. Saint-Marc T, et al. Beneficial effects of intravenous immunoglobulins in AIDS. *Lancet* 1992; **340:** 1347.

MALIGNANCIES. Hypogammaglobulinaemia and the effects of treatment may increase the susceptibility to infection of patients with *chronic lymphocytic leukaemia*.[1] In a study of 81 patients with chronic lymphocytic leukaemia considered to be at an increased risk of infection, intravenous normal immunoglobulin 400 mg per kg body-weight given every 3 weeks for one year reduced the incidence of bacterial infection compared with saline placebo. The incidence of viral and fungal infections was not affected. A study in 34 patients[2] suggested that a dose of normal immunoglobulin 250 mg per kg per month was adequate for routine prophylaxis in most patients. Beneficial effects on infection rates have been reported in patients with *multiple myeloma* receiving normal immunoglobulins.[3]
1. Cooperative Group for the Study of Immunoglobulin in Chronic Lymphocytic Leukemia. Intravenous immunoglobulin for *N Engl J Med* 1988; **319:** 902–7.
2. Chapel H, et al. Immunoglobulin replacement in patients with chronic lymphocytic leukaemia: a comparison of two dose regimes. *Br J Haematol* 1994; **88:** 209–12.
3. Chapel HM, et al. Randomised trial of intravenous immunoglobulin as prophylaxis against infection in plateau-phase multiple myeloma. *Lancet* 1994; **343:** 1059–63.

PRIMARY ANTIBODY DEFICIENCY. There are three major forms of primary antibody deficiency: X-linked agammaglobulinaemia (XLA, Bruton's agammaglobulinaemia), common variable immunodeficiency (CVID) which includes IgG subclass and specific antibody deficiencies, and selective IgA deficiency. The disease is characterised by a wide range of infective complications as well as auto-immune disorders. Management is by replacement therapy with normal immunoglobulin accompanied by appropriate antimicrobial therapy for breakthrough infections. Immunisation against infection is of no value and is contra-indicated for live viral vaccines.

Normal immunoglobulin was traditionally administered by the intramuscular route. However, the maximum dose that can be reasonably given by this route is 25 mg per kg body-weight weekly, and it is therefore only satisfactory for patients with mild disease.[1] The introduction of intravenous preparations of normal immunoglobulin allows high doses to be given to those with severe disease. This route should therefore be used for all patients with XLA and for patients with CVID who have more than mild disease. The use of intravenous normal immunoglobulin in IgG subclass deficiency, with or without IgA deficiency, or in specific antibody deficiency is successful, though less well established. The dose and frequency of administration of intravenous normal immunoglobulin is variable and should be adjusted to prevent breakthrough infection. Most patients require 200 to 600 mg per kg every 2 or 3 weeks to maintain optimum protection.[1] In a recent study,[2] doses of between 260 and 1120 mg per kg every 3 weeks were necessary to maintain residual serum IgG concentrations above 500 mg per dL: these doses were found to be effective in reducing the incidence of severe acute bacterial infections and pulmonary insufficiency in children with XLA. Surgical procedures should be covered with additional normal immunoglobulin and appropriate prophylactic antibacterials. Home treatment with intravenous normal immunoglobulin has been used successfully in several countries in both adults and children.[1,3-6] Adverse reactions have been few and generally mild.[1,4,5] They are most likely to occur during the first infusion and during intercurrent illness, and may be precipitated by a high infusion rate.[6] Long-term treatment of children with antibody deficiencies with intravenous normal immunoglobulin has been shown to lead to normal growth and similar rates of infection to those found in non-immunodeficient children.[7]

Some patients have been successfully treated with subcutaneous infusion of normal immunoglobulin (see Administration, above) and the intraventricular route may be of benefit to some patients with echovirus encephalitis.[1,8]

In a pilot study, normal immunoglobulin given subcutaneously to 10 patients with selective IgA deficiency was safe and reduced the rate of respiratory-tract infections.[9]

1. Spickett GP, et al. Primary antibody deficiency in adults. Lancet 1991; 337: 281–4.
2. Quartier P, et al. Early and prolonged intravenous immunoglobulin replacement therapy in childhood agammaglobulinaemia: a retrospective survey of 31 patients. J Pediatr 1999; 134: 589–96.
3. Ochs HD, et al. Intravenous immunoglobulin home treatment for patients with primary immunodeficiency diseases. Lancet 1986; i: 610–11.
4. Ryan A, et al. Home intravenous immunoglobulin therapy for patients with primary hypogammaglobulinaemia. Lancet 1988; ii: 793.
5. Kobayashi RH, et al. Home self-administration of intravenous immunoglobulin therapy in children. Pediatrics 1990; 85: 705–9.
6. Chapel HM. Consensus on diagnosis and management of primary antibody deficiencies. BMJ 1994; 308: 581–5.
7. Skull S, Kemp A. Treatment of hypogammaglobulinaemia with intravenous immunoglobulin, 1973-93. Arch Dis Child 1996; 74: 527–30.
8. Erlendsson K, et al. Successful reversal of echovirus encephalitis in x-linked hypogammaglobulinemia by intraventricular administration of immunoglobulin. N Engl J Med 1985; 312: 351–30.
9. Gustafson R, et al. Prophylactic therapy for selective IgA deficiency. Lancet 1997; 350: 865.

Inflammatory bowel diseases.
Intravenous normal immunoglobulin may be beneficial[1-3] in inducing remission of Crohn's disease and ulcerative colitis and has been tried[4] in antibiotic-associated colitis.

1. Rohr G, et al. Treatment of Crohn's disease and ulcerative colitis with 7S-immunoglobulin. Lancet 1987; i: 170.
2. Knoflach P, et al. Crohn disease and intravenous immunoglobulin G. Ann Intern Med 1990; 112: 385–6.
3. Körber J, et al. A case of Crohn's disease with increased CD8 T-cell activation and remission during therapy with intravenous immunoglobulins. Scand J Gastroenterol 1998; 33: 1113–17.
4. Leung DYM, et al. Treatment with intravenously administered gamma globulin of chronic relapsing colitis induced by Clostridium difficile toxin. J Pediatr 1991; 118: 633–7.

Kawasaki disease.
Kawasaki disease, also known as mucocutaneous lymph node syndrome of childhood, occurs mainly in children under 5 years of age. It is epidemic and endemic worldwide but is a particular problem in Japan. Kawasaki disease presents with high fever which persists for at least 5 days and may be followed by bilateral conjunctival injection, changes in the oropharyngeal mucosa, signs of vasculitis in the extremities, rash, and cervical lymphadenopathy. The major complications of Kawasaki disease are cardiac effects including coronary artery aneurysm, aortic or mitral incompetence, myocarditis, and pericarditis with effusion. The cause of the disease is unknown, although an infective aetiology has been suggested. Early diagnosis, expert cardiac assessment, and immediate treatment are essential for improved outcome.

Treatment aims to reduce inflammation, particularly in the coronary arterial wall and myocardium, and therefore prevent the development of cardiac complications. Long-term antiplatelet treatment is given as necessary to prevent coronary thrombosis.[1]

Initial treatment is with aspirin and normal immunoglobulin.[2] A decreased incidence of coronary-artery abnormalities has been demonstrated after such a combination as compared with aspirin alone.[3] Normal immunoglobulin has generally been given by intravenous infusion in divided doses over 2 to 5 days, although administration as a single dose is recommended as an alternative,[2,4] and has been associated with a lower incidence of coronary abnormalities after 30 days than multiple-dose treatment.[5] The optimum dosage and duration of treatment with aspirin is not yet established, but the usual practice is to use an anti-inflammatory regimen until the fever has settled and then to convert to an antithrombotic regimen. A few patients fail to respond to treatment with aspirin and normal immunoglobulin. A small study[6] suggested that re-treatment with normal immunoglobulin may be considered for those with persistent or recurring fever. The use of corticosteroids remains controversial.[2] Corticosteroids have not been routinely used in Kawasaki disease since the introduction of immunoglobulin therapy as there is a risk that they may exacerbate coronary artery aneurysms. Nevertheless, they have been used in some centres.[7]

Long-term management. Aspirin should be continued for 6 to 8 weeks after the onset of illness and then discontinued if there are no coronary abnormalities. Some practitioners use aspirin and dipyridamole as antithrombotic therapy although it is not known whether this combination provides benefit over aspirin alone.[1] Dipyridamole may be used as an alternative antithrombotic agent for patients who cannot tolerate aspirin. Aspirin is usually continued for at least one year if coronary abnormalities are present and should be continued indefinitely if coronary aneurysms persist. Anticoagulation with warfarin or heparin in

addition to aspirin may be necessary in some patients such as those with giant or multiple aneurysms.

1. Dajani AS, et al. Guidelines for long-term management of patients with Kawasaki disease: report from the Committee on Rheumatic Fever, Endocarditis, and Kawasaki Disease, Council on Cardiovascular Disease in the Young, American Heart Association. Circulation 1994; 89: 916–22.
2. Onouchi Z, Kawasaki T. Overview of pharmacological treatment of Kawasaki disease. Drugs 1999; 58: 813–22.
3. Newburger JW, et al. The treatment of Kawasaki syndrome with intravenous gamma globulin. N Engl J Med 1986; 315: 341–7.
4. Newburger JW, et al. A single intravenous infusion of gamma globulin as compared with four infusions in the treatment of acute Kawasaki syndrome. N Engl J Med 1991; 324: 1633–9.
5. Durongpisitkul K, et al. The prevention of coronary artery aneurysm in Kawasaki disease: a meta-analysis on the efficacy of aspirin and immunoglobulin treatment. Pediatrics 1995; 96: 1057–61.
6. Sundel RP, et al. Gamma globulin re-treatment in Kawasaki disease. J Pediatr 1993; 123: 657–9.
7. Shinohara M, et al. Corticosteroids in the treatment of the acute phase of Kawasaki disease. J Pediatr 1999; 135: 465–9.

Kidney disorders.
Treatment with normal immunoglobulin has been of benefit in some patients with haemolytic-uraemic syndrome (see under Blood Disorders, above) and with lupus nephritis (see under Musculoskeletal and Nerve Disorders, below). For mention of the use of normal immunoglobulin in IgA nephropathy, see Glomerular Kidney Disease, p.1051.

Musculoskeletal and nerve disorders.
High-dose intravenous normal immunoglobulin has been tried with some benefit in various disorders of the nerves, muscles, joints, and connective tissues which may have an auto-immune basis. These include multiple sclerosis,[1] chronic inflammatory demyelinating polyneuropathy,[2] polymyositis and dermatomyositis,[3-7] myasthenia gravis,[8-11] stiff-man syndrome,[12-15] chronic systemic juvenile arthritis,[16-18] systemic lupus erythematosus[19] including lupus nephritis,[20] Guillain-Barré syndrome (see below), and motor neurone disease (see also below).

1. Fazekas F, et al. Randomised placebo-controlled trial of monthly intravenous immunoglobulin therapy in relapsing-remitting multiple sclerosis. Lancet 1997; 349: 589–93.
2. van Doorn PA, et al. High-dose intravenous immunoglobulin treatment in chronic inflammatory demyelinating polyneuropathy: a double-blind, placebo-controlled, crossover study. Neurology 1990; 40: 209–12.
3. Cherin P, et al. Efficacy of intravenous gammaglobulin therapy in chronic refractory polymyositis and dermatomyositis: an open study with 20 adult patients. Am J Med 1991; 91: 162–8.
4. Lang BA, et al. Treatment of dermatomyositis with intravenous gammaglobulin. Am J Med 1991; 91: 169–72.
5. Dalakas MC, et al. A controlled trial of high-dose intravenous immune globulin infusions as treatment for dermatomyositis. N Engl J Med 1993; 329: 1993–2000.
6. Brownell AKW. Intravenous immune globulin for dermatomyositis. N Engl J Med 1994; 330: 1392.
7. Collet E, et al. Juvenile dermatomyositis: treatment with intravenous gammaglobulin. Br J Dermatol 1994; 130: 231–4.
8. Bassan H, et al. High-dose intravenous immunoglobulin in transient neonatal myasthenia gravis. Pediatr Neurol 1998; 18: 181–3.
9. Jongen JLM, et al. High-dose intravenous immunoglobulin therapy for myasthenia. J Neurol 1998; 245: 26–31.
10. Howard JF. Intravenous immunoglobulin for the treatment of acquired myasthenia gravis. Neurology 1998; 51 (suppl 5): S30–S36.
11. Selcen D, et al. High-dose intravenous immunoglobulin therapy in juvenile myasthenia gravis. Pediatr Neurol 2000; 22: 40–3.
12. Karlson EW, et al. Treatment of stiff-man syndrome with intravenous immune globulin. Arthritis Rheum 1994; 37: 915–18.
13. Amato AA, et al. Treatment of stiff-man syndrome with intravenous immunoglobulin. Neurology 1994; 44: 1652–4.
14. Barker RA, Marsden CD. Successful treatment of stiff man syndrome with intravenous immunoglobulin. J Neurol Neurosurg Psychiatry 1997; 62: 426–7.
15. Khanlou H, Eiger G. Long-term remission of refractory stiff-man syndrome after treatment with intravenous immunoglobulin. Mayo Clin Proc 1999; 74: 1231–2.
16. Groothoff JW, van Leeuwen EF. High dose intravenous gammaglobulin in chronic systemic juvenile arthritis. BMJ 1988; 296: 1362–3.
17. Giannini EH, et al. Intravenous immunoglobulin in the treatment of polyarticular juvenile rheumatoid arthritis: a phase I/II study. J Rheumatol 1996; 23: 919–24.
18. Uziel Y, et al. Intravenous immunoglobulin therapy in systemic onset juvenile rheumatoid arthritis: a followup study. J Rheumatol 1996; 23: 910–18.
19. Francioni C, et al. Long term IV Ig treatment in systemic lupus erythematosus. Clin Exp Rheumatol 1994; 12: 163–8.
20. Lin C-Y, et al. Improvement of histological and immunological change in steroid and immunosuppressive drug-resistant lupus nephritis by high-dose intravenous gamma globulin. Nephron 1989; 53: 303–10.

GUILLAIN-BARRÉ SYNDROME. Guillain-Barré syndrome (acute idiopathic inflammatory polyneuropathy; acute idiopathic demyelinating neuropathy; acute infectious polyneuropathy) may follow an infection or, more rarely, immunisation, but very often no predisposing factor can be identified.[1-4] There may be an association with infection with Campylobacter jejuni.[5] Reversible demyelination results in pain and progressive flaccid paralysis. An auto-immune aetiology seems likely.[6] Severely affected patients require cardiovascular monitoring and respiratory support if respiratory muscles are affected or autonomic instability is present. Corticosteroids have been given[6-9] but are generally considered to be of little value (see Polyneuropathies, p.1057). Plasma exchange (see p.740) is effective if given early,[1,7,10,11] but is not universally available and is not suitable for all patients.[7] Administration of immunoglobulins has been shown to be at least as effective as plasma exchange in a study of 150 patients[12] although the response to plasma exchange in this study was lower than would be expected.[1,7] A more recent

study[13] has confirmed the equivalent efficacy of plasma exchange and immunoglobulins, and has also demonstrated no advantage from combining the two forms of treatment. Deterioration has also been noted in some patients following immunoglobulin therapy[14,15] and further evaluation of the use of immunoglobulins is awaited.

1. Howard RS. Neurology. BMJ 1994; 309: 392–5.
2. Morris K, Rylance G. Guillain-Barré syndrome after measles, mumps, and rubella vaccine. Lancet 1994; 343: 60.
3. Hadden RDM, Hughes RAC. Guillain-Barré syndrome: recent advances. Hosp Med 1998; 59: 55–60.
4. Hahn AF. Guillain-Barré syndrome. Lancet 1998; 352: 635–41.
5. Rees JH, et al. Campylobacter jejuni infection and Guillain-Barré syndrome. N Engl J Med 1995; 333: 1374–9.
6. Anonymous. Guillain-Barré syndrome: immunoglobulins or steroids? WHO Drug Inf 1993; 7: 110–11.
7. Rees J. Guillain-Barré syndrome: the latest on treatment. Br J Hosp Med 1993; 50: 226–9.
8. Guillain-Barré Syndrome Steroid Trial Group. Double-blind trial of intravenous methylprednisolone in Guillain-Barré syndrome. Lancet 1993; 341: 586–90.
9. Korinthenberg R, Mönting JS. Natural history and treatment effects in Guillain-Barré syndrome: a multicentre study. Arch Dis Child 1996; 74: 281–7.
10. The Guillain-Barré Syndrome Study Group. Plasmapheresis and acute Guillain-Barré syndrome. Neurology 1985; 35: 1096–1104.
11. French Cooperative Group on Plasma Exchange in Guillain-Barré syndrome. Efficacy of plasma exchange in Guillain-Barré syndrome: role of replacement fluids. Ann Neurol 1987; 22: 753–61.
12. van der Maché FGA, et al. A randomized trial comparing intravenous immune globulin and plasma exchange in Guillain-Barré syndrome. N Engl J Med 1992; 326: 1123–9.
13. Plasma Exchange/Sandoglobulin Guillain-Barré Syndrome Trial Group. Randomised trial of plasma exchange, intravenous immunoglobulin, and combined treatments in Guillain-Barré syndrome. Lancet 1997; 349: 225–30.
14. Irani DN, et al. Relapse in Guillain-Barré syndrome after treatment with human immune globulin. Neurology 1993; 43: 872–5.
15. Castro LHM, Ropper AH. Human immune globulin infusion in Guillain-Barré syndrome: worsening during and after treatment. Neurology 1993; 43: 1034–6.

MOTOR NEURONE DISEASE. Normal immunoglobulins have been tried in the treatment of multifocal motor neuropathy, a form of motor neurone disease (p.1658) associated with anti-GM$_1$ antibody formation.[1-5]

1. Van den Berg LH, et al. Treatment of multifocal motor neuropathy with high dose intravenous immunoglobulins: a double blind, placebo controlled study. J Neurol Neurosurg Psychiatry 1995; 59: 248–52.
2. Azulay J-P, et al. Long term follow up of multifocal motor neuropathy with conduction block under treatment. J Neurol Neurosurg Psychiatry 1997; 62: 391–4.
3. Meucci N, et al. Long term effect of intravenous immunoglobulins and oral cyclophosphamide in multifocal motor neuropathy. J Neurol Neurosurg Psychiatry 1997; 63: 765–9.
4. Van den Berg LH, et al. The long-term effect of intravenous immunoglobulin treatment in multifocal motor neuropathy. Brain 1998; 121: 421–8.
5. Ellis CM, et al. Use of human intravenous immunoglobulin in lower motor neuron syndromes. J Neurol Neurosurg Psychiatry 1999; 67: 15–19.

Neonatal disorders.
HAEMOLYTIC DISEASE OF THE NEWBORN. For a discussion of haemolytic disease of the newborn and its management, including the use of intravenous immunoglobulin as an alternative to exchange transfusions in affected pregnancies, see p.1532.

NEONATAL SEPSIS. Sepsis is a serious problem in premature infants despite appropriate antimicrobial therapy.[1] Preterm infants are born with low serum-immunoglobulin concentrations which decrease over the next several weeks of life.[1,2] There is also a deficiency of antibodies to specific organisms such as group B streptococci, Staphylococcus epidermidis, and Escherichia coli.[1,2]

Some, but not all, studies suggest that prophylactic administration of intravenous normal immunoglobulin to premature infants shortly after birth can decrease the incidence of septicaemia.[1] Aspects of the methodology of these studies have, however, been criticised.[2] Some benefit has been observed after administration of intravenous immunoglobulin to treat infants with suspected sepsis,[1] and may improve the response to antibacterials[3] although a systematic review[4] found insufficient evidence to support routine treatment in infants with suspected, or subsequently proved, neonatal infection.

The optimum effective dosage of intravenous immunoglobulin is not established. A prophylactic dose of 500 mg per kg body-weight on admission repeated every one to two weeks has been suggested for units where infection is common in very low birth-weight infants.[1] Others have suggested adjusting the dose to maintain a specified serum-immunoglobulin concentration.[5,6] Alternatively, normal immunoglobulin could be administered only to infants with immunoglobulin concentrations below a certain level, or be reserved for immediate use in those who become ill with suspected sepsis.[1]

Normal immunoglobulin cannot protect against all types of infection. Normal immunoglobulin preparations from different manufacturers may demonstrate, for a specific pathogen (group B streptococcus), differing levels of specific antibody and differing levels of functional activity both in vitro and in animals.[7] Lot-to-lot variability in functional activity was also observed for normal immunoglobulin from a specific manufacturer. Such variability, resulting in low concentrations of functional antibodies in the 4 batches of immunoglobulins used in the National Institute of Child Health Study,[8] was held responsible for the lack of demonstrable effectiveness of immunoglobulins in that study, one of the largest to date. It has been suggested[9] that normal immunoglobulin would probably not be effective for the prevention of serious *Herpes simplex* virus infection in neonates at risk.

The use of fresh frozen plasma as an alternative to normal immunoglobulin could not be recommended following a study[10] which showed that it did not produce the beneficial effects on humoral immune markers seen with normal immunoglobulin.

Human immunoglobulin preparations hyperimmune for a specific pathogen[7] or human monoclonal antibody preparations against common perinatal pathogens[1,11] are possible future strategies.

1. Whitelaw A. Treatment of sepsis with IgG in very low birth-weight infants. *Arch Dis Child* 1990; **65**: 347–8.
2. Noya FJD, Baker CJ. Intravenously administered immune globulin for premature infants: a time to wait. *J Pediatr* 1989; **115**: 969–71.
3. Christensen RD, *et al.* Effect on neutrophil kinetics and serum opsonic capacity of intravenous administration of immune globulin to neonates with clinical signs of early-onset sepsis. *J Pediatr* 1991; **118**: 606–14.
4. Ohlsson A, Lacy JB. Intravenous immunoglobulin for suspected or subsequently proven infection in neonates (updated 23 August 2001). Available in The Cochrane Library; Issue 4. Oxford: Update Software; 2001.
5. Clapp DW, *et al.* Use of intravenously administered immune globulin to prevent nosocomial sepsis in low birth weight infants: report of a pilot study. *J Pediatr* 1989; **115**: 973–8.
6. Kyllonen KS, *et al.* Dosage of intravenously administered immune globulin and dosing interval required to maintain target levels of immunoglobulin G in low birth weight infants. *J Pediatr* 1989; **115**: 1013–16.
7. Givner LB. Human immunoglobulins for intravenous use: comparison of available preparations for group B streptococcal antibody levels, opsonic activity, and efficacy in animal models. *Pediatrics* 1990; **86**: 955–62.
8. Fanaroff AA, *et al.* A controlled trial of intravenous immune globulin to reduce nosocomial infections in very-low-birth-weight infants. *N Engl J Med* 1994; **330**: 1107–13.
9. Kohl S, *et al.* Effect of intravenously administered immune globulin on functional antibody to herpes simplex virus in low birth weight neonates. *J Pediatr* 1989; **115**: 135–9.
10. Acunas BA, *et al.* Effect of fresh frozen plasma and gammaglobulin on humoral immunity in neonatal sepsis. *Arch Dis Child* 1994; **70**: F182–7.
11. Weisman LE, *et al.* Comparison of group B streptococcal hyperimmune globulin and standard intravenously administered immune globulin in neonates. *J Pediatr* 1993; **122**: 929–37.

Obsessive-compulsive disorder. Benefit has been demonstrated from plasma exchange and administration of intravenous immunoglobulin in children with exacerbations of obsessive-compulsive disorder or tic disorders including Tourette's syndrome associated with streptococcal infection.[1] These results suggest that these disorders may respond to immunomodulatory therapy in a subgroup of patients with paediatric autoimmune neuropsychiatric disorders associated with streptococcal infections (PANDAS), believed to be due to cross-reaction of antistreptococcal antibodies with neural tissue.

1. Perlmutter SJ, *et al.* Therapeutic plasma exchange and intravenous immunoglobulin for obsessive-compulsive disorder and tic disorders in childhood. *Lancet* 1999; **354**: 1153–8.

Passive immunisation. CYTOMEGALOVIRUS INFECTION. See Bone Marrow Transplantation, under Immunocompromised Patients, above.

HEPATITIS. *Hepatitis A.* With the decreasing incidence of hepatitis A in the UK, a reduction in the concentration of hepatitis A antibodies in normal immunoglobulin has been observed. In the future, normal immunoglobulin could become unsuitable for hepatitis A prophylaxis.[1,2] However, hepatitis A vaccines (p.1541) have been developed and specific hepatitis A immunoglobulins (p.1541) are available in some countries.

1. Higgins G, *et al.* Hepatitis A virus antibody in East Anglian blood donors. *Lancet* 1990; **335**: 1330.
2. Behrens RH, Doherty JF. Severe hepatitis A despite passive immunisation. *Lancet* 1993; **341**: 972.

Hepatitis C. In a randomised, placebo-controlled study[1] in seronegative sexual partners of patients positive for antibody to hepatitis C, normal immunoglobulin administered intramuscularly every 2 months was found to significantly reduce the incidence of subsequent seroconversion. One of 450 subjects who received normal immunoglobulin became seropositive during follow-up compared with 6 of 449 who had received placebo.

1. Piazza M, *et al.* Sexual transmission of the hepatitis C virus and efficacy of prophylaxis with intramuscular immune serum globulin: a randomized controlled trial. *Arch Intern Med* 1997; **157**: 1537–44.

PARVOVIRUS B19 INFECTION. Persistent infection with human parvovirus B19 can cause red-cell aplasia with resultant anaemia particularly in immunocompromised patients. Resolution of anaemia and clearance of parvovirus B19 from the circulation have been reported after administration of normal immunoglobulin to a patient who had had red-cell aplasia for 10 years.[1] Normal immunoglobulin was given by intravenous infusion in a dose of 400 mg per kg body-weight daily for 10 days and then periodically for several months. Successful treatment of anaemia due to parvovirus B19-induced red-cell aplasia with plasmapheresis and intravenous immunoglobulin has been described in a liver transplant recipient.[2] Clearance of parvovirus B19 from the circulation has been reported in patients who also have AIDS, but the presence of concomitant opportunistic infections may prevent resolution of the anaemia.[3,4]

The symbol † denotes a preparation no longer actively marketed

Beneficial responses to intravenous immunoglobulin have also been reported in a few patients with parvovirus B19 infections associated with vasculitic syndromes.[5]

1. Kurtzman G, *et al.* Pure red-cell aplasia of 10 years' duration due to persistent parvovirus B19 infection and its cure with immunoglobulin therapy. *N Engl J Med* 1989; **321**: 519–23.
2. Ramage JK, *et al.* Parvovirus B19-induced red cell aplasia treated with plasmapheresis and immunoglobulin. *Lancet* 1994; **343**: 667–8.
3. Frickhofen N, *et al.* Persistent B19 parvovirus infection in patients infected with human immunodeficiency virus type 1 (HIV-1): a treatable cause of anemia in AIDS. *Ann Intern Med* 1990; **113**: 926–33.
4. Bowman CA, *et al.* Red cell aplasia associated with human parvovirus B19 and HIV infection: failure to respond clinically to intravenous immunoglobulin. *AIDS* 1990; **4**: 1038–9.
5. Finkel TH, *et al.* Chronic parvovirus B19 infection and systemic necrotising vasculitis: opportunistic infection or aetiological agent? *Lancet* 1994; **343**: 1255–8.

RUBELLA. Normal immunoglobulin does not prevent rubella infection but may reduce the likelihood of clinical symptoms in pregnant women exposed to rubella thereby lessening the risk to the fetus; it should be given as soon as possible after exposure.

TOXIC SHOCK SYNDROME. For a discussion of toxic shock syndrome and its treatment, including reference to clinical improvement after administration of intravenous normal immunoglobulins, see p.143.

Skin disorders. Normal immunoglobulins have been tried in a few patients with blistering skin diseases.[1] The usual treatment for pemphigoid is with systemic corticosteroids; normal immunoglobulins in high doses have produced generally transient improvement when used alone,[2] although steroid-sparing effects have been reported.[3] A patient with severe epidermolysis bullosa responded to therapy with high-dose intravenous immunoglobulins.[4] Clinical benefit was noted in 9 of 10 patients with auto-immune chronic urticaria who were given a 5-day course of intravenous immunoglobulins, 2 of whom experienced prolonged remission over 3 years of follow-up.[5] Benefit has also occurred after intravenous immunoglobulin therapy for atopic dermatitis[6] and pyoderma gangrenosum.[7]

1. Harman KE, Black MM. High-dose intravenous immune globulin for the treatment of autoimmune blistering diseases: an evaluation of its use in 14 cases. *Br J Dermatol* 1999; **140**: 865–74.
2. Godard W, *et al.* Bullous pemphigoid and intravenous gammaglobulin. *Ann Intern Med* 1985; **103**: 965.
3. Beckers RCY, *et al.* Adjuvant high-dose intravenous gammaglobulin in the treatment of pemphigus and bullous pemphigoid: experience in six patients. *Br J Dermatol* 1995; **133**: 289–93.
4. Mohr C, *et al.* Successful treatment of epidermolysis bullosa acquisita using intravenous immunoglobulins. *Br J Dermatol* 1995; **132**: 824–6.
5. O'Donnell BF, *et al.* Intravenous immunoglobulin in autoimmune chronic urticaria. *Br J Dermatol* 1998; **138**: 101–6.
6. Jolles S, *et al.* The treatment of atopic dermatitis with adjunctive high-dose intravenous immunoglobulin: a report of three patients and review of the literature. *Br J Dermatol* 2000; **142**: 551–4.
7. Dirschka T, *et al.* Successful treatment of pyoderma gangrenosum with intravenous human immunoglobulin. *J Am Acad Dermatol* 1998; **39**: 789–90.

Spontaneous abortion. Fetal loss has been attributed in some cases to the presence of antiphospholipid antibodies (lupus anticoagulant and anticardiolipin) in the mother. Successful pregnancy outcome has been reported after administration of intravenous normal immunoglobulin during pregnancy to a few such women.[1-5]

1. Carreras LO, *et al.* Lupus anticoagulant and recurrent fetal loss: successful treatment with gammaglobulin. *Lancet* 1988; **ii**: 393–4.
2. Francois A, *et al.* Repeated fetal losses and the lupus anticoagulant. *Ann Intern Med* 1988; **109**: 993–4.
3. Parke A, *et al.* Intravenous gamma-globulin, antiphospholipid antibodies, and pregnancy. *Ann Intern Med* 1989; **110**: 495–6.
4. Katz VL, *et al.* Human immunoglobulin therapy for preeclampsia associated with lupus anticoagulant and anticardiolipin antibody. *Obstet Gynecol* 1990; **76**: 986–8.
5. Mueller-Eckhardt G, *et al.* IVIG to prevent recurrent spontaneous abortion. *Lancet* 1991; **337**: 424–5.

Preparations

Ph. Eur.: Human Normal Immunoglobulin; Human Normal Immunoglobulin for Intravenous Administration;
USP 25: Immune Globulin.

Proprietary Preparations (details are given in Part 3)
Aust.: Beriglobin; Endobulin; Gamma-Venin; Gammabulin†; Gammagard; Gammonativ†; Igabulin†; Intragam; Intraglobin; Octagam; Pentaglobin; Sandoglobulin; Venimmun; **Austral.:** Intragam; Sandoglobulin; **Belg.:** Gammagard; Globuman†; Sandoglobuline; **Braz.:** Armoglobulina; Gama Venina; Sandoglobulina; Veinoglobuline; **Canad.:** Baygam; Gamimune N; Gammagard; Iveegam; **Denm.:** Beriglobin; Endobulin; Gammagard; Gammaglobulin; Gammanorm; Gammonativ; Nordimmun; **Fin.:** Endobulin; Gammagard; Gammaglobulin SPR; Sandoglobulin; Venogamma; **Fr.:** Endobulin; Gammagard; Sandoglobuline; Tegeline; **Ger.:** Alphaglobin†; Beriglobin; Endobulin; Flebogamma; Gamma-Venin; Gammabulin†; Gammagard; Gammonativ; Intraglobin F; Intrimun; Octagam; Pentaglobin; Polyglobin N†; Sandoglobulin; Venimmun; **Hong Kong:** Gamimune N; Gammabulin; Gammagard; Globuman; Intraglobin F; Octagam; Venoglobulin-S; **Irl.:** Gammabulin; Intraglobin; Sandoglobulin; **Israel:** Beriglobin P; Endobulin; Gamimune N; Gamma-Venin; Gammagard; IG Gamma; Omr-IgG; Sandoglobulin; Venoglobulin; **Ital.:** Alphaglobin; Biaven; Endobulin; Flebogamma; Gamma-Venin P; Gammabulin; Gammagard; Globuman; Haimaven; Ig Vena N; Intraglobin; Isiven; Normogamma; Pentaglobin; Sandoglobulina; Uman-Gamma; Venimmun; Venogamma Polivalente; **Mex.:** Beriglobina P; Intac-

globin; Pentaglobin; Sandoglobulina; Seroglubin; **Norw.:** Gammaglobulin; Gammanorm; Gammonativ; Octagam; Sandoglobulin†; **NZ:** Intragam; Sandoglobulin; **Port.:** Globuman; Sandoglobulina; **S.Afr.:** Beriglobin; Endobulin; Globuman; Intragam; Intraglobin F; Pentaglobin; Polygam; Sandoglobulin†; **Singapore:** Gammagard; Intraglobin F; Venoglobulin; **Spain:** Beriglobina P; Endobulin; Flebogamma; Gamma-Venin; Gammagard; Gammaglob; Globuman; Polyglobin; **Swed.:** Beriglobin; Endobulin; Gammabulin†; Gammagard; Gammanorm; Gammonativ; Nordimmun; Octagam; Polyglobin; Sandoglobulin; **Switz.:** Endobulin; Gammagard; Globuman; Intraglobin F; Octagam; Pentaglobin; Sandoglobuline; **Thai.:** Globuman; Intraglobin; Pentaglobin; Venoglobulin-S; **UK:** Endobulin†; Flebogamma; Gamimune N†; Gammabulin; Gammagard; Kabiglobulin; Octagam; Sandoglobulin; Vigam; **USA:** Gamimune N; Gammagard; Gammar-P; Iveegam; Panglobulin; Polygam; Sandoglobulin; Venoglobulin.

Multi-ingredient: Aust.: Histaglobin; **Ger.:** Histadestal; **S.Afr.:** Histaglobin; **Thai.:** Histaglobin.

Pertussis Immunoglobulins (1237-x)

ATC — J06BB13.

Pertussis Immune Globulin (USP 25) is a sterile solution of globulins derived from the plasma of adult human donors who have been immunised with pertussis vaccine. It may contain glycine as a stabilising agent, and a suitable preservative. It should be stored at 2° to 8°.

Adverse Effects and Precautions

As for immunoglobulins in general, p.1529.

Interactions

As for immunoglobulins in general, p.1529.

Uses and Administration

Pertussis immunoglobulins may be used for passive immunisation against pertussis (whooping cough). They have been used to prevent or modify pertussis in susceptible persons who have been exposed to infection.

◊ References.
1. Granström M, *et al.* Specific immunoglobulin for treatment of whooping cough. *Lancet* 1991; **338**: 1230–3.
2. Bruss JB, *et al.* Treatment of severe pertussis: a study of the safety and pharmacology of intravenous pertussis immunoglobulin. *Pediatr Infect Dis J* 1999; **18**: 505–11.

Preparations

USP 25: Pertussis Immune Globulin.

Proprietary Preparations (details are given in Part 3)
Ital.: Haimapertus; Immunopertox; Pertoglobulin; Pertus-Gamma; Tosuman†; **Switz.:** Tosuman†.

Pertussis Vaccines (7985-I)

ATC — J07AJ01; J07AJ02.

Pertussis Vaccine (Ph. Eur.) (Per/Vac; Vaccinum Pertussis; Whooping-cough Vaccine) is a sterile suspension of inactivated whole cells of one or more strains of *Bordetella pertussis* in saline. The estimated potency is not less than 4 international units per dose. It may contain a suitable antimicrobial preservative. It should be stored at 2° to 8°, not be allowed to freeze, and be protected from light.

Pertussis Vaccine (Adsorbed) (Ph. Eur.) (Per/Vac/Ads; Vaccinum Pertussis Adsorbatum) is a sterile suspension of inactivated whole cells of one or more strains of *Bordetella pertussis* in saline to which hydrated aluminium hydroxide, aluminium phosphate, or calcium phosphate has been added. It may contain a suitable antimicrobial preservative. The estimated potency is not less than 4 units per dose. It should be stored at 2° to 8°, not be allowed to freeze, and be protected from light. The BP 2001 directs that when Pertussis Vaccine is prescribed or demanded and the form is not stated, either the plain or the adsorbed vaccine may be dispensed or supplied.

Pertussis Vaccine (Acellular, Component, Adsorbed) (Ph. Eur.) (Adsorbed Pertussis Vaccine (Acellular Component) (BP 2001)) Vaccinum Pertussis sine Cellulis ex Elementis Praeparatum Adsorbatum) is a preparation of individually prepared and purified antigenic components of *Bordetella pertussis* adsorbed on a mineral carrier such as aluminium hydroxide or hydrated aluminium phosphate. It contains either a suitably prepared pertussis toxoid or a pertussis toxin-like protein free from toxic properties produced by expression of a genetically modified form of the corresponding gene. It may also contain filamentous haemagglutinin, pertactin, and other defined antigens such as fimbrial-2 and fimbrial-3 antigens. The final vaccine contains not more than 100 units of bacterial endotoxin per dose. It may contain a suitable antimicrobial preservative. It should be stored at 2° to 8°, not be allowed to freeze, and be protected from light.

Pertussis Vaccine (Acellular, Co-purified, Adsorbed) (Ph. Eur.) (Vaccinum Pertussis Sine Cellulis Copurificatum Adsorbatum) is a preparation of antigenic components of *Bordetella pertussis* adsorbed on a mineral carrier such as aluminium hydroxide or hydrated aluminium phosphate. It should be stored at 2° to 8°, not be allowed to freeze, and be protected from light.

Pertussis Vaccine (USP 25) is a sterile bacterial fraction or suspension of killed *Bordetella pertussis* of a strain or strains selected for high antigenicity. It contains a preservative. It contains 12 protective units per immunising dose. It should be stored at 2° to 8° and not be allowed to freeze.

Pertussis Vaccine Adsorbed (USP 25) is a sterile bacterial fraction or suspension of killed *Bordetella pertussis* of a strain or strains selected for high antigenicity, precipitated or adsorbed by the addition of aluminium hydroxide or aluminium phosphate. It contains a preservative. It contains 12 protective units per immunising dose. It should be stored at 2° to 8° and not be allowed to freeze.

Adverse Effects

As for vaccines in general, p.1529.

Local reactions may occur at the site of injection of pertussis vaccines or pertussis-containing vaccines and administration may be followed by fever and irritability. Local reactions and fever occur less frequently following use of the acellular vaccine than after whole-cell vaccine, especially in children over 6 months of age and adults.

Severe reactions which have been reported include persistent screaming and generalised collapse but these effects were generally associated with an earlier type of vaccine and the reactions are stated to be rarely observed with the currently available vaccines.

Rare neurological adverse reactions have included convulsions and encephalopathy. There has been much debate, however, on the causal role of pertussis vaccine in such reactions (see below for detailed discussion). It should be remembered that neurological complications occur more frequently as a consequence of pertussis infection than in association with vaccination.

Asthma. A higher incidence of asthma was reported in 243 children who had received pertussis vaccine than in 203 children who had not.[1] However, follow-up of a large Swedish study[2] showed no difference in the incidence of wheezing or allergic reactions between children who had received diphtheria, tetanus, and pertussis vaccines and those who had not. A recent prospective study[3] also found no evidence that pertussis vaccination increased the risk of wheezing illness in young children.

1. Odent MR, *et al.* Pertussis vaccination and asthma: is there a link? *JAMA* 1994; **272:** 592–3.
2. Nilsson L, *et al.* Lack of association between pertussis vaccination and symptoms of asthma and allergy. *JAMA* 1996; **275:** 760.
3. Henderson J, *et al.* Pertussis vaccination and wheezing illnesses in young children: prospective cohort study. *BMJ* 1999; **318:** 1173–6.

Effects on the nervous system. There has been continuing debate over several decades concerning the perceived link between pertussis vaccination and brain damage. Anxiety among both the public and health care professionals in the UK in the mid-1970s over the safety of pertussis vaccines led to a fall in the acceptance rates for infant vaccination and major epidemics of pertussis in 1977/79 and 1981/83. Since that time confidence has been restored, and by 1995 94% of infants were receiving the vaccine before their second birthday.

The consensus of opinion now seems to be that there is a temporal, but not necessarily causal, relationship between pertussis vaccine and acute neurological illness which may occasionally lead to long-term dysfunction, and that risks of not immunising are greater than the potential risks associated with the vaccine.

The difficulty in ascertaining whether a causal relationship exists between pertussis vaccine (usually given as diphtheria, tetanus, and pertussis (DTP) vaccine) and acute neurological reactions arises partly because primary vaccination is given at an age when neurological dysfunction with other causes is often first manifested. The observed temporal relationship may be entirely coincidental, may result from indirect factors such as pyrexia following vaccination, or may represent a direct effect of DTP vaccine. Much of the evidence is based on large epidemiological studies,[1-6] in particular the National Childhood Encephalopathy Study (NCES)[7] from the UK and its 10-year follow-up.[8] Serious acute neurological illnesses reported to the NCES[7] were found to be more common in infants immunised within 7 days (relative risk 2.4), and especially within 72 hours of onset, than in unimmunised children. For previously normal children, irrespective of outcome, the risk was estimated as 1 in 110 000 injections. In a subset of cases diagnosed as infantile spasms,[9] no link with vaccination was found overall, but there was a small excess of cases of infantile spasm in previously normal children who had received either DTP or diphtheria and tetanus vaccines during the previous 7 days (relative risk 2.0-2.5) followed by a corresponding deficit during the next 3 weeks. This suggested that vaccination may trigger the onset of spasms in a child with an underlying predisposition.

In 1991, the Institute of Medicine in the USA reviewed the available data, including the NCES results, and concluded that a causal relationship between DTP vaccine and acute encepha-

lopathy probably existed, with an estimated risk of zero to 10.5 per million vaccinations.[10] They concurred with the conclusion that a causal relationship between vaccination and infantile spasm was unlikely.

The NCES 10-year follow-up found that children who had had a serious acute neurological illness (excluding infantile spasms) had an increased risk of death or long-term dysfunction, but the risk was no greater in children who had received DTP vaccine in the 7 days before the original acute illness.[8] The National Vaccines Advisory Committee concluded that the results were insufficient to determine whether DTP vaccine influenced the development of chronic neurological dysfunction, and this conclusion has been accepted by both the Advisory Committee on Immunization Practices[11] and the American Academy of Pediatrics.[12]

1. Pollock TM, Morris J. A 7-year survey of disorders attributed to vaccination in North West Thames Region. *Lancet* 1983; **i:** 753–7.
2. Pollock TM, *et al.* Symptoms after primary immunisation with DTP and with DT vaccine. *Lancet* 1984; **ii:** 146–9.
3. Walker AM, *et al.* Neurologic events following diphtheria-tetanus-pertussis immunization. *Pediatrics* 1988; **81:** 345–9.
4. Shields WD, *et al.* Relationship of pertussis immunization to the onset of neurologic disorders: a retrospective epidemiologic study. *J Pediatr* 1988; **113:** 801–5.
5. Griffin MR, *et al.* Risk of seizures and encephalopathy after immunization with the diphtheria-tetanus-pertussis vaccine. *JAMA* 1990; **263:** 1641–5.
6. Gale JL, *et al.* Risk of serious acute neurological illness after immunization with diphtheria-tetanus-pertussis vaccine: a population-based case-control study. *JAMA* 1994; **271:** 37–41.
7. Miller DL, *et al.* Pertussis immunisation and serious acute neurological illness in children. *BMJ* 1981; **282:** 1595–9.
8. Miller D, *et al.* Pertussis immunisation and serious acute neurological illnesses in children. *BMJ* 1993; **307:** 1171–6.
9. Bellman MH, *et al.* Infantile spasms and pertussis immunisation. *Lancet* 1983; **i:** 1031–4.
10. Howson CP, Fineberg HV. Adverse events following pertussis and rubella vaccines: summary of a report of the Institute of Medicine. *JAMA* 1992; **267:** 392–6.
11. Centers for Disease Control. Update: vaccine side effects, adverse reactions, contraindications, and precautions: recommendations of the Advisory Committee on Immunization Practices (ACIP). *MMWR* 1996; **45** (RR-12): 1–45.
12. Committee on Infectious Disease, American Academy of Pediatrics. The relationship between pertussis vaccine and central nervous system sequelae: continuing assessment. *Pediatrics* 1996; **97:** 279–81.

Precautions

As for vaccines in general, p.1530. Because of the controversy concerning the potential adverse effects, especially neurotoxicity, of pertussis vaccines (see under Adverse Effects, above) the precautions and contra-indications to the use of these vaccines have sometimes been more stringent than is now considered necessary. As with other vaccines, immunisation should not be carried out in individuals with a definite history of a severe local or general reaction to a preceding dose. In children who have a history of less severe general reactions, immunisation may be completed omitting the pertussis component, or, in the case of local reactions or pyrexia, substituting an acellular pertussis vaccine.

Whether children with a personal or family history of convulsions or epilepsy or who have suffered cerebral damage in the neonatal period should receive pertussis vaccines appears to have been the most difficult question to resolve in the past. In the UK the Department of Health now recommends that children with a personal or family history of febrile convulsions and children with a close family history of idiopathic epilepsy should be immunised and children whose epilepsy is well controlled may receive pertussis vaccine; advice on the prevention of fever should be given at the time of immunisation (see Fever and Hyperthermia, p.8 for comments on the prevention of fever following immunisation). Immunisation should also be carried out in children with a history of cerebral damage in the neonatal period unless there is evidence of an evolving neurological abnormality. In children with a neurological problem that is still evolving it is recommended that immunisation should be deferred until the condition is stable.

A personal or family history of hypersensitivity reactions is not generally considered to be a contra-indication to the use of pertussis vaccines, nor are stable neurological conditions such as cerebral palsy or spina bifida.

◊ Although collapse (hypotonic-hyporesponsive episode) after pertussis vaccination remains a contra-indication to further doses of the whole-cell vaccine in the UK, a follow-up study of infants who had experienced such an episode in the Nether-

lands showed a very low incidence of recurrence on second and subsequent doses.[1]

1. Vermeer-de Bondt PE, *et al.* Rate of recurrent collapse after vaccination with whole cell pertussis vaccine: follow up study. *BMJ* 1998; **316:** 902–3.

Interactions

As for vaccines in general, p.1530.

Poliomyelitis vaccines. A diminished immune response to pertussis vaccine was reported in infants given inactivated poliomyelitis vaccine mixed with diphtheria, tetanus, and pertussis vaccine compared with infants given the two vaccines as separate injections on the same visit.[1]

1. Halperin SA, *et al.* Effect of inactivated poliovirus vaccine on the antibody response to Bordetella pertussis antigens when combined with diphtheria-pertussis-tetanus vaccine. *Clin Infect Dis* 1996; **22:** 59–62.

Uses and Administration

Pertussis vaccines are used for active immunisation against pertussis (whooping cough) (p.134).

For primary immunisation combined diphtheria, tetanus, and whole-cell pertussis vaccines (p.1537) have usually been used. For discussion of immunisation schedules, see below. Acellular pertussis vaccines are taking the place of whole-cell vaccines in several countries including the USA and are being incorporated into primary immunisation schedules for infants and children and for reinforcing doses in older children and adults. In the UK a single-component acellular vaccine is available only for use when the pertussis component has been omitted from all or part of the primary immunisation schedule; if doses of diphtheria and tetanus remain to be given, diphtheria, tetanus, and whole-cell pertussis vaccine should be used followed by acellular pertussis at monthly intervals to complete three doses. A primary course may also be given with the pre-school tetanus and diphtheria booster in a similar way. Acellular vaccines may also be substituted in individuals who have a moderate local reaction or pyrexia following diphtheria, tetanus, and whole-cell pertussis vaccine. Acellular vaccines are given in a dose of 0.5 mL by deep subcutaneous or intramuscular injection.

Acellular vaccines. Vaccination using whole-cell pertussis vaccines has been effective but adverse reactions are common (see above). The immunogenicity of the UK whole-cell vaccine is estimated at about 90% using the current accelerated three-dose schedule.[1] Dissatisfaction with whole-cell vaccines in the 1970s led to reduced uptake and a resurgence of pertussis in several countries. In Japan, research into less reactogenic pertussis vaccines resulted in the introduction of acellular vaccines for routine vaccination in the early 1980s.

The antigenic components of acellular pertussis vaccines are pertussis toxin (PT; also formerly known as lymphocytosis-promoting factor, LPF) either alone or more usually in combination with filamentous haemagglutinin (FHA), the 69 kilodalton outer membrane protein pertactin, and/or fimbrial agglutinogens (with 3 major serotypes; also referred to as fimbrial antigens). Adverse reactions to acellular vaccines are less frequent and less severe than those associated with whole-cell vaccines.[2] The acellular vaccines have successfully controlled pertussis infections but formal comparisons of efficacy with whole-cell vaccines have only been reported more recently. For studies of primary immunisation pertussis vaccine is used in combination with diphtheria and tetanus toxoids, and diphtheria and tetanus vaccines are used in the placebo groups. As with whole-cell vaccines,[3,4] acellular vaccines varied in their efficacy. Multivalent vaccines were generally more effective than monovalent vaccines.[5] It has been argued that a monovalent pertussis toxoid, while providing incomplete protection for the individual, may nevertheless produce adequate herd immunity to inhibit disease transmission.[6] However, the use of multivalent vaccines seems preferable.[7,8]

In general, acellular vaccines approached the efficacy of, and were better tolerated than, whole-cell vaccines.[5,9-12] A surprising result of large studies in Sweden[5] and Italy,[10] in which the acellular vaccines were considerably more effective than the whole-cell vaccines, was the low efficacy of the US whole-cell vaccine (less than 50%). This was attributed to a rapidly waning effect after 3 doses given at 2, 4, and 6 months of age, suggesting that the booster doses at age 12 to 18 months and at school entry are essential to the US schedule. The UK whole-cell vaccine was found to be as effective as a pentavalent acellular vaccine and both were more effective than a trivalent vaccine in a large study in Sweden.[13]

In the UK, confidence in the whole-cell vaccine has been largely restored, and uptake of primary immunisation in infants is approximately 90%.[1] Under these circumstances it is unlikely that there would be any benefit from switching to the use of the more expensive acellular vaccines.[14] However, there is some concern over the incidence of pertussis infection in adults[15] and it is possible that acellular vaccines, which are better tolerated in older recipients than whole-cell vaccines, would be more acceptable if booster doses are added at school entry and in school leavers. In the USA, however, acellular pertussis vaccines are now recommended for both primary immunisation in infants and for the booster doses at 12 to 18 months and at school entry.

1. White JM, et al. The effect of an accelerated immunisation schedule on pertussis in England and Wales. Commun Dis Rep 1996; 6 (review 6): R86–R91.
2. Decker MD, et al. Comparison of 13 acellular pertussis vaccines: adverse reactions. Pediatrics 1995; 96 (suppl): 557–66.
3. Edwards KM, et al. Differences in antibody response to whole-cell pertussis vaccines. Pediatrics 1991; 88: 1019–23.
4. Baker JD, et al. Antibody response to Bordetella pertussis antigens after immunization with American and Canadian whole-cell vaccines. J Pediatr 1992; 121: 523–7.
5. Gustafsson L, et al. A controlled trial of a two-component acellular, five-component acellular, and a whole-cell pertussis vaccine. N Engl J Med 1996; 334: 349–55. Correction. ibid.; 1207.
6. Schneerson R, et al. A toxoid vaccine for pertussis as well as diphtheria? Lessons to be relearned. Lancet 1996; 348: 1289–92.
7. Wirsing von König CH, Schmitt HJ. Toxoid vaccine for pertussis. Lancet 1997; 349: 136.
8. He Q, et al. Toxoid vaccine for pertussis. Lancet 1997; 349: 136–7.
9. Schmitt H-J, et al. Efficacy of acellular pertussis vaccine in early childhood after household exposure. JAMA 1996; 275: 37–41.
10. Greco D, et al. A controlled trial of two acellular vaccines and one whole-cell vaccine against pertussis. N Engl J Med 1996; 334: 341–8.
11. Stehr K, et al. A comparative efficacy trial in Germany in infants who received either the Lederle/Takeda acellular pertussis component DTP (DTaP) vaccine, the Lederle whole-cell component DTP vaccine, or DT vaccine. Pediatrics 1998; 101: 1–11.
12. Giuliano M, et al. Antibody responses and persistence in the two years after immunization with two acellular vaccines and one whole-cell vaccine against pertussis. J Pediatr 1998; 132: 983–8.
13. Olin P, et al. Randomised controlled trial of two-component, three-component, and five-component acellular pertussis vaccines compared with whole-cell pertussis vaccine. Lancet 1997; 350: 1569–77. Correction. ibid.; 351: 454.
14. Miller E. Acellular pertussis vaccines. Arch Dis Child 1995; 73: 390–1.
15. Nenning ME. Prevalence and incidence of adult pertussis in an urban population. JAMA 1996; 275: 1672–4.

Immunisation schedules. A review of the epidemiology and control of pertussis.[1] Pertussis is a common, highly infectious, respiratory disease, predominantly affecting children, and for which there is no effective treatment. WHO has estimated that 60 million cases of pertussis occur annually and that the disease is responsible for half a million to one million deaths each year. The highest incidence of pertussis is observed in developing countries where immunisation is low.

A combined adsorbed diphtheria, tetanus, and pertussis vaccine is now used in most countries but both the strength of the pertussis component and production methods vary, leading to vaccines of different potencies.

Depending upon the country, the age at which a child is given the first dose of the combined vaccine varies from 5 weeks to 6 months. (For summaries of immunisation schedules in the UK and USA, see under Vaccines, p.1530.) In countries with a high incidence of pertussis WHO recommends that immunisation should start at 6 weeks of age and that the schedule involve three doses at monthly intervals. A booster dose should be given one year after the end of the primary series of 3 injections and in some countries a second booster at entry to school is given. Several reports have described the use of a two-dose widely-spaced primary immunisation schedule and this would indeed simplify procedures in developing countries; however, the limitation of such a schedule is the long period of risk between doses without adequate protection and unless the interval can be shortened to 4 weeks, the wide use of such a schedule is not advisable in endemic areas.

1. Muller AS, et al. Pertussis: epidemiology and control. Bull WHO 1986; 64: 321–31.

Preparations

Ph. Eur.: Pertussis Vaccine; Pertussis Vaccine (Acellular Component, Adsorbed); Pertussis Vaccine (Acellular, Co-purified, Adsorbed); Pertussis Vaccine (Adsorbed);
USP 25: Pertussis Vaccine; Pertussis Vaccine Adsorbed.

Proprietary Preparations (details are given in Part 3)
Canad.: Acel-P; *Fr.:* Vaxicoq; *Ger.:* Acel-P; Pa-Vaccinol†; Pac Merieux; Pertuvac†; *Ital.:* Acelluvax; *Switz.:* Acel-P; *Thai.:* Acelluvax.

Pigbel Vaccines (16951-w)

Profile
A vaccine against pigbel (necrotising enteritis), a disease occurring predominantly in children in the highlands of Papua New Guinea, is used for active immunisation against the disease. The vaccine consists of an adsorbed *Clostridium perfringens* type C toxoid.

◊ Subsequent to a study indicating that pigbel vaccine could confer protection against the disease, an immunisation programme was introduced in Papua New Guinea in 1980.[1] Pigbel vaccine was given to children at 2, 4, and 6 months of age and, initially, to older children. A survey has shown a sustained overall fall in the incidence of severe pigbel in children coinci-

dent with the increased induced immunity. However, protection may be relatively short-lived and boosters may be necessary for full protection of young children.

1. Lawrence GW, et al. Impact of active immunisation against enteritis necroticans in Papua New Guinea. Lancet 1990; 336: 1165–7.

Plague Vaccines (7987-j)
ATC — J07AK01.

Plague Vaccine (USP 25) is a sterile suspension of formaldehyde-killed *Yersinia pestis* (strain 195/P). It should be stored at 2° to 8° and not be allowed to freeze.

Adverse Effects and Precautions
As for vaccines in general, p.1529.

Interactions
As for vaccines in general, p.1530.

Uses and Administration
Plague vaccines are used for active immunisation against plague in those occupationally exposed to the organism and in some field workers in infected areas. They may reduce morbidity and mortality in bubonic plague but their activity against pneumonic plague is unknown.

A plague vaccine containing 2000 million inactivated *Yersinia pestis* (strain 195/P) per mL is administered by intramuscular injection. The initial dose for adults and children over 10 years of age is usually 1 mL, and is followed by two further doses, each of 0.2 mL, given 1 to 3 months after the first dose and 5 to 6 months after the second respectively. Booster doses of 0.2 mL may be given at 6-monthly intervals; the interval between booster doses may be extended to every 1 to 2 years in persons who have received 3 or more boosters at intervals of 6 months. First, second, third, and booster doses for children have been: under one year of age, 0.2, 0.04, 0.04, and 0.02 to 0.04 mL respectively; aged 1 to 4 years, 0.4, 0.08, 0.08, and 0.04 to 0.08 mL respectively; 5 to 10 years, 0.6, 0.12, 0.12, and 0.06 to 0.12 mL respectively.

Preparations
USP 25: Plague Vaccine.

Pneumococcal Vaccines (7988-z)
ATC — J07AL01; J07AL02.

Pneumococcal Polysaccharide Vaccine (Ph. Eur.) (Pneumo/Vac; Vaccinum Pneumococcale Polysaccharidum) is a mixture of purified polysaccharide capsular antigens from 23 differing serotypes of *Streptococcus pneumoniae*. Each 0.5-mL dose contains 25 μg of each of the 23 polysaccharide types. An antimicrobial preservative may be added. The vaccine has a pH of 4.5 to 7.4. It should be stored at 2° to 8°, not be allowed to freeze, and be protected from light.

Adverse Effects and Precautions
As for vaccines in general, p.1529. Unless otherwise stated, the information below refers to the unconjugated polyvalent vaccine.

Revaccination of adults is not generally recommended because of the increased incidence and severity of adverse reactions. For details of patient groups in whom revaccination may be considered and timings, see under Uses and Administration, below.

Pneumococcal vaccination is relatively ineffective in patients with multiple myeloma, Hodgkin's and non-Hodgkin's lymphoma, especially during treatment, and in chronic alcoholism. In patients with Hodgkin's disease the use of pneumococcal vaccines is not recommended in those who have received extensive chemotherapy or nodal irradiation. Pneumococcal vaccines should be given at least 10 days before starting immunosuppressive therapy or be delayed until at least 6 months after completion of therapy.

A satisfactory response to the unconjugated polyvalent pneumococcal vaccines is not obtained in children less than 2 years of age and therefore immunisation of this age group is not recommended. In the USA, however, a pneumococcal conjugate vaccine is available that may be given to infants from 6 weeks of age.

Effects on the blood. The manufacturer reports that on rare occasions, relapses have occurred in patients with stabilised idiopathic thrombocytopenic purpura at 2 to 14 days after vaccination against pneumococcal infections, lasting for up to 2 weeks. One such case was reported[1] following revaccination less than 2.5 years after an uneventful primary vaccination with pneumococcal vaccine.

1. Neil VS. Long term management after splenectomy: revaccination may cause relapse. BMJ 1994; 308: 339.

Effects on the kidneys. Glomerulonephritis was described[1] in a splenectomised patient following administration of pneumococcal vaccine. It was postulated that high antibody titres from a recent pneumococcal infection could have contributed.

1. Tan SY, Cumming AD. Vaccine related glomerulonephritis. BMJ 1993; 306: 248.

Effect of nutritional status. An impaired antibody response to pneumococcal vaccine was reported[1] in elderly patients with low serum concentrations of vitamin B[12].

1. Fata FT, et al. Impaired antibody responses to pneumococcal polysaccharide in elderly patients with low serum vitamin B12 levels. Ann Intern Med 1996; 124: 299–304.

Interactions
As for vaccines in general, p.1530.

Uses and Administration
Of the many serotypes of *Streptococcus pneumoniae* the 23 from which antigens are obtained for the most commonly available pneumococcal vaccine are considered to cause about 90% of pneumococcal disease.

Pneumococcal vaccines are used for active immunisation in those at increased risk from infection with the types of *Streptococcus pneumoniae* contained in the vaccine. Pneumococcal vaccines may be in the form of a 23-valent polysaccharide vaccine (suitable only for patients over 2 years of age) or as a conjugate vaccine containing 7 serotypes (suitable for infants aged 2 months to 2 years). In the UK it is recommended that immunisation should be considered in persons who have undergone splenectomy and those with splenic dysfunction due to sickle-cell anaemia or other causes; patients with immunodeficiency or immunosuppression due to disease or treatment including HIV infection at all stages; and persons with chronic cardiac, pulmonary, hepatic, or renal impairment including nephrotic syndrome, or diabetes mellitus.

An antibody response develops by the third week, and usually lasts about 5 years. The antibody response is less reliable and declines more rapidly in young children and persons with impaired immune function.

A single dose of 0.5 mL of the 23-valent vaccine, containing 25 μg of each of the 23 polysaccharide types, is given by subcutaneous or intramuscular injection. The vaccine should be given at least 2 weeks before elective splenectomy or chemotherapy. Revaccination is not generally recommended except, after 5 to 10 years, in patients likely to have rapidly declining antibody concentrations; see below for further discussion.

The pneumococcal conjugate vaccine is given by intramuscular injection. In the UK, the Department of Health recommends that infants under 5 months should be given three single doses of 0.5 mL at intervals of 1 month, starting at 2 months of age, while those aged 5 to 24 months should receive 2 doses at least one month apart. All should receive a single dose of the 23-valent vaccine after their second birthday.

In the USA, three doses of the pneumococcal conjugate vaccine are recommended at 2, 4, and 6 months of age, followed by a fourth dose at 12 to 15 months; it is stated that at least 2 months must elapse before the fourth dose is given. Previously unvaccinated infants aged 7 to 11 months are given two doses of 0.5 mL with an interval of at least 1 month between doses. A third dose is recommended in the second year of life; again in the USA a time interval of 2 months is recommended before this third dose. Previously unvaccinated children aged 12 to 23 months are given two doses of 0.5 mL, separated by an interval of at least 2 months. In the USA a single dose is used for children aged 2 to 9 years.

◊ Although pneumococcal vaccines are effective in protecting against *Streptococcus pneumoniae* infection in healthy subjects there has been much debate over their **efficacy** in patients at increased risk of infection.[1-4] There are several frequently-cited studies demonstrating adequate[5-7] and inadequate[8,9] protection in high-risk groups of patients. Most studies used the now discontinued 14-valent pneumococcal vaccine. They have also been criticised for various aspects of their methodology including the suitability of the chosen end-point.[1,4] It has been suggested that the divergent results are a consequence of the varying type and degree of risk of infection in the populations studied.[1] Most[10-13] but not all[14] studies using the current 23-valent pneumococcal vaccines have demonstrated a useful degree of protection against pneumococcal infections in high-risk groups including the elderly.

One major consequence of the doubts over the efficacy and safety of pneumococcal vaccines has been a low **uptake** of vaccination in persons at risk of infection. It has been estimated that as few as 10% of subjects for whom vaccination is recommended have received it,[15] and surveys[16,17] in splenectomised patients in the UK in 1993 showed that, although the situation was improving, vaccine coverage remained inadequate. Doubts are still occasionally expressed[18] over the necessity to vaccinate any but those at highest risk, despite evidence of efficacy of the 23-valent vaccine in all patient groups covered by current recommendations.[19]

The **recommendations** of the Department of Health in the UK are outlined under Uses and Administration, above. Similar recommendations have been made elsewhere. The Advisory Committee on Immunization Practices in the USA (ACIP)[20] and WHO[21] recommend in addition vaccination of all persons aged 65 years or more. Vaccination of the healthy elderly has also been advocated in the UK[22-25] although the topic remains controversial.[26] Pneumococcal vaccine is also recommended for persons living in environments or social settings with an identified increased risk of pneumococcal disease. Pneumococcal vaccine is not indicated for children with recurrent upper respiratory tract disease including otitis media and sinusitis.

Routine **revaccination** of adults with pneumococcal vaccines is not recommended. The ACIP[20] and the Department of Health in the UK suggest that revaccination be considered after 5 to 10 years for individuals likely to have a rapid decline in antibody titre such as asplenic patients or those with dysfunction of the spleen, severely immunosuppressed patients, or those with nephrotic syndrome. However there is some evidence that earlier revaccination may be needed in these groups.[24] Revaccination may be considered after 3 to 5 years for children at highest risk of pneumococcal infection who would be aged 10 years or under at revaccination.[20]

The increase in pneumococci resistant to antibacterials makes the development of vaccines with improved immunogenicity, especially in young children, more important.[27] Of the possible **new vaccines**, conjugate vaccines have now been developed. Technical difficulties in conjugation mean that most conjugate vaccines use only a subset of the 23 serotypes present in the polysaccharide vaccine.[27] Nevertheless clinical studies have shown that conjugate vaccines can produce an immune response in children under 2 years of age,[28-30] but immunogenicity in a group of healthy adults was no better than that obtained with conventional vaccines.[31] A combined schedule of 7-valent pneumococcal conjugate vaccine followed by 23-valent unconjugated vaccine has been shown to elicit an improved immune response in children and young adults with sickle- cell disease[32] and in the USA, such combined vaccination is recommended for children aged 24 to 59 months who are at increased risk of pneumococcal infection (such as those with sickle-cell haemoglobinopathies, HIV infection, or other immunocompromising or chronic medical conditions). These children should be given two doses of the 7-valent pneumococcal conjugate vaccine, 2 months apart, followed by one dose of a 23-valent pneumococcal polysaccharide vaccine given at least 2 months after the second dose of pneumococcal conjugate vaccine.

1. LaForce FM, Eickhoff TC. Pneumococcal vaccine: an emerging consensus. Ann Intern Med 1988; 108: 757–9.
2. Noah ND. Vaccination against pneumococcal infection. BMJ 1988; 297: 1351–2.
3. Anonymous. When to use the new pneumococcal vaccine. Drug Ther Bull 1990; 28: 31–2.
4. Shann F. Modern vaccines: pneumococcus and influenza. Lancet 1990; 335: 898–901.
5. Gaillat J, et al. Essai clinique du vaccin antipneumococcique chez des personnes âgées vivant en institution. Rev Epidemiol Sante Publique 1985; 33: 437–44.
6. Bolan G, et al. Pneumococcal vaccine efficacy in selected populations in the United States. Ann Intern Med 1986; 104: 1–6.
7. Sims RV, et al. The clinical effectiveness of pneumococcal vaccine in the elderly. Ann Intern Med 1988; 108: 653–7.
8. Forrester HL, et al. Inefficacy of pneumococcal vaccine in a high-risk population. Am J Med 1987; 83: 425–30.
9. Simberkoff MS, et al. Efficacy of pneumococcal vaccine in high-risk patients: results of a Veterans Administration Cooperative Study. N Engl J Med 1986; 315: 1318–27.
10. Lee H, et al. Immunogenicity and safety of a 23-valent pneumococcal polysaccharide vaccine in healthy children and in children at increased risk of pneumococcal infection. Vaccine 1995; 13: 1533–8.
11. Farr BM, et al. Preventing pneumococcal bacteremia in patients at risk. Arch Intern Med 1995; 155: 2336–8.
12. Sankilampi U, et al. Antibody response to pneumococcal capsular polysaccharide vaccine in the elderly. J Infect Dis 1996; 173: 387–93.
13. Furth SL, et al. Pneumococcal polysaccharide vaccine in children with chronic renal disease: a prospective study of antibody response and duration. J Pediatr 1996; 128: 99–101.
14. Örtqvist Å, et al. Randomised trial of 23-valent pneumococcal capsular polysaccharide vaccine in prevention of pneumonia in middle-aged and elderly people. Lancet 1998; 351: 399–403.
15. Williams WW, et al. Immunization policies and vaccine coverage among adults: the risk for missed opportunities. Ann Intern Med 1988; 108: 616–25.
16. Kinnersley P, et al. Pneumococcal vaccination after splenectomy: survey of hospital and primary care records. BMJ 1993; 307: 1398–9.
17. Deodhar HA, et al. Increased risk of sepsis after splenectomy. BMJ 1993; 307: 1408–9.
18. Hirschman JV, Lipsky BA. The pneumococcal vaccine after 15 years of use. Arch Intern Med 1994; 154: 373–7.
19. Butler JC, et al. Pneumococcal polysaccharide vaccine efficacy: an evaluation of current recommendations. JAMA 1993; 270: 1826–31.
20. Centers for Disease Control. Prevention of pneumococcal disease: recommendations of the Advisory Committee on Immunization Practices (ACIP). MMWR 1997; 46 (RR-8): 1–24.
21. Fedson D, et al. WHO recommendations on pneumococcal vaccination: immunization of elderly people with polyvalent pneumococcal vaccine. Infection 1989; 17: 437–41.
22. Steven N, Wright P. Pneumococcal immunisation and the healthy elderly. Lancet 1992; 340: 1036–7. Correction. ibid. 1236.
23. Neal K. Pneumococcal immunisation and the healthy elderly. Lancet 1993; 341: 319.
24. Anonymous. The place of pneumococcal vaccination. Drug Ther Bull 1998; 36: 73–6.
25. Stone S. Pneumococcal vaccine and the elderly. Lancet 2000; 355: 578–9.
26. Bruyn GAW. Pneumococcal immunisation and the healthy elderly. Lancet 1992; 340: 1418.
27. Stephenson J. Conjugate vaccines hold hope for countering resistant pneumococcus. JAMA 1995; 274: 1327–8.
28. Anderson EL, et al. Immunogenicity of heptavalent pneumococcal vaccine in infants. J Pediatr 1996; 128: 649–53.
29. King JC, et al. Safety and immunogenicity of three doses of a five-valent pneumococcal vaccine in children younger than two years with and without human immunodeficiency virus infection. Pediatrics 1997; 99: 575–80.
30. Rennels MB, et al. Safety and immunogenicity of heptavalent pneumococcal vaccine conjugated to CRM197 in United States infants. Pediatrics 1998; 101: 604–11.
31. Powers DC, et al. Reactogenicity and immunogenicity of a protein-conjugated pneumococcal oligosaccharide vaccine in older adults. J Infect Dis 1996; 173: 1014–18.
32. Vernacchio L, et al. Combined schedule of 7-valent pneumococcal conjugate vaccine followed by 23-valent pneumococcal vaccine in children and young adults with sickle cell disease. J Pediatr 1998; 133: 275–8.

Preparations

Ph. Eur.: Pneumococcal Polysaccharide Vaccine.

Proprietary Preparations (details are given in Part 3)
Aust.: Pneumo 23; Pneumovax†; *Austral.:* Pneumovax 23; Prevenar; *Belg.:* Pneumovax 23; Pneumune; *Braz.:* Pneumo 23; *Canad.:* Pneumo 23; Pneumovax 23; Pnu-Imune 23; *Denm.:* Pneumovax 23; Pneumovax 23; Pnu-Imune 23; *Fr.:* Pneumo 23; *Ger.:* Pneumopur; Pneumovax 23; Pnu-Imune 23; *Hong Kong:* Pneumovax 23; *Irl.:* Pneumovax II; Pnu-Immune; *Israel:* Pneumo 23 Imovax; Pneumovax 23; *Ital.:* Pneumo 23; *Mex.:* Pnu-Imune 23; Pulmovax; *Neth.:* Pneumovax 23; Pneumune; *Norw.:* Pneumovax; Pnu-Imune; *Port.:* Pneumo 23; Pnu-Imune; *S.Afr.:* Pneumovax 23; Pneumune; *Singapore:* Pneumo 23; Pneumovax 23; *Spain:* Pneumo 23; Pnu-Inmune; *Swed.:* Pneumovax; Pnu-Imune; *Switz.:* Pneumovax 23; Pnu-Imune 23; *Thai.:* Pneumo 23; Pneumovax 23; *UK:* Pneumovax II; Pnu-Imune; Prevenar; *USA:* Pneumovax 23; Pnu-Imune 23; Prevnar.

Poliomyelitis Vaccines (7992-e)

Polio Vaccines; Poliovirus Vaccines.
ATC — J07BF01; J07BF02; J07BF03.

NOTE. Inactivated poliomyelitis vaccines are sometimes termed Salk Vaccine and live (oral) poliomyelitis vaccines are sometimes termed Sabin Vaccine.

Poliomyelitis Vaccine (Inactivated) (Ph. Eur.) (Pol/Vac(Inact); Inactivated Poliomyelitis Vaccine (BP 2001); Vaccinum Poliomyelitidis Inactivatum) is a liquid preparation of suitable strains of poliomyelitis virus, types 1, 2, and 3, grown in suitable cell cultures and inactivated by a suitable method. Permitted antibacterials may be used in its production and it may contain preservatives. It should be stored at 2° to 8° and be protected from light.

Poliovirus Vaccine Inactivated (USP 25) is a sterile aqueous suspension of poliomyelitis virus, types 1, 2, and 3, grown separately in cultures of monkey kidney tissue and inactivated. Suitable antimicrobial agents may be used during production. It should be stored at 2° to 8°.

Poliomyelitis Vaccine (Oral) (Ph. Eur.) (OPV; Pol/Vac (Oral); Poliomyelitis Vaccine, Live (Oral) (BP 2001); Vaccinum Poliomyelitidis Perorale) is a liquid preparation of suitable live attenuated strains of poliomyelitis virus, types 1, 2, or 3, grown in suitable, approved cell cultures; it may contain any one of the 3 virus types or combinations of them. The trivalent vaccine is standardised for virus titre which is not less than 1×10^6 CCID$_{50}$ for type 1, not less than 1×10^5 CCID$_{50}$ for type 2, and not less than $1 \times 10^{5.5}$ CCID$_{50}$ for type 3 per dose. Permitted antibacterials may be used in its production. It should be stored at 2° to 8°, not be allowed to freeze, and be protected from light.

Poliovirus Vaccine Live Oral (USP 25) is a preparation of a combination of the 3 types of suitable live attenuated polioviruses, grown separately in cultures of monkey kidney tissue. It contains not less than $10^{5.4}$ to $10^{6.4}$ virus titre for type 1, not less than $10^{4.5}$ to $10^{5.5}$ for type 2, and not less than $10^{5.2}$ to $10^{6.2}$ for type 3 per dose. It should be stored at 2° to 8° or in the frozen state. The vaccine should not be thawed and refrozen more than 10 times.

Adverse Effects

As for vaccines in general, p.1529.

Vaccine-associated poliomyelitis has been reported in a small number of recipients of oral poliomyelitis vaccines and in contacts of recipients.

Effects on the nervous system. Case reports of the isolation of poliovaccine virus from the CSF after administration of oral poliomyelitis vaccine.

1. Rantala H, et al. Poliovaccine virus in the cerebrospinal fluid after oral polio vaccination. J Infect 1989; 19: 173–6.
2. Gutierrez K, Abzug MJ. Vaccine-associated poliovirus meningitis in children with ventriculoperitoneal shunts. J Pediatr 1990; 117: 424–7.

GUILLAIN-BARRÉ SYNDROME. A small cluster of cases of Guillain-Barré syndrome has been observed[1] in children after a mass poliomyelitis vaccination campaign in Finland in 1985. An increased frequency of Guillain-Barré syndrome was also seen in adults. However, a direct link with poliovaccine virus infection could not be established and no link between Guillain-Barré syndrome and oral polio vaccine was revealed by a subsequent, epidemiological study in California.[2]

1. Uhari M, et al. Cluster of childhood Guillain-Barré cases after an oral poliovaccine campaign. Lancet 1989; ii: 440–1.
2. Rantala H, et al. Epidemiology of Guillain-Barré syndrome in children: relationship of oral polio vaccine administration to occurrence. J Pediatr 1994; 124: 220–3.

PARALYTIC POLIOMYELITIS. A survey of the incidence of paralytic poliomyelitis following vaccination conducted by WHO[1] reported that, in all but one of the 13 participating countries, the risk was 0.03 per million vaccine recipients. The incidence was least with the use of type 1 strains and greatest with type 3 strains. Paralytic poliomyelitis in contacts of vaccine recipients could be further reduced by ensuring that parents without evidence of previous immunisation receive the vaccine at the same time as their children. The risk of vaccine-associated paralytic poliomyelitis may be increased in immunocompromised patients.

Until recently there has been no satisfactory explanation for the high risk of paralytic poliomyelitis found in Romania by the WHO survey.[1] A case-control study[2] identified intramuscular injections given within 30 days of polio vaccination as a risk factor in the development of paralytic poliomyelitis. This phenomenon, known as provocation paralysis or provocation poliomyelitis has been described with the wild virus[3] and more recently has been recognised as a factor in vaccine-associated paralysis in the UK and USA.[4] Romanian children may be further predisposed to vaccine-associated paralysis because the first dose of polio vaccine is delayed until two to seven months of age, by which time they possess little or no residual maternal antibody.[5]

In the USA, where the majority of cases of clinical poliomyelitis are associated with vaccination, there is evidence that the incidence is still falling.[6-8]

1. Esteves K. Safety of oral poliovirus vaccine: results of a WHO enquiry. Bull WHO 1988; 66: 739–46.
2. Strebel PM, et al. Intramuscular injections within 30 days of immunization with oral poliovirus vaccine—a risk factor for vaccine-associated paralytic poliomyelitis. N Engl J Med 1995; 332: 500–6.
3. Anonymous. Provocation paralysis. Lancet 1992; 340: 1005–6.
4. Wyatt HV. Vaccine-associated poliomyelitis. Lancet 1994; 343: 610.
5. Wright PF, Karzon DT. Minimizing the risks associated with the prevention of poliomyelitis. N Engl J Med 1995; 332: 529–30.
6. Nkowane BM, et al. Vaccine-associated paralytic poliomyelitis. United States: 1973 through 1984. JAMA 1987; 257: 1335–40.
7. Centers for Disease Control. Paralytic poliomyelitis—United States, 1980-1994. MMWR 1997; 46: 79–83.
8. Sepkowitz S. Vaccine-associated paralytic poliomyelitis. Pediatrics 1997; 99: 145.

Precautions

As for vaccines in general, p.1530.

Oral poliomyelitis vaccine may contain trace amounts of penicillin, neomycin, polymyxin, and streptomycin and the inactivated vaccine may contain trace amounts of neomycin and polymyxin: both should be used with caution in patients with severe hypersensitivity to these antibacterials.

Oral poliomyelitis vaccines should not be given to patients with diarrhoea or vomiting.

Because the vaccine virus of oral poliomyelitis vaccines is excreted in the faeces for up to 6 weeks, the contacts of recently vaccinated babies and infants should be advised of the need for strict personal hygiene, particularly hand washing after napkin changing, in order to reduce the possibility of infection in unimmunised contacts. Unimmunised adults can be immunised at the same time as their children.

Immunocompromised patients are at increased risk of developing vaccine-associated paralytic poliomyelitis. Oral poliomyelitis vaccines should not be given to immunocompromised patients or their household contacts and in these persons an inactivated vaccine should be used (see Uses and Administration, below). Asymptomatic HIV-positive persons may receive oral poliomyelitis vaccines but faecal excretion of the vaccine virus may continue for longer than in uninfected individuals. For symptomatic HIV-positive persons the use of inactivated poliomyelitis vaccine may be considered.

Intramuscular injections given after the oral vaccine may also increase the risk of vaccine-associated paralytic poliomyelitis (see above).

Pregnancy. Live vaccines such as *oral poliomyelitis vaccines* are generally contra-indicated in pregnancy because of a theoretical risk to the fetus. Population-wide mass vaccination programmes become impossible, however, if pregnant mothers and women of child-bearing age are to be excluded.[1] In February 1985 mass vaccination with live oral poliomyelitis vaccine was started during a poliomyelitis outbreak in Finland.[1] Pregnant women were advised to take the vaccine. An analysis of all reported congenital malformations in the years 1982 to 1986 suggested that oral poliomyelitis vaccine had no harmful effects on fetal development as measured by overall prevalence of malformations or as the incidence of either CNS or orofacial defects. The results do not, however, exclude an effect measurable by other criteria of fetal development; further analysis will examine the possible increase in rare types of congenital defect.

The incidence of spontaneous abortions was measured during a mass poliomyelitis vaccination campaign in Israel.[2] The number of spontaneous abortions did not differ between controls and women vaccinated during the first trimester of pregnancy; the percentage of spontaneous abortions in relation to live births was also similar. Microscopic examination of placentas from spontaneous abortions indicated no effect of oral poliomyelitis vaccine on the frequency or type of pathological changes. In addition, subsequent epidemiological study[3] found no increases in congenital malformations or in premature births during the period of and immediately following the vaccination campaign compared with those born before the campaign.

The Collaborative Perinatal Project in the USA[4] followed up 50 897 pregnancies to examine risk factors for the development of malignancies in offspring born between 1959 and 1966. In 18 342 children whose mothers were vaccinated during pregnancy with *inactivated poliomyelitis vaccines* there were 14 malignancies (7.6 per 10 000) and in 32 555 non-exposed children there were 10 malignancies (3.1 per 10 000). There were 7 tumours derived from neural tissue in the exposed children (3.8 per 10 000) and one in non-exposed children (0.3 per 10 000). Thus there was an excess of neural tumours but not of leukaemias or other malignancies in children exposed *in utero* to inactivated poliomyelitis vaccine. No malignancies occurred among the children born to 3056 women who received oral poliomyelitis vaccine. Serum samples collected from mothers on entry into the Collaborative Perinatal Project and at delivery have subsequently been analysed[5] for the presence of antibodies to Simian virus 40 (SV40). None of the serum samples from 8 mothers of infants with neural tumours had antibodies to SV40. Two of the 7 mothers of infants with leukaemia had SV40 antibodies, but only one had conversion during pregnancy. None of the samples from the 7 mothers of children with other types of cancer had antibodies. Three of 36 controls had antibodies, but in both the first and second samples. The association between administration of inactivated poliomyelitis vaccine to mothers and neural tumours in their offspring could not be attributed to contamination of vaccine with SV40.

1. Harjulehto T, *et al.* Congenital malformations and oral poliovirus vaccination during pregnancy. *Lancet* 1989; i: 771–2.
2. Ornoy A, *et al.* Spontaneous abortions following oral poliovirus vaccination in first trimester. *Lancet* 1990; i: 800.
3. Ornoy A, Ben Ishai P. Congenital anomalies after oral poliovirus vaccination during pregnancy. *Lancet* 1993; 341: 1162.
4. Heinonen OP, *et al.* Immunization during pregnancy against poliomyelitis and influenza in relation to childhood malignancy. *Int J Epidemiol* 1973; 2: 229–35.
5. Rosa FW, *et al.* Absence of antibody response to simian virus 40 after inoculation with killed-poliovirus vaccine of mothers of offspring with neurologic tumors. *N Engl J Med* 1988; 318: 1469.

Interactions

As for vaccines in general, p.1530.

Normal immunoglobulins. Although the concurrent administration of live vaccines and immunoglobulins is generally not recommended, normal immunoglobulin had no effect on the antibody response to oral poliomyelitis vaccine when the 2 preparations were given simultaneously to 50 subjects.[1]

1. Green MS, *et al.* Response to trivalent oral poliovirus vaccine with and without immune serum globulin in young adults in Israel in 1988. *J Infect Dis* 1990; 162: 971–4.

Pertussis vaccines. For a report of a diminished immune response to the pertussis component of diphtheria, tetanus, and pertussis vaccine when mixed with inactivated poliomyelitis vaccine, see Pertussis vaccines, p.1556.

Uses and Administration

Poliomyelitis vaccines are used for active immunisation against poliomyelitis. For discussion of immunisation schedules see under Vaccines, p.1530. Both live (oral) poliomyelitis vaccines and inactivated poliomyelitis vaccines are available. The oral vaccine stimulates the formation of antibodies both in the

blood and in the mucosal tissues of the gastrointestinal tract.

In the UK an oral poliomyelitis vaccine, containing the three types of poliovirus (trivalent), is recommended for the primary immunisation of all age groups, given as a course of 3 doses at intervals of 4 weeks. The dose of the oral poliomyelitis vaccine is dropped directly into the mouth of an infant or given on a sugar lump to older children and adults. For children who received primary immunisation during infancy reinforcing doses of the oral vaccine are recommended at school entry and before leaving school. Further reinforcing doses are necessary only in adults exposed to infection including travellers to countries where poliomyelitis is epidemic or endemic and health care workers in contact with poliomyelitis cases. A single dose is given, repeated every 10 years if necessary.

In the USA, either the oral or the inactivated vaccine may be used for primary immunisation. In 1997, the controversial decision was made to recommend the use of inactivated vaccine for the first two doses given at 2 and 4 months of age, completing immunisation with two doses of oral vaccine given at between 12 and 18 months, and at 4 to 6 years of age. Subsequently, the recommended schedule has been further changed to four doses of inactivated vaccine given at 2 months, 4 months, 6 to 18 months, and 4 to 6 years of age. See Choice of Vaccine, below for further discussion.

On the occurrence of a single case of paralytic poliomyelitis from wild virus, a single dose of the oral vaccine is recommended for all persons in the neighbourhood, regardless of whether they have previously been immunised. A primary course should be completed in previously unimmunised individuals. Immunisation of contacts is unnecessary in the case of vaccine-associated infections.

Inactivated poliomyelitis vaccine is recommended in the UK for the immunisation of persons in whom the use of the live oral vaccine is contra-indicated; inactivated vaccine, rather than the live oral vaccine, is also recommended for contacts of immunosuppressed persons and may be considered for symptomatic HIV-positive individuals. The inactivated vaccine is given by subcutaneous injection in a dose of 0.5 mL using a similar dosage schedule to the oral vaccine.

Choice of vaccine. In the USA, both oral and inactivated poliomyelitis vaccines (OPV and IPV respectively) are available for primary immunisation. Three schedule options, each involving a total of four doses of vaccine at or before school entry, have been available to physicians:[1]

- sequential IPV and OPV (2 doses of IPV at 2 and 4 months of age, followed by 2 doses of OPV at 12 to 18 months and 4 to 6 years) is intended to minimise the risk of vaccine associated paralytic poliomyelitis (VAPP) while producing adequate intestinal immunity
- IPV only (dose intervals as above) is recommended when OPV is contra-indicated and to reduce the risk of VAPP in unimmunised household contacts of the vaccine recipient
- OPV only (when the third dose may be given 2 months after the second dose) is recommended when rapid immunisation is necessary, for example in older children, or in areas where vaccine uptake is low. It also has the advantage of requiring no injections.

In 1996, the Advisory Committee on Immunization Practices (ACIP) of the Centers for Disease Control and Prevention recommended that the sequential IPV and OPV schedule should be preferred on the basis that, while there had been no cases of poliomyelitis from wild poliovirus in the USA since 1979, 8 to 10 cases of VAPP continued to occur each year. This decision was criticised by commentators both in the USA and elsewhere. Objections raised included the lack of experience with the recommended combined schedule, the lack of evidence that it would reduce the incidence of VAPP, and a possible reduction in compliance because of the increased number of injections needed.[2] Added to this was the greater cost of IPV than OPV which may have further reduced compliance and raised doubts over the cost-effectiveness of the strategy.[3,4] Nevertheless, in 1999 both the ACIP and the American Academy of Pediatrics (AAP) issued revised recommendations[5,6] in which they advocated the use of IPV only and recommended that OPV no longer be given for routine immunisation: they recommended that use of OPV be limited to special situations such as mass vaccination campaigns to control outbreaks.

Commentators for WHO[7] stressed the necessity of the continued use of OPV for global eradication of poliomyelitis (see below). WHO was concerned that the change in US policy could be interpreted as implying that OPV alone is ineffective or unsafe, and might lead to the adoption of inappropriate vaccine policies in countries where wild polio still exists. The continued use of OPV for the global eradication strategy was again endorsed by both the ACIP[6] and the AAP.[5]

1. Committee on Infectious Diseases, American Academy of Pediatrics. Poliomyelitis prevention: recommendations for use of inactivated poliovirus vaccine and live oral poliovirus vaccine. *Pediatrics* 1997; 99: 300–305.
2. Judelsohn R. Changing the US polio immunization schedule would be bad public health policy. *Pediatrics* 1996; 98: 115–16.
3. Miller MA, *et al.* Cost-effectiveness of incorporating inactivated poliovirus vaccine into the routine childhood immunization schedule. *JAMA* 1996; 276: 967–71.
4. Schneider S. The new immunization debate. *Pediatrics* 1996; 98: 795.
5. Committee on Infectious Diseases, American Academy of Pediatrics. Prevention of poliomyelitis: recommendations for use of only inactivated poliovirus vaccine for routine immunization. *Pediatrics* 1999; 104: 1404–6.
6. Centers for Disease Control. Recommendations of the Advisory Committee on Immunization Practices: revised recommendations for routine poliomyelitis vaccination. *MMWR* 1999; 48: 590.
7. Hull HF, Lee JW. Sabine, Salk, or sequential? *Lancet* 1996; 347: 630.

Eradication of infection. In 1988, WHO announced[1] their goal of eradicating poliomyelitis by the year 2000 and, while considerable progress was made towards achieving it, sporadic outbreaks of disease do still occur in unimmunised or inadequately immunised populations[2,3] and are reminders of the importance of maintaining the momentum of the WHO campaign. The campaign continues, with the renewed goal of global polio eradication by the year 2005.

The WHO campaign depended on four strategies:[1]

- routine immunisation—although routine immunisation alone cannot eliminate polio, it remains the foundation of eradication policy
- national immunisation days—regular (usually annual) nationwide immunisation of all children under 5 years of age regardless of immunisation history
- immunisation after an outbreak—all children under 5 years of age living in the vicinity of a suspected case receive one dose of oral vaccine
- mopping-up immunisation—house-to-house immunisation of children in high-risk areas to reach children missed during routine immunisation or national immunisation days.

WHO has consistently argued for the continued use of oral poliomyelitis vaccine (OPV) rather than inactivated vaccine (IPV) in immunisation schedules. The main argument must be the proven efficacy of repeated doses of OPV to abort outbreaks[4] and eliminate wild virus entirely, notably in South America.[1] Other advantages include the rapid induction of both humoral and intestinal immunity that is necessary to interrupt wild virus transmission; passive transfer of vaccine virus to non-immunised individuals improving population immunity; ease of administration by non-medical personnel; and the low cost of OPV.[5]

OPV produces a lower rate of seroconversion in developing countries than in developed countries, typically needing at least 5 doses to produce an adequate response.[1] There have been reports of poliomyelitis occurring in children who have completed a three-dose course of OPV.[6-8] Possible reasons for this suboptimal response include high levels of maternal antibodies, inhibition of types 1 and 3 viruses by type 2, interference from competing enteroviruses, and diarrhoea.[1,9] Mass immunisation campaigns are reported to produce a higher immune response than equivalent doses given in the routine schedule, and are seen as an essential adjunct to routine immunisation.[10] Seroconversion rates are highest when the vaccine is administered during mass campaigns in the cool and dry season.[1]

There have been several advocates of IPV either as an alternative or in addition to OPV. Most cite the higher immunogenicity of IPV and its successful use in some (mainly industrialised) countries.[11,12] Combined IPV and OPV schedules have been shown to produce high levels of humoral immunity, with intestinal immunity equivalent to that produced by OPV alone.[13] The use of combined IPV and OPV schedules in countries which have not eliminated the wild virus could improve the effectiveness of routine vaccination schedules.[11,14] In the USA, a combined schedule was previously advocated to reduce vaccine associated paralytic poliomyelitis while still providing protection against transmission of imported wild virus although use of OPV is now no longer recommended for routine immunisation (see Choice of Vaccine, above).

However, most cases of poliomyelitis in endemic countries occur among unimmunised children and the main priority remains to improve vaccine uptake rather than to alter immunisation schedules.[1,15] There is concern that uncertainty fostered by a change in vaccination policy could be interpreted as implying that OPV alone is ineffective or unsafe, and the central message that high uptake of vaccine is essential could be lost.[5]

1. Hull HF, *et al.* Paralytic poliomyelitis: seasoned strategies, disappearing disease. *Lancet* 1994; 343: 1331–7.
2. van Niekerk ABW, *et al.* Outbreak of paralytic poliomyelitis in Namibia. *Lancet* 1994; 344: 661–4.

The symbol † denotes a preparation no longer actively marketed

3. Oostvogel PM, *et al.* Poliomyelitis outbreak in an unvaccinated community in the Netherlands, 1992-93. *Lancet* 1994; **344:** 665–70.
4. Greco D, *et al.* Poliomyelitis vaccination strategies for Europe. *Lancet* 1997; **349:** 437.
5. Hull HF, Lee JW. Sabine, Salk, or sequential? *Lancet* 1996; **347:** 630.
6. Sutter RW, *et al.* Outbreak of paralytic poliomyelitis in Oman: evidence for widespread transmission among fully vaccinated children. *Lancet* 1991; **338:** 715–20.
7. Samuel R, *et al.* Persisting poliomyelitis after high coverage with oral poliovaccine. *Lancet* 1993; **341:** 903.
8. Mudur G. Flawed immunisation policies in India led to polio paralysis. *BMJ* 1998; **316:** 1264.
9. WHO Collaborative Study Group on Oral Poliovirus Vaccine. Factors affecting the immunogenicity of oral poliovirus vaccine: a prospective evaluation in Brazil and the Gambia. *J Infect Dis* 1995; **171:** 1097–1106.
10. Richardson G, *et al.* Immunogenicity of oral poliovirus vaccine administered in mass campaigns versus routine immunization programmes. *Bull WHO* 1995; **73:** 769–77.
11. Patriarca PA, *et al.* Progress in polio eradication. *Lancet* 1993; **342:** 1461–4.
12. Preston NW. Polio eradication. *Lancet* 1994; **344:** 1163
13. WHO Collaborative Study Group on Oral and Inactivated Polio-virus Vaccines. Combined immunization of infants with oral and inactivated poliovirus vaccines: results of a randomized trial in the Gambia, Oman, and Thailand. *Bull WHO* 1996; **75:** 253–68.
14. Moriniere BJ, *et al.* Immunogenicity of a supplemental dose of oral versus inactivated poliomyelitis vaccine. *Lancet* 1993; **341:** 1545–50.
15. Chander J, Subrahmanyan S. Mass polio vaccination. *BMJ* 1996; **312:** 1178–9.

Preparations

Ph. Eur.: Poliomyelitis Vaccine (Inactivated); Poliomyelitis Vaccine (Oral);
USP 25: Poliovirus Vaccine Inactivated; Poliovirus Vaccine Live Oral.

Proprietary Preparations (details are given in Part 3)
Austral.: Enpovax HDC; Ipol; **Belg.:** Imovax Polio; Sabin; **Fin.:** Imovax Polio; **Fr.:** Imovax Polio; **Ger.:** IPV Merieux; IPV-Vire-lon; Oral-Virelon; Polio-Vaccinol†; Virelon C†; **Hong Kong:** Buccapol†; Imovax Polio; **Israel:** Imovax Polio; Polioral; **Ital.:** Imovax Polio; Polio Sabin (Orale); Polioral; Poliovax-IN; **Mex.:** Polio Sabin; **Norw.:** Imovax Polio; **NZ:** Ipol; **S.Afr.:** OPV-Mer-ieux; Polioral; **Singapore:** Buccapol†; Imovax Polio; **Spain:** Vac Antipolio Or; Vac Antipolio Oral†; Vac Polio Sabin; Vac Poli-omielitica; **Swed.:** Imovax Polio; **Switz.:** Poloral†; **Thai.:** Polio Sabin; Polioral; **USA:** Ipol; Orimune.

Pseudomonas Immunoglobulins (11611-t)

Profile
Preparations containing antibodies against *Pseudomonas aeruginosa* have been used in some countries for passive immuni-sation against severe pseudomonal infections.

Pseudomonas Vaccines (7993-l)

Profile
A number of polyvalent *Pseudomonas aeruginosa* conjugate vaccines are under investigation for the prevention of pseu-domonal infections in a variety of disease states.

◊ References.
1. Schaad UB, *et al.* Safety and immunogenicity of Pseudomonas aeruginosa conjugate A vaccine in cystic fibrosis. *Lancet* 1991; **338:** 1236–7.
2. Cryz SJ, *et al.* Immunization of noncolonized cystic fibrosis pa-tients against Pseudomonas aeruginosa. *J Infect Dis* 1994; **169:** 1159–62.
3. Lang AB, *et al.* Effect of high-affinity anti-Pseudomonas aerugi-nosa lipopolysaccharide antibodies induced by immunization on the rate of Pseudomonas aeruginosa infection in patients with cystic fibrosis. *J Pediatr* 1995; **127:** 711–17.
4. Campbell WN, *et al.* Immunogenicity of a 24-valent Klebsiella capsular polysaccharide vaccine and an eight-valent Pseu-domonas O-polysaccharide conjugate vaccine administered to victims of acute trauma. *Clin Infect Dis* 1996; **23:** 179–81.
5. Mansouri E, *et al.* Safety and immunogenicity of a Pseudomonas aeruginosa hybrid outer membrane protein F-I vaccine in human volunteers. *Infect Immun* 1999; **67:** 1461–70.
6. Knapp B, *et al.* A recombinant hybrid outer membrane protein for vaccination against Pseudomonas aeruginosa. *Vaccine* 1999; **17:** 1663–6.
7. Lee NG, *et al.* Immunization of burn-patients with a Pseu-domonas aeruginosa outer membrane protein vaccine elicits an-tibodies with protective efficacy. *Vaccine* 2000; **18:** 1952–61.

Q Fever Vaccines (16972-z)

Profile
A Q fever vaccine consisting of a purified killed suspension of *Coxiella burnetii* is available in Australia. It is prepared from Phase I Henzerling strain of *C. burnetii* grown in the yolk sacs of embryonated eggs. A single 0.5-mL subcutaneous dose is given for active immunisation in individuals at high risk of Q fever. These include abattoir workers, veterinarians, and labo-ratory workers handling potentially infected tissue.

Preparations

Proprietary Preparations (details are given in Part 3)
Austral.: Q-Vax.

Rabies Antisera (7995-j)

ATC — J06AA06.

Antirabies Serum (USP 25) is a sterile solution containing an-tiviral substances obtained from the serum or plasma of a healthy animal, usually the horse, that has been immunised by vaccine against rabies. It contains a suitable antimicrobial agent. It should be stored at 2° to 8°.

Adverse Effects and Precautions
As for antisera in general, p.1529.

A skin test should be carried out before rabies antisera are ad-ministered.

Hypersensitivity. In a retrospective study[1] of 3156 patients who received rabies antisera, 51 (1.6%) developed one or more symptoms or signs characteristic of serum sickness. All pa-tients recovered within 7 days of the onset of the reaction. There was a higher incidence of serum-sickness-like reactions in females and individuals aged over 21 years. An immediate hypersensitivity reaction occurred in only one patient. The low incidence of adverse reactions compared with earlier studies may be attributed to the reduced protein content of the prepara-tion used.
1. Wilde H, *et al.* Purified equine rabies immune globulin: a safe and affordable alternative to human rabies immune globulin. *Bull WHO* 1989; **67:** 731–6.

Uses and Administration
Rabies antisera have been used to provide passive immunisa-tion against rabies but the use of rabies immunoglobulins (see below) is preferred.

Preparations
USP 25: Antirabies Serum.

Rabies Immunoglobulins (1239-f)

ATC — J06BB05.

Human Rabies Immunoglobulin (Ph. Eur.) (Rabies Immu-noglobulin (BP 2001); Immunoglobulinum Humanum Rabi-cum) is a liquid or freeze-dried preparation containing human immunoglobulins, mainly immunoglobulin G (IgG). It is ob-tained from plasma from donors immunised against rabies and contains specific antibodies that neutralise the rabies virus. Normal immunoglobulin may be added. It contains not less than 150 international units per mL. The liquid preparation should be stored, protected from light, in a colourless, glass container. The freeze-dried preparation should be stored, pro-tected from light, in a colourless, glass container, under vacu-um or under an inert gas.

Rabies Immune Globulin (USP 25) is a sterile solution of globulins derived from plasma or serum from selected adult hu-man donors who have been immunised with rabies vaccine and have developed high titres of rabies antibody. It contains 10 to 18% of protein of which not less than 80% is monomeric im-munoglobulin G. It has a potency of 150 international units per mL. It contains glycine as a stabilising agent, and a suitable preservative. A solution diluted to contain 1% of protein has a pH of 6.4 to 7.2. It should be stored at 2° to 8°.

Adverse Effects and Precautions
As for immunoglobulins in general, p.1529.

Uses and Administration
Rabies immunoglobulins are used for passive immunisation against rabies. They are used in conjunction with active immu-nisation with rabies vaccines (see below) as part of the postex-posure treatment for the prevention of rabies in previously unimmunised persons who have been bitten by rabid animals or animals suspected of being rabid. The recommended dose of rabies immunoglobulin is 20 international units per kg body-weight, up to half of which should be infiltrated around the wound with the remainder being given intramuscularly at a dif-ferent site to that at which the vaccine was administered.

Preparations
Ph. Eur.: Human Rabies Immunoglobulin;
USP 25: Rabies Immune Globulin.

Proprietary Preparations (details are given in Part 3)
Aust.: Berirab; Rabuman†; **Austral.:** Imogam; **Canad.:** BayRab; Hyperab†; Imogam; **Fr.:** Imogam Rage; **Ger.:** Berirab; Tollwut-globulin†; **Hong Kong:** BayRab; Rabuman; **Israel:** Hyperab; Im-ogam Rabies; **Ital.:** Haimarab; Rabies Gamma; Rabuman; **Mex.:** BayRab; **S.Afr.:** Rabigam; **Spain:** Imogam Rabia†; Lyssuman†; **Switz.:** Rabuman; **Thai.:** Rabuman; **USA:** BayRab; Imogam Ra-bies.

Rabies Vaccines (7997-c)

ATC — J07BG01.

Rabies Vaccine for Human Use Prepared in Cell Cultures (Ph. Eur.) (Rab/Vac; Rabies Vaccine (BP 2001); Vaccinum Ra-biei ex Cellulis ad Usum Humanum) is a sterile freeze-dried suspension of inactivated rabies virus; a suitable strain is grown in an approved cell culture. The cell-culture medium may con-tain suitable antibacterials at the smallest effective concentra-tion. The vaccine is prepared immediately before use by the addition of a suitable sterile liquid. The estimated potency is

not less than 2.5 international units per dose. The dried vaccine should be stored at 2° to 8° and be protected from light.

Rabies Vaccine (USP 25) is a sterile preparation, in dried or liquid form, of inactivated rabies virus obtained from inoculat-ed diploid cell cultures. It has a potency of not less than 2.5 international units per dose. It should be stored at 2° to 8°.

Adverse Effects and Precautions
As for vaccines in general, p.1529.

Patients may experience pain, erythema, and indura-tion at the injection site after the use of any type of rabies vaccine; nausea, headache, fever, malaise, or myalgia may also occur. Hypersensitivity reactions including anaphylaxis occur more commonly with vaccines prepared from non-human sources than with human diploid-cell vaccine.

Neuroparalytic reactions (transverse myelitis, neu-ropathy, or encephalopathy) have been associated with the use of animal brain-tissue vaccines and, to a lesser extent, with duck-embryo vaccines.

There are only isolated reports of neurological reac-tions after administration of human diploid-cell vac-cines.

Effects on the nervous system. The incidence of neuropar-alytic accidents following a course of nerve-tissue vaccines is known to vary from country to country.[1] The risk of CNS dam-age associated with the use of rabies vaccines prepared in the brains of adult animals has been stated to be about 1 in 2000 doses administered.[2] Paralytic accidents have occurred much less frequently with vaccines produced from brain tissue of mice younger than 9 days of age compared with older animals[1] and a particularly high risk of neurological complications has been observed with a sheep-brain vaccine.[3]

Neuroparalytic reactions occur less frequently with duck-em-bryo than nerve-tissue vaccines.[1] In an estimated 424 000 pa-tients receiving duck-embryo rabies vaccine in the USA from 1958 to 1971 there were 137 reports of minor transient neuro-logical reactions, 4 of transverse myelitis, 5 of neuropathy, and 4 of encephalopathy (2 fatal).[4]

There are only isolated reports of neuroparalytic reactions as-sociated with human diploid-cell vaccines.[5,6]
1. WHO. WHO expert committee on rabies: seventh report. *WHO Tech Rep Ser 709* 1984.
2. WHO. WHO expert committee on biological standardization: thirty-seventh report. *WHO Tech Rep Ser 760* 1987.
3. Swaddiwuthipong W, *et al.* A high rate of neurological compli-cations following Semple anti-rabies vaccine. *Trans R Soc Trop Med Hyg* 1988; **82:** 472–5.
4. Rubin RH, *et al.* Adverse reactions to duck embryo rabies vac-cine: range and incidence. *Ann Intern Med* 1973; **78:** 643–9.
5. Knittel T, *et al.* Guillain-Barré syndrome and human diploid cell rabies vaccine. *Lancet* 1989; **i:** 1334–5.
6. Tornatore CS, Richert JR. CNS demyelination associated with diploid cell rabies vaccine. *Lancet* 1990; **335:** 1346–7.

Hypersensitivity. An analysis[1] based on clinical observation of 108 cases of systemic hypersensitivity reactions following immunisation with human diploid-cell rabies vaccine reported to the Centers for Disease Control in the USA over the period June 1980 to March 1984 revealed 9 cases of presumed type I immediate hypersensitivity (incidence of 1 in 10 000 vac-cinees), 87 cases of presumed type III hypersensitivity (9 in 10 000 vaccinees), and 12 cases of indeterminate type. All the reactions presumed to be type I occurred during either primary pre- or postexposure immunisation whereas 93% of the presumed type III reactions were observed following booster immunisations. Presenting features of the type III reaction included generalised or pruritic rash or urticaria, angioedema, arthralgias, fever, nausea, vomiting, and malaise.
1. Centers for Disease Control. Systemic allergic reactions follow-ing immunization with HDCV. *JAMA* 1984; **251:** 2194–5.

Spongiform encephalopathies. Possible transmission of Creutzfeldt-Jakob disease associated with sheep-brain rabies vaccine has been reported from India.[1] It was suggested that transmission of the abnormal prion protein from sheep with scrapie could be implicated.
1. Arya SC. Acquisition of spongiform encephalopathies in India through sheep-brain rabies vaccination. *Natl Med J India* 1992; **4:** 311–12.

Interactions
As for vaccines in general, p.1530.

Antimalarials. Studies suggesting that continuous antimalar-ial chemoprophylaxis with *chloroquine* during primary immu-nisation with human diploid-cell rabies vaccine administered intradermally for pre-exposure prophylaxis may be associated with a poor antibody response.[1,2]
1. Taylor DN, *et al.* Chloroquine prophylaxis associated with a poor antibody response to human diploid cell rabies vaccine. *Lancet* 1984; **i:** 1405.
2. Pappaioanou M, *et al.* Antibody response to preexposure human diploid-cell rabies vaccine given concurrently with chloroquine. *N Engl J Med* 1986; **314:** 280–4.

Uses and Administration

Rabies vaccines are used for active immunisation against rabies. They are used as part of postexposure treatment to prevent rabies in patients who have been bitten by rabid animals or animals suspected of being rabid. Infection does not take place through unbroken skin but is possible through uninjured mucous membranes and has been reported after the inhalation of virus in the laboratory. Rabies vaccines are also used for pre-exposure prophylaxis against rabies in persons exposed to a high risk of being bitten by rabid or potentially rabid animals.

Schedules for prophylaxis and treatment of rabies are recommended by WHO (see below) and many countries have immunisation schedules based on these.

In the UK a rabies vaccine prepared from inactivated Wistar rabies virus strain PM/WI38 1503-3M cultured on human diploid cells is used. It contains not less than 2.5 international units per mL. The vaccine should be given by deep subcutaneous or intramuscular injection into the deltoid region, or in a child, the anterolateral aspect of the thigh.

For **pre-exposure prophylaxis** against rabies the recommended schedule in the UK for the human diploid-cell vaccine is 3 doses, each of 1 mL, by deep subcutaneous or intramuscular injection on days 0, 7, and 28; alternatively a dose of 0.1 mL has been given intradermally on the same days. Booster doses may be given every 2 to 3 years depending upon the risk of exposure, but where postexposure treatment is readily available booster doses are not normally required in individuals who have received three doses of vaccine.

A 2-dose schedule has also been employed for travellers to enzootic areas who are not animal handlers: doses of 1 mL by deep subcutaneous or intramuscular injection, or 0.1 mL intradermally, are given 4 weeks apart. This schedule is somewhat less effective than the 3-dose schedule and should only be used where postexposure treatment will be readily available.

It has been suggested that rapid immunisation of personnel engaged in the care of a patient with rabies may be achieved by the intradermal administration of 0.1 mL into each limb (total of 0.4 mL) on the first day of exposure to the patient.

For **postexposure treatment**, thorough cleansing of the wound with soap and water is imperative. The recommended schedule in the UK for the human diploid-cell vaccine is 5 doses, each of 1 mL, by deep subcutaneous or intramuscular injection on days 0, 3, 7, 14, and 30. The UK manufacturers also recommend a further dose on day 90. Vaccination should be started as soon as possible after exposure, and may be discontinued if it is proved that the patient was not at risk. In previously unimmunised patients at high risk, rabies immunoglobulin (see above) should also be given at the same time as the first dose of vaccine. A modified course of vaccine administration may be employed in previously immunised persons consisting of 2 doses on day 0 and between days 3 to 7; rabies immunoglobulins are not required in these patients.

Rabies. Rabies is caused by infection with a rhabdovirus of the genus Lyssavirus which also contains a number of related viruses some of which have caused disease in man. The rabies virus is usually transmitted by the bite of an infected animal or contamination of broken skin by saliva. Infection is possible via intact mucous membranes and by aerosol transmission, but infection is unlikely following contamination of intact skin. Other body fluids such as urine and tears should be regarded as potentially infectious.

Human rabies is almost always fatal once symptoms have appeared. After an incubation period of about 30 to 90 days there is a prodrome lasting up to about 10 days of generally non-specific symptoms. This prodrome is followed by the onset of acute neurological symptoms. Periods of hyperexcitability accompanied by severe agitation and bizarre behaviour alternate with periods of lucidity. Severe spasms of the larynx and pharynx may be provoked by attempts at swallowing leading to hydrophobia or by air blown at the face (aerophobia). Other symptoms include hypersalivation, fever, and convulsions. An alternative presentation of nervous system involvement is a progressive flaccid paralysis. Patients not dying through respiratory or cardiac arrest during the acute phase may develop any of a number of complications culminating in coma and death or

The symbol † denotes a preparation no longer actively marketed

(very rarely) recovery; only 3 patients are documented as having survived after the onset of coma, and all had received either pre- or postexposure immunisation.

Rabies has a worldwide distribution, primarily in domesticated and wild dogs but also in bats and other warm-blooded animals, although some countries, including the UK, most of Australasia, and Antarctica are designated as rabies-free areas. National control programmes involve epidemiological surveillance, mass canine immunisation campaigns, and dog population management. The recent development of oral animal vaccines delivered on baited food has met with considerable success in a number of areas and has become an essential tool for eliminating rabies in wild animals. Rigorously applied controls of international transfer of animals including certification of vaccination and quarantine for animals entering rabies-free areas are necessary to prevent re-introduction of rabies.

Although a number of treatments have been tried including various antivirals including interferons, high doses of rabies immunoglobulin, and corticosteroids, none has shown evidence of effectiveness. Avoidance of rabies after contact with a suspected or confirmed rabid animal depends upon prompt and thorough cleansing of the contaminated site and administration of rabies vaccine with or without rabies immunoglobulins immediately. For a brief outline of postexposure treatment, see below; however, readers are strongly advised to consult the complete guidelines published by WHO if they are likely to be involved with the management of patients exposed to rabies.

Prophylaxis is recommended in persons at high risk of exposure, either due to their occupation or those travelling in enzootic areas. The main obstacle to mass pre-exposure vaccination appears to be the high cost of cell culture vaccines. See under Pre-exposure Immunisation (below) for outlines of recommended vaccination schedules.

CHOICE OF VACCINES. Many different rabies vaccines are available for human use: those derived from nerve tissue of animals; those derived from avian tissues (duck embryos); and those prepared in cell cultures. Originally the only source of rabies virus available for vaccine production was infected brain tissue from adult animals; such vaccines contain neuroparalytic and encephalitogenic substances and WHO supports the trend to limit, or abandon completely, their production.[1] Vaccines prepared from virus grown in duck embryos have been developed and a purified duck-embryo vaccine (PDEV) may provide similar efficacy and safety to vaccines produced from cell cultures.[1] Improvements in biotechnology may reduce the costs of cell-culture production. Among the vaccines prepared in this way is one developed from an adapted Pasteur strain of virus grown in a human diploid cell strain (HDCV), a purified chick embryo-cell vaccine (PCECV), and a purified Vero-cell vaccine (PVRV).[2] There appears to be little difference in terms of safety and antigenicity between HDCV, PCECV, PVRV, and PDEV in recommended regimens.[2] The incidence of severe hypersensitivity reactions should, however, be lower with PVRV and PCECV than with HDCV since the purification process removes most human serum albumin in the cell-growth medium before virus inactivation.[2]

There is little data concerning the efficacy of rabies vaccines.[2] It appears that nerve-tissue vaccines afford limited protection after minor exposures to rabies virus, are less effective after head bites, and are of little use after very severe exposures. Failure rates for HDCV, PCECV, and PVRV (including cases with less than the recommended therapy) has been estimated as less than 1 in 80 000 treatments in the USA, Canada, and Europe, 1 in 12 000 to 20 000 in Thailand, and 1 in 30 000 in the remaining tropical countries. Reported failures of these vaccines are often accounted for by deviation from recommendations, incorrect site of vaccine administration, or delay in treatment.

The cost of cell-culture rabies vaccines is prohibitively high in the developing world. Although the adverse effects of nerve-tissue vaccines preclude their use for pre-exposure prophylaxis, they are still used for postexposure prophylaxis.[2] WHO is anxious that nerve-tissue vaccines should be replaced with affordable cell-culture vaccines as soon as possible. Rabies vaccines for veterinary use have been produced in cell culture at low cost and there are moves to apply the advances made in this field to human vaccines.[3] In the meantime, cost-cutting regimens have been devised for use of cell-culture rabies vaccines by the intradermal route. Rapid immunisation is achieved by the use of several sites of injection; fewer injections are required than with traditional intramuscular regimens.[2,4,5]

1. WHO. WHO expert committee on rabies: eighth report. *WHO Tech Rep Ser 824* 1992.
2. Nicholson KG. Modern vaccines: rabies. *Lancet* 1990; **335:** 1201–5. Correction. *ibid.*; 1540.
3. Petricciani JC. Ongoing tragedy of rabies. *Lancet* 1993; **342:** 1067–8.
4. Warrell MJ, *et al.* Economical multiple-site intradermal immunisation with human diploid-cell-strain vaccine is effective for post-exposure rabies prophylaxis. *Lancet* 1985; **i:** 1059–62.
5. Chutivongse S, *et al.* Postexposure prophylaxis for rabies with antiserum and intradermal vaccination. *Lancet* 1990; **335:** 896–8.

PRE-EXPOSURE IMMUNISATION. Pre-exposure prophylaxis with rabies vaccine is generally recommended for use in persons at high risk of infection with rabies virus. Where available, the vaccines produced in cell culture are preferred over the vaccines produced in animal tissues (see under Choice of Vac-

cines, above). WHO recommends[1] pre-exposure prophylaxis for persons regularly at high risk of exposure, such as certain laboratory workers, veterinarians, animal handlers, and wildlife officers, and those living in or travelling to areas where rabies is endemic. The immunisation schedule should preferably consist of 3 injections of a tissue-culture rabies vaccine of potency at least 2.5 international units given on days 0, 7, and 28, but a few days' variation is unimportant. Administration should be into the deltoid area of the arm or for young children into the anterolateral area of the thigh. Titres of virus-neutralising antibodies can be checked in serum samples collected 1 to 3 weeks after the last dose. Those who work with the live virus should have their antibody titres checked every 6 months and if the figure falls below 0.5 IU per mL they should receive a booster. Other individuals at continuing risk should have their titres checked every 12 months and a booster given if the titre is below 0.5 IU per mL.

The intradermal administration of rabies vaccine in doses of 0.1 mL on days 0, 7, and 28 has also been shown to induce seroconversion.

National policies vary somewhat from that of WHO, depending on the local risk of contracting rabies and the vaccines available.

In the UK the schedule for primary immunisation (see Uses and Administration, above) is similar to that recommended by WHO.

In the USA, immunisation with a human diploid cell vaccine, a vaccine adsorbed onto an aluminium salt, or a purified chick embryo cell vaccine is carried out similarly to the WHO schedule, with serum-antibody titres determined at 6 months to 2 years, depending upon the level of exposure, and booster doses given as necessary.[2]

1. WHO. WHO expert committee on rabies: eighth report. *WHO Tech Rep Ser 824* 1992.
2. Centers for Disease Control. Human rabies prevention—United States, 1999: recommendations of the Advisory Committee on Immunization Practices (ACIP). *MMWR* 1999; **48** (RR-1): 1–21.

POSTEXPOSURE TREATMENT. WHO[1] emphasises the importance of prompt local treatment for all bite wounds and scratches that may be contaminated with rabies virus and that, depending on the category of animal contact, rabies vaccine on its own or with rabies immunoglobulin should be given. The combination of these measures immediately after exposure is considered virtually to guarantee complete protection. Pregnancy and infancy are not contra-indications to postexposure vaccination. Also these measures should be instituted in patients who present even months after having been bitten.

First aid or local treatment consists of immediate thorough flushing and washing of the wound with water, or soap and water, or detergent followed by the application of alcohol 70% or tincture or aqueous solution of iodine. Medical care may then consist of the instillation of rabies immunoglobulin into the depth of the wound and infiltration around the wound. Ideally the wound should not be sutured, but if suturing is necessary then it is essential that it be preceded by the administration of rabies immunoglobulin as above.

The administration of rabies vaccine and of rabies immunoglobulin depends on the category of animal contact. WHO classifies the type of contact with a suspect or rabid animal into 3 categories:

- category I covers touching or feeding of animals and licks on intact skin
- category II covers nibbling of uncovered skin, minor scratches or abrasions without bleeding, and licks on broken skin
- category III covers single or multiple transdermal bites or scratches and contamination of mucous membranes with the animal's saliva

Generally no treatment is required for category I contact. Patients who have experienced category II contact should be given rabies vaccine but the course may be stopped if the contact has been with a cat or dog that remains healthy throughout an observation period of 10 days or if postmortem study of the contact animal shows it to be negative for rabies. Patients who have experienced category III contact should also be given rabies vaccine. It should be preceded by rabies immunoglobulin infiltrated around the wound and instilled into it as described above.

The dose for rabies immunoglobulin is 20 international units per kg body-weight; as much as possible of the dose should be infiltrated into and around the wound with the remainder being injected intramuscularly into the gluteal region.

The potency of rabies vaccines should be at least 2.5 international units per single human dose. For intramuscular vaccination schedules one dose should be administered on days 0, 3, 7, 14, and 30 into the deltoid region or, for small children, into the anterolateral area of the thigh. An abbreviated multisite schedule (the 2-1-1 regimen) induces an early antibody response and may be particularly effective when postexposure treatment has not included a rabies immunoglobulin. This schedule consists of one dose given in the right arm and one in the left arm on day 0, and one dose intramuscularly into the deltoid region on days 7 and 21. For intradermal vaccination one dose (0.1 mL) should be given at each of two sites, either the forearm or the upper arm, on days 0, 3, and 7, and one dose at one site on days 30 and 90.

In the UK, rabies immunoglobulin is given if the patient is previously unimmunised and at high risk. Human diploid cell vaccine is given on days 0, 3, 7, 14, and 30 (five doses) in unimmunised persons (although the UK manufacturers also recommend a sixth dose on day 90), and on days 0 and 3 to 7 (two doses) in previously fully immunised persons.

In the USA, a human diploid cell vaccine, an adsorbed rabies vaccine, or a purified chick embryo cell vaccine may be used for postexposure treatment.[2] In previously unimmunised individuals, a 1 mL dose of either vaccine is given intramuscularly on days 0, 3, 7, 14, and 28 together with rabies immunoglobulin as in the WHO schedule. In previously immunised individuals, two doses of vaccine are given on days 0 and 3, and rabies immunoglobulin is not required.

1. WHO. WHO expert committee on rabies: eighth report. *WHO Tech Rep Ser 824* 1992.
2. Centers for Disease Control. Human rabies prevention—United States, 1999: recommendations of the Advisory Committee on Immunization Practices (ACIP). *MMWR* 1999; **48** (RR-1): 1–21.

Preparations

Ph. Eur.: Rabies Vaccine for Human Use Prepared in Cell Cultures;
USP 25: Rabies Vaccine.

Proprietary Preparations (details are given in Part 3)
Aust.: Rabipur; **Canad.:** Imovax Rabies; **Denm.:** Rabies-Imovax; **Fin.:** Rabies-Imovax; **Ger.:** Rabipur; Rabivac; Tollwut-Impfstoff (HDC); **Hong Kong:** Lyssavac N; **Ital.:** Imovax Rabbia; Lyssavac N; Rasilvax; **Norw.:** Rabies-Imovax; **S.Afr.:** Verorab; **Spain:** Vac Antirrabica; **Swed.:** Rabies-Imovax; **Switz.:** Lyssavac N; **Thai.:** Lyssavac N; Rabipur; TRCS-Verorab; **UK:** Merieux Inactivated Rabies Vaccine; Rabipur; **USA:** Imovax Rabies; RabAvert.

Respiratory Syncytial Virus Immunoglobulins (14725-q)

Adverse Effects and Precautions

As for immunoglobulins in general, p.1529.

Uses and Administration

Respiratory syncytial virus immunoglobulin is available in some countries for the passive immunisation of infants against lower respiratory-tract infections caused by respiratory syncytial virus. It is prepared from the pooled plasma of adults selected for high titres of antibodies that neutralise the virus. Each mL of respiratory syncytial virus immunoglobulin contains approximately 50 mg of protein.

In the USA children under 2 years of age with bronchopulmonary dysplasia or a history of premature birth may receive a prophylactic intravenous infusion once a month during the respiratory syncytial virus season (typically November to April). The drug is given in a dose of 750 mg per kg body-weight at an initial rate of 75 mg per kg per hour for 15 minutes, followed by 150 mg per kg per hour for a further 15 minutes, and then 300 mg per kg per hour until the end of the infusion.

A human monoclonal antibody to respiratory syncytial virus (palivizumab) is available in some countries and is used intramuscularly for similar purposes, in a dose of 15 mg per kg monthly.

◊ General references to respiratory syncytial virus immunoglobulins.

1. Wandstrat TL. Respiratory syncytial virus immune globulin intravenous. *Ann Pharmacother* 1997; **31:** 83–8.
2. The Prophylaxis of Respiratory Syncytial Virus in Elevated-Risk Neonates (PREVENT) Study Group. Reduction of respiratory syncytial virus hospitalization among premature infants and infants with bronchopulmonary dysplasia using respiratory syncytial virus immune globulin prophylaxis. *Pediatrics* 1997; **99:** 93–9.
3. Rodriguez WJ, *et al.* Respiratory syncytial virus (RSV) immune globulin intravenous therapy for RSV lower respiratory tract infection in infants and young children at high risk for severe RSV infections. *Pediatrics* 1997; **99:** 454–61.
4. Committee on Infectious Diseases/Committee on Fetus and Newborn of the American Academy of Pediatrics. Respiratory syncytial virus immune globulin intravenous: indications for use. *Pediatrics* 1997; **99:** 645–50.
5. Meissner HC, Groothuis JR. Immunoprophylaxis and the control of RSV disease. *Pediatrics* 1997; **100:** 260–3.
6. Prober CG, Sullender WM. Advances in prevention of respiratory syncytial virus infections. *J Pediatr* 1999; **135:** 546–58.

◊ References to palivizumab.

1. IMpact-RSV Study Group. Palivizumab, a humanized respiratory syncytial virus monoclonal antibody, reduces hospitalization from respiratory syncytial virus infection in high-risk infants. *Pediatrics* 1998; **102:** 531–7.
2. Committee on Infectious Diseases and Committee on Fetus and Newborn, American Academy of Pediatrics. Prevention of respiratory syncytial virus infections: indications for the use of palivizumab and update on the use of RSV-IGIV. *Pediatrics* 1998; **102:** 1211–16.
3. Scott LJ, Lamb HM. Palivizumab. *Drugs* 1999; **58:** 305–11.
4. Meissner HC, *et al.* Immunoprophylaxis with palivizumab, a humanized respiratory syncytial virus monoclonal antibody, for prevention of respiratory syncytial virus infection in high risk infants: a consensus opinion. *Pediatr Infect Dis J* 1999; **18:** 223–31.
5. Russell AB. Palivizumab: an overview. *Hosp Med* 1999; **60:** 873–7.
6. Robinson RF, Nahata MC. Respiratory syncytial virus (RSV) immune globulin and palivizumab for prevention of RSV infection. *Am J Health-Syst Pharm* 2000; **57:** 259–64.

Preparations

Proprietary Preparations (details are given in Part 3)
USA: RespiGam.

Respiratory Syncytial Virus Vaccines (499-e)

Profile

Vaccines containing respiratory syncytial virus protein subunit are being studied for active immunisation.

◊ References.

1. Karron RA, Ambrosino DM. Respiratory syncytial virus vaccines. *Pediatr Infect Dis J* 1998; **17:** 919–20.
2. Gonzalez IM, *et al.* Evaluation of the live attenuated cpts 248/404 RSV vaccine in combination with a subunit RSV vaccine (PFP-2) in healthy young and older adults. *Vaccine* 2000; **18:** 1763–72.

Rheumatoid Arthritis Vaccines (11865-a)

T-Cell Vaccines.

Profile

Vaccines for the management of rheumatoid arthritis are under investigation.

Rift Valley Fever Vaccines (8290-l)

Profile

An inactivated rift valley fever vaccine has been developed for the active immunisation of persons at high risk of contracting the disease.

Rotavirus Vaccines (16981-c)

ATC — J07BH01.

Profile

Several live oral rotavirus vaccines for use in the prevention of childhood diarrhoea have been developed. A live oral tetravalent rotavirus vaccine (RRV-TV) was formerly available in the USA but was withdrawn by the manufacturer in October 1999 following reports of intussusception associated with its use.

◊ Rotaviruses are an important cause of severe diarrhoea in both developed and developing countries (see Viral Gastro-enteritis, p.605), being most prevalent among children 6 to 24 months of age.[1] Human rotavirus diarrhoea is caused by group A, B, or C rotaviruses.[2] Development of a suitable vaccine has been made difficult by the diversity of rotaviruses.[2] Initial attempts at vaccine development used single bovine or rhesus monkey strains but these were associated with variable efficacy and adverse effects.[1,3-5]

To overcome these problems reassortant rotavirus (RRV) strains were constructed. These combined animal rotavirus strains with human rotavirus genes coding for serotype-specific antigens, enabling polyvalent vaccines to be produced against the major rotavirus serotypes causing disease. One of these, a live oral tetravalent vaccine (RRV-TV) became available in the USA in August 1998 but was withdrawn from the market by the manufacturer in October 1999 following reports of intussusception (a condition when part of the intestine prolapses into the lumen of an adjacent part causing an obstruction). From September 1998 until July 1999, 15 patients with intussusception had been reported to the Vaccine Adverse Event Reporting System (VAERS), 12 of whom developed symptoms within a week of vaccination.[6] While this evidence was considered inconclusive, further studies were expected to clarify the risks associated with routine use of this vaccine.

A live attenuated rotavirus known as 89-12 is currently under investigation.[7]

1. Anonymous. Rotavirus vaccines. *Bull WHO* 1989; **67:** 583–4.
2. Anonymous. Puzzling diversity of rotaviruses. *Lancet* 1990; **335:** 573–5.
3. Levine MM. Modern vaccines: enteric infections. *Lancet* 1990; **335:** 958–61.
4. Bernstein DI, *et al.* Evaluation of WC3 rotavirus vaccine and correlates of protection in healthy infants. *J Infect Dis* 1990; **162:** 1055–62.
5. Flores J, *et al.* Protection against severe rotavirus diarrhoea by rhesus rotavirus vaccine in Venezuelan infants. *Lancet* 1987; **i:** 882–4.
6. Centers for Disease Control. Intussusception among recipients of rotavirus vaccine—United States, 1998-1999. *MMWR* 1999; **48:** 577–81.
7. Bernstein DI, *et al.* Efficacy of live, attenuated, human rotavirus vaccine 89-12 in infants: a randomised placebo-controlled trial. *Lancet* 1999; **354:** 287–90.

Preparations

Proprietary Preparations (details are given in Part 3)
USA: RotaShield†.

Rubella Immunoglobulins (11051-m)

ATC — J06BB06.

Human Rubella Immunoglobulin (Ph. Eur.) (Rubella Immunoglobulin (BP 2001); Immunoglobulinum Humanum Rubellae) is a liquid or freeze-dried preparation containing immunoglobulins, mainly immunoglobulin G (IgG). It is obtained from plasma containing specific antibodies against the rubella immunoglobulins. Normal immunoglobulin may be added. It contains not less than 4500 international units per mL. Both the liquid and freeze-dried preparations should be stored, protected from light, in a colourless, glass container. The freeze-dried preparation should be stored under vacuum or under an inert gas.

Adverse Effects and Precautions

As for immunoglobulins in general, p.1529.

Interactions

As for immunoglobulins in general, p.1529.

Uses and Administration

Rubella immunoglobulin may be used for passive immunisation against rubella (German measles). They have been used to prevent or modify rubella in susceptible persons, although if such a measure is used then normal immunoglobulin is often employed instead.

Preparations

Ph. Eur.: Human Rubella Immunoglobulin.

Proprietary Preparations (details are given in Part 3)
Ital.: Immunoros; Rosol-Gamma; Rubeuman†; **S.Afr.:** Rubegam†; **Switz.:** Rubeuman†.

Rubella Vaccines (8001-w)

ATC — J07BJ01.

Rubella Vaccine (Live) (Ph. Eur.) (Rub/Vac (Live); Rubella Vaccine, Live (BP 2001); Vaccinum Rubellae Vivum) is a freeze-dried preparation of a suitable live attenuated strain of rubella virus grown in human diploid cell cultures. It is reconstituted immediately before use. The cell-culture medium may contain a permitted antibacterial at the smallest effective concentration, and a suitable stabiliser may be added to the bulk vaccine. The final vaccine contains not less than 1×10^3 CCID$_{50}$ per dose. The dried vaccine should be stored at 2° to 8° and be protected from light.

Rubella Virus Vaccine Live (USP 25) is a bacterially sterile preparation of a suitable live strain of rubella virus grown in cultures of duck-embryo tissue or human tissue. It contains the equivalent of not less than 1×10^3 TCID$_{50}$ in each immunising dose. It should be stored at 2° to 8° and be protected from light.

Adverse Effects

As for vaccines in general, p.1529.

Generally, side-effects have not been severe. Those occurring most commonly are skin rashes, pharyngitis, fever, and lymphadenopathy; arthralgia and arthritis may also occur and are reported to be more common in women than young girls. Thrombocytopenia and neurological symptoms including neuropathy and paraesthesia have been reported rarely.

Effects on bones and joints. Although acute arthralgia or arthritis occurs in up to 30% of women following rubella vaccination,[1] a retrospective analysis found no evidence of an increased risk of chronic arthropathies.[2]

1. Tingle AJ, *et al.* Randomised double-blind placebo-controlled study on adverse effects of rubella immunisation in seronegative women. *Lancet* 1997; **349:** 1277–81.
2. Ray P, *et al.* Risk of chronic arthropathy among women after rubella vaccination. *JAMA* 1997; **278:** 551–6.

Effects on the nervous system. For a report of optic neuritis in 2 children following administration of measles and rubella vaccine, see under Adverse Effects of Measles and Rubella Vaccines, p.1549.

Precautions

As for vaccines in general, p.1530.

Rubella vaccines should not be given during pregnancy and in the UK it is recommended that patients should be advised not to become pregnant within one month of vaccination. However, no case of congenital rubella syndrome has been reported following the inadvertent administration of rubella vaccines shortly before or during pregnancy and there is no evidence that the vaccines are teratogenic. Inadvertent administration of rubella vaccines during pregnancy should not therefore result in a routine recommendation to terminate the pregnancy. There is no risk to a pregnant woman from contact with recently vaccinated persons as the vaccine virus is not transmitted.

Rubella vaccines are not generally recommended for children below the age of 1 year in whom maternal antibodies might prevent a response.

The vaccine available in the UK contains traces of neomycin and/or polymyxin. Rubella vaccine should therefore not be given to individuals with a history of anaphylaxis to these antibacterials.

Pregnancy. Since 1971 the Centers for Disease Control in the USA has followed up women who received rubella vaccines within 3 months before or after conception.[1] Up to 1979 vaccines containing either the Cendehill or HPV-77 strains of rubella virus were available. None of the 290 infants born to the 538 women who had received these vaccines had defects indicative of congenital rubella syndrome; this included 94 live-born infants of women who were known to be susceptible to rubella before receiving the vaccine. In 1979 a rubella vaccine containing the Wistar RA 27/3 strain was introduced. None of 212 infants born live to 254 women known to be susceptible to rubella and who had received the RA 27/3 rubella vaccine from 1979 to 1988 had defects indicative of congenital rubella syndrome. These results are consistent with experiences in Germany[2] and the UK.[3,4] However, because of evidence that rubella vaccine viruses can cross the placenta and infect the fetus a theoretical risk to the fetus cannot be completely ruled out.[1] Thus in both the UK and USA pregnancy is considered a contra-indication to rubella vaccination. In the UK patients are also advised not to become pregnant within one month of vaccination; in the USA a period of 3 months is advised.[1] However, in neither country is termination of pregnancy routinely recommended if the vaccine is inadvertently administered during pregnancy.

1. Anonymous. Rubella vaccination during pregnancy—United States, 1971–1988. *JAMA* 1989; **261:** 3374–83.
2. Enders G. Rubella antibody titers in vaccinated and nonvaccinated women and results of vaccination during pregnancy. *Rev Infect Dis* 1985; **7** (suppl 1): S103–S107.
3. Sheppard S, *et al.* Rubella vaccination and pregnancy: preliminary report of a national survey. *BMJ* 1986; **292:** 727.
4. Tookey PA, *et al.* Rubella vaccination in pregnancy. *Commun Dis Rep* 1991; **1** (review 7): R86–R88.

Interactions
As for vaccines in general, p.1530.

Uses and Administration
Rubella vaccines are used for active immunisation against rubella (German measles). The symptoms of rubella infection are generally mild except in the early stages of pregnancy when it leads to fetal damage in most infants.

For primary immunisation combined measles, mumps, and rubella vaccine (p.1549) is usually given. For discussion of immunisation schedules see under Vaccines, p.1530.

In the UK administration of a single-antigen rubella vaccine to girls aged 10 to 14 years has been discontinued following the mass immunisation campaign in 1994 and the introduction of a two-dose immunisation schedule in all children. Vaccine should still be given to women of child-bearing age if they are seronegative; women who are found to be seronegative during pregnancy should be vaccinated in the early postpartum period. Effective precautions against pregnancy must be observed for at least one month following vaccination. To avoid the risk of transmitting rubella to pregnant patients, all health service staff, both male and female, should be screened and those found to be seronegative should be vaccinated.

The rubella vaccine available in the UK contains the Wistar RA 27/3 strain and is given by deep subcutaneous or intramuscular injection in a dose of 0.5 mL. The rubella vaccine available in the USA is similar to that used in the UK. Vaccines containing other strains of rubella virus, such as the Cendehill strain, are available in other countries.

Preparations
Ph. Eur.: Rubella Vaccine (Live);
USP 25: Rubella Virus Vaccine Live.

Proprietary Preparations (details are given in Part 3)
Aust.: Ervevax; Rubeaten; *Austral.:* Ervevax; Meruvax II; *Belg.:* Ervevax; Rubeaten; *Braz.:* Meruvax II; Rudivax; *Denm.:* Meruvax; *Fr.:* Rudivax; *Ger.:* Ervevax; Rubellovac; *Hong Kong:* Meruvax II; Rubeaten†; Rudivax; *Irl.:* Almevax†; Ervevax; *Israel:* Rudivax; *Ital.:* Ervevax; Gunevax; Rosovax; Rubeaten†; Rudivax; *Mex.:* Ervevax; *NZ:* Ervevax; *Port.:* Rubeaten; *S.Afr.:* Rubeaten; Rudivax; *Singapore:* Rubeaten; Rudivax; *Spain:* Rubeaten; Vac Antirrubeola; *Swed.:* Almevax†; Ervevax; *Switz.:* Ervevax; Meruvax II; Rubeaten; *Thai.:* Ervevax; Gunevax; Rubeaten; Rudivax; *UK:* Almevax; Ervevax; Rubilin; *USA:* Meruvax II.

Rubella and Mumps Vaccines   (7999-a)
ATC — J07BJ51.

Rubella and Mumps Virus Vaccine Live (USP 25) is a bacterially sterile preparation of a suitable live strain of rubella virus and a suitable live strain of mumps virus. It may contain suitable antimicrobial agents. It should be stored at 2° to 8° and be protected from light.

Adverse Effects and Precautions
As for vaccines in general, p.1529.
See also under mumps vaccines, p.1551, and rubella vaccines, p.1562.

The symbol † denotes a preparation no longer actively marketed

Interactions
As for vaccines in general, p.1530.

Uses and Administration
Rubella and mumps vaccines may be used for active immunisation against mumps and rubella. Vaccination against mumps and rubella is normally performed using a combined measles, mumps, and rubella vaccine (p.1549) but the bivalent rubella and mumps vaccine may be employed when vaccination against measles is not indicated. For discussion of immunisation schedules see under Vaccines, p.1530.

A vaccine used in the USA is prepared from the Wistar RA 27/3 strain of rubella virus and the Jeryl Lynn (B level) strain of mumps virus. It is generally given in a dose of 0.5 mL by subcutaneous injection to infants during the second year of life or to other children or adults considered to be at risk.

Preparations
USP 25: Rubella and Mumps Virus Vaccine Live.

Proprietary Preparations (details are given in Part 3)
USA: Biavax II.

Schistosomiasis Vaccines   (1795-b)
Bilharzia Vaccines.

Profile
Vaccines against schistosomiasis are under development.

◊ References.
1. Anonymous. From Bilharz to B cells. *Lancet* 1991; **337:** 421–2.
2. Cherfas J. New hope for vaccine against schistosomiasis. *Science* 1991; **251:** 630–1.
3. Butterworth AE. Vaccines against schistosomiasis: where do we stand? *Trans R Soc Trop Med Hyg* 1992; **86:** 1–2.
4. Dunne DW, *et al.* Prospects for immunological control of schistosomiasis. *Lancet* 1995; **345:** 1488–92.
5. Waine GJ, McManus DP. Schistosomiasis vaccine development—the current picture. *Bioessays* 1997; **19:** 435–43.
6. Shuxian L, *et al.* Progress in the development of a vaccine against schistosomiasis in China. *Int J Infect Dis* 1998; **2:** 176–80.
7. McManus DP. The search for a vaccine against schistosomiasis—a difficult path but an achievable goal. *Immunol Rev* 1999; **171:** 149–61.

Scorpion Venom Antisera   (8006-z)
Scorpion Antivenins; Scorpion Antivenoms.

Adverse Effects and Precautions
As for antisera in general, p.1529.

Uses and Administration
Some scorpion stings are dangerous and even fatal. The use of a scorpion antiserum suitable for the species of scorpion can prevent symptoms, provided that it is given with the least possible delay; other general supportive measures and symptomatic treatment are also needed. The effectiveness of scorpion venom antisera is disputed by some clinicians.

Scorpion stings. Scorpion stings are common throughout the tropics, but the most dangerous and potentially fatal species are found in India, North Africa and the Middle East, the southern states of North America and Mexico, Latin America and the Caribbean, and southern Africa. Local symptoms following scorpion stings include intense pain and swelling. Systemic symptoms result from excitation of nerve and muscle cells by the venom: the pattern of symptoms depends upon the species of scorpion. Symptoms of parasympathetic stimulation such as dilatation of pupils, hypersalivation, vomiting and diarrhoea are generally followed by adrenergic features, with release of catecholamines producing hypertension, toxic myocarditis, arrhythmias, heart failure, and pulmonary oedema. The cardiotoxic effects are prominent features of stings in India, North Africa and the Middle East. Neurotoxic effects such as fasciculations, spasms, and respiratory paralysis are seen with stings from North American species. Stings by the black scorpion of Trinidad may also produce pancreatitis.

Pain is treated with local infiltration or peripheral nerve block with local anaesthetics; opioid analgesics may be necessary, but are regarded as dangerous following stings by some North American species. An appropriate antiserum should be administered as soon as possible after envenomation, although the effectiveness of some antisera has been questioned. Supportive treatment for cardiotoxic effects includes alpha blockers, calcium-channel blockers, and ACE inhibitors. The use of cardiac glycosides, beta blockers, and atropine is controversial. Phenobarbital has been suggested for neurotoxic effects.

References.
1. el Amin EO, *et al.* Scorpion sting: a management problem. *Ann Trop Paediatr* 1991; **11:** 143–8.
2. Bond GR. Antivenin administration for Centruroides scorpion sting: risks and benefits. *Ann Emerg Med* 1992; **21:** 788–91.
3. Warrell DA, Fenner PJ. Venomous bites and stings. *Br Med Bull* 1993; **49:** 423–39.
4. Müller GJ. Scorpionism in South Africa: a report of 42 serious scorpion envenomations. *S Afr Med J* 1993; **83:** 405–11.
5. Gateau T, *et al.* Response to specific centruroides sculpturatus antivenom in 151 cases of scorpion stings. *Clin Toxicol* 1994; **32:** 165–71.

6. Sofer S, *et al.* Scorpion envenomation and antivenom therapy. *J Pediatr* 1994; **124:** 973–8.
7. Karalliedde L. Animal toxins. *Br J Anaesth* 1995; **74:** 319–27.
8. Abroug F, *et al.* Serotherapy in scorpion envenomation: a randomised controlled trial. *Lancet* 1999; **354:** 906–9.

Preparations
Proprietary Preparations (details are given in Part 3)
Mex.: Alacramyn.

Shigella Vaccines   (19113-t)
Dysentery Vaccines; Shigellosis Vaccines.

Profile
Live attenuated shigella vaccines have been under investigation since the 1960s but early prototypes were unsatisfactory. Live oral vaccines and conjugated vaccines are now also under development.

◊ References.
1. Levine MM. Modern vaccines: enteric infections. *Lancet* 1990; **335:** 958–61.
2. Taylor DN, *et al.* Outpatient studies of the safety and immunogenicity of an auxotrophic Escherichia coli K-12-Shigella flexneri 2a hybrid vaccine candidate, EcSf2a-2. *Vaccine* 1994; **12:** 565–8.
3. Cohen D, *et al.* Safety and immunogenicity of the oral E coli K12-S flexneri 2a vaccine (EcSf2a-2) among Israeli soldiers. *Vaccine* 1994; **12:** 1436–42.
4. Kärnell A, *et al.* Safety and immunogenicity study of the auxotrophic Shigella flexneri 2a vaccine SFL1070 with a deleted aroD gene in adult Swedish volunteers. *Vaccine* 1995; **13:** 88–99.
5. Cohen D, *et al.* Double-blind vaccine-controlled randomised efficacy trial of an investigational Shigella sonnei conjugate vaccine in young adults. *Lancet* 1997; **349:** 155–9.
6. Coster TS, *et al.* Vaccination against shigellosis with attenuated Shigella flexneri 2a strain SC602. *Infect Immun* 1999; **67:** 3437–43.
7. Ashkenazi S, *et al.* Safety and immunogenicity of Shigella sonnei and Shigella flexneri 2a O-specific polysaccharide conjugates in children. *J Infect Dis* 1999; **179:** 1565–8.

Smallpox Vaccines   (8008-k)

Smallpox Vaccine (USP 25) is a suspension or solid containing a suitable strain of the living virus of vaccinia grown in the skin of bovine calves; it may contain a suitable preservative. The liquid vaccine should be stored below 0° and the dried vaccine at 2° to 8°.

Uses and Administration
Following the global eradication of smallpox, vaccination against smallpox (using vaccinia virus) has been indicated only for investigators at special risk such as laboratory workers handling certain orthopoxviruses.

WHO has recommended that all stocks of smallpox (variola) virus be destroyed. Mass vaccination against smallpox is not considered appropriate, although individuals who may be at risk of exposure to smallpox or those with confirmed infection may be vaccinated.

Recombinant vaccinia viruses are being investigated as vectors of foreign antigens, for example in a candidate AIDS vaccine (p.1531).

◊ References.
1. Jezek Z, *et al.* Smallpox and its post-eradication surveillance. *Bull WHO* 1987; **65:** 425–34.
2. Barquet N, Domingo P. Smallpox: the triumph over the most terrible of the ministers of death. *Ann Intern Med* 1997; **127:** 635–42.

Preparations
USP 25: Smallpox Vaccine.

Snake Venom Antisera   (8011-l)
Snake Antivenins; Snake Antivenoms.
ATC — J06AA03.

European Viper Venom Antiserum (Ph. Eur.) (Immunoserum Contra Venena Viperarum Europaearum) is a preparation containing the specific antitoxic globulins that have the power of neutralising the venom of one or more species of viper (*Vipera ammodytes, V. aspis, V. berus,* or *V. ursinii*). The globulins are obtained by fractionation of the serum of animals that have been immunised against the venom or venoms. Each mL neutralises the venoms in not less than 100 mouse LD_{50} of *V. ammodytes,* 100 of *V. aspis,* 50 of *V. berus,* or 50 of *V. ursinii.* It should be stored at 2° to 8°, and not be allowed to freeze.

Antivenin (Crotalidae) Polyvalent (USP 25) is a sterile freeze-dried preparation of specific venom-neutralising globulins obtained from the serum of healthy horses immunised against 4 species of pit vipers, *Crotalus atrox* (western diamondback), *Crotalus adamanteus, Crotalus durissus terrificus* (South American rattlesnake), and *Bothrops atrox* (South American fer de lance). One dose neutralises the venoms in not less than 180 mouse LD_{50} of *C. atrox,* 1320 of *C. durissus terrificus,* and 780 of *B. atrox.* It may contain a suitable preservative. It should be preserved in single-dose containers and stored at a temperature not exceeding 40°.

Antivenin (Micrurus Fulvius) (USP 25) is a sterile freeze-dried preparation of specific venom-neutralising globulins obtained from the serum of healthy horses immunised against venom of *Micrurus fulvius* (eastern coral snake). One dose neutralises the venom in not less than 250 mouse LD$_{50}$ of *M. fulvius*. It may contain a suitable preservative. It should be preserved in single-dose containers and stored at a temperature not exceeding 40°.

Adverse Effects and Precautions

As for antisera in general, p.1529.

Serum sickness is not uncommon and anaphylactic reactions may occur.

◊ A study[1] on the prediction, prevention, and mechanism of early (anaphylactic) snake venom antiserum reactions in victims of snake bites in Nigeria with systemic envenoming by the saw-scaled or carpet viper (*Echis carinatus*) and in Thailand with local or systemic envenoming by green pit vipers (*Trimeresurus albolabris* and *T. macrops*), the monocellate Thai cobra (*Naja kaouthia*), or the Malayan pit viper (*Calloselasma rhodostoma*). Conjunctival or cutaneous (intradermal or subcutaneous) hypersensitivity testing was performed before the administration of the antisera but failed to predict reactions to the antivenom. It was considered that conventional hypersensitivity testing had no predictive value for the occurrence of allergic reactions to antivenom and that it is not justifiable to delay treatment for 20 or 30 minutes to read the results of these tests. It was also considered that although the rate of administration of the antiserum can be more easily controlled by intravenous infusion this method has serious practical disadvantages in the rural tropics where most cases of snake bite occur and that an advantage of the intravenous push injection is that the person administering the antiserum must remain with the patient during the period when most severe anaphylactic reactions develop.

There is some evidence that pretreatment with low-dose subcutaneous adrenaline [epinephrine] may reduce the incidence of anaphylaxis and other acute adverse reactions to the administration of antiserum.[2] However, the use of premedication with adrenaline [epinephrine], antihistamines, and corticosteroids, although widely practiced, is regarded as controversial.

1. Malasit P, *et al.* Prediction, prevention, and mechanism of early (anaphylactic) antivenom reactions in victims of snake bites. *BMJ* 1986; **292**: 17–20.
2. Premawardhena AP, *et al.* Low dose subcutaneous adrenaline to prevent acute adverse reactions to antivenom serum in people bitten by snakes: randomised, placebo controlled trial. *BMJ* 1999; **318**: 1041–3.

Uses and Administration

Venomous snakes comprise the Viperidae (vipers), Elapidae (cobras, kraits, and mambas), and the Hydrophiidae (sea snakes).

The venom of snakes is a complex mixture chiefly of proteins, many of which have enzymatic activity, and may also provoke local inflammatory reactions. The venom may have profound effects on tissue, blood vessels and other organs, blood cells, coagulation, and myotoxic or neurotoxic effects with sensory, motor, cardiac, renal, and respiratory involvement.

Snake venom antisera are the only specific treatment available for venomous snake bites, but can produce severe adverse reactions. They are generally only used if there are clear indications of systemic involvement, severe local involvement, or, in regions where supplies are not limited, in patients at high risk of systemic or severe local involvement. Adrenaline [epinephrine] should be available in case of anaphylactic reactions to the antiserum; premedication with adrenaline [epinephrine], corticosteroids, and/or antihistamines is widely practiced but is regarded as controversial.

In Great Britain the only indigenous poisonous snake is the adder, *Viperus berus*, and European Viper Venom Antiserum (or Zagreb antivenom) may sometimes be indicated as part of the overall treatment. The usual dose for adults and children is 10 mL by intravenous injection over 10 to 15 minutes or by intravenous infusion over 30 minutes after diluting in 5 mL per kg body-weight of sodium chloride 0.9%; the dose may be repeated after about 1 to 2 hours if symptoms of systemic envenoming persist.

In the USA a polyvalent crotalidae antiserum against *Bothrops atrox*, *Crotalus adamanteus*, *C. atrox*, and *C. durissus terrificus*, and an antiserum against the North American coral snake, *Micrurus fulvius*, are available. In Australia polyvalent antisera against the brown snake, death adder, taipan, and tiger snake,

together with either the king brown snake or black snake, are available. A variety of polyvalent and monovalent antisera are also available as appropriate to the indigenous species of snakes in many other countries.

Snake bites. Most snake species are non-venomous and belong to the colubrid family although a few colubrids are technically venomous. The three families of venomous front-fanged snakes are the elapids, vipers, and sea snakes. Elapids include cobras, mambas, kraits, coral snakes, and the Australasian venomous land snakes. Vipers are subdivided into crotalids (pit vipers) and viperids. Viper bites are much more common than elapid bites, except in Australasia, where vipers do not occur naturally. Sea snake bites occur among fishermen of the Asian and western Pacific coastal areas. Although there are some notable exceptions, viper bites tend to cause vasculotoxicity, elapids cause neurotoxicity, and sea snakes cause myotoxicity.

Only a few snakes are known to be of medical importance. Of the vipers these include *Bothrops atrox* (Central and South America), *Bitis arietans* (Africa), *Echis carinatus* (Africa and Asia), *Vipera russelli* (Asia), and *Agkistrodon rhodostoma* (south-east Asia). In a few restricted areas of Africa and Asia, cobra bites are common; bites by mambas (Africa) and kraits (Asia) are rare. The carpet viper, *Echis pyramidum*, and saw-scaled viper, *Echis carinatus*, can justifiably be labelled the most dangerous snakes in the world and they cause more deaths and serious poisoning than any other snake.

Management of snake bite involves general supportive care and monitoring of vital functions but in a systemic snake-bite poisoning, specific snake venom antiserum is the most effective therapeutic agent available. If used correctly, it can reverse systemic poisoning when given hours or even days after the bite. It is highly desirable to wait for clear clinical evidence of systemic poisoning before giving an antiserum and therefore it should not be given routinely in all cases of snake bite. Monospecific antisera are more effective, and less likely to cause reactions, than polyvalent antisera. The dosage of antiserum to be used is dependent on the species of snake and the consequent potency of the requisite antiserum. The antiserum should be given intravenously diluted in isotonic saline, either by infusion or bolus injection (see under Adverse Effects and Precautions, above). First aid measures including incisions and suction to remove the venom and application of tourniquets are generally to be discouraged. In most cases, the bitten limb should be immobilised and the victim transferred to a medical facility, together with the snake if possible. For bites by elapids, when respiratory failure may occur before the patient reaches hospital, a tourniquet may be justified to delay the onset of neurotoxicity. Supportive treatment is necessary even in patients who have received an adequate dose of antiserum. Local pain may be treated with a suitable analgesic. Artificial respiration may be required in patients with symptoms of neurotoxicity. Anticholinesterases may be of benefit against the neurotoxic effects of some snake venoms and it has been recommended that an intravenous test dose of edrophonium preceded by atropine should be tried in patients with severe symptoms of neurotoxicity. For those patients who respond, treatment with neostigmine should be started but anticholinesterases are unlikely to affect outcome in patients who already require assisted respiration. Hypovolaemia should be corrected cautiously with parenteral fluids. Hypotension may be treated with subcutaneous adrenaline [epinephrine] or, in patients bitten by Russell's viper, a response to dopamine has been noted. Patients with impaired renal function may require dialysis if they do not respond to rehydration, diuretics, and dopamine. Broad spectrum antibacterials and tetanus toxoid should be given as prophylactic measures. Surgical decompression and debridement of necrotic tissue may be necessary once normal haemostasis has been restored.

References.

1. Reid HA, Theakston RDG. The management of snake bite. *Bull WHO* 1983; **61**: 885–95.
2. Nelson BK. Snake envenomation: incidence, clinical presentation and management. *Med Toxicol* 1989; **4**: 17–31.
3. Warrell DA. Snake venoms in science and clinical medicine: 1. Russell's viper: biology, venom and treatment of bites. *Trans R Soc Trop Med Hyg* 1989; **83**: 732–40.
4. Theakston RDG. Snakes venoms in science and clinical medicine: 2. applied immunology in snake venom research. *Trans R Soc Trop Med Hyg* 1989; **83**: 741–4.
5. Hulton RA, *et al.* Arboreal green pit vipers (genus Trimeresurus) of South-east Asia: bites by T. albolabris and T. macrops in Thailand and a review of the literature. *Trans R Soc Trop Med Hyg* 1990; **84**: 866–74.
6. Smith TA, Figge HL. Treatment of snakebite poisoning. *Am J Hosp Pharm* 1991; **48**: 2190–6.
7. Warrell DA, Fenner PJ. Venomous bites and stings. *Br Med Bull* 1993; **49**: 423–39.
8. Tibballs J. Premedication for snake antivenom. *Med J Aust* 1994; **160**: 4–7.
9. Caiaffa WT, *et al.* Snake bite and antivenom complications in Belo Horizonate, Brazil. *Trans R Soc Trop Med Hyg* 1994; **88**: 81–5.
10. Trevett AJ, *et al.* The efficacy of antivenom in the treatment of bites by the Papuan taipan (Oxyuranus scutellatus canni). *Trans R Soc Trop Med Hyg* 1995; **89**: 322–5.
11. Jorge MT, *et al.* A randomized 'blinded' comparison of two doses of antivenom in the treatment of Bothrops envenoming in Sao Paulo, Brazil. *Trans R Soc Trop Med Hyg* 1995; **89**: 111–14.

12. Otero R, *et al.* A randomized double-blind clinical trial of two antivenoms in patients bitten by Bothrops atrox in Colombia. *Trans R Soc Trop Med Hyg* 1996; **90**: 696–700.
13. Mead HJ, Jelinek GA. Suspected snakebite in children: a study of 156 patients over 10 years. *Med J Aust* 1996; **164**: 467–70.
14. Paret G, *et al.* Vipera palaestinae snake envenomations: experience in children. *Hum Exp Toxicol* 1997; **16**: 683–7.

Preparations

Ph. Eur.: European Viper Venom Antiserum;
USP 25: Antivenin (Crotalidae) Polyvalent; Antivenin (Micrurus Fulvius).

Proprietary Preparations (details are given in Part 3)
Austral.: Polyvalent Snake Antivenom; Snake Bite; *Canad.:* Antivenin; *Fr.:* Ipser Europe†; Viperfav; *Ital.:* Siero Antiofidico; *Mex.:* Antivipmyn.

Spider Venom Antisera (8035-x)

Spider Antivenins; Spider Antivenoms.

Antivenin (Latrodectus Mactans) (USP 25) a sterile freeze-dried preparation of specific venom-neutralising globulins obtained from the serum of healthy horses immunised against venom of black widow spiders (*Latrodectus mactans*). One dose neutralises the venom in not less than 6000 mouse LD$_{50}$ of *L. mactans*. It contains thiomersal as preservative. It should be preserved in single-dose containers and stored at a temperature not exceeding 40°.

Adverse Effects and Precautions

As for antisera in general, p.1529.

Uses and Administration

The use of a spider venom antiserum suitable for the species of spider can prevent symptoms, provided that it is done with the least possible delay; other general supportive measures and symptomatic treatment may also be needed.

An antiserum against the black widow spider (*Latrodectus mactans*) is available in the USA and the contents of a vial containing at least 6000 antivenin units is the usual dose for adults and children. In severe cases and in children under 12 years of age it is given by intravenous infusion in sodium chloride 0.9% over 15 minutes; in less severe cases, it may be given by intramuscular injection.

An antiserum against the funnel-web spider (*Atrax robustus*) is available in Australia.

Spider bites. Although many species of spider are venomous, relatively few pose a danger to man. Two main clinical syndromes are recognised; necrotic araneism, produced mainly by members of the genus *Loxosceles* which includes the brown recluse spider *L. reclusa*, and neurotoxic araneism produced by members of the genera *Latrodectus* (including the black widow and red-back spiders), *Phoneutria* (South American banana spiders), and *Atrax* (funnel-web spiders).

Necrotic araneism presents as local pain and erythema at the site of the bite, commonly developing into a necrotic lesion with a black eschar which sloughs after a few weeks, sometimes leaving an ulcer which heals gradually. The area affected can be extensive. Rarely, systemic symptoms including intravascular coagulation, haemolytic anaemia, respiratory distress, and renal failure, occur and may be life-threatening. A number of therapies have been suggested, but conservative management is usually adequate with surgical repair of any persistent defects if necessary. Dapsone is reported to produce beneficial effects on healing. Treatment for systemic manifestations is supportive. Antisera are available in some countries.

Neurotoxic araneism may involve severe pain, headache, vomiting, tachycardia, hypertension, muscle spasms, and occasionally pulmonary oedema, and coma, depending upon the species. Antisera are available and reported to be more effective than those for necrotic araneism, but should be reserved for serious envenomation. Intravenous injection of calcium gluconate 10% has been suggested to relieve muscle spasm as an alternative to conventional muscle relaxants.

References.

1. King LE, Rees RS. Dapsone treatment of a brown recluse bite. *JAMA* 1983; **250**: 648.
2. Hartman LJ, Sutherland SK. Funnel-web spider (Atrax robustus) antivenom in the treatment of human envenomation. *Med J Aust* 1984; **141**: 796–9.
3. Rees RS, *et al.* Brown recluse spider bites: a comparison of early surgical excision versus dapsone and delayed surgical excision. *Ann Surg* 1985; **202**: 659–63.
4. Dieckmann J, *et al.* Efficacy of funnel-web spider antivenom in human envenomation by Hadronyche species. *Med J Aust* 1989; **151**: 706–7.
5. Binder LS. Acute arthropod envenomation: incidence, clinical features and management. *Med Toxicol Adverse Drug Exp* 1989; **4**: 163–73.
6. Clark RF, *et al.* Clinical presentation and treatment of black widow spider envenomation: a review of 163 cases. *Ann Emerg Med* 1992; **21**: 782–7.
7. Warrell DA, Fenner PJ. Venomous bites and stings. *Br Med Bull* 1993; **49**: 423–39.

Preparations

USP 25: Antivenin (Latrodectus Mactans).

Proprietary Preparations (details are given in Part 3)
Canad.: Antivenin (Latrodectus Mactans).

Staphylococcal Vaccines (8013-j)

Profile

Staphylococcal vaccines, prepared from inactivated *Staphylococcus* spp. have been used for the prophylaxis and treatment of staphylococcal infections. They have been administered orally, topically, and by injection.

Preparations

Proprietary Preparations (details are given in Part 3)
Braz.: Anatoxina Estafilococica; Estafiloide; *USA:* SPL.

Stone Fish Venom Antisera (12230-j)

Stone Fish Antivenins; Stone Fish Antivenoms.

Adverse Effects and Precautions

As for antisera in general, p.1529.

Uses and Administration

An antiserum for use in the management of stings by the stone fish (*Synanceja trachynis*) is available in Australia. The antiserum is prepared from the serum of horses that have been immunised with the venom of the stone fish. Other symptomatic and supportive treatments are given in addition.

Stone fish venom antiserum may be given by intramuscular injection or, in more severe cases, by intravenous infusion.

◊ References.
1. Sutherland SK. Stone fish bite. *BMJ* 1990; **300:** 679–80.
2. Lehmann DF, Hardy JC. Stonefish envenomation. *N Engl J Med* 1993; **329:** 510–11.

Streptococcus Group B Vaccines (11716-v)

Profile

Vaccines for active immunisation against group B streptococcal infections are being developed. Administration of a vaccine to pregnant women to prevent neonatal infection has been proposed.

◊ References.
1. Baker CJ, *et al.* Immunization of pregnant women with a polysaccharide vaccine of group B streptococcus. *N Engl J Med* 1988; **319:** 1180–5.
2. Coleman RT, *et al.* Prevention of neonatal group B streptococcal infections: advances in maternal vaccine development. *Obstet Gynecol* 1992; **80:** 301–9.
3. Kasper DL, *et al.* Immune response to type III group B streptococcal polysaccharide-tetanus toxoid conjugate vaccine. *J Clin Invest* 1996; **98:** 2308–14.
4. Kotloff KL, *et al.* Safety and immunogenicity of a tetravalent group B streptococcal polysaccharide vaccine in healthy adults. *Vaccine* 1996; **14:** 446–50.

Tetanus Antitoxins (8016-k)

ATC — J06AA02.

Tetanus Antitoxin for Human Use (Ph. Eur.) (Tetanus Antitoxin (BP 2001); Immunoserum Tetanicum ad Usum Humanum; Tet/Ser) is a sterile preparation containing the specific antitoxic globulins that have the power of neutralising the toxin formed by *Clostridium tetani*. It is obtained by fractionation from the serum of horses, or other mammals, that have been immunised against tetanus toxin. For prophylactic use, it has a potency of not less than 1000 international units per mL, and for therapeutic use not less than 3000 international units per mL. It should be stored at 2° to 8°, and not be allowed to freeze.

Tetanus Antitoxin (USP 25) is a sterile solution of the refined and concentrated proteins, chiefly globulins, containing antitoxic antibodies obtained from the serum or plasma of healthy horses that have been immunised against tetanus toxin or toxoid. It contains not less than 400 units per mL. It should be stored at 2° to 8°.

Profile

Tetanus antitoxins neutralise the toxin produced by *Clostridium tetani* and have been used to provide temporary passive immunity against tetanus, but tetanus immunoglobulins (below) are preferred. A test dose of tetanus antitoxin should always be given to identify those who might suffer hypersensitivity reactions.

Whenever a non-immune patient is seen because of injury opportunity should be taken to institute a course of active immunisation (see Tetanus Vaccines, p.1565).

Preparations

Ph. Eur.: Tetanus Antitoxin for Human Use;
USP 25: Tetanus Antitoxin.

Tetanus Immunoglobulins (1241-c)

ATC — J06BB02.

Human Tetanus Immunoglobulin (Ph. Eur.) (Tetanus Immunoglobulin (BP 2001); Immunoglobulinum Humanum Tetanicum) is a liquid or freeze-dried preparation containing immunoglobulins, mainly immunoglobulin G (IgG). It is obtained from plasma containing specific antibodies against the toxin of *Clostridium tetani*. Normal immunoglobulin may be added. It

---

contains not less than 100 international units per mL. Both the liquid and freeze-dried preparations should be stored, protected from light, in a colourless, glass container. The freeze-dried preparation should be stored under vacuum or under an inert gas.

Tetanus Immune Globulin (USP 25) is a sterile solution of globulins derived from the plasma of adult human donors who have been immunised with tetanus vaccine. It contains not less than 50 units of tetanus antitoxin per mL. It contains 10 to 18% of protein of which not less than 90% is gamma globulin. It contains glycine as a stabilising agent, and a suitable preservative. It should be stored at 2° to 8°.

Adverse Effects and Precautions

As for immunoglobulins in general, p.1529.

Interactions

As for immunoglobulins in general, p.1529.

Tetanus immunoglobulins will neutralise tetanus toxoid and should not be injected into the same site or in the same syringe as a tetanus vaccine.

Uses and Administration

Tetanus immunoglobulins are used for passive immunisation against tetanus.

The use of tetanus immunoglobulins is recommended in the UK and the USA as part of the management of tetanus-prone wounds in persons unimmunised or incompletely immunised against tetanus, in persons whose immunisation history is unknown, in persons who received the last dose of tetanus vaccine more than 10 years previously, and in patients with impaired immunity. Active immunisation with a tetanus vaccine (p.1565) should also be started simultaneously, and antibacterials and symptomatic therapy given as appropriate (see p.142 and p.1332). The usual dose of tetanus immunoglobulin is 250 units by intramuscular injection but if more than 24 hours have elapsed since the wound was sustained, if there is a risk of heavy contamination, or following burns 500 units should be given irrespective of the immunisation history.

Tetanus immunoglobulin is also used in the treatment of tetanus, a recommended dose being 150 units per kg body-weight in total, given intramuscularly into multiple sites. Doses in the range 30 to 300 units per kg are suggested by the manufacturer in the UK.

A preparation suitable for intravenous use is available in some countries. It is given for the treatment of tetanus in a dose of 5000 to 10 000 units by intravenous infusion.

Preparations

Ph. Eur.: Human Tetanus Immunoglobulin;
USP 25: Tetanus Immune Globulin.

Proprietary Preparations (details are given in Part 3)
Aust.: Tetabulin; Tetagam; Tetanosimultan; Tetavenin; Tetuman†; *Belg.:* Tetabuline; Tetuman†; *Braz.:* Tetaglobulina; Tetanobulin; Tetanogamma; *Canad.:* BayTet; Hyper-Tet†; *Fr.:* Gammatetanos; *Ger.:* Tetagam N; Tetanobulin; *Hong Kong:* Tetabulin; Tetuman; *Irl.:* Tetabulin; *Israel:* BayTet; Ig Tetano; Tetaglobuline; *Ital.:* Gamma-Tet P; Haima-Tetanus; Igantet; Immunotetan; Imogam Tetano; Tetabulin; Tetagamma; Tetanus-Gamma; Teteven; Tetuman; *Mex.:* BayTet; Probi-Tet; Tetanogamma; *Port.:* Tetuman; *S.Afr.:* Tetagam; Tetuman; *Spain:* Gamma Antitenos; Gamma Antitetanos; Gammaglob Antite; Tetuman; Torlanbulina Antitenani†; *Switz.:* Tetabuline†; Tetuman; *Thai.:* Tetuman; *UK:* Tetabulin; *USA:* BayTet.

Tetanus Vaccines (8020-y)

ATC — J07AM01.

Tetanus Vaccine (BP 2001) (Tet/Vac/FT) is prepared from tetanus toxin produced by the growth of *Clostridium tetani*. The toxin is converted to tetanus formol toxoid by treatment with formaldehyde solution. It contains suitable non-phenolic antimicrobial preservatives. It should be stored at 2° to 8° and be protected from light. The BP 2001 directs that when Tetanus Vaccine is prescribed or demanded and the form is not stated, Adsorbed Tetanus Vaccine may be dispensed or supplied.

Tetanus Vaccine (Adsorbed) (Ph. Eur.) (Tet/Vac/Ads; Adsorbed Tetanus Vaccine (BP 2001); Vaccinum Tetani Adsorbatum) is prepared from tetanus formol toxoid adsorbed on a mineral carrier which may be hydrated aluminium hydroxide, aluminium phosphate, or calcium phosphate. The resulting mixture is isotonic with blood. Suitable antimicrobial preservatives may be added. The antigenic properties are adversely affected by certain antimicrobial preservatives particularly those of the phenolic type and these should not be added to the vac-

---

cine. It contains not less than 40 units per dose. It should be stored at 2° to 8°, not be allowed to freeze, and be protected from light.

Tetanus Toxoid (USP 25) is a sterile solution of the formaldehyde-treated products of growth of *Clostridium tetani*. It contains a non-phenolic preservative. It should be stored at 2° to 8° and not be allowed to freeze.

Tetanus Toxoid Adsorbed (USP 25) is a sterile preparation of plain tetanus toxoid precipitated or adsorbed by alum, aluminium hydroxide, or aluminium phosphate adjuvants. It should be stored at 2° to 8° and not be allowed to freeze.

Adverse Effects and Precautions

As for vaccines in general, p.1529.

Local reactions, usually following the use of adsorbed vaccines, and mild systemic reactions may occur. The incidence and severity of reactions increases with the number of doses given.

Anaphylaxis and neurological reactions have occasionally been reported.

Although vaccination is usually postponed in patients suffering from an acute febrile illness, tetanus vaccine should be given to such patients in the presence of a tetanus-prone wound.

Booster doses of tetanus vaccine should not generally be given at intervals of less than 10 years because of an increased risk of severe local reactions.

Effects of purification. In a double-blind comparative study[1] involving 205 healthy subjects there was no difference in side-effects in those given a standard (commercial) tetanus vaccine and those given an antibody-affinity-purified vaccine. The results confirmed that side-effects to tetanus vaccines are not eliminated by purification.
1. Leen CLS, *et al.* Double-blind comparative trial of standard (commercial) and antibody-affinity-purified tetanus toxoid vaccines. *J Infect* 1987; **14:** 119–24.

Effects on the nervous system. Neuropathies have been reported rarely following tetanus vaccination. Optic neuritis and myelitis occurred[1] in an 11-year-old girl following a routine booster dose. Corticosteroids and immunoglobulin were given, and both vision and muscle power were restored after 11 months. Acute transverse myelitis was reported[2] in a 50-year-old man who received tetanus toxoid and immunoglobulin following an injury. Neurological deficits were unchanged after 1 month despite treatment with corticosteroids. Other causes could not be ruled out in either case. Brachial neuritis which developed in 2 infants following immunisation with diphtheria, tetanus, and pertussis vaccine was attributed to the tetanus component.[3]
1. Topaloglu H, *et al.* Optic neuritis and myelitis after booster tetanus toxoid vaccination. *Lancet* 1992; **339:** 178–9.
2. Read SJ, *et al.* Acute transverse myelitis after tetanus toxoid vaccination. *Lancet* 1992; **339:** 1111–12.
3. Hamati-Haddad A, Fenichel GM. Brachial neuritis following routine childhood immunization for diphtheria, tetanus, and pertussis (DTP): report of two cases and review of the literature. *Pediatrics* 1997; **99:** 602–3.

GUILLAIN-BARRÉ SYNDROME. A possible causal relationship between tetanus-containing vaccines and Guillain-Barré syndrome has been proposed (see Diphtheria and Tetanus Vaccines, p.1537).

Pregnancy. No connection has been found between administration of tetanus toxoid during pregnancy and either congenital malformations[1] or spontaneous abortion.[2]
1. Silveira CM, *et al.* Safety of tetanus toxoid in pregnant women: a hospital-based case-control study of congenital anomalies. *Bull WHO* 1995; **73:** 605–8.
2. Catindig N, *et al.* Tetanus toxoid and spontaneous abortions: is there epidemiological evidence of an association? *Lancet* 1996; **348:** 1098–9.

Interactions

As for vaccines in general, p.1530.

Tetanus immunoglobulins will neutralise tetanus toxoid and should not be injected into the same site or in the same syringe as a tetanus vaccine.

Uses and Administration

Tetanus vaccines are used for active immunisation against tetanus.

For primary immunisation a combined diphtheria, tetanus, and pertussis vaccine (p.1537) or a combined diphtheria and tetanus vaccine (p.1537) is usually used. For discussion of immunisation schedules see under Vaccines, p.1530. In adults requiring primary immunisation, single component adsorbed tetanus vaccine or, if appropriate, combined tetanus and low-dose diphtheria vaccine may be used. The non-adsorbed type of tetanus vaccine is less potent as an antigen than the adsorbed type and the adsorbed vac-

---

The symbol † denotes a preparation no longer actively marketed

cine is generally preferred. The primary immunisation course in the UK consists of 3 doses, each of 0.5 mL, administered at intervals of one month by deep subcutaneous or intramuscular injection. In children who complete the primary course in infancy, reinforcing doses are given at school entry and on leaving school in combination with the appropriate diphtheria vaccine. In adults, a reinforcing dose is desirable 10 years later with a further dose after a further 10 years. Further booster doses are not recommended for adults who have received 5 doses, other than at the time of injury, since they are unnecessary and can cause considerable local reactions. However, in some countries, including the USA, reinforcing doses are given every 10 years.

The need for tetanus vaccines in wound management depends on both the condition of the wound and the patient's immunisation history. If primary immunisation or a reinforcing dose has been given within the last 10 years, tetanus vaccine should not be given but the patient should receive tetanus immunoglobulin if the risk of infection is considered especially high. If more than 10 years has elapsed, a reinforcing dose of adsorbed vaccine should be given. For tetanus-prone wounds tetanus immunoglobulin (see above) may also be required. Tetanus vaccine and tetanus immunoglobulin may be given concomitantly, but not at the same site. In the event of injury in non-immunised persons or if immunisation status is uncertain opportunity is usually taken to initiate a course of primary immunisation. Since this provides no immediate protection, prophylactic treatment with tetanus immunoglobulin is recommended for tetanus-prone wounds. Suitable antibacterial therapy may also be given (see p.142).

Anergy testing. For reference to the use of tetanus vaccines for anergy testing in HIV-positive patients, see Tuberculins, p.1676.

Bone-marrow transplant recipients. In a study[1] of 48 recipients of bone-marrow transplants immunity to tetanus was not transferred from seropositive donors to seronegative patients. An unexpected finding was that pre-transplant antibody level of the patient, and not the donor, strongly influenced the antibody level one year after transplantation. Immunity quickly waned, however, after transplantation. Reimmunisation with tetanus vaccine is therefore required in long-term survivors of bone-marrow transplants. The study suggested that 3 doses are needed to obtain adequate protection. The necessity for further doses requires study.

1. Ljungman P, et al. Response to tetanus toxoid immunization after allogeneic bone marrow transplantation. J Infect Dis 1990; 162: 496–500.

Neonatal tetanus. Responding to an estimated 800 000 deaths of newborn infants from neonatal tetanus each year world-wide (but excluding China), accounting for approximately 50% of all deaths in the neonatal period in developing countries, WHO adopted a resolution in 1989 to eliminate neonatal tetanus. Control of neonatal tetanus may be achieved by ensuring adequate hygiene during delivery and by ensuring protective immunity of the mother in late pregnancy.

Tetanus vaccine is administered to all women of child-bearing age as part of WHO's Expanded Programme on Immunization. For pregnant women, two doses of vaccine, the second dose at least 4 weeks after the first and at least 2 weeks before delivery, provide the newborn infant with approximately 80% protection against tetanus. For all women of child-bearing age, three doses of vaccine, with at least 4 weeks between the first two doses and 6 months between the second and third doses, provide 95% protection for up to 5 years. Fourth and fifth doses, each at least one year after the previous dose, ensure lifelong protection.

Immunisation of pregnant women with tetanus vaccine lags well behind levels achieved for childhood vaccines in the Expanded Programme on Immunization. In June 1987, it was estimated that fewer than 20% of all pregnant women had received two doses of vaccine.[1] By 1993 this had increased to 45%, and the estimated number of deaths had decreased to 515 000 (including 98 000 in China, where immunisation began in 1992).[2]

1. Hayden GF, et al. Progress in worldwide control and elimination of disease through immunization. J Pediatr 1989; 114: 520–7.
2. Centers for Disease Control. Progress toward the global elimination of neonatal tetanus, 1989-1993. MMWR 1994; 43: 885–94.

Reinforcing doses in adults. Although the current recommendation in the UK is that 5 doses of tetanus vaccine (as a 3-dose primary course and 2 reinforcing doses at 10-year intervals) is sufficient to produce life-long immunity to tetanus, there is still concern about immunity in the elderly, and in particular women. Routine primary immunisation against tetanus

was introduced in the UK in 1961, so individuals born before that year would not have been immunised in infancy, and unless they had been in the armed forces, may never have received a full primary course.[1] Unless there is a clear immunisation history immunity to tetanus may be difficult to assess. Studies in the USA,[2] Australia,[3] and Austria[4] have shown that at least half of healthy people over 50 years of age did not have adequate circulating tetanus antibodies. However, the level of circulating antibodies in the absence of an antigen challenge may not be an appropriate measure of the immune status. The low incidence of clinical tetanus in adults provides circumstantial evidence of an adequate inducible antibody response on exposure to tetanus despite a decline in antibody concentrations with increasing age.[5,6] Conversely, there have been reports of tetanus occurring despite high antibody concentrations.[7,8] There have been calls for the introduction of regular booster injections in adults,[4,8-10] as is standard practice in the USA or alternatively a single booster in late middle age[11,12] or administering a primary course to elderly persons who have never received one.[2]

1. Salisbury DM, Begg NT (eds), Joint Committee on Vaccination and Immunisation. Immunisation against infectious disease. London: HMSO, 1996.
2. Gergen PJ, et al. A population-based serologic survey of immunity to tetanus in the United States. N Engl J Med 1995; 332: 761–6.
3. Heath TC, et al. Tetanus immunity in an older Australian population. Med J Aust 1996; 164: 593–6.
4. Steger MM, et al. Vaccination against tetanus in the elderly: do recommended vaccination strategies give sufficient protection? Lancet 1996; 348: 762.
5. Bowie C. Tetanus toxoid for adults—too much of a good thing. Lancet 1996; 348: 1185–6.
6. Baily G. Are the elderly inadequately protected against tetanus? Lancet 1996; 348: 1389–90.
7. Passen EL, Andersen BR. Clinical tetanus despite a 'protective' level of toxin-neutralising antibody. JAMA 1986; 255: 1171–3.
8. Bowman C, et al. Tetanus toxoid for adults. Lancet 1996; 348: 1664.
9. Rethy LA, Rethy L. Can tetanus boosting be rejected? Lancet 1997; 349: 359–60.
10. Sehgal R. Tetanus toxoid for adults. Lancet 1997; 349: 573.
11. Balestra DJ, Littenberg B. Tetanus immunization in adults. JAMA 1994; 272: 1900.
12. Gardner P, LaForce FM. Protection against tetanus. N Engl J Med 1995; 333: 599.

Preparations

BP 2001: Tetanus Vaccine;
Ph. Eur.: Tetanus Vaccine (Adsorbed);
USP 25: Tetanus Toxoid; Tetanus Toxoid Adsorbed.

Proprietary Preparations (details are given in Part 3)
Aust.: T-Immun; Tanrix†; Te Anatoxal; Tetanol; *Austral.:* Tet-Tox; *Belg.:* Anatoxal Te†; Tetamer†; Tevax; *Fr.:* Tetavax†; *Ger.:* T-Immun†; T-Medevax†; Tetamun SSW; Tetanol; Tetasorbat SSW; Tetavax†; *Hong Kong:* Te Anatoxal; Tetavax; *Ital.:* Anatetall; H-Atetal; Imovax Tetano; Tanrix; Tetatox; *Mex.:* Tetinox; Toxanal; *Neth.:* Tetavax; *NZ:* Te Anatoxal; Tet-Tox; *Port.:* Anatoxal Te; *S.Afr.:* Tetavax; *Singapore:* Te Anatoxal; *Spain:* Anatoxal Te; Vac Antitetanica; *Switz.:* Anatoxal Te; *Thai.:* Anatetall; Te Anatoxal; Tetavax; *UK:* Clostet; Tetavax; *USA:* Te Anatoxal.

Tetanus and Influenza Vaccines (13574-d)

Profile

Tetanus and influenza vaccines are available in some countries for active immunisation against tetanus and influenza.

Preparations

Proprietary Preparations (details are given in Part 3)
Fr.: Tetagrip.

Tetanus and Poliomyelitis Vaccines (13575-n)

Profile

Tetanus and poliomyelitis (inactivated) vaccines are available in some countries for active immunisation against tetanus and poliomyelitis.

Preparations

Proprietary Preparations (details are given in Part 3)
Fr.: T. Polio; Vaccin TP.

Tick Venom Antisera (19671-m)

Tick Antivenins; Tick Antivenoms.

Profile

An antiserum is available in Australia for treatment of the neurotoxic effects of envenomation by the tick *Ixodes holocyclus*. The antiserum is prepared from the serum of dogs that have been immunised with tick venom.

Tick venom antiserum is given by slow intravenous infusion.

Trichomoniasis Vaccines (3870-z)

Profile

A trichomoniasis vaccine containing inactivated *Lactobacillus acidophilus* is available in some countries for the prophylaxis of recurrent vaginal trichomoniasis. The vaccine is reported to

stimulate production of antibodies against the aberrant coccoid forms of the lactobacilli associated with trichomoniasis and also, by cross-reaction, against the trichomonads themselves.

Preparations

Proprietary Preparations (details are given in Part 3)
Ger.: Gynatren; *Ital.:* Ginatren†.

Tularaemia Vaccines (1330-k)

Profile

A tularaemia vaccine prepared from a live attenuated strain of *Francisella tularensis* has been used for active immunisation against tularaemia in persons at high risk of contracting the disease.

Typhoid Vaccines (8027-x)

ATC — J07AP01; J07AP02; J07AP03.

Typhoid Vaccine (Ph. Eur.) (Typhoid/Vac; Vaccinum Febris Typhoidi) is a sterile suspension of inactivated *Salmonella typhi* containing not less than 500 million and not more than 1000 million bacteria per dose which does not exceed 1 mL. It is prepared from a suitable strain of *S. typhi* such as Ty 2. The bacteria are inactivated by heat, or by treatment with acetone, formaldehyde, or phenol, or by phenol and heat. It may also be supplied as a freeze-dried vaccine (Dried Typhoid/Vac) which is reconstituted immediately before use by the addition of suitable sterile liquid. Phenol may not be used in the preparation of the dried vaccine. Ph. Eur. includes the dried vaccine as Typhoid Vaccine, Freeze-dried (Vaccinum Febris Typhoidi Cryodesiccatum). Both the liquid vaccine and the dried vaccine should be stored at 2° to 8°, and be protected from light; the liquid vaccine should not be allowed to freeze. Under these conditions the liquid vaccine may be expected to retain its potency for at least 2 years and the dried vaccine for at least 5 years.

Typhoid Vaccine (Live, Oral, Strain Ty 21a) (Ph. Eur.) (Vaccinum Febris Typhoidis Vivum Perorale (Stirpe Ty 21a); Typhoid (Strain Ty 21a) Vaccine, Live (Oral) (BP 2001); Typhoid/Vac(Oral)) is a freeze-dried preparation of live *S. typhi* strain Ty 21a grown in a suitable medium. It contains not less than 2×10^9 bacteria per dose. It should be stored at 2° to 8°, and be protected from light. Under these conditions it may be expected to retain its potency for at least 18 months.

Typhoid Polysaccharide Vaccine (Ph. Eur.) (Typhoid/Vi/Vac; Vaccinum Febris Typhoidis Polysaccharidicum) is a preparation of purified Vi capsular polysaccharide obtained from *S. typhi* Ty2 strain or some other suitable strain that has the capacity to produce Vi polysaccharide. It contains 25 μg of polysaccharide per dose. It should be stored at 2° to 8° and be protected from light.

Typhoid Vaccine (USP 25) is a sterile suspension or solid containing killed typhoid bacilli (*S. typhi*) of the Ty 2 strain. It has a labelled potency of 8 units per mL. Dried vaccine contains no preservative; aqueous vaccine and reconstituting fluid contain a preservative. It should be stored at 2° to 8° and not be allowed to freeze.

Adverse Effects and Precautions

As for vaccines in general, p.1529.

Oral live typhoid and parenteral polysaccharide vaccines have been associated with fewer adverse effects than parenteral killed typhoid vaccines.

Interactions

As for vaccines in general, p.1530. Oral typhoid vaccine should not be given to individuals receiving antibacterials since the development of immunity may be impaired. Individuals receiving mefloquine for malaria prophylaxis should not take oral typhoid vaccine on the same day or, if this is unavoidable, within 12 hours of the mefloquine dose.

Uses and Administration

Typhoid vaccines are used for active immunisation against typhoid fever. As with many vaccines, the efficacy of typhoid vaccine is not complete and the importance of maintaining attention to hygiene should be emphasised to those travelling to endemic areas.

Typhoid vaccination is advised for laboratory workers handling specimens which may contain typhoid organisms and for persons travelling to areas where typhoid fever is endemic. In the UK, vaccination of contacts of a known typhoid carrier is not recommended; in the USA such persons are advised to receive the vaccine. Typhoid vaccine is not useful in controlling outbreaks of the disease.

In the UK two vaccines are available: a capsular polysaccharide vaccine for parenteral use, and a live oral vaccine.

The capsular polysaccharide typhoid vaccine contains 25 µg of the Vi polysaccharide antigen per dose. A single dose of 0.5 mL is given by deep subcutaneous or intramuscular injection. Booster doses may be given every 3 years to those who remain at risk. The response in children under 18 months of age may be suboptimal, and the decision to vaccinate will be governed by the risk of exposure to infection.

The live oral typhoid vaccine contains an attenuated strain of *Salmonella typhi*, Ty 21a, and is administered as enteric-coated capsules containing not less than 2×10^9 bacteria per dose. A primary immunisation schedule of one capsule every other day for 3 doses is given. The capsule should be taken on an empty stomach with a cold or luke-warm drink. This oral vaccine is not considered suitable for children under 6 years of age. Immunity persists for about 3 years under conditions of continuous or repeated exposure. For less frequent visitors to endemic regions, a 3-dose booster may be given annually.

A monovalent whole-cell killed vaccine was also formerly available, and was given parenterally in 2 doses at an interval of 4 to 6 weeks. The first dose was given by intramuscular or deep subcutaneous injection, although subsequent doses could be given intradermally to reduce adverse reactions.

In the USA, whole-cell parenteral, capsular polysaccharide, and live oral vaccines are available. The former is given in a primary course of 2 injections of 0.5 mL, given subcutaneously at an interval of 4 or more weeks to adults and children over 10 years of age; children from 6 months to 10 years may be given 2 doses of 0.25 mL. An additional alternative accelerated schedule of three doses at weekly intervals may be employed, although this may be less effective than the standard 2-dose schedule. Booster doses should be given every 3 years. The capsular polysaccharide vaccine is given intramuscularly similarly to that in the UK, with a booster dose suggested every 2 years. For the oral vaccine, 4 doses on alternate days is recommended for both primary immunisation and boosters, which are given every 5 years if exposure continues.

Immunisation for travellers. In most developed countries where typhoid is not endemic, the major use for typhoid vaccine is for non-immune travellers visiting endemic areas. Doubts have been raised over the necessity for typhoid vaccination for the majority of travellers because of the rarity of the disease in travellers and the unproven efficacy of the available vaccines in this population.[1] The highest incidence of the disease is associated with travel to the Indian subcontinent and parts of tropical South America although immunisation is also recommended for travellers to lower risk areas of Africa, Asia, and south-east Europe.[1,2] By far the most important form of protection against gastrointestinal infection is strict attention to personal, food, and water hygiene, although in practice this advice is often difficult to follow.

None of the vaccines currently available is 100% effective in preventing disease. The effectiveness of the vaccines has generally been assessed in field trials in the populations of endemic areas. Such populations acquire a degree of natural immunity due to continued exposure and it may not be possible to equate protection rates in these populations to non-immune travellers.[1] The whole-cell vaccine has been evaluated in non-immune subjects[3] and was shown to confer partial protection against a relatively low inoculum compared with that likely to be encountered from foodborne transmission.[1] The live oral vaccine has been shown to confer a useful degree of immunity in field trials[4,5] but the dose used may have been insufficient to protect non-immune individuals. The degree of immunity induced may be increased by the use of higher inocula[6] or liquid preparations.[5,7] In addition, compliance with dosing and storage requirements may further limit the effectiveness of this dosage form.[8]

Two large field studies[9,10] have verified the effectiveness of the capsular polysaccharide vaccine but its efficacy has not been assessed in non-immune populations. However, it does have the advantage of being administered as a single dose.

The symbol † denotes a preparation no longer actively marketed

A meta-analysis[11] of randomised studies has concluded that whole-cell vaccines are more efficacious than the capsular polysaccharide and oral vaccines, but are more frequently associated with adverse effects.

For individuals who have previously received the whole-cell vaccine without difficulty, there is no need to change to the newer vaccines, especially since booster doses can be given intradermally to reduce adverse reactions. The single dose required for the capsular polysaccharide vaccine may recommend it for primary immunisation. The oral vaccine may have obvious advantages in patient acceptability but it is expensive and the importance of correct storage and dosing should be stressed.[2]

1. Anonymous. Typhoid vaccination: weighing the options. *Lancet* 1992; **340:** 341–2.
2. Anonymous. Typhoid vaccines—which one to choose? *Drug Ther Bull* 1993; **31:** 9–10.
3. Hornick RB, *et al.* Typhoid fever: pathogenesis and immunologic control, part 2. *N Engl J Med* 1970; **283:** 739–46.
4. Levine MM, *et al.* Large-scale field trial of Ty21a live oral typhoid vaccine in enteric-coated capsule formulation. *Lancet* 1987; **i:** 1049–52.
5. Simanjuntak CH, *et al.* Oral immunisation against typhoid fever in Indonesia with Ty21a vaccine. *Lancet* 1991; **338:** 1055–9.
6. Ferreccio C, *et al.* Comparative efficacy of two, three, or four doses of Ty21a live oral typhoid vaccine in enteric-coated capsules: a field trial in an endemic area. *J Infect Dis* 1989; **159:** 766–9.
7. Levine MM, *et al.* Comparison of enteric-coated capsules and liquid formulation of Ty21a typhoid vaccine in randomised controlled field trial. *Lancet* 1990; **336:** 891–4.
8. Kaplan DT, *et al.* Compliance with live, oral Ty21a typhoid vaccine. *JAMA* 1992; **267:** 1074.
9. Acharya IL, *et al.* Prevention of typhoid fever in Nepal with the Vi capsular polysaccharide of Salmonella typhi: a preliminary report. *N Engl J Med* 1987; **317:** 1101–4.
10. Klugman KP, *et al.* Protective activity of Vi capsular polysaccharide vaccine against typhoid fever. *Lancet* 1987; **ii:** 1165–9.
11. Engels EA, *et al.* Typhoid fever vaccines: a meta-analysis of studies on efficacy and toxicity. *BMJ* 1998; **316:** 110–16.

Preparations

Ph. Eur.: Freeze-dried Typhoid Vaccine; Typhoid Polysaccharide Vaccine; Typhoid Vaccine; Typhoid Vaccine (Live, Oral, Strain Ty 21a);
USP 25: Typhoid Vaccine.

Proprietary Preparations (details are given in Part 3)

Aust.: Typherix; Typhim Vi; Vivotif; ***Austral.:*** Typh-Vax; Typherix; Typhim Vi; ***Belg.:*** Typherix; Typhim Vi; Vivotif; ***Canad.:*** Typhim Vi; Vivotif; ***Denm.:*** Typherix; Typhim Vi; Vivotif; ***Fin.:*** Typherix; Typhim Vi; Vivotif; ***Fr.:*** Typherix; Typhim Vi; ***Ger.:*** Typherix; Typhim Vi; Typhoral L; Vivotif; ***Hong Kong:*** Typhim Vi; Vivotif; ***Irl.:*** Typherix; Typhim Vi; Vivotif; ***Israel:*** Typhim Vi; Vivotif; ***Ital.:*** Enterovaccino ISI (Antitifico); Enterovaccino Nuovo ISM†; Neotyf; Typherix; Typhim Vi; Vivotif; ***Neth.:*** Typhim Vi; ***Norw.:*** Typhim Vi; Vivotif; ***NZ:*** Typh-Vax; Typherix; Typhim Vi; ***Port.:*** Vivotif; ***S.Afr.:*** Typhim Vi; Vivotif; ***Singapore:*** Typhim Vi; Vivotif; ***Spain:*** Typhim Vi; Vac Antitifica Or; Vivotif; ***Swed.:*** Typherix; Typhim Vi; Vivotif; ***Switz.:*** Vaccin Tab†; Vivotif; ***Thai.:*** Typhim Vi; Vivotif; ***UK:*** Typherix; Typhim Vi; Vivotif; ***USA:*** Typhim Vi; Vivotif.

Typhoid and Tetanus Vaccines (8025-a)

Profile
A combined typhoid and tetanus vaccine has been used by subcutaneous injection for primary immunisation against typhoid fever and tetanus and by intramuscular injection to reinforce immunity.

Typhus Vaccines (8034-t)

Profile
Typhus vaccines may be used for active immunisation against louse-borne typhus. Their use may be considered for those living in or visiting the few endemic areas who are likely to have close contact with the indigenous population, including health care workers, and for laboratory workers. They do not provide protection against scrub typhus.

Vaccinia Immunoglobulins (1243-a)
ATC — J06BB07.

Vaccinia Immune Globulin (USP 25) is a sterile solution of globulins derived from the plasma of adult human donors who have been immunised with vaccinia virus (smallpox vaccine). It contains 15 to 18% of protein, of which not less than 90% is gamma globulin. It contains glycine as a stabilising agent, and a suitable antimicrobial agent. It should be stored at 2° to 8°.

Profile
Vaccinia immunoglobulins have been used for the treatment of clinical complications of smallpox vaccination. They are not effective for postviral encephalitis.

Preparations

USP 25: Vaccinia Immune Globulin.

Varicella-Zoster Immunoglobulins
(17024-h)

ATC — J06BB03.

Human Varicella Immunoglobulin (Ph. Eur.) (Varicella Immunoglobulin (BP 2001); Immunoglobulinum Humanum Varicellae) is a liquid or freeze-dried preparation containing immunoglobulins, mainly immunoglobulin G (IgG). It is obtained from plasma from selected donors having specific antibodies against *Herpesvirus varicellae*. Normal immunoglobulin may be added. It contains not less than 100 international units per mL. The liquid and freeze-dried preparations should be stored, protected from light, in a colourless, glass container. The freeze-dried preparation should be stored under vacuum or under inert gas.

Varicella-Zoster Immune Globulin (USP 25) is a sterile solution of globulins derived from the plasma of adult donors selected for high titres of varicella-zoster antibodies. It contains 15 to 18% of globulins, of which not less than 99% is immunoglobulin G with traces of immunoglobulin A and immunoglobulin M. It contains glycine as a stabilising agent and thiomersal as a preservative. It contains not less than 125 units of specific antibody in not more than 2.5 mL of solution. It should be stored at 2° to 8°.

Adverse Effects and Precautions
As for immunoglobulins in general, p.1529.

Interactions
As for immunoglobulins in general, p.1529.

Uses and Administration
Varicella-zoster immunoglobulins are used for passive immunisation against varicella (chickenpox) in susceptible persons considered to be at high risk of developing varicella-associated complications after exposure to varicella or herpes zoster (shingles).

In the UK varicella-zoster immunoglobulins are recommended for individuals who are at high risk of severe varicella and who have no antibodies to varicella-zoster virus and who have significant exposure to chickenpox or herpes zoster. Those at increased risk include immunosuppressed patients, neonates including those whose mothers develop chickenpox (but not herpes zoster) in the period 7 days before to 28 days after delivery, and pregnant women. Varicella-zoster immunoglobulin does not prevent infection when given after exposure but may modify the course of disease. Treatment with antivirals may be necessary in severe disease (see p.608).

The doses, given by deep intramuscular injection, of the varicella-zoster immunoglobulin available in the UK are: 250 mg for children up to 5 years of age; 500 mg for those aged 6 to 10 years; 750 mg for those aged 11 to 14 years; and 1 g for all those 15 years of age or older. A further dose is required if a second exposure occurs more than 3 weeks later. Varicella-zoster immunoglobulin should be given as soon as possible and not later than 10 days after exposure. Preparations of normal immunoglobulin for intravenous use may be used to provide an immediate source of antibody.

Recommendations in the USA are similar to those in the UK. Doses are 125 units per 10 kg body-weight by intramuscular injection up to a maximum of 625 units. Adults may be given 625 units but higher doses may be required in immunocompromised patients. Administration should start within 96 hours of exposure.

Preparations

Ph. Eur.: Human Varicella Immunoglobulin; Human Varicella Immunoglobulin for Intravenous Administration;
USP 25: Varicella-Zoster Immune Globulin.

Proprietary Preparations (details are given in Part 3)

Aust.: Varitect; ***Ger.:*** Varicellon; Varitect; ***Hong Kong:*** Varitect; ***Irl.:*** Varitect; ***Israel:*** Varitect; ***Ital.:*** Haimazig; Immunoendozig; Immunozig; Intrazig; Uman-Vzig; Var-Zeta†; Varitect; ***Port.:*** Varitect; ***S.Afr.:*** Vazigam; ***Singapore:*** Varitect; ***Switz.:*** Varitect; ***Thai.:*** Varitect.

Varicella-Zoster Vaccines (14011-t)

ATC — J07BK01.

Varicella Vaccine (Live) (Ph. Eur.) (Var/Vac (Live); Varicella Vaccine, Live (BP 2001); Vaccinum Varicellae Vivum) is a freeze-dried preparation of the OKA attenuated strain of *Herpesvirus varicellae* grown in cultures of human diploid cells. The culture medium may contain suitable antibiotics at the smallest effective concentration. It is prepared immediately before use by reconstitution from the dried version; it may contain a stabiliser. The vaccine contains not less than 2000 plaque-forming units per dose. The dried vaccine should be stored at 2° to 8°. Protect from light.

Adverse Effects and Precautions

As for vaccines in general, p.1529.

Rashes at the injection site and varicella-like rashes elsewhere have been reported. It is not known whether the virus becomes latent which could result in late development of zoster infections although there are early indications that the incidence of herpes zoster is lower following vaccination than in an unvaccinated population.

◊ General references.
1. Black S, *et al.* Postmarketing evaluation of the safety and effectiveness of varicella vaccine. *Pediatr Infect Dis J* 1999; **18:** 1041–6.

Pregnancy. Transmission of the vaccine strain of varicella virus has been reported from a young child to his pregnant mother.[1] After elective termination of the pregnancy, no virus was detected in the fetus.
1. Salzman MB, *et al.* Transmission of varicella-vaccine virus from a healthy 12-month-old child to his pregnant mother. *J Pediatr* 1997; **131:** 151–4.

Interactions

As for vaccines in general, p.1530.

Uses and Administration

Varicella-zoster vaccines may be used for active immunisation against varicella (chickenpox) in persons considered to be at high risk of either contracting the infection or to be highly susceptible to any complications it may cause; such patients include those with leukaemia or those receiving immunosuppressant therapy.

In the USA, vaccination against varicella is recommended as part of the primary immunisation schedule (see under Vaccines, p.1530). A single dose of 0.5 mL is given subcutaneously at 12 to 18 months of age to healthy children unless there is a reliable history of varicella although children may receive the vaccine at any time during childhood after the first birthday. Persons over the age of 13 years at increased risk of exposure or complications should receive two doses at an interval of 4 to 8 weeks.

◊ Although the results of studies of varicella-zoster vaccines in healthy and leukaemic children have been largely favourable,[1,2] until recently, these vaccines have not been recommended for routine use in the UK or USA. Protective **efficacy** in healthy children appears to be over 90%.[1-4] In healthy adolescents and adults, adding a second dose 4 or 8 weeks after the first increased seroconversion rates from about 70 to 80% to 97% or better.[5] A protective efficacy of about 85% has been reported in leukaemic children given one dose of varicella-zoster vaccine.[6,7] A two-dose regimen (doses separated by 3 months) has been tried. Although a second dose is probably of benefit to those who do not seroconvert after one dose, its additional benefit to those who do seroconvert is doubtful.[7] Interruption of chemotherapy for vaccination does not appear necessary in terms of immunogenicity of the vaccine.[6,8] A higher rate of vaccine-associated rashes has, however, been observed in leukaemic children when chemotherapy was suspended for 2 weeks compared with those whose chemotherapy had previously been terminated; this only occurred with certain lots of vaccine.[6]

The **duration of immunity** after varicella-zoster vaccination is also under debate. Studies indicate that the immunity induced by natural infection with wild type virus is superior to that induced by the vaccine. In one study,[7] about one-quarter of all vaccinees (both leukaemic children and healthy adults) were seronegative one year after a second dose of vaccine, but none were seronegative after up to 6 years after breakthrough varicella infection. However, immunity to varicella-zoster is complex, depending not only on circulating antibody but also on cellular immunity and secretory antibody.[1] Thus, although a person may become seronegative after vaccination, protection from varicella may remain, albeit partial.[6] Both humoral and cell mediated immunity have been shown to persist for up to 20 years after vaccination.[9] Leukaemic children observed up to 6

years after immunisation have continued to be well protected[6] and varicella in previously-vaccinated persons is usually mild.[6,7]

There is some controversy over vaccinating healthy children, mainly due to uncertainties over long-term consequences and the impact vaccination may have on unimmunised members of the population. Two studies[10,11] in the USA have suggested that inclusion of varicella vaccines into routine **immunisation schedules** in infants could be cost effective, particularly if work time lost by parents caring for sick children is included in the calculation. This view has been rigorously opposed by clinicians who think such a step would be premature.[12-14] Nevertheless, the American Academy of Pediatrics Committee on Infectious Diseases recommends universal vaccination of healthy children at age 12 to 18 months, and in susceptible older children and adolescents.[15] Similar recommendations apply to persons with impaired humoral (but not cellular) immunity and some HIV-infected children.[16,17] The US Advisory Committee on Immunization Practices recommends[16] that, in addition, varicella-zoster vaccine be given to all susceptible persons over age 13 who live or work in environments where transmission can or is likely to occur to non-pregnant women of child-bearing age, to those who live in households with children, and to those travelling abroad.

Varicella-zoster vaccine may prevent or modify varicella if given within 3 days of exposure to the infection. In the US, vaccine administration is now recommended in all susceptible persons following exposure to varicella.[16,17] It may be useful as an **adjunct** to varicella-zoster immunoglobulin.[2] The treatment of varicella-zoster infections with antivirals is discussed on p.608.

One concern of varicella-zoster vaccination has been the possibility of an **increased risk of herpes zoster** (shingles) in immunised children. Although herpes zoster has been reported in vaccinated persons, a study involving 346 leukaemic children and 84 matched controls concluded that the incidence of herpes zoster following varicella-zoster vaccine was no greater than that following natural varicella infection.[18] The study did suggest that the risk of herpes zoster may be lowered by vaccination but this must be confirmed by long-term follow-up. Postmarketing surveys[16,19] of almost 90 000 vaccine recipients also showed a low incidence of herpes zoster. The vaccine strain of varicella-zoster virus is transmissible, particularly from vaccinees who develop a rash (see also under Adverse Effects, above).[1] There is no evidence of reversion to virulence of the vaccine strain with secondary transmission.[1]

Another concern is that vaccination of children could result in more severe infections in later life after immunity has waned. However, studies have shown that in general varicella is less severe in previously immunised than in non-immunised patients.[20,21]

1. Isaacs D, Menser M. Modern vaccines: measles, mumps, rubella, and varicella. *Lancet* 1990; **335:** 1384–7.
2. National Institutes of Health Conference. Varicella-zoster virus infections: biology, natural history, treatment, and prevention. *Ann Intern Med* 1988; **108:** 221–37.
3. White CJ, *et al.* Varicella vaccine (Varivax) in healthy children and adolescents: results from clinical trials, 1987 to 1989. *Pediatrics* 1991; **87:** 604–10.
4. Dennehy PH, *et al.* Immunogenicity of subcutaneous versus intramuscular Oka/Merck varicella vaccination in healthy children. *Pediatrics* 1991; **88:** 604–7.
5. Kuter BJ, *et al.* Safety, tolerability, and immunogenicity of two regimens of Oka/Merck varicella vaccine (Varivax) in healthy adolescents and adults. *Vaccine* 1995; **13:** 967 72.
6. Gershon AA, *et al.* Persistence of immunity to varicella in children with leukemia immunized with live attenuated varicella vaccine. *N Engl J Med* 1989; **320:** 892–7.
7. Gershon AA, *et al.* Live attenuated varicella vaccine: protection in healthy adults compared with leukemic children. *J Infect Dis* 1990; **161:** 661–6.
8. Arbeter AM, *et al.* Immunization of children with acute lymphoblastic leukemia with live attenuated varicella vaccine without complete suspension of chemotherapy. *Pediatrics* 1990; **85:** 338–44.
9. Asano Y, *et al.* Experience and reason: twenty-year follow-up of protective immunity of the Oka strain live varicella vaccine. *Pediatrics* 1994; **94:** 524–6.
10. Huse DM, *et al.* Childhood vaccination against chickenpox: an analysis of benefits and costs. *J Pediatr* 1994; **124:** 869–74.
11. Lieu TA, *et al.* Cost-effectiveness of a routine varicella vaccination program for US children. *JAMA* 1994; **271:** 375–81.
12. Bader M, Oswego L. Varicella vaccine. *JAMA* 1994; **271:** 1744–5.
13. Smukler M. Routine childhood varicella vaccination. *JAMA* 1994; **271:** 1906.
14. Ross LF, Lantos JD. Immunisation against chickenpox. *BMJ* 1995; **310:** 2–3.
15. Committee on Infectious Diseases. Recommendations for the use of live attenuated varicella vaccine. *Pediatrics* 1995; **95:** 791–6. Correction. *ibid.*; **96** (1).
16. Centers for Disease Control. Prevention of varicella: updated recommendations of the Advisory Committee on Immunization Practices (ACIP). *MMWR* 1999; **48** (RR-6): 1–5.
17. Committee on Infectious Diseases, American Academy of Pediatrics. Varicella vaccine update. *Pediatrics* 2000; **105:** 136–41.
18. Lawrence R, *et al.* The risk of zoster after varicella vaccination in children with leukemia. *N Engl J Med* 1988; **318:** 543–8.
19. Black S, *et al.* Postmarketing evaluation of the safety and effectiveness of varicella vaccine. *Pediatr Infect Dis J* 1999; **18:** 1041–6.
20. Watson BM, *et al.* Modified chickenpox in children immunized with the Oka/Merck varicella vaccine. *Pediatrics* 1993; **91:** 17–22.
21. Bernstein HH, *et al.* Clinical survey of natural varicella compared with breakthrough varicella after immunization with live attenuated Oka/Merck varicella vaccine. *Pediatrics* 1993; **92:** 833–7.

Preparations

Ph. Eur.: Varicella Vaccine (Live).

Proprietary Preparations (details are given in Part 3)
Aust.: Varicella; Varilrix; *Austral.:* Varilrix; Varivax; *Belg.:* Varilrix; *Canad.:* Varivax; *Denm.:* Varilrix; *Fin.:* Varilrix; *Ger.:* Varilrix; *Hong Kong:* Varilrix; Varivax; *Ital.:* Varilrix; *Mex.:* Varilrix; *Norw.:* Varilrix; *NZ:* Varilrix; *Singapore:* Varilrix; Varivax; *Spain:* Varilrix; *Swed.:* Varilrix; *Switz.:* Varilrix; *Thai.:* Varilrix; *USA:* Varivax.

Yellow Fever Vaccines (8038-d)

ATC — J07BL01.

Yellow Fever Vaccine (Live) (Ph. Eur.) (Yel/Vac; Yellow Fever Vaccine, Live (BP 2001); Vaccinum Febris Flavae Vivum) is a freeze-dried preparation of the 17D strain of yellow fever virus grown in fertilised hen eggs. It is reconstituted immediately before use. It should be stored at 2° to 8° and be protected from light.

Yellow Fever Vaccine (USP 25) is a freeze-dried preparation of a selected attenuated strain of live yellow fever virus cultured in chick embryos. It is reconstituted, just prior to use, by the addition of sodium chloride containing no antimicrobial agent. It should be stored under nitrogen preferably below 0° but not above 5°.

Adverse Effects and Precautions

As for vaccines in general, p.1529.

Local and general reactions are not common after vaccination for yellow fever. Very rarely encephalitis has followed vaccination, generally in infants under 9 months of age. Therefore, yellow fever vaccine is not usually given to infants under 9 months (but see below).

There is as yet insufficient data on the safety of yellow fever vaccine in HIV-positive individuals. In the UK administration of yellow fever vaccine to such individuals is not recommended. WHO advises that the vaccine should be administered to HIV-positive individuals who are asymptomatic if the risk of infection is high.

◊ There have been a few case reports of fatalities resulting from haemorrhagic fever,[1] hepatitis,[2] and multisystem organ failure[3] associated with the use of yellow fever vaccines.
1. Vasconcelos PFC, *et al.* Serious adverse events associated with yellow fever 17DD vaccine in Brazil: a report of two cases. *Lancet* 2001; **358:** 91–7. Corrections. *ibid.:* **336:** *ibid.:* 1018.
2. Chan RC, *et al.* Hepatitis and death following vaccination with 17D-204 yellow fever vaccine. *Lancet* 2001; **358:** 121–2.
3. Martin M, *et al.* Fever and multisystem organ failure associated with 17D-204 yellow fever vaccination: a report of four cases. *Lancet* 2001; **358:** 98–104.

Effects on the nervous system. Encephalitis may occur very rarely following vaccination against yellow fever, but WHO in 1986 stated[1] that not more than 17 cases of encephalitis had been recorded over a period of 40 years and all occurred in children; although it was possible that some cases may have gone unrecorded, the number would be very small in proportion to the tens of millions of immunisations performed without known encephalitic complications. As a precaution against possible encephalitic complications, infants under 9 months of age are not generally immunised but it may be advisable to immunise children at 6 months of age if they live in rural areas with a history of yellow fever epidemics, and even at 4 months in an active epidemic focus; no child less than 4 months old should receive yellow fever vaccine.
1. WHO. *Prevention and control of yellow fever in Africa.* Geneva: WHO, 1986.

Pregnancy. Although yellow fever vaccine has been given to women during pregnancy without adverse effects in the infants,[1] fetal infection has been reported.[2]
1. Nasidi A, *et al.* Yellow fever vaccination and pregnancy: a four-year prospective study. *Trans R Soc Trop Med Hyg* 1993; **87:** 337–9.
2. Tsai TF, *et al.* Congenital yellow fever virus infection after immunization in pregnancy. *J Infect Dis* 1993; **168:** 1520–3.

Interactions

As for vaccines in general, p.1530.

◊ There have been several studies on the combined use of yellow fever vaccine and other vaccines.[1] The administration of measles vaccine and yellow fever vaccine at the same site has resulted in a decrease in the rate of seroconversions to yellow fever but the injection was made intradermally. When given at different sites, and when diphtheria, tetanus, and pertussis vaccine was also added, no interference was shown. Cholera vaccines should not be given together with yellow fever vaccine, or in the preceding 3 weeks, since the yellow fever neutralising antibody response is reduced at least temporarily. Pooled human immunoglobulin given before, at the same time as, or after yellow fever vaccine does not impair the rate of serological conversion. The UK manufacturers do, however, state that it is advisable to avoid administration of yellow fever vaccine within 6 weeks following administration of normal immunoglobulin and, conversely, to avoid administration of normal immunoglobulin for at least 2 weeks after vaccination.

1. WHO. *Prevention and control of yellow fever in Africa.* Geneva: WHO, 1986.

Uses and Administration

Yellow fever vaccines are used for active immunisation against yellow fever. Immunity is usually established within about 10 days of administration and persists for many years. Only one dose is required for immunisation and is given by subcutaneous injection; the dose (0.5 mL) is the volume containing at least 1000 mouse LD_{50} units.

In the UK, immunisation against yellow fever is recommended for laboratory workers handling infected material, for persons travelling through or living in areas of infection, and for travellers entering countries which require an International Certificate of Vaccination. The immunity produced may last for life although officially an International Certificate of Vaccination against yellow fever is valid only for 10 years starting 10 days after the primary immunisation and only if the vaccine used has been approved by WHO and administered at a designated vaccinating centre.

Vaccination under 9 months of age is not generally recommended (see under Adverse Effects and Pre-cautions, above). In the USA vaccination of children aged 6 to 9 months is recommended only for travel to an area of ongoing yellow fever epidemic, or when travel cannot be postponed and a high level of protection against mosquito bites is not feasible. Infants under 4 months of age should not be vaccinated.

◊ General references.

1. Barrett ADT. Yellow fever vaccines. *Biologicals* 1997; **25**: 17–25.

Immunisation schedules. The 17D (Rockefeller) yellow fever vaccine is now the only yellow fever vaccine produced.[1] The quantity available in the world has been limited and its relatively short half-life does not permit the accumulation of large stocks. The demand for the vaccine is also somewhat irregular, being suddenly high during epidemics and low during inter-epidemic periods.

In Africa two different strategies for yellow fever immunisation have been followed.[1] Firstly, an emergency immunisation programme takes place once an outbreak has begun, in an attempt to limit the spread of infection by immunising all persons in the focus, regardless of their former immune status. One disadvantage is that immunity does not appear until 7 days after immunisation and deaths may be expected to occur in the interim period. Secondly, a routine mass immunisation programme for yellow fever is aimed at immunising in advance all populations considered to be at risk. Yellow fever vaccine may be considered for inclusion in a national Expanded Programme on Immunization; there are obvious logistic advantages in administering it at the age of 9 months at the same time as measles vaccine. In rural areas of the endemic zone that are considered at high risk, the minimum age for routine immunisation may be lowered to 6 months (see under Adverse Effects and Precautions, above). Studies have suggested that immunisation with a combined yellow fever and measles vaccine may be possible.[2]

1. WHO. *Prevention and control of yellow fever in Africa.* Geneva: WHO, 1986.
2. Lhuillier M, *et al.* Study of combined vaccination against yellow fever and measles in infants from six to nine months. *J Biol Stand* 1989; **17**: 9–15.

◊ Recommendations of the Advisory Committee on Immunization Practices for the prevention of yellow fever in the USA.[1]

1. Immunization Practices Advisory Committee. Yellow fever vaccine. *MMWR* 1990; **39** (RR-6): 1–6.

Immunisation for travellers. A booklet entitled *International Travel and Health: Vaccination Requirements and Health Advice* is published annually by WHO. Information is provided concerning the countries in Africa and South America where yellow fever is endemic and also countries requiring a traveller to hold a valid vaccination certificate. For some further details, see p.1531.

Preparations

Ph. Eur.: Yellow Fever Vaccine (Live);
USP 25: Yellow Fever Vaccine.

Proprietary Preparations (details are given in Part 3)
Austral.: Stamaril; *Belg.:* Stamaril; *Denm.:* Stamaril; *Fin.:* Stamaril; *Fr.:* Stamaril; *Ger.:* Stamaril; *Irl.:* Arilvax; Stamaril; *Israel:* Arilvax; *Ital.:* Stamaril; *Neth.:* Arilvax; Stamaril; *Norw.:* Stamaril; *S.Afr.:* Arilvax; Stamaril; *Singapore:* Arilvax; Stamaril; *Swed.:* Arilvax; Stamaril; *Switz.:* Arilvax; Stamaril; *UK:* Arilvax; Stamaril; *USA:* YF-Vax.

Part 2

Supplementary Drugs and Other Substances

Abrus (12303-z)

Abrus Seed; Indian Liquorice; Jequirity Bean; Jumble Beads; Prayer Beads; Rosary Beans.

The seeds of *Abrus precatorius* (Leguminosae), one of whose constituents is abrin.

Profile
Abrin is considered responsible for the toxic effects of abrus seeds. It is closely related to ricin. Deaths of children have occurred from eating one or more seeds. Toxicity may be less likely to occur if the seeds are swallowed whole, than if they are chewed, because of the hard seed coat. Toxic effects may occur within a few hours or may be delayed for several days following ingestion and include gastro-enteritis, circulatory collapse, haemorrhages, oliguria, agglutination and haemolysis of the red blood cells with subsequent acute renal failure, and convulsions. Treatment is symptomatic following removal of ingested beans by gastric lavage; activated charcoal may be given.

Abrus has been used in homoeopathic medicine and as an oral contraceptive in herbal medicine.

◊ General references.
1. Aslam M, Shaw JMH. Abrus in Asian medicine. *Pharm J* 1998; **261:** 822–4.

Absinthium (521-c)

Absinthii Herba; Assenzio; Losna; Pelin; Wermutkraut; Wormwood.
CAS — 546-80-5 (α-thujone); 471-15-8 (β-thujone).
Pharmacopoeias. In Eur. (see p.vi) and Pol.

Thujone, related to camphor, is the major constituent of the essential oil derived from absinthium.

Pharmacopoeial description

Ph. Eur.: The leaves or flowering tops, or a mixture of these dried, whole or cut organs of wormwood, *Artemisia absinthium*. It contains not less than 2 mL per kg of essential oil, calculated with reference to the dried drug. Protect from light.

Profile
Absinthium has been used as a bitter. It is also used in small quantities as a flavour in alcoholic beverages, although it is considered in some countries not to be safe for use in foods, beverages, or drugs. Habitual use or large doses cause absinthism, which is characterised by restlessness, vomiting, vertigo, tremors, and convulsions. Absinthium has been used in homoeopathic medicine.

◊ References.
1. Weisbord SD, *et al.* Poison on line—acute renal failure caused by oil of wormwood purchased through the Internet. *N Engl J Med* 1997; **337:** 825–7.

Preparations

Proprietary Preparations (details are given in Part 3)

Multi-ingredient: *Aust.:* Abdomilon; Amara; Amylatin; Aponatura Erkaltungs; Aponatura Galle; Aponatura Leber; Aponatura Verdauungs; Bio-Garten Tee fur Leber und Galle; Bio-Garten Tropfen fur Galle und Leber; Eryval; Felidon neu; Gallogran; Krauterdoktor Gallentreibende Tropfen; Krauterdoktor Verdauungsfordernde Tropfen; Krauterhaus Mag Kottas Tee fur die Verdauung; Krautertee Nr 17; Krautertee Nr 28; Krautertee Nr 30; Leberund Galletee; Magentee EF-EM-ES; Mariazeller; Pepsiton; Sigman-Haustropfen; St Radegunder Verdauungstee; Vinopepsin; Virgilocard; *Braz.:* Camomila; *Fr.:* Tisane Hepatique de Hoerdt; *Ger.:* Abdomilon N; Agrimonas N; Amara-Tropfen; Amara-Tropfen-Pascoe; Anore X N; Aristochol N; Cefagastrin; Chol-Truw S†; Doppelherz Magenstarkung†; Floradix Multipretten; Gallemolan forte; Gallemolan G; Gallexier; Gastralon N; Gastritol; Gastrol S; Hepaticum novo; Hepatofalk Neu; Hevert-Magen-Galle-Leber-Tee†; Leber-Galle-Tropfen 83; Lomatol; Marianon; Montana; Nervosana; Neurochol C; Novo Mandrogallan N†; Pascopankreat novo; Phonix Gastriphon; Presselin Blahungs K 4 N; Presselin Dyspeptikum; rohasal; Stomachysat N; Stovalid N; Stullmaton; Unex Amarum; Ventrimarin novo; *Switz.:* Baume; Kernosan Heidelberger Poudre; Phytomed Hepato.

Acedoben (11903-p)

Acedoben *(pINN)*.
p-Acetamidobenzoic acid.
$C_9H_9NO_3 = 179.2$.
CAS — 556-08-1.

Profile
Acedoben is a component of inosine pranobex (p.627), and has been given by mouth as the potassium salt in the treatment of skin disorders. Acedoben and its sodium salt have been applied topically.

Preparations

Proprietary Preparations (details are given in Part 3)
Spain: Fibroderm.

Multi-ingredient: *Spain:* Amplidermis; Hongosan; Perlinsol Cutaneo†.

Aceglutamide (12306-a)

Aceglutamide *(rINN)*.
N^2-Acetyl-L-glutamine; 2-Acetylamino-L-glutaramic acid.
$C_7H_{12}N_2O_4 = 188.2$.
CAS — 2490-97-3.

Profile
Aceglutamide has been given in an attempt to improve memory and concentration.

Preparations

Proprietary Preparations (details are given in Part 3)

Multi-ingredient: *Ital.:* Acutil Fosforo; Memovisus; Tonoplus; *Spain:* Levaliver; Teovit.

Acemannan (9340-j)

Acemannan *(USAN, rINN)*.
Polymanoacetate.
CAS — 110042-95-0.

Profile
Acemannan is a highly acetylated, polydispersed, linear mannan obtained from the mucilage of *Aloe vera* (=*A. Barbadensis*). It has immunomodulating properties.

Glacial Acetic Acid (1306-k)

Acide Acetique Cristallisable; Acidum Aceticum Glaciale; Concentrated Acetic Acid; E260 (acetic acid); Eisessig; Etanoico; Ethanoic Acid; Glac. Acet. Acid; Konzentrierte Essigsäure.
$C_2H_4O_2 = 60.05$.
CAS — 64-19-7.
Pharmacopoeias. In Chin., Eur. (see p.vi), Jpn, Pol., and US.

Pharmacopoeial description

Ph. Eur.: A crystalline mass or a clear colourless volatile liquid. F.p. not lower than 14.8°. Miscible with water, with alcohol, with dichloromethane, and with ether. Store in airtight containers.

USP 25: A clear colourless liquid with a pungent characteristic odour. B.p. about 118°. Miscible with water, with alcohol, and with glycerol. Store in airtight containers.

Acetic Acid (1305-c)

ATC — G01AD02; S02AA10.

NOTE. The nomenclature of acetic acid often leads to confusion as to whether concentrations are expressed as percentages of glacial acetic acid (acetic acid ($C_2H_4O_2$) or of this diluted form. In *Martindale*, the percentage figures given against acetic acid represent the amount of $C_2H_4O_2$.
Pharmacopoeias. In Aus. (33.7 to 35.5%), Br. (33%), Jpn (30 to 32%), Pol. (30%), and Swiss (30%). Also in USNF (36 to 37%). The following pharmacopoeias include weaker solutions under the titles or synonyms Dilute Acetic Acid or Diluted Acetic Acid: *Aust.* (11.5 to 12.2%), *Br.* (6%), and *It.* (10%).

Pharmacopoeial description

BP 2001: Acetic acid (33%) is a clear colourless liquid with a pungent odour. Miscible with water, with alcohol, and with glycerol.
Acetic acid 6% is prepared by diluting acetic acid 33%.

USNF 20: Acetic acid (36 to 37%) is a clear colourless liquid with a strong characteristic odour. Miscible with water, with alcohol, and with glycerol. Store in airtight containers.

Adverse Effects and Treatment
Local or topical application of acetic acid preparations may produce stinging or burning. Ingestion of glacial acetic acid can produce similar adverse effects to those of hydrochloric acid (p.1621), which may be treated similarly.

Uses and Administration
Glacial acetic acid has been used as an escharotic. Diluted forms have been used as an antibacterial (it is reported to be effective against *Haemophilus* and *Pseudomonas* spp.), antifungal, and antiprotozoal in vaginal gels and douches, irrigations, topical preparations for the skin and nails, and in ear drops. Diluted forms have also been used as an expectorant, an astringent lotion, and as treatments for warts (p.1108), callosities, and for certain jellyfish stings.

A solution containing 4% w/v $C_2H_4O_2$ is known as artificial vinegar or non-brewed condiment. Vinegar is a product of fermentation.

Jellyfish sting. Vinegar or acetic acid 3 to 10% is applied to box jellyfish stings to inactivate any fragments of adherent tentacle[1,2] (see p.1546). Acetic acid solutions have been reported to be useful in stings by related species[3] although they may produce further discharge of venom in some jellyfish.[4]
1. Hartwick RJ, *et al.* Disarming the box jellyfish. *Med J Aust* 1980; **1:** 15–20.
2. Fenner PJ, Williamson JA. Worldwide deaths and severe envenomation from jellyfish stings. *Med J Aust* 1996; **165:** 658–61.
3. Fenner PJ, *et al.* "Morbakka", another cubomedusan. *Med J Aust* 1985; **143:** 550–5.
4. Fenner PJ, Fitzpatrick PF. Experiments with the nematocysts of Cyanea capillata. *Med J Aust* 1986; **145:** 174.

Wounds and burns. Infection of wounds (p.1108) and burns (p.1104) with *Pseudomonas aeruginosa* may delay healing. Acetic acid has been used, in concentrations of up to 5%, to eradicate these infections.[1]
1. Milner SM. Acetic acid to treat Pseudomonas aeruginosa in superficial wounds and burns. *Lancet* 1992; **340:** 61.

Preparations

BP 2001: Strong Ammonium Acetate Solution;
USP 25: Acetic Acid Irrigation; Acetic Acid Otic Solution; Hydrocortisone and Acetic Acid Otic Solution.

Proprietary Preparations (details are given in Part 3)
Austral.: Summers Eve Disposable; *Canad.:* Midol Douche†; *Fr.:* Para Lentes; *Irl.:* Aci-Jel; *Mex.:* Amigdobis; *UK:* Aci-Jel; Ear-Calm; Meltus Baby; *USA:* Feminique; Massengill Disposable; Summers Eve Disposable.

Multi-ingredient: *Aust.:* Onycho Phytex; Phytex; *Austral.:* Aci-Jel; Aquaear; Ear Clear for Swimmer's Ear; *Belg.:* Aporil; *Braz.:* A Curitybina; Kalostop; Lacto Vagin; Lacto-Gin; *Canad.:* SH-206; Viron Wart Lotion; VoSoL; VoSoL HC; *Fr.:* Nitrol; Ysol 206†; *Ger.:* Chol-Truw S†; Gehwol Huhneraugen Tinktur; Solco-Derman; Phytex; *Irl.:* Phytex; *Ital.:* Silvana; *Neth.:* Hexoll†; *NZ:* Aci-Jel; VoSoL; *Port.:* Calicida Indiano; Lecia; *Spain:* Callicida Cor Pik; Callicida Durcall†; Callicida Rojo; Nitroina; Quocin; *Switz.:* Solcoderm; Solcogyn; *Thai.:* Baby Cough Syrup; Baby Cough with Antihistamine; *UK:* Ellimans; Goddards White Oil Embrocation; Phytex; Sanderson's Throat Specific; *USA:* AA-HC Otic†; Acetasol; Acetasol HC; Aci-Jel; Borofair Otic; Burow's; Otic Domeboro; Renalin Dialyzer Reprocessing Concentrate†; Star-Otic; Tridesilon; VoSoL; VoSoL HC.

Acetohydroxamic Acid (12310-j)

Acetohydroxamic Acid *(USAN, rINN)*.
N-Acetyl Hydroxyacetamide; AHA.
$C_2H_5NO_2 = 75.07$.
CAS — 546-88-3.
ATC — G04BX03.
Pharmacopoeias. In US.

Pharmacopoeial description

USP 25: White, slightly hygroscopic, crystalline powder. Freely soluble in water and in alcohol; very slightly soluble in chloroform. Store in airtight containers at a temperature between 8° and 15°.

Adverse Effects and Precautions
Phlebitis, thromboembolism, haemolytic anaemia, and iron-deficiency anaemia have occurred. Other adverse effects include headache, gastrointestinal disturbances, alopecia, rash (particularly following ingestion of alcohol), trembling, and mental symptoms including anxiety and depression. Blood counts and renal function should be monitored regularly during treatment. Patients with acute renal failure should not be given acetohydroxamic acid.

Studies in *animals* indicate that acetohydroxamic acid is teratogenic and may cause bone-marrow depression.

Interactions

Acetohydroxamic acid chelates iron administered orally, resulting in reduced absorption of both. Concomitant consumption of alcohol may precipitate skin rash.

Pharmacokinetics

Acetohydroxamic acid is rapidly absorbed from the gastrointestinal tract with peak serum concentrations being reached within 1 hour. The plasma half-life is reported to be up to 10 hours, but may be longer in patients with impaired renal function. Acetohydroxamic acid is partially metabolised in the liver to acetamide, which is inactive; up to about two-thirds of a dose may be excreted unchanged in the urine.

Uses and Administration

Acetohydroxamic acid acts by inhibiting bacterial urease, thus decreasing urinary ammonia concentrations and alkalinity. It is used in the prophylaxis of renal calculi formed as a result of bacterial urease and as an adjunct in the treatment of chronic urinary-tract infection due to urease-splitting bacteria.

Acetohydroxamic acid is given by mouth in a usual dose of 250 mg three or four times daily. The total dose should not exceed 1.5 g daily. Children aged over 8 years have been given 10 mg per kg body-weight daily in 2 or 3 divided doses.

In patients with renal impairment the dosage interval should be increased to 12 hours and the dose may also need to be reduced.

◊ References.

1. Martelli A, *et al.* Acetohydroxamic acid therapy in infected renal stones. *Urology* 1981; **17**: 320–2.
2. Griffith DP. Infection-induced renal calculi. *Kidney Int* 1982; **21**: 422–30.
3. Rodman JS, *et al.* Partial dissolution of struvite calculus with oral acetohydroxamic acid. *Urology* 1983; **22**: 410–12.
4. Burr RG, Nuseibeh I. The effect of oral acetohydroxamic acid on urinary saturation in stone-forming spinal cord patients. *Br J Urol* 1983; **55**: 162–5.
5. Williams JJ, *et al.* A randomized double-blind study of acetohydroxamic acid in struvite nephrolithiasis. *N Engl J Med* 1984; **311**: 760–4.
6. Smith LH. New treatment for struvite urinary stones. *N Engl J Med* 1984; **311**: 792–4.
7. El Nujumi AM, *et al.* Effect of inhibition of Helicobacter pylori urease activity by acetohydroxamic acid on serum gastrin in duodenal ulcer subjects. *Gut* 1991; **32**: 866–70.
8. Zullo A, *et al.* Helicobacter pylori and plasma ammonia levels in cirrhosis: role of urease inhibition by acetohydroxamic acid. *Ital J Gastroenterol Hepatol* 1998; **30**: 405–9.

Preparations

USP 25: Acetohydroxamic Acid Tablets.

Proprietary Preparations (details are given in Part 3)
Belg.: Uronefrex†; **Fr.:** Uronefrex; **Spain:** Uronefrex; **USA:** Lithostat.

Acetylcarnitine Hydrochloride (3015-f)

Acetyl-L-carnitine Hydrochloride; ST-200. (3-Carboxy-2-hydroxypropyl)trimethylammonium acetate (ester) chloride.

$C_9H_{17}NO_4,HCl = 239.7$.
CAS — 5080-50-2.

Profile

Acetylcarnitine hydrochloride has been given by mouth and by injection in the treatment of cerebrovascular insufficiency and peripheral neuropathies. It is under investigation in Alzheimer's disease (p.1412).

◊ References.

1. Bella R, *et al.* Effect of acetyl-L-carnitine on geriatric patients suffering from dysthymic disorders. *Int J Clin Pharmacol Res* 1990; **10**: 355–60.
2. Thal LJ, *et al.* A 1-year multicenter placebo-controlled study of acetyl-L-carnitine in patients with Alzheimer's disease. *Neurology* 1996; **47**: 705–11.

Preparations

Proprietary Preparations (details are given in Part 3)
Ital.: Acilen; Branigen; Branitil; Nicetile; Normobren; Zibren†.

Acetylleucine (12313-k)

Acetylleucine (*rINN*).

RP-7542. *N*-Acetyl-DL-leucine.
$C_8H_{15}NO_3 = 173.2$.
CAS — 99-15-0.
ATC — N07CA04.

Profile

Acetylleucine has been used in the treatment of vertigo (p.408) in usual doses of up to 2 g daily by mouth, in divided doses, or 1 g daily by slow intravenous injection. Higher doses are occasionally employed.

Preparations

Proprietary Preparations (details are given in Part 3)
Fr.: Tanganil.

Acexamic Acid (12315-t)

Acexamic Acid (*BAN, rINN*).

CY-153; Epsilon Acetamidocaproic Acid. 6-Acetamidohexanoic acid.

$C_8H_{15}NO_3 = 173.2$.
CAS — 57-08-9 (acexamic acid); 70020-71-2 (zinc acexamate).

Pharmacopoeias. Eur. (see p.vi) includes Zinc Acexamate.

Profile

Acexamic acid is related structurally to the antifibrinolytic agent aminocaproic acid (p.724). Acexamic acid, usually as the calcium or sodium salt, has been administered topically or systemically to promote the healing of ulcers and various other skin lesions. Zinc acexamate has been given for peptic ulcer disease.

Preparations

Proprietary Preparations (details are given in Part 3)
Belg.: Plastenan†; **Braz.:** Plastenan; **Fr.:** Plastenan†; **Mex.:** Recoveron; **Port.:** Plastesol; **Spain:** Copinal.

Multi-ingredient: Fr.: Plastenan Neomycine†; Trofoseptine; **Mex.:** Recoveron N; **Port.:** Plastenan Neomicina; **Spain:** Linitul Antibiotico; Plaskine Neomicina; Unitul Complex.

Achillea (4601-h)

Achillée Millefeuille; Milfoil; Millefolii Herba; Schafgarbe; Yarrow.

Pharmacopoeias. In *Eur.* (see p.vi) and *Pol.*

Pharmacopoeial description

Ph. Eur.: The whole or cut, dried flowering tops of yarrow, *Achillea millefolium*. It contains not less than 2 mL per kg of essential oil and not less than 0.02% of proazulenes, expressed as chamazulene ($C_{14}H_{16} = 184.3$), both calculated with reference to the dried drug. Protect from light.

Profile

Achillea has been used mainly in herbal and homoeopathic medicine for a great variety of purposes. It has been stated to have diaphoretic, anti-inflammatory, and other miscellaneous properties. It has been reported to cause contact dermatitis.

◊ References.

1. Phillipson JD, Anderson LA. Herbal remedies used in sedative and antirheumatic preparations: part 2. *Pharm J* 1984; **233**: 111–15.
2. Chandler RF. Yarrow. *Can Pharm J* 1989; **122**: 41–3.

Preparations

Proprietary Preparations (details are given in Part 3)
Ger.: Kneipp Schafgarbe-Pflanzensaft Frauentost N†; Schamill; **Mex.:** Blancaler.

Multi-ingredient: Aust.: Abfuhrtee EF-EM-ES; Aktiv Leber- und Gallentee; Aktiv milder Magen- und Darmtee; Amersan; Bio-Garten Tee gegen Blahungen; Bio-Garten Tee zur Starkung und Kraftigung; Bio-Garten Tropfen fur Galle und Leber; Chol-Grandelat; Citochol; Felidon neu; Gallen- und Lebertee; Gallogran; Krauterdoktor Gallentreibende Tropfen; Krauterhaus Mag Kottas Blutreinigungstee†; Krauterhaus Mag Kottas Fruhjahrs- und Herbstkurtee; Krauterhaus Mag Kottas Magen- und Darmtee; Krauterhaus Mag Kottas Tee gegen Blahungen; Krauterhaus Mag Kottas Wechseltee; Krautertee Nr 124; Krautertee Nr 16; Krautertee Nr 44; Mag Kottas Wechseltee; Magentee; Mariazeller; Menodoron; Sidroga Leber-Galle-Tee; Sidroga Magen-Darm-Tee; Windtreibender Tee; **Austral.:** Crataegus Complex; Flavons; **Fr.:** Cicaderma†; Tisane Digestive Weleda†; Tisane Hepatique de Hoerdt; Tisanes de l' Abbe Hamon no 14†; **Ger.:** Alasenn; Amara-Tropfen; Aristochol N; Befelka-Tinktur†; Cheiranthol; Dr. Hotz Vollbad†; Floradix Multipretten; Gallexier; Hevert-Golf-Rheuma-Tee comp†; Hevert-Magen-Galle-Leber-Tee†; Kamillan plus; Magen-Tee Stada N†; Marianon; Menaven; Salus Leber-Galle-Tee Nr.18†; Salus Rheuma-Tee Krautertee Nr. 12†; Sedovent; Stomachysat N; Tonsilgon N; **Ital.:** Fluiven†; Forticrin; **Port.:** Cicaderma; **Switz.:** Baume; Enveloppements ECR†; Gastrosan; Kernosan Heidelberger Poudre; Tisane hepatique et biliaire; Tisane pour l'estomac; Tisane relaxante; **UK:** Carminative Tea; Catarrh; Catarrh-eeze; Laxadoron; Liverguard†; Menodoron; Rheumatic Pain Remedy; Tabritis; Wellwoman.

Acid Fuchsine (2247-q)

Acid Magenta; Acid Roseine; Acid Rubine; CI Acid Violet 19; Colour Index No. 42685.

The disodium or diammonium salt of the trisulfonic acid of magenta.

Profile

Acid fuchsine is used as a microscopic stain and a pH indicator.

Aconite (12320-c)

Acetylbenzoylaconine (aconitine); Aconit.; Aconit Napel; Aconite Root; Aconiti Tuber; Monkshood Root; Radix Aconiti; Wolfsbane Root. 8-Acetoxy-3,11,18-trihydroxy-16-ethyl-1,6,19-trimethoxy-4-methoxymethylaconitan-10-yl benzoate (aconitine).

$C_{34}H_{47}NO_{11}$ (aconitine) = 645.7 (aconitine).
CAS — 8063-12-5 (aconite); 302-27-2 (aconitine).

NOTE. Wolfsbane is also used as a common name for arnica flower.

Pharmacopoeias. In *Belg.*
Aust. includes aconitine.

The dried tuberous root of *Aconitum napellus* agg. (Ranunculaceae). It contains a number of alkaloids, the main pharmacologically active one being aconitine.

Adverse Effects

Aconite has variable effects on the heart leading to heart failure. It also affects the CNS.

Symptoms of aconite poisoning may appear almost immediately and are rarely delayed beyond an hour; in fatal poisoning death usually occurs within 6 hours, although with larger doses it may be instantaneous.

Moderately toxic doses produce a tingling of the tongue, mouth, stomach, and skin (this is the most important diagnostic feature) followed by numbness and anaesthesia. Other symptoms include gastrointestinal disturbances; irregular pulse; difficult respiration; cold, clammy, and livid skin; muscular weakness, incoordination, and vertigo.

Treatment of aconite poisoning is symptomatic; atropine sulfate may be given in severe cases.

Poisoning. Reports of poisoning with aconite.

1. Kelly SP. Aconite poisoning. *Med J Aust* 1990; **153**: 499.
2. Tai Y-T, *et al.* Cardiotoxicity after accidental herb-induced aconite poisoning. *Lancet* 1992; **340**: 1254–6.
3. Kolev ST, *et al.* Toxicity following accidental ingestion of Aconitum containing Chinese remedy. *Hum Exp Toxicol* 1996; **15**: 839–42.
4. Mak W, Lau CP. A woman with tetraparesis and missed beats. *Hosp Med* 2000; **61**: 438.

Uses and Administration

Aconite liniments have been used in the treatment of neuralgia, sciatica, and rheumatism. Sufficient aconitine may be absorbed through the skin to cause serious poisoning; liniments should never be applied to wounds or abraded surfaces. Aconite should not be used internally because of its low therapeutic index and variable potency; however it is reported to be a common ingredient in traditional Chinese remedies and is also an ingredient of some cough mixtures.

A preparation of aconite is used in homoeopathic medicine.

Preparations

Proprietary Preparations (details are given in Part 3)
Belg.: Bromofotyl†.

Multi-ingredient: Aust.: Rheuma; **Belg.:** Colimax; Eucalyptine Pholcodine Le Brun; Euphon; Folcodex; Gloceda; Sirop Toux du Larynx†; Solucamphre†; **Braz.:** Axol; Broncofenil; Broncotussan; Expectomel; Gotas Nican; Limao Bravo; Melagriao; Pectal; Pinosil; Xarope de Caraguata + Bromoformio; **Fr.:** Broncorinol toux seches; Bronpax†; Euphon†; Gaiarsol; Peter's Sirop†; Pulmonase†; Sedophon; Sirop Boin†; Sirop Pectoral adulte†; **Ital.:** Lactocol; **Port.:** Anti-Gripe; Calmarum; Codoforme; Lactucol; **Spain:** Encilaina; Etermol; Pectoral Brum†.

Acridine Orange (18717-c)

3,6-Bis(dimethylamino)acridine.
$C_{17}H_{19}N_3 = 265.4$.
CAS — 494-38-2.

Profile

Acridine orange is a dye with antiseptic properties. It has been used as a diagnostic stain in microbiology.

For details of the antiseptic properties of acridine derivatives, see p.1130.

Diagnostic use. Acridine orange has been used for the diagnostic staining of malarial parasites.[1] For the quantitative buffy coat method, acridine orange is used to stain the parasites in a blood sample that is then centrifuged, and the area just below the buffy coat is examined under a fluorescence microscope. It has been described as easier and quicker to use than the standard examination of stained blood films. However, this method is not specific for diagnosis of malarial type, gives only a rough indication of infection intensity, and can give false-positive results. Acridine orange has also been tried for the staining of blood slides.[2-5]

1. Warhurst DC, Williams JE. ACP Broadsheet no 148, July 1996, Laboratory diagnosis of malaria. *J Clin Pathol* 1996; **49**: 533–8.
2. Gay F, *et al.* Direct acridine orange fluorescence examination of blood slides compared to current techniques for malaria diagnosis. *Trans R Soc Trop Med Hyg* 1996; **90**: 576–18.
3. Craig MH, Sharp BL. Comparative evaluation of four techniques for the diagnosis of Plasmodium falciparum infections. *Trans R Soc Trop Med Hyg* 1997; **91**: 279–82.

4. Tarimo DS, *et al.* Appraisal of the acridine orange method for rapid malaria diagnosis at three Tanzanian district hospitals. *East Afr Med J* 1998; **75:** 504–7.

5. Lema OE, *et al.* Comparison of five methods of malaria detection in the outpatient setting. *Am J Trop Med Hyg* 1999; **60:** 177–82.

Acrolein   (12322-a)

Acraldehyde; Acrylaldehyde; Acrylic Aldehyde. Prop-2-enal.
$C_3H_4O = 56.06$.
CAS — 107-02-8.

Profile

Acrolein has various industrial uses. It is irritant to the skin and may cause vesiculation. Ingestion of acrolein produces severe gastrointestinal distress. The vapour causes lachrymation and nasal irritation. Inhalation may cause pulmonary oedema, nephritis, or pneumonia.

◊ References.
1. Acrolein. *Environmental Health Criteria 127.* Geneva: WHO, 1992.
2. Acrolein. *IPCS Health and Safety Guide 67.* Geneva: WHO, 1991.

Acrylamide   (12324-x)

Propenamide.
$C_3H_5NO = 71.08$.
CAS — 79-06-1.

Profile

Acrylamide is highly toxic and moderately irritant; it can be absorbed through unbroken skin. Symptoms of poisoning include cold sweating hands and peripheral neuropathies with numbness, paraesthesias and weakness, especially associated with the lower limbs.

Acrylamide has various industrial applications, including use as a plasticiser and a waterproof 'chemical grout'.

◊ References to acrylamide toxicity.
1. Kesson CM, *et al.* Acrylamide poisoning. *Postgrad Med J* 1977; **53:** 16–17.
2. Acrylamide health and safety guide. *IPCS Health and Safety Guide 45.* Geneva: WHO, 1991.

Actinoquinol   (12281-h)

Actinoquinol (*rINN*).
8-Ethoxy-5-quinolinesulphonic acid.
$C_{11}H_{11}NO_4S = 253.3$.
CAS — 15301-40-3 (*actinoquinol*); 7246-07-3 (*actinoquinol sodium*).

NOTE. Actinoquinol Sodium is *USAN*.

Profile

Actinoquinol is administered as an ingredient of eye drop preparations intended to protect eyes from the effects of light. Actinoquinol sodium is also used.

Preparations

Proprietary Preparations (details are given in Part 3)
Aust.: Ultra Augenschutz.

Multi-ingredient: *Fr.:* Uvicol; *Ger.:* duraultra; Idril sine; Tele-Stulln; *Ital.:* Fotofil.

Ademetionine   (12326-f)

Ademetionine (*rINN*).
Ademethionine; S-Adenosyl-L-methionine; Methioninyl adenylate; SAMe. (S)-5′-[(3-Amino-3-carboxypropyl)methylsulphonio]-5′-deoxyadenosine hydroxide, inner salt.
$C_{15}H_{22}N_6O_5S = 398.4$.
CAS — 29908-03-0; 485-80-3; 17176-17-9.
ATC — A16AA02.

Profile

Ademetionine is a naturally occurring molecule found in virtually all body tissues and fluids. It acts as a methyl group donor in many transmethylation reactions and therefore is involved in the synthesis or metabolism of a wide range of compounds that maintain normal cell function. Ademetionine sulfate tosilate and ademetionine butanedisulfonate are stable forms of ademetionine that have been used for the treatment of depression, liver disorders, and osteoarthritis.

◊ Reviews.
1. Friedel HA, *et al.* S-Adenosyl-L-methionine: a review of its pharmacological properties and therapeutic potential in liver dysfunction and affective disorders in relation to its physiological role in cell metabolism. *Drugs* 1989; **38:** 389–416.
2. Bottiglieri T, *et al.* The clinical potential of ademetionine (S-adenosylmethionine) in neurological disorders. *Drugs* 1994; **48:** 137–52.
3. Chavez M. SAMe: S-adenosylmethionine. *Am J Health-Syst Pharm* 2000; **57:** 119–23.

Depression. Ademetionine has been given by mouth or parenterally in the management of depression (p.271). It appears to be of similar efficacy to the tricyclic antidepressants but evidence is limited to small, heterogeneous groups of patients studied over short periods of time.

The symbol † denotes a preparation no longer actively marketed

References.
1. Baldessarini RJ. Neuropharmacology of S-adenosyl-L-methionine. *Am J Med* 1987; **83** (suppl 5A): 95–103.
2. Bressa GM. S-adenosyl-1-methionine (SAMe) as antidepressant: meta-analysis of clinical studies. *Acta Neurol Scand* 1994; **154** (suppl): 7–14.
3. Anonymous. SAMe for depression. *Med Lett Drugs Ther* 1999; **41:** 107–8.

Liver disorders. Administration of ademetionine in doses of 800 mg daily intravenously or 800 mg twice daily by mouth has produced clinical improvement in patients with intrahepatic cholestasis,[1,2] including that associated with pregnancy.[3,4] Pruritus associated with the condition has also been relieved. Other studies,[5,6] however, have not found any benefit. Ademetionine given by intramuscular injection in a dose of 100 mg daily for one month, followed by 100 mg every other day for a further month, produced a good or excellent clinical response in 21 of 28 patients with hepatic steatosis.[7] In a study[8] of patients with alcoholic liver cirrhosis, treated with ademetionine 400 mg three times daily by mouth for two years, there was a trend towards reduced overall mortality or need for liver transplantation, but only in patients with less severe hepatic dysfunction.

1. Frezza M, *et al.* Oral S-adenosylmethionine in the symptomatic treatment of intrahepatic cholestasis: a double-blind, placebo-controlled study. *Gastroenterology* 1990; **99:** 211–15.
2. Almasio P, *et al.* Role of S-adenosyl-L-methionine in the treatment of intrahepatic cholestasis. *Drugs* 1990; **40** (suppl 3): 111–23.
3. Bonfirraro G, *et al.* S-Adenosyl-L-methionine (SAMe)-induced amelioration of intrahepatic cholestasis of pregnancy: results of an open study. *Drug Invest* 1990; **2:** 125–8.
4. Frezza M, *et al.* S-Adenosylmethionine for the treatment of intrahepatic cholestasis of pregnancy: results of a controlled clinical trial. *Hepatogastroenterology* 1990; **37** (suppl 2): 122–5.
5. Ribalta J, *et al.* S-Adenosyl-L-methionine in the treatment of patients with intrahepatic cholestasis of pregnancy: a randomized, double-blind, placebo-controlled study with negative results. *Hepatology* 1991; **13:** 1084–9.
6. Floreani A, *et al.* S-adenosylmethionine versus ursodeoxycholic acid in the treatment of intrahepatic cholestasis of pregnancy: preliminary results of a controlled trial. *Eur J Obstet Gynecol Reprod Biol* 1996; **67:** 109–13.
7. Caballeria E, Moreno J. Therapeutic effects of S-adenosylmethionine (SAMe) in hepatic steatosis. *Acta Ther* 1990; **16:** 253–64.
8. Mato JM, *et al.* S-Adenosylmethionine in alcoholic liver cirrhosis: a randomized, placebo-controlled, double-blind, multicenter clinical trial. *J Hepatol* 1999; **30:** 1081–9.

Osteoarthritis. Ademetionine has been reported to possess therapeutic efficacy in the treatment of osteoarthritis (p.9) and similar conditions[1–4] possibly due to an effect on cartilage metabolism and formation of anti-inflammatory mediators within the cell; it may also inhibit leukotrienes but does not appear markedly to interfere with prostaglandin synthesis.

1. DiPadova C. S-Adenosylmethionine in the treatment of osteoarthritis. *Am J Med* 1987; **83** (suppl 5A): 60–4.
2. Anonymous. Ademetionine—a new approach to the treatment of degenerative joint diseases. *Drugs Today* 1988; **24:** 165–8.
3. Domljan Z, *et al.* A double-blind trial of ademethionine vs naproxen in activated gonarthrosis. *Int J Clin Pharmacol Ther Toxicol* 1989; **27:** 329–33.
4. Bradley JD, *et al.* A randomized, double-blind, placebo controlled trial of intravenous loading with S-adenosylmethionine (SAM) followed by oral SAM therapy in patients with knee osteoarthritis. *J Rheumatol* 1994; **21:** 905–11.

Preparations

Proprietary Preparations (details are given in Part 3)
Ger.: Gumbaral; *Ital.:* Donamet; Samyr; Transmetil; *Mex.:* Samyr; *Spain:* S Amet.

Adenine   (12325-r)

Adeninum; Vitamin B_4. 6-Aminopurine; 1,6-Dihydro-6-iminopurine.
$C_5H_5N_5 = 135.1$.
CAS — 73-24-5.
Pharmacopoeias. In *Eur.* (see p.vi) and *US.*

Pharmacopoeial description

Ph. Eur.: A white powder. Very slightly soluble in water and in alcohol; practically insoluble in ether; dissolves in dilute mineral acids and in dilute solutions of alkali hydroxides.

USP 25: Odourless white crystals or crystalline powder. Very slightly soluble in water; sparingly soluble in boiling water; slightly soluble in alcohol; practically insoluble in chloroform and in ether.

Profile

Adenine is a constituent of coenzymes and nucleic acids and has been used to extend the storage life of whole blood (p.726). It has also been given for the management of white blood cell disorders. Adenine hydrochloride has also been used.

Preparations

USP 25: Anticoagulant Citrate Phosphate Dextrose Adenine Solution.

Proprietary Preparations (details are given in Part 3)
Fr.: Leuco-4.

Multi-ingredient: *Fr.:* TTD-B_3-B_4; *Spain:* Hepacomplet B12 1000†; Hepadif.

Adenosine Phosphate   (9201-m)

Adenosine Phosphate (*BAN, USAN, rINN*).
Adenosine 5′-Monophosphate; Adenosine-5′-(dihydrogen phosphate); Adenosine-5′-phosphoric Acid; 5′-Adenylic Acid; AMP; A-5MP; Monophosadénine; Muscle Adenylic Acid; NSC-20264. 6-Amino-9-β-D-ribofuranosylpurine 5′-(dihydrogen phosphate).
$C_{10}H_{14}N_5O_7P = 347.2$.
CAS — 61-19-8.
Pharmacopoeias. *Ger.* includes the disodium salt ($C_{10}H_{12}N_5Na_2O_7P,xH_2O$).

Profile

Adenosine is an endogenous nucleoside involved in many biological processes. As well as the base it is present as various phosphates. The monophosphate, adenosine phosphate, has been tried in a variety of disorders including the complications of varicose veins, peripheral neuropathies, and inflammation.

Unlike adenosine (p.828) and adenosine triphosphate (below), adenosine phosphate is not used in supraventricular tachycardias.

Preparations

Proprietary Preparations (details are given in Part 3)
Fr.: Adenyl; *Ger.:* Bio-Regenerat S 3.

Multi-ingredient: *Aust.:* Laevadosin; *S.Afr.:* Lipostabil; *Spain:* Artri; Taurobetina.

Adenosine Triphosphate   (9203-v)

Adenosine 5′-Triphosphate; 5′-Adenyldiphosphoric Acid; Adenylpyrophosphoric Acid; ATP; Triphosadénine. Adenosine 5′-(tetrahydrogen triphosphate).
$C_{10}H_{16}N_5O_{13}P_3 = 507.2$.
CAS — 56-65-5.
Pharmacopoeias. *Ger.* includes the disodium salt ($C_{10}H_{14}N_5Na_2O_{13}P_3 = 551.1$).

Profile

Adenosine triphosphate is a nucleotide constituent of animal cells with a fundamental role in biological energy transformations, being concerned with the storage and release of energy; it is converted to adenosine diphosphate, release of energy occurring during the process.

Adenosine triphosphate and its sodium salt are used as a source of nucleotides. The disodium salt has been given in the treatment of supraventricular tachycardia, but adenosine base (p.828) is the form generally used as an antiarrhythmic. The triphosphate is being investigated for use in cystic fibrosis (p.117), control of blood pressure during surgery, pulmonary hypertension, and cachexia in patients with cancer.

◊ Reviews.
1. Agteresch HJ, *et al.* Adenosine triphosphate: established and potential clinical applications. *Drugs* 1999; **58:** 211–32.

Preparations

Proprietary Preparations (details are given in Part 3)
Fr.: Atepadene; Myoviton; *Hong Kong:* Adesinon-P; *Spain:* Atepodin.

Multi-ingredient: *Aust.:* Laevadosin; *Belg.:* Vitathion†; *Canad.:* Vitathion-ATP; *Fr.:* Betriphos-C; RhinATP; Vita-Iodurol ATP†; *Spain:* Refulgin.

Adipic Acid   (12328-n)

Acidum Adipicum; Adipinsäure; Hexanedioic Acid.
$C_6H_{10}O_4 = 146.1$.
CAS — 124-04-9.
Pharmacopoeias. In *Eur.* (see p.vi).

Pharmacopoeial description

Ph. Eur.: A white crystalline powder. Sparingly soluble in water; soluble in boiling water; freely soluble in alcohol and in methyl alcohol; soluble in acetone.

Profile

Adipic acid is an acidifier that is used in foods and may also be included in preparations for the treatment of urinary-tract infections.

Preparations

Proprietary Preparations (details are given in Part 3)
Multi-ingredient: *Ger.:* Extin.

Adonis Vernalis   (5805-f)

Adonide; Adonis; Adoniskraut; False Hellebore; Herba Adonidis; Vernal Pheasant's Eye.
Pharmacopoeias. In *Ger.*

The dried aerial parts of *Adonis vernalis* (Ranunculaceae).

Profile

Adonis vernalis contains cardiac glycosides which have actions similar to those of digoxin (p.870). Adonis vernalis is used in herbal and homoeopathic medicine.

Preparations

Proprietary Preparations (details are given in Part 3)

Multi-ingredient: *Braz.:* Serenus; *Ger.:* Corguttin N plus†; Miroton; Miroton N; Oxacant N; Oxacant-forte N; Oxacant-Khella N; Raufuncton N; Venopyronum N triplex†.

Adrenalone Hydrochloride (1711-q)

Adrenalone Hydrochloride (pINNM).

3′,4′-Dihydroxy-2-(methylamino)acetophenone hydrochloride.
$C_9H_{11}NO_3,HCl = 217.6$.
CAS — 99-45-6 *(adrenalone)*; 62-13-5 *(adrenalone hydrochloride)*.

NOTE. Adrenalone is *USAN*.

Profile

Adrenalone hydrochloride is used as a local haemostatic and vasoconstrictor. It has also been used in combination with adrenaline [epinephrine] as eye drops for glaucoma.

Preparations

Proprietary Preparations (details are given in Part 3)
Denm.: Stryphnon; *Ger.:* Stryphnasal.

Aesculus (12329-h)

Aesculus hippocastanum; Horse-chestnut; Marron d'Inde; Rosskastaniensamen.
CAS — 6805-41-0 *(aescin)*; 11072-93-8 *(β-aescin)*; 531-75-9 *(anhydrous esculoside)*.
Pharmacopoeias. In Fr. and Ger.
Ger. also includes esculoside in the sesquihydrate form.

The horse-chestnut, *Aesculus hippocastanum* (Hippocastanaceae) contains several active principles including esculoside (aesculin or esculin; 6-β-D-glucopyranosyloxy-7-hydroxycoumarin, $C_{15}H_{16}O_9 = 340.3$) and aescin (escin, whic a mixture of saponins.

Profile

Ingestion of the seeds of *Aesculus hippocastanum* (conkers) may cause nausea, vomiting, diarrhoea, abdominal colic, delirium, and with large doses respiratory arrest.

Aescin and esculoside (aesculin or esculin), the major active principles of aesculus, have been used in the prevention and treatment of various peripheral vascular disorders, including haemorrhoids (p.1205). They have been given by mouth, by intravenous injection (in the form of sodium aescinate), by rectal suppository, and applied topically. Aescin has also been administered intravenously in the prevention and treatment of post-operative oedema. The maximum dose for intravenous administration in adults for such conditions has been stated to be 20 mg daily; acute renal failure has been reported in patients given higher doses, sometimes in conjunction with other nephrotoxic drugs. Other derivatives such as sodium aescin polysulfate have also been used.

Aesculus hippocastanum has been used in homoeopathic medicine.

Effects on the kidneys. A report of the incidence of acute renal failure in patients after cardiac surgery and implicating high-dose intravenous aescin therapy.[1] In 70 patients receiving a mean maximum daily dose of 340 μg per kg body-weight, no alteration of renal function was observed; in 16 receiving 360 μg per kg, mild mild renal impairment was observed; and in 40 given 510 μg per kg, acute renal failure developed.

1. Hellberg K, *et al.* Drug induced acute renal failure after heart surgery. *Thoraxchirurgie* 1975; **23:** 396–400.

Effects on the skin. Contact dermatitis[1] to aesculin and contact urticaria[2] to aescin have been reported following the use of topical preparations that contained these extracts. Both reactions were confirmed by positive skin tests.

1. Comaish JS, Kersey PJ. Contact dermatitis to extract of horse chestnut (esculin). *Contact Dermatitis* 1980; **6:** 150–1.
2. Escribano MM, *et al.* Contact urticaria due to aescin. *Contact Dermatitis* 1997; **37:** 233.

Poisoning. There have been reports of poisoning in children from eating the seeds, or drinking infusions made from the leaves and twigs of horse-chestnut trees.[1] The toxic substance is considered to be esculoside. Symptoms of poisoning were muscle twitching, weakness, lack of coordination, dilated pupils, vomiting, diarrhoea, paralysis, and stupor.

1. Nagy M. Human poisoning from horse chestnuts. *JAMA* 1973; **226:** 213.

Preparations

Proprietary Preparations (details are given in Part 3)
Aust.: Reparil; Traumaparil†; Venoplant†; Venosin; Venostasin; *Belg.:* Reparil; *Braz.:* Reparil; Venostasin; *Fr.:* Flogencyl; Hemorrogel†; *Ger.:* Aescorin Forte; Aescusan N; Aescusan; Aescuven; Concentrin; Essaven Mono†; Hamos-Tropfen-S; Hoevenol; Noricaven novo; opino N; Perivar Rosskaven; Plissamur; Provento N; Reparil; Rexiluven S; Sanaven Venentabletten; Vasoforte N; Vasotonin; Venalot novo; Venen-Dragees; Venen-Fluid; Venen-Tabletten; Venen-Tropfen; Venen-Tropfen N; Venentabs; veno-biomo; Venogal; Venoplant; Venopyronum; Venopyronum N; Venostasin; Venotrulan N†; *Hong Kong:* Reparil; *Ital.:* Curaven; Flebostasin; Ginoven†; Reparil; Venoplant†; *Mex.:* Fluxine; Venastat; Verisan; *Neth.:* Venoplant†; *Port.:* Venoparil; *S.Afr.:*

Reparil†; *Spain:* Feparil; Flebostasin; *Switz.:* Aesculaforce; AesculaMed; Phlebostasin; Reparil; Sanhelios Venen; Venastat; *Thai.:* Reparil.

Multi-ingredient: *Aust.:* Aesrutan; Alpha-Apoplectal†; Amphodyn; Apoplectal; Augentropfen Stulln; Dilaescol; Opino; Reparil; Sandoven; Tussimag Codein; Urelium Neu; Venosin; *Austral.:* Bioglan Cirflo; Bioglan Fingers & Toes†; Bioglan Zellulean with Escin; Cirflo†; Extralife Leg-Care; Herbal Capillary Care; Proflo; *Belg.:* Rectovasol; Reparil; *Braz.:* Castanha de India Composta; Digestron; Hemoaenus; Hemorroidex; Hemorrol; Hemosan; Hemovirtu's; Mirorroidin; Novaboin; Novarrutina; Reparil; Varizol; Venocur Triplex; Venofortan; Venostasin Composto; *Canad.:* Pommade Midy; Proctosedyl; Proctosone; *Denm.:* Proctosedyl; *Fin.:* Proctosedyl; *Fr.:* Actisane Hemorroides, Jambes Lourdes; Anti-Hemorroidaires†; Aphloine P; Arterase; Cepevit; Circularine; Climaxol; Creme Rap; Curoveinyl†; Escinogel; Fluon; Fragonal†; Hemoluol†; Hemorrogel; Histo-Fluine P; Intrait de Marron D'Inde P; Mediflor Tisane Circulation du Sang No 12†; P. Veinos†; Phlebocreme; Phlebogel; Phlebosedol; Phlebosup; Phytomelis; Preparation H; Reparil; Sedorrhoide; Veinophytum; Veinostase; Veinotonyl; Vivene; *Ger.:* Aescorin N; Aescusan; Amphodyn; Anisan; Apoplectal N; Arnika plus†; Augentropfen Stulln Mono; Cefadysbasin; Cefasabal; Cycloven Forte N; Diu Venostasin; Essaven; Essaven N; Essaven ultra; Fagorutin Roßkastanien-Balsam F; Hametum-N; Hamos N; Heparin Comp; Heusin; Heweven P 3; Heweven P 7†; Hoevenol A†; Hoevenol†; Intradermi Fluid N; Intradermi N; JuPhlebon S†; Lindigoa S; Nephrubin†; opino N spezial; Pascovenol novo; PC 30 V; Pe-Ce Ven N; Posti N; Rectosellan†; Reparil-Gel N, Reparil-Sportgel; Revicain comp; Revicain comp plus; Salhumin Teilbad N; Salus Venen Krauter Dragees N; Sklerovenol N; Sportupac N; Trauma-cyl; Varicylum-S; Vasesana-Vasoregulans; Vasotonin forte†; Venacton; Venen-Salbe; Venen-Salbe N; Venengel; Veno-Kattwiga N; Venoplant AHS; Venopyronum N triplex†; Venostasin; Weleda Hamorrhoidalzapfchen; *Hong Kong:* Essaven; Proctosedyl; Proctosone; Protozone; Reparil; Roidhemo; *Irl.:* Proctosedyl; *Ital.:* Bres; Castindia; Centella Complex; Centella Complex C; Centeril H; Dermocinetic; Dermoprolyn; Elisir Depurativo Ambrosiano; Essaven; Ginkgo Plus; Hirudex; Nitesco Smagliature; Pomata Midy HC†; Proctosedyl; Recto-Reparil; Reparil; Sedalen Cort; Sedilene Procto; Somatoline; Tioscina†; Varicogel; Venoplant†; Venoplus; Venotrauma; Venovit; *Norw.:* Proctosedyl; *Port.:* Bio-Strath No 1†; Empads; Relmus Compositum; Venoparil; *S.Afr.:* Essaven; Proctosedyl; Reparil; *Singapore:* Proctosedyl; *Spain:* Caprofides Hemostatico; Circovenil; Circovenil Fuerte†; Contusin; Essavenon; Feparil; Flebo Stop; Hemodren Compuesto; Killpan; Liviane Compuesto†; Roidhemo; Urgenin; Venacol; Venoplant; *Swed.:* Proctosedyl; *Switz.:* Augentonicum; Demoven N; Dolo-Veniten; Flavovenyl; Flogecyl; Optazine†; Phlebostasin compositum; Reparil; Reparil N†; Veino-Gouttes-N; Venoplant comp; Venoplant N†; *Thai.:* Essaven; Proctosedyl; Reparil; *UK:* Catarrh Cream.

Aflatoxins (12330-a)

CAS — 1162-65-8 *(aflatoxin B₁)*; 7220-81-7 *(aflatoxin B₂)*; 1165-39-5 *(aflatoxin G₁)*; 7241-98-7 *(aflatoxin G₂)*; 6795-23-9 *(aflatoxin M₁)*; 6885-57-0 *(aflatoxin M₂)*.

Aflatoxins are toxic metabolites produced by many strains of *Aspergillus flavus* and *A. parasiticus*, growing on many vegetable foods, notably maize and peanuts. A number of forms, including aflatoxins B_1, B_2, G_1, and G_2 have been identified. Aflatoxins M_1 and M_2 are metabolites produced by animals following ingestion of aflatoxins B_1 and B_2; they may be detected in cows' milk.

Profile

Aflatoxins are hepatotoxins that can cause hepatitis and cirrhosis. They have been implicated in liver cancer, and may act as co-carcinogens with hepatitis B virus. Aflatoxin B_1 is reported to be one of the most potent carcinogens known in *animals*.

◊ References.

1. Ross RK, *et al.* Urinary aflatoxin biomarkers and risk of hepatocellular carcinoma. *Lancet* 1992; **339:** 943–6.
2. Jackson PE, Groopman JD. Aflatoxin and liver cancer. *Baillieres Best Pract Res Clin Gastroenterol* 1999; **13:** 545–55.
3. Peraica M, *et al.* Toxic effects of mycotoxins in humans. *Bull WHO* 1999; **77:** 754–66.
4. Pitt JI. Toxigenic fungi and mycotoxins. *Br Med Bull* 2000; **56:** 184–92.

Agalsidase Beta (20647-c)

Agalsidase Beta (pINN).
CAS — 104138-64-9 *(protein moiety)*.

Profile

Agalsidase beta is a recombinant form of the endogenous enzyme α-galactosidase. It is used for the treatment of Fabry disease, a genetic disorder of lipid catabolism. Agalsidase alfa is also under investigation.

Preparations

Proprietary Preparations (details are given in Part 3)
UK: Fabrazyme.

Agnus Castus (14089-a)

Keuschlamm; Mönchspfeffer.

The dried fruits of *Vitex agnus castus* (Verbenaceae).

Profile

Agnus castus is reported to affect the secretion of luteinising

hormone, follicle stimulating hormone, and prolactin by the pituitary. Both inhibition and stimulation of prolactin secretion have been reported, and may be dose-dependent. Agnus castus is included in herbal preparations for menstrual and menopausal disorders, but should be avoided in patients receiving exogenous sex hormones, including oral contraceptives.

It is also used in homoeopathic medicine.

◊ References.

1. Houghton P. Agnus castus. *Pharm J* 1994; **253:** 720–1.
2. Christie S, Walker AF. Vitex agnus-castus L.: (1) a review of its traditional and modern therapeutic use; (2) current use from a survey of practitioners. *Eur J Herbal Med* 1997; **3:** 29–45.
3. Schellenberg R. Treatment for the premenstrual syndrome with agnus castus fruit extract: prospective, randomised, placebo controlled study. *BMJ* 2001; **322:** 134–7.

Preparations

Proprietary Preparations (details are given in Part 3)
Aust.: Agnumes; *Ger.:* Agnolyt; Agnucaston; Agnufemil; Biofem; Castufemin N; Cefanorm; Femicur N; Feminon A; Gynocastus; Kytta-Femin; Strotan; *Hong Kong:* Agnucaston; *Switz.:* Agnolyt; Emoton; Evana; PreMens; *UK:* Agnolyt; Herbal Premens.

Multi-ingredient: *Austral.:* Dong Quai Complex; Feminine Herbal Complex; Lifesystem Herbal Formula 4 Women's Formula; PMT Complex; Women's Formula Herbal Formula 3; *Ger.:* Femisana; Presselin Dysmen Olin 3 N.

Agrimony (11738-e)

Agrimoniae Herba; Aigremoine; Odermennigkraut.
Pharmacopoeias. In Eur. (see p.vi).

Pharmacopoeial description

Ph. Eur.: The dried flowering tops of *Agrimonia eupatoria* containing a minimum of 2.0% of tannins expressed as pyrogallol, calculated with reference to the dried drug.

Profile

Agrimony, the aerial parts of *Agrimonia eupatoria* (Rosaceae) or more rarely *A. procera* (*A. odorata*; fragrant agrimony), has astringent and diuretic properties. It is used internally for diarrhoea, biliary and other gastrointestinal disorders, and urinary-tract disorders, and has been used externally for wound healing and skin disorders.

Agrimony is also used in homoeopathic medicine.

Preparations

Proprietary Preparations (details are given in Part 3)
Multi-ingredient: *Aust.:* Amersan; Gallen- und Lebertee; Krauterhaus Mag Kottas Gallen- und Lebertee; Krautertee Nr 28; Novocholin; *Fr.:* Tisane Hepatique de Hoerdt; *Ger.:* Rhoival; Stomasal Med; *Ital.:* Allergenid†; *Switz.:* The Brioni; *UK:* Piletabs.

Alfalfa (12026-w)

Lucerne; Purple medick.

The plant *Medicago sativa* (Leguminosae) which is cultivated as an animal feedstuff.

Profile

The seeds and sprouts of alfalfa contain canavanine (2-amino-4-(guanidinooxy)butyric acid), a toxic amino acid structurally related to arginine; content is reported to represent about 1.5% of the dry weight. A syndrome resembling systemic lupus erythematosus has been recorded in *monkeys* fed alfalfa.

Alfalfa is used in herbal preparations for a variety of disorders and in homoeopathic medicine.

Preparations

Proprietary Preparations (details are given in Part 3)
Ger.: Schneckensirup.

Multi-ingredient: *Austral.:* Neo-Cleanse; Panax Complex; Plantiodine Plus; Zinc Zenith; *UK:* Fat-Solv.

Alglucerase (5252-v)

Alglucerase (BAN, USAN, rINN).
Glucosylceramidase; Macrophage-targeted β-Glucocerebrosidase.
CAS — 143003-46-7.
ATC — A16AB01.

A modified form of human placental β-glucocerebrosidase (ceramide glucosidase; β-D-glucosyl-N-acylsphingosine glucohydrolase). It is a monomeric glycoprotein of 497 amino acids with glycosylation making up about 6% of the molecule.

Imiglucerase (17703-h)

Imiglucerase (BAN, USAN, rINN).
Recombinant Macrophage-targeted β-Glucocerebrosidase; r-GCR.
CAS — 154248-97-2.
ATC — A16AB02.

A recombinant human-derived β-glucocerebrosidase. It is a monomeric glycoprotein of 497 amino acids glycosylated at 4 asparagine residues.

Adverse Effects and Precautions

Fever, chills, pruritus, flushing, and gastrointestinal symptoms, including cramps, diarrhoea, nausea, and vomiting have been reported following administration of alglucerase or imiglucerase. Some of these may be hypersensitivity reactions; other hypersensitivity reactions, including urticaria and angioedema, respiratory symptoms, and hypotension have also occurred. Anaphylactoid reactions have occurred rarely with imiglucerase. Caution is required in patients who have exhibited signs of hypersensitivity; reduction of the rate of infusion, and pretreatment with antihistamines and/or corticosteroids may permit further treatment. Antibodies have developed in about 15% of patients receiving a glucocerebrosidase enzyme during the first year of therapy. Patients who develop antibodies are at increased risk of hypersensitivity reactions and periodic assessment for antibody formation is recommended.

Pain and irritation at the injection site may occur. Other adverse effects reported include fatigue, dizziness, headache, backache, peripheral oedema, mouth ulcers, and disturbances in sense of smell.

Alglucerase is prepared from human placentas and its infusion therefore carries a risk of transmission of infections although this is minimised by the manufacturing process. Chorionic gonadotrophin, a naturally occurring hormone in human placentas, has been detected in alglucerase. The presence of this hormone may produce early virilisation in young boys when high doses of alglucerase are used; also, pregnancy tests that rely on the detection of this hormone may yield false positive results if performed within 48 hours of administration of alglucerase. Alglucerase should be used with caution, if at all, in patients with androgen-sensitive malignancies.

Effects on the lungs. Pulmonary hypertension developed in two patients with Gaucher disease after initiation of treatment with alglucerase.[1] Neither patient had evidence of parenchymal lung infiltration with Gaucher cells.

1. Dawson A, et al. Pulmonary hypertension developing after alglucerase therapy in two patients with type 1 Gaucher disease complicated by the hepatopulmonary syndrome. *Ann Intern Med* 1996; **125**: 901–4.

Pharmacokinetics

Following intravenous infusion, plasma enzymatic activities of alglucerase and imiglucerase decline rapidly from steady state, with an elimination half-life of between 3.6 and 10.4 minutes.

Uses and Administration

Alglucerase and imiglucerase are forms of β-glucocerebrosidase given as enzyme replacement therapy to patients with symptomatic type 1 Gaucher disease (see below). The oligosaccharide chains of the enzyme are modified to terminate with mannose residues to ensure uptake into macrophages.

Alglucerase and imiglucerase are administered by intravenous infusion over 1 to 2 hours. Up to 60 units of alglucerase or imiglucerase per kg body-weight may be given as a single infusion. The frequency of administration depends on the severity of symptoms, and initial doses can vary from 2.5 units per kg three times weekly to 60 units per kg once weekly for alglucerase, or once every two weeks for imiglucerase. Once the patient's condition is stabilised the dose should be reduced at intervals of 3 to 12 months to a maintenance dose.

◊ References.

1. Anonymous. Alglucerase for Gaucher's disease. *Med Lett Drugs Ther* 1991; **33**: 82.
2. Whittington R, Goa KL. Alglucerase; a review of its therapeutic use in Gaucher's disease. *Drugs* 1992; **44**: 72–93.

Gaucher disease. Gaucher disease[1-3] (glucocerebrosidosis) is a rare, autosomal recessive disorder, although it is the commonest lysosomal storage disease. It is caused by a deficiency of the lysosomal enzyme β-glucocerebrosidase (acid β-glucosidase, ceramide glucosidase, β-D-glucosyl-N-acylsphingosine glucohydrolase, or glucosylceramidase) which catalyses the hydrolysis of glucocerebroside, a lipid component of cell membranes, to glucose and ceramide. Deficiency of β-glucocerebrosidase results in accumulation of glucocerebroside in the lysosomes of reticuloendothelial cells, particularly macrophages. These large lipid-laden macrophages (termed Gaucher cells) eventually infiltrate the liver, spleen, bone, and bone marrow leading to hepatomegaly, splenomegaly, splenic infarction, anaemia, thrombocytopenia, leucopenia, and bone disorders including osteoporosis and osteonecrosis. In some cases infiltration of brain tissue also occurs producing neurological impairment and seizures. Rarely, infiltration of lung parenchymal tissue occurs leading to pulmonary infections.

Gaucher disease is classified into three main forms based on clinical signs and symptoms. Hepatosplenomegaly occurs in all forms. Type 1 Gaucher disease (chronic adult non-neuronopathic disease) accounts for 99% of cases and occurs especially in Ashkenazi Jews. The disease follows a chronic course of variable severity and onset, with hepatosplenomegaly and blood and bone disorders being the main features; there is no neurological involvement. In type 2 Gaucher disease (acute infantile neuronopathic disease), neurological involvement predominates. Patients show developmental delay by the age of 6 months, suffer seizures, pulmonary infections, and usually die during the first year of life. Type 3 Gaucher disease (subacute juvenile neuronopathic disease or Norrbotten disease) is a more slowly progressive form that presents later in childhood than type 2 disease and varies in severity. As in type 2 disease, there

is neurological involvement. Patients may survive into early adulthood, although death by age 10 to 15 is frequent.

Treatment of Gaucher disease was previously limited to symptomatic management. In some cases bone-marrow transplantation was required for life-threatening bone-marrow involvement. Preparations of β-glucocerebrosidase, the deficient enzyme, are now available. Due to the rarity of Gaucher disease, clinical studies have been limited mainly to small case series of patients with type 1 disease. Use of alglucerase or imiglucerase has been shown to reverse hepatosplenomegaly and the haematological abnormalities;[4,5] effects may be seen within a few months, although in many the response is poor during the first 6 to 9 months and then improves rapidly.[2] Bone symptoms respond more slowly. Decreases in bone pain during the first year of treatment have been reported although there was no radiological improvement.[5] Normalised growth velocity has been reported in children[6] and radiographical assessments have shown improvements in bone density and mineralisation.[7] Alglucerase has also been tried in rare cases of Gaucher disease affecting the heart[8] or the eye.[9] The efficacy of enzyme replacement therapy in managing neurological symptoms in patients with type 2 or type 3 disease[10] has yet to be established. It is not yet known whether enzyme replacement is able to prevent the development of symptoms in asymptomatic patients.

Various doses have been tried in order to determine the optimal dosage regimen.[11] Doses of alglucerase as low as 2.3 units per kg body-weight three times a week[12] or 1.15 units per kg three times a week[13] may be sufficient to produce improvement, even in patients with severe symptoms. Doses of imiglucerase of 15 units per kg every two weeks or 2.5 units per kg three times a week have produced satisfactory clinical responses.[14] Patients vary considerably in their response to enzyme replacement therapy, and dosages must be individualised. Antibodies to the enzyme do not generally affect enzyme activity; neutralising antibodies have been reported in a very few patients.[2]

Possible future therapies that are under investigation include gene therapy and miglustat (N-butyldeoxynojirimycin; OGT-918; SC-48334). Miglustat reduces the synthesis of glucocerebroside by inhibiting glucosyltransferase, one of the early enzymes in the sphingolipid biosynthetic pathway. Other modified forms of β-glucocerebrosidase are also under investigation to improve uptake into the affected macrophages.

1. NIH Technology Assessment Panel on Gaucher Disease. Gaucher disease: current issues in diagnosis and treatment. *JAMA* 1996; **275**: 548–53.
2. Grabowski GA. Current issues in enzyme therapy for Gaucher disease. *Drugs* 1996; **52**: 159–67.
3. Morales LE. Gaucher's disease: a review. *Ann Pharmacother* 1996; **30**: 381–8.
4. Grabowski GA, et al. Enzyme therapy in type 1 Gaucher disease: comparative efficacy of mannose-terminated glucocerebrosidase from natural and recombinant sources. *Ann Intern Med* 1995; **122**: 33–9.
5. Pastores GM, et al. Enzyme therapy in Gaucher disease type 1: dosage efficacy and adverse effects in 33 patients treated for 6 to 24 months. *Blood* 1993; **82**: 408–16.
6. Kaplan P, et al. Acceleration of retarded growth in children with Gaucher disease after treatment with alglucerase. *J Pediatr* 1996; **129**: 149–53.
7. Rosenthal DI, et al. Enzyme replacement therapy for Gaucher disease: skeletal responses to macrophage-targeted glucocerebrosidase. *Pediatrics* 1995; **96**: 629–37.
8. Spada M, et al. Cardiac response to enzyme-replacement therapy in Gaucher's disease. *N Engl J Med* 1998; **339**: 1165–6.
9. vom Dahl S, et al. Loss of vision in Gaucher's disease and its reversal by enzyme-replacement therapy. *N Engl J Med* 1998; **338**: 1471–2.
10. Bembi B, et al. Enzyme replacement treatment in type 1 and type 3 Gaucher's disease. *Lancet* 1994; **344**: 1679–82.
11. Beutler E. Enzyme replacement therapy for Gaucher's disease. *Baillieres Clin Haematol* 1997; **10**: 751–63.
12. Zimran A, et al. Low-dose enzyme replacement therapy for Gaucher's disease: effects of age, sex, genotype, and clinical features on response to treatment. *Am J Med* 1994; **97**: 3–13.
13. Hollak CEM, et al. Individualised low-dose alglucerase therapy in Gaucher's disease. *Lancet* 1995; **345**: 1474–8.
14. Zimran A, et al. Replacement therapy with imiglucerase for type 1 Gaucher's disease. *Lancet* 1995; **345**: 1479–80.

Preparations

Proprietary Preparations (details are given in Part 3)

Aust.: Cerezyme; *Austral.:* Cerezyme; *Denm.:* Cerezyme; *Fr.:* Cerezyme; *Ger.:* Ceredase†; *Israel:* Ceredase; Cerezyme; *Ital.:* Ceredase†; Cerezyme; *Jpn:* Ceredase; Cerezyme; *Port.:* Cerezyme; *Spain:* Ceredase†; Cerezyme; *Switz.:* Cerezyme; *UK:* Ceredase†; Cerezyme; *USA:* Ceredase; Cerezyme.

Alibendol (18738-r)

Alibendol (rINN).

5-Allyl-N-(2-hydroxyethyl)-3-methoxysalicylamide.

$C_{13}H_{17}NO_4 = 251.3$.

CAS — 26750-81-2.

Profile

Alibendol is a choleretic used in the treatment of gastrointestinal disorders.

Preparations

Proprietary Preparations (details are given in Part 3)

Fr.: Cebera.

Allergen Products (6175-c)

Pharmacopoeias. In Eur. (see p.vi).

Adverse Effects and Treatment

Adverse effects to prepared allergens can range from mild local reactions to severe generalised reactions which may be fatal. Severe reactions may be seen after skin tests in sensitive individuals as well as at any time during hyposensitisation. Aqueous solutions are more likely to provoke systemic reactions than preparations designed to give slower release rates. Severe reactions have been associated with tyrosine-adsorbed vaccines which have a relatively short half-life.

Hypersensitivity reactions may be immediate or delayed. Local reactions are normally limited to swelling and irritation. Systemic reactions include rhinitis, conjunctivitis, urticaria, bronchospasm, laryngeal oedema, generalised anaphylaxis, and shock. Severe reactions normally occur within 30 minutes and should be treated promptly with intramuscular adrenaline [epinephrine] injection 1 in 1000, which should be immediately available when hyposensitising injections are being administered. Full supportive measures should be implemented and treatment with antihistamines and corticosteroids may be required (for a discussion of the treatment of anaphylactic shock, see p.832). Further hyposensitisation should be stopped or continued at reduced dosage depending on the severity of the reaction and in accordance with the manufacturer's recommendations.

◊ In 1986 the UK Committee on Safety of Medicines reported[1] that hyposensitising vaccines have the potential to induce severe bronchospasm and anaphylaxis, and that these reactions had caused 26 deaths in the UK since 1957. The majority of patients had no reaction to previous hyposensitising injections. In 1989 the FDA reported that since 1980, the American Academy of Allergy and Immunology and the FDA had received 14 reports of death following hyposensitisation, and 4 deaths following skin testing for allergies.[2] The most common clinical factor in these patients was a history of asthma.

In view of these and other reports, recommendations have been made to minimise the risks of systemic reactions.[3-5] Hyposensitising vaccines should only be used for seasonal allergic rhinoconjunctivitis not responding to anti-allergic drugs, and for severe hypersensitivity to Hymenoptera stings. In the UK[4] such treatment is usually avoided in patients with asthma (although asthma is not an absolute contra-indication to Hymenoptera hyposensitisation), but elsewhere[3,5] asthmatic patients whose asthma is stable and not severe may be treated. Hyposensitising agents should be used only where facilities for full cardiopulmonary resuscitation are immediately available. The recommended length of time after injection that patients should be kept under medical observation varies from 30 minutes[3] to 1 hour.[4] The observation period should be extended if the patient develops symptoms, even mild, of a general reaction, until they are completely resolved, and for patients at high risk of reactions.

Of twelve samples of *Aspergillus* extract used for hyposensitisation, 4 were found to contain aflatoxin (p.1574), one being highly mutagenic as determined by the Ames' test. The results suggested that careful screening of commercially available mould extracts was warranted.[6]

1. Committee on Safety of Medicines. Desensitising vaccines. *BMJ* 1986; **293**: 948.
2. Food and Drug Administration. Fatality risk with allergenic extract use. *JAMA* 1989; **261**: 3368.
3. Malling H-J, Weeke B, eds. Position paper: Immunotherapy. (EAACI) The European Academy of Allergology and Clinical Immunology. *Allergy* 1993; **48** (suppl 14): 9–35.
4. Committee on Safety of Medicines/Medicines Control Agency. Desensitising vaccines: new advice. *Current Problems* 1994; **20**: 5.
5. Bousquet J, et al. WHO Position Paper: Allergen immunotherapy: therapeutic vaccines for allergic disease. *Allergy* 1998; **53** (suppl 44): 1–42.
6. Legator MS, et al. Aflatoxin B_1 in mould extracts used for desensitisation. *Lancet* 1983; **ii**: 915.

Precautions

Hyposensitising injections should not be given to patients with febrile conditions, serious immunological illness, or acute asthma. Allergen preparations should be avoided during pregnancy because of the risk to the fetus of any systemic reactions. Hyposensitising injections should only be administered where facilities for full cardiopulmonary resuscitation are immediately available. It has been recommended that patients should be observed for at least 1 hour after each injection (see under Adverse Effects, above). Patients with asthma may be more susceptible to hypersensitivity reactions with allergen extracts and, in the UK, it is considered that hyposensitising injections should be avoided in patients with asthma, with the possible exception of those at risk of severe hypersensitivity reactions to Hymenoptera stings. Hyposensitising injections should also be avoided in children under 5 years of age.

Whenever possible, the same batch of allergen should be used throughout the treatment course. Injections should be given subcutaneously and not intravenously or intramuscularly.

Hyposensitising injections should be avoided in patients taking beta blockers since adrenaline [epinephrine] will be ineffective if hypersensitivity reactions occur in these patients. Severe anaphylactoid reactions have been reported in patients undergoing hyposensitisation who are also receiving ACE inhibitors (p.821). Some manufacturers suggest that the reaction could be

---

The symbol † denotes a preparation no longer actively marketed

avoided by temporarily withholding ACE inhibitor therapy during each desensitisation.

Vaccination against infectious diseases should be separated from hyposensitising vaccines by at least 1 week.

Antihistamines should be avoided for at least 24 hours before sensitivity testing is carried out since they may mask skin reactivity; they have been given, during hyposensitisation, to very sensitive patients. Systemic or long-term topical use of potent corticosteroids may also mask skin reactivity.

Uses

Allergen products are used diagnostically in skin tests and provocation tests to confirm the cause of a suspected hypersensitivity reaction. They are also administered for hyposensitisation of certain patients with hypersensitivity reactions, particularly to insect venoms, pollens, or house-dust mite.

Diagnostic use. Sensitivity testing can be used to confirm that suspected allergens are predominantly responsible for the symptoms of a suspected hypersensitivity reaction. However, sensitivity testing should not form the sole basis of the treatment of hypersensitivity reactions.

Type IV (delayed) hypersensitivity reactions such as contact dermatitis are normally diagnosed using patch tests. A number of standard techniques are available, but in general they all involve maintaining a standard amount of the test substance in contact with the skin for 48 to 72 hours. A positive response is shown by erythema, swelling, or vesiculation. The sensitivity of different parts of the body varies, and this should be accounted for in applying test substances and controls. The test results are normally read half to one hour after removal of the patches to allow any pressure effects of the patches to subside. Patch testing with mixtures of allergens may be necessary to diagnose contact dermatitis in patients hypersensitive to multiple allergens.

Type I (immediate) hypersensitivity reactions such as allergic rhinitis, allergic asthma, and insect-sting hypersensitivity are tested using prick or intradermal tests. Since the allergen is introduced through the skin in these tests the risk of systemic reactions is greater, and adrenaline [epinephrine] injection should be kept available. The test involves pricking the skin through a drop of allergen in solution, and comparing the result after 15 to 20 minutes with positive and negative controls. The intradermal test is used if the prick test result does not agree with a strong clinical suspicion. Skin testing is unreliable for evaluating hypersensitivity to drugs, except for penicillins and for certain macromolecules. Skin test titration, that is testing with a series of dilutions, has been used to determine a safe starting dose for hyposensitisation.

Provocation tests are designed to reproduce symptoms of hypersensitivity by controlled exposure to a suspected allergen. Provocation may be by the bronchial, oral, nasal, or ocular routes. Facilities for full cardiopulmonary resuscitation should be immediately available.

In-vitro methods for measuring antigen-specific IgE include the radioallergosorbent test (RAST).

References.
1. VanArsdel PP, Larson EB. Diagnostic tests for patients with suspected allergic disease: utility and limitations. *Ann Intern Med* 1989; **110:** 304–12.
2. VanArsdel PP, Larson EB. Allergy testing. *Ann Intern Med* 1989; **110:** 317–20.
3. McLelland J, Shuster S. Contact dermatitis with negative patch tests: the additive effects of allergens in combination. *Br J Dermatol* 1990; **122:** 623–30.
4. Anonymous. Allergen testing in patients with type I hypersensitivity. *Drug Ther Bull* 1995; **33:** 45–7. Correction. *ibid.:* 55.

Hyposensitisation. Hyposensitisation (desensitisation or allergen immunotherapy) is the administration of gradually increasing quantities of allergen extract in a vaccine to ameliorate the effects of subsequent exposure to the allergen. Such therapy has become less popular following reports of severe and fatal anaphylactic reactions during therapy and should only be carried out in specialist centres. Hyposensitisation with a specific allergen has been found to be useful in hypersensitivities to pollens and insect venom, particularly that of Hymenoptera. For further discussion of the indications of hyposensitisation, see below.

Allergen vaccines are given as aqueous extracts or as depot preparations bound to aluminium or calcium salts or to tyrosine; allergens modified with glutaral to reduce side-effects while retaining immunogenicity have also been used. Whenever possible, the same batch of allergen should be used during a course of treatment because of possible differences in potency between batches. Allergen extracts are given by subcutaneous injection in dosage regimens as recommended by the manufacturers and depending on the sensitivity of the patient. Skin test titration has been used to determine a safe starting dose. In conventional regimens, increasing doses are given once or twice weekly for aqueous extracts, or every one to two weeks for depot preparations until a maintenance dose is reached. Maintenance doses are given every 4 to 6 weeks. Modified dosage schedules have been used where maintenance needs to be achieved more quickly; such regimens may, however, be associated with an increased rate of adverse reactions. Aqueous extracts should be used for modified schedules until the maintenance dose is reached. In rush schedules, several injections are given daily on consecutive days. Semi-rush, modified rush, or

cluster regimens involve the administration of several injections on a single day, separated by an interval of several days. The optimal duration of hyposensitisation therapy is unknown, but a period of 3 to 5 years is usually recommended.

Oral, nasal, sublingual, and bronchial routes of administration have sometimes been used for hyposensitisation.

The use of hyposensitisation has been reviewed[1,2] and various authorities have published recommendations.[3-6] Hyposensitisation is indicated exclusively for Type I (immediate) hypersensitivity reactions mediated by IgE antibodies. It may be used for the treatment of insect sting hypersensitivity, allergic rhinitis and conjunctivitis, and allergic asthma. Reports of severe and sometimes fatal hypersensitivity reactions to allergen preparations have prompted recommendations to reduce the risk of systemic reactions (see under Adverse Effects, above).

Hyposensitisation is used in children[6] and is thought to be more effective than in adults. It has been suggested that the use of hyposensitisation in children with allergic rhinoconjunctivitis may also prevent the development of asthma. Therapy is generally not recommended for children younger than 5 years of age[3,6] because it is less well tolerated, and in this age group the differential diagnosis between allergic rhinitis and viral infection of the respiratory tract may not be clear.[6]

Hyposensitisation is indicated for patients with specific IgE antibodies who have experienced severe anaphylaxis following insect stings, particularly those of Hymenoptera (bees, wasps, and stinging ants).[3,4,6,7] Vaccines containing purified venom are available for most Hymenoptera and have replaced whole body extract preparations, which were generally found to be ineffective. Venom vaccines are not available for stinging ants but whole body extract vaccines may contain sufficient venom antigens to be effective.[2,6]

Hyposensitisation for seasonal allergic rhinitis and conjunctivitis triggered by pollen has generally been reserved for severely affected patients when anti-allergic drugs have failed.[3,6] However, there is some evidence that hyposensitisation for allergies such as rhinitis may prevent the development of asthma and thus earlier use of hyposensitisation may be warranted.[4] Recommendations for the use of hyposensitisation in patients with asthma vary. Guidelines in the UK[3] recommend that asthmatic patients should not be treated with hyposensitisation because they are more likely to develop severe adverse effects (although asthma is not considered a contra-indication to hyposensitisation for anaphylaxis caused by Hymenoptera). Others, including WHO,[4-6] consider that hyposensitisation for allergic rhinoconjunctivitis can be given to patients whose asthma is stable and not severe (FEV$_1$ is not less than 70% of predicted value), when avoidance of allergens has not been sufficient or is not possible, and drug treatment has failed. Hyposensitisation for rhinoconjunctivitis and asthma due to house-dust mite or animal danders can be considered when the allergen is unavoidable.[4-6,8]

Hyposensitisation to a drug may be warranted on the rare occasions when hypersensitivity has developed and continued use is considered essential, possibly with penicillins or insulin.[3,9] Such regimens produce clinical tolerance, lost on cessation of therapy, without immunological change.[4]

Hyposensitisation therapy has also been tried in other disorders such as atopic dermatitis, urticaria, and food allergies, but there is insufficient evidence to support such use.[2,3]

Rush hyposensitisation has been successful in a woman hypersensitive to seminal plasma.[10]

Hyposensitisation with a single intradermal injection of an enzyme-potentiated allergen extract has been tried.[11]

1. Lobjoy RH. Allergen immunotherapy: when is it useful? *Drugs* 1990; **40:** 493–7.
2. Weber RW. Immunotherapy with allergens. *JAMA* 1997; **278:** 1881–7.
3. Frew AJ, British Society for Allergy and Clinical Immunology Working Party. Injection immunotherapy. *BMJ* 1993; **307:** 919–23.
4. Malling H-J, Weeke B, eds. Position paper: Immunotherapy. (EAACI) The European Academy of Allergology and Clinical Immunology. *Allergy* 1993; **48** (suppl 14): 9–35.
5. Thoracic Society of Australia and New Zealand and Australasian Society of Clinical Immunology and Allergy. Specific allergen immunotherapy for asthma. *Med J Aust* 1997; **167:** 540–44.
6. Bousquet J, et al. WHO Position Paper: Allergen immunotherapy: therapeutic vaccines for allergic diseases. *Allergy* 1998; **53** (suppl 44): 1–42.
7. Valentine MD, Lichtenstein LM. Anaphylaxis and stinging insect hypersensitivity. *JAMA* 1987; **258:** 2881–5.
8. Abramson MJ, et al. Is allergen immunotherapy effective in asthma? A meta-analysis of randomized controlled trials. *Am J Respir Crit Care Med* 1995; **151:** 969–74.
9. Anderson JA, Adkinson NF. Allergic reactions to drugs and biologic agents. *JAMA* 1987; **258:** 2891–9.
10. Frisch C, et al. Rush hyposensitisation for allergy to seminal plasma. *Lancet* 1984; **i:** 1073.
11. Fell P, Brostoff J. A single dose desensitization for summer hay fever. *Eur J Clin Pharmacol* 1990; **38:** 77–9.

Preparations

Proprietary Preparations (details are given in Part 3)
Austral.: Albay; Allpyral; *Belg.:* Pharmalgen; Pollinex; *Braz.:* Nikkho Vac; *Canad.:* Pollinex-R; *Denm.:* Alutard SQ; Aquagen SQ; Pharmalgen; Sensitair; Soluprick SQ; True Test; *Fr.:* Albay; Allpyral; Alpha Fraction; Alyostal; ASAD; Candidine†; *Ger.:* ADL; Alk; Allergovit; Allerset; Depot-Hal; Hal-oral; Novo-Helisen; Oralvac; Pollinex Quattro; Purethal; SDL; TA Baumpollen; TA Graserpollen; TA MIX; True Test†; Tyrosin S; Venomil; *Ital.:* Alhydrox; Alpare; Conjuvac; Phostal; Staloral; *Neth.:* Alavac-S; Allergoid-HAL†; Allerset†; Artoid; Depot-Hal; Haloral†; Immu-

novac; Oralgen; Pollalin†; Pollinex Boompollen; Pollinex Graspollen; Purethal; Sublivac B.E.S.T.; *Norw.:* Alutard; *NZ:* Allpyral; True Test; *Port.:* Polagen; *S.Afr.:* Albay; Allpyral Pure Mite; Allpyral Special Grass; Diagnostic Skin Testing Kit†; *Swed.:* Alutard SQ; Aquagen SQ; Pharmalgen†; Soluprick SQ; *Switz.:* Alavac-S; Allergovit; Alutard SQ; Alyostal; ASAD; Novo-Helisen; Pharmalgen; Phostal; Polvac; SDV; Staloral; *UK:* Bencard Skin Testing Solutions; Pharmalgen; Pollinex; *USA:* Albay; Allpyral; Center-Al; Pharmalgen; True Test; Venomil.

Multi-ingredient: *Braz.:* Alergomed; Alergoral; Aminovac; Insuvac; Multigen AL; Multivac VR; Munolan; Rhinovac; Urtivac; Vag Oral; *Fin.:* Alutard SQ; Aquagen SQ; Soluprick SQ; *Ger.:* BU Pangramin SLIT; Sublivac; Venomenhal; *Neth.:* Venomhal†.

Almond Oil (7352-h)

Aceite de Almendra; Amygdalae Oleum Virginum; Bitter Almond Oil; Expressed Almond Oil; Huile d'Amande; Mandelöl; Ol. Amygdal.; Oleo de Amêndoas; Olio di Mandorla; Sweet Almond Oil; Virgin Almond Oil.

Pharmacopoeias. In *Eur.* (see p.vi). Also in *USNF.*
Eur. also includes Refined Almond Oil (Amygdalae Oleum Raffinatum).
Fr. also specifies Huile de Noyaux, an oil obtained from various species of *Prunus.*

Pharmacopoeial description

Ph. Eur.: A yellow, clear, liquid. It is the fatty oil obtained by cold expression from the ripe seeds of *Prunus dulcis* var. *amara* or *P. dulcis* var. *dulcis* or a mixture of both varieties. Slightly soluble in alcohol; miscible with petroleum spirit. Store in well-filled containers. Protect from light.

Refined Almond Oil is the fatty oil obtained by refining and deodorisation of Almond Oil. It may contain a suitable antioxidant. A pale yellow, clear, transparent liquid. Slightly soluble in alcohol; miscible with petroleum spirit. Store in well-filled containers. Protect from light.

USNF 20: The fixed oil expressed from the kernels of varieties of *Prunus amygdalus* [*Prunus dulcis*] (Rosaceae). A clear, colourless or pale straw-coloured, oily liquid with a bland taste. Slightly soluble in alcohol; miscible with chloroform, with ether, with petroleum spirit, and with benzene. Store in airtight containers.

Profile

Almond oil has nutritive and demulcent properties. It is used as an emollient and to soften ear wax. It is also employed as a vehicle in some injections.

Preparations

BP 2001: Almond Oil Ear Drops;
USP 25: Rose Water Ointment.

Proprietary Preparations (details are given in Part 3)
Fr.: Karelyne; *Mex.:* Dermoskin.

Multi-ingredient: *Austral.:* Curash Babycare; *Ital.:* Babysteril; Otosan Gocce Auricolari; Stilomagic; *Mex.:* Caliderm; *NZ:* Am-O-Lin; *Port.:* Cuidaderma; Olidermil; *Spain:* Pasta Lassar Imba; *Switz.:* Antidry; Balmandol; Premandol; Viola; Woloderma; *UK:* Earex; Imuderm; Infaderm; Snor-Away; Snorenz.

Alpha Glucosidase (19670-h)

Profile

Alpha glucosidase is a therapeutic enzyme under investigation for the treatment of glycogen storage disease type II (Pompe's disease).

Preparations

Proprietary Preparations (details are given in Part 3)
Multi-ingredient: *Austral.:* Digestaid; Zinc Zenith.

Alpha$_1$-proteinase Inhibitor (16516-j)

Alpha$_1$ Antitrypsin.
ATC — B02AB02.

Adverse Effects and Precautions

Intravenous administration of alpha$_1$-proteinase inhibitor may produce flu-like symptoms, chills, dyspnoea, hypotension, tachycardia, or rashes. Allergic-type reactions have been reported. Preparations derived from pooled human plasma carry a risk of transmission of infection (see Blood, p.726). Vaccination against hepatitis B is recommended before starting treatment with alpha$_1$-proteinase inhibitor.

Uses and Administration

Endogenous alpha$_1$-proteinase inhibitor is a serum glycoprotein synthesised in the liver that acts as an elastase inhibitor, primarily inhibiting neutrophil elastase. Alpha$_1$-proteinase inhibitor, prepared from pooled human plasma, is used as replacement therapy in patients with emphysema who have congenital alpha$_1$ antitrypsin deficiency (see below). It is given in a dose of 60 mg per kg body-weight once a week by intravenous infusion over about 30 minutes.

A recombinant form of alpha$_1$-proteinase inhibitor is under investigation for nebulised delivery in congenital alpha$_1$ antitrypsin deficiency and cystic fibrosis.

Alpha$_1$-proteinase inhibitor is also under investigation for the prevention of bronchopulmonary dysplasia in preterm neonates.

Alpha$_1$ antitrypsin deficiency. Alpha$_1$ antitrypsin deficiency is a rare genetic disorder characterised by the development of emphysema usually in the third or fourth decade of life. Patients with this disorder lack alpha$_1$-proteinase inhibitor. Alpha$_1$-proteinase inhibitor acts in the lungs as an inhibitor of neutrophil elastase, an enzyme that is released in response to inflammation. A deficiency of this inhibitor thus leaves the lungs vulnerable to destruction by elastase and leads to the development of emphysema (p.759).

Management of alpha$_1$ antitrypsin deficiency involves avoidance of factors (mainly cigarette smoking) that cause pulmonary inflammation, and supportive treatment with bronchodilators and oxygen as appropriate. Replacement therapy with alpha$_1$-proteinase inhibitor by intravenous infusion has been shown to correct the biochemical abnormality[1] and has been recommended in those patients with some deterioration of lung function.[2,3] However, it has not yet been shown that alpha$_1$-proteinase inhibitor can prevent the development of emphysema,[4] and a small placebo-controlled study[5] found that the rate of decline of FEV_1 was not affected in patients treated for at least 3 years. Data[6] from a large registry of patients also suggested that, overall, treatment did not affect the rate of decline of FEV_1, but that it decreased mortality although this may be influenced by other factors. Alpha$_1$-proteinase inhibitor has limited value in patients with very severe emphysema as replacement therapy cannot reverse established lung damage.[2]

A dosage regimen of 250 mg per kg body-weight intravenously once a month produces adequate serum concentrations of alpha$_1$-proteinase inhibitor and may be an alternative to the recommended weekly injections.[7] Recombinant forms of alpha$_1$-proteinase inhibitor[2] and administration by aerosol[8] are also being investigated.

Patients with alpha$_1$ antitrypsin deficiency may also have some liver involvement. This may present as neonatal jaundice or in adults as cirrhosis. The liver disease is managed symptomatically; it does not respond to treatment with alpha$_1$-proteinase inhibitor.

1. Wewers MD, et al. Replacement therapy for alpha$_1$-antitrypsin deficiency associated with emphysema. N Engl J Med 1987; **316:** 1055–62.
2. MacDonald JL, Johnson CE. Pathophysiology and treatment of α$_1$-antitrypsin deficiency. Am J Health-Syst Pharm 1995; **52:** 481–9.
3. American Thoracic Society. Guidelines for the approach to the patient with severe hereditary alpha-1-antitrypsin deficiency. Am Rev Respir Dis 1989; **140:** 1494–7.
4. Burdon JGW, et al. Antiproteinase deficiency, emphysema and replacement therapy. Aust N Z J Med 1996; **26:** 769–71.
5. Dirksen A, et al. A randomized clinical trial of α$_1$-antitrypsin augmentation therapy. Am J Respir Crit Care Med 1999; **160:** 1468–72.
6. The Alpha-1-Antitrypsin Deficiency Registry Study Group. Survival and FEV_1 decline in individuals with severe deficiency of α$_1$-antitrypsin. Am J Respir Crit Care Med 1998; **158:** 49–59.
7. Hubbard RC, et al. Biochemical efficacy and safety of monthly augmentation therapy for α$_1$-antitrypsin deficiency. JAMA 1988; **260:** 1259–64.
8. Hubbard RC, et al. Anti-neutrophil-elastase defenses of the lower respiratory tract in α1-antitrypsin deficiency directly augmented with an aerosol of α1-antitrypsin. Ann Intern Med 1989; **111:** 206–12.

Cystic fibrosis. Some of the inflammatory damage that occurs in the lungs of patients with cystic fibrosis is thought to be caused by excessive amounts of elastase released locally. Alpha$_1$-proteinase inhibitor given by nebuliser is therefore under investigation[1,2] in patients with cystic fibrosis (p.117).

1. McElvaney NG, et al. Aerosol α1-antitrypsin treatment for cystic fibrosis. Lancet 1991; **337:** 392–4.
2. Balfour-Lynn IM. The protease-antiprotease battle in the cystic fibrosis lung. J R Soc Med 1999; **92** (suppl 37): 23–30.

Preparations

Proprietary Preparations (details are given in Part 3)
Canad.: Prolastin; **Ger.:** Prolastin HS; **Hong Kong:** Prolastin; **Ital.:** Prolastina; **Spain:** Prolastina; **USA:** Prolastin.

Althaea (5404-v)

Alteia; Alth.; Althaeae Radix; Eibischwurzel; Marshmallow; Marshmallow Root; Racine de Guimauve; Raiz de Altea.

Pharmacopoeias. In Eur. (see p.vi) and Pol.
Althaea Leaf is also included in Eur. and Pol. and Althaea Flower in Fr.

Pharmacopoeial description

Ph. Eur.: The peeled or unpeeled, whole or cut, dried root of marshmallow, Althaea officinalis. Protect from light.

Profile

Althaea is demulcent and emollient and has been used for irritation and inflammation of the mucous membranes of the mouth and pharynx. It has also been used in traditional remedies for a variety of disorders including gastrointestinal disturbances.

The symbol † denotes a preparation no longer actively marketed

Preparations

Proprietary Preparations (details are given in Part 3)
Ger.: Phytohustil.

Multi-ingredient: Aust.: Aktiv Husten- und Bronchialtee; Anifer Hustentee; Aponatura Hustenlosende; Bio-Garten Tee gegen Erkaltung; Bronchostop; Erkaltungstee; Heumann's Bronchialtee; Krauterhaus Mag Kottas Husten- und Bronchialtee; Krautertee Nr 11; Krautertee Nr 7; Mag Kottas Husten-Bronchialtee; Mediplant Krauter; Paracodin; Sidroga Brust-Husten-Tee; St Radegunder Hustentee; Synpharma Instant-Brust- und Hustentee; The Chambard-Tee; Tuscalman; **Austral.:** Althaea Complex; Cough Relief; Garlic and Horseradish + C Complex; Hydrastis Complex; Respatona Decongestant Complex; Respatona Plus Bronchial Cough Relief; **Belg.:** Eugiron; Paracodine; Tisane Antibiliaire et Stomachique; Tisane Pectorale; Tisane Purgative; **Braz.:** Limao Bravo; Peitoral Angico Pelotense; **Canad.:** Swiss Herb Cough Drops; **Fr.:** Apilaxe; Elixir Contre La Toux Weleda†; Mediflor Tisane No 4 Diuretique; Mediflor Tisane Pectorale d'Alsace; Tisane des Familles; Tisane Grande Chartreuse; **Ger.:** Biotuss N; Em-eukal Husten- und Brusttee; Heumann Bronchialtee Solubifix; Infantussin N†; Junisana; Tonsilgon N; **Ital.:** Cura†; **Switz.:** Malveol; Sirop antitussif Wyss a base de codeine†; Sirop pectoral DP1†; Sirop pectoral DP2, DP3†; Sirop Wyss contre la toux†; Tisane pectorale et antitussive; Tisane pectorale pour les enfants; Tuscalman; **UK:** Biobalm; Cough Elixir; Digest; Garlodex; Gerard House Golden Seal Compound; Herb and Honey Cough Elixir; Herbheal Ointment; Modern Herbals Cold & Catarrh; Potter's Catarrh Pastilles; Sinotar.

Alum (294-r)

Alaun; Allume; Aluin; Alumbre; Alumen; Aluminium Kalium Sulfuricum; Aluminium Potassium Sulphate; Alun; E522; Potash Alum; Potassium Alum. Potassium aluminium sulphate dodecahydrate.

$AlK(SO_4)_2, 12H_2O = 474.4.$
CAS — 7784-24-9 (alum dodecahydrate); 10043-67-1 (anhydrous alum).
ATC — S01XA07.

Pharmacopoeias. In Chin., Eur. (see p.vi), Jpn, Pol., and US.
US also includes the anhydrous form and both anhydrous and dodecahydrated ammonia alum (Ammonium Alum). Belg. and Jpn also include dried alum.

Pharmacopoeial description

Ph. Eur.: Colourless, transparent, crystalline masses or a granular powder. Freely soluble in water; very soluble in boiling water; practically insoluble in alcohol; soluble in glycerol. A 10% solution in water has a pH of 3.0 to 3.5.

USP 25: A white powder or large, colourless crystals or crystalline fragments. It is odourless. Soluble 1 in 7 of water and 1 in 0.3 of boiling water; insoluble in alcohol; freely but slowly soluble in glycerol. Its solutions are acid to litmus.

Adverse Effects

Large doses of alum are irritant and may be corrosive; gum necrosis and gastrointestinal haemorrhage have occurred. Systemic absorption from bladder irrigation solutions can cause acute aluminium toxicity (see under Aluminium below) including encephalopathy.

◊ References.

1. Phelps KR, et al. Encephalopathy after bladder irrigation with alum: case report and literature review. Am J Med Sci 1999; **318:** 181–5.
2. Nakamura H, et al. Acute encephalopathy due to aluminium toxicity successfully treated by combined intravenous deferoxamine and hemodialysis. J Clin Pharmacol 2000; **40:** 296–300.

Uses and Administration

Alum precipitates proteins and is a powerful astringent. It is often included in preparations used as mouthwashes or gargles and in dermatological preparations.

Alum, either as a solid or as a solution, may be used as a haemostatic.

Alum is also used as a mordant in the dyeing industry.

Haemorrhage. Haemorrhage associated with malignant disease can be difficult to control and some success in bladder haemorrhage[1,2] or rectal haemorrhage[3] has been described with the use of an alum 1% solution.

1. Kennedy C, et al. Use of alum to control intractable vesical haemorrhage. Br J Urol 1984; **56:** 673–5.
2. Goel AK, et al. Intravesical irrigation with alum for the control of massive bladder hemorrhage. J Urol (Baltimore) 1985; **133:** 956–7.
3. Paes TRF, et al. Alum solution in the control of intractable haemorrhage from advanced rectal carcinoma. Br J Surg 1986; **73:** 192.

Preparations

Proprietary Preparations (details are given in Part 3)

Multi-ingredient: Aust.: EST; **Austral.:** BFI†; **Braz.:** Higienex; Leucocida; **Canad.:** Fletchers Sore Mouth Medicine; **Fr.:** Denisoline; **Ger.:** Dr. Hotz Vollbad†; Retterspitz Ausserlich†; Retterspitz Gelee†; Retterspitz Innerlich†; Trachitol†; **Ital.:** Emoplast†; Lavanda Sofar; **Kr.:** Grans Remedy; **Spain:** Cloroboral; Co Bucal; Lindemil; **USA:** BFI; Mycinette.

Aluminium (5261-g)

Aluminum; E173.
Al = 26.981538.
CAS — 7429-90-5.
Pharmacopoeias. Br. includes Aluminium Powder.

Aluminium is a malleable and ductile soft silvery-white metal, becoming coated with a thin layer of oxide.

Pharmacopoeial description

BP 2001: Aluminium powder is an odourless or almost odourless, silvery-grey powder. It consists mainly of metallic aluminium in very small flakes, usually with an appreciable quantity of aluminium oxide. It is lubricated with stearic acid to protect the metal from oxidation. Practically insoluble in water and in alcohol; it dissolves in dilute acids and in aqueous solutions of alkali hydroxides, with the evolution of hydrogen.

◊ CAUTION. *Aluminium powder has been used for the illicit preparation of explosives or fireworks; care is required with its supply.*

Incompatibility. Incompatibilities have been reported between aluminium in injection equipment and metronidazole[1,2] and between aluminium and various antineoplastics including cisplatin, daunorubicin, and doxorubicin.[3-6] The suitability of aluminium caps for sugar-containing liquids has also been questioned. Abrasion of the aluminium cap by sugar from Ceporex Syrup has resulted in the formation of a black slime.[7]

1. Schell KH, Copeland JR. Metronidazole hydrochloride-aluminum interaction. Am J Hosp Pharm 1985; **42:** 1040, 1042.
2. Struthers BJ, Parr RJ. Clarifying the metronidazole hydrochloride-aluminum interaction. Am J Hosp Pharm 1985; **42:** 2660.
3. Bohart RD, Ogawa G. An observation on the stability of cis-dichlorodiammineplatinum (II): a caution regarding its administration. Cancer Treat Rep 1979; **63:** 2117–18.
4. Gardiner WA. Possible incompatibility of doxorubicin hydrochloride with aluminum. Am J Hosp Pharm 1981; **38:** 1276.
5. Williamson MJ, et al. Doxorubicin hydrochloride-aluminum interaction. Am J Hosp Pharm 1983; **40:** 214.
6. Ogawa GS, et al. Dispensing-pin problems. Am J Hosp Pharm 1985; **42:** 1042.
7. Tressler LJ. Medicine bottle caps. Pharm J 1985; **235:** 99.

Adverse Effects, Treatment, and Precautions

Aluminium toxicity is well recognised in patients with renal impairment. Patients undergoing dialysis have experienced encephalopathy, osteodystrophy, and anaemia associated with an aluminium salt taken as a phosphate binder or with aluminium present in the water supply. For this reason, aluminium-free phosphate binders are often used in dialysis patients (see Renal Osteodystrophy, p.746); also the concentration of aluminium in dialysis fluid has been limited to not more than 10 µg per litre. Serum-aluminium concentrations should be monitored regularly in patients undergoing dialysis.

Aluminium toxicity has followed the use of parenteral fluids and infant feeds with a high concentration of aluminium.

Aluminium toxicity may be treated by removal of the aluminium with desferrioxamine (p.1004).

The adverse effects of aluminium salts and precautions to be observed are described under Aluminium Hydroxide, p.1210.

◊ A review of aluminium toxicity[1] lists possible sources of aluminium including water, antacids, phosphate-binding gels, total parenteral nutrition solutions, processed human serum albumin, fluids used in infants, and environmental pollution; cooking utensils and beverages such as tea have also been suggested as possible sources of aluminium. Toxicity tends to occur when the gastrointestinal barrier to aluminium absorption is circumvented, as in intravenous fluid administration or dialysis, or if the excretion of aluminium is reduced, as in renal impairment. Infants, especially preterm infants, form a special risk group.[2-5]

Accidental deposition of a large amount of aluminium sulfate in a reservoir in Cornwall in 1988 led to contamination of a nearby town's water supply.[6] Symptoms reported included diarrhoea, mouth ulcers or blisters, malaise, joint symptoms (mainly deterioration of existing symptoms), and memory defects (usually beginning 2 to 3 months after the incident). Although some medical experts considered that no long-term toxic effects were to be expected,[6] aluminium deposits were found in the bones of 2 individuals 6 to 7 months later.[7] In a study[8] undertaken 3 years after the incident, 55 adults who claimed to have suffered cerebral damage performed poorly in psychomotor testing. The authors attributed this to aluminium exposure, but the study's design and conclusions have been criticised.[9-11]

1. Monteagudo FSE, et al. Recent developments in aluminium toxicology. Med Toxicol 1989; **4:** 1–16.
2. Bishop N, et al. Aluminium in infant formulas. Lancet 1989; **i:** 490.
3. Lawson M, et al. Aluminium and infant formulae. Lancet 1989; **i:** 614–15.
4. Anonymous. Aluminium content of parenteral drug products. WHO Drug Inf 1990; **4:** 70.
5. American Academy of Pediatrics Committee on Nutrition. Aluminum toxicity in infants and children. Pediatrics 1996; **97:** 413–16.
6. Anonymous. Camelford two years on. Lancet 1990; **336:** 366.
7. Eastwood JB, et al. Aluminium deposition in bone after contamination of drinking water supply. Lancet 1990; **336:** 462–4.
8. Altmann P, et al. Disturbance of cerebral function in people exposed to drinking water contaminated with aluminium sulphate: retrospective study of the Camelford water incident. BMJ 1999; **319:** 807–11.

9. David A. Cerebral dysfunction after water pollution incident in Camelford: results were biased by self selection of cases. *BMJ* 2000; **320:** 1337.
10. Esmonde TFG. Cerebral dysfunction after water pollution incident in Camelford: study has several methodological errors. *BMJ* 2000; **320:** 1337–8.
11. McMillan TM. Cerebral dysfunction after water pollution incident in Camelford: study may prolong the agony. *BMJ* 2000; **320:** 1338.

Effects on mental function. Encephalopathy with seizures has been associated with the use of aluminium-containing materials used for bone reconstruction.[1,2] In each case, reconstruction of areas of the skull resulted in high concentrations of aluminium in the CSF.

1. Renard JL, *et al.* Post-otoneurosurgery aluminium encephalopathy. *Lancet* 1994; **344:** 63–4.
2. Hantson P, *et al.* Encephalopathy with seizures after use of aluminium-containing bone cement. *Lancet* 1994; **344:** 1647.

ALZHEIMER'S DISEASE. The role of aluminium in the aetiology of Alzheimer's disease (see Dementia, p.1412) is, at best, unclear.[1-4] Circumstantial evidence of a positive association arises from *animal* and *in-vitro* data, together with clinical observations that aluminium is present in senile plaques and neurofibrillary tangles occurring in Alzheimer's disease, that the administration of aluminium chelators to Alzheimer patients may slow the progression of the disease, and that the risk of brain changes is increased in people living in areas with a high aluminium content in the drinking water supply. Some of these findings have been criticised, unconfirmed, or disproved by other workers. Listed below are some of the studies which point to an association between aluminium intake and Alzheimer's disease,[5-8] some criticisms,[9-13] and some negative findings.[14,15]

There does not appear to be a risk of aluminium accumulation from normal use of aluminium-containing antacids by patients with normal renal function; consequently use of these antacids by such patients should not be considered to put them at risk of Alzheimer's disease.[16,17]

1. Crapper McLachlan DR, *et al.* Would decreased aluminum ingestion reduce the incidence of Alzheimer's disease? *Can Med Assoc J* 1991; **145:** 793–804.
2. Anonymous. Is aluminium a dementing ion? *Lancet* 1992; **339:** 713–14.
3. Munoz DG. Is exposure to aluminium a risk factor for the development of Alzheimer disease?—No. *Arch Neurol* 1998; **55:** 737–9.
4. Forbes WF, Hill GB. Is exposure to aluminium a risk factor for the development of Alzheimer disease?—-Yes. *Arch Neurol* 1998; **55:** 740–1.
5. Martyn CN, *et al.* Geographical relation between Alzheimer's disease and aluminium in drinking water. *Lancet* 1989; **i:** 59–62.
6. Crapper McLachlan DR, *et al.* Intramuscular desferrioxamine in patients with Alzheimer's disease. *Lancet* 1991; **337:** 1304–8.
7. Good PF, *et al.* Selective accumulation of aluminum and iron in the neurofibrillary tangles of Alzheimer's disease: a laser microprobe (LAMMA) study. *Ann Neurol* 1992; **31:** 286–92.
8. Harrington CR, *et al.* Alzheimer's-disease-like changes in tau protein processing: association with aluminium accumulation in brains of renal dialysis patients. *Lancet* 1994; **343:** 993–7.
9. Ebrahim S. Aluminium and Alzheimer's disease. *Lancet* 1989; **i:** 267.
10. Schupf N, *et al.* Aluminium and Alzheimer's disease. *Lancet* 1989; **i:** 267.
11. Lindesay J. Aluminium and Alzheimer's disease. *Lancet* 1989; **i:** 268.
12. Birchall JD, Chappell JS. Aluminium, water chemistry, and Alzheimer's disease. *Lancet* 1989; **i:** 953.
13. Whalley LJ, *et al.* Aluminium and dementia. *Lancet* 1992; **339:** 1235–6.
14. Markesbery WR, *et al.* Instrumental neutron activation analysis of brain aluminum in Alzheimer's disease and aging. *Ann Neurol* 1981; **10:** 511–16.
15. Wettstein A, *et al.* Failure to find a relationship between mnestic skills of octogenarians and aluminum in drinking water. *Int Arch Occup Environ Health* 1991; **63:** 97–103.
16. Anonymous. Aluminium salts and Alzheimer's disease. *Pharm J* 1991; **246:** 809.
17. Flaten TP, *et al.* Mortality from dementia among gastroduodenal ulcer patients. *J Epidemiol Community Health* 1991; **45:** 203–6.

Uses and Administration

Aluminium is used in packaging and in injection equipment. The foil is also used as a dressing and for insulation. Aluminium may also be employed as a colouring agent for some foodstuffs. Aluminium powder alone and in paste form with zinc oxide has been used as a dressing. Astringent aluminium salts are used as antiperspirants. Aluminium hydroxide is used as an antacid.

Aluminium is used in homoeopathic medicine.

Preparations

BP 2001: Compound Aluminium Paste.

Proprietary Preparations (details are given in Part 3)
Multi-ingredient: *Braz.:* Belagin.

Aluminium Acetate   (296-d)

Aluminum Acetate.
$C_6H_9AlO_6 = 204.1$.
CAS — 139-12-8.

Pharmacopoeial description

Aluminium acetate is prepared from aluminium sulfate and acetic acid. The BP 2001 includes Aluminium Acetate Ear Drops which correspond to a solution of aluminium acetotartrate in that they are prepared from aluminium sulfate with the aid of acetic acid and tartaric acid. The USP 25 includes

Aluminum Acetate Topical Solution which is prepared from glacial acetic acid and Aluminum Subacetate Topical Solution (which is itself prepared from aluminium sulfate and acetic acid); it does not involve tartaric acid.

Profile

Solutions containing aluminium acetate are astringent. Ear drops containing aluminium acetate reduce oedema and inflammation of the ear by producing an acidic environment hostile to pathogenic bacteria; they are also hygroscopic. Solutions are also used in dermatology as astringent lotions for irritating skin conditions.

Various preparations containing aluminium acetate have been known as Burow's creams, emulsions, lotions, or solutions. Aluminium acetotartrate and aluminium subacetate (basic aluminium acetate) are also used as topical astringents.

Preparations

BP 2001: Aluminium Acetate Ear Drops;
USP 25: Aluminum Subacetate Topical Solution.

Proprietary Preparations (details are given in Part 3)
Aust.: Euceta; *Ger.:* Alsol; Alsol N; Essigsaure Tonerde-Salbe; Essitol; *Ital.:* Euceta†; *Neth.:* Euceta†; *Switz.:* Euceta; *USA:* Bite Rx; Buro-Sol.

Multi-ingredient: *Aust.:* Acetonal; Euceta mit Kamille; Methyment; Nasanal; Neo-Phlogicid; *Austral.:* Xyloproct; *Belg.:* Xyloproct; *Braz.:* Xyloproct; *Canad.:* Buro Derm†; Buro-Sol; *Fin.:* Xyloproct; *Fr.:* Gel a l'Acetotartrate d'Alumine Defresne; *Ger.:* Anisan; *Hong Kong:* Xyloproct; *Israel:* Contra Combustiones; Proctozorin-N; *Ital.:* Betaderm; Micofoot; Neo Zeta-Foot†; Vegetallumina; Xyloproct; *Mex.:* Xyloproct; *Neth.:* Xyloproct; *Norw.:* Xyloproct; *NZ:* Xyloproct; *Singapore:* Xyloproct; *Spain:* Avril; *Swed.:* Xyloproct; *Switz.:* Anginesin; Cetona Plus; Euceta avec camomille et arnica; Euceta Pic; Fortacet; Frigoplasma; Fungex; Mikutan N; Realderm; *Thai.:* Xyloproct; *UK:* Xyloproct; *USA:* Borofair Otic; Burow's; Otic Domeboro; Star-Otic.

Aluminium Lactate   (12347-b)

Tris(lactato)aluminium.
$C_9H_{15}AlO_9 = 294.2$.
CAS — 537-02-0; 18917-91-4.

Profile

Aluminium lactate is used in the local treatment of various disorders of the mouth.

Preparations

Proprietary Preparations (details are given in Part 3)
Fr.: Aluctyl†; *Ital.:* Aluctyl.

Multi-ingredient: *Israel:* Aronal Forte; *Ital.:* Lacalut; *Switz.:* Deaftol avec lidocaine; Gynasol†.

Aluminium Sulfate   (301-b)

Alumnii Sulfas; Aluminium Sulfuricum; Aluminium Sulphate; Aluminium Trisulphate; Aluminum Sulfate; E520.
$Al_2(SO_4)_3, xH_2O = 342.2$ (anhydrous).
CAS — 10043-01-3 (anhydrous aluminium sulfate); 17927-65-0 (aluminium sulfate hydrate).
Pharmacopoeias. In Eur. (see p.vi), Int., Pol., and US.

Pharmacopoeial description

Ph. Eur.: Colourless lustrous crystals or crystalline masses. It contains 51 to 59% of $Al_2(SO_4)_3$. Soluble in cold water; freely soluble in hot water; practically insoluble in alcohol. Store in airtight containers.

USP 25: Contains 54 to 59% of $Al_2(SO_4)_3$. An odourless, white, crystalline powder, shining plates, or crystalline fragments. Soluble 1 in 1 of water; insoluble in alcohol. The pH of a 5% solution in water is not less than 2.9.

Profile

Aluminium sulfate has an action similar to that of alum (p.1577) but is more astringent. A 20% solution is employed for the treatment of envenomation by certain insects and marine organisms. The aluminium may cause precipitation of the proteins contained within the venoms thus reducing local toxicity. Aluminium sulfate is also included in astringent preparations intended to sooth irritating skin conditions.

Aluminium sulfate is also used in the preparation of aluminium acetate solutions.

Adverse effects. Possible adverse effects or toxicity associated with aluminium, or aluminium salts such as aluminium sulfate, in the public water supply are discussed under Aluminium, p.1577.

Preparations

USP 25: Aluminum Subacetate Topical Solution; Aluminum Sulfate and Calcium Acetate Tablets for Topical Solution.

Proprietary Preparations (details are given in Part 3)
Austral.: Stingose; *Hong Kong:* Stingose; *Israel:* Stingose; *NZ:* Stingose; *S.Afr.:* Stingose†; *UK:* Stingose.

Multi-ingredient: *Aust.:* Citoburol; *Ger.:* Schupps Kohlensaurebad; Tannoli; *Ital.:* Cepral†; *Mex.:* Domeboro; *Switz.:* Gynasol†; *USA:* Bluboro; Boropak; Domeboro; Ostiderm; Pedi-Boro Soak Paks.

Ambucetamide   (5227-b)

Ambucetamide (BAN, rINN).
A-16; Dibutamide. 2-Dibutylamino-2-(4-methoxyphenyl)acetamide.
$C_{17}H_{28}N_2O_2 = 292.4$.
CAS — 519-88-0.

Profile

Ambucetamide is used as an antispasmodic and has been given for the relief of dysmenorrhoea. The hydrochloride is also used.

Preparations

Proprietary Preparations (details are given in Part 3)
Multi-ingredient: *Belg.:* Neomeritine†; *Neth.:* Femerital†.

Amikhelline Hydrochloride   (12356-v)

Amikhelline Hydrochloride (rINNM).
9-(2-Diethylaminoethoxy)-4-hydroxy-7-methyl-5*H*-furo[3,2-g][1]benzopyran-5-one hydrochloride.
$C_{18}H_{21}NO_5, HCl = 367.8$.
CAS — 4439-67-2 (amikhelline); 40709-23-7 (amikhelline hydrochloride).

Profile

Amikhelline hydrochloride has been used as an antispasmodic.

Aminohippuric Acid   (2122-k)

p-Aminobenzoylglycine; *p*-Aminohippuric Acid; PAHA; Para-aminohippuric Acid. N-4-Aminobenzoylaminoacetic acid.
$C_9H_{10}N_2O_3 = 194.2$.
CAS — 61-78-9 (aminohippuric acid); 94-16-6 (sodium aminohippurate).
ATC — V04CH30.
Pharmacopoeias. In US.

Pharmacopoeial description

USP 25: A white crystalline powder which discolours on exposure to light. Soluble 1 in 45 of water, 1 in 50 of alcohol, and 1 in 5 of 3N hydrochloric acid; very slightly soluble in carbon tetrachloride, in chloroform, in ether, and in benzene; freely soluble in alkaline solutions with some decomposition, and in diluted hydrochloric acid. Store in airtight containers. Protect from light.

Adverse Effects

Sodium aminohippurate may cause nausea and vomiting, hypersensitivity reactions, vasomotor disturbances, flushing, tingling, cramps, and a feeling of warmth. Patients may develop an urge to urinate or defaecate after infusion.

Interactions

The estimation of sodium aminohippurate may be affected in patients taking procaine, sulfonamides, or thiazosulfone. Probenecid diminishes the excretion of aminohippuric acid. Clearance is also affected by penicillins, salicylates, sulfinpyrazone, and other drugs that compete for the same excretory pathways.

Uses and Administration

Aminohippuric acid is excreted mainly by proximal tubular secretion, with some glomerular filtration. It is given by intravenous infusion, as the sodium salt, sodium aminohippurate (aminohippurate sodium; $C_9H_9N_2NaO_3 = 216.2$), for the estimation of effective renal plasma flow. Doses are aimed at producing a plasma concentration of 20 µg per mL; at these concentrations approximately 90% of aminohippurate is cleared from the renal blood stream in a single circuit in patients with normal renal function. Sodium aminohippurate has also been used for the assessment of the renal tubular secretory mechanism. Doses for this purpose are infused slowly to achieve a plasma concentration of 400 to 600 µg per mL to saturate the tubular secretion. These tests are used mainly in research procedures.

Preparations

USP 25: Aminohippurate Sodium Injection.

Amiprilose Hydrochloride   (1207-j)

Amiprilose Hydrochloride (USAN, rINNM).
SM-1213 (amiprilose). 3-*O*-[3-(Dimethylamino)propyl]-1,2-*O*-isopropylidene-α-D-glucofuranose hydrochloride.
$C_{14}H_{27}NO_6, HCl = 341.8$.
CAS — 56824-20-5 (amiprilose); 60414-06-4 (amiprilose hydrochloride).

Profile

Amiprilose hydrochloride is an immunomodulator that has been investigated in the treatment of rheumatoid arthritis.

Ammi Visnaga Fruit (9204-g)

Khella; Khellah; Picktooth Fruit; Visnaga.

Khellin (9249-t)

Khelline (rINN).

Khelline; Khellinum; Visammin. 4,9-Dimethoxy-7-methyl-5H-furo[3,2-g]chromen-5-one.
$C_{14}H_{12}O_5 = 260.2$.
CAS — 82-02-0.
Pharmacopoeias. In Aust.

Visnadine (9284-f)

Visnadine (BAN, rINN).
10-Acetoxy-9,10-dihydro-8,8-dimethyl-2-oxo-2H,8H-pyrano[2,3-f]chromen-9-yl 2-methylbutyrate.
$C_{21}H_{24}O_7 = 388.4$.
CAS — 477-32-7.
ATC — C04AX24.

Profile

Ammi visnaga fruit is used in herbal and homoeopathic preparations.

Khellin and visnadine are vasodilators obtained from Ammi visnaga fruit or by synthesis. Khellin also has a bronchodilatory action and has been used in angina pectoris and asthma. Visnadine has been used in coronary, cerebral, and peripheral vascular disorders.

Preparations

Proprietary Preparations (details are given in Part 3)
Ger.: Carduben†; Khellangan N; steno-loges N.
Multi-ingredient: Aust.: Urelium Neu; **Ger.:** Aesrutal S; Cefedrin N; Hepatofalk Neu; Hevertopect; Oxacant-Khella N; Salusan†; Stenocrat.

Strong Ammonia Solution (201-d)

Ammoniaca; Ammoniacum; Ammoniae Solutio Concentrata; Ammoniaque Officinale; Concentrated Ammonia Solution; Liquor Ammoniae Fortis; Solutio Ammoniaci Concentrata; Stronger Ammonia Water; Stronger Ammonium Hydroxide Solution.
CAS — 7664-41-7 (NH_3).

NOTE. The food additive number E527 is used for ammonium hydroxide.
Pharmacopoeias. In Chin. (25 to 28%) and Eur. (see p.vi) (25 to 30%). Also in USNF (27 to 31%).

'0.880 ammonia' contains about 35% w/w.

Pharmacopoeial description

Ph. Eur.: Contains between 25% and 30% (w/w) of ammonia, NH_3. A clear colourless liquid. Very caustic. Miscible with water and with alcohol. Store at a temperature not exceeding 20° in airtight containers.

USNF 20: Contains between 27% and 31% (w/w) of NH_3. On exposure to air, it loses ammonia rapidly. A clear colourless liquid with an exceedingly pungent characteristic odour. Store at a temperature not exceeding 25° in airtight containers.

◊ CAUTION. Strong Ammonia Solution should be handled with great care because of the caustic nature of the solution and the irritating properties of the vapour. Cool the container well before opening and avoid inhalation of the vapour.

Dilute Ammonia Solution (202-n)

Ammonia Water; Ammoniaque Officinale Diluée; Ammonium Hydricum Solutum; Diluted Ammonium Hydroxide Solution; Liquor Ammoniae; Liquor Ammoniae Dilutus.
Pharmacopoeias. In Br., Ger., Jpn, Pol., and Swiss (all about 10%); in Aust. (10.2 to 11%).

Pharmacopoeial description

BP 2001: Prepared by diluting Strong Ammonia Solution with freshly boiled and cooled purified water. It contains 9.5 to 10.5% w/w of NH_3.
NOTE. The BP directs that when Ammonia Solution is prescribed or demanded, Dilute Ammonia Solution shall be dispensed or supplied.

Adverse Effects

Ingestion of strong solutions of ammonia causes severe pain in the mouth, throat, and gastrointestinal tract, as well as severe local oedema and salivation, with cough, vomiting, and shock. Burns to the oesophagus and stomach may result in perforation. Stricture formation usually in the oesophagus can occur weeks or months later. Ingestion may also cause oedema of the respiratory tract and pneumonitis, though this may not develop for a few hours.

Inhalation of ammonia vapour causes sneezing and coughing and in high concentration causes pulmonary oedema. Asphyxia has been reported following oedema or spasm of the glottis. Ammonia vapour is irritant to the eyes and causes weeping; there may be conjunctival swelling and temporary blindness. Strong solutions on the conjunctiva cause a severe reaction with conjunctival oedema, corneal damage, and acute glaucoma. Late complications include angle-closure glaucoma,

---

The symbol † denotes a preparation no longer actively marketed

opaque corneal scars, atrophy of the iris, and formation of cataracts.
Ammonia burns have resulted from treating insect bites and stings with the strong solution, and even with the dilute solution, especially if a dressing is subsequently applied.

◊ References.
1. Beare JDL, et al. Ammonia burns of the eye: an old weapon in new hands. BMJ 1988; 296: 590.
2. Payne MP, Delic JI. Ammonia. In: Toxicity Review 24. London: HMSO, 1991: 1–12.
3. Payne MP, et al. Toxicology of substances in relation to major hazards: ammonia. London: HMSO, 1991.
4. Leduc D, et al. Acute and long term respiratory damage following inhalation of ammonia. Thorax 1992; 47: 755–7.
5. Amstel CE, et al. Anhydrous ammonia burns case report and review of the literature. Burns 2000; 26: 493–7.

Treatment of Adverse Effects

Ingestion should not be treated by lavage or emesis. Milk or water have been given as diluents, but small volumes should be used to reduce the risk of inducing emesis. Appropriate measures should be taken to alleviate pain, shock, and pulmonary oedema, and maintain an airway.
Contaminated skin and eyes should be flooded immediately with water and the washing continued for at least 15 minutes. Any affected clothing should be removed while flooding is being carried out.

Uses and Administration

Dilute solutions of ammonia have been used as reflex stimulants either as smelling salts or solutions for oral administration. They have also been used as rubefacients and counter-irritants (see p.4) and to neutralise insect stings. Users should always be aware of the irritant properties of ammonia.
Hartshorn and Oil was sometimes used as a name for an ammonia liniment. Household ammonia and cloudy ammonia have been used as names for cleaning preparations of ammonia with oleic acid or soap respectively.

Stings. Bathers who were stung by Portuguese men-of-war (Physalia physalis) were rapidly and effectively relieved of discomfort, paresis, irritation, and other symptoms by the application of aromatic ammonia spirit compresses.[1]
1. Frohman IG. Treatment of physalia stings. JAMA 1966; 197: 733.

Preparations

BP 2001: Aromatic Ammonia Solution; Aromatic Ammonia Spirit; Strong Ammonium Acetate Solution; White Liniment.
Proprietary Preparations (details are given in Part 3)
Canad.: After Bite; **Israel:** After Bite; **Spain:** After Bite; Calmapica; **UK:** After Bite.
Multi-ingredient: Aust.: Apotheker Bauer's Franzbranntwein-Gel; Rowalind; **Austral.:** Senega and Ammonia; **Canad.:** Bronchex; Bronchisaft†; SJ Liniment; **Ger.:** Laryngsan N; Rowalind†; **Irl.:** Rowalind; **Ital.:** Stilomagic; **Port.:** Broncodiazina; **S.Afr.:** Enterodyne; Famstim; Peter Pote's†; **Spain:** Analgesico Ut Asens Fn†; Licor Amoniacal†; Linimento Sloan; Masagil; **Swed.:** Sloan's liniment†; **UK:** Blisteze; BN; Goddards White Oil Embrocation; Mackenzies Smelling Salts; Pickles Smelling Salts; **USA:** Emergent-Ez.

Ammonium Iodide (4572-y)

Ammonii Iodetum; Ammonii Iodidum; Ammonium Iodatum.
$NH_4I = 144.9$.
CAS — 12027-06-4.

Profile

Ammonium iodide has the actions of iodine and iodides (p.1522). It was formerly included in preparations used as antiseptics and for the local treatment of inflammatory disorders.

Ammonium Phosphate (12369-w)

545 (ammonium polyphosphates); Diammonium Hydrogen Phosphate; Dibasic Ammonium Phosphate. Diammonium hydrogen orthophosphate.
$(NH_4)_2HPO_4 = 132.1$.
CAS — 7783-28-0.
Pharmacopoeias. In USNF.

Pharmacopoeial description

USNF 20: Colourless or white granules or powder. Freely soluble in water; practically insoluble in alcohol and in acetone. A 1% solution in water has a pH of 7.6 to 8.2. Store in airtight containers.

Profile

Ammonium phosphate was formerly used as a diuretic. It may be used as a buffering agent in pharmaceutical preparations.
Ammonium biphosphate (monobasic ammonium phosphate; $(NH_4)H_2PO_4 = 115.0$) has been used to acidify urine and as a phosphate supplement.

Preparations

Proprietary Preparations (details are given in Part 3)
Multi-ingredient: Fr.: Phosphore-Sandoz†.

Amnion (16505-e)

Profile

Human extra-embryonic fetal membranes comprise an inner amniotic membrane, the amnion, and an outer membrane, the chorion. Amnion is used in ocular surgery for a range of conditions. Both amnion and combined membranes have been used as a dressing for raw wounds including chronic ulcers and burns.

Preparations

Proprietary Preparations (details are given in Part 3)
Ital.: Amniex†.

Amylase (3702-f)

Diastase; Glucogenase; Ptyalin.
CAS — 9000-92-4 (amylase); 9000-85-5 (bacterial α-amylase); 9000-90-2 (porcine α-amylase, pancreatic).
ATC — A09AA01.
Pharmacopoeias. In Fr. and Jpn.

An enzyme catalysing the hydrolysis of α-1,4-glucosidic linkages of polysaccharides such as starch, glycogen, or their degradation products. Amylases may be classified according to the manner in which the glucosidic bond is attacked. Endoamylases attack the α-1,4-glucosidic linkage at random. Alpha-amylases are the only types of endoamylases known and yield dextrins, oligosaccharides, and monosaccharides. The more common alpha-amylases include those isolated from human saliva, mammalian pancreas, Bacillus subtilis, Aspergillus oryzae, and barley malt. Exoamylases attack the α-1,4-glucosidic linkage only from the non-reducing outer polysaccharide chain ends. They include beta-amylases and glucoamylases (amyloglucosidases or gamma-amylases) and are of vegetable or microbial origin. Beta-amylases yield beta-limit dextrins and maltose, and glucoamylases yield glucose.

Adverse Effects

Hypersensitivity reactions have been reported.

Hypersensitivity. A report of allergic responses in workers exposed to fungal α-amylase derived from Aspergillus oryzae.[1] These responses were not obtained with α-amylase derived from Bacillus subtilis. These findings have implications for workers in the flour milling and bakery industries.
1. Flindt MLH. Allergy to α-amylase and papain. Lancet 1979; i: 1407–8.

Uses and Administration

Amylase is used in the production of predigested starchy foods and for the conversion of starch to fermentable sugars in the baking, brewing, and fermentation industries.

Amylase from various sources has been used as an ingredient of preparations of digestive enzymes, and has been given by mouth for its supposed activity in reducing respiratory-tract inflammation and local swelling and oedema.

Preparations

Proprietary Preparations (details are given in Part 3)
Fr.: Amylodiastase†; Maxilase; Megamylase; **Port.:** Maxilase; **Spain:** Maxilase†.
Multi-ingredient: Aust.: Festal†; Ozym†; Wobenzym; **Austral.:** Enzyme; **Belg.:** Digestomen; **Braz.:** Digesnorma; Enziprid; Essen; Filogaster; Nompride Enzimatico; Primeral; **Fr.:** Hepatoum; Maxilase-Bacitracine; **Ger.:** Enzym-Wied; **Hong Kong:** Enzyplex; GI; Magesto; **Ital.:** Digestopan; Essen Enzimatico; Luizym†; **Mex.:** Ochozim; Wobenzym; **Port.:** Luizym†; Modulanzime; **Singapore:** Enzyplex; Weisen-U; **Spain:** Demusin; Digestomen Complex; Espasmo Digestomen; Paidozim; Polidasa†; Takadispep Complex†; **Switz.:** Zymoplex; **Thai.:** Diasgest; Digestin; Endogest; Enzyplex; Flatulence Gastulence; Magesto; Papytazyme; Pepsitase; Polyenzyme-I; **UK:** Enzyme Digest; **USA:** Arco-Lase; Arco-Lase Plus; Enzyme; Gustase; Gustase Plus; Ku-Zyme; Kutrase; Papaya Enzyme.

Anagrelide Hydrochloride (12375-p)

Anagrelide Hydrochloride (BANM, USAN, rINNM).
BL-4162A; BL-4162a. 6,7-Dichloro-1,5-dihydroimidazo[2,1-b]quinazolin-2(3H)-one hydrochloride.
$C_{10}H_7Cl_2N_3O,HCl = 292.5$.
CAS — 68475-42-3 (anagrelide); 58579-51-4 (anagrelide hydrochloride).

Adverse Effects

Anagrelide may cause headache, diarrhoea, abdominal pain, nausea, and oedema. Cardiovascular effects include vasodilatation, positive inotropic effects, and palpitations; myocardial infarction and heart failure have also been reported. Anagrelide has been shown to be embryotoxic and fetotoxic in animal studies.

Precautions

Anagrelide should not be used during pregnancy. It should be used with caution in patients with cardiovascular disease. Platelet counts should be monitored closely, especially during the initial stages of treatment (see below). Hepatic and renal function should also be monitored while the platelet count is being lowered.

Pharmacokinetics

Anagrelide is rapidly absorbed from the gastrointestinal tract. It is extensively metabolised before elimination in the urine; less than 1% of a dose is excreted unchanged. The plasma half-life is 1.3 hours, and the terminal elimination half-life has been reported to be about 3 days.

Uses and Administration

Anagrelide reduces platelet production and at higher doses inhibits platelet aggregation. It is used to reduce platelet production in patients with primary (essential) thrombocythaemia and thrombocythaemia secondary to other myeloproliferative disorders (p.486).

Anagrelide is given by mouth as the hydrochloride but doses are expressed in terms of the base. The initial dose is 2 mg daily divided into 2 or 4 doses. After at least a week, the dose is adjusted, by increasing the daily dose by not more than 0.5 mg in any one week, until the platelet count is maintained within the normal range. The usual maintenance dose is 1.5 to 3 mg daily. The dose should not exceed 10 mg per day or 2.5 mg as a single dose.

Platelet counts should be measured every 2 days during the first week of treatment and then at least weekly until the maintenance dose is reached.

◊ References.
1. Anagrelide Study Group. Anagrelide, a therapy for thrombocythemic states: experience in 577 patients. *Am J Med* 1992; **92:** 69–76.
2. Spencer CM, Brogden RN. Anagrelide: a review of its pharmacodynamic and pharmacokinetic properties, and therapeutic potential in the treatment of thrombocythaemia. *Drugs* 1994; **47:** 809–22.
3. Chintagumpala MM, *et al.* Treatment of essential thrombocythemia with anagrelide. *J Pediatr* 1995; **127:** 495–8. [Study in children].
4. Anonymous. Anagrelide for essential thrombocythemia. *Med Lett Drugs Ther* 1997; **39:** 120.
5. Petitt RM, *et al.* Anagrelide for control of thrombocythemia in polycythemia and other myeloproliferative disorders. *Semin Hematol* 1997; **34:** 51–4.
6. Oertel MD. Anagrelide, a selective thrombocytopenic agent. *Am J Health-Syst Pharm* 1998; **55:** 1979–86.
7. Lackner H, *et al.* Treatment of children with anagrelide for thrombocythemia. *J Pediatr Hematol Oncol* 1998; **20:** 469–73.
8. Bellucci S, *et al.* Studies of platelet volume, chemistry and function in patients with essential thrombocythaemia treated with anagrelide. *Br J Haematol* 1999; **104:** 886–92.

Preparations

Proprietary Preparations (details are given in Part 3)
Austral.: Agrylin; *Canad.:* Agrylin; *Israel:* Agrylin; *USA:* Agrylin.

Anethole (4606-q)

Anethol; Anetol; *p*-Propenylanisole. (*E*)-1-Methoxy-4-(prop-1-enyl)benzene.
$C_{10}H_{12}O = 148.2.$
CAS — 104-46-1; 4180-23-8 (E isomer).

NOTE. Distinguish from Anethole Trithione (below).
Pharmacopoeias. In Ger. Also in USNF.

Pharmacopoeial description

USP 25: Obtained from anise oil or other sources or prepared synthetically. At or above 23° anethole is a colourless or faintly yellow liquid with a sweet taste and the aromatic odour of aniseed. Very slightly soluble in water; soluble 1 in 2 by volume of alcohol; readily miscible with chloroform and with ether. Store in airtight containers. Protect from light.

Profile

Anethole has similar properties to anise oil (below).

Preparations

Proprietary Preparations (details are given in Part 3)
Multi-ingredient: *Aust.:* Rowatinex; *Belg.:* Calmant Martou†; *Canad.:* Beech Nut Cough Drops; Bentasil; Bronco Asmol; *Ger.:* Pinimenthol Oral N†; Rowatinex; Tussipect†; *Hong Kong:* Neo-Rowatinex; Rowatinex; *Irl.:* Rowatinex; *Israel:* Rowatinex; *Spain:* Pulmofasa; Pulmofasa Antihist; Rowanefrin; Vicks Formula 44; *Switz.:* Dental-Phenjoca†; Neo-Angin exempt de sucre; Pectocalmine Junior N; Spirogel†; *Thai.:* Rowatinex; *UK:* Rowatinex.

Anethole Trithione (3703-d)

SKF-1717; Trithioparamethoxyphenylpropene. 5-(4-Methoxyphenyl)-3*H*-1,2-dithiole-3-thione.
$C_{10}H_8OS_3 = 240.4.$
CAS — 532-11-6 (anethole trithione).
ATC — A16AX02.

NOTE. Distinguish from Anethole (above).

Profile

Anethole trithione has been given orally in the management of dry mouth (p.1498) and as a choleretic. The usual daily dose is 37.5 to 75 mg, generally in divided doses before meals. Anethole trithione may cause discoloration of the urine.

Preparations

Proprietary Preparations (details are given in Part 3)
Belg.: Sulfarlem S 25; Sulfarlem†; *Canad.:* Sialor; Sulfarlem; *Fr.:* Sulfarlem; *Ger.:* Mucinol; *Hong Kong:* Sulfarlem; *Port.:* Sufralem; *S.Afr.:* Sulfarlem†; *Spain:* Sonicur; *Switz.:* Sulfarlem.

Multi-ingredient: *Belg.:* Sulfarlem Choline.

Angelica (2007-j)

Angelicae Radix; Archangelica.

Pharmacopoeias. In Eur. (see p.vi) and Pol.

Jpn has separate monographs for *Angelica acutiloba* (Japanese Angelica) and *A. dahurica. Chin.* specifies *A. dahurica, A. dahurica* var. *formosana, A. pubescens,* and *A. sinensis.*

Pharmacopoeial description

Ph. Eur.: The whole or cut, carefully dried rhizome and root of *Angelica archangelica* (*Archangelica officinalis*) containing a minimum of 0.2% v/w of essential oil, calculated with reference to the dried drug.

Profile

Angelica is widely used in herbal medicine. The root is used as a bitter to stimulate the appetite. Angelica also has diaphoretic and expectorant properties and has been used for circulatory and respiratory disorders. The stems are candied for use in cooking.

Angelica contains furanocoumarins and may cause photosensitivity reactions.

Other *Angelica* spp. that are employed in herbal medicine include *A. acutiloba* (Japanese angelica), *A. dahurica, A. pubescens,* and *A. sinensis* (Chinese angelica).

Angelica is also used in homoeopathic medicine.

Preparations

Proprietary Preparations (details are given in Part 3)
Ger.: Pascovegeton.

Multi-ingredient: *Aust.:* Abdomilon; Amylatin; Aponatura Verdauungs; Apotheker Bauer's Blahungstee; Apotheker Bauer's Magentee; Bio-Garten Tee fur Leber und Galle; Euflat†; Krauterdoktor Verdauungsfordernde Tropfen; Krautertee Nr 107; Krautertee Nr 28; Krautertee Nr 44; Leber- und Galletee; Magentee; Schwedenjorg mild†; *Austral.:* Infant Tonic; Irontona; Lifesystem Herbal Formula 4 Women's Formula; Medinat Esten; Vitatona; Women's Formula Herbal Formula 3; *Belg.:* Tisane Depurative "les 12 Plantes"; Tisane Diuretique; Tisane Pectorale; Tisane Purgative; *Fr.:* Mediflor Tisane Digestive No 3†; *Ger.:* Abdomilon N; Anore X N; Carvomin; Doppelherz Melissengeist; Euvitan; Gastritol; Iberogast; Infi-tract N; Melissengeist; Schwedentrunk der Echte Elixier; Schwedentrunk mit Ginseng†; Schwedentrunk†; Stovalid N; Ventrimarin novo; *Ital.:* Bitteridina; Florelax; Tisana Arnaldi†; Tonactiv†; *Spain:* Agua del Carmen; *Switz.:* Gastrosan; Iberogast; Phytomed Gastro†; *UK:* Cough Drops; Melissa comp..

Aniracetam (16511-s)

Aniracetam (USAN, rINN).
Ro-13-5057. 1-(4-Methoxybenzoyl)-2-pyrrolidinone.
$C_{12}H_{13}NO_3 = 219.2.$
CAS — 72432-10-1.
ATC — N06BX11.

Profile

Aniracetam is a nootropic drug which has been tried in senile dementia (p.1412). It is given by mouth in usual doses of 1.5 g daily.

◊ References.
1. Lee CR, Benfield P. Aniracetam: an overview of its pharmacodynamic and pharmacokinetic properties, and a review of its therapeutic potential in senile cognitive disorders. *Drugs Aging* 1994; **4:** 257–73.

Preparations

Proprietary Preparations (details are given in Part 3)
Ital.: Ampamet; Draganon; Reset†; *Jpn:* Sarpul.

Aniseed (4607-p)

Anice; Anis Verde; Anis Vert; Anise; Anise Fruit; Anisi Fructus; Fructus Anisi Vulgaris.

NOTE. The names Anís Estrellado, Anis Étoilé, Anisum Badium, Anisum Stellatum, Badiana, Badiane de Chine, Star Anise Fruit, and Sternanis are synonyms for Star Anise.
Pharmacopoeias. In Eur. (see p.vi) and Pol.
Eur. also includes a monograph for Star Anise (Anisi Stellati Fructus).

Pharmacopoeial description

Ph. Eur.: Aniseed is the whole dried fruit of *Pimpinella anisum,* containing not less than 2% v/w of essential oil. It has an odour reminiscent of anethole. Protect from light.

Star anise is the dried composite fruit of *Illicium verum,* containing not less than 7% v/w of essential oil with reference to the anhydrous drug. The fruit carpels are brown and have an odour of anethole. Protect from light.

Profile

Aniseed is carminative and mildly expectorant; it is used mainly as anise oil or as preparations of the oil. It may cause contact dermatitis, probably due to its anethole content.

Aniseed and star anise are the source of anise oil (below).

◊ A brief review of aniseed and anise oil.[1]
1. Chandler RF, Hawkes D. Aniseed—a spice, a flavor, a drug. *Can Pharm J* 1984; **117:** 28–9.

Preparations

Proprietary Preparations (details are given in Part 3)
Multi-ingredient: *Aust.:* Aktiv Husten- und Bronchialtee; Aktiv milder Magen- und Darmtee; Anifer Hustentee; Aponatura Wind; Asthmatee; Brady's-Magentropfen; Euka; Krauterdoktor Krampf- und Reizhustensirup; Krauterhaus Mag Kottas Tee gegen Durchfall; Krautertee Nr 10; Krautertee Nr 107; Krautertee Nr 11; Krautertee Nr 126; Krautertee Nr 211; Krautertee Nr 7; Mag Kottas Husten-Bronchialtee; Nesthakchen; Sidroga Brust-Husten-Tee; Spasmo-Granobil-Krampf- und Reizhusten; Species Carvi comp; Teekanne Husten- und Brusttee; *Austral.:* Neo-Cleanse; *Belg.:* Eugiron; Tisane Antibiliaire et Stomachique; Tisane pour le Foie; Tisane Purgative; *Braz.:* Balsamo Branco; Broncmel; Camomila; Desensibilizante Chauvin; Fargestium; *Canad.:* Pectothymin†; *Fr.:* Elixir Bonjean; Elixir Contre La Toux Weleda†; Herbesan; Mediflor Tisane Digestive No 3†; Mucinum a l'Extrait de Cascara; Mucinum†; Peter's Sirop†; Santane D₅; Soker†; Tisane Clairo†; Tisane des Familles; Tisane Digestive Weleda†; *Ger.:* Echtroferment-N†; Em-eukal; Em-eukal Husten- und Brusttee; Grunlicht Hingfong Essenz; Hevert-Carmin symbio; Kneipp Magen-Tee; Majocarmin-Tee; Ramend Krauter; rohasal; Stovalid N; *Hong Kong:* Mucinum Cascara; *Israel:* Jungborn; *Ital.:* Dicalmir; Florerbe Lassativa; Lassatina; Tisana Kelemata; Tonactiv†; *Spain:* Broncomicin Bals†; Bronquinflamatoria†; Crislaxo; Digestol Sanatorium; Digestovital; Laxante Sanatorium; *Switz.:* Kernosan Elixir; Kernosan Heidelberger Poudre; The Franklin†; Tisane favorisant l'allaitement; Tisane laxative H nouvelle formulation; Tisane laxative Natterman no 13†; *UK:* Carminative Tea; Clairo Tea; Cough Elixir; Laxadoron; Revitonil.

Anise Oil (4609-w)

Aniseed Oil; Anisi Aetheroleum; Esencia de Anís; Essence d'Anis; Oleum Anisi.

Pharmacopoeias. In Chin., Eur. (see p.vi), and Pol.

If the oil has crystallised it should be melted completely and mixed before use.

Pharmacopoeial description

Ph. Eur.: A clear, colourless or pale yellow liquid obtained by steam distillation from aniseed or star anise. Solidifies on cooling; f.p. 15° to 19°. Practically insoluble in water; miscible with alcohol, with dichloromethane, with ether, and with petroleum spirit. Store in airtight well-filled containers. Protect from light and heat.

Incompatibility. PVC bottles softened and distorted fairly rapidly in the presence of anise oil, which should not be stored or dispensed in such bottles.[1]
1. Department of Pharmaceutical Sciences of the Pharmaceutical Society of Great Britain. Plastics medicine bottles of rigid PVC. *Pharm J* 1973; **210:** 100.

Profile

Anise oil is carminative and mildly expectorant and is a common ingredient of cough preparations. It is also a flavour.

It may cause contact dermatitis, probably due to its anethole content.

◊ For a brief review of aniseed and anise oil, see Aniseed, above.

Preparations

BP 2001: Camphorated Opium Tincture; Compound Orange Spirit; Concentrated Anise Water; Concentrated Camphorated Opium Tincture.

Proprietary Preparations (details are given in Part 3)
Multi-ingredient: *Aust.:* Anitos; Bradosol; Bronchostop; Embrocation; Expectal-Tropfen; Expigen; Heumann's Bronchialtee; Luuf-Hustentee; Medizinalbad; Neo-Angin; Nesthakchen; Red Point; SynPharma Bronchial; *Austral.:* Cough Relief; Digestive Aid; Gartech; Respatona Decongestant Formula; Respatona Plus Bronchial Cough Relief; *Canad.:* Babys Own Gripe Water; Beech Nut Cough Drops; Herbal Cough Expectorant; *Fr.:* Paregorique; *Ger.:* Aspasmon N; Benium†; Bronchicum Hustentee†; Bronchocedin N†; Bronchoforton; Em-eukal; Em-eukal Husten- und Brusttee; Ephepect; Floradix Multipretten; Grunlicht Hingfong Essenz; Grunlicht Magenbalsam Tropfen; Heumann Bronchialtee Solubifix; Hevert-Carmin symbio; Hevertopect; Hingfong-Essenz Hofmanns Tropfen; Infantussin N†; Kamillosan Mundspray; Leber-Galle-Tropfen 83; Neo-Ballistol; Pulmocordio mite SL; Pulmotin-N; ratioGast; Repha-Os; Salmiak; Salviathymol N; Sinuforton; *Neth.:* Bronchicum; *Spain:* Carminativo Ibys; Carminativo Juventus; H Tussan; Odontocromil c Sulfamida; *Switz.:* Bronchol N†; Capsules laxatives Nattermann Nr. 13†; Demo pates pectorales†; Endomethasone†; Kamillosan; Liberol Baby N; Makatussin; Makatussin forte; Pastilles pectorales Demo N; *UK:* Hactos; Honey & Molasses; Liqufruta Cough Remedy; Potters Sugar Free Cough Pastilles; Slippery Elm Stomach Tablets; Vegetable Cough Remover; Zubes; Zubes Blackcurrant.

Apis mellifera (12386-e)

The honey bee.

Profile

A preparation containing the venom of *Apis mellifera*, the honey bee, is used in homoeopathic medicine where it is known as Apis mellifica or Apis mel. Apis mellifera is a source of purified honey (p.1366) and royal jelly (p.1659).

◊ For reference to the use of whole body extracts or venom from Hymenoptera spp. in hyposensitisation procedures in allergic subjects, see under Allergen Products, p.1576.

◊ There have been a number of anecdotal reports of successful treatment of chronic inflammatory disease such as arthritis with bee venom.[1] Studies *in vitro* have shown that bee venom has anti-inflammatory activity similar to that of cyclophosphamide. Melittin appears to be the active constituent, and seems to act by interfering with superoxide radical production from human leucocytes.
1. Somerfield SD. Bee venom and arthritis: magic, myth or medicine? *N Z Med J* 1986; **99:** 281–3.

Preparations

Proprietary Preparations (details are given in Part 3)
Multi-ingredient: *Aust.:* Forapin†; *Belg.:* Forapin†; *Ger.:* Forapin E; *Switz.:* Forapin.

Aptiganel (14951-k)

Aptiganel (*pINN*).
CNS-1102 (aptiganel hydrochloride). 1-(*m*-Ethylphenyl)-1-methyl-3-(1-naphthyl)guanidine.
$C_{20}H_{21}N_3 = 303.4$.
CAS — 137159-92-3 (*aptiganel*); 137160-11-3 (*aptiganel hydrochloride*).
NOTE. Aptiganel Hydrochloride is *USAN*.

Profile

Aptiganel is a guanidine derivative which antagonises the effects of the excitatory amino-acid neurotransmitter glutamate at the *N*-methyl D-aspartate (NMDA) receptor. It is under investigation for the prevention of ischaemic brain damage in patients with traumatic head injury or stroke.

◊ References.
1. Muir KW, *et al.* Pharmacological effects of the non-competitive NMDA antagonist CNS 1102 in normal volunteers. *Br J Clin Pharmacol* 1994; **38:** 33–8.
2. Block GA, *et al.* Final results from a dose-escalating safety and tolerance study of the non-competitive NMDA antagonist CNS1102 in patients with acute cerebral ischaemia. *Stroke* 1995; **26:** 185.
3. Dyker AG, *et al.* Safety and tolerability study of aptiganel hydrochloride in patients with an acute ischemic stroke. *Stroke* 1999; **30:** 2038–42.

Arachis Oil (7353-m)

Arachidis Oleum Raffinatum; Earth-nut Oil; Erdnussöl; Groundnut Oil; Huile d'Arachide; Nut Oil; Ol. Arach.; Óleo de Amendoim; Oleum Arachis; Peanut Oil; Refined Arachis Oil.

Pharmacopoeias. In *Eur.* (see p.vi), *Int.*, and *Pol.* Also in *USNF*. *Eur.* also includes Hydrogenated Arachis Oil.

Pharmacopoeial description

Ph. Eur.: Arachis oil is the refined fatty oil obtained from the shelled seeds of *Arachis hypogaea*. A suitable antioxidant may be added. It is a clear, yellowish viscous liquid consisting of glycerides, chiefly of oleic and linoleic acids, with smaller amounts of other acids. It solidifies at about 2°. Very slightly soluble in alcohol; miscible with ether and with petroleum spirit. Store in well-filled containers. Protect from light.

Hydrogenated arachis oil is arachis oil (as above) that has been refined, bleached, hydrogenated, and deodorised. It is a white or faintly yellowish soft mass that melts to a clear pale yellow liquid when heated. Practically insoluble in water; very slightly soluble in alcohol; freely soluble in dichloromethane and in petroleum spirit (b.p. 65° to 70°). Protect from light.

USNF 20: The refined fixed oil obtained from the seed kernels of one or more of the cultivated varieties of *Arachis hypogaea* (Leguminosae). It is a colourless or pale yellow, oily liquid with a bland taste; it may have a characteristic nutty odour. Very slightly soluble in alcohol; miscible with carbon disulfide, with chloroform, and with ether. Store at a temperature not exceeding 40° in airtight containers. Protect from light.

Uses and Administration

Emulsions containing arachis oil are used in nutrition. Arachis oil is given as an enema for softening impacted faeces. It is used in drops for softening ear wax and in emollient creams. Arachis oil is given by mouth, usually with sorbitol, as a gallbladder evacuant prior to cholecystography.

Precautions. It has been suggested that the use during infancy of preparations containing arachis oil, including infant formulae and topical preparations, may be responsible for sensitisation, with a subsequent risk of hypersensitivity reactions.[1,2] However, the arachis oil used in such preparations is refined oil and it has been pointed out that such oil should not

contain the proteins that produce allergic reactions in susceptible people.[3,4]
1. de Montis G, *et al.* Sensitisation to peanut and vitamin D oily preparations. *Lancet* 1993; **341:** 1411.
2. Lever LR. Peanut and nut allergy: creams and ointments containing peanut oil may lead to sensitisation. *BMJ* 1996; **313:** 299.
3. Hourihane J O'B, *et al.* Randomised, double blind, crossover challenge study of allergenicity of peanut oil in subjects allergic to peanuts. *BMJ* 1997; **314:** 1084–8.
4. Committee on Toxicity of chemicals in Food, Consumer Products and the Environment. *Peanut allergy.* London: Department of Health, 1998.

Preparations

BP 2001: Arachis Oil Enema.

Proprietary Preparations (details are given in Part 3)
Austral.: Calogen; *Fin.:* Calogen; *Fr.:* Matiga†; *Ger.:* Olbad Cordes †; *Hong Kong:* Oilatum Cream; *Irl.:* Calogen; Oilatum Cream; *Mex.:* Oilatum Jabon; *NZ:* Calogen; *Singapore:* Oilatum Cream; *UK:* Calogen; Fletchers Arachis Oil Retention Enema.

Multi-ingredient: *Aust.:* Balneum F; *Austral.:* Cerumol; Medevac; *Fr.:* Balneum surgras†; *Ger.:* Balneum F; Dr. Hotz Vollbad†; Hoecutin Olbad F†; Parfenac Basisbad; *Hong Kong:* Cerumol; *Irl.:* Hydromol; *Israel:* Balneum F; *Ital.:* Balneum Hermal Forte; *NZ:* Medevac; *S.Afr.:* Cerumol; *Singapore:* Cerumol; *Switz.:* Balneum Hermal F; *UK:* Cerumol; Earex; Hewletts; Red Oil.

Areca (758-j)

Areca Nuts; Arecae Semen; Arekasame; Betel Nuts; Noix d'Arec.

Pharmacopoeias. In *Jpn.*

Profile

Areca consists of the dried ripe seeds of *Areca catechu* (Palmae) containing the alkaloid arecoline.

Areca is used in eastern countries as a masticatory. It is chewed alone or in a 'betel quid' (betel), which usually consists of areca nut and lime (calcium hydroxide) wrapped in the leaf of the betel pepper (*Piper betle*; unrelated to areca). Other ingredients that might be added to the quid include catechu gum, spices, or tobacco. Areca has sialogogue properties and is chewed for its mild intoxicant and euphoriant effects. Both arecoline and arecaidine (produced by the hydrolysis of arecoline by the lime in betel) have cholinergic activity.

The red juice from the chewed betel stains the saliva, teeth and mucosa. After many years of chewing betel, the stain may become dark-brown or black. Adverse cholinergic effects, including excessive salivation, sweating, lachrymation, urinary incontinence, or diarrhoea may occur with initial or heavy use of areca. An increased incidence of oral submucosal fibrosis, oral leucoplakia, and oral squamous cell carcinoma has been reported in persons in the habit of chewing areca or betel.

Areca was formerly used in the treatment of tapeworm infection, and arecoline has been used in veterinary medicine as a purgative and taenifuge.

◊ General references.
1. Arjungi KN. Areca nut: a review. *Arzneimittelforschung* 1976; **26:** 951–6.
2. Norton SA. Betel: consumption and consequences. *J Am Acad Dermatol* 1998; **38:** 81–8.
3. Nelson BS, Heischober B. Betel nut: a common drug used by naturalized citizens from India, Far East Asia, and the South Pacific Islands. *Ann Emerg Med* 1999; **34:** 238–43.

Carcinogenicity. Precancerous and cancerous conditions of the oral cavity have been attributed to the chewing of 'betel' (above). In betel-chewer's mucosa, the oral mucosa is discoloured and there is desquamation or peeling of the oral epithelium, from the traumatic effect of chewing and possibly a chemical action of betel. This condition may be a precursor of oral submucosal fibrosis, which is considered to be precancerous.[1] Oral leukoplakia is another precancerous condition that is reported in betel chewers. The role of areca in the development of these conditions and oral squamous cell carcinoma has been debated. The effects of betel may be due to the arecaidine content of areca, the alkalinity of the lime, tobacco, or a combination of these.[2,3]
1. Reichart PA, Philipsen HP. Betel chewer's mucosa—a review. *J Oral Pathol Med* 1998; **27:** 239–42.
2. Norton SA. Betel: consumption and consequences. *J Am Acad Dermatol* 1998; **38:** 81–8.
3. Nelson BS, Heischober B. Betel nut: a common drug used by naturalized citizens from India, Far East Asia, and the South Pacific Islands. *Ann Emerg Med* 1999; **34:** 238–43.

Effects on the lungs. Evidence suggesting that there is an association between betel-nut chewing and bronchoconstriction in asthmatic patients.[1,2]
1. Taylor RFH, *et al.* Betel-nut chewing and asthma. *Lancet* 1992; **339:** 1134–6.
2. Kiyingi KS. Betel nut chewing and asthma. *Lancet* 1992; **340:** 59–60.

Effects on the nervous system. Areca-nut (betel-nut) chewing is associated with habituation, addiction, and dependence,[1] and CNS symptoms of withdrawal have been described in 2 patients.[2] Psychosis has also been reported.[1]

It has been suggested that the muscarinic action of areca alkaloids may have a beneficial effect on symptoms of schizophrenia, and a study of such patients in a Micronesian population provides some support for this idea.[3] However, severe extrapyramidal symptoms followed betel-nut chewing in 2 patients

with chronic schizophrenia who were also receiving neuroleptic therapy.[4]
1. Nelson BS, Heischober B. Betel nut: a common drug used by naturalized citizens from India, Far East Asia, and the South Pacific Islands. *Ann Emerg Med* 1999; **34:** 238–43.
2. Wiesner DM. Betel-nut withdrawal. *Med J Aust* 1987; **146:** 453.
3. Sullivan RJ, *et al.* Effects of chewing betel nut (Areca catechu) on the symptoms of people with schizophrenia in Palau, Micronesia. *Br J Psychiatry* 2000; **177:** 174–8.
4. Deahl MP. Psychostimulant properties of betel nuts. *BMJ* 1987; **294:** 841.

Aristolochia (541-x)

Pharmacopoeias. Chin. allows various species of *Aristolochia.*

Serpentary (serpentaria) is the dried rhizome and roots of *Aristolochia serpentaria* (Virginian snakeroot) and of *A. reticulata* (Texan snakeroot) (Aristolochiaceae). Snakeroot is also used as a common name to describe poisonous *Eupatorium* spp.

Chinese medicine has employed various species of Aristolochia including *A. contorta, A. debilis,* and *A. manshuriensis.*

Profile

Aristolochia spp. including *A. clematis* and *A. ringens (A. brasiliensis)* have been used in herbal medicine. Preparations of serpentary have been employed as bitters. The active ingredient is aristolochic acid, which has been tried in a number of inflammatory disorders, mainly in folk medicine. However, there is concern over its use since it has been reported to be carcinogenic and nephrotoxic.

Adverse effects. Progressive interstitial fibrosis of the kidney related to a slimming regimen containing Chinese herbs had been reported in 70 patients in Belgium by 1993; 30 of these patients had terminal renal failure.[1] Renal failure has also been reported[2] in 2 patients in the UK following ingestion of Chinese herbal medicines that were subsequently found to contain aristolochic acid, a known nephrotoxin. This can originate as a result of the substitution of Aristolochia spp. (probably *A. manshuriensis*) for other innocuous herbal substances;[2,3] the Belgian cases were probably as a result of substitution of *A. fangchi* extracts for *Stephania tetrandra*.[1] As a result of these cases, the UK Medicines Control Agency has issued a permanent ban on *Aristolochia* preparations. Examination of 39 patients in Belgium with nephropathy associated with *A. fangchi* ingestion had revealed 18 cases of urothelial carcinoma and evidence of mild to moderate dysplasia in 19 patients.[4] There had appeared to be a higher risk of carcinoma with total doses of *A. fangchi* in excess of 200 g.
1. Vanhaelen M, *et al.* Identification of aristolochic acid in Chinese herbs. *Lancet* 1994; **343:** 174.
2. Lord GM, *et al.* Nephropathy caused by Chinese herbs in the UK. *Lancet* 1999; **354:** 481–2.
3. But PP, Ma S-c. Chinese-herb nephropathy. *Lancet* 1999; **354:** 1731–2.
4. Nortier JL, *et al.* Urothelial carcinoma associated with the use of a chinese herb (Aristolochia fangchi). *N Engl J Med* 2000; **342:** 1686–92.

Arnica (303-g)

Wolfsbane.

NOTE. Wolfsbane is also used as a common name for aconite.
Pharmacopoeias. In *Eur.* (see p.vi) and *Pol.*
Aust. also includes arnica root. *Ger.* allows Arnica montana or A. chamissonis subsp. *foliosa,* or a mixture of both.

Pharmacopoeial description

Ph. Eur.: Arnica Flower (Arnica Flos) consists of the whole or partially broken, dried flowerheads of *Arnica montana*. It contains not less than 0.4% w/w of total lactone sesquiterpenes expressed as helenalin tiglate, calculated with reference to the dried drug. It has an aromatic odour. Protect from light.

Profile

Arnica is generally employed in the form of the flowerheads of *Arnica montana* (Compositae).

Arnica flower is irritant to mucous membranes and when ingested has produced severe symptoms including gastrointestinal and nervous system disturbances, both tachycardia and bradycardia, and collapse. Tincture of arnica may cause dermatitis when applied to the skin of sensitive persons.

Preparations of arnica flower and arnica root are used as astringents for topical application to unbroken skin in conditions such as sprains and bruises; such preparations are not considered suitable for internal use.

Herbal and homoeopathic preparations containing arnica are available for oral use.

Preparations

Proprietary Preparations (details are given in Part 3)
Austral.: Sports Eze Bruising Relief; *Fr.:* Arnican; Pharmadose teinture d'arnica; *Ger.:* Arnica-loges; Arniflor-N; Arnikatinktur; Arthrosenex AR; Doc; Hovenol A†; Hyzum N; Vasotonin; *Ital.:* Venustas Lozione Caduta; *Neth.:* Arniflort†; *Port.:* Arnigel; *UK:* Savlon Natural First Aid for Bruises.

Multi-ingredient: *Aust.:* Arnicet; Asthmatee; Berggeist; Cional; Dynexan; Embrocation; Red Point; Rheuma; Sportino Akut; Varicylum; *Austral.:* Anti-Flamme; Joint & Muscle Relief Cream; *Fr.:* Arnicadol; Carli; Creme Rap; Dermocica; Lelong Contu-

The symbol † denotes a preparation no longer actively marketed

sions†; *Ger.:* ABC Warme-Pflaster N; Arnica Kneipp Salbe; Arnika plus†; Arnikamill; Befelka-Tinktur†; Cefagastrin; Cefawell; Ceprovit†; Combudoron; derma-loges N; Dolo-cyl; Essaven Sport; Fagorutin Roßkastanien-Balsam F; Grunlicht Hingfong Essenz; Heparin Comp; Heusin; Hoevenol A†; Lindofluid N; Rhoival; Sportino Akut; Stullmaton; Trauma-cyl; Varicylum-S; Vasesana-Vasoregulans; Venen-Salbe; Venengel; Vitosal; *Hong Kong:* New Patecs A; *Ital.:* Elisir Depurativo Ambrosiano; Herbavit; *S.Afr.:* Dynexan; *Spain:* Arnicon; Encialina; Killpan; Uralyt†; *Switz.:* Alpina Gel a l'arnica avec spilanthes†; Cetona Plus; Dynexan; Eubucal; Euceta avec camomille et arnica; Fortacet; *UK:* Frost Cream; Hansaplast Herbal Heat Plaster; Savlon Natural First Aid for Insect Bites & Stings; WCS Dusting Powder.

Arsenic Trioxide (12396-y)

Acidum Arsenicosum Anhydricum; Arseni Trioxydum; Arsenic; Arsenicum Album; Arsenious Acid; Arsenous Oxide; White Arsenic.

$As_2O_3 = 197.8$.

CAS — 1327-53-3 (arsenic trioxide); 7784-45-4 (arsenic triiodide).

Pharmacopoeias. In Jpn.

Adverse Effects

The toxicity of inorganic arsenic increases with increasing solubility, and trivalent compounds are considered to be more toxic than pentavalent compounds. The symptoms of **acute poisoning** due to arsenic usually occur within one hour of ingestion but may be delayed for up to 12 hours, especially in the presence of food. In severe poisoning, the principal toxic effect is haemorrhagic gastroenteritis, with acute abdominal pain, severe nausea, vomiting, and diarrhoea, and this can result in profound dehydration, collapse, shock, and death. Cardiac arrhythmias, convulsions, or muscle cramps may also occur. From 70 to 300 mg of arsenic trioxide may be fatal depending on the physical form and the rate of absorption. In the absence of adequate treatment death can occur within one hour but a period of 12 to 48 hours is more usual. Patients who survive the initial effects of arsenic trioxide may develop severe peripheral neuropathies and encephalopathy. Other effects following acute poisoning resemble those seen in chronic poisoning. Acute systemic effects may also be seen following inhalation or contact with the skin. Ingested arsenic salts cause oral irritation and a sensation of burning in the mouth and throat; pulmonary irritation may follow inhalation.

Chronic poisoning or occupational exposure typically produces varied skin disorders, particularly hyperkeratosis, especially affecting the palms and soles, skin pigmentation, eczematous or follicular dermatitis, oedema especially affecting the eyelids, and alopecia. Muscle aching and weakness, and stomatitis may also occur. Gastrointestinal disturbances are generally mild. The breath and perspiration may have an odour of garlic. Patients may also experience excessive salivation, lachrymation, and inflammation of the conjunctiva and nasal mucosa resembling coryza. Chronic inhalation of arsenic salts may result in perforation of the nasal septum. Characteristic deposits of arsenic may appear in the nails 6 weeks after absorption. Obstructive jaundice may occur as a result of hepatomegaly and portal hypertension may eventually develop. Cirrhosis has been reported rarely. Proteinuria, haematuria, and anuria may occur secondary to renal damage. In advanced poisoning neurological effects are prominent. Encephalopathy has been reported but peripheral neuropathies are more common. There is both sensory and motor involvement and patients may at first experience paraesthesia, and numbness and burning in the extremities, but eventually muscular atrophy and paralysis occur. The legs are usually more affected than the arms. Arsenic is toxic to the bone marrow and produces a wide range of blood disorders including leucopenia, thrombocytopenia, and various anaemias.

Chronic exposure to arsenic has been associated with neoplasms of the skin, lungs, and liver and possibly other organs.

Adverse effects that have been reported with the **therapeutic use** of arsenic trioxide in patients with acute promyelocytic leukaemia include leucocytosis, gastrointestinal disturbances, fatigue, oedema, hyperglycaemia, dyspnoea, cough, skin rashes, pruritus, headaches, and dizziness. Prolongation of the QT interval and other cardiac arrhythmias have occurred. A syndrome similar to that observed with tretinoin therapy (see Retinoic Acid Syndrome, p.1126) has developed in some patients. Sudden death has been reported in a few patients.

◊ Reviews.
1. Arsenic. *Environmental Health Criteria 18.* Geneva: WHO, 1981.
2. Health and Safety Executive. Inorganic arsenic compounds. *Toxicity Review 16.* London: HMSO, 1986.
3. Shannon RL, Strayer DS. Arsenic-induced skin toxicity. *Hum Toxicol* 1989; **8:** 99–104.

◊ Arsenical compounds have reportedly been used to "cut" cocaine and symptoms of arsenic poisoning may occur in cocaine abusers.[1] Toxicity due to the presence of arsenic in various ethnic remedies has also been reported.[2]

1. Lombard J, *et al.* Arsenic intoxication in a cocaine abuser. *N Engl J Med* 1989; **320:** 869.
2. Kew J, *et al.* Arsenic and mercury intoxication due to Indian ethnic remedies. *BMJ* 1993; **306:** 506–7.

◊ References to adverse effects in patients receiving arsenic trioxide for the treatment of acute promyelocytic leukaemia,[1-4] including a report of sudden death occurring in 3 patients in a dose-finding study.[5]

1. Huang SY, *et al.* Acute and chronic arsenic poisoning associated with treatment of acute promyelocytic leukaemia. *Br J Haematol* 1998; **103:** 1092–5.
2. Huang CH, *et al.* Complete atrioventricular block after arsenic trioxide treatment in an acute promyelocytic leukemic patient. *Pacing Clin Electrophysiol* 1999; **22:** 965–7.
3. Camacho LH, *et al.* Leukocytosis and the retinoic acid syndrome in patients with acute promyelocytic leukemia treated with arsenic trioxide. *J Clin Oncol* 2000; **18:** 2620–5.
4. Ohnishi K, *et al.* Prolongation of the QT interval and ventricular tachycardia in patients treated with arsenic trioxide for acute promyelocytic leukemia. *Ann Intern Med* 2000; **133:** 881–5.
5. Westervelt P, *et al.* Sudden death among patients with acute promyelocytic leukemia treated with arsenic trioxide. *Blood* 2001; **98:** 266–71.

Treatment of Adverse Effects

Acute poisoning due to the ingestion of arsenic compounds should be treated by immediate gastric lavage if the patient presents within one hour and has not already vomited. Activated charcoal may be of use to reduce absorption. Intravenous replacement of fluids and electrolytes should be undertaken as necessary to correct dehydration and electrolyte imbalance and to prevent shock; pressor agents and oxygen may be required. Morphine may be given for severe abdominal pain but care should be taken that this does not lead to colonic retention of arsenic compounds.

Chelation therapy with intramuscular dimercaprol (p.1007) should be started immediately the cause of poisoning is suspected. Prompt treatment is necessary to prevent or reduce the severity of neuropathy. It has been suggested that administration of dimercaprol should continue until abdominal symptoms subside and the gut is clear of ingested arsenic. Unithiol (p.1025) given intravenously may be used as an alternative. Oral treatment with succimer (p.1024) or penicillamine (p.1019) may then be substituted. A second course of treatment with penicillamine may be required if symptoms recur.

If renal failure occurs haemodialysis may be required to remove any absorbed or chelated arsenic. Exchange blood transfusion may be required for severe liver damage.

Dimercaprol may also be used in the treatment of chronic poisoning, but penicillamine, succimer, or unithiol (all given orally) may be preferred.

Precautions

Arsenic trioxide should be used with caution in renal impairment since renal excretion is the main route of elimination. Patients receiving arsenic trioxide for acute promyelocytic leukaemia should have their ECG monitored weekly; electrolytes, blood count, and coagulation should be checked twice weekly during induction and at least weekly during consolidation.

Pharmacokinetics

Water-soluble arsenic acids and their salts are more rapidly absorbed from the gastrointestinal tract than poorly soluble arsenicals such as arsenic trioxide. The absorption of arsenic trioxide is dependent upon the physical form of the compound and coarsely powdered material may be eliminated in the faeces before significant dissolution and absorption can occur. Soluble arsenic salts may also be absorbed following inhalation and through skin.

Once absorbed, arsenic is stored mainly in the liver, kidneys, heart, and lungs, with smaller amounts in the muscles and nervous tissue. About two weeks after ingestion, arsenic is deposited in the hair and nails and remains fixed to the keratin for years. It is also deposited in the bones and teeth.

Although pentavalent arsenic is reduced to some degree *in vivo* to the more toxic trivalent form, trivalent arsenic is slowly and extensively oxidised to pentavalent arsenic. Both forms are methylated to relatively non-toxic derivatives and excreted in the urine, mainly as dimethylarsinic acid, with smaller amounts appearing as monomethylarsonic acid and inorganic arsenic compounds. Although 50% of a dose may be eliminated in the urine within 3 to 5 days, small amounts may continue to be excreted for several weeks after a single dose. Less significant amounts of arsenic are excreted in the faeces and sweat and via the lungs and skin. It is also distributed into breast milk and readily crosses the placenta.

Uses and Administration

Arsenic trioxide and arsenic triiodide were formerly used internally as solutions or externally as ointments in the treatment of various skin diseases, but such use is generally no longer recommended. Externally, arsenic trioxide has a caustic action.

Arsenic trioxide may have a role in the treatment of some patients with acute promyelocytic leukaemia (see below). It is used for induction of remission and consolidation in patients who are refractory to, or who have relapsed from, conventional therapy with retinoids and antineoplastics. It is given by intravenous infusion over 1 to 2 hours; if acute vasomotor reactions occur, the rate of infusion may be slowed and up to 4 hours may be taken. For induction, a dose of 0.15 mg per kg body-weight is given once daily until remission occurs; no more than 60 doses should be given. The dose for consolidation is 0.15 mg per kg once daily for 25 doses, beginning 3 to 6 weeks after the completion of induction therapy; these doses may be spread over a time period of up to 5 weeks.

Arsenic trioxide is used in homoeopathic medicine and in certain Asian herbal remedies. Arsenic anhydride has also been used.

Arsenic trioxide has been widely employed as a constituent of weedkillers and sheepdips and as a rodenticide.

Acute myeloid leukaemias. Arsenic trioxide has been tried in patients with acute promyelocytic leukaemia (p.485). Remission was achieved in patients who had relapsed despite conventional therapy with retinoids and antineoplastics.[1,2] Treatment was also successful in newly-diagnosed patients but severe liver toxicity occurred in some cases.[2]

For references to adverse effects occurring in patients receiving arsenic trioxide for acute promyelocytic leukaemia, see under Adverse Effects, above.

1. Soignet SL, *et al.* Complete remission after treatment of acute promyelocytic leukemia with arsenic trioxide. *N Engl J Med* 1998; **339:** 1341–8.
2. Niu C, *et al.* Studies on treatment of acute promyelocytic leukemia with arsenic trioxide: remission induction, follow-up, and molecular monitoring in 11 newly diagnosed and 47 relapsed acute promyelocytic leukemia patients. *Blood* 1999; **94:** 3315–24.

Preparations

Proprietary Preparations (details are given in Part 3)
USA: Trisenox.

Arsine (12397-j)

Arsenic Trihydride; Hydrogen Arsenide.
$AsH_3 = 77.95$.
CAS — 7784-42-1.

Profile

Arsine gas has no clinical uses but is an environmental or occupational hazard. It is highly toxic and causes severe haemolysis which may result in acute renal failure. Exposure to as little as 3 ppm may cause symptoms, after a latent period of 2 to 24 hours, including headache, abdominal pain, nausea, vomiting, anorexia, jaundice, haemolytic anaemia, haematuria, oliguria, and anuria. Pulmonary oedema, ECG abnormalities, and neurological disorders have also been reported. Treatment involves exchange transfusions and haemodialysis; dimercaprol has been used but does not prevent haemolysis.

◊ References.
1. Fowler BA, Weissberg JB. Arsine poisoning. *N Engl J Med* 1974; **291:** 1171–4.
2. Hesdorffer CS, *et al.* Arsine gas poisoning: the importance of exchange transfusions in severe cases. *Br J Ind Med* 1986; **43:** 353–5.

Asafetida (272-z)

Asafoetida; Asant; Devil's Dung; Gum Asafetida.
Pharmacopoeias. In Chin.

An oleo-gum-resin obtained from various species of *Ferula* (Umbelliferae).

Profile

Asafetida has been used as a carminative and antispasmodic. It was also formerly used as an expectorant. It is used in cooking and is an ingredient of certain foods.

◊ References.
1. Kelly KJ, *et al.* Methemoglobinemia in an infant treated with the folk remedy glycerited asafoetida. *Pediatrics* 1984; **73:** 717–19.

Preparations

Proprietary Preparations (details are given in Part 3)
Multi-ingredient: *Thai.:* Flatulence Gastulence; *UK:* Daily Tension & Strain Relief.

Asarabacca (12401-k)

Hazelwort; Rhizoma Asari; Wild Nard.

The dried rhizome, roots, and leaves of *Asarum europaeum* (Aristolochiaceae).

Profile

Asarabacca is an ingredient of snuffs. It is also an irritant emetic and has been used in rodent poisons. Asarabacca has been used in homoeopathic medicine and is an ingredient of preparations given for respiratory disorders.

Preparations

Proprietary Preparations (details are given in Part 3)
Ger.: Escarol.

Asbestos (12402-a)

The name asbestos is applied to several naturally occurring and widely distributed fibrous mineral silicates of the serpentine and amphibole groups. They include amosite (brown asbestos), anthophyllite, chrysotile (white asbestos), and crocidolite (blue asbestos).

Profile

Asbestos has properties of heat resistance, insulation, and reinforcement and has been used extensively for heat or electrical insulation, fire protection, in friction materials, and in the construction industry in a wide variety of materials including cement, pipes, and tiles.

When inhaled, asbestos fibres can cause asbestosis (pulmonary fibrosis), lung cancer, and mesothelioma of the pleura and peritoneum. Mesothelioma has been reported in persons exposed to relatively small amounts of asbestos after an average latent period of 30 to 40 years. Occupational exposure has sometimes been associated with an increased incidence of gastrointestinal, laryngeal, and other cancers. Some types of asbestos are more hazardous than others; crocidolite (a member of the amphibole group) is considered to be the most dangerous.

◊ References.
1. Wagner GR. Asbestosis and silicosis. *Lancet* 1997; **349:** 1311–15.
2. Landrigan PJ, *et al.* The hazards of chrysotile asbestos: a critical review. *Ind Health* 1999; **37:** 271–80.

Avena (12408-n)

Aven; Cultivated White Oats; Oatmeal; Oats.

Pharmacopoeias. US includes Colloidal Oatmeal.

The grain of *Avena sativa* (Gramineae).

Pharmacopoeial description

USP 25: Colloidal Oatmeal is the powder resulting from the grinding and further processing of whole oat grain. When dried at 120° for 4 hours it loses not more than 10% of its weight.

Profile

Avena is used in herbal and in homoeopathic medicine and is reputed to have sedative activity.

A colloidal fraction extracted from avena is used in the preparation of emollient dermatological preparations.

Whether avenin, a protein present in oats, is harmful to patients with coeliac disease is controversial.

Preparations

Proprietary Preparations (details are given in Part 3)
Austral.: DermaVeen Bath; DermaVeen Dry Skin; *Canad.:* Aveeno Preparations; *Fr.:* Aveeno Preparations; Emulave; Sensifluid; *Hong Kong:* Sensifluid; Ultra-Rich; *Irl.:* Aveeno; *Israel:* Nutrasoothe; *Ital.:* Avalon; Aveeno Preparations; Emulave; Micaveen; *Port.:* Aveeno Preparations†; Emulave†; *Switz.:* Avenaforce; *UK:* Aveeno Preparations; *USA:* ActiBath.

Multi-ingredient: *Austral.:* Avena Complex; Bioglan The Blue One; Calmo; DermaVeen Acne†; DermaVeen Moisturising; DermaVeen Shower and Bath; Dong Quai Complex; Glycyrrhiza Complex; Pacifenity; Panax Complex; Vitaglow Herbal Stress†; *Canad.:* Aveeno Acne Bar; *Fr.:* Acnaveen; Aveenoderm; Biocarde; Cytelium; Dermalibour; Epitheliale; Eryase; Exomega; Micaveen; Septalibour; *Ger.:* Requiesan; Vollmers praparierter gruner; *Hong Kong:* Aderma Dermalibour; Aderma Epitheliale; Aderma Exomega; Aderma Ultra High Protection; Oat Milk Treatment Cream; *Ital.:* Acnaveen; Sebaveen†; *Port.:* Acnaveen†; Aveenocream†; Aveenoderm†; D'Aveia; Micaveen†; Sebaveen†; *Switz.:* Mucilar Avena; *UK:* Avena sativa comp.; Daily Overwork & Mental Fatigue Relief; Daily Tension & Strain Relief; *USA:* Aveeno Cleansing Bar.

Azadirachta (523-a)

Margosa; Neem.

The dried stem bark, root bark, and leaves of *Azadirachta indica* (=*Melia azadirachta*) (Meliaceae).

Profile

Azadirachta has been used as a bitter. It is widely used in South Asia and has been reported to have insecticidal, antimalarial, and spermicidal properties. Neem oil (margosa oil) expressed from the seeds has also been used.

Poisoning. Severe poisoning in Indian children given neem oil (margosa oil) as a remedy for minor ailments.[1]

1. Sinniah D, Baskaran G. Margosa oil poisoning as a cause of Reye's syndrome. *Lancet* 1981; **i:** 487–9.

Azintamide (4119-z)

Azintamide (*rINN*).

Azinthiamide; ST-9067. 2-[(6-Chloro-3-pyridazinyl)thio]-*N*,*N*-diethylacetamide.
$C_{10}H_{14}ClN_3OS = 259.8$.
CAS — 1830-32-6.

Profile

Azintamide has been used as a choleretic.

Preparations

Proprietary Preparations (details are given in Part 3)
Aust.: Ora-Gallin purum; *Port.:* Colerin.

Multi-ingredient: *Aust.:* Ora-Gallin; *Ger.:* Oragallin S†; *Port.:* Colerin-F; *Spain:* Oragalin Espasmolitico.

The symbol † denotes a preparation no longer actively marketed

Azovan Blue (2123-a)

Azovan Blue (*BAN*).

Azovanum Caeruleum; CI Direct Blue 53; Colour Index No. 23860; Evans Blue; T-1824. Tetrasodium 1,1'-diamino-8,8'-dihydroxy-7,7'-(2,2'-dimethylbiphenyl-4,4'-diylbisdiazo)di-(naphthalene-2,4-disulphonate); Tetrasodium 6,6'-[3,3'-dimethylbiphenyl-4,4'-diylbis(azo)]bis[4-amino-5-hydroxynaphthalene-1,3-disulphonate].
$C_{34}H_{24}N_6Na_4O_{14}S_4 = 960.8$.
CAS — 314-13-6.

Profile

Azovan blue is a dye that has been given intravenously for the determination of blood volume; it is firmly bound to plasma proteins and is slow to leave the circulation. Some patients may experience staining of the skin.

Azulene (1594-a)

Cyclopentacycloheptene.
$C_{10}H_8 = 128.2$.
CAS — 275-51-4.

NOTE. The name 'Azulene' has also been used for a number of derivatives of azulene including azulene sodium sulfonate, chamazulene, guaiazulene, and sodium gualenate.

Profile

Azulene has been used in preparations for anorectal disorders. The sodium sulfonate salt has been used in preparations for oral hygiene and for dyspepsia; sodium gualenate has also been used in gastrointestinal disorders.

Hypersensitivity. Allergic cheilitis occurred in a patient following long-term use of a toothpaste containing azulene.[1]

1. Balato N, *et al.* Allergic cheilitis to azulene. *Contact Dermatitis* 1985; **13:** 39–40.

Preparations

Proprietary Preparations (details are given in Part 3)
Hong Kong: Azunol; *Israel:* Kamil Blue.

Multi-ingredient: *Aust.:* Emser Nasensalbe; *Ger.:* Emser Nasensalbe N; *Israel:* Kamil Blue; *Ital.:* AZ 15 Gengidentifricio; Otazul†.

Bactericidal Permeability Increasing Protein (11623-d)

NOTE. Opebacan is BAN and pINN for a recombinant fragment of bactericidal permeability increasing protein.

Profile

Bactericidal permeability increasing protein is produced by human leucocytes and possesses both bactericidal and endotoxin-neutralising properties. A recombinant fragment of bactericidal permeability increasing protein has been investigated for the treatment of meningococcal septicaemia and for other endotoxin-in-related disorders, including complications of haemorrhagic trauma.

Bactericidal permeability increasing protein also possesses antifungal activity.

◊ References.
1. Giroir BP, *et al.* Preliminary evaluation of recombinant amino-terminal fragment of human bactericidal/permeability-increasing protein in children with severe meningococcal sepsis. *Lancet* 1997; **350:** 1439–43.
2. Levin M, *et al.* Recombinant bactericidal/permeability-increasing protein (rBPI₂₁) as adjunctive treatment for children with severe meningococcal sepsis: a randomised trial. *Lancet* 2000; **356:** 961–7.
3. Levy O. A neutrophil-derived anti-infective molecule: bactericidal/permeability-increasing protein. *Antimicrob Agents Chemother* 2000; **44:** 2925–31.

Barium (5263-p)

Ba = 137.327.
CAS — 7440-39-3.

A soft, highly reactive, silvery-white metal.

Adverse Effects and Treatment

The symptoms of barium poisoning from soluble barium salts arise from stimulation of all forms of muscle and include vomiting, excess salivation, colic, diarrhoea, slow or irregular pulse, hypertension, dysarthria, confusion, somnolence, headache, paraesthesias, tinnitus, giddiness, vertigo, muscle twitching, convulsive tremors, and muscular paralysis. Hypokalaemia is common. A case of renal failure due to barium poisoning has been reported. Death from cardiac or respiratory failure may occur.

Treatment of poisoning with soluble barium salts may involve emptying the stomach by lavage, unless vomiting is severe. Magnesium or sodium sulfate may be given to convert barium to insoluble barium sulfate. Hypokalaemia should be corrected. Assisted ventilation may be necessary. Excretion may be increased by diuresis. Haemodialysis may be used in severe poisoning.

◊ Reports of barium intoxication.
1. Lewi Z, Bar-Khayim Y. Food poisoning from barium carbonate. *Lancet* 1964; **ii:** 342–3.
2. Diengott D, *et al.* Hypokalaemia in barium poisoning. *Lancet* 1964; **ii:** 343–4.
3. Gould DB, *et al.* Barium sulfide poisoning: some factors contributing to survival. *Arch Intern Med* 1973; **132:** 891–4.
4. Berning J. Hypokalaemia of barium poisoning. *Lancet* 1975; **i:** 110.
5. Wetherill SF, *et al.* Acute renal failure associated with barium chloride poisoning. *Ann Intern Med* 1981; **95:** 187–8.
6. Phelan DM, *et al.* Is hypokalaemia the cause of paralysis in barium poisoning? *BMJ* 1984; **289:** 882.
7. Barium. *Environmental Health Criteria 107*. Geneva: WHO, 1990.
8. Sigue G, *et al.* From profound hypokalemia to life-threatening hyperkalemia: a case of barium sulfide poisoning. *Arch Intern Med* 2000; **160:** 548–51.

Uses and Administration

The soluble barium salts are not used in therapeutics but are widely used in industry. Barium sulfide has been used as a depilatory and barium carbonate was used as a rodenticide. The insoluble barium sulfate (p.1032) is used as a contrast medium.

Barium Hydroxide Lime (203-h)

CAS — 17194-00-2 (anhydrous barium hydroxide); 12230-71-6 (barium hydroxide octahydrate).

Pharmacopoeias. In US.

Pharmacopoeial description

USP 25: A mixture of barium hydroxide octahydrate and calcium hydroxide; it may also contain potassium hydroxide. White or greyish-white granules, or coloured with an indicator to show when absorptive power is exhausted. It absorbs not less than 19% of its weight of carbon dioxide. Store in airtight containers.

Profile

Barium hydroxide lime is used similarly to soda lime to absorb carbon dioxide in closed-circuit anaesthetic apparatus. Barium hydroxide lime contains a soluble form of barium and is toxic if swallowed.

Precautions. Excessive drying out of barium hydroxide lime in anaesthetic apparatus, which may occur if oxygen flow through the equipment is left on for prolonged periods, can lead to the production of carbon monoxide and the risk of inducing carboxyhaemoglobinaemia in patients undergoing anaesthesia using the apparatus.[1]

1. Committee on Safety of Medicines/Medicines Control Agency. Safety issues in anaesthesia: volatile anesthetic agents and carboxyhaemoglobinaemia. *Current Problems* 1997; **23:** 7.

Bay Oil (4611-b)

Myrcia Oil; Oleum Myrciae.

NOTE. Distinguish from Laurel Leaf Oil (Bay Leaf Oil) which is obtained from the leaves of *Laurus nobilis* (Lauraceae).

A yellow volatile oil, darkening rapidly on exposure to air, with a pleasant odour and spicy taste, obtained by distillation from the leaves of *Pimenta racemosa* (Myrtaceae) and probably other allied species.

Profile

The principal use of bay oil is in the preparation of bay rum, which is used as a hair lotion and as an astringent application.

Preparations

Proprietary Preparations (details are given in Part 3)
Multi-ingredient: *UK:* Adiantine; Medicated Extract of Rosemary.

Bayberry (305-p)

Bayberry Bark; Candle Berry Bark; Myrica; Wax Myrtle Bark.

Profile

Bayberry, the root bark of *Myrica cerifera* (Myricaceae), is used in upper respiratory-tract disorders and as a gargle for sore throat. It has also been used in gastrointestinal disorders, to treat vaginal discharge, and topically on ulcers and sores.

It is also used in homoeopathic medicine.

Preparations

Proprietary Preparations (details are given in Part 3)
Multi-ingredient: *UK:* EP&C Essence; Peerless Composition Essence.

Bearberry (12420-x)

Bärentraubenblätter; Bearberry Leaves; Busserole; Ptarmiganberry Leaves; Uva Ursi; Uvae Ursi Folium.

Pharmacopoeias. In Eur. (see p.vi) and Jpn.

Pharmacopoeial description

Ph. Eur.: The whole or cut dried leaves of the bearberry, *Arctostaphylos uva-ursi*. It contains not less than 7.0% of anhydrous arbutin, calculated with reference to the dried drug. Protect from light.

Profile
Bearberry has been reported to be a diuretic, bacteriostatic, and astringent and has been used in the treatment of urinary-tract disorders. It has also been used in homoeopathic medicine.

Preparations
Proprietary Preparations (details are given in Part 3)
Ger.: Cystinol Akut; Uvalysat; *Ital.:* Ginocap†.

Multi-ingredient: *Aust.:* Aktiv Blasen- und Nierentee; Apotheker Bauer's Nieren- und Blasentee; Bio-Garten Tee fur Niere und Blase; Blasen- und Nierentee; Blasen-Tee; Krautertee Nr 204; Krautertee Nr 3; Krautertee Nr 31; Mag Kottas Nieren-Blasentee; Sidroga Nieren- und Blasentee; St Radegunder Nierentee; Uropurat; *Austral.:* Althaea Complex; Bioglan Cranbiotic Super; Cranberry Complex; De Witts New Pills; Extralife Fluid-Care; Extralife PMS-Care; Extralife Uri-Care; Fluid Loss; Herbal Diuretic Formula; Medinat PMT-Eze; New De Witt's Pills†; PMT-EZE†; Profluid; Protemp; Urinase; Uva-Ursi Complex; Uva-Ursi Plus; *Belg.:* Tisane Contre la Tension; Tisane Diuretique; *Braz.:* Pilulas De Witt's; *Fr.:* Mediflor Tisane Antirhumatismale No 2†; Mediflor Tisane No 4 Diuretique; Santane O₁; Santane R₈; Tisane Orientale Soker†; Uromil; Urophytum; *Ger.:* Arctuvan N; Cefanephrin; Cystinol; Cysto Fink; Harntee 400; Harntee STADA; Hernia-Tee†; Herniol; Hevert-Blasen- und Nieren- Tee; Prostatin F; Salusan†; Uro Fink†; *Israel:* Jungborn; *NZ:* De Witts Pills; *Port.:* Asic; *Spain:* Genurat; Vegetalin; *Switz.:* Cysto Fink†; Cysto-Caps Chassot†; Demonatur Dragees pour les reins et la vessie; Dragees pour reins et vessie S; Tisane pour les reins et la vessie; Urinex (nouvelle formule); *UK:* Antitis; Backache; Backache Relief; Boldo; Cascade; De Witt's K & B Pills; Diuretabs; Gerard House Buchu Compound; Gerard House Waterlex; HealthAid Boldo-Plus; Hofels White Willow and Burdock; HRI Water Balance; Kas-Bah; Modern Herbals Water Retention; Prementaid; Sciargo; Tabritis; Uvacin; Watershed; Wellwoman†; *USA:* Tri-Aqua†.

Bentiromide (1957-g)

Bentiromide *(BAN, USAN, rINN)*.
BTPABA; BT-PABA; E-2663; PFT; Ro-11-7891. 4-(*N*-Benzoyl-L-tyrosylamino)benzoic acid.
$C_{23}H_{20}N_2O_5 = 404.4$.
CAS — 37106-97-1.
ATC — V04CK03.

Adverse Effects and Precautions
Reported adverse effects of bentiromide include headache, diarrhoea, and other gastrointestinal effects. There may be hypersensitivity and transient increases in the values obtained in liver function studies.

The bentiromide test may give misleading results in patients with gastrointestinal, liver, or kidney disorders, or in patients receiving certain foods or drugs that are excreted as arylamines. Some of these drugs include benzocaine, chloramphenicol, lignocaine [lidocaine], paracetamol, procaine, procainamide, sulfonamides, and some diuretics.

Pharmacokinetics
Following administration by mouth, bentiromide is hydrolysed by chymotrypsin in the gut to release *p*-aminobenzoic acid and benzoyl-tyrosine. The aminobenzoic acid is absorbed, metabolised in the liver, and excreted in the urine as *p*-aminobenzoic acid and metabolites.

Uses and Administration
Bentiromide has been used as a noninvasive test of exocrine pancreatic function, the amount of *p*-aminobenzoic acid and its metabolites excreted in the urine being taken as a measure of the chymotrypsin-secreting activity of the pancreas.

The usual dose has been 500 mg by mouth. Children aged 6 to 12 years have been given 14 mg per kg body-weight up to a maximum dose of 500 mg.

◊ **References.**
1. oek FJ, *et al.* Improved specificity of the PABA test with p-aminosalicylic acid (PAS). *Gut* 1987; **28:** 468–73.
2. Puntis JWL, *et al.* Simplified oral pancreatic function test. *Arch Dis Child* 1988; **63:** 780–4.

Preparations
Proprietary Preparations (details are given in Part 3)
USA: Chymex.

Benzaldehyde (4612-v)

$C_6H_5.CHO = 106.1$.
CAS — 100-52-7.
Pharmacopoeias. In Belg. and Br. Also in USNF.

Pharmacopoeial description
BP 2001: A clear colourless liquid with a characteristic odour of bitter almonds. Slightly soluble in water; miscible with alcohol and with ether. Store at a temperature not exceeding 15° in well-filled containers. Protect from light.

USNF 20: A colourless strongly refractive liquid with an odour resembling that of bitter almond oil and a burning aromatic taste. Slightly soluble in water; miscible with alcohol, with ether, and with fixed and volatile oils. Store in well-filled, airtight containers. Protect from light.

Profile
Benzaldehyde is used as a flavour as an alternative to volatile bitter almond oil. It may cause contact dermatitis.

Preparations
USNF 20: Compound Benzaldehyde Elixir.

Benzyl Isothiocyanate (12434-m)

Benzyl Mustard Oil; Benzylsenföl; Oleum Tropaeoli.
$C_8H_7NS = 149.2$.
CAS — 622-78-6.
Pharmacopoeias. In Fr. which also includes Capucine (Tropaeolum majus).

An oil obtained from *Tropaeolum majus* (Capuchin cress; common nasturtium) (Tropaeolaceae).

Profile
Benzyl isothiocyanate has been given as an antibacterial.
Tropaeolum majus has been used in herbal and in homoeopathic medicine.

Preparations
Proprietary Preparations (details are given in Part 3)
Multi-ingredient: *Ger.:* Angocin Anti-Infekt N; Nephroselect M.

Berberine (524-t)

5,6-Dihydro-9,10-dimethoxybenzo[g]-1,3-benzodioxolo[5,6-a]quinolizinium.
$C_{20}H_{18}NO_4 = 336.4$.
CAS — 2086-83-1 (berberine); 633-65-8 (berberine chloride); 633-66-9 (berberine sulfate).
Pharmacopoeias. Jpn includes berberine chloride and berberine tannate.

A quaternary alkaloid present in hydrastis, in various species of *Berberis*, and in many other plants.

Profile
Berberine has been used as a bitter. It possesses antimicrobial activity and has been tried as various salts in a number of infections. Berberine may also be used as a flavour in food and alcoholic drinks.

◊ **References.**
1. Khin-Maung-U, *et al.* Clinical trial of berberine in acute watery diarrhoea. *BMJ* 1985; **291:** 1601–5.
2. Rabbani GH, *et al.* Randomized controlled trial of berberine sulfate therapy for diarrhea due to enterotoxigenic Escherichia coli and Vibrio cholerae. *J Infect Dis* 1987; **155:** 979–84.
3. Vennerstrom JL, *et al.* Berberine derivatives as antileishmanial drugs. *Antimicrob Agents Chemother* 1990; **34:** 918–21.
4. Phillipson JD, Wright CW. Medicinal plants in tropical medicine: 1 Medicinal plants against protozoal diseases. *Trans R Soc Trop Med Hyg* 1991; **85:** 18–21.

Preparations
Proprietary Preparations (details are given in Part 3)
Austral.: Murine; *NZ:* Murine.

Multi-ingredient: *Braz.:* Lerin; Visolon; *Fr.:* Sedacollyre.

Bergamot Oil (4613-g)

Bergamot Essence; Oleum Bergamottae.
Pharmacopoeias. In Fr.

A greenish or brownish-yellow volatile oil with a characteristic fragrant odour and a bitter aromatic taste, obtained by expression from the fresh peel of fruit of *Citrus bergamia* (Rutaceae). Constituents include linalyl acetate and 5-methoxypsoralen (p.1120).

Profile
Bergamot oil is employed in perfumery. It is also used as a flavour in Earl Grey tea. It has been included in some preparations for upper respiratory-tract disorders. It contains 5-methoxypsoralen (p.1120). Photosensitivity reactions have occurred following the topical use of preparations containing bergamot oil.

Preparations
Proprietary Preparations (details are given in Part 3)
Multi-ingredient: *Fr.:* Ephydrol; *Ital.:* Cura†; Sanaderm†.

Betahistine Hydrochloride (9213-q)

Betahistine Hydrochloride *(USAN, rINNM)*.
Betahistine Dihydrochloride *(BANM)*; PT-9. *N*-Methyl-2-(2-pyridyl)ethylamine dihydrochloride.
$C_8H_{12}N_2,2HCl = 209.1$.
CAS — 5638-76-6 (betahistine); 5579-84-0 (betahistine hydrochloride).

Betahistine Mesilate (10085-v)

Betahistine Mesylate *(BANM, rINNM)*.
Betahistine Mesylate; Betahistini Mesilas. *N*-Methyl-2-(2-pyridyl)ethylamine bismethanesulphonate.
$C_8H_{12}N_2,(CH_4O_3S)_2 = 328.4$.
CAS — 54856-23-4.
Pharmacopoeias. In Eur. (see p.vi) and Jpn.

Pharmacopoeial description
Ph. Eur.: A white, crystalline, very hygroscopic powder. Very soluble in water; freely soluble in alcohol; very slightly soluble in isopropyl alcohol. A 10% solution in water has a pH of 2.0 to 3.0. Store in airtight containers.

Adverse Effects
Gastrointestinal disturbances, headache, skin rashes, and pruritus have been reported.

Precautions
Betahistine should not be given to patients with phaeochromocytoma. It should be given with care to patients with asthma, peptic ulcer disease, or a history of peptic ulcer disease.

Porphyria. Betahistine hydrochloride is considered to be unsafe in patients with porphyria because it has been shown to be porphyrinogenic in *in-vitro* systems.

Uses and Administration
Betahistine is an analogue of histamine and is claimed to improve the microcirculation of the labyrinth resulting in reduced endolymphatic pressure. It is used to reduce the symptoms of vertigo (p.408), particularly in Ménière's disease (p.407). Betahistine is given by mouth as the hydrochloride or mesilate. The usual initial dose (of the hydrochloride) is 16 mg three times daily taken preferably with meals; maintenance doses are generally in the range of 24 to 48 mg daily. Betahistine mesilate is used in similar doses.

◊ **Reviews**
1. James AL, Burton MJ. Betahistine for Ménière's disease or syndrome (updated 16 May 2001). Available in The Cochrane Library; Issue 4. Oxford: Update Software; 2001.

Preparations
Proprietary Preparations (details are given in Part 3)
Aust.: Betaserc; *Austral.:* Serc; *Belg.:* Betaserc; Lobiene; *Canad.:* Serc; *Denm.:* Betaserc; *Fin.:* Betaserc; *Fr.:* Evolis; Extovyl; Lectil; Serc; Vertigirex; *Ger.:* Aequamen; Betavert; Melopat; Ribrain; Vasomotal; *Hong Kong:* Betaserc; Bymeniere; Merislon; *Irl.:* Serc; Vertigon; *Israel:* Agiserc; *Ital.:* Microser; Vertiserc; *Jpn:* Merislon; *Mex.:* Serc; *Neth.:* Betaserc; *NZ:* Serc; *Port.:* Betaserc; *S.Afr.:* Serc; *Singapore:* Betaserc; Merislon; *Spain:* Fidium; Serc; *Switz.:* Betaserc; *Thai.:* Merislon; Serc; *UK:* Serc.

Betaine (16532-j)

Glycine Betaine; Glycocoll Betaine; Lycine; Trimethylglycine. (Carboxymethyl)trimethylammonium hydroxide inner salt.
$C_5H_{11}NO_2 = 117.1$.
CAS — 107-43-7.

Betaine Hydrochloride (1303-j)

Trimethylglycine Hydrochloride. (Carboxymethyl)trimethylammonium hydroxide inner salt hydrochloride.
$C_5H_{11}NO_2,HCl = 153.6$.
CAS — 590-46-5.
ATC — A09AB02.
Pharmacopoeias. In Aust., Belg., and US.

Pharmacopoeial description
USP 25: A 25% solution in water has a pH of 0.8 to 1.2.

Uses and Administration
Betaine is used as a methyl donor to remethylate homocysteine to methionine in the treatment of patients with homocystinuria (p.1350). It is given by mouth in a usual dose of 3 g twice daily. Doses are adjusted according to plasma-homocysteine concentrations; up to 20 g daily has been required in some patients. In children under 3 years old, an initial dose of 100 mg per kg body-weight daily may be used.

Betaine has also been used as a variety of salts in preparations for liver and gastrointestinal disorders. The hydrochloride has been given as a source of hydrochloric acid in the treatment of hypochlorhydria.

Homocystinuria. References.
1. Smolin LA, *et al.* The use of betaine for the treatment of homocystinuria. *J Pediatr* 1981; **99:** 467–72.
2. Wilcken DEL, *et al.* Homocystinuria—the effects of betaine in the treatment of patients not responsive to pyridoxine. *N Engl J Med* 1983; **309:** 448–53.
3. Holme E, *et al.* Betaine for treatment of homocystinuria caused by methylenetetrahydrofolate reductase deficiency. *Arch Dis Child* 1989; **64:** 1061–4.
4. Anonymous. Betaine for homocystinuria. *Med Lett Drugs Ther* 1997; **39:** 12.

Preparations
Proprietary Preparations (details are given in Part 3)
Austral.: Cystadane; *Canad.:* Cystadane; *Israel:* Cystadan; *Ital.:* Somatyl; *USA:* Cystadane.

Multi-ingredient: *Aust.:* CO₂ Granulat; Oroacid; *Austral.:* Bepep; Betaine Digestive Aid; Bioglan Digestive Zyme; Digestaid; *Belg.:* Digestomen; Gastrobul; *Braz.:* Aminotox; Anekron;

Betaliver; Biofigado; Colachofra; Colinvintol; Cynatrop; Epacrosil; Eparex; Epativan B6; Epocler; Eviepar; Figadobil; Hepalin; Hepasedan; Hepatocler; Hepofilina; Hormo Hepatico; Mesitol; Necrohepat; Xantinon Complex; *Fr.:* Citrarginine; Gastrobul; Hepagrume; Nivabetol; Ornitaine; *Ger.:* CO₂ Granulat; Flacar; Unexym MD; *Hong Kong:* Jetepar; *Israel:* Betazim; *Ital.:* Betascor B12†; Citroepatina; Epabetina; Ietepar; *S.Afr.:* Kloref; *Singapore:* Jetepar; *Spain:* Espasmo Digestomen; Levaliver; *UK:* Digezyme; Enzyme Digest; Fat-Solv; Kloref; Kloref-S†.

Bibrocathol   (5267-l)

Bibrocathol *(rINN)*.

Bibrocathin; Bibrokatol; Bismuth Tetrabrompyrocatechinate; Tetrabromopyrocatechol Bismuth. 4,5,6,7-Tetrabromo-2-hydroxy-1,3,2-benzodioxabismole.
$C_6HBiBr_4O_3 = 649.7$.
CAS — 6915-57-7.
ATC — S01AX05.

Profile
Bibrocathol is a bismuth-containing compound that has been applied topically in the treatment of eye disorders, wounds, and burns.

Preparations
Proprietary Preparations (details are given in Part 3)
Ger.: Noviform; Posiformin; *Swed.:* Noviform; *Switz.:* Noviform; Noviforme-Blache.

Multi-ingredient: *Ger.:* Novifort.

Bifemelane   (1962-m)

Bifemelane *(rINN)*.

N-Methyl-4-[(α-phenyl-o-tolyl)oxy]butylamine.
$C_{18}H_{23}NO = 269.4$.
CAS — 90293-01-9.
ATC — N06AX08.

Profile
Bifemelane is a nootropic that has been used in the treatment of senile dementia.

Preparations
Proprietary Preparations (details are given in Part 3)
Jpn: Alnert†.

Bile Acids and Salts   (998-q)

CAS — 81-25-4 (cholic acid); 11006-55-6 (sodium tauroglycocholate).
Pharmacopoeias. Aust. includes cholic acid. Jpn includes bear bile.

Profile
The principal primary bile acids, cholic acid and chenodeoxycholic acid (p.1594), are produced in the liver from cholesterol and are conjugated with glycine or taurine to give glycocholic acid, taurocholic acid, glycochenodeoxycholic acid, and taurochenodeoxycholic acid, before being secreted into the bile where they are present as the sodium or potassium salts (bile salts). Secondary bile acids are formed in the colon by bacterial deconjugation and 7α-dehydroxylation of cholic acid and chenodeoxycholic acid, producing deoxycholic acid and lithocholic acid, respectively. Ursodeoxycholic acid (p.1677) is a minor bile acid in man although it is the principal bile acid in *bears*. Dehydrocholic acid (p.1602) is a semisynthetic bile acid.

The total body pool of bile salts is about 3 g, and most of the secreted bile salts are reabsorbed in a process of enterohepatic recycling, so that only a small fraction of this amount must be synthesised *de novo* each day.

Bile salts are strongly amphiphilic; with the aid of phospholipids they form micelles and emulsify cholesterol and other lipids in bile. Oral administration of chenodeoxycholic acid also reduces the synthesis of cholesterol in the liver, while ursodeoxycholic acid reduces biliary cholesterol secretion apparently by increasing conversion of cholesterol to other bile acids. The bile acids (but not the bile salts) also have a choleretic action, increasing the secretion of bile, when given by mouth.

Chenodeoxycholic acid and ursodeoxycholic acid are given by mouth in the management of cholesterol-rich gallstones (p.1678) in patients unsuited to, or unwilling to undergo, surgery. Ursodeoxycholic acid is also being studied in some liver disorders.

Preparations containing bile salts have been used to assist the emulsification of fats and absorption of fat-soluble vitamins in conditions in which there is a deficiency of bile in the gastrointestinal tract. Ox bile has also been used in the treatment of chronic constipation.

◊ References.
1. Hofmann AF. The continuing importance of bile acids in liver and intestinal disease. *Arch Intern Med* 1999; **159:** 2647–58.

Preparations
Proprietary Preparations (details are given in Part 3)
Austral.: Proslim-Lipid†; *Fr.:* Antimucose†; *Ger.:* Cholecysmon; *S.Afr.:* Bilron.

Multi-ingredient: *Aust.:* Arca-Enzym; Buccalin; Combizym Compositum; Dragees Neunzehn; Euflat†; Festal†; Helopanzym;

Hylakombun; Nutrizym; Ozym†; Pankreon compositum; Peribilan; Silberne; Spasmo Gallosanol†; *Austral.:* Digestaid; Enzyme; Lexat; *Belg.:* Buccaline; Grains de Vals; *Braz.:* Colagolen; Dasc; Digestal; Emagrex; Esbelt; Figatil; Hepatobyl; Macroten; Magroton; Normagrin; Nutrizim; *Canad.:* Aid-Lax†; Alsiline†; Bicholate; Caroid†; Herbalax; Herbalax Forte†; Laxa†; Laxative; Phytolax†; Regubil†; Triolax†; Vesilax†; *Fin.:* Combizym Compositum; *Fr.:* Bilifluine†; Bilkaby†; Mucinum†; Rectopanbiline; *Ger.:* Combizym Compositum; Eupond†; Hepatofalk Neu; Spasmo Gallo Sanol N†; *Hong Kong:* Bilsan; Buccaline; Hepatofalk; *Israel:* Encypalmed; *Ital.:* Bilagar†; Pancreon Compositum†; Reolina†; *Mex.:* Dixiflen; Espaven Enzimatico; Ochozim; *Neth.:* Combizym Compositum†; *NZ:* Combizym Compositum; *Port.:* Byl; Caroid; Combizym Compositum†; Dagragel; Fermetone Composto; Nutrizym†; *Spain:* Espasmo Digestomen; Menabil Complex; *Swed.:* Combizym Compositum; *Switz.:* Buccaline; Combizym Compositum†; Opobyl†; *Thai.:* Buccaline; Combizym Compositum; Papytazyme; Veracolate; *UK:* Digezyme; *USA:* Digepepsin.

Birch Leaf   (9616-m)

Betulae Folium; Birkenblätter; Bouleau; Silver Birch Leaf.
Pharmacopoeias. In Eur. (see p.vi) and Pol.

Pharmacopoeial description
Ph. Eur.: The whole or fragmented dried leaves of *Betula pendula* and/or *B. pubescens* as well as hybrids of both species. It contains not less than 1.5% of flavonoids, calculated as hyperoside, with reference to the dried drug. Protect from light.

Profile
Birch leaf is used in herbal medicine, particularly for urinary-tract disorders.

Preparations
Proprietary Preparations (details are given in Part 3)
Aust.: Bakanasan Entwasserungs; Galama; Sanhelios-Entwasserungsdragees; *Ger.:* Kneipp Birkenblatter Pflanzensaft; Uroflan; Urorenal.

Multi-ingredient: *Aust.:* Aktiv Blasen- und Nierentee; Apotheker Bauer's Nieren- und Blasentee; Bio-Garten Entschlackungstee; Bio-Garten Tee fur Niere und Blase; Bio-Garten Tee zur Erhohung der Harnmenge; Bio-Garten Tropfen fur Niere und Blase; Blasenund Nierentee; Blasentee; Brennesseltonikum; Drogimed; Ehrmann's Entschlackungstee; Entschlackungstee; Fruhjahrs-Elixier ohne Alkohol; Harntreibender Tee; Kneipp Entwasserungstee; Kneipp Nieren- und Blasen-Tee; Krauterdoktor Entwasserungs-Elixier; Krauterhaus Mag Kottas Blasentee; Krauterhaus Mag Kottas Entschlackungstee; Krautertee Nr 19; Krautertee Nr 2; Krautertee Nr 24; Krautertee Nr 25; Krautertee Nr 29; Krautertee Nr 30; Mag Doskar's Nieren- und Blasentonikum; Mag Kottas Entschlackungstee; Rheuma; Sanvita Entschlackungstonikum†; Sidroga Nieren- und Blasentee; Solubitrat; St Radegunder Entwasserungs-Elixier; St Radegunder Entwasserungstee; Synpharma Instant-Blasen-und-Nierentee; Teekanne Blasen- und Nierentee; *Fr.:* B.O.P.; Depuratum; Drainactil; Mediflor Tisane Antirhumatismale No 2†; *Ger.:* Agamadon†; Antihypertonicum S; Befelka-Tinktur†; BioCyst; Blasen-Nieren-Tee Stada†; Canephron novo; Cystinol; Cysto Fink; Discmigon; Dr Wiemanns Rheumatonikum; Etmoren†; Eupond†; Harntee 400; Harntee 450; Harntee STADA; Harntee-Steiner; Heumann Blasen- und Nierentee Solubitrat N; Hevert-Blasen- und -Nierentee; Hevert-Entwasserungs-Tee†; Hevert-Gicht-Rheuma-Tee comp†; Heweberol-Tee; Kneipp Blasen- und Nieren-Tee; Kneipp Entschlackungs-Tee; NB-Tee N†; Nephro-Pasc; Nephronorm med†; Nephropur tri; Nephroselect M; Nephrubin†; Nierentee 2000; Nieron Blasen- und Nieren-Tee VI; Nieron-Tee N; Presseln Nieren-Blasen K 3; Reducelle†; Renob Blasen- und Nierentee; Salus Rheuma-Tee Krautertee Nr. 12†; Ullus Blasen-Nieren-Tee N; Uro Fink†; Urodil Blasen-Nieren Entwasserungstee†; Urodil phyto; Urostei; *Ital.:* Artoxan†; Depurfat†; Fluend†; Ginoday†; Prexene†; SlimLinea†; *Spain:* Genurat; *Switz.:* Nephrosolid N; Phytomed Nephro†; Tisane Diuretique; Tisane pour le coeur et la circulation; Tisane pour les reins et la vessie; Urinex (nouvelle formule); *UK:* Erysidoron 2; Massage Balm Calendula.

Black Nightshade   (12449-w)

Morelle Noire.

The leaves and flowering tops of the black or garden nightshade, *Solanum nigrum* (Solanaceae). It contains solanine and its allied alkaloids.

Profile
Black nightshade is distributed throughout most of the world as a weed of cultivation. It appears to have little medicinal value but was used in liniments, poultices, and decoctions for external application. Ingestion can cause typical antimuscarinic effects that may require treatment as described under Atropine, p.461.

Bladderwrack   (5408-s)

Fucus; Kelpware; Seawrack; Tang.
Pharmacopoeias. In Eur. (see p.vi) and Pol.

Pharmacopoeial description
Ph. Eur.: The fragmented or powdered, dried thallus of *Fucus vesiculosus* or *F. serratus* or *Ascophyllum nodosum*. It contains not less than 0.03% and not more than 0.2% of total iodine, calculated with reference to the dried drug. It has a salty and

mucilaginous taste, and an unpleasant marine odour. Protect from light.

Profile
Bladderwrack, a dried seaweed, is an ingredient of a number of herbal preparations given for various disorders including obesity, constipation, and iodine deficiency. Kelp (p.1625) is another preparation of dried seaweeds.

Bladderwrack is used in homoeopathic medicine.

Preparations
Proprietary Preparations (details are given in Part 3)
Multi-ingredient: *Austral.:* Bioglan Zellulean with Escin; Plantiodine Plus; PMT Complex; *Braz.:* Emagrex; Esbelt; Esbeltrat; Fucus Composto; Macroten; Magroton; Normagrin; Obesidex; Obesifran; *Fr.:* Actisane Minceur; Aminsane†; AMK; Dellova; Dragees Fucus; Obeflorine; Phytotherapie Boribel no 9; Promincil; Tisanes de l'Abbe Hamon no 11; *Ger.:* Krophan N; Viscophyll; *Ital.:* Fave di Fuca; Fitolinea; SlimLinea†; *Spain:* Lipograsil; *UK:* Adios; Boldex; Boldo; HealthAid Boldo-Plus; Heath & Heather Water Relief Tablets; Water Naturtabs; Weight Loss Aid.

Blue Cohosh   (9165-z)

Caulophyllum; Papoose Root; Squaw Root.

Profile
Blue cohosh, the rhizome and roots of *Caulophyllum thalictroides* (Berberidaceae), has uterotonic and antirheumatic properties. It is used for menstrual and other gynaecological disorders.

It is also used in homoeopathic medicine.

Preparations
Proprietary Preparations (details are given in Part 3)
Multi-ingredient: *Austral.:* Lifesystem Herbal Formula 4 Women's Formula; Women's Formula Herbal Formula 3.

Boldo   (2309-v)

Boldo Leaves; Peumus.
CAS — 476-70-0 (boldine); 1398-22-7 (boldoglucin).
Pharmacopoeias. In Eur. (see p.vi).
Fr. also includes Boldine.

Pharmacopoeial description
Ph. Eur.: The whole or fragmented dried leaf of *Peumus boldus*. The whole drug contains not more than 20 mL per kg, and the fragmented drug not more than 15 mL per kg, of essential oil. It contains not less than 0.1% of total alkaloids, expressed as boldine ($C_{19}H_{21}NO_4 = 327.4$), calculated with reference to the anhydrous drug. It has an aromatic odour especially when rubbed. Protect from light.

Profile
Boldo is employed in herbal medicine as a diuretic and in the treatment of gallstones and gastrointestinal disorders such as constipation. The alkaloid boldine is also used.

Boldo is used in homoeopathic medicine.

Preparations
Proprietary Preparations (details are given in Part 3)
Ger.: Cefabol.

Multi-ingredient: *Aust.:* St Bonifatius-Tee; *Austral.:* Berberis Complex; Lexat; *Belg.:* Tisane pour le Foie; *Braz.:* Alcafelol; Atroveran; Atrovex; Boldiman; Boldo Jurubeba; Boldobeba; Boldopeptan; Colachofra; Cynarobil; Dorveran; Epagogo; Eparema; Epatovis; Espasmolex; Figadosan; Figatil; Gotas Digestivas; Gotas Hepaticas; Hepato-Flux; Hepatobyl; Hepatoregius; Hepavirmo; Kop Hepar; Litrison; Metionina Composta; Prinachol; Solvobil; *Canad.:* Alsilax†; *Fr.:* Actisane Digestion†; Aromabyl†; Bolcitol; Boldoflorine; Drainactil; Elixir Spark; Gastralsan†; Grains de Vals; Hepaclem; Hepax; Jecopeptol; Mediflor Tisane Hepatique No 5†; Mucinum a l'Extrait de Cascara; Mucinum†; Neo-Boldolaxine†; Opobyl; Oxyboldine; Palmi†; Petites Pilules Carters; Romarinex-Choline†; Santane C₆; Santane F₁₀; Solution Stago Diluee; Spark†; Tisane des Familles; Tisane Hepatique de Hoerdt; Tisane Mexicaine†; Vegelax; *Ger.:* Cholapret; Cynarzym N; Gallemolan G; Hepatofalk Neu; Heumann Leber- und Gallentee Solu-Hepar NT; Hevert-Gall S; Pankreaticum; *Hong Kong:* Mucinum Cascara; *Ital.:* Amaro Medicinale; Boldina He; Caramelle alle Erbe Digestive; Certobil†; Coladren; Colax; Confetti Lassativi CM; Confetti Lassativi†; Confetto Complex†; Critichol; Digelax; Dis-Cinil Complex; Eparema; Eparema-Levul; Eupatol; Fitodorf Rabarbaro; Florerbe Lassativa; Frangulina; Hepasil Composto; Hepatos; Hepatos B12; Magisbile; Mepalax; Ormobyl†; Raboldo; Schias-Amaro Medicinale; Sintobil†; Solvobil; Tisana Arnaldi†; Vegebyl†; *Mex.:* Chofabol; *Port.:* Solucao Stago; *Spain:* Boldolaxin; Boldosal; Menabil Complex; Nico Hepatocyn; Opobyl; Resolutivo Regium; Sambil†; Sol Schoum; *Switz.:* Boldocynara†; Boldoflorine†; Dragees pour reins et vessie S; Grains de Vals; Laxativum Nouvelle Formule†; Opobyl†; Stago; The Franklin†; Tisane hepatique et biliaire; *UK:* Adios; Boldex; Boldo; HealthAid Boldo-Plus; Weight Loss Aid.

Bone Morphogenetic Proteins   (11757-j)

BMP.

Profile
Bone morphogenetic proteins (BMPs) are growth factors which promote ectopic bone formation and can be extracted

---

The symbol † denotes a preparation no longer actively marketed

from demineralised bone matrix. At least 7 have been identi-fied, including osteogenin (BMP-3) and osteogenic protein 1 (OP-1, BMP-7), and some have been produced by recombinant technology. They are under investigation for use in orthopaedic and reconstructive surgery.

◊ References.
1. Anonymous. New bone? *Lancet* 1992; **339:** 463–4.
2. Reddi AH. Bone morphogenetic proteins, bone marrow stromal cells, and mesenchymal cells: Maureen Owen revisited. *Clin Orthop* 1995; (313): 115–19.
3. Croteau S, *et al.* Bone morphogenetic proteins in orthopedics: from basic science to clinical practice. *Orthopedics* 1999; **22:** 686–95.

Boneset (14033-h)

Feverwort; Thoroughwort.

Profile
Boneset, the aerial parts of *Eupatorium perfoliatum* (Compositae), has diaphoretic and immunostimulant properties and has been used in the treatment of fever, influenza, the common cold, and other upper respiratory-tract disorders.

It is also used in homoeopathic medicine.

Preparations
Proprietary Preparations (details are given in Part 3)
Multi-ingredient: Austral.: Flavons; **UK:** Catarrh Mixture.

Borage (5138-m)

Bourrache.

Pharmacopoeias. Fr. includes monographs for flowers and flowering tops.

Profile
Borage, the aerial parts of *Borago officinalis* (Boraginaceae), has been used in herbal medicine as a demulcent and emollient. However, it contains pyrrolizidine alkaloids which may be toxic and internal use is not recommended.

Borage oil (p.1613) is used as a source of gamolenic and linoleic acids.

Preparations
Proprietary Preparations (details are given in Part 3)
Multi-ingredient: Fr.: Tisanes de l'Abbe Hamon no 15†.

Borax (261-l)

Disodium Tetraborate; E285; Natrii Tetraboras; Natrium Boricum; Purified Borax; Sodium Biborate; Sodium Borate; Sodium Pyroborate; Sodium Tetraborate.
$Na_2B_4O_7,10H_2O = 381.4$.
$CAS — 1330-43-4$; $61028-24-8$ (*both anhydrous borax*); $1303-96-4$ (*borax decahydrate*).
$ATC — S01AX07$.
Pharmacopoeias. In *Chin., Eur.* (see p.vi), *Jpn,* and *Pol.* Also in *USNF.*

For a warning on the supply of preparations of borax, see under Boric Acid, below.

Pharmacopoeial description
Ph. Eur.: Colourless crystals or crystalline masses, or white crystalline powder. It effloresces. Soluble in water; very soluble in boiling water; freely soluble in glycerol. A 4% solution in water has a pH of 9.0 to 9.6.

USNF 20: Odourless transparent colourless crystals or white crystalline powder. Its solutions are alkaline to phenolphthalein. It effloresces in warm dry air. Soluble 1 in 16 of water, 1 in 1 of boiling water, and 1 in 1 of glycerol; insoluble in alcohol. Store in airtight containers.

Boric Acid (260-e)

Acidum Boricum; Boracic Acid; Borsäure; E284; Orthoboric Acid; Sal Sedativa de Homberg.
$H_3BO_3 = 61.83$.
$CAS — 10043-35-3$.
$ATC — S02AA03$.
Pharmacopoeias. In *Chin., Eur.* (see p.vi), *Jpn,* and *Pol.* Also in *USNF.*

It volatilises in steam.
Boric acid forms a complex with glycerol which is a stronger acid than boric acid.

Pharmacopoeial description
Ph. Eur.: Colourless shiny plates greasy to the touch, or white crystals, or white crystalline powder. Soluble in water and in alcohol; freely soluble in boiling water and in glycerol (85%). A 3.3% solution in water has a pH of 3.8 to 4.8.

USNF 20: Odourless, colourless, somewhat pearly lustrous scales, or crystals, or white powder, slightly unctuous to the touch. Soluble 1 in 18 of water, 1 in 4 of boiling water, 1 in 18 of alcohol, 1 in 6 of boiling alcohol, and 1 in 4 of glycerol.

◊ CAUTION. *Pharmacists are advised not to sell boric acid as such for use as a dusting powder. Dusting powders containing*

more than 5% of boric acid should be labelled: 'not to be applied to raw or weeping surfaces'. *Pharmacists are also advised not to supply Borax Glycerin or Honey of Borax, even with an appropriate warning, because of the hazards associated with the use of these preparations in infants.*

Adverse Effects and Treatment
The main symptoms of acute boric acid poisoning are vomiting and diarrhoea, abdominal pain, an erythematous rash involving both skin and mucous membranes, followed by desquamation, and stimulation or depression of the CNS. There may be convulsions and hyperpyrexia. There may also be renal tubular damage. Abnormal liver function and jaundice have been reported rarely. Death, resulting from circulatory collapse and shock, may occur within 3 to 5 days.

The slow excretion of boric acid can lead to cumulative toxicity during repeated use. Symptoms of chronic intoxication include anorexia, gastrointestinal disturbances, debility, confusion, dermatitis, menstrual disorders, anaemia, convulsions, and alopecia.

Fatalities have occurred most frequently in young children after the accidental ingestion of solutions of boric acid or after the application of boric acid powder to abraded skin. The concentration of boric acid in talcs and products for oral hygiene is limited in the UK to 5% and 0.5% respectively and talcs must be labelled 'not to be used for children less than 3 years old'. In the UK, the concentration of boric acid in other cosmetic products is limited to 3%. Topical preparations of boric acid should not be applied to extensive areas of abraded or damaged skin.

Deaths have resulted from absorption following lavage of body cavities with solutions of boric acid, and this practice is no longer recommended.

Inhaled boric acid and borax are pulmonary irritants.

Treatment of poisoning is symptomatic. The stomach should be emptied if the patient presents within 1 hour and a large amount of boric acid has been ingested; activated charcoal is not effective. Peritoneal dialysis or haemodialysis may be of value.

Pharmacokinetics
Boric acid is absorbed from the gastrointestinal tract, from damaged skin, from wounds, and from mucous membranes. It does not readily penetrate intact skin. About 50% of the amount absorbed is excreted in the urine within 12 hours; the remainder is probably excreted over 5 to 7 days.

Uses and Administration
Boric acid possesses weak bacteriostatic and fungistatic properties; it has generally been superseded by more effective and less toxic disinfectants. It is used as a pesticide against ants and cockroaches.

Boric acid is used, usually with borax, as a buffer and antimicrobial in eye drops, and was formerly used as a soluble lubricant in solution-tablets. It is also used as a preservative for urine samples. Boric acid and borax are not used internally.

In the UK, the use of boric acid in cosmetics and toiletries is restricted.

Borax is used similarly to boric acid and has also been used externally as a mild astringent and as an emulsifier in creams. Preparations of borax in glycerol or in honey (Borax Glycerin; Honey of Borax) were formerly used as paints for the throat, tongue, and mouth, but should not be used due to the risk of toxicity.

Other salts of boric acid, including potassium and zinc salts, have been used.

A preparation of borax is used in homoeopathic medicine.

Antimicrobial activity. Evaluation of the antimicrobial activity of 1.22% borate buffer.[1]
1. Houlsby RD, *et al.* Antimicrobial activity of borate-buffered solutions. *Antimicrob Agents Chemother* 1986; **29:** 803–6.

Urine preservation. Boric acid in concentrations of about 2% may be a suitable preservative for urine samples in transit requiring bacteriological examination.[1,2] However, overnight storage of specimens preserved with boric acid may significantly alter culture results.[3]
1. Porter IA, Brodie J. Boric acid preservation of urine samples. *BMJ* 1969; **2:** 353–5.
2. Lum KT, Meers PD. Boric acid converts urine into an effective bacteriostatic transport medium. *J Infect* 1989; **18:** 51–8.
3. Gillespie T, *et al.* The effect of specimen processing delay on borate urine preservation. *J Clin Pathol* 1999; **52:** 95–8.

Vaginitis. Vaginal candidiasis due to *Candida glabrata* and other non-*albicans* frequently respond to topical boric acid.[1,2] Satisfactory clinical and mycological responses to topical boric acid were reported in 2 patients with *Candida glabrata* vaginitis (p.372) who had not responded to repeated courses of azole antifungals.[3]
1. Sobel JD, Chaim W. Treatment of Torulopsis glabrata vaginitis: retrospective review of boric acid therapy. *Clin Infect Dis* 1997; **24:** 649–52.
2. Rex JH, *et al.* Infectious Diseases Society of America. Practice guidelines for the treatment of candidiasis. *Clin Infect Dis* 2000; **30:** 662–78.
3. Redondo-Lopez V, *et al.* Torulopsis glabrata vaginitis: clinical aspects and susceptibility of antifungal agents. *Obstet Gynecol* 1990; **76:** 651–5.

Preparations
BP 2001: Kaolin Poultice;
BPC 1973: Magenta Paint; Surgical Chlorinated Soda Solution;
USP 25: Rose Water Ointment.

Proprietary Preparations (details are given in Part 3)
Canad.: Eye Wash; RO-Eyewash†; **Fr.:** Hydralin; **Port.:** Onycho Phytex†.

Multi-ingredient: Aust.: Coldophthal; Ophtaguttal; Polyrinse-Augenelement; **Austral.:** Floraquin†; **Belg.:** Alcasol; Amazyl†; Baseler Haussalbe†; Boradrine†; Borostyrol; Osmoleine†; **Braz.:** Albicon; Antiphlogistine; Bluderm; Blumen; Boralina; Borato de Sodio; Colpagex N; Dermobion; Dermosed; Dinill; Forsalil; Fungol; Gynaseptol; Gynax-N; Gyrol; Hipoderme; Hipodermon; Hipoglos; Hipoglos com Hidrocortisona; Lavolho; Leucocida; Lisofenicol; Lisoquinol; Lucretin; Novaboin; Oto-Biotic; Oturga; Po Antisseptico; Pomada Blumen; Pomaglos Pomada; Senophile; Topo Worth; Vagitrin-N; Verlin; Visiplex; Visogenul; Visual; Vitacolor; **Canad.:** British Army Foot Powder; Eye Eze; Ingrown Toe Nail Salve†; Thunas Eye Drops; **Fin.:** Otiborin; **Fr.:** Antiseptique-Calmante; Boroclarine; Borostyrol; Dacryoboraline; Dacryoserum; Dacudoses; Dragee Vauban; Eau Precieuse; Genola; Glyco-Thymoline; Gynescal†; Homeoplasmine; Hydralin; Ophtalmine; Paps; Pate a l'Eau Roche-Posay; Phylarm; Sophtal; **Ger.:** Ensinger Schiller-Quelle Heilwasser; Ophtopur-N; **Hong Kong:** Eye Mo; Eye Mo 36; **Irl.:** Phytex; **Israel:** Gargol; **Ital.:** Aquasalina; Bagno Oculare; Boma; Borossigeno Plus Stomatologico†; Fotofil; **Mex.:** Hipoglos Plus; **S.Afr.:** Anugesic; Anusol-HC†; Oestro-Gynedron†; Poly-Gynedron†; Universal Eye Drops; Vagarsol; **Singapore:** Buffelin; Eye Mo; New Daigaku; **Spain:** Acnosan; Banoftal; Boradren; Cloranfe Hemidex; Cloroboral; Coliriocilina Adren Astr; Dermomycose Liquido; Euboral; Fungusol; Lamnotyl; Lema C; Milrosina; Natusan; Oftalmol Dexa†; Oftalmol Ocular; Pomada Infantil Vera; Talquissar†; Topico Denticion Vera; Vaselina Boricada; Zolina; **Swed.:** Antasten-Privin; **Switz.:** Chibro-Boraline; **Thai.:** Eye Mo; Floraquin; Opplin; Opsil; Optal; Quinradon; Quinradon-N; Visotone; **UK:** Oxy Clean Facial Scrub; Phytex; **USA:** Auro-Dri; BFI; Castaderm; Collyrium for Fresh Eyes; Dri/Ear; Ear-Dry; Phylorinol; RA Lotion; Saratoga; Scale's Lotion; Star-Otic; Succus Cineraria Maritima; Trichotine; Trimo-San; Wyanoids†.

Bornyl Acetate (9377-b)

Bornyl Acetate (*USAN*).
Borneol Acetate. 1,7,7-Trimethylbicyclo[2.2.1]heptan-2-ol acetate.
$C_{12}H_{20}O_2 = 196.3$.
$CAS — 76-49-3$.

Profile
Bornyl acetate is a constituent of some essential oils. It has been used in aromatic preparations in the treatment of coughs, other respiratory-tract disorders, and musculoskeletal and joint disorders.

Preparations
Proprietary Preparations (details are given in Part 3)
Multi-ingredient: Ger.: Lindofluid N; **Hong Kong:** Vapex; **Singapore:** Vapex.

Bromelains (3705-h)

Bromelains (*BAN, USAN, rINN*).
Bromelins; Plant Protease Concentrate.
$CAS — 9001-00-7$.
$ATC — B06AA11$.

A concentrate of proteolytic enzymes derived from the pineapple plant, *Ananas comosus* (=*A. sativus*) (Bromeliaceae).

Units
One Rorer unit of protease activity has been defined as that amount of enzyme which hydrolyses a standardised casein substrate at pH 7 and 25° so as to cause an increase in absorbance of 0.00001 per minute at 280 nm.

One FIP unit of bromelain activity is reported to be contained in that amount of a standard preparation, which hydrolyses a suitable preparation of casein (FIP controlled) under the standard conditions at an initial rate such that there is liberated per minute an amount of peptides, not precipitated by a specified protein precipitation reagent which gives the same absorbance as 1 μmol of tyrosine at 275 nm.

Activity has also been described in terms of milk-clotting units.

Adverse Effects
Bromelains may cause nausea, vomiting, and diarrhoea. Metrorrhagia and menorrhagia have occasionally occurred. Hypersensitivity reactions have been reported and have included skin reactions and asthma.

Effects on the respiratory system. Bronchial asthma was experienced by 2 patients after exposure to bromelains.[1] Of 6 workers sensitised to papain, 5 showed positive skin tests to bromelains and 2 of them also showed immediate asthmatic reactions after bronchial challenge with bromelains.[2]
1. Galleguillos F, Rodriguez JC. Asthma caused by bromelin inhalation. *Clin Allergy* 1978; **8:** 21–4.
2. Baur X, Fruhmann G. Allergic reactions, including asthma, to the pineapple protease bromelin following occupational exposure. *Clin Allergy* 1979; **9:** 443–50.

Precautions
Bromelains should be given with care to patients with coagulation disorders or with severe hepatic or renal impairment.

Uses and Administration

Bromelains are used as an adjunct in the treatment of soft-tissue inflammation and oedema associated with trauma and surgery. Bromelains have also been given as an aid to digestion.

Preparations

Proprietary Preparations (details are given in Part 3)
Fr.: Extranase; *Ger.:* Mucozym; Proteozym; Traumanase; *Hong Kong:* Ananase; *Irl.:* Ananase†; *Ital.:* Ananase; *Port.:* Ananase; *S.Afr.:* Ananase; *Switz.:* Traumanase; *USA:* Dayto Anase†.

Multi-ingredient: *Aust.:* Arca-Enzym; Nutrizym; Phlogenzym; Wobenzym; *Austral.:* Bio-Disc; Bioglan Discone; Digestaid; Digestive Aid; Natures Own Digestive Enzymes; Prost-1; Prost-2†; Prozyme; Vita Disc†; *Braz.:* Labfcilina; Monocetin; Nutrizim; Plasil Enzimatico; Sintozima; Vonil Enzimatico; *Ger.:* Enzym-Wied; Esberizym N†; Floradix Multipretten; Mulsal N; Phlogenzym; Wobenzym N; *Ital.:* Bres; Derinase Plus†; *Mex.:* Phlogenzym; Plasil Enzimatico; Wobenzym; *Port.:* Nutrizym†; *S.Afr.:* Haemonase P†; *Spain:* Bequipecto†; Flebo Stop; *UK:* Cardeymin; Digezyme; Enzyme Digest.

Bromides (20799-s)

ATC — N05CM11.

Pharmacopoeias. Chin., Eur.(see p.vi), *Jpn,* and *Pol* include standards for Potassium Bromide and Sodium Bromide. Ammonium Bromide is in *Eur.* and *Pol.* Bromoform is included in *Belg.* Calcium bromide is in *Aust., Belg.,* and *Pol.*

Adverse Effects

During prolonged exposure bromide accumulation may occur giving rise to bromide intoxication or bromism. Symptoms include nausea and vomiting, slurred speech, memory impairment, drowsiness, irritability, ataxia, tremors, hallucinations, mania, delirium, psychoses, stupor, coma, and other manifestations of CNS depression. Skin rashes of various types may occur and toxic epidermal necrolysis has been reported. Death after acute poisoning appears to be rare as vomiting follows the ingestion of large doses.

There have been reports of neonatal bromide intoxication and growth defects associated with maternal bromide ingestion during pregnancy. Symptoms of bromide intoxication have also been reported in breast-fed infants whose mothers were taking bromides.

Treatment of Adverse Effects

In acute poisoning, the stomach should be emptied (if emesis has not already occurred), and sodium chloride should be given by intravenous infusion. Glucose may also be administered and frusemide [furosemide] may be given to aid diuresis.

In chronic poisoning, bromide administration is stopped and sodium chloride is given intravenously or by mouth with adequate amounts of fluid. Ammonium chloride has been given but is no longer recommended as it may precipitate metabolic acidosis. Diuretics are of value. In severe cases of bromide intoxication or when the usual treatments cannot be used, haemodialysis may be of benefit.

Pharmacokinetics

Bromides are readily absorbed from the gastrointestinal tract. They displace chloride in extracellular body fluids and have a half-life in the body of about 12 days. They may be detected in the milk of nursing mothers and in the fetus.

Uses and Administration

Bromides depress the CNS. Potassium bromide has been used as a sedative and anticonvulsant, but has generally been replaced by more effective, less toxic drugs. Ammonium, calcium, sodium, and strontium bromide have been used similarly, as have bromoform and dilute hydrobromic acid. Bromides have also been used in multi-ingredient preparations for the treatment of coughs.

Potassium bromide has been used in homoeopathic medicine.

Preparations

Proprietary Preparations (details are given in Part 3)
Belg.: Bromofotyl†.

Multi-ingredient: *Belg.:* Normogastryl†; *Braz.:* Bromosedan; Broncotussan; Frenotosse; Gotas Nican; Limao Bravo; Naquinto; Tossefedrin; Xarope de Caraguata + Bromoformio; Xarope Peitoral de Ameixa Composto; Xarope Sao Joao; *Fr.:* Dinacode; Eucalyptine Le Brun†; Galirene; Lyptocodine†; Neurocalcium; Pectosan†; Sedatif Tiber; Sirop Pectoral adulte†; Sirop Pectoral enfant†; Sirop Teyssedre; *Ital.:* Fertomcidina-U; Neo Soluzione Sulfo Balsamica†; *Port.:* Lactucol; *S.Afr.:* Bronchicum; *Spain:* Medecitral; Stomosan; Topico Denticion Vera.

Bromine (1022-v)

Bromum.
$Br_2 = 159.808$.
CAS — 7726-95-6.

A dark reddish-brown, heavy, mobile liquid which gives off intensely irritating brown fumes.

Adverse Effects

Bromine is intensely irritating and corrosive to mucous membranes and, even in dilute solution, may cause fatal gastro-enteritis if swallowed. Contact with the skin can produce severe burns and inhalation of the vapour causes violent irritation of the respiratory tract and pulmonary oedema.

The symbol † denotes a preparation no longer actively marketed

Treatment of Adverse Effects

Milk or antacids should be given as soon as possible following ingestion of bromine. Gastric lavage is not recommended. If bromine vapour has been inhaled, oxygen should be administered and assisted ventilation may be necessary. Corticosteroids may be given for laryngeal and pulmonary oedema. Splashes on the skin and eyes should be immediately washed off; washing under running water should continue for at least 15 minutes.

Uses and Administration

Bromine is widely used in industry. It was formerly used, in the form of an adduct with a quaternary ammonium compound, in the treatment of plantar warts.

Bryonia (12460-v)

The root of *Bryonia alba* or *B. dioica* (Cucurbitaceae).

Profile

Bryonia is an ingredient of preparations used in respiratory-tract infections and inflammatory disorders. It is also used in homoeopathic medicine.

Preparations

Proprietary Preparations (details are given in Part 3)

Multi-ingredient: *Austral.:* Cough Relief; Harpagophytum Complex; Joint & Muscle Relief Cream; Respatona Decongestant Formula; Respatona Plus Bronchial Cough Relief; *Fr.:* Homeoplasmine.

Buchu (12461-g)

Bucco; Buchu Leaves; Diosma; Folia Bucco.

Pharmacopoeias. In *Fr.*

The dried leaves of 'short' or 'round' buchu, *Agathosma betulina* (=*Barosma betulina*) (Rutaceae).

Profile

Buchu is a weak diuretic and urinary antiseptic and has been used in multi-ingredient preparations for the treatment of urinary-tract disorders.

Buchu has been used in homoeopathic medicine.

Preparations

Proprietary Preparations (details are given in Part 3)

Multi-ingredient: *Austral.:* Althaea Complex; Bioglan Cranbiotic Super; Cranberry Complex; De Witts New Pills; Extralife Uri-Care; Fluid Loss; Medinat PMT-Eze; New De Witt's Pills†; PMS Support; Serenoa Complex; Urinase; Uva-Ursi Complex; *Canad.:* Herbal Laxative; *Fr.:* Urophytum; *Ger.:* Hevert-Entwasserungs-Tee†; *NZ:* De Witts Pills; *Port.:* Solucao Stago; *S.Afr.:* Docrub; *Switz.:* Urinex (nouvelle formule); *UK:* Antitis; Backache; Backache Relief; De Witt's K & B Pills; Diuretabs; Gerard House Buchu Compound; HRI Water Balance; Kas-Bah; Skin Eruptions Mixture; Watershed; *USA:* Aqua-Rid†; Fluidex†; Tri-Aqua†.

Bucillamine (2897-a)

Bucillamine (*rINN*).

DE-019; SA-96; Tioburtarit. *N*-(2-Mercapto-2-methylpropionyl)-L-cysteine.
$C_7H_{13}NO_3S_2 = 223.3$.
CAS — 65002-17-7.
ATC — M01CC02.

Profile

Bucillamine is structurally related to penicillamine (p.1017) and is reported to be an immunomodulator. It has been used in rheumatoid arthritis.

◊ Bucillamine has been used in rheumatoid arthritis.[1] Pemphigus lesions have been reported in a patient following use for arthralgia.[2]

1. Kim HA, Song YW. A comparison between bucillamine and D-penicillamine in the treatment of rheumatoid arthritis. *Rheumatol Int* 1997; **17:** 5–9.
2. Ogata K, *et al.* Drug-induced pemphigus foliaceus with features of pemphigus vulgaris. *Br J Dermatol* 2001; **144:** 421–2.

Bucladesine Sodium (18881-v)

Bucladesine Sodium (*rINNM*).

DBcAMP (bucladesine); Dibutyryl Cyclic AMP Sodium; DT-5621 (bucladesine). *N*-(9-β-D-Ribofuranosyl-9*H*-purin-6-yl)butyramide cyclic 3′,5′-(hydrogen phosphate) 2′-butyrate sodium.
$C_{18}H_{24}N_5O_8PNa = 492.4$.
CAS — 362-74-3 (bucladesine); 16980-89-5 (bucladesine sodium).

Profile

Bucladesine sodium has been reported to have cardiotonic properties when given intravenously. It has been applied topically for the treatment of bedsores.

Bufotenine (5012-l)

NN-Dimethylserotonin; 5-Hydroxy-*NN*-dimethyltryptamine; Mappine. 3-(2-Dimethylaminoethyl)indol-5-ol.
$C_{12}H_{16}N_2O = 204.3$.
CAS — 487-93-4.

An indole alkaloid obtained from the seeds and leaves of *Piptadenia peregrina,* from which the hallucinogenic snuff cohoba is prepared, and *P. macrocarpa* (Mimosaceae). It was first isolated from the skin glands of toads (*Bufo* spp.) and has also been isolated from species of *Amanita* (Agaricaceae).

Profile

Bufotenine has serotonergic activity and is reported to have hallucinogenic properties. It has no therapeutic use.

Buphenine Hydrochloride (9214-p)

Buphenine Hydrochloride (*BANM*).

Nylidrin Hydrochloride; Nylidrinium Chloride. 1-(4-Hydroxyphenyl)-2-(1-methyl-3-phenylpropylamino)propan-1-ol hydrochloride.
$C_{19}H_{25}NO_2,HCl = 335.9$.
CAS — 447-41-6 (buphenine); 849-55-8 (buphenine hydrochloride).

Adverse Effects and Precautions

For the adverse effects of sympathomimetics in general and precautions for their use, see Adrenaline, p.829.

Uses and Administration

Buphenine produces peripheral vasodilatation through beta-adrenoceptor stimulation and a direct action on the arteries and arterioles of the skeletal muscles.

Buphenine has been used in the treatment of disorders of peripheral and cerebral circulatory insufficiency. It has also been used in preparations for rhinitis and nasal congestion. Doses of buphenine hydrochloride in the range of 3 to 12 mg by mouth three or four times daily have been given, although total daily doses of up to 90 mg have been used.

An intravenous infusion of buphenine hydrochloride has been used to arrest premature labour. It has also been given orally as a prophylactic tocolytic agent.

Preparations

Proprietary Preparations (details are given in Part 3)
Aust.: Dilatol; Dilydrin; *Canad.:* Arlidin; *Mex.:* Arlidin; Nilken; *Spain:* Diatolin; *Switz.:* Dilydrine Retard; Tocodrine.

Multi-ingredient: *Aust.:* Apoplectal; Arbid; Dilaescol; Dilatol-Chinin; Opino; Tropoderm; *Fr.:* Ophtadil; Phlebogel; *Ger.:* Apoplectal N; opino N spezial; *Spain:* Circovenil; Circovenil Fuerte†; *Switz.:* Arbid; Visaline.

Burnet (3890-t)

Garden Burnet; Greater Burnet; Sanguisorba.

Profile

Burnet, the aerial parts and roots of *Sanguisorba officinalis* (*Poterium officinalis*) (Rosaceae), has antihaemorrhagic and astringent properties. It has been used internally to treat menorrhagia and gastrointestinal disorders and is also used topically for eczema, burns, and other skin disorders.

It is also used in homoeopathic medicine.

Burnet is also used as an animal fodder and salad vegetable, and as an ingredient in beer-making.

Preparations

Proprietary Preparations (details are given in Part 3)
Multi-ingredient: *Canad.:* Swiss Herb Cough Drops.

Butinoline Phosphate (11282-a)

Butinoline Phosphate (*rINNM*).

1,1-Diphenyl-4-pyrrolidino-1′-yl but-2-yn-1-ol phosphate.
$C_{20}H_{21}NO,H_3PO_4 = 389.4$.
CAS — 968-63-8 (butinoline); 54118-66-0 (butinoline phosphate).

Profile

Butinoline phosphate is used as an antispasmodic in preparations for gastrointestinal disorders.

Preparations

Proprietary Preparations (details are given in Part 3)
Multi-ingredient: *Aust.:* Spasmo-Solugastril; *Ger.:* Jasicholin N; Spasmo-Nervogastrol; Spasmo-Solugastril.

Butyl Nitrite (12483-l)

$C_4H_9NO_2 = 103.1$.

Profile

Butyl nitrite is not used medicinally but, as with other volatile nitrites, is abused for its vasodilating and related effects following inhalation (see Abuse, under Amyl Nitrite, p.1002).

Cadmium (1596-x)

Cd = 112.411.
CAS — 7440-43-9.

Profile
Cadmium is employed in a wide range of manufacturing processes and cadmium poisoning presents a recognised industrial hazard. Inhalation of cadmium fumes during welding procedures may not produce symptoms until 4 to 10 hours have passed and these symptoms include respiratory distress leading to pulmonary oedema; kidney toxicity is also a feature of acute cadmium poisoning. Ingestion of cadmium or its salts has the additional hazard of severe gastrointestinal effects. Cadmium has a long biological half-life and accumulates in body tissues, particularly the liver and kidneys. Chelation therapy is not generally recommended for cadmium poisoning, although calcium edetate has been used following acute ingestion. However, chelators do not increase cadmium elimination in chronic poisoning and administration of dimercaprol may increase cadmium toxicity and should be avoided. Chronic exposure to cadmium results in progressive renal insufficiency and other effects (see below).

Cadmium sulfide has been used topically in some countries for the treatment of skin conditions. Cadmium sulfate has been included in some preparations for the treatment of eye irritation.

Adverse effects. The toxicity of cadmium has been reviewed.[1] Environmental or occupational exposure to cadmium has been associated with renal dysfunction,[2-4] although this may be reversible if exposure is reduced.[5] A reduction in bone density may also occur.[6] Fatalities due to industrial exposure or self-poisoning have also been reported.[7,8] No effect on testicular endocrine function was observed in 77 industrial workers exposed to cadmium.[3]

An increased incidence of cancer of the prostate has been reported in subjects exposed to high levels of cadmium but the evidence is not conclusive.[9] There may be an association between cadmium exposure and lung cancer, although observations on this type of cancer are difficult to interpret because of exposure to other hazards such as smoking.

1. Fielder RJ, Dale EA. Cadmium and its compounds. *Toxicity Review 7.* London: HMSO, 1983.
2. Buchet JP, *et al.* Renal effects of cadmium body burden of the general population. *Lancet* 1990; **336:** 699–702. Correction. *ibid.* 1991; **337:** 1554.
3. Mason HJ. Occupational cadmium exposure and testicular endocrine function. *Hum Exp Toxicol* 1990; **9:** 91–4.
4. Cai S, *et al.* Renal dysfunction from cadmium contamination of irrigation water: dose-response analysis in a Chinese population. *Bull WHO* 1998; **76:** 153–9.
5. Hotz P, *et al.* Renal effects of low-level environmental cadmium exposure: 5-year follow-up of a subcohort from the Cadmibel study. *Lancet* 1999 **354:** 1508–13.
6. Staessen JA, *et al.* Environmental exposure to cadmium, forearm bone density, and risk of fractures: prospective population study. *Lancet* 1999 **353:** 1140–44.
7. Taylor A, *et al.* Poisoning with cadmium fumes after smelting lead. *BMJ* 1984; **288:** 1270–1.
8. Buckler HM, *et al.* Self poisoning with oral cadmium chloride. *BMJ* 1986; **292:** 1559–60. Correction. *ibid.*; **293:** 236.
9. Bell GM. Carcinogenicity of cadmium and its compounds. *Toxicity Review 24.* London: HMSO, 1991.

Preparations
Proprietary Preparations (details are given in Part 3)
Spain: Biocadmio.

Multi-ingredient: *Aust.:* Ichtho-Cadmin; *Fr.:* Visiolyre.

Cajuput Oil (4616-s)

Cajeput Oil; Cajuput Essence; Oleum Cajuputi.

A volatile oil obtained by distillation from the fresh leaves and twigs of *Melaleuca cajuputi* (*M. leucadendron*) (Myrtaceae). It contains eucalyptol.

Profile
Cajuput oil has been applied externally as a stimulant and mild rubefacient in rheumatism. It is also used with other volatile agents in preparations for the relief of respiratory congestion. It has been given internally as a carminative.

Preparations
Proprietary Preparations (details are given in Part 3)
Multi-ingredient: *Aust.:* Babix; Luuf-Heilpflanzenol; Tiger Balsam Rot; *Austral.:* Breathe Eazy Chest Rub; Capsolin; Goanna Heat Cream; Methyl Salicylate Ointment Compound; Relief Rub; Silver Clove Medicated Balm; Tiger Balm Red†; Tiger Balm White†; *Canad.:* Broncho Rub; Penetrating Rub†; Tiger Balm Red; Tiger Balm White; Youngflex Massage 168; *Fr.:* Phytolithe; Vegebom; *Ger.:* Liniplant; Olbas; Palatol; Palatol N; *Ital.:* Otosan Gocce Auricolari; *Singapore:* Begesic; *Switz.:* Frigoplasma; Olbas; *Thai.:* Begesic; Dexalin; Olympic Balm; *UK:* Olbas; Penetrol†; Tiger Balm Liquid†; Tiger Balm Red; *USA:* Dermal-Rub†.

Calamus (525-x)

Acore Vrai; Calamus Rhizome; Kalmus; Sweet Flag Root.
CAS — 8015-79-0 (calamus oil).
Pharmacopoeias. In *Aust.* and *Swiss.*

The dried rhizome of the sweet flag, *Acorus calamus* (Araceae).

Profile
Calamus has been used as a bitter and carminative; it is also used as a source of calamus oil which is employed in perfumery. In the USA the FDA has prohibited marketing calamus as a food or food additive; the oil (Jammu variety) is reported to be a carcinogen.

Preparations
Proprietary Preparations (details are given in Part 3)
Port.: Cholagutt.

Multi-ingredient: *Aust.:* Abdomilon; Aponatura Starkungs; Bio-Garten Tee fur Leber und Galle; Leber- und Galletee; Mag Kottas Magen-Darmtee; Sidroga Magen-Darm-Tee; *Fr.:* Jouvence de l'Abbe Soury; *Ger.:* Abdomilon N; Gallexier; Gastrol S; Grunlicht Hingfong Essenz; Hevert-Gall S; Hevert-Magen-Galle-Leber-Tee†; Montana; Presselin Blahungs K 4 N; Sedovent; Stomasal Med; Stovalid N; *Israel:* Rekiv; *Ital.:* Frerichs Maldifassi; *Spain:* Caved-S†; Roter Complex†; *Switz.:* Caved-S†; Kernosan Elixir; Tisane pour l'estomac; Urinex (nouvelle formule); *UK:* Pegina.

Calcium Carbimide (2732-x)

Calcium Carbimide (rINN).
Calcium Cyanamide; Cyanamide.
$CCaN_2 = 80.1.$
CAS — 156-62-7 (calcium carbimide); 8013-88-5 (citrated calcium carbimide).
ATC — V03AA02.

NOTE. The name cyanamide is also used to designate carbimide, which is used in veterinary medicine.

Adverse Effects and Precautions
Calcium carbimide may cause drowsiness, dizziness, fatigue, skin rash, tinnitus, depression, impotence, and urinary frequency. There may be a reversible increase in the white cell count. It should be used with caution in patients with asthma, coronary artery disease, or myocardial disease. Calcium carbimide causes a reaction in patients who have consumed alcohol similar to that seen with disulfiram (see p.1605).

Effects on the heart. Hypotension and tachycardia were reported during the carbimide-alcohol reaction.[1]

1. Peachey JE, *et al.* Cardiovascular changes during the calcium carbimide-ethanol interaction. *Clin Pharmacol Ther* 1981; **29:** 40–6.

Effects on the liver. Reports[1,2] of hepatic lesions in patients receiving calcium carbimide.

1. Vázquez JJ, Cervera S. Cyanamide-induced liver injury in alcoholics. *Lancet* 1980; **i:** 361–2.
2. Moreno A, *et al.* Structural hepatic changes associated with cyanamide treatment: cholangiolar proliferation, fibrosis and cirrhosis. *Liver* 1984; **4:** 15–21.

Uses and Administration
Calcium carbimide has actions and uses similar to those of disulfiram (p.1605). It is an aversive agent used as an adjunct in the treatment of chronic alcoholism (p.1131). It is given in a dose of up to 60 mg twice daily by mouth. Citrated calcium carbimide has been used similarly.

◊ References.

1. Peachey JE, *et al.* A comparative review of the pharmacological and toxicological properties of disulfiram and calcium carbimide. *J Clin Psychopharmacol* 1981; **1:** 21–6.

Preparations
Proprietary Preparations (details are given in Part 3)
Aust.: Colme; *Austral.:* Dipsan†; *Canad.:* Temposil†; *Irl.:* Abstem; *Neth.:* Dipsan†; *S.Afr.:* Dipsan†; *Spain:* Colme; *Swed.:* Dipsan†.

Calcium Dihydrogen Phosphate (1167-f)

Acid Calcium Phosphate; Calcium Dihydrogenphosphoricum; E341; Monobasic Calcium Phosphate; Monocalcium Phosphate. Calcium tetrahydrogen diorthophosphate monohydrate.
$Ca(H_2PO_4)_2,H_2O = 252.1.$
CAS — 7758-23-8 (anhydrous calcium dihydrogen phosphate).
Pharmacopoeias. In *Jpn* and *Swiss.*

Profile
Calcium dihydrogen phosphate is used in fertilisers. It is also used as an antoxidant in baking powders and flours and as a source of calcium in some mineral supplement preparations.

Preparations
Proprietary Preparations (details are given in Part 3)
Multi-ingredient: *Braz.:* Salutina; *Fr.:* Marinol; Phosphoneuros.

Calcium Dobesilate (12506-m)

Calcium Dobesilate (rINN).
Calcii Dobesilas; Calcium Doxybenzylate; 205E. Calcium 2,5-dihydroxybenzenesulphonate.
$C_{12}H_{10}CaO_{10}S_2 = 418.4.$
CAS — 88-46-0 (dobesilic acid); 20123-80-2 (calcium dobesilate).
ATC — C05BX01.

Pharmacopoeias. In *Eur.* (see p.vi) which specifies the monohydrate.

Pharmacopoeial description
Ph. Eur.: Calcium dobesilate monohydrate is a white or almost white hygroscopic powder. Very soluble in water; freely soluble in dehydrated alcohol; practically insoluble in dichloromethane; very slightly soluble in isopropyl alcohol. A 10% solution in water has a pH of 4.5 to 6.0. Store in airtight containers. Protect from light.

Profile
Calcium dobesilate is claimed to reduce capillary permeability and has been used in various peripheral circulatory disorders including diabetic retinopathy and haemorrhoids (p.1205). Gastrointestinal disturbances have occurred with its use, and there are also reports of hypersensitivity reactions.

Calcium dobesilate is given by mouth in usual doses of 0.5 to 1g daily in divided doses. It is also given rectally for haemorrhoids and is an ingredient of some preparations given for various skin disorders.

◊ Reviews.

1. Tejerina T, Ruiz E. Calcium dobesilate: pharmacology and future approaches. *Gen Pharmacol* 1998; **31:** 357–60.
2. Berthet P, *et al.* Calcium dobesilate: pharmacological profile related to its use in diabetic retinopathy. *Int J Clin Pract* 1999; **53:** 631–6.

Effects on the blood. Agranulocytosis has been reported[1-3] in a few patients following treatment with calcium dobesilate, and in 2 cases recurred on rechallenge.[1,2]

1. Kulessa W, *et al.* Wiederholte agranulozytose nach einnahme von calciumdobesilat. *Dtsch Med Wochenschr* 1992; **117:** 372–4.
2. Cladera Serra A, *et al.* Agranulocitosis inducida por dobesilato calcico. *Med Clin (Barc)* 1995; **105:** 558–9.
3. García Benayas E, *et al.* Calcium dobesilate-induced agranulocytosis. *Pharm World Sci* 1997; **19:** 251–2.

Preparations
Proprietary Preparations (details are given in Part 3)
Aust.: Doxium; *Belg.:* Doxium; *Braz.:* Doxium; *Ger.:* Dexium; Dobica; *Hong Kong:* Dobesifar; Doxium; *Ital.:* Doxium; *Mex.:* Doxium; *Mon.:* Doxium; *Port.:* Doxi-Om; *Spain:* Doxium; *Switz.:* Doxium.

Multi-ingredient: *Aust.:* Doxiproct; Doxiproct mit Dexamethason; *Braz.:* Proctium; *Ital.:* Doxiproct Plus; *Port.:* Doxiproct; Doxivenil; *Spain:* Acnisdin; Acnisdin Retinoico; Ederal; Proctium; *Switz.:* Doxiproct; Doxiproct Plus; Doxivenil.

Calcium Hopantenate (12509-g)

Calcium Hopantenate (rINNM).
Calcium Homopantothenate. Calcium D-(+)-4-(2,4-dihydroxy-3,3-dimethylbutyramido)butyrate hemihydrate.
$Ca(C_{10}H_{18}NO_5)_2,\frac{1}{2}H_2O = 513.6.$
CAS — 18679-90-8 (hopantenic acid); 17097-76-6 (anhydrous calcium hopantenate); 1990-07-4 (calcium hopantenate hemihydrate).

Profile
Calcium hopantenate is a homologue of pantothenic acid (p.1374) and has been tried in the treatment of various behavioural and extrapyramidal disorders. Its use is limited by severe metabolic side-effects and fatalities have been reported.

Calcium Hydroxide (204-m)

Calcii Hydroxidum; Calcium Hydrate; E526; Slaked Lime.
$Ca(OH)_2 = 74.09.$
CAS — 1305-62-0.
Pharmacopoeias. In *Eur.* (see p.vi), *Jpn*, and *US.*

Pharmacopoeial description
Ph. Eur.: A fine white powder. Practically insoluble in water.

USP 25: A white powder with a slightly bitter alkaline taste. Soluble 1 in 630 of water and 1 in 1300 of boiling water; insoluble in alcohol; soluble in glycerol and in syrup. Store in airtight containers.

Profile
Calcium hydroxide is a weak alkali. It is used in the form of Calcium Hydroxide Solution (lime water) in some skin lotions and oily preparations to form calcium soaps of fatty acids which produce water-in-oil emulsions.

Calcium hydroxide pastes are used in dentistry. A paste made from a mixture of calcium hydroxide and potassium hydroxide and known as Vienna paste was used as an escharotic. Soda lime (p.1665) is a mixture of calcium hydroxide and potassium hydroxide and/or sodium hydroxide.

◊ For the use of disodium edetate in the treatment of calcium hydroxide burns of the eye, see p.1008.

Preparations

BP 2001: Calcium Hydroxide Solution;
USP 25: Calcium Hydroxide Topical Solution.
Proprietary Preparations (details are given in Part 3)
Aust.: Dermi-cyl Allerg; *Ger.:* Dermi-cyl; *Ital.:* Stomidros†; *Mex.:* Lipocal; Oleocal; Oleoderm.
Multi-ingredient: *Belg.:* Oxyplastine†; *Mex.:* Caliderm; Oleoderm Plus; *Spain:* Cremsol; *Swed.:* Calasept†; *Switz.:* Calcipulpe†.

Calcium Oxide (12510-f)

Calcium Oxydatum; Calx; Calx Usta; Chaux Vive; E529; Gebrannter Kalk; Lime; Quicklime.
CaO = 56.08.
CAS — 1305-78-8.
Pharmacopoeias. In Belg., Jpn, Pol., Swiss, and US.

Pharmacopoeial description

USP 25: Hard, odourless, white or greyish-white masses, granules, or powder. When it is moistened with water a reaction occurs, heat being evolved and calcium hydroxide formed. Slightly soluble in water; very slightly soluble in boiling water. Store in airtight containers.

Adverse Effects and Treatment

Calcium oxide may cause burns on contact with moist skin and mucous membranes; it is particularly irritant to the eyes. Washing or flooding of affected areas may need to be prolonged. Pneumonitis may follow inhalation.

◊ For the use of disodium edetate in the treatment of calcium oxide burns of the eye, see p.1008.

Uses and Administration

Calcium oxide has been used in various dermatological preparations. With sulfur it forms sulfurated lime (p.1124). A paste made from a mixture of calcium oxide and sodium hydroxide and known as London paste was used as an escharotic.

Calcium Saccharate (1163-a)

Calcium Saccharate *(rINN).*
Calcii Saccharas; Calcium D-Saccharate. Calcium D-glucarate tetrahydrate.
$C_6H_8CaO_8,4H_2O = 320.3.$
CAS — 5793-88-4 (anhydrous calcium saccharate); 5793-89-5 (calcium saccharate tetrahydrate).
Pharmacopoeias. In US.

Each g represents approximately 3.1 mmol of calcium. Calcium saccharate 8 g is approximately equivalent to 1 g of calcium.

Pharmacopoeial description

USP 25: A white, odourless, crystalline powder. Very slightly soluble in cold water and in alcohol; slightly soluble in boiling water; practically insoluble in chloroform and in ether; soluble in dilute mineral acids and in solutions of calcium gluconate.

Profile

Calcium saccharate is employed as a stabilising agent in solutions of calcium gluconate for injection.

Preparations

Proprietary Preparations (details are given in Part 3)
Aust.: Calcium Fresenius; *Ger.:* Calcium Fresenius.
Multi-ingredient: *Ger.:* Calcitrans†; Calcium Braun; Calcium Truw†; Calcium Verla; *Switz.:* C-Calcium.

Calcium Sulfate (1165-x)

Calcii Sulfas; Calcium Sulphate; E516; Gypsum (calcium sulfate dihydrate).
$CaSO_4 = 136.1.$
CAS — 7778-18-9 (anhydrous calcium sulfate); 10101-41-4 (calcium sulfate dihydrate).
Pharmacopoeias. In Chin., Eur. (see p.vi), Int., and Jpn which specify the dihydrate. Also in USNF which specifies the dihydrate or the anhydrous material.

Pharmacopoeial description

Ph. Eur.: Calcium sulfate dihydrate is a white fine powder. Very slightly soluble in water; practically insoluble in alcohol.
USNF 20: A white to slightly yellow-white odourless fine powder. Soluble 1 in 375 of water and 1 in 485 of boiling water; soluble in 3N hydrochloric acid.

Profile

Calcium sulfate is used as an excipient for the preparation of tablets or capsules.
Calcium sulfate has also been used as a bone graft substitute.

Preparations

Proprietary Preparations (details are given in Part 3)
Austral.: Celloids CS 36.
Multi-ingredient: *UK:* New Era Hymosa†.

Dried Calcium Sulfate (1166-r)

Calcii Sulfas Hemihydricus; Calcined Gypsum; Calcium Sulfuricum ad Usum Chirurgicum; Calcium Sulphuricum Ustum; Dried Calcium Sulphate; Exsiccated Calcium Sulphate; Gebrannter Gips; Gêsso; Gypsum Siccatum; Plaster of Paris; Plâtre Cuit; Sulphate of Lime; Yeso Blanco.
$CaSO_4, \frac{1}{2}H_2O = 145.1.$
CAS — 10034-76-1 (calcium sulfate hemihydrate); 26499-65-0 (calcium sulfate hemihydrate).
Pharmacopoeias. In Aust., Br., Ger., and Jpn.

Pharmacopoeial description

BP 2001: A white or almost white, odourless or almost odourless hygroscopic powder. It may contain suitable setting accelerators or decelerators. Slightly soluble in water; more soluble in dilute mineral acids; practically insoluble in alcohol.

Profile

Dried calcium sulfate is used for the preparation of Plaster of Paris Bandage which is used for the immobilisation of limbs and fractures. It is also employed for making dental casts.

Preparations

Proprietary Preparations (details are given in Part 3)
Fr.: Biplatrix.

Calendula (12116-l)

Gold-bloom; Marigold; Marybud; Pot Marigold; Souci.
Pharmacopoeias. In Eur. (see p.vi).

Profile

Calendula, the flowers of *Calendula officinalis* (Compositae), has antiseptic, anti-inflammatory, and astringent properties. It is used in external preparations for minor skin disorders, and also internally for gastrointestinal and menstrual disorders. Calendula is also included in numerous herbal preparations to improve their appearance.

It is also used in homoeopathic medicine.

Calendula oil is also used.

Preparations

Proprietary Preparations (details are given in Part 3)
Fr.: Calendulene†; *UK:* Calendolon.

Multi-ingredient: *Aust.:* Apotheker Bauer's Magentee; Bio-Garten Entschlackungstee; Dr. Ernst Richter's Abfuhrtee-Filterbeutel; Kneipp Nieren- und Blasen-Tee; Krauterhaus Mag Kottas Blutreinigungstee†; Krauterhaus Mag Kottas Entwasserungstee; Krauterhaus Mag Kottas Fruhjahrs- und Herbstkurtee; Krauterhaus Mag Kottas Gallen- und Lebertee; Krauterhaus Mag Kottas Magen- und Darmtee; Krauterhaus Mag Kottas Nerven- und Schlaftee; Krauterhaus Mag Kottas Tee fur die Verdauung; Krauterhaus Mag Kottas Tee gegen Blahungen; Krauterhaus Mag Kottas Wechseltee; Krautertee Nr 16; Krautertee Nr 2; Krautertee Nr 207; Krautertee Nr 44; Mag Kottas Blahungs-Verdauungstee; Mag Kottas Entschlackungstee; Mag Kottas Entwasserungstee; Mag Kottas Leber-Gallentee; Mag Kottas Magen-Darmtee; Mag Kottas Nerven-Beruhigungstee; Mag Kottas Nieren-Blasentee; Mag Kottas Tee fur stillende Mutter; The Chambard-Tee; *Austral.:* Anti-Flamme; Galium Complex; Nappy Rash Relief Cream; Skin Healing Cream; *Belg.:* Tisane Antibiliaire et Stomachique; Tisane Depurative "les 12 Plantes"; Tisane Diuretique; Tisane Pectorale; Tisane pour le Foie; Tisane Purgative; *Fr.:* Cicaderma†; Hemorrogel; Homeoplasmine; Mediflor Tisane Pectorale d'Alsace; Santane F$_{10}$; Santane H$_7$; Tisanes de l'Abbe Hamon no 14†; Tisanes de l'Abbe Hamon no 6; *Ger.:* Befelka-Oel; bioplant-Kamillenfluid; Cefagastrin; Cefaktivon; Cefaktiven "novum"†; Cefawell; Harntee 400; Hevert-Entwasserungs-Tee†; Hevert-Magen-Galle-Leber-Tee†; JuGrippan†; Nephronorm med†; Salus Abfuhr-Tee Nr. 2†; Salus Bronchial-Tee Nr.8†; Salus Leber-Galle-Tee Nr.18†; Salus Rheuma-Tee Krautertee Nr. 12†; Unguentum lymphaticum; Urodil Blasen-Nieren Arzneitee†; *Ital.:* Alkagin; Babygella; Fluxoten†; Lenirose; Sanaderm†; *Port.:* Cicaderma; *Spain:* Banoftal; *Switz.:* Alpina Gel a la consoude†; Alpina Pommade au souci†; Cetona Plus; Gel a la consoude; Keppur; Pommade Po-Ho N A Vogel; Urinex (nouvelle formule); *UK:* Balsamicum; Massage Balm Calendula; Oleum Rhinale; Savlon Natural First Aid for Burns; Savlon Natural First Aid for Cuts & Sores; Savlon Natural First Aid for Insect Bites & Stings; WCS Dusting Powder; *USA:* Nasal-Ease.

Calumba (526-r)

Calumba Root; Colombo.
Pharmacopoeias. In Jpn.

The dried root of *Jateorhiza palmata* (*=J. columba*) (Menispermaceae).

Profile

Calumba has been used as a bitter and as a flavour.

Preparations

Proprietary Preparations (details are given in Part 3)
Multi-ingredient: *Fr.:* Ducase†; *Ital.:* Bitteridina; *Switz.:* Padma-Lax; *UK:* Appetiser Mixture; Pegina; Travel-Caps.

Camostat Mesilate (3922-e)

Camostat Mesylate *(pINNM).*
Camostat Mesylate; FOY-305. N,N-Dimethylcarbamoylmethyl 4-(4-guanidinobenzoyloxy)phenylacetate methanesulphonate.
$C_{20}H_{22}N_4O_5,CH_4O_3S = 494.5.$
CAS — 59721-28-7 (camostat); 59721-29-8 (camostat mesilate).
Pharmacopoeias. In Jpn.

Profile

Camostat mesilate is a protease inhibitor that has been used in the treatment of pancreatitis (p.1646) and postoperative reflux oesophagitis (p.1204). The usual dose is 100 to 200 mg three times daily by mouth.

Preparations

Proprietary Preparations (details are given in Part 3)
Jpn: Foipan.

Camphor (263-j)

Alcanfor; 2-Camphanone; D-Camphor (natural); Camphora; Camphre Droit (natural); Camphre du Japon (natural); Cânfora; Kamfer. Bornan-2-one; 1,7,7-Trimethylbicyclo[2.2.1]heptan-2-one.
$C_{10}H_{16}O = 152.2.$
CAS — 76-22-2(±); 464-49-3 (+); 464-48-2 (−); 21368-68-3 (±).
ATC — C01EB02.
Pharmacopoeias. In Chin., Eur. (see p.vi), Jpn, Pol., and US; some only describe natural camphor and some only synthetic camphor; Eur. and Jpn have separate monographs for natural and racemic or synthetic camphor.

A liquid or soft mass is formed when camphor is triturated with chloral hydrate, menthol, phenol, and many other substances. Camphor is readily powdered by triturating with a few drops of alcohol, ether, or chloroform.

Pharmacopoeial description

Ph. Eur.: Racemic Camphor is a white crystalline powder or friable crystalline masses, highly volatile even at room temperature. Slightly soluble in water; very soluble in alcohol, in ether, and in petroleum spirit; very slightly soluble in glycerol; freely soluble in fatty oils.
D-Camphor is a white crystalline powder or friable crystalline masses, highly volatile even at room temperature. Slightly soluble in water; very soluble in alcohol and in petroleum spirit; very slightly soluble in glycerol; freely soluble in fatty oils.
USP 25: Camphor is a ketone obtained from *Cinnamomum camphora* (Lauraceae) or produced synthetically. The natural product is dextrorotatory and the synthetic product is optically inactive.
Colourless or white crystals, granules, or crystalline masses, or colourless to white, translucent, tough masses with a penetrating characteristic odour. It slowly volatilises at ordinary temperatures.
Soluble 1 in 800 of water, 1 in 1 of alcohol, 1 in 0.5 of chloroform, and 1 in 1 of ether; freely soluble in carbon disulfide, in petroleum spirit, and in fixed and volatile oils. Store at a temperature not exceeding 40° in airtight containers.

Adverse Effects

In addition to accidental ingestion of preparations containing camphor, poisoning has also occurred after giving camphorated oil (camphor liniment) to children in mistake for castor oil. The symptoms include nausea, vomiting, colic, headache, dizziness, a feeling of warmth, delirium, muscle twitching, epileptiform convulsions, depression of the CNS, and coma. Breathing is difficult and the breath has a characteristic odour; anuria may occur. Death from respiratory failure or status epilepticus may occur; fatalities in children have been recorded from 1 g. There have been reports of instant collapse in infants following the local application of camphor to their nostrils.

Treatment of Adverse Effects

Gastric lavage may be considered if the patient presents within 1 hour of ingestion; any convulsions must be controlled first. Activated charcoal may be given by mouth. Convulsions may be controlled by the slow intravenous administration of diazepam; alternative antiepileptics such as phenobarbital or phenytoin may also be required. Haemodialysis with a lipid dialysate or haemoperfusion have been tried but are of doubtful value.

Precautions

Camphor should not be applied to the nostrils of infants even in small quantities, as this may cause immediate collapse.

◊ The UK Committee on the Review of Medicines[1] recommended that camphor should not be included in products intended for the treatment of hepatic and biliary disorders, gallstones, colic, renal disorders, urinary-tract infections, or ureteral stones. The administration of camphor parenterally or as irrigants was undesirable due to the associated safety hazard.

1. Anonymous. Camphorated oil: licensing authority takes action on camphor products. *Pharm J* 1984; **232:** 792.

Pharmacokinetics

Camphor is readily absorbed from all administration sites. It is hydroxylated in the liver to yield hydroxycamphor metabolites

---

The symbol † denotes a preparation no longer actively marketed

which are then conjugated with glucuronic acid and excreted in the urine. Camphor crosses the placenta.

Uses and Administration
Applied externally, camphor acts as a rubefacient and mild analgesic (see p.4) and is employed in liniments as a counter-irritant in fibrositis, neuralgia, and similar conditions. It is also an ingredient of many inhaled nasal decongestant preparations but it is of doubtful efficacy. The use of camphor liniment (camphorated oil) is discouraged because of its potential toxicity. It has been withdrawn from the market in both the UK and the USA. In the USA the concentration of camphor in preparations for external use may not exceed 11%.

Taken internally camphor has irritant and carminative properties and has been used as a mild expectorant. It has also been used in mixed preparations for cardiovascular disorders.

Preparations
BP 2001: Camphorated Opium Tincture; Concentrated Camphor Water; Concentrated Camphorated Opium Tincture;
USP 25: Camphor Spirit; Camphorated Parachlorophenol; Flexible Collodion.

Proprietary Preparations (details are given in Part 3)
Fr.: Camphrice Du Canada; **Ger.:** Camphoderm N; Divinal Rheumat†; Mulmicor; Pectocor N; Rheunervol N; Trauma-Salbe Rodler 303 N†; **UK:** Zi.

Multi-ingredient: numerous preparations are listed in Part 3.

Camylofin Hydrochloride (5230-f)
Camylofin Hydrochloride (rINNM).
Acamylophenine Hydrochloride; Camylofin Dihydrochloride. Isopentyl 2-(2-diethylaminoethylamino)-2-phenylacetate dihydrochloride.
$C_{19}H_{32}N_2O_2,2HCl = 393.4$.
$CAS — 54-30-8$ (camylofin); 5892-41-1 (camylofin hydrochloride).

Profile
Camylofin is used as an antispasmodic, usually in combination preparations. It is usually used as the hydrochloride; the bis(noramidopyrine mesilate) and the sodium salts have also been used.

Overdosage. Ingestion of large doses of camylofin by two infants produced symptoms similar to those of opioid intoxication.[1] Both infants responded to treatment with naloxone.
1. Schvartsman S, et al. Camylofin intoxication reversed by naloxone. Lancet 1988; ii: 1246.

Preparations
Proprietary Preparations (details are given in Part 3)
Multi-ingredient: Aust.: Avamigran; Spasmo-Urolong†; **Braz.:** Espasmo Silidron; **Fr.:** Avafortan.

Cannabis (842-w)
Cáñamo Indiano; Cannab.; Cannabis Indica; Chanvre; Hanfkraut; Indian Hemp.
$CAS — 8063-14-7$.

NOTE. Cannabis has also been known as: Ait makhlif, Aliamba, Anassa, Anhascha, Assyuni, Bambalacha, Bambia, Bangi-Aku, Bango, Bangue, Bhang, Bhangaku, Canapa, Cangonha, Canhama, Cannacoro, Can-Yac, Caroçuda, Chur ganja, Chutras, Chutsao, Da-boa, Dacha, Dagga, Darakte-Bang, Diamba, Dirijo, Djamba, Djoma, Dokka, Donajuanita, Dormilona, Durijo, Elva, Erva maligna, Erva do norte, Esrar, Fêmea, Fininha, Finote, Fokkra, Fumo brabo, Fumo de caboclo, Gandia, Ganga, Ganja, Ganjila, Gnaoui, Gongo, Gozah, Grahni Sherdool, Greefe, Grifa, Guabza, Guaza, Gunjah, Gunza, Hamp, Haouzi, Hen-Nab, Hursini, Hashish, Igbo, Indischehennepkruid, Indisk hampa, Intianhamppu, Intsangu, Isangu, Janjah, Jatiphaladya churna, Jea, Juana, Kanab, Karpura rasa, Khanh-Chha, Khanje, Kif, Kif Ktami, Kinnab, Liamba, Lianda, Maconha, Maconia, Madi, Magiyam, Makhlif, Malva, Maraguango, Marigongo, Marihuana, Marijuana, Mariquita, Maruamba, Matekwane, Mbanje, Meconha, Misari, Mnoana, Momea, Mota, Mulatinha, Mundyadi vatika, Namba, Ntsangu, Nwonkaka, Peinka, Penek, Penka, Pito, Pot, Pretinha, Rafe, Rafi, Rafo, Riamba, Rongony, Rora, Rosa Maria, Sabsi, Sadda, Siddhi, Soñadora, Soussi, Subji, Summitates cannabis, Suruma, Tahgalim, Takrouri, Tedrika, Teloeut, Teriaki, Tronadora, Umya, Urumogi, Wee, Wewe, Yamba, Yoruba, Zacate chino, Zerouali, and Ziele konopi indyjskich.
Synonyms and approximate synonyms for cannabis resin included: Bheng, Charas, Charris, Chira, Churrus, Chus, Garaouich, Garawiche, Garoarsch, Gauja, Hachiche, Hascisc, Hashish, Hasis, Hasji's, Hasjisj, Haszysz, Haxixe, Heloua, Kamonga, Malak, Manzul, Momeka, N'rama, and Sighirma.
Pharmacoeias. In Chin.

The dried flowering or fruiting tops of the pistillate plant of *Cannabis sativa* (Cannabinaceae). In the UK cannabis is defined by law as any part of any plant of the genus *Cannabis.* *Marihuana* usually refers to a mixture of the leaves and flowering tops. *Bhang, dagga, ganja, kif,* and *maconha* are commonly used in various countries to describe similar preparations. *Hashish* and *charas* are names often applied to the resin, although in some countries *hashish* is applied to any cannabis preparation.

A series of cannabinoids has been extracted from the drug, the most important being Δ^9-tetrahydrocannabinol (dronabinol), Δ^8-tetrahydrocannabinol, Δ^9-tetrahydrocannabinolic acid, cannabinol, and cannabidiol. Cannabinol and cannabidiol may be present in large amounts but have little activity. The amount of Δ^9-tetrahydrocannabinol may average 1, 3, and 5% in marihuana, ganja, and hashish respectively.

Dependence
It has been reported that the prolonged heavy use of cannabis could lead to tolerance and psychological dependence but that physical dependence had not been demonstrated. There have been occasional reports of non-specific symptoms such as anorexia, anxiety, insomnia, irritability, restlessness, sweating, headache, and mild gastrointestinal upsets occurring when cannabis is withdrawn.

Adverse Effects, Treatment, and Precautions
Nausea and vomiting may be the first effects of cannabis taken by mouth. The most frequent physical effects of cannabis intoxication are an increase in heart rate with alterations in blood pressure, conjunctival congestion, dry mouth, and increased appetite. Deterioration in motor coordination is common and cannabis has been reported to affect driving. The psychological effects include elation, distortion of time and space, irritability, and disturbances of memory and judgement. Anxiety or panic reactions may occur, particularly in inexperienced users. These reactions do not usually require specific therapy; diazepam may be necessary for severe reactions. Psychotic episodes of a paranoid or schizophrenic nature, and usually acute, have occurred in subjects taking cannabis, especially in large doses or after the use of varieties bred for a high yield of cannabinoids (so-called skunk).

◊ Some reviews of the adverse effects of cannabis.
1. Nahas GG. Cannabis: toxicological properties and epidemiological aspects. Med J Aust 1986; 145: 82–7.
2. Johnson BA. Psychopharmacological effects of cannabis. Br J Hosp Med 1990; 43: 114–22.
3. American Academy of Pediatrics. Marijuana: a continuing concern for pediatricians. Pediatrics 1991; 88: 1070–2.
4. Wills S. Cannabis and cocaine. Pharm J 1993; 251: 483–5.
5. Hall W, Solowij N. Adverse effects of cannabis. Lancet 1998; 352: 1611–16.
6. Ashton CH. Adverse effects of cannabis and cannabinoids. Br J Anaesth 1999; 83: 637–49.

Coma. Coma, reversed by flumazenil, has been reported in 2 children who had ingested cannabis.[1]
1. Rubio F, et al. Flumazenil for coma reversal in children after cannabis. Lancet 1993; 341: 1028–9.

Effects on the eyes. A report of persistent visual abnormalities in a patient following discontinuation of heavy abuse of hashish.[1] No organic cause for the effects, which were accompanied by less persistent mental changes, could be found.
1. Laffi GL, Safran AB. Persistent visual changes following hashish consumption. Br J Ophthalmol 1993; 77: 601–2.

Hyperthermia. Life-threatening hyperthermia was reported[1] in a 24-year-old man who went jogging after smoking cannabis.
1. Walter FG, et al. Marijuana and hyperthermia. J Toxicol Clin Toxicol 1996; 34: 217–21.

Pregnancy. Cannabis has effects on sperm and can alter reproductive hormonal systems. Infants born to mothers exposed to cannabis during pregnancy tend to have a lower birthweight[1,2] and may suffer from increased excitation in the postnatal period.[3]
1. Zuckerman B, et al. Effects of maternal marijuana and cocaine use on fetal growth. N Engl J Med 1989; 320: 762–8.
2. Frank DA, et al. Neonatal body proportionality and body composition after in utero exposure to cocaine and marijuana. J Pediatr 1990; 117: 622–6.
3. Silverman S. Interaction of drug-abusing mother, fetus, types of drugs examined in numerous studies. JAMA 1989; 261: 1689, 1693.

Psychosis. References to psychosis associated with cannabis.
1. Rottanburg D, et al. Cannabis-associated psychoses with hypomanic features. Lancet 1982; ii: 1364–6.
2. Andréasson S, et al. Cannabis and schizophrenia: a longitudinal study of Swedish conscripts. Lancet 1987; ii: 1483–6.
3. Wylie AS, et al. Psychosis due to "skunk". BMJ 1995; 311: 125.
4. McKay DR, Tennant CC. Is the grass greener? The link between cannabis and psychosis. Med J Aust 2000; 172: 284–6.

Interactions
Cannabis and alcohol have additive effects. The sedative effects of cannabis may be potentiated by other CNS depressants. Additive antimuscarinic effects, for example tachycardia, may occur with concomitant use of drugs such as tricyclic antidepressants. Cannabis induces microsomal enzymes and therefore interactions with a wide range of drugs that are metabolised by these enzymes might be expected (see, for example, Theophylline, p.781).

Disulfiram. Limited evidence indicates that a combination of disulfiram and cannabis may produce a hypomanic state.[1]
1. Lacoursiere RB, Swatek R. Adverse interaction between disulfiram and marijuana: a case report. Am J Psychiatry 1983; 140: 243–4.

Pharmacokinetics
The active principles of cannabis are absorbed from the gastrointestinal tract and the lungs.
About 50% of the Δ^9-tetrahydrocannabinol available in cannabis is present in the smoke inhaled from a whole cannabis cigarette. This produces an effect almost immediately, reaches a peak in 20 to 30 minutes, and is dissipated in about 3 to 4 hours. When cannabis is taken by mouth absorption may be slow and irregular. Effects are not seen for 30 minutes to 1 hour and persist for about 8 hours.
Tetrahydrocannabinol is lipophilic and becomes widely distributed in the body. It crosses the placenta and is distributed into breast milk. It is extensively metabolised, primarily in the liver, to the active 11-hydroxy derivative; both are extensively bound to plasma proteins. It is excreted in the urine and faeces, sometimes over prolonged periods. Excretion may be more rapid in chronic users.

Uses and Administration
Cannabis was formerly employed as a sedative or narcotic. Its main active constituent Δ^9-tetrahydrocannabinol (dronabinol, p.1224) and a synthetic cannabinoid (nabilone, p.1237) are used as antiemetics in patients receiving cancer chemotherapy; they are also being investigated for a number of other potential therapeutic uses. Cannabis has analgesic, muscle relaxant, and appetite stimulant effects and reduces intra-ocular pressure. Anecdotal reports exist of benefit from cannabis in a variety of disorders including glaucoma, multiple sclerosis, and wasting in patients with AIDS and malignant neoplasms.

◊ References to the potential medical uses of cannabis.
1. Doyle E, Spence AA. Cannabis as a medicine? Br J Anaesth 1995; 74: 359–61.
2. Gray C. Cannabis—the therapeutic potential. Pharm J 1995; 254: 771–3.
3. Grinspoon L, Bakalar JB. Marihuana as a medicine: a plea for reconsideration. JAMA 1995; 273: 1875–6.
4. Wills S. The use of cannabis in multiple sclerosis. Pharm J 1995; 225: 237–8.
5. Voth EA, Schwartz RH. Medicinal applications of delta-9-tetrahydrocannabinol and marijuana. Ann Intern Med 1997; 126: 791–8.
6. British Medical Association. Therapeutic uses of cannabis. Amsterdam: Harwood Academic, 1997.
7. Robson P. Cannabis as medicine: time for the phoenix to rise? BMJ 1998; 316: 1034–5.

Canola Oil (17665-l)
Profile
Canola oil is a form of rape oil (p.1657) from strains selected for low erucic acid content. It is used as an edible oil and in pharmaceutical manufacturing and cosmetics.

Cantharides (12517-g)
Blistering Beetle; Cantharis; Insectes Coléoptères Hétéromères; Lytta; Méloides; Russian Flies; Spanish Fly.

The dried beetle *Cantharis vesicatoria* (=*Lytta vesicatoria*) (Meloidae) or other spp., containing not less than 0.6% of cantharidin.

Adverse Effects
Following ingestion of cantharides there is burning pain in the throat and stomach, difficulty in swallowing, nausea, vomiting, haematemesis, abdominal pain, bloody diarrhoea, tenesmus, renal pain, frequent micturition, haematuria, uraemia, severe hypotension, and circulatory failure. Oral doses of cantharidin (the active ingredient of cantharides) of less than 65 mg have been lethal. A dose of 1 mg or contact with one insect can produce distressing symptoms. Skin contact results in blisters.

◊ References.
1. Hundt HKL, et al. Post-mortem serum concentration of cantharidin in a fatal case of cantharides poisoning. Hum Exp Toxicol 1990; 9: 35–40.

Uses and Administration
Preparations of cantharides have been employed externally as rubefacients, counter-irritants, and vesicants. They should not be taken internally or applied over large surfaces owing to the risk of absorption. The use of cantharides in cosmetic products is prohibited in the UK by law.
Cantharides is used in homoeopathic medicine.
Mylabris (Chinese blistering beetle; Chinese cantharides; Indian blistering beetle), the dried beetles of the species *Mylabris sidae* (= *M. phalerata*), *M. cichorii*, and *M. pustulator*, has been used as a substitute for cantharides and as a source of cantharidin (see below) in the East.

Cantharidin (12518-q)
Hexahydro-3aα,7aα-dimethyl-4β,7β-epoxyisobenzofuran-1,3-dione.
$C_{10}H_{12}O_4 = 196.2$.
$CAS — 56-25-7$.

Cantharidin is obtained from cantharides or mylabris (see under Cantharides, above).

Profile
Cantharidin in flexible collodion has been applied for the removal of warts. It has also been used in veterinary medicine. Owing to the high toxicity of cantharidin it has been recommended that preparations containing it should not be used me-

dicinally. Adverse effects are those described for cantharides (see above).

Preparations

Proprietary Preparations (details are given in Part 3)
Canad.: Canthacur; Cantharone; *Singapore:* Canthacur; *USA:* Verr-Canth†.

Multi-ingredient: *Canad.:* Canthacur-PS; Cantharone Plus.

Capsicum (4617-w)

Capsic.; Capsici Fructus; Chillies; Piment Rouge; Pimentão; Spanischer Pfeffer.
CAS — 404-86-4 (capsaicin).

NOTE. Ground cayenne pepper of commerce is normally a blend of varieties of capsicum. Paprika is from *Capsicum annuum* var. *longum*; it is milder than capsicum.
Pharmacopoeias. In Aust., Ger., It., Jpn, Swiss, and US.
US also includes capsicum oleoresin (capsicin).

Pharmacopoeial description

USP 25: The dried ripe fruits of *Capsicum frutescens*, known in commerce as African Chillies, or of *C. annuum* var. *connoides*, known in commerce as Tabasco Pepper, or *C. annuum* var. *longum*, known in commerce as Louisiana Long Pepper, or of a hybrid between the Honka variety of Japanese Capsicum and the Old Louisiana Sport Capsicum, known in commerce as Louisiana Sport Pepper. An off-white powder. M.p. about 65°. Practically insoluble in cold water; soluble in alcohol, in chloroform, and in benzene; slightly soluble in carbon disulfide.

Capsicum Oleoresin is an alcoholic extract of the dried ripe fruits of *Capsicum annum* var. *minimum* and small fruited varieties of *C. fruiscons* (Solanaceae). It contains not less than 8% of total capsaicins. It is a dark red oily liquid. Soluble in alcohol, in acetone, in chloroform, in ether, and in volatile oils; soluble with opalescence in fixed oils. Store in airtight containers.

Profile

Capsicum has a carminative action but it is mainly used externally, often in the form of capsicum oleoresin, as a counter-irritant (see Rubefacients and Topical Analgesia, p.4). It is also included in preparations for the management of cough and cold symptoms. However, preparations of capsicum and capsicum oleoresin can be very irritant. Capsaicin (p.23), the active ingredient of capsicum, is also used in topical preparations in the treatment of painful skin conditions.

Capsicum oleoresin is used in 'pepper sprays' for law enforcement and self defence.

Capsicum is also used in homoeopathic medicine and in cookery.

Effects on the gastrointestinal tract. The initial response to the ingestion of a hot pepper is a hot or burning sensation in the mouth which is attributed to the binding of capsaicin to receptors in the oral cavity.[1] Casein-containing substances such as milk can reverse this burning sensation, apparently by displacing capsaicin due to their lipophilicity.

Spicy meals have long been associated with gastrointestinal discomfort and ingestion of meals containing 1.5 g of red or black pepper has been shown to cause signs of gastric mucosal damage comparable to those caused by a 625-mg dose of aspirin.[2] However, other studies in *animals*[3] and humans[4,5] suggest that capsaicin may have a protective effect on gastric mucosa. Ingestion of approximately 30 g of jalapeño peppers (a capsicum fruit) caused no visible damage to the duodenal or gastric mucosa of 12 healthy subjects[6] and daily ingestion of meals containing a total of 3 g of chilli powder did not affect the clinical progress of patients with duodenal ulcers given antacids.[7]

1. Henkin R. Cooling the burn from hot peppers. *JAMA* 1991; **266:** 2766.
2. Myers BM, *et al.* Effect of red pepper and black pepper on the stomach. *Am J Gastroenterol* 1987; **82:** 211–14.
3. Holzer P. Peppers, capsaicin, and the gastric mucosa. *JAMA* 1989; **261:** 3244.
4. Kang JY, *et al.* Chili—protective factor against peptic ulcer? *Dig Dis Sci* 1995; **40:** 576–9.
5. Yeoh KG, *et al.* Chili protects against aspirin-induced gastroduodenal mucosal injury in humans. *Dig Dis Sci* 1995; **40:** 580–3.
6. Graham DY, *et al.* Spicy food and the stomach: evaluation by videoendoscopy. *JAMA* 1988; **260:** 3473–5.
7. Kumar N, *et al.* Do chillies influence healing of duodenal ulcer? *BMJ* 1984; **288:** 1803–4.

Preparations

Proprietary Preparations (details are given in Part 3)
Aust.: ABC; Capsiplast; *Austral.:* Shingles Pain Relief; *Ger.:* Capsamol; Dolenon; Kneipp Rheuma Salbe; Rheumaplast N; Thermo Burger; *Ital.:* Cerotto Bertelli Arnikos; Dolpyc; Thermogene; *Mex.:* Capsidol; *UK:* Fiery Jack.

Multi-ingredient: *Aust.:* Mayfit chronisch†; Mentopin; Red Point; Salhumin; Trauma-warmend; Traumasalbe; *Austral.:* APR Cream; Bioglan Joint Mobility; Bioglan The Blue One; Capsolin; For Peripheral Circulation Herbal Plus Formula 5; Gingo A; Goanna Heat Cream; Lifesystem Herbal Formula 6 For Peripheral Circulation; Radian-B; Thermalife C†; Valerian; *Belg.:* Dolpyc†; Rado-Salil; Stilene; *Canad.:* Absorbine Athritis; Herbalax Forte†; Phytolax†; Rheumalan; Rhumatisme; *Fr.:* Baume Saint-Bernard†; Capsic; Disalgyl; Dolpyc†; Kamol; Le Thermogene; *Ger.:* ABC Warme-Pflaster N; Caye Balsam; Finalgon N Schmerzpflaster†; Hewedolor; *Israel:* Mento-O-Cap; Radian-B; Rublex Massage Cream; *Ital.:* Capso; Capsolin; Remy; Sloan; *Neth.:* Sloan's

balsem; *Port.:* Balsamo Analgesico; Balsamo Analgesico Sanitas; Caroid; Dologel; Medalginan; *S.Afr.:* Chisi†; Radian†; Sportsman Rub; *Spain:* Balsamo Midalgan; Dolokey; Embrocacion Gras; Killpan; Linimento Klari; Linimento Naion; Linimento Sloan; Pomada Revulsiva†; Termosan; *Swed.:* Sloan's liniment†; *Switz.:* Capsolin†; Embropax; Emplatre Croix D; Incutin; Massorax; Midalgan; Sloan Baume†; Sloan Liniment†; *Thai.:* Flatulence Gastulence; Meloids; Veracolate; *UK:* Algipan; Allcock's Porous Capsicum Plaster; Allens Dry Tickly Cough; Balmosa; Buttercup Syrup; Cremalgin; Fiery Jack; Hactos; Hansaplast Herbal Heat Plaster; Herbal Indigestion Naturtabs; Honey & Molasses; Indian Brandee; Indigestion and Flatulence; Indigestion and Flatulence Tablets; Indigestion Relief; Jamaican Sarsaparilla; Kilkof; Life Drops; Potters Sugar Free Cough Pastilles; Radian-B; Ralgex; Rheumatic Pain Relief; Sanderson's Throat Specific; Vegetable Cough Remover; *USA:* Throat Discs; Veracolate†.

Caraway (4619-l)

Alcaravia; Caraway Fruit; Caraway Seed; Carum; Cumin des Prés; Fructus Carvi; Kümmel.
Pharmacopoeias. In Eur. (see p.vi) and Pol.

Pharmacopoeial description

Ph. Eur.: The whole, dried fruits of *Carum carvi*. It contains not less than 3.0% v/w of essential oil, calculated with reference to the dried drug. It has an odour reminiscent of carvone. Protect from light.

BP 2001: directs that when Powdered Caraway is prescribed or demanded, material complying with the appropriate requirements of the Ph. Eur. monograph for Caraway and containing not less than 2.5% v/w of essential oil shall be dispensed or supplied.

Profile

Caraway is an aromatic carminative, and is used in gastrointestinal disorders and as a flavour. The seeds are used in cookery. It is the source of caraway oil.

Preparations

Proprietary Preparations (details are given in Part 3)
Multi-ingredient: *Aust.:* Abbiofort; Absimed; Aktiv milder Magen- und Darmtee; Aponatura Wind; Apotheker Bauer's Magentee; Bio-Garten Tee fur den Magen; Bio-Garten Tee gegen Blahungen; Bio-Garten Tropfen gegen Blahungen; Carminative; Karvisin; Krauterdoktor Magen-Darmtropfen; Krauterhaus Mag Kottas Babytee; Krauterhaus Mag Kottas Tee fur die Verdauung; Krauterhaus Mag Kottas Tee gegen Blahungen; Krautertee Nr 107; Krautertee Nr 126; Krautertee Nr 14; Krautertee Nr 17; Krautertee Nr 217; Mag Kottas Baby-Tee; Mag Kottas Blahungs-Verdauungstee; Mag Kottas Tee fur stillende Mutter; Magentee; Midro Tee; Montana; Myrtilen; Naturland Verdauungs; Nesthakchen; Sanvita Verdauungstropfen†; Sidroga Leber-Galle-Tee; Species Carvi comp; St Radegunder Blahungstreibender Tee; St Radegunder Verdauungstee; Windtreibender Tee; *Braz.:* Balsamo Branco; *Fr.:* Santane C₆; Santane D₅; Santane F₁₀; Santane O₁; Tisane des Familles; Tisane Digestive Weleda†; *Ger.:* Agamadon N†; Carminativum-Hetterich N; Carminativum-Pascoe; Cholosom-Tee; Divinal Gastro†; Echtroferment-N†; Floradix Multipretten; Gastrol S; Gastrosecur; Hevert-Carmin symbio; Iberogast; Kneipp Flatuol; Kneipp Magen-Tee; Lomatol; Majocarmin-Tee; Meteophyt S; Montana; Presselin Blahungs K 4 N; Presselin Dyspeptikum; Stomachicon N; Stovalid N; *Israel:* Jungborn; Lido Tea; Midro-Tea; *Ital.:* Florelax; Midro; *Switz.:* Adistop Lax†; Ajaka†; Kernosan Heidelberger Poudre; Phytomed Gastro†; Tisane favorisant l'allaitement; Tisane laxative Natterman no 13†; *UK:* Carminative Tea; Laxadoron.

Caraway Oil (4620-v)

Kümmelöl; Oleum Cari; Oleum Carui; Oleum Carvi.
Pharmacopoeias. In Aust., Br., and Ger.

Pharmacopoeial description

BP 2001: A clear, colourless or pale yellow liquid, visibly free from water, with an odour of caraway. It is obtained by distillation from caraway. It contains 53 to 63% w/w of ketones calculated as carvone ($C_{10}H_{14}O$). At 20° it is soluble 1 in 7 of alcohol (80%). Store at a temperature not exceeding 25° in well-filled containers. Protect from light.

Profile

Caraway oil is an aromatic carminative and is used in gastrointestinal disorders and as a flavour. It is also employed as caraway water for infant colic (see Gastrointestinal Spasm, p.1204).

Preparations

BP 2001: Aromatic Cardamom Tincture; Compound Cardamom Tincture.

Proprietary Preparations (details are given in Part 3)
Multi-ingredient: *Aust.:* Nesthakchen; Parodontax†; Pascopankreat; Sanvita Magen; Sigman-Haustropfen; Spasmo Claim; *Ger.:* Aspasmon N; Benium†; Enteroplant; Euflat I; Floradix Multipretten; Galloselect M; Gastricard N; Grunlicht Magenbalsam Tropfen; Hevert-Carmin symbio; Hevert-Gall S; Kneipp Rheuma Stoffwechsel-Bad Heublumen-Aquasan†; Lomatol; Neo-Ballistol; Pascopankreat novo; Pascopankreat S†; ratioGast; Roflatol Phyto (Rowo-146)†; Sirmia Abfuhrkapseln†; *Switz.:* Ajaka†; Capsules laxatives Nattermann Nr. 13†; Flatulex; Huile Po-Ho A. Vogel; *UK:* Atkinson & Barker's Gripe Mixture; Nurse Harvey's Gripe Mixture.

Carbon-13 (18909-n)

CAS — 14762-74-4.

Profile

Carbon-13 is a naturally occurring, non-radioactive, stable isotope of carbon. It has been used to label organic compounds, such as urea (p.1127), for use in diagnostic tests.

Preparations

Proprietary Preparations (details are given in Part 3)
Ital.: Pylobactell; *Spain:* Tau Kit; *Swed.:* Diabact UBT; *UK:* Pylobactell; *USA:* Meretek UBT.

Multi-ingredient: *USA:* Ez-HBT.

Cardamom Fruit (4621-g)

Cardam. Fruit; Cardamom Seed; Cardamomi Fructus.
Pharmacopoeias. In Br. and Jpn.

Pharmacopoeial description

BP 2001: The dried, nearly ripe fruit of *Elettaria cardamomum* var. *minuscula*. Only the seeds are used in making preparations of cardamom and they are used immediately after removal from the fruit. The seeds should not be stored after removal from the fruit. They have a strongly aromatic odour and taste and contain not less than 4% v/w of volatile oil.

Profile

Preparations of cardamom fruit are used as carminatives and as flavours. The seeds are used in cookery.

Cardamom fruit is the source of cardamom oil.

Preparations

Proprietary Preparations (details are given in Part 3)
Multi-ingredient: *Aust.:* Mariazeller; *Austral.:* Peritone; Travelaide; Vitaglow Herbal Laxative†; *Ger.:* Montana; Presselin Dyspeptikum; Schwedentrunk der Echte Elixier; *Ital.:* Sedobex†; *S.Afr.:* Alma; Enterodyne; *Spain:* Digestovital; *Switz.:* Stomacine; *Thai.:* Carmicide; *UK:* Aluminium Free Indigestion†; Indian Brandee; Pegina.

Cardamom Oil (4622-q)

Ol. Cardamom.
Pharmacopoeias. In Br.

Pharmacopoeial description

BP 2001: A clear, colourless or pale yellow liquid, visibly free from water, with an odour of cardamom fruit. It is distilled from crushed cardamom fruit. At 20° it is soluble 1 in 6 of alcohol (70%). Store at a temperature not exceeding 25° in well-filled containers. Protect from light.

Profile

Preparations of cardamom oil are used as carminatives and as flavours.

Preparations

BP 2001: Aromatic Cardamom Tincture; Compound Cardamom Tincture; Compound Rhubarb Tincture.

Carnauba Wax (12527-p)

Caranda Wax; Cera Carnauba; Cera Coperniciae; E903.
CAS — 8015-86-9.
Pharmacopoeias. In Eur. (see p.vi), Int., and Jpn. Also in USNF.

Pharmacopoeial description

Ph. Eur.: It is obtained from the leaves of *Copernicia cerifera*. Pale yellow or yellow powder, flakes, or hard masses. It has a relative density of about 0.97. M.p. 80° to 88°. Practically insoluble in water and in alcohol; soluble in warm ethyl acetate and in warm xylene. Protect from light.

USNF 20: It is obtained from the leaves of *Copernicia cerifera* (Palmae). A light brown to pale yellow, moderately coarse powder or flakes, possessing a characteristic bland odour, and free from rancidity. Sp. gr. about 0.99. M.p. 80° to 86°. Insoluble in water; slightly soluble in boiling alcohol; soluble in warm chloroform and in warm toluene; freely soluble in warm benzene.

Profile

Carnauba wax is used in pharmacy as a coating agent. Various types and grades are used industrially in the manufacture of polishes. Its use is also permitted in certain foods.

Caroverine (19682-g)

Caroverine (pINN).
1-[2-(Diethylamino)ethyl]-3-(p-methoxybenzyl)-2(1H)-quinoxalinone.
$C_{22}H_{27}N_3O_2 = 365.5.$
CAS — 23465-76-1.
ATC — A03AX11.

Profile

Caroverine is a smooth muscle relaxant with calcium-channel blocking and glutamate-antagonist properties. It is used as the

---

The symbol † denotes a preparation no longer actively marketed

base or the hydrochloride in conditions associated with painful smooth muscle spasm. Typical doses (expressed as the base) are 20 to 40 mg by mouth three or four times daily, or 40 to 80 mg by slow intravenous or intramuscular injection, up to a maximum of 200 mg daily; it has also been given rectally. It is also used in cerebral circulatory disorders and in tinnitus.

◊ References.
1. Denk DM, *et al.* Caroverine in tinnitus treatment: a placebo-controlled blind study. *Acta Otolaryngol (Stockh)* 1997; **117**: 825–30.

Preparations
Proprietary Preparations (details are given in Part 3)
Aust.: Spasmium; Tinnitin; *Switz.:* Calmaverine.
Multi-ingredient: *Aust.:* Spagall; Spasmium comp.

Carzenide (11597-j)
Carzenide *(rINN)*.
p-Sulphamoylbenzoic acid.
$C_7H_7NO_4S = 201.2$.
CAS — 138-41-0.

Profile
Carzenide is an antispasmodic which has been used in the treatment of dysmenorrhoea.

Cassia Oil (4624-s)
Chinese Cinnamon Oil; Cinnamomi Cassiae Aetheroleum; Oleum Cassiae; Oleum Cinnamomi; Oleum Cinnamomi Cassiae.
Pharmacopoeias. In Chin., Eur. (see p.vi), and *Jpn.*
Chin. and *Jpn* also include cassia bark which may be known as cinnamon bark. In some countries cassia oil is known as cinnamon oil.

Pharmacopoeial description
Ph. Eur.: The oil obtained by steam distillation of the leaves and young branches of *Cinnamomum cassia (C. aromaticum)*. It contains 70 to 90% of cinnamaldehyde. A clear, mobile, yellow to reddish-brown liquid, with a characteristic odour of cinnamaldehyde. Store in well-filled airtight containers. Protect from light and heat.

Profile
Cassia oil has properties resembling those of cinnamon oil (p.1596) and is used similarly as a carminative and flavour. There have been a number of reports of hypersensitivity to cinnamaldehyde, the main constituent of cassia oil.

Preparations
Proprietary Preparations (details are given in Part 3)
Multi-ingredient: *Austral.:* Tiger Balm Red†; *Ger.:* Grunlicht Hingfong Essenz; *UK:* Dragon Balm.

Castor Oil (7355-v)
Aceite de Ricino; Huile de Ricin; Ol. Ricin.; Oleum Ricini; Ricini Oleum Virginum; Rizinusöl.
ATC — A06AB05.
NOTE. CASOIL is a code approved by the BP 2001 for use on single unit doses of eye drops containing castor oil where the individual container may be too small to bear all the appropriate labelling information.
Pharmacopoeias. In Chin., Eur. (see p.vi), *Jpn*, and *US.*
Eur. and *USNF* also include hydrogenated castor oil.

Pharmacopoeial description
Ph. Eur.: The fatty oil obtained by cold expression from the seeds of *Ricinus communis*. It is a clear, almost colourless or slightly yellow, viscous, hygroscopic liquid. Miscible with alcohol and with glacial acetic acid; slightly soluble in petroleum spirit. Store at a temperature not exceeding 25° in well-filled containers. Protect from light.
Hydrogenated Castor Oil is obtained by hydrogenation of castor oil. It consists mainly of the triglyceride of 12-hydroxystearic acid. Almost white to pale yellow fine powder, masses, or flakes. M.p. 83° to 88°. Practically insoluble in water; very slightly soluble in dehydrated alcohol; freely soluble in dichloromethane; slightly soluble in petroleum spirit. Store in well-filled containers.
USP 25: The fixed oil obtained from the seed of *Ricinus communis* (Euphorbiaceae). It is a pale yellowish or almost colourless, transparent, viscid liquid. Has a faint, mild odour; is free from foreign and rancid odour; and has a bland, characteristic taste. Soluble in alcohol; miscible with dehydrated alcohol, with chloroform, with ether, and with glacial acetic acid. Store in airtight containers at a temperature not exceeding 40°.

Adverse Effects and Precautions
The administration of castor oil by mouth, particularly in large doses, may produce nausea, vomiting, colic, and severe purgation. Castor oil should not be given when intestinal obstruction is present.
The seeds of *Ricinus communis* contain a toxic protein, ricin (p.1658). Allergic reactions have been reported in subjects handling the seeds.

Uses and Administration
Castor oil is used externally for its emollient effect. It has also been used topically to allay irritation due to foreign bodies in the eye. Castor oil may be employed as the solvent in some injections.
Hydrogenated castor oil is used as a stiffening agent. Polyoxyl castor oils (p.1347) are used as emulsifying and solubilising agents.
Castor oil has been used for its laxative action, but such use is obsolete.

Preparations
BP 2001: Chloroxylenol Solution; Flexible Collodion; Zinc and Castor Oil Ointment;
USP 25: Aromatic Castor Oil; Castor Oil Capsules; Castor Oil Emulsion; Flexible Collodion.
Proprietary Preparations (details are given in Part 3)
Canad.: Neoloid; Unisoil†; *Ger.:* Laxopol; *Israel:* Laxopol; *Spain:* Palmil; Ricino Koki; *USA:* Emulsoil; Neoloid; Purge.
Multi-ingredient: *Austral.:* Seda-Rash; *Braz.:* Laxol; Steitonit; *Ital.:* Bal Tar†; Herbatar; *Spain:* Otocerum; *UK:* Exzem Oil; Panda Baby Cream; *USA:* Dermospray; Dr Dermi-Heal; Granulderm; Granulex; GranuMed; Mammol; Medicone Rectal; Proderm.

Catalase (3044-b)
Caperase; Equilase; Optidase.
A protein composed of 4 polypeptide subunits, the precise composition of which varies according to the source, and having a molecular weight of about 240 000.

Profile
Catalase is an enzyme obtained from a wide variety of biological sources including animal liver (hepatocatalase) and certain bacteria and fungi. It has the ability to promote the decomposition of hydrogen peroxide to water and oxygen.
It has been applied to wounds and skin ulcers and has also been used in the treatment of eczema. It has sometimes been used with glucose oxidase (p.1616) in food preservation to break down hydrogen peroxide produced during oxidation of glucose, and is also included in preparations for contact lens care to neutralise hydrogen peroxide.
Catalase is a free-radical scavenger and has been investigated for its ability to limit reperfusion injury thought to be related to free-radical production. Combinations of catalase with superoxide dismutase have also been investigated.

◊ References.
1. Greenwald RA. Superoxide dismutase and catalase as therapeutic agents for human diseases: a critical review. *Free Radic Biol Med* 1990; **8**: 201–9.

Preparations
Proprietary Preparations (details are given in Part 3)
Aust.: Lensan B; Les Yeux 2; Oxysept Quick†; Titmus Losung 2; *Ital.:* Citrizan; *Spain:* Biocatalase.
Multi-ingredient: *Aust.:* Omnicare†; Oxysept Comfort†; Oxysept†; *Belg.:* Pulvo 47; Pulvo Neomycine†; *Canad.:* UltraCare; *Fr.:* Pulvo 47; Pulvo 47 Neomycine; *Ger.:* Oxysept Comfort†; Pulvo; Pulvo Neomycin; *Israel:* Omnicare; Oxysept; *Ital.:* Citrizan Antibiotico; *Neth.:* Rheumajecta; *NZ:* Omnicare 1 Step; *Thai.:* Pulvo 47; *USA:* UltraCare.

Catechu (306-s)
Gambier; Gambir; Pale Catechu.
CAS — 8001-48-7 (catechu); 8001-76-1 (black catechu).
Pharmacopoeias. In Jpn. Also in *BP(Vet).*
Chin. includes Ramulus Uncariae cum Uncis from various species of *Uncaria* and Black Catechu from *Acacia catechu* (Leguminosae).

Pharmacopoeial description
BP(Vet) 2001: A dried aqueous extract of the leaves and young shoots of *Uncaria gambier* occurring as dull pale greyish-brown to dark reddish-brown cubes. Odourless or almost odourless.

Profile
Catechu is an astringent and has been given in preparations for the treatment of diarrhoea and other gastrointestinal disorders.

Preparations
Proprietary Preparations (details are given in Part 3)
Multi-ingredient: *Austral.:* Diarcalm; *Fr.:* Elixir Bonjean; *S.Afr.:* Enterodyne; *UK:* Spanish Tummy Mixture.

CD4 Antibodies (14392-h)
Anti-CD4 Monoclonal Antibodies; CD4mAb; Monoclonal CD4 Antibodies.

Profile
Monoclonal antibodies raised against CD4 receptors are under investigation in the treatment of immunologically mediated disorders, such as rheumatoid arthritis, multiple sclerosis, inflammatory bowel disease, asthma, and various skin disorders, with the aim of decreasing and eliminating circulating helper T

lymphocytes. They have also been tried in transplantation. CD4 antibodies investigated include clenoliximab and keliximab.

◊ References.
1. Mathieson PW, *et al.* Monoclonal-antibody therapy in systemic vasculitis. *N Engl J Med* 1990; **323**: 250–4.
2. Poizot-Martin I, *et al.* Are CD4 antibodies and peptide T new treatments for psoriasis? *Lancet* 1991; **337**: 1477.
3. van der Lubbe PA, *et al.* Anti-CD4 monoclonal antibody for relapsing polychondritis. *Lancet* 1991; **337**: 1349.
4. Prinz J, *et al.* Chimaeric CD4 monoclonal antibody in treatment of generalised pustular psoriasis. *Lancet* 1991; **338**: 320–1.
5. Nicolas JF, *et al.* CD4 antibody treatment of severe psoriasis. *Lancet* 1991; **338**: 321.
6. Choy EHS, *et al.* Chimeric anti-CD4 monoclonal antibody for relapsing polychondritis. *Lancet* 1991; **338**: 450.
7. Heipe F, *et al.* Treatment of severe systemic lupus erythematosus with anti-CD4 monoclonal antibody. *Lancet* 1991; **338**: 1529–30.
8. Horneff G, *et al.* Treatment of rheumatoid arthritis with an anti-CD4 monoclonal antibody. *Arthritis Rheum* 1991; **34**: 129–40.
9. Wendling D, *et al.* Therapeutic use of monoclonal anti-CD4 antibody in rheumatoid arthritis. *J Rheumatol* 1991; **18**: 325–7.
10. Robinet E, *et al.* CD4 monoclonal antibody administration in atopic dermatitis. *J Am Acad Dermatol* 1997; **36**: 582–8.
11. van Oosten BW, *et al.* CD4 antibody treatment in multiple sclerosis with the monoclonal anti-CD4 antibody cM-T412: results of a randomized, double-blind, placebo-controlled, MR-monitored phase II trial. *Neurology* 1997; **49**: 351–7.
12. Stronkhorst A, *et al.* CD4 antibody treatment in patients with active Crohn's disease: a phase I dose finding study. *Gut* 1997; **40**: 320–7.
13. Cooperative Clinical Trials in Transplantation Research Group. Murine OKT4A immunosuppression in cadaver donor renal allograft recipients: a cooperative clinical trials in transplantation pilot study. *Transplantation* 1997; **15**: 1243–51.
14. Kon OM, *et al.* Randomised, dose-ranging, placebo-controlled study of chimeric antibody to CD4 (keliximab) in chronic severe asthma. *Lancet* 1998; **352**: 1109–13.
15. Yocum DE, *et al.* Clinical and immunologic effects of a PRIMATIZED anti-CD4 monoclonal antibody in active rheumatoid arthritis: results of a phase I, single dose, dose escalating trial. *J Rheumatol* 1998; **25**: 1257–62.
16. Wendling D, *et al.* A randomized, double blind, placebo controlled multicenter trial of murine anti-CD4 monoclonal antibody therapy in rheumatoid arthritis. *J Rheumatol* 1998; **25**: 1457–61.
17. Gottlieb AB, *et al.* Anti-CD4 monoclonal antibody treatment of moderate to severe psoriasis vulgaris: results of a pilot, multicenter, multiple-dose, placebo-controlled study. *J Am Acad Dermatol* 2000; **43**: 595–604.

CDP-571 (1460-b)

Profile
CDP-571 is a humanised monoclonal antibody to tumour necrosis factor. It is under investigation in the treatment of Crohn's disease, ulcerative colitis, and rheumatoid arthritis.

◊ References.
1. Rankin EC, *et al.* The therapeutic effects of an engineered human anti-tumour necrosis factor alpha antibody (CDP571) in rheumatoid arthritis. *Br J Rheumatol* 1995; **34**: 334–42.
2. Evans RC, *et al.* Treatment of ulcerative colitis with an engineered human anti-TNF antibody CDP571. *Aliment Pharmacol Ther* 1997; **11**: 1031–5.
3. Stack WA, *et al.* Randomised controlled trial of CDP571 antibody to tumour necrosis factor-α in Crohn's disease. *Lancet* 1997; **349**: 521–4.

Celery (4626-e)
Apium; Celery Fruit; Celery Seed.
CAS — 8015-90-5 (celery oil).
The dried ripe fruits of celery, *Apium graveolens* (Umbelliferae). Other parts of the plant are also used.

Profile
Celery is reported to have diuretic properties and has been included in herbal preparations for rheumatic disorders. Celery oil has also been used as a spasmolytic. Allergic and photoallergic reactions have been reported.
Celery is also used in homoeopathic medicine.

◊ References.
1. Houghton P. Bearberry, dandelion and celery. *Pharm J* 1995; **255**: 272–3.

Interactions. For a report of severe phototoxicity occurring in a patient who had consumed celery soup before undergoing PUVA therapy, see Interactions under Methoxsalen, p.1119.

Preparations
Proprietary Preparations (details are given in Part 3)
Multi-ingredient: *Austral.:* Arthritic Pain Herbal Formula 1; Devils Claw Plus; Fluid Loss; Lifesystem Herbal Formula 1 Arthritic Aid; *Ger.:* Nephrubin†; *UK:* Mixed Vegetable Tablets; Modern Herbals Rheumatic Pain; Rheumatic Pain; Rheumatic Pain Tablets; Vegetex.

Cellobiose (18926-h)
4-O-β-D-Glucopyranosyl-D-glucose.
$C_{12}H_{22}O_{11} = 342.3$.
CAS — 528-50-7.

Profile
Cellobiose is a disaccharide that has been used to assess intes-

tinal permeability. It has been used as an alternative to lactulose in the differential sugar absorption test (p.1230).

◊ References.
1. Hodges S, *et al.* Cellobiose: mannitol differential permeability in small bowel disease. *Arch Dis Child* 1989; **64:** 853–5.
2. Juby LD, *et al.* Cellobiose/mannitol sugar test—a sensitive tubeless test for coeliac disease: results on 1010 unselected patients. *Gut* 1989; **30:** 476–80.

Cellulase (18473-l)

Cellulase (USAN).
CAS — 9012-54-8.

Profile
Cellulase is a concentrate of cellulose-splitting (cellulolytic) enzymes derived from *Aspergillus niger* or other sources. It is used in food processing and has been given by mouth in combination with other digestive enzymes for its supposed benefit in minor digestive disorders such as dyspepsia and flatulence. Hemicellulase has been given for similar purposes.

Preparations
Proprietary Preparations (details are given in Part 3)
Multi-ingredient: *Aust.:* Arca-Enzym; Festal†; Gallo Merz; Ora-Gallin; *Belg.:* Digestomen; *Braz.:* Dasc; Digeplus; Espasmo Novozyme; Essen; Normopride Enzimatico; Sintozima; *Fr.:* Pancrelase; *Ital.:* Digestopan; Essen Enzimatico; Luizym†; *Mex.:* Dixiflen; Espaven Enzimatico; Ochozim; *Port.:* Colerin-F; Espasmo Canulase; *S.Afr.:* Spasmo-Canulase; *Spain:* Digestomen Complex; Espasmo Canulasa†; Espasmo Digestomen; Lidobama Complex†; Paidozim; Polidasa†; *Switz.:* Spasmo-Canulase; Zymoplex†; *Thai.:* Sanzyme-S; *USA:* Arco-Lase; Arco-Lase Plus; Enzyme; Gustase; Gustase Plus.

Centaury (527-f)

Centaurii Minoris Herba; Petite Centaurée; Tausendgüldenkraut.
Pharmacopoeias. In Eur. (see p.vi).

Pharmacopoeial description
Ph. Eur.: The whole or cut dried flowering tops of *Centaurium erythraea* (= *C. minus*; *C. umbellatum*; *Erythraea centaurium*). It has a very bitter taste. Protect from light.

Profile
Centaury is used as a bitter.

Preparations
Proprietary Preparations (details are given in Part 3)
Multi-ingredient: *Aust.:* Amylatin; Aponatura Starkungs; Apotheker Bauer's Magentee; China-Eisenwein; Eryval; Grippogran; Kneipp Verdauungs-Tee; Krauterdoktor Erkaltungstropfen; Krauterdoktor Harnstein- und Nieren-griesstropfen; Krauterdoktor Verdauungsfordernde Tropfen; Krautertee Nr 14; Krautertee Nr 17; Krautertee Nr 20; Krautertee Nr 9; Mag Kottas Blahungs-Schladung-stee; Mag Kottas Magen-Darmtee; Magentee EF-EM-ES; Mariazeller; Sidroga Magen-Darm-Tee; Solisan; St Radegunder Verdauungstee; *Braz.:* Camomila; *Fr.:* Copaltra; Diacure; Tisane Hepatique de Hoerdt; Tisanes de l'Abbe Hamon no 16†; *Ger.:* Alsicur†; Amara-Tropfen; Aranidorm-S†; Canephron N; Cefagastrin; Hevert-Magen-Galle-Leber-Tee†; JuGrippan†; Kneipp Verdauungs-Tee N; Leber-Galle-Tropfen 83; Montana; Nephrubin†; Phonix Gastriphon; Stullmaton; *Hong Kong:* Canephron N; *Ital.:* Fluxoten†; *Spain:* Digestol Sanatorium; *Switz.:* Gastrosan; Phytomed Gastro†; Tisane pour l'estomac; *UK:* Digest; Laxadoron.

Cereus (9194-x)

Night-blooming Cereus.

Profile
Cereus, the flowers and stems of night-blooming cereus (*Selenicereus grandiflorus*; *Cactus grandiflorus*) (Cactaceae), has cardiac stimulant actions and has been used in various cardiovascular disorders. It has also been used as an anthelmintic and in the treatment of rheumatism.

It is also used in homoeopathic medicine.

Preparations
Proprietary Preparations (details are given in Part 3)
Multi-ingredient: *Ger.:* Cardibisana; Oxacant N; Oxacant-forte N; Oxacant-Khella N; *Switz.:* Phytomed Cardio†.

Ceruletide (2124-t)

Ceruletide (BAN, USAN, rINN).
Caerulein.
$C_{58}H_{73}N_{13}O_{21}S_2 = 1352.4$.
CAS — 17650-98-5 (ceruletide); 71247-25-1 (ceruletide diethylamine).
ATC — V04CC04.

NOTE. The name Ceruleinum has been applied to Indigo Carmine (p.1623).

Ceruletide is a decapeptide amide originally isolated from the skin of the Australian frog, *Hyla caerulea*, and other amphibi-

ans. Ceruletide may exist as a salt with 1 to 3 moles of diethylamine (ceruletide diethylamine).

Adverse Effects
Ceruletide stimulates gallbladder contraction and gastrointestinal muscle and may give rise to abdominal discomfort. Hypotensive reactions may also occur.

Uses and Administration
Ceruletide is structurally related to pancreozymin (p.1647) and has similar actions. When administered parenterally it stimulates gallbladder contraction and relaxes the sphincter of Oddi; it also causes an increase in the secretion of pancreatic enzymes and stimulates intestinal muscle.

As ceruletide diethylamine it is used as an aid to diagnostic radiology and in the management of paralytic ileus. It is also used in tests of pancreatic exocrine function, sometimes in combination with secretin (p.1661); these studies generally require duodenal intubation of the patient and examination of duodenal aspirate and are rarely performed.

For most radiographic procedures of the biliary and digestive tracts and for treatment of postoperative ileus, ceruletide diethylamine is given by intramuscular injection in a dose equivalent to 300 nanograms per kg body-weight of ceruletide. Doses equivalent to 1 to 2 nanograms per kg per minute are given by intravenous infusion in pancreatic function tests and in the treatment of other causes of paralytic ileus.

◊ References.
1. Vincent ME, *et al.* Pharmacology, clinical uses, and adverse effects of ceruletide, a cholecystokinetic agent. *Pharmacotherapy* 1982; **2:** 223–34.
2. Gullo L, *et al.* Caerulein induced plasma amino acid decrease: a simple, sensitive, and specific test of pancreatic function. *Gut* 1990; **31:** 926–9.

Preparations
Proprietary Preparations (details are given in Part 3)
Ger.: Takus.

Chamomile (4628-y)

NOTE. The name Chamomile is used for the dried flowerheads from 2 species of *Compositae* having similar medicinal properties:

Chamomile from *Anthemis nobilis* (*Chamaemelum nobile*) is known as **Roman Chamomile Flower** (Ph. Eur.) (Chamomile Flowers, Chamomillae Romanae Flos, or Manzanilla Romana).

Chamomile from *Matricaria recutita* (*Chamomilla recutita*) is known as **Matricaria Flower** (Ph. Eur.) (Camomile Allemande, Camomilla, Chamomilla, Chamomillae Anthodium, Flos Chamomillae, Flos Chamomillae Vulgaris, German Chamomile, Hungarian Chamomile, Kamillenblüten, Manzanilla Ordinaria, or Matricariae Flos).

Pharmacopoeias. Eur. (see p.vi) includes chamomile from *Anthemis nobilis* and *Matricaria recutita. Pol.* and *USNF* include chamomile from *Matricaria recutita.*
Aust. and *Ger.* also include Matricaria Oil.

Pharmacopoeial description
Ph. Eur.: Roman Chamomile Flower consists of the dried flowerheads obtained from the cultivated double variety of *Anthemis nobilis* (= *Chamaemelum nobile*), containing not less than 0.7% v/w of essential oil. It has a strong characteristic odour. Protect from light.

Matricaria Flower consists of the dried flowerheads obtained from *Matricaria recutita* (= *Chamomilla recutita*), containing not less than 0.4% v/w of blue essential oil. It has a characteristic, pleasant and aromatic odour. Protect from light.

USNF 20: The dried flowerheads of *Matricaria recutita* (*Matricaria chamomilla*, *Matricaria chamomilla* var. *courrantiana*, *Chamomilla recutita*) (Asteraceae alt. Compositae). It contains not less than 0.4% of blue volatile oil and not less than 0.3% of apigenin-7-glucoside. Protect from light.

Profile
Chamomile has been applied externally as a poultice in the early stages of inflammation, and ointments containing chamomile or extracts of chamomile have been used for the prevention and treatment of cracked nipples and nappy rash. It is also used in homoeopathic medicine. 'Chamomile tea' is a domestic remedy for indigestion and has also been reported to have hypnotic properties.

There have been reports of contact sensitivity and anaphylaxis.

◊ Reviews.
1. Berry M. The chamomiles. *Pharm J* 1995; **254:** 191–3.

Hypersensitivity. References.
1. Van Ketel WG. Allergy to Matricaria chamomilla. *Contact Dermatitis* 1987; **16:** 50–1.
2. McGeorge BC, Steele MC. Allergic contact dermatitis of the nipple from Roman chamomile ointment. *Contact Dermatitis* 1991; **24:** 139–40.
3. Rodriguez-Serna M, *et al.* Allergic and systemic contact dermatitis from Matricaria chamomilla tea. *Contact Dermatitis* 1998; **39:** 192–3.
4. Jensen-Jarolim E, *et al.* Fatal outcome of anaphylaxis to camomile-containing enema during labor: a case study. *J Allergy Clin Immunol* 1998; **102:** 1041–2.

5. Giordano-Labadie F, *et al.* Allergic contact dermatitis from camomile used in phytotherapy. *Contact Dermatitis* 2000; **42:** 247.
6. Foti C, *et al.* Contact urticaria from Matricaria chamomilla. *Contact Dermatitis* 2000; **42:** 360–1.

Preparations
Ph. Eur.: Matricaria Liquid Extract.

Proprietary Preparations (details are given in Part 3)
Aust.: Kamillat; Kamillen; Kamillomed; Markalakt; *Austral.:* Camoderm; *Belg.:* Kamillosan; *Fr.:* Cefamig; *Ger.:* Azulon; Chamo S; Eukamillat; Galenat Kamill N; Kamillan supra; Kamille N; Kamillen; Kamillencreme N; Kamillenextract; Kamillin; Kamilloderm; Kamillosan; Markalakt; Matmille; PC 30 N; Perkamillon; *Irl.:* Kamillosan; *Ital.:* Ceru Spray; Milla; *Mex.:* Kamillosan; *Neth.:* Kamillosan†; *NZ:* Kamillosan; *Spain:* Kamillosan; *Switz.:* Edmilla; Kamillen-Bad; Kamillofluid; Kamillosan; Perkamillon; *UK:* Ashton & Parsons Infants Powders; Kamillosan.

Multi-ingredient: *Aust.:* Abfuhrtee; Aktiv milder Magen- und Darmtee; Apotheker Bauer's Blahungstee; Bio-Garten Tee fur den Magen; Bio-Garten Tee gegen Blahungen; Bio-Garten Tee gegen Durchfall; Bio-Garten Tee gegen Verstopfung; Bio-Garten Tropfen fur Magen und Darm; Bogumil-tassenfertiger milder Abfurtee; Bronchostop; Carminativum Babynos; Chol-Grandelat; Cional; Dentinox; Diarrhoesan; Dynexan; Ehrmann's Entschlackungstee; Eogran; Euceta mit Kamille; Gastregan; Illings Bozner Maycur-Tee; Karvisin; Kneipp Grippe-Tee; Kneipp Verdauungs-Tee; Krauterhaus Mag Kottas Babytee; Krauterhaus Mag Kottas Entschlackungstee; Krauterhaus Mag Kottas Magen-und Darmtee; Krauterhaus Mag Kottas Tee gegen Durchfall; Krauterhaus Mag Kottas Wechseltee; Krautertee Nr 1; Krautertee Nr 124; Krautertee Nr 17; Krautertee Nr 209; Krautertee Nr 217; Krautertee Nr 311; Krautertee Nr 8; Krautertee Nr 9; Laxalpin; Laxolind†; Mag Doskar's Magentonikum; Mag Doskar's Nerventonikum; Mag Kottas Baby-Tee; Mag Kottas Leber-Gallentee; Mag Kottas Magen-Darmtee; Mag Kottas Wechseltee; Magentee; Mariazeller; May-Cur-Tee; Nesthakchen; Paididont; Paradenton; Parodontax†; Planta Lax; Sidroga Erkaltungstee; Sidroga Kindertee; Sidroga Magen-Darm-Tee; Sigman-Haustropfen; St Radegunder Blahungstreibender Tee; St Radegunder Fiebertee; St Radegunder Reizmildernder Magentee; St Radegunder Tee gegen Durchfall; Sulgan 99; Tee gegen Durchfall; Teekanne Leber- und Galletee; Teekanne Magen- und Darmtee; Windtreibender Tee; *Austral.:* Antassa; Cough Relief; Goodnight Formula; Herbal Anxiety Formula; Hydrastis Complex; Multi-Vitamin Day & Night; Nappy Rash Relief Cream; Respatona Decongestant Formula; Respatona Plus Bronchial Cough Relief; *Belg.:* Tisane pour Dormir; *Braz.:* Camomila; Camomilina C; Dinill; Gotas Digestivas; Matricaria Vitam AED; Nene Dent; Parodontax; Passaneuro; Serenase; Vidcalm; *Fr.:* Activox; Calmiphase; Calmophytum; Dologyne†; Santane A₄; Santane D₅; Santane F₁₀; Solution Stago Diluee; Tisane Digestive Weleda†; *Ger.:* Ad-Muc; Agamadon N†; Agamadon†; Anisan; Aranidorm-S†; Arnikamill; Befelka-Tinktur†; bioplant-Kamillenfluid; Carminativum Babynos; Carminativum-Hetterich N; Carminativum-Pascoe; Cefagastrin; Dentinox N; derma-loges N; Diarrhoesan; Esberigal N†; Gallemolan G; Gallexier; Galloselect M; Gastralon N; Gastrarctin N; Gastricholan-L; Gastritol; Gastrol S; Grunlicht Hingfong Essenz; Gutnacht; Hamo-ratiopharm; Helago-oel N; Hevert-Gall S; Iberogast; JuGrippan†; Kamillan plus; Kamillen-Bad-Robugen; Kamillobad†; Kamillosan Mundspray; Kamistad; Kneipp Verdauungs-Tee N; Magen-Tee Stada N†; Magentee; Majocarmin-Tee; Matmille; Meteophyt S; Myrrhinil-Intest; Nervosana; Odala wern; Parodontal; Pascoletten N; Pascomag; PC 30 V; Presselin Blahungs K 4 N; Presselin Dyspeptikum; Presselin Stoffwechsel-Tee Hapeka 225 N; Roflatol Phyto (Rowo-146)†; Salus Abfuhr-Tee Nr. 2†; Salus Leber-Galle-Tee Nr.18†; Salus Nerven-Schlaf-Tee Nr.22†; Stomachicon N; Stovalid N; Stullmaton; Tonsilgon N; Ulcotruw N†; Ulcu-Pasc; Ullus Kapseln N; Valeriana comp; *Hong Kong:* Camoderm; Kamistad; *Israel:* Derma Care; Gingisan; Jungborn; Kamil Blue; Kamilotract; Kamiltract Baby; Lido Tea; Parodontax; Pedisol; *Ital.:* Babygella; Dicalmir; Donalg; Florelax; Hamamilla; Herbatar; Lycia Luminique; Microclisma Evacuante AD-BB; Nebris; Neutrogena Anti-Acne; Normalax†; Otosan Gocce Auricolari; Parvisedil; Propomill; Relaten†; Sedatol; Senna-Specie Composta; Vegebyl†; Videorelax; *Mex.:* Kamiloderm; *Port.:* Erpecalm; Gabisedil; Solucao Stago; *S.Afr.:* Dynexan; Kamillosan†; *Singapore:* Kamistad; *Spain:* Agua del Carmen; Digestol Sanatorium; Encialina; Ginejuvent; Laxante Sanatorium; *Switz.:* Bain extradoux dermatologique Nouvelle Formule; Bain extra-doux dermatologique†; Beclonarin; Cetona Plus; Dentinox†; Dynexan; Enveloppements ECR†; Eubucal; Euceta avec camomille et arnica; Fortacet; Frigoplasma; Iberogast; Kamillosan; Korodin†; Narifresh; Optilax†; Perkamillon; Phytomed Gastro†; Rhinocure†; Riccomycine†; Riccovitan; Saltrates Rodell; Sulgan; Tavolax†; Tisane antiflatulente pour les enfants; Tisane contre les refroidissements; Tisane pour l'estomac; Tisane pour les enfants†; Tonex; *Thai.:* Kamillosan-M; Kamistad; *UK:* Appetiser Mixture; Carminative Tea; HRI Calm Life; Travel-Caps.

Chaparral (3046-g)

Profile
Chaparral is derived from the leaves of the creosote bush, *Larrea tridentata* (Zygophyllaceae). It has been taken as an ingredient of various herbal preparations but such use has been associated with severe hepatotoxicity. Recommendations that products containing chaparral should not be consumed have been made in several countries.

◊ References.
1. Gordon DW, *et al.* Chaparral ingestion: the broadening spectrum of liver injury caused by herbal medications. *JAMA* 1995; **273:** 489–90.
2. Batchelor WB, *et al.* Chaparral-induced hepatic injury. *Am J Gastroenterol* 1995; **90:** 831–3.
3. Sheikh NM, *et al.* Chaparral-associated hepatotoxicity. *Arch Intern Med* 1997; **157:** 913–19.

The symbol † denotes a preparation no longer actively marketed

Preparations

Proprietary Preparations (details are given in Part 3)
Multi-ingredient: *Austral.:* Proyeast.

Chenodeoxycholic Acid (3706-m)

Chenodeoxycholic Acid (*BAN, rINN*).

Acidum Chenodeoxycholicum; CDCA; Chenic Acid; Chenodiol (*USAN*). 3α,7α-Dihydroxy-5β-cholan-24-oic acid.
$C_{24}H_{40}O_4 = 392.6$.
CAS — 474-25-9.
ATC — A05AA01.
Pharmacopoeias. In *Eur.* (see p.vi).

Pharmacopoeial description

Ph. Eur.: A white or almost white powder. Very slightly soluble in water; freely soluble in alcohol; soluble in acetone; slightly soluble in dichloromethane.

Adverse Effects and Precautions

As for Ursodeoxycholic Acid, p.1677. Diarrhoea may occur more frequently than with ursodeoxycholic acid. A transient rise in liver-function test values and hypercholesterolaemia (low-density lipoprotein) have been reported with chenodeoxycholic acid.

Chenodeoxycholic acid is embryotoxic in some *animals*.

Interactions

As for Ursodeoxycholic Acid, p.1677.

Pharmacokinetics

Chenodeoxycholic acid is absorbed from the gastrointestinal tract and undergoes first-pass metabolism and enterohepatic recycling. It is partly conjugated in the liver before being excreted into the bile and, under the influence of intestinal bacteria, the free and conjugated forms undergo 7α-dehydroxylation to lithocholic acid, some of which is excreted directly in the faeces and the rest absorbed, mainly to be conjugated and sulfated by the liver before excretion in the faeces. Chenodeoxycholic acid also undergoes epimerisation to ursodeoxycholic acid.

◊ References.
1. Crosignani A, *et al.* Clinical pharmacokinetics of therapeutic bile acids. *Clin Pharmacokinet* 1996; **30:** 333–58.

Uses and Administration

Chenodeoxycholic acid is a naturally occurring bile acid (p.1585). When given by mouth it reduces hepatic synthesis of cholesterol and provides additional bile salts to the pool available for solubilisation of cholesterol and lipids. It has been used for the dissolution of cholesterol-rich gallstones (p.1678) in patients with a functioning gallbladder, in usual doses of about 15 mg per kg body-weight daily. The daily dose may be divided unequally and the larger dose given before bedtime to counteract the increase in biliary cholesterol concentrations seen overnight. Treatment may need to be given for up to 2 years, depending on the size of the stone. It should be continued for about 3 months after radiological disappearance of the stones. Chenodeoxycholic acid is also used in reduced doses in combination with ursodeoxycholic acid.

Preparations

Proprietary Preparations (details are given in Part 3)
Aust.: Chenofalk; *Belg.:* Chenofalk; *Braz.:* Fluibil; *Fr.:* Chenodex†; *Ger.:* Chenofalk; *Hong Kong:* Chenofalk; *Irl.:* Chendol†; Chenofalk; *Israel:* Soluston; *Jpn:* Regalen†; *Mex.:* Chenofalk; Sulobil; *Neth.:* Chenofalk; *Port.:* Chebil; *Spain:* Quenobilan; Quenocol; *Switz.:* Chenofalk; *UK:* Chendol†; Chenofalk†.

Multi-ingredient: *Aust.:* Lithofalk; *Ger.:* Lithofalk; Urso Mix; Ursofalk + Chenofalk; *Ital.:* Bilenor; Litobile†; *Switz.:* Lithofalk; *UK:* Combidol†; Lithofalk†.

Chloroacetophenone (12553-w)

CN; Phenacyl Chloride. 2-Chloroacetophenone.
$C_8H_7ClO = 154.6$.
CAS — 532-27-4.

NOTE. The name mace is applied to solutions of chloroacetophenone.

Profile

Chloroacetophenone is a lachrymatory which is irritant to the skin and eyes. It has been used in a riot-control gas.

◊ References.
1. Hu H, *et al.* Tear gas—harassing agent or toxic chemical weapon? *JAMA* 1989; **262:** 660–3.
2. Treudler R, *et al.* Occupational contact dermatitis due to 2-chloroacetophenone tear gas. *Br J Dermatol* 1999; **140:** 531–4.

Chloroplatinic Acid (12555-l)

Kloroplatinasyra. Hexachloroplatinic acid hexahydrate.
$H_2PtCl_6,6H_2O = 517.9$.
CAS — 16941-12-1 (*anhydrous chloroplatinic acid*); 18497-13-7 (*chloroplatinic acid hexahydrate*).

Profile

Aqueous solutions of platinic chloride ($PtCl_4 = 336.9$) are used in corneal tattooing solutions.

Chondroitin Sulfate A (12558-z)

Chondroitin 4-Sulphate; Chondroitin Sulphate A; CSA.
CAS — 24967-93-9 (*chondroitin sulfate A*); 39455-18-0 (*chondroitin sulfate A sodium*).

Profile

Chondroitin sulfate A is an acid mucopolysaccharide which is a constituent of most mammalian cartilaginous tissues. It is a component of the heparinoid danaparoid (p.866). It has been used in osteoporosis, osteoarthritis, ischaemic heart disease, and hyperlipidaemias. It is also used as an adjunct to ocular surgery. A medium containing chondroitin sulfate A has been used to preserve corneas for transplantation. It may also be used as the sodium salt.

Osteoarthritis. A meta-analysis[1] of double-blind, randomised controlled studies concluded that, while there was some evidence for efficacy of chondroitin and glucosamine in the treatment of osteoarthritis, methodological flaws and publication bias had led to exaggeration of their potential benefit.

1. McAlindon TE, *et al.* Glucosamine and chondroitin for treatment of osteoarthritis: a systematic quality assessment and meta-analysis. *JAMA* 2000; **283:** 1469–75.

Preparations

Proprietary Preparations (details are given in Part 3)
Aust.: Condrosulf; *Fr.:* Chondrosulf; Lacrypos; Structum; *Port.:* Ossin; *Spain:* Turkadon†; *Switz.:* Condrosulf; Structum.

Multi-ingredient: *Aust.:* Viscoat†; *Austral.:* Duovisc; Viscoat; *Belg.:* Viscoat†; *Fr.:* Viscoat; *Ger.:* Duovisc; Viscoat; *Hong Kong:* Viscoat; *Ital.:* Viscoat; *NZ:* Viscoat; *S.Afr.:* Viscoat; *Singapore:* Duovisc; Viscoat; *Swed.:* Viscoat†; *Switz.:* Viscoat†; *Thai.:* Duovisc; Viscoat; *UK:* Viscoat; *USA:* Viscoat.

Chrome Alum (12559-c)

Chromium Potassium Sulphate.
$KCr(SO_4)_2,12H_2O = 499.4$.
CAS — 10141-00-1 (*anhydrous chrome alum*).

Profile

Chrome alum is used in tanning, as a mordant in dyeing, and for hardening gelatin in photographic materials. It has been used as a sclerosant in medicine.

Preparations

Proprietary Preparations (details are given in Part 3)
Multi-ingredient: *Fr.:* Scleremo.

Chromium Trioxide (307-w)

Anhídrido Crómico; Chromic Acid; Chromic Anhydride.
$CrO_3 = 99.99$.
CAS — 1333-82-0.

◊ CAUTION. *Chromium trioxide is a powerful oxidising agent and is liable to explode in contact with small quantities of alcohol, ether, glycerol, and other organic substances.*

Profile

Chromium trioxide and other chromium compounds are used in industry. Solutions of chromium trioxide are corrosive, acting by oxidation. Repeated contact with chromium and its salts may cause eczematous dermatitis, particularly in hypersensitive persons and can also cause deep perforating ulcers known as 'chrome holes'. If inhaled, chromic dusts cause rhinitis and painless ulcers which may perforate the nasal septum; inhalation may cause severe lung damage and inflammation of the eyes. There may also be involvement of the CNS and there is an increased risk of lung cancer. Hexavalent chromium compounds are more dangerous than di- or trivalent compounds.

Acute symptoms of poisoning from the ingestion of chromium salts include intense thirst, dizziness, abdominal pain with vomiting and diarrhoea, hepatic injury, anuria or oliguria, and peripheral vascular collapse. Kidney damage may lead to fatal uraemia.

Treatment is symptomatic and supportive. Protective measures should be taken when handling or working with chromium and its salts.

Chromium trioxide was formerly used as a caustic and astringent.

Chromium is an essential trace element as described on p.1357.

Adverse effects. General references[1-3] to chromium toxicity including reports of poisoning with sodium dichromate[4] and potassium dichromate.[5]

1. Chromium. *Environmental Health Criteria 61.* Geneva: WHO, 1988.
2. Health and Safety Executive. The toxicity of chromium and inorganic chromium compounds. *Toxicity Review 21.* London: HMSO, 1989.
3. Barceloux DG. Chromium. *J Toxicol Clin Toxicol* 1999; **37:** 173–94.

4. Ellis EN, *et al.* Effects of hemodialysis and dimercaprol in acute dichromate poisoning. *J Toxicol Clin Toxicol* 1982; **19:** 249–58.
5. Michie CA, *et al.* Poisoning with a traditional remedy containing potassium dichromate. *Hum Exp Toxicol* 1991; **10:** 129–31.

Chromocarb Diethylamine (12561-w)

The diethylamine salt of 4-oxo-4*H*-1-benzopyran-2-carboxylic acid .
$C_{14}H_{17}O_4N = 263.3$.
CAS — 4940-39-0 (*chromocarb*).

NOTE. Chromocarb is *rINN*.

Profile

Chromocarb diethylamine is used to reduce capillary haemorrhage (including conjunctival haemorrhage) associated with various disorders, and for venous insufficiency. It is given by mouth in doses of 0.6 to 1.2 g daily in divided doses. It is also used as eye drops; 1 or 2 drops of a 10% solution have been instilled up to 6 times daily.

Preparations

Proprietary Preparations (details are given in Part 3)
Belg.: Angiophtal†; *Fr.:* Angiophtal; Campel; *Ital.:* Fludarene; *Port.:* Fradilen; *Spain:* Activadone.

Chrysoidine Hydrochloride Citrate (12562-e)

4-Phenylazobenzene-1,3-diamine hydrochloride citrate; Azobenzene-2,4-diamine hydrochloride citrate.
$C_{12}H_{12}N_4,HCl,C_6H_8O_7 = 440.8$.
CAS — 532-82-1 (*chrysoidine hydrochloride*); 5909-04-6 (*chrysoidine hydrochloride citrate*).

Profile

Chrysoidine hydrochloride citrate has been used as a dye but has been associated with tumours of the bladder.

Carcinogenicity. Mention that the development of tumours of the urinary bladder in anglers was possibly associated with the use of chrysoidine hydrochloride (chrysoidine Y; CI Basic Orange 2; Colour Index No. 11270) for colouring the maggots used as bait.[1-3]

1. Searle CE, Teale J. Chrysoidine-dyed bait: a possible carcinogenic hazard to anglers? *Lancet* 1982; **i:** 564.
2. Sole GM. Maggots dyed with chrysoidine: a possible risk to anglers. *BMJ* 1984; **289:** 1043–4.
3. Massey JA, *et al.* Maggots dyed with chrysoidine. *BMJ* 1984; **289:** 1451–2.

Chymopapain (3708-v)

Chymopapain (*BAN, USAN, rINN*).
BAX-1526; NSC-107079; Quimopapaina.
CAS — 9001-09-6.
ATC — M09AB01.

A proteolytic enzyme isolated from the latex of papaya (*Carica papaya*), differing from papain in electrophoretic mobility, solubility, and substrate specificity. Molecular weight approximately 27 000.

Units

One nanokatal (nKat) is defined as the amount of chymopapain which produces 1 nanomole of *p*-nitroaniline per second from DL-benzoylarginine-*p*-nitroanilide substrate at pH 6.4 and 37°.

In some countries CTE units have been used, defined as the amount of chymopapain which produces a hydrolysate from acid-denatured haemoglobin at pH 4.0 in one minute with an optical density at 275 nm equivalent to that of a tyrosine solution 0.0001%.

Adverse Effects

The most important adverse effect of chymopapain is anaphylaxis which can occur in up to about 1% of patients. It has resulted in fatalities and restricts use to a single treatment session per patient. Typical symptoms include angioedema, hypotension, laryngeal oedema and bronchospasm, shock, and cardiac arrest. Allergic skin reactions may also occur. Other reported reactions include headache, nausea and vomiting, paralytic ileus, urinary retention, thrombophlebitis, paraesthesias, footdrop, and discitis. Severe muscle spasm and an increase in back pain are common. Paraplegia, acute transverse myelitis, and intracerebral and subarachnoid haemorrhage have occurred.

◊ In a postmarketing surveillance study on a chymopapain preparation for intradiscal injection (Chymodiactin) data was received on 29 075 patients by January 1984 (representing about 50% of the total number of vials sold by that USA manufacturer to that date).[1] Anaphylactic reactions were confirmed in 194 patients (0.67%), 2 of whom died. The incidence was higher in women than in men. In 52 cases the reaction occurred after the test dose.

Neurological reactions of a serious nature were reported in 22 patients. Six patients had cerebral haemorrhage and 3 died; autopsy revealed that they had underlying cerebrovascular abnormalities. Eleven patients were reported to have developed paraplegia; in 5 of these cases this may have been due to incorrect needle placement. Two patients suddenly developed transverse myelitis with paraplegia after 2 and 3 weeks, with subsequent recovery. Two patients had seizures after the injection of chymopapain, and in another patient this reaction occurred several days after the procedure. Hypersensitivity to the contrast medium and underlying epilepsy may have played a role in 2 of these cases. Twenty-two patients had discitis with severe back pain and spasm. In 9 cases bacteria could be cultured. There were 11 deaths. In addition to the 5 deaths mentioned above, 1 patient developed a fatal *Staphylococcus aureus* meningitis following discitis at the site of injection. Three patients apparently died of an underlying disease and in 2 other cases the relationship to the administration of chymopapain was not clear.

Another review[2] of serious reactions associated with chymopapain administration reported between 1982 and 1991 (including the earlier postmarketing study) found 121 reactions among approximately 135 000 patients. They included fatal anaphylaxis (7), infections (24), haemorrhage (32), and neurological reactions (32).

Both reviews concluded that careful attention to proper patient selection and correct techniques of intradiscal needle placement are the most important factors in avoiding adverse effects with chymopapain.

1. Agre K, *et al.* Chymodiactin postmarketing surveillance: demographic and adverse experience data in 29075 patients. *Spine* 1984; **9:** 479–85.
2. Nordby EJ, *et al.* Safety of chemonucleolysis: adverse effects reported in the United States, 1982–1991. *Clin Orthop* 1993; **293:** 122–34.

Precautions
Chymopapain should not be used in those patients with a known sensitivity to papaya proteins or in patients with progressive paralysis, or tumours of the spinal cord, or lesions of the cauda equina. Severe spondylolisthesis is also a contra-indication. It should not be given to patients with heart failure, coronary artery disease, or respiratory failure who may be at increased risk if anaphylaxis occurs, nor to patients receiving beta blockers.

Care is required in administering chymopapain to ensure that the injection is into the disc and not intrathecal. However, discography is not recommended since the use of contrast media may exacerbate neurotoxicity and may inactivate the enzyme. The risk of allergic reactions associated with chymopapain is so high that no patient should ever receive it more than once. Tests to identify those most at risk and pretreatment with antihistamines (H_1 and H_2) and corticosteroids may be used, but drugs and equipment for the emergency management of anaphylactic reactions should always be to hand when giving patients chymopapain. The risk of anaphylaxis is higher in women.

Injection of more than one disc is associated with an increased frequency of neurological reactions; therefore, such injection should only be carried out following confirmation of definite further disc involvement.

Uses and Administration
Chymopapain is used as an injection into the intervertebral disc in the treatment of sciatic pain secondary to herniation of intervertebral discs of the lumbar spine (chemonucleolysis).

Chymopapain injection should preferably be administered under local anaesthesia rather than under general anaesthesia. The dose for a single intervertebral disc is 2 to 4 nanokatals, with a maximum dose per patient of 8 nanokatals.

Sciatica. The use of chymopapain for the treatment of discogenic sciatica remains controversial. While some clinicians consider it when conservative management of low back pain (p.6) has failed and before proceeding to surgery[1] others are reported to have largely abandoned the technique in view of its serious adverse effects.[2]

1. Williams F. Chemonucleolysis for treating sciatica. *Br J Hosp Med* 1994; **52:** 52.
2. Bush K. Chemonucleolysis for treating sciatica. *Br J Hosp Med* 1994; **52:** 52–3.

Preparations
Proprietary Preparations (details are given in Part 3)
Austral.: Chymodiactin; *Belg.:* Discase; *Canad.:* Chymodiactin; *Fr.:* Chymodiactine; *Irl.:* Chymodiactin†; *Spain:* Chymodiactin; *UK:* Chymodiactin; *USA:* Chymodiactin.

Chymotrypsin (3709-g)
Chymotrypsin (BAN, rINN).
α-Chymotrypsin; Chymotrypsinum; Quimotripsina.
CAS — 9004-07-3.
ATC — B06AA04; S01KX01.
Pharmacopoeias. In *Chin.*, *Eur.* (see p.vi), and *US.*

Pharmacopoeial description
Ph. Eur.: A proteolytic enzyme obtained by the activation of chymotrypsinogen extracted from the pancreas of beef. It contains not less than 5 microkatals in each mg. A white crystalline or amorphous powder; the amorphous form is hygroscopic. Sparingly soluble in water. A 1% solution in water has a pH of 3.0 to 5.0. Solutions have a maximum stability at pH 3 and a maximum activity at about pH 8. Store at 2° to 8° in airtight containers. Protect from light.

USP 25: A proteolytic enzyme crystallised from an extract of the pancreas gland of the ox, *Bos taurus* (Bovidae). It contains not less than 1000 USP units in each mg, calculated on the

dried basis. A white to yellowish-white, crystalline or amorphous, odourless powder. An amount equivalent to 100 000 USP units is soluble in 10 mL of water and in 10 mL of sodium chloride 0.9%. Store in airtight containers at a temperature not exceeding 40°.

Units
Various methods have been used to assay the potency of chymotrypsin. Ph. Eur. expresses activity in terms of microkatals while USP 25 expresses in terms of USP units. Other units that may be encountered are FIP units, Armour units, and Denver (or Wallace or Wampole) units.

Adverse Effects
Chymotrypsin is antigenic and severe allergic reactions have occasionally followed its intramuscular injection; where hypersensitivity is suspected, a sensitivity test should be made before injection.

Increased intra-ocular pressure, corneal oedema, striation, and moderate uveitis have occurred following its use in ophthalmology.

Precautions
It is inadvisable to use chymotrypsin in ocular surgery for patients under 20 years of age or for patients with congenital cataracts or high vitreous pressure and a gaping incisional wound.

Uses and Administration
Chymotrypsin is a proteolytic enzyme that has been used in ophthalmology for the dissection of the zonule of the lens, thus facilitating intracapsular cataract extraction and reducing trauma to the eye. For this purpose a solution of chymotrypsin in a sterile diluent such as sodium chloride 0.9% has been injected to irrigate the posterior chamber.

Chymotrypsin has also been given, usually by mouth or topically, for its supposed action in reducing soft-tissue inflammation and oedema associated with surgery or traumatic injuries, and in patients suffering from upper respiratory-tract disorders.

Preparations
USP 25: Chymotrypsin for Ophthalmic Solution.

Proprietary Preparations (details are given in Part 3)
Fr.: Alphacutanee; *Ger.:* Alpha-Chymocutan†; Alpha-Chymotrase†; *Ital.:* Zonulasi†; *S.Afr.:* Zonulysin†; *Spain:* Quimotrase; *UK:* Zonulysin†.

Multi-ingredient: *Aust.:* Wobenzym; *Braz.:* Parenzyme; Parenzyme Ampicilina; Parenzyme Tetraciclina; Probenzima Ampicilina; Probenzima Analgesico; *Fr.:* Alphintern†; *Ger.:* Enzym-Wied; Wobe-Mugos E; Wobenzym N; *Ital.:* Essen Enzimatico; *Mex.:* Ochozim; Wobenzym; *Port.:* Chimar; *Spain:* Bristaciclina Dental; Dertrase; Dosil Enzimatico; Doxiten Enzimatico; Duo Gobens; Epixian†; Quimodril; Solupen Enzimatico; Terranilo.

Cicloxilic Acid (12569-a)
Cicloxilic Acid (rINN).
cis-2-Hydroxy-2-phenylcyclohexanecarboxylic acid.
$C_{13}H_{16}O_3 = 220.3.$
CAS — 57808-63-6.

Profile
Cicloxilic acid has been used in the treatment of hepatic disorders.

Ciliary Neurotrophic Factor (11770-e)
CNTF.

Profile
Ciliary neurotrophic factor is a nerve growth factor produced in neural tissues and released in response to injury. Recombinant ciliary neurotrophic factor is under investigation in motor neurone disease (p.1658) and peripheral neuropathy.

◊ References.
1. Miller RG, *et al.* A placebo-controlled trial of recombinant human ciliary neurotrophic (rhCNTF) factor in amyotrophic lateral sclerosis. *Ann Neurol* 1996; **39:** 256–60.

Cimicifuga (12570-e)
Black Cohosh; Black Snakeroot.
Pharmacopoeias. Chin. includes the rhizome of *C. heracleifolia, C. dahurica,* and *C. foetida. Jpn* includes the rhizome of *C. simplex* (=*C. foetida*) or other species of the same genus.

The roots of *Cimicifuga racemosa* (Ranunculaceae).

Profile
Cimicifuga is used for menopausal and gynaecological disorders and is included in a number of preparations for coughs. It is reported that it may cause vertigo, headache, prostration, and gastrointestinal irritation when taken in large doses.

It is used in homoeopathic medicine when it is known as Actaea racemosa or Actaea rac.

◊ Reviews.
1. Pepping J. Black cohosh: Cimicifuga racemosa. *Am J Health-Syst Pharm* 1999; **56:** 1400–2.

Preparations
Proprietary Preparations (details are given in Part 3)
Aust.: Agnukliman; *Fr.:* Cimipax; *Ger.:* Cefakliman mono; Cimisan; Cirkufemal; Evalin; Femikliman uno; Femilla N; Feminon C; Herbagyn; Indianische Frauenwurzel Kapseln; Jinda; Klimadynon; Kytta-Kliman; Natu-fem; Remifemin; Valverde Traubensilberkerze; *Hong Kong:* Klimadynon; *Singapore:* Klimadynon; Remifemin; *Switz.:* Cimifemine; Menofem; Remifemin†.

Multi-ingredient: *Austral.:* Dong Quai Complex; Esten†; Extralife Meno-Care; Extralife PMS-Care; Harpagophytum Complex; Herbal PMS Formula; Lifesystem Herbal Formula 4 Women's Formula; Medinat Esten; PMT Complex; Proesten; Salagesic; Soy Forte with Block Cohosh; Viburnum Complex; Women's Formula Herbal Formula 3; *Ger.:* Femisana; Presselin Dysmen Olin 3 N; Remifemin plus; *S.Afr.:* Bronchicough; Bronchicum; *UK:* Biophylin†; Gerard House Helonias Compound; Gerard House Ligvites; Gerard House Reumalex; Modern Herbals Rheumatic Pain; St Johnswort Compound; Super Mega B+C; Vegetable Cough Remover; Vegetex; *USA:* Estrocare.

Cinametic Acid (3711-d)
Cinametic Acid (rINN).
Acidum Cinameticum. 4-(2-Hydroxyethoxy)-3-methoxycinnamic acid.
$C_{12}H_{14}O_5 = 238.2.$
CAS — 35703-32-3.

Profile
Cinametic acid is used as a choleretic in doses of 750 mg daily by mouth in divided doses.

Preparations
Proprietary Preparations (details are given in Part 3)
Fr.: Transoddi.

Cinchona Bark (529-n)
Chinae Cortex; Chinarinde; Cinchona; Cinchonae Cortex; Cinchonae Succirubrae Cortex; Jesuit's Bark; Peruvian Bark; Quina; Quina Vermelha; Quinquina; Quinquina Rouge; Red Cinchona Bark.
Pharmacopoeias. In *Eur.* (see p.vi).

Pharmacopoeial description
Ph. Eur.: The dried bark of *Cinchona pubescens* (=*Cinchona succirubra*) or of its varieties or hybrids. It contains not less than 6.5% of total alkaloids, of which 30 to 60% are quinine-type alkaloids. It has an intensely bitter, somewhat astringent taste. Protect from light and moisture.

Profile
Cinchona contains a number of alkaloids including two pairs of optical isomers quinine (p.445) and quinidine (p.964) and cinchonine and cinchonidine. Cinchona alkaloids have long been used for their antimalarial activity either singly, as quinine or quinidine, or in mixtures, such as totaquine. Quinidine is also used for its antiarrhythmic properties.

Cinchona bark is used as a bitter and is also employed in herbal remedies and in homoeopathic medicine.

Preparations
Proprietary Preparations (details are given in Part 3)
Ital.: Venustas Lozione Antiforfora.

Multi-ingredient: *Aust.:* Amara; Brady's-Magentropfen; China Eisenwein; China-Eisenwein; Ferrovin-Chinaeisenwein; Mariazeller; *Belg.:* Aperop; *Braz.:* Gastrogenol; Vinho Reconstituinte; *Fr.:* Phospharome†; Quintonine; *Ger.:* Amara-Tropfen-Pascoe; Cardibisana; Gastrol S; Hepaticum-Medice H; Hicoton; Sedovent; *Ital.:* Bitteridina; Chinoidina; Crisolax†; Rabarbaroni; *Port.:* Solucao Stago; *Spain:* Pildoras Ferrug Sanatori; *Switz.:* Phytomed Rhino†; Vin Tonique de Vial.

Cinnamaverine (13340-v)
Cinnamaverine (rINN).
2-(Diethylamino)ethyl 2,3-diphenylacrylate.
$C_{21}H_{25}NO_2 = 323.4.$
CAS — 1679-75-0.

Profile
Cinnamaverine has been used for its relaxant effect on smooth muscle. The hydrochloride has been an ingredient in some cough preparations.

Cinnamon (4630-q)
Canela; Canela do Ceilão; Cannelle Dite de Ceylan; Ceylon Cinnamon; Ceylonzimt; Cinnam.; Cinnamomi Cortex; Cinnamon Bark; Zimt.
Pharmacopoeias. In *Eur.* (see p.vi).

Pharmacopoeial description
Ph. Eur.: The dried bark of the shoots of coppiced trees of *Cinnamomum zeylanicum* containing not less than 1.2% v/w of es-

sential oil. It has a characteristic, aromatic odour. Protect from light.

BP 2001: directs that when Powdered Cinnamon is prescribed or demanded, material complying with the appropriate requirements of the Ph. Eur. monograph for Cinnamon and containing not less than 1.0% v/w of essential oil shall be dispensed or supplied.

Profile

Cinnamon is carminative and slightly astringent and is included in some preparations for gastrointestinal disorders. It is also used as a flavour. There have been a number of reports of hypersensitivity to cinnamaldehyde and other constituents of cinnamon oil.

Preparations

Proprietary Preparations (details are given in Part 3)
Multi-ingredient: *Aust.:* Brady's-Magentropfen; China-Eisenwein; Mariazeller; Montana; Teekanne Magen- und Darmtee; *Braz.:* Balsamo Branco; Formitonicum; Licor de Cacau; *Fr.:* Elixir Grez; Quintonine; Santane D₅; Santane F₁₀; Santane R₈; *Ger.:* Amara-Tropfen-Pascoe; Doppelherz Melissengeist; Gastrosecur; Melissengeist; Montana; Schwedentrunk der Echte Elixier; Sedovent; *Hong Kong:* GI; *Ital.:* Dam; *Spain:* Agua del Carmen; Vigortonic; *Switz.:* Baume; *Thai.:* Carmicide; Meloids; *UK:* Aluminium Free Indigestion†; Cough Drops; Melissa comp..

Cinnamon Oil (4631-p)

Aetheroleum Cinnamomi Zeylanici; Ceylon Cinnamon Bark Oil; Cinnam. Oil; Cinnamomi Zeylanicii Corticus Aetheroleum; Esencia de Canela; Essence de Cannelle de Ceylan; Oleum Cinnamomi; Zimtöl.

Pharmacopoeias. In Eur. (see p.vi). Eur. also includes Ceylon Cinnamon Leaf Oil. Jpn specifies oil from either Cinnamomum cassia or Cinnamomum zeylanicum.

Cinnamon oil has been used as the name for cassia oil in some countries.

It contains eugenol.

Pharmacopoeial description

Ph. Eur.: The oil obtained by steam distillation of the bark of the shoots of *Cinnamomum zeylanicum* (*C. verum*). It contains 55 to 75% of cinnamaldehyde. A clear, mobile, light yellow liquid becoming reddish over time, with a characteristic odour of cinnamaldehyde. Store in well-filled airtight containers. Protect from light and heat.

Profile

Cinnamon oil has properties and uses similar to those of cinnamon (above). It is also included in preparations for musculoskeletal and joint disorders and for respiratory-tract disorders. There have been a number of reports of hypersensitivity to cinnamaldehyde and other constituents of cinnamon oil.

Preparations

BP 2001: Aromatic Cardamom Tincture; Compound Cardamom Tincture; Concentrated Cinnamon Water; Tolu-flavour Solution.

Proprietary Preparations (details are given in Part 3)
Multi-ingredient: *Aust.:* Dr Fischers Melissengeist†; Melissengeist; Tiger Balsam Rot; *Belg.:* Calmant Martoul†; *Braz.:* Axol; *Canad.:* Tiger Balm Red; *Fr.:* Aromasol; Gouttes aux Essences; Tigridol; *Ger.:* Amol Heilkrautergeist N; Melissengeist; Salviathymol N; *Hong Kong:* Magesto; *Israel:* Karvol; *NZ:* Karvol; *S.Afr.:* Enterodyne; Karvol; *Singapore:* Karvol; *Spain:* Depurativo Richelet; *Switz.:* Baume de Chine Temple of Heaven blanc; Pirom; Spagyrom; *Thai.:* Magesto; *UK:* Slippery Elm Stomach Tablets; Tiger Balm Liquid†.

Citicoline (12576-k)

Citicoline (pINN).
CDP-Choline; Citidoline; Cytidine Diphosphate Choline; IP-302. Choline cytidine-5′-pyrophosphate.
$C_{14}H_{26}N_4O_{11}P_2 = 488.3$.
CAS — 987-78-0.
ATC — N06BX06.

NOTE. Citicoline Sodium is *USAN.*

Profile

Citicoline is a derivative of choline and cytidine involved in the biosynthesis of lecithin. It is claimed to increase blood flow and oxygen consumption in the brain and has been given in the treatment of cerebrovascular disorders (including ischaemic stroke, p.813), parkinsonism, and head injury. It is given by intravenous or intramuscular injection in doses of up to 1 g daily or by mouth in divided doses of 200 to 600 mg daily.

Citicoline sodium has also been used.

◊ Reviews.
1. Fioravanti M, Yanagi M. Cytidinediphosphocholine (CDP choline) for cognitive and behavioural disturbances associated with chronic cerebral disorders in the elderly (updated 9 May 2001). Available in The Cochrane Library; Issue 4. Oxford: Update Software; 2001.

Preparations

Proprietary Preparations (details are given in Part 3)
Aust.: Startonyl; *Fr.:* Rexort; *Ital.:* Acticolin; Actomin; Brassel; Cebroton; Cidilin; Citidel†; Citifar; Citsav†; Difosfocin; Encelin†; Flussorex; Gerolin; Kemodyn; Link; Logan; Neurex; Neuro-

ton; Nicholin; Nicolsint; Polineural†; Sinkron; Sintoclar; *Jpn:* Nicholin; *Mex.:* Somazina; *Port.:* Hipercol; Somazina; Startonyl; Trausan; *Spain:* Neurodynamicum†; Numatol; Sauran; Somazina.

Citiolone (12577-a)

Citiolone (rINN).
BO-714. N-(Perhydro-2-oxo-3-thienyl)acetamide.
$C_6H_9NO_2S = 159.2$.
CAS — 1195-16-0.
ATC — A05BA04.

Profile

Citiolone has been used in the treatment of hepatic disorders and as a mucolytic. Hypersensitivity reactions have been reported.

◊ References.
1. de Barrio M, *et al.* Recurrent fixed drug eruption caused by citiolone. *J Investig Allergol Clin Immunol* 1997; **7:** 193–4.

Preparations

Proprietary Preparations (details are given in Part 3)
Ital.: Citiolase†; *Spain:* Mucorex.

Multi-ingredient: *Spain:* Hubergrip; Mucorex Ampicilina; Mucorex Ciclin; Sulquibron; Tosdetan†.

Anhydrous Citric Acid (1307-a)

Acidum Citricum Anhydricum; Citronensäure; E330. 2-Hydroxypropane-1,2,3-tricarboxylic acid.
$C_6H_8O_7 = 192.1$.
CAS — 77-92-9.
ATC — A09AB04.

Pharmacopoeias. In Eur. (see p.vi) and Jpn. US allows either the anhydrous or monohydrate form.

Pharmacopoeial description

Ph. Eur.: Colourless crystals or granules or a white crystalline powder. Very soluble in water; freely soluble in alcohol; sparingly soluble in ether.

USP 25: Citric acid is anhydrous or contains one molecule of water of hydration. Colourless, translucent crystals, or a white, granular to fine, crystalline powder. Soluble 1 in 0.5 of water, 1 in 2 of alcohol, and 1 in 30 of ether. Store in airtight containers.

Citric Acid Monohydrate (1308-t)

Acido del Limón; Acidum Citricum Monohydricum; Hydrous Citric Acid.
$C_6H_8O_7,H_2O = 210.1$.
CAS — 5949-29-1.

Pharmacopoeias. In Chin., Eur. (see p.vi), Jpn, and Pol. US allows either the anhydrous or monohydrate form.

Pharmacopoeial description

Ph. Eur.: Efflorescent, colourless crystals or granules, or a white crystalline powder. Very soluble in water; freely soluble in alcohol; sparingly soluble in ether. Store in airtight containers.

USP 25: Citric acid is anhydrous or contains one molecule of water of hydration. Colourless, translucent crystals, or a white, granular to fine, crystalline powder. The hydrous form is efflorescent in dry air. Soluble 1 in 0.5 of water, 1 in 2 of alcohol, and 1 in 30 of ether. Store in airtight containers.

Adverse Effects and Precautions

Citric acid ingested frequently or in large quantities may cause erosion of the teeth and have a local irritant action.

Interactions

Aluminium hydroxide. Intestinal absorption of aluminium ions may be enhanced by concurrent administration of citrates. Caution is needed in patients with chronic renal disease receiving aluminium hydroxide as a phosphate binder who are given a calcium supplement in the form of effervescent tablets which contain citric acid.[1]
1. Mees EJD, Basçi A. Citric acid in calcium effervescent tablets may favour aluminium intoxication. *Nephron* 1991; **59:** 322.

Uses and Administration

Citric acid is used in effervescing mixtures; the monohydrate is used in the preparation of effervescent granules.

Citric acid monohydrate is used as a synergist to enhance the effectiveness of antioxidants.

Preparations containing citric acid are used in the management of dry mouth (p.1498) and to dissolve renal calculi, alkalinise the urine, and prevent encrustation of urinary catheters. Citric acid is an ingredient of citrated anticoagulant solutions. Citric acid has also been used in preparations for the treatment of gastrointestinal disturbances and metabolic acidosis.

Preparations

BP 2001: Lemon Syrup; Paediatric Compound Tolu Linctus; Paediatric Simple Linctus; Potassium Citrate Mixture; Simple Linctus;
Ph. Eur.: Anticoagulant Acid-Citrate-Glucose Solutions (ACD); Anticoagulant Citrate-Phosphate-Glucose Solution (CPD);
USP 25: Anticoagulant Citrate Dextrose Solution; Anticoagulant Citrate Phosphate Dextrose Adenine Solution; Anticoagulant Citrate Phosphate Dextrose Solution; Citric Acid, Magnesium Oxide,

and Sodium Carbonate Irrigation; Magnesium Carbonate and Citric Acid for Oral Solution; Magnesium Citrate Oral Solution; Potassium and Sodium Bicarbonates and Citric Acid Effervescent Tablets for Oral Solution; Potassium Citrate And Citric Acid Oral Solution; Sodium Citrate and Citric Acid Oral Solution; Tricitrates Oral Solution.

Proprietary Preparations (details are given in Part 3)
Ger.: Citrosteril†.

Multi-ingredient: *Aust.:* Alka-Seltzer; Duplotrast Z; Helo-acid; Kalioral; *Austral.:* Alka-Seltzer; Citralite; Citravescent; Durolax X-Pack; Eno; Picolax; Picoprep; Ural; *Belg.:* Alka-Seltzer; Andrews; *Braz.:* Alka-Seltzer; Citrosodine; Estomazil; Licor de Cacau; Otosynalar; Sal de Andrews; Solucao Anticoagulante; Sonrisal; *Canad.:* Alka-Seltzer; Bromo Madelon; Citrocarbonate; PMS-Dicitrate; *Denm.:* Fenwal ACD†; *Fin.:* Alka-Seltzer; *Fr.:* Alka-Seltzer; Citrocholine; Elixir Grez; Foncitril; Gastrilax†; Hepargitol; Ornitine; *Ger.:* Alka-Seltzer; Barilux Brausetabletten; Blemaren N; Citropepsin; Lithurex; Pepzitrat; Retterspitz Ausserlich†; Retterspitz Gelee†; Retterspitz Innerlich†; Unibaryt†; Uronor; *Irl.:* Andrews; Cymalon; Mictral; *Israel:* Eno; Pico-Salax; Urikal; *Ital.:* Alka-Seltzer; Citroepatina; Duogas; Eno†; Gastrovison†; Geffer; Lavanda Sofar; Limonal; Roge; *Mex.:* Corpotasin CL; *Neth.:* Alka-Seltzer; Hexoll†; *Norw.:* Alka-Seltzer†; *NZ:* Alka-Seltzer; Ural; *Port.:* Alka-Seltzer; Creme Laser Hidrante; Eno; Sais Andrews; *S.Afr.:* Adco-Sodasol; Alkafizz; Betasoda; Citro-Soda; Citrocit; Citrovescent†; Effersol; Pneucid; Quatro-Soda; Uri-Alk; *Singapore:* Alka-Seltzer; Dicitrate; *Spain:* Alka-Seltzer; Justegas; Pastillas Antisep Garg L; Sal de Fruta Eno; Salcedogen; Sales de Frutas P G; Sales Örto†; Uralyt Urato; *Swed.:* Alka-Seltzer; Pico-Salax†; Renapur; *Switz.:* Alka-Seltzer; E-Z-Gas II; Pico-Salax†; Siesta-1; Uro-Tainer Solutio R†; Uro-Tainer Suby G†; *Thai.:* Alka-Seltzer; Carmicide; *UK:* Alka-Seltzer; Alka-Seltzer XS; Allens Junior Cough; Andrews; Carbex; Collins Elixir Pastilles†; Cymalon; Dinneford's†; Effercitrate; Eno; Hill's Balsam Chesty Cough for Children; Lemsip Cough & Cold Dry Cough; Melissin; Mictral; Potters Children's Cough Pastilles; Resolve; Throaties Family Cough Linctus†; Uriflex G; Uriflex R; Uro-Tainer Solution R; Uro-Tainer Suby G; Zubes Blackcurrant; Zubes Honey & Lemon; *USA:* Alka-Seltzer Antacid; Alka-Seltzer Effervescent Tablets; Alka-Seltzer with Aspirin; Bicitra; Bromo Seltzer Effervescent Granules; Cytra-2; Cytra-3; Cytra-K; Cytra-LC; Extra Strength Alka-Seltzer Effervescent Tablets; Gold Alka-Seltzer; Oracit; Original Alka-Seltzer Effervescent Tablets; Polycitra; Polycitra-K; Polycitra-LC; Renacidin; Sparkles; Summers Eve Disposable.

Citronella Oil (4633-w)

Citronellae Aetheroleum; Oleum Citronellae.
Pharmacopoeias. In Eur. (see p.vi).

Pharmacopoeial description

Ph. Eur.: The oil obtained by steam distillation from the fresh or partially dried aerial parts of *Cymbopogon winterianus*. It contains 30.0 to 45.0% citronellal, 9.0 to 15.0% citronellol, 2.0 to 4.0% citronellyl acetate, less than 2.0% geranial, 20.0 to 25.0% geraniol, 3.0 to 8.0% geranyl acetate, 1.0 to 5.0% limonene, and less than 2.0% neral. A pale yellow to brownish-yellow liquid with a very strong odour of citronellal. Store in well-filled containers. Protect from light.

Profile

Citronella oil is used as a perfume and insect repellent. Hypersensitivity has been reported.

Preparations

Proprietary Preparations (details are given in Part 3)
Ger.: Kneipp Beruhigungs-Bad spezial; Schupps Melissen Olbad; Valmarin Bad N†; *UK:* Mozzie Patch; Natrapel.

Multi-ingredient: *Aust.:* Dr Fischers Melissengeist†; Embrocation; Medizinalbad; Melissengeist; Red Point; Valin Baldrian; *Fr.:* Ysol 206†; *Ger.:* Kneipp Krauter Taschenkur Nerven und Schlaf N; Melissengeist; Schupps Baldrian Sedativbad†; *Ital.:* Citrosystem; Mistick; Natural Zanzy; Punginot†; *S.Afr.:* No-Bite; *UK:* Snowfire; *USA:* Treo.

Clivers (12130-w)

Cleavers; Galii Aparinis Herba; Galium; Goosegrass.

Profile

Clivers is the dried aerial parts of *Galium aparine* (Rubiaceae). It has been used in herbal medicine, principally as a diuretic.

Preparations

Proprietary Preparations (details are given in Part 3)
Multi-ingredient: *Austral.:* Galium Complex; Herbal Cleanse; Uva-Ursi Complex; *UK:* Antitis; Athera; Backache; Boldo; Cascade; Gerard House Buchu Compound; HealthAid Boldo-Plus; Heath & Heather Water Relief Tablets; Kas-Bah; Modern Herbals Menopause; Modern Herbals Water Retention; Psorasolv; Sciargo; Skin Cleansing; Tabritis; Water Naturtabs; Watershed.

Clove (4634-e)

Caryoph.; Caryophylli Flos; Caryophyllum; Clou de Girofle; Cloves; Cravinho; Cravo-da-Índia; Gewürznelke; Giroflier; Tropical Myrtle.

Pharmacopoeias. In Chin., Eur. (see p.vi), and Jpn.

Pharmacopoeial description

Ph. Eur.: The whole flower buds of *Syzygium aromaticum* (*Eugenia caryophyllus*), containing not less than 15% v/w of volatile oil, dried until they become reddish-brown, and with a characteristic aromatic odour. Protect from light.

BP 2001: directs that when Powdered Clove is prescribed or demanded, material complying with the appropriate requirements of the Ph. Eur. monograph for Clove and containing not less than 12.0% v/w of essential oil shall be dispensed or supplied.

Profile
Clove is a carminative and is used as a flavour. It is the source of clove oil (below).

Clove and clove oil have been abused in the form of cigarettes.

Abuse. Smoking of cigarettes composed of a mixture of tobacco and cloves is a habit which originated in Indonesia and has spread to the USA. There have been a number of reports of severe and sometimes fatal respiratory illness related to smoking clove cigarettes and there is also evidence from *animal* studies that clove cigarette smoke and eugenol (the principal constituent of clove oil) have harmful pulmonary effects. The Council on Scientific Affairs of the American Medical Association considers that in addition to the hazards associated with smoking tobacco, clove cigarettes may also produce severe lung injury in certain susceptible individuals and could also induce pulmonary aspiration in healthy individuals due to diminution of the gag reflex produced by the local anaesthetic action of eugenol.[1] The American Academy of Pediatrics has also alerted paediatricians in the USA to clove-cigarette smoking by young people and warned of the risks.[2]

1. American Medical Association Council on Scientific Affairs. Evaluation of the health hazard of clove cigarettes. *JAMA* 1988; **260:** 3641–4.
2. Committee on Substance Abuse. Hazards of clove cigarettes. *Pediatrics* 1991; **88:** 395–6.

Preparations
Proprietary Preparations (details are given in Part 3)

Multi-ingredient: *Aust.:* Apotheker Bauer's Kindertee; Drovitol; Mariazeller; *Belg.:* Eugiron; *Braz.:* Balsamo Branco; Fargestium; *Fr.:* Tisane Clairo†; *Ger.:* Discmigon; Doppelherz Melissengeist; Inconturina; Melissengeist; *Hong Kong:* GI; *Ital.:* Promix; Saugella Uomo; *Port.:* Midro; *UK:* Aluminium Free Indigestion†; Clairo Tea; Cough Drops; Laxadoron; Melissa comp.; Revitonil.

Clove Oil (4635-l)
Caryophylli Floris Aetheroleum; Esencia de Clavo; Essence de Girofle; Nelkenöl; Ol. Caryoph.; Oleum Caryophylli.

Pharmacopoeias. In *Eur.* (see p.vi) and *Jpn.*

It contains phenolic substances, chiefly eugenol.

Pharmacopoeial description
Ph. Eur.: A clear yellow liquid obtained by steam distillation from clove. It becomes brown on exposure to air. Miscible with dichloromethane, with ether, with toluene, and with fatty oils. Store in well-filled airtight containers. Protect from light and heat.

Incompatibility. PVC bottles softened and distorted fairly rapidly in the presence of clove oil, which should not be stored or dispensed in such bottles.[1]

1. Department of Pharmaceutical Sciences of the Pharmaceutical Society of Great Britain. Plastics medicine bottles of rigid PVC. *Pharm J* 1973; **210:** 100.

Profile
Clove oil is a carminative that is sometimes used in the treatment of flatulent colic. It is also used as a flavour.

Applied externally clove oil is irritant but can produce local anaesthesia. It is used as a domestic remedy for toothache, a plug of cotton wool soaked in the oil being inserted in the cavity of the carious tooth; repeated application may damage the gingival tissues. Mixed with zinc oxide, it is used as a temporary anodyne dental filling, although eugenol (p.1609), one of its constituents, is often preferred.

Eugenol may cause hypersensitivity.

Adverse effects. A report of severe toxicity following ingestion of clove oil in a child.[1] Adverse effects included coma, acidosis, a generalised seizure, disordered blood clotting, and acute liver damage.

For reference to the harmful effects of smoking clove cigarettes, see under Clove, above.

1. Hartnoll G, *et al.* Near fatal ingestion of oil of cloves. *Arch Dis Child* 1993; **69:** 392–3.

Preparations
BP 2001: Aromatic Cardamom Tincture.

Proprietary Preparations (details are given in Part 3)
UK: Dentogen; Soothake Toothache Gel.

Multi-ingredient: *Aust.:* China-Balsam; Dr Fischers Melissengeist†; Fittydent; Melissengeist; Neo-Angin; Parodontax†; Tiger Balsam Rot; *Austral.:* Dentese†; Logicin Chest Rub; Silver Clove Medicated Balm; Tiger Balm Red†; Tiger Balm White†; *Braz.:* Algidente; Anestesiol; *Canad.:* Dentalgar; Gouttes Dentaires; Tiger Balm Red; Tiger Balm White; *Fr.:* Aromasol; Baume Aroma; Gouttes aux Essences; Tigridol; *Ger.:* Amol Heilkrautergeist N; China-Balsam; Erkaltungsbalsam forte Salbe; GA-301-Redskin 301†; Hustagil Erkaltungsbalsam; Hustagil Inhalationsol; Melissengeist; Nur 1 Tropfen intensives Mundwasser; Parodontal F5 med; Repha-Os; Rheuma-Salbe; Salviathymol N; *Hong Kong:* Magesto; *Ital.:* Dentosan Azione Intensiva; Dentosan Mese; Fialetta Odontalgica Dr Knapp; Ondroly-A; *NZ:* Toothache Drops;

S.Afr.: Enterodyne; *Spain:* Dentol Topico; Otogen Calmante; *Switz.:* Baume de Chine Temple of Heaven blanc; Olbas; Osa Gel de dentition aux plantes†; Spagyrom; *Thai.:* Magesto; Masaga; *UK:* Eftab; Hactos; Medicinal Gargle; Nine Rubbing Oils; Olbas; Pickles Toothache Tincture; Potters Sugar Free Cough Pastilles; Red Oil; Snowfire; Teenstick; Tiger Balm Liquid†; Tiger Balm Red; *USA:* Dentapaine; Numzit; Toothache Gel.

Cnicus Benedictus (530-k)
Blessed Thistle; Cardo Santo; Carduus Benedictus; Chardon Bénit; Holy Thistle; Kardobenediktenkraut.

Pharmacopoeias. In *Aust.*

The flowering tops of *Cnicus benedictus* (=*Carbenia benedicta; Carduus benedictus*) (Compositae).

Profile
Cnicus benedictus has been used as a bitter.

Preparations
Proprietary Preparations (details are given in Part 3)

Multi-ingredient: *Aust.:* Aponatura Galle; Mag Kottas Leber-Gallentee; Mariazeller; *Belg.:* Tisane Antibiliaire et Stomachique; *Braz.:* Digestron; *Ger.:* Bomagall forte S†; Carvomin; Cheiranthol; Esberigal N†; Gallexier; Gastritol; Hevert-Gall S; *Switz.:* Gastrosan; *UK:* Bio-Strath Artichoke Formula; Gerard House Gladlax; Sure-Lax (Herbal).

Cobalt Chloride (12597-f)
Cobaltous Chloride.
$CoCl_2,6H_2O = 237.9$.
CAS — 7646-79-9 (anhydrous).
Pharmacopoeias. In *Aust.*

Adverse Effects
Reactions to cobalt have included anorexia, nausea and vomiting, diarrhoea, precordial pain, cardiomyopathy, flushing of the face and extremities, skin rashes, tinnitus, temporary nerve deafness, renal injury, diffuse thyroid enlargement, and hypothyroidism. In large doses it may reduce the production of erythrocytes.

◊ References.
1. Kennedy A, *et al.* Fatal myocardial disease associated with industrial exposure to cobalt. *Lancet* 1981; **i:** 412–4.
2. Cugell DW, *et al.* The respiratory effects of cobalt. *Arch Intern Med* 1990; **150:** 177–83.
3. Evans P, *et al.* Cobalt and cobalt compounds. *Toxicity Review 29.* London: HMSO, 1993.

Uses and Administration
Cobalt chloride, when administered to both normal and anaemic subjects, produces reticulocytosis and a rise in the erythrocyte count. This property suggested its use in the treatment of certain types of anaemia, but its general therapeutic use is, however, unjustified and not without danger.

In veterinary medicine, cobalt chloride has been given as a dietary supplement to ruminants.

Cobalt Oxide (12598-d)
Tricobalt Tetroxide.
$Co_3O_4 = 240.8$.
CAS — 1308-06-1.
Pharmacopoeias. In *BP(Vet).*

Pharmacopoeial description
BP(Vet) 2001: It consists of cobalt (II, III) oxide (tricobalt tetroxide) with a small proportion of cobalt (III) oxide (dicobalt trioxide). A black, odourless or almost odourless, powder. Practically insoluble in water; dissolves in mineral acids and in solutions of alkali hydroxides.

Profile
Cobalt oxide is used in veterinary practice for the prevention of cobalt deficiency in ruminants. The chloride and sulfate have been used similarly. For the adverse effects of cobalt, see Cobalt Chloride, above.

Coccidioidin (7942-n)
Pharmacopoeias. In *US.*

Pharmacopoeial description
USP 25: A sterile solution containing the antigens obtained from the byproducts of mycelial growth or from the spherules of the fungus *Coccidioides immitis*; it contains a suitable antimicrobial. A clear, practically colourless or amber-coloured liquid. Store at 2° to 8°. Any dilutions should be stored at 2° to 8° and used within 24 hours. The expiry date is not later than 3 years (mycelial product) or 18 months (spherule-derived product) after release from the manufacturer's cold storage.

Profile
Coccidioidin is used as an aid to the diagnosis of coccidioidomycosis and, in conjunction with other antigens, to assess the

---

status of cell-mediated immunity. The usual dose is 0.1 mL of a 1 in 100 dilution by intradermal (intracutaneous) injection.

◊ For reference to the use of coccidioidin for anergy testing in HIV-positive patients, see Tuberculins, p.1676.

Preparations
USP 25: Coccidioidin.

Proprietary Preparations (details are given in Part 3)
USA: BioCox; Spherulin.

Co-dergocrine Mesilate (1503-f)
Co-dergocrine Mesylate (BAN); Co-dergocrine Methanesulphonate; Dihydroergotoxine Mesylate; Dihydroergotoxine Methanesulphonate; Dihydrogenated Ergot Alkaloids; Ergoloid Mesylates (USAN); Hydrogenated Ergot Alkaloids.
CAS — 11032-41-0 (co-dergocrine); 8067-24-1 (co-dergocrine mesilate).
ATC — C04AE01.
Pharmacopoeias. In *Br., Fr., Jpn, Swiss,* and *US.*

Pharmacopoeial description
BP 2001: A mixture in equal proportions of dihydroergocornine mesilate ($C_{31}H_{41}N_5O_5,CH_4O_3S = 659.8$), dihydroergocristine mesilate, and dihydroergocryptine mesilate, the dihydroergocryptine being present as both the α and β forms in the ratio 1.5 to 2.5:1. A white to yellowish-white, odourless or almost odourless powder. Sparingly soluble in water; soluble in alcohol and in acetone; slightly soluble in chloroform; practically insoluble in ether. A 0.5% solution in water has a pH of 4.2 to 5.2. Store at a temperature not exceeding 25°. Protect from light.

USP 25: A mixture of the methanesulfonate salts of the three hydrogenated alkaloids, dihydroergocristine, dihydroergocornine, and dihydroergocryptine, in an approximate weight ratio of 1:1:1. Dihydroergocryptine mesilate exists as a mixture of alpha- and beta-isomers. The ratio of alpha- to beta-isomers is not less than 1.5:1.0 and not more than 2.5:1.0.

A white to off-white, microcrystalline or amorphous, practically odourless powder. Slightly soluble in water; soluble in alcohol and in methyl alcohol; sparingly soluble in acetone. A 0.5% solution in water has a pH of 4.2 to 5.2. Store in airtight containers. Protect from light.

Adverse Effects
Side-effects occasionally reported with co-dergocrine mesilate include abdominal cramps, nausea, vomiting, headache, blurred vision, skin rashes, nasal congestion, flushing of the skin, dizziness, bradycardia, and orthostatic hypotension.

Local irritation has been reported following sublingual use.

Effects on the cardiovascular system. Of 8 patients given co-dergocrine mesilate 1.5 mg three times daily for the treatment of dementia, 3 developed severe sinus bradycardia associated with general deterioration in their condition, necessitating withdrawal of the treatment.[1] However, no sinus bradycardia had been observed in 40 elderly patients in whom the dose was built up to 1.5 mg three times daily over 3 weeks.[2]

1. Cayley ACD, *et al.* Sinus bradycardia following treatment with Hydergine for cerebrovascular insufficiency. *BMJ* 1975; **4:** 384–5.
2. Cohen C. Sinus bradycardia following treatment with Hydergine. *BMJ* 1975; **4:** 581.

Precautions
Co-dergocrine mesilate should be used with caution in patients with severe bradycardia.

Pharmacokinetics
Bioavailability of co-dergocrine after administration by mouth is low; this has been attributed to incomplete absorption from the gastrointestinal tract and extensive first-pass metabolism of the portion that is absorbed. Elimination is biphasic with a short half-life of 1.5 to 2.5 hours (α phase) and a longer half-life of 13 to 15 hours (β phase). Co-dergocrine is mainly excreted with bile in the faeces, although small amounts are eliminated in the urine.

Uses and Administration
Unlike the natural ergot alkaloids, co-dergocrine mesilate has only limited vasoconstrictor effects.

It is used with the intention of treating symptoms of mild to moderate dementia in the elderly in doses of 3 or 4.5 mg daily by mouth, preferably before meals. Higher doses have also been used. It is also given sublingually in similar doses. Doses of 300 to 600 µg once or twice daily have been given intramuscularly; it has also been given subcutaneously or by intravenous infusion.

In some countries, co-dergocrine mesilate has been used in the treatment of hypertension (p.802), migraine (p.449), and in peripheral vascular disease (p.809).

Co-dergocrine esilate has been used similarly to the mesilate.

Dementia. Co-dergocrine has been used for many years in dementia (p.1412) but its value is not established.[1-3] Originally its effects were thought to be mediated through peripheral and

---

The symbol † denotes a preparation no longer actively marketed

cerebral vasodilatation but it is now classified as a metabolic enhancer.

1. Wadworth AN, Chrisp P. Co-dergocrine mesylate: a review of its pharmacodynamic and pharmacokinetic properties and therapeutic use in age-related cognitive decline. *Drugs Aging* 1992; **2:** 153–73.
2. Schneider LS, Olin JT. Overview of clinical trials of Hydergine in dementia. *Arch Neurol* 1994; **51:** 787–98.
3. Olin J, *et al.* Hydergine for dementia (updated 6 March 2001). Available in The Cochrane Library; Issue 2. Oxford: Update Software; 2001.

Erectile dysfunction. A cream containing aminophylline, co-dergocrine mesilate, and isosorbide dinitrate produced satisfactory erections following topical application in 21 of 36 men with erectile dysfunction (p.1663) due to various causes.[1] Eight out of 9 men with erectile dysfunction of psychogenic origin reported a satisfactory response. However, another study was abandoned after the cream produced no effect in 10 consecutive patients.[2] The study was subsequently repeated in 14 patients who received a total of 77 applications of the cream, but no benefit was demonstrable over placebo.[3]

1. Gomaa A, *et al.* Topical treatment of erectile dysfunction: randomised double blind placebo controlled trial of cream containing aminophylline, isosorbide dinitrate, and co-dergocrine mesylate. *BMJ* 1996; **312:** 1512–15.
2. Naude JH, Le Roux PJ. Topical treatment of erectile dysfunction did not show results. *BMJ* 1998; **316:** 1318.
3. Le Roux PJ, Naude JH. Topical vasoactive cream in the treatment of erectile failure: a prospective, randomized placebo-controlled trial. *BJU Int* 1999; **83:** 810–11.

Preparations

BP 2001: Co-dergocrine Tablets;
USP 25: Ergoloid Mesylates Capsules; Ergoloid Mesylates Oral Solution; Ergoloid Mesylates Tablets.

Proprietary Preparations (details are given in Part 3)
Aust.: Aramexe; Dorehydrin; Ergomed; Ergoplex†; Hydergin; **Belg.:** Hydergine; Ibexone; Stofilan; **Braz.:** Hydergine; **Canad.:** Hydergine; **Fin.:** Artergin; Hydergin; **Fr.:** Capergyl; Ergodose; Hydergine; Optamine†; Perenan; Zenium; **Ger.:** Circanol; Dacoren; DCCK; Defluina N; Enirant; Ergodesit; ergoplus; ergotox; Hydergin; Hydro-Cebral; Nehydrin N; Orphol; Sponsin; **Hong Kong:** Hydergine; Perenan; Stofilan; **Irl.:** Hydergine; **Israel:** Hydergine; **Ital.:** Hydergina; Ischelium; **Mex.:** Hydergina; Progeril; **Neth.:** Hydergine; Hydroxium†; **Port.:** Hydergine; Redergot†; Secamin; **Singapore:** Hydergine; Perenan; Trigogine; **Spain:** Ergodilat; Hydergina; **Swed.:** Hydergin; **Switz.:** Ergohydrine; Hydergine; Progeril; **Thai.:** Codergine; Coergot; Helcon; Hyceral; Hydergine; Hydrine; Hymed; Naline; Perenan; Redergin; Trigogine; Vaculin; Vasian; **UK:** Hydergine; **USA:** Gerimal; Hydergine.

Multi-ingredient: Aust.: Pontuc; **Braz.:** Vincetron; **Ger.:** Pontuc; Sinedyston†; **Ital.:** Ischelium Papaverina†; Visergil; **Port.:** Euvifor; Projuvex; **Spain:** Clinadil Compositum; Neorgine†; Piracetam Complex; Visergil.

Coenzyme A (12604-v)

CoA; CoASH. 5'-*O*-{3-Hydroxy-3-[2-(2-mercaptoethylcarbamoyl)ethylcarbamoyl]-2,2-dimethylpropyl}adenosine-3'-dihydrogenphosphate-5'-trihydrogendiphosphate.

$C_{21}H_{36}N_7O_{16}P_3S = 767.5$.
CAS — 85-61-0.

Profile
Formed from adenosine triphosphate, cysteine, and pantothenic acid, coenzyme A is involved in the body in many physiological roles, including the formation of citrate, the oxidation of pyruvate, the oxidation and synthesis of fatty acids, the synthesis of triglycerides, cholesterol, and phospholipids, and the acetylation of amines, choline, and glucosamine. It has been given by injection in a variety of metabolic disorders. Coenzyme A is contra-indicated in acute myocardial infarction.

Preparations

Proprietary Preparations (details are given in Part 3)
Ital.: Coalip; **Spain:** Aluzime†.

Multi-ingredient: Ital.: Bio-Biol.

Cogalactoisomerase Sodium (12605-g)

UDPG; Uridine-5'-diphosphoglucose Sodium.
$C_{15}H_{22}N_2Na_2O_{17}P_2,3H_2O = 664.3$.
CAS — 133-89-1 (cogalactoisomerase).

Profile
Cogalactoisomerase sodium is used in various hepatic disorders.

Preparations

Proprietary Preparations (details are given in Part 3)
Ital.: Bivitox; Epatoxil; Liverasi; Toxepasi.

Colforsin (16542-c)

Colforsin *(USAN, rINN)*.

Boforsin; Forscolin; Forskolin; HL-362; L-75-1362B. (3R,4aR,5S,6S,6aS,10S,10aR,10bS)-Dodecahydro-5,6,10,10b-tetrahydroxy-3,4a,7,7,10a-pentamethyl-3-vinyl-1*H*-naphtho[2,1-*b*]pyran-1-one, 5-acetate.
$C_{22}H_{34}O_7 = 410.5$.
CAS — 66575-29-9.

Profile
Colforsin is an adenylate cyclase stimulator derived from *Coleus forskholii* that has been investigated for a number of conditions, including glaucoma and impotence. It is reported to have positive inotropic and bronchodilator effects. It has been used in the form of colforsin daropate hydrochloride.

Preparations

Proprietary Preparations (details are given in Part 3)
Jpn: Adehl.

Collagen (15335-n)

ATC — B02BC07; G04BX11.

A fibrous protein component of mammalian connective tissue making up almost one third of the total body protein.

Profile
Collagen, processed in a variety of ways, has been used in surgery as a haemostatic and as a repair and suture material. For cosmetic purposes it has been injected into the dermis to correct scars and other contour deformities of the skin. Collagen implants have been used to block tear outflow in the management of dry eye (p.1498).

Intraurethral administration of collagen has been used in the treatment of stress incontinence (p.459). There has also been interest in the use of collagen by mouth to suppress the inflammatory process in rheumatoid arthritis (p.9) and scleroderma (p.505).

◊ References.

1. Herschorn S, *et al.* Early experience with intraurethral collagen injections for urinary incontinence. *J Urol (Baltimore)* 1992; **148:** 1797–1800.
2. Sieper J, *et al.* Oral type II collagen treatment in early rheumatoid arthritis: a double-blind, placebo-controlled, randomized trial. *Arthritis Rheum* 1996; **39:** 41–51.
3. Stanton SL, Monga AK. Incontinence in elderly women: is periurethral collagen an advance? *Br J Obstet Gynaecol* 1997; **104:** 154–7.
4. Anonymous. GAX collagen for genuine stress incontinence. *Drug Ther Bull* 1997; **35:** 86–7.

Preparations

Proprietary Preparations (details are given in Part 3)
Aust.: Avitene; Instat; Urgo Pangen†; Zyderm; Zyplast; **Austral.:** Ionil Rinse; Zyderm; Zyplast; **Belg.:** Colgen†; **Fr.:** Collafilm†; Lenidermyl†; Pangen; Zyderm†; Zyplast†; **Ger.:** Opragen; Pangen; Porcoll; Surgicoll†; Tachotop N; TissuVlies†; Tutoplast Dura; Tutoplast Fascia lata; Zyderm; Zyplast; **Hong Kong:** Avitene; Zyderm; Zyplast; **Israel:** Zyderm; Zyplast; **Ital.:** Alfagen; Condress; Idroskin; Instat†; Neopelle; Skinat; Stimtes; **Neth.:** Willospon Forte; **Singapore:** Articolase; Zyderm; Zyplast; **Switz.:** Instat†; Lyostypt†; **UK:** Contigen; Fibracol; Instat; Lyostypt; **USA:** Avitene; Helistat†; Hemotene; Instat†.

Multi-ingredient: Aust.: TachoComb; **Austral.:** John Plunketts Protective Day Cream; John Plunketts Super Wrinkle Cream; **Belg.:** Duracoll; **Ger.:** TachoComb; **Hong Kong:** TachoComb; **Ital.:** Artrodue; Unidermo; **Port.:** Estriagel; **Switz.:** Gorgonium; **Thai.:** TachoComb; **USA:** PDP Liquid Protein.

Collagenase (12606-q)

Clostridiopeptidase A.
CAS — 9001-12-1.

Profile
Collagenase is a proteolytic enzyme with the ability to break down collagen. Preparations containing collagenase are used topically for the debridement of dermal ulcers and burns, and possibly other necrotic lesions, to facilitate granulation and epithelialisation. It has also been given by injection into the intervertebral disc for chemonucleolysis in the treatment of low back pain (p.6).

Hypersensitivity reactions may occur. Local burning, erythema, and pain have been reported at the site of application. It has been suggested that debridement of infected wounds may increase the risk of bacteraemia and that patients should be watched for signs of systemic bacterial infection. The activity of collagenase may be reduced by antiseptics containing detergents, hexachlorophene, and heavy metal ions.

Collagenase potency is expressed in units based on the amount of enzyme required to degrade a standard preparation of undenatured collagen.

Peyronie's disease.
Beneficial effects have been reported with intralesional collagenase in men with Peyronie's disease.[1,2]

1. Gelbard MK, *et al.* The use of collagenase in the treatment of Peyronie's disease. *J Urol (Baltimore)* 1985; **134:** 280–3.
2. Gelbard MK, *et al.* Collagenase versus placebo in the treatment of Peyronie's disease: a double-blind study. *J Urol (Baltimore)* 1993; **149:** 56–8.

Preparations

Proprietary Preparations (details are given in Part 3)
Belg.: Varilisin; **Canad.:** Santyl; **Hong Kong:** Iruxol Mono; **Ital.:** Noruxol; **Neth.:** Novuxol; **Port.:** Ulcerase†; **USA:** Santyl.

Multi-ingredient: Braz.: Gyno Iruxol; Iruxol; **Fin.:** Iruxol; Iruxol Mono; **Ger.:** Iruxol; **Irl.:** Iruxol Mono; **Ital.:** Iruxol; **Mex.:** Ulcoderma; **S.Afr.:** Iruxol Mono; **Spain:** Iruxol Mono; Iruxol Neo; **Switz.:** Iruxol Mono.

Colophony (276-t)

Coloph.; Colophane; Colophonium; Resin; Resina Pini; Resina Terebinthinae; Rosin.

Pharmacopoeias. In Aust., Br., Jpn, Pol., and Swiss.

Pharmacopoeial description

BP 2001: The residue left after distilling the volatile oil from the oleoresin obtained from various species of *Pinus*. Translucent, pale yellow or brownish-yellow, angular, brittle, readily fusible, glassy masses with a faint terebinthinate odour. Practically insoluble in water; soluble in alcohol, in carbon disulfide, and in ether; partially soluble in petroleum spirit (boiling range, 40° to 60°).

Profile
Colophony is an ingredient of some collodions and plastermasses. It has been used as an ingredient of ointments and dressings for wounds and minor skin disorders. Skin sensitisation and allergic respiratory symptoms have been reported.

Hypersensitivity. Reviews.

1. Downs AM, Sansom JE. Colophony allergy: a review. *Contact Dermatitis* 1999; **41:** 305–10.

Preparations

BP 2001: Flexible Collodion.

Proprietary Preparations (details are given in Part 3)

Multi-ingredient: Aust.: Ehrenhofer-Salbe; Vulpuran; **Austral.:** Zam-Buk; **Hong Kong:** Zam-Buk; **Ital.:** Fialetta Odontalgica Dr Knapp; **Singapore:** Zam-Buk; **Spain:** Empapol; **UK:** Herbheal Ointment; Pickles Corn Caps.

Comfrey (12607-p)

Comfrey Root; Consolidae Radix; Symphytum.

The dried root and rhizome of *Symphytum officinale* (Boraginaceae). It contains about 0.7% of allantoin, large quantities of mucilage, and some tannin. It may also contain pyrrolizidine alkaloids.

Profile
Comfrey was formerly used as an application to wounds and ulcers to stimulate healing and was also given systemically for gastric ulceration. It has been applied topically in the treatment of inflammatory disorders. The healing action of comfrey has been attributed to the presence of allantoin (p.1110). Comfrey is used in homoeopathic medicine.

There are reports of hepatotoxicity attributed to pyrrolizidine alkaloids present in comfrey preparations and such preparations have been withdrawn or banned in a number of countries.

Adverse effects. Toxic pyrrolizidine alkaloids have been isolated from several species of comfrey plants including common comfrey (*Symphytum officinale*), prickly comfrey (*S. asperum*), and Russian comfrey (*S. uplandicum*). Ingestion of plants containing pyrrolizidine alkaloids is a common cause of hepatic veno-occlusive disease in developing countries[1] and pyrrolidine alkaloid hepatotoxicity presumably due to comfrey has been reported in North America and Europe.[1,2] Pulmonary endothelial hyperplasia and carcinogenic activity have also been reported in *animals*.[1,2]

1. Ridker PM, McDermott WV. Comfrey herb tea and hepatic veno-occlusive disease. *Lancet* 1989; **i:** 657–8.
2. Bach N, *et al.* Comfrey herb tea-induced hepatic veno-occlusive disease. *Am J Med* 1989; **87:** 97–9.

Preparations

Proprietary Preparations (details are given in Part 3)
Canad.: Procomfrin†; **Ger.:** Kytta-Plasma f; Kytta-Salbe f; Traumaplant.

Multi-ingredient: Fr.: Tisanes de l'Abbe Hamon no 15†; **Ger.:** Kytta-Balsam f; Rhus-Rheuma-Gel N; Syviman N; **Israel:** Comfrey Plus; **Port.:** Solucao Stago; **Switz.:** Alpina Gel a la consoude†; Cetona Plus; Gel a la consoude; Keppur; Kytta Baume†; Kytta Pommade†.

Complement Blockers (12038-j)

Profile
A number of compounds are under investigation for their ability to inhibit activation of the complement system. Such compounds include soluble forms of the complement receptors such as TP-10 (sCR1) or its derivatives, naturally-occurring complement blockers such as CD59, and synthetic complement blockers. The potential clinical applications of such compounds are being investigated in various conditions, including the prevention of acute respiratory distress syndrome, and for the prevention of reperfusion injury following myocardial infarction or lung transplantation.

◊ References.
1. Makrides SC. Therapeutic inhibition of the complement system. *Pharmacol Rev* 1998; **50**: 59–87.
2. McGeer EG, McGeer PL. The future use of complement inhibitors for the treatment of neurological diseases. *Drugs* 1998; **55**: 739–46.

Complement C1 Esterase Inhibitor (16557-d)

C₁ Esterase Inhibitor.

Profile
Complement C1 esterase inhibitor is prepared from human plasma and is used as replacement therapy in the management of life-threatening attacks of hereditary angioedema (p.743).

◊ Complement C1 esterase inhibitor may be effective in both the prevention and treatment of acute hereditary angioedema.[1] It has also been tried in the management of other conditions including sepsis (p.138) and capillary leak syndrome.[2] It is under investigation for the treatment of pancreatitis and for use in allogeneic lung transplantation, thermal injury, and shock.[2]
1. Waytes AT, *et al.* Treatment of hereditary angioedema with a vapor-heated C1 inhibitor concentrate. *N Engl J Med* 1996; **334**: 1630–4.
2. Caliezi C, *et al.* C1-esterase inhibitor: an anti-inflammatory agent and its potential use in the treatment of diseases other than hereditary angioedema. *Pharmacol Rev* 2000; **52**: 91–112.

Preparations
Proprietary Preparations (details are given in Part 3)
Aust.: Berinert; **Fr.:** Esterasine; **Ger.:** Berinert; **Ital.:** C1 Inattivatore Umano; **Switz.:** Berinert HS; **UK:** Berinert P†.

Condurango (531-a)

Condurango Bark; Eagle-vine Bark.
Pharmacopoeias. In Aust., Belg., Jpn, and Swiss.

The dried stem bark of *Marsdenia condurango* (=*Gonolobus condurango*) (Asclepiadaceae).

Profile
Condurango has been used as a bitter. It has also been used in homoeopathic medicine.

Preparations
Proprietary Preparations (details are given in Part 3)
Multi-ingredient: Aust.: Pascopankreat; Sigman-Haustropfen; **Braz.:** Camomila; **Fr.:** Soker†; **Ger.:** Nervogastrol; Pankreaplex Neu; Pascopankreat novo; **Switz.:** Padma-Lax; Stomacine.

Congo Red (2125-x)

CI Direct Red 28; Colour Index No. 22120; Rubrum Congoensis. Disodium 3,3′-[biphenyl-4,4′-diylbis(azo)]bis[4-aminonaphthalene-1-sulphonate].
C₃₂H₂₂N₆Na₂O₆S₂ = 696.7.
CAS — 573-58-0.

Profile
Congo red is used as a stain in the diagnosis of amyloidosis. It causes amyloid in tissue samples to fluoresce under polarised light.

Convallaria (5806-d)

Lily of the Valley; Maiblume; Maiglöckchenkraut; May Lily; Muguet.
CAS — 3253-62-1 (convallatoxol); 13473-51-3 (convalloside); 13289-19-5 (convallatoxoloside); 508-75-8 (convallatoxin).
Pharmacopoeias. In Aust. and Ger. (from C. majalis or closely related species).

The dried flowers, herb, or the rhizomes and roots of lily of the valley, *Convallaria majalis* (Liliaceae). Several crystalline glycosides have been obtained from the plant including convallarin, convalloside, convallatoxoloside, and convallatoxin.

Profile
Convallaria contains cardiac glycosides and has actions on the heart similar to those of digoxin (p.870). Convallaria is used in herbal and homoeopathic medicine.

The symbol † denotes a preparation no longer actively marketed

---

◊ *Convallaria majalis* has been designated unsafe for inclusion in foods, beverages, or drugs by the FDA in the USA.[1]
1. Larkin T. *FDA Consumer* 1983; **17** (Oct.): 5.

Preparations
Proprietary Preparations (details are given in Part 3)
Ger.: Convacard; Valdig-N Burger.
Multi-ingredient: Aust.: Cardiofrik; Omega; **Fr.:** Tisanes de l'Abbe Hamon no 16†; Tisanes de l'Abbe Hamon no 3; **Ger.:** Aesrutal S; Cardibisana; Cefascillan; Convallocor-SL; Convastabil; Cor-loges; Cor-Vel N†; Corguttin N plus†; Goldtropfen-Hetterich; Guttacor; Hypercard; Lacoerdin-N; Miroton; Miroton N; Oxacant N; Oxacant-forte N; Oxacant-Khella N; Raufuncton N; Venopyronum N triplex†; Viscorapas duo; **Spain:** Uralyt†.

Corbadrine (2076-b)

Corbadrine (*rINN*).
l-3,4-Dihydroxynorephedrine; Levonordefrin; *l*-Nordefrin. (−)-2-Amino-1-(3,4-dihydroxyphenyl)propan-1-ol.
C₉H₁₃NO₃ = 183.2.
CAS — 829-74-3 (corbadrine); 6539-57-7 (nordefrin); 61-96-1 (nordefrin hydrochloride).
Pharmacopoeias. In US.
Aust. includes Nordefrin Hydrochloride, which is the salt of the racemic substance.

Pharmacopoeial description
USP 25: A white to buff-coloured, odourless, crystalline solid. Practically insoluble in water; slightly soluble in alcohol, in acetone, in chloroform, and in ether; freely soluble in aqueous solutions of mineral acids.

Profile
Corbadrine is a sympathomimetic (see Adrenaline, p.829) that has been added to local anaesthetic preparations in dentistry to diminish absorption and to localise the effect; a concentration of 1 in 20 000 has been used.

Preparations
USP 25: Mepivacaine Hydrochloride and Levonordefrin Injection; Procaine and Tetracaine Hydrochlorides and Levonordefrin Injection; Propoxycaine and Procaine Hydrochlorides and Levonordefrin Injection.

Proprietary Preparations (details are given in Part 3)
Used as an adjunct in: **S.Afr.:** Carbocaine; **USA:** Carbocaine with Neo-Cobefrin; Isocaine; Polocaine.

Coriander (4637-j)

Coentro; Coriand.; Coriander Fruit; Coriander Seed; Coriandri Fructus; Fruto de Cilantro.
Pharmacopoeias. In Eur. (see p.vi) and Pol.

Pharmacopoeial description
Ph. Eur.: The dried cremocarp of *Coriandrum sativum*, containing not less than 0.3% v/w of essential oil, calculated with reference to the dried substance. Protect from light.

Profile
Coriander is the source of coriander oil. It is a carminative and is used as a flavour.

Preparations
Proprietary Preparations (details are given in Part 3)
Multi-ingredient: Aust.: Apotheker Bauer's Blahungstee; Bio-Garten Tropfen gegen Blahungen; Brady's-Magentropfen; Carminative; Carminativum Babynos; Dr. Ernst Richter's Abfuhrtee-Filterbeutel; Mariazeller; Planta Lax; **Belg.:** Tamarine; **Braz.:** Fitolax; Florlax; Frutalax; Frutovena; Laxarine; Laxtam; Novolax; Tamaril; Tamarine; **Fr.:** Mediflor Tisane Digestive No 3†; Tisane Grande Chartreuse; **Ger.:** Carminativum Babynos; Floradix Multipretten; Gastrol S; Presselin Dyspeptikum; Ramend Krauter; **Ital.:** Dicalmir; Tamarine; Tisana Cisbey†; **Mex.:** Naturetti; **Spain:** Agua del Carmen; Jarabe Manceau; Jarabe Manzanas Siken; Pruina; Vegetalin; **Switz.:** Boldoflorine†; Tamarine†; Tisane laxative Natterman no 13†; **UK:** Cough Drops; Melissa comp..

Coriander Oil (4638-z)

Ol. Coriand; Oleum Coriandri.
Pharmacopoeias. In Br.

Pharmacopoeial description
BP 2001: A clear colourless or pale yellow liquid, visibly free from water, with the characteristic odour and taste of coriander, obtained by distillation from coriander. It contains not less than 65% w/w and not more than 75% w/w of linalol. Soluble 1 in 3 of alcohol. Store in well-filled containers at a temperature not exceeding 25°. Protect from light.

Profile
Coriander oil is aromatic and carminative and is used as a flavour.

Preparations
BP 2001: Compound Orange Spirit; Compound Rhubarb Tincture.
Proprietary Preparations (details are given in Part 3)
Multi-ingredient: Ger.: Floradix Multipretten; Gastricard N.

Corn Silk (3937-a)

Stigma Maydis; Zea.

Profile
Corn silk, the stigma and style of maize (*Zea mays*) (Gramineae), has diuretic properties and is used for urinary-tract disorders including renal calculi.

Maize is widely used as a food and has also been used in herbal medicine.

Preparations
Proprietary Preparations (details are given in Part 3)
Braz.: Insadol; **Fr.:** Insadol; **Switz.:** Insadol.
Multi-ingredient: Austral.: Althaea Complex; Urinase; **Fr.:** Antigoutteux Rezall†; Aromalgyl†; Tisane Orientale Soker†; Tisanes de l'Abbe Hamon no 3; **UK:** Elixir Damiana and Saw Palmetto; Protat; **USA:** Aqua-Rid†; Fluidex†; Tri-Aqua†.

Cottonseed Oil (7358-p)

Aceite de Algodon; Cotton Oil; Ol. Gossyp. Sem.; Oléo de Algodoeiro; Oleum Gossypii Seminis.
Pharmacopoeias. In USNF. Eur. (see p.vi) *includes Hydrogenated Cottonseed Oil.*

Pharmacopoeial description
Ph. Eur.: Hydrogenated Cottonseed Oil is obtained by refining and hydrogenation of oil obtained from seeds of cultivated plants of various varieties of *Gossypium hirsutum* or of other species of *Gossypium*. It consists mainly of triglycerides of palmitic and stearic acids. It is a white mass or powder which melts to a clear pale yellow liquid when heated. M.p. 57° to 70°. Practically insoluble in water; very slightly soluble in alcohol; freely soluble in dichloromethane and in toluene. Protect from light.
USNF 20: Cottonseed Oil is the refined fixed oil obtained from the seed of plants of various varieties of *Gossypium hirsutum* or of other species of *Gossypium* (Malvaceae). It is a pale yellow, oily liquid, odourless or nearly so. Slightly soluble in alcohol; miscible with carbon disulfide, with chloroform, with ether, and with petroleum spirit. Store in airtight containers at a temperature not exceeding 40°. Protect from light. At temperatures below 10° particles of solid fat may separate from the oil and at about 0° to −5° the oil becomes a solid or nearly so.

Profile
Cottonseed oil is used as an oily vehicle.

An extract of cottonseed oil, gossypol (p.1618), has been tried as a contraceptive in males.

Couch-grass (2322-h)

Agropyron; Chiendent; Dogs Grass; Graminis Rhizoma; Quackgrass; Twitch.
Pharmacopoeias. In Eur. (see p.vi) and Pol.

It contains glucose, mannitol, inositol, and triticin (a carbohydrate resembling inulin).

Pharmacopoeial description
Ph. Eur.: The whole or cut, washed and dried rhizome of *Agropyron repens* (*Elymus repens*); the adventitious roots are removed. Protect from light.

Profile
Couch-grass is a mild diuretic which has been used in herbal medicine in the treatment of cystitis.

Preparations
Proprietary Preparations (details are given in Part 3)
Ger.: Acorus.
Multi-ingredient: Aust.: Abfuhrtee; Brostalin; Krauterhaus Mag Kottas Blasentee; Krauterhaus Mag Kottas Entwasserungstee; Krautertee Nr 2; Sidroga Nieren- und Blasentee; **Fr.:** Herbesan; Mediflor Tisane Antirhumatismale No 2†; Mediflor Tisane No 4 Diuretique; Mediflor Tisane Pectorale d'Alsace; Tisane Hepatique de Hoerdt; Tisane Orientale Soker†; Tisanes de l'Abbe Hamon no 11; **Ger.:** Blasen-Nieren-Tee Stada†; Harntee 400; Hevert-Blasen-und Nieren- Tee; Presselin Stoffwechsel-Tee Hapeka 225 N; Renob Blasen- und Nierentee; **Ital.:** Depurativo; Emmenoiasi; Tisana Arnaldi†; Tisana Cisbey†; Tisana Kelemata; **Switz.:** The Franklin†; **UK:** Antitis; Kas-Bah; **USA:** Aqua-Rid†; Fluidex†.

Coumarin (2388-x)

1,2-Benzopyrone; 5,6-Benzo-α-pyrone; Cumarin; Tonka Bean Camphor. 2H-1-Benzopyran-2-one.
C₉H₆O₂ = 146.1.
CAS — 91-64-5.
Pharmacopoeias. In Ger.

Coumarin is the odorous principle of Tonka seed (Tonka or Tonquin bean); it may be prepared synthetically.

Profile
Coumarin has been used in the treatment of lymphoedema. It has also been used as a fixative in perfumery and as a flavour. It is reported to be an immunostimulant and has been tried in the treatment of malignant neoplasms.

Coumarin derivatives are used as anticoagulants.

Effects on the liver. Coumarin has been classified as hepatotoxic based on studies in *animals*. Liver toxicity ranging from elevated liver enzymes to serious organ damage has been reported in humans. Seventeen of 2173 patients enrolled in a clinical/toxicological study of coumarin developed elevated liver enzyme values;[1] the majority of patients were given 100 mg coumarin daily for 1 month followed by 50 mg daily for 2 years. However, none of the patients developed permanent liver damage and liver enzyme values returned to normal in 5 patients who continued taking coumarin. Results from 5 studies supported by the Lymphoedema Association of Australia, in which patients received 400 mg daily for a mean duration of 14.6 months, showed 2 cases of hepatotoxicity among 1106 patients.[2] In the period of 14 months up to May 1995, the Australian Drug Evaluation Committee received 10 reports of suspected adverse reactions to coumarin,[3] including 6 cases of jaundice in women who had taken 400 mg daily for 1 to 4 months. Periportal and lobular necrosis were found on biopsy in 1 case and another had a fatal outcome due to massive hepatic necrosis.

Reports of hepatotoxicity have led to the withdrawal of coumarin in a number of countries.

1. Cox D, *et al*. The rarity of liver toxicity in patients treated with coumarin (1,2-benzopyrone). *Hum Toxicol* 1989; **8**: 501–6.
2. Casley-Smith JR, Casley-Smith JR. Frequency of coumarin hepatotoxicity. *Med J Aust* 1995; **162**: 391.
3. Anonymous. Lodema and the liver. *Aust Adverse Drug React Bull* 1995; **14**: 11.

Lymphoedema. Benzopyrones such as coumarin are reported to reduce excess protein in tissues with high-protein oedema, hence the use of coumarin in lymphoedema of various causes, including postmastectomy, and filarial lymphoedema and elephantiasis.[1-4] Evidence for its efficacy is, however, conflicting;[4,5] at best the action is slow and treatment may need to be continued for 6 months to 2 years before any benefit is seen.

1. Jamal S, *et al*. The effects of 5,6 benzo-[a]-pyrone (coumarin) and DEC on filaritic lymphoedema and elephantiasis in India: preliminary results. *Ann Trop Med Parasitol* 1989; **83**: 287–90.
2. Turner CS. Congenital lymphedema. *JAMA* 1990; **264**: 518.
3. Casley-Smith JR, *et al*. Treatment of lymphedema of the arms and legs with 5,6-benzo-[α]-pyrone. *N Engl J Med* 1993; **329**: 1158–63.
4. Casley-Smith JR, *et al*. Treatment of filarial lymphoedema and elephantiasis with 5,6-benzo-α-pyrone (coumarin). *BMJ* 1993; **307**: 1037–41.
5. Loprinzi CL, *et al*. Lack of effect of coumarin in women with lymphedema after treatment for breast cancer. *N Engl J Med* 1999; **340**: 346–50.

Preparations

Proprietary Preparations (details are given in Part 3)
Austral.: Lodema†; *Fr.:* Lysedem†; *Ger.:* Venalot mono; *Switz.:* Lymphex†; Venalot†; Venium†.

Multi-ingredient: *Braz.:* Venalot; Venalot H; *Ger.:* Caye Balsam; Kneipp Rheuma Stoffwechsel-Bad Heublumen-Aquasan†; Venalot; Venalot N; *Mex.:* Venalot.

Cowberry (308-e)

Red Whortleberry.

Pharmacopoeias. In Aust.

Profile
The leaves of the cowberry, *Vaccinium vitis-idaea* (Ericaceae), have astringent properties and have been used as a domestic remedy for diarrhoea.

Cowslip (2023-j)

Primelwurzel; Primula; Racine de Primevére; Schlüsselblumenwurzel.

Pharmacopoeias. Eur. (see p.vi) includes Primula Root from *Primula veris* or *P. elatior*.

Pharmacopoeial description
Ph. Eur.: Primula Root consists of the whole or cut, dried rhizome and root of *Primula veris* [cowslip] or *P. elatior* [oxlip]. It has a bitter taste. Protect from light.

Profile
Cowslip, the flowers, leaves, and roots of *Primula veris* (*P. officinalis*) (Primulaceae), is widely used in herbal medicine. The flowers have sedative properties and are used for insomnia, hyperactivity, and anxiety disorders. The roots have expectorant properties and are used for cough and other respiratory-tract disorders; the leaves have been used similarly.

It is also used in homoeopathic medicine.

Oxlip root (*P. elatior*) and primrose root (*P. vulgaris*) have also been used.

Preparations

Proprietary Preparations (details are given in Part 3)
Ger.: Ipalat.

Multi-ingredient: *Aust.:* Anifer Hustentropfen; Apotheker Bauer's Brust- und Hustentee; Apotheker Bauer's Grippetee; Cardiodoron; Granobil; Heumann's Bronchialtee; Hustensaft-Dr Schmidgall; Kneipp Husten- und Bronchial-Tee; Hustensaft; Krauterdoktor Hustentropfen; Sinupret; Sinusol; Sinusol-Schleimlosender Tee; St Radegunder Thorasan-Krauterhustensaft;

Synpharma Instant-Brust- und Hustentee; Thymoval; *Canad.:* Pectothymin†; *Ger.:* Bronchicum Elixir N; Bronchicum Elixir Plus; Bronchicum Sekret-Loser; Bronchicum Thymian; Bronchipret; Bronchitten forte K; Brust- und Hustentee; Cardiodoron; Drosithym-N; Ephepect; Equisil; Expectysat N; Guttae 20 Hustentropfen N†; Harzer Hustenloser; Heumann Bronchialtee Solubifix; Ipalat†; JuViton; Kinder Em-eukal Hustensaft; Kneipp Husten- und Bronchial-Tee; Melrosum Hustensirup N; Mintetten Truw†; Perdiphen phyto†; Phytobronchin; Praecipect†; Primotussan; Salus Bronchial-Tee Nr.8†; Sinuforton; Sinupret; Sinupret forte; Tussiflorin Hustensaft; Tussiflorin Hustentropfen; Tussiflorin N; TUSSinfant N; *Hong Kong:* Pectoral; Sinupret; *Neth.:* Abdijsiroop (Akker-Siroop)†; Bronchicum; *Port.:* Bio-Strath No 1†; Bio-Strath No 5†; Codeisan†; Fluidin Infantil; *S.Afr.:* Bronchicough; Bronchicum; *Singapore:* Sinupret; *Switz.:* Demo sirop bronchique N†; DemoPectol; Bronchicum Elixir; Pectoral N; Perpector; Sinupret; Sirop S contre la toux et la bronchite; Tisane pectorale pour les enfants; *Thai.:* Sinupret; Solvopret TP; *UK:* Bio-Strath Willow Formula; Onoporaon Comp B.

CR Gas (12615-p)

EA-3547. Dibenz[*b,f*][1,4]oxazepine.
$C_{13}H_9NO = 195.2$.
CAS — 257-07-8.

Profile
A riot-control gas with properties similar to those of CS gas (p.1601); it is described as a tear gas. CR gas is reported not to be hydrolysed by water and therefore to be suitable for use in water cannons.

Cranberry (9415-k)

Pharmacopoeias. USNF includes Cranberry Liquid Preparation.

The fruit of *Vaccinium macrocarpon*, the American cranberry.

Profile
Cranberry juice has been reported to reduce the incidence of urinary-tract infections.

Urinary-tract infections. Cranberries and cranberry juice have been used widely for many years for both the treatment and prevention of urinary-tract infections. Despite this, there is a lack of well designed, double-blind, randomised studies assessing their efficacy for treatment of urinary-tract infections and a systematic review[1] of available data concluded that there was no good quality evidence to suggest efficacy.

In a further systematic review[2] assessing the effectiveness of cranberry for preventing urinary-tract infections it was concluded that, although some placebo-controlled studies had been conducted and had indicated some efficacy, the quality of these studies was poor and the evidence could not be considered reliable, and therefore cranberry could not be recommended for prevention of urinary-tract infections in the absence of better evidence from further properly designed studies.

1. Jepson RG, *et al*. Cranberries for treating urinary tract infections (updated 15 August 2001). Available in The Cochrane Library; Issue 4. Oxford: Update Software; 2001.
2. Jepson RG, *et al*. Cranberries for preventing urinary tract infections (updated 15 August 2001). Available in The Cochrane Library; Issue 4. Oxford: Update Software; 2001.

Preparations

USNF 20: Cranberry Liquid Preparation.

Proprietary Preparations (details are given in Part 3)
Multi-ingredient: *Austral.:* Bioglan Cranbiotic Super; Cranberry Complex; Extralife Uri-Care; *USA:* Uro-pH Control†.

Crataegus (5807-n)

Aubépine; Biancospino; Crataegus Oxyacantha; English Hawthorn; Haw; Pilriteiro; Weissdorn; Whitethorn.

Pharmacopoeias. In Chin., Eur. (see p.vi), and Pol.

Pharmacopoeial description
Ph. Eur.: Hawthorn Berries consists of the dried false fruits of *Crataegus oxyacantha* (*C. laevigata*), or *C. monogyna*, or their hybrids or a mixture of these false fruits. They contain not less than 1% of procyanidins, calculated as cyanidin chloride ($C_{15}H_{11}ClO_6 = 322.7$) with reference to the dried drug. Protect from light.

Hawthorn Leaf and Flower consists of the whole or cut, dried flower bearing branches of *Crataegus oxyacantha* (*C. laevigata*), or *C. monogyna*, or their hybrids or, more rarely, other European *Crataegus* species including *C. pentagyna*, *C. nigra*, and *C. azarolus*. It contains not less than 1.5% of flavonoids, calculated as hyperoside ($C_{21}H_{20}O_{12} = 464.4$) calculated with reference to the dried drug. Protect from light.

Profile
Crataegus contains flavonoid glycosides with cardiotonic properties similar to those of digoxin (p.870). Crataegus is used in herbal and homoeopathic medicine.

◊ General references.
1. Hamon NW. Hawthorns: the genus Crataegus. *Can Pharm J* 1988; **121**: 708–9 and 724.

Preparations

Proprietary Preparations (details are given in Part 3)
Aust.: Bericard; Cardiphyt; Crataegan; Crataegutt; Esbericard; Neo-Cratylen†; Sanadorn†; Senecard†; Senecard†; *Fr.:* Aubeline; Cardiocalm; Crataegol; Spasmosedine; *Ger.:* Adenylocrat; Arte-Rutin C; Basticrat; Born†; Chronocard N; Cordapur Novo; Corocrat; Coronator†; Craegium; Crataegutt; Crataegysat F; Crataepas; Crataezyma†; Cratamed novo†; Cratecor; Craviscum mono; Esbericard novo; Faros; Herz-Tropfen Eu Rho; Kneipp Pflanzen-Dragees Weissdorn; Kneipp Weissdorn-Pflanzensaft Sebastianeum; Kneipp Weissdorn-Tee; Kyaugutt; Kytta-Cor; Liquicard†; Logomed Herz†; Naranocor†; Neo-Cratylen†; Normotin V1†; Optocor†; Orthangin N; Orthangin novo; Orthocardon-N†; Oxacant-mono; Poikilocard Mono; Regulacor-POS; Rephacratin†; Senicor; Steicorton; Tensitruw†; Tonoplantin Mono†; Vitalin; *Ital.:* Cardiplant†; *Neth.:* Crataegutt†; *Spain:* Crataegutt; Elusanes Espino Albar; *Switz.:* Cardiplant; Crataegisan; Crataegitan; Esbericard†; Eurhyton†; Faros.

Multi-ingredient: *Aust.:* Apotheker Bauer's Grippetee; Biovital Weissdorn; Cardalept; Cardiofrik; Corodyn; Coroverlan†; Doppelherz Tonikum; Heli-Sal; Herz- und Kreislauftonikum Bioflora; Kneipp Herz- und Kreislauf-Unterstutzungs-Tee; Krautertee Nr 20; Krautertee Nr 32; Krautertee Nr 44; Mag Kottas Herz- und Kreislauftee; Naturland Herz-Kreislauf; Omega; Rutiviscal; Sanvita Herz†; Sidroga Herz-Kreislauf-Tee; St Radegunder Herz-Kreislauf-Tonikum; St Radegunder Herz-Kreislauf-unterstutzender Tee; Teekanne Herz- und Kreislauftee; Virgilocard; Wechseltee; *Austral.:* Asa Tones; Bioglan Bioage Peripheral; Crataegus Complex; For Peripheral Circulation Herbal Plus Formula 5; Gingo A; Ginkgo Biloba Plus; Ginkgo Complex; Lifechange Circulation Aid; Lifesystem Herbal Formula 6 For Peripheral Circulation; Multi-Vitamin Day & Night; *Belg.:* Sedinal; Seneuval; Spasmosedine†; Tisane Contre la Tension; Tisane pour Dormir; *Braz.:* Anevrase; Calman; Maracugina Composta; Pasalix; Passicarbone; Passiflorine; Sedalin; Serenus; Sominex; *Fr.:* Actisane Nervosite†; Actisane Troubles du Sommeil; Anxoral; Astressane†; Biocarde; Euphytose; Germose; Lenicalm; Mediflor Tisane Calmante Troubles du Sommeil No 14†; Mediflor Tisane Circulation du Sang No 12†; Natudor; Neurephytum; Neuropax; Neurotensyl†; Nicoprive; Noctisan†; Nocvalene; Nuidort†; Passiflorine; Passinevryl; Phytocalm; Quinisedine; Santane H₇; Santane N₉; Santane V₃; Sedalozia; Sedatif Tiber; Sedatonyl†; Sedibaine†; Sedopal; Serenival†; Spasmidenal; Spasmine; Sympaneurol†; Sympathyl; Sympavagol; Tranquital; Vagostabyl; Vericardine; *Ger.:* Aesrutal S; Antihypertonicum S; Antisklerosin S; Ardeycordal N; Asgoviscum N; Biovital Forte N; Biovital N; Biovital Weissdorn Tonikum; Bomacorin; Cardibisana; Cardio-Longoral; Cefasedativ; Chlorophyl liquid "Schuh"; Convallocor-SL; Convastabil; Cor-Select; Cor-Vel; Corguttin N plus†; Coroverlan; Crataelanat†; Diawern; Dr. Hotz Vollbrad†; Euvalon†; Fovysat; Gastricard N; Ginseng-Complex "Schuh"; Goldtropfen-Hetterich; Guttacor; Herz-Starkung N; Heusin; Ilja Rogoff; JuViton; Kneipp Drei-Pflanzen-Dragees N; Kneipp Herz- und Kreislauf-Tee; Korodin; Kreislauftropen; Lacoerdin-N; Nephrisan P; Nitro-Crataegutt; Nitro-cum; Oxacant N; Oxacant-forte N; Oxacant-Khella N; Oxacant-sedativ; Passin; Passiorin N†; Presselin Arterien K 5 P; Protecor; Rauwoplant; Salus Herz-Schutz-Kapseln; Salusan†; Septacord; Stenocrat; Szillosan forte†; Tornix; Vasesana-Vasoregulans; Viscorapas duo; *Israel:* Nerven-Dragees; Passiflora; *Ital.:* Anevrasi; Bianco Val; Blandonal; Lenicalm; Mirtiros; Nicoprive; Noctis; Parvisedil; Passiflorine; Prexene†; Quietan†; Relaten†; Sedatol; Sedopuer F; Tauma; *Port.:* Calmo; Gabisedil; Neurocardol; *Singapore:* Noricaven; *Spain:* Passiflorine; Sonofit; *Switz.:* Arterosan Plus; Cardiaforce; Dragees pour le coeur et les nerfs; Gouttes pour le coeur et les nerfs Concentrees; Korodin†; Phytomed Cardio†; Sedosan; Sirop Passi-Par; Tai Ginseng N; Tisane pour le coeur et la circulation; Valverde Dragees pour le coeur; Valverde Gouttes pour le coeur; *UK:* Tranquil.

Creatine Phosphate (6828-j)

Creatine Phosphoric Acid; Phosphocreatine. *N*-[Imino(phosphonoamino)-methyl]-*N*-methylglycine.
$C_4H_{10}N_3O_5P = 211.1$.
CAS — 67-07-2 (creatine phosphate); 922-32-7 (creatine phosphate disodium).

Profile
Creatine phosphate is an endogenous substance found mainly in skeletal muscle of vertebrates. It has been tried in the treatment of cardiac disorders and has been added to cardioplegic solutions. Creatine monohydrate has been tried in metabolic disorders and used as a dietary supplement.

◊ References.
1. Pedone V, *et al*. An assessment of the activity of creatine phosphate (Neoton) on premature ventricular beats by continuous ECG monitoring in patients with coronary cardiac disease. *Clin Trials J* 1984; **21**: 91.
2. Ferraro S, *et al*. Acute and short-term efficacy of high doses of creatine phosphate in the treatment of cardiac failure. *Curr Ther Res* 1990; **47**: 917–23.
3. Mastoroberto P, *et al*. Creatine phosphate protection of the ischemic myocardium during cardiac surgery. *Curr Ther Res* 1992; **51**: 37–45.
4. Stöckler S, *et al*. Creatine replacement therapy in guanidinoacetate methyltransferase deficiency, a novel inborn error of metabolism. *Lancet* 1996; **348**: 789–90.
5. Mujika I, Padilla S. Creatine supplementation as an ergogenic aid for sports performance in highly trained athletes: a critical review. *Int J Sports Med* 1997; **18**: 491–6.
6. Juhn MS, Tarnopolsky M. Oral creatine supplementation and athletic performance: a critical review. *Clin J Sport Med* 1998; **8**: 286–97. Correction. *ibid.* 1999; **9**: 62.
7. Kayne S. Creatine: the athlete's wonder supplement? *Pharm J* 1999; **263**: 906–8.

8. Pepping J. Creatine. *Am J Health-Syst Pharm* 1999; **56:** 1608–10.
9. Benzi G. Is there a rationale for the use of creatine either as nutritional supplementation or drug administration in humans participating in a sport? *Pharmacol Res* 2000; **41:** 255–64.

Preparations

Proprietary Preparations (details are given in Part 3)
Ital.: Creatile.

Creatinine   (14445-f)

2-Amino-1-methyl-4-imidazolidinone.
$C_4H_7N_3O = 113.1$.
CAS — 60-27-5.
Pharmacopoeias. In *Ger.* and *USNF.*

Pharmacopoeial description

USNF 20: White, odourless, crystals or crystalline powder. Soluble in water; slightly soluble in alcohol; practically insoluble in acetone, in chloroform, and in ether.

Profile

Creatinine is used as a bulking agent for freeze-drying.
Plasma concentrations or clearance of endogenous creatinine are used as an index of renal function.

Creatinolfosfate Sodium   (12616-s)

Creatinolfosfate Sodium *(rINNM)*.
The sodium salt of 1-(2-hydroxyethyl)-1-methylguanidine *O*-phosphate .
$C_4H_{11}N_3NaO_4P = 219.1$.
CAS — 6903-79-3 *(creatinolfosfate)*.

Profile

Creatinolfosfate has been used as an adjuvant in the treatment of cardiac disorders.

Preparations

Proprietary Preparations (details are given in Part 3)
Ital.: Aplodan; *Spain:* Dragosil†.

Crotalaria   (12021-v)

Profile

Crotalaria spp. have been used in the preparation of herbal teas but liver damage has been reported following their ingestion, possibly due to their content of pyrrolizidine alkaloids.

CS Gas   (12618-e)

CS Spray. α-(*o*-Chlorobenzylidene)malononitrile.
$C_{10}H_5ClN_2 = 188.6$.
CAS — 2698-41-1.

Profile

CS gas has been used as a riot-control gas.
It is known as a tear gas and its toxic effects include irritation of the eyes and nose, with copious lachrymation and rhinorrhoea; a burning sensation of the mouth and throat; pain in the chest, with difficulty in breathing; coughing; an increase in salivation; and retching and vomiting. These effects usually disappear a few minutes after exposure ends. The effects of pre-existing disease of the chest may be exacerbated. Erythema and blistering of the skin may occur.
Exposed persons should be removed to a well ventilated area. Treatment is symptomatic. Contaminated skin may be washed with soap and water, although exposure to water may initially exacerbate symptoms. If contamination of the eyes has been severe they should be irrigated with physiological saline or water and a local anaesthetic instilled to relieve pain.

◊ References.

1. Hu H, *et al.* Tear gas—harassing agent or toxic chemical weapon? *JAMA* 1989; **262:** 660–3.
2. Yih J-P. CS gas injury to the eye. *BMJ* 1995; **311:** 276.
3. Gray PJ. Treating CS gas injuries to the eye: exposure at close range is particularly dangerous. *BMJ* 1995; **311:** 871.
4. Jones GRN. CS sprays: antidote and decontaminant. *Lancet* 1996; **347:** 968–9.
5. Anderson PJ, *et al.* Acute effects of the potent lacrimator o-chlorobenzylidene malonitrile (CS) tear gas. *Hum Exp Toxicol* 1996; **15:** 461–5.
6. Anonymous. "Safety" of chemical batons. *Lancet* 1998; **352:** 159.

Cucurbita   (769-k)

Abóbora; Kürbissamen; Melon Pumpkin Seeds; Pepo; Semence de Courge.
Pharmacopoeias. In *Ger.* which specifies seeds of *Cucurbita pepo.*
The seeds of *Cucurbita pepo* (Cucurbitaceae) or related species.

Profile

Cucurbita was formerly used for the expulsion of tapeworms (*Taenia*).

The symbol † denotes a preparation no longer actively marketed

It is an ingredient of several herbal preparations used in urinary-tract disorders.

Preparations

Proprietary Preparations (details are given in Part 3)
Ger.: Granufink Kurbiskern; Nomon mono; Prosta Fink forte; Prostalog; Turiplex; Uvirgan mono; Vesiherb.
Multi-ingredient: *Austral.:* Lifechange Mens Complex with Saw Palmetto; *Fr.:* Salucur; *Ger.:* Alsicur†; Granufink Kurbiskern N; Prosta Fink N; Prostamed; Prostata-Kurbis S; Uvirgan N; *Port.:* Prostamed; *Switz.:* Cysto-Caps Chassot†; Prosta-Caps Chassot N; Prosta-Caps Fink.

Cusparia   (532-t)

Angostura Bark; Carony Bark; Cusparia Bark.

NOTE. 'Angostura Bitters' (*Dr. J.G.B. Siegert & Sons Ltd*) contain gentian and various aromatic ingredients but no cusparia; they are named after the town in which they were first made.
The bark of *Galipea officinalis* (Rutaceae).

Profile

Cusparia has been used as a bitter.

Cyanoacrylate Adhesives   (12619-l)

CAS — 1069-55-2 (bucrilate); 6606-65-1 (enbucrilate); 137-05-3 (mecrilate).

Profile

A number of cyanoacrylate compounds have been used as surgical tissue adhesives. They include bucrilate (bucrylate; isobutyl 2-cyanoacrylate, $C_8H_{11}NO_2 = 153.2$), enbucrilate (butyl 2-cyanoacrylate, $C_8H_{11}NO_2 = 153.2$), mecrilate (mecrylate; methyl 2-cyanoacrylate, $C_5H_5NO_2 = 111.1$), and ocrilate (ocrylate; octil 2-cyanoacrylate, $C_{12}H_{19}NO_2 = 209.3$). Some cyanoacrylates are used for household purposes and as nail fixatives and others have been investigated as tubal occlusive agents for female sterilisation, for sclerotherapy in bleeding gastric varices (p.1637), and for embolisation of intracranial vascular lesions.
In the event of accidental adhesion of the skin or lips the bonded surfaces should be immersed in warm soapy water, the surfaces peeled or rolled apart with the aid of a spatula, and the adhesive removed from the skin with soap and water; attempts should not be made to pull the surfaces directly apart.
Solvents such as nitromethane, toluene, or xylene may be used to aid skin detachment from solid objects. Eyelids stuck together or bonded to the eyeball should be washed thoroughly with warm water and a gauze patch applied; the eye will open without further action in 1 to 4 days. Manipulative attempts to open the eyes should not be made. Although cyanoacrylate introduced into the eyes may cause double vision and lachrymation there is usually no residual damage. If lips are accidentally stuck together plenty of warm water should be applied and maximum wetting and pressure from saliva inside the mouth encouraged. Lips should be peeled or rolled apart and not pulled. Adhesive introduced into the mouth solidifies and adheres, but saliva will lift the adhesive in ½ to 2 days. Care should be taken to avoid choking.
Heat is evolved on solidification of cyanoacrylate and in rare cases may cause burns.

◊ Reports of inadvertent application of cyanoacrylate adhesives to the eyes,[1,2] mouth,[3] and ears.[4]

1. Lyons C, *et al.* Superglue inadvertently used as eyedrops. *BMJ* 1990; **300:** 328.
2. DeRespinis PA. Cyanoacrylate nail glue mistaken for eye drops. *JAMA* 1990; **263:** 2301.
3. Cousin GCS. Accidental application of cyanoacrylate to the mouth. *Br Dent J* 1990; **169:** 293–4.
4. O'Donnell JJ, *et al.* Cyanoacrylate adhesive mistaken for ear drops. *J Accid Emerg Med* 1997; **14:** 199.

Preparations

Proprietary Preparations (details are given in Part 3)
UK: Histoacryl; Indermil; SuperSkin.

Cyclobutyrol Sodium   (3712-n)

Cyclobutyrol Sodium *(rINNM)*.
Sodium 2-(1-hydroxycyclohexyl)butyrate.
$C_{10}H_{17}NaO_3 = 208.2$.
CAS — 512-16-3 (cyclobutyrol); 1130-23-0 (cyclobutyrol sodium).

Profile

Cyclobutyrol sodium is a choleretic. It has been given by mouth in doses of 0.5 to 1 g daily in divided doses with meals. Cyclobutyrol betaine, cyclobutyrol calcium, and cyclobutyrol nicotinamide have been used similarly.

Preparations

Proprietary Preparations (details are given in Part 3)
Fr.: Hebucol†; *Ital.:* Epa-Bon†.
Multi-ingredient: *Aust.:* Tromgallol†; *Spain:* Hepadigest†; Levaliver; Liberbil†; Lidobama Complex†; Menabil Complex; Prodessal; Salcemetic; Sugarbil.

Cyclodextrins   (16595-g)

NOTE. Alfadex is *rINN* for α-cyclodextrin (alpha cyclodextrin). Betadex is *pINN* for β-cyclodextrin (beta cyclodextrin).
Pharmacopoeias. Eur. (see p.vi) includes alfadex and betadex. *USNF* includes betadex.

Pharmacopoeial description

Ph. Eur.: Alfadex is a white or almost white, amorphous or crystalline powder. Freely soluble in water and in propylene glycol; practically insoluble in dehydrated alcohol and in dichloromethane. Store in airtight containers.
Betadex is a white or almost white, amorphous or crystalline powder. Sparingly soluble in water; practically insoluble in alcohol and in dichloromethane; freely soluble in propylene glycol. Store in airtight containers.
USNF 20: Betadex is a nonreducing cyclic compound composed of seven alpha-(1-4) linked D-glucopyranosyl units. It is a white, practically odourless, fine crystalline powder. Soluble 1 in 54 of water. Store in airtight containers.

Profile

Cyclodextrins, such as alfadex and betadex, are produced by the enzymatic degradation of starch and are used as carrier molecules for drug delivery systems.

◊ References.

1. Ridgway K. Drug release rates: cyclodextrin complexes. *Pharm J* 1990; **245:** 344–5.
2. Szejtli J. Cyclodextrins: properties and applications. *Drug Invest* 1990; **2** (suppl 4): 11–21.
3. El Shaboury MH. Physical properties and dissolution profiles of tablets directly compressed with β-cyclodextrin. *Int J Pharmaceutics* 1990; **63:** 95–100.
4. Stella VJ, Rajewski RA. Cyclodextrins: their future in drug formulation and delivery. *Pharm Res* 1997; **14:** 556–67.
5. Loftsson T, Olafsson JH. Cyclodextrins: new drug delivery systems in dermatology. *Int J Dermatol* 1998; **37:** 241–6.
6. Redenti E, *et al.* Drug/cyclodextrin/hydroxy acid multicomponent systems: properties and pharmaceutical applications. *J Pharm Sci* 2000; **89:** 1–8.

Cyclovalone   (3713-h)

Cyclovalone *(rINN)*.
2,6-Divanillylidenecyclohexanone.
$C_{22}H_{22}O_5 = 366.4$.
CAS — 579-23-7.

Profile

Cyclovalone is a choleretic that has been given by mouth.

Preparations

Proprietary Preparations (details are given in Part 3)
Belg.: Vanidene†; *Fr.:* Vanilone.

Cynara   (3714-m)

Alcachôfra; Artichaut; Artichoke Leaf.
Pharmacopoeias. In *Fr.*
The leaves of the globe artichoke, *Cynara scolymus* (Compositae).

Profile

Cynara is reputed to have diuretic and choleretic properties. It may also have some hypolipidaemic activity.

Preparations

Proprietary Preparations (details are given in Part 3)
Aust.: Cynarix; Hepa-S; *Belg.:* Cynarol; *Braz.:* Chophytol; *Fr.:* Chophytol; Gallexier; Hepanephrol; *Ger.:* Cyna Bilisan; Cynacur; Cynafol; Divinal Galle†; Hekbilin Kapseln†; Hepa-POS†; Hepagallin N; Hepar SL; Hepar-POS; Heparstad; Hewechol Artischockendragees; Losapan; Maquil†; ratioHepar; *Port.:* Hepanephrol; *Switz.:* Chophytol†; Hepa-S.

Multi-ingredient: *Aust.:* Agnuchol; Aponatura Leber; Cynarix comp; Gallesyn neu; Mag Doskar's Leber-Galletonikum; Magentropen N Legastol; Sanvita Leber-Galle; *Austral.:* Extralife Liva-Care; Lifesystem Herbal Formula 7 Liver Tonic; Liver Tonic Herbal Formula 6; *Belg.:* Tisane pour le Foie; *Braz.:* Alcafelol; Boldigan; Chofranina; Colachofra; Cynarobil; Digestron; Epagogo; Epatovis; Figadosan; Figatil; Gotas Hepaticas; Hepasedan; Hepatoregius; Hepavirmo; Kop Hepar; Litrison; Metionina Composta; Necrohepat; Olocynan; Pirinachol; Solvobil; *Fr.:* Actibil; Actisane Digestion†; Aromabyl†; Canol; Elixir Spark; Gastralsan†; Hepaclem; Hepax; Romarinex-Choline†; Tisane des Familles; Vegelax; *Ger.:* Artischocke plus Legastol; Bilicura Forte; Carminagal N; Cynarzym N; Gallexier; Galloselect M; Hepatofalk Neu; Pascobilin novo; Salus Leber-Galle-Tee Nr.18†; Sirmia Artischockenelixier; or Ullus Galle-Tee N; *Hong Kong:* Hepatofalk; *Ital.:* Colax; Digelax; Florerbe Lassativa; Fluend†; Lievistar; Vadolax; Vegebyl†; *Mex.:* Chofabol; *Spain:* Cinaro Bilina†; Cynaro Bilina; Lipograsil; Menabil Complex; Nico Hepatocyn; *Switz.:* Bilifuge; Boldocynara N; Demonatur Gouttes pour le foie et la bile; Phytomed Hepato; Stago; Tisane hepatique et biliaire; *UK:* Bio-Strath Artichoke Formula.

Cynarine (3715-b)

Cynarin; 1,5-Dicaffeoylquinic Acid. 1-Carboxy-4,5-dihydroxy-1,3-cyclohexylene bis(3,4-dihydroxycinnamate).
$C_{25}H_{24}O_{12} = 516.5$.
CAS — 1182-34-9; 1884-24-8.

Profile
Cynarine is an active ingredient of cynara (above). It has been used as a choleretic.

Preparations
Proprietary Preparations (details are given in Part 3)
Braz.: Cynaron.

Multi-ingredient: *Aust.:* Tromgallol†; *Braz.:* Colagolen.

Cytochrome C (12622-q)

Pharmacopoeias. Chin. includes Cytochrome C Solution and preparations for injection.

A haemoprotein occurring in the body and involved in electron and hydrogen transport in biological oxidation processes.

Profile
Cytochrome C has been given intravenously in various hypoxic conditions.

It is an ingredient of some eye drops used for the treatment of cataract but its actions, if any, are unclear.

Preparations
Proprietary Preparations (details are given in Part 3)
Multi-ingredient: *Fr.:* Vitaphakol; *Ger.:* Vitreolent plus; *Port.:* Vitaphakol; *Spain:* Vitaphakol; *Switz.:* Vitaphakol†.

Cytokines (230-v)

Profile
Cytokines are a group of endogenous peptide regulatory molecules with the ability to affect cellular differentiation and/or proliferation. In contrast to peptide hormones, cytokines tend to act locally. Most cytokines are multifunctional molecules with a range of biological effects; they act primarily as mediators of inflammation or as growth factors. Cytokines that are being used clinically include erythropoietin (p.730), thrombopoietin (p.742), granulocyte and granulocyte-macrophage colony-stimulating factors such as filgrastim (p.736) and molgramostim (p.738), interferons (p.628), interleukin-1 (p.1623), interleukin-2 (p.547), interleukin-3 (p.738), oprelvekin (p.739), tumour necrosis factor (p.577), somatomedins (p.1296), and urogastrone (p.1254); those under investigation include fibroblast growth factor, keratinocyte growth factor, nerve growth factor, platelet-derived growth factor, and transforming growth factor. Some cytokines are involved in the pathophysiology of diseases and a number of cytokine antagonists are also being studied.

◊ References.
1. Lambiase A, *et al.* Topical treatment with nerve growth factor for corneal neurotrophic ulcers. *N Engl J Med* 1998; **338:** 1174–80.
2. Fu X, *et al.* Randomised placebo-controlled trial of use of topical recombinant bovine basic fibroblast growth factor for second-degree burns. *Lancet* 1998; **352:** 1661–4.
3. Wieman TJ, *et al.* Efficacy and safety of a topical gel formulation of recombinant human platelet-derived growth factor-BB (becaplermin) in patients with chronic neuropathic diabetic ulcers: a phase III randomized placebo-controlled double-blind study. *Diabetes Care* 1998; **21:** 822–7.
4. Anonymous. Platelet-derived growth factor for diabetic ulcers. *Med Lett Drugs Ther* 1998; **40:** 73–4.
5. Bernabei R, *et al.* Effect of topical application of nerve-growth factor on pressure ulcers. *Lancet* 1999; **354:** 307.
6. Kuter DJ. Future directions with platelet growth factors. *Semin Hematol* 2000; **37:** 41–9.
7. Apfel SC, *et al.* Efficacy and safety of recombinant human nerve growth factor in patients with diabetic polyneuropathy: a randomized controlled trial. *JAMA* 2000; **284:** 2215–21.

Damiana (14088-k)

Turnera.

Profile
Damiana is the dried leaves and stem of *Turnera diffusa* var. *aphrodisiaca* (Turneraceae) and possibly other species of *Turnera*. Damiana is drunk as a tea, and is used in herbal medicine for a variety of indications. It has a reputation as an aphrodisiac, but there is no evidence for this. It is also used in homoeopathic medicine.

Preparations
Proprietary Preparations (details are given in Part 3)
UK: Gerard House Curzon.

Multi-ingredient: *Austral.:* Bioglan Mens Super Soy/Clover; Bioglan The Blue One; Medinat Esten; *Ital.:* Dam; Four-Ton; *UK:* Daily Fatigue Relief; Damiana and Kola Tablets; Elixir Damiana and Saw Palmetto; Regina Royal Concorde; Strength.

Dapiprazole Hydrochloride (19035-r)

Dapiprazole Hydrochloride (*USAN, rINNM*).
AF-2139. 5,6,7,8-Tetrahydro-3-[2-(4-o-tolyl-1-piperazinyl)ethyl]-s-triazolo[4,3-a]pyridine monohydrochloride.
$C_{19}H_{27}N_5,HCl = 361.9$.
CAS — 72822-12-9 (dapiprazole); 72822-13-0 (dapiprazole hydrochloride).

Profile
Dapiprazole hydrochloride is an alpha blocker administered as eye drops to reverse mydriasis; it is also used in some countries in the management of glaucoma. Dapiprazole may also have antipsychotic activity.

Reversal of mydriasis. Dapiprazole is used to reverse the effects of mydriatics (sympathomimetics, and to some extent tropicamide) following surgery or ophthalmoscopic examination (p.1414). It also appears to enhance recovery of accommodation after the use of cycloplegics and may be effective for reversing mydriasis after cataract extraction.

References.
1. Allinson RW, *et al.* Reversal of mydriasis by dapiprazole. *Ann Ophthalmol* 1990; **22:** 131–8.
2. Ponte F, *et al.* Intraocular dapiprazole for the reversal of mydriasis after extracapsular cataract extraction with intraocular lens implantation: Part II: comparison with acetylcholine. *J Cataract Refract Surg* 1991; **17:** 785–9.
3. Johnson ME, *et al.* Efficacy of dapiprazole with hydroxyamphetamine hydrobromide and tropicamide. *J Am Optom Assoc* 1993; **64:** 629–33.
4. Molinari JF, *et al.* Dapiprazole clinical efficacy for counteracting tropicamide 1%. *Optom Vis Sci* 1994; **71:** 319–22.
5. Wilcox CS, *et al.* Comparison of the effects on pupil size and accommodation of three regimens of topical dapiprazole. *Br J Ophthalmol* 1995; **79:** 544–8.

Preparations
Proprietary Preparations (details are given in Part 3)
Aust.: Benglau; *Ger.:* Remydrial; *Israel:* Glamidolo; *Ital.:* Glamidolo; *USA:* Rev-Eyes.

Dehydrocholic Acid (3716-v)

Dehydrocholic Acid (*BAN, rINN*).
Chologon; Triketocholanic Acid. 3,7,12-Trioxo-5β-cholan-24-oic acid.
$C_{24}H_{34}O_5 = 402.5$.
CAS — 81-23-2 (dehydrocholic acid); 145-41-5 (sodium dehydrocholate).
Pharmacopoeias. In Aust., It., Jpn, and US.

Pharmacopoeial description
USP 25: A white, fluffy, odourless powder. Practically insoluble in water; soluble 1 in 100 of alcohol, 1 in 135 of acetic acid at 15°, 1 in 130 of acetone at 15°, 1 in 35 of chloroform, 1 in 2200 of ether at 15°, 1 in 135 of ethyl acetate at 15°, and 1 in 960 of benzene at 15°; solutions in alcohol and in chloroform are usually slightly turbid; soluble in glacial acetic acid and in solutions of alkali hydroxides and carbonates.

Profile
Dehydrocholic acid is a semisynthetic bile acid (p.1585) which is used for its hydrocholeretic properties, increasing the volume and water content of the bile without appreciably altering the content of bile acids. It has been used to improve biliary drainage and has also been given for the temporary relief of constipation. Usual doses of 250 to 500 mg three times daily by mouth after meals have been employed.

Dehydrocholic acid is contra-indicated in complete mechanical biliary obstruction and in severe hepatitis.

Preparations
USP 25: Dehydrocholic Acid Tablets.

Proprietary Preparations (details are given in Part 3)
Braz.: Decholin; *Canad.:* Dycholium†; *USA:* Cholan-HMB†; Decholin.

Multi-ingredient: *Aust.:* Gallo Merz; *Braz.:* Colagolen; Colagotil; Digeplus; Digestron; Dioctosal; Espasmo Novozyme; Essen; Filogaster; Hepatobyl; Plasil Enzimatico; Sintozima; Vonil Enzimatico; *Canad.:* Regubil†; *Fin.:* Fellesan; *Ger.:* Eupond†; *Hong Kong:* Bilsan; *Ital.:* Agarbil†; Certobil†; *Mex.:* Plasil Enzimatico; *Port.:* Drenomade; Espasmo Canulase; *S.Afr.:* Spasmo-Canulase; *Spain:* Espasmo Canulasa†; Nulacin Fermentos; *Swed.:* Fellesan†; *Switz.:* Gillazyme plus†; Gillazyme†; Spasmo-Canulase.

Denatonium Benzoate (533-x)

Denatonium Benzoate (*BAN, USAN, rINN*).
NSC-157658. Benzyldiethyl(2,6-xylylcarbamoylmethyl)ammonium benzoate monohydrate.
$C_{28}H_{34}N_2O_3,H_2O = 464.6$.
CAS — 3734-33-6 (anhydrous denatonium benzoate); 86398-53-0 (denatonium benzoate monohydrate).
Pharmacopoeias. In USNF.

Pharmacopoeial description
USNF 20: Denatonium benzoate, dried at 105° for 2 hours, contains one molecule of water of hydration or is anhydrous. Soluble 1 in 20 of water, 1 in 2.4 of alcohol, 1 in 2.9 of chloroform, and 1 in 5000 of ether; very soluble in methyl alcohol. pH

of a 3% solution in water is between 6.5 and 7.5. Store in airtight containers.

Profile
Denatonium benzoate is used where an intensely bitter taste is required for medicinal or industrial purposes and as a partial denaturant for alcohol in toiletries. It is known commercially as Bitrex.

Deoxyribonucleic Acid (12632-s)

ADN; Animal Nucleic Acid; Desoxypentose Nucleic Acid; Desoxyribonucleic Acid; Desoxyribose Nucleic Acid; DNA; Thymus Nucleic Acid.

A nucleotide polymer, and 1 of the 2 distinct varieties of nucleic acid (p.1642). It is found in the cell nuclei of living tissues.

Profile
Proprietary preparations of deoxyribonucleic acid are marketed in some countries and are advocated for a variety of debilitated and convalescent conditions. The sodium and magnesium salts are also used.

Preparations
Proprietary Preparations (details are given in Part 3)
Ital.: Placentex; Polides†.

Multi-ingredient: *Fr.:* Adena C; Nutrigene†; Osteogen†.

Dexpanthenol (7869-p)

Dexpanthenol (*BAN, USAN, rINN*).
Dexpanthenolum; Dextro-Pantothenyl Alcohol; Pantothenol. (R)-2,4-Dihydroxy-N-(3-hydroxypropyl)-3,3-dimethylbutyramide.
$C_9H_{19}NO_4 = 205.3$.
CAS — 81-13-0.
ATC — A11HA30; D03AX03; S01XA12.
Pharmacopoeias. In Eur. (see p.vi) and US. US also includes a racemic mixture under the title Panthenol.

Pharmacopoeial description
Ph. Eur.: A colourless or slightly yellowish, hygroscopic, viscous liquid, or a white, crystalline powder. Very soluble in water; freely soluble in alcohol; slightly soluble in ether. A 5% solution in water has a pH not greater than 10.5. Store in airtight containers.

USP 25: A clear, viscous, somewhat hygroscopic liquid, having a slight characteristic odour. Some crystallisation may occur on standing. Freely soluble in water, in alcohol, in methyl alcohol, and in propylene glycol; soluble in chloroform and in ether; slightly soluble in glycerol. Store in airtight containers.
Panthenol is a white to creamy white, crystalline powder with a slight, characteristic odoour. Freely soluble in water, in alcohol, and in propylene glycol; soluble in chloroform and in ether; slightly soluble in glycerol. Store in airtight containers.

Adverse Effects and Precautions
There have been a few reports of allergic reactions associated with the administration of dexpanthenol although these have not been confirmed. Dexpanthenol is contra-indicated in haemophiliacs and in patients with ileus due to mechanical obstruction.

Uses and Administration
Dexpanthenol is the alcoholic analogue of D-pantothenic acid (p.1374). It has been given intramuscularly in doses of 250 to 500 mg to prevent or control gastrointestinal atony but its value has not been established. It has also been given by slow intravenous infusion.

Dexpanthenol has been used topically as an ointment, cream, or solution, usually in a strength of 2%, for the treatment of various minor skin disorders.

Dexpanthenol and the racemate panthenol are included in some vitamin preparations.

Preparations
USP 25: Dexpanthenol Preparation.

Proprietary Preparations (details are given in Part 3)
Aust.: Bepanthen; Panthoten; *Belg.:* Bepanthene†; *Braz.:* Bepantol; *Fin.:* Bepanthen; *Fr.:* Bepanthene; *Ger.:* Corneregel; Cutemul†; Dexpanol; Marolderm†; Nasicur; Pan-Ophtal; Panthenol; Panthogenat; Pelina; Ucee D; Urupan; Wund- und Heilsalbe N; *Israel:* Bepanthen; *Ital.:* Bepanten; *NZ:* Bepanthen; *Port.:* Bepanthene; *S.Afr.:* Bepantol; *Spain:* Bepanthene; *Switz.:* Bepanthene; *UAE:* Dexipan; *USA:* Ilopan; Panthoderm.

Multi-ingredient: *Aust.:* Beneuran Vit B-Komplex; Bepanthen; Bepanthen Plus; Colda; Coldistan; Dolobene; Felix; Hermasept†; Keratosis; Keratosis forte; Oleovit; Pelsana Med; Siccaprotect; Sigman-Haustropfen; Sunsan-Heillotion; Venobene; *Austral.:* Egozite Baby Cream; Macro Natural Vitamin E Cream; Sebirinse; Superfade; Z-Acne†; *Braz.:* Angino-Rub; Capel; Naridrin; Nasopan; Nazobio; Nitronasal; Perlax; Rinatrol; Rinozin; Solucao Nasal de Nafazolina; Varizol; *Canad.:* Aquasol A†; Selsun with Provitamin B₅; *Fin.:* Oftan A-Pant; Pantyson; Wicaran; Wicarba; Wicnevit; *Ger.:* Brand- und Wund-Gel Eu Rho; Dispatenol; Dolobene; Essaven Tri-Complex; Hermalind; Hewekzem novo; Hydro Cordes; Lipo Cordes; Lipovitan; Lygal Kopftinktur; mar plus; Nasic; Pantederm; PC 30 V; Remederm; Siccaprotect; Wund- und Brand-Gel Eu Rho; *Hong Kong:* Dolobene; Egozite Baby Cream; *Israel:* Bepanthen Plus; Kamil Blue; Panthisone;

Pedisol; *Ital.:* Alfa Acid; Emazian B12; Emoantitossina; Herbavit; Lenirose; Rinopanteina; *NZ:* Sebirinse; *Port.:* Bepanthene; Bepanthene Plus; Carmitol; Eucerin Pele com tendencia para o acne creme anti-borbulhas; Nutraisdin; Ureadin 10 Plus; *S.Afr.:* Broncol; *Singapore:* Egozite; *Spain:* Anasilpiel; Neo Visage; *Switz.:* Alphastria; Bepanthene Plus; Carbamide + VAS; Carbamide Creme; Cetona Plus; Cortimycine; Demostan N; Dermacalm-d; Dolobene; Galamila; Gorgonium; Hepathrombine; Lyman; Nastop; Pelsano; Pigmanorm; Remexal; Roll-bene; Siccalix; Sportium Emgel; Sportusal; Sportusal Spray sine heparino; Stilex; Turexan Capilla; Turexan Lotion; Unatol; Venucreme; Venugel; *Thai.:* Detuss; Romilar; *UK:* Vipsogal; *USA:* Ilopan-Choline.

Dextran Sulfate (4810-e)

Dextran Sulfate Sodium; Dextran Sulphate; Dextran Sulphate Sodium.
CAS — 9011-18-1.
Pharmacopoeias. In Jpn.

The sodium salt of sulfuric acid esters of dextran.

Profile
Dextran sulfate has been used as an anticoagulant and as a lipid regulating drug, and has been investigated for its antiviral activity. Dextran sulfate potassium has also been used.

Interactions. As mentioned on p.821, anaphylactoid reactions have occurred in patients receiving ACE inhibitors during low-density lipoprotein apheresis using a dextran sulfate-cellulose column.[1,2] Withdrawal of the ACE inhibitor for 1 to 3 days before apheresis may prevent the reaction.[2]

1. Olbricht CJ, *et al.* Anaphylactoid reactions, LDL apheresis with dextran sulphate, and ACE inhibitors. *Lancet* 1992; **340:** 908–9.
2. Agishi T. Anion-blood contact reaction (ABC reaction) in patients treated by LDL apheresis with dextran sulfate-cellulose column while receiving ACE inhibitors. *JAMA* 1994; **271:** 195–6.

Preparations
Proprietary Preparations (details are given in Part 3)
Multi-ingredient: *Austral.:* VR; *Fr.:* Dextrarine Phenylbutazone; *Ger.:* Phlebodril N; *Ital.:* Stranoval; *Port.:* Doxivenil; *Spain:* Fabroven; *Switz.:* Doxivenil.

Dextrorphan (5614-z)

Dextrorphan *(BAN, pINN).*
Ro-01-6794/706 (dextrorphan hydrochloride). (+)-9a-Methyl-morphinan-3-ol.
$C_{17}H_{23}NO = 257.4$.
CAS — 125-73-5 (dextrorphan); 69376-27-8 (dextrorphan hydrochloride).

NOTE. Dextrorphan Hydrochloride is *USAN.*

Profile
Dextrorphan, a metabolite of dextromethorphan (p.1087), is an antagonist of the excitatory neurotransmitter *N*-methyl-D-aspartate (NMDA). It possesses some cough suppressant activity and is under investigation as a neuroprotective agent in the management of stroke.

◊ References.
1. Albers GW, *et al.* Safety, tolerability, and pharmacokinetics of the N-methyl-D-aspartate antagonist dextrorphan in patients with acute stroke. *Stroke* 1995; **26:** 254–8.

Dibutyl Sebacate (11142-g)

$C_{18}H_{34}O_4 = 314.5$.
CAS — 109-43-3.
Pharmacopoeias. In USNF.

Pharmacopoeial description
USNF 20: It consists of esters of *n*-butyl alcohol and saturated dibasic acids, principally sebacic acid. A colourless, oily liquid of very mild odour. Practically insoluble in water and in glycerol; soluble in alcohol, in isopropyl alcohol, and in liquid paraffin; very slightly soluble in propylene glycol. Store in airtight containers.

Profile
Dibutyl sebacate is a plasticiser.

Dichlorodiethylsulfide (1830-j)

Dichlorodiethylsulphide; Mustard Gas; Sulphur Mustard; Yellow Cross Liquid. Bis(2-chloroethyl)sulphide.
$C_4H_8Cl_2S = 159.1$.
CAS — 505-60-2.

Profile
Dichlorodiethylsulfide was developed for use in chemical warfare and has more severe vesicant and irritant properties than its nitrogen analogue, mustine [chlormethine] (p.561). It was formerly used topically in the treatment of psoriasis.

◊ Reviews of the toxicology of dichlorodiethylsulfide,[1,2] and debate on the management of casualties injured by dichlorodiethylsulfide and other chemical warfare agents.[3-9] Most patients exposed to dichlorodiethylsulfide recover completely

and only a small proportion will have long-term eye or lung damage,[10] although death from respiratory, renal, and bonemarrow failure may occur.[9]

Eleven fishermen who accidentally retrieved corroded and leaking gas shells containing dichlorodiethylsulfide from underwater dumps, presented with very inflamed skin, especially in the axillary and genitofemoral regions, yellow blisters on the hands and legs, painful irritation of the eyes, and transient blindness. Two developed pulmonary oedema.[11] There was no evidence of a mutagenic effect and in view of the increased risk of lung cancer in soldiers and workers exposed to the gas it is reasonable to assume that fishermen heavily exposed to dichlorodiethylsulfide also have an increased cancer risk.

1. Smith KJ, *et al.* Sulfur mustard: its continuing threat as a chemical warfare agent, the cutaneous lesions induced, progress in understanding its mechanism of action, its long-term health effects, and new developments for protection and therapy. *J Am Acad Dermatol* 1995; **32:** 765–76.
2. Dacre JC, Goldman M. Toxicology and pharmacology of the chemical warfare agent sulfur mustard. *Pharmacol Rev* 1996; **48:** 289–326.
3. Heyndrickx A, Heyndrickx B. Management of war gas injuries. *Lancet* 1990; **ii:** 1248–9.
4. Fouyn T, *et al.* Management of chemical warfare injuries. *Lancet* 1991; **337:** 121.
5. Willems JL, *et al.* Management of chemical warfare injuries. *Lancet* 1991; **337:** 121–2.
6. Maynard RL, *et al.* Management of chemical warfare injuries. *Lancet* 1991; **337:** 122.
7. Newman-Taylor AJ, Morris AJR. Experience with mustard gas casualties. *Lancet* 1991; **337:** 242.
8. Heyndrickx A. Chemical warfare injuries. *Lancet* 1991; **337:** 430.
9. Rees J, *et al.* Mustard gas casualties. *Lancet* 1991; **337:** 430.
10. Murray VSG, Volans GN. Management of injuries due to chemical weapons. *BMJ* 1991; **302:** 129–30.
11. Wulf HC, *et al.* Sister chromatid exchanges in fishermen exposed to leaking mustard gas shells. *Lancet* 1985; **i:** 690–1.

Digitalin (5811-x)

Amorphous Digitalin; Digitalinum Purum Germanicum.

NOTE. Distinguish from Digitaline Cristallisée (digitoxin, p.869) which is very much more potent.

A standardised mixture of glycosides from *Digitalis purpurea.*

Profile
Digitalin has actions similar to those of digoxin (p.870). Because of its ready solubility in water it was formerly used for the preparation of solutions for injection. It is also present in some ophthalmic preparations.

Preparations
Proprietary Preparations (details are given in Part 3)
Multi-ingredient: *Ger.:* Augentonikum; *Ital.:* Digifar.

Dihydroergocristine Mesilate (12007-q)

Dihydroergocristine Mesilate *(BANM).*
Dihydroergocristine Mesylate; Dihydroergocristine Methanesulphonate; Dihydroergocristini Mesilas. (6aR,9R,10aR)-*N*-[(2R,5S,10aS,10bS)-5-Benzyl-10b-hydroxy-2-isopropyl-3,6-di-oxooctahydro-8*H*-[1,3]oxazolo[3,2-*a*]pyrrolo[2,1-*c*]pyrazin-2-yl]-7-methyl-4,6,6a,7,8,9,10,10a-octahydroindolo[4,3-*fg*]quinoline-9-carboxamide methanesulphonate.
$C_{35}H_{41}N_5O_5,CH_4O_3S = 707.8$.
CAS — 17479-19-5 (dihydroergocristine); 24730-10-7 (dihydroergocristine mesilate).
Pharmacopoeias. In Eur. (see p.vi).

Pharmacopoeial description
Ph. Eur.: A white or almost white, fine crystalline powder. Slightly soluble in water; soluble in methyl alcohol. A 0.5% solution in water has a pH of 4.0 to 5.0. Protect from light.

Profile
Dihydroergocristine mesilate is a component of co-dergocrine mesilate (p.1597) and has similar actions. In some countries it has been given by mouth in the symptomatic treatment of mental deterioration associated with cerebrovascular insufficiency and in peripheral vascular disease. It has also been given by intramuscular injection.

◊ References.
1. Franciosi A, Zavattini G. Dihydroergocristine in the treatment of elderly patients with cognitive deterioration: a double-blind, placebo-controlled, dose-response study. *Curr Ther Res* 1994; **55:** 1391–1401.

Preparations
Proprietary Preparations (details are given in Part 3)
Aust.: Diertina; Nehydrin; *Braz.:* Iskemil; Iskevert; *Ital.:* Defluina; Diertina; Difluid; Ergocris; Gral†; Unergol†; Vasoton; *Mex.:* Decme; *Port.:* Diertina; *Spain:* Diertine; Ergodavur; *Switz.:* Diertina.
Multi-ingredient: *Aust.:* Brinerdin; Defluina; Pressimedin; Sandoven; Supergan; *Braz.:* Isketam; Norogil; Vasofluina; Vertizine D; *Fr.:* Cervilane†; Iskedyl; *Ital.:* Brinerdina; *Mex.:* Cervilan; *Neth.:* Brinerdin†; *Port.:* Brinerdine; Cervilane; *S.Afr.:* Brinerdin; *Spain:* Brinerdina; Clinadil; Diemil; Dipervina; Iskedyl; Isquebral; *Switz.:* Brinerdine; Pressimed†; *Thai.:* Bedin; Brinerdin; Hyperdine.

Dihydroergocryptine Mesilate (12008-p)

Dihydroergocryptine Mesylate; Dihydroergocryptine Methanesulphonate; Dihydroergokryptine Mesylate.
$C_{32}H_{43}N_5O_5,CH_4O_3S = 673.8$.
CAS — 25447-66-9 (dihydroergocryptine, α-isomer); 19467-62-0 (dihydroergocryptine, β-isomer); 14271-05-7 (dihydroergocryptine mesilate, α-isomer); 65914-79-6 (dihydroergocryptine mesilate, β-isomer).
ATC — N04BC03.

Profile
Dihydroergocryptine mesilate is a component of co-dergocrine mesilate (p.1597) and has similar actions. In some countries it has been given by mouth, often in combination with caffeine, in the symptomatic treatment of mental deterioration associated with cerebrovascular insufficiency and in peripheral vascular disease. It has also been used in the management of hyperprolactinaemia and parkinsonism.

◊ References.
1. Faglia G, *et al.* Dihydroergocriptine in management of microprolactinomas. *J Clin Endocrinol Metab* 1987; **65:** 779–84.
2. Martignoni E, *et al.* Dihydroergocryptine in the treatment of Parkinson's disease: a six months' double-blind clinical trial. *Clin Neuropharmacol* 1991; **14:** 78–83.
3. Scarzella L, *et al.* Dihydroergocryptine in the management of senile psycho-organic syndrome. *Int J Clin Pharmacol Res* 1992; **12:** 37–46.
4. Battistin L, *et al.* Alpha-dihydroergocryptine in Parkinson's disease: a multicentre randomized double blind parallel group study. *Acta Neurol Scand* 1999; **99:** 36–42.

Preparations
Proprietary Preparations (details are given in Part 3)
Ger.: Almirid; Cripar; *Ital.:* Daverium; Myrol†.
Multi-ingredient: *Fr.:* Vasobral; *Hong Kong:* Vasobral; *Ital.:* Vasobral.

Dihydroxydibutylether (12654-z)

Hydroxybutyloxide. 4,4'-Oxybis(butan-2-ol).
$C_8H_{18}O_3 = 162.2$.
CAS — 821-33-0.

Profile
Dihydroxydibutylether is a choleretic.

Preparations
Proprietary Preparations (details are given in Part 3)
Fr.: Dyskinebyl†; *Hong Kong:* Diskinebyl; *Ital.:* Dis-Cinil Ilfi†; Diskin.
Multi-ingredient: *Ital.:* Dis-Cinil Complex.

Diiodhydrin (12655-c)

Iodazone; lothion. 1,3-Di-iodopropan-2-ol.
$C_3H_6I_2O = 311.9$.
CAS — 534-08-7.

Profile
Diiodhydrin is an organic iodine-containing compound that has been used with aromatic oils in nose drops for the treatment of rhinitis and pharyngitis.

Diisopropanolamine (206-v)

1,1'-Iminobis(propan-2-ol).
$C_6H_{15}NO_2 = 133.2$.
CAS — 110-97-4.

Profile
Diisopropanolamine is an organic base which is used as a neutralising agent in cosmetics and toiletries.

Dill Oil (4642-e)

European Dill Seed Oil; Oleum Anethi.
CAS — 8016-06-6.
Pharmacopoeias. In Br.

Pharmacopoeial description
BP 2001: A clear colourless or pale yellow liquid, visibly free from water, obtained by distillation from the dried ripe fruits of *Anethum graveolens.* It darkens with age and has a characteristic odour of the crushed fruit. It contains 43 to 63% of carvone. At 20°, soluble 1 in 1 or more of alcohol (90%) and 1 in 10 or more of alcohol (80%). Store at a temperature not exceeding 25° in well-filled containers. Protect from light.

Profile
Dill oil, usually in the form of dill water, is used as an aromatic carminative, although the efficacy of such traditional remedies in infant colic is considered dubious (see Gastrointestinal Spasm, p.1204).

Preparations
Proprietary Preparations (details are given in Part 3)
Multi-ingredient: *Canad.:* Babys Own Gripe Water; Chase Kolik Gripe Water; Woodwards Gripe Water; *Israel:* Dentinox; Nurse Harvey's Gripe Mixture; Woodwards Gripe Water; *Singapore:*

The symbol † denotes a preparation no longer actively marketed

Dentinox; *Thai.*: Baby Gripe; Bebidol; *UK*: Atkinson & Barker's Gripe Mixture; Neo; Nurse Harvey's Gripe Mixture; Woodwards Gripe Water.

Dimethoxymethane (19847-e)

Formal; Formaldehyde Dimethyl Acetal; Methylal.
$CH_2(OCH_3)_2 = 76.09$.
CAS — 109-87-5.

Profile
Dimethoxymethane has been used in perfumery. It has been included in preparations for topical analgesia.

Preparations
Proprietary Preparations (details are given in Part 3)
Multi-ingredient: *UK*: PR Freeze Spray.

Dimethyltryptamine (5013-y)

Businessman's Trip; *N,N*-Dimethyltryptamine; DMT. 3-(2-Dimethylaminoethyl)indole.
$C_{12}H_{16}N_2 = 188.3$.
CAS — 61-50-7.

An active principle obtained from the seeds and leaves of *Piptadenia peregrina* (Mimosaceae) from which the hallucinogenic snuff cohoba is prepared, and other South American plants. It has been reported to be present in the tropical legume *Mucuna pruriens*.

Profile
Dimethyltryptamine produces hallucinogenic and sympathomimetic effects which are similar to those of lysergide (p.1630), but of shorter duration. It has no therapeutic use. Diethyltryptamine (DET) and dipropyltryptamine (DPT) are related synthetic hallucinogens with longer actions but are less potent than dimethyltryptamine.

2,4-Dinitrochlorobenzene (12666-t)

DNCB. 1-Chloro-2,4-dinitrobenzene.
$C_6H_3ClN_2O_4 = 202.6$.
CAS — 97-00-7.

Profile
2,4-Dinitrochlorobenzene is a potent sensitiser and has been applied topically in the evaluation of delayed hypersensitivity. It has also been used as an immunostimulant in various conditions including leprosy, HIV infection, and some forms of cancer, and in the treatment of alopecia and warts.

2,4-Dinitrochlorobenzene has been reported to be mutagenic *in vitro*.

◊ References.
1. Happle R. The potential hazards of dinitrochlorobenzene. *Arch Dermatol* 1985; **121**: 330–2.
2. Stricker RB, Goldberg B. Host-directed therapy for AIDS. *Ann Intern Med* 1995; **123**: 471–2.
3. Todd DJ. Topical treatment with dinitrochlorobenzene. *Lancet* 1995; **346**: 975.
4. Stricker RB, Goldberg B. Safety of topical dinitrochlorobenzene. *Lancet* 1995; **346**: 1293.
5. Strobbe LJ, *et al.* Topical dinitrochlorobenzene combined with systemic dacarbazine in the treatment of recurrent melanoma. *Melanoma Res* 1997; **7**: 507–12.
6. Traub A, *et al.* Topical immune modulation with dinitrochlorobenzene in HIV disease: a controlled trial from Brazil. *Dermatology* 1997; **195**: 369–73.
7. Yoshizawa Y, *et al.* Successful immunotherapy of chronic nodular prurigo with topical dinitrochlorobenzene. *Br J Dermatol* 1999; **141**: 350–92.
8. Yoshizawa Y, *et al.* Topical dinitrochlorobenzene therapy in the treatment of refractory atopic dermatitis: systemic immunotherapy. *J Am Acad Dermatol* 2000; **42**: 258–62.

Diolamine (205-b)

Diolamine (*pINN*).
Diaethanolamin; Diethanolamine. Bis(2-hydroxyethyl)amine; 2,2′-Iminobisethanol.
$C_4H_{11}NO_2 = 105.1$.
CAS — 111-42-2.
Pharmacopoeias. In USNF, which specifies a mixture of ethanolamines consisting largely of diolamine.

Pharmacopoeial description
USNF 20: It is a mixture of ethanolamines, consisting largely of diolamine. White or clear, colourless crystals, deliquescing in moist air, or a colourless liquid. Miscible with water, with alcohol, with acetone, with chloroform, and with glycerol; slightly soluble to insoluble in ether, in petroleum spirit, and in benzene. Store in airtight containers. Protect from light.

Profile
Diolamine is an organic base which is used as an emulsifier and dispersant.

It is used to solubilise fusidic acid and sulfafurazole by the formation of the diolamine salt. It has been used for the preparation of salts of iodinated organic acids used as contrast media. It may be irritating to the skin and mucous membranes.

Preparations
Proprietary Preparations (details are given in Part 3)
Multi-ingredient: *Aust.*: Oleosint; *Hong Kong:* Jetepar; *Ital.*: Ietepar; *Singapore:* Jetepar.

Dioxins (13301-r)

NOTE. The name Dioxin has also been applied to dimethoxane.

The term 'dioxins' encompasses a large group of closely related chemicals known as polychlorinated dibenzo-*p*-dioxins (PCDDs) and polychlorinated dibenzofurans (PCDFs). The most toxic is 2,3,7,8-tetrachlorodibenzo-*p*-dioxin (TCDD).

Profile
Dioxins are byproducts in the manufacture of commercial chemical products such as chlorinated phenols and polychlorinated biphenyls (PCBs), and can also be produced in smaller quantities by combustion processes and industrial waste. They first came to public attention during the Vietnam War, when they were found to be present in the herbicide Agent Orange used as a defoliant. They are incriminated as causing chloracne (a severe and persistent acne caused by chlorinated compounds). They are potent teratogens and carcinogens in *animals*. An increased incidence of cancer at different organs due to dioxins has been claimed but this has not been substantiated by clinical and follow-up studies. An effect on cell-mediated immunity has been observed.

Exposure should be limited to the lowest feasible concentration.

◊ The impact of dioxins in food and the environment has been reviewed.[1-3]

An excess of soft tissue sarcomas was found in workers exposed to chlorophenoxy herbicides including those contaminated with TCDD,[4] but cautious interpretation of these results was advised.[5] In Vietnam veterans the risk of non-Hodgkin's lymphoma was approximately 50% higher than control subjects, but was not related to exposure to Agent Orange, nor was there evidence for an increase in other cancers.[6] Exposure to TCDD was implicated in an increase in cancer mortality in chemical workers,[7,8] but confounding factors such as smoking may have been present.[8,9] Other studies[10,11] have not shown an association between dioxin exposure and an increase in the incidence of human cancer, and epidemiological studies following occupational or accidental exposures have found no clear persistent systemic effects, except for chloracne, and no clear association with carcinogenesis or reproductive disorders.[1,2] In the USA, the National Academy of Sciences' Institute of Medicine is reported to have carried out an evaluation of publications on herbicide exposure, largely in industrial and agricultural workers.[12] They concluded that exposure to herbicides or dioxin was associated with soft-tissue sarcomas, Hodgkin's disease, non-Hodgkin lymphoma, chloracne, and porphyria cutanea tarda, and that there was limited evidence of an association with respiratory and prostate cancers and multiple myeloma. An update to the report has also suggested a link between Agent Orange exposure and spina bifida in veterans' offspring.[13] There is some evidence that exposure of men to TCDD is associated with a decreased male to female sex ratio in their offspring.[14]

1. Polychlorinated dibenzo-para-dioxins and dibenzofurans. *Environmental Health Criteria 88*. Geneva: WHO, 1989.
2. Department of the Environment. Dioxins in the environment. *Pollution Paper 27*. London: HMSO, 1989.
3. MAFF. Dioxins in food. *Food Surveillance Paper 31*. London: HMSO, 1992.
4. Saracci R, *et al.* Cancer mortality in workers exposed to chlorophenoxy herbicides and chlorophenols. *Lancet* 1991; **338**: 1027–32.
5. Peto R. Occupational exposure to chlorophenoxy herbicides and chlorophenols. *Lancet* 1991; **338**: 1392.
6. Suskind R. The association of selected cancers with service in the US military in Vietnam. *Arch Intern Med* 1990; **150**: 2449–50.
7. Manz A, *et al.* Cancer mortality among workers in chemical plant contaminated with dioxin. *Lancet* 1991; **338**: 959–64.
8. Fingerhut MA, *et al.* Cancer mortality in workers exposed to 2,3,7,8-tetrachlorodibenzo-p-dioxin. *N Engl J Med* 1991; **324**: 212–18.
9. Triebig G. Is dioxin carcinogenic? *Lancet* 1991; **338**: 1592.
10. Coggon D, *et al.* Mortality and incidence of cancer at four factories making phenoxy herbicides. *Br J Ind Med* 1991; **48**: 173–80.
11. Green LM. A cohort mortality study of forestry workers exposed to phenoxy acid herbicides. *Br J Ind Med* 1991; **48**: 234–8.
12. McCarthy M. Agent Orange. *Lancet* 1993; **342**: 362.
13. Stephenson J. New IOM report links Agent Orange Exposure to risk of birth defect in Vietnam vets' children. *JAMA* 1996; **275**: 1066–7.
14. Mocarelli P, *et al.* Paternal concentrations of dioxin and sex ratio of offspring. *Lancet* 2000; **355**: 1858–63.

Diphenyl (6644-g)

E230; Phenylbenzene. Biphenyl.
$C_{12}H_{10} = 154.2$.
CAS — 92-52-4.

Profile
Diphenyl is fungistatic against a limited number of moulds and

has been employed for impregnating the material used for wrapping citrus fruits.

Adverse effects. Workers exposed to high concentrations of diphenyl (up to 128 mg per m^3) developed toxic symptoms which included irritation of the throat and eyes, headache, nausea, diffuse abdominal pain, numbness, aching of limbs, and general fatigue.[1] One of the workers, who also had somnolence, icterus, ascites, and oedema of the legs, died; at autopsy, the liver showed necrosis. Chronic hepatitis was reported in a woman exposed over a 25-year period to diphenyl in the paper used to pack citrus fruit.[2]

1. Häkkinen I, *et al.* Diphenyl poisoning in fruit paper production. *Arch Environ Health* 1973; **26**: 70–4.
2. Carella G, Bettolo PM. Reversible hepatotoxic effects of diphenyl: report of a case and a review of the literature. *J Occup Med* 1994; **36**: 575–6.

Dipivefrine Hydrochloride (12670-z)

Dipivefrine Hydrochloride (*BANM, rINNM*).
Dipivalyl Adrenaline Hydrochloride; Dipivalyl Epinephrine Hydrochloride; Dipivefrin Hydrochloride; DPE (dipivefrine). (*RS*)-4-[1-Hydroxy-2-(methylamino)ethyl]-*o*-phenylene dipivalate hydrochloride.
$C_{19}H_{29}NO_5,HCl = 387.9$.
CAS — 52365-63-6 (dipivefrine); 64019-93-8 (dipivefrine hydrochloride).
NOTE. Dipivefrin is *USAN*.
Pharmacopoeias. In Br. and US.

Pharmacopoeial description
BP 2001: A white crystalline powder or small crystals. Freely soluble in water, in alcohol, and in methyl alcohol.
USP 25: White, crystalline powder or small crystals, having a faint odour. Very soluble in water. Store in airtight containers.

Profile
Dipivefrine is an ester and prodrug of adrenaline [epinephrine] (p.829). A 0.1% solution of the hydrochloride is used topically as eye drops to reduce intra-ocular pressure in patients with open-angle glaucoma or ocular hypertension (p.1413).

◊ References.
1. Parrow KA, *et al.* Is it worthwhile to add dipivefrin HCl 0.1% to topical β₁-, β₂-blocker therapy? *Ophthalmology* 1989; **96**: 1338–41.
2. Drake MV, *et al.* Levobunolol compared to dipivefrin in African American patients with open angle glaucoma. *J Ocul Pharmacol* 1993; **9**: 91–5. Correction. *ibid.*; 385.
3. Albracht DC, *et al.* A double-masked comparison of betaxolol and dipivefrin for the treatment of increased intraocular pressure. *Am J Ophthalmol* 1993; **116**: 307–13.
4. Widengard I, *et al.* Effects of latanoprost and dipivefrin, alone or combined, on intraocular pressure and on blood-aqueous barrier permeability. *Br J Ophthalmol* 1998; **82**: 404–6.

Preparations
BP 2001: Dipivefrine Eye Drops;
USP 25: Dipivefrin Hydrochloride Ophthalmic Solution.
Proprietary Preparations (details are given in Part 3)
Aust.: Glaucothil; *Austral.:* Dipoquin; Propine; *Belg.:* Propine; *Braz.:* Propine; *Canad.:* DPE; Propine; *Denm.:* Diprin†; Oftapinex; Propine; *Fin.:* Oftapinex; Propine; *Fr.:* Propine; *Ger.:* d Epifrin; Glaucothil; *Hong Kong:* Propine; *Irl.:* Propine; *Israel:* Difrin; Prodren; Propine; *Ital.:* Propine; *Mex.:* Diopine; *Neth.:* Diopine†; *Norw.:* Oftapinex; *NZ:* Dipoquin; Propine; *Port.:* Propine; *S.Afr.:* Propine; *Singapore:* Propine; *Spain:* Diopine; Glaudrops; *Swed.:* Diprin; Oftapinex; Propine; *Switz.:* Diopine; Diphemin†; *Thai.:* Propine; *UK:* Propine; *USA:* AkPro; Propine.
Multi-ingredient: *Aust.:* Thiloadren; Thilodigon; *Canad.:* Probeta; *Ger.:* Thiloadren N; Thilodigon.

Disodium Guanylate (12675-x)

Disodium Guanosine-5′-monophosphate; E627; Sodium 5′-Guanylate. Guanosine 5′-(disodium phosphate).
$C_{10}H_{12}N_5Na_2O_8P,xH_2O$.
CAS — 5550-12-9 (anhydrous disodium guanylate).

Profile
Disodium guanylate has been used as a flavour enhancer in foods. It has also been used in eye drops containing other nucleosides in the treatment of corneal damage. The term sodium 5′-ribonucleotide has been used to refer to a mixture of disodium guanylate with disodium inosinate (below).

Preparations
Proprietary Preparations (details are given in Part 3)
Multi-ingredient: *Aust.:* Vitasic; *Fr.:* Vitacic.

Disodium Inosinate (12676-r)

Disodium Inosine-5′-monophosphate; E631; Sodium 5′-Inosinate. Inosine 5′-(disodium phosphate).
$C_{10}H_{11}N_4Na_2O_8P,xH_2O$.
CAS — 4691-65-0 (anhydrous disodium inosinate).

Profile
Disodium inosinate has been used as a flavour enhancer in

foods. It has also been given by mouth and been applied topically in the treatment of visual disturbance.

Preparations

Proprietary Preparations (details are given in Part 3)
Fr.: Correctol; *Ger.:* Antikataraktikum N; *Switz.:* Catacol†.

Disulfiram (2731-t)

Disulfiram *(BAN, rINN)*.

Dissulfiramo; Disulfiramum; Éthyldithiourame; TTD. Tetraethylthiuram disulphide; Bis(diethylthiocarbamoyl) disulfide.

$C_{10}H_{20}N_2S_4 = 296.5$.

CAS — 97-77-8.
ATC — P03AA04; V03AA01.

Pharmacopoeias. In Eur. (see p.vi), *Jpn, Pol.,* and *US.*

Pharmacopoeial description

Ph. Eur.: A white or almost white, crystalline powder. M.p. 70° to 73°. Practically insoluble in water; sparingly soluble in alcohol; freely soluble in dichloromethane; soluble in ether. Protect from light.

USP 25: A white to off-white, odourless crystalline powder. M.p. 69° to 72°. Very slightly soluble in water; soluble 1 in 30 of alcohol and 1 in 15 of ether; soluble in acetone, in carbon disulfide, and in chloroform. Store in airtight containers. Protect from light.

Stability. Studies on the stability of disulfiram preparations.

1. Gupta VD. Stability of aqueous suspensions of disulfiram. *Am J Hosp Pharm* 1981; **38:** 363–4.
2. Philips M, *et al.* Stability of an injectable disulfiram formulation sterilized by gamma irradiation. *Am J Hosp Pharm* 1985; **42:** 343–5.

Adverse Effects and Treatment

Drowsiness and fatigue are common during initial treatment with disulfiram. Other side-effects reported include a garlic-like or metallic aftertaste, gastrointestinal upsets, body odour, bad breath, headache, impotence, and allergic dermatitis. Peripheral and optic neuropathies, psychotic reactions, and hepatotoxicity may occur.

Disulfiram-alcohol reaction. The use of disulfiram in the management of alcoholism is based on the extremely unpleasant, but generally self-limiting, systemic effects which occur when a patient receiving the drug ingests alcohol. These effects begin with flushing of the face and, as vasodilatation spreads, throbbing in the head and neck and a pulsating headache may develop. Respiratory difficulties, nausea, copious vomiting, sweating, thirst, chest pain, tachycardia, palpitations, marked hypotension, giddiness, weakness, blurred vision, and confusion may follow. The intensity and duration of symptoms is very variable and even small quantities of alcohol may result in alarming reactions. In addition to the above effects, severe reactions have included respiratory depression, cardiovascular collapse, cardiac arrhythmias, myocardial infarction, acute heart failure, unconsciousness, convulsions, and sudden death. Severe reactions require intensive supportive therapy; oxygen and intravenous fluids may be necessary. Potassium concentrations should be monitored. The intravenous administration of ascorbic acid, ephedrine sulfate, or antihistamines has been suggested, but no benefit has been established.

◊ Reviews.

1. Chick J. Safety issues concerning the use of disulfiram in treating alcohol dependence. *Drug Safety* 1999; **20:** 427–35.

Effects on the blood. There were isolated reports of blood dyscrasias associated with disulfiram in the 1960s. The US manufacturer recommends that blood counts should be performed every 6 months during treatment.

Effects on the liver. A review of 18 cases of hepatitis in patients receiving disulfiram.[1] Symptoms have appeared between 10 days and six months after initiating disulfiram, and clinical improvement has been seen within 2 weeks of discontinuing disulfiram although liver enzyme values may not return to normal for several months. Fatal hepatic coma had been reported in 7 patients. The clinical picture of disulfiram-induced hepatitis is consistent with a hypersensitivity reaction.

1. Mason NA. Disulfiram-induced hepatitis: case report and review of the literature. *DICP Ann Pharmacother* 1989; **23:** 872–4.

Effects on the nervous system. ENCEPHALOPATHY. A 2% incidence of reversible toxic encephalopathy has been reported in patients receiving disulfiram.[1] Onset varies from days to months following the start of therapy and early signs include impaired concentration, memory deficits, anxiety, depression, and somnolence. Confusion and disorientation follow, often accompanied by paranoid delusions and sometimes hallucinations. Other symptoms may include ataxia, loss of fine motor coordination, slurred speech, and intention tremor. The encephalopathy usually resolves within 3 days to 2 weeks of stopping disulfiram, although symptoms may persist for 6 weeks. There are conflicting opinions on whether this psychosis is a toxic reaction to disulfiram or a response to abstinence from alcohol, but the authors suspected that most cases represent a toxic en-

cephalopathy. However, psychosis without any suggestion of encephalopathy has been reported.[2]

1. Hotson JR, Langston JW. Disulfiram-induced encephalopathy. *Arch Neurol* 1976; **33:** 141–2.
2. Rossiter SK. Psychosis with disulfiram prescribed under probation order. *BMJ* 1992; **305:** 763.

PERIPHERAL NEUROPATHY. Reports of peripheral neuropathy associated with disulfiram and reference to previously reported cases.[1,2] Onset of neuropathy varied from days to months after starting disulfiram treatment and could develop with doses of 250 or 500 mg daily. The most common symptom reported was pins and needles, but numbness, pain/burning, and weakness were frequently described; usually both muscle weakness and sensory loss were noted. Optic atrophy has also been described. Although there might be some improvement immediately after disulfiram withdrawal, the neurological deficit only improved slowly and symptoms might persist for as long as 2 years.[1]

1. Watson CP, *et al.* Disulfiram neuropathy. *Can Med Assoc J* 1980; **123:** 123–6.
2. Frisoni GB, Di Monda V. Disulfiram neuropathy: a review (1971–1988) and report of a case. *Alcohol Alcohol* 1989; **24:** 429–37.

Effects on the respiratory tract. Bronchospasm and hypertension were observed in an asthmatic patient taking disulfiram following an alcohol challenge test.[1]

1. Zapata E, Orwin A. Severe hypertension and bronchospasm during disulfiram-ethanol test reaction. *BMJ* 1992; **305:** 870.

Effects on the skin. Orange-coloured palms and soles, provoking an initial diagnosis of jaundice, developed in a 55-year-old man who had been taking disulfiram for about 2 months.[1] It was postulated that the discoloration was due to accumulation of carotenes in the skin as a result of inhibition of vitamin A metabolism by disulfiram. The discoloration disappeared soon after disulfiram was stopped.

1. Santonastaso M, *et al.* Yellow palms with disulfiram. *Lancet* 1997; **350:** 266.

Overdosage. Disulfiram intoxication has been reported in a 6-year-old boy who recovered after receiving disulfiram 250 mg four times daily to a total of 13 doses.[1] Of 6 previous reports one child died and 3 had moderate or severe brain damage. The syndrome of disulfiram intoxication in children is distinct from the disulfiram-alcohol interaction or acute disulfiram intoxication in adults. It is characterised by lethargy or somnolence, weakness, hypotonia, and vomiting, beginning approximately 12 hours after ingestion and progressing to stupor or coma. Dehydration, moderate tachycardia, and marked tachypnoea occur frequently, muscle tone is greatly decreased, and deep-tendon reflexes may be weak or absent.

Severe neurological damage has also been reported[2] in a 5-year-old girl following acute disulfiram intoxication which was initially diagnosed as diabetic ketoacidosis.

1. Benitz WE, Tatro DS. Disulfiram intoxication in a child. *J Pediatr* 1984; **105:** 487–9.
2. Mahajan P, *et al.* Basal ganglion infarction in a child with disulfiram poisoning. *Pediatrics* 1997; **99:** 605–8.

Precautions

Disulfiram is contra-indicated in the presence of cardiovascular disease or psychosis or severe personality disorders, and should not be given to patients known to be hypersensitive to it or to other thiuram compounds, such as those used in rubber vulcanisation or pesticides. It should be used with caution in the presence of diabetes mellitus, epilepsy, impaired hepatic or renal function, respiratory disorders, cerebral damage, or hypothyroidism. Caution is also advised when administering disulfiram to drug addicts. It is probably best avoided in pregnancy.

Disulfiram should not be given until at least 24 hours after the last ingestion of alcohol. Patients beginning therapy should be fully aware of the disulfiram-alcohol reaction and should be warned to avoid alcohol in any form, including alcohol-containing medicines and alcohol-based topical preparations. Reactions to alcohol may occur as long as 2 weeks after the cessation of disulfiram.

The US manufacturers have recommended that regular blood counts and liver function tests should be performed during long-term therapy.

Pregnancy. A report of 2 infants with severe limb-reduction anomalies whose mothers had taken disulfiram during pregnancy.[1] Only 2 similar cases had previously been reported.

1. Nora AH, *et al.* Limb-reduction anomalies in infants born to disulfiram-treated alcoholic mothers. *Lancet* 1977; **ii:** 664.

Interactions

Disulfiram inhibits hepatic enzymes and may interfere with the metabolism of other drugs taken at the same time. It enhances the effects of phenytoin and coumarin anticoagulants and their dosage may need to be reduced. It also inhibits the metabolism and excretion of rifampicin. Toxic reactions have occurred following the concomitant administration of disulfiram and isoniazid or metronidazole. Disulfiram may inhibit the metabolism of paraldehyde leading to an accumulation of acetaldehyde and these drugs should not be given concomitantly.

◊ The potential of disulfiram to impair drug metabolism was demonstrated[1] when it was found to prolong the plasma half-life of *phenazone*, probably by inhibiting the hepatic microsomal mixed function oxidases. It was also suggested[1] that disulfiram alters catecholamine metabolism since urinary excretion of vanilmandelic acid was significantly reduced and that of homovanillic acid was increased.

Although *chlorpromazine* was formerly given to reduce the nausea and vomiting associated with the disulfiram-alcohol reaction,[2] it has been suggested[3] that phenothiazine antiemetics such as chlorpromazine might increase hypotension because of their α-adrenoceptor blocking activity and should therefore be contra-indicated. Clinically serious pharmacodynamic interactions might be anticipated during the disulfiram-alcohol reaction in patients taking other drugs that impair blood pressure regulation, such as alpha blockers, beta blockers, and vasodilators.[4] It was reported[5] that *amitriptyline* appeared to enhance the disulfiram-alcohol reaction. There is the potential for serious interactions during the disulfiram-alcohol reaction with drugs having CNS actions mediated by noradrenaline or dopamine, such as *tricyclic antidepressants* and *phenothiazines*, or those inhibiting the same enzymes as disulfiram, such as *MAOIs*.[4] Conversely, *diazepam* was reported[5] to reduce the intensity of the disulfiram-alcohol reaction.

For a suggestion that a combination of disulfiram and *cannabis* may produce a hypomanic state, see p.1590.

For reference to toxicity associated with *metronidazole* given to alcoholic patients who were also receiving disulfiram, see p.595.

1. Vesell ES, *et al.* Impairment of drug metabolism by disulfiram in man. *Clin Pharmacol Ther* 1971; **12:** 785–92.
2. Cummins JF, Friend DG. Use of chlorpromazine in chronic alcoholics. *Am J Med Sci* 1954; **227:** 561–4.
3. Kwentus J, Major LF. Disulfiram in the treatment of alcoholism: a review. *J Stud Alcohol* 1979; **40:** 428–46.
4. Sellers EM, *et al.* Drugs to decrease alcohol consumption. *N Engl J Med* 1981; **305:** 1255–62.
5. MacCallum WAG. Drug interactions in alcoholism treatment. *Lancet* 1969; **i:** 313.

Pharmacokinetics

Disulfiram is absorbed variably from the gastrointestinal tract and is rapidly reduced to diethyldithiocarbamate (ditiocarb, p.619), principally by the glutathione reductase system in the erythrocytes; reduction may also occur in the liver. Diethyldithiocarbamate is metabolised in the liver to its glucuronide and methyl ester and to diethylamine, carbon disulfide, and sulfate ions. Metabolites are excreted primarily in the urine; carbon disulfide is exhaled in the breath.

◊ There was marked intersubject variability in plasma concentrations of disulfiram and its metabolites in a study of 15 male alcoholics given single 250-mg doses of disulfiram by mouth and repeated dosing with 250 mg daily for 12 days.[1] Variability might result from the marked lipid solubility of disulfiram, differences in plasma protein binding, or enterohepatic cycling. Average times to reach peak plasma concentrations after single or repeated doses were 8 to 10 hours for disulfiram, diethyldithiocarbamate, diethyldithiocarbamate-methyl ester, and diethylamine, and for carbon disulfide in breath; peak plasma concentrations of carbon disulfide occurred after 5 to 6 hours. Plasma concentrations of disulfiram were negligible within 48 hours of a dose, although concentrations of some metabolites were still raised. In urine, 1.7 and 8.3% of a dose was eliminated as diethyldithiocarbamate-glucuronide in the 24 hours after a single and repeated dose respectively, while diethylamine accounted for 1.6 and 5.7%, respectively. In the 24 hours after a single and repeated dose 22.4 and 31.3%, respectively, was eliminated as carbon disulfide in the breath.

1. Faiman MD, *et al.* Elimination kinetics of disulfiram in alcoholics after single and repeated doses. *Clin Pharmacol Ther* 1984; **36:** 520–6.

Uses and Administration

Disulfiram is used as an adjunct in the treatment of chronic alcoholism (p.1131). Disulfiram is not a cure and the treatment is likely to be of little value unless it is undertaken with the willing cooperation of the patient and is employed in conjunction with supportive psychotherapy.

Disulfiram inhibits aldehyde dehydrogenase, the enzyme responsible for the oxidation of acetaldehyde, a metabolite of alcohol. The resulting accumulation of acetaldehyde in the blood is widely believed to be responsible for many of the unpleasant symptoms of the disulfiram-alcohol reaction which occur when alcohol is taken, even in small quantities, after the administration of disulfiram (see Adverse Effects, above). Symptoms can arise within 10 minutes of the ingestion of alcohol and last from half an hour in mild cases to several hours in severe cases. It is advisable to carry out the initial treatment in hospital or in a specialised unit where the patient can be kept under close supervision.

Disulfiram is given by mouth. The dose is 800 mg, taken as a single dose, on the first day of treatment, reduced by 200 mg daily to a maintenance dose which is usually 100 to 200 mg daily. In the USA, where doses above 500 mg daily are not recommended, an initial dose of 500 mg daily for 1 to 2 weeks is given, followed by a maintenance dose of 250 mg daily or within the range of 125 to 500 mg daily. Treatment should be reviewed after no longer than 6 months. Maintenance therapy with disulfiram needs to be continued for months or years, until the patient is fully recovered socially and a basis for permanent self-control has been established.

A test dose of alcohol has been given under close supervision when the patient is receiving maintenance doses of disulfiram, in order to demonstrate the nature of the disulfiram-alcohol reaction. However, these challenge tests are not routinely recommended, and should not in any case be used in patients over 50

The symbol † denotes a preparation no longer actively marketed

years of age. Many authorities consider that an explicit description of the reaction is sufficient.

Disulfiram implants have been used in an attempt to overcome problems of patient compliance but have been largely abandoned due to lack of clinical efficacy.

Alcoholism. References.
1. Wright C, Moore RD. Disulfiram treatment of alcoholism. *Am J Med* 1990; **88**: 647–55.
2. Hughes JC, Cook CCH. The efficacy of disulfiram: a review of outcome studies. *Addiction* 1997; **92**: 381–95.

Preparations
BP 2001: Disulfiram Tablets;
USP 25: Disulfiram Tablets.
Proprietary Preparations (details are given in Part 3)
Aust.: Antabus; *Austral.:* Antabuse; *Belg.:* Antabuse; *Braz.:* Antietanol; *Canad.:* Antabuse; *Denm.:* Antabus; *Fin.:* Antabus; *Fr.:* Esperal; *Ger.:* Antabus; *Irl.:* Antabuse; *Israel:* Antabuse; *Ital.:* Antabuse; Etiltox; *Mex.:* Etabus; *Neth.:* Refusal; *Norw.:* Antabus; *NZ:* Antabuse; *Port.:* Tetradin; *S.Afr.:* Antabuse; *Spain:* Antabus; *Swed.:* Antabus; *Switz.:* Antabus; *Thai.:* Antabuse; Difiram; *UK:* Antabuse; *USA:* Antabuse†.
Multi-ingredient: *Braz.:* Sarcoton; *Fr.:* TTD-B₃-B₄; *Swed.:* Tenutex.

Dizocilpine Maleate (9426-x)

Dizocilpine Maleate (*USAN, rINNM*).
MK-801.   (+)-10,11-Dihydro-5-methyl-5*H*-dibenzo[*a,d*]-cyclohepten-5,10-imine maleate.
$C_{16}H_{15}N,C_4H_4O_4 = 337.4$.
CAS — 77086-21-6 (dizocilpine); 77086-22-7 (dizocilpine maleate).

Profile
Dizocilpine is an antagonist of the excitatory neurotransmitter *N*-methyl-ᴅ-aspartate (NMDA). It has been investigated for its antiepileptic properties as well as for a potential role in various other neurological disorders including the prevention of damage due to cerebral ischaemia.

◊ Dizocilpine has good anticonvulsant activity but as it causes alarming psychotropic effects it had been abandoned as a possible therapy for epilepsy.[1] Interest in its use as a possible therapy for stroke continued.
1. Richens A. New antiepileptic drugs. *Br J Hosp Med* 1990; **44**: 241.

Drosera (12681-a)

Droserae Herba; Herba Rorellae; Rorela; Ros Solis; Sundew.
Pharmacopoeias. In Belg.

The air-dried entire plant *Drosera rotundifolia* (Droseraceae) and other *Drosera* spp.

Profile
Preparations of drosera have been used for its reputed value in respiratory disorders but it is of doubtful value.
It has been used in homoeopathic medicine.

Preparations
Proprietary Preparations (details are given in Part 3)
Ger.: Makatussin Saft Drosera; Makatussin Tropfen Drosera.
Multi-ingredient: *Aust.:* Erkaltungstee; Grippetee Dr Zeidler; Heumann Hustenstiller†; Krauterdoktor Krampf- und Reizhustensirup; Krautertee Nr 211; Pilka; Pilka Forte; *Austral.:* Asa Tones; *Belg.:* Gloceda; Sirop Toux du Larynx†; *Braz.:* Broncotussan; *Fr.:* Pastilles Monleon; Pulmonase†; Sirop Pectoral adulte†; Sirop Pectoral enfant†; Tussidoron†; *Ger.:* Biotuss N; Bronchicum Pflanzlicher; Drosithym-N; Makatussin Tropfen forte; Mintetten Truw†; Tussiflorin Hustenstiller; *Israel:* Pilka; *Neth.:* Abdijsiroop (Akker-Siroop)†; *Port.:* Fluidin Infantil; Lactucol; Pilka F; *Spain:* Broncovital; Mentobox†; Pazbronquial; Pilka; *Switz.:* Bromocod N; Bronchialin†; Bronchofluid†; Demo elixir pectoral N; Demo gouttes contre la toux†; Demo pates pectorales†; Demo sirop contre la toux†; Drosinula N; Escotussin; Famel; Gouttes contre la toux "S"; Makatussin; Makatussin forte; Nican; Pastilles pectorales Demo N; Pastilles pectorales formule 541; Pilka; Sirop S contre la toux et la bronchite; Thymodrosin N; Thymodrosin†; Tussanil Compositum.

Drotaverine (12682-t)

Drotaverine (*rINN*).
1-(3,4-Diethoxybenzylidene)-6,7-diethoxy-1,2,3,4-tetrahydroisoquinoline.
$C_{24}H_{31}NO_4 = 397.5$.
CAS — 14009-24-6.
ATC — A03AD02.
Pharmacopoeias. Pol. includes Drotaverine Hydrochloride.

Profile
Drotaverine is used as an antispasmodic.

◊ References.
1. Bolaji OO, *et al.* Pharmacokinetics and bioavailability of drotaverine in humans. *Eur J Drug Metab Pharmacokinet* 1996; **21**: 217–21.

Porphyria. Drotaverine has been associated with acute attacks of porphyria and is considered unsafe in porphyric patients.

Preparations
Proprietary Preparations (details are given in Part 3)
Hung.: No-Spa; *Thai.:* Deolin; No-Spa; Toverine.
Multi-ingredient: *Hung.:* Bispan; Neotroparin; Quarelin; Triospan.

Dulcamara (12684-r)

Bittersweet; Douce-Amère; Dulcamarae Caulis; Woody Nightshade.

The dried stems and branches of *Solanum dulcamara* (Solanaceae).

Profile
Dulcamara was formerly a popular remedy for chronic rheumatism and skin eruptions and was administered as an infusion. It has been used in homoeopathic medicine.

All parts of the plant are poisonous due to the presence of solanaceous alkaloids. The berries have caused poisoning in children. Adverse effects are treated as described under Atropine, p.461.

Preparations
Proprietary Preparations (details are given in Part 3)
Ger.: Cefabene; Dolexaderm H†.
Multi-ingredient: *Aust.:* Dermatodoron; *Fr.:* Elixir Contre La Toux Weleda†; *Ger.:* Dermatodoron; Kneipp Rheuma Tee N†; *Ital.:* Depurativo; Tisana Arnaldi†; *UK:* Dermatodoron.

Ebselen (2036-t)

Ebselen (*rINN*).
2-Phenyl-1,2-benzisoselenazolin-3-one.
$C_{13}H_9NOSe = 274.2$.
CAS — 60940-34-3.

Profile
Ebselen has antioxidant activity and inhibits lipid peroxidation. It is under investigation as a neuroprotectant in stroke.

◊ References.
1. Yamaguchi T, *et al.* Ebselen is acute ischemic stroke: a placebo-controlled, double-blind clinical trial. *Stroke* 1998; **29**: 12–17.
2. Saito I, *et al.* Neuroprotective effect of an antioxidant, ebselen, in patients with delayed neurologic deficits after aneurysmal subarachnoid hemorrhage. *Neurosurgery* 1998; **42**: 269–78.

Echinacea (7140-y)

Black Sampson; Brauneria; Coneflower; Rudbeckia; Sonnenhutkraut.

The dried roots of *Echinacea angustifolia* (Compositae). *E. pallida* or *E. purpura* are sometimes substituted.

Profile
Echinacea is reported to have immunostimulant properties and is used in herbal preparations for the prophylaxis of bacterial and viral infections. It is also used in homoeopathic medicine.

◊ References.
1. Houghton P. Echinacea. *Pharm J* 1994; **253**: 342–3.
2. Pepping J. Echinacea. *Am J Health-Syst Pharm* 1999; **56**: 121–2.
3. Melchart D, *et al.* Echinacea for preventing and treating the common cold (updated 18 July 2001). Available in The Cochrane Library; Issue 4. Oxford: Update Software; 2001.

Preparations
Proprietary Preparations (details are given in Part 3)
Aust.: Echinacin; Echinaforce; Myo-Echinacin†; *Austral.:* Echinacin; Proechina†; *Canad.:* Echina Pro†; *Ger.:* Berubi; Bilgast echinac†; Cefasept; Cefasept mono; Dore Immun; Echan; Echifit; Echiherb; Echinacin; Echinaforce; Echinapur; Episcorit; Esberitox mono; Fudimun†; Immunopret; Logopharm Immun†; Mentopin Echinacea†; Pascotox forte-Injektopas; Pascotox mono; Resplant; Wiedimmun; *Spain:* Echinacin; *Switz.:* Echinacin; Echinaforce; EchinaMed; *UK:* Benylin Active Response; Echinacea; Echinaforce; Phytocold; Skin Clear.
Multi-ingredient: *Aust.:* Parodontax†; Spasmo-Urgenin; Urgenin; *Austral.:* Cold and Flu Relief; Cough Relief; Echinacea & Antioxidants; Echinacea 4000; Echinacea ACE + Zinc; Echinacea ACE Plus Zinc; Echinacea Complex; Echinacea Herbal Plus Formula†; Echinacea Lozenge; Echinacea Plus; Flavons; Galium Complex; Gartech; Herbal Cleanse; Herbal Cold & Flu Relief; Lifesystem Herbal Plus Formula 8 Echinacea†; Odourless Garlic; Proyeast; Relief Rub; Respatona Plus Bronchial Cough Relief; Sambucus Complex; Urgenin; Urinase; Vita-Minis Cold & Flu; *Belg.:* Urgenin; *Braz.:* Parodontax; *Ger.:* Alsicur†; Bagnisan med Heilbad; Bomagall forte S†; Cefaktivon; Cefaktivon "novum"†; Ermsech; Esberitox N; Hewenephron duo; JuGrippan†; Lymphozil; Pascotox; *Hong Kong:* Urgenin; *Israel:* Parodontax; Urgenin; *Ital.:* Aclon Lievit; Allergenid†; Bodyguard; Enertonic; Probigol; Promix; Promix 3; Ribovir; Sanaderm†; *Port.:* Neo Urgenin†; Spasmo-Urgenin; *S.Afr.:* Spasmo-Urgenin; *Singapore:* Noricaven; *Spain:* Neo Urgenin; Spasmo-Urgenin; Uralyt†; Urgenin; *Switz.:* Alpina Gel a la consoude†; Demonatur Capsules contre les refroidissements; Demonatur Dragees pour les reins et la vessie; Esberitop; Esberitox N†; Gel a la consoude†; Phytomed Prosta; Phytomed Rhino†; Prosta-Caps Chassot N; Spagymun; Spagyrom; Urgenine†; *Thai.:* Spasmo-Urgenin; *UK:* Antifect; Beechams for Natural Relief; Buttercup Pol'N'Count; Catarrh Cream; Cold-eeze; Echinacea; Goodypops; Hay Fever & Sinus Relief; Hayfever & Sinus Relief; Herbal Booster; Kleer; Modern Herbals

Cold & Catarrh; Revitonil; Savlon Natural First Aid for Burns; Savlon Natural First Aid for Insect Bites & Stings; Sinotar; WCS Dusting Powder.

Eledoisin (3898-b)

Eledoisin (*rINN*).
ELD-950.   5-Oxo-Pro-Pro-Ser-Lys-Asp-Ala-Phe-Ile-Gly-Leu-Met-NH₂.
$C_{54}H_{85}N_{13}O_{15}S = 1188.4$.
CAS — 69-25-0.

Profile
Eledoisin is a peptide extracted from the posterior salivary glands of certain small octopuses (*Eledone* spp., Mollusca), or obtained by synthesis. Its actions resemble those of substance P; it is a potent vasodilator and increases capillary permeability. It has been given as eye drops to stimulate lachrymal secretion in Sjögren's syndrome and other dry eye conditions (p.1498).

Preparations
Proprietary Preparations (details are given in Part 3)
Spain: Eloisin.

Entsufon Sodium (3541-r)

Entsufon Sodium (*USAN, rINN*).
Sodium   2-{2-[2-(*p*-1,3,3-tetramethylbutylphenoxy)ethoxy]ethoxy}ethanesulfonate.
$C_{20}H_{33}NaO_6S = 424.5$.
CAS — 55837-16-6 (entsufon); 2917-94-4 (entsufon sodium).

Profile
Entsufon sodium is a detergent used as a soap substitute for cleansing the skin and mucous membranes.

Preparations
Proprietary Preparations (details are given in Part 3)
Hong Kong: pHisoDerm; *USA:* pHisoHex.
Multi-ingredient: *Canad.:* pHisoHex.

Epomediol (12695-n)

1,8-Epoxy-4-isopropyl-1-methylcylohexane-2,6-diol.
$C_{10}H_{18}O_3 = 186.2$.
ATC — A05BA05.

Profile
Epomediol has been given by mouth in the treatment of hepatic disorders.

◊ References.
1. Capurso L, *et al.* Activity of epomediol in the treatment of hepatopathies: a double-blind multi-centre study. *J Int Med Res* 1987; **15**: 134–47.

Preparations
Proprietary Preparations (details are given in Part 3)
Ital.: Clesidren.

Epostane (19144-m)

Epostane (*BAN, USAN, rINN*).
Win-32729.   4α,5α-Epoxy-3,17β-dihydroxy-4β,17α-dimethyl-5α-androst-2-ene-2-carbonitrile.
$C_{22}H_{31}NO_3 = 357.5$.
CAS — 80471-63-2.

Profile
Epostane has antiprogestogenic activity and has been investigated for use in the termination of pregnancy in conjunction with prostaglandins, and as a uterine stimulant for the induction of labour.

◊ References.
1. Webster MA, *et al.* Interruption of first trimester human pregnancy following epostane therapy: effect of prostaglandin E₂ pessaries. *Br J Obstet Gynaecol* 1985; **92**: 963–8.
2. Birgerson L, Odlind V. Early pregnancy termination with antiprogestins: a comparative clinical study of RU 486 given in two dose regimens and epostane. *Fertil Steril* 1987; **48**: 565–70.
3. Crooij MJ, *et al.* Termination of early pregnancy by the 3β-hydroxysteroid dehydrogenase inhibitor epostane. *N Engl J Med* 1988; **319**: 813–17.
4. Webster MA, Gillmer MD. Induction of abortion in early first trimester human pregnancy using epostane. *Br J Obstet Gynaecol* 1989; **96**: 340–5.

Equisetum (12699-v)

Herba Equiseti; Horsetail; Prêle; Schachtelhalmkraut.
Pharmacopoeias. In Aust., Fr., Ger., Pol., and Swiss.

The dried sterile green stems of the common horsetail, *Equisetum arvense* (Equisetaceae).

Profile
Equisetum is an ingredient of herbal preparations that have been used in the treatment of genito-urinary and respiratory

disorders. Similar preparations have been used in the treatment of cardiovascular disorders, rheumatic disorders, liver disorders, constipation, and as a tonic.

Equisetum is used in homoeopathic medicine.

The related species *Equisetum hiemale* is used in China for the treatment of eye disorders.

Preparations

Proprietary Preparations (details are given in Part 3)

Austral.: Bioglan Silica-Vite; *Fr.:* Siliprele; *Ger.:* Biolavant†; Kneipp Zinnkraut-Pflanzensaft; Produiret; Pulvhydrops Mono; Redaxa fit; Salus Zinnkraut; Zinnkraut-Tropfen; *Ital.:* Bioequiseto; Osteosil.

Multi-ingredient: *Aust.:* Bio-Garten Tee fur Niere und Blase; Bio-Garten Tropfen fur Niere und Blase; Blasen- und Nierentee; Blasentee; Bogumil-tassenfertiger milder Abfurtee; Drogimed; Droxitop; Ehrmann's Entschlackungstee; Entschlackender Abfuhrtee; Kneipp Nieren- und Blasen-Tee; Krauterdoktor Entwasserungs-Elixier; Krauterhaus Mag Kottas Entwasserungstee; Krauterhaus Mag Kottas Fruhjahrs- und Herbstkurtee; Krauterhaus Mag Kottas Nierentee; Krautertee Nr 3; Krautertee Nr 32; Krautertee Nr 4; Mag Doskar's Nieren- und Blasentonikum; Mag Kottas Entwasserungstee; Mag Kottas Nieren-Blasentee; Naturland Rheuma-Tee; Nierentee; Pneumopan; St Bonifatius-Tee; St Radegunder Entwasserungs-Elixier; St Radegunder Entwasserungstee; St Radegunder Nierentee; Synpharma Instant-Blasen-und-Nierentee; Teekanne Blasen- und Nierentee; Uropurat; *Austral.:* Cal Alkyline; Extralife Fluid-Care; Medinat Esten; Serenoa Complex; Silicic Complex; *Fr.:* Arterase; Circulatonic; Tisane des Familles; Tisanes de l'Abbe Hamon no 3; *Ger.:* Agamadon†; Cystinol; Equisil; Eviprostat N; Harntee 400; Harntee STADA; Hernia-Tee†; Hevert-Blasen- und Nieren- Tee; Kneipp Blasen-und Nieren-Tee; nephro-loges; Nephroselect M; Nieron-Tee N; Presseln Nieren-Blasen K 3; Presseln Stoffwechsel-Tee Hapeka 225 N; Salus Rheuma-Tee Krautertee Nr. 12†; Salusan†; Solidagoren N; Tonsilgon N; Tussiflorin N; *Hong Kong:* Eviprostat; *Ital.:* Nosenil†; *Singapore:* Eviprostat; *Spain:* Resolutivo Regium; Uralyt†; *Switz.:* Enveloppements ECR†; Eviprostat†; Nephrosolid N; Tisane Diuretique; Urinex (nouvelle formule); *UK:* Antiglan; Antitis; Aqualette; Gerard House Waterlex; Kas-Bah.

Ergometrine Maleate (1506-h)

Ergometrine Maleate *(BANM, rINNM).*

Ergobasine Maleate; Ergometrinhydrogenmaleat; Ergometrini Maleas; Ergonovine Bimaleate; Ergonovine Maleate; Ergostetrine Maleate; Ergotocine Maleate; Maleato de Ergonovina. N-[(S)-2-Hydroxy-1-methylethyl]-D-lysergamide hydrogen maleate; 9,10-Didehydro-N-[(S)-2-hydroxy-1-methylethyl]-6-methylergoline-8β-carboxamide hydrogen maleate.

$C_{19}H_{23}N_3O_2,C_4H_4O_4 = 441.5.$

CAS — 60-79-7 (ergometrine); 129-51-1 (ergometrine maleate).

Pharmacopoeias. In Chin., Eur. (see p.vi), Int., Jpn, and US.

Pharmacopoeial description

Ph. Eur.: A white or slightly coloured crystalline powder. Sparingly soluble in water; slightly soluble in alcohol; practically insoluble in ether. A 1% solution in water has a pH of 3.6 to 4.4. Store in airtight glass containers at a temperature of 2° to 8°. Protect from light.

USP 25: A white to greyish-white or faintly yellow, odourless, microcrystalline powder. It darkens with age and on exposure to light. Sparingly soluble in water; slightly soluble in alcohol; insoluble in chloroform and in ether. Store in airtight containers at a temperature not exceeding 8°. Protect from light.

Stability. Reports of deterioration and degradation of ergometrine-containing injections when exposed to high temperatures in the tropics.[1-3] The mean loss in one study[3] of ergometrine injection under shipment to the tropics was 5.8%, but in some individual samples the loss was more marked: 18 of 80 test samples contained less than 80% of the stated content, and in 3 cases the content was less than 60% of the stated amount. A similar but much less significant pattern was seen with methylergometrine: the content varied from 98.6 to 99.5% of the labelled amount.

1. Walker GJA, *et al.* Potency of ergometrine in tropical countries. *Lancet* 1988; ii: 393.
2. Abu-Reid IO, *et al.* Stability of drugs in the tropics. *Int Pharm J* 1990; **4:** 6–10.
3. Hogerzeil HV, *et al.* Stability of essential drugs during shipment to the tropics. *BMJ* 1992; **304:** 210–12.

Adverse Effects and Treatment

Nausea and vomiting, abdominal pain, diarrhoea, headache, dizziness, tinnitus, chest pain, palpitations, bradycardia and other cardiac arrhythmias, myocardial infarction, dyspnoea, and pulmonary oedema have been reported after administration of ergometrine. Hypertension has occurred, particularly after rapid intravenous administration. Hypersensitivity reactions, including shock, have occurred. Ergometrine shows less tendency to produce gangrene than ergotamine, but ergotism has been reported and symptoms of acute poisoning are similar (see p.452).

Adverse effects should be treated as for ergotamine, p.452.

Effects on the respiratory system. Bronchospasm has been reported after administration of ergometrine.[1] Although studies *in vitro* on *canine* bronchi have suggested a direct ac-

tion on smooth muscle, this could not be confirmed in studies using human bronchi.

1. Hill H, *et al.* Ergometrine and bronchospasm. *Anaesthesia* 1987; **42:** 1115–16.

Overdosage. There have been reports[1-5] of accidental administration of adult doses of ergometrine maleate to neonates, sometimes instead of vitamin K. Symptoms have included peripheral vasoconstriction, encephalopathy, convulsions, respiratory failure, acute renal failure, and temporary lactose intolerance. After administration of ergometrine with oxytocin, water intoxication has also been reported.[1] In all of these cases, recovery occurred after intensive symptomatic treatment including assisted ventilation and anticonvulsants. However, deaths have also been recorded.[5] The long-term outcome of ergometrine overdosage has been reported for 6 infants.[5] Their ages at follow-up ranged from 18 months to 5 years; all had normal physical and behavioural development and neurological outcomes.

1. Whitfield MF, Salfield SAW. Accidental administration of Syntometrine in adult dosage to the newborn. *Arch Dis Child* 1980; **55:** 68–70.
2. Pandey SK, Haines CI. Accidental administration of ergometrine to newborn infant. *BMJ* 1982; **285:** 693.
3. Mitchell AA, *et al.* Accidental administration of ergonovine to a newborn. *JAMA* 1983; **250:** 730–1.
4. Donatini B, *et al.* Inadvertent administration of uterotonics to neonates. *Lancet* 1993; **341:** 839–40.
5. Dargaville PA, Campbell NT. Overdose of ergometrine in the newborn infant: acute symptomatology and long-term outcome. *J Paediatr Child Health* 1998; **34:** 83–9.

Precautions

As for Ergotamine Tartrate, p.452. Ergometrine maleate is contra-indicated for the induction of labour or for use during the first stage of labour. If used at the end of the second stage of labour, prior to delivery of the placenta, there must be expert obstetric supervision. Its use should be avoided in patients with pre-eclampsia, eclampsia, or threatened spontaneous abortion.

Porphyria. Ergometrine maleate has been associated with acute attacks of porphyria and is considered unsafe in porphyric patients.

Interactions

The vasoconstrictor effects of ergometrine are enhanced by sympathomimetics. Halothane has been considered to diminish the effects of ergometrine on the uterus.

Sympathomimetics. Use of *dopamine* in a patient treated with ergometrine was associated with subsequent development of gangrene in both hands and feet.[1]

1. Buchanan N, *et al.* Symmetrical gangrene of the extremities associated with the use of dopamine subsequent to ergometrine administration. *Intensive Care Med* 1977; **3:** 55–6.

Pharmacokinetics

Ergometrine is reported to be rapidly absorbed after administration by mouth and by intramuscular injection, with onset of uterine contractions in about 5 to 15 minutes after an oral dose and 2 to 7 minutes after an intramuscular dose. Elimination appears to be principally by metabolism in the liver.

Uses and Administration

Ergometrine has a much more powerful action on the uterus than most of the other alkaloids of ergot, especially on the puerperal uterus. Its main action is the production of intense contractions, which at higher doses are sustained, in contrast to the more physiological rhythmic uterine contractions induced by oxytocin; its action is more prolonged than that of oxytocin.

Ergometrine maleate is used in the active management of the third stage of labour, and to prevent or treat postpartum or postabortal haemorrhage caused by uterine atony; by maintaining uterine contraction and tone, blood vessels in the uterine wall are compressed, and blood flow reduced.

In the active management of the third stage of labour, ergometrine maleate and oxytocin are administered together under full obstetric supervision. A dose of ergometrine maleate 500 μg and oxytocin 5 units is injected intramuscularly after delivery of the anterior shoulder of the infant; contractions are reported to occur within 2 to 3 minutes. Delivery of the placenta is actively assisted while the uterus is firmly contracted.

In the prevention or treatment of postpartum haemorrhage, a similar dose of ergometrine maleate with oxytocin is given intramuscularly following delivery of the placenta or when bleeding occurs. Intravenous administration of the combined preparation has been used but is no longer recommended. Ergometrine maleate alone is used for prevention or treatment of postpartum or postabortal haemorrhage in a usual intramuscular dose of 200 μg. In emergencies such as excessive uterine bleeding, ergometrine maleate has been given intravenously in a dose of 200 μg. This dose may be repeated every 2 to 4 hours as needed, for up to 5 doses. Single doses of 250 to 500 μg have also been used. Intravenous doses should be administered slowly to reduce the risk of adverse effects, particularly hypertension. Parenteral treatment of haemorrhage may be followed by ergometrine maleate 200 to 400 μg by mouth two to four times daily for up to 7 days, until the danger of atony and haemorrhage has passed.

In the treatment of mild secondary postpartum haemorrhage, ergometrine maleate has been given by mouth in a dose of 500 μg three times daily for 2 to 7 days.

Ergometrine maleate has been administered by the sublingual and rectal routes.

Ergometrine tartrate was formerly used.

Diagnosis and testing. Ergometrine maleate[1-4] or methylergometrine maleate[2,5] have been used in a provocation test for the diagnosis of Prinzmetal's angina (variant angina) (p.791). Ergometrine maleate has also been used in the diagnosis of oesophageal spasm.[6]

1. Waters DD, *et al.* Ergonovine testing in a coronary care unit. *Am J Cardiol* 1980; **46:** 922–30.
2. Anonymous. Provocation of coronary spasm: research or diagnostic test? *Lancet* 1982; ii: 805.
3. Health and Public Policy Committee, American College of Physicians. Performance of ergonovine provocative testing for coronary artery spasm. *Ann Intern Med* 1984; **100:** 151–2.
4. Song J-K, *et al.* Safety and clinical impact of ergonovine stress echocardiography for diagnosis of coronary vasospasm. *J Am Coll Cardiol* 2000; **35:** 1850–6.
5. Bertrand ME, *et al.* Frequency of provoked coronary arterial spasm in 1089 consecutive patients undergoing coronary arteriography. *Circulation* 1982; **65:** 1299–1306.
6. Richter JE, *et al.* Esophageal chest pain: current controversies in pathogenesis, diagnosis, and therapy. *Ann Intern Med* 1989; **110:** 66–78.

Postpartum haemorrhage. In normal labour, once the child is born myometrial retraction and strong uterine contractions cause shortening and kinking of the uterine blood vessels and a retraction of the placental bed: these changes operate to minimise blood loss. However, if the uterus fails to contract adequately (uterine atony) or if retained placental remnants prevent retraction of the placental bed, postpartum haemorrhage may occur. These two causes account for about 80% of cases of postpartum haemorrhage; in the remainder it is usually due to trauma of the genital tract.

Postpartum haemorrhage may be fatal to the mother unless promptly dealt with: management generally involves removal of the placenta if this has not been expelled, the use of oxytocics to contract the uterus, and, if blood loss is severe, transfusion. Prophylactic management is favoured in some countries but in others may be reserved for women at greater risk, including those who have undergone prolonged labour, those who have an overdistended uterus (for example in multiple pregnancy), or after antepartum haemorrhage, or deep general anaesthesia.

Active management of the third stage of labour involves prophylactic administration of an oxytocic, cord clamping before placental delivery, and cord traction. Studies[1,2] and a subsequent meta-analysis[3] including additional trials of actively managed labour found that routine oxytocics (usually with crowning of the head, delivery of the anterior shoulder, or after delivery of the placenta) reduced blood loss, the risk of postpartum haemorrhage, and the risk of prolonged third stage of labour. Comparisons of the efficacy and safety of different oxytocics have been made.[4] Oxytocin and ergot alkaloids may be of similar efficacy in decreasing postpartum haemorrhage, but oxytocin is less likely to predispose to delayed placental delivery and also less likely to cause hypertension. Syntometrine (ergometrine and oxytocin) and ergot alkaloids also appeared to be of similar efficacy, but Syntometrine may be less likely to be associated with a prolonged third stage of labour. Syntometrine may be associated with a reduction in the risk of postpartum haemorrhage compared with oxytocin,[5] but a higher incidence of nausea, vomiting, and hypertension.

Prostaglandins such as carboprost, dinoprostone, or sulprostone are used in the treatment of established postpartum haemorrhage that has not been controlled by oxytocin and ergot preparations. Their role in active management of third stage labour has not been established, although results from small trials suggest that they may be effective for the prevention of postpartum haemorrhage.[6] Prophylactic use of misoprostol, given orally immediately after delivery was effective in one study,[7] and a large international study comparing misoprostol with oxytocin is underway.

1. Prendiville WJ, *et al.* The Bristol third stage trial: active versus physiological management of third stage of labour. *BMJ* 1988; **297:** 1295–1300.
2. Rogers J, *et al.* Active versus expectant management of third stage of labour: the Hinchingbrooke randomised controlled trial. *Lancet* 1998; **351:** 693–9.
3. Prendiville WJ, *et al.* Active versus expectant management in the third stage of labour (updated 1 March 2001). Available in The Cochrane Library; Issue 4. Oxford: Update Software; 2001.
4. Elbourne D, *et al.* Choice of oxytocic preparation for routine use in the management of the third stage of labour: an overview of the evidence from controlled trials. *Br J Obstet Gynaecol* 1988; **95:** 17–30.
5. McDonald S, *et al.* Prophylactic syntometrine versus oxytocin for delivery of the placenta (updated 23 April 2001). Available in The Cochrane Library; Issue 4. Oxford: Update Software; 2001.
6. Gülmezoglu AM. Prostaglandins for prevention of postpartum haemorrhage (updated 29 August 2001). Available in The Cochrane Library; Issue 4. Oxford: Update Software; 2001.
7. El-Refaey H, *et al.* Use of oral misoprostol in the prevention of postpartum haemorrhage. *Br J Obstet Gynaecol* 1997; **104:** 336–9.

Preparations

BP 2001: Ergometrine and Oxytocin Injection; Ergometrine Injection; Ergometrine Tablets;

The symbol † denotes a preparation no longer actively marketed

USP 25: Ergonovine Maleate Injection; Ergonovine Maleate Tablets.

Proprietary Preparations (details are given in Part 3)
Braz.: Ergotrate; **Canad.:** Ergotrate†; **Ger.:** Secalysat EM†; **Mex.:** Ergotrate; **S.Afr.:** Ergotrate†; **Thai.:** Gynaemine; **USA:** Ergotrate.
Multi-ingredient: Austral.: Syntometrine; **Hong Kong:** Syntometrine; **Irl.:** Syntometrine; **Israel:** Syntometrine; **NZ:** Syntometrine; **S.Afr.:** Syntometrine; **UK:** Syntometrine.

Ergot (1501-x)

Secale Cornutum.

Pharmacopoeias. In *Aust.*, which also includes Prepared Ergot.

The sclerotium of the fungus *Claviceps purpurea* (Hypocreaceae) developed in the ovary of the rye, *Secale cereale* (Gramineae), containing not less than 0.15% of total alkaloids, calculated as ergotoxine, and not less than 0.01% of water-soluble alkaloids, calculated as ergometrine. Some authorities have expressed alkaloidal content in terms of ergotamine and ergometrine.

Adverse Effects and Treatment

As for Ergotamine Tartrate, p.452.

Epidemic ergot poisoning, arising from the ingestion of ergotised rye bread, is now seldom seen. Two forms of epidemic toxicity, which rarely occur together, have been described: a gangrenous form characterised by agonising pain of the extremities of the body followed by dry gangrene of the peripheral parts, and a rarer nervous type giving rise to paroxysmal epileptiform convulsions.

Poisoning. A report of an outbreak of ergotism, attributed to the ingestion of infected wild oats (*Avena abyssinica*), in Ethiopia.[1]

1. King B. Outbreak of ergotism in Wollo, Ethiopia. *Lancet* 1979; **ii:** 1411.

Uses and Administration

Ergot has the vasoconstricting and oxytocic actions of its constituent alkaloids, especially ergotamine (p.452) and ergometrine (above). A liquid extract or tablets of prepared ergot were formerly used as an oxytocic. Preparations containing ergot extracts have been promoted for use in dyspepsia and nervous disorders.

Ergotoxine (1509-v)

CAS — 8006-25-5 (ergotoxine); 8047-28-7 (ergotoxine esilate); 8047-29-8 (ergotoxine phosphate); 564-36-3 (ergocornine); 511-08-0 (ergocristine); 511-09-1 (ergocryptine).

A mixture in equal proportions of ergocornine ($C_{31}H_{39}N_5O_5 = 561.7$), ergocristine ($C_{35}H_{39}N_5O_5 = 609.7$), and ergocryptine, as the α- and β-isomers ($C_{32}H_{41}N_5O_5 = 575.7$).

Profile

Ergotoxine is a mixture of naturally occurring ergot alkaloids. The esilate was formerly used as an oxytocic and in the treatment of migraine. Ergotoxine phosphate has also been used.

Preparations

Proprietary Preparations (details are given in Part 3)
Multi-ingredient: Thai.: Belloid.

Etanercept (20283-b)

Etanercept (BAN, USAN, rINN).

rhu-TNFR:Fc. A dimer of 1-235 tumour necrosis factor receptor (human) fusion protein with 236-467-immunoglobulin G1 (human γ1-chain Fc fragment).
CAS — 185243-69-0.
ATC — L04AA11.

Adverse Effects and Precautions

Mild to moderate injection site reactions with symptoms of erythema, itching, pain, or swelling are common with etanercept.

Upper respiratory-tract infections and sinusitis have been reported with etanercept. Serious infections and sepsis, sometimes resulting in death, have also occurred, mainly in patients with underlying conditions predisposing them to infections. Consequently, it is recommended that etanercept should be discontinued if a patient develops a serious infection or sepsis. Likewise etanercept should not be initiated in patients with active infections, including chronic or localized infections; caution is recommended in those with a history of recurrent infections or with underlying conditions that may predispose to infections.

Blood dyscrasias, including pancytopenia and aplastic anaemia, have been reported rarely with etanercept treatment; in some cases the outcome was fatal. Etanercept should be used with caution in patients with a history of blood dyscrasias.

There have also been rare reports of CNS demyelinating disorders such as multiple sclerosis, myelitis, and optic neuritis in patients receiving etanercept and caution is advised when using etanercept in patients with pre-existing or recent-onset CNS demyelinating disorders.

Antinuclear antibody formation has been noted.

Effects on the skin. Discoid lupus and necrotising vasculitis have been reported with etanercept treatment.[1] Urticaria has also been seen in 2 patients receiving etanercept for juvenile idiopathic arthritis.[2]

1. Brion PH, *et al.* Autoimmune skin rashes associated with etanercept for rheumatoid arthritis. *Ann Intern Med* 1999; **131:** 634.
2. Skyttä E, *et al.* Etanercept and urticaria in patients with juvenile idiopathic arthritis. *Clin Exp Rheumatol* 2000; **18:** 533–4.

Pharmacokinetics

After subcutaneous administration of single doses of etanercept the median half-life was 115 hours and the time to maximum concentration was 72 hours. Repeated dosing was noted to result in a two- to fivefold increase in serum levels of etanercept in some patients.

◊ References.

1. Korth-Bradley JM, *et al.* The pharmacokinetics of etanercept in healthy volunteers. *Ann Pharmacother* 2000; **34:** 161–4.

Uses and Administration

Etanercept is a recombinant version of soluble human tumour necrosis factor (TNF) receptor that binds specifically to tumour necrosis factor (p.577) and blocks its interaction with endogenous cell-surface TNF receptors. This interaction prevents the important effect that TNF has in the inflammatory processes of rheumatoid arthritis (p.9). Etanercept is used in the treatment of moderately to severely active rheumatoid arthritis. In the UK, its use is limited to patients who have had an inadequate response to standard disease-modifying antirheumatic drugs; however, in the USA it may be used for treating early rheumatoid arthritis, to reduce the signs and the symptoms and delay structural damage. In both cases, it is given as a subcutaneous injection in a dose of 25 mg twice weekly at intervals of 72 to 96 hours.

Etanercept is also used in the treatment of unresponsive moderate to severe polyarticular juvenile idiopathic arthritis (p.9) in children aged 4 years and over. It is given subcutaneously in a dose of 0.4 mg per kg body-weight (up to a maximum dose of 25 mg) twice weekly at intervals of 72 to 96 hours.

Psoriatic arthritis. Preliminary findings[1] suggest that etanercept may be useful in the treatment of psoriatic arthritis (see Spondyloarthropathies, p.10).

1. Mease PJ, *et al.* Etanercept in the treatment of psoriatic arthritis and psoriasis: a randomised trial. *Lancet* 2000; **356:** 385–90.

Rheumatoid arthritis. Some references to the use of etanercept in rheumatoid arthritis and juvenile idiopathic arthritis.

1. Weinblatt ME, *et al.* A trial of etanercept, a recombinant tumour necrosis factor receptor: Fc fusion protein, in patients with rheumatoid arthritis receiving methotrexate. *N Engl J Med* 1999; **340:** 253–9.
2. Moreland LW, *et al.* Etanercept therapy in rheumatoid arthritis: a randomized, controlled trial. *Ann Intern Med* 1999; **130:** 478–86.
3. Jarvis B, Faulds O. Etanercept: a review of its use in rheumatoid arthritis. *Drugs* 1999; **57:** 945–66.
4. Garrison L, McDonnell ND. Etanercept: therapeutic use in patients with rheumatoid arthritis. *Ann Rheum Dis* 1999; **58** (suppl 1): 165–169.
5. Lovell DJ, *et al.* Etanercept in children with polyarticular juvenile rheumatoid arthritis. *N Engl J Med* 2000; **342:** 763–9.
6. Bathon JM, *et al.* A comparison of etanercept and methotrexate in patients with early rheumatoid arthritis. *N Engl J Med* 2000; **343:** 1586–93. Correction. *ibid.* 2001; **344:** 76.

Preparations

Proprietary Preparations (details are given in Part 3)
UK: Enbrel; **USA:** Enbrel.

Ethaverine Hydrochloride (5232-n)

Ethaverine Hydrochloride (rINNM).

6,7-Diethoxy-1-(3,4-diethoxybenzyl)isoquinoline hydrochloride.
$C_{24}H_{29}NO_4,HCl = 432.0$.
CAS — 486-47-5 (ethaverine); 985-13-7 (ethaverine hydrochloride).

Profile

Ethaverine is the tetraethoxy analogue of papaverine (p.1648) and has been used as the hydrochloride as an antispasmodic in biliary, gastrointestinal, and genito-urinary disorders. It has also been used in vascular disorders and as an antiarrhythmic.

Ethaverine sulfamate has also been used.

Preparations

Proprietary Preparations (details are given in Part 3)
Multi-ingredient: Aust.: Asthma Efeum; Gastripan†; Hylakombun; **Braz.:** Eufermen; **Ger.:** Migrane-Kranit Kombi; **Switz.:** Elzym; **Thai.:** Elzym.

Ethoxyphenyldiethylphenylbutylamine Hydrochloride (11368-n)

1-(4-Ethoxyphenyl)-N,N-diethyl-3-phenylbutylamine hydrochloride.
$C_{22}H_{31}NO,HCl = 361.9$.
CAS — 10535-87-2 (ethoxyphenyldiethylphenylbutylamine hydrochloride); 13988-32-4 (ethoxyphenyldiethylphenylbutylamine).

Profile

Ethoxyphenyldiethylphenylbutylamine hydrochloride has been used as an antispasmodic.

Ethyl Cinnamate (18370-v)

Ethyl (E)-3-phenylprop-2-enoate.
$C_{11}H_{12}O_2 = 176.2$.
CAS — 103-36-6.
Pharmacopoeias. In *Br.*

Pharmacopoeial description

BP 2001: A clear, colourless or almost colourless liquid with a fruity, balsamic odour. Practically insoluble in water; miscible with most organic solvents.

Profile

Ethyl cinnamate is used as a flavour and perfume; it is an ingredient of Tolu-flavour Solution (BP 2001).

Preparations

BP 2001: Tolu-flavour Solution.

Ethyl Oleate (7359-s)

Aethylis Oleas; Ethylis Oleas.
$C_{20}H_{38}O_2 = 310.5$.
CAS — 111-62-6.
Pharmacopoeias. In *Eur.* (see p.vi). Also in *USNF.*

Ethyl oleate dissolves some types of rubber and causes others to swell.

Pharmacopoeial description

Ph. Eur.: A clear, pale yellow or colourless liquid. It consists of the ethyl esters of fatty acids mainly oleic acid. It may contain a suitable antioxidant. Practically insoluble in water; miscible with alcohol, with dichloromethane, and with petroleum spirit (40° to 60°). Protect from light.

USNF 20: It consists of esters of ethyl alcohol and high-molecular-weight fatty acids, principally oleic acid. A mobile, practically colourless liquid. Insoluble in water; miscible with alcohol, with vegetable oils, with liquid paraffin, and with most organic solvents. Store in airtight containers. Protect from light.

Profile

Ethyl oleate is used as an oily vehicle.

Ethyl Vanillin (2393-k)

3-Ethoxy-4-hydroxybenzaldehyde.
$C_9H_{10}O_3 = 166.2$.
CAS — 121-32-4.
Pharmacopoeias. In *USNF.*

Pharmacopoeial description

USNF 20: Fine, white or slightly yellowish crystals with a vanilla-like odour. M.p. is between 76° and 78°. Soluble 1 in 100 of water at 50° and 1 in 2 of alcohol; freely soluble in chloroform, in ether, and in solutions of alkali hydroxides. Its solutions are acid to litmus. Store in airtight containers. Protect from light.

Profile

Ethyl vanillin is used as a flavour and in perfumery to impart the odour and taste of vanilla.

Ethylene Glycol (1907-t)

Ethylene Alcohol; Glycol. Ethane-1,2-diol.
$C_2H_6O_2 = 62.07$.
CAS — 107-21-1.

Adverse Effects

Toxic effects arising from ingestion of ethylene glycol result from its major metabolites: aldehydes, glycolate, lactate, and oxalate. Clinical features may be divided into three stages depending on the time elapsed since ingestion. In the first 12 hours, the patient may show signs of drunkenness and experience nausea and vomiting. Convulsions and neurological defects may occur. From 12 to 24 hours, there may be tachycardia, mild hypertension, pulmonary oedema, and heart failure. Between 24 and 72 hours, patients with severe ethylene glycol poisoning may experience flank pain and renal involvement with associated decreased plasma concentrations of calcium and bicarbonate, metabolic acidosis, deposition of oxalate in tissues and kidney tubules, proteinuria, oxaluria, haematuria, and renal failure. There may be respiratory failure, cardiovascular collapse, and sometimes coma and death. The fatal dose is reported to be about 100 mL.

Skin irritation and penetration have been reported following topical application.

Diethylene glycol produces similar toxicity, except that there is no conversion to oxalate and there is greater nephrotoxicity. Poisoning has followed adulteration of medicinal products with diethylene glycol.

◊ References.
1. Anonymous. Some wine to break the ice. *Lancet* 1985; **ii**: 254.
2. Vale JA, Buckley BM. Metabolic acidosis in diethylene glycol poisoning. *Lancet* 1985; **ii**: 394.
3. Buckley BM, Vale JA. Poisoning by alcohols and ethylene glycol. *Prescribers' J* 1986; **26**: 110–15.
4. Hanif M, et al. Fatal renal failure caused by diethylene glycol in paracetamol elixir: the Bangladesh epidemic. *BMJ* 1995; **311**: 88–91.
5. Lewis LD, et al. Delayed sequelae after acute overdoses or poisonings: cranial neuropathy related to ethylene glycol ingestion. *Clin Pharmacol Ther* 1997; **61**: 692–9.
6. O'Brien KL, et al. Epidemic of pediatric deaths from acute renal failure caused by diethylene glycol poisoning. *JAMA* 1998; **279**: 1175–80.

Treatment of Adverse Effects
The stomach should be emptied by lavage if ingestion of ethylene glycol was within the preceding hour. Severe metabolic acidosis should be corrected with sodium bicarbonate intravenously and hypocalcaemia corrected with calcium gluconate. Haemodialysis or peritoneal dialysis may be of value. Alcohol may be given by mouth or intravenously as it is a competitor of the metabolism of ethylene glycol. Alternatively fomepizole (p.1009), an alcohol-dehydrogenase inhibitor, may be used for the treatment of ethylene glycol poisoning.

◊ References.
1. Vale JA, et al. Treatment of ethylene glycol poisoning with peritoneal dialysis. *BMJ* 1982; **284**: 557.
2. Porter GA. The treatment of ethylene glycol poisoning simplified. *N Engl J Med* 1988; **319**: 109–10.
3. Harry P, et al. Ethylene glycol poisoning in a child treated with 4-methylpyrazole. *Pediatrics* 1998; **102**: E31.
4. Barceloux DG, et al. American Academy of Clinical Toxicology practice guidelines on the treatment of ethylene glycol poisoning. *Clin Toxicol* 1999; **37**: 537–60.
5. Brent J, et al. Fomepizole for the treatment of ethylene glycol poisoning. *N Engl J Med* 1999; **340**: 832–8.
6. Borron SW, et al. Fomepizole in treatment of uncomplicated ethylene glycol poisoning. *Lancet* 1999; **354**: 831.

Pharmacokinetics
Ethylene glycol is absorbed from the gastrointestinal tract and is metabolised, chiefly in the liver, by alcohol dehydrogenase. Its breakdown products account for its toxicity and include aldehydes, glycolate, lactate, and oxalate.

Uses
Ethylene glycol is commonly encountered in antifreeze solutions and has been used illicitly to sweeten some wines. Diethylene glycol has been used similarly.

Ethylenediamine (208-q)
Edamine (USAN, pINN); Ethylenediaminum.
$C_2H_8N_2 = 60.10$.
CAS — 107-15-3 (anhydrous ethylenediamine); 6780-13-8 (ethylenediamine monohydrate).
Pharmacopoeias. In Eur. (see p.vi), Jpn, and US.

Pharmacopoeial description
Ph. Eur.: A clear, colourless or slightly yellow, hygroscopic liquid. On exposure to air, white fumes are evolved. On heating it evaporates completely. Miscible with water and with alcohol; slightly soluble in ether. Store in airtight containers. Protect from light.
USP 25: A clear, colourless or only slightly yellow liquid having an ammonia-like odour. It is strongly alkaline and may readily absorb carbon dioxide from the air to form a non-volatile carbonate. Miscible with water and with alcohol. Store in well-filled, airtight, glass containers.

Adverse Effects
Ethylenediamine is irritant to the skin and to mucous membranes. Severe exfoliative dermatitis has been reported following systemic use of preparations containing ethylenediamine. Hypersensitivity reactions are common. Concentrated solutions cause skin burns. Headache, dizziness, shortness of breath, nausea, and vomiting have also been reported following exposure to fumes. Ethylenediamine splashed onto the skin or eyes should be removed by flooding with water for a prolonged period.

Hypersensitivity. A review of allergy to ethylenediamine and aminophylline.[1]
1. Anonymous. Allergy to aminophylline. *Lancet* 1984; **ii**: 1192–3.

Precautions
Skin reactions may occur in patients given aminophylline after they have become sensitised to ethylenediamine. Cross-sensitivity with edetic acid and with some antihistamines has been reported.

◊ It was reported that some topical corticosteroid creams, including Tri-Adcortyl in the UK,[1] and Kenacomb, Halcicomb, and Viaderm in Canada,[2] contained ethylenediamine and could cause unexpected cross-sensitivity reactions with piperazine[1] or aminophylline.[2]
1. Wright S, Harman RRM. Ethylenediamine and piperazine sensitivity. *BMJ* 1983; **287**: 463–4.
2. Hogan DJ. Excipients in topical corticosteroid preparations in Canada. *Can Med Assoc J* 1989; **141**: 1032.

Uses and Administration
Ethylenediamine or ethylenediamine hydrate forms a stable mixture with theophylline to produce aminophylline or aminophylline hydrate. Ethylenediamine is widely used in the chemical and pharmaceutical industries and as an ingredient of some topical creams.

Preparations
Proprietary Preparations (details are given in Part 3)
Multi-ingredient: *Braz.:* Narizima Adulto.

Eucalyptol (4629-j)
Eucalyptol (USAN).
Cajuputol; Cineol; Cineole. 1,8-Epoxy-p-menthane; 1,3,3-Trimethyl-2-oxabicyclo[2.2.2]octane.
$C_{10}H_{18}O = 154.2$.
CAS — 470-82-6.
Pharmacopoeias. In Belg., Fr., Swiss, and US.

A colourless liquid with an aromatic camphoraceous odour obtained from eucalyptus oil, cajuput oil, and other oils.

Pharmacopoeial description
USP 25: It is obtained from eucalyptus oil and from other sources. Store in airtight containers.

Profile
Eucalyptol has the actions and uses of eucalyptus oil (below). It has been used in counter-irritant ointments and in dentifrices. It has also been used in nasal preparations, but oily solutions inhibit ciliary movement and may cause lipoid pneumonia. Preparations containing eucalyptol with other volatile substances have been used in the treatment of renal and biliary calculi.

Preparations
Proprietary Preparations (details are given in Part 3)
Ger.: Soledum; Soledum Balsam.
Multi-ingredient: numerous preparations are listed in Part 3.

Eucalyptus Oil (4644-y)
Esencia de Eucalipto; Essence d'Eucalyptus Rectifiée; Eucalypti Aetheroleum; Oleum Eucalypti.
Pharmacopoeias. In Chin., Eur. (see p.vi), which also includes Eucalyptus Leaf from E. globulus, Jpn, and Pol.

Pharmacopoeial description
Ph. Eur.: A colourless or pale yellow liquid with a characteristic aromatic camphoraceous odour and a pungent camphoraceous cooling taste. It is obtained by rectifying the oil distilled from the fresh leaves or terminal branches of various species of *Eucalyptus* (*E. globulus*, *E. fructicetorum*, and *E. smithii* are used). It contains not less than 70% w/w of eucalyptol. Soluble 1 in 5 of alcohol (70%). Store in airtight well-filled containers. Protect from heat.

Adverse Effects and Precautions
The symptoms of poisoning with eucalyptus oil include gastrointestinal symptoms such as epigastric burning, nausea and vomiting, and CNS depression, including coma. Cyanosis, ataxia, miosis, pulmonary damage, delirium, and convulsions may occur. Deaths have been reported.
Oily solutions of eucalyptus oil are unsuitable for use in nasal sprays as the vehicle inhibits ciliary movements and may cause lipoid pneumonia.

◊ References.
1. Patel S, Wiggins J. Eucalyptus oil poisoning. *Arch Dis Child* 1980; **55**: 405.
2. Spoerke DG, et al. Eucalyptus oil: 14 cases of exposure. *Vet Hum Toxicol* 1989; **31**: 166–8.
3. Webb NJA, Pitt WR. Eucalyptus oil poisoning in childhood: 41 cases in south-east Queensland. *J Paediatr Child Health* 1993; **29**: 368–71.
4. Tibballs J. Clinical effects and management of eucalyptus oil ingestion in infants and young children. *Med J Aust* 1995; **163**: 177–80.
5. Anpalahan M, Le Couteur DG. Deliberate self-poisoning with eucalyptus oil in an elderly woman. *Aust N Z J Med* 1998; **28**: 58.
6. Darben T, et al. Topical eucalyptus oil poisoning. *Australas J Dermatol* 1998; **39**: 265–7.

Uses and Administration
Eucalyptus oil has been taken by mouth for catarrh and coughs and is an ingredient of many preparations. It has been used as an inhalation often in combination with other volatile substances. Eucalyptus oil has also been applied as a rubefacient and is used as a flavour.

Preparations
Proprietary Preparations (details are given in Part 3)
Austral.: Bosisto's Eucalyptus Spray; **Ger.:** Bronchodurat Eucalyptusol; Bronchomed†; Eucalyptrol L†; Exeu; Nasivin gegen Erkaltung Kinderbad; Pinimenthol Erkaltungskapseln; Tussidermil N.
Multi-ingredient: numerous preparations are listed in Part 3.

Eugenol (4645-j)
4-Allylguaiacol; Eugen.; Eugenic Acid; Eugenolum. 4-Allyl-2-methoxyphenol.
$C_{10}H_{12}O_2 = 164.2$.
CAS — 97-53-0.
Pharmacopoeias. In Eur. (see p.vi), Pol., and US.

Pharmacopoeial description
Ph. Eur.: A colourless or pale yellow liquid with a strong odour of clove. Practically insoluble in water and in glycerol; freely soluble in alcohol (70%); miscible with alcohol, with glacial acetic acid, with dichloromethane, with ether, and with fatty oils. Eugenol darkens in colour on exposure to air. Store in well-filled containers. Protect from light.
USP 25: It is obtained from clove oil or from other sources. A colourless or pale yellow liquid having a strongly aromatic odour of clove. Upon exposure to air, it darkens and thickens. Slightly soluble in water; miscible with alcohol, with chloroform, with ether, and with fixed oils. Store in airtight containers. Protect from light.

Profile
Eugenol is a constituent of clove oil (p.1597) and some other essential oils. It is employed in dentistry, often mixed with zinc oxide, as a temporary anodyne dental filling, and is an ingredient in oral hygiene preparations. Eugenol has been used as a flavour.
Eugenol is an irritant and sensitiser and can produce local anaesthesia. It is reported to inhibit prostaglandin synthesis.
For the pulmonary effects of eugenol inhalation from clove cigarettes, see Abuse, under Clove, p.1597.

Preparations
Proprietary Preparations (details are given in Part 3)
Ital.: Bastoncino†; **USA:** Red Cross Toothache.
Multi-ingredient: *Aust.:* Ledermix; **Belg.:** Calmant Martou†; Dentophar; **Braz.:** Passaja; UM Instante; **Canad.:** Jiffy Toothache Drops; **Denm.:** Ledermix; **Fr.:** Alodont; Pectoderme; **Hong Kong:** Counterpain; **Irl.:** Ledermix; **Israel:** Dentin; **Ital.:** Odongi; **S.Afr.:** Counterpain; Ledermix; **Singapore:** Begesic; Flanil; **Spain:** Alvogil; Neodesfila; Piorlis; Pomada Revulsiva†; Tangenol; Tifell; **Switz.:** Alodont nouvelle formule; Alvogyl; Benzocaine PD; Dental-Phenjoca†; Endomethasone†; Ledermix; Rocanal Permanent Gangrene†; Rocanal Permanent Vital†; Spirogel†; **Thai.:** Begesic; Counterpain; Flanil; Heat Cream; Masa Balm; Muscalax; Neotica; Olympic Balm; Painza; Reduxpain; Stopain; **UK:** Aezodent; Ledermix.

Euphorbia (2013-l)
Pill-bearing Spurge; Snake Weed.
Pharmacopoeias. Chin. includes monographs for Euphorbia humifusa or E. maculata herb and E. pekinensis root.

Profile
Euphorbia, the aerial parts of *Euphorbia hirta* (*E. pilulifera*) (Euphorbiaceae), has sedative and expectorant properties and is used in the treatment of asthma and other respiratory-tract disorders. It has also been used for intestinal amoebiasis.
Other *Euphorbia* spp. are used for a variety of disorders. The seeds and latex of *E. lathyrus* (caper spurge) have been used as a purgative but are too toxic for general use. Many species have been used as arrow poisons.

Preparations
Proprietary Preparations (details are given in Part 3)
Multi-ingredient: *Austral.:* Asa Tones; Euphorbia Complex; Procold; Sambucus Complex; **Belg.:** Gloceda; **Canad.:** Sirop Cocillana Codeine; **Fr.:** Tisanes de l'Abbe Hamon no 14†; **Hong Kong:** Cocillana Compound; **UK:** Antibron.

Euphrasia (12724-y)
Eyebright.

Profile
Euphrasia, the aerial parts of various *Euphrasia* spp. including *E. rostkoviana* and *E. officinalis* (Scrophulariaceae), has been used topically for blepharitis, conjunctivitis, and other eye disorders. However, such use is not generally recommended. Euphrasia has also been used for nasal catarrh and sinusitis.
It is also used in homoeopathic medicine.

Preparations
Proprietary Preparations (details are given in Part 3)
Multi-ingredient: *Austral.:* Bilberry Plus; Eye Health Herbal Plus Formula 4; Lifesystem Herbal Plus Formula 5 Eye Relief; Sambucus Complex; **Switz.:** Collypan; Oculosan†; **UK:** Še-Power; Vital Eyes.

The symbol † denotes a preparation no longer actively marketed

Febuprol (16800-a)

Febuprol (rINN).

1-Butoxy-3-phenoxy-2-propanol.

$C_{13}H_{20}O_3 = 224.3$.

CAS — 3102-00-9.

Profile

Febuprol is a choleretic used in the treatment of biliary-tract disorders in a dose of 100 mg three times daily by mouth.

Preparations

Proprietary Preparations (details are given in Part 3)
Ger.: Valbil; *Port.*: Valbil.

Fenalamide (12731-l)

Fenalamide (USAN, pINN).

Ethyl N-(2-diethylaminoethyl)-2-ethyl-2-phenylmalonamate.

$C_{19}H_{30}N_2O_3 = 334.5$.

CAS — 4551-59-1.

Profile

Fenalamide has been used as an antispasmodic.

Fencibutirol (12735-c)

Fencibutirol (USAN, rINN).

Mg-4833. 2-(1-Hydroxy-4-phenylcyclohexyl)butyric acid.

$C_{16}H_{22}O_3 = 262.3$.

CAS — 5977-10-6.

Profile

Fencibutirol is a choleretic that has been used in the treatment of constipation and hepatic disorders.

Preparations

Proprietary Preparations (details are given in Part 3)
Multi-ingredient: *Ital.*: Hepasil Composto; Magisbile; Neo-Heparbil†; Sintobil†; Verecolene Complesso†.

Fenclonine (12736-k)

Fenclonine (USAN, rINN).

CP-10188; NSC-77370; Parachlorophenylalanine. 2-Amino-3-(4-chlorophenyl)propionic acid; DL-3-(p-Chlorophenyl)alanine.

$C_9H_{10}ClNO_2 = 199.6$.

CAS — 7424-00-2.

Profile

Fenclonine is an inhibitor of the biosynthesis of serotonin. It has been given to patients with carcinoid syndrome and some relief of symptoms, especially of flushing and diarrhoea, has been reported. Hypothermia, bone marrow depression, and psychiatric side-effects such as confusion and depression have occurred during treatment.

Fenipentol (3722-m)

Fenipentol (rINN).

1-Phenylpentan-1-ol; α-Butylbenzyl alcohol.

$C_{11}H_{16}O = 164.2$.

CAS — 583-03-9.

Profile

Fenipentol is a choleretic used in the treatment of hepatic and biliary-tract disorders. The hemisuccinate and sodium hemisuccinate are also used.

Preparations

Proprietary Preparations (details are given in Part 3)
Ger.: Febichol; *Ital.*: Pentabil.

Multi-ingredient: *Ital.*: Critichol; *Port.*: Cholipin; *Spain:* Menabil Complex.

Fennel (4646-z)

Fenchel; Fennel Fruit; Fennel Seed; Fenouil; Fenouil Amer; Foeniculum; Fruto de Hinojo; Funcho.

Pharmacopoeias. In *Chin.*, *Eur.* (see p.vi), *Jpn*, and *Pol.*

Pharmacopoeial description

Ph. Eur.: Bitter Fennel (Foeniculi Amari Fructus) consists of the dry, cremocarps and mericarps of *Foeniculum vulgare*, subsp. *vulgare*, var. *vulgare*. It contains not less than 4.0% v/w of essential oil, calculated with reference to the anhydrous drug. The oil contains not less than 60.0% of anethole and not less than 15.0% of fenchone. Bitter fennel is greenish-brown, brown, or green. Store protected from light and moisture.

Sweet Fennel (Foeniculi Dulcis Fructus) consists of the dry, cremocarps and mericarps of *Foeniculum vulgare*, subsp. *vulgare*, var. *dulce*. It contains not less than 2.0% v/w of essential oil, calculated with reference to the anhydrous drug. The oil contains not less than 80.0% of anethole. Sweet fennel is pale green or pale yellowish-brown. Store protected from light and moisture.

Profile

Fennel is the source of fennel oil (below). It is used as a flavour and carminative, although the efficacy of such traditional remedies in infant colic is considered dubious (see Gastrointestinal Spasm, p.1204). It is also used in herbal remedies for respiratory-tract disorders.

Preparations

Proprietary Preparations (details are given in Part 3)
Ger.: roha-Fenchel-Tee.

Multi-ingredient: *Aust.*: Aktiv Leber- und Gallentee; Aktiv milder Magen- und Darmtee; Anifer Fenchelhonig; Aponatura Wind; Apotheker Bauer's Blahungstee; Apotheker Bauer's Brust-und Hustentee; Apotheker Bauer's Kindertee; Bio-Garten Tee gegen Blahungen; Bio-Garten Tee gegen Verstopfung; Brady's-Magentropfen; Carminativum Babynos; Caved-S†; Euka; Granobil; Illings Bozner Maycur-Tee; Karvisin; Kneipp Husten- und Bronchial-Tee; Kneipp Verdauungs-Tee; Krauterdoktor Hustentropfen; Krauterhaus Mag Kottas Babytee; Krauterhaus Mag Kottas milder Abfuhrtee; Krauterhaus Mag Kottas Tee gegen Blahungen; Krautertee Nr 10; Krautertee Nr 11; Krautertee Nr 126; Krautertee Nr 14; Krautertee Nr 217; Krautertee Nr 8; Krautertee Nr 9; Laxalpin; Mag Kottas Baby-Tee; Mag Kottas Blahungs-Verdauungstee; Mag Kottas Magen-Darmtee; Mag Kottas Tee fur stillende Mutter; May-Cur-Tee; Nesthakchen; Pascopankreat; Planta Lax; Sidroga Kindertee; Sinolax-Milder; Species Carvi comp; St Radegunder Abfuhrtee mild; St Radegunder Blahungstreibender Tee; St Radegunder Bronchialtee; St Radegunder Magenberuhigungstee; St Radegunder Reizmildernder Magentee; St Radegunder Tee gegen Durchfall; Teekanne Herz- und Kreislauftee; Teekanne Husten-und Brusttee; Teekanne Leber- und Galletee; Windtreibender Tee; *Austral.*: Digestive Aid; *Belg.*: Eugiron; Tisane Antibiliaire et Stomachique; Tisane Depurative "les 12 Plantes"; Tisane Diuretique; Tisane Purgative; *Braz.*: Funchicorea; Puersan; Zweca. Thunas Laxative; *Fr.*: Bolcitol; Colominthe†; Mediflor Tisane Contre la Constipation Passagere No 7†; Mediflor Tisane Digestive No 3†; Mediflor Tisane No 4 Diuretique; Santane D₅; Tisane H₇; Tisane des Familles; Tisane Digestive Weleda†; *Ger.*: Brust-und Husten-Tee Stada N†; Carminativum Babynos; Carminativum-Hetterich N; Cefabronchin; Cefagastrin; Divinal Gastro†; Echtroferment-N†; Em-eukal; Em-eukal Husten- und Brusttee; Floradix Maskam†; Floradix Multipretten; Gallexier; Gastricholan-L; Gastrol S; Grunlicht Hingfong Essenz; Harntee 400; Hevert-Magen-Galle-Leber-Tee†; Kneipp Flatuol; Kneipp Husten- und Bronchial-Tee; Kneipp Magen-Tee; Kneipp Verdauungs-Tee N; Leber-Galle-Tropfen 83; Lomatol; Magentee; Majocarmin-Tee; Pascopankreat novo; Presselin Blahungs K 4 N; Presselin Dyspeptikum; Presselin Stoffwechsel-Tee Hapeka 225 N; Ramend Krauter; Salus Abfuhr-Tee Nr. 2†; Salus Bronchial-Tee Nr.8†; Salus Leber-Galle-Tee Nr.18†; Salus Nerven-Schlaf-Tee Nr.22†; Salus Rheuma-Tee Krautertee Nr. 12†; Stovalid N; Ullus Magen-Tee N; Urodil Blasen-Nieren Arzneitee†; *Hong Kong:* GI; *Israel:* Jungborn; *Ital.*: Dicalmir; Normalax†; Senna-Specie Composta; Tisana Cisbey†; Tonactiv†; *Mex.:* Crislaxo; Jarabe Manzanas Siken; *Swed.:* Cavedess†; *Switz.:* Adistop Lax†; Ajaka†; Caved-S†; Kernosan Elixir; Kernosan Heidelberger Poudre; The Brioni; The Franklin†; Tisane antiflatulente pour les enfants; Tisane favorisant l'allaitement; Tisane laxative; Tisane laxative H nouvelle formulation; Tisane laxative Natterman no 13†; Tisane pectorale et antitussive; Tisane pour les enfants†; *UK:* Carminative Tea; Cleansing Herb Tablets; Gerard House Gladlax; Herbal Indigestion Naturtabs; Indigestion and Flatulence; Lion Cleansing Herbs; Lustys Herbalene; Out-of-Sorts; Revitonil; Sure-Lax (Herbal).

Fennel Oil (4647-c)

Aetheroleum Foeniculi; Esencia de Hinojo; Essência de Funcho; Oleum Foeniculi.

Pharmacopoeias. In *Aust.*, *Ger.*, *Jpn*, *Neth.*, and *Swiss.*

A colourless or pale yellow volatile oil with the characteristic aromatic odour and taste of fennel, obtained by distillation from dried ripe fennel fruit. It contains anethole. **Soluble** 1 in 1 of alcohol (90%). If solid matter separates it should be melted and mixed before use. **Store** in airtight containers. Protect from light.

Profile

Fennel oil is used as an aromatic flavour and carminative (but see the comment under Fennel, above). It is also used in herbal remedies for respiratory-tract disorders.

Preparations

Proprietary Preparations (details are given in Part 3)
Aust.: Stern Biene Fenchelhonig; *Ger.:* Fenchelsaft N; Stern Biene Fenchelhonig; Stern Biene Fenchelsirup.

Multi-ingredient: *Aust.:* Eucarbon; Luuf-Hustentee; Nesthakchen; Solubitrat; Spasmo Claim; Thierry; *Belg.:* Eucarbon; *Canad.:* Babys Own Gripe Water; Chase Kolik Gripe Water Alcohol-Free; *Ger.:* Benium†; Bronchicum Hustentee†; Cystium†; Em-eukal Husten- und Brusttee; Ephepect; Euflat I; Floradix Multipretten; Gastricard N; Grunlicht Hingfong Essenz; Grunlicht Magenbalsam Tropfen; Heumann Blasen- und Nierentee Solubitrat N; Hevert-Carmin symbio; Hevertopect; Hingfong-Essenz Hofmanns Tropfen; Infantutus N†; Neo-Lapitrypsin†; Nierentee 2000; Pulmocordio mite SL; ratioGast; Roflatol Phyto (Rowo-146)†; Salviathymol N; *Hong Kong:* Magesto; *Israel:* Novicarbon; *Switz.:* Ajaka†; Eucarbon†; Flatulex; Huile Po-Ho A. Vogel; Lapidar 10 plus†; Laxasan; Pastilles pectorales formule 541; *Thai.:* Magesto; *UK:* Indigestion and Flatulence Tablets.

Fenoverine (12019-e)

Fenoverine (rINN).

10-[(4-Piperonyl-1-piperazinyl)acetyl]phenothiazine.

$C_{26}H_{25}N_3O_3S = 459.6$.

CAS — 37561-27-6.

ATC — A03AX05.

Profile

Fenoverine has been used as an antispasmodic but has been withdrawn in some countries following reports of rhabdomyolysis.

Adverse effects. Reports of rhabdomyolysis associated with fenoverine administration,[1,2] including a fatality.[1] A genetic predisposition has been suggested.[2]

1. Chariot P, et al. Fenoverine-induced rhabdomyolysis. *Hum Exp Toxicol* 1995; **14:** 654–6.
2. Jouglard J, et al. Research into individual predisposition to develop acute rhabdomyolysis attributed to fenoverine. *Hum Exp Toxicol* 1996; **15:** 815–20.

Preparations

Proprietary Preparations (details are given in Part 3)
Ital.: Spasmopriv†; *Mex.:* Spasmopriv; *Singapore:* Spasmopriv; *Thai.:* Spasmopriv.

Fenpipramide Hydrochloride (16444-j)

Fenpipramide Hydrochloride (BANM, rINNM).

2,2-Diphenyl-4-piperidinobutyramide hydrochloride.

$C_{21}H_{26}N_2O,HCl = 358.9$.

CAS — 77-01-0 (fenpipramide); 14007-53-5 (fenpipramide hydrochloride).

Profile

Fenpipramide hydrochloride has been used as an antispasmodic.

Fenpiverinium Bromide (13439-c)

Fenpiverinium Bromide (rINN).

Fenpipramide Methobromide; Fenpipramide Methylbromide. 1-(3-Carbamoyl-3,3-diphenylpropyl)-1-methylpiperidinium bromide; 2,2-Diphenyl-4-piperidinobutyramide methyl bromide.

$C_{22}H_{29}BrN_2O = 417.4$.

CAS — 125-60-0.

Profile

Fenpiverinium bromide has been used as an antispasmodic.

Preparations

Proprietary Preparations (details are given in Part 3)
Multi-ingredient: *S.Afr.:* Baralgan†.

Fenugreek (12748-r)

Bockshornsame; Faenum-Graecum; Semen Foenugraeci; Semen Trigonellae.

Pharmacopoeias. In *Chin.* and *Eur.* (see p.vi).

Pharmacopoeial description

Ph. Eur.: The dried ripe seeds of *Trigonella foenum-graecum*. It has a strong characteristic odour. Protect from light.

Profile

Fenugreek has been used as an appetite stimulant and as an ingredient in preparations for respiratory disorders.

◊ Loss of consciousness occurred in a 5-week-old infant following ingestion of a herbal tea containing fenugreek.[1] On recovery the infant (and a sample of his urine) exuded an aroma characteristic of that found in 'maple syrup urine disease', an inborn condition involving defective metabolism of branched-chain amino acids. Further investigation revealed that the infant did not have the disease; the aroma was due to the presence of sotolone in the fenugreek seeds used to prepare the tea.

1. Sewell AC, et al. False diagnosis of maple syrup urine disease owing to ingestion of herbal tea. *N Engl J Med* 1999; **341:** 769.

Preparations

Proprietary Preparations (details are given in Part 3)
Fr.: Fenugrene.

Multi-ingredient: *Austral.:* Bilberry Plus; Garlic and Horseradish + C Complex; Panax Complex; Sinus and Hayfever; *UK:* Fenulin.

Ferric Chloride (5036-x)

Ferr. Perchlor.; Ferri Chloridum Hexahydricum; Ferrum Sesquichloratum; Iron Chloride; Iron Perchloride; Iron Sesquichloride; Iron Trichloride.

$FeCl_3,6H_2O = 270.3$.

CAS — 7705-08-0 (anhydrous ferric chloride); 10025-77-1 (ferric chloride hexahydrate).

Pharmacopoeias. In *Eur.* (see p.vi).

Pharmacopoeial description

Ph. Eur.: A very hygroscopic, crystalline mass or orange-yellow to brownish-yellow crystals. Very soluble in water and in alcohol; freely soluble in glycerol. Store in airtight containers. Protect from light.

Profile

Ferric chloride has the general properties of iron salts (p.1366) but is exceptionally astringent. It has been used mainly by local application for its styptic and astringent properties. Local application of ferric chloride or other iron salts may cause permanent discoloration of the skin.

Preparations

Proprietary Preparations (details are given in Part 3)
Ital.: Cotone Emostatico.

Multi-ingredient: *Belg.:* Ouate Hemostatique.

Fibronectin (16809-b)

Cold-insoluble Globulin.

Profile

Fibronectin is an endogenous polypeptide with a molecular weight of 440 000 to 550 000 whose roles include attachment of cells to the extracellular matrix and stimulation of phagocytosis. It is used in combination with other blood products in wound-sealant preparations. Infusion of fibronectin or fibronectin-rich plasma has been tried in patients with sepsis, infection, burns or other trauma, or severe malnutrition. Eye drops of fibronectin have been used in the treatment of corneal erosions.

◊ References.
1. Anonymous. Fibronectins and vitronectin. *Lancet* 1989; **i:** 474–6.
2. Gipson IK, *et al.* Corneal wound healing and fibronectin. *Int Ophthalmol Clin* 1993; **33:** 149–63.

Preparations

Ph. Eur.: Fibrin Sealant Kit.

Proprietary Preparations (details are given in Part 3)
Multi-ingredient: *Aust.:* Tissucol; Tissucol Duo Quick; *Canad.:* Tisseel; *Denm.:* Tisseel Duo Quick; *Fin.:* Tisseel Duo Quick; *Fr.:* Biocol; *Ger.:* Tissucol Duo S; Tissucol Fibrinkleber tiefgefroren†; Tissucol-Kit; *Hong Kong:* Tisseel; *Israel:* Tisseel; *Spain:* Tissucol; *Swed.:* Tisseel Duo Quick; *Switz.:* Tissucol; Tissucol Duo S; *UK:* Tisseel.

Flavodate Sodium (12752-k)

Flavodate Disodium. Disodium (4-oxo-2-phenyl-4*H*-chromene-5,7-diyldioxy)diacetate.
$C_{19}H_{12}Na_2O_8 = 414.3$.
CAS — 37470-13-6 (flavodic acid); 13358-62-8 (flavodate disodium).

NOTE. Flavodic Acid is rINN.

Profile

Flavodate is stated to increase the resistance of capillaries and to reduce their permeability. It has been given as the sodium salt in the treatment of vascular disorders in usual doses of 200 to 600 mg daily by mouth. It has also been administered by intravenous or intramuscular injection.

Preparations

Proprietary Preparations (details are given in Part 3)
Fr.: Intercyton; Squad†; *Ital.:* Pericel; *Spain:* Intercyton.

Flavonoid Compounds (7910-c)

Bioflavonoids; Vitamin P Substances.

Benzquercin (12493-j)

Benzquercin *(rINN).*

3,3′,4′,5,7-Pentakis(benzyloxy)flavone.
$C_{50}H_{40}O_7 = 752.8$.
CAS — 13157-90-9.

Diosmin (12667-x)

Diosmin *(BAN, rINN).*

Barosmin; Buchu Resin; Diosmetin 7-Rutinoside; Diosminum. 3′,5,7-Trihydroxy-4′-methoxyflavone 7-[6-*O*-(6-deoxy-α-L-mannopyranosyl)-β-D-glucopyranoside].
$C_{28}H_{32}O_{15} = 608.5$.
CAS — 520-27-4.
ATC — C05CA03.
Pharmacopoeias. In Eur. (see p.vi).

Pharmacopoeial description

Ph. Eur.: A greyish-yellow or light yellow hygroscopic powder. Practically insoluble in water and in alcohol; soluble in dimethyl sulfoxide. It dissolves in dilute solutions of alkali hydroxides. Store in airtight containers.

The symbol † denotes a preparation no longer actively marketed

Ethoxazorutoside (11367-d)

Ethoxazorutoside *(rINN).*

Aethoxazorutin; Aethoxazorutoside; Aethoxazorutin.
$C_{33}H_{41}NO_{17} = 723.7$.
CAS — 30851-76-4.

Hesperidin (12821-j)

5-Hydroxy-2-(3-hydroxy-4-methoxyphenyl)-4-oxo-4*H*-chromen-7-yl rutinoside.
$C_{28}H_{34}O_{15} = 610.6$.
CAS — 520-26-3 (hesperidin); 24292-52-2 (hesperidin methyl chalcone).

A flavonoid isolated from the rind of certain citrus fruits.

Leucocianidol (12894-p)

Leucocianidol *(rINN).*

Leucocyanidin; Leucocyanidol. 2-(3,4-Dihydroxyphenyl)chroman-3,4,5,7-tetrol.
$C_{15}H_{14}O_7 = 306.3$.
CAS — 480-17-1.

Monoxerutin (11467-b)

Monoxerutin *(rINN).*

Monohydroxyethylrutosides. 7-(β-Hydroxyethyl)rutoside.
$C_{29}H_{34}O_{17} = 654.6$.
CAS — 23869-24-1.
ATC — C05CA02.

Oxerutins (12020-b)

Oxerutins *(BAN).*

Hydroxyethylrutosides.

A mixture of 5 different *O*-(β-hydroxyethyl)rutosides, not less than 45% of which is troxerutin (trihydroxyethylrutoside, below), but which also includes monohydroxyethylrutoside, dihydroxyethylrutoside, and tetrahydroxyethylrutoside.

Quercetin (488-p)

3,3′,4′,5,7-Pentahydroxyflavone. 2-(3,4-Dihydroxyphenyl)-3,5,7-trihydroxy-4*H*-1-benzopyran-4-one.
$C_{15}H_{10}O_7 = 302.2$.
CAS — 117-39-5.

Rutoside (15304-k)

Rutoside *(BAN, rINN).*

Rutin. 2-(3,4-Dihydroxyphenyl)-3,5,7-trihydroxy-4-oxo-4*H*-chromen-3-yl rutinoside trihydrate; 2-(3,4-Dihydroxyphenyl)-5,7-dihydroxy-4-oxo-4*H*-chromen-3-yl 6-*O*-(α-L-rhamnosyl)-β-D-glucoside.
$C_{27}H_{30}O_{16},3H_2O = 664.6$.
CAS — 153-18-4 (anhydrous).
ATC — C05CA01.
Pharmacopoeias. In Aust., Fr., Ger., Pol., and Swiss.

A flavonoid obtained from buckwheat, *Fagopyrum esculentum* (Polygonaceae), or from other sources which include the flower buds of the Japanese pagoda-tree, *Sophora japonica*, and the leaves of several species of *Eucalyptus*.

Troxerutin (13386-t)

Troxerutin *(BAN, rINN).*

THR; Trihydroxyethylrutoside; Trioxyethylrutin. 3′,4′,7-Tris[*O*-(2-hydroxyethyl)]rutin; 5-Hydroxy-7-(2-hydroxyethoxy)-2-[3,4-bis(2-hydroxyethoxy)phenyl]-4-oxo-4*H*-chromen-3-yl rutinoside.
$C_{33}H_{42}O_{19} = 742.7$.
CAS — 7085-55-4.
ATC — C05CA04.
Pharmacopoeias. In Ger.

The principal component of oxerutins, above.

Profile

Flavonoids are naturally occurring antioxidants that are widely distributed in plants. Preparations containing natural or semisynthetic flavonoids are thought to improve capillary function by reducing abnormal leakage. They have been given to relieve capillary impairment and venous insufficiency of the lower limbs, and for haemorrhoids.

It has been suggested that flavonoids present in some foods, such as fruit, vegetables, tea, and red wine may protect against the development of atherosclerosis (p.793).

◊ References.
1. Anonymous. Paroven: not much effect in trials. *Drug Ther Bull* 1992; **30:** 7–8.
2. Wadworth AN, Faulds D. Hydroxyethylrutosides: a review of its pharmacology, and therapeutic efficacy in venous insufficiency and related disorders. *Drugs* 1992; **44:** 1013–32.
3. Knekt P, *et al.* Flavonoid intake and coronary mortality in Finland: a cohort study. *BMJ* 1996; **312:** 478–81.
4. Hertog MGL, *et al.* Antioxidant flavonols and coronary heart disease risk. *Lancet* 1997; **349:** 699.

Preparations

Proprietary Preparations (details are given in Part 3)
Aust.: Venoruton; *Austral.:* Paroven; Varemoid†; *Belg.:* Veinamitol; Ven-Detrex; Venoruton; *Braz.:* Daflon; Venoruton; *Denm.:* Venoruton; *Fr.:* Daflon; Diamoril; Dio; Diosmil; Diovenor; Endium; Flavan; Flebosmil; Litosmil†; Mediveine; Preparation H Veinotonic; Relvene; Rheoflux; Veinamitol; Veineva; Venirene; *Ger.:* Drisi-Ven; Pherarutin†; Venoruton†; Venoton; Tovene; Trirutin N†; Troxeven; Vastribil; Veno SL; Venoruton; *Hong Kong:* Venoruton; *Irl.:* Paroven; *Israel:* Novorutin; Venoruton; Vridol; *Ital.:* Alven; Arvenum; Diosven; Doven; Flebil; Venolen; Venoruton; Venosmine; *Mex.:* Sies; Teboven; *Neth.:* Venoruton; *NZ:* Paroven; *Port.:* Fleboton†; Hepacalmina; Venex; Veno-V; Venoruton; Venosmil; Veroven; *S.Afr.:* Paroven; Varemoid†; *Spain:* Daflon; Diosminil; Insuven; Pentovena; Venolep; Venoruton; Venosmil; Viodenum†; *Switz.:* Daflon†; Hemerven; Neorutin; Pur-Rutin; Varemoid†; Veniten†; Venoruton; *Thai.:* Flavon; Heteroid; Varemoid; Venoruton; *UK:* Paroven; *USA:* Citro-Flav.

Multi-ingredient: *Aust.:* Aesrutan; Calcipot C; Daflon; Helopyrin; Influvidon; Phlogenzym; Ruticalzon; Rutiscorbin; Rutiviscal; Sandoven; Sklerovitol; Sterofundin R; Tetesept; Trimedil; Veno; Venotop; Vit-C-Lutsch; Wobenzym; *Austral.:* B-Complex Threshold; Beta A-C; Bio C; Bio-C Complex; Bioglan Cirflo; Bioglan Fingers & Toes†; Bioglan Mega C; Bioglan Super Cal C; Bioglan The Blue One; Bioglan Zellulean with Escin; Bioglan Zn-A-C; Biosor-C; C Supa + Bioflavonoids; Child Chew C; Cirflo†; Cold & Flu Tablets Non Drowsy; Crataegus Complex; Devils Claw Plus; Ethical Nutrients Bioflavonoids Plus; Extralife Leg-Care; Eye Health Herbal Plus Formula 4; Flavonoid C†; Flavonoid Complex†; Flavons; For Peripheral Circulation Herbal Plus Formula 5; Gentle C with Bioflavonoids; Ginkgo ACE†; Hamamelis Complex; Harpagophytum Complex; Lifesystem Herbal Formula 6 For Peripheral Circulation; Lifesystem Herbal Plus Formula 5 Eye Relief; Macro C; Natures Way Total C; Proflo; Rubus Complex; Super Cal-C Bio; Sustained Release Buffered C; Vita-Minis Vitamin C Plus; Z-Acne; *Belg.:* Daflon; Ex'ail†; *Braz.:* Castanha de India Composta; Dactil-OB; Frenovex; Gingilone; Gripen; Hemoaenus; Hemorroidex; Hemorrol; Mirorroidin; Novaboin; Novarrutina; Panvitrop; Trimedal; Varizol; Venalot; Venocur Triplex; *Canad.:* Duo-CVP; *Denm.:* Capiven; *Fr.:* Cemaflavone; Cepevit; Circularine; Cirkan; Cyclo 3 Fort; Ercevit†; Esberiven Forte; Ex'ail; Gel a l'Acetotartrate d'Alumine Defresne; Ginkor; Ginkor Fort; Ophtadil; Rheobral; Solurutine Papaverine F. Retard†; Trisolvit†; Vascocitrol; Veliten; Venyl; Video†; Vincarutine; Vita 3; Vitarutine; Vivene; *Ger.:* Aescorin N; Antihypertonicum S; Antimyopikum; Antisklerosin S; Calcium-Rutinion; Cycloven Forte N; Echtrovit-K†; Emocrat forte; Enzym-Wied; Essaven N; Essaven ultra; Eukalisan forte; Eukalisan N; Euvitan; Fagorutin Buchweizen; Fagorutin Roßkastanien-Balsam F; Intradermi N; Lindigoa S; Movicard; Perivar; Phlebodril; Phlogenzym; Posti N; Ruticalzon VC; Sklerovenol N; Tornix; Vaso-E-Bion; Venalot; Venalot N; Venelbin†; Veno-Hexanicit†; Veno-Tebonin N; Vitosal; Wobenzym N; *Hong Kong:* Daflon; Essaven; Ginkor Fort; Haemosol; *Ital.:* Angioton; Blunorm†; Bo-Gum†; CVP†; Daflon 500; Dermoangiopan; Digifar; Flavone 500†; Fleboside; Ginkoftal; Rutisan CE; Traumal; Venactive; *Mex.:* Daflon; Phlogenzym; Variton; Venalot; Venoruton; *Port.:* Actilamt; Cegripe; Cyclo 3; Daflon; Projuvex; Rutinice Fortissimo; *S.Afr.:* Essaven; *Singapore:* Cyclo 3 Fort; Daflon 500; *Spain:* Caprofides Hemostatico; Circovenil Fuerte†; Citroflavona; Citroflavona Magt; Daflon 500; Epistaxol; Esberiven; Fabroven; Flebeside; Gingilone; Nasopomada; Quercetol Hemostatico; Quercetol K†; Rutice Fuerte; Venosan; Vitaendil C K P†; *Switz.:* Daflon 500; Demoven N; Flavovenyl; No Grip†; Optazine†; Phlebodril N; Phlebodril†; Venosan†; Video-Net; Vita 3†; *Thai.:* Biocalron; Cyclo 3 Fort; Daflon; Essaven; Ginkor Fort; Heroid; Siduol; *UK:* Flavorola C; *USA:* Ak-Biocholine†; Amino-Opti-C; Bio-Acerola C Complex†; C Factors "1000" Plus; C Speridin†; Cholinoid; Citrus-flav C; Ester-C Plus; Ester-C Plus Multi-Mineral; Flavons; Lipoflavonoid; Pan C; Peridin-C; Proflavanol; Pycnogenol Plus; Span C; Super Citro Cee†; Super Complex C†.

Flopropione (5234-m)

Flopropione *(rINN).*

Fluropropiofenone; Phloropropiophenone; RP-13907. 2′,4′,6′-Trihydroxypropiophenone.
$C_9H_{10}O_4 = 182.2$.
CAS — 2295-58-1.
Pharmacopoeias. In Jpn.

Profile

Flopropione has been used as an antispasmodic.

Preparations

Proprietary Preparations (details are given in Part 3)
Hong Kong: Cospanon; *Jpn:* Cospanon†.

Multi-ingredient: *Spain:* Espasmo Digestomen.

Flumecinol (19184-e)

Flumecinol *(rINN).*

RGH-3332. α-Ethyl-3-(trifluoromethyl)benzhydrol.
$C_{16}H_{15}F_3O = 280.3$.
CAS — 56430-99-0.

Profile

Flumecinol has been investigated for treatment of neonatal hyperbilirubinaemia and has been tried for cholestatic pruritus.

◊ References.
1. Turner IB, *et al.* Flumecinol for the treatment of pruritus associated with primary biliary cirrhosis. *Aliment Pharmacol Ther* 1994; **8:** 337–42.

Fluorescein   (2129-n)

Fluorescein (BAN).

3′,6′-Dihydroxyspiro[isobenzofuran-1(3H),9′(9H)xanthen]-3-one.

$C_{20}H_{12}O_5 = 332.3$.
CAS — 2321-07-5.
ATC — S01JA01.
Pharmacopoeias. In US.

Pharmacopoeial description

USP 25: A yellowish-red to red, odourless powder. Insoluble in water; soluble in dilute alkali hydroxides. Store in airtight containers.

Fluorescein Dilaurate   (1956-v)

Fluorescein Dilaurate (BANM).
$C_{44}H_{56}O_7 = 696.9$.
CAS — 7308-90-9.

Fluorescein Sodium   (2130-k)

Fluorescein Sodium (BANM).
CI Acid Yellow 73; Colour Index No. 45350; D & C Yellow No. 8; Fluorescein Natrium; Fluoresceinum Natricum; Obiturin; Resorcinolphthalein Sodium; Sodium Fluorescein; Soluble Fluorescein; Uranin. Disodium fluorescein.
$C_{20}H_{10}Na_2O_5 = 376.3$.
CAS — 518-47-8.

NOTE. FLN is a code approved by the BP 2001 for use on single unit doses of eye drops containing fluorescein sodium where the individual container may be too small to bear all the appropriate labelling information. LIDFLN is a similar code approved for eye drops containing lignocaine [lidocaine] hydrochloride and fluorescein sodium and PROXFLN a code for eye drops containing proxymetacaine hydrochloride and fluorescein sodium.

Pharmacopoeias. In Chin., Eur. (see p.vi), Int., Jpn, and US.

Pharmacopoeial description

Ph. Eur.: An orange-red, fine hygroscopic powder. Freely soluble in water; soluble in alcohol; practically insoluble in dichloromethane and in hexane. A 2% solution in water has a pH of 7.0 to 9.0. Store in airtight containers. Protect from light.

USP 25: An orange-red, hygroscopic, odourless powder. Freely soluble in water; sparingly soluble in alcohol. Store in airtight containers.

Adverse Effects and Precautions

The intravenous injection of fluorescein sodium may produce nausea and vomiting. Extravasation is painful. Hypersensitivity reactions range from urticaria to occasional instances of severe anaphylaxis. Cardiac arrests and fatalities have occurred rarely. Concern that impurities or a defect in manufacturing processes might be responsible for the serious reactions led to a review of the BP specification in the early 1980s and a reduction in the permitted level of impurities.

The skin and urine may be coloured yellow but this is transient. Fluorescein sodium can stain skin, clothing, and soft contact lenses on contact.

Facilities for resuscitation should be available whenever fluorescein sodium is administered intravenously.

Oral fluorescein dilaurate should not be given to patients with acute necrotising pancreatitis. Sulfasalazine may interfere with estimations of fluorescein in the fluorescein dilaurate test.

◊ Two large studies have examined the incidence of adverse reactions following intravenous fluorescein angiography. An international survey[1] collected information concerning 594 687 angiographic procedures; the incidence of serious reactions was 1 in 18 020, and that of fatal reactions, 1 in 49 557. Reactions included anaphylactic shock, cardiac arrest, myocardial infarction, and shock with hypotension or respiratory distress. A USA survey of 221 781 fluorescein angiograms[2] reported frequency rates of 1 in 63 for a moderate reaction (urticaria, syncope, thrombophlebitis, pyrexia, tissue necrosis, or nerve palsy) and 1 in 1900 for severe reactions (respiratory or cardiac events or tonic-clonic seizures); there was one death.

Individual reports of adverse reactions to intravenous fluorescein sodium include pancreatitis,[3] painful crises in patients with sickle-cell disease,[4] psoriasiform drug eruption,[5] and photoallergy[6] and phototoxicity.[7]

1. Zografos L. Enquête internationale sur l'incidence des accidents graves ou fatals pouvant survenir lors d'une angiographie fluoresceinique. J Fr Ophtalmol 1983; 6: 495–506.
2. Yannuzzi LA, et al. Fluorescein angiography complication survey. Ophthalmology 1986; 93: 611–17.
3. Morgan LH, Martin JM. Acute pancreatitis after fluorescein. BMJ 1983; 287: 1596.
4. Acheson R, Serjeant G. Painful crises in sickle cell disease after fluorescein angiography. Lancet 1985; i: 1222.
5. Mayama M, et al. Psoriasiform drug eruption induced by fluorescein sodium used for fluorescein angiography. Br J Dermatol 1999; 140: 982–4.
6. Hochsattel R, et al. Photoallergic reaction to fluorescein. Contact Dermatitis 1990; 22: 42–4.
7. Kearns GL, et al. Fluorescein phototoxicity in a premature infant. J Pediatr 1985; 107: 796–8.

Uses and Administration

Fluorescein sodium stains damaged cornea and ocular fluids and is applied to the eye for the detection of corneal lesions and foreign bodies, as an aid to the fitting of hard contact lenses, and in various other diagnostic ophthalmic procedures. It is applied as a 1 or 2% solution as eye drops or as sterile papers impregnated with fluorescein sodium. It may also be given in combination with a local anaesthetic, typically as a 0.25% solution with oxybuprocaine hydrochloride or proxymetacaine hydrochloride.

Fluorescein sodium may be given by rapid intravenous injection, usually as a solution equivalent to fluorescein 10 or 25% for the examination of the ophthalmic vasculature by retinal angiography. The usual dose is the equivalent of 500 mg of fluorescein. A dose of 7.5 mg per kg body-weight has been suggested for children. The oral route has also been tried for angiography. Other uses of intravenous fluorescein sodium have included the differentiation of healthy from diseased or damaged tissue and visualisation of the biliary tract.

Fluorescein dilaurate is given by mouth for the assessment of exocrine pancreatic function (see below). Pancreatic enzymes hydrolyse the ester and the amount of free fluorescein excreted in the urine can therefore be taken as a measure of pancreatic activity. A dose of 348.5 mg of fluorescein dilaurate, equivalent to 0.5 mmol of fluorescein, is given with a standard meal, and urine collected for the following 10 hours. The manufacturers give instructions concerning the type and amount of liquid and food which may be taken during this period. A control dose of 188.14 mg of fluorescein sodium, also equivalent to 0.5 mmol of fluorescein, is given on the following day under the same conditions.

Pancreatic function test. Studies of the fluorescein dilaurate test have considered it to be a useful noninvasive screening test for the exclusion of pancreatic exocrine failure in outpatients, particularly those presenting with steatorrhoea.[1-3] The need for tests such as the pancreozymin-secretin test, which requires duodenal intubation, may thus be avoided. However, low specificity (a relatively high rate of false-positive responses) has been reported with the fluorescein dilaurate test in some patient populations,[2,4] and the need for careful patient instruction in performance of the test has been emphasised.[3] In order to avoid the prolonged collection of urine necessary in the standard test, serum concentrations of fluorescein may be measured several hours after taking the test substance.[5]

The test has been used successfully in children,[6] particularly when the doses of fluorescein dilaurate and fluorescein sodium are reduced and fluid intake modified,[7] although the manufacturers recommend that the commercially available test is not used for this age group. In children, a simplified, single-day test using dual markers, fluorescein dilaurate and mannitol, has been investigated with encouraging results.[8]

1. Barry RE, et al. Fluorescein dilaurate—tubeless test for pancreatic exocrine failure. Lancet 1982; ii: 742–4.
2. Boyd EJS, et al. Prospective comparison of the fluorescein-dilaurate test with the secretin-cholecystokinin test for pancreatic exocrine function. J Clin Pathol 1982; 35: 1240–3.
3. Gould SR, et al. Evaluation of a tubeless pancreatic function test in patients with steatorrhoea in a district general hospital. J R Soc Med 1988; 81: 270–3.
4. Braganza JM. Fluorescein dilaurate test. Lancet 1982; ii: 927–8.
5. Dimagno EP. A perspective on the use of tubeless pancreatic function tests in diagnosis. Gut 1998; 42: 2–3.
6. Cumming JGR, et al. Diagnosis of exocrine pancreatic insufficiency in cystic fibrosis by use of fluorescein dilaurate test. Arch Dis Child 1986; 61: 573–5.
7. Dalzell AM, Heaf DP. Fluorescein dilaurate test of exocrine pancreatic function in cystic fibrosis. Arch Dis Child 1990; 65: 788–9.
8. Green MR, et al. Dual marker one day pancreolauryl test. Arch Dis Child 1993; 68: 649–52.

Pediculosis. Infestation of the eye lashes or brows with pubic lice (p.1427) has been successfully treated with a single application of a 20% solution of fluorescein.[1]

1. Mathew M, et al. A new treatment of pthiriasis palpebrarum. Ann Ophthalmol 1982; 14: 439–41.

Retinal angiography. Fluorescein is usually given intravenously for retinal angiography, but a study in 20 healthy subjects concluded that an oral dose of fluorescein sodium 25 mg per kg body-weight could produce good quality retinal angiograms in the majority of subjects.[1] This study used specially prepared 500-mg capsules of fluorescein sodium; the authors commented that previous oral studies had used the liquid preparation intended for intravenous use. Only mild reactions, possibly due to hypersensitivity, appear to have been reported with oral fluorescein.

1. Watson AP, Rosen ES. Oral fluorescein angiography: reassessment of its relative safety and evaluation of optimum conditions with use of capsules. Br J Ophthalmol 1990; 74: 458–61.

Preparations

BP 2001: Fluorescein Eye Drops; Fluorescein Injection;
USP 25: Fluorescein Injection; Fluorescein Sodium and Benoxinate Hydrochloride Ophthalmic Solution; Fluorescein Sodium and Proparacaine Hydrochloride Ophthalmic Solution; Fluorescein Sodium Ophthalmic Strips.

Proprietary Preparations (details are given in Part 3)
Aust.: Fluoftal; Austral.: Disclo-Plaque; Canad.: Fluorets; Ful-Glo; Canad.: Diofluor; Fluor-I-Strip AT†; Fluorescite; Fluorets; Funduscein†; Hong Kong: Fluorescite; Fluorets; Irl.: Fluorets; Ital.: Fluoralfa; Pancreolauryl-Test†; Mex.: Optifluor; NZ: Fluorescite; Fluorets; Ful-Glo; S.Afr.: Fluorescite; Fluorets; Sin-

gapore: Fluorescite; Fluorets; Thai.: Fluorescite; UK: Fluorets; USA: Ak-Fluor; Fluor-I-Strip; Fluorescite; Fluorets; Ful-Glo; Funduscein; Ophthifluor.

Multi-ingredient: Aust.: Flurekain; Healonid Yellow†; Pancreolauryl-Test; Austral.: Fluress; Canad.: Fluoracaine; Fluress; Fin.: Oftan Flurekain; Ger.: Pancreolauryl-Test N; Thilorbin; Ital.: Healon Yellow†; NZ: Fluress; Spain: Fluotest†; Swed.: Fluress; Healon Yellow†; UK: Pancreolauryl-Test; USA: Flu-Oxinate†; Fluoracaine; Fluorocaine; Fluorox; Flurate; Fluress; Flurox; Healon Yellow.

Formic Acid   (1309-x)

Ameisensäure; Aminic Acid; E236; E238 (calcium formate); E237 (sodium formate).
$CH_2O_2 = 46.03$.
CAS — 64-18-6.
Pharmacopoeias. In Aust. and Pol.

Profile

Formic acid resembles acetic acid in its properties (see p.1571) but is more irritating and pungent. The acid and its sodium and calcium salts are used as preservatives in food. Solutions containing about 60% formic acid have been marketed for the removal of lime scales from kettles. Formic acid has also been used for the removal of tattoos. It is an ingredient of some external preparations promoted for the relief of musculoskeletal and joint disorders, and has been applied in conjunction with benzyl alcohol to aid the removal of nits.

◊ In a report of 3 patients who swallowed descaling agents containing 40 or 55% formic acid, the major complications included local corrosive effects, metabolic acidosis, derangement of blood-clotting mechanisms, and acute onset of respiratory and renal failure.[1] All 3 patients died between 5 and 14 days after admission to hospital. A further report of 53 cases of formic acid ingestion included 15 fatalities.[2]

1. Naik RB, et al. Ingestion of formic acid-containing agents — report of three fatal cases. Postgrad Med J 1980; 56: 451–6.
2. Rajan N, et al. Formic acid poisoning with suicidal intent: a report of 53 cases. Postgrad Med J 1985; 61: 35–6.

Preparations

Proprietary Preparations (details are given in Part 3)

Multi-ingredient: Aust.: Aciforin; Berggeist; Belg.: Euphon; Fr.: Euphon†; Ger.: Discmigon; Ital.: Rubistenol†; Rubjovit; Switz.: Fortalis; USA: Step 2†.

Fosfocreatinine   (3794-t)

Fosfocreatinine (rINN).
(1-Methyl-4-oxo-2-imidazolidinylidene)phosphoramidic acid.
$C_4H_8N_3O_4P = 193.1$.
CAS — 5786-71-0 (fosfocreatinine); 19604-05-8 (fosfocreatinine sodium).

Profile

Fosfocreatinine or fosfocreatinine sodium has been used in muscle disorders.

Preparations

Proprietary Preparations (details are given in Part 3)
Ital.: Neoton; Sustenium.

Fosforylcholine   (12771-x)

Phosphorylcholine. (2-Hydroxyethyl)trimethylammonium chloride dihydrogen phosphate.
$C_5H_{15}ClNO_4P = 219.6$.
CAS — 107-73-3.

Profile

Fosforylcholine is a choleretic that has been used in the treatment of hepatic disorders. The calcium and magnesium salts have also been used.

Preparations

Proprietary Preparations (details are given in Part 3)
Fr.: Heparexine.

Fumitory   (8880-e)

Erdrauchkraut; Herba Fumariae.
Pharmacopoeias. In Ger.

Profile

Fumitory comprises the dried or fresh flowering plant Fumaria officinalis (Papaveraceae) and is used in herbal medicine. It is an ingredient of preparations used mainly for gastrointestinal and biliary-tract disorders. Fumitory is also used in homoeopathic medicine.

Preparations

Proprietary Preparations (details are given in Part 3)
Aust.: Bilobene; Oddibil; Oddispasmol†; Fr.: Oddibil; Ger.: Bilobene; Bomagall mono; Oddibil; Mex.: Oddibil; Spain: Colambil.

Multi-ingredient: Aust.: Hepabene; Belg.: Tisane Depurative "les 12 Plantes"; Fr.: Actibil; Actisane Digestion†; Bolcitol; Depuratif Parnel; Depuratum; Gastralsan†; Schoum; Ital.: Depurativo; *Soluzione Schoum*; *Spain:* Sol Schoum; *UK:* Echinacea; Skin Cleansing.

Gabexate Mesilate (12777-m)

Gabexate Mesilate *(rINNM)*.

Gabexate Mesylate. Ethyl 4-(6-guanidinohexanoyloxy)benzoate methanesulphonate.

$C_{16}H_{23}N_3O_4,CH_4SO_3 = 417.5$.

CAS — 39492-01-8 (gabexate); 56974-61-9 (gabexate mesilate).

Pharmacopoeias. In Jpn.

Profile

Gabexate mesilate is a proteolytic enzyme inhibitor which has been tried in the treatment of pancreatitis (p.1646), and in the prevention of pancreatitis following endoscopic retrograde cholangiopancreatography. It has also been tried as an anticoagulant for haemodialysis. Hypersensitivity reactions including anaphylaxis have occurred.

◊ References.
1. Scuro LA, *et al.* Gabexate mesilate (Foy) treatment of acute pancreatitis: an Italian multicentre pilot study. *Clin Trials J* 1990; **27:** 39–49.
2. Messori A, *et al.* Effectiveness of gabexate mesilate in acute pancreatitis: a metaanalysis. *Dig Dis Sci* 1995; **40:** 734–8.
3. Cavallini G, *et al.* Gabexate for the prevention of pancreatic damage related to endoscopic retrograde cholangiopancreatography. *N Engl J Med* 1996; **335:** 919–23.
4. Matsukawa Y, *et al.* Anaphylaxis induced by gabexate mesylate. *BMJ* 1998; **317:** 1563.
5. Ranucci M, *et al.* Gabexate mesilate and antithrombin III for intraoperative anticoagulation in heparin pretreated patients. *Perfusion* 1999; **14:** 357–62.

Preparations

Proprietary Preparations (details are given in Part 3)
Ital.: Foy; *Jpn:* Foy.

Gall (310-v)

Aleppo Galls; Blue Galls; Galla; Galläpfel; Galls; Noix de Galle; Nutgall.

Pharmacopoeias. In Aust.

Excrescences on the twigs of *Quercus infectoria* (Fagaceae), resulting from the stimulus given to the tissues of the young twigs by the development of the larvae of the gall-wasp, *Adleria gallae-tinctoriae* (= *Cynips gallae-tinctoriae*) (Cynipidae). It contains about 50 to 70% of gallotannic acid.

Profile

Gall is an astringent and has been used in ointments and suppositories for the treatment of haemorrhoids. It is a source of tannic acid (p.1669).

Preparations

Proprietary Preparations (details are given in Part 3)
Spain: Litiax.

Gamma-aminobutyric Acid (12359-p)

Aminobutyric Acid; GABA; Piperidic Acid. 4-Aminobutyric acid.

$C_4H_9NO_2 = 103.1$.

CAS — 56-12-2.
ATC — N03AG03.

Profile

Gamma-aminobutyric acid is a principal inhibitory neurotransmitter in the CNS. It has been claimed to be of value in cerebral disorders and to have an antihypertensive effect.

Preparations

Proprietary Preparations (details are given in Part 3)
Braz.: Gammar; *Hong Kong:* Gammalon; *Port.:* Mielomade; *Thai.:* Bainto; Gammalon.

Multi-ingredient: *Braz.:* Complevit; Gaba; Gabax; Gabormon; Id Sedin; *Spain:* Cefabol; Gamalate B6.

Gamolenic Acid (11660-v)

Gamolenic Acid *(BAN, rINN)*.

GLA; γ-Linolenic Acid. (Z,Z,Z)-Octadeca-6,9,12-trienoic acid.

$C_{18}H_{30}O_2 = 278.4$.

CAS — 506-26-3.
ATC — D11AX02.

Borage Oil (12114-w)

Starflower Oil.

An oil derived from the seeds of borage (*Borago officinalis*, Boraginaceae).

Evening Primrose Oil (9808-e)

King's Cureall.

A fixed oil obtained from the seeds of *Oenothera biennis* or other spp. (Onagraceae) and containing linoleic acid with some gamolenic acid.

Linoleic Acid (9748-z)

Linolic Acid. (Z,Z)-Octadeca-9,12-dienoic acid.

$C_{18}H_{32}O_2 = 280.4$.

Adverse Effects and Precautions

Evening primrose oil, and presumably other sources of gamolenic and linoleic acids, can produce minor gastrointestinal disturbances and headache. It can precipitate symptoms of undiagnosed temporal lobe epilepsy, and should be used with caution in patients with a history of epilepsy or those taking epileptogenic drugs, in particular phenothiazines. Hypersensitivity reactions may also occur.

Effects on the nervous system. Temporal lobe epilepsy was diagnosed following treatment with evening primrose oil in 3 patients who had previously been diagnosed as schizophrenic.[1] Tonic-clonic (grand mal) seizures occurred in 2 additional schizophrenic patients during treatment with evening primrose oil.[2] All of these patients had received or were taking phenothiazine antipsychotics.
1. Vaddadi KS. The use of gamma-linolenic acid and linoleic acid to differentiate between temporal lobe epilepsy and schizophrenia. *Prostaglandins* 1981; **6:** 375–9.
2. Holman CP, Bell AFJ. A trial of evening primrose oil in the treatment of chronic schizophrenia. *J Orthomol Psychiatry* 1983; **12:** 302–4.

Uses and Administration

Linoleic and gamolenic acid are essential fatty acids of the omega-6 series that act as prostaglandin precursors; endogenous gamolenic acid is derived from linoleic acid which is an essential constituent of the diet. Evening primrose oil, which contains these acids, is used for symptomatic relief of atopic eczema and mastalgia. Typical doses expressed as gamolenic acid are 320 to 480 mg daily in divided doses in eczema, and 240 to 320 mg daily as a single dose or in divided doses for mastalgia. Children aged 1 to 12 years with atopic eczema may be given 80 to 160 mg twice daily. Evening primrose oil has been investigated in a variety of other disorders including multiple sclerosis, rheumatoid arthritis, and the premenstrual syndrome. Mixtures of essential fatty acids (including EF-4, EF-12, and EF-27) derived from evening primrose oil and other oils have also been investigated in various conditions, including diabetic neuropathy, restenosis following angioplasty, and skin damage following radiotherapy.

Other plant oils which have been used similarly to evening primrose oil include black currant seed oil, and borage oil (starflower oil). Products containing gamolenic acid-rich plant oils are promoted in many countries as dietary supplements, often in combination with fish oils or other sources of omega-3 triglycerides (see p.949).

A derivative of gamolenic acid, lithium gamolenate (p.550), has been investigated in pancreatic cancer.

◊ General references.
1. Kleijnen J. Evening primrose oil. *BMJ* 1994; **309:** 824–5.

Eczema. Atopic eczema (p.1105) may be due to a defect in essential fatty acid metabolism[1] and some beneficial symptomatic effects have been reported with evening primrose oil.[1,2] Meta-analysis of 9 studies involving 311 patients[3] has reported improvement in disease symptoms, especially itching, but a subsequent study in 123 patients found no therapeutic effect of evening primrose oil, alone or with fish oil.[4] Although the design and interpretation of this study has been criticised by the manufacturers of evening primrose oil,[5] the authors consider such criticism invalid,[6] and point out that an earlier large study yielded similar results.[7] No difference was found between placebo and evening primrose oil in a further study[8] in children with eczema, and there was also no effect on asthma symptoms in those patients suffering from both disorders. A study of borage oil also found no overall efficacy in adults with atopic eczema, although the authors noted a suggestion of benefit in a subgroup of patients.[9]
Benefit has been reported in infants with seborrhoeic dermatitis from local application of borage oil.[10]
1. Wright S. Essential fatty acids and the skin. *Br J Dermatol* 1991; **125:** 503–15.
2. Rustin MHA. Dermatology. *Postgrad Med J* 1990; **66:** 894–905.
3. Morse PF, *et al.* Meta-analysis of placebo-controlled studies of the efficacy of Epogam in the treatment of atopic eczema: relationship between plasma essential fatty acid changes and clinical response. *Br J Dermatol* 1989; **121:** 75–90.
4. Berth-Jones J, Graham-Brown RAC. Placebo-controlled trial of essential fatty acid supplementation in atopic dermatitis. *Lancet* 1993; **341:** 1557–60. Correction. *ibid.*; **342:** 564.
5. Shield MJ, *et al.* Essential fatty acid supplementation in atopic dermatitis. *Lancet* 1993; **342:** 377.
6. Berth-Jones J, *et al.* Essential fatty acid supplementation in atopic dermatitis. *Lancet* 1993; **342:** 377–8. Correction. *ibid.*; 752.
7. Bamford JTM, *et al.* Atopic eczema unresponsive to evening primrose oil (linoleic and gamma-linolenic acids). *J Am Acad Dermatol* 1985; **13:** 959–65.
8. Hederos C-A, Berg A. Epogam evening primrose oil treatment in atopic dermatitis and asthma. *Arch Dis Child* 1996; **75:** 494–7.

9. Henz BM, *et al.* Double-blind, multicentre analysis of the efficacy of borage oil in patients with atopic eczema. *Br J Dermatol* 1999; **140:** 685–8.
10. Tollesson A, Frithz A. Borage oil, an effective new treatment for infantile seborrhoeic dermatitis. *Br J Dermatol* 1993; **129:** 95.

Mastalgia. Gamolenic acid (usually given in the form of evening primrose oil) has fewer adverse effects than drugs such as danazol or bromocriptine and is sometimes preferred for mastalgia (p.1470), especially in patients with less severe symptoms or those who require prolonged or repeated treatment.

Menopausal disorders. For reference to a study suggesting that evening primrose oil is of no benefit in preventing menopausal vasomotor symptoms, see p.1464.

Multiple sclerosis. There is some evidence that modifying the intake of dietary fats and supplementing the diet with omega-6 polyunsaturated fatty acids, such as linoleic acid, could influence the clinical course of multiple sclerosis (p.633) and many patients practise dietary modification, including taking evening primrose oil. One study[1] has shown a reduction in severity and duration of relapse in patients taking linoleic acid supplements (as sunflower oil), and another[2] has reported benefit in patients who limited their intake of dietary saturated fatty acids and supplemented their diet with polyunsaturated fatty acids. However, the relationship between dietary fat and multiple sclerosis cannot be considered proven.
1. Millar JHD, *et al.* Double-blind trial of linoleate supplementation of the diet in multiple sclerosis. *BMJ* 1973; **1:** 765–8.
2. Swank RL, Dugan BB. Effect of low saturated fat diet in early and late cases of multiple sclerosis. *Lancet* 1990; **336:** 37–9.

Premenstrual syndrome. Progressive improvement in premenstrual syndrome was reported over 5 cycles in an open pilot study in 19 patients receiving evening primrose oil.[1] However, subsequent results have not demonstrated any benefit.[2-4] Evening primrose oil may be considered for cyclical mastalgia associated with premenstrual syndrome, but other drugs are preferred if other symptoms predominate (see p.1475).
1. Larsson B, *et al.* Evening primrose oil in the treatment of premenstrual syndrome: a pilot study. *Curr Ther Res* 1989; **46:** 58–63.
2. Khoo SK, *et al.* Evening primrose oil and treatment of premenstrual syndrome. *Med J Aust* 1990; **153:** 189–92.
3. Collins A, *et al.* Essential fatty acids in the treatment of premenstrual syndrome. *Obstet Gynecol* 1993; **81:** 93–8.
4. Budeiri DJ, *et al.* Is evening primrose oil of value in the treatment of premenstrual syndrome? *Control Clin Trials* 1996; **17:** 60–8.

Rheumatoid arthritis. Patients with rheumatoid arthritis (p.9) taking NSAIDs have shown subjective improvement following 12 months' treatment with evening primrose oil, with or without fish oil, when compared with placebo.[1] A clinically important reduction in signs and symptoms of disease activity has also been seen in patients treated with gamolenic acid in the form of borage oil.[2] It has been demonstrated[3] that during treatment with evening primrose oil patients with rheumatoid arthritis have increased plasma concentrations of gamolenic, dihomo-gamma-linolenic, and arachidonic acids, and decreased plasma concentrations of oleic and eicosapentaenoic acids and apolipoprotein B. The increase in plasma-arachidonic acid and decrease in eicosapentaenoic acid may be unfavourable in patients with rheumatoid arthritis, since arachidonic acid is the precursor of inflammatory prostaglandins and eicosapentaenoic acid may have an anti-inflammatory role.
1. Belch JJF, *et al.* Effects of altering dietary essential fatty acids on requirements for non-steroidal anti-inflammatory drugs in patients with rheumatoid arthritis: a double blind placebo controlled study. *Ann Rheum Dis* 1988; **47:** 96–104.
2. Leventhal LJ, *et al.* Treatment of rheumatoid arthritis with gammalinolenic acid. *Ann Intern Med* 1993; **119:** 867–73.
3. Jäntti J, *et al.* Evening primrose oil in rheumatoid arthritis: changes in serum lipids and fatty acids. *Ann Rheum Dis* 1989; **48:** 124–7.

Preparations

Proprietary Preparations (details are given in Part 3)
Austral.: Bioglan Primrose Micelle; Efamol†; Epogam†; Naudicelle; *Canad.:* Boracelle†; Efalex Focus; Efamol; Gamma Oil; Naudicelle; Onagre; Primanol; *Denm.:* Epogam; *Fr.:* Bioleine; Bionagrol; Gamatol; Omegaline; *Ger.:* Epogam; Gammacur; Linola gamma; Linola-Fett 2000; Neobonsen; Unigamol; *Hong Kong:* Efamast; *Irl.:* Epogam; Naudicelle; *Ital.:* Epogam; Gammavit; Ictage 6; Normogam; *NZ:* Efamol; Epogam; *Port.:* Atopic; *S.Afr.:* Epogam; *Spain:* Epogam; *Switz.:* Cremol-P†; Efamol; Glandol; *UK:* Boracelle; E.P.O. & E; Efamast; Efamol; EPOC†; Epogam; Evening Gold; Evoprim; Floresse; Galanol GLX; Gamma Oil; GammaOil Premium; Naudicelle; PowerLean; Super Galanol; Super GLA; Unigam†.

Multi-ingredient: *Austral.:* Bioglan Arthri Plus; Bioglan E-Plus†; Bioglan Ginger-Vite Forte; Bioglan Primrose-E; Bioglan Zellulean with Escin; Curaderm; Efacal; Efamol Marine†; Epo + Maxepa + Vitamin E Herbal Plus Formula 8†; For Women Multi Plus EPO; Lifesystem Herbal Plus Formula 9 Fatty Acids And Vitamin E†; Maxepa & EPO; Medinat PMT-Eze; Naudicelle Marine; Naudicelle Plus†; PMS Support; *Canad.:* Bionagre plus E; Efamol Fortify; Gamma Oil Marine; GLA-130; Primanol-Borage†; Super Gamma Oil with Vitamin E; *Fr.:* Bionagrol Plus; Elteans; Exomega; Phytophanere; *Ger.:* Linola; Linola-Fett N; *Hong Kong:* Aderma Exomega; *Ital.:* Dermon-Oil; Dermana; Efagel; Errevit Forte Gamma; Granoleina; Topialyse; Trofinerv Antiox; *NZ:* Efacal; Efamast; Efamol Marine; *Port.:* Antiestrias; Geriso; Nutraisdin; Ureadin Facial; *S.Afr.:* Efamol G; *Switz.:* Linola; Linola gras; Linola mi-gras; Linoladiol; Vitafissan; *UK:* Efacal; Efalex; Efamarine; Efamol Plus Coenzyme Q10; Efamol PMP; Efamol Safflower & Linseed; EPOC Marine†; Epopa; Exzem Oil;

The symbol † denotes a preparation no longer actively marketed

Galanol Gold; Galmarin; Gamma Marine; Naudicelle Forte; Naudicelle Plus; PMT Formula; Royal Galanol; Super GammaOil Marine.

Gangliosides (16820-f)

Profile
Gangliosides are endogenous substances present in mammalian cell membranes, especially in the cortex of the brain. They are glycosphingolipids composed of a hydrophilic oligosaccharide chain, characterised by sialic acid residues, attached to a lipophilic moiety. The four major gangliosides found in the mammalian brain are referred to as G_{M1}, G_{D1a}, G_{D1b}, and G_{T1b}. Experimental studies have reported that gangliosides may have a neuroprotective effect on the central and peripheral nervous systems. Preparations of gangliosides from bovine brain were given for peripheral neuropathies and cerebrovascular disorders and their role in spinal cord injury has also been investigated. The modified ganglioside siagoside is being studied in patients with Parkinson's disease.

Concern has been expressed by several authorities about the development of Guillain-Barré syndrome and other motor neurone disorders in some patients and it was suggested that gangliosides were contra-indicated in Guillain-Barré syndrome and all auto-immune disorders. Subsequently these concerns over safety as well as of efficacy led to the withdrawal of ganglioside preparations in many countries.

◊ References.
1. Geisler FH, *et al.* Recovery of motor function after spinal-cord injury—a randomized, placebo-controlled trial with GM-1 ganglioside. *N Engl J Med* 1991; **324:** 1829–38.
2. Raschetti R, *et al.* Guillain-Barré syndrome and ganglioside therapy in Italy. *Lancet* 1992; **340:** 60.
3. Figueras A, *et al.* Bovine gangliosides and acute motor polyneuropathy. *BMJ* 1992; **305:** 1330–1.
4. Roberts JW, *et al.* Iatrogenic hyperlipidaemia with GM-1 ganglioside. *Lancet* 1993; **342:** 115.
5. Landi G, *et al.* Guillain-Barré syndrome after exogenous gangliosides in Italy. *BMJ* 1993; **307:** 1463–4.
6. Nobile-Orazio E, *et al.* Gangliosides: their role in clinical neurology. *Drugs* 1994; **47:** 576–85.
7. Candelise L, Ciccone A. Gangliosides for acute ischaemic stroke (updated 14 August 2001). Available in The Cochrane Library; Issue 4. Oxford: Update Software; 2001.

Preparations
Proprietary Preparations (details are given in Part 3)
Braz.: Sygen; *Thai.:* Cronassial.

Garlic (2014-y)

Aglio; Ail; Ajo; Allium; Knoblauch.
CAS — 8008-99-9 (garlic extract).
Pharmacopoeias. In *USNF*, which also includes Garlic Fluidextract, Powdered Garlic, and Powdered Garlic Extract. *Eur.* (see p.vi) includes Garlic Powder.

Constituents of garlic include alliin, allicin, diallyl disulfide, and ajoene.

Pharmacopoeial description
Ph. Eur.: Garlic Powder is produced from garlic that has been cut, freeze-dried or dried at a temperature not exceeding 65°, and powdered. It contains not less than 0.45% of allicin, calculated with reference to the dried drug. It is a light yellowish powder. Protect from light.

USNF 20: The fresh or dried compound bulbs of *Allium sativum* (Liliaceae). It contains not less than 0.5% of alliin and not less than 0.2% of γ-glutamyl-*(S)*-allyl-L-cysteine, calculated on the dried basis. Store in a dry place at a temperature of 8° to 15°. Protect from light.

Powdered Garlic is produced from garlic that has been cut, freeze-dried or dried at a temperature not exceeding 65°, and powdered. It contains not less than 0.3% of alliin and not less than 0.1% of γ-glutamyl-*(S)*-allyl-L-cysteine, calculated on the dried basis. Store in a dry place at a temperature of 8° to 15°. Protect from light.

Adverse Effects
◊ Reports of burns or skin lesions following topical application of garlic to children,[1,2] and to adults.[3,4]
1. Garty B-Z. Garlic burns. *Pediatrics* 1993; **91:** 658–9.
2. Canduela V, *et al.* Garlic: always good for the health? *Br J Dermatol* 1995; **132:** 161–2.
3. Farrell AM, Staughton RCD. Garlic burns mimicking herpes zoster. *Lancet* 1996; **347:** 1195.
4. Eming SA, *et al.* Severe toxic contact dermatitis caused by garlic. *Br J Dermatol* 1999; **141:** 391–2.

Uses and Administration
Garlic has traditionally been reported to have expectorant, diaphoretic, disinfectant, and diuretic properties. More recently, it has been investigated for antimicrobial, antihypertensive, lipid-lowering, fibrinolytic, antiplatelet, and cancer protective effects. It is used in homoeopathic medicine.

◊ References.
1. Kleijnen J, *et al.* Garlic, onions and cardiovascular risk factors: a review of the evidence from human experiments with emphasis on commercially available preparations. *Br J Clin Pharmacol* 1989; **28:** 535–44.
2. Mansell P, Reckless JPD. Garlic. *BMJ* 1991; **303:** 379–80.

3. McElnay JC, Po ALW. Garlic. *Pharm J* 1991; **246:** 324–6.
4. Kiesewetter H, *et al.* Effect of garlic on platelet aggregation in patients with increased risk of juvenile ischaemic attack. *Eur J Clin Pharmacol* 1993; **45:** 333–6.
5. Deshpande RG, *et al.* Inhibition of Mycobacterium avium complex isolates from AIDS patients by garlic (Allium sativum). *J Antimicrob Chemother* 1993; **32:** 623–6.
6. Dorant E, *et al.* Garlic and its significance for the prevention of cancer in humans: a critical review. *Br J Cancer* 1993; **67:** 424–9.

Hyperlipidaemia. Garlic has been widely promoted for use in the treatment of hyperlipidaemia. Several early placebo-controlled trials[1,2] and meta-analyses[3,4] showed that garlic significantly decreased total serum-cholesterol concentrations. However, more recent data suggest that the effect is at best modest[5] or that there is no significant difference[6-8] when compared with placebo.
1. Jain AK, *et al.* Can garlic reduce levels of serum lipids? A controlled clinical study. *Am J Med* 1993; **94:** 632–5.
2. Kenzelmann R, Kade F. Limitation of the deterioration of lipid parameters by a standardized garlic-ginkgo combination product: a multicenter placebo-controlled double-blind study. *Arzneimittelforschung* 1993; **43:** 978–81.
3. Warshafsky S, *et al.* Effect of garlic on total serum cholesterol: a meta-analysis. *Ann Intern Med* 1993; **119:** 599–605.
4. Silagy C, Neil A. Garlic as a lipid lowering agent—a meta-analysis. *J R Coll Physicians Lond* 1994; **28:** 39–45.
5. Stevinson C, *et al.* Garlic for treating hypercholesterolemia: a meta-analysis of randomized clinical trials. *Ann Intern Med* 2000; **133:** 420–9.
6. Neil HAW, *et al.* Garlic powder in the treatment of moderate hyperlipidaemia: a controlled trial and a meta-analysis. *J R Coll Physicians Lond* 1996; **30:** 329–34.
7. Berthold HK, *et al.* Effect of a garlic oil preparation on serum lipoproteins and cholesterol metabolism: a randomized controlled trial. *JAMA* 1998; **279:** 1900–2.
8. Isaacsohn JL, *et al.* Garlic powder and plasma lipids and lipoproteins: a multicenter, randomized, placebo-controlled trial. *Arch Intern Med* 1998; **158:** 1189–94.

Preparations
Proprietary Preparations (details are given in Part 3)
Aust.: Kwai; *Austral.:* Garlix; Kwai†; Macro Garlic; *Fr.:* Past Ail†; Thirial; *Ger.:* Alliosan; Beni-cur; Carisano; Ilja Rogoff Forte; Kneipp Knoblauch Dragees N; Kneipp Knoblauch-Pflanzensaft; Kwai; Quam; Sapec; Sirmia Knoblauchsaft N†; Strongus; *Ital.:* Kwai; *Port.:* Alho Rogoff; *Switz.:* A Vogel Capsules a l'ail; Kwai; Sanhelios 333; *UK:* Garlimega; Kwai; Kyolic.

Multi-ingredient: *Aust.:* Heli-Sal; Rutiviscal; *Austral.:* Crataegus Complex; Echinacea & Antioxidants; Esten†; Garlic Allium Complex; Garlic and Horseradish + C Complex; Gartech; Herbal Cold & Flu Relief; Horse Radish and Garlic Tablets; Lifesystem Herbal Formula 7 Liver Tonic; Liver Tonic Herbal Formula 6; Macro C + Garlic with Zinc†; Odourless Garlic; Procold; Proesten; Protol; Proyeast; Silybum Complex; *Belg.:* Ex'ail†; *Braz.:* Neo Sativan; *Fr.:* Arterase; Ex'ail; *Ger.:* Asgoviscum N; Discmigon; Ilja Rogoff; Kneipp Drei-Pflanzen-Dragees N; Lipidavit; Presselin Arterien K 5 P; *Ital.:* Prexene†; *Switz.:* Allium Plus; Keli-med; *UK:* Antifect; Beechams for Natural Relief; Brewers Yeast with Garlic; Buttercup Pol'N'Count; Clogar; Coldeeze; Fishogar; Hay Fever & Sinus Relief; Hayfever & Sinus Relief; Kincare.

Gavestinel (3223-q)

Gavestinel *(BAN, USAN, rINN).*
GV-150526X. 4,6-Dichloro-3-[(E)-2-(phenylcarbamoyl)vinyl]indole-2-carboxylic acid.
$C_{18}H_{12}Cl_2N_2O_3 = 375.2.$
CAS — 153436-22-7.

Profile
Gavestinel is a glycine antagonist that has been investigated as a neuroprotectant in stroke.

Stroke. Gavestinel has been tried for its supposed neuroprotective properties in acute stroke, but two major multicentre, randomised controlled studies have failed to demonstrate any benefit over placebo.[1,2]
1. Lees KR, *et al.* Glycine antagonist (gavestinel) in neuroprotection (GAIN International) in patients with acute stroke: a randomised controlled trial. *Lancet* 2000; **355:** 1949–54.
2. Sacco RL, *et al.* Glycine antagonist in neuroprotection for patients with acute stroke: GAIN Americas: a randomized controlled trial. *JAMA* 2001; **285:** 1719–28.

Gelsemium (12781-f)

Gelsemium Root; Jessamine; Yellow Jasmine Root.
CAS — 509-15-9 (gelsemine).

The dried rhizome and roots of *Gelsemium sempervirens* (Loganiaceae). It contains indole alkaloids including gelsemine ($C_{20}H_{22}N_2O_2 = 322.4$).

Profile
Gelsemium depresses the CNS and has been used mainly in neuralgic conditions, particularly trigeminal neuralgia and migraine.

Gelsemium is used in homoeopathic medicine.

Preparations
Proprietary Preparations (details are given in Part 3)
Multi-ingredient: *Fr.:* Coquelusedal; Coquelusedal Paracetamol.

Gene Therapy (10553-k)

Profile
Gene therapy is a product of the increasing knowledge of genetic function and the availability of methods to examine and manipulate the genome. It comprises the administration of exogenous genetic material into body cells (transfection) in such a way that the cells are able to express the products of the new genes. It should be distinguished from the administration of products themselves derived from organisms (usually microorganisms) whose genome has been manipulated by similar recombinant DNA technology, for example the use of recombinant cytokines, monoclonal antibodies, or antisense products.

Gene therapy is under investigation in three main areas:
- the replacement of abnormal or defective genes in patients with inherited disease
- the alteration of the characteristics of cells to change their relative susceptibility to other therapies (for example by making haematopoietic stem cells more resistant to the adverse effects of antineoplastics, or by making tumour cells selectively express an enzyme which converts an otherwise non-toxic prodrug into a cytotoxic agent)
- for localised production of a biologically active substance that cannot be administered directly or would have unacceptable effects following systemic administration.

To date, all gene therapy in humans has been of differentiated somatic cells; alteration of the human genome in a manner transmissible to offspring, either by treating the germ cells or the early embryo, is considered at present to pose insuperable ethical problems.

Various methods for delivery of genetic material have been investigated, none of which is yet completely satisfactory. Although removal of donor cells from the patient followed by *ex vivo* transfer of the new gene (by physical or viral methods) and return of the modified cells may be feasible for modifying haematopoietic stem cells, for most tissues, methods of *in vivo* transfer are required. Modified viruses rendered incapable of replicating have been widely studied as vectors for gene therapy. Retroviruses have the advantage that the DNA they carry is integrated into the host genome, resulting in permanent expression of the gene, but there has been some concern that they may disrupt existing genetic material with possibly oncogenic effect; in addition, their small size limits the size of gene that they can carry, and they are largely ineffective in infecting non-dividing cells. Adenoviruses are more stable and can infect non-dividing as well as dividing cells, but their genetic freight is not integrated into the chromosome and transmitted to the cell's progeny, and the gene products are therefore only expressed transiently; they are also highly immunogenic which limits repeated administration. Some other viral types, including herpes simplex viruses, adeno-associated viruses, and lentiviruses, are also under investigation. Viruses with tropisms for a particular tissue may be useful in producing localised effects.

Chemical or physical methods for DNA delivery have been extensively investigated *in vitro* and in *animals*, and have been studied in small numbers of patients. Such methods include direct injection of DNA, the use of DNA complexes bound to a ligand which can be taken up by cells, formulation of DNA in liposomes which can fuse with cell membranes and allow the DNA to enter the cell, and more exotic methods such as 'gene guns', in which DNA-coated gold particles are fired into the cells. Although gene expression can be achieved following such methods, it is again transient because the new genetic material is not integrated with that of the host, and physical methods are currently less efficient and more limited in scope than viral ones.

Numerous clinical studies are being carried out although, at present, relatively few patients have actually received gene therapy. The first successful therapy was for severe combined immunodeficiency, a single-gene disorder due to deficiency of the enzyme adenosine deaminase. Transfection of the gene for this enzyme into the patient's T-cells *ex vivo* and re-infusion of the modified T-cells has been shown to produce substantial clinical improvement, although therapy must be repeated periodically because of the limited lifespan of the lymphocytes.

Studies in patients with cystic fibrosis have also shown some success, and a number of other single-gene disorders, including alpha$_1$ antitrypsin deficiency, familial hypercholesterolaemia, Gaucher disease, the haemoglobinopathies and haemophilias, and Duchenne muscular dystrophy are being studied or have been proposed as possible candidates.

Gene therapy is also under investigation in various acquired diseases, particularly in the management of various types of cancer. Strategies being studied include modification of tumour cells either to increase their immunogenicity or to render them selectively sensitive to antineoplastics, and transfection of tumour cells with tumour suppressor genes. Other disorders being studied clinically include HIV infection, rheumatoid arthritis, and atherosclerosis.

◊ Some reviews and references concerning gene therapy are listed below. See also under the discussions of individual diseases for comments on gene therapy in the context of their conventional treatment.
1. Coutelle C. Gene therapy approaches for cystic fibrosis. *Biologicals* 1995; **23:** 21–5.

2. Hoeben RC. Gene therapy for the haemophilias: current status. *Biologicals* 1995; **23:** 27–9.
3. Lever AML, Goodfellow P, eds. Gene therapy. *Br Med Bull* 1995; **51:** 1–242.
4. Hanania EG, *et al.* Recent advances in the application of gene therapy to human disease. *Am J Med* 1995; **99:** 537–52.
5. Blau HM, Springer ML. Gene therapy—a novel form of drug delivery. *N Engl J Med* 1995; **333:** 1204–7.
6. Whartenby KA, *et al.* Gene therapy: clinical potential and relationships to drug treatment. *Drugs* 1995; **50:** 951–8.
7. Dorin J. Somatic gene therapy. *BMJ* 1996; **312:** 323–4.
8. Southern KW. Gene therapy for cystic fibrosis: current issues. *Br J Hosp Med* 1996; **55:** 495–9.
9. Weichselbaum RR, Kufe D. Gene therapy of cancer. *Lancet* 1997; **349** (suppl II): 10–12.
10. Alton EWFW, Geddes DM. Prospects for respiratory gene therapy. *Br J Hosp Med* 1997; **58:** 47–9.
11. Knoell DL, Yiu IM. Human gene therapy for hereditary diseases: a review of trials. *Am J Health-Syst Pharm* 1998; **55:** 899–904.
12. Smith AE. Gene therapy—where are we? *Lancet* 1999; **354** (suppl): 1–4.

Gentian   (534-r)

Bitter Root; Enzianwurzel; Gentian Root; Gentiana; Gentianae Radix; Genziana; Raiz de Genciana.

Pharmacopoeias. In *Eur.* (see p.vi), *Jpn*, and *Pol.*
Jpn includes Japanese Gentian, from *G. scabra* and other species.
Chin. also specifies *G. scabra* and other species.

Pharmacopoeial description

Ph. Eur.: The dried underground organs of *Gentiana lutea* yielding not less than 33% of water-soluble extractive. It has a characteristic odour. Protect from light and moisture.

Profile

Gentian is used as a bitter. An alcoholic infusion of gentian, bitter-orange peel, and lemon peel has been used as an ingredient in a number of bitter mixtures.
Gentian has been used in homoeopathic medicine.

Preparations

BP 2001: Acid Gentian Mixture; Alkaline Gentian Mixture; Compound Gentian Infusion; Concentrated Compound Gentian Infusion.

Proprietary Preparations (details are given in Part 3)
Ger.: Digestivum-Hetterich S; Enziagil Magenplus.

Multi-ingredient: *Aust.:* Abdomilon; Amara; Bio-Garten Tee zur Starkung und Kraftigung; Brady's-Magentropfen; China-Eisenwein; Digestol; Krautertee Nr 20; Magentee; Mariazeller; Montana; Naturland Verdauungs; Sanvita Magen; Sanvita Verdauungstropfen†; Schwedenjorg mild†; Sigman-Haustropfen; Sinupret; Sinusol; St Radegunder Verdauungstee; *Austral.:* Calmo; Digestaid; Digestive Aid; Extralife Sleep-Care; Pacifenity; Plantago Complex†; Relaxaplex; Sinulin; *Braz.:* Camomila; Fargestium; Fideine; Formitonicum; Gotas Digestivas; Lactifero; *Canad.:* Herbal Laxative; Herbal Nerve; *Fr.:* Ducase†; Elixir Grez; Palmi†; Phospharome†; Quintonine; Triogene†; *Ger.:* Abdomilon N; Amara-Tropfen; Amara-Tropfen-Pascoe; Anore X N; Discmigon; Dr. Hotz Vollbad†; Gallexier; Gastralon N; Gastricard N; Gastrol S; Gastrosecur; Hepaticum-Medice H; Infi-tract N; Kneipp Flatuol; Leber-Galle-Tropfen 83; Montana; Phonix Gastriphon; Schwedentrunk der Echte Elixier; Schwedentrunk mit Ginseng†; Schwedentrunk†; Sedovent; Sinupret; Stovalid N; Unex Amarum; Ventrimarin novo; *Hong Kong:* Sinupret; *Ital.:* Amaro Medicinale; Amaro Padil; Caramelle alle Erbe Digestive; Chinoidina; Depurativo; Elisir Depurativo Ambrosiano; Frerichs Maldifassi; *Singapore:* Sinupret; *Spain:* Depurativo Richelet; Digestol Sanatorium; *Switz.:* Demonatur Gouttes pour le foie et la bile; Gastrosan; Padma-Lax; Sinupret; *Thai.:* Pepsitase; Sinupret; *UK:* Appetiser Mixture; Indigestion Mixture; Kalms; Quiet Tyme; Scullcap & Gentian Tablets; Stomach Mixture.

Gentisic Acid Ethanolamide   (3272-c)

2,5-Dihydroxybenzoic acid ethanolamine.
$C_9H_{11}NO_4 = 197.2$.

Profile

Gentisic acid ethanolamide has been used as a complexing agent in the manufacture of pharmaceutical preparations.

Geranium Oil   (4652-y)

Aetheroleum Pelargonii; Oleum Geranii; Pelargonium Oil; Rose Geranium Oil.

A volatile oil obtained by distillation from the aerial parts of various species and hybrid forms of *Pelargonium* (Geraniaceae). It contains geraniol. Store in airtight containers. Protect from light.

Profile

Geranium oil is used to perfume various preparations. Hypersensitivity reactions have been associated with geraniol.

Preparations

Proprietary Preparations (details are given in Part 3)
Ital.: Entom Nature.

Multi-ingredient: *Fr.:* Acarcid; Euvanol†; *Ital.:* Dentosan Azione Intensiva; Dentosan Mese; Mistick; Natural Zanzy; Otosan Gocce Auricolari; Sanaderm†; Vapor Flay; *UK:* Medicated Extract of Rosemary; Medicinal Gargle; Nostroline; Teenstick.

Germanium   (5251-b)

Ge = 72.64.
CAS — 7440-56-4.

Profile

Germanium compounds have been used in dietary supplements promoted as beneficial in a wide range of conditions including cancer, chronic fatigue syndrome, and immunodeficiency disorders. However, germanium compounds can produce severe renal damage and their use should be discouraged.
Germanium has also been used in dental alloys and has various industrial uses.

Effects on the kidneys. In the UK the Department of Health has recommended that germanium should not be taken as a dietary supplement due to a significant incidence of renal toxicity. There have been a number of reports of severe renal damage resulting from germanium ingestion.

References.
1. Okada K, *et al.* Renal failure caused by long-term use of a germanium preparation as an elixir. *Clin Nephrol* 1989; **31:** 219–24.
2. van der Spoel JI, *et al.* Dangers of dietary germanium supplements. *Lancet* 1990; **336:** 117. Correction. *ibid.* 1991; **337:** 864.
3. Schauss AG. Nephrotoxicity in humans by the ultratrace element germanium. *Ren Fail* 1991; **13:** 1–4.
4. Hess B, *et al.* Tubulointerstitial nephropathy persisting 20 months after discontinuation of chronic intake of germanium lactate citrate. *Am J Kidney Dis* 1993; **21:** 548–52.
5. Tao SH, Bolger PM. Hazard assessment of germanium supplements. *Regul Toxicol Pharmacol* 1997; **25:** 211–19.

Ginkgo Biloba   (19248-e)

EGB-761; Fossil Tree; GBE-761; Kew Tree; Maidenhair Tree; *Salisburia adiantifolia.*
ATC — N06DX02.
Pharmacopoeias. In *Eur.* (see p.vi). Also in *USNF.*
Chin. includes the seeds.

Pharmacopoeial description

Ph. Eur.: The whole or fragmented dried leaf of *Ginkgo biloba* containing not less than 0.5% of flavonoids, calculated as flavone glycosides with reference to the dried drug. The leaf is greyish or yellowish-green or yellowish-brown.

USNF 20: The dried leaf of *Ginkgo biloba* (Ginkgoaceae). Protect from light and moisture.

Ginkgolides   (3033-n)

Ginkgolides A, B, and C (BN-52020, BN-52021, and BN-52022 respectively) are isolated from *Ginkgo biloba* (Ginkgoaceae) (see above).

Profile

An extract from the leaves of *Ginkgo biloba* has been used in cerebrovascular and peripheral vascular disorders. It is also being investigated in Alzheimer's disease and multi-infarct dementia.
Adverse effects include headaches, dizziness, palpitations, gastrointestinal disturbances, bleeding disorders, and skin hypersensitivity reactions.
Ginkgo biloba is used in homoeopathic medicine.
Ginkgolides are terpenoid molecules isolated from *Ginkgo biloba*, with platelet-activating factor (PAF) antagonist properties. They have been investigated as BN-52063, a mixture of ginkgolides A, B, and C, for asthma and other inflammatory and allergic disorders, and also in immune disorders such as endotoxic shock and graft rejection; ginkgolide B, which has the most potent PAF antagonist properties, has been investigated in similar conditions administered alone.
Other ginkgolides, including ginkgolide M (BN-52023) and ginkgolide J (BN-52024), have also been identified.

◊ References.
1. Braquet P. The ginkgolides: potent platelet- activating factor antagonists isolated from Ginkgo biloba L: chemistry, pharmacology and clinical applications. *Drugs Of The Future* 1987; **12:** 643–99.
2. Chung KF, *et al.* Effect of a ginkgolide mixture (BN 52063) in antagonising skin and platelet responses to platelet activating factor in man. *Lancet* 1987; **i:** 248–51.
3. Roberts NM, *et al.* Effect of a PAF antagonist, BN52063, on PAF-induced bronchoconstriction in normal subjects. *Br J Clin Pharmacol* 1988; **26:** 65–72.
4. Kleijnen J, Knipschild P. Ginkgo biloba. *Lancet* 1992; **340:** 1136–9.
5. Houghton P. Ginkgo. *Pharm J* 1994; **253:** 122–3.

Dementia. *Ginkgo biloba* extracts have been tried in the treatment of dementia including Alzheimer's disease (p.1412). Two meta-analyses[1,2] have found the extracts to be more effective than placebo but the authors of both analyses commented that further investigation is needed to establish any clinical value.
1. Oken BS, *et al.* The efficacy of ginkgo biloba on cognitive function in Alzheimer disease. *Arch Neurol* 1998; **55:** 1409–15.
2. Ernst E, Pittler MH. Ginkgo biloba for dementia: a systematic review of double-blind, placebo-controlled trials. *Clin Drug Invest* 1999; **17:** 301–8.

Preparations

Proprietary Preparations (details are given in Part 3)
Aust.: Ceremin; Tebofortan; Tebonin; *Austral.:* Proginkgo; *Braz.:* Equitam; Tanakan; Tebonin; *Fr.:* Ginkogink; Tanakan; Tramisal; *Ger.:* Duogink; Gingiloba; Gingium; Gingobeta; Gingopret;

Ginkobil; Ginkodilat; Ginkopur; Isoginkgo; Kaveri; Rokan; Tebonin; *Hong Kong:* Exormin; Tanakan; *Ital.:* Ginkoba; Novel Ginkgo; *Mex.:* Tanakan; Tebonin; Vasodil; *Neth.:* Tavonin; *Port.:* Abolibe; Biloban; Gincoben; Vasactife; *Singapore:* Ginexin-F; Ginkapran; Ginkosen; Oxivel; Tanakan; Tebokan; *Spain:* Normocir; Tanakene; *Switz.:* Geriaforce; Gingosol; Ginkoba; Oxivel; Symfona N; Tanakene; Tebofortin; Valverde Vitalite; *Thai.:* Tanakan; *UK:* Ginkovital; Mentor; *USA:* BioGinkgo.

Multi-ingredient: *Austral.:* Bilberry Plus Eye Health; Bioglan Fingers & Toes†; Bioglan Vision-Eze; Bioglan Zellulean with Escin; Extralife Extra-Brite; Extralife Eye-Care; Extralife Leg-Care; Eye Health Herbal Plus Formula 4; For Peripheral Circulation Herbal Plus Formula 5; Gingo A; Ginkgo ACE†; Ginkgo Biloba Plus; Ginkgo Complex; Ginkgo Plus Herbal Plus Formula 10; Ginzing G; Herbal Arthritis Formula; Herbal Capillary Care; Lifechange Circulation Aid; Lifechange Multi Plus Antioxidant; Lifesystem Herbal Plus Formula 6 For Peripheral Circulation; Lifesystem Herbal Plus Formula 11 Ginkgo; Lifesystem Herbal Plus Formula 5 Eye Relief; Prophthal; Vig; *Fr.:* Ginkor; Ginkor Fort; Ginkor Procto†; *Ger.:* Perivar; Veno-Tebonin N; *Hong Kong:* Ginkor Fort; *Ital.:* Alvear Sport†; Enertonic; Forticrin; Ginkgo Plus; Ginkoftal; Memorandum; Nosenil†; Nutrex†; Pik-Gel; Pollingel con Ginkgo Biloba; Vasobrain; *Switz.:* Allium Plus; Arterosan Plus; Gincosan; *Thai.:* Ginkor Fort.

Ginseng   (12784-h)

Ginseng Radix; Jintsam; Ninjin; Panax; Pannag; Schinsent.

Pharmacopoeias. In *Chin.*, *Eur.* (see p.vi), and *Jpn*. Also in *USNF* as Asian Ginseng. *USNF* also includes Powdered Asian Ginseng and Powdered Asian Ginseng Extract. *Jpn* also includes Red Ginseng, the dried root which has been steamed.
Chin. and *Jpn* also include Rhizoma Panacis Japonica from *Panax japonicus*. *Chin.* also includes Radix Notoginseng from *P. notoginseng*, and Rhizoma Panacis Majoris from *P. japonicus* var. *major* and *P. japonicus* var. *bipinnatifidus.*

The dried root of *Panax ginseng* (= *P. schinseng*) (Araliaceae). Other varieties of ginseng include *Panax quinquefolium* (North America) and *P. pseudoginseng*. The root commonly known as Siberian or Russian ginseng belongs to the same family, Araliaceae, but is an entirely different plant, *Eleutherococcus senticosis*. Ginseng contains complex mixtures of saponins termed ginsenosides or panaxosides. At least 13 saponins have been isolated from extracts of *P. ginseng* roots.

Pharmacopoeial description

Ph. Eur.: The whole or cut dried root of *Panax ginseng*. It contains not less than 0.4% of combined ginsenosides, $Rg1$ ($C_{42}H_{72}O_{14}$,$2H_2O = 837.0$) and $Rb1$ ($C_{54}H_{92}O_{23}$,$3H_2O = 1163.3$), calculated with reference to the dried drug. Protect from light.

USNF 20: Asian Ginseng consists of the dried roots of *Panax ginseng* (Araliaceae). Store in a dry place at a temperature of 8° to 15°.

◊ Some material supplied as Siberian ginseng may be *Periploca sepium* (Asclepiadaceae), a plant unrelated to either *Panax ginseng* or *Eleutherococcus senticosis*, due to the similarity of the Chinese names for these plants.[1] Brazilian ginseng is reported to be derived from another unrelated plant, *Pfaffia paniculata*.[2]
1. Awang DVC. Maternal use of ginseng and neonatal androgenization. *JAMA* 1991; **266:** 363.
2. Walker AF. What is in ginseng? *Lancet* 1994; **344:** 619.

Profile

Ginseng is reported to enhance the natural resistance and recuperative power of the body and to reduce fatigue. Its toxicity at usual dosages appears to be low. It is available commercially as roots, powdered roots, tablets, capsules, teas, oils, or extracts. Siberian or Russian ginseng is used similarly.

Adverse effects. A 2-year study[1] of ginseng in 133 subjects who had used a wide variety of commercial preparations including roots, capsules, tablets, teas, extracts, cigarettes, chewing gum, and candies reported that the majority of preparations were taken by mouth, but a few subjects had experimented with intranasal or parenteral routes, and topical preparations had also been used. The stimulant effects of ginseng were confirmed but there was also a high incidence of side-effects including 47 cases of morning diarrhoea, 33 of skin eruptions, 26 of sleeplessness, 25 of nervousness, 22 of hypertension, 18 of euphoria, and 14 of oedema. The 'ginseng abuse syndrome' defined as hypertension together with nervousness, sleeplessness, skin eruptions, and morning diarrhoea was experienced by 14 subjects who took ginseng by mouth in an average daily dose of 3 g. Abrupt withdrawal precipitated hypotension, weakness, and tremor in 1 user. About 50% of the subjects had discontinued the use of ginseng within the 2 years.
Oestrogenic effects have also been reported from the use of ginseng,[2-4] and a case of Stevens-Johnson syndrome has also occurred.[5]
1. Siegel RK. Ginseng abuse syndrome: problems with the panacea. *JAMA* 1979; **241:** 1614–15.
2. Palmer BV, *et al.* Gin Seng and mastalgia. *BMJ* 1978; **1:** 1284.
3. Punnonen R, Lukola A. Oestrogen-like effect of ginseng. *BMJ* 1980; **281:** 1110.
4. Greenspan EM. Ginseng and vaginal bleeding. *JAMA* 1983; **249:** 2018.
5. Dega H, *et al.* Ginseng as a cause for Stevens-Johnson syndrome? *Lancet* 1996; **347:** 1344.

Interactions. For a report of raised serum-digoxin concentrations in a patient taking *digoxin* and Siberian ginseng, see p.872. For details of an interaction between *warfarin* and ginseng, see p.997.

Preparations

Proprietary Preparations (details are given in Part 3)
Aust.: Ginsana; *Austral.:* Ginzing; Herbal Stress Relief; *Braz.:* Ginsana; *Canad.:* Ginsana; *Fr.:* Gerimax; Ginsana; Ginsatonic†; *Ger.:* Ardey-aktiv; Eleu-Kokk; Eleutheroforce; Eleutherokokk; Eleutherokokk-Aktiv-Kapseln SenticoMega†; Gerivit†; Ginroy†; Ginsana; Herz-Punkt Starkungstonikum mit Ginseng N; Hevert-Aktivon Mono†; Kneipp Ginsenetten†; Konstitutin; Lebensenergie-Kapseln; Orgaplasma; Vital-Kapseln; *Ital.:* Gi-Sen; Ginsana; Novel 1000; *Mex.:* Gincaps; *Port.:* Ginsana; Vitalisan†; *S.Afr.:* Ginsana; *Singapore:* Ginsana; *Spain:* Bio Star; Ginsana; *Switz.:* Eleu-Kokk; Ginsana; *Thai.:* Ginsana; Ginsroy; *UK:* Elagen; Korseng; Red Kooga.

Multi-ingredient: *Austral.:* Bioglan Ginsynergy; Extralife Extra-Brite; Gingo A; Ginkgo Biloba Plus; Ginkgo Complex; Ginzing E; Ginzing G; Glycyrrhiza Complex; Infant Tonic; Irontona; Medinat Esten; Nervatona Plus; Panax Complex; Trillium Complex; Tyroseng; Vig; Vitatona; *Fr.:* Actisane Fatigue Passagere†; Tonactil; Tonisan†; *Ger.:* Alsiroyal†; Cardibisana; Ginseng-Complex "Schuh"; Hypercard; Peking Ginseng Royal Jelly N; Schwedentrunk mit Ginseng†; *Ital.:* Apergan; Bio-Real Complex†; Bio-Real Plus†; Bioton; Cocktail Reale; Enertonic; Fitostress; Fon Wan Eleuthero; Fon Wan Ginsenergy; Fon Wan Pocket Energy†; Fon Wan Pollen; Forticrin; Fosfarsile Forte; Four-Ton; Gincola†; Neoplus; Nosenil†; Nutrex†; Ottovis; Vitalmix; *S.Afr.:* Activex 40 Plus; *Spain:* Farmacola; Minadex Mix Ginseng; Ton Was; Vigortonic; *Switz.:* Biorganic Geri; Biovital Ginseng; Gincosan; Imuvit; Tai Ginseng N; Vigoran; *Thai.:* Imugins; Imuvit; Multilim RG; Revitan; *UK:* Red Kooga Co-Q-10 and Ginseng; Regina Royal Concorde.

Glatiramer Acetate (6806-p)

Glatiramer Acetate (BAN, USAN).

COP-1; Copolymer 1. L-Glutamic acid polymer with L-alanine, L-lysine and L-tyrosine, acetate.

CAS — 28704-27-0; 147245-92-9.
ATC — L04AA07.

Adverse Effects and Precautions

The most commonly seen side-effects following injection of glatiramer acetate are chest pain, palpitations or tachycardia, dyspnoea, asthenia, flushing (vasodilatation), nausea, arthralgia, hypertonia, and anxiety. Many of these occur as an immediate post-injection reaction. Convulsions and anaphylactoid reactions have been reported rarely. Antibodies to the drug develop with chronic therapy but are of unknown clinical significance. Pain, erythema, pruritus, and induration may occur at the injection site.

Glatiramer acetate should be given with caution to patients with pre-existing cardiac disorders; such patients should be followed up regularly during treatment.

Effects on the skin. Localised lipoatrophy at the injection site developed in 6 patients receiving glatiramer acetate treatment.[1]

1. Drago F, *et al.* Localized lipoatrophy after glatiramer acetate injection in patients with remitting-relapsing multiple sclerosis. *Arch Dermatol* 1999; **135:** 1277–8.

Interactions

The UK manufacturer reports that an increased incidence of injection-site reactions to glatiramer acetate has been seen in patients receiving corticosteroids concurrently.

Uses and Administration

Glatiramer acetate, a random polymer of L-alanine, L-glutamic acid, L-lysine, and L-tyrosine, is a peptide which has some structural resemblance to myelin basic protein, and is used to reduce the frequency of relapses in the management of relapsing-remitting multiple sclerosis (p.633). It is administered by subcutaneous injection in a dose of 20 mg daily. It should not be given by the intravenous route. An oral formulation is under investigation.

Multiple sclerosis. References.

1. Johnson KP, *et al.* Copolymer 1 reduces relapse rate and improves disability in relapsing-remitting multiple sclerosis: results of a phase III multicenter, double-blind, placebo-controlled study. *Neurology* 1995; **45:** 1268–76.
2. Anonymous. Glatiramer acetate for relapsing multiple sclerosis. *Med Lett Drugs Ther* 1997; **39:** 61–2.
3. Johnson KP, *et al.* Extended use of glatiramer acetate (Copaxone) is well tolerated and maintains its clinical effect on multiple sclerosis relapse rate and degree of disability. *Neurology* 1998; **50:** 701–8.
4. Ge Y, *et al.* Glatiramer acetate (copaxone) treatment in relapsing-remitting MS: quantitative MR assessment. *Neurology* 2000; **54:** 813–17.

Preparations

Proprietary Preparations (details are given in Part 3)
Austral.: Copaxone; *Canad.:* Copaxone; *Israel:* Copaxone; *Switz.:* Copaxone; *UK:* Copaxone; *USA:* Copaxone.

Glicofosfopeptical (3905-w)

Fosfoglicopeptical.

Profile

Glicofosfopeptical is reported to possess immunostimulant properties and has been given in doses of 1 g by mouth every eight hours.

Preparations

Proprietary Preparations (details are given in Part 3)
Mex.: Inmunoferon; Inmunol; *Port.:* Imunoferon; *Spain:* Inmunoferon.

Glucomannan (16823-h)

Konjac Flour; Konjac Mannan.

Profile

Glucomannan, a powdered extract from the tubers of *Amorphophallus konjac,* has been promoted as an anorectic. It has been claimed to reduce the appetite by absorbing liquid in the gastrointestinal tract. It is also used in the treatment of constipation and hyperlipidaemia. Glucomannan has been investigated as a dietary adjunct in the management of diabetes mellitus.

There is a risk of intestinal or oesophageal obstruction and faecal impaction, especially if it is swallowed dry. Therefore, it should always be taken with sufficient fluid and should not be taken immediately before going to bed. It should be avoided in patients who have difficulty swallowing.

◊ References.

1. Henry DA, *et al.* Glucomannan and risk of oesophageal obstruction. *BMJ* 1986; **292:** 591–2.
2. Renard E, *et al.* Noninsulin-dependent diabetes and glucose intolerance: effect of glucomannan fibre on blood glucose and serum insulin. *Sem Hop Paris* 1991; **67:** 153–7.
3. Vuksan V, *et al.* Beneficial effects of viscous dietary fiber from konjac-mannan in subjects with the insulin resistance syndrome: results of a controlled metabolic trial. *Diabetes Care* 2000; **23:** 9–14.
4. Staiano A, *et al.* Effect of the dietary fiber glucomannan on chronic constipation in neurologically impaired children. *J Pediatr* 2000; **136:** 41–5.

Preparations

Proprietary Preparations (details are given in Part 3)
Fr.: Konjax†; Muraligne; *Ital.:* Dicoplus; Dietoman; NormaLine; *Mex.:* Dietoman; Esbeltex; *Port.:* Bioregime; Florilax.

Multi-ingredient: *Fr.:* AMK; *Ital.:* Dimalosio; Ecamannan; Fibrovit; Glucoman; Lacomannan; *Port.:* Bioregime Fort.

Glucosamine (12790-d)

Glucosamine (USAN, rINN).

Chitosamine; NSC-758. 2-Amino-2-deoxy-β-D-glucopyranose.
$C_6H_{13}NO_5 = 179.2$.
CAS — 3416-24-8.
ATC — M01AX05.

Glucosamine is found in chitin, mucoproteins, and mucopolysaccharides; it is isolated from chitin or prepared synthetically.

Profile

Glucosamine is a natural substance found in cartilage, tendons, and ligament tissues; it is also involved in the manufacture of glycosaminoglycan, which forms most of the cartilage tissue. Glucosamine must be synthesised by the body and the ability to do this declines with age. For this reason, its salts, glucosamine sulfate and hydriodide, have been given in the treatment of rheumatic disorders including osteoarthritis (p.9).

Osteoarthritis. A systematic review[1] of the use of glucosamine for osteoarthritis has concluded that it is generally both safe and superior to placebo, but that further research is still necessary to confirm its long-term value, and particularly its long-term toxicity.

1. Towheed TE, *et al.* Glucosamine therapy for treating osteoarthritis (updated 25 April 2001). Available in The Cochrane Library; Issue 4. Oxford: Update Software; 2001.

Preparations

Proprietary Preparations (details are given in Part 3)
Ger.: Dona 200-S; Progona; *Hong Kong:* Viartril; *Ital.:* Dona; Viartril S; *Port.:* Viartril S; *Spain:* Hespercorbin; Xicil; *Thai.:* Viartril.

Multi-ingredient: *Austral.:* Bioglan Joint Mobility; *Ital.:* Artrosan; *Spain:* Anartril†; *UK:* Healtheries Musseltone & Glucosamine.

Glucose Oxidase (10555-t)

Corylophyline; β-D-Glucopyranose aerodehydrogenase; Microcide; Notatin; P-FAD.
CAS — 9001-37-0.

Profile

Glucose oxidase is an enzyme obtained from certain fungi which catalyses the oxidation of glucose to gluconic acid, with the concomitant production of hydrogen peroxide. It is used for its preservative properties as an additive in certain foods, sometimes in combination with catalase (p.1592). It is also used in fertility tests and tests of diabetic control. It has been used as an

ingredient of toothpastes for its supposed benefits in the prophylaxis of dental caries.

Preparations

Proprietary Preparations (details are given in Part 3)
Multi-ingredient: *Singapore:* Biotene.

Glucose Tests (1958-q)

Profile

Several tests are available so that patients with diabetes mellitus (p.315) can monitor their disease. Tests can be employed to detect the presence of glucose in the urine and some of the preparations are used to detect several substances in the urine. These tests are easy to carry out but are not considered reliable enough for insulin-dependent patients who should ideally check their blood-glucose concentrations using one of the available blood tests. Diabetic clinics often measure the degree of haemoglobin glycosylation as an indicator of mean blood-glucose control over a period of weeks.

Urine tests generally employ either the copper-reduction method or the glucose-oxidase method and both methods produce a colour change in the presence of glucose. Blood tests generally employ the glucose-oxidase method; they may be read visually or by means of a meter. A meter gives the more precise reading. Patients should be properly trained in the use of these tests and in the interpretation of the results; they should be aware that concomitant drug therapy might affect the result.

Preparations

USP 25: Glucose Enzymatic Test Strip.

Proprietary Preparations (details are given in Part 3)
Austral.: Accutrend Glucose; Advantage; Betachek; BM-Test BG; BM-Test Glycemie 20-800; Clinistix; Clinitest; Diabur-Test 5000; Diascreen 1G; Diastix; Esprit; Exatech; Excel ET; Glucofilm; Glucometer; Glucostix; Glucostrip; Glucotrend; Medi-Test Glucose; Precision Plus; Tes-Tape; *Braz.:* Glico-Fita; *Canad.:* Accu-Check III/Chemstrip bG†; Accutrend GC; Advantage; Chemstrip bG†; Chemstrip uG; Clinistix†; Clinitest; Companion 2†; Diastix; Easy Strip†; Glucofilm†; Glucostix†; Tes-Tape; *Fr.:* Accu-Chek†; BM-Test Glycemie; Clinistix; Clinitest; Dextrostix†; Glucofilm†; Glucostix†; Glucotide; One Touch; Tracer Glucose†; *Irl.:* BM-Accutest; BM-Test 1-44; Clinistix; Clinitest; Dextrostix†; Diabur-Test 5000; Diastix; Glucomen; Glucostix; Glucotide; Glucotrend; Hypoguard; Medisense; One Touch; PocketScan; Tes-Tape; *Israel:* Clinistix; Clinitest; *Ital.:* Accutrend Glucose; BM-Test BG; Clinistix; Clinitest; Dextrostix†; Diabur-Test 5000; Diastix; Glico Test†; Glico Urine B†; Glucofilm; Glucometer; Glucosan; Glucostix; Glukurtest; Haemoglukotest 20-800; Reflocheck; Tes-Tape; *Mex.:* Accutrend Glucose; Clinitest; Dextrostix; Diabur-Test 5000; Diastix; Glucostix; Glucotide; Haemo-Glukotest 20-800; *NZ:* Accutrend Glucose; Advantage; BM-Test 1-44; Clinistix; Clinitest; Diabur-5000; Diastix; Exatech; Glucocard; Glucofilm; Glucometer Elite; Glucometer Esprit; Glucostix; Precision Plus; Tes-Tape; *Port.:* Clinistix; Elite; Euroflash; Glucostix; Glucotouch; One Touch; *S.Afr.:* Tes-Tape†; *Switz.:* Tes-Tape; *UK:* BM-Accutest; BM-Test 1-44; BM-Test BG; Clinistix; Clinitest; Dextrostix†; Diabur-Test 5000; Diastix; Easistix BG; Easistix UG; Exactech; Glucostix; Glucotide; Hypoguard GA; Medi-Test Glucose; Medi-Test Glycaemie C; Medisense G2; *USA:* Accu-Check Advantage; Biotel diabetes†; Chemstrip bG; Chemstrip uG; Clinistix; Clinitest; Dextrostix; Diascan; Diastix; First Choice; Glucofilm; Glucostix; One Touch; Tracer bG†.

Gluten (12792-h)

A mixture of 2 proteins, gliadin and glutenin, present in wheat flour and to a lesser extent in barley and rye. Gliadin is a prolamine, one of the 2 chief groups of plant proteins, and glutenin belongs to the other main group termed glutelins.

Profile

Gluten is of medicinal and pharmaceutical interest in that patients with coeliac disease (p.1350) are sensitive to the gliadin fraction of gluten contained in the normal diet. Treatment consists of the use of gluten-free diets; gluten-free foods are available.

A gluten-free diet may also be beneficial in patients with dermatitis herpetiformis (p.1104).

Glycerol (1901-y)

Glycerol (rINN).

E422; Glicerol; Glycerin; Glycerine; Glycerolum. Propane-1,2,3-triol.
$C_3H_8O_3 = 92.09$.
CAS — 56-81-5.
ATC — A06AG04; A06AX01.
Pharmacopoeias. In *Chin., Eur.* (see p.vi), *Int., Jpn,* and *US.*
Eur. and *Int.* also include Glycerol (85 per cent).
Pol. includes Glycerol (86 per cent).

Strong oxidising agents form explosive mixtures with glycerol. Black discoloration has been reported with glycerol and bismuth subnitrate or zinc oxide when exposed to light.

Pharmacopoeial description

Ph. Eur.: A clear, colourless or almost colourless, very hygroscopic, syrupy liquid, unctuous to the touch. Miscible with water and with alcohol; slightly soluble in acetone; practically insoluble in ether, in fixed oils, and in essential oils. Store in airtight containers.

USP 25: A clear, colourless, hygroscopic, syrupy liquid. Has not more than a slight characteristic odour, which is neither harsh nor disagreeable. Miscible with water and with alcohol; insoluble in chloroform, in ether, and in fixed and volatile oils. Its solutions are neutral to litmus. Store in airtight containers.

Adverse Effects and Precautions

The adverse effects of glycerol are primarily due to its dehydrating action.

When taken by mouth glycerol may cause headache, nausea, and vomiting; less frequently diarrhoea, thirst, dizziness, and mental confusion can occur. Cardiac arrhythmias have been reported.

Glycerol increases plasma osmolality resulting in the withdrawal of water from the extravascular spaces. The consequent expansion of extracellular fluid, especially if sudden, can lead to circulatory overload, pulmonary oedema, and heart failure; glycerol must therefore be used with caution in patients at risk, such as those with hypervolaemia, cardiac failure, or renal disease. Severe dehydration can occur and glycerol should be used cautiously in dehydrated patients. Patients with diabetes mellitus may additionally develop hyperglycaemia and glycosuria following metabolism of glycerol. Nonketotic hyperosmolar hyperglycaemic coma is rare, but fatalities have been reported.

Haemolysis, haemoglobinuria, and acute renal failure have also been associated with glycerol when administered intravenously (see Raised Intracranial Pressure, below).

Glycerol can cause irritation when given topically or rectally. A local anaesthetic may be used before application of glycerol to the cornea to reduce the likelihood of a painful response.

For incompatibilities with glycerol, including the risk of explosive mixtures, see above.

Effects on the cardiovascular system. A 73-year-old man, free of cardiac complaints but who had previously experienced an acute myocardial infarction, developed severe pulmonary oedema following the administration of glycerol by mouth for elevated intra-ocular pressure.[1] The necessity for detailed cardiac evaluation before the use of oral glycerol was emphasised.

1. Almog Y, et al. Pulmonary edema as a complication of oral glycerol administration. Ann Ophthalmol 1986; 18: 38–9.

Effects on the ears. A report of temporary hearing loss in the noninvolved ear of a 56-year-old man following the ingestion of 100 mL of glycerol and 100 mL of sodium chloride 0,9% as part of a glycerol test for Ménière's disease, and a review of two previous reports associating the glycerol test with a deterioration in hearing.[1]

1. Mattox DE, Goode RL. Temporary loss of hearing after a glycerin test. Arch Otolaryngol 1978; 104: 359–61.

Effects on the eyes. Studies in animals[1] and in man[2] have indicated that the topical application of glycerol to the eye can damage the endothelial cells of the cornea. Caution in applying glycerol to the cornea has been recommended.

1. Sherrard ES. The corneal endothelium in vivo: its response to mild trauma. Exp Eye Res 1976; 22: 347–57.
2. Goldberg MH, et al. The effects of topically applied glycerin on the human corneal endothelium. Cornea 1982; 1: 39–44.

Hyperosmolar nonketotic coma. Hyperosmolar nonketotic coma has been associated with the administration of glycerol by mouth[1] and deaths have occurred.[2] The most susceptible patients are maturity-onset elderly diabetics with acute or chronic disease predisposing to fluid deprivation, and in these patients oral glycerol may be best avoided.[1] If glycerol is used in patients with predisposing conditions, adequate measures should be taken to recognise the development of hyperosmolar nonketotic hyperglycaemia and prevent dehydration.[1,2]

1. Oakley DE, Ellis PP. Glycerol and hyperosmolar nonketotic coma. Am J Ophthalmol 1976; 81: 469–72.
2. Sears ES. Nonketotic hyperosmolar hyperglycemia during glycerol therapy for cerebral edema. Neurology 1976; 26: 89–94.

Pharmacokinetics

Glycerol is readily absorbed from the gastrointestinal tract and undergoes extensive metabolism, principally in the liver; it may be used in the synthesis of lipids, metabolised to glucose or glycogen, or oxidised to carbon dioxide and water. It may also be excreted in the urine unchanged.

◊ References.
1. Nahata MC, et al. Variations in glycerol kinetics in Reye's syndrome. Clin Pharmacol Ther 1981; 29: 782–7.
2. Heinemeyer G. Clinical pharmacokinetic considerations in the treatment of increased intracranial pressure. Clin Pharmacokinet 1987; 13: 1–25.

Uses and Administration

Glycerol is an osmotic dehydrating agent with hygroscopic and lubricating properties. When administered by mouth or parenterally, glycerol increases the plasma osmolality, resulting in the movement of water by osmosis from the extravascular spaces into the plasma.

Glycerol is given by mouth for the short-term reduction of vitreous volume and intra-ocular pressure before and after ophthalmic surgery, and as an adjunct in the management of acute glaucoma (p.1413). Its onset of action is rapid, with a maximal reduction in intra-ocular pressure occurring approximately 1 to 1½ hours after administration; the duration of action is about 5 hours. The usual initial dose of glycerol is 1 to 1.5 g per kg body-weight, administered as a 50% or 75% solution; further

The symbol † denotes a preparation no longer actively marketed

doses of 0.5 g per kg may be given if necessary. There can be problems of palatability when glycerol solutions are given by mouth; chilling or flavouring the solutions may help.

Glycerol may be applied topically to reduce corneal oedema, but as the effect is only transient its use is primarily limited to facilitating ocular examination and diagnosis. Glycerol eye drops can be painful on instillation and the prior application of a local anaesthetic has been recommended.

Glycerol has also been given by mouth or intravenously to reduce intracranial pressure (see below).

Glycerol may be administered rectally as suppositories or a solution in single doses to promote faecal evacuation in the management of constipation (p.1202). It usually acts within 15 to 30 minutes. Glycerol is commonly classified as an osmotic laxative but may act additionally or alternatively through its local irritant effects; it may also have lubricating and faecal softening actions.

Glycerol is used as a demulcent in cough preparations (p.1082).

Glycerol has a wide range of applications in pharmaceutical formulation; these include its use as a vehicle and solvent, as a sweetening agent, as a preservative in some liquid medications, as a plasticiser in tablet film-coating, and as a tonicity adjuster. It is often included in topical preparations such as eye drops, creams, and lotions as a lubricant and also for its moisturising properties since, when absorbed, its hygroscopic action may enhance moisture retention. Ear drops for the removal of ear wax often contain glycerol as a lubricating and softening agent.

Glycerol is also used as a cryoprotectant in cryopreservation.

Diagnosis of Ménière's disease. Glycerol has been used in the diagnosis of Ménière's disease (p.407), although the test can have problems.[1] The aim is to distinguish potentially reversible cochlear dysfunction from the relatively irreversible pathology found in the advanced stages of the disease or to predict the hearing results following endolymphatic sac surgery. The test involves the administration of glycerol by mouth to reduce the endolymphatic fluid volume and pressure and the measurement of any transient improvement in hearing. However, the side-effects of glycerol such as headache, nausea, and vomiting can be a problem and the test has been reported to have low sensitivity and to give false-positive results. See also under Effects on the Ears under Adverse Effects, above.

1. Skalabrin TA, Mangham CA. Analysis of the glycerin test for Meniere's disease. Otolaryngol Head Neck Surg 1987; 96: 282–8.

Raised intracranial pressure. Glycerol has been given intravenously or by mouth for its osmotic diuretic effect to reduce cerebral oedema and hence decrease the intracranial pressure (p.811). It is also reported to be able to increase blood flow to areas of brain ischaemia. It has been used in a variety of clinical conditions[1] including cerebral infarction or stroke,[2] Reye's syndrome,[3] and meningitis;[4] it has been reported to be ineffective in hepatic coma.[5] Some patients have experienced serious adverse effects including haemolysis, haemoglobinuria, and renal failure.[6,7]

1. Frank MSB, et al. Glycerol: a review of its pharmacology, pharmacokinetics, adverse reactions, and clinical use. Pharmacotherapy 1981; 1: 147–60.
2. Righetti E, et al. Glycerol for acute stroke (updated 12 February 2001). Available in The Cochrane Library; Issue 4. Oxford: Update Software; 2001.
3. Nahata MC, et al. Variations in glycerol kinetics in Reye's syndrome. Clin Pharmacol Ther 1981; 29: 782–7.
4. Kilpi T, et al. Oral glycerol and intravenous dexamethasone in preventing neurologic and audiologic sequelae of childhood bacterial meningitis. Pediatr Infect Dis J 1995; 14: 270–8.
5. Record CO, et al. Glycerol therapy for cerebral oedema complicating fulminant hepatic failure. BMJ 1975; ii: 540.
6. Hägnevik K, et al. Glycerol-induced haemolysis with haemoglobinuria and acute renal failure: report of three cases. Lancet 1974; i: 75–7.
7. Welch KMA, et al. Glycerol-induced haemolysis. Lancet 1974; i: 416–17.

Trigeminal neuralgia. Selective destruction of pain-bearing nerves is reserved for patients who do not respond to conventional drug therapy for trigeminal neuralgia (p.8). This may be achieved by the instillation of glycerol among the trigeminal rootlets (percutaneous retrogasserian glycerol rhizolysis).[1-5] The efficacy and safety of this procedure have been debated,[1,4] but some centres report good long-term results in the majority of patients.[5] It has been suggested that variations in viscosity and osmolality may influence results.[2]

1. Sweet WH. The treatment of trigeminal neuralgia (tic douloureux). N Engl J Med 1986; 315: 174–7.
2. Waltz TA, Copeland BR. Treatment of trigeminal neuralgia. N Engl J Med 1987; 316: 693.
3. Young RF. Glycerol rhizolysis for treatment of trigeminal neuralgia. J Neurosurg 1988; 69: 39–45.
4. Burchiel KJ. Percutaneous retrogasserian glycerol rhizolysis in the management of trigeminal neuralgia. J Neurosurg 1988; 69: 361–6.
5. Jho H-D, Lunsford LD. Percutaneous retrogasserian glycerol rhizotomy: current technique and results. Neurosurg Clin N Am 1997; 8: 63–74.

Preparations

BP 2001: Glycerol Suppositories; Phenol and Glycerol Injection; *USP 25:* Calamine Lotion; Glycerin Ophthalmic Solution; Glycerin Oral Solution; Glycerin Suppositories.

Proprietary Preparations (details are given in Part 3)
Aust.: Babylax†; *Austral.:* Bausch & Lomb Computer Eye Drops; *Canad.:* Alpha Keri; Gly-Rectal; *Fr.:* Bebegel; Glycerotone; *Ger.:* Babylax†; Glycerosteril; Glycilax; Milax; Nene-Lax; *Hong Kong:* Glyceol; *Irl.:* Babylax; *Israel:* Minilax; Marco Viti; Microclismi Sella; Verolax; *Jpn:* Glyceol; *Mex.:* BB Fleet; Neutro Bar; Supositorios Senosiain; *Port.:* Bebegel; Rectiole; *S.Afr.:* Regard; *Singapore:* Fleet Babylax; *Spain:* Adulax; Gely; Glicerotens; Supo Gliz; Supo Kristal†; Vitrosups; *Switz.:* Bulboid; Cristal†; Practomil; *Thai.:* Glyceol; Glycerosteril; *UAE:* Laxolyne; *UK:* Neutrogena Norwegian Formula Dermatological Cream; Tixylix Baby Syrup; *USA:* Computer Eye Drops; Dry Eye Therapy†; Eye-Lube-A; Fleet Babylax; Glyrol†; Listermint Arctic Mint Mouthwash; Ophthalgan; Osmoglyn; Sani-Supp.

Multi-ingredient: *Austral.:* Aci-Jel; Anusol; Auralgan; Body Lotion; Cleansing Lotion; Egopsoryl TA; Egozite Baby Cream; Egozite Cream†; Hamilton Dry Skin; Magnoplasm; Murine Contact; Nutrasorb†; *Belg.:* Laxavit; *Braz.:* Bluderm; Narizima Adulto; Narizima Pediatrico; Pasta d'Agua; *Canad.:* Agarol Plain; Agarol†; Auralgan; Bronchex; Bronchisaft†; Collyrium†; Epi-Lyt; Moisture Drops; Rhinedrine Moisturizing; Swim-Ear; Tucks; *Denm.:* Glyoktyl; Pectyl; *Fr.:* Aloplastine; Charlieu Topicrem; Dexeryl; Glyco-Thymoline; Pharmatex; Rectopanbiline; Scleremo; *Ger.:* Lacrisic; Norgalax Miniklistier; Pero; Zinksalbe; *Hong Kong:* Aderma Dermalibour; Aderma Exomega; Baby Cough with Antihistamine; Ego Skin Cream; *Irl.:* Micolette; *Israel:* Kamil Blue; Lubrin; Microlet; Taro Gel; *Ital.:* Dropyal; Evasen Dischetti; Glicerolax; Microclisma Evacuante AD-BB; Naturalass; Novilax; Salviette H; Solecin; *Mex.:* Nutrasorb; *NZ:* Aci-Jel; Karicare Breast Care; Karicare Ointment; Rosken Skin Repair; Silic; *Port.:* Antiacneicos Niacex; Dagragel; Hidratante; Ureadin Facial; Ureadin Maos; *Singapore:* Egozite; Topicrem; Tropex; *Switz.:* Neo-Decongestine; Realderm; *Thai.:* Baby Cough Syrup; Baby Cough with Antihistamine; Tussis; *UK:* Allens Junior Cough; Codella; Collins Elixir Pastilles†; Earex Plus; Honey & Molasses; Imuderm; Jackson's Lemon Linctus; Jackson's Troublesome Coughs; Lemsip Cough & Cold Dry Cough; Lockets; Lockets Medicated Linctus; Melissin; Meltus Honey & Lemon; Micolette; Relaxit; Swim-Ear; Throaties Family Cough Linctus†; *USA:* Aci-Jel; Allergen; Astroglide; Auralgan; Clearasil Antibacterial; Collyrium Fresh; Dermasil†; Entertainer's Secret; Epi-Lyt; Hemorid For Women; Lubrin; Maxilube; Moisture Drops; N'ice; Numzit; Surgel; Swim-Ear; Therevac Plus; Therevac SB; Trimo-San; Triple Care Cleanser†; Tucks.

Glycerophosphoric Acid   (1935-d)

Glycerylphosphoric Acid; Monoglycerylphosphoric Acid.
$C_3H_9O_6P = 172.1$.
CAS — 27082-31-1; 57-03-4 (α-form); 17181-54-3 (β-form); 5746-57-6 (L-α-form); 1509-81-5 (DL-α-form).

Profile
Glycerophosphoric acid and various glycerophosphates have been used in tonics. They were once considered as a suitable means of providing phosphorus. Calcium and magnesium glycerophosphates (see p.1188 and p.1191, respectively) may be considered as a source of calcium or magnesium.

◊ References to the use of sodium glycerophosphate as a source of phosphorus in infant parenteral nutrition.[1]

1. Costello I, et al. Sodium glycerophosphate in the treatment of neonatal hypophosphataemia. Arch Dis Child 1995; 73: F44–5.

Preparations

Proprietary Preparations (details are given in Part 3)
Aust.: Glycophos; *Fin.:* Glycophos; *Neth.:* Glycophos†; *Port.:* Glycophos; *Swed.:* Glycophos; *Switz.:* Glycophos.

Multi-ingredient: *Belg.:* Verrulyse-Methionine†; *Fr.:* Biotone; Ionyl; Phosphore-Sandoz†; Verrulyse-Methionine; *Israel:* Babyzim; *Ital.:* Calciofix; Glicero-Valerovit; Neuroftal; Neurol; *S.Afr.:* Nervade.

Glyceryl Palmitostearate   (17666-y)

A mixture of mono-, di-, and triglycerides of C_{16} and C_{18} fatty acids.
CAS — 8067-32-1.

Profile
Glyceryl palmitostearate is used in pharmaceutical manufacturing as a diluent and lubricant for tablets and capsules.

Gold   (5292-y)

E175.
Au = 196.96655.
CAS — 7440-57-5.

A bright-yellow, malleable, and ductile metal; the finely divided powder may be black, ruby, or purple.

Profile
The main use of metallic gold in health care is now in dentistry. Gold may also be employed as a colouring agent for some foodstuffs. In the treatment of rheumatoid arthritis, gold is used in the form of compounds such as auranofin (p.18), aurothioglucose (p.18), and sodium aurothiomalate (p.82). The radionuclide gold-198 is described in the chapter on radiopharma-

ceuticals (p.1449). There have been rare reports of hypersensitivity reactions to metallic gold.

Gold is used (as Aurum or Aurum Met.) in homoeopathic medicine. Gold salts are also used in homoeopathy.

◊ References.
1. Merchant B. Gold, the noble metal and the paradoxes of its toxicology. *Biologicals* 1998; **26:** 49–59.

Preparations
Proprietary Preparations (details are given in Part 3)
USA: Aurasol†.

Multi-ingredient: *Ger.:* Cefossin H.

Gossypol (12798-p)

2,2′-Bis(1,6,7-trihydroxy-3-methyl-5-isopropylnaphthalene-8-carboxaldehyde).
$C_{30}H_{30}O_8 = 518.6$.
$CAS — 303-45-7$.

Gossypol is a pigment extracted from cottonseed oil (p.1599).

Profile
Gossypol possesses antispermatogenic activity and has been studied, especially in China, as a male contraceptive. It has also been investigated for its antineoplastic, antiprotozoal, antiviral, and spermicidal activity and has been studied in women in the treatment of certain gynaecological disorders.

Side-effects have included fatigue, changes in appetite, gastrointestinal effects, burning sensation of the face and hands, some loss of libido, and persistent oligospermia. Hypokalaemia has occurred.

◊ The pharmacology and therapeutic potential of gossypol have been reviewed.[1] Although controlled studies[2,3] have shown gossypol to be an effective male contraceptive, WHO concluded[4] that gossypol would not be acceptable as a male antifertility drug because of the occurrence of adverse effects such as hypokalaemia and irreversible testicular damage resulting in azoospermia or severe oligozoospermia.

1. Wu D. An overview of the clinical pharmacology and therapeutic potential of gossypol as a male contraceptive agent and in gynaecological disease. *Drugs* 1989; **38:** 333–41.
2. Coutinho EM, *et al.* Antispermatogenic action of gossypol in men. *Fertil Steril* 1984; **42:** 424–30.
3. Liu G, *et al.* Clinical trial of gossypol as a male contraceptive drug part I: efficacy study. *Fertil Steril* 1987; **48:** 459–61.
4. Waites GMH, *et al.* Gossypol: reasons for its failure to be accepted as a safe, reversible male antifertility drug. *Int J Androl* 1998; **21:** 8–12.

Gravel Root (15843-r)

Joe Pye Weed.

Profile
Gravel root is the root of *Eupatorium purpureum* (Compositae) and has diuretic, antilithic, and antirheumatic properties. It is used for renal and urinary calculus and other urinary-tract disorders, and has also been used for gout and rheumatism.

Preparations
Proprietary Preparations (details are given in Part 3)
Multi-ingredient: *UK:* Backache.

Greater Celandine (9145-e)

Chelidonii Herba; Chelidonium; Schöllkraut; Tetterwort.
Pharmacopoeias. In Eur. (see p.vi) and Pol.

Pharmacopoeial description
Ph. Eur.: The dried, whole, or cut aerial parts of *Chelidonium majus* collected during flowering. It contains a minimum of 0.6% of total alkaloids expressed as chelidonine ($C_{20}H_{19}NO_5 = 353.4$), calculated with reference to the dried drug.

Profile
Greater celandine has sedative and spasmolytic properties and is used for liver, biliary, and gastrointestinal disorders, and has also been used for respiratory-tract disorders. The latex has been used externally for warts and other skin conditions.

It is also used in homoeopathic medicine.

Greater celandine has been reported to cause hepatotoxicity.

Effects on the liver. References.
1. Benninger J, *et al.* Acute hepatitis induced by greater celandine (*Chelidonium majus*). *Gastroenterology* 1999; **117:** 1234–7.

Preparations
Proprietary Preparations (details are given in Part 3)
Ger.: Ardeycholan N; Aristochol CC; Chelidophyt; Chol 4000†; Cholarist; Cholspasmin Phyto; Gallopas; Panchelidon N; Siosol; *Port.:* Cholagutt; *Switz.:* Virulex.

Multi-ingredient: *Aust.:* Aristochol; Choleodoron; *Austral.:* Berberis Complex; Extralife Liva-Care; Lexat; *Belg.:* Aporil; *Braz.:* Quelodin; *Fr.:* Nitrol; *Ger.:* Aristochol N; Bilisan C3†; Cefachol; Chol-Kugeletten Neu; Chol-Truw S†; Cholagogum F; Cholagogum N; Cholagutt-N; Cholapret; Cholhepan N; Cholosolm Phyto; Cholosom SL; Cynarzym N; Esberigal N†; Femisana; Gallemolan forte; Gallemolan G; Galloselect M;

Hepar-Pasc N†; Hepaticum-Medice H; Hepatimed N†; Hepatofalk Neu; Heumann Leber- und Gallentee Solu-Hepar NT; Hevert-Gall S; Hevert-Magen-Galle-Leber-Tee†; Horvilan N†; Iberogast; Infi-tract N; JuCholan S†; Legapas comp†; Marianon; Nervogastrol; Neurochol C; Novo Mandrogallan N†; Opobyl-phyto; Pascohepan novo; Paverysat forte; Presselin Hepaticum P; Schwohepan S; spasmo gallo sanol; Steigal; *Hong Kong:* Hepatofalk; Hepatofalk Planta; *Ital.:* Tisana Arnaldi†; *Singapore:* Hepatofalk Planta; *Spain:* Nitroina; *Switz.:* Demonatur Gouttes pour le foie et la bile; Iberogast; Stago.

Green-lipped Mussel (12983-s)

Profile
An extract from the green-lipped mussel *Perna canaliculata* (Mytilidae), stated to contain amino acids, fats, carbohydrates, and minerals, has been promoted for the treatment of rheumatic disorders including rheumatoid arthritis (p.9).

Rheumatic disorders. A review of the investigation of green-lipped mussel in the treatment of arthritis has not revealed conclusive evidence of its usefulness.[1]

1. Li Wan Po A, Maguire T. Green-lipped mussel. *Pharm J* 1990; **244:** 640–1.

Preparations
Proprietary Preparations (details are given in Part 3)
UK: Healtheries Musseltone; Lyprinex; Mobilyzer; Oceantone; Seatone.

Multi-ingredient: *Austral.:* Prost-1; Prost-2†; *UK:* Healtheries Musseltone & Glucosamine.

Grindelia (2015-j)

Gum Plant; Gumweed; Tar Weed.
Pharmacopoeias. In Fr. which allows G. camporum, G. humilis, G. robusta, and G. squarrosa.

Profile
Various *Grindelia* spp. have been included in preparations used for respiratory-tract disorders.

Preparations
Proprietary Preparations (details are given in Part 3)
Multi-ingredient: *Aust.:* Paracodin; *Austral.:* Asa Tones; Breathe Eazy Chest Rub; Euphorbia Complex; *Belg.:* Paracodine; *Braz.:* Broncmel; Broncotussan; Gotas Nican; Limao Bravo; Lobelia Composta; Pectal; Pectoss; Pulmoformil; Xarope de Caraguata + Bromoformio; Xarope de Limao Bravo; Xarope Grindelia de Oliveira Junior; *Canad.:* Herbal Cold Relief; *Fr.:* Coquelusedal; Coquelusedal Paracetamol; Dinacode; Ephydion; Germose; Glottyl; Neo-Codion; Niver; Vegetoserum; *Ger.:* Asthma 6-N; Bronchicum Elixir N; Melrosum Hustensirup N; *Ital.:* Broncosedina; Sedobex†; Tussanyl; *Neth.:* Bronchicum; *Port.:* Lactucol; *S.Afr.:* Bronchicough; Bronchicum; *Spain:* Pazbronquial; *Switz.:* Famel; Neo-Codion N; Nican.

Ground Ivy (13448-k)

Lierre Terrestre.
Pharmacopoeias. In Chin. and Fr.

Profile
Ground ivy, the aerial parts of *Glechoma hederacea* (*Nepeta hederacea*) (Labiatae) has been used for respiratory-tract and gastrointestinal disorders.

It is also used in homoeopathic medicine.

Preparations
Proprietary Preparations (details are given in Part 3)
Multi-ingredient: *Belg.:* Tisane Pectorale; *Fr.:* Mediflor Tisane Pectorale d'Alsace; *Switz.:* Demo gouttes bronchiques†; *UK:* Heath & Heather Water Relief Tablets; Water Naturtabs.

Guaiacum Resin (278-r)

Guaiac; Guaiacum; Guajakharz.

Profile
Guaiacum resin is obtained from guaiacum wood (lignum vitae; *Guaiacum officinale* or *G. sanctum*) and has been used in the treatment of rheumatism. It is used in herbal and homoeopathic medicine.

Guaiacum resin is used in the detection of occult blood in the faeces. The accuracy of the guaiacum test has been questioned and some drugs may interfere with the result.

Preparations
Proprietary Preparations (details are given in Part 3)
Multi-ingredient: *UK:* Gerard House Ligvites; Gerard House Reumalex; Rheumasol; Rheumatic Pain; Rheumatic Pain Relief; Rheumatic Pain Remedy; Rheumatic Pain Tablets.

Guaiazulene (1611-m)

1,4-Dimethyl-7-isopropylazulene.
$C_{15}H_{18} = 198.3$.
$CAS — 489-84-9$.

Profile
Guaiazulene has been reported to have anti-allergic, anti-inflammatory, antipyretic, and antiseptic properties.

Preparations
Proprietary Preparations (details are given in Part 3)
Aust.: Azulen; Azulenal; Garmastan; *Ger.:* Garmastan.

Multi-ingredient: *Aust.:* Piniment; Spasmo Claim; Tampositorien mit Belladonna; Thrombocid; *Fr.:* Cicatryl; Pepsane; *Ger.:* Azupanthenol; Thrombocid; *Hong Kong:* Thrombocid; *Israel:* Aronal Forte; *Ital.:* Collyria; *Port.:* Thrombocid; *Spain:* Anticatarral; Beogel; Nani Pre Dental; Predni Azuleno; *Switz.:* Bain extra-doux dermatologique Nouvelle Formule; Phlogidermil†; Phytoberidin; Thrombocid.

Gutta Percha (12809-a)

Gummi Plasticum; Gutt. Perch.
Pharmacopoeias. In US.

Pharmacopoeial description
USP 25: The coagulated, dried, purified latex of the trees of the genera *Palaquium* and *Payena* and most commonly *Palaquium gutta* (Sapotaceae). It occurs in lumps or blocks of variable size; externally brown or greyish-brown to greyish-white in colour; internally reddish-yellow or reddish-grey and having a laminated or fibrous appearance. It is flexible but only slightly elastic. Has a slight, characteristic odour. Insoluble in water; partly soluble in carbon disulfide, in turpentine oil, and in benzene; about 90% soluble in chloroform. Store under water. Protect from light.

Profile
Gutta percha has been used in various dressings. In dentistry, gutta percha has been used as a filling material and as the basis of compounds for taking dental impressions.

Haematoporphyrin (12811-l)

$C_{34}H_{38}N_4O_6 = 598.7$.
$CAS — 14459-29-1$.

A red pigment, free from iron, obtained from haematin.

Profile
Haematoporphyrin is an ingredient of preparations promoted as tonics, particularly for the elderly, and has been used in the treatment of depression; it has been given by mouth and by intramuscular injection. Derivatives of haematoporphyrin have been used as photosensitisers in the phototherapy of malignant neoplasms (see Porfimer Sodium, p.566).

Preparations
Proprietary Preparations (details are given in Part 3)
Fr.: Hemedonine.

Multi-ingredient: *Aust.:* KH3; *Fr.:* Novitan†; *Ger.:* KH3; Revicain comp plus; *Hong Kong:* KH3; *Ital.:* Porfirin 12; Tonogen; Vit-Porphyrin; *NZ:* KH3; *Port.:* KH3†; *S.Afr.:* Revaton†; *Spain:* Actilevol Orex†; KH3 Powel; *Thai.:* KH3; *UK:* KH3.

Hamamelis (311-g)

Amamelide; Hamamelidis; Witch Hazel.
Pharmacopoeias. In Eur. (see p.vi) and US.

It also contains gallic acid, a bitter principle, and a trace of volatile oil.

Pharmacopoeial description
Ph. Eur.: The whole or cut dried leaves of *Hamamelis virginiana* containing not less than 7% tannins, expressed as pyrogallol ($C_6H_6O_3 = 126.1$), calculated with reference to the dried drug. Protect from light.

USP 25: A clear, colourless distillate prepared from recently cut and partially dried dormant twigs of *Hamamelis virginiana*. pH between 3.0 and 5.0. Store in airtight containers at a temperature not exceeding 40°.

Profile
Hamamelis has astringent properties. It is used in preparations for the symptomatic relief of haemorrhoids (p.1205). Hamamelis water is used as a cooling application and has been applied as a haemostatic.

Hamamelis, from various parts of the plant, is used in herbal or homoeopathic preparations for a variety of disorders.

Preparations
USP 25: Witch Hazel.
Proprietary Preparations (details are given in Part 3)
Aust.: Hametum; *Austral.:* Optrex; Witch Doctor; *Canad.:* Optrex; Preparation H Cleansing Pads; Snap Skin Cleanser Sensitive; *Fr.:* Optrex; *Ger.:* Aescorin N; F 99 Sulgan N†; Haemo Duoform; Hamasana; Hametum; Pellit Sonnenbrand†; Posterine; Tampositorien N; Venoplant top; Virgamelis†; *Irl.:* Optrex; *Ital.:* Acqua Virginiana; Optrex; *Neth.:* Venoplant†; *NZ:* Optrex; *Port.:* Optrex; *Singapore:* Optrex; *Spain:* Optrex; *Switz.:* Hametum-N†;

Hametum†; Optrex; **Thai.:** Hametum; Optrex; **UK:** I-Doc; Optrex; Preparation H Clear Gel; Witch Doctor; Witch Sunsore; **USA:** A-E-R; Fleet Medicated Pads; Mediconet†; Neutrogena Drying.

Multi-ingredient: Aust.: Arnicet; Felix; Inotyol; Mirfulan; St Radegunder Tee gegen Durchfall; Sulgan 99; Tampositorien mit Belladonna; Varicylum; **Austral.:** Anusol; Bioglan Cirflo; Bioglan Fingers & Toes†; Cirflo†; Gentlees; Hamamelis Complex; Hemocane; John Plunketts Vita-Pore; Optrex Medicated; Proflo; **Belg.:** Rectovasol; **Braz.:** Dinill; Hemoaenus; Hemorroidex; Hemorrol; Hemosan; Hemovirtu's; Mirorroidin; Varizol; **Canad.:** Onrectal; Penaten; Pommade Midy; Preparation H Cooling Gel; Snap Skin Cleanser Normal; Tucks; **Fr.:** Aphloine P; Climaxol; Curoveinyl†; Fluon; HEC; Histo-Fluine P; Inotyol; Jouvence de l' Abbe Soury; Mediflor Tisane Circulation du Sang No 12†; Ophtalmine; P. Veinos†; Pastilles Monleon; Phlebosedol; Phytomelis; Sacnel†; Veinostase; Vitalgine; **Ger.:** Aescusan; Anisan; Bagnisan med Heilbad; Chlorophyllin Salbe "Schuh"; derma-loges N; Eulatin NN; Hametum-N; Heusin; Heweven P 3; Heweven P 7†; Leukona-Wundsalbe; Mirfulan; Palatol N; Pascovenol novo; Rheuma-Pasc N†; Sagittaproct; Siozwo N; Trauma-cyl; Varicylum-S; Vasesana-Vasoregulans; Venacton; Venotrulan; Weleda Hamorrhoidalzapfchen; **Hong Kong:** Roidhemo; **Israel:** Aforinol; Derma Care; Inotyol; **Ital.:** Castindia; Centella Complex; Centella Complex C; Centeril H; Dermitina; Dermoprolyn; Elisir Depurativo Ambrosiano; Fluiven†; Ginkgo Plus; Ginoxil Ecoschiuma; Hamamilla; Herbe; Inotyol; Intim; Lycia Luminique; Mirtiros; Neo Topico Giusto†; Nevril; Otazul†; Pomata Midy HC†; Sacnel; Salviette H; Sedalen Cort; Sedilene Procto; Steril Zeta; Stilomagic; Varicogel; Venoplant†; Venoplus; Venotrauma; Venovit; **NZ:** Lacto Calamine; Optrex Red-Eye Relief; **Port.:** Hemofissural; Pruridermase†; **S.Afr.:** Lacto Calamine†; **Singapore:** HEC; **Spain:** Banoftal; Hemodren Compuesto; Hemostatico Antisep Asen†; Lamnotyl; Ojosbel; Ojosbel Azul; Roidhemo; Sol Schoum; Venofit; Venoplant; **Switz.:** Anal-Gen; Collypan; Frigoplasma; Haemocortin; Haemolan; HEC; Oculosan; Oculosan forte; Optazine†; Optrex compresses; Perkamillon; Phlogidermil†; Pommade Po-Ho N A Vogel; Proctalgen; Riccompense†; Riccovitan; Sulgan; **Thai.:** Opplin; **UK:** Adiantine; Eye Dew; Heemex; Kleer Cream; Lacto Calamine; Modern Herbals Pile; Optrex Clear Eyes; Swarm; Tea Tree & Witch Hazel Cream; Varicose Ointment; Vital Eyes; **USA:** Clearasil Double Clear; Preparation H Cooling Gel; Succus Cineraria Maritima; Tucks.

Harmaline (5015-z)

3,4-Dihydroharmine.
$C_{13}H_{14}N_2O = 214.3$.
CAS — 304-21-2.

An alkaloid obtained from peganum, the dried seeds of *Peganum harmala* (Zygophyllaceae).

Harmine (5016-c)

7-Methoxy-1-methyl-9H-pyrido[3,4-b]indole.
$C_{13}H_{12}N_2O = 212.2$.
CAS — 442-51-3.

An alkaloid obtained from peganum, the dried seeds of *Peganum harmala* (Zygophyllaceae).

Harmine is identical with an alkaloid known as banisterine or telepathine obtained from *Banisteria caapi* (Malpighiaceae).

Profile
A hallucinogenic drink which is known in the Western Amazonian regions as 'caapi' (Brazil and Colombia), 'Yagé' (Colombia), and 'ayahuasca' (Ecuador, Peru, and Bolivia), is made from closely related plants of the family Malpighiaceae. The main active principles are harmine and harmaline. It has no therapeutic use.

Helonias (12135-z)

Blazing Star; Chamaelirium; False Unicorn; Starwort.

Profile
Helonias is the root of *Chamaelirium luteum* (*Helonias dioica*) (Liliaceae). It is used in herbal medicine particularly for gynaecological disorders. It is also used in homoeopathic preparations.

Preparations
Proprietary Preparations (details are given in Part 3)
Multi-ingredient: Austral.: Nervatona; Nervatona Plus; **UK:** Gerard House Helonias Compound; Period Pain Relief.

Henna (12817-a)

Henna Leaf; Lawsonia.

The dried leaves of *Lawsonia inermis* (= *L. alba*) (Lythraceae), containing lawsone (p.1627).

Profile
Powdered henna is used for dyeing the hair and skin.

Adverse effects. Allergic skin reactions to henna used to dye the skin have been reported.[1] The authors commented that such reactions were usually due to additives used to shorten the application time of the dye and that allergic reactions to 'plain' henna were rare.

The symbol † denotes a preparation no longer actively marketed

The suggestion that henna may cause neonatal hyperbilirubinaemia is discussed under Lawsone, p.1627.

1. Lestringant GG, *et al.* Cutaneous reactions to henna and associated additives. *Br J Dermatol* 1999; **141:** 598–600.

Heptaminol Hydrochloride (12819-x)

Heptaminol Hydrochloride (BANM, rINNM).

Heptaminoli Hydrochloridum; RP-2831. 6-Amino-2-methylheptan-2-ol hydrochloride.
$C_8H_{19}NO,HCl = 181.7$.
CAS — 372-66-7 (heptaminol); 543-15-7 (heptaminol hydrochloride).
Pharmacopoeias. In *Eur.* (see p.vi).

Pharmacopoeial description
Ph. Eur.: A white or almost white crystalline powder. Freely soluble in water; soluble in alcohol; practically insoluble in dichloromethane.

Profile
Heptaminol hydrochloride is a cardiac stimulant and vasodilator and has been given in the treatment of cardiovascular disorders. Heptaminol and heptaminol adenosine phosphate have also been used.

Preparations
Proprietary Preparations (details are given in Part 3)
Belg.: Hept-A-Myl†; **Fr.:** Ampecyclal; Hept-A-Myl; **Ital.:** Coreptil; **Port.:** Heptylon.

Multi-ingredient: Aust.: Thilocombin; **Fr.:** Debrumyl; Ginkor Fort; **Ger.:** Normotin-R; Perivar; Veno-Hexanicit†; Veno-Tebonin N; **Hong Kong:** Ginkor Fort; **Port.:** Debrumyl; Forticol; **Spain:** Denubil; Largatrex; **Thai.:** Ginkor Fort.

Herniaria (12820-y)

Bruchkraut; Herba Herniariae; Herniary; Rupture-wort.
Pharmacopoeias. In *Aust.*

The dried leaves and flowering tops of various species of rupture-wort, chiefly *Herniaria glabra* and *H. hirsuta* (Caryophyllaceae).

Profile
Herniaria has astringent and diuretic properties and has been given by mouth, usually as an infusion, in urinary-tract disorders.

Preparations
Proprietary Preparations (details are given in Part 3)
Multi-ingredient: Aust.: Blasen-Tee; Blasentee; Krauterhaus Mag Kottas Blasentee; Krauterhaus Mag Kottas Nierentee; Mag Kottas Entwasserungstee; Mag Kottas Nieren-Blasentee; St Radegunder Nierentee; Uropurat; **Ger.:** Hernia-Tee†; Herniol; Nephrubin†.

Hexylene Glycol (18345-b)

2-Methyl-2,4-pentanediol.
$C_6H_{14}O_2 = 118.2$.
CAS — 107-41-5.
Pharmacopoeias. In *USNF.*

Pharmacopoeial description
USNF 20: A clear, colourless, viscous liquid. Absorbs moisture when exposed to moist air. Miscible with water and with many organic solvents including alcohol, acetone, chloroform, ether, and hexanes. Store in airtight containers.

Profile
Hexylene glycol has properties similar to those of propylene glycol (p.1655). It is used as a pharmaceutical aid.

Histamine (2132-t)

2-(Imidazol-4-yl)ethylamine.
$C_5H_9N_3 = 111.1$.
CAS — 51-45-6.
ATC — V04CG03.

Histamine Hydrochloride (2133-x)

Histamine Dihydrochloride (USAN); Histamini Dihydrochloridum.
$C_5H_9N_3,2HCl = 184.1$.
CAS — 56-92-8.
Pharmacopoeias. In *Eur.* (see p.vi).

Histamine hydrochloride 1.66 mg is approximately equivalent to 1 mg of histamine.

Pharmacopoeial description
Ph. Eur.: Hygroscopic, colourless crystals or white crystalline powder. Very soluble in water; soluble in alcohol; practically insoluble in ether. A 5% solution in water has a pH of 2.85 to 3.60. Protect from light.

Histamine Phosphate (2134-r)

Histamine Acid Phosphate; Histamine Diphosphate; Histamini Phosphas.
$C_5H_9N_3,2H_3PO_4,H_2O = 325.2$.
CAS — 51-74-1 (anhydrous histamine phosphate).
Pharmacopoeias. In *Eur.* (see p.vi). *US* specifies the anhydrous substance.

Histamine phosphate (anhydrous) 2.76 mg or histamine phosphate monohydrate 2.93 mg is approximately equivalent to 1 mg of histamine.

Pharmacopoeial description
Ph. Eur.: Colourless, long prismatic crystals. Freely soluble in water; slightly soluble in alcohol. A 5% solution in water has a pH of 3.75 to 3.95. Protect from light.

USP 25: Anhydrous histamine phosphate occurs as colourless, odourless, long prismatic crystals. Is stable in air but is affected by light. Soluble 1 in 4 of water. Its solutions are acid to litmus. Store in airtight containers. Protect from light.

Stability. A study concluded that solutions of histamine phosphate could be sterilised by heating in an autoclave with little degradation.[1] Autoclaved solutions could be stored for a minimum of 4 months.

1. McDonald C, *et al.* Stability of solutions of histamine acid phosphate after sterilization by heating in an autoclave. *J Clin Pharm Ther* 1990; **15:** 41–4.

Adverse Effects and Treatment
Injection of histamine salts can produce a range of adverse effects that includes headache, flushing of the skin, general vasodilatation with a fall in blood pressure, tachycardia, bronchial constriction and dyspnoea, visual disturbances, vomiting, diarrhoea, and other gastrointestinal effects. These reactions may be serious and excessive dosage can produce collapse and shock, and may be fatal. Reactions may occur at the injection site.

Some of these effects may be relieved by an antihistamine, but adrenaline [epinephrine] may be required and should always be available.

Precautions
Histamine salts should be used with care in patients with asthma or other hypersensitivity disorders, in elderly patients, and in patients with cardiovascular disorders.

Pharmacokinetics
Histamine salts exert a rapid, though transient, effect when given parenterally. Histamine is rapidly metabolised by methylation and oxidation; the metabolites are excreted in the urine.

Uses and Administration
Histamine causes stimulation of smooth muscle, especially of the bronchioles, and lowers blood pressure by dilating the arterioles and capillaries. It also stimulates exocrine gland secretion, especially the gastric glands.

Intradermal injection of histamine produces the characteristic 'triple response' of erythema, flare, and wheal. This is utilised as a control response in skin testing for hypersensitivity. Also, since it is mediated in part by axon reflexes, it has been used to test the integrity of sensory nerves, for example in leprosy.

Inhalation of histamine causes bronchoconstriction and is used as a test of bronchial reactivity.

Histamine has also been given subcutaneously to identify the causes of achlorhydria and intravenously in the diagnosis of phaeochromocytoma, but safer tests are generally preferred.

Histamine is included in some combination topical preparations for musculoskeletal disorders.

Histamine hydrochloride is under investigation as an adjunct in the management of acute myeloid leukaemia and malignant melanoma. It has also been tried as an adjunct to interferons and other drugs in the management of hepatitis C.

Preparations
USP 25: Histamine Phosphate Injection.

Proprietary Preparations (details are given in Part 3)
Mex.: Destamin.

Multi-ingredient: Aust.: Histaglobin; **Braz.:** Infrarub; **Canad.:** Midalgan; **Fr.:** Algipan; Pneumoplasme a l'Histamine†; **Ger.:** GA-301-Redskin 301†; Histadestal; Midysalb†; **Port.:** Midalgan; **S.Afr.:** Histaglobin; **Switz.:** Midalgan; Radalgin; **Thai.:** Histaglobin.

Histoplasmin (8040-k)

Pharmacopoeias. In *US.*

Pharmacopoeial description
USP 25: A clear, colourless, sterile solution containing standardised culture filtrates of *Histoplasma capsulatum* grown on liquid synthetic medium. It may contain a suitable antimicrobial. Store at 2° to 8°. The expiry date is not later than 2 years after release from the manufacturer's cold storage.

Profile
Histoplasmin, in an intradermal (intracutaneous) dose of 0.1 mL of a 1 in 100 dilution, may be used as an aid to the diagnosis of histoplasmosis. However, the diagnostic value of the test has been questioned and it may interfere with serological tests for histoplasmosis.

Histoplasmin has also been used, in conjunction with other antigens, to assess cell-mediated immunity.

◊ For reference to the use of histoplasmin for anergy testing in HIV-positive patients, see Tuberculins, p.1676.

Preparations

USP 25: Histoplasmin.

Proprietary Preparations (details are given in Part 3)
USA: Histolyn-CYL.

Horseradish   (12119-z)

Armoracia.

Profile

Horseradish, the root of *Cochlearia armoracia* (*Armoracia rusticana*; *Nasturtium armoracia*; *Radicula armoracia*) (Cruciferae), has diuretic and antiseptic properties and stimulates the digestion. It is used in gastrointestinal, respiratory-tract, and urinary-tract disorders, and has also been used externally.

It is also used in homoeopathic medicine.

Horseradish is widely used as a food flavouring and condiment.

Preparations

Proprietary Preparations (details are given in Part 3)
Multi-ingredient: *Austral.:* Garlic and Horseradish + C Complex; Garlic, Horseradish, A & C Capsules; Horse Radish and Garlic Tablets; Procold; Sinus and Hayfever; *Ger.:* Angocin Anti-Infekt N; *Switz.:* Kernosan Elixir; *UK:* Mixed Vegetable Tablets.

Hyaluronic Acid   (19888-x)

Hyaluronic Acid (BAN).
(1→3)-O-(2-Acetamido-2-deoxy-β-D-glucopyranosyl)-(1→4)-O-β-D-glucopyranosiduronan.
CAS — 9004-61-9.
ATC — D03AX05; M09AX01; S01KA01.

NOTE. The term Hyaluronan is used to cover both hyaluronic acid and sodium hyaluronate.

Sodium Hyaluronate   (13251-b)

Sodium Hyaluronate (BANM).
Hyaluronate Sodium (USAN); Natrii Hyaluronas.
CAS — 9067-32-7.
Pharmacopoeias. In *Eur.* (see p.vi).

Pharmacopoeial description

Ph. Eur.: The sodium salt of hyaluronic acid, a glycosaminoglycan consisting of D-glucuronic acid and N-acetyl-D-glucosamine disaccharide units. It is extracted from cocks' combs or obtained by fermentation from streptococci, (Lancefield Groups A and C). A white or almost white, very hygroscopic powder or a fibrous aggregate. Sparingly soluble to soluble in water; practically insoluble in dehydrated alcohol, in acetone, and in ether. A 0.5% solution in water has a pH of 5.0 to 8.5. Store in airtight containers. Protect from light and humidity.

Adverse Effects

There have been reports of a transient rise in intra-ocular pressure following the administration of sodium hyaluronate into the eye. When administered to the knee, pain and inflammation may occur at the injection site. There have also been occasional reports of hypersensitivity, including, rarely, anaphylaxis.

Effects on the eyes. Crystalline deposits on intra-ocular lenses have been reported in patients following the use of a high viscosity sodium hyaluronate preparation during cataract surgery.[1]

1. Jensen MK, *et al.* Crystallization on intraocular lens surfaces associated with the use of Healon GV. *Arch Ophthalmol* 1994; **112:** 1037–42.

Inflammatory reaction. Severe peritoneal inflammation has been reported[1] following use of a sodium hyaluronate-based bioresorbable membrane to prevent postoperative adhesion formation.

1. Klingler PJ, *et al.* Seprafilm®-induced peritoneal inflammation: a previously unknown complication: report of a case. *Dis Colon Rectum* 1999; **42:** 1639–43.

Uses and Administration

Hyaluronic acid is widely distributed in body tissues and intracellular fluids, including the aqueous and vitreous humour, and synovial fluid; it is a component of the ground substance or tissue cement surrounding cells.

A viscous solution of sodium hyaluronate is used during surgical procedures on the eye, for example for cataract extraction. Introduction of the solution into the anterior or posterior chamber via a fine cannula or needle allows tissues to be separated during surgery and protects them from trauma. Sodium hyaluronate is also given by intra-articular injection in the treatment of osteoarthritis of the knee. Doses vary according to the preparation used, but are of the order of 20 mg once weekly for 5 weeks or up to 30 mg once weekly for 3 weeks; it is generally recommended that the treatment course for any individual joint should not be repeated within 6 months.

Hyaluronic acid is applied topically to promote wound healing. Zinc hyaluronate has also been used. A film containing sodium hyaluronate and carmellose is used to prevent surgical adhesion.

Hylans, which are polymers derived from hyaluronic acid, are used similarly.

Sodium hyaluronate instilled intravesically has been used as a temporary replacement of the glycosaminoglycan layer in the bladder for the symptomatic treatment of interstitial cystitis.

Topical formulations of diclofenac in hyaluronic acid (CT-1101, AT-2101) are under investigation in the treatment of actinic keratoses.

◊ Reviews.
1. Goa KL, Benfield P. Hyaluronic acid: a review of its pharmacology and use as a surgical aid in ophthalmology, and its therapeutic potential in joint disease and wound healing. *Drugs* 1994; **47:** 536–66.
2. Adams ME, *et al.* A risk-benefit assessment of injections of hyaluronan and its derivatives in the treatment of osteoarthritis of the knee. *Drug Safety* 2000; **23:** 115–30.

Actinic keratoses. For references to the use of diclofenac in a hyaluronic acid gel in the treatment of actinic keratoses, see p.32.

Dry eye. The usual management of dry eye (p.1498) is with artificial tears. Sodium hyaluronate has also been reported to be of some benefit. Alleviation of symptoms[1-3] and an increase in tear film stability[1,2] has been demonstrated following the topical application of sodium hyaluronate solution (0.1 or 0.2%) compared with saline-based placebo solutions. However, another study[4] failed to demonstrate any advantage over placebo, although it was suggested that sodium hyaluronate might play a role in maintaining a healthy corneal epithelium.

1. Mengher LS, *et al.* Effect of sodium hyaluronate (0.1%) on break-up time (NIBUT) in patients with dry eyes. *Br J Ophthalmol* 1986; **70:** 442–7.
2. Sand BB, *et al.* Sodium hyaluronate in the treatment of keratoconjunctivitis sicca: a double masked clinical trial. *Acta Ophthalmol (Copenh)* 1989; **67:** 181–3.
3. Condon PI, *et al.* Double blind, randomised, placebo controlled, crossover, multicentre study to determine the efficacy of a 0.1% (w/v) sodium hyaluronate solution (Fermavisc) in the treatment of dry eye syndrome. *Br J Ophthalmol* 1999; **83:** 1121–4.
4. Shimmura S, *et al.* Sodium hyaluronate eyedrops in the treatment of dry eyes. *Br J Ophthalmol* 1995; **79:** 1007–11.

Osteoarthritis. In osteoarthritis, the size and concentration of hyaluronic acid molecules naturally present in synovial fluid is reduced. Thus, one approach in the management of osteoarthritis (p.9) of the knee is viscosupplementation of the synovial fluid by the intra-articular injection of hyaluronic acid or its derivatives. This may be an effective option for patients who are unable to take oral NSAIDs or have regular intra-articular corticosteroids, and who are unsuitable candidates for joint replacement surgery.

References.
1. Altman RD, Moskowitz R. Intraarticular sodium hyaluronate (Hyalgan) in the treatment of patients with osteoarthritis of the knee: a randomized clinical trial. *J Rheumatol* 1998; **25:** 2203–12. Correction. *ibid.* 1999; **26:** 1216.
2. Anonymous. Hyaluronan or hylans for knee osteoarthritis? *Drug Ther Bull* 1999; **37:** 71–2.
3. Huskisson EC, Donnelly S. Hyaluronic acid in the treatment of osteoarthritis of the knee. *Rheumatology* 1999; **38:** 602–7.
4. Wobig M, *et al.* The role of elastoviscosity in the efficacy of viscosupplementation for osteoarthritis of the knee: a comparison of hylan G-F 20 and a lower-molecular-weight hyaluronan. *Clin Ther* 1999; **21:** 1549–62.

Wound healing. Hyaluronic acid has been used to aid wound healing,[1,2] the overall management of which is discussed on p.1108.

1. Soldati D, *et al.* Mucosal wound healing after nasal surgery: a controlled clinical trial on the efficacy of hyaluronic acid containing cream *Drugs Exp Clin Res* 1999; **25:** 253–61.
2. Harris PA, *et al.* Use of hyaluronic acid and cultured autologous keratinocytes and fibroblasts in extensive burns. *Lancet* 1999; **353:** 35–6.

Preparations

Proprietary Preparations (details are given in Part 3)
Aust.: Amvisc; Artzal; Connettivina; Etamucin; Healonid; Hyalgan; Provisc†; *Austral.:* AMO Vitrax; Fermathron; Healon; Ophthalin; Provisc; Synvisc; Vismed; *Belg.:* Healon; Provisc†; *Braz.:* Polireumin; *Canad.:* Biolon; Cystistat; Eyestil; Healon; Hylashield†; Suplasyn; Synvisc; Vismed; *Denm.:* Artz; Hyalgan; *Fin.:* Artzal; Healon; Hyalgan; *Fr.:* Arthrum H; Healon†; Hyalgan†; Hyalofill; Provisc; Synvisc; Vismed; Vitrax†; *Ger.:* Biolon; Dispasan; Healon; Hy-GAG; Hya-ject; Hya-Ophtal; Hyalart; Hylaform; Hylo-Comod; Jossalind†; Laservis; Orthovisc; Ostenil; Provisc; Synvisc; Vislube; Vismed; *Hong Kong:* Connettivina; Healon; Hialid; Hyalgan; Ial; Ophthalin; Provisc; Synvisc; Vislube; *Irl.:* Healonid; Hyalgan; *Israel:* Adant; Amvisc; Biolon; Healon; Orthovisc; Synvisc; *Ital.:* Artz; Biolon†; Connettivina; Dropstar; Healon†; Hy-Drop; Hyalart; Hyalgan; Hyalistil; Ial; Ialum; Ialurex; Ocustil; Ophthalin; Otoial; Provisc; Synvisc; *Jpn:* Hyalein; *Mex.:* Biolon; *Neth.:* Healon†; *Norw.:* Healon†; *NZ:* AMO Vitrax; Healon; Ophthalin; Provisc; Synvisc; *Port.:* Gengigel; *S.Afr.:* AMO Vitrax; Amvisc; Biolone; Healon; Provisc; Synvisc; *Singapore:* AMO Vitrax; Healon; Ophthalin; Provisc; Synvisc; *Spain:* liyalgon; *Swed.:* AMO Vitrax†; Amvisc†; Artzal; Healon†; Hyalgan; Synvisc; *Switz.:* AMO Vitrax†; Biolon; Healon; Ial; Ialugen; Laservis; Ostenil; Rhinogen; Vislube; Vismed; *Thai.:* AMO Vitrax; Connettivina; Healon; Ial; Ophthalin; Provisc; *UK:* Cystistat; Fermathron; Gengigel; Healonid; Hyalgan; Hyalofill; Ophthalin;

Orthovisc; Provisc; Supartz; Suplasyn; Synvisc; *USA:* AMO Vitrax; Amvisc; Healon; Hyalgan; Synvisc.

Multi-ingredient: *Aust.:* Healonid Yellow†; Viscoat†; *Austral.:* Duovisc; Viscoat; *Belg.:* Viscoat†; *Fr.:* Hyalogran; Viscoat; *Ger.:* Duovisc; Viscoat; *Hong Kong:* Viscoat; *Ital.:* Connettivina Plus; Dropyal; Healon Yellow†; Trofo 5; Viscoat; *NZ:* Viscoat; *Port.:* Synchrorose; *S.Afr.:* Viscoat; *Singapore:* Duovisc; Viscoat; *Swed.:* Healon Yellow†; Viscoat; *Switz.:* Alphastria; Ialugen Plus; Viscoat†; *Thai.:* Duovisc; Viscoat; *UK:* Gelclair; Seprafilm; Viscoat; *USA:* Healon Yellow; Viscoat.

Hyaluronidase   (3724-v)

Hyaluronidase (BAN, rINN).
Hyaluronidasum.
CAS — 9001-54-1.
ATC — B06AA03.
Pharmacopoeias. In *Chin.* and *Eur.* (see p.vi). US includes as an injectable form.

Pharmacopoeial description

Ph. Eur.: An enzyme capable of hydrolysing mucopolysaccharides of the hyaluronic acid type. It is prepared from the testes of mammals by a method that has been shown to reduce contamination by known infectious agents to acceptable limits; a suitable stabilising agent may be added to the purified preparation. A white or yellowish-white, amorphous powder; it contains not less than 300 international units of hyaluronidase activity per mg, calculated with reference to the dried substance. Soluble in water; practically insoluble in alcohol, in acetone, and in ether. A 0.3% solution in water has a pH of 4.5 to 7.5. Store at 2° to 8° in airtight containers.

Units

The international and USP 25 units are equivalent. One international or USP 25 unit is equivalent to one turbidity-reducing unit or about 3.3 viscosity-reducing units.

Adverse Effects and Precautions

Sensitivity to hyaluronidase occasionally occurs. Hyaluronidase should be administered with caution to patients with infections; because of the danger of spreading infection, the enzyme generally should not be injected into or around an infected area. It has been suggested that the presence of malignancy may similarly be a contra-indication to the use of hyaluronidase. It should not be administered by intravenous injection nor should it be used for anaesthetic procedures in cases of unexplained premature labour. Hyaluronidase should not be applied directly to the cornea. It should not be used to reduce the swelling of bites or stings.

Uses and Administration

Hyaluronidase is an enzyme that reversibly depolymerises hyaluronic acid, a component of the ground substance or tissue cement surrounding cells, thereby temporarily reducing its viscosity and rendering the tissues more readily permeable to injected fluids.

Therapeutically, hyaluronidase is employed to increase the speed of absorption and to diminish discomfort due to subcutaneous or intramuscular injection of fluids, to promote resorption of excess fluids and extravasated blood in the tissues, and to increase the effectiveness of local anaesthesia.

In the UK, the usual dose of hyaluronidase to facilitate subcutaneous or intramuscular injection is 1500 units, added directly to the injection. To aid the dispersal of extravasated fluids or blood, the same dose is given in 1 mL of Water for Injections or 0.9% sodium chloride into the affected area. Lower doses of hyaluronidase are used in some countries; in the USA, the usual dose is one-tenth the UK dose, i.e. 150 units.

In hypodermoclysis, hyaluronidase is used to aid the subcutaneous administration of relatively large volumes of fluids, especially in infants and young children, where intravenous injection is difficult. Care should be taken in the treatment of children to control the speed and total volume administered and to avoid overhydration. Hyaluronidase may be added to the injection fluid or may be injected into the site before the fluid is given. In the UK, 1500 units of hyaluronidase is generally used for each 500 to 1000 mL of fluid for subcutaneous administration, but again, in the USA, 150 units of hyaluronidase is considered adequate for each litre of hypodermoclysis solution.

The diffusion of local anaesthetics is accelerated by the addition of 1500 units (in the USA, 150 units) of hyaluronidase to the anaesthetic solution. This is of value in the reduction of fractures and in pudendal block in midwifery. It has also been used in ophthalmology as an aid to local anaesthesia at recommended doses of 15 units per mL of local anaesthetic solution. Intravitreal hyaluronidase injection is under investigation in the management of vitreous haemorrhage.

Hyalosidase (GL enzyme) is a highly purified form of hyaluronidase that has been studied in the treatment of myocardial infarction but without much apparent success.

◊ General references.
1. Watson D. Hyaluronidase. *Br J Anaesth* 1993; **71:** 422–5.

Ophthalmic surgery. In a study[1] involving 150 consecutive patients undergoing surgery for senile cataract, retrobulbar anaesthesia with lignocaine [lidocaine] 2% solution plus adrenaline [epinephrine] 1:100 000 and hyaluronidase 15 units per mL produced successful anaesthesia in 69 of 75 cases (92%),

which was significantly better than 42 of 75 treated with lignocaine [lidocaine] plus adrenaline [epinephrine] alone. Although poor results have been reported from hyaluronidase and
a local anaesthetic without adrenaline [epinephrine] to restrict
local anaesthetic absorption, the use of the enzyme and adrenaline [epinephrine] was recommended as an aid to achieving
complete ocular akinesia and anaesthesia in cataract surgery.
Hyaluronidase has also been used in conjunction with a mixture of bupivacaine and lignocaine [lidocaine] for peribulbar
anaesthesia, but conflicting results have been reported. In a
study[2] in 50 patients, addition of hyaluronidase 25 units per mL
of local anaesthetic mixture had no significant effect on time to
satisfactory anaesthesia. However, in a second study[3] involving
200 patients, addition of hyaluronidase 50 or 300 units per mL
improved the quality of the peribulbar block and, in the case of
the higher concentration, also increased the speed of onset.

1. Thomson I. Addition of hyaluronidase to lignocaine with adrenaline for retrobulbar anaesthesia in the surgery of senile cataract.
   Br J Ophthalmol 1988; **72:** 700–2.
2. Prosser DP, *et al.* Re-evaluation of hyaluronidase in peribulbar
   anaesthesia. *Br J Ophthalmol* 1996; **80:** 827–30.
3. Dempsey GA, *et al.* Hyaluronidase and peribulbar block. *Br J
   Anaesth* 1997; **78:** 671–4.

Preparations

BP 2001: Hyaluronidase Injection;
USP 25: Hyaluronidase for Injection; Hyaluronidase Injection.

Proprietary Preparations (details are given in Part 3)
Aust.: Neopermease; Permease; **Austral.:** Hyalase; **Braz.:** Hyalozima; **Canad.:** Wydase; **Ger.:** Hylase; **Israel:** Hyalase; **Ital.:** Jaluran; **Neth.:** Hyason; **NZ:** Hyalase; **S.Afr.:** Hyalase; **UK:** Hyalase;
USA: Wydase.

Multi-ingredient: Aust.: Lemuval; **Austral.:** Lasonil; **Belg.:** La-
sonil; **Braz.:** Oto Xilodase; Xilodase; **Fr.:** Lasonil†; **Israel:** La-
sonil; **Ital.:** Jalovis†; Lasonil†; Lasoproct†; Lido-Hyal; **NZ:** La-
sonil; **Spain:** Lasonil; Oto Difusor; **Switz.:** Lido-Hyal.

Hydrangea   (12136-c)

Seven Barks; Smooth Hydrangea; Wild Hydrangea.

Profile
Hydrangea, the root of *Hydrangea arborescens* (Hydrangeace-
ae), has diuretic and litholytic properties and is used for genito-
urinary disorders including renal and urinary calculi.

Preparations
Proprietary Preparations (details are given in Part 3)
Multi-ingredient: UK: Antiglan; Backache; **USA:** Aqua-Rid†;
Fluidex†.

Hydrastine Hydrochloride   (12828-r)

6,7-Dimethoxy-3-(5,6,7,8-tetrahydro-6-methyl-1,3-dioxo-
lo[4,5-g]isoquinolin-5-yl)isobenzofuran-1(3H)-one hydrochloride.
$C_{21}H_{21}NO_6,HCl = 419.9$.
*CAS — 118-08-1 (hydrastine); 5936-28-7 (hydrastine hy-
drochloride).*

Profile
Hydrastine hydrochloride, the hydrochloride of an alkaloid obtained from *Hydrastis canadensis* (Ranunculaceae), has been
reputed to cause uterine contractions and arrest uterine haemorrhage but it is of doubtful value. It was also formerly used in
gastrointestinal disorders. Toxic doses are reported to cause
strychnine-like convulsions and relaxation of the gut.

Hydrastis   (12830-z)

Golden Seal; Hidraste; Hydrast.; Idraste; Yellow Root.
Pharmacopoeias. In Fr.

The dried rhizome and roots of golden seal, *Hydrastis canadensis* (Ranunculaceae), containing not less than 1.5% of hydrastine (above); it also contains the alkaloids berberine
(p.1584) and canadine.

Profile
Hydrastis was formerly used to arrest excessive uterine haemorrhage. It is included in some herbal preparations for gastrointestinal disorders and peripheral vascular disorders. It is used in
homoeopathic medicine.

Preparations
Proprietary Preparations (details are given in Part 3)
Ger.: Gingivitol N.

Multi-ingredient: Austral.: Bilberry Plus; Herbal Cleanse; Hy-
drastis Complex; Sambucus Complex; Trillium Complex; Urapro;
Urinase; **Braz.:** Uterovarol; **Fr.:** Climaxol; Curoveinyl†; **Ger.:**
Hepatimed N†; **Spain:** Sol Schoum; **UK:** Digestive; Fenulin; Ger-
ard House Golden Seal Compound; HRI Golden Seal Digestive;
Papaya Plus; Wind & Dyspepsia Relief.

Hydrazine Sulfate   (12831-c)

Hydrazine Sulphate.
$H_6N_2O_4S = 130.1$.
*CAS — 302-01-2 (hydrazine); 10034-93-2 (hydrazine sul-
fate).*

Profile
Hydrazine sulfate is employed in various industrial processes.
It is used in the preparation of hydrazine hydrate which is ap-
plied after a solution of platinic chloride for corneal tattooing.
It has been tried, but with little if any benefit, in the manage-
ment of cancer-related anorexia and cachexia.

Adverse effects and treatment. References to adverse effects resulting from exposure to hydrazine.[1-5] Pyridoxine has
been used in the management of hydrazine intoxication.[6-8]

1. Albert DM, Puliafito CA. Choroidal melanoma: possible exposure to industrial toxins. *N Engl J Med* 1977; **296:** 634–5.
2. Durant PJ, Harris RA. Hydrazine and lupus. *N Engl J Med* 1980;
   303: 584–5.
3. Hydrazine. *Environmental Health Criteria 68.* Geneva: WHO,
   1987.
4. Hydrazine health and safety guide. *IPCS Health and Safety
   Guide 56.* Geneva: WHO, 1991.
5. Hainer MI, *et al.* Fatal hepatorenal failure associated with hydrazine sulfate. *Ann Intern Med* 2000; **133:** 877–80.
6. Kirklin JK, *et al.* Treatment of hydrazine-induced coma with pyridoxine. *N Engl J Med* 1976; **294:** 938–9.
7. Harati Y, Niakan E. Hydrazine toxicity, pyridoxine therapy, and
   peripheral neuropathy. *Ann Intern Med* 1986; **104:** 728–9.
8. Nagappan R, Riddell T. Pyridoxine therapy in a patient with severe hydrazine sulfate toxicity. *Crit Care Med* 2000; **28:**
   2116–18.

Anorexia and cachexia. References[1-3] to the use of hydrazine sulfate in patients with anorexia or cachexia associated
with cancer.

1. Tayek JA, *et al.* Effect of hydrazine sulphate on whole-body protein breakdown measured by ¹⁴C-lysine metabolism in lung cancer patients. *Lancet* 1987; **ii:** 241–4.
2. Loprinzi CL, *et al.* Cancer-associated anorexia and cachexia: implications for drug therapy. *Drugs* 1992; **43:** 499–506.
3. Kaegi E. Unconventional therapies for cancer: hydrazine sulfate.
   Can Med Assoc J 1998; **158:** 1327–30.

Hydrochloric Acid   (1301-l)

Acidum Hydrochloricum; Acidum Hydrochloricum Concentratum; Concentrated Hydrochloric Acid; E507; Salzsäure.
$HCl = 36.46$.
CAS — 7647-01-0.
ATC — A09AB03; B05XA13.
Pharmacopoeias. In Chin., Eur. (see p.vi), Int., and Jpn (all specify
approximately 35 to 39% w/w). USNF specifies 36.5 to
38.0% w/w. Swiss also has Acidum Hydrochloricum 25%. Aust.
also has Acidum Hydrochloricum (19 to 21%). The impure acid
of commerce is known as Spirits of Salt and as Muriatic Acid.

Pharmacopoeial description
Ph. Eur.: It contains 35.0 to 39.0% w/w of HCl. A clear, colourless, fuming liquid. Miscible with water. Store below 30° in
stoppered containers of glass or other inert material.
USNF 20: It contains 36.5 to 38.0% w/w of HCl. A colourless,
fuming liquid having a pungent odour. It ceases to fume when
it is diluted with 2 volumes of water. Store in airtight containers.

Dilute Hydrochloric Acid   (1302-y)

Acidum Hydrochloricum Dilutum; Diluted Hydrochloric Acid;
Verdünnte Salzsäure.
Pharmacopoeias. In Eur. (see p.vi), Int., Jpn, and Pol. (all approxi-
mately 9.5 to 10.5% w/w). Also in USNF (9.5 to 10.5% w/v).

Pharmacopoeial description
Ph. Eur.: It contains 9.5 to 10.5% w/w of HCl prepared by
mixing hydrochloric acid 274 g with water 726 g.
USNF 20: It contains 9.5 to 10.5% w/v of HCl and may be
prepared by mixing hydrochloric acid 226 mL with sufficient
water to make 1000 mL. A colourless, odourless liquid. Store
in airtight containers.

Adverse Effects
Hydrochloric acid is highly irritant and corrosive and ingestion
has proved fatal. The corrosive effect causes severe pain. There
may be violent vomiting, haematemesis, and circulatory collapse; acids can also produce intravascular coagulation and
haemolysis. Ulceration may lead to perforation and patients
can suffer strictures and pyloric stenosis. Asphyxiation may result from laryngeal oedema. Inhalation of acid fumes or aspiration of ingested acids may cause pneumonitis.

◊ References.
1. Chlorine and hydrogen chloride. *Environmental Health Criteria
   21.* Geneva: WHO, 1982.

Treatment of Adverse Effects
Treatment following ingestion is mainly symptomatic. Gastric
lavage and activated charcoal are not generally appropriate and
emetics must *not* be used. Small amounts of water or milk may
be given to dilute the acid but larger volumes may increase the
risk of emesis and hence of further damage. Some recommend
the use of antacids such as aluminium hydroxide for neutralisation, but carbonates and bicarbonates should not be used as re-

lease of carbon dioxide distends the stomach. Opioid analgesia
may be required for pain. Endoscopy should be performed and
surgical intervention may be necessary. There is little evidence
to support the value of corticosteroids in preventing stricture
formation.
Acid burns of the skin should be flooded immediately with water and the washing should be copious and prolonged. Any affected clothing should be removed while flooding is being carried out. For burns in the eye, the lids should be kept open and
the eye flushed with a steady stream of water or sodium chloride 0.9%. A few drops of a local anaesthetic solution will relieve lid spasm and facilitate irrigation.

Uses and Administration
Hydrochloric acid has been used as an escharotic. It has been
used in the diluted form for the treatment of achlorhydria and
other gastrointestinal disorders. It has been given intravenously in the management of metabolic alkalosis (p.1180). An
acid perfusion test using hydrochloric acid has been used in the
diagnosis of oesophageal disorders. When taken orally, it
should be sipped through a straw to protect the teeth.
Hydrochloride acid (muriaticum acidum) is used in homoeopathic medicine.

Diagnosis and testing. References and comments on the use
of an acid perfusion test in the diagnosis of oesophageal disorders,[1-5] such as gastro-oesophageal reflux disease (p.1204) and
oesophageal motility disorders (p.1208). The test involves in-
tra-oesophageal perfusion of 0.1M hydrochloric acid; subsequent development of pain indicates an acid-sensitive oesophagus. This test has also been used in the differential diagnosis of
angina.[2]

1. Sladen GE, *et al.* Oesophagoscopy, biopsy, and acid perfusion
   test in diagnosis of "reflux oesophagitis". *BMJ* 1975; **1:** 71–6.
2. Anonymous. Angina and oesophageal disease. *Lancet* 1986; **i:**
   191–2.
3. Hewson EG, *et al.* Acid perfusion test: does it have a role in the
   assessment of non cardiac chest pain? *Gut* 1989; **30:** 305–10.
4. de Caestecker JS, Heading RC. Acid perfusion in the assessment
   of non-cardiac chest pain. *Gut* 1989; **30:** 1795–7.
5. Howard PJ, *et al.* Acid perfusion is a good screening test for
   symptomatic oesophageal reflux. *Gut* 1989; **30:** A1445.

Pregnancy. Heartburn during pregnancy may be due to reflux
of alkaline duodenal contents. A dilute solution of hydrochloric
acid (pH 2) taken after meals and at bedtime produced improvements in heartburn in pregnant women.[1]

1. Anonymous. Heartburn in pregnancy. *Drug Ther Bull* 1990; **28:**
   11–12.

Preparations
Proprietary Preparations (details are given in Part 3)
Multi-ingredient: Ital.: Gastro-Pepsin.

Hydrofluoric Acid   (1311-j)

Fluohydric Acid; Fluoric Acid.
$HF = 20.01$.
CAS — 7664-39-3.

A solution of hydrogen fluoride in water. Various strengths are
used. It attacks glass strongly.

Adverse Effects
As for Hydrochloric Acid, above. Although the corrosive effects of hydrofluoric acid tend to predominate, absorption may
produce systemic fluoride poisoning as described under Sodium Fluoride, p.1375.
The pain from contact with weak solutions may be delayed, so
that the patient is not aware of being burnt until some hours
later, when the area begins to smart; intense pain then sets in
and this may persist for several days. Destruction of tissue proceeds under the toughened coagulated skin, so that the ulcers
extend deeply, heal slowly, and leave a scar.
The fumes of hydrofluoric acid are highly irritant.

Treatment of Adverse Effects
The initial treatment of poisoning following oral exposure to
hydrofluoric acid is similar to that described for hydrochloric
acid, see above. Calcium gluconate should also be given intravenously to correct known or suspected hypocalcaemia. Burns
in the eye are also managed as for hydrochloric acid, although
irrigation of the eye may be continued with calcium gluconate
solution 2% after initial flood with water or sodium chloride
0.9%.
In the event of skin burns with hydrofluoric acid, contaminated
clothing or articles should be removed and the skin washed
with copious cold water or sodium chloride 0.9%. Irrigation
with a solution of a calcium salt, e.g. 1% calcium gluconate, is
carried out to convert the fluoride to an insoluble form and so
prevent absorption. Milk may be tried if such solutions are not
available. A calcium gluconate gel is sometimes used and it
may be necessary to infiltrate the affected areas with calcium
gluconate intradermally or subcutaneously. Hydrofluoric acid
passes through finger- and toe-nails without causing any apparent damage; nails will therefore have to be removed or perforated to be able to treat the underlying tissues. Other first-aid
measures reported to be effective include prolonged soaks in
iced solutions of benzalkonium chloride or benzethonium chloride; iced water has sometimes been used as has iced magnesium sulfate solution. Local, or even general, anaesthesia may be
needed. Burn eschars should be excised and necrotic tissue de-

brided. Absorption may lead to systemic fluoride toxicity and the need for intravenous calcium gluconate to manage hypocalcaemic symptoms.

◊ References to the treatment of hydrofluoric acid burns.
1. Browne TD. The treatment of hydrofluoric acid burns. *J Soc Occup Med* 1974; **24:** 80–9.
2. MacKinnon MA. Hydrofluoric acid burns. *Dermatol Clin* 1988; **6:** 67–74.
3. McIvor ME. Acute fluoride toxicity: pathophysiology and management. *Drug Safety* 1990; **5:** 79–85.
4. Kirkpatrick JJR, *et al.* Hydrofluoric acid burns: a review. *Burns* 1995; **21:** 483–93.

Uses
Hydrofluoric acid is used in industry. Its main use has been for the production of fluorocarbons for use as refrigerants and propellants. It has also been used as an ingredient of preparations for glass etching and rust removal.

Hydrofluoric acid (fluoricum acidum) is used in homoeopathic medicine.

Hydroquinine Hydrobromide (7850-x)
Dihydrochinin Hydrobromide; Dihydroquinine Hydrobromide; Hydrochinin Hydrobromide; Methylhydrocupreine Hydrobromide. 8α,9R-10,11-Dihydro-6′-methoxycinchonan-9-ol hydrobromide.
$C_{20}H_{26}N_2O_2,HBr = 407.3$.
CAS — 522-66-7 (hydroquinine).

NOTE. Do not confuse with Hydroquinone (p.1115).

Profile
Hydroquinine is a derivative of quinine (p.445) used similarly in the treatment of nocturnal muscle cramps. It is given as the hydrobromide in a dose of 200 mg with the evening meal and a further 100 mg at bedtime for 14 days.

Muscle spasm. Quinine and its derivatives such as hydroquinine have traditionally been used for the prevention of nocturnal cramps (p.1322) but there has been concern over their efficacy and potential for adverse effects, especially in the elderly. References.
1. Jansen PHP, *et al.* Randomised controlled trial of hydroquinine in muscle cramps. *Lancet* 1997; **349:** 528–32.
2. van Kan HJM, *et al.* Hydroquinine pharmacokinetics after oral administration in adult patients with muscle cramps. *Eur J Clin Pharmacol* 2000; **56:** 263–7.

Preparations
Proprietary Preparations (details are given in Part 3)
Neth.: Inhibin.

Hydroxyamfetamine Hydrobromide
(2067-m)
Hydroxyamfetamine Hydrobromide (BANM, rINNM).
Bromhidrato de Hidroxianfetamina; Hydroxyamphetamine Hydrobromide; Oxamphetamine Hydrobromide. (±)-4-(2-Aminopropyl)phenol hydrobromide.
$C_9H_{13}NO,HBr = 232.1$.
CAS — 103-86-6 (hydroxyamfetamine); 1518-86-1 ((±)-hydroxyamfetamine); 306-21-8 (hydroxyamfetamine hydrobromide); 140-36-3 ((±)-hydroxyamfetamine hydrobromide).
Pharmacopoeias. In US.

Pharmacopoeial description
USP 25: A white, crystalline powder. Freely soluble in water and in alcohol; slightly soluble in chloroform; practically insoluble in ether. Its solutions in water are slightly acid to litmus, having a pH of about 5. Protect from light.

Profile
Hydroxyamfetamine hydrobromide is a sympathomimetic with an action similar to that of ephedrine (p.1090), but it has little or no stimulant effect on the CNS. It was formerly used as a vasopressor and in the management of some cardiac disorders.

In ophthalmology, hydroxyamfetamine hydrobromide has been used in a 1% solution as a mydriatic and in the diagnosis of Horner's syndrome.

Preparations
USP 25: Hydroxyamphetamine Hydrobromide Ophthalmic Solution.

Proprietary Preparations (details are given in Part 3)
USA: Paredrine.
Multi-ingredient: *USA:* Paremyd.

Hydroxyapatite (1168-d)
Hydroxyapatite (BAN).
542 (edible bone phosphate); Durapatite (USAN); Hydroxylapatite; Win-40350. Decacalcium dihydroxide hexakis(orthophosphate).
$3Ca_3(PO_4)_2,Ca(OH)_2 = 1004.6$.
CAS — 1306-06-5.

A natural mineral with composition similar to that of the mineral in bone.

Profile
Hydroxyapatite for therapeutic purposes is prepared from bovine bone and contains, in addition to calcium and phosphate, trace elements, fluoride and other ions, proteins, and glycosaminoglycans. It is administered by mouth to patients requiring both calcium and phosphorus supplementation in typical doses of about 3 to 7 g daily in divided doses. Hydroxyapatite with tricalcium phosphate has been used in bone grafts.

Hydroxyapatite derived from marine coral has been used in the construction of orbital implants for use following surgical removal of the eye.

Adverse effects. Reference to problems associated with the use of coral-derived orbital implants.[1]
1. Shields CL, *et al.* Problems with the hydroxyapatite orbital implant: experience with 250 consecutive cases. *Br J Ophthalmol* 1994; **78:** 702–6.

Uses. A mixture of calcium phosphates with calcium carbonate could be combined to form a paste which could be injected into acute fractures;[1] under physiological conditions the paste hardened within minutes, due to the formation of dahllite, a carbonated apatite, and held the bones in place as it was progressively replaced by living bone.
1. Constanz BR, *et al.* Skeletal repair by in situ formation of the mineral phase of bone. *Science* 1995; **267:** 1796–9.

Preparations
Proprietary Preparations (details are given in Part 3)
Aust.: Ossopan; Osteogenon; *Braz.:* Ossopan; *Fr.:* Ossopan; *Ger.:* Ossopan; *Irl.:* Ossopan; *Ital.:* Apagen; *Mex.:* Ossopan; *Port.:* Ossopan; *Singapore:* Ossopan; *Spain:* Osteopor; *Switz.:* Ossopan; *Thai.:* Ossopan; *UK:* Ossopan; Osteo Support.

Hydroxymethylnicotinamide (12835-x)
N-Hydroxymethylnicotinamide; Nicotinylmethylamide. N-Hydroxymethylpyridine-3-carboxamide.
$C_7H_8N_2O_2 = 152.2$.
CAS — 3569-99-1.
Pharmacopoeias. In Pol.

Profile
Hydroxymethylnicotinamide is a cholagogue and has been used in the treatment of various disorders of the gallbladder.

Preparations
Proprietary Preparations (details are given in Part 3)
Multi-ingredient: *Spain:* Sambil†.

Hydroxyquinoline Sulfate (1614-g)
Chinosolum; Hydroxyquinoline Sulphate; Oxichinolini Sulfas; Oxine Sulphate; Oxyquinol; Oxyquinoline Sulfate (USAN); Sulfate d'Orthoxyquinoléine. Quinolin-8-ol sulphate; 8-Quinolinol sulphate.
$(C_9H_7NO)_2,H_2SO_4 = 388.4$.
CAS — 148-24-3 (hydroxyquinoline); 134-31-6 (hydroxyquinoline sulfate).
Pharmacopoeias. In Fr. and Swiss. Also in USNF.

Pharmacopoeial description
USNF 20: A yellow powder. Very soluble in water; slightly soluble in alcohol; practically insoluble in acetone and in ether; freely soluble in methyl alcohol.

Profile
Hydroxyquinoline sulfate has properties similar to those of potassium hydroxyquinoline sulfate (p.1654) and has been used similarly in the topical treatment of skin, oropharyngeal, and vaginal disorders.

Hydroxyquinoline salicylate, hydroxyquinoline benzoate, hydroxyquinoline borate, hydroxyquinoline hydrofluoride, hydroxyquinoline iodochloride, and hydroxyquinoline silicofluoride have been used similarly.

Preparations
Proprietary Preparations (details are given in Part 3)
Braz.: Oto-Cer; *Ger.:* Leioderm; *Ital.:* Aftir Shampoo; *Neth.:* Superol.

Multi-ingredient: *Aust.:* Racestyptin; *Austral.:* Aci-Jel; *Braz.:* Andolba; Cerumin; Colpolase; Gynaseptol; Higienex; Lacto Vagin; Lacto-Gin; Leucocida; Lisofenicol; Lisoquinol; Nestosyl; Pan-Emecort; Predmicin; Senol; Varigerm; *Canad.:* Dermoplast†; *Fr.:* Chromargon; Dermacide; Nestosyl; *Ger.:* Chinosol; Chinosol S Vaseline†; Leioderm P; *Ital.:* Leucorsan†; Ustiosan; Viderm; *NZ:* Aci-Jel; *Spain:* Neodesfila; *Switz.:* Benzocaine PD; Nasellot†; Racestyptine; *USA:* Aci-Jel; Analgesic Otic Solution†; Medicone Derma; Medicone Dressing†; Medicone Rectal; Oxyzal; Stypto-Caine; Trimo-San; Triv.

Hymecromone (3725-g)
Hymecromone (BAN, USAN, rINN).
Hymecromonum; Imecromone; LM-94. 7-Hydroxy-4-methyl-coumarin.
$C_{10}H_8O_3 = 176.2$.
CAS — 90-33-5.
ATC — A05AX02.
Pharmacopoeias. In Eur. (see p.vi) and Jpn.

Pharmacopoeial description
Ph. Eur.: An almost white crystalline powder. Very slightly soluble in water; slightly soluble in dichloromethane; sparingly soluble in methyl alcohol. It dissolves in dilute solutions of ammonia. Protect from light.

Profile
Hymecromone is a choleretic and biliary antispasmodic. It has been given in doses of 400 mg three times daily before meals. It has also been given as the sodium salt by slow intravenous injection as an adjunct to diagnostic procedures. Diarrhoea may occasionally occur.

Preparations
Proprietary Preparations (details are given in Part 3)
Aust.: Cholonerton; Unichol; *Belg.:* Cantabiline; *Fr.:* Bilicante; Cantabiline; *Ger.:* Chol-Spasmoletten; Cholspasmin; Gallo Merz Spasmo; Logomed Galle-Dragees†; *Ital.:* Cantabilin; *Spain:* Bilicanta.

Hypoglycin A (12837-f)
L-2-Amino-3-(2-methylenecyclopropyl)propionic acid.
$C_7H_{11}NO_2 = 141.2$.
CAS — 156-56-9.

A toxic substance present in the arillus of unripe ackee (akee), the fruit of *Blighia sapida* (Sapindaceae).

Profile
Hypoglycin A is responsible for Jamaican vomiting sickness, with symptoms of acute and severe vomiting, hypoglycaemia, muscular weakness, CNS depression, convulsions, and coma, frequently fatal. Glycine (p.1365) has been suggested for the management of hypoglycin A toxicity.

Hypophosphorous Acid (1936-n)
Acidum Hypophosphorosum; Phosphinic Acid.
$H_3PO_2 = 66.0$.
CAS — 6303-21-5; 14332-09-3.
Pharmacopoeias. In USNF.

Pharmacopoeial description
USNF 20: It contains 30 to 32% of H_3PO_2. A colourless or slightly yellow, odourless liquid. Store in airtight containers.

Profile
Hypophosphorous acid is used as an antioxidant. Hypophosphates were used in tonics; like the glycerophosphates they are not a suitable source of phosphorus.

Ibogaine (17207-s)
NIH-10567.

Profile
Ibogaine is a hallucinogenic indole alkaloid extracted from the West African shrub *Tabernanthe iboga* (Apocynaceae). It has been investigated as an aid to withdrawal from drug addiction.

◊ References.
1. Popik P, *et al.* 100 years of ibogaine: neurochemical and pharmacological actions of a putative anti-addictive drug. *Pharmacol Rev* 1995; **47:** 235–53.
2. Alper KR, *et al.* Treatment of acute opioid withdrawal with ibogaine. *Am J Addict* 1999; **8:** 234–42.

Idazoxan Hydrochloride (16846-s)
Idazoxan Hydrochloride (BANM, pINNM).
RX-781094. 2-(2,3-Dihydro-1,4-benzodioxin-2-yl)-2-imidazoline hydrochloride.
$C_{11}H_{12}N_2O_2,HCl = 240.7$.
CAS — 79944-58-4 (idazoxan); 79944-56-2 (idazoxan hydrochloride).

Profile
Idazoxan hydrochloride is an alpha$_2$-adrenoceptor antagonist that has been investigated in neurological disorders including depression, dementia, and parkinsonism.

◊ References.
1. Ghika J, *et al.* Idazoxan treatment in progressive supranuclear palsy. *Neurology* 1991; **41:** 986–91.
2. Litman RE, *et al.* Idazoxan, an alpha2 antagonist, augments fluphenazine in schizophrenic patients: a pilot study. *J Clin Psychopharmacol* 1993; **13:** 264–7.

3. Grossman F, *et al.* A double-blind study comparing idazoxan and bupropion in bipolar depressed patients. *J Affect Disord* 1999; **56:** 237–43.
4. Manson AJ, *et al.* Idazoxan is ineffective for levodopa-induced dyskinesias in Parkinson's disease. *Mov Disord* 2000; **15:** 336–7.

Idebenone (19336-e)

Idebenone (rINN).

CV-2619. 2-(10-Hydroxydecyl)-5,6-dimethoxy-3-methyl-*p*-benzoquinone.
$C_{19}H_{30}O_5 = 338.4$.
CAS — 58186-27-9.
ATC — N06BX13.

Profile
Idebenone has been used in the treatment of mental impairment associated with cerebrovascular disorders. A dose of 90 mg daily, in divided doses after food, has been given by mouth. Idebenone has also been tried in Alzheimer's disease.

◊ References.
1. Weyer G, *et al.* Efficacy and safety of idebenone in the long-term treatment of Alzheimer's disease: a double-blind, placebo controlled multicentre study. *Hum Psychopharmacol Clin Exp* 1996; **11:** 53–65.

Preparations
Proprietary Preparations (details are given in Part 3)
Ital.: Daruma; Mnesis; *Jpn:* Avan†; *Port.:* Cerestabon; Idecortex.

Ilodecakin (17460-f)

Ilodecakin (USAN, rINN).
Sch-52000.
CAS — 149824-15-7.

Profile
Ilodecakin is a recombinant human interleukin-10. It is under investigation for its anti-inflammatory properties in several diseases including psoriasis, inflammatory bowel disease, and hepatitis C.

Indeloxazine Hydrochloride (15324-r)

Indeloxazine Hydrochloride (USAN, rINNM).
CI-874. (±)-2-[(Inden-7-yloxy)methyl]morpholine hydrochloride.
$C_{14}H_{17}NO_2,HCl = 267.8$.
CAS — 60929-23-9 (indeloxazine); 65043-22-3 (indeloxazine hydrochloride).

Profile
Indeloxazine hydrochloride has been reported to improve cerebral function. It has been promoted for the treatment of hypobulia (a lack of volition or drive) and for emotional disturbances associated with cerebrovascular disorders.

Preparations
Proprietary Preparations (details are given in Part 3)
Jpn: Elen†.

Indigo Carmine (2135-f)

Blue X; Ceruleinum; CI Food Blue 1; Colour Index No. 73015; Disodium Indigotin-5,5'-disulphonate; E132; FD & C Blue No. 2; Indicarminum; Indigotindisulfonate Sodium; Indigotine; Sodium Indigotindisulphonate. Disodium 3,3'-dioxo-2,2'-bi-indolinylidene-5,5'-disulphonate.
$C_{16}H_8N_2Na_2O_8S_2 = 466.4$.
CAS — 483-20-5 (indigotin-5,5'-disulphonic acid); 860-22-0 (indigo carmine).
ATC — V04CH02.

NOTE. The name Caerulein has been applied to Ceruletide (p.1593).
Pharmacopoeias. In Fr., It., Jpn, and US.

Pharmacopoeial description
USP 25: A dusky, purplish-blue powder, or blue granules having a coppery lustre. Soluble 1 in 100 of water; slightly soluble in alcohol; practically insoluble in most other organic solvents. Its solutions have a blue or bluish-purple colour. Store in airtight containers. Protect from light.

Adverse Effects and Precautions
Indigo carmine may cause nausea, vomiting, hypertension, and bradycardia, and occasionally, hypersensitivity reactions such as skin rash, pruritus, and bronchoconstriction. Skin discoloration may occur following administration of large parenteral doses.

Hypersensitivity. Cardiac arrest following the administration of indigo carmine 80 mg intravenously resulted in the deaths of 2 elderly patients.[1] Both had a history of asthmatic bronchitis. A life-threatening anaphylactoid reaction associated with indi-

go carmine use has also been reported, although the authors commented that such events are rare.[2]
1. Voiry AM, *et al.* Deux accidents mortels lors d'une injection peropératoire de carmin d'indigo. *Ann Med Nancy* 1976; **15:** 413–19.
2. Gousse AE, *et al.* Life-threatening anaphylactoid reaction associated with indigo carmine intravenous injection. *Urology* 2000; **56:** 508.

Uses and Administration
Following intravenous injection indigo carmine is rapidly excreted, principally by the kidneys. It has been used in a test of renal function, but has largely been replaced by agents which give more precise results. It is used as a marker dye, particularly in urological procedures, when it is administered in a usual dose of 40 mg, preferably by intravenous injection but sometimes intramuscularly. It has also been used as a marker dye in amniocentesis.

Indigo carmine has been used as a blue dye in medicinal preparations but it is relatively unstable. It is used as a food colour.

Preparations
USP 25: Indigotindisulfonate Sodium Injection.

Indocyanine Green (2136-d)

Sodium 2-{7-[1,1-dimethyl-3-(4-sulphobutyl)benz[e]indolin-2-ylidene]hepta-1,3,5-trienyl}-1,1-dimethyl-1H-benz[e]indolio-3-(butyl-4-sulphonate).
$C_{43}H_{47}N_2NaO_6S_2 = 775.0$.
CAS — 3599-32-4.
Pharmacopoeias. In US.

Pharmacopoeial description
USP 25: An olive-brown, dark green, blue-green, dark blue, or black powder. Is odourless or has a slight odour. It contains not more than 5.0% of sodium iodide, calculated on the dried basis. Soluble in water and in methyl alcohol; practically insoluble in most other organic solvents. Its solutions are deep emerald-green in colour. pH of a 0.5% solution in water is about 6. Its aqueous solutions are stable for about 8 hours.

Adverse Effects and Precautions
Indocyanine green is reported to be well tolerated. Solutions contain a small amount of sodium iodide and should be used with caution in patients hypersensitive to iodine. Clearance of indocyanine green may be altered by drugs that interfere with liver function.

Hypersensitivity. A report of anaphylactoid reactions to indocyanine green in 3 patients.[1] The authors commented that of 20 reactions that had been reported 9 involved anaphylactoid shock (with 2 subsequent deaths) and 11 involved hypotension or bronchospasm; they suggested that such reactions were dose-dependent and had a non-immune mechanism.
1. Speich R, *et al.* Anaphylactoid reactions after indocyanine-green administration. *Ann Intern Med* 1988; **109:** 345–6.

Pharmacokinetics
After intravenous injection indocyanine green is almost completely bound to plasma protein. It is taken up by the liver and is rapidly excreted unchanged into the bile.

Uses and Administration
Indocyanine green is an indicator dye used for assessing cardiac output and liver function, and for examining the choroidal vasculature in ophthalmic angiography. It is also used to assess blood flow and haemodynamics in various organs including the liver.

The usual dose for cardiac assessment is 5 mg injected rapidly via a cardiac catheter. A suggested dose for children is 2.5 mg, and for infants 1.25 mg. Several doses need to be given to obtain a number of dilution curves. However, the total dose should not exceed 2 mg per kg body-weight.

The usual dose of indocyanine green for testing liver function is 500 µg per kg intravenously.

Diagnostic use. Indocyanine green has been employed to assess blood flow to various organs and in other haemodynamic studies. However, some methods of determination of indocyanine green clearance as a measure of liver blood flow have been questioned on the grounds that extraction of the dye by the liver is not complete as is often assumed.[1] Interindividual variability in indocyanine clearance may introduce further error.[2] There have been reports of the use of indocyanine green to assess cerebral blood flow in children during cardiopulmonary bypass[3] and to measure plasma volume in neonates.[4] In ophthalmology, indocyanine green angiography is used to visualise the choroidal circulation.[5]
1. Skak C, Keiding S. Methodological problems in the use of indocyanine green to estimate hepatic blood flow and ICG clearance in man. *Liver* 1987; **7:** 155–62.
2. Bauer LA, *et al.* Variability of indocyanine green pharmacokinetics in healthy adults. *Clin Pharm* 1989; **8:** 54–5.
3. Roberts I, *et al.* Estimation of cerebral blood flow with near infrared spectroscopy and indocyanine green. *Lancet* 1993; **342:** 1425.
4. Anthony MY, *et al.* Measurement of plasma volume in neonates. *Arch Dis Child* 1992; **67:** 36–40.
5. Owens SL. Indocyanine green angiography. *Br J Ophthalmol* 1996; **80:** 263–6.

Preparations
USP 25: Indocyanine Green for Injection.
Proprietary Preparations (details are given in Part 3)
Ger.: Cardio-Green†; ICG-Pulsion; *Israel:* ICG-Pulsion; *USA:* Cardio-Green; IC Green.

Inhibin (19345-l)

Profile
Inhibin is a glycoprotein secreted by the testes and ovaries which has been investigated as a potential contraceptive in both men and women, because of its ability to suppress secretion of follicle-stimulating hormone by the pituitary.

Inosine (12852-r)

Inosine (rINN).
Hypoxanthine Riboside. 6,9-Dihydro-9-β-D-ribofuranosyl-1H-purin-6-one.
$C_{10}H_{12}N_4O_5 = 268.2$.
CAS — 58-63-9.
ATC — D06BB05; G01AX02; S01XA10.

Profile
Inosine has been used in the treatment of anaemias and cardiovascular, liver, and skin disorders and has been used as a tonic.

Preparations
Proprietary Preparations (details are given in Part 3)
Braz.: Troficardil; *Spain:* Tebertin†.
Multi-ingredient: *Aust.:* Laevadosin; *Ital.:* For Liver†; Fruttocal; Neo-Eparbiol; *Spain:* Boldosal; Nutracel; Rubrocortin.

Inositol (7877-p)

i-Inositol; meso-Inositol. myo-Inositol.
$C_6H_{12}O_6 = 180.2$.
CAS — 87-89-8.
Pharmacopoeias. In Aust., Belg., and Fr.

Profile
Inositol, an isomer of glucose, has traditionally been considered to be a vitamin B substance although it has an uncertain status as a vitamin and a deficiency syndrome has not been identified in man. Sources of inositol include whole-grain cereals, fruits, and plants, in which it occurs as the hexaphosphate, phytic acid. It also occurs in both vegetables and meats in other forms. The usual daily intake of inositol from the diet is about 1 g. It is an ingredient of numerous vitamin preparations and dietary supplements, and of preparations promoted for a wide variety of disorders.
Inositol appears to be involved physiologically in lipid metabolism and has been tried, with little evidence of efficacy, in disorders associated with fat transport and metabolism. It has been investigated in the treatment of depression and anxiety, in diabetic neuropathy, and in neonatal respiratory distress syndrome and retinopathy of prematurity.

Neonatal respiratory distress syndrome. Inositol supplementation has been tried in premature infants with respiratory distress syndrome. A meta-analysis[1] found that infants given inositol had improved survival and lower rates of bronchopulmonary dysplasia and retinopathy of prematurity than those given placebo.
1. Howlett A, Ohlsson A. Inositol for respiratory distress syndrome in preterm infants (updated 27 February 2001). Available in The Cochrane Library; Issue 4. Oxford: Update Software; 2001.

Preparations
Proprietary Preparations (details are given in Part 3)
Hong Kong: Inositab.
Multi-ingredient: *Aust.:* Aslavital; Lemazol; *Austral.:* Ginkgo ACE†; Hair and Skin Formula; Liv-Detox; *Braz.:* Hepatogenol; Hormo Hepatico; Metiocolin B12; Metiocolin Composto; Metionina Composta; Necrohepat; Xantina B12; Xantinon B12; Xantinon Complex; *Canad.:* Amino-Cerv; *Fr.:* Hepagrume; *Ger.:* Hepalipon N†; Lipovitan; *Hong Kong:* Bilsan; Lipochol; *Ital.:* Digelax; Hepatos B12; Porfirin 12; *Port.:* Metionina; *S.Afr.:* Hepavite; Prohep; *Spain:* Complidermol; Dertrase; Policolinosil; Tri Hachemina; *Thai.:* Lipochol; Liporon; Proheparum; *UK:* Fat-Solv; Lipotropic Factors; *USA:* Amino-Cerv.

Interleukin-1 (16853-p)

Catabolin; Endogenous Pyrogen; Haematopoietin-1; IL-1; Leucocyte Endogenous Mediator; Lymphocyte Activating Factor.

A protein produced by monocytes and a variety of other cell types *in vivo* and which may also be produced by recombinant DNA technology.

Two distinct forms, interleukin-1α and interleukin-1β, are known to exist, which interact with the same receptor and appear to have similar biological activities.

Profile
Interleukin-1 is one of a number of polypeptides produced by lymphocytes, monocytes, and other cells which are involved in the complex hormonal regulation of immune response, and

The symbol † denotes a preparation no longer actively marketed

which are known collectively as cytokines. The term lymphokines has also been used to describe these compounds but is more properly restricted to products of the various lymphocyte subsets, such as interleukin-2.

It has been suggested that interleukin-1 may be of value in a wide variety of conditions including burn and wound healing, as an adjuvant to enhance the response to vaccines, and as an adjunct to cancer chemotherapy or radiotherapy for its haematopoietic and possible antitumour activity. Adverse effects include fever, chills, headache, gastrointestinal disturbances, local erythema at the injection site, hypotension, and CNS effects.

Interleukin-2 is described in the chapter on Antineoplastics and Immunosuppressants (p.547). Other interleukins under investigation include interleukin-3 (p.738) as a haematopoietic; interleukin-4 (IL-4) and interleukin-6 (IL-6) for malignant neoplasms and thrombocytopenia; interleukin-10 for inflammatory disorders; and interleukin-12 for malignant neoplasms and infections. Oprelvekin (p.739) is a recombinant interleukin-11 used in thrombocytopenia.

◊ Pharmacokinetics of some interleukins.
1. Bocci V. Interleukins: clinical pharmacokinetics and practical implications. *Clin Pharmacokinet* 1991; **21:** 274–84.

Interleukin-1 Receptor Antagonists (19857-y)

IL-1ra; IL-1i; Interleukin-1 Inhibitors.

Anakinra (10702-j)

Anakinra (BAN, USAN, rINN).
rhIL-1ra.
CAS — 143090-92-0.

Profile
Antagonism of interleukin-1 is under investigation in a range of disorders where interleukin-1 is thought to play a role. A recombinant interleukin-1 receptor antagonist, anakinra, is used in rheumatoid arthritis in a dose of 100 mg daily by subcutaneous injection. It has also been suggested for the management of graft-versus-host disease in transplant recipients. It was tried in septic shock, but results were disappointing.

Anakinra has been associated with an increased incidence of serious infections. It should not be given to patients with active infections and its use should be discontinued in those who develop a serious infection during treatment.

◊ References.
1. Fisher CJ, Recombination human interleukin 1 receptor antagonist in the treatment of patients with sepsis syndrome: results from a randomized, double-blind, placebo-controlled trial. *JAMA* 1994; **271:** 1836–43.
2. Bresnihan B, *et al.* Treatment of rheumatoid arthritis with recombinant human interleukin-1 receptor antagonist. *Arthritis Rheum* 1998; **41:** 2196–2204.

Preparations
Proprietary Preparations (details are given in Part 3)
USA: Kineret.

Interleukin-2 Fusion Toxins (19769-y)

Profile
Recombinant technology has permitted the production of a number of products in which protein sequences from natural growth factors or cytokines are combined with a toxin. Such products include fusion toxins in which the receptor binding domain of diphtheria toxin is replaced with sequences from interleukin-2, thus producing specific cytotoxicity in cells expressing the interleukin-2 receptor. The interleukin-2 fusion toxin denileukin diftitox (p.533) is used in the treatment of cutaneous T-cell lymphoma, and both this and the related compound DAB_{486} interleukin-2 have been investigated in a variety of disorders including diabetes mellitus, psoriasis, rheumatoid arthritis, cutaneous T-cell lymphoma and other malignancies, and HIV infection.

Inulin (2137-n)

Inulin (BAN).
Alant Starch.
CAS — 9005-80-5.
Pharmacopoeias. In Br. and US.

Crystals of inulin may be deposited on storage of the injection; they should be dissolved by heating for not more than 15 minutes before use and the injection cooled to a suitable temperature before administration.

Pharmacopoeial description
BP 2001: A polysaccharide obtained from the tubers of *Dahlia variabilis, Helianthus tuberosus,* and other genera of the family Compositae. It is a white, odourless or almost odourless, hygroscopic, amorphous, granular powder. Slightly soluble in cold water, but freely soluble in hot water; slightly soluble in organic solvents.

USP 25: A polysaccharide which, on hydrolysis, yields mainly fructose. A white, friable, chalk-like, amorphous, odourless powder. Soluble in hot water; slightly soluble in cold water and in organic solvents. A 10% solution in water has a pH of 4.5 to 7.0.

Pharmacokinetics
Inulin is rapidly removed from the circulation following intravenous administration but is not metabolised. A trace may be found in the bile and may cross the placenta, but it is predominantly eliminated in the urine by glomerular filtration without secretion or reabsorption in the renal tubule.

Uses and Administration
Inulin is used intravenously as a diagnostic agent to measure the glomerular filtration rate. Although an accurate test, it is complex to perform and is generally reserved for research purposes.

Polyfructosan, an inulin analogue of lower average molecular weight, has been used similarly.

Preparations
BP 2001: Inulin Injection;
USP 25: Inulin in Sodium Chloride Injection.
Proprietary Preparations (details are given in Part 3)
Aust.: Inutest; *Swed.:* Inutest†; *Switz.:* Inutest†.
Multi-ingredient: *Ital.:* Lactolas; Naturalass.

Iris Versicolor (14052-v)

Blue Flag; Iris Virginica.

Profile
The rhizomes of *Iris versicolor* (Iridaceae) are used in herbal and homoeopathic medicine.

Preparations
Proprietary Preparations (details are given in Part 3)
Multi-ingredient: *UK:* Blue Flag Root Compound; Catarrh Mixture; HRI Clear Complexion; Skin Eruptions Mixture.

Isometheptene Hydrochloride (2072-d)

Isometheptene Hydrochloride (BANM, rINNM).
1,5,N-Trimethylhex-4-enylamine hydrochloride; 1,5-Dimethylhex-4-enyl(methyl)amine hydrochloride.
$C_9H_{19}N,HCl = 177.7$.
CAS — 503-01-5 (isometheptene); 6168-86-1 (isometheptene hydrochloride).

Isometheptene Mucate (2073-n)

Isometheptene Mucate (BANM, rINNM).
Isometheptene galactarate.
$(C_9H_{19}N)_2,C_6H_{10}O_8 = 492.6$.
CAS — 7492-31-1.
Pharmacopoeias. In Br. and US.

Pharmacopoeial description
BP 2001: A white crystalline powder. Very soluble in water; slightly soluble in dehydrated alcohol; very slightly soluble in chloroform; practically insoluble in ether. A 5% solution in water has a pH of 5.4 to 6.6. Store in airtight containers. Protect from light.

USP 25: A white crystalline powder. Freely soluble in water; soluble in alcohol; practically insoluble in chloroform and in ether. pH of a 5% solution in water is between 6.0 and 7.5.

Adverse Effects and Precautions
For the adverse effects of sympathomimetics, and precautions to be observed, see under Adrenaline, p.829.

Porphyria. Isometheptene mucate has been associated with acute attacks of porphyria and is considered unsafe in porphyric patients.

Interactions
For the interactions of sympathomimetics in general, see under Adrenaline, p.830. Isometheptene has been reported to produce severe hypertensive reactions in patients receiving MAOIs.

◊ For a report of hypertension and life-threatening complications following concomitant use of isometheptene and *bromocriptine*, see under Sympathomimetics, p.1166.

Uses and Administration
Isometheptene is an indirect-acting sympathomimetic (see under Adrenaline, p.831). It is included for its vasoconstrictor effect, usually as the mucate, in some analgesic combination products used to treat acute migraine attacks (p.449). Typical doses of isometheptene mucate in migraine are 130 mg at the beginning of an attack, with 65 mg hourly thereafter as necessary, up to a total maximum dose of 325 mg in a 12-hour period.

Isometheptene hydrochloride is also used in the management of migraine and smooth muscle spasm. Usual doses are 75 to 100 mg by mouth 3 or 4 times daily, although higher doses have been given. It is also given by intramuscular, or occasionally, or slow intravenous, injection. The mucate has also been used in the management of muscle spasms.

Preparations
USP 25: Isometheptene Mucate, Dichloralphenazone, and Acetaminophen Capsules.
Proprietary Preparations (details are given in Part 3)
Braz.: Cefaldina; *Switz.:* Octinum.
Multi-ingredient: *Braz.:* Neosaldina; Sulindor; *Hong Kong:* Midrid; *UK:* Midrid; *USA:* Duradrin; Isocom; Isopap; Midchlor†; Midrin; Migralam†; Migratine.

Isospaglumic Acid (2547-t)

Isospaglumic Acid (rINN).
N-(N-Acetyl-L-α-aspartyl)-L-glutamic acid.
$C_{11}H_{16}N_2O_8 = 304.3$.
CAS — 3106-85-2.

Profile
Isospaglumic acid is used as the sodium or the magnesium salt in eye drops for allergic eye conditions and in nasal solutions for allergic rhinitis.

Preparations
Proprietary Preparations (details are given in Part 3)
Aust.: Rhinaaxia; *Braz.:* Naaxia; *Fr.:* Naabak; Naaxia; Rhinaaxia; *Ger.:* Naaxia†; *Spain:* Naaxia; *Switz.:* Rhinaaxia.
Multi-ingredient: *S.Afr.:* Naaxia; *Switz.:* Naaxia.

Isoxsuprine Hydrochloride (9246-c)

Isoxsuprine Hydrochloride (BANM, rINNM).
Caa-40; Isoxsuprini Hydrochloridum; Phenoxyisopropylnorsuprifen. 1-(4-Hydroxyphenyl)-2-(1-methyl-2-phenoxyethylamino)propan-1-ol hydrochloride.
$C_{18}H_{23}NO_3,HCl = 337.8$.
CAS — 395-28-8 (isoxsuprine); 579-56-6 (isoxsuprine hydrochloride).
Pharmacopoeias. In Eur. (see p.vi) and US.

Pharmacopoeial description
Ph. Eur.: A white or almost white crystalline powder. Sparingly soluble in water and in alcohol; practically insoluble in dichloromethane and in ether. A 1% solution in water has a pH of 4.5 to 6.0. Protect from light.

USP 25: A white, odourless, crystalline powder. Soluble 1 in 500 of water, 1 in 100 of alcohol and of 0.1N sodium hydroxide solution, and 1 in 2500 of 0.1N hydrochloric acid; practically insoluble in chloroform and in ether. pH of a 1% solution in water is between 4.5 and 6.0. Store in airtight containers.

Adverse Effects
Isoxsuprine may cause transient flushing, hypotension, tachycardia, rashes, and gastrointestinal disturbances. Maternal pulmonary oedema and fetal tachycardia have been reported following intravenous administration in premature labour.

Pulmonary oedema. Pulmonary oedema has been reported in mothers given isoxsuprine for premature labour.[1,2]
1. Nagey DA, Crenshaw MC. Pulmonary complications of isoxsuprine therapy in the gravida. *Obstet Gynecol* 1982; **59** (suppl): 38S–42S.
2. Nimrod C, *et al.* Pulmonary edema associated with isoxsuprine therapy. *Am J Obstet Gynecol* 1984; **148:** 625–9.

Precautions
Isoxsuprine is contra-indicated after recent arterial haemorrhage. It should not be given immediately post partum, nor should it be used for premature labour if there is infection.

In women being treated for premature labour, the risk of pulmonary oedema means that extreme caution is required and the precautions and risk factors discussed under Salbutamol Sulfate, p.771, apply.

Pregnancy. Ileus was found to be more common in the offspring of mothers who received isoxsuprine than in matched controls.[1] The incidence of respiratory distress syndrome also rose as the isoxsuprine concentration in cord blood exceeded 10 nanograms per mL; likewise the incidence of hypocalcaemia and hypotension rose progressively with increasing concentrations. The cord concentrations correlated inversely with the drug-free interval before delivery and it was suggested that with frequent assessment of uterine response it should be possible to avoid delivering infants at a time when they have high plasma-isoxsuprine concentrations.[1]

In another study[2] of the association between ruptured membranes, beta-adrenergic therapy, and respiratory distress syndrome, it was found that both therapy with isoxsuprine and premature rupture of membranes were individually associated with a lowered incidence of respiratory distress syndrome, but when present together they resulted in an increased risk of respiratory distress syndrome. It was suggested that therapy with beta-adrenergic drugs including isoxsuprine should be restricted to patients with intact membranes.[1]
1. Brazy JE, *et al.* Isoxsuprine in the perinatal period II: relationships between neonatal symptoms, drug exposure, and drug concentration at the time of birth. *J Pediatr* 1981; **98:** 146–51.
2. Curet LB, *et al.* Association between ruptured membranes, tocolytic therapy, and respiratory distress syndrome. *Am J Obstet Gynecol* 1984; **148:** 263–8.

Pharmacokinetics

Isoxsuprine hydrochloride is well absorbed from the gastrointestinal tract. The peak plasma concentration occurs about 1 hour after administration by mouth. A plasma half-life of 1.5 hours has been reported. Isoxsuprine is excreted in the urine mainly as conjugates.

Uses and Administration

Isoxsuprine is a vasodilator which also stimulates beta-adrenergic receptors. It causes direct relaxation of vascular and uterine smooth muscle and its vasodilating action is greater on the arteries supplying skeletal muscles than on those supplying skin. Isoxsuprine also produces positive inotropic and chronotropic effects.

Isoxsuprine hydrochloride has been used to arrest premature labour (p.773), but drugs with a more selective action on beta$_2$ receptors, such as ritodrine, are now preferred. It has also been given in the treatment of cerebral and peripheral vascular disease.

For use as a vasodilator, isoxsuprine hydrochloride is given by mouth in doses of 10 to 20 mg 3 or 4 times daily.

To arrest premature labour, isoxsuprine hydrochloride is given initially by intravenous infusion in doses of 200 to 500 µg per minute, adjusted according to the patient's response, until control is achieved. It is now common practice to administer beta agonists by syringe pump when using them to delay premature labour. Maternal blood pressure and hydration, and maternal and fetal heart rates should be monitored during the infusion. Subsequent treatment when labour has been arrested consists of intramuscular injections of 10 mg every 3 to 8 hours for several days. Prophylaxis may be continued by mouth with 30 to 90 mg daily in divided doses.

The resinate has also been used similarly.

Preparations

USP 25: Isoxsuprine Hydrochloride Injection; Isoxsuprine Hydrochloride Tablets.

Proprietary Preparations (details are given in Part 3)
Aust.: Xuprin; **Austral.:** Duvadilan†; **Belg.:** Duvadilan; **Braz.:** Inibina; **Fr.:** Duvadilan†; **Hong Kong:** Duvadilan; **Irl.:** Duvadilan; **Israel:** Vasolan; **Ital.:** Duvadilan†; Fenam†; Vasosuprina Ilfi; **Mex.:** Vadosilan; **Neth.:** Duvadilan; **Port.:** Dilum; **Spain:** Duvadilan†; **Thai.:** Duvadilan; **USA:** Vasodilan; Voxsuprine.

Jamaica Dogwood   (5135-d)

Fish Poison Bark.

Profile
Jamaica dogwood, the root bark of *Piscidia erythrina* (*P. piscipula*; *Ichthyomethia piscipula*) (Leguminosae), has analgesic, antispasmodic, and sedative properties. It is mainly used for insomnia due to neuralgia or nervous tension. The bark and twigs of Jamaica dogwood have been used as a fish poison.

Preparations

Proprietary Preparations (details are given in Part 3)
Multi-ingredient: Braz.: Regran; **Fr.:** Bronpax†; Jouvence de l'Abbe Soury; Schoum; **Ital.:** Sedatol; Soluzione Schoum; **Spain:** Sol Schoum; **UK:** Anased; Biophylin†; Gerard House Valerian Compound; HRI Calm Life; Nodoff; Nytol Herbal; Slumber.

Java Tea   (11483-b)

Orthosiphonblätter; Orthosiphonis Folium.
Pharmacopoeias. In *Eur.* (see p.vi).

Pharmacopoeial description
Ph. Eur.: The fragmented, dried leaves and tops of stems of *Orthosiphon stamineus* (*O. aristatus*; *O. spicatus*). Protect from light.

Profile
Java tea is used in herbal medicine.

Preparations

Proprietary Preparations (details are given in Part 3)
Aust.: Carito mono; **Fr.:** Urosiphon; **Ger.:** Aquacaps†; Carito mono; Nephronorm med; Orthosiphonblatter Indischer Nierentee; Repha Orphon.

Multi-ingredient: Aust.: Apotheker Bauer's Harntreibender Tee; Apotheker Bauer's Nieren- und Blasentee; Blasen- und Nierentee; Droxitop; Krauterhaus Mag Kottas Blasentee; Krauterhaus Mag Kottas Nierentee; Krautertee Nr 31; Mag Kottas Entwasserungstee; Mag Kottas Nieren-Blasentee; Sidroga Nieren- und Blasentee; Solubitrat; **Belg.:** Tisane Contre la Tension; **Fr.:** Actisane Minceur; Aminsane†; Aromalgyl†; Dellova; Promincil; Tealine; **Ger.:** Aqualibra; BioCyst; Canephron novo; Cysto Fink; Etmoren†; Harntee 400; Harntee 450; Harntee STADA; Harntee-Steiner; Heumann Blasen- und Nierentee Solubitrat N; Hevert-Blasen- und Nieren- Tee; Heweberberol-Tee; NB-Tee N†; Nephro-Pasc; Nephronorm med†; Nephropur tri; Nephrubin†; Nierentee 2000; Nieron Blasen- und Nieren-Tee VI; Presselin Arterien K 5 P; Presselin Nieren-Blasen K 3; Uro Fink†; Urodil Blasen-Nieren Arzneitee†; Urodil phyto; Urostei; **Switz.:** Bilifuge; Demonatur Dragees pour les reins et la vessie; Dragees pour reins et vessie S; Phytomed Nephro†; Prosta-Caps Chassot N; Tisane pour les reins et la vessie.

Jin Bu Huan   (17753-l)

Profile
Jin bu huan is a traditional Chinese remedy used as a sedative and analgesic and variously stated to contain *Lycopodium serratum* or *Polygala chinensis*. Adverse effects including CNS depression and acute hepatotoxicity have been attributed to its alkaloidal content of L-tetrahydropalmatine.

Adverse effects. Acute hepatitis has been reported in 7 previously healthy patients following ingestion of jin bu huan; symptoms occurred again in 2 following re-use.[1] It was noted that the content of plant material did not seem to correspond to the labelled species. Hepatitis and extreme fatigue have also been reported in 3 adults after taking jin bu huan for periods ranging from 6 days to 6 months.[2]

Accidental ingestion of jin bu huan by 3 children[2] produced profound lethargy and muscle weakness. Two of the children also developed respiratory depression and bradycardia.

1. Woolf GM, *et al.* Acute hepatitis associated with the Chinese herbal product jin bu huan. *Ann Intern Med* 1994; **121:** 729–35.
2. Horowitz RS, *et al.* The clinical spectrum of jin bu huan toxicity. *Arch Intern Med* 1996; **156:** 899–903.

Juniper   (4654-z)

Baccae Juniperi; Genièvre; Juniper Berry; Juniper Fruit; Juniperi Fructus; Juniperi Galbulus; Juniperi Pseudo-fructus; Wacholderbeeren; Zimbro.
Pharmacopoeias. In *Eur.* (see p.vi).

Pharmacopoeial description
Ph. Eur.: The dried ripe cone berry of *Juniperus communis*. It contains not less than 1% v/w of essential oil, calculated with reference to the anhydrous drug. It has a strongly aromatic odour, especially if crushed. Protect from light.

Profile
Juniper is the source of juniper oil (below). It has carminative, diuretic, antiseptic, and anti-inflammatory properties. It is used in herbal and homoeopathic medicine and as a flavour in gin.

Preparations

Proprietary Preparations (details are given in Part 3)
Ger.: Kneipp Wacholderbeer-Pflanzensaft†.

Multi-ingredient: Aust.: Aktiv Blasen- und Nierentee; Aponatura Entwasserungs; Apotheker Bauer's Harntreibender Tee; Blasen-Tee; Kneipp Entwasserungstee; Krautertee Nr 18; Krautertee Nr 19; Krautertee Nr 29; Krautertee Nr 30; Krautertee Nr 4; Mariazeller; St Bonifatius-Tee; **Austral.:** Arthritic Pain Herbal Formula 1; Fluid Loss; Lifesystem Herbal Formula 1 Arthritic Aid; PMT-EZE†; Profluid; Protemp; **Belg.:** Tisane Diuretique; **Braz.:** Pilulas De Witt's; **Canad.:** Arthrisan†; Herbal Laxative; **Fr.:** Depuratum; Mediflor Tisane Antirhumatismale No 2†; Santane A₄; Santane R₈; **Ger.:** Amara-Tropfen; Befelka-Tinktur†; Discmigon; Gastrol S; Harntee 400; Hevert-Entwasserungs-Tee†; Hevert-Gicht-Rheuma-Tee comp†; Imbak; Junisana; Kneipp Entschlackungs-Tee; Kneipp Rheuma Tee N†; Montana; Presselin Stoffwechsel-Tee Hapeka 225 N; Salus Rheuma-Tee Krautertee Nr. 12†; **Ital.:** Broncosedina; Depurfat†; **Switz.:** Ajaka†; Kernosan Heidelberger Poudre; Phytomed Nephro†; Tisane laxative Natterman no 13†; Tisane pour les reins et la vessie; **UK:** Backache; Watershed.

Juniper Oil   (4655-c)

Essence de Genièvre; Juniper Berry Oil; Juniperi Aetheroleum; Oleum Juniperi; Wacholderöl.
Pharmacopoeias. In *Eur.* (see p.vi) and *Pol.*

Pharmacopoeial description
Ph. Eur.: The essential oil obtained by steam distillation from the ripe, non-fermented berry cones of *Juniperus communis*. A suitable antioxidant may be added. A mobile, colourless to yellowish liquid with a characteristic odour. Store in well-filled airtight containers at a temperature not exceeding 25°. Protect from light.

Profile
Juniper oil has been used as a carminative and as an ingredient of herbal remedies for urinary-tract disorders and muscle and joint pain. Prolonged use may cause gastrointestinal irritation and there may be a risk of renal damage from high doses.

Preparations

Proprietary Preparations (details are given in Part 3)
Ger.: Leukona-Stoffwechsel-Bad; Roleca Wacholder; **Switz.:** Roleca-S.

Multi-ingredient: Aust.: Apotheker Bauer's Inhalationsmischung; Berggeist; **Austral.:** Medinat PMT-Eze; **Ger.:** Dolo-cyl; GA-301-Redskin 301†; Kneipp Rheuma-Bad; Neo-Lapitrypsin†; Nierentee 2000; Nieroxin N; Olbas; Schupps Heilkrauter Rheumabad; Schupps Latschenkiefer Olbad†; **Ital.:** Otosan Gocce Auricolari; **Spain:** Emolytar; Polytar; **Switz.:** Ajaka†; Baby Liberol†; Caprisana†; Demo pommade contre les refroidissements pour bebes; Huile Po-Ho A. Vogel; Liberol Baby N; Olbas; Spagyrom; **UK:** Diuretabs; HealthAid Boldo-Plus; Juno Junipah; Olbas; Sciargo; St Johnswort Compound; Watershed.

Kallidinogenase   (9248-a)

Kallidinogenase *(BAN, rINN)*.
Callicrein; Kalléone; Kallikrein.
CAS — 9001-01-8.
ATC — C04AF01.
Pharmacopoeias. In *Jpn.*

An enzyme isolated from the pancreas and urine of mammals.

Profile
Kallidinogenase converts kininogen into the kinin, kallidin. It is used in male infertility (p.1275) since the kallikrein-kinin system has a physiological role in the male genital tract. It also has vasodilating properties and has been used in the treatment of peripheral vascular disease (p.809).

Preparations

Proprietary Preparations (details are given in Part 3)
Aust.: Padutin; **Ger.:** Padutin.

Kava   (12878-p)

Kava-Kava.
CAS — 500-64-1 (kawain); 495-85-2 (methysticin); 500-62-9 (yangonin).

The rhizome of *Piper methysticum* (Piperaceae), a shrub indigenous to islands of the South Pacific. It contains pyrones including kawain, methysticin, and yangonin.

Profile
Kava has been used in the South Pacific to produce an intoxicating beverage used for recreational purposes and during convalescence. It is reported to have sedative, skeletal muscle relaxant, and anaesthetic properties. It is given in some anxiety- and stress-related disorders. It was formerly used as an antiseptic and diuretic in inflammatory conditions of the genito-urinary tract in the form of a liquid extract. Kawain has also been used.

A characteristic rash resembling that of pellagra occurs in some heavy consumers of kava. Extrapyramidal effects and cases of hepatitis have been reported.

◊ **References.**
1. Anonymous. Kava. *Lancet* 1988; **ii:** 258–9.
2. Anonymous. Tonga trouble. *Pharm J* 1990; **245:** 288.
3. Ruze P. Kava-induced dermopathy: a niacin deficiency? *Lancet* 1990; **335:** 1442–5.
4. Schelosky L, *et al.* Kava and dopamine antagonism. *J Neurol Neurosurg Psychiatry* 1995; **58:** 639–40.
5. Spillane PK, *et al.* Neurological manifestations of kava intoxication. *Med J Aust* 1997; **167:** 172–3.
6. Pepping J. Kava: piper methysticum. *Am J Health-Syst Pharm* 1999; **56:** 957–60.
7. Anonymous. Kava extract linked to hepatitis. *WHO Drug Inf* 2000; **14:** 98.
8. Escher M, *et al.* Hepatitis associated with kava, a herbal remedy for anxiety. *BMJ* 2001; **322:** 139.

Preparations

Proprietary Preparations (details are given in Part 3)
Aust.: Largon; **Ger.:** Aigin; Antares; Ardeydystin; Cefakava; Eukavan; Jakava; Kava-Phyton; Kavacur; Kavaform N; Kavasedon; Kavatino; Kavosporal forte; Kytta-Kava; Laitan; Limbao; Maoni; Nervonocton N; Neuronika; Sedalint Kava; **Mex.:** Laiken; **Switz.:** Kavasedon; Kavasol; Laitan; Songha Day.

Multi-ingredient: Aust.: Kavaform; Kavavit; **Ger.:** Bilicura Forte; Cysto Fink; Hewepsychon duo; Hyposedon N; Kavain Harras Plus; Kavosporal comp; Somnuvis S; Valeriana comp; **Ital.:** Ansidem; **Spain:** Bleukawine†; **Switz.:** Cysto Fink†; Cysto-Caps Chassot†; Kawaform; Yakona N†; **UK:** Antiglan; GB Tablets; Protat.

Kelp   (12137-k)

Profile
Kelp is a preparation of dried seaweed of various species that is present as an ingredient of several dietary supplements and herbal preparations. It has been used as a source of iodine.

◊ Kelp can concentrate various heavy metals; auto-immune thrombocytopenic purpura with dyserythropoiesis occurring in a patient who had been taking kelp tablets for 6 weeks was attributed to the arsenic content of the preparation.[1]

Clinical hyperthyroidism has also been reported in patients taking kelp-containing preparations as part of a slimming regimen[2] or a dietary supplement.[3]

The FDA has advised that preparations containing compounds such as kelp, which may be taken by mouth in bulk laxatives or weight-control preparations, should be taken with a full glass of water or, if the patient has difficulty in swallowing, they should be avoided. Such compounds swell into masses that may obstruct the oesophagus if not taken with sufficient water.

1. Pye KG, *et al.* Severe dyserythropoiesis and autoimmune thrombocytopenia associated with ingestion of kelp supplements. *Lancet* 1992; **339:** 1540.
2. de Smet PA, *et al.* Hyperthyreoidie tijdens het gebruik van kelp tabletten. *Ned Tijdschr Geneeskd* 1990; **134:** 1058–9.
3. Eliason BC. Transient hyperthyroidism in a patient taking dietary supplements containing kelp. *J Am Board Fam Pract* 1998; **11:** 478–80.

The symbol † denotes a preparation no longer actively marketed

Preparations

Proprietary Preparations (details are given in Part 3)
UK: Phytoslim.

Multi-ingredient: *S.Afr.:* Activex 40 Plus; *UK:* Fat-Solv; Kelp Plus 3; *USA:* KLB6.

Keracyanin (12879-s)

Keracyanin (*rINN*).

3-[6-O-(6-Deoxy-α-L-mannopyranosyl)-β-D-glucopyranosyloxy]-3′,4′,5,7-tetrahydroxyflavylium chloride.

$C_{27}H_{31}ClO_{15}$ = 631.0.
CAS — 18719-76-1.

Profile

Keracyanin is claimed to improve visual function in poor light conditions. It has been given by mouth in usual doses of 400 to 600 mg daily.

Preparations

Proprietary Preparations (details are given in Part 3)
Fr.: Meralops†; *Ital.:* Meralop; *Spain:* Meralop.

Keratinase (7377-e)

CAS — 9025-41-6.

Profile

Keratinase is a proteolytic enzyme that has been obtained from cultures of *Streptomyces fradiae*. It can digest keratin, which is resistant to most proteolytic enzymes, in the presence of trace amounts of metal ions. It is used in the commercial separation of hair from animal hides, and has been tried as a depilatory; it has also been included in some topical antibacterial ointments, presumably to aid penetration of the active substances.

Preparations

Proprietary Preparations (details are given in Part 3)
Multi-ingredient: *Spain:* Deltasiton†.

Kinkeliba (12883-v)

Combreti Folium.

Pharmacopoeias. In *Fr.*

The dried leaves of *Combretum micranthum* (=*C. altum*; *C. raimbaultii*) (Combretaceae), a shrub indigenous to West Africa.

Profile

Kinkeliba has been used as an ingredient of herbal remedies given for the treatment of biliary, liver, and gastrointestinal disorders. Other species of *Combretum* are also used.
Kinkeliba is used in homoeopathic medicine.

Preparations

Proprietary Preparations (details are given in Part 3)
Multi-ingredient: *Belg.:* Tisane pour le Foie; *Fr.:* Hepaclem; Hepax; Jecopeptol; Mediflor Tisane Hepatique No 5†; Palmi†; Romarene; Romarinex; Romarinex-Choline†; Solution Stago Diluee; Uremiase†; *Switz.:* Bilifuge.

Klebsiella pneumoniae Glycoprotein

(3028-b)
RU-41740.

Profile

Klebsiella pneumoniae glycoprotein has been used for its immunomodulating activity in the management of respiratory-tract infections, wounds, burns, and soft-tissue disorders. It has also been used in immunotherapy.

Preparations

Proprietary Preparations (details are given in Part 3)
Braz.: Biostim; *Fr.:* Biostim; *Ital.:* Acintor; Biostim; *Mex.:* Biostim; *Port.:* Biostim; *S.Afr.:* Biostim†.

Krebiozen (12884-g)

CAS — 9008-19-9.

Profile

Krebiozen is the name of a preparation that was formerly promoted as a 'cancer cure' in the USA, but totally discredited by the FDA. It was stated to be obtained from the blood of horses previously injected with an extract of *Actinomyces bovis*.

Kveim Antigen (12885-q)

Profile

Kveim antigen is a fine suspension in physiological saline of sarcoid tissue prepared from spleens taken from patients with active sarcoidosis. It is used as an intradermal injection in the Kveim-Siltzbach test for the diagnosis of sarcoidosis (p.1058).

◊ References.

1. James DG, Williams WJ. Kveim-Siltzbach test revisited. *Sarcoidosis* 1991; **8:** 6–9.

◊ The safety of the Kveim test has been questioned, particularly with reference to the risk of transmission of sarcoidosis, and of hepatitis B, human immunodeficiency virus, and Creutzfeldt-Jakob disease.[1] However, the procedure to identify acceptable sarcoid spleens and the method of preparation were considered sufficient to reduce the risk of transmission of infections[2] and of Creutzfeldt-Jakob disease.[3]

1. Wigly RD. Moratorium on Kveim tests. *Lancet* 1993; **341:** 1284.
2. du Bois RM, *et al.* Moratorium on Kveim tests. *Lancet* 1993; **342:** 173.
3. de Silva RN, Will RG. Moratorium on Kveim tests. *Lancet* 1993; **342:** 173.

Laburnum (12886-p)

Golden Chain; Golden Rain.

Laburnum anagyroides (=*L. vulgare*; *Cytisus laburnum*) (Leguminosae).

Profile

All parts of laburnum are toxic. The toxic principle is cytisine which has actions similar to nicotine.

Lactic Acid (1312-z)

Acidum Lacticum; E270; E326 (potassium lactate); Milchsäure. 2-Hydroxypropionic acid.

$C_3H_6O_3$ = 90.08.
CAS — 50-21-5; 79-33-4 (+); 10326-41-7 (–); 598-82-3 (±).
ATC — G01AD01.

Pharmacopoeias. In *Chin., Int., Jpn, Pol.,* and *US.*
Eur. (see p.vi) includes monographs for the racemate and the (*S*)-enantiomer.

Pharmacopoeial description

Ph. Eur.: A colourless or slightly yellow, syrupy liquid. It consists of a mixture of lactic acid, its condensation products such as lactoyl-lactic acid and other polylactic acids, and water. Miscible with water and with alcohol.

Lactic Acid is usually the racemate (*RS*-lactic acid), and contains the equivalent of 88 to 92% w/w of $C_3H_6O_3$.

(*S*)-Lactic Acid contains the equivalent of 88 to 92% w/w of $C_3H_6O_3$, of which not less than 95% is the (*S*)-enantiomer.

USP 25: A mixture of lactic acid and lactic acid lactate equivalent to a total of 88 to 92% w/w of $C_3H_6O_3$. It is obtained by the lactic fermentation of sugars or is prepared synthetically. Lactic acid obtained by fermentation of sugars is laevorotatory, while that prepared synthetically is racemic.

A colourless or yellowish, hygroscopic, practically odourless, syrupy liquid. When it is concentrated by boiling, lactic acid lactate is formed. Miscible with water, with alcohol, and with ether; insoluble in chloroform. Store in airtight containers.

Adverse Effects, Treatment, and Precautions

As for Hydrochloric Acid, p.1621, although in the concentrations used it is less corrosive.

Neonates. There was evidence that neonates had difficulty in metabolising *R*-(–)-lactic acid and this isomer and the racemate should not be used in foods for infants less than 3 months old.[1]

1. FAO/WHO. Toxicological evaluation of certain food additives with a review of general principles and of specifications: seventeenth report of the joint FAO/WHO expert committee on food additives. *WHO Tech Rep Ser 539* 1974.

Uses and Administration

Lactic acid has actions similar to those of acetic acid (p.1571) and has been used similarly in the treatment of infective skin and vaginal disorders. It has been used in the preparation of lactate injections and infusions to provide a source of bicarbonate for the treatment of metabolic acidosis (for the problems of using lactate in metabolic acidosis, see p.1180). It is also employed topically in the treatment of warts (p.1108), often in combination with salicylic acid, and in emollient creams. Other uses include the treatment of severe aphthous stomatitis in terminally ill, immunocompromised patients.

Lactic acid is also used as a food preservative and as an ingredient of cosmetics.

◊ References to the use of lactic acid in the treatment of bacterial vaginosis,[1,2] warts,[3] and dry[4,5] or photodamaged[6] skin.

1. Andersch B, *et al.* Treatment of bacterial vaginosis with an acid cream: a comparison between the effect of lactate-gel and metronidazole. *Gynecol Obstet Invest* 1986; **21:** 19–25.
2. Holst E, Brandberg Å. Treatment of bacterial vaginosis in pregnancy with a lactate gel. *Scand J Infect Dis* 1990; **22:** 625–6.
3. Bunney MH, *et al.* An assessment of methods of treating viral warts by comparative treatment trials based on a standard design. *Br J Dermatol* 1976; **94:** 667–79.
4. Dahl MV, Dahl AC. 12% Lactate lotion for the treatment of xerosis: a double-blind clinical evaluation. *Arch Dermatol* 1983; **119:** 27–30.
5. Rogers RS, *et al.* Comparative efficacy of 12% ammonium lactate lotion and 5% lactic acid lotion in the treatment of moderate to severe xerosis. *J Am Acad Dermatol* 1989; **21:** 714–16.
6. Stiller MJ, *et al.* Topical 8% glycolic acid and 8% L-lactic acid creams for the treatment of photodamaged skin: a double-blind vehicle-controlled clinical trial. *Arch Dermatol* 1996; **132:** 631–6.

Preparations

BP 2001: Lactic Acid Pessaries;
USP 25: Compound Clioquinol Topical Powder.

Proprietary Preparations (details are given in Part 3)
Aust.: Espritin; Warzin; *Austral.:* Avecyde; *Belg.:* Lacta-Gynecogel; *Canad.:* Calmurid†; Lubriderm AHA; Penederm; *Ger.:* Lactisan; Lactisol; RMS; Tampovagan c Acid lact; Unguentum Lactisol†; *Irl.:* Relact; *Ital.:* Unigyn; *Mex.:* Acid-Lac; *Neth.:* Calmurid; *NZ:* BK; *Singapore:* Avecyde; Lachydrin; *Spain:* Keratisdin; *Swed.:* Calmuril; *Switz.:* Vagoclyss; *USA:* Lactinol.

Multi-ingredient: *Aust.:* Anthozym; Apotheker Bauer's Huhneraugentinktur; Calmurid; Calmurid HC; Duofilm; Helo-acid; Hylak; Hylak forte; Lavagin; *Austral.:* Aussie Tan Skin Moisturiser; Calmurid; Cornkil; Dermadrate; Dermatech Wart Treatment; Duofilm; Lacticare†; *Belg.:* Aporil; Calmurid; *Braz.:* Calope; Colpacid; Colpolase; Dermacyd; Higienex; Kalostop; Lacto Vagin; Lacto-Gin; Tirakallos; Varigerm; Verrux; Vulgix; *Canad.:* Calmurid HC†; Cuplex; Duofilm; Duoplant; Epi-Lyt; Lacticare; Penederm; Tiacid; Viron Wart Lotion; *Denm.:* Verucid; *Fin.:* Calmuril; Wicnelact; *Fr.:* Duofilm; Geliofil; Kerafilm; Lactacyd; Lacticare; Propy-Lacticare; Verrufilm; Verrupan; *Ger.:* Aknederm N; Anthozym N†; Calmurid; Calmurid HC; Collomack; Dr. Hotz Vollbad†; Duofilm; Efasit N†; Gehwol Huhneraugenpflaster; Gelum-Tropfen; Kneipp Milch-Molke-Bad†; Petrasch-Anthozym N; Sagrosept; Solco-Derman; Vagisan; W-Tropfen; Warzen-Alldahin; *Hong Kong:* Collomack; Duofilm; Lactacyd; Lacticare; Roidhemo; Solcoderm; Verrufilm; *Irl.:* Calmurid; Calmurid HC; Cuplex; Duofilm; Lacticare; Salactol; Salatac; *Israel:* Babyzim; Calmurid; Calmurid HC; Salatac; U-Lactin Foot Cream; U-Lactin Forte; *Ital.:* Aflogine†; Bruciaporri; Duofilm; Eudermico; Gastro-Pepsin; Geroderm Zolfo; Lactacyd Derma; Lactacyd Intimo; Lactocol; Pluriderm†; Saugella Salviettine; Sensigel; Unidermo; Verel; Verucid; Verunec 3; Violgen; *Mex.:* Duofilm; Lacticare; *Neth.:* Tintorine; *Norw.:* Verucid; *NZ:* Calmurid; Duofilm; *Port.:* Calmurid; Creme Laser Hidrante; Duofilm; Hidro-Lact; Lactacyd; Lecia; Pansebase Composto†; Pansebase†; Secpel; Secpel Composto; Ureadin Maos; Verrucare; Verrufilm; *S.Afr.:* Duofilm; *Singapore:* Collomack; Duofilm; High Potency Lightening Serum; Lactacyd; Lacticare; *Spain:* Antiverrugas; Callicida Brujo; Callicida Cor Pik; Callicida Durcall†; Callicida D; Cusiter†; Euzymina Lisina I; Ginejuvent; Roidhemo; Unguento Callicida Naion; Verufil; *Swed.:* Lactal†; Vartmedel†; *Switz.:* Acne Lotion; Calmurid; Calmurid HC; Clabin; Duofilm; Elle-care; Solcoderm; Vin Tonique de Vial; Warz-ab Extor; *Thai.:* Collomack; Duofilm; Lactacyd; Lacticare; *UK:* Bazuka; Calmurid; Calmurid HC; Cuplex; Duofilm; Lacticare; Salactol; Salatac Gel; Tampovagan; *USA:* Epi-Lyt; Feminique; Lacticare; Lactinol-E; Massengill; Massengill Disposable; SLT.

Lactic-acid-producing Organisms (1313-c)

Profile

Lactic-acid-producing organisms were introduced as therapeutic agents with the idea of acidifying the intestinal contents and thus preventing the growth of putrefactive organisms. *Lactobacillus bulgaricus*, which occurs in naturally soured milk, was the organism originally used but it can be difficult to obtain growth of this organism in the intestines and *L. acidophilus*, which is an inhabitant of the human intestine, is preferred by many.

Preparations containing various *Lactobacillus* spp. and other lactic-acid-producing organisms have been used in the treatment of vaginal and gastrointestinal disorders but evidence to support this use is limited. Other organisms which have been tried include *Bifidobacterium bifidum*, *Enterococcus* and *Streptococcus* spp., and the yeast *Saccharomyces boulardii*. Natural yogurt is a common source of lactic-acid-producing organisms.

A vaccine produced from strains of lactobacillus found in women with trichomoniasis has been used in the prophylaxis of recurrent trichomoniasis (see p.1566).

◊ Reviews[1-4] concerning the use of lactic-acid-producing organisms including *Lactobacillus* spp., *Bifidobacterium bifidum*, and *Streptococcus thermophilus* have been published. However, some preparations have been found to contain smaller quantities or different species of organisms to those specified on the label.[5]

Metabolic acidosis has occurred following use of tablets containing *Lactobacillus acidophilus*.[6] Fungaemia associated with the use of *Saccharomyces boulardii* has also been reported.[7]

1. Scott E, Li Wan Po A. Lactobacillus. *Pharm J* 1990; **245:** 698–9.
2. Fuller R. Probiotics in human medicine. *Gut* 1991; **32:** 439–42.
3. Drutz DJ. Lactobacillus prophylaxis for Candida vaginitis. *Ann Intern Med* 1992; **116:** 419–20.
4. Roffe C. Biotherapy for antibiotic-associated and other diarrhoeas. *J Infect* 1996; **32:** 1–10.
5. Hamilton-Miller JMT, *et al.* "Probiotic" remedies are not what they seem. *BMJ* 1996; **312:** 55–6.
6. Oh MS, *et al.* D-lactic acidosis in a man with short-bowel syndrome. *N Engl J Med* 1979; **301:** 249–52.
7. Piarroux R, *et al.* Are live saccharomyces yeasts harmful to patients? *Lancet* 1999; **353:** 1851–2.

Preparations

Proprietary Preparations (details are given in Part 3)
Aust.: Antibiophilus; Bioflorin; Doederlein; Symbioflor 1; *Austral.:* Acidophilus Tablets; Bioglan Acidophilus; Bioglan Superdophilus; Ethical Nutrients Inner Health Powder; Ethical Nutri-

ents Maxi Bifidus; Ethical Nutrients Maxi Dophilus; Mega Acidophilus; **Belg.:** Lacteol; Perenterol; **Braz.:** Bac Resistente; Camboacy; Floratil; Leiba; **Canad.:** Bacid; **Denm.:** Paraghurt; Precosa; **Fin.:** Lactophilus; Precosa; **Fr.:** Bacilor; Diarlac; Lacteol; Lyo-Bifidus; Rhino-Lacteol†; Ultra-Levure; Ultraderme; **Ger.:** Acidophilus; Diarrhoesan SC; Hamadin; Hylak N; Omniflora Akut; Omnisept; Paidoflor; Perenterol; Perocur; Santax S; Symbioflor 1; Vagiflor; **Hong Kong:** Lacteol; Solco-Trichovac; **Ital.:** Biofiorin; Codex; Dicoflor; Ecoflorina; Hygine In†; Inulac; Lab/A; Lacteol; Ramno-Flor; Regolact Plus; **Mex.:** Floratil; Lacteol Fort; Sinuberase; **Norw.:** Precosa; **Port.:** Antibiophilus; Enterol; Lacteol; UL 250; **S.Afr.:** Actiflora†; Inteflora; **Singapore:** Lacteol; **Spain:** Lacteol; Lactofilus; Lactoliofil; Ultra-Levura; **Swed.:** Precosa; Trevis†; **Switz.:** Bioflorin; Fiormil; Lacteol; Lactoferment; Perenterol; Solco-Trichovac; Ultra-Levure; Ventrux; **Thai.:** Lacbon; Lacteol; **UK:** Bio Acidophilus; Biodophilus; Culturelle LCG; **USA:** Bacid; Kala; Lactinex; MoreDophilus; Pro-Bionate; Superdophilus.

Multi-ingredient: Aust.: Gynoflor; Hylak; Hylak forte; Hylakombun; Infloran; Omniflora; Prosymbioflor; **Austral.:** Acidophilus Bifidus; Acidophilus Complex; Acidophilus Plus; Cyto-Bifidus; Enterocare; Lactobac; Natures Own Acidophilus Plus; Natures Way Acidophilus Plus; Ultra Strength Megadophilus; **Belg.:** Gynoflor; **Braz.:** Lactipan; **Canad.:** Fermalac; Fermalac Vaginal; **Fr.:** Ampho-Vaccin intestinal†; Biolactyl; Florgynal; Imudon; IRS 19; Trophigil; **Ger.:** Antiprurit; Eksalb; Eksalb Simplex; Gynoflor; Hylak forte N; Imbak; IRS 19; Pro-Symbioflor; **Hong Kong:** Gynoflor E; Infloran; Shin-Bioformin S; **Ital.:** Al-Flor; Alvear Complex†; Bifilact; Bifilact 6; Biolactine; Coli-Fagina S; Ecoendocilli Testimonia†; Ecofermenti; Fermenturto-Lio; Flar; Florbiox; Florelax; Giflorex; Infloran; Lactipan; Lactisporin; Lactivis; Lactogermine; Lactolife; Lactonorm; Lactovit†; Liozim; Neo Lactoflorene; Pentaglucano; Probiox; Prontomixin; Vaxitiol; Yovis†; **Mex.:** Neo-Panlacticos; Neo-Panlacticos Plus; **Port.:** Benflorene; Coli-Fagina S; Infloran; **Spain:** Antibiofilus; Infloran; **Switz.:** Gynoflor; Infloran; Ribolac; **Thai.:** Infloran; **UK:** Acidophilus Plus; Natudophilus; **USA:** Entrin Acidophilus†; Entrin Bifidus†.

Laetrile (12887-s)

CAS — 1332-94-1 (laetrile); 29883-15-6 (amygdalin).

The term laetrile is used for a product consisting chiefly of amygdalin, which is the major cyanogenic glycoside of apricot kernels. Amygdalin is R-α-cyanobenzyl-6-O-β-D-glucopyranosyl-β-D-glucopyranoside ($C_{20}H_{27}NO_{11}$ = 457.4). Laetrile is also used as a term for R-α-cyanobenzyl-6-O-β-D-glucopyranosiduronic acid ($C_{14}H_{15}NO_7$ = 309.3).

Profile
Laetrile was claimed to be preferentially hydrolysed in cancer cells by β-glucosidases to benzaldehyde and hydrogen cyanide, which killed the cell, but amygdalin does not appear to be absorbed from the gastrointestinal tract, and both normal and malignant cells contain only traces of β-glucosidases. Laetrile has also been claimed to be 'vitamin B_{17}', the deficiency of which is said to result in cancer; there is no evidence for accepting this view and laetrile is of no known value in human nutrition.

There have been several reports of cyanide poisoning and other adverse reactions associated with the use of laetrile, especially when taken by mouth.

◊ A review of the sources, chemistry, metabolism, claims for efficacy, and toxicity of laetrile.[1]

1. Chandler RF, *et al.* Controversial laetrile. *Pharm J* 1984; **232:** 330–2.

Laminaria (12888-w)

Stipites Laminariae; Styli Laminariae; Thallus Eckloniae; Thallus Laminariae.

Pharmacopoeias. In *Chin.*

The dried stalks of the seaweeds *Laminaria japonica, L. digitata,* and possibly other species of *Laminaria.*

Profile
Laminaria stalks swell in water to about 6 times their volume and have been used surgically to dilate cavities and to dilate the cervix in labour or abortion induction.

An extract of laminaria has been used as a dietary supplement.

Adverse effects. Anaphylaxis has been reported following the insertion of laminaria for cervical dilatation.[1,2]

1. Nguyen MT, Hoffman DR. Anaphylaxis to laminaria. *J Allergy Clin Immunol* 1995; **95:** 138–9.
2. Cole DS, Bruck LR. Anaphylaxis after laminaria insertion. *Obstet Gynecol* 2000; **95:** 1025.

Preparations

Proprietary Preparations (details are given in Part 3)
Multi-ingredient: Ger.: Cetraria Salbe.

Lappa (12889-e)

Bardanae Radix; Bardane (Grande); Burdock; Burdock Root; Lappa Root.

Pharmacopoeias. In *Fr.*
Chin. includes the fruits.

The dried root of the great burdock, *Arctium lappa* (=*A. majus*), and other species of *Arctium* (Compositae).

Profile
Lappa was formerly used in the form of a decoction as a diuretic and diaphoretic but there is little evidence of its efficacy. Herbal preparations containing lappa have been used in the treatment of skin, musculoskeletal, and gastrointestinal disorders. The leaves and fruits of *Arctium* spp. have also been used.

Lappa is used in homoeopathic medicine.

Preparations

Proprietary Preparations (details are given in Part 3)
Fr.: Anthraxivore†.

Multi-ingredient: Austral.: Acne Oral Spray; Herbal Cleanse; Trifolium Complex; **Belg.:** Stanno-Bardane†; Tisane Depurative "les 12 Plantes"; **Fr.:** Arbum; Aromabyl†; Depuratif Parnel; Fitacnol; Tisanes de l'Abbe Hamon no 16†; **Ital.:** Depurativo; **Port.:** Erpecalm; **UK:** Backache; Blue Flag Root Compound; Cascade; Catarrh Mixture; GB Tablets; Heath & Heather Skin Tablets; Heath & Heather Water Relief Tablets; Hofels White Willow and Burdock; HRI Clear Complexion; Kleer; Modern Herbals Water Retention; Rheumatic Pain Remedy; Skin Cleansing; Skin Eruptions Mixture; Tabritis; Water Naturtabs.

Lavender Oil (4659-x)

English Lavender Oil; Esencia de Alhucema; Esencia de Espliego; Essência de Alfazema; Foreign Lavender Oil; Huile Essentielle de Lavande; Lavandulae Aetheroleum; Lavendelöl; Lavender Flower Oil; Oleum Lavandulae.

Pharmacopoeias. In *Eur.* (see p.vi) and *Pol.* Some pharmacopoeias include Lavender Flower.

Pharmacopoeial description
Ph. Eur.: A colourless or pale yellow clear liquid with a characteristic odour, obtained by steam distillation from the fresh flowering tops of *Lavandula angustifolia* (=*L. officinalis*). Miscible with alcohol (90%), with ether, and with fatty oils. Store in well-filled airtight containers. Protect from light and heat.

Profile
Lavender oil has been used as a carminative and as a flavour. It is sometimes applied externally as an insect repellent. Its chief use is in perfumery and it is occasionally used in ointments and other pharmaceutical preparations to cover disagreeable odours. It has been suggested that lavender oil may have sedative properties following inhalation.

Lavender oil has been reported to produce nausea, vomiting, headache, and chills when inhaled or absorbed through the skin. It may cause contact allergy and phototoxicity.

Adverse effects. There have been reports of contact dermatitis associated with lavender oil in a shampoo,[1] and facial dermatitis following application of the oil to pillows for its sedative properties.[2]

1. Brandão FM. Occupational allergy to lavender oil. *Contact Dermatitis* 1986; **15:** 249–50.
2. Coulson IH, Khan ASA. Facial 'pillow' dermatitis due to lavender oil allergy. *Contact Dermatitis* 1999; **41:** 111.

Insomnia. Ambient exposure to lavender oil produced similar sleep patterns to conventional sedatives in 4 elderly patients.[1]

1. Hardy M, *et al.* Replacement of drug treatment for insomnia by ambient odour. *Lancet* 1995; **346:** 701.

Preparations

Proprietary Preparations (details are given in Part 3)
Port.: Rowalind.

Multi-ingredient: Aust.: Baldrian-Krautertonikum; Berggeist; Beruhigungstee; Bio-Garten Tee zur Beruhigung; Euka; Herz- und Kreislauftonikum Bioflora; Inno Rheuma; Krautertee Nr 1; Krautertee Nr 141; Krautertee Nr 201; Mentopin; Rowalind; St Radegunder Herz-Kreislauf-unterstutzender Tee; Teekanne Schlaf- und Nerventee; **Austral.:** Neutralice; **Braz.:** Analgen; Balsamo Branco; Benegel; Gelflex; Gelofrix; Gelol; Geloneval; Rinofen; Traumac; Vulgix; Yatropan; **Fr.:** Aromasol; Balsofumine; Balsofumine Mentholee; Bronchospray†; Citrosil; Ephydrol; Gouttes aux Essences; Mediflor Tisane Digestive No 3†; Paps; Pectoderme; Perubore; Santane N₄; Santane R₈; Tisane Sedative Weleda†; **Ger.:** Amol Heilkrautergeist N; Aranidorm-S†; Dolo-cyl; Euviterin†; Leber-Galle-Tropfen 83; Presselin Dyspeptikum; Rowalind†; Salus Nerven-Schlaf-Tee Nr.22†; **Irl.:** Rowalind; **Ital.:** Citrosystem; Mistick; Natural Zanzy; Sanaderm†; **Port.:** Erpecalm; Solubeol; Vaporil; **Singapore:** Vapex; **Spain:** Dolokey; Linimento Naion; Termosan; **Switz.:** Baume du Chalet; Demo baume†; Dolo-Arthrosenex sine Heparino; Dolorex†; Embropax; Hygiodermil; Kernosan Huile de Massage†; Kytta Pommade†; Liberol Bain; Lyman; Massorax; Muco-Sana; Nasobol; Oculosan; Perubare; Phlogidermil†; Saltrates; Seracalm†; Spagyrom; Tisane relaxante; **UK:** Larch Resin comp.; Massage Balm Arnica; Massage Balm Calendula; Medicinal Gargle; Migrastick; Penetrol†; Vital Eyes; **USA:** Nasal Jelly.

Lawsone (9307-y)

2-Hydroxy-1,4-naphthoquinone.
$C_{10}H_6O_3$ = 174.2.
CAS — 83-72-7.

Lawsone is a dye present in henna (p.1619), the leaves of *Lawsonia* spp., and may also be prepared synthetically.

Profile
Lawsone has been used with dihydroxyacetone in sunscreen preparations. There appears to be no evidence that it has any sunscreening properties when used alone.

Adverse effects. Observation that lawsone causes oxidative damage to red blood cells *in vitro* supported a suggestion that percutaneous absorption of henna could contribute to unexplained neonatal hyperbilirubinaemia in countries where the ceremonial use of henna is widespread.[1]

1. Zinkham WH, Oski FA. Henna: a potential cause of oxidative hemolysis and neonatal hyperbilirubinemia. *Pediatrics* 1996; **97:** 707–9.

Lead (5298-t)

Pb = 207.2.
CAS — 7439-92-1.

A grey, malleable and ductile metal.

Adverse Effects
Lead poisoning (plumbism) may be due to inorganic or organic lead and may be acute or, more often, chronic. It has followed exposure to a wide range of compounds and objects from which lead may be absorbed following ingestion or inhalation. Some of those incriminated include paint, pottery glazes, crystal glassware, domestic water supplies, petrol and poteen, cosmetics, herbal or folk remedies, newsprint, and even bullets. Children are often the victims of accidental poisoning and may be vulnerable to chronic exposure to lead from environmental pollution.

Acute effects of lead poisoning include metallic taste, abdominal pain, diarrhoea, vomiting, hypotension, muscle weakness, fatigue, abnormal liver function tests, and acute interstitial nephritis. Encephalopathy may occur and is more common in children. Symptoms of chronic poisoning with inorganic lead include anorexia, colic, constipation, anaemia, peripheral neuropathy, and encephalopathy with convulsions and coma. There may be kidney damage and impairment of mental function. Children with elevated lead concentrations may be asymptomatic apart from intellectual deficits and behavioural disorders.

Organic lead poisoning produces mainly CNS symptoms; there can be gastrointestinal and cardiovascular effects, and renal and hepatic damage.

◊ General references.

1. WHO. Recommended health-based limits in occupational exposure to heavy metals: report of a WHO study group. *WHO Tech Rep Ser* 647 1980.
2. Ibels LS, Pollock CA. Lead intoxication. *Med Toxicol* 1986; **1:** 387–410.
3. Lead—environmental aspects. *Environmental Health Criteria* 85. Geneva: WHO, 1989.
4. Inorganic lead. *Environmental Health Criteria* 165. Geneva: WHO, 1995.

Acute poisoning. Acute lead intoxication following the intravenous injection of lead acetate.[1]

1. Sixel-Dietrich F, *et al.* Acute lead intoxication due to intravenous injection. *Hum Toxicol* 1985; **4:** 301–9.

Treatment of Adverse Effects
Treatment of lead poisoning is aimed at controlling symptoms and reducing the concentration of lead in the body with chelators. Sodium calcium edetate (p.1022) in conjunction with dimercaprol (p.1007) is given for the initial management of symptomatic lead poisoning. Sodium calcium edetate, succimer (p.1024), or penicillamine (p.1017) are used for chelation therapy in asymptomatic patients.

◊ Treatment of lead poisoning is aimed primarily at alleviating acute symptoms, and then at reducing the body-lead stores.[1] Initial therapy of acute symptomatic poisoning entails supportive therapy including intravenous fluids and antiepileptics if necessary. Encephalopathy is rare in adults but more common in children and requires urgent treatment; combined therapy with sodium calcium edetate in combination with dimercaprol has substantially reduced mortality rates.[2] In this case, only the minimum fluid should be administered to avoid overload. Chelation therapy with both sodium calcium edetate and dimercaprol should be continued for 5 days and may be repeated if necessary.[1,4] For symptomatic patients without encephalopathy it may be possible to discontinue the dimercaprol after 3 days. Patients who are asymptomatic may be treated with sodium calcium edetate alone[1,3,4] or succimer.[4] Penicillamine may be used as an alternative.[4] Long-term management involves eliminating environmental exposure.[5] Continued chelation with oral penicillamine may be necessary until the desired tissue levels are achieved.[2,3]

A provocation test that measures urinary excretion of lead following administration of a standard dose of sodium calcium edetate has been widely used as a means of assessing the need for therapy. However, sodium calcium edetate is associated with nephrotoxicity and the test is cumbersome to perform, thus guidelines recommend blood-lead concentrations as a guide to treatment.[4]

Finally, it should be noted that chelation therapy is not a substitute for environmental controls in those suffering occupational exposure.[6] Chelation therapy is generally not appropriate for long-term lead exposure in asymptomatic individuals in whom a significant proportion of the total body lead is tightly bound to compact bone and brain. A provocation test may be useful in

---

The symbol † denotes a preparation no longer actively marketed

identifying patients with mild symptoms who may respond to chelation therapy.[6]

1. Ibels LS, Pollock CA. Lead intoxication. *Med Toxicol* 1986; **1:** 387–410.
2. Chisholm JJ. The use of chelating agents in the treatment of acute and chronic lead intoxication in childhood. *J Pediatr* 1968; **73:** 1–38.
3. Chisholm JJ, Barltrop D. Recognition and management of children with increased lead absorption. *Arch Dis Child* 1979; **54:** 249–62.
4. Committee on Drugs of the American Academy of Pediatrics. Treatment guidelines for lead exposure in children. *Pediatrics* 1995; **96:** 155–60.
5. Committee on Environmental Health of the American Academy of Pediatrics. Lead poisoning: from screening to primary prevention. *Pediatrics* 1993; **92:** 176–83.
6. Rempel D. The lead-exposed worker. *JAMA* 1989; **262:** 532–4.

Lead in the Environment
Many countries have taken action to reduce lead exposure from environmental sources, including food, paint, and petrol, by limiting or banning altogether the use of lead compounds in such sources. Such measures have been of value in reducing childhood exposure to lead. Screening of all children to detect those at risk of chronic lead poisoning and developmental deficit has been advocated, but selective screening in areas perceived as high risk may be appropriate in countries where the overall level of lead contamination is low.

Pharmacokinetics
Lead is absorbed from the gastrointestinal tract. It is also absorbed by the lungs from dust particles or fumes.

Inorganic lead is not absorbed through intact skin, but organic lead compounds may be absorbed rapidly.

Lead is distributed in the soft tissues, with higher concentrations in the liver and kidneys. In the blood it is associated with the erythrocytes. Over a period of time lead accumulates in the body and is deposited in calcified bone, hair, and teeth. Lead crosses the placental barrier. It is excreted in the faeces, urine, and sweat, and also appears in breast milk.

Uses and Administration
Lead compounds were formerly employed as astringents, but the medicinal use of preparations containing lead is no longer recommended. The lead salts or compounds that have been used have included lead acetate and lead subacetate (for lead lotion, still known sometimes as lotio plumbi), lead carbonate, lead monoxide, and lead oleate (for lead plaster-mass).

Preparations
Proprietary Preparations (details are given in Part 3)
Aust.: Pasta Plumbi†.
Multi-ingredient: *Aust.:* Vulpuran.

Lecithin (596-l)
E322.
Pharmacopoeias. In Aust. and Ger. Also in USNF.

Pharmacopoeial description
USNF 20: A complex mixture of acetone-insoluble phosphatides, which consist chiefly of phosphatidyl choline, phosphatidyl ethanolamine, phosphatidyl serine, and phosphatidyl inositol, combined with various amounts of other substances such as triglycerides, fatty acids, and carbohydrates, as separated from the crude vegetable oil source. It contains not less than 50% of acetone-insoluble matter.

The consistency of both natural grades and refined grades of lecithin may vary from plastic to fluid, depending upon the content of free fatty acid and oil, and upon the presence or absence of other diluents. Its colour varies from light yellow to brown, depending on the source, on crop variations, and on whether it is bleached or unbleached.

It is odourless or has a characteristic, slight nutlike odour. It is partially soluble in water, but readily hydrates to form emulsions. The oil-free phosphatides are soluble in fatty acids, but are practically insoluble in fixed oils. When all phosphatide fractions are present, lecithin is partially soluble in alcohol and practically insoluble in acetone.

Profile
Lecithin is an emulsifying and stabilising agent used in both the pharmaceutical and the food industries.

Lecithin has also been used as a source of choline and tried in the treatment of dementia (p.1412) but with little evidence of clinical benefit. It has also been tried in various extrapyramidal disorders. Phosphatidyl serine (p.1651) has been used similarly. Other constituents of lecithin such as phosphatidyl ethanolamine and phosphatidyl inositol may be found in natural pulmonary surfactants (p.1655).

◊ References.
1. Higgins JPT, Flicker L. Lecithin for dementia and cognitive impairment (updated 30 August 2000). Available in The Cochrane Library; Issue 4. Oxford: Update Software; 2001.

Preparations
Proprietary Preparations (details are given in Part 3)
Aust.: Buerlecithin Compact; Dermo WAS; *Austral.:* Buerlecithin; *Ger.:* Buerlecithin; *Ital.:* Misura; *Mex.:* Leciderm; *Switz.:* Buerlecithin Compact.
Multi-ingredient: *Aust.:* Aponatura Leber; Bilatin; Buerlecithin; Colagain†; Lecikur; Lecivital; Sanvita Enerlecit-Tonikum mit

Rosmarin†; *Austral.:* Berberis Complex; Bioglan E-Plus†; Bioglan Zellulean with Escin; Esten†; Extralife Arthri-Care; Extralife Extra-Brite; Extralife Liva-Care; ML 20; Plantiodine Plus; *Canad.:* Complex 15; *Fr.:* Arkotonic†; Cholegene†; *Ger.:* Balneoconzen; Haut-Vital N; Hicoton; Kola-Dallmann mit Lecithin†; Lipidavit; Vita Buerlecithin; *Hong Kong:* Wari-Procomil; *Ital.:* Lemivit; Nutrigel; Ottovis; Solecin; Tricortin; *Port.:* Pansebase Composto†; Pansebase†; Secpel; Secpel Composto; *Switz.:* Biovital Ginseng; Vita Buerlecithin; *Thai.:* Wari-Procomil; *UK:* All In One Plus Grapefruit; Kelp Plus 3; Naudicelle SL; S.P.H.P.; *USA:* KLB6.

Leishmanin (4333-r)
Profile
Leishmanin is a suspension of *Leishmania* promastigotes used in an intradermal test to indicate previous exposure to leishmanial antigens. Its chief use is in epidemiological studies of leishmaniasis (p.584). The leishmanin skin test has also been known as the Montenegro test.

Lemon Grass Oil (4661-j)
Essência de Capim-Limão; Indian Melissa Oil; Indian Verbena Oil; Lemongrass Oil; Oleum Graminis Citrati.

The volatile oil is obtained by distillation from *Cymbopogon flexuosus* or *C. citratus* (Gramineae). It contains citral and citronellal. Store in airtight containers. Protect from light.

Profile
Lemon grass oil was formerly given as a carminative. It has been used in perfumery and as a flavour.

Preparations
Proprietary Preparations (details are given in Part 3)
Multi-ingredient: *Ger.:* Kneipp Krauter Taschenkur Nerven und Schlaf N.

Lemon Oil (4662-z)
Aetheroleum Citri; Citronenöl; Esencia de Cidra; Essence de Citron; Essência de Limão; Limonis Aetheroleum; Ol. Limon.; Oleum Citri; Oleum Limonis.
Pharmacopoeias. In Eur. (see p.vi).
Br. also includes a monograph on dried lemon peel; Fr. also includes fresh lemon peel.

Pharmacopoeial description
Ph. Eur.: The essential oil obtained by suitable mechanical means without the aid of heat from the fresh peel of *Citrus limon*. It contains a maximum of 0.5% β-caryophyllene, 0.5 to 2.3% geranial, 0.1 to 0.8% geranyl acetate, 56.0 to 78.0% limonene, 0.3 to 1.5% neral, 0.2 to 0.9% neryl acetate, 7.0 to 17.0% β-pinene, 1.0 to 3.0% sabinene, 6.0 to 12.0% γ-terpinene, and a maximum of 0.6% α-terpineol.

A clear mobile pale yellow to greenish-yellow liquid with a characteristic odour. It may become cloudy at low temperatures. Store in well-filled airtight containers at a temperature not exceeding 25°. Protect from light. Where applicable the label should state that the contents are Italian-type lemon oil.

Profile
Lemon oil is chiefly used in perfumery and as a flavour. It is used in the preparation of terpeneless lemon oil (below). It has also been used with other volatile agents in rubefacient preparations and preparations for respiratory-tract disorders. Photosensitivity reactions and contact dermatitis have been reported.

Preparations
BP 2001: Aromatic Ammonia Spirit.
Proprietary Preparations (details are given in Part 3)
Multi-ingredient: *Aust.:* Spasmo Claim; *Austral.:* Austral-Balm; Genuine Australian Eucalyptus Drops; *Fr.:* Citrosil; Ephydrol; *Ger.:* Amol Heilkrautergeist N; Babix-Wundsalbe N; Ceprovit†; Melissengeist; Tachynerg N; *Israel:* Garonsept; *Switz.:* Neo-Angin au miel et citron; Pommade Po-Ho N A Vogel; *UK:* Collins Elixir Pastilles†; Cough Drops; Famel Catarrh & Throat Pastilles†; Melissa comp.; Throaties Catarrh Pastilles†; *USA:* Mexsana.

Terpeneless Lemon Oil (4663-c)
Oleum Limonis Deterpenatum.
Pharmacopoeias. In Br.

Pharmacopoeial description
BP 2001: A clear colourless or pale yellow liquid, visibly free from water, with the characteristic odour and taste of lemon, prepared by concentrating lemon oil under reduced pressure until most of the terpenes have been removed, or by solvent partition. It contains not less than 40% w/w of aldehydes calculated as citral. Soluble 1 in 1 of alcohol (80%). Store in well-filled containers at a temperature not exceeding 25°. Protect from light.

Profile
Terpeneless lemon oil is used as a flavour. It has the advantages of being stronger in taste and odour and more readily soluble

than the natural oil and is used in the preparation of lemon spirit and lemon syrup. Photosensitivity is associated with citrus oils.

Preparations
BP 2001: Compound Orange Spirit; Lemon Spirit; Lemon Syrup.
Proprietary Preparations (details are given in Part 3)
Multi-ingredient: *UK:* Lemsip Cough & Cold Dry Cough; Meltus Honey & Lemon; Throaties Family Cough Linctus†.

Lemon Verbena (14059-l)
Herba Lippiae Citriodorae; Herba Verbenae Odoratae; Verveine Odorante.

Profile
Lemon verbena, the leaves of *Lippia citriodora* (*Aloysia triphylla*; *Verbena triphylla*) (Verbenaceae) has antispasmodic and sedative actions and has been used for gastrointestinal disorders and as a tonic. It is most commonly used as an ingredient of herbal teas.

Preparations
Proprietary Preparations (details are given in Part 3)
Multi-ingredient: *Fr.:* Tisanes de l'Abbe Hamon no 14†; *Spain:* Agua del Carmen.

Lentinan (19404-q)
LC-33.
ATC — L03AX01.

A glucan extracted from the mushroom *Lentinus edodes*.

Profile
Lentinan appears to act as an immunostimulant. It has been tried in the treatment of malignant neoplasms and in HIV infection.

Lepromin (12892-g)
Profile
Lepromin is a suspension of killed *Mycobacterium leprae* prepared from the skin of heavily infected patients suffering from lepromatous leprosy (lepromin H) or from armadillo tissue infected with *M. leprae* (lepromin A). It is used in an intradermal skin test for the classification of leprosy (p.126) and the assessment of immune responsiveness to *M. leprae*. The test is not diagnostic for leprosy.

◊ The original lepromin (of Mitsuda and Hayashi), a suspension of the whole autoclaved homogenised leproma including some tissue elements, is sometimes called integral lepromin, whereas purified bacillary suspensions are sometimes called bacillary lepromins.[1] Leprolins are the soluble proteins of the bacilli with or without proteins of the lepra, not coagulated by heating, and do not elicit the early reaction. The Dharmendra antigen is neither a lepromin nor a leprolin and is used especially for testing the early reactions; it gives only a weak late reaction. Purified protein derivatives of *Mycobacterium leprae*, such as leprosin A,[2] have also been developed.

1. Abe M, *et al.* Immunological problems in leprosy research. *Lepr Rev* 1974; **45:** 244–72.
2. Stanford JL. Skin testing with mycobacterial reagents in leprosy. *Tubercle* 1984; **65:** 63–74.

Leptin (1669-r)
Profile
Leptin is an endogenous protein that is involved in the control of body-weight. A recombinant form is under investigation in the management of obesity (p.1505).

Obesity. Leptin is a 167-amino acid peptide hormone, secreted by adipose tissue, that acts either directly or via specific receptors in the CNS to decrease food intake, increase energy expenditure, and influence glucose and fat metabolism and neuroendocrine function. Although there is some evidence that subcutaneous administration results in loss of body fat it is not clear whether leptin will prove a suitable treatment for most obese patients.

References.
1. Auwerx J, Staels B. Leptin. *Lancet* 1998; **351:** 737–42.
2. Mantzoros CS. The role of leptin in human obesity and disease: a review of current evidence. *Ann Intern Med* 1999; **130:** 671–80.
3. Heymsfield SB, *et al.* Recombinant leptin for weight loss in obese and lean adults: a randomized, controlled, dose-escalation trial. *JAMA* 1999; **282:** 1568–75.
4. Hukshorn CJ, *et al.* Weekly subcutaneous pegylated recombinant native human leptin (PEG-OB) administration in obese men. *J Clin Endocrinol Metab* 2000; **85:** 4003–4009.

Levomenol (9734-s)

Levomenol (rINN).

(−)-α-Bisabolol. (−)-6-Methyl-2-(4-methyl-3-cyclohexen-1-yl)-5-hepten-2-ol.

$C_{15}H_{26}O = 222.4$.
CAS — 23089-26-1.

Profile
Levomenol has been tried as a transepidermal penetration enhancer and is present in many emollient preparations.

◊ References.
1. Kadir R, Barry BW. α-Bisabolol, a possible safe penetration enhancer for dermal and transdermal therapeutics. Int J Pharmaceutics 1991; 70: 87–94.

Preparations
Proprietary Preparations (details are given in Part 3)
Multi-ingredient: Fr.: Apaisance; Dermophil Indien; Ger.: Mirfulan Spray N; Sensicutan; Hong Kong: Camoderm; Kamillosan; Oat Milk Treatment Cream; Ital.: Broxo al Fluoro; Intim; Port.: Lactonico; Switz.: Antidry; Dermophil Indien; Thai.: Kamillosan.

Lexipafant (15459-y)

Lexipafant (BAN, USAN, rINN).

BB-882; DO-6. Ethyl N-methyl-N-[α-(2-methylimidazo[4,5-c]pyridin-1-yl)tosyl]-L-leucinate.

$C_{23}H_{30}N_4O_4S = 458.6$.
CAS — 139133-26-9.

Profile
Lexipafant is a platelet-activating factor antagonist that is being investigated in the prevention of neurological and renal complications following cardiac surgery. It has also been studied for possible applications in asthma, sepsis, and pancreatitis.

Linseed (5441-w)

Flaxseed; Leinsamen; Lin; Linho; Lini Semen; Lini Semina; Linum; Semilla de Lino.

ATC — A06AC05.
Pharmacopoeias. In Chin., Eur. (see p.vi), and Pol.

Pharmacopoeial description
Ph. Eur.: The dried ripe seeds of Linum usitatissimum. Protect from light.

Profile
Preparations of linseed have been administered for their demulcent action. Crushed linseed has been used as a poultice. See also Linseed Oil, below.

Preparations
Proprietary Preparations (details are given in Part 3)
Aust.: Linusit Gold; Ger.: Linusit Creola†; Linusit Darmaktiv Leinsamen†.
Multi-ingredient: Ger.: Dralinsa†; Duoventrin; Pascomag; Switz.: Enveloppements ECR†; Linoforce; Optilax†.

Linseed Oil (7360-h)

Aceite de Linaza; Flaxseed Oil; Huile de Lin; Leinöl; Oleum Lini.
Pharmacopoeias. In Aust., Br., Pol., and Swiss.

Pharmacopoeial description
BP 2001: The fixed oil expressed from the ripe seeds of linseed (p.1629), Linum usitatissimum. A clear, yellowish-brown oil with a characteristic odour. Gradually thickens on exposure to air forming, when spread in a thin film, a hard transparent varnish. Slightly soluble in alcohol; miscible with chloroform, with ether, and with petroleum spirit. Store in well-filled containers.

Profile
Linseed oil is used in veterinary medicine as a purgative for horses and cattle. In man, linseed oil is included in topical preparations for a variety of skin disorders. It has been tried as a vegetable source of omega-3 fatty acids (p.949).

Boiled linseed oil ('boiled oil') is linseed oil heated with litharge, manganese resinate, or other driers, to a temperature of about 150° so that metallic salts of the fatty acids are formed and cause the oil to dry more rapidly. It must not be used for medicinal purposes.

Preparations
Proprietary Preparations (details are given in Part 3)
Multi-ingredient: Aust.: Dermowund; Fr.: Huile de Haarlem†; Switz.: Malvedrin; UK: Efamol Safflower & Linseed; Nine Rubbing Oils.

Lithium Benzoate (2337-s)

$C_7H_5LiO_2 = 128.1$.
CAS — 553-54-8.

Each g represents 7.8 mmol of lithium.

Profile
Lithium benzoate has been used as a diuretic and urinary disinfectant. Its use cannot be recommended because of the pharmacological effect of the lithium ion (p.292).

Preparations
Proprietary Preparations (details are given in Part 3)
Multi-ingredient: Fr.: Antigoutteux Rezall†; Port.: Urocrasina.

Lobenzarit Sodium (16879-a)

Lobenzarit Sodium (USAN, rINNM).

CCA. 4-Chloro-2,2′-iminodibenzoate disodium.

$C_{14}H_8ClNNa_2O_4 = 335.7$.
CAS — 63329-53-3 (lobenzarit); 64808-48-6 (lobenzarit sodium).

Profile
Lobenzarit sodium has been used as an immunomodulator in rheumatoid arthritis.

Preparations
Proprietary Preparations (details are given in Part 3)
Jpn: Carfenil†.

Lorenzo's Oil (14102-f)

Profile
Lorenzo's oil is a liquid containing glyceryl trierucate (a source of erucic acid) and glyceryl trioleate (a source of oleic acid), in the ratio one part to four parts respectively. It has been used in conjunction with dietary modification for the treatment of adrenoleucodystrophy, a genetic disorder characterised by demyelination, adrenal cortical insufficiency, and accumulation of saturated 'very-long-chain fatty acids'.

Adrenoleucodystrophy. Adrenoleucodystrophy is a rare X-linked metabolic disorder in which accumulation of saturated very-long-chain fatty acids results in diffuse and multifocal demyelination of the nervous system and adrenocortical insufficiency. The most common form usually affects children and is characterised primarily by cerebral demyelination; it is usually fatal within a few years. In the adult variant, called adrenomyeloneuropathy, demyelination of the spinal cord and peripheral neuropathy progress slowly over many years.[1]

There appears to be no effective treatment for adrenoleucodystrophy or its variants. A high dietary intake of long-chain monounsaturated fatty acids, as provided by the mixture Lorenzo's oil (glyceryl trierucate with glyceryl trioleate), has been tried, the idea being to monopolise the specific enzyme involved in the conversion of long-chain fatty acids to very-long-chain fatty acids. Although dietary therapy with Lorenzo's oil has reduced plasma concentrations of saturated very-long-chain fatty acids, there is no evidence that this improves or delays progression of adrenoleucodystrophy or adrenomyeloneuropathy.[2-5] However, it has been suggested that these disorders may not respond to correction of the biochemical abnormality once neurological damage has occurred.[4] The effectiveness of treatment before the appearance of neurological symptoms is currently being studied.[1,6] There is some evidence to suggest that the childhood form may have an immunological component, but results using immunosuppressants or immunoglobulins have been reported to be disappointing.[4] Bone marrow transplants may improve symptoms but should only be tried in those with mild cerebral involvement.[1] Lovastatin can also reduce plasma concentrations of very-long-chain fatty acids.[7]

1. van Geel BM, et al. X linked adrenoleukodystrophy: clinical presentation, diagnosis, and therapy. J Neurol Neurosurg Psychiatry 1997; 63: 4–14.
2. Aubourg P, et al. A two-year trial of oleic and erucic acids ("Lorenzo's oil") as treatment for adrenomyeloneuropathy. N Engl J Med 1993; 329: 745–52.
3. Kaplan PW, et al. Visual evoked potentials in adrenoleukodystrophy: a trial with glyceryl trioleate and Lorenzo oil. Ann Neurol 1993; 34: 169–74.
4. Rizzo WB. Lorenzo's oil—hope and disappointment. N Engl J Med 1993; 329: 801–2.
5. van geel BM, et al. Progression of abnormalities in adrenomyeloneuropathy and neurologically asymptomatic X-linked adrenoleukodystrophy despite treatment with "Lorenzo's oil". J Neurol Neurosurg Psychiatry 1999; 67: 290–9.
6. Moser HW. Treatment of X-linked adrenoleukodystrophy with Lorenzo's oil. J Neurol Neurosurg Psychiatry 1999; 67: 279–80.
7. Pari GS, et al. Lovastatin therapy for X-linked adrenoleukodystrophy: clinical and biochemical observations on 12 patients. Mol Genet Metab 2000; 69: 312–22.

Adverse effects. Thrombocytopenia has been reported in patients receiving Lorenzo's oil, although patients are often asymptomatic.[1] It is possible that giant platelets which retain most of their function are produced and that these are not counted by automatic counting procedures giving a false impression of thrombocytopenia.[2]

Lymphocytopenia with an increased incidence of infection has also been reported in few patients.[3]

1. Zinkham WH, et al. Lorenzo's oil and thrombocytopenia in patients with adrenoleukodystrophy. N Engl J Med 1993; 328: 1126–7.
2. Stöckler S, et al. Giant platelets in erucic acid therapy for adrenoleukodystrophy. Lancet 1993; 341: 1414–15.
3. Unkrig CJ, et al. Lorenzo's oil and lymphocytopenia. N Engl J Med 1994; 330: 577.

Preparations
Proprietary Preparations (details are given in Part 3)
Multi-ingredient: UK: Lorenzo's Oil.

Lovage Root (11834-e)

Levistici Radix.
Pharmacopoeias. In Eur. (see p.vi) and Pol.

Pharmacopoeial description
Ph. Eur.: The whole or cut, dried rhizome and root of Levisticum officinale. The whole drug contains not less than 0.4% v/w of essential oil and the cut drug not less than 0.3% v/w of essential oil, calculated with reference to the anhydrous drug. Protect from light.

Profile
Lovage root is used in herbal medicine for gastrointestinal and urinary-tract disorders.

Preparations
Proprietary Preparations (details are given in Part 3)
Multi-ingredient: Aust.: Aponatura Entwasserungs; Aponatura Verdauungs; Ehrenhofer-Salbe; Kneipp Stoffwechsel-Unterstutzungs-Tee; Krautertee Nr 19; Krautertee Nr 2; Krautertee Nr 31; Ger.: Canephron N; Hevert-Entwasserungs-Tee†; Nephroselect M; Presselin Nieren-Blasen K 3; Hong Kong: Canephron N; Switz.: Tisane pour les reins et la vessie; UK: Fragador.

Lupulus (535-f)

Hop Strobile; Hopfenzapfen; Hops; Houblon; Humulus; Lupuli Flos; Lupuli Strobulus; Strobili Lupuli.
Pharmacopoeias. In Eur. (see p.vi).

Pharmacopoeial description
Ph. Eur.: The dried, generally whole, female inflorescences (strobiles) of the hop plant Humulus lupulus. It has a characteristic aromatic odour. Protect from light.

Profile
Lupulus has been used as a bitter, and supplies the characteristic flavour of beers. It is used in herbal and folk medicine as a sedative. It is also used in homoeopathic medicine.

Preparations
Proprietary Preparations (details are given in Part 3)
Aust.: Zirkulin Beruhigungs-Tee; Ger.: Bonased-L†; Lactidorm.

Multi-ingredient: Aust.: Aktiv Nerven- und Schlaftee; Aponatura Beruhigungs; Aponatura Einschlaf; Bakanasan Einschlaf; Baldracin; Baldrian AMA; Baldrian Dispert Compositum; Baldrian-Elixier; Baldrian-Krautertonikum; Baldriparan Beruhigungs; Beruhigungskapseln; Beruhigungstee; Bio-Garten Tee zur Beruhigung; Bio-Garten Tropfen zur Beruhigung; Biogelat Schlaf; Doppelherz Tonikum; Einschlafkapseln; Hova; Krauterdoktor Beruhigungstropfen; Krauterdoktor Entspannungs- und Einschlaftropfen; Krauterdoktor Nerven-Tonikum; Krauterhaus Mag Kottas Nerven- und Schlaftee; Krautertee Nr 141; Krautertee Nr 16; Krautertee Nr 201; Luvased; Mag Doskar's Nerventonikum; Mag Kottas Krauterexpress-Nerven-Schlaf-Tee; Mag Kottas Schlaftee; Montana; Nervendragees; Nervenruh; Nerventee; Nervifloran; Phytogran; Sanhelios Einschlaf; Seda-Grandelat; Sedogelat; Sidroga Nerven- und Schlaftee; St Radegunder Beruhigungs- und Einschlaftee; St Radegunder Nerven-Tonikum; St Radegunder Nerventee; Vivinox; Wechseltee; Austral.: Extralife Sleep-Care; Pacifenity; Passiflora Complex; Passionflower Plus; Prosed-X; ReDormin; Relaxaplex; Vitaglow Executive Anti Stress†; Vitaglow Herbal Stress†; Canad.: Herbal Sleep Aid; Relax and Sleep; Fr.: Santane D₅; Santane N₉; Ger.: Aranidorm-S†; Ardeysedon N; Avedorm; Avedorm N; Baldrian-Dispert Nacht; Baldrianox S†; Baldriparan N; Baldriparan stark N; Biosedon S; Boxocalm; Cefasedativ; Cysto Fink; Discmigon; Dormeasan; Dormoverlan; Einschlaf-Kapseln biologisch; Dutmcht; Hicoton; Hovaletten N†; Ilja Rogoff; Ivel Schlaf; JuDorm; JuNeuron S†; Kneipp Baldrian + Hopfen; Kytta-Sedativum†; Leukona-Sedativ-Bad; Leukona-Sedativ-Bad sine Chloralhydrat; Luvased; Luvased-Tropfen N; Moradorm S; Nervendragees; Nervinetten†; Nervinfant N; Nervoregin forte; Pascosedon; Phytogran; Presselin Nerven K 1 N; Salus Nerven-Schlaf-Tee Nr.22†; Salusan†; Schlafund Nerventee; Schupps Baldrian Sedativbad†; Seda Kneipp N†; Seda-Plantina; Sedacur; Sedahopf†; Sedaselect N; Sedasyx; Sedatruw S†; Selon; Sensinerv forte; Somnuvis S; Stomasal Med; Valdispert comp; Valeriana comp; Valeriana forte; Valeriana mild; Visinal†; Vivinox N; Vivinox-Schlafdragees†; Israel: Nerven-Dragees; Ital.: Emmenoiasi; Melissa Specie Composta; Mex.: Ivel; Switz.: Baldriparan; Cysto Fink†; Cysto-Caps Chassot†; Dicalm; Dormeasan N; Dragees pour le coeur et les nerfs; Dragees pour le sommeil nouvelle formule; Hova; Hyperiforce comp; Phytoberidin; Phytomed Somni; ReDormin; Soporin; Tisane calmante pour les enfants; Tisane pour le sommeil et les nerfs; Valverde Dragees pour le coeur; Valverde Dragees pour le sommeil; UK: Anased; Avena sativa comp.; Gerard 99; Gerard House Serenity; Gerard House Somnus; Gerard House Valerian Compound; Heath & Heather Becalm; Heath & Heather Quiet Night; HRI Calm Life; HRI Night; Kalms; Newrelax; Night Time; Nodoff; Nytol Herbal; Quiet Days; Quiet Life; Quiet Nite; Quiet Tyme; Relax B†; Slumber; Super Mega B+C; Valerina Night-Time.

The symbol † denotes a preparation no longer actively marketed

Lysergide (5011-e)

Lysergide (BAN, rINN).

LSD; LSD-25; Lysergic Acid Diethylamide. (+)-NN-Diethyl-D-lysergamide; (6aR,9R)-NN-Diethyl-4,6,6a,7,8,9-hexahydro-7-methylindolo[4,3-fg]quinoline-9-carboxamide.
$C_{20}H_{25}N_3O = 323.4$.
CAS — 50-37-3.

Profile

Lysergide was formerly used therapeutically but is now encountered as a drug of abuse for its hallucinogenic and psychedelic properties.

There is considerable variation in individual reaction to lysergide. Disorders of visual perception are among the first and most constant reactions to lysergide. Subjects may be hypersensitive to sound. Extreme alterations of mood, depression, distortion of body image, depersonalisation, disorders of thought and time sense, and synaesthesias may be experienced. Anxiety, often amounting to panic, may occur (a 'bad trip'). The effects of lysergide may recur months after ingestion of lysergide; the recurrence or 'flashback' may be spontaneous or induced by alcohol, other drugs, stress, or fatigue.

The subjective effects of lysergide may be preceded or accompanied by somatic effects which are mainly sympathomimetic in nature and include mydriasis, tremor, hyperreflexia, hyperthermia, piloerection, muscle weakness, and ataxia. There may be nausea and vomiting and increased heart rate and blood pressure. Derangement of blood clotting mechanisms has been described. In addition, respiratory arrest, convulsions, and coma may result from overdoses. There is no evidence of fatal reactions to lysergide in man, although accidental deaths, suicides, and homicides have occurred during lysergide intoxication.

Tolerance develops to the behavioural effects of lysergide after several days and may be lost over a similar period. There is cross-tolerance between lysergide, mescaline, and psilocybine and psilocin, but not to amfetamine or to cannabis.

Physical dependence on lysergide does not seem to occur.

Mace Oil (4667-x)

NOTE. Mace has also been used as a name for a tear gas.

A volatile oil obtained by distillation from mace, the arillus of the seed of Myristica fragrans (Myristicaceae). Store in airtight containers. Protect from light.

Nutmeg (p.1643) is the dried kernel of the seed of M. fragrans.

Profile

Mace is used as a flavour and carminative similarly to nutmeg (p.1643). It has also been used with herbal substances and other volatile agents in preparations for musculoskeletal and respiratory-tract disorders. As with nutmeg, large doses of mace may cause epileptiform convulsions and hallucinations.

Macrogols (1922-a)

Macrogols (BAN, rINN).

Macrogola; PEGs; Polyethylene Glycols; Polyoxyethylene Glycols.

$CH_2(OH)(CH_2OCH_2)_mCH_2OH$. Alternatively some authorities use the general formula $H(OCH_2CH_2)_nOH$ when the number assigned to n for a specified macrogol is 1 more than that of m in the first formula.
CAS — 25322-68-3 (macrogols); 37361-15-2 (macrogol 300).

Pharmacopoeias. Macrogols of various molecular weights are included in many pharmacopoeias.
Eur. (see p.vi) specifies macrogol 300, 400, 600, 1000, 1500, 3000, 3350, 4000, 6000, 8000, 20 000, and 35 000. USNF has a general monograph describing Polyethylene Glycol which requires that it be labelled with the average nominal molecular weight as part of the official title.

Macrogols are condensation polymers of ethylene oxide and water. Each macrogol name is followed by a number indicating its approximate average molecular weight; thus macrogol 300 has an average molecular weight of about 300 (m = 5 or 6 giving a molecular weight of 282.3 or 326.4).

Macrogols with an average molecular weight of 200 to 600 are clear to slightly hazy, colourless or almost colourless, viscous liquids with a slight characteristic odour; those with an average molecular weight of more than 1000 are white to off-white solids, also with a slight characteristic odour, which vary in consistency between soft unctuous pastes and hard waxy flakes, beads, or powder. Viscosity increases with increasing molecular weight, but hygroscopicity decreases and, at average molecular weights above 4000, hygroscopicity is low.

Macrogols can demonstrate oxidising activity leading to incompatibilities. The activity of bacitracin or benzylpenicillin may be reduced in a macrogol base. Some plastics are softened by macrogols.

Aqueous solutions can be sterilised by autoclaving or filtration.

Pharmacopoeial description

Ph. Eur.: Mixtures of polymers with the general formula $H(OCH_2CH_2)_nOH$, corresponding to an average relative molecular mass of the labelled nominal value (n). A suitable stabiliser may be added.

Macrogol 300, 400, and 600 are clear, viscous, colourless or almost colourless, hygroscopic liquids. Miscible with water; very soluble in alcohol, in acetone, and in dichloromethane.

Macrogol 1000 is a white or almost white, hygroscopic solid with a waxy or paraffin-like appearance. Very soluble in water; freely soluble in alcohol and in dichloromethane.

Macrogol 1500 is a white or almost white solid with a waxy or paraffin-like appearance. Very soluble in water and in dichloromethane; freely soluble in alcohol.

Macrogol 3000 and 3350 are white or almost white solids with a waxy or paraffin-like appearance. Very soluble in water and in dichloromethane; very slightly soluble in alcohol.

Macrogol 4000, 6000, and 8000 are white or almost white solids with a waxy or paraffin-like appearance. Very soluble in water and in dichloromethane; practically insoluble in alcohol.

Macrogol 20 000 and 35 000 are white or almost white solids with a waxy or paraffin-like appearance. Very soluble in water; practically insoluble in alcohol; soluble in dichloromethane.

All macrogols are practically insoluble in fatty oils and in mineral oils.

USNF 20: Macrogols are addition polymers of ethylene oxide and water, represented by the formula $H(OCH_2CH_2)_nOH$, in which n represents the average number of oxyethylene groups. Each macrogol is usually designated by a number that corresponds approximately to its average molecular weight. As the average molecular weight increases, the water solubility, hygroscopicity, and solubility in organic solvents decrease, while the viscosity increases.

Liquid grades occur as clear to slightly hazy, colourless or practically colourless, slightly hygroscopic, viscous liquids, having a slight, characteristic odour. Solid grades occur as practically odourless, white, waxy, plastic material having a consistency similar to beeswax, or as creamy-white flakes, beads, or powders. Liquid grades are miscible with water; solid grades are freely soluble in water; all grades are soluble in alcohol, in acetone, in chloroform, in ethoxyethanol, in ethyl acetate, and in toluene; all grades are insoluble in ether and in hexane. The pH of a 5% solution of a macrogol in water is between 4.5 and 7.5.

Store in airtight containers.

Adverse Effects and Precautions

Macrogols appear to have relatively low toxicity, although any toxicity appears to be greatest with the macrogols of low molecular weight. They may cause stinging when administered topically, especially to mucous membranes, and have been associated with hypersensitivity reactions such as urticaria. Hyperosmolality, metabolic acidosis, and renal failure have been reported following the topical application of macrogols to burn patients. Topical preparations with a macrogol base should therefore be used with caution in patients with renal impairment and/or large areas of raw surfaces, burns, or open wounds.

Patients undergoing bowel cleansing with mixtures of macrogols (3350 or 4000) and electrolytes commonly experience local gastrointestinal discomfort, bloating, and nausea. Abdominal cramps, vomiting, and anal irritation may also occur and there have been rare reports of possible hypersensitivity reactions. These colonic lavage solutions are contra-indicated in gastrointestinal obstruction or perforation, ileus, gastric retention, peptic ulcer disease, and toxic megacolon; caution is advisable in patients with ulcerative colitis. Since aspiration may be a problem, they should be used with caution in patients with an impaired gag reflex, reflux oesophagitis, or diminished levels of consciousness. They should be given with caution to diabetic patients. Drugs taken within one hour of starting colonic lavage with an orally administered macrogol and electrolyte mixture may be flushed from the gastrointestinal tract unabsorbed.

Effects on the kidneys. Macrogol 400 which was present in a lorazepam injection could have contributed to renal damage suggestive of acute tubular necrosis in a patient who received large doses (averaging lorazepam 95 mg daily) for 43 days.[1] The cumulative dose of macrogol 400 during this period was about 220 mL.

1. Laine GA, et al. Polyethylene glycol nephrotoxicity secondary to prolonged high-dose intravenous lorazepam. Ann Pharmacother 1995; 29: 1110–14.

Fluid and electrolyte homoeostasis. A syndrome of elevated total serum calcium (with a concomitant decrease in ionised calcium), hyperosmolality, metabolic acidosis, and renal failure has been observed in animals[1] and in burn patients[2] following the topical application of preparations with a macrogol base. The FDA has recommended that topical preparations containing macrogols should be used with caution in burn patients with known or suspected renal impairment, as macrogols absorbed through denuded skin and not excreted normally by a compromised kidney could lead to symptoms of progressive renal impairment.[3]

The use of macrogol and electrolyte solutions for bowel preparation has also been associated with sodium and water retention, resulting in exacerbation of heart failure in a patient with

diabetic gastroparesis,[4] and with the development of pulmonary oedema possibly due to aspiration in a child without cardiac or renal disease.[5]

1. Herold DA, et al. Toxicity of topical polyethylene glycol. Toxicol Appl Pharmacol 1982; 65: 329–35.
2. Bruns DE, et al. Polyethylene glycol intoxication in burn patients. Burns 1982; 9: 49–52.
3. Anonymous. Topical PEG in burn ointments. FDA Drug Bull 1982; 12: 25–6.
4. Granberry MC, et al. Exacerbation of congestive heart failure after administration of polyethylene glycol-electrolyte lavage solution. Ann Pharmacother 1995; 29: 1232–5.
5. Paap CM, Ehrlich R. Acute pulmonary edema after polyethylene glycol intestinal lavage in a child. Ann Pharmacother 1993; 27: 1044–7.

Hypersensitivity. Hypersensitivity to macrogols is uncommon but both immediate urticarial reactions and delayed allergic contact dermatitis have been reported following the topical application of preparations with a macrogol vehicle or base.[1] An anaphylactic reaction has been associated with the ingestion of macrogols in a multivitamin tablet.[2] The manufacturers of preparations containing macrogols and electrolytes for bowel cleansing have reported isolated instances of skin reactions and rhinorrhoea.

1. Fisher AA. Immediate and delayed allergic contact reactions to polyethylene glycol. Contact Dermatitis 1978; 4: 135–8.
2. Kwee YN, Dolovich J. Anaphylaxis to polyethylene glycol (PEG) in a multivitamin tablet. J Allergy Clin Immunol 1982; 69: 138.

Overdosage. Ingestion of 2 litres of a colonic lavage solution containing macrogol 400 instead of macrogol 4000 resulted in a patient developing severe metabolic acidosis and rapidly becoming comatose due to systemic absorption of the macrogol.[1] The patient was successfully treated with intravenous bicarbonate and dialysis.

1. Bélaïche J, et al. Coma acidosique après préparation colique par du polyèthylglycol. Gastroenterol Clin Biol 1983; 7: 426–7.

Pharmacokinetics

Liquid macrogols may be absorbed when taken by mouth but macrogols of high molecular weight, such as macrogol 3350, are not significantly absorbed from the gastrointestinal tract. There is evidence of absorption of macrogols when applied to damaged skin. Macrogols entering the systemic circulation are predominantly excreted unchanged in the urine; low-molecular-weight macrogols may be partly metabolised.

◊ References.

1. DiPiro JT, et al. Absorption of polyethylene glycol after administration of a PEG-electrolyte lavage solution. Clin Pharm 1986; 5: 153–5.

Uses and Administration

Macrogols are relatively stable, non-toxic compounds which have a range of properties depending on their molecular weight. They are widely used in pharmaceutical manufacturing as water-soluble bases for topical preparations and suppositories, as solvents and vehicles, and as solubilising agents, tablet binders, plasticisers in film coating, and tablet lubricants. They have also been reported to have antibacterial properties.

A mixture of macrogol 3350 or 4000 with electrolytes is used to empty the bowel before colonoscopy, radiological procedures, or surgery. These preparations have been formulated so that the osmotic activity of the macrogol and concentrations of the electrolytes result in a minimum net effect on the fluid and electrolyte balance. Adults are given 200 to 300 mL of reconstituted aqueous solution (containing about 59 or 60 g or 105 g of the macrogol per litre), which they have to swallow rapidly, and this is repeated every 10 to 15 minutes until the rectal effluent is clear, or until a total of 4 litres of the solution has been consumed. A dose for children is 25 to 40 mL per kg body-weight per hour. Bowel evacuation usually begins about 1 hour after starting administration and is complete in about 4 hours. Patients should fast for at least 2 or 3 hours before drinking the solution. Flavours such as clear fruit cordials may be added, or palatability may be improved by chilling the solution, but sugar or other sweeteners should not be added. If distension or pain occur, administration should be temporarily stopped or the interval between drinks extended. For administration by nasogastric tube, a rate of 20 to 30 mL per minute has been used. Similar preparations are used as routine laxatives in a usual dose of 125 mL of a solution containing 105 g of the macrogol per litre two or three times daily.

Macrogols of high molecular weight such as macrogol 4000 have been used as inert markers in studies on intestinal absorption and excretion.

Pegylation of drugs and therapeutic proteins by conjugation with macrogols has been tried in an attempt to improve their pharmacokinetic profiles and to reduce their adverse effects. Pegylation may also reduce the immunogenicity of therapeutic proteins. Examples of pegylated proteins include pegademase (p.1649), pegaspargase (p.508), and peginterferon alfa (p.630).

Drug delivery systems. References to the use of macrogols in delivery systems for drugs and proteins.

1. Reddy KR. Controlled-release, pegylation, liposomal formulations: new mechanisms in the delivery of injectable drugs. Ann Pharmacother 2000; 34: 915–23.
2. Harris JM, et al. Pegylation: a novel process for modifying pharmacokinetics. Clin Pharmacokinet 2001; 40: 539–51.

Phenol poisoning. Washing with liquid macrogols has been recommended in the emergency treatment of skin contamination with phenol, see p.1153.

Preparations

BP 2001: Macrogol Ointment;
USP 25: PEG 3350 and Electrolytes for Oral Solution.

Proprietary Preparations (details are given in Part 3)
Canad.: Visatear†; Visine True Tears; *Fr.:* Forlax; *Ger.:* Forlax; *Hong Kong:* Forlax; *Thai.:* Forlax; *USA:* MiraLax.

Multi-ingredient: *Aust.:* Klean-Prep; Movicol; *Austral.:* Colonlytely; Colonprep; Glycoprep; Glycoprep-C; GoLytely; Movicol; Visine Advanced Relief; Visine Revive; *Belg.:* Colopeg; Klean-Prep; Movicol; Precosol; Transipeg; *Braz.:* Blinkene; *Canad.:* Aquasite; CoLyte; GoLytely; Klean-Prep; Peglyte; Pro-Lax†; Rhinaris; Salinol; Secaris; Visine Moisturizing; *Denm.:* Klean-Prep; Ledermix; Movicol; *Fin.:* Colonsteril; Klean-Prep; Movicol; *Fr.:* Colopeg; Fortrans; Klean-Prep; Movicol; Transipeg; *Ger.:* Delcoprep; Endofalk; Isomol; Klean-Prep; Lens Fresh†; Movicol; Oralav; *Hong Kong:* Fortrans; Hypotears; Klean-Prep; Movicol; *Irl.:* Klean-Prep; Movicol; *Israel:* Hypotears PF; Lubrin; Meroken New; *Ital.:* Agena†; Gofreely; Hypotears; Isocolan; Macro-P; Movicol; Selg; Selg-Esse; *Mex.:* NuLytely; Transipeg; Visine Extra; *Neth.:* Klean-Prep; Movicolon; *Norw.:* Klean-Prep; Laxabon; *NZ:* Glycoprep; GoLytely; Klean-Prep; Revive; *Port.:* Klean-Prep; *S.Afr.:* GoLytely; Klean-Prep; Movicol; *Singapore:* Fortrans; Klean-Prep; Movicol; *Spain:* Evacuante; Movicol; *Swed.:* Klean-Prep; Laxabon; Movicol; *Switz.:* Colo-Sol; Cololyt; Fordtran; Gleitmittel; Hypotears; Isocolan; Klean-Prep; Movicol; Tracheo Fresh; Transipeg; *Thai.:* Unison Enema; *UK:* Hypotears; Klean-Prep; Movicol; SST; *USA:* Advanced Relief Visine; Aquasite; Co-Lav†; Colovage†; CoLyte; Go-Evact†; GoLytely; Hypotears; Nu-Tears II; NuLytely; OCL; Tetrasine Extra; Visine Moisturizing.

Magnesium Ferulate   (12908-r)

Magnesium 4-hydroxy-3-methoxycinnamate.
$(C_{10}H_9O_4)_2Mg = 410.7$.
CAS — 32179-46-7.

Profile
Magnesium ferulate has been used as a choleretic.

Magnesium Glutamate Hydrobromide
(12910-z)

Magnesium α-Aminoglutarate Hydrobromide; Magnesium Bromoglutamate.
$(C_5H_8NO_4)_2Mg,HBr = 397.5$.

Profile
Magnesium glutamate hydrobromide has been used as a sedative and hypnotic in the treatment of insomnia, neuroses, and behavioural disorders.

Preparations
Proprietary Preparations (details are given in Part 3)
Multi-ingredient: *Spain:* Cefabol; Gamalate B6; Psicosoma Solucion.

Maleic Acid   (1314-k)

Acidum Maleicum; Toxilic Acid. *cis*-Butenedioic acid.
$C_2H_2(CO_2H)_2 = 116.1$.
CAS — 110-16-7.
Pharmacopoeias. In *Eur.* (see p.vi).

Pharmacopoeial description
Ph. Eur.: A white crystalline powder. Freely soluble in water and in alcohol; sparingly soluble in ether. A 5% solution in water has a pH of less than 2. Store in glass containers. Protect from light.

Profile
Maleic acid is used in the preparation of Ergometrine Injection (BP 2001) and Ergometrine and Oxytocin Injection (BP 2001).

Malic Acid   (1315-a)

Apple Acid; E296; Hydroxysuccinic Acid. Hydroxybutanedioic acid.
$C_4H_6O_5 = 134.1$.
CAS — 6915-15-7; 636-61-3 ((+)-form); 97-67-6 ((−)-form); 617-48-1 ((±)-form).
Pharmacopoeias. In *Ger.* Also in *USNF.*

Pharmacopoeial description
USNF 20: A white or practically white, crystalline powder or granules. Very soluble in water; freely soluble in alcohol.

Profile
Malic acid is used in pharmaceutical formulations as an acidifier, flavour, and as an alternative to citric acid in effervescent powders. It is used in combination with butylated hydroxytoluene as an antioxidant in vegetable oils. It is used topically in combination with benzoic acid and salicylic acid for deslough-

ing of ulcers, burns, and wounds, and systemically in combination with arginine (p.1353) in preparations for the treatment of liver disorders. Pastilles containing malic acid are also used in the management of dry mouth (p.1498).

Preparations
Proprietary Preparations (details are given in Part 3)
Multi-ingredient: *Aust.:* Acerbine; Leberinfusion; Rocmaline; *Fin.:* Xerodent; *Fr.:* Rocmaline; *Ger.:* Infumal; *Port.:* Hyfac AHA; Squaphane; *S.Afr.:* Acerbine; *Spain:* Acerbiol; *Swed.:* Salivin†; Xerodent; *Switz.:* Acerbine; *UK:* Aserbine; Salivix; SST; *USA:* Super Malic†.

Malotilate   (17039-s)

Malotilate (USAN, rINN).
NKK-105. Diisopropyl 1,3-dithiole-$\Delta^{2,\alpha}$-malonate.
$C_{12}H_{16}O_4S_2 = 288.4$.
CAS — 59937-28-9.

Profile
Malotilate has been investigated for its reported protective effects on liver function in patients with chronic hepatic disease.

◊ References.
1. A European Multicentre Study Group. The results of a randomized double blind controlled trial evaluating malotilate in primary biliary cirrhosis. *J Hepatol* 1993; **17:** 227–35.

Mammalian Tissue Extracts   (12913-a)

Profile
Many medicinal preparations with definite pharmacological activity and valid clinical uses are of mammalian origin and are described under their appropriate monographs—for example, calcitonin, corticotropin, hydrocortisone (cortisol), some enzymes, heparin, insulin, parathyroid hormone, pituitary hormones, some sex hormones, and thyroid.

Many other preparations of animal origin have been promoted for a wide variety of disorders. Evidence of pharmacological activity is often lacking, and such preparations are often of doubtful benefit.

Preparations
Proprietary Preparations (details are given in Part 3)
Aust.: Cerebrolysin; Epiphysan; *Ger.:* Cerebrolysin; *Hong Kong:* Cerebrolysin; *Ital.:* Liposom; *Thai.:* Cerebrolysin.

Multi-ingredient: *Canad.:* Revitonus C; *Fr.:* Pro-Nat†; *Ger.:* AntiFocal; NeyChondrin N (Revitorgan-Dilutionen N Nr 68); NeyTumorin N (Revitorgan-Dilutionen N Nr 66); NeyTumorin-Tropfen (Revitorgan-Lingual Nr 66); Ribo-Wied; *UK:* S.P.H..

Mastic   (280-z)

Almáciga; Mastiche; Mastix.
Pharmacopoeias. In *Aust.* and *Swiss.*

A resinous exudation from certain forms or varieties of *Pistacia lentiscus* (Anacardiaceae).

Profile
Solutions of mastic in alcohol, chloroform, or ether have been used, applied on cotton wool, as temporary fillings for carious teeth. Compound Mastic Paint (BP 1980) was formerly used as a protective covering for wounds and to hold gauze in position.

Mastic may be effective in the treatment of peptic ulcer disease possibly due to an antibacterial action on *Helicobacter pylori.* However, further investigation is needed.

◊ References.
1. Huwez FU, *et al.* Mastic gum kills Helicobacter pylori. *N Engl J Med* 1998; **339:** 1946. Correction. *ibid.:* **340:** 576 [dose].

Preparations
Proprietary Preparations (details are given in Part 3)
UK: Mastika.

Meadowsweet   (13569-m)

Reine des Prés; Spiraeae Herba; Ulmaria.

Profile
Meadowsweet comprises the dried, aerial flowering parts of *Filipendula ulmaria* (*Spiraea ulmaria*) (Rosaceae). It is used in herbal medicine as a diuretic and in gastrointestinal and rheumatic disorders. It is also used in homoeopathic medicine.

Preparations
Proprietary Preparations (details are given in Part 3)
Multi-ingredient: *Belg.:* Tisane Diuretique; *Fr.:* Actisane Douleurs Articulaires†; Actisane Minceur; Aminsane†; Artrosan†; Mediflor Tisane Antirhumatismale No 2†; Mediflor Tisane No 4 Diuretique; Mediflor Tisane Pectorale d'Alsace; Polypirine; Santane A$_4$; Santane O$_1$; Santane R$_8$; Tisane des Familles; Tisane Tou-

raine†; Tisanes de l'Abbe Hamon no 3; *Ital.:* Artoxan†; Sambuco (Specie Composta); *Switz.:* Urinex (nouvelle formule); *UK:* Acidosis; Indigestion Mixture; Natraleze; *USA:* Amerigel.

Meclofenoxate Hydrochloride   (1429-v)

Meclofenoxate Hydrochloride (BANM, rINNM).
Centrophenoxine Hydrochloride; Clofenoxine Hydrochloride; Clophenoxate Hydrochloride; Deanol 4-Chlorophenoxyacetate Hydrochloride; Meclofenoxane Hydrochloride. 2-Dimethylaminoethyl 4-chlorophenoxyacetate hydrochloride.
$C_{12}H_{16}ClNO_3,HCl = 294.2$.
CAS — 51-68-3 (meclofenoxate); 3685-84-5 (meclofenoxate hydrochloride).
Pharmacopoeias. In *Jpn.*

Profile
Meclofenoxate hydrochloride has been claimed to aid cellular metabolism in the presence of diminished oxygen concentrations. It has been given mainly for mental changes in the elderly, or following strokes or head injury.

Preparations
Proprietary Preparations (details are given in Part 3)
Aust.: Lucidril; *Fr.:* Lucidril; *Ger.:* Cerutil; Helfergin.

Meglumine   (209-p)

Meglumine (BAN, rINN).
N-Methylglucamine; 1-Methylamino-1-deoxy-D-glucitol.
$C_7H_{17}NO_5 = 195.2$.
CAS — 6284-40-8.
Pharmacopoeias. In *Br., Chin., Fr., Int., Jpn,* and *US.*

Pharmacopoeial description
BP 2001: A white microcrystalline powder with a slight odour. Freely soluble in water; slightly soluble in alcohol; practically insoluble in chloroform and in ether.

USP 25: White to faintly yellowish-white, odourless crystals or powder. Freely soluble in water; sparingly soluble in alcohol.

Profile
Meglumine is an organic base used for the preparation of salts of organic acids including many used as contrast media.

Melaleuca Oil   (4669-f)

Australian Tea Tree Oil; Melaleucae Aetheroleum; Oleum Melaleucae; Tea Tree Oil.
CAS — 68647-73-4; 8022-72-8.
NOTE. Though the synonym Ti-tree Oil has been used for melaleuca oil (e.g. in BPC 1949), the name Ti-tree is also applied to species of *Cordyline* (Liliaceae) indigenous to New Zealand.
Pharmacopoeias. In *Eur.* (see p.vi).

Pharmacopoeial description
Ph. Eur.: The essential oil obtained by steam distillation from the foliage and terminal branchlets of *Melaleuca alternifolia, M. linariifolia, M. dissitiflora,* and/or other species of *Melaleuca.* It contains less than 7.0% aromadendrene, less than 15% cineole, 0.5 to 12.0% p-cymene, 0.5 to 4.0% limonene, 1.0 to 6.0% α-pinene, less than 3.5% sabinene, 5.0 to 13.0% α-terpinene, 10.0 to 28.0% γ-terpinene, minimum of 30% terpinen-4-ol, 1.5 to 8.0% α-terpineol, and 1.5 to 5.0% terpinolene.

A clear, mobile, colourless to pale yellow liquid with a characteristic odour. Store in well-filled airtight containers at a temperature not exceeding 25°. Protect from light.

Profile
Melaleuca oil has been reported to have bactericidal and fungicidal properties and is used topically for various skin disorders.

◊ References.
1. Altman PM. Australian tea tree oil. *Aust J Pharm* 1988; **69:** 276–8.
2. Altman PM. Australian tea tree oil—a natural antiseptic. *Aust J Biotechnol* 1989; **3:** 247–8.
3. Bassett IB, *et al.* A comparative study of tea-tree oil versus benzoylperoxide in the treatment of acne. *Med J Aust* 1990; **153:** 455–8.
4. Blackwell AL. Tea tree oil and anaerobic (bacterial) vaginosis. *Lancet* 1991; **337:** 300.
5. Carson CF, *et al.* Susceptibility of methicillin-resistant Staphylococcus aureus to the essential oil of melaleuca alternifolia. *J Antimicrob Chemother* 1995; **35:** 421–4.
6. Carson CF, *et al.* Efficacy and safety of tea tree oil as a topical antimicrobial agent. *J Hosp Infect* 1998; **40:** 175–8.

Preparations
Proprietary Preparations (details are given in Part 3)
Austral.: Clean Skin Anti Acne; Rapaid First Aid; *Fr.:* Myleuca; *UK:* Amber Gold; Burnshield Gel; Savlon Natural Antiseptic.

Multi-ingredient: *Austral.:* APR Cream; Austral-Balm; Burnaid First Aid Burn Gel; Clean Skin Face Wash; Curaderm; Neutralice; Rapaid Medicated; Relief Rub; SP Cream; VR; *Fr.:* Dermocica; *Port.:* Emopads; Mycogel; Peliphane†; *UK:* Kleer Cream; Skin Clear; Tea Tree & Witch Hazel Cream; Teenstick.

The symbol † denotes a preparation no longer actively marketed

Melatonin (12924-r)

N-Acetyl-5-methoxytryptamine. N-[2-(5-Methoxyindol-3-yl)ethyl]acetamide.

$C_{13}H_{16}N_2O_2 = 232.3$.

CAS — 73-31-4.

Profile

Melatonin is a hormone produced in the pineal gland from the amino acid tryptophan. Results mainly from *animal* studies indicate that melatonin increases the concentration of aminobutyric acid and serotonin in the midbrain and hypothalamus and enhances the activity of pyridoxal-kinase, an enzyme involved in the synthesis of aminobutyric acid, dopamine, and serotonin. Melatonin is involved in the inhibition of gonadal development and in the control of oestrus. It is also involved in protective changes in skin coloration. There appears to be a diurnal rhythm of melatonin secretion; it is secreted during hours of darkness and may affect sleep pattern. Because of its possible role in influencing circadian rhythm, melatonin has been tried in the alleviation of jet lag and other disorders resulting from delay of sleep. It has also been studied in various depressive disorders including seasonal affective disorder, and in large doses for its contraceptive activity.

A number of melatonin analogues are being developed.

Adverse effects. An increase in seizure activity was noted in 4 of 6 children with severe neurological deficits during treatment with melatonin for sleep disorders.[1] Seizure activity returned to baseline values when melatonin was stopped and recurred on rechallenge.

1. Sheldon SH. Pro-convulsant effects of oral melatonin in neurologically disabled children. *Lancet* 1998; **351:** 1254.

Uses. Melatonin has been tried in a number of disorders[1] including, in large doses, as an adjunct to conventional chemotherapy for malignant neoplasms[2,3] and, in combination with norethisterone, as a contraceptive.[4] It is possible that contraceptive use of melatonin may be associated with a reduced risk of breast cancer.[5] (For mention of response to melatonin in 2 patients with sarcoidosis, see p.1058.) However, the effects of long-term administration have yet to be assessed. Preliminary studies have also suggested that melatonin may be beneficial in hyperlipidaemias,[6] cluster headaches,[7] and tinnitus.[8] Claims for its value as an anti-ageing treatment and for use in conditions such as Alzheimer's disease and AIDS are unfounded.[2,9]

1. Wetterberg L. Melatonin and clinical application. *Reprod Nutr Dev* 1999; **39:** 367–82.
2. Pepping J. Melatonin. *Am J Health-Syst Pharm* 1999; **56:** 2520–7.
3. Lissoni P, *et al.* Decreased toxicity and increased efficacy of cancer chemotherapy using the pineal hormone melatonin in metastatic solid tumour patients with poor clinical status. *Eur J Cancer* 1999; **35:** 1688–92.
4. Short RV. Melatonin. *BMJ* 1993; **307:** 952–3.
5. Cohen M, *et al.* Hypotheses: melatonin/steroid combination contraceptives will prevent breast cancer. *Breast Cancer Res Treat* 1995; **33:** 257–64.
6. Pittalis S, *et al.* Effect of a chronic therapy with the pineal hormone melatonin on cholesterol levels in idiopathic hypercholesterolemic patients. *Recenti Prog Med* 1997; **88:** 401–2.
7. Leone M, *et al.* Melatonin versus placebo in the prophylaxis of cluster headache; a double-blind pilot study with parallel groups. *Cephalalgia* 1996; **16:** 494–6.
8. Rosenberg SI, *et al.* Effect of melatonin on tinnitus. *Laryngoscope* 1998; **108:** 305–10.
9. Brzezinski A. Melatonin in humans. *N Engl J Med* 1997; **336:** 186–95.

INSOMNIA. Although melatonin is considered[1-6] to be potentially useful in the management of various forms of insomnia (p.652), especially those associated with circadian rhythm disturbances, there is little evidence of efficacy from large studies and its long-term safety remains to be established. In healthy subjects melatonin has been reported[7,8] to reduce the time to onset of sleep and to increase the time spent asleep. Whether this is due to adjustment of the 'body clock' or any hypnotic action of melatonin is unclear. Improved quality of sleep has been reported in elderly patients treated with melatonin for insomnia,[9] and it might be of use in delayed sleep phase syndrome[10] and insomnia in shift workers and totally blind people, although some[11,12] have found no beneficial effects of melatonin in night shift workers or emergency medicine employees. There has also been a report[13] of a patient with somnolence associated with melatonin deficiency after pinealectomy who responded to treatment with melatonin. A preliminary report[14] has suggested that use of melatonin may enable benzodiazepine therapy for insomnia to be discontinued without impairing the quality of sleep. However, melatonin might have a deleterious effect on sleep patterns in some circumstances.[15]

1. Haimov I, Lavie P. Potential of melatonin replacement therapy in older patients with sleep disorders. *Drugs Aging* 1995; **7:** 75–8.
2. Brown GM. Melatonin in psychiatric and sleep disorders: therapeutic implications. *CNS Drugs* 1995; **3:** 209–26.
3. Anonymous. Melatonin. *Med Lett Drugs Ther* 1995; **37:** 111–12.
4. Arendt J. Melatonin. *BMJ* 1996; **312:** 1242–3.
5. Lamberg L. Melatonin potentially useful but safety, efficacy remain uncertain. *JAMA* 1996; **276:** 1011–14.
6. Skene DJ, *et al.* Use of melatonin in the treatment of phase shift and sleep disorders. *Adv Exp Med Biol* 1999; **467:** 79–84.
7. Zhdanova IV, *et al.* Sleep-inducing effects of low doses of melatonin ingested in the evening. *Clin Pharmacol Ther* 1995; **57:** 552–8.

8. Attenburrow MEJ, *et al.* Low dose melatonin improves sleep in middle-aged subjects. *Psychopharmacology (Berl)* 1996; **126:** 179–81.
9. Garfinkel D, *et al.* Improvement of sleep quality in elderly people by controlled-release melatonin. *Lancet* 1995; **346:** 541–4.
10. Nagtegaal JE, *et al.* Effects of melatonin on the quality of life in patients with delayed sleep phase syndrome. *J Psychosom Res* 2000; **48:** 45–50.
11. Wright SW, *et al.* Randomized clinical trial of melatonin after night-shift work: efficacy and neuropsychologic effects. *Ann Emerg Med* 1998; **32:** 334–40.
12. Jockovich M, *et al.* Effect of exogenous melatonin on mood and sleep efficiency in emergency medicine residents working night shifts. *Acad Emerg Med* 2000; **7:** 955–8.
13. Lehmann ED, *et al.* Somnolence associated with melatonin deficiency after pinealectomy. *Lancet* 1996; **347:** 323.
14. Garfinkel D, *et al.* Facilitation of benzodiazepine discontinuation by melatonin: a new clinical approach. *Arch Intern Med* 1999; **159:** 2456–60.
15. Middleton BA, *et al.* Melatonin and fragmented sleep patterns. *Lancet* 1996; **348:** 551–2.

JET LAG. Melatonin has been reported to alleviate jet lag following long flights.[1-3] The most appropriate dosing schedule has yet to be determined but will depend on both the direction of travel and the distance travelled. A systematic review[4] has concluded that melatonin is effective in preventing or reducing jet lag in those travelling across 2 to 5 time zones, particularly in an easterly direction, and especially if jet lag has been experienced previously.

1. Waterhouse J, *et al.* Jet-lag. *Lancet* 1997; **350:** 1611–16.
2. Arendt J. Jet-lag. *Lancet* 1998; **351:** 293–4.
3. Arendt J. Jet-lag and shift work: (2) therapeutic use of melatonin. *J R Soc Med* 1999; **92:** 402–5.
4. Herxheimer A, Petrie KJ. Melatonin for the prevention and treatment of jet lag (updated 11 May 2001). Available in The Cochrane Library; Issue 4. Oxford: Update Software; 2001.

Preparations

Proprietary Preparations (details are given in Part 3)

Hong Kong: HT903; Melapure; *Mex.:* Cronocaps; *USA:* Transzone.

Multi-ingredient: *UK:* Rapi-snooze; *USA:* Bevitamel; Melagesic PM.

Melissa (4670-z)

Balm; Lemon Balm; Melissae Folium; Melissenblatt.

Pharmacopoeias. In *Eur.* (see p.vi) and *Pol.*

The chief constituent is citral.

Pharmacopoeial description

Ph. Eur.: The dried leaf of *Melissa officinalis*. It contains not less than 4% of total hydroxycinnamic derivatives expressed as rosmarinic acid ($C_{18}H_{16}O_8 = 360.3$), calculated with reference to the dried drug. It has an odour reminiscent of lemon. Protect from light.

Profile

Melissa has been used as a carminative and sedative. It is an ingredient of herbal remedies used for a variety of disorders. It is also reported to have virustatic activity. Hypersensitivity reactions have been reported.

◊ References.

1. Wölbling RH, Milbradt R. Klinik und therapie des Herpes simplex: vorstellung eines neuen phytotherapeutischen wirkstoffes. *Therapiewoche* 1984; **34:** 1193–1200.

Preparations

Proprietary Preparations (details are given in Part 3)

Aust.: Lomaherpan; *Ger.:* Gastrovegetalin; Kneipp Melisse Pflanzensaft; Lomaherpan; *Switz.:* Valverde boutons de fievre creme.

Multi-ingredient: *Aust.:* Abdomilon; Absimed; Aktiv Nerven- und Schlaftee; Aponatura Beruhigungs; Aponatura Einschlaf; Baldracin; Baldrian-Elixier; Baldrian-Krautertonikum; Baldriparan Beruhigungs; Beruhigungstee; Bio-Garten Tee zur Beruhigung; Bio-Garten Tropfen zur Beruhigung; Cardalept; Doppelherz Tonikum; Gastregan; Herz- und Kreislauftonikum Bioflora; Kneipp Nerven- und Schlaf-Tee; Krauterdoktor Beruhigungstropfen; Krauterdoktor Entspannungs- und Einschlaftropfen; Krauterdoktor Magen-Darmtropfen; Krauterdoktor Nerven-Tonikum; Krauterdoktor Rosmarin-Wein; Krauterhaus Mag Kottas Babytee; Krauterhaus Mag Kottas Magen- und Darmtee; Krauterhaus Mag Kottas Nerven- und Schlaftee; Krauterhaus Mag Kottas Wechseltee; Krautertee Nr 1; Krautertee Nr 141; Krautertee Nr 16; Krautertee Nr 201; Krautertee Nr 209; Krautertee Nr 9; Mag Doskar's Magentonikum; Mag Doskar's Nerventonikum; Mag Kottas Beruhigungstee; Mag Kottas Krauterexpress-Nerven-Schlaf-Tee; Mag Kottas Magen-Darmtee; Mag Kottas Nerven-Beruhigungstee; Mag Kottas Schlaftee; Mag Kottas Tee fur stillende Mutter; Mag Kottas Wechseltee; Mariazeller; Nervendragees; Nervifloran; Passedan; Passelyt; Phytogran; Seda-Grandelat; Sidroga Herz-Kreislauf-Tee; Sidroga Kindertee; Sidroga Magen-Darm-Tee; Sidroga Nerven- und Schlaftee; Species nervinae; St Radegunder Beruhigungs- und Einschlaftee; St Radegunder Fiebertee; St Radegunder Herz-Kreislauf-Tonikum; St Radegunder Herz-Kreislauf-unterstutzender Tee; St Radegunder Magenberuhigungstee; St Radegunder Nerven-Tonikum; St Radegunder Nervetee; St Radegunder Reizmildernder Magentee; St Radegunder Rosmarin-Wein; Synpharma Instant-Nervetee; Teekanne Magen- und Darmtee; Teekanne Schlaf- und Nervetee; The Chambard-Tee; Wechseltee; *Belg.:* Tisane pour le Foie; Tisane Purgative; *Braz.:* Anevrase; Balsamo Branco; Camomila; Especies Calmantes; Fargestium; Passiflora Composta; Sedantol; *Canad.:* Nyrene†; *Fr.:* Biocarde; Colominthe†; Elixir Bonjean; Mediflor Tisane Calmante Tisane du Sommeil No 14†; Mediflor Tisane Circulation du Sang No 12†; Mediflor Tisane Pectorale d'Alsace; Santane D_5; Santane N_9; Tisane des Familles; Tisane Grande Chartreuse; Ti-

sane Touraine†; Vagostabyl; *Ger.:* Abdomilon N; Aranidorm-S†; Avedorm; Baldriparan stark N; Befelka-Tinktur†; Doppelherz Melissengeist; Dormarist; Euvegal Entspannungs- und Einschlafdragees; Euvegal forte†; Euvegal N; Euviterin†; Gastrol S; Gutnacht; Heumann Beruhigungstee Tenerval N; Iberogast; Ju-Dorm; JuNeuron S†; Kneipp Krauter Taschenkur Nerven und Schlaf N; Kneipp Nerven- und Schlaf-Tee N; Lindofluid N; Luvased-Tropfen N; Melissengeist; Nerven-Tee Stada N†; Nervosana; Oxacant N; Oxacant-sedativ; Pascosedon; Phytonoctu; Plantival novo; Presselin Blahungs K 4 N; Pronervon Phyto; RubieSed; Salus Nerven-Schlaf-Tee Nr.22†; Salusan†; Schlaf- und Nerventee; Seda-Plantina; Sedacur; Sedariston; Sedaselect N; Sedasyx; Sedatruw S†; Sedinfant N; Sirmiosta Nervenelixier N†; Stullmaton; SX Valeriana comp; *Ital.:* Cura†; Emmenoiasi; Fluxoten†; Melissa Specie Composta; Sedatol; Tisana Arnaldi†; Tisana Cisbey†; Tisana Kelemata; *Mex.:* Plantival; *Port.:* Songha; *Spain:* Agua del Carmen; Caramelos Agua del Carmen; Digestol Sanatorium; Resolutivo Regium; Sol Schoum; *Switz.:* Arterosan Plus; Baldriparan; Cardiaforce; Dormiplant†; Dragees pour la detente nerveuse; Gastrosan; Hyperiforce comp; Iberogast; Melissa Tonic†; Phytoberidin; Relax; Seracalm†; Songha Night; Soporin; The Brioni; The Franklin†; Tisane antiflatulente pour les enfants; Tisane calmante pour les enfants; Tisane favorisant l'allaitement; Tisane pour l'estomac; Tisane pour le coeur et la circulation; Tisane pour le sommeil et les nerfs; Tisane pour les enfants†; Tisane relaxante; Valverde Dragees pour la detente; *UK:* Cough Drops; Melissa comp.; Melissin; Valerina Day Time; Valerina Night-Time.

Menbutone (12927-n)

Menbutone (*BAN, rINN*).

SC-1749 (menbutone sodium). 4-(4-Methoxy-1-naphthyl)-4-oxobutyric acid.

$C_{15}H_{14}O_4 = 258.3$.

CAS — 3562-99-0.

Profile

Menbutone is used as a choleretic to stimulate gastrointestinal function in veterinary medicine.

Menthol (266-k)

Hexahydrothymol; Mentholum; Mentol. *p*-Menthan-3-ol; 2-Isopropyl-5-methylcyclohexanol.

$C_{10}H_{20}O = 156.3$.

CAS — 89-78-1; 1490-04-6; 15356-60-2 (+); 2216-51-5 (−); 15356-70-4 (±).

NOTE. Levomenthol and racementhol are both *rINN* and *BAN*.

Pharmacopoeias. In *Chin., Eur.* (see p.vi), *Jpn, Pol.,* and *US.*

Eur. and *Jpn* have separate monographs for laevo-menthol (levomenthol) and racemic menthol (racementhol).

Natural laevo-menthol obtained from the volatile oils of various species of *Mentha* (Labiatae) or synthetic laevo-menthol or racemic menthol. A liquid or soft mass is formed when menthol is triturated with camphor, cloral hydrate, phenol, and many other substances.

Pharmacopoeial description

Ph. Eur.: Levomenthol occurs as colourless, acicular or prismatic shiny crystals. M.p. about 43°. Practically insoluble in water; very soluble in alcohol, in ether, and in petroleum spirit; freely soluble in fatty oils and in liquid paraffin; very slightly soluble in glycerol. Store at 8° to 15°.

Racemic menthol occurs as colourless, acicular or prismatic shiny crystals or as a free-flowing or agglomerated crystalline powder. M.p. about 34°. Practically insoluble in water; very soluble in alcohol, in ether, and in petroleum spirit; freely soluble in fatty oils and in liquid paraffin; very slightly soluble in glycerol. Store at 8° to 15°.

USP 25: An alcohol obtained from diverse mint oils or prepared synthetically. It may be laevorotatory (*l*-menthol), from natural or synthetic sources, or racemic (*dl*-menthol). It occurs as colourless, hexagonal crystals, usually needle-like, or in fused masses, or crystalline powder. Has a pleasant, peppermint-like odour. M.p. of *l*-menthol 41° to 44°. Slightly soluble in water; very soluble in alcohol, in chloroform, in ether, and in petroleum spirit; freely soluble in glacial acetic acid, in fixed and volatile oils, and in liquid paraffin. Store in airtight containers preferably at a temperature of 15° to 30°.

Adverse Effects

Menthol may give rise to hypersensitivity reactions including contact dermatitis. There have been reports of apnoea and instant collapse in infants following the local application of menthol to their nostrils. Ingestion of menthol is reported to cause severe abdominal pain, nausea, vomiting, vertigo, ataxia, drowsiness, and coma.

◊ Instillation of decongestant preparations containing menthol directly into the nostrils of infants and young children has resulted in acute respiratory distress with cyanosis[1] and respiratory arrest.[2] In one case,[1] nasal application was associated with concurrent chemical conjunctivitis.

1. Wyllie JP, Alexander FW. Nasal instillation of 'Olbas Oil' in an infant. *Arch Dis Child* 1994; **70:** 357–8.
2. Blake KD. Dangers of common cold treatments in children. *Lancet* 1993; **341:** 640.

Effects on the nervous system. Ataxia, confusion, euphoria, nystagmus, and diplopia developed in a 13-year-old boy following the inhalation of 5 mL of Olbas oil instead of the recommended few drops.[1] It was considered probable that the menthol in the preparation was responsible for the symptoms; the amount of menthol inhaled was approximately 200 mg.

1. O'Mullane NM, *et al.* Adverse CNS effects of menthol-containing Olbas oil. *Lancet* 1982; **i:** 1121.

Treatment of Adverse Effects and Precautions
As for Camphor, p.1589.

Pharmacokinetics
After absorption, menthol is excreted in the urine and bile as a glucuronide.

Uses and Administration
Menthol is chiefly used to relieve symptoms of bronchitis, sinusitis, and similar conditions. For this purpose it may be used as an inhalation, usually with benzoin or eucalyptus oil, as pastilles, or as an ointment with camphor and eucalyptus oil for application to the chest or nostrils (but see Adverse Effects above). However, as mentioned under the section on the management of cough (p.1082), the use of menthol in inhalations is unlikely to provide any additional benefit to that from the steam inhalation.

When applied to the skin menthol dilates the blood vessels, causing a sensation of coldness followed by an analgesic effect. It relieves itching and is used in creams, lotions, or ointments in pruritus and urticaria.

In small doses by mouth menthol has a carminative action.

Action. It has been suggested that the apparent benefits of menthol in nasal congestion may be due to an effect on calcium channels of sensory nerves.[1] This mechanism has also been implicated in its muscle relaxant action (as peppermint oil) on the gastrointestinal tract (p.1243).

1. Anonymous. How does menthol work? *Pharm J* 1993; **251:** 480.

Preparations
BP 2001: Menthol and Benzoin Inhalation;
USP 25: Benzocaine and Menthol Topical Aerosol; Menthol Lozenges; Tetracaine and Menthol Ointment.

Proprietary Preparations (details are given in Part 3)
Aust.: Nifint; Wick Vapo Sirup; *Austral.:* Dencorub Arthritis Ice; Ice Gel; Kaz†; Vicks Throat Drops; Vicks Vapodrops with Butter and Menthol; *Canad.:* Absorbine Jr; Absorbine Power Gel; Antiphlogistine Rub A-535 Ice; Ben-Gay Ice; Big V Cough Lozenge†; Celestial Seasonings; Certified Ice; Cough Drops; Deep Cold; Direct Formulary Cough Lozenges†; Fisherman's Friend; Flex-All; Honey Lemon Cough Lozenges; Ice Gel; Ice Gel Therapy; Ice Therapy†; Life Brand Cough Lozenges†; Meggezones; Myoflex Ice†; No Name Cough Lozenge†; Obus Form Therapeutic Ice; Physiomenthol; Polar Ice; Safeway Cough Lozenges†; Vicks Throat Drops; Vicks Vaposyrup; *Fr.:* Matiga†; *Ger.:* Nifint; Novopin MIG†; Wick Vaposyrup†; *Hong Kong:* Perskindol; *Spain:* Icespray; Prulit; *Switz.:* Perskindol†; *Thai.:* Counterpain Cool; Stopain; *UK:* Avoca Menthol Cone; Deep Freeze Cold Gel; Happinose; Ice Cool Stress & Tension Relief; Meggezones; Quool; Vicks Vaposyrup for tickly coughs; *USA:* Absorbine Jr; Absorbine Power Gel†; Ben-Gay Vanishing†; Blue Gel Muscular Pain Reliever†; Extra Strength Vicks Cough Drops; Halls-Plus Maximum Strength; Kof-Eze; N'ice†; N'ice 'n Clear; Pain Gel Plus†; Pain Patch†; Sportscreme Ice; Therapeutic Mineral Ice; Vicks Cough Drops; Wonder Ice.

Multi-ingredient: numerous preparations are listed in Part 3.

Menyanthes (537-n)

Bitterklee; Bogbean; Buckbean; Folia Trifoli Fibrini; Marsh Trefoil; Menyanthidis Trifoliatae Folium; Trèfle d'Eau.

Pharmacopoeias. In *Eur.* (see p.vi) and *Pol.*

Pharmacopoeial description
Ph. Eur.: The dried, entire or fragmented leaf of *Menyanthes trifoliata*. It has a very bitter and persistent taste.

Profile
Menyanthes has been used as a bitter. It is used in herbal medicine for rheumatic disorders. It is also used in homoeopathic and folk medicine.

Preparations
Proprietary Preparations (details are given in Part 3)
Multi-ingredient: *Aust.:* Krauterhaus Mag Kottas Gallen- und Lebertee; Krautertee Nr 9; Mag Kottas Leber-Gallentee; Magentee; Mariazeller; *Fr.:* Tisane Hepatique de Hoerdt; *Ger.:* Cefaktivon; Cefaktivon "novum"†; Gallexier; Montana; *UK:* Modern Herbals Rheumatic Pain; Rheumatic Pain; Rheumatic Pain Relief; Rheumatic Pain Remedy; Rheumatic Pain Tablets; Vegetex.

Mercaptamine (20830-z)

Mercaptamine (*BAN, rINN*).

Cysteamine (*USAN*); L-1573; MEA; Mercamine. 2-Aminoethanethiol.
$C_2H_7NS = 77.15$.
CAS — 60-23-1.

Mercaptamine Bitartrate (3575-p)

Mercaptamine Bitartrate (*BANM, rINNM*).
Cysteamine Bitartrate.
$C_2H_7NS, C_4H_6O_6 = 227.2$.
CAS — 27761-19-9.

Mercaptamine Hydrochloride (1041-p)

Mercaptamine Hydrochloride (*BANM, rINNM*).
Cl-9148; Cysteamine Hydrochloride (*USAN*).
$C_2H_7NS,HCl = 113.6$.
CAS — 156-57-0.

Adverse Effects and Precautions
When taken by mouth mercaptamine can be unpalatable and may cause breath and body odour. It may cause gastrointestinal side-effects including anorexia, nausea, vomiting, diarrhoea, and abdominal pain; rarely, there may be gastrointestinal ulceration or bleeding. Other side-effects may include drowsiness, malaise, rashes, fever, flushing, and ventricular tachycardia. Mercaptamine may cause increases in liver enzyme values and precipitate hepatic coma in patients with overt hepatic damage. Interstitial nephritis has also occurred rarely. Nervousness, depression, and, rarely, hallucinations, have been reported.

◊ Three patients with nephropathic cystinosis developed fever, maculopapular eruption, leucopenia, or headache within 2 weeks of starting mercaptamine at doses of 53, 67, and 75 mg per kg body-weight daily by mouth,respectively.[1] These side-effects resolved within 48 hours of drug withdrawal and all 3 patients were able to tolerate mercaptamine when restarted at a dose of 10 mg per kg daily, slowly increased to therapeutic levels over 2 to 3 months. Higher doses of mercaptamine had been associated with lethargy and seizures.

1. Schneider JA, *et al.* Cysteamine therapy in nephropathic cystinosis. *N Engl J Med* 1981; **304:** 1172.

Uses and Administration
Mercaptamine reduces intracellular cystine levels and is given by mouth as the bitartrate in the treatment of cystinosis (see below); it has also been given as the hydrochloride. Doses are expressed in terms of the base. Mercaptamine bitartrate is given in an initial dose that is one-sixth to one-quarter of the expected maintenance dose, and is then increased gradually over 4 to 6 weeks. The usual maintenance dose in adults is 2 g daily in 4 divided doses with or after food. Children up to 12 years of age are given 1.3 g per m² body-surface daily in 4 divided doses. Doses are given in conjunction with monitoring of leucocyte-cystine levels which should be kept below 1 nanomol of hemicystine per mg of protein.

Phosphocysteamine, a phosphorothioester of mercaptamine, is more palatable being odourless and tasteless, and is used similarly.

Mercaptamine facilitates glutathione synthesis and was formerly used intravenously in the treatment of severe paracetamol poisoning to prevent hepatic damage, but other forms of treatment are now preferred (see p.71).

Cystinosis. Mercaptamine and phosphocysteamine (which appears to be rapidly hydrolysed to mercaptamine after administration) have been reported to be of benefit in children with cystinosis, a rare autosomal recessive metabolic disorder characterised by the intracellular accumulation of cystine. Cystinosis is marked by growth retardation, rickets, Fanconi syndrome, and renal failure; acute episodes of acidosis and dehydration may develop, and there may be photophobia associated with deposition of cystine in the eye. Treatment, which results in a reduction in the concentrations of cystine in leucocytes, has been shown to be effective in controlling many of the symptoms,[1-3] especially if begun early, although it is not clear from the present contradictory results[3,4] how much benefit is seen on renal function. Compliance may be a problem, due to the unpalatable taste and odour of mercaptamine, and the more palatable prodrug phosphocysteamine has been developed as an alternative;[5,6] more palatable formulations of mercaptamine are also being investigated. Mercaptamine eye drops are reportedly of benefit in reversing or preventing deposition of corneal cystine crystals.[7]

1. Yudkoff M, *et al.* Effects of cysteamine therapy in nephropathic cystinosis. *N Engl J Med* 1981; **304:** 141–5.
2. Gahl WA, *et al.* Cysteamine therapy for children with nephropathic cystinosis. *N Engl J Med* 1987; **316:** 971–7.
3. Reznik VM, *et al.* Treatment of cystinosis with cysteamine from early infancy. *J Pediatr* 1991; **119:** 491–3.
4. Markello TC, *et al.* Improved renal function in children with cystinosis treated with cysteamine. *N Engl J Med* 1993; **328:** 1157–62.
5. Gahl WA, *et al.* Cystinosis: progress in a prototypic disease. *Ann Intern Med* 1988; **109:** 557–69.
6. van't Hoff WG, *et al.* Effects of oral phosphocysteamine and rectal cysteamine in cystinosis. *Arch Dis Child* 1991; **66:** 1434–7.
7. Kaiser-Kupfer MI, *et al.* A randomized placebo-controlled trial of cysteamine eye drops in nephropathic cystinosis. *Arch Ophthalmol* 1990; **108:** 689–93.

Preparations
Proprietary Preparations (details are given in Part 3)
Austral.: Cystagon; *Denm.:* Cystagon; *Fin.:* Cystagon; *Fr.:* Cystagon; *Swed.:* Cystagon; *UK:* Cystagon.

Mercuric Chloride (5307-b)

Bicloruro de Mercurio; Cloreto Mercúrico; Corrosive Sublimate; Hydrarg. Perchlor.; Hydrargyri Dichloridum; Hydrargyri Perchloridum; Hydrargyrum Bichloratum; Mercuric Chlor.; Mercurique (Chlorure); Mercury Bichloride; Mercury Perchloride; Quecksilberchlorid.
$HgCl_2 = 271.5$.
CAS — 7487-94-7.
ATC — D08AK03.
Pharmacopoeias. In *Eur.* (see p.vi).

Pharmacopoeial description
Ph. Eur.: A white crystalline powder, or colourless or white crystals or heavy crystalline masses. Soluble in water, in ether, and in glycerol; freely soluble in alcohol. Protect from light.

Profile
The use of mercuric chloride as an antibacterial substance is limited by its toxicity, its precipitating action on proteins, its irritant action on raw surfaces, its corrosive action on metals, and by the fact that its activity is greatly reduced in the presence of excreta or body fluids.

Details of the adverse effects of inorganic mercury compounds are provided under Mercury, below.

Preparations
Proprietary Preparations (details are given in Part 3)
Multi-ingredient: *Spain:* Oxido Amari; Pantenil.

Yellow Mercuric Oxide (5311-d)

Gelbes Quecksilberoxyd; Hydrargyri Oxidum Flavum; Hydrargyri Oxydum Flavum; Mercurique (Oxyde) Jaune; Oxido Amarillo de Mercurio; Yellow Precipitate.
$HgO = 216.6$.
CAS — 21908-53-2.
Pharmacopoeias. In *Belg., Fr.,* and *It.*

Profile
Yellow mercuric oxide has been used in eye ointments for the local treatment of minor infections including the eradication of pubic lice from the eyelashes. Absorption can occur and produce the adverse effects of inorganic mercury (see Mercury, below).

Porphyria. Mercuric oxide has been associated with acute attacks of porphyria and is considered unsafe in porphyric patients.

Pediculosis. Yellow mercuric oxide 1% eye ointment was considered to be a safe and effective treatment in pediculosis (p.1427) of the eyelashes caused by pubic lice (pthiriasis palpebrarum).[1]

1. Ashkenazi I, *et al.* Yellow mercuric oxide: a treatment of choice for phthiriasis palpebrarum. *Br J Ophthalmol* 1991; **75:** 356–8.

Preparations
Proprietary Preparations (details are given in Part 3)
Austral.: Golden Eye Ointment; *Fr.:* Pommade Maurice; *USA:* Stye.

Multi-ingredient: *Spain:* Oxido Amari.

Mercurous Chloride (5314-m)

Calomel; Calomelanos; Cloreto Mercuroso; Hydrarg. Subchlor.; Hydrargyri Subchloridum; Hydrargyrosi Chloridum; Hydrargyrum Chloratum (Mite); Mercureux (Chlorure); Mercurius Dulcis; Mercury Monochloride; Mercury Subchloride; Mild Mercurous Chloride; Protocloruro de Mercurio; Quecksilberchlorür.
$HgCl = 236.0$.
CAS — 7546-30-7 (HgCl); 10112-91-1 (Hg_2Cl_2).
Pharmacopoeias. In *Chin.*

Some pharmacopoeias also include Precipitated Mercurous Chloride (Hydrargyri Subchloridum Praecipitatum), a white amorphous powder, to which the synonym 'White Precipitate' (Praecipitatum Album) may be applied. White Precipitate has also been used as a name for Ammoniated Mercury.

Profile
Mercurous chloride was formerly given as a laxative and was applied topically as an antibacterial. It was one of the mercury compounds employed in the management of syphilis in the pre-antibiotic era.

The mercurous form of mercury does not possess the corrosive properties of the mercuric form and is not absorbed to any great extent. However, the mercurous form can be converted to the mercuric with consequent toxicity as described under Mercury (see below).

The symbol † denotes a preparation no longer actively marketed

Mercury (5306-m)

Hydrarg.; Hydrargyrum; Hydrargyrum Depuratum; Mercure; Mercurio; Quecksilber; Quicksilver.
Hg = 200.59.
CAS — 7439-97-6.
ATC — D08AK05.
Pharmacopoeias. In Aust. and Fr.

A shining, silvery white, very mobile liquid, easily divisible into globules, which readily volatilises on heating.

Adverse Effects
Poisoning with liquid mercury or inorganic mercury salts has arisen from a variety of sources such as batteries, cosmetics, dental materials, medical equipment, and jewellery manufacture. Barometers, sphygmomanometers, and thermometers are still sources of liquid mercury. Trace amounts of organic and inorganic mercury may also be ingested in the diet.

Liquid mercury if ingested is poorly absorbed and, unless there is aspiration or pre-existing gastrointestinal disorders, is not considered to be a severe toxicological hazard. The greatest dangers from liquid mercury arise from the inhalation of mercury vapour. On *acute* exposure, it can cause various gastrointestinal effects including nausea, vomiting, and diarrhoea; more importantly it is toxic to the respiratory system and this effect can be fatal. Some CNS involvement has also been reported. Liquid mercury is also not without its dangers when injected and there have been a number of reports of accidental or intentional parenteral administration. *Inorganic salts* such as mercuric chloride are corrosive when ingested causing severe nausea, vomiting, pain, bloody diarrhoea, and necrosis. The kidney is also involved and tubular necrosis may develop. Mercurous salts are considered to be less hazardous, but the mercurous form can be converted to the mercuric. *Organic mercurial compounds* produce similar toxic effects to inorganic compounds, but they have a more selective action on the CNS that has proved difficult to treat. The degree of toxicity varies with the different groups of organic mercurials; those used as preservatives or disinfectants being less toxic than the ethyl or methyl compounds that are not used pharmaceutically or clinically. Methylmercury is notorious for its toxicity; there have been cases of fetal neurotoxicity during outbreaks of methylmercury poisoning.

Chronic mercury poisoning may result from inhalation of mercury vapour, skin contact with mercury or mercury compounds, or ingestion of mercury salts over prolonged periods. It is characterised by many symptoms including tremor, motor and sensory disturbances, mental deterioration, gastrointestinal symptoms, dermatitis, kidney damage, salivation, and loosening of teeth. A blue line may be present on the gums. There is little difference between acute and chronic poisoning with organic mercurials.

The syndrome of acrodynia (pink disease), with symptoms of sweat, rash, oedema of the extremities, photophobia, wasting, weakness, hypertension, tachycardia, and diminished reflexes, occurred in children given mercury in teething powders or in ointments or dusting powders. Such preparations have long since been withdrawn from use. However, the syndrome is still a feature of mercury poisoning from other sources.

Hypersensitivity to mercury and mercurial compounds has been reported.

Mercurialentis has been reported in patients treated with eye drops containing an organomercurial preservative.

◊ Acute *occupational exposure* to mercury vapour in 53 men resulted in an initial phase described as metal fume fever, an intermediate phase of severe symptoms with CNS, gastrointestinal, respiratory, and urological involvement, and a late phase with persistent CNS symptoms, dysuria, and pain on ejaculation.[1,2] Although persistent hyperchloraemia was noted in the 11 patients with the highest mercury levels, renal impairment tended to be temporary.[2] Long-term follow-up of a patient who had an intravenous injection of mercury 12 years previously also revealed no persistent renal impairment,[3] despite the presence of mercury microemboli in lungs, kidneys, liver, and subcutaneous tissues and high concentrations in the urine. At this time, the patient had residual reductions in respiratory function, polyneuropathy, and marked asthenozoospermia. Spermatozoal abnormalities may also have contributed to his wife's miscarriage.

Fetal neurotoxicity following *maternal exposure* to methylmercury is well recognised, and has been shown to cause delays in neurological development in affected children up to the age of 7 years.[4]

There has been considerable concern over the systemic absorption of mercury from *dental amalgam*, which typically contains between 40 and 70% of mercury. However, the quantities absorbed from amalgam fillings is reported to be relatively small[5,6] and current evidence suggests that the use of dental amalgam for tooth restoration is both safe and effective.[7,8] The main risks appear to be occupational exposure of dental staff and environmental concerns. Some patients with hypersensitivity to mercury (manifest most commonly as local lichenoid reactions) may benefit from removal of amalgam fillings.[9,10]

The symptoms of *acrodynia* have sometimes been mistaken for those of phaeochromocytoma.[11-14]

1. Bluhm RE, *et al.* Elemental mercury vapour toxicity, treatment, and prognosis after acute, intensive exposure in chloralkali plant workers part I: history, neuropsychological findings and chelator effects. *Hum Exp Toxicol* 1992; **11**: 201–10.
2. Bluhm RE, *et al.* Elemental mercury vapour toxicity, treatment, and prognosis after acute, intensive exposure in chloralkali plant workers part II: hyperchloraemia and genitourinary symptoms. *Hum Exp Toxicol* 1992; **11**: 211–15.
3. dell'Omo M, *et al.* Long-term toxicity of intravenous mercury injection. *Lancet* 1996; **348**: 64.
4. Grandjean P, *et al.* Cognitive deficit in 7-year-old children with prenatal exposure to methylmercury. *Neurotoxicol Teratol* 1997; **19**: 417–28.
5. Eley BM. The future of dental amalgam: a review of the literature. Part 3: mercury exposure from amalgam restorations in dental patients. *Br Dent J* 1997; **182**: 333–8.
6. Eley BM. The future of dental amalgam: a review of the literature. Part 4: mercury exposure hazards and risk assessment. *Br Dent J* 1997; **182**: 373–81.
7. FDI/WHO. Consensus statement on dental amalgam. *FDI World* 1995; 4 (July/Aug): 9–10.
8. Eley BM. The future of dental amalgam: a review of the literature. Part 6: possible harmful effects of mercury from dental amalgam. *Br Dent J* 1997; **182**: 455–9.
9. Ibbotson SH, *et al.* The relevance and effect of amalgam replacement in subjects with oral lichenoid reactions. *Br J Dermatol* 1996; **134**: 420–3.
10. McGivern B, *et al.* Delayed and immediate hypersensitivity reactions associated with the use of amalgam. *Br Dent J* 2000; **188**: 73–6.
11. Henningsson C, *et al.* Acute mercury poisoning (acrodynia) mimicking pheochromocytoma in an adolescent. *J Pediatr* 1993; **122**: 252–3.
12. Velzeboer SCJM, *et al.* A hypertensive toddler. *Lancet* 1997; **349**: 1810.
13. Wößmann W, *et al.* Mercury intoxication presenting with hypertension and tachycardia. *Arch Dis Child* 1999; **80**: 556–7.
14. Torres AD, *et al.* Mercury intoxication and arterial hypertension: report of two patients and review of the literature. Abstract: *Pediatrics* 2000; **105**: 627. Full version: http://www.pediatrics.org/cgi/content/full/105/3/e34

Effects on the kidneys. The kidneys are one of the primary sites for the accumulation of mercury in the body. All forms of mercury (liquid mercury, inorganic mercury, and organic mercury) may be toxic to the kidney although the inorganic forms are the most nephrotoxic.[1]

1. Zalups RK. Molecular interactions with mercury in the kidney. *Pharmacol Rev* 2000; **52**: 113–43.

Treatment of Adverse Effects
The treatment of **acute** mercury toxicity depends on the form of mercury, the route of exposure, and the dose. Supportive measures may be needed with all types of toxicity. Ingestion of liquid mercury seldom requires active treatment since it is poorly absorbed by this route. Acute oral poisoning due to other inorganic mercury sources should be treated if appropriate by activated charcoal or gastric lavage to reduce absorption. Acute exposure via inhalation or injection mainly requires supportive therapy although excision of the affected area has been recommended following subcutaneous administration. In severe cases chelation therapy may be required to facilitate the removal of mercury from the body. Chelating agents that may be used include dimercaprol (p.1007), penicillamine (p.1019), succimer (p.1025), or unithiol (p.1026). Some centres institute haemodialysis at the beginning of treatment; others wait until renal failure develops when either haemodialysis or peritoneal dialysis is used.

Poisoning due to organic mercury is difficult to treat. The same measures as above should be adopted, except that it is recommended by some that dimercaprol should not be used since *animal* evidence indicates that it may increase the brain concentrations of mercury. An additional measure that has been tried is the administration of a thiol resin complex to prevent the reabsorption of mercury from the bile.

Mercurials on the skin should be removed by copious washing with soap and water.

The management of **chronic** toxicity is generally symptomatic although chelation therapy has been used in some patients.

◊ References.
1. Kostyniak PJ, *et al.* Extracorporeal regional complexing haemodialysis treatment of acute inorganic mercury intoxication. *Hum Toxicol* 1990; **9**: 137–41.
2. Ferguson L, Cantilena LR. Enhanced mercury clearance during hemodialysis with chelating agents. *Clin Pharmacol Ther* 1991; **49**: 131.
3. Florentine MJ, Sanfilippo DJ. Elemental mercury poisoning. *Clin Pharm* 1991; **10**: 213–21.
4. Bluhm RE, *et al.* Elemental mercury vapour toxicity, treatment, and prognosis after acute, intensive exposure in chloralkali plant workers part I: history, neuropsychological findings and chelator effects. *Hum Exp Toxicol* 1992; **11**: 201–10.
5. Toet AE, *et al.* Mercury kinetics in a case of severe mercuric chloride poisoning treated with dimercapto-1-propane sulphonate (DMPS). *Hum Exp Toxicol* 1994; **13**: 11–16.
6. Houeto P, *et al.* Elemental mercury vapour toxicity: treatment and levels in plasma and urine. *Hum Exp Toxicol* 1994; **13**: 848–52.
7. Aaseth J, *et al.* Treatment of mercury and lead poisonings with dimercaptosuccinic acid and sodium dimercaptopropanesulfonate: a review. *Analyst* 1995; **120**: 853–4.
8. Isik S, *et al.* Subcutaneous metallic mercury injection: early, massive excision. *Ann Plast Surg* 1997; **38**: 645–8.
9. Baum CR. Treatment of mercury intoxication. *Curr Opin Pediatr* 1999; **11**: 265–8.

Pharmacokinetics
There is little absorption of liquid mercury from globules in the gastrointestinal tract. The main hazard of liquid mercury is from absorption following inhalation of mercury vapour; this mercury is widely distributed before being oxidised to the mercuric form. Concentrations can be detected in the brain.

Soluble inorganic mercuric salts are absorbed from the gastrointestinal tract and can also be absorbed through the skin. The mercury is distributed throughout the soft tissues with high concentrations in the kidneys; it is mainly excreted in the urine and through the colon with an elimination half-life of about 60 days, although it may take years to eliminate mercury from the brain; elimination from other tissues may take several months.

Organic alkyl mercury compounds are more readily absorbed from both the gastrointestinal and the respiratory tracts. They are widely distributed and can produce high concentrations in the brain. Alkyl mercury compounds are excreted in urine and in the faeces with extensive enterohepatic recycling. The biological half-life varies but is longer than that of inorganic mercury.

Organic mercury, and to some extent inorganic mercury, diffuse across the placenta and are distributed into breast milk.

Uses and Administration
The hazards associated with mercury generally outweigh any therapeutic benefit and its clinical use has largely been abandoned. The use of mercurial diuretics such as mersalyl (p.926) has generally been superseded by other diuretics. Ointments containing mercurials, such as ammoniated mercury (p.1118) have also generally been replaced by less toxic preparations. Mercurials were formerly used as spermicides.

Some ionisable inorganic mercury salts and certain organic compounds of mercury have been used as disinfectants, and some mercury salts are effective parasiticides and fungicides. Organic mercurials such as phenylmercuric acetate, borate, and nitrate are also used as preservatives (p.1153). Mercury is a component of dental amalgams.

Other mercury salts which have been used for their antibacterial activity include mercuric chloride, yellow mercuric oxide, and mercurous chloride (above).

Some mercury compounds have been used in homoeopathic medicine.

Preparations
Proprietary Preparations (details are given in Part 3)
Ger.: Farco-Oxicyanid-Tupfer.

Multi-ingredient: *Aust.:* Coldophthal; *Spain:* Oftalmol Dexa†; Oftalmol Ocular.

Mescaline (5017-k)

3,4,5-Trimethoxyphenethylamine.
$C_{11}H_{17}NO_3 = 211.3.$
CAS — 54-04-6.

An alkaloid obtained from the cactus *Lophophora williamsii* (=*Anhalonium williamsii* =*A. lewinii*) (Cactaceae), which grows in the northern regions of Mexico. The cactus is known in those areas by the Aztec name 'peyote' or 'peyotl' and dried slices of the cactus are called 'mescal buttons'.

Profile
Mescaline produces hallucinogenic and sympathomimetic effects similar to those produced by lysergide (see p.1630), but it is less potent. Its effects last for up to 12 hours. It has no therapeutic use. Both Mexican and North American Indians have used peyote in religious ceremonies on account of its hallucinogenic activity.

◊ Peyote consumed during a ceremonial ritual was believed to have caused botulism in three men.[1] The sample was found to contain type B botulinum toxin when assayed.

1. Hashimoto H, *et al.* Botulism from peyote. *N Engl J Med* 1998; **339**: 203–4.

Mesoglycan Sodium (14224-s)

A mucopolysaccharide complex (glycosaminoglycan) extracted from calf aorta.

Profile
Mesoglycan sodium has been claimed to have antithrombotic, antiplatelet, and antihyperlipidaemic properties.

◊ References.
1. Forconi S, *et al.* A randomized, ASA-controlled trial of mesoglycan in secondary prevention after cerebral ischemic events. *Cerebrovasc Dis* 1995; **5**: 334–41.

Preparations
Proprietary Preparations (details are given in Part 3)
Ital.: Perclar; Prisma; *Port.:* Prisma.

Metamfepramone Hydrochloride (1476-l)

Metamfepramone Hydrochloride (rINNM).
Dimepropion Hydrochloride (BANM); Metamfepyramone Hydrochloride. 2-Dimethylaminopropiophenone hydrochloride.
$C_{11}H_{15}NO,HCl = 213.7.$
CAS — 15351-09-4 (metamfepramone); 10105-90-5 (metamfepramone hydrochloride).

Profile
Metamfepramone, the dimethyl analogue of diethylpropion (p.1508), is a sympathomimetic that has been used as the hydrochloride in the treatment of hypotension and in preparations for the symptomatic relief of the common cold. It was formerly used as an anorectic agent.

Preparations
Proprietary Preparations (details are given in Part 3)
Multi-ingredient: *Ger.:* Tempil N.

Metescufylline (12934-d)
Metescufylline (*rINN*).
7-(2-Diethylaminoethyl)theophylline (7-hydroxy-4-methyl-2-oxo-2*H*-1-benzopyran-6-yloxy)acetate.
$C_{25}H_{31}N_5O_8 = 529.5$.
CAS — 15518-82-8.

Profile
Metescufylline is a compound of metesculetol (below) and etamiphylline (p.764) that has been given by mouth for its reputed vasoprotectant effect.

Metesculetol Sodium (13490-t)
Metesculetol Sodium (*rINNM*).
[(7-Hydroxy-4-methyl-2-oxo-2*H*-1-benzopyran-6-yl)oxy]acetate sodium.
$C_{12}H_9NaO_6 = 272.2$.
CAS — 52814-39-8 (metesculetol); 53285-61-3 (metesculetol sodium).

Profile
Metesculetol is contained in preparations for peripheral vascular disorders and haemorrhoids.

Preparations
Proprietary Preparations (details are given in Part 3)
Multi-ingredient: *Fr.:* Fluon; Intrait de Marron D'Inde P; Veinotonyl.

Metallibure (12935-n)
Metallibure (*BAN, rINN*).
AY-61122; ICI-33828; Methallibure (*USAN*); NSC-69536. 1-Methyl-6-(1-methylallyl)-2,5-dithiobiurea.
$C_7H_{14}N_4S_2 = 218.3$.
CAS — 926-93-2.

Profile
Metallibure has the property of modifying certain hypothalamic and anterior pituitary functions. It has been used in veterinary medicine.

Methiosulfonium Chloride (12939-v)
Methylmethionine Sulfonium Chloride; Vitamin U. (3-Amino-3-carboxypropyl)dimethylsulphonium chloride.
$C_6H_{14}ClNO_2S = 199.7$.
CAS — 1115-84-0.
ATC — A02BX04.

Profile
Methiosulfonium chloride has been used for its reputed protective effect on the liver and gastrointestinal mucosa.

Preparations
Proprietary Preparations (details are given in Part 3)
Multi-ingredient: *Hong Kong:* Crema-U; RUDD-U; *Singapore:* Weisen-U.

Methyl Fluorosulfate (12951-n)
Methyl Fluorosulphate; Methyl Fluorosulphonate.
$CH_3O.SO_2F = 114.1$.

Profile
Methyl fluorosulfate has been used as a laboratory methylating agent. Pulmonary oedema has occurred after inhalation, and concern has been expressed concerning possible carcinogenicity.

Methylergometrine Maleate (1512-d)
Methylergometrine Maleate (*BANM, rINNM*).
Methylergobasine Maleate; Methylergonovine Maleate. N-[(S)-1-(Hydroxymethyl)propyl]-D-lysergamide hydrogen maleate; 9,10-Didehydro-N-[(S)-1-(hydroxymethyl)propyl]-6-methylergoline-8β-carboxamide hydrogen maleate.
$C_{20}H_{25}N_3O_2,C_4H_4O_4 = 455.5$.
CAS — 113-42-8 (methylergometrine); 57432-61-8 (methylergometrine maleate).
Pharmacopoeias. In Jpn and US.

The symbol † denotes a preparation no longer actively marketed

Pharmacopoeial description
USP 25: A white to pinkish-tan, odourless, microcrystalline powder. Soluble 1 in 100 of water, 1 in 175 of alcohol, 1 in 1900 of chloroform, and 1 in 8400 of ether. pH of a 0.02% solution in water is between 4.4 and 5.2. Store in airtight containers at a temperature not exceeding 8°. Protect from light.

Stability. For mention of slight variations in the methylergometrine content of the injection following transport to a tropical climate, see under Ergometrine Maleate, p.1607.

Adverse Effects, Treatment, and Precautions
As for Ergometrine Maleate, p.1607.

Pharmacokinetics
Methylergometrine maleate is reported to be rapidly absorbed after administration by mouth and by intramuscular injection. Oral bioavailability may show considerable interindividual variation. It undergoes extensive first-pass hepatic metabolism and only small amounts of unchanged drug are excreted in the urine. The elimination half-life is reported to be about 2 to 3 hours.

◊ The pharmacokinetics of methylergometrine maleate has been studied following oral administration in healthy subjects[1,2] and in postpartum women.[3] Small amounts of methylergometrine have been detected in breast milk.[4]

1. Mäntylä R, *et al.* Methylergometrine (methylergonovine) concentrations in the human plasma and urine. *Int J Clin Pharmacol Biopharm* 1978; **16:** 254–7.
2. de Groot ANJA, *et al.* Comparison of the bioavailability and pharmacokinetics of oral methylergometrine in men and women. *Int J Clin Pharmacol Ther* 1995; **33:** 328–32.
3. Allonen H, *et al.* Methylergometrine: comparison of plasma concentrations and clinical response of two brands. *Int J Clin Pharmacol Biopharm* 1978; **16:** 340–2.
4. Erkkola R, *et al.* Excretion of methylergometrine (methylergonovine) into the human breast milk. *Int J Clin Pharmacol Biopharm* 1978; **16:** 579–80.

Uses and Administration
Methylergometrine maleate has an action on the uterus similar to that of ergometrine maleate (p.1607) and is used similarly in the prevention and treatment of postpartum haemorrhage. It is given after delivery of the anterior shoulder or on completion of the third stage of labour in a dose of 200 µg intramuscularly, repeated for up to 5 doses if necessary at intervals of 2 to 4 hours. In emergencies 200 µg may be given by slow intravenous injection over at least 60 seconds. In the USA its use before delivery of the placenta is not generally recommended. During the puerperium 200 µg has been given by mouth 3 or 4 times daily for up to 7 days.
Methylergometrine is a metabolite of methysergide (p.454).

Diagnosis and testing. For reference to the use of methylergometrine maleate in the diagnosis of variant angina, see Ergometrine Maleate, p.1607.

Preparations
USP 25: Methylergonovine Maleate Injection; Methylergonovine Maleate Tablets.
Proprietary Preparations (details are given in Part 3)
Aust.: Methergin; *Belg.:* Methergin; *Braz.:* Methergin; *Denm.:* Methergin; *Fin.:* Methergin; *Fr.:* Methergin; *Ger.:* Methergin; Methylergobrevin; *Hong Kong:* Methergin; *Israel:* Methergin; *Ital.:* Methergin; *Mex.:* Methergin; *Neth.:* Methergin; *Norw.:* Methergin†; *Port.:* Methergin; *Spain:* Methergin; *Swed.:* Methergin; *Switz.:* Methergin; *Thai.:* Ergotyl; Metrine; Nathergen; *USA:* Methergine.

Multi-ingredient: *Ger.:* Syntometrin.

Methylhydroxyquinoline Metilsulfate
(12949-q)
Methylhydroxyquinoline Methylsulphate. 1-Methyl-8-hydroxyquinolinium methyl sulphate.
$C_{10}H_{10}NO,CH_3O_4S = 271.3$.

Profile
Methylhydroxyquinoline metilsulfate has been used topically to treat eye irritation.

Preparations
Proprietary Preparations (details are given in Part 3)
Belg.: Uvestat†; *Fr.:* Uveline; *Spain:* Chibro Uvelina.

Methylmethacrylate (12950-d)
Methyl 2-methylacrylate; Methyl 2-methylpropenoate.
$C_5H_8O_2 = 100.1$.
CAS — 80-62-6.

Adverse Effects
Occupational exposure to methylmethacrylate monomer vapour during preparation of the bone cement may irritate the respiratory tract, eyes, and skin. Cases of occupational asthma have been reported. Contact dermatitis, dizziness, nausea and vomiting may also occur. Methylmethacrylate monomer may be harmful to the liver.
Methylmethacrylate monomer acts as a peripheral vasodilator and has caused hypotension and, rarely, cardiac arrest and death when absorbed during the use of polymethylmethacr-

ylate (PMMA) as a bone cement during orthopaedic surgery. Other adverse effects associated with the use of polymethylmethacrylate as a bone cement include thrombophlebitis, pulmonary embolism, haemorrhage, haematoma, short-term irregularities in cardiac conduction, and cerebrovascular accident.

Effects on the nervous system. Sensory polyneuropathy has been reported in a dental technician following occupational exposure to methylmethacrylate monomer.[1]

1. Sadoh DR, *et al.* Occupational exposure to methyl methacrylate monomer induces generalised neuropathy in a dental technician. *Br Dent J* 1999; **186:** 380–1.

Uses and Administration
Methylmethacrylate forms the basis of acrylic bone cements used in orthopaedic surgery. A liquid consisting chiefly of methylmethacrylate monomer with a polymerisation initiator is mixed with a powder consisting of polymethylmethacrylate (PMMA) or a methylmethacrylate ester copolymer. The reaction is exothermic. Barium sulfate or zirconium dioxide may be added as a contrast medium. Beads of polymethylmethacrylate containing gentamicin have been implanted in the prophylaxis and treatment of bone infections and some soft-tissue infections. Bone cements containing antibacterials such as gentamicin or erythromycin are also available.
Polymethylmethacrylate has also been used as a material for intra-ocular lenses, for denture bases, as a cement for dental prostheses, and in composite resins for dental restoration.
A number of polymers based on methacrylic acid are used in pharmaceutical technology mainly as film coating agents and binders. The Ph. Eur. includes Methacrylic Acid-Methyl Methacrylate Copolymer (1:1), Methacrylic Acid-Ethyl Acrylate Copolymer (1:1), Methacrylic Acid-Ethyl Acrylate Copolymer (1:1) Dispersion 30 per cent, Methacrylic Acid-Methyl Methacrylate Copolymer (1:2), and Polyacrylate Dispersion 30 per cent (a dispersion of an ethylacrylate-methyl methacrylate copolymer in water). USNF 20 includes Methacrylic Acid Copolymer (a copolymer of methacrylic acid and an acrylic or methacrylic ester) and Ammonio Methacrylate Copolymer (a copolymer of acrylic and methacrylic acid esters).

Bone disorders. Percutaneous vertebral injection of methylmethacrylate bone cement has been used successfully to relieve the pain of metastatic vertebral bone lesions (p.490) and vertebral compression fractures due to osteoporosis (p.745).[1,2]

1. Kaemmerlen P, *et al.* Percutaneous injection of orthopedic cement in metastatic vertebral lesions. *N Engl J Med* 1989; **321:** 121.
2. Barr JD, *et al.* Percutaneous vertebroplasty for pain relief and spinal stabilization. *Spine* 2000; **25:** 923–8.

Preparations
Proprietary Preparations (details are given in Part 3)
Aust.: Knochenzement; Sulfix; *Ger.:* flint; Hansaplast Spruhpflaster; Palacos R; *Neth.:* Palacos; *Port.:* Palacos R†; *Singapore:* Palacos R; *Switz.:* Palacos†; *Thai.:* Palacos R; *UK:* Palacos R.
Multi-ingredient: *Aust.:* AKZ; Refobacin-Palacos R; Septopal; *Austral.:* Palacos E with Garamycin; Palacos R with Garamycin; Septopal; *Belg.:* Palacos R avec Gentamicine; Septopal; *Braz.:* Septopal; *Denm.:* Antibiotic Simplex†; Palacos cum Gentamicin; Septopal; *Fin.:* Palacos R cum Gentamicin; Septopal; *Fr.:* Palacos LV avec Gentamicine; Palacos R avec Gentamicine; *Ger.:* Refobacin-Palacos R; Septopal; *Hong Kong:* Septopal; *Irl.:* Palacos R with Gentamicin; Septopal; *Neth.:* Palacos met gentamicine; Septopal; *Norw.:* Palacos cum Gentamicin†; Septopal; *NZ:* Palacos with Garamycin; *Port.:* Palacos R com Gentamicina†; *S.Afr.:* Palacos R with Garamycin; Septopal; *Singapore:* Refobacin-Palacos R; Septopal; *Swed.:* Palacos cum gentamicin†; Septopal; *Switz.:* AKZ†; Palacos avec Garamycin†; Septopal; *Thai.:* Refobacin-Palacos R; Septopal; *UK:* Epiglu; Palacos LV with Gentamicin; Palacos R with Gentamicin; Septopal.

Metochalcone (3727-p)
Metochalcone (*rINN*).
CB1314; Methochalcone; Trimethoxychalcone. 2',4,4'-Trimethoxychalcone.
$C_{18}H_{18}O_4 = 298.3$.
CAS — 18493-30-6.

Profile
Metochalcone has been used as a choleretic.

Preparations
Proprietary Preparations (details are given in Part 3)
Multi-ingredient: *Spain:* Neocolan.

Metyrapone (2139-m)
Metyrapone (*BAN, USAN, rINN*).
Su-4885 (metyrapone tartrate). 2-Methyl-1,2-di(3-pyridyl)propan-1-one.
$C_{14}H_{14}N_2O = 226.3$.
CAS — 54-36-4.
ATC — V04CD01.
Pharmacopoeias. In Br., Jpn, and US.

Pharmacopoeial description
BP 2001: A white to light amber crystalline powder with a characteristic odour. M.p. 50° to 53°. Sparingly soluble in

water; freely soluble in alcohol and in chloroform; it dissolves in dilute mineral acids. Protect from light.

USP 25: A white to light amber, fine, crystalline powder, having a characteristic odour. It darkens on exposure to light. Sparingly soluble in water; soluble in chloroform and in methyl alcohol; forms water-soluble salts with acids. Store in airtight containers. Protect from heat and light.

Adverse Effects
Metyrapone may give rise to nausea and vomiting, abdominal pain, headache, sedation, dizziness, hypotension, and hypersensitivity rashes. Hypoadrenalism, hirsutism, and bone marrow depression may occur rarely. Long-term use of metyrapone can cause hypertension.

Alopecia. Reports of alopecia[1,2] associated with administration of metyrapone for Cushing's syndrome.
1. Harris PL. Alopecia associated with long-term metyrapone use. *Clin Pharm* 1986; **5:** 66–8.
2. Harries-Jones R, Overstall P. Metyrapone-induced alopecia. *Postgrad Med J* 1990; **66:** 584.

Precautions
Metyrapone should be used with extreme caution, if at all, in patients with gross hypopituitarism or with reduced adrenal secretory activity because of the risk of precipitating acute adrenal failure. Thyroid dysfunction or liver cirrhosis may alter the response to metyrapone.

Porphyria. Metyrapone is considered to be unsafe in patients with porphyria because it has been shown to be porphyrinogenic in *in-vitro* systems.

Interactions
Phenytoin is reported to increase the metabolism of metyrapone; doubling the dose of metyrapone may counteract the interaction. However, as many other drugs may interfere with the steroid assessment, medication is best avoided where possible during the metyrapone test. Drugs reported to interfere with the metyrapone test include antidepressants such as amitriptyline, antithyroid drugs, antipsychotics such as chlorpromazine, barbiturates, corticosteroids, cyproheptadine, and hormones that affect the hypothalamic-pituitary axis such as oestrogens and progestogens.

Pharmacokinetics
Metyrapone is rapidly absorbed from the gastrointestinal tract. It is metabolised by rapid reduction to metyrapol and excreted in the urine as glucuronide conjugates of metyrapone and metyrapol.

Uses and Administration
Metyrapone inhibits the enzyme 11β-hydroxylase responsible for the synthesis of the glucocorticoids cortisone and hydrocortisone (cortisol) as well as aldosterone from their precursors. The consequent fall in the plasma concentrations of circulating glucocorticoids stimulates the anterior pituitary gland to produce more corticotropin. This, in turn, stimulates the production of more 11-deoxycortisol and other precursors which are metabolised in the liver and excreted in the urine where they can be measured. Metyrapone is therefore used as a test of the feedback hypothalamic-pituitary mechanism in the diagnosis of Cushing's syndrome, although the dexamethasone suppression test (p.1068) may be preferred.

After demonstration of the responsiveness of the adrenal cortex, metyrapone is given by mouth, usually in a dose of 750 mg every 4 hours for 6 doses. Administration with milk or after a meal may minimise the gastrointestinal side-effects of metyrapone. A suggested dose by mouth for children is 15 mg per kg body-weight, with a minimum dose of 250 mg, every 4 hours for 6 doses. In patients with a normally functioning pituitary gland excretion of 17-hydroxycorticosteroids is increased two- to fourfold and that of 17-ketosteroids about twofold.

Metyrapone is also used in the management of Cushing's syndrome (p.1272) when doses may range from 250 mg to 6 g daily.

Since metyrapone inhibits the synthesis of aldosterone it has been used to treat some cases of resistant oedema; it is given in conjunction with a glucocorticoid to suppress the normal corticotropin response to low plasma concentrations of glucocorticoids. The suggested usual dosage of metyrapone in resistant oedema is 3 g daily in divided doses.

Metyrapone tartrate has also been used.

◊ References.
1. Atkinson AB. The treatment of Cushing's syndrome. *Clin Endocrinol (Oxf)* 1991; **34:** 507–13.
2. Avgerinos PC, *et al.* The metyrapone and dexamethasone suppression tests for the differential diagnosis of the adrenocorticotropin-dependent Cushing syndrome: a comparison. *Ann Intern Med* 1994; **121:** 318–27.
3. Avgerinos PC, *et al.* A comparison of the overnight and the standard metyrapone test for the differential diagnosis of adrenocorticotrophin-dependent Cushing's syndrome. *Clin Endocrinol (Oxf)* 1996; **45:** 483–91.

Preparations
BP 2001: Metyrapone Capsules;
USP 25: Metyrapone Tablets.

Proprietary Preparations (details are given in Part 3)
Austral.: Metopirone; *Fr.:* Metopirone; *Irl.:* Metopirone; *Neth.:* Metopiron; *Norw.:* Metopiron†; *NZ:* Metopirone; *Swed.:* Metopiron; *Switz.:* Metopirone; *UK:* Metopirone; *USA:* Metopirone.

Dementholised Mint Oil (3268-x)
Menthae Arvensis Aetheroleum Partim Mentholi Privum.
Pharmacopoeias. In *Eur.* (see p.vi).
Mint oil or Mentha oil is in *Ger.* and *Jpn.*

Pharmacopoeial description
Ph. Eur.: The essential oil obtained by steam distillation from the fresh, flowering aerial parts, recently gathered from *Mentha canadensis* (=*M. arvensis* var. *glabrata*; *M. arvensis* var. *piperascens*) followed by partial separation of menthol by crystallisation. A colourless or pale yellow to greenish-yellow liquid with a characteristic odour. Store in well-filled airtight containers at a temperature not exceeding 25°. Protect from light.

Profile
Dementholised mint oil is used as a flavour. *Mentha arvensis* is used in herbal medicine as a febrifuge and for rheumatic disorders. Peppermint oil (p.1243) and spearmint oil (p.1666) are used as carminatives and flavours.

Preparations
Proprietary Preparations (details are given in Part 3)
Aust.: Physiomint; *Ger.:* Japanol; JHP Rodler Tropfen; Kneipp Minzol Trost Tropfen.

Multi-ingredient: *Aust.:* Parodontax†; *Austral.:* Tiger Balm White†; *Belg.:* Calmant Martou†; *Ger.:* Dreierlei; Parodontal F5 med; Trachiform; *Ital.:* Broncosedina; *Switz.:* Acidodermil†; Huile analgesique "Polar-Bar"; Kernosan Huile de Massage†; Lapidar 10 plus†; Malveol; Neo-Angin au miel et citron; Neo-Angin exempt de sucre; Onguent nasal Ruedi; Osa Gel de dentition aux plantes†; Pastilles pectorales Demo N; Pommade nasale Ruedi†; Roliwol†; Tonex; Tyrothricin; *UK:* Olbas.

Miracle Fruit (12965-q)
The fruit of *Synsepalum dulcificum* (=*Richardella dulcifica*) (Sapotaceae).

Profile
Miracle fruit contains a glycoprotein 'miraculin' with no apparent taste of its own but which is able to make sour substances taste sweet and to improve the flavour of foods. Its activity is reduced by heating.

Mistletoe (885-r)
European Mistletoe; Gui; Mistelkraut; Tallo de Muérdago; Visci Caulis; Viscum; Viscum Album.
Pharmacopoeias. In *Ger.*

The dried, evergreen, dioecious semi-parasite, *Viscum album* (Loranthaceae), which grows on the branches of deciduous trees, chiefly apple, poplar, and plum. It occurs as a mixture of broken stems and leaves and occasional fruits.

Profile
Mistletoe has a vasodilator action and has been used in herbal preparations for hypertension and cardiovascular disorders although its activity when taken orally is questionable. It has also been used in nervous disorders and in homoeopathic medicine. Mistletoe contains lectins with cytotoxic and immunomodulatory actions *in vitro* and preparations have been given by injection in a number of neoplastic diseases. Ingestion of the berries and other parts has been reported to cause nausea, vomiting, diarrhoea, and bradycardia.

◊ A review of mistletoe.[1] There are about 1300 species of mistletoe representing 36 genera of the Loranthaceae, and what is called the "common mistletoe" varies from country to country: in Europe the term describes *Viscum album* while in the USA it describes *Phoradendron flavescens*. The toxicity of aqueous extracts of mistletoe has been found to depend upon the nature of the host plant. Three classes of cytotoxic compounds are present in the leaves and stems of *V. album* although the berries are generally considered to be the most toxic part of the plant. These are alkaloids, viscotoxins, and lectins. The viscotoxins have been shown to cause hypotension, bradycardia, arterial vasoconstriction, and a negative inotropic effect, and may act as acetylcholine agonists. The lectins show toxic effects in *animals* similar to those seen with ricin.
1. Anderson LA, Phillipson JD. Mistletoe—the magic herb. *Pharm J* 1982; **229:** 437–9.

◊ Reports of hepatitis following the ingestion of herbal remedies containing mistletoe.[1,2]
1. Harvey J, Colin-Jones DG. Mistletoe hepatitis. *BMJ* 1981; **282:** 186–7.
2. Weeks GR, Proper JS. Herbal medicines—gaps in our knowledge. *Aust J Hosp Pharm* 1989; **19:** 155–7.

Preparations
Proprietary Preparations (details are given in Part 3)
Aust.: Apotheker Bauer's Misteltinktur; Eurixor; Helixor; Iscador; Isorel; Isugran; *Ger.:* Abnobaviscum; Cefalektin; Eurixor; Helixor; Iscador; Kneipp Mistel-Pflanzensaft; Kneipp Pflanzen-Dragees Mistel; Lektinol; Mistel Curarina; Mistel-Krautertabletten; Mistelol-Kapseln; Misteltropfen 11; Misteltropfen Hofmanns; Plenosol N†; Salus Mistel-Tropfen; Viscysat; Vysorel.

Multi-ingredient: *Aust.:* Heli-Sal; Herz- und Kreislauftonikum Bioflora; Krautertee Nr 20; Krautertee Nr 22; Mag Kottas Nerven-Beruhigungstee; Rutiviscal; Vivinox; Wechseltee; *Austral.:* Calmo; Pacifenity; Vitaglow Herbal Stress†; *Belg.:* Tisane Contre la

Tension; *Fr.:* Mediflor Tisane Circulation du Sang No 12†; Santane H₇; Tisanes de l'Abbe Hamon no 6; *Ger.:* Antihypertonicum S; Antisklerosin S; Asgoviscum N; Heusin; Hypercard; Ilja Rogoff; Kneipp Drei-Pflanzen-Dragees N; Presselin Arterien K 5 P; Salusan†; Syviman N; Vasesana-Vasoregulans; Viscophyll.

Monoctanoin (12794-b)
Monoctanoin (*BAN, USAN*).
Monooctanoin; Mono-octanoin.
CAS — 26402-26-6 (glyceryl mono-octanoate).

A semisynthetic mixture of glycerol esters, containing 80 to 85% of glyceryl mono-octanoate ($C_{11}H_{22}O_4 = 218.3$), 10 to 15% of glyceryl mono-decanoate ($C_{13}H_{26}O_4 = 246.3$) and glyceryl di-octanoate ($C_{19}H_{36}O_5 = 344.5$), and a maximum of 2.5% of free glycerol ($C_3H_8O_3 = 92.09$).

Adverse Effects and Precautions
Abdominal pain, nausea, vomiting, and diarrhoea may occur particularly if monoctanoin is infused rapidly or in large doses; it has been recommended that perfusion pressure should not exceed 20 cm of water. Minor irritation of the gastric and duodenal mucosa has been reported. Acidosis may occur, particularly in patients with impaired hepatic function, and leucopenia has been reported. Monoctanoin should not be administered to patients with hepatic impairment, biliary tract infection, cholestatic jaundice, jejunitis, duodenal ulcer, or pancreatitis. It should not be given by the intravenous or intramuscular routes.

◊ Side-effects[1] occurred in 67% of 343 patients treated with monoctanoin perfusion, with multiple side-effects in 41%. Abdominal pain was the most common adverse effect occurring in 40% of patients. Nausea, vomiting, and diarrhoea were usually dose related, occurring in 25%, 15%, and 16% of patients respectively. Fever, attributed to cholangitis, was noted in 5%. Severe side-effects occurred in 12 patients; a patient with cirrhosis developed acidosis and encephalopathic signs.
1. Palmer KR, Hofmann AF. Intraductal mono-octanoin for the direct dissolution of bile duct stones: experience in 343 patients. *Gut* 1986; **27:** 196–202.

Uses and Administration
Monoctanoin is used to dissolve cholesterol gallstones (p.1678) retained following cholecystectomy. It is administered by continuous perfusion through a catheter inserted directly into the common bile duct at a rate of 3 to 5 mL per hour at a pressure of 10 cm of water. Perfusion may be suspended during meals. The solution should be warmed prior to perfusion, and the temperature should be maintained at 37° during administration. Treatment is continued for 2 to 10 days. If no reduction in the size of the stones is detectable after 7 to 10 days of treatment, further treatment is unlikely to be effective.

◊ References.
1. Palmer KR, Hofmann AF. Intraductal mono-octanoin for the direct dissolution of bile duct stones: experience in 343 patients. *Gut* 1986; **27:** 196–202.
2. Stock SE, *et al.* Treatment of common bile duct stones using mono-octanoin. *Br J Surg* 1992; **79:** 653–4.

Preparations
Proprietary Preparations (details are given in Part 3)
USA: Moctanin.

Monoethanolamine Oleate (207-g)
Monoethanolamine Oleate (*rINN*).
Aethanolaminum; Ethanolamine Oleate (*USAN*). 2-Hydroxyethylamine compound with oleic acid; 2-Aminoethanol compound with oleic acid.
$C_2H_7NO,C_{18}H_{34}O_2 = 343.5$.
CAS — 141-43-5 (monoethanolamine); 2272-11-9 (monoethanolamine oleate).
ATC — C05BB01.
Pharmacopoeias. *Aust.*, *Br.*, and *USNF* include monographs for monoethanolamine.

Pharmacopoeial description
BP 2001: Ethanolamine is a clear, colourless, or pale yellow liquid with a slight odour. It is alkaline to litmus. Miscible with water and with alcohol; slightly soluble in ether.

USNF 20: Monoethanolamine is a clear, colourless, moderately viscous liquid having a distinctly ammoniacal odour. Miscible with water, with alcohol, with acetone, with chloroform, and with glycerol; immiscible with ether, with petroleum spirit, and with fixed oils, although it dissolves many essential oils. Store in airtight containers. Protect from light.

Adverse Effects and Precautions
Monoethanolamine oleate is irritant to skin and mucous membranes. Local injection may cause sloughing, ulceration, and, in severe cases, necrosis. Pain may occur at the site of injection. Patients receiving treatment for oesophageal varices may develop pleural effusion or infiltration. Hypersensitivity reactions have been reported.

When used to treat varicose veins of the legs, monoethanolamine oleate and other sclerotherapeutic agents should not be used in patients with thrombosis and a tendency to thrombosis, or with acute phlebitis, marked arterial, cardiac, or renal disease, local or systemic infections, or uncontrolled metabolic disorders such as diabetes mellitus.

Effects on the kidneys. Acute renal failure, which cleared spontaneously within 3 weeks, occurred in 2 obese women given sclerosing injections of 15 to 20 mL of a solution containing monoethanolamine oleate 5% and benzyl alcohol 2%.[1]

1. Maling TJB, Cretney MJ. Ethanolamine oleate and acute renal failure. *N Z Med J* 1975; **82:** 269–70.

Uses and Administration
Monoethanolamine oleate is used as a sclerosant in the treatment of varicose veins and oesophageal varices. For sclerotherapy of varicose veins, 2 to 5 mL of a 5% solution of monoethanolamine oleate is injected slowly into empty isolated sections of vein, divided between 3 or 4 sites. Injection into full veins is also possible. For sclerotherapy of oesophageal varices, the dose is 1.5 to 5 mL of a 5% solution per varix to a maximum total dose of 20 mL per treatment session. Treatment may be given in the initial management of bleeding varices, then repeated at intervals until the varices are occluded.

Variceal haemorrhage. Portal hypertension may occur in many conditions that affect the liver, and leads to the development of collateral channels linking the portal and systemic circulations. Enlargement of such blood vessels beneath the oesophageal and gastric mucosa produces varices which have about a 30% risk of rupture and bleeding. Oesophageal varices are more often a cause of haemorrhage than gastric varices. Capillaries and veins in the gastric mucosa may also become swollen, a condition known as portal hypertensive gastropathy, and clinically important bleeding may occur in severe cases.

Variceal haemorrhage is usually severe, with mortality as high as 50% for the initial episode, and the recurrence rate as high as 100% within two years. Bleeding stops spontaneously in many patients, but in those who continue to bleed, control of haemorrhage is difficult and patients should be referred to a centre with appropriate specialist facilities. Treatment to stabilise the patient may be necessary before they can be safely transferred.

Acute management. Initial treatment is supportive and requires measures to prevent aspiration and maintain a clear airway, and volume replacement with colloid and blood. Emergency endoscopy should be performed to establish the site of haemorrhage and exclude non-variceal sources of bleeding. The choice of treatment depends on the site of haemorrhage.[1-7] *Endoscopic methods* are favoured for initial management with injection sclerotherapy or banding ligation being used in bleeding oesophageal varices. The optimum management of bleeding gastric varices remains to be defined. Injection sclerotherapy is a suitable method for controlling bleeding from varices on the lesser curve of the stomach or within a hiatus hernia, but is not as effective in haemorrhaging fundal gastric varices. Intravariceal injection of bovine or human thrombin, or cyanoacrylate tissue adhesives, has been used in gastric varices. Where the source of haemorrhage is non-variceal and due to gastropathy, portal decompressive surgery is effective, although it is associated with a high incidence of encephalopathy in cirrhotic patients. Small studies have shown propranolol to be effective in arresting haemorrhage.[8]

Injection sclerotherapy for variceal haemorrhage may be performed during the emergency endoscopy procedure. Intravariceal injection, paravariceal injection, or a combination of the two have been used. The most widely used sclerosants are monoethanolamine oleate and sodium tetradecyl sulfate for intravariceal injection and lauromacrogol 400 for paravariceal injection. Sclerotherapy controls bleeding in up to 95% of cases. Ulceration and stricture formation occur frequently following injection sclerotherapy.

An alternative technique is *endoscopic banding ligation*, where elastic bands are placed around the varices. The tissue subsequently necroses to leave a superficial ulcer. This technique has a similar efficacy to injection sclerotherapy, but may be more difficult to perform if active bleeding is occurring. Procedures may be repeated if bleeding continues or restarts.

Where endoscopy is unavailable, drug therapy or balloon tamponade may be used until the patient can be transferred to a specialist centre. These techniques may also have a role when sclerotherapy fails. *Drug therapy* is aimed at controlling portal venous pressure, although it is ineffective in massive haemorrhage and its effects cease once the drug is stopped. Drugs that are used include vasopressin and its analogue terlipressin and, more recently, somatostatin and its analogue octreotide. Vasopressin controls haemorrhage in about 50% of patients. It is given by continuous intravenous infusion, together with glyceryl trinitrate, which counteracts the adverse cardiac effects of vasopressin, while potentiating its reduction of portal pressure. Terlipressin has the advantage of a longer therapeutic action, enabling bolus doses to be given. A comparison of terlipressin and sclerotherapy found them to be equally effective for the control of acute variceal bleeding.[9] However, somatostatin, and particularly octreotide, which may be given by bolus injection, are now generally preferred as they have similar efficacy to vasopressin but fewer side-effects.[2] Octreotide is as effective as injection sclerotherapy in the control of acute variceal bleeding.[10] Octreotide[11] or somatostatin[12] may also have a role as adjuncts to sclerotherapy or ligation, but no mortality benefit has yet been shown.

Balloon tamponade controls bleeding by direct pressure on the varices. Although it is a very effective means of controlling haemorrhage, there is a high incidence of rebleeding once pressure is removed and the incidence of complications is high. It is useful in cases of massive haemorrhage when drug therapy is ineffective and sclerotherapy is difficult.

Surgery, such as the formation of a shunt or oesophageal transection, may be necessary if the above measures fail to control the bleeding. However, such techniques have been associated with high mortality in some series. Formation of a transjugular intrahepatic portal-systemic shunt is now generally preferred.[4] It may be particularly useful in candidates for liver transplantation.

Short-term *antibacterial prophylaxis* has been proposed[13] for cirrhotic patients with gastrointestinal bleeding, including variceal bleeding, because reduced rates of infection and improved short-term survival have been reported in a few studies.

Long-term management. Once the acute bleeding has been controlled measures are needed to prevent rebleeding. Endoscopic therapy is widely used, with injection sclerotherapy or banding ligation being repeated until the varices are obliterated. Banding ligation is now the treatment of choice; it eradicates varices in fewer treatment sessions than injection sclerotherapy and reduces the risk of ulceration and stricture formation.[14] Sucralfate has been given following sclerotherapy as it may reduce the frequency of stricture formation and reduce bleeding from treatment-related ulcers. It seems to have no influence on ulcer healing following banding ligation.[15] Some practitioners carry out regular endoscopic checks and repeat sclerotherapy or banding ligation when varices reappear, although this approach is no more effective in terms of improving survival than giving treatment once bleeding occurs. Drug therapy is an alternative to endoscopic methods. Beta blockers (mainly propranolol) reduce the incidence of recurrent variceal bleeding and may improve survival.[16] A combination of nadolol with isosorbide mononitrate has been reported to reduce the risk of rebleeding more than repeated sclerotherapy, although there was no significant effect on mortality.[17] Drug therapy has also been used as an adjunct to endoscopic methods to control rebleeding in the period before variceal obliteration has occurred, or for long-term management following endoscopic therapy. Long-term octreotide therapy following sclerotherapy has also been investigated and may reduce recurrent variceal bleeding.[18] Several studies[19-21] have compared transjugular intrahepatic portosystemic shunting with endoscopic treatment, but no clear benefit has been demonstrated and there may be an increased risk of encephalopathy with the use of shunts. Surgery, including liver transplantation, should be considered in patients with recurrent life-threatening haemorrhage. Propranolol may also have a role in patients with portal hypertensive gastropathy. In a controlled study, propranolol reduced the incidence of recurrent bleeding from portal hypertensive gastropathy in patients with cirrhosis.[22]

Prophylaxis of a first bleed in patients with portal hypertension is controversial since about 70% of patients who have varices will never bleed, but should probably be given to patients with cirrhosis and varices thought to be at high risk of bleeding. A reliable system that will identify those at high risk of haemorrhage has yet to be devised. The NIEC (North Italian Endoscopic Club) system is probably the best so far.[23] Sclerotherapy had been considered as a method of prophylaxis, but its value has not been clearly established. Studies show that beta blockers decrease the incidence of a first bleed[24] and are probably the treatment of choice if prophylaxis is to be given. Banding ligation may be a suitable alternative for patients who are unable to take beta blockers.[25]

It is postulated that a reduction in portal pressure to below 12 mmHg is necessary to reduce the incidence of variceal bleeding and that treatment with beta blockers alone does not achieve this. More effective drugs are being sought, and isosorbide mononitrate[26,27] (as adjunctive therapy with a beta blocker) and clonidine[28] are under investigation for the prophylaxis of a first bleed and prevention of recurrent haemorrhage in patients with portal hypertension.

1. Williams SGJ, Westaby D. Management of variceal haemorrhage. *BMJ* 1994; **308:** 1213–17.
2. Roberts LR, Kamath PS. Pathophysiology and treatment of variceal haemorrhage. *Mayo Clin Proc* 1996; **71:** 973–83.
3. Sung JJY. Non-surgical treatment of variceal haemorrhage. *Br J Hosp Med* 1997; **57:** 162–6.
4. Stanely AJ, Haynes PC. Portal hypertension and variceal haemorrhage. *Lancet* 1997; **350:** 1235–9.
5. McCormack G, McCormick PA. A practical guide to the management of oesophageal varices. *Drugs* 1999; **57:** 327–35.
6. Dagher L, *et al.* Management of oesophageal varices. *Hosp Med* 2000; **61:** 711–17.
7. Anonymous. Early management of bleeding oesophageal varices. *Drug Ther Bull* 2000; **38:** 37–40.
8. Anonymous. Portal hypertensive gastropathy. *Lancet* 1991; **338:** 1045–6.
9. Escorsell À, *et al.* Multicenter randomized controlled trial of terlipressin versus sclerotherapy in the treatment of acute variceal bleeding: the TEST study. *Hepatology* 2000; **32:** 471–6.
10. Jenkins SA, *et al.* A multicentre randomised trial comparing octreotide and injection sclerotherapy in the management and outcome of acute variceal haemorrhage. *Gut* 1997; **41:** 526–33.
11. Sung JJY, *et al.* Prospective randomised study of effect of octreotide on rebleeding from oesophageal varices after endoscopic ligation. *Lancet* 1995; **346:** 1666–9.

12. Avgerinos A, *et al.* Early administration of somatostatin and efficacy of sclerotherapy in acute oesophageal variceal bleeds: the European Acute Bleeding Oesophageal Variceal Episodes (ABOVE) randomised trial. *Lancet* 1997; **350:** 1495–9.
13. Bernard B, *et al.* Antibiotic prophylaxis for the prevention of bacterial infections in cirrhotic patients with gastrointestinal bleeding: a meta-analysis. *Hepatology* 1999; **29:** 1655–61.
14. Laine L, Cook D. Endoscopic ligation compared with sclerotherapy for treatment of esophageal variceal bleeding: a meta-analysis. *Ann Intern Med* 1995; **123:** 280–7.
15. Nijhawan S, Rai RR. Does post-ligation oesophageal ulcer healing require treatment? *Lancet* 1994; **343:** 116–17.
16. Bernard B, *et al.* Beta-adrenergic antagonists in the prevention of gastrointestinal rebleeding in patients with cirrhosis: a meta-analysis. *Hepatology* 1997; **25:** 63–70.
17. Villanueva C, *et al.* Nadolol plus isosorbide mononitrate compared with sclerotherapy for the prevention of variceal rebleeding. *N Engl J Med* 1996; **334:** 1624–9.
18. Jenkins SA, *et al.* Randomised trial of octreotide for long term management of cirrhosis after variceal haemorrhage. *BMJ* 1997; **315:** 1338–41.
19. Sanyal AJ, *et al.* Transjugular intrahepatic portosystemic shunts compared with endoscopic sclerotherapy for the prevention of recurrent variceal hemorrhage: a randomized, controlled trial. *Ann Intern Med* 1997; **126:** 849–57.
20. Cello JP, *et al.* Endoscopic sclerotherapy compared with percutaneous transjugular intrahepatic portosystemic shunt after initial sclerotherapy in patients with acute variceal hemorrhage: a randomized, controlled trial. *Ann Intern Med* 1997; **126:** 858–65.
21. Rössle M, *et al.* Randomised trial of transjugular-intrahepatic-portosystemic shunt versus endoscopy plus propranolol for prevention of variceal rebleeding. *Lancet* 1997; **349:** 1043–9.
22. Pérez-Ayuso RM, *et al.* Propranolol in prevention of recurrent bleeding from severe portal hypertensive gastropathy in cirrhosis. *Lancet* 1991; **337:** 1431–4.
23. The North Italian Endoscopic Club for the Study and Treatment of Esophageal Varices. Prediction of the first variceal hemorrhage in patients with cirrhosis of the liver and esophageal varices: a prospective multicenter study. *N Engl J Med* 1988; **319:** 983–9.
24. Pagliaro L, *et al.* Prevention of first bleeding in cirrhosis: a meta-analysis of randomised trials of nonsurgical treatment. *Ann Intern Med* 1992; **117:** 59–70.
25. Burroughs AK, Patch D. Primary prevention of bleeding from esophageal varices. *N Engl J Med* 1999; **340:** 1033–5.
26. Angelico M, *et al.* Isosorbide-5-mononitrate versus propranolol in the prevention of first bleeding in cirrhosis. *Gastroenterology* 1993; **104:** 1460–5.
27. Merkel C, *et al.* Randomised trial of nadolol alone or with isosorbide mononitrate for primary prophylaxis of variceal bleeding in cirrhosis. *Lancet* 1996; **348:** 1677–81.
28. Blendis LM. Clonidine for portal hypertension: a sympathetic solution? *Ann Intern Med* 1992; **116:** 515–17.

Varicose veins. Varicose veins are tortuous, protruding veins in the legs, that occur when weak vein walls and valve incompetence result in venous reflux and dilatation. Symptoms associated with varicose veins include heaviness, tension, aching, and itching of the legs. Complications include oedema, thrombophlebitis, deep venous thrombosis, lipodermatosclerosis, and venous ulceration. Risk factors for varicose veins include increasing age, pregnancy, and occupations that involve prolonged standing.

Conservative management using compression hosiery may be effective for relief of symptoms in some patients. Surgery or sclerotherapy are other treatment options, depending on the veins affected. In sclerotherapy, a sclerosant is injected into the affected vein where it irritates and damages the lining of the vein causing local thrombosis, fibrosis, and stenosis. Graduated compression dressings are usually applied after sclerotherapy to minimise the time taken for the surrounding tissue to absorb the damaged segment of vein. Compression may also help to reduce complications of sclerotherapy including hyperpigmentation, oedema, aching, thrombophlebitis, and deep venous thrombosis. Various agents have been used as sclerosants: detergent sclerosants include monoethanolamine oleate, sodium tetradecyl sulfate, lauromacrogol 400, and sodium morrhuate; osmotic sclerosants include hypertonic sodium chloride solutions, and hypertonic mixtures of sodium chloride and glucose; caustic sclerosants include chromated glycerol, and a mixture of iodine and sodium iodide.

References.

1. Drake LA, *et al.* Guidelines of care for sclerotherapy treatment of varicose veins and telangiectatic leg veins. *J Am Acad Dermatol* 1996; **34:** 523–8.
2. Green D. Sclerotherapy for the permanent eradication of varicose veins: theoretical and practical considerations. *J Am Acad Dermatol* 1998; **38:** 461–75.
3. London NJ, Nash R. ABC of arterial and venous disease: varicose veins. *BMJ* 2000; **320:** 1391–4.

Preparations

BP 2001: Ethanolamine Oleate Injection.

Proprietary Preparations (details are given in Part 3)

Austral.: Ethamolin†; *Braz.:* Ethamolin; *Canad.:* Ethamolin†; *Jpn:* Oldamin; *USA:* Ethamolin.

Motherwort (11430-j)

Herba Leonuri Cardiacae; Leonurus; Motherwort Herb.

Pharmacopoeias. In Ger.

Profile
Motherwort is the dried aerial parts of *Leonurus cardiaca* (Labiatae). It is given in herbal medicine for nervous and cardiac disorders; it is also used in products promoted for mild hyperthyroidism.

Preparations

Proprietary Preparations (details are given in Part 3)
Ger.: Thyreogutt mono.

Multi-ingredient: *Aust.:* Thyreogutt; *Austral.:* Pacifenity; Valerian; *Canad.:* Thunas Tab for Menstrual Pain; *Fr.:* Biocarde; *Ger.:* Biovital N; Biovital Weissdorn Tonikum; Kneipp Herz- und Kreislauf-Tee; Mutellon; Oxacant N; Oxacant-sedativ; *Switz.:* Tisane pour le coeur et la circulation; *UK:* Daily Menopause Relief; Gerard House Motherwort Compound; Modern Herbals Stress; Period Pain Relief; Prementaid; Quiet Life; SuNerven; Wellwoman.

Moxaverine Hydrochloride (5237-g)

Moxaverine Hydrochloride (BANM, rINNM).

Meteverine Hydrochloride. 1-Benzyl-3-ethyl-6,7-dimethoxyisoquinoline hydrochloride.
$C_{20}H_{21}NO_2,HCl = 343.8$.
CAS — 10539-19-2 (moxaverine); 1163-37-7 (moxaverine hydrochloride).

Profile
Moxaverine hydrochloride has a similar structure to papaverine (p.1648) and has been given by mouth and injection as an antispasmodic and in vascular disorders. The base is also used as an antispasmodic.

Doses of moxaverine hydrochloride of up to 300 mg three times daily by mouth have been suggested for the treatment of vasospastic disorders, although much lower doses are recommended for the treatment of gastrointestinal and biliary-tract spasm.

Preparations

Proprietary Preparations (details are given in Part 3)
Ger.: Certonal; Kollateral.

Multi-ingredient: *Aust.:* Hedonin; *Ger.:* Kollateral A + E.

Mumps Skin Test Antigen (7980-q)

Pharmacopoeias. In US.

Pharmacopoeial description
USP 25: A sterile suspension of formalin-inactivated mumps virus prepared from the extra-embryonic fluid of virus-infected chick embryos, concentrated and purified by differential centrifugation, and diluted with isotonic sodium chloride solution. It contains a preservative and glycine as a stabilising agent. Each mL contains not less than 20 complement-fixing units. It should be stored at 2° to 8°. The expiry date is not later than 18 months after date of manufacture or of release from manufacturer's cold storage.

Profile
Recovery from mumps produces skin hypersensitivity to mumps virus. Mumps skin test antigen, 0.1 mL intradermally (intracutaneously), is used in conjunction with other antigens to assess the status of cell-mediated immunity. A positive reaction may indicate previous infection with mumps virus but it is not considered to be very reliable. It should not be given to patients hypersensitive to egg protein.

◊ For reference to the use of mumps skin test antigen for anergy testing in HIV-positive patients, see Tuberculins, p.1676.

Preparations

USP 25: Mumps Skin Test Antigen.

Proprietary Preparations (details are given in Part 3)
USA: MSTA.

Muramidase Hydrochloride (11469-g)

N-Acetylmuramide Glycanohydrolase Hydrochloride; E1105 (muramidase); Globulin G₁ Hydrochloride; Lysozyme Hydrochloride.

Profile
Muramidase is a mucopolysaccharidase which is active against Gram-positive bacteria, possibly by transforming the insoluble polysaccharides of the cell wall to soluble mucopeptides. It is also thought to be active against some viruses and some Gram-negative bacteria.

Muramidase has been given, usually as the hydrochloride, to patients with herpes zoster and other painful viral infections, and for mouth and respiratory-tract disorders. It has been used in combination with antibacterials in an attempt to enhance their activity. Sensitivity reactions have been reported.

◊ A report[1] of a toxic epidermal necrolysis-type drug eruption in a patient who took an oral cold preparation containing muramidase chloride, which was considered to be the probable cause. The patient's condition improved following intravenous corticosteroid therapy.

1. Kobayashi M, *et al.* A case of toxic epidermal necrolysis-type drug eruption induced by oral lysozyme chloride. *J Dermatol* 2000; **27:** 401–4.

Preparations

Proprietary Preparations (details are given in Part 3)
Belg.: Murazyme; *Braz.:* Murazyme; *Hong Kong:* Flemizyme; Jemizym; Neuzym; *Ital.:* Immunozima†; *Jpn:* Leftose; Neuzym; *Singapore:* Leftose; Lyzyme; Neuzyme; *Thai.:* Leftose.

Multi-ingredient: *Aust.:* Sanoral; Tongill; *Braz.:* Cifrantil; Colpistar; Eritrosima; Floregin; Floregin Composto; Lisofenicol; Lisoquinol; Munolan; Narizima Adulto; Narizima Pediatrico; Trinotrex; Trisdazol; Vagi Biotic; Velutrix; *Fr.:* Cantalene; Glossithiase; Hexalyse; Lyso-6; Lysocalm; Lysopaine; Oroseptol Lysozyme; *Ger.:* Frubienzym; *Hong Kong:* Haemosol; Hexalyse; Quadezyme; *Ital.:* Narlisim; *Port.:* Narizima; *Singapore:* Biotene; *Spain:* Anticatarral; Egarone; Espectral; Espectral Balsamico; Inexfal; Lizipaina; Lysokana†; Normo Nar; Pulmotropic; Rino Dexa; Trofalgon; *Switz.:* Arbid-top; Lyso-6; Lysopaine; Sangerol; *Thai.:* Siduol.

Poisonous Mushrooms or Toadstools

(12350-f)

CAS — 23109-05-9 (α-amanitin); 21150-22-1 (β-amanitin); 21150-23-2 (γ-amanitin); 58919-61-2 (coprine); 16568-02-8 (gyromitrin); 2552-55-8 (ibotenic acid); 60-34-4 (methylhydrazine); 300-54-9 (muscarine); 2763-96-4 (muscimol); 37338-80-0 (orellanine); 17466-45-4 (phalloidin); 28227-92-1 (phallon); 39412-56-1 (phallolysin).

This monograph describes poisonous mushrooms often known as toadstools, their toxins, toxic effects, and the treatment of those effects. Their only use is in homoeopathic medicine which employs *Amanita muscaria* as Agaricus muscarius. *A. muscaria* and *Psilocybe* spp. are abused for their psychoactive properties (see also Psilocin, p.1655).

Mushrooms can be classified into 8 groups according to their principal toxins and toxic effects:

- *Group I.* Most deaths due to mushroom poisoning follow the ingestion of mushrooms containing cyclopeptides and among these mushrooms *Amanita phalloides* ('death cap') has been reported to be responsible for 90% of all mushroom fatalities. The cyclopeptides are a group of heat-stable cyclic polypeptides with molecular weights ranging from 800 to 1100 and include the amatoxins (α-, β-, γ-amanitin) and phallotoxins (phalloidin, phaloin, phallolysin). Other mushrooms containing cyclopeptides include *A. verna* ('deadly agaric', fool's mushroom'), *A. virosa*, ('destroying angel') and *A. bisporigera* ('white destroying angel'), and *Galerina autumnalis*, *G. marginata*, and *G. venenata*.
- *Group II.* Although *A. muscaria* ('fly agaric') and *A. pantherina* ('panther cap', 'false blusher') may contain small amounts of muscarine, the antimuscarinic effects of the hallucinogenic agent muscimol and the insecticidal agent ibotenic acid usually predominate.
- *Group III.* Many species of *Gyromitra* contain toxins known as gyromitrins that decompose to release methylhydrazine (monomethylhydrazine; MMH) an inhibitor of the coenzyme pyridoxal phosphate.
- *Group IV.* Mushrooms whose principal toxin is muscarine include many of the *Clitocybe* and *Inocybe* spp. *A. muscaria* and *A. pantherina* (see above) may also contain small amounts.
- *Group V.* *Coprinus atramentarius* ('ink cap') contains the compound coprine, one of whose metabolites is an inhibitor of acetaldehyde dehydrogenase and it may therefore produce 'disulfiram-like' symptoms after drinking alcohol.
- *Group VI.* Mushrooms which may contain the hallucinogenic indoles psilocin and psilocybine include species of *Psilocybe*, *Panaeolus*, *Gymnopilus*, *Stropharia*, and *Conocybe*.
- *Group VII.* Many mushrooms which only act as gastrointestinal irritants and do not produce systemic effects are included in this group.
- *Group VIII.* A further group has sometimes been used to classify some species of *Cortinarius* that contain a renal toxin thought by some to be orellanine, but whose exact nature remains to be determined.

Adverse Effects
The clinical course of poisoning due to mushrooms is related to their principal toxins:

- *Group I.* The manifestations of poisoning with mushrooms containing cyclopeptides may be divided into three phases. Initial symptoms may occur 4 to 24 hours after ingestion and usually consist of gastrointestinal effects such as abdominal pain, nausea, severe vomiting, and profuse diarrhoea similar to that in cholera. The patient may then appear to recover and be symptom-free for 2 to 3 days, but liver-enzyme values may be increasing. Following this phase, the more serious toxic effects of the amatoxins become apparent and there are signs of liver, renal, cardiac, and CNS toxicity. Symptoms include jaundice, oliguria, anuria, hypoglycaemia, coagulopathies, circulatory collapse, convulsions, and coma. The mortality rate is high in this phase with death usually being due to liver failure following hepatic necrosis. Up to 90% of untreated patients may die, though the rate may be as low as 15 to 30% following treatment.
- *Group II.* The adverse effects of mushrooms containing ibotenic acid and muscimol usually occur within 2 hours of ingestion. Symptoms may include ataxia, euphoria, delirium, and hallucinations associated with other antimuscarinic effects. Fatalities are rare.
- *Group III.* Patients who have ingested mushrooms containing gyromitrins usually develop symptoms of poisoning within 6 to 24 hours. These consist initially of nausea, vomiting, abdominal pain, and muscle cramps, headache, dizziness and fatigue. Delirium, convulsions, coma, methaemoglobinaemia and haemolysis may also occur. Occasionally jaundice and hepatic necrosis may lead to hepatic failure and death. Up to 40% of patients may die.
- *Group IV.* Symptoms typical of 'cholinergic crisis' (see Neostigmine Metilsulfate, p.1420) may appear about 30 minutes to 2 hours after ingestion of mushrooms containing muscarine. These may include bradycardia, bronchospasm, salivation, perspiration, lachrymation, rhinorrhoea, involuntary urination and defaecation, and diarrhoea. Miosis, hypotension, and cardiac arrhythmias may also occur. Rarely death may follow due to cardiac arrest or respiratory-tract obstruction.
- *Group V.* Since one of the metabolites of coprine is an acetaldehyde dehydrogenase inhibitor, drinking alcohol, even up to several days after ingestion of mushrooms containing this compound, will produce symptoms similar to those of the 'disulfiram-alcohol' interaction (see Disulfiram, Adverse Effects, p.1605). Fatalities are rare.
- *Group VI.* The adverse effects of ingestion of mushrooms containing psilocin and psilocybine are similar to those described under Lysergide (p.1630). Symptoms usually occur within about 30 minutes to 2 hours. Fatalities are rare.
- *Group VII.* Generally no treatment is required for adverse gastrointestinal effects seen with this group of mushrooms.
- *Group VIII.* There may be a delay of as long as 14 to 20 days before symptoms of poisoning due to *Cortinarius* appear. Patients will develop an intense thirst. Other symptoms usually include nausea, vomiting, diarrhoea, and anorexia. Muscle aching and spasms and a feeling of coldness may also occur. In severe cases renal failure may lead to death. It has been reported that up to 15% of patients may die.

Pregnancy. α-Amanitine does not appear to cross the placental barrier, even during the acute phase of intoxication.[1]

1. Belliardo F, *et al.* Amatoxins do not cross the placental barrier. *Lancet* 1983; **i:** 1381.

Treatment of Adverse Effects
As there are no specific antidotes for the majority of cases of mushroom poisoning and which species is involved is often unknown, treatment consists primarily of symptomatic and supportive measures. The stomach may be emptied by gastric lavage if the patient has not already vomited spontaneously. However, if presentation is delayed because of the slow onset of symptoms seen with some types of mushrooms measures to empty the stomach are unlikely to be productive. An exception is poisoning with group I mushrooms when gastric lavage may be of benefit for up to 12 hours post-ingestion. Activated charcoal may be of use in binding toxins in the gastrointestinal tract and preventing absorption. Determining the interval between ingestion and the onset of symptoms often helps to identify the type of mushrooms ingested. If possible specimens of the mushrooms or a sample of the stomach contents should be sent to an expert mycologist for identification. Particular attention should be paid to intravenous replacement of fluids and electrolytes especially if vomiting and diarrhoea are severe. If the ingestion of hepatotoxic or nephrotoxic mushrooms is suspected liver and renal function should be monitored.

Since some mushrooms contain a wide range of toxins and patients may have ingested more than one species, specific therapy should only be instituted following positive identification.

- *Group I.* There is little clinical evidence to support the efficacy of specific agents or treatments used in the management of cyclopeptide poisoning. A variety of agents including benzylpenicillin and silymarin or silybin (silibinin) have been administered to try to protect the liver against the hepatotoxic effects of the amatoxins. Exchange transfusions, haemodialysis, or charcoal haemoperfusion have been tried to facilitate amatoxin removal. The removal of bile via a duodenal tube left *in situ* has been suggested to reduce enterohepatic circulation of amatoxins. Forced diuresis has also been advocated by some for amatoxin poisoning. Liver transplantation may be required in patients with progressive liver failure. A radio-immunoassay for the detection of amatoxins is available in some countries to confirm a diagnosis of cyclopeptide poisoning.
- *Group II.* Specific treatment is usually only required if symptoms are severe. Physostigmine should only be used if definite antimuscarinic symptoms are present. As mushrooms containing ibotenic acid and muscimol may also contain small amounts of muscarine, atropine may be required to control muscarinic symptoms.
- *Group III.* Pyridoxine hydrochloride 25 mg per kg bodyweight given as an intravenous infusion and repeated as required has been recommended as specific therapy to overcome the inhibition of pyridoxal phosphate by methylhydrazine. However, concern has been expressed that the use of such large doses of pyridoxine can itself produce adverse neurological effects. Methylene blue [methylthioninium chloride] may be required if methaemoglobinaemia is severe.

- *Group IV.* Atropine sulfate may be required to control the symptoms of muscarine poisoning but it should only be used if definite muscarinic symptoms are present.
- *Group V.* There is no specific treatment for the 'disulfiram-alcohol' reaction except for the maintenance of blood pressure.
- *Group VI.* If symptoms are severe some patients may require sedation with diazepam.

◊ General reviews.
1. Köppel C. Clinical symptomatology and management of mushroom poisoning. *Toxicon* 1993; **31:** 1513–40.

Amanita phalloides. The use of specific antidotes in the treatment of poisoning due to *Amanita phalloides* remains controversial. Benzylpenicillin, sulfamethoxazole, thioctic acid, cytochrome C, ascorbic acid, insulin, growth hormone, silymarin or silybin, and corticosteroids have all been used or suggested. However, at present there is limited clinical evidence to support the use of only benzylpenicillin and silymarin or silybin.[1,2] Liver transplantation should be considered in patients with progressive liver failure.[2]
1. Floersheim GL. Treatment of human amatoxin mushroom poisoning: myths and advances in therapy. *Med Toxicol* 1987; **2:** 1–9.
2. Klein AS, *et al.* Amanita poisoning: treatment and the role of liver transplantation. *Am J Med* 1989; **86:** 187–93.

Musk (12982-p)

Almíscar; Deer Musk; Mosc.; Moschus.
CAS — 541-91-3 (muskone).
Pharmacopoeias. In Chin.

The dried secretions from the preputial follicles of the musk deer, *Moschus moschiferus* or some other spp. of *Moschus* (Cervidae).

Profile

Musk is used as a fragrance and fixative in perfumery.

A series of nitrated tertiary butyl toluenes or xylenes, or related compounds, are used as artificial musks. Musk ambrette, a synthetic nitromusk compound used in perfumery and as a food flavour, has been reported to cause contact dermatitis and photosensitivity.

Musk is used in homoeopathic medicine.

◊ References.
1. Golightly LK, *et al.* Pharmaceutical excipients: adverse effects associated with inactive ingredients in drug products (part I). *Med Toxicol* 1988; **3:** 128–65.

Black Mustard (4672-k)

Graine de Moutarde Noire; Mostarda Preta; Moutarde Jonciforme; Schwarzer Senfsame; Semen Sinapis; Semilla de Mostaza; Sinapis Nigra.
Pharmacopoeias. In Aust. and Swiss.
Swiss allows B. nigra, B. juncea, and other species.

The dried ripe seeds of *Brassica nigra* (= *B. sinapioides*) (Cruciferae).

White Mustard (4673-a)

Sinapis Alba.
Pharmacopoeias. Chin. allows B. alba or B. juncea under the title Semen Sinapis.

The dried ripe seeds of *Brassica alba* (Cruciferae).

Volatile Mustard Oil (4675-x)

Allylsenföl; Essence of Mustard; Oleum Sinapis Volatile.
CAS — 57-06-7 (allyl isothiocyanate).

NOTE. Allyl Isothiocyanate is *USAN.*
Pharmacopoeias. In Aust. and Pol.
Fr. and US include allyl isothiocyanate.

Pharmacopoeial description

USP 25: Allyl isothiocyanate ($C_4H_5NS = 99.15$) is a colourless to pale yellow, very refractive, liquid with a pungent, irritating odour and an acrid taste. Slightly soluble in water; miscible with alcohol, with carbon disulfide, and with ether. Store in airtight containers.

◊ CAUTION. *Allyl isothiocyanate is a potent lachrymator, with a pungent irritating odour. Care should be taken to protect the eyes, to prevent inhalation of fumes, and to avoid tasting.*

Profile

Black and white mustard seeds have been used as emetics, in counter-irritant and rubefacient preparations, and as a condiment. Volatile mustard oil, a fixed oil largely composed of allyl isothiocyanate, is an extremely powerful irritant that has been used as a counter-irritant and rubefacient. Expressed mustard oil contains a smaller proportion of volatile oil and was used as a less powerful counter-irritant.

Adverse effects. A report of 2 cases of IgE-mediated anaphylaxis to mustard condiment.[1]
1. Vidal C, *et al.* Anaphylaxis to mustard. *Postgrad Med J* 1991; **67:** 404.

The symbol † denotes a preparation no longer actively marketed

Preparations

Proprietary Preparations (details are given in Part 3)
Fr.: Autoplasme Vaillant; Pneumoplasme†; Sinapisme Rigollot.

Multi-ingredient: *Aust.:* Red Point; *Braz.:* Analgen; Benegel; Gelflex; Gelofrix; Gelol; Geloneval; *Canad.:* Kinot; Penetrating Rub†; Rheumalan; *Fr.:* Pneumoplasme a l'Histamine†; *Ger.:* CorSelect; *Spain:* Dolokey; *Switz.:* Liberol†; *UK:* Nine Rubbing Oils; Red Oil; *USA:* Dermolin; Methalgen; Musterole Extra.

Myristyl Alcohol (7190-d)

1-Tetradecanol.
$C_{14}H_{30}O = 214.4.$

Profile

Myristyl alcohol is used as an oleaginous vehicle. Contact dermatitis has been associated with its use.

Myrrh (281-c)

Gum Myrrh; Myrrha.
Pharmacopoeias. In Eur. (see p.vi) and US.

Pharmacopoeial description

Ph. Eur.: A gum-resin, hardened in air, obtained from the stem and branches of *Commiphora molmol* and/or other species of *Commiphora.* Protect from light.

USP 25: The oleo-gum resin obtained from the stems and branches of *Commiphora molmol* and other related species of *Commiphora* (Burseraceae) other than *C. mukul.* Store in airtight containers in a dry place.

Profile

Myrrh is astringent to mucous membranes; the tincture is used in mouthwashes and gargles for inflammatory disorders of the mouth and pharynx. It has also been used as a carminative.

Preparations

USP 25: Myrrh Topical Solution.

Proprietary Preparations (details are given in Part 3)
Ger.: Inspirol P; Lomasatin M.

Multi-ingredient: *Aust.:* Brady's-Magentropfen; Dentinox; Drovitol; Paradenton; Parodontax†; *Braz.:* Malvosulfam; Nene Dent; Parodontax; *Canad.:* Chase Coldsorex; Cold Sore Lotion†; Lotion pour Feux Sauvages; *Denm.:* Dolodent; *Ger.:* Ad-Muc; Infi-tract N; Mint-Lysoform; Myrrhinil-Intest; Repha-Os; Schwedentrunk mit Ginseng†; Schwedentrunk†; *Israel:* Parodontax; *Ital.:* Gengivario; *Spain:* Buco Regis; Nani Pre Dental; Regal†; *Switz.:* Baume; Eubucal; *UK:* Allcock's Porous Capsicum Plaster; Herbal Indigestion Naturtabs; HRI Golden Seal Digestive; Indigestion and Flatulence; Medicinal Gargle; Vocalzone; Wind & Dyspepsia Relief; *USA:* Astring-O-Sol†.

Myrtillus (12987-y)

Baccae Myrtilli; Bilberry; Blaeberry; Heidelbeere; Huckleberry; Hurtleberry; Myrtilli Fructus; Whortleberry.
Pharmacopoeias. In Eur. (see p.vi).

Pharmacopoeial description

Ph. Eur.: The ripe fruit of *Vaccinium myrtillus.* The dried fruit contains a minimum of 1.0% of tannins, expressed as pyrogallol, calculated with reference to the dried drug. The fresh or frozen fruit contains a minimum of 0.30% of anthocyanins, expressed as cyanidin-3-glucoside chloride (chrysanthemin, $C_{21}H_{21}ClO_{11}$=484.8), calculated with reference to the dried drug. The frozen fruit should be stored at or below −18°.

Profile

Myrtillus has diuretic and astringent properties. It has been used for ophthalmic and circulatory disorders and for non-specific diarrhoea.

Myrtillus is used in homoeopathic medicine.

Preparations

Proprietary Preparations (details are given in Part 3)
Austral.: Herbal Eye Care Formula; *Ger.:* Difrarel; *Ital.:* Alcodin; Angiorex; Antocin; Mirtilene Forte; Retinol; Tegens; *Port.:* Difrarel; Varison; *Spain:* Difrarel; Largitor; *Switz.:* Myrtaven.

Multi-ingredient: *Aust.:* Amersan; Aponatura Durchfall; Krauterhaus Mag Kottas Tee gegen Durchfall; Myrtilen; *Austral.:* Bilberry Plus; Bilberry Plus Eye Health; Bioglan Pygno-Vite; Bioglan Vision-Eze; Extralife Eye-Care; Extralife Sleep-Care; Herbal PMS Formula; Pine OPC; Prophthal; Pykno; St Mary's Thistle Plus; *Braz.:* Antomiopic; *Fr.:* Diacure; Difrarel; Difrarel E; Santane H_7; *Ger.:* Salus Augenschutz-Kapseln N; *Ital.:* Alvear Sport†; Api Baby; Bebimix; Biolactine; Biophil; Fluiven†; Lactovit†; Memovisus; Mirtilene; Mirtiros; Neomyrt Plus; Nerex; Promix 3; Tussol; Ultravisin; Vitalmix; *Spain:* Antomiopic; Difrarel E; Mirtillus; *UK:* Se-Power.

Nadide (12991-s)

Nadide *(BAN, USAN, rINN).*
Codehydrogenase I; Coenzyme I; Co-I; Diphosphopyridine Nucleotide; DPN; NAD; Nicotinamide Adenine Dinucleotide; NSC-20272. 1-(3-Carbamoylpyridinio)-β-D-ribofuranoside 5-(adenosine-5'-pyrophosphate).
$C_{21}H_{27}N_7O_{14}P_2 = 663.4.$
CAS — 53-84-9.

Profile

Nadide is a naturally occurring coenzyme claimed to be of value in the treatment of alcohol and opioid addiction. The reduced form of nadide, NADH, has been used in the management of chronic fatigue syndrome.

Parkinsonism. The reduced form of nadide, NADH (β-NADH; reduced DPN) and its phosphate derivative (NADPH) have been given in the management of Parkinson's disease in an attempt to enhance endogenous dopamine synthesis by stimulating the enzyme tyrosine hydroxylase. Although some beneficial effects have been reported in several case series, a placebo-controlled study failed to find any evidence of efficacy and the routine use of NADH has not been recommended.[1]
1. Swerdlow RH. Is NADH effective in the treatment of Parkinson's disease? *Drugs Aging* 1998; **13:** 263–8.

Preparations

Proprietary Preparations (details are given in Part 3)
S.Afr.: DPN; *Spain:* Nad; *UK:* Enada.

Nafamostat (1775-d)

Nafamostat *(rINN).*
FUT-175 (nafamostat mesilate). 6-Amidino-2-naphthyl *p*-guanidinobenzoate.
$C_{19}H_{17}N_5O_2 = 347.4.$
CAS — 81525-10-2 (nafamostat); 82956-11-4 (nafamostat mesilate).

NOTE. Nafamostat Mesylate is *USAN.*

Profile

Like aprotinin (p.725) nafamostat is a proteolytic enzyme inhibitor. It has been used as the mesilate in the treatment of acute pancreatitis and disseminated intravascular coagulation, and as an anticoagulant in haemodialysis.

Hyperkalaemia has been reported.

◊ References.
1. Yanamoto H, *et al.* Therapeutic trial of cerebral vasospasm with the serine protease inhibitor, FUT-175, administered in the acute stage after subarachnoid hemorrhage. *Neurosurgery* 1992; **30:** 358–63.
2. Akizawa T, *et al.* Nafamostat mesilate: a regional anticoagulant for haemodialysis in patients at high risk for bleeding. *Nephron* 1993; **64:** 376–81.
3. Miyata T, *et al.* Effectiveness of nafamostat mesilate on glomerulonephritis in immune-complex diseases. *Lancet* 1993; **341:** 1353.
4. Murase M, *et al.* Nafamostat mesilate reduces blood loss during open heart surgery. *Circulation* 1993; **88:** 432–6.
5. Kitagawa H, *et al.* Hyperkalaemia due to nafamostat mesylate. *N Engl J Med* 1995; **332:** 687.

Nafiverine Hydrochloride (12994-l)

Nafiverine Hydrochloride *(rINNM).*
DA-914 (base). *NN'*-Bis{2-[2-(1-naphthyl)propionyloxy]ethyl}piperazine dihydrochloride.
$C_{34}H_{38}N_2O_4,2HCl = 611.6.$
CAS — 5061-22-3 (nafiverine); 5051-16-1 (nafiverine hydrochloride).

Profile

Nafiverine hydrochloride has been used as an antispasmodic.

Naphthylacetic Acid (14833-e)

1-Naphthaleneacetic Acid; 1-Naphthylacetic Acid.
$C_{12}H_{10}O_2 = 186.2.$
CAS — 86-87-3.

Profile

Naphthylacetic acid has been used as a choleretic.

Preparations

Proprietary Preparations (details are given in Part 3)
Multi-ingredient: *Aust.:* Galle-Donau; Spagall; *Switz.:* Bilipax.

Nebracetam (6489-e)

Nebracetam *(rINN).*
WEB-1881-FU. (±)-4-(Aminomethyl)-1-benzyl-2-pyrrolidinone.
$C_{12}H_{16}N_2O = 204.3.$
CAS — 116041-13-5.

Profile
Nebracetam acts on the CNS and has been investigated as a cognition adjuvant in the treatment of Alzheimer's disease.

Nefiracetam (15298-l)
Nefiracetam (rINN).
DM-9384; DZL-221. 2-Oxo-1-pyrrolidineaceto-2′,6′-xylidide.
$C_{14}H_{18}N_2O_2 = 246.3$.
CAS — 77191-36-7.

Profile
Nefiracetam acts on the CNS and has been described as a 'nootropic'. It has been investigated in some cerebrovascular disorders and for the treatment of Alzheimer's disease.

Neroli Oil (4676-r)
Aurantii Amari Floris Aetheroleum; Bitter-Orange Flower Oil; Esencia de Azahar; Essência de Flor de Laranjeira; Oleum Neroli; Orange Flower Oil; Orange-flower Oil.
Pharmacopoeias. In Eur. (see p.vi).
Aust. also includes a monograph on the dried flowers.

Pharmacopoeial description
Ph. Eur.: A clear, pale yellow or dark yellow liquid with a characteristic odour reminiscent of bitter-orange flowers, obtained by steam distillation from the fresh flowers of Citrus aurantium subsp. aurantium (=C. aurantium subsp. amara). Miscible with alcohol, with ether, with liquid paraffin, with petroleum spirit, and with fatty oils. Store in well-filled airtight containers. Protect from light and heat.

Profile
Neroli oil is used as a flavour and in perfumery. Photosensitivity reactions have been reported.

Preparations
Proprietary Preparations (details are given in Part 3)
Multi-ingredient: Braz.: Thiodeol; Switz.: Hygiodermil; Kemeol; Kemerhine; Oculosan; Seracalm†.

Nerve Agents (15575-k)

Sarin (8370-l)
GB. Isopropyl methylphosphonofluoridate.
$C_4H_{10}FO_2P = 140.1$.
CAS — 107-44-8.

Soman (11059-e)
GD. Pinacolyl methylphosphonofluoridate.
$C_7H_{16}FO_2P = 182.2$.
CAS — 96-64-0.

Tabun (11062-g)
GA. Ethyl N-dimethylphosphoramidocyanidate.
$C_5H_{11}N_2O_2P = 162.1$.
CAS — 77-81-6.

VX (11080-p)
Methylphosphonothioic acid S-{2-[bis(1-methylethyl)amino]ethyl} O-ethyl ester.
$C_{11}H_{26}NO_2PS = 267.4$.
CAS — 50782-69-9.

Profile
The nerve agents, sarin, soman, tabun, and vx (also referred to as 'nerve gases') used in chemical warfare are extremely potent inhibitors of cholinesterase. The effects of poisoning due to these agents, and their treatment, are similar to those for organophosphorus insecticides (p.1435) but as the nerve agents have a much greater intrinsic toxicity the symptoms of poisoning are more severe. Pyridostigmine has been administered prophylactically to personnel at risk from exposure to nerve agents (see p.1424).

◊ References.
1. Ministry of Defence. Medical manual of defence against chemical agents. London: HMSO, 1987. (JSP312).
2. World MJ. Toxic gas trauma. Lancet 1995; 346: 260–1.
3. Nozaki H, et al. A case of VX poisoning and the difference from sarin. Lancet 1995; 346: 698–9.
4. Okumura T, et al. Report on 640 victims of the Tokyo subway sarin attack. Ann Emerg Med 1996; 28: 129–35.
5. Suzuki J, et al. Eighteen cases exposed to sarin in Matsumoto, Japan. Intern Med 1997; 36: 466–70.
6. Holstege CP, et al. Chemical warfare: nerve agent poisoning. Crit Care Clin 1997; 13: 923–42.
7. Weinbroum AA, et al. Anaesthesia and critical care considerations in nerve agent warfare trauma casualties. Resuscitation 2000; 47: 113–23.

Neutral Red (13005-y)
CI Basic Red 5; Colour Index No. 50040; Neutral Red Chloride; Nuclear Fast Red; Toluylene Red. 3-Amino-7-dimethylamino-2-methylphenazine hydrochloride.
$C_{15}H_{16}N_4,HCl = 288.8$.
CAS — 553-24-2.

Profile
Neutral red is used as an indicator for alkalinity and for preparing neutral-red paper. It is also used as a stain in microscopy. It is a photoactive dye that has been tried in photodynamic therapy of recurrent herpes simplex infections with limited success.

Niaouli Oil (4677-f)
Essence de Niaouli.
Pharmacopoeias. In Fr. and Neth.

A volatile oil, obtained by distillation from the fresh leaves of Melaleuca viridiflora or Melaleuca quinquenervia (Myrtaceae).

Profile
Niaouli oil contains eucalyptol and has similar actions to eucalyptus oil (p.1609). It is an ingredient of many preparations. Typical indications include respiratory tract congestion. Cajuput oil (p.1588) and tea tree oil (see Melaleuca Oil, p.1631) are also prepared from Melaleuca spp.

Preparations
Proprietary Preparations (details are given in Part 3)
Fr.: Gomenol; Gomenoleo; Huile Gomenolee.
Multi-ingredient: Aust.: Expigen; Medizinalbad; Red Point; Belg.: Beogaze†; Braz.: Benzotal Balsamico; Binotine Balsamico; Canfomenol; Cortagrip; Durapen Balsamico; Gripefago C; Gripomatine; Griponia; Gripsay; Inalobel; Inatrex Balsamico; Killgrip; Optacilin Balsamico; Ozonyl; Plenogripe; Pulmogripe; Soma Balsamico; Canad.: Balminil Suppositories; Fr.: Balsolene; Biogaze; Coquelusedal; Coquelusedal Paracetamol; Dinacode; Euvanol†; Gomenol-Syner-Penicilline†; Hexaguine; Terpone; Thiopon Balsamique†; Vapo-Myrtol†; Vaseline Gomenolee; Ger.: Palatol; Palatol N; Ital.: Broncopulmin†; Paidorinovit; Rinantipiol; Rinobalsamiche; Rinofomentil; Rinopaidolo; Rinovit; Rinovit Nube†; Port.: Creodermol; Recto Bronco Tosse†; Rectopulmo Adultos; Rectopulmo Infantil; Spain: Brisfirina Balsamica†; Broncovital; Bronquimar Vit A†; Bronquimar†; Brota Rectal Bals; Dimayon†; Diminex Balsamico†; Edusan Fte Rectal; Electopen Balsam Retard; Etro Balsamico; Maboterpen†; Neumobiot†; Pastillas Pectoral Kely; Pulmo Grey Balsam†; Pulmonilo Synergium†; Rinobanedif; Sanaden Reforzado; Ultrabion Balsamico; Vapores Pyt; Vitavox Pastillas; Xibornol Prodes; Switz.: Bisolvex; Demo baume†; Liberol Bain; Resorbane.

Nicaraven (10338-w)
Nicaraven (rINN).
(±)-N,N′-Propylenebis[nicotinamide].
$C_{15}H_{16}N_4O_2 = 284.3$.
CAS — 79455-30-4.

Profile
Nicaraven is under investigation as a cerebral vasodilator.

Nicergoline (1514-h)
Nicergoline (BAN, USAN, rINN).
FI-6714. 10α-Methoxy-1,6-dimethylergolin-8β-ylmethyl 5-bromonicotinate.
$C_{24}H_{26}BrN_3O_3 = 484.4$.
CAS — 27848-84-6.
ATC — C04AE02.
Pharmacopoeias. In Fr.

Adverse Effects and Precautions
Adverse effects which may occur after nicergoline include gastrointestinal disturbances and, particularly after parenteral administration, hypotension.

◊ Of 359 patients with cerebrovascular insufficiency treated with nicergoline for 1 month[1] toxicity occurred in 25, necessitating withdrawal of therapy in 11. The reactions included 6 cases of hot flushes, 8 of general malaise, 2 of agitation, 3 of hyperacidity, 1 of nausea, 3 of diarrhoea, and 2 of dizziness and somnolence.
1. Dauverchain J. Bedeutung von Nicergolin bei der symptomatischen Behandlung des arteriellen Hochdrucks und der chronischen zerebro-vaskulären Insuffizienz. Arzneimittelforschung 1979; 29: 1308–10.

Porphyria. Nicergoline is considered to be unsafe in patients with porphyria because it has been shown to be porphyrinogenic in in-vitro systems, although there is conflicting evidence of porphyrinogenicity.

Interactions
◊ For a study indicating that nicergoline enhances the cardiac depressant action of propranolol, see Beta Blockers, p.847.

Uses and Administration
Nicergoline is an ergot derivative. It has been used similarly to co-dergocrine mesilate (p.1597) to treat symptoms of mental deterioration associated with cerebrovascular insufficiency (see Dementia, p.1412) and has been used in peripheral vascular disease (p.809). Nicergoline has been given in doses of up to 60 mg daily by mouth in divided doses, and by intramuscular injection in doses of 2 to 4 mg twice daily; 4 to 8 mg has been given by slow intravenous infusion. Nicergoline tartrate has been used in preparations for parenteral administration.

◊ References.
1. Ronchi F, et al. Symptomatic treatment of benign prostatic obstruction with nicergoline: a placebo controlled clinical study and urodynamic evaluation. Urol Res 1982; 10: 131–4.
2. Bousquet J, et al. Double-blind, placebo-controlled study of nicergoline in the treatment of pruritus in patients receiving maintenance hemodialysis. J Allergy Clin Immunol 1989; 83: 825–8.
3. Saletu B, et al. Nicergoline in senile dementia of Alzheimer type and multi-infarct dementia: a double-blind, placebo-controlled, clinical and EEG/ERP mapping study. Psychopharmacology (Berl) 1995; 117: 385–95.
4. Herrmann WM, et al. A multicenter randomized double-blind study on the efficacy and safety of nicergoline in patients with multi-infarct dementia. Dementia Geriatr Cogn Disord 1997; 8: 9–17.

Preparations
Proprietary Preparations (details are given in Part 3)
Aust.: Ergotop; Sermion; Braz.: Sermion; Fr.: Sermion; Ger.: Circo-Maren; duracebrol; ergobel; Memoq; Nicergobeta; Nicerium; Sermion; Hong Kong: Sermion; Ital.: Cebran; Ergolin; Neugent†; Nicer; Sermion; Mex.: Sermion; Port.: Erg XXI†; Sermion; Spain: Fisifax; Sermion; Varson; Switz.: Sermion; Thai.: Sermion.

Nicofetamide (3938-t)
C-1065. N-(1,2-Diphenylethyl)-3-pyridinecarboxamide.
$C_{20}H_{18}N_2O = 302.4$.
CAS — 553-06-0.
ATC — A03AC04.

Profile
Nicofetamide has been used as an antispasmodic.

Nicotine (15303-c)
Nicotinum. (S)-3-(1-Methylpyrrolidin-2-yl)pyridine.
$C_{10}H_{14}N_2 = 162.2$.
CAS — 54-11-5 (nicotine); 65-31-6 (anhydrous nicotine tartrate).
ATC — N07BA01.

NOTE. Nicotine Bitartrate is USAN.
Pharmacopoeias. In Eur. (see p.vi) and US.
US also includes Nicotine Polacrilex (a complex of nicotine with a methacrylic acid polymer).

A liquid alkaloid obtained from the dried leaves of the tobacco plant, Nicotiana tabacum and related species (Solanaceae). Tobacco leaves contain 0.5 to 8% of nicotine combined as malate or citrate.

Pharmacopoeial description
Ph. Eur.: A colourless or brownish, volatile, hygroscopic, viscous liquid. Soluble in water; miscible with dehydrated alcohol. Store under nitrogen in airtight containers. Protect from light.
USP 25: Store under nitrogen at a temperature below 25°. Protect from light and moisture.

Nicotine Polacrilex is a weak carboxylic cation-exchange resin prepared from methacrylic acid and divinylbenzene, in complex with nicotine. Stored in airtight containers.

Dependence and Withdrawal
Nicotine dependence is most commonly associated with cigarette smoking. It is characterised by a strong desire to continue taking the agent, a physical and psychological need for it, and a characteristic abstinence syndrome on withdrawal. Common symptoms seen on nicotine withdrawal include irritability, anxiety, depression, restlessness, poor concentration, increased appetite, weight gain, and insomnia. The management of smoking cessation is discussed under Uses and Administration, below.

Mild withdrawal symptoms have been reported from nicotine replacement preparations used to aid smoking cessation.

◊ References.
1. Hatsukami D, et al. Physical dependence on nicotine gum: effect of duration of use. Psychopharmacology (Berl) 1993; 111: 449–56.
2. Benowitz NL, Henningfield JE. Establishing a nicotine threshold for addiction: the implications for tobacco regulation. N Engl J Med 1994; 331: 123–5.
3. Keenan RM, et al. Pharmacodynamic effects of cotinine in abstinent cigarette smokers. Clin Pharmacol Ther 1994; 55: 581–90.
4. Slade J, et al. Nicotine and addiction: the Brown and Williamson documents. JAMA 1995; 274: 225–33.
5. Kessler DA. Nicotine addiction in young people. N Engl J Med 1995; 333: 186–9.
6. Doll R, Crofton J, eds. Tobacco and health. Br Med Bull 1996; 52: 1–223.
7. Benowitz NL. Nicotine addiction. Prim Care 1999; 26: 611–31.

8. Colby SM, et al. Are adolescent smokers dependent on nicotine? A review of the evidence. Drug Alcohol Depend 2000; 59 (suppl 1): S83–S95.
9. Royal College of Physicians. Nicotine addiction in Britain: a report of the Tobacco Advisory Group of the Royal College of Physicians. London: Royal College of Physicians, 2000.
10. West R, et al. A comparison of the abuse liability and dependence potential of nicotine patch, gum, spray and inhaler. Psychopharmacology (Berl) 2000; 149: 198–202.

Adverse Effects and Treatment

Nicotine is a highly toxic substance and in acute poisoning death may occur within a few minutes due to respiratory failure arising from paralysis of the muscles of respiration. The fatal dose of nicotine for an adult is from 30 to 60 mg.

Less severe poisoning causes initial stimulation followed by depression of the autonomic nervous system. Typical symptoms include burning of the mouth and throat, nausea and salivation, abdominal pain, vomiting, diarrhoea, dizziness, hypertension followed by hypotension, mental confusion, headache, disturbed hearing and vision, dyspnoea, faintness, convulsions, sweating, and prostration. Transient cardiac standstill or paroxysmal atrial fibrillation may occur.

Nicotine is rapidly absorbed through the skin or by inhalation as well as by ingestion and nicotine poisoning may occur due to careless handling when it is employed as a horticultural insecticide.

Prompt treatment of nicotine poisoning is essential. If contact was with the skin, contaminated clothing should be removed and the skin washed thoroughly with cold water without rubbing. If the patient has swallowed nicotine, gastric lavage and administration of activated charcoal may be beneficial. Treatment is supportive and includes support of respiration and control of convulsions. Atropine may be used to suppress features of parasympathomimetic stimulation.

Apart from effects such as dizziness, headache, and gastrointestinal disturbances mentioned above, adverse effects associated with nicotine replacement preparations have also included cold and flu-like symptoms, palpitations, insomnia, vivid dreams, myalgia, chest pain, blood pressure changes, anxiety, irritability, somnolence, and dysmenorrhoea. Allergic reactions have been reported. Adverse effects associated with specific preparations include skin reactions with transdermal patches; nasal irritation, epistaxis, lachrymation, and sensations in the ear with the nasal spray; throat irritation with the spray, inhalator, sublingual tablets, or chewing gum; aphthous ulceration with the inhalator, sublingual tablets, or chewing gum; increased salivation and sometimes swelling of the tongue with chewing gum; cough, rhinitis, stomatitis, sinusitis, and dry mouth with the inhalator; and unpleasant taste with the sublingual tablets. Excessive swallowing of nicotine released from oral replacement preparations may cause hiccups in the first few days of treatment.

◊ References.
1. Greenland S, et al. A meta-analysis to assess the incidence of adverse effects associated with the transdermal nicotine patch. Drug Safety 1998; 18: 297–308.
2. Gourlay SG, et al. Predictors and timing of adverse experiences during transdermal nicotine therapy. Drug Safety 1999; 20: 545–55.

◊ Vasculitis occurring in 2 patients was associated with transdermal nicotine patches.[1] Hyperinsulinaemia and insulin resistance have been associated with long-term use of nicotine gum.[2]
1. van der Klauw MM, et al. Vasculitis attributed to the nicotine patch (Nicotinell). Br J Dermatol 1996; 134: 361–4.
2. Eliasson B, et al. Long-term use of nicotine gum is associated with hyperinsulinemia and insulin resistance. Circulation 1996; 94: 878–81.

Adverse effects of tobacco products. Chronic use of tobacco is linked to a variety of diseases. By the mid-1960s, epidemiological data established tobacco smoking as a cause of lung cancer. Smoking is also associated with cancers of the larynx, mouth, cervix, bladder, pancreas, oesophagus, stomach, and kidneys, and with leukaemia.[1] Smoking is a risk factor in cardiovascular, respiratory, and peripheral and cerebral vascular diseases.[1,2] Smoking also increases the risk of developing peptic ulcer disease and may affect other gastrointestinal disorders.

Maternal smoking in pregnancy is associated with low birthweight infants and increased risk of abortion, still-birth, and neonatal death.

Passive smoking refers to inhalation of secondhand tobacco smoke or environmental tobacco smoke. Risks to health from passive exposure are lower than those from active smoking. However, studies have established passive smoking as a cause of lung cancer;[3] passive smoking is also associated with increased risk of heart disease[4] and chronic respiratory disease.[5,6] Smokeless tobacco products also carry risks to health, for example the association of cancers of the head and neck (see p.494) with the use of snuff or chewing tobacco.
1. Wald NJ, Hackshaw AK. Cigarette smoking: an epidemiological overview. Br Med Bull 1996; 52: 3–11.
2. Ashton H. Adverse effects of nicotine. Adverse Drug React Bull 1991; 149: 560–3.
3. Lam TH. Passive smoking in perspective. Med Toxicol Adverse Drug Exp 1989; 4: 153–62.
4. Steenland K. Passive smoking and the risk of heart disease. JAMA 1992; 267: 94–9.

5. Law MR, Hackshaw AK. Environmental tobacco smoke. Br Med Bull 1996; 52: 22–34.
6. DiFranza JR, Lew RA. Mortality and morbidity in children associated with the use of tobacco products by other people. Pediatrics 1996; 97: 560–8.

Effects on the cardiovascular system. As mentioned above, nicotine from tobacco products is associated with increased risk of cardiovascular disease. It would not be surprising, therefore, if nicotine replacement preparations were also associated with cardiovascular adverse effects, and there are anecdotal reports of cardiovascular events, including myocardial infarction,[1,2] stroke,[3] and cerebral haematoma,[4] associated with use of such products. However, in studies in patients with cardiovascular disease, 5- or 10-week courses of transdermal nicotine were not associated with an increase in cardiovascular events compared with placebo.[5,6]
1. Warner JG, Little TC. Myocardial infarction in a patient who smoked while wearing a nicotine patch. Ann Intern Med 1994; 120: 695.
2. Arnaot MR. Nicotine patches may not be safe. BMJ 1995; 310: 663–4.
3. Pierce JR. Stroke following application of a nicotine patch. Ann Pharmacother 1994; 28: 402.
4. Riche G, et al. Intracerebral haematoma after application of nicotine patch. Lancet 1995; 346: 777–8.
5. Working Group for the Study of Transdermal Nicotine in Patients with Coronary Artery Disease. Nicotine replacement therapy for patients with coronary artery disease. Arch Intern Med 1994; 154: 989–95.
6. Joseph AM. The safety of transdermal nicotine as an aid to smoking cessation in patients with cardiac disease. N Engl J Med 1996; 335: 1792–8.

Precautions

Nicotine preparations should not be used in patients who have experienced recent cerebrovascular accident. They should be used with caution in patients with cardiovascular disease and should be avoided in severe cardiovascular disease, including during the immediate postmyocardial infarction period, and in patients with severe arrhythmias or unstable angina pectoris. They should be used with caution in those with peripheral vascular disease, in endocrine disorders including phaeochromocytoma, hyperthyroidism, and diabetes mellitus, in peptic ulcer disease, or renal or hepatic impairment. Their use is contra-indicated during pregnancy or breast feeding.

Nicotine preparations should not be used in patients who continue to smoke. Combined use of different preparations is not recommended (but see under Smoking Cessation, below).

Skin patches should not be used on broken skin.

Exercise. Physical exercise increased mean peak plasma concentrations of nicotine in 8 healthy subjects treated with a transdermal nicotine patch.[1] The effect was thought to be most likely due to increased skin perfusion resulting in increased uptake.
1. Klemsdal TO, et al. Physical exercise increases plasma concentrations of nicotine during treatment with a nicotine patch. Br J Clin Pharmacol 1995; 39: 677–9.

Myasthenia gravis. A patient with myasthenia gravis noted worsening of his symptoms following application of transdermal nicotine patches, the effects being most severe about 1 hour after application, and resolving within 3 hours once the patch was removed.[1] Previous heavy smoking had not produced similar adverse effects, despite the fact that blood-nicotine concentrations are typically higher just after finishing a cigarette than when using the patch.[2]
1. Moreau T, et al. Nicotine-sensitive myasthenia gravis. Lancet 1994; 344: 548–9.
2. Pethica D. Nicotine-sensitive myasthenia gravis. Lancet 1994; 344: 961.

Interactions

Tobacco smoking induces hepatic metabolic enzymes and the pharmacokinetics of many drugs are altered, as discussed under their individual monographs. Drugs such as methoxsalen which inhibit the cytochrome P450 isoenzyme CYP2A6 may decrease the metabolism of nicotine, resulting in increased plasma concentrations.

◊ References.
1. Miller LG. Cigarettes and drug therapy: pharmacokinetic and pharmacodynamic considerations. Clin Pharm 1990; 9: 125–35.
2. Zevin S, Benowitz NL. Drug interactions with tobacco smoking: an update. Clin Pharmacokinet 1999; 36: 425–38.
3. Sellers EM, et al. Inhibition of cytochrome P450 2A6 increases nicotine's oral bioavailability and decreases smoking. Clin Pharmacol Ther 2000; 68: 35–43.

Nicotinic acid. As described on p.1373, a possible interaction between nicotinic acid and nicotine from a transdermal patch has been reported.

Pharmacokinetics

Nicotine is readily absorbed through mucous membranes and the skin; bioavailability of oral nicotine is low due to extensive first-pass metabolism. Nicotine is widely distributed; it crosses the placenta and is found in breast milk. The elimination half-life is about 1 to 2 hours. Nicotine is metabolised mainly in the liver via the cytochrome P450 isoenzyme CYP2A6 to cotinine and nicotine-N-oxide. Nicotine and its metabolites are excreted in the urine.

◊ References.
1. Gorsline J, et al. Steady-state pharmacokinetics and dose relationship of nicotine delivered from Nicoderm (nicotine transdermal system). J Clin Pharmacol 1993; 33: 161–8.

2. Gupta SK, et al. Bioavailability and absorption kinetics of nicotine following application of a transdermal system. Br J Clin Pharmacol 1993; 36: 221–7.
3. Schneider NG, et al. Clinical pharmacokinetics of nasal nicotine delivery: a review and comparison to other nicotine systems. Clin Pharmacokinet 1996; 31: 65–80.
4. Benowitz NL, et al. Sources of variability in nicotine and cotinine levels with the use of nicotine nasal spray, transdermal nicotine and cigarette smoking. Br J Clin Pharmacol 1997; 43: 259–67.
5. Zins BJ, et al. Pharmacokinetics of nicotine tartrate after single-dose liquid enema, oral, and intravenous administration. J Clin Pharmacol 1997; 37: 426–36.

Uses and Administration

The main physiological action of nicotine is paralysis of all autonomic ganglia, preceded by stimulation. Centrally, small doses cause respiratory stimulation, while larger doses produce convulsions of the medullary type and cause arrest of respiration. The effects on skeletal muscle are similar to those on ganglia.

Nicotine chewing gum, transdermal patches, lozenges, sublingual tablets, a nasal spray, or inhalator are used as aids to giving up smoking. *Chewing gum* is available in strengths of 2 mg and 4 mg; the nicotine may be present in the gum in the form of a complex with methacrylic acid polymer (nicotine polacrilex). Individuals who smoke 20 cigarettes or less a day should start with the 2-mg strength gum chewed slowly over about 30 minutes when the urge to smoke occurs. Those who smoke over 20 cigarettes a day or require more than 15 pieces daily of the 2-mg gum should receive the 4-mg strength. Not more than 15 pieces should be used per day.

Sublingual tablets containing the equivalent of 2 mg of nicotine as a β-cyclodextrin complex may also be used: the recommended dose is 1 or 2 tablets sublingually every hour, increased to a maximum of 40 tablets daily if necessary, for at least 3 months. The dose should then be gradually reduced until it can be withdrawn.

Lozenges containing 1 mg of nicotine (as the tartrate) are also available although they may not be suitable for individuals with a strong nicotine dependence or those who have failed to stop smoking with the aid of other nicotine replacement preparations. The initial dose is 1 lozenge every 1 to 2 hours increased to a maximum of 25 lozenges daily. Treatment should continue for at least 3 months, after which the dose should be gradually reduced and then withdrawn.

Adhesive *transdermal patches* are designed to be worn for 16 or 24 hours and are available in different strengths which deliver from 5 to 22 mg during the recommended wearing time. One patch should be applied daily to the hip, trunk, or upper arm, usually beginning with the highest strength or with a dose determined by the previous daily consumption of cigarettes. A different site of application should be used each day with several days elapsing before the patch is applied to the same area of skin. Treatment is usually withdrawn gradually by reducing the dose every 2 to 8 weeks.

A suggested initial dosage for a *nasal spray* containing 500 µg per spray is one spray administered into each nostril up to twice hourly as required up to a maximum of 80 sprays daily for the first 8 weeks and reduced gradually thereafter.

Nicotine *inhalator cartridges* contain nicotine 10 mg for use in an appropriate inhaler mouthpiece. The initial dose is 6 to 16 cartridges daily for up to 12 weeks and is reduced gradually over a further 6 to 12 weeks.

It has been recommended that the use of nicotine therapy for smoking cessation should be reviewed if abstinence has not been achieved in 3 months.

Nicotine has been used as a horticultural insecticide either as a vapour or as a spray.

Alzheimer's disease. The use of nicotine as a cholinergic agonist is one of a number of methods being studied[1] to overcome brain cholinergic deficits in patients with Alzheimer's disease (see Dementia, p.1412). Preliminary studies[2,3] using nicotine patches have been of limited duration and are inconclusive.
1. Baldinger SL, Schroeder DJ. Nicotine therapy in patients with Alzheimer's disease. Ann Pharmacother 1995; 29: 314–15.
2. Wilson AL, et al. Nicotine patches in Alzheimer's disease: pilot study on learning, memory, and safety. Pharmacol Biochem Behav 1995; 51: 509–14.
3. Snaedal J, et al. The effects of nicotine in dermal plaster on cognitive functions in patients with Alzheimer's disease. Dementia 1996; 7: 47–52.

Blepharospasm. Nicotine nasal spray was reported to be of benefit in a patient with blepharospasm (p.1325) refractory to botulinum A toxin.[1]
1. Dursun SM, et al. Treatment of blepharospasm with nicotine nasal spray. Lancet 1996; 348: 60.

Extrapyramidal disorders. Nicotine transdermal patches have been reported to produce beneficial effects[1] in schizophrenic patients with antipsychotic-induced akathisia (p.662).
1. Anfang MK, Pope HG. Treatment of neuroleptic-induced akathisia with nicotine patches. Psychopharmacology (Berl) 1997; 134: 153–6.

Skin disorders. There have been anecdotal reports of nicotine producing beneficial effects in various skin disorders, includ-

The symbol † denotes a preparation no longer actively marketed

ing pyoderma gangrenosum,[1] and dermatitis due to fluorouracil therapy.[2]

1. Kanekura T, et al. Nicotine for pyoderma gangrenosum. Lancet 1995; 345: 1058.
2. Kingsley EC. 5-Fluorouracil dermatitis prophylaxis with a nicotine patch. Ann Intern Med 1994; 120: 813.

Smoking cessation. Smoking is the single most important cause of preventable illness and premature death in the UK and USA; it is estimated that around 1 in 5 deaths are due to smoking-related illnesses. The financial burden of smoking-related diseases on health care providers is also substantial. As such many governments have undertaken initiatives to promote smoking cessation.

Nicotine dependence and the development of a characteristic withdrawal syndrome (see Dependence, above) make stopping smoking very difficult. Many individuals relapse when trying to give up or need several attempts before successfully stopping. Both nonpharmacological and pharmacological treatments can improve the abstinence rate and are most effective when the two approaches are combined.[1-8]

Nonpharmacological methods include counselling, training in coping skills, and support groups; although the abstinence rate increases with the intensity of the support, even brief advice is effective in encouraging cessation.

The first-line pharmacological intervention is *nicotine replacement therapy* (NRT) which is an effective treatment for reducing the cravings associated with stopping smoking. NRT is available in numerous formulations: chewing gum, transdermal patches, inhalators, and nasal spray and, more recently, sublingual tablets and lozenges. A systematic review[8] of NRT found abstinence was approximately doubled when compared with controls, regardless of the intensity of any additional nonpharmacological support. Choice of formulation is based on patient preference, tolerance, and previous treatments, if any. The transdermal patch is easiest to use and compliance is greatest with this route but local effects may be troublesome. The gum has an unpleasant taste initially and some find the chewing action difficult. The sublingual tablet may be useful for those who have difficulty chewing the gum. The nasal spray has a fast onset of action but may cause local irritation. The inhalator has the advantage of simulating cigarette smoking but may cause local irritation of the mouth and throat. The lozenge has the advantage that it can be sucked discreetly. Patients who are unable to tolerate one type of NRT may benefit from a course of an alternative NRT preparation.

Combination therapy with different types of NRT (patches with either the nasal spray, inhalator, or chewing gum) has also been tried as a means of increasing efficacy although combination therapy is not recommended by the manufacturers of NRT preparations.

NRT is usually continued for about 3 months before being withdrawn. Although the manufacturers advise gradual withdrawal, others[4,6] have found that this offers no advantage and recommend abrupt withdrawal. NRT has also been used long-term and may be of particular benefit in those patients who feel they would relapse if NRT was stopped or in those who have persistent withdrawal symptoms.

There has been concern over the use of NRT in patients with cardiovascular disease (see above) but clinical experience and studies have shown that NRT can be used with caution in these patients. The use of NRT in those who have suffered a recent myocardial infarction or those with severe arrhythmias or unstable angina is, however, contra-indicated as such patients have not been adequately studied.

A number of other drugs have also been used to achieve abstinence from smoking. *Bupropion* is effective and recommended by some as a first-line alternative to NRT; its action is said to be independent of its antidepressant activity. Bupropion in combination with NRT has been used successfully. *Clonidine* is also effective but adverse effects limit its usefulness and it is reserved as a second-line treatment. The antidepressant *nortriptyline* is another second-line drug. There is little or no evidence to support the efficacy of other treatments such as *silver acetate, mecamylamine, lobeline,* or *anxiolytics* such as *buspirone,* and their use is not recommended.

1. American Society of Health-System Pharmacists. ASHP therapeutic position statement on smoking cessation. Am J Health-Syst Pharm 1999; 56: 460–4.
2. Anonymous. Nicotine replacement to aid smoking cessation. Drug Ther Bull 1999; 37: 52–4.
3. West R, et al. Smoking cessation guidelines for health professionals: an update. Thorax 2000; 55: 987–99.
4. Royal College of Physicians. Nicotine addiction in Britain: a report of the Tobacco Advisory Group of the Royal College of Physicians. London: Royal College of Physicians, 2000.
5. Fiore MC, et al. A clinical practice guideline for treating tobacco use and dependence: a US public health service report. JAMA 2000; 283: 3244–54.
6. Simpson D. Smoking cessation. In: Doctors and tobacco: medicine's big challenge. London: Tobacco Control Resource Centre, British Medical Association, 2000. Available at: http://www.tobacco-control.org/tcrc.nsf/htmlpagesvw/resourcesfrm (accessed 31/08/00).
7. Covey LS, et al. Advances in non-nicotine pharmacotherapy for smoking cessation. Drugs 2000; 59: 17–31.
8. Silagy C, et al. Nicotine replacement therapy for smoking cessation (updated 22 May 2001). Available in The Cochrane Library; Issue 3. Oxford: Update Software; 2001.

Spasticity. There have been anecdotal reports[1] of beneficial responses to nicotine in spastic dystonia.

1. Vaughan CJ, et al. Treatment of spastic dystonia with transdermal nicotine. Lancet 1997; 350: 565.

Tics. Tourette's syndrome (p.650) is characterised by motor and vocal tics and behavioural disturbances. Nicotine[1-4] has been reported to be of benefit when used alone or with the more usual treatment of haloperidol in patients with Tourette's syndrome whose symptoms were not satisfactorily controlled with haloperidol alone. It is hoped that the use of transdermal nicotine patches will avoid the reported problems of compliance associated with the taste and gastrointestinal effects of nicotine gum.

1. McConville BJ, et al. The effects of nicotine plus haloperidol compared to nicotine only and placebo nicotine only in reducing tic severity and frequency to Tourette's disorder. Biol Psychiatry 1992; 31: 832–40.
2. Silver AA, Sanberg PR. Transdermal nicotine patch and potentiation of haloperidol in Tourette's syndrome. Lancet 1993; 342: 182.
3. Dursun SM, et al. Longlasting improvement of Tourette's syndrome with transdermal nicotine. Lancet 1994; 344: 1577.
4. Sanberg PR, et al. Nicotine for the treatment of Tourette's syndrome. Pharmacol Ther 1997; 74: 21–5.

Ulcerative colitis. Investigation of the use of nicotine in ulcerative colitis (see Inflammatory Bowel Disease, p.1205) has been prompted by the observation that this condition is rare in smokers.[1] Results from 2 studies[2,3] suggested that transdermal nicotine added to conventional therapy could improve symptoms in active disease. However another study[4] found that transdermal nicotine was no more effective than placebo in maintaining disease remission. Some consider[5] that the adverse effects of nicotine are likely to limit its use in some patients, particularly those who have never smoked. Local delivery to the colon, in the form of enemas[6] and oral modified-release capsules,[7] is under investigation as a means of reducing the adverse effects of nicotine.

1. Guslandi M. Nicotine treatment for ulcerative colitis. Br J Clin Pharmacol 1999; 48: 481–4.
2. Pullan RD, et al. Transdermal nicotine for active ulcerative colitis. N Engl J Med 1994; 330: 811–15.
3. Sandborn WJ, et al. Transdermal nicotine for mildly to moderately active ulcerative colitis: a randomized, double-blind, placebo-controlled trial. Ann Intern Med 1997; 126: 364–71.
4. Thomas GAO, et al. Transdermal nicotine as maintenance therapy for ulcerative colitis. N Engl J Med 1995; 332: 988–92.
5. Rhodes J, Thomas G. Nicotine treatment in ulcerative colitis. Drugs 1995; 49: 157–60.
6. Sandborn WJ, et al. Nicotine tartrate liquid enemas for mildly to moderately active left-sided ulcerative colitis unresponsive to first-line therapy: a pilot study. Aliment Pharmacol Ther 1997; 11: 663–71.
7. Green JT, et al. An oral formulation of nicotine for release and absorption in the colon: its development and pharmacokinetics. Br J Clin Pharmacol 1999; 48: 485–93.

Preparations

USP 25: Nicotine Polacrilex Gum; Nicotine Transdermal System.

Proprietary Preparations (details are given in Part 3)

Aust.: Nicolan; Nicorette; Nicotinell; Nicotrol; *Austral.:* Nicabate; Nicorette; Nicotinell; Prostep†; *Belg.:* Nicorette; Nicotinell; NiQuitin; *Braz.:* Nicolan; Nicotinell TTS; *Canad.:* Habitrol; Nicoderm; Nicorette; Nicotrol; Prostep†; *Denm.:* Nicorette; Nicotinell; NiQuitin; *Fin.:* Nicorette; Nicotinell; *Fr.:* Nicogum; Nicopatch; Nicorette; NiQuitin; *Ger.:* Nicorette; Nicotinell; nikofrenon; *Hong Kong:* Nicorette; Nicotinell; *Irl.:* Nicontinell; Nicorette; Nicotinell; *Israel:* Nicorette; Nicotinell; Nicorette; Nicotinell TTS; Nicotrans†; *Mex.:* Nicorette; Nicotinell TTS; *Neth.:* Nicorette; Nicotinell; *Norw.:* Nicorette; Nicotinell; *NZ:* Nicabate; Nicorette; Nicotinell; *Port.:* Nicorette; Nicotinell TTS; *S.Afr.:* Nicorette; Nicotinell TTS; Quit; *Singapore:* Nicorette; Nicotinell; *Spain:* Nicodisc†; Nicomax; Nicorette; Nicotinell; Nicotrans†; Nicotrol; *Swed.:* Nicolan†; Nicorette; Nicotinell; Nikotugg; NiQuitin; Quitt†; *Switz.:* Nicorette; Nicostop TTS†; Nicotinell; *Thai.:* Nicorette; Nicotinell; *UK:* Niconil†; Nicorette; Nicotinell; NiQuitin; Stoppers; Stubit†; *USA:* Habitrol; Nicoderm; Nicorette; Nicotrol; Prostep.

Multi-ingredient: *UK:* Resolution.

Nitisinone (20114-w)

Nitisinone (rINN).

NTBC. 2-(α,α,α-Trifluoro-2-nitro-p-toluoyl)-1,3-cyclohexanedione.

$C_{14}H_{10}F_3NO_5 = 329.2$.
CAS — 104206-65-7.

Profile

Nitisinone is a 4-hydroxyphenylpyruvate dioxygenase inhibitor that is used in the management of hereditary tyrosinaemia.

◊ References.

1. Holme E, Lindstedt S. Tyrosinaemia type I and NTBC (2-(2-nitro-4-trifluoromethylbenzoyl)-1,3-cyclohexanedione). J Inherit Metab Dis 1998; 21: 507–17.
2. Ros J, et al. NTBC as palliative treatment in chronic tyrosinaemia type I. J Inherit Metab Dis 1999; 22: 665–6.

Nitric Acid (1318-r)

Acidum Nitricum; Aqua Fortis; Azotic Acid; Nit. Acid; Salpetersäure.

$HNO_3 = 63.01$.
CAS — 7697-37-2.

Pharmacopoeias. In Eur. (see p.vi) (68 to 70%) and *Pol.* (10%). Also in *USNF* (69 to 71%).

Pharmacopoeial description

Ph. Eur.: A clear, colourless to almost colourless liquid. Miscible with water. It contains 68.0 to 70.0% w/w of HNO_3. Protect from light.

USNF 20: A highly corrosive fuming liquid, having a characteristic, highly irritating odour. It contains 69.0 to 71.0% w/w of HNO_3. Store in airtight containers.

Adverse Effects and Treatment

As for Hydrochloric Acid, p.1621.
There may be methaemoglobinaemia. Nitric acid stains the skin yellow.

Effects on the respiratory system. Respiratory failure due to pulmonary oedema occurred in a 56-year-old man after inhaling nitric acid which he had used as a metal cleaner.[1] The man died despite extensive ventilatory support.

1. Bur A, et al. Fatal pulmonary edema after nitric acid inhalation. Resuscitation 1997; 35: 33–6.

Uses and Administration

Nitric acid has a powerful corrosive action and has been used to remove warts (p.1108), but it should be applied with caution, and less corrosive substances are available. It has also been used for the removal of tattoos.

Preparations

Proprietary Preparations (details are given in Part 3)

Multi-ingredient: *Ger.:* Solco-Derman; *Hong Kong:* Solcoderm; *Switz.:* Solcoderm; Solcogyn.

Nitrobenzene (13025-k)

Nitrobenzol; Oil of Mirbane.

$C_6H_5NO_2 = 123.1$.
CAS — 98-95-3.

Adverse Effects

Nitrobenzene is highly toxic and the ingestion of 1 g may be fatal. Toxic effects from ingestion are usually delayed for several hours and may include nausea, prostration, burning headache, methaemoglobinaemia with cyanosis, haemolytic anaemia, vomiting (with characteristic odour), convulsions, and coma, ending in death after a few hours. Poisoning may also occur from absorption through the skin, or by inhalation.

Treatment of Adverse Effects

After ingestion of nitrobenzene the stomach should be emptied. Methaemoglobinaemia may be treated with methylene blue [methylthioninium chloride]. Blood transfusions or haemodialysis may be necessary. Oxygen should be given if cyanosis is severe.

If the skin or eyes are splashed with nitrobenzene, contaminated clothing should be removed immediately and the affected areas washed with running water for at least 15 minutes.

Uses

Nitrobenzene is used in the manufacture of aniline, as a preservative in polishes, and in perfumery and soaps.

Nizofenone (19584-b)

Nizofenone (rINN).

Y-9179. 2′-Chloro-2-[2-[(diethylamino)methyl]imidazol-1-yl]-5-nitrobenzophenone.

$C_{21}H_{21}ClN_4O_3 = 412.9$.
CAS — 54533-85-6.
ATC — N06BX10.

Profile

Nizofenone has been investigated for its nootropic actions.

Nucleic Acid (15306-t)

Acide Zymonucléique; Acidum Nucleicum; Nucleinic Acid.

A complex mixture of phosphorus-containing organic acids present in living cells.

Profile

Nucleic acids are of 2 types, ribonucleic acids (RNA, see p.1657) and deoxyribonucleic acids (DNA, see p.1602). They are composed of chains of nucleotides (phosphate esters of purine or pyrimidine bases and pentose sugars).

Since the administration of nucleic acid gives rise to a marked temporary leucocytosis (usually preceded by a short period of leucopenia) it was formerly used in the treatment of a variety of bacterial infections in the hope of enhancing the natural defence mechanisms. Its therapeutic value, however, was never established.

Nutmeg (4679-n)

Muscade; Myristica; Noz Moscada; Nuez Moscada; Nux Moschata.

Pharmacopoeias. In Chin.

The dried kernels of the seeds of *Myristica fragrans* (Myristicaceae), containing not less than 5% v/w of volatile oil; the powdered drug contains not less than 4% v/w. Mace (p.1630) is the dried arillus of the seed of *M. fragrans.*

Adverse Effects

Nutmeg, taken in large doses, may cause nausea and vomiting, flushing, dry mouth, tachycardia, stimulation of the CNS possibly with epileptiform convulsions, miosis or occasionally mydriasis, euphoria, and hallucinations. Myristicin and elimicin are thought to be the constituents responsible for the psychotic effects of nutmeg, possibly following metabolism to amfetamine-like compounds.

◊ Some references to the adverse effects of nutmeg.
1. Panayotopoulos DJ, Chisholm DD. Hallucinogenic effect of nutmeg. *BMJ* 1970; **1:** 754.
2. Venables GS, *et al.* Nutmeg poisoning. *BMJ* 1976; **1:** 96.
3. Dietz WH, Stuart MJ. Nutmeg and prostaglandins. *N Engl J Med* 1976; **294:** 503.
4. Faguet RA, Rowland KF. "Spice cabinet" intoxication. *Am J Psychiatry* 1978; **135:** 860–1.
5. Abernethy MK, Becker LB. Acute nutmeg intoxication. *Am J Emerg Med* 1992; **10:** 429–30.
6. Brenner N, *et al.* Chronic nutmeg psychosis. *J R Soc Med* 1993; **86:** 179–80.
7. Quin GI, *et al.* Nutmeg intoxication. *J Accid Emerg Med* 1998; **15:** 287–8.

Uses and Administration

Nutmeg is the source of nutmeg oil (below). It is aromatic and carminative and is used as a flavour. Nutmeg has been reported to inhibit prostaglandin synthesis.

It is used in homoeopathic medicine.

Preparations

Proprietary Preparations (details are given in Part 3)
Multi-ingredient: *Aust.:* Mariazeller; Schwedenjorg mild†; ***Ger.:*** Doppelherz Melissengeist; Melissengeist; ***Spain:*** Agua del Carmen; Vicks Vaporub; ***UK:*** Aluminium Free Indigestion†; Cough Drops; Melissa comp..

Nutmeg Oil (4678-d)

Átherisches Muskatöl; Esencia de Nuez Moscada; Essence de Muscade; Essência de Moscada; Myristica Oil; Myristicae Fragrantis Aetheroleum; Oleum Myristicae.

Pharmacopoeias. In Eur. (see p.vi).

Pharmacopoeial description

Ph. Eur.: The oil obtained by steam distillation of the dried and crushed kernels of *Myristica fragrans.* A colourless to pale yellow liquid with a spicy odour. Store in well-filled, airtight containers. Protect from light and heat.

Profile

Nutmeg oil is aromatic and carminative and is used as a flavour. Nutmeg oil and expressed nutmeg oil, a solid fat, are rubefacient.

Preparations

BP 2001: Aromatic Ammonia Spirit.

Proprietary Preparations (details are given in Part 3)
Multi-ingredient: *Aust.:* Dr Fischers Melissengeist†; Emser Nasensalbe; Expectal-Balsam; Melissengeist; Pe-Ce; Wick Vaporub; ***Austral.:*** Vicks Vaporub; ***Belg.:*** Vicks Vaporub; ***Braz.:*** Vick Vaporub; ***Canad.:*** Vaporizing Ointment; ***Fr.:*** Vegebom; Vicks Vaporub; ***Ger.:*** Emser Nasensalbe N; ***NZ:*** Vicks Vaporub; ***S.Afr.:*** Enterodyne; ***Swed.:*** Vicks Vaporub; ***Switz.:*** Roliwol†; Vicks Vaporub N; ***Thai.:*** Tiffyrub; ***UK:*** Dragon Balm; No-Sor Vapour Rub.

Nux Vomica (538-h)

Brechnuss; Neuz Vómica; Noce Vomica; Noix Vomique; Strychni Semen.

CAS — 357-57-3 (anhydrous brucine).

Pharmacopoeias. In Aust., Chin., Fr., and Jpn.
Chin. and Fr. also include Powdered Nux Vomica.
Chin. also allows Strychnos pierriana.

The dried ripe seeds of *Strychnos nux-vomica* (Loganiaceae).

Profile

Nux vomica has the actions of strychnine (see p.1667). As well as containing strychnine, nux vomica contains brucine which has similar properties.

Nux vomica (Nux vom.) is used in herbal and homoeopathic medicine for a wide variety of disorders including those of digestion or debility. Ignatia, the dried seed of *Strychnos ignatii,* is also used in homoeopathic medicine where it is known as Ignatia amara or Iamara.

The symbol † denotes a preparation no longer actively marketed

Preparations

Proprietary Preparations (details are given in Part 3)
Multi-ingredient: *Belg.:* Aperop; Sanicolax†; ***Braz.:*** Fargestium; Gotas Digestivas; Kola Fosfatada Soel; ***Fr.:*** Curoveinyl†; ***Ital.:*** Lassatina; ***S.Afr.:*** Peter Pote's†; ***Spain:*** Alofedina; ***Switz.:*** Padma-Lax; ***Thai.:*** Flatulence Gastulence.

Oak Bark (317-l)

Common Oak; Durmast Oak; Écorce de Chêne; Eichenrinde; Quercus; Quercus Cortex.

Pharmacopoeias. In Eur. (see p.vi) and Pol.

Pharmacopoeial description

Ph. Eur.: The cut and dried bark from the fresh young branches of *Quercus robur, Q. petraea,* and *Q. pubescens.* It contains a minimum of 3.0% of tannins, expressed as pyrogallol, calculated with reference to the dried drug.

Profile

Oak bark contains quercitannic acid. It has astringent properties and is used in some herbal and homoeopathic preparations for a variety of disorders. It was formerly used for haemorrhoids and as a gargle.

Preparations

Proprietary Preparations (details are given in Part 3)
Ger.: Traxaton; ***Singapore:*** Urocalun; ***USA:*** Amerigel.
Multi-ingredient: *Aust.:* Menodoron; ***Fr.:*** Tisanes de l'Abbe Hamon no 14†; ***Ger.:*** Tonsilgon N; ***Switz.:*** Kernosan Elixir; ***UK:*** Conchae comp.; Menodoron; Peerless Composition Essence; ***USA:*** Amerigel.

Octanoic Acid (2597-g)

Octanoic Acid (USAN, rINN).
Acidum Caprylicum; Caprylic Acid.
$CH_3.(CH_2)_6.CO_2H = 144.2.$
CAS — 124-07-2.
Pharmacopoeias. In Eur. (see p.vi).

Pharmacopoeial description

Ph. Eur.: A clear, colourless or slightly yellowish, oily liquid. Very slightly soluble in water; very soluble in alcohol and in acetone. It dissolves in dilute solutions of alkali hydroxides.

Sodium Octanoate (3004-t)

Natrii Caprylas; Sodium Caprylate.
$C_8H_{15}NaO_2 = 166.2.$
CAS — 1984-06-1.
Pharmacopoeias. In Eur. (see p.vi).

Pharmacopoeial description

Ph. Eur.: A white crystalline powder. Very soluble or freely soluble in water; sparingly soluble in alcohol; freely soluble in acetic acid; practically insoluble in acetone. A 10% solution in water has a pH of 8.0 to 10.5.

Profile

Octanoic acid and its salts have antifungal activity.
Sodium octanoate is used to stabilise albumin solution against the effects of heat. Octanoic acid labelled with carbon-13 has been used in a breath test to measure‡ gastric emptying.

Preparations

Proprietary Preparations (details are given in Part 3)
Canad.: Capricin†.
Multi-ingredient: *Austral.:* Caprilate.

Octaverine Hydrochloride (13037-r)

Octaverine Hydrochloride (BANM, rINNM).
6,7-Dimethoxy-1-(3,4,5-triethoxyphenyl)isoquinoline hydrochloride.
$C_{23}H_{27}NO_5,HCl = 433.9.$
CAS — 549-68-8 (octaverine); 6775-26-4 (octaverine hydrochloride).

Profile

Octaverine hydrochloride is an analogue of papaverine (p.1648) that has been used as an antispasmodic.

Olaquindox (16936-e)

Olaquindox (BAN, rINN).
Bay-Va-9391. 2-(2-Hydroxyethylcarbamoyl)-3-methylquinoxaline 1,4-dioxide.
$C_{12}H_{13}N_3O_4 = 263.2.$
CAS — 23696-28-8.

Profile

Olaquindox is an antibacterial added to animal feedstuffs as a growth promotor. Photoallergic reactions in animal handlers have been reported following exposure to olaquindox.

Oleander (16134-d)

Common Oleander; Oleanderblätter; Oleandri Folium; Rose Bay.

Profile

Oleander is the dried leaves of the shrub *Nerium oleander* (Apocynaceae), which contain cardioactive glycosides, including oleandrin. It has been used in the treatment of heart disorders. The flowers and bark have been used similarly. Toxicity, similar to that seen with digoxin, may occur following ingestion of any part of the plant; fatalities have been reported. Yellow oleander (*Thevetia peruviana*) also contains cardiac glycosides and exhibits similar toxicity to oleander.

Oleander has also been used in homoeopathic medicine.

◊ References to the treatment of oleander poisoning or yellow oleander poisoning with digoxin-specific antibody fragments (p.1006).
1. Shumaik GM, *et al.* Oleander poisoning: treatment with digoxin-specific Fab antibody fragments. *Ann Emerg Med* 1988; **17:** 732–5.
2. Safadi R, *et al.* Beneficial effect of digoxin-specific Fab antibody fragments in oleander intoxication. *Arch Intern Med* 1995; **155:** 2121–5.
3. Eddleston M, *et al.* Anti-digoxin Fab fragments in cardiotoxicity induced by ingestion of yellow oleander: a randomised controlled trial. *Lancet* 2000; **355:** 967–72.

Preparations

Proprietary Preparations (details are given in Part 3)
Multi-ingredient: *Ger.:* Miroton; Venopyronum N triplex†.

Olive Oil (7363-v)

Azeite; Olivae Oleum.

Pharmacopoeias. In Jpn. Also in USNF. Fr. also includes olive leaves. Eur. (see p.vi) includes monographs for Virgin Olive Oil and Refined Olive Oil.

Pharmacopoeial description

Ph. Eur.: Virgin olive oil is the fatty oil obtained by cold expression or other suitable mechanical means from the ripe drupes of *Olea europaea.* It is a clear, yellow or greenish-yellow, transparent liquid with a characteristic odour. When cooled it begins to become cloudy at 10° and becomes a butter-like mass at 0°. Practically insoluble in alcohol; miscible with petroleum spirit (50° to 70°). Store in well-filled containers at a temperature not exceeding 25°. Protect from light.

Refined olive oil is the fatty oil obtained by refining of crude olive oil. A suitable antioxidant may be added. It is a clear, colourless, or greenish-yellow, transparent liquid. When cooled it begins to become cloudy at 10° and becomes a butter-like mass at about 0°. Practically insoluble in alcohol; miscible with petroleum spirit (50° to 70°). Store in well-filled containers at a temperature not exceeding 25°. Protect from light. Store under an inert gas if intended for use in the manufacture of parenteral dosage forms.

USNF 20: Olive oil is the fixed oil obtained from the ripe fruits of *Olea europaea* (Oleaceae). It is a pale yellow, or light greenish-yellow, oily liquid, having a slight characteristic odour. Slightly soluble in alcohol; miscible with carbon disulfide, with chloroform, and with ether. Store in airtight containers at a temperature not exceeding 40°.

Profile

When taken internally, olive oil is nutrient, demulcent, and mildly laxative. It may also be given rectally (100 to 500 mL warmed to about 32°) to soften impacted faeces (p.1202).

Externally, olive oil is emollient and soothing to inflamed surfaces, and is employed to soften the skin and crusts in eczema (p.1105) and psoriasis (p.1106), and as a lubricant for massage. It is used to soften ear wax.

Olive oil is used in the preparation of liniments, ointments, plasters, and soaps; it is also used as a vehicle for oily suspensions for injection.

Epidemiological evidence points to the cardiovascular benefits of olive oil in the diet.

Preparations

BP 2001: Olive Oil Ear Drops.

Proprietary Preparations (details are given in Part 3)
Multi-ingredient: *Austral.:* Egozite Cream†; ***Belg.:*** Clinoleic; ***Braz.:*** Quelodin; Steitonit; ***Denm.:*** Clinoleic; ***Fin.:*** Clinoleic; ***Fr.:*** Clinoleic; ***Ger.:*** Baran-mild N; Befelka-Oel; Clinoleic; Dr. Hotz Vollbad†; ***Ital.:*** Clinoleic; Prexene†; ***Spain:*** Aceite Acalorico; Clinoleic; ***UK:*** Clinoleic; Exzem Oil; Snor-Away; Snorenz.

Ololiuqui (5018-a)

CAS — 2889-26-1 (isoergine); 478-94-4 (ergine); 2390-99-0 (chanoclavine); 548-43-6 (elymoclavine); 602-85-7 (lysergol).

The seeds of *Rivea corymbosa* or *Ipomoea tricolor* (= *I. violacea*) both convolvulaceous plants similar to the garden plant 'morning glory', *Ipomoea purpurea.* The brown seeds of *R. corymbosa* are known as 'badoh' and the black seeds of *I. tricolor* as 'badoh negro'.

Profile

Ololiuqui has hallucinogenic properties and is considered to be sacred by some Mexican Indians. Alkaloidal fractions contain at least 5 closely related individual components, viz. D-isolysergic acid amide (isoergine), D-lysergic acid amide (ergine), chanoclavine, elymoclavine, and lysergol.

The name 'ololiuqui' has been erroneously applied to seeds of *Datura meteloides* (Solanaceae).

Onion (13040-c)

The bulb of *Allium cepa* (Liliaceae).

Profile

Onion has been reported to reduce platelet aggregation, lower serum cholesterol, and to enhance fibrinolysis. It has been used in preparations for the treatment of urinary-tract disorders and in topical preparations for scars and contractures.

Onion is used in homoeopathic medicine.

Cardiovascular disease. A review of controlled studies purporting to show beneficial effects of garlic and/or onion on cardiovascular risk factors found those studies to have severe methodological failings.[1]

1. Kleijnen J, *et al.* Garlic, onions and cardiovascular risk factors: a review of the evidence from human experiments with emphasis on commercially available preparations. *Br J Clin Pharmacol* 1989; **28**: 535–44.

Stings. An onion bulb was used to treat the wound caused by a blue-spotted stingray (*Dasyatis kuhlii*).[1] Pain relief occurred within 30 minutes.

1. Whiting SD, Guinea ML. Treating stingray wounds with onions. *Med J Aust* 1998; **168**: 584.

Preparations

Proprietary Preparations (details are given in Part 3)
USA: Mederma.

Multi-ingredient: *Aust.:* Contractubex; *Austral.:* Garlic Allium Complex; *Belg.:* Pelvo Magnesium; *Ger.:* Contractubex; *Hong Kong:* Contractubex; *Switz.:* Contractubex.

Ononis (13041-k)

Arrête-Boeuf; Hauhechelwurzel; Racine de Bugrane; Radix Ononidis; Restharrow Root; Spiny Restharrow.
Pharmacopoeias. In *Eur.* (see p.vi).

Pharmacopoeial description

Ph. Eur.: The whole or cut, dried root of *Ononis spinosa*.

Profile

Ononis has diuretic activity and has been used in herbal preparations for the treatment of oedema, urinary-tract disorders, rheumatic disorders, and constipation.

Preparations

Proprietary Preparations (details are given in Part 3)

Multi-ingredient: *Aust.:* Aktiv Blasen- und Nierentee; Aponatura Entwasserungs; Bio-Garten Tee zur Erhohung der Harnmenge; Blasen-Tee; Harntreibender Tee; Kneipp Nieren- und Blasen-Tee; Krauter Hustensaft; Krauterdoktor Harnstein- und Nierengriesstropfen; Krauterhaus Mag Kottas Blasentee; Krauterhaus Mag Kottas Entschlackungstee; Krauterhaus Mag Kottas Nierentee; Krautertee Nr 18; Krautertee Nr 204; Krautertee Nr 25; Krautertee Nr 30; Mag Kottas Nieren-Blasentee; Naturland Entschlackung; Nierentee; Sanvita Entschlackungstonikum†; Solisan; St Radegunder Entwasserungstee; St Radegunder Nierentee; Teekanne Blasen- und Nierentee; Uropurat; *Fr.:* Schoum; *Ger.:* Alasenn; Aqualibra; Befelka-Tinktur†; Blasen-Nieren-Tee Stada†; Eupond†; Harntee 400; Hevert-Blasen- und Nieren- Tee; Hevert-Entwasserungs-Tee†; Hevert-Gicht-Rheuma-Tee comp†; Heweberberol-Tee; Kneipp Blasen- und Nieren-Tee; nephro-loges; Nephronorm med†; Nephroselect M; Nieron Blasen- und Nieren-Tee VI; Nieron-Tee N; Presselin Nieren-Blasen K 3; Reducelle†; Renob Blasen- und Nierentee; Ullus Blasen-Nieren-Tee N; Urodil Blasen-Nieren Arzneitee†; Uvirgan N; *Ital.:* Soluzione Schoum; *Switz.:* Demonatur Dragees pour les reins et la vessie; Dragees pour reins et vessie S; Nephrosolid N; Phytomed Nephro†; Prosta-Caps Chassot N.

Orange Oil (4680-k)

Arancia Dolce Essenza; Essence of Orange; Essence of Portugal; Essência de Laranja; Sweet Orange Oil.

NOTE. The oil from the flowers of *Citrus aurantium* var. *amara* is known as neroli oil or orange flower oil (p.1640).
Pharmacopoeias. In *Br.*, *Fr.*, *It.*, and *Jpn.*

Pharmacopoeial description

BP 2001: A yellow to yellowish-brown liquid, visibly free from water, with an odour of orange, obtained by mechanical means from the fresh peel of the sweet orange *Citrus sinensis*, containing not less than 1% w/w of aldehydes, calculated as decanal ($C_{10}H_{20}O$). Soluble 1 in 7 of alcohol (90%). Store in well-filled containers at a temperature not exceeding 25°. Protect from light.

Profile

Orange oil is used as a flavour and in perfumery. It is used in

the preparation of terpeneless orange oil. Photosensitivity reactions have been reported with citrus oils.

Preparations

Proprietary Preparations (details are given in Part 3)
Multi-ingredient: *Hong Kong:* Magesto; *Switz.:* Pinimenthol; *Thai.:* Magesto.

Terpeneless Orange Oil (4681-a)

Oleum Aurantii Deterpenatum.
Pharmacopoeias. In *Br.*

It consists chiefly of the free alcohols (+)-linalol and (+)-terpineol.

Pharmacopoeial description

BP 2001: A clear yellow or orange-yellow liquid, visibly free from water, with the odour and taste of orange, prepared by concentrating orange oil under reduced pressure until most of the terpenes have been removed, or by solvent partition. It contains not less than 18% w/w of aldehydes calculated as decanal, $C_{10}H_{20}O$. Soluble 1 in 1 of alcohol (90%). Store in well-filled containers at a temperature not exceeding 25°. Protect from light.

Profile

Terpeneless orange oil is used as a flavour. It is stronger in flavour and more readily soluble than the natural oil. Photosensitivity is associated with citrus oils.

Preparations

BP 2001: Compound Orange Spirit.

Dried Bitter-Orange Peel (4682-t)

Aurantii Amari Cortex; Aurantii Cortex Siccatus; Corteza de Naranja Amarga; Écorce de Bigaradier; Flavedo Aurantii Amara; Pericarpium Aurantii; Pomeranzenschale.
Pharmacopoeias. In *Eur.* (see p.vi) and *Jpn.*

Pharmacopoeial description

Ph. Eur.: The dried epicarp and mesocarp of the ripe fruit of *Citrus aurantium*, partly freed from the white spongy tissue of the mesocarp and endocarp, containing a minimum of 2.0% v/w of essential oil, calculated with reference to the anhydrous drug. It has an aromatic odour and a spicy bitter taste.

Profile

Dried bitter-orange peel is used as a flavour and for its bitter and carminative properties. Photosensitivity is associated with citrus oils.

◊ *Citrus aurantium* was one of the most frequently used herbal remedies in Puerto Rico.[1] Indications included sleep disorders, gastrointestinal disorders, respiratory ailments, and raised blood pressure.
The volatile oil of dried bitter-orange peel has shown antifungal activity.[2]

1. Hernández L, *et al.* Use of medicinal plants by ambulatory patients in Puerto Rico. *Am J Hosp Pharm* 1984; **41**: 2060–4.
2. Ramadan W, *et al.* Oil of bitter orange: new topical antifungal agent. *Int J Dermatol* 1996; **35**: 448–9.

Preparations

BP 2001: Concentrated Compound Gentian Infusion; Concentrated Orange Peel Infusion; Orange Peel Infusion; Orange Syrup; *Ph. Eur.:* Bitter-Orange-Epicarp and Mesocarp Tincture.

Proprietary Preparations (details are given in Part 3)
Ger.: Carvomin Magentropfen mit Pomeranze.

Multi-ingredient: *Aust.:* Aponatura Starkungs; Bio-Garten Tee zur Starkung und Kraftigung; Bronchiplant; Bronchiplant light; China-Eisenwein; Digestol; Ferrovin-Eisenelixier; Krauterdoktor Entschlackungs-Elixier; Krauterhaus Mag Kottas Tee fur die Verdauung; Krauterhaus Mag Kottas Tee gegen Durchfall; Krautertee Nr 210; Krautertee Nr 217; Mariazeller; Montana; Sigman-Haustropfen; St Radegunder Entschlackungs-Elixier; St Radegunder Verdauungstee; *Belg.:* Aperop; *Braz.:* Catuaba; *Fr.:* Antigoutteux Rezall†; Élixir Bonjean; Elixir Grez; Mediflor Tisane Calmante Troubles du Sommeil No 14†; Quintonine; Santane V₃; *Ger.:* Carminativum-Hetterich N; Doppelherz Melissengeist; Gastrosecur; Meteophyt S; Montana; Salusan†; Sedovent; Stomachicon N; Valeriana comp; *Ital.:* Depurativo; Rabarbaroni; *Spain:* Agua del Carmen; *Switz.:* Pastilles pectorales Demo N.

Orazamide (13042-a)

Orazamide (*rINN*).
AICA Orotate; Oroxamide. 5-Aminoimidazole-4-carboxamide orotate dihydrate.
$C_9H_{10}N_6O_5,2H_2O = 318.2$.
CAS — 2574-78-9 (anhydrous orazamide); 60104-30-5 (orazamide dihydrate).

Profile

Orazamide has been given by mouth in the treatment of liver disorders. AICA riboside, a ribonucleoside analogue, has been investigated for its cardioprotective activity.

◊ References.
1. Dixon R, *et al.* AICA-riboside: safety, tolerance, and pharmacokinetics of a novel adenosine-regulating agent. *J Clin Pharmacol* 1991; **31**: 342–7.

Preparations

Proprietary Preparations (details are given in Part 3)
Belg.: Aicamin†; *Port.:* Aicamin.
Multi-ingredient: *Port.:* Oraica.

Orlistat (10352-p)

Orlistat (*BAN, USAN, rINN*).
Orlipastat; Ro-18-0647; Ro-18-0647/002; Tetrahydrolipstatin. N-Formyl-L-leucine, ester with (3S,4S)-3-hexyl-4-[(2S)-2-hydroxytridecyl]-2-oxetanone; (S)-1-[(2S,3S)-3-Hexyl-4-oxo-oxetan-2-ylmethyl]dodecyl N-formyl-L-leucinate.
$C_{29}H_{53}NO_5 = 495.7$.
CAS — 96829-58-2.
ATC — A08AB01.

Adverse Effects

Gastrointestinal disturbances, including faecal urgency and incontinence, flatulence, and fatty stools or discharge, are the most frequently reported adverse effects during treatment with orlistat. They may be minimised by limiting the amount of fat in the diet. Other reported side-effects have included headache, anxiety, fatigue, and menstrual irregularities. There have been concerns about an increased risk of breast cancer in patients taking orlistat but the manufacturers consider that there is no evidence of a causal link.

Effects on the cardiovascular system. A report of hypertension associated with orlistat therapy.[1] Blood pressure decreased on discontinuing orlistat and increased again on rechallenge. The authors noted that 13 cases of hypertension associated with orlistat had been reported to the manufacturers.

1. Persson M, *et al.* Orlistat associated with hypertension. *BMJ* 2000; **321**: 87.

Precautions

Orlistat should not be given to patients with chronic malabsorption syndrome or cholestasis and should be given with caution to diabetic patients. Supplements of fat-soluble vitamins may be necessary during long-term therapy, but they should be taken at least 2 hours before or after an orlistat dose or at bedtime.

Interactions

Orlistat may reduce the absorption of fat-soluble vitamins. The manufacturer recommends that concomitant administration with acarbose or anorectic drugs should be avoided. In patients receiving warfarin, international normalised ratio should be monitored during treatment with orlistat. A reduction in ciclosporin concentrations to subtherapeutic levels has been reported in transplant recipients following concomitant administration of orlistat (see p.522). Orlistat has been reported to elevate plasma concentrations of pravastatin, and monitoring has therefore been recommended to avoid a potential increase in adverse effects of the latter.

Pharmacokinetics

Orlistat is minimally absorbed following oral administration.

Uses and Administration

Orlistat is a gastric and pancreatic lipase inhibitor that limits the absorption of dietary fat. It is used in conjunction with dietary modification in the management of obesity (p.1505), i.e. in patients with a body mass index of 30 kg per m² or greater. It may also be used in overweight patients with a body mass index of 28 kg per m² or more if there are associated risk factors. Treatment with orlistat should only be started once the patient has achieved a weight loss of at least 2.5 kg over 4 consecutive weeks as a result of diet alone. Orlistat is given in a usual dose of 120 mg by mouth three times daily, immediately before, during, or up to 1 hour after meals. If a meal is missed or contains no fat, the dose should be omitted. Orlistat therapy should be discontinued if the patient does not lose at least 5% of their body-weight during the first 12 weeks of therapy. Long-term therapy should not continue beyond 2 years.

◊ References.
1. Davidson MH, *et al.* Weight control and risk factor reduction in obese subjects treated for 2 years with orlistat: a randomized controlled trial. *JAMA* 1999; **281**: 235–42. Correction. *ibid.*; 1174.
2. Hvizdos KM, Markham A. Orlistat: a review of its use in the management of obesity. *Drugs* 1999; **58**: 743–60.
3. Heymsfield SB, *et al.* Effects of weight loss with orlistat on glucose tolerance and progression to type 2 diabetes in obese adults. *Arch Intern Med* 2000; **160**: 1321–6.
4. Finer N, *et al.* One-year treatment of obesity: a randomized, double-blind, placebo-controlled, multicentre study of orlistat, a gastrointestinal lipase inhibitor. *Int J Obes Relat Metab Disord* 2000; **24**: 306–13.
5. Rossner S, *et al.* Weight loss, weight maintenance, and improved cardiovascular risk factors after 2 years treatment with orlistat for obesity. *Obes Res* 2000; **8**: 49–61.
6. Heck AM, *et al.* Orlistat, a new lipase inhibitor for the management of obesity. *Pharmacotherapy* 2000; **20**: 270–9.

Preparations

Proprietary Preparations (details are given in Part 3)
Aust.: Xenical; *Austral.:* Xenical; *Belg.:* Xenical; *Canad.:* Xenical; *Denm.:* Xenical; *Fin.:* Xenical; *Fr.:* Xenical; *Ger.:* Xenical; *Irl.:* Xenical; *Ital.:* Xenical; *Mex.:* Xenical; *Neth.:* Xenical; *NZ:*

Xenical; *Port.*: Xenical; *S.Afr.*: Xenical; *Singapore:* Xenical; *Spain:* Xenical; *Swed.*: Xenical; *Switz.*: Xenical; *Thai.*: Xenical; *UK:* Xenical; *USA:* Xenical.

Ornicarbase (13044-x)

Ornithine Carbamoyltransferase.
CAS — 9001-69-8.

Profile
Ornicarbase has been used in hepatic disorders. Hypersensitivity reactions have occurred occasionally.

Orotic Acid (13045-r)

Orotic Acid *(BAN, pINN)*.
Animal Galactose Factor; Uracil-6-carboxylic Acid; Whey Factor. 1,2,3,6-Tetrahydro-2,6-dioxopyrimidine-4-carboxylic acid.
$C_5H_4N_2O_4 = 156.1$.
CAS — 65-86-1 (anhydrous orotic acid); 50887-69-9 (orotic acid monohydrate).

Profile
Orotic acid occurs naturally in the body; it is found in milk. It is an intermediate in the biosynthesis of pyrimidine nucleotides. Orotic acid and its calcium, choline, lithium, lysine, magnesium, and potassium salts have been used in liver disorders. Some of these salts, chromium orotate, cyproheptadine orotate, and deanol orotate, have been given as tonics or dietary supplements. Magnesium and ferrous orotates have been used as mineral sources.

Preparations
Proprietary Preparations (details are given in Part 3)
Ger.: magnerot Classic; Magnesorot; Power Orot.

Multi-ingredient: *Aust.:* Kavaform; Lemazol; Prospervital†; *Austral.:* Bioglan Bioage Peripheral; Mag-Oro; Magnesium Plus; *Ger.:* Antisklerosin S; Hepatofalk; Hepatofalk Neu; Neuro-Wied; *Hong Kong:* Hepatofalk; Lipochol; Tres Orix Forte; *Ital.:* Epa-Treis; Oro B12; *Mex.:* Lipovitasi-Or; *Port.:* Oraica; *S.Afr.:* Hepabionta; *Spain:* Antibiofilus; Hepadif; Hepato Fardi; Tres Orix Forte; *Switz.:* Kawaform; Magnesium Complexe; Vigoran; *Thai.:* Lipochol; *UK:* Cardeymin; Sugar Bloc.

Orthodichlorobenzene (3598-z)

1,2-Dichlorobenzene.
$C_6H_4Cl_2 = 147.0$.
CAS — 95-50-1.

Profile
Orthodichlorobenzene has been used as a wood and furniture preservative. It has also been used as an ingredient of solutions for dissolving ear wax. It is an irritant volatile liquid; lens opacities have occurred.

Preparations
Proprietary Preparations (details are given in Part 3)
Multi-ingredient: *Austral.:* Cerumol; *Switz.:* Cerumenol.

Oryzanol (13046-f)

Gamma Oryzanol; γ-Oryzanol; γ-OZ. Triacontanyl 3-(4-hydroxy-3-methoxyphenyl)prop-2-enoate.
$C_{40}H_{58}O_4 = 602.9$.
CAS — 11042-64-1.

A substance extracted from rice bran oil and rice embryo bud oil.

Profile
Oryzanol has been given by mouth in the treatment of hyperlipidaemias. It has also been used for its supposed effects on autonomic and endocrine function.

◊ References.
1. Yoshino G, *et al.* Effects of gamma-oryzanol on hyperlipidemic subjects. *Curr Ther Res* 1989; **45:** 543–52.
2. Yoshino G, *et al.* Effects of gamma-oryzanol and probucol on hyperlipidemia. *Curr Ther Res* 1989; **45:** 975–82.

Preparations
Proprietary Preparations (details are given in Part 3)
Hong Kong: Gammariza; *Jpn:* Hi-Z†.

Multi-ingredient: *Ital.:* Lenirose; Mavipiu.

Osalmid (3729-w)

Osalmid *(rINN)*.
L-1718; Oxaphenamide. 4′-Hydroxysalicylanilide.
$C_{13}H_{11}NO_3 = 229.2$.
CAS — 526-18-1.

Profile
Osalmid is a choleretic.

The symbol † denotes a preparation no longer actively marketed

Preparations
Proprietary Preparations (details are given in Part 3)
Belg.: Driol†.

Otilonium Bromide (13048-n)

Otilonium Bromide *(BAN, rINN)*.
SP-63. Diethylmethyl{2-[4-(2-octyloxybenzamido)benzoyloxy]ethyl}ammonium bromide.
$C_{29}H_{43}BrN_2O_4 = 563.6$.
CAS — 26095-59-0.
ATC — A03AB06.

Profile
Otilonium bromide is used in the symptomatic treatment of gastrointestinal disorders associated with smooth muscle spasms in doses up to 120 mg daily by mouth. It has also been administered rectally and by nebuliser.

◊ References.
1. Battaglia G, *et al.* Otilonium bromide in irritable bowel syndrome: a double-blind, placebo-controlled, 15-week study. *Aliment Pharmacol Ther* 1998; **12:** 1003–10.

Preparations
Proprietary Preparations (details are given in Part 3)
Belg.: Spasmomen; *Hong Kong:* Spasmomen; *Ital.:* Spasen; Spasmomen; *Spain:* Spasmoctyl.

Multi-ingredient: *Ital.:* Spasen; Spasen Somatico; Spasmomen Somatico.

Oxaceprol (13051-t)

Oxaceprol *(rINN)*.
Acetylhydroxyproline; C061. (–)-1-Acetyl-4-hydroxy-L-proline.
$C_7H_{11}NO_4 = 173.2$.
CAS — 33996-33-7.
ATC — D11AX09; M01AX24.

Profile
Oxaceprol is reported to affect connective-tissue metabolism and has been used in dermatology, to promote wound healing, and in rheumatic disorders. Adverse effects have included gastric pain, nausea, diarrhoea, dizziness, headache, and skin rashes.

◊ References.
1. Bauer HW, *et al.* Oxaceprol is as effective as diclofenac in the therapy of osteoarthritis of the knee and hip. *Clin Rheumatol* 1999; **18:** 4–9.
2. Herrmann G, *et al.* Oxaceprol is a well-tolerated therapy for osteoarthritis with efficacy equivalent to diclofenac. *Clin Rheumatol* 2000; **19:** 99–104.

Preparations
Proprietary Preparations (details are given in Part 3)
Fr.: Jonctum; *Ger.:* AHP 200; *Spain:* Tejuntivo.
Multi-ingredient: *Spain:* Robervital.

Oxalic Acid (1320-z)

$HO_2C,CO_2H,2H_2O = 126.1$.
CAS — 144-62-7 (anhydrous oxalic acid); 6153-56-6 (oxalic acid dihydrate).

Adverse Effects
Following ingestion, severe gastroenteritis is produced by the corrosive action of oxalic acid and its soluble salts on the gastrointestinal tract. Burning of the mouth, throat, and oesophagus with ulceration may also occur. Hypoxia may occur in the presence of laryngeal oedema, and shock and hypotension may arise in severe cases. Oxalates can chelate body calcium following systemic absorption, and may produce symptoms of hypocalcaemia such as tetany, convulsions, and, in some cases, ventricular fibrillation. Oxalate crystals may be deposited in the blood vessels, heart, liver, and lungs; deposition in the renal tubules leads to acute renal failure. The mean fatal dose of oxalates has been reported to be about 15 to 30 g, although death has occurred with much lower doses. Death may occur within a few hours of ingestion.

◊ Fatalities have resulted from intravenous administration of sodium oxalate[1] or ingestion of oxalic acid.[2]
Crystals of calcium oxalate present in the sap of daffodils have been reported[3] to contribute to the rash experienced by commercial pickers.
1. Dvořáčková I. Tödliche Vergiftung nach intravenöser Verabreichung von Natriumoxalat. *Arch Toxikol* 1966; **22:** 63–7.
2. Farré M, *et al.* Fatal oxalic acid poisoning from sorrel soup. *Lancet* 1989; **ii:** 1524.
3. Julian CG, Bowers PW. The nature and distribution of daffodil pickers' rash. *Contact Dermatitis* 1997; **37:** 259–62.

Treatment of Adverse Effects
Following ingestion of oxalic acid, a dilute solution of any soluble calcium salt should be given to precipitate the oxalate; alternatively milk may be given. Oral activated charcoal has also been suggested if ingestion has occurred within 1 hour. Gastric lavage is contra-indicated by some centres given the corrosive nature of oxalic acid. However, others have recommended that if mucosal corrosion has not occurred the stomach may be care-

fully emptied by lavage using large quantities of diluted lime water or dilute solutions of other calcium salts. Calcium gluconate 10% should be given intravenously in doses of 10 mL to prevent tetany. Acute renal failure should be anticipated in surviving patients and calls for careful fluid management. Haemodialysis or peritoneal dialysis have also been suggested for the removal of oxalate in primary oxalosis in an attempt to prevent acute renal failure and correct hypocalcaemia.

Uses
Oxalic acid has varied industrial uses and has been used in escharotic preparations. Oxalic acid salts have been administered by mouth and the urinary excretion of oxalate used as a screening test for lipid malabsorption.

Diagnostic use. References.
1. Rampton DS, *et al.* Screening for steatorrhoea with an oxalate loading test. *BMJ* 1984; **288:** 1419. Correction. *ibid.*; 1728.
2. Sangaletti O, *et al.* Urinary oxalate recovery after oral oxalic acid load: an alternative method to the quantitative determination of stool fat for the diagnosis of lipid malabsorption. *J Int Med Res* 1989; **17:** 526–31.

Preparations
Proprietary Preparations (details are given in Part 3)
Multi-ingredient: *Ger.:* Solco-Derman; *Hong Kong:* Solcoderm; *Switz.:* Solcoderm; Solcogyn.

Oxiracetam (16922-v)

Oxiracetam *(BAN, rINN)*.
CGP-21690E; ISF-2522. 4-Hydroxy-2-oxo-1-pyrrolidineacetamide.
$C_6H_{10}N_2O_3 = 158.2$.
CAS — 62613-82-5.
ATC — N06BX07.

Profile
Oxiracetam has been used as a nootropic in organic brain syndromes and senile dementia.

Dementia. Clinical benefit has been reported in patients with dementia (p.1412) given oxiracetam,[1] but in the USA it was withdrawn from phase II clinical studies in patients with Alzheimer's disease due to lack of efficacy.[2]
1. Maina G, *et al.* Oxiracetam in the treatment of primary degenerative and multi-infarct dementia: a double-blind, placebo-controlled study. *Neuropsychobiology* 1990; **21:** 141–5.
2. Parnetti L. Clinical pharmacokinetics of drugs for Alzheimer's disease. *Clin Pharmacokinet* 1995; **29:** 110–29.

Preparations
Proprietary Preparations (details are given in Part 3)
Ital.: Neuractiv†; Neuromet.

Oxybromonaftoic Acid (13069-g)

4-Bromo-3-hydroxy-2-naphthoic acid.
$C_{11}H_7BrO_3 = 267.1$.
CAS — 2208-15-3.

Profile
Oxybromonaftoic acid has been given by mouth in hepatic disorders.

Ozagrel (19602-y)

Ozagrel *(rINN)*.
OKY-046 (hydrochloride). (E)-p-(imidazol-1-ylmethyl)cinnamic acid.
$C_{13}H_{12}N_2O_2 = 228.2$.
CAS — 82571-53-7.

Profile
Ozagrel is a thromboxane synthetase inhibitor which has been used as the hydrochloride and as the sodium salt in the treatment of asthma and of cerebrovascular disorders.

◊ References.
1. Nagatsuka K, *et al.* A new approach to antithrombotic therapy—evaluation of combined therapy of thromboxane synthetase inhibitor and very low dose of aspirin. *Stroke* 1985; **16:** 806–9.
2. Fujimura M, *et al.* Effects of aerosol administration of a thromboxane synthetase inhibitor (OKY-046) on bronchial responsiveness to acetylcholine in asthmatic subjects. *Chest* 1990; **98:** 276–9.
3. Fujimura M, *et al.* Attenuating effect of a thromboxane synthetase inhibitor (OKY-046) on bronchial responsiveness to methacholine is specific to bronchial asthma. *Chest* 1990; **98:** 656–60.
4. Oishi M, *et al.* Effects of sodium ozagrel on hemostatic markers and cerebral blood flow in lacunar infarction. *Clin Neuropharmacol* 1996; **19:** 526–31.
5. Kato H, *et al.* Treatment of branch retinal arterial occlusion with sodium ozagrel, a thromboxane A2 synthetase inhibitor. *J Int Med Res* 1997; **25:** 108–11.
6. Kunitoh H, *et al.* A double-blind, placebo-controlled trial of the thromboxane synthetase blocker OKY-046 on bronchial hypersensitivity in bronchial asthma patients. *J Asthma* 1998; **35:** 355–60.
7. Seki H, *et al.* Trial of prophylactic administration of TXA2 synthetase inhibitor, ozagrel hydrochloride, for preeclampsia. *Hypertens Pregnancy* 1999; **18:** 157–64.

Preparations

Proprietary Preparations (details are given in Part 3)
Jpn: Cataclot†; Domenan; Vega†; Xanbon.

Palmidrol (14843-y)

Palmidrol *(rINN)*.
N-(2-Hydroxyethyl)palmitamide.
$C_{18}H_{37}NO_2 = 299.5$.
CAS — 544-31-0.

Profile
Palmidrol is a naturally occurring lipid compound which has been used as an immunostimulant. It is given by mouth for the treatment of respiratory-tract infections.

Pancreatin (3731-b)

Pancreatin *(BAN)*.
Pancreatinum.
CAS — 8049-47-6.
Pharmacopoeias. In *Chin.*, *Eur.* (see p.vi), *Jpn*, and *US* as pancreatin or another pancreatic extract or both.

Pharmacopoeial description
Ph. Eur.: Pancreas Powder (Pancreatis Pulvis) is prepared from the fresh or frozen pancreases of mammals. It contains various enzymes having proteolytic, lipolytic, and amylolytic activities. Each mg of pancreas powder contains not less than 1 Ph. Eur. unit of total proteolytic activity, not less than 15 Ph. Eur. units of lipolytic activity, and not less than 12 Ph. Eur. units of amylolytic activity. A slightly brown, amorphous powder. Partly soluble in water; practically insoluble in alcohol and in ether. Store in airtight containers at a temperature not exceeding 15°.

BP 2001: Pancreatin is a preparation of mammalian pancreas containing enzymes having protease, lipase, and amylase activity. Each mg of pancreatin contains not less than 1.4 FIP units of free protease activity, not less than 20 FIP units of lipase activity, and not less than 24 FIP units of amylase activity. It may contain sodium chloride. A white or buff amorphous powder, free from unpleasant odour. Soluble or partly soluble in water forming a slightly turbid solution; practically insoluble in alcohol and in ether. Store at a temperature not exceeding 15°.

USP 25: A substance containing enzymes, principally amylase, lipase, and protease, obtained from the pancreas of the hog or of the ox. It is a cream-coloured, amorphous powder, having a faint, characteristic, but not offensive odour. Its greatest activities are in neutral or faintly alkaline media; more than traces of mineral acids or large amounts of alkali hydroxides make it inert. An excess of alkali carbonate also inhibits its action.
Pancreatin contains, in each mg, not less than 25 USP units of amylase activity, not less than 2 USP units of lipase activity, and not less than 25 USP units of protease activity. Pancreatin of a higher digestive power may be labelled as a whole-number multiple of the 3 minimum activities, or may be diluted with lactose, or with sucrose containing not more than 3.25% of starch, or with pancreatin of lower digestive power. Store in airtight containers at a temperature not exceeding 30°.

Units
The Ph. Eur. and USP 25 units of protease activity depend upon the rate of hydrolysis of casein, those of lipase activity depend upon the rate of hydrolysis of olive oil, and those of amylase activity depend upon the rate of hydrolysis of starch. Because of differences in the assay conditions, the Ph. Eur. and USP 25 units are not readily comparable.

FIP units of protease, lipase, and amylase activity are equivalent to Ph. Eur. units.

Adverse Effects and Precautions
Pancreatin commonly causes gastrointestinal side-effects such as abdominal discomfort and nausea and vomiting. It may also cause buccal and perianal soreness, particularly in infants. Colonic strictures (fibrosing colonopathy) have occurred, mainly in children with cystic fibrosis receiving high doses of pancreatin preparations; the use of high doses in patients with cystic fibrosis should preferably be avoided (see Effects on the Gastrointestinal Tract, below). Adequate hydration should be maintained at all times in patients receiving higher strength preparations.

Hypersensitivity reactions have been reported; these may be sneezing, lachrymation, or skin rashes. Hyperuricaemia or hyperuricosuria have occurred with high doses. There have been occasional reports of the contamination of pancreatin preparations with *Salmonella* spp.

Effects on folic acid. Pancreatic extract significantly inhibited folate absorption in healthy subjects and in pancreatic insufficient patients.[1] Testing *in vitro* showed that pancreatic extract formed insoluble complexes with folate. Patients being treated for pancreatic insufficiency should be monitored for folate status or given folic acid supplementation, particularly if pancreatic enzymes and bicarbonate (or cimetidine) were being used together in the treatment regimen.

1. Russell RM, *et al.* Impairment of folic acid absorption by oral pancreatic extracts. *Dig Dis Sci* 1980; **25:** 369–73.

Effects on the gastrointestinal tract. FIBROSING COLONOPATHY. Following the introduction of high-strength pancreatic enzyme preparations, there were a number of reports[1-6] of colonic strictures in children with cystic fibrosis who received these formulations, and the problem was reviewed.[7,8] The pathogenesis and aetiology of this condition, which has since been termed fibrosing colonopathy, still remain unclear. Dose-related thickening of the colon wall has been described,[9] and an inflammatory or immune-mediated mechanism has been suggested.[10,11] It has been suggested that the presence of intact enteric-coated granules in the colon[12] and possibly a direct effect of components of the methylacrylic acid copolymer (MAC) used in the enteric coating could be responsible[12,13] but at least one case of fibrosing colonopathy has been reported in a child receiving a standard strength preparation which did not contain this coating material.[14] An analysis[15] of cases of fibrosing colonopathy occurring in the UK between 1984 and 1994 demonstrated that there was a dose-related association between the high-strength preparations and this adverse effect, and the results were confirmed by a case-control study[16] of patients in the US presenting between 1990 and 1994. However, re-analysis[17] of the UK data found a highly statistically significant association with the intake of MAC-coated preparations, but no evidence that a high intake of lipase in the absence of MAC was a risk factor for the disease. As a result of these problems, high-strength preparations were withdrawn in the USA, while in the UK, the Committee on Safety of Medicines recommended[18] that unless special reasons exist, patients with cystic fibrosis should not use high-strength pancreatin preparations, and that all patients treated with these products should be monitored carefully for gastrointestinal obstruction. The Committee subsequently elaborated on these recommendations:[19] they advised that Nutrizym 22, Pancrease HL, and Panzytrat 25 000 should not be used in children with cystic fibrosis who were aged 15 years or less; that the total daily dose of pancreatic enzyme supplements for patients with cystic fibrosis should not exceed 10 000 units of lipase activity per kg body-weight; and that patients on any pancreatin preparation should be reviewed to exclude colonic damage if new abdominal symptoms or a change in symptoms occurred. The US Cystic Fibrosis Foundation has made recommendations for the management of patients who do not respond adequately to moderate doses of pancreatic enzymes,[20] and similar recommendations have been made in the UK.[21] Fibrosing colonopathy has also been reported[22] in an adult who was not thought to have cystic fibrosis, but who had been taking high doses of pancreatic enzyme supplements following surgical removal of the pancreas, including two with MAC coatings, for five years.

1. Smyth RL, *et al.* Strictures of ascending colon in cystic fibrosis and high-strength pancreatic enzymes. *Lancet* 1994; **343:** 85–6.
2. Oades PJ, *et al.* High-strength pancreatic enzyme supplements and large-bowel stricture in cystic fibrosis. *Lancet* 1994; **343:** 109.
3. Campbell CA, *et al.* High-strength pancreatic enzyme supplements and large-bowel stricture in cystic fibrosis. *Lancet* 1994; **343:** 109–110.
4. Mahony MJ, Corcoran M. High-strength pancreatic enzymes. *Lancet* 1994; **343:** 599–600.
5. Knabe N, *et al.* Extensive pathological changes of the colon in cystic fibrosis and high-strength pancreatic enzymes. *Lancet* 1994; **343:** 1230.
6. Pettei MJ, *et al.* Pancolonic disease in cystic fibrosis and high-dose pancreatic enzyme therapy. *J Pediatr* 1994; **125:** 587–9.
7. Taylor CJ. Colonic strictures in cystic fibrosis. *Lancet* 1994; **343:** 615–16. Correction. *ibid.;* 1108.
8. Taylor CJ. The problems with high dose pancreatic enzyme preparations. *Drug Safety* 1994; **11:** 75–9.
9. MacSweeney EJ, *et al.* Relationship of thickening of colon wall to pancreatic-enzyme treatment in cystic fibrosis. *Lancet* 1995; **345:** 752–6.
10. Croft NM, *et al.* Gut inflammation in children with cystic fibrosis on high-dose enzyme supplements. *Lancet* 1995; **346:** 1265–7.
11. Lee J, *et al.* Is fibrosing colonopathy an immune mediated disease? *Arch Dis Child* 1997; **77:** 66–70.
12. Jones R, *et al.* Colonic strictures in children with cystic fibrosis on low-strength pancreatic enzymes. *Lancet* 1995; **346:** 499.
13. van Velzen D. Colonic strictures in children with cystic fibrosis on low-strength pancreatic enzymes. *Lancet* 1995; **346:** 499–500.
14. Taylor CJ, Steiner GM. Fibrosing colonopathy in a child on low-dose pancreatin. *Lancet* 1995; **345:** 1106–7.
15. Smyth RL. Fibrosing colonopathy in cystic fibrosis: results of a case-control study. *Lancet* 1995; **346:** 1247–51.
16. FitzSimmons SC, *et al.* High-dose pancreatic-enzyme supplements and fibrosing colonopathy in children with cystic fibrosis. *N Engl J Med* 1997; **336:** 1283–9.
17. Prescott P, Bakowski MT. Pathogenesis of fibrosing colonopathy: the role of methacrylic acid copolymer. *Pharmacoepidemiol Drug Safety* 1999; **8:** 377–84.
18. Committee on Safety of Medicines/Medicines Control Agency. Update: bowel strictures and high-potency pancreatins. *Current Problems* 1994; **20:** 13.
19. Committee on Safety of Medicines/Medicines Control Agency. Fibrosing colonopathy associated with pancreatic enzymes. *Current Problems* 1995; **21:** 11.
20. Borowitz DS, *et al.* Use of pancreatic enzyme supplements for patients with cystic fibrosis in the context of fibrosing colonopathy. *J Pediatr* 1995; **127:** 681–4.
21. Littlewood JM. Fibrosing colonopathy in cystic fibrosis: commentary, implications of the Committee on Safety of Medicines 10 000 IU lipase/kg/day recommendation for use of pancreatic enzymes in cystic fibrosis. *Arch Dis Child* 1996; **74:** 466–8.
22. Bansi DS, *et al.* Fibrosing colonopathy in an adult owing to over use of pancreatic enzyme supplements. *Gut* 2000; **46:** 283–5.

MOUTH ULCERATION. In 3 children taking preparations of pancreatic extracts (Pancrex V powder, Pancrex V Forte), severe mouth ulceration and angular stomatitis, causing dysphagia,

loss of weight, and pyrexia, were attributed to digestion of the mucous membrane due to retention of the preparations in the mouth before swallowing.[1]

1. Darby CW. Pancreatic extracts. *BMJ* 1970; **2:** 299–300.

Hypersensitivity. A successful desensitisation regimen has been described[1] for a child with cystic fibrosis who vomited within 1 to 2 hours after ingestion of pancreatic enzymes, suggestive of a type I hypersensitivity reaction.

1. Chamarthy LM, *et al.* Desensitization to pancreatic enzyme intolerance in a child with cystic fibrosis. Abstract: *Pediatrics* 1998; **102:** 134–5. Full version: http://www.pediatrics.org/cgi/content/full/102/1/e13

Uses and Administration
Pancreatin hydrolyses fats to glycerol and fatty acids, breaks down protein into peptides, proteoses and derived substances, and converts starch into dextrins and sugars. It is given by mouth in conditions of pancreatic exocrine deficiency such as pancreatitis and cystic fibrosis. It is available in the form of powder, capsules containing powder or enteric-coated granules (which may be opened before use and the contents sprinkled on the food), enteric-coated tablets, or granules. If pancreatin is mixed with liquids or food the resulting mixture should not be allowed to stand for more than 1 hour prior to use. Histamine H_2-receptor antagonists, such as cimetidine or ranitidine, have been given an hour before administration of pancreatin in an attempt to lessen destruction of pancreatin by the gastric acids; alternatively, antacids may be administered concurrently.

The dose of pancreatin is adjusted according to the needs of the individual patient and will also depend on the dosage form. In the UK doses of up to about 56 000 units of lipase activity (with varying proportions of protease and amylase activity, depending on the preparation) have been given with each meal. In the USA doses providing up to 45 000 USP units of lipase activity have been given with each meal. So called high-strength or high-potency preparations are available for those receiving high doses, but their use has been associated with the development of fibrosing colonopathy in children with cystic fibrosis (see above). Such preparations are consequently not recommended for children in the UK and authorities there consider the total daily dose of pancreatic supplements for patients with cystic fibrosis should not exceed 10 000 units of lipase activity per kg body-weight.

Pancreatin is also used to remove protein deposits from the surface of soft contact lenses (p.1129).

Cystic fibrosis. Patients with cystic fibrosis (p.117) suffer from pancreatic insufficiency and consequent malabsorption. Pancreatin or pancrelipase may therefore play a role in the management of the disorder, being taken before or with each meal or snack.

Pancreatitis. Pancreatitis is an inflammatory process affecting the pancreas. Acute pancreatitis comprises necrosis of pancreatic tissue occurring in an otherwise healthy gland, whereas chronic pancreatitis is the manifestation of pathological processes resulting in inflammation and progressive fibrosis of pancreatic tissue. Acute disease may be superimposed on a background of chronic pancreatitis.

Acute pancreatitis is frequently associated with either biliary tract disorders (such as gallstones or cholecystitis) or the intake of large amounts of alcohol, or less frequently with abdominal surgery, pancreatic trauma, hyperparathyroidism, hyperlipidaemia, infection, or the adverse effects of drugs. Symptoms include pain, which ranges from mild to extremely severe and which typically persists for several days, nausea and vomiting, ileus, and hypovolaemic shock. In severe disease, pulmonary, renal, and hepatic failure, encephalopathy, and death may ensue. A mortality rate of about 10% has been reported.

The management of acute disease is essentially supportive. Adequate analgesia for pain is important (see Pancreatic Pain, p.7); in mild cases, analgesia, adequate hydration, and temporary interruption of oral intake of food to 'rest' the pancreas may be adequate. Since most patients suffer from hypoxaemia it has been recommended that they should receive additional humidified oxygen by mask, with mechanical ventilation if blood gases indicate the development of severe pulmonary failure. Shock should be managed with blood or plasma, and electrolyte solutions, while insulin may be required for disturbances of glucose homoeostasis.

The value of other interventions is mostly doubtful. As an extension of the concept of 'pancreatic rest' inhibitors of pancreatic secretion such as somatostatin or octreotide have been tried but without significant effect, while protease inhibitors such as aprotinin or gabexate mesilate have also proven disappointing,[1] perhaps because activation of pancreatic proteases (thought to play a significant role in pathogenesis) has already taken place by the time therapy is begun.[1] Preliminary studies of the platelet-activating factor antagonist lexipafant have been more promising. Although prophylactic antibacterials are often given, there has been some uncertainty about their value.[2] However, a study in patients with acute necrotising pancreatitis indicated markedly reduced mortality in those given prophylactic antibacterials (initially cefuroxime),[3] and a retrospective study[4] reported a reduction in the incidence, but not in the time of onset, of infection in those receiving such drugs. In a review[5] of the treatment of acute necrotising pancreatitis, it was pointed out that early studies that failed to demonstrate any benefit of prophylactic antibacterials had also included patients with interstitial oedematous acute pancreatitis. The authors emphasised that the prevention of infection is critical in acute necrotising pancreatitis, since the development of infected necrosis substantially increases mortality, and concluded that use of antibacterials is the mainstay of management in such patients. Peritoneal dialysis reduces early complications of acute pancreatitis but increases the risk of subsequent infection and has no overall effect on survival.[2] The role of surgery continues to be somewhat controversial; it is accepted for complications or when a potential surgical emergency exists. Surgery to remove gallstones may be carried out once pancreatitis has resolved, but surgical intervention during acute episodes may increase morbidity and mortality. Early endoscopic decompression of the obstructed bile duct may be beneficial in patients with cholangitis or progressive jaundice but not in those without biliary obstruction.[6]

Chronic pancreatitis is frequently associated with high alcohol-intake although a tropical form, associated with malnutrition, also exists, and some cases are idiopathic. Symptoms include recurrent episodes of pain (often less excruciating and of shorter duration than in acute pancreatitis) which normally become less severe and frequent over the years with the inexorable progression of fibrosis. Loss of exocrine tissue eventually leads in many patients to pancreatic exocrine insufficiency, with maldigestion and steatorrhoea, and in some to diabetes mellitus due to islet cell loss. Other symptoms may include cholestatic jaundice, fatty degeneration of the liver, stenosis of the bile duct, and hepatic cirrhosis (although this may also be due to alcohol intake). It has been estimated that more than 50% of patients die within 20 years of diagnosis, with those who continue to drink alcohol being at greatest risk.

Adequate analgesia with opioids is essential (see Pancreatic Pain, p.7). Nerve blocks of the coeliac plexus with phenol or alcohol may be helpful, and there is a report of a response to danazol.[7] Patients should be advised to abstain from alcohol, which can exacerbate the frequency and severity of painful episodes. Steatorrhoea requires replacement of pancreatic enzymes with preparations of pancreatin or pancrelipase. Because the enzymes are inactivated by gastric acid they may be taken after histamine H_2 antagonists or with a sodium-containing antacid such as sodium bicarbonate (magnesium-, calcium-, and, according to some authorities, aluminium-containing antacids may further interfere with fat absorption). Alternatively, enteric-coated enzyme preparations may be used. In some patients with mild disease pancreatic enzyme replacement may also improve pain. Supplements of fat-soluble vitamins are not normally necessary, but may be given intravenously if required. Diabetes should be managed appropriately once steatorrhoea is under control.

Surgery, up to and including total pancreatectomy, has an important role in the relief of intractable pain, and may also be necessary for the management of complications. Endoscopic decompression using contrast media containing prednisolone and ulinastatin has been reported to produce beneficial responses.[8] Anecdotal results suggest that some patients with pancreatic pseudocysts, which usually require surgical drainage, may respond to octreotide.[9]

1. Steinberg W, Tenner S. Acute pancreatitis. *N Engl J Med* 1994; **330:** 1198–1210.
2. Fernández-del Castillo C, *et al.* Acute pancreatitis. *Lancet* 1993; **342:** 475–9.
3. Sainio V, *et al.* Early antibiotic treatment in acute necrotising pancreatitis. *Lancet* 1995; **346:** 663–7.
4. Ho HS, Frey CF. The role of antibiotic prophylaxis in severe acute pancreatitis. *Arch Surg* 1997; **132:** 487–93.
5. Baron TH, Morgan DE. Acute necrotizing pancreatitis. *N Engl J Med* 1999; **340:** 1412–17. Correction. *ibid.* **341:** 460.
6. Baillie J. Treatment of acute biliary pancreatitis. *N Engl J Med* 1997; **336:** 286–7.
7. Hardo PG, Axon ATR. Danazol improves chronic pancreatic pain. *J R Soc Med* 1993; **86:** 359.
8. Ohwada M, *et al.* New endoscopic treatment for chronic pancreatitis, using contrast media containing ulinastatin and prednisolone. *J Gastroenterol* 1997; **32:** 216–21.
9. Gullo L, Barbara L. Treatment of pancreatic pseudocysts with octreotide. *Lancet* 1991; **338:** 540–1.

Preparations

BP 2001: Pancreatin Granules; Pancreatin Tablets;
USP 25: Pancreatin Tablets.

Proprietary Preparations (details are given in Part 3)
Aust.: Kreon; Opti-Free; Pancrin; Pankreon forte; Panzynorm; Polyzym; **Austral.:** Bioglan Panazyme; Creon; Opti-Free Enzymatic; Opti-Plus; Pancenz; Polyzym; Viokase; **Belg.:** Creon; **Braz.:** Cotazym; Pankreon; Panzytrat; Polyzym; **Canad.:** Creon; Opti-Zyme; **Denm.:** Creon; **Fin.:** Pankreon; **Fr.:** Creon; Licrease; Opti-Plus†; Pancreal Kirchner; Polyzym; **Ger.:** Bilipeptal Mono; Carzodelan; Cholspasminase N; Cotazym; Euflat-E; Hevertozym; Kreon; Lipazym; Meteophyt forte; Mezym F; Nutrizym N; Ozym; Pancholtruw N†; Pangrol; Pankreatan; Pankreon; Panpeptal N; Panpur; Panzynorm forte-N; Panzytrat; Tryptoferm; Unexym mono; **Hong Kong:** Creon; **Irl.:** Creon; Nutrizym; Pancrease; Pancrex; Panzytrat; **Israel:** Creon; **Ital.:** Creon; Enzipan; Festal N†; Pancreon; Pancrex; Pancrin; Pancrotanort†; **Mex.:** Creon; Polyzym; Selecto; **Neth.:** Creon; Pancrease HL; Panzytrat; **Norw.:** Pankreon; **NZ:** Creon; Pancrex; Panzytrat; Viokase; **Port.:** Kreon; **S.Afr.:** Creon; Viokase; **Spain:** Kreon; Pankreon†; **Swed.:** Pankreon; **Switz.:** Creon; Panzytrat; **UK:** Clen-Zym; Creon; Nutrizym; Pancrease HL; Panzytrat; **USA:** Creon; Donnazyme; Enzymatic Cleaner; Opti-Zyme; Viokase; Vision Care Enzymatic Cleaner.

Multi-ingredient: Aust.: Arca-Enzym; Aristochol; Combizym; Combizym Compositum; Digestif Rennie; Enzyflat; Euflat†; Gal-

lo Merz; Helopanflat; Helopanzym; Intestinol; Nutrizym; Ora-Gallin; Ozym†; Pankreoflat; Pankreon compositum; Paspertase; Recessan†; Wobenzym; **Austral.:** Digestaid; Enzyme; Lexat; Natures Own Digestive Enzymes; Prozyme; **Belg.:** Combizym†; Digestomen; **Braz.:** Digecap-Zimatico; Digeplus; Digestal; Elozima; Espasmo Novozyme; Essen; Filogaster; Hepatoregius; Nutrizim; Pankreoflat; Peptopancreasi; Plasil Enzimatico; Sintozima; Vonil Enzimatico; **Canad.:** Alsilax†; Vesilax†; **Fin.:** Combizym; Combizym Compositum; **Fr.:** Hepatoum; Pancrelase; **Ger.:** Arbuz; Chol-Arbuz N; Combizym; Combizym Compositum; Enzym-Lefax; Enzym-Wied; Esberizym N†; Fermento duodenal; Helopanflat N; Hevert Enzym Novot†; Meteozym; Pankreoflat; Pascopankreat novo; Paspertase; Stacho-Zym N†; Unexym MD; Ventracid N; Wobenzym N; **Hong Kong:** Combizym; Pankreoflat; **Israel:** Encypalmed; Pankreoflat; **Ital.:** Combizym; Digestopan; Ede 6; Eudigestio; Pancreoflat; Pancreon Compositum†; Pancresil; Pepto-Pancreasi; Taka-Diastase†; **Mex.:** Dixiflen; Espaven Enzimatico; Pancreoflat; Plasil Enzimatico; Selecto-D; Wobenzym; **Neth.:** Combizym; Combizym Compositum†; Wobenzym; **Norw.:** Combizym; **NZ:** Combizym; Combizym Compositum; **Port.:** Colerin-F; Combizym; Combizym Compositum†; Espasmo Canulase; Fermetone Composto; Helopanflat; Nutrizym†; Pankreoflat; **S.Afr.:** Pankreoflat; Spasmo-Canulase; **Spain:** Digestomen Complex; Edym Sedante†; Espasmo Canulasa†; Espasmo Digestomen; Lidobama Complex†; Nulacin Fermentos; Paigastrol†; Pankreoflat; Takadispep Complex†; Wobenzimal; **Swed.:** Combizym; Combizym Compositum; **Switz.:** Combizym; Combizym Compositum†; Fermento duodenal; Gillazyme plus†; Gillazyme†; Helopanflat; Spasmo-Canulase; **Thai.:** Combizym; Combizym Compositum; Enzymet; Gaszym; Papytazyme; Pepsitase; Polyenzyme-I; Polyenzyme-N; Proctase-P; Sanzyme-S; **USA:** Digepepsin; Hi-Vegi-Lip; Pancrezyme 4X.

Pancrelipase (3732-v)

Pancrelipase (USAN).
CAS — 53608-75-6.
Pharmacopoeias. In US.

Pharmacopoeial description

USP 25: A substance containing enzymes, principally lipase, with amylase and protease, obtained from the pancreas of the hog. It is a cream-coloured, amorphous powder having a faint characteristic, but not offensive odour. Its greatest activities are in neutral or faintly alkaline media; more than traces of mineral acids or large amounts of alkali hydroxides make it inert. An excess of alkali carbonate also inhibits its action. Pancrelipase contains, in each mg, not less than 24 USP units of lipase activity, not less than 100 USP units of amylase activity, and not less than 100 USP units of protease activity. Store in airtight containers preferably at a temperature not exceeding 25°.

Units

See Pancreatin, p.1646.

Uses and Administration

Pancrelipase has the actions and uses of pancreatin (see p.1646). Various doses are employed. In the USA the equivalent of 4000 to 48 000 USP 25 units of lipase activity may be given with each meal or snack, adjusted according to the patient's needs. In the UK a preparation may be used that provides 5000 Ph. Eur. units of lipase activity in each capsule; one to three capsules may be given with each meal.

◊ Three patients with cystic fibrosis whose gastrointestinal symptoms had been well controlled with pancrelipase developed symptoms following substitution of generic pancrelipase for their previous brand.[1] The generic product had a different lipase content and was almost inactive at stomach pH *in vitro*, apparently because of a defective enteric coating. Different brands of pancrelipase may not be therapeutically equivalent and should not be routinely substituted.

1. Hendeles L, *et al.* Treatment failure after substitution of generic pancrelipase capsules: correlation with in vitro lipase activity. *JAMA* 1990; **263:** 2459–61.

Preparations

USP 25: Pancrelipase Capsules; Pancrelipase Delayed-release Capsules; Pancrelipase Tablets.

Proprietary Preparations (details are given in Part 3)
Aust.: Prolipase; **Austral.:** Cotazym S Forte; Pancrease; **Belg.:** Pancrease; Viokase†; **Canad.:** Cotazym; Digess†; Pancrease; Ultrase; Viokase; **Denm.:** Pancrease; **Fin.:** Pancrease; **Fr.:** Eurobiol; **Israel:** Pancrease; **Ital.:** Krebsilasi; Luitase; Pancrease; Pankreaden; **Mex.:** Pancrease; **Neth.:** Pancrease; **Norw.:** Pancrease; **NZ:** Cotazym; Pancrease; **S.Afr.:** Pankrease; **Spain:** Pancrease; **Swed.:** Pancrease; **Switz.:** Prolipase; **UK:** Pancrease; **USA:** Cotazym; Ilozyme; Ku-Zyme HP; Lipram; Pancrease; Protilase; Ultrase; Zymase.

Multi-ingredient: Belg.: Digestomen; **Braz.:** Dasc; **UK:** Digezyme; **USA:** Hi-Vegi-Lip; Pancrezyme 4X.

Pancreozymin (2141-x)

Pancreozymin (BAN).
CCK-PZ.
ATC — V04CK02.

NOTE. The endogenous hormone is known as cholecystokinin (CCK).

Units

The potency of pancreozymin may be expressed as Crick-Harper-Raper units based on the pancreatic secretion in *cats* or as Ivy *dog* units based on the increase in gallbladder pressure.

One Ivy dog unit is considered to be approximately equivalent to 1 Crick-Harper-Raper unit.

Adverse Effects

Flushing of the skin and other vasomotor effects may occur, particularly after rapid intravenous injection of pancreozymin. Hypersensitivity reactions may occasionally occur. Gallbladder contraction may give rise to abdominal discomfort.

Uses and Administration

Pancreozymin is a polypeptide hormone prepared from the duodenal mucosa of *pigs*. When administered by intravenous injection it causes an increase in the secretion of pancreatic enzymes and stimulates gallbladder contraction.

Pancreozymin has been used, usually in conjunction with secretin, as a test for exocrine pancreatic function and in the diagnosis of biliary-tract disorders; these tests generally involved duodenal intubation of the patient and examination of duodenal aspirate. Pancreozymin has also been used as an adjunct to cholecystography.

The dose of pancreozymin used has varied, but a dose of 1 to 2 Crick-Harper-Raper units per kg body-weight has commonly been given by slow intravenous injection.

◊ It was concluded that cholecystokinin provocation testing was ineffective in predicting which patients with acalculous biliary pain would receive symptomatic relief from cholecystectomy in a study involving 58 patients.[1]

1. Smythe A, *et al.* A requiem for the cholecystokinin provocation test? *Gut* 1998; **43:** 571–4.

Pangamic Acid (13074-m)

The name pangamic acid has been applied variously to gluconic acid 6-[bis(diisopropylamino)acetate] ($C_{20}H_{40}N_2O_8 = 436.5$), gluconic acid, 6-ester with N,N-dimethylglycine ($C_{10}H_{19}NO_8 = 281.3$), gluconic acid, 6-ester with N,N-diisopropylglycine ($C_{14}H_{27}NO_8 = 337.4$), and a substance or mixture of substances isolated from apricot kernels and rice bran. It has also been known as vitamin B_{15} although there is no evidence that pangamic acid is a vitamin. Preparations containing the vasoactive substance di-isopropylammonium dichloroacetate (p.874) have sometimes been described as pangamic acid or vitamin B_{15}. There is much uncertainty about the identity of products sold in health food stores as 'vitamin B_{15}', pangamic acid, or sodium or calcium pangamate and different brands have been reported to have completely different compositions.

Profile

Claims for the activity of pangamic acid as a promotor of tissue oxygenation and its alleged value in numerous disorders have not been substantiated. There is no evidence that pangamic acid is a vitamin.

Preparations

Proprietary Preparations (details are given in Part 3)
Ger.: Oyo.
Multi-ingredient: Spain: Policolinosil.

Papain (3733-g)

Papayotin.
CAS — 9001-73-4.
Pharmacopoeias. In US.

Pharmacopoeial description

USP 25: A purified proteolytic substance derived from *Carica papaya* (Caricaceae). It contains not less than 6000 USP units per mg. A white to light tan, amorphous powder. Soluble in water, the solution being colourless to light yellow and more or less opalescent; practically insoluble in alcohol, in chloroform, and in ether. pH of a 2% solution in water is between 4.8 and 6.2. Store in airtight containers at a temperature of 8° to 15°. Protect from light.

Units

USP 25 defines the USP unit of papain activity as the activity that releases the equivalent of 1 μg of tyrosine from a specified casein substrate under the conditions of the assay, using the enzyme concentration that liberates 40 μg of tyrosine per mL of test solution.

One FIP unit of papain is defined as the enzyme activity which under specified conditions hydrolyses 1 μmol of N-benzoyl-L-arginine ethyl ester per minute.

The Warner-Chilcott unit, based on the quantity of enzyme required to clot 2.64 μL of milk substrate in 2 minutes at 40°, under specified conditions, has also been used for papain.

Adverse Effects

Hypersensitivity reactions have occurred.

Effects on the eyes. Ocular and periorbital angioedema occurring within 4 hours of use of a contact lens cleansing solution containing papain has been reported.[1]

1. Bernstein DI, *et al.* Local ocular anaphylaxis to papain enzyme contained in a contact lens cleansing solution. *J Allergy Clin Immunol* 1984; **74:** 258–60.

Oesophageal perforation. Extensive destruction of the oesophageal wall, with perforation, resulted from the use of a papain suspension given to treat an obstruction caused by impacted meat.[1] The patient had been given 1.2 g of papain over a 12-hour period. Ten days after a thoracotomy, the descending thoracic aorta ruptured, and she died from haemorrhage.

1. Holsinger JW, *et al.* Esophageal perforation following meat impaction and papain ingestion. *JAMA* 1968; **204:** 734–5.

Uses and Administration
Papain consists chiefly of a mixture of papain and chymopapain, proteolytic enzymes which hydrolyse polypeptides, amides, and esters, especially at bonds involving basic amino acids, or leucine or glycine, yielding peptides of lower molecular weight. It is used as a topical debriding agent in conjunction with urea. It is also used for the removal of protein deposits from the surface of soft contact lenses (p.1129).

Preparations of papain, alone or combined with antibacterial agents and/or other substances, have been taken by mouth for their supposed anti-inflammatory properties, and it has also been used as an ingredient of various mixtures claimed to aid digestion.

Papain is widely used as a meat tenderiser and in the clarification of beverages.

◊ Papain has been included in proteolytic enzyme preparations used in oncology to reduce the adverse effects of chemotherapy and radiotherapy. Although the number of clinical studies on which to judge efficacy is limited, a review[1] of such studies suggested that systemic enzyme therapy might be beneficial. Clinical studies have used a preparation containing papain, trypsin, and chymotrypsin in a weight ratio of 5:2:2, and the beneficial effect seems to be based on its anti-inflammatory potential.

1. Leipner J, Saller R. Systemic enzyme therapy in oncology: effect and mode of action. *Drugs* 2000; **59:** 769–80.

Preparations
USP 25: Papain Tablets for Topical Solution.

Proprietary Preparations (details are given in Part 3)
Austral.: Hydrocare Enzymatic Protein Remover; Stop Itch; *Canad.:* Hydrocare Protein Remover; Solarcaine Stop Itch; *Ger.:* Verizym; *NZ:* Hydrocare Fizzy Protein Remover; *S.Afr.:* Tromasin SA†; *Spain:* Cacital†; *USA:* Allergan Enzymatic; ProFree.

Multi-ingredient: *Aust.:* Digestif Rennie; Ozym†; Wobe-Mugos; Wobenzym; *Austral.:* Betaine Digestive Aid; Bio-Disc; Bioglan Discone; Digestaid; Digestive Aid; Enzyme; Natures Own Digestive Enzymes; Prost-1; Prost-2†; Prozyme; Vita Disc†; *Belg.:* Digestomen; *Braz.:* Fideine; Filogaster; *Canad.:* Herbalax Forte†; Phytolax†; Vesilax†; *Ger.:* Arbuz; Chol-Arbuz N; Enzym-Wied; Mulsal N; Unexym MD; Wobe-Mugos E; Wobe-Mugos Th; Wobenzym N; *Ital.:* Digestopan; *Mex.:* Digenor Plus; Wobenzym; *Port.:* Caroid; *Spain:* Digestomen Complex; Espasmo Digestomen; Lizipaina; Lysokana†; Nasotic Oto; Takadispep Complex†; *Switz.:* Lysopaine; *Thai.:* Papytazyme; Pepsitase; Polyenzyme-1; *UK:* Enzyme Digest; Herbal Indigestion Naturtabs; Indigestion and Flatulence; Papaya Plus; *USA:* Accuzyme; Panafil; Panafil-White; Papaya Enzyme.

Papaverine (5221-r)
Papaverine *(BAN).*
6,7-Dimethoxy-1-(3,4-dimethoxybenzyl)isoquinoline.
$C_{20}H_{21}NO_4 = 339.4.$
$CAS — 58-74-2.$
$ATC — A03AD01; G04BE02.$

NOTE. Papaverine should not be confused with papaveretum (p.70).

Papaverine Hydrochloride (5224-n)
Papaverine Hydrochloride *(BAN).*
Papaverini Hydrochloridum; Papaverinii Chloridum; Papaverinium Chloride. 6,7-Dimethoxy-1-(3,4-dimethoxybenzyl)isoquinoline hydrochloride.
$C_{20}H_{21}NO_4,HCl = 375.8.$
$CAS — 63817-84-5$ (papaverine cromesilate); $61-25-6$ (papaverine hydrochloride); $39024-96-9$ (papaverine monophosadenine); $2053-26-1$ (anhydrous papaverine sulfate).
Pharmacopoeias. In *Chin., Eur.* (see p.vi), *Int., Jpn, Pol.,* and *US.*

Pharmacopoeial description
Ph. Eur.: White or almost white crystals or crystalline powder. Sparingly soluble in water; slightly soluble in alcohol; practically insoluble in ether. A 2% solution in water has a pH of 3.0 to 4.0.

USP 25: White crystals or white, crystalline powder. Is odourless. Soluble 1 in 30 of water and 1 in 120 of alcohol; soluble in chloroform; practically insoluble in ether. pH of a 2% solution in water is between 3.0 and 4.5. Store in airtight containers. Protect from light.

Adverse Effects
Side-effects of papaverine given by mouth include gastrointestinal disturbance, flushing of the face, headache, malaise, drowsiness, skin rash, sweating, orthostatic hypotension, and dizziness. Jaundice, eosinophilia, and signs of altered liver function may occur, sometimes due to hypersensitivity. In addition parenteral administration of high doses can result in cardiac arrhythmias; a slow rate of intravenous or intramuscular administration is recommended. Thrombosis has been reported at the injection site.

Intracavernosal injection can cause dose-related priapism and local fibrosis has been reported following long-term therapy.

◊ Systemic adverse effects occurring after intracavernosal injection of papaverine are infrequent but include dizziness and syncope,[1,2] probably related to the hypotensive effects of papaverine, and abnormal liver function test results.[1-3]

The most serious acute adverse effect is priapism[1,2,4] and patients should be instructed to seek medical help if an erection lasts for more than 4 hours. Detumescence can be effected by aspiration of blood from the corpus or by local injection of an alpha-adrenergic agonist such as adrenaline [epinephrine], metaraminol, or phenylephrine (see Priapism under Alprostadil, p.1440). Other local effects include haematoma, infection, and, on long-term therapy, fibrosis and penile distortion.[1,2]

Dispensing errors have resulted in inadvertent injection of *papaveretum* with potentially fatal consequences.[2,5,6]

1. Krane RJ, *et al.* Impotence. *N Engl J Med* 1989; **321:** 1648–59.
2. Bénard F, Lue TF. Self-administration in the pharmacological treatment of impotence. *Drugs* 1990; **39:** 394–8.
3. Levine SB, *et al.* Side effects of self-administration of intracavernous papaverine and phentolamine for the treatment of impotence. *J Urol (Baltimore)* 1989; **141:** 54–7.
4. Virag R. About pharmacologically induced prolonged erection. *Lancet* 1985; **i:** 519–20.
5. Robinson LQ, Stephenson TP. Self injection treatment for impotence. *BMJ* 1989; **299:** 1568.
6. Gregoire A. Self injection treatment for impotence. *BMJ* 1990; **300:** 537.

Precautions
Papaverine should be given with caution to patients with reduced gastrointestinal motility. Caution is also advisable in the presence of cardiac conduction disorders or unstable cardiovascular disease, especially when papaverine is administered parenterally. Intravenous administration is contra-indicated in patients with complete atrioventricular block.

Glaucoma. There appeared to be no basis for the manufacturers' recommendation that papaverine be used with caution in patients with glaucoma.[1] There was no obvious mechanism for such a warning and only 1 report of an adverse reaction had been received by the FDA. The author had given papaverine intracavernosally to patients with glaucoma and had observed no deterioration.

1. Swartz DA, Todd MW. Intracavernous papaverine and glaucoma. *JAMA* 1990; **264:** 570.

Interactions
Levodopa. For a report of papaverine decreasing the effectiveness of levodopa, see p.1172.

Pharmacokinetics
The biological half-life of papaverine given by mouth is reported to be between one and two hours, but there is wide interindividual variation. It is extensively bound (about 90%) to plasma proteins.

Papaverine is mainly metabolised in the liver and excreted in the urine, almost entirely as glucuronide-conjugated phenolic metabolites.

The reports of infrequent systemic effects following intracavernosal injection of papaverine indicate that there is some distribution to the systemic circulation from the corpus cavernosus.

Uses and Administration
Papaverine is an alkaloid present in opium, although it is not related chemically or pharmacologically to the other opium alkaloids. Papaverine has a direct relaxant effect on smooth muscle which is attributed in part to its ability to inhibit phosphodiesterase. It has been given in the management of cerebral, peripheral, and coronary vascular disorders; it is also given as an antispasmodic for gastrointestinal disorders and coughs. However, there is little evidence to justify its clinical use in these conditions.

Papaverine has been given by mouth as the hydrochloride in doses of up to 600 mg daily. Sustained-release preparations have been used. The codecarboxylate, cromesilate, hydrobromide, monophosadenine, nicotinate, sulfate, and teprosilate have also been used. Papaverine hydrochloride has also been given in doses of 30 to 120 mg by slow intramuscular or intravenous injection (but see Adverse Effects, above).

Papaverine hydrochloride has been given by injection into the corpus cavernosus of the penis for the diagnosis and treatment of erectile dysfunction (p.1663). Phentolamine may be added if the response is inadequate. It has been recommended that such injections should not be given more than three times each week or on two successive days.

Preparations
USP 25: Papaverine Hydrochloride Injection; Papaverine Hydrochloride Tablets.

Proprietary Preparations (details are given in Part 3)
Fr.: Albatran†; Oxadilene; *UK:* Papaverine Hydrochloride; *USA:* Genabid†; Pavabid; Pavarine†; Pavatine†; Paverolan†.

Multi-ingredient: *Aust.:* Androskat; Asthma; Euflat†; Myocardon; Normensan; Ora-Gallin compositum; Perphyllon; *Braz.:* Angalgosedan; Antispasmin; Atroveran; Atrovex; Calmovarin; Diarona; Espasmalgin; Espasmobel; Espasmocron; Espasmolex; Espasmosan; Espasmosan Composto; Gaba; Melpaz; Metilsedor; Monotrean; Nicopaverina; Nicopaverina B6; Plenocedan; Regran; Sedalene; Somasedin; Spasmotropin; Tebasedan; Uroseptin; Vagostesyl; *Fr.:* Acticarbine; Solurutine Papaverine F. Retard†; *Hong Kong:* Codoplex; Metoplex; *Israel:* Patropin; Spasmalgin;

Ital.: Antispasmina Colica; Farmospasmina; Ischelium Papaverina†; Monotrean; *Mex.:* Ayoral; *Neth.:* Androskat; *Port.:* Antispasmina Colica; Cosmaxil†; *Spain:* Aletor Compositum†; Analgilasa†; Angiosedante; Rubia Paver; Sulmetin Papaver; Sulmetin Papaverina; *Swed.:* Spasmofen; *Switz.:* Dolopyrine†; Spasmosol.

Paradichlorobenzene (3599-c)
Dichlorbenzol. 1,4-Dichlorobenzene.
$C_6H_4Cl_2 = 147.0.$
$CAS — 106-46-7.$

Profile
Paradichlorobenzene has general properties similar to those of orthodichlorobenzene (see p.1645) but is considered to be less toxic. It is present in several preparations intended for the removal of ear wax (see p.1223). It has been used as a furniture preservative and in mothballs and lavatory deodorant blocks. Abuse of preparations containing paradichlorobenzene has been reported.

Preparations
Proprietary Preparations (details are given in Part 3)
Multi-ingredient: *Austral.:* Cerumol; *Canad.:* Cerumol; *Hong Kong:* Cerumol; *Irl.:* Cerumol†; *Israel:* Cerumol; *Port.:* Otoceril; *S.Afr.:* Cerumol; *Singapore:* Cerumol; *Switz.:* Cerumenol; *UK:* Cerumol.

Paraphenylenediamine (13078-q)
$C_6H_4(NH_2)_2 = 108.1.$
$CAS — 106-50-3.$

NOTE. Commonly known in the hairdressing trade as 'para'.

Profile
Paraphenylenediamine is used in hair colour preparations.

It is estimated that about 4% of apparently normal subjects are sensitive to paraphenylenediamine, and 1% acutely sensitive; oedema and severe dermatitis may follow application in such persons. Effects on the eye may include chemosis, lachrymation, exophthalmos, and sometimes permanent blindness.

Following ingestion, severe angioedema-like symptoms with respiratory difficulty and dyspnoea may occur and may require emergency tracheostomy; vomiting, massive oedema, gastritis, rise in blood pressure, vertigo, tremors, convulsions, and coma have been reported.

Some studies have linked hair dyes with mutagenicity and carcinogenicity, although such findings have often been refuted.

Paratoluenediamine (13080-n)
2-Methyl-1,4-phenylenediamine.
$C_7H_{10}N_2 = 122.2.$
$CAS — 95-70-5.$

Profile
Paratoluenediamine is used in hair colour preparations.

Like paraphenylenediamine, above, paratoluenediamine may be associated with sensitivity reactions.

Parsley (4686-d)
Persil; Petroselinum.

Profile
Parsley (*Petroselinum crispum*, Umbelliferae) is used in herbal medicine, where it is mainly given as a diuretic. It is also used as a culinary herb and flavour.

Preparations
Proprietary Preparations (details are given in Part 3)
Ger.: Kneipp Petersilie N.

Multi-ingredient: *Aust.:* Apotheker Bauer's Harntreibender Tee; Blasen-Tee; Krauterhaus Mag Kottas Entwasserungstee; Krautertee Nr 126; Krautertee Nr 18; Krautertee Nr 25; Krautertee Nr 3; Krautertee Nr 4; Magentee; Naturland Entschlackung; Sanvita Entschlackungstonikum†; *Austral.:* Extralife Fluid-Care; Fluid Loss; Medinat PMT-Eze; Odourless Garlic; PMT-EZE†; Uva-Ursi Plus; *Braz.:* Tintura de Salsa Caroba e Manaca; *Canad.:* Herbal Throat; *Ger.:* Asparagus-P; Eupond†; nephro-loges; Nephrubin†; *UK:* Athera; Digest; Fre-bre; Garlodex; Gerard House Helonias Compound; Kincare; Mixed Vegetable Tablets; Modern Herbals Menopause.

Parsley Piert (3895-n)
Aphanes.
Pharmacopoeias. Eur. (see p.vi) includes *Alchemilla vulgaris* (*A. xanthochlora*).

Profile
Parsley piert, the aerial parts of *Aphanes arvensis* (*Alchemilla arvensis*) (Rosaceae) has astringent, diuretic, and demulcent properties. It is used for urinary-tract disorders, including renal and urinary calculi.

The related species *Alchemilla vulgaris* (lady's mantle) has been used similarly.

Preparations

Proprietary Preparations (details are given in Part 3)
Multi-ingredient: *Austral.:* Feminine Herbal Complex; Profluid; Protemp; *Canad.:* Swiss Herb Cough Drops; *Fr.:* Phlebosedol; *UK:* Backache Relief; Diuretabs; HRI Water Balance; Period Pain Relief; Watershed.

Passion Flower (13086-q)

Grenadille; May-pop; Pasionari; Passiflora; Passiflorae Herba.
CAS — 486-84-0 (harman).
Pharmacopoeias. In *Eur.* (see p.vi).

The dried aerial parts of *Passiflora incarnata* (Passifloraceae) containing flavonoids and varying quantities of harman alkaloids.

Pharmacopoeial description

Ph. Eur.: The fragmented or cut, dried aerial parts of *Passiflora incarnata*; it may also contain flowers and/or fruits. It contains not less than 1.5% of total flavonoids expressed as vitexin ($C_{21}H_{20}O_{10}$ = 432.4), calculated with reference to the dried drug. Protect from light.

Profile

Passion flower is reputed to have antispasmodic and sedative properties and has been used as an ingredient of herbal remedies, chiefly in the form of a liquid extract tincture.
Passion flower is also used in homoeopathic medicine.

Preparations

Proprietary Preparations (details are given in Part 3)
Aust.: Passiflorin; *Ger.:* Passiflora Curarina; *UK:* Modern Herbals Sleep Aid; Natracalm; Naturest; Nodoff; Phytocalm.

Multi-ingredient: *Aust.:* Nervenruh; Passedan; Passelyt; Sedogelat; Sedogelat forte; Wechseltee; *Austral.:* Calmo; Esten†; Euphorbia Complex; Executive B; Extralife Sleep-Care; Goodnight Formula; Herbal Anxiety Formula; Infant Calm; Lifesystem Herbal Plus Formula 2 Valerian; Multi-Vitamin Day & Night; Naturest; Nervatona; Nervatona Plus; Pacifenity; Passiflora Complex; Passionflower Plus; Proesten; Prosed-X; Relaxaplex; Tranquiplex†; Valerian Plus Herbal Plus Formula 12; Vitaglow Executive Anti Stress†; Vitaglow Herbal Stress†; *Belg.:* Sedinal; Senuval; Tisane Contre la Tension; *Braz.:* Anevrase; Bronquiogen; Calman; Elixir de Maracuja Composto; Especies Calmantes; Gotas Nican; Maracugina Composta; Pasalix; Passaneuro; Passicarbone; Passiflora Composta; Passiflorine; Sedalin; Sedantol; Serenase; Serenus; Sominex; Vagostesyl; Vidcalm; *Canad.:* Herbal Sleep Aid; Relax and Sleep; *Fr.:* Actisane Nervosite†; Anxoral; Astressane†; Biocarde; Euphytose; Mediflor Tisane Calmante Troubles du Sommeil No 14†; Natisedine†; Natudor; Neuroflorine; Neuropax; Neurotensyl†; Nocvalene; Nuidor†; Panxeol; Passiflorine; Passinevryl; Phytocalm; Phytotherapie Boribel no 8; Sedatif Tiber; Serenival†; Sympaneurol†; Sympavagol; Tisanes de l'Abbe Hamon no 6; *Ger.:* Aranidorm-S†; Avedorm; Biosedon S; Biral; Dormo-Sern; Dormoverlan; Euvegal N; Gutnacht; Habstal-Nerv N; Hyposedon N; JuNeuron S†; Kytta-Sedativum f; Luvased-Tropfen N; Moradorm; Moradorm S; Nerven-Tee Stada N†; Nervendragees; Nervinfant N; Nervoregin forte; Neurapas; Passin; Passiorin N†; Phytonoctu; Presselin Nerven K 1 N; Pronervon Phyto; RubieSed; Salusan†; Seda-Plantina; Sedaselect N; Sedinfant N; Sirmiosta Nervenelixier N†; Sonnuvis S; Tornix; Valena N; Valeriana mild; Visinal†; Vivinox N; *Hong Kong:* Epizon; *Israel:* Calmanervin; Nerven-Dragees; Passiflora; Passiflora Compound; *Ital.:* Anevrasi; Bio-Strath; Blandonal; Fitosonno; Noctis; Parvisedil; Passiflorine; Quietan†; Reve; Sedatol; Sedopuer F; Tauma; Val-Plus; *Port.:* Bio-Strath No 8†; Calmo; Gabisedil; Neurocardol; Valesono; *S.Afr.:* Biral; *Spain:* Baldrian; Brevilon†; Passiflorine; Sonofit; *Switz.:* Dicalm; Dragees antirhumatismales; Dragees pour la detente nerveuse; Dragees pour le coeur et les nerfs; Gouttes pour le coeur et les nerfs Concentrees; Melissa Tonic†; Phytoberidin; Phytomed Cardio†; Phytomed Somni; Plantival†; Relax; Sedosan; Sirop Passi-Par; Soporin; Tisane antirhumatismale; Tisane calmante pour les enfants; Tisane relaxante; Valverde Dragees pour la detente; Valverde Dragees pour le coeur; Valverde Gouttes pour le coeur; *UK:* Anased; Avena sativa comp.; Bio-Strath Valerian Formula; Daily Tension & Strain Relief; Gerard 99; Gerard House Motherwort Compound; Gerard House Serenity; Gerard House Valerian Compound; Heath & Heather Becalm; Heath & Heather Quiet Night; Herbal Pain Relief; HRI Night; Modern Herbals Stress; Night Time; Nodoff; Nytol Herbal; PMT Formula; Quiet Life; Quiet Nite; Quiet Tyme; Relax B⁺; Slumber; SuNerven; Super Mega B+C.

Patent Blue V (2142-r)

Acid Blue 3; CI Food Blue 5; Colour Index No. 42051; E131.
Calcium α-(4-diethylaminophenyl)-α-(4-diethyliminiocyclohexa-2,5-dienylidene)-5-hydroxytoluene-2,4-disulphonate.
$(C_{27}H_{31}N_2O_7S_2)_2Ca$ = 1159.4.
CAS — 3536-49-0.

NOTE. The name Patent Blue V is also used as a synonym for Sulphan Blue (CI No. 42045) (see p.1668).
Pharmacopoeias. In *Fr.*

Adverse Effects and Precautions

Hypersensitivity reactions may occur immediately or a few minutes after injection of patent blue V; on rare occasions they may be severe and include shock, dyspnoea, laryngeal spasm, and oedema. Nausea, hypotension, and tremor have been reported.

Administration of a small dose to test for hypersensitivity has been suggested.

The symbol † denotes a preparation no longer actively marketed

---

Hypersensitivity. An urticarial rash occurred in a 5-year-old girl after use of tablets containing patent blue V to disclose the presence of dental plaque.[1] Anaphylactic shock has been reported[2] in sentinel lymph node biopsy procedure.

1. Chadwick BL, *et al.* Allergic reaction to the food dye patent blue. *Br Dent J* 1990; **168:** 386–7.
2. Woltsche-Kahr I, *et al.* Anaphylactic shock following peritumoral injection of patent blue in sentinel lymph node biopsy procedure. *Eur J Surg Oncol* 2000; **26:** 313–14.

Uses and Administration

Patent blue V is injected subcutaneously to colour the lymph vessels so that they can be injected with a contrast medium. A dose of 0.25 mL of the 2.5% solution diluted with an equal volume of sodium chloride 0.9% or lignocaine [lidocaine] hydrochloride 1% injected subcutaneously in each interdigital web space has been used. Additional injections at different sites may be required when the lower limbs are to be examined. The bluish skin colour which may develop after injection usually disappears after 24 to 48 hours.

Patent blue V is used as a food colour.

◊ Intradermal injection of patent blue V at the site of a primary breast tumour has been used to identify the associated lymph nodes,[1] but concern has been expressed regarding possible long-term staining of the skin.[2]

1. Borgstein PJ, *et al.* Intradermal blue dye to identify sentinel lymphnode in breast cancer. *Lancet* 1997; **349:** 1668–9.
2. Giuliano AE. Intradermal blue dye to identify sentinel lymph node in breast cancer. *Lancet* 1997; **350:** 958.

Pegademase (14397-q)

Pegademase *(rINN)*.
PEG-ADA; PEG-Adenosine Deaminase.
ATC — L03AX04.
NOTE. Pegademase Bovine is *USAN*.

Profile

Pegademase is a conjugate of adenosine deaminase, an endogenous enzyme which converts adenosine to inosine, with a macrogol (polyethylene glycol). Pegademase bovine is used in the treatment of severe combined immunodeficiency disease (SCID) associated with a deficiency of adenosine deaminase in patients who are not suitable for bone-marrow transplantation or in whom the transplantation has failed. It is administered by intramuscular injection once every 7 days in an initial dose of 10 units per kg body-weight; increments of 5 units per kg are then given weekly up to a weekly maintenance dose of 20 units per kg. A single dose of 30 units per kg should not be exceeded. Pegademase should be administered with caution to patients with thrombocytopenia and avoided if the latter is severe.
Gene therapy (p.1614) has also been tried successfully in this deficiency syndrome.

◊ References.

1. Hershfield MS, *et al.* Treatment of adenosine deaminase deficiency with polyethylene glycol-modified adenosine deaminase. *N Engl J Med* 1987; **316:** 589–96.
2. Anonymous. Pegademase. *Med Lett Drugs Ther* 1990; **32:** 87–8.
3. Lee CR, *et al.* Pegademase bovine: replacement therapy for severe combined immunodeficiency disease. *DICP Ann Pharmacother* 1991; **25:** 1092–5.
4. Shovlin CL, *et al.* Adult presentation of adenosine deaminase deficiency. *Lancet* 1993; **341:** 1471.
5. Hershfield MS. Adenosine deaminase deficiency: clinical expression, molecular basis, and therapy. *Semin Hematol* 1998; **35:** 291–8.

Preparations

Proprietary Preparations (details are given in Part 3)
USA: Adagen.

Penicilloyl-polylysine (2143-f)

Benzylpenicilloyl-polylysine; PO-PLL; PPL.
CAS — 53608-77-8.
Pharmacopoeias. US includes Benzylpenicilloyl Polylysine Concentrate.

A polypeptide compound formed by the interaction of a penicillanic acid and polylysine of an average degree of polymerisation of 20 lysine residues per molecule.

Adverse Effects and Precautions

Severe hypersensitivity reactions have occasionally been reported following administration of penicilloyl-polylysine; a scratch test is recommended before intradermal administration.

Uses and Administration

Penicilloyl-polylysine is used to detect penicillin hypersensitivity. It is generally indicated only for adults with a history of penicillin hypersensitivity. After a preliminary scratch test it is given by intradermal injection. The development, usually within 5 to 15 minutes, of a wheal, erythema, and pruritus is generally judged a positive reaction. The incidence of penicillin hypersensitivity is stated to be less than 5% in patients showing a negative reaction. Penicilloyl-polylysine does not detect those liable to suffer late reactions or reactions due to minor antigen determinants; these reactions require other tests. False-positive reactions to penicilloyl-polylysine also occur.

Preparations

USP 25: Benzylpenicilloyl Polylysine Injection.
Proprietary Preparations (details are given in Part 3)
Canad.: Pre-Pen; *Swed.:* Pre-Pen; *USA:* Pre-Pen.

Pentagastrin (2144-d)

Pentagastrin *(BAN, USAN, rINN)*.
AY-6608; ICI-50123. *tert*-Butyloxycarbonyl-[β-Ala¹³]gastrin-(13-17)-pentapeptide amide; Boc-βAla-Trp-Met-Asp-Phe—NH_2.
$C_{37}H_{49}N_7O_9S$ = 767.9.
CAS — 5534-95-2.
ATC — V04CG04.
Pharmacopoeias. In *Br.*

Pharmacopoeial description

BP 2001: A white or almost white powder. Practically insoluble in water; slightly soluble in alcohol; soluble in dimethylformamide and in 5M ammonia. Protect from light.

Adverse Effects

Pentagastrin may cause a number of gastrointestinal effects including nausea and abdominal cramps. Cardiovascular effects including flushing of the skin, tachycardia, bradycardia, and hypotension have occasionally been reported. There may be headache, drowsiness, dizziness, and altered sensations in the extremities. Hypersensitivity reactions are rare.

◊ Some individual reports of adverse effects of pentagastrin.

1. Drucker D. Atrial fibrillation after administration of calcium and pentagastrin. *N Engl J Med* 1981; **304:** 1427–8.
2. Goldman M. Acute interstitial nephritis after administration of pentagastrin. *BMJ* 1984; **289:** 470.
3. Arnved J, *et al.* Pentagastrin-induced thrombocytopenia. *Lancet* 1985; **ii:** 1068–9.

Precautions

Pentagastrin should be given with care to patients with acute peptic ulceration or with active pancreatic, hepatic, or biliary-tract disease.

Uses and Administration

Pentagastrin is a synthetic pentapeptide which is not active when given by mouth but when given parenterally has effects similar to those of natural gastrin. Since it stimulates the secretion of gastric acid, pepsin, and intrinsic factor, it is used as a diagnostic agent to test the secretory action of the stomach. It has been used to diagnose disorders associated with increased or decreased gastric acid secretion and in the evaluation of gastric acid secretion following vagotomy or gastric resection. The usual dose is 6 μg per kg body-weight by subcutaneous injection; by intravenous infusion the dose is 0.6 μg per kg per hour, in sodium chloride 0.9%. It has also been given intramuscularly and by nasal inhalation.
Pentagastrin stimulates the secretion of pancreatic enzymes and thus has been used as a test for pancreatic function. It has also been tried in the diagnosis of medullary carcinoma of the thyroid.

Preparations

BP 2001: Pentagastrin Injection.
Proprietary Preparations (details are given in Part 3)
Aust.: Peptavlon†; *Canad.:* Peptavlon†; *Fr.:* Peptavlon; *Swed.:* Peptavlon†; *Switz.:* Peptavlon†; *UK:* Peptavlon; *USA:* Peptavlon†.

Pepsin (3736-s)

Pepsina; Pepsini Pulvis.
CAS — 9001-75-6.
ATC — A09AA03.
Pharmacopoeias. In *Eur.* (see p.vi). In *Chin.* and *Jpn* as Saccharated Pepsin.

Pharmacopoeial description

Ph. Eur.: Pepsin powder is prepared from the gastric mucosa of pigs, cattle, or sheep. It contains gastric proteinases active in acid medium (pH 1 to 5). It has an activity of not less than 0.5 Ph. Eur. units per mg, calculated with reference to the dried substance. A hygroscopic, white or slightly yellow, crystalline or amorphous powder. Soluble in water; practically insoluble in alcohol and in ether. A solution in water may be slightly opalescent with a weak acidic reaction. Store at 2° to 8° in airtight containers. Protect from light.

Uses and Administration

Pepsin contains proteolytic enzymes secreted by the stomach, which control the degradation of proteins into proteases and peptones. It hydrolyses polypeptides including those with bonds adjacent to aromatic or dicarboxylic L-amino-acid residues.

Pepsin has been given with dilute hydrochloric acid, or with substances such as glutamic acid hydrochloride, or betaine hydrochloride, as an adjunct in the treatment of gastric hypochlorhydria, or to treat deficiencies of digestive enzyme secretion. It has also been given for its supposed benefit as an ingredient of mixtures for dyspepsia and other gastrointestinal disorders.

Preparations

Proprietary Preparations (details are given in Part 3)
Canad.: Fermentol.

Multi-ingredient: *Aust.:* Everon; Helo-acid; Helopanzym; Oroacid; Pansan; Pepsiton; Vinopepsin; *Austral.:* Bepep; Betaine Digestive Aid; Bioglan Digestive Zyme; Digestaid; Enzyme; Natures Own Digestive Enzymes; Prozyme; *Belg.:* Digestomen; *Braz.:* Digeplus; Espasmo Novozyme; Essen; Filogaster; Hepatoregius; Pantopept; Peptopancreasi; Primeral; *Fr.:* Hepatoum; *Ger.:* Citropepsin; Pepzitrat; *Israel:* Babyzim; Betazim; *Ital.:* Digestomen; Essen Enzimatico; Eudigestio; Gastro-Pepsin; Pepto-Pancreasi; Taka-Diastase†; *Mex.:* Ochozim; *Port.:* Espasmo Canulase; Modulanzime; *S.Afr.:* Peter Pote's†; Spasmo-Canulase; *Spain:* Digestomen Complex; Espasmo Canulasa†; Digestomen; Euzymina Lisina I; Euzymina Lisina II; Paigastrol†; Troforex Pepsico; *Switz.:* Spasmo-Canulase; Stomacine; *Thai.:* Papytazyme; Pepsitase; *UK:* Digezyme; *USA:* Digepepsin.

Perflubron (15914-x)

Perflubron *(USAN, rINN)*.

Perfluorooctylbromide; PFOB. 1-Bromoheptadecafluorooctane.

$C_8BrF_{17} = 499.0$.
CAS — 423-55-2.
ATC — V08CX01.
Pharmacopoeias. In *US.*

Pharmacopoeial description

USP 25: A clear, colourless, practically odourless liquid. Store in airtight containers. Protect from light.

Profile

Perfluorocarbons (fluorocarbons) can absorb, transport, and release oxygen and carbon dioxide. Perflubron is a perfluorocarbon tried as an alternative to red blood cell preparations to improve gaseous transport, in particular oxygen supply, to the tissues. It is also under investigation for direct administration to the lungs for use in partial liquid ventilation as an adjunct to mechanical ventilation in patients with respiratory failure.

Perflubron is in clinical trials for use as an intravenous contrast medium to enhance imaging with computed tomography and ultrasound. It has been investigated for the detection of primary and metastatic cancer and other pathological conditions. It has also been given by mouth to enhance delineation of the bowel during magnetic resonance imaging.

Other perfluorocarbons have also been used. A mixture of perfluamine (perfluorotripropylamine) and perflunafene (perfluorodecahydronaphthalene, perfluorodecalin) has been used to prevent myocardial ischaemia during percutaneous transluminal coronary angioplasty.

Perfluorocarbons have been used in eye surgery.

Blood substitutes. References to the use of perflubron and other perfluorocarbons as blood substitutes.

1. Garrelts JC. Fluosol: an oxygen-delivery fluid for use in percutaneous transluminal coronary angioplasty. *DICP Ann Pharmacother* 1990; **24:** 1105–12.
2. Ravis WR, *et al.* Perfluorochemical erythrocyte substitutes: disposition and effects on drug distribution and elimination. *Drug Metab Rev* 1991; **23:** 375–411.
3. Urbaniak SJ. Artificial blood. *BMJ* 1991; **303:** 1348–50.
4. Jones JA. Red blood cell substitutes: current status. *Br J Anaesth* 1995; **74:** 697–703.
5. Remy B, *et al.* Red blood cell substitutes: fluorocarbon emulsions and haemoglobin solutions. *Br Med Bull* 1999; **55:** 277–98.
6. Lowe KC. Perfluorinated blood substitutes and artificial oxygen carriers. *Blood Rev* 1999; **13:** 171–84.
7. Prowse CV. Alternatives to standard blood transfusion: availability and promise. *Transfus Med* 1999; **9:** 287–99.

Respiratory distress syndrome. References to the use of perfluorocarbons, including perflubron, for partial liquid ventilation in neonatal respiratory distress syndrome (p.1055) and acute respiratory distress syndrome (p.1046).

1. Hirschl RB, *et al.* Liquid ventilation in adults, children, and full-term neonates. *Lancet* 1995; **346:** 1201–2.
2. Leach CL, *et al.* Partial liquid ventilation with perflubron in premature infants with severe respiratory distress syndrome. *N Engl J Med* 1996; **335:** 761–7.
3. Hirschl RB, *et al.* Initial experience with partial liquid ventilation in adult patients with acute respiratory distress syndrome. *JAMA* 1996; **275:** 383–9.
4. Wolfson MR, Shaffer TH. Liquid assisted ventilation update. *Eur J Pediatr* 1999; **158:** S27–S31.
5. Davies M. Liquid ventilation. *J Paediatr Child Health* 1999; **35:** 434–7.
6. Weis CM, Fox WW. Current status of liquid ventilation. *Curr Opin Pediatr* 1999; **11:** 126–32.

Preparations

Proprietary Preparations (details are given in Part 3)
Israel: Adato-Deca.

Persic Oil (7364-g)

Oleum Persicorum; Peach or.

Pharmacopoeias. Chin. and Jpn include Peach Kernel (Persicae Semen) and also Apricot Kernel (Armeniacae Semen).

The fixed oil expressed from the kernels of varieties of *Prunus persica* (peach) or *P. armeniaca* (apricot) (Rosaceae).

Profile

Persic oil closely resembles almond oil (p.1576) in its general characteristics and is used as an oily vehicle.

Peru Balsam (282-k)

Bals. Peruv.; Balsamum Pieruvianum; Baume du Pérou; Baume du San Salvador; Peruvian Balsam.

Pharmacopoeias. In *Eur.* (see p.vi).

Pharmacopoeial description

Ph. Eur.: The balsam obtained from the scorched and wounded trunk of *Myroxylon balsamum* var. *pereirae.* It contains not less than 45.0% w/w and not more than 70.0% w/w of esters, mainly benzyl benzoate and benzyl cinnamate.

A dark brown, viscous liquid which is not sticky, is non-drying, and does not form threads. It is transparent and yellowish-brown when viewed in a thin layer. Practically insoluble in water, freely soluble in dehydrated alcohol; not miscible with fatty oils except for castor oil. Protect from light.

Profile

Peru balsam has a very mild antiseptic action by virtue of its content of cinnamic and benzoic acids. Diluted with an equal part of castor oil, it has been used as an application to bedsores and chronic ulcers; it has also been used in topical preparations for the treatment of superficial skin lesions and pruritus. It is an ingredient of some rectal preparations used for the symptomatic relief of haemorrhoids (see p.1205). Peru balsam is an ingredient of some preparations used in the treatment of respiratory congestion.

Skin sensitisation has been reported.

Preparations

Proprietary Preparations (details are given in Part 3)
Aust.: Perudent; *Belg.:* Tulle Gras Lumiere†; *Fr.:* Tulle Gras Lumiere; *Ger.:* Branolind N; Tulle Gras Lumiere†; *USA:* Flanders Buttocks.

Multi-ingredient: *Aust.:* Mamellin; Pudan-Lebertran-Zinksalbe; Pulmex; Rombay; Vulpuran; *Austral.:* Anusol; Ayrton's Chilblain; *Belg.:* Oxyplastine†; Perubore; Pulmex; Pulmex Baby; Rectovasol; *Braz.:* Anusol-HC; Calminex S; Claudemor; *Canad.:* Derat†; *Fr.:* Agathol; Anaxeryl; Balsofumine; Balsofumine Mentholee; Brulex; Dermophil Indien; Oxyperol; Perubore; Pommade Lelong†; Pulmax†; *Ger.:* Anusol; derma-loges N; Ekzevowen; Peru-Lenicet; *Hong Kong:* Anusol; Anusol-HC; Cortison-Kemicetine; *Irl.:* Anugesic-HC; Anusol; Anusol-HC; *Israel:* Anusol; Contra Combustiones; Hemo; Pulmex; *Ital.:* Anusol; Fomentil; *NZ:* Anusol; *Port.:* Anucet; Claudemor; *S.Afr.:* Anugesic; Anusol-HC†; Rectosan 'A'†; Ung Vernleigh; *Singapore:* Anusol; *Spain:* Antigrietun; Cicatral; Grietalgen; Kneipp Balsamo; Linitul; Vapores Pyt; Vitamina F99 Topica; *Swed.:* Anusol†; *Switz.:* Anginol; Anusol†; Demo pommade contre les refroidissements; Demo pommade contre les refroidissements pour bebes; Dermophil Indien; Furodermil†; Haemocortin; Haemolan; HEC; Nasobol; Perubare; Pulmex; Pulmex Baby; Rapura; *Thai.:* Anusol; *UK:* Anugesic-HC; Anusol; Anusol-HC, Plus HC; Balsamicum; Dragon Balm; Frost Cream; *USA:* Anumed; Anumed HC; Balmex Baby; Dermuspray; Dr Dermi-Heal; Granulderm; Granulex; GranuMed; Hemril; Mammol; Medicone Rectal; Proderm; Rectagene II†; Saratoga; Wyanoids†.

Phencyclidine Hydrochloride (13100-l)

Phencyclidine Hydrochloride *(BANM, USAN, rINNM)*.

CI-395; CN-25253-2; GP-121; NSC-40902; PCP. 1-(1-Phenylcyclohexyl)piperidine hydrochloride.

$C_{17}H_{25}N,HCl = 279.8$.
CAS — 77-10-1 *(phencyclidine);* 956-90-1 *(phencyclidine hydrochloride).*

NOTE. The name PCP has also been used as a synonym for pentachlorophenol.

Phencyclidine used illicitly has been known as: angel dust, angel hair, angel mist, crystal, cyclone, dust, elephant tranquilliser, embalming fluid, goon, hog, horse tranquilliser, killer weed, KW, mint weed, mist, monkey dust, monkey gland, peace pills, peace weed, rocket fuel, scuffle, sheets, super weed, surfer, and T.

Adverse Effects and Treatment

Phencyclidine can induce a psychosis clinically indistinguishable from schizophrenia. Adverse effects reported include bizarre and violent behaviour, hallucinations, euphoria, agitation, catatonic rigidity, disorientation, incoordination, nystagmus, hypersalivation, vomiting, convulsions, numbness, hypertension, tachycardia, rhabdomyolysis leading to renal failure, acidosis, and, occasionally, malignant hyperthermia. Severe intoxication may result in respiratory depression, coma, and death.

Treatment of the adverse effects of phencyclidine is symptomatic; if agitated the patient should be kept quiet in a darkened room, and diazepam given if necessary. Hyperthermia should be treated. Activated charcoal should preferably be given within 1 hour of ingestion; multiple doses may be of benefit since phencyclidine is actively secreted into the gastrointestinal tract. Renal excretion should be promoted by hydration and use of diuretics if necessary. Acidification of the urine is no longer recommended since acidosis may be exacerbated and renal failure precipitated. Haloperidol or a similar butyrophenone

may be preferable to chlorpromazine in the management of psychotic symptoms.

Uses and Administration

Phencyclidine is related chemically to ketamine (see p.1262) and is a potent analgesic and anaesthetic. It was formerly given intravenously to produce an amnesic trance-like state, with analgesia, but severe adverse effects, especially postoperative psychoses, precluded its use. It was formerly used in veterinary medicine as an immobilising agent. Phencyclidine is widely abused in some countries for its hallucinogenic effects and has been taken by mouth, sniffed, injected or smoked.

Numerous analogues of phencyclidine have been similarly abused and include PHP (rolicyclidine; 1-(1-phenylcyclohexyl)pyrrolidine), PCC (1-piperidinocyclohexanecarbonitrile), PCE (*N*-ethyl-1-phenylcyclohexylamine), and TCP (1-[1-(2-thienyl)cyclohexyl]piperidine).

Phenolsulfonphthalein (2145-n)

Fenolsolfonftaleina; Phenol Red; Phenolsulphonphthaleinum; Phenolsulphonphthalein *(BAN);* PSP. 4,4'-(3H-2,1-Benzoxathiol-3-ylidene)diphenol S,S-dioxide.

$C_{19}H_{14}O_5S = 354.4$.
CAS — 143-74-8.
ATC — V04CH03.
Pharmacopoeias. In *Chin., Eur.* (see p.vi), and *Jpn.*

Pharmacopoeial description

Ph. Eur.: A bright to dark red, crystalline powder. Very slightly soluble in water; slightly soluble in alcohol.

Adverse Effects and Precautions

Hypersensitivity reactions to phenolsulfonphthalein may occasionally occur. Excretion may be altered in patients with gout.

Interactions

Excretion of phenolsulfonphthalein may be affected in patients taking aminohippuric acid, atropine, contrast media, diuretics, penicillin, probenecid, salicylates, sulfinpyrazone, or some sulfonamides.

Pharmacokinetics

After intravenous injection, phenolsulfonphthalein is in part bound to plasma proteins, and in a patient with normal kidney function is rapidly excreted, mainly in the urine; some is excreted by the liver. Renal clearance is predominantly by tubular secretion, only a small amount being eliminated by glomerular filtration.

Uses and Administration

Phenolsulfonphthalein has been used as a test of renal function by estimating the rate of urinary excretion after intravenous administration. It has also been given intramuscularly.

Alkaline urine is coloured red to violet.

Phenolsulfonphthalein has also been used as a drug ingestion indicator, a marker in drug absorption studies, and in a test of residual urine.

Phenylpropanol (3737-w)

Ethyl Phenyl Carbinol; α-Hydroxypropylbenzene; SH-261. 1-Phenylpropan-1-ol; α-Ethylbenzyl alcohol.

$C_9H_{12}O = 136.2$.
CAS — 93-54-9.
Pharmacopoeias. In *Chin.*

Profile

Phenylpropanol is a choleretic.

Preparations

Proprietary Preparations (details are given in Part 3)
Aust.: Gallenperlen.

Multi-ingredient: *Aust.:* Hedonin; *Braz.:* Quelodin.

Phloroglucinol (13104-c)

Phloroglucin. Benzene-1,3,5-triol.

$C_6H_6O_3 = 126.1$.
CAS — 108-73-6.
Pharmacopoeias. In *Fr.*

Profile

Phloroglucinol is used as an antispasmodic sometimes in combination with trimethylphloroglucinol.

Preparations

Proprietary Preparations (details are given in Part 3)
Fr.: Spasfon-Lyoc; Spassirex; *Ital.:* Spasmex.

Multi-ingredient: *Belg.:* Spasfon; *Fr.:* Meteoxane; Spasfon; *Ital.:* Spasmex; *Mex.:* Panclasa.

Phosgene (13105-k)

Carbonic Dichloride; Carbonyl Chloride; Chloroformyl Chloride.
$COCl_2 = 98.92$.
CAS — 75-44-5.

Adverse Effects

Poisoning may occur from industrial use or from the generation of phosgene from chlorinated compounds such as dichloromethane, chloroform, or carbon tetrachloride in the presence of heat. Symptoms of poisoning, which may be delayed for up to 24 hours, include burning of the eyes and throat, cough, dyspnoea, cyanosis, and pulmonary congestion and oedema. Death may result from anoxia. Exposure to 50 ppm may be rapidly fatal. Massive exposure may cause intravascular haemolysis, thrombus formation, and immediate death. Generalised weakness may persist for months after non-fatal exposure.

Treatment of Adverse Effects

After inhalation of phosgene or absorption from the skin, treatment consists of complete rest and the administration of oxygen. The mouth, eyes, nose, and skin should be irrigated with copious amounts of water. Corticosteroids may reduce tissue damage. Antibacterials may reduce respiratory infections. Further treatment is symptomatic.

Uses and Administration

Phosgene is used in the chemical industry. It has been used as a war gas.

Phosphatidyl Choline (11497-w)

Phosphatidylcholine.

Profile

Phosphatidyl choline is a phospholipid and a constituent of lecithin (p.1628). Phosphatidyl choline is an ingredient of preparations that have been promoted for liver disorders, peripheral vascular disorders, and hyperlipidaemias.

Preparations

Proprietary Preparations (details are given in Part 3)
Ital.: Essentiale; Lipostabil; *USA:* PhosChol.
Multi-ingredient: *Austral.:* Tyroseng; *Ital.:* Essaven.

Phosphatidyl Serine (3918-z)

Phosphatidylserine.

Profile

Phosphatidyl serine is a phospholipid which has been tried in the treatment of organic psychiatric syndromes and investigated as a cognition adjuvant. Phosphatidyl serine is a constituent of lecithin (p.1628).

◊ References.
1. Pepping J. Phosphatidylserine. *Am J Health-Syst Pharm* 1999; **56:** 2038, 2043–4.

Preparations

Proprietary Preparations (details are given in Part 3)
Braz.: Bros; *Ital.:* Senefort†; *UK:* Cognito.
Multi-ingredient: *Ital.:* Neobros; Neobros 10.

Phosphoric Acid (1321-c)

Acido Fosfórico; Acidum Phosphoricum Concentratum; Concentrated Phosphoric Acid; E338; Orthophosphoric Acid; Phosph. Acid; Phosphorsäure.
$H_3PO_4 = 98.00$.
CAS — 7664-38-2.
Pharmacopoeias. In *Eur.* (see p.vi) (84 to 90%). Also in *USNF* (85 to 88%).

Pharmacopoeial description

Ph. Eur.: It contains 84 to 90% w/w of H_3PO_4. A clear, colourless, corrosive, syrupy liquid. When stored at a low temperature it may solidify, forming a mass of colourless crystals which do not melt until the temperature reaches 28°. Miscible with water and with alcohol. Store in glass containers.
USNF 20: It contains 85 to 88% w/w H_3PO_4. A colourless, odourless liquid of syrupy consistency. Miscible with water and with alcohol. Store in airtight containers.

Dilute Phosphoric Acid (1322-k)

Acidum Phosphoricum Dilutum; Diluted Phosphoric Acid.
Pharmacopoeias. In *Eur.* (see p.vi) and *Pol.* Also in *USNF.*

Pharmacopoeial description

Ph. Eur.: It contains 9.5 to 10.5% w/w H_3PO_4 and is prepared by mixing phosphoric acid 115 g with water 885 g.
USNF 20: It contains 9.5 to 10.5% w/v H_3PO_4 and may be prepared by mixing phosphoric acid 69 mL with purified water to 1000 mL. A clear, colourless, odourless liquid. Store in airtight containers.

Adverse Effects and Treatment

As for Hydrochloric Acid, p.1621.

The symbol † denotes a preparation no longer actively marketed

Uses and Administration

Phosphoric acid has industrial uses. Dilute phosphoric acid has been used well diluted in preparations intended for the management of nausea and vomiting (p.1206). Phosphoric acid is used in dentistry to etch tooth enamel.
Phosphoric acid is used in homoeopathic medicine.

Preparations

USP 25: Sodium Fluoride and Phosphoric Acid Gel; Sodium Fluoride and Phosphoric Acid Topical Solution.
Proprietary Preparations (details are given in Part 3)
Fr.: Phosoforme.
Multi-ingredient: *Austral.:* Emetrol; Floraquin†; *Braz.:* Biotonico Fontoura; Teutonico; Tonico No 1; *Fr.:* Acti 5†; Actiphos; Biotone; Ionyl; Marinol; Phosphoneuros; *S.Afr.:* Emetrol; Emex; *Switz.:* Frubiose Calcium†; *Thai.:* Floraquin; Quinradon; Quinradon-N; *USA:* Emecheck†; Emetrol; Formula EM; Naus-A-Way†.

Phosphorus (13106-a)

Fósforo; White Phosphorus; Yellow Phosphorus.
$P = 30.973761$.
CAS — 7723-14-0.

It is unstable in air and should be stored under water.

◊ WARNING. *Phosphorus has been used for the illicit preparation of explosives or fireworks; care is required with its supply.*

Adverse Effects

Acute poisoning by phosphorus, a general protoplasmic poison, occurs in three distinct stages. The first stage represents local gastrointestinal irritation with intense thirst, pain, nausea, vomiting, and diarrhoea. The breath may smell of garlic and vomitus and excreta are luminescent. Shock, delirium, convulsions, coma, and death may occur. In patients who survive, a second, asymptomatic stage may be present lasting for up to several days. The third stage represents systemic toxicity and is characterised by hepatic and renal damage, haemorrhage due to hypoprothrombinaemia and low fibrinogen concentrations, cardiovascular collapse, and CNS involvement including confusion, convulsions, and coma. Death may occur during either the first or third stages.
The fatal dose is about 1 mg per kg body-weight.
Symptoms of chronic poisoning are very slow in onset and are associated with lowered resistance to infection and defective tissue repair. They include periostitis and necrosis of the mandible ('phossy jaw').
Externally, phosphorus causes severe burns to the skin. Phosphorus is absorbed following skin contamination and systemic symptoms may occur.

Treatment of Adverse Effects

After ingestion of phosphorus the stomach should be washed out with copious amounts of water; alternatives that have been suggested include potassium permanganate solution 1 in 5000, copper sulfate solution 0.2%, or hydrogen peroxide 2%.
Liquid paraffin or a solution of sodium sulfate may be introduced into the stomach following lavage and left there. Activated charcoal may be given by mouth. The use of digestible fats and oils should be avoided.
Further treatment is symptomatic and supportive and may include: fluid and electrolyte replacement; blood transfusion or vitamin K to correct coagulation disorders; and management of convulsions and renal and hepatic dysfunctions. Contaminated areas on skin should be immersed in water or irrigated with copious amounts of warm water; warm solutions of sodium bicarbonate 1% or copper sulfate 1% have also been suggested. It is essential that all particles of unoxidised phosphorus are removed from the skin.

Uses and Administration

Elemental phosphorus is no longer used in medicine. Inorganic phosphates are given in deficiency states and bone diseases (see Sodium Phosphate, p.1194). Phosphorus has been used in the manufacture of rat and cockroach poisons.
It is used in homoeopathic medicine.

Physalis (13109-r)

Alkekengi; Bladder Cherry; Chinese Lantern; Ground Cherry; Strawberry Tomato; Winter Cherry.
Pharmacopoeias. In *Chin.*

Profile

The berries of *Physalis alkekengi* (Solanaceae) are reputed to have diuretic properties.
Cape gooseberry is the edible fruit of *P. peruviana.*

Picibanil (19659-q)

OK-432.

Profile

Picibanil, which is derived from *Streptococcus pyogenes,* is an immunomodulator that has been tried in the treatment of malignant neoplasms and viral infections.

◊ References.
1. Shirai M, *et al.* Intratumoural injection of OK-432 and lymphokine-activated killer activity in peripheral blood of patients with hepatocellular carcinoma. *Eur J Cancer* 1990; **26:** 965–9.
2. Imarura T, *et al.* Intrapericardial OK-432 instillation for the management of malignant pericardial effusion. *Cancer* 1991; **68:** 259–63.
3. Tanaka N, *et al.* Intratumoral injection of a streptococcal preparation, OK-432, before surgery for gastric cancer: a randomized trial. *Cancer* 1994; **74:** 3097–3103.
4. Katano M, Morisaki T. The past, the present and future of the OK-432 therapy for patients with malignant effusions. *Anticancer Res* 1998; **18:** 3917–25.
5. Luzzatto C, *et al.* Sclerosing treatment of lymphangiomas with OK-432. *Arch Dis Child* 2000; **82:** 316–18.

Pidotimod (14649-e)

Pidotimod (*rINN*).
(*R*)-3-[(*S*)-5-Oxoprolyl]-4-thiazolidinecarboxylic acid.
$C_9H_{12}N_2O_4S = 244.3$.
CAS — 121808-62-6.
ATC — L03AX05.

Profile

Pidotimod is an immunostimulant used in patients with cell-mediated immunodepression during respiratory- and urinary-tract infections. It is given by mouth in usual doses of 800 mg twice daily.

◊ References.
1. Various. Pidotimod: a new biological response modifier. *Arzneimittelforschung* 1994; **44** (12a): 1399–1530.
2. Guerra B, *et al.* Pidotimod in the management of vulvar papillomatosis: double-blind clinical trial versus placebo. *Am J Ther* 1998; **5:** 147–52.

Preparations

Proprietary Preparations (details are given in Part 3)
Ital.: Onaka; Pigitil; Polimod; *Mex.:* Adimod.

Pilewort (16571-r)

Ficaire; Ficaria Ranunculoides; Ficaria Verna; Lesser Celandine.
Pharmacopoeias. In *Fr.*

Profile

Pilewort, the aerial parts of *Ranunculus ficaria* (Ranunculaceae), has astringent and demulcent properties and is used topically for the treatment of haemorrhoids.

Preparations

Proprietary Preparations (details are given in Part 3)
Multi-ingredient: *Fr.:* Avenoc†; Hemorrogel; *UK:* Piletabs; Pilewort Compound.

Pinaverium Bromide (13119-d)

Pinaverium Bromide (*rINN*).
4-(6-Bromoveratryl)-4-{2-[2-(6,6-dimethyl-2-norpinyl)ethoxy]ethyl}morpholinium bromide.
$C_{26}H_{41}Br_2NO_4 = 591.4$.
CAS — 59995-65-2 (pinaverium); 53251-94-8 (pinaverium bromide).

Profile

Pinaverium bromide is a calcium-channel blocker with some antimuscarinic-like effects. It is used as an antispasmodic in the gastrointestinal tract in usual doses of 50 mg by mouth three times daily at mealtimes.

◊ Two patients experienced heartburn and dysphagia after taking pinaverium bromide by mouth between meals; endoscopy revealed acute oesophageal ulceration which healed on discontinuation of treatment.[1] The manufacturer's recommendation to take pinaverium bromide during meals was emphasised.
1. André J-M, *et al.* Ulcères oesophagiens après prise de bromure de pinaverium. *Acta Endosc* 1980; **10:** 289–91.

Preparations

Proprietary Preparations (details are given in Part 3)
Aust.: Dicetel; *Belg.:* Dicetel; *Braz.:* Dicetel; *Canad.:* Dicetel; *Fr.:* Dicetel; *Hong Kong:* Dicetel; *Ital.:* Dicetel; *Mex.:* Dicetel; *Neth.:* Dicetel†; *Port.:* Dicetel; *Spain:* Eldicet; *Switz.:* Dicetel; *Thai.:* Dicetel.

Pipoxolan (5240-n)

Pipoxolan (*BAN, pINN*).
5,5-Diphenyl-2-(2-piperidinoethyl)-1,3-dioxolan-4-one.
$C_{22}H_{25}NO_3 = 351.4$.
CAS — 23744-24-3 (pipoxolan); 18174-58-8 (pipoxolan hydrochloride).
NOTE. Pipoxolan Hydrochloride is *USAN.*

Profile

Pipoxolan is used as a smooth muscle relaxant in usual doses of 10 to 30 mg by mouth three times daily. Pipoxolan hydrochloride has also been used.

Preparations

Proprietary Preparations (details are given in Part 3)
Ger.: Rowapraxin; *Hong Kong*: Rowapraxin; *Irl.*: Rowapraxin.
Multi-ingredient: *Irl.*: Migranat.

Piprozolin (3738-e)

Piprozolin (USAN, rINN).
Gö-919; W-3699. Ethyl (3-ethyl-4-oxo-5-piperidinothiazolidin-2-ylidene)acetate.
$C_{14}H_{22}N_2O_3S = 298.4$.
CAS — 17243-64-0.
ATC — A05AX01.

Profile
Piprozolin has been used as a choleretic.

Piracetam (13124-x)

Piracetam (BAN, USAN, rINN).
CI-871; Pyrrolidone Acetamide; UCB-6215. 2-(2-Oxopyrrolidin-1-yl)acetamide.
$C_6H_{10}N_2O_2 = 142.2$.
CAS — 7491-74-9.
ATC — N06BX03.
Pharmacopoeias. In Fr.

Adverse Effects and Precautions
Piracetam is reported to produce insomnia or somnolence, weight gain, hyperkinesia, nervousness, and depression. Diarrhoea and rashes may occur at a lower frequency. Piracetam should not be given to patients with hepatic impairment or severe renal impairment; dosage reductions are recommended for patients with lesser degrees of renal impairment. Therapy with piracetam should not be withdrawn abruptly.

Interactions
Anticoagulants. For reference to the effect of piracetam on warfarin, see p.997.

Uses and Administration
Piracetam acts on the CNS and has been described as a 'nootropic'; it is said to protect the cerebral cortex against hypoxia. It is also reported to inhibit platelet aggregation and reduce blood viscosity at high doses. Piracetam is used as an adjunct in the treatment of myoclonus of cortical origin. It has also been used in dementia. Other disorders or states in which it has been tried (on the basis of a supposed 'cerebrocortical insufficiency' responsive to piracetam) include alcoholism, vertigo, cerebrovascular accidents, behavioural disorders in children, and after trauma or surgery.

In cortical myoclonus, piracetam is given in doses of 7.2 g daily increasing by 4.8 g per day every 3 or 4 days up to a maximum of 20 g daily. It is given by mouth in 2 or 3 divided doses. Once the optimal dose of piracetam has been established, attempts should be made to reduce the dose of concurrent therapy. Dosage should be reduced in patients with mild to moderate renal impairment: a reduction to half the usual dose is recommended where creatinine clearance is between 60 and 40 mL per minute, and to one-quarter of the usual dose if creatinine clearance is between 40 and 20 mL per minute.

Piracetam has been given for various other disorders in doses of 0.8 to 1 g three times daily by mouth. In severe disorders it has been given by intramuscular or intravenous injection.

Dementia. Although piracetam is used in some countries in the management of cognitive impairment and dementia (p.1412), a recent systematic review[1] concluded that the evidence from the published literature did not support this use.

1. Flicker L, Grimley Evans J. Piracetam for dementia or cognitive impairment (updated 20 May 2001). Available in The Cochrane Library; Issue 4. Oxford: Update Software; 2001.

Myoclonus. A review[1] of 62 case reports, 3 open studies, and 2 double-blind studies concluded that piracetam is beneficial in the treatment of disabling myoclonus (p.342), either as adjunctive treatment or as monotherapy. Similar conclusions were made in another review[2] in which experience of 12 patients with progressive myoclonus epilepsy, 8 of whom benefited from piracetam in doses of up to 45 g daily without significant adverse effects, was described.

1. Van Vleymen B, Van Zandijcke M. Piracetam in the treatment of myoclonus: an overview. *Acta Neurol Belg* 1996; **96**: 270–80.
2. Genton P, et al. Piracetam in the treatment of cortical myoclonus. *Pharmacopsychiatry* 1999; **32** (suppl): 49–53.

Stroke. Piracetam did not influence the outcome if given within 12 hours of the onset of acute ischaemic stroke in a multicentre, randomised, double-blind trial,[1] although post hoc analyses suggested that it might confer benefit when given within 7 hours of onset, particularly in patients with stroke of moderate to severe degree. Further analyses of the same data concluded that piracetam did not produce significant adverse effects when given in high doses to patients with acute stroke,[2] and significantly more patients had recovered from aphasia on piracetam than placebo.[3] The results of two further randomised, double-blind, placebo-controlled trials supporting the role of piracetam as an adjunct to intensive speech therapy in improving aphasia following stroke were also reported.[3] In contrast, a review of

the first study considered that the trend towards an increased risk of early death in patients allocated to piracetam was of concern, and concluded that the data did not support routine use of piracetam in acute ischaemic stroke.[4]

1. De Deyn PP, et al. Treatment of acute and ischemic stroke with piracetam. *Stroke* 1997; **28**: 2347–52.
2. De Reuck J, Van Vleyman B. The clinical safety of high-dose piracetam—its use in the treatment of acute stroke. *Pharmacopsychiatry* 1999; **32** (suppl 1): 33–7.
3. Huber W. The role of piracetam in the treatment of acute and chronic aphasia. *Pharmacopsychiatry* 1999; **32** (suppl 1): 38–43.
4. Ricci S, et al. Piracetam for acute ischaemic stroke (updated 21 February 2000). Available in The Cochrane Library; Issue 4. Oxford: Update Software; 2001.

Vertigo. Piracetam has been reported to be of benefit in patients with vertigo (p.408) of both central or peripheral origin.[1]

1. Oosterveld WJ. The effectiveness of piracetam in vertigo. *Pharmacopsychiatry.* 1999; **32** (suppl 1): 54–60.

Preparations
Proprietary Preparations (details are given in Part 3)
Aust.: Cerebryl; Nootropil; Novocephal; Pirabene; *Belg.*: Braintop; Geratam; Noodis; Nootropil; *Braz.*: Cintilan; Nootron; Nootropil; *Fin.*: Nootropil; *Fr.*: Axonyl; Gabacet; Geram; Nootropyl; *Ger.*: Avigilen; Cerebroforte; Cerepar N; Cuxabrain; durapitrop; Encetrop; Memo-Puren; Nootrop; Normabrain; Novocetam; Piracebral; Piracetrop; Sinapsan; *Hong Kong*: Nootropil; *Ital.*: Cerebropan; Cleveral; Flavis; Nootropil; Norzetam; Psycoton; *Mex.*: Dinagen; Nootropil; *Neth.*: Nootropil; *Port.*: Acetar; Noostan; Nootropil; Oxibran; Stimubral; *S.Afr.*: Nootropil; *Singapore*: Cebrotonin; Nootropil; Piratam; Racetam; *Spain*: Ciclofalina; Genogris; Nootropil; *Swed.*: Nootropil; *Switz.*: Nootropil; Pirax; *Thai.*: Embol; Memphil; Noocetam; Nootropil; *UK*: Nootropil.
Multi-ingredient: *Braz.*: Energivit; Exit; Isketam; Psicoglut; Vincetron; *Port.*: Anacervix; Centracetam; Euvifor; Stimilfar; *Spain*: Anacervix; Devincal; Diemil; Memorino; Piracetam Complex.

Pirenoxine Sodium (13131-t)

Pirenoxine Sodium (rINNM).
Catalin Sodium; Pirfenoxone Sodium. Sodium 1-hydroxy-5-oxo-5H-pyrido[3,2-a]phenoxazine-3-carboxylate.
$C_{16}H_7N_2NaO_5 = 330.2$.
CAS — 1043-21-6 (pirenoxine); 51410-30-1 (pirenoxine sodium).
Pharmacopoeias. Jpn includes Pirenoxine.

Profile
Pirenoxine sodium is used in the treatment of cataracts, usually as 0.005% eye drops.

Preparations
Proprietary Preparations (details are given in Part 3)
Ger.: Clarvisor; *Hong Kong*: Catalin; *Ital.*: Clarvisan; Pirfalin; *Mex.*: Clarvisan; *Port.*: Clarvisan; *Singapore*: Catalin; *Spain*: Clarvisan.

Pirfenidone (6383-n)

Pirfenidone (USAN, rINN).
AMR-69. 5-Methyl-1-phenyl-2(1H)-pyridone.
$C_{12}H_{11}NO = 185.2$.
CAS — 53179-13-8.

Profile
Pirfenidone is an antifibrotic drug under investigation in fibrosing disorders such as idiopathic pulmonary fibrosis.

◊ References.
1. Nicod LP. Pirfenidone in idiopathic pulmonary fibrosis. *Lancet* 1999; **354**: 268–9.

Pirglutargine (13132-x)

Arginine Pidolate; Arginine Pyroglutamate. L-Arginine DL-pyroglutamate.
$C_{11}H_{21}N_5O_5 = 303.3$.
CAS — 64855-91-0.

Profile
Pirglutargine has been used for its reputed cerebral stimulant effect.

Preparations
Proprietary Preparations (details are given in Part 3)
Ital.: Adiuvant.
Multi-ingredient: *Ital.*: Detoxergon†; *Port.*: Detoxergon.

Piridoxilate (13133-r)

Piridoxilate (BAN, rINN).
Pyridoxine α_5-Hemiacetal Glyoxylate; Pyridoxylate. The reciprocal salt of 2-(5-hydroxy-4-hydroxymethyl-6-methyl-3-pyridylmethoxy)glycolic acid with 2-[4,5-bis(hydroxymethyl)-2-methyl-3-pyridyloxy]glycolic acid (1:1).
$C_{10}H_{13}NO_6, C_{10}H_{13}NO_6 = 486.4$.
CAS — 24340-35-0.

Profile
Piridoxilate was formerly used in the treatment of various circulatory disorders.

Pirisudanol Maleate (13192-s)

Pirisudanol Maleate (rINNM).
Pyrisuccideanol Maleate. 2-Dimethylaminoethyl 5-hydroxy-4-hydroxymethyl-6-methyl-3-pyridylmethyl succinate maleate.
$C_{16}H_{24}N_2O_6, (C_4H_4O_4)_2 = 572.5$.
CAS — 33605-94-6 (pirisudanol); 53659-00-0 (pirisudanol maleate).

Pirisudanol is the succinic acid ester of pyridoxine and of deanol.

Profile
Pirisudanol has been given as the maleate in the treatment of cerebrovascular and similar disorders in doses of up to 1200 mg daily.

Preparations
Proprietary Preparations (details are given in Part 3)
Belg.: Nadex†; *Fr.*: Stivane†; *Ital.*: Mentium; *Port.*: Pridana; *Spain*: Mentis; *Switz.*: Nadex.

Pitofenone Hydrochloride (5241-h)

Pitofenone Hydrochloride (rINNM).
Methyl 2-[4-(2-piperidinoethoxy)benzoyl]benzoate hydrochloride.
$C_{22}H_{25}NO_4, HCl = 403.9$.
CAS — 54063-52-4 (pitofenone); 1248-42-6 (pitofenone hydrochloride).

Profile
Pitofenone hydrochloride has been used as an antispasmodic.

Preparations
Proprietary Preparations (details are given in Part 3)
Multi-ingredient: *Fin.*: Litalgin; *S.Afr.*: Baralgan†.

Plantain (5448-k)

Pharmacopoeias. In Chin. and Jpn., which also have separate monographs for the seed. Chin also permits P. depressa. Fr. includes the leaves.

The seeds or leaves of *Plantago major* var. *asiatica*.

Profile
Plantain is reported to possess diuretic and antihaemorrhagic properties. It is used in homoeopathic medicine and various forms of traditional medicine.

Preparations
Proprietary Preparations (details are given in Part 3)
Fr.: Sensivision au plantain.
Multi-ingredient: *Austral.*: Hamamelis Complex; *Fr.*: Ephydrol; *Port.*: Erpecalm; *Switz.*: Kernosan Elixir; Pastilles pectorales Demo N; Pectoral N; Sirop pectoral DP1†; Sirop pectoral DP2, DP3†; Tisane pectorale pour les enfants.

Plastics (13141-r)

Pharmacopoeias. Many pharmacopoeias include standards for plastic containers and closures.

Adverse Effects
Plastic materials used in medicine and pharmacy may give rise to various adverse effects, either by direct contact of the plastic with tissues or by indirect contact (for example, when a solution stored in a plastic container, such as a disposable syringe, is injected). Adverse effects may also arise among workers through handling the materials or by inhaling fumes during manufacture.

Pure polymeric plastics appear to be of low toxicity, though carcinogenic effects have been produced by some on prolonged implantation. However, some monomers are toxic, as may be substances added during manufacture to impart specific physical properties. These additives include plasticisers added to reduce brittleness, ultraviolet-ray absorbers to prevent degradation by light, and antioxidants and lubricants which are sometimes needed for satisfactory processing. Monomer residues or additives can leach out from the finished plastic materials and have been the main causes of adverse effects. These may include haemolysis of blood cells, thrombosis, hypersensitivity reactions, precancerous changes, and local tissue necrosis. Silicone particles have been shed from dialysis tubing resulting in hypersplenism, pancytopenia, and occasionally in the production of a granulomatous hepatitis.

See also under Vinyl Chloride, p.1680, Methylmethacrylate, p.1635, and Polytef, below.

Pleurisy Root   (12110-g)

Butterfly Weed.

Profile

The root of *Asclepias tuberosa* (Asclepiadaceae) has traditionally been used for pleurisy and other respiratory-tract disorders.

Preparations

Proprietary Preparations (details are given in Part 3)

Multi-ingredient: *Austral.:* Verbascum Complex; *UK:* Antibron; Chest Mixture; Horehound and Aniseed Cough Mixture; Vegetable Cough Remover.

Pokeroot   (13111-z)

Poke Root.

Pharmacopoeias. In Chin.

Profile

Pokeroot, the root of *Phytolacca decandra* (*P. americana*) (Phytolaccaceae) has emetic, purgative, anti-inflammatory, and anti-infective actions. It has been used for rheumatic and arthritic disorders, and for respiratory-tract infections, but is highly toxic in large doses and is not generally recommended. It has also been used externally for skin disorders.

It is also used in homoeopathic medicine.

The related species, *P. dodecandra*, is the source of the molluscicide endod (p.1432).

Preparations

Proprietary Preparations (details are given in Part 3)

Multi-ingredient: *Braz.:* Fucus Composto; *Fr.:* Homeoplasmine; *UK:* Psorasolv.

Polacrilin Potassium   (5006-j)

Polacrilin Potassium (USAN, rINNM).

Polacrilinum Kalii.

CAS — 54182-62-6 (polacrilin); 50602-21-6 (polacrilin).

Pharmacopoeias. In USNF.

Pharmacopoeial description

USNF 20: The potassium salt of a unifunctional low-cross-linked carboxylic cation-exchange resin prepared from methacrylic acid and divinylbenzene. A white to off-white, free-flowing powder. Has a faint odour or is odourless. Insoluble in water and in most liquids.

Profile

Polacrilin potassium is used as a tablet and capsule disintegrant.

Poly A.poly U   (13143-d)

Polyadenylic-polyuridylic Acid.

CAS — 24936-38-7.

Profile

Poly A.poly U is a double-stranded polyribonucleotide comprising polyadenylic and polyuridylic acids, and is believed to be a stimulant of the immune system. It has been studied as an adjuvant in the management of operable solid tumours.

Poly I.poly C   (13144-n)

Polyinosinic-polycytidylic Acid.

CAS — 24939-03-5.

Poly I.poly C is a synthetic double-stranded polyribonucleotide complex of equimolar concentrations of polyinosinic and polycytidylic acids, described as a mismatched double-strand RNA.

Profile

Poly I.poly C and the complex of poly I.poly C stabilised with poly-L-lysine in carmellose (carboxymethylcellulose) [poly(ICLC)] have been found to induce the production of interferon and have been investigated in the treatment of malignant neoplasms and viral infections. Poly I.poly C has been investigated for the treatment of AIDS, chronic fatigue syndrome, renal cell carcinoma, and invasive metastatic melanoma, and poly(ICLC) for the treatment of primary brain tumours.

Preparations

Proprietary Preparations (details are given in Part 3)

USA: Ampligen.

Polysaccharide-K   (3850-e)

PSK; PS-K.

Profile

Polysaccharide-K is a protein-bound polysaccharide isolated from a fungus. It is claimed to have immunostimulant and antineoplastic properties.

The symbol † denotes a preparation no longer actively marketed

---

◊ References.

1. Tsukagoshi S, *et al.* Krestin (PSK). *Cancer Treat Rev* 1984; **11:** 131–55.
2. Go P, Chung C-H. Adjuvant PSK immunotherapy in patients with carcinoma of the nasopharynx. *J Int Med Res* 1989; **17:** 141–9.
3. Torisu M, *et al.* Significant prolongation of disease-free period gained by oral polysaccharide K (PSK) administration after curative surgical operation of colorectal cancer. *Cancer Immunol Immunother* 1990; **31:** 261–8.
4. Nakazato H, *et al.* Efficacy of immunochemotherapy as adjuvant treatment after curative resection of gastric cancer. *Lancet* 1994; **343:** 1122–6.
5. Hayakawa K, *et al.* Effect of Krestin as adjuvant treatment following radical radiotherapy in non-small cell lung cancer patients. *Cancer Detect Prev* 1997; **21:** 71–7.

Polytef   (13150-f)

Polytef (USAN).

Politef (pINN); PTFE. Poly(tetrafluoroethylene).

$(C_2F_4)_n$.

CAS — 9002-84-0.

Profile

Polytef has numerous industrial applications. As 'Teflon' it is used on 'non-stick' cooking utensils.

A paste of polytef has been used for a variety of purposes including the treatment of aphonia, for replacement grafts in vascular surgery, and in the correction of some forms of urinary incontinence (p.459). The main concern with these procedures is migration of polytef particles. It has also been applied to the skin as a barrier paste with perfluoroalkylpolyether to reduce exposure to chemical warfare agents.

Adverse effects. Brain injury in a child was possibly associated with migration of polytef particles from a periureteral injection performed 1 year earlier.[1] Three cases of polytef adenopathy and one case of giant granuloma have been reported[2] in children who had previously undergone subureteral polytef injection for the treatment of vesicoureteral reflux.

1. Borgatti R, *et al.* Brain injury in a healthy child one year after periureteral injection of Teflon. *Pediatrics* 1996; **98:** 290–1.
2. Aragona F, *et al.* Polytetrafluoroethylene giant granuloma and adenopathy: long-term complications following subureteral polytetrafluoroethylene injection for the treatment of vesicoureteral reflux in children. *J Urol (Baltimore)* 1997; **158:** 1539–42.

Uses. References.

1. Kidson IG. Prosthetic implants: arterial prostheses. *Br J Hosp Med* 1983; **30:** 248–54.
2. Schulman CC, *et al.* Endoscopic injections of Teflon to treat urinary incontinence in women. *BMJ* 1984; **288:** 192.
3. O'Donnell B, Puri P. Endoscopic correction of primary vesicoureteric reflux: results in 94 ureters. *BMJ* 1986; **293:** 1404–6.
4. Polley JW, *et al.* The use of Teflon in orbital floor reconstruction following blunt facial trauma: a 20-year experience. *Plast Reconstr Surg* 1987; **79:** 39–43.
5. Puri P. Endoscopic correction of primary vesicoureteric reflux by subureteric injection of polytetrafluoroethylene. *Lancet* 1990; **335:** 1320–2.
6. Maskell R, *et al.* Correction of vesicoureteric reflux by endoscopic injection. *Lancet* 1991; **338:** 1460–1.
7. Anonymous. Use of Teflon preparations for urinary incontinence and vesicoureteral reflux. *JAMA* 1993; **269:** 2975–80.
8. Duckett JRA. The use of periurethral injectables in the treatment of genuine stress incontinence. *Br J Obstet Gynaecol* 1998; **105:** 390–6.
9. Su TH, *et al.* Injection therapy for stress incontinence in women. *Int Urogynecol J* 1999; **10:** 200–6.

Poplar Buds   (8199-k)

Balm of Gilead Buds.

Profile

The buds of various species of *Populus*, including *P. nigra, P. candicans, P. gileadensis*, and *P. tacamahacca* (*P. balsamifera*) have been used for the analgesic properties conveyed by their salicin content, as well as in preparations for a variety of other disorders. They also contain volatile oil, resin, and other substances. The resin from poplar buds is one of the major sources of propolis (p.1655).

Preparations

Proprietary Preparations (details are given in Part 3)

Multi-ingredient: *Aust.:* Phytodolor; Prostagutt; *Austral.:* Valerian; *Braz.:* Eviprostat; *Canad.:* Mielocol; Wampole Bronchial Cough Syrup; *Ger.:* Eviprostat N; Phytodolor; Prostamed; *Hong Kong:* Eviprostat; *Port.:* Prostamed; *Singapore:* Eviprostat; *Switz.:* Eviprostat†; Phytomed Prosta; *UK:* Balm of Gilead; Gerard House Ligvites; Gerard House Reumalex; Hofels White Willow and Burdock; Peerless Composition Essence; Tabritis.

Poppy-seed Oil   (7365-q)

Huile d'Oeillette; Maw Oil; Oleum Papaveris; Oleum Papaveris Seminis.

The fixed oil expressed from the ripe seeds of the opium poppy, *Papaver somniferum* (Papaveraceae)

Profile

Poppy-seed oil is used as a substitute for olive oil for culinary and pharmaceutical purposes. It is also used in the preparation

---

of Iodised Oil Fluid Injection (BP 2001). Commercial grades are used in making soaps, paints, and varnishes.

Potassium Aminobenzoate   (7872-m)

Aminobenzoate Potassium. Potassium 4-aminobenzoate.

$C_7H_6KNO_2 = 175.2$.

CAS — 138-84-1.

Pharmacopoeias. In US.

Pharmacopoeial description

USP 25: A white crystalline powder. Very soluble in water; soluble in alcohol; practically insoluble in ether. A 1% solution in water has a pH of about 7, while a 5% solution has a pH of 8.0 to 9.0.

Adverse Effects and Precautions

Anorexia, nausea, fever, and skin rash have been reported. Potassium aminobenzoate should be given with caution to patients with renal impairment. The manufacturers recommend that treatment should be interrupted during periods of fasting, anorexia, or low food intake, to avoid the possible development of hypoglycaemia.

Interactions

Potassium aminobenzoate will inactivate sulfonamides given concurrently.

Uses and Administration

Potassium aminobenzoate has been used in the treatment of various disorders associated with excessive fibrosis, such as scleroderma (p.505) and Peyronie's disease, in usual doses of 12 g daily by mouth in 4 to 6 divided doses.

Peyronie's disease. Variable results have been reported with potassium aminobenzoate in the treatment of Peyronie's disease,[1-3] but evidence from well controlled trials is lacking. It has been suggested that a successful response is more likely if treatment is commenced in the acute stage.[2]

1. Gingell JC, Desai KM. Peyronie's disease. *BMJ* 1988; **298:** 1489–90.
2. Mohanty KC, Strachan RG. Peyronie's disease. *BMJ* 1989; **298:** 254.
3. Carson CC. Potassium aminobenzoate for the treatment of Peyronie's disease: is it effective? *Tech Urol* 1997; **3:** 135–9.

Preparations

USP 25: Aminobenzoate Potassium Capsules; Aminobenzoate Potassium for Oral Solution; Aminobenzoate Potassium Tablets.

Proprietary Preparations (details are given in Part 3)

Aust.: Potaba; *Canad.:* Potaba; *Ger.:* Potaba; *Hong Kong:* Potaba; *Mex.:* Potabex; *Switz.:* Potaba; *UK:* Potaba; *USA:* Potaba.

Potassium Borotartrate   (13152-n)

Potassium Sodium Borotartrate; Soluble Cream of Tartar.

Profile

Potassium borotartrate is reported to have similar properties to those of bromides. It has been used in nervous disorders and has been used in photography as a retarder for alkaline developers. Chronic boron poisoning (see under Boric Acid, p.1586) has been reported following the use of potassium borotartrate internally.

Preparations

Proprietary Preparations (details are given in Part 3)

Multi-ingredient: *Fr.:* Dinacode.

Potassium Bromate   (13153-h)

924.

$KBrO_3 = 167.0$.

CAS — 7758-01-2.

Adverse Effects

Nausea, vomiting, severe abdominal pains, diarrhoea, and lethargy are common symptoms following the ingestion of potassium bromate.

Ototoxicity and nephrotoxicity are the major toxic effects of potassium bromate poisoning, and may be irreversible. Acute renal failure arising from tubular necrosis usually presents with oliguria or anuria within 1 to 3 days of significant ingestion, and is the most frequent cause of death. Ototoxicity may present as tinnitus or hearing loss within hours of ingestion, and can progress to sensorineural deafness in some patients.

Potassium bromate poisoning may also produce myocarditis, hepatitis, and encephalopathy characterised by agitation, delirium, convulsions, and coma. Microangiopathic anaemia has also been reported.

Potassium bromate is carcinogenic in *animals*.

◊ Reports of bromate poisoning.

1. Lue JN, *et al.* Bromate poisoning from ingestion of professional hair-care neutralizer. *Clin Pharm* 1988; **7:** 66–70.
2. Lichtenberg R, *et al.* Bromate poisoning. *J Pediatr* 1989; **114:** 891–4.
3. De Vriese A, *et al.* Severe acute renal failure due to bromate intoxication: report of a case and discussion of management guidelines based on a review of the literature. *Nephrol Dial Transplant* 1997; **12:** 204–9.

Treatment of Adverse Effects

After the ingestion of potassium bromate the stomach should be emptied by lavage; use of a 2 to 5% solution of sodium bicarbonate has been suggested to reduce bromate absorption and prevent hydrobromic acid production. Administration of activated charcoal has also been recommended as an adsorbent. Attention to the patient's fluid, acid-base, and electrolyte status is important, particularly in the presence of acute renal failure. Pain is relieved by the injection of pethidine. An intravenous infusion of 100 to 500 mL of a 1% sodium thiosulfate solution has sometimes been given. Oxygen may be indicated. The prompt use of haemodialysis or peritoneal dialysis has been suggested.

◊ Although the use of intravenous sodium thiosulfate is an accepted practice in the treatment of bromate poisoning, convincing evidence that it reduces bromate to bromide is lacking.[1,2] Oral sodium thiosulfate solutions have also been used but are no longer recommended because hydrogen sulfide, itself a powerful irritant and toxic agent, may be evolved in the presence of hydrochloric acid.[2]

1. McElwee NE, Kearney TE. Sodium thiosulfate unproven as bromate antidote. *Clin Pharm* 1988; **7:** 570–2.
2. De Vriese A, *et al.* Severe acute renal failure due to bromate intoxication: report of a case and discussion of management guidelines based on a review of the literature. *Nephrol Dial Transplant* 1997; **12:** 204–9.

Uses

Potassium bromate is an oxidising agent. It has no therapeutic uses but it has been widely used as the 'neutraliser' of thioglycollate hair-waving lotions. It has been used in the preparation of barley malt for beer. It has also been used as a flour-maturing agent but such use is no longer considered appropriate and is prohibited in some countries.

◊ Potassium bromate is a genotoxic carcinogen and should not be present in foods as consumed. Its use for the treatment of flour for bread-making is not appropriate.

1. FAO/WHO. Evaluation of certain food additives and contaminants: forty-fourth report of the joint FAO/WHO expert committee on food additives. *WHO Tech Rep Ser* 859 1995.

Potassium Chlorate (318-y)

Kalium Chloricum; Potassii Chloras.
$KClO_3 = 122.5$.
CAS — 3811-04-9.
Pharmacopoeias. In *Belg.* and *Swiss.*

◊ CAUTION. *Potassium chlorate is unstable and, in contact with organic or readily oxidisable substances such as charcoal, phosphorus, or sulfur it is liable to explode especially if heated or subjected to friction or percussion. It should not be allowed to come into contact with matches or surfaces containing phosphorus compounds. Reasonable steps should be taken before supplying potassium chlorate to ensure that it will not be used for the illicit preparation of explosives or fireworks.*

Profile

Potassium chlorate has been used as an astringent, usually as a mouthwash or gargle. Concentrated solutions are irritant.

Acute poisoning from ingestion requires prompt symptomatic treatment. Symptoms include nausea, vomiting, diarrhoea, abdominal pain, haemolytic anaemia, haemorrhage, methaemoglobinaemia, hyperkalaemia, and renal failure. There may be liver damage and central effects with convulsions and coma.

If methaemoglobinaemia is severe, patients may require exchange transfusion with whole blood. Several authorities consider that methylene blue [methylthioninium chloride] should be given intravenously if methaemoglobinaemia is greater than 30%, although the UK manufacturers of the injection advise against its use in chlorate poisoning for fear of converting chlorate to the more toxic hypochlorite.

Preparations

Proprietary Preparations (details are given in Part 3)
Multi-ingredient: *Canad.:* Fletchers Sore Mouth Medicine; *Ger.:* Gargarisma†; *Spain:* Cloroboral; Edifaringen; Solurrinol; Tyroneomicin†.

Potassium Hydroxide (211-h)

Ätzkali; Caustic Potash; E525; Kalii Hydroxidum; Kalii Hydroxydum; Kalium Hydroxydatum; Potash Lye.
$KOH = 56.11$.
CAS — 1310-58-3.
Pharmacopoeias. In *Eur.* (see p.vi) and *Jpn.* Also in *USNF.*

Pharmacopoeial description

Ph. Eur.: White, crystalline, hard masses, supplied as sticks, pellets, or irregularly shaped pieces; it is deliquescent in air, hygroscopic, and absorbs carbon dioxide. Very soluble in water; freely soluble in alcohol. Store in airtight, non-metallic containers.

USNF 20: It contains not less than 85% of total alkali, calculated as KOH, including not more than 3.5% of K_2CO_3. White or practically white, fused masses, or small pellets, or flakes, or sticks, or other forms. It is hard and brittle and shows a crystalline fracture. Exposed to air, it rapidly absorbs carbon dioxide

and moisture, and deliquesces. Soluble 1 in 1 of water, 1 in 3 of alcohol, and 1 in 2.5 of glycerol; very soluble in boiling alcohol. Store in airtight containers.

Adverse Effects and Treatment

As for Sodium Hydroxide, p.1665.

Uses and Administration

Potassium hydroxide is a powerful caustic which has been used to remove warts (p.1108). A 2.5% solution in glycerol has been used as a cuticle solvent. An escharotic preparation of potassium hydroxide and calcium hydroxide was known as Vienna paste.

Preparations

BP 2001: Chloroxylenol Solution; Potassium Hydroxide Solution.
Proprietary Preparations (details are given in Part 3)
Spain: Cerumenol; Kuson.

Multi-ingredient: *Aust.:* Leberinfusion; *Ger.:* Acarex; Glutarsin E; Kalium-Magnesium-Asparaginat; KMA; Sekudrill; *Ital.:* Sekudrill; *S.Afr.:* Peter Pote's†.

Potassium Hydroxyquinoline Sulfate

(1630-g)

Oxyquinol Potassium; Potassii Hydroxyquinolini Sulphas; Potassium Hydroxyquinoline Sulphate; Potassium Oxyquinoline Sulphate.
Pharmacopoeias. In *Aust., Br., Fr.,* and *Ger.*

Pharmacopoeial description

BP 2001: An equimolecular mixture of potassium sulfate and quinolin-8-ol sulfate monohydrate. It contains 50.6 to 52.6% of quinolin-8-ol and 29.5 to 32.5% of potassium sulfate, calculated with reference to the anhydrous substance. A pale yellow, odourless or almost odourless, microcrystalline powder. Freely soluble in water; insoluble in ether. On extraction with hot dehydrated alcohol a residue of potassium sulfate and a solution of quinolin-8-ol sulfate are obtained.

Profile

Potassium hydroxyquinoline sulfate has antibacterial, antifungal, and deodorant properties and is used, often in conjunction with benzoyl peroxide, in the topical treatment of fungal infections, minor bacterial infections, and acne.

Preparations

BP 2001: Potassium Hydroxyquinoline Sulphate and Benzoyl Peroxide Cream.
Proprietary Preparations (details are given in Part 3)
Multi-ingredient: *Belg.:* Aseptosyl; *Irl.:* Quinocort; Quinoderm; Valderma; *S.Afr.:* Auralgicin; Oto-Phen Forte; Quinoderm; Quinoderm-H†; Universal Earache Drops; *Spain:* Stoma Anestesia Dental; *Switz.:* Quinoderm†; Rectoseptal-Neo bismuthe; Rectoseptal-Neo simple; *UK:* Quinocort; Quinoderm; Quinoped; Valderma.

Potassium Metaphosphate (1182-r)

E450(c); Potassium Kurrol's Salt; Potassium Polymetaphosphate.
$(KPO_3)_x$.
CAS — 7790-53-6.
Pharmacopoeias. In *USNF.*

Pharmacopoeial description

USNF 20: A straight-chain polyphosphate, having a high degree of polymerisation. It contains the equivalent of 59 to 61% of P_2O_5. A white, odourless powder. Insoluble in water; soluble in dilute solutions of sodium salts.

Profile

Potassium metaphosphate is used as a buffer.

Pramiracetam Sulfate (16967-a)

Pramiracetam Sulfate (USAN, rINNM).
Amacetam Sulphate; CI-879; Pramiracetam Sulphate. *N*-[2-(Diisopropylamino)ethyl]-2-oxo-1-pyrrolidineacetamide sulphate.
$C_{14}H_{27}N_3O_2,H_2SO_4 = 367.5$.
CAS — 68497-62-1 (pramiracetam); 72869-16-0 (pramiracetam sulfate).

Profile

Pramiracetam sulfate is used in age-related memory impairment and senile dementia (p.1412), in doses equivalent to 600 mg of pramiracetam twice daily by mouth. It has also been tried, without much success, as an adjunct to electroconvulsive therapy in severe depression.

◊ References.
1. Chang T, *et al.* Pharmacokinetics of oral pramiracetam in normal volunteers. *J Clin Pharmacol* 1985; **25:** 291–5.
2. Dejong R. Safety of pramiracetam. *Curr Ther Res* 1987; **41:** 254–7.
3. Scarpazza P, *et al.* Multicenter evaluation of pramiracetam for the treatment of memory impairment of probable vascular origin. *Adv Therapy* 1993; **10:** 217–25.

Preparations

Proprietary Preparations (details are given in Part 3)
Ital.: Neupramir; Pramistar; Remen†.

Pramiverine Hydrochloride (5242-m)

Pramiverine Hydrochloride (BANM, rINNM).
EMD-9806 (pramiverine); HSP-2986 (pramiverine). *N*-Isopropyl-4,4-diphenylcyclohexylamine hydrochloride.
$C_{21}H_{27}N,HCl = 329.9$.
CAS — 14334-40-8 (pramiverine); 14334-41-9 (pramiverine hydrochloride).

Profile

Pramiverine hydrochloride has been used as an antispasmodic.

Pregnancy and Fertility Tests (1959-p)

Profile

There are a number of kits available for simple pregnancy and fertility testing. A common method of detecting pregnancy is to use specific antibodies to measure the increase in chorionic gonadotrophin in the urine. The period of ovulation can be detected by measuring luteinising hormone excretion in similar ways.

These tests can give false results. Those carrying out the tests should be aware of this and of problems such as contaminated specimens, concomitant drug therapy, or other factors that could affect the result.

Preparations

Proprietary Preparations (details are given in Part 3)
Austral.: Answer; Clearblue One Step; Clearplan One Step; Clearview HCG; Clinitek HCG; Discover Onestep; Discover Onestep Ovulation Prediction; Dotest; Easy hCG†; Evaplan; Evatest One Step; First Response†; Fortel One Step; Neo-Planotest Duoclon†; Neo-Pregnosticon†; Nimbus; Ovuplan; Predictor†; Pregnosis; UCG-Beta†; UCG-Slide†; *Braz.:* Predictor; *Canad.:* Answer Now; Clearblue; Clearplan; Conceive†; Confidelle; Confirm; Fact Plus; First Response; Simplicity; *Fr.:* Bluetest†; Clearblue; Clearplan; G.Test; Indicatest; Predictor; Primacard; Primastick; Primatime; Revelatest; *Irl.:* Fertility Score; Testpack hCG-Urine; Uni-Gold hCG; *Israel:* Clearblue; Gravindex; Predictor; Pregnosticon; Preprurex; *Ital.:* Advisor; Clearplan; Confidelle Progress; Diagnosis; PG 53†; Predictor; Rivela; *NZ:* Cards HCG-Urine; Clearblue; Clearplan; LH Predict; *Port.:* Bluetest†; Clearview HCG†; *Switz.:* Clearplan; *UK:* Auratek hCG; Clearblue; Clearplan; Clearview HCG; Concept Blue; Concise†; Discover; Early Bird; First Response; Neo-Planotest; Ovukit; Ovuquick; Predictor; Pregna-Cert; Pregna-Sure HCG; Pregnospia Duoclon; Preprurex; Ramp; Reveal; Tandem Icon; Test Pack Plus; *USA:* Advance; Answer; Clearblue Easy; Clearplan Easy; Clearview HCG; Conceive Ovulation Predictor; Conceive Pregnancy; Daisy†; ept Stick Test; Fact Plus; First Response; Fortel; Nimbus; OvuGen; Ovukit; Ovuquick; Pregnosis; QTest; QTest Ovulation; QuickVue; RapidVue; TestPack Plus hCG-Urine; UCG-Slide; Unistep hCG.

Prenylamine Lactate (9275-r)

Prenylamine Lactate (BANM, rINNM).
B-436 (prenylamine); Hoechst-12512 (prenylamine); Prenylaminii Lactas. 2-Benzhydrylethyl(α-methylphenethyl)amine lactate.
$C_{24}H_{27}N,C_3H_6O_3 = 419.6$.
CAS — 69-43-2 (prenylamine lactate); 390-64-7 (prenylamine).
NOTE. Prenylamine is USAN
Pharmacopoeias. In *Pol.*

Profile

Prenylamine depletes myocardial catecholamine stores and has some calcium-channel blocking activity. It was formerly used in the treatment of angina pectoris but has been superseded by less toxic drugs. Administration of prenylamine has been associated with the development of ventricular arrhythmias and ECG abnormalities. Tremor and extrapyramidal symptoms have also occurred.

Porphyria. Prenylamine is considered to be unsafe in patients with porphyria because it has been shown to be porphyrinogenic in *in-vitro* systems.

Proadifen Hydrochloride (13169-w)

Proadifen Hydrochloride (USAN, rINNM).
NSC-39690; Propyladiphenine Hydrochloride; RP-5171; SKF-525A; SKF-525-A. 2-Diethylaminoethyl 2,2-diphenylvalerate hydrochloride.
$C_{23}H_{31}NO_2,HCl = 390.0$.
CAS — 302-33-0 (proadifen); 62-68-0 (proadifen hydrochloride).

Profile

Proadifen has been found to enhance the effects of a large number of drugs, possibly by inhibiting metabolism.

Procodazole (13172-v)

Procodazole (rINN).

Propazol; Propazole. 3-(Benzimidazol-2-yl)propionic acid.
$C_{10}H_{10}N_2O_2 = 190.2.$
CAS — 23249-97-0 (procodazole); 6315-23-7 (procodazole ethyl ester); 59345-72-1 (procodazole sodium).

Profile
Procodazole is reported to have immunostimulant properties. It is given as the ethyl ester. The sodium salt has also been used.

Preparations
Proprietary Preparations (details are given in Part 3)
Spain: Estimulocel†.

Promelase (8399-h)

Promelase (pINN).

Seaprose S.
CAS — 9074-07-1.

Profile
Promelase is an alkaline protease derived from *Aspergillus melleus*. It has been taken by mouth in doses of 30 to 90 mg daily for its supposed benefit in oedema and inflammation associated with trauma, infection, and surgical procedures.

Preparations
Proprietary Preparations (details are given in Part 3)
Ital.: Altan; Flaminase; Mezen; *Jpn:* Onoprose†; *Port.:* Onoprose; *Thai.:* Korynase.

Propolis (8226-b)

Bee Glue.

Profile
Propolis is a resinous substance collected by bees, primarily, at least in Europe, from poplar buds (see also p.1653), and used by them to seal their hives. It has been traditionally used for a wide variety of disorders, in cosmetics, and for the varnishing of Stradivarius violins. Propolis has been reported to have anti-inflammatory and antimicrobial properties. It has been used as an ointment for the relief of symptoms of herpes labialis. Hypersensitivity reactions have been reported.

◊ References.
1. Grange JM, Davey RW. Antibacterial properties of propolis (bee glue). *J R Soc Med* 1990; **83:** 159–60.
2. Krol W, *et al.* Synergistic effect of ethanolic extract of propolis and antibiotics on the growth of Staphylococcus aureus. *Arzneimittelforschung* 1993; **43:** 607–9.
3. Volpert R, Elstner EF. Interactions of different extracts of propolis with leukocytes and leukocytic enzymes. *Arzneimittelforschung* 1996; **46:** 47–51.
4. Murray MC, *et al.* A study to investigate the effect of a propolis-containing mouthrinse on the inhibition of de novo plaque formation. *J Clin Periodontol* 1997; **24:** 796–8.
5. Burdock GA. Review of the biological properties and toxicity of bee propolis (propolis). *Food Chem Toxicol* 1998; **36:** 347–63.

Preparations
Proprietary Preparations (details are given in Part 3)
Austral.: Helastop; *Ger.:* Propolisept-Salbe; *Ital.:* Golapiol; Pro-30C; Pro-Gola; Propolcream; *UK:* Buttercup Lozenges; *USA:* Probax.

Multi-ingredient: *Fr.:* Pollen Royal; Propargile; *Ital.:* Apistress; Biogreen; Bodyguard; Cocktail Reale; Fosfarsile Forte; Keratolip; Neo-Stomygen; Orostick; Probigol; Promix; Promix 3; Propast; Propomill; *Switz.:* Osa Gel de dentition aux plantes†; *UK:* Beeline.

Propylene Glycol (1908-x)

E1518; Glicol Propilênico; Propilenoglicol; Propylenglycolum.
(±)-Propane-1,2-diol.
$C_3H_8O_2 = 76.09.$
CAS — 57-55-6 ((±)-propylene glycol); 4254-16-4 ((±)-propylene glycol); 4254-14-2 ((−)-propylene glycol); 4254-15-3 ((+)-propylene glycol);.
Pharmacopoeias. In *Eur.* (see p.vi), *Jpn, Pol.,* and *US.*

Pharmacopoeial description
Ph. Eur.: A clear, colourless, viscous, hygroscopic liquid. Miscible with water and with alcohol. Store in airtight containers.

USP 25: A clear, colourless, practically odourless, viscous liquid. It absorbs moisture when exposed to moist air. Miscible with water, with acetone, and with chloroform; soluble in ether; will dissolve in many essential oils but is immiscible with fixed oils. Store in airtight containers.

Adverse Effects and Precautions
Systemic toxicity of propylene glycol is considered to be low following oral administration unless large quantities have been ingested, or when preparations containing propylene glycol are administered to neonates or to patients in renal failure. Systemic toxicity is manifested most commonly by CNS depression, especially in neonates and children. Other reported adverse effects include hepatic or renal impairment, intravascular haemolysis, seizures, coma, arrhythmias, and cardiorespiratory arrest. Hyperosmolality has occurred, particularly in small infants and

in patients with renal impairment; lactic acidosis may also be a greater problem in the latter group.

Following topical administration, propylene glycol may produce some local irritation, particularly if applied under occlusive dressings or to mucous membranes; toxicity may occur following application to burns. Hypersensitivity reactions have also been reported. Local sensitivity has been reported following administration of ear drops containing propylene glycol as the vehicle. Injections of preparations containing high concentrations of propylene glycol may produce pain or irritation.

Interactions
Anticoagulants. Propylene glycol has been reported to decrease the effect of *heparin*.[1]
1. Col J, *et al.* Propylene glycol-induced heparin resistance during nitroglycerin infusion. *Am Heart J* 1985; **110:** 171–3.

Pharmacokinetics
Propylene glycol is rapidly absorbed from the gastrointestinal tract. There is evidence of topical absorption when applied to damaged skin.

It is extensively metabolised in the liver primarily by oxidation to lactic and pyruvic acid and is also excreted in the urine unchanged.

◊ References.
1. Yu DK, *et al.* Pharmacokinetics of propylene glycol in humans during multiple dosing regimens. *J Pharm Sci* 1985; **74:** 876–9.
2. Speth PAJ, *et al.* Propylene glycol pharmacokinetics and effects after intravenous infusion in humans. *Ther Drug Monit* 1987; **9:** 255–8.

Uses and Administration
Propylene glycol is widely used in pharmaceutical manufacturing as a solvent and vehicle especially for drugs unstable or insoluble in water. It may also be employed as a stabiliser in vitamin preparations, as a plasticiser, and as a preservative. Propylene glycol is also used extensively in foods and cosmetics.

Propylene glycol has humectant properties and is used similarly to glycerol in topical moisturising preparations.

Propylene glycol is used in veterinary medicine as a glucose precursor.

Preparations
Proprietary Preparations (details are given in Part 3)
Multi-ingredient: *Aust.:* Acerbine; *Austral.:* Dermatech Liquid; *Canad.:* Episec; Gyne-Moistrin; Rhinaris; Rhinedrine Lubricant; Rhinedrine Moisturizing; Salinol; Secaris; *Fr.:* Intrasite; Propy-Lacticare; *Ger.:* Sekudrill; *Israel:* Taro Gel; *Ital.:* Dopo Pik; Sekudrill; *Port.:* Emopads; *S.Afr.:* Aserbine; *Spain:* Acerbiol; *Switz.:* Acerbine; *UK:* Aserbine; *USA:* Astroglide; Gyne-Moistrin†; Massengill Disposable; Surgel; Zonite.

Protoporphyrin IX Disodium (5575-n)

Protoporphyrin Disodium. Disodium 7,12-diethenyl-3,8,13,17-tetramethyl-21H,23H-porphine-2,18-dipropanoate.
$C_{34}H_{32}N_4Na_2O_4 = 606.6.$
CAS — 50865-01-5 (protoporphyrin IX disodium); 553-12-8 (protoporphyrin IX).

Profile
Protoporphyrin IX disodium has been given by mouth for the treatment of impaired hepatic function associated with gallstones and cholecystitis.

Preparations
Proprietary Preparations (details are given in Part 3)
Hong Kong: Prolmon.

Proxazole Citrate (5243-b)

Proxazole Citrate (USAN, rINNM).

AF-634; Propaxoline Citrate; PZ-17105. NN-Diethyl-3-(1-phenylpropyl)-1,2,4-oxadiazole-5-ethanamine citrate.
$C_{17}H_{25}N_3O, C_6H_8O_7 = 479.5.$
CAS — 5696-09-3 (proxazole); 132-35-4 (proxazole citrate).

Profile
Proxazole citrate is used as an antispasmodic and in vascular disorders and has been used in veterinary medicine.

Preparations
Proprietary Preparations (details are given in Part 3)
Ital.: Toness.

Prozapine Hydrochloride (3740-v)

Prozapine Hydrochloride (rINNM).

Hexadiphane Hydrochloride. 1-(3,3-Diphenylpropyl)cyclohexamethyleneimine hydrochloride.
$C_{21}H_{27}N, HCl = 329.9.$
CAS — 3426-08-2 (prozapine); 13657-24-4 (prozapine hydrochloride).

Profile
Prozapine hydrochloride is an antispasmodic used with sorbitol

in biliary and gastrointestinal disorders. It has been given in doses of 2 to 6 mg daily taken in water before meals.

Preparations
Proprietary Preparations (details are given in Part 3)
Multi-ingredient: *Fr.:* Norbiline; *Ital.:* Norbiline.

Psilocin (5019-t)

4-Hydroxy-NN-dimethyltryptamine; Psilocyn. 3-(2-Dimethylaminoethyl)indol-4-ol.
$C_{12}H_{16}N_2O = 204.3.$
CAS — 520-53-6.

An indole alkaloid obtained from the sacred Mexican mushroom (Teonanácatl), *Psilocybe mexicana* (Agaricaceae).

Psilocybine (5020-l)

Psilocybine (BAN, rINN).

CY-39; 4-Phosphoryloxy-NN-dimethyltryptamine; Psilocybin. 3-(2-Dimethylaminoethyl)indol-4-yl dihydrogen phosphate.
$C_{12}H_{17}N_2O_4P = 284.2.$
CAS — 520-52-5.

The main indole alkaloid present in the sacred Mexican mushroom (Teonanácatl), *Psilocybe mexicana* (Agaricaceae). In the UK, psilocybine is present in the indigenous mushroom *Psilocybe semilanceata* (magic mushroom; liberty cap). Psilocybine is also present in other species of mushrooms including *Stropharia cubensis* and *Conocybe* spp.

Profile
Psilocybine has hallucinogenic and sympathomimetic properties similar to those of lysergide (p.1630). It is less potent than lysergide and its hallucinogenic effects last for up to 6 hours. There is evidence to suggest that psilocybine is converted to the active form psilocin in the body. It has no therapeutic use.

Pulegium Oil (4696-h)

Pennyroyal Oil.

A volatile oil distilled from pennyroyal herb, *Mentha pulegium* (Labiatae), containing pulegone ($C_{10}H_{16}O = 260.3$).

Profile
Pulegium oil was formerly used as an emmenagogue. Severe toxic effects have followed its use as an abortifacient with convulsions, hepatotoxicity, and death. It is reported to have insect repellent activity.

◊ Severe hepatotoxicity accompanied by seizures occurred in 2 infants each of whom had received herbal teas containing pulegium oil.[1] In one of the infants multiple organ failure developed, and fulminant hepatic failure with hepatocellular necrosis and cerebral oedema proved fatal. A further 4 cases of toxicity associated with ingestion of pulegium oil have been reported;[2] three of the cases were adult patients who had ingested either herbal teas to induce menses (2 cases) or a herbal extract as an abortifacient (1 fatality), and the fourth was a 22-month old child who had ingested the oil.
1. Bakerink JA, *et al.* Multiple organ failure after ingestion of pennyroyal oil from herbal tea in two infants. *Pediatrics* 1996; **98:** 944–7.
2. Anderson IB, *et al.* Pennyroyal toxicity: measurement of toxic metabolite levels in two cases and review of the literature. *Ann Intern Med* 1996; **124:** 726–34.

Preparations
Proprietary Preparations (details are given in Part 3)
Multi-ingredient: *Fr.:* Santane O₁.

Pulmonary Surfactants (15937-b)

Pulmonary surfactants are used to replace deficient endogenous lung surfactants. A number of preparations have been studied including: natural human surfactant obtained from amniotic fluid or biosynthetic material; natural animal-derived surfactants, which are bovine or porcine lung extracts that may be modified by the addition of synthetic surfactants, as in the case of beractant, or unmodified, as in the case of bovactant and calfactant; and synthetic or semisynthetic preparations, which often contain colfosceril palmitate, a major constituent of natural lung surfactants, in combination with other surfactants which aid spreading and absorption.

Beractant (11625-h)

Beractant (BAN, USAN).

A-60386X.
CAS — 108778-82-1.

NOTE. The term Surfactant TA has been applied to a modified bovine lung surfactant.

Beractant is a modified bovine lung extract containing mostly phospholipids, modified by the addition of colfosceril palmitate, palmitic acid, and tripalmitin.

The symbol † denotes a preparation no longer actively marketed

Bovactant (15942-n)

Bovactant (BAN).
SF-RI1.

Bovactant is an extract of bovine lung containing about 92% of phospholipids, 3.2% of cholesterol, 0.6% of surfactant-associated hydrophobic proteins, and 0.4% of free fatty acid.

Calfactant (19960-l)

Calfactant (BAN, USAN).
CAS — 183325-78-2.

Calfactant is an unmodified calf lung extract that includes mostly phospholipids and hydrophobic surfactant-specific proteins (SP-B and SP-C).

Colfosceril Palmitate (13779-y)

Colfosceril Palmitate (BAN, USAN, rINN).
Dipalmitoylphosphatidylcholine; DPPC; 129Y83. 1,2-Dipalmitoyl-sn-glycero(3)phosphocholine.
$C_{40}H_{80}NO_8P = 734.0$.
CAS — 63-89-8.
ATC — R07AA01.

Colfosceril palmitate is a phospholipid which forms an important constituent of natural and many synthetic pulmonary surfactant compounds.

Poractant Alfa (17490-v)

Poractant Alfa (BAN).
CAS — 129069-19-8.

Poractant alfa is an extract of porcine lung containing not less than 90% of phospholipids, about 1% of hydrophobic proteins (SP-B and SP-C), and about 9% of other lipids.

Pumactant (11043-m)

Pumactant (BAN).
Artificial Lung Expanding Compound.

Pumactant is a mixture of colfosceril palmitate and phosphatidyl glycerol (2-oleoyl-1-palmitoyl-sn-glycero(3)phospho(1)-sn-glycerol) in the proportion 7:3.

Adverse Effects and Precautions

Surfactant therapy may be associated with an increased risk of pulmonary haemorrhage, especially in more premature infants. Therapy should only be given where there are adequate facilities for ventilation and monitoring. Rapid chest expansion and improvement of oxygenation may follow successful treatment, and peak ventilatory pressure and inspired oxygen concentration may need to be reduced promptly to avoid the risk of pneumothorax and hyperoxaemia. A transient decrease in brain electrical activity has been reported in neonates given surfactant but its significance is unknown. Administration of surfactant has occasionally been associated with obstruction of the endotracheal tube by mucus.

◊ While surfactant therapy is clearly associated with an increased risk of pulmonary haemorrhage,[1-4] meta-analysis suggests that the risk is small compared with the benefits of therapy.[1] However, neonates who do develop moderate or severe pulmonary haemorrhage following surfactant therapy are at increased risk of death or short-term morbidity.[5] Haemodynamic changes associated with surfactant therapy or consequent pulmonary haemorrhage may also predispose premature infants to intracranial (periventricular) haemorrhage.[5,6] Early preventive use of surfactant in very low birth-weight infants may be associated with a poorer long-term neurodevelopmental outcome,[7] although the significance of this finding is as yet uncertain. Decreased brain electrical activity has been reported following surfactant treatment.[8]

The rate of instillation of surfactant may be significant: one study,[9] in which the apparatus was adapted so that mechanical ventilation could continue during administration of surfactant, found that rapid instillation over a 5-minute period provoked a transient increase in cerebral blood flow velocity associated with an increase in carbon dioxide tension, compared with slow instillation over 15 minutes. Although the authors acknowledged that such changes are likely to be related to several factors, particularly the type of surfactant, they recommended that, until further data are available, instillation should take place slowly, over at least 15 to 20 minutes.

1. Raju TNK, Langenberg P. Pulmonary hemorrhage and exogenous surfactant therapy: a metaanalysis. J Pediatr 1993; 123: 603–10.
2. Majeed-Saidan MA, et al. Pulmonary haemorrhage in low-birthweight babies. Lancet 1993; 341: 120.
3. Rogers D. Pulmonary haemorrhage, surfactant, and low-birthweight babies. Lancet 1993; 341: 698.
4. Pappin A, et al. Extensive intraalveolar pulmonary hemorrhage in infants dying after surfactant therapy. J Pediatr 1994; 124: 621–6.
5. Pandit PB, et al. Outcome following pulmonary haemorrhage in very low birthweight neonates treated with surfactant. Arch Dis Child Fetal Neonatal Ed 1999; 81: F40–F44.
6. Gunkel JH, Banks PLC. Surfactant therapy and intracranial hemorrhage: review of the literature and results of new analyses. Pediatrics 1993; 92: 775–86.

7. Vaucher YE, et al. Outcome at twelve months of adjusted age in very low birthweight infants with lung immaturity: a randomized placebo-controlled trial of human surfactant. J Pediatr 1993; 122: 126–32.
8. Hellström-Westas L, et al. Cerebroelectrical depression following surfactant treatment in preterm neonates. Pediatrics 1992; 89: 643–7.
9. Saliba E, et al. Instillation rate effects of Exosurf on cerebral and cardiovascular haemodynamics in preterm neonates. Arch Dis Child 1994; 71: F174–8.

Uses and Administration

Pulmonary surfactants are compounds with surface active properties similar to those natural substances in the lung which help to maintain the patency of the airways by reducing the surface tension of pulmonary fluids. Exogenous pulmonary surfactants are used in the treatment of neonatal respiratory distress syndrome in premature infants, and may also be given for prevention in infants considered to be at risk of developing the syndrome. Doses vary: most pulmonary surfactants are given in recommended doses of 100 to 200 mg phospholipids per kg birth-weight, although a suggested dose for colfosceril palmitate is 67.5 mg per kg. For the treatment of overt neonatal respiratory distress syndrome, the initial dose is given as soon as possible after diagnosis, while for prevention it is given as soon as possible after birth. Administration is as a suspension via an endotracheal tube to intubated neonates receiving mechanical ventilation. Manufacturers may recommend regimens with or without disconnection from the ventilator. Repeat doses may be given if necessary, although the number of doses and the dosage interval varies.

Pulmonary surfactants have also been tried in acute respiratory distress syndrome and for meconium aspiration syndrome. A pulmonary surfactant containing the peptide sinapultide is also under investigation for acute respiratory distress syndrome and for meconium aspiration in neonates. A similar compound, lusupultide, is also under investigation for acute respiratory distress syndrome.

Acute respiratory distress syndrome. Pulmonary surfactants have been investigated in the management of acute respiratory distress syndrome (p.1046). In adults, they have been given by intratracheal instillation[1] or nebulisation[2-4] but results have been largely disappointing. Sequential bronchopulmonary segmental lavage with a synthetic surfactant has also been tried[5] and appeared to be well tolerated. Endotracheal administration of poractant alfa moderately improved oxygenation in some children with severe acute respiratory distress syndrome secondary to pulmonary or systemic disease.[6]

1. Haslam PL, et al. Surfactant replacement therapy in late-stage adult respiratory distress syndrome. Lancet 1994; 343: 1009–11.
2. do Campo JL, et al. Natural surfactant aerosolisation in adult respiratory distress syndrome. Lancet 1994; 344: 413–14.
3. Weg JG, et al. Safety and potential efficacy of an aerosolized surfactant in human sepsis-induced adult respiratory distress syndrome. JAMA 1994; 272: 1433–8.
4. Anzueto A, et al. Aerosolized surfactant in adults with sepsis-induced respiratory distress syndrome. N Engl J Med 1996; 334: 1417–21.
5. Wiswell TE, et al. Bronchopulmonary segmental lavage with Surfaxin (KL$_4$-Surfactant) for acute respiratory distress syndrome. Am J Respir Crit Care Med 1999; 160: 1188–95.
6. López-Herce J, et al. Surfactant treatment for acute respiratory distress syndrome. Arch Dis Child 1999; 80: 248–52.

Drowning. Reference to the use of colfosceril palmitate in the management of a 9-year-old rescued after near drowning.[1]

1. McBrien M, et al. Artificial surfactant in the treatment of near drowning. Lancet 1993; 342: 1485–6.

Meconium aspiration syndrome. Results from a pilot study[1] of beractant as a tracheobronchial lavage fluid for the treatment of infants with severe meconium aspiration syndrome were promising. Meta-analysis[2] of two randomised controlled trials evaluating the effect of intratracheal administration of beractant also produced encouraging results, although comparison with other established treatments for meconium aspiration syndrome remains to be done.

1. Lam BCC, Yeung CY. Surfactant lavage for meconium aspiration syndrome: a pilot study. Pediatrics 1999; 103: 1014–18.
2. Soll RF, Dargaville P. Surfactant for meconium aspiration syndrome in full term infants (updated 27 February 2001). Available in The Cochrane Library; Issue 4. Oxford: Update Software, 2001.

Neonatal respiratory distress syndrome. Surfactants are effective in the treatment of neonatal respiratory distress syndrome. The merits of initiating preventive treatment in all neonates thought to be at risk or only in those with established disease, or whether any one preparation is better than another, or whether surfactants of natural origin are superior to synthetic ones, are discussed on p.1055.

Preparations

Proprietary Preparations (details are given in Part 3)
Aust.: Alveofact; Curosurf; Exosurf; Survanta; *Austral.:* Exosurf; Survanta; *Belg.:* Alvofact; Exosurf; Survanta; *Braz.:* Alveofact; Curosurf; Exosurf; Survanta; *Canad.:* Exosurf; Survanta; *Denm.:* Curosurf; Exosurf†; *Fin.:* Curosurf; Surfexo Neonatal; *Fr.:* Curosurf; Survanta; *Ger.:* Alveofact; Curosurf; Exosurf; Survanta; *Hong Kong:* Exosurf; Survanta; *Irl.:* Curosurf; Exosurf; *Israel:* Curosurf; Survanta; *Ital.:* Alveofact†; Curosurf; Exosurf; *Jpn:* Surfacten; *Mex.:* Exosurf; Survanta; *Neth.:* Alvofact; Curosurf; Exosurf; Survanta; *Norw.:* Curosurf; Survanta-Vent; *NZ:* Survanta; *Port.:* Curosurf; Exosurf; Survanta; *S.Afr.:* Exosurf; Survanta; *Singapore:* Exosurf; Survanta; *Spain:* Curosurf; Exosurf; Survanta; *Swed.:*
Curosurf; Exosurf; Survanta-Vent; *Switz.:* Curosurf; Exosurf; Survanta; *Thai.:* Alvofact; Exosurf; Survanta; *UK:* Alec†; Curosurf; Exosurf; Survanta; *USA:* Curosurf; Exosurf; Infasurf; Survanta.

Pulsatilla (13187-l)

Meadow Anemone; Pasque Flower.
CAS — 62887-80-3.

The whole flowering plant of *Pulsatilla vulgaris* (*Anemone pulsatilla*) or *Pulsatilla pratensis* (Ranunculaceae).

Profile

Pulsatilla has been used in herbal preparations for the treatment of a wide variety of conditions including nervous disorders, circulatory disorders, and gynaecological disorders and is used in homoeopathic medicine.

Preparations

Proprietary Preparations (details are given in Part 3)
USA: Yeast-X.

Multi-ingredient: *Austral.:* Bioglan Cirflo; Calmo; Cirflo†; Lifesystem Herbal Formula 4 Women's Formula; Proflo; Viburnum Complex; Women's Formula Herbal Formula 3; *Braz.:* Eviprostat; *Fr.:* Cicaderma†; Hepatoum; Histo-Fluine P; *Ger.:* Eviprostat N; *Hong Kong:* Eviprostat; *Singapore:* Eviprostat; *Switz.:* Eviprostat†; *UK:* Anased; Daily Menopause Relief; Nytol Herbal; Period Pain Relief; Prementaid.

Pumilio Pine Oil (4697-m)

Dwarf Pine Needle Oil; Essence de Pin de Montagne; Latschenöl; Oleum Pini Pumilionis; Olio di Mugo.
CAS — 8016-46-4.
Pharmacopoeias. In Aust. and Swiss.

A volatile oil obtained by distillation from the fresh leaves of *Pinus mugo* var. *pumilio* (Pinaceae).

Profile

Pumilio pine oil has been inhaled with steam, sometimes with other essential oils, to relieve cough and nasal congestion and has been applied externally as a rubefacient. It has also been used as a perfume.

Preparations

Proprietary Preparations (details are given in Part 3)
Ital.: Recto Mugolio†.

Multi-ingredient: *Aust.:* Allgauer; Anifer Hustenbalsam; Anifer Krauterol; Apotheker Bauer's Inhalationsmischung; Babix; Berggeist; Bronchostop; Colda; Emser Nasensalbe; Erkaltungsbad; Erkaltungsbalsam; Expectal-Balsam; Jopinol†; Leukona-Rheuma-Bad; Luuf Balsam; Luuf-Erkaltungsol; Makatussin†; Mentopin; Nasanal; Opino; Piniment; Resol; Tetesept; *Austral.:* Analgesic Rub†; Biosal; Goanna Heat Cream; Goanna Liniment; Goanna Salve; Karvol; Menalation; Vicks Inhaler; *Canad.:* Vap Air†; *Ger.:* Aerosol Spitzner N; Cefarheumin N; Dolo-cyl; Emeukal; Emser Erkaltungsgel; Emser Nasensalbe N; Euflux-N; Hevertopect; Hustagil Inhalationsol; Inspirol Mundwasser konzentrat†; Ipalat; Klosterfrau Franzbranntwein Latschenkiefer; Kneipp Erkaltungs-Balsam N; Kneipp Krauter Hustensaft N Kneipp Tannolsaft; Nasentropfen-ratiopharm; Neo-Lapitrypsin†; Nervfluid S; Nettinerv; Night-Care†; Pinimenthol Oral N†; Pumilen-N†; Retterspitz Aerosol†; Retterspitz Heilsalbe†; Rosarthron; Schupps Latschenkiefer Olbad†; Thrombocid; *Irl.:* Karvol; *Israel:* Karvol; Mentholatum Balm; *Ital.:* Abiostil; Antipulmina; Broncosedina; Pinedrin; *Neth.:* Bronchoforton†; *NZ:* Vicks Inhaler; *Port.:* Thrombocid; *Switz.:* Baby Liberol†; Eau-de-vie de France avec huile de pin nain du Tirol; Liberol Baby N; Liberol Bain; Liberol N; Liberol†; Makatussin; Pinimenthol; Thrombocid; *UK:* Boots Vapour Rub; Catarrh Pastilles; Karvol; Mentholatum Rub; Nasal Inhaler; Original Cabdrivers Expectorant; Potter's Catarrh Pastilles.

Punarnava (13188-y)

Punarnaba.

The fresh or dried plant *Boerhaavia diffusa* (= B. repens) (Nyctaginaceae), containing an alkaloid, punarnavine.

Profile

Punarnava has been used in India as a diuretic and for liver disorders, usually in the form of a liquid extract.

Pyricarbate (13191-p)

Pyricarbate (rINN).
Pyridinolcarbamate. 2,6-Pyridinediyldimethylene bis(methylcarbamate).
$C_{11}H_{15}N_3O_4 = 253.3$.
CAS — 1882-26-4.
Pharmacopoeias. In Fr. and Pol.

Profile

Pyricarbate has been given by mouth in the treatment of atherosclerosis and other vascular disorders, hyperlipidaemias, and thromboembolic disorders. Adverse effects have included gastrointestinal disturbances and liver damage.

Preparations

Proprietary Preparations (details are given in Part 3)
Hong Kong: Anginin; *Ital.:* Cicloven; *Jpn:* Anginin†; *Port.:* Anginin†; *Spain:* Colesterinex; Esterbiol; *Thai.:* Anginin.

Multi-ingredient: *Braz.:* Davistar.

Pyritinol Hydrochloride   (13194-e)

Pyritinol Hydrochloride (*BANM, rINNM*).
Pyrithioxine Hydrochloride. 5,5-Dihydroxy-6,6-dimethyl-3,3-dithiodimethylenebis(4-pyridylmethanol) dihydrochloride monohydrate.
$C_{16}H_{20}N_2O_4S_2,2HCl,H_2O = 459.4$.
CAS — 1098-97-1 (pyritinol); 10049-83-9 (anhydrous pyritinol hydrochloride).
Pharmacopoeias. In Pol.

Profile

Pyritinol hydrochloride has been described as a nootropic which promotes the uptake of glucose by the brain and has been used in the treatment of various cerebrovascular and mental function disorders. It has been given by mouth in a usual dose of 600 mg daily. Pyritinol hydrochloride has also been given as an alternative to penicillamine in rheumatoid arthritis.

◊ References.
1. Knezevic S, *et al.* Pyritinol treatment of SDAT patients: evaluation by psychiatric and neurological examination, psychometric testing and rCBF measurements. *Int Clin Psychopharmacol* 1989; **4:** 25–38.
2. Lemmel EM. Comparison of pyritinol and auranofin in the treatment of rheumatoid arthritis. *Br J Rheumatol* 1993; **32:** 375–82.
3. Straumann A, *et al.* Acute pancreatitis due to pyritinol: an immune-mediated phenomenon. *Gastroenterology* 1998; **115:** 452–4.

Preparations

Proprietary Preparations (details are given in Part 3)
Aust.: Encephabol; *Braz.:* Encefabol; *Fr.:* Encephabol; *Ger.:* Ardeyceryl P; Encephabol; Logomed Neuro-Aktiv-Tabletten†; *Hong Kong:* Encephabol; *Ital.:* Encefabol; *Mex.:* Bonifen; Encephabol; *Port.:* Bonifen; Cerbon; *S.Afr.:* Encephabol; *Singapore:* Encephabol; *Thai.:* Encephabol; Memonol; Pyritil.

Multi-ingredient: *Spain:* Memorino; Refulgin; Viadetres.

Quassia   (539-m)

Bitter Wood; Leño de Cuasia; Quassia Wood; Quassiae Lignum; Quassiaholz.
CAS — 76-78-8 (quassin); 76-77-7 (neoquassin).
ATC — P03AX04.
Pharmacopoeias. In Jpn.

The dried stem wood of Jamaica quassia, *Picrasma excelsa* (=*Aeschrion excelsa; Picraena excelsa*) (Simaroubaceae) or of Surinam quassia, *Quassia amara* (Simaroubaceae).

Profile

Quassia has been used as a bitter. It was formerly given as an enema for the expulsion of threadworms and was applied for pediculosis. It may also be used as a flavour in food, drinks, and confectionery. Extracts of quassia or preparations containing its triterpenoid bitter principle quassin are used to denature alcohol.

Preparations

Proprietary Preparations (details are given in Part 3)
Multi-ingredient: *Braz.:* Camomila; Fargestium; *Fr.:* Ducase†; Quintonine; Spevin; *Ital.:* Cura†; Dekar 2; *Switz.:* Stomacine; *UK:* Sanderson's Throat Specific.

Quinine and Urea Hydrochloride   (13201-k)

Carbamidated Quinine Dihydrochloride; Chininum Dihydrochloricum Carbamidatum; Urea-Quinine.
$C_{20}H_{24}N_2O_2,CH_4N_2O,2HCl,5H_2O = 547.5$.
CAS — 549-52-0 (anhydrous quinine and urea hydrochloride).

Profile

Quinine and urea hydrochloride is used for the treatment of haemorrhoidal bleeding and anal fissure. It was formerly used as a local anaesthetic and for the therapeutic actions of quinine.

Preparations

Proprietary Preparations (details are given in Part 3)
Fr.: Kinurea H.

Quinine Ascorbate   (13202-a)

Quinine Ascorbate (*USAN*).
Quinine Biascorbate.
$C_{20}H_{24}N_2O_2,2C_6H_8O_6 = 676.7$.
CAS — 146-40-7.

A compound (2 : 1) of ascorbic acid with quinine.

Profile

Quinine ascorbate has been used as an ingredient of preparations promoted as smoking deterrents.

The symbol † denotes a preparation no longer actively marketed

Preparations

Proprietary Preparations (details are given in Part 3)
Multi-ingredient: *Fr.:* Paranico†; *Ital.:* Nicoprive.

Rape Oil   (7366-p)

Colza Oil; Oleum Rapae; Rapeseed Oil.
Pharmacopoeias. In Eur. (see p.vi), *Jpn,* and *Pol.*

Pharmacopoeial description

Ph. Eur.: The fatty oil obtained from the seeds of *Brassica napus* and *Brassica campestris* by mechanical expression or extraction and then refined. A suitable antioxidant may be added. It contains not more than 2% of erucic acid. A clear light yellow liquid. Practically insoluble in water and in alcohol; miscible with petroleum spirit. Store in well-filled airtight containers. Protect from light.

Profile

Rape oil has been used in liniments in place of olive oil. It is used in some countries as an edible oil but the erucic acid ($C_{22}H_{42}O_2 = 338.6$) content of the oil has been implicated in muscle damage. The erucic acid content of oils and fats intended for human consumption and of foodstuffs containing oil or fat is subject to legal control. Contaminated rape oil was the cause of the toxic oil syndrome that affected thousands of Spanish citizens following its distribution in early 1981. Rape oil is also used in industrial manufacturing.

There has been some debate whether increased frequencies of allergic respiratory symptoms occur in sensitive individuals in areas in which oilseed rape is cultivated.

Raspberry Leaf   (13207-d)

Rubi Idaei Folium.

The dried leaflets of *Rubus idaeus* (Rosaceae).

Profile

Raspberry leaf contains a principle, readily extracted with hot water, which relaxes the smooth muscle of the uterus and intestine of some *animals*.

Raspberry 'tea' has been a traditional remedy for painful and profuse menstruation and for use before and during labour. The infusion has also been used as an astringent gargle.

◊ References.
1. Parsons M, *et al.* Raspberry leaf and its effect on labour: safety and efficacy. *J Aust Coll Midwives* 1999; **12:** 20–5.

Preparations

Proprietary Preparations (details are given in Part 3)
Multi-ingredient: *Aust.:* Bio-Garten Tee gegen Durchfall; Tee gegen Durchfall; *Austral.:* Rubus Complex; *Belg.:* Eugiron; *Ger.:* Salus Bronchial-Tee Nr.8†; *UK:* Gerard House Helonias Compound.

Red Clover   (12167-d)

Cow Clover; Meadow Clover; Purple Clover; Trefoil.

Profile

The flowerheads of red clover, *Trifolium pratense* (Leguminosae), have been used in herbal medicine. The isoflavones present in red clover have been investigated, similarly to other phyto-oestrogens, for their potential endocrine effects.

Preparations

Proprietary Preparations (details are given in Part 3)
Austral.: Promensil.

Multi-ingredient: *Austral.:* Bioglan Mens Super Soy/Clover; Bioglan Soy Power Plus; Lifechange Menopause Formula; Trifolium Complex.

Relaxin   (13208-n)

CAS — 9002-69-1.

A polypeptide hormone that has been extracted from the corpus luteum of the ovaries of pregnant sows, although a human recombinant form is also now available. It is reported to be related structurally to insulin and has a molecular weight of about 6000.

Profile

Relaxin is secreted by the human corpus luteum during pregnancy and is thought to interact with other reproductive hormones. It acts on connective tissue, including collagen, and causes relaxation of the pubic symphysis and softening of the uterine cervix. In many *animal* species relaxin appears to play a major part in cervical ripening before parturition; significant species difference is shown. It has been studied for cervical ripening in humans. Recombinant human relaxin has been investigated in scleroderma (p.505).

◊ References.
1. Seibold JR, *et al.* Safety and pharmacokinetics of recombinant human relaxin in systemic sclerosis. *J Rheumatol* 1998; **25:** 302–7.

2. Seibold JR, *et al.* Recombinant human relaxin in the treatment of scleroderma: a randomized, double-blind, placebo-controlled trial. *Ann Intern Med* 2000; **132:** 871–9.
3. Kelly AJ, *et al.* Relaxin for cervical ripening and induction of labour (updated 26 February 2001). Available in The Cochrane Library; Issue 4. Oxford: Update Software; 2001.

Rhamnose   (3921-w)

L-Rhamnose. 6-Deoxy-L-mannose.
$C_6H_{12}O_5 = 164.2$.
CAS — 3615-41-6.

Profile

Rhamnose is a monosaccharide used to assess intestinal permeability.
For reference to the use of rhamnose in the differential sugar absorption test, see Lactulose, p.1230.

◊ References.
1. van Nieuwenhoven MA, *et al.* The sensitivity of the lactulose/rhamnose gut permeability test. *Eur J Clin Invest* 1999; **29:** 160–5.
2. Haase AM, *et al.* Dual sugar permeability testing in diarrheal disease. *J Pediatr* 2000; **136:** 232–7.
3. van Nieuwenhoven MA, *et al.* Effects of pre- and post-absorptive factors on the lactulose/rhamnose gut permeability test. *Clin Sci* 2000; **98:** 349–53.

Rhatany Root   (319-j)

Krameria; Krameria Root; Ratanhiae Radix.
Pharmacopoeias. In Eur. (see p.vi).

Pharmacopoeial description

Ph. Eur.: The dried, usually fragmented, underground organs of *Krameria triandra*. It contains not less than 5% of tannins, expressed as pyrogallol, calculated with reference to the dried drug. It is known as Peruvian rhatany. Protect from light.

Profile

Rhatany root has astringent properties and is used in herbal and homoeopathic preparations for a variety of disorders, including oropharyngeal inflammation.

Preparations

Proprietary Preparations (details are given in Part 3)
Ger.: ratioSept; Salvibest.

Multi-ingredient: *Aust.:* Parodontax†; *Braz.:* Parodontax; *Ger.:* Repha-Os; *Israel:* Parodontax; *Ital.:* Gengivario; *Spain:* Encialina; Regal†; *Switz.:* Eubucal; *UK:* Medicinal Gargle.

Rhus   (13210-a)

Sumach Berries.

The dried fruits of the smooth or Pennsylvanian sumach, *Rhus glabra* (Anacardiaceae).

Profile

Rhus has astringent and reputed diuretic properties. *Rhus aromatica* has been used similarly to *R. glabra*. Poison ivy (*R. radicans*) and poison oak (*R. toxicodendron*), species growing in the USA, contain irritant poisons such as urushiol, producing severe contact dermatitis. Extracts of poison ivy and poison oak have been used for the prophylaxis of poison ivy dermatitis but their effectiveness has not been proved.
Some *Rhus* spp. are used in homoeopathic medicine.

Preparations

Proprietary Preparations (details are given in Part 3)
Multi-ingredient: *Ger.:* Cysto Fink; Hewedolor; Hicoton; Rhus-Rheuma-Gel N; *Switz.:* Cysto Fink†; Cysto-Caps Chassot†.

Ribonuclease   (13211-t)

RNase.
CAS — 9001-99-4.

An enzyme present in most mammalian tissue.

Profile

Ribonuclease is involved in the catalytic cleavage of ribonucleic acid. It has been applied, alone or in combination with other drugs, for its supposed anti-inflammatory properties.

Preparations

Proprietary Preparations (details are given in Part 3)
Mex.: Cro 50.

Multi-ingredient: *Fr.:* Ribatran; *Mex.:* Ridasa.

Ribonucleic Acid   (15326-d)

ARN; Plant Nucleic Acid; Ribose Nucleic Acid; RNA; Yeast Nucleic Acid.

Profile

Ribonucleic acid is a nucleotide polymer, and 1 of the 2 distinct varieties of nucleic acid (see p.1642). It is found in the cytoplasm and in small amounts in the cell nuclei of living tissues and is directly involved in protein synthesis. It can be extracted from beer or bread yeast. Therapeutically, it has been tried in the treatment of mental retardation and to improve memory in senile dementia, and proprietary preparations containing various salts of ribonucleic acid have been advocated for a variety of asthenic and convalescent conditions. Ribonucleic acid may have a role in enteral feeds under some circumstances.

Immune RNA (extracted from the spleens and lymph nodes of immunised animals) has been tried in the immunotherapy of hepatitis and cancer.

Preparations

Proprietary Preparations (details are given in Part 3)

Ger.: AU 4 Regeneresen; Osteochondrin S; RN13 Regeneresen.

Multi-ingredient: *Fr.:* Megasthenyl†; Nutrigene†; *Spain:* Dertrase; Nucleserina; Policolinosil.

Ricin (13213-r)

NOTE. The title ricin is used for the castor seed in *Chin.* and *Fr.*

A highly toxic lectin present in castor seeds, the seeds of *Ricinus communis* (Euphorbiaceae).

Profile

Ricin is extremely toxic when administered parenterally. The toxicity of orally ingested beans depends on how thoroughly they are chewed since the hard seed coat prevents absorption. Ingestion of up to 3 castor seeds by a child and 8 by an adult may be fatal; signs and symptoms of poisoning are similar to those described for abrus seeds (p.1571).

After expression of the oil from castor seeds (see p.1592), the ricin remaining in the seed cake or 'pomace' is destroyed by steam treatment. The detoxified pomace is used as a fertiliser.

Ricin conjugated with monoclonal or polyclonal antibodies is being studied in the treatment of cancers; zolimomab aritox (p.581) is an example of such a conjugate. Some of these conjugates have been investigated for various malignancies, particularly leukaemias and lymphomas.

Toxicity. A report of ricin toxicity following partial chewing and ingestion of 10 to 15 castor oil seeds.[1]
1. Aplin PJ, Eliseo T. Ingestion of castor oil plant seeds. *Med J Aust* 1997; **167:** 260–1.

Uses. References to the use of ricin conjugates with monoclonal antibodies in the treatment of cancer.
1. Byers VS, *et al.* Phase I study of monoclonal antibody-ricin A chain immunotoxin XomaZyme-791 in patients with metastatic colon cancer. *Cancer Res* 1989; **49:** 6153–60.
2. Oratz R, *et al.* Antimelanoma monoclonal antibody-ricin A chain immunoconjugate (XMMME-001-RTA) plus cyclophosphamide in the treatment of metastatic malignant melanoma: results of a phase II trial. *J Biol Response Mod* 1990; **9:** 345–54.
3. Anonymous. Application considered for immunotoxin in treatment of graft-vs-host disease. *JAMA* 1991; **265:** 2041–2.
4. Amlot PL, *et al.* A phase I study of an anti-CD22-deglycosylated ricin A chain immunotoxin in the treatment of B-cell lymphomas resistant to conventional therapy. *Blood* 1993; **81:** 2624–33.
5. Senderowicz AM, *et al.* Complete sustained response of a refractory, post-transplantation, large B-cell lymphoma to an anti-CD22 immunotoxin. *Ann Intern Med* 1997; **126:** 882–5.
6. Multani PS, *et al.* Phase II clinical trial of bolus infusion anti-B4 blocked ricin immunoconjugate in patients with relapsed B-cell non-Hodgkin's lymphoma. *Clin Cancer Res* 1998; **4:** 2599–2604.

Ricinoleic Acid (1323-a)

A mixture of fatty acids obtained by the hydrolysis of castor oil.

Profile

Ricinoleic acid is an ingredient of some proprietary vaginal jellies used to maintain or restore normal vaginal acidity.

Preparations

Proprietary Preparations (details are given in Part 3)

Multi-ingredient: *Austral.:* Aci-Jel; *Israel:* Glovan; *NZ:* Aci-Jel; *USA:* Aci-Jel.

Riluzole (10406-g)

Riluzole (BAN, USAN, rINN).

PK-26124; RP-54274. 2-Amino-6-(trifluoromethoxy) benzothiazole; 6-Trifluoromethoxy-1,3-benzothiazol-2-ylamine.

$C_8H_5F_3N_2OS = 234.2.$
CAS — 1744-22-5.
ATC — N07XX02.

Adverse Effects and Treatment

Adverse effects associated most commonly with riluzole are asthenia, nausea, elevations in liver enzyme values, headache, and abdominal pain. Other gastrointestinal effects may include diarrhoea or constipation, anorexia, and vomiting. There may be tachycardia, dizziness, vertigo, or somnolence. Circumoral paraesthesia has been reported and decreased lung function and rhinitis may occur. Anaphylactoid reactions, angioedema, pancreatitis, and neutropenia have all been reported rarely.

Effects on the blood. See under Overdosage, below.

Effects on the kidneys. A 44-year-old patient developed renal tubular impairment 3 months after starting riluzole treatment for amyotrophic lateral sclerosis.[1] Tubular function recovered 1 month after discontinuation of riluzole.
1. Poloni TE, *et al.* Renal tubular impairment during riluzole therapy. *Neurology* 1999; **52:** 670.

Effects on the liver. Icteric toxic hepatitis manifested by jaundice and elevated liver enzyme values has been reported[1] in an elderly woman receiving riluzole for amyotrophic lateral sclerosis (ALS). Acute hepatitis developed in 2 patients several weeks after starting therapy with riluzole for ALS.[2] Liver histology showed hepatocellular damage with inflammatory infiltration and microvesicular steatosis without fibrosis. Symptoms of hepatotoxicity were reversed in all these cases following discontinuation of riluzole.
1. Castells LI, *et al.* Icteric toxic hepatitis associated with riluzole. *Lancet* 1998; **351:** 648.
2. Remy A-J, *et al.* Acute hepatitis after riluzole administration. *J Hepatol* 1999; **30:** 527–30.

Effects on the pancreas. Riluzole was cited[1] as the most likely cause of severe pancreatitis that developed in a 77-year-old woman 6 months after starting therapy for sporadic amyotrophic lateral sclerosis; pancreatic symptoms improved on discontinuation of riluzole.
1. Drory VE, *et al.* Riluzole-induced pancreatitis. *Neurology* 1999; **52:** 892–3.

Overdosage. Severe neutropenia developed in a 63-year-old woman receiving riluzole for amyotrophic lateral sclerosis 10 days after inadvertent dose escalation to 200 mg daily (twice the standard recommended dose).[1]

Methaemoglobinaemia has been reported[2] in a 43-year-old patient with amyotrophic lateral sclerosis following intentional overdose with 2.8 g of riluzole. The patient was treated with gastric lavage followed by administration of activated charcoal; intravenous methylene blue [methylthioninium chloride] successfully reversed the methaemoglobinaemia. However, the patient died of respiratory failure related to her underlying disease 7 days after the overdose.
1. North WA, *et al.* Reversible granulocytopenia in association with riluzole therapy. *Ann Pharmacother* 2000; **34:** 322–4.
2. Viallon A, *et al.* Methemoglobinemia due to riluzole. *N Engl J Med* 2000; **343:** 665–6.

Precautions

Riluzole is contra-indicated in patients with hepatic disease or markedly raised liver enzyme values. Liver function tests should be performed before and throughout treatment with riluzole. Extreme caution should be exercised in patients with renal impairment or those with a history of liver disorders. Patients or their carers should be told how to recognise signs of neutropenia and should be advised to seek immediate medical attention if symptoms such as fever develop; white blood cell counts should be determined in febrile illness and riluzole discontinued if neutropenia occurs. Riluzole may cause dizziness or vertigo and patients should be warned not to drive or operate machinery if these symptoms occur.

Riluzole has been reported to impair fertility in *animals*.

Pharmacokinetics

Riluzole is rapidly absorbed from the gastrointestinal tract following oral administration with peak plasma concentrations occurring after 1 to 1½ hours. The rate and extent of absorption are decreased when riluzole is administered with a high-fat meal. Riluzole is widely distributed throughout the body and is approximately 97% bound to plasma proteins. It crosses the blood-brain barrier. Riluzole is extensively metabolised to several metabolites in the liver, mainly by the cytochrome P450 isoenzyme CYP1A2, and subsequent glucuronidation. Riluzole is excreted mainly in the urine predominantly as glucuronides with an elimination half-life of about 12 hours. Approximately 2% is excreted unchanged in the urine. Small amounts are excreted in faeces. There is some evidence that clearance of riluzole might be reduced in Japanese patients.

◊ References.
1. Le Liboux A, *et al.* Single- and multiple-dose pharmacokinetics of riluzole in white subjects. *J Clin Pharmacol* 1997; **37:** 820–7.
2. Le Liboux A, *et al.* A comparison of the pharmacokinetics and tolerability of riluzole after repeat dose administration in healthy elderly and young volunteers. *J Clin Pharmacol* 1999; **39:** 480–6.

Uses and Administration

Riluzole is a glutamate antagonist used in the management of amyotrophic lateral sclerosis, a form of motor neurone disease. Riluzole is indicated to slow progression of early disease but efficacy has not been demonstrated in its late stages. The precise mechanism of action is unknown but it may inhibit presynaptic glutamate release and interfere with its postsynaptic effects. The usual adult dose of riluzole is 50 mg twice daily by mouth on an empty stomach.

Motor neurone disease. Motor neurone disease (motoneuron disease) represents a group of fatal progressive degenerative disorders that affect upper and/or lower motor neurones in the brain and spinal cord. The most common form of motor neurone disease is amyotrophic lateral sclerosis (known in the USA as Lou Gehrig's disease), which involves both upper and lower motor neurones. It produces muscular atrophy and weakness and symptoms of progressive bulbar palsy such as slowness of movement and speech disturbances. Most patients die within 2 to 5 years of disease onset, usually from respiratory failure. There is no completely effective treatment and management remains largely supportive with appropriate symptomatic management of spasticity (p.1322), neuropathic pain (p.7), and sialorrhoea. Tricyclic antidepressants are widely used for their multiple beneficial effects. Occupational and speech therapy also play a crucial role in maximising function. Pathological crying or laughing (pseudobulbar affect) may occur in as many as 50% of patients and has been treated with amitriptyline or fluvoxamine. Dysphagia may eventually compromise food and fluid intake necessitating enteral nutrition as an alternative or supplemental route for oral nutrition. Respiratory support will ultimately be necessary, initially with non-invasive ventilation but progressing eventually to tracheostomy.

Although the pathogenesis of motor neurone disease is still uncertain, it is thought that accumulation of the excitatory neurotransmitter glutamate in the CNS may be involved. Clinical studies have shown riluzole, a glutamate antagonist, to be modestly effective in prolonging survival and delaying the time to use of tracheostomy. However, there is still insufficient data to be able to assess which patients would derive greatest benefit. Additionally, questions have been raised about the clinical usefulness of riluzole in terms of cost-benefit, and there are concerns about adverse effects, notably hepatotoxicity.

Also under study for the treatment of motor neurone disease are somatomedins, in particular mecasermin (insulin-like growth factor I). Neurotrophic factors have been investigated including brain-derived neurotrophic factor (BDNF) and recombinant ciliary neurotrophic factor (CNTF), but results have been generally inconclusive. Glial-cell-derived neurotrophic factor (GDNF) is also under investigation. There has also been some interest in the antiepileptic drug gabapentin, which may inhibit glutamate formation in the CNS from branched-chain amino acids. Lamotrigine has also been tried but with disappointing results. Dextromethorphan has also been studied in amyotrophic lateral sclerosis. Immunoglobulins have been tried in some forms of motor neurone disease such as multifocal motor neuropathy.

A small percentage of patients with familial amyotrophic lateral sclerosis have been shown to have a mutation in the gene encoding for the enzyme copper-zinc superoxide dismutase but there has been no consensus as to whether patients with this mutation should be given superoxide dismutase supplements.

References.
1. Bryson HM, *et al.* Riluzole: a review of its pharmacodynamic and pharmacokinetic properties and therapeutic potential in amyotrophic lateral sclerosis. *Drugs* 1996; **52:** 549–63.
2. Wagner ML, Landis BE. Riluzole: a new agent for amyotrophic lateral sclerosis. *Ann Pharmacother* 1997; **31:** 738–44.
3. Anonymous. Riluzole for amyotrophic lateral sclerosis. *Drug Ther Bull* 1997; **35:** 11–12.
4. Quality Standards Subcommittee of the American Academy of Neurology. Practice advisory on the treatment of amyotrophic lateral sclerosis with riluzole: report of the Quality Standards Subcommittee of the American Academy of Neurology. *Neurology* 1997; **49:** 657–9.
5. Walling AD. Amyotrophic lateral sclerosis: Lou Gehrig's disease. *Am Fam Physician* 1999; **59:** 1489–96.
6. Mackin GA. Optimizing care of patients with ALS: steps to early detection and improved quality of life. *Postgrad Med* 1999; **105:** 143–56.
7. Parton MJ, *et al.* Motor neuron disease and its management. *J R Coll Physicians Lond* 1999; **33:** 212–8.
8. Miller RG, *et al.* Practice parameter: the care of the patient with amyotrophic lateral sclerosis (an evidence-based review): report of the Quality Standards Subcommittee of the American Academy of Neurology. *Neurology* 1999; **52:** 1311–23.
9. Shaw PJ. Motor neurone disease. *BMJ* 1999; **318:** 1118–21.
10. Ludolph AC, Riepe MW. Do the benefits of currently available treatments justify early diagnosis and treatment of amyotrophic lateral sclerosis? — Arguments against. *Neurology* 1999; **53** (suppl 5): S46–S49.
11. Cashman NR. Do the benefits of currently available treatments justify early diagnosis and announcement? — Arguments for. *Neurology* 1999; **53** (suppl 5): S50–S52.
12. Miller RG, *et al.* Riluzole for amyotrophic lateral sclerosis (ALS)/motor neuron disease (MND) (updated 29 August 2001). Available in The Cochrane Library; Issue 4. Oxford: Update Software; 2001.
13. Rowland LP, Shneider NA. Amyotrophic lateral sclerosis. *N Engl J Med* 2001; **344:** 1688–1700.

Movement disorders. Beneficial results have been obtained with riluzole in small studies of patients with Huntington's chorea[1] and levodopa-induced dyskinesias in Parkinson's disease.[2]
1. Rosas HD, *et al.* Riluzole therapy in Huntington's disease (HD). *Mov Disord* 1999; **14:** 326–30.
2. Merims D, *et al.* Riluzole for levodopa-induced dyskinesias in advanced Parkinson's disease. *Lancet* 1999; **353:** 1764–5.

Preparations

Proprietary Preparations (details are given in Part 3)

Aust.: Rilutek; *Belg.:* Rilutek; *Denm.:* Rilutek; *Fin.:* Rilutek; *Fr.:* Rilutek; *Ger.:* Rilutek; *Hong Kong:* Rilutek; *Irl.:* Rilutek; *Israel:* Rilutek; *Ital.:* Rilutek; *Jpn:* Rilutek; *Mex.:* Rilutek; *Neth.:* Rilutek; *Norw.:* Rilutek; *Port.:* Rilutek; *S.Afr.:* Rilutek; *Singapore:* Rilutek; *Spain:* Rilutek; *Swed.:* Rilutek; *Switz.:* Rilutek; *Thai.:* Rilutek; *UK:* Rilutek; *USA:* Rilutek.

Ritodrine Hydrochloride (2103-j)

Ritodrine Hydrochloride (BANM, USAN, rINNM).

DU-21220 (ritodrine). erythro-2-(4-Hydroxyphenethylamino)-1-(4-hydroxyphenyl)propan-1-ol hydrochloride.

$C_{17}H_{21}NO_3,HCl = 323.8$.

CAS — 26652-09-5 (ritodrine); 23239-51-2 (ritodrine hydrochloride).

Pharmacopoeias. In Br. and US.

Pharmacopoeial description

BP 2001: A white or almost white, crystalline powder. Freely soluble in water; soluble in dehydrated alcohol; practically insoluble in acetone and in ether. A 2% solution in water has a pH of 4.5 to 6.0. Store in airtight containers.

USP 25: A white to nearly white, odourless or practically odourless, crystalline powder. Freely soluble in water and in alcohol; practically insoluble in ether; soluble in propyl alcohol. pH of a 2% solution in water is between 4.5 and 6.0. Store in airtight containers.

Adverse Effects and Precautions

As for Salbutamol Sulfate, p.770. Leucopenia or agranulocytosis has been reported occasionally in association with prolonged intravenous administration of ritodrine.

In women being treated for premature labour, the risk of pulmonary oedema means that extreme caution is required and the precautions and risk factors discussed under Salbutamol Sulfate, p.771, apply.

Effects on the eyes. Ritodrine and to a lesser extent salbutamol have been implicated in retinopathy in the premature infant when used for premature labour.[1]

1. Michie CA, et al. Do maternal β-sympathomimetics influence the development of retinopathy in the premature infant? Arch Dis Child 1994; **71:** F149.

Effects on the heart. Myocardial ischaemia or signs of myocardial ischaemia have been reported in patients given ritodrine.[1,2]

1. Brosset P, et al. Cardiac complications of ritodrine in mother and baby. Lancet 1982; **i:** 1468.
2. Ben-Shlomo I, et al. Myocardial ischaemia during intravenous ritodrine treatment: is it so rare? Lancet 1986; **ii:** 917–18.

Pulmonary oedema. Several cases of pulmonary oedema have been reported in patients given a beta$_2$ agonist, including ritodrine, for premature labour.[1-4] In 1995 the UK Committee on Safety of Medicines[4] (CSM) commented that it had received 10 reports of pulmonary oedema, fatal in 2 patients. The CSM considered that fluid overload was the most important predisposing factor. Other risk factors included multiple pregnancies, a history of cardiac disease, and maternal infection. For further discussion of the precautions necessary in the use of beta$_2$ agonists to treat premature labour, and the risk factors involved, see p.771.

1. Hawker F. Pulmonary oedema associated with β$_2$-sympathomimetic treatment of premature labour. Anaesth Intensive Care 1984; **12:** 143–51.
2. Pisani RJ, Rosenow EC. Pulmonary edema associated with tocolytic therapy. Ann Intern Med 1989; **110:** 714–18.
3. Clesham GJ, et al. β Adrenergic agonists and pulmonary oedema in preterm labour. BMJ 1994; **308:** 260–2.
4. Committee on Safety of Medicines/Medicines Control Agency. Reminder: ritodrine and pulmonary oedema. Current Problems 1995; **21:** 7.

Interactions

As for Salbutamol Sulfate, p.771.

Pharmacokinetics

Ritodrine is rapidly absorbed from the gastrointestinal tract but is subject to fairly extensive first-pass metabolism; about 30% of an oral dose is bioavailable. It is metabolised in the liver primarily by conjugation with glucuronic acid or sulfate and excreted in urine as unchanged drug and metabolites. About 70 to 90% of a dose is reported to be excreted in the urine within 10 to 12 hours. It crosses the placenta.

◊ References.

1. Gandar R, et al. Serum level of ritodrine in man. Eur J Clin Pharmacol 1980; **17:** 117–22.
2. Gross AS, Brown KF. Plasma protein binding of ritodrine at parturition and in nonpregnant women. Eur J Clin Pharmacol 1985; **28:** 479–81.
3. Pacifici GM, et al. Sulphation and glucuronidation of ritodrine in human foetal and adult tissues. Eur J Clin Pharmacol 1993; **44:** 259–64.
4. Pacifici GM, et al. Ritodrine sulphation in the human liver and duodenal mucosa: interindividual variability. Eur J Drug Metab Pharmacokinet 1998; **23:** 67–74.

Uses and Administration

Ritodrine hydrochloride is a direct-acting sympathomimetic with predominantly beta-adrenergic activity and a selective action on beta$_2$ receptors (a beta$_2$ agonist). It has general properties similar to those of salbutamol (see p.772). It decreases uterine contractility and is used to arrest premature labour (p.773). Ritodrine hydrochloride is given by intravenous infusion, preferably with the aid of a syringe pump, when the concentration should be 3 mg per mL, using glucose 5% as the diluent. A recommended initial rate of infusion is 50 µg per minute increased at intervals of 10 minutes by 50-µg increments until there is evidence of patient response, which is usually at a rate of 150 to 350 µg per minute, the latter figure being the maximum recommended rate. The maternal pulse should be monitored throughout the infusion and the rate adjusted to avoid a

maternal heart rate of more than 140 beats per minute. A close watch should also be kept on the patient's state of hydration since fluid overload is considered to be a key risk factor for pulmonary oedema. The infusion should be continued for 12 to 48 hours after the contractions have stopped. Ritodrine hydrochloride may subsequently be given by mouth in an initial dose of 10 mg every 2 hours for 24 hours, starting 30 minutes before the end of the intravenous infusion. Thereafter, 10 to 20 mg may be given every 4 to 6 hours according to the patient's response. The total daily dose by mouth should not exceed 120 mg.

If no syringe pump is available then the infusion may be made using a controlled infusion device to deliver a more dilute solution of 300 µg per mL, with glucose 5% being used once again as the diluent. The same dose is employed as with the syringe pump. If intravenous infusion is inappropriate, 10 mg may be given intramuscularly every 3 to 8 hours and continued for 12 to 48 hours after the contractions have stopped.

Preparations

BP 2001: Ritodrine Injection; Ritodrine Tablets;
USP 25: Ritodrine Hydrochloride Injection; Ritodrine Hydrochloride Tablets.

Proprietary Preparations (details are given in Part 3)
Austral.: Yutopar; **Belg.:** Pre-Par; **Braz.:** Miodrina; **Canad.:** Yutopar; **Fr.:** Pre-Par; **Ger.:** Pre-Par†; **Hong Kong:** Yutopar; **Irl.:** Yutopar; **Israel:** Ritopar; **Ital.:** Miolene; **Neth.:** Pre-Par; **Port.:** Pre-Par; **Singapore:** Yutopar; **Spain:** Pre-Par; **Thai.:** Yutopar; **UK:** Yutopar; **USA:** Yutopar.

Rociverine (13217-h)

Rociverine (rINN).

LG-30158. 2-Diethylamino-1-methylethyl cis-1-hydroxy(bicyclohexyl)-2-carboxylate.

$C_{20}H_{37}NO_3 = 339.5$.

CAS — 53716-44-2.

ATC — A03AA06.

Profile

Rociverine is an antispasmodic that has been given by mouth in doses of 30 to 40 mg or rectally in doses of 50 to 75 mg daily. It has also been given by injection.

Preparations

Proprietary Preparations (details are given in Part 3)
Ital.: Rilaten.

Rose Bengal Sodium (2146-h)

CI Acid Red 94; Colour Index No. 45440; Rose Bengal; Sodium Rose Bengal. The disodium salt of 4,5,6,7-tetrachloro-2',4',5',7'-tetraiodofluorescein .

$C_{20}H_2Cl_4I_4Na_2O_5 = 1017.6$.

CAS — 11121-48-5 (rose bengal); 632-69-9 (rose bengal disodium).

ATC — S01JA02.

NOTE. The name Rose Bengale has been applied to the substance described in this monograph as well as to dichlorotetraiodofluorescein (CI Acid Red 93; Ext. D & C Reds Nos. 5 and 6; Colour Index No. 45435), a compound used as its disodium or dipotassium salt as a colouring agent.

ROS is a code approved by the BP 2001 for use on single unit doses of eye drops containing rose bengal sodium where the individual container may be too small to bear all the appropriate labelling information.

Profile

Rose bengal sodium stains devitalised conjunctival and corneal epithelial cells as well as mucus and is used as an aid in the diagnosis of dry eye. It is used to detect or assess ocular damage resulting from Sjögren's syndrome or from ill-fitting contact lenses, and for keratitis, squamous cell carcinomas, and detection of foreign bodies. Rose bengal sodium is applied as 1% eye drops or as sterile papers impregnated with the dye.

Instillation of this dye may be painful, especially in dry eyes. Rose bengal sodium can stain exposed skin, clothing, and soft contact lenses.

Rose bengal sodium is taken up by the liver and excreted in the bile; the iodine-131-labelled compound (p.1450) has been used as a diagnostic aid in the determination of hepato-biliary function.

Preparations

Proprietary Preparations (details are given in Part 3)
Canad.: Ak-Rose; **USA:** Rosets.

Rose Oil (4699-v)

Attar of Rose; Esencia de Rosa; Oleum Rosae; Otto of Rose.

Pharmacopoeias. In USNF.

It contains citronellol.

Pharmacopoeial description

USNF 20: A volatile oil distilled with steam from the fresh flowers of Rosa gallica, R. damascena, R. alba, R. centifolia, and varieties of these species (Rosaceae). It is a colourless or yellow liquid, having the characteristic odour of rose. At 25° it

is a viscous liquid. On gradual cooling, it changes to a translucent, crystalline mass, easily liquefied by warming. Miscible with an equal volume of chloroform. Store in well-filled airtight containers.

Profile

Rose oil is largely employed in perfumery and toilet preparations and has been used as a flavour. Hypersensitivity reactions have been reported.

Preparations

USNF 20: Stronger Rose Water;
USP 25: Rose Water Ointment.

Rosemary Oil (4700-v)

Esencia de Romero; Essence de Romarin; Essência de Alecrim; Oleum Roris Marini; Oleum Rosmarini; Rosmarini Aetheroleum; Rosmarinöl.

Pharmacopoeias. In Eur. (see p.vi) and Pol.

Pharmacopoeial description

Ph. Eur.: The essential oil obtained by steam distillation from the flowering aerial parts of Rosmarinus officinalis. It is available as Spanish type rosemary oil and Moroccan and Tunisian type rosemary oil. Spanish type rosemary oil contains 2.0 to 4.5% borneol, 0.5 to 2.5% bornyl acetate, 8.0 to 12.0% camphene, 13.0 to 21.0% camphor, 13.0 to 25.0% cineole, 1.0 to 2.2% p-cymene, 2.5 to 5.0% limonene, 1.5 to 5.0% β-myrcene, 18 to 26% α-pinene, 2.0 to 6.0% β-pinene, 1.0 to 3.5% α-terpineol, and 0.7 to 2.5% verbenone. Moroccan and Tunisian type rosemary oil contains 1.5 to 5.0% borneol, 0.1 to 1.5% bornyl acetate, 2.5 to 6.0% camphene, 5.0 to 15.0% camphor, 38.0 to 55.0% cineole, 0.8 to 2.5% p-cymene, 1.5 to 4.0% limonene, 1.0 to 2.0% β-myrcene, 9.0 to 14.0% α-pinene, 4.0 to 9.0% β-pinene, 1.0 to 2.6% α-terpineol, and a maximum of 0.4% verbenone.

A clear, mobile, colourless to pale yellow liquid with a characteristic odour. Store in well-filled airtight containers at a temperature not exceeding 25°. Protect from light.

Profile

Rosemary oil is carminative and mildly irritant. It is used in perfumery and as a flavour and has been employed in hair lotions, inhalations, and liniments.

Preparations

Proprietary Preparations (details are given in Part 3)
Ger.: Perozon Rosmarin-Olbad mono.

Multi-ingredient: **Aust.:** Berggeist; Bronchiplant; Carl Baders Divinal; Criniton; Dracodermalin; Embrocation; Inno Rheuma; Medizinalbad; Opino; Pulmex; Red Point; Rheuma; Rowalind; Salhumin; Tetesept; **Austral.:** Bioglan E-Plus†; Bioglan Fingers & Toes†; Euky Bearub; Tixylix Chest Rub; **Belg.:** Perubore; Pulmex; Pulmex Baby; **Braz.:** Analgen; Benegel; Gelflex; Gelofrix; Gelol; Geloneval; **Fr.:** Aromasol; Dinacode; Perubore; Pulmax†; **Ger.:** Arthrodeformat P; Arthrodynat P; Balnostim Bad N†; Cefarheumin N; Cor-Vel; Criniton; Dolexamed N†; Dolo-cyl; Dr. Hotz Vollbad†; Eucafluid N; Fagorutin Roßkastanien-Balsam F; Grunlicht Hingfong Essenz; Guttacor-Balsam N; Hingfong-Essenz Hofmanns Tropfen; Histajodol N; Kneipp Erkaltungs-Balsam N; Kneipp Herzsalbe Unguentum Cardiacum Kneipp; Kneipp Kreislauf-Bad Rosmarin-Aquasan†; Leukona-Kreislauf-Bad; Leukona-Rheumasalbe; Retterspitz Ausserlich†; Retterspitz Gelee†; Retterspitz Quick†; Rheuma-Pasc N†; Rosarthron; Rosarthron forte; Rowalind†; Schupps Heilkrauter Rheumabad; thermo-loges; Thrombocid; Togal Mobil Rheuma-Bad; Vaxicum N†; Weleda-Rheumasalbe M; **Irl.:** Rowalind; **Ital.:** Calyptol; **Mon.:** Calyptol; **NZ:** Tixylix Chest Rub; **Port.:** Thrombocid; **Spain:** Calyptol Inhalante; Dolokey; Linimento Klari; Masagil; **Switz.:** Acidodermil†; Caprisanat†; Frigoplasma; Incutin; Kernosan Huile de Massage†; Liberol Bain; Perubore; Pulmex; Pulmex Baby; Spagyrom; Thrombocid; **UK:** Adiantine; Frost Cream; Massage Balm Arnica; Medicated Extract of Rosemary.

Roxarsone (13220-x)

Roxarsone (BAN, USAN, rINN).

NSC-2101. 4-Hydroxy-3-nitrophenylarsonic acid.

$C_6H_6AsNO_6 = 263.0$.

CAS — 121-19-7.

Pharmacopoeias. In US for veterinary use only.

Pharmacopoeial description

USP 25: A pale yellow, crystalline powder. Slightly soluble in cold water; soluble in boiling water; freely soluble in dehydrated alcohol, in acetic acid, in acetone, in methyl alcohol, and in alkalis; insoluble in ether and in ethyl acetate; sparingly soluble in dilute mineral acids. It puffs up and deflagrates on heating.

Profile

Roxarsone has been used as a growth promotor in animal feeds.

Royal Jelly (13221-r)

Queen Bee Jelly.

A milky-white viscid secretion from the salivary glands of the worker honey bee, Apis mellifera (Apidae); it is essential for the development of queen bees.

Profile
Royal jelly has been used as a general 'tonic', to ward off the effects of old age, and to ease sufferers from chronic degenerative diseases, but of the many and diverse claims made for the therapeutic value of the jelly, none has been substantiated.

Royal jelly is also incorporated in some cosmetic preparations for its supposed beneficial effect on skin tissue.

Hypersensitivity. There have been a number of cases of anaphylactoid reactions and acute severe exacerbations of asthma[1-4] (one fatal[2]) in atopic individuals who took royal jelly.

1. Thien FCK, *et al.* Royal jelly-induced asthma. *Med J Aust* 1993; **159:** 639.
2. Bullock RJ, *et al.* Fatal royal jelly-induced asthma. *Med J Aust* 1994; **160:** 44.
3. Peacock S, *et al.* Respiratory distress and royal jelly. *BMJ* 1995; **311:** 1472.
4. Thien FCK, *et al.* Asthma and anaphylaxis induced by royal jelly. *Clin Exp Allergy* 1996; **26:** 216–22.

Preparations
Proprietary Preparations (details are given in Part 3)
Fr.: Apiserum; *Ital.:* Alvear; Biogel; Biovital; Clinvit; Gelamel; Natura Viva; Novel Jelly; Opalia†; Pa-Real; Ritmogel; Roburvit; Telergon II; Theogel†; Trefovital†; Trofomed†; *UK:* Regina Royal One Hundred; Rojema.

Multi-ingredient: *Fr.:* Arkotonic†; Pollen Royal; *Ger.:* Alsiroyal†; Peking Royal Jelly N; *Ital.:* Alvear Complex†; Alvear Sport†; Apergan; Api Baby; Apiserum con Telergon 1; Apistress; Bebimix; Bio-200; Bio-Real Complex†; Bio-Real Plus†; Bio-Real†; Bioton; Biotrefon Plus; Biovigor†; Cocktail Redic; Eurogel; Fon Wan Ginsenergy; Fon Wan Pollen; Fosfarsile Forte; Fosfarsile Yunior; Four-Ton; Granvit; Longevital; Miegel†; Mnemo Organico†; Neoplus; Nerex; Novogel; Nutrex†; Nutrigel; Ottovis; Pollingel; Provitamin A-E; Ribovir; Royal E; Vigogel†; Vitalmix; *Thai.:* Multilim RG; *UK:* Arthrotone; Beeline; Regina Royal Concorde; Regina Royal Five; Royal Galanol.

Rubber (12519-p)
Caoutchouc; India-Rubber.

Profile
Rubber consists of the prepared latex of *Hevea brasiliensis* and other species of *Hevea* (Euphorbiaceae). It is used as a component of many medical devices such as catheters, syringes, enema tips, ostomy bags, balloons, and surgical gloves. Hypersensitivity reactions have occurred after direct contact of skin and mucous membranes with rubber components of such products and also after indirect contact with preparations stored in or administered by them; deaths have been reported. Reactions have been attributed either to protein components of the rubber or to additives such as preservatives or vulcanisation accelerators. For references to glove starch powder as a possible risk factor in the development of rubber latex allergy, see p.1380. Cross-sensitivity between rubber proteins and those of certain fruits, including bananas and chestnuts, has been reported.

◊ References.
1. Landwehr LP, Boguniewicz M. Current perspectives on latex allergy. *J Pediatr* 1996; **128:** 305–12.
2. Senst BL, Johnson RA. Latex allergy. *Am J Health-Syst Pharm* 1997; **54:** 1071–5.
3. Woods JA, *et al.* Natural rubber latex allergy: spectrum, diagnostic approach, and therapy. *J Emerg Med* 1997; **15:** 71–85.
4. Zaidi T, *et al.* Latex allergy: a life-threatening complication. *Hosp Med* 1998; **59:** 505–7.
5. Smith CC. Risk of latex allergy from medication vial closures. *Ann Pharmacother* 1999; **33:** 373–4.
6. Wakelin SH, White IR. Natural rubber latex allergy. *Clin Exp Dermatol* 1999; **24:** 245–8.
7. Bowyer RVStL. Latex allergy: how to identify it and the people at risk. *J Clin Nurs* 1999; **8:** 144–9.

Rubidium Iodide (11529-h)
RbI = 212.4.
CAS — 7790-29-6.

Profile
Rubidium iodide has the actions of iodine and the iodides (see p.1522). It is an ingredient of several proprietary ophthalmic preparations promoted for the treatment of eye disorders.

Preparations
Proprietary Preparations (details are given in Part 3)
Multi-ingredient: *Ital.:* Facovit; Jodo-Calcio-Vitaminico; Polijodurato; Rubidiosin Composto; Rubistenol†; Rubjovit.

Rue Oil (4702-q)
Oleum Rutae.

A volatile oil obtained from rue, *Ruta graveolens* (Rutaceae).

Profile
Rue oil and infusions of rue were formerly used as antispasmodics and emmenagogues and are reported to have abortifacient properties. Rue is a photosensitiser and the oil is a powerful local irritant.

Rue (Ruta grav.) is used in homoeopathic medicine.

Preparations
Proprietary Preparations (details are given in Part 3)
Multi-ingredient: *Austral.:* Joint & Muscle Relief Cream; *Singapore:* Noricaven.

Ruscogenin (3913-w)
(25R)-Spirost-5-ene-1β,3β-diol.
$C_{27}H_{42}O_4$ = 430.6.
CAS — 472-11-7.

A sapogenin obtained from butcher's broom, *Ruscus aculeatus* (Liliaceae).

Profile
Ruscogenin has been applied in the local treatment of haemorrhoids as rectal ointment or suppositories. It has also been tried in peripheral vascular disorders.

Preparations
Proprietary Preparations (details are given in Part 3)
Ger.: Ruscorectal; *Spain:* Hemodren Simple†; Ruscorectal.

Multi-ingredient: *Fr.:* Calmoroide†; Proctolog; *Ital.:* Ruscoroid; *Port.:* Proctolog; *Singapore:* Proctolog; *Spain:* Abrasone Rectal; Hemodren Compuesto; Neo Analsona; Proctolog; Ruscus; Venacol.

Sabeluzole (2980-y)
Sabeluzole (BAN, USAN, rINN).
R-58735. (±)-4-(2-Benzothiazolylmethylamino)-α-[(4-fluorophenoxy)methyl]-1-piperidineethanol.
$C_{22}H_{26}FN_3O_2S$ = 415.5.
CAS — 104153-38-0.

Profile
Sabeluzole is a benzothiazole derivative with anticonvulsant and antihypoxic properties. It has been investigated in the treatment of Alzheimer's disease and of sleep apnoea.

Sacrosidase (19809-v)
Sacrosidase (USAN).
CAS — 85897-35-4.

Profile
Sacrosidase is a therapeutic enzyme used for sucrase replacement therapy in congenital sucrase-isomaltase deficiency.

◊ References.
1. Treem WR, *et al.* Sacrosidase therapy for congenital sucrase-isomaltase deficiency. *J Pediatr Gastroenterol Nutr* 1999; **28:** 137–42.

Preparations
Proprietary Preparations (details are given in Part 3)
USA: Sucraid.

Sage (4704-s)
Feuilles de Sauge; Salbeiblätter; Salvia.

Pharmacopoeias. In *Eur.* (see p.vi) and *Pol. Eur.* also includes Sage Leaf, Three-lobed.

The oil of Greek sage (*Salvia triloba*), which is sometimes employed as an adulterant, has a lower thujone content than sage leaf oil.

Pharmacopoeial description
Ph. Eur.: The whole or cut dried leaves of *Salvia officinalis*. The whole drug contains not less than 1.5% v/w and the cut drug not less than 1.0% v/w of essential oil, both calculated with reference to the anhydrous drug. Sage leaf oil is rich in thujone. Protect from light.

Sage Leaf, Three-lobed consists of the whole or cut, dried leaves of *Salvia fructicosa* (*S. triloba*). The whole drug contains not less than 1.8% v/w of essential oil, and the cut drug not less than 1.2% v/w of essential oil, both calculated with reference to the anhydrous drug. It has a spicy odour when ground, similar to eucalyptus oil. Protect from light.

Profile
Sage has carminative, antispasmodic, antiseptic, and astringent properties and is used as a flavour. It is used in preparations for a wide variety of purposes, including respiratory-tract disorders, gastrointestinal disorders, and in mouthwashes and gargles for disorders of the mouth and throat. It is also used in homoeopathic medicine.

Sage oil has also been used.

Preparations
Proprietary Preparations (details are given in Part 3)
Aust.: Salvysat; *Ger.:* Aperisan; Buchol†; Fichtensirup N; Salbei Curarina; Salvysat; Sweatosan N; Viru-Salvysat.

Multi-ingredient: *Aust.:* Anifer Hustenbalsam; Apotheker Bauer's Blahungstee; Bronchostop; Cional; Colda; Coldistan; Dynexan; Fittydent; Krauterhaus Mag Kottas Wechseltee; Krautertee Nr 10; Krautertee Nr 107; Krautertee Nr 16; Krautertee Nr 311; Kra-

---

utertee Nr 8; Mentopin; Paradenton; Parodontax†; Piniment; Salbei-Halspastillen; Teekanne Husten- und Brusttee; Tetesept; *Austral.:* Feminine Herbal Complex; *Belg.:* Tisane pour Dormir; *Fr.:* Bolcitol; Santane V₃; Tisane Hepatique de Hoerdt; Tisanes de l'Abbe Hamon no 6; *Ger.:* Agamadon†; Amara-Tropfen; Dr. Hotz Vollbad†; Helago-oel N; Hoemarin Derma; Kneipp Rheuma Stoffwechsel-Bad Heublumen-Aquasan†; Leber-Galle-Tropfen 83; Melissengeist; Mycatox; Odala wern; Parodontal; Parodontal F5 med; Pernionin N; Polypharm-Zahnungsgel N†; Presselin Blahungs K 4 N; Presselin Dyspeptikum; Salviathymol N; Schupps Heilkrauter Rheumabad; Trauma-cyl; Varicylum-S; Vitosal; *Israel:* Kamilotract; Kamiltract Baby; Parodontax; *Ital.:* Donalg; Pluriderm†; Saugella Salviettine; *Port.:* Emopads; *S.Afr.:* Dynexan; *Spain:* Vegetalin; *Switz.:* Anginesin; Bismorectal; Demo pommade contre les refroidissements pour bebes; Dynexan; Kernosan Huile de Massage†; Osa Gel de dentition aux plantes†; Pastilles pectorales formule 541; Tisane pectorale et antitussive; Tonex; *UK:* Catarrh; Fragador; Medicinal Gargle.

Salverine Hydrochloride (19696-l)
Salverine Hydrochloride (rINNM).
M-811 (salverine). 2-[2-(Diethylamino)ethoxy]-benzanilide hydrochloride.
$C_{19}H_{24}N_2O_2,HCl$ = 348.9.
CAS — 6376-26-7 (salverine).

Profile
Salverine hydrochloride has been used as an antispasmodic in combination preparations for the treatment of biliary-tract disorders, respiratory-tract disorders, and pain.

Preparations
Proprietary Preparations (details are given in Part 3)
Multi-ingredient: *Aust.:* Cynarix comp; Montamed; Novipec.

Sambucus (320-q)
Elder Flowers; Fleurs de Sureau; Holunderblüten; Sabugueiro; Sambuc.; Sambuci Flos.

Pharmacopoeias. In *Eur.* (see p.vi) and *Pol.*

Pharmacopoeial description
Ph. Eur.: The dried flowers of *Sambucus nigra*. It contains not less than 0.8% of flavonoids, calculated as isoquercitroside with reference to the dried drug. Protect from light.

Profile
Sambucus has astringent, diaphoretic, and anticatarrhal properties and is used in herbal and homoeopathic preparations for a variety of disorders, particularly respiratory-tract disorders. Elder-flower water has been used as a vehicle for eye and skin lotions. Elder-flower ointment has been used as a basis for pomades and cosmetic ointments.

Preparations
Proprietary Preparations (details are given in Part 3)
Port.: Sambucol.

Multi-ingredient: *Aust.:* Apotheker Bauer's Grippetee; Bio-Garten Entschlackungstee; Bogumil-tassenfertiger milder Abfurtee; Entschlackender Abfuhrtee; Grippetee Dr Zeidler; Grippetee EF-EM-ES; Grippogran; Krauter Hustensaft; Krauterdoktor Erkaltungstropfen; Krauterhaus Mag Kottas Grippetee; Krautertee Nr 10; Krautertee Nr 2; Krautertee Nr 210; Laxalpin; Mag Kottas Grippe-Tee; Sidroga Erkaltungstee; Sinupret; Sinusol-Schleimlosender Tee; St Radegunder Fiebertee; Teekanne Erkaltungstee; Tuscalman; *Austral.:* Sambucus Complex; *Fr.:* Tisane des Familles; *Ger.:* Hevert-Erkaltungs-Tee†; Hevert-Gicht-Rheuma-Tee comp†; Kneipp Erkaltungs-Tee; Kneipp Rheuma Tee N†; Nephrubin†; Sinupret; *Hong Kong:* Sinupret; *Ital.:* Sambuco (Specie Composta); *Singapore:* Sinupret; *Switz.:* Sinupret; The Brioni; Tisane contre les refroidissements; Tisane laxative H nouvelle formulation; *Thai.:* Sinupret; *UK:* EP&C Essence; Hay Fever & Sinus Relief; Hayfever & Sinus Relief; Herb and Honey Cough Elixir; Life Drops; Lifedrops; Lion Cleansing Herbs; Lustys Herbalene; Modern Herbals Cold & Catarrh; Sinotar; Tabritis.

Sanguinaria (739-e)
Bloodroot; Red Puccoon; Sanguinaria canadensis; Sanguinarine canadensis; Sanguinaris canadensis.

The dried rhizome of *Sanguinaria canadensis* (Papaveraceae).

Profile
Sanguinarine, an alkaloid extracted from *Sanguinaria canadensis*, has been used as an antiplaque agent in toothpaste and mouthwash preparations. Sanguinaria was formerly used as an expectorant but fell into disuse because of its toxicity. Sanguinaria has also been classified by the FDA as a herb that is unsafe for use in foods, beverages, or drugs.

Sanguinaria is used in homoeopathic medicine.

◊ Reviews.
1. Karlowsky JA. Bloodroot: Sanguinaria canadensis L. *Can Pharm J* 1991; **124:** 260, 262–3, 267.
2. Grenby TH. The use of sanguinarine in mouthwashes and toothpaste compared with some other antimicrobial agents. *Br Dent J* 1995; **178:** 254–8.
3. Tenenbaum H, *et al.* Effectiveness of a sanguinarine regimen after scaling and root planing. *J Periodontol* 1999; **70:** 307–11.

Preparations

Proprietary Preparations (details are given in Part 3)
Canad.: Viadent; *Ital.:* Periogard; *Port.:* Periogard†.
Multi-ingredient: *Austral.:* Lexat; *Canad.:* Mielocol; Viadent; Wampole Bronchial Cough Syrup; *Ital.:* Dentosan Carie & Alito; Eudent con Glysan; Periogard; *Port.:* Periogard†.

Sapropterin Hydrochloride (13781-q)

Sapropterin Hydrochloride (rINNM).
Dapropterin Hydrochloride; SUN-0588 (sapropterin or sapropterin hydrochloride); (6*R*)-5,6,7,8-Tetrahydrobiopterin Hydrochloride. (−)-(6*R*)-2-Amino-6-[(1*R*,2*S*)-1,2-dihydroxypropyl]- 5,6,7,8-tetrahydro-4(3*H*)-pteridinone dihydrochloride.
$C_9H_{15}N_5O_3,2HCl = 314.2$.
CAS — 62989-33-7 (sapropterin); 69056-38-8 (sapropterin hydrochloride).

Profile
Sapropterin, the active form of tetrahydrobiopterin, has been tried as the hydrochloride to correct the hyperphenylalaninaemia which may be responsible for neurological symptoms seen in patients receiving treatment for leukaemia, and in other conditions associated with tetrahydrobiopterin (BH_4) deficiency.

◊ References.
1. Blau N, *et al.* Hyperphenylalaninemia caused by dihydropteridine reductase deficiency in children receiving chemotherapy for acute lymphoblastic leukemia. *J Pediatr* 1989; **115:** 661–2.
2. Hyland K, *et al.* *J Pediatr* 1989; **115:** 662.
3. Ueda S, *et al.* Tetrahydrobiopterin restores endothelial function in long-term smokers. *J Am Coll Cardiol* 2000; **35:** 71–5.
4. Thony B, *et al.* Tetrahydrobiopterin biosynthesis, regeneration and functions. *Biochem J* 2000; **347:** 1–16.

Sarsaparilla (2408-p)

Salsaparilha; Salsepareille; Sarsa; Sarsaparilla Root; Smilacis Rhizoma.
Pharmacopoeias. In *Chin.* and *Jpn.* which specify *Smilax glabra.*
The dried root of various species of *Smilax* (Liliaceae).

Profile
Sarsaparilla, usually in the form of a decoction or extract, has been used as a vehicle and flavour for medicaments. It is also an ingredient of herbal and homoeopathic preparations.

Preparations

Proprietary Preparations (details are given in Part 3)
Ger.: Sarsapsor†.
Multi-ingredient: *Austral.:* Esten†; Herbal Cleanse; Proesten; *Belg.:* Tisane Depurative "les 12 Plantes"; *Braz.:* Elixir de Marinheiro; Licor de Tayuya; Tintura de Salsa Caroba e Manaca; *Ger.:* Montana; Pankreaplex Neu; *Ital.:* Depurativo; Tisana Kelemata; *Port.:* Solucao Stago; *UK:* Blue Flag Root Compound; Gerard House Ligvites; Gerard House Reumalex; HRI Clear Complexion; Jamaican Sarsaparilla; Skin Eruptions Mixture.

Sassafras Oil (4708-y)

Oleum Sassafras.
A volatile oil distilled from the root or root bark of *Sassafras albidum* (Lauraceae), or from the wood of certain species of *Ocotea* (Lauraceae). It contains safrole.

Profile
Sassafras oil has rubefacient properties and was formerly used as a pediculicide. Neither sassafras nor the oil should be taken internally; the use of herb teas of sassafras may lead to a large dose of safrole. The use of safrole in foods has been banned because of carcinogenic and hepatotoxic risks. The use of safrole in toilet preparations is also controlled.

Poisoning. A 47-year-old woman experienced 'shakiness', vomiting, anxiety, tachycardia, and raised blood pressure following ingestion of a potentially fatal dose of sassafras oil (5 mL). Treatment was symptomatic following the use of activated charcoal.[1]
1. Grande GA, Dannewitz SR. Symptomatic sassafras oil ingestion. *Vet Hum Toxicol* 1987; **29:** 447.

Preparations

Proprietary Preparations (details are given in Part 3)
Multi-ingredient: *Austral.:* Zam-Buk; *Fr.:* Vegebom; *S.Afr.:* Zam-Buk†; *Spain:* Inhalador†; Linimento Klari.

Saxitoxin (746-w)

Profile
Saxitoxin is a neurotoxin associated with paralytic shellfish poisoning. It is an endotoxin produced by species of dinoflagellate plankton present in infected molluscs.

◊ References.
1. Halstead BW, Schantz EJ. *Paralytic shellfish poisoning.* Geneva: WHO, 1984.
2. Aquatic (marine and freshwater) biotoxins. *Environmental Health Criteria 37.* Geneva: WHO, 1984.

The symbol † denotes a preparation no longer actively marketed

---

3. Hartigan-Go K, Bateman DN. Redtide in the Philippines. *Hum Exp Toxicol* 1994; **13:** 824–30.
4. Gessner BD, *et al.* Hypertension and identification of toxin in human urine and serum following a cluster of mussel-associated paralytic shellfish poisoning outbreaks. *Toxicon* 1997; **35:** 711–22.
5. de Carvalho M, *et al.* Paralytic shellfish poisoning: clinical and electrophysiological observations. *J Neurol* 1998; **245:** 551–4.

Schick Test (8005-j)

Pharmacopoeias. *Br.* and *US* include standards for Schick test toxin and control.

Pharmacopoeial description
BP 2001: Schick Test Toxin is prepared from a toxigenic strain of *Corynebacterium diphtheriae.* It contains a suitable antimicrobial preservative. Store at 2° to 8°.
Schick Control is Schick Test Toxin that has been heated at a temperature not lower than 70° and not higher than 85° for not less than 5 minutes. It is prepared from the same batch of Schick Test Toxin as that with which it is to be used. Store at 2° to 8°.
USP 25: Diphtheria Toxin for Schick Test is a sterile solution of the diluted, standardised toxic products of the growth of the diphtheria bacillus (*Corynebacterium diphtheriae*). Store at 2° to 8°.
Schick Test Control is Diphtheria Toxin for Schick Test that has been inactivated by heat. Store at 2° to 8°.

Profile
The Schick test has been used for the diagnosis of susceptibility to diphtheria and, more importantly, to detect patients who might experience an adverse reaction to diphtheria vaccines. Children up to the age of about 8 to 10 years rarely suffer from such reactions following diphtheria vaccination and therefore the Schick test is not usually performed in this age group. In older children and adults a Schick test was formerly used before the use of standard diphtheria vaccines. However, diphtheria vaccines for use in adults and adolescents (p.1536) are now formulated with lesser amounts of toxoid so that the need for prior Schick testing is unnecessary.
A dose of 0.2 mL of the Schick toxin was administered intradermally (intracutaneously) into the flexor surface of the forearm. A similar dose of Schick control was injected into the other forearm. The reaction to the injections was read after 24 to 48 hours, and again after 5 to 7 days to detect late reactors and to confirm a reading taken earlier.
A *negative reaction*, indicating that the patient is immune to diphtheria, occurs when there is no redness at either injection site. A *positive reaction*, indicating susceptibility to diphtheria, occurs as a red flush about 10 mm or more in diameter at the site of injection of the test dose with no reaction to the control injection. A *negative-and-pseudo reaction*, also indicating immunity, is shown by a flush which develops rapidly at each injection site but the reaction fades more rapidly than a positive reaction; the reaction is due to non-specific constituents of the injection. A *combined* or *positive-and-pseudo reaction*, also indicating susceptibility, is shown by a flush which develops rapidly at each injection site, but as it fades a positive reaction develops at the site of the test dose.

Preparations
BP 2001: Schick Control; Schick Test Toxin;
USP 25: Diphtheria Toxin for Schick Test; Schick Test Control.

Scoparium (13224-n)

Broom Tops; Genêt; Genêt à Balai; Planta Genista; Scoparii Cacumina.
Pharmacopoeias. In *Fr.*
The dried tops of broom, *Sarothamnus scoparius* (=*Cytisus scoparius*) (Leguminosae).

Profile
Scoparium is a mild diuretic, haemostatic, and vasoconstrictor and has been administered as a decoction or infusion. It has oxytocic properties and should be avoided in pregnancy. It contains sparteine (p.1666).

Preparations

Proprietary Preparations (details are given in Part 3)
Ger.: Cefacor; Repowine†; Spartiol.
Multi-ingredient: *Fr.:* Creme Rap; Curoveinyl†; Santane H₇; Santane R₈; Santane V₃; Tisanes de l'Abbe Hamon no 16†; *Ger.:* Goldtropfen-Hetterich; Intradermi N; JuPhlebon S†; Oxacant N; Venacton.

Secretin (2147-m)

Secretin (BAN, rINN).
CAS — 17034-35-4.
ATC — V04CK01.
Pharmacopoeias. In *Jpn.*

Units
The potency of secretin may be expressed as Crick-Harper-Raper (CHR) units based on the pancreatic secretion in *cats* or

---

as Clinical units, the value of which was amended in the 1960s. One Clinical unit is considered to be approximately equivalent to 4 CHR units.

Adverse Effects
Hypersensitivity reactions may occasionally occur. Diarrhoea has occurred in patients given high doses by intravenous infusion.

Precautions
The secretin test should be avoided in patients with acute pancreatitis. Administration of a test dose has been suggested for patients at particular risk of hypersensitivity reactions.

Uses and Administration
Secretin is a polypeptide hormone involved in the regulation of gastric function; it is prepared from the duodenal mucosa of *pigs.* Following administration by intravenous injection it causes an increase in the secretion by the pancreas of water and bicarbonate into the duodenum. It is used alone, or in conjunction with pancreozymin or other cholecystokinetic agents such as ceruletide (p.1593) or sincalide (p.1664), as a test for exocrine pancreatic function. The test usually involves duodenal intubation of the patient and examination of duodenal aspirate. The dose of secretin used has varied but common doses have been 1 Clinical unit per kg body-weight given by slow intravenous injection.
Patients with the Zollinger-Ellison syndrome (p.1209) show an increase in gastrin following the administration of secretin; this is in contrast to a small change or no effect in subjects without the disorder. The usual dose of secretin for the diagnosis of Zollinger-Ellison syndrome is 2 Clinical units per kg by slow intravenous injection. Serum-gastrin concentrations are measured for up to 30 minutes following the test dose.

Autism. There have been anecdotal reports of improvement in behaviour in autistic children after administration of porcine secretin. However, a double-blind placebo-controlled study[1] involving 60 children with autism or pervasive developmental disorder noted no benefit over 4 weeks following a single infusion of 400 µg per kg body-weight of synthetic human secretin. A randomised, placebo-controlled study[2] in 64 children with autism has similarly found no evidence of efficacy from 2 repeated doses of porcine secretin.
1. Sandler AD, *et al.* Lack of benefit of a single dose of synthetic human secretin in the treatment of autism and pervasive developmental disorder. *N Engl J Med* 1999; **341:** 1801–6.
2. Roberts W, *et al.* Repeated doses of porcine secretin in the treatment of autism: a randomized, placebo-controlled trial. Abstract: *Pediatrics* 2001; **107:** e71. Full version: http://www.pediatrics.org/cgi/content/full/107/5/e71

Preparations

Proprietary Preparations (details are given in Part 3)
Ger.: Secrelux; Sekretolin†.

Selfotel (17312-w)

Selfotel (USAN, rINN).
CGS-19755. *cis*-4-(Phosphonomethyl)pipecolic acid.
$C_7H_{14}NO_5P = 223.2$.
CAS — 110347-85-8.

Profile
Selfotel is an *N*-methyl-D-aspartate (NMDA) antagonist which has been investigated for use in ischaemic stroke and head trauma.

◊ References.
1. Davis SM, *et al.* Termination of acute stroke studies involving selfotel treatment. *Lancet* 1997; **349:** 32.
2. Yenari MA, *et al.* Dose escalation safety and tolerance study of the competitive NMDA antagonist selfotel (CGS 19755) in neurosurgery patients. *Clin Neuropharmacol* 1998; **21:** 28–34.
3. Stewart L, *et al.* First observations of the safety and tolerability of a competitive antagonist to the glutamate NMDA receptor (CGS 19755) in patients with severe head injury. *J Neurotrauma* 1999; **16:** 843–50.
4. Morris GF, *et al.* Failure of the competitive N-methyl-D-aspartate antagonist Selfotel (CGS 19755) in the treatment of severe head injury: results of two phase III clinical trials. *J Neurosurg* 1999; **91:** 737–43.
5. Davis SM, *et al.* Selfotel in acute ischemic stroke: possible neurotoxic effects of an NMDA antagonist. *Stroke* 2000; **31:** 347–54.

Senecio (13229-g)

Profile
The ragwort, *Senecio jacobaea,* and, in the USA, the golden ragwort (golden senecio; lifereot; squaw weed) *S. aureus,* have been used in the form of extracts as emmenagogues but are of doubtful value. Ragwort, in the form of a decoction or ointment, has also been applied externally to aid wound healing and in the treatment of peripheral vascular disorders. *S. aureus* is also used in homoeopathic preparations.
Many species of the genus *Senecio* (Compositae), which includes the ragworts and groundsels, are poisonous and have been found to contain pyrrolizidine alkaloids which produce hepatic necrosis. The ragwort, *S. jacobaea,* which is abundant throughout the British Isles, is poisonous to livestock when eat-

en in quantity. Poisoning has also been reported in humans following ingestion of herbal teas containing pyrrolizidine alkaloids.

Preparations

Proprietary Preparations (details are given in Part 3)

Multi-ingredient: *Canad.:* Thunas Tab for Menstrual Pain; *Ger.:* Senecion†; *USA:* Succus Cineraria Maritima.

Sepia (13230-f)

Profile
Sepia is the dried inky secretion of the cuttle fish. It is used in homoeopathic medicine.

Serotonin (15305-a)

Enteramine; 5-HT; 5-Hydroxytryptamine. 3-(2-Aminoethyl)-1*H*-indol-5-ol.

$C_{10}H_{12}N_2O = 176.2$.

CAS — 50-67-9.

Serotonin is widely distributed in the body; it also occurs in stinging nettles (*Urtica dioica*), bananas, and other fruit, and in the stings of wasps and scorpions.

Profile
Serotonin is found in the brain, blood platelets, and throughout the gastrointestinal tract and its roles include involvement in CNS neurotransmission, haemostasis, vascular spasm, and gastrointestinal motility. Many drugs have some action on serotonin receptors. Several types and subtypes of serotonin receptors have been identified and drugs with serotonin-agonist activity and those displaying serotonin-antagonist activity may both be used to treat the same condition, as in migraine or depression.

Serotonin itself may be of value in the treatment of posthypoxic myoclonus (p.342). Serotonin *precursors* have been given for the treatment of depression (see Oxitriptan, p.302 and Tryptophan, p.311). *Selective serotonin reuptake inhibitors* are used in depression (see Fluoxetine Hydrochloride, p.284); also *MAOIs* and *tricyclic antidepressants* have some serotonin-agonist activity. *Sumatriptan* (p.456) is an agonist used in migraine. The *dopaminergic ergot derivatives* such as bromocriptine (p.1164), lisuride (p.1174), and pergolide (p.1175) are partial serotonin agonists.

Among the drugs exhibiting serotonin-antagonist activity are the antimigraine *ergot alkaloids*; *antihistamines* such as cyproheptadine (p.414), and pizotifen (p.455); *antihypertensives* such as ketanserin (p.917); and *antiemetics* such as ondansetron (p.1241). *Other drugs* with recognised serotonin-antagonist activity include fenclonine (p.1610), dexfenfluramine (p.1508), fenfluramine (p.1510), chlorpromazine (p.660), and the tetracyclic antidepressant mianserin (p.298).

◊ References.
1. Hindle AT. Recent developments in the physiology and pharmacology of 5-hydroxytryptamine. *Br J Anaesth* 1994; **73:** 395–407.
2. Hoyer D, *et al.* International Union of Pharmacology classification of receptors for 5-hydroxytryptamine (serotonin). *Pharmacol Rev* 1994; **46:** 157–203.

Serrapeptase (13233-h)

Serrapeptase (*rINN*).

Serratia Extracellular Proteinase; Serratiopeptidase.

CAS — 37312-62-2.

A proteolytic enzyme derived from *Serratia* spp.

Profile
Serrapeptase has been taken by mouth for its supposed action in relieving inflammation and oedema associated with trauma, infection, or chronic venous insufficiency, in usual doses of 5 to 10 mg (10 000 to 20 000 units) up to three times daily.

◊ References.
1. Tachibana M, *et al.* A multi-centre, double-blind study of serrapeptase versus placebo in post-antrotomy buccal swelling. *Pharmatherapeutica* 1984; **3:** 526–30.
2. Paparella P, *et al.* Serratia peptidase and acute phase protein behavior following vaginal hysterectomy: results of a randomized double-blind, placebo-controlled trial. *Curr Ther Res* 1989; **45:** 664–76.
3. Shimizu H, *et al.* A case of serratiopeptidase-induced subepidermal bullous dermatosis. *Br J Dermatol* 1999; **141:** 1139–40.

Preparations

Proprietary Preparations (details are given in Part 3)

Braz.: Danzen; *Fr.:* Dazen; *Ger.:* Aniflazym; *Hong Kong:* Danzen; *Ital.:* Danzen; *Jpn:* Dasen; *Mex.:* Danzen; *Port.:* Aniflazime; *Singapore:* Danzen; Korzen; Septirose; Serrazyme; Unizen; *Thai.:* Dailat; Danzen; Denzo; Medizyme; Podase; Rodase; Seramed; Serradase; Serrano; Serrao; Serrapep; Serrason; Sumidin; Unizen.

Sesame Oil (7368-w)

Aceite de Ajonjoli; Benne Oil; Gingelly Oil; Oleum Sesami; Refined Sesame Oil; Teel Oil.

Pharmacopoeias. In Chin., Eur. (see p.vi), and Jpn. Also in USNF.

Pharmacopoeial description
Ph. Eur.: Refined Sesame Oil is the fatty oil obtained from the ripe seeds of *Sesamum indicum* by expression or extraction and subsequent refining. It may contain a suitable antioxidant. It is a clear, light yellow, almost colourless liquid. It solidifies to a soft mass at about −4°. Practically insoluble in alcohol; miscible with petroleum spirit. Store in well-filled, airtight containers. Protect from light. Refined sesame oil for use in the manufacture of parenteral dosage forms should be stored under an inert gas in airtight containers.

USNF 20: The refined fixed oil obtained from the seed of one or more cultivated varieties of *Sesamum indicum* (Pedaliaceae). A pale yellow, practically odourless, oily liquid. Slightly soluble in alcohol; miscible with carbon disulfide, with chloroform, with ether, and with petroleum spirit. Store in airtight containers at a temperature not exceeding 40°. Protect from light.

Profile
Sesame oil has been used in the preparation of liniments, plasters, ointments, and soaps. Because it is relatively stable, it is a useful solvent and vehicle for parenteral products. Hypersensitivity reactions have been observed.

◊ Reports of hypersensitivity reactions[1-4] and subcutaneous nodules[5] associated with sesame administration.
1. Kanny G, *et al.* Sesame seed and sesame seed oil contain masked allergens of growing importance. *Allergy* 1996; **51:** 952–7.
2. Stern A, Wuthrich B. Non-IgE-mediated anaphylaxis to sesame. *Allergy* 1998; **53:** 325–6.
3. Pecquet C, *et al.* Immediate hypersensitivity to sesame in foods and cosmetics. *Contact Dermatitis* 1998; **39:** 313.
4. Asero R, *et al.* A case of sesame seed-induced anaphylaxis. *Allergy* 1999; **54:** 526–7.
5. Darsow U, *et al.* Subcutaneous oleomas induced by self-injection of sesame seed oil for muscle augmentation. *J Am Acad Dermatol* 2000; **42:** 292–4.

Preparations

Proprietary Preparations (details are given in Part 3)

Multi-ingredient: *UK:* Snor-Away; Snorenz.

Shellac (285-x)

E904; Gomme Laque; Lacca; Lacca in Tabulis; Schellack.

Pharmacopoeias. In Eur. (see p.vi). Also in USNF.
Jpn includes Purified Shellac and White Shellac (Bleached).

Pharmacopoeial description
Ph. Eur.: Shellac is obtained by purification of the resinous secretion of the female insect *Kerria lacca* (Kerr) Lindinger (*Laccifer lacca* Kerr). There are 4 types of shellac depending on the nature of the treatment of crude secretion (seedlac): Wax-containing Shellac; Bleached Shellac; Dewaxed Shellac; and Bleached, Dewaxed Shellac.

Brownish-orange or yellow, shining, translucent, hard or brittle more or less thin flakes (Wax-containing Shellac; Dewaxed Shellac), or a creamy-white or brownish-yellow powder (Bleached Shellac; Bleached, Dewaxed Shellac).

Practically insoluble in water; partly soluble in ether. With dehydrated alcohol it gives a more or less opalescent solution (Wax-containing Shellac; Bleached Shellac) or a clear solution (Dewaxed Shellac; Bleached, Dewaxed Shellac). When warmed, it is sparingly soluble or soluble in alkaline solutions. Protect from light. Store Bleached Shellac and Bleached, Dewaxed Shellac at a temperature not exceeding 15°.

USNF 20: Shellac is obtained by purification of lac, the resinous secretion of the insect *Laccifer lacca kerr* (Coccidae). There are 4 varieties: Orange Shellac, Dewaxed Orange Shellac, Regular Bleached (White) Shellac, and Refined Bleached Shellac. Orange Shellac occurs as thin, hard, brittle, transparent, pale lemon-yellow to brownish-orange flakes, having little or no odour. Bleached Shellac occurs as opaque, amorphous, cream to yellow granules or coarse powder, having little or no odour.

Insoluble in water; very slowly soluble in alcohol, 85 to 95% (w/w); soluble in ether, 13 to 15%, in petroleum spirit, 2 to 6%, in benzene, 10 to 20%, and in aqueous solutions of ethanolamines, alkalis, and borax; sparingly soluble in turpentine oil. Store preferably at a temperature not exceeding 8°.

Profile
Shellac is used as an enteric coating for pills and tablets, but disintegration time has been reported to increase markedly on storage.

Preparations

USNF 20: Pharmaceutical Glaze.

Shepherd's Purse (11290-a)

Capsella; Herba Bursae Pastoris; Shepherds Burse Herb.

Pharmacopoeias. In Fr.

Profile
Shepherd's purse, the aerial parts of *Capsella bursa-pastoris* (*Thlaspi bursa-pastoris*) (Cruciferae) has antihaemorrhagic and astringent properties. It is used to prevent or arrest bleeding, and has been specifically used for menorrhagia. It is also used for urinary-tract disorders and diarrhoea.

It is also used in homoeopathic medicine.

Preparations

Proprietary Preparations (details are given in Part 3)

Ger.: Styptysat.

Multi-ingredient: *Aust.:* Menodoron; *Fr.:* Hemoluol†; Histo-Fluine P; Tisanes de l'Abbe Hamon no 14†; *Ger.:* Bomagall forte S†; Presselin Dysmen Olin 3 N; Rhoival; *UK:* Antitis; Menodoron; Sciargo.

Siam Benzoin (273-c)

Benjoin du Laos; Benzoe Tonkinensis.

Pharmacopoeias. In Aust., Chin., Fr., It., and Swiss. Also in many pharmacopoeias under the title benzoin and should not be confused with Sumatra benzoin. Jpn and US allow both Siam benzoin and Sumatra benzoin under the title Benzoin.

Pharmacopoeial description
USP 25: A balsamic resin from *Styrax tonkinensis*, or other species of the *Anthostyrax* section of the genus *Styrax* (Styracaceae). It yields not less than 90% of alcohol-soluble extractive. It occurs as pebble-like tears of variable size and shape, compressed, yellowish-brown to rusty brown externally, milky white on fracture, separate or very slightly agglutinated, hard and brittle at ordinary temperatures but softened by heat. It has an agreeable, balsamic, vanilla-like odour.

Profile
Siam benzoin has been used similarly to Sumatra benzoin (p.1668). It has also been used as a preservative and was formerly used in the preparation of benzoinated lard.

Preparations

USP 25: Compound Benzoin Tincture; Podophyllum Resin Topical Solution.

Proprietary Preparations (details are given in Part 3)

Multi-ingredient: *Canad.:* Cold Sore Lotion†; *Fr.:* Balsolene; Borostyrol; Homeoplasmine; Inotyol; *Israel:* Inotyol; Kank-A; *Ital.:* Ondroly-A; *Switz.:* Borostyrol N.

Sildenafil Citrate (17680-e)

Sildenafil Citrate (*BANM, USAN, rINNM*).

UK-92480-10. 5-[2-Ethoxy-5-(4-methylpiperazin-1-ylsulfonyl)phenyl]-1,6-dihydro-1-methyl-3-propylpyrazolo[4,3-*d*]pyrimidin-7-one citrate; 1-{[3-(6,7-Dihydro-1-methyl-7-oxo-3-propyl-1*H*-pyrazolo[4,3-*d*]pyrimidin-5-yl)-4-ethoxyphenyl]sulfonyl}-4-methylpiperazone citrate.

$C_{22}H_{30}N_6O_4S,C_6H_8O_7 = 666.7$.

CAS — 139755-83-2 (sildenafil); 171599-83-0 (sildenafil citrate).

Adverse Effects
Adverse effects most commonly reported from sildenafil are headache, flushing, and dyspepsia. There may be visual disturbances, dizziness, and nasal congestion. Other adverse effects reported include diarrhoea, muscle pain, skin rashes, and urinary- or respiratory-tract infection. Priapism has also occurred. There have also been reports of serious cardiovascular events, including sudden cardiac death, associated with the use of sildenafil.

Effects on the cardiovascular system. There has been considerable uncertainty about the potential cardiovascular risk associated with sildenafil treatment. Minor effects associated with vasodilatation, such as headache and flushing are relatively common, but in patients without pre-existing cardiovascular risk factors the risk of serious cardiovascular events associated with the drug appears to be low. However, there has been a report of myocardial infarction in a patient without apparent risk factors,[1] and a consensus document issued by the American College of Cardiology and the American Heart Association (ACC/AHA) has pointed out that patients with erectile dysfunction are mostly over 45 years of age and are more likely to have risk factors predisposing them to cardiovascular disease.[2] As of August 1998, there had been 69 deaths in patients taking sildenafil reported to the FDA; 2 of these were due to stroke and 46 to some other cardiovascular event.[3] The nature of the relationship between drug and event was considered unclear, but some of these patients were also receiving nitrates, a combination now contra-indicated because of the greatly increased risk of potentially life-threatening hypotension.[2]

It is still uncertain whether patients with **pre-existing** cardiovascular disease are at increased risk when taking sildenafil without concomitant nitrates. The ACC/AHA consensus statement noted that the evidence was scanty and suggested that sildenafil could be used, but with caution, in patients with stable coronary artery disease provided that nitrates were not taken.[2] An open-label, uncontrolled assessment of the haemodynamic effects of sildenafil in 14 men with coronary artery disease found no evidence of adverse effects on coronary blood flow, resistance, or flow reserve.[4] Evidence to assess the risk in other cardiovascular disorders is even less extensive, although a case report of a patient with hypertrophic cardiomyopathy who experienced cardiovascular adverse effects following a dose of sildenafil suggested that the drug may precipitate an unstable haemodynamic state in this condition.[5]

1. Feenstra J, *et al.* Acute myocardial infarction associated with sildenafil. *Lancet* 1998; **352:** 957–8.
2. Cheitlin MD, *et al.* Use of sildenafil (Viagra) in patients with cardiovascular disease. ACC/AHA Expert Consensus Document. *J Am Coll Cardiol* 1999; **33:** 273–82. Correction. *ibid.*; **34:** 1850.
3. Anonymous. Sildenafil for erectile dysfunction. *Drug Ther Bull* 1998; **36:** 81–4.
4. Herrmann HC, *et al.* Hemodynamic effects of sildenafil in men with severe coronary artery disease. *N Engl J Med* 2000; **342:** 1622–6.
5. Stauffer J-C, *et al.* Subaortic obstruction after sildenafil in a patient with hypertrophic cardiomyopathy. *N Engl J Med* 1999; **341:** 700–701.

Effects on the eyes. A bluish tinge or haze to vision and some increased light sensitivity has been reported by a significant percentage of patients taking sildenafil, with the percentage of reports increasing with increasing dose.[1] The visual symptoms usually peak after 1 to 2 hours following ingestion and resolve about 3 to 4 hours later. The effects of a single dose of sildenafil 100 mg were studied in 5 healthy volunteers.[2] Electroretinogram measurements showed significant changes that correlated well with plasma-sildenafil concentrations, peaking at 1 hour after administration and showing complete recovery at the 6-hour measurements. Inhibition of phosphodiesterase type-6 in rod photoreceptors is the most likely mechanism of sildenafil-associated retinal dysfunction. However, there is as yet no clear evidence of retinal toxic effects or whether repeated dosing with sildenafil causes prolonged or further retinal dysfunction.[1,2] Likewise, it remains to be determined whether recovery of function as plasma-sildenafil concentrations subside also occurs in older patients or those with retinal degenerative disorders such as retinitis pigmentosa. Other visual disturbances reported in patients taking sildenafil have included temporary loss of vision and increased intra-ocular pressure.[3] A 69-year-old man who experienced permanent loss of vision in one eye a few hours after taking sildenafil 100 mg was found to have an occlusion in a retinal artery.[4]

1. Marmor MF. Sildenafil (Viagra) and ophthalmology. *Arch Ophthalmol* 1999; **117:** 518–19.
2. Vobig MA, *et al.* Retinal side-effects of sildenafil. *Lancet* 1999; **353:** 375.
3. Committee on Safety of Medicines/Medicines Control Agency. Sildenafil (Viagra). *Current Problems* 1999; **25:** 16.
4. Tripathi A, O'Donnell N. Branch retinal artery occlusion; another complication of sildenafil. *Br J Ophthalmol* 2000; **84:** 934–5.

Precautions
The cardiovascular risks of sexual activity should be considered before beginning therapy with sildenafil; in some patients, sexual activity may be inadvisable. Caution is required in patients with hepatic or severe renal impairment, and dosage reduction may be necessary. Care is also needed in patients with anatomical or haematological disorders which may predispose them to priapism. Patients who experience dizziness or visual disturbances should not drive or operate hazardous machinery.

The safety of sildenafil is uncertain in patients with severe hepatic impairment, bleeding disorders, active peptic ulceration, hypotension, a recent history of stroke, myocardial infarction, or life-threatening arrhythmia, unstable angina, heart failure, or retinal disorders such as retinitis pigmentosa (a minority of whom have genetic disorders of retinal phosphodiesterases). The manufacturers advise that it should not be used in these groups.

Cardiovascular disease. For mention of a consensus statement on the use of sildenafil in patients with cardiovascular disease, see above.

Interactions
Sildenafil may potentiate the hypotensive effects of organic nitrates, and is therefore contra-indicated in patients receiving such drugs. Concomitant administration of sildenafil with drugs that inhibit the cytochrome P450 isoenzyme CYP3A4, such as cimetidine, erythromycin, itraconazole, ketoconazole, and HIV-protease inhibitors may reduce sildenafil clearance necessitating a reduction in dosage. However, plasma concentrations of sildenafil are significantly increased by ritonavir, requiring even greater dosage reduction, and it is therefore strongly recommended that these two drugs are not given together.

Antivirals. Rises in sildenafil concentrations following concomitant administration of *saquinavir* or *ritonavir* were consistent[1] with inhibition of metabolism mediated by the cytochrome P450 isoenzyme CYP3A4. The larger increases seen with ritonavir may be due to its additional inhibition of the isoenzyme CYP2C9. Death following myocardial infarction has been reported[2] in a 47-year-old patient who took sildenafil 25 mg concomitantly with ritonavir and saquinavir.

1. Muirhead GJ, *et al.* Pharmacokinetic interactions between sildenafil and saquinavir/ritonavir. *Br J Pharmacol* 2000; **50:** 99–107.
2. Hall MCS, Ahmad S. Interaction between sildenafil and HIV-1 combination therapy. *Lancet* 1999; **353:** 2071–2.

Nitrates. Administration of sildenafil 50 mg to patients receiving isosorbide mononitrate, or sublingual administration of glyceryl trinitrate 1 hour after sildenafil, resulted in substantially greater decreases in blood pressure than when the nitrate was administered alone in 2 crossover studies in patients with angina.[1] Treatment-related adverse effects were reported in 8 of 16 patients who took sildenafil with isosorbide mononitrate and 3 of 15 who received sildenafil with glyceryl trinitrate. The authors confirmed that sildenafil should not be taken concomitantly with nitrates.

1. Webb DJ, *et al.* Sildenafil citrate potentiates the hypotensive effects of nitric oxide donor drugs in male patients with stable angina. *J Am Coll Cardiol* 2000; **36:** 25–31.

Pharmacokinetics
Sildenafil is rapidly absorbed following administration by mouth, with a bioavailability of approximately 40%. Peak plasma concentrations are attained within 30 to 120 minutes; the rate of absorption is reduced when sildenafil is administered with food.

Sildenafil is widely distributed into tissues and is approximately 96% bound to plasma proteins. It is metabolised in the liver primarily by cytochrome P450 isoenzymes CYP3A4 (the major route) and CYP2C9. The major metabolite, *N*-desmethyl-sildenafil, also has some activity. The terminal half-lives of sildenafil and the *N*-desmethyl metabolite are about 4 hours.

Sildenafil is excreted, predominantly as metabolites, in the faeces, and to a lesser extent the urine. Clearance may be reduced in the elderly and in patients with hepatic or severe renal impairment.

◊ References.
1. Muirhead GJ, *et al.* Pharmacokinetics of sildenafil (VIAGRA™), a selective cGMP PDE5 inhibitor, after single oral doses in fasted and fed healthy volunteers. *Br J Clin Pharmacol* 1996; **42:** 268P.

Uses and Administration
Sildenafil is a phosphodiesterase type-5 inhibitor used in the management of erectile dysfunction (see below). It is given by mouth as the citrate although doses are expressed in terms of the base. The usual dose is 50 mg about one hour before sexual intercourse. The dose may be increased or decreased depending on response. The maximum recommended dose is 100 mg, and sildenafil should not be taken more often than once in 24 hours. An initial dose of 25 mg is recommended in elderly patients and in those with hepatic impairment or renal impairment (creatinine clearance less than 30 mL per minute). An initial dose of no more than 25 mg daily is also advised in patients taking sildenafil concomitantly with inhibitors of cytochrome P450 isoenzyme CYP3A4; the manufacturers advise that the dose should not exceed 25 mg every 48 hours in the case of co-administration with ritonavir, although such a combination is best avoided entirely (see under Interactions, above).

◊ References.
1. Goldstein I, *et al.* Oral sildenafil in the treatment of erectile dysfunction. *N Engl J Med* 1998; **338:** 1397–1404. Correction. *ibid.*; **339:** 59.
2. Anonymous. Sildenafil: an oral drug for impotence. *Med Lett Drugs Ther* 1998; **40:** 51–2.
3. Anonymous. Sildenafil for erectile dysfunction. *Drug Ther Bull* 1998; **36:** 81–4.
4. Derry FA, *et al.* Efficacy and safety of oral sildenafil (Viagra) in men with erectile dysfunction caused by spinal cord injury. *Neurology* 1998; **51:** 1629–33.
5. Langtry HD, Markham A. Sildenafil: a review of its use in erectile dysfunction. *Drugs* 1999; **57:** 967–89.
6. Montorsi F, *et al.* Efficacy and safety of fixed-dose oral sildenafil in the treatment of erectile dysfunction of various etiologies. *Urology* 1999; **53:** 1011–18.
7. Rendell MS, *et al.* Sildenafil for treatment of erectile dysfunction in men with diabetes: a randomized controlled trial. *JAMA* 1999; **281:** 421–6.
8. Kedia S, *et al.* Treatment of erectile dysfunction with sildenafil citrate (Viagra) after radiation therapy for prostate cancer. *Urology* 1999; **54:** 308–12.
9. Zippe CD, *et al.* Role of Viagra after radical prostatectomy. *Urology* 2000; **55:** 241–5.

Erectile dysfunction. Erectile dysfunction (impotence) signifies inability of a male to achieve satisfactory erection of the penis during sexual intercourse. Estimates of prevalence depend to some extent upon the definitions that are used, and are in any case difficult to come by, but the problem is thought to be not uncommon, particularly in older men.

In a normal erection parasympathetic stimulation, usually initiated by the CNS and enhanced by sensory stimuli from the penis, dilates penile arteries and relaxes trabecular smooth muscle via a second messenger, probably nitric oxide. This favours flow of blood into the spaces of the corpora cavernosa, increasing pressure in the penis and leading to tumescence. The increased pressure compresses the venules against the fibrous tissue layer called the tunica albuginea, thus preventing outflow of the blood and leading to rigidity.

The causes of erectile dysfunction may be psychological, organic, or a combination of both. Psychological factors include stress, mental depression, and anxieties about sexual performance. Organic causes include androgen deficiency as a result of hypogonadism, neurological dysfunction (including central or peripheral lesions due to malignancy or trauma), peripheral vascular disorders, and penile abnormalities such as Peyronie's disease or microphallus. Sometimes organic dysfunction may be secondary to another disease, such as diabetes mellitus in which neurological and vascular damage lead to erectile dys-

function in over one-third of all patients. In addition, erectile dysfunction may be drug-induced.

Approaches to the management of erectile dysfunction depend to some extent upon the causative factors.

In those few patients in whom erectile dysfunction is secondary to androgen deficiency in hypogonadism, androgen replacement, preferably by the intramuscular injection or transdermal application of a suitable testosterone ester, may be of value. Androgen replacement therapy is inappropriate in patients with normal testosterone concentrations and may carry significant health risks. In patients with hypogonadism secondary to hyperprolactinaemia addition of bromocriptine is often effective in improving sexual function.

Psychotherapy or behavioural therapy alone may be adequate in patients in whom no organic cause is detected, but even when organic factors play a role psychosocial factors are also important and should be addressed by appropriate counselling.

When causes of erectile dysfunction are partly or primarily organic, the main options in common use are: use of a vacuum pump to induce erection by negative pressure, followed by constriction of the base of the penis with a band to maintain tumescence; oral therapy; injection of vasoactive substances into the corpora cavernosa; or transurethral administration of vasoactive substances. Implantation of a penile prosthesis is generally reserved for patients in whom other therapy has failed or is refused, but it may also be a suitable first-line choice for some patients. Vascular surgery has a limited application, in vasogenic dysfunction, but its role is not clearly defined and there are some doubts about its long-term effectiveness.

Oral therapy for erectile dysfunction has had a chequered history, and most of the drugs tried have proved little more effective than placebo. However, with the advent of sildenafil, the place of oral therapy in the treatment of erectile dysfunction has altered. Sildenafil, a selective inhibitor of phosphodiesterase type-5, is probably now the drug of first-choice in many cases of erectile dysfunction. Data from randomised controlled trials have shown efficacy in erectile dysfunction compared with placebo, including men with diabetes mellitus and spinal-cord injury; it has no effect on the penis in the absence of sexual stimulation. It is generally more effective in erectile dysfunction of psychogenic origin and in mild to moderate cases of organic origin. There has, however, been concern about cardiac-related deaths associated with the use of sildenafil, although causality has not yet been firmly established. Visual disturbances have also been reported. Other phosphodiesterase type-5 inhibitors being investigated include tadalafil and vardenafil. Other drugs that have been tried as oral therapy with mixed results. Yohimbine, an α_2-adrenoceptor antagonist, may have some benefit, although more in erectile dysfunction of psychological than organic origin. Oral phentolamine is available for the treatment of erectile dysfunction in some countries and has been reported to be of benefit. Apomorphine, a dopaminergic (D_1 or D_2) agonist has also demonstrated efficacy in clinical trials when given sublingually, but nausea may be a problem. Trazodone, a serotonin antagonist and reuptake inhibitor used in the treatment of depression, may rarely cause priapism and has therefore been investigated for the treatment of erectile dysfunction. Beneficial effects have been reported either alone or in combination with yohimbine. Orally administered L-arginine, the precursor of nitric oxide, has also shown some promise in studies.

Intracavernosal injection therapy is the most effective pharmacological method of treating erectile dysfunction and, until the advent of an effective oral therapy, was the most widely used. Unfortunately, one major disadvantage of this method is the need for repeated self-injection of the penis, and studies suggest that the long-term drop-out rate is high. However, it is still a valuable option in men unresponsive to, or unable to take, oral therapy. The drugs most commonly used for intracavernosal injection therapy are alprostadil, papaverine, and phentolamine. Alprostadil is the preferred drug because it is superior in efficacy to papaverine (with or without phentolamine), and is associated with a lower incidence of priapism and fibrosis. However, the erection is frequently painful. Papaverine, a non-specific phosphodiesterase inhibitor, has been used alone or in combination with phentolamine, an α-adrenoceptor antagonist. Erectile dysfunction of neurogenic or psychogenic origin generally responds better to papaverine than dysfunction of vascular origin. However, long-term use of intracavernosal papaverine may result in fibrosis, and it has been suggested that it should not be used more than three times a week or on two successive days. Priapism may also be a problem. Triple therapy, involving the combination of alprostadil, papaverine, and phentolamine, has been reported to be effective and to have a relatively low incidence of adverse effects. Other drugs that have been used for intracavernosal therapy include aviptadil, a smooth muscle relaxant used with phentolamine in some countries, and ketanserin used in combination with alprostadil. Thymoxamine [moxisylyte] has also been tried.

Transurethral administration is a less invasive but also less effective option than intracavernosal therapy. Transurethral administration of a pellet of alprostadil is reported to be effective, although efficacy is inconsistent; common side-effects include penile pain and urethral pain or burning.

A number of studies have also investigated **transcutaneous** administration. Results from pilot studies investigating transcutaneous delivery of glyceryl trinitrate, papaverine, minoxidil, or alprostadil from creams, gels, or pastes have been variable.

References.
1. Dinsmore W, Evans C. ABC of sexual health: Erectile dysfunction. *BMJ* 1999; **318:** 387–90.
2. Burnett AL. Oral pharmacotherapy for erectile dysfunction: current perspectives. *Urology* 1999; **54:** 392–400.
3. Meinhardt W, *et al.* Comparative tolerability and efficacy of treatments for impotence. *Drug Safety* 1999; **20:** 133–46.
4. Langford N. Adverse reactions to drugs used for erectile dysfunction. *Adverse Drug React Bull* 1999; (Apr): 743–6.
5. Nehra A, *et al.* Pharmacotherapeutic advances in the treatment of erectile dysfunction. *Mayo Clin Proc* 1999; **74:** 709–21.
6. Cummings MH, Alexander WD. Erectile dysfunction in patients with diabetes. *Hosp Med* 1999; **60:** 638–44.
7. Morgentaler A. Male impotence. *Lancet* 1999; **354:** 1713–18.
8. Williams G. Male erectile dysfunction. *Prescribers' J* 2000; **40:** 49–58.
9. Lue TF. Erectile dysfunction. *N Engl J Med* 2000; **342:** 1802–13.

Preparations

Proprietary Preparations (details are given in Part 3)
Aust.: Viagra; **Austral.:** Viagra; **Belg.:** Viagra; **Canad.:** Viagra; **Denm.:** Viagra; **Fin.:** Viagra; **Fr.:** Viagra; **Ger.:** Viagra; **Hong Kong:** Viagra; **Irl.:** Viagra; **Israel:** Viagra; **Ital.:** Viagra; **Mex.:** Viagra; **Norw.:** Viagra; **NZ:** Viagra; **Port.:** Viagra; **S.Afr.:** Viagra; **Singapore:** Viagra; **Spain:** Viagra; **Swed.:** Viagra; **Switz.:** Viagra; **Thai.:** Viagra; **UK:** Viagra; **USA:** Viagra.

Silver   (5316-v)

E174.
Ag = 107.8682.
CAS — 7440-22-4.
ATC — D08AL30.

Pharmacopoeias. In Swiss.

A pure white, malleable and ductile metal.

Profile
Silver possesses antibacterial properties and is used topically either as the metal or as silver salts. It is not absorbed to any great extent and the main problem associated with the metal is argyria, a grey discoloration of the tissues. Silver is also present as the core in some copper-wound plastic intra-uterine contraceptive devices. Silver is used as a colouring agent for some types of confectionery. It is also used as Argentum Metallicum in homoeopathy.

Numerous salts or compounds of silver have been employed for various therapeutic purposes, including silver acetate (p.1664), silver allantoinate, silver zinc allantoinate, silver borate, silver carbonate, silver chloride, silver chromate, silver glycerolate, colloidal silver iodide, silver lactate, silver manganite, silver nitrate (p.1664), silver-nylon polymers, silver protein (p.1664), and sulfadiazine silver (p.251).

◊ The benefits of silver coated or impregnated catheters in preventing or reducing urinary-tract infection are uncertain, and studies have provided conflicting evidence. Some[1] consider that the benefits are statistically insignificant. However, a meta-analysis[2] involving 8 trials with a total of 2355 patients concluded, despite some concerns about the quality and heterogeneity of the studies, that there was a benefit, but that silver alloy coated catheters were significantly more effective in preventing urinary-tract infections than were those coated with silver oxide.

1. Reiche T, *et al.* A prospective, controlled, randomized study of the effect of a slow-release silver device on the frequency of urinary tract infection in newly catheterized patients. *BJU Int* 2000; **85:** 54–9.
2. Saint S, *et al.* The efficacy of silver alloy-coated urinary catheters in preventing urinary tract infection: a meta-analysis. *Am J Med* 1998; **105:** 236–41.

Preparations

Proprietary Preparations (details are given in Part 3)
Austral.: Micropur†; **Braz.:** Ultradina; **Denm.:** CuNova T; **Fr.:** Micropur†; **Ital.:** Katomed; **UK:** Avance.

Multi-ingredient: Canad.: Nova-T; **Fr.:** Actisorb Plus; Nova-T; **Ger.:** Actisorb 3; Grune Salbe "Schmidt" N†; Nova-T; **Hong Kong:** Nova-T; **Irl.:** Actisorb Plus; **Israel:** Nova-T; **Ital.:** Actisorb Plus; Agipiu; Katoxyn; Nova-T; **Mex.:** Nova-T; **Neth.:** Nova-T; **NZ:** Nova-T; **S.Afr.:** Nova-T; **Singapore:** Nova-T; **Spain:** Argentocromo; **Switz.:** Nova-T; **Thai.:** Nova-T; **UK:** Actisorb Plus; Nova-T.

Silver Acetate   (5319-p)

Argenti Acetas.
$C_2H_3AgO_2 = 166.9.$
CAS — 563-63-3.

Pharmacopoeias. In Aust.

Profile
Silver acetate has been used similarly to silver nitrate as an antiseptic. It has also been used in antismoking preparations.

Smoking cessation. References.
1. Lancaster T, Stead LF. Silver acetate for smoking cessation (update 30 August 2000). Available in The Cochrane Library; Issue 4. Oxford: Update Software; 2001.

Preparations

Proprietary Preparations (details are given in Part 3)
Canad.: Smokerette†.

Silver Nitrate   (5321-h)

Argenti Nitras; Nitrato de Plata; Nitrato de Prata.
$AgNO_3 = 169.9.$
CAS — 7761-88-8.
ATC — D08AL01.

Pharmacopoeias. In Eur. (see p.vi), Int., Jpn, Pol., and US.

Silver nitrate is incompatible with a range of substances. Although it is unlikely that there will be a need to add any of the interacting substances to silver nitrate solutions considering its current uses, pharmacists should be aware of the potential for incompatibility.

Pharmacopoeial description
Ph. Eur.: A white crystalline powder or transparent colourless crystals. Very soluble in water; soluble in alcohol. Store in non-metallic containers. Protect from light.

USP 25: Colourless or white crystals. On exposure to light in the presence of organic matter, it becomes grey or greyish-black. Soluble 1 in 0.4 of water, 1 in 0.1 of boiling water, 1 in 30 of alcohol, and 1 in 6.5 of boiling alcohol; slightly soluble in ether. Its solutions in water have a pH of about 5.5. Store in airtight containers. Protect from light.

Incompatibility. The reported yellow-brown discoloration of samples of silver nitrate bladder irrigation (1 in 10 000) probably arose from the reaction of the silver nitrate with alkali released from the glass bottle which appeared to be soda-glass.[1]

1. *PSGB Lab Report P/80/6* 1980.

Adverse Effects
Symptoms of poisoning stem from the corrosive action of silver nitrate and include pain in the mouth, sialorrhoea, diarrhoea, vomiting, coma, and convulsions.

Short-term mild conjunctivitis is common in infants given silver nitrate eye drops; repeated use or the use of high concentrations produces severe damage and even blindness. Chronic application to the conjunctiva, mucous surfaces, or open wounds leads to argyria (see Silver, above), which though difficult to treat is mainly a cosmetic hazard.

Although silver nitrate is not readily absorbed, absorption of nitrite following reduction of nitrate may cause methaemoglobinaemia. There is also a risk of electrolyte disturbances.

Effects on the eyes. Silver nitrate from a stick containing 75% was applied to the eyes of a newborn infant instead of a 1% solution.[1] After 1 hour there was a thick purulent secretion, the eyelids were red and oedematous, and the conjunctiva markedly injected. The corneas had a blue-grey bedewed appearance with areas of corneal opacification. After treatment by lavage and topical application of antibacterials and homatropine 2% there was a marked improvement and after 1 week topical application of corticosteroids was started. Residual damage was limited to slight corneal opacity.

1. Hornblass A. Silver nitrate ocular damage in newborns. *JAMA* 1975; **231:** 245.

Uses and Administration
Silver nitrate possesses antiseptic properties and is used in many countries as a 1% solution for the prophylaxis of gonococcal ophthalmia neonatorum (see Neonatal Conjunctivitis, p.130). However, as it can cause irritation, other drugs are often used.

In stick form it has been used as a caustic to destroy warts (p.1108) and other small skin growths. Compresses soaked in a 0.5% solution of silver nitrate have been applied to severe burns to reduce infection. Solutions have also been used as topical antiseptics and astringents in other conditions.

Silver nitrate (Argentum Nitricum; Argent. Nit.) is used in homoeopathic medicine. It has also been used in cosmetics to dye eyebrows and eye lashes.

Preparations

BP 2001: Sterile Silver Nitrate Solution;
USP 25: Silver Nitrate Ophthalmic Solution; Toughened Silver Nitrate.

Proprietary Preparations (details are given in Part 3)
Denm.: Helvedstensstifter; **Ger.:** Mova Nitrat; **Spain:** Argenpal.

Multi-ingredient: Austral.: Super Banish; **Hong Kong:** Biscasil; **Spain:** Argentofenol; **Switz.:** Grafco batonnets de bois; **UK:** Avoca.

Silver Protein   (5322-m)

Albumosesilber; Argentoproteinum; Argentum Proteinicum; Protargolum; Proteinato de Plata; Proteinato de Prata; Strong Protargin; Strong Protein Silver; Strong Silver Protein.
CAS — 9007-35-6 (colloidal silver).

NOTE. Synonyms for mild silver protein include: Argentoproteinum Mite; Argentum Vitellinicum; Mild Protargin; Mild Silver Proteinate; Silver Nucleinate; Silver Vitellin; Vitellinato de Plata and Vitelinato de Prata.

Pharmacopoeias. In Aust., Belg., Fr., It., Jpn, and Pol. Many of these pharmacopoeias include monographs on mild silver protein as well as on colloidal silver.

Profile
Silver protein solutions have antibacterial properties, due to the presence of low concentrations of ionised silver, and have been used as eye drops and for application to mucous membranes. The mild form of silver protein is considered to be less irritating, but less active.

Colloidal silver, which is also a preparation of silver in combination with protein, has also been used topically for its antibacterial activity.

Preparations

Proprietary Preparations (details are given in Part 3)
Braz.: Colirio de Argyrol; **Fr.:** Stillargol; Vitargenol†.

Multi-ingredient: Aust.: Coldargan; **Ital.:** Arscolloid; Bio-Arscolloid; Corti-Arscolloid; Rinantipiol; Rinofomentil; Rinovit Nube†; **Port.:** Naso-Calma.

Sincalide   (2148-b)

Sincalide (BAN, USAN, rINN).
CCK-OP;   SQ-19844.   De-1-(5-oxo-L-proline)-de-2-L-glutamine-5-methionine-caerulein.
$C_{49}H_{62}N_{10}O_{16}S_3 = 1143.3.$
CAS — 25126-32-3.
ATC — V04CC03.

Pharmacopoeias. US includes Sincalide for Injection.

Adverse Effects
Sincalide stimulates gallbladder contraction and gastrointestinal muscle and may give rise to abdominal discomfort. Dizziness, nausea, and flushing may also occur.

Uses and Administration
Sincalide is the synthetic C-terminal octapeptide of cholecystokinin (pancreozymin, p.1647) and when administered by intravenous injection it stimulates gallbladder contraction; it also stimulates intestinal muscle.

Sincalide is used for testing gallbladder function and as an adjunct to cholecystography. It is usually given in doses of 20 nanograms per kg body-weight by intravenous injection over 30 to 60 seconds. It is also used as a diagnostic agent, often in conjunction with secretin (p.1661), for testing the functional capacity of the pancreas; this test generally requires duodenal intubation of the patient and examination of duodenal aspirate. A suggested procedure is to give a 1-hour intravenous infusion of secretin, and 30 minutes after starting this infusion, to infuse sincalide 20 nanograms per kg over a 30-minute period.

Preparations

USP 25: Sincalide for Injection.

Proprietary Preparations (details are given in Part 3)
Canad.: Kinevac; **USA:** Kinevac.

Skullcap   (847-z)

Scullcap; Scutellaria.

Pharmacopoeias. Chin. includes Scutellariae Darbatae (Barbated Skullcap Herb; Scutellaria barbata) and Radix Scutellariae (Baical Skullcap Root; S. baicalensis) Jpn includes Scutellaria Root (S. baicalensis).

Profile
Skullcap, the aerial parts of *Scutellaria lateriflora* (Labiatae) and other *Scutellaria* spp., has sedative and antispasmodic properties. It is used as a nerve tonic, and for insomnia and menstrual disorders.

Baical skullcap (*S. baicalensis*) is used in Chinese herbal medicine.

Preparations

Proprietary Preparations (details are given in Part 3)
Multi-ingredient: Austral.: Calmo; Feminine Herbal Complex; Goodnight Formula; Lifesystem Herbal Formula 12 Willowbark†; Naturest; Pacifenity; Passiflora Complex; Passionflower Plus; Relaxaplex; Tranquiplex†; Valerian; Vitaglow Executive Anti Stress†; Vitaglow Herbal Stress†; Willowbark Plus Herbal Formula 11†; **Canad.:** Herbal Nerve; **UK:** Biophylin†; Gerard House Valerian Compound; Herbal Indigestion Naturtabs; HRI Calm Life; Newrelax; Nodoff; Quiet Days; Quiet Tyme; Scullcap & Gentian Tablets; St Johnswort Compound; Super Mega B+C; Vegetable Cough Remover; Wellwoman.

Skunk Cabbage   (3990-d)

Skunkweed.

Profile
Skunk cabbage, the root and rhizome of *Symplocarpus foetidus* (*Dracontium foetidum*) (Araceae), has expectorant properties and is used in respiratory-tract disorders.

Preparations
Proprietary Preparations (details are given in Part 3)
Multi-ingredient: *UK:* Horehound and Aniseed Cough Mixture; Vegetable Cough Remover.

Slippery Elm (5458-t)
Elm Bark; Slippery Elm Bark; Ulmus; Ulmus Fulva.
Pharmacopoeias. In *US.*

Pharmacopoeial description
USP 25: The dried inner bark of *Ulmus rubra* (=*U. fulva*) (Ulmaceae). Store in a dry place at a temperature of 8° to 15°.

Profile
Slippery elm contains a considerable amount of mucilage and has been used as a demulcent.

Preparations
Proprietary Preparations (details are given in Part 3)
Multi-ingredient: *Austral.:* Bioglan Psylli-Mucil Plus; Cal Alkyline; Digestive Aid; Enterocare; Herbal Cleanse; PC Regulax; Travelaide; *Canad.:* Herbal Cough Expectorant; Herbal Throat; *UK:* Biobalm; Fenulin; Modern Herbals Pile; Natraleze; Papaya Plus; Pileabs; Slippery Elm Stomach Tablets.

Soda Lime (212-m)
Cal Sodada; Calcaria absorbens; Calcaria Compositio; Calx Sodica; Chaux Sodée.
CAS — 8006-28-8.
Pharmacopoeias. In *Br.* Also in *USNF.*

Incompatible with trichloroethylene.

Pharmacopoeial description
BP 2001: A mixture of sodium hydroxide, or sodium hydroxide and potassium hydroxide, with calcium hydroxide. White or greyish-white granules, or it may be coloured with an indicator to show when its absorptive capacity is exhausted. It absorbs about 20% of its weight of carbon dioxide. Partially soluble in water; almost completely soluble in 1M acetic acid. A suspension in water is strongly alkaline to litmus.
USNF 20: A mixture of calcium hydroxide and sodium or potassium hydroxide or both. It may contain an indicator that is inert and that changes colour when the soda lime can no longer absorb carbon dioxide. White or greyish-white granules. May have a colour if an indicator is added.

Profile
Soda lime is used to absorb carbon dioxide, for instance in closed-circuit anaesthetic apparatus, and in the determination of the basal metabolic rate. Limits are specified for particle size, and particles should be free from dust.
Soda lime must not be used with trichloroethylene, since this is decomposed by warm alkali to produce a toxic end product that gives rise to lesions of the nervous system.
Soda lime is irritating and corrosive to skin, mucous membranes, and eyes.

Sodium Arsenate (13242-m)
Natrium Arsenicicum; Sodium Arseniate.
$Na_2HAsO_4,7H_2O = 312.0.$
CAS — 7778-43-0 (anhydrous sodium arsenate); 10048-95-0 (sodium arsenate heptahydrate).

Profile
Sodium arsenate was formerly used in the treatment of chronic skin diseases, in parasitic diseases of the blood, and in some forms of anaemia. It has the adverse effects of Arsenic Trioxide, p.1582.

Preparations
Proprietary Preparations (details are given in Part 3)
Multi-ingredient: *Fr.:* Aromabyl†.

Sodium Carbonate Anhydrous (213-b)
Cenizas de Soda; E500; Exsiccated Sodium Carbonate; Natrii Carbonas Anhydricus; Natrium Carbonicum Calcinatum; Natrium Carbonicum Siccatum.
$Na_2CO_3 = 106.0.$
CAS — 497-19-8.
NOTE. Soda ash is a synonym for the technical grade of sodium carbonate anhydrous.
Pharmacopoeias. In *Eur.* (see p.vi), *Jpn,* and *Pol. USNF* allows the anhydrous substance or the monohydrate.

Pharmacopoeial description
Ph. Eur.: A white or almost white, slightly granular, hygroscopic powder. Freely soluble in water; practically insoluble in alcohol. A 10% solution in water is strongly alkaline. Store in airtight containers.
USNF 20: Colourless crystals, or white, crystalline powder or granules. Soluble 1 in 3 of water and 1 in 1.8 of boiling water.

The symbol † denotes a preparation no longer actively marketed

Sodium Carbonate Decahydrate (214-v)
Cristales de Sosa; E500; Natrii Carbonas; Natrii Carbonas Decahydricus; Natrium Carbonicum Crystallisatum.
$Na_2CO_3,10H_2O = 286.1.$
CAS — 6132-02-1.
NOTE. Washing soda is a synonym for the technical grade of sodium carbonate decahydrate.
Pharmacopoeias. In *Eur.* (see p.vi), *Jpn,* and *Pol.*

Pharmacopoeial description
Ph. Eur.: Colourless, efflorescent, transparent crystals or white crystalline powder. Freely soluble in water; practically insoluble in alcohol. A 10% solution in water is strongly alkaline. Store in airtight containers.

Sodium Carbonate Monohydrate (215-g)
E500; Natrii Carbonas Monohydricus.
$Na_2CO_3,H_2O = 124.0.$
CAS — 5968-11-6.
Pharmacopoeias. In *Eur.* (see p.vi). *USNF* allows the anhydrous substance or the monohydrate.

Pharmacopoeial description
Ph. Eur.: A white, crystalline powder or colourless crystals. Freely soluble in water; practically insoluble in alcohol. A 10% solution in water is strongly alkaline. Store in airtight containers.
USNF 20: Colourless crystals, or white, crystalline powder or granules. When exposed to dry air above 50°, it effloresces and at 100° it becomes anhydrous. Soluble 1 in 3 of water and 1 in 1.8 of boiling water.

Profile
Sodium carbonate is used in antacid preparations. Anhydrous sodium carbonate and the monohydrate are also used as reagents. The decahydrate has been used in alkaline baths. Sodium carbonate in its anhydrous or hydrated form is also used as a water softener.
Sodium carbonate may be irritating or mildly corrosive to skin, mucous membranes, and eyes.

Preparations
BPC 1973: Surgical Chlorinated Soda Solution;
USP 25: Citric Acid, Magnesium Oxide, and Sodium Carbonate Irrigation.
Proprietary Preparations (details are given in Part 3)
Multi-ingredient: *Austral.:* Eno; *Braz.:* Albicon; Estomazil; Sal de Fruta Eno; Sonrisal; *Fr.:* Bactident; Hydralin; *Irl.:* Cymalon; *Israel:* Urikal; *Ital.:* Eno†; *Port.:* Eno; Sais de Frutos; Sais Zitos†; *Spain:* Cloritines; Sal de Fruta Eno; Tanasid; *Switz.:* Saltrates Rodell; *UK:* Cymalon; Eno; Resolve.

Sodium Chlorate (321-p)
Natrium Chloricum; Sodii Chloras.
$NaClO_3 = 106.4.$
CAS — 7775-09-9.

Profile
Sodium chlorate closely resembles potassium chlorate (p.1654) in its properties and has been used as an astringent. Its main use is as a weedkiller and it is therefore a common household chemical. Poor storage conditions can lead to explosions.

Preparations
Proprietary Preparations (details are given in Part 3)
Multi-ingredient: *Spain:* Co Bucal.

Sodium Dichloroacetate (13247-p)
Sodium Dichloroacetate (*USAN*).
CPC-211; DCA.
$C_2HCl_2NaO_2 = 150.9.$
CAS — 2156-56-1 (sodium dichloroacetate); 79-43-6 (dichloroacetic acid).

Profile
Dichloroacetic acid activates pyruvate dehydrogenase, a mitochondrial enzyme which catalyses metabolism of pyruvate and lactate, and it inhibits glycolysis. It also stimulates myocardial contractility. Sodium dichloroacetate has been used for the treatment of congenital lactic acidosis, lactic acidosis in patients with severe malaria, homozygous familial hypercholesterolaemia, and for severe brain injury. It is also under investigation for stroke.

Adverse effects. Adverse effects reported to date with sodium dichloroacetate have mainly involved the central and peripheral nervous systems.[1] Anxiolytic or sedative effects are common. Reversible polyneuropathy has been reported after chronic use, as has asymptomatic elevation of serum transaminases. Reduced urate clearance and elevated serum urate levels have been reported in patients with type 2 diabetes mellitus.

1. Stacpoole PW, *et al.* Pharmacokinetics, metabolism, and toxicology of dichloroacetate. *Drug Metab Rev* 1998; **30:** 499–539.

Pharmacokinetics. References.
1. Henderson GN, *et al.* Pharmacokinetics of dichloroacetate in adult patients with lactic acidosis. *J Clin Pharmacol* 1997; **37:** 416–25.
2. Shangraw RE, Fisher DM. Pharmacokinetics and pharmacodynamics of dichloroacetate in patients with cirrhosis. *Clin Pharmacol Ther* 1999 **66:** 380–90.

Use in metabolic acidosis. In a study[1] in 29 patients with lactic acidosis (p.1180), sodium dichloroacetate 50 mg per kg body-weight given by intravenous infusion over 30 minutes, followed by a second dose 2 hours after beginning the first infusion, produced a metabolic response in 23 patients with a short-term increase in survival. However, a subsequent study[2] found that, while dichloroacetate infusion did reduce blood-lactate concentrations, it did not alter haemodynamics or survival in patients with severe lactic acidosis. A review[3] of the treatment of children with dichloroacetate for congenital lactic acidosis hypothesised that it might improve quality of life by reducing the frequency of acid-base decompensations, improving neurological function, and stimulating linear growth, and noted that a controlled clinical trial was underway.

1. Stacpoole PW, *et al.* Dichloroacetate in the treatment of lactic acidosis. *Ann Intern Med* 1988; **108:** 58–63.
2. Stacpoole PW, *et al.* A controlled clinical trial of dichloroacetate for treatment of lactic acidosis in adults. *N Engl J Med* 1992; **327:** 1564–9.
3. Stacpoole PW, *et al.* Treatment of congenital lactic acidosis with dichloroacetate. *Arch Dis Child* 1997; **77:** 535–41.

Sodium Dithionite (13248-s)
Sodium Hydrosulfite; Sodium Hydrosulphite; Sodium Sulphoxylate.
$Na_2S_2O_4 = 174.1.$
CAS — 7775-14-6.
NOTE. The name sodium hydrosulfite is also applied to $NaHSO_2 = 88.06.$
Pharmacopoeias. In *Pol.*

Profile
Sodium dithionite is used as a reducing agent. It may be used in the form of a simple urine test in the detection of paraquat poisoning. A 0.25% solution has been used to remove phenazopyridine stains from fabric. It is irritant to the skin.

Sodium Gluconate (3942-z)
E576. Monosodium D-gluconate.
$C_6H_{11}NaO_7 = 218.1.$
CAS — 527-07-1.
Pharmacopoeias. In *US.*

Profile
Sodium gluconate is a food additive.
Gluconates act as acceptors of hydrogen ions produced by metabolic processes and are an indirect source of bicarbonate ions.

Sodium Hydroxide (216-q)
Ätznatron; Caustic Soda; E524; Hidróxido de Sódio; Natrii Hydroxidum; Natrium Hydricum; Natrium Hydroxydatum; Soda Lye.
$NaOH = 40.00.$
CAS — 1310-73-2.
Pharmacopoeias. In *Chin., Eur.* (see p.vi), *Int., Jpn,* and *Pol.* Also in *USNF.*

Strongly alkaline and corrosive, and rapidly destroys organic tissues.

Pharmacopoeial description
Ph. Eur.: White, crystalline masses supplied as pellets, sticks, or slabs. It is deliquescent and readily absorbs carbon dioxide. Very soluble in water; freely soluble in alcohol. A 0.01% solution in water has a pH of not less than 11.0. Store in airtight, non-metallic containers.
USNF 20: White or practically white fused masses, small pellets, flakes, sticks, or other forms. It is hard and brittle and shows a crystalline fracture. When exposed to air it rapidly absorbs moisture and carbon dioxide. Soluble 1 in 1 of water; freely soluble in alcohol. Store in airtight containers.

Adverse Effects
The ingestion of caustic alkalis causes immediate burning pain in the mouth, throat, substernal region, and epigastrium, and the lining membranes become swollen and detached. There is dysphagia, hypersalivation, vomiting with the vomitus becoming blood-stained, diarrhoea, and shock. In severe cases, asphyxia due to oedema of the glottis, circulatory failure, oesophageal or gastric perforation, peritonitis, or pneumonia may occur. Stricture of the oesophagus can develop weeks or months later.
Caustic alkalis on contact with the eyes cause conjunctival oedema and corneal destruction.

Treatment of Adverse Effects
Ingestion should not be treated by lavage or emesis. Copious drinks of water should be given and followed by milk. The airway should be maintained and shock and pain alleviated.

Contaminated skin and eyes should be flooded immediately with water and the washing continued for about 30 minutes. Any affected clothing should be removed while flooding is being carried out.

Uses and Administration
Sodium hydroxide is a powerful caustic. A 2.5% solution in glycerol has been used as a cuticle solvent. An escharotic preparation of sodium hydroxide and calcium oxide was known as London paste. Sodium hydroxide is also used for adjusting the pH of solutions.

Disinfection. For reference to the possible use of sodium hydroxide for the disinfection of material contaminated by the agent causing Creutzfeldt-Jakob disease, see p.1129.

Preparations
Proprietary Preparations (details are given in Part 3)
Multi-ingredient: *Aust.*: Leberinfusion; Sulfo-Schwefelbad; *Ger.*: Glutarsin E; Infumal; *Switz.*: Saltrates.

Sodium Iodoheparinate (4820-y)
Iodoheparinate Sodium.

Profile
Sodium iodoheparinate is a derivative of heparin (p.902) used topically for the treatment of corneal burns and ulceration.

Preparations
Proprietary Preparations (details are given in Part 3)
Fr.: Dioparine†; *Switz.*: Dioparine.

Sodium Methylarsinate (13253-g)
Natrium Methylarsonicum; Sodium Metharsinite. Disodium monomethylarsonate hexahydrate.
$CH_3AsNa_2O_3,6H_2O = 292.0$.
CAS — 5967-62-4.

Profile
Sodium methylarsinate is an organic arsenic compound with adverse effects similar to those of arsenic trioxide (p.1582). It was formerly included in some vitamin and mineral preparations. It has also been used as a herbicide.

Preparations
Proprietary Preparations (details are given in Part 3)
Multi-ingredient: *Braz.*: Carneferrol; Thiodeol.

Sodium Morrhuate (9845-c)
Sodium Morrhuate (rINN).
Morrhuate Sodium.
CAS — 8031-09-2.
Pharmacopoeias. US includes Morrhuate Sodium Injection.

Profile
Sodium morrhuate consists of the sodium salts of the fatty acids of cod-liver oil. It is a sclerosant that has been used in the treatment of varicose veins (p.1637). Usual doses are 50 to 100 mg for small or medium veins or 150 to 250 mg for large veins given as a 5% solution by intravenous injection.

Preparations
USP 25: Morrhuate Sodium Injection.
Proprietary Preparations (details are given in Part 3)
USA: Scleromate.

Sodium Phenylacetate (16986-r)
Sodium Phenylacetate (USAN).
$C_8H_7NaO_2 = 158.1$.
CAS — 114-70-5.

Profile
Sodium phenylacetate is used for hyperammonaemia in patients with enzymatic deficiencies in the urea cycle (p.1354). Sodium phenylbutyrate (see below) is a prodrug for sodium phenylacetate.

◊ **References.**
1. The Urea Cycle Disorders Conference Group. Consensus statement from a conference for the management of patients with urea cycle disorders. *J Pediatr* 2001; **138** (suppl 1): S1–S5.
2. Summar M. Current strategies for the management of neonatal urea cycle disorders. *J Pediatr* 2001; **138** (suppl 1): S30–S39.
3. Batshaw ML, *et al.* Alternative pathway therapy for urea cycle disorders: twenty years later. *J Pediatr* 2001; **138** (suppl 1): S46–S55.

Preparations
Proprietary Preparations (details are given in Part 3)
Fr.: Ammonaps; *UK*: Ammonaps; *USA*: Buphenyl.
Multi-ingredient: *USA*: Ucephan.

Sodium Phenylbutyrate (17130-b)
Sodium Phenylbutyrate (BAN, USAN).
Sodium 4-Phenylbutyrate.
$C_{10}H_{11}NaO_2 = 186.2$.
CAS — 1716-12-7.
ATC — A16AX03.

Profile
Sodium phenylbutyrate is a prodrug for sodium phenylacetate (see above) and is used in the treatment of hyperammonaemia in patients with urea cycle disorders (p.1354). It is given by mouth in equally divided doses with meals. The total daily dose for patients weighing under 20 kg is 450 to 600 mg per kg body-weight, and for those weighing over 20 kg, 9.9 to 13.0 g per m² body-surface.

Sodium phenylbutyrate is also under investigation for the treatment of some sickle-cell disorders (p.717) and for use as an adjunct in the treatment of patients with primary or recurrent malignant glioma (see under Malignant Neoplasms of the Brain, p.490).

◊ **References.**
1. Batshaw ML, *et al.* Alternative pathway therapy for urea cycle disorders: twenty years later. *J Pediatr* 2001; **138** (suppl 1): S46–S55.

Preparations
Proprietary Preparations (details are given in Part 3)
Fr.: Ammonaps; *UK*: Ammonaps; *USA*: Buphenyl.

Sodium Polymetaphosphate (1640-p)
E450(c) (sodium polyphosphates).
CAS — 50813-16-6.
NOTE. Although Sodium Hexametaphosphate has been used as a synonym for the polymetaphosphate, the latter also exists in much higher degrees of polymerisation.

Profile
Sodium polymetaphosphate has been used as a 5% dusting powder in hyperhidrosis and bromhidrosis, and as a prophylactic against athlete's foot.

Sodium polymetaphosphate combines with calcium and magnesium ions to form complex soluble compounds and is used as a water softener.

Sodium Pyruvate (8584-m)
Sodium α-ketopropionate; sodium 2-oxopropanoate.
$C_3H_4NaO_3 = 111.1$.
CAS — 127-17-3 (pyruvic acid); 113-24-6 (sodium pyruvate).

Profile
Sodium pyruvate has been administered intravenously in the diagnosis of disorders of pyruvate metabolism.

◊ Relative serum concentrations of lactate and pyruvate following a 10-minute intravenous infusion of sodium pyruvate 500 mg per kg body-weight have been used as an aid to the diagnosis of disorders of pyruvate metabolism.[1] Death shortly after pyruvate loading in a 9-year-old child with restrictive cardiomyopathy suggests that the test should not be performed when cardiac function is decreased.[2]
1. Dijkstra U, *et al.* Friedreich's ataxia: intravenous pyruvate load to demonstrate a defect in pyruvate metabolism. *Neurology* 1984; **34**: 1493–7.
2. Matthys D, *et al.* Fatal outcome of pyruvate loading test in child with restrictive cardiomyopathy. *Lancet* 1991; **338**: 1020–1.

Sodium Silicate (13260-v)
Soluble Glass; Water Glass.
CAS — 1344-09-8.

Profile
Concentrated aqueous solutions of sodium silicate are commercially available and have many industrial uses. The solutions vary in composition, viscosity, and density; the greater the ratio of Na_2O to SiO_2 the more tacky and alkaline the solution.

Sodium Succinate (13261-g)
E363 (succinic acid); E363 (succinic acid).
$C_4H_4Na_2O_4,6H_2O = 270.1$.
CAS — 150-90-3 (anhydrous sodium succinate); 6106-21-4 (sodium succinate hexahydrate).

Profile
Sodium succinate is an ingredient of topical preparations tried for the treatment of cataract. It is also used as a food additive.

Preparations
Proprietary Preparations (details are given in Part 3)
Multi-ingredient: *Fr.*: Cristopal; Vitaphakol; *Port.*: Vitaphakol; *Spain*: Vitaphakol; *Switz.*: Vitaphakol†.

Sparteine Sulfate (13264-s)
Sparteine Sulfate (USAN, rINNM).
Spart. Sulph.; Sparteine Sulphate; (−)-Sparteine Sulphate; *l*-Sparteine Sulphate; Sparteinum Sulfuricum; Sulfato de Esparteina. Dodecahydro-7,14-methano-2H,6H-dipyrido[1,2-a:1′,2′-e][1,5]diazocine sulphate pentahydrate.
$C_{15}H_{26}N_2,H_2SO_4,5H_2O = 422.5$.
CAS — 90-39-1 (sparteine); 299-39-8 (anhydrous sparteine sulfate); 6160-12-9 (sparteine sulfate pentahydrate).
Pharmacopoeias. In Fr.

Sparteine sulfate is a salt of the dibasic alkaloid, sparteine, which is obtained from scoparium (p.1661).

Profile
Sparteine sulfate has been reported to lessen the irritability and conductivity of cardiac muscle and has been used in the treatment of cardiac arrhythmias. Small doses stimulate and large doses paralyse the autonomic ganglia. Peripherally, it has a fairly strong curare-like action, arresting respiration by paralysing the phrenic endings.

The metabolic oxidation of sparteine exhibits genetic polymorphism and this property has been exploited in *in-vitro* screening tests to identify other drugs that may be subject to similar genetic variations in their metabolism.

Precautions. Concern has been expressed that sparteine present in a herbal slimming preparation may cause adverse effects in slow metabolisers if excessive doses are ingested; pregnant women may be particularly at risk.[1]
1. Galloway JH, *et al.* Potentially hazardous compound in a herbal slimming remedy. *Lancet* 1992; **340**: 179.

Preparations
Proprietary Preparations (details are given in Part 3)
Multi-ingredient: *Braz.*: Belacodid; Bromosedan.

Spearmint (4712-s)
Mentha Viridis; Menthae Crispae Folium; Mint.

The dried leaves and flowering tops of common spearmint, *Mentha spicata* (= *M. viridis*) or of scotch spearmint (*M. cardiaca*) (Labiatae).

Profile
Spearmint is the source of spearmint oil. It has carminative properties and is used as a flavour.

Preparations
Proprietary Preparations (details are given in Part 3)
Multi-ingredient: *Aust.*: Carminative; Mag Kottas Baby-Tee; Mag Kottas Beruhigungstee; Sidroga Herz-Kreislauf-Tee; Sidroga Magen-Darm-Tee; Sidroga Nerven- und Schlaftee; Sidroga Stoffwechseltee; Teekanne Herz- und Kreislauftee; *Fr.*: Mediflor Tisane Digestive No 3†; Tisanes de l'Abbe Hamon no 17†; *Switz.*: Alpina Gel a la consoude†; Gel a la consoude; Tisane antirhumatismale; Tisane laxative H nouvelle formulation); Tisane pour l'estomac; Tisane pour le coeur et la circulation; Tisane pour le sommeil et les nerfs.

Spearmint Oil (4713-w)
Huile Essentielle de Menthe Crépue; Oleum Menthae Crispae; Oleum Menthae Viridis.
Pharmacopoeias. In Br. and Fr.

It is obtained by distillation from the overground parts of fresh flowering common spearmint (*Mentha spicata*) or scotch spearmint (*Mentha cardiaca* or *Mentha × cardiaca*) (Labiatae).

Pharmacopoeial description
BP 2001: Spearmint oil is obtained by distillation from fresh flowering plants of *Mentha spicata* or *Mentha × cardiaca* (Gray) Bak. A clear colourless, pale yellow or greenish-yellow liquid when freshly distilled, visibly free from water and with the odour of spearmint. It becomes darker and viscous on keeping. It contains not less than 55% w/w of carvone. Soluble in 1 of alcohol (80%) at 20°; the solution may become cloudy when diluted. Store at a temperature not exceeding 25° in well-filled containers. Protect from light.

Profile
Spearmint oil has similar properties to peppermint oil and is used as a carminative and as a flavour.

Allergy. Allergic contact cheilitis in a patient has been attributed to the spearmint oil present in tooth paste.[1]
1. Skrebova N, *et al.* Allergic contact cheilitis from spearmint oil. *Contact Dermatitis* 1998; **39**: 35.

Preparations
Proprietary Preparations (details are given in Part 3)
Multi-ingredient: *Aust.*: Euka; *Ital.*: Dentosan Azione Intensiva; Dentosan Mese; *Switz.*: Alvogyl; *UK*: Eftab; Fre-bre.

Spike Lavender Oil (4660-y)

Huile Essentielle d'Aspic; Ol. Lavand. Spic.; Oleum Lavandulae Spicatae; Spicae Aetheroleum; Spike Oil.

Pharmacopoeias. In Fr.

The volatile oil from *Lavandula latifolia* (= *L. spica*) (Labiatae).

Profile

Spike lavender oil resembles lavender oil (p.1627) in its properties and is mainly used in perfumery. Hypersensitivity reactions may occur.

Preparations

Proprietary Preparations (details are given in Part 3)
Aust.: Tavipec; *Ger.:* Bronchobest; *Thai.:* Tavipec.

Multi-ingredient: *Aust.:* Novipec; Tussamag; *Ger.:* Neo-Lapitrypsin†; *Switz.:* Baume du Chalet.

Spirulina (8599-w)

Profile

Spirulina is a species of blue-green algae that has been promoted as an anorectic, but there is no convincing evidence that it is safe or effective for this indication.

◊ References.
1. Popovich NG. Spirulina. *Am Pharm* 1982; **NS22** (June): 8–10.

Preparations

Proprietary Preparations (details are given in Part 3)
UK: Biolina.

Multi-ingredient: *Austral.:* Cal Alkyline; Rubus Complex; *UK:* Herbal Booster.

Stearic Acid (1324-t)

Acido Esteárico; Acidum Stearicum; Octadecanoic Acid; Stearinsäure.

CAS — 57-11-4 (stearic acid); 57-10-3 (palmitic acid).

NOTE. Stearic acid is sometimes incorrectly called 'stearine' in commerce.

Pharmacopoeias. In Chin., Eur. (see p.vi), Jpn, and Pol. Also in US-NF.

USNF also includes Purified Stearic Acid.

Pharmacopoeial description

Ph. Eur.: Stearic acid is obtained from fat or oils from a vegetable or animal source and is a mixture consisting mainly of stearic acid ($C_{18}H_{36}O_2 = 284.5$) and palmitic acid ($C_{16}H_{32}O_2 = 256.4$). Stearic Acid 50 contains 40 to 60% stearic acid, the sum of the contents of stearic and palmitic acids being a minimum 90%. Stearic Acid 70 contains 60 to 80% stearic acid, the sum of the contents of stearic and palmitic acids being a minimum 90%. Stearic Acid 95 contains a minimum of 90% stearic acid, the sum of the contents of stearic and palmitic acids being a minimum 96%. White, waxy, flaky crystals, white hard masses, or a white or yellowish-white powder. Practically insoluble in water; soluble in alcohol and in petroleum spirit (50° to 70°).

USNF 20: Stearic acid is a mixture of stearic acid and palmitic acid, the content of stearic acid being not less than 40%, and the sum of the two not less than 90%. Congealing point not lower than 54°. Hard, white or faintly yellowish, somewhat glossy and crystalline solid, or white or yellowish-white powder, with a slight odour, suggesting tallow. Practically insoluble in water; soluble 1 in 20 of alcohol, 1 in 2 of chloroform, and 1 in 3 of ether.

Purified stearic acid contains not less than 90% stearic acid and not less than 96% of stearic and palmitic acids. Congealing point 66° to 69°.

Profile

Stearic acid is used as a lubricant in making tablets and capsules. It is also used as an emulsifying and solubilising agent. Various stearates are also used as pharmaceutical aids (see Nonionic Surfactants, p.1344, and Soaps and other Anionic Surfactants, p.1496).

Stone Root (9172-j)

Collinsonia; Hardhack; Heal-all; Knob Root.

Profile

Stone root, the root and rhizome of *Collinsonia canadensis* (Labiatae), has diuretic and litholytic properties and is used in the treatment of renal and urinary calculi. It is also used as an astringent for gastrointestinal disorders.

It is also used in homoeopathic medicine.

Preparations

Proprietary Preparations (details are given in Part 3)
Multi-ingredient: *Austral.:* Hamamelis Complex; *UK:* Piletabs.

Storax (286-r)

Balsamum Styrax Liquidus; Estoraque Líquido; Liquid Storax; Styrax.

Pharmacopoeias. In Chin. and US.

Pharmacopoeial description

USP 25: The balsam obtained from the trunk of *Liquidambar orientalis* (Levant storax) or *L. styraciflua* (American storax) (Hamamelidaceae). It is a semiliquid greyish to greyish-brown, sticky, opaque mass depositing on standing a heavy dark brown layer (Levant storax), or semisolid, sometimes a solid mass, softened by gently heating (American storax). It is transparent in thin layers, has a characteristic odour, and is more dense than water.

Insoluble in water; soluble, usually incompletely, in an equal weight of warm alcohol; soluble in acetone, in carbon disulfide, and in ether, some insoluble residue usually remaining.

Profile

Storax has actions similar to those of Peru balsam (p.1650). Purified storax or prepared storax was formerly applied as an ointment in the treatment of parasitic skin diseases. Storax has a mild antiseptic action and is an ingredient of some preparations for upper respiratory-tract disorders and for application to skin and mucous membranes. Skin sensitisation has been reported.

Preparations

BP 2001: Benzoin Inhalation; Compound Benzoin Tincture;
BPC 1954: Compound Iodoform Paint;
USP 25: Compound Benzoin Tincture.

Proprietary Preparations (details are given in Part 3)
Multi-ingredient: *Ital.:* Lacrime; *UK:* Frador.

Streptodornase (3745-w)

Streptodornase (BAN, rINN).
Streptococcal Deoxyribonuclease.

CAS — 37340-82-2.

An enzyme obtained from cultures of various strains of *Streptococcus haemolyticus.*

Profile

Streptodornase catalyses the depolymerisation of polymerised deoxyribonucleoproteins. It liquefies the viscous nucleoprotein of dead cells; it has no effect on living cells. It is used in combination with streptokinase in the topical treatment of lesions, wounds, and other conditions that require the removal of clots or purulent matter; the combination may also be used to dissolve clots in the bladder or in urinary catheters.

It has also been given by mouth with streptokinase and sometimes with antibacterials, for its supposed benefit in reducing oedema and inflammation associated with trauma and infection.

Preparations

Proprietary Preparations (details are given in Part 3)
Multi-ingredient: *Aust.:* Varidase; *Austral.:* Varidase; *Belg.:* Varidase; *Denm.:* Varidase; *Fin.:* Varidase; *Ger.:* Varidase; *Irl.:* Varidase; *Israel:* Varidase; *Ital.:* Varidase; *Mex.:* Varidasa; *Neth.:* Varidase; *Norw.:* Varidase; *NZ:* Varidase; *Port.:* Varidase; *S.Afr.:* Varidase; *Spain:* Ernodasa; Varibiotic; Varidasa; *Swed.:* Varidase; *UK:* Varidase.

Strontium Chloride (13270-q)

$SrCl_2,6H_2O = 266.6.$
CAS — 10476-85-4 (anhydrous strontium chloride).

Profile

Strontium chloride is used as a 10% toothpaste for the relief of dental hypersensitivity.

Preparations

Proprietary Preparations (details are given in Part 3)
Aust.: Sensodyne med; *Canad.:* Sensodyne; *Switz.:* Sensodent; *USA:* Original Sensodyne; Sensodyne-SC.

Strychnine (542-r)

Estricnina; Strychnina. Strychnidin-10-one.
$C_{21}H_{22}N_2O_2 = 334.4.$
CAS — 57-24-9.

An alkaloid obtained from the seeds of nux vomica (p.1643) and other species of *Strychnos.*

Strychnine Hydrochloride (543-f)

Strych. Hydrochlor.; Strychninae Hydrochloridum.
$C_{21}H_{22}N_2O_2,HCl,2H_2O = 406.9.$
CAS — 1421-86-9 (anhydrous strychnine hydrochloride); 6101-04-8 (strychnine hydrochloride dihydrate).

Strychnine Nitrate (544-d)

Azotato de Estricnina; Nitrato de Estricnina; Strychninae Nitras; Strychninum Nitricum.
$C_{21}H_{22}N_2O_2,HNO_3 = 397.4.$
CAS — 66-32-0.
Pharmacopoeias. In Aust. and Belg.

Strychnine Sulfate (546-h)

Strychninae Sulphas; Strychnine Sulphate; Strychninum Sulfuricum; Sulfato de Estricnina.
$(C_{21}H_{22}N_2O_2)_2,H_2SO_4,5H_2O = 857.0.$
CAS — 60-41-3 (anhydrous strychnine sulfate); 60491-10-3 (strychnine sulfate pentahydrate).
Pharmacopoeias. In Fr.

Adverse Effects

The symptoms of strychnine poisoning are mainly those arising from stimulation of the CNS. Early signs occurring within 15 to 30 minutes of ingestion include tremors, slight twitching, and stiffness of the face and limbs. Painful convulsions develop and may be triggered by minor sensory stimuli; since consciousness is not impaired patients may be extremely distressed. All forms of sensation are heightened. The body becomes arched backwards in hyperextension with the head retracted, arms and legs extended, fists clenched, and the feet turned inward. The jaw is rigidly clamped and contraction of the facial muscles produces a characteristic grinning expression known as 'risus sardonicus'. The convulsions may recur repeatedly and are interspersed with periods of relaxation. If not treated adequately, few patients survive more than 5 episodes of convulsions, death usually occurring due to respiratory arrest. Fatalities have occurred with doses as little as 16 mg.

Secondary effects arising from the severe spasms include lactic acidosis, rhabdomyolysis, renal failure, hyperthermia, hyperkalaemia, and dehydration.

Poisoning. References.
1. O'Callaghan WG, *et al.* Unusual strychnine poisoning and its treatment: report of eight cases. *BMJ* 1982; **285:** 478.
2. Blain PG, *et al.* Strychnine poisoning: abnormal eye movements. *J Toxicol Clin Toxicol* 1982; **19:** 215–17.
3. Boyd RE, *et al.* Strychnine poisoning: recovery from profound lactic acidosis, hyperthermia, and rhabdomyolysis. *Am J Med* 1983; **74:** 507–12.
4. Burn DJ, *et al.* Strychnine poisoning as an unusual cause of convulsions. *Postgrad Med J* 1989; **65:** 563–4.
5. Yamarick W, *et al.* Strychnine poisoning in an adolescent. *J Toxicol Clin Toxicol* 1992; **30:** 141–8.
6. Heiser JM, *et al.* Massive strychnine intoxication: serial blood levels in a fatal case. *J Toxicol Clin Toxicol* 1992; **30:** 269–83.
7. Nishiyama T, Nagase M. Strychnine poisoning: natural course of a nonfatal case. *Am J Emerg Med* 1995; **13:** 172–3.
8. Katz J, *et al.* Strychnine poisoning from a Cambodian traditional remedy. *Am J Emerg Med* 1996; **14:** 475–7.
9. Hernandez AF, *et al.* Acute chemical pancreatitis associated with nonfatal strychnine poisoning. *J Toxicol Clin Toxicol* 1998; **36:** 67–71.

Treatment of Adverse Effects

The main object of therapy in strychnine poisoning is the prompt prevention or control of convulsions and asphyxia. Patients should be given activated charcoal. Convulsions should be controlled or prevented by diazepam. Should diazepam fail then muscle relaxants should be tried together with intubation and assisted respiration. All unnecessary external stimuli should be avoided and if possible the patient should be kept in a quiet darkened room. Patients should be monitored for any secondary effects from the convulsions so that appropriate symptomatic treatment can be given.

Uses and Administration

Strychnine competes with glycine which is an inhibitory neurotransmitter; it thus exerts a central stimulant effect through blocking an inhibitory activity.

Strychnine was formerly used as a bitter and analeptic but is now mainly used under strict control as a rodenticide, or as a mole poison. It has been used in multi-ingredient preparations for the treatment of ophthalmic and urinary-tract disorders. It has also been tried in the treatment of nonketotic hyperglycinaemia.

Nonketotic hyperglycinaemia. Nonketotic hyperglycinaemia is an inborn defect in the enzyme system responsible for the metabolism of glycine. It is characterised by raised concentrations of glycine in plasma, CSF, and urine. Symptoms of glycine accumulation include respiratory distress, muscular hypotonia, seizures, vomiting, and extreme lethargy. Mental retardation and early infant death are common.

Sodium benzoate has been reported to be effective in reducing plasma-glycine concentrations to near normal but is relatively ineffective in reducing CSF levels or in preventing mental retardation.[1] Strychnine, a glycine antagonist, has been of some benefit in counteracting the effects of high concentrations of glycine in the CNS.[2-4] However, some reports suggest that even concomitant treatment with sodium benzoate and strychnine may be ineffective in severe forms[5] and may ultimately have little effect on the course of the disease.[6] The combination of strychnine and ketamine (an *N*-methyl-D-aspartate receptor antagonist) was of some benefit in a newborn infant with severe nonketotic hyperglycinaemia.[7] Addition of low-dose dextromethorphan to treatment with sodium benzoate, arginine, carnitine, diazepam, and phenobarbital in an infant with nonketotic hyperglycinaemia[8] was associated with resolution of nystagmus and improvement in eye contact and interactive behaviour, without altering serum- or CSF-glycine concentrations. Dextromethorphan with sodium benzoate alone may also be helpful, although the combination is not uniformly effective.[9] Treatment with sodium benzoate and dextromethorphan was beneficial in a 6-month-old child with mild atypical nonketotic hyperglycinaemia,[10] although it was later shown that it was sodium benzoate that had the greatest effect on EEG and behavioural changes. A partial response to low-protein diet and sodium benzoate was demonstrated in a patient with late-onset nonketotic hyperglycinaemia; there was a more dramatic response when imipramine was added to therapy.[11]

1. Krieger I, et al. Cerebrospinal fluid glycine in nonketotic hyperglycinemia: effect of treatment with sodium benzoate and a ventricular shunt. Metabolism 1977; 26: 517–24.
2. Ch'ien LT, et al. Glycine encephalopathy. N Engl J Med 1978; 298: 687.
3. Gitzelmann R, et al. Strychnine for the treatment of nonketotic hyperglycinaemia. N Engl J Med 1978; 298: 1424.
4. Arneson D, et al. Strychnine therapy in nonketotic hyperglycinemia. Pediatrics 1979; 63: 369–73.
5. Sankaran K, et al. Glycine encephalopathy in a neonate. Clin Pediatr (Phila) 1982; 21: 636–7.
6. MacDermot KD, et al. Attempts at use of strychnine sulfate in the treatment of nonketotic hyperglycinemia. Pediatrics 1980; 65: 61–4.
7. Tegtmeyer-Metzdorf H, et al. Ketamine and strychnine treatment of an infant with nonketotic hyperglycinaemia. Eur J Pediatr 1995; 154: 649–53.
8. Alemzadeh R, et al. Efficacy of low-dose dextromethorphan in the treatment of nonketotic hyperglycinemia. Pediatrics 1996; 97: 924–6.
9. Hamosh A, et al. Long-term use of high-dose benzoate and dextromethorphan for the treatment of nonketotic hyperglycinemia. J Pediatr 1998; 132: 709–13.
10. Neuberger JM, et al. Effect of sodium benzoate in the treatment of atypical nonketotic hyperglycinaemia. J Inherit Metab Dis 2000; 23: 22–6.
11. Wiltshire EJ, et al. Treatment of late-onset nonketotic hyperglycinaemia: effectiveness of imipramine and benzoate. J Inherit Metab Dis 2000; 23: 15–21.

Preparations

Proprietary Preparations (details are given in Part 3)

Multi-ingredient: *Aust.:* Dysurgal; *Israel:* Tesopalmed Forte cum Yohimbine; *Ital.:* Neuroftal; *Thai.:* Hemo-Cyto-Serum.

Suanzaorentang (985-h)

Ziziphus Soup.

Profile
Suanzaorentang is an ancient Chinese remedy for anxiety and insomnia. It contains five herbs: suanzaoren (*Ziziphus spinosus* of the Rhamnaceae), fuling (*Poria cocos* of the Polyporaceae), gancao (*Glycyrrhiza uralensis* of the Leguminosae), zhimu (*Anemarrhena asphodeloides* of the Liliaceae), and chuanxiong (*Ligusticum chuanxiong* of the Umbelliferae).

Succinimide (13271-p)

Butanimide. Pyrrolidine-2,5-dione.
$C_4H_5NO_2 = 99.09$.
CAS — 123-56-8.
ATC — G04BX10.

Profile
Succinimide has been claimed to inhibit the formation of oxalic acid calculi in the kidney and to reduce hyperoxaluria.

Preparations

Proprietary Preparations (details are given in Part 3)
Spain: Orotric†.

Sucrose Octa-acetate (13273-w)

Sucrose Octaacetate.
$C_{28}H_{38}O_{19} = 678.6$.
CAS — 126-14-7.
Pharmacopoeias. In USNF.

Pharmacopoeial description
USNF 20: A white, practically odourless, hygroscopic powder. M.p. not lower than 78°. Soluble 1 in 1100 of water, 1 in 11 of alcohol, 1 in 0.3 of acetone, 1 in 0.5 of toluene, and 1 in 0.6 of benzene; very soluble in chloroform and in methyl alcohol; soluble in ether. Store in airtight containers.

Profile
Sucrose octa-acetate has been used as an alcohol denaturant. It is also incorporated into preparations intended to deter nail biting.

Preparations

Proprietary Preparations (details are given in Part 3)
Multi-ingredient: *Spain:* Morde X; *USA:* Don't†.

Sulfobromophthalein Sodium (2151-f)

Bromsulfophthalein Sodium; Bromsulphthalein Sodium; BSP; SBP; Sodium Sulfobromophthalein; Sulphobromophthalein Sodium (BANM). Disodium 4,5,6,7-tetrabromophenolphthalein-3′,3″-disulphonate; Disodium 5,5′-(4,5,6,7-tetrabromophthalidylidene)bis(2-hydroxybenzenesulphonate).
$C_{20}H_8Br_4Na_2O_{10}S_2 = 838.0$.
CAS — 297-83-6 (sulfobromophthalein); 71-67-0 (sulfobromophthalein sodium).
Pharmacopoeias. In It. and Jpn.

Profile
In patients with normal hepatic function sulfobromophthalein sodium is rapidly extracted, conjugated, and excreted in bile. It was formerly used intravenously as a diagnostic agent for testing the functional capacity of the liver but may cause severe hypersensitivity reactions.

Sulfuric Acid (1325-x)

Acid. Sulph. Conc.; Acidum Sulfuricum; E513; Oil of Vitriol; Schwefelsäure; Sulphuric Acid.
$H_2SO_4 = 98.08$.
CAS — 7664-93-9.
Pharmacopoeias. In Eur. (see p.vi). Also in USNF.

Concentrated oil of vitriol of commerce, 'COV', contains about 95 to 98% w/w, and brown oil of vitriol, 'BOV', contains 75 to 85% w/w of H_2SO_4. Nordhausen or fuming sulfuric acid, 'Oleum', is sulfuric acid containing SO_3; battery or accumulator acid is sulfuric acid diluted with distilled water to a specific gravity of 1.2 to 1.26.

Pharmacopoeial description
Ph. Eur.: A colourless, very hygroscopic, oily liquid. Miscible with water and with alcohol producing intense heat. Store in airtight containers.
USNF 20: A clear, colourless, oily liquid. Is very caustic and corrosive. Miscible with water and with alcohol with the generation of much heat. Store in airtight containers.

◊ CAUTION. *When sulfuric acid is mixed with other liquids, it should always be added slowly, with constant stirring, to the diluent.*

Dilute Sulfuric Acid (1326-r)

Acid. Sulph. Dil.; Dilute Sulphuric Acid; Verdünnte Schwefelsäure.
Pharmacopoeias. In Aust. (9.1 to 9.4%), Br. (9.5 to 10.5%), and Pol. (15.5 to 16.3%).

Pharmacopoeial description
BP 2001: It contains 9.5 to 10.5% w/w of H_2SO_4 and is prepared by adding 104 g of sulfuric acid to 896 g of water, with constant stirring and cooling.

Adverse Effects and Treatment
As for Hydrochloric Acid, p.1621.

Uses and Administration
Sulfuric acid has various industrial uses. Dilute sulfuric acid has been used as an astringent in diarrhoea and it has occasionally been prescribed in mixtures with vegetable bitters to stimulate appetite.

Preparations

Proprietary Preparations (details are given in Part 3)
Multi-ingredient: *USA:* Debacterol.

Sulphan Blue (2150-r)

Sulphan Blue (BAN).
Blue VRS; Isosulfan Blue (USAN); P-1888; P-4125; Sulfan Blue. Sodium α-(4-diethylaminophenyl)-α-(4-diethyliminiocyclohexa-2,5-dienylidene)toluene-2,5-disulfonate.
$C_{27}H_{31}N_2NaO_6S_2 = 566.7$.
CAS — 68238-36-8 (2,5-disulfonate isomer); 129-17-9 (2,4-disulfonate isomer).

NOTE. Sulphan blue was formerly described in *BPC 1954* as the 2,4-disulfonate isomer and the following synonyms have been applied to this 2,4-isomer: Acid Blue 1; Alphazurine 2G; Colour Index No. 42045; Patent Blue V; Sulphanum Caeruleum. The name Patent Blue V, however, is mainly used for CI No. 42051 (p.1649).

Profile
Intravenous administration of sulphan blue produces staining of the skin and has been used as a direct visual test of the state of the circulation in healthy and damaged tissues, particularly in assessing tissue viability in burns and soft-tissue trauma. It has also been used subcutaneously in lymphangiography to outline the lymph vessels.

Hypersensitivity reactions including anaphylaxis and attacks of asthma have been reported with sulphan blue. It has also been reported to interfere with blood tests for protein and iron.

Preparations

Proprietary Preparations (details are given in Part 3)
USA: Lymphazurin.

Sumatra Benzoin (274-k)

Benjoim; Benzoë; Benzoin; Gum Benjamin; Gum Benzoin.
CAS — 9000-05-9 (.
Pharmacopoeias. In Br. and Jpn.
US allows both Siam benzoin and Sumatra benzoin under the title Benzoin.

Pharmacopoeial description
BP 2001: A balsamic resin obtained from the incised stem of *Styrax benzoin* and of *S. paralleloneurus*. It contains not less than 25% of total balsamic acids, calculated as cinnamic acid and with reference to the dried material, and not more than 20% of alcohol (90%)-insoluble matter.

Hard brittle masses of whitish tears embedded in a greyish-brown to reddish-brown translucent matrix, known in commerce as block benzoin. It also occurs in the form of tears with cream-coloured surfaces and, when broken, exhibiting surfaces having a milky-white colour. It has an agreeable balsamic odour. Store at a temperature not exceeding 25°. Protect from light.

USP 25: A balsamic resin from *Styrax paralleloneurus* or *S. benzoin* (Styracaceae). It yields not less than 75% of alcohol-soluble extractive. It occurs as blocks or lumps of variable size made up of tears, compacted together, with a reddish-brown, reddish-grey, or greyish-brown resinous mass. The tears are externally yellowish or rusty brown, milky white on fresh fracture, hard and brittle at ordinary temperatures but softened by heat. It has an aromatic and balsamic odour. When heated it does not emit a pinaceous odour. When digested with boiling water, the odour suggests cinnamates or storax.

Profile
Sumatra benzoin is an ingredient of inhalations which are used in the treatment of catarrh of the upper respiratory tract. Sumatra benzoin is also used in topical preparations for its antiseptic and protective properties. Skin sensitisation has been reported.

Preparations

BP 2001: Benzoin Inhalation; Compound Benzoin Tincture; **BPC 1954:** Compound Iodoform Paint; **USP 25:** Compound Benzoin Tincture; Podophyllum Resin Topical Solution.

Proprietary Preparations (details are given in Part 3)
Multi-ingredient: *Austral.:* Nappy-Mate; Nyal Cold Sore†; **Belg.:** Borostyrol; **Braz.:** Axol; Inalobel; Micotissim; Micoz; Rinofen; Yatropan; **Canad.:** Chase Coldsorex; Cold Sore Lotion; Lotion pour Feux Sauvages; **Fr.:** Balsofumine; Balsofumine Mentholee; **Ger.:** Nur 1 Tropfen medizinisches Mundwasser; **Ital.:** Citrosil Nubesan; Fomentil; **NZ:** Cold Sore; **Port.:** Kemphor; Vaporil; **Switz.:** Baume; UK: Allens Dry Tickly Cough; Frador; Kilkof; Potters Sugar Free Cough Pastilles; Snowfire; Sunspot; **USA:** Pfeiffer's Cold Sore.

Surgibone (13290-e)

Surgibone (USAN).

Profile
Surgibone is sterile, specially processed mature bovine bone, that has been used for grafting procedures in orthopaedic and reconstructive surgery.

Sutilains (3748-y)

Sutilains (BAN, USAN, rINN).
BAX-1515.
CAS — 12211-28-8.

Profile
Sutilains contains enzymes derived from *Bacillus subtilis*. It has proteolytic actions in most conditions, and has been used for the debridement of wounds, burns, and decubitus ulcers.

Tadalafil (20267-b)

Tadalafil (USAN).
IC-351. (6R,12aR)-2,3,6,7,12,12a-Hexahydro-2-methyl-6-[3,4-(methylenedioxy)phenyl]pyrazino[1′,2′:1,6]pyrido[3,4-b]indole-1,4-dione.
$C_{22}H_{19}N_3O_4 = 389.4$.
CAS — 171596-29-5.

Profile
Tadalafil is a phosphodiesterase type-5 inhibitor given by mouth and is under investigation for the management of erectile dysfunction.

Tannic Acid (322-s)

Acidum Tannicum; Gallotannic Acid; Gerbstoff; Tanin; Tann. Acid; Tannin; Tanninum.
CAS — 1401-55-4.

NOTE. In pharmaceutical literature, the name digallic acid is frequently confused with tannic acid.

Pharmacopoeias. In *Eur.* (see p.vi), *Jpn*, *Pol.*, and *US*.

Commercial grades of tannic acid may contain gallic acid and being less soluble are not suitable for medicinal use.

Pharmacopoeial description

Ph. Eur.: A mixture of esters of glucose with gallic acid and 3-galloylgallic acid. A yellowish-white or slightly brown amorphous light powder or shiny plates. Very soluble in water; freely soluble in alcohol, in acetone, and in glycerol (85%); practically insoluble in dichloromethane. Protect from light.

USP 25: A tannin usually obtained from nutgalls, the excrescences produced on the young twigs of *Quercus infectoria* and allied species of *Quercus*, from the seed pods of tara (*Caesalpinia spinosa*), or from the nutgalls or leaves of sumac (any of a genus *Rhus*).

Amorphous powder, glistening scales, or spongy masses, varying in colour from yellowish-white to light brown. Is odourless or has a faint, characteristic odour. Very soluble in water, in alcohol, and in acetone; freely soluble in diluted alcohol; slightly soluble in dehydrated alcohol; practically insoluble in chloroform, in ether, in petroleum spirit, and in benzene; soluble 1 in about 1 of warm glycerol. Store in airtight containers. Protect from light.

Profile

Tannic acid has been used as an astringent for the mucous membranes of the mouth and throat. Suppositories containing tannic acid have been used in the treatment of haemorrhoids. It is an ingredient in a number of dermatological preparations.

Former uses of tannic acid include application to burns, addition to barium sulfate enemas to improve the quality of radiological pictures of the colon, and as an ingredient of 'Universal Antidote'. However, tannic acid has been associated with liver toxicity, sometimes fatal.

◊ Although tannic acid may be used by plastic surgeons and dermatologists to produce a controlled partial-thickness burn in tattoo removal[1] it has been pointed out that in unskilled or amateur hands this procedure has resulted in full thickness burns requiring skin grafting to obtain satisfactory healing.[2]

1. Mercer NSG, Davies DM. Tattoos. *BMJ* 1991; **303:** 380.
2. Scott M, Ridings P. Tattoos. *BMJ* 1991; **303:** 720.

Preparations

Proprietary Preparations (details are given in Part 3)
Ger.: Tannosynt; *USA:* Zilactin.

Multi-ingredient: *Aust.:* Haemanal; Onycho Phytex; Paradenton; Phytex; Tebege-Tannin; *Austral.:* SM-33; *Belg.:* Aperop; *Braz.:* Anapyon; Boralina; Lacto Vagin; Lacto-Gin; *Canad.:* Bunion Salve†; Outgro†; Tanac; *Fr.:* Allerbiocid S; Eau Precieuse; HEC; Marinol; *Ger.:* Bioget; Tannolil; *Hong Kong:* Cortison-Kemicetine; *Irl.:* Phytex; *Israel:* Rectozorin; *Ital.:* Blefarolin; Neo-Emocicatrol; *S.Afr.:* Burn-A-Sept; *Singapore:* HEC; *Spain:* Antihemorroidal; Depurativo Richelet; Queratil; Sabanotropico; Talkosona†; Talquissar†; Tangenol; *Switz.:* HEC; *UK:* Colsor; Phytex; TCP; *USA:* Dermasept Antifungal; Orasept; Outgro; Tanac; Tanac Dual Core.

Tansy (19673-v)

Profile

Tansy, the flowering tops of *Tanacetum vulgare* (*Chrysanthemum vulgare*) (Compositae), has been used as an anthelmintic and to stimulate menstruation. The oil is highly toxic and use of tansy is generally not recommended.

Preparations

Proprietary Preparations (details are given in Part 3)
Multi-ingredient: *Austral.:* Calmo.

Taraxacum (547-m)

Dandelion Root; Löwenzahnwurzel; Pissenlit; Taraxacum Root.
Pharmacopoeias. In *Aust.* and *Pol.*

Chin. specifies Taraxacum Herb from other species of *Taraxacum*.

The fresh or dried root of the common dandelion, *Taraxacum officinale* (Compositae).

Profile

Taraxacum has been used as a bitter, as a diuretic, and as a mild laxative. It has also been used in homoeopathic medicine.

◊ References.
1. Houghton P. Bearberry, dandelion and celery. *Pharm J* 1995; **255:** 272–3.

Preparations

Proprietary Preparations (details are given in Part 3)
Ger.: Carvicum; Galleb S†; Justogen mono; Kneipp Lowenzahn-Pflanzensaft; Taraleon.

Multi-ingredient: *Aust.:* Agnuchol; Bio-Garten Entschlackungstee; Bio-Garten Tee zur Erhohung der Harnmenge; Bio-Garten

Tropfen fur Galle und Leber; Brennnesseltonikum; Citochol; Digestol; Ehrmann's Entschlackungstee; Entschlackungstee; Felidon neu; Fruhjahrs-Elixier ohne Alkohol; Gallen- und Lebertee; Gallesyn neu; Gallogran; Harntreibender Tee; Kneipp Galle- und Leber-Tee; Kneipp Stoffwechsel-Unterstutzungs-Tee; Krauterdoktor Entschlackungs-Elixier; Krauterdoktor Gallentreibende Tropfen; Krauterdoktor Harnstein- und Nieren-griesstropfen; Krauterhaus Mag Kottas Blutreinigungstee†; Krauterhaus Mag Kottas Entschlackungstee; Krauterhaus Mag Kottas Gallen- und Lebertee; Krautertee Nr 17; Krautertee Nr 20; Krautertee Nr 25; Krautertee Nr 29; Mag Doskar's Leber-Galletonikum; Mag Kottas Entschlackungstee; Mag Kottas Entwasserungstee; Mag Kottas Leber-Gallentee; Magentee EF-EM-ES; Magentropen N Legastol; Montana; Naturland Rheuma-Tee; Sanvita Leber-Galle; Sidroga Leber-Galle-Tee; Sidroga Stoffwechseltee; Solisan; St Radegunder Entschlackungs-Elixier; St Radegunder Leber-Galle-Tee; Teekanne Leber- und Galletee; Urelium Neu; *Austral.:* Berberis Complex; Bioglan Cranbiotic Super; Extralife Fluid-Care; Extralife Liva-Care; Feminine Herbal Complex; Fluid Loss; Glycoplex; Herbal Cleanse; Herbal Diuretic Formula; Lifesystem Herbal Formula 7 Liver Tonic; Liver Tonic Herbal Formula 6; Profluid; Silybum Complex; St Mary's Thistle Plus; Trifolium Complex; Uva-Ursi Complex; Uva-Ursi Plus; *Fr.:* Diacure; Lithiabyl†; Romarene; Romarinex-Choline†; *Ger.:* Agrimonas N; Alasenn; Amara-Tropfen; Aristochol N; Artischocke plus Legastol; Cefachol; Cholosolm Phyto; Cholosom SL; Cholosom-Tee; Gallemolan forte; Gallemolan G; Gallexier; Galloselect M; Hepatofalk Neu; Hevert-Entwasserungs-Tee†; Hevert-Gall S; JuCholan S†; Kneipp Galle-und Leber-Tee N; Legapas comp†; Neurochol C; Nieron S; Nieron-Tee N; Novo Mandrogallan N†; Pascobilin novo; Pascohepan novo; Presselin Hepaticum P; Salus Leber-Galle-Tee Nr.18†; Salus Rheuma-Tee Krautertee Nr 12†; Sirmia Artischockenelixier N; Tonsilgon N; Ullus Galle-Tee N; Uro-Pasc; *Hong Kong:* Hepatofalk; *Ital.:* Depurfast†; *Switz.:* Boldocynara N; Demonatur Gouttes pour le foie et la bile; Gastrosan; Phytomed Hepato; Phytomed Nephro†; Tisane hepatique et biliaire; *UK:* Adios; Aqualette; Backache; Boldex; Boldo; Califig; Cleansing Herb Tablets; Gerard House Buchu Compound; Gerard House Golden Seal Compound; Gerard House Waterlex; HealthAid Boldo-Plus; Herbulax; HRI Water Balance; Natural Herb Tablets; Out-of-Sorts; Rheumatic Pain; Stomach Mixture; Uvacin; Weight Loss Aid; Wind & Dyspepsia Relief.

Targinine (3222-g)

Targinine (BAN, pINN).

BW-546C88; 546C88; N^G-Monomethyl-L-arginine; L-NMMA. N^ω-Methyl-L-arginine.
$C_7H_{16}N_4O_2 = 188.2.$
CAS — 17035-90-4.

Profile

Targinine is a nitric oxide synthase inhibitor under investigation in the treatment of septic shock and migraine.

◊ References.
1. Lassen LH, *et al.* Nitric oxide synthase inhibition in migraine. *Lancet* 1997; **349:** 401–2.
2. Hussein Z, *et al.* Pharmacokinetics of the nitric oxide synthase inhibitor L-N^G-methylarginine hydrochloride in patients with septic shock. *Clin Pharmacol Ther* 1999; **65:** 1–9.

Tartaric Acid (1327-f)

Acidum Tartaricum; E334; E353 (metatartaric acid); Tart. Acid; Tartrique (Acide); Weinsäure. (+)-L-Tartaric acid; (2R,3R)-2,3-Dihydroxybutane-1,4-dioic acid.
$C_4H_6O_6 = 150.1.$
CAS — 87-69-4; 526-83-0.

Pharmacopoeias. In *Eur.* (see p.vi), *Jpn*, and *Pol.* Also in *USNF*.

Pharmacopoeial description

Ph. Eur.: A white or almost white, crystalline powder or colourless crystals. Very soluble in water; freely soluble in alcohol.

USNF 20: Colourless or translucent crystals or a white, fine to granular, crystalline powder. Is odourless. Soluble 1 in 0.8 of water, 1 in 0.5 of boiling water, 1 in 3 of alcohol, 1 in 250 of ether, and 1 in 1.7 of methyl alcohol.

Adverse Effects

Strong solutions of tartaric acid are mildly irritant and if ingested undiluted may cause violent vomiting and diarrhoea, abdominal pain, and thirst. Cardiovascular collapse or acute renal failure may follow.

Pharmacokinetics

Tartaric acid is absorbed from the gastrointestinal tract but up to 80% of an ingested dose is probably destroyed by microorganisms in the lumen of the intestine before absorption occurs. Absorbed tartaric acid is excreted unchanged in the urine.

Uses and Administration

Tartaric acid is used in the preparation of effervescent powders, granules, and tablets, as an ingredient of cooling drinks, and as a saline purgative. If not neutralised, it must be taken well diluted. Tartaric acid or metatartaric acid are used in wine-making as de-acidifying agents to assist in the removal of excess malic acid by forming an insoluble double salt with calcium carbonate.

Preparations

Proprietary Preparations (details are given in Part 3)
Multi-ingredient: *Aust.:* Helo-acid; Lactolavol; *Austral.:* Dexsal; Salvital; Ural; *Belg.:* Zoru; *Canad.:* E-Z-Gas II; Unik-Zoru†; *Fr.:* Dermacide; Zeniac LP Fort; *Ger.:* Bourget†; Retterspitz Ausserlich†; Retterspitz Gelee†; Retterspitz Innerlich†; *Hong Kong:* Floxil; *Israel:* Eno; *Ital.:* Geffer; Magnesia Effervescente Sella; Non Acid†; *NZ:* Solucol; Ural; *Port.:* Sais de Frutos; Sais Zitos†; *S.Afr.:* Adco-Sodasol; Alkafizz; Citro-Soda; Citrovescent†; Quatro-Soda; Uri-Alk; *Spain:* Hectonona; Mucorex Ciclin; Salcedol; Sales de Frutas P G; Sales Fruta Mag Viviar; Sales Orto†; Salmagne; Starlep; *Swed.:* Gastroluft†; *Switz.:* Gastroluft†; Gynasol†; Siesta-1; *UK:* Bioglan Effervescent Granules†; Bioglan Effervescent Tablets†; Jaaps Health Salt; *USA:* Baros.

Taurine (13299-x)

Taurine (rINN).
2-Aminoethanesulphonic acid.
$C_2H_7NO_3S = 125.1.$
CAS — 107-35-7.

Profile

Taurine is an amino acid known to be involved in bile acid conjugation as well as other physiological functions. It has been included in preparations for parenteral nutrition of low-birth-weight infants and in infant formulas but its role as an essential nutrient has not been established.

Taurine is included in some preparations for cardiovascular and metabolic disorders.

Preparations

Proprietary Preparations (details are given in Part 3)
Ital.: O-Due.

Multi-ingredient: *Braz.:* Clarvisol; *Ital.:* Detoxergon†; *Port.:* Detoxergon; *Spain:* Taurobetina.

Terpineol (4715-l)

$C_{10}H_{18}O = 154.2.$
CAS — 8000-41-7 (terpineol); 98-55-5 (α-terpineol).
Pharmacopoeias. In *Br.*

Pharmacopoeial description

BP 2001: A mixture of structural isomers in which α-terpineol predominates. It is a colourless, slightly viscous liquid which may deposit crystals; it has a pleasant characteristic odour. Very slightly soluble in water; freely soluble in alcohol (70%); soluble in ether.

Profile

Terpineol has disinfectant and solvent properties. It is used with other volatile agents in preparations for respiratory-tract disorders.

Preparations

BP 2001: Chloroxylenol Solution.

Proprietary Preparations (details are given in Part 3)
Multi-ingredient: *Aust.:* Resol; Tineafax†; *Austral.:* Karvol; Tixylix Chest Rub; *Belg.:* Balsoclase; *Braz.:* Eucaliptol Composto; Mentolatun; Napiro; Penetro; Tabletes Valda; *Canad.:* Iba-Cide†; *Fr.:* Pectoderme; Valda; *Hong Kong:* Valda; *Irl.:* Karvol; Valda; *Israel:* Gargol; Karvol; Rexitol; *Ital.:* Calyptol; Rikospray; *Mon.:* Calyptol; *Neth.:* Rhinocaps†; *NZ:* Tixylix Chest Rub; *Port.:* Valda; *S.Afr.:* AF; Karvol; *Singapore:* Karvol; *Spain:* Caltoson Balsamico; Calyptol Inhalante; Empapol; Eupnol; Pastillas Juanola; *Swed.:* Munvatten†; *Switz.:* Sedotussin; *UK:* Biocream; Chymol; Karvol; Valda†; Waxwane.

Tetrabenazine (7109-j)

Tetrabenazine (BAN, rINN).
Ro-1-9569. 1,3,4,6,7,11b-Hexahydro-3-isobutyl-9,10-dimethoxybenzo-[a]quinolizin-2-one.
$C_{19}H_{27}NO_3 = 317.4.$
CAS — 58-46-8.
ATC — N05AK01.

Adverse Effects

Drowsiness is the most frequent side-effect of tetrabenazine. Orthostatic hypotension, symptoms of extrapyramidal dysfunction, gastrointestinal disturbances, and depression may also occur. Neuroleptic malignant syndrome and parkinsonism have been reported rarely. Overdosage has produced sedation, sweating, hypotension, and hypothermia.

Extrapyramidal disorders. Dysphagia and choking were associated with tetrabenazine in the treatment of Huntington's chorea.[1] Fatal pneumonia, probably as a consequence of aspiration, had also been reported.

1. Snaith RP, Warren H de B. Treatment of Huntington's chorea with tetrabenazine. *Lancet* 1974; **i:** 413–14.

Overdosage. A patient who swallowed approximately 1 g (40 tablets) of tetrabenazine became drowsy 2 hours later and marked sweating occurred.[1] Her state of consciousness improved after 24 hours and she talked rationally and gained full control of micturition after 72 hours.

1. Kidd DW, McLellan DL. Self-poisoning with tetrabenazine. *Br J Clin Pract* 1972; **26:** 179–80.

The symbol † denotes a preparation no longer actively marketed

Precautions

Tetrabenazine may exacerbate the symptoms of parkinsonism. It may cause drowsiness; affected patients should not drive or operate machinery.

Interactions

Tetrabenazine has been reported to block the action of reserpine. It may also diminish the effects of levodopa and exacerbate the symptoms of parkinsonism. Use of tetrabenazine immediately following a course of an MAOI may lead to a state of confusion, restlessness, and disorientation; tetrabenazine should not be given with, or within 14 days of discontinuation of, such therapy.

Pharmacokinetics

Absorption of tetrabenazine is poor and erratic following oral administration. It appears to be extensively metabolised by first-pass metabolism. Its major metabolite, hydroxytetrabenazine, which is formed by reduction, is reported to be as active as the parent compound. It is excreted in the urine mainly in the form of metabolites.

Uses and Administration

Tetrabenazine is used in the management of movement disorders including chorea (p.650), ballism (p.650), dystonias (p.1173), tardive dyskinesia (p.662), and similar symptoms of CNS dysfunction.

For the treatment of chorea, ballism, and other organic CNS movement disorders, a starting dose of 25 mg three times daily by mouth has been recommended, although a dose of 12.5 mg twice daily may be more appropriate initially as it is less likely to cause excessive sedation. The dose may be gradually increased according to response up to a maximum of 200 mg daily. If the patient does not respond within 7 days of receiving the maximum dose further treatment with tetrabenazine is unlikely to be of benefit. An initial starting dose of 12.5 mg daily has been suggested for elderly patients.

For moderate to severe tardive dyskinesia, a dose of 12.5 mg daily is recommended initially, subsequently titrated according to response.

Extrapyramidal disorders. In a long-term study[1] of the use of tetrabenazine in 400 patients with various movement disorders, those disorders which appeared to respond best to tetrabenazine included tardive dyskinesia, tardive dystonia, and Huntington's disease but benefit was also obtained in some patients with idiopathic dystonia, segmental myoclonus, and Tourette's syndrome. Others have commented that in severe dystonia unresponsive to other drugs a combination of tetrabenazine with benzhexol [trihexyphenidyl] and pimozide is sometimes effective.[2]

1. Jankovic J, Beach J. Long-term effects of tetrabenazine in hyperkinetic movement disorders. *Neurology* 1997; **48:** 358–62.
2. Marsden CD, Quinn NP. The dystonias. *BMJ* 1990; **300:** 139–44.

Preparations

Proprietary Preparations (details are given in Part 3)

Austral.: Nitoman†; **Canad.:** Nitoman; **Denm.:** Nitoman; **UK:** Xenazine.

Tetrachlorodecaoxide (1145-c)

Oxoferin; TCDO; Tetrachlorodecaoxygen Anion Complex.

$Cl_4O_{10} = 301.8$.

CAS — 92047-76-2.

Profile

Tetrachlorodecaoxide is a water-soluble anion complex containing oxygen in a chlorite matrix. Active oxygen is only released in the presence of biological material. It has been applied as a solution for the stimulation of wound healing.

Wounds. Tetrachlorodecaoxide was reported to promote wound healing compared with saline in a double-blind study of 271 patients,[1] but a smaller study failed to show any benefit over glycerol.[2]

1. Hinz J, *et al.* Rationale for and results from a randomised, double-blind trial of tetrachlorodecaoxygen anion complex in wound healing. *Lancet* 1986; **i:** 825–8.
2. Hughes LE, *et al.* Failure of tetrachlorodecaoxygen anion complex to assist wound healing. *Lancet* 1989; **ii:** 1271.

Preparations

Proprietary Preparations (details are given in Part 3)

Aust.: Oxilium; **Switz.:** Oxilium; **Thai.:** Immunokine; Oxoferin.

Tetramethylammonium Iodide (13313-h)

$C_4H_{12}IN = 201.0$.

CAS — 75-58-1.

Profile

Tetramethylammonium iodide is a quaternary ammonium compound that has been used for the emergency disinfection of drinking water. It has also been employed for its ganglion-blocking properties.

Thalidomide (13316-v)

Thalidomide (BAN, USAN, rINN).

K-17; NSC-66847. 2-Phthalimidoglutarimide.

$C_{13}H_{10}N_2O_4 = 258.2$.

CAS — 50-35-1.

ATC — L04AX02.

Pharmacopoeias. In US.

Pharmacopoeial description

USP 25: A white to off-white powder. Sparingly soluble in water, in dehydrated alcohol, in acetone, in butyl acetate, in ethyl acetate, in glacial acetic acid, and in methyl alcohol; practically insoluble in chloroform, in ether, and in benzene; very soluble in dimethylformamide, in dioxan, and in pyridine.

Adverse Effects and Precautions

Thalidomide was withdrawn from use as a hypnotic in the early 1960s after it was discovered that it produced teratogenic effects when administered to women in early pregnancy. These effects involved mainly malformations of the limbs and defects of the ears, eyes, and internal organs, and could develop following a single dose. Further abnormalities and problems, including effects on the CNS, developed in later life.

In consequence, thalidomide should not be used in women of child-bearing potential, or if such use is absolutely essential then stringent contraceptive measures, including the simultaneous use of 2 reliable forms, and regular pregnancy testing are mandatory. If pregnancy occurs during thalidomide therapy the drug must be discontinued immediately and the patient given appropriate evaluation and counselling. Although it is unclear if thalidomide is present in semen, male patients receiving thalidomide should use barrier methods of contraception if their partner is of child-bearing potential. Patients should not donate blood or sperm during thalidomide therapy.

The other major adverse effect of thalidomide is peripheral neuropathy, which can be severe and irreversible. Concomitant administration of other drugs that have the potential to produce peripheral neuropathy should therefore be undertaken cautiously.

Other common adverse effects include constipation, dizziness, and orthostatic hypotension. Drowsiness or somnolence occur frequently and, if affected, patients should not drive or operate machinery. An erythematous macular rash may develop, usually 2 to 10 days after initiation of therapy. Stevens-Johnson syndrome has also been reported, and therefore thalidomide should be discontinued if any skin rash develops and only reinstated after appropriate clinical evaluation. Thalidomide therapy should not be resumed if the rash is exfoliative, purpuric, or bullous, or if Stevens-Johnson syndrome or toxic epidermal necrolysis is suspected. Bradycardia, neutropenia, and an increase in the viral load in HIV-infected patients have also been reported. Hypersensitivity reactions have occurred.

◊ **Reviews.**
1. Günzler V. Thalidomide in human immunodeficiency virus (HIV) patients: a review of safety considerations. *Drug Safety* 1992; **7:** 116–34.
2. Clark TE, *et al.* Thalomid® (thalidomide) capsules: a review of the first 18 months of spontaneous postmarketing adverse event surveillance, including off-label prescribing. *Drug Safety* 2001; **24:** 87–117.

Effects on the skin. Toxic epidermal necrolysis has been reported[1] in a 62-year-old woman approximately 5 weeks after starting thalidomide therapy for the treatment of a glioblastoma. Although the patient was taking several other drugs, including dexamethasone, thalidomide was considered responsible since its administration had the closest temporal relationship to the adverse effect. Toxic epidermal necrolysis has also been reported[2] in a 64-year-old patient 24 days after initiation of thalidomide and dexamethasone therapy for myeloma. The authors in this case postulated that there may be an adverse interaction between thalidomide and dexamethasone.

Thalidomide had previously been investigated in a randomised placebo-controlled trial[3] for the treatment of toxic epidermal necrolysis, but the trial was prematurely terminated because of significantly higher mortality in the thalidomide group; the causes of death were those usually attributed to the disease itself. Thalidomide had been chosen as an investigative drug because it is a potent inhibitor of tumour necrosis factor (TNF)-α, which has been implicated in the pathogenesis of this condition. However, the authors noted that there was a tendency for plasma concentrations of TNF-α to increase after treatment with thalidomide compared with the placebo group, and postulated that thalidomide might paradoxically enhance TNF-α production in these patients.

1. Horowitz SB, Stirling AL. Thalidomide-induced toxic epidermal necrolysis. *Pharmacotherapy* 1999; **19:** 1177–80.
2. Rajkumar SV, *et al.* Life-threatening toxic epidermal necrolysis with thalidomide therapy for myeloma. *N Engl J Med* 2000; **343:** 972–3.
3. Wolkenstein P, *et al.* Randomised comparison of thalidomide versus placebo in toxic epidermal necrolysis. *Lancet* 1998; **352:** 1586–9.

Migraine. Migraine attacks were associated with thalidomide administration in a 36-year-old man.[1]

1. García-Albea E, *et al.* Jaqueca típica y talidomida. *Med Clin (Barc)* 1993; **100:** 557.

Mutagenicity. Reports of the birth of 3 malformed infants to parents who had themselves been exposed to thalidomide *in*

utero[1,2] have provoked fears that thalidomide may be a mutagen. However, the limb malformations seen in the infants are not typical of mutagenesis[3] and the teratogenic effect of thalidomide is likely to be associated with interference with angiogenesis in the fetus rather than mutation.[4]

1. McBride WG. Thalidomide may be a mutagen. *BMJ* 1994; **308:** 1635–6.
2. Tenconi R, *et al.* Amniotic band sequence in child of thalidomide victim. *BMJ* 1994; **309:** 1442.
3. Read AP. Thalidomide may be a mutagen. *BMJ* 1994; **308:** 1636.
4. D'Amato RJ, *et al.* Thalidomide is an inhibitor of angiogenesis. *Proc Natl Acad Sci U S A* 1994; **91:** 4082–5.

Interactions

The sedative activity of barbiturates, alcohol, chlorpromazine, and reserpine has been reported to be enhanced by thalidomide.

Corticosteroids. For reference to a possible interaction between thalidomide and *dexamethasone*, see under Effects on the Skin in Adverse Effects, above.

Hormonal contraceptives. Thalidomide does *not* alter the metabolism of ethinylestradiol and norethisterone,[1,2] and so the efficacy of oral contraceptives should not be affected by concomitant thalidomide therapy. Nevertheless, 2 reliable forms of contraception should always be used simultaneously when taking thalidomide (see under Adverse Effects and Precautions, above), bearing in mind that the reliability of hormonal contraceptives may be compromised by the concomitant administration of drugs other than thalidomide (see p.1458).

1. Trapnell CB, *et al.* Thalidomide does not alter the pharmacokinetics of ethinyl estradiol and norethindrone. *Clin Pharmacol Ther* 1998; **64:** 597–602.
2. Scheffler MR, *et al.* Thalidomide does not alter estrogen-progesterone hormone single-dose pharmacokinetics. *Clin Pharmacol Ther* 1999; **65:** 483–90.

Pharmacokinetics

◊ **References.**
1. Chen T-L, *et al.* Plasma pharmacokinetics and urinary excretion of thalidomide after oral dosing in healthy male volunteers. *Drug Metab Dispos* 1989; **17:** 402–5.
2. Piscitelli SC, *et al.* Single-dose pharmacokinetics of thalidomide in human immunodeficiency virus-infected patients. *Antimicrob Agents Chemother* 1997; **41:** 2797–9.
3. Teo SK, *et al.* Single-dose oral pharmacokinetics of three formulations of thalidomide in healthy male volunteers. *J Clin Pharmacol* 1999; **39:** 1162–8.
4. Figg WD, *et al.* Pharmacokinetics of thalidomide in an elderly prostate cancer population. *J Pharm Sci* 1999; **88:** 121–5.

Uses and Administration

Thalidomide has immunomodulating activity. It should always be administered under appropriately supervised and controlled conditions because of the teratogenic risks and other potential adverse effects (see under Adverse Effects and Precautions, above).

Thalidomide is used for the treatment of acute cutaneous manifestations of moderate to severe type 2 (erythema nodosum leprosum) lepra reactions (see Leprosy, p.126), but should not be given as monotherapy if moderate to severe neuritis is present. It may also be used for maintenance therapy for prevention and suppression of the cutaneous manifestations of recurrent type 2 lepra reactions. Thalidomide is of no value in type 1 lepra reactions. It is given by mouth in usual doses of 100 to 300 mg once daily, preferably at bedtime. In severe cases up to 400 mg daily may be given. The dose should be reduced gradually by 50 mg every 2 to 4 weeks once a satisfactory response has been achieved.

Thalidomide has been used in several other conditions whose aetiology may involve the immune system, such as treatment and prevention of graft-versus-host disease, treatment and prevention of recurrent aphthous stomatitis in severely and terminally immunocompromised patients, treatment of the clinical manifestations of both tuberculous and non-tuberculous mycobacterial infection, and treatment of HIV-associated wasting syndrome, Kaposi's sarcoma, and Crohn's disease. It has also been used in the treatment of primary brain malignancies. Thalidomide is also being investigated in some other malignancies.

◊ **Guidelines on the clinical use of thalidomide.**
1. Powell RJ, Gardner-Medwin JMM. Guideline for the clinical use and dispensing of thalidomide. *Postgrad Med J* 1994; **70:** 901–4.
2. Lary JM, *et al.* The return of thalidomide: can birth defects be prevented? *Drug Safety* 1999; **21:** 161–9.

Action. The mechanism of action of thalidomide is not completely understood, although investigations have shown that it has various anti-inflammatory and immunomodulating effects, including inhibition of the synthesis of tumour necrosis factor (TNF)-α. However, this inhibition is incomplete and selective, and increased plasma-TNF-α concentrations have been observed in some patient groups. Other immunomodulatory and anti-inflammatory properties include inhibition of leucocyte chemotaxis into the site of inflammation and reduction of phagocytosis by polymorphonuclear leucocytes. Thalidomide also appears to modulate interleukins, although results of investigations into its effect on specific interleukins and interferon gamma have so far been equivocal. Effects on CD4+ cells and variable effects on other mediators of intercellular reactions have also been implicated. Thalidomide also inhibits angiogenesis, which may have implications in solid tumours and other diseases.

References.
1. Schuler U, Ehninger G. Thalidomide: rationale for renewed use in immunological disorders. *Drug Safety* 1995; **12**: 364–9.
2. Calabrese L, Fleischer AB. Thalidomide: current and potential clinical applications. *Am J Med* 2000; **108**: 487–95.
3. Peuckmann V, *et al.* Potential novel uses of thalidomide: focus on palliative care. *Drugs* 2000; **60**: 273–92.

Behçet's syndrome. Thalidomide was effective for the treatment of oral and genital ulceration and follicular lesions in a randomised, double-blind, placebo-controlled trial[1] in 96 male patients with Behçet's syndrome (p.1047). It was also noted that the development of new oral and genital ulcers was prevented. Thalidomide has also been reported[2,3] to be of benefit for severe oral and genital ulceration in children with Behçet's syndrome unresponsive to other treatments.

1. Hamuryudan V, *et al.* Thalidomide in the treatment of the mucocutaneous lesions of the Behçet syndrome: a randomized, double-blind, placebo-controlled trial. *Ann Intern Med* 1998; **128**: 443–50.
2. Shek LP-C, *et al.* Thalidomide responsiveness in an infant with Behçet's syndrome. *Pediatrics* 1999; **103**: 1295–7.
3. Kari JA, *et al.* Thalidomide use in childhood Behçet's syndrome. *Arch Dis Child* 2000; **82** (suppl 1): A46.

Graft-versus-host disease. Beneficial responses to thalidomide have been reported[1-6] in graft-versus-host disease (p.502) in bone marrow transplant recipients, including children.

1. Lim SH, *et al.* Successful treatment with thalidomide of acute graft-versus-host disease after bone-marrow transplantation. *Lancet* 1988; **i**: 117.
2. McCarthy DM, *et al.* Thalidomide for graft-versus-host disease. *Lancet* 1988; **i**: 1135.
3. Heney D, *et al.* Thalidomide for chronic graft-versus-host disease in children. *Lancet* 1988; **ii**: 1317.
4. Vogelsang GB, *et al.* Thalidomide for the treatment of chronic graft-versus-host disease. *N Engl J Med* 1992; **326**: 1055–8.
5. Cole CH, *et al.* Thalidomide in the management of chronic graft-versus-host disease in children following bone marrow transplantation. *Bone Marrow Transplant* 1994; **14**: 937–42.
6. Mehta P, *et al.* Thalidomide in children undergoing bone marrow transplantation: series at a single institution and review of the literature. Abstract: *Pediatrics* 1999; **103**: 806. Full version: http://www.pediatrics.org/cgi/content/full/103/4/e44

HIV-associated complications. It has been proposed that thalidomide's inhibitory activity against tumour necrosis factor (TNF)-α may explain its anti-HIV effect. However, there are conflicting reports as both decreased and increased TNF-α levels, as well as unchanged levels, have been observed in HIV-patients. Nevertheless, thalidomide has shown some promise as a therapeutic agent for some AIDS-related diseases. It is an effective treatment for severe ulceration of the mouth (p.1206), oropharynx, and oesophagus in patients with HIV-infection.[2-4] It has also proved to be of benefit in HIV-associated wasting[5] (p.610), and has shown promise in high doses for the treatment of Kaposi's sarcoma[6] (p.501). However, of concern is the finding that modest increases in plasma HIV RNA levels have been observed in some patients, which correlated with increases in TNF-α levels.[2,4]

1. Ravot E, *et al.* New uses for old drugs in HIV infection: the role of hydroxyurea, cyclosporin and thalidomide. *Drugs* 1999; **58**: 953–63.
2. Jacobson JM, *et al.* Thalidomide for the treatment of oral aphthous ulcers in patients with human immunodeficiency virus infection. *N Engl J Med* 1997; **336**: 1487–93.
3. Ramirez-Amador VA, *et al.* Thalidomide as therapy for human immunodeficiency virus-related oral ulcers: a double-blind placebo-controlled clinical trial. *Clin Infect Dis* 1999; **28**: 892–4.
4. Jacobson JM, *et al.* Thalidomide for the treatment of esophageal aphthous ulcers in patients with human immunodeficiency virus infection. *J Infect Dis* 1999; **180**: 61–7.
5. Reyes-Terán G, *et al.* Effects of thalidomide on HIV-associated wasting syndrome: a randomized, double-blind, placebo-controlled trial. *AIDS* 1996; **10**: 1501–7.
6. Little RF, *et al.* Activity of thalidomide in AIDS-related Kaposi's sarcoma. *J Clin Oncol* 2000; **18**: 2593–2602.

Inflammatory bowel disease. Preliminary data from 2 open-label trials demonstrated efficacy of thalidomide in patients with refractory Crohn's disease (see under Inflammatory Bowel Disease, p.1205).[1,2] In those patients already receiving corticosteroids the dosage could be reduced in most and in some corticosteroids could be withdrawn completely.

1. Ehrenpreis ED, *et al.* Thalidomide therapy for patients with refractory Crohn's disease: an open-label trial. *Gastroenterology* 1999; **117**: 1271–7.
2. Vasiliauskas EA, *et al.* An open-label pilot study of low-dose thalidomide in chronically active, steroid-dependent Crohn's disease. *Gastroenterology* 1999; **117**: 1278–87.

Kaposi's sarcoma. See under HIV-associated complications, above.

Lupus erythematosus. Thalidomide has been found to be of benefit in lupus erythematosus, including chronic discoid lupus erythematosus,[1] lupus erythematosus profundus,[2] systemic lupus erythematosus[3] (p.1059), and cutaneous lupus erythematosus.[4-6]

1. Knop J, *et al.* Thalidomide in the treatment of sixty cases of chronic discoid lupus erythematosus. *Br J Dermatol* 1983; **108**: 461–6.
2. Burrows NP, *et al.* Lupus erythematosus profundus with partial C4 deficiency responding to thalidomide. *Br J Dermatol* 1991; **125**: 62–7.
3. Bessis D, *et al.* Thalidomide for systemic lupus erythematosus. *Lancet* 1992; **339**: 549–50.
4. Atra E, Sato EI. Treatment of the cutaneous lesions of systemic lupus erythematosus with thalidomide. *Clin Exp Rheumatol* 1993; **11**: 487–93.

5. Stevens RJ, *et al.* Thalidomide in the treatment of the cutaneous manifestations of lupus erythematosus: experience in sixteen consecutive patients. *Br J Rheumatol* 1997; **36**: 353–9.
6. Duong DJ, *et al.* American experience with low-dose thalidomide therapy for severe cutaneous lupus erythematosus. *Arch Dermatol* 1999; **135**: 1079–87.

Malignant neoplasms. Thalidomide has been investigated in patients with recurrent high-grade gliomas[1] (p.490) and in patients with relapsed advanced myeloma[2,3] (p.489) with encouraging results.

1. Fine HA, *et al.* Phase II trial of the antiangiogenic agent thalidomide in patients with recurrent high-grade gliomas. *J Clin Oncol* 2000; **18**: 708–15.
2. Singhal S, *et al.* Antitumor activity of thalidomide in refractory multiple myeloma. *N Engl J Med* 1999; **341**: 1565–71.
3. Rajkumar SV, *et al.* Thalidomide in the treatment of relapsed multiple myeloma. *Mayo Clin Proc* 2000; **75**: 897–901.

Mouth ulceration. See under Behçet's syndrome and under HIV-associated complications, above.

Oesophageal ulceration. Thalidomide has been shown to be of benefit in the treatment of idiopathic oesophageal ulcers in patients with AIDS (see under HIV-associated complications, above). Thalidomide has also been reported[1] to have healed an oesophageal ulcer refractory to other treatments in an immunocompetent patient.

1. Ollivier S, *et al.* Idiopathic giant oesophageal ulcer in an immunocompetent patient: the efficacy of thalidomide treatment. *Gut* 1999; **45**: 463–4.

Rheumatic disorders. Beneficial responses to thalidomide have been reported in the treatment of refractory rheumatoid arthritis[1] and adult-onset Still's disease.[2]

1. Gutiérrez-Rodríguez O, *et al.* Treatment of refractory rheumatoid arthritis—the thalidomide experience. *J Rheumatol* 1989; **16**: 158–63.
2. Stambe C, Wicks IP. TNFα and response of treatment-resistant adult-onset Still's disease to thalidomide. *Lancet* 1998; **352**: 544–5.

Sarcoidosis. Beneficial responses to thalidomide have been reported[1] in the treatment of sarcoidosis.

1. Carlesimo M, *et al.* Treatment of cutaneous and pulmonary sarcoidosis with thalidomide. *J Am Acad Dermatol* 1995; **32**: 866–9.

Skin disorders. Beneficial responses to thalidomide have been reported in a variety of dermatological disorders, including erythema multiforme[1,2] (p.1105), pruritus associated with uraemia,[3] Langerhans cell histiocytosis,[4] epidermolysis bullosa,[5] prurigo nodularis,[6] and pyoderma gangrenosum[7] (p.1107).

1. Bahmer FA, *et al.* Thalidomide treatment of recurrent erythema multiforme. *Acta Derm Venereol (Stockh)* 1982; **62**: 449–50.
2. Moisson YF, *et al.* Thalidomide for recurrent erythema multiforme. *Br J Dermatol* 1992; **126**: 92–3.
3. Silva SRB, *et al.* Thalidomide for the treatment of uremic pruritus: a crossover randomized double-blind trial. *Nephron* 1994; **67**: 270–3.
4. Meunier L, *et al.* Adult cutaneous Langerhans cell histiocytosis: remission with thalidomide treatment. *Br J Dermatol* 1995; **132**: 168.
5. Goulden V, *et al.* Linear prurigo simulating dermatitis artefacta in dominant dystrophic epidermolysis bullosa. *Br J Dermatol* 1993; **129**: 443–6.
6. Ferrándiz C, *et al.* Sequential combined therapy with thalidomide and narrow-band (TL01) UVB in the treatment of prurigo nodularis. *Dermatology* 1997; **195**: 359–61.
7. Federman GL, Federman DG. Recalcitrant pyoderma gangrenosum treated with thalidomide. *Mayo Clin Proc* 2000; **75**: 842–4.

Preparations

USP 25: Thalidomide Capsules.

Proprietary Preparations (details are given in Part 3)
USA: Thalomid.

Thallium Acetate (15328-h)

Thallous Acetate.
$C_2H_3O_2Tl = 263.4$.
CAS — 563-68-8.

Adverse Effects

Thallium salts are toxic when inhaled, ingested, or absorbed through the skin. Symptoms of poisoning may appear within 12 to 24 hours of a single toxic dose and include severe abdominal pain, nausea and vomiting, diarrhoea, gastrointestinal haemorrhage, salivation, metallic taste, paralytic ileus, pancreatic damage, and in severe cases cardiovascular collapse, tremors, delirium, convulsions, paralysis, and coma, leading to death in 1 to 2 days. However, the acute reaction may subside, to be followed within about 10 days by the development of neurological effects including paraesthesia, myalgia, myopathy, motor neuropathy, and visual disturbances due to optic neuropathy, psychosis, delirium, convulsions, and other signs of encephalopathy, tachycardia, hypertension, skin eruptions, and hepatorenal injury. Recovery from neurological damage is slow and may be incomplete. Alopecia occurs within 15 to 20 days; stomatitis and a bluish line in the gums may also develop. Death may result from respiratory failure; patients are also predisposed for several weeks to cardiac arrhythmias and sudden death. Fatalities have occurred after ingestion of 1 g or less in adults, although the UK Poisons Information Service consider the usual lethal dose by ingestion to be in the range 3 to 10 g in adults.

Smaller repeated doses are also toxic, with symptoms appearing over several weeks. Constipation is a common feature of less severe poisoning.

Poisoning. References.

1. Moeschlin S. Thallium poisoning. *Clin Toxicol* 1980; **17**: 133–46.
2. Heyl T, Barlow RJ. Thallium poisoning: a dermatological perspective. *Br J Dermatol* 1989; **121**: 787–92.
3. Luckit J, *et al.* Thrombocytopenia associated with thallium poisoning. *Hum Exp Toxicol* 1990; **9**: 47–8.
4. Moore D, *et al.* Thallium poisoning. *BMJ* 1993; **306**: 1527–8.
5. Tabandeh H, Thompson GM. Visual function in thallium toxicity. *BMJ* 1993; **307**: 324.
6. Questel F, *et al.* Thallium-contaminated heroin. *Ann Intern Med* 1996; **124**: 616.
7. Tromme I, *et al.* Skin signs in the diagnosis of thallium poisoning. *Br J Dermatol* 1998; **138**: 321–5.

Treatment of Adverse Effects

After the acute ingestion of thallium, gastric lavage should be considered within 1 hour of ingestion; a saline purgative such as magnesium sulfate may be given. Intensive supportive therapy is necessary.

Various methods have been employed in an attempt to increase the faecal and urinary excretion of thallium. A suspension of activated charcoal has been given to reduce intestinal absorption and enteric recycling, but is less successful than Prussian blue (p.1021) administered by mouth or duodenal tube. The administration of potassium chloride by mouth may mobilise thallium from the tissues but is hazardous, especially if given during the early stage; signs of poisoning may be transiently aggravated.

Haemoperfusion or haemodialysis combined with forced diuresis are reported to be effective in eliminating absorbed thallium if given within 48 hours of ingestion.

Uses and Administration

Thallium acetate was formerly used by mouth for depilation in ringworm and as an ingredient of depilatory creams but, owing to numerous fatalities following both systemic and local treatments, it is no longer used for such purposes. It has also been used as a rodenticide and insecticide, although its use is strictly regulated in many countries. However, it is used in industry and is therefore still a hazard. Cases of malicious poisoning are still encountered occasionally.

Theobroma (2412-b)

Cacao or Cocoa Powder; Non-alkalised Cocoa Powder; Theobrom.

The roasted seed of theobroma, *Theobroma cacao* (Sterculiaceae), deprived of most of the shell, pressed to remove a portion of its fat, and finely ground.

Profile

Prepared theobroma is used as a flavoured basis for tablets and lozenges. Theobroma oil (p.1410) is used as a basis for suppositories.

Preparations

Proprietary Preparations (details are given in Part 3)
Multi-ingredient: *Aust.:* Asthmatee; *Braz.:* Licor de Cacau.

Theodrenaline Hydrochloride (13321-h)

Theodrenaline Hydrochloride (BANM, rINNM).

H-8352; Noradrenaline Theophylline Hydrochloride. 7-[2-(3,4,β-Trihydroxyphenethylamino)ethyl]theophylline hydrochloride.
$C_{17}H_{21}N_5O_5,HCl = 411.8$.
CAS — 13460-98-5 (theodrenaline); 2572-61-4 (theodrenaline hydrochloride).

Profile

Theodrenaline is mainly used as the hydrochloride in preparations with cafedrine promoted for the treatment of hypotension.

Preparations

Proprietary Preparations (details are given in Part 3)
Multi-ingredient: *Aust.:* Akrinor; *Fr.:* Praxinor; *Ger.:* Akrinor; *S.Afr.:* Akrinor; *Spain:* Bifort; *Switz.:* Akrinor†.

Thioctic Acid (13325-g)

Lipoic Acid. 5-(1,2-Dithiolan-3-yl)valeric acid.
$C_8H_{14}O_2S_2 = 206.3$.
CAS — 62-46-4.

Profile

Thioctic acid is used for its antioxidant effects in the treatment of diabetic neuropathy. It has been tried in the treatment of liver dysfunction and in subacute necrotising encephalopathy. Beneficial results have been claimed in amanitin poisoning following ingestion of the mushroom *Amanita phalloides*, but its use is controversial (see under Poisonous Mushrooms or Toadstools, p.1639). Ethylenediamine thioctate, sodium thioctate, and thioctic acid amide (thioctamide) have been used similarly.

Diabetic neuropathy. Some studies[1,2] have suggested that thioctic acid may be of benefit in diabetic neuropathy although further work is still needed.

1. Ziegler D, *et al.* Effects of treatment with the antioxidant α-lipoic acid on cardiac autonomic neuropathy in NIDDM patients: a 4-month randomized controlled multicenter trial (DEKAN study). *Diabetes Care* 1997; **20:** 369–73.
2. Ziegler D, *et al.* Treatment of symptomatic diabetic polyneuropathy with the antioxidant α-lipoic acid: a 7-month multicenter randomized controlled trial (ALADIN III study). *Diabetes Care* 1999; **22:** 1296–1301.

Preparations

Proprietary Preparations (details are given in Part 3)
Aust.: Tioctan; *Ger.:* Alpha-Lipon; alpha-Vibolex; Alphaflam; Azulipont; Berlithion; Biomo-lipon; duralipon; espa-lipon; Fenint; Neurium; Neurothioct; Pleomix-Alpha; Thioctacid; Thiogamma; Tromlipon; Verla-Lipon; *Hong Kong:* Lipoicin; *Ital.:* Tioctidasi†; *Jpn:* Tioctan; *Thai.:* Lipoicin.
Multi-ingredient: *Hong Kong:* Lipochol; *Ital.:* Byodinoral; Tiobec; *Spain:* Policolinosil; Sugarceton†; *Thai.:* Lipochol.

Thiomucase (3903-p)

C-84-04; Chondroitinsulphatase.

Profile
Thiomucase is a mucopolysaccharidase with general properties similar to those of hyaluronidase, p.1620, but which also depolymerises chondroitin sulfate. It has been given to assist the diffusion of local anaesthetic injections.

Thiram (13330-m)

Thiram (*USAN, rINN*).
NSC-1771; SQ-1489; TMT; TMTD. Tetramethylthiuram disulphide.
$C_6H_{12}N_2S_4 = 240.4$.
CAS — 137-26-8.
ATC — P03AA05.

Profile
Thiram, the methyl analogue of disulfiram (p.1605), has antibacterial and antifungal activity. It is applied topically as an aerosol in the treatment of wounds and other skin disorders. It has been used as a fungicide in agriculture, and in industry as a rubber accelerator. Occupational exposure to thiram may cause irritation of mucous membranes and skin.

Preparations

Proprietary Preparations (details are given in Part 3)
Belg.: Nobecutane†; *Ger.:* Nobecutan.
Multi-ingredient: *Spain:* Sulfiselen.

Thorium Dioxide (13332-v)

Thorium Oxide.
$ThO_2 = 264.0$.
CAS — 1314-20-1.

Profile
Colloidal solutions of thorium dioxide were formerly used as X-ray contrast media for examination of the liver and spleen, for arteriography, and occasionally for outlining the cerebral ventricles. Its elimination is very slow and incomplete. It accumulates in the reticuloendothelial system, especially in the liver and spleen. As it is radioactive (half-life: 1.41×10^{10} years), this accumulation is dangerous and there is strong evidence that the ensuing prolonged exposure to its radiation is a contributing factor in the development of malignant diseases and blood disorders often 20 to 30 years after its administration.

Thuja (13333-g)

The fresh leaves and twigs of *Thuja occidentalis* (Coniferae).

Profile
Thuja is included in some topical preparations for warts and in herbal antiseptic preparations. It is also used in homoeopathic medicine.

Preparations

Proprietary Preparations (details are given in Part 3)
Multi-ingredient: *Belg.:* Aporil; *Braz.:* Calope; *Fr.:* Nitrol; Verrupan; *Ger.:* Esberitox N; *Port.:* Erpecalm; *Spain:* Nitroina; *Switz.:* Esberitop; Esberitox N†.

Thymalfasin (1233-c)

Thymalfasin (*USAN, rINN*).
Thymosin α1.
CAS — 62304-98-7; 69521-94-4.

Profile
Thymalfasin is a thymus hormone (p.1672); it is a component of thymosin fraction 5 (a crude thymus gland extract), which has been synthesised. Thymalfasin is used alone or in combination with interferon as an immunomodulator for the treat-

ment of chronic hepatitis B and C (p.605). It is given by subcutaneous injection in a dose of 1.6 mg twice weekly for up to 12 months. It is also used to enhance the effectiveness of influenza vaccines in immunocompromised or elderly patients and of influenza and hepatitis B vaccines in chronic haemodialysis patients.

Thymalfasin is under investigation for a number of other diseases, including hepatitis D, hepatocellular carcinoma, non-small cell lung cancer, melanoma, and HIV infection and AIDS.

◊ References.
1. Garaci E, *et al.* Sequential chemoimmunotherapy for advanced non-small cell lung cancer using cisplatin, etoposide, thymosin-α1 and interferon-α2a. *Eur J Cancer* 1995; **31** 2403–5.
2. Rasi G, *et al.* Combination thymosin α1 and lymphoblastoid interferon treatment in chronic hepatitis C. *Gut* 1996; **39:** 679–83.
3. Zavaglia C, *et al.* A pilot study of thymosin-α1 therapy for chronic hepatitis D. *J Clin Gastroenterol* 1996; **23:** 162–3.
4. Andreone P, *et al.* A randomized controlled trial of thymosin-α1 versus interferon alfa treatment in patients with hepatitis B e antigen antibody- and hepatitis B virus DNA-positive chronic hepatitis B. *Hepatology* 1996; **24:** 774–7.
5. Sherman KE, *et al.* Combination therapy with thymosin α1 and interferon for the treatment of chronic hepatitis C infection: a randomized, placebo-controlled double-blind trial. *Hepatology* 1998; **27:** 1128–35.
6. Chien R-N, *et al.* Efficacy of thymosin α1 in patients with chronic hepatitis B: a randomized, controlled trial. *Hepatology* 1998; **27:** 1383–7.
7. Rasi G, *et al.* Combined treatment with thymosin-α1 and low dose interferon-α after dacarbazine in advanced melanoma. *Melanoma Res* 2000; **10:** 189–92.

Preparations

Proprietary Preparations (details are given in Part 3)
Ital.: Timosin†; Zadaxin; *Singapore:* Zadaxin.

Thyme (4716-y)

Common Thyme; Garden Thyme; Rubbed Thyme; Thymi Herba; Timo.

Pharmacopoeias. In *Eur.* (see p.vi) and *Pol.*

Pharmacopoeial description
Ph. Eur.: The whole leaves and flowers separated from the previously dried stems of *Thymus vulgaris*, or *T. zygis*, or a mixture of both species. It contains not less than 12 mL per kg of essential oil, of which a minimum of 40% is thymol and carvacrol, both calculated with reference to the anhydrous drug. It has a strong aromatic odour reminiscent of thymol.

Profile
Thyme is the source of thyme oil. It has carminative, antiseptic, antitussive, and expectorant properties and is used chiefly in preparations for respiratory-tract disorders and as a flavour.

Preparations

Proprietary Preparations (details are given in Part 3)
Aust.: Heumann's Bronchial†; Scottopect; *Ger.:* Anastil; Antussan†; Aspecton; Bronchipret; Bronchitten; Expectal N†; Fichten-sirup N; Makatussil Thymian-Hustensaft; Hustagil Thymiantropfen; Husties; Isephca S; Kolton bronchiale Erkaltungssaft†; Makatussin Saft; Melrosum Hustensirup Forte; Menthymin mono; Mirfusot; Nimopect; Schneckensirup; Soledum Hustensaft; Soledum Hustentropfen; Thymi-Fips†; Thymipin N; Thymiverlan; Tussamag Hustensaft N; Tussamag Hustentropfen N; *Israel:* Thymi Syrup; *Neth.:* Daro Thijm†.
Multi-ingredient: *Aust.:* Aktiv Husten- und Bronchialtee; Anifer Hustentee; Anifer Hustentropfen; Anitos; Aponatura Hustenstillende; Apotheker Bauer's Brust- und Hustentee; Bio-Garten Tee gegen Erkaltung; Bio-Garten Tropfen gegen Husten; Bronchiplant; Bronchiplant light; Bronchostop; Brust- und Hustentee; Codelum; Codipront cum Expectorans†; Erkaltungstee; Expectal-Tropfen; Granobil; Grippetee Dr Zeidler; Heumann Hustenstiller†; Hustensaft-Dr Schmidgall; Jutussin neo; Kneipp Grippe-Tee; Kneipp Husten- und Bronchial-Tee; Krauter Hustensaft; Krauterdoktor Hustentropfen; Krauterdoktor Krampf- und Reizhustensirup; Krauterhaus Mag Kottas Husten- und Bronchialtee; Krautertee Nr 10; Krautertee Nr 126; Krautertee Nr 211; Krautertee Nr 311; Krautertee Nr 7; Luuf-Hustentee; Mag Kottas Husten-Bronchialtee; Mediplant Krauter; Paracodin; Pilka; Pilka Forte; Pneumopan; Pneumopect; Purianta†; Scottopect; Sidroga Brust-Husten-Tee; Spasmo-Granobil-Krampf- und Reizhusten; St Radegunder Brusttee; St Radegunder Thorasan-Krauterhustensaft; Synpharma Instant-Brust- und Hustentee; Teekanne Erkaltungstee; Teekanne Husten- und Brusttee; Thymoval; Tussamag; Tussimont; *Austral.:* Bronchilin; Cough Relief; Euphorbia Complex; Respatona Decongestant Formula; Respatona Plus Bronchial Cough Relief; *Belg.:* Balsoclase; Colimax; *Braz.:* Broncmel; Pectoss; *Canad.:* Herbal Throat; Pectothymin†; Swiss Herb Cough Drops; *Fin.:* Katapekt; *Fr.:* Depuratum; Elixir Contre La Toux Weleda†; Germose; Niver; Santane D₅; Santane R₈; Tussidoron; *Ger.:* Anastil N; Aspecton N; Biotuss N; Bronchialtee N; Bronchicum Elixir N; Bronchicum Elixir Plus; Bronchicum Hustentee†; Bronchicum Pflanzlicher; Bronchicum Sekret-Loser; Bronchicum Thymian; Bronchicum Tropfen N; Bronchipret; Bronchitten forte K; Bronchosyx N; Brust- und Husten-Tee Stada N†; Brust- und Hustentee; Cefabronchin; Cefedrin N; Cito-Guakalin; Drosithym-N; Em-eukal; Ephepect; Equisil; Eucabal†; Eupatal; Expectysat N; Guttae 20 Hustentropfen N†; Harzer Hustenloser; Hevert-Erkaltungs-Tee†; Hevert-Magen-Galle-Leber-Tee†; Hevertopect; Infantussin N†; Ipalat†; Junisana; Kinder Em-eukal Hustensaft; Kneipp Erkaltungs-Tee; Kneipp Husten- und Bronchial-Tie; Kneipp Krauter Hustensaft N Kneipp Tannolsaft; Makatussin Tropfen; Melissengeist; Melrosum Hustensirup N; Mintetten Truw†; Perdiphen phyto†; Phytobronchin; Praecipect†; Primotussan; Pulmocordio forte; Pulmocordio mite SL; Pulmotin;

Salus Bronchial-Tee Nr.8†; Schneckensaft N†; Sedotussin Expectorans†; Sinuforton; Thymipin N; Tussiflorin forte; Tussiflorin Hustenstiller; TUSSinfant N; Tussipect†; *Hong Kong:* Pectoral; *Israel:* Pilka; *Ital.:* Broncosedina; Fluend†; Pinedrin; Piodermina; Pluriderm†; Sciroppo Merck all'Efetonina; Tussol; *Neth.:* Balsoclase Compositum; Bronchicum; *Port.:* Calmarum; Fluidin Antiasmatico; *S.Afr.:* Bronchicough; Bronchicum; *Switz.:* Mentobox†; Pazbronquial; Pilka; Wobenzimal; *Switz.:* Bronchalin†; Bronchofluid†; Bronchosan; Codipront cum Expectorans; Demo gouttes bronchiques†; Demo sirop bronchique N†; Demo sirop contre la toux†; DemoPectol; Dinacode N; Dragees contre la toux no 536; Expectoran Codein; Liberol Dragees contre la toux; Liberol Pastilles contre la toux; Liberol Sirop contre la toux; Makatussin forte; Nican; Pastilles pectorales formule 541; Pectoral N; Pilka; Sedotussin; Sirop pectoral DP1†; Sirop pectoral DP2, DP3†; Thymodrosin N; Thymodrosin†; Tisane pectorale et antitussive; Tisane pectorale pour les enfants; *Thai.:* Solvopret; Solvopret TP; *UK:* Cough Elixir; Herb and Honey Cough Elixir; Snowfire.

Thyme Oil (4717-j)

Esencia de Tomillo; Essência de Tomilho; Ol. Thym.; Oleum Thymi.

Pharmacopoeias. In *Eur.* (see p.vi) and *Pol.*

Pharmacopoeial description
Ph. Eur.: The essential oil obtained by steam distillation from the fresh flowering aerial parts of *Thymus vulgaris*, *T. zygis*, or a mixture of both species. A clear, yellow or very dark reddish-brown, mobile liquid with a characteristic aromatic, spicy odour, reminiscent of thymol. Miscible with dehydrated alcohol and with petroleum spirit. It contains between 36 and 55% of thymol. Store in well-filled, airtight containers at a temperature not exceeding 25°. Protect from light.

Profile
Thyme oil is used similarly to thyme (above).

Preparations

Proprietary Preparations (details are given in Part 3)
Ger.: Bronchicum Medizinal-Bad; Fichtensirup N; Kneipp Erkaltungs-Bad; Penaten; Thymian Erkaltungs-Bad.
Multi-ingredient: *Aust.:* Bronchostop; Expectal-Balsam; Expigen; Heumann's Bronchialtee; Luuf-Hustentee; Makatussin†; Medizinalbad; Perozon Heublumen; Red Point; Sanvita Bronchial; Scottopect; SynPharma Bronchial; *Austral.:* Breathe Eazy Chest Rub; Relief Rub; Tixylix Chest Rub; Zam-Buk; *Belg.:* Perubore; *Fr.:* Acarcid; Balsofumine; Balsofumine Mentholee; Biogaze; Citrosil; Gouttes aux Essences; Otylol; Perubore; Vapo-Myrtol†; *Ger.:* Antitussivum Burger N; Aspecton-Balsam; Em-eukal; Engelin Hingfong Essenz; Heumann Bronchialtee Solubifix; Hoepixin N; Hustagil Erkaltungsbalsam; Hustagil Inhalationsol; Kneipp Erkaltungs-Balsam N; Kneipp Rheuma Stoffwechsel-Bad Heublumen-Aquasan†; Makatussin Balsam mit Menthol; Melrosum Medizinalbad; Nasivin gegen Erkaltung N; Nasivin Intensiv-Bad N; Nasulind; Night-Care†; Pulmotin-N; Retterspitz Aerosol†; Retterspitz Innerlich†; Schupps Heilkrauter Erkaltungsbad; *Hong Kong:* Zam-Buk; *Ital.:* Calyptol; Fomentil; Neo Zeta-Foot†; Sanaderm†; Vegetallumina; *Mon.:* Calyptol; *NZ:* Tixylix Chest Rub; *Port.:* Creodermol; Erpecalm; Vaporil; *S.Afr.:* Zam-Buk; *Singapore:* Zam-Buk; *Spain:* Calyptol Inhalante; H Tussan; Termosan; *Switz.:* Brosol; Caprisana†; Demo gouttes contre la toux†; Demo pommade contre les refroidissements; Demo pommade contre les refroidissements pour bebes; Demonatur Capsules contre les refroidissements; Dolo-Arthrosenex sine Heparino; Dolorex†; Frigoplasma; Kernosan Huile de Massage†; Liberol Bain; Liberol N; Liberol†; Makatussin; Perubare; Sedasept; Spagyrom; *Thai.:* St Luke's Oil; *UK:* Catarrh Cream; Efalex; Nine Rubbing Oils; Snowfire; Snufflebabe; *USA:* Maximum Strength Flexall 454; Unguentine.

Thymidine (13334-q)

NSC-21548; Thymine 2-Desoxyriboside. 1-(2-Deoxy-β-D-ribofuranosyl)-5-methyluracil; 1-(2-Deoxy-β-D-ribofuranosyl)-1,2,3,4-tetrahydro-5-methylpyrimidine-2,4-dione.
$C_{10}H_{14}N_2O_5 = 242.2$.
CAS — 50-89-5.

Profile
Thymidine is a nucleoside constituent of cells. It was formerly given by intravenous infusion to modulate the toxicity of methotrexate; it may also have an antineoplastic action of its own. Thymidine is not considered to be a substitute for calcium folinate.

Thymidine is given topically with other nucleosides in preparations for the treatment of corneal damage.

Preparations

Proprietary Preparations (details are given in Part 3)
Multi-ingredient: *Aust.:* Vitasic; *Fr.:* Vitacic.

Thymus Hormones (13335-p)

CAS — 69558-55-0 (thymopentin); 60529-76-2 (thymopoietin); 63340-72-7 (thymic humoral factor).

Profile
The thymus gland controls the development of T-lymphocytes and thereby plays a central role in cell-mediated immunity and the regulation of immune responses. It secretes hormones although the multiplicity of factors isolated has led to some con-

fusion. Several polypeptides characterised in the thymus or serum are able to induce lymphocyte differentiation *in vitro* and *in vivo*. They include: thymalfasin (p.1672); thymosin fraction 5, a crude thymus gland extract; thymic humoral factor (THF), isolated from crude thymic extract dialysate; nonathymulin (thymulin, serum thymic factor, Facteur Thymique Serique, FTS), a synthetic nonapeptide; thymomodulin, a partially purified extract from calf thymus; thymogene A, extracted from calf thymus; thymopoietin, a polypeptide of known amino acid sequence; thymopentin (thymopoietin pentapeptide, TP-5) a fragment of thymopoietin with 5 amino acids; and thymostimulin (TP-1), extracted from calf thymus.

Various preparations, including crude extracts from calf thymus gland, thymopentin, and thymostimulin have been tried as immunomodulators in auto-immune and immunodeficiency disorders and as adjuncts in the treatment of malignant disease.

◊ Thymus hormones have been tried in the treatment of numerous conditions including rheumatoid arthritis,[1-4]diabetes mellitus,[5,6] immunodeficiency disorders,[7-12] skin disorders[13-16] (for mention of their use in scleroderma, see p.505), malignant neoplasms,[17-19] and some infections.[20,21]

1. Amor B, *et al.* Nonathymulin in rheumatoid arthritis: two double blind, placebo controlled trials. *Ann Rheum Dis* 1987; **46**: 549–54.
2. Lemmel EM, *et al.* Immunomodulating therapy in chronic polyarthritis with thymopentin: a multicenter placebo-controlled study of 119 patients. *Dtsch Med Wochenschr* 1988; **113**: 172–6.
3. Kantharia BK, *et al.* Thymopentin (TP-5) in the treatment of rheumatoid arthritis. *Br J Rheumatol* 1989; **23**: 118–23.
4. Sundal E, Bertelletti D. Thymopentin treatment of rheumatoid arthritis. *Arzneimittelforschung* 1994; **44**: 1145–9.
5. Giordano C, *et al.* Early administration of an immunomodulator and induction of remission in insulin-dependent diabetes mellitus. *J Autoimmun* 1990; **3**: 611–17.
6. Moncada E, *et al.* Insulin requirements and residual beta-cell function 12 months after concluding immunotherapy in type I diabetic patients treated with combined azathioprine and thymostimulin administration for one year. *J Autoimmun* 1990; **3**: 625–38.
7. Terrizzi A, *et al.* Thymomodulin prevents post-operative immunodepression measured by means of skin tests. *Int J Immunother* 1988; **4**: 193–8.
8. Skotnicki AB. Thymic hormones and lymphokines. *Drugs Today* 1989; **25**: 337–62.
9. Beyer WEP, *et al.* Effect of immunomodulator thymopentin on impaired seroresponse to influenza vaccine in patients on haemodialysis. *Nephron* 1990; **54**: 296–301.
10. Beall G, *et al.* A double-blind, placebo-controlled trial of thymostimulin in symptomatic HIV-infected patients. *AIDS* 1990; **4**: 679–81.
11. Brivio F, *et al.* Effect of thymopentin administered perioperatively on the surgery-induced increase in soluble interleukin-2 receptor blood levels in colon cancer patients. *Curr Ther Res* 1991; **50**: 293–7.
12. Hassner A, Adelman DC. Biologic response modifiers in primary immunodeficiency disorders. *Ann Intern Med* 1991; **115**: 294–307.
13. David TJ. Recent developments in the treatment of childhood atopic eczema. *J R Coll Physicians Lond* 1991; **25**: 95–101.
14. Harper JI, *et al.* A double-blind placebo-controlled study of thymostimulin (TP-1) for the treatment of atopic eczema. *Br J Dermatol* 1991; **125**: 368–72.
15. Giordano N, *et al.* Efficacy and safety of thymopentin in patients suffering from progressive systemic sclerosis. *Curr Ther Res* 1991; **49**: 731–9.
16. Hsieh K-H, *et al.* Thymopentin treatment in severe atopic dermatitis—clinical and immunological evaluations. *Arch Dis Child* 1992; **67**: 1095–1102.
17. Cascinelli N, *et al.* Perinodular injection of thymopentine (TP5) in cutaneous and subcutaneous metastases of melanoma. *Melanoma Res* 1993; **3**: 471–6.
18. Pavesi L, Italian Cooperative Trials Group. Fluorouracil (F), with and without high dose folinic acid (HDFA) plus epirubicin (E) and cyclophosphamide (C): FEC versus HDFA-FEC plus or minus thymostimulin (TS) in metastatic breast cancer: results of a multicenter study. *Eur J Cancer* 1993; **29A**: S77.
19. Mustacchi G, Italian Cooperative Trials Group. High dose folinic acid (HDFA) and fluorouracil (Fu) plus or minus thymostimulin (TS) for treatment of metastatic colorectal cancer (MCRC): a randomized multicentric study. *Eur J Cancer* 1993; **29A**: S89.
20. Periti P, *et al.* Antimicrobial chemoimmunoprophylaxis in colorectal surgery with cefotetan and thymostimulin: prospective, controlled multicenter study. *J Chemother* 1993; **5**: 37–42.
21. Sundal E, Bertelletti D. Management of viral infections with thymopentin. *Arzneimittelforschung* 1994; **44**: 866–71.

Preparations

Proprietary Preparations (details are given in Part 3)
Braz.: Leucogen; Timosan; TP-1; *Ital.:* Leucotrofina†; Sintomodulina; Timunox; TP-1†; *Mex.:* Himus; Leucotrofina; *Spain:* TP-1.

Tibezonium Iodide (13341-g)

Tibezonium Iodide *(rINN)*.
Rec-15/0691.   Diethylmethyl{2-[4-(4-phenylthiophenyl)-3*H*-1,5-benzodiazepin-2-ylthio]ethyl}ammonium iodide.
$C_{28}H_{32}IN_3S_2 = 601.6$.
CAS — 54663-47-7.
ATC — A01AB15.

Profile
Tibezonium iodide has been used in the treatment of infections of the mouth and throat.

Preparations

Proprietary Preparations (details are given in Part 3)
Ital.: Antoral; *Mex.:* Maxoral; *Port.:* Maxius.

Tilactase (12779-v)

Tilactase *(rINN)*.
β-D-Galactosidase; Lactase.
CAS — 9031-11-2.
ATC — A09AA04.
Pharmacopoeias. In US.

Pharmacopoeial description
USP 25: A hydrolytic enzyme derived from *Aspergillus oryzae*. Each g contains not less than 30 000 USP units. Store in airtight containers at room temperature.

Profile
Tilactase hydrolyses lactose into glucose and galactose. It has been added to milk and milk products, or taken by mouth before a meal containing dairy products, in order to prevent the symptoms of lactose intolerance (p.1370) in persons deficient in the endogenous enzyme.

Preparations

Proprietary Preparations (details are given in Part 3)
Austral.: Lact-Easy; Lactaid; *Canad.:* Dairyaid; Lactaid; Lactrase; *Irl.:* Colief; Lactaid†; *Ital.:* Lactaid†; Silact; *Jpn:* Galantase; *Port.:* Lisolac; *S.Afr.:* Galantase†; *Switz.:* Lacdigest; *UK:* Colief; Lactaid†; *USA:* Dairy Ease; Lactaid; Lactrase; SureLac.

Multi-ingredient: *Spain:* Lactored†; Polidasa†.

Tilia (323-w)

Lime Flower; Linden; Tiliae Flos; Tilleul; Tilo.
Pharmacopoeias. In Eur. (see p.vi) and Pol.

Pharmacopoeial description
Ph. Eur.: The whole dried inflorescences of *Tilia cordata*, *Tilia platyphyllos*, *Tilia × vulgaris*, or a mixture of these species. It has a faint aromatic odour. Protect from light.

Profile
Tilia is mildly astringent and is reputed to have antispasmodic and diaphoretic properties. Lime-flower 'tea' is a traditional domestic remedy.

Various species of tilia are used in herbal and homoeopathic preparations for a variety of disorders.

Preparations

Proprietary Preparations (details are given in Part 3)
Belg.: Vibtil; *Canad.:* Hepamig; *Fr.:* Vibtil.

Multi-ingredient: *Aust.:* Aponatura Erkaltungs; Apotheker Bauer's Grippetee; Bogumil-tassenfertiger milder Abfurtee; Grippefloran; Grippetee Dr Zeidler; Grippetee EF-EM-ES; Grippogran; Kneipp Grippe-Tee; Krauterdoktor Erkaltungstropfen; Krauterhaus Mag Kottas Grippetee; Krautertee Nr 10; Krautertee Nr 210; Mag Kottas Grippe-Tee; Sidroga Erkaltungstee; Sidroga Kindertee; St Bonifatius-Tee; St Radegunder Fiebertee; Teekanne Erkaltungstee; *Austral.:* Crataegus Complex; *Belg.:* Eugiron; Tisane Antibiliaire et Stomachique; Tisane Pectorale; Tisane pour le Foie; *Fr.:* Actisane Troubles du Sommeil; Apaisance; Assagix†; Calmophytum; Lenicalm; Mediflor Tisane Antirhumatismale No 2†; Mediflor Tisane Calmante Troubles du Sommeil No 14†; Noctisan†; Phytotherapie Boribel no 8; Santane N₀; Santane O₁; Tisane des Familles; Tisanes de l'Abbe Hamon no 6; Vigilia; *Ger.:* Grunlicht Hingfong Essenz; Hevert-Blasen- und Nieren- Tee; Kneipp Erkaltungs-Tee; Nephrובin†; Nervosana; Salus Bronchial-Tee Nr.8†; *Israel:* Jungborn; *Ital.:* Alkagin; Fluend†; Lenicalm; Sambuco (Specie Composta); Tussol; Videorelax; *Switz.:* Tisane antiflatulente pour les enfants; Tisane contre les refroidissements; Tisane pour les enfants†; *UK:* Daily Menopause Relief; Gerard House Motherwort Compound; Tranquil; Wellwoman.

Timonacic (3749-j)

Timonacic *(rINN)*.
ATC; NSC-25855; Thioproline. Thiazolidine-4-carboxylic acid.
$C_4H_7NO_2S = 133.2$.
CAS — 444-27-9.

NOTE. The name ATC has also been used for a combination of paracetamol and trichloroethanol (4-acetamidophenyl 2,2,2-trichloroethyl carbonate).

Profile
Timonacic is used as an adjuvant in the treatment of acute and chronic hepatic disorders.

Timonacic methyl hydrochloride (carbolidine hydrochloride) has been used as a mucolytic.

Preparations

Proprietary Preparations (details are given in Part 3)
Ital.: Ciliar; Muvial; Tiazolidin†; *Switz.:* Heparegen.

Tin (5326-q)

Sn = 118.71.
CAS — 7440-31-5.

A silver-white, lustrous, malleable, ductile metal.

Profile
Owing to their low solubility, tin and tin oxide are very poorly absorbed from the gastrointestinal tract and are not toxic. Chronic inhalation causes a benign form of pneumoconiosis.

Organic compounds of tin are highly toxic and may cause liver and kidney damage as well as severe neurological damage associated with oedema of the white matter of the brain. Treatment has been symptomatic. Contamination of the skin with organic tin compounds can cause severe burning; suitable precautions should be taken to prevent absorption of organic tin compounds through the skin.

Tin and tin oxide have been given in the treatment of boils, but there is little evidence of effectiveness; they were also formerly used in some countries for the treatment of tapeworm. Organic tin compounds, especially tributyltin oxide (TBTO), are used as molluscicides; they are highly toxic.

◊ Excess amounts of tin in food tend to arise from tin-coated cans, especially unlacquered ones, and may produce gastric irritation. It appears likely that infants and small children consume proportionally greater amounts of tin than adults. Consumers should be advised not to store foods in opened cans.

Concentrations as low as 150 μg per gram in canned beverages and 250 μg per gram in other canned foods have produced adverse effects in certain individuals, but some foods containing up to 700 μg per gram have not produced any detectable effects. Further studies were required to identify the chemical forms of tin that cause acute gastric irritation and any possible potentiating or moderating factors.

The previously recommended acceptable daily intake for chronic exposure to tin was re-affirmed as a provisional tolerable weekly intake of 14 mg per kg body-weight.[1]

1. FAO/WHO. Evaluation of certain food additives and contaminants: thirty-third report of the joint FAO/WHO expert committee on food additives. *WHO Tech Rep Ser 776* 1989.

Preparations

Proprietary Preparations (details are given in Part 3)
Multi-ingredient: *Belg.:* Stanno-Bardane†.

Tin-protoporphyrin (1896-s)

(Sn)-protoporphyrin.

Profile
Tin-protoporphyrin and the related compound tin-mesoporphyrin are metalloporphyrins which inhibit haem oxygenase, an enzyme involved in the breakdown of haem to bile pigments. They have been investigated as inhibitors of bilirubin production in hyperbilirubinaemia of various causes, and have been tried in porphyria (p.1011).

◊ References.
1. Rubaltelli FF, *et al.* Tin-protoporphyrin in the management of children with Crigler-Najjar disease. *Pediatrics* 1989; **84**: 728–31.
2. McDonagh AF. Tin-protoporphyrin in the management of children with Crigler-Najjar disease. *Pediatrics* 1990; **86**: 151–2.
3. Berglund L, *et al.* Studies with the haeme oxygenase inhibitor Sn-protoporphyrin in patients with primary biliary cirrhosis and idiopathic haemochromatosis. *Gut* 1990; **31**: 899–904.
4. Dover SB, *et al.* Tin-protoporphyrin combined with haem arginate—an improved treatment for acute hepatic porphyria. *Gut* 1991; **32**: A597.
5. Dover SB, *et al.* Haem-arginate plus tin-protoporphyrin for acute hepatic porphyria. *Lancet* 1991; **338**: 263.
6. Kappas A, *et al.* Direct comparison of Sn-mesoporphyrin, an inhibitor of bilirubin production, and phototherapy in controlling hyperbilirubinemia in term and near-term newborns. *Pediatrics* 1995; **95**: 468–74.
7. Rubaltelli FF, *et al.* Congenital nonobstructive, nonhemolytic jaundice: effect of tin-mesoporphyrin. *Pediatrics* 1995; **95**: 942–4.
8. Valaes T, *et al.* Control of hyperbilirubinemia in glucose-6-phosphate dehydrogenase-deficient newborns using an inhibitor of bilirubin production, Sn-mesoporphyrin. Abstract: *Pediatrics* 1998; **101**: 915. Full version: http://www.pediatrics.org/cgi/content/full/101/5/e1
9. Martinez JC, *et al.* Control of severe hyperbilirubinemia in full-term newborns with the inhibitor of bilirubin production Sn-mesoporphyrin. *Pediatrics* 1999; **103**: 1–5.

Tiquizium Bromide (1276-b)

Tiquizium Bromide *(pINN)*.
HSR-902. *trans*-3-(Di-2-thienylmethylene)octahydro-5-methyl-2*H*-quinolizinium bromide.
$C_{19}H_{24}BrNS_2 = 410.4$.
CAS — 71731-58-3.

Profile
Tiquizium bromide is used as an antispasmodic.

Preparations

Proprietary Preparations (details are given in Part 3)
Jpn: Thiaton†.

Tiropramide Hydrochloride (17012-r)

Tiropramide Hydrochloride *(rINNM)*.
DL-α-Benzamido-*p*-[2-(diethylamino)ethoxy]-*N*,*N*-dipropylhydrocinnamamide hydrochloride.
$C_{28}H_{41}N_3O_3,HCl = 504.1$.
CAS — 55837-29-1 (tiropramide); 57227-16-4 (tiropramide hydrochloride).

Profile

Tiropramide hydrochloride is used as an antispasmodic. Doses of 100 mg have been given two or three times daily by mouth. It has also been given rectally and parenterally.

Preparations

Proprietary Preparations (details are given in Part 3)
Ger.: Alfospas; *Ital.:* Alfospas; Maiorad; *Port.:* Maiorad; *Thai.:* Maiorad.

Titanium (13355-l)

Ti = 47.867.
CAS — 7440-32-6.

Profile

Titanium has been used in the repair of skull damage and for implantation in dental surgery.

◊ References.
1. Brown D. All you wanted to know about titanium, but were afraid to ask. *Br Dent J* 1997; **182:** 393–4.

Tolonium Chloride (2152-d)

Tolonium Chloride (rINN).

Cl Basic Blue 17; Colour Index No. 52040; Toluidine Blue O. 3-Amino-7-dimethylamino-2-methylphenazathionium chloride.
$C_{15}H_{16}ClN_3S = 305.8$.
CAS — 92-31-9.

NOTE. Distinguish from Toluidine Blue, Colour Index No. 63340.

Profile

Tolonium chloride is a thiazine dye chemically related to methylene blue [methylthioninium chloride] (p.1012). It has been used to stain oral and gastric neoplasms and was given intravenously to stain the parathyroid glands. Other uses have included the treatment of menstrual disorders and methaemoglobinaemia.

Tolonium chloride should be avoided in patients with glucose-6-phosphate dehydrogenase deficiency as haemolysis may occur.

Preparations

Proprietary Preparations (details are given in Part 3)
Canad.: Orascan; *Ger.:* Toluidinblau.

Tolynol (13362-e)

1-(p-Tolyl)ethanol; p,α-Dimethylbenzyl alcohol.
$C_9H_{12}O = 136.2$.
CAS — 536-50-5.

Profile

Tolynol has been used as a choleretic in the treatment of hepatic disorders and is an ingredient of preparations for gastrointestinal disorders. Tolynol nicotinate has also been used.

Preparations

Proprietary Preparations (details are given in Part 3)
Multi-ingredient: *Aust.:* Claim; Galle-Donau; Spagall; Spasmo Claim.

Tonzonium Bromide (13331-b)

Tonzonium Bromide (rINN).

NC-1264; NSC-5648; Thonzonium Bromide (USAN). Hexadecyl[2-(N-p-methoxybenzyl-N-pyrimidin-2-ylamino)ethyl]dimethylammonium bromide.
$C_{32}H_{55}BrN_4O = 591.7$.
CAS — 553-08-2.

Profile

Tonzonium bromide is a cationic surfactant. As an additive in ear drops and aerosol sprays it has been claimed to promote tissue contact by dispersion and penetration of cellular debris and exudate.

Preparations

Proprietary Preparations (details are given in Part 3)
Multi-ingredient: *Ital.:* Rinedrone†; *NZ:* Coly-Mycin S Otic; *USA:* Coly-Mycin S Otic; Cortisporin-TC.

Tormentil (324-e)

Consolda Vermelha; Erect Cinquefoil; Tormentillae Rhizoma.
Pharmacopoeias. In Eur. (see p.vi) and *Pol.*

Pharmacopoeial description

Ph. Eur.: Tormentil consists of the whole or cut, dried rhizome, freed from the roots, of *Potentilla erecta* (*P. tormentilla*). It contains not less than 7% of tannins expressed as pyrogallol, calculated with reference to the dried drug. Protect from light.

Profile

Tormentil has astringent properties and is used in herbal preparations for diarrhoea and other indications.

Preparations

Proprietary Preparations (details are given in Part 3)
Ger.: Herbatorment†; ratioGast.

Multi-ingredient: *Aust.:* Aponatura Durchfall; Bio-Garten Tee gegen Durchfall; Drovitol; Eogran; Krauterhaus Mag Kottas Tee gegen Durchfall; Tee gegen Durchfall; *Ger.:* Mundra; Repha-Os; *Switz.:* Baume.

Transfer Factor (13365-j)

Profile

Transfer factor can passively transfer cell-mediated immunity from a sensitised donor to a non-sensitised recipient. It is a peptide constituent of dialysable leucocyte extracts prepared from the leucocytes of the donor, whose sensitivity may have been demonstrated by skin tests.

Transfer factor has been suggested for use in infections due to bacteria, fungi, and viruses, inflammatory disorders, nervous system disorders, immunodeficiency diseases, and malignancies, although the response when it has been tried in some of these conditions has not always been satisfactory.

◊ References.
1. Attallah AM, *et al.* Biological response modifiers and their promise in clinical medicine. *Pharmacol Ther* 1983; **19:** 435–54.
2. Gibson J, *et al.* Clinical use of transfer factor: 25 years on. *Clin Immunol Allergy* 1983; **3:** 331–57.
3. Fudenberg HH. "Transfer factor": an update. *Proc Soc Exp Biol Med* 1985; **178:** 327–32.
4. Tsang KY, Fudenberg HH. Transfer factor and other T cell products. *Springer Semin Immunopathol* 1986; **9:** 19–32.
5. Carey JT, *et al.* Augmentation of skin test reactivity and lymphocyte blastogenesis in patients with AIDS treated with transfer factor. *JAMA* 1987; **257:** 651–5.
6. Anonymous. Zidovudine and other drugs against HIV. *Drug Ther Bull* 1988; **26:** 101–4.
7. Fudenberg HH, Fudenberg HH. Transfer factor: past, present and future. *Annu Rev Pharmacol Toxicol* 1989; **29:** 475–516.
8. AUSTIMS Research Group. Interferon-α and transfer factor in the treatment of multiple sclerosis: a double-blind, placebo-controlled trial. *J Neurol Neurosurg Psychiatry* 1989; **52:** 566–74.
9. McBride SJ, McCluskey DR. Treatment of chronic fatigue syndrome. *Br Med Bull* 1991; **47:** 895–907.
10. Hassner A, Adelman DC. Biologic response modifiers in primary immunodeficiency disorders. *Ann Intern Med* 1991; **115:** 294–307.

Trepibutone (13369-a)

Trepibutone (rINN).

AA-149; Trepionate. 3-(2,4,5-Triethoxybenzoyl)propionic acid.
$C_{16}H_{22}O_6 = 310.3$.
CAS — 41826-92-0.
ATC — A03AX09.
Pharmacopoeias. In Jpn.

Profile

Trepibutone has been reported to have spasmolytic and choleretic activity and is used in biliary-tract disorders and pancreatitis.

Preparations

Proprietary Preparations (details are given in Part 3)
Port.: Choliatron.

Tribenoside (13374-z)

Tribenoside (USAN, rINN).

21401-Ba; Ba-21401. Ethyl 3,5,6-tri-O-benzyl-D-glucofuranoside.
$C_{29}H_{34}O_6 = 478.6$.
CAS — 10310-32-4.
ATC — C05AX05; C05CX01.

Profile

Tribenoside has been used in inflammatory and varicose disorders of the veins, including haemorrhoids (p.1205). It has been given by mouth in usual doses of 800 mg daily. It has also been administered rectally and topically.

Preparations

Proprietary Preparations (details are given in Part 3)
Aust.: Glyvenol; *Belg.:* Glyvenol; *Braz.:* Glyvenol; *Hong Kong:* Glyvenol; *Ital.:* Venalisin; Venodin†; *Mex.:* Glyvenol; *Switz.:* Glyvenol; *Thai.:* Glyvenol.

Multi-ingredient: *Aust.:* Procto-Glyvenol; *Braz.:* Procto-Glyvenol; Rectanus; *Israel:* Procto-Glyvenol; *Mex.:* Procto-Glyvenol; *Port.:* Procto-Glyvenol; *Switz.:* Procto-Glyvenol; *UAE:* Haemoproct.

Tricarbaurinium (13376-k)

Aluminon; Triammonium Aurintricarboxylate. 3-(3,3'-Dicarboxy-4,4'-dihydroxybenzhydrylidene)-6-oxocyclohexa-1,4-diene-1-carboxylic acid, triammonium salt.
$C_{22}H_{23}N_3O_9 = 473.4$.
CAS — 569-58-4.

Profile

Tricarbaurinium has been used topically in the treatment of oropharyngeal disorders.

Trichloroacetic Acid (1328-d)

Acidum Trichloraceticum; Trichloracetic Acid; Trichloressigsäure.
$C_2HCl_3O_2 = 163.4$.
CAS — 76-03-9.
Pharmacopoeias. In Eur. (see p.vi) and *Pol.*

Pharmacopoeial description

Ph. Eur.: A very deliquescent white crystalline mass or colourless crystals. Very soluble in water, in alcohol, and in dichloromethane. Store in airtight containers.

Adverse Effects and Treatment

As for Hydrochloric Acid, p.1621.

Uses and Administration

Trichloroacetic acid is caustic and astringent. It is used as a quick escharotic for warts. It is applied as a strong solution, prepared by adding 10% by weight of water [e.g. trichloroacetic acid 10 g plus water 1 g]; the surrounding parts are usually protected. It has also been used for the removal of tattoos.

Tattoo removal. References to the use of trichloroacetic acid in the removal of tattoos.
1. Hall-Smith P, Bennett J. Tattoos: a lasting regret. *BMJ* 1991; **303:** 397.

Warts. References to the use of trichloroacetic acid in the treatment of genital warts (p.1108).
1. Godley MJ, *et al.* Cryotherapy compared with trichloroacetic acid in treating genital warts. *Genitourin Med* 1987; **63:** 390–2.
2. Davis AJ, Emans SJ. Human papilloma virus infection in the pediatric and adolescent patient. *J Pediatr* 1989; **115:** 1–9.
3. Boothby RA, *et al.* Single application treatment of human papillomavirus infection of the cervix and vagina with trichloroacetic acid: a randomized trial. *Obstet Gynecol* 1990; **76:** 278–80.

Preparations

Proprietary Preparations (details are given in Part 3)
Ital.: Averuk Bruciaporri; CL tre; Porriver; Verrupor; *USA:* Tri-Chlor.

Multi-ingredient: *Spain:* Callicida Brum.

Triethyl Citrate (18351-h)

E1505; Triethylis Citras. 2-Hydroxy-1,2,3-propanetricarboxylic acid triethyl ester.
$C_{12}H_{20}O_7 = 276.3$.
CAS — 77-93-0.
Pharmacopoeias. In Eur. (see p.vi). Also in *USNF.*

Pharmacopoeial description

Ph. Eur.: A clear, viscous, colourless or almost colourless, hygroscopic liquid. Soluble in water; miscible with alcohol and with ether; slightly soluble in fatty oils. Store in airtight containers.

USNF 20: A practically colourless oily liquid. Soluble in water; miscible with alcohol and with ether. Store in airtight containers.

Profile

Triethyl citrate is a plasticiser used in pharmaceutical manufacturing and in the food and cosmetics industries.

Trilostane (13380-y)

Trilostane (BAN, USAN, pINN).

Win-24540. 4α,5α-Epoxy-17β-hydroxy-3-oxoandrostane-2α-carbonitrile.
$C_{20}H_{27}NO_3 = 329.4$.
CAS — 13647-35-3.
ATC — H02CA01.

Adverse Effects

Side-effects associated with trilostane have included flushing, nausea, vomiting, diarrhoea, rhinorrhoea, and oedema of the palate. Skin rashes may occur and, rarely, granulocytopenia in immunocompromised patients.

Precautions

Trilostane is contra-indicated in pregnancy and should be used with caution in patients with renal or hepatic impairment. Circulating corticosteroids and blood electrolytes should be monitored. During severe stress, the drug may have to be discontinued and corticosteroid supplements may be required.

Interactions

Trilostane may interfere with the activity of oral contraceptives. Hyperkalaemia may occur if trilostane is given concurrently with potassium-sparing diuretics.

Uses and Administration

Trilostane is an adrenocortical suppressant which inhibits the enzyme system essential for the production of glucocorticoids and mineralocorticoids. It has been used in the treatment of Cushing's syndrome (p.1272) and primary aldosteronism.

The usual dose is 240 mg by mouth in divided doses for at least 3 days and then adjusted, according to the patient's response, within the range of 120 to 480 mg daily. Doses of 960 mg daily have been given.

Trilostane with concurrent glucocorticoid replacement therapy has also been used in postmenopausal women with breast cancer who relapse following initial oestrogen receptor antagonist therapy. In these patients, the maintenance dose is 960 mg daily, or 720 mg daily if side-effects occur.

Preparations

Proprietary Preparations (details are given in Part 3)
UK: Modrenal.

Trimebutine Maleate (13381-j)

Trimebutine Maleate (BANM, rINNM).
2-Dimethylamino-2-phenylbutyl 3,4,5-trimethoxybenzoate hydrogen maleate.
$C_{22}H_{29}NO_5,C_4H_4O_4 = 503.5$.
CAS — 39133-31-8 (trimebutine); 34140-59-5 (trimebutine maleate).

Profile

Trimebutine maleate has been used as an antispasmodic in gastrointestinal disorders in doses of up to 600 mg daily by mouth. It has also been given by injection and rectally. Trimebutine base has also been used.

Irritable bowel syndrome. Trimebutine has been reported[1,2] to be effective in the treatment of irritable bowel syndrome (p.1206) although a considerable placebo response has been observed.[1] Some[2] consider that the effectiveness of trimebutine might be related to its action on opioid receptors in the gastrointestinal tract.

1. Ghidini O, *et al.* Single drug treatment for irritable colon: rociverine versus trimebutine maleate. *Curr Ther Res* 1986; **39:** 541–8.
2. Schaffstein W, *et al.* Comparative safety and efficacy of trimebutine versus mebeverine in the treatment of irritable bowel syndrome. *Curr Ther Res* 1990; **47:** 136–45.

Preparations

Proprietary Preparations (details are given in Part 3)
Aust.: Debridat; *Braz.:* Debridat; *Canad.:* Modulon; *Fr.:* Debridat; Modulon; Transacalm; *Hong Kong:* Cerekinon; *Ital.:* Debridat; Digerent; Kalius†; Trimedat; *Jpn:* Cerekinon; *Mex.:* Debridat; Espabion; Libertrim; Prescol; *Port.:* Debridat; *Singapore:* Cerekinon; Debridat; *Spain:* Polibutin; *Switz.:* Debridat; *Thai.:* Cerekinon.

Multi-ingredient: *Fr.:* Modulite†; Proctolog; *Ital.:* Debrum; *Port.:* Proctolog; *Singapore:* Proctolog; *Spain:* Proctolog.

Trinitrophenol (2288-c)

Carbazotic Acid; Picric Acid; Picrinic Acid. 2,4,6-Trinitrophenol.
$C_6H_3N_3O_7 = 229.1$.
CAS — 88-89-1.
Pharmacopoeias. In Fr.

Trinitrophenol should be stored in a cool place, mixed with an equal weight of water. It must not be stored in glass-stoppered bottles.

◊ CAUTION. *Trinitrophenol burns readily and explodes when heated rapidly or when subjected to percussion. For safety in handling it is usually supplied mixed with not less than half its weight of water. It combines with metals to form salts, some of which are very explosive.*

Profile

Trinitrophenol has disinfectant properties and was formerly used in the treatment of burns. It is now chiefly used in manufacturing and as a laboratory reagent.

Dermatitis, skin eruptions, severe itching, and yellow staining of the skin may occur following contact with trinitrophenol. Systemic toxicity may follow ingestion or absorption through the skin or lungs; symptoms may include vomiting, pain, and diarrhoea, progressing to haemolysis, hepatitis, anuria, convulsions, unconsciousness, and death. The metabolic rate is increased, causing pyrexia.

It has been used in homoeopathy.

Preparations

Proprietary Preparations (details are given in Part 3)
Multi-ingredient: *Spain:* Oftalmol Dexa†; Oftalmol Ocular; Queratil.

Trolamine (218-s)

Trolamine (pINN).
Triethanolamine; Trolaminum.
CAS — 102-71-6.
Pharmacopoeias. In Eur. (see p.vi). Also in USNF.

A variable mixture of bases containing mainly 2,2′,2′′-nitrilotriethanol (trolamine (CH$_2$OH.CH$_2$)$_3$N), together with 2,2′-iminobisethanol (diolamine) and smaller amounts of 2-aminoethanol (monoethanolamine).

The symbol † denotes a preparation no longer actively marketed

Pharmacopoeial description

Ph. Eur.: A clear, viscous, colourless or slightly yellow, very hygroscopic liquid. Miscible with water and with alcohol; soluble in dichloromethane; slightly soluble in ether. Store in airtight containers. Protect from light.

USNF 20: A mixture of alkanolamines consisting largely of trolamine containing some diolamine and monoethanolamine. A colourless to pale yellow, viscous, hygroscopic liquid having a slight ammoniacal odour. Miscible with water and with alcohol; soluble in chloroform. Store in airtight containers. Protect from light.

Adverse Effects

Trolamine salts may be irritating to the skin and mucous membranes. Contact dermatitis has been reported following the use of ear drops containing trolamine polypeptide oleate-condensate.

◊ Following concern about the possible production of carcinogenic nitrosamines in the stomach, the Swiss authorities restricted the use of trolamine to preparations for external use.[1]

1. Anonymous. Trolamine: concerns regarding potential carcinogenicity. *WHO Drug Inf* 1991; **5:** 9.

Uses and Administration

Trolamine is used combined with fatty acids such as stearic and oleic acids as an emulsifier and as an alkalinising agent. It has also been used to reduce dithranol-induced staining of the skin. Ear drops containing trolamine polypeptide oleate-condensate 10% are used for the removal of impacted ear wax.
Trolamine salicylate (p.90) has also been used.

Preparations

Proprietary Preparations (details are given in Part 3)
Belg.: Xerumenex; *Canad.:* Cerumenex; *Fr.:* Biafine; *Ger.:* Cerumenex N; *Israel:* Biafine; *Ital.:* Cerumenex†; *Neth.:* Xerumenex; *S.Afr.:* Cerumenex; *Switz.:* Cerumenex; *USA:* Cerumenex; Curastain†.

Multi-ingredient: *Austral.:* Neutrogena; *Braz.:* Benzilol; Cerumin; Paraqueimol; *Canad.:* Soropon; *Ital.:* Dopo Pik; *Port.:* Biafine; Transbronquina; *USA:* Maxilube.

Trometamol (2360-p)

Trometamol (BAN, rINN).
NSC-6365; THAM; Trihydroxymethylaminomethane; TRIS; Tris(hydroxymethyl)aminomethane; Trometamolum; Tromethamine (USAN). 2-Amino-2-(hydroxymethyl)propane-1,3-diol.
$C_4H_{11}NO_3 = 121.1$.
CAS — 77-86-1.
ATC — B05BB03; B05XX02.
Pharmacopoeias. In Eur. (see p.vi) and US.

Pharmacopoeial description

Ph. Eur.: A white crystalline powder or colourless crystals. Freely soluble in water; sparingly soluble in alcohol; very slightly soluble in ethyl acetate. A 5% solution in water has a pH of 10.0 to 11.5.

USP 25: A white, crystalline powder having a slight characteristic odour. Soluble 1 in 1.8 of water and 1 in 45.5 of alcohol; freely soluble in low-molecular-weight aliphatic alcohols, practically insoluble in carbon tetrachloride, in chloroform, and in benzene. pH of a 5% solution in water is between 10.0 and 11.5. Store in airtight containers.

Adverse Effects and Precautions

Great care must be taken to avoid extravasation at the injection site as solutions may cause tissue damage. Local irritation may follow administration and venospasm and phlebitis have occurred.

Respiratory depression and hypoglycaemia may occur and mechanical ventilation may be required. Trometamol is contra-indicated in anuria and uraemia, and should be administered cautiously in patients with renal impairment as hyperkalaemia has been reported in such patients. Trometamol is not recommended for use in patients with respiratory acidosis alone. If it is used in patients with respiratory acidosis accompanying metabolic acidosis, ventilation should be maintained mechanically. Trometamol is contra-indicated in chronic respiratory acidosis.

Blood concentrations of bicarbonate, glucose, and electrolytes, partial pressure of carbon dioxide, and blood pH should be monitored during infusion of trometamol.

Uses and Administration

Trometamol is an organic amine proton acceptor which is used as an alkalinising agent in the treatment of metabolic acidosis (p.1180). It also acts as a weak osmotic diuretic. Trometamol is mainly used during cardiac bypass surgery and during cardiac arrest. It may also be used to reduce the acidity of citrated blood for use in bypass surgery.

The dose used should be the minimum required to increase the pH of the blood to within normal limits and is based on the body-weight and the base deficit. Trometamol is administered by slow intravenous infusion as a 0.3M solution.

Trometamol citrate is given by mouth for the management of urinary calculi and acidosis.

Trometamol acephyllinate and trometamol thioctate have also been used.

◊ References.

1. Nahas GG, *et al.* Guidelines for the treatment of acidaemia with THAM. *Drugs* 1998; **55:** 191–224.

Preparations

USP 25: Tromethamine for Injection.

Proprietary Preparations (details are given in Part 3)
Aust.: Tris; *Austral.:* Tham; *Fr.:* Thamacetat†; *Ger.:* Pleomix-Alpha; Tham; Thiectacid; Tris; Tromlipon; *Ital.:* Thamesol; *Swed.:* Addex-THAM.

Multi-ingredient: *Fr.:* Alcaphor; *Ger.:* Complete†; *Israel:* Complete All-In-One; *Norw.:* Tribonat; *Spain:* Sugarceton†; *Swed.:* Tribonat; *Switz.:* Saltrates.

Trypsin (3751-p)

Trypsin (BAN).
CAS — 9002-07-7.
ATC — B06AA07; D03BA01.
Pharmacopoeias. In Chin., Eur. (see p.vi), and US.

Pharmacopoeial description

Ph. Eur.: A proteolytic enzyme obtained by the activation of trypsinogen extracted from mammalian pancreas. It has an activity of not less than 0.5 microkatals per mg, calculated with reference to the dried substance. A white or almost white, crystalline or amorphous powder; the amorphous form is hygroscopic. Sparingly soluble in water. A 1% solution in water has a pH of 3.0 to 6.0. Solutions have a maximum stability at pH 3 and a maximum activity at pH 8. Store at 2° to 8° in airtight containers. Protect from light.

USP 25: A proteolytic enzyme crystallised from an extract of the pancreas gland of the ox. It contains not less than 2500 USP units in each mg, calculated on the dried basis. A white to yellowish-white, odourless, crystalline or amorphous powder. Store in airtight containers at temperature not exceeding 40°.

Profile

Trypsin is a proteolytic enzyme that has been applied for the debridement of wounds. It has also been taken by mouth, usually in combination with chymotrypsin (p.1595), and sometimes with antibacterial or other drugs, for its supposed benefit in relieving oedema and inflammation associated with infection or trauma. Trypsin solutions have been inhaled for the liquefaction of viscous sputum, and trypsin is also an ingredient of mixtures intended to relieve various gastrointestinal disorders. Trypsin has been used in oncology in a combination preparation with chymotrypsin and papain (see under Uses and Administration of Papain, p.1648).

Hypersensitivity reactions may occasionally occur.

Preparations

USP 25: Crystallized Trypsin for Inhalation Solution.

Proprietary Preparations (details are given in Part 3)
Multi-ingredient: *Aust.:* Leukase; Leukase-Kegel; Phlogenzym; Wobenzym; *Braz.:* Parenzyme; Parenzyme Ampicilina; Parenzyme Tetraciclina; Probenzima Ampicilina; Probenzima Analgesico; *Fr.:* Alphintern†; Ribatran; *Ger.:* Enzym-Wied; Hevert Enzym Novo†; Mulsal N; Phlogenzym; Wobe-Mugos E; Wobe-Mugos Th; Wobenzym N; *Ital.:* Essen Enzimatico; *Mex.:* Ochozim; Phlogenzym; Wobenzym; *Port.:* Chimar; *Spain:* Bristaciclina Dental; Dertrase; Dosil Enzimatico; Doxiten Enzimatico; Duo Gobens; Epixian†; Kanapomada; Naso Pekamin; Oxidermiol Enzima; Quimodril; Solupen Enzimatico; *USA:* Dermuspray; Granulderm; Granulex; GranuMed.

Tuberculins (8024-k)

Pharmacopoeias. In Eur. (see p.vi) and US.

Pharmacopoeial description

Ph. Eur.: Old Tuberculin for Human Use consists of a filtrate, concentrated by heating, containing the soluble products of the culture and lysis of one or more strains of *Mycobacterium tuberculosis* and/or *M. bovis*. It contains a suitable preservative that does not give rise to false-positive reactions. In concentrated form, it is a transparent, viscous, yellow or brown liquid. Protect from light.

Tuberculin Purified Protein Derivative for Human Use is a preparation obtained by precipitation from the heated products of the culture and lysis of *Mycobacterium tuberculosis* and/or *M. bovis*. It contains a suitable preservative that does not give rise to false-positive reactions. It is a colourless or pale yellow liquid; the diluted preparation may be a freeze-dried powder which upon dissolution gives a colourless or pale yellow liquid. Protect from light.

USP 25: Tuberculin is a sterile solution derived from the concentrated, soluble products of growth of the tubercle bacillus (*Mycobacterium tuberculosis* or *M. bovis*) prepared in a special medium. It is provided either as Old Tuberculin, a culture filtrate adjusted to the standard potency by the addition of glycerol and isotonic sodium chloride solution, or as Purified Protein Derivative (PPD), a further purified protein fraction. Store at 2° to 8°.

Adverse Effects

Pain and pruritus may occur at the injection site, occasionally with vesiculation, ulceration, or necrosis in highly sensitive persons. Granuloma has been reported.

Nausea, headache, dizziness, malaise, rash, urticaria, oedema, and pyrexia have been reported occasionally. There have been rare reports of lymphangitis.

Hypersensitivity. There are rare reports,[1-3] occasionally fatal,[1] of severe anaphylactic or anaphylactoid reactions to tuberculin.

1. DiMaio VJM, Froede RC. Allergic reactions to the tine test. *JAMA* 1975; **233**: 769.
2. Spiteri MA, *et al.* Life threatening reaction to tuberculin testing. *BMJ* 1986; **293**: 243–4.
3. Wright DN, *et al.* Systemic and local allergic reactions to the tine test purified protein derivative. *JAMA* 1989; **262**: 2999–3000.

Lymphangitis. Lymphangitis has been reported on 5 occasions after the Mantoux test and on 7 occasions after the Heaf test.[1] However, it was noted that performance of a tuberculin test may have been inappropriate in some of these patients, particularly older subjects and those with evidence of healed tuberculous lesions.[2]

1. Morrison JB. Lymphangitis after tuberculin tests. *BMJ* 1984; **289**: 413.
2. Festenstein F. Lymphangitis after tuberculin tests. *BMJ* 1984; **289**: 625–6.

Precautions
Tuberculin should be given with caution to patients who have, or are suspected of having, active tuberculosis; it has been suggested that severe local reactions may occur in patients with active tuberculosis, whereas sensitivity to tuberculin may be diminished in patients with severe overwhelming infection. Sensitivity to tuberculin may also be diminished in the following conditions: viral or severe bacterial infection including HIV infection and infectious mononucleosis; neoplastic disease particularly lymphoma; sarcoidosis; corticosteroid or immunosuppressive therapy; recent administration of live virus vaccines; ultraviolet light treatment; chronic renal failure; dehydration; and malnutrition.

Tuberculins may be adsorbed onto the surface of syringes and should therefore be administered immediately.

Uses and Administration
Tuberculin skin tests are used to detect tuberculoprotein hypersensitivity when BCG vaccination is being considered or as an aid to diagnosis of tuberculosis. A person showing a specific sensitivity to tuberculin is considered to have been infected with the tubercle bacillus, though the infection may be inactive. Administration of tuberculin for sensitivity testing is by intradermal injection (as in the Mantoux test) or by multiple-puncture devices (such as the Heaf test or tine tests). The term tine test is generally used for disposable multiple-puncture devices coated with dried old tuberculin or purified protein derivative. However, some consider tine tests to be unreliable and they are not recommended for use in the UK.

In the UK, it is recommended that tuberculin testing should always be performed, except in neonates, when BCG vaccination is being considered; either the Mantoux test or the Heaf test is recommended.

For a routine **Mantoux** test, 0.1 mL (10 units) of a diluted solution of tuberculin purified protein derivative (PPD), containing 100 units per mL, is injected intradermally. A positive and a strongly positive result are considered to consist of palpable induration of at least 5 mm and 15 mm respectively in diameter; the results should be read after 48 to 72 hours but may, if necessary, be read for up to 96 hours after the test. If a patient is suspected of having tuberculosis or is known to be hypersensitive to tuberculin, 0.1 mL (1 unit) of a solution of tuberculin PPD containing 10 units per mL should be used. A solution containing 1000 units per mL is also available; it may be used if there is doubt about interpretation when the 100 units per mL solution is used.

For the **Heaf** test, a solution of tuberculin purified protein derivative, containing 100 000 units per mL, is used. The solution is applied to the forearm and a multiple-puncture gun (Heaf gun) is used; a puncture of 1 mm depth is recommended for children under 2 years of age and a puncture of 2 mm for older children and adults. Results may be read 3 to 10 days after the test and the reaction graded 0 to 4 according to the degree of induration. No induration at the puncture sites (grade 0) or discrete induration at 4 or more needle sites (grade 1) indicate a negative reaction. Positive results are: an indurated ring formed by confluent papules with a clear centre (grade 2); one uniform circle of induration 5 to 10 mm wide (grade 3); solid induration over 10 mm wide, possibly with accompanying vesiculation or ulceration (grade 4). Grade 3 and 4 reactions are regarded as strongly positive equivalent to an induration of 15 mm or more in the Mantoux test. In individuals with grade 1 reactions who have not previously received BCG vaccination, the reaction is not usually related to infection with *Mycobacterium tuberculosis* and these patients may be offered BCG vaccination. Patients with a grade 2 reaction or more (or an induration of 5 to 14 mm in the Mantoux test) are considered to be hypersensitive to tuberculoprotein and should not be vaccinated. Investigation for the presence of active tuberculosis is generally only indicated for patients showing a strongly positive reaction to a Mantoux or Heaf test. However, there are many factors that should be considered when interpreting the results of a tuberculin skin test; in addition to those listed under Precautions (see above), there are the effects of previous BCG vaccination, repeated tuberculin testing, and age. In some areas, a positive reaction may

be a result of cross-sensitivity of the test to non-tuberculous mycobacteria (see below).

In some other countries the population tested, the procedures used, and grading of reactions may differ slightly from that outlined above.

Tuberculins are also used, in conjunction with other antigens, to assess the status of cell-mediated immunity (see Anergy Testing, below).

Anergy testing. Patients with HIV infection are at an increased risk of developing tuberculosis but often show a diminished reactivity to antigens (anergy), making the interpretation of negative tuberculin skin tests difficult. Anergy testing has therefore been recommended in patients with HIV infection when tuberculin testing is used in the diagnosis of tuberculosis. However, the Centers for Disease Control (CDC) in the USA[1] no longer recommend routine anergy testing in HIV patients because of problems with standardisation and reproducibility of the test, amongst other factors limiting the test's usefulness. They do suggest, however, that anergy testing may be of benefit in guiding individual therapeutic decisions in selected situations. In general, the CDC recommend two additional skin test antigens, *Candida* and mumps, in conjunction with tuberculin purified protein derivative. The test antigens are given concurrently with tuberculin, usually by the Mantoux method (see above). Other antigens may be administered, and tetanus antigens are frequently used for anergy testing. In some cases more than two control antigens may be required to avoid misclassifying immunocompetent patients as anergic. Variations on the usual definitions of positive and negative response to the Mantoux test have also been employed.

1. Centers for Disease Control. Anergy skin testing and preventive therapy for HIV-infected persons: revised recommendations. *MMWR* 1997; **46** (RR-15): 1–10.

Non-tuberculous mycobacterial infection. The tuberculin skin test is not specific for *Mycobacterium tuberculosis*, but can also represent a cross-reaction caused by antigens on other non-tuberculous mycobacteria. Re-examination[1] of results from children with non-tuberculous mycobacterial infection concluded that the avian Mantoux test (avian tuberculin purified protein derivative (PPD) prepared from *M. avium*) was more sensitive than the human Mantoux test (tuberculin PPD prepared from *M. tuberculosis*) in the detection of non-tuberculous mycobacteria in regions with a low incidence of tuberculosis, and may be a useful aid to differential diagnosis in areas where tuberculosis is prevalent.

1. Daley AJ, Isaacs D. Differential avian and human tuberculin skin testing in non-tuberculous mycobacterial infection. *Arch Dis Child* 1999; **80**: 377–9.

Malignant disease. Benefit has been reported[1] in 2 patients with adult T-cell leukaemia/lymphoma predominantly involving the skin following local treatment with tuberculin purified protein derivative.

1. Kanekura T, *et al.* Purified protein derivative treatment for skin lesions of adult T-cell leukaemia/lymphoma. *Br J Dermatol* 1999; **140**: 767–8.

Preparations
Ph. Eur.: Old Tuberculin for Human Use; Tuberculin Purified Protein Derivative for Human Use;
USP 25: Tuberculin.

Proprietary Preparations (details are given in Part 3)
Aust.: Monotest; *Belg.:* Monovacc-Test; *Braz.:* Multitest; *Canad.:* Tubersol; *Fr.:* Monotest; Neotest†; *Ger.:* Tubergen-Test; *Ital.:* Biocine-Test PPD; Monotest; *NZ:* Tubersol; *S.Afr.:* Biocine Test; Japan Freeze-Dried Tuberculin; Monotest; PPD Tine Test†; *Spain:* Tubersol PPD; *Swed.:* Monotest; Rhoditest-Tuberkulin†; *USA:* Aplisol; Aplitest; Mono-Vacc Test (O.T.); Tine Test PPD; Tubersol.

Multi-ingredient: *Aust.:* Immognost†; Multitest; *Austral.:* Multitest CMI; *Belg.:* Multitest†; *Canad.:* Multitest CMI; *Fr.:* Multitest IMC; *Ger.:* Immognost†; Multitest; *Israel:* Multitest CMI; *Ital.:* Multitest IMC; *Neth.:* Multitest CMI; *NZ:* Multitest CMI; *S.Afr.:* Multitest CMI; *Spain:* Multitest IMC; *USA:* Multitest CMI†.

Tucaresol (11118-g)
Tucaresol (BAN, rINN).

BW-589C; 589C; 589C80. α-(2-Formyl-3-hydroxyphenoxy)-*p*-toluic acid.
$C_{15}H_{12}O_5 = 272.3$.
CAS — 84290-27-7.

Profile
Tucaresol is reported to interact with haemoglobin to increase oxygen affinity. It has been investigated as an oral drug for the treatment of sickle-cell disease (p.717). Tucaresol is also reported to have immunostimulant properties and is under investigation in HIV infection and hepatitis B. Hypersensitivity reactions have occurred.

◊ References.
1. Rolan PE, *et al.* The pharmacokinetics, tolerability and pharmacodynamics of tucaresol (589C80; 4[2-formyl-3-hydroxyphenoxymethyl]benzoic acid), a potential anti-sickling agent, following oral administration to healthy subjects. *Br J Clin Pharmacol* 1993; **35**: 419–25.

2. Rolan PE, *et al.* Pharmacokinetics and pharmacodynamics of tucaresol, an antisickling agent, in healthy volunteers. *Br J Clin Pharmacol* 1995; **39**: 375–80.
3. Peck RW, *et al.* Effect of food and gender on the pharmacokinetics of tucaresol in healthy volunteers. *Br J Clin Pharmacol* 1998; **46**: 83–6.

Tuftsin (1329-n)
N^2-[1-(N^2-L-threonyl-L-lysyl)-L-prolyl]-L-arginine.
$C_{21}H_{40}N_8O_6 = 500.6$.
CAS — 9063-57-4.

Profile
Tuftsin is a naturally occurring tetrapeptide and has been investigated as the acetate for its immunostimulant activity.

Turpentine Oil (4720-s)
Aetheroleum Terebinthinae; Esencia de Trementina; Essence de Térébenthine; Oleum Terebinthinae; Oleum Terebinthinae Depuratum; Rectified Turpentine Oil; Spirits of Turpentine.
Pharmacopoeias. In *Aust., Br., Chin., Fr., Jpn,* and *Swiss.*

Pharmacopoeial description
BP 2001: A clear bright colourless liquid, visibly free from water, with a characteristic odour, obtained by distillation from the oleoresin obtained from various species of *Pinus* and rectified. Soluble 1 in 7 of alcohol (90%) and 1 in 3 of alcohol (96%). Store in well-filled containers at a temperature not exceeding 25°. Protect from light.

Adverse Effects
In poisoning with turpentine oil there may be local burning and gastrointestinal upset, coughing and choking, pulmonary oedema, excitement, coma, fever, tachycardia, liver damage, haematuria, and albuminuria. Fatalities have occurred.

The application to the skin of liniments containing turpentine oil may cause irritation and absorption of large amounts may cause some of the effects listed above. Hypersensitivity reactions and local irritation have been reported.

Uses and Administration
Turpentine oil is widely used as a solvent. It is applied topically as a rubefacient. It is an ingredient of many preparations used in respiratory-tract disorders, but is now judged to be neither safe nor effective.

Preparations
BP 2001: White Liniment.

Proprietary Preparations (details are given in Part 3)
Fr.: Ozothine; *Ger.:* Terpestrol H.

Multi-ingredient: *Aust.:* Aciforin; Baby Luuf; Bronchostop; Carl Baders Divinal; Dolex; Dracodermalin; Emser Nasensalbe; Ilon Abszess†; Kinder Erkaltungsbalsam; Kinder Luuf; Leukona-Rheuma-Bad; Luuf Balsam; Makatussin†; Mayfit chronisch†; Pe-Ce; Piniment; Rubriment; Salhumin; Scottopect; Tetesept; Trauma-warmend; Traumasalbe; Tussamag; Vulpuran; Wick Vaporub; *Austral.:* Capsolin; Goanna Heat Cream; Goanna Liniment; Goanna Salve; Logicin Chest Rub; Relief Rub; Turpentine White Liniment; Vicks Vaporub; *Belg.:* Reflexspray; Vicks Vaporub; *Braz.:* A Curitybina; Analgen; Benegel; Frixopel; Gelflex; Gelofrix; Gelogel; Gelol; Geloneveral; Massageol; Massubal; Mialgex; Oleo Eletrico; Prontoalivio; Salimetin; Sanador; Traumac; Traumagel; Vick Vaporub; *Canad.:* Cal Mo Dol; Cerumol; *Fin.:* Vicks Vaporub; *Fr.:* Dinacode; Huile de Haarlem†; Lao-Dal†; Lumbalgine; Ozothine; Ozothine a la Diprophylline; Vicks Vaporub; *Ger.:* Angocin percutan; Bartelin N; Cuxaflex N†; Divinal-Broncho-Balsam†; Em-eukal; Emser Nasensalbe N; Erkaltungsbalsam-ratiopharm E Salbe; Fibraflex†; Hevertopect; Hoemarin Rheuma†; Ilon Abszess; Kneipp Erkaltungs-Balsam N; Kneipp Tonikum-Bad Fichtennadel-Aquasan†; Leukona-Rheuma-Bad N; Leukona-Rheumasalbe; Logomed Erkaltungs-Balsam†; Ozothin; Plantmobil; Rheumaliment N; Schupps Latschenkiefer Olbad†; Trauma-Salbe Rodler 302 N; Wick Vaporub; *It.:* Cerumol†; Vicks Vaporub†; *Israel:* Cerumol; Deep Heat Rub; Mento-O-Cap†; *Ital.:* Capsolin; Vicks Vaporub; *Neth.:* Vicks Vaporub; *NZ:* Vicks Vaporub; *Port.:* Freimax; Lauromentol; Lecia; Linimento de Sloan; *S.Afr.:* Chisit†; Respisniffers; Warm-Up†; *Spain:* Dologex; Embrocacion Gras; Killpan; Linimento Klari; Linimento Sloan; Masagil; Otocerum; Pomada Revulsiva†; Reflex; Termosan; *Swed.:* Sloan's liniment†; Vicks Vaporub; *Switz.:* Alginex; Artragel; Baume du Chalet; Caprisana†; Capsolin†; Cerumenol; Embropax; Kernosan Huile de Massage†; Liberol†; Makatussin; Massorax; Olbas; Pinimenthol; Roliwol†; Schwefelbad Dr Klopfer†; Sloan Baume†; Sloan Liniment†; Tumarol; Vicks Vaporub N; *Thai.:* Stopain; Tiffyrub; *UK:* BN; Boots Vapour Rub; Deep Heat Rub; Dragon Balm; Ellimans; Goddards White Oil Embrocation; Gonne Balm; Modern Herbals Muscular Pain; Nasciodine; Nine Rubbing Oils; Tixycolds Cold and Hayfever; Vicks Vaporub; Waxwane; Woodwards Baby Chest Rub.

Tyramine Hydrochloride (2153-n)
p-Tyramine Hydrochloride; Tyrosamine Hydrochloride. 4-Hydroxyphenethylamine hydrochloride; 4-(2-Aminoethyl)phenol hydrochloride.
$C_8H_{11}NO,HCl = 173.6$.
CAS — 51-67-2 (tyramine); 60-19-5 (tyramine hydrochloride).

Profile
Tyramine hydrochloride is a sympathomimetic with indirect ef-

fects on adrenergic receptors. It has been given by mouth or injection in the tyramine pressor test in the investigation of monoamine oxidase inhibitory activity or of amine uptake blocking activity as well as of various physiological and diseased states.

It has also been tried in the diagnosis of migraine and phaeochromocytoma.

The hazards of taking foods rich in tyramine while under treatment with MAOIs are described in the chapter on Antidepressants (see Phenelzine, p.305).

Preparations
Proprietary Preparations (details are given in Part 3)
Multi-ingredient: Ger.: Mydrial-Atropin.

Ubidecarenone (14000-c)
Ubidecarenone (BAN, rINN).

Coenzyme Q10; Ubidecarenonum; Ubiquinone-10. 2-Deca(3-methylbut-2-enylene)-5,6-dimethoxy-3-methyl-p-benzoquinone.
$C_{59}H_{90}O_4 = 863.3$.
CAS — 303-98-0.
ATC — C01EB09.
Pharmacopoeias. In Eur. (see p.vi) and Jpn. Also in USNF.

Pharmacopoeial description
Ph. Eur.: A yellow or orange crystalline powder. It gradually decomposes and darkens on exposure to light. M.p. about 48°. Practically insoluble in water; very slightly soluble in dehydrated alcohol; soluble in acetone. Store in airtight containers. Protect from light.

USNF 20: A yellow to orange, crystalline powder. M.p. about 48°. Practically insoluble in water; very slightly soluble in dehydrated alcohol; soluble in ether.

Profile
Ubidecarenone is a naturally occurring coenzyme involved in electron transport in the mitochondria. It is claimed to be a free radical scavenger and to have antioxidant and membrane stabilising properties. It has been given by mouth, in conjunction with standard treatment, in cardiovascular disorders including mild or moderate heart failure. It has also been tried in other conditions associated with coenzyme deficiency. Ubidecarenone is under investigation for the management of Huntington's chorea.

◊ For a report of the use of ubidecarenone in muscle weakness, see Effects on Skeletal Muscle, under Lovastatin, p.923.

◊ References.
1. Greenberg S, Frishman WH. Co-enzyme Q10: a new drug for cardiovascular disease. *J Clin Pharmacol* 1990; **30**: 596–608.
2. Spigset O. Reduced effect of warfarin caused by ubidecarenone. *Lancet* 1994; **344**: 1372–3.
3. Garcia Silva MT, et al. Improvement of refractory sideroblastic anaemia with ubidecarenone. *Lancet* 1994; **343**: 1039.
4. Gattermann N, et al. No improvement of refractory sideroblastic anaemia with ubidecarenone. *Lancet* 1995; **345**: 1121–2.
5. Nagao T, et al. Treatment of warfarin-induced hair loss with ubidecarenone. *Lancet* 1995; **346**: 1104–5.
6. Pepping J. Coenzyme Q10. *Am J Health-Syst Pharm* 1999; **56**: 519–21.
7. Khatta M, et al. The effect of coenzyme Q10 in patients with congestive heart failure. *Ann Intern Med* 2000; **132**: 636–40.

Preparations
USNF 20: Ubidecarenone Capsules; Ubidecarenone Tablets.

Proprietary Preparations (details are given in Part 3)
Hong Kong: Eiquinon; Salcotan; **Ital.:** Caomet; Cardioton; Coedieci; Decafar; Decorenone; Dymion†; Iuvacor; Miodene; Miotyn; Mitocor; Roburis; Ubicarden†; Ubicardio; Ubicor; Ubidenone; Ubidex; Ubifactor; Ubilab†; Ubimaior; Ubisint†; Ubiten; Ubivis; **Jpn.:** Neuquinon; **Port.:** Q 10; Ubenzima; Ubicondrial; **Thai.:** BioQuinone; Decaquinon; **UK:** Co-Q-10; **USA:** Co-Q-10; CoQuinone.

Multi-ingredient: Ital.: Agedin Plus; Ener-E; **UK:** Efamol Plus Coenzyme Q10; Red Kooga Co-Q-10 and Ginseng.

Ulinastatin (2998-d)
Ulinastatin (rINN).
Pharmacopoeias. In Jpn.

Profile
Ulinastatin is a glycoprotein proteolytic enzyme inhibitor isolated from human urine. It has been given by injection in acute pancreatitis (p.1646) and in acute circulatory insufficiency.

◊ References.
1. Ohwada M, et al. New endoscopic treatment for chronic pancreatitis, using contrast media containing ulinastatin and prednisolone. *J Gastroenterol* 1997; **32**: 216–21.

Preparations
Proprietary Preparations (details are given in Part 3)
Jpn.: Miraclid.

Urazamide (14003-t)
5-Aminoimidazole-4-carboxamide ureidosuccinate.
$C_9H_{14}N_6O_6 = 302.2$.

Profile
Urazamide has been used in the treatment of hepatic disorders in doses of 400 to 800 mg daily by mouth. It has also been administered by intramuscular and intravenous injection.

Preparations
Proprietary Preparations (details are given in Part 3)
Ital.: Carbaica.

Uridine (14004-x)
Uracil Riboside. 1-β-D-Ribofuranosyluracil; 1-β-D-Ribofuranosylpyrimidine-2,4(1H,3H)-dione.
$C_9H_{12}N_2O_6 = 244.2$.
CAS — 58-96-8.

Profile
Uridine is one of the four nucleosides present in ribonucleic acid. Uridine has been used in patients with hereditary orotic aciduria.

◊ References.
1. Girot R, et al. Cellular immune deficiency in two siblings with hereditary orotic aciduria. *N Engl J Med* 1983; **308**: 700–4.
2. Becroft DMO, et al. Absence of immune deficiency in hereditary orotic aciduria. *N Engl J Med* 1984; **310**: 1333–4.

Preparations
Proprietary Preparations (details are given in Part 3)
Multi-ingredient: Aust.: Laevadosin; Vitasic; **Fr.:** Vitacic; **Ital.:** Centrum; Cituridina; For Liver†; **Spain:** Inexfal; Prodessal.

Uridine Triphosphate (14005-r)
Uridine Triphosphoric Acid; UTP. Uridine 5'-(tetrahydrogen triphosphate).
$C_9H_{15}N_2O_{15}P_3 = 484.1$.
CAS — 63-39-8.

Profile
Uridine triphosphate has been investigated for the treatment of cystic fibrosis (p.117). It has also been claimed to be of value in muscular atrophy and muscular weakness.

◊ Uridine triphosphate has been reported to be effective in stimulating chloride secretion in the nasal epithelium of patients with cystic fibrosis.[1] It has been suggested that correction of the ion-transport abnormalities in cystic fibrosis patients may reduce the viscosity of the secretions in the early stages of the disease,[2] and selected nucleotides such as uridine triphosphate should be investigated as therapeutic agents.[1]

The suggestion that uridine might produce improvement in patients with galactosaemia has not been confirmed.[3]

1. Knowles MR, et al. Activation by extracellular nucleotides of chloride secretion in the airway epithelia of patients with cystic fibrosis. *N Engl J Med* 1991; **325**: 533–8.
2. Davis PB. Cystic fibrosis from bench to bedside. *N Engl J Med* 1991; **325**: 575–77.
3. Holton JB, Leonard JV. Clouds still gathering over galactosaemia. *Lancet* 1994; **344**: 1242–3.

Preparations
Proprietary Preparations (details are given in Part 3)
Multi-ingredient: Ital.: Fosfoutipi Vitaminico; **Spain:** Taurobetina.

Ursodeoxycholic Acid (3753-w)
Ursodeoxycholic Acid (BAN, rINN).
Acidum Ursodeoxycholicum; UDCA; Ursodesoxycholic Acid; Ursodiol (USAN). 3α,7β-Dihydroxy-5β-cholan-24-oic acid.
$C_{24}H_{40}O_4 = 392.6$.
CAS — 128-13-2.
ATC — A05AA02.
Pharmacopoeias. In Chin., Eur. (see p.vi), Jpn, and US.

Pharmacopoeial description
Ph. Eur.: A white or almost white powder. Very slightly soluble in water; freely soluble in alcohol; slightly soluble in acetone and in dichloromethane.

USP 25: A white or almost white, crystalline powder. Practically insoluble in water; freely soluble in alcohol and in glacial acetic acid; sparingly soluble in chloroform; slightly soluble in ether. Store in airtight containers.

Stability. References.
1. Mallett MS, et al. Stability of ursodiol 25 mg/mL in an extemporaneously prepared oral liquid. *Am J Health-Syst Pharm* 1997; **54**: 1401–4.

Adverse Effects and Precautions
Ursodeoxycholic acid may cause nausea, vomiting, and other gastrointestinal disturbances but diarrhoea is reported to occur less frequently than with chenodeoxycholic acid. Increased liver enzyme values are also less likely. Pruritus may occur. Treatment with ursodeoxycholic acid may cause more calcification of cholesterol stones than chenodeoxycholic acid.

Ursodeoxycholic acid should not be administered to patients with chronic liver disease, peptic ulcer disease, or inflammatory bowel disease. It is ineffective for the dissolution of calcified and pigment gallstones and is of no value in patients without a patent and functioning gallbladder. Its use should be avoided in pregnancy.

Interactions
Ursodeoxycholic acid should not be used with drugs, such as oestrogenic hormones, that increase bile cholesterol. Concomitant administration with bile-acid binding drugs including antacids, charcoal, and colestyramine should be avoided since this may reduce the effectiveness of therapy with ursodeoxycholic acid.

Pharmacokinetics
Ursodeoxycholic acid is absorbed from the gastrointestinal tract and undergoes enterohepatic recycling. It is partly conjugated in the liver before being excreted into the bile. Under the influence of intestinal bacteria the free and conjugated forms undergo 7α-dehydroxylation to lithocholic acid, some of which is excreted directly in the faeces and the rest absorbed and mainly conjugated and sulfated by the liver before excretion in the faeces. However, in comparison with chenodeoxycholic acid, less ursodeoxycholic acid undergoes such bacterial degradation.

◊ References.
1. Crosignani A, et al. Clinical pharmacokinetics of therapeutic bile acids. *Clin Pharmacokinet* 1996; **30**: 333–58.

Uses and Administration
Ursodeoxycholic acid is a naturally occurring bile acid (see p.1585) present in small quantities in human bile. Ursodeoxycholic acid suppresses the synthesis and secretion of cholesterol by the liver and inhibits intestinal absorption of cholesterol. It is used for the dissolution of cholesterol-rich gallstones in patients with functioning gallbladders (see below). The usual dose is 6 to 12 mg per kg body-weight daily as a single bedtime dose or in 2 or 3 divided doses; obese patients may require up to 15 mg per kg daily. The daily dose may be divided unequally and the larger dose given before bedtime to counteract the increase in biliary cholesterol concentration seen overnight. The time required for dissolution of gallstones is likely to be between 6 and 24 months depending on stone size and composition. Treatment should be continued for 3 to 4 months after radiological disappearance of the stones. Ursodeoxycholic acid has also been given in reduced doses in combination with chenodeoxycholic acid (p.1594).

Ursodeoxycholic acid is also used in primary biliary cirrhosis. The usual dose is 10 to 15 mg per kg daily in 2 to 4 divided doses.

Ursodeoxycholic acid has been tried in the treatment of primary sclerosing cholangitis.

The more hydrophilic derivative, tauroursodeoxycholic acid, has also been used.

Chronic liver disease. The use of ursodeoxycholic acid in chronic liver diseases has been summarised.[1-3] Although used to slow disease progression in primary biliary cirrhosis (p.501) there have been differing opinions as to its value, with a meta-analysis[4] failing to show any reduction in the rate of liver transplantation or death with ursodeoxycholic acid therapy. Response has also been reported in liver disease in cystic fibrosis,[5-7] cholestasis associated with pregnancy,[8] sclerosing cholangitis,[9] chronic active hepatitis,[10] and viral hepatitis.[11,12] Ursodeoxycholic acid has also shown some promise in the treatment of nonalcoholic steatohepatitis,[13] but randomised, controlled studies are required to confirm this. There has also been some interest in the use of ursodeoxycholic acid to treat refractory graft-versus-host disease of the liver in transplant patients,[14] and possibly as an adjuvant to immunosuppressant therapy[15-17] after orthotopic liver transplantation (p.504).

1. de Caestecker JS, et al. Ursodeoxycholic acid in chronic liver disease. *Gut* 1991; **32**: 1061–5.
2. Rubin RA, et al. Ursodiol for hepatobiliary disorders. *Ann Intern Med* 1994; **121**: 207–18.
3. Kowdley KV. Ursodeoxycholic acid therapy in hepatobiliary disease. *Am J Med* 2000; **108**: 481–6.
4. Goulis J, et al. Randomised controlled trials of ursodeoxycholic-acid therapy for primary biliary cirrhosis: a meta-analysis. *Lancet* 1999; **354**: 1053–60.
5. Colombo C, et al. Effects of ursodeoxycholic acid therapy for liver disease associated with cystic fibrosis. *J Pediatr* 1990; **117**: 482–9.
6. Cotting J, et al. Effects of ursodeoxycholic acid treatment on nutrition and liver function in patients with cystic fibrosis and longstanding cholestasis. *Gut* 1990; **31**: 918–21.
7. Scher H, et al. Ursodeoxycholic acid improves cholestasis in infants with cystic fibrosis. *Ann Pharmacother* 1997; **31**: 1003–5.
8. Palma J, et al. Ursodeoxycholic acid in the treatment of cholestasis of pregnancy: a randomized, double-blind study controlled with placebo. *J Hepatol* 1997; **27**: 1022–8.
9. Lindor KD, et al. Ursodiol for primary sclerosing cholangitis. *N Engl J Med* 1997; **336**: 691–5.
10. Rolandi E, et al. Effects of ursodeoxycholic acid (UDCA) on serum liver damage indices in patients with chronic active hepatitis: a double-blind controlled study. *Eur J Clin Pharmacol* 1991; **40**: 473–6.
11. Puoti C, et al. Ursodeoxycholic acid and chronic hepatitis C infection. *Lancet* 1993; **341**: 1413–14.
12. Angelico M, et al. Recombinant interferon-α and ursodeoxycholic acid versus interferon-α alone in the treatment of chronic hepatitis C: a randomized clinical trial with long-term follow-up. *Am J Gastroenterol* 1995; **90**: 263–9.

The symbol † denotes a preparation no longer actively marketed

13. Laurin J, *et al.* Ursodeoxycholic acid or clofibrate in the treatment of non-alcohol-induced steatohepatitis: a pilot study. *Hepatology* 1996; **23:** 1464–7.
14. Fried RH, *et al.* Ursodeoxycholic acid treatment of refractory chronic graft-versus-host disease of the liver. *Ann Intern Med* 1992; **116:** 624–9.
15. Persson H, *et al.* Ursodeoxycholic acid for prevention of acute rejection in liver transplant recipients. *Lancet* 1990; **ii:** 52–3.
16. Friman S, *et al.* Adjuvant treatment with ursodeoxycholic acid reduces acute rejection after liver transplantation. *Transplant Proc* 1992; **24:** 389–90.
17. Clavien P-A, *et al.* Evidence that ursodeoxycholic acid prevents steroid-resistant rejection in adult liver transplantation. *Clin Transplant* 1996; **10:** 658–62.

Gallstones. Gallstones (cholelithiasis) occur when mechanisms for the solubilisation of cholesterol or bilirubin fail or are overcome. They may be divided into those formed of pure cholesterol, which are usually solitary; pigment stones, largely made up of bilirubin or its derivatives; and mixed stones of cholesterol, bile pigment, and calcium salts, which form the great majority of cases seen in the West.

Gallstones are generally more common in women than in men. The prevalence also increases with age and obesity, although rapid weight loss as a result of dieting or surgery is associated with an increased risk.

As many as two-thirds of patients with gallstones are asymptomatic. Symptoms, when present, usually relate to the site of the stone although biliary colic is often present regardless of whether the stone is in the gallbladder or biliary tract. If the stone blocks the exit from the gallbladder, inflammation and bacterial infection may follow (acute cholecystitis), sometimes leading to perforation and subsequent peritonitis. Less commonly, obstruction of the common bile duct by gallstones (choledocholithiasis) may lead to cholestasis and jaundice; infection of the bile ducts and septicaemia may follow. Pancreatitis may also be associated with gallstone disease, and there may be an increased risk of developing malignant neoplasms of the gallbladder.

Treatment. Asymptomatic gallstones discovered during other investigations should not be treated, and even mildly symptomatic patients may be managed with analgesics and subsequent observation. More potent analgesics such as pethidine may be required in more severe cases (see Biliary and Renal Colic, p.5). In symptomatic patients the preferred treatment for gallstones is surgical removal of the gallbladder; 'keyhole surgery' (laparoscopic cholecystectomy) is associated with less postoperative morbidity than open surgery, and has largely replaced other methods of treatment.

In patients unsuited to, or unwilling to undergo, surgery for gallbladder stones, drug therapy, alone or in combination with lithotripsy, may be considered.

Administration of exogenous bile acids has been tried in an attempt to dissolve the cholesterol component of gallstones. Ursodeoxycholic acid is the drug of choice since it is more effective and is associated with fewer adverse effects than chenodeoxycholic acid. Combination therapy has also been tried but this is no more effective than ursodeoxycholic acid alone. Dissolution of gallstones is slow but can be achieved in about one-third of cases with the best results seen with small stones. However, about half of all successfully treated patients will develop further gallstones within 10 years. Studies of prophylactic bile acid therapy have mostly yielded disappointing results, although such therapy may be of benefit in patients on very-low-calorie diets, after surgery for weight loss, and in those receiving treatment with octreotide.

Somewhat larger stones may respond to extracorporeal shock-wave lithotripsy, or fluoroscopically guided laser lithotripsy, which may be more effective. Subsequent treatment with oral bile acids should be given to dissolve the stone fragments.

Another method is the direct instillation of a solvent (usually methyl *tert*-butyl ether) into the gallbladder. This dissolves stones within a matter of hours, and is effective against almost all cholesterol-based stones regardless of size and number. Care is required to avoid overflow of the solvent into the common bile duct or the duodenum, where it may cause inflammation. Other solvents, such as ethyl propionate have been investigated as potentially less toxic alternatives, and edetic acid has been suggested as a possible solvent for non-cholesterol gallstones. As with all non-surgical methods, recurrence is likely.

Patients with **stones in the common bile duct** or **acute cholecystitis** require prompt therapy because of the risk of serious complications; endoscopic sphincterotomy and physical retrieval of the stones with a basket or balloon appears to be the preferred treatment, with open surgery as an alternative. The insertion of a biliary stent to allow bile flow around the stone has been used as a temporary measure in patients with stones too large to remove by endoscopic sphincterotomy. Lithotripsy or infusion of a solvent such as monoctanoin or methyl *tert*-butyl ether are possible alternatives in patients unfit for surgery.

In patients who develop cholecystitis or cholangitis antibacterial therapy may be required (see p.115).

References.

1. Johnston DE, Kaplan MM. Pathogenesis and treatment of gallstones. *N Engl J Med* 1993; **328:** 412–21.
2. Ransohoff DF, Gracie WA. Treatment of gallstones. *Ann Intern Med* 1993; **119:** 606–19.
3. American College of Physicians. Guidelines for the treatment of gallstones. *Ann Intern Med* 1993; **119:** 620–2.
4. May GR, *et al.* Efficacy of bile acid therapy for gallstone dissolution: a meta-analysis of randomized trials. *Aliment Pharmacol Ther* 1993; **7:** 139–48.
5. Hofmann AF, *et al.* Pathogenesis and treatment of gallstones. *N Engl J Med* 1993; **328:** 1854–5.
6. Anonymous. Managing patients with gallstones. *Drug Ther Bull* 1994; **32:** 33–5.
7. Lanzini A, Northfield TC. Pharmacological treatment of gallstones: practical guidelines. *Drugs* 1994; **47:** 458–70.
8. Tait N, Little JM. The treatment of gall stones. *BMJ* 1995; **311:** 99–105.
9. Jakobs R, *et al.* Fluoroscopically guided laser lithotripsy versus extracorporeal shock wave lithotripsy for retained bile duct stones: a prospective randomised study. *Gut* 1997; **40:** 678–82.
10. Toouli J, Wright TA. Gallstones. *Med J Aust* 1998; **169:** 166–71.
11. Bateson MC. Gallbladder disease. *BMJ* 1999; **318:** 1745–8.
12. Ahmed A, *et al.* Management of gallstones and their complications. *Am Fam Physician* 2000; **61:** 1673–80.

Preparations

BP 2001: Ursodeoxycholic Acid Capsules; Ursodeoxycholic Acid Tablets;
USP 25: Ursodiol Capsules.

Proprietary Preparations (details are given in Part 3)

Aust.: Ursofalk; *Austral.:* Ursofalk; *Belg.:* Ursochol; Ursofalk; *Braz.:* Ursacol; *Canad.:* Urso; Ursofalk†; *Fin.:* Adursal; *Fr.:* Arsacol†; Delursan; Destolit†; Ursolvan; *Ger.:* Cholacid†; Cholit-Ursan; Cholofalk; UDC; Urso; Ursochol; Ursofalk; *Hong Kong:* Ursofalk; Ursolvan; Ursosan; *Irl.:* Ursofalk; *Israel:* Ursolit; *Ital.:* Biliepar; Coledos; Desocol; Desoxil; Deursil; Fraurs; Galmax; Lentorsil; Litoff; Litursol; Tauro; Tudcabil; Urdes; Ursacol; Ursilon; Ursobil; Ursodamor; Ursodiol; Ursofalk; Ursoflor; Ursolac; Ursolisin; Urson; Ursoproge; *Jpn:* Urso†; *Mex.:* Ursofalk; *Neth.:* Ursochol; Ursofalk; *NZ:* Actigall; Destolit; Ursofalk; *Port.:* Destolit; Ursofalk; *S.Afr.:* Ursotan; *Singapore:* Ursofalk; Ursolvan; *Spain:* Ursobilane; Ursochol; Ursolite; *Swed.:* Deursil; Ursochol; Ursofalk; *Switz.:* Deursil; Ursofalk; *Thai.:* Ursofalk; *UK:* Destolit; Urdox; Ursofalk; Ursogal; *USA:* Actigall; Urso.

Multi-ingredient: *Aust.:* Lithofalk; *Ger.:* Urso Mix; Ursofalk + Chenofalk; *Ital.:* Bilenor; Litobile†; *Switz.:* Lithofalk; *UK:* Combidol†; Lithofalk†.

Urtica (18427-g)

Stinging Nettle.

Pharmacopoeias. Ger. includes monographs for the leaves and root of *U. dioica*. Swiss includes a monograph for Urtica Herba.

Profile

Urtica is the dried aerial parts, leaves, or root of the stinging nettle, *Urtica dioica* (Urticaceae). It has been used in herbal medicine, mainly for urinary-tract and rheumatic disorders. *Urtica urens* has been used similarly.

Preparations

Proprietary Preparations (details are given in Part 3)

Aust.: Urtica Plus; *Braz.:* Bazoton; *Ger.:* Arthrodynat N; Bazoton; Cirkuprostan†; Cletan†; Dr Grandel Brennessel Vital Tonikum; Hostid; Kneipp Brennesselkraut Pflanzensaft Kneippianum; Kneipp Pflanzen-Dragees Brennessel; Logomed Prostata-Kapseln†; Prostaforton; Prostagalen; Prostaherb N; Prostaneurin; Prostata; Prostawern; Reumaless†; Rheuma-Hartkapseln; Rheuma-Hekt; Serless; Uriginex Urtica†; Uro-POS; Urtica Plus N†; Urticaprostat uno; Urticur†; Urtipret; Urtivit; utk; *Ital.:* Venustas Shampoo per Capelli con Forfora e/o Grassi; *Switz.:* Simic†; Valverde prostate capsules; *Thai.:* Urtipret.

Multi-ingredient: *Aust.:* Anaemodoron; Apotheker Bauer's Harntreibender Tee; Apotheker Bauer's Nieren- und Blasentee; Berggeist; Bio-Garten Tee zur Erhohung der Harnmenge; Bogumil-tassenfertiger milder Abfurtee; Brennesseltonikum; Brostalin; Ehrmann's Entschlackungstee; Florissamol; Fruhjahrs-Elixier ohne Alkohol; Harntreibender Tee; Krauterdoktor Entwasserungs-Elixier; Krauterhaus Mag Kottas Blutreinigungstee†; Krauterhaus Mag Kottas Entschlackungstee; Krauterhaus Mag Kottas Entwasserungstee; Krauterhaus Mag Kottas Fruhjahrs- und Herbstkurtee; Krautertee Nr 19; Krautertee Nr 8; Mag Doskar's Nieren-und Blasentonikum; Mag Kottas Entschlackungstee; Menodoron; Mentopin; Naturland Rheuma-Tee; Prostagutt; Prostatonin; Sidroga Stoffwechseltee; Species Carvi comp; St Radegunder Entwasserungs-Elixier; St Radegunder Entwasserungstee; Synpharma Instant-Blasen-und-Nierentee; *Austral.:* Cough Relief; Extralife Flow-Care; Infant Tonic; Irontona; Respatona Decongestant Formula; Respatona Plus Bronchial Cough Relief; Urapro; Vitatona; *Braz.:* Lactifero; Prostem Plus; *Fr.:* Lithiabyl†; Salucur; *Ger.:* Befelka-Tinktur†; Combudoron; Presselin Nieren-Blasen K 3; Prostagutt forte; Prostatin F; Salus Rheuma-Tee Krautertee Nr. 12†; Uvirgan N; Vollmers praparierter gruner; Winar; *Ital.:* Herbavit; Nosenil†; Omadine; Shamday Antiforfora; *Switz.:* Prostagutt-F; Prostatonin; Tisane Diuretique; *UK:* Fragador; Kleer; Menodoron; Savlon Natural First Aid for Burns.

Usnea Barbata (14006-f)

CAS — 125-46-2 (usnic acid).

Usnea barbata is a lichen.

Profile

Usnea barbata contains usnic acid, which is reported to have antimicrobial activity. *Usnea barbata* extract, usnic acid, and copper usnate have been used in topical preparations.

Preparations

Proprietary Preparations (details are given in Part 3)
Ger.: Dr Grandel Granobil; *Ital.:* Vidermina; Zeta N.
Multi-ingredient: *Ital.:* Aseptil; Foot Zeta; Micofoot; Neo Zeta-Foot†; Steril Zeta.

Valepotriates (14008-n)

CAS — 18296-45-2 (didrovaltrate); 18296-44-1 (valtrate); 25161-41-5 (acevaltrate).

NOTE. Acevaltrate and didrovaltrate are *rINN*; valtrate is *pINN*.

Epoxy-iridoid esters, isolated from valerian (see below). They include *didrovaltrate* (6-acetoxy-1,4a,5,6,7,7a-hexahydro-1-isovaleryloxy-4-isovaleryloxymethylcyclopenta[*c*]pyran-7-spiro-2′-oxiran, $C_{22}H_{32}O_8 = 424.5$), *valtrate* (4-acetoxymethyl-1,6-di-isovaleryloxy-1,6,7,7a-tetrahydrocyclopenta[*c*]pyran-7-spiro-2′-oxiran, $C_{22}H_{30}O_8 = 422.5$), and *acevaltrate* (4-acetoxymethyl-(1 or 6)-3-(acetoxy-3-methylbutyryloxy)-1,6,7,7a-tetrahydro-(6 or 1)-isovaleryloxy-cyclopenta[*c*]pyran-7-spiro-2′-oxiran, $C_{24}H_{32}O_{10} = 480.5$). On prolonged storage and drying they are hydrolysed to yield isovaleric acid.

Profile

A mixture stated to contain didrovaltrate, valtrate, and acevaltrate has been used as a sedative and as an anxiolytic. Concern has been expressed over the potential toxicity of valepotriates which have been reported to have cytotoxic properties *in vitro*.

Preparations

Proprietary Preparations (details are given in Part 3)
Aust.: Nervipane†; Valmane; *Braz.:* Valmane.

Valerian (14009-h)

Baldrianwurzel; Valer; Valerian Rhizome; Valerian Root; Valerianae Radix.
CAS — 8057-49-6 (valerian extract).
ATC — N05CM09.
Pharmacopoeias. In *Eur.* (see p.vi) and *Pol.* Also in *USNF*, which also includes Powdered Valerian Extract. *Jpn* has Japanese Valerian from *V. fauriei*.

Pharmacopoeial description

Ph. Eur.: The yellowish-grey to pale brownish-grey whole underground parts of *Valeriana officinalis*, including the rhizome surrounded by the roots and stolons, or by fragments of these parts. It contains not less than 0.5% v/v of essential oil for the whole drug and not less then 0.3% v/v for the cut drug, both calculated with reference to the dried drug. Protect from light.

USNF 20: The subterranean parts of *Valeriana officinalis* (Valerianaceae), including the rhizome, roots, and stolons. It contains not less than 0.5% of volatile oil and not less than 0.05% of valerenic acid, calculated on the dried basis. Store in airtight containers. Protect from light.

Profile

Valerian has sedative properties and is used as an extract, infusion, or tincture, or occasionally as the dried root, in preparations for anxiety states. It has also been used as a carminative. The odour of valerian may be removed from the skin and from hard surfaces with sodium bicarbonate.

◊ Reviews.

1. Houghton P. Valerian. *Pharm J* 1994; **253:** 95–6.
2. Houghton PJ. The scientific basis for the reputed activity of valerian. *J Pharm Pharmacol* 1999; **51:** 505–12.
3. Plushner SL. Valerian: valeriana officinalis. *Am J Health-Syst Pharm* 2000; **57:** 328–35.

Adverse effects. Four cases of liver damage[1] were reported in patients who took herbal remedies that contained valerian for stress. Cardiac complications and delirium in a 58-year-old man may have been caused by the withdrawal of prolonged therapy with a valerian root extract preparation.[2]

1. MacGregor FB, *et al.* Hepatotoxicity of herbal remedies. *BMJ* 1989; **299:** 1156–7.
2. Garges HP, *et al.* Cardiac complications and delirium associated with valerian root withdrawal. *JAMA* 1998; **280:** 1566–7.

Preparations

USNF 20: Valerian Tablets.

Proprietary Preparations (details are given in Part 3)
Aust.: Baldrinetten; Cirkulin Baldrian; Gewusst wie Beruhigungst†; *Austral.:* Herbal Sleep Formula; *Belg.:* Relaxine; Valdispert; Valerial†; *Canad.:* Nytol Natural Source; Sleep-Eze V Natural; Unisom Natural Source; *Fin.:* Valrian; *Fr.:* Relaxine; *Ger.:* Baldrianetten N†; Baldrisedon Monot†; Benedorm†; Hewedormir; Kneipp Baldrian; Kneipp Baldrian Pflanzensaft Nerventrost; Melival; Nervipan†; Recvalysat; Sedalint Baldrian; Sedonium; Valdispert; Valmane; *Israel:* Valeton; *Ital.:* Ticalma; Val-Uno; *Neth.:* Valdispert; Valmane†; *Port.:* Valdispert; *S.Afr.:* Calmettes; *Spain:* Cirkused; Tauval; Valdispert; Valeriana Orto; *Swed.:* Baldrian-Dispert; Neurol; Valerecen; *Switz.:* Baldrisedon; ReDormin; Sirop pour le sommeil; Valdispert; Valverde Sirop pour le sommeil.

Multi-ingredient: *Aust.:* Absimed; Aktiv Nerven- und Schlaftee; Aponatura Einschlaf; Bakanasan Einschlaf; Baldracin; Baldrian AMA; Baldrian Dispert Compositum; Baldrian-Elixier; Baldrian-Dispert Compositum; Baldrian-Elixier; Baldrian-Dispert Compositum; Baldriparan Beruhigungs; Beruhigungskapseln; Beruhigungstee; Bio-Garten Tee fur den Magen; Bio-Garten Tee zur Beruhigung; Bio-Garten Tropfen fur Magen und Darm; Biogelat Schlaf; Cardiofrik; Einschlafkapseln; Eryval; Hova; Kneipp Nerven- und Schlaf-Tee; Krauterdoktor Entspannungs- und Einschlaftropfen; Krauterdoktor Magen-Darmtropfen; Krauterdoktor Nerven-Tonikum; Krauterhaus Mag Kottas Nerven- und Schlaftee; Krauterhaus Mag Kottas Wechseltee; Krauterdoktor Nerven Nr 1; Krautertee Nr 124; Krautertee Nr 141; Krautertee Nr 9; Luvased; Mag Doskar's Nerventonikum; Mag Kottas Beruhigungstee; Mag Kottas Krauterexpress-Nerven-Schlaf-Tee; Mag Kottas Nerven-Beruhigungstee; Mag Kottas Schlaftee; Mag Kottas Wechseltee; Magentee; Nervendragees; Nervenruh; Nerventee; Nervifloran; Phytogran; Psychobald; Sanhelios Einschlaf; Sedogelat; Sedogelat forte; Sidroga Nerven- und Schlaftee; Species nervinae; St Bonifatius-Tee; St Radegunder Beruhigungs- und Einschlaftee; St Radegunder Nerven-Tonikum; St Radegunder Nerventee; Synpharma Instant-Nerventee; Teekanne Schlaf- und Nervantee; Thymoval; Valin Baldrian; Vivinox; Wechseltee; *Austral.:* Calmo; Executive B; Extralife Sleep-Care; Goodnight Formula; Lifesystem Herbal Plus Formula 2 Valerian; Macro Anti-Stress; Multi-Vitamin Day & Night; Naturest; Pacifenity; Passiflora Complex; Passionflower Plus; Prosed-X; ReDormin; Relaxaplex; Tranquiplex†; Valerian; Valerian Plus Herbal Plus Formula 12; Vitaglow Herbal Stress†; *Belg.:* Seneuval; *Braz.:* Anevrase; Antispasmin; Regran; Sedantol; Sominex; Uterovarol; Vidcalm; *Canad.:* Herbal Nerve; Herbal Sleep Aid; Nyrene†; Relax and Sleep; *Fr.:* Actisane Troubles du Sommeil; Anxoral; Biocarde; Euphytose; Mediflor Tisane Calmante Troubles du Sommeil No 14†; Mediflor Tisane Circulation du Sang No 12†; Neuroflorine; Neurotensyl†; Noctisan†; Palpipax; Passinevryl; Phytocalm; Phytotherapie Boribel no 8; Sedalozia; Sedibaine†; Serenival†; Spasmidenal; Spasmine; Sympaneurol†; Tisane Sedative Weleda†; Tranquital; Valerbe; *Ger.:* Aranidorm-S†; Ardeysedon N; Avedorm; Baldrian-Dispert Nacht; Baldrianox S†; Baldriparan N; Baldriparan stark N; Biosedon S; Biral; Boxocalm; Cefasedativ; Cor-Select; Diawern; Dormarist; Dormeasan; Dormo-Sern; Dormoverlan; Dreierlei; Einschlaf-Kapseln biologisch; Euvalon†; Euvegal Entspannungs- und Einschlafdragees; Euvegal forte†; Euvegal N; Euvitan; Goldtropfen-Hetterich; Grunlicht Dreierlei Tropfen; Grunlicht Hingfong Essenz; Gutnacht; Guttacor; Habstal-Nerv N; Heumann Beruhigungstee Tenerval N; Hingfong-Essenz Hofmanns Tropfen; Hovaletten N†; Hyperesa; Ivel Schlaf; JuDorm; JuNeuron S†; Kavosporal comp; Kneipp Baldrian + Hopfen; Kneipp Krauter Taschenkur Nerven und Schlaf N; Kneipp Nerven- und Schlaf-Tee N; Kytta-Sedativum f; Leukona-Sedativ-Bad; Leukona-Sedativ-Bad sine Chloralhydrat; Luvased; Luvased-Tropfen N; Montana; Moradorm; Moradorm S; Mutellon; Nerven-Tee Stada N†; Nervendragees; Nervinetten†; Nervoregin forte; Nervosana; Neurapas; Nitrangin compositum; Nitro-cum; Oxacant N; Oxacant-sedativ; Pascoseodon; Phytonoctu; Plantival novo; Presselin Nerven K 1 N; Pronervon Phyto; Psychotonin-sed; Rhoival; RubieSed; Salusan†; Schlaf- und Nerventee; Schupps Baldrian Sedativbad†; Schwedentrunk der Echte Elixier; Seda Kneipp N†; Seda-Plantina; Sedacur; Sedahopf†; Sedariston; Sedariston Konzentrat; Sedaselect N; Sedasyx; Sedatruw S†; Sedinfant N; Selon; Sesinerv forte; Sirmiosta Nervenelixier N†; Somnuvis S; SX Valeriana comp; Tornix; Valdispert comp; Valena N; Valeriana comp; Valeriana forte; Valeriana mild; Visinal†; Vivinox N; Vivinox-Schlafdragees†; *Hong Kong:* Epizon; *Israel:* Calmanervin; Nerven-Dragees; Passiflora; Passiflora Compound; *Ital.:* Anevrasi; Bianco Val; Bio-Strath; Bitteridina; Fitosonno; Florelax; Glicero-Valerovit; Melissa Sedse Composta; Noctis; Parvisedil; Quietan†; Reve; Sedatol; Sedopuer F; Val-Plus; *Mex.:* Ivel; Plantival; *Port.:* Antispasmina Colica; Bio-Strath No 8†; Gabisedil; Neurocardol; Songha; Valesono; *S.Afr.:* Biral; Restin; *Spain:* Baldrian; Brevilon†; *Switz.:* Baldriparan; Dicalm; Dormeasan N; Dormiplant†; Dragees pour la detente nerveuse; Dragees pour le coeur et les nerfs; Dragees pour le sommeil nouvelle formule; Hova; Melissa Tonic†; Perpector; Phytoberidin; Phytomed Somni; Plantival†; ReDormin; Relax; Seracalm†; Songha Night; Soporin; Tisane calmante pour les enfants; Tisane pour le sommeil et les nerfs; Tisane relaxante; Valverde Dragees pour la detente; Valverde Dragees pour le coeur; Valverde Dragees pour le sommeil; *UK:* Avena sativa comp.; Bio-Strath Valerian Formula; Biophylin†; Daily Menopause Relief; Daily Tension & Strain Relief; Digestive; Gerard 99; Gerard House Gladlax; Gerard House Serenity; Gerard House Somnus; Gerard House Valerian Compound; Heath & Heather Becalm; Heath & Heather Quiet Night; Herbal Indigestion Naturtabs; Herbal Pain Relief; HRI Calm Life; HRI Golden Seal Digestive; HRI Night; Indigestion and Flatulence; Kalms; Laxative Tablets; Modern Herbals Stress; Natrasleep; Natural Herb Tablets; Newrelax; Night Time; Nodoff; Period Pain Relief; PMT Formula; Prementaid; Quiet Days; Quiet Life; Quiet Nite; Quiet Tyme; Rapi-snooze; Relax B†; Scullcap & Gentian Tablets; SuNerven; Super Mega B+C; Sure-Lax (Herbal); Valerina Day Time; Valerina Night-Time; Vegetable Cough Remover; Wellwoman; Wind & Dyspepsia Relief.

Vanilla (2416-p)

Baunilha; Vainilla; Vanilla Beans; Vanilla Pods.

The cured, fully grown, unripe fruit of Madagascar, Mexican, or Bourbon vanilla, *Vanilla planifolia*, or of Tahiti vanilla, *V. tahitensis* (Orchidaceae). Its odour and flavour are not entirely due to vanillin (see below) but depend on the presence of other aromatic substances. Vanilla which has become brittle should not be used.

Profile
Vanilla is used as a flavour and in perfumery.

Vanillin (2417-s)

Vainillina; Vanillic Aldehyde; Vanillinum. 4-Hydroxy-3-methoxy-benzaldehyde.
$C_8H_8O_3 = 152.1$.
CAS — 121-33-5.
Pharmacopoeias. In Eur. (see p.vi) and Pol. Also in USNF.

The symbol † denotes a preparation no longer actively marketed

Pharmacopoeial description
Ph. Eur.: White or slightly yellowish crystalline needles or powder. M.p. 81° to 84°. Slightly soluble in water; freely soluble in alcohol and in methyl alcohol; soluble in ether; it dissolves in dilute solutions of alkali hydroxides. Protect from light.

USNF 20: Fine, white to slightly yellow crystals, usually needle-like, having an odour and taste suggestive of vanilla. M.p. 81° to 83°. Soluble 1 in 100 of water at 25°, 1 in 20 of water at 80°, 1 in 20 of glycerol; freely soluble in alcohol, in chloroform, in ether, and in solutions of fixed alkali hydroxides. Its solutions are acid to litmus. Store in airtight containers. Protect from light.

Profile
Vanillin is used as a flavour and in perfumery.

Preparations
BP 2001: Tolu-flavour Solution.

Vardenafil (20645-j)

Vardenafil *(rINN)*.
1-{[3-(3,4-Dihydro-5-methyl-4-oxo-7-propylimidazo[5,1-*f*]-as-triazin-2-yl)-4-ethoxyphenyl]sulfonyl}-4-ethylpiperazine.
$C_{23}H_{32}N_6O_4S = 488.6$.
CAS — 224785-90-4.

Profile
Vardenafil is a phosphodiesterase type-5 inhibitor given by mouth and is under investigation for the management of erectile dysfunction.

Vasoactive Intestinal Peptide (17025-m)

VIP.
CAS — 37221-79-7.

Aviptadil (20746-t)

Aviptadil *(BAN, rINN)*.
Vasoactive Intestinal Octacosapeptide (Swine).
$C_{147}H_{238}N_{44}O_{42}S = 3325.8$.
CAS — 40077-57-4.

Profile
Vasoactive intestinal peptide acts as a hormone and neurotransmitter in various parts of the body; it is a potent relaxant of smooth muscle and has vasodilator and bronchodilator properties as well as stimulating the gastrointestinal tract to increased secretion. Its analogue aviptadil has been tried in combination with phentolamine for erectile dysfunction (p.1663). It also has been used in the management of acute oesophageal food impaction.

Hydrogenated Vegetable Oil (7371-v)

Pharmacopoeias. In Br. and Jpn. Also in USNF.

Refined, bleached, hydrogenated, and deodorised vegetable oil stearins consisting mainly of the triglycerides of stearic and palmitic acids.

Pharmacopoeial description
BP 2001: A mixture of triglycerides of fatty acids of vegetable origin. An almost white, fine powder at room temperature and a pale yellow, oily liquid above its m.p. of 57° to 70°. Practically insoluble in water; soluble in chloroform, in hot isopropyl alcohol, and in petroleum spirit. Store at a temperature of 8° to 25°.

USNF 20: Type 1 Hydrogenated Vegetable Oil occurs as a fine, white powder, beads, or small flakes; m.p. 57° to 85°. Type 2 Hydrogenated Vegetable Oil occurs as a plastic (semi-solid) or flakes, having a softer consistency than Type 1; m.p. 20° to 50°. Insoluble in water; soluble in chloroform, in hot isopropyl alcohol, and in petroleum spirit. Store in airtight containers at a temperature of 8° to 15°.

Profile
Hydrogenated vegetable oil is used as a tablet lubricant and as an ointment basis.

Preparations
Proprietary Preparations (details are given in Part 3)
Spain: Blodex.

Veratrine (14013-r)

Veratrine.
CAS — 8051-02-3 (mixture).

NOTE. Veratrine should be distinguished from protoveratrines obtained from veratrum.

A mixture of alkaloids from the dried ripe seeds of *Schoeno-caulon officinale* (Liliaceae) (sabadilla).

Adverse Effects, Treatment, and Precautions
Veratrine resembles aconite (p.1572) in its action on the peripheral nerve endings and poisoning should be treated similarly. It

is an intense local irritant and has a powerful direct stimulating action on all muscle tissues. It has a violent irritant action on mucous membranes, even in minute doses, and must be handled with great care. When ingested it causes violent vomiting, purging, an intense burning sensation in the mouth and throat, and general muscular weakness.

Uses and Administration
Veratrine should not be used internally. It was formerly applied externally for its analgesic properties and as a parasiticide, especially for head lice, but even when used in this way there is danger of systemic poisoning from absorption.

Green Veratrum (913-s)

American Hellebore; American Veratrum; Green Hellebore; Green Hellebore Rhizome; Veratro Verde; Veratrum Viride.
CAS — 8002-39-9.

White Veratrum (914-w)

European Hellebore; Veratrum Album; White Hellebore; White Hellebore Rhizome.

Green veratrum consists of the dried rhizome and roots of *Veratrum viride* (Liliaceae) from which are derived the alkaloidal mixtures alkavervir and cryptenamine.

White veratrum consists of the dried rhizome and roots of *Veratrum album* (Liliaceae) from which are derived the alkaloids protoveratrine A and B.

Adverse Effects
Veratrum alkaloids may cause nausea and vomiting at conventional therapeutic doses. Other adverse effects include epigastric and substernal burning, sweating, mental confusion, cardiac arrhythmias, dizziness, and hiccup. Profound hypotension and respiratory depression can occur at high doses.

◊ Various symptoms of intoxication occurred in 7 patients due to the use of a sneezing powder containing white veratrum alkaloids.[1]

1. Fogh A, *et al.* Veratrum alkaloids in sneezing-powder: a potential danger. *J Toxicol Clin Toxicol* 1983; **20:** 175–9.

Treatment of Adverse Effects
Following oral ingestion of veratrum alkaloids the stomach should be emptied by aspiration and lavage. Excessive hypotension with bradycardia or cardiac arrhythmias can be treated with atropine by intramuscular injection. The patient should be placed in a supine position with the feet raised.

Uses and Administration
White and green veratrum contain a number of pharmacologically active alkaloids that produce centrally mediated peripheral vasodilatation and bradycardia. They have been used in the treatment of hypertension but are generally considered to produce an unacceptably high incidence of adverse effects and have largely been replaced by less toxic antihypertensives.
Both green and white veratrum have also been used as insecticides.
White veratrum has been used, as Veratrum Album, in homoeopathy.

Vervain (11587-l)

Herba Columbariae; Herba Verbenae; Shop Vervain Wort.
Pharmacopoeias. In Chin.

Profile
Vervain, the aerial parts of *Verbena officinalis* (Verbenaceae), has been used for a wide range of disorders. It is a bitter and has been used for digestive disorders. It also has sedative properties and has been used for anxiety disorders and as a tonic during convalescence from chronic illness.

Preparations
Proprietary Preparations (details are given in Part 3)
Multi-ingredient: *Aust.:* Sinupret; Sinusol; Sinusol-Schleimlosender Tee; *Austral.:* Avena Complex; Calmo; Naturest; *Belg.:* Tisane pour le Foie; *Fr.:* Calmophytum; Santane A_4; Santane C_6; Santane H_7; Tisane des Familles; Tisane Touraine†; Vigilia; *Ger.:* Sinupret; *Hong Kong:* Sinupret; *Singapore:* Sinupret; *Switz.:* Sinupret; Tisane antiflatulente pour les enfants; Tisane pour les enfants†; *Thai.:* Sinupret; *UK:* Athera; Catarrh; HRI Night; Modern Herbals Menopause; Modern Herbals Stress; Newrelax; Period Pain Relief; Prementaid; Scullcap & Gentian Tablets; SuNerven.

Vetrabutine Hydrochloride (12663-c)

Vetrabutine Hydrochloride *(BANM, rINNM)*.
Dimophebumine Hydrochloride; Sp-281. N,N-Dimethyl-α-(3-phenylpropyl)veratrylamine hydrochloride.
$C_{20}H_{27}NO_2,HCl = 349.9$.
CAS — 3735-45-3 (vetrabutine); 5974-09-4 (vetrabutine hydrochloride).

Profile
Vetrabutine hydrochloride is used as a uterine relaxant in veterinary medicine.

Vinburnine (14014-f)

Vinburnine (rINN).

CH-846; (−)-Eburnamonine; 3α,16α-Eburnamonine; Vincamone. (3α,16α)-Eburnamenin-14(15H)-one.
$C_{19}H_{22}N_2O = 294.4$.
CAS — 4880-88-0.
ATC — C04AX17.

Profile
Vinburnine is an alkaloid related to vincamine (below) and has been used in conditions associated with cerebral circulatory insufficiency.

Vinburnine phosphate has been used similarly.

Preparations
Proprietary Preparations (details are given in Part 3)
Fr.: Cervoxan; *Ital.:* Eburnal; Scleramin; Tensiplex; *Port.:* Cervoxan; *Spain:* Cervoxan; Eburnoxin†.

Vincamine (14015-d)

Vincamine (BAN, rINN).

Methyl (3α,16α)-14,15-dihydro-14β-hydroxyeburnamenine-14-carboxylate.
$C_{21}H_{26}N_2O_3 = 354.4$.
CAS — 1617-90-9.
ATC — C04AX07.
Pharmacopoeias. In Belg. and Fr.

An alkaloid obtained from *Vinca minor* (Apocynaceae).

Profile
Vincamine is claimed to increase cerebral circulation and utilisation of oxygen and has been used in a variety of cerebral disorders. Vincamine may have adverse effects on the cardiovascular system and care should be taken in patients with hypertension or cardiac dysfunction.

Vincamine salts including vincamine hydrochloride, oxoglurate, teprosilate, and hydrogen tartrate have also been used.

Preparations
Proprietary Preparations (details are given in Part 3)
Aust.: Aethroma†; Cetal; Oxygeron†; *Belg.:* Cerebroxine; *Braz.:* Vincagil; *Fr.:* Pervincamine†; Vinca; Vincafor; Vincimax†; *Ger.:* Cetal; Equipur†; Ophdilvas N; Vinca-Tablinen†; Vincapront†; *Hong Kong:* Aethroma; *Ital.:* Anasclerol†; Ausomina†; Vasonett; Vinca-Ri; Vinca-Treis; Vincadar; Vincafolina†; Vinsal; Vraap; *Mex.:* Cetovinca; Vincapan; *Port.:* Arteriovinca; Cervinca; Vincagil; *Spain:* Arteriovinca; Cetovinca; Dilarterial†; Tefavinca; Vadicate; Vincacen; Vincaminol; *Switz.:* Aethroma; Cetal; Oxygeron; *Thai.:* Oxygeron.
Multi-ingredient: *Fr.:* Rheobral; Vincarutine; *Port.:* Anacervix; Centracetam; Stimilfar; *Spain:* Anacervix; Arteriobrate†; Devincal; Dipervina.

Vinpocetine (14016-n)

Vinpocetine (USAN, rINN).

AY-27255; Ethyl Apovincaminate; Ethyl Apovincaminoate; RGH-4405. Ethyl (3α,16α)-eburnamenine-14-carboxylate.
$C_{22}H_{26}N_2O_2 = 350.5$.
CAS — 42971-09-5.
ATC — N06BX18.

Profile
Vinpocetine is a derivative of vincamine (above). It has been used in cerebrovascular and cognitive disorders in doses of 15 to 30 mg daily by mouth in divided doses.

◊ **References.**
1. Grandt R, *et al.* Vinpocetine pharmacokinetics in elderly subjects. *Arzneimittelforschung* 1989; **39:** 1599–1602.
2. Blaha L, *et al.* Clinical evidence of the effectiveness of vinpocetine in the treatment of organic psychosyndrome. *Hum Psychopharmacol Clin Exp* 1989; **4:** 103–11.
3. Bereczki D, Fekete I. A systematic review of vinpocetine therapy in acute ischaemic stroke. *Eur J Clin Pharmacol* 1999; **55:** 349–52.

Preparations
Proprietary Preparations (details are given in Part 3)
Ger.: Cavinton; *Jpn:* Calan; *Mex.:* Cavinton; *Port.:* Cavinton; DC Vin; Ultra-Vinca; Vipocem; *Singapore:* Cavinton; *Thai.:* Cavinton.

Vinyl Chloride (14017-h)

VCM; Vinyl Chloride Monomer. Chloroethylene.
$C_2H_3Cl = 62.50$.
CAS — 75-01-4.

Profile
Vinyl chloride is used in the manufacture of polyvinyl chloride (PVC) and other vinyl polymers. Occupational exposure to vinyl chloride in polymerisation plants has been associated with acro-osteolysis, especially in the terminal phalanges of the fingers, a condition resembling Raynaud's phenomenon, and sclerodermatous skin changes. Liver damage and hepatic angiosarcoma, splenomegaly, thrombocytopenia, impaired respiratory function, and chromosomal abnormalities have also occurred.

◊ **References.**
1. Infante PF, *et al.* Genetic risks of vinyl chloride. *Lancet* 1976; **i:** 734–5.
2. Black CM, *et al.* Genetic susceptibility to scleroderma-like syndrome induced by vinyl chloride. *Lancet* 1983; **i:** 53–5.
3. Piratsu R, *et al.* La mortalità dei produttori di cloruro di vinile in Italia. *Med Lav* 1991; **82:** 388–423.
4. Riordan SM, *et al.* Vinyl chloride related hepatic angiosarcoma in a polyvinyl chloride autoclave cleaner in Australia. *Med J Aust* 1991; **155:** 125–8.
5. Mur JM, *et al.* Spontaneous abortion and exposure to vinyl chloride. *Lancet* 1992; **339:** 127–8.
6. McLaughlin JK, Lipworth L. A critical review of the epidemiologic literature on health effects of occupational exposure to vinyl chloride. *J Epidemiol Biostat* 1999; **4:** 253–75.

Viquidil Hydrochloride (14019-b)

Viquidil Hydrochloride (rINNM).

LM-192; Mequiverine Hydrochloride; Quinicine Hydrochloride. 1-(6-Methoxy-4-quinolyl)-3-(3-vinyl-4-piperidyl)propan-1-one hydrochloride.
$C_{20}H_{24}N_2O_2,HCl = 360.9$.
CAS — 84-55-9 (viquidil); 52211-63-9 (viquidil hydrochloride).

Profile
Viquidil hydrochloride has been used in various cerebrovascular disorders.

Preparations
Proprietary Preparations (details are given in Part 3)
Ger.: Desclidium†.

Water (7700-g)

Aqua; Aqua Communis; Aqua Fontana; Aqua Potabilis; Eau Potable; Wasser.
$H_2O = 18.02$.
CAS — 7732-18-5.

Purified Water (7701-q)

Aqua Purificata; Purified water.
Pharmacopoeias. In Chin., Eur. (see p.vi), Int., Jpn, Pol., and US. Eur. also includes Highly Purified Water. US also includes Sterile Purified Water.

Some pharmacopoeias only include distilled water or have additional monographs for demineralised water or distilled water.

PREPARATION BY DEIONISATION. By passing potable water through columns of anionic and cationic ion-exchange resins, ionisable substances can be removed, producing a water of high specific resistance. Colloidal and non-ionisable impurities such as pyrogens may not be removed by this process.

PREPARATION BY DISTILLATION. In this process water is separated as vapour from non-volatile impurities and is subsequently condensed. In practice, non-volatile impurities may be carried into the distillate by entrainment unless a suitable baffle is fitted to the still.

Pharmacopoeial description
Ph. Eur.: Purified Water is water for the preparation of medicines other than those that are required to be both sterile and apyrogenic, unless otherwise justified and authorised. It is prepared from suitable potable water either by distillation, by ion exchange, or by any other suitable method. Store in conditions designed to prevent growth of micro-organisms and to avoid any other contamination. Sub-monographs cover Purified Water in Bulk and Purified Water in Containers.

Highly Purified Water is water intended for the preparation of medicinal products where water of high biological quality is needed, except where Water for Injections is required.

USP 25: Purified Water is prepared from potable water by a suitable process.

Water for Injections (7702-p)

Aq. pro Inj.; Aqua ad Iniectabilia; Aqua ad Injectionem; Aqua Injectabilis; Aqua pro Injectione; Aqua pro Injectionibus; Eau pour Préparations Injectables; Wasser für Injektionszwecke; Water for Injection.
Pharmacopoeias. In Chin., Eur. (see p.vi), Int., Jpn, Pol., and US. US also includes Sterile Water for Injection, Sterile Water for Inhalation, Sterile Water for Irrigation, and Bacteriostatic Water for Injection.

Pharmacopoeial description
Ph. Eur.: Water for Injections is water for the preparation of medicines for parenteral administration when water is used as the vehicle, and for dissolving or diluting substances or preparations for parenteral administration. It is prepared by distillation of potable water or purified water from a neutral glass, quartz, or suitable metal still fitted with an effective device for preventing the entrainment of droplets; the first portion of the distillate is discarded and the remainder collected. Store in conditions designed to prevent growth of micro-organisms and to avoid any other contamination. Sub-monographs cover Water for Injections in Bulk and Sterilised Water for Injections.

USP 25: Water for Injection is purified by distillation or by reverse osmosis. When used for the preparation of parenteral solutions it should be sterilised first or the final preparation should be sterilised after preparation. Sterile Water for Injection, Inhalation, or Irrigation and Bacteriostatic Water for Injection are the subjects of separate monographs.

Profile
There are international standards for the quality of water intended for human consumption. Toxic substances such as arsenic, barium, cadmium, chromium, copper, cyanide, lead, and selenium may constitute a danger to health if present in drinking water in excess of the recommended concentrations. Waterborne infections are also a hazard.

Fluoride is regarded as an essential constituent of drinking water but may endanger health if present in excess—see Sodium Fluoride, p.1375. Ingestion of water containing large amounts of nitrates may cause methaemoglobinaemia in infants; many countries have standards for nitrates in water.

The use of tap water containing metal ions (such as aluminium, copper, and lead), fluoride, or tosylchloramide sodium, for dialysis may be hazardous.

Hard water contains soluble calcium and magnesium salts, which form scale and sludge in boilers, water pipes, and autoclaves; they also cause the precipitation of soap and prevent its lathering. Temporary hardness in water is due to the presence of bicarbonates which are converted to insoluble carbonates on heating. Permanent hardness is due to dissolved chlorides, nitrates, and sulfates, which do not form a precipitate on heating. The presence or absence of such salts can play a part in cardiovascular health.

Without further purification, potable water may be unsuitable for certain pharmaceutical purposes. In such instances, purified water should always be used. Most pharmacopoeias include monographs on various preparations of water, such as water suitable for injections. Potable water should not be used when such preparations are specified.

Excessive ingestion of water can lead to water intoxication with disturbances of the electrolyte balance.

Preparations
Proprietary Preparations (details are given in Part 3)
Fin.: Aquasteril; *Switz.:* Replens; *UK:* Aquasol; Sterac; Uriflex W.

Wild Carrot (13990-c)

Dauci Herba; Daucus.
Pharmacopoeias. In Chin.

Profile
The fruits of the wild carrot, *Daucus carota* (Umbelliferae) have been used as a diuretic and anthelmintic, and are included in herbal preparations for various indications. Other parts of the plant have been used in folk medicine. The root of the cultivated form is a culinary item and a source of carotenoids in the diet.

Preparations
Proprietary Preparations (details are given in Part 3)
Multi-ingredient: *Ital.:* Pluriderm†; *UK:* Sciargo; Watershed.

Wild Cherry Bark (2418-w)

Prunus Serotina; Virginian Prune; Virginian Prune Bark; Wild Black Cherry Bark; Wild Cherry.

The dried bark of the wild or black cherry, *Prunus serotina* (Rosaceae), known in commerce as Thin Natural Wild Cherry Bark, containing not less than 10% of water-soluble extractive. It has a slight odour and an astringent, aromatic, bitter taste, recalling that of bitter almonds. It contains (+)-mandelonitrile glucoside (prunasin) and an enzyme system, which interact in the presence of water yielding benzaldehyde, hydrocyanic acid, and glucose.

Profile
Wild cherry bark, in the form of the syrup, has been used in the treatment of cough but it has little therapeutic value. It has also been used as a flavour.

Preparations
Proprietary Preparations (details are given in Part 3)
Multi-ingredient: *Canad.:* Mielocol; Rophelin; Wampole Bronchial Cough Syrup; *UK:* Potters Day & Night Cough Pastilles.

Wild Lettuce (19394-r)

Herba Lactucae Virosae.

Profile
The wild lettuce, *Lactuca virosa* (Compositae), has been given in herbal medicine as a sedative and antitussive. The dried sap (lactucarium; lettuce opium) is also used.

Preparations
Proprietary Preparations (details are given in Part 3)
Multi-ingredient: *Canad.:* Sirop Cocillana Codeine; *UK:* Anased; Antibron; Gerard House Somnus; Gerard House Valerian

Compound; HRI Night; Nytol Herbal; Quiet Life; Quiet Nite; Slumber.

Xanthine-containing Beverages (3874-t)

Adverse Effects
The adverse effects of xanthine-containing beverages are largely due to their caffeine (p.761), theophylline (p.777), and theobromine (p.777) content. Common side-effects are sleeplessness, anxiety, tremor, palpitations, and withdrawal headache.

Effects on the heart. A meta-analysis of published studies found no evidence of an association between coffee consumption and the development of coronary heart disease,[1] and a large cohort study in women also found no evidence of a link.[2] Expert opinion in the UK[3] is that the evidence that caffeine or coffee consumption contributes to its development is inconsistent. Coffee prepared by boiling, as is the practice in Scandinavia for example, does raise serum cholesterol concentrations due to the presence of the diterpenes cafestol and kahweol, and coffee made in a cafetière has a similar effect, but filtered coffee does not, as the hypercholesterolaemic fraction does not pass a paper filter.[4] Others have raised concern that the potential pressor effect of caffeine itself may be a cardiovascular risk factor,[5] but as mentioned above there is little evidence for this. Tea drinking has not been associated with increased cardiovascular risk[3]—indeed, its polyphenol content has been suggested to have beneficial antoxidant effects.[6,7]

1. Myers MG, Basinski A. Coffee and coronary heart disease. *Arch Intern Med* 1992; **152:** 1767–72.
2. Willett WC, *et al.* Coffee consumption and coronary heart disease in women: a ten-year follow-up. *JAMA* 1996; **275:** 458–62.
3. Department of Health. Nutritional aspects of cardiovascular disease. Report of the cardiovascular review group committee on medical aspects of food policy. Report on health and social subjects no. 46. London: HMSO, 1994.
4. Urgert R, *et al.* Comparison of effect of cafetière and filtered coffee on serum concentrations of liver aminotransferases and lipids: six month randomised controlled trial. *BMJ* 1996; **313:** 1362–6.
5. James JE. Is habitual caffeine use a preventable cardiovascular risk factor? *Lancet* 1997; **349:** 279–81.
6. Luo M, *et al.* Inhibition of LDL oxidation by green tea extract. *Lancet* 1997; **349:** 360–1.
7. Geleijnse JM, *et al.* Tea flavonoids may protect against atherosclerosis. *Arch Intern Med* 1999; **159:** 2170–4.

Effects on the muscles. Severe myositis in an elderly man who drank around 14 litres of tea daily was attributed to hypokalaemia produced by the xanthine content of the beverage.[1] The patient improved following intravenous potassium replacement and subsequently remained well following a reduction in tea intake.

1. Trewby PN, *et al.* Teapot myositis. *Lancet* 1998; **351:** 1248.

Malignant neoplasms. A review of available data did not suggest a clinically significant association between the regular use of coffee and the development of cancer of the lower urinary tract in men or women.[1]

1. Viscoli CM, *et al.* Bladder cancer and coffee drinking: a summary of case-control research. *Lancet* 1993; **341:** 1432–7.

Interactions
The possibility of synergistic effects in patients receiving xanthines who consume large amounts of xanthine-containing beverages should be borne in mind.

Antipsychotics. Xanthine-containing beverages have been reported to precipitate some antipsychotic drugs from solution *in vitro*, but do not appear to alter antipsychotic concentrations *in vivo*. For references, see p.665.

Uses and Administration
Xanthine-containing beverages including chocolate, coffee, cocoa, cola, maté, and tea are widely consumed and have a mild stimulant effect on the CNS. The primary xanthine constituent is caffeine but other xanthine derivatives may also be present; cocoa and chocolate contain significant amounts of theobromine.

Coffee is the kernel of the dried ripe seeds of *Coffea arabica*, *C. liberica*, *C. canephora* (robusta coffee), and other species of *Coffea* (Rubiaceae), roasted until it acquires a deep brown colour and a pleasant characteristic aroma. It contains about 1 to 2% of caffeine. Coffee has been used in the form of an infusion or decoction as a stimulant and as a flavour in some pharmaceutical preparations. A decoction is used as a beverage containing up to about 100 mg of caffeine per 100 mL. Preparations of instant coffee may contain up to 40% less caffeine while decaffeinated preparations may contain only up to about 3 mg per 100 mL.

Kola (cola, cola seeds, kola nuts) is the dried cotyledons of *Cola nitida* and *C. acuminata* (Sterculiaceae), containing up to about 2.5% of caffeine and traces of theobromine. Kola is used in the preparation of cola drinks which may contain up to 20 mg of caffeine per 100 mL. Kola has been used to treat migraine in homoeopathic medicine.

Maté (Paraguay Tea) is the dried leaves of *Ilex paraguensis* (Aquifoliaceae), containing 0.2 to 2% of caffeine. Maté is less astringent than tea and is extensively used as a beverage in South America.

Tea (thea, thé, tee) is the prepared young leaves and leafbuds of *Camellia sinensis* (=*C. thea*) (Theaceae). It contains 1 to 5% of caffeine and up to 24% of tannin. Tea is used in an infusion as a beverage containing up to about 60 mg of caffeine per 100 mL.

Guarana consists of the crushed seeds of *Paullinia cupana* var *sorbilis*. Caffeine appears to be its major active ingredient which was once termed guaranine. Herbal preparations include a beverage or liquid extract and may contain 5% caffeine.

Preparations

Proprietary Preparations (details are given in Part 3)
Fr.: Camiline; Exolise; *Ger.:* Bioday; Carbo Konigsfeld; *UK:* Yariba; *USA:* Tegreen.

Multi-ingredient: *Aust.:* Aponatura Kreislauf; Blasen- und Nierentee; Colagin†; Euflat†; Kneipp Herz- und Kreislauf-Unterstutzungs-Tee; Mag Kottas Herz- und Kreislauftee; *Austral.:* Avena Complex; Bioglan 3B Beer Belly Buster; Infant Tonic; Irontona; T & T Antioxidant; Vig; Vig Recovery; Vitatona; *Belg.:* Aperop; *Braz.:* Catuaba; Catuama; Gastogenol; Geripan; Iofoscal; Kola Fosfatada Soel; Salutina; *Fr.:* Actisane Fatigue Passagere†; Biotone; Euphytose; Kola Astier; Mincifit; Phospharome†; Promincil; Quintonine; Santane V₃; Tealine; Tonactil; Tonisan†; Triogene†; Uromil; YSE; *Ger.:* Cardibisana; Kola-Dallmann mit Lecithin†; Kola-Dallmann†; Myrrhinil-Intest; Nieroxin N; Ramend Krauter; Repursan ST; *Hong Kong:* Wari-Procomil; *Ital.:* Chinoidina; Dam; Enertonic; Fitostress; Four-Ton; Gincola†; Memorandum; Nosenil†; *Spain:* Elingrip†; Fitosvelt; Rimagrip; Vigortonic; *Switz.:* Dragees contre les maux de tete; Ganavit; *Thai.:* Wari-Procomil; *UK:* Chlorophyll; Daily Fatigue Relief; Damiana and Kola Tablets; Herbal Booster; Koladex; Labiton; Lion Cleansing Herbs; S.P.H.P.; Strength.

Xantofyl Palmitate (14020-x)

Xantofyl Palmitate *(rINN)*.
Heleniene; Xanthophyl Dipalmitate. β,ε-Carotene-3,3′-diyl dipalmitate.
$C_{72}H_{116}O_4 = 1045.7$.
$CAS — 547-17-1$.

Profile
Xantofyl palmitate has been used by mouth in the treatment of some visual disturbances.

Xylazine (14023-d)

Xylazine *(BAN, rINN)*.
N-(5,6-Dihydro-4H-1,3-thiazin-2-yl)-2,6-xylidine.
$C_{12}H_{16}N_2S = 220.3$.
$CAS — 7361-61-7$.
Pharmacopoeias. In US.

Pharmacopoeial description
USP 25: Colourless to white crystals. Sparingly soluble in acetone, in chloroform, and in dilute acid; insoluble in dilute alkali. Store in airtight containers.

Xylazine Hydrochloride (20663-c)

Xylazine Hydrochloride *(BANM, USAN, rINNM)*.
Bay-Va-1470.
$C_{12}H_{16}N_2S, HCl = 256.8$.
$CAS — 23076-35-9$.
Pharmacopoeias. In Eur. (see p.vi) for veterinary use only. Also in US.

Pharmacopoeial description
Ph. Eur.: A white or almost white, crystalline, hygroscopic powder. Freely soluble in water and in dichloromethane; very soluble in methyl alcohol. Store in airtight containers. Protect from light.

USP 25: Colourless to white crystals. Sparingly soluble in acetone, in methyl alcohol, and in dilute acid; insoluble in dilute alkali. A 1% solution in water has a pH of 4.0 to 6.0. Store in airtight containers.

Profile
Xylazine is a sedative, analgesic, and muscle relaxant used in veterinary medicine. The hydrochloride is used similarly.

Adverse effects. Bradycardia, hypotension, and coma was associated with the self-administration of 200 mg of xylazine. Treatment was supportive.[1]

1. Samanta A, *et al.* Accidental self administration of xylazine in a veterinary nurse. *Postgrad Med J* 1990; **66:** 244–5.

Xylose (2154-h)

Wood Sugar; D-Xylose; Xylosum. α-D-Xylopyranose.
$C_5H_{10}O_5 = 150.1$.
$CAS — 58-86-6; 6763-34-4$.
Pharmacopoeias. In Eur. (see p.vi) and US.

Pharmacopoeial description
Ph. Eur.: Colourless needles or a white crystalline powder. Freely soluble in water; soluble in hot alcohol.

USP 25: Odourless, colourless needles or white crystalline powder. Very soluble in water; slightly soluble in alcohol. Store in airtight containers at a temperature of 15° to 30°.

Adverse Effects and Precautions
Xylose may cause some gastrointestinal discomfort with large doses. Other drugs may affect the absorption of xylose and interfere with the xylose test.

Pharmacokinetics
Xylose is incompletely absorbed from the gastrointestinal tract. Part of the absorbed xylose is metabolised in the body mainly to carbon dioxide and water. In the absence of malabsorption, about 35% of a 5-g oral dose and about 25% of a 25-g oral dose are reported to be excreted in the urine within 5 hours.

Uses and Administration
Xylose is used for the investigation of absorption from the gastrointestinal tract. It is given by mouth, usually in a dose of either 5 or 25 g, with up to 700 mL of water. The amount recovered in the urine is estimated over a certain period and that figure can be used to assess any malabsorption. Adjustment may have to be made for renal impairment.

The test has been adapted to use blood-xylose concentrations.

◊ References.

1. Craig RM, Ehrenpreis ED. D-xylose testing. *J Clin Gastroenterol* 1999; **29:** 143–50.

Preparations

Proprietary Preparations (details are given in Part 3)
Canad.: Xylo-Pfan†; *UK:* Xylose-BMS; *USA:* Xylo-Pfan†.

Yellow Dock (12157-r)

Curly Dock.

Profile
Yellow dock, the root of *Rumex crispus* (Polygonaceae) has laxative and choleretic properties. It is used for constipation, jaundice, and chronic skin disorders.

It is also used in homoeopathic medicine.

Sorrel (*R. acetosa*; sorrel dock) has been used for respiratory-tract disorders.

Preparations

Proprietary Preparations (details are given in Part 3)
Multi-ingredient: *Aust.:* Sinupret; *Austral.:* Herbal Cleanse; Trifolium Complex; *Canad.:* Herborex; *Fr.:* Tisanes de l'Abbe Hamon no 11; *Ger.:* Sinupret; *Hong Kong:* Sinupret; *Singapore:* Sinupret; *Switz.:* Sinupret; *Thai.:* Sinupret; *UK:* Herbal Booster; Savlon Natural First Aid for Insect Bites & Stings; Skin Eruptions Mixture.

Yohimbine Hydrochloride (14024-n)

Yohimbine Hydrochloride *(rINNM)*.
Aphrodine Hydrochloride; Chlorhydrate de Québrachine; Corynine Hydrochloride. Methyl 17α-hydroxy-yohimban-16α-carboxylate hydrochloride.
$C_{21}H_{26}N_2O_3, HCl = 390.9$.
$CAS — 146-48-5$ (yohimbine); $65-19-0$ (yohimbine hydrochloride).
Pharmacopoeias. In Aust. and US.

The hydrochloride of the principal alkaloid of the bark of the yohimbe tree, *Pausinystalia yohimbe* (=*Corynanthe yohimbi*) (Rubiaceae).

Pharmacopoeial description
USP 25: A white to yellow powder. Slightly soluble in water and in alcohol; soluble in boiling water. Store in airtight containers.

Profile
Yohimbine is an α₂-adrenoceptor blocker with a short duration of action. It has an antidiuretic effect and produces increases in heart rate and blood pressure, and orthostatic hypotension. It has been reported to cause anxiety and manic reactions. It has been given by mouth in the treatment of erectile dysfunction (p.1663) and for its alleged aphrodisiac properties but convincing evidence of such an effect is lacking. It is contra-indicated in renal or hepatic disease.

Adverse effects. A warning as to the potential adverse effects, including anxiety, manic reactions, bronchospasm and a lupus-like syndrome, associated with yohimbine taken in health food products.[1] Interactions with tricyclic antidepressants and with phenothiazines might also occur.

1. De Smet PAGM, Smeets OSNM. Potential risks of health food products containing yohimbe extracts. *BMJ* 1994; **309:** 958.

Uses. References to the use of yohimbine in erectile dysfunction.

1. Ernst E, Pittler MH. Yohimbine for erectile dysfunction: a systematic review and meta-analysis of randomised clinical trials. *J Urol (Baltimore)* 1998; **159:** 433–6.

Preparations

USP 25: Yohimbine Injection.

Proprietary Preparations (details are given in Part 3)
Aust.: Yocon; *Braz.:* Yohydrol; Yomax; *Canad.:* Yocon; *Fr.:* Yocoral; *Ger.:* Pluriviron mono; Yocon; *Hong Kong:* Yocon; *Port.:* Zumba; *Singapore:* Urobine; *UK:* Prowess Plain; *USA:* Aphrodyne; Dayto Himbin; Yocon; Yohimex.

Multi-ingredient: *Aust.:* Pasuma-Dragees†; *Braz.:* Geravitine; Gerosenil; Ioimbina Composta; Lupercaina; Sexomrom; Testofran; Tonaton; *Fin.:* Potentol; *Hong Kong:* Wari-Procomil; *Israel:*

The symbol † denotes a preparation no longer actively marketed

Tesopalmed Forte cum Yohimbine; *Thai.:* Wari-Procomil; *UK:* Prowess.

Yucca (14092-y)

Profile

Various species of *Yucca* (Liliaceae), including Mohave yucca (*Y. schidigera*; *Y. mohavensis*), the Joshua tree (*Y. brevifolia*; *Y. arborescens*), and bear grass (*Y. filamentosa*) have been used in herbal medicine and as foods.

Preparations

Proprietary Preparations (details are given in Part 3)
Multi-ingredient: *Austral.:* Prost-1; *Braz.:* Bronquiogen.

Zanthoxylum Fruit (14025-h)

Prickly Ash Berries.

Pharmacopoeias. In *Jpn.*

The pericarp of the ripe fruit of *Zanthoxylum piperitum* (=*Xanthoxylum piperitum*) (Rutaceae) or other species of *Zanthoxylum*. It contains about 3.3% v/w of essential oil.

Zanthoxylum (BPC 1934) (Toothache Bark; Xanthoxylum) is the dried bark of the northern prickly ash, *Z. americanum*, or the southern prickly ash, *Z. clavaherculis*. Both varieties contain a complex mixture of components, including benzophenanthridine alkaloids; northern prickly ash also contains coumarins.

Profile

Zanthoxylum fruit has carminative properties and has been used for rheumatic disorders. Zanthoxylum bark has been used similarly, but there is some concern about the potential toxicity of the benzophenanthridine alkaloids which it contains, and some authorities consider that it should not be recommended.

Preparations

Proprietary Preparations (details are given in Part 3)
Multi-ingredient: *Austral.:* For Peripheral Circulation Herbal Plus Formula 5; Lifesystem Herbal Formula 6 For Peripheral Circulation; Uva-Ursi Plus; *UK:* Daily Overwork & Mental Fatigue Relief; Hofels White Willow and Burdock; Peerless Composition Essence; Rheumasol; Tabritis.

Zein (3925-j)

Pharmacopoeias. In *USNF.*

Pharmacopoeial description

USNF 20: A prolamine derived from corn, *Zea mays* (Gramineae). A white to yellow powder. Insoluble in water and in acetone; readily soluble in acetone-water mixtures between the limits of 60% and 80% of acetone by volume; soluble in aqueous alcohols, in ethoxyethanol; in glycols, in furfuryl alcohol, in tetrahydrofurfuryl alcohol, and in aqueous alkaline solutions of pH 11.5 and above; insoluble in all anhydrous alcohols except methyl alcohol. Store in airtight containers.

Profile

Zein is used as a tablet binder and coating agent for pharmaceutical preparations and foodstuffs. It has been used as a substitute for shellac.

Zirconium (15965-p)

Zr = 91.224.
CAS — 7440-67-7.

Profile

Zirconium and its compounds e.g. zirconium dioxide, zirconium lactate, and zirconium oxychloride, have been used in deodorant preparations; the dioxide is also used in dentistry. There have been reports of hypersensitivity reactions with granulomas. Zirconium dioxide has also been used as a contrast medium.

Adverse effects. A report[1] of pulmonary fibrosis associated with inhalation of a polishing agent containing mainly zirconium dioxide with quartz.

1. Bartter T, *et al.* Zirconium compound-induced pulmonary fibrosis. *Arch Intern Med* 1991; **151:** 1197–1201.

Part 3

Preparations

This part of Martindale contains brief details of proprietary preparations available in a number of countries and includes those supplied on prescription as well as those sold directly to the public. They are provided to help the reader identify preparations and to suggest their uses. Inclusion is not an endorsement of the activity of any ingredient nor of the preparation's indications.

For this edition we have covered Australia, Austria, Belgium, Brazil, Canada, Denmark, Finland, France, Germany, Hong Kong, Ireland, Israel, Italy, Mexico, the Netherlands, Norway, New Zealand, Portugal, Singapore, South Africa, Spain, Sweden, Switzerland, Thailand, the United Arab Emirates, UK, and USA. We have also included some proprietary preparations from Japan. Generally each entry consists of: the proprietary name; manufacturer or source of supply and country; ingredients usually listed by the manufacturer as being active; and a guide to the manufacturer's indications. Where possible, entries from different countries but with the same name and active ingredients have been amalgamated for clarity.

An entry may cover a range of dosage forms and strengths. Dosage forms are only specified when different forms have the same proprietary name but different active ingredients. Specifying all dosage forms and the quantity of each active ingredient would have vastly increased the number of entries. Furthermore, Part 3 is not intended as a guide to prescribing; where a preparation is to be

supplied the dose should be appropriate for that preparation and that particular patient, and authoritative local sources should be consulted.

With the exception of homoeopathic preparations the names of the ingredients have been translated into English. Almost all the ingredients listed are described in the monographs in Parts 1 and 2, and readers are directed to an appropriate monograph by the page number provided after the ingredient.

We have tried to include preparations that were available in the last few years since they may still be in circulation and their names may still be referred to in the literature and in practice. Such preparations that have been withdrawn from the market or are no longer being actively marketed may be identified by the symbol †. Readers should be aware that since Part 3 was prepared other preparations are likely to have been withdrawn or introduced; also ingredients may change, as may indications.

The manufacturer's full name and address can be found in the Directory of Manufacturers.

Each preparation title is also listed in the General Index. Where thought helpful, preparation titles have also been listed at the end of the relevant monograph. However, it should be noted that the absence of such a list at the end of a monograph is no indication as to the availability of a substance as many drugs are marketed as generic or unbranded preparations.

50:50 *BCM, UK.*
White soft paraffin (p.1407·3); liquid paraffin (p.1407·1).
Dry skin.

217 *Frosst, Canad.†.*
Aspirin (p.14·2); caffeine citrate (p.761·3).
Fever; inflammation; pain.

222 *Johnson & Johnson, Canad.*
Aspirin (p.14·2); caffeine citrate (p.761·3); codeine phosphate (p.25·2).
Fever; inflammation; pain.

282 *Lioh, Canad.*
Aspirin (p.14·2); caffeine citrate (p.761·3); codeine phosphate (p.25·2).
Fever; inflammation; pain.

292 *Lioh, Canad.*
Aspirin (p.14·2); caffeine citrate (p.761·3); codeine phosphate (p.25·2).
Fever; inflammation; pain.

642 *Lioh, Canad.*
Dextropropoxyphene hydrochloride (p.27·1).
Pain.

692 *Frosst, Canad.†.*
Dextropropoxyphene hydrochloride (p.27·1); aspirin (p.14·2); caffeine (p.761·3).
Pain.

3-A *Sophia, Mex.*
Diclofenac sodium (p.30·3).
Pain and inflammation associated with eye surgery; prevention of cystoid macular oedema; prevention of miosis during cataract surgery.

A-200 *Shalpharm, Israel; Hogil, USA†.*
Pyrethrins; piperonyl butoxide (p.1436·2).
Pediculosis.

A 313 *Pharmadeveloppement, Fr.*
Capsules: Vitamin A palmitate (p.1383·2).
Vitamin A deficiency.
Ointment: Vitamin A (p.1382·1).
Formerly contained vitamin A and tyrothricin.
Dermatitis.

A + B Balsam N *Mickan, Ger.*
Menthol (p.1632·3); camphor (p.1589·3); eucalyptus oil (p.1609·2).
Respiratory-tract disorders.

A and D Medicated *Schering-Plough, USA.*
Zinc oxide (p.1128·2); cod-liver oil (p.1357·2); vitamin A (p.1382·1); vitamin D (p.1391·1).
Nappy rash.

A + D + E-Vicotrat *Heyl, Ger.*
Vitamin A palmitate (p.1383·2); colecalciferol (p.1391·1); alpha tocoferil acetate (p.1394·1).
Deficiency of fat-soluble vitamins.

A Curitybina *Uniao Quimica, Braz.*
Paste; plaster: Salicylic acid (p.1122·3).
Topical liquid: Salicylic acid (p.1122·3); glacial acetic acid (p.1571·2); turpentine oil (p.1676·3).
Keratinisation disorders.

A & D Ointment *Schering-Plough, Canad.; National Care, Canad.*
Vitamin A (p.1382·1); vitamin D (p.1391·1).
Minor skin disorders.

A + D₃-Vicotrat *Heyl, Ger.†.*
Vitamin A palmitate (p.1383·2); colecalciferol (p.1391·1).
Vitamin A and D₃ deficiency.

A + E Thilo *Alcon-Thilo, Ger.*
Vitamin A acetate (p.1383·2); alpha tocoferil acetate (p.1394·1).
Vitamin A and E deficiency.

A Grin *Grin, Mex.*
Vitamin A palmitate (p.1383·2).
Vitamin A deficiency.

A Vogel Capsules a l'ail *Bioforce, Switz.*
Garlic (p.1614·1).
Cerebrovascular disorders.

A Vogel Capsules polyvitaminees *Bioforce, Switz.*
Halibut-liver oil (p.1366·1); rose fruit (p.1389·3); red cherry (p.1029·1); dried yeast (p.1398·1); safflower oil (p.1375·1).
Tonic.

A to Z Centabs *Hall, Canad.*
Multivitamin and mineral preparation (p.1350·1).

AA Cold *General Drugs, Thai.*
Brompheniramine maleate (p.410·2); phenylephrine hydrochloride (p.1097·1); phenylpropanolamine hydrochloride (p.1098·1).
Nasal congestion.

AAA
Note.This name is used for preparations of different composition.
Rhone-Poulenc Rorer, Irl.†.
Benzocaine (p.1306·2); cetylpyridinium chloride (p.1138·1).
Mouth and throat disorders.

Roche, S.Afr.
Benzocaine (p.1306·2); cetalkonium chloride (p.1137·1).
Mouth and throat disorders.

Manx, UK.
Benzocaine (p.1306·2).
Sore throat.

Aacidexam *Aaciphar, Belg.*
Dexamethasone sodium phosphate (p.1067·1).
Corticosteroid.

Aacifemine *Aaciphar, Belg.*
Estriol (p.1475·3).
Oestrogen deficiency.

AA-HC Otic *Schein, USA†.*
Hydrocortisone (p.1073·3); glacial acetic acid (p.1571·2); propylene glycol diacetate (p.1348·2); benzethonium chloride (p.1134·2).
Ear infection.

Aarane *Sanova, Aust.; Rhone-Poulenc Rorer, Switz.*
Sodium cromoglicate (p.774·3); reproterol hydrochloride (p.770·2).
Obstructive airways disease.

Aarane N *Rhone-Poulenc Rorer, Ger.*
Sodium cromoglicate (p.774·3); reproterol hydrochloride (p.770·2).
Obstructive airways disease.

AAS *Sanofi Winthrop, Braz.; Sterling, Port.; Sanofi Synthelabo, Spain.*
Aspirin (p.14·2).
Fever; inflammation; pain; thromboembolism prophylaxis.

AB FE *Camps, Spain.*
Aspirin (p.14·2); caffeine (p.761·3); phenazone (p.77·2).
Fever; pain.

Abacateirol *Regius, Braz.*
Persea persea; sodium salicylate (p.84·2); methenamine (p.223·1); theophylline (p.777·2).
Kidney disorders.

Abacin *Benedetti, Ital.*
Co-trimoxazole (p.193·3).
Bacterial infections; Pneumocystis carinii pneumonia.

Abactrim *Andreu, Spain†.*
Co-trimoxazole (p.193·3).
Bacterial infections; Pneumocystis carinii pneumonia.

Abacus *Pharmaland, Thai.*
Hydroxyzine hydrochloride (p.419·1).
Anxiety; hypersensitivity reactions; pruritus; tension.

Abaktal *Hind Wing, Hong Kong; Lek, Thai.*
Pefloxacin mesilate (p.234·3).
Bacterial infections.

Abalgin *Nycomed, Denm.; Nycomed, Fin.*
Dextropropoxyphene hydrochloride (p.27·1).
Musculoskeletal and joint disorders; pain.

Abaprim *Gentili, Ital.†.*
Trimethoprim (p.264·2).
Bacterial infections.

Abbiofort *Synpharma, Aust.*
Caraway (p.1591·2); psyllium seed (p.1229·1).
Constipation; stool softener.

Abbocillin-V *Abbott, Austral.*
Benzathine phenoxymethylpenicillin (p.157·1).
Bacterial infections.

Abbocillin-VK *Abbott, Austral.*
Phenoxymethylpenicillin potassium (p.235·1).
Bacterial infections.

Abbodop *Abbott, Denm.; Abbott, Fin.; Abbott, Norw.; Abbott, Swed.*
Dopamine hydrochloride (p.881·3).
Heart failure; oliguria; shock.

Abbokinase *Abbott, Aust.; Abbott, Canad.; Abbott, Israel; Abbott, Spain†; Abbott, Swed.; Abbott, USA.*
Urokinase (p.988·1).
Intra-ocular haemorrhage; thromboembolic disorders; to restore patency of intravenous shunts.

Abbolipid *Abbott, Ger.*
Safflower oil (p.1375·1); soya oil (p.1378·1).
Lipid infusion for parenteral nutrition.

Abbopen *Abbott, Swed.†.*
Phenoxymethylpenicillin potassium (p.235·1).
Bacterial infections.

Abboplegisol *Abbott, Spain.*
Electrolyte infusion (p.1180·1).
Adjunct to open-heart surgery.

Abboticin
Abbott, Denm.; Abbott, Fin.; Abbott, Norw.; Abbott, Swed.
Erythromycin (p.201·2), erythromycin ethyl succinate
(p.201·2), erythromycin lactobionate (p.201·3), or
erythromycin stearate (p.201·3).
Bacterial infections.

Abboticine *Abbott, Fr.*
Erythromycin ethyl succinate (p.201·2).
Bacterial infections.

Abbottselsun *Abbott, Spain.*
Selenium sulfide (p.1123·1).
Scalp disorders.

Abburic *Quick-Med, S.Afr.†.*
Allopurinol (p.397·2).
Gout; hyperuricaemia.

Abbutamol *Norton, S.Afr.†.*
Salbutamol (p.770·3).
Obstructive airways disease.

ABC *Beiersdorf, Aust.*
Capsicum (p.1591·1).
Muscle and joint pain.

ABC Warme-Pflaster N *Beiersdorf, Ger.*
Arnica flowers (p.1581·3); cayenne pepper (p.1591·1).
Musculoskeletal and joint disorders.

ABC Warme-Pflaster Sensitive *Beiersdorf, Ger.*
Nonivamide (p.63·1).
*Musculoskeletal, joint, peri-articular, and soft-tissue
disorders.*

ABC Warme-Salbe *Beiersdorf, Ger.*
Diethylamine salicylate (p.32·2); benzyl nicotinate
(p.20·2); nonivamide (p.63·1).
*Musculoskeletal, joint, and soft-tissue disorders; neu-
ralgia.*

ABC to Z *Nature's Bounty, USA.*
Ferrous fumarate (p.1360·1); folic acid (p.1361·1);
multivitamins and minerals (p.1350·1).
Iron-deficiency anaemias.

ABCDin *Ferrosan, Denm.*
Multivitamin preparation (p.1350·1).

Abdijsiroop (Akker-Siroop) *Alfaco, Neth.†.*
Belladonna tincture (p.463·1); drosera (p.1606·1); ipecacuanha tincture (p.1093·1); cowslip tincture
(p.1600·1); ephedrine hydrochloride (p.1090·1).
Coughs.

Abdomilon *Caesaro, Aust.*
Absinthium (p.1571·1); angelica (p.1580·2); calamus
(p.1588·1); frangula bark (p.1227·1); gentian
(p.1615·1); melissa (p.1632·2); rhubarb (p.1248·1).
Dyspepsia.

Abdomilon N *Cesra, Ger.*
Absinthium (p.1571·1); angelica root (p.1580·2); calamus root (p.1588·1); gentian root (p.1615·1); melissa
leaves (p.1632·2).
Dysmenorrhoea; gastrointestinal disorders.

Abdominol *Medea, Spain.*
Atropine methobromide (p.460·3); caffeine (p.761·3);
propyphenazone (p.80·2).
Pain due to smooth muscle spasm.

Abdoscan
*Nycomed, Aust.; Nycomed Imaging, Denm.; Nycomed, Fin.; Ny-
comed, Ger.; Nycomed Imaging, Norw.; Nycomed, Spain; Nycomed
Amersham, Swed.; Nycomed, Switz.; Nycomed Amersham, UK.*
Ferristene (p.1032·2).
Contrast medium for magnetic resonance imaging.

Abelcet
*Liposome Company, Aust.; Amgen, Austral.; Liposome Company,
Denm.; Wyeth Lederle, Fin.; Wyeth Lederle, Fr.; Liposome Company,
Hong Kong; Liposome Company, Irl.; Liposome Company, Ital.; Lipo-
some Company, Norw.; Liposome Company, Singapore; Pensa, Spain;
Wyeth Lederle, Swed.; Liposome Company, Switz.; Elan, UK; Lipo-
some Company, USA.*
Amphotericin B phospholipid complex (p.377·2).
Fungal infections.

Abenol *SmithKline Beecham, Canad.*
Paracetamol (p.71·2).
Fever; pain.

Abentel *Atlantic, Thai.*
Albendazole (p.95·2).
Worm infections.

Aberel *Janssen-Cilag, Fr.*
Tretinoin (p.1126·2).
Keratinisation disorders.

Aberela
Janssen-Cilag, Norw.; Janssen-Cilag, Swed.
Tretinoin (p.1126·2).
Acne; photoageing of the skin.

Abesira *Clariana, Spain.*
Vitamin B substances and amino acids (p.1350·1).
Anaemias; metabolic disorders; tonic.

Abetol *CT, Ital.†.*
Labetalol hydrochloride (p.918·1).
Hypertension.

Abflex *Xeragen, S.Afr.*
Paracetamol (p.71·2); doxylamine succinate (p.417·1);
caffeine (p.761·3); codeine phosphate (p.25·2).
Pain with tension.

Abfuhrdragees *Sanochemia, Aust.*
Aloes (p.1210·1); phenolphthalein (p.1244·1); hard
soap (p.1496·2).
Bowel evacuation; constipation.

Abfuhrdragees mild *Sanochemia, Aust.*
Aloes (p.1210·1); frangula bark (p.1227·1); hard soap
(p.1496·2).
Constipation.

Abfuhrtee *Sanochemia, Aust.*
Couch-grass (p.1599·3); chamomile (p.1593·2); centaurea cyanus; frangula bark (p.1227·1); rhubarb
(p.1248·1); senna (p.1248·2).
Constipation.

Abfuhrtee EF-EM-ES *Smetana, Aust.*
Achillea (p.1572·2); peppermint leaf (p.1243·2); senna
(p.1248·2).
Formerly contained frangula bark, hypericum, pepper-
mint leaf, and senna.
Constipation.

Abfuhrtee N *Bad Heilbrunner, Ger.*
Senna (p.1248·2).
Constipation.

Abfuhrtropfen *Ratiopharm, Ger.*
Sodium picosulfate (p.1249·3).
Constipation.

Abidec
*Warner-Lambert, Irl.; Teofarma, Ital.; Parke, Davis, S.Afr.†; Warner-
Lambert, UK.*
Multivitamin preparation (p.1350·1).

Abiocef *NCSN, Ital.*
Cefonicid sodium (p.168·1).
Lignocaine [lidocaine] hydrochloride (p.1313·2) is in-
cluded in this preparation to alleviate the pain of injec-
tion.
Bacterial infections.

Abiostil *Deca, Ital.*
Neomycin sulfate (p.228·1); eucalyptol (p.1609·2);
pumilio pine oil (p.1656·3); camphor (p.1589·3); menthol (p.1632·3).
Nasopharyngeal infections.

Abiplatin
Sanova, Aust.; Abic, Israel; Teva, S.Afr.; Abic, Thai.
Cisplatin (p.525·1).
Malignant neoplasms.

Abiposid *Sanova, Aust.*
Etoposide (p.538·1).
Malignant neoplasms.

Abitren
Teva, Hong Kong; Biogal, Israel; Abic, Thai.
Diclofenac sodium (p.30·3).
*Gout; inflammation; musculoskeletal, joint, peri-artic-
ular, and soft-tissue disorders; pain.*

Abitrexate
*Sanova, Aust.; Abic, Israel; Teva, S.Afr.; Abic, Thai.; International Phar-
maceutical, Ital†.*
Methotrexate sodium (p.553·2).
Malignant neoplasms; psoriasis; rheumatoid arthritis.

Abnobaviscum *Abnoba, Ger.*
Mistletoe (p.1636·2).
Malignant neoplasms.

Abolibe *Asta Medica, Port.*
Ginkgo biloba (p.1615·2).
Mental function disorders; vascular disorders.

Abopur *Norton Healthcare, Denm.*
Allopurinol (p.397·2).
Gout.

Abrasone *Seid, Spain.*
Fluocinolone acetonide (p.1071·1); framycetin sulfate
(p.208·2).
Infected skin disorders.

Abrasone Rectal *Seid, Spain.*
Fluocinonide acetonide; hexetidine (p.1146·3); rusco-
genin (p.1660·2).
Anorectal disorders.

Abreva *SmithKline Beecham Consumer, USA.*
Docosanol (p.619·3).
Herpes labialis.

Abrinac *Boots, Neth.†.*
Pirenzepine hydrochloride (p.472·2).
Peptic ulcer; Zollinger-Ellison syndrome.

Abrol *Rekah, Israel.*
Paracetamol (p.71·2).
Fever; pain.

Abrolet *Rekah, Israel.*
Paracetamol (p.71·2).
Fever; pain.

Absenor
Orion, Fin.; Orion, Swed.
Sodium valproate (p.366·3).
Epilepsy.

Absimed *Synpharma, Aust.*
Caraway (p.1591·2); melissa (p.1632·2); valerian
(p.1678·3).
Gastrointestinal disorders.

Absint *Medochemie, Hong Kong.*
Flunitrazepam (p.683·2).
Insomnia.

Absorbase *Carolina, USA.*
Vehicle for topical preparations.

Absorber HFV *Arteva, Ger.*
Dimethicone (p.1249·2).
Reduction of gastrointestinal gas.

Absorbine Analgesic *Young, Canad.*
Methyl salicylate (p.55·1); camphor (p.1589·3); menthol (p.1632·3); eucalyptus oil (p.1609·2).

Absorbine Antifungal
Young, Canad.†; Young, USA†.
Tolnaftate (p.395·2).
Fungal skin infections.

Absorbine Antifungal Foot Powder *Young, USA.*
Miconazole nitrate (p.391·1).
Fungal skin infections.

Absorbine Athletes Foot Care *Young, USA.*
Tolnaftate (p.395·2); menthol (p.1632·3).
Fungal infections.

Absorbine Athritis *Young, Canad.*
Menthol (p.1632·3); capsicum (p.1591·1).

Absorbine Jr
Young, Canad.; Young, USA.
Menthol (p.1632·3).
Muscle, joint, and soft-tissue pain; neuralgia.

Absorbine Jr Antifungal *Young, Canad.*
Tolnaftate (p.395·2); menthol (p.1632·3).
Tinea pedis.

Absorbine Power Gel
Young, Canad.; Young, USA†.
Menthol (p.1632·3).
Muscular aches.

Absorlent *Esteve, Spain.*
Estradiol (p.1473·1).
Menopausal disorders; osteoporosis.

Absorlent Plus *Esteve, Spain.*
Patch A, estradiol (p.1473·1); patch B, estradiol; nore-
thisterone acetate (p.1485·1).
Menopausal disorders.

Abstem *Wyeth, Irl.*
Calcium carbimide (p.1588·2).
Alcoholism.

Absten S *Medley, Braz.*
Mazindol (p.1510·3).
Obesity.

Abtrim *Ashbourne, UK.*
Clotrimazole (p.382·1).
Fungal skin infections; vaginal candidiasis.

Abufene *Doms-Adrian, Fr.*
Beta-alanine.
Menopausal disorders.

Abutol *Nettopharma, Denm.†.*
Acebutolol hydrochloride (p.825·1).
Angina pectoris; arrhythmias; hypertension.

AC & C *WestCan, Canad.*
Aspirin (p.14·2); caffeine (p.761·3); codeine phosphate
(p.25·2).
Fever; inflammation; pain.

AC Vax *SmithKline Beecham, UK.*
A meningococcal vaccine (groups A and C) (p.1550·1).
Active immunisation.

Aca *Atlantic, Thai.*
Benzhexol [trihexyphenidyl] hydrochloride (p.463·3).
Parkinsonism.

Acabel
Euro-Labor, Port.; Grunenthal, Port.; Grunenthal, Spain.
Lornoxicam (p.50·2).
*Inflammation; osteoarthritis; pain; rheumatoid arthri-
tis.*

Acadione *Cassenne, Fr.*
Tiopronin (p.1025·1).
Cystinuric lithiasis; polyarthritis.

A-Caine *AVP, USA†.*
Diperodon hydrochloride (p.1311·3); mepyramine
maleate (p.421·1); phenylephrine hydrochloride
(p.1097·1); bismuth subcarbonate (p.1213·1); zinc oxide (p.1128·2).
Anorectal disorders.

Acalka
Helsinn, Port.; Robert, Spain.
Potassium citrate (p.1186·1).
Alkalinisation of urine; renal calculi.

Acamed *Medifive, Thai.*
Benzhexol [trihexyphenidyl] hydrochloride (p.463·3).
Parkinsonism.

Acamol *Teva, Israel.*
Paracetamol (p.71·2).
Fever; pain.

Acamoli *Teva, Israel.*
Paracetamol (p.71·2).
Fever; pain.

Acarcid *Pierre Fabre Sante, Fr.*
Acetamide; crotamiton (p.1112·3); benzalkonium
chloride (p.1133·2); thyme oil (p.1672·3); geranium oil
(p.1615·1); myrtle oil.
Elimination of house dust mites.

Acarcid perles *Pierre Fabre Sante, Fr.*
Piperonyl butoxide (p.1436·2); permethrin (p.1436·1);
carbaryl (p.1429·2); methoprene (p.1434·3).
Acaricide.

Acardi *Boehringer Ingelheim, Jpn.*
Pimobendan (p.955·3).
Heart failure.

Acardust
Pharmygiene, Fr.; Scot, Israel; Geymonat, Ital.; SCAT, Switz.†.
Esdepallethrine (p.1432·2); piperonyl butoxide
(p.1436·2).
Acaricide.

Acarex *Allergopharma, Ger.*
Potassium hydroxide (p.1654·1); methyl alcohol
(p.1404·2).
Test for detection of house dust mite excretae.

Acaril *Allergopharma, Ger.*
Benzyl benzoate (p.1428·2).
Elimination of house dust mites.

Acarilbial *Bial, Port.*
Benzyl benzoate (p.1428·2).

Acarosan *Allergopharma, Ger.*
Benzyl benzoate (p.1428·2).
Elimination of house-dust mites.

Acarsan *Biosintetica, Braz.*
Benzyl benzoate (p.1428·2).
Pediculosis; scabies.

Acatar *SMB, Belg.*
Dextromethorphan hydrobromide (p.1087·3); guaifen-
esin (p.1092·2).
Coughs.

ACB
Pacific, NZ; Alphapharm, Singapore; Merck, Singapore.
Acebutolol (p.825·2) or acebutolol hydrochloride
(p.825·1).
Angina pectoris; arrhythmias; hypertension.

ACC
Hexal, Aust.; Hexal, Ger.; Hexal, S.Afr.; Ecosol, Switz.
Acetylcysteine (p.1082·3) or acetylcysteine sodium
(p.1083·1).
*Paracetamol overdosage; respiratory-tract disorders
with increased or viscous mucus.*

Accolate
*Zeneca, Austral.; Zeneca, Belg.; AstraZeneca, Canad.; AstraZeneca,
Fin.; Zeneca, Hong Kong; Zeneca, Irl.; Zeneca, Mex.; Zeneca, Port.;
AstraZeneca, Singapore; Zeneca, Spain; Zeneca, Switz.; AstraZene-
ca, Thai.; AstraZeneca, UK; AstraZeneca, USA.*
Zafirlukast (p.785·3).
Asthma.

Accoleit *Zeneca, Ital.*
Zafirlukast (p.785·3).
Asthma.

Accomin *Whitehall, Austral.*
Vitamin B substances with lysine and iron (p.1350·1).

Accomin Centrum *Whitehall, Austral.*
Capsules†: Multivitamin and mineral preparation with
lysine (p.1350·1).
Oral liquid: Vitamin B substances with lysine and iron
(p.1350·1).

Accomin Vitamin *Whitehall, Austral.†.*
Amino-acid, vitamin, and iron preparation (p.1350·1).

Accu-Check Advantage *Boehringer Mannheim, USA.*
Test for glucose in blood (p.1616·3).

Accu-Check III/Chemstrip bG *Boehringer Mannheim, Canad.†.*
Test for glucose in blood (p.1616·3).

Accu-Chek *Boehringer Mannheim, Fr.†.*
Test for glucose in blood (p.1616·3).

Accuneb *Dey, USA.*
Salbutamol sulfate (p.770·3).
Asthma.

Accupaque *Nycomed, Ger.*
Iohexol (p.1035·1).
Radiographic contrast medium.

Accupep *Sherwood, USA.*
Preparation for enteral nutrition (p.1350·1).
Gastrointestinal disorders.

Accupril
*Parke, Davis, Austral.; Parke, Davis, Belg.; Parke, Davis, Canad.;
Parke, Davis, Hong Kong; Parke, Davis, NZ; Parke, Davis, S.Afr.;
Parke, Davis, Singapore; Warner-Lambert, Thai.; Parke, Davis, USA.*
Quinapril hydrochloride (p.963·3).
Heart failure; hypertension.

Accuprin *Parke, Davis, Ital.*
Quinapril hydrochloride (p.963·3) or quinaprilat
(p.964·1).
Heart failure; hypertension.

Accupro
*Parke, Davis, Aust.; Parke, Davis, Denm.; Parke, Davis, Fin.; Godecke,
Ger.; Parke, Davis, Ger.; Parke, Davis, Irl.; Parke, Davis, Swed.; Warn-
er-Lambert, Switz.; Parke, Davis, UK.*
Quinapril hydrochloride (p.963·3) or quinaprilat
(p.964·1).
Heart failure; hypertension.

Accupro Comp
Parke, Davis, Fin.; Parke, Davis, Swed.
Quinapril hydrochloride (p.963·3); hydrochlorothi-
azide (p.907·3).
Hypertension.

Accurbron *Marion Merrell Dow, USA.*
Theophylline (p.777·2).
Asthma; bronchospasm.

Accure *Alphapharm, Austral.*
Isotretinoin (p.1115·3).
Acne.

Accuretic
*Parke, Davis, Belg.; Parke, Davis, Canad.; Parke, Davis, Irl.; Parke,
Davis, Ital.; Parke, Davis, S.Afr.; Warner-Lambert, Switz.; Parke, Dav-
is, UK; Parke, Davis, USA.*
Quinapril hydrochloride (p.963·3); hydrochlorothi-
azide (p.907·3).
Hypertension.

AccuSite *Matrix, UK†.*
Fluorouracil (p.540·2).
Adrenaline [epinephrine] (p.829·1) is included in this
preparation as a vasoconstrictor to diminish absorption
and localise the effect of the antineoplastic.
Genital warts.

Accutane
Roche, Canad.; Roche, USA.
Isotretinoin (p.1115·3).
Acne.

Accutest Fecal *Marco, Austral.*
Test for haemoglobin in faeces.

Accutest Multi-Drug *Marco, Austral.*
Test for amfetamine, benzoylecgonine, methamfeta-
mine, morphine, or THC in urine.

Accutrend Cholesterol
Roche Diagnostics, Ital.; Boehringer Mannheim Diagnostics, UK.
Test for cholesterol in blood.

Accutrend Colesterol Lakeside, Mex.
Test for cholesterol in blood.

Accutrend GC Roche, Canad.
Test for glucose and cholesterol in blood (p.1616·3).

Accutrend Glucose
Roche Diagnostics, Austral.; Roche Diagnostics, Ital.; Roche Diagnostics, NZ.
Test for glucose in blood (p.1616·3).

Accuvit Ache, Braz.
Multivitamin preparation (p.1350·1).

Accuzide
Parke, Davis, Aust.; Godecke, Ger.; Parke, Davis, Ger.
Quinapril hydrochloride (p.963·3); hydrochlorothiazide (p.907·3).
Hypertension.

Accuzyme Healthpoint, USA.
Papain (p.1647·3); urea (p.1127·3).
Debridement of necrotic tissue.

Ac-De Lemery, Mex.
Dactinomycin (p.532·2).
Malignant neoplasms.

Aceclofar Julphar, UAE.
Aceclofenac (p.11·1).
Musculoskeletal and joint disorders; pain.

Acecol Sankyo, Jpn.
Temocapril hydrochloride (p.979·3).
Hypertension.

Acecomb Zeneca, Aust.
Hydrochlorothiazide (p.907·3); lisinopril (p.921·1).
Hypertension.

Acecor SPA, Ital.
Acebutolol hydrochloride (p.825·1).
Arrhythmias; heart failure; hypertension.

Acecromol Wolff, Ger.
Sodium cromoglicate (p.774·3).
Asthma.

Acedicone Boehringer Ingelheim, Belg.
Thebacon hydrochloride (p.1101·3).
Coughs.

Acediur
Note. This name is used for preparations of different composition.
Menarini, Ital.
Captopril (p.853·3); hydrochlorothiazide (p.907·3).
Hypertension.

Sigma-Tau, Spain.
Enalapril maleate (p.883·3); hydrochlorothiazide (p.907·3).
Hypertension.

Acef Eurofarmaco, Ital.
Cefazolin sodium (p.164·3).
Bacterial infections.

ACE-Hemmer Ratiopharm, Ger.
Captopril (p.853·3).
Heart failure; hypertension.

Aceite Acalorico Ordesa, Spain.
Olive oil (p.1643·3); betacarotene (p.1355·3); liquid paraffin (p.1407·1).
Constipation; obesity.

Aceite Geve Concentrado Teofarma, Spain.
Cod-liver oil (p.1357·2).
Deficiency of vitamins A and D.

Acekapton Strallhofer, Aust.
Aspirin (p.14·2).
Fever; pain.

Acel-Imune Lederle, Switz.; Wyeth-Ayerst, USA†.
A diphtheria, tetanus, and acellular pertussis vaccine (p.1537·3).
Active immunisation of infants and young children.

Acelluvax Chiron, Ital.; Chiron, Thai.
An acellular pertussis vaccine (p.1555·3).
Active immunisation.

Acelluvax DTP Chiron, Thai.
A diphteria, tetanus, and acellular pertussis vaccine (p.1537·3).
Active immunisation of infants and young children.

Acel-P
Wyeth-Ayerst, Canad.; Lederle, Ger.; Lederle, Switz.
An adsorbed acellular pertussis vaccine (p.1555·3).
Active immunisation.

Acemetadoc Docpharm, Ger.
Acemetacin (p.11·2).
Gout; inflammation; musculoskeletal, joint, and peri-articular disorders.

Acemin Zeneca, Aust.
Lisinopril (p.921·1).
Heart failure; hypertension; myocardial infarction.

Acemix Bioprogress, Ital.
Acemetacin (p.11·2).
Musculoskeletal and joint disorders.

Acemuc Betapharm, Ger.
Acetylcysteine (p.1082·3).
Respiratory-tract disorders with viscous mucus.

Acemucol Streuli, Switz.
Acetylcysteine (p.1082·3).
Respiratory-tract disorders associated with excess or viscous mucus.

Acenorm
Alphapharm, Austral.; Azupharma, Ger.
Captopril (p.853·3).
Diabetic nephropathy; heart failure; hypertension; myocardial infarction.

Acenorm HCT Azupharma, Ger.
Captopril (p.853·3); hydrochlorothiazide (p.907·3).
Hypertension.

Acenterine Christiaens, Belg.
Aspirin (p.14·2).
Musculoskeletal and joint disorders.

Aceomel Clonmel, Irl.
Captopril (p.853·3).
Heart failure; hypertension.

Aceon Solvay, USA.
Perindopril erbumine (p.953·2).
Hypertension.

Aceoto Zambon, Spain.
Ciprofloxacin (p.182·3).
Otitis externa; otitis media.

Acephen G & W, USA.
Paracetamol (p.71·2).
Pain.

Acephlogont Azupharma, Ger.
Acemetacin (p.11·2).
Gout; inflammation, musculosketal, joint, and soft-tissue disorders.

Aceplus
Bristol-Myers Squibb, Ital.; Bristol-Myers Squibb, Neth.
Captopril (p.853·3); hydrochlorothiazide (p.907·3).
Hypertension.

Acepress Bristol-Myers Squibb, Ital.
Captopril (p.853·3).
Diabetic nephropathy; heart failure; hypertension; myocardial infarction.

Acepril
Note. This name is used for preparations of different composition.
United Nordic, Denm.
Lisinopril (p.921·1).
Heart failure; hypertension.

Spirig, Switz.
Enalapril maleate (p.883·3).
Heart failure; hypertension.

Squibb, UK.
Captopril (p.853·3).
Diabetic nephropathy; heart failure; hypertension; myocardial infarction.

Acequide Recordati, Ital.
Quinapril hydrochloride (p.963·3); hydrochlorothiazide (p.907·3).
Hypertension.

Acequin Recordati, Ital.
Quinapril hydrochloride (p.963·3) or quinaprilat (p.964·1).
Heart failure; hypertension.

Aceratun Delta, Braz.
Urea hydrogen peroxide (p.1159·3).
Cleansing of external ear.

Acerbine
Note. This name is used for preparations of different composition.
Montavit, Aust.
Benzoic acid (p.1134·2); malic acid (p.1631·1); propylene glycol (p.1655·1); propylene glycol malate (p.1655·2); salicylic acid (p.1122·3).
Bruises; burns; sunburn; ulcers; wounds.

Interdelta, Switz.
Ointment: Benzoic acid (p.1134·2); malic acid (p.1631·1); salicylic acid (p.1122·3); propylene glycol (p.1655·1); propylene glycol malate (p.1655·2); hexachlorophene (p.1146·1).
Topical solution; topical gel: Benzoic acid (p.1134·2); malic acid (p.1631·1); salicylic acid (p.1122·3); propylene glycol (p.1655·1); propylene glycol malate (p.1655·2).
Burns; wounds.

Acerbiol Vitafarma, Spain.
Benzyl alcohol (p.1135·2); benzoic acid (p.1134·2); malic acid (p.1631·1); propylene glycol (p.1655·1); propylene glycol (p.1655·1); salicylic acid (p.1122·3).
Burns; skin ulcers; wounds.

Acerbon Zeneca, Ger.
Lisinopril (p.921·1).
Heart failure; hypertension.

Acercomp
AstraZeneca, Fin.; Zeneca, Ger.
Lisinopril (p.921·1); hydrochlorothiazide (p.907·3).
Hypertension.

Aceren Nycomed, Denm.
Enalapril maleate (p.883·3).
Heart failure; hypertension.

Aceril Dexcel, Israel.
Captopril (p.853·3).
Diabetic nephropathy; heart failure; hypertension; myocardial infarction.

Acertil Servier, Hong Kong.
Perindopril (p.953·2).
Heart failure; hypertension.

Acertol Lacer, Spain.
Paracetamol (p.71·2).
Fever; pain.

Aces Carlson, USA.
Betacarotene; calcium ascorbate; d-alpha tocoferol; selenomethionine (p.1350·1).
Nutritional supplement.

Acesal
OPW, Ger.; Roland, Ger.; Geymonat, Ital.
Aspirin (p.14·2).
Fever; musculoskeletal, joint, and soft-tissue disorders; pain.

Acesal Calcium OPW, Ger.†; Roland, Ger.†.
Aspirin (p.14·2).
Calcium carbonate (p.1215·1) is included in this preparation in an attempt to limit adverse effects on the gastrointestinal mucosa.
Fever; pain; rheumatism; thromboembolic disorders.

Acesistem Sigma-Tau, Ital.
Enalapril maleate (p.883·3); hydrochlorothiazide (p.907·3).
Hypertension.

Acestrol Probios, Port.
Megestrol acetate (p.1481·2).
Malignant neoplasms.

Acet
Pharmascience, Canad.; Pharmascience, Singapore.
Paracetamol (p.71·2).
Fever; pain.

Acet-2, Acet-3 Pharmascience, Canad.†.
Paracetamol (p.71·2); codeine phosphate (p.25·2); caffeine (p.761·3).
Fever; pain.

Acet Codeine Pharmascience, Canad.†.
Paracetamol (p.71·2); codeine phosphate (p.25·2).
Fever; pain.

Aceta Century, USA.
Paracetamol (p.71·2).
Fever; pain.

Aceta with Codeine Century, USA.
Paracetamol (p.71·2); codeine phosphate (p.25·2).
Pain.

Acetab Romilo, Canad.
Paracetamol (p.71·2).
Fever; pain.

Acetabs Krewel, Ger.
Acetylcysteine (p.1082·3).
Respiratory-tract disorders.

Acetacol PP Lab, Thai.
Paracetamol (p.71·2); phenylpropanolamine hydrochloride (p.1098·1); chlorpheniramine [chlorphenamine] maleate (p.412·1).
Cold symptoms; hay fever; nasal congestion.

Acetadiazol Grin, Mex.
Acetazolamide (p.826·1).
Epilepsy; glaucoma; oedema.

Acetafen Rayere, Mex.
Paracetamol (p.71·2).
Fever; pain.

Aceta-Gesic Rugby, USA.
Phenyltoloxamine citrate (p.423·1); paracetamol (p.71·2).
Upper respiratory-tract symptoms.

Acetalgine Streuli, Switz.
Paracetamol (p.71·2).
Fever; pain.

Acetaminophen with Codeine Pharmascience, Canad.
Paracetamol (p.71·2); caffeine (p.761·3); codeine phosphate (p.25·2).
Coughs; fever; pain.

Acetamol
Bergamo, Braz.; Abiogen, Ital.
Paracetamol (p.71·2).
Fever; pain.

Acetan Kwizda, Aust.
Lisinopril (p.921·1).
Heart failure; hypertension; myocardial infarction.

Aceta-P PP Lab, Thai.
Paracetamol (p.71·2).
Fever; pain.

Acetapon Pharmagen, S.Afr.†.
Aspirin (p.14·2); paracetamol (p.71·2); codeine phosphate (p.25·2).
Fever; pain.

Acetapyrin-C PP Lab, Thai.
Paracetamol (p.71·2); chlorpheniramine [chlorphenamine] maleate (p.412·1).
Cold symptoms; hay fever.

Acetar
Note. This name is used for preparations of different composition.
Clintex, Port.
Piracetam (p.1652·1).
Cerebrovascular disorders; chronic alcoholism; mental function impairment; Raynaud's syndrome.

Thai Otsuka, Thai.
Electrolyte infusion with or without glucose (p.1180·1).
Carbohydrate source; fluid and electrolyte disorders.

Acetard Nycomed, Denm.†.
Aspirin (p.14·2).
Fever; inflammation; pain.

Acetasil Silom, Thai.
Paracetamol (p.71·2).
Fever; pain.

Acetasol Barre-National, USA.
Acetic acid (p.1571·3); propylene glycol acetate (p.1348·2); benzethonium chloride (p.1134·2).
Ear infection.

Acetasol HC Barre-National, USA.
Hydrocortisone (p.1073·3); acetic acid (p.1571·3); propylene glycol diacetate (p.1348·2); benzethonium chloride (p.1134·2).
Ear infection.

Acetat-Haemodialyse Alte Kreis, Aust.
Sodium chloride; potassium chloride; magnesium chloride; calcium chloride; sodium acetate; with or without glucose (p.1184·1).
Haemodialysis solutions.

Acetazone Forte Technilab, Canad.
Chlorzoxazone (p.1327·3); paracetamol (p.71·2).
Pain; skeletal muscle spasm.

Acetazone Forte C8 Technilab, Canad.
Chlorzoxazone (p.1327·3); paracetamol (p.71·2); codeine phosphate (p.25·2).
Pain; skeletal muscle spasm.

Acetensil Andromaco, Spain.
Enalapril maleate (p.883·3).
Heart failure; hypertension.

Acetensil Plus Andromaco, Spain.
Enalapril maleate (p.883·3); hydrochlorothiazide (p.907·3).
Hypertension.

Acetest
Bayer, Canad.; Bayer Diagnostics, Fr.; Bayer Diagnostics, Irl.; Bayer Diagnostics, Mex.; Bayer Diagnostics, UK; Bayer, USA.
Test for ketones in urine, blood, plasma, or serum.
In the UK these are described in the Drug Tariff as Nitroprusside Reagent Tablets (Rothera's Tablets).

Aceticil Cazi, Braz.
Aspirin (p.14·2).
Fever; inflammation; pain; thromboembolism prophylaxis.

Acetif Novag, Mex.
Paracetamol (p.71·2).
Fever; pain.

Acetin
Note. This name is used for preparations of different composition.
Millet Roux, Braz.
Aspirin (p.14·2).
Fever; inflammation; pain; thromboembolism prophylaxis.

LBS, Thai.
Acetylcysteine (p.1082·3).
Respiratory-tract disorders.

Acetocaustin Asta Medica, Ger.
Monochloroacetic acid.
Verrucas.

Acetocaustine Asta Medica, Switz.
Monochloroacetic acid.
Warts.

Acetofen Medley, Braz.
Paracetamol (p.71·2).
Fever; pain.

Acetolyt Madaus, Aust.; Madaus, Ger.
Calcium-sodium-hydrogencitrate.
Metabolic acidosis.

Acetonal Brady, Aust.
Aluminium acetotartrate (p.1578·2); trichlorisobutyl salicylate.
Anorectal disorders.

Acetopt
Sigma, Austral.; Sigma, NZ.
Sulfacetamide sodium (p.250·3).
Bacterial eye infections.

Acetosal Rekah, Israel.
Aspirin (p.14·2).
Fever; inflammation; pain.

Acetoxyl
Stiefel, Canad.; Stiefel, UK†.
Benzoyl peroxide (p.1111·1).
Acne.

Acetuber
Note. This name is used for preparations of different composition.
ICN, Spain†.
Injection: Pituitary extract (p.1295·2).
Acetonaemia; vomiting in pregnancy.

Teofarma, Spain.
Suppositories: Cocarboxylase (p.1385·2); dimenhydrinate (p.415·2); glucose (p.1364·2); pyridoxine (p.1387·1); potassium chloride (p.1194·3); dibasic sodium phosphate (p.1193·2).
Acetonaemia; vomiting in pregnancy.

Acetylcodone Bios, Belg.
Acetyldihydrocodeine hydrochloride (p.1084·2).
Coughs.

Acetylin Bristol-Myers Squibb, Ger.
Aspirin (p.14·2).
Fever; pain.

Acetyst Pharbita, Thai.
Acetylcysteine (p.1082·3).
Respiratory-tract disorders associated with increased or viscous mucus.

Acezide Squibb, UK.
Captopril (p.853·3); hydrochlorothiazide (p.907·3).
These ingredients can be described by the British Approved Name Co-zidocapt.
Hypertension.

AC-FA Pharmasant, Thai.
Ketoconazole (p.389·1).
Fungal skin infections.

Acfol
Cazi, Braz.; Italfarmaco, Spain.
Folic acid (p.1361·1).
Folic acid deficiency; prevention of neural tube defects in pregnancy.

Aches/Pains Homeocan, Canad.
Homoeopathic preparation.

Achromide Propan, S.Afr.
Merbromin (p.1150·1); acriflavinium chloride (p.1130·2); sulfanilamide (p.256·2); zinc oxide (p.1128·2); cod-liver oil (p.1357·2).
Burns; ulcers; wounds.

The symbol † denotes a preparation no longer actively marketed

Achromycin *Wyeth Lederle, Aust.; Lederle, Austral.; Wyeth-Ayerst, Canad.†; Wyeth Lederle, Denm.†; Lederle, Ger.; Lederle, Irl.; Lederle, S.Afr.†; Wyeth Lederle, Swed.; Wyeth-Ayerst, Thai.; Wyeth, UK.*
Tetracycline hydrochloride (p.258·3).
Amoebiasis; bacterial infections.

Achromycin V *Lederle, Austral.; Wyeth-Ayerst, Canad.†; Lederle, Hong Kong; Lederle, USA.*
Tetracycline hydrochloride (p.258·3).
Bacterial infections.

Achromycine *Lederle, Switz.†*
Tetracycline hydrochloride (p.258·3).
Bacterial infections.

Aciben *Mavi, Mex.*
Aspirin (p.14·2).

Acic *Hexal, Ger.*
Aciclovir (p.612·3) or aciclovir sodium (p.612·3).
Herpesvirus infections.

Aciclin *Fidia, Ital.*
Aciclovir (p.612·3).
Herpesvirus infections.

Aciclobene *Ratiopharm, Aust.*
Aciclovir (p.612·3).
Herpesvirus infections.

Aciclobeta *Betapharm, Ger.*
Aciclovir (p.612·3).
Herpesvirus infections.

Aciclodan *Pharmacodane, Denm.*
Aciclovir (p.612·3).
Herpesvirus infections.

Aciclosina *Cipan, Port.*
Aciclovir (p.612·3).
Herpesvirus infections.

Aciclostad *Stada, Ger.; Ciclum, Spain.*
Aciclovir (p.612·3).
Herpesvirus infections.

Aciclotyrol *Tyrol, Aust.*
Aciclovir (p.612·3).
Herpes simplex infections; varicella zoster infections.

Acic-Ophtal *Winzer, Ger.*
Aciclovir (p.612·3).
Herpes simplex eye infections.

Acid A Vit *Pierre Fabre, Neth.†*
Tretinoin (p.1126·2).
Acne.

Acid Control *Novapharm, Canad.; Stanley, Canad.*
Famotidine (p.1225·3).

Acid Halt *Wampole, Canad.*
Famotidine (p.1225·3).

Acid Mantle *Sandoz Consumer, USA.*
An ointment base.

Acidac *Pfizer Consumer, Spain†.*
Aluminium hydroxide (p.1210·3); dimethicone (p.1249·2); magnesium carbonate (p.1232·3); magnesium hydroxide (p.1233·1).
Flatulence; hyperchlorhydria.

Acide acetylsalicylique comp. "Radix" *Streuli, Switz.†.*
Aspirin (p.14·2); paracetamol (p.71·2); codeine hydrochloride (p.25·2); lignocaine [lidocaine] hydrochloride (p.1313·2).
Fever; pain.

Acidern *Sanval, Braz.*
Undecenoic acid (p.395·3); triacetin (p.395·3); lignocaine [lidocaine] hydrochloride (p.1313·2).
Fungal skin infections.

Acidex
Note.This name is used for preparations of different composition.
Heralds, Braz.
Aluminium hydroxide (p.1210·3); magnesium hydroxide (p.1233·1); aluminium hydroxide-magnesium carbonate co-dried gel (p.1211·2); dimethicone (p.1249·2).
Flatulence; gastrointestinal hyperacidity.

Pinewood, Irl.; Pinewood, UK.
Sodium alginate (p.1498·3); sodium bicarbonate (p.1186·2); calcium carbonate (p.1215·1).
Dyspepsia; gastro-oesophageal reflux; heartburn.

Salters, S.Afr.
Aluminium hydroxide gel (p.1210·3).
Dyspepsia; heartburn.

Acid-Eze *Norton, UK.*
Cimetidine (p.1216·3).
Dyspepsia; heartburn.

Acidion *Inibsa, Spain.*
Aluminium hydroxide (p.1210·3); dimethicone (p.1249·2); magnesium carbonate (p.1232·3); magnesium hydroxide (p.1233·1).
Dyspepsia; flatulence; gastrointestinal hyperacidity.

Acidix *Solfran, Mex.*
Nalidixic acid (p.227·1).
Urinary-tract infections.

Acid-Lac *Mex-America, Mex.*
Lactic acid (p.1626·2).
Maintenance of normal skin pH.

Acidodermil *Vifor, Switz.†.*
Bornyl salicylate (p.20·3); mint oil (p.1636·3); rosemary oil (p.1659·3).
Skin disorders.

Acidophilus *Novartis Consumer, Ger.*
Lactobacillus acidophilus (p.1626·3).
Gastrointestinal disorders.

Acidophilus Bifidus *Blackmores, Austral.*
Lactobacillus acidophilus (p.1626·3); Bifidobacterium bifidum (p.1626·3).
Maintenance of normal gastrointestinal flora.

Acidophilus Complex *Neo-Life, Austral.*
Lactobacillus acidophilus (p.1626·3); Lactobacillus bulgaricus (p.1626·3); Bifidobacterium bifidum (Bacillus bifidus) (p.1626·3).
Digestive disorders.

Acidophilus Plus
GNLD, Austral.
Lactobacillus acidophilus (p.1626·3); Bifidobacterium bifidum (p.1626·3); Lacotbacillus bulgaricus (p.1626·3); Lactobacillus casei; Streptococcus thermophilus (p.1626·3).
Digestive disorders.

Quest, UK.
Lactobacillus acidophilus (p.1626·3); Lactobacillus rhamnosus (p.1626·3); Bifidobacterium bifidum (p.1626·3); Enterococcus faecium (p.1626·3).

Acidophilus Tablets *Vitaglow, Austral.*
Lactobacillus acidophilus (p.1626·3).
Digestive disorders.

Acidosis *Potter's, UK.*
Meadowsweet (p.1631·2); vegetable charcoal (p.1000·3); rhubarb (p.1248·1).
Dyspepsia; gastric hyperacidity; heartburn.

Acidovert *Klein, Ger.*
Calcium citrate (p.1188·1); magnesium citrate (p.1232·3).
Acid-base regulation; metabolic acidosis.

Acidown *Brunel, S.Afr.†.*
Cimetidine (p.1216·3).
Gastrointestinal disorders.

Acidrina *Solvay, Spain.*
Aluminium hydroxide (p.1210·3); dimethicone (p.1249·2); magnesium hydroxide (p.1233·1).
Dyspepsia; flatulence; gastrointestinal hyperacidity.

Acidrine
Solvay, Aust.; Solvay, Belg.; Solvay, Fr.; Solvay, Ger.; Teofarma, Ital.
Myrtecaine laurilsulfate (p.1317·3); aluminium glycinate (p.1210·3); galactase sulfate.
Gastrointestinal disorders.

Acidum phosphoricum Med Complex *Dynamit, Aust.*
Homoeopathic preparation.

Acidum picrinicum Med Complex *Dynamit, Aust.*
Homoeopathic preparation.

Acid-X *BDI, USA.*
Paracetamol (p.71·2); calcium carbonate (p.1215·1).
Gastrointestinal disorders.

Acidylina *Fermenti, Ital.†.*
Ascorbic acid (p.1389·3).

Aciflux *SmithKline Beecham, Neth.*
Cimetidine (p.1216·3); alginic acid (p.1498·3).
Gastro-oesophageal reflux.

Aciforin *Pharmonta, Aust.*
Formic acid (p.1612·3); methyl salicylate (p.55·1); turpentine oil (p.1676·3).
Musculoskeletal pain.

Acifugan
Henning, Ger.; Jaba, Port.; Lacer, Spain; Synthelabo, Switz.
Allopurinol (p.397·2); benzbromarone (p.399·3).
Gout; hyperuricaemia.

Acifur *Fustery, Mex.*
Aciclovir (p.612·3).
Herpesvirus infections.

Acihexal *Hexal, Austral.*
Aciclovir (p.612·3).
Herpesvirus infections.

Aci-Jel
Note.This name is used for preparations of different composition.
Janssen-Cilag, Austral.; Janssen-Cilag, NZ; Ortho McNeil, USA.
Glacial acetic acid (p.1571·2); hydroxyquinoline sulfate (p.1622·2); ricinoleic acid (p.1658·1); glycerol (p.1616·3).
Maintenance of vaginal acidity.

Janssen-Cilag, Irl.; Janssen-Cilag, UK.
Acetic acid (p.1571·2).
Maintenance of vaginal acidity.

Acilac *Technilab, Canad.*
Lactulose (p.1230·1).
Constipation; hepatic encephalopathy.

Acilen *IFI, Ital.*
Acetylcarnitine or acetylcarnitine hydrochloride (p.1572·1).
Cerebrovascular disorders; peripheral neuropathy.

Aciloc
Note.This name is used for preparations of different composition.
Orion, Denm.; Orion, Swed.
Cimetidine (p.1216·3).
Acid aspiration; gastro-oesophageal reflux; gastrointestinal haemorrhage; peptic ulcer; Zollinger-Ellison syndrome.

Cadila, Thai.
Ranitidine hydrochloride (p.1245·2).
Gastro-oesophageal reflux; peptic ulcer; Zollinger-Ellison syndrome.

Acimax *PMC, Austral.*
Omeprazole (p.1239·1) or omeprazole magnesium (p.1239·1).
Gastro-oesophageal reflux; peptic ulcer; Zollinger-Ellison syndrome.

Aci-Med *Triomed, S.Afr.*
Cimetidine (p.1216·3).
Gastro-oesophageal reflux; peptic ulcer; upper gastrointestinal haemorrhage; Zollinger-Ellison syndrome.

Acimethin *Madaus, Aust.; Gry, Ger.; Gry, Switz.*
Methionine (p.1012·2).
Adjunct in antibiotic therapy; paracetamol overdosage; renal calculi; urinary-tract disorders.

Acimetten *Pharmonta, Aust.†*
Aspirin (p.14·2).
Fever; pain.

Acimox *Diba, Mex.*
Amoxicillin trihydrate (p.149·2).
Bacterial infections.

Acimox-Ex *Diba, Mex.*
Amoxicillin trihydrate (p.149·2); ambroxol hydrochloride (p.1084·3).
Respiratory-tract infections.

Acimpil *Farcoral, Mex.*
Ampicillin (p.150·3).
Bacterial infections.

Acinal *Tegur, Mex.*
Nalidixic acid (p.227·1).

Acinil
Gea, Denm.; Gea, Norw.; Gea, Swed.
Cimetidine (p.1216·3).
Acid aspiration; gastro-oesophageal reflux; gastrointestinal haemorrhage; peptic ulcer; Zollinger-Ellison syndrome.

Acintor *Hoechst Marion Roussel, Ital.*
Klebsiella pneumoniae glycoprotein (p.1626·1).
Respiratory-tract infections.

Acipem *Caber, Ital.*
Pipemidic acid (p.236·1).
Urinary-tract infections.

Acipen *Yamanouchi, Neth.*
Phenoxymethylpenicillin potassium (p.235·1).
Bacterial infections.

Acipen-V *Yamanouchi, Neth.*
Phenoxymethylpenicillin (p.235·1).
Bacterial infections.

Aciphex *Eisai, USA; Janssen, USA.*
Rabeprazole sodium (p.1245·1).
Gastro-oesophageal reflux; peptic ulcer; Zollinger-Ellison syndrome.

Aciril *Molteni, Ital.*
Ibuprofen lysine (p.44·1).
Musculoskeletal and joint disorders.

Acirufan *Madaus, Ger.*
Homoeopathic preparation.

Aci-Sanorania *Sanorania, Ger.†.*
Aciclovir (p.612·3).
Herpesvirus infections.

Acistin *Piam, Ital.*
Infant feed (p.1350·1).
Cystinosis.

Acitak *Opus, UK.*
Cimetidine (p.1216·3).
Acid aspiration; gastro-oesophageal reflux; peptic ulcer; Zollinger-Ellison syndrome.

Acitra *Procter & Gamble, Braz.*
Benzethonium chloride (p.1134·2); vitamin C (p.1389·3).
Mouth disinfection.

Acivir *Curasan, Ger.*
Aciclovir sodium (p.612·3).
Herpes simplex infections.

Aclacin *Medac, UK.*
Aclarubicin hydrochloride (p.505·3).
Acute myeloid leukaemia.

Aclaplastin *Ebewe, Aust.; Medac, Ger.*
Aclarubicin hydrochloride (p.505·3).
Now known as Aclarubicin in Aust.
Acute myeloid leukaemia; thyroid cancer.

Aclimafel *AF, Mex.*
Veralipride (p.711·2).
Menopausal disorders.

Aclin *Alphapharm, Austral.; Alphapharm, Hong Kong.*
Sulindac (p.85·3).
Musculoskeletal and joint disorders; pain with inflammation.

Aclinda *Azupharma, Ger.*
Clindamycin hydrochloride (p.188·1).
Bacterial infections.

Aclon Lievit *Geymonat, Ital.*
Dried yeast (p.1398·1); vitamins (p.1350·1); echinacea (p.1606·2); betacarotene (p.1355·1).
Acne; seborrhoea.

Aclonium *SmithKline Beecham, Ital.*
Gabapentin (p.350·2).
Epilepsy.

Aclophen *Nutripharm, USA.*
Phenylephrine hydrochloride (p.1097·1); paracetamol (p.71·2); chlorpheniramine [chlorphenamine] maleate (p.412·1).
Upper respiratory-tract symptoms.

Acloral *Liomont, Mex.*
Ranitidine hydrochloride (p.1245·2).
Acid aspiration; gastro-oesophageal reflux; gastrointestinal haemorrhage; peptic ulcer; Zollinger-Ellison syndrome.

Aclorisan *Dovalle, Braz.*
Aluminium hydroxide (p.1210·3); magnesium hydroxide (p.1249·2).
Flatulence; gastrointestinal hyperacidity.

Aclosone *Schering-Plough, Fr.; Schering-Plough, Neth.; Schering-Plough, S.Afr.*
Alclometasone dipropionate (p.1061·1).
Skin disorders.

Aclotan *Piam, Ital.*
Dermatan sodium sulfate (p.867·1).
Thrombosis prophylaxis.

Aclotine *Lab Francais du Fractionnement, Fr.*
Antithrombin (human) (p.725·2).
Thromboembolic disorders.

Aclovate *Glaxo Wellcome, USA.*
Alclometasone dipropionate (p.1061·1).
Skin disorders.

Aclovir *Medinovum, Fin.*
Aciclovir (p.612·3).
Herpes simplex infections; varicella-zoster infections.

ACM 20 *Paraphar, Fr.*
Multivitamin, mineral, and amino-acid preparation (p.1350·1).

Acnacyl
Rosken, Hong Kong; Rosken, Singapore.
Benzoyl peroxide (p.1111·1).
Acne.

Acnase *Zurita, Braz.*
Benzoyl peroxide (p.1111·1); sulfur (p.1123·3).
Acne.

Acnaveen
Note.This name is used for preparations of different composition.
Rydelle, Fr.; Dermoteca, Port.†.
Avena (p.1583·1); salicylic acid (p.1122·3); carbocisteine (p.1086·3).
Acne; seborrhoea.

Johnson & Johnson, Ital.
Avena (p.1583·1); salicylic acid (p.1122·3).
Acne; seborrhoea.

Bioglan, UK.
Sulfur (p.1123·3); salicylic acid (p.1122·3).
Acne.

Acne *Homeocan, Canad.*
Homoeopathic preparation.

Acne Blemish Cream *Bonne Bell, Canad.†*
Sulfur (p.1123·3).
Acne.

Acne Complex *Brauer, Austral.†*
Homoeopathic preparation.

Acne Creme *Widmer, Switz.*
Salicylic acid (p.1122·3); colloidal sulfur (p.1123·3); colloidal silicon dioxide (p.1503·3); triclosan (p.1159·2).
Acne.

Acne Creme Plus *Widmer, Switz.*
Benzoyl peroxide (p.1111·1); miconazole nitrate (p.391·1).
Acne.

Acne Derm *Fischer, Israel.*
Benzoyl peroxide (p.1111·1).
Acne.

Acne Gel *Widmer, Switz.*
Colloidal sulfur (p.1123·3); pyridoxine hydrochloride (p.1386·3); triclosan (p.1159·2); urea (p.1127·3).
Acne.

Acne Lotion *Widmer, Switz.*
Salicylic acid (p.1122·3); lactic acid (p.1626·2); triclosan (p.1159·2); zinc sulfate (p.1398·2); magnesium sulfate dihydrate (p.1191·2).
Acne.

Acne Lotion 10 *C & M, USA.*
Sulfur (p.1123·3).
Acne.

Acne Mask *Neutrogena, Israel.*
Benzoyl peroxide (p.1111·1).
Acne.

Acne Oral Spray *Brauer, Austral.*
Lappa (p.1627·1); artemisia abrotanum; bellis perennis; fumaria; hepar sulf; juglans reg.; kali brom.; nat. mur.; rhus ven.; saponaria; selenium; sulfur; sulfur iod.; viola tric.
Acne.

Acne & Pimple Gel *Curacel, Austral.*
Sulfur (p.1123·3); allantoin (p.1110·1); zinc oxide (p.1128·2); resorcinol (p.1122·2).
Acne.

Acne Plus *Widmer, Ger.*
Miconazole nitrate (p.391·1); benzoyl peroxide (p.1111·1).
Acne.

Acne-Aid
Note.This name is used for preparations of different composition.
Stiefel, Austral.; Stiefel, Canad.; Stiefel, Hong Kong; Stiefel, Israel; Stiefel, Mex.; Stiefel, Singapore; Stiefel, Thai.; Stiefel, USA†.
Skin cleanser.
Acne.

Stiefel, Canad.†.
Topical gel: Sulfur (p.1123·3); resorcinol (p.1122·2); chloroxylenol (p.1142·1).
Acne.

Stiefel, Hong Kong; Stiefel, Singapore.
Cream: Sulfur (p.1123·3); resorcinol (p.1122·2); chloroxylenol (p.1142·1).
Acne.

Acnecide *Galderma, Irl.; Galderma, UK.*
Benzoyl peroxide (p.1111·1).
Acne.

Acneclear *Janpharm, S.Afr.*
Cleansing bar: Triclosan (p.1159·2).
Cream: Miconazole nitrate (p.391·1); benzoyl peroxide (p.1111·1).
Acne.

Acnecolor *Spirig, Switz.*
Clotrimazole (p.382·1).
Acne.

Acnecure *Taxandria, Neth.*
Miconazole nitrate (p.391·1); benzoyl peroxide (p.1111·1).
Acne.

Acne-Cy-Clean *Brovar, S.Afr.†.*
Doxycycline hyclate (p.200·1).
Acne.

Acnederm
Note.This name is used for preparations of different composition.
Ego, Austral.; Ego, Hong Kong; Ego, Singapore.
Sulfur (p.1123·3); ichthammol (p.1115·2); undecylenic alkanolamide (p.396·1); zinc oxide (p.1128·2).
Acne.

Ego, NZ.
Sulfur (p.1123·3); ammoniumsulfobitol (p.1115·2); undecylenic alkanolamide (p.396·1); zinc oxide (p.1128·2); alcloxa (p.1109·3).
Acne.

Acnederm Wash
Note.This name is used for preparations of different composition.
Ego, Austral.; Ego, Singapore.
Cetrimide (p.1137·1).
Acne.

Ego, NZ.
Cetrimide (p.1137·1); chlorhexidine gluconate (p.1138·2); propylene phenoxetol.
Acne.

Acnefuge *Spirig, Switz.*
Benzoyl peroxide (p.1111·1).
Acne.

Acneryne *Galderma, Belg.*
Erythromycin (p.201·2).
Acne.

Acnesan
Note.This name is used for preparations of different composition.
QIF, Braz.
Benzoyl peroxide (p.1111·1).
Acne.

Novogaleno, Ital.
Sulfur (p.1123·3); zinc sulfate (p.1398·2); glycolic acid (p.1115·1); enoxolone (p.34·3).
Seborrhoea.

Acnestrol *Poirier, Fr.†.*
Broparestrol (p.1465·3); pyridoxine (p.1387·1); hexachlorophene (p.1146·1).
Acne.

Acnetrim *Trima, Israel; Trima, Singapore; Unipharm, Singapore.*
Erythromycin (p.201·2).
Acne.

Acnex
Note.This name is used for preparations of different composition.
Dermtek, Canad.
Salicylic acid (p.1122·3).
Acne.

Rafa, Israel.
Hexachlorophene (p.1146·1); tyrothricin (p.267·1); resorcinol (p.1122·2); sulfur (p.1123·3); zinc oxide (p.1128·2).
Acne; dermatitis; eczema.

Acnezaic *Pfizer Consumer, Ital.*
Azelaic acid (p.1110·3).
Acne.

Acnidazil *Janssen-Cilag, Aust.; Janssen-Cilag, Belg†; Janssen-Cilag, Denm.†; Janssen-Cilag, Ger.†; Italchimici, Ital.; Janssen-Cilag, Neth.; Janssen-Cilag, Switz.†; Johnson & Johnson MSD Consumer, UK†.*
Miconazole nitrate (p.391·1); benzoyl peroxide (p.1111·1).
Acne.

Acnisal *Dermapharm, Irl.; Dermapharm, UK.*
Salicylic acid (p.1122·3).
Acne.

Acnisdin *Isdin, Spain.*
Sulfur (p.1123·3); calcium dobesilate (p.1588·3); resorcinol (p.1122·2).
Acne.

Acnisdin Retinoico *Isdin, Spain.*
Calcium dobesilate (p.1588·3); tretinoin (p.1126·2).
Acne; psoriasis.

Acno *Baker Cummins, USA.*
Sulfur (p.1123·3); salicylic acid (p.1122·3).
Acne.

Acno Cleanser *Baker Cummins, USA.*
Skin cleanser.

Acnomel
Note.This name is used for preparations of different composition.
Chattem, Canad.
Cream: Resorcinol (p.1122·2); sulfur (p.1123·3); isopropyl alcohol (p.1149·2).
Acne.

Vanishing cream: Resorcinol (p.1122·2); sulfur (p.1123·3).
Acne.

SmithKline Beecham Consumer, USA.
Resorcinol (p.1122·2); sulfur (p.1123·3); titanium dioxide (p.1126·1).
Acne.

Acnomel Acne Mask *Chattem, Canad.*
Resorcinol (p.1122·2); sulfur (p.1123·3).
Formerly contained salicylic acid.
Acne.

Acnomel BP 5 *Chattem, Canad.†.*
Benzoyl peroxide (p.1111·1).
Acne.

Acnosan *Bescansa, Spain.*
Camphor (p.1589·3); boric acid (p.1586·1); resorcinol (p.1122·2); salicylic acid (p.1122·3); undecenoic acid (p.395·3); zinc sulfate (p.1398·2); copper sulfate (p.1358·1).
Acne.

Acnosil *Heralds, Braz.*
Benzoyl peroxide (p.1111·1); sulfur (p.1123·3).
Acne.

Acnotex *C & M, USA.*
Sulfur (p.1123·3); salicylic acid (p.1122·3); methyl-benzethonium chloride (p.1150·3).
Acne.

ACNU *Asta Medica, Ger.; Asta Medica, Neth.; Asta Medica, Switz.*
Nimustine hydrochloride (p.562·3).
Malignant neoplasms.

Acobiotic *Heralds, Braz.*
Tetracycline hydrochloride (p.258·3); thiamphenicol (p.261·3).
Bacterial infections.

Acodon *Nakorn, Thai.*
Dipyrone (p.34·1).
Fever; pain.

Acoflam *Goldshield, UK.*
Diclofenac sodium (p.30·3).
Gout; inflammation; musculoskeletal, joint, and peri-articular disorders; pain.

Acoin *Combustin, Ger.*
Amethocaine [tetracaine] hydrochloride (p.1305·2); lauromacrogol 400 (p.1345·2).
Local anaesthesia.

Acomin *ACO, Swed.†.*
A range of vitamin preparations (p.1350·1).

Acon *Rhone-Poulenc Rorer, Mex.*
Vitamin A palmitate (p.1383·2).
Vitamin A deficiency.

Aconeurin *Heralds, Braz.*
Vitamin B substances (p.1350·1).
Vitamin B deficiency.

Aconex *Agepha, Aust.*
Naphazoline hydrochloride (p.1095·1).
Conjunctivitis.

Aconit-Nervenol *Wala, Ger.*
Homoeopathic preparation.

Aconitum *Truw, Ger.†; Weleda, Ger.*
Homoeopathic preparation.

Aconitum Med Complex *Dynamit, Aust.*
Homoeopathic preparation.

Acordin
Note.This name is used for preparations of different composition.
Kwizda, Aust.†.
Isosorbide dinitrate (p.915·2); diazepam (p.674·3).
Angina pectoris.

Mepha, Switz.
Isosorbide dinitrate (p.915·2).
Angina pectoris; heart failure; myocardial infarction.

Acorus *Zeppenfeldt, Ger.*
Couch-grass (p.1599·3).
Urinary-tract disorders.

Acovil *Hoechst Marion Roussel, Spain.*
Ramipril (p.966·3).
Heart failure following myocardial infarction; hypertension.

Acqua di Sirmione *Terme Sirmione, Ital.*
Sulfurous thermal water (p.1123·3).
Catarrh; cold symptoms; rhinitis; sinusitis.

Acqua Virginiana *Kelemata, Ital.*
Hamamelis virginiana (p.1618·3).
Skin irritation.

Acridin *Legrand, Braz.*
Acriflavinium chloride (p.1130·2); methenamine (p.223·1); methylene blue [methylthioninium chloride] (p.1012·3); belladonna (p.463·1).
Urinary-tract infections.

Acriflex *SSL, UK.*
Chlorhexidine gluconate (p.1138·2).
Burns; scalds; wounds.

Acrisuxin *Chemomedica, Aust.; Geistlich, Switz.†.*
Ethosuximide (p.348·1); mepacrine hydrochloride (p.593·1).
Absence seizures.

Acromax *Agepha, Aust.*
Sodium cromoglicate (p.774·3).
Allergic conjunctivitis; allergic rhinitis.

Acromicina *Cyanamid, Ital.†; Wyeth, Mex.*
Tetracycline hydrochloride (p.258·3).
Bacterial infections.

Acrosin *Climax, Braz.*
Liver extract.
Liver disorders.

Acroxil *Sons, Mex.*
Amoxicillin trihydrate (p.149·2).
Bacterial infections.

Acsacea *Chemomedica, Aust.*
Metronidazole (p.594·1).
Rosacea.

Acset *Bio-Transfusion, Fr.†.*
Activated factor VII (p.733·3).
Haemophilias A and B.

ACT
Note. A similar name is used for preparations of different composition (see below).
Johnson & Johnson Medical, USA.
Sodium fluoride (p.1375·3).
Dental caries prophylaxis.

ACT-3
Note. A similar name is used for preparations of different composition (see above).
Whitehall, Austral.; Whitehall, NZ.
Ibuprofen (p.43·2).
Fever; inflammation; musculoskeletal, joint, and soft-tissue disorders; pain.

Acta
Jean-Marie, Hong Kong; Jean-Marie, Singapore.
Tretinoin (p.1126·2).
Acne.

Actacode *Sigma, Austral.*
Codeine phosphate (p.25·2).
Coughs.

Actagen *Goldline, USA.*
Pseudoephedrine hydrochloride (p.1099·2); triprolidine hydrochloride (p.427·2).
Upper respiratory-tract symptoms.

Actagen-C Cough *Goldline, USA.*
Pseudoephedrine hydrochloride (p.1099·2); codeine phosphate (p.25·2); triprolidine hydrochloride (p.427·2).
Coughs and cold symptoms.

Actal
Note.This name is used for preparations of different composition.
ICN, Hong Kong; SmithKline Beecham, Irl.; ICN, Singapore; ICN, Thai.
Alexitol sodium (p.1209·3).
Gastric hyperacidity; peptic ulcer.

Merck Consumer, UK.
Pastilles: Hydrotalcite (p.1228·1).
Dyspepsia; heartburn.
Tablets: Alexitol sodium (p.1209·3).
Dyspepsia; gastric hyperacidity.

Actal Plus *ICN, Hong Kong.*
Aluminium hydroxide (p.1210·3); magnesium hydroxide (p.1233·1); simeticone (p.1249·2).
Gastrointestinal hyperacidity; peptic ulcer.

Actan *Restan, S.Afr.*
Alexitol sodium (p.1209·3).
Hyperchlorhydria; peptic ulcer, gastro-oesophageal reflux.

Actapulgite *Ipsen, Belg.; Beaufour, Fr.; Beaufour, Switz.*
Attapulgite (p.1212·1).
Gastrointestinal disorders.

Actebral *Menarini, Belg.; Biologiques de l'Ile-de-France, Fr.†.*
Cyprodenate (p.1507·2) or cyprodenate maleate (p.1507·2).
Cerebral disorders; tonic.

Acthar *Rhone-Poulenc Rorer, Austral.†; Rorer, Irl.; Roche, S.Afr.†; Rorer, UK; Rhone-Poulenc Rorer, USA.*
Corticotropin (p.1280·2).
Available on a named-patient basis only in the UK.
Corticosteroid release stimulant; diagnostic testing of adrenocortical function.

Act-HIB *Pasteur Merieux, Aust.; Pasteur Merieux, Belg.; Pasteur Merieux, Braz.; Connaught, Canad.; Pasteur Merieux, Denm.; Pasteur Merieux, Fr.; Pasteur Merieux, Ger.; Pasteur Merieux, Hong Kong; Aventis, Irl.; Pasteur Merieux, Israel; Pasteur Merieux, Ital.; Pasteur Merieux, Neth.; Pasteur Merieux, Norw.; Aventis, S.Afr.; Pasteur Merieux, Spain; Pasteur Merieux, Swed.; Pro Vaccine, Switz.; Pasteur Merieux, Thai.; Pasteur Merieux, UK; Pasteur Merieux, USA.*
A haemophilus influenzae conjugate vaccine (tetanus toxoid conjugate) (p.1540·2).
Active immunisation.

Act-HIB DTP *Pasteur Merieux, UK.*
A diphtheria, tetanus, pertussis, and haemophilus influenzae vaccine (p.1538·3).
Active immunisation.

Act-HIB plus DPT *Pasteur Merieux, Aust.*
Haemophilus influenzae conjugate vaccine (tetanus toxoid conjugate); diphtheria, tetanus, and pertussis vaccine (p.1538·3).
Active immunisation.

Act-HIB Polio *Pasteur Merieux, Swed.*
A haemophilus influenzae conjugate vaccine (tetanus toxoid conjugate) and an injectable inactivated poliomyelitis vaccine (types I, II and III).
Active immunisation.

Acthrel *Ferring, USA.*
Corticorelin triflutate (p.1280·2).
Determination of ACTH production in Cushing's syndrome.

Acti 5 *Pierre Fabre, Fr.*
Syrup†: Deanol glutamate; lysine hydrochloride (p.1370·3); calcium gluconogluceptate; phosphoric acid (p.1651·1).
Oral liquid: Deanol glutamate; sodium ascorbate (p.1390·1); magnesium aminobenzoate.
Formerly contained deanol glutamate, sodium ascorbate, magnesium aminobenzoate, and hesperidin methyl chalcone.
Tonic.

Acti-B₁₂ *Technilab, Canad.*
Hydroxocobalamin (p.1388·1); amino acids (p.1350·1).
Anaemia.

ActiBath *Jergens, USA.*
Avena (p.1583·1).
Dry skin; pruritus.

Actibil *Arkopharma, Fr.*
Cynara (p.1601·3); fumitory (p.1612·3).
Gastrointestinal and urinary-tract disorders.

Actibrush *Colgate-Palmolive, UK†.*
Triclosan (p.1159·2); gantrez.
Dental hygiene.

Acticalcin *TRB, Braz.*
Salcatonin (p.749·3).
Hypercalcaemia; osteoporosis; Paget's disease of bone.

Acticarbine *Elerte, Fr.*
Papaverine hydrochloride (p.1648·1); activated charcoal (p.1000·2).
Gastrointestinal disorders.

Actichlor *Adams, Hong Kong.*
Sodium dichloroisocyanurate (p.1156·1).
Disinfection of surfaces and equipment.

Acticillin *British Dispensary, Thai.*
Amoxicillin trihydrate (p.149·2).
Bacterial infections.

Acticin
Note.This name is used for preparations of different composition.
Penederm, UK.
Tretinoin (p.1126·2).
Acne.

Penederm, USA; Alpharma, USA.
Permethrin (p.1436·1).
Scabies.

Acticinco *Robapharm, Spain.*
Calcium gluceptate (p.1188·1); lysine hydrochloride (p.1370·3); deanol pyroglutamate (p.1507·2).
Tonic.

Acticolin *Upsamedica, Ital.*
Citicoline sodium (p.1596·1).
Cerebrovascular disorders; parkinsonism.

Acticort *Baker Cummins, USA.*
Hydrocortisone (p.1073·3).
Skin disorders.

Acticrom *Francia, Ital.*
Sodium cromoglicate (p.774·3).
Allergic conjunctivitis; keratoconjunctivitis.

Actidil *Glaxo Wellcome, Aust.; Warner-Lambert, Ital.*
Triprolidine hydrochloride (p.427·2).
Hypersensitivity reactions.

Actidine *Daewon, Hong Kong.*
Famotidine (p.1225·3).
Gastro-oesophageal reflux; gastrointestinal haemorrhage; peptic ulcer; Zollinger-Ellison syndrome.

Actidose with Sorbitol *Paddock, USA.*
Activated charcoal (p.1000·2); sorbitol (p.1377·2).
Emergency treatment of poisoning.

Actidose-Aqua *Cambridge, UK; Paddock, USA.*
Activated charcoal (p.1000·2).
Emergency treatment of poisoning.

Actidox *Saninter, Port.*
Doxycycline (p.200·1).
Bacterial infections.

Actidue *Warner-Lambert, Ital.*
Yellow tablets (daytime), paracetamol (p.71·2); phenylpropanolamine hydrochloride (p.1098·1); blue tablets (night-time) paracetamol; diphenhydramine hydrochloride (p.416·1).
Cold and influenza symptoms.

Actifed
Note.This name is used for preparations of different composition.
Warner-Lambert, Austral.; Glaxo Wellcome, Belg.; Warner-Lambert, Canad.; Warner-Lambert, Ger.†; Glaxo Wellcome, Hong Kong; Warner-Lambert, Irl.; Glaxo Wellcome, Israel; Warner-Lambert, Ital.; Warner-Lambert, NZ; Warner-Lambert Consumer, Port.; Glaxo Wellcome, S.Afr.; Glaxo Wellcome, Singapore; Glaxo Wellcome, Thai.; Warner-Lambert, UK; Wellcome, UK.
Triprolidine hydrochloride (p.427·2); pseudoephedrine hydrochloride (p.1099·2).
Upper respiratory-tract congestion.

Glaxo Wellcome, Hong Kong.
Syrup: Triprolidine hydrochloride (p.427·2); codeine phosphate (p.25·2); pseudoephedrine hydrochloride (p.1099·2); guaifenesin (p.1092·2).
Coughs.

Warner-Lambert, Fr.
Triprolidine hydrochloride (p.427·2); pseudoephedrine hydrochloride (p.1099·2); paracetamol (p.71·2).
Cold symptoms; upper respiratory-tract congestion.

Actifed Allergy *Wellcome, USA.*
White daytime caplets, pseudoephedrine (p.1099·2); blue night time caplets, pseudoephedrine; diphenhydramine hydrochloride (p.416·1).

The symbol † denotes a preparation no longer actively marketed

Actifed Anaesthetic Warner-Lambert, Austral.†
Lignocaine [lidocaine] hydrochloride (p.1313·2); dichlorobenzyl alcohol (p.1143·2); cetylpyridinium chloride (p.1138·1).
Sore throat.

Actifed CC Chesty Warner-Lambert, NZ.
Capsules: Guaifenesin (p.1092·2); pseudoephedrine hydrochloride (p.1099·2).
Linctus: Guaifenesin (p.1092·2); pseudoephedrine hydrochloride (p.1099·2); triprolidine hydrochloride (p.427·2).
Coughs and cold symptoms.

Actifed CC Dry Warner-Lambert, NZ.
Capsules: Dextromethorphan hydrobromide (p.1087·3); pseudoephedrine hydrochloride (p.1099·2).
Linctus: Dextromethorphan hydrobromide (p.1087·3); pseudoephedrine hydrochloride (p.1099·2); triprolidine hydrochloride (p.427·2).
Coughs.

Actifed CC Junior Warner-Lambert, Austral.; Warner-Lambert, NZ.
Dextromethorphan hydrobromide (p.1087·3); triprolidine hydrochloride (p.427·2).
Coughs.

Actifed Chesty
Note.This name is used for preparations of different composition.
Warner-Lambert, Austral.
Guaifenesin (p.1092·2); pseudoephedrine hydrochloride (p.1099·2).
Actifed CC Chesty Elixir formerly contained guaifenesin, pseudoephedrine hydrochloride, and triprolidine hydrochloride.
Coughs; respiratory-tract congestion.

Warner-Lambert, Irl.
Triprolidine hydrochloride (p.427·2); pseudoephedrine hydrochloride (p.1099·2); guaifenesin (p.1092·2).
Formerly known as Actifed Expectorant.
Coughs; upper respiratory-tract congestion.

Actifed Co Glaxo Wellcome, S.Afr.
Triprolidine hydrochloride (p.427·2); pseudoephedrine hydrochloride (p.1099·2); codeine phosphate (p.25·2).
Coughs.

Actifed with Codeine Glaxo Wellcome, USA†.
Codeine phosphate (p.25·2); triprolidine hydrochloride (p.427·2); pseudoephedrine hydrochloride (p.1099·2).
Coughs and cold symptoms.

Actifed Cold & Allergy Warner-Lambert, USA.
Triprolidine hydrochloride (p.427·2); pseudoephedrine hydrochloride (p.1099·2).
Upper respiratory-tract congestion.

Actifed Cold & Sinus Warner-Lambert, USA.
Triprolidine hydrochloride (p.427·2); pseudoephedrine hydrochloride (p.1099·2); paracetamol (p.71·2).
Cold symptoms.

Actifed Composto Warner-Lambert, Ital.
Triprolidine hydrochloride (p.427·2); pseudoephedrine hydrochloride (p.1099·2); dextromethorphan hydrobromide (p.1087·3).
Coughs; respiratory tract congestion.

Actifed Compound
Note.This name is used for preparations of different composition.
Glaxo Wellcome, Hong Kong; Glaxo Wellcome, Israel; Glaxo Wellcome, Singapore; Glaxo Wellcome, Thai.
Triprolidine hydrochloride (p.427·2); pseudoephedrine hydrochloride (p.1099·2); codeine phosphate (p.25·2).
Coughs; upper respiratory-tract congestion.

Warner-Lambert, Irl.; Warner-Lambert, UK.
Triprolidine hydrochloride (p.427·2); pseudoephedrine hydrochloride (p.1099·2); dextromethorphan hydrobromide (p.1087·3).
Coughs; upper respiratory-tract congestion.

Actifed DM Warner-Lambert, Canad.; Glaxo Wellcome, Hong Kong; Glaxo Wellcome, Israel; Glaxo Wellcome, S.Afr.; Glaxo Wellcome, Singapore; Glaxo Wellcome, Thai.
Triprolidine hydrochloride (p.427·2); pseudoephedrine hydrochloride (p.1099·2); dextromethorphan hydrobromide (p.1087·3).
Coughs and cold symptoms.

Actifed Dry Warner-Lambert, Austral.
Pseudoephedrine hydrochloride (p.1099·2); dextromethorphan hydrobromide (p.1087·3).
Actifen CC Dry Syrup formerly contained pseudoephedrine hydrochloride, dextromethorphan hydrobromide, and triprolidine hydrochloride.
Upper respiratory-tract disorders.

Actifed Expectorant
Note.This name is used for preparations of different composition.
Warner-Lambert, Fr.
Carbocisteine (p.1086·3).
Respiratory-tract disorders.

Glaxo Wellcome, Israel; Glaxo Wellcome, Singapore; Warner-Lambert, UK.
Triprolidine hydrochloride (p.427·2); pseudoephedrine hydrochloride (p.1099·2); guaifenesin (p.1092·2).
Coughs; upper respiratory-tract congestion.

Actifed jour et nuit Warner-Lambert, Fr.
Yellow tablets, paracetamol (p.71·2); phenylpropanolamine hydrochloride (p.1098·1); blue tablets, paracetamol; diphenhydramine hydrochloride (p.416·1).
Rhinitis.

Actifed Nasale Warner-Lambert, Ital.
Oxymetazoline hydrochloride (p.1096·2).
Nasal congestion.

Actifed Plus Warner-Lambert, Canad; Wellcome, USA.
Triprolidine hydrochloride (p.427·2); pseudoephedrine hydrochloride (p.1099·2); paracetamol (p.71·2).
Cold symptoms.

Actifed Sinus Daytime Wellcome, USA.
Pseudoephedrine hydrochloride (p.1099·2); paracetamol (p.71·2).
Upper respiratory-tract symptoms.

Actifed Sinus Nighttime Wellcome, USA.
Pseudoephedrine hydrochloride (p.1099·2); diphenhydramine hydrochloride (p.416·1); paracetamol (p.71·2).
Upper respiratory-tract symptoms.

Actifed Toux Seche Warner-Lambert, Fr.
Triprolidine hydrochloride (p.427·2); dextromethorphan hydrobromide (p.1087·3).
Coughs.

Actifedrin Glaxo Wellcome, Braz.
Triprolidine (p.427·2); pseudoephedrine hydrochloride (p.1099·2).
Hypersensitivity.

Actifen Gebro, Aust.
Dexibuprofen (p.44·1).
Fever; inflammation; pain.

Actiferrine Mepha, Switz.
Ferrous sulfate (p.1360·3); DL-serine.
Iron deficiency; iron-deficiency anaemia.

Actiferrine-F Nouvelle formule Mepha, Switz.
Ferrous sulfate (p.1360·3); DL-serine; folic acid (p.1361·1).
Pregnancy- or lactation-induced anaemia.

Actiferro Lampugnani, Ital.
Ferric sodium gluconate (p.1360·2).
Iron-deficiency disorders.

Actiflora Brovar, S.Afr.†
Lactobacillus acidophilus (p.1626·3).
Restoration of a normal gastrointestinal flora.

Actifluor Byk Gulden, Ital.
Sodium fluoride (p.1375·3); stannous fluoride (p.1379·3).
Dental caries prophylaxis.

Actigall Novartis, NZ; Novartis, USA.
Ursodeoxycholic acid (p.1677·2).
Gallstones; primary biliary cirrhosis; primary sclerosing cholangitis.

Actigesic Glaxo Wellcome, S.Afr.
Triprolidine hydrochloride (p.427·2); pseudoephedrine hydrochloride (p.1099·2); paracetamol (p.71·2).
Cold and influenza symptoms.

Actigrip Warner-Lambert, Ital.
Triprolidine hydrochloride (p.427·2); pseudoephedrine hydrochloride (p.1099·2); paracetamol (p.71·2).
Influenza symptoms; respiratory tract congestion.

Actihaemyl Solco, Ger.; Stulln, Ger.
Protein-free bovine blood extract.
Burns; ophthalmic disorders; peripheral and cerebral vascular disorders; wounds.

Actil Masa, Thai.
Triprolidine hydrochloride (p.427·2); pseudoephedrine hydrochloride (p.1099·2).
Allergic rhinitis; cold symptoms; hay fever; nasal congestion.

Actilam Sofex, Port.†
Hesperidin (p.1611·2); deanol acetamidobenzoate (p.1507·2); magnesium glycerophosphate (p.1191·1).
Mental function disorders; vascular disorders.

Actilax Alphapharm, Austral.
Lactulose (p.1230·1).
Constipation; hepatic encephalopathy.

Actilevol Orex Wasserman, Spain†.
Vitamins (p.1350·1); carnosine; cyproheptadine hydrochloride (p.414·2); haematoporphyrin hydrochloride (p.1618·3).
Tonic.

Actilife Lifeplan, UK.
Vitamins, minerals, fish oils, ginseng, and betacarotene (p.1350·1).
Nutritional supplement.

Actilis Pautrat, Fr.
Barrier cream.

Actilyse Boehringer Ingelheim, Aust.; Boehringer Ingelheim, Austral.; Boehringer Ingelheim, Belg.; Boehringer Ingelheim, Canad.; Boehringer de Angeli, Braz.; Boehringer Ingelheim, Denm.; Boehringer Ingelheim, Fin.; Boehringer Ingelheim, Fr.; Boehringer Ingelheim, Hong Kong; Boehringer Ingelheim, Irl.; Boehringer Ingelheim, Israel; Boehringer Ingelheim, Ital.; Promeco, Mex.; Boehringer Ingelheim, Neth.; Boehringer Ingelheim, NZ; Boehringer Ingelheim, Port.; Boehringer Ingelheim, S.Afr.; Boehringer Ingelheim, Singapore; Boehringer Ingelheim, Swed.; Boehringer Ingelheim, Switz.; Boehringer Ingelheim, Thai.; Boehringer Ingelheim, UK.
Alteplase (p.833·3).
Myocardial infarction; pulmonary embolism.

Actimag Vita, Ital.; Iquinosa, Spain.
Magnesium pidolate (p.1191·1).
Magnesium depletion.

Actimidol Sterling Health, Spain.
Ibuprofen (p.43·2).
Fever; musculoskeletal and joint disorders; pain.

Actimmune Genentech, USA.
Interferon gamma-1b (p.634·1).
Infections in chronic granulomatous disease; osteopetrosis.

Actimoxi Clariana, Spain.
Amoxicillin trihydrate (p.149·2).
Bacterial infections.

Actin The Forty-Two, Thai.
Co-trimoxazole (p.193·3).
Bacterial infections.

Actinac Hoechst Marion Roussel, Canad.; Hoechst Marion Roussel, Irl.; Peckforton, UK.
Chloramphenicol (p.179·1); hydrocortisone acetate (p.1073·3); nicoboxil (p.62·2); allantoin (p.1110·1); precipitated sulfur (p.1123·3).
Acne.

Actinex Schwarz, USA†.
Masoprocol (p.551·1).
Solar keratoses.

Actino-Hermal Hermal, Ger.
Fluorouracil (p.540·2).
Skin cancer.

Action Sante Naturelle, Canad.
Ascorbic acid (p.1389·3).

Action Chewable Bayer, Austral.
Chlorpheniramine [chlorphenamine] maleate (p.412·1); phenylephrine tartrate (p.1097·1).
Cold symptoms; hay fever.

Action Cold & Flu Bayer, Austral.
Chlorpheniramine [chlorphenamine] maleate (p.412·1); phenylephrine acid tartrate (p.1097·1); aspirin (p.14·2); ascorbic acid (p.1389·3).
Cold and influenza symptoms.

Actiphos Teofarma, Fr.
Phosphoric acid salts (p.1651·1).
Tonic.

Actiplas Dompe Biotec, Ital.
Alteplase (p.833·3).
Myocardial infarction.

Actiprofen SmithKline Beecham Consumer, Austral.; Sanofi Winthrop, Braz.; Bayer, Canad.; SmithKline Beecham, Irl.†.
Ibuprofen (p.43·2).
Fever; inflammation; pain.

Actiq Elan, UK; Cephalon, USA.
Fentanyl citrate (p.37·1).
Pain.

Actiquim Quimica y Farmacia, Mex.
Naproxen (p.60·3).
Inflammation; musculoskeletal and joint disorders.

Actireuma Farmila, Ital.
Multivitamin preparation with omega-3 and omega-6 triglycerides and herbal extracts (p.1350·1).
Nutritional supplement in joint disorders.

Actisane Constipation Occasionnelle Dolisos, Fr.†
Senna (p.1248·2); tamarind (p.1253·2).
Constipation.

Actisane Digestion Dolisos, Fr.†.
Cynara (p.1601·3); boldo (p.1585·3); fumitory (p.1612·3).
Biliary-tract disorders.

Actisane Douleurs Articulaires Dolisos, Fr.†
Devil's claw root (p.26·3); meadowsweet (p.1631·2).
Joint disorders.

Actisane Fatigue Passagere Dolisos, Fr.†
Ginseng (p.1615·3); tea (p.1681·1).
Tonic.

Actisane Hemorroides, Jambes Lourdes Dolisos, Fr.
Aesculus (p.1574·1); melilotus officinalis; red vine.
Haemorrhoids; venous insufficiency.

Actisane Minceur Dolisos, Fr.
Bladderwrack (p.1585·2); java tea (p.1625·1); meadowsweet (p.1631·2).
Obesity.

Actisane Nervosite Dolisos, Fr.†
Crataegus (p.1600·2); red-poppy petal (p.1029·1); passion flower (p.1649·1).
Cardiac disorders.

Actisane Troubles du Sommeil Dolisos, Fr.
Crataegus (p.1600·2); tilia (p.1673·2); valerian (p.1678·3).
Formerly known as Achisane Troubles du Sommeil.
Insomnia.

Actisite Willvonseder, Aust.; Meda, Denm.†; Wybert, Ger.; Dental Trey, Ital.; Dentaid, Spain; Solco, Swed.; Alza, Switz.; Alza, USA.
Tetracycline hydrochloride (p.258·3).
Bacterial mouth infections.

Actiskenan UPSA, Fr.
Morphine sulfate (p.56·1).
Pain.

Actisorb Johnson & Johnson Medical, Fr.†.
Activated charcoal (p.1000·2).
Infected wounds.

Actisorb 3 Johnson & Johnson, Ger.
Activated charcoal (p.1000·2); silver (p.1664·1).
Infected wounds; ulcers.

Actisorb Plus Johnson & Johnson Medical, Fr.; Johnson & Johnson, Irl.; Ethicon, Ital.; Johnson & Johnson Medical, UK.
Activated charcoal (p.1000·2); silver (p.1664·1).
Infected or malodorous wounds.

Actisoufre Grimberg, Fr.
Sodium sulfate (p.1250·1); dried yeast (p.1398·1).
Rhinitis; upper respiratory-tract inflammation.

Actisson Urgo, Fr.†.
Dietary fibre preparation (p.1350·1).
Constipation.

Actithiol Almirall, Spain.
Carbocisteine (p.1086·3).
Respiratory-tract disorders.

Actithiol Antihist Almirall, Spain.
Carbocisteine (p.1086·3); promethazine hydrochloride (p.423·2).
Respiratory-tract disorders.

Actitonic Amido, Fr.
Solution for adults: Amino-acid and mineral preparation (p.1350·1).
Solution for children†: Amino-acid preparation (p.1350·1).
Tonic.

Activadone Alcon Cusi, Spain.
Eye drops: Chromocarb diethylamine (p.1594·3).
Adjunct in eye surgery; conjunctival capillary fragility.

Thea, Spain.
Capsules: Chromocarb diethylamine (p.1594·3).
Capillary haemorrhage; venous insufficiency.

Activarol Merck-Belgolabo, Belg.†
Ascorbic acid; haematoporphyrin; glycine; vitamin B₁₂; dried yeast (p.1350·1).
Tonic.

Monot, Fr.†
Glycine; arginine (p.1350·1).
Tonic.

Carlo Erba OTC, Ital.
Haematoporphyrin hydrochloride; glycine; cyanocobalamin; calcium gluconate (p.1350·1).
Tonic.

Azevedos, Port.†
Haematoporphyrin hydrochloride; glycine; cyanocobalamin (p.1350·1).
Tonic.

Activase Roche, Canad.; Genentech, USA.
Alteplase (p.833·3).
Myocardial infarction; pulmonary embolism; stroke.

Active Dry Lotion Norwood, Canad.
SPF 15†: Octinoxate (p.1517·3); oxybenzone (p.1518·1).
SPF 30: Octinoxate (p.1517·3); oxybenzone (p.1518·1); octisalate (p.1518·1).
Sunscreen.

Active Multi Quest, Canad.
Multivitamin and mineral preparation (p.1350·1).

Activella Pharmacia Upjohn, USA.
Estradiol (p.1473·1); norethisterone acetate (p.1485·1).
Menopausal disorders; osteoporosis.

Activelle Novo Nordisk, Aust.; Novo Nordisk, Belg.; Novo Nordisk, Denm.; Novo Nordisk, Fin.; Novo Nordisk, Fr.; Novo Nordisk, Ger.; Novo Nordisk, Ital.; Novo Nordisk, Neth.; Novo Nordisk, Norw.; Novo Nordisk, Singapore; Isdin, Spain; Novo Nordisk, Swed.; Novo Nordisk, Switz.
Estradiol (p.1473·1); norethisterone acetate (p.1485·1).
Menopausal disorders; osteoporosis.

Activex 40 Plus Mer-National, S.Afr.; Propan, S.Afr.
Ginseng (p.1615·3); muira puama; vitamins (p.1350·1); minerals; kelp (p.1625·3); lysine hydrochloride.

Activir Glaxo Wellcome, Aust.; Glaxo Wellcome, Fr.; Glaxo Wellcome, S.Afr.
Aciclovir (p.612·3).
Herpes labialis.

Activital ECR, Switz.
Arginine aspartate (p.1354·1); calcium gluconate (p.1188·2); magnesium gluconate (p.1190·3).
Tonic.

Activon Bayer, Switz.
Etofenamate (p.35·3).
Soft-tissue disorders.

Activox Arkopharma, Fr.
Erysimum; chamomile (p.1593·2).
Mouth and throat disorders.

Actizyme Willvonseder, Aust.
Subtilisin-A; poloxamer 338 (p.1347·1) (p.1129·2).
Cleaning of contact lenses.

Actocortina Byk Leo, Spain.
Hydrocortisone sodium phosphate (p.1074·1).
Corticosteroid.

Actol Mayrhofer, Aust.; Fournier, Ger.†.
Niflumic acid (p.62·3).
Inflammation; pain.

Actomin GNR, Ital.
Citicoline sodium (p.1596·1).
Cerebrovascular disorders; parkinsonism.

Actomite Ceuta, UK.
Bioallethrin (p.1428·3).
Elimination of house dust mite.

Actonel Aventis, Austral.; Procter & Gamble, Fr.; Aventis, Irl.; Aventis, UK; Procter & Gamble, UK; Procter & Gamble, USA.
Risedronate sodium (p.755·2).
Osteoporosis; Paget's disease of bone.

Actonorm Wallace Mfg Chem., UK.
Oral gel: Aluminium hydroxide (p.1210·3); magnesium hydroxide (p.1233·1); simeticone (p.1249·2).
Dyspepsia; flatulence; gastric hyperacidity.

Oral powder: Magnesium carbonate (p.1232·3); aluminium hydroxide (p.1210·3); atropine sulfate (p.461·1); calcium carbonate (p.1215·1); magnesium trisilicate (p.1233·3); sodium bicarbonate (p.1186·2); peppermint oil (p.1243·3).
Dyspepsia; flatulence; gastric hyperacidity; gastrointestinal spasm.

Actophlem *Covan, S.Afr.*
Theophylline (p.777·2); etofylline (p.765·1); diphenylpyraline hydrochloride (p.417·1); ammonium chloride (p.1085·2); sodium citrate (p.1186·2).
Coughs.

Actopril *Ergha, Irl.*
Captopril (p.853·3).
Heart failure; hypertension.

Actos
Lilly, Austral.; Takeda, UK; Takeda, USA; Lilly, USA.
Pioglitazone hydrochloride (p.333·3).
Diabetes mellitus.

Actosolv
Hoechst Marion Roussel, Aust.; Aventis, Belg.; Hoechst, Fr.; Hoechst Marion Roussel, Ger.; Hoechst Marion Roussel, Israel; Hoechst Marion Roussel, Ital.
Urokinase (p.988·1).
Thromboembolic disorders.

Actovegin
Nycomed, Aust.; Nycomed, Ger.; Nycomed, Hong Kong; Hafslund Nycomed, Thai.
Protein-free bovine blood extract.
Burns; cerebral circulatory and metabolic disorders; peripheral vascular disorders; ulcers; wounds.

Actraphane 10/90, 20/80, 30/70, 40/60, 50/50
Novo Nordisk, Ital.
Mixtures of neutral insulin injection (human, monocomponent) and isophane insulin injection (human, monocomponent) respectively in the proportions indicated (p.324·1).
Diabetes mellitus.

Actraphane HM *Novo Nordisk, S.Afr.*
Mixture of soluble insulin injection (human, biosynthetic) 30% and isophane insulin injection (human, biosynthetic) 70% (p.324·1).
Diabetes mellitus.

Actraphane HM 10/90, 20/80, 30/70, 40/60, 50/50 *Novo Nordisk, Ger.*
Mixture of insulin injection (human) and isophane insulin injection (human) respectively in the proportions indicated (p.324·1).
Diabetes mellitus.

Actrapid
Novo Nordisk, Austral.; Novo Nordisk, Denm.; Novo Nordisk, Fin.; Novo Nordisk, Irl.; Novo Nordisk, Ital.; Novo Nordisk, Neth.; Novo Nordisk, Norw.; Novo Nordisk, NZ; Novo Nordisk, Port.; Novo Nordisk, Singapore; Novo Nordisk, Spain; Novo Nordisk, Swed.
Insulin injection (human, monocomponent) (p.324·1).
Formerly known as Human Actrapid in *Irl.*
Diabetes mellitus.

Actrapid HM
Novo Nordisk, Aust.; Novo Nordisk, Belg.; Novo Nordisk, Fr.; Novo Nordisk, Ger.; Novo Nordisk, Hong Kong; Novo Nordisk, S.Afr.; Novo Nordisk, Switz.; Novo Nordisk, Thai.
Neutral insulin injection (human, monocomponent) (p.324·1).
Diabetes mellitus.

Actrapid MC
Novo Nordisk, Denm.; Novo Nordisk, Hong Kong; Novo Nordisk, Switz.
Insulin injection (porcine, monocomponent) (p.324·1).
Diabetes mellitus.

Actron
Note. This name is used for preparations of different composition.
Bayer, Aust.; Bayer, USA†.
Ketoprofen (p.47·3).
Fever; musculoskeletal and joint disorders; pain.

Bayer, Fr.
Aspirin (p.14·2); paracetamol (p.71·2); caffeine (p.761·3).
Fever; pain.

Bayer, Spain.
Paracetamol (p.71·2).
Fever; pain.

Actron Compuesto *Bayer, Spain.*
Aspirin (p.14·2); caffeine (p.761·3); paracetamol (p.71·2).
Fever; pain.

Actroneffix *Bayer, Fr.*
Ketoprofen (p.47·3).
Fever; pain.

Actuss *Sigma, Austral.*
Pholcodine (p.1099·1).
Coughs.

Acuatim *Otsuka, Jpn.*
Nadifloxacin (p.226·3).
Acne.

Acubiron *Bohm, Spain.*
Pygeum africanum (p.1490·3).
Benign prostatic hyperplasia.

Acucil *Apotex, S.Afr.†.*
Amoxicillin trihydrate (p.149·2).
Bacterial infections.

Acuco *Apotex, S.Afr.†.*
Co-trimoxazole (p.193·3).
Bacterial infections.

Acudor *Ferring, Port.*
Etodolac (p.35·2).
Gout; musculoskeletal, joint, and peri-articular disorders; pain.

ACU-dyne *Acme, USA.*
Povidone-iodine (p.1155·1).
Skin disinfection; vaginal disorders.

Acu-Erylate S *Apotex, S.Afr.†.*
Erythromycin estolate (p.201·2).
Bacterial infections.

Acuflex *Apotex, S.Afr.†.*
Indometacin (p.44·3).
Gout; musculoskeletal and joint disorders.

Acuflu-P *Apotex, S.Afr.†.*
Triprolidine hydrochloride (p.427·2); pseudoephedrine hydrochloride (p.1099·2); paracetamol (p.71·2).
Cold and influenza symptoms.

Acugesil *Apotex, S.Afr.†.*
Paracetamol (p.71·2); codeine phosphate (p.25·2); caffeine (p.761·3); meprobamate (p.691·1).
Pain with tension.

Acugest *Apotex, S.Afr.*
Triprolidine hydrochloride (p.427·2); pseudoephedrine hydrochloride (p.1099·2).
Cold and influenza symptoms.

Acugest Co *Apotex, S.Afr.*
Triprolidine hydrochloride (p.427·2); pseudoephedrine hydrochloride (p.1099·2); codeine phosphate (p.25·2).
Coughs.

Acugest Expect *Apotex, S.Afr.*
Triprolidine hydrochloride (p.427·2); pseudoephedrine hydrochloride (p.1099·2); guaifenesin (p.1092·2).
Coughs.

Acuilix *Parke, Davis, Fr.*
Hydrochlorothiazide (p.907·3); quinapril hydrochloride (p.963·3).
Hypertension.

Acuitel *Parke, Davis, Fr.*
Quinapril hydrochloride (p.963·3).
Heart failure; hypertension.

Acular
Allergan, Aust.; Allergan, Austral.; Allergan, Canad.; Allergan, Denm.; Allergan, Fin.; Allergan, Fr.; Allergan, Ger.; Allergan, Hong Kong; Allergan, Irl.; Allergan, Ital.; Allergan, Neth.†; Allergan, NZ; Allergan, Port.; Allergan, S.Afr.; Allergan, Singapore; Allergan, Spain; Allergan, Switz.; Allergan, UK; Allergan, USA.
Ketorolac trometamol (p.48·2).
Allergic conjunctivitis; cystoid macular oedema; inflammation, pain, and photophobia following ocular surgery.

Aculare *Allergan, Belg.*
Ketorolac trometamol (p.48·2).
Ocular inflammation following cataract surgery.

Acularen *Allergan, Mex.*
Ketorolac trometamol (p.48·2).
Allergic conjunctivitis; postoperative ocular inflammation.

Aculfin *Apsen, Braz.*
Sulfasalazine (p.1251·1).
Ankylosing spondylitis; rheumatoid arthritis; ulcerative colitis.

Aculoid *Apotex, S.Afr.†.*
Cyclizine hydrochloride (p.414·1).
Nausea; vestibular disorders; vomiting.

Acumet *Apotex, S.Afr.†.*
Metoclopramide hydrochloride (p.1235·2).
Gastrointestinal disorders.

Acumod *Apotex, S.Afr.†.*
Amiloride hydrochloride (p.835·1); hydrochlorothiazide (p.907·3).
Hypertension; oedema.

Acunaso *Apotex, S.Afr.*
Pseudoephedrine hydrochloride (p.1099·2).
Upper respiratory-tract congestion.

Acuolens *Alcon Cusi, Spain.*
Hypromellose (p.1501·3).
Dry eyes.

Acu-Oxytet *Apotex, S.Afr.†.*
Oxytetracycline hydrochloride (p.234·1).
Bacterial infections.

Acupan
3M, Belg.; Biocodex, Fr.; 3M, Irl.; 3M, Israel; 3M, NZ; 3M, S.Afr.†; CEPA, Spain†; 3M, Switz.; 3M, UK.
Nefopam hydrochloride (p.62·1).
Pain.

Acuphlem *Apotex, S.Afr.†.*
Carbocisteine (p.1086·3).
Respiratory-tract disorders with excess mucus.

Acupillin *Apotex, S.Afr.†.*
Ampicillin trihydrate (p.151·1).
Bacterial infections.

Acuprel *Parke, Davis, Spain.*
Quinapril hydrochloride (p.963·3).
Heart failure; hypertension.

Acupril
Parke, Davis, Mex.; Parke, Davis, Neth.; Parke, Davis, Port.
Quinapril hydrochloride (p.963·3) or quinaprilat (p.964·1).
Heart failure; hypertension.

Acurate *Apotex, S.Afr.†.*
Paracetamol (p.71·2); doxylamine succinate (p.417·1); caffeine (p.761·3); codeine phosphate (p.25·2).
Pain with tension.

Acuretic
Parke, Davis, Port.; Parke, Davis, Spain.
Quinapril hydrochloride (p.963·3); hydrochlorothiazide (p.907·3).
Hypertension.

Acusprain *Apotex, S.Afr.†.*
Naproxen (p.60·3).
Dysmenorrhoea; gout; musculoskeletal and joint disorders.

Acustop *Apotex, S.Afr.†.*
Paracetamol (p.71·2); codeine phosphate (p.25·2); promethazine hydrochloride (p.423·2).
Fever; pain.

AcuTect *Diatide, USA.*
Technetium-99m apcitide (p.1451·1).
Scintigraphic imaging of acute venous thrombosis.

Acutil Fosforo *Angelini, Ital.*
Aceglutamide (p.1571·2) or levoglutamide (p.1365·2); L-asparagine; DL-phosphoserine; pyridoxine (p.1387·1) or pyridoxine hydrochloride (p.1386·3).
Tonic.

Acutrim *Ciba, USA†; Heritage Consumer, USA†.*
Phenylpropanolamine hydrochloride (p.1098·1).
Obesity.

Acutussive *Apotex, S.Afr.*
Triprolidine hydrochloride (p.427·2); pseudoephedrine hydrochloride (p.1099·2); guaifenesin (p.1092·2); codeine phosphate (p.25·2).
Coughs.

Acuzide *Parke, Davis, Neth.*
Quinapril hydrochloride (p.963·3); hydrochlorothiazide (p.907·3).
Hypertension.

Acuzole *Apotex, S.Afr.†.*
Metronidazole (p.594·1).
Anaerobic bacterial infections; protozoal infections.

ACV *Greater Pharma, Thai.*
Aciclovir (p.612·3).
Herpes simplex infections.

ACWY Vax *SmithKline Beecham, UK.*
A meningococcal vaccine (groups A, C, W_{135}, and Y) (p.1550·1).
Active immunisation.

ACY *Ecobi, Ital.*
Aciclovir (p.612·3).
Herpesvirus infections of the skin and mucous membranes.

Acyclostad *Berner, Fin.*
Aciclovir (p.612·3).
Herpesvirus infections.

Acyclo-V *Alphapharm, Austral.*
Aciclovir (p.612·3).
Herpesvirus infections; HIV infection.

Acylene *UCB, Spain.*
Aluminium hydroxide (p.1210·3); magnesium hydroxide (p.1233·1); aluminium hydroxide-magnesium carbonate co-dried gel (p.1211·2).
Gastrointestinal hyperacidity.

Acyrax *Orion, Fin.*
Aciclovir (p.612·3).
Herpesvirus infections.

Acyvir
Glaxo Allen, Ital.; Pharmasant, Thai.
Aciclovir (p.612·3).
Herpesvirus infections.

AD Pabyrn *LPB, Ital.*
Vitamin A palmitate (p.1383·2); colecalciferol (p.1391·1).
Formerly contained vitamin A palmitate and ergocalciferol.
Vitamin A and D deficiency.

AD Til *Byk, Braz.*
Colecalciferol (p.1391·1); vitamin A acetate (p.1383·2).
Vitamin deficiencies.

ADA *Estedi, Spain.*
Phenylephrine hydrochloride (p.1097·1).
Nasal congestion; sinus congestion.

Adaferin
Galderma, Israel; Alcon, Mex.
Adapalene (p.1109·3).
Acne.

Adagen *Enzon, USA.*
Pegademase bovine (p.1649·2).
Adenosine deaminase deficiency.

Adalat
Bayer, Aust.; Bayer, Austral.; Bayer, Belg.; Bayer, Braz.; Bayer, Canad.; Bayer, Denm.; Bayer, Fin.; Bayer, Ger.; Bayer, Hong Kong; Bayer, Irl.; Bayer, Ital.; Bayer, Mex.; Bayer, Neth.; Bayer, Norw.; Bayer, NZ; Bayer, Port.; Bayer, S.Afr.; Bayer, Singapore; Bayer, Spain; Bayer, Swed.; Bayer, Switz.; Bayer, Thai.; Bayer, UK; Bayer, USA.
Nifedipine (p.940·1).
Angina pectoris; coronary spasm; hypertension; Raynaud's syndrome.

Adalate *Bayer, Fr.*
Nifedipine (p.940·1).
Angina pectoris; hypertension; Raynaud's syndrome.

Adalgur *Roussel, Spain.*
Paracetamol (p.71·2); thiocolchicoside (p.1330·2).
Painful skeletal muscle spasm.

Adalgur N *Roussel, Spain.*
Paracetamol (p.71·2); thiocolchicoside (p.1330·2).
Musculoskeletal and joint pain.

Adalken *Kendrick, Mex.*
Penicillamine (p.1017·1).
Heavy metal poisoning; Wilson's disease.

Adamon *Asta Medica, Thai.*
Ciclonium bromide (p.465·1).
Dysmenorrhoea; gastro-intestinal, biliary, and urinary-tract spasm.

Adancor *Lipha Sante, Fr.*
Nicorandil (p.939·2).
Angina pectoris.

Adant *Tedec Meiji, Israel.*
Sodium hyaluronate (p.1620·1).
Osteoarthritis of the knee; shoulder pain.

Adapettes
Alcon, Braz.; Alcon, Mex.; Alcon, USA.
Range of solutions for contact lenses (p.1129·2).

Adapine *Amrad, Austral.*
Nifedipine (p.940·1).
Hypertension.

Adapt *Alcon, USA†.*
Wetting solution for hard contact lenses (p.1129·2).

Adasept *Odan, Canad.*
Cleanser: Triclosan (p.1159·2).
Skin cleanser.

Topical gel: Triclosan (p.1159·2); salicylic acid (p.1122·3); sodium thiosulfate (p.1024·2).
Acne.

Adato-Cel *Chiron, Israel.*
Hypromellose (p.1501·3) in sodium chloride.
Aid in eye surgery and gonioscopy.

Adato-Deca *Chiron, Israel.*
Perflunafene (p.1650·1).
Aid in eye surgery.

Adato-Octa *Chiron, Israel.*
Perfluoro-octa.
Aid in eye surgery.

Adato-Sil Ol *Chiron, Israel.*
Dimethicone (p.1410·1).
Aid in eye surgery.

Adavite *Hudson, USA.*
A range of vitamin preparations (p.1350·1).

Adcal *Strakan, UK.*
Calcium carbonate (p.1215·1).
Calcium supplement; hyperphosphataemia; osteoporosis.

Adcal-D$_3$ *Strakan, UK.*
Calcium carbonate (p.1215·1); colecalciferol (p.1391·1).
Calcium and vitamin D deficiency; osteoporosis.

Adco-Dol *Adcock Ingram Generics, S.Afr.*
Paracetamol (p.71·2); codeine phosphate (p.25·2); caffeine (p.761·3); doxylamine succinate (p.417·1).
Fever; pain.

Adco-Flupain *Adcock Ingram Generics, S.Afr.*
Triprolidine hydrochloride (p.427·2); pseudoephedrine hydrochloride (p.1099·2); paracetamol (p.71·2).
Cold and influenza symptoms.

Adco-Linctopent *Adcock Ingram, S.Afr.*
Bromhexine hydrochloride (p.1085·3); orciprenaline sulfate (p.769·1).
Coughs.

Adco-Loten *Adcock Ingram, S.Afr.*
Atenolol (p.841·3); chlortalidone (p.857·1).
Hypertension.

Adco-Muco Expect *Adcock Ingram Generics, S.Afr.†.*
Triprolidine hydrochloride (p.427·2); pseudoephedrine hydrochloride (p.1099·2); guaifenesin (p.1092·2).
Coughs.

Adco-Phenobarbitone Vitalet *Adcock Ingram, S.Afr.*
Phenobarbital (p.355·1); vitamin B substances (p.1350·1).
Epilepsy; insomnia; sedative.

Adco-Retic *Adcock Ingram Generics, S.Afr.*
Amiloride hydrochloride (p.835·1); hydrochlorothiazide (p.907·3).
Hypertension; oedema.

Adcortyl
Bristol-Myers Squibb, Irl.; Bristol-Myers Squibb, Israel; Bristol-Myers Squibb, UK.
Triamcinolone acetonide (p.1080·1).
Inflammatory disorders; musculoskeletal, joint, and peri-articular disorders; skin disorders.

Adcortyl with Graneodin *Bristol-Myers Squibb, UK†.*
Triamcinolone acetonide (p.1080·1); neomycin sulfate (p.228·1); gramicidin (p.213·3).
Infected skin disorders.

Adcortyl in Orabase
Bristol-Myers Squibb, Irl.; Bristol-Myers Squibb, UK.
Triamcinolone acetonide (p.1080·1).
Inflammatory disorders of the mouth; lesions of the oral mucosa.

Adco-Sinal Co *Adcock Ingram Generics, S.Afr.*
Paracetamol (p.71·2); phenylpropanolamine hydrochloride (p.1098·1); phenyltoloxamine citrate (p.423·1); codeine phosphate (p.25·2).
Cold and influenza symptoms.

Adco-Sodasol *Adcock Ingram, S.Afr.*
Sodium citrate (p.1186·2); sodium bicarbonate (p.1186·2); anhydrous citric acid (p.1596·2); tartaric acid (p.1669·2).
Gastric hyperacidity; urinary alkalinisation.

Adco-Sufedrin *Adcock Ingram Generics, S.Afr.*
Pseudoephedrine hydrochloride (p.1099·2).
Upper respiratory-tract congestion.

Adco-Tussend *Adcock Ingram Generics, S.Afr.*
Triprolidine hydrochloride (p.427·2); pseudoephedrine hydrochloride (p.1099·2); codeine phosphate (p.25·2).
Coughs.

The symbol † denotes a preparation no longer actively marketed

Addamel Kabi Pharmacia, NZ; Baxter, NZ; Pharmacia, S.Afr.†; Fresenius Kabi, Spain.
Electrolyte (p.1180·1) and trace-element preparation (p.1350·1).
Parenteral nutrition.

Addamel N Pharmacia Upjohn, Hong Kong; Pharmacia Upjohn, Israel; Fresenius Kabi, Ital.; Pharmacia Upjohn, Neth.; Fresenius Kabi, Port.; Fresenius Kabi, Singapore; Fresenius Kabi, Switz.; Pharmacia Upjohn, Thai.
Electrolyte (p.1180·1) and trace element preparation (p.1350·1).
Parenteral nutrition.

Addamel Novum Pharmacia Upjohn, Belg.†.
Electrolyte (p.1180·1) and trace element (p.1350·1) preparation.
Parenteral nutrition.

Addel N Pharmacia Upjohn, Ger.
Electrolyte (p.1180·1) and trace element (p.1350·1) preparation.
Parenteral nutrition.

Addera Semper, Fin.
Nutritional supplement (p.1350·1).

Adderall Shire Richwood, USA.
Dexamfetamine sulfate (p.1507·3); dexamfetamine saccharate (p.1508·2); amfetamine sulfate (p.1506·3); amfetamine aspartate (p.1506·3).
Formerly known as Obetrol.
Attention deficit hyperactivity disorder; narcoleptic syndrome.

Addex Fresenius Kabi, Fin.; Fresenius Kabi, Norw.; Fresenius Kabi, Swed.
A range of electrolyte preparations (p.1180·1).

Addex-THAM Fresenius Kabi, Swed.
Trometamol (p.1675·2).
Acute metabolic acidosis; acute respiratory acidosis.

Addi-K Leo, Hong Kong; Leo, Singapore; Leo, Thai.
Potassium chloride (p.1194·3).
Hypokalaemia.

Addiphos Fresenius Kabi, Denm.; Pharmacia Upjohn, Irl.; Pharmacia Upjohn, Neth.; Fresenius Kabi, Swed.; Fresenius, UK.
Electrolyte preparation (p.1180·1).
Parenteral nutrition.

Additene Novartis, Fin.
Nutritional supplement (p.1350·1).

Additrace Pharmacia, Irl.; Fresenius Kabi, S.Afr.; Fresenius, UK.
Trace element preparation (p.1350·1).
Parenteral nutrition.

ADE 2 Prodotti, Braz.
Vitamin A (p.1382·1); vitamin D (p.1391·1).
Vitamin A and D deficiencies.

Adecaps Sanova, Aust.
Cod-liver oil (p.1357·2).
Vitamin A and D deficiency.

Adecur Asofarma, Mex.
Terazosin hydrochloride (p.980·1).
Benign prostatic hyperplasia; hypertension.

Adecut Takeda, Jpn.
Delapril hydrochloride (p.867·1).
Hypertension.

Adeflor M Upjohn, USA.
Multivitamin and mineral preparation with fluoride (p.1375·3) and iron (p.1350·1).
Dental caries prophylaxis; dietary supplement.

Adegrip Herald, Braz.
Dipyrone (p.34·1); caffeine (p.761·3); guaifenesin (p.1092·2) ascorbic acid (p.1389·3).
Cold and influenza symptoms.

Adegripan Herald, Braz.
Dipyrone (p.34·1); sodium camsilate; guaifenesin (p.1092·2); vitamin C (p.1389·3); mepyramine maleate (p.421·1).
Cold and influenza symptoms.

Adehl Kayaku, Jpn.
Colforsin daropate hydrochloride (p.1598·2).

Adek Falk, Ger.
Multivitamin preparation (p.1350·1).

Adekin Desitin, Ger.
Amantadine hydrochloride (p.1161·2).
Influenza A; parkinsonism.

Adekon Rhone-Poulenc Rorer, Mex.
Vitamin A palmitate (p.1383·2); ergocalciferol (p.1391·2).
Vitamin A and D deficiency.

Adekon C Rhone-Poulenc Rorer, Mex.
Vitamin A palmitate (p.1383·2); ergocalciferol (p.1391·2); ascorbic acid (p.1389·3).
Vitamin A, D, and C deficiency.

Adeks Axcan, Canad.
Multivitamin preparation with zinc (p.1350·1).

Scandipharm, USA.
Multivitamin and mineral preparation (p.1350·1).

Adel Senosiain, Mex.
Clarithromycin (p.186·2).
Bacterial infections.

Ad-Element Darrow, Braz.
Trace-element preparation (p.1350·1).
Parenteral nutrition.

Adelfan-Esidrex Novartis, Braz.; Novartis, Spain.
Reserpine (p.967·3); dihydralazine sulfate (p.874·2); hydrochlorothiazide (p.907·3).
Hypertension.

Adelheid-Jodquelle, Tolzer Jodquellen, Ger.
Sodium iodide (p.1522·3); potassium; sodium; ammonium; calcium; magnesium; iron; chloride; sodium bromide; bicarbonate.
Iodine-deficiency disorders.

Adeloren Loren, Mex.
Vitamin A (p.1382·1); colecalciferol (p.1391·1).

Adelphane-Esidrex Novartis, Hong Kong; Ciba-Geigy, S.Afr.†.
Reserpine (p.967·3); dihydralazine sulfate (p.874·2); hydrochlorothiazide (p.907·3).
Hypertension.

Adelphan-Esidrex Novartis, Aust.; Novartis, Switz.
Reserpine (p.967·3); dihydralazine sulfate (p.874·2); hydrochlorothiazide (p.907·3).
Hypertension.

Adelphan-Esidrix Novartis, Ger.
Reserpine (p.967·3); dihydralazine sulfate (p.874·2); hydrochlorothiazide (p.907·3).
Hypertension.

Adena C Innothera, Fr.
Pink tablets, deoxyribonucleic acid (p.1602·3); white tablets, ascorbic acid (p.1389·3).
Tonic.

Adenas Eagle, Austral.
Vitamins; minerals; ginseng; eleutherococcus senticosis root (p.1350·1).
Tonic.

Adenobeta Salus, Ital.
Cocarboxylase chloride (p.1385·2); cyanocobalamin (p.1388·1).
Neuritis.

Adenocard Libbs, Braz.; Fujisawa, Canad.; Fujisawa, USA.
Adenosine (p.828·2).
Diagnosis of arrhythmias; paroxysmal supraventricular tachycardia.

Adenocor Sanofi Synthelabo, Austral.; Sanofi Synthelabo, Belg.; Sanofi Winthrop, Denm.; Sanofi Winthrop, Fin.; Sanofi Winthrop, Irl.; Sanofi Winthrop, Israel; Sanofi Synthelabo, Neth.; Sanofi Winthrop, Norw.; Sanofi Winthrop, NZ; Sanofi Synthelabo, Port.; Sanofi Synthelabo, S.Afr.; Sanofi Synthelabo, Singapore; Sanofi Synthelabo, Spain; Sanofi Winthrop, Swed.†; Sanofi Synthelabo, Thai.; Sanofi Winthrop, UK.
Adenosine (p.828·2).
Diagnosis of arrhythmias; paroxysmal supraventricular tachycardia.

Adenoplex Forte Scharper, Ital.
Cocarboxylase (p.1385·2); pyridoxine hydrochloride (p.1386·3); cyanocobalamin (p.1388·1).
Neuritis.

Adenoprostal IBSA, Switz.
Pollen extract.
Micturition disorders associated with benign prostatic hyperplasia.

Adenoscan Sanofi Synthelabo, Austral.; Sanofi Winthrop, Fin.; Sanofi Winthrop, Fr.; Sanofi Synthelabo, Ger.; Sanofi Synthelabo, Ital.; Sanofi Synthelabo, Neth.; Sanofi Synthelabo, Spain; Sanofi Winthrop, UK; Fujisawa, USA.
Adenosine (p.828·2).
Coronary vasodilator during radionuclide myocardial perfusion imaging.

Adenovit Nuovo, Ital.
Cyanocobalamin (p.1388·1); cocarboxylase hydrochloride (p.1385·2); pyridoxine hydrochloride (p.1386·3).
Neuropathies.

Adenyl Ferlux, Fr.
Adenosine phosphate (p.1573·3).
Haemorrhoids; venous insufficiency.

Adenylocrat Godecke, Ger.
Crataegus (p.1600·2).
Cardiac disorders.

Adepal Wyeth Lederle, Fr.
Levonorgestrel (p.1486·2); ethinylestradiol (p.1476·2).
Biphasic oral contraceptive.

Adepril
Note.This name is used for preparations of different composition.
Teofarma, Ital.
Amitriptyline hydrochloride (p.273·3).
Depression.

Wayne, Mex.
Carbamazepine (p.342·2).

Adepsique Psicofarma, Mex.
Amitriptyline hydrochloride (p.273·3); diazepam (p.674·3); perphenazine (p.699·1).
Insomnia; mixed anxiety depressive states.

Adept ML Laboratories, UK.
Icodextrin (p.1359·1).
Prevention of surgical adhesions.

Adeptolon Godecke, Ger.†.
Prednisolone (p.1077·3); N-(4-bromobenzyl)-N'-ethyl-N'-methyl-N-(2-pyridyl)ethylenediamine maleate.
Hypersensitivity disorders; pruritus.

Aderma Dermalibour Pierre Fabre, Hong Kong.
Avena (p.1583·1); zinc oxide (p.1128·2); zinc sulfate (p.1398·2); copper sulfate (p.1358·1); glycerol (p.1616·3).
Dry skin; eczema; nappy rash.

Aderma Epitheliale Pierre Fabre, Hong Kong.
Avena (p.1583·1); vitamin A (p.1382·1); vitamin E (p.1393·3).
Skin abrasions; sunburn; wounds.

Aderma Exomega Pierre Fabre, Hong Kong.
Avena (p.1583·1); omega 6 fatty acids (p.1613·3); glycerol (p.1616·3).
Eczema.

Aderma Ultra High Protection Pierre Fabre, Hong Kong.
Titanium dioxide (p.1126·1); zinc oxide (p.1128·2); avena (p.1583·1).
Sunscreen.

Adermykon Terramin, Aust.
Chlorphenesin (p.381·3).
Fungal and bacterial infections.

Adermykon-C Allergan-Frumtost, Braz.
Chlorphenesin (p.381·3); chloramphenicol (p.179·1); lignocaine [lidocaine] (p.1313·2).
Ear infections.

Aderofix D3 Precifarma, Braz.
Vitamin A (p.1382·1); colecalciferol (p.1391·1).
Vitamin deficiencies.

Aderogil D3 Hoechst Marion Roussel, Braz.
Colecalciferol (p.1391·1); vitamin A acetate (p.1383·2).
Vitamin deficiencies.

Aderplus spezial Dr Hagedorn Naturarzneimittel, Ger.
Homoeopathic preparation.

Adesinon-P Wakamoto, Hong Kong.
Adenosine triphosphate, disodium salt (p.1573·3).
Cardiac disorders; cerebral disorders; deafness; eczema; eye strain; muscle weakness.

Adesipress-TTS Pharmacia Upjohn, Ital.
Clonidine (p.861·1).
Hypertension.

Adesitrin Pharmacia Upjohn, Ital.
Glyceryl trinitrate (p.897·3).
Angina pectoris.

Adex Dexxon, Israel.
Ibuprofen (p.43·2).
Musculoskeletal and joint disorders; pain.

Adexolin Seven Seas, UK†.
Multivitamin preparation (p.1350·1).

Adexone Rekah, Israel.
Dexamethasone (p.1067·1); salicylic acid (p.1122·3).
Skin disorders.

Adfen Adcock Ingram Self Medication, S.Afr.†.
Ibuprofen (p.43·2).
Fever; inflammation; musculoskeletal and joint disorders; pain.

Adgyn Combi Strakan, UK.
16 Tablets, estradiol (p.1473·1); 12 tablets, estradiol; norethisterone (p.1485·1).
Menopausal disorders.

Adgyn Estro Strakan, UK.
Estradiol (p.1473·1).
Menopausal disorders.

Adgyn Medro Strakan, UK.
Medroxyprogesterone acetate (p.1480·1).
Adjunct in hormone replacement therapy; amenorrhoea; dysfunctional uterine bleeding; endometriosis.

Adhaegon Ratiopharm, Aust.
Dihydroergotamine mesilate (p.450·3).
Chronic venous insufficiency; hypotension; migraine; varicose veins.

Adiantine Potter's, UK.
Hamamelis (p.1618·3); rosemary oil (p.1659·3); bay oil (p.1583·3).
Scalp disorders.

Adiaril Gallia, Fr.
Glucose; sucrose; potassium gluconate; sodium bicarbonate; sodium chloride (p.1185·2).
Diarrhoea; oral rehydration therapy.

Adiazine Doms-Adrian, Fr.
Sulfadiazine (p.251·1).
Nocardiosis; toxoplasmosis.

Adibal Diba, Mex.
Vitamin A palmitate (p.1383·2); ergocalciferol (p.1391·2).
Vitamin A and D deficiency.

Adiboran AD Eurospital, Ital.
Vitamin A palmitate (p.1383·2); colecalciferol (p.1391·1).
Vitamin A and D deficiency.

Adiclair Ardeypharm, Ger.
Nystatin (p.392·2).
Fungal infections.

Adiefim Calcium Francia, Ital.
Calcium carbonate; fluorine; colecalciferol; malt (p.1350·1).
Nutritional supplement.

Adifteper ISM, Ital.
A diphtheria, tetanus, and pertussis vaccine (p.1537·3).
Active immunisation.

Adinol Teva, Israel.
Zinc oxide (p.1128·2); Burrow's solution; wool alcohols (p.1410·3); silicon dioxide (p.1503·3).
Barrier preparation; eczema; nappy rash; skin irritation.

Adiod Teofarma, Spain.
Colecalciferol (p.1391·1); vitamin A (p.1382·1); iodine (p.1522·3).
Deficiency of vitamins A and D.

Adios Dendron, UK.
Bladderwrack (p.1585·2); boldo (p.1585·3); butternut; taraxacum (p.1669·1).
Obesity.

Adipex Gerot, Aust.†; Gerot, Switz.
Phentermine polystyrene sulfonate (p.1514·1).
Obesity.

Adipex-P Gate, USA.
Phentermine hydrochloride (p.1514·1).
Obesity.

Adipine Trinity, UK.
Nifedipine (p.940·1).
Angina pectoris; hypertension.

Adipodiet Frandiet, Fr.
Nutritional supplement (p.1350·1).

Adiporell Sanorell, Ger.
Homoeopathic preparation.

Adiporetic Frandiet, Fr.
Nutritional supplement (p.1350·1).

Adipost Ascher, USA†.
Phendimetrazine tartrate (p.1513·3).
Obesity.

Adiro Bayer, Mex.; Bayer, Spain.
Aspirin (p.14·2).
Fever; inflammation; musculoskeletal and joint disorders; pain; thromboembolism prophylaxis.

Adisterolo Abiogen, Ital.
Vitamin A (p.1382·1); colecalciferol (p.1391·1).
Vitamin A and D deficiency.

Adistop Phyteia, Switz.
Cathine hydrochloride (p.1507·1).
Obesity.

Adistop Lax Phyteia, Switz.†.
Frangula (p.1227·1); aloes (p.1210·1); senna (p.1248·2); peppermint leaf (p.1243·2); caraway (p.1591·2); fennel (p.1610·1).
Constipation.

Adiugrip Chiron, Ital.
An influenza vaccine (p.1544·3).
Active immunisation.

Adiuvant Manetti Roberts, Ital.
Pirglutargine (p.1652·2).
Mental function disorders.

Adivon Ederka, Mex.
Ibuprofen (p.43·2).

Adizem Napp, Irl.; Rafa, Israel; Napp, UK.
Diltiazem hydrochloride (p.874·3).
Angina pectoris; hypertension.

Adizem-XL Plus Napp, UK†.
Diltiazem hydrochloride (p.874·3); hydrochlorothiazide (p.907·3).
Hypertension.

ADL Bencard, Ger.
Allergen extracts (p.1575·3).
Hyposensitisation.

Adlone UAD, USA†.
Methylprednisolone acetate (p.1076·1).

Admag TP, Thai.
Aluminium hydroxide (p.1210·3); magnesium hydroxide (p.1233·1); simeticone (p.1249·2).
Flatulence; gastric hyperacidity.

Admag-M TP, Thai.
Dried aluminium hydroxide gel (p.1210·3); magnesium trisilicate (p.1233·3).
Gastric hyperacidity; gastritis; peptic ulcer.

Admon Esteve, Spain.
Nimodipine (p.946·1).
Mental function impairment; neurological deficit following subarachnoid haemorrhage.

Ad-Muc Merz, Ger.
Chamomile (p.1593·2); myrrh (p.1639·2).
Inflammatory disorders of the mouth and gums.

Adnax Newlab, Braz.
Naphazoline hydrochloride (p.1095·1); diphenhydramine hydrochloride (p.416·1).
Nasal congestion.

Adnemic Nakorn, Thai.
Multivitamin and mineral preparation with ferrous fumarate (p.1360·1) (p.1350·1).
Iron-deficiency anaemia; vitamin deficiency.

Adnemic F Nakorn, Thai.
Multivitamin and mineral preparation with ferrous fumarate (p.1360·1) and folic acid (p.1361·1) (p.1350·1).
Iron-deficiency anaemia; vitamin deficiency.

Ado C Kwizda, Aust.
Paracetamol (p.71·2); ascorbic acid (p.1389·3).
Fever; pain.

Adocante Docura Bravir, Braz.
Sodium cyclamate (p.1358·3); saccharin (p.1374·3).
Sugar substitute.

Adocomp TAD, Ger.
Captopril (p.853·3); hydrochlorothiazide (p.907·3).
Hypertension.

Adocor TAD, Ger.
Captopril (p.853·3).
Heart failure; hypertension.

Adocyl C *Virtus, Braz.*
Sodium cyclamate (p.1358·3); saccharin (p.1374·3).
Sugar substitute.

Adofen *Ferrer, Spain.*
Fluoxetine hydrochloride (p.284·2).
Bulimia nervosa; depression; obsessive-compulsive disorder.

Adol *Julphar, UAE.*
Paracetamol (p.71·2).
Fever; pain.

Adol Allergy Sinus *Julphar, UAE.*
Paracetamol (p.71·2); pseudoephedrine hydrochloride (p.1099·2); chlorpheniramine [chlorphenamine] (p.412·2).
Hay fever; sinusitis; upper respiratory-tract disorders.

Adol Cold *Julphar, UAE.*
Paracetamol (p.71·2); pseudoephedrine hydrochloride (p.1099·2); dextromethorphan hydrobromide (p.1087·3).
Cold and influenza symptoms.

Adol Compound *Julphar, UAE.*
Salicylamide (p.82·1); paracetamol (p.71·2); caffeine (p.761·3); codeine phosphate (p.25·2).
Fever; pain.

Adol Extra *Julphar, UAE.*
Paracetamol (p.71·2); caffeine (p.761·3).
Fever; pain.

Adol PM *Julphar, UAE.*
Paracetamol (p.71·2); diphenhydramine hydrochloride (p.416·1).
Fever; insomnia; pain.

Adol Sinus *Julphar, UAE.*
Paracetamol (p.71·2); pseudoephedrine hydrochloride (p.1099·2).
Nasal congestion; sinusitis.

Adolan *Abic, Israel.*
Methadone hydrochloride (p.53·1).
Opioid withdrawal syndrome; pain.

Adolkin *Prodes, Spain†.*
Metamizole magnesium (p.34·2).
Fever; pain.

Adolonta *Grunenthal, Spain.*
Tramadol hydrochloride (p.89·1).
Pain.

Adolorin *Kwizda, Aust.*
Propyphenazone (p.80·2); paracetamol (p.71·2); caffeine (p.761·3).
Fever; pain.

Adolphs Salt Substitute *Adolphs, USA.*
Sodium-free dietary salt substitute (p.1350·1).

Adoluron CC *Kwizda, Aust.*
Propyphenazone (p.80·2); paracetamol (p.71·2); codeine hydrochloride (p.25·2).
Fever; pain.

Adomed *Kwizda, Aust.†.*
Bupranolol hydrochloride (p.852·3).
Hypertension.

Adona *Tanabe, Hong Kong; SIT, Ital.; Tanabe, Jpn.*
Carbazochrome sodium sulfonate (p.728·1).
Haemorrhagic disorders.

Adovit C *Kwizda, Aust.*
Aspirin (p.14·2); ascorbic acid (p.1389·3).
Fever; pain.

Adoxa *Bioglan, USA.*
Doxycycline (p.200·1).
Bacterial infections.

Adprin-B *Pfeiffer, USA.*
Aspirin (p.14·2).
Calcium carbonate (p.1215·1), magnesium carbonate (p.1232·3), and magnesium oxide (p.1233·2) are included in this preparation in an attempt to limit adverse effects on the gastrointestinal mucosa.
Pain.

Adrectal *Vifor, Switz.†.*
Ointment: Ephedrine hydrochloride (p.1090·1); lignocaine [lidocaine] hydrochloride (p.1313·2); peppermint oil (p.1243·3); thymol (p.1158·3); zinc stearate (p.1497·3).
Suppositories: Ephedrine hydrochloride (p.1090·1); lignocaine [lidocaine] hydrochloride (p.1313·2); amethocaine [tetracaine] hydrochloride (p.1305·2); peppermint oil (p.1243·3); thymol (p.1158·3); zinc stearate (p.1497·3).
Anorectal disorders.

Adreject *ALK, Spain.*
Adrenaline [epinephrine] hydrochloride (p.829·2).
Anaphylaxis; asthma; bronchospasm; circulatory collapse; hypotension; shock; Stokes-Adams attacks.

Adrekar *Sanofi Winthrop, Aust.†; Sanofi Synthelabo, Ger.*
Adenosine (p.828·2).
Tachycardia.

Adrenam *NAM, Ger.*
Etilefrine hydrochloride (p.888·1).
Hypotension.

Adrenoplasma *Climax, Braz.*
Carbazochrome (p.728·1).
Haemorrhage.

Adrenor *Llorens, Spain†.*
Noradrenaline [norepinephrine] acid tartrate (p.948·2).
Glaucoma.

Adrenoxil *Climax, Braz.; CPH, Port.*
Carbazochrome (p.728·1).
Haemorrhagic disorders.

Adrenoxyl *Sanofi Synthelabo, Ger.*
Carbazochrome (p.728·1).
Haemorrhage.

Adreson *Organon, Belg.*
Cortisone acetate (p.1065·3).
Corticosteroid.

Adrevil *Novartis Consumer, Ger.*
Butalamine hydrochloride (p.853·1).
Peripheral and cerebral vascular disorders.

Adrexan *Mayoly-Spindler, Fr.*
Propranolol hydrochloride (p.962·3).
Cardiovascular disorders.

Adrezon *Ono, Hong Kong.*
Carbazochrome (p.728·1).
Haemorrhage.

Adriablastin *Pharmacia Upjohn, Aust.; Pharmacia Upjohn, Ger.; Pharmacia Upjohn, Switz.*
Doxorubicin hydrochloride (p.534·3).
Malignant neoplasms.

Adriablastina *Pharmacia Upjohn, Belg.; Pharmacia Upjohn, Braz.; Farmitalia, Israel; Pharmacia Upjohn, Israel; Pharmacia Upjohn, Ital.; Pharmacia Upjohn, Mex.; Pharmacia Upjohn, Neth.; Pharmacia Upjohn, Port.; Pharmacia Upjohn, S.Afr.; Pharmacia Upjohn, Thai.*
Doxorubicin hydrochloride (p.534·3).
Malignant neoplasms.

Adriblastine *Pharmacia Upjohn, Fr.*
Doxorubicin hydrochloride (p.534·3).
Malignant neoplasms.

Adrigyl *Doms-Adrian, Fr.*
Colecalciferol (p.1391·1).
Vitamin D deficiency.

Adrim *Dabur, Thai.*
Doxorubicin hydrochloride (p.534·3).
Malignant neoplasms.

Adrimedac *Medac, Ger.*
Doxorubicin hydrochloride (p.534·3).
Malignant neoplasms.

Adrinex *Medical, Port.*
Adrenaline [epinephrine] (p.829·1); benzyl nicotinate (p.20·2).
Musculoskeletal, joint, peri-articular, and soft-tissue disorders.

Adrocil *Oftalder, Port.*
Trifluridine (p.642·2).
Viral eye infections.

Adro-derm *Adroka, Switz.*
Propyl alcohol (p.1155·3); alcohol (p.1130·3); chlorhexidine gluconate (p.1138·2).
Skin disinfection.

Adronat *Neopharmed, Ital.; Tecnifar, Port.*
Alendronate sodium (p.747·3).
Osteoporosis.

Adrucil *Pharmacia Upjohn, Canad.; Adria, USA.*
Fluorouracil (p.540·2).
Malignant neoplasms.

Adrusen *SIFI, Singapore.*
Food supplement with vitamins and minerals (p.1350·1).

Ad-Sorb *Key, Austral.*
Activated charcoal (p.1000·2).
Flatulence.

Adsorbed DT Coq *Pasteur Merieux, Hong Kong.*
An adsorbed diphtheria, tetanus, and pertussis vaccine (p.1537·3).
Active immunisation.

Adsorbed DT Vax *Pasteur Merieux, Hong Kong.*
An adsorbed diphtheria and tetanus vaccine (p.1537·1).
Active immunisation.

Adsorbocarpine *Alcon, USA.*
Pilocarpine hydrochloride (p.1422·3).
Glaucoma; raised intra-ocular pressure; reversal of mydriasis.

Adsorbonac *Alcon, Ger.; Alcon, Hong Kong; Alcon, Ital.; Alcon, Singapore; Alcon, USA.*
Sodium chloride (p.1196·1).
Corneal oedema.

Adsorbotear *Alcon, USA†.*
Hyetellose (p.1501·1); povidone (p.1503·2).
Dry eyes.

ADT
Note. This name is used for preparations of different composition.
CSL, NZ.
An adsorbed diphtheria and tetanus vaccine (p.1537·1).
Active immunisation.
Zimaia, Port.
Amitriptyline hydrochloride (p.273·3).
Depression; nocturnal enuresis.

ADT Vaccine *CSL, Austral.*
An adsorbed diphtheria and tetanus vaccine (p.1537·1).
Active immunisation.

Aducin *Nettopharma, Denm.*
Ranitidine hydrochloride (p.1245·2).
Acid aspiration; gastro-oesophageal reflux; peptic ulcer; Zollinger-Ellison syndrome.

Adulax *Casen Fleet, Spain.*
Glycerol (p.1616·3).
Constipation.

Adult Ideal Quota *Larkhall Laboratories, UK.*
Multivitamin and mineral preparation (p.1350·1).

Adult Meltus for Chesty Coughs & Catarrh *SSL, UK.*
Guaifenesin (p.1092·2); cetylpyridinium chloride (p.1138·1); honey (p.1366·2).
Catarrh; coughs.

Adumbran *Boehringer Ingelheim, Aust.; Boehringer Ingelheim, Ger.; Boehringer Ingelheim, Switz.*
Oxazepam (p.697·1).
Anxiety; insomnia.

Adurix *Nycomed, Denm.*
Clopamide (p.863·1).
Diabetes insipidus; hypertension; oedema.

Adursal *Leiras, Fin.*
Ursodeoxycholic acid (p.1677·2).
Biliary-tract disorders; chronic active hepatitis; gallstones.

Advair *Glaxo Wellcome, Canad.; Glaxo Wellcome, USA.*
Fluticasone propionate (p.1072·2); salmeterol xinafoate (p.773·3).
Asthma.

Advance *Advanced Care, USA.*
Pregnancy test (p.1654·3).

Advanced Antioxidants Formula *Solgar, UK.*
Multivitamin and mineral preparation with superoxide dismutase inducers and proanthocyanidin complex (p.1350·1).
Dietary supplement.

Advanced Formula Di-Gel *Schering-Plough, USA.*
Magnesium hydroxide (p.1233·1); calcium carbonate (p.1215·1); simeticone (p.1249·2).
Hyperacidity.

Advanced Formula Multibionta *Seven Seas, UK.*
Vitamins; minerals; *Lactobacillus acidophilus; Bifidobacterium bifidum; Bifidobacterium longum* (p.1350·1).
Tonic.

Advanced Formula Plax *Pfizer, USA.*
Sodium pyrophosphate.

Advanced Formula Tegrin *Block, USA.*
Coal tar (p.1125·1).
Scalp disorders.

Advanced Formula Zenate *Solvay, USA.*
Multivitamin and mineral preparation with iron and folic acid (p.1350·1).
Formerly called Zenate.
Nutritional supplement in pregnancy and lactation.

Advanced Relief Visine *Pfizer Consumer, USA.*
Tetryzoline hydrochloride (p.1101·2); macrogol 400 (p.1630·3); povidone (p.1503·2); dextran 70 (p.729·2).
Dry eyes; eye irritation.

Advantage
Note. A similar name is used for preparations of different composition (see below).
Allergan, Austral.†; Allergan, Canad.
Subtilisin (p.1129·2).
Protein and lipid remover for contact lenses.
Roche Diagnostics, Austral.; Roche, Canad.; Roche Diagnostics, NZ.
Test for glucose in blood (p.1616·3).

Advantage 24
Note. A similar name is used for preparations of different composition (see above).
Roberts, Canad.; Lake, USA.
Nonoxinol 9 (p.1346·1).
Contraceptive.

Advantan *Schering, Aust.; CSL, Austral.; Schering, Belg.; Schering, Fin.; Schering, Ger.; Schering, Hong Kong; Schering, Ital.; Schering, Mex.; CSL, NZ; Schering, Port.; Schering, S.Afr.; Lederle, Switz.*
Methylprednisolone aceponate (p.1076·2).
Skin disorders.

Adventan *Schering, Spain.*
Methylprednisolone aceponate (p.1076·2).
Skin disorders.

Advera *Abbott, Austral.; Abbott, Canad.†; Abbott, Fin.; Abbott, Fr.; Abbott, Ital.; Ross, USA.*
Preparation for enteral nutrition in immunocompromised patients (p.1350·1).

Adversuten *Asta Medica, Ger.*
Prazosin hydrochloride (p.958·1).
Heart failure; hypertension; Raynaud's syndrome.

Advil *Whitehall, Braz.; Whitehall-Robins, Canad.; Whitehall, Fr.; Whitehall, Hong Kong; Whitehall-Robins, Irl.; Wyeth, Mex.; Whitehall, Neth.; Wyeth, Spain; Whitehall, UK; Wyeth-Ayerst, USA; Whitehall, USA.*
Ibuprofen (p.43·2).
Fever; osteoarthritis; pain; rheumatoid arthritis.

Advil Cold & Flu *Whitehall, Irl.*
Ibuprofen (p.43·2); pseudoephedrine (p.1099·2).
Cold and influenza symptoms.

Advil Cold & Sinus *Whitehall-Robins, Canad.; Whitehall, UK; Whitehall, USA.*
Ibuprofen (p.43·2); pseudoephedrine hydrochloride (p.1099·2).
Formerly known as Coadvil in the USA.
Cold and influenza symptoms; sinusitis.

Advil CS *Whitehall, S.Afr.*
Ibuprofen (p.43·2); pseudoephedrine hydrochloride (p.1099·2).
Cold and influenza symptoms.

Advil Mono *Whitehall, Belg.*
Ibuprofen (p.43·2).
Fever; pain.

Advil NS *Akromed, S.Afr.†.*
Oxymetazoline hydrochloride (p.1096·2).
Nasal congestion.

Advisor *Abbott, Ital.*
Pregnancy test (p.1654·3).

AD-vitamin *ACO, Swed.*
Vitamin A palmitate (p.1383·2); colecalciferol (p.1391·1).
Vitamin supplement.

Ad-Vitan *Janssen-Cilag, Belg.†.*
Vitamin A acetate (p.1383·2); colecalciferol (p.1391·1).
Osteomalacia; rickets; vitamin A and D deficiency.

Adyston *Krewel, Ger.*
Pholedrine sulfate (p.955·2); norfenefrine hydrochloride (p.949·1).
Hypotension.

Aedolac *Guieu, Fr.†; Guieu, Ital.*
Emollient.
Dry skin; eczema.

Aegrosan *Opfermann, Ger.*
Dimethicone (p.1249·2).
Reduction of gastrointestinal gas.

A-E-Mulsin *Mucos, Aust.; Mucos, Ger.*
Vitamin A palmitate (p.1383·2); alpha tocoferil acetate (p.1394·1).
Vitamin A and E deficiency.

Aequalyre *Boehringer Ingelheim, Fr.*
Sodium chloride (p.1196·1).
Conjunctival irrigation; eyelid cleansing.

Aequamen *Byk Gulden, Ger.*
Betahistine mesilate (p.1584·3).
Ménière's syndrome; vestibular disorders.

Aequifusine *Braun, Switz.*
Electrolyte infusion with glucose (p.1180·1).
Fluid and electrolyte disorders.

Aequiseral *Streuli, Switz.*
Electrolyte and glucose solution (p.1180·1).
Dehydration.

Aequiton-P *Sudmedica, Ger.*
Phenazone (p.77·2).
Fever; pain.

A-E-R *Birchwood, USA.*
Hamamelis (p.1618·3).
Anorectal disorders; vaginal irritation.

Aero Plus *Upsamedica, Spain.*
Dimethicone (p.1249·2); metoclopramide hydrochloride (p.1235·2).
Aerophagia; delayed gastric emptying.

Aero Red *Upsamedica, Spain.*
Dimethicone (p.1249·2).
Flatulence.

Aero Red Antiacido *Upsamedica, Spain.*
Calcium carbonate (p.1215·1); dimethicone (p.1249·2); magnesium hydroxide (p.1233·1).
Flatulence; gastrointestinal hyperacidity.

Aero Red Complex *Upsamedica, Spain.*
Dimethicone (p.1249·2); lipolytic enzymes; amylolytic enzymes; proteolytic enzymes; cellulolytic enzymes.
Formerly known as Aero Red Eupeptico.
Digestive system disorders.

Aeroaid *Health & Medical, USA; Graham-Field, USA.*
Thiomersal (p.1158·2).
Skin disinfection; wounds.

AeroBec *3M, Denm.; 3M, Fin.; 3M, Ger.; Asta Medica, Ger.; 3M, Irl.; Riker, Mex.; 3M, Neth.; 3M, S.Afr.; 3M, UK.*
Beclometasone dipropionate (p.1061·2).
Obstructive airways disease.

AeroBid *Forest Pharmaceuticals, USA.*
Flunisolide (p.1070·3).
Asthma.

Aerobin *Farmasan, Ger.; Farmasan, Thai.; TTN, Thai.*
Theophylline (p.777·2) or theophylline sodium glycinate (p.783·2).
Obstructive airways disease.

Aerocaine *Aeroceuticals, USA.*
Benzocaine (p.1306·2); benzethonium chloride (p.1134·2).
Skin disorders.

Aerocef *Klinge, Aust.*
Cefixime (p.166·2).
Bacterial infections.

Aerocid *Aerocid, Fr.*
Pancreas powder (porcine); simeticone (p.1249·2).
Formerly contained adrenaline [epinephrine], pancreatin, liver extract, and ergot.
Dyspepsia.

Aero-Clenil *Farmalab, Braz.*
Salbutamol (p.770·3).
Obstructive airways disease.

Aerocrom *Rhone-Poulenc Rorer, Mex.; Castlemead, UK.*
Sodium cromoglicate (p.774·3); salbutamol sulfate (p.770·3).
Asthma.

Aeroderm *Seid, Spain.*
Lignocaine [lidocaine] hydrochloride (p.1313·2).
Burns; insect stings; skin irritation.

Aerodesin *Lysoform, Ger.*
Propyl alcohol (p.1155·3); alcohol (p.1130·3); glutaral (p.1145·2).
Surface disinfection.

The symbol † denotes a preparation no longer actively marketed

Aerodine *Graham-Field, USA.*
Povidone-iodine (p.1155·1).
Skin disinfection.

Aerodiol *Servier, UK.*
Estradiol (p.1473·1).
Menopausal disorders.

Aerodur *Stern, Ger.; Astra, Ger.*
Terbutaline sulfate (p.776·2).
Obstructive airways disease.

Aerodyne *Klinge, Aust.*
Theophylline (p.777·2) or theophylline sodium glycinate (p.783·2).
Obstructive airways disease.

Aerofagil *Geymonat, Ital.*
Sodium citrate (p.1186·2); dimethicone (p.1249·2).
Aerophagia; meteorism.

Aeroflat *Biosarto, Spain.*
Dimethicone (p.1249·2); metoclopramide (p.1236·3).
Aerophagia; delayed gastric emptying.

Aeroflux *Glaxo Wellcome, Mex.*
Salbutamol sulfate (p.770·3); ambroxol hydrochloride (p.1084·3).
Asthma; bronchitis; respiratory-tract disorders with increased mucus.

Aeroflux Edulito *Glaxo Wellcome, Braz.*
Salbutamol (p.770·3); guaifenesin (p.1092·2); sodium citrate (p.1186·2).
Obstructive airways disease.

Aerofreeze *Graham-Field, USA.*
Dichlorodifluoromethane (p.1199·1); trichlorofluoromethane (p.1199·1).
Topical anaesthesia.

Aerogel *Upsamedica, Spain.*
Aluminium hydroxide (p.1210·3); dimethicone (p.1249·2).
Dyspepsia; flatulence; gastrointestinal hyperacidity.

Aerolate *Fleming, USA.*
Theophylline (p.777·2).
Obstructive airways disease.

Aerolin
Glaxo Wellcome, Braz.; 3M, Irl.; 3M, Israel; 3M, Neth.; 3M, UK.
Salbutamol sulfate (p.770·3).
Obstructive airways disease.

Aerolind *TAD, Ger.*
Salbutamol (p.770·3).
Obstructive airways disease.

Aeromax *Cascan, Ger.; Cascapharm, Ger.; Glaxo Wellcome, Ger.; Asta Medica, Ger.*
Salmeterol xinafoate (p.773·3).
Obstructive airways disease.

Aeromuc *Klinge, Aust.*
Acetylcysteine (p.1082·3).
Otitis media; respiratory-tract disorders.

Aero-Om *OM, Port.*
Simeticone (p.1249·2).
Adjunct in radiology; aerophagia; gasto-intestinal distension; infant colic; meteorism.

Aeropax
Orion, Denm.; Ercopharm, Switz.†.
Dimethicone (p.1249·2).
Aid in radiography and gastroscopy; infant colic; meteorism.

Aeroseb-Dex *Allergan Herbert, USA.*
Dexamethasone (p.1067·1).
Skin disorders.

Aeroseb-HC *Allergan Herbert, USA†.*
Hydrocortisone (p.1073·3).
Skin disorders.

Aerosol Spitzner N *Spitzner, Ger.*
Oleum pini sylvestris; pumilio pine oil; eucalyptus oil (p.1609·2); siberian fir oil; noble pine oil.
Respiratory-tract disorders.

Aerosporin
Glaxo Wellcome, Canad.†; Glaxo Wellcome, USA†.
Polymyxin B sulfate (p.238·1).
Gram-negative infections.

Aerotec *Sanofi Synthelabo, Ital.*
Salbutamol sulfate (p.770·3).
Obstructive airways disease.

Aerotherm *Aeroceuticals, USA.*
Benzocaine (p.1306·2); benzethonium chloride (p.1134·2).
Skin disorders.

Aerotide *Glaxo Wellcome, Braz.*
Beclometasone dipropionate (p.1061·2); salbutamol (p.770·3).
Asthma.

Aerotrat *Cazi, Braz.*
Salbutamol sulfate (p.770·3).
Obstructive airways disease.

Aerovacuna *Nezel, Spain†.*
Lysates of *diplococcus; streptococcus; Micrococcus pyogenes; Gaffkya anaerobia; Neisseria; Haemophilus influenzae; Klebsiella pneumoniae; Moraxella.*
Respiratory-tract infections.

Aerovent *Teva, Israel.*
Ipratropium bromide (p.766·1).
Obstructive airways disease.

Aerozoin *Graham-Field, USA.*
Compound benzoin tincture.
Barrier preparation.

AErrane
Zeneca, Austral.; Pharmacia Upjohn, Belg.; Pharmacia Upjohn, Irl.; Zeneca, Israel; Pharmacia Upjohn, Ital.; Pharmacia Upjohn, Neth.;
AstraZeneca, NZ; Zeneca, S.Afr.; Pharmacia Upjohn, Spain; Astra-Zeneca, Thai.; Baxter, UK.
Isoflurane (p.1261·1).
General anaesthesia.

Aescorin Forte *Steigerwald, Ger.*
Aesculus (p.1574·1).
Soft-tissue injury; venous insufficiency.

Aescorin N *Steigerwald, Ger.*
Injection: Rutoside sodium sulfate (p.1611·2); esculoside (p.1574·1).
Ointment: Aesculus (p.1574·1); hamamelis (p.1618·3).
Haemorrhoids; vascular disorders.

Aesculaforce *Bioforce, Switz.*
Aesculus (p.1574·1).
Venous insufficiency.

Aesculaforce N *Bioforce, Switz.*
Homoeopathic preparation.
Venous insufficiency.

AesculaMed *Bioforce, Switz.*
Aesculus (p.1574·1).
Venous insufficiency.

Aesculo Gel L *Engelhard, Ger.*
Coconut oil (p.1409·1).
Pediculosis.

Aesculus Med Complex *Dynamit, Aust.*
Homoeopathic preparation.

Aescusan *Jenapharm, Ger.*
Note.This name is used for preparations of different composition.
Jenapharm, Ger.
Tablets; oral liquid: Aesculus (p.1574·1).
Soft-tissue inflammation; venous insufficiency.
LAW, Ger.
Cream: Aesculus (p.1574·1); hamamelis (p.1618·3).
Soft-tissue inflammation; venous insufficiency.

Aescuven *Cesra, Ger.*
Aesculus (p.1574·1).
Soft-tissue inflammation; venous insufficiency.

Aesol *Leiras, Fin.*
Vitamin A palmitate (p.1383·2); alpha tocoferil acetate (p.1394·1).
Vitamins A and E deficiency; vitamins A and E supplement.

Aesrutal S *Steigerwald, Ger.*
Convallaria (p.1599·1); crataegus (p.1600·2); ammi visnaga fruit (p.1579·1).
Circulatory insufficiency; heart failure.

Aesrutan *Engelshof, Aust.*
Rutoside (p.1611·2); aesculus (p.1574·1).
Chronic venous insufficiency; haemorrhoids.

Aethoxysklerol
Nycomed, Aust.; Codali, Belg.; Kreussler, Denm.; Kreussler, Fin.; Kreussler, Ger.; Novartis, Neth.; Inverdia, Swed.; Kreussler, Switz.; Kreussler, Thai.
Lauromacrogol 400 (p.1345·2).
Dilated cutaneous veins; haemorrhoids; varices.

Aethroma *Ratiopharm, Aust.†; Mepha, Hong Kong; Mepha, Switz.*
Vincamine (p.1680·1).
Cerebrovascular disorders.

Aetoxisclerol *Kreussler, Fr.*
Lauromacrogol 400 (p.1345·2).
Formerly known as Veinosclerol.
Varices.

Aezodent *Associated Dental, UK.*
Chlorobutanol (p.1141·2); methyl salicylate (p.55·1); benzocaine (p.1306·2); menthol (p.1632·3); eugenol (p.1609·3).
Denture irritation.

AF
Note.This name is used for preparations of different composition.
Valdecasas, Mex.
Folic acid (p.1361·1).
Folic acid deficiency.

Aspen Consumer, S.Afr.
Zinc undecenoate (p.395·3); undecenoic acid (p.395·3); terpineol (p.1669·3).
Fungal skin infections.

222 AF *Johnson & Johnson, Canad.*
Paracetamol (p.71·2).
Fever; pain.

AF Anacin *Whitehall-Robins, Canad.†.*
Paracetamol (p.71·2).
Fever; pain.

Afazol *Grin, Mex.*
Naphazoline hydrochloride (p.1095·1).
Eye irritation.

Afazol Z *Grin, Mex.*
Naphazoline hydrochloride (p.1095·1); zinc sulfate (p.1398·2).
Eye disorders.

Afebrin *Legrand, Braz.*
Note.This name is used for preparations of different composition.
Legrand, Braz.
Phenylpropanolamine hydrochloride (p.1098·1); phenylephrine hydrochloride (p.1097·1); phenyltoloxamine citrate (p.423·1); carbinoxamine maleate (p.411·1).
Cold and influenza symptoms.
Westmont, Hong Kong.
Paracetamol (p.71·2).
Fever; pain.
Inkeysa, Spain†.
Dipyrone (p.34·1).
Fever; pain.

Afebryl
SMB, Belg.†; Galephar, Fr.; Azevedos, Port.†.
Aspirin (p.14·2); paracetamol (p.71·2); ascorbic acid (p.1389·3).
Fever; inflammation; pain.

Afeksin *United Nordic, Denm.*
Fluoxetine hydrochloride (p.284·2).
Bulimia; depression.

Aferadol *Oberlin, Fr.†.*
Paracetamol (p.71·2).
Fever; pain.

Affectine *Taro, Israel.*
Fluoxetine hydrochloride (p.284·2).
Depression; obsessive-compulsive disorder.

Affex *Klinge, Irl.*
Fluoxetine (p.288·2).
Bulimia; depression; obsessive-compulsive disorder.

AFI-B₆ *Nycomed, Norw.*
Pyridoxine hydrochloride (p.1386·3).
Peripheral neuritis; pyridoxine deficiency; sideroblastic anaemia.

AFI-B-Total *Nycomed, Norw.*
Vitamin B substances (p.1350·1).
Vitamin B deficiency.

AFI-C *Nycomed, Norw.*
Ascorbic acid (p.1389·3).
Vitamin C deficiency.

AFI-D₂ *Nycomed, Norw.*
Ergocalciferol (p.1391·2).
Hypoparathyroid tetany.

Afid Plus *Fresenius Kabi, Ger.*
Bis(3-aminopropyl)-dodecylamine; cocospropylenediamineguanidinium diacetate.
Instrument disinfection.

AFI-E *Nycomed, Norw.*
Alpha tocoferil acetate (p.1394·1).
Vitamin E deficiency.

A-Fil *GenDerm, USA.*
Methyl anthranilate; titanium dioxide (p.1126·1).
Sunscreen.

Afipran *Nycomed, Norw.*
Metoclopramide (p.1236·3) or metoclopramide hydrochloride (p.1235·2).
Gastrointestinal disorders.

Aflamin *Hexal, S.Afr.*
Indometacin (p.44·3).
Gout; musculoskeletal and joint disorders.

Aflamina *Boehringer Ingelheim, Mex.*
Phenylbutazone piperazine (p.78·3).

Afloben *Esseti, Ital.*
Benzydamine hydrochloride (p.20·1).
Inflammation; pain.

Aflodac *Biotekfarma, Ital.†.*
Sulindac (p.85·3).
Gout; musculoskeletal and joint disorders.

Aflogine *Deverge, Ital.†.*
Cetrimonium tosilate (p.1137·3); allantoin (p.1110·1); lactic acid (p.1626·2); sodium adipate.
Personal hygiene; vaginal douche.

Aflogos *Biomedica, Ital.*
Diflunisal arginine (p.33·1).
Pain.

Afloxan
Rotta, Hong Kong; Rotta, Ital.; Rotta, Thai.
Proglumetacin dimaleate (p.80·1).
Gout; inflammation; musculoskeletal, joint, and peri-articular disorders; pain.

Afloyan *Farmabion, Spain†.*
Etofibrate (p.888·2).
Hyperlipidaemias.

Aflubin *Bittner, Aust.*
Homoeopathic preparation.

Aflukin C *IPS, Neth.†.*
Quinine sulfate (p.445·1); ascorbic acid (p.1389·3).
Cold and influenza symptoms.

Aflumycin *Agis, Israel.*
Prednisolone (p.1077·3); gentamicin sulfate (p.210·1).
Infected skin disorders.

Afluon *Asta Medica, Spain.*
Azelastine hydrochloride (p.409·3).
Allergic conjunctivitis; allergic rhinitis.

Afluvit *IPS, Neth.†.*
Paracetamol (p.71·2); ascorbic acid (p.1389·3).
Cold and influenza symptoms.

Afongan
Galderma, Ital.; Alcon, Mex.; Galderma, Port.†; Galderma, Spain†.
Omoconazole nitrate (p.393·1).
Fungal infections of the skin and mucous membranes.

Afonilum *Knoll, Ger.*
Controlled-release capsules; oral drops: Theophylline (p.777·2).
Obstructive airways disease.

Afonilum novo *Knoll, Ger.*
Theophylline sodium glycinate (p.783·2).
Obstructive airways disease.

Afonina *Farmatrading, Port.*
Benzocaine (p.1306·2); tyrothricin (p.267·1).
Mouth and throat disorders.

Aforinol *Rekah, Israel.*
Mepyramine maleate (p.421·2); xylometazoline hydrochloride (p.1102·2); hamamelis (p.1618·3).
Nasal congestion.

Afos *Salus, Ital.*
Tablets: Fosfomycin calcium (p.208·2).
Bacterial infections.

afpred-DEXA *Hefa, Ger.*
Dexamethasone sodium metasulfobenzoate (p.1067·1).
Formerly known as afpred-1.
Obstructive airways disease.

afpred-THEO *Hefa, Ger.*
Theophylline (p.777·2).
Formerly known as afpred-2.
Cor pulmonale; neonatal apnoea; obstructive airways disease.

Afrazine *Schering-Plough, UK.*
Oxymetazoline hydrochloride (p.1096·2).
Nasal congestion.

African Gold *Strickland, Canad.*
Hydroquinone (p.1115·1).

Afrin
Note.This name is used for preparations of different composition.
Schering-Plough, Braz.; Schering-Plough, Hong Kong; Schering-Plough, Mex.; Schering-Plough, S.Afr.†; Schering-Plough, Singapore.
Oxymetazoline hydrochloride (p.1096·2).
Ear disorders; nasal congestion; ocular congestion.
Schering-Plough, USA.
Nasal drops; nasal spray: Oxymetazoline hydrochloride (p.1096·2).
Tablets: Pseudoephedrine sulfate (p.1099·3).
Nasal congestion.

Afrin Moisturizing Saline Mist *Schering-Plough, USA.*
Sodium chloride (p.1196·1).
Formerly called Afrin Saline Mist.
Inflammation and dryness of nasal membranes.

Afrinex *Schering-Plough, Mex.*
Brompheniramine maleate (p.410·2); pseudoephedrine sulfate (p.1099·3).
Nasal congestion.

Afrinex Infantil *Schering-Plough, Mex.*
Aspirin (p.14·2); phenylephrine hydrochloride (p.1097·1); chlorpheniramine [chlorphenamine] maleate (p.412·1).
Allergic rhinitis; fever; nasal congestion; pain.

Afrodor *Farco, Ger.*
Quebracho; accearbromal; vitamin E (p.1350·1).
Tonic.

Afrolate *Bayer, Spain†.*
Etofenamate (p.35·3).
Peri-articular disorders; soft-tissue disorders.

Aftab
Rottapharm, Fin.; Opfermann, Ger.; Rottapharm, Ital.
Triamcinolone acetonide (p.1080·1).
Aphthous ulcer; gingivitis; stomatitis.

Aftach *Helsinn, Port.*
Triamcinolone acetonide (p.1080·1).
Aphthous ulcer.

Af-Taf *Sam-On, Israel.*
Phenylephrine hydrochloride (p.1097·1).
Nasal congestion.

Aftagel *Cooperation Pharmaceutique, Fr.*
Lignocaine [lidocaine] hydrochloride (p.1313·2); zinc sulfate (p.1398·2).
Inflammatory mouth disorders.

Aftajuventus *Ern, Spain.*
Benzalkonium chloride (p.1133·2); hydrocortisone hydrogen succinate (p.1074·1).
Formerly known as Afta.
Stomatitis.

Aftasone *Vinas, Spain.*
Hydrocortisone hydrogen succinate (p.1074·1).
Mouth ulcers.

Aftasone B C *Vinas, Spain.*
Ascorbic acid (p.1389·3); hydrocortisone hydrogen succinate (p.1074·1); pyridoxine (p.1387·1); riboflavin (p.1386·1).
Formerly known as Oralsone B C.
Mouth ulcers.

Aftate
Schering-Plough, Hong Kong; Schering-Plough, USA.
Tolnaftate (p.395·2).
Fungal skin infections.

After Bite
Tender, Canad.; Tender, Israel; Pensa, Spain; De Witt, UK.
Ammonia (p.1579·1).
Insect bites; stings.

Afterburn *Tender, Canad.*
Lignocaine [lidocaine] hydrochloride (p.1313·2).

After-Work *Hamilton, Austral.*
Emollient.
Dry skin.

Aftir Gel *Biochimici, Ital.*
Malathion (p.1434·2).
Pediculosis.

Aftir Shampoo *Biochimici, Ital.*
Hydroxyquinoline sulfate (p.1622·2).
For use after Aftir Gel; pediculosis.

Aftsinun *Sam-On, Israel.*
Diphenhydramine hydrochloride (p.416·1); pseudoephedrine hydrochloride (p.1099·2).
Cold symptoms; coughs; nasal congestion; sinusitis.

Aftsinun Veshiul *Sam-On, Israel.*
Diphenhydramine hydrochloride (p.416·1); pseudoephedrine hydrochloride (p.1099·2); codeine phosphate (p.25·2).
Cold symptoms; coughs; nasal congestion; sinusitis.

Afungil *Senosiain, Mex.*
Fluconazole (p.383·2).
Fungal infections.

Agaffin *Merck, Aust.*
Sodium picosulfate (p.1249·3).
Bowel evacuation; constipation.

Agamadon *Agamadon, Ger.†*
Aquilegia; sedi telephii; teucrii scor; equisetum (p.1606·3); sanicula; chamomile (p.1593·2); sage (p.1660·2); birch leaves (p.1585·2).
Gastrointestinal disorders.

Agamadon N *Agamadon, Ger.†*
Chamomile (p.1593·2); peppermint leaf (p.1243·2); caraway (p.1591·2).
Dyspepsia.

Agapurin *Medphano, Ger.*
Oxpentifylline [pentoxifylline] (p.950·3).
Circulatory disorders.

Agarbil *Ottolenghi, Ital.†.*
Agar (p.1498·3); phenolphthalein (p.1244·1); sodium dehydrocholate (p.1602·2).
Constipation.

Agarol
Note.This name is used for preparations of different composition.
Parke, Davis, Austral.
Liquid paraffin (p.1407·1).
Formerly contained liquid paraffin and phenolphthalein.
Constipation.

Warner-Lambert Consumer, Belg.†; Ache, Braz.; Warner-Lambert, Irl.†; Warner-Lambert, Ital.†; Warner-Lambert, Neth.†; Aspen Consumer, S.Afr.; Warner-Lambert Consumer, Switz.†; Warner-Lambert, UK.
Liquid paraffin (p.1407·1); phenolphthalein (p.1244·1); agar (p.1498·3).
Constipation.

Warner-Lambert, Canad.†
Liquid paraffin (p.1407·1); glycerol (p.1616·3); phenolphthalein (p.1244·1); agar (p.1498·3).
Constipation.

Warner-Lambert, Hong Kong.
Liquid paraffin (p.1407·1).
Constipation.

Warner-Lambert, Spain†; Warner-Lambert, Thai.
Liquid paraffin (p.1407·1); phenolphthalein (p.1244·1).
Constipation.

Agarol CM *Warner-Lambert, Ital.*
Liquid paraffin (p.1407·1).
Constipation.

Agarol N *Warner-Lambert, Ger.*
Liquid paraffin (p.1407·1).
Agarol formerly contained liquid paraffin and phenolphthalein.
Constipation.

Agarol Plain *Numark, Canad.*
Liquid paraffin (p.1407·1); glycerol (p.1616·3).
Constipation.

Agarol Soft *Warner-Lambert Consumer, Switz.*
Fig (p.1227·1); sorbitol (p.1377·3).
Constipation.

Agaroletten *Warner-Lambert, Ger.*
Bisacodyl (p.1212·2).
Bowel evacuation; constipation.

Agasten *Novartis, Braz.*
Clemastine fumarate (p.413·2).
Hypersensitivity.

Agastrin *Rottapharm, Ital.*
Trihydroxyaluminium magnesium carbonate.
Gastrointestinal disorders associated with hyperacidity.

Agathol *Iderne, Fr.*
Zinc oxide (p.1128·2); titanium dioxide (p.1126·1); peru balsam (p.1650·2).
Formerly contained zinc oxide, titanium dioxide, peru balsam, and cresol.
Skin disorders.

Age Block *Avon, Canad.*
Avobenzone (p.1517·1); octinoxate (p.1517·3); oxybenzone (p.1518·1).
Sunscreen.

Agedin Plus *GD, Ital.*
Eicosapentaenoic acid (p.949·3); ubidecarenone (p.1677·1); methionine (p.1012·2); betacarotene (p.1355·1).
Nutritional supplement.

A-Gel *Pharmatel, Austral.*
Lubricant gel.

Agelan *Antigen, Hong Kong; Antigen, Irl.*
Indapamide (p.913·1).
Hypertension.

A-gen 53
Note.This name is used for preparations of different composition.
Solco, Aust.
Polysaccharide polysulfuric acid ester.
Contraceptive.

Herbrand, Ger.; Chefaro, Ger.
Cellulose poly(sulfuric acid ester), trisodium salt; nonoxinol 9 (p.1346·1).
Contraceptive.

Agena *Lusofarmaco, Ital.†.*
Vaginal gel: Benzalkonium chloride (p.1133·2); nonoxinol (p.1346·1); ethylene glycol monolaurate; carmellose sodium (p.1499·3).

Vaginal tablets: Benzalkonium chloride (p.1133·2); nonoxinol (p.1346·1); ethylene glycol monolaurate; macrogol (p.1630·1).
Contraceptive; vaginal disinfection.

Agenerase *Glaxo Wellcome, Fr.; Glaxo Wellcome, Switz.; Glaxo Wellcome, UK; Glaxo Wellcome, USA.*
Amprenavir (p.616·1).
HIV infection.

Ageroplas *Farma Lepori, Spain.*
Ditazole (p.880·1).
Thromboembolism prophylaxis.

Agerpen *I Farmacologia, Spain.*
Amoxicillin trihydrate (p.149·2).
Bacterial infections.

Agerpen Mucolitico *I Farmacologia, Spain.*
Amoxicillin trihydrate (p.149·2); bromhexine hydrochloride (p.1085·3).
Respiratory-tract infections.

Agevit *Stafford-Miller, Fr.*
A range of vitamin and mineral supplements (p.1350·1).

Aggrastat *Merck Sharp & Dohme, Austral.; Merck Sharp & Dohme, Belg.; Merck Sharp & Dohme, Denm.; Merck Sharp & Dohme, Fin.; Merck Sharp & Dohme, Ger.; Merck Sharp & Dohme, Irl.; Merck Sharp & Dohme, Ital.; Merck Sharp & Dohme, Neth.; Merck Sharp & Dohme, NZ; Merck Sharp & Dohme, Singapore; Merck Sharp & Dohme, Swed.; Merck Sharp & Dohme, Switz.; Merck Sharp & Dohme, UK; Merck, USA.*
Tirofiban hydrochloride (p.983·2).
Myocardial infarction; prevention of ischaemic cardiac compliations during angioplasty or atherectomy; unstable angina.

Aggrastet *Merck Sharp & Dohme, S.Afr.*
Tirofiban hydrochloride (p.983·2).
Prevention of cardiac ischaemia in angioplasty or atherectomy.

Aggrenox *Boehringer Ingelheim, Belg.; Boehringer Ingelheim, USA.*
Dipyridamole (p.877·2); aspirin (p.14·2).
Cerebrovascular ischaemia; thrombosis prophylaxis.

Agilan *Klinge, Aust.*
Dihydroergotamine mesilate (p.450·3); etilefrine hydrochloride (p.888·1).
Hypotension.

Agilisin *Luitpold, Braz.*
Indometacin (p.44·3).
Fever; gout; musculoskeletal, joint, and peri-articular disorders; pain.

Aginax *Biogyne, Fr.*
Soap substitute.
Skin irritation.

Agiobulk *Byk Madaus, S.Afr.*
Ispaghula (p.1229·1).
Constipation.

Agiocur *Madaus, Aust.; Madaus, Fin.; Madaus, Ger.; Madaus, Hong Kong; Madaus, Israel; Neo-Farmaceutica, Port.; Madaus, Thai.*
Ispaghula (p.1229·1).
Colostomy management; constipation; diarrhoea; inflammatory bowel disease; irritable bowel syndrome; stool softener.

Agiofibe *Knoll, Austral.*
Ispaghula (p.1229·1).
Dietary fibre supplement.

Agiofibra *Byk Gulden, Mex.*
Ispaghula (p.1229·1).
Constipation; dietary fibre supplement.

Agiolax *Madaus, Aust.; Knoll, Austral.; Madaus, Belg.; Byk, Braz.; Madaus, Fin.; Madaus, Fr.; Madaus, Ger.; Madaus, Hong Kong; Madaus, Israel; Madaus, Ital.; Byk Gulden, Mex.; Madaus, Neth.; Neo-Farmaceutica, Port.; Byk Madaus, S.Afr.; Madaus, Spain; Madaus, Switz.; Madaus, Thai.*
Ispaghula (p.1229·1); senna (p.1248·2).
Formerly contained ispaghula, senna, and guaiazulene in Belg.
Bowel evacuation; constipation; stool softener.

Agiolax Ballast *Madaus, Ger.*
Ispaghula (p.1229·1).
Constipation; stool softener.

Agiolax mite *Madaus, Switz.*
Ispaghula (p.1229·1).
Constipation; irritable bowel syndrome; stool softener.

Agiolax Pico *Madaus, Ger.*
Sodium picosulfate (p.1249·3).
Constipation.

Agiolind *Madaus, Aust.†.*
Ispaghula (p.1229·1).
Constipation; stool softener.

AgioPico Plus *Madaus, Ger.*
Sodium picosulfate (p.1249·3).
Constipation.

Agipiu *Candioli, Ital.*
Silver carbonate (p.1664·3); alkylbenzyldimethylammonium saccharinate (p.1133·3).
Wound disinfection.

Agiserc *Agis, Israel.*
Betahistine (p.1584·3).
Vestibular disorders.

Agisolvan *Agis, Israel.*
Acetylcysteine (p.1082·3).
Respiratory-tract disorders associated with viscous mucus.

Agispor *Agis, Israel.*
Bifonazole (p.381·1).
Fungal skin infections; seborrhoeic dermatitis.

Agispor Onychoset *Agis, Israel.*
Bifonazole (p.381·1); urea (p.1127·3).
Fungal nail infections.

Agisten *Agis, Israel.*
Clotrimazole (p.382·1).
Fungal skin infections; vaginitis.

Agit *Sanol, Ger.*
Dihydroergotamine mesilate (p.450·3).
Hypotension; migraine and other vascular headaches; varices.

Agit plus *Sanol, Ger.*
Dihydroergotamine mesilate (p.450·3); etilefrine hydrochloride (p.888·1).
Hypotension.

Aglucil *Elofar, Braz.*
Glibenclamide (p.321·3).
Diabetes mellitus.

Aglutella *Gentili, Ital.*
Range of gluten-free food for special diets (p.1350·1).

Ultrapharm, UK.
Low-protein food for special diets (p.1350·1).

Agnesin *Hevert, Ger.*
Homoeopathic preparation.

Agnolyt *Madaus, Ger.; Madaus, Switz.; Natural Touch, UK.*
Vitex agnus castus (p.1574·2).
Premenstrual syndrome.

Agnucaston *Bionorica, Ger.; Bionorica, Hong Kong.*
Vitex agnus castus (p.1574·2).
Mastalgia; menstrual disorders.

Agnuchol *Smetana, Aust.*
Cynara (p.1601·3); taraxacum (p.1669·1); peppermint leaf (p.1243·2).
Digestive disorders; gallbladder disorders.

Agnufemil *Steigerwald, Ger.*
Agnus castus (p.1574·2).
Mastalgia; premenstrual syndrome.

Agnukliman *Smetana, Aust.*
Cimicifuga (p.1595·2).
Menopausal disorders.

Agnumens *Smetana, Aust.*
Agnus castus (p.1574·2).
Menstrual disorders; premenstrual syndrome.

Agnurell *Sanorell, Ger.*
Homoeopathic preparation.

Agnus castus *Hevert, Ger.*
Homoeopathic preparation.

Agofell *Janssen-Cilag, S.Afr.*
Diisopromine hydrochloride (p.1222·2); sorbitol (p.1377·3).
Biliary-tract disorders.

Agofenac *Ogera, Switz.*
Diclofenac sodium (p.30·3).
Gout; inflammation; musculoskeletal and joint disorders; pain.

Agon *Therapharm, Austral.; Aventis, NZ.*
Felodipine (p.888·3).
Angina pectoris; hypertension.

Agoprim *Ogera, Switz.*
Co-trimoxazole (p.193·3).
Bacterial infections; Pneumocystis carinii pneumonia.

Agopton *Takeda, Aust.; Takeda, Ger.; Takeda, Switz.*
Lansoprazole (p.1230·3).
Gastro-oesophageal reflux; gastrointestinal hyperacidity; peptic ulcer; Zollinger-Ellison syndrome.

Agoral *Warner-Lambert, USA.*
Liquid paraffin (p.1407·1); phenolphthalein (p.1244·1); agar (p.1498·3).
Constipation.

Agoral Plain *Warner-Lambert, USA†.*
Liquid paraffin (p.1407·1).
Constipation.

Agorex *Ogera, Switz.*
Amiloride hydrochloride (p.835·1); hydrochlorothiazide (p.907·3).
Hypertension; oedema.

Agorhino *Ogera, Switz.*
Phenylephrine hydrochloride (p.1097·1); dimenhydrinate (p.415·2); caffeine (p.761·3).
Cold symptoms; nasal and sinus congestion; rhinitis.

A/G-Pro *Miller, USA.*
Multivitamin, mineral, and amino-acid preparation (p.1350·1).

Agradil *Sanofi Synthelabo, Ital.*
Veralipride (p.711·2).
Menopausal disorders.

A-Gram *Inava, Fr.*
Amoxicillin trihydrate (p.149·2) or amoxicillin sodium (p.149·2).
Bacterial infections.

Agrastat *Merck Sharp & Dohme-Chibret, Fr.; Merck Sharp & Dohme, Mex.; Merck Sharp & Dohme, Spain.*
Tirofiban hydrochloride (p.983·2).
Ischaemic heart disease; myocardial infarction.

Agreal *Sanofi Synthelabo, Belg.; Synthelabo, Braz.; Synthelabo, Fr.; Synthelabo, Hong Kong; Sanofi Synthelabo, Port.; Synthelabo, Spain.*
Veralipride (p.711·2).
Menopausal disorders.

Agre-Gola *Vernedia, Neth.*
Cetylpyridinium chloride (p.1138·1); phenol (p.1152·3); menthol (p.1632·3).
Sore throat.

Agremol *Eurodrug, Thai.*
Dipyridamole (p.877·2).
Angina pectoris; thromboembolic disorders.

Agrimonas N *Niedermaier, Ger.*
Taraxacum (p.1669·1); celandine; absinthium (p.1571·1).
Dyspepsia.

Agrippal *Chiron, Ital.; Biovac, S.Afr.; Chiron, Thai.; Wyeth, UK.*
An inactivated influenza vaccine (p.1544·3).
Active immunisation.

Agrumina *Also, Ital.*
Ascorbic acid (p.1389·3).
Vitamin C deficiency; vitamin C supplement.

Agruvit *Hoechst Marion Roussel, Ital.*
Ascorbic acid (p.1389·3); calcium ascorbate dihydrate (p.1389·3) or sodium ascorbate (p.1390·1).
Vitamin C deficiency; vitamin C supplement.

Agrylin *Orphan, Austral.; Roberts, Canad.; Roberts, Israel; Roberts, USA.*
Anagrelide hydrochloride (p.1579·3).
Essential thrombocythaemia.

Agua del Carmen *Fardi, Spain.*
Coriander seeds (p.1599·2); matricaria (p.1593·2); melissa (p.1632·2); dried bitter-orange peel (p.1644·2); lemon verbena (p.1628·3); cinnamon (p.1595·3); angelica (p.1580·2); nutmeg (p.1643·1); hyssopus officinalis.
Hyperactivity; nervous disorders; pain.

Agua Inglesa *Catarinense, Braz.*
Cassau; chamomile; broom; cinnamon; centaury; bitter orange; absinthium; cinchona.

Agudil *Sigma-Tau, Spain.*
Levoglutamide (p.1365·2); asparagine; pyridoxine hydrochloride (p.1386·3); phosphoserine.
Tonic.

Agyrax *Darci, Belg.*
Meclozine hydrochloride (p.420·3).
Formerly contained buclizine hydrochloride, hydroxyzine hydrochloride, and buphenine hydrochloride.
Hearing disorders; tinnitus; vertigo.

Vedim, Fr.
Meclozine hydrochloride (p.420·3).
Formerly contained buphenine hydrochloride, meclozine hydrochloride, and hydroxyzine hydrochloride.
Motion sickness; vertigo.

AH 3 N *Rodleben, Ger.*
Hydroxyzine hydrochloride (p.419·1).
Pruritus.

AHA Skin Lightening Gel *Therapeutic-Ocean, Singapore.*
Kojic acid; hydroquinone (p.1115·1); glycolic acid (p.1115·1).
Skin hyperpigmentation.

AH-chew *WE, USA.*
Phenylephrine hydrochloride (p.1097·1); chlorpheniramine [chlorphenamine] maleate (p.412·1); hyoscine methonitrate (p.468·2).
Upper respiratory-tract symptoms.

AH-chew D *WE, USA.*
Phenylephrine hydrochloride (p.1097·1).
Nasal congestion.

AHD 2000 *Lysoform, Ger.*
Alcohol (p.1130·3).
Hand disinfection; skin disinfection.

Ahecan *Marrero, Spain.*
Hydrogen peroxide (p.1147·1).
Epistaxis; mouth, skin, and wound disinfection.

AHF *CSL, Austral.; CSL, NZ.*
A factor VIII preparation (p.734·1).
Factor VIII deficiency; von Willebrand's disease.

Ahiston *Teva, Israel.*
Chlorpheniramine [chlorphenamine] maleate (p.412·1).
Hypersensitivity reactions.

Ahiston Compound *Teva, Israel.*
Chlorpheniramine [chlorphenamine] maleate (p.412·1); phenylephrine hydrochloride (p.1097·1).
Hypersensitivity reactions.

AHP 200 *Chephasaar, Ger.*
Oxaceprol (p.1645·2).
Musculoskeletal, joint, peri-articular, and soft-tissue disorders.

A-Hydrocort *Abbott, Canad.; Abbott, USA.*
Hydrocortisone sodium succinate (p.1074·1).
Corticosteroid.

Aicamin *Sanofi Winthrop, Belg.†; Esfar, Port.*
Orazamide (p.1644·2).
Liver disorders.

Aid III MSUD *SHS, Fr.*
Food for special diets (p.1350·1).
Leucinosis.

The symbol † denotes a preparation no longer actively marketed

Aida *Paraphar, Fr.; Paraphar, Singapore.*
Hydroquinone (p.1115·1).
Skin hyperpigmentation.

Aid-Lax *Nobel, Canad.†*
Aloin (p.1210·2); cascara (p.1216·1); phenolphthalein (p.1244·1); bile salts (p.1585·1).

Aigin *Hevert, Ger.*
Kava (p.1625·3).
Nervous disorders.

Aiglonyl *Fumouze, Fr.*
Sulpiride (p.706·1).
Neuroses.

Ailax *Galen, Irl.; Galen, UK.*
Dantron (p.1221·3); poloxamer 188 (p.1347·1).
These ingredients can be described by the British Approved Name Co-danthramer.
Constipation.

Aima-Calcin *ISI, Ital.†*
Elcatonin (p.749·2).
Hypercalcaemia; osteoporosis; Paget's disease of bone; reflex sympathetic dystrophy.

Aimafix *ISI, Ital.*
Factor IX (p.735·1).
Haemorrhagic disorders.

Ainex *Promeco, Mex.*
Ibuprofen (p.43·2).

Ainscrid *Ethypharm, Fr.†*
Indometacin (p.44·3).
Fever; inflammation.

Aircort *Italchimici, Ital.*
Budesonide (p.1064·2).
Asthma.

Airest *Caber, Ital.*
Bamifylline hydrochloride (p.761·2).
Asthma; bronchospasm.

Airet *Medeva, Ital.*
Salbutamol sulfate (p.770·3).
Obstructive airways disease.

Airol *Roche, Aust.†; Pierre Fabre, Ger.; Roche, Israel; Pierre Fabre, Ital.; Roche, Mex.; Orient, Singapore; Pierre Fabre, Singapore; Pierre Fabre, Switz.*
Tretinoin (p.1126·2).
Acne.

Airomet *Masa, Thai.*
Omeprazole (p.1239·1).
Peptic ulcer; Zollinger-Ellison syndrome.

Airomir *3M, Austral.; 3M, Belg.; 3M, Canad.; 3M, Denm.; 3M, Fin.; 3M, Fr.; 3M, Irl.; 3M, Neth.; 3M, Norw.; 3M, NZ; 3M, S.Afr.; 3M, Singapore; 3M, Swed.; 3M, Switz.; 3M, Thai.; 3M, UK.*
Salbutamol sulfate (p.770·3) or salbutamol sulfate (p.770·3).
Obstructive airways disease.

Air-Tal *Sintesa, Belg.*
Aceclofenac (p.11·1).
Inflammation; musculoskeletal, joint, and peri-articular disorders.

Airtal *Rowex, Irl.†; Probios, Port.; Almirall, Spain.*
Aceclofenac (p.11·1).
Gout; musculoskeletal, joint, and peri-articular disorders; pain.

Airtal Difucrem *Almirall, Spain.*
Aceclofenac (p.11·1).
Peri-articular and soft-tissue disorders.

Airvitess *Farmasan, Ger.*
Ketotifen fumarate (p.767·2).
Asthma; hypersensitivity disorders.

Air-X *RX, Thai.*
Simeticone (p.1249·2).
Aid to gastroscopy and X-ray examination; flatulence.

Ajaka *Streuli, Switz.†*
Aloes (p.1210·1); aloin (p.1210·2); belladonna (p.463·1); caraway (p.1591·2); fennel (p.1610·1); juniper (p.1625·2); caraway oil (p.1591·2); fennel oil (p.1610·2); juniper oil (p.1625·2).
Constipation.

Ajan *3M, Ger.*
Nefopam hydrochloride (p.62·1).
Pain.

Akabar *AF, Mex.*
Nifuroxazide (p.230·2).
Bacterial infections of the gastrointestinal tract.

Akacin *Diba, Mex.; Atlantic, Thai.*
Amikacin sulfate (p.148·1).
Gram-negative bacterial infections.

Akamin *Alphapharm, Austral.*
Minocycline hydrochloride (p.224·3).
Bacterial infections.

Akamon *Medochemie, Hong Kong.*
Bromazepam (p.656·3).
Anxiety.

Akarin *Nycomed, Denm.*
Citalopram hydrobromide (p.281·2) or citalopram hydrochloride (p.281·2).
Depression; panic attacks.

Akarpine *Akorn, USA.*
Pilocarpine hydrochloride (p.1422·3).
Glaucoma; raised intra-ocular pressure; reversal of mydriasis.

Akatinol *Merz, Ger.*
Memantine hydrochloride (p.1174·3).
Mental function impairment; parkinsonism; spasticity.

Ak-Beta *Akorn, USA.*
Levobunolol hydrochloride (p.920·3).
Glaucoma; ocular hypertension.

Ak-Biocholine *Akorn, USA†.*
Choline bitartrate (p.1356·3); citrus bioflavonoid complex (p.1611·1).

Ak-Chlor *Akorn, USA.*
Chloramphenicol (p.179·1).
Eye infections.

Ak-Cide *Akorn, USA.*
Prednisolone acetate (p.1078·1); sulfacetamide sodium (p.250·3).
Infected eye disorders.

Ak-Con *Akorn, Canad.; Akorn, USA.*
Naphazoline hydrochloride (p.1095·1).
Minor eye irritation.

Ak-Con-A *Akorn, USA†.*
Naphazoline hydrochloride (p.1095·1); pheniramine maleate (p.422·3).
Eye irritation.

Ak-Dex *Akorn, USA.*
Dexamethasone sodium phosphate (p.1067·1).
Eye inflammation.

Ak-Dilate *Akorn, USA.*
Phenylephrine hydrochloride (p.1097·1).
Funduscopy; open-angle glaucoma; ophthalmic examination; pupil dilatation during surgery; refraction without cycloplegia; uveitis.

Ak-Fluor *Akorn, USA.*
Fluorescein sodium (p.1612·1).
Ophthalmic diagnostic agent.

Akicin *General Drugs, Thai.*
Amikacin sulfate (p.148·1).
Bacterial infections.

Akila mains et peau *Adam, Mon.†*
Chlorhexidine gluconate (p.1138·2); hydrogen peroxide (p.1147·1); propyl alcohol (p.1155·3).
Skin disinfection.

Akila spray *Adam, Mon.†*
Glutaral (p.1145·2); benzalkonium chloride (p.1133·2); bromonitrodioxan; alcohol (p.1130·3); propyl alcohol (p.1155·3).
Surface disinfection.

Akildia *Asepta, Mon.*
Centella (p.1112·3); karite.
Moisturiser and barrier cream for foot disorders.

Akileine *Asepta, Mon.*
A range of preparations for foot disorders.

Akilen *Medochemie, Hong Kong.*
Verapamil hydrochloride (p.989·1).
Angina pectoris; arrhythmias; heart failure.

Akindex *Fournier, Belg.†; Urgo, Fr.; Freda, Port.†*
Dextromethorphan hydrobromide (p.1087·3).
Coughs.

Akindol *Fournier, Spain†.*
Paracetamol (p.71·2).
Fever; pain.

Akineton *Ebewe, Aust.; Knoll, Austral.; Knoll, Belg.; Knoll, Braz.; Knoll, Canad.; Knoll, Denm.; Knoll, Fin.; Knoll, Fr.; Knoll, Ger.; Knoll, Irl.; Ravizza, Ital.; Knoll, Mex.; Knoll, Neth.; Knoll, Norw.; Knoll, Port.; Knoll, S.Afr.; Knoll, Singapore; Knoll, Spain; Knoll, Swed.; Knoll, Switz.; Knoll, Thai.; Knoll, UK; Knoll, USA.*
Biperiden (p.464·2), biperiden hydrochloride (p.464·2), or biperiden lactate (p.464·2).
Bronchospasm; drug-induced extrapyramidal disorders; head injury; nicotine poisoning; parkinsonism; phosphorus poisoning; spasticity; trigeminal neuralgia.

Akinspray *Fournier, Belg.*
Benzalkonium chloride (p.1133·2); lignocaine [lidocaine] hydrochloride (p.1313·2).
Mouth and throat disorders.

Akipic *Asepta, Mon.*
Insect repellent.

Akistin *Nycomed, Aust.*
Diethylamine salamidacetate (p.81·3).
Musculoskeletal and joint disorders; neuralgias.

Aklonin *Wernigerode, Ger.*
Phenamazide hydrochloride (p.472·1).
Smooth muscle cramp; vomiting.

Ak-Mycin *Akorn, USA†.*
Erythromycin (p.201·2).
Eye infections.

Ichthyol, Switz.
Sodium bituminosulfonate (p.1115·3); salicylic acid (p.1122·3).
Acne.

Aknilox *Drossapharm, Switz.*
Erythromycin (p.201·2).
Acne.

Aknin *Sanofi Synthelabo, Ger.*
Lotion: Erythromycin (p.201·2).
Ointment: Sulfur (p.1123·3); salicylic acid (p.1122·3).
Acne.

Aknin-Mino *Sanofi Synthelabo, Ger.*
Minocycline hydrochloride (p.224·3).
Acne.

Aknin-N *Sodip, Switz.*
Minocycline hydrochloride (p.224·3).
Acne.

Aknoral *IBSA, Switz.*
Minocycline hydrochloride (p.224·3).
Acne.

Aknosan *Hermal, Ger.*
Minocycline hydrochloride (p.224·3).
Acne.

Akorazol *Collins, Mex.*
Ketoconazole (p.389·1).
Fungal infections.

Ak-Pentolate *Akorn, USA.*
Cyclopentolate hydrochloride (p.465·2).
Production of mydriasis and cycloplegia.

Ak-Poly-Bac *Akorn, USA.*
Polymyxin B sulfate (p.238·1); bacitracin zinc (p.155·2).
Eye infections.

Ak-Pred *Akorn, USA.*
Prednisolone sodium phosphate (p.1078·1).
Eye inflammation.

AkPro *Akorn, USA.*
Dipivefrine hydrochloride (p.1604·3).
Glaucoma.

Akrinor *Asta Medica, Aust.; Asta Medica, Ger.; Adcock Ingram, S.Afr.; Asta Medica, Switz.†.*
Cafedrine hydrochloride (p.853·1); theodrenaline hydrochloride (p.1671·3).
Circulatory disorders; hypotension.

Ak-Rinse *Akorn, USA.*
Electrolytes (p.1180·1).
Eye irrigation.

Ak-Rose *Akorn, Canad.*
Rose bengal sodium (p.1659·2).
Ophthalmic diagnostic agent.

Akrotherm *Gepepharm, Ger.*
Benzyl nicotinate (p.20·2); nonivamide (p.63·1).
Peripheral vascular disorders; soft-tissue injury.

Ak-Spore *Akorn, USA.*
Eye drops: Polymyxin B sulfate (p.238·1); neomycin sulfate (p.228·1); gramicidin (p.213·3).
Eye ointment: Polymyxin B sulfate (p.238·1); neomycin sulfate (p.228·1); bacitracin zinc (p.155·2).
Eye infections.

Ak-Spore HC *Akorn, USA.*
Ear drops: Hydrocortisone (p.1073·3); neomycin sulfate (p.228·1); polymyxin B (p.238·3).
Bacterial ear infections.
Eye drops; eye ointment: Polymyxin B sulfate (p.238·1); neomycin sulfate (p.228·1); hydrocortisone (p.1073·3).
Eye inflammation with bacterial infection.

Ak-Sulf *Akorn, USA.*
Sulfacetamide sodium (p.250·3).
Eye infections.

Ak-Taine *Akorn, Canad.; Akorn, USA.*
Proxymetacaine hydrochloride (p.1320·1).
Local anaesthesia.

Ak-T-Caine *Akorn, USA†.*
Amethocaine [tetracaine] hydrochloride (p.1305·2).

Aktiferrin *Ratiopharm, Aust.*
Ferrous sulfate (p.1360·3); DL-serine.
Iron deficiency; iron deficiency anaemia.

Aktiferrin compositum *Ratiopharm, Aust.*
Ferrous sulfate (p.1360·3); DL-serine; folic acid (p.1361·2); cyanocobalamin (p.1388·1).
Iron deficiency anaemia with folic acid deficiency.

Aktiferrin N *Merckle, Ger.*
Ferrous sulfate (p.1360·3).
Iron deficiency.

Aktiferrin-F *Mepha, Israel.*
Ferrous sulfate (p.1360·3); folic acid (p.1361·1); DL-serine.
Iron and folic acid deficiency.

Aktipar *Orion, Fin.*
Levodopa (p.1169·2); benserazide hydrochloride (p.1164·2).
Parkinsonism.

Aktiv Blasen- und Nierentee *Krug, Aust.*
Silver birch (p.1585·2); juniper (p.1625·2); ononis (p.1644·1); bearberry (p.1583·3); peppermint leaf (p.1243·2).
Renal and urinary-tract disorders.

Aktiv Husten- und Bronchialtee *Krug, Aust.*
Plantago lanceolata; aniseed (p.1580·2); thyme (p.1672·2); althaea (p.1577·1).
Catarrh; coughs.

Ak-NaCl *Akorn, USA.*
Sodium chloride (p.1196·1).
Corneal oedema.

Akne *Ichthyol, Aust.*
Erythromycin (p.201·2).
Acne.

Akne Cordes *Ichthyol, Ger.*
Erythromycin (p.201·2).
Acne.

Aknecin *Dermopen, Braz.*
Salicylic acid (p.1122·3); sulfur (p.1123·3).
Acne.

Aknederm Ery *Gepepharm, Ger.*
Erythromycin (p.201·2).
Acne.

Aknederm N *Gepepharm, Ger.*
Salicylic acid (p.1122·3); lactic acid (p.1626·2).
Skin disorders.

Aknederm Neu *Gepepharm, Ger.*
Ictasol (p.1115·3); zinc oxide (p.1128·2).
Skin disorders.

Aknederm Oxid *Gepepharm, Ger.*
Benzoyl peroxide (p.1111·1).
Acne.

Ak-Nefrin *Akorn, USA.*
Phenylephrine hydrochloride (p.1097·1).
Minor eye irritation.

Aknefug simplex *Wolff, Ger.*
Hexachlorophene (p.1146·1).
Acne; rosacea.

Aknefug-EL *Wolff, Ger.*
Erythromycin (p.201·2).
Acne.

Aknefug-Emulsion *Wolff, Ger.*
Estradiol (p.1473·1); hexachlorophene (p.1146·1).
Acne.

Aknefug-liquid *Wolff, Ger.*
Salicylic acid (p.1122·3).
Acne; eczema; seborrhoea.

Aknefug-oxid *Wolff, Ger.*
Benzoyl peroxide (p.1111·1).
Acne.

aknemago *Strathmann, Ger.*
Erythromycin (p.201·2).
Acne.

Aknemin
Merck, Neth.†; Crookes Healthcare, UK.
Minocycline hydrochloride (p.224·3).
Bacterial infections.

Aknemycin
Note. This name is used for preparations of different composition.
Hermal, Aust.; Boots Healthcare, Belg.; Hermal, Ger.; Hermal, Hong Kong; Boots Healthcare, Neth.; Hermal, Port.; Hermal, Singapore; Boots Healthcare, Switz.; Healthpoint, USA.
Erythromycin (p.201·2).
Acne.
Hermal, Ger.; Hermal, Israel; Boots Healthcare, Switz.
Topical emulsion: Erythromycin (p.201·2); ichthammol (p.1115·2).
Acne.

Aknemycin compositum *Hermal, Aust.*
Erythromycin (p.201·2); light ammonium bituminosulfonate (p.1115·2).
Acne.

Aknemycin Plus
Hermal, Ger.; Crookes Healthcare, UK.
Erythromycin (p.201·2); tretinoin (p.1126·2).
Acne.

Ak-Neo-Dex *Akorn, USA.*
Neomycin sulfate (p.228·1); dexamethasone sodium phosphate (p.1067·1).
Eye inflammation with bacterial infection.

Akne-Puren *Isis Puren, Ger.*
Minocycline hydrochloride (p.224·3).
Acne.

Aknereduct *Azupharma, Ger.†.*
Minocycline hydrochloride (p.224·3).
Acne.

Akneroxid
Hermal, Ger.; Boots Healthcare, Belg.; Hermal, Ger.; Boots Healthcare, Neth.; Boots Healthcare, Switz.
Benzoyl peroxide (p.1111·1).
Acne.

Aknex *Gebro, Switz.*
Benzoyl peroxide (p.1111·1).
Acne.

Aknicare
General Topics, Ital.; Dermoteca, Port.
Pyruvic acid; triclosan (p.1159·2).
Soap substitute for acne-prone skin.

Aknichthol *Ichthyol, Aust.*
Ictasol (p.1115·3); salicylic acid (p.1122·3); colloidal sulfur (p.1123·3).
Acne.

Aknichthol Creme *Ichthyol, Ger.*
Ictasol (p.1115·3).
Acne.

Aknichthol N
Note. This name is used for preparations of different composition.
Ichthyol, Ger.
Ictasol (p.1115·3); salicylic acid (p.1122·3).
Acne; rosacea.

Aktiv Leber- und Gallentee *Krug, Aust.*
Peppermint leaf (p.1243·2); achillea (p.1572·2); fennel (p.1610·1); turmeric (p.1029·3).
Liver and gallbladder disorders.

Aktiv milder Magen- und Darmtee *Krug, Aust.*
Aniseed (p.1580·2); fennel (p.1610·1); caraway (p.1591·2); chamomile (p.1593·2); achillea (p.1572·2).
Gastrointestinal disorders.

Aktiv Nerven- und Schlaftee *Krug, Aust.*
Lupulus (p.1629·3); valerian (p.1678·3); melissa (p.1632·2); peppermint leaf (p.1243·2); orange flowers.
Nervous disorders; sleep disorders.

Aktivakid *Hoechst Marion Roussel, S.Afr.†.*
Liver extracts; vitamin B₁₂; yeast extract; ferric glycerophosphate; lysine (p.1350·1).
Tonic.

Aktivanad
Ebewe, Aust.
Oral liquid: Liver extract; yeast; rose fruit; caffeine (p.1350·1).
Syrup: Liver extract; yeast; rose fruit; ferric glycerophosphate; lysine (p.1350·1).
Tonic.
Aventis, S.Afr.
Syrup: Haematoporphyrin; liver extracts; caffeine; yeast extract (p.1350·1).
Tablets: Haematoporphyrin; liver extracts; amino acids; vitamins; caffeine; yeast extract; ferric glycerophosphate (p.1350·1).
Tonic.

Aktivanad-N *Knoll, Ger.*
Oral liquid: Liver extract; yeast extract; caffeine (p.1350·1).
Tablets: Vitamins; caffeine (p.1350·1).
Tonic.

Aktiv-Puder *Klosterfrau, Ger.*
Colloidal silicon dioxide (p.1503·3).
Burns; skin disorders.

AkTob *Akorn, USA.*
Tobramycin (p.263·3).

Akton *Exel, Belg.*
Cloxazolam (p.671·2).
Anxiety; premedication; sleep disorders.

Ak-Tracin *Akorn, USA.*
Bacitracin (p.155·2).
Eye infections.

Aktren *Bayer, Ger.*
Ibuprofen (p.43·2).
Fever; pain.

Ak-Trol *Akorn, USA.*
Dexamethasone (p.1067·1); neomycin sulfate (p.228·1); polymyxin B sulfate (p.238·1).
Eye inflammation with bacterial infection.

Akudol *Wassermann, Ital.*
Naproxen sodium (p.61·1).
Fever; musculoskeletal and joint disorders; pain.

Ak-Vernacon *Akorn, Canad.*
Pheniramine maleate (p.422·3); phenylephrine hydrochloride (p.1097·1).
Antihistamine; decongestant.

Akwa Tears
Note. This name is used for preparations of different composition.
Akorn, Canad.; Akorn, USA.
Eye ointment: White soft paraffin (p.1407·3); liquid paraffin (p.1407·1); wool fat (p.1410·3).
Dry eyes.
Akorn, USA.
Eye drops: Polyvinyl alcohol (p.1503·1).
Dry eyes.

AKZ
Pfizer, Aust.; Howmedica, Switz.†.
Polymethylmethacrylate/methylmethacrylate copolymer (p.1635·2); erythromycin gluceptate (p.201·3); colistimethate sodium (p.192·3).
Bone cement for orthopaedic surgery.

al 110
Nestlé, Fr.; Nestlé, Ital.; Nestlé, Port.; Nestlé, Switz.†; Nestlé, UK.
Food for special diets (p.1350·1).
Lactose intolerance.

Alacetan *Riemser, Ger.*
Aspirin (p.14·2); paracetamol (p.71·2); caffeine (p.761·3).
Fever; inflammation; pain.

Alacor *Durascan, Denm.*
Enalapril maleate (p.883·3).
Heart failure; hypertension.

Ala-Cort *Del-Ray, USA.*
Hydrocortisone (p.1073·3).
Skin disorders.

Alacramyn *Bioclon, Mex.*
Scorpion venom antisera (p.1563·2).
Scorpion stings.

Alacta-NF *Mead Johnson Nutritionals, Thai.*
Food supplement with vitamins and minerals (p.1350·1).

Alamag *Goldline, USA.*
Aluminium hydroxide (p.1210·3); magnesium hydroxide (p.1233·1).
Hyperacidity.

Alamag Plus *Goldline, USA.*
Aluminium hydroxide (p.1210·3); magnesium hydroxide (p.1233·1); simeticone (p.1249·2).
Hyperacidity.

Alamast *Santen, USA.*
Pemirolast potassium (p.769·3).
Allergic conjunctivitis.

Alanase *Pacific, NZ.*
Beclometasone dipropionate (p.1061·2).
Nasal polyps; rhinitis.

Alandiem *Zimaia, Port.*
Diltiazem hydrochloride (p.874·3).
Angina pectoris; hypertension.

Alantomicina *Cantabria, Spain†.*
Allantoin (p.1110·1); bacitracin (p.155·2); neomycin (p.228·1); zinc oxide (p.1128·2).
Skin infections.

Alantomicina Complex *Cantabria, Spain†.*
Allantoin (p.1110·1); bacitracin (p.155·2); hydrocortisone acetate (p.1073·3); neomycin (p.228·1); zinc oxide (p.1128·2).
Infected skin disorders.

Alapren *Chibret, Denm.†.*
Enalapril (p.883·3) or enalapril maleate (p.883·3).
Heart failure; hypertension.

Alapril *Mediolanum, Ital.*
Lisinopril (p.921·1).
Heart failure; hypertension; myocardial infarction.

Alapryl *Menarini, Spain.*
Halazepam (p.686·2).
Anxiety.

Ala-Quin *Del-Ray, USA†.*
Hydrocortisone (p.1073·3); clioquinol (p.190·2).
Skin disorders.

Alasenn *Schworer, Ger.*
Senna (p.1248·2); ononis (p.1644·1); achillea (p.1572·2); taraxacum (p.1669·1).
Constipation.

Alasulf *Major, USA.*
Sulfanilamide (p.256·2); aminoacridine hydrochloride (p.1130·2); allantoin (p.1110·1).
Vaginal infections.

Alatone *Major, USA.*
Spironolactone (p.973·2).
Hyperaldosteronism; hypertension; hypokalaemia; oedema.

Alavac-S
Artu, Neth.; Teomed, Switz.
Allergen extracts (p.1575·3).
Hyposensitisation.

Alaxa *Angelini, Ital.*
Bisacodyl (p.1212·2).
Constipation.

Alaxan *Great Eastern, Thai.; Therapharma, Thai.*
Carisoprodol (p.1327·1); phenylbutazone calcium (p.78·3).
Musculoskeletal and joint disorders.

Alba *SNBTS, UK.*
Albumin (p.724·1).
Plasma volume expansion.

Alba-3
Note. This name is used for preparations of different composition.
IQB, Braz.
Albendazole (p.95·2).
Worm infections.
Alba, USA†.
Eye drops: Polymyxin B sulfate (p.238·1); neomycin sulfate (p.228·1) l gramicidin (p.213·3).
Eye ointment: Polymyxin B sulfate (p.238·1); neomycin sulfate (p.228·1); bacitracin zinc (p.155·2).
Ointment: Polymyxin B sulfate (p.238·1); neomycin sulfate (p.228·1); bacitracin (p.155·2).

Alba CE *Alba, USA†.*
Ascorbic acid (p.1389·3).

Alba Dex *Alba, USA†.*
Dexamethasone sodium phosphate (p.1067·1).
Corticosteroid.

Alba Gyn *Alba, USA†.*
Sulfathiazole (p.257·1); sulfacetamide (p.250·3); sulfabenzamide (p.250·2).

Alba Lybe *Alba, USA†.*
Vitamin B substances with lysine (p.1350·1).

Albaform HC *Alba, USA†.*
Hydrocortisone (p.1073·3); clioquinol (p.190·2).

Albafort *Alba, USA†.*
Vitamin B substances with iron (p.1350·1).

Albalon
Allergan, Austral.; Allergan, Belg.; Allergan, Canad.; Allergan, Hong Kong; Allergan, NZ; Allergan, S.Afr.; Allergan, Switz.; Allergan, Thai.; Allergan, USA.
Naphazoline hydrochloride (p.1095·1).
Eye irritation.

Albalon Liquifilm *Allergan, Neth.†.*
Naphazoline hydrochloride (p.1095·1).
Conjunctival congestion; eye irritation.

Albalon Relief
Allergan, Austral.; Allergan, NZ.
Phenylephrine hydrochloride (p.1097·1).
Eye irritation.

Albalon-A
Allergan, Austral.; Allergan, NZ; Allergan, S.Afr.
Naphazoline hydrochloride (p.1095·1); antazoline phosphate (p.408·3).
Allergic inflammatory eye conditions; eye irritation.

Albalon-A Liquifilm *Allergan, Canad.*
Naphazoline hydrochloride (p.1095·1); antazoline phosphate (p.408·3).
Antihistamine; decongestant.

Albamycin *Upjohn, USA†.*
Novobiocin sodium (p.232·2).
Bacterial infections.

Albassol *Allergan-Frumtost, Braz.*
Antazoline phosphate (p.408·3); naphazoline hydrochloride (p.1095·1).
Ocular congestion.

Albatel *TO-Chemicals, Thai.*
Albendazole (p.95·2).
Worm infections.

AlbaTemp *Alba, USA†.*
Paracetamol (p.71·2).
Fever; pain.

Albatran *Beaufour, Fr.†.*
Papaverine codecarboxylase derivative (p.1648·2).
Peripheral and cerebral vascular disorders.

Albatussin *Alba, USA†.*
Guaifenesin (p.1092·2); dextromethorphan hydrobromide (p.1087·3); phenylephrine hydrochloride (p.1097·1).
Coughs.

Albatussin NN *Alba, USA†.*
Dextromethorphan hydrobromide (p.1087·3); mepyramine maleate (p.421·1); sulfogaiacol (p.1101·1); phenylephrine hydrochloride (p.1097·1).
Coughs.

Albatussin Pediatric *Alba, USA†.*
Dextromethorphan hydrobromide (p.1087·3); phenylephrine hydrochloride (p.1097·1).
Coughs.

Albay
Bayer, Austral.; Dome-Hollister-Stier, Fr.; Bayer, NZ; Bayer, S.Afr.; Miles, USA.
Venoms of bee, wasp, hornet, yellow jacket, and mixed vespids (p.1575·3).
Diagnosis of hypersensitivity to insect stings; hyposensitisation to insect stings.

Albego *Daker Farmasimes, Spain†.*
Camazepam (p.659·1).
Anxiety; insomnia.

Alben
Infabra, Braz.; Biolab, Thai.
Albendazole (p.95·2).
Worm infections.

Albenda
Milano, Thai.; Julphar, UAE.
Albendazole (p.95·2).
Worm infections.

Albensil *Arlex, Mex.*
Albendazole (p.95·2).

Albenza *SmithKline Beecham, USA.*
Albendazole (p.95·2).
Cysticercosis; echinococcosis.

Alber T *Unison, Thai.*
Tolnaftate (p.395·2); triacetin (p.395·3).
Fungal skin infections.

Albert Tiafen *Albert, Canad.*
Tiaprofenic acid (p.88·1).
Osteoarthritis; rheumatoid arthritis.

Albetol *Leiras, Fin.*
Labetalol hydrochloride (p.918·1).
Angina pectoris; hypertension.

Albicansan *Sanum-Kehlbeck, Ger.*
Homoeopathic preparation.

Albicon *Farmalab, Braz.*
Borax (p.1586·1); potassium chloride (p.1194·3); benzocaine (p.1306·2); sodium carbonate (p.1665·1).
Local disinfection and anaesthesia.

Albicort
Sanofi Synthelabo, Belg.; Sanofi Synthelabo, Neth.
Triamcinolone acetonide (p.1080·1).
Corticosteroid.

Albicort Compositum
Sanofi Synthelabo, Belg.; Sanofi Synthelabo, Neth.
Triamcinolone acetonide (p.1080·1); salicylic acid (p.1122·3).
Keratinisation disorders; psoriasis.

Albicort Oticum *Sanofi Synthelabo, Belg.*
Triamcinolone acetonide (p.1080·1); salicylic acid (p.1122·3).
Otitis externa.

Albintil *Solvay, Spain.*
Multivitamin preparation (p.1350·1).

Albiotic *Pharmacia Upjohn, Ger.*
Lincomycin hydrochloride (p.219·2).
Bacterial infections.

Albistat *Janssen-Cilag, Belg.*
Miconazole nitrate (p.391·1).
Vulvovaginal yeast infections.

Albital *Biagini, Ital.*
Albumin (p.724·1).
Cerebral oedema; hyperbilirubinaemia; hypoproteinaemia; shock.

Albocresil *Byk, Braz.*
Policresulen.
Vaginal infections.

Alboral *Silanes, Mex.*
Diazepam (p.674·3).
Alcohol withdrawal syndrome; anxiety disorders; epilepsy; insomnia; premedication; skeletal muscle spasm; tetany.

Albothyl
Byk Gulden, Ger.; Byk Gulden, Hong Kong; Byk Gulden, Mex.; Byk Gulden, Singapore; Pasture, Singapore; Byk Gulden, Thai.
Metacresolsulfonic acid-formaldehyde (p.738·3).
Gynaecological disorders; skin and mucous membrane disorders.

Albraton *Steigerwald, Ger.*
Homoeopathic preparation.

Albucid
Chauvin ankerpharm, Ger.; Schering-Plough, S.Afr.†.
Sulfacetamide sodium (p.250·3).
Chlamydial eye infections.

Albumaid Preparations *Scientific Hospital Supplies, UK.*
A range of amino-acid preparations for special diets (p.1350·1).
Homocystinuria; phenylketonuria; protein malabsorption syndromes.

Albuman
Berna, Belg.†; Berna, Ital.; Berna, Switz.; Berna, Thai.
Albumin (p.724·1).
Burns; hypoalbuminaemia; hypovolaemic shock.

Albumarc *American Red Cross, USA.*
Albumin (p.724·1).

Albumex
CSL, Austral.; CSL, NZ.
Albumin (p.724·1).
Adult respiratory distress syndrome; burns; cardiopulmonary bypass surgery; haemodialysis; hypoproteinaemia; hypovolaemia; plasma exchange; shock.

Albuminar
Centeon, Irl.; Centeon, Israel; Centeon, Swed.†; Centeon, UK†; Centeon, USA.
Albumin (p.724·1).
Burns; hypoproteinaemia; hypovolaemic shock; neonatal hyperbilirubinaemia; plasma volume expansion.

Albumyn *Bioclon, Mex.*
Albumin (p.724·1).
Hypoproteinaemia; plasma volume expansion.

Albunex *Mallinckrodt, USA†.*
Albumin (p.724·1).
Burns; hypoproteinaemia; shock.

Alburone
Nestle, Fr.; Roussel, S.Afr.†.
Food for special diets (p.1350·1).
Protein supplement.

Albusol *NBI, S.Afr.*
Albumin (p.724·1).
Hypoproteinaemia; hypovolaemia.

Albustix
Bayer, Austral.†; Bayer Diagnostics, Fr.; Bayer Diagnostics, Irl.; Bayer Diagnostici, Ital.; Bayer, NZ; Bayer Diagnostics, UK; Bayer, USA.
Test for protein in urine.

Albutein
Alpha, Hong Kong; Grifols, Ital.; Alpha Therapeutic, Singapore; Alpha Therapeutic, Thai.; Alpha Therapeutic, UK; Alpha Therapeutic, USA.
Albumin (p.724·1).
Burns; cardiopulmonary bypass procedures; hyperbilirubinaemia; hypoalbuminaemia; shock.

Albyl *Leo, Denm.†.*
Aspirin (p.14·2).
Fever; inflammation; pain.

Albyl minor *Recip, Swed.*
Aspirin (p.14·2).
Fever; pain.

Albyl-E *Nycomed, Norw.*
Aspirin (p.14·2).
Magnesium oxide (p.1233·2) is included in this preparation in an attempt to limit adverse effects on the gastrointestinal mucosa.
Fever; pain; thrombosis prophylaxis.

Albym-Test
Boehringer Mannheim Diagnostics, Irl.†; Roche Diagnostics, NZ; Roche Diagnostics, UK†.
Test for protein in urine.

Alca-C *Novartis Consumer, Switz.*
Carbasalate calcium (p.23·3); ascorbic acid (p.1389·3).
Cold symptoms.

Alcacyl *Novartis Consumer, Switz.*
Carbasalate calcium (p.23·3).
Aluminium hydroxide (p.1210·3) is included in this preparation in an attempt to limit adverse effects on the gastrointestinal mucosa.
Fever; inflammation; pain.

Alcacyl instant *Novartis Consumer, Switz.*
Lysine aspirin (p.50·3).
Fever; inflammation; pain.

Alcafelol *Luper, Braz.*
Choline citrate (p.1356·3); cynara (p.1601·3); boldo (p.1585·3); magnesium sulfate (p.1191·1).
Liver disorders.

Alcaine
Alcon, Austral.; Alcon, Canad.; Alcon, Hong Kong; Alcon, Mex.; Alcon, Norw.; Alcon, Singapore; Alcon, Switz.; Alcon, USA.
Proxymetacaine hydrochloride (p.1320·1).
Local anaesthesia.

Alcalinos Gelos *Gelos, Spain.*
Calcium carbonate (p.1215·1); magnesium hydroxide (p.1233·1); sodium bicarbonate (p.1186·2); dibasic sodium phosphate (p.1193·2).
Gastrointestinal hyperacidity.

Alcalinos Vita *Vita, Spain.*
Aluminium hydroxide (p.1210·3); calcium carbonate (p.1215·1); magnesium hydroxide (p.1233·1).
Gastrointestinal hyperacidity.

The symbol † denotes a preparation no longer actively marketed

Alcalone Plus *Bunker, Braz.*
Magnesium hydroxide (p.1233·1); aluminium hydroxide (p.1210·3); simeticone (p.1249·2).
Flatulence; gastrointestinal hyperacidity.

Alcalosio *SIT, Ital.*
Anhydrous glucose (p.1364·1); potassium citrate (p.1186·1); pyridoxine hydrochloride (p.1386·3); sodium bicarbonate (p.1186·2); sodium citrate (p.1186·2).
Electrolyte disorders; gastrointestinal disorders.

Alca-Luftal *Bristol-Myers Squibb, Braz.*
Simeticone (p.1249·2); magnesium hydroxide (p.1233·1); aluminium hydroxide (p.1210·3).
Flatulence; gastrointestinal hyperacidity.

Alcamag *Laborsil, Braz.*
Aluminium hydroxide (p.1210·3); magnesium hydroxide (p.1233·1); calcium carbonate (p.1215·1).
Gastrointestinal hyperacidity.

Alcan *Sons, Mex.*
Chloramphenicol (p.179·1).
Bacterial infections.

Alcaphor *Pharmadeveloppement, Fr.*
Trometamol citrate (p.1675·2); sodium acid citrate (p.1186·2); dipotassium citrate.
Metabolic acidosis; renal calculi.

Alcare *Calgon Vestal, Belg.*
Alcohol (p.1130·3).
Antiseptic.

Alcasedine *Will-Pharma, Neth.*
Algeldrate (p.1210·3); magnesium trisilicate (p.1233·3).
Dyspepsia; heartburn.

Alcasol *Asta Medica, Belg.*
Sodium bicarbonate (p.1186·2); borax (p.1586·1); sodium chloride (p.1196·1).
Eye disorders.

Alcaten *Ariston, Braz.*
Fentetramin.
Sympathomimetic.

Alcatex *Medix, Mex.*
Cimetidine (p.1216·3).

Alcelam *Pharmasant, Thai.*
Alprazolam (p.654·2).
Anxiety; insomnia.

Alchera *Aspen, S.Afr.*
Zopiclone (p.713·1).
Insomnia.

Alcinal *Rekah, Israel.*
Dextromethorphan hydrobromide (p.1087·3); guaifenesin (p.1092·2); chlorpheniramine [chlorphenamine] maleate (p.412·1); phenylpropanolamine hydrochloride (p.1098·1).
Coughs and cold symptoms.

Alcinal Plus *Rekah, Israel.*
Dextromethorphan hydrobromide (p.1087·3); guaifenesin (p.1092·2); chlorpheniramine [chlorphenamine] maleate (p.412·1); phenylpropanolamine hydrochloride (p.1098·1); paracetamol (p.71·2).
Coughs and cold symptoms.

Alcis *Wasserman, Spain.*
Estradiol (p.1473·1).
Menopausal disorders; osteoporosis.

Alclox *Alphapharm, Austral.†*
Cloxacillin sodium (p.192·1).
Bacterial infections.

Alcobon *Roche, Irl.; ICN, NZ; Pacific, NZ.*
Flucytosine (p.385·2).
Fungal infections.

Alcoderm
Note.This name is used for preparations of different composition.
Galderma, Irl.
Liquid paraffin (p.1407·1).
Dry skin.

Galderma, UK.
Moisturiser.
Dry skin.

Alcodin *Alcon, Ital.*
Myrtillus (p.1639·2).
Capillary fragility; eye disorders.

Alco-Gel *Tweezerman, USA†.*
Alcohol (p.1130·3).
Disinfection of hands.

Alcohcan *Marrero, Spain.*
Alcohol (p.1130·3); benzalkonium chloride (p.1133·2).
Skin and wound disinfection.

Alcohocel *Calmante Vitaminado, Spain.*
Alcohol (p.1130·3); cetylpyridinium chloride (p.1138·1).
Skin disinfection.

Alcohol Benzalconio *Viviar, Spain.*
Alcohol (p.1130·3); benzalkonium chloride (p.1133·2).
Skin, wound, and surface disinfection.

Alcohol Cetil *Noriega, Spain.*
Alcohol (p.1130·3); cetylpyridinium chloride (p.1138·1).
Skin disinfection.

Alcohol CL Benz *Betamadrileno, Spain.*
Alcohol (p.1130·3); benzalkonium chloride (p.1133·2).
Skin, wound, and surface disinfection.

Alcohol Poten *Maxfarma, Spain.*
Alcohol (p.1130·3); benzethonium chloride (p.1134·2).
Skin, wound, and surface disinfection.

Alcohol Potenciado *Viviar, Spain.*
Alcohol (p.1130·3); benzalkonium chloride (p.1133·2).
Skin, wound, and surface disinfection.

Alcohol Reforzado *PQS, Spain.*
Alcohol (p.1130·3); benzalkonium chloride (p.1133·2).
Skin, wound, and surface disinfection.

Alcohol Sanit Cuve *Calmante Vitaminado, Spain.*
Alcohol (p.1130·3); cetylpyridinium chloride (p.1138·1).
Skin disinfection.

Alcohten *Marrero, Spain.*
Alcohol (p.1130·3).
Skin disinfection.

Alcojel *Roberts, Canad.*
Isopropyl alcohol (p.1149·2).
Skin disorders.

Alcomicin *Alcon, Canad.*
Gentamicin sulfate (p.210·1).
Eye infections.

Alcon Adequad *Alcon, Belg.*
Dextran 70 (p.729·2); hypromellose (p.1501·3).
Dry eyes.

Alcon Eye Gel *Alcon, Belg.*
Carbomer (p.1499·2).
Dry eyes.

Alconefrin *PolyMedica, USA.*
Phenylephrine hydrochloride (p.1097·1).
Nasal congestion.

Alcopac Reforzado *Agua del Carmen, Spain.*
Alcohol (p.1130·3); benzalkonium chloride (p.1133·2).
Skin, wound, and surface disinfection.

Alcophyllex *Propan, S.Afr.*
Theophylline (p.777·2); etofylline (p.765·1); diphenhydramine hydrochloride (p.416·1); ammonium chloride (p.1085·2); sodium citrate (p.1186·2).
Bronchospasm.

Alcophyllin *Propan, S.Afr.*
Theophylline (p.777·2).
Obstructive airways disease.

Alcos-Anal
Note.This name is used for preparations of different composition.
Bristol-Myers Squibb, Ger.; Meda, Norw.
Sodium oleate (p.1497·1); lauromacrogol 400 (p.1345·2); chlorocarvacrol.
Anorectal disorders.

Meda, Swed.
Sodium oleate (p.1497·1); 2-hydroxy-5-chlorothymol.
Anorectal disorders.

Alco-Screen *Marco, Austral.*
Test for alcohol in saliva.

Alcover *CT, Ital.*
Sodium oxybate (p.1268·2).
Alcohol withdrawal syndrome.

Alcowipe *SSL, UK.*
Isopropyl alcohol (p.1149·2).
Hard surface disinfection.

Alcoxidine *Vitamed, Israel.*
Chlorhexidine gluconate (p.1138·2).
Skin disinfection.

Alcusal *Alcusal, Austral.*
Copper (p.1357·3); salicylic acid (p.1122·3).
Musculoskeletal and joint disorders; sports injuries.

Alcusal Sport *Alcusal, Austral.†.*
Copper (p.1357·3); methyl salicylate (p.55·1); menthol (p.1632·3); camphor (p.1589·3); eucalyptus oil (p.1609·2).
Pain and inflammation due to sports injuries.

Alda *Nakorn, Thai.*
Albendazole (p.95·2).
Worm infections.

Aldactacine *Monsanto, Spain.*
Altizide (p.835·1); spironolactone (p.973·2).
Ascites; hypertension; oedema.

Aldactazide
Searle, Canad.; SPA, Ital.; Searle, USA.
Spironolactone (p.973·2); hydrochlorothiazide (p.907·3).
Heart failure; hypertension; liver cirrhosis with oedema and/or ascites; nephrotic syndrome.

Aldactazine
Searle, Belg.; Monsanto, Fr.; Monsanto, Port.
Altizide (p.835·1); spironolactone (p.973·2).
Hypertension; oedema.

Aldactide
Searle, Irl.; Pharmacia, UK.
Spironolactone (p.973·2); hydroflumethiazide (p.911·3).
These ingredients can be described by the British Approved Name Co-flumactone.
Heart failure.

Aldactone
Roche, Aust.; Searle, Austral.; Searle, Belg.; Searle, Braz.; Searle, Canad.; Searle, Fin.; Monsanto, Fr.; Boehringer Mannheim, Ger.; Searle, Hong Kong; Searle, Irl.; Searle, Israel; Lepetit, Ital.; Searle, Mex.; Searle, Neth.; Searle, Norw.; Searle, NZ; Monsanto, Port.; Searle, S.Afr.; Searle, Singapore; Monsanto, Spain; Searle, Swed.; Searle, Switz.; Searle, Thai.; Pharmacia, UK; Searle, USA.
Potassium canrenoate (p.957·1) or spironolactone (p.973·2).
Heart failure; hirsutism in females; hyperaldosteronism; hypertension; hypokalaemia; hypomagnesaemia; liver cirrhosis with ascites or oedema; myasthenia gravis; nephrotic syndrome; oedema.

Aldactone Saltucin
Roche, Aust.; Boehringer Mannheim, Ger.
Spironolactone (p.973·2); butizide (p.853·1).
Heart failure; hyperaldosteronism; hypertension; liver cirrhosis and ascites; oedema.

Aldalix *Monsanto, Fr.*
Spironolactone (p.973·2); frusemide [furosemide] (p.893·1).
Heart failure.

Aldar *Mavi, Mex.*
Nifedipine (p.940·1).

Aldara
3M, Austral.; 3M, Belg.; 3M, Canad.; 3M, Denm.; 3M, Fin.; 3M, Fr.; 3M, Ger.; 3M, Hong Kong; 3M, Irl.; 3M, Ital.; 3M, Neth.; 3M, Norw.; 3M, NZ; 3M, S.Afr.; 3M, Singapore.; 3M, Spain; 3M, Swed.; 3M, Thai.; 3M, UK; 3M, USA.
Imiquimod (p.625·2).
Anogenital warts.

Aldazida *Searle, Braz.*
Spironolactone (p.973·2); hydrochlorothiazide (p.907·3).
Hypertension; oedema.

Aldazide *Searle, S.Afr.*
Spironolactone (p.973·2); butizide (p.853·1).
Glomerular kidney disease; hypertension; oedema.

Aldazine
Alphapharm, Austral.; Pacific, NZ.
Thioridazine hydrochloride (p.708·1).
Agitation; anxiety; behavioural disorders; mixed anxiety depressive states; pain; psychoses; sleep disorders.

Aldecin
Schering-Plough, Austral.; Byk, Belg.†; Schering-Plough, Denm.; Schering-Plough, Hong Kong; Byk, Neth.†; Schering-Plough, NZ; Byk, Switz.†.
Beclometasone dipropionate (p.1061·2).
Allergic rhinitis; nasal polyps; obstructive airways disease.

Aldecina
Schering-Plough, Braz.; Byk, Port.
Beclometasone dipropionate (p.1061·2).
Obstructive airways disease; rhinitis.

Aldic *Shiwa, Thai.*
Frusemide [furosemide] (p.893·1).
Barbiturate poisoning; hypertension; oedema; renal impairment.

Al-Dim *Francia, Ital.*
Citric acid; chromium picolinate (p.1350·1).
Nutritional supplement.

Aldipin *Helvepharm, Switz.*
Nifedipine (p.940·1).
Angina pectoris; hypertension; Raynaud's syndrome.

Aldira *Novartis Consumer, Spain.*
Terfenadine (p.424·3).
Hypersensitivity reactions.

Aldo Asma *Aldo, Spain.*
Ascorbic acid; phenylephrine hydrochloride (p.1097·1); isoprenaline hydrochloride (p.914·3).
Obstructive airways disease.

Aldo Otico *Aldo, Spain.*
Framycetin sulfate (p.208·2); lignocaine [lidocaine] hydrochloride (p.1313·2); triamcinolone acetonide (p.1080·1); choline salicylate (p.24·3).
External ear disorders; otitis media.

Aldoacne *Aldo, Spain.*
Benzoyl peroxide (p.1111·1).
Acne.

Aldobronquial *Aldo, Spain.*
Salbutamol sulfate (p.770·3).
Obstructive airways disease.

Aldoclor *Merck, USA.*
Methyldopa (p.927·3); chlorothiazide (p.856·3).
Hypertension.

Aldocumar *Aldo, Spain.*
Warfarin sodium (p.992·2).
Thromboembolic disorders; thrombosis prophylaxis.

Aldoderma *Aldo, Spain.*
Framycetin sulfate (p.208·2); triamcinolone acetonide (p.1080·1).
Infected skin disorders.

Aldoleo *Byk Leo, Spain.*
Chlortalidone (p.857·1); spironolactone (p.973·2).
Hypertension; oedema.

Aldolor *CTI, Israel.*
Paracetamol (p.71·2).
Fever; pain.

Aldomet
Merck Sharp & Dohme, Austral.; Merck Sharp & Dohme, Belg.; Prodome, Braz.; Merck Frosst, Canad.; Merck Sharp & Dohme, Denm.; Merck Sharp & Dohme-Chibret, Fr.; Merck Sharp & Dohme, Hong Kong; Merck Sharp & Dohme, Irl.; Merck Sharp & Dohme, Ital.; Merck Sharp & Dohme, Norw.; Merck Sharp & Dohme, NZ; Merck Sharp & Dohme, Port.; Merck Sharp & Dohme, S.Afr.; Merck Sharp & Dohme, Singapore; Merck Sharp & Dohme, Swed.; Merck Sharp & Dohme, Switz.; Merck Sharp & Dohme, Thai.; Merck Sharp & Dohme, UK; Merck, USA.
Methyldopa (p.927·3) or methyldopate hydrochloride (p.927·3).
Hypertension.

Aldometil *Merck Sharp & Dohme, Aust.*
Methyldopa (p.927·3).
Hypertension.

Aldomin *Merck Sharp & Dohme, Israel.*
Methyldopa (p.927·3).
Hypertension.

Aldonar *Upsifarma, Port.*
Spironolactone (p.973·2).
Hypertension.

Aldopren *Amrad, Austral.*
Methyldopa (p.927·3).
Hypertension.

Aldopur *Kwizda, Aust.; Hormosan, Ger.†.*
Spironolactone (p.973·2).
Cor pulmonale; heart failure; hyperaldosteronism; hypertension; liver cirrhosis with ascites and oedema; nephrotic syndrome.

Aldoretic
Merck Sharp & Dohme, Aust.; Chibret, Port.†; Merck Sharp & Dohme, S.Afr.; Merck Sharp & Dohme, Switz.
Amiloride hydrochloride (p.835·1); hydrochlorothiazide (p.907·3); methyldopa (p.927·3).
Hypertension.

Aldoril *Merck Sharp & Dohme, Canad.†; Merck, USA.*
Methyldopa (p.927·3); hydrochlorothiazide (p.907·3).
Hypertension.

Aldosomnil *Aldo, Spain.*
Lormetazepam (p.689·3).
Insomnia.

Aldospirone *Teva, Israel.*
Spironolactone (p.973·2).
Heart failure; hyperaldosteronism; hypertension; hypokalaemia; liver cirrhosis; oedema.

Aldospray Analgesico *Aldo, Spain.*
Mabuprofen (p.44·1).
Peri-articular and soft-tissue disorders.

Aldozone *Searle, Switz.*
Spironolactone (p.973·2); butizide (p.853·1).
Heart failure; hypertension; liver cirrhosis with ascites; nephrotic syndrome; oedema.

Aldrox *Whitehall, Braz.*
Aluminium hydroxide (p.1210·3).
Gastrointestinal hyperacidity.

Alec *Britannia Pharmaceuticals, UK†.*
Pumactant (p.1656·1).
Respiratory distress syndrome.

Aledin *Nestle, Switz.†.*
Preparation for enteral nutrition (p.1350·1).
Coeliac disease; diarrhoea.

Aleevex *Food Supplement, UK.*
Eucalyptus oil (p.1609·2); camphor (p.1589·3); menthol (p.1632·3).
Cold symptoms.

Alegysal *Mitsubishi-Tokyo, Jpn.*
Pemirolast potassium (p.769·3).
Allergic rhinitis; asthma.

Alembicol D *Alembic Products, UK.*
Fractionated coconut oil (p.1372·1).
Food for special diets; malabsorption syndromes.

Al-En *Francia, Ital.*
Creatine; carnitine bitartrate; magnesium oxide; vitamins (p.1350·1).
Nutritional supplement.

Alendros *Abiogen, Ital.*
Alendronate sodium (p.747·2).
Osteoporosis.

Alenic Alka *Rugby, USA.*
Oral liquid: Aluminium hydroxide (p.1210·3); magnesium carbonate (p.1232·3).

Tablets: Aluminium hydroxide (p.1210·3); magnesium trisilicate (p.1233·3); sodium bicarbonate (p.1186·2).
Hyperacidity.

Aleot *Apomedica, Aust.*
Chlorphenesin (p.381·3); diphenhydramine hydrochloride (p.416·1); chlorobutanol (p.1141·2); benzalkonium chloride (p.1133·2); urea (p.1127·3).
Ear disorders.

Alepa *Duopharm, Ger.*
Silybum marianum (p.1021·3).
Liver disorders.

Alepam *Alphapharm, Austral.*
Oxazepam (p.697·1).
Alcohol withdrawal syndrome; anxiety.

Alepsal
Note.This name is used for preparations of different composition.
Genevrier, Fr.
Phenobarbital (p.355·1); caffeine (p.761·3).
Epilepsy; febrile convulsions.

Rudefsa, Mex.
Phenobarbital (p.355·1).

Alercrom *Grin, Mex.*
Sodium cromoglicate (p.774·3).
Allergic conjunctivitis.

Alerdil *Diba, Mex.*
Chlorpheniramine [chlorphenamine] (p.412·2).
Hypersensitivity.

Aler-Dryl *Reese, USA.*
Diphenhydramine hydrochloride (p.416·1).

Alerfrin *Allergan, Spain.*
Oxymetazoline hydrochloride (p.1096·2).
Ocular congestion and irritation.

Alergibon
Galderma, Braz.; Galderma, Mex.
Emollient; soap substitute.
Barrier preparation; dry skin.

Alergical
Note.This name is used for preparations of different composition.
Iquinosa, Spain.
Cream: Betamethasone valerate (p.1063·2); fluocinolone acetonide (p.1071·1).
Skin disorders.

Llorente, Spain.
Syrup: Chlorpheniramine [chlorphenamine] maleate (p.412·1); prednisolone metasulfobenzoate sodium (p.1078·1).

Tablets: Ascorbic acid (p.1389·3); chlorpheniramine [chlorphenamine] maleate (p.412·1); prednisolone (p.1077·3).
Hypersensitivity reactions; skin disorders.

Alergical Expect *Llorente, Spain.*
Chlorpheniramine [chlorphenamine] maleate (p.412·1); diprophylline (p.764·1); guaifenesin (p.1092·2); paracetamol (p.71·2).
Bronchospasm; fever; pain.

Alergiftalmina *Davi, Port.*
Antazoline phosphate (p.408·3); naphazoline hydrochloride (p.1095·1).
Conjunctivitis.

Alergist *Almirall, Spain.*
Terfenadine (p.424·3).
Hypersensitivity reactions.

Alergo Filinal *Eurofarma, Braz.*
Diphenhydramine hydrochloride (p.416·1); aminophylline (p.760·1); guaifenesin (p.1092·2); pyridoxine hydrochloride (p.1386·3).
Respiratory-tract disorders.

Alergo Glucalbet *Dansk-Flama, Braz.*
Mepyramine maleate (p.421·1); pentoxyverine citrate (p.1096·3); calcium gluconate (p.1188·2); ammonium chloride (p.1085·2).
Coughs.

Alergocrom *Aldo, Spain.*
Sodium cromoglicate (p.774·3).
Asthma; bronchospasm.

Alergoftal *Cusi, Singapore; Alcon Cusi, Spain.*
Antazoline phosphate (p.408·3); naphazoline hydrochloride (p.1095·1).
Eye irritation.

Alergogel *Laborsil, Braz.*
Diphenhydramine hydrochloride (p.416·1); ammonium chloride (p.1085·2).
Respiratory-tract congestion.

Alergomed *Alergomed, Braz.*
Allergen preparation (p.1575·3).
Hyposensitisation.

Alergoral *Darrow, Braz.*
Allergen preparation (p.1575·3).
Hyposensitisation.

Alergotox *Makros, Braz.*
Diphenhydramine hydrochloride (p.416·1); theophylline (p.777·2); aminophylline (p.760·1).
Hypersensitivity.

Alergotox Efedrina *Makros, Braz.*
Diphenhydramine hydrochloride (p.416·1); ephedrine hydrochloride (p.1090·1); liver antitoxin.
Hypersensitivity.

Alergotox Expectorante *Makros, Braz.*
Diphenhydramine hydrochloride (p.416·1); guaifenesin (p.1092·2); aminophylline (p.760·1); liver antitoxin.
Respiratory-tract congestion.

Alergotox Nasal *Makros, Braz.*
Diphenhydramine hydrochloride (p.416·1); naphazoline hydrochloride (p.1095·1).
Nasal congestion.

Alergotox Pastilhas *Makros, Braz.*
Diphenhydramine hydrochloride (p.416·1); cetylpyridinium chloride (p.1138·1); benzocaine (p.1306·2).
Mouth and throat disorders.

Alerid *Asche, Ger.*
Cetirizine hydrochloride (p.411·2).
Hypersensitivity reactions.

Alerjon *Oftalder, Port.*
Oxymetazoline hydrochloride (p.1096·2).
Eye irritation.

Alerken *Kener, Mex.*
Astemizole (p.409·1).

Alerlisin *Menarini, Spain.*
Cetirizine hydrochloride (p.411·2).
Hypersensitivity reactions.

Alermizol *Septa, Spain.*
Astemizole (p.409·1).
Hypersensitivity reactions.

Aler-Releaf *Reese, USA†.*
Chlorpheniramine [chlorphenamine] maleate (p.412·1); phenylpropanolamine hydrochloride (p.1098·1).

Alersan *QIF, Braz.*
Mepyramine maleate (p.421·1); magnesium thiosulfate (p.1024·2).
Hypersensitivity.

Alersule *Misemer, USA†.*
Phenylephrine hydrochloride (p.1097·1); chlorpheniramine [chlorphenamine] maleate (p.412·1).
Upper respiratory-tract symptoms.

Alertal *Sintofarma, Braz.*
Loratadine (p.420·1).
Hypersensitivity.

Alertec *Draxis, Canad.*
Modafinil (p.1512·3).
Narcoleptic syndrome.

Alertonic
Hoechst Marion Roussel, Austral.
Pipradrol hydrochloride (p.1514·1); vitamin B substances; minerals; trace elements (p.1350·1).
Tonic.
Hoechst Marion Roussel, Canad.
Pipradrol hydrochloride (p.1514·1); vitamin B substances (p.1350·1).
Tonic.

Mer-National, S.Afr.
Pipradrol hydrochloride (p.1514·1); vitamin B substances (p.1350·1); minerals.
Tonic.

Alertrin *Helsinn, Port.†*
Loratadine (p.420·1).
Allergic rhinitis; eye irritation; urticaria.

Alesion *Boehringer Ingelheim, Jpn†.*
Epinastine hydrochloride (p.417·3).
Allergic rhinitis; asthma; pruritus.

Alesse
Wyeth-Ayerst, Canad.; Wyeth-Ayerst, USA.
Levonorgestrel (p.1486·2); ethinylestradiol (p.1476·2).
28-Day packs also contain 7 inert tablets.
Combined oral contraceptive.

Aletor Compositum *Cantabria, Spain†.*
Bromhexine (p.1085·3); codeine acephyllinate (p.26·1); diphenhydramine hydrochloride (p.416·1); papaverine teprosilate (p.1648·2); pyridofylline (p.770·2).
Upper-respiratory-tract disorders.

Aletris Oligoplex *Madaus, Ger.*
Homoeopathic preparation.

Aleudrina *Boehringer Ingelheim, Spain.*
Isoprenaline sulfate (p.914·3).
Cardiac disorders; shock.

Aleve
Roche, Austral.; Nicholas, Fr.; Roche Nicholas, Ger.; Roche, Ital.; Roche Consumer, Neth.; Roche, S.Afr.; Roche, Spain; Procter & Gamble, USA.
Naproxen sodium (p.61·1).
Fever; gout; musculoskeletal and joint disorders; pain.

Aleviatin *Dainippon, Jpn†.*
Phenytoin sodium (p.357·2).
Epilepsy.

Alexan
Pfizer, Aust.; Pharmacia Upjohn, Braz.; Mack, Illert., Ger.; Mack, Hong Kong; Pharmacia Upjohn, Mex.; Ferraz, Lynce, Port.†; Intramed, S.Afr.; Mack, Singapore; Nycomed, Swed.†; Mack, Switz.†; Mack, Thai.
Cytarabine (p.530·1).
Leukaemias; non-Hodgkins lymphomas.

Aleztem *Rayere, Mex.*
Astemizole (p.409·1).
Hypersensitivity.

Alfa *Pfizer Consumer, Spain.*
Naphazoline nitrate (p.1095·1).
Eye irritation.

Alfa Acid *Erredici, Ital.*
Ammonium lactate (p.1110·3); salicylic acid (p.1122·3); dexpanthenol (p.1602·3).
Scalp disorders.

Alfa C *Bracco, Ital.*
Benzalkonium chloride (p.1133·2).
Eye irritation.

Alfa Kappa *Biagini, Ital.*
Amino-acid preparation (p.1350·1).
Nutritional supplement in renal failure.

Alfabetal *Mitim, Ital.†.*
Labetalol hydrochloride (p.918·1).
Hypertension.

Alfabios *Biotekfarma, Ital.†.*
Fluocinolone acetonide (p.1071·1).
Corticosteroid.

Alfacid *Grunenthal, Ger.*
Rifabutin (p.242·1).
Mycobacterium-avium complex infections in AIDS patients; tuberculosis.

Alfacort *Julphar, UAE.*
Hydrocortisone (p.1073·3).
Skin disorders.

Alfacortone *Spirig, Switz.*
Hydrocortisone acetate (p.1073·3).
Skin disorders.

Alfad
Byk Gulden, Mex.; Berk, UK.
Alfacalcidol (p.1391·1).
Hyperparathyroidism; hypoparathyroidism; osteomalacia; osteoporosis; renal osteodystrophy; rickets.

Alfadelta *Farmacusi, Braz.*
Alfacalcidol (p.1391·1).
Hypoparathyroidism; osteomalacia; renal osteodystrophy; vitamin D deficiency.

Alfadil *Pfizer, Swed.*
Doxazosin mesilate (p.883·2).
Benign prostatic hyperplasia; hypertension.

Alfaferone *Wassermann, Ital.*
Interferon alfa (p.628·1).
Malignant neoplasms; viral infections.

Alfaflor *INTES, Ital.*
Betamethasone sodium phosphate (p.1063·2); naphazoline nitrate (p.1095·1); tetracycline hydrochloride (p.258·3).
Inflammatory eye and ear disorders.

Alfa-Fluorone *New Farma, Ital.*
Lotion: Fluocinolone acetonide (p.1071·1).
Skin disorders.
Vaginal solution: Fluocinolone acetonide (p.1071·1); benzalkonium chloride (p.1133·2).
Vulvovaginal infections.

Alfagamma *Humana, Ital.*
Essential fatty acids; vitamin E; vitamin B₆ (p.1350·1).
Nutritional supplement.

Alfagen *Wassermann, Ital.*
Collagen (p.1598·2).
Ulcers; wounds.

Alfakinasi *Wassermann, Ital.*
Urokinase (p.988·1).
Thromboembolic disorders.

Alfalfa Tonic
Boiron, Canad.; Homeocan, Canad.
Homoeopathic preparation.

Alfamox *Teofarma, Ital.*
Amoxicillin trihydrate (p.149·2).
Bacterial infections.

Alfan *Alpharma, Mex.*
Dextromethorphan hydrobromide (p.1087·3); chlorpheniramine [chlorphenamine] maleate (p.412·1); ephedrine hydrochloride (p.1090·1).
Coughs; nasal congestion.

Alfare
Nestle, Austral.; Nestle, Fr.; Nestle, Ital.; Nestle, Mex.; Nestle, Port.; Nestle, Switz.; Nestle, UK.
Preparation for enteral nutrition (p.1350·1).
Cow's milk and soya intolerance; diarrhoea; malabsorption disorders.

Alfarol
Chugai, Hong Kong; Chugai, Jpn.
Alfacalcidol (p.1391·1).
Hypoparathyroidism; osteomalacia; osteoporosis; renal failure; rickets.

Alfason *Yamanouchi, Ger.*
Hydrocortisone butyrate (p.1073·3).
Skin disorders.

Alfater *Sclavo, Ital.*
Interferon alfa (p.628·1).
Genital warts; hepatitis B; hepatitis non-A non-B; malignant neoplasms.

Alfatil *Lilly, Fr.*
Cefaclor (p.161·1).
Bacterial infections.

Alfavir *Medgenix, Belg.*
Ephedrine tartrate (p.1090·3); vitamins (p.1350·1).
Tonic.

Alfazina *Salus, Ital.*
Propyphenazone (p.80·2); caffeine (p.761·3).
Fever; pain.

Alfenta
Janssen-Ortho, Canad.; Taylor, USA.
Alfentanil hydrochloride (p.11·3).
Analgesia during anaesthesia.

Alferm *Schoning-Berlin, Ger.†*
Ointment: Prednisolone (p.1077·3); thymol (p.1158·3); allantoin (p.1110·1).
Suppositories: Prednisolone (p.1077·3); thymol (p.1158·3); menthol (p.1632·3).
Anorectal disorders.

Alferon *Cryopharma, Mex.*
Interferon alfa-2a (recombinant) (p.628·1).
Hepatitis B; malignant neoplasms.

Alferon N *Interferon Sciences, USA.*
Interferon alfa-n3 (p.628·1).
Genital warts.

Alferos *Berenguer Infale, Spain†.*
Azelastine hydrochloride (p.409·3).
Allergic rhinitis.

Alfetim *Beecham, Spain.*
Alfuzosin hydrochloride (p.833·2).
Benign prostatic hyperplasia.

Al-Flor *Francia, Ital.*
Lactic-acid producing bacteria (p.1626·3); yeast; anise; lime; vitamin C; vitamin B substances (p.1350·1).
Restoration of gastrointestinal flora.

Alfospas
Opfermann, Ger.; Rottapharm, Ital.
Tiropramide hydrochloride (p.1673·3).
Smooth muscle spasm.

Algafan *Darrow, Braz.*
Dextropropoxyphene (p.27·1); paracetamol (p.71·2).
Pain.

Alganex *Roche, Swed.*
Tenoxicam (p.87·2).
Dysmenorrhoea; inflammation; musculoskeletal and joint disorders; postoperative pain.

Algedrox *De Mayo, Braz.*
Aluminium hydroxide (p.1210·3); magnesium hydroxide (p.1233·1); dimethicone (p.1249·2).
Flatulence; gastrointestinal hyperacidity.

Algefit *Medicopharm, Aust.*
Diclofenac sodium (p.30·3).
Soft-tissue and peri-articular disorders.

Algenac *Ofimex, Mex.*
Diclofenac (p.30·2).

Algesal
Note. This name is used for preparations of different composition.
Solvay, Aust.; Solvay, Ger.; Solvay, Port.; Solvay, Spain; Solvay, Switz.
Diethylamine salicylate (p.32·2); myrtecaine (p.1317·3) or myrtecaine laurilsulfate (p.1317·3).
Musculoskeletal, joint, peri-articular, and soft-tissue disorders; neuralgia.
Solvay, Belg.
Diethylamine salicylate (p.32·2).
Algesal cream formerly contained diethylamine salicylate and myrtecaine.
Musculoskeletal, joint, peri-articular, and soft-tissue disorders; neuralgias.
Solvay, Canad.†; Solvay, Fin.; Solvay, Ital.; LTM, Neth.; Nycomed, Norw.; Solvay, Swed.; Solvay, UK.
Diethylamine salicylate (p.32·2).
Musculoskeletal, joint, and soft-tissue disorders.

Algesal Forte *LTM, Neth.*
Diethylamine salicylate (p.32·2); myrtecaine (p.1317·3).
Muscle and joint pain.

Algesal Suractive *Solvay, Fr.*
Diethylamine salicylate (p.32·2); myrtecaine (p.1317·3).
Soft-tissue disorders.

Algesalona *Solvay, Ger.; Solvay, Switz.*
Diethylamine salicylate (p.32·2); myrtecaine (p.1317·3); flufenamic acid (p.41·1).
Musculoskeletal, joint, and soft-tissue disorders.

Algesalona E *Solvay, Ger.*
Etofenamate (p.35·3).
Musculoskeletal, joint, peri-articular, and soft-tissue disorders.

Algexin *Honorterapica, Braz.*
Hyoscine butylbromide (p.468·2).
Smooth muscle spasm.

Algho *Rhone-Poulenc Rorer, Spain†.*
Aspirin (p.14·2).
Fever; inflammation; pain; thromboembolism prophylaxis.

Algi *Mabo, Spain.*
Metamizole magnesium (p.34·2).
Fever; pain.

Algiasdin *Isdin, Spain.*
Ibuprofen (p.43·2).
Fever; inflammation; musculoskeletal, joint, and peri-articular disorders; pain.

Algice *Cazi, Braz.*
Dipyrone (p.34·1); eucalyptol (p.1609·2); vitamin C (p.1389·3); guaifenesin (p.1092·2).
Cold and influenza symptoms.

Algicon
Note. This name is used for preparations of different composition.
Rhone-Poulenc Rorer, Austral.†; Rhone-Poulenc Rorer, Irl.; Rhone-Poulenc Rorer, Neth.
Oral suspension: Magnesium alginate (p.1499·1); aluminium hydroxide-magnesium carbonate co-dried gel (p.1211·2); magnesium carbonate (p.1232·3); potassium bicarbonate (p.1186·1); calcium carbonate (p.1215·1).
Gastro-oesophageal reflux.
Rhone-Poulenc Rorer, Austral.†; Rhone-Poulenc Rorer, Irl.†; Rhone-Poulenc Rorer, Neth.; Rhone-Poulenc Rorer, Norw.†; Rhone-Poulenc Rorer, UK.
Oral suspension; tablets: Aluminium hydroxide-magnesium carbonate co-dried gel (p.1211·2); magnesium alginate (p.1499·1); magnesium carbonate (p.1232·3); potassium bicarbonate (p.1186·1).
Gastric hyperacidity; gastro-oesophageal reflux.
Rhone-Poulenc Rorer, Mex.
Magnesium alginate (p.1499·1); aluminium hydroxide-magnesium carbonate co-dried gel (p.1211·2); magnesium carbonate (p.1232·3); calcium carbonate (p.1215·1).
Gastrointestinal disorders.

Algicote *Rhodia, Braz.*
Aluminium hydroxide-magnesium carbonate co-dried gel (p.1211·2); magnesium alginate (p.1499·1); magnesium carbonate (p.1232·3).
Gastrointestinal hyperacidity.

Algi-Danilon *Allergan-Frumtost, Braz.*
Ibuprofen (p.43·2); paracetamol (p.71·2).
Fever; inflammation; pain.

Algidente *Sedabel, Braz.*
Chloroform (p.1256·3); phenol (p.1152·3); procaine hydrochloride (p.1319·1); clove oil (p.1597·1).
Mouth disorders.

Algiderma *Davi, Port.*
Diethylamine salicylate (p.32·2).
Musculoskeletal, joint, and soft-tissue disorders.

Algidol
Note. This name is used for preparations of different composition.
Sintesa, Belg.; Almirall, Spain.
Paracetamol (p.71·2); codeine phosphate (p.25·2); ascorbic acid (p.1389·3).
Fever; pain.
Vitae, Mex.
Ibuprofen (p.43·2).
Pain.

Algifen *Sintofarma, Braz.*
Ibuprofen (p.43·2); paracetamol (p.71·2).
Fever; inflammation; pain.

Algifene
Note. This name is used for preparations of different composition.
Nicholas, Fr.
Ibuprofen (p.43·2).
Fever; pain.
Ferraz, Lynce, Port.
Injection: Dextropropoxyphene hydrochloride (p.27·1).
Tablets: Dextropropoxyphene (p.27·1); paracetamol (p.71·2).
Pain.

Algiflamanil *Neo Quimica, Braz.*
Oxyphenbutazone (p.71·1); paracetamol (p.71·2).
Fever; inflammation; pain.

Algiflan *Teuto, Braz.*
Phenylbutazone (p.78·1); paracetamol (p.71·2).
Fever; inflammation; pain.

Algiflex *Gilton, Braz.*
Orphenadrine (p.471·1); dipyrone (p.34·1); caffeine (p.761·3).
Skeletal muscle spasm.

Algifor Vifor, Switz.
Ibuprofen (p.43·2) or ibuprofen lysine (p.44·1).
Fever; pain.

Algik Azevedos, Port.
Paracetamol (p.71·2); caffeine (p.761·3).
Fever; pain.

Algikey Inkeysa, Spain.
Ketorolac trometamol (p.48·2).
Pain.

Algimate Bonafarma, Port.
Clonixin lysine (p.25·1).
Pain.

Algimesil Francia, Ital.
Nimesulide (p.62·3).
Musculoskeletal and joint disorders.

Alginex Sanopharm, Switz.
Ethyl salicylate (p.35·1); camphor (p.1589·3); menthol (p.1632·3); turpentine oil (p.1676·3).
Musculoskeletal, joint, and peri-articular disorders; sports injuries.

Alginor Boehringer Ingelheim, Ital.
Cimetropium bromide (p.465·1).
Adjunct in gastrointestinal examinations and surgical procedures; gastrointestinal disorders.

Algiospray
Note. This name is used for preparations of different composition.
Novag, Mex.
Peridilmethylamine.

Robert, Spain†.
Picolamine salicylate (p.78·3).
Peri-articular disorders; soft-tissue disorders.

Algipan
Note. This name is used for preparations of different composition.
Qualiphar, Belg.
Methyl nicotinate (p.55·1); glycol salicylate (p.42·2); mephenesin (p.1329·2).
Musculoskeletal pain; skeletal muscle spasm.

Darci, Fr.
Mephenesin (p.1329·2); methyl nicotinate (p.55·1); glycol salicylate (p.42·2); histamine hydrochloride (p.1619·2).
Formerly contained mephenesin, methyl nicotinate, glycol salicylate, histamine hydrochloride, and capsicum oleoresin.
Muscle pain.

Whitehall, Irl.
Methyl nicotinate (p.55·1); glycol salicylate (p.42·2); capsaicin (p.23·1).
Musculoskeletal and joint pain.

Whitehall, UK.
Methyl nicotinate (p.55·1); glycol salicylate (p.42·2); capsicum oleoresin (p.1591·1).
Muscle and joint pain.

Algi-Peralgin Infabra, Braz.
Oxyphenbutazone (p.71·1); paracetamol (p.71·2).
Fever; inflammation; pain.

Algiprofen Eurofarma, Braz.
Ketoprofen (p.47·3).
Gout; musculoskeletal, joint, and peri-articular disorders; pain.

Algi-Reumac Windson, Braz.
Oxyphenbutazone (p.71·1); paracetamol (p.71·2).
Fever; inflammation; pain.

Algisan Prodes, Spain†.
Ibuprofen (p.43·2).
Fever; inflammation; musculoskeletal and joint disorders; pain.

Algisedal Asta Medica, Fr.
Paracetamol (p.71·2); codeine phosphate (p.25·2).
Pain.

Algist Hoechst Marion Roussel, S.Afr.†
Paracetamol (p.71·2); caffeine (p.761·3); chlorpheniramine [chlorphenamine] maleate (p.412·1); phenylephrine hydrochloride (p.1097·1).
Cold symptoms.

Algistat Convatec, UK†.
Calcium alginate (p.728·1).
Haemostatic dressing.

Algitec
SmithKline Beecham, Irl.; SmithKline Beecham, UK†.
Alginic acid (p.1498·3) or sodium alginate (p.1498·3); cimetidine (p.1216·3).
Gastro-oesophageal reflux.

Algizolin Luper, Braz.
Oxyphenbutazone (p.71·1); paracetamol (p.71·2).
Fever; inflammation; pain.

Algobene Ratiopharm, Aust.
Aspirin (p.14·2).
Fever; pain.

Algocetil Francia, Ital.†.
Sulindac sodium (p.86·2).
Gout; musculoskeletal, joint, and peri-articular disorders; neuritis.

Algocor Teofarma, Ital.
Gallopamil hydrochloride (p.896·2).
Ischaemic heart disease; myocardial infarction.

Algoderm Inibsa, Spain†.
Diethylamine salicylate (p.32·2).
Peri-articular and soft-tissue disorders.

Algofen Pfizer Consumer, Ital.
Ibuprofen (p.43·2).
Pain.

Algoflex Same Savorna, Ital.†.
Diethylamine salicylate (p.32·2).
Musculoskeletal and joint disorders.

Algogen Nakorn, Thai.
Paracetamol (p.71·2).
Pain.

Algolider Garant, Ital.
Nimesulide (p.62·3).
Fever; inflammation; pain.

Algolisina Celsius, Ital.
Pridinol mesilate (p.1330·1); benzydamine hydrochloride (p.20·1); lignocaine [lidocaine] hydrochloride (p.1313·2).
Formerly contained pridinol mesilate, benzydamine hydrochloride, cinchocaine hydrochloride, and hyaluronidase.
Musculoskeletal, joint, and soft-tissue disorders.

Algolysin Teva, Israel.
Dextropropoxyphene hydrochloride (p.27·1); paracetamol (p.71·2).
Pain.

Algo-Nevriton Sciencex, Fr.
Acetiamine hydrochloride (p.1384·3); aspirin (p.14·2).
Musculoskeletal and joint disorders; neuralgia; pain.

Algophene SMB, Belg.
Paracetamol (p.71·2); dextropropoxyphene hydrochloride (p.27·1).
Pain.

Algophytum Herbaxt, Fr.†.
Devil's claw root (p.26·3).
Joint pain.

Algopirina Medisint, Ital.
Aspirin (p.14·2); paracetamol (p.71·2).
Cold and influenza symptoms; pain.

Algoplaque Urgo, Fr.
A hydrocolloid dressing.
Burns; ulcers; wounds.

Algopriv Interdelta, Switz.
Diproqualone camsilate (p.34·1); ethenzamide (p.35·1).
Inflammation; pain.

Algo-Prolixan Jacoby, Aust.
Azapropazone (p.19·1); dextropropoxyphene hydrochloride (p.27·1).
Musculoskeletal and joint disorders.

Algostase SMB, Belg.
Paracetamol (p.71·2); caffeine (p.761·3).
Fever; pain.

Algosteril Brothier, Fr.; Johnson & Johnson, Ger.; Johnson & Johnson, Ital.; Beiersdorf, UK.
Calcium alginate (p.728·1).
Haemostatic dressing.

Algotropyl Alpharma, Fr.
Paracetamol (p.71·2); promethazine hydrochloride (p.423·2).
Cold symptoms.

Alho Rogoff Crefar, Port.
Garlic (p.1614·1).
Cardiovascular disorders; rheumatic disorders; senility; stress.

Alho-Arthrosan N Wiedemann, Ger.
Homoeopathic preparation.

Alho-Sedosan Wiedemann, Ger.
Homoeopathic preparation.

Alhydrate
Nestle, Fr.; Nestle, Ital.
Maltodextrin; sucrose; sodium chloride; citric acid; potassium citrate (p.1185·2).
Diarrhoea; oral rehydration therapy.

Alhydrox Stallergenes, Ital.
An allergen extract (p.1575·3).
Hyposensitisation.

Ali Veg SmithKline Beecham, Spain.
Cimetidine (p.1216·3).
Acid aspiration; gastro-oesophageal reflux; gastrointestinal haemorrhage; gastrointestinal hyperacidity; peptic ulcer; short-bowel syndrome; Zollinger-Ellison syndrome.

A-Lices Hoe, Singapore.
Malathion (p.1434·2).
Pediculosis.

Alicura Catarinense, Braz.
Aspirin (p.14·2); caffeine (p.761·3).
Fever; pain.

Alidol Syntex, Mex.
Ketorolac trometamol (p.48·2).
Pain.

Alidor Hoechst Marion Roussel, Braz.
Aspirin (p.14·2).
Fever; inflammation; pain; thromboembolism prophylaxis.

Aligest Schering-Plough, Spain†.
Aluminium hydroxide (p.1210·3); dimethicone (p.1249·2); magnesium hydroxide (p.1233·1).
Gastrointestinal hyperacidity and flatulence.

Aligest Plus Schering-Plough, Spain.
Aluminium hydroxide (p.1210·3); calcium carbonate (p.1215·1); magnesium hydroxide (p.1233·1); simeticone (p.1249·2).
Flatulence; gastrointestinal hyperacidity.

Alimentum
Ross, Canad.; Abbott, Canad.; Abbott, Fin.; Ross, USA.
Protein hydrolysate infant feed (p.1350·1).
Fat malabsorption; food hypersensitivity; protein maldigestion; protein sensitivity.

Alimix
Janssen-Cilag, Ger.; JC Healthcare, Ital.; Janssen, UK†.
Cisapride (p.1220·1).
Gastric motility disorders; gastro-oesophageal reflux.

Alin
Note. This name is used for preparations of different composition.
Millet Roux, Braz.
Albendazole (p.95·2).
Worm infections.

Chinoin, Mex.
Dexamethasone (p.1067·1), dexamethasone isonicotinate (p.1067·1), or dexamethasone sodium phosphate (p.1067·1).
Corticosteroid.

Alin Nasal Chinoin, Mex.
Dexamethasone sodium phosphate (p.1067·1); neomycin sulfate (p.228·1); phenylephrine hydrochloride (p.1097·1).
Rhinitis; sinusitis.

Alin Oftalmico Chinoin, Mex.
Dexamethasone sodium phosphate (p.1067·1); neomycin sulfate (p.228·1).
Eye disorders.

Alinamin B12
Takeda, Singapore.
Fursultiamine (p.1384·3); vitamin B₁₂ (p.1388·1).
Procaine hydrochloride (p.1319·1) is included in this preparation to alleviate the pain of injection.
Anaemias; neuritis.

Takeda, Thai.
Fursultiamine hydrochloride (p.1384·3); vitamin B₁₂ (p.1388·1).
Macrocytic anaemia; megaloblastic anaemia; neuritis.

Alinamin-F
Note. This name is used for preparations of different composition.
Takeda, Hong Kong; Takeda, Singapore.
Fursultiamine (p.1384·3); riboflavin (p.1386·1).
Arthralgia; beri-beri; CNS disorders; gastrointestinal motility disorders; myalgia; myocardial metabolic disorders; neuralgia; peripheral nerve paralysis; peripheral neuritis; vitamin B₁ deficiency; Wernicke's encephalopathy.

Takeda, Jpn.
Fursultiamine hydrochloride (p.1384·3).
Vitamin B₁ deficiency; vitamin B₁ supplement.

Takeda, Thai.
Injection: Fursultiamine hydrochloride (p.1384·3).
Tablets: Fursultiamine hydrochloride (p.1384·3); riboflavin (p.1386·1).
Vitamin B₁ deficiency.

Alindrin Astra, Swed.
Ibuprofen (p.43·2).
Fever; pain.

Alinol Pharmasant, Thai.
Allopurinol (p.397·2).
Gout; hyperuricaemia; renal calculi.

Alinor Alpharma, Norw.
Atenolol (p.841·3).
Angina pectoris; arrhythmias; hypertension; hyperthyroidism; migraine; myocardial infarction.

Alipase Janssen-Cilag, Fr.
Pancrelipase (p.1647·2).
Pancreatic insufficiency.

Aliseum Formenti, Ital.
Diazepam (p.674·3).
Anxiety disorders; epilepsy; insomnia.

Alitraq
Abbott, Austral.; Abbott, Fin.; Abbott, Hong Kong; Abbott, Irl.; Ross, Israel; Abbott, NZ; Abbott, Singapore; Abbott Nutrition, UK.
Preparation for enteral nutrition (p.1350·1).

Aliviador Biologia, Braz.
Methyl salicylate (p.55·1); camphor (p.1589·3); menthol (p.1632·3).
Musculoskeletal and joint disorders.

Aliviaderm QIF, Braz.
Nitrofurazone (p.231·3).
Infected burns; skin infections.

Aliviomas Alacan, Spain.
Naproxen (p.60·3).
Fever; gout; musculoskeletal and joint disorders; pain.

Aliviosin Alacan, Spain.
Indometacin (p.44·3).
Gout; inflammation; musculoskeletal, joint, and peri-articular disorders; pain.

Alk Scherax, Ger.
A range of allergen extracts (p.1575·3).
Hyposensitisation.

Alkaban Quad, USA†.
Vinblastine sulfate (p.577·3).
Malignant neoplasms.

Alkafizz Xeragen, S.Afr.
Sodium citrate (p.1186·2); sodium bicarbonate (p.1186·2); anhydrous citric acid (p.1596·2); tartaric acid (p.1669·2).
Gastric hyperacidity; urinary alkalinisation.

Alkagin Ganassini, Ital.
Calendula (p.1589·2); mallow; tilia (p.1673·2).
Personal hygiene.

Alkala T Sanum-Kehlbeck, Ger.
Sodium bicarbonate (p.1186·2).
Metabolic acidosis.

Alkalite D Aspen Consumer, S.Afr.
Dicyclomine [dicycloverine] hydrochloride (p.466·1); dried aluminium hydroxide gel (p.1210·3); light magnesium oxide (p.1233·2).
Gastric hyperacidity.

Alkamine ANB, Thai.
Aluminium hydroxide gel (p.1210·3); magnesium trisilicate (p.1233·3); kaolin (p.1229·3); atropine sulfate (p.461·1).
Gastric hyperacidity; peptic ulcer.

Alka-Mints Bayer, USA.
Calcium carbonate (p.1215·1).
Hyperacidity.

Alka-Seltzer
Note. This name is used for preparations of different composition.
Bayer, Aust.; Bayer, Austral.; Bayer, Belg.; Bayer, Braz.; Bayer, Canad.; Bayer, Fin.; Bayer, Fr.; Bayer, Ger.; Bayer, Ital.; Bayer, Neth.; Bayer, NZ; Bayer Consumer, Singapore; Bayer, Swed.; Bayer, Switz.; Bayer, Thai.; Bayer Consumer, UK.
Aspirin (p.14·2); citric acid (p.1596·2); sodium bicarbonate (p.1186·2).
Dyspepsia; fever; pain.

Agis, Israel.
Aspirin (p.14·2).
Fever; musculoskeletal and joint pain; pain; thrombosis prophylaxis.

Bayer, Port.; Bayer, Spain.
Aspirin (p.14·2); calcium phosphate (p.1188·3); citric acid (p.1596·2); sodium bicarbonate (p.1186·2).
Dyspepsia; fever; pain.

Alka-Seltzer Antacid Miles Consumer Healthcare, USA.
Sodium bicarbonate (p.1186·2); citric acid (p.1596·2); potassium bicarbonate (p.1186·1).
Gastrointestinal disorders.

Alka-Seltzer with Aspirin Miles Consumer Healthcare, USA.
Aspirin (p.14·2); citric acid (p.1596·2); sodium bicarbonate (p.1186·2).
Arthritis; fever; gastrointestinal disorders; myocardial infarction; pain.

Alka-Seltzer Effervescent Tablets Miles, USA.
Sodium bicarbonate (p.1186·2); citric acid (p.1596·2); aspirin (p.14·2).
Hyperacidity.

Alka-Seltzer Plus Cold
Note. This name is used for preparations of different composition.
Bayer, Canad.†.
Aspirin (p.14·2); phenylpropanolamine bitartrate (p.1098·3); chlorpheniramine [chlorphenamine] maleate (p.412·1).
Cold symptoms.

Miles Consumer Healthcare, USA.
Capsules: Chlorpheniramine [chlorphenamine] maleate (p.412·1); pseudoephedrine hydrochloride (p.1099·2); paracetamol (p.71·2).
Tablets†: Phenylpropanolamine bitartrate (p.1098·3); chlorpheniramine [chlorphenamine] maleate (p.412·1); aspirin (p.14·2).
Cold symptoms; nasal congestion.

Alka-Seltzer Plus Cold & Cough
Miles, USA†.
Tablets: Phenylpropanolamine bitartrate (p.1098·3); chlorpheniramine [chlorphenamine] maleate (p.412·1); dextromethorphan hydrobromide (p.1087·3); aspirin (p.14·2).
Coughs and cold symptoms.

Miles Consumer Healthcare, USA.
Capsules: Dextromethorphan (p.1087·3); pseudoephedrine hydrochloride (p.1099·2); chlorpheniramine [chlorphenamine] maleate (p.412·1); paracetamol (p.71·2).
Coughs and cold symptoms.

Alka-Seltzer Plus Cold & Sinus
Bayer, USA.
Capsules: Pseudoephedrine hydrochloride (p.1099·2); paracetamol (p.71·2).
Effervescent tablets†: Aspirin (p.14·2); phenylpropanolamine bitartrate (p.1098·3).
Cold symptoms; nasal congestion.

Alka-Seltzer Plus Night-Time Cold Miles Consumer Healthcare, USA.
Capsules: Doxylamine succinate (p.417·1); dextromethorphan (p.1087·3); pseudoephedrine hydrochloride (p.1099·2); paracetamol (p.71·2).
Tablets†: Phenylpropanolamine bitartrate (p.1098·3); brompheniramine maleate (p.410·2); dextromethorphan hydrobromide (p.1087·3); aspirin (p.14·2).
Coughs and cold symptoms.

Alka-Seltzer Plus Sinus Bayer, USA†.
Phenylpropanolamine tartrate (p.1098·3); aspirin (p.14·2).
Upper-respiratory tract congestion.

Alka-Seltzer Plus Sinus Allergy Miles, USA†.
Phenylpropanolamine bitartrate (p.1098·3); brompheniramine maleate (p.410·2); aspirin (p.14·2).
Upper respiratory-tract symptoms.

Alka-Seltzer XS Bayer Consumer, UK.
Aspirin (p.14·2); paracetamol (p.71·2); caffeine (p.761·3); citric acid (p.1596·2); sodium bicarbonate (p.1186·2).
Gastric discomfort; pain.

Alkasid
Leo, Denm.; Julphar, UAE.
Aluminium magnesium silicate (p.1499·1); simeticone (p.1249·2).
Gastritis; gastro-oesophageal reflux; peptic ulcer.

Alkasolve Sam-On, Israel.
Potassium citrate (p.1186·1); sodium citrate (p.1186·2).
Diabetic acidosis; urinary alkalisation.

Alkavite Vitality, USA.
A multivitamin and mineral preparation (p.1350·1).

Alkenide Medeva, Fr.
Poloxamer 188 (p.1347·1).
Skin cleanser.

Alkeran
Glaxo Wellcome, Aust.; Glaxo Wellcome, Austral.; Glaxo Wellcome, Belg.; Glaxo Wellcome, Braz.; Glaxo Wellcome, Canad.; Glaxo Well-

come, Denm.; Glaxo Wellcome, Fin.; Glaxo Wellcome, Fr.; Glaxo Wellcome, Ger.; Glaxo Wellcome, Hong Kong; Wellcome, Irl.; Glaxo Wellcome, Israel; Glaxo Wellcome, Ital.; Glaxo Wellcome, Mex.; Glaxo Wellcome, Neth.; Glaxo Wellcome, Norw.; Glaxo Wellcome, NZ; Wellcome, Port.; Glaxo Wellcome, S.Afr.; Glaxo Wellcome, Singapore; Glaxo Wellcome, Swed.; Wellcome, Switz.; Glaxo Wellcome, Thai.; Glaxo Wellcome, UK; Glaxo Wellcome, USA.
Melphalan (p.551·2) or melphalan hydrochloride (p.551·3).
Malignant neoplasms; polycythaemia vera.

Alket Ripari-Gero, Ital.
Ketoprofen (p.47·3).
Gout; musculoskeletal, joint, peri-articular, and soft-tissue disorders; pain; phlebitis.

Alkets Roberts, USA; Hauck, USA.
Calcium carbonate (p.1215·1).
Hyperacidity.

Alko Isol Marc-O, Canad.
Isopropyl alcohol (p.1149·2).

Alkocean Proceane, Fr.
Shark-liver oil.
Tonic.

Alkyloxan Choongwae, Singapore.
Cyclophosphamide (p.527·3).
Malignant neoplasms.

All Clear Bausch & Lomb, USA.
Naphazoline hydrochloride (p.1095·1).
Eye irritation.

All In One Plus Grapefruit Solgar, UK.
Soya lecithin (p.1628·1); grapefruit powder concentrate; cider vinegar.
Dietary supplement.

All Pecium Dermoteca, Port.
Pyrithione zinc (p.1122·1); sulfur (p.1123·3).
Seborrhoeic dermatitis.

Allamin Kyorin, Thai.
Amino-acid preparation (p.1350·1).
Nutritional supplement.

Allbece Whitehall, Swed.†.
Vitamin B and C preparation (p.1350·1).

Allbee Robins, USA.
A range of vitamin preparations (p.1350·1).

Allbee with C
Whitehall, Austral.†; Whitehall-Robins, Canad.; Whitehall, Irl.
Vitamin B substances with ascorbic acid (p.1350·1).

Allbee C-550 Whitehall-Robins, Canad.
Vitamin B substances with ascorbic acid (p.1350·1).

Allbee C-800 Whitehall-Robins, Canad.
Vitamin B substances, ascorbic acid, and vitamin E (p.1350·1).

Allbee C-800 plus Iron Whitehall-Robins, Canad.
Vitamin B substances, ascorbic acid, vitamin E, folic acid, and iron (p.1350·1).

Allcock's Porous Capsicum Plaster Richards & Appleby, UK.
Burgundy pitch; frankincense; orris; capsicum (p.1591·1); camphor (p.1589·3); elemi; myrrh (p.1639·2).

Allegra
Hoechst Marion Roussel, Canad.; Hoechst Marion Roussel, Mex.; Hoechst Marion Roussel, USA.
Fexofenadine hydrochloride (p.417·3).
Allergic rhinitis; allergic skin disorders; eye irritation.

Allegra-D
Hoechst Marion Roussel, Canad.; Aventis Pharma, USA.
Fexofenadine hydrochloride (p.417·3); pseudoephedrine hydrochloride (p.1099·2).
Allergic rhinitis.

Allegron
Dista, Austral.; Lilly, NZ; Dista, UK.
Nortriptyline hydrochloride (p.301·3).
Depression; nocturnal enuresis.

Allens Chesty Cough Allens, UK.
Ammonium chloride (p.1085·2); tolu tincture (p.1101·3); squill tincture (p.1100·3); menthol (p.1632·3); marrubium (p.1094·2).
Coughs.

Allens Dry Tickly Cough Allens, UK.
Benzoin tincture (p.1668·3); ipecacuanha tincture (p.1093·1); capsicum tincture (p.1591·1); cetylpyridinium chloride (p.1138·1).
Coughs.

Allens Junior Cough Allens, UK.
Glycerol (p.1616·3); anhydrous citric acid (p.1596·2).
Coughs; sore throat.

Allens Pine & Honey Allens, UK.
Ipecacuanha (p.1093·1); liquorice (p.1231·3); squill oxymel.
Coughs; cold symptoms; bronchitis.

Allent Ascher, USA.
Brompheniramine maleate (p.410·2); pseudoephedrine hydrochloride (p.1099·2).
Allergic rhinitis; nasal congestion.

Aller-Aide Technilab, Canad.
Diphenhydramine hydrochloride (p.416·1).

Allerbiocid S Allerbio, Fr.
Benzyl benzoate (p.1428·2); tannic acid (p.1669·1).
Insecticide for bedding and upholstery.

Allercalm Amnol, Ital.
Zinc orotate; vitamin A (p.1350·1).
Nutritional supplement.

Aller-Chlor Rugby, USA.
Chlorpheniramine [chlorphenamine] maleate (p.412·1).
Hypersensitivity reactions.

Allercon Parmed, USA.
Pseudoephedrine hydrochloride (p.1099·2); triprolidine hydrochloride (p.427·2).
Upper respiratory-tract symptoms.

Allercreme Carme, USA.
Emollient and moisturiser.

Allercrom Rhone-Poulenc Rorer, Aust.
Sodium cromoglicate (p.774·3).
Allergic conjunctivitis; allergic rhinitis.

Allerdine LBS, Thai.
Loratadine (p.420·1).
Allergic rhinitis; allergic skin disorders.

Allerdryl ICN, Canad.
Diphenhydramine hydrochloride (p.416·1).
Hypersensitivity.

Allerest Fisons, USA.
Naphazoline hydrochloride (p.1095·1).
Minor eye irritation.

Allerest Headache Strength Ciba, USA.
Pseudoephedrine hydrochloride (p.1099·2); chlorpheniramine [chlorphenamine] maleate (p.412·1); paracetamol (p.71·2).
Upper respiratory-tract symptoms.

Allerest 12 Hour Ciba, USA†.
Phenylpropanolamine hydrochloride (p.1098·1); chlorpheniramine [chlorphenamine] maleate (p.412·1).
Upper respiratory-tract symptoms.

Allerest 12 Hour Nasal Ciba Consumer, USA.
Oxymetazoline hydrochloride (p.1096·2).
Nasal congestion.

Allerest Maximum Strength Ciba, USA.
Pseudoephedrine hydrochloride (p.1099·2); chlorpheniramine [chlorphenamine] maleate (p.412·1).
Upper respiratory-tract symptoms.

Allerest Sinus Pain Formula Ciba, USA.
Pseudoephedrine hydrochloride (p.1099·2); chlorpheniramine [chlorphenamine] maleate (p.412·1); paracetamol (p.71·2).
Upper respiratory-tract symptoms.

Aller-eze Novartis Consumer, UK.
Cream: Diphenhydramine hydrochloride (p.416·1).
Tablets†: Clemastine hydrogen fumarate (p.413·2).
Hypersensitivity reactions; insect bites and stings.

Aller-eze Clear Novartis Consumer, UK†.
Terfenadine (p.424·3).
Hay fever; urticaria.

Aller-eze Plus Novartis Consumer, UK†.
Clemastine hydrogen fumarate (p.413·2); phenylpropanolamine hydrochloride (p.1098·1).
Hay fever.

Allerfen Sella, Ital.
Promethazine hydrochloride (p.423·2).
Hypersensitivity reactions; insomnia.

Allerfre Boots Healthcare, Neth.
Loratadine (p.420·1).
Allergic rhinitis; urticaria.

Allerfrim Rugby, USA.
Pseudoephedrine hydrochloride (p.1099·2); triprolidine hydrochloride (p.427·2).
Upper respiratory-tract symptoms.

Allerfrim with Codeine Rugby, USA.
Pseudoephedrine hydrochloride (p.1099·2); codeine phosphate (p.25·2); triprolidine hydrochloride (p.427·2).
Coughs and cold symptoms.

Allergan Bouty, Ital.
Diphenhydramine hydrochloride (p.416·1).
Insect bites; pruritus; sunburn.

Allergan Enzymatic Allergan, USA.
Papain (p.1647·3) (p.1129·2).
Cleansing solution for soft contact lenses.

Allergefon Lafon, Fr.
Carbinoxamine maleate (p.411·1).
Hypersensitivity reactions.

Allergen Goldline, USA.
Benzocaine (p.1306·3); phenazone (p.77·2); glycerol (p.1616·3).
Ear pain.

Allergenid Herbaline, Ital.†.
Agrimony (p.1574·3); black currant (p.1389·3); echinacea (p.1606·2).
Hypersensitivity reactions.

Allergex Propan, S.Afr.
Chlorpheniramine [chlorphenamine] maleate (p.412·1).
Hypersensitivity reactions.

Allergie-Injektopas Pascoe, Ger.
Homoeopathic preparation.

Allergies Homeocan, Canad.
Homoeopathic preparation.

Allergin
Note. This name is used for preparations of different composition.
Propan, S.Afr.
Diphenhydramine hydrochloride (p.416·1); ammonium chloride (p.1085·2); sodium citrate (p.1186·2); menthol (p.1632·3).
Coughs.
PP Lab, Thai.
Chlorpheniramine [chlorphenamine] maleate (p.412·1).
Hypersensitivity.

Allergipuran N Scheurich, Ger.†.
Bufexamac (p.20·3).
Inflammatory skin disorders.

Allergo-COMOD Ursapharm, Ger.
Sodium cromoglicate (p.774·3).
Allergic conjunctivitis; allergic rhinitis.

Allergocrom
Ursapharm, Ger.; Ursapharm, Neth.†.
Sodium cromoglicate (p.774·3).
Allergic conjunctivitis; allergic rhinitis.

Allergodil
Asta Medica, Aust.; Asta Medica, Belg.; Asta, Denm.; Asta Medica, Fr.; Asta Medica, Ger.; Asta Medica, Ital.; Asta Medica, Neth.; Asta Medica, Port.; Asta Medica, Switz.
Azelastine hydrochloride (p.409·3).
Allergic conjunctivitis; allergic rhinitis.

Allergodose Europhta, Mon.
Sodium cromoglicate (p.774·3).
Allergic eye disorders.

Allergoid-HAL Hal, Neth.†.
Aluminium hydroxide adsorbed modified allergens (p.1575·3).
Hyposensitisation.

Allergokatt Kattwiga, Ger.
Homoeopathic preparation.

Allergopos N Ursapharm, Ger.
Antazoline phosphate (p.408·3); tetryzoline hydrochloride (p.1101·2).
Eye disorders.

Allergospasmin
Asta Medica, Aust.; Asta Medica, Ger.
Sodium cromoglicate (p.774·3); reproterol hydrochloride (p.770·2).
Obstructive airways disease.

Allergospasmine Asta Medica, Switz.
Sodium cromoglicate (p.774·3); reproterol hydrochloride (p.770·2).
Obstructive airways disease.

Allergosyx Syxyl, Ger.
Homoeopathic preparation.

Allergovit
Allergopharma, Ger.; Allergopharma, Switz.
Allergen extracts (p.1575·3).
Hyposensitisation.

Allergy Parmed, USA.
Chlorpheniramine [chlorphenamine] maleate (p.412·1).

Allergy Cold Geneva, USA†.
Pseudoephedrine hydrochloride (p.1099·2); triprolidine hydrochloride (p.427·2).
Upper respiratory-tract symptoms.

Allergy Drops
Bausch & Lomb, Canad.; Bausch & Lomb, USA.
Naphazoline hydrochloride (p.1095·1).
Eye irritation.

Allergy Elixir Tanta, Canad.
Diphenhydramine hydrochloride (p.416·1).

Allergy Eyes Abbott, Austral.
Antazoline sulfate (p.408·3); xylometazoline hydrochloride (p.1102·2).
Allergic and inflammatory eye disorders.

Allergy Formula Stanley, Canad.
Diphenhydramine hydrochloride (p.416·1).

Allergy Relief
Note. This name is used for preparations of different composition.
Brauer, Austral.
Homoeopathic preparation.
Formerly known as Allergy Symptoms Relief.
JCP, Canad.†.
Terfenadine (p.424·3).
Unichem, UK.
Chlorpheniramine [chlorphenamine] maleate (p.412·1).
Hypersensitivity reactions.

Allergy Relief Medicine Rugby, USA†.
Phenylpropanolamine hydrochloride (p.1098·1); chlorpheniramine [chlorphenamine] maleate (p.412·1).
Upper respiratory-tract symptoms.

Allergy Sinus WestCan, Canad.
Pseudoephedrine hydrochloride (p.1099·2); chlorpheniramine [chlorphenamine] maleate (p.412·1); paracetamol (p.71·2).

Allergy Tablets Tanta, Canad.
Diphenhydramine hydrochloride (p.416·1).

Allerhist Propan, S.Afr.†.
Chlorpheniramine [chlorphenamine] maleate (p.412·1).
Hypersensitivity reactions.

Allerin
United American, Singapore; Great Eastern, Thai.; United American, Thai.
Diphenhydramine hydrochloride (p.416·1); guaifenesin (p.1092·2); sodium citrate (p.1186·2); phenylpropanolamine hydrochloride (p.1098·1).
Coughs and cold symptoms.

AllerMax
Note. This name is used for preparations of different composition.
Schering-Plough, Austral.
Mometasone furoate (p.1077·2).
Hay fever.
Pfeiffer, USA.
Diphenhydramine hydrochloride (p.416·1).
Insomnia; motion sickness; parkinsonism.

Allermed Murdock, USA.
Pseudoephedrine hydrochloride (p.1099·2).
Nasal congestion.

Allernix Technilab, Canad.
Diphenhydramine hydrochloride (p.416·1).
Antihistamine.

Allerphed Great Southern, USA.
Pseudoephedrine hydrochloride (p.1099·2); triprolidine hydrochloride (p.427·2).
Upper respiratory-tract symptoms.

Allerphen MPF, Singapore.
Chlorpheniramine [chlorphenamine] maleate (p.412·1).
Hay fever; hypersensitivity reactions; insect bites; pruritus.

Allerplus Astra, Ital.†.
Terfenadine (p.424·3).
Hypersensitivity reactions.

Allerset Hal, Ger.
Allergen extracts of pollen, fungi, house dust mites, and skin (p.1575·3).
Hyposensitisation.
Hal, Neth.†.
Aqueous allergen extracts (p.1575·3).
Hyposensitisation.

Allersil Silom, Thai.
Loratadine (p.420·1).
Allergic rhinitis; allergic skin disorders; hay fever.

Allersol Ocusoft, USA.
Naphazoline hydrochloride (p.1095·1).

Aller-Tab Silom, Thai.
Loratadine (p.420·1).
Allergic rhinitis; allergic skin disorders; hay fever.

Allertac Propan, S.Afr.
Atropine sulfate (p.461·1); hyoscine hydrobromide (p.468·2); hyoscyamine sulfate (p.469·3); phenylpropanolamine hydrochloride (p.1098·1); pheniramine maleate (p.422·3); chlorpheniramine [chlorphenamine] maleate (p.412·1).
Congestion and hypersecretion of the nasal and paranasal sinuses.

AlleRx Adams, USA.
AM Tablets, pseudoephedrine hydrochloride (p.1099·2); hyoscine methonitrate (p.468·2); PM tablets, chlorpheniramine [chlorphenamine] maleate (p.412·1); hyoscine methonitrate.
Cold symptoms; rhinitis; sinusitis.

Allerzil Bruno, Ital.
Terfenadine (p.424·3).
Allergic conjunctivitis; allergic rhinitis; allergic skin disorders.

Allevyn
Smith & Nephew, Irl.; Smith & Nephew, UK.
Hydrophilic polyurethane dressing.
Ulcers; wounds.

Allgauer Allga, Aust.
Pumilio pine oil (p.1656·3); eucalyptus oil (p.1609·2); peppermint oil (p.1243·3).
Cold and influenza symptoms.

Alliosan Allmedica, Ger.
Garlic (p.1614·1).
Atherosclerosis; hyperlipidaemias.

Allium Cepa Compose Boiron, Fr.
Homoeopathic preparation.

Allium Plus Zeller, Switz.
Ginkgo biloba (p.1615·2); garlic (p.1614·1).
Cerebrovascular disorders; tonic.

All-Nite Cold Formula Major, USA.
Pseudoephedrine hydrochloride (p.1099·2); dextromethorphan hydrobromide (p.1087·3); doxylamine succinate (p.417·1); paracetamol (p.71·2).
Coughs and cold symptoms.

Allo CT, Ger.; ABZ, Ger.
Allopurinol (p.397·2).
Gout; hyperuricaemia; renal calculi.

allo-basan Schonenberger, Switz.
Allopurinol (p.397·2).
Gout; hyperuricaemia; renal calculi.

Allobenz Merck, Aust.; Arcana, Aust.
Allopurinol (p.397·2); benzbromarone (p.399·3).
Gout; hyperuricaemia; renal calculi.

Allobeta Betapharm, Ger.
Allopurinol (p.397·2).
Gout; hyperuricaemia; renal calculi.

Allochrysine
Solvay, Belg.; Solvay, Fr.
Aurotioprol (p.19·1).
Rheumatoid arthritis.

Allo.comp. Ratiopharm, Ger.
Allopurinol (p.397·2); benzbromarone (p.399·3).
Gout; hyperuricaemia.

Allo-Efeka Wyeth, Ger.
Allopurinol (p.397·2).
Gout; hyperuricaemia; renal calculi.

Alloferin
Roche, Austral.; ICN, Ger.; ICN, Hong Kong; Roche, Israel; Roche, Neth.†; Pharmaco, S.Afr.; ICN, Singapore; ICN, Thai.
Alcuronium chloride (p.1332·3).
Competitive neuromuscular blocker.

Alloferine Roche, Braz.
Alcuronium chloride (p.1332·3).
Competitive neuromuscular blocker.

Allohexal Hexal, Austral.; Hexal, Ger.†.
Allopurinol (p.397·2).
Gout; hyperuricaemia; renal calculi.

The symbol † denotes a preparation no longer actively marketed

Allomaron *Rhone-Poulenc Rorer, Ger.; Aventis, S.Afr.; Rhone-Poulenc Rorer, Thai.*
Allopurinol (p.397·2); benzbromarone (p.399·3).
Gout; hyperuricaemia.

Allonol *Medinovum, Fin.*
Allopurinol (p.397·2).
Gout; hyperuricaemia; uric acid nephropathy.

Allopin *General Drugs, Thai.*
Allopurinol (p.397·2).
Gout; hyperuricaemia.

Allopur *Nycomed, Norw.; Gea, Switz.*
Allopurinol (p.397·2).
Gout; hyperuricaemia; renal calculi; uric acid nephropathy.

Allo-Puren *Isis Puren, Ger.*
Allopurinol (p.397·2).
Gout; hyperuricaemia; renal calculi.

Alloril *Dexxon, Israel.*
Allopurinol (p.397·2).
Gout; hyperuricaemia; renal calculi; uric acid nephropathy.

Allorin *Douglas, Austral.; Douglas, Hong Kong; Douglas, NZ; Douglas, Singapore; Douglas, Thai.; TTN, Thai.*
Allopurinol (p.397·2).
Gout; hyperuricaemia; renal calculi.

Allostad *Stada, Aust.*
Allopurinol (p.397·2).
Gout; hyperuricaemia; renal calculi; uric acid nephropathy.

Allo-300-Tablinen *Sanorania, Ger.†*
Allopurinol (p.397·2).
Gout; hyperuricaemia; renal calculi.

Allotyrol *Tyrol, Aust.*
Allopurinol (p.397·2).
Hyperuricaemia.

Allpargin *Merz, Ger.*
Allopurinol (p.397·2).
Gout; hyperuricaemia.

All-Pro *Solgar, UK.*
Amino-acid preparation (p.1350·1).

Allpyral *Bayer, Austral.; Dome-Hollister-Stier, Fr.; Bayer, NZ.; Miles, USA.*
Range of allergen extracts (p.1575·3).
Hyposensitisation.

Allpyral Pure Mite *Bayer, S.Afr.*
D. pteronyssinus extracts(p.1575·3).
Hyposensitisation.

Allpyral Special Grass *Bayer, S.Afr.*
Grass pollen extracts(p.1575·3).
Hyposensitisation.

Allsan *Biomed, Switz.*
A range of vitamin preparations with or without minerals (p.1350·1).

Alltotal *Allergan, Aust.*
Cleaning, wetting, and storage solution for hard and gas permeable contact lenses (p.1129·2).

Allergan, Ger.†
Polyvinyl alcohol (p.1503·1) (p.1129·2).
Storage and wetting solution for contact lenses.

Alltracel P *Synapse, Irl.*
Calcium cellulose.
Haemorrhage.

Alltracel S *Synapse, Irl.*
Calcium cellulose; chlorhexidine (p.1138·2).
Haemorrhage.

Allural *Britisfarma, Spain.*
Allopurinol (p.397·2).
Gout; hyperuricaemia; renal calculi; uric acid nephropathy.

Allurit *Rhone-Poulenc Rorer, Ital.*
Allopurinol (p.397·2).
Gout; hyperuricaemia.

Allvoran *TAD, Ger.*
Diclofenac sodium (p.30·3).
Inflammation; musculoskeletal, joint, and soft-tissue disorders; pain.

ALLYA *Pascoe, Ger.*
Injection: Homoeopathic preparation.
Tablets: Devil's claw root (p.26·3).
Musculoskeletal and joint disorders.

Alma *Restan, S.Afr.*
Peppermint oil (p.1243·3); cardamom (p.1591·3).
Carminative.

Almac *Hovid, Singapore.*
Aluminium hydroxide (p.1210·3); magnesium hydroxide (p.1233·1); simeticone (p.1249·2).
Dyspepsia; flatulence; gastric hyperacidity; heartburn.

Almacone *Rugby, USA.*
Aluminium hydroxide (p.1210·3); magnesium hydroxide (p.1233·1); simeticone (p.1249·2).
Hyperacidity.

Almag *CT, Ger.*
Algeldrate (p.1210·3); magnesium hydroxide (p.1233·1) or magnesium trisilicate (p.1233·3).
Gastrointestinal hyperacidity; hyperphosphataemia.

Hua, Thai.
Aluminium hydroxide (p.1210·3); magnesium hydroxide (p.1233·1) or magnesium trisilicate (p.1233·3).
Gastric hyperacidity; gastritis; peptic ulcer.

Almagel *Atlas, Canad.*
Aluminium hydroxide (p.1210·3); magnesium hydroxide (p.1233·1).

Almagel Plus *Atlas, Canad.*
Aluminium hydroxide (p.1210·3); magnesium hydroxide (p.1233·1); simeticone (p.1249·2).

Almarion *Chew, Thai.*
Theophylline (p.777·2).
Obstructive airways disease.

Almarl *Sumitomo, Jpn.*
Arotinolol hydrochloride (p.841·3).
Angina pectoris; hypertension; tachycardia; tremor.

Almarytm *3M, Ital.*
Flecainide acetate (p.890·1).
Arrhythmias.

Almasal *Chew, Thai.*
Theophylline (p.777·2); salbutamol sulfate (p.770·3).
Obstructive airways disease.

Almax *Almirall, Spain.*
Almagate (p.1209·3).
Dyspepsia; gastritis; gastro-oesophageal reflux; peptic ulcer.

Almaxane *Siam Bheasach, Thai.*
Suspension: Dried aluminium hydroxide gel (p.1210·3); magnesium hydroxide (p.1233·1); simeticone (p.1249·2).
Tablets: Dried aluminium hydroxide gel (p.1210·3); aluminium magnesium silicate (p.1499·1); magnesium hydroxide (p.1233·1); simeticone (p.1249·2).
Flatulence; gastric hyperacidity; peptic ulcer.

Almay Total Sunbloc *Revlon, UK†.*
Cream: Padimate O (p.1518·2); oxybenzone (p.1518·1); titanium dioxide (p.1126·1).
Lip balm: Padimate O (p.1518·2); oxybenzone (p.1518·1).
Sunscreen.

Almebex Plus B₁₂ *Dayton, USA.*
Vitamin B substances (p.1350·1).

Almevax *Wellcome, Irl.†; SBL, Swed.†; Medeva, UK.*
A rubella vaccine (Wistar RA 27/3 strain) (p.1562·3).
Active immunisation.

Almide *Alcon, Fr.*
Lodoxamide trometamol (p.768·1).
Allergic eye disorders.

Almigastrico *Labesfal, Port.*
Aluminium hydroxide (p.1210·3).
Antacid.

Almigripe *Labesfal, Port.*
Paracetamol (p.71·2); caffeine (p.761·3).
Fever; pain.

Alminox *Nycomed, Denm.*
Aluminium glycinate (p.1210·3); magnesium oxide (p.1233·2).
Gastritis; gastro-oesophageal reflux; peptic ulcer.

Almiral *Medochemie, Hong Kong; Medochemie, Singapore; Medochemie, Thai.*
Diclofenac diethylamine (p.30·2) or diclofenac sodium (p.30·3).
Gout; inflammation; musculoskeletal, joint, and periarticular disorders; pain.

Almirid *Desitin, Ger.*
Dihydroergocryptine mesilate (p.1603·3).
Parkinsonism.

Almiron *Nutricia, Thai.*
Infant feed (p.1350·1).
Lactase deficiency; lactose intolerance.

Almiron Pepti *Nutricia, Fin.*
Infant feed (p.1350·1).
Cow's milk and soya protein allergy.

Almitil *Almirall, Spain.*
Enoxacin (p.201·1).
Urinary-tract infections.

Almodan *Berk, Irl.†; Berk, UK.*
Amoxicillin (p.149·2) or amoxicillin sodium (p.149·2).
Bacterial infections.

Almogran *Lundbeck, UK.*
Almotriptan malate (p.450·2).
Migraine.

Almora *Forest Pharmaceuticals, USA.*
Magnesium gluconate (p.1190·3).
Dietary supplement.

Alna *Boehringer Ingelheim, Aust.; Boehringer Ingelheim, Ger.*
Tamsulosin hydrochloride (p.978·3).
Benign prostatic hyperplasia.

Alnase *Taro, Israel.*
Phenylephrine hydrochloride (p.1097·1); naphazoline hydrochloride (p.1095·1); mepyramine maleate (p.421·1).
Cold symptoms; rhinitis; sinusiti.

Alnax *Masa, Thai.*
Alprazolam (p.654·2).
Anxiety; mixed anxiety depressive states.

Alnert *Mitsubishi, Jpn†.*
Bifemelane hydrochloride (p.1585·1).
Cerebrovascular disorders.

Alnex *Pisa, Mex.*
Dipyrone (p.34·1).
Fever; pain.

Alocril *Allergan, USA.*
Nedocromil sodium (p.768·3).
Allergic conjunctivitis.

Alodan *Gerot, Aust.*
Pethidine hydrochloride (p.75·1).
Pain.

Alodont *Warner-Lambert, Fr.*
Cetylpyridinium chloride (p.1138·1); chlorobutanol (p.1141·2); eugenol (p.1609·3).
Mouth and throat infections.

Alodont nouvelle formule *Parke, Davis, Switz.*
Cetylpyridinium chloride (p.1138·1); chlorobutanol (p.1141·2); eugenol (p.1609·3).
Mouth and throat disorders.

Alodorm *Alphapharm, Austral.*
Nitrazepam (p.695·2).
Insomnia.

Aloe Complex *Dolisos, Canad.*
Homoeopathic preparation.

Aloe Grande *Gordon, USA.*
Vitamin A (p.1382·1); vitamin E (p.1393·3); aloe vera (p.1110·1).
Skin disorders.

Aloe Vera Plus *GNLD, Austral.*
Aloe vera (p.1110·1); ascorbic acid; chamomile; eleutherococcus senticosis; passion flower (p.1350·1).
Digestive disorders; tonic.

Aloe Vesta *Calgon Vestal, USA.*
Skin cleanser.

Alofedina *Coll, Spain.*
Aloin (p.1210·2); belladonna (p.463·1); phenolphthalein (p.1244·1); ipecacuanha (p.1093·1); nux vomica (p.1643·1); podophyllum (p.1121·1).
Constipation.

Aloid *Cilag, Mex.*
Miconazole nitrate (p.391·1).
Fungal skin and nail infections.

Aloinophen *Streuli, Switz.†*
Aloes (p.1210·1); belladonna (p.463·1); bisacodyl (p.1212·2); ipecacuanha (p.1093·1).
Constipation.

Alomen *Benedetti, Ital.*
Ceftezole sodium (p.176·1).
Bacterial infections.

Alomide *Alcon, Belg.; Alcon, Braz.; Alcon, Canad.; Alcon, Denm.; Alcon, Fin.; Alcon, Ger.; Alcon, Hong Kong; Galen, Irl.†; Alcon, Israel; Alcon, Ital.; Alcon, Mex.; Alcon, Norw.; Alcon, Port.; Alcon, S.Afr.; Alcon, Singapore; Alcon Cusi, Spain; Alcon, Switz.; Alcon, Thai.; Alcon, UK; Alcon, USA.*
Lodoxamide trometamol (p.768·1).
Allergic conjunctivitis.

Alonet *Pharbita, Singapore.*
Atenolol (p.841·3).
Angina pectoris; arrhythmias; hypertension; myocardial infarction.

Alongamicina Balsa *Synthelabo, Spain.*
Ampicillin sodium (p.150·3); ampicillin benzathine (p.151·3); bromhexine hydrochloride (p.1085·3); guaifenesin (p.1092·2).
Respiratory-tract infections.

Alopam *Alpharma, Denm.; Alpharma, Fin.; Alpharma, Norw.; Dumex-Alpharma, Swed.†*
Oxazepam (p.697·1).
Anxiety; insomnia; restlessness.

Alopate *Wolfs, Belg.*
Zinc oxide (p.1128·2); titanium oxide (p.1126·1); kaolin (p.1229·3).
Skin disorders.

Alopexy *Pierre Fabre, Fr.; Pierre Fabre, Switz.*
Minoxidil (p.934·2).
Alopecia androgenetica.

Alophen *Warner-Lambert, Irl.†; Warner-Lambert, UK.*
Phenolphthalein (p.1244·1); aloin (p.1210·2).
Formerly contained phenolphthalein, aloin, belladonna, and ipecacuanha.
Constipation.

Alophen Pills *Warner-Lambert, USA†.*
Phenolphthalein (p.1244·1).
Formerly called Alophen Pills No. 973.
Constipation.

Aloplastine
Note.This name is used for preparations of different composition.
Wolfs, Belg.
Zinc oxide (p.1128·2); purified talc (p.1124·2).
Skin disorders.

Biologiques de l'Ile-de-France, Fr.
Zinc oxide (p.1128·2); glycerol (p.1616·3); purified talc (p.1124·2).
Eczema; napkin rash.

Alopon *Resinag, Switz.*
Aluminium chlorohydrate (p.1110·2).
Anorectal disorders.

Alopresin *Synthelabo, Spain.*
Captopril (p.853·3).
Diabetic nephropathy; heart failure; hypertension; myocardial infarction.

Alopresin Diu *Synthelabo, Spain.*
Hydrochlorothiazide (p.907·3); captopril (p.853·3).
Hypertension.

Aloprim *Nabi, USA.*
Allopurinol sodium (p.398·3).
Hyperuricaemia during cancer chemotherapy.

Alor *Atley, USA.*
Hydrocodone tartrate (p.42·2); aspirin (p.14·2).
Pain.

Alora *Procter & Gamble, USA.*
Estradiol (p.1473·1).
Menopausal disorders; oestrogen deficiency.

Aloral *Lagap, UK†.*
Allopurinol (p.397·2).
Gout; hyperuricaemia.

Alorin *Schering-Plough, Ital.*
Loratadine (p.420·1).
Allergic rhinitis; allergic skin disorders.

Alosfar *Esfar, Port.*
Allopurinol (p.397·2).
Gout; hyperuricaemia; renal calculi.

Alostil *Pharmacia Upjohn, Fr.*
Minoxidil (p.934·2).
Alopecia androgenetica.

Alovir *Caber, Ital.*
Aciclovir (p.612·3).
Herpesvirus infections.

Aloxan Derma *Resinag, Israel.*
Aluminium chlorohydrate (p.1110·2).
Burns; skin disorders; skin ulceration; wounds.

Aloxidil *IDI, Ital.*
Minoxidil (p.934·2).
Alopecia androgenetica.

Al-Oxin *Francia, Ital.*
Carnitine; betacarotene; sodium glutathione; ginkgo; yeast; vitamin C; vitamin E (p.1350·1).
Nutritional supplement.

Alpadinal *Alpharma, Mex.*
Naphazoline (p.1095·1).
Nasal congestion.

Alpagelle *Pharmadeveloppement, Fr.*
Miristalkonium chloride (p.1151·2).
Contraceptive.

Alpare *Stallergenes, Ital.*
An allergen extract (p.1575·3).
Hyposensitisation.

I-Alpha *Leo, Belg.*
Alfacalcidol (p.1391·1).
Hypoparathyroidism; osteoporosis; renal osteodystrophy; rickets.

Alpha VIII *Alpha Therapeutic, UK†.*
A factor VIII preparation (p.734·1).
Formerly known as Profilate HT and Profilate-SD.
Factor VIII deficiency.

Alpha Cade *Dermoteca, Port.*
Salicylic acid (p.1122·3); cade oil (p.1124·3); cedar oil.
Psoriasis; seborrhoeic dermatitis.

Alpha D3 *Teva, Hong Kong; Teva, Israel; Teva, Ital.; Teva, Singapore; Teva, Thai.*
Alfacalcidol (p.1391·1).
Hyperparathyroidism; hypoparathyroidism; neonatal hypocalcaemia; osteomalacia; osteoporosis; renal osteodystrophy; rickets.

Alpha Fraction *Dome-Hollister-Stier, Fr.*
Modified coca extract (p.1575·3).
Hyposensitisation.

Alpha Keri
Note.This name is used for preparations of different composition.
Bristol-Myers, Austral.; Bristol-Myers Squibb, Canad.; Bristol-Myers Squibb, Hong Kong; Bristol-Myers Squibb, NZ; Westwood, Singapore; Bristol-Myers Squibb, UK; Westwood, USA.
Bath oil: Liquid paraffin (p.1407·1); lanolin oil (p.1410·3).
Bath additive; dry skin disorders; pruritus.

Bristol-Myers Squibb, Canad.
Soap: Glycerol (p.1616·3).

Alpha Keri Silky Smooth *Bristol-Myers, Austral.†*
Vitamin E (p.1393·3).
Emollient.

Alpha Keri Tar *Bristol-Myers.*
Bath oil: Coal tar (p.1125·1); oil-soluble, dewaxed lanolin fraction (p.1410·3); liquid paraffin (p.1407·1).
Bath additive; skin disorders.
Shampoo: Coal tar (p.1125·1); salicylic acid (p.1122·3); sulfur (p.1123·3).
Scalp disorders.
Topical gel: Coal tar (p.1125·1).
Skin disorders.

Alpha Septol *Dermoteca, Port.*
Pyrithione zinc (p.1122·1); piroctone olamine (p.1121·1); salicylic acid (p.1122·3).
Seborrhoeic dermatitis.

Alpha UV *LED, Fr.*
SPF 15; SPF 30: Butyl methoxycinnamate methane (p.1516·3); octinoxate (p.1517·3); titanium dioxide (p.1126·1).
Sunscreen.

Alpha-Amoxyclav *Alpha, NZ.*
Amoxicillin trihydrate (p.149·2); potassium clavulanate (p.187·2).
Bacterial infections.

Alpha-Apoplectal *Klinge, Aust.†*
Sodium aescinate (p.1574·1); etofylline (p.765·1).
Cerebrovascular disorders.

Alphacaine *SPAD, Fr.*
Articaine hydrochloride (p.1306·1).
Adrenaline [epinephrine] hydrochloride (p.829·2) is included in this preparation as a vasoconstrictor to diminish absorption and localise the effect of the local anaesthetic.
Local anaesthesia.

Alpha-Chymocutan *Strathmann, Ger.†*
Chymotrypsin (p.1595·1).
Soft tissue inflammation and oedema.

Alpha-Chymotrase Strathmann, Ger.†
Chymotrypsin (p.1595·1).
Respiratory-tract disorders; soft tissue inflammation and oedema.

Alphacin Alphapharm, Austral.
Ampicillin trihydrate (p.151·1).
Bacterial infections.

Alphacortison Procter & Gamble, Neth.†
Hydrocortisone (p.1073·3); urea (p.1127·3).
Skin disorders.

Alphacutanee Leurquin, Fr.
Chymotrypsin (p.1595·1).
Oedema.

Alpha-Depressan OPW, Ger.†
Urapidil (p.987·3).
Hypertension.

Alphaderm
Procter & Gamble, Belg.†; Procter & Gamble, Irl.; Procter & Gamble, UK.
Hydrocortisone (p.1073·3); urea (p.1127·3).
Skin disorders.

Alphadrate Procter & Gamble, Neth.†
Urea (p.1127·3).
Dry skin disorders.

Alphaflam Lichtenstein, Ger.
Thioctic acid (p.1671·3).
Diabetic polyneuropathy.

Alphagan
Allergan, Aust.; Allergan, Austral.; Allergan, Belg.; Allergan, Canad.; Allergan, Denm.; Allergan, Fin.; Allergan, Fr.; Allergan, Ger.; Allergan, Hong Kong; Allergan, Irl.; Allergan, Israel; Allergan, Ital.; Allergan, Mex.; Allergan, NZ; Allergan, Port.; Allergan, S.Afr.; Allergan, Singapore; Allergan, Spain; Allergan, Swed.; Allergan, Switz.; Allergan, Thai.; Allergan, UK; Allergan, USA.
Brimonidine tartrate (p.851·2).
Glaucoma; ocular hypertension.

Alphaglobin
Alpha Therapeutic, Ger.†; Grifols, Ital.
A normal immunoglobulin (p.1551·3).
Chronic lymphocytic leukaemia; idiopathic thrombocytopenic purpura; immunodeficiencies; passive immunisation.

Alphakinase Alpha Therapeutic, Ger.†
Urokinase (p.988·1).
Thromboembolic disorders.

Alpha-Lipon Stada, Ger.
Thioctic acid (p.1671·3).
Diabetic polyneuropathy.

Alphamex Pharmagen, S.Afr.†
Methyldopa (p.927·3).
Hypertension.

Alphamox Alphapharm, Austral.
Amoxicillin trihydrate (p.149·2).
Bacterial infections.

Alphanate
Alpha, Hong Kong; Grifols, Ital.; Alpha Therapeutic, Singapore; Alpha Therapeutic, Thai.; Alpha Therapeutic, UK; Alpha Therapeutic, USA.
A factor VIII preparation (p.734·1).
Haemorrhagic disorders.

Alphane Bailleul, Fr.†
Zinc sulfate (p.1398·2); pyridoxine hydrochloride (p.1386·3).
Seborrhoea.

Alphanine
Alpha Therapeutic, Ger.†; Grifols, Ital.; Alpha Therapeutic, Singapore; Alpha Therapeutic, UK; Alpha Therapeutic, USA.
Factor IX (p.735·1).
Factor IX deficiency.

Alphaparin Grifols, UK.
Certoparin sodium (p.856·2).
Venous thromboembolism prophylaxis.

Alphapress
Alphapharm, Austral.; Unipharm, Israel.
Hydralazine hydrochloride (p.905·3).
Hypertension.

Alphapril Alphapharm, Austral.
Enalapril maleate (p.883·3).
Heart failure; hypertension.

Alphastria Inpharzam, Switz.
Sodium hyaluronate (p.1620·1); vitamin A palmitate (p.1383·2); alpha tocoferil acetate (p.1394·1); dexpanthenol (p.1602·3); allantoin (p.1110·1); camphor (p.1589·3); menthol (p.1632·3).
Prevention of skin striae.

Alphatrex Savage, USA.
Betamethasone dipropionate (p.1063·2).
Skin disorders.

Alphavase Ashbourne, UK.
Prazosin hydrochloride (p.958·1).

alpha-Vibolex Chephasaar, Ger.
Thioctic acid (p.1671·3).
Diabetic polyneuropathy.

Alphexine Lilly, Fr.
Cefaclor (p.161·1).
Bacterial infections.

Alphintern Leurquin, Fr.†
Chymotrypsin (p.1595·1); trypsin (p.1675·3).
Oedema.

Alphosyl
Note.This name is used for preparations of different composition.
Sanova, Aust.; Block, Aust.; Stafford-Miller, Austral.; Stafford-Miller Continental, Belg.†; Reed & Carnrick, Canad.; Stafford-Miller, Fin.; Stafford-Miller, Fr.; Stafford-Miller, Irl.; Stafford-Miller, Israel; Stafford-

Miller, Port.; Searle, S.Afr.; Stafford-Miller, Spain; Meda, Swed.; Stafford-Miller, Switz.; Stafford-Miller, UK.
Allantoin (p.1110·1); coal tar (p.1125·1).
Psoriasis.

Stafford-Miller, Austral.; Stafford-Miller, Spain.
Shampoo: Coal tar (p.1125·1).
Scalp disorders.

Alphosyl 2 in 1
Stafford-Miller, Israel; Stafford-Miller, UK.
Coal tar (p.1125·1).
Scalp disorders.

Alphosyl HC
Stafford-Miller, Irl.; Stafford-Miller, Israel; Stafford-Miller, Port.; Stafford-Miller, UK.
Allantoin (p.1110·1); coal tar (p.1125·1); hydrocortisone (p.1073·3).
Psoriasis.

Alphosyle Monsanto, Ital.
Allantoin (p.1110·1); coal tar (p.1125·1).
Psoriasis.

Alpicort
Note.This name is used for preparations of different composition.
Montavit, Aust.
Prednisolone (p.1077·3); salicylic acid (p.1122·3); coal tar (p.1125·1); colloidal sulfur (p.1123·3); thymol (p.1158·3).
Scalp disorders.

Cimex, Switz.
Prednisolone (p.1077·3); salicylic acid (p.1122·3).
Scalp disorders.

Alpicort F Cimex, Switz.
Prednisolone (p.1077·3); salicylic acid (p.1122·3); estradiol benzoate (p.1473·1).
Scalp disorders.

Alpicort F neu Wolff, Ger.
Prednisolone (p.1077·3); salicylic acid (p.1122·3); estradiol benzoate (p.1473·1).
Hair loss.

Alpicort N Wolff, Ger.
Prednisolone (p.1077·3); salicylic acid (p.1122·3).
Scalp disorders.

Alpin Arlex, Mex.
Hyoscine butylbromide (p.468·2).

Alpina Gel a la consoude Alpinamed, Switz.†
Comfrey (p.1598·3); hypericum (p.290·2); calendula (p.1589·2); spearmint (p.1666·3); echinacea purpurea (p.1606·2).
Soft-tissue injury.

Alpina Gel a l'arnica avec spilanthes Alpinamed, Switz.†
Arnica (p.1581·3); spilantes oleracea.
Musculoskeletal and joint pain; soft-tissue disorders.

Alpina Pommade au souci Alpinamed, Switz.†
Calendula (p.1589·2); calendula oil (p.1589·2).
Burns; wounds.

Alpirex Berman, Mex.
Paracetamol (p.71·2).
Fever; pain.

Alpoxen
Alpharma, Denm.; Alpharma, Fin.; Alpharma, Norw.; Dumex-Alpharma, Swed.
Naproxen (p.60·3).
Fever; gout; inflammation; musculoskeletal and joint disorders; pain.

Alpralid
CTI, Israel; Dumex-Alpharma, Swed.†
Alprazolam (p.654·2).
Anxiety; panic disorders.

Alpraz SMB, Belg.
Alprazolam (p.654·2).
Anxiety disorders; depression; nervous tension.

Alpress Pfizer, Fr.
Prazosin hydrochloride (p.958·1).
Hypertension.

Alprim
Alphapharm, Austral.; Alphapharm, Singapore; Merck, Singapore.
Trimethoprim (p.264·2).
Bacterial infections of the urinary tract.

Alpronax Merck, Port.†
Alprazolam (p.654·2).
Anxiety disorders.

Alprostar Recordati, Ital.
Alprostadil alfadex (p.1440·1).
Thromboangiitis obliterans.

Alprox
Orion, Denm.; Orion, Fin.; Orion, Irl.; Orion, Israel.
Alprazolam (p.654·2).
Alcohol withdrawal syndrome; anxiety; panic attacks.

Alquen Allen, Spain.
Ranitidine hydrochloride (p.1245·2).
Acid aspiration; gastro-oesophageal reflux; peptic ulcer; Zollinger-Ellison syndrome.

Alrac Euroforma, Braz.
Aluminium hydroxide (p.1210·3); magnesium hydroxide (p.1233·1).
Gastrointestinal hyperacidity.

Alramucil Alra, USA†.
Psyllium hydrophilic mucilloid (p.1229·1).
Constipation.

Alramucil Instant Mix Alra, USA†.
Ispaghula (p.1229·1).

Alrex Bausch & Lomb, USA.
Loteprednol etabonate (p.1075·3).
Allergic conjunctivitis.

Alrheumun Logosys, Ger.†
Ketoprofen (p.47·3).
Gout; inflammation; musculoskeletal and joint disorders; pain.

Alrin Teva, Israel.
Oxymetazoline hydrochloride (p.1096·2).
Nasal congestion.

Alserine Samakeephaesaj, Thai.
Cimetidine (p.1216·3).
Gastric hyperacidity; gastro-oesophageal reflux; peptic ulcer; Zollinger-Ellison syndrome.

Alsicur Alsitan, Ger.†
Cucurbita (p.1601·1); cucurbita oil; pollen; centaury (p.1593·1); echinacea (p.1606·2); vitamin E (p.1393·3).
Urinary-tract disorders.

Alsidexten Lemery, Mex.
Diclofenac sodium (p.30·3).
Inflammation; pain.

Alsidrine Alsi, Canad.
Ammonium chloride (p.1085·2); cocillana (p.1087·2).

Alsilax Alsi, Canad.†
Magnesium sulfate (p.1191·1); cascara (p.1216·1); boldo (p.1585·3); pancreatin (p.1646·1); peptone.

Alsiline Alsi, Canad.
Aloin (p.1210·2); cascara (p.1216·1); phenolphthalein (p.1244·1); bile salts (p.1585·1).

Alsimine with Vitamins A & D Alsi, Canad.
Multivitamins with calcium and iron (p.1350·1).

Alsiphene Alsi, Canad.
Paracetamol (p.71·2).

Alsiroyal Alsitan, Ger.†
Royal jelly (p.1659·3); vitamin E (p.1393·3); ginseng (p.1615·3).
Tonic.

Alsirub Alsi, Canad.
Methyl salicylate (p.55·1); menthol (p.1632·3); eucalyptol (p.1609·2).

Alsogil Also, Ital.
Suppositories†: Aspirin (p.14·2); paracetamol (p.71·2).
Tablets: Aspirin (p.14·2); paracetamol (p.71·2); caffeine (p.761·3).
Cold symptoms; pain.

Alsol
Note.This name is used for preparations of different composition.
Athenstaedt, Ger.
Topical solution: Basic aluminium acetotartrate (p.1578·2).
Hyperhidrosis; soft-tissue injury.

Also, Ital.†
Cetylpyridinium chloride (p.1138·1).
Formerly contained bisdequalinium diacetate.
Mouth and throat infections.

Alsol N Athenstaedt, Ger.
Basic aluminium acetotartrate (p.1578·2).
Napkin rash; skin disorders; wounds.

Alsoy
Nestle, Braz.; Nestle, Canad.; Nestle, Ital.; Nestle, Thai.
Soya infant feed (p.1350·1).
Cow's milk intolerance; lactose intolerance.

Alsucral Orion, Fin.
Sucralfate (p.1250·2).
Gastro-oesophageal reflux; peptic ulcer.

Altace
Hoechst Marion Roussel, Canad.; Monarch, USA.
Ramipril (p.966·3).
Heart failure following myocardial infarction; hypertension; primary prophylaxis of atherosclerotic complications.

Altacet Hoechst Marion Roussel, Swed.†
Hydrotalcite (p.1228·1).
Gastrointestinal disorders.

Altacite
Hoechst Marion Roussel, Irl.†; Hoechst Marion Roussel, S.Afr.†; Peckforton, UK†.
Hydrotalcite (p.1228·1).
Gastrointestinal hyperacidity.

Altacite Plus
Hoechst Marion Roussel, Irl.†; Peckforton, UK.
Hydrotalcite (p.1228·1); simeticone (p.1249·2).
These ingredients can be described by the British Approved Name Co-simalcite.
Gastrointestinal disorders.

Altan Rottapharm, Ital.
Promelase (p.1655·1).
Respiratory-system disorders.

Altat Teikoku, Jpn.
Roxatidine acetate hydrochloride (p.1248·1).
Gastritis; gastro-oesophageal reflux; gastrointestinal haemorrhage; peptic ulcer; premedication; Zollinger-Ellison syndrome.

Altemol Andromaco, Mex.
Interferon alfa-n3 (p.628·1).
Anogenital warts.

Alten
Medochemie, Hong Kong; Medochemie, Singapore.
Tretinoin (p.1126·2).
Acne.

Alteporina Alter, Spain.
Cefminox sodium (p.167·3).
Bacterial infections.

Alter-H$_2$ Carter-Wallace, Mex.
Ranitidine hydrochloride (p.1245·2).
Gastro-oesophageal reflux; peptic ulcer; Zollinger-Ellison syndrome.

Alrheumun — see above column.

Alterna GEL J&J-Merck, USA.
Dried aluminium hydroxide gel (p.1210·3).
Hyperacidity symptoms.

Altesona Farmabion, Spain.
Cortisone acetate (p.1065·3).
Corticosteroid.

Althaea Complex Blackmores, Austral.
Maize (p.1599·3); althaea (p.1577·1); buchu (p.1587·2); bearberry (p.1583·3); d-alpha tocoferil acid succinate (p.1394·1); vitamin A acetate (p.1383·2).
Urinary-tract disorders.

Altiazem
Lusofarmaco, Hong Kong; Lusofarmaco, Ital.; Menarini, Singapore; Menarini, Thai.
Diltiazem hydrochloride (p.874·3).
Angina pectoris; hypertension; myocardial infarction.

Alti-CPA Altimed, Canad.
Cyproterone acetate (p.1467·3).

Altim Roussel Diamant, Fr.
Cortivazol (p.1066·1).
Corticosteroid.

Alti-MPA Altimed, Canad.
Medroxyprogesterone acetate (p.1480·1).

Altinac Upsher-Smith, USA.
Tretinoin (p.1126·2).
Acne.

Altior Pensa, Spain.
Ibuprofen (p.43·2).
Fever; pain.

Altocel Irex, Fr.
Loperamide hydrochloride (p.1231·3).
Diarrhoea.

Altodor OM, Ger.
Etamsylate (p.732·2).
Haemorrhagic disorders.

Altone Pharmasant, Thai.
Spironolactone (p.973·2).
Heart failure; liver cirrhosis with ascites; oedema.

Altosone Formenti, Ital.; Essex, Ital.
Mometasone furoate (p.1077·2).
Skin disorders.

Altracart II Althin, Swed.†
Sodium bicarbonate (p.1184·1).
Haemodialysis.

Altramet
Asta Medica, Ger.; Lek, Hong Kong.
Cimetidine (p.1216·3) or cimetidine hydrochloride (p.1218·3).
Aspiration syndromes; gastro-oesophageal reflux; gastrointestinal hyperacidity; gastrointestinal haemorrhage; hypersensitivity reactions; peptic ulcer; Zollinger-Ellison syndrome.

Altruline Pfizer, Mex.
Sertraline hydrochloride (p.308·3).
Depression; mixed anxiety depressive states; obsessive-compulsive disorder.

Alu-3 Germania, Aust.
Aluminium tyrosinate.
Gastrointestinal disorders; hyperphosphataemia.

Alubifar Rottapharm, Spain.
Almasilate (p.1210·1).
Dyspepsia; gastritis; gastro-oesophageal reflux; peptic ulcer.

Alubron-Saar CPF, Ger.
Aluminium chloride (p.1110·2).
Mouth and throat inflammation.

Alu-Cap
3M, Israel; 3M, UK; 3M, USA.
Aluminium hydroxide (p.1210·3).
Gastric hyperacidity; hyperphosphataemia; peptic ulcer.

Alucid Labima, Belg.
Aluminium glycinate (p.1210·3); calcium carbonate (p.1215·1); magnesium trisilicate (p.1233·3); sodium bicarbonate (p.1186·2).
Gastrointestinal disorders.

Alucol
Sanova, Aust.; Novartis Consumer, Switz.
Dried aluminium hydroxide gel (p.1210·3); magnesium hydroxide (p.1233·1).
Gastric hyperacidity; gastric irritation; gastro-oesophageal reflux.

Alucol Silicona Novartis Consumer, Spain†.
Aluminium hydroxide (p.1210·3); dimethicone (p.1249·2); magnesium hydroxide (p.1233·1).
Gastrointestinal hyperacidity and flatulence.

Aluctyl Monal, Fr.†; Yamanouchi, Ital.
Aluminium lactate (p.1578·2).
Mouth and throat disorders.

Aludrox
Note.This name is used for preparations of different composition.
Wyeth, Ger.; Pfizer Consumer, Irl.; Pfizer Consumer, UK.
Aluminium hydroxide (p.1210·3).
Gastritis; gastrointestinal hyperacidity; heartburn; hyperphosphataemia; peptic ulcer.

Pfizer Consumer, UK.
Tablets: Aluminium hydroxide-magnesium carbonate co-dried gel (p.1211·2); magnesium hydroxide (p.1233·1).
Dyspepsia; hyperphosphataemia.

Wyeth-Ayerst, USA.
Aluminium hydroxide (p.1210·3); magnesium hydroxide (p.1233·1); simeticone (p.1249·2).
Hyperacidity.

Alugel *Atlas, Canad.; Pharmacia Upjohn, Spain.*
Aluminium hydroxide (p.1210·3).
Formerly known as Alugelibys in *Spain.*
Dyspepsia; gastritis; gastro-oesophageal reflux; gastrointestinal hyperacidity; hyperphophataemia.

Alugel Magnesiado *Pharmacia Upjohn, Spain.*
Chewable tablets: Aluminium hydroxide (p.1210·3); magnesium oxide (p.1233·2).
Oral suspension: Aluminium hydroxide (p.1210·3); magnesium hydroxide (p.1233·1).
Formerly known as Alugelibys Magnesiado.
Dyspepsia; gastrointestinal hyperacidity.

Alukon *Apotex, S.Afr.†.*
Aluminium hydroxide (p.1210·3).
Gastric hyperacidity.

Alum Milk *Hoechst Marion Roussel, Thai.*
Aluminium hydroxide (p.1210·3); magnesium hydroxide (p.1233·1).
Dyspepsia; peptic ulcer.

Alumadrine *Fleming, USA†.*
Phenylpropanolamine hydrochloride (p.1098·1); chlorpheniramine [chlorphenamine] maleate (p.412·1); paracetamol (p.71·2).
Upper respiratory-tract symptoms.

Alu-Mag *Kanda, Braz.*
Aluminium hydroxide (p.1210·3); magnesium hydroxide (p.1233·1).
Gastrointestinal hyperacidity.

Alumag *Trianon, Canad.; Teva, Israel.*
Aluminium hydroxide (p.1210·3); magnesium hydroxide (p.1233·1).
Flatulence; gastrointestinal hyperacidity; peptic ulcer.

Alumagall *Interdelta, Switz.*
Dried aluminium hydroxide gel (p.1210·3); magnesium hydroxide (p.1233·1); allantoin (p.1110·1).
Gastric hyperacidity.

Aluminium Free Indigestion *Larkhall Laboratories, UK†.*
Calcium carbonate (p.1215·1); cinnamon (p.1595·3); nutmeg (p.1643·1); clove (p.1596·3); cardamom seed (p.1591·3).

Alumite *Xixia, S.Afr.*
Dicyclomine [dicycloverine] hydrochloride (p.466·1); aluminium hydroxide (p.1210·3); magnesium oxide (p.1233·2).
Gastrointestinal disorders.

Alupent *Boehringer Ingelheim, Aust.; Boehringer Ingelheim, Austral.; Boehringer Ingelheim, Belg.†; Boehringer Ingelheim, Canad.; Boehringer Ingelheim, Fr.†; Boehringer Ingelheim, Ger.; Boehringer Ingelheim, Irl.; Boehringer Ingelheim, Ital.; Promeco, Mex.; Boehringer Ingelheim, Neth.†; Boehringer Ingelheim, NZ; Boehringer Ingelheim, S.Afr.; Boehringer Ingelheim, Spain; Boehringer Ingelheim, Switz.†; Boehringer Ingelheim, Thai.; Boehringer Ingelheim, UK; Boehringer Ingelheim, USA.*
Orciprenaline sulfate (p.769·1).
Arrhythmias; beta blocker overdosage; digitalis intoxication; obstructive airways disease; Stokes-Adams syndrome.

Alupent Expectorant *Boehringer Ingelheim, Irl.*
Orciprenaline sulfate (p.769·1); bromhexine hydrochloride (p.1085·3).
Obstructive airways disease.

Alupir *Pharma Line, Ital.*
Aluminium aspirin (p.13·3).
Cold symptoms; musculoskeletal disorders; neuritis.

Aluprim *Zimaia, Port.†.*
Aluminium aspirin (p.13·3).
Fever; pain.

Alurate *Roche, USA†.*
Aprobarbital (p.656·1).
Insomnia; sedative.

Alusil *Salters, S.Afr.*
Magnesium trisilicate (p.1233·3); aluminium hydroxide (p.1210·3).
Gastrointestinal hyperacidity.

Alusorb *DHA, Singapore.*
Dried aluminium hydroxide gel (p.1210·3); simeticone (p.1249·2).
Flatulence; gastric hyperacidity; heartburn; peptic ulcer.

Alu-Tab *3M, Austral.; 3M, Canad.; 3M, Hong Kong; 3M, Singapore; 3M, USA.*
Aluminium hydroxide (p.1210·3).
Gastric hyperacidity; hyperphosphataemia; peptic ulcer.

Alutabs *3M, NZ.*
Aluminium hydroxide (p.1210·3).
Gastric hyperacidity; hyperphosphataemia; peptic ulcer.

Alutard *ALK, Norw.*
Allergen extracts from timothy (*Phleum pratense*) or birch (*Betula verrucosa*) (p.1575·3).
Hyposensitisation.

Alutard SQ
ALK, Denm.; ALK, Fin.; ALK, Swed.; Trimedal, Switz.
Allergen extracts (p.1575·3).
Hyposensitisation.

Alutop *General Drugs, Thai.*
Oral gel: Dried aluminium hydroxide gel (p.1210·3); magnesium hydroxide (p.1233·1); simeticone (p.1249·2).
Flatulence; gastric hyperacidity; peptic ulcer.

Tablets: Dried aluminium hydroxide gel (p.1210·3); magnesium hydroxide (p.1233·1).
Gastric hyperacidity; peptic ulcer.

Aluzime *Alter, Spain†.*
Coenzyme A (p.1598·1).
Glomerular kidney disease; metabolic disorders.

Alvadermo Fuerte *Inexfa, Spain.*
Fluocinolone acetonide (p.1071·1).
Skin disorders.

Alvear *Whitehall, Ital.*
Royal jelly (p.1659·3).
Nutritional supplement.

Alvear Complex *Whitehall, Ital.*
Royal jelly (p.1659·3); pollen; dried yeast (p.1398·1); lactic-acid-producing organisms (p.1626·3).
Nutritional supplement.

Alvear Sport *Whitehall, Ital.†.*
Yellow capsules: royal jelly (p.1659·3); pollen; red capsules: ginkgo biloba (p.1615·2); myrtillus (p.1639·2); tablets: glucose (p.1364·1); royal jelly.
Nutritional supplement.

Alvedon *Astra, Norw.†; Astra, Swed.; Novex Pharma, UK.*
Paracetamol (p.71·2).
Fever; pain.

Alven *Wassermann, Ital.*
Diosmin (p.1611·1).
Peripheral vascular disorders.

Alveofact
Boehringer Ingelheim, Aust.; Boehringer de Angeli, Braz.; Boehringer Ingelheim, Ger.; Boehringer Ingelheim, Ital.†.
Bovactant (p.1656·1).
Neonatal respiratory distress syndrome.

Alveolex *Klinge, Irl.*
Acetylcysteine (p.1082·3).
Cystic fibrosis; respiratory-tract disorders with excess or viscous mucus.

Alveoten *Ibi, Ital.*
Neltenexine (p.1095·3).
Respiratory-tract disorders.

Alvercol
Norgine, Austral.; Norgine, Hong Kong; Norgine, Irl.; Norgine, S.Afr.
Sterculia (p.1250·2); alverine citrate (p.1211·3).
Formerly known as Normacol Antispasmodic in *S.Afr.*
Hypertonic constipation; irritable bowel syndrome.

Alvesin *Berlin-Chemie, Ger.*
Amino-acid and electrolyte infusion (p.1350·1).
Parenteral nutrition.

Alvidina *Farcoral, Mex.*
Ranitidine hydrochloride (p.1245·2).
Peptic ulcer; Zollinger-Ellison syndrome.

Alvityl *Solvay, Fr.*
Multivitamin preparation (p.1350·1).

Alvofact
Boehringer Ingelheim, Belg.; Boehringer Ingelheim, Neth.; Boehringer Ingelheim, Thai.
Bovactant (p.1656·1).
Neonatal respiratory distress syndrome.

Alvogil *Prats, Spain.*
Butyl aminobenzoate (p.1308·2); eugenol (p.1609·3); iodoform (p.1149·1).

Alvogyl *Septodont, Switz.*
Butyl aminobenzoate (p.1308·2); iodoform (p.1149·1); eugenol (p.1609·3); spearmint oil (p.1666·3); penghawar djambi fibra.
Pain following tooth extraction.

Alxen *Ofimex, Mex.*
Naproxen (p.60·3).

Alymphon *Iso, Ger.*
Homoeopathic preparation.

Alyostal *Stallergenes, Fr.; Stallergenes, Switz.*
A range of allergan extracts (p.1575·3).
Diagnosis of hypersensitivity; hyposensitisation.

Alyrane
Zeneca, Austral.; Pharmacia Upjohn, Belg.; Pharmacia Upjohn, Denm.†; Zeneca, Israel; Pharmacia Upjohn, Neth.; Zeneca, S.Afr.; Pharmacia Upjohn, Swed.†; Baxter, UK.
Enflurane (p.1258·1).
General anaesthesia.

Alzam *Parke-Med, S.Afr.*
Alprazolam (p.654·2).
Anxiety disorders.

Alzental *Shin Poong, Singapore.*
Albendazole (p.95·2).
Worm infections.

Alzol *Pharmasant, Thai.*
Albendazole (p.95·2).
Worm infections.

Alzolam *Sun, Singapore.*
Alprazolam (p.654·2).
Anxiety; mixed anxiety depressive states; panic disorders; phobias.

Alzomed-F *Farcoral, Mex.*
Benzonatate (p.1085·3).
Coughs.

AM Treatment *Avon, Canad.*
SPF 15: Octinoxate (p.1517·3); oxybenzone (p.1518·1).
Sunscreen.

Ama *Atlantic, Thai.*
Chlorpromazine hydrochloride (p.660·2); amobarbital (p.655·2).
Anxiety; psychoses; tension.

Amabagyl *Hoechst Marion Roussel, Mex.*
Diiodohydroxyquinoline (p.590·2).

Amacin *Asian Pharm, Thai.*
Amoxicillin trihydrate (p.149·2).
Bacterial infections.

Amacodone *Trimen, USA†.*
Hydrocodone tartrate (p.42·2); paracetamol (p.71·2).
Pain.

Amacone *Hua, Thai.*
Aluminium hydroxide (p.1210·3); magnesium hydroxide (p.1233·1) or magnesium trisilicate (p.1233·3); simeticone (p.1249·2).
Flatulence; gastric hyperacidity; peptic ulcer.

Amadol *TAD, Ger.; Asta Medica, Ger.*
Tramadol hydrochloride (p.89·1).
Pain.

Amagesan *PB, Ger.*
Amoxicillin trihydrate (p.149·2).
Bacterial infections.

Amalium *Janssen-Cilag, Aust.*
Flunarizine hydrochloride (p.418·1).
Migraine; vertigo.

Aman *Hexal, Ger.*
Amantadine (p.1162·2).
Drug-induced extrapyramidal disorders; influenza A; parkinsonism.

Amanta *ABZ, Ger.; Azupharma, Ger.*
Amantadine hydrochloride (p.1161·2) or amantadine sulfate (p.1161·2).
Influenza A; parkinsonism.

Amantagamma *Worwag, Ger.*
Amantadine hydrochloride (p.1161·2).
Drug-induced exptrapyramidal disorders; parkinsonism.

Amantan *Byk, Belg.*
Amantadine hydrochloride (p.1161·2).
Influenza A; parkinsonism.

Amaphen *Trimen, USA†.*
Paracetamol (p.71·2); caffeine (p.761·3); butalbital (p.658·3).
Pain.

Amaphen with Codeine *Trimen, USA.*
Codeine phosphate (p.25·2); paracetamol (p.71·2); caffeine (p.761·3); butalbital (p.658·3).
Pain.

Amara *Koch, Aust.*
Gentian tincture (p.1615·1); cinchona bark tincture (p.1595·3); absinthium tincture (p.1571·1).
Gastrointestinal disorders.

Amara-Tropfen *Weleda, Ger.*
Absinthium (p.1571·1); centaury (p.1593·1); gentian (p.1615·1); imperatoria; juniper (p.1625·2); achillea (p.1572·2); sage (p.1660·2); taraxacum (p.1669·1).
Gastrointestinal disorders.

Amara-Tropfen-Pascoe *Pascoe, Ger.*
Gentian (p.1615·1); cinchona bark (p.1595·3); absinthium (p.1571·1); cinnamon bark (p.1595·3).
Gastrointestinal disorders.

Amarel *Hoechst, Fr.*
Glimepiride (p.322·3).
Diabetes mellitus.

Amaro Medicinale *Giuliani, Ital.*
Rhubarb (p.1248·1); cascara (p.1216·1); gentian (p.1615·1); boldo (p.1585·3).
Gastrointestinal disorders.

Amaro Padil *Pfizer, Ital.*
Cascara (p.1216·1); gentian (p.1615·1).
Constipation.

Amaryl
Hoechst Marion Roussel, Aust.; Aventis, Austral.; Aventis, Denm.; Hoechst Marion Roussel, Fin.; Hoechst Marion Roussel, Ger.; Hoechst Marion Roussel, Hong Kong; Hoechst Marion Roussel, Irl.; Hoechst Marion Roussel, Ital.; Hoechst Marion Roussel, Mex.; Hoechst Marion Roussel, Neth.; Hoechst Marion Roussel, Norw.; Aventis, Port.; Aventis, S.Afr.; Hoechst Marion Roussel, Singapore; Hoechst Marion Roussel, Spain; Hoechst Marion Roussel, Swed.; Hoechst Marion Roussel, Switz.; Hoechst Marion Roussel, Thai.; Hoechst Marion Roussel, UK; Hoechst Marion Roussel, USA.
Glimepiride (p.322·3).
Diabetes mellitus.

Amarylle *Aventis, Belg.*
Glimepiride (p.322·3).
Diabetes mellitus.

Amasulin *Takeda, Jpn.*
Carumonam sodium (p.161·1).
Mepivacaine hydrochloride (p.1317·1) is included in the intramuscular injection to alleviate the pain of injection.
Bacterial infections.

Amatine *Roberts, Canad.*
Midodrine hydrochloride (p.933·3).
Idiopathic orthostatic hypotension.

Amazyl *Christiaens, Belg.†.*
Bismuth subnitrate (p.1213·2); magnesium trisilicate (p.1233·3); borax (p.1586·1).
Cracked nipples.

Ambacamp *Pharmacia Upjohn, Ger.*
Bacampicillin hydrochloride (p.155·1).
Bacterial infections.

Ambatrol *SmithKline Beecham, Fr.†.*
Nifuroxazide (p.230·2).
Diarrhoea.

Ambaxin *Pharmacia Upjohn, UK†.*
Bacampicillin hydrochloride (p.155·1).
Bacterial infections.

Ambaxino *Pharmacia Upjohn, Spain.*
Bacampicillin hydrochloride (p.155·1).
Bacterial infections.

Ambe 12 *Merckle, Ger.*
Cyanocobalamin (p.1388·1).
Vitamin B_{12} deficiency.

Amben *Medochemie, Hong Kong.*
Cefadroxil (p.161·2).
Bacterial infections.

Ambenat *Ratiopharm, Aust.*
Glycol salicylate (p.42·2); benzyl nicotinate (p.20·2); heparin sodium (p.902·1).
Muscle, nerve, and joint pain.

Ambene
Note.This name is used for preparations of different composition.
Ratiopharm, Aust.
Ampoule A, phenylbutazone sodium (p.78·3); sodium salamidacetate (p.81·3); dexamethasone (p.1067·1); ampoule B, cyanocobalamin (p.1388·1).
Lignocaine [lidocaine] hydrochloride (p.1313·2) is included in both ampoules to alleviate the pain of injection.
Arthritis; degenerative spinal disorders; neuralgias; neuritis.

Merckle, Ger.
Phenylbutazone (p.78·1) or phenylbutazone sodium (p.78·3).
Lignocaine [lidocaine] hydrochloride (p.1313·2) is included in the injection to alleviate the pain of injection.
Gout; musculoskeletal and joint disorders.

Ambene Comp *Merckle, Ger.*
Ampoule 1, phenylbutazone sodium (p.78·3); ampoule 2, cyanocobalamin (p.1388·1).
Lignocaine [lidocaine] hydrochloride (p.1313·2) is included in each ampoule to alleviate the pain of injection.
Gout; musculoskeletal and joint-disorders.

Ambene N
Note.This name is used for preparations of different composition.
Ratiopharm, Aust.
Suppositories: Phenylbutazone (p.78·1); cyanocobalamin (p.1388·1).
Tablets: Phenylbutazone (p.78·1); thiamine hydrochloride (p.1385·1); cyanocobalamin (p.1388·1).
Aluminium glycinate (p.1210·3) is included in this preparation in an attempt to limit adverse effects on the gastrointestinal mucosa.
Gout; musculoskeletal, joint, soft-tissue, and peri-articular disorders; neuritis; superficial thrombophlebitis.

Merckle, Ger.
Glycol salicylate (p.42·2); benzyl nicotinate (p.20·2).
Musculoskeletal, joint, and soft-tissue disorders.

Ambenyl *Parke, Davis, Canad.†.*
Codeine phosphate (p.25·2); bromazine hydrochloride (p.410·1); diphenhydramine hydrochloride (p.416·1); ammonium chloride (p.1085·2); sulfogaiacol (p.1101·1).
Coughs.

Ambenyl Cough Syrup *Forest Pharmaceuticals, USA.*
Codeine phosphate (p.25·2); bromazine hydrochloride (p.410·1).
Allergic upper respiratory symptoms; coughs and cold symptoms.

Ambenyl-D *Forest Pharmaceuticals, USA.*
Guaifenesin (p.1092·2); pseudoephedrine hydrochloride (p.1099·2); dextromethorphan hydrobromide (p.1087·3).
Coughs; nasal congestion.

Amber Gold *Larkhall Laboratories, UK.*
Melaleuca oil (p.1631·3).

Amberin *ACO, Swed.†.*
Hydrocortisone (p.1073·3).
Anogenital pruritus; eczema.

Ambezetal *Honorterapica, Braz.*
Ampicillin benzathine (p.151·2); ampicillin sodium (p.150·3).
Bacterial infections.

Ambi 10 *Kiwi, USA.*
Cream: Benzoyl peroxide (p.1111·1).
Acne.
Soap: Triclosan (p.1159·2).

Ambi Skin Tone *Kiwi, USA.*
Hydroquinone (p.1115·1); padimate O (p.1518·2).
Hyperpigmentation.

Ambien *Searle, USA.*
Zolpidem tartrate (p.712·2).
Insomnia.

Ambilan *Orion, Fin.*
Emollient.

Ambiosol *Solfran, Mex.*
Ampicillin (p.150·3).
Bacterial infections.

AmBisome
Fresenius Kabi, Aust.; Nexstar, Austral.; Nexstar, Belg.†; Nexstar, Denm.; Orphan, Fin.; Nexstar, Fr.; Nexstar, Ger.; Nexstar, Hong Kong; Nexstar, Irl.; Nexstar, Israel; Nexstar, Ital.; Baxter, NZ; Nexstar, Spain; Swedish Orphan, Swed.; Fresenius Kabi, Switz.; Nexstar, Thai.; Nexstar, UK; Fujisawa, USA.
Liposomal amphotericin B (p.377·2).
Fungal infections; leishmaniasis.

Ambi-Wolff *Wolff, Ger.*
Barrier cream.

Ambodil *Arlex, Mex.*
Ambroxol (p.1084·3).

Amboneural *Merck, Aust.; Arcana, Aust.*
Selegiline hydrochloride (p.1177·2).
Parkinsonism.

Ambotetra *Gilag, Mex.*
Tetracycline hydrochloride (p.258·3).
Bacterial infections.

Ambra Med Complex *Dynamit, Aust.*
Homoeopathic preparation.

Ambral *Beige, S.Afr.*
Metronidazole (p.594·1).
Amoebiasis; anaerobic bacterial infections; giardiasis; trichomoniasis.

Ambramicina *Scharper, Ital.; Marion Merrell, Spain†.*
Tetracycline hydrochloride (p.258·3).
Bacterial infections.

Ambra-Sinto T *Medley, Braz.*
Tetracycline hydrochloride (p.258·3).
Bacterial infections.

Ambre Solaire *Garnier, UK.*
Avobenzone (p.1517·1); enzacamene (p.1517·2); terephthalylidene dicamphor sulfonic acid; titanium dioxide (p.1126·1).
Sunscreen.

Ambredin *Solco, Aust.*
Theophylline (p.777·2); aceverine hydrochloride; octodrine phosphate (p.949·2).
Obstructive airways disease.

Ambril *Cascan, Ger.; Glaxo Wellcome, Ger.*
Ambroxol hydrochloride (p.1084·3).
Respiratory-tract disorders associated with increased or viscous mucus.

Ambritan *Daker Farmasimes, Spain†.*
Cobamamide (p.1388·3).
Tonic.

Ambro *ABZ, Ger.*
Ambroxol hydrochloride (p.1084·3).
Respiratory-tract disorders with viscous mucus.

Ambrobene *Ratiopharm, Aust.*
Ambroxol hydrochloride (p.1084·3).
Respiratory-tract disorders with viscous mucus.

Ambrobeta *Betapharm, Ger.*
Ambroxol hydrochloride (p.1084·3).
Respiratory-tract disorders with viscous mucus.

Ambrodoxy *Hexal, Ger.*
Doxycycline hyclate (p.200·1); ambroxol hydrochloride (p.1084·3).
Respiratory-tract infections with increased or viscous mucus.

Ambrofur *Fustery, Mex.*
Ambroxol hydrochloride (p.1084·3).
Respiratory-tract disorders with viscous mucus.

Ambrohexal *Hexal, Ger.*
Ambroxol hydrochloride (p.1084·3).
Respiratory-tract disorders associated with increased or viscous mucus.

Ambrol *Shiwa, Thai.*
Ambroxol hydrochloride (p.1084·3).
Respiratory-tract disorders associated with increased or viscous mucus.

Ambrolan *Lannacher, Aust.*
Ambroxol hydrochloride (p.1084·3).
Respiratory-tract disorders.

Ambrolitic *Wasserman, Spain.*
Ambroxol hydrochloride (p.1084·3).
Respiratory-tract disorders.

Ambrolos *Hexal, Ger.*
Ambroxol hydrochloride (p.1084·3).
Respiratory-tract disorders.

Ambrolytic *Samakeephaesaj, Thai.*
Ambroxol hydrochloride (p.1084·3).
Respiratory-tract disorders associated with increased or viscous mucus.

Ambromucil *Malesci, Ital.*
Ambroxol acefyllinate (p.1084·3).
Obstructive airways disease.

Ambropp *Pulmopharm, Ger.*
Ambroxol hydrochloride (p.1084·3).
Respiratory-tract disorders with increased or viscous mucus.

Ambro-Puren *Isis Puren, Ger.*
Ambroxol hydrochloride (p.1084·3).
Respiratory-tract disorders with viscous mucus.

Ambroten *Marjan, Braz.*
Ambroxol (p.1084·3).
Respiratory-tract congestion.

Ambrowel *Welfer, Mex.*
Ambroxol (p.1084·3).

Ambrox *Nakorn, Thai.*
Ambroxol hydrochloride (p.1084·3).
Respiratory-tract disorders associated with increased or viscous mucus.

Ambroxol AL comp *Aliud, Ger.*
Ambroxol hydrochloride (p.1084·3); doxycycline hyclate (p.200·1).
Respiratory-tract infections.

Ambroxol comp *Ratiopharm, Ger.*
Ambroxol hydrochloride (p.1084·3); doxycycline hyclate (p.200·1).
Respiratory-tract infections.

Amchafibrin *Fides Rottapharm, Spain.*
Tranexamic acid (p.742·2).
Haemorrhage; hereditary angioedema.

Amciderm *Hermal, Ger.; Pharmasant, Thai.*
Amcinonide (p.1061·2).
Skin disorders.

Amcillin *Dumex, Thai.*
Ampicillin sodium (p.150·3) or ampicillin trihydrate (p.151·1).
Bacterial infections.

Amcinil *Crosara, Ital.*
Amcinonide (p.1061·2).
Skin disorders.

Amco *Polipharm, Thai.*
Magnesium trisilicate (p.1233·3); aluminium hydroxide (p.1210·3); magnesium hydroxide (p.1233·1); simeticone (p.1249·2).
Dyspepsia; flatulence; gastric hyperacidity; peptic ulcer.

Amcoral *Meiji, Jpn†.*
Amrinone (p.839·2).
Heart failure.

Amcort *Keene, USA.*
Triamcinolone diacetate (p.1080·2).
Corticosteroid.

Amc-Puren *Isis Puren, Ger.*
Amoxicillin trihydrate (p.149·2).
Bacterial infections.

AMD *Seroyal, Canad.*
Trace element preparation with vitamin C (p.1350·1).

AMD *NBF-Lanes, Ital.*
Lutein; betacarotene; vitamin C; vitamin E; nicotinic acid; licopene; carrot extract (p.1350·1).
Macular degeneration in the elderly.

Amdox-Puren *Isis Puren, Ger.*
Doxycycline hyclate (p.200·1); ambroxol hydrochloride (p.1084·3).
Respiratory-tract infections with increased or viscous mucus.

Ameblin *Degorts, Mex.*
Metronidazole benzoate (p.594·1).
Amoebiasis; anaerobic bacterial infections; giardiasis; trichomoniasis.

Amebysol *Rayere, Mex.*
Tinidazole (p.603·3).
Amoebiasis; giardiasis; trichomoniasis.

Amefin *Searle, Mex.*
Quinfamide.
Amoebiasis.

Amefur *Fustery, Mex.*
Quinfamide.
Amoebiasis.

Amekrin *Parke, Davis, Denm.; Parke, Davis, Fin.; Warner-Lambert, Norw.; Parke, Davis, Swed.*
Amsacrine (p.507·3).
Acute leukaemias.

Amen *Carnrick, USA.*
Medroxyprogesterone acetate (p.1480·1).
Abnormal uterine bleeding; secondary amenorrhoea.

Amender *Serral, Mex.*
Methyldopa (p.927·3).
Hypertension.

Amenox *Sanofi Winthrop, Mex.*
Quinfamide.
Amoebiasis.

Amerge *Glaxo Wellcome, Canad.; Glaxo Wellcome, USA.*
Naratriptan hydrochloride (p.454·3).
Migraine.

Americaine *Novartis Consumer, USA.*
Benzocaine (p.1306·2).
Anorectal disorders.

Americaine Anesthetic *Fisons, USA.*
Benzocaine (p.1306·2).
Local anaesthesia; lubrication.

Americaine First Aid *Fisons, USA.*
Benzocaine (p.1306·2); benzethonium chloride (p.1134·2).
Skin disorders.

Americaine Otic *Fisons, USA.*
Benzocaine (p.1306·2).
Pain and pruritus in otitis.

Ameride *Du Pont, Spain.*
Amiloride hydrochloride (p.835·1); hydrochlorothiazide (p.907·3).
Hepatic cirrhosis; hypertension; oedema.

Amerigel *Amerx, USA.*
Lotion: Oak (p.1643·2).
Nappy rash.
Ointment: Oak bark (p.1643·2); meadowsweet (p.1631·2); zinc acetate (p.1398·1).
Skin disorders.

Amermycin *Unison, Thai.*
Doxycycline (p.200·1).
Bacterial infections.

Amersan *Australpam, Aust.*
Agrimony herb (p.1574·3); achillea (p.1572·2); peppermint oil (p.1243·3); rose fruit (p.1389·3); berberis; black currant (p.1389·3); myrtillus (p.1639·3).
Liver and biliary tract disorders.

Amerscan DMSA *Nycomed Amersham, UK.*
Technetium-99m succimer (p.1451·1).
Radionuclide imaging of the kidney.

Amerscan Hepatate *Nycomed Amersham, UK.*
Technetium-99m colloidal tin (p.1451·1).
Radionuclide imaging of the liver and spleen.

Amerscan Medronate *Nycomed Amersham, UK.*
Technetium-99m medronate (p.1451·1).
Bone scintigraphy.

Amerscan Pentetate *Nycomed Amersham, UK.*
Technetium-99m pentetate (p.1451·1).
Assessment of renal function; radionuclide imaging of the brain and lungs; studies of gastro-oesophageal reflux and gastric emptying.

Amerscan Pulmonate *Nycomed Amersham, UK.*
Technetium-99m (p.1451·1) labelled albumin aggregates.
Scintigraphic imaging of the lung.

Amerscan Stannous *Nycomed Amersham, UK.*
Technetium-99m stannous medronate (p.1451·1).
Red blood cell labelling for blood pool scintigraphy.

Amertec *Nycomed Amersham, UK.*
Technetium-99m (p.1451·1) as sodium pertechnetate.
Radionuclide imaging.

Amesec *Lilly, S.Afr.†.*
Aminophylline hydrate (p.760·1); ephedrine hydrochloride (p.1090·1); amobarbital (p.655·2).
Asthma.

A-Methapred *Abbott, Israel; Abbott, USA.*
Methylprednisolone (p.1076·1) or methylprednisolone sodium succinate (p.1076·1).
Corticosteroid.

Ametic *Aspen, S.Afr.*
Metoclopramide hydrochloride (p.1235·2).
Gastrointestinal disorders.

Ametionin *Piam, Ital.*
Food for special diets (p.1350·1).
Homocystinuria.

Ametop *Smith & Nephew, Canad.; Smith & Nephew, NZ; Smith & Nephew, S.Afr.; Smith & Nephew Healthcare, UK.*
Amethocaine [tetracaine] (p.1305·2) or amethocaine [tetracaine] hydrochloride (p.1305·2).
Local anaesthesia.

Ametricid *Medix, Mex.*
Tinidazole (p.603·3).
Amoebiasis; giardiasis; trichomoniasis.

Ametycine *Sanofi Winthrop, Fr.; Biosyn, Ger.*
Mitomycin (p.558·1).
Malignant neoplasms.

Ameu *Democal, Switz.*
Omega-3 triglycerides (p.949·2).
Hyperlipidaemias.

Amfamox *Amrad, Austral.*
Famotidine (p.1225·3).
Gastro-oesophageal reflux; peptic ulcer; Zollinger-Ellison syndrome.

Amfipen *Yamanouchi, Irl.; Yamanouchi, UK.*
Ampicillin (p.150·3).
Bacterial infections.

Amfostat *Bristol-Myers Squibb, Mex.*
Amphotericin B (p.377·2).
Fungal infections.

Amgenal Cough *Goldline, USA.*
Bromazine hydrochloride (p.410·1); codeine phosphate (p.25·2).
Coughs and cold symptoms.

Amias *AstraZeneca, UK; Takeda, UK.*
Candesartan cilexetil (p.853·2).
Hypertension.

Amicaliq *Tanabe, Jpn.*
Amino-acid, carbohydrate, and electrolyte infusion (p.1350·1).
Parenteral nutrition.

Amicar *Lederle, Austral.; Wyeth-Ayerst, Canad.; Wyeth, Mex.; Wyeth, NZ; Wyeth, S.Afr.; Immunex, USA.*
Aminocaproic acid (p.724·3).
Fibrinolysis.

Amicasil *Pharmatex, Ital.*
Amikacin sulfate (p.148·1).
Bacterial infections.

Amicel *Salus, Ital.†.*
Econazole nitrate (p.382·3).
Fungal infections.

Amicic *Ciba Vision, Fr.; Ciba Vision, Switz.†.*
Amino-acid preparation (p.1350·1).
Corneal ulcers.

Amicla *Wyeth Lederle, Belg.; Wyeth, Neth.†.*
Amcinonide (p.1061·2).
Skin disorders.

Amiclair *Abatron, UK.*
Contact lens cleanser (p.1129·2).

Amiclav *Ashbourne, UK.*
Amoxicillin trihydrate (p.149·2); potassium clavulanate (p.187·2).
These ingredients can be described by the British Approved Name Co-amoxiclav.
Bacterial infections.

Amico *SIT, Ital.*
Amino-acid preparation with cobamamide (p.1350·1).
Tonic.

Amico-L *TO-Chemicals, Thai.*
Aluminium hydroxide (p.1210·3); magnesium hydroxide (p.1233·1); simeticone (p.1249·2).
Dyspepsia; flatulence; gastric hyperacidity; peptic ulcer.

Amicrobin *Quimifar, Spain.*
Norfloxacin (p.232·1).
Genito-urinary tract infections.

Amidal *Douglas, Austral.†.*
Amiloride hydrochloride (p.835·1).
Hepatic cirrhosis with ascites; hypertension; oedema.

Amidalin *QIF, Braz.*
Tyrothricin (p.267·1); benzocaine (p.1306·2).
Mouth and throat disorders.

Amidate *Abbott, USA.*
Etomidate (p.1259·2).
General anaesthesia.

Amidonal *PCR, Ger.*
Aprindine hydrochloride (p.841·1).
Arrhythmias.

Amidox *Berk, UK.*
Amiodarone hydrochloride (p.836·1).
Arrhythmias.

Amidrin *Fardi, Spain.*
Xylometazoline hydrochloride (p.1102·2).
Formerly contained ephedrine hydrochloride and sulfanilamide.
Nasal congestion; sinus congestion.

Ami-Drix *Amide, USA†.*
Pseudoephedrine sulfate (p.1099·3); dexbrompheniramine maleate (p.410·2).
Upper respiratory-tract symptoms.

Amiduret *Trommsdorff, Ger.†.*
Amiloride hydrochloride (p.835·1); hydrochlorothiazide (p.907·3).
Ascites; hypertension; oedema.

Amigdagen *Prodotti, Braz.*
Neomycin (p.228·1); tyrothricin (p.267·1); benzocaine (p.1306·2); menthol (p.1632·3).
Mouth and throat disorders.

Amigdalol *Delta, Braz.*
Tyrothricin (p.267·1); cetrimonium bromide (p.1137·3); vitamin C (p.1389·1); lignocaine [lidocaine] (p.1313·2).
Mouth and throat disorders.

Amigdamicin *Sedabel, Braz.*
Neomycin sulfate (p.228·1); tyrothricin (p.267·1); benzocaine (p.1306·2); menthol (p.1632·3).
Mouth and throat disorders.

Amigdobis *Chinoin, Mex.*
Acetic acid (p.1571·2).

Amigesic *Amide, USA.*
Salsalate (p.82·2).
Fever; inflammation; pain.

Amikafur *Fustery, Mex.*
Amikacin sulfate (p.148·1).
Bacterial infections.

Amikal *Gea, Denm.; Selena, Swed.†.*
Amiloride hydrochloride (p.835·1).
Hypertension; liver cirrhosis with ascites; oedema.

Amikalem *Lemery, Mex.*
Amikacin sulfate (p.148·1).
Bacterial infections.

Amikan *SoSe, Ital.*
Amikacin sulfate (p.148·1).
Bacterial infections.

Amikasol *Samakeephaesaj, Thai.*
Amikacin sulfate (p.148·1).
Bacterial infections.

Amikason's *Sons, Mex.*
Amikacin sulfate (p.148·1).
Bacterial infections.

Amikavi *Mavi, Mex.*
Amikacin sulfate (p.147·3).
Bacterial infections.

Amikayect *Grossman, Mex.*
Amikacin sulfate (p.148·1).
Bacterial infections.

Amikin *Bristol-Myers Squibb, Austral.; Cibran, Braz.; Bristol, Canad.; Bristol-Myers Squibb, Hong Kong; Bristol-Myers Squibb, Irl.; Bristol-Myers Squibb, Israel; Mead Johnson, Mex.; Bristol-Myers Squibb, NZ; Bristol-Myers Squibb, S.Afr.; Bristol-Myers Squibb, Singapore; Bristol-Myers Squibb, Thai.; Bristol-Myers Squibb, UK; Apothecon, USA.*
Amikacin sulfate (p.148·1).
Bacterial infections.

Amikine *Bristol-Myers Squibb, Switz.*
Amikacin sulfate (p.148·1).
Bacterial infections.

Amiklin *Bristol-Myers Squibb, Fr.*
Amikacin sulfate (p.148·1).
Bacterial infections.

Amilamont *Rosemont, UK.*
Amiloride hydrochloride (p.835·1).
Heart failure; hepatic cirrhosis with ascites; hypertension.

Amilco *Nycomed, Denm.; Baker Norton, Hong Kong; Baker Norton, Irl.; Baker Norton, UK.*
Amiloride hydrochloride (p.835·1); hydrochlorothiazide (p.907·3).
These ingredients can be described by the British Approved Name Co-amilozide.
Ascites; heart failure; hepatic cirrhosis; hypertension.

Amilhydrozide *Douglas, Thai.; TTN, Thai.*
Amiloride hydrochloride (p.835·1); hydrochlorothiazide (p.907·3).
Hepatic cirrhosis with ascites and oedema; hypertension; oedema.

The symbol † denotes a preparation no longer actively marketed

Amilide *Ranbaxy, Thai.*
Amiloride hydrochloride (p.835·1); hydrochlorothiazide (p.907·3).
Heart failure; hypertension.

Amilin *Hua, Thai.*
Ampicillin trihydrate (p.151·1).
Bacterial infections.

Amilit-IFI *IFI, Ital.*
Amitriptyline hydrochloride (p.273·3).
Depression.

Amilmaxco *Ashbourne, UK.*
Amiloride hydrochloride (p.835·1); hydrochlorothiazide (p.907·3).
These ingredients can be described by the British Approved Name Co-amilozide.
Ascites; heart failure; hypertension.

Amilo-basan *Schonenberger, Switz.*
Amiloride hydrochloride (p.835·1); hydrochlorothiazide (p.907·3).
Hypertension; liver cirrhosis with ascites; oedema.

Amilocomp beta *Betapharm, Ger.*
Amiloride hydrochloride (p.835·1); hydrochlorothiazide (p.907·3).
Hypertension; oedema.

Amiloferm *Nordic, Swed.*
Amiloride hydrochloride (p.835·1); hydrochlorothiazide (p.907·3).
Hypertension; liver cirrhosis with ascites; oedema.

Amilohyd *Gerard, Denm.†*
Amiloride (p.835·3); hydrochlorothiazide (p.907·3).
Hypertension; oedema.

Amiloretic *Aspen, S.Afr.*
Amiloride hydrochloride (p.835·1); hydrochlorothiazide (p.907·3).
Hypertension; oedema.

Amiloretik *Hexal, Aust.; Hexal, Ger.*
Amiloride hydrochloride (p.835·1); hydrochlorothiazide (p.907·3).
Hypertension; liver cirrhosis with ascites; oedema.

Amilorid comp *Genericon, Aust.; Heumann, Ger.; Ratiopharm, Ger.; Upsamedica, Switz.†.*
Amiloride hydrochloride (p.835·1); hydrochlorothiazide (p.907·3).
Hypertension; liver cirrhosis with ascites; oedema.

Amiloride Composto *Ratiopharm, Port.*
Amiloride hydrochloride (p.835·1); hydrochlorothiazide (p.907·3).

Amilorid/HCT *Aliud, Ger.; Atid, Ger.; Maurer, Ger.*
Amiloride hydrochloride (p.835·1); hydrochlorothiazide (p.907·3).
Hypertension; oedema.

Amilospare *Ashbourne, UK†.*
Amiloride hydrochloride (p.835·1).
Ascites; heart failure; hypertension.

Amilostad HCT *Stada, Aust.*
Amiloride hydrochloride (p.835·1); hydrochlorothiazide (p.907·3).
Hypertension; liver cirrhosis with ascites; oedema.

Amilothiazid *Isis Puren, Ger.†*
Amiloride hydrochloride (p.835·1); hydrochlorothiazide (p.907·3).
Hypertension; oedema.

Amilozid *CT, Ger.*
Amiloride hydrochloride (p.835·1); hydrochlorothiazide (p.907·3).
Hypertension; oedema.

Amimox *Tika, Norw.†; Tika, Swed.*
Amoxicillin (p.149·2) or amoxicillin trihydrate (p.149·2).
Bacterial infections; peptic ulcer associated with Helicobacter pylori.

Amin 21 *Italfarmacia, Ital.*
Amino-acid preparation with potassium (p.1350·1).
Nutritional supplement.

Amin-Aid *McGaw, NZ; R&D, USA.*
Preparation for enteral nutrition in renal failure (p.1350·1).

Amindan *Desitin, Ger.*
Selegiline hydrochloride (p.1177·2).
Parkinsonism.

Aminess
Recip, Denm.†; Pharmacia Upjohn, Neth.†; Clintec, USA.
Amino-acid infusion (p.1350·1).
Parenteral nutrition in renal impairment.

Pharmacia Upjohn, Hong Kong; Recip, Norw.; Recip, Swed.
Amino-acid preparation (p.1350·1).
Nutritional supplement in renal failure.

Aminess-N *Recip, Fin.; Pharmacia, Neth.†*
Amino-acid preparation (p.1350·1).
Dietary supplement.

Amineurin *Hexal, Ger.*
Amitriptyline hydrochloride (p.273·3).
Depression; pain.

Amino 3 *Fiori, Ital.*
Amino-acid preparation (p.1350·1).

Amino MS *Larkhall Laboratories, UK.*
Alanine (p.1353·3); lysine hydrochloride (p.1370·3); glutamic acid hydrochloride (p.1365·2); tyrosine (p.1381·3).

Amino PG *Cantassium Co., UK.*
Amino-acid and zinc preparation (p.1350·1).

Aminoblastin *Pharmacia, S.Afr.†.*
Aminoglutethimide (p.506·3).
Adrenocortical adenoma; breast cancer; Cushing's syndrome.

Amino-Cerv
Milex, Canad.; Milex, USA.
Cystine (p.1359·1); inositol (p.1623·3); methionine (p.1012·2); sodium propionate (p.393·2); urea (p.1127·3).
Cervicitis; post cauterisation; post conisation; post cryosurgery; postpartum cervical tears.

Aminocid *Faria, Braz.*
Dipyrone (p.34·1); thiamine (p.1385·2); pyridoxine (p.1387·1); cyanocobalamin (p.1388·1).
Neuritis.

Aminocont *Mundipharma, Fin.*
Aminophylline hydrate (p.760·1).
Obstructive airways disease.

Aminoefedrison NF *Columbia, Mex.*
Theophylline (p.777·2); ambroxol hydrochloride (p.1084·3).
Respiratory-tract disorders with viscous mucus.

Aminoflex *Braun, Switz.*
Amino-acid and electrolyte infusion (p.1350·1).
Parenteral nutrition.

Aminofluid *Otsuka, Jpn.*
Amino-acid, carbohydrate, and electrolyte infusion (p.1350·1).
Parenteral nutrition.

Aminofusin Hepar *Pharmacia Upjohn, Ger.*
Amino-acid and electrolyte infusion (p.1350·1).
Parenteral nutrition in liver disorders.

Aminofusin L kohlenhydratfrei *Fresenius Kabi, Aust.*
Amino-acid, electrolyte, and pyridoxine hydrochloride infusion (p.1350·1).
Parenteral nutrition.

Aminofusin N *Pharmacia Upjohn, Ger.*
Amino-acid, xylitol, and electrolyte infusion (p.1350·1).
Parenteral nutrition.

Aminofusin 10% Plus *Pharmacia Upjohn, Ger.*
Amino-acid and electrolyte infusion (p.1350·1).
Parenteral nutrition.

Aminogran
Faulding, Austral.; UCB, Irl.; Eurospital, Ital.; Pharmabroker, NZ; UCB, Swed.; UCB, UK.
Food for special diets (p.1350·1).
Phenylketonuria.

Aminogran Mineral Mixture
Faulding, Austral.; UCB, Irl.
Mineral preparation (p.1350·1).
Mineral supplement; phenylketonuria (in conjunction with Aminogran).

Aminoleban
Otsuka, Jpn; Thai Otsuka, Thai.
Amino-acid infusion (p.1350·1).
Chronic liver impairment; hepatic encephalopathy.

Aminoleban EN
Otsuka, Hong Kong; Otsuka, Jpn; Thai Otsuka, Thai.
Preparation for enteral nutrition (p.1350·1).
Hepatic encephalopathy; liver failure.

Aminolete *Tyson, USA†.*
Amino acid preparation (p.1350·1).

Aminomal
Malesci, Ital.
Elixir: Theophylline (p.777·2).

Tablets; injection; suppositories: Aminophylline (p.760·1).
Lignocaine [lidocaine] hydrochloride (p.1313·2) is included in the intramuscular injection to alleviate the pain of injection; lignocaine [lidocaine] (p.1313·2) is also included in the suppositories.
Obstructive airways disease.

Menarini, Switz.
Aminophylline (p.760·1).
Obstructive airways disease.

Aminomega *Larkhall Laboratories, UK.*
Amino-acid preparation (p.1350·1).

Aminomel *Baxter, Ger.*
Amino-acid infusion (p.1350·1).
Parenteral nutrition.

Amino-Mel baby *Leopold, Aust.†.*
Amino-acid infusion (p.1350·1).
Parenteral nutrition.

Aminomel E *Baxter, Ger.*
Amino-acid and electrolyte infusion (p.1350·1).
Parenteral nutrition.

Amino-Mel G *Fresenius Kabi, Aust.*
Amino-acid, electrolyte, and glucose infusion (p.1350·1).
Parenteral nutrition.

Amino-Mel hepa *Fresenius Kabi, Aust.*
Amino-acid and electrolyte infusion (p.1350·1).
Parenteral nutrition in liver disease.

Amino-Mel nephro *Fresenius Kabi, Aust.*
Amino-acid infusion (p.1350·1).
Parenteral nutrition in renal disease.

Aminomel nephro *Baxter, Ger.*
Amino-acid infusion (p.1350·1).
Parenteral nutrition in renal disease.

Amino-Mel optimal *Leopold, Aust.†.*
Amino-acid, carbohydrate, and electrolyte infusion (p.1350·1).
Parenteral nutrition.

Aminomel X-E *Baxter, Ger.*
Amino-acid, carbohydrate, and electrolyte infusion (p.1350·1).
Parenteral nutrition.

Amino-Min-D *Tyson, USA.*
Calcium with vitamin D and minerals (p.1350·1).
Calcium deficiency; dietary supplement.

Aminomine *Tyson, USA†.*
Amino acid preparation (p.1350·1).

Aminomix
Fresenius Kabi, Aust.; Fresenius Kabi, Fr.; Fresenius-Klinik, Ger.; Fresenius Kabi, Spain; Meda, Swed.†; Fresenius Kabi, Switz.
A range of amino-acid and carbohydrate infusions with or without electrolytes (p.1350·1).
Parenteral nutrition.

Fresenius Kabi, Neth.
Amino-acid and electrolyte infusion (p.1350·1).
Parenteral nutrition.

Amino-Opti-C *Tyson, USA.*
Lemon bioflavonoids (p.1611·1); rutoside (p.1611·2); hesperidin (p.1611·2); vitamin C (p.1389·3); rose hips (p.1389·3).
Capillary bleeding.

Amino-Opti-E *Tyson, USA†.*
Vitamin E (p.1393·3).
Vitamin E deficiency.

Aminopad
Fresenius Kabi, Aust.; Pharmacia Upjohn, Ger.
Amino-acid infusion (p.1350·1).
Parenteral nutrition.

Aminopan *UCB, Ger.*
Somatostatin acetate (p.1297·3).
Gastrointestinal haemorrhage; postoperative pancreatic disorders.

Aminoped *Fresenius, Braz.*
Amino-acid infusion (p.1350·1).
Parenteral nutrition.

Aminoplasmal
Braun, Aust.; Braun, Denm.; Braun, Fin.; Braun, Ger.; Braun, Hong Kong; Braun, Irl.†; Braun, Israel; Braun Melsungen, Ital.; Braun, Norw.; Braun, Port.; Braun, Singapore; Braun, Spain; Braun, Swed.; Braun, Thai.; Braun, UK.
A range of amino-acid infusions with or without electrolytes and glucose (p.1350·1).
Parenteral nutrition.

Aminoplex *Tyson, USA†.*
Amino acid preparation (p.1350·1).

Aminoplex 12 *Geistlich, UK.*
Amino acid and electrolyte infusion (p.1350·1).
Parenteral nutrition.

Aminoplex 24 *Geistlich, UK.*
Amino-acid infusion with or without electrolytes (p.1350·1).
Parenteral nutrition.

Aminopt *Sigma, Austral.*
Aminoacridine hydrochloride (p.1130·2).
Eye infections.

Aminoram *Torre, Ital.*
Food for special diets (p.1350·1).
Liver disorders.

Aminorell *Sanorell, Ger.†.*
Amino-acid and trace element preparation (p.1350·1).

Aminosol
Abbott, Mex.; Thai Otsuka, Thai.
Amino-acid infusion with or without electrolytes (p.1350·1).
Parenteral nutrition.

Aminostab *Fresenius Kabi, Fr.*
Amino-acid infusion (p.1350·1).
Parenteral nutrition.

Aminostasis *Tyson, USA†.*
Amino acid preparation (p.1350·1).

Aminosteril
Fresenius Kabi, Aust.; Fresenius, Braz.; Fresenius Kabi, Denm.; Orion, Fin.; Fresenius Kabi, Ger.; Alpha, Mex.; Mein, Spain; Fresenius Kabi, Switz.; Fresenius, Thai.; Fresenius, UK†.
A range of amino-acid infusions with or without carbohydrate or electrolytes (p.1350·1).
Parenteral nutrition.

Aminostress *Lofarе, Ital.*
Nutritional supplement (p.1350·1).

Aminosyn
Abbott, Canad.†; Abbott, USA.
A range of amino-acid infusions with or without glucose and electrolytes (p.1350·1).
Parenteral nutrition.

Aminotate *Tyson, USA†.*
Amino acid preparation (p.1350·1).

Aminotool *Volchem, Ital.*
Amino-acid preparation (p.1350·1).

Aminotox *Teuto, Braz.*
Adenosine (p.828·2); methionine (p.1012·2); betaine hydrochloride (p.1584·3); choline (p.1356·3); pyridoxine (p.1387·1).
Liver disorders.

Aminotrans *GHP, Thai.*
Amino-acid infusion (p.1350·1).
Parenteral nutrition.

Aminotril *Progest, Ital.*
Lotion: Triaminodil; vitamin A palmitate (p.1383·2).

Shampoo: Pyrithione zinc (p.1122·1); Triaminodil.
Hair loss; seborrhoeic dermatitis.

Aminotripa *Otsuka, Jpn.*
Amino-acid, carbohydrate, and electrolyte infusion (p.1350·1).
Parenteral nutrition.

Aminovac *Nikkho, Braz.*
Allergen preparation (p.1575·3).
Hyposensitisation.

Aminoveinte *Madariaga, Spain.*
Multivitamin and amino-acid preparation (p.1350·1).
Tonic.

Aminoven *Fresenius Kabi, Port.*
Amino-acid infusion (p.1350·1).
Parenteral nutrition.

Aminoven Infant
Fresenius Kabi, Ger.; Fresenius Kabi, Switz.
Amino-acid infusion (p.1350·1).
Formerly known as Aminovenos Pad and Aminovenos Infant in *Switz.*
Parenteral nutrition.

Aminovenos N-Pad *Fresenius, Thai.*
Amino-acid infusion (p.1350·1).
Parenteral nutrition.

Aminovenos Pad
Fresenius, Belg.†; Fresenius-Klinik, Ger.†.
Amino-acid infusion (p.1350·1).
Parenteral nutrition.

Aminovit con Carnosina *FAMA, Ital.†.*
Carbohydrate, amino acids, minerals, and vitamins (p.1350·1).
Nutritional supplement.

Aminoxin *Tyson, USA†.*
Pyridoxal phosphate (p.1387·1).

Aminozim *Searle, Ital.*
Amino-acid preparation (p.1350·1).
Tonic.

Aminsane *Dolisos, Fr.†.*
Bladderwrack (p.1585·2); java tea (p.1625·1); meadowsweet (p.1631·2).
Obesity.

Aminsolut *Delta, Ger.*
Amino-acid, carbohydrate, and electrolyte infusion (p.1350·1).
Parenteral nutrition.

Amiobeta *Betapharm, Ger.*
Amiodarone hydrochloride (p.836·1).
Arrhythmias.

Amiodacore *CTI, Israel.*
Amiodarone hydrochloride (p.836·1).
Arrhythmias; heart failure.

Amiodar *Sigma-Tau, Ital.*
Amiodarone hydrochloride (p.836·1).
Angina pectoris; arrhythmias.

Amiodarex *Sanofi Synthelabo, Ger.*
Amiodarone hydrochloride (p.836·1).
Arrhythmias.

Amiogamma *Worwag, Ger.*
Amiodarone hydrochloride (p.836·1).
Arrhythmias.

Amiohexal *Hexal, Ger.*
Amiodarone hydrochloride (p.836·1).
Arrhythmias.

Amiopia *Medical, Spain.*
Vitamins, minerals, amino acids (p.1350·1); isoniazid (p.215·3).
Eye disorders.

Amioxid *Neuraxpharm, Ger.*
Amitriptylinoxide (p.278·1).
Depression.

Amipaque *Winthrop, USA†.*
Metrizamide (p.1037·3).
Radiographic contrast medium.

Amiparen
Otsuka, Jpn; Thai Otsuka, Thai.
Amino-acid infusion (p.1350·1).
Parenteral nutrition.

Amipress *Salus, Ital.*
Labetalol hydrochloride (p.918·1).
Hypertension.

Amirone *Julphar, UAE.*
Amiodarone hydrochloride (p.836·1).
Arrhythmias.

Amisol *Dong, Singapore.*
Clobetasone butyrate (p.1065·2).
Skin disorders.

Amitacon *Egis, Thai.*
Glyceryl trinitrate (p.897·3).
Angina pectoris.

Ami-Tex LA *Amide, USA†.*
Phenylpropanolamine hydrochloride (p.1098·1); guaifenesin (p.1092·2).
Coughs.

Amithiazide *Jean-Marie, Hong Kong.*
Amiloride hydrochloride (p.835·1); hydrochlorothiazide (p.907·3).
Hypertension; oedema.

Amitone *Menley & James, USA.*
Calcium carbonate (p.1215·1).
Hyperacidity.

Amitrex *Sanofi Synthelabo, Port.*
Amisulpride (p.655·1).
Schizophrenia.

Amitrid *Leiras, Fin.*
Amiloride hydrochloride (p.835·1); hydrochlorothiazide (p.907·3).
Heart failure; hypertension; oedema.

Amitrip *Pacific, NZ.*
Amitriptyline hydrochloride (p.273·3).
Depression; nocturnal enuresis.

Amitrol *Douglas, Austral.†*
Amitriptyline hydrochloride (p.273·3).
Depression; nocturnal enuresis.

Amitron *Torlan, Spain.*
Amoxicillin sodium (p.149·2) or amoxicillin trihydrate (p.149·2).
Bacterial infections.

Amix *Ashbourne, UK.*
Note. A similar name is used for preparations of different composition (see below).
Amoxicillin trihydrate (p.149·2).
Bacterial infections.

Amixx *Krewel, Ger.*
Note. A similar name is used for preparations of different composition (see below).
Amantadine hydrochloride (p.1161·2).
Drug-induced extrapyramidal disorders; parkinsonism.

Amiyodazol *Rimsa, Mex.*
Metronidazole (p.594·1).

Amiyu *Hoechst Marion Roussel, Thai.*
Amino-acid preparation (p.1350·1).
Renal failure.

Amizet 10 *Tanabe, Jpn.*
Amino-acid infusion (p.1350·1).
Parenteral nutrition.

Amizet 10X *Tanabe, Jpn.*
Amino-acid and carbohydrate infusion (p.1350·1).
Parenteral nutrition.

Amizide
Alphapharm, Austral.; Pacific, NZ; Rolab, S.Afr.
Amiloride hydrochloride (p.835·1); hydrochlorothiazide (p.907·3).
Now known as Rolab Amiloride HCl/Hydrochlorothiazide in S.Afr.
Cardiac oedema; hepatic cirrhosis with ascites; hypertension.

AMK
Note. This name is used for preparations of different composition.
Plantes Tropicales, Fr.
Glucomannan (p.1616·2); bladderwrack (p.1585·2).
Slimming aid.

Pisa, Mex.
Amikacin sulfate (p.148·1).
Bacterial infections.

Amlactin *Upsher-Smith, USA.*
Ammonium lactate (p.1110·3).
Dry skin.

Amlodin *Sumitomo, Jpn†.*
Amlodipine besilate (p.838·3).
Angina pectoris; hypertension.

Amlor
Roerig, Belg.; Pfizer, Fr.
Amlodipine besilate (p.838·3).
Angina pectoris; heart failure; hypertension.

Ammeltz *Kobayashi, Thai.*
Methyl salicylate (p.55·1); menthol (p.1632·3); camphor (p.1589·3).
Musculoskeletal pain; soft-tissue disorders.

Ammonaps
Orphan, Fr.; Orphan, UK.
Sodium phenylbutyrate (p.1666·2).
Urea cycle disorders.

Amniex *Mastelli, Ital.†.*
Amniotic membrane (human) (p.1579·3).
Skin substitute.

Amniolina *Reig Jofre, Spain.*
Talc (p.1124·2); zinc oxide (p.1128·2).
Nappy rash.

Amnivent *Ashbourne, UK.*
Aminophylline (p.760·1).
Bronchospasm.

AMO Endosol
Allergan, Austral.; Allergan, USA.
Electrolytes (p.1180·1).
Irrigation solution during surgery.

Amo Resan *Alacan, Spain.*
Amoxicillin trihydrate (p.149·2); bromhexine hydrochloride (p.1085·3).
Respiratory-tract infections.

AMO Vitrax
Allergan, Austral.; Allergan, NZ; Allergan, S.Afr.; Allergan, Singapore; Allergan, Swed.†; Allergan, Switz.†; Allergan, Thai.; Allergan, USA.
Sodium hyaluronate (p.1620·1).
Aid in ophthalmic surgery.

Amobronc *Ist. Chim. Inter., Ital.*
Ambroxol hydrochloride (p.1084·3).
Respiratory-system disorders.

Amocid *Lysoform, Ger.*
Orthophenylphenol (p.1152·1).
Surface disinfection.

Amocillin *Caps, S.Afr.*
Amoxicillin sodium (p.149·2).
Bacterial infections.

Amoclan *Hexal, Austral.*
Amoxicillin trihydrate (p.149·2); potassium clavulanate (p.187·2).
Bacterial infections.

Amoclav *Hexal, Ger.*
Amoxicillin trihydrate (p.149·2); potassium clavulanate (p.187·2).
Bacterial infections.

Amoclavam *Merck, Port.*
Amoxicillin trihydrate (p.149·2); potassium clavulanate (p.187·2).
Bacterial infections.

Amoclave *Bial-Aristegui, Spain.*
Amoxicillin trihydrate (p.149·2); potassium clavulanate (p.187·2).
Bacterial infections.

Amodex *Bouchara, Fr.*
Amoxicillin trihydrate (p.149·2) or amoxicillin sodium (p.149·2).
Bacterial infections.

Amofat *Protein, Mex.*
Famotidine (p.1225·3).

Amofil *Veripalvelu, Fin.*
A factor VIII preparation (p.734·1).
Factor VIII deficiency; haemophilia A.

Amoflamisan *Beecham, Spain.*
Amoxicillin trihydrate (p.149·2).
Bacterial infections.

Amoflux *Lampugnani, Ital.*
Amoxicillin trihydrate (p.149·2).
Bacterial infections.

Amohexal *Hexal, Austral.*
Amoxicillin trihydrate (p.149·2).
Bacterial infections.

Amoksiklav
Lek, Hong Kong; Lek, Thai.
Amoxicillin trihydrate (p.149·2); potassium clavulanate (p.187·2).
Bacterial infections.

Amol Heilkräutergeist N *Roland, Ger.*
Melissa oil; clove oil (p.1597·1); cinnamon oil (p.1596·1); lemon oil (p.1628·2); peppermint oil (p.1243·3); lavender oil (p.1627·2); menthol (p.1632·3).
Colds; coughs; gastrointestinal disorders; neuralgia; rheumatoid disorders; sore throat.

Amolgen *Solfran, Mex.*
Paracetamol (p.71·2).
Fever; pain.

Amolin *Ergha, Irl.*
Note. A similar name is used for preparations of different composition (see below).
Atenolol (p.841·3).
Angina pectoris; arrhythmias; hypertension; myocardial infarction.

Am-O-Lin *Bayer, NZ.*
Note. A similar name is used for preparations of different composition (see above).
Almond oil (p.1576·3); calamine (p.1111·3); salicylic acid (p.1122·3).
Nappy rash; skin irritation.

Amopen *Yorkshire Pharmaceuticals, UK.*
Amoxicillin (p.149·2).
Bacterial infections.

Amophar *Irex, Fr.*
Amoxicillin trihydrate (p.149·2).
Bacterial infections.

Amoram *Eastern Pharmaceuticals, UK.*
Amoxicillin (p.149·2).
Bacterial infections.

Amorion *Orion, Fin.*
Amoxicillin trihydrate (p.149·2).
Bacterial infections.

Amosan
Note. This name is used for preparations of different composition.
Oral-B, Austral.
Sodium perborate (p.1156·3); sodium bitartrate.
Inflammation of the oral cavity.

Oral-B, Canad.; Oral-B, Switz.
Sodium perborate (p.1156·3).
Oral lesions.

Oral-B, Mex.
Urea hydrogen peroxide (p.1159·3).

Amosyt *Abigo, Swed.*
Dimenhydrinate (p.415·2).
Ménière's syndrome; nausea; vertigo.

Amotein *Wasserman, Spain.*
Metronidazole (p.594·1).
Amoebiasis; anaerobic bacterial infections; dracunculiasis; trichomoniasis.

Amox
Salus, Ital.; Berenguer Infale, Spain†; SM, Thai.
Amoxicillin trihydrate (p.149·2).
Bacterial infections.

Amoxa
Atlantic, Hong Kong; Atlantic, Singapore; Atlantic, Thai.
Amoxicillin trihydrate (p.149·2).
Bacterial infections.

Amoxapen
Remedica, Hong Kong; Remedica, Singapore.
Amoxicillin (p.149·2).
Bacterial infections.

Amoxaren *Areu, Spain.*
Amoxicillin trihydrate (p.149·2).
Bacterial infections.

Amoxi
SMB, Belg.; CT, Ger.; BASF, Ger.; ABZ, Ger.; Schwarz, Ger.; Sanol, Ger.; Generics, Israel.
Amoxicillin trihydrate (p.149·2).
Bacterial infections.

Amoxi Gobens *Normon, Spain.*
Amoxicillin sodium (p.149·2) or amoxicillin trihydrate (p.149·2).
Bacterial infections.

Amoxi Gobens Mucol *Normon, Spain.*
Amoxicillin trihydrate (p.149·2); bromhexine hydrochloride (p.1085·3).
Respiratory-tract infections.

Amoxibacter *Rubio, Spain.*
Amoxicillin trihydrate (p.149·2).
Bacterial infections.

amoxi-basan *Schonenberger, Switz.*
Amoxicillin (p.149·2).
Bacterial infections.

Amoxibeta *Betapharm, Ger.*
Amoxicillin trihydrate (p.149·2).
Bacterial infections.

Amoxibiocin *Orion, Ger.*
Amoxicillin (p.149·2).
Bacterial infections.

Amoxibron *Sanfer, Mex.*
Amoxicillin trihydrate (p.149·2); bromhexine hydrochloride (p.1085·3).
Respiratory-tract infections.

Amoxicap *Hovid, Singapore.*
Amoxicillin trihydrate (p.149·2).
Bacterial infections.

Amoxiclav *Columbia, Mex.*
Amoxicillin trihydrate (p.149·2); potassium clavulanate (p.187·2).
Bacterial infections.

Amoxi-Clavulan *Stada, Ger.*
Amoxicillin trihydrate (p.149·2); potassium clavulanate (p.187·2).
Bacterial infections.

Amoxi-Cophar *Cophar, Switz.*
Amoxicillin trihydrate (p.149·2).
Bacterial infections.

Amoxid *Kwizda, Aust.*
Amoxicillin trihydrate (p.149·2).
Bacterial infections.

Amoxidel *Synthelabo, Spain.*
Amoxicillin trihydrate (p.149·2).
Bacterial infections.

Amoxidel Bronquial *Synthelabo, Spain.*
Amoxicillin trihydrate (p.149·2); brovanexine hydrochloride (p.1086·1).
Respiratory-tract infections.

Amoxi-Diolan
Engelhard, Ger.; Brahms, Ger.
Amoxicillin trihydrate (p.149·2).
Bacterial infections.

Amoxidura *Merck dura, Ger.*
Amoxicillin trihydrate (p.149·2); potassium clavulanate (p.187·2).
Bacterial infections.

Amoxifar *Farmoquimica, Braz.*
Amoxicillin (p.149·2).
Bacterial infections.

Amoxifar Balsamico *Farmoquimica, Braz.*
Amoxicillin (p.149·2); bromhexine (p.1085·3).
Bacterial infections.

Amoxiferm *Fermenta, Swed.†.*
Amoxicillin trihydrate (p.149·2).
Bacterial infections.

Amoxifur *Fustery, Mex.*
Amoxicillin trihydrate (p.149·2).
Bacterial infections.

Amoxigran *Hovid, Singapore.*
Amoxicillin trihydrate (p.149·2).
Bacterial infections.

Amoxi-Hefa *Hefa, Ger.*
Amoxicillin trihydrate (p.149·2).
Bacterial infections.

Amoxihexal
Hexal, Aust.; Hexal, Ger.
Amoxicillin trihydrate (p.149·2).
Bacterial infections.

Amoxil
SmithKline Beecham, Austral.; SmithKline Beecham, Braz.; Wyeth-Ayerst, Canad.; SmithKline Beecham, Hong Kong; SmithKline Beecham, Irl.; Sanfer, Mex.; SmithKline Beecham, NZ; SmithKline Beecham, S.Afr.; SmithKline Beecham, Singapore; SmithKline Beecham, Thai.; Bencard, UK; SmithKline Beecham, USA.
Amoxicillin (p.149·2), amoxicillin sodium (p.149·2), or amoxicillin trihydrate (p.149·2).
Bacterial infections.

Amoxilan *Lannacher, Aust.*
Amoxicillin trihydrate (p.149·2).
Bacterial infections.

Amoxillat *Azupharma, Ger.*
Amoxicillin trihydrate (p.149·2).
Bacterial infections.

Amoxillat-Clav *Azupharma, Ger.*
Amoxicillin trihydrate (p.149·2); potassium clavulanate (p.187·2).
Bacterial infections.

Amoxillin
Esseti, Ital.; Alpharma, Norw.
Amoxicillin trihydrate (p.149·2).
Bacterial infections.

Amoximedical *Medical, Spain.*
Amoxicillin trihydrate (p.149·2).
Bacterial infections.

Amoxi-Mepha *Mepha, Switz.*
Amoxicillin trihydrate (p.149·2).
Bacterial infections.

Amoximerck *Merck dura, Ger.*
Amoxicillin trihydrate (p.149·2).
Bacterial infections.

Amoximex *Cimex, Switz.*
Amoxicillin trihydrate (p.149·2).
Bacterial infections.

Amoxin *Medinovum, Fin.*
Amoxicillin trihydrate (p.149·2).
Bacterial infections.

Amoxin Comp *Medinovum, Fin.*
Amoxicillin trihydrate (p.149·2); potassium clavulanate (p.187·2).
Bacterial infections.

Amoxina *Aesculapius, Ital.*
Amoxicillin trihydrate (p.149·2).
Bacterial infections.

Amoxinovag *Novag, Mex.*
Amoxicillin trihydrate (p.149·2).
Bacterial infections.

Amoxipen *Metapharma, Ital.*
Amoxicillin trihydrate (p.149·2).
Bacterial infections.

Amoxi-Puren *Isis Puren, Ger.*
Amoxicillin trihydrate (p.149·2).
Bacterial infections.

Amoxisol *Rimsa, Mex.*
Amoxicillin trihydrate (p.149·2).
Bacterial infections.

Amoxistad *Stada, Aust.*
Amoxicillin trihydrate (p.149·2).
Bacterial infections.

Amoxitab *Hovid, Singapore.*
Amoxicillin trihydrate (p.149·2).
Bacterial infections.

Amoxi-Tablinen *Lichtenstein, Ger.*
Amoxicillin trihydrate (p.149·2).
Bacterial infections.

Amoxivet *ICN, Mex.*
Amoxicillin trihydrate (p.149·2).
Bacterial infections.

Amoxi-Wolff *Wolff, Ger.*
Amoxicillin trihydrate (p.149·2).
Bacterial infections.

Amoxtiol *Daker Farmasimes, Spain.*
Amoxicillin trihydrate (p.149·2); carbocisteine (p.1086·3).
Respiratory-tract infections.

Amoxyfizz *Schwulst, S.Afr.†.*
Amoxicillin (p.149·2).
Bacterial infections.

Amoxylin *Biomedis, Thai.; Great Eastern, Thai.*
Amoxicillin trihydrate (p.149·2).
Bacterial infections.

Amoxypen *Grunenthal, Ger.*
Amoxicillin trihydrate (p.149·2).
Bacterial infections.

Amoxyplus *Novag, Spain.*
Amoxicillin trihydrate (p.149·2); potassium clavulanate (p.187·2).
Bacterial infections.

Ampamet *Menarini, Ital.*
Aniracetam (p.1580·2).
Mental function impairment.

Ampat *Asian Pharm, Thai.*
Ampicillin trihydrate (p.151·1).
Bacterial infections.

Ampavit *ANB, Thai.*
Vitamin B₁₂ (p.1388·1).
Megaloblastic anaemia.

Ampecyclal *Sarget, Fr.; Asta Medica, Fr.*
Heptaminol adenosine phosphate (p.1619·2).
Haemorrhoids; metrorrhagia; peripheral vascular disorders.

Ampexin
Note. This name is used for preparations of different composition.
Amrad, Austral.†.
Amoxicillin trihydrate (p.149·2).
Bacterial infections.

Biolab, Thai.
Ampicillin trihydrate (p.151·1).
Bacterial infections.

Amphisept *Goldschmidt, Switz.*
Alcohol (p.1130·3).
Hand disinfection.

Amphisept E *Bode, Ger.*
Alcohol (p.1130·3).
Hand disinfection.

Amphocil
Torrex, Aust.; Alza, Denm.; Alza, Irl.; Sequus, Israel; Zeneca, Ital.; Lemery, Mex.; Zeneca, Neth.; Zeneca, Port.†; Sequus, Singapore; Almirall, Spain; Zeneca, Swed.; Cambridge, UK.
Amphotericin B-sodium cholesteryl sulfate complex (p.377·3).
Fungal infections; leishmaniasis.

Amphocycline *Bristol-Myers Squibb, Fr.*
Amphotericin B (p.377·2); tetracycline (p.258·3) or tetracycline hydrochloride (p.258·3).
Bacterial and fungal infections.

Amphodyn
Klinge, Aust.
Etilefrine hydrochloride (p.888·1); aescin (p.1574·1).
Circulatory disorders; hypotension.

Klinge, Ger.
Etilefrine hydrochloride (p.888·1); aesculus (p.1574·1).
Circulatory disorders; hypotension.

Amphodyn mono Klinge, Aust.†
Etilefrine hydrochloride (p.888·1).
Hypotension.

Amphojel
Whitehall, Austral.†; Axcan, Canad.; Whitehall, NZ; Aspen Consumer, S.Afr.; Wyeth-Ayerst, USA.
Aluminium hydroxide (p.1210·3).
Gastrointestinal hyperacidity.

Amphojel 500 Axcan, Canad.†
Aluminium hydroxide (p.1210·3); magnesium hydroxide (p.1233·1).
Antacid.

Amphojel Plus Axcan, Canad.†
Oral liquid: Aluminium hydroxide (p.1210·3); magnesium hydroxide (p.1233·1); simeticone (p.1249·2).
Tablets: Aluminium hydroxide-magnesium carbonate co-dried gel (p.1211·2); magnesium hydroxide (p.1233·1); simeticone (p.1249·2).
Antacid; flatulence.

Ampholysine Plus Peters, Fr.
Polihexanide (p.1154·2); mixed amphoteric and quaternary ammonium salts.
Instrument disinfection.

Ampho-Moronal
Bristol-Myers Squibb, Aust.; Bristol-Myers Squibb, Ger.; Bristol-Myers Squibb, Switz.
Amphotericin B (p.377·2).
Fungal infections.

Ampho-Moronal V Bristol-Myers Squibb, Ger.
Amphotericin B (p.377·2); triamcinolone acetonide (p.1080·1).
Fungal skin infections.

Ampho-Moronal V L Bristol-Myers Squibb, Ger.
Amphotericin B (p.377·2); triamcinolone acetonide (p.1080·1).
Formerly known as Ampho-Moronal V N.
Skin disorders with fungal infection.

Amphosca a l'orchitine Lehning, Fr.
Homoeopathic preparation.

Amphosca a l'ovarine Lehning, Fr.
Homoeopathic preparation.

Amphosca Orchitine Homeocan, Canad.
Homoeopathic preparation.

Amphosca Ovarine Homeocan, Canad.
Homoeopathic preparation.

Amphosept BV Anios, Fr.†
Didecyldimethylammonium chloride (p.1143·2); alkylbenzylammonium chloride; alkylethylbenzylammonium chloride; alkylaminoalkyl glycine.
Instrument disinfection.

Amphotec Sequus, USA.
Amphotericin B (p.377·2).
Aspergillosis.

Ampho-Vaccin intestinal Sanofi Winthrop, Fr.†
Bifidobacterium bifidum (p.1626·3); Escherichia coli; Enterococcus faecalis (p.1626·3); Proteus vulgaris; Pseudomonas aeruginosa.
Diarrhoea.

Ampi ABZ, Ger.
Ampicillin trihydrate (p.151·1).
Bacterial infections.

Ampicap Hovid, Singapore.
Ampicillin trihydrate (p.151·1).
Bacterial infections.

Ampicil Medley, Braz.
Ampicillin (p.150·3).
Bacterial infections.

Ampicilase Teuto, Braz.
Ampicillin (p.150·3).
Bacterial infections.

Ampicin Bristol, Canad.
Ampicillin sodium (p.150·3).
Bacterial infections.

Ampicler Herald's, Braz.
Ampicillin trihydrate (p.151·1).
Bacterial infections.

Ampicler com Probenecide Herald's, Braz.
Ampicillin (p.150·3).
Probenecid (p.401·3) is included in this preparation to reduce renal tubular excretion of the antibiotic.
Bacterial infections.

Ampiclox
SmithKline Beecham, Hong Kong; SmithKline Beecham, Irl.; SmithKline Beecham, S.Afr.; SmithKline Beecham, Thai.; SmithKline Beecham, UK†.
Ampicillin (p.150·3), ampicillin sodium (p.150·3), or ampicillin trihydrate (p.151·1); cloxacillin (p.192·1) or cloxacillin sodium (p.192·1).
Bacterial infections.

Ampiclox-D Sanfer, Mex.
Ampicillin (p.150·3); dicloxacillin (p.199·1).
Bacterial infections.

Ampicrom Brasifa, Braz.
Ampicillin (p.150·3).
Bacterial infections.

Ampicyn
Rhone-Poulenc Rorer, Austral.; IBI, Thai.
Ampicillin (p.150·3) or ampicillin sodium (p.150·3).
Bacterial infections.

Ampifar Farmoquimica, Braz.
Ampicillin (p.150·3).
Bacterial infections.

Ampifar Balsamico Farmoquimica, Braz.
Ampicillin sodium (p.150·3); ampicillin benzathine (p.151·3).
Lignocaine [lidocaine] hydrochloride (p.1313·2) is included in this preparation to alleviate the pain of injection.
Bacterial infections.

Ampifen MPF, Singapore.
Ibuprofen (p.43·2).
Musculoskeletal, joint, and soft-tissue disorders; pain.

Ampilin
Atlantic, Hong Kong; Atlantic, Singapore; Atlantic, Thai.
Ampicillin sodium (p.150·3) or ampicillin trihydrate (p.151·1).
Bacterial infections.

Ampilisa Lisapharma, Ital.
Ampicillin (p.150·3) or ampicillin sodium (p.150·3).
Bacterial infections.

Ampillin PP Lab, Thai.
Ampicillin trihydrate (p.151·1).
Bacterial infections.

Ampilux Tubilux, Ital.
Ampicillin sodium (p.150·3).
Eye infections.

Ampimax Hexal, S.Afr.
Ampicillin trihydrate (p.151·1).
Bacterial infections.

Ampimex Arlex, Mex.
Ampicillin (p.150·3).
Bacterial infections.

Ampipen Caps, S.Afr.
Ampicillin (p.150·3).
Bacterial infections.

Ampiplus
Note.This name is used for preparations of different composition.
Menarini, Ital.†.
Ampicillin (p.150·3) or ampicillin sodium (p.150·3); dicloxacillin sodium (p.199·1).
Bacterial infections.

Tecefarma, Spain.
Ampicillin trihydrate (p.151·1).
Bacterial infections.

Ampiplus Simplex Menarini, Ital.†
Ampicillin sodium (p.150·3).
Bacterial infections.

Ampi-Quim Quimica y Farmacia, Mex.
Ampicillin (p.150·3).
Bacterial infections.

Ampiretard Cibran, Braz.
Benzathine benzylpenicillin (p.156·2).
Bacterial infections.

Ampi-Rol Rolab, S.Afr.
Ampicillin trihydrate (p.151·1).
Bacterial infections.

Ampisalt Propan, S.Afr.†
Ampicillin trihydrate (p.151·1).
Bacterial infections.

Ampispectrin QIF, Braz.
Ampicillin (p.150·3).
Bacterial infections.

Ampisuspen Medifarma, Mex.
Ampicillin (p.150·3).
Bacterial infections.

Ampitab Hovid, Singapore.
Ampicillin trihydrate (p.151·1).
Bacterial infections.

Ampi-Tecno Tecnofarma, Mex.
Ampicillin (p.150·3).
Bacterial infections.

Ampitotal Eurofarma, Braz.
Ampicillin (p.150·3).
Bacterial infections.

Ampizan Allergan-Frumtost, Braz.
Ampicillin benzathine (p.151·3); ampicillin sodium (p.150·3).
Bacterial infections.

Amplacilina Wyeth, Braz.
Ampicillin sodium (p.150·3).
Bacterial infections.

Amplamox Tecnifar, Port.
Amoxicillin trihydrate (p.149·2).
Bacterial infections.

Amplavit Honorterapica, Braz.
Multivitamin preparation (p.1350·1).

Amplexol Sanofi Synthelabo, Braz.
Isosorbide mononitrate (p.916·2).
Angina pectoris; heart failure; myocardial infarction.

Amplictil Rhodia, Braz.
Chlorpromazine (p.660·2).
Nausea and vomiting; premedication; psychoses; tetanus.

Amplidermis Medea, Spain.
Acedoben (p.1571·1); allantoin (p.1110·1); chlorquinaldol (p.182·1); dexamethasone (p.1067·1); mepyramine maleate (p.421·1); vitamin F.
Infected burns, skin ulcers, and wounds; infected skin disorders.

Amplifar Tecnifar, Port.
Ampicillin trihydrate (p.151·1).
Bacterial infections.

Ampligen
Note.This name is used for preparations of different composition.
Natus, Braz.
Gentamicin (p.212·1).
Bacterial infections.

HemispheRx, USA.
Poly I.poly C (p.1653·1).
AIDS and HIV infection; chronic fatigue syndrome; invasive metastatic melanoma; renal cell carcinoma.

Amplimed Medquimica, Braz.
Ampicillin (p.150·3).
Bacterial infections.

Ampliron Rhein, Mex.
Amoxicillin trihydrate (p.149·2).
Bacterial infections.

Amplital Pharmacia Upjohn, Ital.
Ampicillin (p.150·3), ampicillin sodium (p.150·3), or ampicillin trihydrate (p.151·1).
Bacterial infections.

Amplitor Cibran, Braz.
Ampicillin (p.150·3).
Bacterial infections.

Amplium
Note.This name is used for preparations of different composition.
Farmasa, Braz.
Tinidazole (p.603·3).
Anaerobic bacterial infections; protozoal infections.

Sigma-Tau, Ital.
Ampicillin sodium (p.150·3) or ampicillin trihydrate (p.151·1); cloxacillin sodium (p.192·1).
Bacterial infections.

Amplium-G Farmasa, Braz.
Tinidazole (p.603·3); miconazole (p.391·1).
Vulvovaginal infections.

Amplizer OFF, Ital.
Ampicillin trihydrate (p.151·1).
Bacterial infections.

Amplofen Merck, Braz.
Ampicillin (p.150·3).
Bacterial infections.

Amplomicina Cibran, Braz.
Gentamicin sulfate (p.210·1).
Bacterial infections.

Amplotal Medley, Braz.
Ampicillin benzathine (p.151·3); ampicillin sodium (p.150·3).
Bacterial infections.

Amplozol Novaquimica, Braz.
Albendazole (p.95·2).
Worm infections.

Ampra M & H, Thai.
Ampicillin sodium (p.150·3) or ampicillin trihydrate (p.151·1).
Bacterial infections.

Amprace Amrad, Austral.
Enalapril maleate (p.883·3).
Heart failure; hypertension.

Amprexyl Unison, Thai.
Ampicillin (p.150·3).
Bacterial infections.

Ampro Nakorn, Thai.
Ampicillin trihydrate (p.151·1).
Bacterial infections.

Amrit BHR, UK†.
Amoxicillin trihydrate (p.149·2).
Bacterial infections.

AMS Salters, S.Afr.
Sulfanilamide (p.256·2); acriflavinium chloride (p.1130·2); merbromin (p.1150·1).
Wounds.

Amsa P-D Parke, Davis, Canad.
Amsacrine (p.507·3).
Acute leukaemias.

Amsapen Antibioticos, Mex.
Ampicillin sodium (p.150·3).
Bacterial infections.

Amsidine
Parke, Davis, Belg.; Parke, Davis, Fr.†; Parke, Davis, Irl.; Parke, Davis, Neth.; Goldshield, UK.
Amsacrine (p.507·3).
Acute leukaemias.

Amsidyl
Parke, Davis, Austral.; Godecke, Ger.; Parke, Davis, NZ; Warner-Lambert, Switz.
Amsacrine (p.507·3).
Acute leukaemias.

Amuchina Pisa, Mex.
Sodium hypochlorite (p.1156·2); sodium chloride (p.1196·1).
Mucous membrane, skin, surface, and wound disinfection.

Amukin
Bristol-Myers Squibb, Belg.; Bristol-Myers Squibb, Neth.
Amikacin sulfate (p.148·1).
Bacterial infections.

Amukine Gifrer Barbezat, Fr.
Sodium hypochlorite (p.1156·2); sodium chloride (p.1196·1).
Skin, mucous membrane and wound cleansing.

Amukine Med Amuchina, Ital.
Sodium hypochlorite (p.1156·2).
Disinfection of skin, wounds, and mucous membranes.

A-Mulsin Mucos, Ger.
Vitamin A palmitate (p.1383·2).
Adjunct in cytotoxic therapy or radiotherapy; keratinisation disorders; vitamin A deficiency.

A-Mulsion Seroyal, Canad.
Vitamin A palmitate (p.1383·2).

Amuno Merck Sharp & Dohme, Ger.
Indometacin (p.44·3).
Gout; inflammation; musculoskeletal, joint, peri-articular, and soft-tissue disorders; pain.

Amunovax Pasteur Merieux, Spain†.
A measles vaccine (Schwarz strain) (p.1547·1).
Active immunisation.

Amvisc
Johnson & Johnson, Aust.; Iolab, Israel; MCM, S.Afr.; Johnson & Johnson, Swed.†; Bausch & Lomb, USA.
Sodium hyaluronate (p.1620·1).
Aid in ophthalmic surgery.

AMX
Pisa, Mex.; Brovar, S.Afr.†.
Amoxicillin (p.149·2) or amoxicillin trihydrate (p.149·2).
Bacterial infections.

Amxol
Biolab, Hong Kong; Biolab, Singapore; Biolab, Thai.
Ambroxol hydrochloride (p.1084·3).
Respiratory-tract disorders associated with increased or viscous mucus.

Amycil Rimsa, Mex.
Mebendazole (p.102·2).

Amycor Lipha Sante, Fr.
Bifonazole (p.381·1).
Fungal skin infections.

Amycor Onychoset Lipha Sante, Fr.
Bifonazole (p.381·1); urea (p.1127·3).
Fungal nail infections.

Amydramine Julphar, UAE.
Diphenhydramine hydrochloride (p.416·1); ammonium chloride (p.1085·2); sodium citrate (p.1186·2); menthol (p.1632·3).
Coughs; upper respiratory-tract congestion.

Amydramine II Julphar, UAE.
Diphenhydramine hydrochloride (p.416·1).
Cold symptoms; coughs.

Amydramine Paediatric Julphar, UAE.
Diphenhydramine hydrochloride (p.416·1); sodium citrate (p.1186·2); menthol (p.1632·3).
Coughs; upper respiratory-tract congestion.

Amygdol Knoll, Fr.
Chlorhexidine gluconate (p.1138·2); amylocaine hydrochloride (p.1306·1).
Mouth and throat disorders.

Amygdorectol
Monot, Fr.; Merck-Clevenot, Switz.
Bismuth camphocarbonate (p.1214·1).
Mouth and throat disorders.

Amygdospray Monot, Fr.†.
Hexamidine isetionate (p.1146·2); amethocaine [tetracaine] hydrochloride (p.1305·2).
Mouth and throat disorders.

Amykon Engelhard, Ger.
Miconazole nitrate (p.391·1).
Fungal skin infections.

Amylatin Synpharma, Aust.
Angelica (p.1580·2); century (p.1593·1); absinthium (p.1571·1).
Gastrointestinal disorders.

Amylodiastase Thepenier, Fr.†.
Amylase (cereal extract) (p.1579·3).
Dyspepsia.

Amytal
Lilly, Austral.; Lilly, Canad.; Flynn, Irl.; Flynn, UK; Lilly, USA.
Amobarbital (p.655·2) or amobarbital sodium (p.655·2).
Insomnia; sedative; status epilepticus.

AN 1 Krugmann, Ger.
Amfetaminil (p.1506·3).
Narcoleptic syndrome.

Anabact
Bioglan, Irl.; Bioglan, Singapore; Bioglan, Thai.; Cambridge Healthcare, UK.
Metronidazole (p.594·1).
Malodorous fungating tumours; malodorous skin ulcers; rosacea.

Anabar Lunsco, USA.
Paracetamol (p.71·2); salicylamide (p.82·1); phenyltoloxamine citrate (p.423·1).

Anabol British Dispensary, Thai.
Methandienone (p.1482·2).
Anabolic.

Anabol-Hevert Hevert, Ger.
Homoeopathic preparation.

anabol-loges Loges, Ger.
Alpha tocoferil acetate (p.1394·1); magnesium hydrogen phosphate; potassium chloride; terra silicea; hypericum (p.290·2).
Bone and connective tissue disorders.

Anabron Millet Roux, Braz.
Ambroxol (p.1084·3).
Respiratory-tract congestion.

Anacal
Note.This name is used for preparations of different composition.
Sankyo, Port.
A heparinoid (p.905·2); lauromacrogol 400 (p.1345·2); prednisolone (p.1077·3); hexachlorophene (p.1146·1).
Anorectal disorders.

Sankyo, UK.
A heparinoid (p.905·2); lauromacrogol 400 (p.1345·2).
Formerly contained a heparinoid, prednisolone, lauromacrogol 400, and hexachlorophene.
Anorectal disorders.

Anacalcit *Belmac, Spain.*
Sodium cellulose phosphate (p.1022·3).
Hypercalcaemia; hypercalciuria; osteopetrosis; vitamin D intoxication.

Anacervix *Lepori, Port.; Farma Lepori, Spain.*
Piracetam (p.1652·1); vincamine (p.1680·1).
Cerebral trauma; cerebrovascular disorders.

Anacidol
Note. This name is used for preparations of different composition.
Menarini, Ital.
Aluminium hydroxide (p.1210·3); magnesium hydroxide (p.1233·1); dimethicone (p.1249·2); milk powder.
Gastrointestinal disorders.

Spirig, Switz.
Calcium carbonate (p.1215·1); aluminium hydroxide-magnesium carbonate co-dried gel (p.1211·2).
Gastric disorders.

Anacidron *Bergamo, Braz.*
Dicyclomine [dicycloverine] hydrochloride (p.466·1); magnesium hydroxide (p.1233·1); aluminium hydroxide (p.1210·3); simeticone (p.1249·2).
Flatulence; gastrointestinal disorders.

Anacidron-H *Bergamo, Braz.*
Aluminium hydroxide (p.1210·3).
Gastrointestinal hyperacidity.

Anacin *Whitehall-Robins, Canad.; Whitehall, Hong Kong; Whitehall, Israel; ICC, Israel; Whitehall, Singapore; Robins, USA.*
Aspirin (p.14·2); caffeine (p.761·3).
Fever; pain.

Anacin with Codeine *Whitehall-Robins, Canad.†*
Aspirin (p.14·2); caffeine (p.761·3); codeine phosphate (p.25·2).
Fever; pain.

Anaclosil *Antibioticos, Spain.*
Cloxacillin sodium (p.192·1).
Bacterial infections.

Anacrodyne *Rekah, Israel.*
Vitamin B₆ (p.1386·3).
Vitamin B₆ deficiency.

Anacyclin *Novartis, Braz.; Geigy, Ger.†*
Lynestrenol (p.1480·1); ethinylestradiol (p.1476·2).
28-Day packs also contain 6 inert tablets.
Combined oral contraceptive.

Anadent *Taro, Israel.*
Topical gel: Benzocaine (p.1306·2).
Topical solution: Benzocaine (p.1306·2); phenylephrine hydrochloride (p.1097·1).
Mouth disorders.

Anadermin *Ecobi, Ital.*
Chlorhexidine gluconate (p.1138·2); precipitated sulfur (p.1123·3).
Skin disinfection.

Anadin
Note. This name is used for preparations of different composition.
Whitehall, Irl.
Aspirin (p.14·2); caffeine (p.761·3); quinine sulfate (p.445·1).
Cold symptoms; pain.

Whitehall, UK.
Aspirin (p.14·2); caffeine (p.761·3).
Fever; pain.

Anadin Cold Control *Whitehall, UK.*
Paracetamol (p.71·2); caffeine (p.761·3); phenylephrine hydrochloride (p.1097·1).
Cold and influenza symptoms.

Anadin Cold Control Flu Strength *Whitehall, UK.*
Paracetamol (p.71·2); phenylephrine hydrochloride (p.1097·1).
Cold and influenza symptoms.

Anadin Extra *Whitehall, Irl.; Whitehall, Port.; Whitehall, UK.*
Aspirin (p.14·2); paracetamol (p.71·2); caffeine (p.761·3).
Fever; pain.

Anadin Ibuprofen *Whitehall, UK.*
Ibuprofen (p.43·2).
Fever; pain.

Anadin Paracetamol *Whitehall, UK.*
Paracetamol (p.71·2).
Fever; pain.

Anadin Ultra *Whitehall, UK.*
Ibuprofen (p.43·2).
Fever; pain.

Anadol *TO-Chemicals, Thai.*
Tramadol hydrochloride (p.89·1).
Pain.

Anador *Boehringer de Angeli, Braz.*
Dipyrone (p.34·1).
Fever; pain.

Anadrol *Unimed, USA.*
Oxymetholone (p.1487·3).
Anaemias.

Anadur *Pharmacia Upjohn, Aust.†*
Nandrolone hexyloxyphenylpropionate (p.1484·3).
Anabolic; chronic renal and intestinal disorders; osteoporosis; radiation and chemotherapy induced myelosuppression.

Anadvil *Whitehall, Fr.*
Ibuprofen (p.43·2).
Fever; pain.

Anaemodoron *Weleda, Aust.*
Fragaria vesca; urtica dioica (p.1678·2).
Iron-deficiency anaemia.

Anaerobex *Gerot, Aust.*
Metronidazole (p.594·1).
Anaerobic bacterial infections; Helicobacter pylori infections.

Anaerobyl *Searle, S.Afr.†*
Metronidazole (p.594·1).
Anaerobic bacterial infections; protozoal infections.

Anaeromet *Glaxo Wellcome, Belg.*
Metronidazole (p.594·1).
Anaerobic bacterial infections; protozoal infections.

Anaestalgin *Streuli, Switz.*
Procaine hydrochloride (p.1319·1); caffeine (p.761·3).
Pain.

Anaesthecomp N *Ritsert, Ger.*
Lignocaine [lidocaine] hydrochloride (p.1313·2); diphenhydramine hydrochloride (p.416·1).
Allergic rashes; insect stings; sunburn.

Anaestherit *Sanova, Aust.*
Benzocaine (p.1306·2).
Anorectal disorders; skin disorders.

Anaesthesin *Ritsert, Ger.*
Benzocaine (p.1306·2).
Coughs and associated throat disorders; haemorrhoids; skin disorders; wounds.

Anaesthesin N *Ritsert, Ger.*
Benzocaine (p.1306·2).
Haemorrhoids; skin disorders; wounds.

Anaesthesin-Rivanol *Ritsert, Ger.*
Benzocaine (p.1306·2); ethacridine lactate (p.1130·3).
Painful throat infections.

Anaesthesulf *Ritsert, Ger.*
Lauromacrogol 400 (p.1345·2).
Formerly known as Anaesthesulf P and contained lauromacrogol 400 and zinc oxide.
Pruritic skin disorders.

Anaesthetic Ear Drops *Vitamed, Israel.*
Amethocaine [tetracaine] (p.1305·2); phenazone (p.77·2).
Otitis.

Anaesthol *Merz, Ger.†*
Lignocaine [lidocaine] hydrochloride (p.1313·2). Adrenaline [epinephrine] (p.829·1) and noradrenaline [norepinephrine] (p.948·2) are included in this preparation as vasoconstrictors to diminish absorption and localise the effect of the local anaesthetic.
Local anaesthesia.

Anafen
Note. This name is used for preparations of different composition.
Pacific, NZ.
Ibuprofen (p.43·2).
Musculoskeletal, joint, peri-articular, and soft-tissue disorders; pain.

TO-Chemicals, Thai.
Tiaprofenic acid (p.88·1).
Pain.

Anafertin *Armstrong, Mex.*
Algestone acetophenide (p.1465·1); estradiol enantate (p.1473·2).
Injectable contraceptive; menstrual disorders.

Ana-Flex *Gunther, Braz.*
Note. A similar name is used for preparations of different composition (see below).
Diclofenac sodium (p.30·3).
Gout; inflammation; musculoskeletal, joint, and peri-articular disorders; pain.

Anaflex
Note. A similar name is used for preparations of different composition (see below).
Chemomedica, Aust.†; Geistlich, Singapore; Geistlich, UK.
Polynoxylin (p.1154·2).
Skin infections.

Anaflin *Ehlinger, Mex.*
Naproxen (p.60·3).

Anafranil *Novartis, Aust.; Novartis, Austral.; Novartis, Belg.; Novartis, Braz.; Novartis, Canad.; Novartis, Denm.; Novartis, Fin.; Novartis, Fr.; Novartis, Ger.; Du Pont, Ger.; Novartis, Hong Kong; Novartis, Irl.; Novartis, Israel; Novartis, Ital.; Novartis, Mex.; Novartis, Neth.; Novartis, Norw.; Novartis, NZ; Novartis, Port.; Novartis, Swed.; Novartis, Switz.; Novartis, Thai.; Novartis, USA.*
Clomipramine hydrochloride (p.282·1).
Depression; narcoleptic syndrome; nocturnal enuresis; obsessive-compulsive disorder; pain syndromes; panic attacks; phobic states.

Anagastra *Madaus, Spain.*
Pantoprazole sodium (p.1243·2).
Gastro-oesophageal reflux; peptic ulcer.

Anagen *Rydelle, Fr.†*
Amino-acid, vitamin, and mineral preparation (p.1350·1).
Hair and nail disorders.

Anagregal *Gentili, Ital.*
Ticlopidine hydrochloride (p.981·1).
Thrombosis prophylaxis.

Ana-Guard *Bayer, S.Afr.*
Adrenaline [epinephrine] hydrochloride (p.829·2).
Anaphylaxis.

Anahelp *Stallergenes, Fr.*
Adrenaline [epinephrine] (p.829·1).
Anaphylaxis.

Anakit *Dome-Hollister-Stier, Fr.*
Adrenaline [epinephrine] (p.829·1).
Anaphylaxis.

Ana-Kit *Bayer, Canad.; Bayer, NZ; Bayer, USA.*
Combination pack: Injection, adrenaline [epinephrine] hydrochloride (p.829·2); 4 chewable tablets, chlorpheniramine [chlorphenamine] maleate (p.412·1).
Anaphylaxis.

Analfin *Tecnofarma, Mex.*
Morphine sulfate (p.56·1).
Pain.

Analgen
Note. A similar name is used for preparations of different composition (see below).
Johnson & Johnson, Braz.
Turpentine oil (p.1676·3); methyl salicylate (p.55·1); camphor (p.1589·3); mustard oil (p.1639·1); rosemary oil (p.1659·3); lavender oil (p.1627·2); menthol (p.1632·3).
Musculoskeletal and joint disorders.

Aventis, S.Afr.
Aspirin (p.14·2); paracetamol (p.71·2); codeine phosphate (p.25·2); caffeine (p.761·3).
Fever; pain.

Anal-Gen *BCL, Switz.*
Note. A similar name is used for preparations of different composition (see below).
Hamamelis water (p.1618·3); melissa oil.
Anogenital skin disorders.

Analgen-SA *Aventis, S.Afr.*
Aluminium aspirin (p.13·3); paracetamol (p.71·2); codeine phosphate (p.25·2); caffeine (p.761·3); chlorphenoxamine hydrochloride (p.412·3); phenobarbital (p.355·1); ascorbic acid (p.1389·3).
Fever; pain.

Analgesia Creme *Rugby, USA.*
Trolamine salicylate (p.90·1).
Muscle, joint, and soft-tissue pain; neuralgia.

Analgesic Balm
Note. This name is used for preparations of different composition.
Drug Trading, Canad.†
Menthol (p.1632·3); methyl salicylate (p.55·1); cloral hydrate (p.669·3).

Stanley, Canad.
Menthol (p.1632·3); methyl salicylate (p.55·1); eucalyptus oil (p.1609·2); guaiacol (p.1092·1).

Warner-Lambert, Canad.; Goldline, USA; Major, USA; URL, USA.
Menthol (p.1632·3); methyl salicylate (p.55·1).
Muscle, joint, and soft-tissue pain; neuralgia.

Analgesic Otic Solution *Akorn, USA†.*
Phenazone (p.77·2); benzocaine (p.1306·2); hydroxyquinoline sulfate (p.1622·2).
Earache.

Analgesic Rub *McGloin, Austral.†*
Menthol (p.1632·3); camphor (p.1589·3); eucalyptus oil (p.1609·2); methyl salicylate (p.55·1); pumilio pine oil (p.1656·3).
Muscle and joint pain.

Analgesico Ut Asens Fn *Asens, Spain†.*
Camphor (p.1589·3); alcohol (p.1130·3); ammonia (p.1579·1); menthol (p.1632·3).
Soft-tissue disorders.

Analgex *Uniao Quimica, Braz.*
Dipyrone (p.34·1).
Fever; pain.

Analgex C *Uniao Quimica, Braz.*
Injection: Ampoule 1, dipyrone (p.34·1); guaifenesin (p.1092·2); caffeine (p.761·3); mepyramine maleate (p.421·1); ampoule 2, vitamin C (p.1389·3).
Lignocaine [lidocaine] hydrochloride (p.1313·2) is included in this preparation to alleviate the pain of injection.
Tablets: Green tablets, dipyrone (p.34·1); caffeine (p.761·3); mepyramine maleate (p.421·1); orange tablets, vitamin C (p.1389·3).
Cold and influenza symptoms.

Analgi *Azevedos, Port.*
Methyl salicylate (p.55·1); menthol (p.1632·3); camphor (p.1589·3); guaiacol (p.1092·1).
Musculoskeletal and joint disorders.

Analgilasa *Ipsen, Spain.*
Tablets: Caffeine (p.761·3); codeine phosphate (p.25·2); paracetamol (p.71·2).
Suppositories†: Caffeine (p.761·3); codeine phosphate (p.25·2); papaverine hydrochloride (p.1648·1); paracetamol (p.71·2).
Pain.

Analgin
Note. This name is used for preparations of different composition.
Medphano, Ger.
Dipyrone (p.34·1).
Fever; pain.

Sam-On, Israel.
Aspirin (p.14·2); codeine phosphate (p.25·2).
Influenza symptoms; pain.

Analgin C-R *EMS, Braz.*
Dipyrone (p.34·1); chlorpheniramine [chlorphenamine] maleate (p.412·1); vitamin C (p.1389·3).
Cold and influenza symptoms.

Analgina *Apsen, Braz.*
Dipyrone (p.34·1).
Fever; pain.

Analgiol *Abello, Spain.*
Codeine phosphate (p.25·2).
Pain.

Analgit *Krewel, Ger.†*
Dipyrone (p.34·1).
Fever; pain.

Analgosedan *Brasmedica, Braz.*
Dipyrone (p.34·1); homatropine methylbromide (p.468·1); adiphenine; papaverine hydrochloride (p.1648·1).
Smooth muscle spasm.

Analip *Iketon, Ital.†*
Pantethine (p.952·1).
Hyperlipidaemias.

Analmex *Ofimex, Mex.*
Paracetamol (p.71·2).
Fever; pain.

Analog LCP *Scientific Hospital Supplies, Irl.*
Food for special diets (p.1350·1).
Formerly known as Analog XP.
Phenylketonuria.

Analog MSUD *SHS, Fr.; Scientific Hospital Supplies, UK.*
Food for special diets (p.1350·1).
Maple syrup urine disease.

Analog RVHB *Scientific Hospital Supplies, UK.*
Food for special diets (p.1350·1).
Homocystinuria; hypermethioninaemia.

Analog XLEU *SHS, Fr.*
Food for special diets (p.1350·1).
Isovaleric acidaemia.

Analog XLYS *SHS, Fr.*
Food for special diets (p.1350·1).
Hyperlysinaemia.

Analog XLYS Low Try *SHS, Fr.*
Food for special diets (p.1350·1).
Glutaric aciduria.

Analog XMET *SHS, Fr.*
Food for special diets (p.1350·1).
Homocystinuria.

Analog XMET, Cys *SHS, Fr.*
Food for special diets (p.1350·1).
Sulfite oxidase deficiency.

Analog Xmet, Thre, Val, Isoleu *Scientific Hospital Supplies, UK.*
Food for special diets (p.1350·1).
Methylmalonic or propionic acidaemia.

Analog XMTVI *SHS, Fr.*
Food for special diets (p.1350·1).
Methylmalonic or propionic acidaemia.

Analog XP *SHS, Fr.; Scientific Hospital Supplies, UK.*
Food for special diets (p.1350·1).
Phenylketonuria.

Analog Xphen, Tyr *SHS, Fr.; Scientific Hospital Supplies, UK.*
Food for special diets (p.1350·1).
Tyrosinaemia.

Analog XPTM *SHS, Fr.*
Food for special diets (p.1350·1).
Tyrosinaemia.

Analpan *Duopharma, Hong Kong.*
Diclofenac sodium (p.30·3).
Inflammation; musculoskeletal and joint disorders; pain.

Analpram-HC *Ferndale, USA.*
Hydrocortisone acetate (p.1073·3); pramocaine hydrochloride (p.1318·2).
Anorectal disorders.

Analter *Alter, Spain.*
Paracetamol (p.71·2).
Fever; pain.

Analtrix *Faria, Braz.*
Oxyphenbutazone (p.71·1); paracetamol (p.71·2).
Aluminium hydroxide (p.1210·3) is included in this preparation in an attempt to limit adverse effects on the gastrointestinal mucosa.
Fever; inflammation; pain.

Analux *Cusi, Hong Kong; Cusi, Singapore; Alcon Cusi, Spain.*
Phenylephrine hydrochloride (p.1097·1).
Eye irritation.

Analverin *Dovalle, Braz.*
Hyoscyamine hydrobromide (p.469·3); dipyrone (p.34·1).
Pain; smooth muscle spasm.

Anamai *Nakorn, Thai.*
21 Tablets, norethisterone (p.1485·1); mestranol (p.1482·1); 7 tablets, inert.
Combined oral contraceptive.

Anamine *Mayrand, USA.*
Pseudoephedrine hydrochloride (p.1099·2); chlorpheniramine [chlorphenamine] maleate (p.412·1).
Cold symptoms.

Anamorph *Fawns & McAllan, Austral.*
Morphine sulfate (p.56·1).
Pain.

Ananase *Rhone-Poulenc Rorer, Hong Kong; Rhone-Poulenc Rorer, Irl.†; Rottapharm, Ital.; Delta, Port.; Aventis, S.Afr.*
Bromelains (p.1586·3).
Skin disorders; skin ulceration; soft-tissue inflammation and oedema.

Anandron *Hoechst Marion Roussel, Austral.; Hoechst Marion Roussel, Braz.; Hoechst Marion Roussel, Canad.; Aventis, Denm.; Hoechst Marion Roussel, Fin.; Cassenne, Fr.; Hoechst Marion Roussel, Neth.; Hoechst Marion Roussel, Norw.; Roussel, Port.; Hoechst Marion Roussel, Swed.*
Nilutamide (p.562·3).
Prostatic cancer.

Anapen
Note.This name is used for preparations of different composition.
Allerbio, Fr.; Decomed, Port.; Lincoln, UK.
Adrenaline [epinephrine] (p.829·1).
Anaphylaxis.

CEPA, Spain†.
Benzylpenicillin sodium (p.157·2); clemizole penicillin (p.188·1).
Bacterial infections.

Anapenil Grossman, Mex.
Injection: Clemizole penicillin (p.188·1); benzylpenicillin sodium (p.157·2).
Tablets; oral solution: Phenoxymethylpenicillin potassium (p.235·1).
Bacterial infections.

Anaphase Ducray, Fr.
Tocoferil nicotinate (p.984·3); vitamin B substances (p.1350·1).
Hair disorders.

Anaphyl Sam-On, Israel.
Chlorpheniramine [chlorphenamine] maleate (p.412·1).
Hypersensitivity reactions.

Anaphylaxie-Besteck Bencard, Ger.
Adrenaline [epinephrine] hydrochloride (p.829·2).
Anaphylactic shock.

Anapirol Dinafarma, Braz.
Dipyrone (p.34·1); caffeine (p.761·3); orphenadrine citrate (p.470·3).
Smooth muscle spasm.

Anaplex Medi-Plex, USA†.
Pseudoephedrine hydrochloride (p.1099·2); chlorpheniramine [chlorphenamine] maleate (p.412·1).
Cold symptoms.

Anaplex DM ECR, USA.
Dextromethorphan hydrobromide (p.1087·1); brompheniramine maleate (p.410·2); pseudoephedrine hydrochloride (p.1099·2).
Coughs.

Anaplex HD ECR, USA.
Hydrocodone tartrate (p.42·2); pseudoephedrine hydrochloride (p.1099·2); brompheniramine maleate (p.410·2).
Formerly contained hydrocodone tartrate, phenylephrine hydrochloride, and chlorpheniramine [chlorphenamine] maleate.
Coughs and cold symptoms.

Anapolon Roche, S.Afr.†; Syntex, UK†.
Oxymetholone (p.1487·3).
Anaemias.

Anapres Lemery, Mex.
Prazosin (p.958·1).
Hypertension.

Anapril Berlin Pharm, Singapore; Berlin Pharm, Thai.
Enalapril maleate (p.883·3).
Heart failure; hypertension.

Anaprol Provit, Mex.
Dipyrone (p.34·1).
Fever; inflammation; pain.

Anaprox Syntex, Austral.; Roche, Canad.; Roche, Spain; Roche, USA.
Naproxen sodium (p.61·2).
Fever; inflammation; musculoskeletal, joint, and periarticular disorders; pain.

Anapsique Psicofarma, Mex.
Amitriptyline hydrochloride (p.273·3).
Depression; hyperactivity in children; nocturnal enuresis.

Anapyon Dorsay, Braz.
Tyrothricin (p.267·1); chlorophyll (p.1028·1); tannic acid (p.1669·1).
Mouth and throat infections.

Anara Chinoin, Mex.
Sodium picosulfate (p.1249·3).
Bowel evacuation; constipation.

Anarex Beacons, Singapore.
Orphenadrine citrate (p.470·3); paracetamol (p.71·2).
Skeletal muscle spasm.

Anargil Medochemie, Hong Kong; Medochemie, Thai.
Danazol (p.1468·3).
Benign breast disorders; endometriosis; female infertility; gynaecomastia; hereditary angioedema; menorrhagia; precocious puberty.

Anaribes Farmachimici, Ital.
Black currant; betacarotene; vitamin E (p.1350·1).
Nutritional supplement.

Anartril Farma Lepori, Spain†.
Glucosamine sulfate (p.1616·2); glucosamine hydroiodide (p.1616·2).
Inflammation; osteomyelitis.

Anartrit QIF, Braz.
Piroxicam (p.79·1).
Dysmenorrhoea; gout; musculoskeletal, joint, and peri-articular disorders.

Anasclerol Expharma, Ital.†.
Vincamine hydrochloride (p.1680·1).
Cerebrovascular disorders.

Anased Potter's, UK.
Lupulus (p.1629·3); Jamaica dogwood (p.1625·1); wild lettuce (p.1680·3); passion flower (p.1649·1); pulsatilla (p.1656·3).
Pain; tension.

Anaseptil Sanofi Winthrop, Braz.
Polymyxin B sulfate (p.238·1); neomycin sulfate (p.228·1); zinc peroxide (p.1159·3); zinc oxide (p.1128·2).
Bacterial skin infections.

Anasilpiel Euroexim, Spain.
Ointment: Dexpanthenol (p.1602·3); neomycin undecenoate (p.228·1); triamcinolone acetonide (p.1080·1).
Topical aerosol: Neomycin undecenonate (p.228·1); triamcinolone acetonide (p.1080·1).
Infected skin disorders.

Anaspaz Ascher, USA.
Hyoscyamine sulfate (p.469·3).
Smooth muscle spasm.

Anasten Errekappa, Ital.
Magnesium; potassium; carnitine; ubidecarenone; vitamin C (p.1350·1).
Nutritional supplement.

Anastil Eberth, Ger.
Injection: Guaiacol (p.1092·1).
Bronchitis; pneumonia.
Lozenges: Thyme (p.1672·2).
Bronchitis; catarrh.

Anastil N Eberth, Ger.
Thyme (p.1672·2); camphor (p.1589·3); guaifenesin (p.1092·2).
Bronchitis; catarrh; coughs.

Anatac UCB, Spain.
Carbocisteine (p.1086·3).
Respiratory-tract disorders.

Anatensol Bristol-Myers Squibb, Austral.; Bristol-Myers Squibb, Braz.; Mead Johnson, Ital.; Bristol-Myers Squibb, Neth.; Bristol-Myers Squibb, Port.
Fluphenazine decanoate (p.684·3), fluphenazine enantate (p.684·3), or fluphenazine hydrochloride (p.684·3).
Psychoses.

Anatetall Chiron, Ital.; Chiron, Thai.
An adsorbed tetanus vaccine (p.1565·2).
Active immunisation.

Anatopic Martin, Spain†.
Fluocinolone acetonide (p.1071·1).
Skin disorders.

Anatoxal Di Berna, Switz.
An adsorbed diphtheria vaccine (p.1536·2).
Active immunisation.

Anatoxal Di Te Kwizda, Aust.; Berna, Belg.†; Berna, Ital.; Berna, Port.; Berna, Spain; Berna, Switz.
An adsorbed diphtheria and tetanus vaccine (p.1537·1). Separate preparations are available for infants and young children and for older children and adults.
Active immunisation.

Anatoxal Di Te Per Kwizda, Aust.; Berna, Belg.†; Berna, Ital.†; Berna, Port.†; Berna, Spain†; Berna, Switz.†.
An adsorbed diphtheria, tetanus, and pertussis vaccine (p.1537·3).
Active immunisation of infants and young children.

Anatoxal Te Berna, Belg.†; Berna, Port.; Berna, Spain; Berna, Switz.
An adsorbed tetanus vaccine (p.1565·2).
Active immunisation.

Anatoxal Te Di Berna, Spain.
A diphtheria and tetanus vaccine (p.1537·1).
Active immunisation of children and adults.

Anatoxina Estafilococica Butantan, Braz.
A staphylococcal vaccine (p.1565·1).
Active immunisation.

Anatrast Lafayette, USA.
Barium sulfate (p.1032·1).
Contrast medium for gastrointestinal radiography.

Anatuss Mayrand, USA†.
Syrup: Phenylpropanolamine hydrochloride (p.1098·1); dextromethorphan hydrobromide (p.1087·3); guaifenesin (p.1092·2).
Tablets: Phenylpropanolamine hydrochloride (p.1098·1); dextromethorphan hydrobromide (p.1087·3); guaifenesin (p.1092·2); paracetamol (p.71·2).
Coughs.

Anatuss DM Merz, USA.
Guaifenesin (p.1092·2); pseudoephedrine hydrochloride (p.1099·2); dextromethorphan hydrobromide (p.1087·3).
Coughs.

Anatuss LA Merz, USA.
Guaifenesin (p.1092·2); pseudoephedrine hydrochloride (p.1099·2).
Coughs.

Anatyl Sanval, Braz.
Paracetamol (p.71·2).
Fever; pain.

Anauran Zambon, Ital.
Polymyxin B sulfate (p.238·1); neomycin sulfate (p.228·1); lignocaine [lidocaine] hydrochloride (p.1313·2).
Formerly contained polymyxin B sulfate, neomycin sulfate, lignocaine [lidocaine] hydrochloride, betamethasone, and furaltadone hydrochloride.
External ear disorders.

Anausin Asta Medica, Fr.
Metoclopramide hydrochloride (p.1235·2).
Nausea and vomiting.

Anax Whan In, Singapore.
Naproxen sodium (p.61·2).
Gout; musculoskeletal, joint, and peri-articular disorders; pain.

Anaxeryl Bailly, Fr.
Dithranol (p.1113·3); ichthammol (p.1115·2); salicylic acid (p.1122·3); resorcinol (p.1122·2); peru balsam (p.1650·2).
Formerly contained dithranol, ichthammol, salicylic acid, resorcinol, peru balsam, and birch tar oil.
Alopecia; psoriasis.

Anazo Progress, Thai.
Phenazopyridine hydrochloride (p.77·3).
Urinary-tract pain.

Anbesol
Note.This name is used for preparations of different composition.
Whitehall-Robins, Canad.; Whitehall, USA.
Topical gel: Benzocaine (p.1306·2); phenol (p.1152·3).
Minor skin abrasions; mouth pain.

Whitehall-Robins, Canad.
Topical liquid: Benzocaine (p.1306·2); phenol (p.1152·3); camphor (p.1589·3); menthol (p.1632·3).
Minor skin abrasions; mouth pain.

Whitehall, USA.
Topical liquid: Benzocaine (p.1306·2); phenol (p.1152·3); menthol (p.1632·3); camphor (p.1589·3); povidone-iodine (p.1155·1).
Mouth and throat disorders.

Seton, Irl.; SSL, UK.
Cetylpyridinium chloride (p.1138·1); chlorocresol (p.1141·3); lignocaine [lidocaine] hydrochloride (p.1313·2).
Oral pain and irritation.

Anbesol Baby Whitehall-Robins, Canad.
Benzocaine (p.1306·2).
Teething.

Anbikan ANB, Thai.
Kanamycin (p.218·2).
Gram-negative bacterial infections.

Anbikin ANB, Thai.
Amikacin sulfate (p.148·1).
Bacterial infections.

Anbin Grifols, Ital.
Antithrombin III (p.725·2).
Antithrombin III deficiency.

Anbycin ANB, Thai.
Lincomycin (p.219·3).
Gram-positive bacterial infections.

Ancamin PP Lab, Thai.
Calamine (p.1111·3); zinc oxide (p.1128·2); chlorpheniramine [chlorphenamine] maleate (p.412·1).
Pruritus; skin irritation.

Ancef SmithKline Beecham, Canad.; SmithKline Beecham, USA.
Cefazolin sodium (p.164·3).
Bacterial infections.

Anceron Schering-Plough, S.Afr.
Beclometasone dipropionate (p.1061·2).
Rhinitis.

Ancet C & M, USA.
Skin cleanser.

Ancid Hexal, Ger.
Hydrotalcite (p.1228·1).
Gastrointestinal hyperacidity; heartburn; peptic ulcer.

Anco BASF, Ger.
Ibuprofen (p.43·2).
Inflammation; musculoskeletal, joint, and soft-tissue disorders; pain.

Ancobon ICN, USA.
Flucytosine (p.385·2).
Candidiasis; cryptococcosis.

Ancopir Grossmann, Hong Kong; Grossmann, Switz.
Vitamin B substances (p.1350·1).
Lignocaine [lidocaine] hydrochloride (p.1313·2) is included in the intramuscular injection to alleviate the pain of injection.
Adjuvant in radiation therapy; alcoholism; lumbago; neuralgia; neuritis; sciatica; vitamin B deficiency.

Ancoren Sanitas, Port.
Atenolol (p.841·3).
Angina pectoris; arrhythmias; hypertension; myocardial infarction.

Ancoron Libbs, Braz.
Amiodarone hydrochloride (p.836·1).
Arrhythmias.

Ancotil Roche, Aust.; Dermatech, Austral.; Roche, Braz.; Medilink, Denm.; CSP, Fr.; ICN, Ger.; ICN, Hong Kong; ICN, Irl.; ICN, Ital.; ICN, Neth.†; Medilink, Norw.†; ICN, Singapore; Medilink, Swed.; ICN, Switz.; CN, UK.
Flucytosine (p.385·2).
Formerly known as Alcobon in the UK.
Fungal infections.

Andante Boehringer Ingelheim, Ger.
Bunazosin hydrochloride (p.852·3).
Hypertension.

Andantol Asta Medica, Belg.; Asta Medica, Braz.; Sanfer, Mex.
Isothipendyl hydrochloride (p.419·2).
Allergic skin disorders.

Andapsin Orion, Swed.
Sucralfate (p.1250·2).
Gastrointestinal haemorrhage; peptic ulcer.

Andehist Cypress, USA.
Oral drops: Carbinoxamine maleate (p.411·1); pseudoephedrine hydrochloride (p.1099·2).
Rhinitis.
Syrup: Pseudoephedrine hydrochloride (p.1099·2); brompheniramine maleate (p.410·2).
Upper respiratory-tract disorders.

Andehist DM Cypress, USA.
Oral drops: Carbinoxamine maleate (p.411·1); pseudoephedrine hydrochloride (p.1099·2); dextromethorphan hydrobromide (p.1087·3).
Coughs and cold symptoms.
Syrup: Pseudoephedrine hydrochloride (p.1099·2); brompheniramine maleate (p.410·2); dextromethorphan hydrobromide (p.1087·3).
Coughs.

Andergin Searle, Ital.†.
Miconazole nitrate (p.391·1).
Fungal infections.

Andion Gea, Denm.†.
Beclometasone dipropionate (p.1061·2).
Asthma.

Andociclina Balsamica Andromaco, Mex.
Oxytetracycline (p.234·1); guaifenesin (p.1092·2); eucalyptol (p.1609·2).
Lignocaine [lidocaine] (p.1313·2) is included in this preparation to alleviate the pain of injection.
Respiratory-tract disorders.

Andolba Whitehall, Braz.
Benzocaine (p.1306·2); benzethonium chloride (p.1134·2); menthol (p.1632·3); hydroxyquinoline benzoate (p.1622·2).
Gynaecological disorders.

Andolex 3M, Denm.; 3M, S.Afr.; 3M, Swed.
Benzydamine hydrochloride (p.20·1).
Mouth and throat disorders.

Andolex-C 3M, S.Afr.
Benzydamine hydrochloride (p.20·1); chlorhexidine gluconate (p.1138·2).
Inflammation and infection of the mouth and throat.

Andolor Krewel, Ger.
Tilidate hydrochloride (p.88·2); naloxone hydrochloride (p.1014·3).
Pain.

Andopan Atlantis, Mex.
Paracetamol (p.71·2).
Fever; pain.

Andox Atlantis, Mex.
Paracetamol (p.71·2).
Fever; pain.

Andractim Piette, Belg.; Besins-Iscovesco, Fr.; Piette, Thai.
Androstanolone (p.1465·2).
Gynaecomastia; lichen; male hypogonadism.

Andreafol Andreabal, Switz.
Folic acid (p.1361·1).
Neural tube defect prophylaxis.

Andrews SmithKline Beecham, Belg.; SmithKline Beecham Consumer, Irl.; SmithKline Beecham Consumer, UK.
Citric acid (p.1596·2); magnesium sulfate (p.1191·1); sodium bicarbonate (p.1186·2).
Constipation; dyspepsia.

Andrews Answer SmithKline Beecham Consumer, UK.
Paracetamol (p.71·2); caffeine (p.761·3).
Dyspepsia; headache.

Andrews Antacid SmithKline Beecham Consumer, Irl.; SmithKline Beecham Consumer, UK.
Calcium carbonate (p.1215·1); magnesium carbonate (p.1232·3).
Dyspepsia.

Andrews Tums Antacid SmithKline Beecham Consumer, Austral.
Calcium carbonate (p.1215·1).
Calcium supplement; dyspepsia; heartburn.

Andriodermol Cypress, USA.
Undecenoic acid (p.395·3); propionic acid (p.393·2); hexylresorcinol (p.1146·3).
Skin infections.

Andriol Organon, Aust.; Organon, Austral.; Organon, Canad.; Organon, Ger.; Organon, Hong Kong; Organon, Ital.; Organon, Mex.; Organon, Neth.; Organon, Port.; Organon, Singapore; Organon, Switz.; Organon, Thai.
Testosterone undecylate (p.1492·2).
Delayed puberty; primary and hypogonadotrophic hypogonadism; testosterone deficiency.

Andro Forest Pharmaceuticals, USA†.
Testosterone enantate (p.1492·2).
Breast cancer; delayed puberty (males); male hypogonadism.

Androcur Schering, Aust.; Schering, Austral.; Schering, Belg.; Schering, Braz.; Berlex, Canad.; Schering, Denm.; Schering, Fin.; Schering, Fr.; Schering, Ger.; Schering, Hong Kong; Schering, Irl.; Schering, Israel; Schering, Ital.; Schering, Mex.; Schering, Neth.; Schering, Norw.; Schering, NZ; Schering, Port.; Schering, S.Afr.; Schering, Singapore; Schering, Spain; Schering, Swed.; Schering, Switz.; Schering, Thai.; Schering, UK.
Cyproterone acetate (p.1467·3).
Androgen-dependent hirsutism, alopecia, acne, and seborrhoea in females; male sexual deviation; male virilisation; prostatic cancer.

Androderm Faulding, Austral.; Astra, Ger.; Promed, Ger.; Schwarz, Ital.; Astra, Switz.; SmithKline Beecham, USA.
Testosterone (p.1492·1).
Testosterone deficiency.

Andro-Diane Schering, Aust.
Cyproterone acetate (p.1467·3).
Androgen-dependent hirsutism, alopecia, acne, and seborrhoea in females.

Androfemon *Jenapharm, Ger.*
Estradiol valerate (p.1473·2); testosterone enantate (p.1492·2).
Menopausal disorders.

AndroGel *Unimed, USA.*
Testosterone (p.1492·1).
Hypogonadism.

Android *ICN, USA.*
Methyltestosterone (p.1482·3).
Breast cancer; cryptorchidism; male hypogonadism.

Androlone-D *Keene, USA.*
Nandrolone decanoate (p.1484·2).
Anaemia in renal disease.

Andropatch *SmithKline Beecham, Irl.; SmithKline Beecham, UK.*
Testosterone (p.1492·1).
Testosterone deficiency.

Andropository *Rugby, USA†.*
Testosterone enantate (p.1492·2).
Breast cancer; delayed puberty (males); male hypogonadism.

Androskat *Byk, Aust.; Byk, Neth.*
Papaverine hydrochloride (p.1648·1); phentolamine mesilate (p.954·3).
Erectile dysfunction.

Androtardyl *Schering, Fr.*
Testosterone enantate (p.1492·2).
Male hypogonadism.

Androvite *Optimox, USA.*
Multivitamin and mineral preparation with iron and folic acid (p.1350·1).

Androxicam *Andromaco, Mex.*
Piroxicam (p.79·1).
Gout; musculoskeletal, joint and peri-articular disorders; pain.

Androxon *Akzo, Braz.; Organon, Israel; Organon, Norw.; Donmed, S.Afr.*
Testosterone undecylate (p.1492·2).
Male hypogonadism.

Androxyl *Duopharma, Hong Kong.*
Cefadroxil (p.161·2).
Bacterial infections.

Andrumin *Janssen-Cilag, Austral.†.*
Dimenhydrinate (p.415·2).
Motion sickness; vestibular disorders.

Andursil *Novartis, Braz.; Sanopharm, Switz.*
Aluminium hydroxide-magnesium carbonate co-dried gel (p.1211·2); simeticone (p.1249·2).
Flatulence; gastro-oesophageal reflux; gastrointestinal hyperacidity.

Andursil N *Zyma, Ger.†.*
Heavy magnesium carbonate (p.1232·3); dried aluminium hydroxide gel (p.1210·3).
Gastrointestinal disorders.

Anebron *Protein, Mex.*
Salbutamol (p.770·3).

Anectine *Glaxo Wellcome, Canad.; Wellcome, Irl.; Glaxo Wellcome, Mex.; Wellcome, Spain; Glaxo Wellcome, UK; Glaxo Wellcome, USA.*
Suxamethonium chloride (p.1340·1).
Depolarising neuromuscular blocker.

Anekron *EMS, Braz.*
Choline citrate (p.1356·3); betaine hydrochloride (p.1584·3); methionine (p.1012·2); adenosine (p.828·2); vitamin B₆ (p.1386·3); sorbitol (p.1377·3).
Liver disorders.

Anemagen *Ethex, USA.*
Ferrous fumarate (p.1360·1); cyanocobalamin (p.1388·1); stomach extract.
Ascorbic acid (p.1389·3) is included in this preparation to increase the absorption and availability of iron.
Anaemias.

Anemagen OB *Ethex, USA.*
Ferrous fumarate (p.1360·1); calcium; vitamins (p.1350·1).
Docusate sodium (p.1223·1) is included in this preparation to reduce the constipating effects of iron.

Anemet *Hoechst Marion Roussel, Ger.*
Dolasetron mesilate (p.1223·3).
Nausea and vomiting induced by cytotoxic therapy; postoperative nausea and vomiting.

Anemital *Basi, Port.*
Ferrous gluconate (p.1360·1).
Anaemias.

Anemofer *Marjan, Braz.*
Cyanocobalamin (p.1388·1); ferrous sulfate (p.1360·3); folic acid (p.1361·1).
Anaemias.

Anemokol *Biologia, Braz.*
Liver extract; malt extract (p.1371·1); ferric ammonium citrate (p.1359·2).
Anaemias.

Anemul mono *Medopharm, Ger.†.*
Dexamethasone (p.1067·1).
Skin disorders.

Anerex *AF, Mex.*
Vitamin B substances with iron (p.1350·1).
Anaemias; tonic.

Anergan *Forest Pharmaceuticals, USA.*
Promethazine hydrochloride (p.423·2).
Hypersensitivity reactions; motion sickness; nausea; postoperative pain (adjunct); sedative; vomiting.

Anervan *Recip, Fin.; Recip, Norw.; Recip, Swed.*
Ergotamine tartrate (p.452·1); chlorcyclizine hydrochloride (p.411·3); caffeine (p.761·3); meprobamate (p.691·1).
Cluster headache; migraine.

Anesdente do Bebe *Lopes, Braz.*
Amethocaine [tetracaine] hydrochloride (p.1305·2); menthol (p.1632·3).
Teething pain.

Anespas *Rudefsa, Mex.*
Prifinium bromide (p.473·1).
Muscle spasm; pain.

Anest Compuesto *Llorens, Spain†.*
Amethocaine [tetracaine] (p.1305·2).
Naphazoline nitrate (p.1095·1) is included in this preparation as a vasoconstrictor to diminish absorption and localise the effect of the local anaesthetic.
Local anaesthesia.

Anestacon *PolyMedica, USA.*
Lignocaine [lidocaine] hydrochloride (p.1313·2).
Urethral pain.

Anestalcon *Alcon, Braz.*
Proxymetacaine hydrochloride (p.1320·1).
Local anaesthesia.

Anestesia Loc Braun C/A *Braun, Spain.*
Procaine hydrochloride (p.1319·1).
Adrenaline [epinephrine] (p.829·1) is included in this preparation as a vasoconstrictor to diminish absorption and localise the effect of the local anaesthetic.
Local anaesthesia.

Anestesia Loc Braun S/A *Braun, Spain.*
Cinchocaine (p.1309·1); procaine hydrochloride (p.1319·1).
Local anaesthesia.

Anestesia Topi Braun C/A *Braun, Spain.*
Amethocaine [tetracaine] hydrochloride (p.1305·2).
Adrenaline [epinephrine] (p.829·1) is included in this preparation as a vasoconstrictor to diminish absorption and localise the effect of the local anaesthetic.
Local anaesthesia.

Anestesico *Allergan-Frumtost, Braz.; Alcon, Port.; Alcon Cusi, Spain.*
Amethocaine [tetracaine] (p.1305·2) or amethocaine [tetracaine] hydrochloride (p.1305·2).
Naphazoline hydrochloride (p.1095·1) or phenylephrine hydrochloride (p.1097·1) is included in this preparation as a vasoconstrictor to diminish absorption and localise the effect of the local anaesthetic.
Local anaesthesia.

Anestesiol *Lopes, Braz.*
Thymol (p.1158·3); menthol (p.1632·3); camphor (p.1589·3); amethocaine [tetracaine] hydrochloride (p.1305·2); phenazone (p.77·2); clove oil (p.1597·1).
Mouth disorders.

Anesthesique Double *Asta Medica, Belg.†.*
Oxybuprocaine hydrochloride (p.1318·1); amethocaine [tetracaine] hydrochloride (p.1305·2).
Local anaesthesia.

Anesti Doble *Alcon Cusi, Spain.*
Oxybuprocaine hydrochloride (p.1318·1); amethocaine [tetracaine] hydrochloride (p.1305·2).
Local anaesthesia.

Anestina Braun *Polex, Spain†.*
Lignocaine [lidocaine] hydrochloride (p.1313·2); procaine hydrochloride (p.1319·1); amethocaine [tetracaine] hydrochloride (p.1305·2).
Local anaesthesia.

Anestocil *Oftalder, Port.*
Oxybuprocaine hydrochloride (p.1318·1).
Local anaesthesia.

Anethaine *Rhone-Poulenc Rorer, S.Afr.; Torbet Laboratories, UK.*
Amethocaine [tetracaine] hydrochloride (p.1305·2).
Local anaesthesia.

Anetin *Ibirn, Ital.*
Carnitine (p.1356·1).
Carnitine deficiency; myocardial ischaemia.

Aneural *Merck dura, Ger.*
Maprotiline hydrochloride (p.297·2).
Depression.

Aneurin *Teva, Ger.*
Thiamine hydrochloride (p.1385·1).
Vitamin B deficiency.

Aneurol
Note. This name is used for preparations of different composition.
Sanico, Belg.†.
Thiamine hydrochloride (p.1385·1).
Neurogenic pain; rheumatic pain; vitamin B₁ deficiency.

Lacer, Spain.
Diazepam (p.674·3).
Contains pyridoxine hydrochloride.
Alcohol withdrawal syndrome; anxiety; febrile convulsions; insomnia; skeletal muscle spasm.

Anevrase *Cazi, Braz.*
Amethocaine [tetracaine] hydrochloride (p.1305·2); phenylephrine hydrochloride (p.1097·1); passion flower (p.1649·1); erythrina verna; valerian (p.1678·3); hyoscyamus (p.470·1); crataegus (p.1600·2); melissa (p.1632·2).
Sedative.

Anevrasi *Donini, Ital.*
Passion flower (p.1649·1); crataegus (p.1600·2); valerian (p.1678·3).
Insomnia.

Anew *Avon, Canad.*
SPF 15 eye cream: Octinoxate (p.1517·3); titanium dioxide (p.1126·1).

SPF 8; SPF 15 cream; SPF 15 lotion: Octinoxate (p.1517·3); oxybenzone (p.1518·1).
Sunscreen.

Anexate *Roche, Aust.; Roche, Austral.; Roche, Belg.; Roche, Canad.; Roche, Fr.; Roche, Ger.; Roche, Hong Kong; Roche, Irl.; Roche, Israel; Roche, Ital.; Roche, Neth.; Roche, Norw.; Roche, NZ; Roche, Port.; Roche, S.Afr.; Roche, Singapore; Roche, Spain; Roche, Switz.; Roche, Thai.; Roche, UK.*
Flumazenil (p.1008·3).
Benzodiazepine overdosage; reversal of benzodiazepine-induced sedation.

Anexsia *Mallinckrodt, USA.*
Hydrocodone tartrate (p.42·2); paracetamol (p.71·2).
Pain.

Anfenax *Douglas, NZ.*
Diclofenac sodium (p.30·3).
Osteoarthritis; rheumatoid arthritis.

Anfertil *Wyeth, Braz.*
Norgestrel (p.1486·1); ethinylestradiol (p.1476·2).
Combined oral contraceptive.

Anflat *Cazi, Braz.*
Simeticone (p.1249·2).
Flatulence.

Anfocort *Bristol-Myers Squibb, Ital.*
Halcinonide (p.1073·2); amphotericin B (p.377·2).
Formerly contained halcinonide, neomycin sulfate, and amphotericin B.
Infected skin disorders.

Anfomicin *Windson, Braz.*
Neomycin sulfate (p.228·1); sulfadiazine (p.251·1); tyrothricin (p.267·1); benzocaine (p.1306·2).
Mouth and throat disorders.

Angass *Medice, Ger.*
Bismuth subnitrate (p.1213·2); bismuth aluminate (p.1213·1).
Peptic ulcer.

Angass S *Medice, Ger.*
Bismuth subnitrate (p.1213·2).
Peptic ulcer.

Angettes *Bristol-Myers Squibb, UK.*
Aspirin (p.14·2).
Cardiovascular disorders.

Angeze *Opus, UK.*
Isosorbide mononitrate (p.916·2).
Angina pectoris.

Angiact *Nycomed, Denm.*
Diltiazem hydrochloride (p.874·3).
Angina pectoris; hypertension.

Angicontin *Norpharma, Denm.*
Diltiazem hydrochloride (p.874·3).
Angina pectoris; hypertension.

Angicor *Aventis, Denm.*
Nicorandil (p.939·2).
Angina pectoris.

Angidil *Errekappa, Ital.†.*
Diltiazem hydrochloride (p.874·3).
Angina pectoris; hypertension.

Angidine *Vifor, Switz.*
Gramicidin (p.213·3); benzethonium chloride (p.1134·2); amethocaine [tetracaine] hydrochloride (p.1305·2).
Mouth and throat disorders.

Angifebrine *Pharmacal, Switz.†.*
Propyphenazone (p.80·2); paracetamol (p.71·2).
Fever; pain.

Angifonil *Diviser Aquilea, Spain.*
Cetylpyridinium chloride (p.1138·1).
Bacterial mouth infections.

Angileptol *Sigma-Tau, Spain.*
Enoxolone (p.34·3); benzocaine (p.1306·2); chlorhexidine hydrochloride (p.1138·2).
Formerly contained enoxolone, benzocaine, and sulfaguanidine.
Mouth and throat disorders.

Angilol *Douglas, Hong Kong; Douglas, NZ; DDSA Pharmaceuticals, UK.*
Propranolol hydrochloride (p.962·3).
Angina pectoris; arrhythmias; hypertension; hyperthyroidism; migraine; myocardial infarction; obstructive cardiomyopathy; tremor.

Angimon *Dexcel, USA.*
Verapamil hydrochloride (p.989·1).
Angina pectoris; hypertension.

Angina MCC *Streuli, Switz.*
Cetylpyridinium chloride (p.1138·1); lignocaine [lidocaine] hydrochloride (p.1313·2); menthol (p.1632·3).
Mouth and throat disorders.

Angina-Gastreu N R1 *Reckeweg, Ger.*
Homoeopathic preparation.

Anginamide *Medgenix, Belg.*
Sulfacetamide sodium (p.250·3).
Infections of the mouth and throat.

Anginasin N *Opfermann, Ger.*
Hexetidine (p.1146·3); camphor (p.1589·3); menthol (p.1632·3).
Mouth and throat disorders.

Anginesin *Grossmann, Switz.*
Aluminium acetotartrate (p.1578·2); sage (p.1660·2).
Mouth and throat pain.

Anginin *Banyu, Hong Kong; Banyu, Jpn†; Delta, Port.†; Banyu, Thai.*
Pyricarbate (p.1656·3).
Thromboembolic disorders; vascular disorders.

Anginine *Glaxo Wellcome, Austral.; Glaxo Wellcome, NZ.*
Glyceryl trinitrate (p.897·3).
Angina pectoris.

Angino Tricin *Sanval, Braz.*
Neomycin (p.228·1); tyrothricin (p.267·1); benzocaine (p.1306·2); sodium perborate (p.1156·3).
Mouth and throat disorders.

Anginol
Note. This name is used for preparations of different composition.
Labima, Belg.
Dequalinium chloride (p.1143·1).
Mouth and throat disorders.

Streuli, Switz.
Ethacridine lactate (p.1130·3); levomenthol (p.1632·3); camphor (p.1589·3); peru balsam (p.1650·2).
Mouth and throat disorders.

Anginol-Lidocaine *Labima, Belg.*
Dequalinium chloride (p.1143·1); lignocaine [lidocaine] hydrochloride (p.1313·2).
Mouth and throat disorders.

Anginomycin *MIP, Ger.*
Tyrothricin (p.267·1); bacitracin (p.155·2).
Mouth and throat infections.

Anginor *Vesta, S.Afr.†.*
Nifedipine (p.940·1).
Angina pectoris; hypertension.

Angino-Rub *Eurofarma, Braz.*
Naphazoline (p.1095·1); chlorobutanol (p.1141·2); dexpanthenol (p.1602·3).
Nasal congestion.

Anginova *Medinova, Port.*
Dequalinium chloride (p.1143·1); benzocaine (p.1306·2).
Mouth and throat disorders.

Anginova Nouvelle formule *Medinova, Switz.*
Dequalinium chloride (p.1143·1); lignocaine [lidocaine] hydrochloride (p.1313·2).
Mouth and throat disorders.

Anginovag *Novag, Spain.*
Dequalinium chloride (p.1143·1); enoxolone (p.34·3); hydrocortisone acetate (p.1073·3); lignocaine [lidocaine] hydrochloride (p.1313·2); tyrothricin (p.267·1).
Mouth and throat disorders.

Anginovin H *Pfluger, Ger.*
Homoeopathic preparation.

Anginozetes *Gilton, Braz.*
Tyrothricin (p.267·1); benzocaine (p.1306·2).
Mouth and throat disorders.

Angiocardyl N *Rhenomed, Ger.†.*
Atropine sulfate (p.461·1); glyceryl trinitrate (p.897·3); theobromine and sodium salicylate (p.777·2).
Formerly contained atropine sulfate, glyceryl trinitrate, phenobarbital, and theobromine and sodium salicylate.
Cardiac disorders.

Angiocine *Wolfs, Belg.*
Lignocaine [lidocaine] hydrochloride (p.1313·2); chlorhexidine hydrochloride (p.1138·2).
Mouth and throat disorders.

Angio-Conray *Bracco, Ital.†; Mallinckrodt, USA†.*
Sodium iothalamate (p.1036·2).
Radiographic contrast medium.

Angiodarona *Cazi, Braz.*
Amiodarone (p.838·1).
Arrhythmias.

Angiodrox *Solvay, Spain.*
Diltiazem hydrochloride (p.874·3).
Angina pectoris; hypertension.

Angioflux *Mitim, Ital.*
A heparinoid (p.905·2).
Thrombosis prophylaxis.

Angiografin *Schering, Aust.†; Schering, Ger.; Schering, Neth.; Schering, S.Afr.*
Meglumine amidotrizoate (p.1031·2).
Radiographic contrast medium.

Angiografine *Schering, Fr.†.*
Meglumine amidotrizoate (p.1031·2).
Radiographic contrast medium.

Angiolong *Carlo Erba, Braz.*
Diltiazem hydrochloride (p.874·3).
Angina pectoris; arrhythmias; hypertension.

Angiomax *Medicines Company, USA.*
Bivalirudin (p.850·2).
Thromboembolism prophylaxis in patients with unstable angina undergoing coronary angioplasty.

Angionorm *Farmasan, Ger.*
Dihydroergotamine mesilate (p.450·3).
Chronic venous insufficiency; hypotension; migraine and other vascular headache.

Angiopas *Pascoe, Ger.*
Homoeopathic preparation.

Angiophtal *Bournonville, Belg.†; Merck Sharp & Dohme-Chibret, Fr.*
Chromocarb diethylamine (p.1594·3).
Capillary fragility in the eye; subconjunctival haemorrhage.

Angiopine *Ashbourne, UK.*
Nifedipine (p.940·1).
Angina pectoris; hypertension; Raynaud's syndrome.

Angiorex *Lampugnani, Ital.*
Myrtillus (p.1639·2).
Capillary disorders.

The symbol † denotes a preparation no longer actively marketed

Angiosedante *Unifarma, Spain.*
Aminophylline (p.760·1); papaverine hydrochloride (p.1648·1).
Biliary colic; cardiac stimulation; obstructive airways disease.

Angioton *GD, Ital.*
Centella (p.1112·2); rutoside (p.1611·2); vitamins (p.1350·1).
Venous disorders.

Angioton S *DHU, Ger.*
Homoeopathic preparation.

Angiotrofin *Armstrong, Mex.*
Diltiazem hydrochloride (p.874·3).
Angina pectoris; hypertension.

Angiovist 282 *Berlex, USA†.*
Meglumine amidotrizoate (p.1031·2).
Radiographic contrast medium.

Angiovist 292, Angiovist 370 *Berlex, USA†.*
Meglumine amidotrizoate (p.1031·2); sodium amidotrizoate (p.1031·2).
Radiographic contrast medium.

Angiozem *Ashbourne, UK.*
Diltiazem hydrochloride (p.874·3).
Angina pectoris; hypertension.

Angipress
Note. This name is used for preparations of different composition.
Biosintetica, Braz.
Atenolol (p.841·3).
Angina pectoris; arrhythmias; hypertension; myocardial infarction.
Crinos, Ital.
Diltiazem hydrochloride (p.874·3).
Hypertension; ischaemic heart disease.

Angisan *Sanabo, Aust.†.*
Chlorhexidine gluconate (p.1138·2).
Mouth disorders.

Angised
Glaxo Wellcome, Hong Kong; Wellcome, Irl.; Glaxo Wellcome, Israel; Glaxo Wellcome, S.Afr.; Glaxo Wellcome, Singapore; Glaxo Wellcome, Thai.
Glyceryl trinitrate (p.897·3).
Angina pectoris.

Angispray *Monot, Fr.†.*
Note. A similar name is used for preparations of different composition (see below).
Hexetidine (p.1146·3); propionic acid (p.393·2); chlorobutanol (p.1141·2).
Mouth and throat disorders.

Angi-Spray *Aspen, S.Afr.*
Note. A similar name is used for preparations of different composition (see above).
Isosorbide dinitrate (p.915·2).
Angina pectoris; heart failure; myocardial infarction.

Angitak *Eastern Pharmaceuticals, UK.*
Isosorbide dinitrate (p.915·2).
Angina pectoris.

Angitil *Trinity, UK.*
Diltiazem hydrochloride (p.874·3).
Angina pectoris; hypertension.

Angitrate *Aspen, S.Afr.*
Isosorbide mononitrate (p.916·2).
Angina pectoris.

Angitrit *Ranbaxy, Thai.*
Isosorbide dinitrate (p.915·2).
Angina pectoris.

Angizem
Inverni della Beffa, Ital.; Sun, Singapore; Sun, Thai.
Diltiazem hydrochloride (p.874·3).
Angina pectoris; hypertension.

Anglix *Novartis, Mex.*
Glyceryl trinitrate (p.897·3).
Angina pectoris.

Anglopen *Liomont, Mex.*
Ampicillin (p.150·3), ampicillin sodium (p.150·3), or ampicillin trihydrate (p.151·1).
Bacterial infections.

Angocin Anti-Infekt N *Repha, Ger.*
Tropaeolum majus (p.1584·2); horseradish (p.1620·1).
Respiratory-tract infections; urinary-tract infections.

Angocin Bronchialtropfen *Repha, Ger.*
Marrubium vulgare (p.1094·2).
Catarrh.

Angocin percutan *Repha, Ger.*
Camphor (p.1589·3); eucalyptus oil (p.1609·2); turpentine oil (p.1676·3).
Muscle and joint pain; respiratory-tract disorders.

Angstrom Corpo *Pfizer Consumer, Ital.*
Octinoxate (p.1517·3); avobenzone (p.1517·1).
Sunscreen.

Angstrom Viso/Labbra Alta Protezione *Pfizer Consumer, Ital.*
Cream: Octinoxate (p.1517·3); avobenzone (p.1517·1); vitamin E acetate (p.1394·1); dimethicone (p.1410·1); betacarotene (p.1355·1); allantoin (p.1110·1); sodium pidolate (p.1123·3); triclosan (p.1159·2).
Stick: Octinoxate (p.1517·3); avobenzone (p.1517·1); vitamin E acetate (p.1394·1); betacarotene (p.1355·1).
Barrier preparation; sunscreen.

Angurate Magentee *Alsitan, Ger.*
Mentzelia cordifolia.
Gastrointestinal disorders.

Anhisnon *Polipharm, Thai.*
Astemizole (p.409·1).
Hypersensitivity reactions.

Anhydrol Forte
Dermal Laboratories, Irl.; Dermal, Israel; Dermal Laboratories, UK.
Aluminium chloride (p.1110·2).
Hyperhidrosis.

Anhypen *Yamanouchi, Denm.†.*
Ampicillin sodium (p.150·3).
Bacterial infections.

Anidrosan *Cesam, Port.*
Aluminium chloride (p.1110·2).
Hyperhidrosis.

Anifed *Formenti, Ital.†.*
Nifedipine (p.940·1).
Hypertension; ischaemic heart disease.

Anifer Fenchelhonig *Hofmann, Aust.*
Fennel (p.1610·1); honey (p.1366·2).
Coughs and cold symptoms.

Anifer Hustenbalsam *Hofmann, Aust.*
Eucalyptus oil (p.1609·2); pumilio pine oil (p.1656·3); sage oil (p.1660·2).
Respiratory-tract disorders.

Anifer Hustentee *Anifer, Aust.*
Althaea (p.1577·1); aniseed (p.1580·2); thyme (p.1672·2); plantago lanceolata leaf; mallow flowers.
Respiratory-tract disorders.

Anifer Hustentropfen *Hofmann, Aust.*
Thyme (p.1672·2); cowslip rhizome (p.1600·1).
Coughs.

Anifer Krauterol *Hofmann, Aust.*
Eucalyptus oil (p.1609·2); oleum pini sylvestris; pumilio pine oil (p.1656·3).
Respiratory-tract disorders.

Aniflazime *Seber, Port.*
Serrapeptase (p.1662·1).
Inflammation; respiratory-tract congestion.

Aniflazym *Takeda, Ger.*
Serrapeptase (p.1662·1).
Inflammation.

Anilid *Kener, Mex.*
Chlortalidone (p.857·1).

Anilusin *Cryopharma, Mex.*
Insulin (p.324·1).
Diabetes mellitus.

Animal Shapes *Major, USA.*
Multivitamin preparation (p.1350·1).

Animal Shapes + Iron *Major, USA.*
Multivitamin preparation with iron (p.1350·1).

Animine
Note. This name is used for preparations of different composition.
McGloin, Argent.
Cream: Benzocaine (p.1306·2); benzalkonium chloride (p.1133·2).
Lotion: Lignocaine [lidocaine] hydrochloride (p.1313·2); benzalkonium chloride (p.1133·2); calamine (p.1111·3).
Bites; pruritus; stings.
Sanofi Synthelabo, Belg.
Trimethylxanthine sodium alphanaphthylacetate.
Mental function impairment; tonic.

Anionen-Spurenelement *Fresenius Kabi, Aust.*
Electrolytes for infusion (p.1180·1).
Parenteral nutrition.

Aniospray *Anios, Fr.*
Formaldehyde (p.1144·2); glyoxal (p.1145·3); glutaral (p.1145·2); didecyldimethylammonium chloride (p.1143·2).
Disinfection of instruments and surfaces.

Anisan *Pascoe, Ger.*
Menthol (p.1632·3); bismuth subgallate (p.1213·2); aluminium acetate tartrate (p.1578·2); hypericum oil (p.290·3); aesculus (p.1574·1); chamomile (p.1593·2); hamamelis (p.1618·3); liver oil.
Anorectal disorders.

Anistal *Silanes, Mex.*
Ranitidine hydrochloride (p.1245·2).
Acid aspiration; gastro-oesophageal reflux; gastrointestinal haemorrhage; peptic ulcer; Zollinger-Ellison syndrome.

Anitos *Bittner, Aust.*
Senega (p.1100·2); plantago lanceolata; thyme (p.1672·2); anise oil (p.1580·3).
Coughs and cold symptoms.

Anitrim *Italmex, Mex.*
Co-trimoxazole (p.193·3).
Bacterial infections.

Anivy *Roberts, Canad.†.*
Chlorphenesin (p.381·3); benzocaine (p.1306·2).
Insect bites; poison ivy; skin irritation.

Anna *Nakorn, Thai.*
21 Tablets, levonorgestrel (p.1486·2); ethinylestradiol (p.1476·2); 7 tablets, inert.
Combined oral contraceptive.

Annadine *Unison, Thai.*
Povidone-iodine (p.1155·1).
Skin disinfection.

Anningzochin *Laves, Ger.†.*
Mycobacterium chelonae subsp. chelonae.
Immunotherapy.

Annoxen *Siam Bheasach, Thai.*
Naproxen (p.60·3) or naproxen sodium (p.61·1).
Acute gout; musculoskeletal, joint, and peri-articular disorders.

Anoclor *Rolab, S.Afr.*
Chloroquine phosphate (p.432·3).
Now known as Rolab-Chloroquin Phosphate.
Malaria.

Anodan-HC *Odan, Canad.*
Hydrocortisone acetate (p.1073·3); zinc sulfate (p.1398·2).
Anorectal disorders.

Anodesyn *SSL, UK.*
Lignocaine [lidocaine] hydrochloride (p.1313·2); allantoin (p.1110·1).
Anorectal disorders.

Anodynos *Buffington, USA†.*
Aspirin (p.14·2); salicylamide (p.82·1); caffeine (p.761·3).
Pain.

Anolor *Blansett, USA.*
Butalbital (p.658·3); paracetamol (p.71·2); caffeine (p.761·3).
Pain.

Anoquan *Roberts, USA†.*
Paracetamol (p.71·2); caffeine (p.761·3); butalbital (p.658·3).
Pain.

Anoran *Labima, Belg.*
Phendimetrazine hydrochloride (p.1513·3).
Obesity.

Anore Dolor *Schwarzwalder, Ger.*
Homoeopathic preparation.

Anore rheumatic N *Schwarzwalder, Ger.*
Homoeopathic preparation.

Anore X N *Schwarzwalder, Ger.*
Absinthium (p.1571·1); gentian (p.1615·1); angelica (p.1580·2).
Appetite loss; dyspepsia; meteorism.

Anoreine
Note. This name is used for preparations of different composition.
Janssen-Cilag, Aust.
Carrageenan (p.1500·1); titanium dioxide (p.1126·1); zinc oxide (p.1128·2).
Anorectal disorders.
Martin, Fr.
Carrageenan (p.1500·1); bismuth subgallate (p.1213·2); zinc oxide (p.1128·2).
Anorectal disorders.

Anoreine mit Lidocain *Janssen-Cilag, Aust.*
Carrageenan (p.1500·1); titanium dioxide (p.1126·1); zinc oxide (p.1128·2); lignocaine [lidocaine] (p.1313·2).
Anorectal disorders.

Anorex *Dunhall, USA†.*
Phendimetrazine tartrate (p.1513·3).
Obesity.

Anorfin *Gea, Denm.*
Buprenorphine hydrochloride (p.21·1).
Pain.

Anorsia *Asian Pharm, Thai.*
Pizotifen malate (p.455·1).
Anorexia; vascular headache.

Anosedil *Heralds, Braz.*
Lorazepam (p.688·3).
Alcohol withdrawal syndrome; anxiety; epilepsy; insomnia; nausea and vomiting; premedication.

Anoxant *Eagle, Austral.*
A vitamin, mineral. amino-acid, and herbal antioxidant preparation (p.1350·1).

Anoxid *Volchem, Ital.*
Vitamins A, C, and E (p.1350·1).
Formerly contained vitamins A, C, and E with selenium.
Nutritional supplement.

Anpec *Alphapharm, Austral.*
Verapamil hydrochloride (p.989·1).
Angina; arrhythmias; hypertension.

Anplag *Mitsubishi, Jpn.*
Sarpogrelate hydrochloride (p.969·1).
Thromboembolic disorders.

Anpress *Condrugs, Thai.*
Alprazolam (p.654·2).
Anxiety; mixed anxiety depressive states.

Anquil
Janssen-Cilag, Irl.; Janssen-Cilag, UK.
Benperidol (p.656·2).
Deviant sexual behaviour.

Ansaid
Pharmacia Upjohn, Canad.; Pharmacia Upjohn, Mex.; Upjohn, USA.
Flurbiprofen (p.41·2).
Gout; inflammation; musculoskeletal, joint, and peri-articular disorders; pain.

Ansar *Bioclon, Mex.*
Benzyl benzoate (p.1428·2).
Pediculosis; scabies.

Ansatipin
Pharmacia Upjohn, Fin.; Kenforma, Spain; Pharmacia Upjohn, Swed.
Rifabutin (p.242·1).
Opportunistic mycobacterial infections; tuberculosis.

Ansatipine *Pharmacia Upjohn, Fr.*
Rifabutin (p.242·1).
Mycobacterial infections; tuberculosis.

Anselol
Douglas, Austral.; Douglas, NZ.
Atenolol (p.841·3).
Angina pectoris; arrhythmias; hypertension; myocardial infarction.

Anseren *Novartis, Ital.*
Ketazolam (p.688·2).
Anxiety disorders.

Ansiderm *IDI, Ital.*
Magnesium (p.1190·3); kava (p.1625·3).
Nutritional supplement.

Ansilive *Libbs, Braz.*
Diazepam (p.674·3).
Alcohol withdrawal syndrome; anxiety; epilepsy; insomnia; premedication; sedative; skeletal muscle spasm.

Ansilor *Produfarma, Port.*
Lorazepam (p.688·3).
Anxiety; insomnia.

Ansimar *ABC, Ital.*
Doxofylline (p.764·2).
Obstructive airways disease.

Ansiolin *Hoechst Marion Roussel, Ital.*
Diazepam (p.674·3).
Anxiety; epilepsy; insomnia.

Ansitec *Libbs, Braz.*
Buspirone (p.657·2).
Anxiety.

Ansiten *Azevedos, Port.*
Buspirone hydrochloride (p.657·2).
Anxiety disorders.

Ansium *Vita Elan, Spain.*
Diazepam (p.674·3); sulpiride (p.706·1).
Anxiety.

Ansiven *Abbott, Switz.*
Propofol (p.1265·3).
General anaesthesia; sedative.

Anso
Lacer, Hong Kong; Lacer, Spain.
Hexetidine (p.1146·3); lignocaine [lidocaine] hydrochloride (p.1313·2); triamcinolone acetonide (p.1080·1); pentosan polysulfate (p.953·1) or pentosan polysulfate sodium (p.953·1).
Anorectal disorders.

Ansudor *Galderma, Ger.*
Aluminium chlorohydrate (p.1110·2); triclocarban (p.1159·2).
Hyperhidrosis; intertrigo; wound exudate.

Answer
Carter-Wallace, Austral.; Carter-Wallace, USA.
Fertility test or pregnancy test (p.1654·3).

Answer Now *Carter Horner, Canad.*
Pregnancy test (p.1654·3).

Anta *Pharmasant, Thai.*
Lorazepam (p.688·3).
Anxiety; epilepsy; insomnia; muscle relaxation.

Antabus
Chemomedica, Aust.; Dumex-Alpharma, Denm.; Dumex-Alpharma, Fin.; Byk Gulden, Ger.; Byk Tosse, Ger.; Dumex, Norw.; Bohm, Spain; Dumex-Alpharma, Swed.; Dumex, Switz.
Disulfiram (p.1605·1).
Chronic alcoholism.

Antabuse
Orphan, Austral.; Sanofi Synthelabo, Belg.; Wyeth-Ayerst, Canad.; Dumex, Irl.; Wyeth-Ayerst, Israel; Crinos, Ital.; CSL, NZ; Dumex, NZ; Aspen, S.Afr.; Dumex, Thai.; Dumex, UK; Odyssey, USA†.
Disulfiram (p.1605·1).
Chronic alcoholism.

Antacal *Errekappa, Ital.*
Amlodipine besilate (p.838·3).
Angina pectoris; hypertension.

Antacia *The Forty-Two, Thai.*
Aluminium hydroxide (p.1210·3); magnesium hydroxide (p.1233·1); simeticone (p.1249·2).
Flatulence; gastric hyperacidity; gastritis; peptic ulcer.

Antacid
Note. This name is used for preparations of different composition.
Geneva, USA.
Oral suspension: Aluminium hydroxide (p.1210·3); magnesium hydroxide (p.1233·1).
Hyperacidity.
Goldline, USA.
Tablets: Calcium carbonate (p.1215·1).
Hyperacidity.

Antacid Chewable Tablets *Vitelle, Austral.*
Calcium carbonate (p.1215·1); magnesium carbonate (p.1232·3).
Dyspepsia; gastro-oesophageal reflux; heartburn.

Antacid Liquid *Shoppers Drug Mart, Canad.†.*
Aluminium hydroxide (p.1210·3); magnesium hydroxide (p.1233·1); simeticone (p.1249·2).

Antacid Plus Antiflatulant *Stanley, Canad.*
Aluminium hydroxide (p.1210·3); magnesium hydroxide (p.1233·1); simeticone (p.1249·2).

Antacid Suspension *Pharmel, Canad.*
Aluminium hydroxide (p.1210·3); magnesium hydroxide (p.1233·1).

Antacid Tablet
Note. This name is used for preparations of different composition.
Stanley, Canad.
Aluminium hydroxide (p.1210·3); magnesium hydroxide (p.1233·1); simeticone (p.1249·2).
Swiss Herbal, Canad.
Magnesium hydroxide (p.1233·1); calcium carbonate (p.1215·1).

Antacide Suspension *Therapex, Canad.*
Aluminium hydroxide (p.1210·3); magnesium hydroxide (p.1233·1).

Antacide Suspension avec Antiflatulent *Therapex, Canad.*
Aluminium hydroxide (p.1210·3); magnesium hydroxide (p.1233·1); simeticone (p.1249·2).

Antacidum *Pfizer, Aust.*
Dihydroxyaluminum sodium carbonate (p.1222·1).
Dyspepsia; hyperacidity; peptic ulcer.

Antacidum OPT *Optimed, Ger.†*
Aluminium hydroxide (p.1210·3).
Gastric hyperacidity; hyperphosphaturia.

Antacidum Rennie *Roche, Aust.*
Calcium carbonate (p.1215·1); magnesium carbonate (p.1232·3).
Hyperacidity.

Antacil *Nakorn, Thai.*
Oral suspension: Aluminium hydroxide gel (p.1210·3); magnesium hydroxide (p.1233·1); simeticone (p.1249·2).
Flatulence; gastric hyperacidity; peptic ulcer.
Tablets: Magnesium trisilicate (p.1233·3); dried aluminium hydroxide gel (p.1210·3); kaolin (p.1229·3).
Gastric hyperacidity; peptic ulcer.

Antacsal *Alpharma, Mex.*
Aspirin (p.14·2).
Fever; pain; thromboembolism prophylaxis.

Antaderm *Darier, Mex.*
Allantoin (p.1110·1); coal tar (p.1125·1).
Psoriasis; seborrhoeic dermatitis.

Antadine *Boots, S.Afr.†*
Amantadine hydrochloride (p.1161·2).
Drug-induced extrapyramidal disorders; influenza A; parkinsonism.

Antadys *Theramex, Mon.*
Flurbiprofen (p.41·2).
Dysmenorrhoea; musculoskeletal and joint disorders.

Antafit *Polipharm, Thai.*
Carbamazepine (p.342·2).
Epilepsy; trigeminal neuralgia.

Antagon
Note.This name is used for preparations of different composition.
Ativus, Braz.
Ranitidine (p.1246·3).
Gastro-oesophageal reflux; gastrointestinal haemorrhage; peptic ulcer; Zollinger-Ellison syndrome.

Organon, USA.
Ganirelix acetate (p.1283·3).
Inhibition of premature luteinising hormone surges in controlled ovarian hyperstimulation.

Antagon I *Liomont, Mex.*
Astemizole (p.409·1).
Hypersensitivity.

Antagonil *Novartis, Ger.*
Nicardipine hydrochloride (p.938·3).
Angina pectoris; hypertension.

Antagosan
Hoechst, Fr.; Hoechst Marion Roussel, Ger.; Hoechst Marion Roussel, Ital.†
Aprotinin (p.725·3).
Haemorrhagic disorders; shock.

Antak *Glaxo Wellcome, Braz.*
Ranitidine hydrochloride (p.1245·2).
Acid aspiration; gastro-oesophageal reflux; gastrointestinal haemorrhage; peptic ulcer; Zollinger-Ellison syndrome.

Antalgic *Caps, S.Afr.*
Paracetamol (p.71·2).
Fever; pain.

Antalgil *Janssen-Cilag, Ital.*
Ibuprofen (p.43·2).
Pain.

Antalgin
Note.This name is used for preparations of different composition.
Medix, Mex.
Indometacin (p.44·3).
Inflammation; musculoskeletal, joint and peri-articular disorders; pain.

Roche, Spain.
Naproxen sodium (p.61·1).
Fever; gout; musculoskeletal and joint disorders; pain.

Antalgo *Selvi, Ital.*
Nimesulide (p.62·3).
Fever; inflammation; pain.

Antalisin *Merck Sharp & Dohme, Ital.*
Ibuprofen lysine (p.44·1).
Fever; pain.

Antalon *Dresden, Ger.†*
Pimozide (p.699·3).
Schizophrenia.

Antalvic *Aventis, Fr.†*
Dextropropoxyphene hydrochloride (p.27·1).
Pain.

Antalyre *Boehringer Ingelheim, Fr.*
Chlorhexidine gluconate (p.1138·2); oxedrine tartrate (p.950·3).
Conjunctival irritation.

Antanazol *Shin Poong, Singapore.*
Ketoconazole (p.389·1).
Fungal infections; seborrhoeic dermatitis.

Antanidina *Bergamo, Braz.*
Ranitidine (p.1246·3).
Gastro-oesophageal reflux; gastrointestinal haemorrhage; peptic ulcer; Zollinger-Ellison syndrome.

Antarene *Elerte, Fr.†*
Ibuprofen (p.43·2).
Fever; pain.

Antares *Krewel, Ger.*
Kava (p.1625·3).
Anxiety; nervous disorders.

Antarol *Antigen, Hong Kong.*
Propranolol hydrochloride (p.962·3).
Angina pectoris; anxiety; arrhythmias; hypertension; hyperthyroidism; migraine; myocardial infarction.

Antassa *Medical Industries, Austral.*
Calcium carbonate (p.1215·1); chamomile (p.1593·2).
Gastrointestinal hyperacidity.

Antasten-Privin *Ciba Vision, Swed.*
Antazoline sulfate (p.408·3); naphazoline nitrate (p.1095·1); boric acid (p.1586·1); borax (p.1586·1).
Allergic conjunctivitis.

Antaxone
Zambon, Ital.; Zambon, Port.; Pharmazam, Spain.
Naltrexone hydrochloride (p.1016·1).
Alcohol withdrawal syndrome; opioid withdrawal.

Antazallerge *Siam Bheasach, Thai.*
Antazoline hydrochloride (p.408·3); tetryzoline hydrochloride (p.1101·2).
Conjunctivitis.

Antazoline-V *Rugby, USA.*
Naphazoline hydrochloride (p.1095·1); antazoline phosphate (p.408·3).
Eye irritation.

Antebor *Wolfs, Belg.; Biologiques de l'Ile-de-France, Fr.*
Sulfacetamide sodium (p.250·3).
Skin infections.

Antebor B₆ *Biologiques de l'Ile-de-France, Fr.†*
Sulfacetamide sodium (p.250·3); pyridoxine hydrochloride (p.1386·3).
Bacterial skin infections.

Antebor N *Sodip, Switz.*
Chlorhexidine (p.1138·2); triclosan (p.1159·2).
Acne.

Antelepsin *Desitin, Ger.*
Clonazepam (p.347·1).
Epilepsy.

Antelmina *Gerda, Fr.†*
Piperazine hydrate (p.106·1).
Intestinal nematode infections.

Antemesyl *Molteni, Ital.*
Injection: Mepyramine hydrochloride (p.421·1); pyridoxine hydrochloride (p.1386·3).
Suppositories: Mepyramine hydrochloride (p.421·1).
Nausea and vomiting.

Antemin *Streuli, Switz.*
Dimenhydrinate (p.415·2).
Nausea and vomiting.

Antemin compositum *Streuli, Switz.*
Dimenhydrinate (p.415·2); caffeine (p.761·3); pyridoxine hydrochloride (p.1386·3).
Nausea and vomiting.

Anten *Pacific, NZ.*
Doxepin hydrochloride (p.283·3).
Depression.

Antenex *Alphapharm, Austral.*
Diazepam (p.674·3).
Alcohol withdrawal syndrome; anxiety; skeletal muscle spasm; spasticity.

Antepan *Mayrhofer, Aust.; Henning, Ger.*
Protirelin (p.1295·3).
Assessment of pituitary and thyroid function.

Antepar *Glaxo Wellcome, Thai.*
Piperazine hydrate (p.106·1).
Ascariasis; enterobiasis.

Antepsin *Whitehall, Braz.; Orion, Denm.; Orion, Fin.; Wyeth, Irl.; Baldacci, Ital.; Orion, Norw.; Chugai, UK.*
Sucralfate (p.1250·2).
Gastritis; gastrointestinal haemorrhage; gastro-oesophageal reflux; peptic ulcer.

Antergan *Nakorn, Thai.*
Hydrocortisone acetate (p.1073·3); mepyramine maleate (p.421·1).
Pruritus; skin irritation.

Anthel
Note.This name is used for preparations of different composition.
Alphapharm, Austral.
Pyrantel embonate (p.108·1).
Worm infections.

Shiwa, Thai.
Albendazole (p.95·2).
Worm infections.

Anthelios
Note.This name is used for preparations of different composition.
Cosmair, Canad.
Avobenzone (p.1517·1); enzacamene (p.1517·2); terephthalylidene dicamphor sulfonic acid; titanium dioxide (p.1126·1).
Sunscreen.

Roche-Posay, Fr.
SPF 10: Octocrilene (p.1518·1); avobenzone (p.1517·1).
SPF 20; SPF 30; SPF 40; SPF 50; SPF 60;: Octocrilene (p.1518·1); titanium dioxide (p.1126·1); avobenzone (p.1517·1).
Sunscreen.

Roche-Posay, Irl.
Octocrilene (p.1518·1); avobenzone (p.1517·1); terephthalylidene dicamphor sulfonic acid; titanium dioxide (p.1126·1).
Sunscreen.

Anthelios Stick *Cosmair, Canad.†*
Avobenzone (p.1517·1); enzacamene (p.1517·2).
Sunscreen.

Anthelios T *Roche-Posay, Fr.*
SPF10: Titanium dioxide (p.1126·1).
Sunscreen.

Antherpos
Roche-Posay, Fr.; Roche-Posay, Irl.
Enzacamene (p.1517·2); avobenzone (p.1517·1); titanium dioxide (p.1126·1).
Sunscreen.

Anthex *Rolab, S.Afr.*
Mebendazole (p.102·2).
Worm infections.

Anthisan
Rhone-Poulenc Rorer, Austral.†; Rhone-Poulenc Rorer, Hong Kong; Rhone-Poulenc Rorer, Irl.; Aventis, NZ; Aventis, S.Afr.; Rhone-Poulenc Rorer, UK.
Mepyramine maleate (p.421·1).
Allergic skin disorders; insect bites and stings.

Anthisan Plus *Rhone-Poulenc Rorer, UK.*
Mepyramine maleate (p.421·1); benzocaine (p.1306·2).
Bites and stings.

Anthozym *Petrasch, Aust.*
Beta vulgaris; lactic acid (p.1626·2); ferrous lactate (p.1360·2); ascorbic acid (p.1389·3); calcium lactate (p.1188·2); potassium aspartate (p.1195·2); magnesium aspartate (p.1190·3); black currant juice (p.1389·3).
Tonic.

Anthozym N *Reith & Petrasch, Ger.†*
Beetroot; lactic acid (p.1626·2).
Tonic.

Anthraderm *Gerot, Aust.*
Note. A similar name is used for preparations of different composition (see below).
Dithranol (p.1113·3); salicylic acid (p.1122·3).
Psoriasis.

Anthra-Derm *Dermik, USA.*
Note. A similar name is used for preparations of different composition (see above).
Dithranol (p.1113·3).
Psoriasis.

Anthraforte *Medican, Canad.*
Dithranol (p.1113·3).
Psoriasis.

Anthranol
Medican, Canad.; Stiefel, Mex.; Stiefel, S.Afr.†; Stiefel, Spain.
Dithranol (p.1113·3).
Psoriasis.

Anthrascalp *Medican, Canad.*
Dithranol (p.1113·3).
Psoriasis.

Anthraxivore *Picot, Fr.†*
Arctium lappa (p.1627·1).
Skin infections.

Anti Anorex Triple *Lesvi, Spain.*
Cyproheptadine hydrochloride (p.414·2); deanol aceglumate (p.1507·2); metoclopramide hydrochloride (p.1235·2).
Tonic.

Anti CD3 *Butantan, Braz.*
Muromonab-CD3 (p.560·3).
Transplant rejection.

Anti Itch
Medibrands, Israel; Blistex, USA†.
Pramocaine hydrochloride (p.1318·2).
Pruritus; skin irritation.

Anti-Ac *Clement, Fr.*
Pyrimiphos methyl; permethrin (p.1436·1); piperonyl butoxide (p.1436·2).
House dust mite acaricide.

Antiacide *Marc-O, Canad.*
Aluminium hydroxide (p.1210·3); magnesium hydroxide (p.1233·1).

Anti-Acido *Giuliani, Ital.*
Aluminium hydroxide dried gel (p.1210·3); magnesium hydroxide (p.1233·1); dimethicone (p.1249·2).
Aerophagia; gastric hyperacidity; meteorism.

Antiacido Eno *SmithKline Beecham, Spain.*
Calcium carbonate (p.1215·1); magnesium carbonate (p.1232·3).
Gastrointestinal hyperacidity.

Antiacido Salud *Boots Healthcare, Spain.*
Aluminium hydroxide (p.1210·3); calcium carbonate (p.1215·1); magnesium hydroxide (p.1233·1).
Gastrointestinal hyperacidity.

Anti-Acne
Note.This name is used for preparations of different composition.
LPB, Canad.
Sublimed sulfur (p.1123·3); meclocycline sulfosalicylate (p.222·1); nicoboxil (p.62·2).
Formerly contained sulfur, nicoboxil, chloramphenicol, hydrocortisone acetate, and titanium dioxide.
Acne.

Byk Leo, Spain.
Alcohol; sulfur (p.1123·3); resorcinol (p.1122·2); triclosan (p.1159·2).
Acne.

Anti-Acne Control Formula *Clinique, Canad.*
Salicylic acid (p.1122·3).
Acne.

Anti-Acne Formula for Men *Clinique, Canad.†*
Salicylic acid (p.1122·3); sulfur (p.1123·3).
Acne.

Anti-Acne Spot Treatment *Clinique, Canad.*
Salicylic acid (p.1122·3).
Acne.

Antiacneicos Ac-Sal *Isdin, Port.*
Salicylic acid (p.1122·3); triclosan (p.1159·2); aloe vera (p.1110·1); polyglyceryl methacrylate.
Acne.

Antiacneicos Niacex *Isdin, Port.*
Niseiramida; glycerol (p.1616·3); sodium carbomer.
Acne.

Antiadipositum X-112 *Hanseler, Switz.*
Cathine hydrochloride (p.1507·1).
Obesity.

Antiadipositum X-112 S *Hanseler, Ger.*
Cathine hydrochloride (p.1507·1).
Obesity.

Antiadiposo *Teofarma, Ital.*
Iodocasein (p.1523·2); thiamine nitrate (p.1385·1).
Metabolic activator.

Anti-Ageing Kalmia *Homeocan, Canad.*
Homoeopathic preparation.

Anti-Algos *Truw, Ger.†*
Paracetamol (p.71·2).
Fever; pain.

Anti-Asmatico *CPH, Port.*
Aminophylline (p.760·1); phenobarbital (p.355·1); ephedrine hydrochloride (p.1090·1).
Asthma.

Antibio-Aberel *Janssen-Cilag, Fr.*
Tretinoin (p.1126·2); erythromycin (p.201·2).
Acne.

Antibiocin *Orion, Ger.†*
Phenoxymethylpenicillin potassium (p.235·1).
Bacterial infections.

Antibiofilus *Llorente, Spain.*
Lactobacillus acidophilus (p.1626·3); choline orotate (p.1645·1); vitamins (p.1350·1).
Gastrointestinal disorders; restoration of the gastrointestinal flora.

Antibiopen *Antibioticos, Spain.*
Ampicillin sodium (p.150·3) or ampicillin trihydrate (p.151·1).
Bacterial infections.

Antibiophilus *Germania, Aust.; Azevedos, Port.*
Lactobacillus rhamnosus (p.1626·3).
Gastrointestinal disorders.

Antibioptal *Farmila, Ital.*
Chloramphenicol (p.179·1); neomycin sulfate (p.228·1).
Bacterial eye infections.

Antibio-Synalar *Cassenne, Fr.†*
Fluocinolone acetonide (p.1071·1); polymyxin B sulfate (p.238·1); neomycin sulfate (p.228·1).
Otitis.

Antibi-Otic *Seng, Thai.*
Note. A similar name is used for preparations of different composition (see below).
Chloramphenicol (p.179·1).
Bacterial ear infections.

AntibiOtic *Parnell, USA.*
Note. A similar name is used for preparations of different composition (see above).
Hydrocortisone (p.1073·3); neomycin sulfate (p.228·1); polymyxin B (p.238·3).
Bacterial ear infections.

Antibiotic Cold Sore Ointment *Novartis Consumer, Canad.*
Polymyxin B sulfate (p.238·1); tyrothricin (p.267·1); camphor (p.1589·3); menthol (p.1632·3); benzocaine (p.1306·2).
Herpes labialis.

Antibiotic Cream *Technilab, Canad.*
Gramicidin (p.213·3); polymyxin B sulfate (p.238·1).

Antibiotic Ointment *Stanley, Canad.; Technilab, Canad.*
Bacitracin (p.155·2); polymyxin B sulfate (p.238·1).

Antibiotic Simplex *Pfizer, Denm.†.*
Erythromycin gluceptate (p.201·3); colistimethate sodium (p.192·3); polymethylmethacrylate/methylmethacrylate copolymer (p.1635·2).
Bone cement for orthopaedic surgery.

Antibiotique Onguent *Prodemdis, Canad.*
Bacitracin (p.155·2); polymyxin B sulfate (p.238·1).

Antibiotrex *Stiefel, Fr.*
Isotretinoin (p.1115·3); erythromycin (p.201·2).
Acne.

Antibiotulle Lumiere
Solvay, Fr.; Hefa, Ger.
Neomycin sulfate (p.228·1); polymyxin B sulfate (p.238·1).
Infected leg ulcers; infected wounds and burns.

Antiblef Eczem *Ciba Vision, Spain.*
Clioquinol (p.190·2); hydrocortisone acetate (p.1073·3).
Infected eye disorders.

Antiblefarica *Ciba Vision, Spain.*
Bismuth loretinate; chlortetracycline hydrochloride (p.182·1); cortisone acetate (p.1065·3).
Eye disorders.

Antibron *Potter's, UK.*
Lobelia (p.1510·2); wild lettuce (p.1680·3); coltsfoot (p.1087·2); euphorbia (p.1609·3); pleurisy root (p.1653·1); senega (p.1100·2).
Coughs.

Anticatarral *Edigen, Spain.*
Chlorpheniramine [chlorphenamine] maleate (p.412·1); phenylephrine hydrochloride (p.1097·1); guaiazulene (p.1618·3); muramidase hydrochloride (p.1638·1); paracetamol (p.71·2).
Cold and influenza symptoms.

The symbol † denotes a preparation no longer actively marketed

Anticerumen Liade, Spain.
Sodium laurilsulfate (p.1496·3).
Removal of ear wax.

Antichloric Bio-Therabel, Belg.
Calcium carbonate (p.1215·1); heavy magnesium carbonate (p.1232·3).
Formerly contained light calcium carbonate, heavy magnesium carbonate, belladonna, and liquorice.
Peptic ulcer.

Anticholium Kohler, Aust.; Kohler, Ger.
Physostigmine salicylate (p.1421·3).
Alcohol withdrawal syndrome; antimuscarinic poisoning; central anticholinergic syndrome.

Anticon Uniderm, Israel.
Copper-wound plastic (p.1357·3).
Intra-uterine contraceptive device.

Anticongestiva Synthelabo, Spain.
Zinc oxide (p.1128·2).
Skin irritation.

Anticorizza Ogna, Ital.
Paracetamol (p.71·2); salicylamide (p.82·1); caffeine (p.761·3); tripelennamine hydrochloride (p.427·1).
Cold and influenza symptoms.

Anticude UCB, Spain.
Edrophonium bromide (p.1418·2).
Diagnosis of myasthenia gravis; reversal of competitive neuromuscular blockade.

Anti-Dandruff Shampoo Avant Garde, Canad.
Pyrithione zinc (p.1122·1).

Antidep Torrent, Thai.
Imipramine hydrochloride (p.291·1).
Depression; nocturnal enuresis.

Antidia Daewon, Hong Kong.
Nifuroxazide (p.230·2).
Diarrhoea.

Antidiar Aerocid, Fr.
Loperamide hydrochloride (p.1231·3).
Diarrhoea.

Anti-Diarrheal Stanley, Canad.
Loperamide hydrochloride (p.1231·3).

Antidifar Alpharma, Mex.
Diiodohydroxyquinoline (p.590·2).
Amoebiasis.

Antidol
Note.This name is used for preparations of different composition.
Gerbex, Canad.
Aspirin (p.14·2); caffeine (p.761·3).

Quimica y Farmacia, Mex.; Cinfa, Spain.
Paracetamol (p.71·2).
Fever; pain.

Antidoloroso Rudol Areu, Spain.
Aspirin (p.14·2); caffeine (p.761·3).
Fever; pain.

Antidot zu Arwin Knoll, Ger.†.
Ancrod antisera.
Overdosage with or adverse effects of ancrod.

Antidote Anti-Digitale BM Roche, Switz.
Digoxin-specific antibody fragments (p.1006·3).
Digitalis poisoning.

Antidoto Arvin Knoll, Spain†.
Ancrod antisera.
Overdosage with ancrod.

Antidotum Thallii-Heyl Heyl, Ger.
Prussian blue (p.1021·2).
Thallium poisoning.

Antidrasi Visufarma, Ital.
Diclofenamide (p.869·1) or diclofenamide sodium (p.869·1).
Control of intra-ocular pressure during eye surgery; glaucoma.

Antidry Adroka, Switz.
Bath oil: Liquid paraffin (p.1407·1); almond oil (p.1576·3).
Ointment: Pansy; zinc oxide (p.1128·2); almond oil (p.1576·3).
Shower oil: Liquid paraffin (p.1407·1); soya oil (p.1378·1); levomenol (p.1629·1).
Topical lotion: Sodium lactate (p.1186·2); almond oil (p.1576·3).
Skin disorders.

Antiedema Alcon Cusi, Spain.
Sodium chloride (p.1196·1).
Corneal oedema.

Antiemorroidali Ogna, Ital.; AFOM, Ital.
Ichthammol (p.1115·2); zinc oxide (p.1128·2); bismuth subgallate (p.1213·2); belladonna (p.463·1).
Haemorrhoids.

Antiestrias Isdin, Port.
Centella (p.1112·2); borage oil (p.1613·1); *dl*-alpha tocoferil acetate (p.1394·1); jojoba oil.
Firming cream.

Antietanol Hoechst Marion Roussel, Braz.
Disulfiram (p.1605·1).
Chronic alcoholism.

Antifect
Note.This name is used for preparations of different composition.
Schulke & Mayr, Ger.†.
Alcohol (p.1130·3); propyl alcohol (p.1155·3); glyoxal (p.1145·3).
Surface disinfection.

Potter's, UK.
Garlic (p.1614·1); garlic oil; echinacea (p.1606·2).
Catarrh; nasal congestion; rhinitis.

Antiflam Rolab, S.Afr.
Ibuprofen (p.43·2).
Now known as Rolab-Ibuprofen.
Fever; musculoskeletal, joint, peri-articular, and soft-tissue disorders; pain.

Anti-Flamme Natures Kiss, Austral.
Arnica (p.1581·3); calendula (p.1589·2); hypericum (p.290·2); peppermint oil (p.1243·3).
Local pain and injury.

Antiflog FIRMA, Ital.
Piroxicam (p.79·1).
Rheumatic disorders.

Antiflogil Farmasa, Braz.
Nimesulide (p.62·3).
Fever; inflammation; pain.

Antifloxil Alter, Spain.
Nimesulide (p.62·3).
Fever; inflammation; pain.

Antiflu
Note.This name is used for preparations of different composition.
Byk Gulden, Ital.
Paracetamol (p.71·2); chlorpheniramine [chlorphenamine] maleate (p.412·1); caffeine (p.761·3).
Cold and influenza symptoms.

Pharmco, S.Afr.
Paracetamol (p.71·2); mepyramine maleate (p.421·1); diphenhydramine hydrochloride (p.416·1); caffeine (p.761·3); codeine phosphate (p.25·2); phenylephrine hydrochloride (p.1097·1).
Cold and influenza symptoms.

Antiflu Forte Synco, Hong Kong.
Paracetamol (p.71·2); salicylamide (p.82·1); phenylpropanolamine hydrochloride (p.1098·1); phenylephrine hydrochloride (p.1097·1); chlorpheniramine [chlorphenamine] maleate (p.412·1); caffeine (p.761·3).
Cold and influenza symptoms; rhinitis.

Antiflu-Des Chinoin, Mex.
Amantadine hydrochloride (p.1161·2); chlorpheniramine [chlorphenamine] maleate (p.412·1); phenylpropanolamine hydrochloride (p.1098·1); paracetamol (p.71·2).
Influenza symptoms.

Antiflu-N-Forte Synco, Hong Kong.
Paracetamol (p.71·2); salicylamide (p.82·1); ephedrine hydrochloride (p.1090·1); phenylephrine hydrochloride (p.1097·1); dexchlorpheniramine maleate (p.412·1); caffeine (p.761·3).
Cold and influenza symptoms; rhinitis.

AntiFocal Vitorgan, Ger.
Animal tissue extract: diencephalon; cerebellum (p.1631·2); cort. cerebri; cerebrum fet.; medulla spinal; hepar.; pancreas; lien; thyreoidea (p.1526·2); thymus juv.; placenta; mucosa misc.
Nervous system disorders.

AntiFocal N Vitorgan, Ger.
Metenolone acetate (p.1482·2); liothyronine hydrochloride (p.1524·3); chorionic gonadotrophin (p.1279·2); pyridoxine hydrochloride (p.1386·3); cyanocobalamin (p.1388·1).
Nervous system disorders.

Antifohnon-N Sudmedica, Ger.
Ephedrine hydrochloride (p.1090·1); ethenzamide (p.35·1).
Circulatory disorders.

Antifungal Foot Deodorant Or-Dov, Austral.
Tolnaftate (p.395·2).
Tinea pedis.

Antifungol Hexal, Ger.
Clotrimazole (p.382·1).
Fungal infections of the skin and genito-urinary tract.

Anti-Gas Antacid Invamed, USA†.
Calcium carbonate (p.1215·1); magnesium hydroxide (p.1233·1); simeticone (p.1249·2).

Antigeron Farmasa, Braz.
Cinnarizine (p.413·1).
Peripheral vascular disorders; vestibular disorders.

Anti-Geruchs Twardy, Ger.
Chlorophyllin (p.1028·1).
Body odour; metabolic disorders.

Antiglan Potter's, UK.
Kava (p.1625·3); saw palmetto (p.1491·2); equisetum (p.1606·3); hydrangea (p.1621·1).
Bladder discomfort.

Antigoutteux Rezall Medecine Vegetale, Fr.†.
Lithium benzoate (p.1629·1); lithium salicylate (p.50·1); colchicum (p.401·2); maize (p.1599·3); bitter-orange (p.1644·2).
Gout; rheumatism.

Antigreg Piam, Ital.; Piam, Singapore.
Ticlopidine hydrochloride (p.981·1).
Thrombosis prophylaxis.

Antigrietun Casen Fleet, Spain.
Allantoin (p.1110·1); aminoacridine (p.1130·3); peru balsam (p.1650·2); prednisolone (p.1077·3).
Allergic skin disorders; cracked nipples; mastitis; superficial burns.

Anti-Gripe Plough, Port.
Aconite (p.1572·3); belladonna (p.463·1); codeine (p.25·2); caffeine (p.761·3); paracetamol (p.71·2).
Cold symptoms; fever; pain.

Antigripina Sanofi Winthrop, Braz.
Paracetamol (p.71·2); caffeine (p.761·3); cresotamide.
Cold and influenza symptoms.

Antigrippine
Note.This name is used for preparations of different composition.
SmithKline Beecham Consumer, Neth.
Paracetamol (p.71·2); caffeine (p.761·3); ascorbic acid (p.1389·3).
Fever; pain.

Sterling, Port.
Aspirin (p.14·2); codeine phosphate (p.25·2); vitamin C (p.1389·3).
Fever; pain.

SmithKline Beecham Consumer, Switz.
Paracetamol (p.71·2); ascorbic acid (p.1389·3).
Cold symptoms.

Antigrippine a l'Aspirine SmithKline Beecham Sante, Fr.
Aspirin (p.14·2); ascorbic acid (p.1389·3); caffeine hydrate (p.761·3).
Fever; pain.

Antigrippine Midy SmithKline Beecham, Belg.
Paracetamol (p.71·2); 3-methylsalicylamide; codeine phosphate (p.25·2); caffeine (p.761·3); ascorbic acid (p.1389·3).
Cold symptoms.

Anti-H Amido, Fr.
Aluminium sodium silicate (p.1211·3); kaolin (p.1229·3); sodium bicarbonate (p.1186·2); calcium carbonate (p.1215·1).
Flatulence; gastrointestinal pain.

Anti-Hemorroidaires Aventis, Fr.†.
Rectal ointment: Hydrocortisone (p.1073·3); cinchocaine hydrochloride (p.1309·1).
Suppositories: Hydrocortisone acetate (p.1073·3); esculoside (p.1574·1); benzocaine (p.1306·2).
Formerly contained hydrocortisone acetate, benzocaine, esculoside, framycetin sulfate, heparin, and butyl amino benzoate.
Anorectal disorders.

Antihemorroidal
Note.This name is used for preparations of different composition.
Cinfa, Spain.
Benzocaine (p.1306·2); hydrocortisone acetate (p.1073·3); neomycin sulfate (p.228·1); tannic acid (p.1669·1).
Anorectal disorders.

ICN, Spain.
Ointment: Hydrocortisone acetate (p.1073·3); neomycin sulfate (p.228·1); promethazine hydrochloride (p.423·2); vitamin A (p.1382·1).
Suppositories: Hydrocortisone acetate (p.1073·3); promethazine hydrochloride (p.423·2); vitamin A (p.1382·1).
Anorectal disorders.

Anti-Hist Clonmel, Irl.†.
Note. A similar name is used for preparations of different composition (see below).
Chlorpheniramine [chlorphenamine] maleate (p.412·1).
Hypersensitivity reactions.

Antihist-I Goldline, USA; Major, USA; Rugby, USA.
Note. A similar name is used for preparations of different composition (see above).
Clemastine fumarate (p.413·2).

Antihistamine Forte Unichem, UK.
Terfenadine (p.424·3).
Hay fever; hypersensitivity reactions.

Antihistaminico Llorens, Spain.
Chlorpheniramine [chlorphenamine] maleate (p.412·1).
Hypersensitivity reactions of the eye.

Antihist-D Goldline, USA†.
Clemastine fumarate (p.413·2); phenylpropanolamine hydrochloride (p.1098·1).
Upper-respiratory-tract disorders.

Anti-Homocysteine Factor Eagle, Austral.
Amino acids, vitamin B substances; minerals (p.1350·1).
Elevated homocysteine levels.

Antihydral Schmidgall, Aust.; Robugen, Ger.; Medipharm, Switz.
Methenamine (p.223·1).
Fungal skin infections; hyperhidrosis; wounds.

Antihydral M Schmidgall, Aust.; Robugen, Ger.; Robugen, Hong Kong; Medipharm, Switz.
Methenamine (p.223·1); sulfur (p.1123·3).
Fungal skin infections; hyperhidrosis.

Antihypertonicum S Schuck, Ger.
Betula (p.1585·2); crataegus (p.1600·2); mistletoe (p.1636·2); olive; rhododendron leaf; rutoside (p.1611·2); proxyphylline (p.770·1).
Arteriosclerosis; hypertension.

Antihypertonicum-Weliplex Weber & Weber, Ger.†.
Homoeopathic preparation.

Antihypertonikum-Tropfen N Schuck, Ger.
Homoeopathic preparation.

Anti-inhibitor Coagulant Complex Baxter, UK.
A factor VIII inhibitor bypassing fraction (p.734·3).
Haemorrhage in patients with inhibitors to factor VIII.

Anti-Inhibitor Coagulant Complex (Autoplex T) Baxter, Israel.
A factor VIII inhibitor bypassing fraction (p.734·3).
Haemorrhage in patients with inhibitors to factor VIII.

Anti-Kalium Medice, Ger.
Calcium polystyrene sulfonate (p.1002·3).
Hyperkalaemia.

Antikataraktikum N Ursapharm, Ger.
Disodium inosinate (p.1604·3).
Visual disturbances.

Antikataraktikum N oral Ursapharm, Ger.
Disodium uridine 5'-monophosphate.
Cataracts.

Antikeloides Creme Widmer, Switz.
Dexamethasone (p.1067·1); urea (p.1127·3); vitamin A palmitate (p.1383·2).
Scars.

Antil Carnot, Mex.
Cimetidine (p.1216·3).

Antilirium Forest Pharmaceuticals, USA.
Physostigmine salicylate (p.1421·3).
Reversal of drug-induced CNS antimuscarinic effects.

Antimast N Selz, Ger.
Homoeopathic preparation.

Antimast T Selz, Ger.
Homoeopathic preparation.

Antimet
Note.This name is used for preparations of different composition.
Antigen, Irl.
Metoclopramide hydrochloride (p.1235·2).
Gastrointestinal disorders.

Rolab, S.Afr.
Cinnarizine (p.413·1).
Now known as Rolab-Cinnarizine.
Nausea; vertigo.

Antimicotico
Note.This name is used for preparations of different composition.
IFI, Ital.
Ointment: Benzoxiquine; dexamethasone (p.1067·1); pyridoxine (p.1387·1); polyenacid.
Fungal skin infections.

Savoma, Ital.
Cream: Clotrimazole (p.382·1).
Fungal infections.

Antimigrin Gebro, Aust.
Naratriptan hydrochloride (p.454·3).
Migraine.

Antiminth Pfizer, USA.
Pyrantel embonate (p.108·1).
Worm infections.

Antimucose Promedica, Fr.†.
Ox bile extract (p.1585·1).
Bowel evacuation; constipation.

Antimyk Pfleger, Ger.
Clotrimazole (p.382·1).
Fungal infections.

Antimyopikum Ursapharm, Ger.
Troxerutin (p.1611·2); alpha tocoferil acetate (p.1394·1).
Progressive shortsightedness.

Antinal Roques, Fr.†.
Nifuroxazide (p.230·2).
Diarrhoea.

Antinaus Pacific, NZ.
Prochlorperazine maleate (p.701·2).
Anxiety; nausea and vomiting; psychoses; vertigo.

Anti-Nauseant Stanley, Canad.
Dimenhydrinate (p.415·2).
Nausea.

Antinephrin M Hanosan, Ger.
Homoeopathic preparation.

Antinerveux Lesourd Lesourd, Fr.
Lotus petal; melilot.
Insomnia; irritability.

Antineuralgica Alpharma, Norw.
Caffeine (p.761·3); phenazone (p.77·2).
Pain.

Antineuralgicum (Rowo-633) Pharmakon, Ger.†.
Homoeopathic preparation.
Lignocaine [lidocaine] hydrochloride (p.1313·2) is included in this preparation to alleviate the pain of injection.

Antineurina Mabo, Spain.
Cyanocobalamin (p.1388·1); pyridoxine hydrochloride (p.1386·3); thiamine hydrochloride (p.1385·1).
Neuralgia; neuritis; peripheral neuropathy; vitamin B deficiency.

Antinevralgico Dr Knapp Montefarmaco, Ital.
Paracetamol (p.71·2); aspirin (p.14·2); caffeine (p.761·3).
Fever; pain.

Antinevralgico Penegal FAMA, Ital.†.
Paracetamol (p.71·2); aspirin (p.14·2).
Fever; pain.

Antinicoticum sine (Rowo-100) Pharmakon, Ger.
Homoeopathic preparation.

Antiobes Novartis Consumer, Spain.
Fenproporex hydrochloride (p.1510·2).
Obesity.

Antiotic Grossmann, Switz.
Amoxicillin trihydrate (p.149·2).
Bacterial infections.

Antiox Mayrand, USA.
Betacarotene (p.1355·2); ascorbic acid (p.1389·3).

Antioxidans E Hevert, Ger.
dl-Alpha tocoferil acetate (p.1394·1).
Vitamin E deficiency.

Antioxidant Forte Tablets Vitelle, Austral.
Betacarotene (p.1355·1); riboflavin (p.1386·1); ascorbic acid (p.1389·3); sodium ascorbate (p.1390·1); *d*-alpha tocoferil acid succinate (p.1394·1); zinc amino

acid chelate (p.1398·3); folic acid (p.1361·1); silybum marianum (p.1021·3); vitis vinifera.
Anti-oxidant; vitamin A, C, E, and B₂, folic acid, and zinc deficiencies.

Antioxidant Nutrients *Solgar, UK.*
Multivitamin preparation with amino acids and zinc (p.1350·1).
Dietary supplement.

Antioxidant Tablets *Cenovis, Austral.; Vitelle, Austral.*
Ascorbic acid (p.1389·3); sodium ascorbate (p.1390·1); betacarotene (p.1355·1); d-alpha tocoferil acid succinate (p.1394·2); zinc amino acid chelate (p.1398·3); riboflavin (p.1386·1).
Anti-oxidant; vitamin A, C, E, B₂, and zinc deficiencies.

Antioxirell *Sanorell, Ger.†*
Vitamin C; vitamin E; betacarotene; vitamin A; selenium (p.1350·1).
Dietary supplement.

Antipanin N *Michallik, Ger.*
Paracetamol (p.71·2).
Formerly contained ethenzamide and paracetamol.
Pain.

Antipanin P *Michallik, Ger.*
Paracetamol (p.71·2).
Pain.

Antiparkin *Asta Medica, Ger.*
Selegiline hydrochloride (p.1177·2).
Formerly known as Movergan.
Parkinsonism.

Antipen *Biochemie, Aust.†.*
Clemizole penicillin (p.188·1); benzylpenicillin sodium (p.157·2).
Lignocaine [lidocaine] hydrochloride (p.1313·2) is included in the highest strength injections to alleviate the pain of injection.
Bacterial infections.

Antipeol
Note.This name is used for preparations of different composition.
Restan, S.Afr.
Zinc oxide (p.1128·2); ichthammol (p.1115·2); salicylic acid (p.1122·3).
Skin disorders.

Medico-Biological Laboratories, UK.
Zinc oxide (p.1128·2); ichthammol (p.1115·2); salicylic acid (p.1122·3); urea (p.1127·3).
Skin disorders.

Antiphlebin *Sudmedica, Ger.†.*
Quinine hydrochloride (p.445·1); lignocaine [lidocaine] hydrochloride (p.1313·2).
Haemorrhoids.

Antiphlogistine
Note.This name is used for preparations of different composition.
CIF, Braz.
Boric acid (p.1586·1); salicylic acid (p.1122·3); iodine (p.1522·3); peppermint oil (p.1243·3); sweet birch oil (p.55·2); eucalyptus oil (p.1609·2).
Inflammation.

Fumouze, Fr.
Kaolin (p.1229·3); salicylic acid (p.1122·3).
Muscle and connective tissue pain.

Carter-Wallace, Switz.
Salicylic acid (p.1122·3); methyl salicylate (p.55·1); eucalyptus oil (p.1609·2); peppermint oil (p.1243·3).
Inflammation; pain.

Antiphlogistine Rub A-535 *Carter Horner, Canad.*
Methyl salicylate (p.55·1); camphor (p.1589·3); menthol (p.1632·3); eucalyptus oil (p.1609·2).
Musculoskeletal pain.

Antiphlogistine Rub A-535 Capsaicin *Carter Horner, Canad.*
Capsaicin (p.23·1).
Musculoskeletal and joint disorders.

Antiphlogistine Rub A-535 Ice *Carter Horner, Canad.*
Menthol (p.1632·3).
Musculoskeletal pain.

Antiphlogistine Rub A-535 No Odour *Carter Horner, Canad.*
Trolamine salicylate (p.90·1).
Musculoskeletal pain.

Anti-Phosphat
Brady, Aust.; Gry, Ger.
Aluminium hydroxide (p.1210·3).
Hyperphosphataemia.

Anti-Phosphate *Bichsel, Switz.*
Dried aluminium hydroxide (p.1210·3).
Hyperphosphataemia.

Anti-Plaque Chewing Gum *Or-Dov, Austral.*
Chlorhexidine acetate (p.1138·2).
Dental plaque.

Antipressan
Teva, Hong Kong; Berk, Irl.†; Berk, UK.
Atenolol (p.841·3).
Angina pectoris; arrhythmias; hypertension; myocardial infarction.

Antiprotin *Julphar, UAE.*
Bromocriptine mesilate (p.1164·3).
Acromegaly; benign breast disorders; female infertility; hyperprolactinaemia; menstrual disorders; parkinsonism.

Antiprurit *Kade, Ger.*
Cell components and metabolic products of *Staphylococcus aureus*; *Enterococcus faecalis* (p.1626·3); *Pseudomonas aeruginosa*; and *Escherichia coli*; hydrocortisone (p.1073·3).
Skin disorders.

Antipulmina *Lisapharma, Ital.*
Peppermint oil (p.1243·3); pumilio pine oil (p.1656·3); eucalyptus oil (p.1609·2).
Respiratory-tract disorders.

Antipyn *Aspen Consumer, S.Afr.*
Paracetamol (p.71·2); codeine phosphate (p.25·2); caffeine (p.761·3).
Fever; pain.

Antipyn Forte *Aspen Consumer, S.Afr.*
Paracetamol (p.71·2); codeine phosphate (p.25·2); caffeine (p.761·3); meprobamate (p.691·1).
Pain associated with tension.

Antireumina *ISI, Ital.*
Aspirin (p.14·2); paracetamol (p.71·2); caffeine (p.761·3).
Fever; pain.

Antirrinum *Reig Jofre, Spain.*
Oxymetazoline hydrochloride (p.1096·2); chlorhexidine gluconate (p.1138·2).
Nasal congestion; sinus congestion.

Anti-rugas C *Dermoteca, Port.*
Ascorbic acid (p.1389·3).
Sun-induced skin damage.

Antiscabbia Candioli al DDT Terapeutico
Candioli, Ital.
Benzyl benzoate (p.1428·2); benzocaine (p.1306·2); clofenotane (p.1430·1).
Scabies.

Antiscabiosum *Strathmann, Ger.*
Benzyl benzoate (p.1428·2).
Scabies.

Antisept *Salud, Spain.*
Chlorhexidine gluconate (p.1138·2).
Skin and wound disinfection.

Antiseptic Foot Balm *Scholl, Israel; Scholl, UK.*
Menthol (p.1632·3); halquinol (p.214·1); methyl salicylate (p.55·1).
Sore feet.

Antiseptic Lozenges *Mentholatum, UK.*
Menthol (p.1632·3); eucalyptus oil (p.1609·2); amylmetacresol (p.1133·2).
Cold symptoms; coughs; nasal congestion; sore throat.

Antiseptic Mouthwash *Scott, Canad.; Sutton, Canad.*
Eucalyptol (p.1609·2); menthol (p.1632·3); thymol (p.1158·3).
Sore throat.

Antiseptic Ointment *National Care, Canad.*
Chloroxylenol (p.1142·1).
Skin protection.

Antiseptic Skin Cream
Note.This name is used for preparations of different composition.
National Care, Canad.
Benzalkonium chloride (p.1133·2).

National Care, Canad.
Benzethonium chloride (p.1134·2); vitamin A (p.1382·1); vitamin D (p.1391·1).
Ostomy care; skin irritation.

Antiseptic Throat Lozenges
Note.This name is used for preparations of different composition.
Sutton, Canad.
Hexylresorcinol (p.1146·3).
Formerly known as Antiseptic Sore Throat Lozenges.

Ernest Jackson, UK†.
Amylmetacresol (p.1133·2); dichlorobenzyl alcohol (p.1143·2).
Sore throat.

Unichem, UK.
Amylmetacresol (p.1133·2).
Sore throat.

Antiseptic Throat Pastilles *Ernest Jackson, UK†.*
Menthol (p.1632·3); camphor (p.1589·3); benzoic acid (p.1134·2).
Sore throat.

Antiseptique Pastilles *Prodemdis, Canad.*
Domiphen bromide (p.1143·3).

Antiseptique-Calmante *Chauvin, Fr.*
Methylene blue [methylthioninium chloride] (p.1012·3); methylrosanilinium chloride (p.1150·3); boric acid (p.1586·1); procaine hydrochloride (p.1319·1).
Eye disorders.

Antisettico Astringente Sedativo *Bruschettini, Ital.*
Zinc phenolsulfonate (p.1128·3); sulfacetamide sodium (p.250·3); naphazoline hydrochloride (p.1095·1); lignocaine [lidocaine] hydrochloride (p.1313·2).
Conjunctivitis.

Antisklerosin S *Medopharm, Ger.*
Crataegus (p.1600·2); mistletoe (p.1636·3); nicotinic acid (p.1372·3); magnesium orotate (p.1645·1); rutoside (p.1611·2).
Arteriosclerosis; circulatory disorders; hyperlipidaemias.

Anti-Smoking Tablets *Potter's, UK.*
Lobelia (p.1510·2).
Aid to smoking withdrawal.

Antispa *TP, Thai.*
Hyoscine butylbromide (p.468·2).
Gastric hyperacidity; motion sickness; urinary-tract spasm; vomiting.

Antispas *Keene, USA.*
Dicyclomine [dicycloverine] hydrochloride (p.466·1).
Functional bowel syndrome; irritable bowel syndrome.

Antispasmin *QIF, Braz.*
Belladonna (p.463·1); papaverine hydrochloride (p.1648·1); valerian (p.1678·3).
Smooth muscle spasm.

Antispasmina Colica
Note.This name is used for preparations of different composition.
Recordati, Ital.
Papaverine hydrochloride (p.1648·1); belladonna (p.463·1); hyoscyamine (p.469·3).
Gastrointestinal spasm.

Lepori, Port.
Papaverine (p.1648·1); belladonna (p.463·1); valerian (p.1678·3).
Smooth muscle spasm.

Antispasmodic Elixir *Morton Grove, USA.*
Phenobarbital (p.355·1); hyoscyamine sulfate (p.469·3); atropine sulfate (p.461·1); hyoscine hydrobromide (p.468·2).
Gastrointestinal spasm.

Antistax
Note.This name is used for preparations of different composition.
Pharmaton, Ger.; Boehringer Ingelheim, UK.
Red vine leaf.
Venous insufficiency.

Pharmaton, Switz.†.
Proanthocyanidins.
Chronic venous insufficiency.

Antistina-Privin *Ciba Vision, Denm.*
Antazoline sulfate (p.408·3); naphazoline nitrate (p.1095·1).
Conjunctivitis.

Antistine-Privine *Ciba Vision, Austral.*
Antazoline sulfate (p.408·3); naphazoline nitrate (p.1095·1).
Allergic conjunctivitis; eye irritation.

Antistin-Privin
Ciba Vision, Fin.; Ciba Vision, Ger.; Ciba Vision, Israel; Novartis, S.Afr.; Ciba Vision, Singapore; Ciba Vision, Switz.
Antazoline sulfate (p.408·3); naphazoline nitrate (p.1095·1).
Allergic conjunctivitis.

Antistin-Privina *Ciba Vision, Ital.*
Antazoline sulfate (p.408·3); naphazoline nitrate (p.1095·1).
Allergic conjunctivitis.

Antitis *Potter's, UK.*
Buchu leaf (p.1587·2); clivers (p.1596·3); couch-grass (p.1599·3); equisetum (p.1606·3); shepherd's purse (p.1662·3); bearberry (p.1583·3).
Cystitis; urinary or bladder discomfort.

Antitoxikon *Synthelabo, Braz.*
Liver extract.
Liver disorders.

Antituss *Pharmco, S.Afr.†.*
Note. A similar name is used for preparations of different composition (see below).
Promethazine hydrochloride (p.423·2); codeine phosphate (p.25·2); ephedrine hydrochloride (p.1090·1).
Cold symptoms; coughs.

Anti-Tuss *Century, USA.*
Note. A similar name is used for preparations of different composition (see above).
Guaifenesin (p.1092·2).
Coughs.

Antitussive Decongestant Antihistamine Syrup *Prodemdis, Canad.†.*
Phenylpropanolamine hydrochloride (p.1098·1); pheniramine maleate (p.422·3); mepyramine maleate (p.421·1); dextromethorphan hydrobromide (p.1087·3).

Antitussivum Burger *Ysatfabrik, Ger.*
Codeine phosphate (p.25·2).
Coughs.

Antitussivum Burger N *Ysatfabrik, Ger.*
Dihydrocodeine tartrate (p.33·1); thyme oil (p.1672·3).
Catarrh; coughs.

Antivenin *Wyeth-Ayerst, Canad.*
Crotalidae antiserum (p.1563·3).
Snake envenomation.

Antivenin (Latrodectus Mactans) *Merck Frosst, Canad.*
Black widow spider antiserum (p.1564·3).
Black widow spider bite.

Antiverrugas *Isdin, Spain.*
Lactic acid (p.1626·2); salicylic acid (p.1122·3).
Warts.

Antivert
Pfizer, Canad.; Pfizer, USA.
Meclozine hydrochloride (p.420·3).
Motion sickness; radiation sickness; vascular headaches; vertigo.

Antivipmyn *Bioclon, Mex.*
Polyvalent crotalidae antiserum (p.1563·3).
Snake envenomation.

Antizid *Lilly, S.Afr.*
Nizatidine (p.1238·1).
Heartburn; hyperacidity.

Antizine *Pharmasant, Thai.*
Hydroxyzine hydrochloride (p.419·1).
Hypersensitivity reactions; sedative.

Antizol
Orphan Medical, Israel; Cambridge, UK; Orphan Medical, USA.
Fomepizole (p.1009·3).
Available on a named patient basis only in the UK.
Ethylene glycol poisoning; methanol poisoning.

Antizona *Alonga, Spain†.*
Idoxuridine (p.625·1) in dimethyl sulfoxide.
Herpesvirus skin infections.

Antocin *Tubilux, Ital.*
Myrtillus (p.1639·2).
Capillary disorders.

Antomiopic
Allergan-Frumtost, Braz.; Ciba Vision, Spain.
Vitamins and amino acids (p.1350·1); myrtillus (p.1639·2).
Eye disorders.

Antopal *Bama, Spain.*
Binifibrate (p.850·1).
Hyperlipidaemias.

Antopar *Lek, Hong Kong.*
Benzoyl peroxide (p.1111·1).
Acne.

Antoral *Recordati, Ital.*
Tibezonium iodide (p.1673·2).
Mouth and throat disinfection.

Antoxymega *Larkhall Laboratories, UK.*
Multivitamin and mineral preparation (p.1350·1).

Antra
Astra, Aust.; Astra, Ger.; Astra, Ital.; Astra, Switz.
Omeprazole (p.1239·1), omeprazole magnesium (p.1239·1), or omeprazole sodium (p.1239·1).
Acid aspiration; gastro-oesophageal reflux; peptic ulcer; Zollinger-Ellison syndrome.

Antral *Carnot, Mex.*
Metronidazole (p.594·1).
Amoebiasis; giardiasis; trichomoniasis.

Antramups *Astra, Switz.*
Omeprazole magnesium (p.1239·1).
Gastro-oesophageal reflux; peptic ulcer; Zollinger-Ellison syndrome.

Antran *Solfran, Mex.*
Multivitamin and mineral preparation (p.1350·1).

Antranol *Stiefel, Ger.*
Dithranol (p.1113·3).
Psoriasis.

Antrex *Orion, Fin.*
Calcium folinate (p.1363·1).
Adjunct to fluorouracil in colorectal cancer; megaloblastic leukaemia; reduction of methotrexate toxicity.

Antrimox *Antigen, Irl.†.*
Co-trimoxazole (p.193·3).
Bacterial infections.

Antrizine *Major, USA.*
Meclozine hydrochloride (p.420·3).
Motion sickness; vertigo.

Antrocol *Poythress, USA.*
Atropine sulfate (p.461·1); phenobarbital (p.355·1).
Gastrointestinal disorders.

Antroquoril *Schering-Plough, Austral.*
Betamethasone valerate (p.1063·2).
Skin disorders.

Anturan
Novartis, Aust.; Novartis, Austral.; Novartis, Canad.†; Novartis, Israel; Novartis, NZ; Ciba-Geigy, S.Afr.†; Geigy, Switz.†; Sovereign, UK.
Sulfinpyrazone (p.402·2).
Gout; hyperuricaemia; myocardial infarction; thromboembolic disorders.

Anturane *Novartis, USA.*
Sulfinpyrazone (p.402·2).
Gouty arthritis.

Antussan *Dolorgiet, Ger.†.*
Oral drops; oral liquid: Thyme (p.1672·2).
Formerly contained menthol, camphor, benzoic acid, ephedrine hydrochloride, sodium dibunate, thyme, and primula rhizome.
Catarrh; coughs.

Tablets: Ambroxol hydrochloride (p.1084·3).
Respiratory-tract disorders with increased or viscous mucus.

Antussia *Asian Pharm, Thai.*
Capsules: Dextromethorphan hydrobromide (p.1087·3); guaifenesin (p.1092·2); pseudoephedrine hydrochloride (p.1099·2); diphenhydramine hydrochloride (p.416·1).

Syrup: Dextromethorphan hydrobromide (p.1087·3); guaifenesin (p.1092·2); phenylpropanolamine hydrochloride (p.1098·1); phenylephrine hydrochloride (p.1097·1).

Hypersensitivity reactions.

Antust *Progress, Thai.*
Dextromethorphan hydrobromide (p.1087·3); chlorpheniramine [chlorphenamine] maleate (p.412·1); terpin hydrate (p.1101·2).
Coughs.

Anu-Aide *Technilab, Canad.*
Zinc sulfate (p.1398·2).
Haemorrhoids.

Anucet *Sanobia, Port.*
Ointment: Hydrocortisone acetate (p.1073·3); phenylephrine hydrochloride (p.1097·1); lignocaine [lidocaine] hydrochloride (p.1313·2); belladonna (p.463·1); peru balsam (p.1650·2).

Suppositories: Hydrocortisone acetate (p.1073·3); phenylephrine hydrochloride (p.1097·1); lignocaine [lidocaine] hydrochloride (p.1313·2); amethocaine [tetracaine] hydrochloride (p.1305·2); belladonna (p.463·1).

Anorectal disorders.

Anucort-HC *G & W, USA.*
Hydrocortisone acetate (p.1073·3).

Anugesic *Parke, Davis, USA.*
Ointment: Pramocaine hydrochloride (p.1318·2).

Suppositories: Bismuth subgallate (p.1213·2); bismuth oxide (p.1213·1); resorcinol (p.1122·3); bismuth oxyiodide (p.1214·1); peru balsam (p.1650·2); benzyl ben-

---

The symbol † denotes a preparation no longer actively marketed

zoate (p.1428·2); zinc oxide (p.1128·2); boric acid (p.1586·1); pramocaine hydrochloride (p.1318·2).
Anorectal disorders.

Anugesic-HC
Note.This name is used for preparations of different composition.
Parke, Davis, Canad.
Pramocaine hydrochloride (p.1318·2); hydrocortisone acetate (p.1073·3); zinc sulfate (p.1398·2).
Anorectal disorders.

Parke, Davis, Irl.
Cream: Pramocaine hydrochloride (p.1318·2); hydrocortisone acetate (p.1073·3); zinc oxide (p.1128·2); peru balsam (p.1650·2); benzyl benzoate (p.1428·2); bismuth oxide (p.1213·1); resorcinol (p.1122·2).
Anorectal disorders.

Parke, Davis, UK.
Cream: Pramocaine hydrochloride (p.1318·2); hydrocortisone acetate (p.1073·3); bismuth oxide (p.1213·1); peru balsam (p.1650·2); zinc oxide (p.1128·2); benzyl benzoate (p.1428·2).
Anorectal disorders.

Parke, Davis, Irl.; Parke, Davis, UK.
Suppositories: Pramocaine hydrochloride (p.1318·2); hydrocortisone acetate (p.1073·3); zinc oxide (p.1128·2); bismuth subgallate (p.1213·2); bismuth oxide (p.1213·1); Peru balsam (p.1650·2); benzyl benzoate (p.1428·2).
Anorectal disorders.

Anumed *Major, USA.*
Bismuth subgallate (p.1213·2); bismuth resorcinol compound (p.1214·1); benzyl benzoate (p.1428·2); zinc oxide (p.1128·2); peru balsam (p.1650·2).
Anorectal disorders.

Anumed HC *Major, USA.*
Hydrocortisone acetate (p.1073·3); bismuth subgallate (p.1213·2); bismuth resorcinol compound (p.1214·1); benzyl benzoate (p.1428·2); peru balsam (p.1650·2); zinc oxide (p.1128·2).
Anorectal disorders.

Anumedin *Kade, Ger.*
Prednisolone acetate (p.1078·1); cinchocaine hydrochloride (p.1309·1).
Anorectal disorders.

Anurin *Abbott, Mex.*
Pipemidic acid (p.236·1).

Anusept *Lichtenstein, Ger.†*
Bismuth subnitrate (p.1213·2); zinc oxide (p.1128·2); benzocaine (p.1306·2).
Anorectal disorders.

Anusol
Note.This name is used for preparations of different composition.
Parke, Davis, Austral.; Warner-Lambert, NZ.
Suppositories; ointment: Zinc oxide (p.1128·2); peru balsam (p.1650·2); benzyl benzoate (p.1428·2).
Anorectal disorders.

Parke, Davis, Austral.
Wipes: Hamamelis water (p.1618·3); glycerol (p.1616·3).
Anorectal irritation.

Warner-Lambert, Canad.
Zinc sulfate (p.1398·2).
Anorectal disorders.

Warner-Lambert, Fr.; Parke, Davis, S.Afr.
Ointment; suppositories: Bismuth subgallate (p.1213·2); bismuth oxide (p.1213·1); zinc oxide (p.1128·2).
Anorectal disorders.

Warner-Lambert, Ger.
Bismuth oxide-bismuthoxyiodide-1,3-bis-(ammoniumoxy)-benzol-4,5-(bismuthylsulfonate); zinc oxide (p.1128·2); peru balsam (p.1650·2).

Warner-Lambert, Hong Kong; Warner-Lambert, Irl.; Parke, Davis, Israel; Warner-Lambert, UK.
Ointment; suppositories: Bismuth subgallate (p.1213·2); bismuth oxide (p.1213·1); peru balsam (p.1650·2); zinc oxide (p.1128·2).
Anorectal disorders.

Warner-Lambert, Irl.; Warner-Lambert, UK.
Cream: Bismuth oxide (p.1213·1); peru balsam (p.1650·2); zinc oxide (p.1128·2).
Anorectal disorders.

Warner-Lambert, Ital.
Resorcinol (p.1122·2); yellow bismuth oxide (p.1213·1); bismuth subgallate (p.1213·2); bismuth oxyiodide (p.1214·1); peru balsam (p.1650·2); zinc oxide (p.1128·2).
Anorectal disorders.

Warner-Lambert, Neth.
Bismuth subgallate (p.1213·2); zinc oxide (p.1128·2).
Anorectal disorders.

Parke, Davis, Singapore.
Ointment: Peru balsam (p.1650·2); benzyl benzoate (p.1428·2); bismuth oxide (p.1213·1); bismuth subgallate (p.1213·2); bismuth oxyiodide (p.1214·1); resorcinol (p.1122·2).
Haemorrhoids.

Parke, Davis, Singapore; Warner-Lambert, Thai.
Suppositories: Peru balsam (p.1650·2); benzyl benzoate (p.1428·2); bismuth oxide (p.1213·1); bismuth subgallate (p.1213·2); resorcinol (p.1122·2); zinc oxide (p.1128·2).
Haemorrhoids.

Lundbeck, Swed.†
Bismuth oxyiodoresorcinsulfonate; zinc oxide (p.1128·2); peru balsam (p.1650·2).
Anorectal disorders.

Warner-Lambert Consumer, Switz.†
Bismuth oxide (p.1213·1); bismuth subgallate (p.1213·2); bismuth oxyiodide (p.1214·1); peru balsam (p.1650·2); benzyl benzoate (p.1428·2); zinc oxide (p.1128·2).
Anorectal disorders.

Warner-Lambert, USA.
Ointment: Zinc oxide (p.1128·2); pramocaine hydrochloride (p.1318·2).
Suppositories: Benzyl alcohol (p.1135·2); soybean oil (p.1378·1); tocoferil acetate (p.1394·1).
Formerly contained bismuth subgallate, bismuth resorcinol compound, benzyl benzoate, zinc oxide, and peru balsam.
Anorectal disorders.

Anusol Antifungal Foot Powder *Young, USA†.*
Miconazole nitrate (p.391·1).
Fungal infections.

Anusol Plus *Warner-Lambert, Canad.*
Pramocaine hydrochloride (p.1318·2); zinc sulfate (p.1398·2).
Anorectal disorders.

Anusol-HC
Note.This name is used for preparations of different composition.
Warner-Lambert, Braz.
Hydrocortisone acetate (p.1073·3); bismuth resorcinol compound (p.1214·1); zinc oxide (p.1128·2); bismuth subgallate (p.1213·2); peru balsam (p.1650·2); benzyl benzoate (p.1428·2).
Anorectal disorders.

Parke, Davis, Canad.
Zinc sulfate (p.1398·2); hydrocortisone acetate (p.1073·3).
Anorectal disorders.

Warner-Lambert, Hong Kong.
Ointment: Peru balsam (p.1650·2); benzyl benzoate (p.1428·2); bismuth oxide (p.1213·1); bismuth subgallate (p.1213·2); zinc oxide (p.1128·2); hydrocortisone acetate (p.1073·3).
Anorectal disorders.

Warner-Lambert, Hong Kong.
Suppositories: Peru balsam (p.1650·2); benzyl benzoate (p.1428·2); bismuth subgallate (p.1213·2); zinc oxide (p.1128·2); hydrocortisone acetate (p.1073·3).
Anorectal disorders.

Parke, Davis, Irl.
Hydrocortisone acetate (p.1073·3); benzyl benzoate (p.1428·2); bismuth subgallate (p.1213·2); bismuth oxide (p.1213·1); peru balsam (p.1650·2); zinc oxide (p.1128·2); resorcinol (p.1122·2).
Anorectal disorders.

Parke, Davis, S.Afr.†
Bismuth subgallate (p.1213·2); bismuth oxide (p.1213·1); bismuth oxyiodide (p.1214·1); resorcinol (p.1122·2); peru balsam (p.1650·2); benzyl benzoate (p.1428·2); zinc oxide (p.1128·2); boric acid (p.1586·1); hydrocortisone acetate (p.1073·3).
Anorectal disorders.

Monarch, USA.
Hydrocortisone acetate (p.1073·3).
Anorectal disorders; skin disorders.

Anusol-HC, Plus HC *Warner-Lambert, UK.*
Bismuth subgallate (p.1213·2); bismuth oxide (p.1213·1); peru balsam (p.1650·2); zinc oxide (p.1128·2); hydrocortisone acetate (p.1073·3); benzyl benzoate (p.1428·2).
Anusol HC formerly contained bismuth subgallate, bismuth oxide, peru balsam, zinc oxide, hydrocortisone acetate, benzyl benzoate, and resorcinol.
Anorectal disorders.

Anuzinc
Note.This name is used for preparations of different composition.
Technilab, Canad.
Zinc sulfate (p.1398·2).
Anorectal disorders.

Technilab, Hong Kong.
Ointment: Zinc sulfate (p.1398·2).
Suppositories: Bismuth oxide (p.1213·1); bismuth subgallate (p.1213·2); zinc oxide (p.1128·2).
Anorectal disorders.

Anvitoff
Knoll, Ger.; Knoll, Switz.
Tranexamic acid (p.742·2).
Haemorrhagic disorders.

Anvitol *Azevedos, Port.*
Haematoporphyrin hydrochloride; glycine; cyanocobalamin (p.1350·1).
Tonic.

Anxanil *Econo Med, USA†.*
Hydroxyzine hydrochloride (p.419·1).
Anxiety; hypersensitivity reactions.

Anxer *Unison, Thai.*
Cefalexin (p.161·3).
Bacterial infections.

Anxicalm *Clonmel, Irl.*
Diazepam (p.674·3).
Anxiety; epilepsy; insomnia; premedication; skeletal muscle spasm.

Anxiety/Stress L72 *Homeocan, Canad.*
Homoeopathic preparation.

Anxiolan *Medochemie, Thai.*
Buspirone hydrochloride (p.657·2).
Anxiety.

Anxiolit
Gerot, Aust.; Medichemie, Switz.
Oxazepam (p.697·1).
Anxiety disorders; insomnia.

Anxiolit plus *Gerot, Aust.*
Oxazepam (p.697·1); methylbenactyzium bromide (p.470·2).
Anxiety disorders.

Anxipress-D *Pharmaland, Thai.*
Perphenazine (p.699·1); amitriptyline hydrochloride (p.273·3).
Depression.

Anxira *Condrugs, Thai.*
Lorazepam (p.688·3).
Anxiety.

Anxirid *Aspen, S.Afr.*
Alprazolam (p.654·2).
Anxiety disorders; mixed anxiety depressive states.

Anxoral *IPRAD, Fr.*
Phenobarbital (p.355·1); crataegus (p.1600·2); passion flower (p.1649·1); valerian (p.1678·3).
Formerly contained crataegus, passion flower, valerian, sparteine sulfate, phenobarbital, and papaverine hydrochloride.
Anxiety; insomnia.

Anxyrex *Irex, Fr.*
Bromazepam (p.656·3).
Alcohol withdrawal syndrome; anxiety.

Any *Homme de Fer, Fr.*
Mequinol (p.1118·2).
Hyperpigmentation.

Anzatax
Faulding, Austral.; Faulding, Hong Kong; Faulding, Singapore; DBL, Thai.; Faulding, Thai.
Paclitaxel (p.563·2).
Breast cancer; non-small cell lung cancer; ovarian cancer.

Anzem *Rolab, S.Afr.*
Diltiazem hydrochloride (p.874·3).
Angina pectoris; hypertension.

Anzemet
Hoechst Marion Roussel, Aust.; Hoechst Marion Roussel, Austral.; Hoechst Marion Roussel, Canad.; Roussel Diamant, Fr.; Hoechst Marion Roussel, Ital.; Hoechst Marion Roussel, Mex.; Hoechst Marion Roussel, USA.
Dolasetron mesilate (p.1223·3).
Nausea and vomiting.

Aodrops *Ciba Vision, Canad.*
Lubricant for contact lenses (p.1129·2).

Aoflow *Ciba Vision, Canad.*
Cleansing solution for contact lenses (p.1129·2).

A-O-Q10 MaxiPower Formula *Solgar, UK.*
Multivitamin and mineral preparation with amino acids, coenzyme Q-10, and fibre (p.1350·1).
Dietary supplement.

Aorinyl *Progress, Thai.*
Phenylephrine hydrochloride (p.1097·1); brompheniramine maleate (p.410·2); phenylpropanolamine hydrochloride (p.1098·1).
Allergic respiratory-tract disorders; nasal congestion.

Aosept
Novartis, Aust.; Ciba Vision, Austral.; Ciba Vision, Canad.; Ciba Vision, NZ; Ciba Vision, USA.
Hydrogen peroxide (p.1147·1) (p.1129·2).
Disinfection and storage of contact lenses.

Aotal *Lipha Sante, Fr.*
Acamprosate calcium (p.653·3).
Alcoholism.

APA
Note.This name is used for preparations of different composition.
Lannacher, Aust.
Suppositories: Paracetamol (p.71·2); propyphenazone (p.80·2).
Tablets: Paracetamol (p.71·2); dextropropoxyphene hydrochloride (p.27·1).
Pain.

Merck, Hong Kong.
Paracetamol (p.71·2); propyphenazone (p.80·2).
Fever; pain.

APAC Improved *Vortech, USA†.*
Aspirin (p.14·2); caffeine (p.761·3).
Pain.

Apacef
Zeneca, Belg.; AstraZeneca, Fr.
Cefotetan disodium (p.170·3).
Lignocaine [lidocaine] hydrochloride (p.1313·2) is included in the intramuscular injection to alleviate the pain of injection.
Bacterial infections.

Apacet
Merck, Aust.; Parmed, USA.
Paracetamol (p.71·2).
Fever; pain.

Apagen *Stomygen, Ital.*
Hydroxyapatite (p.1622·1).
Dental disorders.

Apain *AstraZeneca, Denm.*
Ibuprofen (p.43·2).
Pain.

Apaisac *Saninter, Port.*
Emollient.

Apaisance *Lierac, Fr.*
Tilia (p.1673·2); levomenol (p.1629·1).
Hypersensitive skin.

Apaisyl *Monot, Fr.†.*
Isothipendyl hydrochloride (p.419·2).
Hypersensitivity.

Apamid
Parke, Davis, Fin.; Weifa, Norw.; Parke, Davis, Swed.
Glipizide (p.322·3).
Diabetes mellitus.

Apamox *F5 Profas, Spain.*
Amoxicillin trihydrate (p.149·2).
Bacterial infections.

Apap
CPC, Hong Kong; Cypress, USA.
Paracetamol (p.71·2).
Fever; pain.

A-Par
Note.This name is used for preparations of different composition.
Pharmygiene, Fr.
Esdepallethrine (p.1432·2); piperonyl butoxide (p.1436·2).
Destruction of scabies mite, fleas and lice in textiles and adjunct to treatment.

SCAT, Switz.†.
Pyrethrum (p.1436·3); piperonyl butoxide (p.1436·2).
Pediculosis.

A-Parkin *Dexxon, Israel.*
Amantadine sulfate (p.1161·2).
Influenza A; parkinsonism.

Aparoxal *Veyron-Froment, Fr.*
Phenobarbital (p.355·1).
Epilepsy.

Aparsonin N *Merckle, Ger.*
Bromhexine hydrochloride (p.1085·3).
Respiratory-tract disorders associated with increased mucus.

Apatate *Kenwood, USA.*
Vitamin B complex (p.1350·1).

Apatate with Fluoride *Kenwood, USA.*
Vitamin B substances (p.1350·1) with sodium fluoride (p.1375·3).

Apatef
Lederle, Austral.; Zeneca, Ital.; Lederle, NZ; Zeneca, Port.
Cefotetan disodium (p.170·3).
Bacterial infections.

Apatite *Weleda, UK.*
Homoeopathic preparation.

Apefer *Teuta, Braz.*
Ferrous gluconate (p.1360·1); vitamins (p.1350·1).
Ascorbic acid (p.1389·3) is included in this preparation to increase the absorption and availability of iron.
Anaemias.

Apegmone *Lipha Sante, Fr.*
Tioclomarol (p.983·1).
Thromboembolic disorders.

Apekumarol *Pharmacia Upjohn, Swed.†.*
Dicoumarol (p.869·1).
Thromboembolic disorders.

A-Pen *Orion, Fin.*
Note. A similar name is used for preparations of different composition (see below).
Ampicillin sodium (p.150·3).
Bacterial infections.

Apen *Xixia, S.Afr.*
Note. A similar name is used for preparations of different composition (see above).
Ampicillin (p.150·3); cloxacillin (p.192·1).
Bacterial infections.

Aperamid *Ardeypharm, Ger.†.*
Loperamide hydrochloride (p.1231·3).
Diarrhoea.

Aperdan *ABC, Ital.*
Naproxen cetrimonium (p.61·3).
Formerly contained dequalinium chloride, crotamiton, undecenoic acid diethanolamide, thymol, and phenoxyethanol.
Vulvovaginal disorders.

Apergan *Panzera, Ital.*
Royal jelly (p.1659·3); glucose (p.1364·1); ginseng (p.1615·3).
Nutritional supplement.

Aperisan *Dentinox, Ger.*
Sage (p.1660·2).
Mouth and throat inflammation.

Aperop *Pharmacobel, Belg.*
Nux vomica (p.1643·1); kola (p.1681·1); orange peel (p.1644·2); cinchona bark (p.1595·3); haemoglobin (p.738·1); iodine (p.1522·3); tannic acid (p.1669·1); calcium phosphate hydrochloride.
Tonic.

Apetibe *Luper, Braz.*
Buclizine (p.411·1); amino acids; vitamins (p.1350·1).
Reduced appetite; tonic.

Apetil
Note.This name is used for preparations of different composition.
Bunker, Braz.
Buclizine hydrochloride (p.411·1); amino acids; vitamin B substances (p.1350·1).
Reduced appetite; tonic.

Ram, USA.
Multivitamin and mineral preparation (p.1350·1).

Apetin *Gilton, Braz.*
Carnitine; vitamin B subsances (p.1350·1).
Reduced appetite; tonic.

Apetinil-Depo *Syntex, Switz.†.*
Etilamfetamine hydrochloride.
Obesity.

Apevitin BC *EMS, Braz.*
Cyproheptadine hydrochloride (p.414·2); vitamin B substances; ascorbic acid (p.1350·1).
Reduced appetite; tonic.

APF *Cypress, USA.*
Sodium fluoride (p.1375·3).
Dental caries prophylaxis.

Aphenylbarbit *Streuli, Switz.*
Phenobarbital (p.355·1).
Epilepsy; febrile convulsions; sedative.

Aphilan *Darci, Fr.*
Buclizine hydrochloride (p.411·1).
Allergic conjunctivitis; allergic rhinitis; pruritus.

Aphloine P *DB, Fr.*
Aphloia; hamamelis (p.1618·3); viburnum; esculoside
(p.1574·1).
Formerly contained aphloia, hamamelis, hydrastis, pis-
cidia, viburnum, and esculoside.
Haemorrhoids; peripheral vascular insufficiency.

Aphrodyne *Star, USA.*
Yohimbine hydrochloride (p.1681·3).

Aphthasol *Block, USA.*
Amlexanox (p.760·3).
Aphthous ulcers.

Aphtiria *Debat, Fr.†*
Lindane (p.1434·1).
Disinfection of clothes and bedding; pediculosis.

Aphtoral *Pierre Fabre Sante, Fr.*
Chlorhexidine gluconate (p.1138·2); amethocaine [tet-
racaine] hydrochloride (p.1305·2); ascorbic acid
(p.1389·3).
Formerly known as Eludril.
Mouth and throat disorders.

Api Baby *Sanitalia, Ital.*
Pollen; royal jelly (p.1659·3); fructose; myrtillus
(p.1639·2).
Nutritional supplement.

Apifortyl *Mack, Thai.*
Multivitamin and mineral preparation (p.1350·1).

Apihepar *Asta Medica, Aust.*
Silybum marianum (p.1021·3).
Liver disorders.

Apilaxe *Cooperation Pharmaceutique, Fr.*
Sorbitol (p.1377·3); althaea leaf (p.1577·1).
Constipation.

Apimid *Apogepha, Ger.*
Flutamide (p.542·3).
Prostatic cancer.

Apiocolina *Bruschettini, Ital.*
Escherichia coli lysate.
Anorectal inflammation.

Apir Clorurado *Antibioticos, Spain.*
Sodium chloride (p.1196·1).
Fluid and electrolyte disorders.

Apir Cloruro Amonico *Antibioticos, Spain.*
Ammonium chloride (p.1085·2).
Hypochloraemia; metabolic alkalosis.

Apir Glucoibys *Pharmacia Upjohn, Spain†.*
Glucose (p.1364·2).
Carbohydrate source; fluid and electrolyte disorders.

Apir Glucopotasico *Antibioticos, Spain.*
Glucose (p.1364·2); potassium chloride (p.1194·3).
Hypokalaemia.

Apir Glucosado *Antibioticos, Spain.*
Glucose (p.1364·2).
Fluid and electrolyte disorders; parenteral nutrition.

Apir Glucosalino *IPS, Spain.*
Glucose (p.1364·2); sodium chloride (p.1196·1).
Fluid and electrolyte disorders.

Apir Ringer *Antibioticos, Spain.*
Electrolyte infusion (p.1180·1).
Fluid and electrolyte depletion.

Apir Ringer Lactato *Antibioticos, Spain.*
Electrolyte infusion with sodium lactate (p.1180·1).
Fluid and electrolyte depletion.

Apiretal *Ern, Spain.*
Paracetamol (p.71·2).
Fever; pain.

Apiretal Codeina *Ern, Spain.*
Paracetamol (p.71·2); codeine (p.25·2).
Pain.

Apiroflex Clorurado *IPS, Spain.*
Sodium chloride (p.1196·1).
Fluid and electrolyte disorders.

Apiroflex Glucosada *Antibioticos, Spain.*
Glucose (p.1364·2).
Fluid and electrolyte disorders; parenteral nutrition.

Apiroflex Glucosalina *IPS, Spain.*
Glucose (p.1364·2); sodium chloride (p.1196·1).
Fluid and electrolyte disorders.

Apirol *Merck Sharp & Dohme, Israel.*
Norfloxacin (p.232·1).
Bacterial infections.

Apis *Brauer, Austral.*
Homoeopathic preparation.

Apiserum *DB, Fr.*
Royal jelly (p.1659·3).
Tonic.

Apiserum con Telergon I *Codit, Ital.*
Wine; acacia honey (p.1366·2); royal jelly (p.1659·3).
Nutritional supplement.

Apisgel *Dolisos, Canad.*
Homoeopathic preparation.

Apistress *Sanitalia, Ital.*
Royal jelly (p.1659·3); pollen; propolis (p.1655·1).
Nutritional supplement.

APL
Wyeth-Ayerst, Austral.; Wyeth-Ayerst, Canad.; Aspen, S.Afr.; Wyeth-Ayerst, USA.
Chorionic gonadotrophin (p.1279·2).
*Cryptorchidism; male and female infertility; male hy-
pogonadism; pituitary dwarfism; recurrent miscar-
riage.*

Aplace *Kyorin, Jpn.*
Troxipide (p.1254·2).
Gastritis; peptic ulcer.

Aplactin *Mead Johnson, Ital.*
Pravastatin sodium (p.957·3).
Arteriosclerosis; hyperlipidaemias.

Aplaket *Rottapharm, Ital.; Rotta, Singapore; Rotta, Thai.*
Ticlopidine hydrochloride (p.981·1).
Thrombosis prophylaxis.

A-Plex *Lemery, Mex.*
Tretinoin (p.1126·2).

Aplexil *Rhone-Poulenc Rorer, Aust.*
Oxomemazine (p.422·2); guaifenesin (p.1092·2); para-
cetamol (p.71·2); sodium benzoate (p.1134·3).
Respiratory-tract disorders.

Apligraf *Novartis, Aust.*
Bioengineered human skin equivalent (p.1123·2).
Diabetic foot ulcers; venous leg ulcers.

Aplisol *Parkedale, USA.*
Tuberculin purified protein derivative (p.1675·3).
Diagnosis of tuberculosis.

Aplitest *Parke, Davis, USA.*
Tuberculin purified protein derivative (p.1675·3).
Diagnosis of tuberculosis.

Aplodan *Astra, Ital.*
Creatinolfosfate (p.1601·1).
Muscle disorders.

Aplona *Athenstaedt, Ger.*
Apple powder; colloidal silicon dioxide (p.1503·3).
Diarrhoea.

Ap-Napro-Na *Apotex, Hong Kong.*
Naproxen sodium (p.61·1).
Musculoskeletal and joint disorders; pain.

Apnol *Pharmaland, Thai.*
Allopurinol (p.397·2).
Gout; hyperuricaemia.

Apoacor *Curex, Israel.*
Verapamil hydrochloride (p.989·1).
Angina pectoris; arrhythmias; hypertension.

Apo-Alpraz *Apotex, Canad.; Apotex, Singapore.*
Alprazolam (p.654·2).
Anxiety.

Apo-Amilzide *Apotex, Canad.; Apotex, Hong Kong; Apotex, Singapore.*
Amiloride hydrochloride (p.835·1); hydrochlorothi-
azide (p.907·3).
Hepatic cirrhosis with ascites; hypertension; oedema.

Apo-Amoxi *Apotex, Canad.; Apotex, Hong Kong; Apotex, NZ; Apotex, Singapore.*
Amoxicillin (p.149·2) or amoxicillin trihydrate
(p.149·2).
Bacterial infections.

Apo-Ampi *Apotex, Canad.*
Ampicillin trihydrate (p.151·1).
Bacterial infections.

Apo-Atenol *Apotex, Canad.; Apotex, Hong Kong; Apotex, Singapore.*
Atenolol (p.841·3).
Angina pectoris; arrhythmias; hypertension.

Apobase *Alpharma, Fin.*
Emollient.

Apo-C *Apotex, Canad.*
Ascorbic acid (p.1389·3).
Vitamin supplement.

Apo-Cal *Apotex, Canad.*
Calcium carbonate (p.1215·1).
Calcium supplement.

Apocanda *Apogepha, Ger.†*
Clotrimazole (p.382·1).
Fungal infections.

Apocapen *Curex, Israel.*
Captopril (p.853·3).
*Diabetic nephropathy; heart failure; hypertension;
myocardial infarction.*

Apo-Capto *Apotex, Canad.; Apotex, Hong Kong; Apotex, Singapore.*
Captopril (p.853·3).
Heart failure; hypertension.

Apocard *3M, Port.†; 3M, Spain.*
Flecainide acetate (p.890·1).
Arrhythmias.

Apo-Cepalex *Apotex, Hong Kong.*
Cefalexin (p.161·3).
Bacterial infections.

Apo-Cephalex *Apotex, Canad.*
Cefalexin (p.161·3).
Bacterial infections.

Apo-Chlorax *Apotex, Canad.; Apotex, Singapore.*
Chlordiazepoxide hydrochloride (p.659·2); clidinium
bromide (p.465·1).
Gastrointestinal disorders with associated anxiety.

Apociclina *Protein, Mex.*
Doxycycline (p.200·1).

Apocillin *Alpharma, Norw.*
Phenoxymethylpenicillin potassium (p.235·1).
Bacterial infections.

Apo-Cloxi *Apotex, Canad.; Apotex, Hong Kong.*
Cloxacillin sodium (p.192·1).
Bacterial infections.

Apocort *Alpharma, Fin.*
Hydrocortisone acetate (p.1073·3).
Skin disorders.

Apocortal *Alpharma, Norw.*
Hydrocortisone acetate (p.1073·3).
Skin disorders.

Apo-Cromolyn *Apotex, Canad.*
Sodium cromoglicate (p.774·3).
Allergic rhinitis; asthma.

Apocyclin *Alpharma, Fin.*
Tetracycline hydrochloride (p.258·3).
Bacterial infections.

Apoderm *Nycomed, Aust.*
Deproteinised derivative of calf blood.
Burns; ulcers; wounds.

Apo-Diclo *Apotex, Canad.; Apotex, Hong Kong; Apotex, NZ.*
Diclofenac (p.30·2) or diclofenac sodium (p.30·3).
*Inflammation; musculoskeletal and joint disorders;
pain.*

Apo-Diltiaz *Apotex, Canad.; Apotex, Hong Kong.*
Diltiazem hydrochloride (p.874·3).
Angina pectoris; hypertension.

Apodorm *Alpharma, Denm.; Alpharma, Norw.; Dumex-Alpharma, Swed.*
Nitrazepam (p.695·2).
Epilepsy; infantile spasm; insomnia.

Apodoxin *Alpharma, Fin.*
Doxycycline (p.200·1).
Bacterial infections.

Apodoxy *Curex, Israel.*
Doxycycline (p.200·1).
Bacterial infections; malaria.

Apo-Doxy *Apotex, Canad.; Apotex, Singapore.*
Doxycycline (p.200·1) or doxycycline hyclate
(p.200·1).
Bacterial infections.

Apo-Erythro *Apotex, Canad.; Apotex, Hong Kong.*
Erythromycin (p.201·2), erythromycin ethyl succinate
(p.201·2), or erythromycin stearate (p.201·3).
Bacterial infections.

Apo-Feno *Apotex, Canad.*
Fenofibrate (p.889·1).
Hyperlipidaemias.

Apofin *Chiesi, Ital.*
Apomorphine hydrochloride (p.1163·1).
Parkinsonism.

Apo-Gain *Apotex, Canad.; Apotex, Hong Kong; Apotex, NZ.*
Minoxidil (p.934·2).
Alopecia androgenetica.

Apogastine *Curex, Israel.*
Famotidine (p.1225·3).
*Gastro-oesophageal reflux; peptic ulcer; Zollinger-El-
lison syndrome.*

APO-go *Britannia Pharmaceuticals, UK.*
Apomorphine hydrochloride (p.1163·1).
Parkinsonism.

Apohair *Curex, Israel.*
Minoxidil (p.934·2).
Alopecia.

Apo-Hepat *Pekana, Ger.*
Homoeopathic preparation.

Apo-Hexa *Apotex, Canad.*
Multivitamin preparation (p.1350·1).

Apo-Hydro *Apotex, Canad.; Apotex, Singapore.*
Hydrochlorothiazide (p.907·3).
Hypertension; oedema.

Apo-Infekt *Pekana, Ger.*
Homoeopathic preparation.

Apo-Ipravent *Apotex, Canad.*
Ipratropium bromide (p.766·1).
Bronchodilator.

Apo-ISDN *Apotex, Canad.; Apotex, Singapore.*
Isosorbide dinitrate (p.915·2).
Angina pectoris.

Apo-K *Apotex, Canad.; Apotex, Hong Kong.*
Potassium chloride (p.1194·3).
Potassium depletion.

Apo-Keto *Apotex, Canad.; Apotex, Hong Kong; Apotex, Singapore.*
Ketoprofen (p.47·3).
Musculoskeletal, joint, and peri-articular disorders.

Apokinon *Aguettant, Fr.*
Apomorphine hydrochloride (p.1163·1).
Parkinsonism.

Apolar *Alpharma, Fin.; Alpharma, Norw.; Dumex-Alpharma, Swed.*
Desonide (p.1066·2).
Skin disorders.

Apolar med dekvalon *Alpharma, Norw.*
Desonide (p.1066·2); dequalinium chloride (p.1143·1).
Infected skin disorders.

Apo-Levocarb *Apotex, Canad.; Apotex, Hong Kong; Apotex, NZ.*
Levodopa (p.1169·2); carbidopa (p.1168·2).
Parkinsonism.

Apolide *Protein, Mex.*
Nimesulide (p.62·3).

Apo-Methazide *Apotex, Canad.*
Methyldopa (p.927·3); hydrochlorothiazide (p.907·3).
Hypertension.

Apo-Metoclop *Apotex, Canad.; Apotex, Hong Kong.*
Metoclopramide hydrochloride (p.1235·2).
Gastrointestinal disorders; nausea and vomiting.

Apomex *Curex, Israel.*
Selegiline hydrochloride (p.1177·2).
Parkinsonism.

Apomine *Faulding, Austral.; Baxter, NZ; Faulding, NZ.*
Apomorphine hydrochloride (p.1163·1).
Parkinsonism.

Apominolin *Curex, Israel.*
Minocycline hydrochloride (p.224·3).
Bacterial infections.

Apomoxyn *Curex, Israel.*
Amoxicillin (p.149·2).
Bacterial infections.

Aponacin *Curex, Israel.*
Naproxen (p.60·3).
Musculoskeletal and joint disorders; pain.

Apo-Nadol *Apotex, Canad.; Apotex, Hong Kong.*
Nadolol (p.937·1).
Angina pectoris; hypertension.

Aponal *Roche, Ger.; Dresden, Ger.*
Doxepin hydrochloride (p.283·3).
Anxiety; depression; insomnia; withdrawal syndromes.

Apo-Napro-Na *Apotex, Canad.; Apotex, Singapore.*
Naproxen sodium (p.61·1).
Inflammation; pain.

Aponatura Beruhigungs *Terralife, Aust.*
Lupulus (p.1629·3); melissa (p.1632·2) with or without
vitamin C (p.1389·3).
Sedative.

Aponatura Durchfall *Terralife, Aust.*
Capsule: Tormentil (p.1674·1); myrtillus (p.1639·2).
Oral drops: Tormentil (p.1674·1); myrtillus
(p.1639·2); strawberry leaf.
Diarrhoea.

Aponatura Einschlaf *Terralife, Aust.*
Valerian (p.1678·3); lupulus (p.1629·3); melissa
(p.1632·2).
Sleep disorders.

Aponatura Entwasserungs *Terralife, Aust.*
Capsules: Juniper (p.1625·2); ononis (p.1644·1).
Oral drops: Juniper (p.1625·2); ononis (p.1644·1);
lovage (p.1629·3).
Urinary-tract disorders.

Aponatura Erkaltungs *Terralife, Aust.*
Tilia (p.1673·2); absinthium (p.1571·1); vitamin C
(p.1389·3).
Cold and influenza symptoms.

Aponatura Galle *Terralife, Aust.*
Absinthium (p.1571·1); peppermint leaf (p.1243·2);
cnicus benedictus (p.1597·2).
Gallbladder disorders.

Aponatura Hustenlosende *Terralife, Aust.*
Althaea (p.1577·1); mallow leaf; ammonium chloride
(p.1085·2).
Coughs.

Aponatura Hustenstillende *Terralife, Aust.*
Plantago lanceolata; thyme (p.1672·2); wild thyme.
Coughs.

Aponatura Kreislauf *Terralife, Aust.*
Rosemary; maté (p.1681·3).
Circulatory disorders.

Aponatura Leber *Terralife, Aust.*
Lecithin (p.1628·1); cynara (p.1601·3); absinthium
(p.1571·1).
Liver disorders.

Aponatura Nieren- und Blasen *Terralife, Aust.*
Java tea; peppermint leaf (p.1243·2).
Kidney and bladder disorders.

Aponatura Starkungs *Terralife, Aust.*
Centaury (p.1593·1); bitter orange peel (p.1644·2); ca-
lamus root (p.1588·1).
Tonic.

Aponatura Verdauungs *Terralife, Aust.*
Capsules: Angelica (p.1580·2); absinthium (p.1571·1).
Oral drops: Angelica (p.1580·2); absinthium
(p.1571·1); lovage (p.1629·3).
Gastrointestinal disorders.

Aponatura Wind *Terralife, Aust.*
Aniseed (p.1580·2); fennel (p.1610·1); caraway
(p.1591·2).
Gastrointestinal disorders.

Apo-Nifed *Apotex, Canad.; Apotex, Singapore.*
Nifedipine (p.940·1).
Angina pectoris; hypertension.

The symbol † denotes a preparation no longer actively marketed

Aponil Glaxo Allen, Ital.
Lacidipine (p.919·1).
Hypertension.

Apo-Norflox Apotex, Canad.
Norfloxacin (p.232·1).
Urinary-tract infections.

Aponorm Curex, Israel.
Atenolol (p.841·3).
Angina pectoris; hyertension.

Apo-Oflox Apotex, Canad.
Ofloxacin (p.232·3).
Bacterial infections.

Apo-Paradex Apotex, NZ.
Paracetamol (p.71·2); dextropropoxyphene napsilate (p.27·1).
Pain.

Apo-Pen-VK Apotex, Canad.
Phenoxymethylpenicillin potassium (p.235·1).
Bacterial infections.

Apophage Curex, Israel.
Metformin hydrochloride (p.332·3).
Diabetes mellitus.

Apo-Pindol Apotex, Canad.
Pindolol (p.955·3).
Angina pectoris; hypertension.

Apopiran Protein, Mex.
Piroxicam (p.79·1).

Apoplectal Klinge, Aust.
Etofylline (p.765·1); aesculus (p.1574·1); buphenine hydrochloride (p.1587·3).
Cerebrovascular disorders.

Apoplectal N Klinge, Ger.
Aesculus (p.1574·1); buphenine hydrochloride (p.1587·3).
Formerly contained aesculus, buphenine hydrochloride, and etofylline.
Cerebrovascular disorders.

Apo-Prazo
Apotex, Canad.; Apotex, Hong Kong.
Prazosin hydrochloride (p.958·1).
Hypertension.

Apoprin Protein, Mex.
Ranitidine (p.1246·3).

Apo-Pulm Pekana, Ger.
Homoeopathic preparation.

A-Por Quatromed, S.Afr.
Clotrimazole (p.382·1).
Fungal skin infections; vulvovaginal fungal infections.

Aporex Alpharma, Norw.
Dextropropoxyphene hydrochloride (p.27·1); paracetamol (p.71·2).
Pain.

Aporil Qualiphar, Belg.
Salicylic acid (p.1122·3); acetic acid (p.1571·2); lactic acid (p.1626·2); thuja (p.1672·1); greater celandine (p.1618·1).
Warts.

Apo-Salvent
Apotex, Canad.; Apotex, Hong Kong.
Salbutamol (p.770·3) or salbutamol sulfate (p.770·3).
Obstructive airways disease.

Apo-Sulfatrim
Apotex, Canad.; Apotex, Hong Kong; Apotex, NZ; Apotex, Singapore.
Co-trimoxazole (p.193·3).
Bacterial infections; Pneumocystis carinii pneumonia.

Apo-Sulin Apotex, Canad.
Sulindac (p.85·3).
Inflammation; pain.

Apo-Tamox
Apotex, Canad.; Apotex, Hong Kong; Apotex, Singapore.
Tamoxifen citrate (p.571·1).
Anovulatory infertility; breast cancer; endometrial cancer.

Apoterfin Curex, Israel.
Terfenadine (p.588·2).
Allergic rhinitis; allergic skin disorders.

Apo-Tetra
Apotex, Canad.; Apotex, Hong Kong.
Tetracycline hydrochloride (p.258·3).
Bacterial infections.

Apotheker Bauer's Blahungstee Jauntal, Aust.
Angelica (p.1580·2); fennel (p.1610·1); chamomile (p.1593·2); coriander (p.1599·2); sage (p.1660·2).
Flatulence.

Apotheker Bauer's Brust- und Hustentee
Jauntal, Aust.
Fennel (p.1610·1); Iceland moss; cowslip flowers (p.1600·1); thyme leaf (p.1672·2); verbascum flowers.
Catarrh.

Apotheker Bauer's Franzbranntwein-Gel
Jauntal, Aust.
Brandy (p.1130·3); concentrated ammonia (p.1579·1).
Insect bites; minor injuries.

Apotheker Bauer's Grippetee Jauntal, Aust.
Cowslip rhizome (p.1600·1); pimpinella; sambucus (p.1660·3); tilia (p.1673·2); crataegus (p.1600·2).
Cold and influenza symptoms.

Apotheker Bauer's Harntreibender Tee
Jauntal, Aust.
Urtica (p.1678·2); java tea (p.1625·1); parsley root (p.1648·3); solidago virgaurea; juniper (p.1625·2).
Renal calculi.

Apotheker Bauer's Huhneraugentinktur
Jauntal, Aust.
Salicylic acid (p.1122·3); lactic acid (p.1626·2); resorcinol (p.1122·2); flexible collodion.
Corns and calluses.

Apotheker Bauer's Inhalationsmischung
Jauntal, Aust.
Eucalyptus oil (p.1609·2); juniper oil (p.1625·2); pumilio pine oil (p.1656·3).
Respiratory-tract disorders.

Apotheker Bauer's Kindertee Jauntal, Aust.
Orange flowers; fennel (p.1610·1); clove (p.1596·3); hibiscus flowers; pansy.
Gastrointestinal disorders.

Apotheker Bauer's Magentee Jauntal, Aust.
Angelica (p.1580·2); caraway (p.1591·2); mallow leaf; rosemary leaf; centaury (p.1593·1); calendula (p.1589·2).
Gastrointestinal disorders.

Apotheker Bauer's Misteltinktur Jauntal, Aust.
Mistletoe (p.1636·2).
Circulatory disorders.

Apotheker Bauer's Nieren- und Blasentee
Jauntal, Aust.
Silver birch leaves (p.1585·2); urtica (p.1678·2); java tea (p.1625·1); solidago virgaurea; bearberry (p.1583·3).
Kidney and bladder disorders.

Apo-Theo
Apotex, Canad.; Apotex, Hong Kong; Apotex, Singapore.
Theophylline (p.777·2).
Obstructive airways disease.

Apotil Curex, Israel.
Timolol maleate (p.982·1).
Glaucoma; ocular hypertension.

Apo-Timol
Apotex, Canad.; Apotex, NZ.
Timolol maleate (p.982·1).
Angina pectoris; arrhythmias; hypertension; migraine; myocardial infarction.

Apo-Timop
Apotex, Canad.; Apotex, Hong Kong.
Timolol maleate (p.982·1).
Glaucoma; ocular hypertension.

Apo-Triazide
Apotex, Canad.; Apotex, Hong Kong; Apotex, Singapore.
Hydrochlorothiazide (p.907·3); triamterene (p.986·1).
Hypertension; oedema.

Apo-Triazo Apotex, Canad.
Triazolam (p.709·3).
Insomnia.

Apo-Trihex
Apotex, Canad.; Apotex, Hong Kong; Apotex, Singapore.
Benzhexol [trihexyphenidyl] hydrochloride (p.463·3).
Drug-induced extrapyramidal disorders; parkinsonism.

Apo-Trimip
Apotex, Canad.; Apotex, Hong Kong.
Trimipramine maleate (p.311·2).
Depression.

Apotrin Ridupharm, Switz.
Betacarotene (p.1355·1); canthaxanthin (p.1027·2).
Photodermatoses; protoporphyria.

Apo-Tuss Pekana, Ger.
Homoeopathic preparation.

Apoven Douglas, Austral.
Ipratropium bromide (p.766·1).
Obstructive airways disease.

Apovent Curex, Israel.
Ipratropium bromide (p.766·1).
Obstructive airways disease.

Apo-Verap Apotex, Canad.
Verapamil hydrochloride (p.989·1).
Angina; arrhythmias; hypertension.

Apox Curex, Israel.
Alprazolam (p.654·2).
Anxiety; panic disorders.

Apozan Curex, Israel.
Ranitidine hydrochloride (p.1245·2).
Gastro-oesophageal reflux; gastrointestinal hyperacidity; peptic ulcer; zollinger Ellison syndrome.

Apozepam
Alpharma, Denm.; Dumex-Alpharma, Swed.
Diazepam (p.674·3).
Alcohol withdrawal syndrome; anxiety; insomnia; premedication; restlessness; skeletal muscle spasm.

Appedrine
Note. This name is used for preparations of different composition.
Stella, Austral.
Benzocaine (p.1306·2); ferrous fumarate (p.1360·1); carmellose sodium (p.1499·3); vitamins (p.1350·1).
Obesity.

Thompson, USA†.
Phenylpropanolamine hydrochloride (p.1098·1); multivitamins and minerals.

Appelin-B12 Pharos, Singapore.
Benzoic acid; inositol; lysine; sorbitol; vitamin B_{12}; vitamin C (p.1350·1).
Tonic.

Appetiser Mixture Potter's, UK.
Chamomile (p.1593·2); calumba (p.1589·2); compound gentian infusion (p.1615·1).
Flatulence; tonic.

Appetrol Covan, S.Afr.
Cathine hydrochloride (p.1507·1).
Obesity.

Applicaine
Note. This name is used for preparations of different composition.
Carter-Wallace, Austral.; ICN, NZ.
Oral gel: Choline salicylate (p.24·3).
Oral pain; teething.

Carter-Wallace, Austral.; ICN, NZ.
Topical liquid: Benzocaine (p.1306·2).
Mouth ulcers; oral pain; teething.

APR Cream Curacel, Austral.
Methyl salicylate (p.55·1); camphor (p.1589·3); menthol (p.1632·3); capsicum oleoresin (p.1591·1); copper sulfate (p.1358·1); eicosapentaenoic acid (p.949·3); melaleuca oil (p.1631·3); zinc sulfate (p.1398·2).
Musculoskeletal and joint disorders.

Apracur
Note. This name is used for preparations of different composition.
Schering, Aust.
Paracetamol (p.71·2); clemizole hydrochloride (p.413·3); phenylephrine hydrochloride (p.1097·1).
Cold and influenza symptoms.

Virtus, Braz.
Chlorpheniramine [chlorphenamine] maleate (p.412·1); ascorbic acid (p.1389·3); dipyrone (p.34·1).
Cold and influenza symptoms.

Apra-Gel Roche, Belg.
Naproxen (p.60·3).
Musculoskeletal, joint, and peri-articular disorders.

Apranax
Roche, Belg.; Roche, Fr.; Syntex, Ger.†; Roche, Ger.†; Roche, Switz.
Naproxen (p.60·3) or naproxen sodium (p.61·1).
Gout; inflammation; musculoskeletal, joint, and peri-articular disorders; pain.

Aprednislon Merck, Aust.
Prednisolone (p.1077·3).
Corticosteroid.

Apresazide Novartis, USA.
Hydralazine hydrochloride (p.905·3); hydrochlorothiazide (p.907·3).
Hypertension.

Apresolin
Novartis, Denm.; Novartis, Norw.; Novartis, Swed.
Hydralazine hydrochloride (p.905·3).
Heart failure; hypertension.

Apresolina Novartis, Braz.
Hydralazine hydrochloride (p.905·3).
Heart failure; hypertension.

Apresoline
Novartis, Austral.; Novartis, Canad.; Novartis, Hong Kong; Novartis, Irl.; Novartis, Neth.; Novartis, NZ; Novartis, S.Afr.; Novartis, Thai.; Sovereign, UK; Novartis, USA.
Hydralazine hydrochloride (p.905·3).
Heart failure; hypertension.

Apri Duramed, USA.
Desogestrel (p.1470·3); ethinylestradiol (p.1476·2).
28-Day packs also contain 7 inert tablets.
Combined oral contraceptive.

Aprical
Fuisz, Ger.; Rentschler, Israel.
Nifedipine (p.940·1).
Angina pectoris; hypertension; Raynaud's syndrome.

Aprinox
Knoll, Austral.; Waymade, UK.
Bendrofluazide [bendroflumethiazide] (p.844·1).
Hypertension; oedema; suppression of lactation.

Aprodine Major, USA.
Pseudoephedrine hydrochloride (p.1099·2); triprolidine hydrochloride (p.427·2).
Upper respiratory-tract symptoms.

Aprodine with Codeine Major, USA.
Pseudoephedrine hydrochloride (p.1099·2); codeine phosphate (p.25·2); triprolidine hydrochloride (p.427·2).
Coughs and cold symptoms.

Aprofen Progress, Thai.
Ibuprofen (p.43·2).
Fever; musculoskeletal and joint disorders; pain.

Aproten
Diet Erba, NZ; Ultrapharm, UK.
Low-protein, gluten-free foods for special diets (p.1350·1).

Aprovel
Sanofi Synthelabo, Belg.; Sanofi, Denm.; Sanofi Winthrop, Fin.; Bristol-Myers Squibb, Fin.; Bristol-Myers Squibb, Fr.; Sanofi Synthelabo, Ger.; Sanofi Winthrop, Hong Kong; Sanofi Winthrop, Irl.; Bristol-Myers Squibb, Irl.; Sanofi Synthelabo, Ital.; Sanofi Winthrop, Mex.; Sanofi Winthrop, Neth.; Bristol-Myers Squibb, Neth.; Sanofi Winthrop, Norw.; Bristol-Myers Squibb, Norw.; Bristol-Myers Squibb, Port.; Sanofi Winthrop, Port.; Sanofi Synthelabo, Singapore; Sanofi Synthelabo, Spain; Sanofi Winthrop, Swed.; Bristol-Myers Squibb, Swed.; Sanofi Synthelabo, Switz.; Bristol-Myers Squibb, Switz.; Sanofi Synthelabo, Thai.; Sanofi Winthrop, UK; Bristol-Myers Squibb, UK.
Irbesartan (p.914·2).
Hypertension.

APS Balneum APS, Ger.†
Chamomile oil.
Bath additive; skin disorders.

Apsifen Approved Prescription Services, UK†.
Ibuprofen (p.43·2).
Fever; inflammation; pain; rheumatoid arthritis.

Apsin VK Approved Prescription Services, UK†.
Phenoxymethylpenicillin potassium (p.235·1).
Bacterial infections.

Apsolol Approved Prescription Services, UK†.
Propranolol hydrochloride (p.962·3).
Angina pectoris; anxiety; arrhythmias; essential tremor; hypertension; hyperthyroidism; migraine; myocardial infarction.

Apsolox Approved Prescription Services, UK†.
Oxprenolol hydrochloride (p.951·3).
Angina pectoris; arrhythmias; hypertension; hypertrophic obstructive cardiomyopathy.

Apsomol Farmasan, Ger.
Salbutamol sulfate (p.770·3).
Obstructive airways disease.

Apsor
Note. This name is used for preparations of different composition.
Lipha Sante, Fr.
Tacalcitol (p.1124·2).
Psoriasis.

IDI, Ital.†
Betamethasone valero-acetate (p.1063·3); tretinoin (p.1126·2); salicylic acid (p.1122·3).
Formerly contained betamethasone valero-acetate, tretinoin, precipitated sulfur, salicylic acid, camphor, and allantoin.
Psoriasis.

Apstil Approved Prescription Services, UK†.
Diethylstilbestrol (p.1471·2).
Breast cancer; prostatic cancer.

Aptamil HA Milupa, Port.
Infant feed (p.1350·1).
Milk intolerance.

Aptamil HA 2 Milupa, Ital.
Infant feed (p.1350·1).
Cow's milk intolerance.

Aptamil HA con LCP Milupan Milupa, Ital.
Infant feed (p.1350·1).
Milk intolerance.

Aptin
Astra, Austral.†; Astra, Denm.†; Astra, Ger.; Astra, Norw.†.
Alprenolol benzoate (p.833·3) or alprenolol hydrochloride (p.833·3).
Angina pectoris; arrhythmias; heart failure; hypertension; myocardial infarction.

Aptin N Hassle, Swed.†.
Alprenolol benzoate (p.833·3).
Angina pectoris; arrhythmias; hypertension; myocardial infarction.

Aptine
Astra, Belg.†; Astra, Neth.†.
Alprenolol benzoate (p.833·3).
Angina pectoris; arrhythmias; hypertension; myocardial infarction.

Aptodin Plus GD, Ital.
Vitamin, mineral, and amino-acid preparation (p.1350·1).

Apton Delta, Port.
Pantoprazole (p.1243·1).
Gastro-oesophageal reflux; peptic ulcer.

Apurin
Fresenius Kabi, Aust.; Gea, Denm.; Gea, Fin.
Allopurinol (p.397·2) or allopurinol sodium (p.398·3).
Gout; hyperuricaemia; renal calculi.

Apurol Siegfried, Thai.
Allopurinol (p.397·2).
Gout; hyperuricaemia.

Apurone
3M, Austral.†; 3M, Fr.
Flumequine (p.207·3).
Bacterial infections of the urinary tract.

Apydan
Desitin, Denm.; Desitin, Fin.
Oxcarbazepine (p.354·1).
Epilepsy.

Apyrol Salusif, Port.
Sodium hydroxyquinoline sulfate; camphor (p.1589·3).
Muscular pain; wounds.

Aqium Active Defence Ego, Austral.†.
Barrier cream and emollient.

Aqsia Chauvin, UK.
Electrolyte solution (p.1180·1).
Eye irrigation.

Aqua Ban
Thompson, USA; Thompson, USA.
Ammonium chloride (p.1085·2); caffeine (p.761·3).
Premenstrual water retention.

Aqua Ban Plus Thompson, USA.
Ammonium chloride (p.1085·2); caffeine (p.761·3); ferrous sulfate (p.1360·3).
Premenstrual water retention.

Aqua Emoform Byk Gulden, Ital.
Sodium monofluorophosphate (p.1377·2); sodium fluoride (p.1375·3).
Gingival inflammation; oral hygiene.

Aqua Lub Probifasa, Mex.
Lubricant for vaginal and rectal use.

Aqua Soap Mex-America, Mex.
Soap substitute.

Aquabase
Westbrook, UK.
A non ionic emulsifying wax.

Paddock, USA.
Vehicle for topical preparations.

Aquacaps Muller Goppingen, Ger.†.
Java tea (p.1625·1).
Urinary-tract disorders.

Aquacare
Allergan, UK; Menley & James, USA.
Urea (p.1127·3).
Dry skin; hyperkeratosis.

Aquacare-HP *Allergan, Austral.*
Urea (p.1127·3).
Eczema; skin disorders.

Aquacel
Convatec, Fr.; Convatec, Port.
Carmellose sodium (p.1499·3).
Burns; ulcers; wounds.

Aquachloral *PolyMedica, USA.*
Cloral hydrate (p.669·3).
Sedative.

Aquacort *Spectropharm, Canad.*
Hydrocortisone (p.1073·3).
Skin disorders.

Aquaderm
Note.This name is used for preparations of different composition.
Baker Cummins, Canad.
Emollient.

Baker Cummins, Canad.
SPF 15: Octisalate (p.1518·1); avobenzone (p.1517·1);
octinoxate (p.1517·3); titanium dioxide (p.1126·1).

SPF 30: Avobenzone (p.1517·1); octocrilene
(p.1518·1); octinoxate (p.1517·3); titanium dioxide
(p.1126·1).
Sunscreen.

Baker Cummins, USA.
SPF 15: Octinoxate (p.1517·3); oxybenzone
(p.1518·1).
Sunscreen.

Aquadon *Rekah, Israel.*
Chlortalidone (p.857·1).
Hypertension; oedema.

Aquadrate
Procter & Gamble, Austral.†; Procter & Gamble, Irl.; Procter & Gam-
ble, UK.
Urea (p.1127·3).
Dry skin disorders.

Aquadrex *Parke-Med, S.Afr.†.*
Amiloride (p.835·3); hydrochlorothiazide (p.907·3).
Hypertension; oedema.

Aquae
Hamilton, Austral.; Hamilton, Hong Kong.
Carmellose sodium (p.1499·3); sorbitol (p.1377·3);
electrolytes (p.1180·1).
Artificial saliva.

Aquaear *Whitehall, Austral.*
Glacial acetic acid (p.1571·2); isopropyl alcohol
(p.1149·2).
Prevention of otitis externa.

Aquafor *Asta Medica, Ital.*
Xipamide (p.999·2).
Hypertension.

Aquaform *Scimat, UK.*
Hydrogel dressing.
Ulcers; wounds.

Aquagel *Adams, Hong Kong.*
Lubricating jelly.

Aquagen SQ
ALK, Denm.; ALK, Fin.; ALK, Swed.
Allergen extracts (p.1575·3).
Diagnosis of hypersensitivity; hyposensitisation.

Aqualan *Orion, Fin.*
Emollient.

Aqualarm *Chauvin, Fr.*
Carbomer 980 (p.1499·2).
Dry eyes.

Aqualcium *Aqualab, Fr.*
Mineral preparation (p.1350·1).
Calcium deficiency.

Aqualette *Lichtwer, UK.*
Taraxacum (p.1669·1); equisetum (p.1606·3).

Aqualibra *Medice, Ger.*
Ononis (p.1644·1); java tea (p.1625·1); solidago.
Urinary-tract disorders.

Aquamag *Aqualab, Fr.*
Mineral preparation (p.1350·1).
Magnesium deficiency.

Aquamephyton *Merck, USA†.*
Phytomenadione (p.1396·1).
Coagulation disorders associated with vitamin K defi-
ciency, due to faulty formation of factors II, VII, IX, and
X.

Aquamycetin-N *Winzer, Ger.*
Chloramphenicol (p.179·1).
Bacterial eye infections.

Aquanil
Note.This name is used for preparations of different composition.
Ciba Vision, Denm.; Ciba Vision, Fin.; Ciba Vision, Norw.; Ciba Vision,
Swed.
Timolol maleate (p.982·1).
Glaucoma; ocular hypertension.

Darier, Mex.
Sodium laurilsulfate (p.1496·3).
Skin disorders.

Person & Covey, USA.
Emollient and moisturiser.

Aquanil HC
Darier, Mex.; Person & Covey, USA.
Hydrocortisone (p.1073·3).
Skin disorders.

Aquaphilic *Medco, USA.*
Vehicle for topical preparations.

Aquaphor
Note.This name is used for preparations of different composition.
Smith & Nephew, Canad.
White soft paraffin (p.1407·3).
Dry skin; ointment base.

Lilly, Ger.
Xipamide (p.999·2).
Hypertension; oedema.

Beiersdorf, USA.
Yellow soft paraffin; liquid paraffin; mineral wax; wool
wax alcohol.
Barrier ointment; ointment base.

Aquaphor Antibiotic *Beiersdorf, USA†.*
Polymyxin B sulfate (p.238·1); bacitracin zinc
(p.155·2).

Aquaphor Healing Ointment *Beiersdorf, USA.*
Soft paraffin; liquid paraffin; ceresin; wool alcohols;
panthenol; bisabolol.
Dry skin disorders.

Aquaphoril *Asta Medica, Aust.*
Xipamide (p.999·2).
Oedema.

Aquaphyllin *Ferndale, USA.*
Theophylline (p.777·2).
Asthma; bronchospasm.

Aquapred *Winzer, Ger.*
Chloramphenicol hydrogen succinate (p.181·1); pred-
nisolone hemisuccinate (p.1078·1).
Inflammatory disorders and infections of the eye.

Aquareduct *Azupharma, Ger.*
Spironolactone (p.973·2).
Ascites; hyperaldosteronism; oedema.

Aquaretic *Azupharma, Ger.*
Amiloride hydrochloride (p.835·1); hydrochlorothi-
azide (p.907·3).
Hypertension; oedema.

Aquarhine *Monot, Fr.*
Sodium chloride (p.1196·1).

Aquarid *Alliance, S.Afr.*
Note. A similar name is used for preparations of different composition
(see below).
Frusemide [furosemide] (p.893·1).
Oedema.

Aqua-Rid *Goldline, USA†.*
Note. A similar name is used for preparations of different composition
(see above).
Buchu (p.1587·2); couch-grass (p.1599·3); corn silk
(p.1599·3); hydrangea (p.1621·1).
Premenstrual water retention.

Aquasalina *Bruschettini, Ital.*
Sodium chloride (p.1196·1); borax (p.1586·1); boric
acid (p.1586·1).
Eye and nasal irrigation.

Aquasept *SSL, UK.*
Triclosan (p.1159·2).
Skin disinfection.

Aquasite
Note.This name is used for preparations of different composition.
Ciba Vision, Canad.
Macrogol 400 (p.1630·3); dextran 70 (p.729·2).

Ciba Vision, USA.
Macrogol 400 (p.1630·3); dextran 70 (p.729·2); poly-
carbophil (p.1244·2).
Dry eyes.

Aquasol *SSL, UK.*
Purified water (p.1680·2).

Aquasol A
Note.This name is used for preparations of different composition.
Dermik, Canad.†.
Cream: Vitamin A palmitate (p.1383·2); dexpanthenol
(p.1602·3).
Skin disorders.

Rhone-Poulenc Rorer, Hong Kong; Astra, USA.
Vitamin A (p.1382·1).
Vitamin A deficiency.

Aquasol E
Novartis Consumer, Canad.; Astra, USA†.
Alpha tocoferil acetate (p.1393·3).
Vitamin supplement.

Aquasport *Also, Ital.*
Mineral preparation (p.1350·1).

Aquasteril *Orion, Fin.*
Water for injections (p.1680·2).

Aquasun *Pfizer, NZ.*
SPF 4; SPF 8; SPF 15; SPF 18; SPF 30: Octinoxate
(p.1517·3); avobenzone (p.1517·1).
Sunscreen.

Aquasun Sports *Pfizer, NZ.*
SPF 15: Octinoxate (p.1517·3); avobenzone
(p.1517·1); oxybenzone (p.1518·1); octil triazone.
Sunscreen.

Aquasun Stick *Pfizer, NZ.*
SPF 15: Octinoxate (p.1517·3); avobenzone
(p.1517·1); oxybenzone (p.1518·1); octil triazone.
Sunscreen.

Aquatab C *Adams, USA†.*
Guaifenesin (p.1092·2); phenylpropanolamine hydrochloride (p.1098·2); dextromethorphan hydrobromide
(p.1087·3).
Coughs.

Aquatab D *Adams, USA†.*
Guaifenesin (p.1092·2); phenylpropanolamine hydro-
chloride (p.1098·1).
Nasal congestion.

Aquatab DM *Adams, USA.*
Guaifenesin (p.1092·2); dextromethorphan hydrobro-
mide (p.1087·3).
Coughs.

Aquatabs
Medentech, Irl.†; Rudefsa, Mex.
Sodium dichloroisocyanurate (p.1156·1).
Water purification.

Aquatain
Whitehall, Austral.†; Whitehall-Robins, Canad.
Emollient.

AquaTar *Allergan Herbert, USA.*
Coal tar (p.1125·1).
Skin disorders.

Aquatensen *Wallace, USA.*
Methyclothiazide (p.927·3).
Hypertension; oedema.

Aquavit-E *Cypress, USA.*
dl-Alpha tocoferil acetate (p.1394·1).
Vitamin E deficiency.

Aqua-Vite Super Kelp *Bio-Health, UK.*
Multivitamins; ascophyllum nodosum (p.1350·1).

Aqucilina *Antibioticos, Spain.*
Procaine penicillin [procaine benzylpenicillin]
(p.239·2).
Bacterial infections.

Aqucilina D A *Antibioticos, Spain.*
Benzylpenicillin potassium (p.157·1); procaine peni-
cillin [procaine benzylpenicillin] (p.239·2).
Bacterial infections.

Aqudux *Sanofi Synthelabo, Port.*
Frusemide [furosemide] (p.893·1).
Hypertension; oedema.

Aqueous Charcodote *Pharmascience, Singapore.*
Activated charcoal (p.1000·2).
Emergency treatment of poisoning.

Aquest *Dunhall, USA†.*
Estrone (p.1476·1).

Aquim *Ego, NZ.*
Dimethicone (p.1410·1).
Barrier preparation.

Aquitol *Teva, Israel.*
Vitamin A palmitate (p.1383·2); ergocalciferol
(p.1391·2).
Vitamin A and D supplement.

Aquo-Cytobion *Merck, Ger.*
Hydroxocobalamin acetate (p.1388·3).
Vitamin B₁₂ deficiency.

Aquomin *Belmac, Spain.*
Ciclopirox olamine (p.382·1).
Fungal skin and nail infections.

Aquo-Trinitrosan *Merck, Ger.*
Glyceryl trinitrate (p.897·3).
Cardiovascular disorders.

Aqupla *Shionogi, Jpn.*
Nedaplatin (p.562·3).
Malignant neoplasms.

Arabine
Faulding, Denm.; Baxter, Fin.; Baxter, Swed.
Cytarabine (p.530·1).
Acute leukaemias.

Aracaf *Nakorn, Thai.*
Diphenhydramine hydrochloride (p.416·1); ammoni-
um chloride (p.1085·2); sodium citrate (p.1186·2).
Cold symptoms; cough; nasal congestion.

ARA-cell *Cell Pharm, Ger.*
Cytarabine (p.530·1).
Malignant neoplasms.

Aracytin
Pharmacia Upjohn, Braz.; Pharmacia Upjohn, Ital.
Cytarabine (p.530·1).
Leukaemias; lymphomas; myelodysplastic syndrome.

Aracytine *Pharmacia Upjohn, Fr.*
Cytarabine (p.530·1).
Leukaemias; myelodysplasia.

Aragest *Dexxon, Israel.*
Medroxyprogesterone acetate (p.1480·1).
Endometriosis; menstrual disorders.

Aralen
Sanofi Synthelabo, Canad.; Sanofi Winthrop, Israel; Sanofi Winthrop,
Mex.; Sanofi Winthrop, USA.
Chloroquine (p.432·2), chloroquine hydrochloride
(p.432·2), or chloroquine phosphate (p.432·3).
Amoebiasis; malaria.

Aralia Med Complex *Dynamit, Aust.*
Homoeopathic preparation.

Aramexe *Ratiopharm, Aust.*
Co-dergocrine mesilate (p.1597·3).
Cerebrovascular disorders; cervical syndrome; hyper-
tension; migraine; peripheral vascular disease.

Aramin *Cristalia, Braz.*
Metaraminol tartrate (p.926·3).
Hypotension.

Aramine
Merck Sharp & Dohme, Austral.; Merck Sharp & Dohme, Belg.; Mer-
ck Sharp & Dohme, Hong Kong; Merck Sharp & Dohme, Norw.; Mer-
ck Sharp & Dohme, NZ; Merck Sharp & Dohme, Thai.; Merck Sharp
& Dohme, UK; Merck, USA.
Metaraminol tartrate (p.926·3).
Hypotension; shock.

Aranesp
Amgen, Austral.; Amgen, UK; Amgen, USA.
Darbepoetin alfa (p.728·2).
Anaemia in renal failure.

Aranidorm-S *Weber & Weber, Ger.†*
Centaury (p.1593·1); chamomile (p.1593·1); passion
flower (p.1649·1); valerian (p.1678·3); lavender
(p.1627·2); lupulus (p.1629·3); melissa (p.1632·2); atropa bellad.; avena sat.; coffeinum; datura stram.;
eschscholtzia calif.; hyoscyamus nig.; lactuca vir.; papaver dub.; zincum isovalerianicum.
Hyperactivity; insomnia.

Araniforce-forte *Weber & Weber, Ger.*
Homoeopathic preparation.

Aranisan-N *Weber & Weber, Ger.†.*
Homoeopathic preparation.

Arasena-A *Mochida, Jpn†.*
Vidarabine (p.643·2).
Herpesvirus infections.

Aratac
Alphapharm, Austral.; Pacific, NZ; Alphapharm, Singapore; Merck,
Singapore; Merck, Thai.
Amiodarone hydrochloride (p.836·1).
Arrhythmias.

Arava
Hoechst Marion Roussel, Austral., Aventis, Denm.; Hoechst Marion
Roussel, Fin.; Roussel Diamant, Fr.; Hoechst Marion Roussel, Ger.;
Aventis, Irl.; Hoechst Marion Roussel, Neth.; Hoechst Marion Roussel,
Swed.; Hoechst Marion Roussel, Switz.; Aventis, UK; Hoechst Marion
Roussel, USA.
Leflunomide (p.549·3).
Rheumatoid arthritis.

Arbe-Plus *Helfarma, Port.*
Arginine hydrochloride; vitamin B substances
(p.1350·1).
Tonic.

Arbid
Kolassa, Aust.; Medichemie, Switz.
Buphenine hydrochloride (p.1587·3); diphenylpraline
hydrochloride (p.417·1).
Rhinitis; sinusitis.

Arbid N *Gepepharm, Ger.*
Diphenylpyraline hydrochloride (p.417·1).
Cold symptoms.

Arbid-top *Medichemie, Switz.*
Phenylephrine hydrochloride (p.1097·1); dequalinium
chloride (p.1143·1); muramidase hydrochloride
(p.1638·1).
Nasal congestion.

Arbralene *Berk, UK.*
Metoprolol tartrate (p.931·2).
Angina pectoris; arrhythmias; hypertension; hyperthy-
roidism; migraine; myocardial infarction.

Arbum *Jaldes, Fr.*
Lappa (p.1627·1); zinc gluconate (p.1398·2); pyridox-
ine hydrochloride (p.1386·3); biotin (p.1355·3).
Formerly contained lappa, cystine, zinc gluconate, py-
ridoxine hydrochloride, and biotin.
Seborrhoea.

Arbuz *Bittermedizin, Ger.*
Papain (p.1647·3); pancreatin (p.1646·1).
Digestive disorders.

Arca-Be *Arcana, Aust.*
Thiamine disulfide (p.1385·2); pyridoxine hydrochlo-
ride (p.1386·3); cyanocobalamin (p.1388·1).
Neuralgia; neuritis.

Arcablock *Arcana, Aust.*
Atenolol (p.841·3).
Angina pectoris; arrhythmias; hypertension; myocar-
dial infarction.

Arcablock comp *Arcana, Aust.*
Atenolol (p.841·3); chlortalidone (p.857·1).
Hypertension.

Arcadipin *Merck, Aust.†.*
Nilvadipine (p.946·1).
Hypertension.

Arca-Enzym *Arcana, Aust.*
Pancreatin (p.1646·1); cellulase (p.1593·1); ox bile
(p.1585·1); bromelains (p.1586·3).
Digestive disorders.

Arcafen *Merck, Hong Kong.*
Clomifene citrate (p.1465·3).
Anovulatory infertility.

Arcalion
Servier, Braz.; Therval, Fr.; Servier, Hong Kong; Servier, Port.; Servier,
Singapore; Servier, Spain; Servier, Switz.; Servier, Thai.
Sulbutiamine (p.1385·1).
Asthenia.

Arcana Cough Linctus *Arcana, S.Afr.*
Triprolidine hydrochloride (p.427·2); pseudoephedrine
hydrochloride (p.1099·2); codeine phosphate (p.25·2).
Coughs.

Arcana Expectorant *Arcana, S.Afr.†.*
Triprolidine hydrochloride (p.427·2); pseudoephedrine
hydrochloride (p.1099·2); codeine phosphate (p.25·2);
guaifenesin (p.1092·2).
Coughs.

Arcanacillin *Arcana, S.Afr.†.*
Amoxicillin trihydrate (p.149·2).
Bacterial infections.

Arcanacycline *Arcana, S.Afr.†.*
Tetracycline hydrochloride (p.258·3).
Bacterial infections.

Arcanacysteine *Arcana, S.Afr.†.*
Carbocisteine (p.1086·3).
Respiratory-tract disorders with increased or viscous
mucus.

Arcanadopa *Arcana, S.Afr.†.*
Methyldopa (p.927·3).
Hypertension.

Arcanafed Arcana, S.Afr.†
Triprolidine hydrochloride (p.427·2); pseudoephedrine hydrochloride (p.1099·2).
Cold and influenza symptoms.

Arcanafenac Arcana, S.Afr.†
Diclofenac sodium (p.30·3).
Gout; inflammation; musculoskeletal and joint disorders; pain.

Arcanaflex Arcana, S.Afr.†
Paracetamol (p.71·2); chlormezanone (p.660·1).
Pain with tension.

Arcanaflu Arcana, S.Afr.†
Capsules: Paracetamol (p.71·2); vitamin C (p.1389·3); phenylephrine hydrochloride (p.1097·1); chlorphenramine [chlorphenamine] maleate (p.412·1); caffeine (p.761·3).
Syrup: Paracetamol (p.71·2); phenylpropanolamine hydrochloride (p.1098·1); dextromethorphan hydrobromide (p.1087·3).
Cold and influenza symptoms.

Arcanagesic Arcana, S.Afr.†
Syrup: Paracetamol (p.71·2).
Tablets: Paracetamol (p.71·2); codeine phosphate (p.25·2).
Fever; pain.

Arcanamide Arcana, S.Afr.†
Frusemide [furosemide] (p.893·1).
Ascites; hypertension; oedema.

Arcanamycin Arcana, S.Afr.†
Erythromycin estolate (p.201·2) or erythromycin stearate (p.201·3).
Bacterial infections.

Arcanaprim Arcana, S.Afr.†
Co-trimoxazole (p.193·3).
Bacterial infections.

Arcanaretic Arcana, S.Afr.†
Amiloride hydrochloride (p.835·1); hydrochlorothiazide (p.907·3).
Hypertension; oedema.

Arcasin
Note.This name is used for preparations of different composition.
Engelhard, Ger.; Brahms, Ger.; Cimex, Switz.†
Phenoxymethylpenicillin potassium (p.235·1).
Bacterial infections.

Esteve, Spain.
Cisapride (p.1220·1).
Gastro-oesophageal reflux; gastroparesis.

Arcavit A Merck, Aust.
Vitamin A acetate (p.1383·2).
Vitamin A deficiency.

Arcavit A/E Arcana, Aust.
Vitamin A palmitate (p.1383·2); dl-alpha tocoferil acetate (p.1394·1).
Vitamin A and E deficiency.

Arcental Martin, Spain.
Ketoprofen (p.47·3).
Gout; inflammation; musculoskeletal, joint, peri-articular, and soft-tissue disorders; pain.

Arcental Topica F5 Profas, Spain.
Ketoprofen (p.47·3).
Musculoskeletal, joint, peri-articular, and soft-tissue disorders.

Arcet Econo Med, USA†
Butalbital (p.658·3); paracetamol (p.71·2); caffeine (p.761·3).

Archidex TP, Thai.
Dexamethasone phosphate (p.1067·1); neomycin (p.228·1).
Infected eye or ear disorders.

Archifen Archifar, Thai.
Ear drops: Chloramphenicol (p.179·1); lignocaine [lidocaine] hydrochloride (p.1313·2).
Bacterial ear infections.
Eye drops: Chloramphenicol (p.179·1).
Bacterial eye infections.

Architex Cooperation Pharmaceutique, Fr.
Sodium monofluorophosphate (p.1377·2); calcium carbonate (p.1215·1).
Osteoporosis.

Arclonac Condrugs, Thai.
Diclofenac sodium (p.30·3).
Musculoskeletal and joint disorders.

Arco Pain Romilo, Canad.
Aspirin (p.14·2); caffeine citrate (p.761·3).

Arcobee with C Nature's Bounty, USA.
Vitamin B substances with vitamin C (p.1350·1).

Arcoiran Alter, Spain.
Sumatriptan succinate (p.456·1).
Cluster headache; migraine.

Arcolan Galderma, Braz.
Ketoconazole (p.389·1).
Seborrhoeic dermatitis.

Arco-Lase Arco, USA.
Amylolytic enzymes (p.1579·3); proteolytic enzymes; cellulolytic enzymes (p.1593·1); lipase.
Digestion disorders.

Arco-Lase Plus Arco, USA.
Amylolytic enzymes (p.1579·3); proteolytic enzymes; cellulolytic enzymes (p.1593·1); lipase; hyoscyamine sulfate (p.469·3); atropine sulfate (p.461·1); phenobarbital (p.355·1).
Gastrointestinal disorders.

Arcosal Rosco, Denm.
Tolbutamide (p.336·3).
Diabetes mellitus.

Arcostrong Arcolab, Switz.
Vitamins; minerals; ginseng; lecithin; choline; inositol; methionine (p.1350·1).
Tonic.

Arctuvan N Klinge, Ger.
Bearberry leaves (p.1583·3).
Formerly contained methenamine, salol, and bearberry leaves.
Urinary-tract infections.

Ardey-aktiv Ardeypharm, Ger.
Ginseng (p.1615·3).
Tonic.

Ardeyceryl P Ardeypharm, Ger.
Pyritinol hydrochloride (p.1657·1).
Mental function disorders.

Ardeycholan N Ardeypharm, Ger.
Greater celandine (p.1618·1).
Smooth muscle spasm.

Ardeycordal N Ardeypharm, Ger.
Crataegus (p.1600·2); potassium aspartate (p.1195·2); magnesium aspartate (p.1190·3).
Formerly contained etheverine, crataegus, valerian, potassium aspartate, magnesium aspartate, and sparteine sulfate.
Arrhythmias.

Ardeydystin Ardeypharm, Ger.
Kava (p.1625·3).
Formerly contained valerian root, kavain, and crataegus.
Nervous disorders.

Ardeyhepan N Ardeypharm, Ger.
Silybum marianum (p.1021·3).
Liver disorders.

Ardeysedon N Ardeypharm, Ger.
Valerian root (p.1678·3); lupulus (p.1629·3).
Nervous disorders; sleep disorders.

Ardeytropin Ardeypharm, Ger.
Tryptophan (p.311·3).
Depression; sleep disorders.

Ardine
Columbia, Mex.; Antibioticos, Spain.
Amoxicillin trihydrate (p.149·2).
Bacterial infections.

Ardine Bronquial Antibioticos, Spain.
Amoxicillin trihydrate (p.149·2); bromhexine hydrochloride (p.1085·3).
Respiratory-tract infections.

Ardinex
Knoll, Fin.; Mundipharma, Swed.
Ibuprofen (p.43·2); codeine phosphate (p.25·2).
Pain.

Arduan
Organon Teknika, Ital.†; Organon, USA.
Pipecuronium bromide (p.1339·1).
Competitive neuromuscular blocker.

Aredia
Novartis, Aust.; Novartis, Austral.; Novartis, Belg.; Novartis, Braz.; Novartis, Canad.; Novartis, Denm.; Novartis, Fin.; Novartis, Fr.; Novartis, Ger.; Novartis, Hong Kong; Novartis, Irl.; Novartis, Israel; Novartis, Ital.; Novartis, Neth.; Novartis, Norw.; Novartis, NZ; Novartis, Port.; Novartis, S.Afr.; Novartis, Singapore; Novartis, Spain; Novartis, Swed.; Novartis, Switz.; Novartis, Thai.; Novartis, UK; Novartis, USA.
Disodium pamidronate (p.754·2).
Hypercalcaemia of malignancy; osteolytic lesions and bone pain in multiple myeloma and in bone metastases associated with breast cancer; Paget's disease of bone.

Arelcant Boehringer Ingelheim, Aust.
Fenoterol hydrobromide (p.765·1); ipratropium bromide (p.766·1).
Obstructive airways disease.

Arelix
Hoechst Marion Roussel, Aust.; Hoechst Marion Roussel, Braz.; Hoechst Marion Roussel, Ger.; Hoechst Marion Roussel, Irl.; Sanofi Synthelabo, S.Afr.; Hoechst Marion Roussel, Switz.; Hoechst Marion Roussel, UK†.
Piretanide (p.956·2) or piretanide sodium (p.956·2).
Forced diuresis; heart failure; hypertension; oedema; renal failure.

Arelix ACE Hoechst Marion Roussel, Ger.
Piretanide (p.956·2); ramipril (p.966·3).
Hypertension.

Arem Aspen, S.Afr.
Nitrazepam (p.695·2).
Insomnia.

Aremin Boniscontro & Gazzone, Ital.
Suleparoid (p.978·2).
Thromboembolic disorders.

Aremis Esteve, Spain.
Sertraline hydrochloride (p.308·3).
Depression; obsessive-compulsive disorder; panic attacks.

Arestal
Janssen-Cilag, Aust.; Janssen-Cilag, Fr.; Norgine, Neth.
Loperamide oxide (p.1232·1).
Diarrhoea.

Arestin OraPharma, USA.
Minocycline hydrochloride (p.224·3).
Periodontitis.

Areuma Ecobi, Ital.
Nimesulide (p.62·3).
Fever; inflammation; pain.

Areuzolin Areu, Spain.
Cefazolin sodium (p.164·3).
Bacterial infections.

Arfen
Note.This name is used for preparations of different composition.
Medochemie, Hong Kong.
Paracetamol (p.71·2).
Fever; pain.

Lisapharma, Ital.
Ibuprofen lysine (p.44·1).
Arthritic disorders; gynaecological disorders; radiculitis.

Medinfar, Port.
Ibuprofen (p.43·2).
Fever; inflammation; musculoskeletal, joint, peri-articular, and soft-tissue disorders; pain.

Arfloxina Arlex, Mex.
Ciprofloxacin (p.182·3).
Bacterial infections.

Arfonad Cambridge, UK.
Trimetaphan camsilate (p.987·2).
Now known as Trimetaphan Camsilate Ampoules.
Induction of controlled hypotension.

Argatroban® SmithKline Beecham, USA.
Argatroban (p.841·3).
Heparin-induced thrombocytopenia.

Argenpal Braun, Spain.
Silver nitrate (p.1664·2).
Skin disorders; verrucas.

Argental Liferpal, Mex.
Sulfadiazine silver (p.251·3).

Argent-Eze Lennon, S.Afr.†
Sulfadiazine silver (p.251·3).
Burns.

Argentocromo Bucca, Spain.
Merbromin (p.1150·1); silver (p.1664·1).
Gingivitis; mouth infection.

Argentofenol Bucca, Spain.
Phenol (p.1152·3); methylene blue [methylthioninium chloride] (p.1012·3); silver nitrate (p.1664·2).
Aphthous stomatitis; oral bleeding; tonsillitis.

Argentum Med Complex Dynamit, Aust.
Homoeopathic preparation.

Argesic Econo Med, USA.
Methyl salicylate (p.55·1).
Muscle, joint, and soft-tissue pain; neuralgia.

Argesic-SA Econo Med, USA.
Salsalate (p.82·2).
Fever; inflammation; pain.

Argicilline Monot, Fr.†
Gramicidin (p.213·3).
Formerly contained methocidin and cetylpyridinium chloride.
Nose and throat infections.

Argin Volchem, Ital.
Protein supplement (p.1350·1).
Arginine deficiency.

Arginotri-B
Bouchara, Fr.
Arginine hydrochloride (p.1353·3); thiamine hydrochloride; pyridoxine hydrochloride (p.1350·1).
Formerly contained arginine hydrochloride, thiamine hydrochloride, pyridoxine hydrochloride, and hydroxocobalamin.
Tonic.

Bouchara, Switz.
Arginine hydrochloride (p.1353·3); vitamin B substances (p.1350·1).
Pain; vitamin B deficiency.

Argirofedrina Vaillant, Ital.
Ephedrine sulfate (p.1090·2); anhydrous sodium sulfate (p.1250·1); mild silver protein (p.1664·2).
Nasal congestion.

Argirol Allergan-Frumtost, Braz.
Mild silver protein (p.1664·2).
Eye infections.

Argisone Teofarma, Ital.
Hydrocortisone acetate (p.1073·3); mild silver protein (p.1664·2).
Bacterial eye infections.

Argobase Westbrook, UK.
A range of emulsifying product bases.

Argotone Lipha, Ital.
Ephedrine hydrochloride (p.1090·1); mild silver protein (p.1664·2).
Nasal congestion.

Argun Merckle, Ger.
Lonazolac calcium (p.50·2).
Inflammation; musculoskeletal, joint, and soft-tissue disorders; pain.

Argyrophedrine
Note.This name is used for preparations of different composition.
Merck-Belgolabo, Belg.
Ephedrine levulinate (p.1090·1); mild silver protein (p.1664·2).
Respiratory-tract congestion.

Synthelabo, Braz.
Ephedrine sulfate (p.1090·2); mild silver protein (p.1664·2); sodium sulfate (p.1250·1).
Nasal congestion.

Lipha Sante, Fr.†
Ephedrine levulinate (p.1090·1); mild silver protein (p.1664·2); sodium levulinate; calcium levulinate (p.1188·3).
Nasal congestion.

Arhemapectine Antihemorragique Aerocid, Fr.
Pectin (p.1502·3).
Haemorrhage.

Aria Lichtwer, UK.
Soya isoflavones; calcium; folic acid; B vitamins; selenium (p.1350·1).
Nutritional supplement.

Arial Dompe, Ital.
Salmeterol xinafoate (p.773·3).
Obstructive airways disease.

Aricept
Pfizer, Aust.; Pfizer, Austral.; Pfizer, Belg.; Pfizer, Canad.; Pfizer, Denm.; Pfizer, Fin.; Eisai, Fr.; Eisai, Ger.; Pfizer, Ger.; Eisai, Hong Kong; Pfizer, Irl.; Pfizer, Israel; Roerig, Ital.; Pfizer, Norw.; Douglas, NZ; Pfizer, Port.; Pfizer, S.Afr.; Eisai, Singapore; Pfizer Consumer, Spain; Pfizer, Swed.; Pfizer, Switz.; Eisai, Thai.; Eisai, UK; Eisai, USA; Pfizer, USA.
Donepezil hydrochloride (p.1417·2).
Alzheimer's disease.

Aricodil Menarini, Ital.
Dextromethorphan hydrobromide (p.1087·3).
Coughs.

Aridil CP Pharmaceuticals, UK.
Frusemide [furosemide] (p.893·1); amiloride hydrochloride (p.835·1).
These ingredients can be described by the British Approved Name Co-amilofruse.
Ascites; oedema.

Arilin
Wolff, Ger.; Cimex, Switz.
Metronidazole (p.594·1).
Amoebiasis; anaerobic bacterial infections; trichomoniasis.

Ariline Montavit, Aust.†
Metronidazole (p.594·1).
Anaerobic bacterial infections; protozoal infections.

Arilvax
Medeva, Irl.; Evans Medical, Israel; Evans, Neth.; Medpro, S.Afr.; Medeva, Singapore; SBL, Swed.; Medeva, Switz.; Evans, UK.
A yellow fever vaccine (17D strain) (p.1568·3).
Active immunisation.

Arima Alphapharm, Austral.
Moclobemide (p.299·3).
Depression.

Arimidex
Zeneca, Aust.; AstraZeneca, Austral.; Zeneca, Belg.; AstraZeneca, Canad.; AstraZeneca, Denm.; AstraZeneca, Fin.; AstraZeneca, Fr.; Zeneca, Ger.; Zeneca, Hong Kong; Zeneca, Irl.; Zeneca, Israel; Zeneca, Ital.; Zeneca, Mex.; Zeneca, Port.; Zeneca, S.Afr.; AstraZeneca, Singapore; Zeneca, Spain; Zeneca, Swed.; Zeneca, Switz.; AstraZeneca, Thai.; AstraZeneca, UK; AstraZeneca, USA.
Anastrozole (p.508·1).
Breast cancer.

Aristo Steiner, Ger.
Hypericum (p.290·2).
Depression; nervous disorders.

Aristo L Steiner, Ger.†
Aloes (p.1210·1).
Constipation.

Aristochol
Note.This name is used for preparations of different composition.
Linobion, Aust.
Greater celandine (p.1618·1); curcuma zanthorrhiza; silybum marianum (p.1021·3); aloes (p.1210·1); pancreatin (p.1646·1).

Steiner, Ger.
Greater celandine (p.1618·1); cape aloe (p.1210·1).
Constipation.

Aristochol CC Steiner, Ger.
Greater celandine (p.1618·1); turmeric (p.1029·3).
Gastrointestinal spasm.

Aristochol N Steiner, Ger.
Greater celandine (p.1618·1); achillea (p.1572·2); taraxacum (p.1669·1); gnaphalii flowers; absinthium (p.1571·1).
Biliary disorders.

Aristocomb Lederle, Austral.†
Triamcinolone acetonide (p.1080·1); neomycin sulfate (p.228·1); gramicidin (p.213·3); nystatin (p.392·2).
Infected skin disorders.

Aristocor Kiwizda, Aust.
Flecainide acetate (p.890·1).
Arrhythmias.

Aristocort
Lederle, Austral.; Stiefel, Canad.; Lederle, Hong Kong; Wyeth, NZ; Wyeth-Ayerst, Thai.; Fujisawa, USA.
Triamcinolone (p.1080·1), triamcinolone acetonide (p.1080·1), or triamcinolone diacetate (p.1080·2).
Corticosteroid.

Aristoforat Steiner, Ger.
Hypericum (p.290·2).
Depression; nervous disorders.

Aristospan
Stiefel, Canad.; Fujisawa, USA.
Triamcinolone hexacetonide (p.1080·2).
Corticosteroid.

Aritmina Solvay, Ital.†
Ajmaline (p.833·1).
Arrhythmias.

Ariven Beiersdorf-Lilly, Ger.†
Heparin sodium (p.902·1).
Skin trauma.

Arkin-Z Otsuka, Jpn†.
Vesnarinone (p.992·2).
Heart failure.

Arkocapsulas Carbon Veg Arkochim, Spain.
Activated charcoal (p.1000·2).
Diarrhoea.

Arkocapsulas Hiperico *Arkochim, Spain.*
Hypericum (p.290·2).
Tonic.

Arkogelules *Arkopharma, Fr.*
A range of herbal preparations.

Arkonsol *Romilo, Canad.*
Benzalkonium chloride (p.1133·2).

Arkonutril MM *Arkopharma, Fr.†*
Preparation for enteral nutrition (p.1350·1).

Arkophytum *Arkopharma, Fr.*
Devil's claw root (p.26·3); black currant (p.1389·3); salix (p.82·1).
Painful joint disorders.

Arkotonic *Arkopharma, Fr.†*
Pollen; carnitine (p.1356·1); vitamin E (p.1393·3); ascorbic acid (p.1389·3); royal jelly (p.1659·3); soya lecithin (p.1628·1).
Tonic.

Arkovital *Arkopharma, Fr.†*
A range of vitamin, mineral, and trace element supplements (p.1350·1).

Arkovital C *Arkopharma, Fr.†*
Ascorbic acid (p.1389·3).
Cold symptoms; tonic; vitamin C deficiency.

Arlevert *Hennig, Ger.*
Cinnarizine (p.413·1); dimenhydrinate (p.415·2).
Vertigo.

Arlexicam *Arlex, Mex.*
Piroxicam (p.79·1).

Arlidin
Rhone-Poulenc Rorer, Canad.; Grossman, Mex.
Buphenine hydrochloride (p.1587·3).
Organic mental disorders; peripheral vascular disorders.

Arlitene *Asta Medica, Ital.†*
Thymoxamine [moxisylyte] hydrochloride (p.980·2).
Cardiovascular disorders.

ARM *Ascher, USA†.*
Phenylpropanolamine hydrochloride (p.1098·1); chlorpheniramine [chlorphenamine] maleate (p.412·1).
Upper respiratory-tract symptoms.

Armaya *Centrum, Spain.*
Polypodium leucotomos.
Eczema; psoriasis.

Armil *Squibb, Spain.*
Benzalkonium chloride (p.1133·2).
Skin and mucous membrane disinfection.

Arminol *Krewel, Ger.*
Sulpiride (p.706·1).
Depression; schizophrenia; vestibular disorders.

Armocur *Agis, Israel.*
Cyproterone acetate (p.1467·3).
Prostatic cancer; sexual disorders.

Armoglobulina *Centeon, Braz.*
A normal immunoglobulin (p.1551·3).
Hypogammaglobulinaemia; idiopathic thrombocytopenic purpura; passive immunisation.

Armonil *Recordati, Ital.*
Estradiol (p.1473·1).
Menopausal disorders; osteoporosis.

Arnica comp *DHU, Ger.*
Homoeopathic preparation.

Arnica comp/Apis Salbe *Weleda, Ger.*
Homoeopathic preparation.

Arnica Kneipp Salbe *Kneipp, Ger.*
Arnica oil (p.1581·3); heparin (p.902·1).
Peripheral vascular disorders; skin trauma.

Arnica Komplex *Richter, Aust.*
Homoeopathic preparation.

Arnica Med Complex *Dynamit, Aust.*
Homoeopathic preparation.

Arnica Oligoplex *Madaus, Ger.*
Homoeopathic preparation.

Arnica Plus *Homeocan, Canad.*
Homoeopathic preparation.

Arnicadol *Phytomedica, Fr.*
Arnica (p.1581·3); menthol (p.1632·3).
Soft-tissue injury.

Arnicaid *Hylands, Canad.*
Homoeopathic preparation.

Arnicalm *Boiron, Canad.*
Homoeopathic preparation.

Arnica-loges *Loges, Ger.*
Arnica (p.1581·3).
Boils; insect bites; musculoskeletal, joint, and soft-tissue disorders; superficial phlebitis.

Arnican *Cooperation Pharmaceutique, Fr.*
Arnica (p.1581·3).
Soft-tissue disorders.

Arnicet *Metochem, Aust.*
Arnica (p.1581·3); hamamelis (p.1618·3).
Muscle pain; skin irritation; soft-tissue disorders.

Arnicon *Pan Quimica, Spain.*
Arnica (p.1581·3); methyl salicylate (p.55·1); menthol (p.1632·3).
Musculoskeletal and joint pain.

Arniflor *VSM, Neth.†*
Arnica (p.1581·3).
Bruising; haematoma; muscle pain; sprain.

Arniflor-N *Spitzner, Ger.; Schwabe, Ger.*
Arnica (p.1581·3).
Boils; insect bites; musculoskeletal and joint disorders; superficial phlebitis; wounds.

Arnigel *Boiron, Port.*
Arnica (p.1581·3).
Muscle pain; soft-tissue injuries.

Arnika plus *Ratiopharm, Ger.†*
Arnica (p.1581·3); heparin sodium (p.902·1); aesculus (p.1574·1).
Soft-tissue injury; venous disorders.

Arnikamill *Biomo, Ger.*
Chamomile (p.1593·2); arnica flowers (p.1581·3).
Haemorrhoids; skin disorders; soft-tissue inflammation; wounds.

Arnikatinktur *Hetterich, Ger.*
Arnica (p.1581·3).
Inflammation; musculoskeletal, joint, and soft-tissue disorders.

Arnilose *AJC, Fr.†*
Arginine hydrochloride (p.1353·3); ornithine hydrochloride (p.1374·1); sorbitol (p.1377·3); fructose (p.1363·3).
Dyspepsia.

Arobon
Sanova, Aust.; Nestle, Ital.; Nestle, Norw.; Nestle, UK†.
Ceratonia (p.1500·3).
Diarrhoea.

Arocin *Modern Health Products, UK.*
Betacarotene (p.1355·1).

Arola Rosebalm *Pharmaceutical Enterprises, S.Afr.*
Bismuth subnitrate (p.1213·2); dimethicone (p.1410·1); allantoin (p.1110·1); zinc oxide (p.1128·2).
Skin disorders.

Arolac *IPRAD, Fr.*
Lisuride maleate (p.1174·1).
Hyperprolactinaemia; lactation inhibition.

Aromabyl *Plantes et Medecines, Fr.†*
Cynara (p.1601·3); lappa (p.1627·1); cascara (p.1216·1); juglans regia; sodium salicylate (p.84·2); sodium arsenate (p.1665·1); boldo (p.1585·3).
Constipation; dyspepsia.

Aromalgyl *Plantes et Medecines, Fr.†*
Maize (p.1599·3); methenamine (p.223·1); fleabane; java tea (p.1625·1); ash.
Rheumatism.

Aromasin
Pharmacia Upjohn, Austral.; Pharmacia Upjohn, Denm.; Pharmacia Upjohn, Fin.; Pharmacia Upjohn, Ger.; Pharmacia Upjohn, Irl.; Pharmacia Upjohn, Ital.; Pharmacia Upjohn, Neth.; Pharmacia Upjohn, Port.; Pharmacia Upjohn, Swed.; Pharmacia, UK; Pharmacia Upjohn, USA.
Exemestane (p.539·1).
Breast cancer.

Aromasol *Dolisos, Fr.*
Clove oil (p.1597·1); peppermint oil (p.1243·3); pine oil; lavender oil (p.1627·2); cinnamon oil (p.1596·1); rosemary oil (p.1659·3); wild thyme oil.
Respiratory-tract congestion.

Aronal Forte *Teva, Israel.*
Vitamin A (p.1382·1); guaiazulene (p.1618·3); aluminium lactate (p.1578·2); aldioxa (p.1109·3).
Sensitive gums; toothpaste.

Aropax
SmithKline Beecham, Austral.; SmithKline Beecham, Belg.; SmithKline Beecham, Braz.; Novartis, Mex.; SmithKline Beecham, NZ; SmithKline Beecham, S.Afr.
Paroxetine hydrochloride (p.302·3).
Depression; obsessive-compulsive disorder; panic disorder; social phobias.

Arovit
Roche, Braz.; Bio-Sante, Canad.; Roche, Fr.; Roche, Ital.; Roche, S.Afr.; Roche, Swed.; Roche, Switz.
Vitamin A (p.1382·1), vitamin A acetate (p.1383·2), or vitamin A palmitate (p.1383·2).
Keratinisation disorders; vitamin A deficiency.

Aroxin
DHA, Hong Kong; DHA, Singapore.
Amoxicillin trihydrate (p.149·2).
Bacterial infections.

Arpamyl LP *GNR, Fr.*
Verapamil hydrochloride (p.989·1).
Hypertension.

Arpha *Urgo, Fr.†*
Paracetamol (p.71·2); chlorpheniramine [chlorphenamine] maleate (p.412·1).
Cold symptoms.

Arpha Hustensirup *Fournier, Ger.*
Dextromethorphan hydrobromide (p.1087·3).
Coughs.

Arphos *Fournier, Fr.*
Calcium glycerophosphate; magnesium gluconate (p.1350·1).
Formerly contained cyanocobalamin, phosphoric acid, and calcium gluceptate.
Tonic.

Arpicolin *Rosemont, UK.*
Procyclidine hydrochloride (p.473·1).
Drug-induced extrapyramidal disorders; parkinsonism.

Arpilon
Enzypharm, Aust.; Organon Teknika, Neth.†
Pipecuronium bromide (p.1339·1).
Competitive neuromuscular blocker.

Arpimycin *Rosemont, UK.*
Erythromycin ethyl succinate (p.201·2).
Bacterial infections.

Arrestin *Vortech, USA†.*
Trimethobenzamide hydrochloride (p.426·3).
Nausea and vomiting.

Arret
Janssen-Cilag, Irl.; Johnson & Johnson MSD Consumer, UK.
Loperamide hydrochloride (p.1231·3).
Diarrhoea.

Arretin *ICN, Mex.*
Tretinoin (p.1126·2).
Acne.

Arritlan *QIF, Braz.*
Endralazine mesilate (p.885·1).
Hypertension.

Arsacol *Zambon, Fr.†*
Ursodeoxycholic acid (p.1677·2).
Gallstones.

Arscolloid *SIT, Ital.*
Dichlorobenzyl alcohol (p.1143·2); silver protein (p.1664·2).
Oral disinfection.

Arsiquinoforme *Synthelabo, Fr.†*
Quinine acetarsolate (p.447·1); quinine formate (p.447·1).
Malaria.

Arsobal *Rhone-Poulenc Rorer, S.Afr.†*
Melarsoprol (p.593·1).
African trypanosomiasis.

Art *Negma, Fr.; NSID, Israel.*
Diacerein (p.28·3).
Osteoarthritis.

Artagen *Ranbaxy, Thai.*
Naproxen (p.60·3).
Dysmenorrhoea; gout; musculoskeletal, joint, and soft-tissue disorders.

Artal *Leiras, Fin.*
Oxpentifylline [pentoxifylline] (p.950·3).
Peripheral and cerebral vascular disorders; vascular eye disorders.

Artamin
Biochemie, Aust.†; Biochemie, Singapore.
Penicillamine (p.1017·1).
Benign hyperglobulinaemic purpura; chronic active hepatitis; cystinosis; cystinuria; heavy metal poisoning; primary biliary cirrhosis; rheumatoid arthritis; scleroderma; Wilson's disease.

Artandyl *Synco, Hong Kong.*
Benzhexol [trihexyphenidyl] hydrochloride (p.463·3).
Drug-induced extrapyramidal disorders; parkinsonism.

Artane
Wyeth Lederle, Aust.; Lederle, Austral.; Wyeth Lederle, Belg.; Wyeth, Braz.; Wyeth-Ayerst, Canad.†; Lederle, Fin.; Rhone-Poulenc Rorer, Fr.; Lederle, Ger.; Lederle, Hong Kong; Lederle, Irl.; Lederle, Israel; Wyeth Lederle, Ital.; Wyeth, Mex.; Lederle, Neth.; Wyeth Lederle, Port.; Wyeth, S.Afr.; Cyanamid, Spain; Lederle, Switz.; Wyeth-Ayerst, Thai.; Wyeth, UK†; Lederle, USA†.
Benzhexol [trihexyphenidyl] hydrochloride (p.463·3).
Drug-induced extrapyramidal disorders; parkinsonism.

Artaxan *Malesci, Ital.*
Nabumetone (p.59·3).
Musculoskeletal, joint, peri-articular, and soft-tissue disorders.

Arte Rautin forte S *Maurer, Ger.*
Rauwolfia serpentina (p.967·2).
Formerly contained rauwolfia serpentina, olive leaf, crataegus, mistletoe, juniper, valerian, rutoside, and etofylline.
Anxiety disorders; hypertension.

Artedin *GD, Ital.*
Garlic; ginkgo biloba; vitamin C; vitamin E (p.1350·1).

Artelac
Riel, Aust.; Tramedico, Belg.; Santen, Fin.; Mann, Ger.; Mann, Irl.; Santen, Swed.; Nucare, UK.
Hypromellose (p.1501·3).
Dry eyes.

Arteolol *Lacer, Spain.*
Carteolol hydrochloride (p.855·1).
Angina pectoris; arrhythmias; hypertension.

Arteoptic
Ciba Vision, Denm.; Ciba Vision, Fin.; Ciba Vision, Ger.; Otsuka, Hong Kong; OM, Port.; Ciba Vision, Swed.; Chauvin Novopharma, Switz.; Otsuka, Thai.
Carteolol hydrochloride (p.855·1).
Glaucoma; ocular hypertension.

Arterase *Clement, Fr.*
Equisetum (p.1606·3); garlic (p.1614·1); cupressus sempervirens; aesculus (p.1574·1).
Formerly contained equisetum, garlic, cupressus sempervirens, aesculus, mistletoe, magnesium thiosulfate, and sodium citrate.
Capillary fragility; venous insufficiency.

Arterenol *Hoechst Marion Roussel, Ger.*
Noradrenaline [norepinephrine] hydrochloride (p.948·2).
Hypotension.

Artergin *Orion, Fin.*
Co-dergocrine mesilate (p.1597·3).
Mental function disorders in the elderly.

Arteria-cyl Ho-Len-Complex *Liebermann, Ger.*
Homoeopathic preparation.

Arteriobrate *Farma Lepori, Spain†.*
Aluminium clofibrate (p.859·1); vincamine (p.1680·1).
Exudative diabetic retinopathy; hyperlipidaemias.

Arterioflexin *Lannacher, Aust.*
Clofibrate (p.859·1).
Hyperlipidaemias.

Arteriovinca *Lepori, Port.; Farma Lepori, Spain.*
Vincamine (p.1680·1) or vincamine hydrochloride (p.1680·1).
Cerebral trauma; cerebrovascular disorders; circulatory disorders of the eye, ear, nose, and throat; vestibular disorders.

Arterium *Llorens, Spain†.*
Nicofibrate hydrochloride (p.939·2).
Hyperlipidaemias.

Arterodiet *Yves Ponroy, Fr.*
Fish oil (p.1350·1).
Nutritional supplement.

Arterosan Plus *Mavena, Switz.*
Crataegus (p.1600·2); melissa (p.1632·2); garlic oil; ginkgo biloba (p.1615·2).
Cerebrovascular disorders.

Arte-Rutin C *Maurer, Ger.*
Crataegus (p.1600·2).
Formerly contained rutoside, crataegus, olive leaf, valerian, lupulus, and mistletoe.
Heart failure.

Arteven *Boehringer Ingelheim, Ital.*
Suleparoid (p.978·2).
Thrombosis prophylaxis.

Artex
Servier, Belg.†; Therval, Fr.; Servier, Neth.; Servier, Port.
Tertatolol hydrochloride (p.980·2).
Hypertension.

Artexal
Servier, Denm.; Servier, Irl.
Tertatolol hydrochloride (p.980·2).
Hypertension.

Arth-A Oligocan *Homeocan, Canad.*
Homoeopathic preparation.

Artha-G *Williams, USA.*
Salsalate (p.82·2).
Fever; inflammation; pain.

Arthaxan *SmithKline Beecham, Ger.†*
Nabumetone (p.59·3).
Musculoskeletal and joint disorders.

Arth-B Oligocan *Homeocan, Canad.*
Homoeopathic preparation.

Arthotec *Heumann, Ger.; Hoechst Marion Roussel, Ger.*
Diclofenac sodium (p.30·3).
Misoprostol (p.1446·1) is included in this preparation in an attempt to limit adverse effects on the gastrointestinal mucosa.
Musculoskeletal and joint disorders.

Arthrabas *Tosse, Ger.†*
Chloroquine phosphate (p.432·3).
Arthritis; lupus erythematosus.

Arthrex *BASF, Ger.*
Diclofenac sodium (p.30·3).
Gout; inflammation; musculoskeletal, joint, and soft-tissue disorders; pain.

Arthrex Duo *BASF, Ger.*
Diclofenac sodium (p.30·3).
Gout; inflammation; musculoskeletal, joint, and soft-tissue disorders; pain.

Arthrexin
Alphapharm, Austral.; Pacific, NZ; Aspen, S.Afr.
Indometacin (p.44·3).
Gout; inflammation; musculoskeletal, joint, peri-articular, and soft-tissue disorders; pain.

Arthribosan B 31 *Bock, Ger.†*
Homoeopathic preparation.

Arthricare Double Ice *Del, USA; Commerce, USA.*
Menthol (p.1632·3); camphor (p.1589·3).
Muscle and joint pain.

Arthricare Odor Free
Del, Canad.; Del, USA; Commerce, USA.
Menthol (p.1632·3); methyl nicotinate (p.55·1); capsaicin (p.23·1).
Muscle and joint pain.

Arthricare Triple Medicated
Del, Canad.; Del, USA; Commerce, USA.
Methyl salicylate (p.55·1); menthol (p.1632·3); methyl nicotinate (p.55·1).
Muscle and joint pain.

Arthricare Ultra *Del, Canad.*
Menthol (p.1632·3); capsaicin (p.23·1).

Arthrifid S *Fides, Ger.†*
Homoeopathic preparation.

Arthriforte *Blackmores, Austral.*
Fish oil (p.949·3); eicosatetraenoic acid (p.949·3); vitamin A (p.1382·1); turmeric (p.1029·3); devil's claw root (p.26·3); celery seed oil; vitamin E (p.1393·3).
Arthritis; inflammation; rheumatism.

Arthrirub *Slimax, Austral.*
Camphor (p.1589·3); eucalyptus (p.1609·2); methyl salicylate (p.55·1); menthol (p.1632·3); alisma plantago aquatica oil.
Cold symptoms; hay fever; headache; musculoskeletal and joint disorders.

Arthrisan *Planta, Canad.†*
Capsules: Salix (p.82·1); juniper (p.1625·2).
Oral drops: Salix (p.82·1); juniper (p.1625·2); solidago canadensis.
Arthritis.

Arthritic Pain *Homeocan, Canad.*
Homoeopathic preparation.

Arthritic Pain Herbal Formula I *Vitelle, Austral.*
Celery (p.1592·3); juniper (p.1625·2); devil's claw root (p.26·3); salix alba (p.82·1).
Arthritis; rheumatism.

The symbol † denotes a preparation no longer actively marketed

Arthritic Pain L10 *Homeocan, Canad.*
Homoeopathic preparation.

Arthritic Pain Relief *Mentholatum, Canad.*
Capsaicin (p.23·1).

Arthritis Foundation Ibuprofen *McNeil Consumer, USA†.*
Ibuprofen (p.43·2).
Fever; osteoarthritis; pain; rheumatoid arthritis.

Arthritis Foundation Nighttime *McNeil Consumer, USA†.*
Paracetamol (p.71·2); diphenhydramine hydrochloride (p.416·1).
Insomnia associated with pain.

Arthritis Foundation Pain Reliever *McNeil Consumer, USA†.*
Aspirin (p.14·2).
Fever; musculoskeletal and joint disorders; myocardial infarction; pain; transient ischaemic attacks.

Arthritis Foundation Pain Reliever, Aspirin Free *McNeil Consumer, USA†.*
Paracetamol (p.71·2).
Fever; musculoskeletal and joint disorders; pain.

Arthritis Hot Creme *Thompson, USA.*
Methyl salicylate (p.55·1); menthol (p.1632·3).
Muscle, joint, and soft-tissue pain; neuralgia.

Arthritis Pain Formula *Whitehall, USA.*
Aspirin (p.14·2).
Aluminium hydroxide (p.1210·3) and magnesium hydroxide (p.1233·1) are included in this preparation in an attempt to limit adverse effects on the gastrointestinal mucosa.
Arthritis; fever; pain.

Arthritis Pain Formula Aspirin Free *Whitehall, USA.*
Paracetamol (p.71·2).
Fever; pain.

Arthritis Pain Tablets *Invamed, USA†.*
Aspirin (p.14·2).
Calcium carbonate (p.1215·1), magnesium carbonate (p.1232·3), and magnesium oxide (p.1233·2) are included in this preparation in an attempt to limit adverse effects on the gastrointestinal mucosa.

Arthritis Relief *Brauer, Austral.*
Homoeopathic preparation.

Arthrixyl N *Syxyl, Ger.*
Homoeopathic preparation.

arthro akut *Byk Tosse, Ger.; Byk Gulden, Ger.*
Lonazolac calcium (p.50·2).
Inflammation; musculoskeletal and joint disorders; pain.

Arthrocine *Merck Sharp & Dohme-Chibret, Fr.*
Sulindac (p.85·3).
Musculoskeletal, joint, and peri-articular disorders.

Arthrodeformat P *Ziethen, Ger.*
Pituitary extract (p.1080·1); rosemary oil (p.1659·3).
Rheumatic disorders.

Arthrodestal N *Krugmann, Ger.*
Glycol salicylate (p.42·2); camphor (p.1589·3); benzyl nicotinate (p.20·2).
Nerve, joint, and muscle pain.

Arthrodont *Veyron-Froment, Fr.*
Enoxolone (p.34·3).
Gum disorders.

Arthrodynat N *Ziethen, Ger.*
Urtica (p.1678·2).
Rheumatic disorders.

Arthrodynat P *Ziethen, Ger.*
Rosemary oil (p.1659·3); camphor (p.1589·3); hypericum oil (p.290·3).
Rheumatic disorders.

Arthrofen *Ashbourne, UK.*
Ibuprofen (p.43·2).
Inflammation; musculoskeletal and joint disorders; pain.

Arthrokehlan A *Sanum-Kehlbeck, Ger.*
Formoltoxoid from *Corynebacterium parvum* (p.527·2).
Musculoskeletal and joint disorders.

Arthrokehlan U *Sanum-Kehlbeck, Ger.*
Formol toxoid from Corynebacterium spp.
Tonic.

Arthropan *Purdue Frederick, USA.*
Choline salicylate (p.24·3).
Fever; inflammation; pain.

Arthropas K *Pascoe, Ger.*
Homoeopathic preparation.

Arthrorell *Sanorell, Ger.*
Homoeopathic preparation.

Arthrose-Echtroplex *Weber & Weber, Ger.*
Homoeopathic preparation.

Arthrose-Gastreu R73 *Reckeweg, Ger.*
Homoeopathic preparation.

Arthrosenex AR *Brenner-Efeka, Ger.; LAW, Ger.; Hotz, Ger.*
Arnica (p.1581·3).
Muscular and joint disorders.

Arthrosetten H *Hotz, Ger.*
Devil's claw root (p.26·3).
Musculoskeletal and joint disorders.

Arthrosin *Ashbourne, UK.*
Naproxen (p.60·3).
Dysmenorrhoea; gout; musculoskeletal and joint disorders.

Arthrotabs *Duopharm, Ger.*
Devil's claw root (p.26·3).
Musculoskeletal and joint disorders.

Arthrotec
Sanova, Aust.; Searle, Austral.; Searle, Canad.; Searle, Denm.; Searle, Fin.; Searle, Hong Kong; Searle, Irl.; Searle, Israel; Searle, Neth.; Searle, Norw.; Monsanto, Port.; Searle, S.Afr.; Searle, Singapore; Searle, Swed.; Searle, Switz.; Searle, Thai.; Pharmacia, UK; Searle, USA.
Diclofenac sodium (p.30·3).
Misoprostol (p.1446·1) is included in this preparation in an attempt to limit adverse effects on the gastrointestinal mucosa.
Osteoarthritis; rheumatoid arthritis.

Arthrotone *Pharmadass, UK.*
Devil's claw root (p.26·3); royal jelly (p.1659·3).

Arthroxen *CP Pharmaceuticals, UK.*
Naproxen (p.60·3).
Musculoskeletal and joint disorders.

Arthrum H *LCA, Fr.*
Sodium hyaluronate (p.1620·1).
Joint disorders.

Arthryl *Rottapharm, Fin.*
Glucosamine sulfate.
Musculoskeletal and joint disorders.

Articolase *SIRC, Singapore.*
Collagen (p.1598·2).
Peri-articular disorders.

Articulan *Tecnimede, Port.*
Etodolac (p.35·2).
Musculoskeletal and joint disorders.

Articulen *Rolab, S.Afr.*
Indometacin (p.44·3).
Now known as Rolab-Indometacin.
Dysmenorrhoea; gout; musculoskeletal and joint disorders.

Articulose-50 *Seatrace, USA†.*
Prednisolone acetate (p.1078·1).
Corticosteroid.

Articulose LA *Seatrace, USA†.*
Triamcinolone diacetate (p.1080·2).
Corticosteroid.

Articurell *Sanorell, Ger.*
Homoeopathic preparation.

Artificial Tears
Note.This name is used for preparations of different composition.
Rivex, Canad.
Polyvinyl alcohol (p.1503·1).
Dry eyes.

Bausch & Lomb, USA.
Hypromellose (p.1501·3).
Dry eyes.

Artiflam *Tramedico, Belg.*
Tiaprofenic acid (p.88·1) or tiaprofenic acid, trometamol salt (p.88·2).
Inflammation.

Artin *Sanova, Aust.*
Aloes (p.1210·1); frangula bark (p.1227·1).
Constipation; stool softener.

Artinor *ICN, Mex.*
Piroxicam (p.79·1).
Gout; inflammation; musculoskeletal, joint, peri-articular, and soft-tissue disorders; pain.

Artischocke plus Legastol *Twardy, Ger.*
Peppermint leaf (p.1243·2); cynara (p.1601·3); taraxacum (p.1669·1).
Biliary disorders.

Artisial
Note.This name is used for preparations of different composition.
Jouveinal, Canad.†.
Electrolyte preparation (p.1180·1).
Saliva substitute.

Parke, Davis, Fr.; Cell Pharm, Ger.†.
Electrolytes (p.1180·1); carmellose sodium (p.1499·3); sorbitol (p.1377·3).
Saliva substitute.

Artistry *Amway, Canad.*
SPF 8; SPF 15: Octinoxate (p.1517·3); oxybenzone (p.1518·1).
Sunscreen.

Artocoron *Knoll, Ger.*
Naftidrofuryl oxalate (p.937·3).
Peripheral vascular disorders.

Artofen *Biogal, Israel.*
Ibuprofen (p.43·2).
Musculoskeletal and joint disorders; pain.

Artoid *Artu, Neth.*
Pollen extracts (p.1575·3).
Hyposensitisation.

Artonil *Gea, Swed.*
Ranitidine hydrochloride (p.1245·2).
Gastro-oesophageal reflux; peptic ulcer; Zollinger-Ellison syndrome.

Artosin
Boehringer Mannheim, Ger.†; Boehringer Mannheim, Neth.†.
Tolbutamide (p.336·3).
Diabetes mellitus.

Artotec *Monsanto, Fr.*
Diclofenac sodium (p.30·3).
Misoprostol (p.1446·1) is included in this preparation in an attempt to limit adverse effects on the gastrointestinal mucosa.
Musculoskeletal and joint disorders.

Artoxan *Herbaline, Ital.†.*
Devil's claw root (p.26·3); silver birch (p.1585·2); fraxinus excelsior; meadowsweet (p.1631·2).
Musculoskeletal, joint, and peri-articular disorders; myalgia.

Artracin *Trinity, UK.*
Indometacin (p.44·3).
Inflammation; musculoskeletal, joint, and peri-articular disorders; pain.

Artragel *Interdelta, Switz.*
Glycol salicylate (p.42·2); benzyl nicotinate (p.20·2); camphor (p.1589·3); levomenthol (p.1632·3); turpentine oil (p.1676·3).
Musculoskeletal and joint pain.

Artragil *Iquinosa, Spain.*
Piroxicam (p.79·1).
Gout; musculoskeletal, joint, and peri-articular disorders; pain.

Artralgon *Saunier-Daguin, Fr.†.*
Amylocaine hydrochloride (p.1306·1); glycol orthocresotinate; guaiacyl nicotinate.
Soft-tissue disorders.

Artren *Merck, Braz.*
Diclofenac sodium (p.30·3).
Gout; inflammation; musculoskeletal, joint, and peri-articular disorders; pain.

Artrenac *Merck, Mex.*
Diclofenac sodium (p.30·3).
Inflammation; musculoskeletal and peri-articular disorders; pain.

Artrenac Pro *Merck, Mex.*
Diclofenac sodium (p.30·3).
Misoprostol (p.1446·1) is included in this preparation in an attempt to limit adverse effects on the gastrointestinal mucosa.
Osteoarthritis; rheumatoid arthritis.

Artrex *AyurCore, Singapore.*
Withania somnifera; boswellia serrata; turmeric (p.1029·3); ginger (p.1227·2).
Musculoskeletal, joint, and soft-tissue disorders.

Artri *Medical, Spain.*
Adenosine phosphate (p.1573·3); indometacin (p.44·3).
Fever; inflammation; pain.

Artribid *Merck Sharp & Dohme, Port.*
Sulindac (p.85·3).
Gout; musculoskeletal, joint, and peri-articular disorders.

Artriden *Degorts, Mex.*
Mefenamic acid (p.51·2).
Inflammation; pain.

Artridol *Merck, Port.*
Hydroxymethoxy ethyl benzoate; phenylpropyl salicylate.
Musculoskeletal, joint, peri-articular, and soft-tissue disorders.

Artril *Farmasa, Braz.*
Ibuprofen (p.43·2).
Fever; inflammation; pain.

Artrinid *Uniao Quimica, Braz.*
Ketoprofen (p.47·3).
Gout; musculoskeletal, joint, and peri-articular disorders; pain.

Artrinovo *Llorens, Spain.*
Indometacin (p.44·3).
Gout; inflammation; musculoskeletal, joint, and peri-articular disorders; pain.

Artritol *Bio-Sante, Canad.*
Capsules: Paracetamol (p.71·2).
Cream: Methyl salicylate (p.55·1); menthol (p.1632·3).

Artriunic *Novag, Spain.*
Tenoxicam (p.87·2).
Musculoskeletal, joint and peri-articular disorders.

Artrocaptin *Estedi, Spain.*
Tolmetin sodium (p.88·3).
Musculoskeletal, joint, and peri-articular disorders; pain.

Artrocur *Wyeth Lederle, Ital.*
A heparinoid (p.905·2); aminopropylone (p.13·3).
Muscle and joint pain.

Artrodar *Ecupharma, Ital.†.*
Diacerein (p.28·3).
Osteoarthritis.

Artrodesmol Extra *Reig Jofre, Spain.*
Dimethyl sulfoxide (p.1402·2); phenylbutazone (p.78·1); fluocinolone acetonide (p.1071·1); methyl salicylate (p.55·1).
Soft-tissue disorders.

Artrodol *AGIPS, Ital.*
Diflunisal (p.32·2).
Pain.

Artrodue *MDM, Ital.*
Collagen (p.1598·2); mucopolysaccharides; vitamins; copper (p.1350·1).
Joint disorders.

Artrofene *Sankyo, Port.*
Ketoprofen lysine (p.48·1).
Musculoskeletal, joint, peri-articular, and soft-tissue disorders; neuralgia.

Artrogota *Teofarma, Spain.*
Diethylamine salicylate (p.32·2).
Peri-articular and soft-tissue disorders.

Artrolyt *Neo-Farmaceutica, Port.*
Diacerein (p.28·3).
Osteoarthrosis.

Artromed *Medosan, Ital.*
Amtolmetin guacil (p.14·1).
Musculoskeletal and joint disorders; pain.

Artron *Liomont, Mex.*
Naproxen (p.60·3).
Musculoskeletal, joint, and peri-articular disorders; pain.

Artroreuma *Teofarma, Ital.*
Tiaprofenic acid (p.88·1).
Inflammation; pain.

Artrosal *OTC, Spain.*
Ethyl vanillin; phenylpropanol salicylate.
Rheumatic and muscle pain.

Artrosan
Note.This name is used for preparations of different composition.
Dolisos, Spain.
Devil's claw root (p.26·3); meadowsweet (p.1631·2).
Joint disorders.

Provita, Spain.
Multivitamin and mineral preparation with glucosamine sulfate (p.1616·2) (p.1350·1).
Joint disorders.

Artrosilene *Dompe, Ital.*
Ketoprofen lysine (p.48·1).
Musculoskeletal, joint, and peri-articular disorders.

Artrotec
Monsanto, Ital.; Searle, Mex.; Monsanto, Spain.
Diclofenac sodium (p.30·3).
Misoprostol (p.1446·1) is included in this preparation in an attempt to limit adverse effects on the gastrointestinal mucosa.
Ankylosing spondylitis; osteoarthritis; rheumatoid arthritis.

Artroxen *Errekappa, Ital.†.*
Naproxen (p.60·3).
Musculoskeletal and joint disorders.

Artroxicam *Fonten, Ital.*
Piroxicam (p.79·1).
Musculoskeletal, joint, peri-articular, and soft-tissue disorders.

Arturic *Alpharma, Fin.; Alpharma, Norw.*
Allopurinol (p.397·2).
Gout; hyperuricaemia; renal calculi; uric acid nephropathy.

Artyflam *Rayere, Mex.*
Piroxicam (p.79·1).
Inflammation; musculoskeletal and joint disorders.

Artz
Astra, Denm.; Sankyo, Ital.
Sodium hyaluronate (p.1620·1).
Osteoarthritis.

Artzal
Sankyo, Aust.; AstraZeneca, Fin.; Astra, Swed.
Sodium hyaluronate (p.1620·1).
Arthrosis of the knee.

Aru C *Chauvin ankerpharm, Ger.*
Clotrimazole (p.382·1).
Corynebacterium skin infections; fungal skin infections.

Arubendol
Note.This name is used for preparations of different composition.
Isis, Ger.
Terbutaline sulfate (p.776·2).
Obstructive airways disease.

Klinge, Ger.
Salbutamol (p.770·3).
Obstructive airways disease.

Aruclonin *Chauvin ankerpharm, Ger.*
Clonidine hydrochloride (p.860·1).
Glaucoma; ocular hypertension.

Arufil *Chauvin ankerpharm, Ger.*
Povidone (p.1503·2).
Dry eyes.

Arutimol *Chauvin ankerpharm, Ger.*
Timolol maleate (p.982·1).
Glaucoma; ocular hypertension.

Arutrin *Chauvin ankerpharm, Ger.*
Triamcinolone acetonide (p.1080·1).
Skin disorders.

Arvenum *Stroder, Ital.*
Diosmin (p.1611·1).
Peripheral vascular disorders.

Arvin
Knoll, Canad.†; Knoll, Spain†; Knoll, UK†.
Ancrod (p.839·3).
Thrombosis.

Arvin Antidote *Knoll, UK†.*
Ancrod antisera.
Overdosage with or adverse effects of ancrod.

Arwin
Ebewe, Aust.†; Knoll, Ger.†.
Ancrod (p.839·3).
Peripheral vascular disorders.

Arythmol
Knoll, Irl.; Knoll, UK.
Propafenone hydrochloride (p.961·3).
Arrhythmias.

Arzepam *Solfran, Mex.*
Diazepam (p.674·3).

Arzimol *Belmac, Spain.*
Cefprozil (p.173·2).
Bacterial infections.

AS/85 *Aesculapius, Ital.*
Naproxen aminobutanol (p.61·3).
Gynaecological disorders.

AS Cor *SmithKline Beecham, Mex.*
Norfenefrine hydrochloride (p.949·1).
Hypotension.

AS 101 VA N *Staufen, Ger.*
Homoeopathic preparation.

ASA *Liomont, Mex.*
Aspirin (p.14·2).
Fever; pain; thromboembolism prophylaxis.

Asa Right Powder *Eagle, Austral.*
Vitamin and mineral preparation with equisetum and ginger (p.1350·1).
Respiratory congestion.

Asa Tones *Eagle, Austral.*
Grindelia camporum (p.1618·2); hedera helix; potassium iodide (p.1522·3); crataegus (p.1600·2); euphorbia hirta (p.1609·3); liquorice (p.1231·2); polygala tenuifolia (p.1100·2); drosera longifolia (p.1606·1).
Upper respiratory-tract symptoms.

Asacol *Byk, Belg.; Procter & Gamble, Canad.; Leiras, Denm.; Leiras, Fin.; Tillotts, Hong Kong; Tillotts, Israel; Giuliani, Ital.; Byk, Neth.; Leiras, Norw.; Baxter, NZ; Tillotts, NZ; Helsinn, Port.; Aventis, S.Afr.; Tillotts, Singapore; Schering, Swed.; Synthelabo, Switz.; Tillotts, Thai.; Smith-Kline Beecham, UK; Procter & Gamble, USA.*
Mesalazine (p.1234·1).
Inflammatory bowel disease.

Asacolitin *Henning, Ger.*
Mesalazine (p.1234·1).
Ulcerative colitis.

Asacolon *Medeva, Irl.*
Mesalazine (p.1234·1).
Proctitis; proctosigmoiditis; ulcerative colitis.

ASAD *Stallergenes, Fr.; Stallergenes, Switz.*
A range of allergen extracts (p.1575·3).
Hyposensitisation.

Asafen *Sanofi Winthrop, Braz.*
Paracetamol (p.71·2); ephedrine hydrochloride (p.1090·1); thenyldiamine (p.425·3); caffeine (p.761·3).
Cold and influenza symptoms.

Asaflow *Sandipro, Belg.*
Aspirin (p.14·2).
Cardiovascular and cerebrovascular disorders.

Asalen *Covan, S.Afr.*
Phenylephrine hydrochloride (p.1097·1); chlorpheniramine [chlorphenamine] maleate (p.412·1); paracetamol (p.71·2); caffeine (p.761·3).
Formerly contained phenylephrine hydrochloride, thenyldiamine hydrochloride, paracetamol, and caffeine.
Cold symptoms.

Asalex *Chiesi, Ital.*
Mesalazine (p.1234·1).
Inflammatory bowel disease.

Asalit *Merck, Braz.*
Mesalazine (p.1234·1).
Inflammatory bowel disease.

Asaphen *Pharmascience, Canad.*
Aspirin (p.14·2).
Fever; inflammation; pain.

Asarid *Boehringer Ingelheim, Belg.*
Aspirin (p.14·2).
Cardiovascular disorders; fever; pain.

Asarum Med Complex *Dynamit, Aust.*
Homoeopathic preparation.

Asasantin *Boehringer Ingelheim, Aust.; Boehringer Ingelheim, Austral.; Boehringer Ingelheim, Fin.; Boehringer Ingelheim, Ger.; Boehringer Ingelheim, Mex.; Boehringer Ingelheim, Neth.; Boehringer Ingelheim, Norw.; Boehringer Ingelheim, S.Afr.; Boehringer Ingelheim, Spain; Boehringer Ingelheim, Swed.; Boehringer Ingelheim, UK.*
Aspirin (p.14·2); dipyridamole (p.877·2).
Thromboembolism prophylaxis.

Asasantine *Boehringer Ingelheim, Canad.; Boehringer Ingelheim, Fr.; Boehringer Ingelheim, Switz.*
Dipyridamole (p.877·2); aspirin (p.14·2).
Thromboembolic disorders.

ASAtard *Boehringer Ingelheim, S.Afr.*
Aspirin (p.14·2).
Thrombosis prophylaxis.

Asaurex *Cryopharma, Mex.*
Cimetidine (p.1216·3).

Asawin *Sanofi Winthrop, Mex.*
Aspirin (p.14·2).

Asazine *Tillotts, Switz.*
Mesalazine (p.1234·1).
Ulcerative colitis.

Asba *Medirel, Switz.†*
Calcium carbonate (p.1215·1); camphor (p.1589·3); peppermint oil (p.1243·3).
Mouth and throat disorders.

Ascabiol
Note.This name is used for preparations of different composition.
Rhone-Poulenc Rorer, Austral.; Rhone-Poulenc Rorer, Irl.; Aspen Consumer, S.Afr.; Rhone-Poulenc Rorer, UK.
Benzyl benzoate (p.1428·2).
Pediculosis; scabies.

Medeva, Fr.
Benzyl benzoate (p.1428·2); sulfiram (p.1437·2).
Scabies.

Ascal
Asta Medica, Neth.; Asta Medica, Spain.
Carbasalate calcium (p.23·3).
Fever; pain; thromboembolism prophylaxis.

Ascarical *Farmoquimica, Braz.*
Pyrantel embonate (p.108·1).
Worm infections.

Ascaridil *Cilag, Braz.*
Levamisole hydrochloride (p.101·2).
Ascariasis.

Ascarient *Propan, S.Afr.†*
Piperazine citrate (p.105·3).
Enterobiasis; roundworm infections.

Ascarin *Iodo Suma, Braz.*
Piperazine hydrate (p.106·1).
Ascariasis; enterobiasis.

Ascariobel *Sedabel, Braz.*
Mebendazole (p.102·2).
Worm infections.

Ascaritor *Kanda, Braz.*
Mebendazole (p.102·2).
Worm infections.

Ascarobex *Opofarm, Braz.*
Mebendazole (p.102·2).
Worm infections.

Ascarotrat *Medley, Braz.*
Tetramisole hydrochloride (p.108·3).
Nematode infections.

Ascaverm *Gemballa, Braz.*
Tetramisole (p.108·3).
Nematode infections.

Ascencyl *Theraplix, Fr.†*
Adenosine phosphate; cyanocobalamin; magnesium aspartate; manganese gluconate (p.1350·1).
Tonic.

Ascocid *Volchem, Ital.*
Peptide, lipid, and carbohydrate preparation with vitamin C (p.1350·1).
Nutritional supplement.

Ascodyne *Chemedica, Switz.*
Multivitamin preparation with amino acids (p.1350·1).
Tonic.

Ascofer
Desbergers, Canad.; Gerda, Fr.
Ferrous ascorbate (p.1359·3).
Iron-deficiency anaemias.

Ascold *Propan, S.Afr.†*
Phenylephrine hydrochloride (p.1097·1); salicylamide (p.82·1); mepyramine maleate (p.421·1); caffeine (p.761·3); ascorbic acid (p.1389·3).
Cold and influenza symptoms.

Ascomed *Ripari-Gero, Ital.†*
Ascorbic acid (p.1389·3).
Vitamin C deficiency.

Ascorbex *Sante Naturelle, Canad.*
Ascorbic acid (p.1389·3).

Ascorbicap *ICN, USA†.*
Ascorbic acid (p.1389·3).
Scurvy; vitamin C deficiency.

Ascorbin
Montavit, Aust.; Orion, Fin.; Leiras, Fin.; Orion, Singapore.
Ascorbic acid (p.1389·3) or sodium ascorbate (p.1390·1).
Vitamin C deficiency.

Ascorbisal *Lannacher, Aust.*
Aspirin (p.14·2); ascorbic acid (p.1389·3).
Fever; musculoskeletal and joint disorders; pain.

Ascorell *Sanorell, Ger.*
Ascorbic acid (p.1389·3).
Vitamin C deficiency.

Ascortil *UCI, Braz.*
Vitamin C (p.1389·3).
Vitamin C supplement.

Ascortonyl *Gerda, Fr.†.*
Ascorbic acid (p.1389·3); magnesium potassium aspartate.
Formerly contained ascorbic acid, magnesium potassium aspartate, and cyanocobalamin.
Tonic.

Ascorvit *Jenapharm, Ger.*
Ascorbic acid (p.1389·3).
Vitamin C deficiency.

Ascotodin *Bruschettini, Ital.*
Mebechinium metilsulfate; thonzylamine hydrochloride (p.426·2).
Eye disorders.

AscoTop *Zeneca, Ger.*
Zolmitriptan (p.458·1).
Migraine.

Ascoxal
Astra, Austral.; AstraZeneca, Fin.; Astra, Mex.; AstraZeneca, Norw.; Astra, Swed.
Ascorbic acid (p.1389·3); sodium percarbonate; copper sulfate (p.1358·1).
Mouth and throat disorders.

Ascredar *Roche, Aust.*
Disodium clodronate (p.751·2).
Hypercalcaemia of malignancy; osteolytic bone metastases; Paget's disease of bone.

Ascriptin
Rhone-Poulenc Rorer, Hong Kong; Rhone-Poulenc Rorer, Irl.†; Rhone-Poulenc Rorer, Israel; Rhone-Poulenc Rorer, Ital.; Rhone-Poulenc Rorer, Mex.
Aspirin (p.14·2).
Aluminium hydroxide (p.1210·3) and magnesium hydroxide (p.1233·1) are included in this preparation in

an attempt to limit adverse effects on the gastrointestinal mucosa.
Fever; inflammation; pain; thromboembolic disorders.

Rhone-Poulenc Rorer, USA.
Aspirin (p.14·2).
Aluminium hydroxide (p.1210·3), calcium carbonate (p.1215·1), and magnesium hydroxide (p.1233·1) are included in this preparation in an attempt to limit adverse effects on the gastrointestinal mucosa.
Fever; inflammation; myocardial infarction; pain; transient ischaemic attacks.

Asdron *Marjan, Braz.*
Ketotifen fumarate (p.767·2).
Allergic conjunctivitis; allergic rhinitis; asthma; urticaria.

Aselli *Weifa, Norw.*
Cream: Cetylpyridinium chloride (p.1138·1); zinc tannate.
Minor skin disorders; skin disinfection; sunburn.
Ointment: Zinc tannate; zinc oxide (p.1128·2); titanium dioxide (p.1126·1); cod-liver oil (p.1357·2).
Minor skin disorders.

Asendin *Wyeth-Ayerst, Canad.; Wyeth, NZ; Lederle, USA.*
Amoxapine (p.279·2).
Depression.

Asendis *Wyeth, Irl.; Wyeth, UK.*
Amoxapine (p.279·2).
Depression.

Asenlix *Hoechst Marion Roussel, Mex.*
Clobenzorex hydrochloride (p.1507·2).
Obesity.

ASEP *Galen, UK.*
Glutaral (p.1145·2).
Instrument disinfection.

Asepsal *Magis, Ital.†.*
Ibuprofen isobutanolammonium (p.44·1).
Gynaecological disorders.

Aseptiderm *Pharmethic, Belg.*
Cetrimonium bromide (p.1137·3).
Disinfection of skin and instruments.

Aseptil *SmithKline Beecham, Ital.*
Copper usnate (p.1678·2); diazolidinyl urea; zinc oxide (p.1128·2); alcloxa (p.1109·3).
Skin and wound disinfection.

Aseptisol *Bode, Ger.*
Glutaral (p.1145·2); formaldehyde (p.1144·2); didecylmethyloxyethylammonium propionate.
Instrument disinfection.

Aseptoman *Geistlich, Switz.†.*
Isopropyl alcohol (p.1149·2); 1,3-butanediol.
Hand disinfection.

Aseptone 1 *Rougier, Canad.*
Clorophene sodium (p.1142·3); sodium o-phenylphenol (p.1152·1).
Surface disinfection for clean surfaces.

Aseptone 2 *Rougier, Canad.*
Clorophene sodium (p.1142·3); sodium o-phenylphenol (p.1152·1); sodium lauril ether sulfate (p.1496·3).
Surface disinfection.

Aseptone 5 *Rougier, Canad.*
Clorophene sodium (p.1142·3); sodium o-phenylphenol (p.1152·1); sodium alkyl-polyether sulfate.
Surface disinfection.

Aseptone Quat *Rougier, Canad.*
n-Alkyldimethylbenzylammonium chlorides (p.1133·2); n-alkyldimethylethylbenzylammonium chlorides; octaxinols (p.1346·3).
Surface disinfection.

Aseptosyl *Sanofi Synthelabo, Belg.*
Potassium hydroxyquinoline sulfate (p.1654·2); lignocaine [lidocaine] hydrochloride (p.1313·2).
Mouth and throat disorders.

Aserbine
Pharmaco, S.Afr.; Forley, UK.
Benzoic acid (p.1134·2); malic acid (p.1631·1); salicylic acid (p.1612·2); propylene glycol (p.1655·1).
Burns; skin ulcers; wounds.

Asercit *Serono, Mex.*
Dacarbazine (p.531·2).

Aseroprim *Serono, Mex.*
Azathioprine (p.509·3).

Asfeina *Bial, Port.*
Aspirin (p.14·2); caffeine (p.761·3).
Fever; pain.

Asgoviscum N *Rhein-Pharma, Ger.*
Mistletoe (p.1636·2); crataegus (p.1600·2); garlic (p.1614·1).
Cardiac disorders.

Ashton & Parsons Infants Powders *SSL, UK.*
Matricaria tincture (p.1593·2).
Colic; teething.

Asialax *Asian Pharm, Thai.*
Carisoprodol (p.1327·1); phenylbutazone (p.78·1).
Musculoskeletal and joint disorders.

Asialum *Asian Pharm, Thai.*
Aluminium hydroxide (p.1210·3); magnesium hydroxide (p.1233·1).
Dyspepsia; gastric hyperacidity; peptic ulcer.

Asiamox *Asian Pharm, Thai.*
Amoxicillin trihydrate (p.149·2).
Bacterial infections.

Asianbron *Asian Pharm, Thai.*
Theophylline (p.777·2); guaifenesin (p.1092·2).
Obstructive airways disease.

Asiatapp *Asian Pharm, Thai.*
Brompheniramine maleate (p.410·2); phenylephrine hydrochloride (p.1097·1); phenylpropanolamine hydrochloride (p.1098·1).
Asthma; cold symptoms.

Asiazole *Asian Pharm, Thai.*
Metronidazole (p.594·1).
Amoebiasis; trichomoniasis.

Asiazole-TN *Asian Pharm, Thai.*
Tinidazole (p.603·3).
Amoebiasis; giardiasis; trichomoiasis.

Asic
Note.This name is used for preparations of different composition.
Cesam, Braz.
Bearberry (p.1583·3); carboxyethylgermanium; titanium dioxide (p.1126·1); methoxycinnamate.
Hyperpigmentation.

Pharmaceutical Enterprises, S.Afr.
Dicyclomine [dicycloverine] hydrochloride (p.466·1); doxylamine succinate (p.417·1); pyridoxine hydrochloride (p.1386·3).
Nausea and vomiting in pregnancy.

Asig *Sigma, Austral.*
Quinapril hydrochloride (p.963·3).
Heart failure; hypertension.

Asilone
Note.This name is used for preparations of different composition.
Sanofi Winthrop, Braz.; Knoll, Irl.; Roche, S.Afr.; SSL, UK.
Oral suspension; oral gel: Aluminium hydroxide (p.1210·3); ; magnesium hydroxide (p.1233·1) or magnesium oxide (p.1233·2); simeticone (p.1249·2).
Dyspepsia; flatulence; gastritis; gastro-oesophageal reflux; hiatus hernia; peptic ulcer.

Sanofi Winthrop, Braz.; Knoll, Irl.; Roche, S.Afr.; SSL, UK.
Tablets: Aluminium hydroxide (p.1210·3); simeticone (p.1249·2).
Dyspepsia; flatulence; gastritis; gastro-oesophageal reflux; hiatus hernia; peptic ulcer.

Asilone Heartburn *SSL, UK.*
Alginic acid (p.1498·3) or sodium alginate (p.1498·3); aluminium hydroxide (p.1210·3); magnesium trisilicate (p.1233·3); sodium bicarbonate (p.1186·2).
Dyspepsia; heartburn.

Asilone Windcheaters *SSL, UK.*
Simeticone (p.1249·2).
Flatulence.

Asimil B12 *Torlan, Spain.*
Mecobalamin (p.1388·3).
Vitamin B12 deficiency.

Asinis *Bittner, Aust.*
Homoeopathic preparation.

Askina
Note.This name is used for preparations of different composition.
Braun, Fr.
Hydrogel dressing.
Ulcers; wounds.

Braun, UK.
Sodium chloride (p.1196·1).
Wound cleansing and irrigation.

Askina Biofilm *Braun, Fr.*
Carmellose (p.1499·3).
Wounds.

Askit *Askit, UK.*
Aspirin (p.14·2); aloxiprin (p.13·2); caffeine citrate (p.761·3).
Fever; pain.

ASL *Normon, Spain.*
Lysine aspirin (p.50·3).
Fever; inflammation; pain; thromboembolism prophylaxis.

Aslavital *Sanova, Aust.*
Injection: Procaine hydrochloride (p.1319·1); glutamic acid (p.1365·2).
Tablets: Procaine hydrochloride (p.1319·1); pyridoxine hydrochloride (p.1386·3); inositol (p.1623·3).
Tonic.

Asmabec *Medeva, Fr.; Medeva, Irl.; Medeva, UK.*
Beclometasone dipropionate (p.1061·2).
Asthma.

Asmacortone *Nuovo, Ital.*
Methylprednisolone sodium hemisuccinate (p.1076·1).
Corticosteroid.

Asmafen
Xepa-Soul Pattinson, Hong Kong; Pacific, NZ; Xepa-Soul Pattinson, Singapore.
Ketotifen (p.767·2) or ketotifen fumarate (p.767·2).
Allergic bronchitis; allergic conjunctivitis; allergic rhinitis; allergic skin disorders; asthma; hay fever.

Asmafort *Julphar, UAE.*
Ketotifen fumarate (p.767·2).
Allergic conjunctivitis; allergic rhinitis; asthma; urticaria.

Asmalene *FIRMA, Ital.*
Bitolterol mesilate (p.761·2).
Obstructive airways disease.

Asmalergin *Merck, Braz.*
Ketotifen fumarate (p.767·2).
Allergic conjunctivitis; allergic rhinitis; asthma; urticaria.

Asmaline *Polipharm, Thai.*
Terbutaline sulfate (p.776·2).
Obstructive airways disease.

Asmaliv *Legrand, Braz.*
Salbutamol sulfate (p.770·3).
Obstructive airways disease.

Asmalix *Century, USA.*
Theophylline (p.777·2).
Obstructive airways disease.

Asmanoc *Shiwa, Thai.*
Ketotifen fumarate (p.767·2).
Asthma; bronchitis; hay fever.

Asmaral-K *Serral, Mex.*
Ketotifen (p.767·2).
Asthma.

Asmasal
Medeva, Fr.; Medeva, Irl.; Silom, Thai.; Celltech, UK.
Salbutamol (p.770·3) or salbutamol sulfate (p.770·3).
Obstructive airways disease.

Asmasal Expectorant *Silom, Thai.*
Salbutamol (p.770·3); guaifenesin (p.1092·2).
Bronchospasm associated with respiratory-tract congestion.

Asmasolon *Great Eastern, Thai.; Westmont, Thai.*
Theophylline (p.777·2).
Obstructive airways disease.

Asmatil *Alter, Port.*
Fluticasone propionate (p.1072·2).
Asthma.

Asmaven *Berk, UK.*
Salbutamol sulfate (p.770·3).
Obstructive airways disease; premature labour.

Asmavent *Technilab, Canad.*
Salbutamol sulfate (p.770·3).
Obstructive airways disease.

Asmax *Ativus, Braz.*
Ketotifen fumarate (p.767·2).
Allergic conjunctivitis; allergic rhinitis; asthma; urticaria.

Asmen *Farmalab, Braz.*
Ketotifen fumarate (p.767·2).
Allergic conjunctivitis; allergic rhinitis; asthma; urticaria.

Asmeton
Sankyo, Hong Kong; Sankyo, Thai.
Methoxyphenamine hydrochloride (p.1094·3); aminophylline (p.760·1); chlorpheniramine [chlorphenamine] maleate (p.412·1); noscapine (p.1096·1).
Asthma; bronchitis; coughs.

Asmo *ICN, Spain†.*
Theophylline (p.777·2).
Heart failure; obstructive airways disease; paroxysmal dyspnoea.

Asmodrin *Sanval, Braz.*
Aminophylline (p.760·1).
Obstructive airways disease.

Asmol
Alphapharm, Austral.; Pacific, NZ.
Salbutamol (p.770·3) or salbutamol sulfate (p.770·3).
Obstructive airways disease.

Asmo-Lavi *Vitoria, Port.*
Fluticasone propionate (p.1072·2).
Asthma.

Asmosterona *Zambon, Braz.*
Prednisolone (p.1077·3); tripelennamine hydrochloride (p.427·1); ephedrine hydrochloride (p.1090·1).
Asthma.

Asodal *Sandipro, Belg.*
Paracetamol (p.71·2); codeine phosphate (p.25·2); caffeine (p.761·3); tiemonium iodide (p.474·2).
Colic; muscle spasm and pain.

Asonacor *Ebewe, Aust.†.*
Propafenone hydrochloride (p.961·3).
Arrhythmias.

Asotax *Asofarma, Mex.*
Paclitaxel (p.563·2).
Malignant neoplasms.

Asovon *Progress, Thai.*
Bromhexine hydrochloride (p.1085·3).
Respiratory-tract disorders associated with increased or viscous mucus.

ASP *Merck, Port.*
Aspirin (p.14·2).
Fever; pain.

Aspac *Inexfa, Spain.*
Paracetamol (p.71·2).
Fever; pain.

Aspalgin *Fawns & McAllan, Austral.*
Aspirin (p.14·2); codeine phosphate (p.25·2).
Fever; inflammation; pain.

Asparagus-P *Plantina, Ger.*
Asparagus; parsley (p.1648·3).
Oedema; renal calculi.

Aspartamins *Solgar, UK.*
Mineral aspartate preparation (p.1350·1).

Aspartatol *Eagle, Austral.*
Potassium aspartate (p.1195·2); magnesium aspartate (p.1190·3); levoglutamide (p.1365·2).
Tonic.

Asparten *Euro-Labor, Port.*
Arginine aspartate (p.1354·1).
Fatigue.

Aspartina *Bouty, Ital.*
Aspartame (p.1354·3).
Sugar substitute.

Aspartono *Medix, Spain.*
Adenosine triphosphate; glucose; magnesium aspartate; potassium aspartate.
Cardiopathies; liver disorders; muscular dystrophies; tonic.

A-Spas *Hyrex, USA.*
Hyoscyamine sulfate (p.469·3).
Gastrointestinal disorders.

Aspaserine B6 Tranq *UCB, Spain.*
Diazepam (p.674·3).
Contains pyridoxine.
Alcohol withdrawal syndrome; anxiety; febrile convulsions; insomnia; skeletal muscle spasm.

Aspasmon N *Norgine, Ger.*
Peppermint oil (p.1243·3); anise oil (p.1580·3); caraway oil (p.1591·2).
Asthma; gastrointestinal disorders.

Aspav *Cox, UK.*
Aspirin (p.14·2); papaveretum (p.70·1).
Pain.

Aspec *PSM, NZ.*
Aspirin (p.14·2).
Fever; inflammation; pain.

Aspecton *Krewel, Ger.*
Thyme (p.1672·2).
Catarrh; coughs.

Aspecton N *Krewel, Ger.*
Thyme (p.1672·2); gypsophila saponins.
Respiratory-tract disorders.

Aspecton-Balsam *Krewel, Ger.*
Camphor (p.1589·3); thyme oil (p.1672·3); eucalyptus oil (p.1609·2).
Cold symptoms; coughs.

Aspectonetten N *Krewel, Ger.*
Gypsophila saponins.
Formerly contained butetamate citrate.
Respiratory-tract catarrh.

Aspegic
Sanofi Synthelabo, Belg.; Synthelabo, Fr.; Sanofi Synthelabo, Ital.; Sanofi Synthelabo, Neth.; Sanofi Synthelabo, Port.; Cantabria, Spain†; Synthelabo, Switz.
Lysine aspirin (p.50·3).
Fever; inflammation; musculoskeletal and joint disorders; pain; thromboembolism prophylaxis.

Aspellin *Fisons, UK.*
Methyl salicylate (p.55·1); ethyl salicylate (p.35·1); ammonium salicylate (p.14·1); menthol (p.1632·3); camphor (p.1589·3).
Pain.

Aspent *Ranbaxy, Thai.*
Aspirin (p.14·2).
Myocardial infarction; osteoarthritis; rheumatoid arthritis; transient ischaemic attacks.

Aspercreme
Note. This name is used for preparations of different composition.
Stella, Canad.; Thompson, USA.
Trolamine salicylate (p.90·1).
Muscle, joint, and soft-tissue pain; neuralgia.

Roche, Ital.†.
Diethylamine salicylate (p.32·2); methyl nicotinate (p.55·1).
Musculoskeletal disorders.

Aspergum
Schering-Plough, Canad.; Schering-Plough, USA.
Aspirin (p.14·2).
Fever; inflammation; myocardial infarction; pain; transient ischaemic attacks.

Aspex *Rekah, Israel.*
Aspirin (p.14·2); caffeine (p.761·3).
Fever; pain.

Asphaline *Galenica, Switz.*
Camphor (p.1589·3); thymol (p.1158·3); paraformaldehyde (p.1152·2); zinc oxide (p.1128·2).
Root canal infections.

Aspi-C *Eurofarma, Braz.*
Aspirin (p.14·2); ascorbic acid (p.1389·3).
Fever; pain.

Aspidol *Piam, Ital.*
Lysine aspirin (p.50·3).
Pain.

Aspiglicina *Antonetto, Ital.*
Aspirin (p.14·2).
Glycine (p.1365·3) is included in this preparation in an attempt to limit adverse effects on the gastrointestinal mucosa.
Neuralgia.

Aspilets *United American, Hong Kong.*
Aspirin (p.14·2).
Fever; pain.

Aspinfantil *Diviser Aquilea, Spain.*
Aspirin (p.14·2).
Fever; musculoskeletal, joint, and peri-articular disorders; pain; thromboembolism prophylaxis.

Aspiricor *Bayer, Aust.*
Aspirin (p.14·2).
Migraine; thromboembolism prophylaxis.

Aspirin Backache *Bayer, Canad.*
Aspirin (p.14·2); methocarbamol (p.1329·3).
Back pain.

Aspirin C
Bayer, Fin.; Bayer, Israel.
Aspirin (p.14·2); ascorbic acid (p.1389·3).
Fever; musculoskeletal and joint disorders; pain; thrombosis prophylaxis.

Aspirin + C *Bayer, Aust.*
Aspirin (p.14·2); ascorbic acid (p.1389·3).
Fever; pain.

Aspirin Cardio *Bayer, Fin.*
Aspirin (p.14·2).
Thromboembolism prophylaxis.

Aspirin forte *Bayer, Ger.*
Aspirin (p.14·2); caffeine (p.761·3).
Inflammation; pain.

Aspirin Free Anacin *Robins, USA.*
Paracetamol (p.71·2).
Formerly known as Anacin-3.

Aspirin Free Anacin PM *Whitehall, USA.*
Paracetamol (p.71·2); diphenhydramine hydrochloride (p.416·1).
Insomnia; pain.

Aspirin Free Excedrin *Bristol-Myers Squibb, USA.*
Paracetamol (p.71·2); caffeine (p.761·3).
Pain.

Aspirin Free Excedrin Dual *Bristol-Myers Squibb, USA†.*
Paracetamol (p.71·2); calcium carbonate (p.1215·1); magnesium carbonate (p.1232·3); magnesium oxide (p.1233·2).

Aspirin Free Pain Relief *Hudson, USA.*
Paracetamol (p.71·2).
Fever; pain.

Aspirin Plus *Invamed, USA†.*
Paracetamol (p.71·2); aspirin (p.14·2); caffeine (p.761·3).

Aspirin plus C *Bayer, Ger.*
Aspirin (p.14·2); ascorbic acid (p.1389·3).
Cold symptoms; fever; pain.

Aspirin with Stomach Guard *Bayer, Canad.*
Aspirin (p.14·2).
Calcium carbonate (p.1215·1), magnesium carbonate (p.1232·3), and magnesium oxide (p.1233·2) are included in this preparation in an attempt to limit adverse effects on the gastrointestinal mucosa.
Fever; inflammation; pain.

Aspirina
Bayer, Braz.; Bayer, Ital.; Bayer, Mex.; Bayer, Port.; Bayer, Spain.
Aspirin (p.14·2).
Calcium carbonate (p.1215·1) may be included in the chewable tablets in an attempt to limit adverse effects on the gastrointestinal mucosa.
Fever; musculoskeletal, joint, and peri-articular disorders; pain; thromboembolism prophylaxis.

Aspirina 03 and 05 *Bayer, Ital.*
Aspirin (p.14·2).
Magnesium hydroxide (p.1233·1) and aluminium glycinate (p.1210·3) are included in this preparation in an attempt to limit adverse effects on the gastrointestinal mucosa.
Fever; pain.

Aspirina 05 *Bayer, Ital.*
Aspirin (p.14·2).
Calcium carbonate (p.1215·1) is included in this preparation in an attempt to limit adverse effects on the gastrointestinal mucosa.
Fever; pain.

Aspirina C
Bayer, Braz.; Bayer, Ital.; Bayer, Port.; Bayer, Spain.
Aspirin (p.14·2); ascorbic acid (p.1389·3).
Fever; musculoskeletal disorders; pain.

Aspirina Complex *Bayer, Spain.*
Aspirin (p.14·2); phenylpropanolamine tartrate (p.1099·3); chlorpheniramine [chlorphenamine] maleate (p.412·1).
Cold and influenza symptoms.

Aspirina Forte *Bayer, Spain.*
Aspirin (p.14·2); caffeine (p.761·3).
Fever; pain.

Aspirine
Bayer, Belg.; Bayer, Fr.; Bristol-Myers Squibb, Fr.
Aspirin (p.14·2).
Fever; pain; thromboembolism prophylaxis.

Aspirine C
Bayer, Belg.; Bayer, Neth.
Aspirin (p.14·2); ascorbic acid (p.1389·3).
Fever; pain.

Aspirine pH8 *3M, Fr.*
Aspirin (p.14·2).
Fever; pain.

Aspirine Protect *Bayer, Neth.*
Aspirin (p.14·2).
Thrombosis prophylaxis.

Aspirine vitamine C *Bayer, Fr.; Oberlin, Fr.; UPSA, Fr.*
Aspirin (p.14·2); ascorbic acid (p.1389·3).
Fever; pain.

Aspirinetta *Bayer, Ital.*
Aspirin (p.14·2).
Fever; inflammation; pain.

Aspirinetta C *Bayer, Ital.*
Aspirin (p.14·2); ascorbic acid (p.1389·3).
Fever; inflammation; pain.

Aspirin-Free Bayer Select Allergy Sinus *Sterling Health, USA.*
Pseudoephedrine hydrochloride (p.1099·2); chlorpheniramine [chlorphenamine] maleate (p.412·1); paracetamol (p.71·2).

Aspirin-Free Bayer Select Head & Chest Cold *Sterling Health, USA.*
Pseudoephedrine hydrochloride (p.1099·2); dextromethorphan hydrobromide (p.1087·3); guaifenesin (p.1092·2); paracetamol (p.71·2).

Aspirin-Free Bayer Select Headache *Sterling Health, USA†.*
Paracetamol (p.71·2); caffeine (p.761·3).

Aspirisan *Sanval, Braz.*
Aspirin (p.14·2); caffeine (p.761·3).
Fever; pain.

Aspirisucre *Arkomedika, Fr.*
Aspirin (p.14·2).
Fever; pain.

Aspisin *Farmasa, Braz.*
Aspirin (p.14·2).
Fever; inflammation; pain; thromboembolism prophylaxis.

Aspisol *Bayer, Ger.*
Lysine aspirin (p.50·3).
Fever; pain; rheumatism; thromboembolic disorders.

Asplin *Diafarm, Spain†.*
Paracetamol (p.71·2).
Fever; pain.

Asporin 0.5 *MC, Ital.†.*
Sodium phenolate; glutaral (p.1145·2).
Instrument sterilisation.

Asporin 2 *MC, Ital.†.*
Glutaral (p.1145·2).
Instrument sterilisation.

Asprimox *Invamed, USA.*
Aspirin (p.14·2).
Aluminium hydroxide (p.1210·3), calcium carbonate (p.1215·1), and magnesium hydroxide (p.1233·1) are included in this preparation in an attempt to limit adverse effects on the gastrointestinal mucosa.

Aspro
Roche, Aust.; Roche Consumer, Austral.; Roche, Belg.; Roche Nicholas, Fr.; Roche Nicholas, Ger.; Roche, Hong Kong; Roche Consumer, Irl.; Roche, Ital.; Roche Consumer, Neth.; Roche, NZ; Roche, Port.; Roche, S.Afr.†; Roche Consumer, Singapore; Roche Nicholas, Spain†; Roche, Switz.; Roche Consumer, UK.
Aspirin (p.14·2).
Fever; inflammation; pain; thromboembolism prophylaxis.

Aspro C
Roche, Aust.; Roche, Ital.; Roche, Switz.†
Aspirin (p.14·2); ascorbic acid (p.1389·3).
Fever; pain.

Aspro + C *Roche, Belg.*
Aspirin (p.14·2); ascorbic acid (p.1389·3).
Fever; pain.

Aspro vitamine C *Roche Nicholas, Fr.*
Aspirin (p.14·2); ascorbic acid (p.1389·3).
Fever; pain.

Asproaccel *Roche Nicholas, Fr.*
Aspirin (p.14·2); caffeine (p.761·3).
Fever; pain.

Aspylin *QIF, Braz.*
Aspirin (p.14·2).
Fever; inflammation; pain; thromboembolism prophylaxis.

ASS
Genericon, Aust.; Aspro-Nicholas, Aust.; Roche, Aust.; Hexal, Ger.; CT, Ger.; Ratiopharm, Ger.; Stada, Ger.; Worwag, Ger.; Azupharma, Ger.; Heumann, Ger.; Aliud, Ger.; Merck dura, Ger.; Atid, Ger.; Isis, Ger.; RAN, Ger.; Mepha, Switz.
Aspirin (p.14·2).
Fever; inflammation; pain; rheumatism; thromboembolic disorders.

ASS + C *Ratiopharm, Ger.; Hexal, Ger.*
Aspirin (p.14·2); ascorbic acid (p.1389·3).
Cold symptoms; fever; pain.

ASS OPT *Optimed, Ger.†.*
Aspirin (p.1389·3).
Fever; musculoskeletal and joint disorders; pain; thromboembolic disorders.

Assagix *Plantes et Medecines, Fr.†*
Tilia (p.1673·2); calcium bromolactobionate (p.659·1).
Insomnia.

Assal *Salus, Mex.*
Salbutamol (p.770·3).

Assalix *Plantina, Ger.*
Salix (p.82·1).
Fever; pain; rheumatism.

Assan *Permamed, Switz.*
Flufenamic acid (p.41·1); glycol salicylate (p.42·2); heparin sodium (p.902·1).
Musculoskeletal and joint pain; peripheral vascular disorders; soft-tissue injury.

Assan-Thermo *Permamed, Switz.*
Flufenamic acid (p.41·1); glycol salicylate (p.42·2); benzyl nicotinate (p.20·2); heparin sodium (p.902·1).
Musculoskeletal and joint disorders.

Assepium *Gross, Braz.*
Co-trimoxazole (p.193·3).
Bacterial infections; Pneumocystis carinii pneumonia; protozoal infections.

Assepium Balsamico *Gross, Braz.*
Co-trimoxazole (p.193·3); guaifenesin (p.1092·2); ammonium chloride (p.1085·2).
Bacterial infections.

Asseptobron *Eurofarma, Braz.*
Oxytetracycline (p.234·1); sodium camsilate; guaifenesin (p.1092·2).
Bacterial infections.

Assist Energetico *Ledi, Ital.*
Vitamin preparation (p.1350·1).

Assist Reintegratore *Ledi, Ital.*
Nutritional supplement (p.1350·1).
Fluid and electrolyte imbalance.

Assival *Biogal, Israel.*
Diazepam (p.674·3).
Anxiety; epilepsy; insomnia; skeletal muscle spasm.

ASS-Kombi Ratiopharm, Ger.†
Paracetamol (p.71·2); aspirin (p.14·2); ascorbic acid (p.1389·3).
Pain.

ASS-Kreuz RAN, Ger.
Aspirin (p.1389·3).
Fever; musculoskeletal and joint disorders; pain; thromboembolic disorders.

Assocort Bristol-Myers Squibb, Ital.
Triamcinolone acetonide (p.1080·1); nystatin (p.392·2).
Formerly contained triamcinolone acetonide, neomycin sulfate, gramicidin, and nystatin.
Infected skin disorders.

Assogen Metapharma, Ital.
Cloricromen hydrochloride (p.863·2).
Thrombosis prophylaxis.

Assoral Savio, Ital.
Roxithromycin (p.247·2).
Bacterial infections.

Assplant Robugen, Ger.
Salix (p.82·1).
Rheumatism.

Astahis Siam Bheasach, Thai.
Astemizole (p.409·1).
Hypersensitivity reactions.

Astat Tsumura, Jpn.
Lanoconazole (p.390·3).
Fungal skin infections.

Astec Gebro, Aust.†
Salbutamol sulfate (p.770·3).
Obstructive airways disease.

Astelin
Sanfer, Mex.; Wallace, USA.
Azelastine hydrochloride (p.409·3).
Allergic rhinitis.

Astem Asian Pharm, Thai.
Astemizole (p.409·1).
Hypersensitivity reactions.

Astemina Diba, Mex.
Astemizole (p.409·1).
Hypersensitivity.

Astenolit Byk Leo, Spain.
Vitamin, mineral and amino-acid preparation (p.1350·1).
Tonic.

Astesen Senosiain, Mex.
Astemizole (p.409·1).
Allergic conjunctivitis; allergic rhinitis; urticaria.

Asthamsian Asian Pharm, Thai.
Terbutaline sulfate (p.776·2).
Obstructive airways disease.

Asthavent Cipla-Medpro, S.Afr.
Salbutamol (p.770·3).
Obstructive airways disease.

Asthenal Grossmann, Switz.
Sodium dimethyl aminophenylphosphinate; glutamic acid; thiamine hydrochloride; ascorbic acid (p.1350·1).
Tonic.

Asthenopin Mann, Ger.†
Pilocarpine hydrochloride (p.1422·3).
Eye disorders.

Asthma Disperga, Aust.
Papaverine hydrochloride (p.1648·1); ephedrine hydrochloride (p.1090·1); propyphenazone (p.80·2); hyoscine hydrobromide (p.468·2).
Obstructive airways disease.

Asthma & Catarrh Relief Herbal Concepts, UK.
Ipecacuanha (p.1093·1); lobelia (p.1510·2); marrubium (p.1094·2); liquorice (p.1231·2).
Asthma; catarrh.

Asthma Efeum Apomedica, Aust.
Proxyphylline (p.770·1); phenazone (p.77·2); ethaverine sulfamate (p.1608·2); ephedrine hydrochloride (p.1090·1); diphenhydramine hydrochloride (p.416·1).
Obstructive airways disease.

Asthma H Pflüger, Ger.
Homoeopathic preparation.

Asthma 6-N Hobein, Ger.
Ephedrine hydrochloride (p.1090·1); grindelia (p.1618·2); senega root (p.1100·2).
Obstructive airways disease.

Asthma T Sam-On, Israel.
Theophylline (p.777·2).
Asthma.

Asthma-Bisolvon Boehringer Ingelheim, Aust.†
Bromhexine hydrochloride (p.1085·3); ephedrine hydrochloride (p.1090·1); theophylline (p.777·2).
Obstructive airways disease.

Asthma-Bomin H Pflüger, Ger.
Homoeopathic preparation.

Asthma-Frenon Richter, Aust.†
Guaifenesin (p.1092·2); caffeine (p.761·3); phenazone (p.77·2); potassium thiocyanate; ephedrine hydrochloride (p.1090·1); monobenzylphthalate; menthol (p.1632·3); eucalyptol (p.1609·2); camphor (p.1589·3).

AsthmaHaler Mist Numark, USA.
Adrenaline [epinephrine] acid tartrate (p.829·2).
Bronchospasm.

Asthma-Hilfe Agepha, Aust.
Aminophylline (p.760·1); theobromine (p.777·2); ephedrine hydrochloride (p.1090·1); sulfogaiacol (p.1101·1).
Obstructive airways disease.

Asthmakehll N Steigerwald, Ger.
Homoeopathic preparation.

Asthmalgine Cochon, Fr.†
Sodium benzoate (p.1134·3); ephedrine hydrochloride (p.1090·1); caffeine (p.761·3); hyoscyamus (p.470·1).
The oral solution also contains Desessartz syrup.
Asthma.

Asthmalitan MIT, Ger.
Salbutamol sulfate (p.770·3).
Obstructive airways disease.

Asthmalyticum-Ampullen N (Rowo-210)
Pharmakon, Ger.†
Homoeopathic preparation.
Lignocaine [lidocaine] hydrochloride (p.1313·2) is included in this preparation to alleviate the pain of injection.

AsthmaNefrin Menley & James, USA.
Racepinefrine hydrochloride (p.831·1).
Obstructive airways disease.

Asthma-Spray CT, Ger.
Salbutamol (p.770·3).
Obstructive airways disease.

Asthmatee Smetana, Aust.
Enulae root; marrubium vulgare (p.1094·2); origanum; aniseed (p.1580·2); arnica (p.1581·3); cacao husk (p.1671·3).
Obstructive airways disease.

Asthmavowen-N Weber & Weber, Ger.
Homoeopathic preparation.

Asthmaxine Synco, Hong Kong.
Bromhexine hydrochloride (p.1085·3).
Respiratory-tract congestion.

Asthmo-Kranit Mono Krewel, Ger.
Terbutaline sulfate (p.776·2).
Formerly contained ethaverine hydrochloride, ephedrine hydrochloride, phenobarbital, and theophylline.
Obstructive airways disease.

Asthmolin Pharmasant, Thai.
Salbutamol sulfate (p.770·3).
Obstructive airways disease.

Asthmolysin Kade, Ger.†
Diprophylline (p.764·1).
Asthma; bronchial disorders.

Asthmoprotect Azupharma, Ger.
Terbutaline sulfate (p.776·2).
Obstructive airways disease.

Astho-Med Schonenberger, Switz.
Diphenhydramine hydrochloride (p.416·1); diprophylline (p.764·1); guaifenesin (p.1092·2); phenylpropanolamine hydrochloride (p.1098·1).
Bronchitis; coughs.

Asticol Clinced, Aust.
Paracetamol nicotinate (p.73·3); propyphenazone (p.80·2); caffeine (p.761·3).

Astidin Piam, Ital.
Infant feed (p.1350·1).
Histidinaemia.

Astifat Fatol, Ger.
Ketotifen fumarate (p.767·2).
Asthma; bronchitis; hypersensitivity reactions.

Astmazol Pharmasant, Thai.
Astemizole (p.409·1).
Hypersensitivity reactions.

Astomin Yamanouchi, Jpn†.
Dimemorfan phosphate (p.1089·1).
Coughs.

Astone Ramelca, Canad.†.
Aspirin (p.14·2); caffeine (p.761·3).

Astonin Merck, Spain.
Fludrocortisone (p.1070·1).
Adrenocortical insufficiency; hypotonia.

Astonin H
Merck, Aust.; Merck, Ger.
Fludrocortisone (p.1070·1).
Adrenocortical insufficiency; congenital adrenal hyperplasia; hypotension; peripheral perfusion disorders.

Astracaine AstraZeneca, Canad.
Articaine hydrochloride (p.1306·1).
Adrenaline [epinephrine] (p.829·1) is included in this preparation as a vasoconstrictor to diminish absorption and localise the effect of the local anaesthetic.
Local anaesthesia.

Astramorph PF Astra, USA.
Morphine sulfate (p.56·1).
Pain.

Astratonil Astra, Swed.
Multivitamin preparation (p.1350·1).

Astreptine Darci, Belg.†
Sulfanilamide (p.256·2).
Infected wounds.

Astressane Dolisos, Fr.†
Crataegus (p.1600·2); red-poppy petal (p.1029·1); passion flower (p.1649·1).
Cardiac irritability.

Astrexine Darci, Belg.
Chlorhexidine hydrochloride (p.1138·2).
Wounds and skin disinfection.

Astriderm Mex-America, Mex.
Resorcinol (p.1612·2).
Seborrhoeic dermatitis.

Astrin Vita Elan, Spain.
Fluoxetine hydrochloride (p.284·2).
Bulimia nervosa; depression; obsessive-compulsive disorder.

Astring-O-Sol Mentholatum, USA†.
Methyl salicylate (p.55·1); myrrh (p.1639·2); zinc chloride (p.1398·1).
Mouthwash.

Astrix
Faulding, Austral.; Faulding, Hong Kong; Faulding, Singapore.
Aspirin (p.14·2).
Thromboembolic disorders.

Astroglide Biofilm, USA.
Glycerol (p.1616·3); propylene glycol (p.1655·1); polyquaternium-5.
Vaginal lubricant.

Astronautal Strallhofer, Aust.
Diphenylpyraline hydrochloride (p.417·1); pyridoxine hydrochloride (p.1386·3).
Motion sickness; nausea; vertigo.

Astudal Almirall, Spain.
Amlodipine besilate (p.838·3).
Angina pectoris; hypertension.

Astyl Laphal, Fr.
Deanol bisorcate (p.1507·2).
Tonic.

Asvelik Medinsa, Spain†.
Tipepidine hibenzate (p.1101·3).
Coughs.

Asverin Tanabe, Jpn.
Tipepidine hibenzate (p.1101·3).
Coughs.

AT III Baxter, Ger.
Antithrombin III (p.725·2).
Antithrombin III deficiency.

AT 10
Merck, Aust.; Sanofi Synthelabo, Austral.†; Merck-Belgolabo, Belg.; Bayer, Ger.; Sanofi Winthrop, Irl.†; Bayer, S.Afr.†; Bayer, Switz.; Intrapharm, UK.
Dihydrotachysterol (p.1391·2).
Hypoparathyroidism with hypocalcaemia; osteomalacia; renal osteodystrophy; tetany; vitamin D-resistant rickets.

Atacand
Astra, Aust.; Astra, Austral.; Astra, Belg.; AstraZeneca, Canad.; Astra-Zeneca, Denm.; AstraZeneca, Fin.; AstraZeneca, Fr.; Astra, Ger.; Promed, Ger.; AstraZeneca, Irl.; Teva, Israel; Astra, Mex.; Astra, Neth.; AstraZeneca, Norw.; AstraZeneca, NZ; Astra, Port.; Astra, S.Afr.; AstraZeneca, Singapore; Astra, Spain; Hassle, Swed.; Astra, Switz.; ZLB, Switz.
Candesartan cilexetil (p.853·2).
Hypertension.

Atacand HCT AstraZeneca, USA.
Candesartan cilexetil (p.853·2); hydrochlorothiazide (p.907·3).
Hypertension.

Atacand Plus
AstraZeneca, Austral.; AstraZeneca, Irl.; Hassle, Swed.
Candesartan cilexetil (p.853·2); hydrochlorothiazide (p.907·3).
Hypertension.

Ataclor Errekappa, Ital.
Atenolol (p.841·3); chlortalidone (p.857·1).
Hypertension.

Atacoly Profarb, Braz.
Neomycin sulfate (p.228·1); clioquinol (p.190·2); attapulgite (p.1212·1); pectin (p.1502·3).
Diarrhoea.

Atagripe Windson, Braz.
Aspirin (p.14·2); mepyramine maleate (p.421·1); caffeine (p.761·3); vitamin C (p.1389·3).
Cold and influenza symptoms.

Atalin Gembolla, Braz.
Kaolin (p.1229·3); pectin (p.1502·3).
Diarrhoea.

Ataline
Medochemie, Hong Kong; Medochemie, Singapore; Medochemie, Thai.
Terbutaline sulfate (p.776·2).
Obstructive airways disease.

Atamet Athena Neurosciences, USA.
Carbidopa (p.1168·2); levodopa (p.1169·2).
Parkinsonism.

Atamir Biochemie, Denm.
Penicillamine (p.1017·1).
Cystinuria; heavy metal poisoning; rheumatoid arthritis; Wilson's disease.

Atano Milano, Thai.
Hydroxyzine hydrochloride (p.419·1).
Anxiety disoders; hypersensitivity reactions; pruritus.

Atapec Gembolla, Braz.
Homatropine methylbromide (p.468·1); furazolidone (p.592·1); pectin (p.1502·3).
Diarrhoea.

Atapryl Athena Neurosciences, USA.
Selegiline hydrochloride (p.1177·2).

Atarax
UCB, Austral.; Pfizer, Austral.; UCB, Belg.; Pfizer, Canad.; UCB, Denm.; UCB, Fin.; UCB, Fr.; UCB, Ger.; Rodleben, Ger.; Vedim, Ger.; UCB, Hong Kong; Pfizer, Irl.; UCB, Ital.; Riker, Mex.; UCB, Neth.; UCB, Norw.; UCB, Port.; UCB, Singapore; UCB, Swed.; UCB, Switz.; UCB, Thai.; Pfizer, UK; Pfizer, USA.
Hydroxyzine embonate (p.419·1) or hydroxyzine hydrochloride (p.419·1).
Alcohol withdrawal syndrome; anxiety disorders; hypersensitivity reactions; insomnia; nausea and vomiting; premedication; pruritus; urticaria.

Atarin Leiras, Fin.
Amantadine hydrochloride (p.1161·2).
Influenza A; parkinsonism.

Atarone Vinas, Spain†.
Pantethine (p.952·1).
Hyperlipidaemias.

Atasol Carter Horner, Canad.
Paracetamol (p.71·2).
Fever; pain.

Atasol-8, -15, -30 Carter Horner, Canad.
Paracetamol (p.71·2); codeine phosphate (p.25·2); caffeine citrate (p.761·3).
Fever; pain.

Atassol Solfran, Mex.
Dextromethorphan (p.1087·3).

Atatosse Balsamico Windson, Braz.
Potassium iodide (p.1522·3); menthol (p.1632·3).
Respiratory-tract congestion.

Atd Biolab, Thai.
Fluoxetine hydrochloride (p.284·2).
Depression.

Ate ABZ, Ger.
Atenolol (p.841·3).
Angina pectoris; arrhythmias; hypertension.

Ate Lich Lichtenstein, Ger.
Atenolol (p.841·3).
Angina pectoris; arrhythmias; hypertension; myocardial infarction.

Ate Lich comp Lichtenstein, Ger.
Atenolol (p.841·3); chlortalidone (p.857·1).
Hypertension.

Atebemyxine Chauvin, Fr.
Neomycin sulfate (p.228·1); polymyxin B sulfate (p.238·1).
Bacterial eye infections.

Atebeta Betapharm, Ger.
Atenolol (p.841·3).
Angina pectoris; arrhythmias; hypertension.

Atecor Rowex, Irl.
Atenolol (p.841·3).
Angina pectoris; arrhythmias; hypertension; myocardial infarction.

Atedurex Ecosol, Switz.
Atenolol (p.841·3); chlortalidone (p.857·1).
Hypertension.

Atehexal
Hexal, Aust.; Hexal, Austral.; Hexal, Ger.
Atenolol (p.841·3).
Angina pectoris; arrhythmias; hypertension; myocardial infarction.

Atehexal comp Hexal, Ger.
Atenolol (p.841·3); chlortalidone (p.857·1).
Hypertension.

Atel Betapharm, Ger.
Atenolol (p.841·3); chlortalidone (p.857·1).
Hypertension.

Atem Chiesi, Ital.
Ipratropium bromide (p.766·1).
Obstructive airways disease.

Atemaron N R30 Reckeweg, Ger.
Homoeopathic preparation.

Atemperator Armstrong, Mex.
Magnesium valproate (p.368·3).
Epilepsy; migraine.

Atemur Glaxo Wellcome, Ger.; Asta Medica, Ger.
Fluticasone propionate (p.1072·2).
Asthma.

Atenase UCI, Braz.
Niclosamide (p.104·2).
Cestode infections.

Atenativ
Pharmacia Upjohn, Aust.; Pharmacia Upjohn, Denm.; Pharmacia Upjohn, Fin.; Pharmacia Upjohn, Ger.; Pharmacia Upjohn, Neth.; Pharmacia Upjohn, Norw.; Pharmacia Upjohn, Spain; Pharmacia Upjohn, Swed.; ZLB, Switz.
Antithrombin III (p.725·2).
Antithrombin III deficiency.

Atenblock Pharmacia Upjohn, Fin.
Atenolol (p.841·3).
Angina pectoris; arrhythmias; hypertension; hyperthyroidism; myocardial infarction.

Atendol Pohl, Ger.
Atenolol (p.841·3).
Acute myocardial infarction; arrhythmias; hypertension; ischaemic heart disease.

Atenet Nettopharma, Denm.
Atenolol (p.841·3).
Angina pectoris; arrhythmias; hypertension; myocardial infarction.

Atenetic Gerard, Irl.
Atenolol (p.841·3); chlortalidone (p.857·1).
Hypertension.

Ateni Gerard, Irl.
Atenolol (p.841·3).
Angina pectoris; arrhythmias; hypertension; myocardial infarction.

AteNif beta Betapharm, Ger.
Atenolol (p.841·3); nifedipine (p.940·1).
Hypertension.

Ate-Nife Rowex, Irl.
Atenolol (p.841·3); nifedipine (p.940·1).
Angina pectoris; hypertension.

Atenigron Mitim, Ital.
Atenolol (p.841·3); chlortalidone (p.857·1).
Hypertension.

The symbol † denotes a preparation no longer actively marketed

Atenil Ecosol, Switz.
Atenolol (p.841·3).
Angina pectoris; arrhythmias; hypertension; myocardial infarction.

Atenix Ashbourne, UK.
Atenolol (p.841·3).
Angina pectoris; arrhythmias; hypertension.

AtenixCo Ashbourne, UK.
Atenolol (p.841·3); chlortalidone (p.857·1).
These ingredients can be described by the British Approved Name Co-tenidone.
Hypertension.

Ateno
Isis Puren, Ger.; Jean-Marie, Hong Kong.
Atenolol (p.841·3).
Alcohol withdrawal syndrome; angina pectoris; arrhythmias; hypertension; hyperthyroidism; migraine; myocardial infarction.

Ateno comp Isis Puren, Ger.
Atenolol (p.841·3); chlortalidone (p.857·1).
Hypertension.

ateno-basan Schonenberger, Switz.
Atenolol (p.841·3).
Angina pectoris; arrhythmias; hypertension; myocardial infarction.

ateno-basan comp. Schonenberger, Switz.
Atenolol (p.841·3); chlortalidone (p.857·1).
Hypertension.

Atenobene Ratiopharm, Aust.
Atenolol (p.841·3).
Angina pectoris; arrhythmias; hypertension; myocardial infarction.

Atenoblok Triomed, S.Afr.
Atenolol (p.841·3).
Angina pectoris; hypertension; myocardial infarction.

Atenoblok Co Triomed, S.Afr.
Atenolol (p.841·3); chlortalidone (p.857·1).
Hypertension.

Atenodan Pharmacodane, Denm.
Atenolol (p.841·3).
Angina pectoris; arrhythmias; hypertension; myocardial infarction.

Atenogamma Worwag, Ger.
Atenolol (p.841·3).
Angina pectoris; arrhythmias; hypertension.

Atenogamma comp Worwag, Ger.
Atenolol (p.841·3); chlortalidone (p.857·1).
Hypertension.

Atenogen Antigen, Irl.
Atenolol (p.841·3).
Angina pectoris; arrhythmias; hypertension; myocardial infarction.

Atenol
Zeneca, Braz.; Searle, Fin.; CT, Ital.; TO-Chemicals, Thai.
Atenolol (p.841·3).
Angina pectoris; arrhythmias; hypertension; hyperthyroidism; migraine; myocardial infarction.

Atenolan Lannacher, Aust.
Atenolol (p.841·3).
Angina pectoris; arrhythmias; hypertension; myocardial infarction.

Atenolan comp Lannacher, Aust.
Atenolol (p.841·3); chlortalidone (p.857·1).
Hypertension.

Atenolol AL comp Aliud, Ger.
Atenolol (p.841·3); chlortalidone (p.857·1).
Hypertension.

Atenolol comp
Genericon, Aust.; Ratiopharm, Ger.; CT, Ger.; Heumann, Ger.; Stada, Ger.
Atenolol (p.841·3); chlortalidone (p.857·1).
Hypertension.

Atenomel Clonmel, Irl.
Atenolol (p.841·3).
Angina pectoris; arrhythmias; hypertension; myocardial infarction.

Atenomerck Merck, Ger.†.
Atenolol (p.841·3).
Angina pectoris; arrhythmias; hypertension.

Atenomerck comp Merck, Ger.†.
Atenolol (p.841·3); chlortalidone (p.857·1).
Hypertension.

Atenor Durascan, Denm.
Atenolol (p.841·3).
Angina pectoris; arrhythmias; hypertension; myocardial infarction.

Atenos
UCB, Ger.; Vedim, Ger.; Rodleben, Ger.; UCB, Port.
Tulobuterol hydrochloride (p.785·2).
Asthma; bronchitis; bronchospastic disorders.

Atens Farmasa, Braz.
Enalapril maleate (p.883·3).
Heart failure; hypertension.

Atens H Farmasa, Braz.
Enalapril maleate (p.883·3); hydrochlorothiazide (p.907·3).
Hypertension.

Atensin Medochemie, Thai.
Propranolol hydrochloride (p.962·3).
Angina pectoris; arrhythmias; hypertension.

Atensina Boehringer de Angeli, Braz.
Clonidine hydrochloride (p.860·1).
Diagnosis of phaeochromocytoma; dysmenorrhoea; hypertension; menopausal disorders; migraine; opioid withdrawal syndrome; Tourette's syndrome.

Atepadene Mayoly-Spindler, Fr.
Adenosine triphosphate disodium (p.1573·3).
Pain.

Atepodin Medix, Spain.
Adenosine triphosphate sodium (p.1573·3).
Arrhythmias; muscular dystrophies; prevention of anoxia.

Ateran Eurofarmaco, Ital.
A heparinoid (p.905·2).
Thrombosis prophylaxis.

Aterax UCB, S.Afr.
Hydroxyzine hydrochloride (p.419·1).
Anxiety; hypersensitivity reactions; premedication.

Atereal Realpharma, Ger.†.
Atenolol (p.841·3).
Angina pectoris; arrhythmias; hypertension; myocardial infarction.

Ateren Rolab, S.Afr.
Atenolol (p.841·3); chlortalidone (p.857·1).
Hypertension.

Aterina Tedec Meiji, Spain.
Sulodexide (p.978·3).
Arteriosclerosis; atherosclerosis; thromboembolic disorders.

Atermin Magis, Ital.
Atenolol (p.841·3).
Angina pectoris; arrhythmias; hypertension; myocardial infarction.

Ateroclar Medibase, Ital.
Heparin sodium (p.902·1).
Thromboembolic disorders.

Ateroid Crinos, Ital.
A heparinoid (p.905·2).
Thrombosis prophylaxis.

Ateroide Breves, Braz.
Ointment: A heparinoid (p.905·2); methyl nicotinate (p.55·1).
Inflammation.
Tablets: A heparinoid (p.905·2).
Hyperlipidaemias.

Aterol Rolab, S.Afr.
Atenolol (p.841·3).
Now known as Rolab-Atenolol.
Angina pectoris; hypertension.

Ateroxide Ripari-Gero, Ital.
A heparinoid (p.905·2).
Thrombosis prophylaxis.

Atesifar Siphar, Switz.
Atenolol (p.841·3).
Angina pectoris; arrhythmias; hypertension.

ATG
Serotherapeutisches, Aust.†.
Antithymocyte immunoglobulin (horse) (p.508·2).
Transplant rejection.

Aventis, Belg.; Fresenius, Hong Kong; Fresenius Kabi, Switz.; Fresenius, Thai.
Antithymocyte immunoglobulin (rabbit) (p.508·2).
Graft-versus-host disease; transplant rejection.

Atgam
Pharmacia Upjohn, Austral.; Pharmacia Upjohn, Belg.; Pharmacia Upjohn, Canad.; Pharmacia Upjohn, Hong Kong; Pharmacia Upjohn, Israel; Pharmacia Upjohn, NZ; Pharmacia Upjohn, S.Afr.; Pharmacia Upjohn, Singapore; Pharmacia Upjohn, Spain†; Pharmacia Upjohn, Switz.; Upjohn, USA.
Antithymocyte immunoglobulin (horse) (p.508·2).
Aplastic anaemia; renal transplant rejection.

ATG-S Fresenius, Israel.
Antithymocyte immunoglobulin (rabbit) (p.508·2).
Transplant rejection.

Athelmin Apsen, Braz.
Mebendazole (p.102·2).
Worm infections.

Athera Lane, UK.
Parsley (p.1648·3); vervain (p.1679·3); senna leaf (p.1248·2); clivers (p.1596·3).
Menopausal symptoms.

Athero Ono, Hong Kong.
Choline bitartrate (p.1356·3); carbazochrome; rutoside; linoleic acid; vitamin A; vitamin B$_6$; vitamin E.
Hyperlipidaemias.

Athimbin P Centeon, Aust.
Antithrombin III (p.725·2).
Antithrombin III deficiency.

Athletes Foot Scholl, Israel.
Tolnaftate (p.395·2).
Tinea pedis.

Athletes Foot Antifungal Pedi-Pak, Canad.†.
Aluminium chlorohydrate (p.1110·2); undecenoic acid (p.395·3); zinc undecenoate (p.395·3).
Tinea pedis.

Athletes Foot Cream Wallis, UK.
Clotrimazole (p.382·1).
Tinea pedis.

Athos Medix, Mex.
Dextromethorphan hydrobromide (p.1087·3).
Coughs.

Athru-Derm Meyer Zall, S.Afr.
Diclofenac sodium (p.30·3).
Inflammation; pain.

Athymil Organon, Fr.
Mianserin hydrochloride (p.298·1).
Depression.

Atiflan Ederka, Mex.
Naproxen (p.60·3).

Atilan Zambon, Braz.
Fentiazac (p.40·2).
Musculoskeletal and joint disorders.

Atinorm Bioprogress, Ital.
Atenolol (p.841·3); indapamide (p.913·1).
Hypertension.

Atiramin Juste, Spain.
Azatadine maleate (p.409·2); pseudoephedrine sulfate (p.1099·3).
Allergic rhinitis.

Atirosin Piam, Ital.
Infant feed (p.1350·1).
Tyrosinaemia.

Atisuril Byk Gulden, Mex.
Allopurinol (p.397·2).
Gout; hyperuricaemia; renal calculi.

Atiten Bayer, Ital.
Dihydrotachysterol (p.1391·2).
Formerly known as AT 10.
Hypoparathyroidism; pseudohypoparathyroidism.

Ativan
Wyeth, Austral.; Wyeth-Ayerst, Canad.; Wyeth-Ayerst, Hong Kong; Wyeth, Irl.; Wyeth, Mex.; Wyeth, NZ; Aspen, S.Afr.; Wyeth, Singapore; Wyeth-Ayerst, Thai.; Wyeth, UK; Wyeth-Ayerst, USA.
Lorazepam (p.688·3).
Anxiety; insomnia; mania; nausea and vomiting; premedication; status epilepticus.

Ativit Heralds, Braz.
Cyproheptadine (p.414·3); vitamins and minerals (p.1350·1).
Reduced appetite; tonic.

Atkinson & Barker's Gripe Mixture Torbet Laboratories, UK.
Sodium bicarbonate (p.1186·2); caraway oil (p.1591·2); dill oil (p.1603·3).
Formerly contained light magnesium carbonate, sodium bicarbonate, fennel oil, and dill oil.
Infant colic.

Atlansil Sanofi Winthrop, Braz.
Amiodarone hydrochloride (p.836·1).
Arrhythmias.

Atmocol Thackray, UK.
A deodorant spray for use with colostomies and ileostomies.

Atmos
AstraZeneca, Denm.; AstraZeneca, Fin.; AstraZeneca, Norw.; Astra, Swed.
Testosterone (p.1492·1).
Erectile dysfunction; hypogonadism; osteoporosis.

ATnativ Hyland, USA†.
Antithrombin III (p.725·2).
Antithrombin III deficiency.

Atock Yamanouchi, Jpn.
Eformoterol [formoterol] fumarate (p.764·2).
Obstructive airways disease.

Atodel Remedica, Thai.
Prazosin hydrochloride (p.958·1).
Heart failure; hypertension; Raynaud's syndrome.

Atoderm Polaris, Ital.
Emollient.
Dry skin disorders.

Atolant SS, Jpn.
Neticonazole hydrochloride (p.392·2).
Fungal skin infections.

Atolone Major, USA.
Triamcinolone (p.1080·1).
Corticosteroid.

Atomase
Douglas, Hong Kong; Douglas, NZ; Douglas, Singapore; Douglas, Thai.; TTN, Thai.
Beclometasone dipropionate (p.1061·2).
Nasal polyps; rhinitis.

Atomic Enema Health Chemical, Hong Kong.
Sodium chloride (p.1196·1).
Constipation.

Atomide Douglas, NZ.
Beclometasone dipropionate (p.1061·2).
Obstructive airways disease.

Atomolan Kyowa, Jpn†.
Glutathione (p.1010·3).
Corneal injury; drug and metal poisoning; liver disorders; radiation-induced inflammation of oral mucosa; radiation-induced leucopenia; skin disorders; vomiting.

Atopic Dermoteca, Port.
Evening primrose oil (p.1613·2).
Eczema.

Atosil Bayer, Ger.
Promethazine hydrochloride (p.423·2).
Gastrointestinal disorders; hypersensitivity reactions; insomnia; motion sickness; nausea and vomiting; premedication; psychiatric disorders; respiratory disorders.

Atossion Elofar, Braz.
Dropropizine (p.1089·3).
Coughs.

Atossisclerol Kreussler Also, Ital.
Lauromacrogol 400 (p.1345·2).
Sclerotherapy of varices.

Atrac-Tain Sween, USA†.
Urea (p.1127·3).
Dry skin.

Atractil
Trenker, Belg.; Trenker, Thai.
Diethylpropion (p.1508·3).
Obesity.

Atralcilina Atral, Port.
Benzylpenicillin potassium (p.157·1); procaine penicillin [procaine benzylpenicillin] (p.239·2).
Bacterial infections.

Atralidon Atral, Port.
Paracetamol (p.71·2).
Fever; pain.

Atralmicina Atral, Port.
Benethamine penicillin (p.156·2); benzylpenicillin sodium (p.157·2).
Bacterial infections.

Atretol Athena Neurosciences, USA.
Carbamazepine (p.342·2).
Epilepsy; trigeminal neuralgia.

Atrican Innotech, Fr.
Tenonitrozole (p.603·2).
Urogenital trichomoniasis.

Atridox Atrix, UK.
Doxycycline hyclate (p.200·1).
Bacterial mouth infections.

Atrilon Byk, Port.
Lonazolac calcium (p.50·2).
Musculoskeletal, joint, and peri-articular disorders; pain.

Atrisol Química y Farmacia, Mex.
Captopril (p.853·3).
Hypertension.

Atrium
Riom, Fr.†.
Febarbamate (p.683·2); difebarbamate (p.682·1); phenobarbital (p.355·1).
Alcohol withdrawal syndrome.

Roche, Switz.†.
Tetrabamate, a complex of febarbamate (p.683·2), difebarbamate (p.682·1), and phenobarbital (p.355·1).
Anxiety disorders; tremor.

Atro Grin Grin, Mex.
Atropine (p.460·3).
Production of mydriasis.

Atrobel Fawns & McAllan, Austral.
Belladonna herb (p.463·1).
Peptic ulcer; reduction of secretions; smooth muscle spasm.

Atrodual Boehringer Ingelheim, Fin.
Ipratropium bromide (p.766·1); salbutamol sulfate (p.770·3).
Obstructive airways disease.

Atrohist Pediatric Medeva, USA.
Capsules: Pseudoephedrine hydrochloride (p.1099·2); chlorpheniramine [chlorphenamine] maleate (p.412·1).
Formerly contained brompheniramine maleate, phenyltoxamine citrate and phenylephrine hydrochloride.
Allergic rhinitis; cold symptoms; sinusitis.
Oral suspension: Chlorpheniramine [chlorphenamine] tannate (p.412·2); phenylephrine tannate (p.1097·3); mepyramine tannate (p.421·1).
Cold symptoms; nasal congestion.

Atrohist Plus Medeva, USA†.
Phenylpropanolamine hydrochloride (p.1098·1); phenylephrine hydrochloride (p.1097·1); chlorpheniramine [chlorphenamine] maleate (p.412·1); hyoscyamine sulfate (p.469·3); atropine sulfate (p.461·1); hyoscine hydrobromide (p.468·2).
Upper respiratory-tract symptoms.

Atrombin Leiras, Fin.
Dipyridamole (p.877·2).
Thromboembolic disorders.

Atromidin
Zeneca, Belg.†; Zeneca, Denm.†; Zeneca, Swed.†.
Clofibrate (p.859·1).
Hyperlipidaemias; prophylaxis of ischaemic heart disease in high-risk patients.

Atromid-S
ICI, Austral.†; Wyeth-Ayerst, Canad.; Zeneca, Hong Kong; Zeneca, Irl.; Zeneca, Mex.; AstraZeneca, NZ; Zeneca, Port.; Zeneca, S.Afr.†; AstraZeneca, UK†; Wyeth-Ayerst, USA.
Clofibrate (p.859·1).
Hyperlipidaemias.

Atronase
Boehringer Ingelheim, Aust.; Boehringer Ingelheim, Belg.; Boehringer Ingelheim, S.Afr.†.
Ipratropium bromide (p.766·1).
Rhinitis.

AtroPen Survival Technology, USA.
Atropine sulfate (p.461·1).
Organophosphorus or carbamate pesticide poisoning.

Atropine and Demerol Sanofi Winthrop, USA.
Atropine sulfate (p.461·1); pethidine hydrochloride (p.75·1).
Sedative.

Atropinol Winzer, Ger.
Atropine (p.460·3).
Eye disorders.

Atropisol
Ciba Vision, Canad.; Ciba Vision, USA.
Atropine sulfate (p.461·1).
Production of mydriasis and cycloplegia.

Atropocil Oftalder, Port.
Atropine sulfate (p.461·1).
Production of mydriasis and cycloplegia.

Atropt
Sigma, Austral.; Pharmaco, NZ.
Atropine sulfate (p.461·1).
Production of cycloplegia and mydriasis.

Atrosept *Geneva, USA.*
Methenamine (p.223·1); salol (p.82·2); atropine sulfate (p.461·1); hyoscyamine sulfate (p.469·3); benzoic acid (p.1134·2); methylene blue [methylthioninium chloride] (p.1012·3).
Urinary-tract infections.

Atrospan *Fischer, Israel.*
Atropine sulfate (p.461·1).
Production of cycloplegia and mydriasis.

Atrovent *Boehringer Ingelheim, Aust.; Boehringer Ingelheim, Austral.; Boehringer Ingelheim, Belg.; Boehringer de Angeli, Braz.; Boehringer Ingelheim, Canad.; Boehringer Ingelheim, Denm.; Boehringer Ingelheim, Fin.; Boehringer Ingelheim, Fr.; Boehringer Ingelheim, Ger.; Boehringer Ingelheim, Hong Kong; Boehringer Ingelheim, Irl.; Boehringer Ingelheim, Ital.; Boehringer Ingelheim, Mex.; Boehringer Ingelheim, Neth.; Boehringer Ingelheim, Norw.; Boehringer Ingelheim, NZ; Boehringer Ingelheim, Port.; Boehringer Ingelheim, S.Afr.; Boehringer Ingelheim, Singapore; Boehringer Ingelheim, Spain; Boehringer Ingelheim, Swed.; Boehringer Ingelheim, Switz.; Boehringer Ingelheim, Thai.; Boehringer Ingelheim, UK; Boehringer Ingelheim, USA.*
Ipratropium bromide (p.766·1).
Obstructive airways disease; rhinitis.

Atrovent Beta *Boehringer Ingelheim, S.Afr.*
Ipratropium bromide (p.766·1); fenoterol hydrobromide (p.765·1).
Obstructive airways disease.

Atrovent Comp *Boehringer Ingelheim, Fin.*
Ipratropium bromide (p.766·1); fenoterol hydrobromide (p.765·1).
Obstructive airways disease.

Atroveran *Virtus, Braz.*
Oral solution: Papaverine hydrochloride (p.1648·1); belladonna (p.463·1); star anise; hyoscyamus (p.470·1); boldo (p.1585·3).
Smooth muscle spasm.
Tablets: Papaverine hydrochloride (p.1648·1); aspirin (p.14·2); belladonna (p.463·1).
Pain; smooth muscle spasm.

Atrovex *Medquimica, Braz.*
Papaverine (p.1648·1); belladonna (p.463·1); star anise; hyoscyamus (p.470·1); boldo (p.1585·3).
Smooth muscle spasm.

ATS *Hoechst Marion Roussel, USA.*
Erythromycin (p.201·2).
Acne.

Atta *Ranbaxy, Thai.*
Activated attapulgite (p.1212·1).
Diarrhoea.

Attafur *Ranbaxy, Thai.*
Activated attapulgite (p.1212·1); furazolidone (p.592·1).
Diarrhoea.

Attain *Sherwood, USA.*
Lactose-free preparation for enteral nutrition (p.1350·1).

Attenta *Alphapharm, Austral.*
Methylphenidate hydrochloride (p.1511·3).
Attention-deficit hyperactivity disorder; narcoleptic syndrome.

Attenuvax *Merck Sharp & Dohme, Aust.†; Prodome, Braz.; Pasteur Merieux, Denm.; Pasteur Merieux, Ital.†; Merck Sharp & Dohme, Neth.†; Pro Vaccine, Switz.; Merck, USA.*
A live measles vaccine (more attenuated Enders' Edmonston strain) (p.1547·1).
Active immunisation.

Aturgyl
Note.This name is used for preparations of different composition.
SmithKline Beecham, Braz.
Fenoxazoline (p.1091·3).
Nasal congestion.

Synthelabo, Fr.
Oxymetazoline hydrochloride (p.1096·2).
Formerly contained fenoxazoline hydrochloride.
Rhinopharyngeal congestion.

Atus *Metapharma, Ital.*
Ambroxol hydrochloride (p.1084·3).
Respiratory-tract disorders.

Atuss DM *Atley, USA.*
Dextromethorphan hydrobromide (p.1087·3); phenylephrine hydrochloride (p.1097·1); chlorpheniramine [chlorphenamine] maleate (p.412·1).
Coughs and associated respiratory-tract disorders.

Atuss EX *Atley, USA.*
Hydrocodone tartrate (p.42·2); guaifenesin (p.1092·2).
Coughs and associated respiratory-tract disorders.

Atuss G *Atley, USA.*
Hydrocodone tartrate (p.42·2); phenylephrine hydrochloride (p.1097·1); guaifenesin (p.1092·2).
Coughs and associated respiratory-tract disorders.

Atuss HD *Atley, USA.*
Hydrocodone tartrate (p.42·2); phenylephrine hydrochloride (p.1097·1); chlorpheniramine [chlorphenamine] maleate (p.412·1).
Coughs and associated respiratory-tract disorders.

Atuxane *Monot, Fr.†*
Dextromethorphan hydrobromide (p.1087·3).
Coughs.

AU 4 Regeneresen *Dyckerhoff, Ger.*
Ribonucleic acid (p.1657·3).
Ear disorders.

Aubeline *Arkopharma, Fr.*
Crataegus (p.1600·2).
Cardiac disorders; nervous disorders.

Audax *Mundipharma, Ger.; Seton, Irl.; Ethimed, S.Afr.†; SSL, UK.*
Choline salicylate (p.24·3).
Aid to ear wax removal; earache.

Audazol *Lesvi, Spain.*
Omeprazole (p.1239·1) or omeprazole sodium (p.1239·1).
Gastro-oesophageal reflux; peptic ulcer; Zollinger-Ellison syndrome.

Audicort
Lederle, Irl.; Wyeth, UK.
Neomycin undecenoate (p.228·1); triamcinolone acetonide (p.1080·1).
Formerly contained benzocaine, triamcinolone acetonide, and neomycin undecenoate in the UK.
Inflammatory ear disorders with bacterial infection.

Audifluor *Diba, Mex.*
Sodium fluoride (p.1375·3).
Otosclerosis.

Audione *Serra Pamies, Spain.*
Vitamins (p.1350·1); potassium iodide (p.1522·3).
Ear disorders; eye disorders.

Audispray *Diepha, Fr.*
Sea water.
External ear hygiene.

Auditol *Synthelabo, Braz.*
Phenazone (p.77·2); procaine (p.1319·2).
Inflammatory ear disorders.

Augenkraft *Twardy, Ger.*
Vitamin A (p.1382·1).
Night-blindness.

Augentonicum *Stulln, Switz.*
Digitalis (p.869·1); digitoxin (p.869·2); esculoside (p.1574·1).
Eye disorders.

Augentonikum *Stulln, Ger.*
Digitalin (p.1603·2); vitamin A palmitate (p.1383·2).
Eyestrain.

Augentropfen Mucokehl D5 *Sanum-Kehlbeck, Ger.*
Homoeopathic preparation.

Augentropfen Stulln *Sanova, Aust.*
Digitalis (p.869·1); esculoside (p.1574·1).

Augentropfen Stulln Mono *Stulln, Ger.*
Digitalis leaf (p.869·1); esculoside (p.1574·1).
Eyestrain.

Augmaxil *Triomed, S.Afr.*
Amoxicillin (p.149·2); clavulanic acid (p.187·2).
Bacterial infections.

Augmentan *SmithKline Beecham, Ger.*
Amoxicillin sodium (p.149·2) or amoxicillin trihydrate (p.149·2); potassium clavulanate (p.187·2).
Bacterial infections.

Augmentin *SmithKline Beecham, Aust.; SmithKline Beecham, Austral.; SmithKline Beecham, Belg.; SmithKline Beecham, Braz.; SmithKline Beecham, Fin.; SmithKline Beecham, Fr.; SmithKline Beecham, Hong Kong; SmithKline Beecham, Irl.; SmithKline Beecham, Israel; SmithKline Beecham, Ital.; SmithKline Beecham, Mex.; SmithKline Beecham, Neth.; SmithKline Beecham, NZ; Beecham, Port.; SmithKline Beecham, S.Afr.; SmithKline Beecham, Singapore; SmithKline Beecham, Switz.; SmithKline Beecham, Thai.; SmithKline Beecham, UK; SmithKline Beecham, USA.*
Amoxicillin sodium (p.149·2) or amoxicillin trihydrate (p.149·2); potassium clavulanate (p.187·2).
These ingredients can be described by the British Approved Name Co-amoxiclav.
Bacterial infections.

Augmentin-Duo *SmithKline Beecham, UK.*
Amoxicillin trihydrate (p.149·2); potassium clavulanate (p.187·2).
These ingredients can be described by the British Approved Name Co-amoxiclav.

Augmentine *SmithKline Beecham, Spain.*
Amoxicillin sodium (p.149·2) or amoxicillin trihydrate (p.149·2); potassium clavulanate (p.187·2).
Bacterial infections.

Aulcer *Alacan, Spain.*
Omeprazole (p.1239·1).
Gastro-oesophageal reflux; peptic ulcer; Zollinger-Ellison syndrome.

Aulin *Helsinn Birex, Irl.; Roche, Ital.; Helsinn, Port.; Roche, Switz.*
Nimesulide (p.62·3).
Fever; inflammation; musculoskeletal, joint, and periarticular disorders; pain.

Aunativ
Pharmacia Upjohn, Aust.; Pharmacia Upjohn, Denm.; Pharmacia Upjohn, Ger.†; Pharmacia Upjohn, Norw.; Pharmacia Upjohn, Swed.
A hepatitis B immunoglobulin (p.1542·1).
Passive immunisation.

Auralgan
Note.This name is used for preparations of different composition.
Whitehall, Austral.; Whitehall-Robins, Canad.; Wyeth-Ayerst, USA.
Benzocaine (p.1306·2); phenazone (p.77·2); glycerol (p.1616·3).
Acute otitis media; ear wax removal.

Wyeth-Ayerst, Thai.
Benzocaine (p.1306·2); phenazone (p.77·2).
Ear wax removal; otitis media.

Auralgicin *Roche, S.Afr.*
Ephedrine hydrochloride (p.1090·1); phenazone (p.77·2); benzocaine (p.1306·2); potassium hydroxyquinoline sulfate (p.1654·2).
Otitis media.

Auralyt *Whitehall-Robins, Mex.*
Benzocaine (p.1306·2).

Auramin *Solco, Aust.*
Minocycline hydrochloride (p.224·3).
Bacterial infections.

Aurantin *Parke, Davis, Ital.*
Phenytoin sodium (p.357·2).
Arrhythmias; epilepsy.

Auraphene-B *Reese, USA.*
Urea hydrogen peroxide (p.1159·3).

Aurasept *Restan, S.Afr.*
Benzocaine (p.1306·2); phenazone (p.77·2).
Otitis.

Aurasol *Optimax, USA†.*
Colloidal gold (p.1617·3).

Auratek hCG *Organon, UK.*
Pregnancy test (p.1654·3).

Aurecil *Oftalder, Port.*
Chlortetracycline hydrochloride (p.182·1).
Bacterial eye infections.

Aureocort *Wyeth Lederle, Aust.; Wyeth Lederle, Fin.; Wyeth, Irl.; Teofarma, Ital.; Wyeth, UK.*
Chlortetracycline hydrochloride (p.182·1); triamcinolone acetonide (p.1080·1).
Infected skin disorders.

Aureodelf *Lederle, Ger.*
Chlortetracycline hydrochloride (p.182·1); triamcinolone acetonide (p.1080·1).
Infected skin disorders.

Aureodermil *Oftalder, Port.*
Chlortetracycline hydrochloride (p.182·1).
Bacterial skin infections.

Aureomicina *Wyeth Lederle, Ital.; Wyeth, Mex.; Alcon, Port.†; Alcon Cusi, Spain; Ciba Vision, Spain.*
Chlortetracycline hydrochloride (p.182·1).
Bacterial infections.

Aureomix *SIT, Ital.*
Chlortetracycline hydrochloride (p.182·1); sulfacetamide sodium (p.250·3).
Ear, nose, throat, and eye infections.

Aureomycin *Wyeth Lederle, Aust.; Lederle, Austral.; Wyeth Lederle, Belg.; Wyeth-Ayerst, Canad.; Wyeth Lederle, Denm.†; Wyeth Lederle, Fin.; Lederle, Ger.; Lederle, Hong Kong; Wyeth, Irl.; Lederle, Israel; Lederle, Neth.; Wyeth Lederle, Norw.; Wyeth, NZ; Wyeth, S.Afr.; Wyeth Lederle, Swed.; Wyeth-Ayerst, Thai.; Wyeth, UK.*
Chlortetracycline (p.182·1) or chlortetracycline hydrochloride (p.182·1).
Bacterial infections.

Aureomycin N *Lederle, Ger.*
Chlortetracycline hydrochloride (p.182·1); nystatin (p.392·2).
Vaginal infections.

Aureomycine *Asta Medica, Belg.; Medeva, Fr.; Lederle, Switz.*
Chlortetracycline hydrochloride (p.182·1).
Bacterial eye, skin, and mouth infections.

Aureotan *Tosse, Ger.†.*
Aurothioglucose (p.18·3).
Chronic polyarthritis; psoriatic arthritis.

Auricularum *Grimberg, Fr.; Serolam, Israel.*
Oxytetracycline hydrochloride (p.234·1); polymyxin B sulfate (p.238·1); dexamethasone sodium phosphate (p.1067·1); nystatin (p.392·2).
Otitis.

Auricum *Dolisos, Canad.*
Homoeopathic preparation.

Aurigoutte *Monot, Fr.*
Hexamidine isetionate (p.1146·2); lignocaine [lidocaine] hydrochloride (p.1313·2).
Ear disorders.

Aurisan *Nadeau, Canad.*
Benzocaine (p.1306·2); camphor (p.1589·3); chlorobutanol (p.1141·2).
Ear ache.

Auristan *Monin, Fr.*
Phenylephrine hydrochloride (p.1097·1).
Otitis externa.

Auritricin *Delta, Braz.*
Tyrothricin (p.267·1); etyl metaborate; chlorobutanol (p.1141·2).
Ear infections.

Auro *Del, USA.*
Urea hydrogen peroxide (p.1159·3).
Ear wax removal.

Auroanalin *Hevert, Ger.*
Glycol salicylate (p.42·2); benzyl nicotinate (p.20·2).
Inflammation; rheumatism.

Auroclim *Juste, Spain.*
16 Tablets, estradiol valerate (p.1473·2); 12 tablets, estradiol valerate; levonorgestrel (p.1486·2).
Menopausal disorders; osteoporosis.

Auro-Dri *Del, USA.*
Isopropyl alcohol (p.1149·2); boric acid (p.1586·1).
Ear disorders.

Aurolate *Pasadena, USA.*
Sodium aurothiomalate (p.82·3).

Auromyose *Nourypharma, Neth.*
Aurothioglucose (p.18·3).
Rheumatoid arthritis.

Aurone *Aspen Consumer, S.Afr.*
Phenazone (p.77·2).
Earache.

Aurone Forte *Aspen Consumer, S.Afr.*
Phenazone (p.77·2); benzocaine (p.1306·2).
Earache.

Auroplatin *Steigerwald, Ger.*
Homoeopathic preparation.

Aurorex *Roche, Mex.*
Moclobemide (p.299·3).
Depression; phobias.

Aurorix *Roche, Aust.; Roche, Austral.; Roche, Belg.; Roche, Braz.; Roche, Denm.; Roche, Fin.; Roche, Ger.; Roche, Hong Kong; Roche, Ital.; Roche, Neth.; Roche, Norw.; Roche, NZ; Roche, Port.; Roche, S.Afr.; Roche, Singapore; Roche, Swed.; Roche, Switz.; Roche, Thai.*
Moclobemide (p.299·3).
Depression; phobias.

Aurosulfo *Geymonat, Ital.†.*
Colloidal gold sulfide.
Rheumatoid arthritis.

Aurosyx N *Syxyl, Ger.*
Homoeopathic preparation.

Auroto *Barre-National, USA.*
Benzocaine (p.1306·2); phenazone (p.77·2).
Earache.

Aurum-Gastreu N R2 *Reckeweg, Ger.*
Homoeopathic preparation.

Auscap *Sigma, Austral.*
Fluoxetine hydrochloride (p.284·2).
Depression; obsessive-compulsive disorder.

Auscard *Sigma, Austral.*
Diltiazem hydrochloride (p.874·3).
Angina pectoris.

Ausclav *Sigma, Austral.*
Amoxicillin trihydrate (p.149·2); potassium clavulanate (p.187·2).
Bacterial infections.

Ausgem *Sigma, Austral.*
Gemfibrozil (p.896·2).
Hyperlipidaemias.

Ausobronc *Biotekfarma, Ital.†.*
Mesna (p.1011·3).
Respiratory-tract disorders.

Ausomina *Biotekfarma, Ital.†.*
Vincamine (p.1680·1).
Cerebrovascular disorders.

Ausran *Sigma, Austral.*
Ranitidine hydrochloride (p.1245·2).
Gastro-oesophageal reflux; peptic ulcer; Zollinger-Ellison syndrome.

Aussie Tan *Or-Dov, Austral.*
SPF 4: Octinoxate (p.1517·3); avobenzone (p.1517·1).
SPF 7: Octinoxate (p.1517·3); avobenzone (p.1517·1); oxybenzone (p.1518·1).
SPF 15 Lotion: Octinoxate (p.1517·3); avobenzone (p.1517·1); oxybenzone (p.1518·1).
SPF 15 Topical gel: Octinoxate (p.1517·3); avobenzone (p.1517·1).
Sunscreen.

Aussie Tan Pre-Tan *Or-Dov, Austral.*
Tyrosine (p.1381·3); tyrosinase.
To accelerate tanning.

Aussie Tan Skin Moisturiser *Or-Dov, Austral.*
Urea (p.1127·3); lactic acid (p.1626·2).

Aussie Tan Sunstick *Or-Dov, Austral.*
Salol (p.82·2).
Sunscreen.

Austral-Balm *Nutri-Pharm, Austral.*
Melaleuca oil (p.1631·3); eucalyptus oil (p.1609·2); sweet birch oil (p.55·2); emu oil; lemon oil (p.1628·2); peppermint oil (p.1243·3).
Musculoskeletal and joint pain.

Austrapen *CSL, Austral.*
Ampicillin sodium (p.150·3).
Bacterial infections.

Austrialens *Austroflex, Aust.*
Cleaning, wetting, and storage solutions for hard and gas-permeable contact lenses (p.1129·2).

Austroflex *Austroflex, Aust.*
Range of contact lens solutions (p.1129·2).

Austrophyllin *Petrasch, Aust.*
Diprophylline (p.764·1).

Austrorinse *Austroflex, Aust.*
Rinsing solution for contact lenses (p.1129·2).

Austrosept *Austroflex, Aust.*
Hydrogen peroxide (p.1147·1) (p.1129·2).
Disinfecting solution for soft contact lenses.

Austyn *Faulding, Austral.; Faulding, Singapore.*
Theophylline (p.777·2).
Obstructive airways disease.

Autan *Bayer, Ger.†.*
Diethyltoluamide (p.1431·2).
Insect repellent.

Autonic *Acusan, Ger.†.*
Caffeine (p.761·3).
Fatigue.

Autoplasme Vaillant *Chefaro Ardeval, Fr.*
Black mustard (p.1639·1).
Respiratory-tract congestion.

Autoplex *Baxter-Hyland, Ger.; Baxter, Swed.; Travenol, UK.*
A factor VIII inhibitor bypassing fraction (p.734·3).
Haemorrhage in patients with inhibitors to factor VIII.

Autoplex T *Baxter, Belg.†; Baxter, Singapore; Baxter, Spain†; Nabi, USA.*
A factor VIII inhibitor bypassing fraction (p.734·3).
Haemorrhage in patients with inhibitor to factor VIII.

The symbol † denotes a preparation no longer actively marketed

Autosterile *Allergan, Aust.*
Contact lens cleaner (p.1129·2).

Autrin
Wyeth, Mex.
Ferrous fumarate (p.1360·1); folic acid; vitamin B₁₂; ascorbic acid; vitamin E (p.1350·1).
Anaemias.

Wyeth, S.Afr.
Ferrous fumarate (p.1360·1); folic acid; vitamin B₁₂; intrinsic factor; vitamin C (p.1350·1).
Anaemias.

Autritis *Tecnimede, Port.*
Indometacin (p.44·3).

Auxergyl D₃ *Roussel Diamant, Fr.; Roussel, Port.*
Vitamin A (p.1382·1); colecalciferol (p.1391·1).
Vitamin A and D deficiency.

Auxiloson *Boehringer Ingelheim, Ger.*
Dexamethasone isonicotinate (p.1067·1).
Respiratory-tract disorders.

Auxina A + E *Alcala, Spain.*
Vitamin A palmitate (p.1383·2); tocoferil acetate (p.1394·1).
Deficiency of vitamins A and E; eye disorders; infertility; recurrent miscarriage; skin disorders.

Auxina A Masiva *Alcala, Spain.*
Vitamin A palmitate (p.1383·2).
Vitamin A deficiency.

Auxina Complejo B *Alcala, Spain.*
Vitamin B substances (p.1350·1).

Auxina E *Alcala, Spain.*
Tocoferil acetate (p.1394·1).
Biliary-tract disorders; cystic fibrosis; hypoproteinaemia; prevention of intraventricular haemorrhage in premature neonates; vitamin E deficiency.

Auxisone *Boehringer Ingelheim, Fr.†.*
Dexamethasone isonicotinate (p.1067·1).
Obstructive airways disease.

Auxitrans *Alpharma, Fr.*
Pentaerythritol (p.1243·2).
Constipation.

Avafontan *Alpharma, Mex.*
Dipyrone (p.34·1).
Fever; pain.

Avafortan *Therabel, Fr.*
Camylofin hydrochloride (p.1590·1) or camylofin noramidopyrine mesilate (p.1590·1); dipyrone (p.34·1).
Pain; smooth muscle spasm.

Avail *Menley & James, USA.*
Multivitamin and mineral preparation with iron and folic acid (p.1350·1).

Avalide *Bristol-Myers Squibb, USA.*
Irbesartan (p.914·2); hydrochlorothiazide (p.907·3).
Hypertension.

Avalin *Piam, Ital.*
Infant feed (p.1350·1).
Maple syrup urine disease.

Avallone *Novartis, Aust.*
Ibuprofen (p.43·2).
Inflammation; musculoskeletal and joint disorders; pain.

Avalon *Difa, Ital.*
Avena (p.1583·1).
Emollient skin cleanser.

Avalox *Bayer, Ger.*
Moxifloxacin hydrochloride (p.225·3).
Bacterial infections.

Avamigran
Note.This name is used for preparations of different composition.
Asta Medica, Aust.
Ergotamine tartrate (p.452·1); mecloxamine citrate (p.470·2); camylofin hydrochloride (p.1590·1); caffeine (p.761·3); propyphenazone (p.80·2).
Cluster headache; migraine.

Asta Medica, Port.
Ergotamine tartrate (p.452·1); propyphenazone (p.80·2).
Formerly contained ergotamine tartrate, propyphenazone, caffeine, camylofin hydrochloride, and mecloxamine citrate.
Cluster headache; vascular headache.

Asta Medica, Thai.
Ergotamine tartrate (p.452·1); caffeine (p.761·3).
Migraine and related vascular headaches.

Avamigran N *Asta Medica, Ger.*
Ergotamine tartrate (p.452·1); propyphenazone (p.80·2).
Cluster headache; migraine.

Avan *Takeda, Jpn†.*
Idebenone (p.1623·1).
Cerebrovascular disorders.

Avance *SSL, UK.*
Hydropolymer wound dressing containing silver (p.1664·1).
Exuding wounds.

Avancort *Farmades, Ital.*
Methylprednisolone aceponate (p.1076·2).
Skin disorders.

Avandia
SmithKline Beecham, Austral.; SmithKline Beecham, Irl.; SmithKline Beecham, Thai.; SmithKline Beecham, UK; SmithKline Beecham, USA.
Rosiglitazone maleate (p.334·2).
Diabetes mellitus.

Avant Garde Shampoo *Avant Garde, Canad.*
Pyrithione zinc (p.1122·1).

Avantrin *UCB, Ital.*
Trapidil (p.986·1).
Ischaemic heart disease.

Avanza *British Pharmaceuticals, Austral.*
Mirtazapine (p.299·1).
Depression.

Avapena *Novartis, Mex.*
Chloropyramine hydrochloride (p.412·1).
Hypersensitivity.

Avapro
Bristol-Myers Squibb, Austral.; Bristol-Myers Squibb, Canad.; Sanofi Synthelabo, Canad.; Bristol-Myers Squibb, Mex.; Sanofi Winthrop, USA; Bristol-Myers Squibb, USA.
Irbesartan (p.914·2).
Hypertension.

Avapro HCT *Bristol-Myers Squibb, Austral.*
Irbesartan (p.914·2); hydrochlorothiazide (p.907·3).
Hypertension.

Avaxim
Pasteur Merieux, Aust.; Aventis, Austral.; Pasteur Merieux, Denm.†; Pasteur Vaccins, Fr.; Pasteur Merieux, Hong Kong; Pasteur Merieux, Israel; Pasteur Merieux, Ital.; Aventis, S.Afr.; Pasteur Merieux, Neth.; Pasteur Merieux, Singapore; Pasteur Merieux, Spain; Pasteur Merieux, Swed.†; Pasteur Merieux, UK.
An inactivated hepatitis A vaccine (GBM strain) (p.1541·1).
Active immunisation.

Avazinc *Rekah, Israel.*
Zinc sulfate (p.1398·2).
Zinc deficiency.

AVC
Hoechst Marion Roussel, Canad.; Hoechst Marion Roussel, USA†.
Sulfanilamide (p.256·2).
Vulvovaginal candidiasis.

Avecyde
Note.This name is used for preparations of different composition.
3M, Austral.; 3M, Singapore.
Lactic acid (p.1626·2).
Skin irritation; soap substitute.

Galderma, Mex.
Soap substitute.
Skin cleansing.

Avedorm *Eberth, Ger.*
Oral liquid: Valerian (p.1678·3); melissa (p.1632·2); passion flower (p.1649·1).
Tablets: Valerian (p.1678·3); lupulus (p.1629·3).
Agitation; sleep disorders.

Avedorm N *Eberth, Ger.*
Lupulus (p.1629·3); passiflora; zinc valerianic.
Nervous disorders.

Aveeno
Note.This name is used for preparations of different composition.
Bioglan, Irl.
Avena (p.1583·1).
Dry skin.

Rydelle, USA.
Soap-free skin cleanser; emollient and moisturiser.

Aveeno Acne Bar *Johnson, Canad.*
Avena (p.1583·1); salicylic acid (p.1122·3).
Acne.

Aveeno Anti-Itch
Note.This name is used for preparations of different composition.
Johnson, Canad.
Calamine (p.1111·3); pramocaine hydrochloride (p.1318·2).
Aveeno Anti-Itch cream formerly contained calamine, pramocaine hydrochloride, and camphor.
Skin disorders.

Rydelle, USA.
Calamine (p.1111·3); pramocaine hydrochloride (p.1318·2); camphor (p.1589·3).
Minor skin irritation.

Aveeno Cleansing Bar *Rydelle, USA.*
Sulfur (p.1123·3); salicylic acid (p.1122·3); colloidal oatmeal (p.1583·1).
Acne.

Aveeno Preparations
Johnson, Canad.; Rydelle, Fr.; Johnson & Johnson, Ital.; Dermoteca, Port.†; Bioglan, UK.
A range of preparations containing avena (p.1583·1).
Dry skin disorders; skin care.

Aveenocream *Dermoteca, Port.†.*
Avena (p.1583·1); allantoin (p.1110·1).
Dry skin disorders.

Aveenoderm
Rydelle, Fr.; Dermoteca, Port.†.
Avena (p.1583·1); zinc oxide (p.1128·2); allantoin (p.1110·1).
Barrier cream.

Avelox
Bayer, Austral.; Bayer, Fin.; Bayer, Irl.; Bayer, Swed.; Bayer, USA.
Moxifloxacin hydrochloride (p.225·3).
Bacterial infections.

Avena Complex *Blackmores, Austral.*
Rosemary; avena (p.1583·1); vervain (p.1679·3); kola (p.1681·1); vitamin B substances (p.1350·1).
Tonic.

Avena Med Complex *Dynamit, Aust.*
Homoeopathic preparation.

Avena Rihom Komplex *Richter, Aust.*
Homoeopathic preparation.

Avena sativa comp. *Weleda, UK.*
Avena (p.1583·1); lupulus (p.1629·3); passion flower (p.1649·1); valerian root (p.1678·3); coffea tosta.
To aid relaxation.

Avenaforce *Bioforce, Switz.*
Avena (p.1583·1).
Insomnia; nervousness.

Avene Ecran *Avene, Fr.*
SPF 12; cream SPF 20; SPF 60: Cinnamate; titanium dioxide (p.1126·1); zinc oxide (p.1128·2).
SPF 20; SPF 60: Cinnamate; titanium dioxide (p.1126·1).
SPF 25; SPF 50: Titanium dioxide (p.1126·1); zinc oxide (p.1128·2).
Sunscreen.

Avenoc
Note.This name is used for preparations of different composition.
Boiron, Canad.; Boiron, Fr.†; Boiron, Port.
Homoeopathic preparation.

Boiron, Fr.†.
Ointment: Pilewort (p.1651·3); paeonia officinalis; adrenaline [epinephrine]; amylocaine hydrochloride (p.1306·1).
Anorectal disorders; haemorrhoids.

Aventyl
Lilly, Canad.; Lilly, Irl.; Aspen, S.Afr.; Lilly, USA.
Nortriptyline hydrochloride (p.301·3).
Depression; nocturnal enuresis.

Averpan *Natus, Braz.*
Mebendazole (p.102·2).
Worm infections.

Averuk Bruciaporri *Boots Healthcare, Ital.*
Trichloroacetic acid (p.1674·3).
Verrucas; warts.

Aviane *Duramed, USA.*
21 Tablets, levonorgestrel (p.1486·2); ethinylestradiol (p.1476·2); 7 tablets, inert.
Combined oral contraceptive.

Avibon *Theraplix, Fr.*
Vitamin A (p.1382·1) or vitamin A palmitate (p.1383·2).
Skin disorders; vitamin A deficiency.

A-Vicotrat *Heyl, Ger.*
Vitamin A palmitate (p.1383·2).
Vitamin A deficiency.

Avigilen
Note.This name is used for preparations of different composition.
Sanova, Aust.
Alpha tocoferil acetate (p.1394·1).
Intermittent claudication; muscle and connective tissue disorders.

Wyeth, Ger.
Piracetam (p.1652·1).
Mental function disorders.

Avil
Hoechst Marion Roussel, Aust.; Hoechst Marion Roussel, Austral.; Hoechst Marion Roussel, Belg.†; Hoechst Marion Roussel, Ger.; Aventis, NZ; Albert, S.Afr.†.
Pheniramine maleate (p.422·1).
Hypersensitivity reactions; motion sickness; pruritus; rhinitis; vestibular disorders.

Avil Decongestant *Hoechst Marion Roussel, Austral.*
Pheniramine maleate (p.422·3); ammonium chloride (p.1085·2); menthol (p.1632·3).
Bronchial and nasal congestion; coughs.

Avilac *Agis, Israel.*
Lactulose (p.1230·1).
Constipation; hepatic coma.

Avinal-Ex *Sons, Mex.*
Vitamin A (p.1382·1).
Vitamin A deficiency.

Avintac *Mavi, Mex.*
Ranitidine (p.1246·3).

Avipur *Taro, Israel.*
Vitamin A (p.1382·1).
Vitamin A deficiency.

Aviral *Medley, Braz.*
Aciclovir (p.612·3).
Herpesvirus infections.

Avirase *Lampugnani, Ital.*
Aciclovir (p.612·3).
Herpesvirus infections.

Avirax *Fabrigen, Canad.*
Aciclovir (p.612·3).
Herpesvirus infections.

Avirex *Tecnofarma, Mex.*
Aciclovir (p.612·3).
Herpesvirus infections.

Avirin *Eurofarmaco, Ital.*
Inosine pranobex (p.627·2).
Viral infections.

Avishot *Kanebo, Jpn.*
Naftopidil (p.938·1).

A-Vita *Leiras, Fin.*
Note. A similar name is used for preparations of different composition (see below).
Vitamin A palmitate (p.1383·2); menthol (p.1632·3).
Nasal disorders.

Avita *Penederm, USA.*
Note. A similar name is used for preparations of different composition (see above).
Tretinoin (p.1126·2).
Acne.

A-Vitamiini *Leiras, Fin.*
Vitamin A (p.1382·1).
Scalp and skin disorders.

A-vitamin *Medic, Denm.*
Vitamin A (p.1382·1).
Vitamin A deficiency.

Avitcid *Orion, Fin.*
Tretinoin (p.1126·2).
Acne; keratinisation disorders.

A-Vite *Neves, Port.*
Vitamin A (p.1382·1).
Vitamin A deficiency.

Avitene
Agepha, Aust.; Medchem, Hong Kong; Shionogi, USA.
Collagen (p.1598·2).
Haemostasis in surgery.

A-Vitex *Sophia, Mex.*
Vitamin A (p.1382·1).

Avitol *Lannacher, Aust.*
Vitamin A acetate (p.1383·2).
Vitamin A deficiency.

Avitracid *Adroka, Switz.*
Isopropyl alcohol (p.1149·2).
Hand disinfection.

Avix *Ibirn, Ital.*
Aciclovir (p.612·3).
Herpesvirus infections.

Avlocardyl *AstraZeneca, Fr.*
Propranolol hydrochloride (p.962·3).
Cardiovascular disorders; migraine; oesophageal varices; tremor.

Avloclor
Zeneca, Irl.; Zeneca, Israel; AstraZeneca, Singapore; AstraZeneca, UK.
Chloroquine phosphate (p.432·3).
Hepatic amoebiasis; lupus erythematosus; malaria; rheumatoid arthritis.

Avlosulfon
Wyeth-Ayerst, Canad.; Wyeth-Ayerst, Israel.
Dapsone (p.196·1).
Actinomycotic mycetoma; dermatitis herpetiformis; leprosy.

Avoca *Bray, UK.*
Silver nitrate (p.1664·2); potassium nitrate (p.1154·3).
Warts.

Avoca Menthol Cone *Bray, UK.*
Menthol (p.1632·3).
Headache.

Avocin *Wyeth Lederle, Ital.*
Piperacillin sodium (p.236·1).
Lignocaine [lidocaine] hydrochloride (p.1313·2) is included in this preparation to alleviate the pain of injection.
Bacterial infections.

Avomine
Rhone-Poulenc Rorer, Austral.; Rhone-Poulenc Rorer, Hong Kong; Rhone-Poulenc Rorer, Irl.†; Aventis, NZ; Aspen Consumer, S.Afr.; Manx, UK.
Promethazine teoclate (p.423·2).
Motion sickness; nausea and vomiting; vertigo.

Avon Footworks *Avon, Canad.*
Tolnaftate (p.395·2).
Fungal skin infections.

Avon Techniques Anti-Dandruff *Avon, Canad.*
Pyrithione zinc (p.1122·1).
Dandruff.

Avonex
Biogen, Aust.; CSL, Austral.; Biogen, Canad.; Biogen, Denm.; Biogen, Fin.; Biogen, Fr.; Biogen, Ger.; Biogen, Irl.; Biogen, Israel; Dompe Biotec, Ital.; Biogen, Neth.; Biogen, Norw.; Biogen, NZ; CSL, NZ; Schering-Plough, Port.; Schering Plough, Spain; Biogen, Swed.; Dompe Biogen, Switz.; Biogen, UK; Biogen, USA.
Interferon beta-1a (p.632·2).
Multiple sclerosis.

Avorax
Xepa-Soul Pattinson, Hong Kong; Xepa-Soul Pattinson, Singapore.
Aciclovir (p.612·3).
Herpesvirus infections.

Avril *Teofarma, Spain.*
Cod-liver oil (p.1357·2); aluminium acetotartrate (p.1578·2); benzalkonium chloride (p.1133·2); zinc oxide (p.1128·2).
Burns; wounds.

Avyclor *Uno, Ital.*
Aciclovir (p.612·3).
Herpesvirus infections.

Avyplus *Epifarma, Ital.*
Aciclovir (p.612·3).
Herpesvirus infections.

Avysal *Selvi, Ital.*
Aciclovir (p.612·3).
Herpesvirus infections.

Axacef
Durascan, Denm.; Tika, Swed.
Cefuroxime sodium (p.178·2).
Bacterial infections.

Axal *Randall, Mex.*
Aspirin (p.14·2).

Axcil *Ofimex, Mex.*
Amoxicillin (p.149·2).
Bacterial infections.

Axepim *Bristol-Myers Squibb, Fr.*
Cefepime hydrochloride (p.165·3).
Bacterial infections.

Axer *Wassermann, Ital.*
Naproxen sodium (p.61·1).
Inflammation; pain.

Axert *Pharmacia, USA.*
Almotriptan malate (p.450·2).
Migraine.

Axetine *Medochemie, Thai.*
Cefuroxime sodium (p.178·2).
Bacterial infections.

Axid
Lilly, Braz.; Lilly, Canad.; Lilly, Hong Kong; Lilly, Irl.; Lilly, Mex.; Dista, Neth.; Lilly, Neth.; Lilly, S.Afr.†; Lilly, Thai.; Lilly, UK; Lilly, USA; Whitehall-Robins, USA.
Nizatidine (p.1238·1).
Dyspepsia; gastro-oesophageal reflux; heartburn; peptic ulcer.

Axistal *Asian Pharm, Thai.*
Bromhexine hydrochloride (p.1085·3).
Respiratory-tract disorders associated with increased or viscous mucus.

Axocet *Savage, USA.*
Butalbital (p.658·3); paracetamol (p.71·2).
Pain.

Axocillin *MPF, Singapore.*
Cloxacillin sodium (p.192·1).
Bacterial infections.

Axofor *Hoechst Marion Roussel, Mex.*
Hydroxocobalamin acetate (p.1388·3).
Anaemias; neuralgias; neuritis; neuropathies; vitamin B₁₂ deficiency.

Axol *Veritas, Braz.*
Iodine (p.1522·3); phenol (p.1152·3); thymol (p.1158·3); menthol (p.1632·3); methyl salicylate (p.55·1); guaiacol (p.1092·1); procaine (p.1319·2); eucalyptol (p.1609·2); cinnamon oil (p.1596·1); aconite (p.1572·3); cariniana brasiliensis; sumatra benzoin (p.1668·3); eucalyptus (p.1609·2).
Mouth disorders.

Axonyl *Parke, Davis, Fr.*
Piracetam (p.1652·1).
Cerebrovascular insufficiency; mental function disorders; vertigo.

Axoren *Glaxo Wellcome, Ital.*
Buspirone hydrochloride (p.657·2).
Anxiety.

Axotal *Adria, USA†.*
Butalbital (p.658·3); aspirin (p.14·2).
Tension headache.

Axotide *Glaxo Wellcome, Switz.*
Fluticasone propionate (p.1072·2).
Asthma.

Axsain *GenDerm, Canad.†; Elan, Irl.; Bioglan, UK.*
Capsaicin (p.23·1).
Diabetic neuropathy; neuralgia.

Axyol *Richard, Fr.†*
Iodine (p.1522·3).
Burns; leg ulcers; wounds.

Aydolid *Farma Lepori, Spain.*
Fosfosal (p.42·1).
Fever; musculoskeletal, joint, peri-articular, and soft-tissue disorders; pain.

Aydolid Codeina *Farma Lepori, Spain.*
Codeine phosphate (p.25·2); fosfosal (p.42·1).
Pain.

Ayercillin *Wyeth-Ayerst, Canad.†.*
Procaine penicillin [procaine benzylpenicillin] (p.239·2).
Bacterial infections.

Aygestin *ESI, USA.*
Norethisterone acetate (p.1485·1).
Abnormal uterine bleeding; endometriosis; secondary amenorrhoea.

Ayoral *Rayere, Mex.*
Dipyrone (p.34·1); papaverine (p.1648·1).
Fever; muscle spasm; pain.

Ayoral F *Rayere, Mex.*
Dipyrone (p.34·1).
Fever; pain.

Ayr Saline *Ascher, USA.*
Sodium chloride (p.1196·1).
Nasal irritation.

Ayrton's Antiseptic *McGloin, Austral.*
Zinc oxide (p.1128·2); dichlorobenzyl alcohol (p.1143·2).
Superficial skin infections.

Ayrton's Chilblain *McGloin, Austral.*
Camphor (p.1589·3); benzocaine (p.1306·2); peru balsam (p.1650·2); phenol (p.1152·3).
Chilblains.

Ayrton's Iodised *McGloin, Austral.†.*
Iodine (p.1522·3); phenol (p.1152·3); menthol (p.1632·3).
Sore throat.

Aywet *Willvonseder, Aust.*
Wetting solution for hard and soft contact lenses (p.1129·2).

Az *Sophia, Mex.*
Azelastine hydrochloride (p.409·3).
Allergic conjunctivitis.

AZ 15 Gengidentifricio *Procter & Gamble, Ital.*
Sodium chloride (p.1196·1); benzalkonium chloride (p.1133·2); azulene (p.1583·2).
Gum protection; oral hygiene.

AZ Junior *Procter & Gamble, Ital.†.*
Sodium fluoride (p.1375·3); mica-titanium dioxide complex.
Dental caries prophylaxis.

AZ Protezione Completa *Procter & Gamble, Ital.*
Triclosan (p.1159·2); sodium fluoride (p.1375·3).
Dental caries prophylaxis.

AZ Protezione Gengive *Procter & Gamble, Ital.*
Triclosan (p.1159·2); pyrophosphate; sodium fluoride (p.1375·3).
Gum disorders.

Azactam
Bristol-Myers Squibb, Aust.; Bristol-Myers Squibb, Austral.; Bristol-Myers Squibb, Belg.; Bristol-Myers Squibb, Braz.; Bristol-Myers Squibb, Denm.; Bristol-Myers Squibb, Fin.; Sanofi Winthrop, Fr.; Bristol-Myers Squibb, Ger.; Bristol-Myers Squibb, Hong Kong; Bristol-Myers Squibb, Irl.; Bristol-Myers Squibb, Israel; Bristol-Myers Squibb, Ital.; Eisai, Jpn†; Bristol-Myers Squibb, Neth.; Bristol-Myers Squibb, Norw.; Bristol-Myers Squibb, NZ; Bristol-Myers Squibb, Port.; Bristol-Myers Squibb, S.Afr.; Bristol-Myers Squibb, Singapore; Squibb, Spain; Bristol-Myers Squibb, Swed.; Bristol-Myers Squibb, Switz.; Bristol-Myers Squibb, Thai.; Squibb, UK; Bristol-Myers Squibb, USA.
Aztreonam (p.154·2).
Gram-negative bacterial infections.

Azadose *Pfizer, Fr.*
Azithromycin (p.153·1).
Opportunistic mycobacterial infections.

Azafalk *Falk, Ger.*
Azathioprine (p.509·3).
Auto-immune disorders; organ transplantation.

Azahexal *Hexal, Austral.*
Azathioprine (p.509·3).

Azamedac *Medac, Ger.*
Azathioprine sodium (p.510·2).
Auto-immune disorders; organ transplantation.

Azameno *Wyeth Lederle, Aust.†; Wyeth, Switz.*
Omoconazole nitrate (p.393·1).
Fungal and Gram-positive bacterial vaginal infections; fungal infections.

Azamun *Douglas, Austral.; Leiras, Fin.; Douglas, NZ.*
Azathioprine (p.509·3).
Auto-immune disorders; transplant rejection.

Azamune *Penn, UK†.*
Azathioprine (p.509·3).
Auto-immune disorders; organ transplantation.

Azanplus *Glaxo Wellcome, Mex.*
Ranitidine bismuth citrate (p.1247·2).
Peptic ulcer.

Azantac
Glaxo Wellcome, Fr.; Glaxo Wellcome, Mex.
Ranitidine hydrochloride (p.1245·2).
Acid aspiration; gastritis; gastro-oesophageal reflux; peptic ulcer; Zollinger-Ellison syndrome.

Azapress *Intramed, S.Afr.*
Azathioprine (p.509·3).
Transplant rejection.

Azaron
Note. This name is used for preparations of different composition.
Sanova, Aust.; Chefaro, Ger.; Chefaro, Neth.†; Chefaro, Spain.
Tripelennamine hydrochloride (p.427·1).
Bites and stings; hypersensitivity reactions.
Chefaro, Belg.
Diphenhydramine hydrochloride (p.416·1).
Pruritus; skin irritation.

Azatrilem *Lemery, Mex.*
Azathioprine (p.509·3).
Immunosuppressant.

Azedavit *Whitehall, Fr.*
Multivitamin and mineral preparation (p.1350·1).

Azelan *Schering, Braz.*
Azelaic acid (p.1110·3).
Acne.

Azelcream *Crinos, Ital.*
Azelaic acid (p.1110·3).
Acne.

Azelex *Allergan, USA.*
Azelaic acid (p.1110·3).
Acne.

Azenil *Teva, Israel.*
Azithromycin (p.153·1).
Bacterial infections.

Azep
Asta Medica, Hong Kong; Probios, Port.†; Asta Medica, Singapore; Asta Medica, Thai.
Azelastine hydrochloride (p.409·3).
Allergic rhinitis.

Azeptin *Eisai, Jpn†.*
Azelastine hydrochloride (p.409·3).
Allergic rhinitis; asthma; pruritus.

Azerodol *Edmond Pharma, Ital.†.*
Salicylamide (p.82·1); propyphenazone (p.80·2); caffeine (p.761·3).
Pain.

Azerty *AstraZeneca, Fr.*
Nalbuphine hydrochloride (p.60·1).
Pain.

Aziac *Infabra, Braz.*
Aluminium hydroxide (p.1210·3); magnesium hydroxide (p.1233·1).
Gastrointestinal hyperacidity.

Aziclav *Spirig, Switz.*
Amoxicillin trihydrate (p.149·2); potassium clavulanate (p.187·2).
Bacterial infections.

Azilline *Spirig, Switz.*
Amoxicillin trihydrate (p.149·2).
Bacterial infections.

Azimax *Almirall, Spain.*
Zafirlukast (p.785·3).
Asthma.

Azinc
Arkopharma, Fr.; Arkochim, Spain.
A range of vitamin and mineral preparations (p.1350·1).

Azinc Complex *Arkopharma, UK.*
Multivitamin and mineral preparation (p.1350·1).

Azitrocin
Bioindustria, Ital.; Pfizer, Mex.
Azithromycin (p.153·1).
Bacterial infections.

Azitromax *Pfizer, Norw.; Pfizer, Swed.*
Azithromycin (p.153·1).
Bacterial infections.

Azitromin *Farmasa, Braz.*
Azithromycin (p.153·1).
Bacterial infections.

Azmacort *Rhone-Poulenc Rorer, Canad.; Rhone-Poulenc Rorer, USA.*
Triamcinolone acetonide (p.1080·1).
Asthma.

AZM-Tab *Alra, USA†.*
Acetazolamide (p.826·1).

Azodine *Propan, S.Afr.†.*
Phenazopyridine hydrochloride (p.77·3).
Urinary-tract pain.

Azol
Note. This name is used for preparations of different composition.
Alphapharm, Austral.; Alphapharm, Singapore; Merck, Singapore.
Danazol (p.1468·3).
Endometriosis; hereditary angioedema; mastalgia; menorrhagia.
Roche, Spain.
Sulfanilamide (p.256·2).
Skin infections.

Azoline *Fischer, Israel.*
Tetryzoline hydrochloride (p.1101·2).
Allergic conjunctivitis; eye irritation.

Azolmen *Menarini, Ital.*
Bifonazole (p.381·1).
Fungal skin infections.

Azo-Mandelamine *Parke, Davis, S.Afr.†.*
Methenamine mandelate (p.223·1); phenazopyridine hydrochloride (p.77·3).
Urinary-tract infections.

Azomid *Propan, S.Afr.*
Acetazolamide (p.826·1).
Glaucoma.

Azomycin *Julphar, UAE.*
Azithromycin (p.153·1).
Bacterial infections.

Azona
Note. This name is used for preparations of different composition.
Orion, Fin.
Trazodone hydrochloride (p.310·1).
Depression; insomnia; psychoses.
Keton, Mex.
Dexamethasone (p.1067·1).
Corticosteroid.

Azonutril
Pharmacia Upjohn, Fr.†; Rhone-Poulenc Rorer, Spain†.
Amino-acid infusion (p.1350·1).
Parenteral nutrition.

Azopi *Generics, Israel.*
Azathioprine (p.509·3).
Auto-immune disorders; transplant rejection.

Azopine *Pinewood, Irl.*
Azathioprine (p.509·3).
Auto-immune disorders; organ transplantation.

Azopt
Alcon, Austral.; Alcon, Canad.; Alcon, Denm.; Alcon, Fin.; Alcon, Irl.; Alcon, Singapore; Alcon, Thai.; Alcon, UK; Alcon, USA.
Brinzolamide (p.851·3).
Glaucoma; ocular hypertension.

Azor *Aspen, S.Afr.*
Alprazolam (p.654·2).
Anxiety; mixed anxiety depressive states.

Azo-Standard *PolyMedica, USA.*
Phenazopyridine hydrochloride (p.77·3).
Urinary-tract pain.

Azostix
Bayer, Austral.; Miles, Canad.†; Bayer Diagnostics, Irl.; Bayer, NZ; Ames, S.Afr.; Bayer Diagnostics, UK; Bayer, USA.
Test for urea in blood.

Azo-Wintomylon
Sanofi Winthrop, Braz.; Sanofi Winthrop, Mex.
Nalidixic acid (p.227·1); phenazopyridine hydrochloride (p.77·3).
Urinary-tract infections.

Aztemin *Protein, Mex.*
Astemizole (p.409·1).

Azuben *Ipsen, Spain.*
Pefloxacin mesilate (p.234·3).
Bacterial infections.

Azubronchin *Azupharma, Ger.*
Acetylcysteine (p.1082·3).
Respiratory-tract disorders associated with increased or viscous mucus.

Azucalcit *Azupharma, Ger.*
Salcatonin (p.749·3).
Hypercalcaemia; osteoporosis; Paget's disease of bone; reflex sympathetic dystrophy.

Azucaps *Medix, Mex.*
Phenformin (p.333·2).

Azucimet *Azupharma, Ger.*
Cimetidine (p.1216·3).
Aspiration syndromes; gastro-oesophageal reflux; gastrointestinal haemorrhage; peptic ulcer; Zollinger-Ellison syndrome.

Azuder *Mex-America, Mex.*
Sulfur (p.1123·3).

Azudoxat *Azupharma, Ger.*
Doxycycline hyclate (p.200·1).
Bacterial infections.

Azudoxat comp *Azupharma, Ger.*
Doxycycline hyclate (p.200·1); ambroxol hydrochloride (p.1084·3).
Respiratory-tract infections.

Azufibrat
Azupharma, Ger.; Azupharma, Hong Kong.
Bezafibrate (p.849·1).
Hyperlipidaemias.

Azuglucon *Azupharma, Ger.*
Glibenclamide (p.321·3).
Diabetes mellitus.

Azul Metile *Ciba Vision, Spain†.*
Methylene blue [methylthioninium chloride] (p.1012·3).
Ophthalmic diagnostic agent.

Azulen *Provita, Aust.*
Guaiazulene (p.1618·3).
Hypersensitivity and inflammatory disorders.

Azulenal *Agepha, Aust.*
Guaiazulene (p.1618·3).
Hypersensitivity disorders; mucus membrane inflammation; skin disorders.

Azulfidine
Pharmacia Upjohn, Ger.; Pharmacia Upjohn, USA.
Sulfasalazine (p.1251·1).
Inflammatory bowel diseases; rheumatoid arthritis.

Azulfin *Apsen, Braz.*
Sulfasalazine (p.1251·1).
Rheumatoid arthritis; ulcerative colitis.

Azulina *Llorens, Spain.*
Methylene blue [methylthioninium chloride] (p.1012·3); tetryzoline hydrochloride (p.1101·2).
Eye disorders.

Azulipont *Azupharma, Ger.*
Thioctic acid (p.1671·3).
Diabetic polyneuropathy.

Azulon *Asta Medica, Ger.*
Chamomile (p.1593·2).
Skin disorders.

Azumetop *Azupharma, Ger.*
Metoprolol tartrate (p.931·2).
Angina pectoris; arrhythmias; hypertension; migraine; myocardial infarction.

Azumetop HCT *Azupharma, Ger.*
Metoprolol tartrate (p.931·2); hydrochlorothiazide (p.907·3).
Hypertension.

Azunaftil *Azupharma, Ger.*
Naftidrofuryl oxalate (p.937·3).
Peripheral vascular disorders.

Azunol *Shinyaku, Hong Kong.*
Azulene sodium sulfonate (p.1583·2).
Gastric ulcer; gastritis; mouth disorders.

Azupamil *Azupharma, Ger.*
Verapamil hydrochloride (p.989·1).
Angina pectoris; arrhythmias; hypertension.

Azupanthenol *Parke, Davis, Ger.*
Guaiazulene (p.1618·3); sodium pantothenate (p.1374·2).
Gastrointestinal disorders.

Azupentat *Azupharma, Ger.*
Oxpentifylline [pentoxifylline] (p.950·3).
Peripheral vascular disorders.

Azuperamid *Azupharma, Ger.*
Loperamide hydrochloride (p.1231·3).
Diarrhoea.

Azuprostat M *Azupharma, Ger.*
Sitosterol (p.970·3).
Benign prostatic hyperplasia.

Azur *Steiner, Ger.*
Paracetamol (p.71·2); caffeine (p.761·3).
Pain.

Azur compositum *Steiner, Ger.*
Paracetamol (p.71·2); caffeine (p.761·3); codeine phosphate (p.25·2).
Pain.

Azur compositum SC *Steiner, Ger.*
Paracetamol (p.71·2); codeine phosphate (p.25·2).
Pain.

Azuranit *Azupharma, Ger.*
Ranitidine hydrochloride (p.1245·2).
Aspiration syndromes; gastro-oesophageal reflux; gastrointestinal haemorrhage; peptic ulcer; Zollinger-Ellison syndrome.

Azutranquil *Azupharma, Ger.*
Oxazepam (p.697·1).
Insomnia.

Azutrimazol *Azupharma, Ger.*
Clotrimazole (p.382·1).
Fungal skin and genito-urinary tract infections.

Azym *Laphal, Fr.*
Magnesium hydroxide (p.1233·1); magnesium carbonate (p.1232·3); anhydrous sodium sulfate (p.1250·1); dibasic sodium phosphate (p.1193·2); calcium carbonate (p.1215·1); sodium bicarbonate (p.1186·2).
Gastrointestinal disorders.

The symbol † denotes a preparation no longer actively marketed

3B
Atlantic, Hong Kong; Atlantic, Singapore; Atlantic, Thai.
Vitamin B₁ (p.1385·2); vitamin B₆ (p.1387·1); vitamin B₁₂ (p.1388·1).
Anaemias; neural disorders.

B₁₂ Ankermann *Worwag, Ger.*
Cyanocobalamin (p.1388·1).
Vitamin B₁₂ deficiency.

B Chabre *AJC, Fr.*
Vitamin B substances (p.1350·1).

B Complex
Jamieson, Canad.; Sante Naturelle, Canad.; Shaklee, Canad.; CTI, Israel.
Vitamin B substances (p.1350·1).
Vitamin B deficiency.

Phillips Yeast, UK.
Yeast (p.1398·1); vitamin B substances (p.1350·1).

B-100 Complex *TP, Thai.*
Vitamin B substances (p.1350·1).

B Complex 500 *Nobel, Canad.†*
Vitamin B substances and vitamin C (p.1350·1).

B Complex with C *Everest, Canad.*
Vitamin B substances and vitamin C (p.1350·1).

B Complex C 550 *Adams, Canad.*
Vitamin B substances and vitamin C (p.1350·1).

B Complex Fosforilado *Alter, Spain†*
Vitamin B substances (p.1350·1).

B Complex plus C *Jamieson, Canad.*
Vitamin B substances and vitamin C (p.1350·1).

B₁₂ Compositum *Helvepharm, Switz.*
Cyanocobalamin; iron sucrose; calcium glycerophosphate (p.1350·1).
Tonic.

B Compound *Swiss Herbal, Canad.*
Vitamin B substances (p.1350·1).

B₁₂ Depot-Hevert *Hevert, Ger.*
Hydroxocobalamin acetate (p.1388·3).
Vitamin B₁₂ deficiency.

B12 Depot-Rotexmedica *Rotexmedica, Ger.*
Hydroxocobalamin acetate (p.1388·3).
Vitamin B₁₂ deficiency.

B₁₂ Depot-Vicotrat *Heyl, Ger.*
Hydroxocobalamin (p.1388·1).
Vitamin B₁₂ deficiency.

B₁/₆ Effekton *Brenner-Efeka, Ger.†*
Thiamine hydrochloride (p.1385·1); pyridoxine hydrochloride (p.1386·3).
Neurological disorders.

B12 Ehrl *Hormosan, Ger.†*
Cyanocobalamin (p.1388·1).
Vitamin B₁₂ deficiency.

B₁₂ Fol-Vicotrat *Heyl, Ger.*
Cyanocobalamin (p.1388·1); folic acid (p.1361·1).
Vitamin B₁₂ and folic acid deficiency.

B Forte *Bio-Health, UK.*
Vitamin B preparation (p.1350·1).

B 12-L 90 *Loges, Ger.*
Cyanocobalamin (p.1388·1).
Anaemias; tonic; vitamin B deficiency.

B & O Supprettes No. 15A *PolyMedica, USA.*
Prepared opium (p.69·3); powdered belladonna extract (p.463·1).
Ureteral spasm pain.

B & O Supprettes No. 16A *PolyMedica, USA.*
Prepared opium (p.69·3); powdered belladonna extract (p.463·1).
Ureteral spasm pain.

B plus C *Novopharm, Canad.*
Vitamin B substances and vitamin C (p.1350·1).

B Six *Sam-On, Israel.*
Vitamin B₆ (p.1386·3).
Vitamin B₆ deficiency.

B Stress C plus Iron & Vitamins *Stanley, Canad.*
Vitamin preparation with iron (p.1350·1).

B Stress Select *Sisu, Canad.*
Vitamin B substances (p.1350·1).

B Totum *Desbergers, Canad.*
Vitamin B substances and vitamin C (p.1350·1).

B₁ Vicotrat *Heyl, Ger.*
Thiamine nitrate (p.1385·1).
Vitamin B deficiency.

B₆ Vicotrat *Heyl, Ger.*
Pyridoxine hydrochloride (p.1386·3).
Premenstrual syndrome; vitamin B deficiency.

B₁₂ Vicotrat *Heyl, Ger.*
Cyanocobalamin (p.1388·1).
Vitamin B deficiency.

B Virol *Rolmex, Canad.*
Multivitamin preparation (p.1350·1).

Babcon *Eisai, Thai.; Toho, Thai.*
Dimethicone (p.1249·2).
Excess gastrointestinal gas; preparation for gastrointestinal examinations.

Babee *Pfeiffer, USA.*
Benzocaine (p.1306·2); cetalkonium chloride (p.1137·1); camphor (p.1589·3); menthol (p.1632·3); eucalyptol (p.1609·2).
Oral lesions.

Babic *Abic, Israel.*
Sodium bicarbonate (p.1186·2).
Infant colic.

Babiforton *Sanofi Synthelabo, Ger.*
Eucalyptus oil (p.1609·2); pine needle oil; peppermint oil (p.1243·3).
Nasal congestion.

Babigoz Crema Protettiva *Guigoz, Ital.*
Zinc oxide (p.1128·2); magnesium silicate (p.1502·1); wheat-germ oil.
Nappy rash.

Babix *Madaus, Aust.*
Cajuput oil (p.1588·1); pumilio pine oil (p.1656·3); eucalyptus oil (p.1609·2).
Respiratory-tract disorders.

Babix-Inhalat N *Mickan, Ger.*
Eucalyptus oil (p.1609·2); Norway spruce oil.
Respiratory-tract disorders.

Babix-Wundsalbe N *Mickan, Ger.*
Zinc oxide (p.1128·2); lemon oil (p.1628·2); chamomile oil.
Skin disorders.

Baby AF *Sam-On, Israel.*
Sodium chloride (p.1196·1).
Nasal congestion.

Baby Agisten *Agis, Israel.*
Clotrimazole (p.382·1).
Fungal skin infections.

Baby Anbesol *Whitehall, USA.*
Benzocaine (p.1306·2).
Teething pain.

Baby Block *Estee Lauder, Canad.*
SPF 25: Titanium dioxide (p.1126·1).
Sunscreen.

Baby Cough *Greater Pharma, Thai.*
Ammonium chloride (p.1085·2); sodium citrate (p.1186·2).
Coughs.

Baby Cough with Antihistamine
Atlantic, Hong Kong; Atlantic, Thai.
Acetic acid (p.1571·2); ammonium chloride (p.1085·2); sodium citrate (p.1186·2); glycerol (p.1616·3); tolu syrup (p.1101·3); chlorpheniramine [chlorphenamine] maleate (p.412·1).
Coughs.

Baby Cough Syrup *Atlantic, Thai.*
Acetic acid (p.1571·2); ammonium chloride (p.1085·2); glycerol (p.1616·3); sodium citrate (p.1186·2); tolu syrup (p.1101·3).
Coughs.

Baby Gel *Medibrands, Israel.*
Benzocaine (p.1306·2).
Teething pain.

Baby Gripe *TO-Chemicals, Thai.*
Dill oil (p.1603·3); sodium bicarbonate (p.1186·2).
Flatulence; infant bloating.

Baby Liberol *Galactina, Switz.†*
Hyoscyamus (p.470·1); eucalyptus oil (p.1609·2); pumilio pine oil (p.1656·3); star anise oil; juniper oil (p.1625·2); methyl salicylate (p.55·1).
Cold symptoms.

Baby Luuf *Apomedica, Aust.*
Camphor (p.1589·3); eucalyptus oil (p.1609·2); turpentine oil (p.1676·3); majoram oil.
Respiratory-tract disorders.

Baby Orajel
Del, Canad.; Del, USA.
Benzocaine (p.1306·2).
Teething pain.

Baby Orajel Tooth and Gum Cleanser *Del, USA.*
Poloxamer 407 (p.1347·1); simeticone (p.1249·2).
Dental hygiene.

Baby Paste *Vitamed, Israel.*
Zinc oxide (p.1128·2); starch (p.1379·3).
Nappy rash; skin irritation.

Baby Rinol *Marion Merrell, Spain†.*
Chlorpheniramine [chlorphenamine] maleate (p.412·1); phenylpropanolamine hydrochloride (p.1098·1); paracetamol (p.71·2).
Upper-respiratory-tract disorders.

Baby Sebamed *Sebapharma, Thai.*
A range of skin cleansers and emollients.

Baby Shield *Hoe, Singapore.*
Barrier preparation.
Nappy rash.

Babycare *Trima, Israel.*
Barrier preparation.

Babyfort *QIF, Braz.*
Multivitamin preparation (p.1350·1).

Babygella *Guieu, Ital.*
Cream: Calendula (p.1589·2); chamomile (p.1593·2); zinc oxide (p.1128·2).

Topical paste: Squalane; sweet almond oil; lactic acid; zinc oxide (p.1128·2).
Barrier preparation.

Babygencal *Qualiphar, Belg.*
Amylocaine hydrochloride (p.1306·1); potassium bromide; cloral hydrate (p.669·3).
Teething pain.

Babylax
Byk, Aust.†; Mann, Ger.†; Mann, Irl.
Glycerol (p.1616·3).
Constipation.

Baby-Line *Cesam, Port.*
Barrier preparation.

Baby-Rinolo *Lepetit, Ital.*
Phenylpropanolamine hydrochloride (p.1098·1); chlorpheniramine [chlorphenamine] maleate (p.412·1); paracetamol (p.71·2).
Respiratory-tract disorders.

Babys Own Gripe Water *Block, Canad.*
Anise oil (p.1580·3); dill oil (p.1603·3); fennel oil (p.1610·2); sodium bicarbonate (p.1186·2).
Gastrointestinal disorders.

Babys Own Infant Drops *Block, Canad.*
Simeticone (p.1249·2).
Infant colic, bloating, and flatulence.

Babys Own Ointment *Block, Canad.*
Zinc oxide (p.1128·2).
Nappy rash.

Babys Own Teething Gel *Block, Canad.*
Benzyl alcohol (p.1135·2).
Teething pain.

Babysiton *Faes, Spain†.*
Cetylpyridinium chloride (p.1138·1); zinc oxide (p.1128·2).
Skin disorders.

Babysteril *Eurospital, Ital.*
Zinc oxide (p.1128·2); almond oil (p.1576·3); wheatgerm oil; vitamin A (p.1382·1); vitamin E (p.1393·3). Formerly contained zinc oxide, silicon, and wool fat, and was known as Pastasil.
Napkin rash.

Baby-Transpulmin *Asta Medica, Ger.†.*
Eucalyptus oil (p.1609·2); pine needle oil.
Cold symptoms.

Babyzim *Sam-On, Israel.*
Pepsin (p.1649·3); lactic acid (p.1626·3); sodium glycerophosphate (p.1617·3); nicotinic acid (p.1372·3).
Gastrointestinal disorders.

B-A-C *Mayrand, USA.*
Butalbital (p.658·3); aspirin (p.14·2); caffeine (p.761·3).
Tension headache.

Bac Resistente *Sanus, Braz.*
Lactobacillus acidophilus (p.1626·3).
Diarrhoea; restoration of gastrointestinal flora.

Bac Septin *Gilton, Braz.*
Co-trimoxazole (p.193·3).
Bacterial infections; Pneumocystis carinii pneumonia; protozoal infections.

Bacacil *Roerig, Ital.*
Bacampicillin hydrochloride (p.155·1).
Bacterial infections.

Bacagen *Boniscontro & Gazzone, Ital.*
Bacampicillin hydrochloride (p.155·1).
Bacterial infections.

Bacampicin
Pharmacia Upjohn, Belg.; Pharmacia Upjohn, Port.; Pharmacia Upjohn, Switz.
Bacampicillin hydrochloride (p.155·1).
Bacterial infections.

Bacampicine *Pharmacia Upjohn, Fr.*
Bacampicillin hydrochloride (p.155·1).
Bacterial infections.

Bacard *Chew, Thai.*
Chlorhexidine gluconate (p.1138·2); cetrimide (p.1137·1).
Skin, wound, and instrument disinfection.

Bacard Antiseptic *Chew, Thai.*
Chlorhexidine gluconate (p.1138·2).
Skin, hand, and wound disinfection.

Bacasint *Piam, Ital.*
Bacampicillin hydrochloride (p.155·1).
Bacterial infections.

Baccalin *Bode, Ger.*
Benzalkonium chloride (p.1133·2); didecyldimethylammonium chloride (p.1143·2).
Disinfection.

Baccidal
Kyorin, Jpn; Knoll, Spain.
Norfloxacin (p.232·1).
Bacterial infections.

Bacfar *Elofar, Braz.*
Co-trimoxazole (p.193·3).
Bacterial infections; Pneumocystis carinii pneumonia; protozoal infections.

Bacfar Balsamico *Elofar, Braz.*
Co-trimoxazole (p.193·3); guaifenesin (p.1092·2); ammonium chloride (p.1085·2).
Bacterial infections.

Bacgen *Uniao Quimica, Braz.*
Co-trimoxazole (p.193·3).
Bacterial infections; Pneumocystis carinii pneumonia; protozoal infections.

Bacgen Balsamico *Uniao Quimica, Braz.*
Co-trimoxazole (p.193·3); guaifenesin (p.1092·2); ammonium chloride (p.1085·2).
Bacterial infections.

Bach Rescue Remedy *Bach, UK.*
Homoeopathic preparation.

Bacibact *Orion, Fin.*
Bacitracin (p.155·2); neomycin sulfate (p.228·1).
Infected skin disorders.

Bacicoline *Merck Sharp & Dohme-Chibret, Fr.*
Bacitracin (p.155·2); colistimethate (p.193·1); hydrocortisone acetate (p.1073·3).
Eye infections.

Bacicoline-B *Chibret, Neth.†*
Colistimethate sodium (p.192·3); bacitracin (p.155·2); hydrocortisone acetate (p.1073·3).
Inflammatory ear infections.

Bacid
Note. This name is used for preparations of different composition.
Rhone-Poulenc Rorer, Canad.; Ciba, USA.
Lactobacillus acidophilus (p.1626·3).
Diarrhoea; stomatitis.

Uno, Ital.
Cefonicid sodium (p.168·1).
Lignocaine [lidocaine] hydrochloride (p.1313·2) is included in this preparation to alleviate the pain of injection.
Bacterial infections.

Baciderma *Confar, Port.*
Bacitracin (p.155·2); neomycin (p.228·1).

Bacifurane *Melisana, Belg.*
Nifuroxazide (p.230·2).
Diarrhoea.

Bacigem *Cazi, Braz.*
Neomycin (p.228·1); bacitracin (p.155·2).
Skin infections.

Baciguent
Johnson & Johnson, Canad.; Upjohn, USA.
Bacitracin (p.155·2).
Bacterial skin infections.

Baciguent Plus Pain Reliever *McNeil Consumer, Canad.†*
Bacitracin (p.155·2); lignocaine [lidocaine] (p.1313·2).
Pain and infection in burns and wounds.

Baci-IM *Pharma Tek, USA.*
Bacitracin (p.155·2).
Bacterial infections.

Bacillin *Lafare, Ital.*
Bacampicillin hydrochloride (p.155·1).
Bacterial infections.

Bacillocid rasant *Bode, Ger.*
Glutaral (p.1145·2); benzalkonium chloride (p.1133·2); didecyldimethylammonium chloride (p.1143·2).
Surface disinfection.

Bacillocid Spezial *Bode, Ger.*
1,6-Dihydroxy-2,5-dioxahexan; glutaral (p.1145·2); benzalkonium chloride (p.1133·2); cocosguanidinium chloride.
Surface disinfection.

Bacillol *Bode, Ger.*
Propyl alcohol (p.1155·3); isopropyl alcohol (p.1149·2); alcohol (p.1130·3); 1,6-dihydroxy-2,5-dioxahexan; mecetronium etilsulfate (p.1150·1).
Surface disinfection.

Bacillol AF *Bode, Ger.*
Propyl alcohol (p.1155·3); isopropyl alcohol (p.1149·2); alcohol (p.1130·3).
Surface disinfection.

Bacillol plus *Bode, Ger.*
Propyl alcohol (p.1155·3); isopropyl alcohol (p.1149·2); glutaral (p.1145·2).
Surface disinfection.

Bacillotox *Bode, Ger.†*
Chlorocresol (p.1141·3); orthophenylphenol (p.1152·1); chloroxylenol (p.1142·1); clorophene (p.1142·3).
Disinfection.

Bacilor *Lyocentre, Fr.*
Lactobacillus casei var rhamnosus (p.1626·3).
Formerly known as Antiobiophilus.
Diarrhoea.

Bacimex *Alter, Spain.*
Injection: Ampicillin sodium (p.150·3); sulbactam sodium (p.250·1).
Lignocaine [lidocaine] hydrochloride (p.1313·2) is included in the intramuscular injection to alleviate the pain of injection.

Tablets†; oral suspension†: Sultamicillin tosilate (p.257·2).
Bacterial infections.

Bacimycin
Note. This name is used for preparations of different composition.
Grossmann, Hong Kong.
Bacitracin (p.155·2); neomycin (p.228·1).
Burns; infected skin disorders; wounds.

Alpharma, Norw.
Bacitracin zinc (p.155·2); chlorhexidine acetate (p.1138·2).
Bacterial infections of the skin.

Bacimycine *Grossmann, Switz.*
Bacitracin (p.155·2); neomycin sulfate (p.228·1).
Infected skin disorders.

Bacimyxin *Pharmascience, Canad.*
Polymyxin B sulfate (p.238·1); bacitracin (p.155·2).
Bacterial infections.

Bacin
Atlantic, Hong Kong; Atlantic, Singapore; Atlantic, Thai.
Co-trimoxazole (p.193·3).
Bacterial infections.

Bacisporin *Wellcome, Spain.*
Bacitracin zinc (p.155·2); hydrocortisone (p.1073·3); neomycin sulfate (p.228·1); polymyxin B sulfate (p.238·1).
Infected skin disorders.

Bacitin
Pharmascience, Canad.; Pharmascience, Hong Kong.
Bacitracin (p.155·2).
Bacterial infections of the skin.

Bacitracina-Neo *Zimaia, Port.*
Bacitracin (p.155·2); neomycin (p.228·1).

Backache *Potter's, UK.*
Oral mixture: Bearberry (p.1583·3); juniper (p.1625·2); clivers (p.1596·3); taraxacum (p.1669·1); lappa (p.1627·1).
Tablets: Gravel root (p.1618·1); hydrangea root (p.1621·1); buchu (p.1587·2); bearberry (p.1583·3).
Backache.

Backache Ledum *Homeocan, Canad.*
Homoeopathic preparation.

Backache Maximum Strength Relief *Bristol-Myers Squibb, USA.*
Magnesium salicylate (p.50·3).

Backache Relief *Herbal Concepts, UK.*
Buchu (p.1587·2); bearberry (p.1583·3); parsley piert (p.1648·3).
Back pain.

Back-Aid *Technilab, Canad.*
Paracetamol (p.71·2); chlorzoxazone (p.1327·3).

Back-Ese M *Dannorth, Canad.*
Magnesium salicylate (p.50·3).

Baclohexal *Hexal, Austral.*
Baclofen (p.1322·3).
Skeletal muscle spasm.

Baclon *Leiras, Fin.*
Baclofen (p.1322·3).
Spasticity.

Baclopar *Pharmacia Upjohn, Fin.*
Baclofen (p.1322·3).
Spasticity.

Baclosal *Unipharm, Israel.*
Baclofen (p.1322·3).
Spasticity.

Baclospas *Ashbourne, UK.*
Baclofen (p.1322·3).
Skeletal muscle spasm or spasticity.

Bacmin *Marnel, USA.*
Multivitamin and mineral preparation with iron and folic acid (p.1350·1).

Bacocil *Roerig, Belg.*
Bacampicillin hydrochloride (p.155·1).
Bacterial infections.

Bacotan *TO-Chemicals, Thai.*
Hyoscine butylbromide (p.468·2).
Smooth muscle spasm.

Bacpiryl *Parggon, Mex.*
Co-trimoxazole (p.193·3).
Bacterial infections.

Bacris *Cristalia, Braz.*
Co-trimoxazole (p.193·3).
Bacterial infections; Pneumocystis carinii pneumonia; protozoal infections.

Bacta *Masa, Thai.*
Co-trimoxazole (p.193·3).
Bacterial infections.

Bactelan *Quimica y Farmacia, Mex.*
Co-trimoxazole (p.193·3).
Bacterial infections.

Bacteomycine *Monot, Fr.*
Neomycin sulfate (p.228·1).
Formerly contained bacitracin and neomycin sulfate.
Infected skin disorders.

Bacteracin *Teuto, Braz.*
Co-trimoxazole (p.193·3).
Bacterial infections; Pneumocystis carinii pneumonia; protozoal infections.

Bacteracin Balsamico *Teuto, Braz.*
Co-trimoxazole (p.193·3); guaifenesin (p.1092·2); ammonium chloride (p.1085·2).
Bacterial infections.

Bacterial *CT, Ital.†*
Co-trimoxazole (p.193·3).
Bacterial infections.

Bacterianos D *Anios, Fr.*
Formaldehyde (p.1144·2); glyoxal (p.1145·3); glutaral (p.1145·2); didecyldimethylammonium chloride (p.1143·2).
Disinfection of surfaces.

Bacterinil *Luper, Braz.*
Ampicillin (p.150·3).
Bacterial infections.

Bacterion *Opofarm, Braz.*
Ampicillin (p.150·3).
Bacterial infections.

Bacternil *Maffioli, Ital.*
Sulfadiazine silver (p.251·3).
Infected burns and ulcers.

Bacticil *Continentales, Mex.*
Ampicillin (p.150·3).
Bacterial infections.

Bacti-Cleanse *Pedinol, USA.*
Benzalkonium chloride (p.1133·2).
Skin cleanser.

Bacticort *Rugby, USA†.*
Hydrocortisone (p.1073·3); neomycin sulfate (p.228·1); polymyxin B sulfate (p.238·1).
Eye inflammation with bacterial infection.

Bactidan *Pierre Fabre, Ital.*
Enoxacin (p.201·1).
Urinary-tract and respiratory-tract infections.

Bactident *Oberlin, Fr.*
Sodium perborate (p.1156·3); sodium carbonate (p.1665·1); sodium phosphate (p.1193·2); sodium laurilsulfate (p.1496·3).
False teeth hygiene.

Bactidol *Warner-Lambert, Hong Kong; Parke, Davis, Singapore.*
Hexetidine (p.1146·3).
Mouth and throat disorders.

Bactidox *TAD, Ger.*
Doxycycline (p.200·1).
Bacterial infections.

Bactidron *Aventis, S.Afr.*
Enoxacin (p.201·1).
Cystitis; gonorrhoea.

Bactifor *Andromaco, Spain†.*
Co-trimoxazole (p.193·3).
Bacterial infections; Pneumocystis carinii pneumonia.

Bactigras *Smith & Nephew, Austral.; Smith & Nephew, Canad.; Braun, Ger.; Smith & Nephew, Hong Kong; Smith & Nephew, S.Afr.; Smith & Nephew, Thai.; Smith & Nephew, UK.*
Chlorhexidine acetate (p.1138·2).
Burns; skin infections; ulcers; wounds.

Bactilen *Cryopharma, Mex.*
Co-trimoxazole (p.193·3).
Bacterial infections.

Bactine
Note. This name is used for preparations of different composition.
Bayer, Canad.
Benzalkonium chloride (p.1133·2); lignocaine [lidocaine] hydrochloride (p.1313·2).
Skin disorders; wound cleansing.

Miles, USA.
Hydrocortisone (p.1073·3).
Skin disorders.

Bactine Antiseptic *Miles, USA.*
Lignocaine [lidocaine] (p.1313·2); benzalkonium chloride (p.1133·2).
Skin disorders.

Bactine First Aid Antibiotic Plus Anesthetic *Miles Laboratories, USA†.*
Polymyxin B sulfate (p.238·1); bacitracin (p.155·2); neomycin sulfate (p.228·1); diperodon hydrochloride (p.1311·3).
Bacterial skin infections.

Bactisubtil *Sanofi Synthelabo, Belg.; Aventis, Fr.†; Cassella-med, Ger.; Marion Merrell Dow, Port.; Leti, Spain†.*
Bacillus cereus IP 5832 or Bacillus subtilis.
Restoration of the gastrointestinal flora.

Bactiver *Maver, Mex.*
Co-trimoxazole (p.193·3).
Bacterial infections.

Bactocef *Aspen, S.Afr.*
Cefradine (p.173·3).
Bacterial infections.

Bactocill *SmithKline Beecham, USA.*
Oxacillin sodium (p.233·2).
Bacterial infections.

Bactocin
Note. This name is used for preparations of different composition.
Proge, Ital.
Lactobacillus plantarum.
Vulvovaginitis.

Hormona, Mex.
Ofloxacin (p.232·3).
Bacterial infections.

Bactoderm *Agis, Israel.*
Mupirocin (p.226·1).
Bacterial skin infections.

Bactofen *Rusch, Ital.*
Benzoxonium chloride (p.1135·2).
Instrument disinfection; skin and mucous membrane disinfection.

Bactoflox *Probios, Port.*
Ofloxacin (p.232·3).
Bacterial infections.

Bactopumon *Cinfa, Spain.*
Tolu balsam (p.1101·3); bromhexine hydrochloride (p.1085·3); co-trimoxazole (p.193·3).
Respiratory-tract infections.

Bactoreduct *Azupharma, Ger.*
Co-trimoxazole (p.193·3).
Bacterial infections; Pneumocystis carinii pneumonia.

Bactoscrub *Vitamed, Israel.*
Chlorhexidine gluconate (p.1138·2).
Skin cleansing; skin disinfection.

Bactosept *Vitamed, Israel.*
Chlorhexidine gluconate (p.1138·2).
Burns; disinfection of instruments and skin; skin cleansing; wounds.

BactoShield *Amsco, USA.*
Chlorhexidine gluconate (p.1138·2); isopropyl alcohol (p.1149·2).
Skin disinfection.

Bactosone Retard *Belmac, Spain.*
Ampicillin sodium (p.150·3); ampicillin benzathine (p.151·3); bromhexine hydrochloride (p.1085·3); guaifenesin (p.1092·2).
Lignocaine [lidocaine] hydrochloride (p.1313·2) is included in this preparation to alleviate the pain of injection.
Respiratory-tract infections.

Bactox
Note. This name is used for preparations of different composition.
Windson, Braz.
Co-trimoxazole (p.193·3).
Bacterial infections; Pneumocystis carinii pneumonia; protozoal infections.

Innotech, Fr.
Amoxicillin sodium (p.149·2) or amoxicillin trihydrate (p.149·2).
Bacterial infections.

Bactox Balsamico *Windson, Braz.*
Co-trimoxazole (p.193·3); guaifenesin (p.1092·2).
Bacterial infections.

Bactracid *Apogepha, Ger.*
Norfloxacin (p.232·1).
Urinary-tract infections.

Bactrazine *Smith & Nephew, S.Afr.*
Sulfadiazine silver (p.251·3).
Infected ulcers and burns.

Bactren *Sanval, Braz.*
Co-trimoxazole (p.193·3).
Bacterial infections; Pneumocystis carinii pneumonia; protozoal infections.

Bactrex *Sintoforma, Braz.*
Co-trimoxazole (p.193·3); guaifenesin (p.1092·2); ammonium chloride (p.1085·2).
Bacterial infections.

Bactrian *Loveridge, UK.*
Cetrimide (p.1137·1).
Skin infections.

Bactricin *Marjan, Braz.*
Co-trimoxazole (p.193·3).
Bacterial infections; Pneumocystis carinii pneumonia; protozoal infections.

Bactricin Balsamico *Marjan, Braz.*
Co-trimoxazole (p.193·3); guaifenesin (p.1092·2); ammonium chloride (p.1085·2).
Bacterial infections.

Bactrim *Roche, Arg.; Roche, Austral.; Roche, Belg.; Roche, Braz.; Roche, Canad.; Roche, Denm.; Roche, Fr.; Roche, Ger.†; Roche, Irl.; Roche, Ital.; Roche, Mex.; Roche, Norw.; Roche, NZ; Roche, Port.; Roche, S.Afr.; Roche, Singapore; Roche, Swed.; Roche, Switz.; Roche, Thai.; Roche, UK†; Roche, USA.*
Co-trimoxazole (p.193·3).
Bacterial infections; Pneumocystis carinii pneumonia; protozoal infections.

Bactrim Compositum *Roche, Mex.*
Co-trimoxazole (p.193·3); guaifenesin (p.1092·2).
Respiratory-tract infections.

Bactrimel *Roche, Neth.*
Co-trimoxazole (p.193·3).
Bacterial infections; Pneumocystis carinii pneumonia.

Bactrisan *Sanval, Braz.*
Co-trimoxazole (p.193·3).
Bacterial infections; Pneumocystis carinii pneumonia; protozoal infections.

Bactrisan Balsamico *Sanval, Braz.*
Co-trimoxazole (p.193·3); guaifenesin (p.1092·2); ammonium chloride (p.1085·2).
Bacterial infections.

Bactroban *SmithKline Beecham, Aust.; SmithKline Beecham, Austral.; SmithKline Beecham, Belg.; SmithKline Beecham, Braz.; SmithKline Beecham, Canad.; SmithKline Beecham, Denm.; SmithKline Beecham, Fin.; SmithKline Beecham, Fr.; SmithKline Beecham, Hong Kong; SmithKline Beecham, Irl.; SmithKline Beecham, Israel.; SmithKline Beecham, Ital.; SmithKline Beecham, Jpn; SmithKline Beecham, Mex.; SmithKline Beecham, Neth.; SmithKline Beecham, NZ; SmithKline Beecham, S.Afr.; SmithKline Beecham, Singapore; SmithKline Beecham, Spain; SmithKline Beecham, Swed.; SmithKline Beecham, Switz.; SmithKline Beecham, Thai.; SmithKline Beecham, UK; SmithKline Beecham, USA.*
Mupirocin (p.226·1) or calcium mupirocin (p.226·2).
Bacterial skin infections; elimination of nasal staphylococci.

Bactropin *Cimed, Braz.; Sons, Mex.*
Co-trimoxazole (p.193·3).
Bacterial infections; Pneumocystis carinii pneumonia; protozoal infections.

Bactropin Balsamico *Cimed, Braz.*
Co-trimoxazole (p.193·3); guaifenesin (p.1092·2); ammonium chloride (p.1085·2).
Bacterial infections.

Bactylisine *Peters, Fr.*
Mixed quaternary ammonium salts; polyalkylamine.
Surface disinfection.

Bac-Xolid *Ofimex, Mex.*
Ceftriaxone (p.177·1).
Bacterial infections.

Bac-Zidim *Ofimex, Mex.*
Ceftazidime (p.174·3).
Bacterial infections.

Baczole *Nakornpatana, Thai.*
Co-trimoxazole (p.193·3).
Bacterial infections.

Badeol *Agepha, Aust.*
Sulfur (p.1123·3); soya oil (p.1378·1).

Bafucin *Pharmacia Upjohn, Fin.; Pharmacia Upjohn, Swed.*
Benzocaine (p.1306·2); gramicidin (p.213·3); cetylpyridinium chloride (p.1138·1); dichlorobenzyl alcohol (p.1143·2).
Mouth and throat disorders.

Bagnisan med Heilbad *Klemenz, Ger.*
Echinacea purpurea (p.1606·2); hamamelis (p.1618·3); chlorophyllin (p.1028·1).
Bath additive; circulatory disorders; deodorant; nervous disorders; neuralgia; neuritis; skin disorders.

Bagno Oculare *Ogna, Ital.; AFOM, Ital.*
Zinc sulfate (p.1398·2); boric acid (p.1586·1); borax (p.1586·1).
Eye irritation.

Bagren *Serono, Braz.*
Bromocriptine mesilate (p.1164·3).
Acromegaly; hyperprolactinaemia; lactation inhibition; male infertility; neuroleptic malignant syndrome; parkinsonism.

Baicurina *Regius, Braz.*
Paracetamol (p.71·2).
Dysmenorrhoea.

Bain de Bouche Lipha *Monot, Fr.*
Veratrol; menthol (p.1632·3); resorcinol (p.1122·2) cloral hydrate (p.669·3).
Mouthwash.

Bain de Soleil
Note. This name is used for preparations of different composition.
Canderm, Canad.
SPF 4 gel: Octinoxate (p.1517·3); octisalate (p.1518·1).
SPF 4 lotion; SPF 8: Octocrilene (p.1518·1); octinoxate (p.1517·3); titanium dioxide (p.1126·1).
SPF 15; SPF 30: Octocrilene (p.1518·1); octinoxate (p.1517·3); oxybenzone (p.1518·1); titanium dioxide (p.1126·1).
Sunscreen.

Procter & Gamble, USA.
SPF 4: Octinoxate (p.1517·3); octisalate (p.1518·1).
Sunscreen.

Bain de Soleil All Day *Procter & Gamble, USA.*
SPF 4; SPF 8: Octinoxate (p.1517·3); octocrilene (p.1518·1); titanium dioxide (p.1126·1).
SPF 15; SPF 30: Octinoxate (p.1517·3); octocrilene (p.1518·1); oxybenzone (p.1518·1); titanium dioxide (p.1126·1).
Sunscreen.

Bain de Soleil Color *Procter & Gamble, USA.*
SPF 8+: Octinoxate (p.1517·3); octocrilene (p.1518·1).
SPF 15+; SPF 30+: Octinoxate (p.1517·3); octocrilene (p.1518·1); oxybenzone (p.1518·1).
Sunscreen.

Bain de Soleil Mega Tan *Canderm, Canad.*
SPF 4: Octocrilene (p.1518·1); octinoxate (p.1517·3).
Sunscreen.

Bain de Soleil Mega Tanning *Canderm, Canad.*
SPF 30: Octocrilene (p.1518·1); octinoxate (p.1517·3); oxybenzone (p.1518·1).
Sunscreen.

Bain de Soleil Protection *Canderm, Canad.*
SPF 15: Avobenzone (p.1517·1); enzacamene (p.1517·2); octisalate (p.1518·1); titanium dioxide (p.1126·1).
SPF 25: Titanium dioxide (p.1126·1); zinc oxide (p.1128·2).
Sunscreen.

Bain de Soleil Sport
Note. This name is used for preparations of different composition.
Canderm, Canad.
SPF 8: Octocrilene (p.1518·1); octinoxate (p.1517·3); titanium dioxide (p.1126·1).
Sunscreen.

Charton, Canad.
SPF 15: Octocrilene (p.1518·1); octinoxate (p.1517·3); oxybenzone (p.1518·1); titanium dioxide (p.1126·1).
Sunscreen.

Bain extra-doux dermatologique *Widmer, Switz.†*
Coal tar (p.1125·1); chamomile (p.1593·2).
Skin disorders.

Bain extra-doux dermatologique Nouvelle Formule *Widmer, Switz.*
Ichthammol (p.1115·2); chamomile (p.1593·2); guaiazulene (p.1618·3).
Skin disorders.

Bainto *TP, Thai.*
Gamma-aminobutyric acid (p.1613·1).
Amnesia; hypertension; mental function impairment; palsy; speech disorders.

Bakanasan Einschlaf *Bregenzer, Aust.*
Valerian (p.1678·3); lupulus (p.1629·3).
Anxiety; sleep disorders.

Bakanasan Entwasserungs *Bregenzer, Aust.*
Silver birch (p.1585·2).
Urinary-tract disorders.

Bakanasan Leber-Galle *Bregenzer, Aust.*
Silybum marianum (p.1021·3); turmeric (p.1029·3).
Gastrointestinal disorders; liver and gallbladder disorders.

Baknyl *Ariston, Braz.*
Erythromycin (p.201·2); bromhexine hydrochloride (p.1085·3).
Bacterial infections.

Bakteriostat "Herbrand" *Herbrand, Ger.†*
Dequalinium chloride (p.1143·1); ascorbic acid (p.1389·3).
Mouth and throat disorders.

Baktobod Bode, Ger.
Glutaral (p.1145·2); glyoxal (p.1145·3); benzalkonium chloride (p.1133·2).
Surface disinfection.

Baktobod N Bode, Ger.†
Glyoxal (p.1145·3); benzalkonium chloride (p.1133·2).
Surface disinfection.

Baktonium Bode, Ger.
Benzalkonium chloride (p.1133·2).
Hand and skin disinfection.

Bal Tar Euroderm, Ital.†
Castor oil (p.1592·1); ichthammol (p.1115·2).
Seborrhoeic dermatitis.

Balad Korean Drug, Singapore.
Sodium fusidate (p.208·3).
Bacterial skin infections.

Balance ACE Pharmavite, Canad.
Betacarotene; vitamin C; vitamin E; minerals (p.1350·1).

Balanced B Adams, Canad.; Hall, Canad.; Pharmavite, Canad.; Stanley, Canad.; General Nutrition, Canad.
Vitamin B substances (p.1350·1).

Balanced B Complex plus Vitamins C & E Pharmavite, Canad.
Vitamin B substances, vitamin C, and Vitamin E (p.1350·1).

Balanced C Complex Jamieson, Canad.
Ascorbic acid (p.1389·3).

Balanced E Jamieson, Canad.
Vitamin C, vitamin E, and selenium (p.1350·1).

Balanced Irrigating Salt Solution Teva, Israel.
Electrolyte solution (p.1180·1).
Irrigation of eyes, ears, nose, and throat.

Balanced Ratio Cal-Mag Quest, UK.
Calcium, magnesium, and vitamin D preparation (p.1350·1).

Balanced Salt Solution
Alcon, Denm.†; Alcon, NZ; Alcon, UK; Pharmacia, UK; Abbott, USA; Bausch & Lomb, USA; Akorn, USA.
Electrolyte solution (p.1180·1).
Eye irrigation.

Balancid AstraZeneca, Norw.
Magnesium carbonate (p.1232·3); aluminium hydroxide (p.1210·3).
Gastrointestinal disorders associated with hyperacidity.

Balancid Novum
AstraZeneca, Denm.; AstraZeneca, Fin.
Calcium carbonate (p.1215·1); magnesium hydroxide (p.1233·1).
Gastritis; gastro-oesophageal reflux; peptic ulcer.

Balbek Provit, Mex.
Dextromethorphan (p.1087·3).
Coughs.

Balcor
Baldacci, Braz.; Baldacci, Port.
Diltiazem hydrochloride (p.874·3).
Angina pectoris; arrhythmias; hypertension.

Balcoran Whitehall-Robins, Mex.
Vancomycin (p.269·1).

Baldracin Austroplant, Aust.
Valerian (p.1678·3); peppermint leaf (p.1243·2); melissa (p.1632·2); lupulus (p.1629·3).
Nervous disorders; sleep disorders.

Baldrian Solvay, Spain.
Passion flower (p.1649·1); valerian (p.1678·3).
Insomnia; nervous disorders.

Baldrian AMA Kwizda, Aust.
Valerian (p.1678·3); lupulus (p.1629·3).
Nervous disorders; sleep disorders.

Baldrian Dispert Compositum Solvay, Aust.
Valerian (p.1678·3); lupulus (p.1629·3).
Nervous disorders; sleep disorders.

Baldrian-Dispert Solvay, Swed.
Valerian (p.1678·3).
Anxiety; sleep disorders.

Baldrian-Dispert Nacht Solvay, Ger.
Valerian (p.1678·3); lupulus (p.1629·3).
Insomnia.

Baldrian-Elixier Ehrmann, Aust.
Valerian (p.1678·3); lupulus (p.1629·3); melissa (p.1632·2).
Nervous disorders; sleep disorders.

Baldrianetten N Eu Rho, Ger.†
Valerian (p.1678·3).
Anxiety disorders; sleep disorders.

Baldrian-Krautertonikum Bioflora, Aust.
Melissa (p.1632·2); valerian (p.1678·3); lupulus (p.1629·3); orange flowers; lavender flowers (p.1627·2).
Nervous disorders; sleep disorders.

Baldrianox S Hermes, Ger.†
Valerian (p.1678·3); lupulus (p.1629·3).
Nervous and sleep disorders.

Baldrinetten Solvay, Aust.
Valerian (p.1678·3).
Sedative.

Baldriparan Whitehall-Robins, Switz.
Valerian (p.1678·3); melissa (p.1632·2); lupulus (p.1629·3).
Nervous disorders.

Baldriparan Beruhigungs Sanova, Aust.; Wyeth Lederle, Aust.
Valerian (p.1678·3); lupulus (p.1629·3); melissa (p.1632·2).
Nervous disorders; sleep disorders.

Baldriparan N Whitehall-Much, Ger.
Valerian (p.1678·3); lupulus (p.1629·3).
Nervous disorders; sleep disorders.

Baldriparan stark N Whitehall-Much, Ger.
Valerian (p.1678·3); lupulus (p.1629·3); melissa (p.1632·2).
Nervous disorders; sleep disorders.

Baldrisedon Wild, Switz.
Valerian (p.1678·3).
Anxiety; sleep disorders.

Baldrisedon Mono Much, Ger.†
Valerian (p.1678·3).
Nervous disorders; sleep disorders.

Balgifen Berk, UK.
Baclofen (p.1322·3).
Skeletal muscle spasm or spasticity.

Balin
Atlantic, Singapore; Atlantic, Thai.
Sulfadiazine (p.251·1); trimethoprim (p.264·2).
Bacterial infections.

Balisa Hexal, Ger.
Urea (p.1127·3).
Keratinisation disorders.

Balisa VAS Hexal, Ger.
Urea (p.1127·3); tretinoin (p.1126·2).
Keratinisation disorders.

Balkis Dolorgiet, Ger.
Capsules: Phenylephrine hydrochloride (p.1097·1); chlorpheniramine [chlorphenamine] maleate (p.412·1). Formerly contained etilefrine polistirex and chlorpheniramine [chlorphenamine] polistirex.
Colds; hay fever.
Nasal drops; nasal spray: Xylometazoline hydrochloride (p.1102·2).
Nasal congestion.

Balkis Spezial Dolorgiet, Ger.†
Terfenadine (p.424·3).
Allergic rhinitis.

Balm of Gilead
Note.This name is used for preparations of different composition.
Healthcrafts, UK†.
Pastilles: Balm of Gilead (p.1653·2); squill (p.1100·3); lobelia (p.1510·2).
Catarrh; coughs.

Potter's, UK.
Oral mixture: Balm of Gilead (p.1653·2); squill (p.1100·3); lobelia (p.1510·2); lungwort.
Coughs.

Balmandol Spirig, Switz.
Almond oil (p.1576·3); light liquid paraffin (p.1407·2).
Skin disorders.

Balmex
Stafford-Miller, Fr.
Zinc oxide (p.1128·2); liquid paraffin (p.1407·1); beeswax (p.1408·2); silicone (p.1409·3).
Nappy rash.

Stafford-Miller, Port.
Zinc oxide (p.1128·2); liquid paraffin (p.1407·1); beeswax (p.1408·2); dimethicone (p.1410·1).
Nappy rash.

Balmex Baby Macsil, USA.
Zinc oxide (p.1128·2); peru balsam (p.1650·2); corn starch (p.1379·3); calcium carbonate (p.1215·1).
Nappy rash.

Balmex Emollient Block, USA.
Emollient and moisturiser.

Balminil Elfar, Spain.
Nitrendipine (p.947·1).
Angina pectoris; hypertension; Raynaud's syndrome.

Balminil Camphorub Rougier, Canad.
Camphor (p.1589·3); menthol (p.1632·3); eucalyptol (p.1609·2).
Pain.

Balminil Decongestant
Rougier, Canad.; Rougier, Hong Kong.
Pseudoephedrine hydrochloride (p.1099·2).
Nasal and sinus congestion.

Balminil DM
Rougier, Canad.; Rougier, Hong Kong.
Dextromethorphan hydrobromide (p.1087·3).
Coughs.

Balminil DM D Rougier, Canad.
Pseudoephedrine hydrochloride (p.1099·2); dextromethorphan hydrobromide (p.1087·3).
Congestion; coughs.

Balminil DM D E Rougier, Canad.
Dextromethorphan hydrobromide (p.1087·3); pseudoephedrine hydrochloride (p.1099·2); guaifenesin (p.1092·2).
Congestion; cough.

Balminil DM E Rougier, Canad.
Dextromethorphan hydrobromide (p.1087·3); guaifenesin (p.1092·2).
Coughs.

Balminil Expectorant Rougier, Canad.
Guaifenesin (p.1092·2).
Coughs.

Balminil Lozenges Rougier, Canad.
Cetylpyridinium chloride (p.1138·1); benzocaine (p.1306·2).
Mouth and throat disorders.

Balminil Nasal Ointment Rougier, Canad.
Camphor (p.1589·3); menthol (p.1632·3); eucalyptol (p.1609·2); chlorobutanol (p.1141·2); ephedrine hydrochloride (p.1090·1).
Nasal congestion.

Balminil Suppositories Rougier, Canad.
Eucalyptus oil (p.1609·2); niaouli oil (p.1640·2); menthol (p.1632·3); sodium dibunate (p.1100·3).
Coughs.

Balmosa Pharmax, UK.
Methyl salicylate (p.55·1); menthol (p.1632·3); camphor (p.1589·3); capsicum oleoresin (p.1591·1).
Pain.

Balmox
Yamanouchi, Port.; SmithKline Beecham, Switz.
Nabumetone (p.59·3).
Musculoskeletal, joint, peri-articular, and soft-tissue disorders.

Balneoconzen S & K, Ger.
Soya oil (p.1378·1); lecithin (p.1628·1).
Skin disorders.

Balneogel Boots Healthcare, Spain.
Allantoin (p.1110·1); chlorophyllin (p.1028·1); guaiazulene (p.1618·3); lauril polyoxyethylene sulfate; riboflavin sodium phosphate (p.1386·1).
Skin disorders; soap substitute.

Balneol Solvay, USA.
Skin cleanser.

Balneovit Biocur, Ger.
Soya oil (p.1378·1).
Bath additive; skin disorders.

Balnetar
Westwood-Squibb, Canad.; Westwood-Squibb, USA.
Coal tar (p.1125·1).
Dermatitis; psoriasis.

Balneum
Hermal, Aust.; Hermal, Ger.; Boots Healthcare, Irl.; Hermal, Israel; Hermal, Port.†; Crookes Healthcare, UK.
Soya oil (p.1378·1).
Bath additive; dry skin.

Balneum F
Hermal, Aust.; Hermal, Ger.; Hermal, Israel.
Arachis oil (p.1581·1); light liquid paraffin (p.1407·2).
Bath additive; skin disorders.

Balneum Hermal
Hermal, Hong Kong; Boots Healthcare, Ital.; Boots Healthcare, Switz.
Soya oil (p.1378·1).
Bath additive; skin disorders.

Balneum Hermal F Boots Healthcare, Switz.
Arachis oil (p.1581·1); liquid paraffin (p.1407·1).
Skin disorders.

Balneum Hermal Forte Boots Healthcare, Ital.
Liquid paraffin (p.1407·1); arachis oil (p.1581·1).
Bath additive; skin disorders.

Balneum Hermal Plus Boots Healthcare, Switz.
Soya oil (p.1378·1); macrogol lauril ethers (p.1345·2).
Skin disorders.

Balneum mit Teer Hermal, Aust.
Soya oil (p.1378·1); coal tar (p.1125·1).
Skin disorders.

Balneum Plus
Note.This name is used for preparations of different composition.
Hermal, Aust.; Hermal, Ger.; Boots Healthcare, Irl.; Hermal, Israel; Crookes Healthcare, UK.
Soya oil (p.1378·1); lauromacrogol 400 (p.1345·2).
Bath additive; dry skin; pruritus.

Crookes Healthcare, UK.
Cream: Lauromacrogol (p.1345·2); urea (p.1127·3).
Skin disorders.

Balneum surgras Merck-Clevenot, Fr.†
Arachis oil (p.1581·1); liquid paraffin (p.1407·1).
Bath additive; skin disorders.

Balneum with Tar
E. Merck, Irl.; E. Merck, UK†.
Soya oil (p.1378·1); coal tar (p.1125·1).
Bath additive; skin disorders.

Balnostim Bad N Hoernecke, Ger.†
Pine needle oil; rosemary oil (p.1659·3).
Musculoskeletal, joint, and soft-tissue disorders.

Balodin Ferrer, Spain.
Dirithromycin (p.199·2).
Bacterial infections.

Balpril Baldacci, Port.
Enalapril maleate (p.883·3).
Heart failure; hypertension.

Balsabit Pensa, Spain.
Pramocaine hydrochloride (p.1318·2).
Burns; insect bites; pruritus.

Balsacetil Biotekfarma, Ital.†
Guacetisal (p.1092·1).
Respiratory-tract disorders.

Balsamicum Weleda, Ger.
Calendula (p.1589·2); mercurialis perennis; peru balsam (p.1650·2); stibium metallicum praeparatum.
Minor wounds; nappy rash.

Balsamina Kroner Ceccarelli, Ital.
Sulfogaiacol (p.1101·1); mepyramine maleate (p.421·1).
Formerly contained sulfogaiacol, mepyramine, hedera, and cherry-laurel.
Coughs.

Balsamo Analgesic Karmel Agua del Carmen, Spain†.
Camphor (p.1589·3); beleo; stramonium (p.474·1); amyl salicylate (p.14·1); menthol (p.1632·3).

Formerly known as Karmel Balsamo.
Rheumatic and muscle pain.

Balsamo Analgesico
Note.This name is used for preparations of different composition.
Basi, Port.; Upsifarma, Port.
Salicylic acid (p.1122·3); menthol (p.1632·3); methyl salicylate (p.55·1).

Medical, Port.
Salicylic acid (p.1122·3); capsicum (p.1591·1); menthol (p.1632·3).

Balsamo Analgesico Labesfal Labesfal, Port.
Methyl salicylate (p.55·1).
Formerly contained salicylic acid, menthol, methyl salicylate, belladonna, and capsicum.

Balsamo Analgesico Sanitas Upsifarma, Port.
Methyl salicylate (p.55·1); salicylic acid (p.1122·3); menthol (p.1632·3); capsicum (p.1591·1).
Formerly contained methyl salicylate, salicylic acid, menthol, belladonna, and capsicum.
Musculoskeletal and joint pain.

Balsamo Branco Catarinense, Braz.
Lavender (p.1627·2); melissa (p.1632·2); caraway (p.1591·2); aniseed (p.1580·2); cinnamon (p.1595·3); clove (p.1596·3); lemon.
Dyspepsia.

Balsamo Italstadium Falqui, Ital.
Methyl salicylate (p.55·1); menthol (p.1632·3); camphor (p.1589·3).
Musculoskeletal and joint pain.

Balsamo Midalgan Sanofi Synthelabo, Spain.
Capsicum (p.1591·1); methyl nicotinate (p.55·1); methyl salicylate (p.55·1).
Rheumatic and muscle pain.

Balsamo Sifcamina Teoforma, Ital.
Methyl nicotinate (p.55·1); glycol salicylate (p.42·2).
Musculoskeletal disorders.

Balsamorhinol Etris, Fr.
Chlorobutanol (p.1141·2); menthol (p.1632·3).
Nose and throat infections.

Balsandin Dinafarma, Braz.
Co-trimoxazole (p.193·3).
Bacterial infections; Pneumocystis carinii pneumonia; protozoal infections.

Balsatux Edmond Pharma, Ital.
Sulfogaiacol (p.1101·1); dextromethorphan hydrobromide (p.1087·3).
Coughs.

Balsi-Bron Liferpal, Mex.
Ambroxol (p.1084·3).

Balsiprin Eurofarma, Braz.
Co-trimoxazole (p.193·3); guaifenesin (p.1092·2); ammonium chloride (p.1085·2).
Bacterial infections.

Balsoclase
Note.This name is used for preparations of different composition.
Bios, Belg.
Oral drops: Pentoxyverine citrate (p.1096·3); guaifenesin (p.1092·2); eucalyptol (p.1609·2); terpin hydrate (p.1101·2); thymol (p.1158·3).
Oral solution: Pentoxyverine citrate (p.1096·3); terpin hydrate (p.1101·2).
Suppositories: Pentoxyverine citrate (p.1096·3); guaifenesin (p.1092·2); eucalyptol (p.1609·2); terpineol (p.1669·3); terpin hydrate (p.1101·2).
Syrup: Pentoxyverine citrate (p.1096·3); eucalyptol (p.1609·2); terpin hydrate (p.1101·2); thyme (p.1672·2).
Coughs.

UCB, Neth.
Pentoxyverine citrate (p.1096·3).
Coughs.

Balsoclase Compositum UCB, Neth.
Pentoxyverine citrate (p.1096·3); cineole (p.1609·2); sodium citrate (p.1186·2); terpin hydrate (p.1101·2); thyme (p.1672·2).
Coughs.

Balsoclase-E UCB, Neth.
Pentoxyverine citrate (p.1096·3); cineole (p.1609·2).
Coughs.

Balsofumine Sanofi Winthrop, Fr.
Peru balsam (p.1650·2); sumatra benzoin (p.1668·3); eucalyptus (p.1609·2); lavender oil (p.1627·2); thyme oil (p.1672·3).
Respiratory-tract congestion.

Balsofumine Mentholee Sanofi Winthrop, Fr.
Peru balsam (p.1650·2); sumatra benzoin (p.1668·3); eucalyptus (p.1609·2); lavender oil (p.1627·2); thyme oil (p.1672·3); menthol (p.1632·3).
Respiratory-tract congestion.

Balsolene Cooperation Pharmaceutique, Fr.
Eucalyptus oil (p.1609·2); niaouli oil (p.1640·2); menthol (p.1632·3); siam benzoin (p.1662·3).
Respiratory-tract congestion.

Balsoprim Juste, Spain.
Bromhexine hydrochloride (p.1085·3); co-trimoxazole (p.193·3).
Respiratory-tract infections.

Balta Intimo Soluzione Lutsia, Ital.†
Menthol (p.1632·3); eucalyptol (p.1609·2); Iceland moss; undecenoic acid (p.395·3).
Personal hygiene.

Balta-Crin Tar Boots Healthcare, Ital.
Tar (p.1125·1); allantoin (p.1110·1).
Seborrhoeic dermatitis.

Baltar
E. Merck, Irl.; E. Merck, UK†.
Coal tar (p.1125·1).
Scalp disorders.

Balto Foot Balm Lane, UK.
Camphor (p.1589·3); menthol (p.1632·3); zinc oxide (p.1128·2); precipitated sulfur (p.1123·3).
Aching feet; excessive perspiration; hard skin.

Balurol Baldacci, Braz.
Pipemidic acid (p.236·1).
Urinary-tract infections.

Bamalite Tecnobio, Spain.
Lansoprazole (p.1230·3).
Gastro-oesophageal reflux; peptic ulcer.

Bambec
Astra, Aust.; AstraZeneca, Denm.; Stern, Ger.; Astra, Ger.; Astra, Hong Kong; Astra, Ital.; AstraZeneca, Norw.; AstraZeneca, NZ; AstraZeneca, Singapore; Astra, Spain; Draco, Swed.; Astra, Switz.; AstraZeneca, Thai.; AstraZeneca, UK.
Bambuterol hydrochloride (p.761·1).
Obstructive airways disease.

Bamifix
Farmalab, Braz.; Chiesi, Ital.
Bamifylline hydrochloride (p.761·2).
Obstructive airways disease.

Bamixol Pulitzer, Ital.
Bamifylline hydrochloride (p.761·2).
Asthma; bronchospasm.

Bamycor
AstraZeneca, Norw.; Hassle, Swed.
Aspirin (p.14·2).
Cardiovascular and cerebrovascular disorders.

Bamyl Hassle, Swed.
Aspirin (p.14·2).
Fever; inflammation; pain.

Bamyl koffein Hassle, Swed.
Aspirin (p.14·2); caffeine (p.761·3).
Fever; pain.

Bamyl S Hassle, Swed.
Aspirin (p.14·2).
Fever; pain.

Bamyl S koffein Hassle, Swed.
Aspirin (p.14·2); caffeine (p.761·3).
Fever; pain.

Bamyxin Rekah, Israel.
Bacitracin (p.155·2); neomycin sulfate (p.228·1); polymyxin B sulfate (p.238·1).
Bacterial eye infections.

Ban Pain Triomed, S.Afr.
Syrup: Paracetamol (p.71·2); codeine phosphate (p.25·2); promethazine hydrochloride (p.423·2).
Fever; pain.
Tablets: Paracetamol (p.71·2); codeine phosphate (p.25·2); caffeine (p.761·3); meprobamate (p.691·1).
Pain with tension.

Banadyne-3 Norstar, USA.
Lignocaine [lidocaine] (p.1313·2); menthol (p.1632·3); alcohol (p.1630·3).
Herpes labialis.

Banalg Forest Pharmaceuticals, USA.
Methyl salicylate (p.55·1); camphor (p.1589·3); menthol (p.1632·3).
Muscle, joint, and soft-tissue pain; neuralgia.

Banan
Sankyo, Hong Kong; Sankyo, Jpn; Sankyo, Thai.
Cefpodoxime proxetil (p.172·3).
Bacterial infections.

Banana Boat Action Sport Banana Boat, Canad.
SPF 25: Homosalate (p.1517·2); octinoxate (p.1517·3); octisalate (p.1518·1); oxybenzone (p.1518·1).
Sunscreen.

Banana Boat Active Kids Banana Boat, Canad.
SPF 30: Octinoxate (p.1517·3); octisalate (p.1518·1); oxybenzone (p.1518·1); titanium dioxide (p.1126·1).
SPF 50: Octocrilene (p.1518·1); octinoxate (p.1517·3); octisalate (p.1518·1); oxybenzone (p.1518·1).
Sunscreen.

Banana Boat Aloe Vera Lip Balm Sunblock Banana Boat, Canad.
SPF 30†: Padimate O (p.1518·2); octinoxate (p.1517·3); oxybenzone (p.1518·1).
SPF 30: Padimate O (p.1518·2); octinoxate (p.1517·3); oxybenzone (p.1518·1); homosalate (p.1517·2).
Sunscreen.

Banana Boat Baby Sunblock Banana Boat, Canad.
SPF 50: Octinoxate (p.1517·3); octisalate (p.1518·1); oxybenzone (p.1518·1); titanium dioxide (p.1126·1). Formerly contained octocrilene, octinoxate, octisalate, and oxybenzone.
Sunscreen.

Banana Boat Bite Block Banana Boat, Canad.
SPF 15: Octinoxate (p.1517·3); oxybenzone (p.1518·1).
SPF 30: Homosalate (p.1517·2); octinoxate (p.1517·3); octisalate (p.1518·1); oxybenzone (p.1518·1).
Sunscreen.

Banana Boat Cool Coloring Banana Boat, Canad.
SPF 30: Homosalate (p.1517·2); octinoxate (p.1517·3); octisalate (p.1518·1); oxybenzone (p.1518·1); titanium dioxide (p.1126·1).
Sunscreen.

Banana Boat Cool Colorz Banana Boat, Canad.
Homosalate (p.1517·2); octinoxate (p.1517·3); octisalate (p.1518·1); oxybenzone (p.1518·1); titanium dioxide (p.1126·1).
Sunscreen.

Banana Boat Dark Tanning Banana Boat, Canad.
Lotion SPF 4: Padimate O (p.1518·2).
Oil SPF 4: Padimate O (p.1518·2); octinoxate (p.1517·3).
Sunscreen.

Banana Boat Faces Plus Banana Boat, Canad.
SPF 23: Octinoxate (p.1517·3); octisalate (p.1518·1); oxybenzone (p.1518·1); homosalate(p.1517·2); titanium dioxide (p.1126·1). Formerly contained octinoxate, octisalate, and oxybenzone.
SPF 31†: Octinoxate (p.1517·3); octisalate (p.1518·1); oxybenzone (p.1518·1); titanium dioxide (p.1126·1).
Sunscreen.

Banana Boat Funky Fruit Lip Balm Banana Boat, Canad.
SPF 15: Padimate O (p.1518·2); homosalate (p.1517·2); octinoxate (p.1517·3); oxybenzone (p.1518·1).
Sunscreen.

Banana Boat Oil Free Banana Boat, Canad.
SPF 30: Octinoxate (p.1517·3); octisalate (p.1518·1); oxybenzone (p.1518·1); homosalate (p.1517·2); titanium dioxide (p.1126·1). Formerly contained octinoxate, octisalate, and oxybenzone.
Sunscreen.

Banana Boat Quik Blok Banana Boat, Canad.
SPF 15; SPF 25: Homosalate (p.1517·2); octinoxate (p.1517·3); octisalate (p.1518·1); oxybenzone (p.1518·1); titanium dioxide (p.1126·1).
Sunscreen.

Banana Boat Sooth-A-Caine Banana Boat, Canad.
Menthol (p.1632·3); lignocaine [lidocaine] (p.1313·2).

Banana Boat Sport Banana Boat, Canad.
SPF 15: Octinoxate (p.1517·3); octisalate (p.1518·1); oxybenzone (p.1518·1).
SPF 30: Octinoxate (p.1517·3); octisalate (p.1518·1); oxybenzone (p.1518·1); titanium dioxide (p.1126·1).
SPF 50†: Octinoxate (p.1517·3); octisalate (p.1518·1); oxybenzone (p.1518·1); octocrilene (p.1518·1).
Sunscreen.

Banana Boat Sunblock Banana Boat, Canad.
SPF 15: Octinoxate (p.1517·3); octisalate (p.1518·1); oxybenzone (p.1518·1).
Sunscreen.

Banana Boat Sunless Tanning Banana Boat, Canad.
SPF 8: Octinoxate (p.1517·3); oxybenzone (p.1518·1).
Sunscreen.

Banana Boat Sunscreen Banana Boat, Canad.
SPF 8: Padimate O (p.1518·2); oxybenzone (p.1518·1).
Sunscreen.

Banana Boat Ultra Banana Boat, Canad.
SPF 30: Octinoxate (p.1517·3); octisalate (p.1518·1); oxybenzone (p.1518·1); titanium dioxide (p.1126·1).
Sunscreen.

Banana Boat Ultra Plus Banana Boat, Canad.
SPF 50: Octinoxate (p.1517·3); octisalate (p.1518·1); oxybenzone (p.1518·1); octocrilene (p.1518·1).
Sunscreen.

Banana Boat Vitamin E Lip Balm Sunblock Banana Boat, Canad.
SPF 30: Octinoxate (p.1517·3); homosalate (p.1517·2); oxybenzone (p.1518·1); padimate O (p.1518·2). Formerly contained octinoxate, octocrilene, oxybenzone, and padimate O.

Bancap HC Forest Pharmaceuticals, USA.
Hydrocodone tartrate (p.42·2); paracetamol (p.71·2).
Pain.

Band Aid Sprufplaster Johnson & Johnson, Ger.
Cellaburat; octyldiphenylphosphate.
Skin ulcers; wounds.

Band-Aid Antibiotic Johnson & Johnson, Canad.
Bacitracin zinc (p.155·2); polymyxin B sulfate (p.238·1).

Bandol Pharmacia Upjohn, Spain.
Paracetamol (p.71·2).
Fever; pain.

Banedif Maxfarma, Spain.
Bacitracin (p.155·2); neomycin sulfate (p.228·1); zinc oxide (p.1128·2).
Infected skin disorders.

Baneocin
Biochemie, Aust.; Biochemie, Singapore.
Bacitracin (p.155·2) or bacitracin zinc (p.155·2); neomycin sulfate (p.228·1).
Bacterial infections.

Baneopol Streuli, Switz.
Bacitracin (p.155·2); polymyxin B sulfate (p.238·1); neomycin sulfate (p.228·1).
Infected eye and skin disorders.

Banflex Forest Pharmaceuticals, USA.
Orphenadrine citrate (p.470·3).
Musculoskeletal pain.

Banholeum Sofex, Port.†.
Soya oil (p.1378·1).
Skin disorders.

Banholeum Composto Sofex, Port.†.
Soya oil (p.1378·1); coal tar (p.1125·1).
Skin disorders.

Banholeum Gel Sofex, Port.†.
Soya oil (p.1378·1); liquid paraffin (p.1407·1).
Skin disorders.

Banimax SmithKline Beecham, UK.
Aspirin (p.14·2); paracetamol (p.71·2).

Banish II Smith & Nephew, Austral.
Zinc ricinoleate; dipropylene glycol.
Colostomy and ileostomy odour.

Banishing Cream Avon, Canad.
Hydroquinone (p.1115·1).

Banlice Pfizer, Austral.
Pyrethrins; piperonyl butoxide (p.1436·2).
Pediculosis.

Banocin Nakornpatana, Thai.
Ointment: Neomycin sulfate (p.228·1); polymyxin B sulfate (p.238·1); bacitracin zinc (p.155·2).
Topical powder: Clioquinol (p.190·2); bacitracin (p.155·2); neomycin sulfate (p.228·1); zinc stearate (p.1497·3).
Burns; ulcers; wounds.

Banoftal Alcon Cusi, Spain.
Boric acid (p.1586·1); calendula (p.1589·2); hamamelis (p.1618·3); borax (p.1586·1).
Eye disorders.

Banophen Allergy Major, USA.
Diphenhydramine hydrochloride (p.416·1).
Hypersensitivity reactions; insomnia; motion sickness.

Banophen Decongestant Major, USA.
Diphenhydramine hydrochloride (p.416·1); pseudoephedrine hydrochloride (p.1099·2).
Hypersensitivity reactions; insomnia; motion sickness.

BanSmoke Thompson, USA†.
Benzocaine (p.1306·2).
Aid to smoking withdrawal.

Ban-Sol Mex-America, Mex.
SPF 15; SPF 30: Avobenzone (p.1517·1); octinoxate (p.1517·3).
Sunsreen.

Bansor Thornton & Ross, UK.
Cetrimide (p.1137·1).
Sore gums.

Bantel Nakorn, Thai.
Pyrantel embonate (p.108·1).
Worm infections.

Bantenol Abello, Spain.
Mebendazole (p.102·2).
Worm infections.

Banthine Schiapparelli Searle, USA†.
Methanthelinium bromide (p.470·2).
Adjunct in peptic ulcer; neurogenic bladder.

Bantron DEP, USA†.
Lobeline sulfate (p.1510·3).
Aid to smoking withdrawal.

Baralgan Albert, S.Afr.†.
Dipyrone (p.34·1); pitofenone hydrochloride (p.1652·3); fenpiverinium bromide (p.1610·3).
Colic; genital-tract spasm.

Baralgin Hoechst Marion Roussel, Ger.
Dipyrone (p.34·1).
Colic; pain.

Baralgin M Hoechst Marion Roussel, Braz.
Dipyrone (p.34·1).
Fever; pain.

Baran-mild N Mickan, Ger.
Benzocaine (p.1306·2); olive oil (p.1643·3); zinc oxide (p.1398·1).
Skin disorders; wounds.

Baratol
Shire, Irl.; Aspen, S.Afr.; Shire, UK.
Indoramin hydrochloride (p.913·3).
Hypertension.

Barazan Dieckmann, Ger.
Norfloxacin (p.232·1).
Bacterial infections of the urinary tract.

Barbamin Streuli, Switz.†.
Propyphenazone (p.80·2); diphenhydramine hydrochloride (p.416·1).
Fever; pain.

Barbidonna Wallace, USA.
Atropine sulfate (p.461·1); hyoscine hydrobromide (p.468·2); hyoscyamine hydrobromide (p.469·3) or hyoscyamine sulfate (p.469·3); phenobarbital (p.355·1).
Gastrointestinal disorders.

Barbloc Alphapharm, Austral.
Pindolol (p.955·3).
Angina pectoris; arrhythmias; hypertension.

Barc Del, USA.
Pyrethrins; piperonyl butoxide (p.1436·2).
Pediculosis.

Barcan
UCB, Denm.; UCB, Fin.; UCB, Norw.; UCB, Swed.
Aceclofenac (p.11·1).
Inflammation; musculoskeletal and joint disorders.

Bareon Hokuriku, Jpn†.
Lomefloxacin hydrochloride (p.220·1).
Bacterial infections.

Barexal Ipsen, Belg.
Smectite; aluminium hydroxide-magnesium carbonate co-dried gel (p.1211·2).
Diarrhoea.

Baricon Lafayette, USA.
Barium sulfate (p.1032·1).
Contrast medium for gastrointestinal radiography.

Baridium Pfeiffer, USA.
Phenazopyridine hydrochloride (p.77·3).
Irritation of the lower urinary tract.

Barigraf Juste, Spain.
Barium sulfate (p.1032·1).
Contrast medium for gastrointestinal radiography.

Barigraf Tac Juste, Spain.
Barium sulfate (p.1032·1).
Simeticone (p.1249·2) is included in this preparation to eliminate gas from the gastrointestinal tract before tomography.
Contrast medium for gastrointestinal computerised axial tomography.

Barilux
Waldheim, Aust.
Barium sulfate (p.1032·1).
Contrast medium for colon radiography.
Goldham, Ger.
Barium sulfate (p.1032·1).
Formerly known as Falibaryt.
Radiographic contrast medium.
Goldham, Ger.
Barium sulfate (p.1032·1).
Formerly known as Unibaryt.
Contrast medium for gastrointestinal radiography.

Barilux Brausetabletten Goldham, Ger.
Sodium bicarbonate (p.1186·2); citric acid (p.1596·2); dimethicone (p.1249·2).
Adjunct in gastrointestinal radiography.

Bario Dif Rovi, Spain.
Barium sulfate (p.1032·1).
Dimethicone (p.1249·2) is included in this preparation to eliminate gas from the gastrointestinal tract before radiography.
Contrast medium for gastrointestinal radiography.

Bario Faes Faes, Spain†.
Barium sulfate (p.1032·1).
Dimethicone (p.1249·2) is included in this preparation to eliminate gas from the gastrointestinal tract before radiography.
Contrast medium for gastrointestinal radiography.

Bario Faes Ultra Faes, Spain†.
Barium sulfate (p.1032·1).
Contrast medium for gastrointestinal radiography.

Bario Llorente Llorente, Spain.
Barium sulfate (p.1032·1).
Contrast medium for gastrointestinal radiography.

Bariogel Cristalia, Braz.
Barium sulfate (p.1032·1).
Contrast medium for gastrointestinal radiography.

Bariopacin Serra Pamies, Spain.
Barium sulfate (p.1032·1).
Contrast medium for gastrointestinal radiography.

Bariotest Schering, Braz.
Barium sulfate (p.1032·1).
Contrast medium for gastrointestinal radiography.

Baripril Lesvi, Spain.
Enalapril maleate (p.883·3).
Heart failure; hypertension.

Baripril Diu Lesvi, Spain.
Enalapril maleate (p.883·3); hydrochlorothiazide (p.907·3).
Hypertension.

Baritop Bioglan, UK.
Barium sulfate (p.1032·1).
Contrast medium for gastrointestinal tract radiography.

Barium Med Complex Dynamit, Aust.
Homoeopathic preparation.

Barmicil Sons, Mex.
Gentamicin sulfate (p.210·1).
Bacterial infections.

Barnes-Hind Cleaning and Soaking Solution
Allergan, Austral.†.
Cleansing and storage solution for hard contact lenses (p.1129·2).

Barnes-Hind Wetting Solution Allergan, Austral.†.
Polyvinyl alcohol (p.1503·1)(p.1129·2).
Wetting solution for hard contact lenses.

Barnetil
Sanofi Synthelabo, Belg.; Synthelabo, Fr.; Synthelabo, Port.†.
Sultopride hydrochloride (p.707·1).
Psychoses.

Barnotil Sanofi Synthelabo, Ital.
Sultopride hydrochloride (p.707·1).
Psychoses.

Baro-cat Lafayette, USA.
Barium sulfate (p.1032·1).
Contrast medium for gastrointestinal radiography.

Baroflave Lannett, USA†.
Barium sulfate (p.1032·1).
Contrast medium for gastrointestinal radiography.

Barokaton Sanova, Aust.
Injection: 1-(β-Diethylaminoethyl)-theobromin-ethylbromide; 2-diethylaminoethanol hydrochloride (p.1508·3).
Tablets: 1-(β-Diethylaminoethyl)-theobromin-ethylbromide.
Asthma; cardiovascular disorders.

Baropac Darrow, Braz.
Barium sulfate (p.1032·1).
Contrast medium for gastrointestinal radiography.

The symbol † denotes a preparation no longer actively marketed

Baros *Lafayette, USA.*
Sodium bicarbonate (p.1186·2); tartaric acid (p.1669·2); simeticone (p.1249·2).
Adjunct in gastrointestinal radiography.

Barosperse *Lafayette, USA.*
Barium sulfate (p.1032·1).
Contrast medium for gastrointestinal radiography.

Barotonal *Dumex, Ger.*
Hydrochlorothiazide (p.907·3); reserpine (p.967·3).
Hypertension.

Barpil *Biolab, Thai.*
Buspirone hydrochloride (p.657·2).
Anxiety.

Barrier Cream *National Care, Canad.*
Dimethicone (p.1410·1).
Skin disorders.

Barriere *Roberts, Canad.*
Dimethicone (p.1410·1).
Skin disorders.

Barriere-HC *Roberts, Canad.*
Hydrocortisone (p.1073·3).
Skin disorders.

Barrycidal *Barry, Ital.*
Alkylbenzyldimethylammonium chloride (p.1133·2); benzethonium chloride (p.1134·2); diisobutylcresoxyethoxyethyl-benzyldimethylammonium chloride.
Instrument disinfection.

Bartelin N *OTW, Ger.*
Diethylamine salicylate (p.32·2); camphor (p.1589·3); turpentine oil (p.1676·3).
Musculoskeletal and joint disorders; neuralgia; neuritis.

Bartelin nico *OTW, Ger.*
Diethylamine salicylate (p.32·2); benzyl nicotinate (p.20·2); oleum pini sylvestris.
Musculoskeletal and joint disorders; neuralgia; neuritis.

Barytgen *Fuji, Swed.†.*
Barium sulfate (p.1032·1).
Contrast medium for gastrointestinal radiography.

B₁₂-AS *Teva, Ger.*
Cyanocobalamin (p.1388·1).
Vitamin B₁₂ deficiency.

Basal-H-Insulin *Hoechst, Ger.†.*
Isophane insulin (human) (p.324·1).
Diabetes mellitus.

Basaljel
Note. This name is used for preparations of different composition.
Axcan, Canad.
Aluminium hydroxide (p.1210·3).
Hyperphosphataemia.

Wyeth-Ayerst, USA.
Dried basic aluminium carbonate gel (p.1210·2).
Hyperacidity; hyperphosphataemia.

Basan *Leiras, Fin.*
Basis for topical preparations.

Bascardial *Bastian, Ger.*
Potassium aspartate (p.1195·2); magnesium aspartate (p.1190·3).
Coronary circulation disorders with magnesium and potassium deficiency.

Basdene *Doms-Adrian, Fr.*
Benzylthiouracil (p.1521·1).
Hyperthyroidism.

Bas-Dextrano *Braun, Port.*
Dextran 40 (p.728·3) in glucose or sodium chloride.
Plasma volume expansion; thromboembolic disorders.

Baseler Haussalbe *Sanico, Belg.†.*
Zinc oxide (p.1128·2); zinc stearate (p.1497·3); bismuth subnitrate (p.1213·2); titanium dioxide (p.1126·1); borax (p.1586·1); sodium salicylate (p.84·2); purified talc (p.1124·2).
Barrier cream; skin disorders.

Basen
Takeda, Jpn; Takeda, Thai.
Voglibose (p.337·3).
Diabetes mellitus.

Basicaina *Senese, Ital.*
Lignocaine [lidocaine] hydrochloride (p.1313·2).
Local anaesthesia.

Basilan *Baldacci, Braz.*
Arginine; calcium inositol hexaphosphate; magnesium inositol hexaphosphate; pyridoxine (p.1350·1).
Nutritional supplement.

Basinal *Basi, Port.*
Naltrexone hydrochloride (p.1016·1).
Opioid withdrawal syndrome.

Basireuma *Basi, Port.*
Phenylbutazone (p.78·1).

Basiron
Galderma, Denm.; Galderma, Fin.; Galderma, Norw.; Galderma, Swed.; Basotherm, Switz.†.
Benzoyl peroxide (p.1111·1).
Acne.

Basiter *Galderma, Ger.*
Coal tar (p.1125·1).
Eczema; psoriasis.

B1-Asmedic *Dyckerhoff, Ger.*
Thiamine nitrate (p.1385·1).
Vitamin B₁ deficiency.

B2-Asmedic *Dyckerhoff, Ger.*
Riboflavin (p.1386·1).
Riboflavin deficiency.

B6-Asmedic *Dyckerhoff, Ger.*
Pyridoxine hydrochloride (p.1386·3).
Vitamin B₆ deficiency.

Basocef *Curasan, Ger.*
Cefazolin sodium (p.164·3).
Bacterial infections.

Basocin *Galderma, Ger.*
Clindamycin phosphate (p.188·2).
Acne.

Basodexan
Procter & Gamble, Aust.; Hermal, Ger.
Urea (p.1127·3).
Skin disorders.

Basoplex *Riemser, Ger.*
Paracetamol (p.71·2); phenylpropanolamine hydrochloride (p.1098·1); dextromethorphan hydrobromide (p.1087·3).
Coughs and cold symptoms.

Basotar *Galderma, Denm.*
Coal tar (p.1125·1).
Psoriasis; seborrhoeic dermatitis.

Bassado *Monsanto, Ital.*
Doxycycline hyclate (p.200·1).
Bacterial infections.

Basti-Cal *Bastian, Ger.*
Calcium carbonate (p.1215·1).
Calcium deficiency; osteoporosis.

Basticrat *Bastian, Ger.*
Crataegus (p.1600·2).
Cardiac disorders.

Basti-Mag *Bastian, Ger.*
Magnesium aspartate (p.1190·3).
Magnesium deficiency.

Bastiverit *Bastian, Ger.*
Glibenclamide (p.321·3).
Diabetes mellitus.

Bastoncino *Whitehall, Ital.†.*
Eugenol (p.1609·3).
Oral hygiene; temporary dental filling.

Bat *Zeta, Ital.*
Cetylpyridinium chloride (p.1138·1).
Disinfection of wounds and burns.

Bateral *Allen, Mex.*
Co-trimoxazole (p.193·3).
Bacterial infections.

Bath E45 *Crookes Healthcare, UK.*
Bath additive.
Dry skin.

Batmen *Menarini, Spain.*
Prednicarbate (p.1077·3).
Skin disorders.

Batrafen
Hoechst Marion Roussel, Aust.; Hoechst Marion Roussel, Ger.; Hoechst Marion Roussel, Hong Kong; Hoechst Marion Roussel, Irl.; Hoechst Marion Roussel, Israel; Aventis, Ital.; Aventis, NZ; Hoechst Marion Roussel, Spain; Knoll, Switz.
Ciclopirox (p.382·1) or ciclopirox olamine (p.382·1).
Fungal skin, nail, and vulvovaginal infections.

Batramycin *Geistlich, Singapore.*
Bacitracin (p.155·2); neomycin sulfate (p.228·1).
Bacterial skin infections.

Batramycine *Geistlich, Switz.*
Nasal ointment: Bacitracin (p.155·2); neomycin sulfate (p.228·1); octacaine hydrochloride (p.1317·3).
Bacterial nasal infections.

Ointment; topical powder: Bacitracin (p.155·2); neomycin sulfate (p.228·1).
Infected wounds or burns.

Batrax *Gewo, Ger.*
Nasal ointment: Bacitracin (p.155·2); neomycin sulfate (p.228·1); octacaine hydrochloride (p.1317·3).
Nasal infections.

Ointment; topical powder: Bacitracin (p.155·2); neomycin sulfate (p.228·1).
Bacterial skin infections.

Batrizol *Medimport, Mex.*
Co-trimoxazole (p.193·3).
Bacterial infections.

Baudry *Boiron, Canad.*
Homoeopathic preparation.

Baume *Zeller, Switz.*
Achillea (p.1572·2); absinthin (p.1571·1); poppy flowers (p.1029·1); guaiacum wood; tormentil root (p.1674·1); cinnamon bark (p.1595·3); benzoin (p.1668·3); myrrh (p.1639·2); tolu balsam (p.1101·3).
Gastrointestinal disorders.

Baume Analgesique *Multi-Pro, Canad.*
Methyl salicylate (p.55·1); camphor (p.1589·3).

Baume Analgesique Medicamente *Prodemdis, Canad.*
Methyl salicylate (p.55·1); camphor (p.1589·3); menthol (p.1632·3); eucalyptus oil (p.1609·2).

Baume Aroma *Mayoly-Spindler, Fr.*
Clove oil (p.1597·1); capsicum oil; methyl salicylate (p.55·1).
Formerly contained juniper oil, clove oil, capsicum oil, amyl salicylate, and salicylic acid.
Muscle and joint pain.

Baume Bengue *URPAC, Fr.*
Methyl salicylate (p.55·1); menthol (p.1632·3).
Muscle and joint pain.

Baume Dalet
Note. This name is used for preparations of different composition.
COB, Belg.†.
Menthol (p.1632·3); guaiacol (p.1092·1); chloroform (p.1256·3); methyl salicylate (p.55·1); belladonna (p.463·1).
Bunions.

Phygiene, Fr.†.
Hyoscyamus oil (p.470·1); amyl salicylate (p.14·1); guaiacol (p.1092·1); menthol (p.1632·3); chloroform (p.1256·3).
Calluses; corns.

Baume de Chine Temple of Heaven blanc *Panax, Switz.*
Menthol (p.1632·3); camphor (p.1589·3); peppermint oil (p.1243·3); eucalyptus oil (p.1609·2); clove oil (p.1597·1); cinnamon oil (p.1596·1).
Musculoskeletal and joint disorders; soft-tissue injury.

Baume du Chalet *Plan, Switz.*
Lavender oil (p.1627·2); melissa oil; spike lavender oil (p.1667·1); terebinthin (p.1676·3).
Skin disorders; wounds.

Baume Esco *Streuli, Switz.*
Salicylic acid (p.1122·3); menthol (p.1632·3); methyl salicylate (p.55·1).
Musculoskeletal and joint pain.

Baume Esco Forte *Streuli, Switz.*
Salicylic acid (p.1122·3); menthol (p.1632·3); methyl salicylate (p.55·1); ethyl nicotinate (p.35·1).
Musculoskeletal and joint pain.

Baume Saint-Bernard *Monot, Fr.†.*
Salicylic acid (p.1122·3); menthol (p.1632·3); camphor (p.1589·3); methyl salicylate (p.14·1); capsicum (p.1591·1); benzylidene acetone.
Muscle and joint pain.

Bausch & Lomb Computer Eye Drops *Bausch & Lomb, Austral.*
Glycerol (p.1616·3).
Dry eyes; eye irritation.

Bausch & Lomb Concentrated Cleaner *Bausch & Lomb, Austral.*
Cleansing solution for gas permeable and hard contact lenses (p.1129·2).

Bausch & Lomb Conditioning Solution *Bausch & Lomb, Austral.*
Disinfecting and storage solution for gas permeable and hard contact lenses (p.1129·2).

Bausch & Lomb ReNu *Bausch & Lomb, Austral.*
A range of solutions for soft contact lens care (p.1129·2).

Bausch & Lomb Saline Plus *Bausch & Lomb, Austral.†.*
Sodium chloride (p.1196·1) (p.1129·2).
Solution for soft contact lenses.

Bausch & Lomb Sensitive Eyes Daily Cleaner *Bausch & Lomb, Austral.*
Cleansing solution for soft contact lenses (p.1129·2).

Bausch & Lomb Sensitive Eyes Lens Lubricant *Bausch & Lomb, Austral.†.*
Povidone (p.1503·2); hypromellose (p.1501·3)(p.1129·2).
Wetting solution for contact lenses.

Bausch & Lomb Sensitive Eyes Protein Removal *Bausch & Lomb, Austral.*
Proteolytic enzyme (p.1129·2).
Cleanser for soft contact lenses.

Bausch & Lomb Sensitive Eyes Saline *Bausch & Lomb, Austral.*
Sodium chloride (p.1196·1) (p.1129·2).
Saline solution for soft contact lenses.

Bausch & Lomb Sensitive Eyes Thermal Protein Removal *Bausch & Lomb, Austral.†.*
Proteolytic enzyme (p.1129·2).
Cleanser for soft contact lenses.

Baxan *Bristol-Myers Squibb, UK.*
Cefadroxil (p.161·2).
Bacterial infections.

Baxapril *Brasmedica, Braz.*
Co-trimoxazole (p.193·3).
Bacterial infections; Pneumocystis carinii pneumonia; protozoal infections.

Baxedin *Luvabec, Canad.†.*
Chlorhexidine gluconate (p.1138·2).
Disinfection and antisepsis.

Baxidin *Pierrel, Ital.*
Cetrimide (p.1137·1); chlorhexidine gluconate (p.1138·2).
Disinfection of wounds and burns.

Baxo *Toyama, Jpn.*
Piroxicam (p.79·1).
Inflammation; musculoskeletal, joint, and peri-articular disorders; pain.

Baycaron
Bayer, Denm.; Bayer, Ger.†; Bayer, Irl.; Bayer, Neth.; Bayer, Norw.†; Bayer, UK†.
Mefruside (p.926·1).
Diabetes insipidus; hypertension; oedema.

Baycidal *Bayer, Ital.*
Triflumuron (p.1437·3).
Insecticide.

Baycillin *Bayer, Ger.*
Propicillin potassium (p.239·3).
Bacterial infections.

Baycip *Bayer, Spain.*
Ciprofloxacin hydrochloride (p.182·3) or ciprofloxacin lactate (p.182·3).
Bacterial infections.

Baycol
Bayer, Canad.†; Bayer, S.Afr.†; Bayer, USA†.
Cerivastatin sodium (p.856·1).
Hypercholesterolaemia.

Baycuten
Bayer, Braz.; Bayer, Ger.; Bayer, Port.
Clotrimazole (p.382·1); dexamethasone (p.1067·1) or dexamethasone acetate (p.1067·1).
Fungal skin infections.

Baycuten N *Bayer, Mex.*
Clotrimazole (p.382·1); dexamethasone acetate (p.1067·1); neomycin sulfate (p.228·1).
Infected skin disorders.

Bayer Low Adult Strength *Sterling Health, USA.*
Aspirin (p.14·2).

Bayer Select Chest Cold *Sterling Health, USA.*
Dextromethorphan hydrobromide (p.1087·3); paracetamol (p.71·2).

Bayer Select Flu Relief *Sterling Health, USA.*
Paracetamol (p.71·2); pseudoephedrine hydrochloride (p.1099·2); dextromethorphan hydrobromide (p.1087·3); chlorpheniramine [chlorphenamine] maleate (p.412·1).

Bayer Select Head Cold *Sterling Health, USA.*
Pseudoephedrine hydrochloride (p.1099·2); paracetamol (p.71·2).

Bayer Select Maximum Strength Backache *Sterling Health, USA.*
Magnesium salicylate (p.50·3).

Bayer Select Maximum Strength Headache *Sterling Health, USA†.*
Paracetamol (p.71·2); caffeine (p.761·3).

Bayer Select Maximum Strength Menstrual *Sterling Health, USA†.*
Paracetamol (p.71·2); pamabrom (p.952·1).

Bayer Select Maximum Strength Night Time Pain Relief *Sterling Health, USA.*
Paracetamol (p.71·2); diphenhydramine hydrochloride (p.416·1).
Insomnia; pain.

Bayer Select Maximum Strength Sinus Pain Relief *Sterling Health, USA.*
Paracetamol (p.71·2); pseudoephedrine hydrochloride (p.1099·2).
Nasal congestion; pain.

Bayer Select Night Time Cold *Sterling Health, USA.*
Paracetamol (p.71·2); pseudoephedrine hydrochloride (p.1099·2); dextromethorphan hydrobromide (p.1087·3); triprolidine hydrochloride (p.427·2).

Bayer Select Pain Relief Formula *Sterling Health, USA†.*
Ibuprofen (p.43·2).

Baygam *Bayer, Canad.*
A normal immunoglobulin (p.1551·3).
Passive immunisation.

Baygon N *Bayer, Ital.*
Propoxur (p.1436·3); tetramethrin (p.1437·3); piperonyl butoxide (p.1436·2).
Insecticide.

BayHep *Bayer, Israel.*
A hepatitis B immunoglobulin (p.1542·1).
Passive immunisation.

BayHep B
Bayer, Canad.; Bayer Biological, Hong Kong; Bayer, USA.
A hepatitis B immunoglobulin (p.1542·1).
Formerly known as HyperHep in the USA.
Passive immunisation.

Baymycard *Bayer, Ger.; Zeneca, Ger.*
Nisoldipine (p.946·3).
Angina pectoris; hypertension.

Bayolin *Bayer, Aust.*
A heparinoid (p.905·2); glycol salicylate (p.42·2); benzyl nicotinate (p.20·2).
Bruises; haematomas; musculoskeletal and joint disorders; neuralgia.

Bayoline *Bayer, Fr.†.*
A heparinoid (p.905·2); glycol salicylate (p.42·2); benzyl nicotinate (p.20·2).
Muscle and joint pain.

Bayotensin *Bayer, Ger.*
Nitrendipine (p.947·1).
Hypertension.

Baypen
Bayer, Aust.; Bayer, Fr.; Bayer, Ger.; Bayer, Israel; Bayer, Ital.; Bayer, Spain.
Mezlocillin sodium (p.224·1).
Bacterial infections.

Baypresol *Prevision, Spain.*
Nitrendipine (p.947·1).
Angina pectoris; hypertension; Raynaud's syndrome.

Baypress
Bayer, Aust.; Bayer, Belg.; Bayer, Denm.; Bayer, Fr.; Bayer, Hong Kong; Bayer, Ital.; Bayer, Mex.; Bayer, Neth.; Bayer, Switz.; Bayer, Thai.
Nitrendipine (p.947·1).
Hypertension.

BayRab
Bayer, Canad.; Bayer Biological, Hong Kong; Probifasa, Mex.; Bayer, USA.
A rabies immunoglobulin (p.1560·2).
Formerly known as HyperRab in the USA.
Passive immunisation.

BayRho-D
Bayer Biological, Hong Kong; Bayer, Israel; Probifasa, Mex.; Bayer, USA.
An anti-D immunoglobulin (p.1532·1).

Formerly known as HypRho-D in the *USA*.
Prevention of rhesus sensitisation.

Bayro *Bayer, Braz.; Bayer, Ital.; Bayer, Mex.; Bayer, Spain.*
Etofenamate (p.35·3).
Musculoskeletal, joint, peri-articular and soft-tissue disorders.

BayTet *Bayer, Canad.; Bayer, Israel; Probifasa, Mex.; Bayer, USA.*
A tetanus immunoglobulin (p.1565·1).
Formerly known as Hyper-Tet in the *USA*.
Passive immunisation.

Baythion EC *Bayer, Ital.*
Phoxim (p.1436·2).
Insecticide.

Bazalin *Yamanouchi, Spain.*
Coal tar (p.1125·1); fluocinolone acetonide (p.1071·1); salicylic acid (p.1122·3).
Keratinisation disorders; psoriasis.

Bazoton *Schering-Plough, Braz.; Kanoldt, Ger.*
Urtica root (p.1678·2).
Benign prostatic hyperplasia.

Bazuka *Dendron, UK.*
Salicylic acid (p.1122·3); lactic acid (p.1626·2).
Calluses; corns; verrucas; warts.

BB Fleet *Pisa, Mex.*
Glycerol (p.1616·3).

BB-K8 *Bristol-Myers Squibb, Ital.*
Amikacin sulfate (p.148·1).
Bacterial infections.

BC *Block, USA.*
Aspirin (p.14·2); salicylamide (p.82·1); caffeine (p.761·3).
Pain.

BC 500 *Whitehall, Irl.; Whitehall, UK†.*
Vitamin B substances and vitamin C (p.1350·1).
Vitamin supplement.

BC Cold-Sinus *Block, USA†.*
Phenylpropanolamine hydrochloride (p.1098·1); aspirin (p.14·2).
Upper respiratory-tract symptoms.

BC 500 with Iron *Whitehall, Irl.*
Ferrous fumarate (p.1360·1); vitamin B and C substances (p.1350·1).
Dietary supplement; vitamin B and C and iron deficiencies.

BC Multi Symptom Cold Powder *Block, USA†.*
Phenylpropanolamine hydrochloride (p.1098·1); chlorpheniramine [chlorphenamine] maleate (p.412·1); aspirin (p.14·2).
Upper respiratory-tract symptoms.

BCAD 2 *Mead Johnson Nutritionals, USA.*
Food for special diets (p.1350·1).
Maple syrup urine disease.

B-C-Bid *Roberts, USA.*
Vitamin B complex with vitamin C (p.1350·1).

BCM *Pfizer, Austral.*
Vitamin B substances; minerals (p.1350·1).
Tonic.

B-Combin *Nycomed, Denm.†.*
Vitamin B substances (p.1350·1).

B-Complex *Bristol-Myers Squibb, Thai.*
Vitamin B substances (p.1350·1).

B-Complex Plus *Vitaglow, Austral.†.*
Vitamin B substances and vitamin C (p.1350·1).

B-Complex Threshold *GNLD, Austral.*
Vitamin B substances (p.1350·1); rutoside (p.1611·2).
Vitamin B deficiencies.

B-Cool *Julphar, UAE.*
Oxybuprocaine hydrochloride (p.1318·1); cetylpyridinium chloride (p.1138·1); tyrothricin (p.267·1).
Throat disorders.

Beactafed *Beacons, Singapore.*
Codeine phosphate (p.25·2); pseudoephedrine hydrochloride (p.1099·2); triprolidine (p.427·2).
Allergic rhinitis; cold symptoms; nasal congestion; respiratory-tract congestion; sinusitis.

Beaflu *Beacons, Singapore.*
Chlorpheniramine [chlorphenamine] maleate (p.412·1); paracetamol (p.71·2); phenylpropanolamine hydrochloride (p.1098·1).
Fever; hypersenitivity reactions; pain; respiratory-tract congestion.

Beamat *Italmex, Mex.*
Cimetidine (p.1216·3).
Peptic ulcer.

Beamoken A *Kendrick, Mex.*
Dexamethasone (p.1067·1).
Corticosteroid.

Be-Ampicil *Be-Tabs, S.Afr.*
Ampicillin trihydrate (p.151·1).
Bacterial infections.

Beano *Block, Canad.; Stafford-Miller, UK; AkPharma, USA.*
α-D-Galactosidase.
Gas/bloating from ingestion of raffinose, stachyose, or verbascose.

Beaphenicol *Beacons, Singapore.*
Chloramphenicol (p.179·1).
Eye infections.

Bear Essentials *Hall, Canad.†.*
Multivitamin preparation with glucose (p.1350·1).

Bearax *Beacons, Singapore.*
Aciclovir (p.612·3).
Herpesvirus infections.

Beathricin *Beacons, Singapore.*
Lignocaine [lidocaine] hydrochloride (p.1313·2); tyrothricin (p.267·1).
Mouth and throat infections.

Bebedermis *Abbott, Ital.†.*
Glycerol; wool fat; vegetable oil; zinc oxide (p.1128·2).
Barrier cream.

Bebegel *Sarget, Fr.; Dagra, Port.*
Glycerol (p.1616·3).
Bowel evacuation; constipation.

Beben *Parke, Davis, Canad.†; Parke, Davis, Ital.*
Betamethasone benzoate (p.1063·1).
Skin disorders.

Beben Clorossina *Parke, Davis, Ital.*
Betamethasone benzoate (p.1063·1); chloroxine (p.214·1).
Infected skin disorders.

Bebesales *Pharmacia Upjohn, Spain.*
Calcium lactate pentahydrate; citric acid monohydrate; magnesium sulfate; potassium chloride; sodium bicarbonate; sodium chloride; glucose (p.1185·2).
Oral rehydration therapy.

Bebia *Stiefel, Canad.†; Stiefel, Fr.†.*
Zinc oxide (p.1128·2); talc (p.1124·2); heavy kaolin (p.1229·3).
Skin disorders.

Bebidol *Nakorn, Thai.*
Dill oil (p.1603·3); sodium bicarbonate (p.1186·2).
Flatulence; infant bloating.

Bebimix *Sella, Ital.*
Honey (p.1366·2); royal jelly (p.1659·3); myrtillus (p.1639·2).
Nutritional supplement.

Bebulin *Immuno, Braz.*
A factor IX preparation (p.735·1).
Haemorrhagic disorders.

Bebulin S-TIM 4 *Immuno, Aust.†.*
A factor IX preparation (p.735·1).
Factor IX deficiency.

Bebulin TIM 3 *Immuno, Ital.†.*
Factor IX (p.735·1).
Factor IX deficiency; haemophilia B.

Bebulin TIM 4 *Omnimed, S.Afr.†; Baxter, Spain.*
Factor IX (p.735·1).
Factor IX deficiency.

Bebulin VH *Immuno, USA.*
A factor IX preparation (p.735·1).
Haemophilia B.

Bebyderm *QIF, Braz.*
Betamethasone (p.1063·1).
Skin disorders.

Bec *Maruko, Jpn.*
Aranidipine (p.841·2).
Hypertension.

Becaltrin *Natus, Braz.*
Co-trimoxazole (p.193·3).
Bacterial infections; Pneumocystis carinii pneumonia; protozoal infections.

Becantex
Note.This name is used for preparations of different composition.
SmithKline Beecham, Belg.
Sodium dibunate (p.1100·3); guaifenesin (p.1092·2).
Coughs.
CPH, Port.; Sanofi Synthelabo, Thai.
Sodium dibunate (p.1100·3).
Coughs.

Becantosse *Dinafarma, Braz.*
Sodium dibunate (p.1100·3); potassium iodide (p.1522·3).
Coughs.

Becaps *Novaquimica, Braz.*
Thiamine nitrate (p.1385·1).
Vitamin B₁ supplement.

Because *Schering, USA.*
Nonoxinol 9 (p.1346·1).
Contraceptive.

Bece *Codilab, Port.*
Vitamin B substances; vitamin C (p.1350·1).
Vitamin supplement.

Becenun *Bristol-Myers Squibb, Braz.; Bristol-Myers Squibb, Denm.†; Bristol-Myers Squibb, Norw.†; Bristol-Myers Squibb, Swed.†.*
Carmustine (p.516·1).
Malignant neoplasms.

Becetamol *Gebro, Switz.*
Paracetamol (p.71·2).
Fever; pain.

Beceze *Norton, S.Afr.; Norton, UK†.*
Beclometasone dipropionate (p.1061·2).
Allergic rhinitis; asthma.

Bechilar *Montefarmaco, Ital.*
Dextromethorphan hydrobromide (p.1087·3).
Coughs.

Bechlomin *Jean-Marie, Hong Kong.*
Betamethasone (p.1063·1); dexchlorpheniramine maleate (p.412·1).
Hypersensitivity reactions; inflammatory eye disorders.

Becilan *DB, Fr.*
Pyridoxine hydrochloride (p.1386·3).
Vitamin B₆ deficiency.

Beclase *De Mayo, Braz.*
Sodium dibunate (p.1100·3); mepyramine maleate (p.421·1); ephedrine hydrochloride (p.1090·1).
Coughs.

Beclate *Cipla-Medpro, S.Afr.*
Beclometasone dipropionate (p.1061·2).
Allergic rhinitis; asthma.

Beclazone *Norton Waterford, Irl.; Baker Norton, Singapore; Norton Healthcare, Singapore; Baker Norton, UK.*
Beclometasone dipropionate (p.1061·2).
Asthma.

Beclo Aqua *Galen, UK.*
Beclometasone dipropionate (p.1061·2).
Rhinitis.

Beclo Asma *Aldo-Union, Hong Kong; Aldo, Spain.*
Beclometasone dipropionate (p.1061·2).
Asthma.

Beclo Rino *Aldo, Spain.*
Beclometasone dipropionate (p.1061·2).
Nasal polyps; rhinitis.

Beclodisk *Glaxo Wellcome, Canad.*
Beclometasone dipropionate (p.1061·2).
Asthma.

Becloforte *Allen & Hanburys, Austral.; Glaxo Wellcome, Canad.; Glaxo Wellcome, Denm.†; Glaxo Wellcome, Hong Kong; Glaxo Wellcome, Israel; Glaxo Wellcome, Neth.; Glaxo Wellcome, NZ; Glaxo Wellcome, S.Afr.; Glaxo Wellcome, Singapore; Allen, Spain; Glaxo Wellcome, Switz.; Glaxo Wellcome, Thai.; Allen & Hanburys, UK.*
Beclometasone dipropionate (p.1061·2).
Asthma.

Beclogen *Generics, UK.*
Beclometasone dipropionate (p.1061·2).
Rhinitis.

Beclojet *Chiesi, Fr.*
Beclometasone dipropionate (p.1061·2).
Asthma.

Beclomet *Lannacher, Aust.; Orion, Denm.; Orion, Fin.; Orion, Ger.; Orion, Norw.; Orion, Singapore; Orion, Swed.; Orion, Switz.; Orion, Thai.*
Beclometasone dipropionate (p.1061·2).
Asthma; rhinitis.

Beclomin *Jean-Marie, Hong Kong.*
Betamethasone (p.1063·1); dexchlorpheniramine maleate (p.412·1).
Hypersensitivity reactions; inflammatory eye disorders.

Beclonarin *Rappai, Switz.*
Beclometasone dipropionate (p.1061·2); chamomile (p.1593·2).
Allergic rhinitis; polyps.

Beclonasal *Orion, Fin.*
Beclometasone dipropionate (p.1061·2).
Nasal polyps; rhinitis.

Beclone *Leurquin, Fr.*
Beclometasone dipropionate (p.1061·2).
Obstructive airways disease.

Beclo-Rhino *Asta Medica, Fr.; Goldshield, Irl.*
Beclometasone dipropionate (p.1061·2).
Rhinitis.

Beclorhinol *Lindopharm, Ger.*
Beclometasone dipropionate (p.1061·2).
Allergic rhinitis; nasal polyps.

Beclosol *Glaxo Wellcome, Braz.*
Beclometasone dipropionate (p.1061·2).
Asthma; nasal polyps; rhinitis.

Beclosona *Spyfarma, Spain.*
Beclometasone dipropionate (p.1061·2).
Skin disorders.

Beclotaide *Glaxo Wellcome, Port.*
Beclometasone dipropionate (p.1061·2).
Asthma.

Becloturmant *Lindopharm, Ger.*
Beclometasone dipropionate (p.1061·2).
Obstructive airways disease.

Beclovent *Glaxo Wellcome, Canad.; Glaxo Wellcome, USA.*
Beclometasone dipropionate (p.1061·2).
Asthma.

Beco *Mepha, Switz.*
Vitamin B substances (p.1350·1).
Alcoholism; liver disorders; neuropathies; vitamin B deficiency.

Becocent *Glaxo Wellcome, Denm.†.*
Beclometasone dipropionate (p.1061·2).
Asthma.

Becodisk *Glaxo Wellcome, NZ; Glaxo Wellcome, Switz.; Glaxo Wellcome, Thai.*
Beclometasone dipropionate (p.1061·2).
Asthma.

Becodisks *Glaxo Wellcome, Hong Kong; Allen & Hanburys, Irl.; Glaxo Wellcome, S.Afr.; Allen & Hanburys, UK.*
Beclometasone dipropionate (p.1061·2).
Asthma.

Becof *Compu, S.Afr.†.*
Diphenhydramine hydrochloride (p.416·1); ammonium chloride (p.1085·2); sodium citrate (p.1186·2).
Coughs.

Becolim *Atlantic, Hong Kong.; Atlantic, Singapore; Atlantic, Thai.*
Vitamin B substances (p.1350·1).
Vitamin B deficiency.

Becombion *Merck, Singapore.*
Vitamin B substances (p.1350·1).

Becomplex *Dumex-Alpharma, Singapore.*
Vitamin B substances (p.1350·1).
Vitamin B deficiency.

Beconase *Glaxo Wellcome, Aust.; Allen & Hanburys, Austral.; Glaxo Wellcome, Belg.; Glaxo Wellcome, Canad.; Glaxo Wellcome, Denm.; Glaxo Wellcome, Fin.; Glaxo Wellcome, Fr.; Glaxo Wellcome, Hong Kong; Allen & Hanburys, Irl.; Glaxo Wellcome, Mex.; Glaxo Wellcome, Neth.; Glaxo Wellcome, NZ; Glaxo Wellcome, Port.; Glaxo Wellcome, S.Afr.; Glaxo Wellcome, Singapore; Allen, Spain; Glaxo Wellcome, Switz.; Glaxo Wellcome, Thai.; Allen & Hanburys, UK; Glaxo Wellcome, USA.*
Beclometasone dipropionate (p.1061·2).
Nasal polyps; rhinitis.

Beconase Aquosum *Glaxo Wellcome, Ger.*
Beclometasone dipropionate (p.1061·2).
Allergic rhinitis; nasal polyps.

Beconasol *Glaxo Wellcome, Switz.*
Beclometasone dipropionate (p.1061·2).
Nasal polyps; rhinitis.

Becoplex Ido *Novo Nordisk, S.Afr.*
Vitamin B substances (p.1350·1).

Becosol *GHP, Thai.*
Vitamin B substances, glucose, and sodium chloride infusion (p.1350·1).
Parenteral nutrition.

Becosym *Roche Consumer, Irl.; Roche Consumer, UK.*
Vitamin B substances (p.1350·1).
Vitamin B deficiency.

Becotal *Streuli, Switz.*
Vitamin B substances (p.1350·1).
Neuropathies; vitamin B deficiency.

Becotide *Glaxo Wellcome, Aust.; Allen & Hanburys, Austral.; Glaxo Wellcome, Belg.; Glaxo Wellcome, Denm.†; Glaxo Wellcome, Fin.; Glaxo Wellcome, Fr.; Glaxo Wellcome, Hong Kong; Allen & Hanburys, Irl.; Glaxo Wellcome, Israel; Glaxo Wellcome, Ital.; Glaxo Wellcome, Mex.; Glaxo Wellcome, Neth.; Glaxo Wellcome, Norw.; Glaxo Wellcome, NZ; Glaxo Wellcome, S.Afr.; Glaxo Wellcome, Singapore; Glaxo Wellcome, Spain; Glaxo Wellcome, Swed.; Glaxo Wellcome, Switz.; Glaxo Wellcome, Thai.; Allen & Hanburys, UK.*
Beclometasone dipropionate (p.1061·2).
Asthma; nasal polyps; rhinitis.

Becotide A *Glaxo Wellcome, Ital.*
Beclometasone dipropionate (p.1061·2).
Formerly known as Inalone A.
Nasal disorders; obstructive airways disease.

Becovit *Julphar, UAE.*
Vitamin B substances (p.1350·1).
Vitamin B deficiency; vitamin B supplement.

Becovitan *Janssen-Cilag, Belg.†.*
Vitamin B substances (p.1350·1).
Dietary supplementation; digestive disorders; nervous disorders; skin disorders; vitamin B deficiency.

Becozym *Roche, Aust.; Roche, Israel; Roche, Ital.; Roche, Swed.*
Vitamin B substances (p.1350·1).
Alcoholism; neuropathies; vitamin B deficiency.

Becozyme *Roche, Belg.; Roche, Fr.; Roche, Port.; Roche Nicholas, Spain; Roche, Switz.*
Vitamin B substances (p.1350·1).
Alcoholism; liver disorders; nausea and vomiting in pregnancy; neuritis; neuropathies; vitamin B deficiency.

Becozyme C *Roche, Port.*
Vitamin B substances; vitamin C (p.1350·1).
Vitamin B and C deficiency.

Becozyme C Forte *Roche Nicholas, Spain.*
Vitamin B substances and vitamin C (p.1350·1).

Bed Wetting *Hylands, Canad.*
Homoeopathic preparation.

Bed Wetting Relief *Brauer, Austral.*
Homoeopathic preparation.

Bedelix *Beaufour, Fr.*
Montmorillonite beidellitique.
Gastrointestinal disorders.

Bedin *Pharmasant, Thai.*
Dihydroergocristine mesilate (p.1603·2); clopamide (p.863·1); reserpine (p.967·3).
Hypertension.

Bedodeka *Biogal, Israel.*
Vitamin B₁₂ (p.1388·1).
Anaemias; vitamin B₁₂ deficiency.

Bedodeka Antineuralgica *Biogal, Israel.*
Procaine hydrochloride (p.1319·1); vitamin B substances (p.1350·1).
Arthralgia; neuralgia.

The symbol † denotes a preparation no longer actively marketed

Bedorma Nouvelle formulation *Singer, Switz.*
Diphenhydramine hydrochloride (p.416·1).
Sleep disorders.

Bedoxine *Meuse, Belg.*
Pyridoxine hydrochloride (p.1386·3).
Vitamin B₆ deficiency.

Bedoyecta *Grossman, Mex.*
Calcium ascorbate; vitamin B substances; inositol; rutoside (p.1350·1).

Bedoz *Nadeau, Canad.*
Cyanocobalamin (p.1388·1).

Bedoze *Merck, Port.*
Cyanocobalamin (p.1388·1).
Megaloblastic anaemia; neuralgias; neuritis.

Bedozil *Bunker, Braz.*
Cyanocobalamin (p.1388·1).
Megaloblastic anaemia; vitamin B₁₂ supplement.

Bedranol *Lagap, UK.*
Propranolol hydrochloride (p.962·3).
Angina pectoris; hypertension.

Beech Nut Cough Drops *Beta, Canad.*
Black: Menthol (p.1632·3); anise oil (p.1580·3).

Honey-Lemon; wild cherry: Menthol (p.1632·3); eucalyptus (p.1609·2).

Menthol: Menthol (p.1632·3); anethole (p.1580·1); eucalyptus oil (p.1609·2).

Beecham Flu Plus *SmithKline Beecham Consumer, Irl.*
Paracetamol (p.71·2); ascorbic acid (p.1389·3); caffeine (p.761·3); phenylephrine hydrochloride (p.1097·1).
Cold and flu symptoms.

Beecham Lemon *SmithKline Beecham, Spain.*
Ascorbic acid (p.1389·3); phenylephrine hydrochloride (p.1097·1); paracetamol (p.71·2).
Cold symptoms.

Beecham Lemon Miel *SmithKline Beecham, Spain†.*
Paracetamol (p.71·2); caffeine (p.761·3); ascorbic acid (p.1389·3).
Cold symptoms; fever; pain.

Beechams All-In-One *SmithKline Beecham Consumer, UK.*
Paracetamol (p.71·2); guaifenesin (p.1092·2); phenylephrine hydrochloride (p.1097·1).
Cold and influenza symptoms.

Beechams Cold & Flu *SmithKline Beecham Consumer, UK.*
Paracetamol (p.71·2); phenylephrine hydrochloride (p.1097·1); ascorbic acid (p.1389·3).
Cold and influenza symptoms.

Beechams Cold Relief *SmithKline Beecham Consumer, Irl.*
Paracetamol (p.71·2); caffeine (p.761·3); phenylephrine hydrochloride (p.1097·1).
Cold symptoms.

Beechams Flu-Plus *SmithKline Beecham Consumer, UK.*
Oral liquid: Paracetamol (p.71·2); phenylephrine hydrochloride (p.1097·1); vitamin C (p.1389·3).
Tablets: Paracetamol (p.71·2); phenylephrine hydrochloride (p.1097·1); caffeine (p.761·3).
Cold and influenza symptoms.

Beechams Hot Lemon Decongestant *SmithKline Beecham Consumer, Irl.*
Paracetamol (p.71·2); ascorbic acid (p.1389·3); phenylephrine hydrochloride (p.1097·1).
Cold symptoms.

Beechams Hot Remedies *SmithKline Beecham Consumer, Irl.*
Paracetamol (p.71·2); ascorbic acid (p.1389·3).
Cold symptoms.

Beechams Lemon Tablets *SmithKline Beecham Consumer, UK.*
Aspirin (p.14·2).
Glycine (p.1365·3) is included in this preparation in an attempt to limit adverse effects on the gastrointestinal mucosa.
Cold and influenza symptoms; pain.

Beechams for Natural Defence *SmithKline Beecham Consumer, UK.*
Ascorbic acid (p.1389·3) with zinc.

Beechams for Natural Relief *SmithKline Beecham Consumer, UK.*
Echinacea (p.1606·2); garlic (p.1614·1).
Catarrh; cold and influenza symptoms; coughs; rhinitis.

Beechams Pills *SmithKline Beecham Consumer, UK†.*
Aloin (p.1210·2).
Constipation.

Beechams Powders *SmithKline Beecham Consumer, UK.*
Aspirin (p.14·2); caffeine (p.761·3).
Cold and influenza symptoms; pain.

Beechams Powders Capsules *SmithKline Beecham Consumer, UK.*
Paracetamol (p.71·2); caffeine (p.761·3); phenylephrine hydrochloride (p.1097·1).
Cold and influenza symptoms.

Beechams Remedy *SmithKline Beecham, Israel.*
Paracetamol (p.71·2); ascorbic acid (p.1389·3).
Fever; pain.

Beechams Throat-Plus *SmithKline Beecham Consumer, UK.*
Benzalkonium chloride (p.1133·2); hexylresorcinol (p.1146·3).
Sore throat.

Beeline *Lifeplan, UK.*
Propolis (p.1655·1); pollen; royal jelly (p.1659·3).
Nutritional supplement.

Beelith *Beach, USA.*
Pyridoxine hydrochloride (p.1386·3); magnesium oxide (p.1233·2).
Dietary supplement.

Beepen-VK *SmithKline Beecham, USA.*
Phenoxymethylpenicillin potassium (p.235·1).
Bacterial infections.

Beesix *SA Druggists, S.Afr.†.*
Pyridoxine hydrochloride (p.1386·3).
Vitamin B₆ deficiencies.

Beespan *Aspen Consumer, S.Afr.*
Vitamin B substances (p.1350·1).
Vitamin B deficiencies.

Bee-Zee *Rugby, USA.*
Multivitamin and mineral preparation (p.1350·1).

Befact *SMB, Belg.*
Vitamin B substances (p.1350·1).
Neuritis; vitamin B deficiency.

Befelka-Oel *Befelka, Ger.*
Hypericum oil (p.290·3); calendula oil (p.1589·2); chamomile oil; olive oil (p.1643·3); viola tricoloris oil; liquid paraffin (p.1407·1).
Skin disorders.

Befelka-Tinktur *Befelka, Ger.†.*
Aloes (p.1210·1); achillea (p.1572·2); melissa (p.1632·2); juniper fruit (p.1625·2); ononis (p.1644·1); betula (p.1585·2); urtica (p.1678·2); chamomile (p.1593·2); arnica (p.1581·3); pimpinella; turiones pini; liquorice (p.1582·1).
Circulatory disorders; metabolic disorders; skin disorders.

Befibrat *Hennig, Ger.*
Bezafibrate (p.849·1).
Hyperlipidaemias.

Befizal *Roche, Fr.*
Bezafibrate (p.849·1).
Hyperlipidaemias.

Beflavine *Roche, Fr.*
Riboflavin (p.1386·1).
Vitamin B deficiency.

Beforplex *Bournonville, Belg.†.*
Vitamin B substances (p.1350·1).
Digestive disorders; neuritis; skin disorders; vitamin B deficiency.

Begesic *Berlin Pharm, Singapore.; Berlin Pharm, Thai.*
Methyl salicylate (p.55·1); menthol (p.1632·3); eugenol (p.1609·3); cajuput oil (p.1588·1).
Muscle pain; musculoskeletal and joint disorders.

Beglan *Faes, Spain.*
Salmeterol xinafoate (p.773·3).
Asthma; bronchitis.

Beglunina *Llorens, Spain†.*
Pyridoxine (p.1387·1).
Alcohol intoxication; vitamin B₆ deficiency.

Begrivac *Chiron, Aust.; Chiron, Denm.†; Chiron Behring, Fin.; Chiron Behring, Ger.; Chiron, Ital.; Chiron Behring, Norw.; Meda, Swed.; Wyeth, UK.*
An inactivated influenza vaccine (p.1544·3).
Active immunisation.

Begrocit *Grossmann, Switz.*
Vitamin and mineral preparation (p.1350·1).

Behepan
Note. This name is used for preparations of different composition.
Pharmacia Upjohn, Denm.
Cyanocobalamin (p.1388·1).
Megaloblastic anaemia.

Pharmacia Upjohn, Swed.
Injection: Hydroxocobalamin acetate (p.1388·3).
Megaloblastic anaemia; Schilling test; sprue; vitamin B₁₂ deficiency.
Tablets: Cyanocobalamin (p.1388·1).
Megaloblastic anaemia; sprue; vitamin B₁₂ deficiency.

Behexine *Osotspa, Thai.*
Bromhexine hydrochloride (p.1085·3).
Respiratory-tract disorders associated with increased or viscous mucus.

Beiklin *Scherer, Singapore.*
Multivitamin and mineral preparation (p.1350·1).

Bekfan *Arlex, Mex.*
Dextromethorphan (p.1087·3).
Coughs.

Bekidiba *Diba, Mex.*
Dextromethorphan hydrobromide (p.1087·3); guaifenesin (p.1092·2).
Coughs.

Bekidiba Dex *Diba, Mex.*
Dextromethorphan hydrobromide (p.1087·3).
Coughs.

Beknol *Kener, Mex.*
Benzonatate (p.1085·3).

Beko *Orion, Fin.*
Vitamin B substances (p.1350·1).
Vitamin B deficiency; vitamin B supplement.

Bekunis
Note. This name is used for preparations of different composition.
Schulke & Mayr, Aust.; Roha, Irl.†; Roha, Israel; Roha, Port.†.
Senna (p.1248·2).
Constipation.

Roha, Port.†; Roha, Switz.
Senna (p.1248·2); bisacodyl (p.1212·2).
Constipation.

Bekunis Bisacodyl *Roha, Ger.*
Bisacodyl (p.1212·2).
Constipation.

Bekunis Complex *Diafarm, Spain.*
Bisacodyl (p.1212·2); senna (p.1248·2).
Constipation.

Bekunis Fibra *Roha, Port.†.*
Ispaghula (p.1229·1).
Constipation.

Bekunis Herbal Tea *Polcopharma, Austral.*
Senna (p.1248·2).
Constipation.

Bekunis Instant *Polcopharma, Austral.; Roha, Ger.*
Senna (p.1248·2).
Constipation.

Bekunis Leicht *Roha, Ger.†.*
Ispaghula (p.1229·1).
Constipation.

Bekunis Plantago Granule *Roha, Switz.†.*
Ispaghula (p.1229·1).
Constipation; diarrhoea; irritable bowel; obesity; stool softener.

Bekunis-Krautertee N *Roha, Ger.*
Senna (p.1248·2).
Constipation.

Belacid *Nakornpatana, Thai.*
Charcoal (p.1000·2); magnesium hydroxide (p.1233·1); belladonna (p.463·1); peppermint oil (p.1243·3).
Gastric hyperacidity.

Belacodid *Climax, Braz.*
Injection: Codeine (p.25·2); sparteine sulfate (p.1666·3); homatropine (p.468·1).
Smooth muscle spasm.

Oral drops: Codeine (p.25·2); phenethylamine citrate; pentetrazol (p.1513·2); methyl homatropine.
Coughs.

Syrup: Codeine phosphate (p.25·2); phenethylamine citrate; trolamine thymolsulfonate; pentetrazol (p.1513·2); homatropine methonitrate (p.468·1).
Coughs.

Belagin *IMA, Braz.*
Copper sulfate (p.1358·1); zinc sulfate (p.1398·2); aluminium (p.1577·3); menthol (p.1632·3); benzalkonium chloride (p.1133·2).
Gynaecological infections.

Belara *Grunenthal, Ger.*
Ethinylestradiol (p.1476·2); chlormadinone acetate (p.1465·3).
Combined oral contraceptive.

Belcid *Biolab, Thai.*
Aluminium oxide (p.1108·3); magnesium hydroxide (p.1233·1); simeticone (p.1249·2).
Dyspepsia; flatulence; gastric hyperacidity; peptic ulcer.

Belcomycine *Rhone-Poulenc Rorer, Neth.*
Colistin sulfate (p.192·3).
Bacterial infections.

Belep *Lepori, Port.*
Ibuprofen guaiacol (p.44·1).
Fever; pain.

Belexa *Abbott, Braz.*
Vitamin B substances (p.1350·1).

Belidral *Sintesa, Belg.*
Amiloride hydrochloride (p.835·1); hydrochlorothiazide (p.907·3).
Ascites; heart failure; hypertension; oedema.

Belisina *CPH, Port.*
Lysine hydrochloride; vitamin B substances (p.1350·1).
Tonic.

Belivon *Organon, Aust.; Organon, Ital.*
Risperidone (p.704·1).
Schizophrenia.

Belix *Halsey, USA†.*
Diphenhydramine hydrochloride (p.416·1).
Insomnia; motion sickness; parkinsonism.

Bellacane *Treiner, USA.*
Hyoscyamine sulfate (p.469·3); phenobarbital (p.355·1).
Gastrointestinal disorders.

BellaCarotin mono *3M, Ger.*
Betacarotene (p.1355·1).
Sunburn.

Belladol *Dolisos, Canad.*
Homoeopathic preparation.

Belladonna Med Complex *Dynamit, Aust.*
Homoeopathic preparation.

Belladonnysat Burger *Ysatfabrik, Ger.*
Belladonna (p.463·1).
Smooth muscle spasms.

Bellafit N *Streuli, Switz.*
Atropine sulfate (p.461·1).
Colic; hyperhidrosis; sialorrhoea.

Bellafoline *Novartis, USA†.*
Belladonna (p.463·1).
Asthma; dysmenorrhoea; gastrointestinal disorders; motion sickness; nocturnal enuresis; parkinsonism; renal colic; vagal inhibition.

Bellagotin *Streuli, Switz.*
Belladonna (p.463·1); diphenhydramine hydrochloride (p.416·1); ergotamine tartrate (p.452·1).
Nervous disorders.

Bellanorm *Rosch & Handel, Aust.*
Belladonna (p.463·1).
Bronchospasm; gastrointestinal disorders; motion sickness; night sweats.

Bellanox *Bios, Belg.†.*
Brallobarbital (p.656·3); amobarbital (p.655·2); secobarbital (p.705·2).
Insomnia.

Bell/ans *Dent, USA.*
Sodium bicarbonate (p.1186·2).
Hyperacidity.

Bellasthman *Petrasch, Aust.†.*
Ephedrine hydrochloride (p.1090·1); belladonna (p.463·1); theophylline (p.777·2); caffeine (p.761·3); phenazone (p.77·2).

Bellatal *Richwood, USA.*
Phenobarbital (p.355·1); hyoscyamine sulfate (p.469·3); atropine sulfate (p.461·1); hyoscine hydrobromide (p.468·2).
Hypnotic; sedative.

Bellatard *Propan, S.Afr.*
Phenobarbital (p.355·1); atropine sulfate (p.461·1); hyoscine hydrobromide (p.468·2); hyoscyamine sulfate (p.469·3).
Smooth muscle spasm.

Bellavern *Propan-Vernleigh, S.Afr.†.*
Hyoscyamine sulfate (p.469·3); atropine sulfate (p.461·1); hyoscine hydrobromide (p.468·2); phenobarbital (p.355·1).
Smooth muscle spasm.

Bellergal *Novartis, Canad.; Novartis, S.Afr.†; Novartis, Switz.; Novartis, Thai.*
Belladonna alkaloids (p.463·1); ergotamine tartrate (p.452·1); phenobarbital (p.355·1).
Cardiovascular disorders; endocrine disorders; gastrointestinal disorders; menopausal disorders; nervous system disorders.

Bellergal-S *Novartis, USA.*
Laevorotatory alkaloids of belladonna (Bellafoline) (p.463·1); ergotamine tartrate (p.452·1); phenobarbital (p.355·1).
Cardiovascular disorders; gastrointestinal disorders; menopausal disorders; recurrent throbbing headache.

Bellergil *Sandoz, Ital.†.*
Belladonna alkaloids (p.463·1); ergotamine tartrate (p.452·1); phenobarbital (p.355·1).
Dystonias.

Bellocarb *Sinclair, UK†.*
Belladonna (p.463·1); magnesium carbonate (p.1232·3); magnesium trisilicate (p.1233·3).
Gastrointestinal disorders.

Belloform nouvelle formule *Tentan, Switz.*
Cathine hydrochloride (p.1507·1).
Obesity.

Belloid *Gedeon Richter, Thai.*
Hyoscyamine sulfate (p.469·3); ergotoxine (p.1608·1); butobarbital (p.659·1).
Central vegetative disorder; dystonias; migraine.

Belmacina *CEPA, Spain.*
Ciprofloxacin hydrochloride (p.182·3).
Bacterial infections.

Belmalax *Belmac, Spain.*
Lactulose (p.1230·1).
Constipation; hepatic encephalopathy.

Belmazol *Belmac, Spain.*
Omeprazole (p.1239·1).
Gastro-oesophageal reflux; peptic ulcer; Zollinger-Ellison syndrome.

Belnif *Promed, Ger.; Astra, Ger.*
Metoprolol tartrate (p.931·2); nifedipine (p.940·1).
Angina pectoris; hypertension.

Beloc *Astra, Aust.; Astra, Ger.*
Metoprolol tartrate (p.931·2).
Angina pectoris; arrhythmias; heart failure; hypertension; hyperthyroidism; migraine; myocardial infarction.

Beloc comp *Astra, Aust.; Astra, Ger.†.*
Metoprolol tartrate (p.931·2); hydrochlorothiazide (p.907·3).
Hypertension.

Beloc COR *Astra, Switz.*
Metoprolol tartrate (p.931·2).
Heart failure.

Beloc-Zok *Astra, Ger.; Promed, Ger.; Astra, Switz.*
Metoprolol succinate (p.932·1).
Arrhythmias; hypertension; ischaemic heart disease; migraine; myocardial infarction.

Beloc-Zok comp *Astra, Ger.; Promed, Ger.*
Metoprolol succinate (p.932·1); hydrochlorothiazide (p.907·3).
Hypertension.

Belpen *Dermopen, Braz.*
Cyclamic acid (p.1358·3); saccharin (p.1374·3).
Sugar substitute.

Bel-Phen-Ergot S *Goldline, USA.*
Phenobarbital (p.355·1); ergotamine tartrate (p.452·1); belladonna (p.463·1).

Beltop *Janssen-Cilag, Aust.†.*
Ketoconazole (p.389·1).
Dandruff.

Belustine *Bellon, Fr.†; Rhone-Poulenc Rorer, Hong Kong; Rhone-Poulenc Rorer, Ital.†; Rhone-Poulenc Rorer, Spain†.*
Lomustine (p.550·2).
Malignant neoplasms.

Bemedrex *Orion, Fr.*
Beclometasone dipropionate (p.1061·2).
Asthma.

Bemetrazole Be-Tabs, S.Afr.
Metronidazole (p.594·1).
Anaerobic bacterial infections; protozoal infections.

Bemetson Orion, Fin.
Betamethasone valerate (p.1063·2).
Skin disorders.

Beminal
Whitehall, Braz.; Whitehall-Robins, Canad.; Whitehall, USA.
Vitamin B substances with vitamin C (p.1350·1).

Beminal C Fortis Whitehall-Robins, Canad.
Vitamin B substances with ascorbic acid (p.1350·1).

Beminal Fortis Whitehall-Robins, Canad.
Vitamin B substances (p.1350·1).

Beminal with Iron and Liver Whitehall-Robins, Canad.†.
Vitamin B substances with ferrous sulfate and liver (p.1350·1).

Beminal Z Whitehall-Robins, Canad.†.
Multivitamins (p.1350·1); zinc sulfate (p.1398·2).

Bemofil Veripalvelu, Fin.
A factor IX preparation (p.735·1).

Bemolan Roche, Spain.
Magaldrate (p.1232·2).
Dyspepsia; gastro-oesophageal reflux; gastrointestinal hyperacidity.

Bemon Hexal, Ger.
Betamethasone valerate (p.1063·2).
Skin disorders.

Benacne Whitehall, Port.
Benzoyl peroxide (p.1111·1).
Acne.

Benactiv Boots Healthcare, Ital.
Flurbiprofen (p.41·2).
Mouth and throat pain and inflammation.

Benaderma Confar, Port.
Diphenhydramine (p.416·1).
Formerly contained ammonium chloride, diphenhydramine, and menthol.

Benaderma com Calamina Confar, Port.
Calamine (p.1111·3); camphor (p.1589·3); diphenhydramine hydrochloride (p.416·1).

Benadon
Roche, Austral.; Roche Consumer, Irl.; Roche, Ital.; Roche, Mex.; Roche, Port.; Roche Nicholas, Spain; Roche, Swed.; Roche, Switz.; Roche Consumer, UK†.
Pyridoxine hydrochloride (p.1386·3).
Vitamin B₆ deficiency; vomiting.

Benadryl
Note. This name is used for preparations of different composition.
Parke, Davis, Aust.
Capsules†: Diphenhydramine hydrochloride (p.416·1); codeine phosphate (p.25·2).
Coughs.
Oral liquid; oral drops: Diphenhydramine hydrochloride (p.416·1); ammonium chloride (p.1085·2); menthol (p.1632·3); sodium citrate (p.1186·2).
Cold and influenza symptoms; coughs.
Parke, Davis, Austral.†; Warner-Lambert, Canad.; Warner-Lambert, Hong Kong; Warner-Lambert, Spain; Warner-Lambert, Thai.; Warner-Lambert, USA; Parke, Davis, USA.
Diphenhydramine (p.416·1) or diphenhydramine hydrochloride (p.416·1).
Hypersensitivity reactions; minor skin irritation; motion sickness; parkinsonism; sedative.
Ache, Braz.
Diphenhydramine hydrochloride (p.416·1); ammonium chloride (p.1085·2); sodium citrate (p.1186·2); menthol (p.1632·3).
Coughs.
Warner-Lambert, Denm.; Warner-Lambert, UK.
Acrivastine (p.408·2).
Formerly contained diphenhydramine hydrochloride in the UK.
Hypersensitivity reactions.
Warner-Lambert, Ital.
Cream†; elixir†; capsules†: Diphenhydramine hydrochloride (p.416·1).
Hypersensitivity reactions.
Syrup: Diphenhydramine hydrochloride (p.416·1); ammonium chloride (p.1085·2); sodium citrate (p.1186·2); menthol (p.1632·3).
Coughs.

Benadryl Allergy/Cold Warner-Lambert, USA.
Diphenhydramine hydrochloride (p.416·1); pseudoephedrine hydrochloride (p.1099·2); paracetamol (p.71·2).

Benadryl Allergy/Congestion Warner-Lambert, USA.
Diphenhydramine hydrochloride (p.416·1); pseudoephedrine hydrochloride (p.1099·2).

Benadryl Allergy/Sinus Headache Warner-Lambert, USA.
Diphenhydramine hydrochloride (p.416·1); pseudoephedrine hydrochloride (p.1099·2); paracetamol (p.71·2).

Benadryl Allergy/Sinus/Headache Warner-Lambert, Canad.
Diphenhydramine hydrochloride (p.416·1); pseudoephedrine hydrochloride (p.1099·2); paracetamol (p.71·2).
Eye irritation; headache; upper respiratory-tract disorders.

Benadryl CD
Note. This name is used for preparations of different composition.
Parke, Davis, Singapore.
Diphenhydramine hydrochloride (p.416·1); codeine phosphate (p.25·2); ammonium chloride (p.1085·2).
Cold symptoms; coughs.
Warner-Lambert, Thai.
Diphenhydramine hydrochloride (p.416·1); codeine phosphate (p.25·2); ammonium chloride (p.1085·2); sodium citrate (p.1186·2); menthol (p.1632·3).
Coughs.

Benadryl Chesty Cough Warner-Lambert, NZ.
Guaifenesin (p.1092·2); pseudoephedrine hydrochloride (p.1099·2).
Coughs.

Benadryl Cold Nighttime Formula Parke, Davis, USA.
Pseudoephedrine hydrochloride (p.1099·2); diphenhydramine hydrochloride (p.416·1); paracetamol (p.71·2).
Upper respiratory-tract symptoms.

Benadryl Complex Warner-Lambert, Ital.
Diphenhydramine hydrochloride (p.416·1); dextromethorphan hydrobromide (p.1087·3); pseudoephedrine hydrochloride (p.1099·2); ammonium chloride (p.1085·2); sodium citrate (p.1186·2); menthol (p.1632·3).
Coughs.

Benadryl Cough
Note. This name is used for preparations of different composition.
Parke, Davis, Singapore.
Diphenhydramine hydrochloride (p.416·1); ammonium chloride (p.1085·2); menthol (p.1632·3).
Cold symptoms; coughs.
Warner-Lambert, Thai.
Diphenhydramine hydrochloride (p.416·1); ammonium chloride (p.1085·2); sodium citrate (p.1186·2); menthol (p.1632·3).
Coughs; nasal congestion; sneezing.

Benadryl Day & Night Warner-Lambert, NZ.
Day formula, daytime: dextromethorphan hydrobromide (p.1087·3); pseudoephedrine hydrochloride (p.1099·2); night formula, dextromethorphan hydrobromide; pseudoephedrine hydrochloride; diphenhydramine hydrochloride (p.416·1).
Coughs and cold symptoms.

Benadryl Decongestant Warner-Lambert, Canad.†; Warner-Lambert, Thai.; Parke, Davis, USA.
Diphenhydramine hydrochloride (p.416·1); pseudoephedrine hydrochloride (p.1099·2).
Upper respiratory-tract symptoms.

Benadryl DMP Warner-Lambert, Thai.
Diphenhydramine hydrochloride (p.416·1); dextromethorphan hydrobromide (p.1087·3); phenylephrine hydrochloride (p.1097·1); ammonium chloride (p.1085·2); sodium citrate (p.1186·2).
Coughs; respiratory-tract congestion.

Benadryl Dry Cough Warner-Lambert, NZ.
Dextromethorphan hydrobromide (p.1087·3); pseudoephedrine hydrochloride (p.1099·2); diphenhydramine hydrochloride (p.416·1).
Coughs.

Benadryl Expectorante Warner-Lambert, Spain.
Ammonium chloride (p.1085·2); diphenhydramine hydrochloride (p.416·1); sodium citrate (p.1186·2); menthol (p.1632·3).
Respiratory-tract disorders.

Benadryl for the Family Chesty Warner-Lambert, Austral.
Guaifenesin (p.1092·2); pseudoephedrine hydrochloride (p.1099·2).
Formerly known as Benadryl Cough Medicine for Chesty Coughs.
Coughs.

Benadryl for the Family Dry Warner-Lambert, Austral.
Dextromethorphan hydrobromide (p.1087·3); pseudoephedrine hydrochloride (p.1099·2); diphenhydramine hydrochloride (p.416·1).
Coughs and cold symptoms.

Benadryl for the Family Dry Forte Pfizer, Austral.
Dextromethorphan hydrobromide (p.1087·3).
Coughs.

Benadryl for the Family Original Warner-Lambert, Austral.
Diphenhydramine hydrochloride (p.416·1); ammonium chloride (p.1085·2); sodium citrate (p.1186·2).
Formerly known as Benadryl Cough Medicine.
Allergic rhinitis; cough and cold symptoms.

Benadryl Itch Warner-Lambert, USA.
Cream; topical spray; topical stick: Diphenhydramine hydrochloride (p.416·1); zinc acetate (p.1398·1).
Hypersensitivity reactions.
Topical gel: Diphenhydramine hydrochloride (p.416·1).
Pruritus.

Benadryl mit Codein Parke, Davis, Aust.
Oral drops†: Codeine phosphate (p.25·2); diphenhydramine hydrochloride (p.416·1); ammonium chloride (p.1085·2).
Oral liquid: Codeine phosphate (p.25·2); diphenhydramine hydrochloride (p.416·1); ammonium chloride (p.1085·2); menthol (p.1632·3); sodium citrate (p.1186·2).
Coughs.

Benadryl N Warner-Lambert, Ger.
Diphenhydramine hydrochloride (p.416·1).
Coughs, colds and associated respiratory-tract disorders.

Benadryl Original Warner-Lambert, NZ.
Diphenhydramine hydrochloride (p.416·1); ammonium chloride (p.1085·2); sodium citrate (p.1186·2).
Coughs.

Benadryl Plus Warner-Lambert, UK.
Acrivastine (p.408·2); pseudoephedrine (p.1099·2).
Allergic rhinitis.

Benadryl Skin Allergy Relief Warner-Lambert, UK.
Diphenhydramine hydrochloride (p.416·1); camphor (p.1589·3); zinc oxide (p.1128·2).
Allergic skin disorders; skin irritation.

Benagol Boots Healthcare, Ital.
Dichlorobenzyl alcohol (p.1143·2); amylmetacresol (p.1133·2).
Oral hygiene.

Benagol Collutorio Boots Healthcare, Ital.†.
Amylmetacresol (p.1133·2).
Oral hygiene.

Benagol Mentolo-Eucaliptolo Boots Healthcare, Ital.
Dichlorobenzyl alcohol (p.1143·2); amylmetacresol (p.1133·2); menthol (p.1632·3).
Oral hygiene.

Benagol Vitamina C Boots Healthcare, Ital.
Dichlorobenzyl alcohol (p.1143·2); amylmetacresol (p.1133·2); sodium ascorbate (p.1390·1); ascorbic acid (p.1389·3).
Adjunct in cold symptoms; oral hygiene.

Benal-500 Berman, Mex.
Thiamine (p.1385·2).

Benalapril Berlin-Chemie, Ger.
Enalapril maleate (p.883·3).
Heart failure; hypertension.

Benalet Ache, Braz.
Diphenhydramine hydrochloride (p.416·1); ammonium chloride (p.1085·2); sodium citrate (p.1186·2).

Ben-Allergin Dunhall, USA†.
Diphenhydramine hydrochloride (p.416·1).
Motion sickness; parkinsonism.

Benapen Sanus, Braz.
Procaine penicillin [procaine benzylpenicillin] (p.239·2); benzylpenicillin potassium (p.157·1).
Bacterial infections.

Ben-Aqua Syosset, USA†.
Benzoyl peroxide (p.1111·1).
Acne.

Be-Natal Be-Tabs, S.Afr.†.
Multivitamin and mineral preparation (p.1350·1).

Benatoss Herus, Braz.
Ambroxol hydrochloride (p.1084·3).
Respiratory-tract congestion.

Benaxima Fustery, Mex.
Cefotaxime sodium (p.169·1).
Bacterial infections.

Benaxona Fustery, Mex.
Ceftriaxone sodium (p.177·1).
Bacterial infections.

Bencard Skin Testing Solutions Allergy Therapeutics, UK.
Allergen extracts (single and mixed) (p.1575·3).
Diagnosis of hypersensitivity.

Bencelin Antibioticos, Mex.
Benzathine benzylpenicillin (p.156·2).
Bacterial infections.

Bencelin Combinado Antibioticos, Mex.
Benzathine benzylpenicillin (p.156·2); procaine penicillin [procaine benzylpenicillin] (p.239·2); benzylpenicillin (p.157·1).
Bacterial infections.

Bencid Pharmaland, Thai.
Probenecid (p.401·3).
Gout; gouty arthritis.

Benclamin Polipharm, Thai.
Glibenclamide (p.321·3).
Diabetes mellitus.

Bencole Propan, S.Afr.
Co-trimoxazole (p.193·3).
Bacterial infections.

Benda Nakorn, Thai.
Mebendazole (p.102·2).
Worm infections.

Bendalina Angelini, Ital.; Lepori, Port.
Bendazac lysine (p.19·3).
Cataracts.

Bendapar Fustery, Mex.
Albendazole (p.95·2).
Worm infections.

Bendex Cipla-Medpro, S.Afr.
Albendazole (p.95·2).
Giardiasis; worm infections.

Bendigon N Gepepharm, Ger.
Mefruside (p.926·1); reserpine (p.967·3).
Hypertension.

Bendogen Lagap, UK†.
Betanidine sulfate (p.848·2).
Hypertension.

Bendracol Synco, Hong Kong.
Diphenhydramine hydrochloride (p.416·1); ammonium chloride (p.1085·2); sulfogaiacol (p.1101·1); sodium citrate (p.1186·2); terpin hydrate (p.1101·2); menthol (p.1632·3).
Coughs; respiratory-tract congestion.

Bendrax Haller, Braz.
Mebendazole (p.102·2).
Worm infections.

Benecid Valdecasas, Mex.
Probenecid (p.401·3).
Adjunct to beta-lactam antibacterials; gout.

Benectrin Legrand, Braz.
Co-trimoxazole (p.193·3).
Bacterial infections; pneumocystits carinii pneumonia; protozoal infections.

Benectrin Balsamico Legrand, Braz.
Co-trimoxazole (p.193·3); guaifenesin (p.1092·2); ammonium chloride (p.1085·2).
Bacterial infections.

Benecut Sanova, Aust.
Naftifine hydrochloride (p.392·1).
Fungal skin infections.

Benedaxol Liomont, Mex.
Mebendazole (p.102·2).

Benedorm Dresden, Ger.†.
Valerian (p.1678·3).
Anxiety disorders; insomnia.

Benefiber Novartis Consumer, Austral.
Guar gum (p.323·3).
Constipation.

Benefix
Genetics Institute, Aust.; Wyeth, Austral.; Baxter, Belg.; Genetics Institute, Denm.; Baxter, Fr.; Baxter, Ger.; Baxter, Ital.; Baxter, Spain; Baxter, Swed.; Baxter, Switz.; Baxter, UK; Genetics Institute, USA.
A factor IX preparation (recombinant DNA) (p.735·1).
Factor IX deficiency.

Beneflur Schering, Spain.
Fludarabine phosphate (p.539·3).
Chronic lymphocytic leukaemia.

Benegel Legrand, Braz.
Methyl salicylate (p.55·1); camphor (p.1589·3); menthol (p.1632·3); rosemary oil (p.1659·3); lavender oil (p.1627·2); turpentine oil (p.1676·3); mustard oil (p.1639·1).
Musculoskeletal and joint disorders.

Benegrip Newlab, Braz.
Salicylamide (p.82·1); chlorpheniramine [chlorphenamine] (p.412·2); caffeine (p.761·3); vitamin C (p.1389·3).
Cold and influenza symptoms.

Benemid
Merck Sharp & Dohme, Austral.; Merck Frosst, Canad.; Merck Sharp & Dohme, Irl.; Merck Sharp & Dohme, Neth.†; Merck Sharp & Dohme, NZ; Merck Sharp & Dohme, S.Afr.†; Merck Sharp & Dohme, Switz.; Merck Sharp & Dohme, Thai.; Merck Sharp & Dohme, UK†; Merck, USA.
Probenecid (p.401·3).
Adjunct to beta-lactam antibacterials; gout; hyperuricaemia.

Benemide Doms-Adrian, Fr.
Probenecid (p.401·3).
Adjunct to beta-lactam antibacterials; gout; hyperuricaemia.

Benera TO-Chemicals, Thai.
Belladonna alkaloids (p.463·1); ergotamine tartrate (p.452·1); phenobarbital (p.355·1).
Menopausal disorders; migraine; neurocirculatory asthenia; psychosomatic disorders.

Beneroc Roche, Aust.
Multivitamin and mineral preparation (p.1350·1).

Benerva
Roche Consumer, Belg.; Roche, Braz.; Roche, Fr.; Roche Consumer, Irl.; Roche, Ital.; Roche, Mex.; Roche, Spain; Roche, Swed.; Roche, Switz.; Roche Consumer, UK.
Thiamine hydrochloride (p.1385·1).
Alcoholism; beri beri; neuropathies; vitamin B₁ deficiency; Wernicke's encephalopathy.

Benestan
Vita, Ital.; Sanofi Synthelabo, Port.; Synthelabo, Spain.
Alfuzosin hydrochloride (p.833·2).
Benign prostatic hyperplasia.

Benetoss Heralds, Braz.
Ambroxol (p.1084·3).
Respiratory-tract congestion.

Benetussin Janssen-Cilag, Port.
Ammonium chloride (p.1085·2); diphenhydramine (p.416·1); menthol (p.1632·3).
Coughs.

Beneuran Nycomed, Aust.
Thiamine hydrochloride (p.1385·1).
Vitamin B₁ deficiency.

Beneuran compositum Nycomed, Aust.
Thiamine hydrochloride (p.1385·1); pyridoxine hydrochloride (p.1386·3); folic acid (p.1361·1); cyanocobalamin (p.1388·1).
Cervical syndrome; funicular myelosis; herpes zoster infection; nervous exhaustion; neuralgia; neuritis; pregnancy induced vomiting.

Beneuran Vit B-Komplex Nycomed, Aust.
Riboflavin sodium phosphate (p.1386·1); pyridoxine hydrochloride (p.1386·3); dexpanthenol (p.1602·3); thiamine hydrochloride (p.1385·1); nicotinamide (p.1372·3).
Eye disorders; gastrointestinal disorders; liver disorders; mouth and throat disorders; neurological disorders; obstetric disorders; skin disorders; vitamin deficiency.

Beneurol Meuse, Belg.
Thiamine hydrochloride (p.1385·1).
Beri-beri; dietary supplementation; digestive disorders; neuritis.

Benevran Legrand, Braz.
Diclofenac potassium (p.30·2).
Gout; inflammation; musculoskeletal, joint, and periarticular disorders; pain.

The symbol † denotes a preparation no longer actively marketed

Benexol *Roche, Switz.*
Vitamin B substances (p.1350·1).
Alcoholism; neuropathies; vitamin B deficiency.

Benexol B12
Note.This name is used for preparations of different composition.
Roche, Ital.
Injection: Cocarboxylase (p.1385·2); pyridoxine hydrochloride (p.1386·3); hydroxocobalamin (p.1388·1).
Tablets: Thiamine hydrochloride (p.1385·1); pyridoxine hydrochloride (p.1386·3); cyanocobalamin (p.1388·1).
Neuropathies; vitamin B₁, B₆, and B₁₂ deficiency; vomiting.

Roche, Mex.
Thiamine hydrochloride (p.1385·1); pyridoxine hydrochloride (p.1386·3); cyanocobalamin (p.1388·1).
Megaloblastic and sideroblastic anaemias; neuritis; vitamin B deficiencies.

Benexol B1 B6 B12 *Roche, Spain.*
Cyanocobalamin (p.1388·1); pyridoxine hydrochloride (p.1386·3); thiamine hydrochloride (p.1385·1).
Vitamin B deficiency.

Benfast *Novel, Ital.*
Ibuprofen sodium (p.44·1).
Fever; pain.

Benflogin
Note.This name is used for preparations of different composition.
Asta Medica, Braz.
Benzydamine hydrochloride (p.20·1).
Fever; inflammation; pain.

Angelini, Ital.
Ibuprofen guaiacol ester (p.44·1).
Fever; inflammation; pain.

Benflorene *Farmalight, Port.*
Lactic-acid-producing organisms (p.1626·3); dried yeast; vitamin B substances (p.1350·1).
Dietary supplement.

Benflux *Atral, Port.*
Ambroxol hydrochloride (p.1084·3).
Respiratory-tract congestion.

Benfofen *Sanofi Synthelabo, Ger.*
Diclofenac sodium (p.30·3).
Gout; inflammation; musculoskeletal, joint, and soft-tissue disorders; pain.

Ben-Gay
Pfizer, Israel; Pfizer Consumer, Singapore; Pfizer, USA.
Methyl salicylate (p.55·1); menthol (p.1632·3).
Muscle, joint, and soft-tissue pain; neuralgia.

Ben-Gay Ice *Pfizer Consumer, Canad.*
Menthol (p.1632·3).
Muscle and joint pain.

Ben-Gay No Odor *Pfizer Consumer, Canad.*
Trolamine salicylate (p.90·1).
Muscle and joint pain.

Ben-Gay Original, Ben-Gay Extra Strength
Pfizer Consumer, Canad.
Methyl salicylate (p.55·1); menthol (p.1632·3).
Muscle and joint pain.

Ben-Gay Ultra
Pfizer Consumer, Canad.; Pfizer, Israel; Pfizer, USA.
Methyl salicylate (p.55·1); menthol (p.1632·3); camphor (p.1589·3).
Muscle, joint, and soft-tissue pain; neuralgia.

Ben-Gay Vanishing *Pfizer, USA†.*
Menthol (p.1632·3).
Muscle, joint, and soft-tissue pain; neuralgia.

Benglau *CSC, Aust.*
Dapiprazole hydrochloride (p.1602·2).
Reversal of mydriasis.

Bengue's Balsam
Bengue, Irl.; Pfizer, UK†.
Menthol (p.1632·3); methyl salicylate (p.55·1).
Chilblains; cough and cold symptoms; rheumatic and muscular pain.

Benhex *PSM, NZ.*
Lindane (p.1434·1).
Scabies.

Benical *Roche, Switz.*
Dextromethorphan hydrobromide (p.1087·3); pseudoephedrine hydrochloride (p.1099·2); chlorpheniramine [chlorphenamine] maleate (p.412·1).
Coughs.

Beni-cur *Biocur, Ger.*
Garlic (p.1614·1).
Vascular disorders.

Benium *Merckle, Ger.†.*
Anise oil (p.1580·3); fennel oil (p.1610·2); caraway oil (p.1591·2).
Flatulence; gastrointestinal cramp.

Benn *Silom, Thai.*
Betamethasone valerate (p.1063·2); neomycin (p.228·1).
Bacterial skin infections.

Bennasone *Silom, Thai.*
Betamethasone valerate (p.1063·2).
Skin disorders.

Bennatuss *Hoe, Singapore.*
Diphenhydramine hydrochloride (p.416·1); ammonium chloride (p.1085·2); sodium citrate (p.1186·2).
Coughs; nasal congesion.

Benocten *Medinova, Switz.*
Diphenhydramine hydrochloride (p.416·1).
Sleep disorders.

Benodent *IMS, Ital.*
Sodium fluoride (p.1375·3); chlorhexidine (p.1138·2).
Dental caries prophylaxis; dental hygiene.

Benodent CLX *IMS, Ital.*
Chlorhexidine gluconate (p.1138·2).
Dental disorders.

Benoquin
ICN, Canad.; ICN, USA†.
Monobenzone (p.1120·3).
Skin hyperpigmentation.

Benoral
Note.This name is used for preparations of different composition.
Sanofi Winthrop, Irl.; Sanofi Winthrop, UK.
Benorilate (p.19·3).
Fever; inflammation; musculoskeletal and joint disorders; pain.

Reig Jofre, Spain.
Benzathine phenoxymethylpenicillin (p.157·1).
Bacterial infections.

Benormal *Cristalia, Braz.*
Vitamin B substances with calcium (p.1350·1).
Nutritional supplement.

Benosid *Farmasan, Ger.*
Budesonide (p.1064·2).
Obstructive airways disease.

Benoxid *Yamanouchi, Ital.*
Benzoyl peroxide (p.1111·1).
Acne; skin disinfection.

Benoxinat SE *Alcon, Ger.*
Oxybuprocaine hydrochloride (p.1318·1).
Local anaesthesia.

Benoxinato *Cusi, Spain†.*
Oxybuprocaine hydrochloride (p.1318·1).
Local anaesthesia.

Benoxygel
Stiefel, Port.; Stiefel, Spain.
Benzoyl peroxide (p.1111·1).
Acne.

Benoxyl
Stiefel, Canad.; Stiefel, Irl.†; Stiefel, Mex.; Sparks, NZ; Aspen Consumer, S.Afr.; Stiefel, UK; Stiefel, USA.
Benzoyl peroxide (p.1111·1).
Acne.

Benpen
CSL, Austral.; CSL, NZ.
Benzylpenicillin sodium (p.157·2).
Bacterial infections.

Benpine
Atlantic, Singapore; Atlantic, Thai.
Chlordiazepoxide hydrochloride (p.659·2).
Alcohol withdrawal syndrome; anxiety; skeletal muscle spasm.

Bens *Ardern, UK.*
Diethyltoluamide (p.1431·2).
Insect repellent.

Bensal HP *7 Oaks, USA.*
Benzoic acid (p.1134·2); salicylic acid (p.1122·3).
Fungal skin infections.

Bensolmin *Continentales, Mex.*
Mebendazole (p.102·2).

Bensulfoid *ECR, USA.*
Colloidal sulfur (p.1123·3); resorcinol (p.1122·2).
Acne.

Bentasil *Carter Horner, Canad.*
Green lozenges: Anethole (p.1580·1); eucalyptol (p.1609·2); menthol (p.1632·3).
Nasal congestion.

Red lozenges; yellow lozenges: Anethole (p.1580·1); menthol (p.1632·3).
Coughs; sore throats.

Bentelan *Glaxo Wellcome, Ital.*
Betamethasone disodium phosphate (p.1063·2).
Corticosteroid.

Bentiamin *Haller, Braz.*
Albendazole (p.95·2).
Worm infections.

Bentos
Ciba Vision, Fr.; Kaken, Hong Kong; Kaken, Jpn†.
Befunolol hydrochloride (p.843·2).
Glaucoma; ocular hypertension.

Bentyl
Medley, Braz.; Hoechst Marion Roussel, Mex.; Lakeside, USA†.
Dicyclomine [dicycloverine] hydrochloride (p.466·1).
Functional bowel syndrome; irritable bowel syndrome.

Bentylol
Hoechst Marion Roussel, Canad.; Marion Merrell, Spain†.
Dicyclomine [dicycloverine] hydrochloride (p.466·1).
Adjunct in peptic ulcer; irritable bowel syndrome; smooth muscle spasm.

Benur *Bioindustria, Ital.*
Doxazosin mesilate (p.883·2).
Benign prostatic hyperplasia.

Benuride *Roche, Switz.†.*
Pheneturide (p.354·3).
Epilepsy.

Ben-u-ron
Sigmapharm, Aust.; Bene, Ger.; Bene-Chemie, Hong Kong; Neo-Farmaceutica, Port.; Milupa, Switz.
Paracetamol (p.71·2).
Fever; pain.

Benuryl *ICN, Canad.*
Probenecid (p.401·3).
Hyperuricaemia.

Beny-Caps a la codeine *Warner-Lambert Consumer, Switz.†.*
Codeine phosphate (p.25·2); diphenhydramine hydrochloride (p.416·1).
Coughs.

Benylan
Note.This name is used for preparations of different composition.
Warner-Lambert, Denm.
Diphenhydramine hydrochloride (p.416·1); ammonium chloride (p.1085·2); menthol (p.1632·3).
Coughs; hypersensitivity.

Parke, Davis, Fin.; Parke, Davis, Swed.†.
Diphenhydramine hydrochloride (p.416·1).
Hypersensitivity reactions.

Benylin
Note.This name is used for preparations of different composition.
Warner-Lambert Consumer, Port.
Diphenhydramine hydrochloride (p.416·1); menthol (p.1632·3).
Formerly contained diphenhydramine hydrochloride, ammonium chloride, and menthol.
Coughs.

Parke, Davis, S.Afr.; Warner-Lambert Consumer, Switz.
Diphenhydramine hydrochloride (p.416·1); ammonium chloride (p.1085·2).
Coughs.

Benylin a la codeine *Warner-Lambert Consumer, Switz.*
Diphenhydramine hydrochloride (p.416·1); codeine phosphate (p.25·2); ammonium chloride (p.1085·2).
Coughs.

Benylin Active Response *Warner-Lambert, UK.*
Echinacea purpurea (p.1606·2).
Upper respiratory-tract infections.

Benylin Adult *Warner-Lambert, USA.*
Dextromethorphan hydrobromide (p.1087·3).
Formerly called Benylin Cough Syrup and contained diphenhydramine hydrochloride.
Coughs.

Benylin Antihistaminicum *Warner-Lambert Consumer, Belg.*
Diphenhydramine hydrochloride (p.416·1).
Hypersensitivity reactions.

Benylin Antitusivo *Warner-Lambert, Spain.*
Dextromethorphan hydrobromide (p.1087·3).
Coughs.

Benylin Antitussivum *Warner-Lambert Consumer, Belg.†.*
Dextromethorphan hydrobromide (p.1087·3).
Coughs.

Benylin (Benylin Original) *Warner-Lambert, Irl.*
Diphenhydramine hydrochloride (p.416·1); menthol (p.1632·3).
Coughs; hypersensitivity reactions.

Benylin CD *Warner-Lambert, Hong Kong.*
Diphenhydramine hydrochloride (p.416·1); codeine phosphate (p.25·2); ammonium chloride (p.1085·2); sodium citrate (p.1186·2); menthol (p.1632·3).
Coughs.

Benylin Chesty *Parke, Davis, S.Afr.*
Orciprenaline sulfate (p.769·1); bromhexine hydrochloride (p.1085·3).
Coughs.

Benylin Chesty Cough Original *Warner-Lambert, UK.*
Diphenhydramine hydrochloride (p.416·1); menthol (p.1632·3).
Coughs.

Benylin Chesty Coughs Non-Drowsy *Warner-Lambert, UK.*
Guaifenesin (p.1092·2); menthol (p.1632·3).
Coughs.

Benylin Childrens Chesty Coughs *Warner-Lambert, UK.*
Guaifenesin (p.1092·2).
Coughs.

Benylin Childrens Cough *Warner-Lambert, Irl.*
Diphenhydramine hydrochloride (p.416·1); sodium citrate (p.1186·2); menthol (p.1632·3).
Coughs.

Benylin Childrens Coughs & Colds *Warner-Lambert, UK.*
Dextromethorphan hydrobromide (p.1087·3); triprolidine hydrochloride (p.427·2).
Coughs and cold symptoms.

Benylin Childrens Dry Coughs *Warner-Lambert, UK.*
Pholcodine (p.1099·1).
Coughs.

Benylin Childrens Night Coughs *Warner-Lambert, UK.*
Diphenhydramine hydrochloride (p.416·1); menthol (p.1632·3).
Coughs; hypersensitivity symptoms of the respiratory tract.

Benylin Codeine *Warner-Lambert, Canad.*
Codeine phosphate (p.25·2); pseudoephedrine hydrochloride (p.1099·2); guaifenesin (p.1092·2).
Coughs; nasal congestion.

Benylin with Codeine
Note.This name is used for preparations of different composition.
Warner-Lambert, Irl.; Warner-Lambert, UK.
Diphenhydramine hydrochloride (p.416·1); codeine phosphate (p.25·2); menthol (p.1632·3).
Coughs.

Parke, Davis, Israel.
Diphenhydramine hydrochloride (p.416·1); codeine phosphate (p.25·2); sodium citrate (p.1186·2); menthol (p.1632·3).
Coughs.

Parke, Davis, S.Afr.
Diphenhydramine hydrochloride (p.416·1); codeine phosphate (p.25·2); ammonium chloride (p.1085·2).
Coughs.

Benylin Cold *Warner-Lambert, NZ.*
Paracetamol (p.71·2); pseudoephedrine hydrochloride (p.1099·2); dextromethorphan hydrobromide (p.1087·3).
Coughs and cold symptoms.

Benylin Cough *Warner-Lambert, Hong Kong.*
Diphenhydramine hydrochloride (p.416·1); ammonium chloride (p.1085·2); sodium citrate (p.1186·2); menthol (p.1632·3).
Cold symptoms; coughs.

Benylin Cough & Congestion *Warner-Lambert, UK.*
Diphenhydramine hydrochloride (p.416·1); menthol (p.1632·3); dextromethorphan hydrobromide (p.1087·3); pseudoephedrine hydrochloride (p.1099·2).
Coughs and cold symptoms.

Benylin Day & Night
Warner-Lambert, Ital.†; Parke, Davis, S.Afr.†; Warner-Lambert, UK.
Day tablets, paracetamol (p.71·2); phenylpropanolamine hydrochloride (p.1098·1); night tablets, paracetamol (p.71·2); diphenhydramine hydrochloride (p.416·1).
Cold and influenza symptoms.

Benylin Decongestant *Parke, Davis, USA†.*
Diphenhydramine hydrochloride (p.416·1); pseudoephedrine hydrochloride (p.1099·2).
Upper respiratory-tract symptoms.

Benylin Descongestivo *Warner-Lambert, Spain.*
Dextromethorphan hydrobromide (p.1087·3); pseudoephedrine hydrochloride (p.1099·2).
Coughs; nasal congestion.

Benylin DM
Warner-Lambert, Canad.; Parke, Davis, USA.
Dextromethorphan hydrobromide (p.1087·3).
Coughs.

Benylin DM-D
Warner-Lambert, Canad.; Parke, Davis, S.Afr.
Dextromethorphan hydrobromide (p.1087·3); pseudoephedrine hydrochloride (p.1099·2).
Coughs; nasal congestion.

Benylin DM-D-E *Warner-Lambert, Canad.*
Dextromethorphan hydrobromide (p.1087·3); pseudoephedrine hydrochloride (p.1099·2); guaifenesin (p.1092·2).
Coughs; nasal congestion.

Benylin DM-E *Warner-Lambert, Canad.*
Dextromethorphan hydrobromide (p.1087·3); guaifenesin (p.1092·2).
Coughs.

Benylin Dry Cough
Note.This name is used for preparations of different composition.
Warner-Lambert, Irl.
Diphenhydramine hydrochloride (p.416·1); dextromethorphan hydrobromide (p.1087·3); sodium citrate (p.1186·2); menthol (p.1632·3).
Coughs.

Parke, Davis, S.Afr.
Dextromethorphan hydrobromide (p.1087·3).
Formerly known as Benylin DM.
Coughs.

Benylin Dry Cough Original *Warner-Lambert, UK.*
Diphenhydramine hydrochloride (p.416·1); dextromethorphan hydrobromide (p.1087·3); menthol (p.1632·3).
Coughs.

Benylin Dry Coughs Non-Drowsy *Warner-Lambert, UK.*
Dextromethorphan hydrobromide (p.1087·3).
Coughs.

Benylin Expectorant *Warner-Lambert, USA.*
Dextromethorphan hydrobromide (p.1087·3); guaifenesin (p.1092·2).
Coughs.

Benylin 4 Flu
Note.This name is used for preparations of different composition.
Warner-Lambert, Canad.
Dextromethorphan hydrobromide (p.1087·3); pseudoephedrine hydrochloride (p.1099·2); guaifenesin (p.1092·2); paracetamol (p.71·2).
Coughs and cold symptoms.

Warner-Lambert, UK.
Hot drink: Diphenhydramine hydrochloride (p.416·1); paracetamol (p.71·2); phenylephrine hydrochloride (p.1097·1).
Oral liquid; tablets: Diphenhydramine hydrochloride (p.416·1); paracetamol (p.71·2); pseudoephedrine hydrochloride (p.1099·2).
Cold and influenza symptoms.

Benylin Mentholated Linctus *Warner-Lambert, UK†.*
Diphenhydramine hydrochloride (p.416·1); dextromethorphan hydrobromide (p.1087·3); pseudoephedrine hydrochloride (p.1099·2); menthol (p.1632·3).
Coughs.

Benylin Multi-Symptom *Warner-Lambert, USA.*
Dextromethorphan hydrobromide (p.1087·3); pseudoephedrine hydrochloride (p.1099·2); guaifenesin (p.1092·2).
Cough and cold symptoms.

Benylin Non-Drowsy Chesty Coughs *Warner-Lambert, Irl.*
Guaifenesin (p.1092·2); menthol (p.1632·3).
Coughs.

Benylin Non-Drowsy Dry Coughs *Warner-Lambert, Irl.*
Dextromethorphan hydrobromide (p.1087·3).
Coughs.

Benylin Paediatric
Note. This name is used for preparations of different composition.
Parke, Davis, Israel.
Sugar/colour-free syrup: Diphenhydramine hydrochloride (p.416·1); menthol (p.1632·3).
Syrup: Diphenhydramine hydrochloride (p.416·1); sodium citrate (p.1186·2); menthol (p.1632·3).
Coughs.
Warner-Lambert Consumer, Switz.†.
Diphenhydramine hydrochloride (p.416·1).
Coughs.

Benylin Pediatric Warner-Lambert, USA.
Dextromethorphan hydrobromide (p.1087·3).
Coughs.

Benylin Solid Parke, Davis, S.Afr.†.
Dextromethorphan hydrobromide (p.1087·3).
Coughs.

Benylin Sore Throat Lozenge Warner-Lambert, UK.
Hexylresorcinol (p.1146·3).
Sore throat.

Benylin-Dextromethorfanhydrobromide
Warner-Lambert, Neth.†.
Dextromethorphan hydrobromide (p.1087·3).
Coughs.

Benylin-Difenhydraminehydrochloride Warner-Lambert, Neth.†.
Diphenhydramine hydrochloride (p.416·1).
Coughs.

Benylin-E Warner-Lambert, Canad.
Guaifenesin (p.1092·2).
Coughs.

Benyphed Parke, Davis, S.Afr.†.
Diphenhydramine hydrochloride (Benadryl) (p.416·1); dextromethorphan hydrobromide (p.1087·3); phenylephrine hydrochloride (p.1097·1).
Coughs.

Benza Century, USA.
Benzalkonium chloride (p.1133·2).
Eye, bladder, urethra, and body cavity irrigation; skin, mucous membrane, and wound disinfection; vaginal douching.

Benzac
Galderma, Austral.; Galderma, Belg.; Galderma, Braz.; Galderma, Canad.; Galderma, Ital.; Galderma, Mex.; Galderma, Neth.; Galderma, NZ; Galderma, Port.; Galderma, Singapore; Galderma, Switz.; Galderma, Thai.; Galderma, USA.
Benzoyl peroxide (p.1111·1).
Acne.

Benzac-AC
Galderma, Braz.; Galderma, Hong Kong; Galderma, Israel; Galderma, S.Afr.
Benzoyl peroxide (p.1111·1).
Acne.

BenzaClin Dermik, USA.
Clindamycin (p.189·3); benzoyl peroxide (p.1111·1).
Acne.

Benzaderm Mex-America, Mex.
Soap.
Skin cleansing.
Topical gel: Benzoyl peroxide (p.1111·1).
Acne.

Benzagel
Darrow, Braz.; Novartis Consumer, Canad.; Dermik, Canad.; Dermik, USA.
Benzoyl peroxide (p.1111·1).
Acne.

Benzaknen
AB-Consult, Aust.; Galderma, Ger.
Benzoyl peroxide (p.1111·1).
Acne.

Benzalc Asens, Spain†.
Benzalkonium chloride (p.1133·2).
Skin and mucous membrane disinfection.

Benzamycin
Trenker, Belg.; Dermik, Canad.; Dermik, Hong Kong; Bioglan, Irl.; Dermik, Israel; Darier, Mex.; Dermik, Singapore; Bioglan, UK; Dermik, USA.
Benzoyl peroxide (p.1111·1); erythromycin (p.201·2).
Acne.

Benzamycine UCB, S.Afr.
Benzoyl peroxide (p.1111·1); erythromycin (p.201·2).
Acne.

Benzanil Compuesto Lakeside, Mex.
Benzathine benzylpenicillin (p.156·2); procaine penicillin [procaine benzylpenicillin] (p.239·2); benzylpenicillin sodium (p.157·2).
Bacterial infections.

Benzanil Simple Lakeside, Mex.
Benzathine benzylpenicillin (p.156·2).
Bacterial infections.

Benzantine H Rekah, Israel.
Diphenhydramine hydrochloride (p.416·1); hydrocortisone (p.1073·3).
Skin disorders; skin irritation.

Benzashave Medicis, USA.
Benzoyl peroxide (p.1111·1).
Acne.

Benzatec Caps, S.Afr.
Benzylpenicillin sodium (p.157·2).
Bacterial infections.

Benzedrex Ascher, USA.
Propylhexedrine (p.1514·2).
Nasal congestion.

Benzemul McGloin, Austral.
Benzyl benzoate (p.1428·2).
Pediculosis; scabies.

Benzet Covan, S.Afr.
Cetrimide (p.1137·1); benzocaine (p.1306·2).
Mouth and throat disorders.

Benzetacil
Wyeth, Braz.; Wyeth, Mex.; Antibioticos, Spain.
Benzathine benzylpenicillin (p.156·2).
Bacterial infections.

Benzetacil Combinado Wyeth, Mex.
Benzathine benzylpenicillin (p.156·2); benzylpenicillin potassium (p.157·1); procaine penicillin [procaine benzylpenicillin] (p.239·2).
Bacterial infections.

Benzetacil Compuesta Antibioticos, Spain.
Benzylpenicillin potassium (p.157·1); procaine penicillin [procaine benzylpenicillin] (p.239·2); benzathine benzylpenicillin (p.156·2).
Bacterial infections.

Benzevit Elofar, Braz.
Nystatin (p.392·2); zinc oxide (p.1128·2).
Skin infections.

Benzibel Lusofarmaco, Ital.†.
Methylbenzethonium chloride (p.1150·3).
Barrier preparation; skin irritation and infection.

Benziflex EMS, Braz.
Benzydamine hydrochloride (p.20·1).
Fever; inflammation; pain.

Benzilol Bunker, Braz.
Benzyl benzoate (p.1428·2); trolamine (p.1675·1).
Pediculosis; scabies.

Benzirin Fater, Ital.
Benzydamine hydrochloride (p.20·1).
Inflammatory mouth disorders.

Benzitrat Searle, Braz.
Benzydamine hydrochloride (p.20·1).
Fever; inflammation; pain.

Benzocaine PD Produits Dentaires, Switz.
Benzocaine (p.1306·2); hydroxyquinoline sulfate (p.1622·2); eugenol (p.1609·3).
Dental pain.

Benzodent Procter & Gamble, USA.
Benzocaine (p.1306·2).
Oral lesions.

Benzoderm Myco Athenstaedt, Ger.
Clotrimazole (p.382·1).
Fungal skin infections.

Benzogen Ferri Cos Farma, Ital.
Benzalkonium chloride (p.1133·2); sodium nitrite (p.1023·1); acetone (p.1400·1).
Instrument disinfection.

Benzo-Ginestryl Hoechst Marion Roussel, Mex.
Estradiol benzoate (p.1473·1).
Lactation inhibition; menopausal disorders; menstrual disorders; osteoporosis.

Benzo-Ginoestril Hoechst Marion Roussel, Braz.
Estradiol hexahydrobenzoate (p.1473·2).
Menopausal disorders; osteoporosis.

Benzo-Gynoestryl Roussel, Fr†.
Estradiol benzoate (p.1473·1) or estradiol hexahydrobenzoate (p.1473·2).
Oestrogen deficiency.

Benzomix Savoma, Ital.†.
Benzoyl peroxide (p.1111·1).
Acne; skin disinfection.

Benzonal Cryopharma, Mex.
Benzonatate (p.1085·3).
Coughs.

Benzopin Alliance, S.Afr.
Diazepam (p.674·3).
Alcohol withdrawal syndrome; anxiety; premedication.

Benzotal Biosintetica, Braz.
Ampicillin benzathine (p.151·3); ampicillin sodium (p.150·3).
Bacterial infections.

Benzotal Balsamico Biosintetica, Braz.
Ampicillin benzathine (p.151·3); ampicillin sodium (p.150·3); guaifenesin (p.1092·2); niaouli oil (p.1640·2); eucalyptol (p.1609·2).
Bacterial infections.

Benzotic Alba, USA†.
Phenazone (p.77·2); benzocaine (p.1306·2).

Benzotran Pacific, NZ.
Oxazepam (p.697·1).
Anxiety.

Benzoyt Hexal, Ger.
Benzoyl peroxide (p.1111·1).
Acne.

Benztrone Amsa, Ital.
Estradiol benzoate (p.1473·1).
Now known as Estradiolo Amsa.
Labour induction; menstrual disorders.

Benzum Lepori, Port.
Bendazac (p.19·3).
Skin disorders.

Benzyme Collins, Mex.
Diazepam (p.674·3).

Beocid Puroptal Metochem, Aust.†.
Sulfacetamide sodium (p.250·3).
Bacterial eye infections.

Beofenac
UCB, Aust.; UCB, Ger.; Rodleben, Ger.; Vedim, Ger.
Aceclofenac (p.11·1).
Musculoskeletal and joint disorders.

Beofta Novag, Mex.
Betaxolol (p.848·3).

Beogaze Hoechst Marion Roussel, Belg.†.
Gauze impregnated with camphor (p.1589·3) and niaouli oil (p.1640·2).
Burns; wounds.

Be-Oxytet Be-Tabs, S.Afr.
Oxytetracycline hydrochloride (p.234·1).
Bacterial infections.

Bepanten Roche, Ital.
Dexpanthenol (p.1602·3).
Intestinal atony.

Bepanthen
Note. This name is used for preparations of different composition.
Roche, Aust.; Roche, Fin.; Roche Nicholas, Ger.; Roche, Israel; Roche, NZ.
Dexpanthenol (p.1602·3) or panthenol (p.1602·3).
Conjunctivitis; dexpanthenol deficiency disorders; gastrointestinal disorders; respiratory-tract disorders; skin disorders.
Roche, Aust.
Solution: Dexpanthenol (p.1602·3); domiphen bromide (p.1143·3).
Gastrointestinal disorders; mouth and throat disorders; nasal disorders; respiratory tract disorders; skin damage.
Roche Consumer, Austral.
Benzalkonium chloride (p.1133·2).
Formerly contained panthenol.
Minor skin lesions; skin irritation.

Bepanthen Plus
Roche, Aust.; Roche, Israel.
Dexpanthenol (p.1602·3); chlorhexidine hydrochloride (p.1138·2).
Dry skin; wounds.

Bepanthene
Note. This name is used for preparations of different composition.
Roche, Belg.†.
Panthenol (p.1602·3).
Hepatitis; intestinal atony; muscular cramps; respiratory-tract disorders; skin disorders.
Roche, Fr.; Roche, Port.; Roche Nicholas, Spain; Roche, Switz.
Dexpanthenol (p.1602·3).
Alopecia; gastrointestinal disorders; mouth and throat disorders; nasal disorders; respiratory-tract disorders; skin disorders; wounds.
Roche, Port.
Lotion: Dexpanthenol (p.1602·3); chlorhexidine hydrochloride (p.1138·2).
Skin disorders; wounds.

Bepanthene Plus
Roche, Port.; Roche, Switz.
Dexpanthenol (p.1602·3); chlorhexidine hydrochloride (p.1138·2).
Skin disorders; wounds.

Bepantol
Roche, Braz.; Roche, S.Afr.
Dexpanthenol (p.1602·3).
Skin disorders.

Bepeno-G Milano, Thai.
Phenylpropanolamine hydrochloride (p.1098·1); phenylephrine hydrochloride (p.1097·1); brompheniramine maleate (p.410·2); guaifenesin (p.1092·2).
Coughs; respiratory-tract congestion.

Bepep Nutrition Care, Austral.
Betaine hydrochloride (p.1584·3); pepsin (p.1649·3).
Digestive disorders.

Bephen Thilo, Hong Kong.
Trifluridine (p.642·2).
Herpes simplex eye infections.

Beplex-Zee Anglo-French Drugs, Thai.
Multivitamin preparation with zinc (p.1350·1).

Beprogel Hoe, Singapore.
Betamethasone dipropionate (p.1063·2).
Skin disorders.

Beprogent Hoe, Singapore.
Betamethasone dipropionate (p.1063·2) gentamicin sulfate (p.210·1).
Infected skin disorders.

Beprogenta Chew, Thai.
Betamethasone dipropionate (p.1063·2); gentamicin sulfate (p.210·1).
Infected inflammatory skin disorders.

Beprosalic Hoe, Singapore.
Betamethasone dipropionate (p.1063·2); salicylic acid (p.1122·3).
Skin disorders.

Beprosone
Hoe, Singapore; Chew, Thai.
Betamethasone dipropionate (p.1063·2).
Skin disorders.

Bequidril Teuto, Braz.
Diphenhydramine hydrochloride (p.416·1); ammonium chloride (p.1085·2); sodium citrate (p.1186·2).
Coughs.

Bequipecto Llorens, Spain†.
Bromelains (p.1586·3); bromhexine (p.1085·3); oxolamine citrate (p.1096·2).
Respiratory-tract disorders.

Beracal Noristan, S.Afr.†.
Diphenhydramine hydrochloride (p.416·1); calamine (p.1111·3); benzocaine (p.1306·2).
Skin disorders.

Beramicina Berman, Mex.
Gentamicin sulfate (p.210·1).
Bacterial infections.

Beramikin Berman, Mex.
Amikacin (p.147·3).
Bacterial infections.

Beramin Hoechst Marion Roussel, S.Afr.†.
Diphenhydramine hydrochloride (p.416·1); ammonium chloride (p.1085·2).
Coughs.

Berazole Hoechst Marion Roussel, S.Afr.†.
Metronidazole (p.594·1).
Anaerobic bacterial infections; protozoal infections.

Berberell Sanorell, Ger.
Homoeopathic preparation.

Berberil N Mann, Ger.
Tetryzoline hydrochloride (p.1101·2).
Eye disorders.

Berberis Complex Blackmores, Austral.
Berberis vulgaris; taraxacum (p.1669·1); greater celandine (p.1618·1); boldo (p.1585·3); lecithin (p.1628·1); methionine (p.1012·2); thiamine hydrochloride (p.1385·1).
Constipation; dyspepsia; liver disorders.

Berberis Med Complex Dynamit, Aust.
Homoeopathic preparation.

Berberis Oligoplex Madaus, Ger.
Homoeopathic preparation.

Berciclina Enzimatica Berman, Mex.
Tetracycline (p.258·3).
Bacterial infections.

Berclomine Polipharm, Thai.
Dicyclomine [dicycloverine] hydrochloride (p.466·1); simeticone (p.1249·2).
Gastrointestinal colic and spasm.

Berex Leiras, Fin.
Vitamin B substances (p.1350·1).
Vitamin B deficiency; vitamin B supplement.

Bergamon Sapone Bergamon, Ital.
Tribromsalan (p.1136·1).
Skin cleansing.

Berggeist Kur und Stadtapotheke, Aust.
Arnica tincture (p.1581·3); urtica tincture (p.1678·2); formic acid (p.1612·3); menthol (p.1632·3); methyl nicotinate (p.55·1); juniper oil (p.1625·2); lavender oil (p.1627·2); eucalyptus oil (p.1609·2); rosemary oil (p.1659·3); pumilio pine oil (p.1656·3).
Bruising; musculoskeletal and joint disorders; neuralgia.

Beriate Centeon, Aust.
A factor VIII preparation (p.734·1).
Factor VIII deficiency.

Beriate P
Centeon, Ger.; Centeon, Ital.; Centeon, Spain; Centeon, Swed.; Aventis Behring, UK.
A factor VIII preparation (p.734·1).
Haemorrhagic disorders.

Bericard Provita, Aust.
Crataegus (p.1600·2).
Cardiovascular disorders.

Beriglobin
Centeon, Aust.; Centeon, Denm.; Chiron Behring, Ger.; Centeon, Ger.; Mirren, S.Afr.; Centeon, Swed.
A normal immunoglobulin (p.1551·3).
Hypogammaglobulinaemia; passive immunisation.

Beriglobin P Centeon, Israel.
A normal immunoglobulin (p.1551·3).
Hypogammaglobulinaemia; passive immunisation.

Beriglobina Anti D-P Centeon, Spain†.
An anti-D immunoglobulin (p.1532·1).
Prevention of rhesus sensitisation.

Beriglobina P
Centeon, Mex.; Centeon, Spain.
A normal immunoglobulin (p.1551·3).
Hypogammaglobulinaemia; passive immunisation.

Berinert
Centeon, Aust.; Centeon, Ger.
Complement C1 esterase inhibitor (p.1599·1).
Hereditary angioedema.

Berinert HS Centeon, Switz.
Complement C1 esterase inhibitor (p.1599·1).
Hereditary angioedema.

Berinert P Centeon, UK†.
Complement C1 esterase inhibitor (p.1599·1).
Hereditary angioedema.

Berinin Centeon, Ger.
A factor IX preparation (p.735·1).
Factor IX deficiency; haemophilia B.

Berinin HS Centeon, Switz.
A factor IX preparation (p.735·1).
Haemophilia B.

Berinin P Centeon, Mex.
A factor IX preparation (p.735·1).
Factor IX deficiency; haemophilia B.

Beriplast
Centeon, Aust.; Centeon, Fin.; Centeon, Fr.; Centeon, Ger.; Centeon, Hong Kong.
1 ampoule: fibrinogen (p.736·1); factor XIII (p.735·3); 1 ampoule: aprotinin (p.725·3); 1 ampoule: thrombin (p.741·3); 1 ampoule: calcium chloride (p.1188·1)
On mixing this forms a fibrin glue (p.735·3).
Haemorrhage; wounds.

Beriplast P
Centeon, Israel; Centeon, Mex.
1 Ampoule, fibrinogen (p.736·1); Factor XIII (p.735·3); 1 ampoule, aprotinin (p.725·3); 1 ampoule, thrombin (p.741·3); 1 ampoule, calcium chloride (p.1188·1)
On mixing this forms a fibrin glue (p.735·3).
Haemorrhage; wounds.

The symbol † denotes a preparation no longer actively marketed

Beriplex *Centeon, Aust.*
A factor IX preparation (p.735·1).
Factor II, VII, IX, and X deficiency; haemorrhagic disorders.

Beriplex PN
Centeon, Ger.; Centeon, UK.
A factor IX preparation (p.735·1).
Anticoagulant overdose; haemorrhagic disorders.

Berirab
Centeon, Aust.; Chiron Behring, Ger.; Centeon, Ger.
A rabies immunoglobulin (p.1560·2).
Passive immunisation.

Berirubin *Ebewe, Aust.*
Pirarubicin hydrochloride (p.565·1).
Now known as Pirarubicin.
Malignant neoplasms.

Berivine *Meuse, Belg.*
Riboflavin (p.1386·1).
Dietary supplement; nocturnal cramps; vitamin B₂ deficiency.

Berkamil
Berk, Irl.†; Berk, UK.
Amiloride (p.835·3).
Heart failure; hepatic cirrhosis with ascites; hypertension.

Berkaprine *Berk, UK†*
Azathioprine (p.509·3).
Auto-immune disorders; organ transplantation.

Berkatens
Berk, Irl.†; Berk, UK†.
Verapamil hydrochloride (p.989·1).
Angina; arrhythmias; hypertension.

Berkmycen
Berk, Irl.†; Berk, UK†.
Oxytetracycline (p.234·1).
Bacterial infections.

Berkolol
Rhone-Poulenc Rorer, Hong Kong; Berk, Irl.†; Berk, UK†.
Propranolol hydrochloride (p.962·3).
Angina pectoris; anxiety; arrhythmias; essential tremor; hypertension; hyperthyroidism; migraine; myocardial infarction.

Berkozide *Berk, UK†*
Bendrofluazide [bendroflumethiazide] (p.844·1).
Heart failure; hypertension; oedema; suppression of lactation.

Berlactone *Berlin Pharm, Thai.*
Spironolactone (p.973·2).
Hypertension; oedema and ascites of heart failure; primary aldosteronism.

Berlicetin
Note.This name is used for preparations of different composition.
Berlin-Chemie, Ger.†.
Chloramphenicol (p.179·1), chloramphenicol palmitate (p.179·2), or chloramphenicol sodium succinate (p.179·2).
Bacterial infections.

Chauvin ankerpharm, Ger.
Azidamfenicol (p.152·3).
Bacterial eye infections.

Berlicetin-Ohrentropfen *Wernigerode, Ger.*
Chloramphenicol (p.179·1); prednisolone (p.1077·3).
Bacterial ear infections with inflammation.

Berlicort *Berlin-Chemie, Ger.*
Triamcinolone (p.1080·1) or triamcinolone acetonide (p.1080·1).
Corticosteroid.

Berlinsulin H 10/90, 20/80, 30/70, 40/60, 50/50 *Berlin-Chemie, Ger.*
Mixtures of insulin injection (human, prb) and isophane insulin injection (human, prb) respectively in the proportions indicated (p.324·1).
Diabetes mellitus.

Berlinsulin H Basal *Berlin-Chemie, Ger.*
Isophane insulin injection (human, prb) (p.324·1).
Diabetes mellitus.

Berlinsulin H Normal *Berlin-Chemie, Ger.*
Insulin injection (human, prb) (p.324·1).
Diabetes mellitus.

Berlison *Schering, Braz.*
Hydrocortisone acetate (p.1073·3).
Skin disorders.

Berlithion *Berlin-Chemie, Ger.*
Thioctic acid (p.1671·3) or ethylenediamine thioctate (p.1671·3).
Diabetic polyneuropathy.

Berlocid *Berlin-Chemie, Ger.*
Co-trimoxazole (p.193·3).
Bacterial infections; Pneumocystis carinii pneumonia.

Berlocombin *Berlin-Chemie, Ger.*
Trimethoprim (p.264·2); sulfamerazine (p.253·3).
Bacterial infections.

Berlosin *Berlin-Chemie, Ger.*
Dipyrone (p.34·1).
Fever; pain.

Berlthyrox *Berlin-Chemie, Ger.*
Thyroxine [levothyroxine] sodium (p.1526·2).
Hypothyroidism.

Bernadine *Shiwa, Thai.*
Povidone-iodine (p.1155·1).
Disinfection of skin, wounds, burns, and mucous membranes; mouth and throat inflammation.

Berniter *Galderma, Ger.*
Coal tar (p.1125·1).
Scalp disorders.

Berocca
Roche Consumer, Austral.; Roche, Fin.; Roche Nicholas, Fr.; Roche, Hong Kong; Roche, Mex.; Roche, NZ; Roche Consumer, Singapore; Roche Consumer, UK.
Vitamin B substances; vitamin C; minerals (p.1350·1).

Roche, Ital.; Roche, USA.
Vitamin B substances with vitamin C (p.1350·1).

Berocca Calcium
Roche, Aust.; Roche, S.Afr.
Vitamin B substances with vitamin C and calcium (p.1350·1).

Berocca Calcium and Magnesium *Roche, Israel.*
Vitamin B substances with vitamin C, calcium, and magnesium (p.1350·1).
Nutritional supplement.

Berocca calcium, magnesium + zinc *Roche, Switz.*
Vitamin B substances; vitamin C; calcium; magnesium; zinc (p.1350·1).
Alcoholism; vitamin deficiency.

Berocca Calmag *Roche, S.Afr.*
Vitamin B substances; vitamin C; calcium; magnesium (p.1350·1).

Berocca Plus
Note.This name is used for preparations of different composition.
Roche, Aust.
Vitamin B substances with vitamin C, calcium, and magnesium (p.1350·1).

Roche, USA.
Ferrous fumarate (p.1360·1); folic acid (p.1361·1); multivitamins and minerals (p.1350·1).
Iron-deficiency anaemias.

Berodual
Boehringer Ingelheim, Aust.; Boehringer Ingelheim, Denm.; Boehringer Ingelheim, Ger.; Boehringer Ingelheim, Hong Kong; Boehringer Ingelheim, Neth.; Boehringer Ingelheim, Port.; Boehringer Ingelheim, Singapore; Boehringer Ingelheim, Spain; Boehringer Ingelheim, Switz.; Boehringer Ingelheim, Thai.
Fenoterol (p.765·2) or fenoterol hydrobromide (p.765·1); ipratropium bromide (p.766·1).
Obstructive airways disease.

Berodualin *Boehringer Ingelheim, Aust.*
Fenoterol hydrobromide (p.765·1); ipratropium bromide (p.766·1).
Obstructive airways disease.

Berofor
Boehringer Ingelheim, Aust.
Eye drops: Interferon alfa-2 (p.628·1).
Herpes simplex virus keratitis.

Injection: Interferon alfa-2c (p.628·1).
Anogenital warts; chronic active hepatitis; herpes infections; malignant neoplasms.

Beromin *Condrugs, Thai.*
Vitamin B₁ (p.1385·2); vitamin B₆ (p.1387·1); vitamin B₁₂ (p.1388·1).
Neuritis; vitamin B deficiency.

Beromun
Boehringer Ingelheim, Neth.†; Boehringer Ingelheim, Spain; Boehringer Ingelheim, Swed.
Tasonermin (p.577·1).
Soft-tissue sarcoma.

Berotec
Boehringer Ingelheim, Aust.; Boehringer Ingelheim, Austral.; Boehringer Ingelheim, Belg.; Boehringer de Angeli, Braz.; Boehringer Ingelheim, Canad.; Boehringer Ingelheim, Denm.; Boehringer Ingelheim, Fin.; Boehringer Ingelheim, Fr.; Boehringer Ingelheim, Ger.; Boehringer Ingelheim, Hong Kong; Boehringer Ingelheim, Irl.; Boehringer Ingelheim, Mex.; Boehringer Ingelheim, Neth.; Boehringer Ingelheim, Norw.; Boehringer Ingelheim, NZ; Boehringer Ingelheim, Port.; Boehringer Ingelheim, S.Afr.; Boehringer Ingelheim, Singapore; Boehringer Ingelheim, Spain; Boehringer Ingelheim, Swed.; Boehringer Ingelheim, Switz.; Boehringer Ingelheim, Thai.; Boehringer Ingelheim, UK†.
Fenoterol (p.765·2) or fenoterol hydrobromide (p.765·1).
Obstructive airways disease.

Berotec solvens *Boehringer Ingelheim, Ger.†.*
Fenoterol hydrobromide (p.765·1); bromhexine hydrochloride (p.1085·3).
Bronchiectasis; bronchitis; emphysema; interstitial lung disease.

Berplex *Schein, USA†.*
Ferrous fumarate (p.1360·1); folic acid (p.1361·1); multivitamins and minerals (p.1350·1).
Iron-deficiency anaemias.

Bertocil *Oftalder, Port.*
Betaxolol hydrochloride (p.848·3).
Glaucoma; ocular hypertension.

Berubi *Redel, Ger.*
Echinacea (p.1606·2).
Formerly contained cyanocobalamin.
Cold and influenza symptoms.

Beruhigungskapseln *Klosterfrau, Aust.*
Valerian (p.1678·3); lupulus (p.1629·3).
Nervous disorders; sleep disorders.

Beruhigungstee *Sanova, Aust.*
Valerian (p.1678·3); melissa (p.1632·2); lupulus (p.1629·3); lavender flower (p.1627·2); orange flowers.
Anxiety; sleep disturbances.

Besaprin *Sanofi Winthrop, Braz.*
Chlormezanone (p.660·1); aspirin (p.14·2).
Muscle spasm.

Besedan *Wyeth, Braz.*
Butamirate citrate (p.1086·2).
Coughs.

Besemax *Covan, S.Afr.*
Orphenadrine citrate (p.470·3); paracetamol (p.71·2).
Musculoskeletal spasm; pain.

Besenol *Covan, S.Afr.†*
Paracetamol (p.71·2); chlormezanone (p.660·1).
Fever; pain; skeletal muscle spasm.

Beserol *Sanofi Winthrop, Braz.*
Chlormezanone (p.660·1); dipyrone (p.34·1).
Muscle spasm.

Besitran *Pfizer Consumer, Spain.*
Sertraline hydrochloride (p.308·3).
Depression; obsessive-compulsive disorder; panic disorder.

Besone
Atlantic, Singapore; Atlantic, Thai.
Betamethasone valerate (p.1063·2).
Skin disorders.

Besone-N
Atlantic, Singapore; Atlantic, Thai.
Betamethasone valerate (p.1063·2); neomycin sulfate (p.228·1).
Infected skin disorders.

Besopartin *Boehringer Ingelheim, Aust.*
Alteplase (p.833·3).
Myocardial infarction; peripheral arterial thromboembolism; pulmonary embolism.

Bespar *Bristol-Myers Squibb, Ger.*
Buspirone hydrochloride (p.657·2).
Anxiety.

Bessasone *Pharmaland, Thai.*
Betamethasone valerate (p.1063·2).
Skin disorders.

Best EPA *Contassium Co., UK.*
Fish oil (eicosapentaenoic acid, and docosahexaenoic acid) (p.949·3).

Bestatin *Kayaku, Jpn†.*
Ubenimex (p.577·1).
Prophylaxis following the induction of remission against adult acute nonlymphoid leukaemias.

Bestcall *Takeda, Jpn.*
Cefmenoxime hydrochloride (p.167·1).
Mepivacaine hydrochloride (p.1317·1) is included in the intramuscular injection to alleviate the pain of injection.
Bacterial infections.

Bester Complex *Salvat, Spain.*
Benfotiamine (p.1384·3); hydroxocobalamin acetate (p.1388·3); pyridoxine hydrochloride (p.1386·3).
Vitamin B deficiency.

Bestron *Senju, Jpn.*
Cefmenoxime hydrochloride (p.167·1).
Bacterial eye infections.

Be-Supra *Sanofi Synthelabo, Port.*
Vitamin B substances and vitamin C (p.1350·1).

Beta *Chew, Thai.*
Betamethasone valerate (p.1063·2).
Skin disorders.

Beta-2 *Nephron, USA†.*
Isoetarine hydrochloride (p.767·1).
Asthma; bronchospasm.

Beta 21 *IDI, Ital.*
Betamethasone valero-acetate (p.1063·3).
Skin disorders.

Beta A-C *Eagle, Austral.*
Oral powder: Ascorbic acid (p.1389·3); sodium ascorbate (p.1390·1); calcium ascorbate (p.1389·3); dl-alpha-tocoferil acetate (p.1394·1); rutoside (p.1611·2); zinc amino acid chelate (p.1398·3); betacarotene (p.1355·1).
Tablets: Ascorbic acid (p.1389·3); sodium ascorbate (p.1390·1); calcium ascorbate (p.1389·3); dl-alpha-tocoferil acetate (p.1394·1); rutoside (p.1611·2); zinc amino acid chelate (p.1398·3); betacarotene (p.1355·1); bioflavonoids (p.1611·1).
Vitamin supplement.

Beta C E with Selenium *Stanley, Canad.*
Betacarotene, selenium, vitamin C, and vitamin E (p.1350·1).

Beta Micoter *Farmacusi, Spain.*
Betamethasone dipropionate (p.1063·2); clotrimazole (p.382·1).
Fungal skin infections.

Beta plus Vitamins C, E & Selenium *Quest, Canad.*
Betacarotene, selenium, vitamin C, and vitamin E (p.1350·1).

Beta Prostate *Young Again Products, USA.*
Sitosterol (p.970·3); zinc citrate.
Dietary supplement.

Beta Scalp *Pacific, NZ.*
Betamethasone valerate (p.1063·2).
Scalp disorders.

Beta-Ace Tablets *Vitaglow, Austral.*
Betacarotene (p.1355·1); ascorbic acid (p.1389·3); d-alpha tocoferil acid succinate (p.1394·1); zinc amino acid chelate (p.1398·3).
Dietary supplement.

Beta-Adalat
Bayer, Aust.; Bayer, Belg.; Bayer, Fin.; Bayer, Irl.; Bayer, Switz.; Bayer, UK.
Atenolol (p.841·3); nifedipine (p.940·1).
Angina pectoris; hypertension.

Beta-Adalate *Bayer, Fr.*
Atenolol (p.841·3); nifedipine (p.940·1).
Hypertension.

Betabactyl *SmithKline Beecham, Ger.†.*
Ticarcillin sodium (p.262·3); potassium clavulanate (p.187·2).
Bacterial infections.

Betabion
Merck, Ger.; Bracco, Ital.; Merck, Swed.
Thiamine hydrochloride (p.1385·1).
Vitamin B₁ deficiency.

Betabioptal *Farmila, Ital.*
Betamethasone (p.1063·1); chloramphenicol (p.179·1).
Infected eye disorders.

Betabiotic *Esseti, S.Afr.*
Flucloxacillin sodium (p.207·1).
Lignocaine [lidocaine] hydrochloride (p.1313·2) is included in the intramuscular injection to alleviate the pain of injection.
Bacterial infections.

Be-Tabs Antacid *Be-Tabs, S.Afr.*
Magnesium trisilicate (p.1233·3); light magnesium carbonate (p.1232·3); sodium bicarbonate (p.1186·2).
Gastrointestinal disorders associated with hyperacidity.

Beta-C *Chew, Thai.*
Betamethasone valerate (p.1063·2); clioquinol (p.190·2).
Infected skin disorders.

Betacap
Dermal Laboratories, Irl.; Dermal Laboratories, UK.
Betamethasone valerate (p.1063·2).
Scalp disorders.

Beta-Cardone *Celltech, UK.*
Sotalol hydrochloride (p.972·2).
Arrhythmias.

Betacarpin *Riel, Aust.*
Pilocarpine hydrochloride (p.1422·3); metipranolol hydrochloride (p.930·2).
Glaucoma.

Betacef
Note.This name is used for preparations of different composition.
FIRMA, Ital.
Cefoxitin sodium (p.171·2).
Bacterial infections.

Be-Tabs, S.Afr.
Cefalexin (p.161·3).
Bacterial infections.

Betacept *Wampole, Canad.*
Vitamin C, vitamin E, and betacarotene (p.1350·1).

Betachek *National Diagnostic, Austral.*
Test for glucose in blood (p.1616·3).

Betachron *Inwood, USA†.*
Propranolol hydrochloride (p.962·3).

Betacin *Be-Tabs, S.Afr.*
Indometacin (p.44·3).
Gout; musculoskeletal and joint disorders.

Betaclar *Angelini, Ital.*
Befunolol hydrochloride (p.843·2).
Glaucoma.

Betaclomin *Be-Tabs, S.Afr.*
Dicyclomine [dicycloverine] hydrochloride (p.466·1); dried aluminium hydroxide gel (p.1210·3); light magnesium oxide (p.1233·2).
Gastrointestinal hyperacidity.

Betaclopramide *Be-Tabs, S.Afr.*
Metoclopramide hydrochloride (p.1235·2).
Gastrointestinal disorders.

Betacod *Be-Tabs, S.Afr.†.*
Paracetamol (p.71·2); codeine phosphate (p.25·2).
Fever; pain.

Betacomplesso *Medosan, Ital.*
Vitamin B substances (p.1350·1).
Tonic; vitamin B deficiency.

Betacort *ICN, Canad.†.*
Betamethasone valerate (p.1063·2).
Scalp disorders.

Betacorten
Trima, Israel; Trima, Singapore; Unipharm, Singapore.
Betamethasone valerate (p.1063·2).
Skin and scalp disorders.

Betacorten-G *Trima, Israel.*
Betamethasone valerate (p.1063·2); gentamicin sulfate (p.210·1).
Infected skin disorders.

Betacortone *Spirig, Switz.*
Cream: Halcinonide (p.1073·2); urea (p.1127·3).
Topical solution: Halcinonide (p.1073·2).
Skin disorders.

Betacortone S *Spirig, Switz.*
Halcinonide (p.1073·2); salicylic acid (p.1122·3).
Skin disorders.

BetaCreme *Lichtenstein, Ger.*
Betamethasone valerate (p.1063·2).
Skin disorders.

Betaderm
Note.This name is used for preparations of different composition.
Stiefel, Braz.; Taro, Canad.
Betamethasone valerate (p.1063·2).
Scalp disorders; skin disorders.

Beta, Ital.
Salicylic acid (p.1122·3); aluminium acetate (p.1578·1); zinc oxide (p.1128·2).
Skin disinfection.

Betadermic *Hexal, Ger.*
Betamethasone dipropionate (p.1063·2); salicylic acid (p.1122·3).
Skin disorders.

Betades *Formades, Ital.*
Sotalol hydrochloride (p.972·2).
Angina pectoris; arrhythmias; hypertension.

Betadine
Faulding, Austral.; Purdue Frederick, Canad.; Leiras, Fin.; Asta Medica, Fr.; Mundipharma, Hong Kong; Seton, Irl.; Rafa, Israel; Asta Medica, Ital.; Asta Medica, Neth.; Baxter, NZ; Faulding, NZ; Asta Medica, Port.; Adcock Ingram, S.Afr.; Restan, S.Afr.; Asta Medica, Spain; Mundipharma, Switz.; Mundipharma, Thai.; SSL, UK; Purdue Frederick, USA.
Povidone-iodine (p.1155·1).
Burns; disinfection of the skin, hands, wounds, oropharynx, and vagina; infections of the skin, wounds, oropharynx, and vagina.

Betadine First Aid Antibiotics + Moisturizer
Purdue Frederick, USA†.
Polymyxin B sulfate (p.238·1); bacitracin zinc (p.155·2).
Minor cuts and burns.

Betadine Plus First Aid Antibiotics & Pain Reliever *Purdue Frederick, USA.*
Polymyxin B sulfate (p.238·1); bacitracin zinc (p.155·2); pramocaine hydrochloride (p.1318·2).
Minor cuts and burns.

Betadipresan *Fides Rottapharm, Spain.*
Hydralazine hydrochloride (p.905·3); propranolol hydrochloride (p.962·3).
Hypertension.

Betadipresan Diu *Fides Rottapharm, Spain.*
Bendrofluazide [bendroflumethiazide] (p.844·1); hydralazine hydrochloride (p.905·3); propranolol hydrochloride (p.962·3).
Hypertension.

Betadiur *Siphar, Switz.*
Amiloride hydrochloride (p.835·1); hydrochlorothiazide (p.907·3).
Hypertension; liver failure with ascites; oedema.

Betadorm-A *Woelm, Ger.*
Diphenhydramine hydrochloride (p.416·1); 8-chlorotheophylline.
Sleep disorders.

Betadrenol *Schwarz, Ger.*
Bupranolol hydrochloride (p.852·3).
Hypertension; ischaemic heart disease; myocardial infarction.

Betadur CR *Monmouth, UK.*
Propranolol hydrochloride (p.962·3).
Angina pectoris; anxiety; essential tremor; hypertension; migraine; variceal haemorrhage.

Betaeffe Plus *Mavi, Ital.*
Betacarotene, vitamin E, and selenium preparation (p.1350·1).
Nutritional supplement.

Betafed *Be-Tabs, S.Afr.*
Triprolidine hydrochloride (p.427·2); pseudoephedrine hydrochloride (p.1099·2).
Nasal congestion.

Betaferon
Schering, Aust.; Schering, Austral.; Schering, Belg.; Schering, Braz.; Schering, Denm.; Schering, Fin.; Schering, Fr.; Schering, Ger.; Schering, Irl.; Schering, Israel; Farmades, Ital.; Schering, Mex.; Schering, Neth.; Schering, Norw.; Schering, NZ; Schering, Port.; Schering, S.Afr.; Schering, Singapore; Schering, Spain; Schering, Swed.; Schering, Switz.; Schering, UK.
Interferon beta-1b (p.632·2).
Multiple sclerosis.

Betaflex *Mer-National, S.Afr.†.*
Paracetamol (p.71·2); chlormezanone (p.660·1).
Pain and associated tension.

Betaform Habitat *Cos Farma, Ital.*
Benzalkonium chloride (p.1133·2); a nonoxinol (p.1346·1).
Surface and room disinfection.

Betagalen *Pharmagalen, Ger.*
Betamethasone valerate (p.1063·2).
Skin disorders.

Betagan
Allergan, Austral.; Allergan, Belg.; Allergan-Frumtost, Braz.; Allergan, Canad.; Allergan, Denm.; Allergan, Fr.; Allergan, Hong Kong; Allergan, Irl.; Allergan, Israel; Allergan, Mex.; Allergan, Neth.†; Allergan, NZ; Allergan, Port.; Allergan, S.Afr.; Allergan, Singapore; Allergan, Spain; Allergan, Swed.†; Allergan, Thai.; Allergan, UK; Allergan, USA.
Levobunolol hydrochloride (p.920·3).
Glaucoma; ocular hypertension.

Betagard *GNLD, Austral.*
Vitamin, mineral, and amino-acid preparation (p.1350·1).

Betagentam *Winzer, Ger.*
Betamethasone sodium phosphate (p.1063·2); gentamicin sulfate (p.210·1).
Infected eye disorders.

Betagesic *Restan, S.Afr.*
Ibuprofen (p.43·2).
Fever; musculoskeletal and joint disorders; pain.

Betagon *Schering, Ital.*
Mepindolol sulfate (p.926·2).
Angina pectoris; cardiac hyperkinesis; hypertension.

Betaimune *Pharmadass, UK.*
Vitamins A, C, and E; selenium; zinc (p.1350·1).

Betaine Digestive Aid *GNLD, Austral.*
Betaine hydrochloride (p.1584·3); pepsin (p.1649·3); papain (p.1647·3); pectin (p.1502·3); natural dried beet; rhubarb (p.1248·1); liquorice (p.1231·2).
Digestive disorders.

Betaisodona
Mundipharma, Aust.; Mundipharma, Ger.
Povidone-iodine (p.1155·1).
Burns; mouth and throat infections; skin and mucous membrane disinfection; skin disorders; skin ulcers; vaginal infections; wounds.

Beta-Isoket *Gebro, Aust.*
Bupranolol hydrochloride (p.852·3); isosorbide dinitrate (p.915·2).
Angina pectoris; myocardial infarction.

Betaject *Sabex, Canad.*
Betamethasone sodium phosphate (p.1063·2); betamethasone acetate (p.1063·1).
Corticosteroid.

Betalgil *Whitehall, Port.*
Aluminium hydroxide (p.1210·3); magnesium hydroxide (p.1233·1); oxetacaine (p.1317·3).
Gastrointestinal disorders.

Betalin *Be-Tabs, S.Afr.*
Diphenhydramine hydrochloride (p.416·1); ammonium chloride (p.1085·2); sodium citrate (p.1186·2); menthol (p.1632·3).
Coughs.

Betaliver *Luper, Braz.*
Methionine (p.1012·2); adenosine (p.828·2); betaine hydrochloride (p.1584·3); pyridoxine hydrochloride (p.1386·3); choline citrate (p.1356·3).
Liver disorders.

Betalix *Be-Tabs, S.Afr.*
Chlorpheniramine [chlorphenamine] maleate (p.412·1); phenylpropanolamine hydrochloride (p.1100·1); phenylephrine hydrochloride (p.1097·1).
Nasal congestion.

Betaloc
Astra, Austral.; AstraZeneca, Canad.; Astra, Hong Kong; Astra, Irl.; AstraZeneca, NZ; AstraZeneca, Singapore; AstraZeneca, Thai.; AstraZeneca, UK.
Metoprolol succinate (p.932·1) or metoprolol tartrate (p.931·2).
Angina pectoris; arrhythmias; hypertension; hyperthyroidism; migraine; myocardial infarction.

Betaloc Comp *Astra, Hong Kong.*
Metoprolol tartrate (p.931·2); hydrochlorothiazide (p.907·3).
Hypertension.

Betalol *Berlin Pharm, Thai.*
Propranolol hydrochloride (p.962·3).
Angina pectoris; anxiety disorders; arrhythmias; hypertension; tremor.

Betama-EN *Samakeephaesaj, Thai.*
Betamethasone valerate (p.1063·2); neomycin sulfate (p.228·1).
Infected skin disorders.

Betamann *Mann, Ger.*
Metipranolol hydrochloride (p.930·2).
Glaucoma; ocular hypertension.

Betamatil *Inibsa, Spain.*
Betamethasone valerate (p.1063·2).
Skin disorders.

Betamatil con Neomicina *Inibsa, Spain.*
Betamethasone valerate (p.1063·2); neomycin sulfate (p.228·1).
Infected skin disorders.

Betamaze *Pfizer, Fr.†.*
Sulbactam sodium (p.250·1).
Bacterial infections.

Betamed *Kwizda, Aust.*
Bupranolol hydrochloride (p.852·3); diazepam (p.674·3).
Anxiety disorders.

Betamesol *Proge, Ital.*
Betamethasone dipropionate (p.1063·2).
Skin disorders.

Betametagen *Kinder, Braz.*
Dexamethasone (p.1067·1).
Skin disorders.

Betameth *Osoth, Thai.*
Betamethasone valerate (p.1063·2).
Skin disorders.

Betamethason Plus *Heumann, Ger.*
Betamethasone dipropionate (p.1063·2); salicylic acid (p.1122·3).
Skin disorders.

Betamican *Alter, Spain.*
Salmeterol xinafoate (p.773·3).
Obstructive airways disease.

Betamida *Alcon Cusi, Spain.*
Betamethasone sodium phosphate (p.1063·2); sulfacetamide sodium (p.250·3).
Eye disorders.

Betamin *Rhone-Poulenc Rorer, Austral.*
Thiamine hydrochloride (p.1385·1).
Vitamin B₁ deficiency.

Betamine *Wolfs, Belg.*
Thiamine hydrochloride (p.1385·1).
Alcoholic polyneuropathy; beri-beri; neuralgia.

Betam-Ophtal *Winzer, Ger.*
Betamethasone sodium phosphate (p.1063·2).
Eye disorders.

Betamox
Note. This name is used for preparations of different composition.
Duopharma, Hong Kong; Be-Tabs, S.Afr.
Amoxicillin trihydrate (p.149·2).
Bacterial infections.
Cipan, Port.
Amoxicillin trihydrate (p.149·2); potassium clavulanate (p.187·2).
Bacterial infections.

Betamycin *Be-Tabs, S.Afr.*
Erythromycin estolate (p.201·2).
Bacterial infections.

Beta-N *Chew, Thai.*
Betamethasone valerate (p.1063·2); neomycin sulfate (p.228·1).
Infected skin disorders.

Beta-Nephral *Pfleger, Ger.†.*
Propranolol hydrochloride (p.962·3); triamterene (p.986·1); hydrochlorothiazide (p.907·3).
Hypertension.

Betanoid *Aspen, S.Afr.*
Betamethasone (p.1063·1).
Corticosteroid.

Betanol *Europhta, Mon.*
Metipranolol (p.930·2).
Glaucoma; ocular hypertension.

Betantrone *Italfarmaco, Ital.†.*
Interferon beta (p.632·2).
Hepatitis; malignant neoplasms; viral infections.

Beta-Ophtiole
Riel, Aust.; Tramedico, Belg.; Mann, Neth.; Lepori, Port.; Bausch & Lomb, S.Afr.; Mann, Singapore; Bausch & Lomb, Thai.; Mann, Thai.
Metipranolol hydrochloride (p.930·2).
Glaucoma; ocular hypertension.

Betapace *Berlex, USA.*
Sotalol hydrochloride (p.972·2).
Arrhythmias.

Betapam *Be-Tabs, S.Afr.*
Diazepam (p.674·3).
Alcohol withdrawal syndrome; anxiety; premedication.

Betapect *Be-Tabs, S.Afr.*
Light kaolin (p.1229·3); apple pectin (p.1502·3).
Diarrhoea.

Betapen *Be-Tabs, S.Afr.*
Phenoxymethylpenicillin potassium (p.235·1).
Bacterial infections.

Betapen-VK *Apothecon, USA†.*
Phenoxymethylpenicillin potassium (p.235·1).
Bacterial infections.

Betaperamide *Restan, S.Afr.*
Loperamide hydrochloride (p.1231·3).
Diarrhoea.

Betaphlem *Be-Tabs, S.Afr.*
Carbocisteine (p.1086·3).
Respiratory-tract disorders.

Betapindol *Helvepharm, Switz.*
Pindolol (p.955·3).
Angina pectoris; arrhythmias; hypertension.

Betapred
Glaxo Wellcome, Fin.; Glaxo Wellcome, Swed.
Betamethasone sodium phosphate (p.1063·2).
Corticosteroid.

Betapresin *Hoechst Marion Roussel, Mex.*
Penbutolol sulfate (p.952·2).

Betapress *Polipharm, Thai.*
Propranolol hydrochloride (p.962·3).
Angina pectoris; arrhythmias; hypertension; tremor.

Betapressin
Hoechst Marion Roussel, Aust.†; Hoechst Marion Roussel, Ger.
Penbutolol sulfate (p.952·2).
Arrhythmias; hypertension; ischaemic heart disease; myocardial infarction.

Betapressine *Roussel Diamant, Fr.†.*
Penbutolol sulfate (p.952·2).
Angina pectoris; hypertension.

Betaprofen *Be-Tabs, S.Afr.*
Ibuprofen (p.43·2).
Musculoskeletal and joint disorders.

Beta-Prograne *Tillomed, UK.*
Propranolol hydrochloride (p.962·3).
Angina pectoris; anxiety; essential tremor; hypertension; hyperthyroidism; migraine; prophylaxis of upper gastrointestinal bleeding.

Betaprol *Helvepharm, Switz.*
Propranolol hydrochloride (p.962·3).
Angina pectoris; arrhythmias; hypertension; migraine; phaeochromocytoma.

Betapyn *Restan, S.Afr.*
Paracetamol (p.71·2); codeine phosphate (p.25·2); doxylamine succinate (p.417·1); caffeine (p.761·3).
Fever; muscular tension; pain.

Betapyr *Wolfs, Belg.*
Thiamine hydrochloride (p.1385·1); pyridoxine hydrochloride (p.1386·3).
Alcoholic polyneuritis; prophylaxis during isoniazid therapy; vitamin B₁ and/or B₆ deficiency.

Betarelix *Hoechst Marion Roussel, Ger.*
Penbutolol sulfate (p.952·2); piretanide (p.956·2).
Hypertension.

Betaren *Dexxon, Israel.*
Diclofenac sodium (p.30·3).
Inflammation; musculoskeletal and joint disorders; pain.

Betaretic *Be-Tabs, S.Afr.*
Amiloride hydrochloride (p.835·1); hydrochlorothiazide (p.907·3).
Hypertension; oedema.

Betartrinovo *Llorens, Spain†.*
Betamethasone phosphate (p.1063·3); indometacin (p.44·3).
Musculoskeletal and joint disorders; peri-articular disorders.

Beta-S *Chew, Thai.*
Betamethasone valerate (p.1063·2); salicylic acid (p.1122·3).
Skin disorders.

BetaSalbe *Lichtenstein, Ger.*
Betamethasone valerate (p.1063·2).
Skin disorders.

Betasan *Mundipharma, Aust.*
Povidone-iodine (p.1155·1).
Mouth and throat infections; wounds.

Betascor B12 *Manetti Roberts, Ital.†.*
Betaine ascorbate (p.1584·3); cyanocobalamin (p.1388·1).
Vitamin C deficiency.

Betasedar *Sedar, Braz.*
Vitamin B substances (p.1350·1).
Vitamin supplement.

Betaselen *Arkopharma, Fr.*
Multivitamin and mineral preparation (p.1350·1).
Tonic.

Betasemid *Hoechst Marion Roussel, Ger.*
Penbutolol sulfate (p.952·2); frusemide [furosemide] (p.893·1).
Hypertension.

Betasept *Purdue Frederick, USA.*
Chlorhexidine gluconate (p.1138·2).
Skin and wound disinfection.

Betaseptic
Note. This name is used for preparations of different composition.
Mundipharma, Aust.; Asta Medica, Ital.
Povidone-iodine (p.1155·1).
Medicated dressing; skin disinfection.
Mundipharma, Ger.; Mundipharma, Switz.
Povidone-iodine (p.1155·1); isopropyl alcohol (p.1149·2); alcohol (p.1130·3).
Skin and hand disinfection.

Betaserc
Solvay, Aust.; Solvay, Belg.; Solvay, Denm.; Solvay, Fin.; Solvay, Hong Kong; Solvay, Neth.; Solvay, Port.; Solvay, Singapore; Solvay, Switz.
Betahistine hydrochloride (p.1584·2).
Ménière's disease; vestibular disorders.

Betaseron
Berlex, Canad.; Berlex, USA.
Interferon beta-1b (p.632·2).
Multiple sclerosis.

Betasit Plus *Ferrer, Spain†.*
Chlortalidone (p.857·1); atenolol (p.841·3).
Hypertension.

Betasleep *Restan, S.Afr.*
Diphenhydramine hydrochloride (p.416·1).
Insomnia.

Betasoda *Restan, S.Afr.*
Citric acid (p.1596·2); sodium bicarbonate (p.1186·2).
Urinary alkalinisation.

Beta-Sol *Fawns & McAllan, Austral.*
Note. A similar name is used for preparations of different composition (see below).
Thiamine hydrochloride (p.1385·1).
Symptoms of vitamin B₁ deficiency.

Betasol *Chew, Thai.*
Note. A similar name is used for preparations of different composition (see above).
Clobetasol propionate (p.1065·2).
Skin disorders.

Betasone
DHA, Hong Kong; Julphar, UAE.
Betamethasone valerate (p.1063·2).
Skin disorders.
Julphar, UAE.
Tablets: Betamethasone (p.1063·1).
Corticosteroid.

Beta-Stulln *Stulln, Ger.*
Betamethasone sodium phosphate (p.1063·2).
Inflammatory eye disorders.

Betasyn *Jacoby, Aust.*
Atenolol (p.841·3).
Angina pectoris; arrhythmias; hypertension; myocardial infarction.

Beta-Tablinen *Lichtenstein, Ger.*
Propranolol hydrochloride (p.962·3).
Angina pectoris; anxiety; arrhythmias; essential tremor; hypertension; migraine.

Betathiazid *Henning, Ger.*
Propranolol hydrochloride (p.962·3); triamterene (p.986·1); hydrochlorothiazide (p.907·3).
Hypertension.

Betathiazid A *Henning, Ger.*
Propranolol hydrochloride (p.962·3); hydrochlorothiazide (p.907·3).
Hypertension.

Beta-Tim *Ciba Vision, Canad.†.*
Timolol maleate (p.982·1).
Glaucoma.

Betatop *EG, Fr.*
Atenolol (p.841·3).
Angina pectoris; hypertension; myocardial infarction.

Betatrex *Savage, USA.*
Betamethasone valerate (p.1063·2).
Skin disorders.

Betatul *Asta Medica, Spain.*
Povidone-iodine (p.1155·1).
Infected skin disorders; skin disinfection.

Beta-Turfa *Worwag, Ger.*
Propranolol hydrochloride (p.962·3); triamterene (p.986·1); hydrochlorothiazide (p.907·3).
Hypertension.

Beta-Val *Lemmon, USA.*
Betamethasone valerate (p.1063·2).
Skin disorders.

The symbol † denotes a preparation no longer actively marketed

Betavert Hennig, Ger.
Betahistine mesilate (p.1584·3).
Vertigo.

Betaxin Sanofi Synthelabo, Canad.
Thiamine hydrochloride (p.1385·1).

Betaxina Terapeutico, Ital.
Nalidixic acid (p.227·1).
Gram-negative genito-urinary tract infections.

Betaxon Alcon, USA.
Levobetaxolol hydrochloride (p.920·2).
Glaucoma; ocular hypertension.

Betazim Sam-On, Israel.
Betaine hydrochloride (p.1584·3); pepsin (p.1649·3).
Anorexia; diarrhoea; gastritis; gastrointestinal hypoacidity.

Betazok Astra, Irl.
Metoprolol succinate (p.932·1).
Angina pectoris; hypertension.

Betazon Bergamo, Braz.
Betamethasone (p.1063·1); phenylbutazone (p.78·1); aluminium glycinate (p.1210·3).

BETE Laevosan, Aust.
Benzatropine hydrochloride (p.463·2).
Pain with spasmodic disorders.

Bethacil Bioindustria, Ital.
Injection: Sulbactam sodium (p.250·1); ampicillin sodium (p.150·3).
Lignocaine [lidocaine] hydrochloride (p.1313·2) is included in the intramuscular injection to alleviate the pain of injection.
Oral suspension†: Sultamicillin (p.257·2).
Tablets†: Sultamicillin tosilate (p.257·2).
Bacterial infections.

Bethasone Greater Pharma, Thai.
Betamethasone (p.1063·1).
Skin disorders.

Bethasone-N Greater Pharma, Thai.
Betamethasone (p.1063·1); neomycin sulfate (p.228·1).
Infected skin disorders.

Betim Leo, Norw.†; ICN, UK.
Timolol maleate (p.982·1).
Angina pectoris; hypertension; hyperthyroidism; migraine; myocardial infarction.

Betimol Ciba Vision, USA.
Timolol (p.982·2).
Glaucoma; ocular hypertension.

Betinex Berk, UK.
Bumetanide (p.852·1).
Oedema.

Betinjectol INQ, Braz.
Vitamin B₁₂ (p.1388·1); vitamin B₁ (p.1385·2); vitamin B₆ (p.1387·1).
Anaemias; vitamin B deficiency.

Betitotal Propan, S.Afr.
Multivitamin and mineral preparation (p.1350·1).

Betnasol Glaxo Wellcome, Port.†
Betamethasone (p.1063·1).
Corticosteroid.

Betnelan
Glaxo Wellcome, Braz.; Evans Medical, Irl.; Glaxo Wellcome, Neth.; Glaxo Wellcome, S.Afr.†; Celltech, UK.
Betamethasone (p.1063·1) or betamethasone valerate (p.1063·2).
Corticosteroid.

Betnelan Clioquinol Glaxo Wellcome, Neth.†.
Betamethasone valerate (p.1063·2); clioquinol (p.190·2).
Infected skin disorders.

Betnelan Neomycine Glaxo Wellcome, Neth.†.
Betamethasone valerate (p.1063·2); neomycin sulfate (p.228·1).
Infected skin disorders.

Betnelan-V Glaxo Wellcome, Belg.
Betamethasone valerate (p.1063·2).
Skin disorders.

Betnelan-VC Glaxo Wellcome, Belg.
Betamethasone valerate (p.1063·2); clioquinol (p.190·2).
Infected skin disorders.

Betnelan-VN Glaxo Wellcome, Belg.†
Betamethasone valerate (p.1063·2); neomycin sulfate (p.228·1).
Infected skin disorders.

Betnesalic
Glaxo Wellcome, Fr.; Glaxo Wellcome, Ger.; Cascan, Ger.; Glaxo Wellcome, Hong Kong; Glaxo Wellcome, Switz.; Glaxo Wellcome, Thai.
Betamethasone valerate (p.1063·2); salicylic acid (p.1122·3).
Skin disorders.

Betnesol
Glaxo Wellcome, Aust.; Glaxo Wellcome, Belg.; Roberts, Canad.; Glaxo Wellcome, Fr.; Glaxo Wellcome, Ger.; Evans Medical, Irl.; Glaxo Wellcome, Israel; Glaxo Wellcome, Neth.; Glaxo Wellcome, NZ; Allen & Hanburys, S.Afr.; Glaxo Wellcome, Switz.; Celltech, UK.
Betamethasone sodium phosphate (p.1063·2).
Corticosteroid; inflammatory disorders of the eye, ear, or nose.

Betnesol Aqueous Glaxo Wellcome, NZ.
Betamethasone sodium phosphate (p.1063·2); naphazoline nitrate (p.1095·2).
Nasal congestion and inflammation.

Betnesol-N
Glaxo Wellcome, Aust.; Evans Medical, Irl.; Glaxo Wellcome, Israel; Glaxo Wellcome, NZ; Allen & Hanburys, S.Afr.; Celltech, UK.
Betamethasone sodium phosphate (p.1063·2); neomycin sulfate (p.228·1).
Infected eye, ear or nose disorders.

Betnesol-V Glaxo Wellcome, Ger.; Cascan, Ger.
Betamethasone valerate (p.1063·2).
Scalp disorders; skin disorders.

Betneval Glaxo Wellcome, Fr.
Betamethasone valerate (p.1063·2).
Mouth disorders; skin disorders.

Betneval-Neomycine Glaxo Wellcome, Fr.
Betamethasone valerate (p.1063·2); neomycin sulfate (p.228·1).
Infected skin disorders.

Betnovat
Glaxo Wellcome, Denm.; Glaxo Wellcome, Fin.; Glaxo Wellcome, Norw.; Glaxo Wellcome, Swed.
Betamethasone valerate (p.1063·2).
Otitis externa; skin disorders.

Betnovat Comp Glaxo Wellcome, Fin.
Betamethasone valerate (p.1063·2); phenylephrine hydrochloride (p.1097·1); lignocaine [lidocaine] hydrochloride (p.1313·2).
Anorectal disorders.

Betnovat med Chinoform
Glaxo Wellcome, Denm.; Glaxo Wellcome, Norw.; Glaxo Wellcome, Swed.
Betamethasone valerate (p.1063·2); clioquinol (p.190·2).
Infected skin disorders.

Betnovat med Neomycin Glaxo Wellcome, Swed.
Betamethasone valerate (p.1063·2); neomycin sulfate (p.228·1).
Infected skin disorders.

Betnovat Rektal Glaxo Wellcome, Denm.
Betamethasone valerate (p.1063·2); lignocaine [lidocaine] hydrochloride (p.1313·2); phenylephrine hydrochloride (p.1097·1).
Anorectal disorders.

Betnovat-C Glaxo Wellcome, Fin.
Betamethasone valerate (p.1063·2); clioquinol (p.190·2).
Infected skin disorders.

Betnovate
Glaxo Wellcome, Aust.; Glaxo Wellcome, Austral.; Glaxo Wellcome, Braz.; Roberts, Canad.; Glaxo Wellcome, Hong Kong; Glaxo Wellcome, Irl.; Glaxo Wellcome, Israel; Glaxo Wellcome, Mex.; Glaxo Wellcome, NZ; Glaxo Wellcome, Port.; Allen & Hanburys, S.Afr.; Glaxo Wellcome, Singapore; Medeva, Spain; Glaxo Wellcome, Switz.; Glaxo Wellcome, Thai.; Glaxo Wellcome, UK.
Betamethasone valerate (p.1063·2).
Skin and scalp disorders.

Betnovate RD (Ready Diluted) Glaxo Wellcome, UK.
Betamethasone valerate (p.1063·2).
Skin disorders.

Betnovate Rectal Ointment Glaxo Wellcome, UK.
Betamethasone valerate (p.1063·2); lignocaine [lidocaine] hydrochloride (p.1313·2); phenylephrine hydrochloride (p.1097·1).
Anorectal disorders.

Betnovate-C
Note.This name is used for preparations of different composition.
Glaxo Wellcome, Aust.; Glaxo Wellcome, Hong Kong; Glaxo Wellcome, Irl.; Glaxo Wellcome, Israel; Glaxo Wellcome, NZ; Allen & Hanburys, S.Afr.; Glaxo Wellcome, Singapore; Glaxo Wellcome, Switz.; Glaxo Wellcome, Thai.; Glaxo Wellcome, UK.
Betamethasone valerate (p.1063·2); clioquinol (p.190·2).
Infected skin disorders.

Glaxo Wellcome, Port.
Betamethasone dipropionate (p.1063·2); clioquinol (p.190·2).
Infected skin disorders.

Betnovate-GM Glaxo Wellcome, Singapore.
Betamethasone valerate (p.1063·2); miconazole nitrate (p.391·1); gentamicin sulfate (p.210·1).
Infected skin disorders.

Betnovate-M Glaxo Wellcome, Singapore.
Betamethasone valerate (p.1063·2); miconazole nitrate (p.391·1).
Infected skin disorders.

Betnovate-N
Note.This name is used for preparations of different composition.
Glaxo Wellcome, Aust.; Glaxo Wellcome, Austral.; Glaxo Wellcome, Hong Kong; Glaxo Wellcome, Irl.; Glaxo Wellcome, Israel; Allen & Hanburys, S.Afr.; Glaxo Wellcome, Singapore; Glaxo Wellcome, Switz.; Glaxo Wellcome, Thai.; Glaxo Wellcome, UK.
Betamethasone valerate (p.1063·2); neomycin sulfate (p.228·1).
Infected skin disorders.

Glaxo Wellcome, Port.
Betamethasone dipropionate (p.1063·2); neomycin sulfate (p.228·1); clioquinol (p.190·2).
Infected skin disorders.

Betnovate-Q Glaxo Wellcome, Braz.
Betamethasone valerate (p.1063·2); clioquinol (p.190·2).
Infected skin disorders.

Betoid Yamanouchi, Denm.; Yamanouchi, Norw.; Yamanouchi, Swed.
Betamethasone valerate (p.1063·2).
Skin disorders.

Betolvex
Dumex-Alpharma, Denm.; Dumex-Alpharma, Fin.; Alpharma, Norw.; Lagamed, S.Afr.†; Dumex-Alpharma, Swed.; Dumex, Switz.
Cyanocobalamin (p.1388·1) or cyanocobalamin tannate (p.1388·3).
Megaloblastic anaemia; vitamin B₁₂ deficiency.

Betoptic
Alcon, Aust.; Alcon, Austral.; Alcon, Belg.; Alcon, Braz.; Alcon, Canad.; Alcon, Denm.; Alcon, Fin.; Alcon, Fr.; Alcon, Hong Kong; Alcon, Irl.; Alcon, Israel; Alcon, Ital.; Alcon, Mex.; Alcon, Neth.†; Alcon, Norw.; Alcon, NZ; Alcon, Port.; Alcon, S.Afr.; Alcon, Singapore; Alcon Cusi, Spain; Alcon, Swed.; Alcon, Thai.; Alcon, UK; Alcon, USA.
Betaxolol hydrochloride (p.848·3).
Glaucoma; ocular hypertension.

Betoptic-S Alcon, Switz.
Betaxolol hydrochloride (p.848·3).
Glaucoma; ocular hypertension.

Betoptima Alcon, Ger.
Betaxolol hydrochloride (p.848·3).
Glaucoma; ocular hypertension.

Betoquin Ioquin, Austral.
Betaxolol hydrochloride (p.848·3).
Glaucoma; ocular hypertension.

Betosalic TO-Chemicals, Thai.
Betamethasone valerate (p.1063·2); salicylic acid (p.1122·3).
Skin disorders.

Betosone TO-Chemicals, Thai.
Betamethasone valerate (p.1063·2).
Skin disorders.

Betosone-CE TO-Chemicals, Thai.
Betamethasone valerate (p.1063·2); clioquinol (p.190·2).
Infected skin disorders.

Be-Total Carlo Erba OTC, Ital.
Vitamin B substances (p.1350·1).
Vitamin B deficiency.

Betozone De Mayo, Braz.
Capsules; oral solution: Ferrous fumarate (p.1360·1); folic acid (p.1361·1); ascorbic acid; vitamin B substances (p.1350·1).
Injection: Vitamin B substances (p.1350·1); liver extract.
Oral liquid: Ferrous sulfate (p.1360·3); vitamin B substances; lysine hydrochloride (p.1350·1).
Anaemias.

Betriphos-C Schwarz, Fr.
Adenosine triphosphate sodium (p.1573·3); vitamin B substances (p.1350·1); ascorbic acid.
Tonic.

Betrivit Biogal, Israel.
Hydroxocobalamin (p.1388·1); pyridoxine hydrochloride (p.1386·3); thiamine nitrate (p.1385·1).
Lignocaine [lidocaine] hydrochloride (p.1313·2) is included in this preparation to alleviate the pain of injection.
Metabolic disorders; neuropathies.

Betron R Italfarmaco, Ital.
Interferon beta (human, recombinant) (p.632·2).
Malignant neoplasms; viral infections.

Betsol Z Zafiro, Mex.
Sodium bicarbonate (p.1186·2).
Metabolic acidosis.

Betsuril Almirall, Spain.
Beclometasone dipropionate (p.1061·2).
Asthma.

Bettamousse
Medeva, Denm.; Vitaflo, Fin.; Medeva, Irl.; Mipharm, Ital.; Medeva, Spain; Vitaflo, Swed.; Celltech, UK.
Betamethasone valerate (p.1063·2).
Scalp disorders.

Betulac Meda, Swed.†
Lactulose (p.1230·1).
Constipation; hepatic encephalopathy.

Betuline Ferndale, USA.
Methyl salicylate (p.55·1); camphor (p.1589·3); menthol (p.1632·3).
Muscle, joint, and soft-tissue pain; neuralgia.

Be-Uric Be-Tabs, S.Afr.
Allopurinol (p.397·2).
Gout; hyperuricaemia.

Beurises Be-Tabs, S.Afr.
Frusemide [furosemide] (p.893·1).
Hypertension; oedema.

Bevicomplex INQ, Braz.
Vitamin B substances (p.1350·1).
Vitamin supplement.

Beviplex Meuse, Belg.
Vitamin B substances (p.1350·1).
Neuritis; vitamin B deficiency.

Beviplex forte Abigo, Swed.
Vitamin B substances (p.1350·1).
Alcoholism; neuropathies; vitamin B deficiency.

Bevispas Aspen, S.Afr.
Mebeverine hydrochloride (p.1233·3).
Irritable bowel syndrome.

Bevit Forte Biocur, Ger.
Thiamine hydrochloride (p.1385·1); pyridoxine hydrochloride (p.1386·3).
Nervous system disorders.

Be-Vital Be-Tabs, S.Afr.†
Multivitamin and mineral preparation (p.1350·1).

Bevitamel Westlake, USA.
Melatonin (p.1632·1); vitamin B₁₂ (p.1388·1); folic acid (p.1361·1).
Aid in homocysteine metabolism; sleep disorders.

Bevitin Abbott, Ital.
Vitamin B substances (p.1350·1).
Vitamin B deficiency.

Bevitine DB, Fr.
Thiamine hydrochloride (p.1385·1).
Beri beri; neuritis; vitamin B deficiency.

Bevitol Lannacher, Aust.
Thiamine hydrochloride (p.1385·1).
Vitamin B₁ deficiency.

Bevitotal comp Astra, Swed.
Vitamin B substances with vitamin C (p.1350·1).
Alcoholism; neuropathies; vitamin B and C deficiency.

Bevoren Sintesa, Belg.
Glibenclamide (p.321·3).
Diabetes mellitus.

Bewon Charton, Canad.†.
Thiamine hydrochloride (p.1385·1).

Bex
Note.This name is used for preparations of different composition.
Roche Consumer, Austral.
Aspirin (p.14·2).
Fever; pain.

Lalco, Canad.†.
Vitamin B substances and vitamin C (p.1350·1).

Bex-Hepar Reuffer, Mex.
Betaxolol (p.848·3).

Bexicortil Isdin, Spain.
Fluorometholone (p.1072·1); miconazole nitrate (p.391·1); neomycin sulfate (p.228·1).
Infected skin disorders.

Bexidermil Isdin, Spain.
Trolamine salicylate (p.90·1).
Peri-articular disorders; soft-tissue disorders.

Bexine Spirig, Switz.
Dextromethorphan hydrobromide (p.1087·3).
Coughs.

Bexinor Beacons, Singapore.
Norfloxacin (p.232·1).
Bacterial infections.

Bextra Pharmacia, USA.
Valdecoxib (p.90·2).
Dysmenorrhoea; osteoarthritis; rheumatoid arthritis.

Beza CT, Ger.; ABZ, Ger.
Bezafibrate (p.849·1).
Hyperlipidaemias.

Bezabeta Betapharm, Ger.
Bezafibrate (p.849·1).
Hyperlipidaemias.

Bezacur Hexal, Ger.
Bezafibrate (p.849·1).
Hyperlipidaemias.

Bezafisal Cryopharma, Mex.
Bezafibrate (p.849·1).
Hyperlipidaemias.

Bezagen Generics, UK.
Bezafibrate (p.849·1).
Hyperlipidaemias.

Beza-Lande Sanofi Synthelabo, Ger.
Bezafibrate (p.849·1).
Hyperlipidaemias.

Bezalip
Roche, Aust.; Roche, Canad.; Roche, Denm.; Roche, Fin.; Roche, Hong Kong; Boehringer Mannheim, Israel; Roche, Ital.; Boehringer Mannheim, Jpn†; Lakeside, Mex.; Roche, Neth.; Roche, NZ; Roche, Port.; Roche, S.Afr.; Roche, Singapore; Roche, Swed.; Roche, Thai.; Roche, UK.
Bezafibrate (p.849·1).
Hyperlipidaemias.

Bezalip Mono Roche, UK.
Bezafibrate (p.849·1).
Hyperlipidaemias.

Bezamerck Merck dura, Ger.
Bezafibrate (p.849·1).
Hyperlipidaemias.

Bezamil Milano, Thai.
Bezafibrate (p.849·1).
Hyperlipidaemias.

Beza-Puren Isis Puren, Ger.
Bezafibrate (p.849·1).
Hyperlipidaemias.

B-Feron Greater Pharma, Thai.
Multivitamin and mineral preparation (p.1350·1).

BFI
Note.This name is used for preparations of different composition.
SmithKline Beecham Consumer, Austral.†.
Bismuth-formic-iodide (p.1214·1); zinc p-phenolsulfonate (p.1128·3); alum (p.1577·2); bismuth subgallate (p.1213·2); menthol (p.1632·3); eucalyptol (p.1609·2); thymol (p.1158·3); magnesium carbonate (p.1232·3); pentyloxyphenol.
Damaged skin; pruritus.

Menley & James, USA.
Bismuth-formic-iodide (p.1214·1); zinc phenolsulfonate (p.1128·3); alum (p.1577·2); bismuth subgallate (p.1213·2); boric acid (p.1586·1); menthol (p.1632·3); eucalyptol (p.1609·2); thymol (p.1158·3).
Antiseptic.

Bgramin Douglas, Austral.
Amoxicillin trihydrate (p.149·2).
Bacterial infections.

B-Hex Xepa-Soul Pattinson, Singapore.
Benzhexol [trihexyphenidyl] hydrochloride (p.463·3).
Drug-induced extrapyramidal disorders; parkinsonism.

B12-Horfervit *Arteva, Ger.*
Cyanocobalamin (p.1388·1).
Vitamin B₁₂ deficiency.

Biactol Antibacterial Facewash *Procter & Gamble, Irl.†.*
Phenoxypropanol (p.1153·3).
Acne.

Biactol Liquid *Procter & Gamble (H&B Care), UK.*
Phenoxypropanol (p.1153·3).
Acne.

Biaferone *Biagini, Ital.*
Interferon alfa (p.628·1).
Hepatitis; malignant neoplasms; viral infections.

Biafine
Medix, Fr.; Medix, Israel; Upsifarma, Port.
Trolamine (p.1675·1).
Burns; wounds.

Biaflu *Biagini, Ital.*
An adsorbed inactivated influenza vaccine (p.1544·3).
Active immunisation.

Biaflu-Zonale SU *Biagini, Ital.*
An influenza vaccine (p.1544·3).
Active immunisation.

Bi-Aglut
Distriborg, Fr.; Novartis Nutrition, UK.
Gluten-free foods (p.1350·1).
Gluten intolerance.

Plasmon, Ital.
A range of gluten-free and lactose-reduced foods (p.1350·1).
Gluten and lactose intolerance.

Bialcol *Novartis Consumer, Ital.*
Benzoxonium chloride (p.1135·2).
Disinfection of skin, wounds, burns, and surfaces.

Bialerge *Elofar, Braz.*
Phenylephrine (p.1097·1); brompheniramine (p.410·3).
Nasal congestion.

Bialminal *Bial, Port.*
Phenobarbital (p.355·1).
Epilepsy; sedative.

Bialzepam *Medibial, Port.*
Diazepam (p.674·3).
Alcohol withdrawal syndrome; anxiety; epilepsy; insomnia; premedication; skeletal muscle spasm.

Biamotil *Allergan-Frumtost, Braz.*
Ciprofloxacin hydrochloride (p.182·3).
Bacterial eye and ear infections.

Biamotil-D *Allergan-Frumtost, Braz.*
Ciprofloxacin hydrochloride (p.182·3); dexamethasone (p.1067·1).
Infected eye disorders.

Bianco Val *Edmond Pharma, Ital.*
Valerian (p.1678·3); crataegus (p.1600·2).
Hyperexcitability; insomnia.

Biarison *Biochemie, Aust.†.*
Proquazone (p.80·3).
Gout; musculoskeletal, joint, peri-articular, and soft tissue disorders.

Biartac *Merck Sharp & Dohme, Belg.*
Diflunisal (p.32·2).
Arthrosis; polyarthritis.

Biavax II *Merck Sharp & Dohme, USA.*
A rubella and mumps vaccine (Wistar RA 27/3 and Jeryl Lynn (B level) strains respectively) (p.1563·1).
Active immunisation.

Biaven *Biagini, Ital.*
A normal immunoglobulin (p.1551·3).
Hypogammaglobulinaemia; idiopathic thrombocytopenic purpura; immunodeficiency.

Biaxin
Note. This name is used for preparations of different composition.
Sigma, Austral.†.
Roxithromycin (p.247·2).
Bacterial infections.

Abbott, Canad.; Abbott, Ger.; Abbott, USA.
Clarithromycin (p.186·2).
Bacterial infections.

Biaxsig *Sigma, Austral.*
Roxithromycin (p.247·2).
Bacterial infections.

Biazolina *Fermenti, Ital.†.*
Cefazolin sodium (p.164·3).
Bacterial infections.

Bibivit Light *Lampugnani, Ital.*
Multivitamin and carbohydrate preparation with fruit and plant extracts (p.1350·1).
Nutritional supplement.

Bicain *Orion, Fin.*
Bupivacaine hydrochloride (p.1306·3).
Local anaesthesia.

Bicam *Biolab, Thai.*
Piroxicam (p.79·1).
Musculoskeletal and joint disorders.

Bicarnat *Pisa, Mex.*
Sodium bicarbonate (p.1186·2).

BiCart *Gambro, Swed.†.*
Concentrates for haemodialysis solutions: Sodium chloride; potassium chloride; magnesium chloride; calcium chloride glacial acetic acid (p.1184·1).
To be used with BiCart powder.

Powder for haemodialysis solutions: Sodium bicarbonate (p.1184·1).
To be used with BiCart concentrates.

Bicavine *Cazi, Braz.*
Dipyrone (p.34·1); vitamin B substances (p.1350·1).
Neuritis; pain.

Bicbag
Fresenius, Denm.; Dicamed, Swed.†.
Sodium bicarbonate (p.1184·1).
Haemodialysis.

Bicetil *Menarini, Spain.*
Quinapril hydrochloride (p.963·3); hydrochlorothiazide (p.907·3).
Hypertension.

Bicholate *Sabex, Canad.*
Bile salts (p.1585·1); cascara (p.1216·1); aloin (p.1210·2); bisacodyl (p.1212·2).
Formerly contained bile salts, cascara, phenolphthalein, aloin.
Constipation.

Bicide *Fischer, Israel.*
Lindane (p.1434·1).
Scabies.

Bicillin *Yamanouchi, UK†.*
Procaine penicillin [procaine benzylpenicillin] (p.239·2); benzylpenicillin sodium (p.157·2).
Bacterial infections.

Bicillin All Purpose *Wyeth, Austral.†.*
Benzathine benzylpenicillin (p.156·2); procaine penicillin [procaine benzylpenicillin] (p.239·2); benzylpenicillin potassium (p.157·1).
Bacterial infections.

Bicillin A-P *Wyeth-Ayerst, Canad.†.*
Benzathine benzylpenicillin (p.156·2); procaine penicillin [procaine benzylpenicillin] (p.239·2); benzylpenicillin potassium (p.157·1).
Bacterial infections.

Bicillin C-R *Monarch, USA.*
Benzathine benzylpenicillin (p.156·2); procaine penicillin [procaine benzylpenicillin] (p.239·2).
Bacterial infections.

Bicillin L-A
Lederle, Austral.; Wyeth-Ayerst, Canad.; Wyeth, NZ; Akromed, S.Afr.†; Wyeth-Ayerst, USA.
Benzathine benzylpenicillin (p.156·2).
Bacterial infections.

Bicilline *Yamanouchi, Neth.†.*
Procaine penicillin [procaine benzylpenicillin] (p.239·2); benzylpenicillin sodium (p.157·2).
Bacterial infections.

Biciron *Alcon, Ger.*
Tramazoline hydrochloride (p.1102·1).
Eye disorders.

Bicitra *Alza, USA.*
Sodium citrate (p.1186·2); citric acid monohydrate (p.1596·2).
Chronic metabolic acidosis; urine alkalinising agent.

Bi-Citrol
Pharmethic, Belg.†; Diepha, Fr.
Monosodium citrate; sodium citrate (p.1186·2).
Dyspepsia.

Biclar *Abbott, Belg.*
Clarithromycin (p.186·2).
Bacterial infections.

Biclin
Bristol-Myers Squibb, Mex.; Bristol-Myers Squibb, Port.; Bristol-Myers, Spain.
Amikacin sulfate (p.148·1).
Bacterial infections.

Biclinocilline *Sanofi Winthrop, Fr.*
Benethamine penicillin (p.156·2); benzylpenicillin sodium (p.157·2).
Bacterial infections.

Biclopan *Pharbita, Singapore.*
Diclofenac sodium (p.30·3).
Gout; inflammation; musculoskeletal, joint, peri-articular, and soft-tissue disorders; pain.

BiCNU
Bristol-Myers Squibb, Austral.; Bristol, Canad.; Bristol-Myers Squibb, Fr.; Bristol-Myers Squibb, Hong Kong; Bristol-Myers Squibb, Irl.; Bristol-Myers Squibb, Israel; Bristol-Myers Squibb, Mex.; Bristol-Myers Squibb, NZ; Bristol-Myers Squibb, S.Afr.; Bristol-Myers Squibb, Singapore; Bristol-Myers Squibb, Thai.; Bristol-Myers Squibb, UK; Bristol-Myers Squibb Oncology, USA.
Carmustine (p.516·1).
Malignant neoplasms.

Bicobon *PP Lab, Thai.*
Sodium bicarbonate (p.1186·2); activated charcoal (p.1000·2); peppermint oil (p.1243·3).
Diarrhoea; flatulence; gastrointestinal disorders.

Bicold *Labima, Belg.*
Diphenylpyraline hydrochloride (p.417·1); phenylephrine hydrochloride (p.1097·1).
Upper respiratory-tract congestion.

Bicomplex *ABC, Ital.*
Vitamin B substances (p.1350·1).
Vitamin B deficiency.

Biconcor *Merck, Mex.*
Bisoprolol fumarate (p.850·1); hydrochlorothiazide (p.907·3).
Hypertension.

Bicozene *Novartis, USA.*
Benzocaine (p.1306·2); resorcinol (p.1122·2).
Local anaesthesia.

Bidiabe *Sanofi Synthelabo, Ital.*
Chlorpropamide (p.321·1); phenformin hydrochloride (p.333·2).
Diabetes mellitus.

Bidien *IDI, Ital.*
Budesonide (p.1064·2).
Skin disorders.

Bidocef *Bristol-Myers Squibb, Ger.†.*
Cefadroxil (p.161·2).
Bacterial infections.

Bidor *Weleda, UK.*
Ferrous sulfate (p.1360·3); silica (p.1503·3).
Headaches; migraine.

Bidrolar *Spyfarma, Spain.*
Pygeum africanum (p.1490·3).
Benign prostatic hyperplasia.

Bienfait Total *Lancome, Canad.*
SPF 15: Octinoxate (p.1517·3); ensulizole (p.1517·2).
Sunscreen.

Bienterico *Caldeira & Marques, Port.*
Streptomycin sulfate (p.249·1); neomycin sulfate (p.228·1).
Bowel sterilisation; diarrhoea; hepatic coma.

Bi-Euglucon *Roche, Ital.*
Glibenclamide (p.321·3); phenformin hydrochloride (p.333·2).
Diabetes mellitus.

Bi-Euglucon M
Roche, Ital.; Lakeside, Mex.
Glibenclamide (p.321·3); metformin hydrochloride (p.332·3).
Diabetes mellitus.

Bifardol S *Liferpal, Mex.*
Naproxen sodium (p.61·1); paracetamol (p.71·2).
Fever; pain.

Bifazol *Bayer, Ital.*
Bifonazole (p.381·1).
Fungal skin infections.

Bifebral *Rhone-Poulenc Rorer, Mex.*
Ketoprofen sodium (p.48·1); paracetamol (p.71·2).
Fever; pain.

Bifen *DHA, Singapore.*
Ibuprofen (p.43·2).
Fever; musculoskeletal and joint disorders; pain.

Bifenabid *Marion Merrell, Spain†.*
Probucol (p.959·2).
Hyperlipidaemias.

Bifenac *Pharmacia Upjohn, Mex.*
Tolfenamic acid (p.88·3).
Fever; gout; inflammation; musculoskeletal, joint and peri-articular disorders; pain.

Bifilact *Fidia, Ital.*
Lactobacillus acidophilus (p.1626·3); Lactobacillus lactis (p.1626·3); Lactobacillus bulgaricus (p.1626·3); Streptococcus thermophilus (p.1626·3); Bifidobacterium bifidum (p.1626·3); Lactobacillus sporogenes; vitamin B substances.
Maintenance of normal gastrointestinal flora.

Bifilact 6 *Fidia, Ital.*
Lactic-acid-producing organisms (p.1626·3); yeast (p.1398·1); vitamins (p.1350·1).
Maintenance of normal gastrointestinal flora.

Bifinorma *Merckle, Ger.*
Lactulose (p.1230·1).
Constipation; hepatic encephalopathy; salmonella enteritis.

Bifiteral
Solvay, Aust.; Solvay, Belg.; Solvay, Ger.
Lactulose (p.1230·1).
Constipation; hepatic encephalopathy; salmonella enteritis.

Bifix *Roche Nicholas, Fr.*
Nifuroxazide (p.230·2).
Diarrhoea.

Bifluorid *Voco, Denm.*
Calcium fluoride (p.1356·1); sodium fluoride (p.1375·3).
Dental caries prophylaxis.

Bifluorid 12 *Meda, Swed.*
Sodium fluoride (p.1375·3); calcium fluoride (p.1356·1).
Dental caries prophylaxis.

Bifokey *Inkeysa, Spain.*
Bifonazole (p.381·1).
Fungal skin and nail infections.

Bifomyk *Hexal, Ger.*
Bifonazole (p.381·1).
Fungal skin infections.

Bifon *Dermapharm, Ger.*
Bifonazole (p.381·1).
Fungal skin infections.

Bifort *Merck, Spain.*
Cafedrine hydrochloride (p.853·1); theodrenaline hydrochloride (p.1671·3).
Hypotension.

Big V *Tanning Research, Canad.†.*
SPF 15: Octinoxate (p.1517·3); oxybenzone (p.1518·1).

SPF 30: Homosalate (p.1517·2); octinoxate (p.1517·3); octilsalate (p.1518·1); oxybenzone (p.1518·1).
Sunscreen.

Big V Baby *Tanning Research, Canad.†.*
SPF 30: Homosalate (p.1517·2); octinoxate (p.1517·3); octilsalate (p.1518·1); oxybenzone (p.1518·1).
Sunscreen.

Big V Cough Lozenge *Sutton, Canad.†.*
Menthol (p.1632·3).

Big V Kids *Tanning Research, Canad.†.*
Octinoxate (p.1517·3); octocrilene (p.1518·1); octilsalate (p.1518·1); oxybenzone (p.1518·1).
Sunscreen.

Bigasan *Phyteia, Switz.†.*
Aluminium hydroxide (p.1210·3); magnesium hydroxide (p.1233·1); magnesium oxide (p.1233·2); magnesium silicate (p.1502·1); mannitol (p.924·3).
Gastric hyperacidity.

Bigonist *Cassenne, Fr.*
Buserelin acetate (p.1278·1).
Prostatic cancer.

Bigpen *Fides Rottapharm, Spain.*
Amoxicillin trihydrate (p.149·2); potassium clavulanate (p.187·2).
Bacterial infections.

Bikalm *Byk Gulden, Ger.*
Zolpidem tartrate (p.712·2).
Sleep disorders.

Biklin
Bristol-Myers Squibb, Aust.; Bristol-Myers Squibb, Denm.†; Bristol-Myers Squibb, Fin.; Bristol-Myers Squibb, Ger.; Bristol-Myers Squibb, Swed.
Amikacin sulfate (p.148·1).
Bacterial infections.

Bilagar *SIT, Ital.†.*
Phenolphthalein (p.1244·1); ox bile extract (p.1585·1).
Constipation.

Bilagit Mono *Temmler, Ger.*
Curcuma zanthorrhiza.
Dyspepsia.

Bilagol *Janssen-Cilag, Belg.†.*
Diisopromine hydrochloride (p.1222·2); sorbitol (p.1377·3).
Constipation; hepatobiliary disorders.

Bilan *Biocur, Ger.*
Haronga.
Digestive disorders.

Bilatin *Stada, Aust.*
Lecithin (p.1628·1); liver extract.
Tonic.

Bilatin Fischol *Stada, Ger.*
Marine triglycerides (p.949·3).
Hyperlipidaemias.

Bilberry Plus *Eagle, Austral.*
Myrtillus (p.1639·2); euphrasia (p.1609·3); fenugreek (p.1610·3); hydrastis (p.1621·1).
Eye fatigue.

Bilberry Plus Eye Health *Cenovis, Austral.*
Myrtillus (p.1639·2); ginkgo biloba (p.1615·2); tagetes erecta; riboflavin; dl-alpha tocoferil acetate; ascorbic acid; zinc gluconate; betacarotene (p.1350·1).
Eye fatigue; eye irritation.

Bilem *Lemery, Mex.*
Tamoxifen (p.572·2).

Bilenor *Schwarz, Ital.*
Magnesium trihydrate sait of chenodeoxycholic and ursodeoxycholic acids (p.1594·1) (p.1677·2).
Biliary dyspepsia; gallstones.

Bilgast echinac *Bilgast, Ger.†.*
Echinacea purpurea (p.1606·2).
Respiratory- and urinary-tract infections.

Bilicanta *Roche, Spain.*
Hymecromone (p.1622·3).
Biliary-tract disorders.

Bilicante *Monot, Fr.*
Hymecromone (p.1622·3).

Bilicura Forte *Muller Goppingen, Ger.*
Kava (p.1625·3); cynara (p.1601·3).
Biliary disorders; dyspepsia.

Biliepar *Ibirn, Ital.*
Ursodeoxycholic acid (p.1677·2).
Biliary dyspepsia; gallstones.

Bilifluine *Promedica, Fr.†.*
Depigmented and decholesterolised ox bile (p.1585·1); sodium oleate (p.1497·1).
Constipation; dyspepsia.

Biliflux *Eurofarma, Braz.*
Diisopromine hydrochloride (p.1222·2); sorbitol (p.1377·3).
Liver disorders.

Bilifuge *Plan, Switz.*
Cynara (p.1601·3); berberis vulgaris; java tea (p.1625·1); kinkeliba (p.1626·1).
Digestive disorders.

Biligrama *Schering, Braz.*
Meglumine ioglicate (p.1034·3).
Contrast medium for biliary-tract radiography.

Bili-Labstix
Bayer Diagnostics, Irl.†; Bayer Diagnostici, Ital.; Bayer Diagnostics, UK†; Bayer, USA.
Test for pH, protein, glucose, ketones, bilirubin, and blood in urine.

Bilina *Esteve, Spain.*
Levocabastine hydrochloride (p.419·3).
Allergic conjunctivitis; allergic rhinitis.

Bilipax *Taphlan, Switz.*
Naphthylacetic acid (p.1639·3); methylphenylethyl nicotinate.
Adjuvant in cholangiography; digestive disorders.

Bilipeptal Mono *Evisco, Ger.*
Pancreatin (p.1646·1).
Pancreatic disorders.

The symbol † denotes a preparation no longer actively marketed

Bilisan C3 Repha, Ger.†
Silybum marianum (p.1021·3); greater celandine (p.1618·1); curcuma zanthorrhiza.
Biliary disorders; gallstones; liver disorders.

Bilisan Duo Repha, Ger.
Silybum marianum (p.1021·3); curcuma zanthorrhiza.
Biliary-tract disorders; dyspepsia; liver disorders.

Biliscopin Schering, Aust.; Schering, Braz.; Schering, Ger.; Schering, Neth.†; Schering, NZ; Schering, Swed.; Schering, Switz.; Schering, UK.
Meglumine iotroxate (p.1036·3).
Contrast medium for biliary-tract radiography.

Bilisegrol Schering, Spain.
Meglumine iotroxate (p.1036·3).
Contrast medium for biliary-tract radiography.

Bilivist Berlex, USA†.
Sodium iopodate (p.1036·1).
Radiographic contrast medium for cholecystography.

Bilkaby Bailly, Fr.†.
Menadione (p.1395·3); bile salts (p.1585·1).
Haemorrhagic disorders due to vitamin K deficiency.

Billerol Lehning, Fr.
Homoeopathic preparation.

Biloban Cipan, Port.
Ginkgo biloba (p.1615·2).
Vascular disorders.

Bilobene Ratiopharm, Aust.; Merckle, Ger.
Fumitory (p.1612·3).
Biliary-tract disorders.

Bilopaque Nycomed, USA†.
Sodium tyropanoate (p.1038·3).
Radiographic contrast medium for cholecystography.

Biloptin Schering, Aust.; Schering, Ger.; Schering, Port.; Schering, S.Afr.; Schering, Switz.†; Schering, UK.
Sodium iopodate (p.1036·1).
Contrast medium for biliary-tract radiography.

Bilron Aspen, S.Afr.
Iron bile salts (p.1585·1).
Bile salt deficiency; biliary-tract disorders.

Bilsan Abbott, Hong Kong.
Choline bicitrate (p.1356·3); inositol (p.1623·3); methionine (p.1012·2); vitamin B substances (p.1350·1); dehydrocholic acid (p.1602·2); ox bile (p.1585·1).
Biliary disorders; liver disorders.

Biltricide Bayer, Austral.; Bayer, Canad.; Bayer, Fr.; Bayer, Ger.; Bayer, Hong Kong; Bayer, Israel; Bayer, Neth.; Bayer, S.Afr.; Bayer, Thai.; Bayer, USA.
Praziquantel (p.106·3).
Worm infections.

Bilugen Roche Diagnostics, Austral.; Roche Diagnostics, UK.
Test for urobilinogen and bilirubin in urine.

Bilugen-Test Boehringer Mannheim Diagnostics, Irl.†.
Test for urobilinogen and bilirubin in urine.

Bimixin Sanofi Synthelabo, Ital.
Bacitracin (p.155·2); neomycin sulfate (p.228·1).
Enteric infections.

Bi-Myconase Yamanouchi, Neth.†.
Glucamylase; invertase.
Diarrhoea due to amylase, isomaltase, or invertase deficiency.

Binaldan Vifor, Switz.
Loperamide hydrochloride (p.1231·3).
Diarrhoea.

Bi-Nerisona
Schering, Braz.; Schering, Mex.
Diflucortolone (p.1069·3) or diflucortolone valerate (p.1069·3); chlorquinaldol (p.182·1).
Infected skin disorders.

Biniwas Wasserman, Spain.
Binifibrate (p.850·1).
Hyperlipidaemias.

Binoctrin Cazi, Braz.
Co-trimoxazole (p.193·3).
Bacterial infections; Pneumocystis carinii pneumonia; protozoal infections.

Binodian Schering, Mex.
Estradiol valerate (p.1473·2); prasterone enantate (p.1488·2).
Menopausal disorders.

Binopen Cazi, Braz.
Ampicillin (p.150·3).
Bacterial infections.

Binordiol
Wyeth Lederle, Belg.; Wyeth, Neth.; Wyeth, Switz.
Levonorgestrel (p.1486·2); ethinylestradiol (p.1476·2).
Biphasic oral contraceptive; menstrual disorders.

Binotal
Bayer, Aust.†; Bayer, Braz.; Grunenthal, Ger.; Bayer, Mex.
Ampicillin (p.150·3), ampicillin sodium (p.150·3), or ampicillin trihydrate (p.151·1).
Bacterial infections.

Binotine Farmalab, Braz.
Ampicillin benzathine (p.151·3); ampicillin sodium (p.150·3).
Bacterial infections.

Binotine Balsamico Farmalab, Braz.
Ampicillin benzathine (p.151·3); sodium camsilate; guaifenesin (p.1092·2); eucalyptol (p.1609·2); niaouli oil (p.1640·2).
Bacterial infections.

Binovum
Janssen-Cilag, Irl.; Janssen-Cilag, UK.
Norethisterone (p.1485·1); ethinylestradiol (p.1476·2).
Biphasic oral contraceptive.

B-Insulin Berlin-Chemie, Ger.
Insulin injection (pork) (p.324·1).
Diabetes mellitus.

Bio² Bio2, Fr.†.
Protein, fibre, and vitamin preparation (p.1350·1).
Low body weight.

Bio-200 Dermoforma, Ital.
Royal jelly (p.1659·3); pollen.
Nutritional supplement.

Bio Ace Blackmores, Austral.
Betacarotene; ascorbic acid; d-alpha tocoferil acid succinate; vitamin B₁; calcium pantothenate; vitamin B₆; vitamin K₃; zinc; ginseng; garlic (p.1350·1).
Tonic.

Bio Ace Excell Blackmores, Austral.
Vitis vinifera; silybum marianum; betacarotene; vitamin C; d-alpha tocopherol; calcium pantothenate; vitamin B₆; zinc; vitamin B₁₂; folic acid thiamine nitrate (p.1350·1).
Tonic.

Bio Acidophilus Bioceuticals, UK.
Lactobacillus acidophilus (p.1626·3).

Bio C Blackmores, Austral.
Ascorbic acid (p.1389·3); sodium ascorbate (p.1390·1); calcium ascorbate (p.1389·3); bioflavonoids (p.1611·1); rutoside (p.1611·2); rose fruit (p.1389·3); red cherry (p.1029·1).
Vitamin C supplement.

Bio E
Blackmores, Austral.; Bio-Health, UK.
Vitamin E (p.1393·3).

Bio Enhaced Natural E Nutrition Care, Austral.
d-Alpha tocopherol (p.1393·3).
Vitamin E deficiency.

Bio Espectrum Centrum, Spain.
Ampicillin sodium (p.150·3); ampicillin benzathine (p.151·3); bromhexine (p.1085·3).
Lignocaine [lidocaine] hydrochloride (p.1313·2) is included in this preparation to alleviate the pain of injection.
Respiratory-tract infections.

Bio Eutrical Crinos, Ital.
An amino-acid preparation with vitamins and minerals (p.1350·1).
Nutritional supplement.

Bio Exazol Leti, Spain†.
Erythromycin ethyl succinate (p.201·2) or erythromycin propionate (p.201·3).
Bacterial infections.

Bio Hubber ICN, Spain†.
Streptomycin sulfate (p.249·1); neomycin sulfate (p.228·1); pectin (p.1502·3); sulfadiazine (p.251·1); menadione sodium bisulfite; nicotinamide.
Gastrointestinal infections.

Bio Hubber Fuerte ICN, Spain†.
Bacitracin zinc (p.155·2); streptomycin sulfate (p.249·1); menadione sodium bisulfite; neomycin sulfate (p.228·1); nicotinamide; pectin (p.1502·3); sulfadiazine (p.251·1).
Gastrointestinal infections.

Bio Magnesium Blackmores, Austral.
Magnesium (p.1190·3); calcium ascorbate (p.1389·3); vitamin B₆ (p.1386·3); colecalciferol (p.1391·1); manganese (p.1371·3).
Muscle cramps.

Bio Star Novag, Spain.
Ginseng (p.1615·3).
Tonic.

Bio Zinc Blackmores, Austral.
Multivitamin and mineral preparation (p.1350·1).
Skin disorders; wounds.

Bio-Acerola C Complex
Solgar, UK.
Vitamin C with bioflavonoids (p.1350·1).

Solgar, USA†.
Vitamin C (p.1389·3); citrus bioflavonoids complex (p.1611·1); rutoside (p.1611·2); red cherry (p.1029·1); rose hips (p.1389·3).
Capillary bleeding.

Bioagil Merck, Aust.
Ascorbic acid (p.1389·3).
Vitamin C deficiency.

Bioarginina Damor, Ital.
Arginine hydrochloride (p.1353·3).
Asthenia; hyperammonaemia.

Bio-Arscolloid SIT, Ital.
Dichlorobenzyl alcohol (p.1143·2); silver protein (p.1664·2); tyrothricin (p.267·1).
Bacterial mouth infections.

Bio-Ascorbate Solgar, UK.
Vitamin C with bioflavonoids (p.1350·1).

Biobalm Modern Health Products, UK.
Slippery elm bark (p.1665·1); althaea root (p.1577·1); chondrus (p.1500·1).
Gastrointestinal disorders.

Bioband Corbridge, Austral.
Triclosan (p.1159·2).
Medicated bandage; ulcers; wounds.

Biobase Odan, Canad.
Alcohol (p.1130·3); (+)-cetyl steryl ethylene oxide.
Antiseptic vehicle for topical preparations.

Bio-Biol Searle, Ital.
Vitamin B substances (p.1350·1); coenzyme A (p.1598·1).
Vitamin deficiency.

Bio-C Pharma Nord, Thai.
Calcium ascorbate (p.1389·3).

Bio-C A Vogel Bioforce, Switz.
Vitamin C preparation (p.1350·1).

Bio-C Complex Blackmores, Austral.
Ascorbic acid (p.1389·3); sodium ascorbate (p.1390·1); calcium ascorbate (p.1389·3); lemon bioflavonoids (p.1611·1); rutoside (p.1611·2); hesperidin (p.1611·2); red cherry (p.1029·1).
Vitamin C preparation.

Biocadmio Uriach, Spain.
Cadmium sulfide (p.1588·1).
Skin and scalp disorders.

Biocalcin Esseti, Ital.
Salcatonin (p.749·3).
Hypercalcaemia; osteoporosis; Paget's disease of bone; sympathetic pain syndrome.

Biocalcio Sedabel, Braz.
Calcium phosphate; cyanocobalamin; ergocalciferol; sodium fluoride; sodium iodide (p.1350·1).
Vitamin and mineral supplement.

Biocalcium Bioprogress, Ital.
Calcium carbonate (p.1215·1).
Calcium deficiency.

Bio-Calcium + D₃ Pharma Nord, Irl.
Calcium (p.1187·3); magnesium (p.1190·3); colecalciferol (p.1391·1).
Calcium deficiency.

Bio-Calcium + D₃ + K Pharma Nord, Irl.
Calcium (p.1187·3); colecalciferol (p.1391·1); vitamin K (p.1395·3).

Biocalm Biolab, Thai.
Tolperisone hydrochloride (p.1330·3).
Obliterative vascular diseases; parkinsonism; skeletal muscle spasticity and spasm.

Biocalron Biomedis, Thai.; Great Eastern, Thai.
Calcium lactate (p.1188·2); ferrous fumarate (p.1360·1); vitamin C (p.1389·3); rutoside (p.1611·2).

Biocalyptol
Laphal, Fr.
Pholcodine (p.1099·1); eucalyptol (p.1609·2); guaiacol (p.1092·1).
The syrup formerly contained pholcodine, eucalyptol, guaiacol, belladonna, and sodium camsilate. The suppositories formerly contained pholcodine, eucalyptol, guaiacol, and sodium camsilate.
Coughs.

Laphal, Hong Kong.
Pholcodine (p.1099·1); eucalyptol (p.1609·2); guaiacol (p.1092·1).
Coughs.

Bio-Caps
Infabra, Braz.; Bio-Health, UK.
Multivitamin and mineral preparation (p.1350·1).

Biocarde Lehning, Fr.
Crataegus (p.1600·2); passion flower (p.1649·2); avena (p.1583·1); valerian (p.1678·3); melissa (p.1632·2); motherwort (p.1637·3).
Formerly contained pulsatilla, crataegus, passion flower, convallaria, strophanthus, avena, valerian, cereus grandiflorus, camphor, and colloidal gold.
Insomnia; nervous disorders.

Biocarn Medice, Ger.
Levocarnitine (p.1356·1).
Carnitine deficiency.

Biocarnil Abiogen, Ital.
Carnitine hydrochloride (p.1356·2); L-lysine hydrochloride (p.1370·3).
Nutritional supplement.

Biocarotine Bioceuticals, UK.
Betacarotene (p.1355·1).

Biocatalase Fournier SA, Spain.
Catalase (p.1592·2).
Burns; skin disorders; ulcers; wounds.

Bioceanat Plantes Tropicales, Fr.
Sea water; copper gluconate (p.1357·3).
Nasal irrigation.

Biocebe Nutergia, Fr.
Vitamin, bioflavonoid, and zinc preparation (p.1350·1).
Nutritional supplement.

Biocef
Note. This name is used for preparations of different composition.
Biochemie, Aust.
Cefpodoxime proxetil (p.172·3).
Bacterial infections.

Zambon, Spain.
Ceftibuten (p.176·1).
Bacterial infections.

International Ethical, USA.
Cefalexin (p.161·3).
Bacterial infections.

Biochetasi Sigma-Tau, Ital.
Injection; suppositories: Vitamin B substances and electrolytes (p.1350·1).
Oral granules: Vitamin B substances, electrolytes, and carbohydrate (p.1350·1).
Fluid and electrolyte disorders; liver disorders.

Bio-Chrome Herbaxt, Fr.†.
Chromium (p.1357·1) from *Saccharomyces cerevisiae*; nicotinamide (p.1372·3).
Nutritional supplement.

Bio-Chromium Blackmores, Austral.
Dried yeast (p.1398·1); chromium amino acid chelate (p.1357·1); manganese amino acid chelate; nicotinamide (p.1372·3); magnesium phosphate (p.1191·1); dibasic potassium phosphate (p.1193·1); zinc amino acid chelate (p.1398·3).
Alcoholism; hyperglycaemia; hypoglycaemia; sugar cravings.

Bio-Ci Ceccarelli, Ital.
Ascorbic acid (p.1389·3).

Biociclin Francia, Ital.
Cefuroxime sodium (p.178·2).
Bacterial infections.

Biocidan Menarini, Fr.
Eye drops: Cethexonium bromide (p.1137·1).
Minor eye infections.
Nasal spray: Cethexonium bromide (p.1137·1); phenyltoloxamine citrate (p.423·1).
Nose and throat disorders.

Biocil
Note. This name is used for preparations of different composition.
Ibirn, Ital.
Cefonicid sodium (p.168·1).
Lignocaine [lidocaine] hydrochloride (p.1313·2) is included in this preparation to alleviate the pain of injection.
Formerly known as Cefid.
Bacterial infections.

Formula, NZ.
Povidone-iodine (p.1155·1).
Herpes labialis; minor cuts and burns; skin disinfection.

Biocin
Note. This name is used for preparations of different composition.
Ibirn, Ital.
Fosfomycin calcium (p.208·2).
Bacterial infections.

Atral, Port.
Doxycycline (p.200·1).
Bacterial infections.

Biocine Test Biovac, S.Afr.
Tuberculin (p.1675·3).
Diagnosis of tuberculosis.

Biocine-Test PPD Chiron, Ital.
Tuberculin purified protein derivative (p.1675·3).
Test for hypersensitivity to tubercle bacillus.

Bioclate
Centeon, Denm.; Centeon, Ger.; Centeon, Spain†; Centeon, UK; Armour, USA.
A factor VIII preparation (p.734·1).
Haemophilia A.

Biocobal Lemery, Mex.
Hydroxocobalamin (p.1388·1).

Biocodone Bios, Belg.
Hydrocodone bitartrate (p.42·2).
Coughs.

Biocol Bio-Transfusion, Fr.
1 Vial, fibrinogen (p.736·1); fibronectin (p.1611·1); factor XIII (p.735·3); 1 syringe, aprotinin (p.725·3); 1 vial, thrombin (p.741·3); calcium chloride (p.1188·1)
On mixing this forms a fibrin glue (p.735·3).
Haemorrhage.

Bioconseils Yves Ponroy, Fr.†.
A range of herbal preparations.

Biocord Biosintetica, Braz.
Nifedipine (p.940·1).
Angina pectoris; hypertension; Raynaud's syndrome.

Biocort Salters, S.Afr.
Hydrocortisone acetate (p.1073·3).
Skin disorders.

Biocoryl Uriach, Spain.
Procainamide hydrochloride (p.960·1).
Arrhythmias.

Biocos APS, Ger.
Metformin hydrochloride (p.332·3).
Diabetes mellitus.

BioCox Iatric, USA.
Coccidioidin (p.1597·2).
Skin test for coccidioidomycosis.

Biocream BritHealth, UK.
Tissue salts; terpineol (p.1669·3); germall.
Skin disorders.

Bio-Cuivre Herbaxt, Fr.
Copper pidolate; manganese pidolate (p.1350·1).
Nutritional supplement.

Bio-C-Vitamin Pharma Nord, Fin.
Calcium ascorbate (p.1389·3).
Vitamin C deficiency; vitamin C supplement.

Biocyclin Biochemie, Aust.†.
Doxycycline hyclate (p.200·1).
Bacterial and protozoal infections.

BioCyst CytoChemia, Ger.
Birch leaf (p.1585·2); solidago virgaurea; java tea (p.1625·1).
Urinary-tract disorders.

Biodalgic Biocodex, Fr.
Tramadol hydrochloride (p.89·1).
Pain.

Biodan Biomedis, Thai.; Great Eastern, Thai.
Sulfaguanidine (p.1000·2); activated charcoal (p.1000·2); bismuth subcarbonate (p.1213·1); pectin (p.1502·3); dicyclomine [dicycloverine] hydrochloride (p.466·1).
Diarrhoea.

Bioday *Biocur, Ger.*
Guarana (p.1681·1).
Fatigue.

Bio-Delta Cortilen *SIFI, Ital.*
Prednisolone acetate (p.1078·1); neomycin sulfate (p.228·1).
Eye infections.

Bioderm *Odan, Canad.*
Polymyxin B sulfate (p.238·1); bacitracin (p.155·2).
Bacterial infections.

Biodermatin *Lafare, Ital.*
Biotin (p.1355·3).
Skin disorders.

Biodexan *Sophia, Mex.*
Dexamethasone sodium phosphate (p.1067·1); neomycin sulfate (p.228·1); polymyxin B sulfate (p.238·1); phenylephrine hydrochloride (p.1097·1).
Eye disorders.

Biodezil *Bioresearch, Mex.*
Captopril (p.853·3).
Hypertension.

Biodine *Major, USA.*
Povidone-iodine (p.1155·1).
Skin disinfection.

Bio-Disc *Blackmores, Austral.*
Minerals; vitamins (p.1350·1); silicon dioxide (p.1503·3); bromelains (p.1586·3); papain (p.1647·3).
Delayed bone healing; muscular and joint pain.

Biodone *McGaw Biomed, NZ.*
Methadone hydrochloride (p.53·1).
Opioid withdrawal syndrome.

Biodone Forte *McGaw Biomed, Austral.*
Methadone hydrochloride (p.53·1).
Opioid dependence.

Biodophilus *Bioceuticals, UK.*
Lactobacillus acidophilus (p.1626·3).

Biodramina *Uriach, Spain.*
Dimenhydrinate (p.415·2).
Motion sickness.

Biodramina Cafeina *Uriach, Spain.*
Caffeine (p.761·3); dimenhydrinate (p.415·2); pyridoxine hydrochloride (p.1386·3).
Motion sickness; vertigo.

Biodroxil
Biochemie, Aust.†; Biochemie, Hong Kong; Biochemie, Singapore.
Cefadroxil (p.161·2).
Bacterial infections.

Bio-E *Pharma Nord, Thai.*
d-Alpha tocoferil acetate (p.1394·1).

Bio-Energol Plus *Yamanouchi, Port.*
Arginine aspartate (p.1354·1).
Tonic.

Bioenterine *DB, Fr.*
Nutritional supplement (p.1350·1).
Maintenance of gastrointestinal flora.

Bioequiseto *Ghimas, Ital.*
Equisetum (p.1606·3).
Nutritional supplement.

Bioesse *Mavi, Ital.*
L-Cystine, L-methionine, zinc, and copper (p.1350·1).
Nutritional supplement.

Bio-E-Vitamin
Pharma Nord, Fin.; Pharma Nord, Norw.
d-Alpha tocoferol (p.1393·3).
Vitamin E deficiency.

Biofanal *Pfleger, Ger.*
Nystatin (p.392·2).
Candidiasis.

Biofaxil *Lepori, Port.*
Cefadroxil (p.161·2).
Bacterial infections.

Biofem *Biocur, Ger.*
Vitex agnus castus (p.1574·2).
Mastalgia; menstrual disorders.

Biofenac
Note.This name is used for preparations of different composition.
UCB, Belg.; UCB, Neth.; UCB, Port.
Aceclofenac (p.11·1).
Inflammation; musculoskeletal, joint, and peri-articular disorders.
Ache, Braz.
Diclofenac diethylamine (p.30·2), diclofenac resinate (p.31·3), or diclofenac sodium (p.30·3).
Gout; inflammation; musculoskeletal, joint, and peri-articular disorders; pain.

Bio-Fer *Herbaxt, Fr.*
Iron pidolate; folic acid; ascorbic acid (p.1350·1).
Nutritional supplement.

Bioferina *Bioresearch, Mex.*
Phenazopyridine (p.78·1).
Pain; urinary-tract infections.

Bioferon *Bio Sidus, Thai.*
Interferon alfa-2b (p.628·1).
Anogenital warts; hepatitis; malignant neoplasms.

Biofibra *Pfizer Consumer, Spain.*
Wheat bran; pectins; oligo-fructose (p.1350·1).
Dietary fibre supplement.

Biofigado *Simoes, Braz.*
Adenosine (p.828·2); methionine (p.1012·2); betaine sodium (p.1584·3); choline citrate (p.1356·2); pyridoxine hydrochloride (p.1386·3); sorbitol (p.1377·3).
Liver disorders.

Biofilm *CliniMed, UK.*
Hydrocolloid dressing.
Ulcers; wounds.

Biofim *Uniao Quimica, Braz.*
14 Tablets, mestranol (p.1482·1); 7 tablets, norethisterone (p.1485·1); mestranol; 7 tablets, inert.
Biphasic oral contraceptive.

Bioflorin
Note.This name is used for preparations of different composition.
Sanova, Aust.
Live *Enterococcus faecium* (p.1626·3).
Gastrointestinal disorders.
Bracco, Ital.; Synthelabo, Switz.
Lactic-acid-producing enterococci (p.1626·3).
Gastrointestinal disorders.

Bioflox *Bioresearch, Mex.*
Ciprofloxacin (p.182·3).
Bacterial infections.

Biofluor *Distrifarma, Port.*
Chlorhexidine gluconate (p.1138·2); sodium fluoride (p.1375·3).
Oral hygiene.

Biofluor Sensitive *Distrifarma, Port.*
Potassium nitrate (p.1154·3); cetylpyridinium chloride (p.1138·1); sodium fluoride (p.1375·3).
Gingivitis; sensitive teeth.

Bioflusin *Bioresearch, Mex.*
Chlorpheniramine [chlorphenamine] (p.412·2).
Hypersensitivity.

Bioflutin-N *Sudmedica, Ger.*
Etilefrine hydrochloride (p.888·1).
Hypotension.

Biofolic *Esseti, Ital.*
Calcium methyltetrahydrofolate (p.1363·2).
Antidote to folic acid antagonists; folic acid deficiency; reduction of aminopterin and methotrexate toxicity.

Bioform *Salters, S.Afr.*
Clioquinol (p.190·2).
Fungal and bacterial skin infections.

Biofructose *Bunker, Braz.*
Vitamin B substances, ascorbic acid, and fructose (p.1350·1).

Biofurex *KBR, Ital.*
Cefuroxime sodium (p.178·2).
Bacterial infections.

Biofurin *Bioresearch, Mex.*
Nitrofurantoin (p.230·3).
Urinary-tract infections.

Biofuroso *Bioresearch, Mex.*
Ferrous fumarate (p.1360·1).
Iron deficiency anaemia.

Biogam *Biogam, Switz.*
Trace element preparations (p.1350·1).

Biogardol *Biophytarom, Fr.†.*
Vitamin E; betacarotene; vitamin C (p.1350·1).

Bio-Garten Entschlackungstee *Bio-Garten, Aust.*
Silver birch (p.1585·2); taraxacum leaf (p.1669·1); prunus spinosa; rose fruit (p.1389·3); sambucus (p.1660·3); calendula (p.1589·2).
Herbal preparation.

Bio-Garten Tee fur den Magen *Bio-Garten, Aust.*
Chamomile (p.1593·2); peppermint leaf (p.1243·2); caraway (p.1591·2); valerian (p.1678·3).
Gastrointestinal disorders.

Bio-Garten Tee fur Leber und Galle *Bio-Garten, Aust.*
Absinthium (p.1571·1); calamus (p.1588·1); angelica (p.1580·2); peppermint leaf (p.1243·2); bitter-orange leaf.
Liver and gallbladder disorders.

Bio-Garten Tee fur Niere und Blase *Bio-Garten, Aust.*
Bearberry (p.1583·3); equisetum (p.1606·3); sliver birch (p.1585·2).
Kidney and bladder disorders.

Bio-Garten Tee gegen Blahungen *Bio-Garten, Aust.*
Fennel (p.1610·1); chamomile (p.1593·2); caraway (p.1591·2); achillea (p.1572·2); peppermint leaf (p.1243·2).
Flatulence.

Bio-Garten Tee gegen Durchfall *Bio-Garten, Aust.*
Tormentil (p.1674·1); chamomile (p.1593·2); strawberry leaf; blackberry leaf; raspberry leaf (p.1657·2).
Diarrhoea.

Bio-Garten Tee gegen Erkaltung *Bio-Garten, Aust.*
Thyme (p.1672·2); althaea (p.1577·1); verbascum flowers; plantago lanceolata leaf.
Catarrh; cold symptoms.

Bio-Garten Tee gegen Verstopfung *Bio-Garten, Aust.*
Prunus spinosa; peppermint leaf (p.1243·2); chamomile (p.1593·2); fennel (p.1610·1).
Constipation.

Bio-Garten Tee zur Beruhigung *Bio-Garten, Aust.*
Valerian (p.1678·3); melissa (p.1632·2); lupulus (p.1629·3); lavender flowers (p.1627·1); orange flowers.
Anxiety; insomnia.

Bio-Garten Tee zur Erhohung der Harnmenge *Bio-Garten, Aust.*
Urtica (p.1678·2); silver birch (p.1585·2); taraxacum leaf (p.1669·1); prunus spinosa; ononis (p.1644·1).
Diuretic.

Bio-Garten Tee zur Starkung und Kraftigung *Bio-Garten, Aust.*
Achillea (p.1572·2); bitter-orange peel (p.1644·2); gentian (p.1615·1); rosemary leaf; rose fruit (p.1389·3).
Tonic.

Bio-Garten Tropfen fur Galle und Leber *Bio-Garten, Aust.*
Absinthium (p.1571·1); achillea (p.1572·2); taraxacum (p.1669·1).
Liver and gallbladder disorders.

Bio-Garten Tropfen fur Magen und Darm *Bio-Garten, Aust.*
Peppermint (p.1243·2); valerian (p.1678·3); chamomile (p.1593·2).
Gastrointestinal disorders.

Bio-Garten Tropfen fur Niere und Blase *Bio-Garten, Aust.*
Silver birch (p.1585·2); equisetum (p.1606·3).
Kidney and bladder disorders.

Bio-Garten Tropfen gegen Blahungen *Bio-Garten, Aust.*
Caraway (p.1591·2); coriander (p.1599·2); peppermint (p.1243·2).
Flatulence.

Bio-Garten Tropfen gegen Husten *Bio-Garten, Aust.*
Thyme (p.1672·2); plantago lanceolata.
Catarrh; coughs.

Bio-Garten Tropfen zur Beruhigung *Bio-Garten, Aust.*
Lupulus (p.1629·3); melissa (p.1632·2).
Nervous disorders.

Biogaze *Medeva, Fr.*
Niaouli oil (p.1640·2); thyme oil (p.1672·3).
Burns.

Biogel *Ghimas, Ital.*
Royal jelly (p.1659·3).

Biogelat Erkaltungs & Grippe *Metochem, Aust.†.*
Salix (p.82·1).
Cold and flu symptoms; pain.

Biogelat Leberschutz *Metochem, Aust.*
Silybum marianum (p.1021·3).
Liver disorders.

Biogelat Schlaf *Metochem, Aust.*
Valerian (p.1678·3); lupulus (p.1629·3).
Sleep disorders.

Biogena Dermo *Biogena, Ital.*
Soap substitute.

Biogenis *Bayer, Ger.†.*
dl-Alpha tocoferil acetate (p.1394·1); magnesium oxide (p.1233·2).
Vitamin E or magnesium deficiency.

Biogenis One-a-Day *Bayer, Ger.*
d-Alpha tocoferol (p.1393·3).
Vitamin E deficiency.

Biogesic
Biomedis, Hong Kong; Biomedis, Singapore; Biomedis, Thai.; Great Eastern, Thai.
Paracetamol (p.71·2).
Fever; pain.

Bioget *Michallik, Ger.*
Tannic acid (p.1669·1); cetylpyridinium chloride (p.1138·1).
Burns; wounds.

BioGinkgo *Pharmanex, USA.*
Ginkgo biloba (p.1615·2).
Nutritional supplement.

Bioglan Acidophilus *Bioglan, Austral.*
Lactobacillus acidophilus (p.1626·3).
Diarrhoea; restoration of gastrointestinal flora.

Bioglan Arthri Plus *Bioglan, Austral.*
Celery seed oil; evening primrose oil (p.1613·2); fish oil (p.949·3); devil's claw root (p.26·3); salix (p.82·1).
Arthritis; rheumatism; sports injuries.

Bioglan 3B Beer Belly Buster *Bioglan, Austral.*
Garcinia; chromium trichloride (p.1357·1); pectin (p.1502·3); methylcellulose (p.1502·2); guarana (p.1681·1); hypericum (p.290·2).
Obesity.

Bioglan Bioage Peripheral *Bioglan, Austral.*
Viola tricolor; crataegus (p.1600·2); olive; magnesium orotate (p.1645·1); d-alpha tocoferil acid succinate (p.1394·1).
Peripheral circulatory disorders.

Bioglan The Blue One *Bioglan, Austral.*
Avena (p.1583·1); gokhru; damiana (p.1602·1); capsicum (p.1591·1); eschscholtzia californica; zinc amino acid chelate (p.1398·3); rutoside (p.1611·2).
Tonic for males.

Bioglan Cal C *Bioglan, Austral.*
Calcium ascorbate (p.1389·3).
Vitamin C supplement.

Bioglan Cirflo *Bioglan, Austral.*
Rutoside (p.1611·2); bioflavonoids (p.1611·1); nicotinic acid (p.1372·3); calcium ascorbate (p.1389·3); calcium gluconate (p.1188·2); aesculus (p.1574·1); hamamelis (p.1618·3); pulsatilla (p.1656·3); ruscus aculeatus.
Peripheral circulatory disorders.

Bioglan Cranbiotic Super *Bioglan, Austral.*
Cranberry (p.1600·2); taraxacum (p.1669·1); bearberry (p.1583·3); buchu (p.1587·2); solidago virgaurea.
Cystitis.

Bioglan Daily Plus *Bioglan, Austral.*
Vitamin and mineral preparation (p.1350·1).

Bioglan Daily Plus Max *Bioglan, Austral.*
Ginseng; garlic; silybum marianum; bladderwrack; lecithin; vitamins; minerals (p.1350·1).
Tonic.

Bioglan Digestive Zyme *Bioglan, Austral.*
Betaine hydrochloride (p.1584·3); glutamic acid (p.1365·2); pepsin (p.1649·3).
Achlorhydria; hypochlorhydria.

Bioglan Discone *Bioglan, Austral.*
Vitamin and mineral preparation (p.1350·1) with bromelain (p.1586·3) and papain (p.1647·3).
Arthritis; rheumatism; sports injuries.

Bioglan Easy Bronz *Bioglan, Austral.*
Lycopersicon esculatum.
Skin tanning.

Bioglan E-Plus *Bioglan, Austral.†.*
d-Alpha tocoferol (p.1393·3); fish oil (p.949·3); evening primrose oil (p.1613·2); rosemary oil (p.1659·3); lecithin (p.1628·1).
Aid in skin tissue repair; antioxidant.

Bioglan Fingers & Toes *Bioglan, Austral.†.*
Calcium ascorbate (p.1389·3); d-alpha tocoferil acid succinate (p.1394·1); rutoside (p.1611·2); bioflavonoids (p.1611·1); nicotinic acid (p.1372·3); aesculus (p.1574·1); hamamelis (p.1618·3); ginkgo biloba (p.1615·2); rosemary oil (p.1659·3).
Peripheral vascular disorders.

Bioglan Formula Four *Bioglan, Austral.*
Vitamin and mineral preparation (p.1350·1).

Bioglan Ginger-Vite Forte *Bioglan, Austral.*
Ginger oil; ginger (p.1227·2); evening primrose oil (p.1613·2).
Arthritis; rheumatism; sports injuries.

Bioglan Ginsynergy *Bioglan, Austral.*
Ginseng (p.1615·3); eleutherococcus senticosis root (p.1615·3); withania somnifera; panax quinquefolium.
Tonic.

Bioglan Hemo Factor *Bioglan, Austral.*
Vitamin preparation with iron and folic acid (p.1350·1).
Anaemia.

Bioglan Joint Mobility *Bioglan, Austral.*
Glucosamine sulfate (p.1616·2); turmeric (p.1029·3); boswellia serrata; capsicum (p.1591·1); zinc gluconate (p.1398·2); manganese amino acid chelate.
Musculoskeletal and joint disorders.

Bioglan Liver-Vite *Bioglan, Austral.*
Silybum marianum (p.1021·3).
Liver disorders.

Bioglan Maxepa *Bioglan, Austral.*
Fish oil (p.949·3); d-alpha tocoferil acetate (p.1394·1).
Atherosclerosis; hypertriglyceridaemia.

Bioglan Mega C *Bioglan, Austral.*
Ascorbic acid (p.1389·3); rose fruit (p.1389·3); hesperidin (p.1611·2).
Vitamin C supplement.

Bioglan Mens Super Soy/Clover *Bioglan, Austral.*
Red clover (p.1657·2); soya bean (p.1378·1); saw palmetto (p.1491·2); damiana (p.1602·1); calcium hydrogen phosphate (p.1188·2).
Male menopausal disorders.

Bioglan Micelle A plus E *Bioglan, Austral.*
Vitamin A (p.1382·1); d-alpha tocoferil acetate (p.1394·1).
Fat malabsorption syndromes; vitamin A and E supplement.

Bioglan Micelle E *Bioglan, Austral.*
d-Alpha tocoferil acetate (p.1394·1).
Vitamin E supplement.

Bioglan Natural E *Bioglan, Austral.*
d-Alpha tocoferol (p.1393·3).
Vitamin E deficiency; vitamin E supplement.

Bioglan Neo Stress *Bioglan, Austral.*
Multivitamin, mineral, and amino-acid preparation (p.1350·1).

Bioglan Organic Mineral *Bioglan, Austral.*
Mineral supplement (p.1350·1).

Bioglan Panazyme *Bioglan, Austral.*
Pancreatin (p.1646·1).
Digestive enzyme supplement.

Bioglan PMT-Eze *Bioglan, Austral.*
Multivitamin and mineral preparation with herbs (bladderwrack, juniper, alchemilla, bearberry, viburnum opulus, vitex agnus castus) (p.1350·1).
Menstrual disorders.

Bioglan Primrose Micelle *Bioglan, Austral.*
Evening primrose oil (p.1613·2).
Eczema; mastalgia.

Bioglan Primrose-E *Bioglan, Austral.*
Evening primrose oil (p.1613·2); d-alpha tocoferol (p.1393·3).
Premenstrual syndrome.

Bioglan Pro-Guard *Bioglan, Austral.*
Saw palmetto (p.1491·2).
Benign prostatic hyperplasia

Bioglan Psylli-Mucil Plus *Bioglan, Austral.*
Ispaghula (p.1229·1); slippery elm (p.1665·1); peppermint leaf (p.1243·2); ginger (p.1227·2); pectin (p.1502·3).
Bowel cleanser.

Bioglan Pygno-Vite *Bioglan, Austral.*
Vitis vinifera; myrtillus (p.1639·2).
Peripheral circulatory disorders.

Bioglan Silica-Vite *Bioglan, Austral.*
Equisetum (p.1606·3).
Skin disorders; wounds.

Bioglan Soy Power Plus *Bioglan, Austral.*
Red clover (p.1657·2); isoflavones; soya bean (p.1378·1); dioscorea villosa; calcium hydrogen phosphate (p.1188·2).
Isoflavone and calcium supplement.

Bioglan Stress-Relax *Bioglan, Austral.*
Hypericum (p.290·2).
Anxiety; nervous disorders.

Bioglan Sucro *Bioglan, Austral.*
Vitamin and mineral preparation (p.1350·1).

Bioglan Super Cal C *Bioglan, Austral.*
Calcium ascorbate (p.1611·1); citrus bioflavonoids (p.1611·1); hesperidin (p.1611·2); rutoside (p.1611·2); rose fruit (p.1389·3).
Vitamin C supplement.

Bioglan Supercarotene C&E *Bioglan, Austral.*
Betacarotene; *d*-alpha tocoferil acid succinate; ascorbic acid (p.1350·1).
Tonic.

Bioglan Superdophilus *Bioglan, Austral.*
Lactobacillus acidophilus (p.1626·3).
Diarrhoea; restoration of gastrointestinal flora.

Bioglan Synergy B *Bioglan, Austral.*
Vitamin B substances with vitamin C and magnesium (p.1350·1).

Bioglan Vision-Eze *Bioglan, Austral.*
Myrtillus (p.1639·2); ginkgo biloba (p.1615·2).
Eye fatigue; peripheral circulatory disorders; poor night vision.

Bioglan Water Soluble E *Bioglan, Austral.*
d-Alpha tocopherol (p.1393·3).
Vitamin E supplement.

Bioglan Zellulean with Escin *Bioglan, Austral.*
Aesculus (p.1574·1); ginkgo biloba (p.1615·2); vitis vinifera; bladderwrack (p.1585·2); bioflavonoids (p.1611·1); lecithin (p.1628·1); pectin (p.1502·3); tyrosine (p.1381·3); evening primrose oil (p.1613·2); omega-3 marine triglycerides (p.949·3); yellow sweet clover.
Aid to skin tissue repair; obesity.

Bioglan Zinc Chelate *Bioglan, Austral.*
Zinc amino acid chelate (p.1398·3).
Zinc deficiency.

Bioglan Zn-A-C *Bioglan, Austral.*
Ascorbic acid (p.1389·3); vitamin A (p.1382·1); zinc amino acid chelate (p.1398·3); calcium pantothenate (p.1374·1); rutoside (p.1611·2).
Vitamin and mineral supplement.

Biogreen *Euro-Pharma, Ital.*
Sodium monofluorophosphate (p.1377·2); propolis (p.1655·1); tabebuia; plant extracts.
Mouth disorders.

Biogyl *Biolab, Thai.*
Metronidazole (p.594·1).
Anaerobic bacterial infections.

Biohisdex DM *Everest, Canad.*
Dextromethorphan hydrobromide (p.1087·3); phenylephrine hydrochloride (p.1097·1); diphenylpyraline hydrochloride (p.417·1).
Coughs; respiratory congestion.

Biohisdine DM *Everest, Canad.*
Dextromethorphan hydrobromide (p.1087·3); phenylephrine hydrochloride (p.1097·1); diphenylpyraline hydrochloride (p.417·1).
Coughs; respiratory congestion.

Biohist *Propan, S.Afr.*
Diphenhydramine hydrochloride (p.416·1); zinc oxide (p.1128·2); calamine (p.1111·3); phenol (p.1152·3).
Skin disorders.

Biohist-LA *Wakefield, USA.*
Chlorpheniramine [chlorphenamine] maleate (p.412·1); pseudoephedrine hydrochloride (p.1099·2). Formerly contained carbinoxamine maleate and pseudoephedrine hydrochloride.
Cold symptoms.

Bio-H-Tin
e+b, Aust.; e+b, Ger.; Gebro, Switz.
Biotin (p.1355·3).
Biotin deficiency.

Biohulin 70/30 and 80/20 *Biobras, Braz.*
A mixture of isophane insulin injection(human, monocomponent) and insulin injection (human, monocomponent) (p.324·1) in the proportions indicated.
Diabetes mellitus.

Biohulin L *Biobras, Braz.*
Insulin zinc suspension (human, monocomponenet) (p.324·1).
Diabetes mellitus.

Biohulin NPH *Biobras, Braz.*
Isophane insulin injection (human, monocomponent) (p.324·1).
Diabetes mellitus.

Biohulin R *Biobras, Braz.*
Insulin injection (human, monocomponenet) (p.324·1).
Diabetes mellitus.

Biohulin Ultralenta *Biobras, Braz.*
Insulin zinc suspension (crystalline) (human, monocomponenet) (p.324·1).
Diabetes mellitus.

Bio-Insulin 10/90, 20/80, 30/70, 40/60, and 50/50 *Guidotti, Ital.*
Mixtures of insulin injection (human, biosynthetic) and isophane insulin injection (human, biosynthetic) respectively in the proportions indicated (p.324·1).
Diabetes mellitus.

Bio-Insulin I *Guidotti, Ital.*
Isophane insulin (human, biosynthetic) (p.324·1).
Diabetes mellitus.

Bio-Insulin L *Guidotti, Ital.*
Insulin zinc suspension (human, biosynthetic) (p.324·1).
Diabetes mellitus.

Bio-Insulin R *Guidotti, Ital.*
Insulin (human, biosynthetic) (p.324·1).
Diabetes mellitus.

Bio-Insulin U *Guidotti, Ital.*
Insulin zinc suspension (crystalline) (human, biosynthetic) (p.324·1).
Diabetes mellitus.

Bioiodine *Bioceuticals, UK.*
Potassium iodate (p.1525·1).

Biojad *Roche, Aust.*
Multivitamin and iron preparation (p.1350·1).
Tonic.

Biokids *Biotherm, Canad.*
SPF 35: Avobenzone (p.1517·1); enzacamene (p.1517·2); octocrilene (p.1518·1); terephthalylidene dicamphor sulfonic acid; titanium dioxide (p.1126·1).
Sunscreen.

Biokur *Biocur, Ger.*
Biotin (p.1355·3).
Biotin deficiency.

Biolac EPS *Angelini, Ital.; Bioprogress, Ital.*
Lactulose (p.1230·1).
Hepatic cirrhosis; hepatic encephalopathy.

Biolactine *Sella, Ital.*
Vitamin B substances (p.1350·1), lactic-acid-producing organisms (p.1626·3); myrtillus (p.1639·2).
Nutritional supplement.

Biolactyl *DB, Fr.*
Lactobacillus acidophilus (p.1626·3); *Lactobacillus casei var rhamnosus* (p.1626·3).
Maintenance of gastrointestinal flora.

Biolan Tar *Biopha, Fr.†.*
Coal tar (p.1125·1); piroctone olamine (p.1121·1); salicylic acid (p.1122·3).
Seborrhoeic dermatitis.

Bioleine *Nutergia, Fr.*
Evening primrose oil (p.1613·2).
Nutritional supplement.

Biolina *Bioceuticals, UK.*
Spirulina (p.1667·1).

Bio-Logos *Sigma-Tau, Switz.*
Hydroxocobalamin; amino acids (p.1350·1).
Tonic.

Biolon
Ophtapharma, Canad.; Stulln, Ger.; Biotechnology, Israel; SIFI, Ital.†; Cryopharma, Mex.; Chauvin Novopharma, Switz.
Sodium hyaluronate (p.1620·1).
Aid in ophthalmic surgery.

Biolone *Pharmafrica, S.Afr.*
Sodium hyaluronate (p.1620·1).
Aid in eye surgery.

Biolucchini *Geymonat, Ital.†.*
Proteins (mol. wt 30-300 kD).
Tissue repair.

Biomag
Note.This name is used for preparations of different composition.
Homeocan, Canad.; Lehning, Fr.
Homoeopathic preparation.
Pulitzer, Ital.
Cimetidine (p.1216·3).
Gastrointestinal disorders associated with hyperacidity.

Biomagnesin *Madaus, Ger.*
Dibasic magnesium phosphate; dibasic magnesium citrate.
Magnesium deficiency.

Bio-Magnesium *Phytomed, Switz.*
Homoeopathic preparation.

Biometalle II-Heyl *Heyl, Ger.†.*
Mineral preparation (p.1350·1).
Correction of metal balance following penicillamine therapy.

Biometalle III-Heyl *Heyl, Ger.†.*
Mineral preparation (p.1350·1).
Correction of metal balance following penicillamine therapy.

Biomina *Precimex, Mex.*
Albumin (human) (p.724·1).

Biomineral *Biochimici, Ital.*
Mineral preparation with cystine (p.1350·1).
Nutritional supplement.

Bio-Mineral Formula *Blackmores, Austral.*
Mineral preparation (p.1350·1).

Biomineral Plus *Biochimici, Ital.*
Multivitamin and mineral preparation with cystine and methionine (p.1350·1).
Nutritional supplement.

Biomineral Unghie *Biochimici, Ital.*
Amino-acid preparation with vitamins and minerals (p.1350·1).
Nail disorders.

Biominol A *Alter, Spain.*
Vitamin A palmitate (p.1383·2).
Vitamin A deficiency.

Biominol A D *Alter, Spain.*
Vitamin A palmitate (p.1383·2); ergocalciferol (p.1391·2).
Deficiency of vitamins A and D.

Biomo-lipon *Biomo, Ger.*
Thioctic acid (p.1671·3).
Diabetic polyneuropathy.

Biomona *Bioresearch, Mex.*
Metronidazole (p.594·1).
Vaginitis.

Biomox *Biolab, Thai.; International Ethical, USA†.*
Amoxicillin (p.149·2) or amoxicillin trihydrate (p.149·2).
Bacterial infections.

Biomunil *Lusofarmaco, Ital.*
Klebsiella pneumoniae ribosomes and membrane fraction; *Streptococcus pneumoniae* ribosomes; *Streptococcus pyogenes* ribosomes; *Haemophilus influenzae* ribosomes.
Immunostimulant.

Bion Tears *Alcon, Austral.; Alcon, Canad.; Alcon, Singapore; Alcon, Swed.; Alcon, Thai.; Alcon, USA.*
Dextran 70 (p.729·2); hypromellose (p.1501·3).
Dry eyes.

Bionagre plus E *Bio-Sante, Canad.*
Linoleic acid (p.1613·2); linolenic acid; vitamin E (p.1393·3).

Bionagrol *Biophytarom, Fr.*
Evening primrose oil (p.1613·2).
Nutritional supplement.

Bionagrol Plus *Biophytarom, Fr.*
Evening primrose oil (p.1613·2); omega-3 fatty acids (p.949·2).
Nutritional supplement.

Bionet *Carter Horner, Canad.*
Benzocaine (p.1306·2); cetalkonium chloride (p.1137·1).
Mouth disorders.

Bionicard *Rottapharm, Ital.*
Nicardipine hydrochloride (p.938·3).
Angina pectoris; hypertension.

Bionif *Bioprogress, Ital.*
Nifedipine (p.940·1).
Angina pectoris; hypertension.

Bionocalcin
Delta, Port.†; Ipsen, Spain.
Salcatonin (p.749·3).
Hypercalcaemia; metastatic bone pain; osteoporosis; Paget's disease of bone.

Bionolip *Bioresearch, Mex.*
Bezafibrate (p.849·1).
Hyperlipidaemias.

Bionorm *Merck, Braz.*
Amino acids and vitamin B substances (p.1350·1).
Nutritional supplement.

Bionoxol *Bioresearch, Mex.*
Ambroxol (p.1084·3).
Respiratory-tract disorders.

Bionutrin *Biomedis, Thai.; Great Eastern, Thai.*
Multivitamin and mineral preparation (p.1350·1).

Biopasal Fibra *Synthelabo, Spain.*
Ispaghula (p.1229·1).
Constipation.

Biopatch *Johnson & Johnson Medical, USA†.*
Chlorhexidine gluconate (p.1138·2).
Wound dressing.

Biopental *OM, Port.*
Lysates of *Streptococcus pneumoniae; Neisseria catarrhalis; Staphylococcus aureus; Klebsiella pneumoniae; Haemophilus influenzae; Streptococcus pyogenes.*
Respiratory-tract infections.

Bioperazone *Biopharma, Ital.*
Cefoperazone sodium (p.168·2).
Bacterial infections.

Bioperidolo *FIRMA, Ital.*
Haloperidol (p.686·3).
Psychoses.

Biophenicol *Biochemie, Aust.†.*
Chloramphenicol (p.179·1) or chloramphenicol sodium succinate (p.179·2).
Bacterial infections.

Biophil *Kemiprogress, Ital.*
Vitamin B substances (p.1350·1); myrtillus (p.1639·2).
Disturbances of the gastrointestinal flora.

Biophylin *Gerard House, UK†.*
Note. A similar name is used for preparations of different composition (see below).
Valerian (p.1678·3); skullcap (p.1664·3); Jamaica dogwood (p.1625·1); cimicifuga (p.1595·2).
Tenseness, restlessness, nervous irritability.

Biophyllin *Propan, S.Afr.†.*
Note. A similar name is used for preparations of different composition (see above).
Theophylline (p.777·2).
Obstructive airways disease.

Biopim *Kemyos, Ital.†.*
Pipemidic acid (p.236·1).
Urinary-tract infections.

Bioplak *Almirall, Spain.*
Aspirin (p.14·2).
Thromboembolism prophylaxis.

bioplant-Kamillenfluid *Serum-Werk Bernburg, Ger.*
Chamomile (p.1593·2); calendula (p.1589·2).
Bedsores; inflammation of the oral cavity; skin inflammation.

Bioplasma FDP *NBI, S.Afr.*
Plasma protein fraction (p.740·2).
Fluid depletion; haemorrhagic disorders.

Bioplex
Note.This name is used for preparations of different composition.
Sante Naturelle, Canad.
Vitamin B substances (p.1350·1).
Fresenius Kabi, Ital.
A range of amino-acid infusions (p.1350·1).
Parenteral nutrition.
Cortecs, UK.
Carbenoxolone sodium (p.1215·3).
Mouth ulcers.

Bioplus *Covan, S.Afr.*
Caffeine; vitamin B substances; calcium citrate; calcium gluconate (p.1350·1).
Tonic.

Biopram *Bioresearch, Mex.*
Metoclopramide (p.1236·3).
Nausea and vomiting.

Bioprim *Bioresearch, Mex.*
Co-trimoxazole (p.193·3).
Bacterial infections.

Bioptimum *Boiron, Port.*
A range of amino-acid, vitamin and mineral preparations (p.1350·1).

Biopto-E *Jenapharm, Ger.*
d-Alpha tocopherol (p.1393·3).
Tonic; vitamin E deficiency.

Biopyn *Laser, S.Afr.†.*
Paracetamol (p.71·2); codeine phosphate (p.25·2); caffeine (p.761·3).
Fever; pain.

Biopyr *Madaus, Ger.*
Homoeopathic preparation.

Bioquidan *Bioresearch, Mex.*
Dextromethorphan (p.1087·3).
Coughs.

Bioquil *Atral, Port.*
Ofloxacin (p.232·3).
Bacterial infections.

Bio-Quinone *Pharma Nord, Thai.*
Ubidecarenone (p.1677·1).

Bioral
Smith & Nephew, Austral.; SmithKline Beecham, Irl.†; Roche, S.Afr.†; Merck Consumer, UK.
Carbenoxolone sodium (p.1215·3).
Mouth ulcers.

Bio-Real *Farmetrusca, Ital.†.*
Royal jelly (p.1659·3); yeast (p.1398·1).

Bio-Real Complex *Farmetrusca, Ital.†.*
Royal jelly (p.1659·3); ginseng (p.1615·3).

Bio-Real Plus *Farmetrusca, Ital.†.*
Royal jelly (p.1659·3); ginseng (p.1615·3).

Bio-Regenerat S 3 *Dibropharm, Ger.*
Adenosine phosphate disodium (p.1573·3).
Psoriasis.

Bioregime *Azevedos, Port.*
Glucomannan (p.1616·2).
Obesity.

Bioregime Fort *Azevedos, Port.*
Glucomannan (p.1616·2); yeast (p.1398·1).
Obesity.

Biorenal *Pharmalink, Swed.†.*
Anhydrous glucose; sodium chloride; sodium lactate; calcium chloride; magnesium chloride (p.1184·1).
Peritoneal dialysis.

Biorenyn *Bioresearch, Mex.*
Salbutamol (p.770·3).

Bioreucam *Helforma, Port.*
Tenoxicam (p.87·2).
Gout; musculoskeletal, joint, and peri-articular disorders.

Biorganic Geri *Gisand, Switz.*
Vitamin, mineral, and amino-acid preparation (p.1350·1) with ginseng (p.1615·3).
Dietary supplement; tonic.

Biorinil *Farmila, Ital.*
Betamethasone (p.1063·1); tetryzoline hydrochloride (p.1101·2). Formerly contained betamethasone, chlorpheniramine [chlorphenamine] maleate, kanamycin sulfate, and tetryzoline hydrochloride.
Rhinitis; rhinopharyngitis; sinusitis.

Bio-Ritmo *Medinfar, Port.*
Arginine aspartate; pyridoxine (p.1350·1).
Tonic.

Biormon *Amsa, Ital.*
Estradiol benzoate (p.1473·1); progesterone (p.1488·3).
Amenorrhoea; oligomenorrhoea.

Biorphen *Alliance, UK.*
Orphenadrine hydrochloride (p.470·3).
Drug-induced extrapyramidal disorders; parkinsonism.

Biortho *Nutergia, Fr.*
Vitamin and mineral preparation (p.1350·1).
Nutritional supplement.

Biosal
Note. This name is used for preparations of different composition.
Yauyip, Austral.
Methyl salicylate (p.55·1); menthol (p.1632·3); camphor (p.1589·3); eucalyptus oil (p.1609·2); pumilio pine oil (p.1656·3).
Arthritis pain.

Bioprogress, Ital.
Nimesulide (p.62·3).
Fever; inflammation; pain.

Biosan E *Biocur, Ger.*
dl-Alpha tocopherol (p.1394·1) or dl-alpha tocoferil acetate (p.1394·1).
Vitamin E deficiency.

Bioscalin *Giuliani, Ital.*
Multivitamin and mineral preparation (p.1350·1).
Hair and nail disorders.

Bioscefal *Unibios, Spain.*
Cefalexin (p.161·3).
Bacterial infections.

Bioscina *Biochimico, Braz.*
Hyoscine butylbromide (p.468·2); dipyrone (p.34·1).
Smooth muscle spasm.

Biosedon S *Biocur, Ger.*
Valerian (p.1678·3); passion flower (p.1649·1); lupulus (p.1629·3).
Anxiety disorders; insomnia.

Bio-Selenium *Herbaxt, Fr.*
Selenium (p.1375·2) from *Saccharomyces cerevisiae*; alpha tocoferil acetate (p.1394·1); wheat-germ oil.
Muscular disorders; skin disorders.

Bioselenium *Uriach, Spain.*
Selenium sulfide (p.1123·1).
Skin disorders.

Biosint *Liomont, Mex.*
Cefotaxime sodium (p.169·1).
Bacterial infections.

Biosol A *Pharmalink, Swed.†*
Sodium chloride; potassium chloride; magnesium chloride; calcium chloride; acetic acid; with or without glucose (p.1184·1).
Haemodialysis.

Biosol B *Pharmalink, Swed.†*
Sodium bicarbonate (p.1184·1).
Haemodialysis.

Biosorb *Nutricia, Port.†*
Preparation for enteral nutrition (p.1350·1).

Biosorbin MCT *Nutricia, Fin.*
Preparation for enteral nutrition (p.1350·1).

Biosor-C *Hamilton, Austral.*
Hesperidin methyl chalcone (p.1611·2); hesperidin (p.1611·2); ascorbic acid (p.1389·3).
Gingivitis; herpes labialis.

Biostan *Bioresearch, Mex.*
Astemizole (p.409·1).

Biostatine *Almirall, Spain.*
Somatostatin acetate (p.1297·3).
Pancreatic fistulae; variceal haemorrhage.

Biostim
Hoechst Marion Roussel, Braz.; Cassenne, Fr.; Hoechst Marion Roussel, Ital.; Hoechst Marion Roussel, Mex.; Roussel, Port.; Roussel, S.Afr.†
Klebsiella pneumoniae glycoprotein (p.1626·1).
Burns; prophylaxis of respiratory-tract infections; ulcers; wounds.

Bio-Strath
Note. This name is used for preparations of different composition.
Lizoform, Ital.
Valerian (p.1678·3); passion flower (p.1649·1); peppermint leaf (p.1243·2).
Insomnia; sedative.

Crefar, Port.
Amino-acid, vitamin, and mineral preparation (p.1350·1).
Tonic.

Cedar Health, UK.
Saccharomyces cerevisiae (p.1398·1).

Bio-Strath Artichoke Formula *Cedar Health, UK.*
Cynara (p.1601·3); thistle seeds (p.1597·2); peppermint leaf (p.1243·2); yeast plasmolysate (p.1398·1).
Dyspepsia.

Bio-Strath No 1 *Crefar, Port.†*
Aesculus (p.1574·1); cowslip root (p.1600·1).
Peripheral vascular disorders; venous disorders.

Bio-Strath No 5 *Crefar, Port.†*
Salix (p.82·1); cowslip root (p.1600·1).
Musculoskeletal and joint disorders.

Bio-Strath No 8 *Crefar, Port.†*
Valerian (p.1678·3); passion flower (p.1649·1); peppermint leaf (p.1243·2).
Anxiety; insomnia.

Bio-Strath Valerian Formula *Cedar Health, UK.*
Valerian (p.1678·3); passion flower (p.1649·1); peppermint leaf (p.1243·2); yeast plasmolysate (p.1398·1).
Insomnia; irritability; tension.

Bio-Strath Willow Formula *Cedar Health, UK.*
Salix (p.82·1); cowslip root (p.1600·1); yeast plasmolysate (p.1398·1).
Musculoskeletal and joint pain.

Biosun *Banana Boat, Canad.†*
SPF 25; SPF 30: Octinoxate (p.1517·3); octisalate (p.1518·1); oxybenzone (p.1518·1); titanium dioxide (p.1126·1).
SPF 45: Octinoxate (p.1517·3); octisalate (p.1518·1); oxybenzone (p.1518·1); octocrilene (p.1518·1).
Sunscreen.

Bio-Tab *International Ethical, USA.*
Doxycycline hyclate (p.200·1).

Biotamin *Sankyo, Jpn†.*
Benfotiamine (p.1384·3).
Vitamin B1 deficiency.

Biotassina *Teofarma, Ital.*
Amino acids; vitamin B substances (p.1350·1); calcium gluconate (p.1188·2).
Lignocaine [lidocaine] hydrochloride (p.1313·2) is included in the intramuscular injection to alleviate the pain of injection.
Asthenia.

Biotazol *Bioresearch, Mex.*
Metronidazole (p.594·1).
Amoebiasis; giardiasis; trichomoniasis.

Biotel diabetes *Biotel, USA†.*
Test for glucose in urine (p.1616·3).

Biotel kidney *Biotel, USA.*
Test for haemoglobin, red blood cells, and albumin in urine.

Biotene *Laclede, Singapore.*
Glucose oxidase (p.1616·2); lactoperoxidase; muramidase (p.1638·1); lactoferrin.
Mouth disorders.

Biotens *Kernyos, Ital.†*
Labetalol hydrochloride (p.918·1); chlortalidone (p.857·1).
Hypertension.

Biotherm *Biotherm, Canad.*
SPF 15; SPF 25; SPF 30: Avobenzone (p.1517·1); enzacamene (p.1517·2); terephthalylidene dicamphor sulfonic acid; titanium dioxide (p.1126·1).
Sunscreen.

Biotherm Gelee Bronzante *Biotherm, Canad.†.*
SPF 8: Octinoxate (p.1517·3); octisalate (p.1518·1); oxybenzone (p.1518·1).
Sunscreen.

Biotherm Gelee Fraiche *Biotherm, Canad.*
SPF 8: Octinoxate (p.1517·3); enzacamene (p.1517·2); terephthalylidene dicamphor sulfonic acid; titanium dioxide (p.1126·1).
Sunscreen.

Biotherm Lait Bronzant *Biotherm, Canad.*
SPF 8: Octinoxate (p.1517·3); terephthalylidene dicamphor sulfonic acid; titanium dioxide (p.1126·1).
Sunscreen.

Biotherm Lait Protecteur *Biotherm, Canad.*
SPF 15: Octinoxate (p.1517·3); terephthalylidene dicamphor sulfonic acid; titanium dioxide (p.1126·1).
Sunscreen.

Biotherm Soin des Levres *Biotherm, Canad.*
SPF 8: Octinoxate (p.1517·3).
Sunscreen.

Biotherm Soin Solaire *Biotherm, Canad.*
SPF 8: Octinoxate (p.1517·3); terephthalylidene dicamphor sulfonic acid; titanium dioxide (p.1126·1).
Sunscreen.

Biotherm Soin Solaire Autobronzant *Biotherm, Canad.*
SPF 8: Avobenzone (p.1517·1); enzacamene (p.1517·2); terephthalylidene dicamphor sulfonic acid.
Sunscreen.

Biotherm Stick Ecran *Biotherm, Canad.*
SPF 20: Avobenzone (p.1517·1); octocrilene (p.1518·1); titanium dioxide (p.1126·1).
Sunscreen.

Biothymus *Biochimica, Ital.*
Thymus gland extract.
Prevention of hair loss.

Biothymus F Urto *Biochimici, Ital.*
Thymus gland extract; paeonia suffruticosa.
Prevention of hair loss.

Biothymus M Urto *Biochimici, Ital.*
Thymus gland extract; paeonia suffruticosa; saw palmetto (p.1491·2).
Prevention of hair loss.

Biotin-Asmedic *Dyckerhoff, Ger.*
Biotin (p.1355·3).
Biotin deficiency.

Bioton *Sella, Ital.*
Honey (p.1366·2); ginseng (p.1615·3); royal jelly (p.1659·3).
Nutritional supplement.

Biotone *Laphal, Fr.*
Kola (p.1681·1); phosphoric acid (p.1651·1); inositol calcium; manganese glycerophosphate (p.1617·3).
Tonic.

Biotonico Fontoura *Newlab, Braz.*
Ferrous sulfate (p.1360·3); phosphoric acid (p.1651·1); plant extracts.
Anaemias.

Biototal *Kanda, Braz.*
Dried yeast; malt; honey (p.1350·1).
Nutritional supplement.

Biotrefon Plus *Whitehall, Ital.*
Pollen; royal jelly (p.1659·3); liver extract.

Biotrefon-L *Italmex, Mex.*
Cobamamide (p.1388·3).
Tonic.

Biotricina *Bioresearch, Mex.*
Tetracycline (p.258·3).
Bacterial infections.

Biotril *Bioresearch, Mex.*
Erythromycin (p.201·2).
Bacterial infections.

Biotrixina *Benedetti, Ital.*
Cefatrizine (p.164·3).
Bacterial infections.

Biotron *Covan, S.Afr.*
Multivitamin and mineral preparation (p.1350·1).

Biotropic *Madaus, Spain†.*
Guar gum (p.323·3).
Diabetes mellitus.

Bio-Tropin *Biotechnology, Israel; Cryopharma, Mex.*
Somatropin (p.1286·1).
Growth disorders in renal failure; growth hormone deficiency; Turner's syndrome.

Biotuss N *Spitzner, Ger.*
Thyme (p.1672·2); althaea (p.1577·1); drosera (p.1606·1).
Catarrh; coughs.

Biotyage *Bionatec, Fr.*
Nutritional supplement (p.1350·1).

Bio-Vagin *Elofar, Braz.*
Metronidazole (p.594·1); nystatin (p.392·2).
Gynaecological infections.

Biovelbin *Biogalenica, Spain†.*
Vinorelbine tartrate (p.580·2).
Breast cancer; lung cancer.

Biovigor
Note. This name is used for preparations of different composition.
Biotrading, Ital.†.
Royal jelly (p.1659·3); honey (p.1366·2).
Nutritional supplement.

IBSA, Switz.
Hydroxocobalamine chloride; amino acids (p.1350·1).
Tonic.

Biovit *Roche, Aust.*
Multivitamin preparation with iron (p.1350·1).

Biovit-A *Bioceuticals, UK.*
Vitamin A (p.1382·1).

Biovital
Note. This name is used for preparations of different composition.
EMS, Braz.
Multivitamin and mineral preparation (p.1350·1).

Rhone-Poulenc Rorer, Irl.†; Roche Consumer, UK.
Vitamin B substances; vitamin C; iron; manganese (p.1350·1).

Lampugnani, Ital.
Royal jelly (p.1659·3).
Nutritional supplement.

Biovital Forte N *Schieffer, Ger.*
Crataegus (p.1600·2); caffeine citrate (p.761·3); ferrous gluconate (p.1360·1); vitamins.
Tonic.

Biovital Ginseng *Roche, Switz.*
Ginseng (p.1615·3); caffeine (p.761·3); lecithin (p.1628·1); vitamins and minerals (p.1350·1).
Tonic.

Biovital N *Schieffer, Ger.*
Oral liquid: Crataegus (p.1600·2); motherwort (p.1637·3); ferric sodium citrate; vitamins.
Tablets: Crataegus (p.1600·2); motherwort (p.1637·3); ferrous sulfate (p.1360·3); ferric sodium citrate; vitamins.
Tonic.

Biovital Weissdorn *Roche, Aust.*
Crataegus (p.1600·2); magnesium citrate (p.1232·3); ascorbic acid (p.1389·3).
Tonic.

Biovital Weissdorn Tonikum *Schieffer, Ger.*
Crataegus (p.1600·2); motherwort (p.1637·3); vitamins.
Nervous disorders.

Bio-Vitas *Kyorin, Thai.*
Chlorpheniramine [chlorphenamine] maleate (p.412·1); DL-methionine (p.1012·2); vitamin B substances (p.1350·1).
Skin disorders.

Bioxan *Bioresearch, Mex.*
Naproxen (p.60·3).
Inflammation; musculoskeletal and joint disorders.

Bioxel *Bioresearch, Mex.*
Fluconazole (p.383·2).
Fungal infections.

Bioxidona *Faes, Spain†.*
Amoxicillin trihydrate (p.149·2).
Bacterial infections.

Bioxima *Kemyos, Ital.†.*
Cefuroxime sodium (p.178·2).
Bacterial infections.

Bioximicina *Bioresearch, Mex.*
Doxycycline (p.200·1).
Bacterial infections.

Bioximil *Bioresearch, Mex.*
Piroxicam (p.79·1).
Inflammation; musculoskeletal and joint disorders.

Bioxtra Programme *Pamex, Irl.*
Artificial saliva, toothpaste, and mouthrinse.
Dry mouth.

Bioxyol *Richard, Fr.*
Zinc oxide (p.1128·2); zinc peroxide (p.1159·3); titanium dioxide (p.1126·1).
Burns; ulcers; wounds.

Bioyetin *Probiomed, Mex.*
Erythropoietin (p.730·2).
Anaemias.

Bio-Zinc *Herbaxt, Fr.*
Zinc pidolate; vitamin A; vitamin B6 (p.1350·1).
Nutritional supplement.

Biozole *Biolab, Thai.*
Fluconazole (p.383·2).
Fungal infections.

Biozolene *Bioindustria, Ital.*
Fluconazole (p.383·2).
Fungal infections.

Bipasmin *Boehringer de Angeli, Braz.; Promeco, Mex.*
Pargeverine hydrochloride.
Smooth muscle spasm.

Bipasmin Composto *Boehringer de Angeli, Braz.*
Pargeverine hydrochloride; metamizole magnesium (p.34·2).
Smooth muscle spasm.

Bipasmin Compuesto *Promeco, Mex.*
Pargeverine hydrochloride; metamizole magnesium (p.34·2).
Smooth muscle pain and spasm.

Bipectinol *Propan, S.Afr.*
Kaolin (p.1229·3); pectin (p.1502·3); electrolytes (p.1180·1).
Diarrhoea.

Bipensaar *Rosen, Ger.*
Benzylpenicillin sodium (p.157·1); procaine penicillin [procaine benzylpenicillin] (p.239·2).
Lignocaine [lidocaine] hydrochloride (p.1313·2) is included in this preparation to alleviate the pain of injection.
Bacterial infections.

Biphasil *Wyeth, Austral.; Wyeth, NZ; Aspen, S.Afr.*
Levonorgestrel (p.1486·2); ethinylestradiol (p.1476·2).
28-Day packs also contain 7 inert tablets.
Biphasic oral contraceptive; menstrual disorders.

Biphaston *Agis, Israel.*
Dydrogesterone (p.1472·3).
Infertility; menorrhagia; menstrual disorders.

Biplatrix *Smith & Nephew, Fr.*
Dried calcium sulfate (p.1589·2).
External splinting.

Bipranix *Ashbourne, UK.*
Bisoprolol fumarate (p.850·1).
Angina pectoris; hypertension.

Bipreterax *Therval, Fr.*
Perindopril erbumine (p.953·2); indapamide (p.913·1).
Hypertension.

Bipro *Kenyaku, Thai.*
Betamethasone valerate (p.1063·2).
Skin disorders.

Bi-Profenid *Rhone-Poulenc Rorer, Fr.*
Ketoprofen (p.47·3).
Musculoskeletal, joint and peri-articular disorders.

Bipronyl *Pharbita, Singapore.*
Naproxen (p.60·3).
Gout; musculoskeletal, joint, peri-articular, and soft-tissue disorders.

Biquin *AstraZeneca, Canad.*
Quinidine bisulfate (p.964·2).
Arrhythmias.

Biquinate *Rhone-Poulenc Rorer, Austral.*
Quinine bisulfate (p.445·1).
Diagnosis of myasthenia gravis; malaria; muscle cramps; myotonia congenita.

Bi-Qui-Nol *Monot, Fr.†.*
Eucalyptol (p.1609·2); guaiacol (p.1092·1); camphor (p.1589·3); bismuth succinate (p.1214·1).
Formerly contained eucalyptol, guaiacol, camphor, bismuth succinate, and quinine sulfate.
Mouth and throat disorders.

Biral *Madaus, Ger.; Byk Madaus, S.Afr.*
Valerian (p.1678·3); passion flower (p.1649·1).
Anxiety; minor nervous disorders.

Birley's *Torbet Laboratories, UK.*
Dried aluminium hydroxide (p.1210·3); magnesium trisilicate (p.1233·3); light magnesium carbonate (p.1232·3).
Dyspepsia; flatulence; gastric hyperacidity; heartburn.

Birobin *Novartis, Aust.*
Metolazone (p.930·3).
Hypertension; oedema.

Birodogyl *Rhone-Poulenc Rorer, Fr.*
Spiramycin (p.248·3); metronidazole (p.594·1).
Bacterial mouth infections.

Birofenid *Aventis, Belg.†.*
Ketoprofen (p.47·3).
Inflammation; musculoskeletal, joint, and peri-articular disorders; oedema; pain.

Biron *Lincoln, NZ.*
Buspirone hydrochloride (p.657·2).
Anxiety.

The symbol † denotes a preparation no longer actively marketed

Biroxol *Salus, Ital.*
Ciclopirox olamine (p.382·1).
Fungal infections.

Bisac-Evac *G & W, USA†.*
Bisacodyl (p.1212·2).
Constipation.

Bisacolax *ICN, Canad.*
Bisacodyl (p.1212·2).
Constipation.

Bisalax *Rhone-Poulenc Rorer, Austral.*
Bisacodyl (p.1212·2).
Bowel evacuation; constipation.

Biscasil *Weimer, Hong Kong.*
Bismuth aluminate (p.1213·1); bismuth subgallate
(p.1213·2); bismuth subnitrate (p.1213·2); calcium carbonate (p.1215·1); sodium bicarbonate (p.1186·2);
peppermint oil (p.1243·3); silver nitrate (p.1664·2);
charcoal (p.1000·2); magnesium phosphate (p.1191·1);
silica (p.1503·3).
Gastrointestinal disorders.

Bisco-Lax *Raway, USA†.*
Bisacodyl (p.1212·2).
Constipation.

Biscotto Plasmon *Plasmon, Ital.*
Protein, carbohydrate, and lipid preparation with min-
erals and vitamins (p.1350·1).
Nutritional supplement.

Bisco-Zitron *Biscova, Ger.*
Bisacodyl (p.1212·2).
Constipation.

Biseko
Note.This name is used for preparations of different composition.
Biotest, Aust.; Biotest, Ger.; Biotest, Thai.
A plasma protein fraction (p.740·2).
*Haemodilution; hypoalbuminaemia; hypogammglob-
ulinaemia; hypoproteinaemia; hypovoalaemia; pas-
sive immunisation.*

Biotest, Hong Kong.
Albumin (p.724·1).
*Hypoproteinaemia; hypovolaemia; passive immunisa-
tion.*

Biselic *ICN, Mex.*
Tripotassium dicitratobismuthate (p.1213·2).
*Dyspepsia; gastritis; gastro-oesophageal reflux; peptic
ulcer.*

Biseptine *Nicholas, Fr.*
Chlorhexidine gluconate (p.1138·2); benzalkonium
chloride (p.1133·2); benzyl alcohol (p.1135·2).
Skin and wound disinfection.

Biseptol simplex *Winzer, Ger.†.*
Ethacridine (p.1130·3).
Antiseptic; eye infections.

Biserirte Magnesia *Whitehall, Norw.†.*
Magnesium subcarbonate (p.1232·3); sodium bicarbonate (p.1186·2); bismuth subcarbonate (p.1213·1).
*Gastrointestinal disorders associated with hyperacidi-
ty.*

Biserol-Potassium *Bichsel, Switz.*
Electrolyte infusion with glucose (p.1180·1).
Fluid and electrolyte disorders.

Biskapect *Propan, S.Afr.*
Light kaolin (p.1229·3); apple pectin (p.1502·3); bis-
muth subcarbonate (p.1213·1).
Diarrhoea.

Bislan *Yung Shin, Thai.*
Bromhexine hydrochloride (p.1085·3).
*Respiratory-tract disorders associated with increased
or viscous mucus.*

Bismag *Whitehall, Singapore; Whitehall, UK†.*
Heavy magnesium carbonate (p.1232·3); light magne-
sium carbonate (p.1232·3); sodium bicarbonate (p.1186·2).
Dyspepsia; gastric hyperacidity.

Bisma-Rex *3M, UK.*
Bismuth subcarbonate (p.1213·1); calcium carbonate
(p.1215·1); magnesium trisilicate (p.1233·3); magnesium carbonate (p.1232·3); peppermint oil (p.1243·3).
Dyspepsia; flatulence.

Bismatrol *Major, USA.*
Bismuth salicylate (p.1213·1).
Diarrhoea; dyspepsia; nausea.

Bismed *Technilab, Canad.*
Oral liquid: Bismuth salicylate (p.1213·1).
Tablets†: Bismuth salicylate (p.1213·1); calcium car-
bonate (p.1215·1).
Diarrhoea; dyspepsia.

Bismofalk *Falk, Ger.; Falk, Hong Kong.*
Bismuth subgallate (p.1213·2); bismuth subnitrate
(p.1213·2).
Gastrointestinal disorders.

Bismofarma *Farmasa, Mex.*
Tripotassium dicitratobismuthate (p.1213·2).
Peptic ulcer.

Bismolan *Bittermedizin, Ger.*
Bismuth subnitrate (p.1213·2); butoxycaine hydrochlo-
ride (p.1308·2); zinc oxide (p.1128·2).
Anorectal disorders.

Bismolan H Corti *Bittermedizin, Ger.*
Prednisolone acetate (p.1078·1); bismuth oxychloride
(p.1214·1); zinc oxide (p.1128·2).
Anorectal disorders.

Bismopepsin *Wiener, Mex.*
Tripotassium dicitratobismuthate (p.1213·2).

Bismorectal *Vifor, Switz.*
Bismuth succinate (p.1214·1); bismuth hydroxyquinoline (p.1214·1); eucalyptus oil (p.1609·2); sage oil
(p.1660·2).
Mouth and throat disorders.

Bismubell *Sanval, Braz.*
Magnesium (p.1190·3); sodium bicarbonate
(p.1186·2); acetylmethionine; belladonna (p.463·1).
Gastrointestinal hyperacidity.

Bismu-Jet *Legrand, Braz.*
Neomycin (p.228·1); bismuth sodium tartrate; menthol
(p.1632·3); procaine (p.1319·2).
Mouth and throat disorders.

Bismurectol *Knoll, Fr.*
Bismuth succinate (p.1214·1); eucalyptol (p.1609·2);
camphor (p.1589·3).
Upper respiratory-tract congestion.

Bismutal *Technilab, Canad.*
Bismuth camphocarbonate (p.1214·1); guaifenesin
(p.1092·2).
Sore throat.

Bismuth Tulasne *Rhone-Poulenc Rorer, Switz.*
Bismuth subnitrate (p.1213·2).
Dyspepsia; peptic ulcer.

Bismylate *Stanley, Braz.*
Bismuth salicylate (p.1213·1).

Bisobloc *Azupharma, Ger.; Lederle, Neth.*
Bisoprolol fumarate (p.850·1).
Angina pectoris; hypertension.

Bisocor *United Nordic, Denm.*
Bisoprolol fumarate (p.850·1).
Angina pectoris; hypertension.

Bisodol
Note.This name is used for preparations of different composition.
Whitehall, Irl.; Whitehall, UK.
Oral powder: Heavy magnesium carbonate (p.1232·3);
light magnesium carbonate; sodium bicarbonate
(p.1186·2).
*Dyspepsia; flatulence; gastric hyperacidity; heart-
burn.*

Whitehall, Irl.; Whitehall, Port.; Whitehall, UK.
Tablets: Calcium carbonate (p.1215·1); light magnesium carbonate (p.1232·3); sodium bicarbonate
(p.1186·2).
*Dyspepsia; flatulence; gastric hyperacidity; heart-
burn.*

Bisodol Heartburn Relief *Whitehall, UK.*
Alginic acid (p.1498·3); magaldrate (p.1232·2); sodi-
um bicarbonate (p.1186·2).
Dyspepsia; heartburn.

Bisodol Wind Relief *Whitehall, UK.*
Calcium carbonate (p.1215·1); light magnesium carbonate (p.1232·3); sodium bicarbonate (p.1186·2);
simeticone (p.1249·2).
Formerly known as Bisodol Extra.
*Dyspepsia; flatulence; gastric hyperacidity; heart-
burn.*

Bisolapid *Boehringer Ingelheim, Switz.*
Acetylcysteine (p.1082·3).
Excess respiratory mucus.

Bisolax *Seng, Thai.*
Bisacodyl (p.1212·2); docusate sodium (p.1223·1);
carmellose sodium (p.1499·3).
Constipation.

Bisolbruis *Boehringer Ingelheim, Neth.*
Acetylcysteine (p.1082·3).
*Respiratory-tract disorders associated with increased
mucus.*

Bisolgrip *Fher, Spain.*
Chlorpheniramine [chlorphenamine] maleate
(p.412·1); phenylephrine hydrochloride (p.1097·1); paracetamol (p.71·2).
Catarrh; cold symptoms.

Bisolgrip T *Boehringer Ingelheim, Port.*
Aspirin (p.14·2); paracetamol (p.71·2); caffeine
(p.761·3).
Fever; inflammation; pain.

Bisolnasal *Boehringer Ingelheim, Neth.*
Tramazoline hydrochloride (p.1102·1).
Nasal congestion.

Bisolspray *Boehringer Ingelheim, Port.*
Fenoxazoline hydrochloride (p.1091·3).
Upper respiratory-tract congestion and inflammation.

Bisoltus *Boehringer Ingelheim, Spain.*
Codeine hydrochloride (p.25·2).
Cough; diarrhoea; pain.

Bisolvex *Boehringer Ingelheim, Switz.*
Eucalyptol (p.1609·2); camphor (p.1589·3); niaouli oil
(p.1640·2).
Cold symptoms.

Bisolvomycin
*Boehringer Ingelheim, Aust.†; Boehringer Ingelheim, Ger.; Boehringer
Ingelheim, S.Afr.*
Bromhexine hydrochloride (p.1085·3); oxytetracycline
hydrochloride (p.234·1).
Bacterial infections of the respiratory tract.

Bisolvon
*Boehringer Ingelheim, Aust.; Boehringer Ingelheim, Belg.; Boehringer
de Angeli, Braz.; Boehringer Ingelheim, Denm.; Boehringer Ingelheim,
Fin.; Boehringer Ingelheim, Ger.; Boehringer Ingelheim, Gr.; Boehringer
Ingelheim, Hong Kong; Boehringer Ingelheim, Irl.; Boehringer Ingelhe-
im; Promeco, Mex.; Boehringer Ingelheim, NZ; Boehringer In-
gelheim, Norw.; Boehringer Ingelheim, Philipp.; Boehringer Ingelheim,
Port.; Boehringer Ingelheim, S.Afr.; Boehringer Ingelheim, Singapore;*

*Fher, Spain; Boehringer Ingelheim, Swed.; Boehringer Ingelheim,
Switz.*
Bromhexine hydrochloride (p.1085·3).
*Respiratory-tract disorders associated with increased
or viscous mucus.*

Bisolvon AM *Thomae, Ger.†.*
Ambroxol hydrochloride (p.1084·3).
*Respiratory-tract disorders associated with increased
or viscous mucus.*

Bisolvon Amoxicilina *Fher, Spain.*
Amoxicillin trihydrate (p.149·2); bromhexine hydro-
chloride (p.1085·3).
Respiratory-tract infections.

Bisolvon Chesty *Boehringer Ingelheim, Austral.*
Bromhexine hydrochloride (p.1085·3).
Respiratory-tract congestion.

Bisolvon Complex *Boehringer de Angeli, Braz.*
Bromhexine hydrochloride (p.1085·3); orciprenaline
sulfate (p.769·1); doxylamine succinate (p.417·1).
Respiratory-tract disorders.

Bisolvon Compositum *Fher, Spain.*
Bromhexine hydrochloride (p.1085·3); codeine hydrochloride (p.25·2); diphenhydramine hydrochloride
(p.416·1); ephedrine hydrochloride (p.1090·1).
Respiratory-tract disorders.

Bisolvon Dry *Boehringer Ingelheim, Austral.*
Dextromethorphan hydrobromide (p.1087·3).
Coughs.

Bisolvon Linctus *Boehringer Ingelheim, Switz.*
Bromhexine hydrochloride (p.1085·3); ammonium
chloride (p.1085·2).
Respiratory-tract disorders.

Bisolvon Linctus DA *Boehringer Ingelheim, S.Afr.*
Bromhexine hydrochloride (p.1085·3); orciprenaline
sulfate (p.769·1).
Cough associated with wheeziness.

Bisolvon NAC *Thomae, Ger.†.*
Acetylcysteine (p.1082·3).
Bronchitis.

Bisolvon Sinus
Boehringer Ingelheim, Austral.; Boehringer Ingelheim, NZ.
Bromhexine hydrochloride (p.1085·3); pseudoephe-
drine hydrochloride (p.1099·2).
Respiratory-tract congestion.

Bisolvonamid *Boehringer Ingelheim, Aust.†.*
Bromhexine hydrochloride (p.1085·3); sulfadiazine
(p.251·1).
Bacterial respiratory-tract infections.

Bisolvonat *Boehringer Ingelheim, Ger.*
Bromhexine hydrochloride (p.1085·3); erythromycin
ethyl succinate (p.201·2).
Bacterial respiratory-tract infections.

Bisolvonat Mono *Thomae, Ger.†.*
Erythromycin (p.201·2) or erythromycin ethyl succi-
nate (p.201·2).
Bacterial infections.

Bisolvotin *Boehringer Ingelheim, Aust.†.*
Bromhexine hydrochloride (p.1085·3); ammonium
chloride (p.1085·2); benzoic acid (p.1134·2).
Coughs.

Bisomerck *Merck dura, Ger.*
Bisoprolol fumarate (p.850·1).
Angina pectoris; hypertension.

Bisopine *Pinewood, Irl.*
Bisoprolol fumarate (p.850·1).
Angina pectoris; hypertension.

Biso-Puren *Isis Puren, Ger.*
Bisoprolol fumarate (p.850·1).
Angina pectoris; hypertension.

Bispan *Chinoin, Hung.*
Isopropamide iodide (p.470·1); drotaverine hydrochlo-
ride (p.1606·1).
Peptic ulcer; smooth muscle spasm.

Bisphonal *Yamanouchi, Jpn.*
Disodium incadronate (p.753·3).
Hypercalcaemia of malignancy.

Bisrenin *Winzer, Ger.†.*
Bismuth subgallate (p.1213·2); naphazoline hydro-
chloride (p.1095·1).
Eye disorders.

Bistatin *Bioresearch, Mex.*
Nystatin (p.392·2).
Fungal infections.

Bisteron *Jenapharm, Hong Kong.*
Estradiol valerate (p.1473·2).
Menopausal disorders; osteoporosis.

Bisuisan *Luper, Braz.*
Sodium bicarbonate (p.1186·2); calcium carbonate
(p.1215·1); magnesium carbonate (p.1232·3); bismuth
subcarbonate (p.1213·1); belladonna (p.463·1); rhubarb (p.1248·1); menthol (p.1632·3).
Gastrointestinal hyperacidity.

Bite & Itch Lotion *Reese, USA.*
Diphenhydramine hydrochloride (p.416·1); pramo-
caine hydrochloride (p.1318·2).
Insect bites.

Bite Rx *International Lab Tech, USA.*
Aluminium acetate (p.1578·1).
Insect bites.

Bitensil *UCB, Spain.*
Enalapril maleate (p.883·3).
Heart failure; hypertension.

Bitensil Diu *UCB, Spain.*
Enalapril maleate (p.883·3); hydrochlorothiazide
(p.907·3).
Hypertension.

Bi-Tildiem *Synthelabo, Fr.*
Diltiazem hydrochloride (p.874·3).
Angina pectoris.

Bitteridina *AFOM, Ital.*
Cinchona calisaya (p.1595·3); calumba (p.1589·2); angelica (p.1580·2); cascara (p.1216·1); valerian
(p.1678·3).
Constipation.

Bituelve *Opofarm, Braz.*
Cyanocobalamin (p.1388·1); thiamine hydrochloride
(p.1385·1).
Anaemias; vitamin B₁ and B₁₂ deficiency.

Bivacyn
Medphano, Ger.; Lek, Hong Kong.
Neomycin sulfate (p.228·1); bacitracin (p.155·2).
*Burns; ear inflammation; eye disorders; skin disor-
ders; urinary-tract infections; wounds.*

Bivalem *Bergamo, Braz.*
Mebendazole (p.102·2).
Worm infections.

Bi-Vaspit *Asche, Ger.*
Fluocortin butyl (p.1071·3); isoconazole nitrate
(p.387·2).
Nappy rash.

Bivate *Douglas, NZ.*
Betamethasone valerate (p.1063·2).
Skin disorders.

Biviol *Nourypharma, Ger.*
Desogestrel (p.1470·3); ethinylestradiol (p.1476·2).
Biphasic oral contraceptive.

Biviraten
Swisspharm, S.Afr.; Berna, Switz.†.
A measles and mumps vaccine (p.1548·3).
Active immunisation.

Bivitasi *ISI, Ital.*
Cocarboxylase (p.1385·2).
Vitamin B₁ deficiency.

Bivitox *Terapeutico, Ital.*
Cogalactoisomerase disodium (p.1598·1).
Liver disorders.

B-Ject *Hyrex, USA.*
Vitamin B substances (p.1350·1).
Parenteral nutrition.

BK *3M, NZ.*
Bath oil; lotion: Liquid paraffin (p.1407·1); oil-soluble
dewaxed lanolin fraction (p.1410·3).
Dry skin disorders.

Liquid soap: Lactic acid (p.1626·2).
Soap substitute in skin disorders.

BK HC *3M, NZ.*
Hydrocortisone (p.1073·3).
Skin disorders.

B-kombin
Leiras, Fin.; ACO, Swed.
Vitamin B substances (p.1350·1).
Vitamin B deficiency.

Black Seeds *Be-Tabs, S.Afr.*
Nutritional supplement (p.1350·1).

Black-Draught *Chattem, USA.*
Syrup: Casanthranol (p.1216·1); senna (p.1248·2); rhubarb (p.1248·1).

Tablets; oral granules: Senna (p.1248·2).
Constipation.

**Blackmores Pregnancy & Breastfeeding
Formula** *Blackmores, Austral.*
Omega-3 marine triglycerides; dunaliella salina; min-
erals; vitamins (p.1350·1).
Dietary supplement.

Blackmores for Women Bio Iron *Blackmores, Austral.*
Ferrous fumarate (p.1360·1); folic acid; vitamin C; vitamin B₁₂; urtica (p.1350·1).
Iron deficiency.

Blackmores for Women PMT *Blackmores, Austral.*
Vitamins; minerals; viburnum; ginseng; bladderwrack
(p.1350·1).
Premenstrual syndrome.

Blackmores for Women Total Calcium *Blackmores, Austral.*
Calcium citrate (p.1188·1); calcium phosphate
(p.1188·3); calcium amino acid chelate; minerals; vitamins (p.1350·1).
Calcium deficiency.

Blackoids du Docteur Meur *SERP, Mon.*
Menthol (p.1632·3); liquorice (p.1231·2).
Sore throat.

Bladder Irritation *Hylands, Canad.*
Homoeopathic preparation.

Bladderon *Shinyaku, Jpn.*
Flavoxate hydrochloride (p.467·1).
Pollakisuria.

Bladuril *Hoechst Marion Roussel, Mex.*
Flavoxate hydrochloride (p.467·1).
Urinary-tract disorders.

Blairex Lens Lubricant *Blairex, USA.*
Range of solutions for soft contact lenses (p.1129·2).

Blancaler *Galderma, Mex.*
Cream: Titanium dioxide (p.1126·1).

Topical gel: Achillea (p.1572·2).

Skin hyperpigmentation.

Blandonal *Falqui, Ital.*
Passion flower (p.1649·1); crataegus (p.1600·2).
Insomnia.

Blanoxan *Bristol-Myers Squibb, Mex.*
Bleomycin sulfate (p.511·3).
Malignant neoplasms.

Blasen- und Nierentee
Note.This name is used for preparations of different composition.
Sanova, Aust.
Bearberry (p.1583·3); equisetum (p.1606·3); birch leaf (p.1585·2).
Kidney and bladder disorders.

Sanova, Aust.
Bearberry (p.1583·3); equisetum (p.1606·3); birch leaf (p.1585·2); java tea (p.1625·1); maté leaf (p.1681·1).
Kidney and bladder disorders.

Blasen-Nieren-Tee Stada *Stada, Ger.†.*
Couch-grass (p.1599·3); ononis (p.1644·1); solidago virgaurea; liquorice (p.1231·2); betulae (p.1585·2).
Urinary-tract infections.

Blasen-Tee *Mayrhofer, Ger.*
Bearberry (p.1583·3); herniaria (p.1619·2); juniper (p.1625·2); ononis (p.1644·1); parsley root (p.1648·3); peppermint leaf (p.1243·2).
Kidney and bladder disorders.

Blasentee *Smetana, Aust.*
Birch leaf (p.1585·2); herniaria (p.1619·2); equisetum (p.1606·3); calluna vulgaris.
Kidney and bladder disorders.

Blastocarb *Lemery, Mex.*
Carboplatin (p.515·1).
Malignant neoplasms.

Blastoestimulina *Almirall, Spain.*
Eye drops: Centella (p.1112·2).
Eye disorders.

Ointment; medicated dressing: Centella (p.1112·2); neomycin sulfate (p.228·1).
Burns; skin infections; ulcers; wounds.

Pessaries: Centella (p.1112·2); clodantoin (p.382·1); metronidazole (p.594·1); neomycin sulfate (p.228·1); polymyxin B sulfate (p.238·1).
Vulvovaginal infections.

Topical aerosol: Centella (p.1112·2); amethocaine [tetracaine] (p.1305·2).
Burns; ulcers; wounds.

Blastolem *Lemery, Mex.*
Cisplatin (p.525·1).
Malignant neoplasms.

Blaston *Lacer, Spain.*
Cinitapride acid tartrate (p.1220·1).
Gastro-oesophageal reflux; gastroparesis.

Blastovin *Teva, Israel.*
Vinblastine sulfate (p.577·3).
Malignant neoplasms.

Bledilait *Bledina, Fr.*
A range of infant feeds (p.1350·1).
Allergic disorders; diarrhoea; regurgitation.

Blef-10 *Allergan, Mex.*
Sulfacetamide sodium (p.250·3).
Eye infections.

Blefamide SF *Allergan, Mex.*
Sulfacetamide sodium (p.250·3); prednisolone acetate (p.1078·1).
Eye disorders.

Blefarida *Alcon, Port.†; Alcon Cusi, Spain.*
Chloramphenicol (p.179·1); cortisone acetate (p.1065·3).
Infected eye disorders.

Blefarolin *Bruschettini, Ital.*
Tannic acid (p.1669·1); resorcinol (p.1122·2); menthol (p.1632·3).
Eye disorders.

Blefcon
Note.This name is used for preparations of different composition.
Alcon, Ger.
Sulfacetamide sodium (p.250·3); prednisolone acetate (p.1078·1).
Allergic and inflammatory disorders of the eye.

Allergan, Swed.†.
Sulfacetamide sodium (p.250·3); prednisolone acetate (p.1078·1); phenylephrine hydrochloride (p.1097·1).
Blepharitis.

Blemaren N *Esparma, Ger.*
Citric acid (p.1596·2); anhydrous sodium citrate (p.1186·2); potassium bicarbonate (p.1186·1).
Hyperuricaemia; porphyria cutanea tarda; renal calculi.

Blemerase *Young, USA.*
Benzoyl peroxide (p.1111·1).
Acne.

Bleminol *Gepepharm, Ger.*
Allopurinol (p.397·2).
Gout; hyperuricaemia; renal calculi.

Blemish Control *Kay, Canad.*
Salicylic acid (p.1122·3).
Acne.

Blemix *Ashbourne, UK.*
Minocycline hydrochloride (p.224·3).
Bacterial infections.

Blendox *Degorts, Mex.*
Chlorpheniramine [chlorphenamine] (p.412·2).

Blenox *Antibioticos, Spain.*
Amoxicillin (p.149·2).
Probenecid (p.401·3) is included in this preparation to reduce renal tubular excretion of amoxicillin.
Bacterial infections.

Blenoxane
Bristol-Myers Squibb, Austral.; Bristol-Myers Squibb, Braz.; Bristol, Ca-

---

nad.; Bristol-Myers Squibb, NZ; Bristol-Myers Squibb, S.Afr.; Bristol-Myers Squibb Oncology, USA.
Bleomycin sulfate (p.511·3).
Malignant neoplasms.

Bleo
Kayaku, Jpn; Kyowa, UK.
Bleomycin hydrochloride (p.512·3) or bleomycin sulfate (p.511·3).
Malignant neoplasms.

Bleo-cell *Cell Pharm, Ger.*
Bleomycin sulfate (p.511·3).
Malignant neoplasms.

Bleolem
Lemery, Mex.; Lemery, Thai.
Bleomyin sulfate (p.511·3).
Malignant neoplasms.

Bleo-S *Kayaku, Jpn.*
Bleomycin sulfate (p.511·3).
Skin cancer.

Bleph-10
Allergan, Austral.; Allergan, Hong Kong; Allergan, NZ; Allergan, S.Afr.; Allergan, Thai.; Allergan, USA.
Sulfacetamide sodium (p.250·3).
Eye infections.

Bleph-10 Liquifilm *Allergan, Canad.†.*
Sulfacetamide sodium (p.250·3).
Eye infections.

Blephagel
Thea, Fr.; Pharmacia Upjohn, Singapore.
Eyelid cleanser.

Blephamide
Note.This name is used for preparations of different composition.
Allergan, Austral.; Allergan, Austral.; Allergan, Hong Kong; Allergan, Israel; Allergan, NZ; Allergan, S.Afr.; Allergan, Singapore.
Eye drops: Sulfacetamide sodium (p.250·3); prednisolone acetate (p.1078·1); phenylephrine hydrochloride (p.1097·1).
Blepharitis; conjunctivitis.

Allergan, Canad.; Allergan, Ger.; Allergan, Israel; Allergan, NZ; Allergan, Switz.; Allergan, USA.
Eye drops; eye ointment: Sulfacetamide sodium (p.250·3); prednisolone acetate (p.1078·1).
Formerly contained sulfacetamide sodium, phenazone, sodium thiosulfate, prednisolone acetate, and phenylephrine hydrochloride in *Switz.*
Blepharitis; conjunctivitis.

Bleukawine *Ern, Spain†.*
Homatropine methylbromide (p.468·1); kava (p.1625·3); methylene blue [methylthioninium chloride] (p.1012·3).
Urinary-tract infections.

Blifamol *Allergan, Port.*
Sulfacetamide sodium (p.250·3); prednisolone acetate (p.1078·1); phenylephrine hydrochloride (p.1097·1).
Infected eye disorders.

Blinkene *Allergan-Frumtost, Braz.*
Polyoxyl 40; macrogol 300 (p.1630·3) (p.1129·2).
Cleansing solution for contact lens.

Blinx *Pilkington Barnes-Hind, USA.*
Electrolytes (p.1180·1).
Eye irrigation.

Blio *Faulding, Port.*
Bleomycin sulfate (p.511·3).

BlisterGard *Medtech, USA.*
Topical barrier preparation.

Blistex *Blistex, USA.*
Camphor (p.1589·3); phenol (p.1152·3); allantoin (p.1110·1).
Oral lesions.

Blistex Aloe & Vitamin E *Key, Austral.†.*
Padimate O (p.1518·2); vitamin E acetate (p.1394·1); aloe vera (p.1110·1).
Dry lips; sunscreen.

Blistex DCT Lip Balm *Blistex, Canad.*
SPF 15: Padimate O (p.1518·2); oxybenzone (p.1518·1); menthol (p.1632·3); phenol (p.1152·3); camphor (p.1589·3).
Chapped lips; sunscreen.

Blistex Faceblock *Key, Austral.†.*
SPF15+: Octinoxate (p.1517·3); meradimate (p.1517·3); oxybenzone (p.1518·1).
Sunscreen.

Blistex Lip Balm
Note.This name is used for preparations of different composition.
Blistex, Canad.
SPF 10: Padimate O (p.1518·2); oxybenzone (p.1518·1); dimethicone (p.1410·1).
Chapped lips; sunscreen.

Blistex, USA.
SPF 10: Camphor (p.1589·3); phenol (p.1152·3); allantoin (p.1110·1); dimethicone (p.1410·1); padimate O (p.1518·2); oxybenzone (p.1518·1).
Chapped lips; sunscreen.

Blistex Lip Ointment
Note.This name is used for preparations of different composition.
Blistex, Canad.
Allantoin (p.1110·1); camphor (p.1589·3); phenol (p.1152·3).
Chapped lips; herpes labialis.

Blistex, Hong Kong.
Allantoin (p.1110·1); camphor (p.1589·3); phenol (p.1152·3); menthol (p.1632·3).
Chapped lips; herpes labialis.

Blistex Lip Revitalizer *Key, Austral.*
SPF 15: Octinoxate (p.1517·3); oxybenzone (p.1518·1).
Dry lips; sunscreen.

Blistex Lip Tone
Note.This name is used for preparations of different composition.
Key, Austral.
SPF 18: Octinoxate (p.1517·3); oxybenzone (p.1518·1).
Dry lips; sunscreen.

Blistex, Canad.
SPF 15: Padimate O (p.1518·2); meradimate (p.1517·3); dimethicone (p.1410·1).
Chapped lips; sunscreen.

Blistex Medicated Lip Balm *Key, Austral.*
SPF 16: Padimate O (p.1518·2); oxybenzone (p.1518·1).
Dry lips; sunscreen.

Blistex Medicated Lip Conditioner *Key, Austral.*
SPF 15+†: Yellow soft paraffin (p.1407·3); padimate O (p.1518·2); oxybenzone (p.1518·1).

SPF 20: Octinoxate (p.1517·3); oxybenzone (p.1518·1).
Dry lips; sunscreen.

Blistex Medicated Lip Conditioner Jar *Blistex, Canad.*
SPF15: Camphor (p.1589·3); menthol (p.1632·3); meradimate (p.1517·3); padimate O (p.1518·2); phenol (p.1152·3).
Chapped lips; herpes labialis.

Blistex Medicated Lip Conditioner Tube *Blistex, Canad.*
SPF 15: Padimate O (p.1518·2); oxybenzone (p.1518·1); camphor (p.1589·3).
Sunscreen.

Blistex Medicated Lip Ointment *Key, Austral.*
SPF 15: Padimate O (p.1518·2); oxybenzone (p.1518·1); allantoin (p.1110·1); camphor (p.1589·3).
Dry lips; sunscreen.

Blistex Ultra *Blistex, USA.*
SPF 30: Octinoxate (p.1517·3); oxybenzone (p.1518·1); octisalate (p.1518·1); methyl anthranilate; homosalate (p.1517·2).
Sunscreen.

Blistex Ultra Lip Balm
Key, Austral.; Blistex, Canad.
SPF 30: Octinoxate (p.1517·3); oxybenzone (p.1518·1); octisalate (p.1518·1); meradimate (p.1517·3); homosalate (p.1517·2).
Chapped lips; sunscreen.

Blisteze *DDD, UK.*
Strong ammonia solution (p.1579·1); ammonia solution aromatic; phenol (p.1152·3).
Chapped and cracked lips; herpes labialis.

Blis-To-Sol *Chattem, USA.*
Topical liquid: Tolnaftate (p.395·2).

Topical powder: Zinc undecenoate (p.395·3).
Formerly contained benzoic acid and salicylic acid.
Fungal skin infections.

Blocadren
Merck Sharp & Dohme, Aust.; Frosst, Austral.†; Merck Sharp & Dohme, Belg.; Merck Frosst, Canad.; Merck Sharp & Dohme, Hong Kong; Merck Sharp & Dohme, Irl.†; Merck Sharp & Dohme, Ital.; Merck Sharp & Dohme, Mex.; Merck Sharp & Dohme, Neth.†; Merck Sharp & Dohme, Norw.; Merck Sharp & Dohme, Port.; Merck Sharp & Dohme, S.Afr.; Merck Sharp & Dohme, Swed.; Merck Sharp & Dohme, Switz.; Merck Sharp & Dohme, UK†; Merck, USA.
Timolol maleate (p.982·1).
Angina pectoris; arrhythmias; glaucoma; hypertension; migraine; myocardial infarction; ocular hypertension.

Blocan *Grossman, Mex.*
Cimetidine (p.1216·3).

Blocanol *Merck Sharp & Dohme, Fin.*
Timolol maleate (p.982·1).
Angina pectoris; glaucoma; hypertension; migraine; myocardial infarction; ocular hypertension.

Blocatril *Tecnofarma, Mex.*
Enalapril (p.883·3).
Hypertension.

Blocotenol *Azupharma, Ger.*
Atenolol (p.841·3).
Angina pectoris; arrhythmias; hypertension.

Blocotenol comp *Azupharma, Ger.*
Atenolol (p.841·3); chlortalidone (p.857·1).
Hypertension.

Blodex *Estedi, Spain.*
Vegetable oil (p.1679·2).
Adjunct in cholecystography and cholangiography.

Blokium
Sintesa, Belg.; Probios, Port.; Almirall, Spain.
Atenolol (p.841·3).
Angina pectoris; arrhythmias; hypertension; myocardial infarction.

Blokium Diu
Probios, Port.; Almirall, Spain.
Chlortalidone (p.857·1); atenolol (p.841·3).
Hypertension.

Bloktus *Pisa, Mex.*
Benzonatate (p.1085·3).

Blopress
Takeda, Aust.; Takeda, Ger.; Takeda, Ital.; Seber, Port.; Takeda, Switz.; Takeda, Thai.
Candesartan cilexetil (p.853·2).
Hypertension.

Bluboro *Allergan Herbert, USA.*
Aluminium sulfate (p.1578·2); calcium acetate (p.1187·3).
Bruises; skin inflammation.

Bluco *Hua, Thai.*
Codeine phosphate (p.25·2); brompheniramine maleate (p.410·2); pseudoephedrine hydrochloride (p.1099·2).
Coughs.

Bluderm *Quimioterapica, Braz.*
Boric acid (p.1586·1); glycerol (p.1616·3); quillaia (p.1348·2).
Skin disinfection.

Blue *Ambix, UK; Moore, USA.*
Pyrethrins; piperonyl butoxide (p.1436·2).
Pediculosis.

Blue Collyrium *Sabex, Canad.†.*
Methylene blue [methylthioninium chloride] (p.1012·3); naphazoline hydrochloride (p.1095·1).
Eye irritation.

Blue Flag Root Compound *Gerard House, UK.*
Blue flag root (p.1624·2); lappa (p.1627·1); sarsaparilla (p.1661·1).
Minor skin disorders.

Blue Gel Muscular Pain Reliever *Rugby, USA†.*
Menthol (p.1632·3).

Bluesteril *IMS, Ital.*
Benzalkonium chloride (p.1133·2).
Instrument disinfection.

Bluetest
Quidel, Fr.†; Farmatrading, Port.†.
Pregnancy or fertility test (p.1654·3).

Blumen *Luper, Braz.*
Cod-liver oil (p.1357·2); boric acid (p.1586·1); zinc oxide (p.1128·2).
Barrier preparation; skin disorders.

Blunorm *Pharma-Natura, Ital.*
Hesperidin (p.1611·2); diosmin (p.1611·1); vitamin C (p.1389·3).
Nutritional supplement in vascular disorders.

Blutal *Dainippon, Jpn†.*
Chondroitin sulfate-iron colloid (p.1357·1).
Iron-deficiency anaemia.

Blutquick Forte *Duopharm, Ger.*
Ferrous gluconate (p.1360·2); vitamin B substances (p.1350·1).
Iron deficiency; tonic.

Blutquick Forte S *Duopharm, Ger.*
Ferrous fumarate (p.1360·1); ferric sodium citrate; ferrous gluconate (p.1360·1).
Iron-deficiency anaemia.

BM-Accutest
Roche Diagnostics, Irl.; Roche Diagnostics, UK.
Test for glucose in blood (p.1616·3).
For use with Accutrend blood glucose meters.

BM-Hopitest *Roche Diagnostics, UK.*
Test for protein, glucose, ketones, and blood in urine.

BM-Test 1-44
Roche Diagnostics, Irl.; Roche Diagnostics, NZ; Roche Diagnostics, UK.
Test for glucose in blood (p.1616·3).
Formerly known as BM-Test Glycemie 1-44 in the *UK.*

BM-Test 3
Boehringer Mannheim Diagnostics, Irl.†; Roche Diagnostics, UK.
Test for pH, protein, and glucose in urine.

BM-Test 4
Boehringer Mannheim Diagnostics, Irl.†; Roche Diagnostics, UK.
Test for pH, protein, glucose, and nitrite in urine.

BM-Test 7
Boehringer Mannheim Diagnostics, Irl.†; Roche Diagnostics, UK.
Test for pH, protein, glucose, ketones, urobilinogen, bilirubin, and blood in urine.

BM-Test 8
Boehringer Mannheim Diagnostics, Irl.†; Roche Diagnostics, UK.
Test for nitrite, pH, protein, glucose, ketones, urobilinogen, bilirubin, and blood in urine.

BM-Test BG
Roche Diagnostics, Austral.; Roche Diagnostics, Ital.; Roche Diagnostics, UK.
Test for glucose in blood (p.1616·3).

BM-Test Glycemie *Roche Diagnostics, Fr.*
Test for glucose in blood (p.1616·3).

BM-Test Glycemie 20-800 *Roche Diagnostics, Austral.*
Test for glucose in blood (p.1616·3).

BM-Test GP
Roche Diagnostics, Austral.; Roche Diagnostics, UK.
Test for glucose and protein in urine.

BM-Test 5L
Boehringer Mannheim Diagnostics, Irl.†; Roche Diagnostics, UK.
Test for pH, protein, glucose, ketones, and blood in urine.

BM-Test LN *Roche Diagnostics, Fr.*
Test for leucocytes and nitrites in urine.

BM-Test Meconium *Roche Diagnostics, UK.*
Test for cystic fibrosis by detection of albumin in the meconium.

BN *3M, UK.*
Turpentine oil (p.1676·3); strong ammonia (p.1579·1); ammonium chloride (p.1085·2).
Musculoskeletal and joint disorders; pain.

BN 53 *Staufen, Ger.*
Homoeopathic preparation.

BNIL *Masa, Thai.*
Glibenclamide (p.321·3).
Diabetes mellitus.

Bo-Cal *Fibertone, USA.*
Calcium with vitamins B and D, and magnesium (p.1350·1).

The symbol † denotes a preparation no longer actively marketed

Bocasan Oral-B, Irl.†; Oral-B, UK.
Sodium perborate (p.1156·3).
Oral hygiene.

Bocytin Asian Pharm, Thai.
Carbocisteine (p.1086·3).
Respiratory-tract disorders.

Bodaril Byk Elmu, Spain.
Inosine pranobex (p.627·2).
Viral infections.

Bodigarde Lifeplan, UK.
Vitamins, fish oils, borage oil, and garlic oil (p.1350·1).
Nutritional supplement.

Bodisan Medinfar, Port.†
Amoxicillin trihydrate (p.149·2).
Bacterial infections.

Bodivitin Hua, Thai.
Multivitamin preparation with calcium (p.1350·1).

Body Progest, Ital.
Barrier gel.

Body Lotion Hamilton, Austral.
Chlorhexidine gluconate (p.1138·2); glycerol (p.1616·3); light liquid paraffin (p.1407·2).
Emollient.

Body Wash Hamilton, Hong Kong.
Light liquid paraffin (p.1407·2).
Skin disorders.

Bodyguard Sanitalia, Ital.
Echinacea (p.1606·2); salix (p.82·1); devil's claw root (p.26·3); propolis (p.1655·1).
Nutritional supplement.

Boflavin Milano, Thai.
Riboflavin (p.1386·1).
Vitamin B2 deficiency.

Bogil Llorente, Spain.
Aminohydroxybutyric acid (p.342·2).
Behaviour disorders; emotional disorders; epilepsy.

Bo-Gum Solvay, Ital.†
Cetylpyridinium chloride (p.1138·1); sorbic acid (p.1157·1); bioflavonoids (p.1611·1).
Oral hygiene.

Bogumil-tassenfertiger milder Abfurtee Enzypharm, Aust.
Sambucus (p.1660·3); equisetum (p.1606·3); urtica (p.1678·2); chamomile (p.1593·2); tilia (p.1673·2).
Constipation; dyspepsia; flatulence.

Boi K BOI, Spain.
Potassium ascorbate (p.1195·2).
Potassium depletion.

Boi K Aspartico BOI, Spain.
Potassium ascorbate (p.1195·2).
Potassium depletion.

Boil Ease
Note. This name is used for preparations of different composition.
Del, Canad.
Benzocaine (p.1306·2); ichthammol (p.1115·2); sulfur (p.1123·3); cade oil (p.1124·3); camphor (p.1589·3); phenol (p.1152·3); zinc oxide (p.1128·2); thymol (p.1158·3).
Del, USA; Commerce, USA.
Benzocaine (p.1306·2); ichthammol (p.1115·2); sulfur (p.1123·3); cade oil (p.1124·3); camphor (p.1589·3); phenol (p.1152·3); zinc oxide (p.1128·2); thymol (p.1158·3); menthol (p.1632·3); eucalyptus oil (p.1609·2).
Boils.

Bok-C-Lin Brovar, S.Afr.†
Doxycycline hyclate (p.200·1).
Bacterial infections.

Bolchipen Cruz, Spain.
Amoxicillin trihydrate (p.149·2).
Bacterial infections.

Bolcitol Lesourd, Fr.
Fumitory (p.1612·3); boldo (p.1585·3); sage (p.1660·2); fennel (p.1610·1).
Biliary disorders; gastrointestinal disorders; kidney disorders.

Boldex Potter's, UK.
Taraxacum (p.1669·1); butternut bark; boldo (p.1585·3); bladderwrack (p.1585·2).
Formerly called Boldo.
Slimming aid.

Boldigan UCI, Braz.
Acetylmethionine; cynara (p.1601·3); solanum paniculatum; boldo (p.1585·3); liver extract.
Liver disorders.

Boldina He Teofarma, Ital.
Boldine (p.1585·3); aloin (p.1210·2).
Constipation.

Boldo Larkhall Laboratories, UK.
Boldo (p.1585·3); clivers (p.1596·3); bearberry (p.1583·3); bladderwrack (p.1585·2); taraxacum (p.1669·1).

Boldo Jurubeba Prima, Braz.
Boldo (p.1585·3); solanum paniculatum.
Liver disorders.

Boldo N "Hanosan" Hanosan, Ger.†
Homoeopathic preparations.

Boldobeba Medquimica, Braz.
Cascara (p.1216·1); boldo (p.1585·3); solanum paniculatum; choline (p.1356·2); vitamin B1 (p.1385·2).
Liver disorders.

Boldocynara N Bioforce, Switz.
Cynara (p.1601·3); silybum marianum (p.1021·3); taraxacum (p.1669·1); boldo (p.1585·3); peppermint leaf (p.1243·2).
Digestive disorders.

Boldoflorine
Note. This name is used for preparations of different composition.
Exflora, Fr.; Exflora, Switz.†
Tablets: Boldine (p.1585·3); senna (p.1248·2); frangula bark (p.1227·1); rosemary.
Constipation.
Exflora, Switz.†
Herbal tea: Senna (p.1248·2); boldo (p.1585·3); rosemary; peppermint leaf (p.1243·2); fraxinus excelsior; corylus avellana leaf; castanea vulgaris; frangula bark (p.1227·1); apple; coriander (p.1599·2); elecampane (p.1089·3); liquorice (p.1231·2).
Constipation.

Boldolaxin Diviser Aquilea, Spain.
Belladonna (p.463·1); bisacodyl (p.1212·2); boldo leaves (p.1585·3); calcium phosphate (p.1188·3); docusate sodium (p.1223·1).
Bowel evacuation; constipation.

Boldopeptan Neo Quimica, Braz.
Cascara (p.1216·1); boldo (p.1585·3); rhubarb (p.1248·1); liver extract.
Liver disorders.

Boldosal Ern, Spain.
Boldine (p.1585·3); inosine (p.1623·3); magnesium sulfate (p.1191·1); sodium bicarbonate (p.1186·2); dibasic sodium phosphate (p.1193·2); sodium sulfate (p.1250·1).
Constipation; hepatobiliary disorders.

Bolinan Nicholas, Fr.
Povidone (p.1503·2).
Gastrointestinal disorders.

Bolo Eagle, Austral.†
Vitamin, mineral and amino-acid preparation with eleutherococcus senticosis (p.1350·1).
Tonic.

Boltin Organon, Spain.
Tibolone (p.1495·3).
Menopausal disorders.

Bolus Eucalypti Comp
Weleda, Aust.; Weleda, UK.
Homoeopathic preparation.

Bolutol ICN, Spain.
Gemfibrozil (p.896·2).
Hyperlipidaemias.

Bolvidon Organon, Israel.
Mianserin hydrochloride (p.298·1).
Depression.

B-OM OM, Switz.
Cyanocobalamin; sorbitol; yeast (p.1350·1).
Tonic.

B-OM Forte OM, Switz.
Cyanocobalamin; nicotinamide; sorbitol; yeast (p.1350·1).
Tonic.

Boma Ogna, Ital.
Borax (p.1586·1); benzocaine (p.1306·2).
Nausea; oral hygiene.

Bomacorin Hevert, Ger.
Crataegus (p.1600·2).
Cardiac disorders.

Bomagall forte S Hevert, Ger.†
Ammi visnaga; atropin sulf.; carduus marianus; taraxacum; shepherd's purse (p.1662·3); cnicus benedictus (p.1597·2); herb. chelidonii; echinacea; echinaceae pallidea (p.1606·2).
Painful and spastic biliary disorders.

Bomagall mono Hevert, Ger.
Fumitory (p.1612·3).
Smooth muscle spasm.

Bomaklim Hevert, Ger.
Homoeopathic preparation.

Bomapect Hevert, Ger.†
Homoeopathic preparation.

Bomix Bode, Ger.
Clorophene (p.1142·3); orthophenylphenol (p.1152·1); chlorocresol (p.1141·3).
Instrument disinfection.

Bonactin Almed, Switz.†
Zinc sulfate (p.1398·2); heparin sodium (p.902·1).
Herpesvirus infections.

Bonadoxina Pfizer, Mex.
Meclozine hydrochloride (p.420·3); pyridoxine hydrochloride (p.1386·3).
Nausea and vomiting; vertigo.

Bonalfa Schering-Plough, Mex.; Isdin, Spain.
Tacalcitol (p.1124·2).
Psoriasis.

Bonamine Pfizer, Canad.; Pfizer, Ger.†; Pfizer, Thai.
Meclozine hydrochloride (p.420·3).
Motion sickness; vestibular disorders.

Bonasanit Biokanol, Ger.
Pyridoxine hydrochloride (p.1386·3).
Vitamin B deficiency.

Bonased-L Dolorgiet, Ger.†
Lupulus (p.1629·3).
Nervous disorders; sleep disorders.

Bonavit QIF, Braz.
Multivitamin and mineral preparation (p.1350·1).

Bonceur Rolab, S.Afr.
Verapamil hydrochloride (p.989·1).
Angina; arrhythmias.

Bondil Vivus, Norw.; Astra, Swed.
Alprostadil (p.1439·3).
Erectile dysfunction.

Bondiol Gry, Ger.
Alfacalcidol (p.1391·1).
Osteomalacia; osteoporosis; renal osteodystrophy.

Bondormin Rafa, Israel.
Brotizolam (p.657·2).
Insomnia.

Bondronat Boehringer Mannheim, Aust.; Roche, Denm.; Roche, Fin.; Roche, Fr.; Roche, Ger.; Roche Diagnostics, Spain; Roche, Swed.; Roche, Switz.; Roche, Thai.
Sodium ibandronate (p.753·2).
Hypercalcaemia of malignancy; osteolytic bone metastases.

Bone Plus Tishcon, Hong Kong.
Calcium carbonate (p.1215·1); ergocalciferol (p.1391·2).
Calcium supplement.

Bo-Ne-Ca ST, Thai.
Calcium carbonate (p.1215·1).
Calcium deficiency.

Bonefos Fresenius Kabi, Aust.; Rhone-Poulenc Rorer, Austral.; UCB, Belg.; Rhodia, Braz.; Rhone-Poulenc Rorer, Canad.; AstraZeneca, Denm.; Leiras, Fin.; Astra, Ger.; Medac, Ger.; Boehringer Ingelheim, Irl.; Leiras, Israel; Schering, Neth.; Leiras, Norw.; Schering, Port.; Schering, Singapore; Schering, Spain; Astra, Swed.; Astra, Switz.; Schering, Thai.; Boehringer Ingelheim, UK.
Disodium clodronate (p.751·2).
Hypercalcaemia of malignancy; osteolysis of malignancy.

Bongreen Korea Green Pharm, Singapore.
Alfacalcidol (p.1391·1).
Osteoporosis; vitamin D metabolic disorders.

Boniderma Bioethical, Ital.
Fluocinolone acetonide (p.1071·1).
Skin disorders.

Bonidon Mepha, Singapore; Mepha, Switz.
Indometacin (p.66·1).
Aluminium glycinate (p.1210·3) may be included in the tablets in an attempt to limit adverse effects on the gastrointestinal mucosa.
Gout; inflammation; musculoskeletal, joint, and periarticular disorders; pain.

Bonifen Merck, Mex.; Merck, Port.
Pyritinol hydrochloride (p.1657·1).
Cerebrovascular disorders; mental function disorders.

Bonine Pfizer Consumer, USA.
Meclozine hydrochloride (p.420·3).
Motion sickness; vertigo.

Bonjela
Note. This name is used for preparations of different composition.
Reckitt & Colman, Austral.; Reckitt & Colman, Hong Kong; Reckitt Benckiser, Irl.; Reckitt & Colman, Israel; Reckitt Benckiser, NZ; Reckitt Benckiser, S.Afr.; Reckitt & Colman, Singapore; Reckitt & Colman, Thai.; Reckitt & Colman, UK.
Oral gel: Choline salicylate (p.24·3); cetalkonium chloride (p.1137·1).
Oral pain and irritation.
Reckitt & Colman, UK.
Pastilles: Lignocaine [lidocaine] hydrochloride (p.1313·2); aminoacridine hydrochloride (p.1130·2).
Mouth ulcers.

Bonlax Synthelabo, Ital.†
Cascara (p.1216·1).
Constipation.

Bonningtons Irish Moss
Note. This name is used for preparations of different composition.
SmithKline Beecham Consumer, Austral.
Carrageenan (p.1500·1); camphor (p.1589·3); menthol (p.1632·3).
Coughs; sore throat.
SmithKline Beecham, NZ.
Menthol (p.1632·3); camphor (p.1589·3); liquorice (p.1231·2); carrageenan (p.1500·1).
Coughs.

Bonomint Intercare, UK.
Yellow phenolphthalein (p.1244·1).
Constipation.

Bon-One Teijin, Thai.
Alfacalcidol (p.1391·1).
Chronic renal failure; hypoparathyroidism; osteomalacia; osteoporosis; rickets.

Bonserin Rafa, Israel.
Mianserin hydrochloride (p.298·1).
Depression.

Bontril Carnrick, USA.
Phendimetrazine tartrate (p.1513·3).
Obesity.

Bonyl Orion, Denm.
Naproxen (p.60·3).
Inflammation; musculoskeletal and joint disorders; pain.

Boost Mead Johnson Nutritionals, USA.
Preparation for enteral nutrition (p.1350·1).

Boostrix GlaxoSmithKline, Austral.; SmithKline Beecham, Ger.
An adsorbed diphtheria, tetanus, and pertussis vaccine (p.1537·3).
Active immunisation.

Boots Covering Cream Boots, UK†.
A covering cream.
Concealment of birth marks, scars, and disfiguring skin disease.

Boots Dental Pain Relief Boots, UK.
Paracetamol (p.71·2); dihydrocodeine tartrate (p.33·1).
Dental pain.

Boots Hayfever Relief Antihistamine Boots, UK.
Terfenadine (p.424·3).
Formerly known as One-a-Day Antihistamine.
Hypersensitivity reactions.

Boots Medicated Pain Relief Plaster Boots, UK.
Camphor (p.1589·3); methyl salicylate (p.55·1); menthol (p.1632·3).
Muscle and soft-tissue pain.

Boots Tension Headache Relief Boots, UK.
Paracetamol (p.71·2); doxylamine succinate (p.417·1); caffeine (p.761·3); codeine phosphate (p.25·2).
Tension headache.

Boots Vapour Rub Boots, UK.
Eucalyptus oil (p.1609·2); camphor (p.1589·3); turpentine oil (p.1676·3); menthol (p.1632·3); thymol (p.1158·3); pumilio pine oil (p.1656·3).

B.O.P. Pautrat, Fr.
Olive leaf; birch leaf (p.1585·2).
Oedema.

Boracelle Swiss Herbal, Canad.†; Bio-Oil Research, UK.
Borage oil (p.1613·1).
Dietary supplement.

Boradren Ciba Vision, Spain.
Boric acid (p.1586·1); phenylephrine hydrochloride (p.1097·1); borax (p.1586·1).
Eye irritation.

Boradrine
Note. This name is used for preparations of different composition.
Bournonville, Belg.†
Borax (p.1586·1); boric acid (p.1586·1); phenylephrine hydrochloride (p.1097·1).
Eye irritation.
Bournonville, Neth.†
Phenylephrine hydrochloride (p.1097·1).
Congestion.

Boralina Veritas, Braz.
Tannic acid (p.1669·1); iodine (p.1522·3); thymol (p.1158·3); salicylic acid (p.1122·3); borax (p.1586·1); boric acid (p.1586·1).
Skin disorders.

Boraline Abello, Spain.
Phenylephrine hydrochloride (p.1097·1).
Eye irritation.

Borato de Sodio Eurofarma, Braz.
Zinc sulfate (p.1398·2); boric acid (p.1586·1); naphazoline hydrochloride (p.1095·1).
Ocular congestion.

Borbalan Spyfarma, Spain.
Amoxicillin trihydrate (p.149·2).
Bacterial infections.

Borea Roche, Spain.
Megestrol acetate (p.1481·2).
Breast cancer; endometrial cancer.

Born Lichtwer, Ger.†
Crataegus (p.1600·2).
Cardiac disorders.

Bornilene Euphar, Ital.
Xibornol (p.270·1).
Mouth and throat infections.

Borocaina Wassermann, Ital.
Benzyl alcohol (p.1135·2); sodium benzoate (p.1134·3).
Mouth and throat disinfection.

Borocaina Gola Wassermann, Ital.
Cetylpyridinium chloride (p.1138·1).
Mouth and throat disinfection.

Borocarpin-S Winzer, Ger.
Pilocarpine hydrochloride (p.1422·3).
Glaucoma; production of miosis.

Borocell Neutron Technology, USA.
Sodium monomercaptoundecahydro-closo-dodecaborate.
Glioblastoma multiforme.

Boroclarine Ciba Vision, Fr.
Borax (p.1586·1); boric acid (p.1586·1); phenylephrine hydrochloride (p.1097·1).
Conjunctivitis.

Borofair Otic Major, USA.
Acetic acid (p.1571·2); aluminium acetate (p.1578·1).

Borofax Warner-Wellcome, USA.
Zinc oxide (p.1128·2).
Formerly contained boric acid.
Skin irritation.

Boropak Glenwood, USA.
Aluminium sulfate (p.1578·2); calcium acetate (p.1187·3).
Inflammatory skin disorders.

Boro-Scopol Winzer, Ger.
Hyoscine borate (p.469·1).
Eye disorders; production of mydriasis.

Borossigeno Plus Stomatologico *Warner-Lambert, Ital.†.*
Sodium perborate (p.1156·3); benzethonium chloride (p.1134·2); borax (p.1586·1); boric acid (p.1586·1).
Oral hygiene.

Borostyrol
Note.This name is used for preparations of different composition.
ACP, Belg.
Ointment†: Thymol (p.1158·3); benzophenol salicylate; menthol (p.1632·3); boric acid (p.1586·1).
Burns; skin disorders; wounds.
Topical solution: Thymol (p.1158·3); benzophenol salicylate; menthol (p.1632·3); boric acid (p.1586·1); benzoin (p.1668·3).
Mouth disorders.

Mayoly-Spindler, Fr.
Cream: Thymol (p.1158·3); salol (p.82·2); menthol (p.1632·3).
Minor burns.
Topical solution: Thymol (p.1158·3); salol (p.82·2); menthol (p.1632·3); boric acid (p.1586·1); siam benzoin (p.1662·3).
Insect stings; minor skin and mouth disorders.

Borostyrol N *Uhlmann-Eyraud, Switz.*
Thymol (p.1158·3); salol (p.82·2); menthol (p.1632·3); Siam benzoin (p.1662·3).
Mouth disorders.

Borraginol-N *Takeda, Hong Kong.*
Benzocaine (p.1306·2); cinchocaine hydrochloride (p.1309·1); diphenhydramine hydrochloride (p.416·1); cetrimide (p.1137·1); lithiospermi radix.
Anorectal disorders.

Bosisto's Eucalyptus Inhalant *Felton, Austral.*
Eucalyptus oil (p.1609·2); menthol (p.1632·3).
Cold symptoms.

Bosisto's Eucalyptus Rub *Felton, Austral.*
Eucalyptus oil (p.1609·2); menthol (p.1632·3); methyl salicylate (p.55·1).
Muscular aches and pains.

Bosisto's Eucalyptus Spray *Felton, Austral.*
Eucalyptus oil (p.1609·2).
Muscular aches and pains.

Bosporon *Grunenthal, Spain.*
Lornoxicam (p.50·2).
Musculoskeletal and joint disorders; pain.

Boston
Polymer Technology, Canad.; Bausch & Lomb, Fr.†; Polymer Technology, USA.
Range of solutions for contact lenses (p.1129·2).

Boston Advance *Essilor, Aust.*
Storage solution for hard and gas permeable contact lens (p.1129·2).

Botox
Allergan, Aust.; Allergan, Austral.; Allergan, Belg.; Allergan-Frumtost, Braz.; Allergan, Canad.; Allergan, Denm.; Allergan, Fin.; Allergan, Ger.; Merz, Ger.; Allergan, Irl.; Allergan, Israel; Allergan, Ital.; Allergan, Jpn; Allergan, Mex.; Allergan, Norw.; Allergan, NZ; Allergan, S.Afr.; Allergan, Singapore; Allergan, Spain; Allergan, Swed.; Allergan, Switz.; Allergan, Thai.; Allergan, UK; Allergan, USA.
Botulinum A toxin (p.1324·2).
Blepharospasm; foot spasticity associated with paediatric cerebral palsy; hemifacial spasm; hyperhidrosis; spasmodic torticollis; strabismus.

Botropase *Ravizza, Ital.*
Batroxobin (p.726·3).
Haemorrhagic disorders.

Bottom Better *InnoVisions, USA.*
Yellow soft paraffin (p.1407·3); wool fat (p.1410·3).
Nappy rash.

Bouillet *Dietetique et Sante, Fr.*
Potassium chloride; calcium glutamate; adipic acid; glutamic acid; magnesium carbonate (p.1350·1).
Dietary salt substitute.

Bounty Bears *Nature's Bounty, USA.*
A range of vitamin preparations (p.1350·1).

Bourget *Medipharma, Ger.†.*
Sodium citrate (p.1186·2); sodium bicarbonate (p.1186·2); tartaric acid (p.1669·2).
Gastrointestinal tract disorders.

Bovisan D5 *Sanum-Kehlbeck, Ger.*
Homoeopathic preparation.

Bowa *Nakorn, Thai.*
Aluminium hydroxide gel (p.1210·3); magnesium hydroxide (p.1233·1); simeticone (p.1249·2).
Flatulence; gastric hyperacidity; peptic ulcer.

Boxazin plus C *Boehringer Ingelheim, Ger.*
Aspirin (p.14·2); ascorbic acid (p.1389·3).
Cold symptoms; fever; inflammation; pain.

Boxocalm *Boxo, Ger.*
Valerian (p.1678·3); lupulus (p.1629·3).
Anxiety; insomnia.

Boxol *Rovi, Spain.*
Dalteparin sodium (p.865·3).
Deep vein thrombosis; thrombosis prophylaxis.

Boxolip *Boxo, Ger.*
Loperamide hydrochloride (p.1231·3).
Diarrhoea.

Boyol Salve *Pfeiffer, USA.*
Ichthammol (p.1115·2); benzocaine (p.1306·2).
Skin disorders.

B-Plex *Stanley, Canad.*
Vitamin B substances (p.1350·1).

B-Plex C *Stanley, Canad.*
Vitamin B substances and vitamin C (p.1350·1).

B-Plus
Volchem, Ital.
Multivitamin preparation (p.1350·1).
Nutritional supplement.

Biolab, Thai.
Vitamin B substances (p.1350·1).

Braccopiral *Rhone-Poulenc Rorer, Mex.*
Pyrazinamide (p.240·1).

Brachialin percutan N *Steigerwald, Ger.†.*
Diethylamine salicylate (p.32·2); benzyl nicotinate (p.20·2); methyl salicylate (p.55·1).
Bruising; lumbago; neuralgia; rheumatism; sciatica; sports injuries.

Brachiapas S *Pascoe, Ger.*
Homoeopathic preparation.

Brachont *Azupharma, Ger.†.*
Glycol salicylate (p.42·2); benzyl nicotinate (p.20·2).
Bruising; muscle and joint disorders.

Bradelmin *Degorts, Mex.*
Albendazole (p.95·2).
Worm infections.

Bradimox *Yamanouchi, Ital.*
Amoxicillin trihydrate (p.149·2).
Bacterial infections.

Bradoral *Novartis Consumer, Ital.*
Domiphen bromide (p.1143·3).
Mouth and throat disinfection.

Bradosol
Note.This name is used for preparations of different composition.
Novartis Consumer, Aust.
Domiphen bromide (p.1143·3); peppermint oil (p.1243·3); eucalyptus oil (p.1609·2); anise oil (p.1580·3).
Sore throat.

Novartis Consumer, Canad.
Hexylresorcinol (p.1146·3).
Sore throat.

Novartis Consumer, UK.
Benzalkonium chloride (p.1133·2).
Formerly contained domiphen bromide.
Sore throat.

Bradosol Plus *Novartis Consumer, UK.*
Domiphen bromide (p.1143·3); lignocaine [lidocaine] hydrochloride (p.1313·2).
Sore throat.

Bradyl *Lafon, Fr.*
Nadoxolol hydrochloride (p.937·2).
Arrhythmias.

Brady's-Magentropfen *Brady, Aust.*
Cinchona bark (p.1595·3); cinnamon (p.1595·3); aniseed (p.1580·2); coriander (p.1599·2); fennel (p.1610·1); myrrh (p.1639·2); santalum album; gentian (p.1615·1); zedoary.
Gastrointestinal disorders.

Bragg's *Brogg, UK.*
Activated charcoal (p.1000·2).
Dyspepsia; flatulence; heartburn.

Brainal *Andromaco, Spain.*
Nimodipine (p.946·1).
Mental function impairment; neurological deficit following subarachnoid haemorrhage.

Brainox *Euro-Labor, Port.*
Nimodipine (p.946·1).
Cerebral ischaemia due to ruptured cerebral aneurism.

Braintop *Exel, Belg.*
Piracetam (p.1652·1).
Alcohol withdrawal syndrome; mental function disorders.

Bralix *Remedica, Hong Kong.*
Chlordiazepoxide (p.659·2); clidinium bromide (p.465·1).
Dysmenorrhoea; gastrointestinal disorders; nocturnal enuresis; ureteral spasm.

Bramin-hepa *Merz, Ger.*
Isoleucine (p.1370·1); leucine (p.1370·3); valine (p.1381·3); pyridoxine hydrochloride (p.1386·3).
Hepatic encephalopathy.

BranchAmin *Clintec, USA.*
Amino-acid infusion (p.1350·1).
Parenteral nutrition in hepatic encephalopathy.

Brand- u. Wundgel-Medice N *Medice, Ger.*
Benzethonium chloride (p.1134·2); lauromacrogol 400 (p.1345·2); urea (p.1127·3).
Burns; insect stings; skin disorders; wounds.

Brand- und Wund-Gel Eu Rho *Eu Rho, Ger.*
Lignocaine [lidocaine] hydrochloride (p.1313·2); allantoin (p.1110·1); cetylpyridinium chloride (p.1138·1); dexpanthenol (p.1602·3).
Burns; insect stings; skin disorders; wounds.

Brandiazin *Medphano, Ger.*
Sulfadiazine silver (p.251·3).
Burns.

Branigen *Glaxo Wellcome, Ital.*
Acetylcarnitine hydrochloride (p.1572·1).
Cerebrovascular disorders; diabetic neuropathy; peripheral nerve disorders.

Branitil *OFF, Ital.*
Acetylcarnitine hydrochloride (p.1572·1).
Carnitine deficiency.

Branolind N *Hartmann, Ger.*
Peru balsam (p.1650·2).
Burns; skin disorders; wounds.

Brasivil *Stiefel, Ger.*
Aluminium oxide (p.1108·3).
Acne.

Brasivol
Stiefel, Austral.; Stiefel, Canad.; Stiefel, Fr.; Stiefel, Hong Kong; Stiefel, Irl.; Stiefel, UK; Stiefel, USA†.
Aluminium oxide (p.1108·3).
Acne.

Brassel *Searle, Ital.*
Citicoline sodium (p.1596·1).
Cerebrovascular disorders; parkinsonism.

Bratenol *Byk Elmu, Spain.*
Pirifibrate (p.956·3).
Arteriosclerosis; hyperlipidaemias.

Braudeide *Braun, Braz.*
Glutaral (p.1145·2).
Instrument disinfection.

Braunoderm
Note.This name is used for preparations of different composition.
Braun, Aust.; Braun, Belg.; Braun, Ger.; Braun, Irl.†; Braun, Ital.; Braun, Switz.
Povidone-iodine (p.1155·1); isopropyl alcohol (p.1149·2).
Skin disinfection; wounds.

Braun, Braz.; Braun, Spain.
Povidone-iodine (p.1155·1).
Skin and mucous membrane disinfection; wounds.

Braunol
Braun, Aust.; Braun, Belg.; Braun, Braz.; Braun, Ger.; Braun, Irl.†; Braun, Ital.; Braun, Spain; Braun, Switz.
Povidone-iodine (p.1155·1).
Skin, mucous membrane, and wound disinfection.

Braunosan
Braun, Irl.†; Braun, Switz.
Povidone-iodine (p.1155·1).
Hand and wound disinfection.

Braunosan H Plus *Braun, Switz.*
Povidone-iodine (p.1155·1).
Hand and skin disinfection.

Braunovidon
Sanova, Aust.; Braun, Ger.; Braun, Irl.†; Braun, Switz.
Povidone-iodine (p.1155·1).
Burns; infected skin disorders; skin ulcers; vaginal infections; wounds.

Braxan *Armstrong, Mex.*
Amiodarone hydrochloride (p.836·1).
Angina pectoris; arrhythmias.

Brazepam *Aspen, S.Afr.*
Bromazepam (p.656·3).
Anxiety.

Breacol *ICN, Hong Kong.*
Guaifenesin (p.1092·2).
Coughs; sore throat.

Breathe Eazy Chest Rub *Breathe Eazy, Austral.*
Adult formula: Grindelia (p.1618·2); cajuput oil (p.1588·1); thyme oil (p.1672·3); peppermint oil (p.1243·3); eucalyptus oil (p.1609·2).
Childrens formula: Grindelia (p.1618·2); cajuput oil (p.1588·1); thyme oil (p.1672·3); peppermint oil (p.1243·3).
Respiratory-tract congestion.

Breathe Free *Thompson, USA.*
Sodium chloride (p.1196·1).
Inflammation and dryness of nasal membranes.

Breatheze *Rolab, S.Afr.†.*
Salbutamol (p.770·3).
Now known as Rolab-Salbutamol.
Bronchospasm.

Bredon *Organon, Mex.*
Oxolamine citrate (p.1096·2).
Coughs.

Breezee Mist Antifungal *Pedinol, USA.*
Miconazole nitrate (p.391·1).
Fungal infections.
Tolnaftate (p.395·2).
Formerly contained aluminium chlorohydrate, menthol, and undecenoic acid.
Fungal skin infections.

Brefar *Forcaral, Mex.*
Paracetamol (p.71·2); phenylephrine hydrochloride (p.1097·1); chlorpheniramine [chlorphenamine] maleate (p.412·1).
Cold symptoms.

Brelomax *Abbott, Ger.*
Tulobuterol hydrochloride (p.785·2).
Obstructive airways disease.

Bremagen Flu *Promeco, Mex.*
Guaifenesin (p.1092·2); phenylephrine hydrochloride (p.1097·1); chlorpheniramine [chlorphenamine] maleate (p.412·1); paracetamol (p.71·2).
Respiratory-tract disorders.

Bremax
Abbott, Aust.; Abbott, Mex.
Tulobuterol hydrochloride (p.785·2).
Obstructive airways disease.

Bremide *AstraZeneca, Norw.*
Amoxicillin trihydrate (p.149·2); potassium clavulanate (p.187·2).
Otitis media.

Bremon *Pensa, Spain.*
Clarithromycin (p.186·2).
Bacterial infections.

Brenazol *Durascan, Denm.*
Miconazole nitrate (p.391·1).
Fungal infections.

Brenda-35 ED *Alphapharm, Austral.*
21 Tablets, cyproterone acetate (p.1467·3); ethinylestradiol (p.1476·2); 7 inert tablets.
Androgenisation in females; combined oral contraceptive.

Brennesseltonikum *Bioflora, Aust.*
Urtica (p.1678·2); taraxacum (p.1669·1); silver birch (p.1585·2).
Diuretic.

Brenoxil *Tecnofarma, Mex.*
Amoxicillin (p.149·2).
Bacterial infections.

Brentacort *Janssen-Cilag, Denm.*
Hydrocortisone (p.1073·3); miconazole nitrate (p.391·1).
Skin disorders with fungal infection.

Brentan
Note.This name is used for preparations of different composition.
Janssen-Cilag, Denm.
Miconazole (p.391·1) or miconazole nitrate (p.391·1).
Fungal infections.

Esteve, Spain.
Hydrocortisone (p.1073·3); miconazole nitrate (p.391·1).
Fungal infections with inflammation.

Breonesin *Sanofi Winthrop, USA.*
Guaifenesin (p.1092·2).
Coughs.

Bres *Farmacologico Milanese, Ital.*
Bromelains (p.1586·3); aescin (p.1574·1).
Peripheral vascular disorders.

Bresal *Berman, Mex.*
Phenylbutazone (p.78·1).

Bresben *Novartis, Ger.*
Atenolol (p.841·3); nifedipine (p.940·1).
Hypertension.

Brethaire *Novartis, USA†.*
Terbutaline sulfate (p.776·2).
Asthma; bronchospasm.

Brethine *Novartis, USA.*
Terbutaline sulfate (p.776·2).
Obstructive airways disease.

Bretylate
Glaxo Wellcome, Belg.; Glaxo Wellcome, Canad.; Wellcome, Irl.; Glaxo Wellcome, Israel; Glaxo Wellcome, UK†.
Bretylium tosilate (p.851·1).
Ventricular arrhythmias.

Bretylol
Boots, S.Afr.†; Du Pont, USA†.
Bretylium tosilate (p.851·1).
Ventricular arrhythmias.

Breva *Valeas, Ital.*
Salbutamol (p.770·3); ipratropium bromide (p.766·1).
Obstructive airways disease.

Brevibloc
Torrex, Aust.; Boots, Austral.; Baxter, Belg.; AstraZeneca, Canad.; Leiras, Denm.; Leiras, Fin.; Sigma-Tau, Fr.; Baxter, Ger.; Baxter, Hong Kong; Baxter, Irl.; Du Pont, Israel; Rhone-Poulenc Rorer, Mex.; Boots, NZ; Probios, Port.; Boots, S.Afr.; Du Pont, Singapore; Almirall, Spain; Schering, Swed.; Baxter Healthcare, Switz.; Baxter, UK; Ohmeda, USA.
Esmolol hydrochloride (p.887·1).
Hypertension; tachycardia.

Brevicon
Searle, Canad.; Searle, USA.
Norethisterone (p.1485·1); ethinylestradiol (p.1476·2).
28-Day packs also contain 7 inert tablets.
Combined oral contraceptive.

Brevilon *Roche Nicholas, Spain†.*
Passion flower (p.1649·1); valerian (p.1678·3).
Sedative.

Brevimytal *Lilly, Ger.*
Methohexital sodium (p.1263·2).
General anaesthesia.

Brevinaze *Intramed, S.Afr.*
Ketamine hydrochloride (p.1262·2).
General anaesthesia.

Brevinor
Searle, Austral.; Searle, Hong Kong; Searle, Irl.; Searle, NZ; Searle, S.Afr.†; Pharmacia, UK.
Norethisterone (p.1485·1); ethinylestradiol (p.1476·2).
28-Day packs also contain 7 inert tablets.
Combined oral contraceptive.

Brevital *Lilly, USA.*
Methohexital sodium (p.1263·2).
General anaesthesia.

Brevoxyl
Sanova, Aust.; Stiefel, Austral.; Stiefel, Fin.; Stiefel, Fr.; Stiefel, Ger.; Stiefel, Hong Kong; Stiefel, Irl.; Stiefel, NZ; Stiefel, Singapore; Sylak, Swed.; Stiefel, Thai.; Stiefel, UK; Stiefel, USA.
Benzoyl peroxide (p.1111·1).
Acne.

Brewers Yeast
Note.This name is used for preparations of different composition.
Jamieson, Canad.; Nature's Bounty, USA.
Vitamin B substances (p.1350·1).

Greater Pharma, Thai.
Dried yeast (p.1398·1).
Vitamin B deficiency.

Phillips Yeast, UK.
Yeast (p.1398·1); vitamin B substances (p.1350·1).

Brewers Yeast with Garlic *Phillips Yeast, UK.*
Yeast (p.1398·1); garlic (p.1614·1); vitamin B substances (p.1350·1).

The symbol † denotes a preparation no longer actively marketed

Brexecam Mer-National, S.Afr.
Piroxicam betadex (p.79·1).
Gout; musculoskeletal and joint disorders.

Brexicam Pharmacia Upjohn, Mex.
Piroxicam betadex (p.79·1).
Gout; inflammation; musculoskeletal, joint, and peri-articular disorders; pain.

Brexidol
Crystaal, Canad.; Nycomed, Denm.; Nycomed, Fin.; Pharmacia Upjohn, Ger.; Nycomed, Norw.; Nycomed, Swed.; Chiesi, Switz.; Trinity, UK.
Piroxicam betadex (p.79·1).
Gout; musculoskeletal, joint, and peri-articular disorders; pain.

Brexin
Note. A similar name is used for preparations of different composition (see below).
Pharmacia Upjohn, Aust.; Farmalab, Braz.; Robapharm, Fr.; Chiesi, Hong Kong; Chiesi, Ital.; Grunenthal, Port.; Chiesi, Singapore; Chiesi, Thai.
Piroxicam betadex (p.79·1).
Gout; inflammation; musculoskeletal, joint, and peri-articular disorders; pain.

Brexin LA Savage, USA.
Note. A similar name is used for preparations of different composition (see above).
Chlorpheniramine [chlorphenamine] maleate (p.412·1); pseudoephedrine hydrochloride (p.1099·2).
Cold symptoms.

Brexine
Christiaens, Belg.; Christiaens, Neth.
Piroxicam betadex (p.79·1).
Gout; musculoskeletal and joint disorders; pain.

Brexinil Andromaco, Spain.
Piroxicam betadex (p.79·1).
Gout; musculoskeletal, joint, and peri-articular disorders; pain.

Brexivel Master Pharma, Ital.
Piroxicam (p.79·1).
Musculoskeletal and joint disorders.

Brezal Novartis, Ital.
Choline alfoscerate (p.1416·2).
Mental function impairment in the elderly.

Briaziide Pierre Fabre, Fr.
Benazepril hydrochloride (p.843·2); hydrochlorothiazide (p.907·3).
Hypertension.

Bricalin Teva, Israel.
Terbutaline sulfate (p.776·2).
Obstructive airways disease.

Bricanyl
Astra, Aust.; Astra, Austral.; Astra, Belg.; Astra, Braz.; AstraZeneca, Canad.; AstraZeneca, Denm.; AstraZeneca, Fin.; AstraZeneca, Fr.; Stern, Ger.; Astra, Hong Kong; Astra, Irl.; Astra, Ital.; Astra, Mex.; Astra, Neth.; AstraZeneca, Norw.; AstraZeneca, NZ; Astra, Port.; AstraZeneca, Thai.; AstraZeneca, UK; Hoechst Marion Roussel, USA.
Terbutaline sulfate (p.776·2).
Obstructive airways disease; premature labour.

Bricanyl comp
Astra, Aust.; Astra, Ger.
Terbutaline sulfate (p.776·2); guaifenesin (p.1092·2).
Obstructive airways disease.

Bricanyl Composto Astra, Braz.
Terbutaline sulfate (p.776·2); guaifenesin (p.1092·2).
Obstructive airways disease.

Bricanyl EX Astra, Mex.
Terbutaline sulfate (p.776·2); guaifenesin (p.1092·2).
Obstructive airways disease.

Bricanyl Expectorant
Astra, Hong Kong; Astra, Irl.; AstraZeneca, Thai.
Terbutaline sulfate (p.776·2); guaifenesin (p.1092·2).
Obstructive airways disease.

Bridotrim Quimifar, Spain.
Co-trimoxazole (p.193·3).
Bacterial infections; Pneumocystis carinii pneumonia.

Briem Pierre Fabre, Fr.
Benazepril hydrochloride (p.843·2).
Hypertension.

Brietal
Lilly, Aust.; Lilly, Austral.; Lilly, Canad.; Lilly, Denm.†; Lilly, Irl.; Lilly, Israel; Lilly, Neth.; Lilly, Norw.†; Lilly, NZ; Aspen, S.Afr.; Lilly, Singapore; Lilly, Swed.; Lilly, Switz.; Lilly, UK†.
Methohexital sodium (p.1263·2).
General anaesthesia.

Brinaldix Novartis, Ger.
Clopamide (p.863·1).
Hypertension; oedema.

Brinerdin
Novartis, Aust.; Wander, Neth.†; Novartis, S.Afr.; Novartis, Thai.
Clopamide (p.863·1); dihydroergocristine mesilate (p.1603·2); reserpine (p.967·3).
Hypertension.

Brinerdina
Novartis, Ital.; Padro, Spain.
Clopamide (p.863·1); dihydroergocristine mesilate (p.1603·2); reserpine (p.967·3).
Hypertension.

Brinerdine
Novartis, Port.; Novartis, Switz.
Clopamide (p.863·1); dihydroergocristine mesilate (p.1603·2); reserpine (p.967·3).
Hypertension.

Brintoverilte Nycomed, Denm.
Hydrogen peroxide (p.1147·1).
Mouth infections; oral disinfection.

Briocor Upsamedica, Ital.
Carnitine (p.1356·1).
Carnitine deficiency; myocardial ischaemia.

Briofil Teofarma, Ital.
Bamifylline hydrochloride (p.761·2).
Bronchospasm.

Briogen ABC, Ital.
Levoglutamide (p.1365·2); DL-phosphoserine; cyanocobalamin (p.1388·1).
Tonic.

Brionil Vita, Spain.
Nedocromil sodium (p.768·3).
Asthma.

Brioschi Brioschi, Canad.
Sodium bicarbonate (p.1186·2).

Briovitan Montefarmaco, Ital.
Multivitamin and mineral preparation with flavonoids (p.1350·1).
Nutritional supplement.

Briscocough Quatromed, S.Afr.†
Diphenhydramine hydrochloride (p.416·1); ammonium chloride (p.1085·2); sodium citrate (p.1186·2).
Coughs.

Briscopyn Quatromed, S.Afr.†
Paracetamol (p.71·2); caffeine (p.761·3); meprobamate (p.691·1); codeine phosphate (p.25·2).
Formerly contained paracetamol, caffeine, and meprobamate.
Pain with tension.

Briscotrim Brissenco, S.Afr.†
Co-trimoxazole (p.193·3).
Bacterial infections.

Briserin N Novartis, Ger.
Clopamide (p.863·1); reserpine (p.967·3).
Hypertension.

Brisfirina Bristol-Myers, Spain.
Cefapirin sodium (p.164·2).
Lignocaine [lidocaine] (p.1313·2) is included in the intramuscular injection to alleviate the pain of injection.
Bacterial infections.

Brisfirina Balsamica Bristol-Myers, Spain†.
Cefapirin (p.164·2); niaouli oil (p.1640·2); guaifenesin (p.1092·2).
Respiratory-tract infections.

Brismucol Bristol-Myers Squibb, Mex.
Acebrophylline.
Respiratory-tract disorders.

Brisoral Bristol-Myers, Spain.
Cefprozil (p.173·2).
Bacterial infections.

Brisovent Bialfar, Port.
Fluticasone propionate (p.1072·2).
Asthma.

Brispen Bristol-Myers Squibb, Mex.
Dicloxacillin (p.199·1).
Bacterial infections.

Bristaciclina Pharmacia Upjohn, Spain†.
Tetracycline hydrochloride (p.258·3).
Bacterial infections.

Bristaciclina Dental Pharmacia Upjohn, Spain.
Benzydamine hydrochloride (p.20·1); chymotrypsin (p.1595·1); tetracycline hydrochloride (p.258·3); trypsin (p.1675·3).
Mouth and upper respiratory-tract infections.

Bristacol Bristol-Myers, Spain.
Pravastatin sodium (p.957·3).
Hypercholesterolaemia; myocardial infarction.

Bristaflam Bristol-Myers Squibb, Mex.
Aceclofenac (p.11·1).
Inflammation; musculoskeletal, joint and peri-articular disorders; pain.

Bristamox
Bristol-Myers Squibb, Fr.; Bristol-Myers Squibb, Swed.†
Amoxicillin (p.149·2) or amoxicillin trihydrate (p.149·2).
Bacterial infections.

BrisTaxol Bristol-Myers Squibb, Mex.
Paclitaxel (p.563·2).
Breast cancer; ovarian cancer.

Bristopen Bristol-Myers Squibb, Fr.
Oxacillin sodium (p.233·2).
Bacterial infections.

Britacil Wyeth Lederle, Port.
Ampicillin (p.150·3).
Bacterial infections.

Britaject
Lilly, Neth.; Britannia Pharmaceuticals, UK.
Apomorphine hydrochloride (p.1163·1).
Parkinsonism.

Britane Martin, Fr.
Miconazole nitrate (p.391·1).
Fungal infections.

Britapen SmithKline Beecham, Spain.
Ampicillin sodium (p.150·3) or ampicillin trihydrate (p.151·1).
Bacterial infections.

Britiazim Thames, UK†.
Diltiazem hydrochloride (p.874·3).
Angina pectoris.

British Army Foot Powder Regal, Canad.
Boric acid (p.1586·1); formaldehyde (p.1144·2); salicylic acid (p.1122·3); zinc oxide (p.1128·2).
Tinea pedis.

Britlofex Britannia Pharmaceuticals, UK.
Lofexidine hydrochloride (p.1011·3).
Opioid withdrawal symptoms.

Brizolina Bristol-Myers, Spain.
Cefazolin sodium (p.164·3).
Lignocaine [lidocaine] (p.1313·2) is included in the intramuscular injection to alleviate the pain of injection.
Bacterial infections.

Broad Spectrum Sunblock Avon, Canad.
SPF15: Avobenzone (p.1517·1); octinoxate (p.1517·3); oxybenzone (p.1518·1).
Sunscreen.

Brochoprex Expectorant Kenyaku, Thai.
Diphenhydramine hydrochloride (p.416·1); guaifenesin (p.1092·2); bromhexine hydrochloride (p.1085·3).
Coughs.

Brocil Berman, Mex.
Chloramphenicol (p.179·1).
Bacterial infections.

Brocolan Berman, Mex.
Dextromethorphan (p.1087·3).

Brodil Ofimex, Mex.
Salbutamol (p.770·3).

Brofed Marnel, USA.
Pseudoephedrine hydrochloride (p.1099·2); brompheniramine maleate (p.410·2).
Upper respiratory-tract symptoms.

Broflex Alliance, UK.
Benzhexol [trihexyphenidyl] hydrochloride (p.463·3).
Drug-induced extrapyramidal disorders; parkinsonism.

Brogal Compositum Rayere, Mex.
Ambroxol hydrochloride (p.1084·3); clenbuterol hydrochloride (p.763·3).
Respiratory-tract disorders.

Brogal-T Rayere, Mex.
Ambroxol hydrochloride (p.1084·3); dextromethorphan hydrobromide (p.1087·3).
Coughs.

Brolene
Rhone-Poulenc Rorer, Austral.; Rhone-Poulenc Rorer, Irl.; Aventis, NZ; Genop, S.Afr.; Rhone-Poulenc Rorer, UK.
Dibromopropamidine isetionate (p.1143·1) or propamidine isetionate (p.1155·3).
Eye infections.

Brol-eze Rhone-Poulenc Rorer, UK.
Sodium cromoglicate (p.774·3).
Allergic conjunctivitis.

Brolin UCB, Spain.
Famotidine (p.1225·3).
Gastro-oesophageal reflux; peptic ulcer; Zollinger-Ellison syndrome.

Broluidan Kenfarma, Spain.
Letosteine (p.1094·1).
Respiratory-tract disorders.

Bromadine-DM Cypress, USA.
Brompheniramine hydrochloride; dextromethorphan hydrobromide (p.1087·3).
Coughs.

Bromalex Vitoria, Port.
Bromazepam (p.656·3).
Anxiety.

Bromalgina Climax, Braz.
Codeine diethylbarbiturate; dipyrone (p.34·1); methylhomatropine.
Painful muscle spasm.

Bromaline Rugby, USA†.
Phenylpropanolamine hydrochloride (p.1098·1); brompheniramine maleate (p.410·2).
Upper respiratory-tract symptoms.

Bromaline Plus Rugby, USA†.
Phenylpropanolamine hydrochloride (p.1098·1); brompheniramine maleate (p.410·2); paracetamol (p.71·2).
Upper respiratory-tract symptoms.

Bromam Durascan, Denm.
Bromazepam (p.656·3).
Anxiety.

Bromanate Alpharma, Singapore; Barre-National, USA†.
Phenylpropanolamine hydrochloride (p.1098·1); brompheniramine maleate (p.410·2).
Nasal congestion; sinusitis.

Bromarest DX Warner Chilcott, USA.
Brompheniramine maleate (p.410·2); pseudoephedrine hydrochloride (p.1099·2); dextromethorphan hydrobromide (p.1087·3).
Coughs and cold symptoms.

Bromatane DX Goldline, USA.
Pseudoephedrine hydrochloride (p.1099·2); brompheniramine maleate (p.410·2); dextromethorphan hydrobromide (p.1087·3).
Coughs.

Bromatapp Copley, USA†.
Phenylpropanolamine hydrochloride (p.1098·1); brompheniramine maleate (p.410·2).
Upper respiratory-tract symptoms.

Bromavon Hua, Thai.
Brompheniramine maleate (p.410·2); phenylephrine hydrochloride (p.1097·1); phenylpropanolamine hydrochloride (p.1098·1).
Nasal congestion.

Bromax Helfarma, Port.
Ambroxol hydrochloride (p.1084·3).
Respiratory-tract congestion.

Bromazanil Hexal, Ger.
Bromazepam (p.656·3).
Anxiety; insomnia; tension.

Bromaze Hexal, S.Afr.
Bromazepam (p.656·3).
Anxiety.

Bromazep CT, Ger.
Bromazepam (p.656·3).
Anxiety; insomnia.

Bromazolo Baldacci, Ital.
Methimazole [thiamazole] (p.1525·1); dibromotyrosine (p.1522·2).
Hyperthyroidism.

Bromed Kolassa, Aust.
Bromocriptine mesilate (p.1164·3).
Acromegaly; parkinsonism.

Bromergon Gea, Denm.; Lek, Thai.
Bromocriptine mesilate (p.1164·3).
Acromegaly; galactorrhoea; hypogonadism; lactation inhibition; mastalgia; menstrual disorders; parkinsonism; prolactinoma.

Bromesep Elixir Siam Bheasach, Thai.
Brompheniramine maleate (p.410·2); phenylephrine hydrochloride (p.1097·1); phenylpropanolamine hydrochloride (p.1098·1).
Hypersensitivity reactions of the respiratory tract.

Bromesep Expectorant Siam Bheasach, Thai.
Brompheniramine maleate (p.410·2); phenylephrine hydrochloride (p.1097·1); phenylpropanolamine hydrochloride (p.1098·1); guaifenesin (p.1092·2).
Coughs; hypersensitivity reactions of the respiratory tract.

Bromex
Qualiphar, Belg.; PP Lab, Thai.
Bromhexine hydrochloride (p.1085·3).
Bronchiectasis; obstructive bronchopneumonopathies; respiratory-tract disorders associated with increased mucus; sinusitis; Sjögren's syndrome.

Bromfed Muro, USA.
Brompheniramine maleate (p.410·2); pseudoephedrine hydrochloride (p.1099·2).
Allergic rhinitis; nasal congestion.

Bromfed-DM Muro, USA.
Brompheniramine maleate (p.410·2); pseudoephedrine hydrochloride (p.1099·2); dextromethorphan hydrobromide (p.1087·3).
Allergic rhinitis; coughs; vasomotor rhinitis.

Bromfed-PD Muro, USA.
Brompheniramine maleate (p.410·2); pseudoephedrine hydrochloride (p.1099·2).
Allergic rhinitis; nasal congestion rhinitis.

Bromfenex Ethex, USA.
Brompheniramine maleate (p.410·2); pseudoephedrine hydrochloride (p.1099·2).
Respiratory-tract disorders.

Bromidem Sandipro, Belg.
Bromazepam (p.656·3).
Anxiety; insomnia.

Bromidol Janssen-Cilag, Denm.†.
Bromperidol (p.657·1).
Psychoses.

Bromi-Lotion Gordon, USA.
Aluminium chlorohydrate (p.1110·2).
Bromidrosis; hyperhidrosis.

Bromo Madelon St Laurent, Canad.
Sodium bicarbonate (p.1186·2); citric acid (p.1596·2).

Bromo Seltzer
Note. This name is used for preparations of different composition.
Warner-Lambert, Canad.
Sodium citrate (p.1186·2).
Dyspepsia; gastric hyperacidity.

Warner-Lambert, USA.
Paracetamol (p.71·2).
Fever; pain.

Bromo Seltzer Effervescent Granules Warner-Lambert, USA.
Sodium bicarbonate (p.1186·2); paracetamol (p.71·2); citric acid (p.1596·2).
Hyperacidity.

Bromocod N Streuli, Switz.
Codeine phosphate (p.25·2); belladonna (p.463·3); drosera (p.1606·1); ipecacuanha (p.1093·1); opium (p.69·3); terpin hydrate (p.1101·2).
Coughs.

Bromocrel Hexal, Ger.
Bromocriptine mesilate (p.1164·3).
Acromegaly; hyperprolactinaemia; lactation inhibition; parkinsonism.

Bromofotyl Centrapharm, Belg.†
Pholcodine (p.1099·1); bromoform (p.1587·1); aconite (p.1572·3); cherry-laurel water; ipecacuanha (p.1093·1); tolu (p.1101·3).
Respiratory-tract disorders.

Bromohexal Hexal, Austral.
Bromocriptine mesilate (p.1164·3).
Acromegaly; hyperprolactinaemia; lactation inhibition; parkinsonism.

Bromo-Kin Irex, Fr.
Bromocriptine mesilate (p.1164·3).
Hyperprolactinaemia; parkinsonism.

Bromolactin *Sigma, Austral.*
Bromocriptine mesilate (p.1164·3).
Acromegaly; hyperprolactinaemia; lactation inhibition; parkinsonism.

Bromopar *Merck, Denm.*
Bromocriptine mesilate (p.1164·3).
Acromegaly; galactorrhoea; hypogonadism; lactation inhibition; mastalgia; menstrual disorders; parkinsonism; prolactinoma.

Bromophar *Qualiphar, Belg.*
Codeine phosphate (p.25·2).
Coughs.

Bromophen TD *Rugby, USA†.*
Phenylpropanolamine hydrochloride (p.1098·1); phenylephrine hydrochloride (p.1097·1); brompheniramine maleate (p.410·2).
Upper respiratory-tract symptoms.

Bromopirin *Novaquimica, Braz.*
Bromazepam (p.656·3); sulpiride (p.706·1).
Depression.

Bromosedan *Dovalle, Braz.*
Calcium bromide (p.1587·1); sodium bromide (p.1587·1); sparteine sulfate (p.1666·3); phenobarbital (p.355·1); belladonna (p.463·1).
Sedative.

Bromoson *Unison, Thai.*
Bromhexine hydrochloride (p.1085·3).
Respiratory-tract disorders associated with increased or viscous mucus.

Bromotiren *Baldacci, Ital.*
Dibromotyrosine (p.1522·2).
Hyperthyroidism.

Bromotuss with Codeine *Rugby, USA.*
Bromazine hydrochloride (p.410·1); codeine phosphate (p.25·2).
Coughs and cold symptoms.

Bromped *Hua, Thai.*
Brompheniramine maleate (p.410·2); phenylephrine hydrochloride (p.1097·1); phenylpropanolamine hydrochloride (p.1098·1).
Nasal congestion.

Bromphen *Schein, USA†.*
Phenylpropanolamine hydrochloride (p.1098·1); brompheniramine maleate (p.410·2).
Upper respiratory-tract symptoms.

Bromphen DX Cough *Muro, USA.*
Pseudoephedrine hydrochloride (p.1099·2); brompheniramine maleate (p.410·2); dextromethorphan hydrobromide (p.1087·3).
Coughs and cold symptoms.

Bromphenex *Ethex, Hong Kong.*
Brompheniramine maleate (p.410·2); pseudoephedrine hydrochloride (p.1099·2).
Rhinitis.

Brompheniramine Cough *Geneva, USA.*
Pseudoephedrine hydrochloride (p.1099·2); brompheniramine maleate (p.410·2); dextromethorphan hydrobromide (p.1087·3).
Coughs and cold symptoms.

Brompheniramine DC Cough *Geneva, USA†.*
Phenylpropanolamine hydrochloride (p.1098·1); codeine phosphate (p.25·2); brompheniramine maleate (p.410·2).
Coughs and cold symptoms.

Brom-PP *Jean-Marie, Hong Kong.*
Brompheniramine maleate (p.410·2); phenylephrine hydrochloride (p.1097·1); phenylpropanolamine hydrochloride (p.1098·1).
Respiratory-tract disorders.

Brom-Ramine Compound *Universal, Hong Kong.*
Brompheniramine maleate (p.410·2); phenylephrine hydrochloride (p.1097·1); phenylpropanolamine hydrochloride (p.1098·1).
Repiratory-tract disorders.

Bromselon *Tecnobio, Spain.*
Ebastine (p.417·2).
Hypersensitivity reactions.

Bromso *TO-Chemicals, Thai.*
Bromhexine hydrochloride (p.1085·3).
Respiratory-tract disorders associated with increased or viscous mucus.

Bromtine *Duopharma, Hong Kong.*
Bromocriptine (p.1166·2).
Acromegaly; hyperprolactinaemia; parkinsonism.

Bromtussia *Asian Pharm, Thai.*
Guaifenesin (p.1092·2); brompheniramine maleate (p.410·2); phenylpropanolamine hydrochloride (p.1098·1).
Nasal congestion.

Bromtussia DC *Asian Pharm, Thai.*
Guaifenesin (p.1092·2); brompheniramine maleate (p.410·2); phenylephrine hydrochloride (p.1097·1); codeine phosphate (p.25·2).
Coughs; nasal congestion.

Bromtussin *Shiwa, Thai.*
Brompheniramine maleate (p.410·2); phenylephrine hydrochloride (p.1097·1); phenylpropanolamine hydrochloride (p.1098·1).
Cold symptoms.

Bromuc *Klinge, Ger.*
Acetylcysteine (p.1082·3).
Respiratory-tract disorders associated with increased or viscous mucus.

Bromurex *Pisa, Mex.*
Pancuronium bromide (p.1338·2).
Competitive neuromuscular blocker.

Bromxin *Masa, Thai.*
Bromhexine hydrochloride (p.1085·3).
Respiratory-tract disorders.

Bromxine
Atlantic, Hong Kong; Atlantic, Singapore; Atlantic, Thai.; General Drugs, Thai.
Bromhexine hydrochloride (p.1085·3).
Respiratory-tract disorders associated with increased or viscous mucus.

Bron 6 *Capo Sole, Ital.*
Chestnut honey; propolis; althaea; erisimo; thyme; wild rose; niaouli oil (p.1350·1).
Food supplement; tonic.

Bronalide *Boehringer Ingelheim, Canad.†.*
Flunisolide (p.1070·3).
Asthma.

Bronalin Decongestant *SSL, UK.*
Pseudoephedrine hydrochloride (p.1099·2).
Nasal and sinus congestion.

Bronalin Dry Cough *SSL, UK.*
Dextromethorphan hydrobromide (p.1087·3); pseudoephedrine hydrochloride (p.1099·2).
Coughs.

Bronalin Expectorant *SSL, UK.*
Diphenhydramine hydrochloride (p.416·1); sodium citrate (p.1186·2); ammonium chloride (p.1085·2).
Coughs.

Bronalin Junior *SSL, UK.*
Diphenhydramine hydrochloride (p.416·1); sodium citrate (p.1186·2).
Formerly known as Bronalin Paediatric.
Coughs.

Broncal
Note. This name is used for preparations of different composition.
Pharmacobel, Belg.
Pholcodine (p.1099·1); ephedrine hydrochloride (p.1090·1); chlorpheniramine [chlorphenamine] maleate (p.412·1); sulfogaiacol (p.1101·1).
Coughs.

Novel, Ital.
Dextromethorphan hydrobromide (p.1087·3); sulfogaiacol (p.1101·1).
Coughs.

Broncalene *Martin, Fr.*
Pholcodine (p.1099·1); chlorpheniramine [chlorphenamine] maleate (p.412·1); sodium benzoate (p.1134·3).
Coughs.

Broncalene Nourisson *Martin, Fr.*
Chlorpheniramine [chlorphenamine] maleate (p.412·1); sodium benzoate (p.1134·3); tolu balsam (p.1101·3).
Coughs.

Broncasma
Berna, Belg.†; Berna, Hong Kong†; Berna, Port.†; Berna, Switz.†; Berna, Thai.
Pneumococcus I, II, III; Streptococcus; Staphylococcus; Moraxella catarrhalis; Gaffkya tetragena; Pseudomonas aeruginosa; Klebsiella pneumoniae (Friedlander); Haemophilus influenzae.
Chronic bronchitis; respiratory-tract infections.

Broncasmin Composto *Opofarm, Braz.*
Terbutaline sulfate (p.776·2); guaifenesin (p.1092·2).
Obstructive airways disease.

Broncaspin *Bayer, Ital.†.*
Guacetisal (p.1092·1).
Respiratory-tract disorders.

Broncatar
Note. This name is used for preparations of different composition.
Cazi, Braz.
Bromhexine hydrochloride (p.1085·3); thiocol.
Respiratory-tract congestion.

Kramer, Switz.
Carbocisteine (p.1086·3); promethazine hydrochloride (p.423·2).
Coughs; respiratory-tract congestion.

Broncelix *Warner-Lambert, NZ.*
Choline theophyllinate (p.763·3); guaifenesin (p.1092·2).
Coughs.

Bronch Eze *Pharmavite, Canad.*
Ephedrine hydrochloride (p.1090·1); ammonium chloride (p.1085·2).

Bronchalene
Aventis, Belg.
Syrup for adults and children: Pholcodine (p.1099·1); chlorpheniramine [chlorphenamine] maleate (p.412·1).

Rhone-Poulenc Rorer, Belg.†
Syrup for infants: Chlorpheniramine [chlorphenamine] maleate (p.412·1).
Coughs.

Bronchalin *Gubler, Switz.†.*
Ephedrine hydrochloride (p.1090·1); guaifenesin (p.1092·2); hyoscyamine sulfate (p.469·3); castanea vulgaris; drosera (p.1606·1); liquorice (p.1231·2); psyllium seed (p.1229·1); thyme (p.1672·2); belladonna (p.463·1); ipecacuanha (p.1093·1); sodium benzoate (p.1134·3).
Respiratory-tract disorders.

Bronchathiol
Aventis, Belg.; Martin, Fr.
Carbocisteine (p.1086·3).
Respiratory-tract disorders.

Bronchenolo *Maggioni, Ital.*
Pastilles: Cetylpyridinium chloride (p.1138·1).
Mouth and throat disinfection.

Syrup: Dextromethorphan hydrobromide (p.1087·3); sulfogaiacol (p.1101·1); ammonium acetate (p.1085·1).
Coughs.

Tablets: Dextromethorphan hydrobromide (adsorbed onto magnesium trisilicate) (p.1087·3).
Coughs.

Bronchenolo Antiflu *SmithKline Beecham, Ital.*
Paracetamol (p.71·2); ascorbic acid (p.1389·3).
Fever; pain.

Bronchex *Hilarys, Canad.*
Ammonium chloride (p.1085·2); ammonia (p.1579·1); ammonium carbonate (p.1085·2); glycerol (p.1616·3); liquorice (p.1231·2); menthol (p.1632·3); siberian fir oil; white pine compound.

Bronchial *Theralab, Canad.*
Ammonium chloride (p.1085·2); senega (p.1100·2); white pine compound.

Bronchial Mixture *Torbet Laboratories, UK.*
Squill (p.1100·3); ipecacuanha tincture (p.1093·1); ammonium bicarbonate (p.1085·1).
Coughs.

Bronchialbalsam *Ratiopharm, Ger.*
Pine needle oil; eucalyptus oil (p.1609·2).
Catarrh.

Bronchialtee N *TAD, Ger.*
Thyme (p.1672·2); hedera helix.
Bronchitis; catarrh.

Bronchiase *Lafare, Ital.*
Dextromethorphan hydrobromide (p.1087·3); sulfogaiacol (p.1101·1).
Coughs.

Bronchicough *Aventis, S.Afr.*
Cimicifuga (p.1595·2); pimpinella (p.1618·2); cowslip (p.1600·1); quebracho; thyme (p.1672·2); ephedrine hydrochloride (p.1090·1); menthol (p.1632·3); eucalyptus oil (p.1609·2); saponin.
Coughs.

Bronchicum
Note. This name is used for preparations of different composition.
Rhone-Poulenc Rorer, Neth.
Thyme (p.1672·2); cowslip root (p.1600·1); grindelia (p.1618·2); pimpinella root; anise oil (p.1580·3); eucalyptus oil (p.1609·2); menthol (p.1632·3); saponin.
Formerly marketed as Bronchicum Hoestsiroop.
Coughs.

Aventis, S.Afr.
Cimicifuga (p.1595·2); grindelia (p.1618·2); pimpinella; cowslip (p.1600·1); quebracho; thyme (p.1672·2); ephedrine hydrochloride (p.1090·1); menthol (p.1632·3); sodium bromide (p.1587·1); eucalyptus oil (p.1609·2); saponin.
Bronchitis.

Bronchicum Balsam mit Eukalyptusol *Rhone-Poulenc Rorer, Ger.*
Eucalyptus oil (p.1609·2); camphor (p.1589·3); oleum pini sylvestris.
Catarrh; cold symptoms.

Bronchicum Elixir N *Rhone-Poulenc Rorer, Ger.*
Grindelia (p.1618·2); pimpinella; cowslip root (p.1600·1); quebracho; thyme (p.1672·2).
Bronchial congestion; coughs.

Bronchicum Elixir Plus *Rhone-Poulenc Rorer, Ger.*
Thyme (p.1672·2); plantago lanceolata; cowslip root (p.1600·1).
Bronchial congestion; coughs.

Bronchicum Extra Sterk *Rhone-Poulenc Rorer, Neth.*
Ephedrine hydrochloride (p.1090·1); codeine phosphate (p.25·2); vegetable extracts.
Coughs.

Bronchicum Hustentee *Nattermann, Ger.†.*
Thyme (p.1672·2); fennel oil (p.1610·2); anise oil (p.1580·3); saponaria; liquorice (p.1231·2).
Coughs and cold symptoms; sore throat.

Bronchicum Medizinal-Bad *Rhone-Poulenc Rorer, Ger.*
Thyme oil (p.1672·3).
Bath additive; respiratory-tract disorders.

Bronchicum Mono Codein *Rhone-Poulenc Rorer, Ger.*
Codeine phosphate (p.25·2).
Coughs.

Bronchicum Pflanzlicher *Rhone-Poulenc Rorer, Ger.*
Thyme (p.1672·2); drosera (p.1606·1).
Cold symptoms; coughs.

Bronchicum Sekret-Loser *Rhone-Poulenc Rorer, Ger.*
Eucalyptus oil (p.1609·2); cowslip root (p.1600·1); thyme (p.1672·2).
Upper respiratory-tract disorders with viscous mucus.

Bronchicum Thymian *Rhone-Poulenc Rorer, Ger.*
Cowslip root (p.1600·1); thyme (p.1672·2).
Bronchitis; coughs.

Bronchicum Tropfen N *Rhone-Poulenc Rorer, Ger.*
Quebracho; saponaria; thyme (p.1672·2).
Bronchitis.

Bronchi-Do *Grasler, Ger.*
Homoeopathic preparation.

Bronchiflu *Aventis, S.Afr.*
Mepyramine maleate (p.421·1); menthol (p.1632·3); ammonium chloride (p.1085·2); paracetamol (p.71·2); phenylpropanolamine hydrochloride (p.1098·1).
Cold symptoms; coughs.

Bronchil *Siam Bheasach, Thai.*
Guaifenesin (p.1092·2); theophylline (p.777·2).
Obstructive airways disease.

Bronchilin *Flordis, Austral.*
Primrose; thyme (p.1672·2).
Coughs.

Bronchi-Pertu *Pekana, Ger.*
Homoeopathic preparation.

Bronchiplant
Note. This name is used for preparations of different composition.
Apotheke Heiligen Josef, Aust.
Balsam: Eucalyptus oil (p.1609·2); rosemary oil (p.1659·3); camphor (p.1589·3).
Coughs and cold symptoms.

Rosch & Handel, Aust.
Oral liquid; syrup: Thyme (p.1672·2); iceland moss; senega root (p.1100·2); bitter-orange peel (p.1644·2).
Catarrh; coughs.

Bronchiplant light *Rosch & Handel, Aust.*
Iceland moss; senega root (p.1100·2); thyme (p.1672·2); bitter-orange peel (p.1644·2).
Catarrh; coughs.

Bronchipret *Bionorica, Ger.*
Oral drops; oral liquid: Thyme (p.1672·2); hedera helix.
Bronchitis.
Pastilles: Thyme (p.1672·2).
Bronchitis; cold symptoms; coughs.
Tablets: Cowslip root (p.1600·1); thyme (p.1672·2).
Bronchitis.

Bronchisaft *Hilarys, Canad.†.*
Ammonia (p.1579·1); glycerol (p.1616·3); ipecacuanha (p.1093·1); menthol (p.1632·3); sodium citrate (p.1186·2).

Bronchisan *Disperga, Aust.*
Theophylline (p.777·2); ephedrine hydrochloride (p.1090·1).
Obstructive airways disease.

Bronchiselect *Dreluso, Ger.*
Homoeopathic preparation.

Bronchistop *Rhone-Poulenc Rorer, S.Afr.†.*
Pholcodine (p.1099·1); ephedrine hydrochloride (p.1090·1); mepyramine maleate (p.421·1); menthol (p.1632·3); cetrimide (p.1137·1).
Coughs.

Bronchitten *Medopharm, Ger.*
Thyme (p.1672·2).
Bronchial catarrh; bronchitis; coughs.

Bronchitten forte K *Medopharm, Ger.*
Thyme (p.1672·2); cowslip root (p.1600·1).
Upper respiratory-tract disorders with thickened secretions.

Broncho D *Sam-On, Israel.*
Diphenhydramine hydrochloride (p.416·1); ammonium chloride (p.1085·2).
Coughs; respiratory-tract congestion.

Broncho Fertiginhalat *Klinge, Ger.*
Salbutamol sulfate (p.770·3).
Obstructive airways disease.

Broncho Inhalat *Klinge, Ger.*
Salbutamol sulfate (p.770·3).
Obstructive airways disease.

Broncho Munal *Medice, Ger.; Abiogen, Ital.*
Lysates of Haemophilus infuenzae; Streptococcus pneumoniae; Klebsiella pneumoniae; Klebsiella ozaenae; Staphylococcus aureus; Streptococcus pyogenese; Streptococcus viridans; Moraxella catarrhalis.
Respiratory-tract infections.

Broncho Rub *Mathieu, Canad.*
Camphor (p.1589·3); menthol (p.1632·3); cajuput oil (p.1588·1); turpentine.

Broncho Saline *Blairex, USA.*
Sodium chloride (p.1196·1).
Diluent for bronchodilator solutions for inhalation.

Bronchobactan *Klinge, Ger.*
Lysate of: Staphylococcus aureus; Streptococcus mitis; Streptococcus pyogenes; Streptococcus pneumoniae; Klebsiella pneumoniae; Moraxella catarrhalis; Haemophilus influenzae.
Respiratory-tract infections.

Bronchobel *Pharmethic, Belg.*
Codeine (p.25·2); ephedrine hydrochloride (p.1090·1); sulfogaiacol (p.1101·1); sodium benzoate (p.1134·3).
Coughs.

Bronchobest *CT, Ger.*
Spike lavender oil (p.1667·1).
Bronchitis.

Bronchocal *Sam-On, Israel.*
Guaifenesin (p.1092·2).
Coughs.

Bronchocedin N *Strathmann, Ger.†.*
Anise oil (p.1580·3); eucalyptus oil (p.1609·2); peppermint oil (p.1243·3).
Catarrh.

Bronchocodin *Grossmann, Switz.†.*
Codeine phosphate (p.25·2); sodium benzoate (p.1134·3); tolu balsam (p.1101·3); senega root (p.1100·2); menthol (p.1632·3); star anise; peppermint oil (p.1243·3); liquorice (p.1231·2).
Coughs.

Bronchocort *Klinge, Ger.*
Beclometasone dipropionate (p.1061·2).
Obstructive airways disease.

Bronchocux *TAD, Ger.*
Budesonide (p.1064·2).
Asthma; bronchitis.

Bronchocyst *SmithKline Beecham, Fr.†.*
Carbocisteine (p.1086·3).
Respiratory-tract disorders associated with increased or viscous mucus.

The symbol † denotes a preparation no longer actively marketed

Bronchodermine Tissot, Fr.
Ointment: Eucalyptol (p.1609·2); guaiacol (p.1092·1); pine oil.
Formerly contained eucalyptol, guaiacol, pine oil, terpin hydrate, and terpineol.

Suppositories: Amylocaine hydrochloride (p.1306·1); eucalyptol (p.1609·2); guaiacol (p.1092·1); pine oil.
Formerly contained amylocaine hydrochloride, eucalyptol, guaiacol, and terpin hydrate.
Respiratory disorders.

Bronchodex D Prodemdis, Canad.†
Phenylpropanolamine hydrochloride (p.1098·1); chlorpheniramine [chlorphenamine] maleate (p.412·1); pheniramine maleate (p.422·3).

Bronchodex DM Prodemdis, Canad.†
Mepyramine maleate (p.421·1); dextromethorphan hydrobromide (p.1087·3); ammonium chloride (p.1085·2); menthol (p.1632·3); sodium citrate (p.1186·2).

Bronchodex Pastilles Prodemdis, Canad.
Domiphen bromide (p.1143·3).

Bronchodex Pastilles Antiseptiques Prodemdis, Canad.
Hexylresorcinol (p.1146·3).

Bronchodex Pediatrique Therapex, Canad.†
Pseudoephedrine hydrochloride (p.1099·2); pheniramine maleate (p.422·3); dextromethorphan hydrobromide (p.1087·3); guaifenesin (p.1092·2).

Bronchodex Vapo Theralab, Canad.
Camphor (p.1589·3); eucalyptus oil (p.1609·2); menthol (p.1632·3).

Bronchodil Asta Medica, UK†.
Reproterol hydrochloride (p.770·2).
Bronchospasm.

Bronchodine Pharmethic, Belg.
Codeine phosphate (p.25·2).
Coughs.

Bronchodual Boehringer Ingelheim, Fr.
Fenoterol hydrobromide (p.765·1); ipratropium bromide (p.766·1).
Obstructive airways disease.

Bronchodurat Eucalyptusol Pohl, Ger.
Eucalyptus oil (p.1609·2).
Bronchitis; cold symptoms.

Bronchodurat N Pohl, Ger.
Eucalyptus oil (p.1609·2); menthol (p.1632·3).
Bronchitis; cold symptoms.

Broncho-Euphyllin Byk Gulden, Ger.
Theophylline (p.777·2); ambroxol hydrochloride (p.1084·3).
Obstructive airways disease.

Broncho-Fips Lichtenstein, Ger.†
Acetylcysteine (p.1082·3).
Respiratory-tract disorders with viscous mucus.

Bronchofluid DP-Medica, Switz.†
Baby: Codeine phosphate (p.25·2); ephedrine hydrochloride (p.1090·1); guaifenesin (p.1092·2); belladonna (p.463·1); drosera (p.1606·1); hedera helix; plantago lanceolata; senega root (p.1100·2); thyme (p.1672·2).
Infant; Adult: Codeine phosphate (p.25·2); ephedrine hydrochloride (p.1090·1); guaifenesin (p.1092·2); belladonna (p.463·1); ipecacuanha (p.1093·1); drosera (p.1606·1); hedera helix; plantago lanceolata; senega root (p.1100·2); thyme (p.1672·2); cherry-laurel.
Coughs; laryngitis; sore throat.

Bronchoforton
Note. This name is used for preparations of different composition.
Sanofi Winthrop, Aust.; Plantorgan, Neth.†; Sodip, Switz.†.
Eucalyptus oil (p.1609·2); pine oil; peppermint oil (p.1243·3).
Cold and influenza symptoms.

Sanofi Synthelabo, Ger.
Capsules: Eucalyptus oil (p.1609·2); anise oil (p.1580·3); peppermint oil (p.1243·3).
Bronchitis; catarrh; sinusitis; throat disorders.

Ointment: Eucalyptus oil (p.1609·2); Norway spruce oil; peppermint oil (p.1243·3).
Catarrh; cold symptoms.

Oral liquid; oral drops: Hedera helix.
Bronchitis; sinusitis.

Bronchoforton Kinderbalsam Sanofi Synthelabo, Ger.
Eucalyptus oil (p.1609·2); pine needle oil.
Respiratory-tract disorders.

Bronchoforton-Solinat Sanofi Synthelabo, Ger.
Cations: sodium, potassium, magnesium, calcium; anions: chloride, sulfate, bicarbonate.
Respiratory-tract disorders.

Broncho-Grippol-DM Charton, Canad.
Dextromethorphan hydrobromide (p.1087·3).
Coughs.

Bronchokod Biogalenique, Fr.
Carbocisteine (p.1086·3).
Respiratory-tract disorders associated with increased or viscous mucus.

Bronchol Streuli, Switz.
Guaifenesin (p.1092·2).
Upper-respiratory-tract disorders.

Bronchol N DP-Medica, Switz.†
Guaifenesin (p.1092·2); ephedrine hydrochloride (p.1090·1); codeine phosphate (p.25·2); camphor (p.1589·1); eucalyptol (p.1609·2); anise oil (p.1580·3).
Coughs.

Broncholate
Note. This name is used for preparations of different composition.
Sam-On, Israel.
Diphenhydramine hydrochloride (p.416·1); phenylpropanolamine hydrochloride (p.1098·1).
Respiratory-tract disorders.

Sanofi Winthrop, USA.
Ephedrine hydrochloride (p.1090·1); guaifenesin (p.1092·2).
Coughs.

Broncholate Forte Sam-On, Israel.
Diphenhydramine hydrochloride (p.416·1); phenylpropanolamine hydrochloride (p.1098·1); codeine phosphate (p.25·2).
Respiratory-tract disorders.

Broncholate Plus Sam-On, Israel.
Diphenhydramine hydrochloride (p.416·1); phenylpropanolamine hydrochloride (p.1098·1); paracetamol (p.71·2).
Cold and influenza symptoms; rhinitis; sinusitis.

Broncholine TO-Chemicals, Thai.
Terbutaline sulfate (p.776·2).
Obstructive airways disease.

Bronchomed Pohl, Ger.†.
Eucalyptus oil (p.1609·2).
Bronchitis; cold symptoms.

Bronchopan DM Atlas, Canad.
Dextromethorphan hydrobromide (p.1087·3).

Bronchoparat Klinge, Ger.
Theophylline sodium glycinate (p.783·2).
Obstructive airways disease.

Broncho-pectoralis Medgenix, Belg.
Pholcodine (p.1099·1); diphenhydramine hydrochloride (p.416·1); ephedrine sulfate (p.1090·2); sulfogaiacol (p.1101·1); Desessartz fluidextract; red-poppy petal fluidextract.
Coughs and nasal congestion.

Bronchoped Adcock Ingram, S.Afr.
Terbutaline sulfate (p.776·2); ammonium chloride (p.1085·2); sodium citrate (p.1186·2).
Coughs with bronchospasm.

Bronchophen Rolab, S.Afr.
Theophylline (p.777·2).
Obstructive airways disease.

Bronchophylline Sam-On, Israel.
Theophylline (p.777·2); guaifenesin (p.1092·2).
Respiratory-tract disorders.

Bronchoprex Kenyaku, Thai.
Diphenhydramine hydrochloride (p.416·1); sodium citrate (p.1186·2); dextromethorphan hydrobromide (p.1087·3).
Respiratory-tract disorders.

Bronchopront Mack, Illert., Ger.; Mack, Hong Kong; Ferraz, Lynce, Port.; Mack, Singapore; Mack, Thai.
Ambroxol hydrochloride (p.1084·3).
Respiratory-tract disorders associated with increased or viscous mucus.

Bronchorectine au Citral Mayoly-Spindler, Fr.
Citral; guaiacol (p.1092·1); terpin hydrate (p.1101·2); oleum pini sylvestris; wild thyme oil.
Formerly contained citral, benzyl cinnamate, guaiacol, terpin hydrate, oleum pini sylvestris, and wild thyme oil.
Respiratory disorders.

Bronchoretard Klinge, Ger.
Theophylline (p.777·2).
Obstructive airways disease.

Broncho-Rivo Rivopharm, Switz.
Adult: Diphenhydramine hydrochloride (p.416·1); ammonium chloride (p.1085·2); sodium citrate (p.1186·2); menthol (p.1632·3).
Paediatric: Diphenhydramine hydrochloride (p.416·1); sodium citrate (p.1186·2); menthol (p.1632·3).
Coughs.

Bronchosan Bioforce, Switz.
Hedera helix; thyme (p.1672·2); pimpinella sax.; horehound (p.1094·2); liquorice (p.1231·2).
Bronchitis; coughs; influenza.

Bronchosedal Janssen-Cilag, Belg.
Oral liquid: Dextromethorphan hydrobromide (p.1087·3).

Syrup: Codeine phosphate (p.25·2).
Formerly contained cherry-laurel water, aconite tincture, codeine phosphate, and sodium benzoate.
Coughs.

Broncho-Sern Serturner, Ger.
Plantago lanceolata.
Coughs; inflammation of mouth and throat; respiratory catarrh.

Bronchosirum Bronchosirum, Canad.†
Phenylpropanolamine hydrochloride (p.1098·1); pheniramine maleate (p.422·3); mepyramine maleate (p.421·1); dextromethorphan hydrobromide (p.1087·3).

Bronchospasmin
Asta Medica, Aust.; Asta Medica, Ger.
Reproterol hydrochloride (p.770·2).

Bronchospasmine Asta Medica, Switz.
Reproterol hydrochloride (p.770·2).
Obstructive airways disease.

Bronchospray
Note. This name is used for preparations of different composition.
Tissot, Fr.†.
Guethol nicotinate (p.1092·3); guaifenesin (p.1092·2); eucalyptol (p.1609·2); pine oil; lavender oil (p.1627·2).
Formerly contained guethol nicotinate, guaifenesin, terpineol, eucalyptol, pine oil, and lavender oil.
Respiratory disorders.

Parke-Med, S.Afr.
Salbutamol (p.770·3).
Obstructive airways disease.

Bronchospray Novo Klinge, Ger.
Salbutamol (p.770·3).
Obstructive airways disease.

Bronchostop Metochem, Aust.
Capsules: Mentholum valerianicum; guaifenesin (p.1092·2); eucalyptus oil (p.1609·2); camphor (p.1589·3).
Formerly known as Nicogelat.
Coughs.

Ointment: Camphor (p.1589·3); menthol (p.1632·3); eucalyptus oil (p.1609·2); turpentine oil (p.1676·3); pumilio pine oil (p.1656·3); thyme oil (p.1672·3).
Catarrh; colds; cough; sore throat.

Oral drops: Guaifenesin (p.1092·2); thyme (p.1672·2); chamomile (p.1593·2); anise oil (p.1580·3).
Coughs.

Oral liquid: Ascorbic acid (p.1389·3); thyme (p.1672·2); althaea syrup (p.1577·1).
Catarrh; colds; cough; sore throat.

Spray: Sage tincture (p.1660·2); thyme tincture (p.1672·2); peppermint leaf tincture (p.1243·2).
Mouth and throat inflammation.

Bronchosyl Pharmalab, Canad.†
Ammonium chloride (p.1085·2); cocillana (p.1087·2).

Bronchosyx N Syxyl, Ger.
Liquorice (p.1231·2); thyme (p.1672·2).
Cold symptoms.

Broncho-Tulisan Eucalyptol Logeais, Fr.†.
Noscapine camsilate (p.1096·2); aspirin (p.14·2); eucalyptol (p.1609·2).
Coughs.

Bronchotussine Medichemie, Switz.
Butetamate citrate (p.1086·2); codeine phosphate (p.25·2).
Coughs.

Broncho-Tyrosolvetten Tosse, Ger.; Roland, Ger.; Byk Gulden, Ger.
Cetylpyridinium chloride (p.1138·1); ammonium chloride (p.1085·2); liquorice (p.1231·2).
Mouth and throat infections; respiratory-tract catarrh.

Broncho-Vaxom
Byk, Aust.; Fournier, Belg.; Byk Gulden, Ger.; Byk Gulden, Ital.; Knoll, Mex.; OM, Port.; OM, Switz.
Lysate of: *Haemophilus influenzae; Streptococcus pneumoniae; Klebsiella pneumoniae; Klebsiella ozaenae; Staphylococcus aureus; Streptococcus pyogenes; Streptococcus viridans; Moraxella catarrhalis.*
Respiratory-tract infections.

Bronchowern Wernigerode, Ger.
Ambroxol hydrochloride (p.1084·3).
Respiratory-tract disorders with viscous mucus.

Bronchozone Drug Trading, Canad.†
Ammonium chloride (p.1085·2); ammonium carbonate (p.1085·1); liquorice (p.1231·2); menthol (p.1632·3); senega (p.1100·2).
Coughs.

Bronchyteine Knoll, Fr.†
Carbocisteine (p.1086·3).
Coughs.

Bronchytuc Knoll, Fr.†
Dextromethorphan hydrobromide (p.1087·3).
Formerly known as Bronchydex.
Coughs.

Broncivent Boehringer Ingelheim, Spain.
Beclometasone dipropionate (p.1061·2).
Asthma.

Bronclear Polipharm, Thai.
Bromhexine hydrochloride (p.1085·3).
Respiratory-tract disorders associated with increased or viscous mucus.

Broncleer Adcock Ingram, S.Afr.
Diphenhydramine hydrochloride (p.416·1); ammonium chloride (p.1085·2); sodium citrate (p.1186·2).
Coughs.

Broncleer with Codeine Adcock Ingram, S.Afr.; Propan, S.Afr.
Codeine phosphate (p.25·2); diphenhydramine hydrochloride (p.416·1); ammonium chloride (p.1085·2); sodium citrate (p.1186·2).
Coughs.

Broncmel La-Sante, Braz.
Grindelia (p.1618·2); aniseed (p.1580·2); senega (p.1100·2); rosa gallica (p.1029·1); thyme (p.1672·2); honey (p.1366·2).
Coughs.

Bronco Aseptilex Wasserman, Spain†.
Sulfadiazine (p.251·1); guaiacol cinnamate (p.1092·1).

Bronco Aseptilex Fuerte Wasserman, Spain.
Bromhexine hydrochloride (p.1085·3); co-trimoxazole (p.193·3); guaiacol cinnamate (p.1092·1).
Respiratory-tract infections.

Bronco Asmol Herbes Universelles, Canad.
Ammonium bicarbonate (p.1085·1); anethole (p.1580·1); tolu balsam (p.1101·3); camphor (p.1589·3); squill (p.1100·3).

Bronco Bactifor Andromaco, Spain.
Bromhexine (p.1085·3); co-trimoxazole (p.193·3).
Respiratory-tract infections.

Bronco Cilimox Baldassari, Braz.
Amoxicillin (p.149·2); bromhexine hydrochloride (p.1085·3).
Bacterial infections.

Bronco Lizom Pensa, Spain†.
Haemophilus influenzae; Klebsiella pneumoniae; Staphylococcus aureus; Streptococcus pyogenes; Streptococcus pneumoniae; Moraxella catarrhalis.
Respiratory-tract infections.

Bronco Medical Medical, Spain.
Sulfogaiacol (p.1101·1); dextromethorphan hydrobromide (p.1087·3).
Coughs.

Bronco Pensusan Wasserman, Spain†.
Ampicillin sodium (p.150·3); ampicillin benzathine (p.151·3); bromhexine hydrochloride (p.1085·3).
Lignocaine [lidocaine] hydrochloride (p.1313·2) is included in this preparation to alleviate the pain of injection.
Respiratory-tract infections.

Bronco Sergo Inexfa, Spain.
Tolu balsam (p.1101·3); bromhexine hydrochloride (p.1085·3); sodium benzoate (p.1134·3); co-trimoxazole (p.193·3).
Respiratory-tract infections.

Bronco Tonic Vir, Spain.
Amoxicillin trihydrate (p.149·2); bromhexine (p.1085·3).
Respiratory-tract infections.

Bronco-Amoxil SmithKline Beecham, Braz.
Amoxicillin (p.149·2); bromhexine hydrochloride (p.1085·3).
Bacterial infections.

Broncoclar Oberlin, Fr.
Granules for oral solution: Acetylcysteine (p.1082·3).

Syrup: Carbocisteine (p.1086·3).
Respiratory-tract disorders associated with increased or viscous mucus.

Bronco-Dex Pastor Farina, Ital.
Dextromethorphan hydrobromide (p.1087·3); sulfogaiacol (p.1101·1).
Coughs.

Broncodiazina Vitoria, Port.
Ammonia solution (p.1579·1); pentetrazol (p.1513·2); sodium benzoate (p.1134·3); sulfadiazine (p.251·1).
Respiratory-tract disorders.

Broncodil
Note. This name is used for preparations of different composition.
Infabra, Braz.
Salbutamol sulfate (p.770·3).
Obstructive airways disease.

Epifarma, Ital.†.
Clenbuterol hydrochloride (p.763·3).
Asthma.

Broncofenil Zurita, Braz.
Guaifenesin (p.1092·2); lobelia (p.1510·2); aconite (p.1572·3).
Coughs.

Broncofisin Luper, Braz.
Tolu balsam (p.1101·3); potassium iodide (p.1522·3); sulfogaiacol (p.1101·1).
Coughs.

Broncofluid Pharmarecord, Ital.
Prenoxdiazine hibenzate (p.1099·2); carbocisteine (p.1086·3).
Coughs.

Broncoformo Muco Dexa Edigen, Spain.
Dexamethasone (p.1067·1); dextromethorphan hydrobromide (p.1087·3); guaifenesin (p.1092·2); sodium benzoate (p.1134·3).
Respiratory-tract disorders.

Broncokin Geymonat, Ital.
Bromhexine hydrochloride (p.1085·3).
Respiratory-tract disorders.

Broncol
Note. This name is used for preparations of different composition.
Crown, S.Afr.
Dextromethorphan hydrobromide (p.1087·3); ammonium chloride (p.1085·2); panthenol (p.1602·3).
Coughs.

Pharmaland, Thai.
Ambroxol hydrochloride (p.1084·3).
Respiratory-tract disorders associated with increased or viscous mucus.

Broncolex Legrand, Braz.
Guaifenesin (p.1092·2); etafedrine hydrochloride (p.1091·2); bufylline (p.761·3); doxylamine succinate (p.417·1).
Coughs.

Broncoliber Tecnimede, Port.
Ambroxol hydrochloride (p.1084·3).
Respiratory-tract disorders.

Broncolin Heralds, Braz.
Salbutamol sulfate (p.770·3).
Obstructive airways disease.

Broncomed Liomont, Mex.
Dextromethorphan (p.1087·3); guaifenesin (p.1092·2).
Coughs.

Broncomicin Bals Edigen, Spain†.
Tolu balsam (p.1101·3); sodium benzoate (p.1134·3); ammoniacal aniseed (p.1580·2); sulfadiazine (p.251·1).
Respiratory-tract infections.

Broncomnes Bracco, Ital.
Ambroxol acefyllinate (p.1084·3).
Bronchospasm.

Broncomucil SmithKline Beecham, Ital.
Carbocisteine (p.1086·3).
Respiratory-tract disorders associated with excess or viscous mucus.

Bronconait SmithKline Beecham, Ital.
Paracetamol (p.71·2); promethazine hydrochloride (p.423·2); dextromethorphan hydrobromide (p.1087·3).
Coughs and cold symptoms.

Bronconovag Novag, Spain.
Amoxicillin trihydrate (p.149·2); bromhexine hydrochloride (p.1085·3).
Respiratory-tract infections.

Bronco-Ped Stiefel, Braz.
Etafedrine hydrochloride (p.1091·2); bufylline (p.761·3); doxylamine succinate (p.417·1); guaifenesin (p.1092·2).
Coughs.

Broncopinol Luper, Braz.
1 Ampoule, dipyrone (p.34·1); sodium camsilate; guaifenesin (p.1092·2); myrtol; suprarenal cortex (p.1080·1); chlorophyllin copper complex potassium (p.1028·1); eucalyptol (p.1609·2); 1 ampoule, chlorpheniramine [chlorphenamine] maleate (p.412·1); vitamin C (p.1389·3).
Cold and influenza symptoms.

Broncoplus Sigma-Tau, Ital.†.
Stepronin sodium (p.1101·1).
Respiratory-tract disorders.

Bronco-Polimoxil Legrand, Braz.
Amoxicillin (p.149·2); bromhexine (p.1085·3).
Bacterial infections.

Broncopulmin Ecobi, Ital.†.
Camphor (p.1589·3); niaouli oil (p.1640·2); eucalyptol (p.1609·2); menthol (p.1632·3).
Respiratory-tract disorders.

Broncopulmo Merck, Port.
Sobrerol (p.1100·3).
Coughs.

Broncoral Ferrer, Spain.
Eformoterol [formoterol] fumarate (p.764·2).
Obstructive airways disease.

Broncorema Septa, Spain†.
Guaifenesin (p.1092·2); co-trimoxazole (p.193·3).
Respiratory-tract infections.

Broncorinol etats grippaux Roche Nicholas, Fr.†.
Paracetamol (p.71·2); pseudoephedrine hydrochloride (p.1099·2); chlorpheniramine [chlorphenamine] maleate (p.412·1).
Cold symptoms.

Broncorinol Expectorant Roche Nicholas, Fr.
Carbocisteine (p.1086·3).
Viscous bronchial secretions.

Broncorinol maux de gorge Roche Nicholas, Fr.
Cetylpyridinium chloride (p.1138·1); amethocaine [tetracaine] hydrochloride (p.1305·2); ascorbic acid (p.1389·3).
Sore throat.

Broncorinol rhinites Roche Nicholas, Fr.
Cetrimide (p.1137·1); tyrothricin (p.267·1).
Formerly contained paracetamol and pseudoephedrine hydrochloride.
Upper respiratory-tract infections.

Broncorinol rhume Roche Nicholas, Fr.
Paracetamol (p.71·2); pseudoephedrine hydrochloride (p.1099·2).
Cold symptoms.

Broncorinol toux seches Roche Nicholas, Fr.
Pholcodine (p.1099·1); sodium benzoate (p.1134·3); aconite (p.1572·3); hyoscyamus (p.470·1); lobelia (p.1510·2); senega (p.1100·2); eucalyptus (p.1609·2).
Coughs.

Broncort
Boehringer Ingelheim, Belg.; Boehringer Ingelheim, Switz.
Flunisolide (p.1070·3).
Obstructive airways disease.

Broncosedina FAMA, Ital.
Cocillana (p.1087·2); eriodictyon (p.1091·2); marrubium (p.1094·2); grindelia (p.1618·2); juniper (p.1625·2); compound thyme (p.1672·2); pumilio pine oil (p.1656·3); mint oil (p.1636·2).
Respiratory-tract disorders.

Broncosedol QIF, Braz.
Salbutamol sulfate (p.770·3).
Obstructive airways disease.

Broncosil Basi, Port.
Camphor (p.1589·3); quinine (p.445·1).

Broncospasmin Merck, Spain†.
Reproterol hydrochloride (p.770·2).
Obstructive airways disease.

Broncospasmine Asta Medica, Ital.
Reproterol hydrochloride (p.770·2).
Asthma.

Broncostat Rhone-Poulenc Rorer, Austral.†.
Haemophilus influenzae killed cells.
Oral prophylaxis against bronchitis.

Broncostyl Robert, Spain†.
Adamexine (p.1084·2).
Respiratory-tract disorders.

Broncosyl Homberger, Switz.
Homoeopathic preparation.

Broncoten Farmion, Braz.
Ketotifen fumarate (p.767·2).
Allergic conjunctivitis; allergic rhinitis; asthma; urticaria.

Broncoterol Quimedical, Port.
Clenbuterol hydrochloride (p.763·3).
Obstructive airways disease.

Bronco-Turbinal Valeas, Ital.
Beclometasone dipropionate (p.1061·2).
Bronchospasm.

Broncotussan INQ, Braz.
Noscapine (p.1096·1); ammonium benzoate; sulfogaiacol (p.1101·1); bromoform (p.1587·1); lobelia (p.1510·2); drosera (p.1606·1); grindelia (p.1618·2); aconite (p.1572·3).
Coughs.

Broncovaleas Valeas, Ital.
Salbutamol (p.770·3).
Bronchospasm.

Broncovanil Pharmafar, Ital.
Guaifenesin (p.1092·2).
Respiratory-tract disorders.

Broncovir Vir, Spain.
Co-trimoxazole (p.193·3); sulfogaiacol (p.1101·1).
Respiratory-tract infections.

Broncovital Puerto Galiano, Spain.
Eucalyptol (p.1609·2); codeine phosphate (p.25·2); ephedrine hydrochloride (p.1090·1); niaouli oil (p.1640·2); sodium benzoate (p.1134·3); sulfogaiacol (p.1101·1); belladonna (p.463·1); drosera (p.1606·1); quebracho; senega (p.1100·2).
Respiratory-tract disorders.

Brondecon Parke, Davis, NZ.
Choline theophyllinate (p.763·3); guaifenesin (p.1092·2).
Obstructive airways disease.

Brondecon Elixir Parke, Davis, Austral.
Choline theophyllinate (p.763·3).
Obstructive airways disease.

Brondecon Expectorant Parke, Davis, Austral.
Choline theophyllinate (p.763·3); guaifenesin (p.1092·2).
Obstructive airways disease.

Brondil Great Eastern, Thai.; Therapharma, Thai.
Ephedrine hydrochloride (p.1090·1); theophylline (p.777·2); guaifenesin (p.1092·2).
Obstructive airways disease.

Brondilat Ache, Braz.
Acebrofylline.
Obstructive airways disease.

Brondix Pentafarm, Spain.
Amoxicillin trihydrate (p.149·2).
Bacterial infections.

Brongenit Elfar, Spain.
Co-trimoxazole (p.193·3).
Bacterial infections; Pneumocystis carinii pneumonia.

Bronica Takeda, Jpn.
Seratrodast (p.774·2).
Asthma.

Bronilide Cassenne, Fr.
Flunisolide (p.1070·3).
Asthma.

Bronitin Mist Whitehall, USA†.
Adrenaline [epinephrine] acid tartrate (p.829·2).
Bronchospasm.

Bronkaid Sanofi Synthelabo, Canad.
Adrenaline [epinephrine] (p.829·1).
Asthma.

Bronkaid Dual Action Sterling, USA.
Ephedrine sulfate (p.1090·2); guaifenesin (p.1092·2).

Bronkaid Mist Sterling Health, USA†.
Adrenaline [epinephrine] nitrate (p.831·1); adrenaline [epinephrine] hydrochloride (p.829·2).
Asthma.

Bronkese Aspen Consumer, S.Afr.
Bromhexine hydrochloride (p.1085·3).
Respiratory-tract disorders.

Bronkese Compound Aspen Consumer, S.Afr.
Bromhexine hydrochloride (p.1085·3); orciprenaline sulfate (p.769·1).
Respiratory-tract disorders.

Bronkirex Irex, Fr.
Carbocisteine (p.1086·3).
Respiratory-tract disorders.

Bronkometer Sanofi Winthrop, USA†.
Isoetarine mesilate (p.767·1).
Asthma; reversible bronchospasm.

Bronkosol Sanofi Winthrop, USA†.
Isoetarine hydrochloride (p.767·1).

Bronkotrat QIF, Braz.
Ammonium chloride (p.1085·2); sulfogaiacol (p.1101·1).
Respiratory-tract congestion.

Bronkotuss Expectorant Hyrex, USA.
Ephedrine sulfate (p.1090·2); chlorpheniramine [chlorphenamine] maleate (p.412·1); guaifenesin (p.1092·2).
Coughs.

Bronkyl Weifa, Norw.
Acetylcysteine (p.1082·3).
Chronic bronchitis; cystic fibrosis.

Bronmycin
Biolab, Singapore; Biolab, Thai.
Doxycycline hyclate (p.200·1).
Bacterial infections.

Bronolban Sons, Mex.
Ambroxol (p.1084·3).

Bro-N-Pain Brovar, S.Afr.†.
Paracetamol (p.71·2); codeine phosphate (p.25·2).
Fever; pain.

Bronpax Biocodex, Fr.†.
Paediatric syrup: Sulfogaiacol (p.1101·1); sodium benzoate (p.1134·3); piscidia (p.1625·1); aconite (p.1572·3); belladonna (p.463·1); pine buds; frangula (p.1227·1); tolu balsam (p.1101·3); terpin hydrate (p.1101·2); liquorice (p.1231·2).
Respiratory disorders.

Pastilles: Tyrothricin (p.267·1); ethylmorphine hydrochloride (p.35·2); sodium benzoate (p.1134·3); menthol (p.1632·3); glycyrrhizinic acid; sulfogaiacol (p.1101·1); terpin hydrate (p.1101·2).
Coughs.

Syrup: Codeine (p.25·2); sulfogaiacol (p.1101·1); sodium benzoate (p.1134·3); piscidia (p.1625·1); aconite (p.1572·3); belladonna (p.463·1); pine buds; Desessartz syrup; tolu balsam (p.1101·3); terpin hydrate (p.1101·2); liquorice (p.1231·2).
Coughs.

Bronpect Kenyaku, Thai.
Codeine phosphate (p.25·2); guaifenesin (p.1092·2); phenylpropanolamine hydrochloride (p.1098·1).
Coughs; nasal congestion.

Bronpect-D Kenyaku, Thai.
Dextromethorphan hydrobromide (p.1087·3); guaifenesin (p.1092·2).
Coughs.

Bronquial OM, Port.
Carbocisteine (p.1086·3); sobrerol (p.1100·3).
Respiratory-tract congestion.

Bronquiasma Heralds, Braz.
Theophylline (p.777·2).
Obstructive airways disease.

Bronquiasmol Confar, Port.
Ephedrine (p.1090·1); ethylmorphine (p.35·2); sodium benzoate (p.1134·3).
Coughs.

Bronquicisteina Iquinosa, Spain.
Carbocisteine (p.1086·3); co-trimoxazole (p.193·3).
Respiratory-tract infections.

Bronquico Zimaia, Port.
Camphor (p.1589·3); quinine (p.445·1).

Bronquidex Farmalab, Braz.
Potassium iodide (p.1522·3); guaifenesin (p.1092·2); diphenhydramine hydrochloride (p.416·1); sodium benzoate (p.1134·3); ammonium chloride (p.1085·2); belladonna (p.463·1); lobelia (p.1510·2).
Respiratory-tract congestion.

Bronquidiazina CR Faes, Spain.
Tolu balsam (p.1101·3); bromhexine (p.1085·3); sodium benzoate (p.1134·3); co-trimoxazole (p.193·3).
Respiratory-tract infections.

Bronquimar Cruz, Spain.
Oral suspension: Guaifenesin (p.1092·2); sodium benzoate (p.1134·3); co-trimoxazole (p.193·3).
Respiratory-tract infections.

Suppositories†: Camphor (p.1589·3); eucalyptol (p.1609·2); niaouli oil (p.1640·2); guaiacol (p.1092·1); propyphenazone (p.80·2); menthol (p.1632·3).
Upper-respiratory-tract disorders.

Bronquimar Vit A Cruz, Spain†.
Camphor (p.1589·3); eucalyptol (p.1609·2); niaouli oil (p.1640·2); guaiacol (p.1092·1); vitamin A (p.1382·1); menthol (p.1632·3).
Respiratory-tract disorders.

Bronquimucil
Note.This name is used for preparations of different composition.
Dansk-Flama, Braz.; Prospa, Port.†.
Brovanexine hydrochloride (p.1086·1).
Respiratory-tract congestion.

Uriach, Spain.
Brovanexine hydrochloride (p.1086·1); co-trimoxazole (p.193·3).
Respiratory-tract infections.

Bronquinflamatoria Faes, Spain†.
Bromhexine hydrochloride (p.1085·3); tetracycline phosphate (p.259·1); ammoniacal aniseed (p.1580·2).
Respiratory-tract infection.

Bronquiogen Prodotti, Braz.
Yucca (p.1682·1); rorippa nasturtium aquaticum; mikania glomerata; lantana camara; passion flower (p.1649·1); erva silvina; oleo vermelho; sodium benzoate (p.1134·3).
Respiratory-tract disorders.

Bronquitos Legrand, Braz.
Diphenhydramine hydrochloride (p.416·1); guaifenesin (p.1092·2); theophylline (p.777·2); vitamin B6 (p.1386·3).
Obstructive airways disease.

Bronquium Ferrer, Spain.
Bromhexine hydrochloride (p.1085·3); co-trimoxazole (p.193·3).
Respiratory-tract infections.

Bronquium Amoxicilina Ferrer, Spain†.
Amoxicillin trihydrate (p.149·2); bromhexine hydrochloride (p.1085·3).
Respiratory-tract infections.

Bronsal UCB, Spain.
Betamethasone sodium phosphate (p.1063·2); diprophylline (p.764·1); guaifenesin (p.1092·2).
Respiratory-tract disorders.

Bronsema Leti, Spain.
Erythromycin ethyl succinate (p.201·2).
Bacterial infections.

Bronsema Expectorante Leti, Spain.
Erythromycin ethyl succinate (p.201·2); guaifenesin (p.1092·2).
Respiratory-tract disorders.

Bronteril Manetti Roberts, Ital.
Guaimesal (p.1092·3).
Respiratory-tract disorders.

Brontex Procter & Gamble, USA.
Codeine phosphate (p.25·2); guaifenesin (p.1092·2).
Coughs.

Brontin Formenti, Ital.†.
Deptropine citrate (p.415·1).
Respiratory-tract disorders.

Brontonyl Rhone-Poulenc Rorer, Mex.
Paracetamol (p.71·2).
Fever; pain.

Bronx Lisapharma, Ital.
Carbocisteine (p.1086·3).
Formerly contained zipeprol hydrochloride.
Respiratory-tract disorders.

Bronze 8882 Juvex, Fr.†.
Octinoxate (p.1517·3); oxybenzone (p.1518·1); avobenzone (p.1517·1); mica-titanium dioxide complex (p.1126·1).
Sunscreen.

Brooklax Intercare, UK.
Yellow phenolphthalein (p.1244·1).
Constipation.

Bropantil Mavi, Mex.
Propantheline (p.473·3).
No indications.

Bros TRB, Braz.
Phosphatidyl serine (p.1651·1).
Cerebrovascular disorders.

Brosol Mepha, Switz.
Codeine phosphate (p.25·2); diprophylline (p.764·1); atropine methobromide (p.460·3); thyme oil (p.1672·3).
Coughs.

Brosoline-Rectocaps Mepha, Switz.
Noscapine hydrochloride (p.1096·1); guaifenesin (p.1092·2).
Bronchial disorders.

Brostalin Synpharma, Aust.
Urtica root and leaves (p.1678·2); couch-grass (p.1599·3).
Urinary-tract disorders.

Brota Rectal Bals Escaned, Spain.
Camphor (p.1589·3); eucalyptol (p.1609·2); ephedrine hydrochloride (p.1090·1); niaouli oil (p.1640·2); quinine sulfate (p.445·1); sulfogaiacol (p.1101·1).
Respiratory-tract disorders.

Brotazona Escaned, Spain.
Feprazone (p.40·3).
Gout; musculoskeletal and joint disorders.

B12-Rotexmedica Rotexmedica, Ger.
Cyanocobalamin (p.1388·1).
Vitamin B12 deficiency.

Brovaflamp Brovar, S.Afr.†.
Diclofenac sodium (p.30·3).
Gout; inflammation; musculoskeletal and joint disorders.

Brown Mixture British Dispensary, Thai.
Liquorice fluid extract (p.1231·2); antimony potassium tartrate (p.97·1); camphorated opium tincture.
Coughs.

Broxil SmithKline Beecham, Neth.
Pheneticillin potassium (p.235·1).
Bacterial infections.

Broxine MPF, Singapore.
Bromhexine hydrochloride (p.1085·3).
Respiratory-tract disorders associated with increased or viscous mucus.

Broxo al Fluoro SIT, Ital.
Levomenol (p.1629·1); sodium fluoride (p.1375·3); sodium monofluorophosphate (p.1377·2).
Gum disorders; halitosis.

Broxodin SIT, Ital.
Chlorhexidine gluconate (p.1138·2).
Oral hygiene.

Broxofar Farcoral, Mex.
Ambroxol hydrochloride (p.1084·3).

Broxofar Compuesto Farcoral, Mex.
Ambroxol hydrochloride (p.1084·3); clenbuterol hydrochloride (p.763·3).
Respiratory-tract disorders with viscous mucus.

Broxol
Mundipharma, Aust.; Pulitzer, Ital.; Carnot, Mex.; Masa, Thai.
Ambroxol hydrochloride (p.1084·3).
Respiratory-tract disorders associated with increased or viscous mucus.

Broxol Plus Carnot, Mex.
Ambroxol hydrochloride (p.1084·3); clenbuterol hydrochloride (p.763·3).
Respiratory-tract disorders with viscous mucus.

Broxolan Collins, Mex.
Ambroxol (p.1084·3).

Broxsa Silom, Thai.
Ambroxol hydrochloride (p.1084·3).
Respiratory-tract disorders associated with increased or viscous mucus.

Brozam Rolab, S.Afr.
Bromazepam (p.656·3).
Nos known as Rolab-Bromazepam.
Anxiety.

The symbol † denotes a preparation no longer actively marketed

Brozepax Biosintetica, Braz.
Bromazepam (p.656·3).
Anxiety.

Bruciaporri Giovanardi, Ital.
Salicylic acid (p.1122·3); lactic acid (p.1626·2).
Verrucas; warts.

Brufen
Ebewe, Aust.; Knoll, Austral.; Knoll, Belg.; Knoll, Denm.; Knoll, Fin.;
Knoll, Fr.; Kanoldt, Ger.; Boots, Hong Kong; Knoll, Irl.; GNR, Ital.;
Knoll, Neth.; Knoll, Norw.; Knoll, NZ; Knoll, Port.; Knoll, S.Afr.; Knoll,
Singapore; Knoll, Swed.; Knoll, Switz.; Boots, Thai.; Knoll, UK.
Ibuprofen (p.43·2) or ibuprofen sodium (p.44·1).
*Fever; gout; inflammation; musculoskeletal, joint,
peri-articular, and soft-tissue disorders; pain.*

Brufort Lampugnani, Ital.
Ibuprofen (p.43·2).
*Inflammation; musculoskeletal and joint disorders;
pain.*

Brugesic Aspen Consumer, S.Afr.
Ibuprofen (p.43·2).
Fever; muscle pain; pain.

Bruiseze Bayer Consumer, UK.
A heparinoid (p.905·2).
Soft-tissue injury.

Brulamycin
Torrex, Aust.; Medphano, Ger.
Tobramycin sulfate (p.263·3).
Bacterial infections.

Brulex Bailly, Fr.
Phenazone (p.77·2); zinc oxide (p.1128·2); peru balsam (p.1650·2); phenol (p.1152·3); sodium salicylate
(p.84·2).
Formerly contained phenazone, zinc oxide, peru balsam, phenosalyl, and bismuth subgallate.
Burns; sunburn.

Brulidine
Rhone-Poulenc Rorer, Austral.; Rhone-Poulenc Rorer, Hong Kong;
Rhone-Poulenc Rorer, Irl.; Rhone-Poulenc Rorer, Norw.; Aventis, NZ;
Manx, UK.
Dibrompropamidine isetionate (p.1143·1).
Burns; napkin rash; skin abrasions; skin infections.

Brulstop Agepharm, Fr.
Hydrocolloid dressing.
Burns.

Brumed LSP, Thai.
Ibuprofen (p.43·2).
Fever; pain.

Brumetidina Bruschettini, Ital.
Cimetidine (p.1216·3).
*Gastrointestinal disorders associated with hyperacidi-
ty.*

Brumeton Colloidale S Bruschettini, Ital.
Betamethasone (p.1063·1); sulfacetamide sodium
(p.250·3).
Eye and ear disorders.

Brumixol Bruschettini, Ital.
Ciclopirox olamine (p.382·1).
Fungal skin and vulvovaginal infections.

Brunac Bruschettini, Ital.
Acetylcysteine (p.1082·3).
Eye disorders.

Brunacod Brunel, S.Afr.
Promethazine hydrochloride (p.423·2); ephedrine hy-
drochloride (p.1090·1); codeine phosphate (p.25·2).
Coughs.

Brunazine Brunel, S.Afr.
Promethazine hydrochloride (p.423·2).
*Hypersensitivity reactions; motion sickness; nausea;
vomiting.*

Brunocillin Mepha, Switz.
Phenoxymethylpenicillin potassium (p.235·1).
Bacterial infections.

Brunomol Brunel, S.Afr.
Paracetamol (p.71·2).
Fever; pain.

Bruprin Condrugs, Thai.
Ibuprofen (p.43·2).
Musculoskeletal and joint disorders.

Brush Off SSL, UK.
Povidone-iodine (p.1155·1).
Herpes labialis.

Brushtox Dentox, UK.
Denatured alcohol (p.1130·3); hydroxybenzoate esters
(p.1148·1); zinc chloride (p.1398·1).
Disinfection of toothbrushes.

Brusil Silom, Thai.
Ibuprofen (p.43·2).
Fever; musculoskeletal and joint disorders; pain.

Brust- und Hustentee
Note.This name is used for preparations of different composition.
Smetana, Aust.
Castanea vulgaris; plantago lanceolata; verbascum
leaf; thyme (p.1672·2); rad. enulae.
Respiratory-tract disorders.

Bad Heilbrunner, Ger.
Thyme (p.1672·2); cowslip root (p.1600·1).
Respiratory-tract disorders with viscous mucus.

Brust- und Husten-Tee Stada N Stada, Ger.†.
Plantago lanceolata; thyme (p.1672·2); fennel
(p.1610·1); liquorice (p.1231·2).
Bronchitis; tracheitis.

Brustan Ranbaxy, Thai.
Ibuprofen (p.43·2); paracetamol (p.71·2).
*Musculoskeletal, joint, peri-articular, and soft-tissue
disorders.*

Brustol Vifor, Switz.†.
Dextromethorphan hydrobromide (p.1087·3); phenylephrine hydrochloride (p.1097·1); chlorpheniramine
[chlorphenamine] maleate (p.412·1).
Coughs.

Bruvac Nikkho, Braz.
A brucellosis vaccine (p.1535·1).
Active immunisation.

Bruxicam Bruschettini, Ital.
Piroxicam (p.79·1).
*Musculoskeletal, joint, peri-articular, and soft-tissue
disorders.*

Brylcreem Anti-Dandruff SmithKline Beecham Con-
sumer, Canad.
Pyrithione zinc (p.1122·1).
Dandruff.

Bryonon B-Komplex Protina, Ger.
Vitamin B substances (p.1350·1).
Vitamin B deficiency.

Bryonon N Protina, Ger.
Vitamin B substances (p.1350·1).
Vitamin B deficiency.

Bryorheum DHU, Ger.
Homoeopathic preparation.

BS
Xepa-Soul Pattinson, Hong Kong; Xepa-Soul Pattinson, Singapore.
Co-trimoxazole (p.193·3).
Bacterial infections.

B-Salt Forte Akorn, USA.
Electrolytes (p.1180·1); glucose (p.1364·1); oxigluta-
tione.
Eye irrigation.

B-Scorbic Pharmics, USA†.
Vitamin C and vitamin B substances (p.1350·1).

BS-ratiopharm Ratiopharm, Ger.
Hyoscine butylbromide (p.468·2).
Smooth muscle spasm.

BSS
Alcon, Aust.; Alcon, Austral.; Alcon, Belg.†; Alcon, Braz.; Alcon, Ca-
nad.; Alcon, Fr.; Alcon, Ger.; Pharmacia Upjohn, Ger.; Alcon, Hong
Kong; Alcon, Irl.; Alcon, Israel; Alcon, S.Afr.; Alcon, Singapore; Alcon
Cusi, Spain; Alcon, Switz.; Alcon, Thai.; Alcon, USA.
Electrolyte solution (p.1180·1).
Eye irrigation; irrigation of ear, nose, and throat.

BSS Compose Alcon, Fr.
Electrolytes (p.1180·1); glucose (p.1364·1); oxigluta-
tione.
Eye irrigation.

BSS Plus
Alcon, Aust.; Alcon, Austral.; Alcon, Belg.†; Alcon, Canad.; Alcon, Ger.;
Alcon, Hong Kong; Alcon, Israel; Alcon, Singapore; Alcon, Switz.; Al-
con, Thai.; Alcon, UK; Alcon, USA.
Electrolytes (p.1180·1); glucose (p.1364·1); oxigluta-
tione.
Eye irrigation.

B12-Steigerwald Steigerwald, Ger.
Cyanocobalamin (p.1388·1).
Vitamin B$_{12}$ deficiency.

B-Tasone-G Beacons, Singapore.
Betamethasone valerate (p.1063·2); gentamicin sulfate
(p.210·1).
Infected skin disorders.

B-Tene Vitaglow, Austral.
Betacarotene (p.1355·1).
*Photosensitivity reactions in patients with erythropoi-
etic protoporphyria.*

B-Tonin Nycomed, Norw.
Vitamin B substances (p.1350·1); caffeine (p.761·3).
Tonic; vitamin B deficiency.

BU Pangramin SLIT Scherax, Ger.
Allergen extracts (p.1575·3).
Hyposensitisation.

Bucagel Asta Medica, Port.
Choline salicylate (p.24·3); cetalkonium chloride
(p.1137·1).
Mouth disorders.

Bucain
Curasan, Aust.; Curasan, Ger.
Bupivacaine hydrochloride (p.1306·3).
Local anaesthesia.

Bucaril Pharmaland, Thai.
Terbutaline sulfate (p.776·2).
Obstructive airways disease.

Bucasept Aerocid, Fr.
Chlorhexidine gluconate (p.1138·2).
Mouth and throat disorders.

Buccalin
Note.This name is used for preparations of different composition.
Kwizda, Aust.
Haemophilus influenzae; pneumococci; streptococci;
staphylococci; ox bile extract (p.1585·1).
*Prophylaxis of bacterial infections in patients with
colds.*

Berna, Ital.
Streptococcus pneumoniae I, II, and III; Streptococcus
haemolyticus; Staphylococcus aureus; Haemophilus
influenzae.
*Prophylaxis of bacterial infections in patients with in-
fluenza.*

Buccalin Complet Berna, Spain†.
Pneumococcus; streptococcus; staphylococcus; Hae-
mophilus influenzae.
Respiratory-tract infections.

Buccaline
Note.This name is used for preparations of different composition.
Berna, Belg.; Berna, Hong Kong; Berna, Switz.; Berna, Thai.
Pneumococcus I, II, III; streptococcus; staphylococc-
us; Haemophilus influenzae; ox bile (p.1585·1).
Prophylaxis of colds.

Pharmabroker, NZ.
Pneumococcus; streptococcus; staphylococcus; Hae-
mophilus influenzae.
Common cold prophylaxis.

Buccalsone
Will-Pharma, Belg.; Will-Pharma, Neth.
Hydrocortisone sodium succinate (p.1074·1).
Aphthous stomatitis.

Buccapol
Berna, Hong Kong†; Berna, Singapore†.
An oral poliomyelitis vaccine (p.1558·2).
Active immunisation.

Buccard AstraZeneca, Denm.
Glyceryl trinitrate (p.897·3).
Angina pectoris; heart failure.

Buccastem
Reckitt Benckiser, Irl.; Reckitt Benckiser, NZ; Reckitt & Colman, UK.
Prochlorperazine maleate (p.701·2).
Migraine; nausea; vertigo; vomiting.

Buccawalter SmithKline Beecham, Fr.
Lignocaine [lidocaine] hydrochloride (p.1313·2); cetrimide (p.1137·1); sodium salicylate (p.84·2); phenol
(p.1152·3).
Formerly contained amylocaine hydrochloride, cloral
hydrate, phenosalyl, and borax.
Mouth and throat disorders.

Buccosan Warner-Lambert Consumer, Belg.
Dequalinium chloride (p.1143·1); lignocaine [lido-
caine] hydrochloride (p.1313·2).
Mouth and throat disorders.

Bucco-Spray Warner-Lambert Consumer, Belg.
Dequalinium chloride (p.1143·1); lignocaine [lido-
caine] hydrochloride (p.1313·2).
Mouth and throat disorders.

Bucco-Tantum Roche, Switz.
Benzydamine hydrochloride (p.20·1).
Mouth and throat inflammation.

Bucet UAD, USA†.
Butalbital (p.658·3); paracetamol (p.71·2).

Buchol Palmicol, Ger.†.
Sage oil (p.1660·2).
Hyperhidrosis.

Bucin Masa, Thai.
Indometacin (p.44·3).
Musculoskeletal, joint, and peri-articular disorders.

Buckley's Bedtime Buckley, Canad.
Diphenhydramine hydrochloride (p.416·1); menthol
(p.1632·3).
Cold symptoms; coughs.

Buckley's DM Buckley, Canad.
Dextromethorphan hydrobromide (p.1087·3).
Dry cough.

Buckley's DM Decongestant Buckley, Canad.
Pseudoephedrine hydrochloride (p.1099·2); dex-
tromethorphan hydrobromide (p.1087·3).
Coughs and cold symptoms.

Buckley's Mixture Buckley, Canad.
Ammonium carbonate (p.1085·1); potassium bicarbonate (p.1186·1); menthol (p.1632·3); camphor
(p.1589·3).
Cough.

Buckleys Pain Relief Buckley, Canad.
Methyl salicylate (p.55·1); menthol (p.1632·3).
Muscle and joint pain.

Buckley's White Rub Buckley, Canad.
Menthol (p.1632·3); camphor (p.1589·3); methyl sali-
cylate (p.55·1); thymol (p.1158·3).
Cold symptoms; muscle and joint pain.

Bucladin-S Softab Stuart, USA.
Buclizine hydrochloride (p.411·1).
Motion sickness.

Buclamin Teuto, Braz.
Buclizine (p.411·1); tryptophan; lysine; pyridoxine;
cyanocobalamin (p.1350·1).
Reduced appetite; tonic.

Bucliamin Baldassari, Braz.
Buclizine hydrochloride (p.411·1); tryptophan hydrochloride; carnitine hydrochloride; lysine hydrochloride; vitamin B$_6$; vitamin B$_{12}$ (p.1350·1).
Reduced appetite; tonic.

Buclifen-Vit Profarb, Braz.
Buclizine hydrochloride (p.411·1); lysine; vitamin B$_{12}$
(p.1350·1).
Reduced appetite; tonic.

Buclina
Sanofi Winthrop, Braz.; Vedim, Port.
Buclizine (p.411·1) or buclizine hydrochloride
(p.411·1).
Motion sickness; reduced appetite.

Bucliplex Dovalle, Braz.
Buclizine hydrochloride (p.411·1); vitamin B sub-
stances (p.1350·1).
Reduced appetite; tonic.

Buclitina Herolds, Braz.
Buclizine (p.411·1); carnitine; gamma-aminobutyric
acid; lysine; vitamin B substances (p.1350·1).
Reduced appetite; tonic.

Buco Regis Ramon Sala, Spain.
Ipecacuanha (p.1093·1); methyl salicylate (p.55·1);
myrrh (p.1639·2); sulfanilamide (p.256·2); zinc chloride (p.1398·1); menthol (p.1632·3).
Mouth and throat inflammation; pyorrhoea.

Bucodrin Fardi, Spain.
Chlorhexidine hydrochloride (p.1138·2); benzocaine
(p.1306·2).
Formerly contained ephedrine ricinoleate, ethacridine
lactate, and sulfathiazole.
Mouth and throat disorders.

Bucometasana Solvay, Spain.
Chlorhexidine hydrochloride (p.1138·2); benzocaine
(p.1306·2); tyrothricin (p.267·1).
Mouth and throat disorders.

Buconif Terrapharm, Aust.
Nifedipine (p.940·1).
*Hypertension; ischaemic heart disease; Raynaud's
syndrome.*

Bucort Orion, Fin.
Hydrocortisone butyrate (p.1073·3).
Skin disorders.

Bucospray Solvay, Spain.
Chlorhexidine gluconate (p.1138·2); benzocaine
(p.1306·2).
Mouth and throat disorders.

Bucovacuna Nezel, Spain†.
Streptococcus pneumoniae; Micrococcus pyogenes;
Haemophilus influenzae(p.0·0); Gaffkya tetragena;
Moraxella catarrhalis; Klebsiella pneumoniae;
Moraxella.
Prophylaxis of respiratory-tract infections.

Budamax PMC, Austral.
Budesonide (p.1064·2).
Allergic rhinitis.

Budapp Pulmopharm, Ger.
Budesonide (p.1064·2).
Obstructive airways disease.

Budecort Klinge, Ger.
Budesonide (p.1064·2).
Obstructive airways disease.

Budefat Fatol, Ger.
Budesonide (p.1064·2).
Obstructive airways disease.

Budeflam Cipla-Medpro, S.Afr.
Budesonide (p.1064·2).
Allergic rhinitis; asthma.

Budenofalk
Falk, Ger.; Phardi, Switz.; Cortecs, UK.
Budesonide (p.1064·2).
Crohn's disease.

Budepur E BASF, Ger.
Budesonide (p.1064·2).
Obstructive airways disease.

Budes Hexal, Ger.
Budesonide (p.1064·2).
Obstructive airways disease.

Budeson Rafa, Israel.
Budesonide (p.1064·2).
Crohn's disease.

Budicort Teva, Israel.
Budesonide (p.1064·2).
Asthma.

Budon Lindopharm, Ger.
Budesonide (p.1064·2).
Obstructive airways disease.

Budo-san Merck, Aust.
Budesonide (p.1064·2).
Crohn's disease.

Buenoson N Zilly, Ger.
Hypericum oil; wheat-germ oil; avocado oil; birch tar
oil; thiamine hydrochloride; dilute formic acid; garlic
juice; birch leaf; juniper berry; gentian root; lupulus;
clove; male fern leaf.
Herbal preparation.

Buer Vitamin E + Magnesium Roland, Ger.
α-Tocoferil acetate (p.1394·1); magnesium oxide
(p.1233·2).
Muscle weakness.

Buerlecithin
Roland, Aust.; Polcopharma, Austral.; Roland, Ger.
Lecithin (p.1628·1) with or without vitamins
(p.1350·1).
Tonic.

Buerlecithin Compact
Roland, Aust.; Byk Roland, Switz.
Lecithin (p.1628·1).
Tonic.

Bufal Pierre Fabre, Fr.†.
Bufexamac (p.20·3).
Inflammatory skin disorders.

Buf-Bar 3M, USA†.
Sulfur (p.1123·3); titanium dioxide (p.1126·1).
Acne.

Bufederm Galen, Ger.
Bufexamac (p.20·3).
Skin disorders.

Bufedil
Abbott, Braz.; Abbott, Ger.
Buflomedil hydrochloride (p.851·3).
Peripheral vascular disorders.

Bufedon Byk, Belg.†.
Ibuprofen (p.43·2).
*Gout; musculoskeletal, joint, and peri-articular disor-
ders; pain.*

Bufene *Ist. Chim. Inter., Ital.†.*
Buflomedil hydrochloride (p.851·3).
Vascular disorders.

Bufeno *Helvepharm, Switz.†.*
Ibuprofen (p.43·2).
Musculoskeletal and joint disorders.

Bufeproct *Hexal, Ger.†.*
Bufexamac (p.20·3); lignocaine [lidocaine] hydrochloride (p.1313·2); bismuth subgallate (p.1213·2); titanium dioxide (p.1126·1).
Haemorrhoids.

Buferin *Bristol-Myers Squibb, Braz.*
Aspirin (p.14·2).
Fever; inflammation; pain; thromboembolism prophylaxis.

Bufexan *Lannacher, Aust.*
Bufexamac (p.20·3).
Inflammatory skin disorders.

Bufexine *Continental Pharma, Belg.*
Bufexamac (p.20·3).
Arthritis; peri-articular inflammation.

Buffelin *Opto-Pharm, Singapore.*
Boric acid (p.1586·1); sodium chloride (p.1196·1).
Eye irritation.

Buffered C *Quest, UK.*
Calcium ascorbate (p.1389·3).

Buffered C 500 *Bio-Health, UK.*
Calcium ascorbate (p.1389·3).

Bufferin
Bristol-Myers Squibb, Canad.
Aspirin (p.14·2).
Aluminium glycinate (p.1210·3) and magnesium carbonate (p.1232·3) are included in this preparation in an attempt to limit adverse effects on the gastrointestinal mucosa.
Fever; pain.

Bristol-Myers Squibb, Ital.; Bristol-Myers Products, USA.
Aspirin (p.14·2).
Calcium carbonate (p.1215·1), magnesium carbonate (p.1232·3), and magnesium oxide (p.1233·2) are included in this preparation in an attempt to limit adverse effects on the gastrointestinal mucosa.
Fever; inflammation; myocardial infarction; pain; transient ischaemic attacks.

Bufferin AF Nite Time *Bristol-Myers Squibb, USA.*
Diphenhydramine citrate (p.416·1); paracetamol (p.71·2).
Insomnia.

Buffets II *JMI, USA†.*
Paracetamol (p.71·2); aspirin (p.14·2); caffeine (p.761·3).
Aluminium hydroxide (p.1210·3) is included in this preparation in an attempt to limit adverse effects on the gastrointestinal mucosa.
Pain.

Buffex *Roberts, USA.*
Aspirin (p.14·2).
Aluminium glycinate (p.1210·3) and magnesium carbonate (p.1232·3) are included in this preparation in an attempt to limit adverse effects on the gastrointestinal mucosa.
Fever; inflammation; myocardial infarction; pain; transient ischaemic attacks.

Bufigen
Note.This name is used for preparations of different composition.
Antigen, Irl.
Ibuprofen (p.43·2).
Musculoskeletal, joint, and peri-articular disorders; pain; soft-tissue injuries.

Pisa, Mex.
Nalbuphine hydrochloride (p.60·1).
Pain.

Bufilem *Lemery, Mex.*
Nalbuphine (p.60·2).
Pain.

Buflan *Fournier, Ital.*
Buflomedil hydrochloride (p.851·3).
Vascular disorders.

Buflo *ABZ, Ger.*
Buflomedil hydrochloride (p.851·3).
Peripheral vascular disorders.

Buflocit *CT, Ital.*
Buflomedil hydrochloride (p.851·3).
Cerebral and peripheral vascular disorders.

Buflofar *Upsamedica, Ital.*
Buflomedil hydrochloride (p.851·3).
Cerebral and peripheral vascular disorders.

Buflohexal
Hexal, Aust.; Hexal, Ger.
Buflomedil hydrochloride (p.851·3).
Peripheral vascular disorders.

Buflo-POS *Ursapharm, Ger.*
Buflomedil hydrochloride (p.851·3).
Peripheral vascular disorders.

Buflo-Puren *Isis Puren, Ger.*
Buflomedil hydrochloride (p.851·3).
Peripheral vascular disorders.

Buflo-Reu *Reusch, Ger.†.*
Buflomedil hydrochloride (p.851·3).
Peripheral vascular disorders.

Bufoxin *Fulton, Ital.†.*
Buflomedil pyridoxal phosphate compound (p.852·1).
Cerebral and peripheral vascular disorders.

Bug Guards *Go Travel, UK.*
Diethyltoluamide (p.1431·2).
Insect repellent.

Bug Proof *Nomad, UK.*
Permethrin (p.1436·1).
Insect repellent for clothing.

Bugs Bunny
Bayer, Canad.; Bayer Consumer, Singapore; Miles, USA.
Multivitamins or multivitamins with minerals (p.1350·1).

Bulboid *Novartis Consumer, Switz.*
Glycerol (p.1616·3).
Bowel evacuation; constipation.

Bulboshap *Farmagan, Ital.*
Shampoo containing achillea, chamomile, cinchona, cornflower, gentian, lilly, and almond.
Seborrhoeic dermatitis.

Bulk *Agepha, Aust.*
Methylcellulose (p.1502·2).
Constipation.

Bullfrog *Chattem, USA.*
Gel SPF 18: Oxybenzone (p.1518·1); octocrilene (p.1518·1); octinoxate (p.1517·3).
Stick SPF 18: Oxybenzone (p.1518·1); octinoxate (p.1517·3).
SPF 36: Oxybenzone (p.1518·1); octocrilene (p.1518·1); octinoxate (p.1517·3).
Sunscreen.

Bullfrog for Kids *Chattem, USA.*
SPF 18: Octocrilene (p.1518·1); octinoxate (p.1517·3) octisalate (p.1518·1).
Sunscreen.

Bullfrog Sport *Chattem, USA.*
SPF 18: Oxybenzone (p.1518·1); octocrilene (p.1518·1); octinoxate (p.1517·3) octisalate (p.1518·1); titanium dioxide (p.1126·1).
Sunscreen.

Bullrich Salz *Mundipharma, Aust.*
Sodium bicarbonate (p.1186·2).
Dyspepsia.

Bumed *Medifive, Thai.*
Ibuprofen (p.43·2).
Inflammation; musculoskeletal and joint disorders; pain.

Bumedyl *Atlantis, Mex.*
Bumetanide (p.852·1).
Cirrhosis with ascites; heart failure; hypertension; oedema.

Bumex *Roche, USA.*
Bumetanide (p.852·1).
Oedema.

Buminate
Baxter-Hyland, Hong Kong; Baxter, Singapore; Baxter, Thai.; Baxter, USA.
Albumin (p.724·1).
Hypoalbuminaemia; hypovolaemia; neonatal hyperbilirubinaemia.

Bumps 'n Falls *Dermamend, UK.*
Benzalkonium chloride (p.1133·2); oxyesterified triglycerides.
Cuts; soft-tissue injury.

Bunil *Dumex, Port.*
Melperone (p.690·3).
Agitation; alcohol withdrawal syndrome; confusion; insomnia; psychoses.

Bunion Salve *Cress, Canad.†.*
Camphor (p.1589·3); menthol (p.1632·3); phenol (p.1152·3); tannic acid (p.1669·1).

Bupap *ECR, USA.*
Butalbital (p.658·3); paracetamol (p.71·2).
Pain.

Buphenyl *Ucyclyd, USA.*
Sodium phenylbutyrate (p.1666·2).
Urea cycle disorders.

Bupiforan *Clarmed, Ital.*
Bupivacaine hydrochloride (p.1306·3).
Adrenaline [epinephrine] acid tartrate (p.829·2) is included in some injections as a vasoconstrictor to diminish absorption and localise the effect of the local anaesthetic.
Local anaesthesia.

Buprenex *Reckitt & Colman, USA.*
Buprenorphine hydrochloride (p.21·1).
Pain.

Buprex
Schering-Plough, Port.; Schering-Plough, Spain.
Buprenorphine hydrochloride (p.21·1).
Pain.

Buprine *Siam Bheasach, Thai.*
Buprenorphine hydrochloride (p.21·1).
Pain.

Bupyl *Molteni, Ital.*
Bupivacaine hydrochloride (p.1306·3).
Adrenaline [epinephrine] acid tartrate (p.829·2) is included in some injections as a vasoconstrictor to diminish absorption and localise the effect of the local anaesthetic.
Local anaesthesia.

Buram
Leo, Denm.; Leo, Irl.
Amiloride hydrochloride (p.835·1); bumetanide (p.852·1).
Oedema.

Burana *Orion, Fin.*
Ibuprofen (p.43·2).
Gout; inflammation; musculoskeletal, joint, and peri-articular disorders; pain.

Burana-C *Orion, Fin.*
Ibuprofen (p.43·2); ascorbic acid (p.1389·3).
Influenza symptoms.

Buraton 10 F *Schülke & Mayr, Ger.*
Glyoxal (p.1145·3); formaldehyde (p.1144·2); glutaral (p.1145·2); ethylhexanal.
Surface disinfection.

Burgerstein Geriatrikum *Antistress, Switz.*
Multivitamin and mineral preparation (p.1350·1).
Tonic.

Burgerstein S *Antistress, Switz.*
Vitamin and mineral preparation (p.1350·1).
Liver disorders.

Burgodin
Janssen-Cilag, Belg.†; Janssen-Cilag, Neth.†.
Bezitramide (p.20·2).
Pain.

Burinax *Sintofarma, Braz.*
Bumetanide (p.852·1).
Hypercalcaemia; hypertension; oedema.

Burinex
Leo, Aust.; Astra, Austral.; Leo, Belg.; Leo, Canad.; Leo, Denm.; Leo, Fin.; Leo, Fr.; Leo, Ger.; Leo, Hong Kong; Leo, Irl.; Leo, Neth.; Leo, Norw.; CSL, NZ; Adcock Ingram, S.Afr.; Leo, Singapore; Leo, Swed.; Leo, Switz.; Leo, Thai.; Leo, UK.
Bumetanide (p.852·1).
Forced diuresis; heart failure; hypertension; oedema; renal failure; sodium retention.

Burinex A *Leo, UK.*
Bumetanide (p.852·1); amiloride hydrochloride (p.835·1).
Oedema.

Burinex K
Leo, Hong Kong; Leo, Irl.; Leo, Norw.; Leo, Singapore; Leo, UK.
Bumetanide (p.852·1); potassium chloride (p.1194·3).
Oedema.

Burinex med kaliumklorid *Leo, Denm.*
Bumetanide (p.852·1); potassium chloride (p.1194·3).
Hypertension; oedema.

Burmicin *I Farmacologia, Spain.*
Amoxicillin trihydrate (p.149·2); potassium clavulanate (p.187·3).
Bacterial infections.

Burn Healing Cream *Brauer, Austral.*
Homoeopathic preparation.

Burnaid First Aid Burn Gel *Rye, Austral.*
Melaleuca oil (p.1631·3); triclosan (p.1159·2).
Burns.

Burn-A-Sept *Salters, S.Afr.*
Tannic acid (p.1669·1); phenol (p.1152·3).
Burns.

Burneze *SSL, UK.*
Benzocaine (p.1306·2).
Burns; scalds.

Burnocaine *Salters, S.Afr.*
Benzocaine (p.1306·2); chlorhexidine acetate (p.1138·2); cetrimide (p.1137·1); benzyl alcohol; vitamin A palmitate; castor oil.
Burns.

Burnol *Boots, Singapore.*
Aminoacridine hydrochloride (p.1130·2); cetrimide (p.1137·1).
Burns; insect bites; rash; wounds.

Burnol Plus *Boots, Thai.*
Aminoacridine hydrochloride (p.1130·2); cetrimide (p.1137·1); thymol (p.1158·3).
Burns; insect bites; skin rashes; wounds.

Burns Ointment *Nelson, UK.*
Homoeopathic preparation.

Burnshield Gel *Ferno, UK.*
Melaleuca oil (p.1631·3).
Burns; scalds.

Buro Derm *Trans Canaderm, Canad.†.*
Aluminium acetate (p.1578·1); benzethonium chloride (p.1134·2).

Buronil
Lundbeck, Aust.; Lundbeck, Belg.; Lundbeck, Denm.; Lundbeck, Fin.; Lundbeck, Norw.; Lundbeck, Swed.
Melperone hydrochloride (p.690·3).
Anxiety disorders; dementia; drug and alcohol withdrawal syndromes; pain; psychoses; sleep disorders.

Buro-Sol
Note.This name is used for preparations of different composition.
Trans Canaderm, Canad.
Aluminium acetate (p.1578·1); benzethonium chloride (p.1134·2).
Ear disorders; skin disorders.

Doak, USA.
Aluminium acetate (p.1578·1).
Skin inflammation.

Burow's *Rugby, USA.*
Acetic acid (p.1571·2); aluminium acetate (p.1578·1).
Ear infections.

Busala *Selz, Ger.†.*
Dimethicone (p.1249·2).
Gastrointestinal disorders.

Busansil *Lepori, Port.*
Buspirone hydrochloride (p.657·2).
Anxiety.

Buscalma *Euro-Labor, Port.*
Buspirone hydrochloride (p.657·2).
Anxiety.

Buscapina
Boehringer Ingelheim, Mex.; Boehringer Ingelheim, Spain.
Hyoscine butylbromide (p.468·2).
Adjuvant in gastrointestinal radiography; gastrointestinal spasm.

Buscapina Compositum
Boehringer Ingelheim, Mex.; Boehringer Ingelheim, Spain.
Hyoscine butylbromide (p.468·2); dipyrone (p.34·1).
Gastrointestinal spasm; pain.

Buscapina Compositum N *Boehringer Ingelheim, Mex.*
Hyoscine butylbromide (p.468·2); paracetamol (p.71·2).
Painful smooth muscle spasm.

Buscolysin *Medphano, Ger.*
Hyoscine butylbromide (p.468·2).
Smooth muscle spasm.

Busconet *Sons, Mex.*
Hyoscine butylbromide (p.468·2); dipyrone (p.34·1).
Painful smooth muscle spasm.

Buscono *Milano, Thai.*
Hyoscine butylbromide (p.468·2).
Smooth muscle spasm.

Buscopamol *Boehringer Ingelheim, Aust.*
Hyoscine butylbromide (p.468·2); paracetamol (p.71·2).
Pain; smooth muscle spasm.

Buscopan
Boehringer Ingelheim, Aust.; Boehringer Ingelheim, Austral.; Boehringer Ingelheim, Belg.; Boehringer de Angeli, Braz.; Boehringer Ingelheim, Canad.; Boehringer Ingelheim, Denm.; Boehringer Ingelheim, Fin.; Boehringer Ingelheim, Ger.; Boehringer Ingelheim, Hong Kong; Boehringer Ingelheim, Irl.; Boehringer Ingelheim, Ital.; Boehringer Ingelheim, Neth.; Boehringer Ingelheim, Norw.; Boehringer Ingelheim, NZ; Boehringer Ingelheim, Port.; Boehringer Ingelheim, S.Afr.; Boehringer Ingelheim, Singapore; Boehringer Ingelheim, Swed.; Boehringer Ingelheim, Switz.; Boehringer Ingelheim, Thai.; Boehringer Ingelheim, UK.
Hyoscine butylbromide (p.468·2).
Diagnostic aid in radiology or endoscopy; smooth muscle spasm.

Buscopan Compositum
Note.This name is used for preparations of different composition.
Boehringer Ingelheim, Aust.; Boehringer Ingelheim, Belg.; Boehringer Ingelheim, S.Afr.
Hyoscine butylbromide (p.468·2); dipyrone (p.34·1).
Smooth muscle spasm and pain.

Boehringer Ingelheim, Ital.
Hyoscine butylbromide (p.468·2); paracetamol (p.71·2).
Formerly contained hyoscine butylbromide and dipyrone.
Smooth muscle spasm.

Buscopan Compositum N *Boehringer Ingelheim, Port.*
Hyoscine butylbromide (p.468·2); paracetamol (p.71·2).
Smooth muscle spasm.

Buscopan Composto *Boehringer de Angeli, Braz.*
Hyoscine butylbromide (p.468·2); dipyrone (p.34·1).
Smooth muscle spasm.

Buscopan Plus
Boehringer de Angeli, Braz.; Boehringer Ingelheim, Ger.; Boehringer Ingelheim, Thai.
Hyoscine butylbromide (p.468·2); paracetamol (p.71·2).
Smooth muscle spasm.

Bush Formula *Or-Dov, Austral.*
Chlorhexidine gluconate (p.1138·2).
Acne; skin rashes.

Busina *Jofrain, Mex.*
Hyoscine butylbromide (p.468·2).

Busopin *Jean-Marie, Hong Kong.*
Hyoscine butylbromide (p.468·2).
Smooth muscle spasm.

Busp *Hexal, Ger.*
Buspirone hydrochloride (p.657·2).
Anxiety disorders.

Buspanil *Novartis, Braz.*
Buspirone hydrochloride (p.657·2).
Anxiety.

Buspar
Bristol-Myers Squibb, Aust.; Bristol-Myers Squibb, Austral.; Bristol-Myers Squibb, Belg.; Bristol-Myers Squibb, Braz.; Bristol, Canad.; Bristol-Myers Squibb, Denm.; Orion, Fin.; Bristol-Myers Squibb, Fin.; UPSA, Fr.; Bristol-Myers Squibb, Hong Kong; Bristol-Myers Squibb, Irl.; Mead Johnson, Ital.; Mead Johnson, Mex.; Bristol-Myers Squibb, Neth.; Bristol-Myers Squibb, Norw.; Bristol-Myers Squibb, NZ; Bristol-Myers Squibb, Port.; Bristol-Myers Squibb, S.Afr.; Bristol-Myers Squibb, Singapore; Bristol-Myers, Spain; Bristol-Myers Squibb, Swed.; Bristol-Myers Squibb, Switz.; Bristol-Myers Squibb, UK; Bristol-Myers Squibb, USA.
Buspirone hydrochloride (p.657·2).
Anxiety.

Buspimen *Menarini, Ital.*
Buspirone hydrochloride (p.657·2).
Anxiety.

Buspirex *Technilab, Canad.*
Buspirone hydrochloride (p.657·2).
Anxiety.

Buspirol *Bristol-Myers Squibb, Israel.*
Buspirone hydrochloride (p.657·2).
Anxiety.

Buspisal *Lesvi, Spain†.*
Buspirone hydrochloride (p.657·2).
Anxiety.

Buspril *Sintofarma, Braz.*
Buspirone hydrochloride (p.657·2).
Anxiety.

Busprina *Farcoral, Mex.*
Hyoscine butylbromide (p.468·2); dipyrone (p.34·1).
Smooth muscle spasm and pain.

The symbol † denotes a preparation no longer actively marketed

Bustab *ICN, Canad.*
Buspirone hydrochloride (p.657·2).
Anxiety.

Busulfex *Orphan Medical, Canad.; Orphan Medical, USA.*
Busulfan (p.513·3).
Malignant neoplasms.

Buta *PD, Thai.*
Phenylbutazone sodium (p.78·3).
Lignocaine [lidocaine] hydrochloride (p.1313·2) is included in this preparation to alleviate the pain of injection.
Gout; musculoskeletal and joint disorders.

Buta Pee Dee *PD, Thai.*
Phenylbutazone (p.78·1); methyl salicylate (p.55·1).
Musculoskeletal and joint disorders.

Butacort *Pacific, NZ.*
Budesonide (p.1064·2).
Nasal polyps; rhinitis.

Butacortelone *Riker, Mex.*
Ibuprofen (p.43·2).
Inflammation; musculoskeletal and joint disorders; pain.

Butacote *Novartis, UK.*
Phenylbutazone (p.78·1).
Ankylosing spondylitis.

Butadion *Streuli, Switz.*
Phenylbutazone (p.78·1) or phenylbutazone sodium (p.78·3).
Lignocaine [lidocaine] hydrochloride (p.1313·2) is included in the intramuscular injection to alleviate the pain of injection.
Gout; musculoskeletal and joint disorders; phlebitis; soft-tissue disorders.

Butafen *Tocogino, Mex.*
Oxyphenbutazone (p.71·1).

Butahale *Reddy, Singapore.*
Salbutamol sulfate (p.770·3).
Obstructive airways disease.

Butalin *Julphar, UAE.*
Salbutamol sulfate (p.770·3).
Obstructive airways disease; premature labour.

Butaliret *Fatol, Ger.*
Terbutaline sulfate (p.776·2).
Obstructive airways disease.

Butalitab *Fatol, Ger.*
Terbutaline sulfate (p.776·2).
Obstructive airways disease.

Butamine *Taro, Israel.*
Dobutamine hydrochloride (p.880·2).
Heart failure.

Butamol *Pharmaland, Thai.*
Salbutamol sulfate (p.770·3).
Obstructive airways disease; premature labour.

Butaparin *Streuli, Switz.*
Heparin sodium (p.902·1); phenylbutazone (p.78·1); thymol (p.1158·3).
Peripheral vascular disorders.

Butapirin *IQB, Braz.*
Phenylbutazone calcium (p.78·3); paracetamol (p.71·2).
Fever; inflammation; pain.

Butarion *Chew, Thai.*
Phenylbutazone (p.78·1); dipyrone (p.34·1).
Gout; musculoskeletal and joint disorders.

Butazil *Neo Quimica, Braz.*
Phenylbutazone (p.78·1); paracetamol (p.71·2).
Fever; inflammation; pain.

Butazolidin
Note.This name is used for preparations of different composition.
Novartis, Aust.; Novartis, Austral.; Novartis, Belg.; Novartis, Ger.; Novartis, Neth.
Phenylbutazone (p.78·1) or phenylbutazone sodium (p.78·3).
Cinchocaine (p.1309·1) is included in the injection to alleviate the pain of injection.
Acute ankylosing spondylitis; gout; osteoarthritis; rheumatoid arthritis.

Butazolidina
Novartis, Braz.; Novartis, Mex.; Padro, Spain.
Phenylbutazone (p.78·1).
Lignocaine [lidocaine] (p.1313·2) is included in the intramuscular injection to alleviate the pain of injection.
Ankylosing spondylitis; arthrosis; gout; rheumatoid arthritis.

Butazolidine
Novartis, Fr.; Geigy, Switz.†.
Phenylbutazone (p.78·1) or phenylbutazone sodium (p.78·3).
Cinchocaine (p.1309·1) is included in the intramuscular injection to alleviate the pain of injection.
Ankylosing spondylitis; arthrosis; gout; rheumatoid arthritis.

Butazolon *Dovalle, Braz.*
Phenylbutazone (p.78·1).
Aluminium hydroxide (p.1210·3) is included in this preparation in an attempt to reduce adverse effects on the gastrointestinal tract.
Gout; musculoskeletal, joint, and peri-articular disorders.

Butazona *Boehringer de Angeli, Braz.*
Phenylbutazone calcium (p.78·3).
Gout; musculoskeletal, joint, and peri-articular disorders.

Butazone *DDSA Pharmaceuticals, UK.*
Phenylbutazone (p.78·1).

Butazonil *Teuto, Braz.*
Phenylbutazone (p.78·1).
Gout; musculoskeletal, joint, and peri-articular disorders.

Buteridol *Lundbeck, Ger.*
Haloperidol (p.686·3).
Anxiety; behaviour disorders; movement disorders; pain; psychoses; stuttering; vomiting.

Butesin Picrate
Note.This name is used for preparations of different composition.
Abbott, Austral.
Butyl aminobenzoate picrate (p.1308·2); nitromersol (p.1151·2).
Burns; skin abrasions.

Abbott, USA.
Butyl aminobenzoate picrate (p.1308·2).
Burns.

Butibel *Wallace, USA.*
Belladonna (p.463·1); secbutabarbital sodium (p.705·2).
Gastrointestinal disorders.

Buticina *Rudefsa, Mex.*
Hyoscine butylbromide (p.468·2).

Butiral *Rayere, Mex.*
Hyoscine butylbromide (p.468·2).
Muscle spasm.

Butiran *Ecobi, Ital.*
Butamirate citrate (p.1086·2).
Coughs.

Butisol
Carter Horner, Canad.†; Wallace, USA.
Secbutabarbital sodium (p.705·2).
Insomnia; sedative.

Buti-Spirobene *Ratiopharm, Aust.*
Butizide (p.853·1); spironolactone (p.973·2).
Aldosteronism; oedema.

Butix *Pierre Fabre, Fr.*
Tablets†: Mequitazine (p.421·2).
Hypersensitivity disorders; skin disorders.
Topical gel: Diphenhydramine hydrochloride (p.416·1).
Insect stings; pruritus; urticaria.

Buto Asma
Aldo-Union, Hong Kong; Aldo, Spain.
Salbutamol (p.770·3) or salbutamol sulfate (p.770·3).
Obstructive airways disease.

Butohaler *Chiesi, Switz.†.*
Salbutamol (p.770·3).
Bronchospasm.

Butosol *Aldo, Spain.*
Beclometasone dipropionate (p.1061·2); salbutamol (p.770·3).
Obstructive airways disease.

Butotal *Kener, Mex.*
Salbutamol (p.770·3).

Butovent
Siphar, Switz.; Chiesi, Thai.
Salbutamol (p.770·3).
Obstructive airways disease.

Butrex *Pharmalab, S.Afr.†.*
Phenylbutazone (p.78·1).
Lignocaine [lidocaine] (p.1313·2) is included in the injection to alleviate the pain of injection.
Ankylosing spondylitis.

Buttercup Lozenges *LRC Products, UK.*
Bee propolis (p.1655·1).
Coughs.

Buttercup Pol'N'Count *LRC Products, UK.*
Echinacea (p.1606·2); garlic (p.1614·1).
Hay fever.

Buttercup Syrup *Pfizer Consumer, UK.*
Squill liquid extract (p.1100·3); capsicum tincture (p.1591·1).
Coughs.

Buttercup Syrup (Blackcurrant flavour) *Pfizer Consumer, UK†.*
Ipecacuanha (p.1093·1); glucose (p.1364·2); menthol (p.1632·3).
Coughs.

Buttercup Syrup (Honey and Lemon flavour) *Pfizer Consumer, UK.*
Ipecacuanha (p.1093·1); glucose (p.1364·2); menthol (p.1632·3); honey (p.1366·2).
Coughs.

Butt-Out *Paradise, Canad.*
Lobelia (p.1510·2).
Aid to smoking withdrawal.

Butyl *Masa, Thai.*
Hyoscine butylbromide (p.468·2).
Smooth muscle spasm.

Butylin *Hovid, Singapore.*
Terbutaline sulfate (p.776·2).
Obstructive airways disease.

Buvacaina *Pisa, Mex.*
Bupivacaine hydrochloride (p.1306·3).
Adrenaline [epinephrine] acid tartrate (p.829·2) is included in some injections as a vasoconstrictor to diminish absorption and localise the effect of the local anaesthetic.
Local anaesthesia.

Buventol
Lannacher, Aust.; Orion, Denm.; Orion, Fin.; Orion, Fr.; Orion, Norw.; Orion, Singapore; Orion, Swed.; Orion, Switz.; Orion, Thai.
Salbutamol (p.770·3) or salbutamol sulfate (p.770·3).
Obstructive airways disease.

Buzpel *Torbet Laboratories, UK.*
Pyrethrins; piperonyl butoxide (p.1436·2).
Insect repellent.

B-Vasc *Aspen, S.Afr.*
Atenolol (p.841·3).
Angina pectoris; hypertension.

BVK Roche plus C *Roche Nicholas, Ger.*
Vitamin B substances with ascorbic acid (p.1350·1).
Vitamin B and C deficiency.

Byclomine *Major, USA.*
Dicyclomine [dicycloverine] hydrochloride (p.466·1).
Functional bowel/irritable bowel syndrome.

Bydramine Cough *Major, USA†.*
Diphenhydramine hydrochloride (p.416·1).
Coughs.

Bye Bye Bite *Daniels, Canad.†.*
Diphenhydramine hydrochloride (p.416·1); menthol (p.1632·3); benzocaine (p.1306·2).
Bites and stings.

Bye Bye Burn *Daniels, Canad.†.*
Benzocaine (p.1306·2); cetrimonium bromide (p.1137·3); allantoin (p.1110·1); vitamin E (p.1393·3).
Burns.

Bykomycin
Byk, Aust.; Byk Gulden, Ger.
Neomycin sulfate (p.228·1).
Hepatic coma.

Byl *Medical, Port.*
Agar (p.1498·3); ox bile (p.1585·1); phenolphthalein (p.1244·1).
Gastrointestinal disorders; liver disorders.

Bymeniere *Toho, Hong Kong.*
Betahistine mesilate (p.1584·3).
Ménière's disease.

By-Mycin *Ergha, Irl.*
Doxycycline hyclate (p.200·1).
Bacterial infections.

Byodin *Lucchini, Ital.†.*
Proteins (mol. wt 30-300 kD).
Tissue repair.

Byodinoral *MDM, Ital.*
Multivitamin preparation with thiotic acid (p.1671·3) (p.1350·1).
Neuropathies.

C-20 *Osoth, Thai.*
Chlorhexidine gluconate (p.1138·2).
Mouth infections.

C500 *Rekah, Israel.*
Vitamin C (p.1389·3).
Vitamin C deficiency; vitamin C supplement.

C-1000
Seroyal, Canad.; Richlife, Hong Kong.
Ascorbic acid (p.1389·3).

C-3000 *Seroyal, Canad.*
Ascorbic acid (p.1389·3).

C Calcio *EMS, Braz.*
Vitamins C, D, and B$_6$ with calcium carbonate (p.1350·1).
Nutritional supplement.

C2 with Codeine *Wampole, Canad.*
Aspirin (p.14·2); caffeine (p.761·3); codeine phosphate (p.25·2).
Aluminium hydroxide (p.1210·3) and magnesium hydroxide (p.1233·1) are included in this preparation in an attempt to limit adverse effects on the gastrointestinal mucosa.
Cardiovascular disorders; fever; inflammation; pain.

C Factors "1000" Plus *Solgar, USA.*
Vitamin C (p.1389·3); rose hips (p.1389·3); citrus bioflavonoids complex (p.1611·1); rutoside (p.1611·2); hesperidin (p.1611·2).
Capillary bleeding.

C Forte *Frega, Canad.†.*
Ascorbic acid (p.1389·3).

C1 Inattivatore Umano *Immuno, Ital.*
Complement C1 esterase inhibitor (p.1599·1).
Hereditary angioedema.

C Mon *PP Lab, Thai.*
Ascorbic acid (p.1389·3).
Scurvy.

C Monovit *Esseti, Ital.*
Sodium ascorbate (p.1390·1).
Vitamin C deficiency.

C Pal
Eagle, Austral.†.
Vitamin and mineral preparation (p.1350·1).

Eagle, Austral.
Vitamin and mineral preparation with lysine (p.1350·1).

C Plus E Natural *Larkhall Laboratories, UK.*
Vitamin C and E preparation (p.1350·1).

C Rose Hips *Richlife, Hong Kong.*
Vitamin C (p.1389·3).

C Speridin *Marlyn, USA†.*
Hesperidin (p.1611·2); lemon bioflavonoids (p.1611·1); ascorbic acid (p.1389·3).
Capillary bleeding.

C Supa + Bioflavonoids *Vitaplex, Austral.*
Calcium ascorbate (p.1389·3); citrus bioflavonoids (p.1611·1); hesperidin (p.1611·2); rutoside (p.1611·2); rose fruit (p.1389·3).
Vitamin C deficiency.

Caas *EMS, Braz.*
Aspirin (p.14·2).
Fever; inflammation; pain; thromboembolism prophylaxis.

Cabaser
Pharmacia Upjohn, Austral.; Pharmacia Upjohn, Denm.; Pharmacia Upjohn, Fin.; Pharmacia Upjohn, Norw.; Pharmacia Upjohn, Swed.; Pharmacia Upjohn, Switz.; Pharmacia, UK.
Cabergoline (p.1167·3).
Parkinsonism.

Cabaseril *Pharmacia Upjohn, Ger.*
Cabergoline (p.1167·3).
Parkinsonism.

Cabdrivers Sugar-Free Linctus *Seven Seas, UK†.*
Ephedrine hydrochloride (p.1090·1); dextromethorphan hydrobromide (p.1087·3).
Coughs.

Cabral *Solvay, Ger.†.*
Fenyramidol hydrochloride (p.40·3).
Muscle relaxant.

Ca-C
Note.This name is used for preparations of different composition.
Novartis Consumer, Belg.; Novartis, Hong Kong; Sandoz, Neth.†; Novartis Consumer, Port.; Novartis Consumer, S.Afr.†; Novartis Nutrition, Singapore; Novartis Consumer, Switz.; Novartis, Thai.
Vitamin C (p.1389·3); calcium carbonate (p.1215·1); calcium lactate gluconate (p.1188·3).
Calcium and vitamin C deficiency.

Novartis, Fr.
Ascorbic acid (p.1389·3); calcium lactate gluconate (p.1188·3).
Asthenia.

Cachexon *Telluride, USA.*
Glutathione (p.1010·3).
AIDS-associated cachexia.

Cacit
Procter & Gamble, Belg.; Procter & Gamble, Fr.; Procter & Gamble, Irl.; Procter & Gamble, Ital.; Procter & Gamble, Neth.; Procter & Gamble, UK.
Calcium carbonate (p.1215·1).
Calcium deficiency; osteoporosis.

Cacit D3 *Procter & Gamble, Irl.*
Calcium carbonate (p.1215·1); colecalciferol (p.1391·1).
Calcium and vitamin D deficiency; osteoporosis.

Cacit Vitamina D3 *Procter & Gamble, Ital.*
Calcium carbonate (p.1215·1); colecalciferol (p.1391·1).
Calcium and vitamin D deficiency; osteoporosis.

Cacit Vitamine D$_3$
Procter & Gamble, Belg.; Procter & Gamble, Fr.
Calcium carbonate (p.1215·1); colecalciferol (p.1391·1).
Calcium and vitamin D deficiency; osteoporosis.

Cacital *Parke, Davis, Spain†.*
Papain (p.1647·3).
Hypersensitivity reactions; tissue injury.

Cactus compositum *Peithner, Aust.*
Homoeopathic preparation.

Cadens *Laphal, Fr.*
Salcatonin (p.749·3).
Hypercalcaemia; hyperphosphataemia; osteoporosis; Paget's disease of bone; reflex sympathetic dystrophy.

Cadex *Israel.*
Doxazosin mesilate (p.883·2).
Benign prostatic hyperplasia; hypertension.

Cadexcin-N *Nakorn, Thai.*
Dexamethasone phosphate (p.1067·1); neomycin sulfate (p.228·1).
Bacterial eye and ear infections.

Cadicon *Pharmasant, Thai.*
Gliclazide (p.322·2).
Diabetes mellitus.

Cadimasol *Asta Medica, Ital.*
Vitamin D and mineral preparation (p.1350·1).

Cadinyl *Medifive, Thai.*
Diphenhydramine hydrochloride (p.416·1); calamine (p.1111·3); zinc oxide (p.1128·2).
Skin irritation.

Caditar *IPRAD, Fr.*
Cade oil (p.1124·3).
Skin disorders.

Cadramine *Vana, Thai.*
Calamine (p.1111·3); zinc oxide (p.1128·2); diphenhydramine hydrochloride (p.416·1); camphor (p.1589·3); menthol (p.1632·3).
Skin irritation.

Cadramine-V *Atlantic, Hong Kong.*
Calamine (p.1111·3); zinc oxide (p.1128·2); diphenhydramine hydrochloride (p.416·1); camphor (p.1589·3); menthol (p.1632·3).
Skin disorders.

Cadraten *SmithKline Beecham, Ital.*
Cadralazine (p.853·1).
Hypertension.

Cadrilan *Ciba, Ital.†.*
Cadralazine (p.853·1).
Hypertension.

Cadrox *Dinafarma, Braz.*
Calcium carbonate (p.1215·1); aluminium hydroxide (p.1210·3).
Gastrointestinal hyperacidity.

Cadyoil *Cady, Ital.*
Emollient.

C-A-E *Seroyal, Canad.†.*
Vitamins A, C, and E (p.1350·1).

Caedax *Aesca, Aust.; Schering-Plough, Port.*
Ceftibuten (p.176·1).
Bacterial infections.

Caelyx *Sequus, Aust.; Schering-Plough, Austral.; Schering-Plough, Belg.; Schering, Canad.; Schering-Plough, Denm.; Schering-Plough, Fin.; Schering-Plough, Fr.; Essex, Ger.; Schering-Plough, Hong Kong; Sequus, Israel; Schering-Plough, Ital.; Schering-Plough, Mex.; Schering-Plough, Neth.; Schering-Plough, Norw.; Schering-Plough, Port.; Schering-Plough, S.Afr.; Schering-Plough, Singapore; Schering-Plough, Spain; Schering-Plough, Swed.; Essex, Switz.; Schering-Plough, UK.*
Liposomal doxorubicin hydrochloride (p.534·3).
Kaposi's sarcoma; ovarian cancer.

Cafadol *Typharm, UK.*
Paracetamol (p.71·2); caffeine (p.761·3).
Fever; pain.

Cafalena *Dinafarma, Braz.*
Dipyrone (p.34·1); sodium camsilate.
Cold and influenza symptoms.

Cafatine *Major, USA.*
Ergotamine tartrate (p.452·1); caffeine (p.761·3).
Migraine.

Cafatine-PB *Major, USA.*
Ergotamine tartrate (p.452·1); caffeine (p.761·3); belladonna (p.463·1); pentobarbital sodium (p.698·2).
Migraine.

Cafcit *Roxane, USA.*
Caffeine citrate (p.761·3).
Apnoea of prematurity.

Cafergot *Novartis, Aust.; Novartis, Austral.; Novartis, Belg.; Novartis, Braz.; Novartis, Canad.; Novartis, Hong Kong; Novartis, Irl.; Novartis, Israel; Novartis, Ital.; Novartis, Mex.; Novartis, Neth.; Novartis, Norw.†; Novartis, NZ; Novartis, S.Afr.; Novartis, Singapore; Novartis, Spain; Novartis, Swed.; Novartis, Switz.; Novartis, Thai.; Alliance, UK; Novartis, USA.*
Ergotamine tartrate (p.452·1); caffeine (p.761·3).
Migraine and related vascular headache.

Cafergot Comp *Novartis, Norw.†.*
Ergotamine tartrate (p.452·1); caffeine (p.761·3); belladonna alkaloids (p.463·1); butalbital (p.658·3).
Migraine and related vascular headache.

Cafergot N *Novartis, Ger.*
Ergotamine tartrate (p.452·1); caffeine (p.761·3).
Headache including migraine.

Cafergot-PB
Note.This name is used for preparations of different composition.
Novartis, Canad.
Ergotamine tartrate (p.452·1); caffeine (p.761·3); laevorotatory alkaloids of belladonna (p.463·1); pentobarbital (p.698·2).
Migraine and related vascular headache.

Novartis, S.Afr.; Novartis, Spain; Novartis, Switz.
Ergotamine tartrate (p.452·1); caffeine (p.761·3); belladonna alkaloids (p.463·1); butalbital (p.658·3).
Migraine and related vascular headache.

Cafetrate *Schein, USA†.*
Ergotamine tartrate (p.452·1); caffeine (p.761·3).
Migraine.

Caffalgina *Whitehall, Ital.*
Propyphenazone (p.80·2); caffeine (p.761·3).
Pain.

Caffedrine *Thompson, USA.*
Caffeine (p.761·3).
Fatigue.

Caffeine Withdrawal Support *Homeocan, Canad.*
Homoeopathic preparation.

Cafiaspirina *Bayer, Ital.†; Bayer, Port.; Bayer, Spain.*
Aspirin (p.14·2); caffeine (p.761·3).
Fever; pain.

Cafinitrina *Almirall, Spain.*
Caffeine citrate (p.761·3); glyceryl trinitrate (p.897·3).
Angina pectoris; biliary-tract spasm; vasospasm.

Cal-500 *Pro Doc, Canad.*
Calcium carbonate (p.1215·1).

Cal Alkyline *Eagle, Austral.*
Calcium carbonate (p.1215·1); slippery elm (p.1665·1); glycine (p.1365·3); equisetum (p.1606·3); dibasic sodium phosphate (p.1193·2); spirulina (p.1667·1); magnesium carbonate (p.1232·3); ginger (p.1227·2).
Gastric hyperacidity.

Cal Carb-HD *Konsyl, USA†.*
Calcium carbonate (p.1215·1).
Calcium deficiency; dietary supplement.

Cal D *Pro Doc, Canad.*
Calcium carbonate (p.1215·1); vitamin D (p.1391·1).

Cal Gel *Lalco, Canad.†.*
Calcium phosphate (p.1188·3).

Cal Mag plus Vitamin D *Quest, Canad.*
Calcium, magnesium, and vitamin D (p.1350·1).

Cal Mo Dol *Herbes Universelles, Canad.*
Methyl salicylate (p.55·1); camphor (p.1589·3); menthol (p.1632·3); eucalyptol (p.1609·2); turpentine oil (p.1676·3); peppermint oil (p.1243·3).

Calaband *Seton Scholl, Austral.; SSL, UK.*
Calamine (p.1111·3); zinc oxide (p.1128·2).
Eczema; leg ulcers; medicated bandage.

Calabren *Teva, Hong Kong; Berk, UK.*
Glibenclamide (p.321·3).
Diabetes mellitus.

Caladerm *Heralds, Braz.; Klinger, Braz.*
Diphenhydramine (p.416·1) or diphenhydramine hydrochloride (p.416·1); calamine (p.1111·3); camphor (p.1589·3).
Pruritus; skin irritation.

Caladryl
Note.This name is used for preparations of different composition.
Parke, Davis, Aust.†; Warner-Lambert, Spain; Warner-Lambert Consumer, Switz.; Warner-Lambert, UK.
Diphenhydramine hydrochloride (p.416·1); zinc oxide (p.1128·2); camphor (p.1589·3).
Formerly contained diphenhydramine hydrochloride, calamine, and camphor in the UK.
Skin irritation; urticaria.

Warner-Lambert, Austral.†.
Lignocaine [lidocaine] (p.1313·2) or lignocaine [lidocaine] hydrochloride (p.1313·2); calamine (p.1111·3); camphor (p.1589·3).
Pruritus; skin irritation.

Ache, Braz.; Warner-Lambert, Hong Kong; Warner-Lambert, Irl.; Warner-Lambert Consumer, Port.; Parke, Davis, S.Afr.; Warner-Lambert, Spain; Warner-Lambert, Thai.
Diphenhydramine hydrochloride (p.416·1); calamine (p.1111·3); camphor (p.1589·3).
Pruritus; skin irritation.

Warner-Lambert, Canad.; Warner-Lambert, Neth.
Diphenhydramine hydrochloride (p.416·1); calamine (p.1111·3).
Insect bites; stings.

Warner-Lambert, USA.
Pramocaine hydrochloride (p.1318·2); calamine (p.1111·3).

Caladryl Clear *Warner-Lambert, USA.*
Pramocaine hydrochloride (p.1318·2); zinc acetate (p.1398·1).

Cala-gen *Goldline, USA.*
Diphenhydramine hydrochloride (p.416·1); camphor (p.1589·3).
Pruritus.

Calais *Mead Johnson Nutritionals, Canad.*
Calcium glycerophosphate hydroxide (p.1188·2).

Calamatum *Blair, USA.*
Calamine (p.1111·3); zinc oxide (p.1128·2); menthol (p.1632·3); camphor (p.1589·3); benzocaine (p.1306·2).
Minor skin irritation.

Calamina *Dermopen, Braz.*
Diphenhydramine hydrochloride (p.416·1); calamine (p.1111·3).
Pruritus; skin irritation.

Calamina Composta
Note.This name is used for preparations of different composition.
Neo Quimica, Braz.
Calamine (p.1111·3); diphenhydramine (p.416·1); camphor (p.1589·3).
Pruritus; skin irritation.

QIF, Braz.
Diphenhydramine hydrochloride (p.416·1); calamine (p.1111·3).
Pruritus; skin irritation.

Calamine Antihistamine *Stanley, Canad.*
Calamine (p.1111·3); diphenhydramine hydrochloride (p.416·1).
Pruritus.

Calamine Lotion
Note.This name is used for preparations of different composition.
McGloin, Austral.
Calamine (p.1111·3); zinc oxide (p.1128·2); phenol (p.1152·3).
Insect bites; skin irritation; sunburn.

Sam-On, Israel; Vitamed, Israel.
Calamine (p.1111·3); zinc oxide (p.1128·2).
Pruritus.

Calamox *Hauck, USA.*
Calamine (p.1111·3).
Minor skin irritation.

Calamycin *Pfeiffer, USA.*
Zinc oxide (p.1128·2); calamine (p.1111·3); benzocaine (p.1306·2); chloroxylenol (p.1142·1); mepyramine maleate (p.421·1).
Pruritus.

Calan
Note.This name is used for preparations of different composition.
Takeda, Jpn.
Vinpocetine (p.1680·1).
Cerebrovascular disorders.

Searle, USA.
Verapamil hydrochloride (p.989·1).
Angina pectoris; arrhythmias; hypertension.

Calanda *Atlantis, Mex.*
Multivitamin and mineral preparation (p.1350·1).

Calanif *Berk, UK.*
Nifedipine (p.940·1).
Angina pectoris; hypertension; Raynaud's syndrome.

Calanol *Nakornpatana, Thai.*
Diphenhydramine hydrochloride (p.416·1); calamine (p.1111·3).
Skin irritation.

Cal-Antagon *Ferring, Port.*
Diltiazem hydrochloride (p.874·3).
Angina pectoris; arrhythmias; hypertension.

Calapro *Progress, Thai.*
Calamine (p.1111·3); diphenhydramine hydrochloride (p.416·1).
Skin irritation.

Calasept *Scania, Swed.†.*
Calcium hydroxide (p.1588·3); sodium chloride; potassium chloride; calcium chloride; sodium bicarbonate.
Dental cavities.

Calasthetic *Restan, S.Afr.*
Calamine (p.1111·3); benzocaine (p.1306·2); pheniramine maleate (p.422·3); phenol (p.1152·3).
Skin disorders.

Calatrim *Trima, Israel.*
Calamine (p.1111·3); zinc oxide (p.1128·2).
Sunburn; urticaria.

Calatrim cum Sulphur *Trima, Israel.*
Calamine (p.1111·3); zinc oxide (p.1128·2); sulfur (p.1123·3).
Pruritus.

Calax *Odan, Canad.*
Docusate calcium (p.1222·3).
Constipation.

Calazem *Berk, UK†.*
Diltiazem hydrochloride (p.874·3).
Angina pectoris.

Calbion *Merck, Spain†.*
Calcium pidolate (p.1188·3).
Hypocalcaemia; osteoporosis.

Calcanate *ST, Thai.*
Calcium carbonate (p.1215·1).
Calcium deficiency.

Cal-Car *Selvi, Ital.*
Calcium carbonate (p.1215·1).
Calcium deficiency; calcium supplement.

Calcarb with Vitamin D *Zenith Goldline, USA.*
Calcium carbonate (p.1215·1); vitamin D (p.1391·1).

Calcascorbin *Pharmonta, Aust.*
Calcium ascorbate (p.1389·3).
Vitamin C deficiency.

Calcchew *Ranbaxy, Thai.*
Calcium carbonate (p.1215·1); calcium gluconate (p.1188·2).
Calcium supplement; hypocalcaemia.

Calcedon *Worwag, Ger.†.*
Calcium carbonate (p.1215·1).
Calcium deficiency.

Calceos *Provalis, UK.*
Calcium carbonate (p.1215·1); colecalciferol (p.1391·1).
Calcium and vitamin D deficiency.

Calcet *Mission Pharmacal, USA.*
Calcium lactate (p.1188·2); calcium gluconate (p.1188·2); calcium carbonate (p.1215·1); vitamin D (p.1391·1).
Calcium supplement.

Calcet Plus *Mission Pharmacal, USA.*
Multivitamin and mineral preparation with iron and folic acid (p.1350·1).
Low-calcium leg cramping; nursing mothers; osteoporosis; patients with milk allergies; pre- and postoperative patients.

Calcetat *Giovanardi, Ital.*
Calcium acetate (p.1187·3).
Calcium supplement.

Calcette *Ashbourne, UK†.*
Calcium carbonate (p.1215·1).
Calcium supplement; hyperphosphataemia; osteoporosis.

Calcevita
Roche Consumer, Neth.; Roche, Swed.
Multivitamin preparation with calcium (p.1350·1).
Calcium and vitamin deficiency.

Calci *Hexal, Ger.*
Salcatonin (p.749·3).
Hypercalcaemia; osteolysis; osteoporosis; Paget's disease of bone; reflex sympathetic dystrophy.

Calcia *Peter Black, UK.*
Calcium carbonate (p.1215·1) with vitamins and iron (p.1350·1).

Calciben *FIRMA, Ital.*
Salcatonin (p.749·3).
Hypercalcaemia; osteoporosis; Paget's disease of bone; prevention of fracture in osteoporosis; reflex sympathetic dystrophy.

Calcibind *Mission Pharmacal, USA.*
Sodium cellulose phosphate (p.1022·3).
Ion exchange resin binding calcium.

Calcibon *Masa, Thai.*
Calcium citrate (p.1188·1).
Calcium deficiency.

Calcibronat *Novartis, Fr.; Novartis, Ital.; Novartis, Mex.*
Calcium bromolactobionate (p.659·1).
Sedative.

CalciCaps *Nion, USA.*
Calcium with vitamin D and phosphorus (p.1350·1).
Calcium deficiency; dietary supplement.

CalciCaps with iron *Nion, USA.*
Calcium with vitamin D, phosphorus, and iron (p.1350·1).
Calcium deficiency; dietary supplement.

CalciCaps M-Z *Nion, USA.*
Calcium with vitamins A and D, and minerals (p.1350·1).

Calcicard
Note.This name is used for preparations of different composition.
Parke-Med, S.Afr.
Verapamil hydrochloride (p.989·1).
Angina pectoris; arrhythmias; hypertension.

Norton, UK.
Diltiazem hydrochloride (p.874·3).
Angina pectoris; hypertension.

Calci-Chew *Piette, Belg.; Christiaens, Neth.; R&D, USA.*
Calcium carbonate (p.1215·1).
Calcium deficiency; calcium supplement; hyperphosphataemia; osteoporosis.

Calcichew *Nycomed, Fin.; Nycomed, Hong Kong; Shire, Irl.; Shire, UK.*
Calcium carbonate (p.1215·1).
Calcium deficiency; hyperphosphataemia; osteoporosis.

Calcichew D₃ *Nycomed, Denm.; Nycomed, Fin.; Nycomed, Hong Kong; Shire, Irl.; Nycomed, Swed.; Shire, UK.*
Calcium carbonate (p.1215·1); colecalciferol (p.1391·1).
Calcium and vitamin D deficiency; osteomalacia; osteoporosis.

Calciday *Nature's Bounty, USA.*
Calcium carbonate (p.1215·1).
Calcium deficiency; dietary supplement.

Calcidia *Nicholas, Fr.*
Calcium carbonate (p.1215·1).
Hypocalcaemia and hyperphosphoraemia related to kidney disorders; renal osteodystrophy.

Calcidon *Roche, Ital.*
Calcium carbonate (p.1215·1); colecalciferol (p.1391·1).
Calcium and vitamin D deficiency.

Calcidose *Opocalcium, Fr.*
Calcium carbonate (p.1215·1).
Calcium deficiency; osteoporosis.

Calcidose Vitamine D *Opocalcium, Fr.*
Calcium carbonate (p.1215·1); colecalciferol (p.1391·1).
Calcium and vitamin D deficiency; osteoporosis.

Calcidrine *Abbott, USA.*
Codeine (p.25·2); calcium iodide (p.1086·2).
Coughs.

Calcidrink *Shire, UK.*
Calcium carbonate (p.1215·1).
Calcium deficiency; osteoporosis.

Calcifar *Farcoral, Mex.*
Calcium carbonate (p.1215·1).

Calciferol
Note.This name is used for preparations of different composition.
Delta, Braz.
Ergocalciferol; vitamin B₁₂; calcium gluconate; calcium phosphate; sodium fluoride (p.1350·1).
Vitamin and mineral supplement.

EMS, Braz.
Ergocalciferol; vitamin B₁₂; calcium chloride; calcium phosphate; sodium fluoride (p.1350·1).
Vitamin and mineral supplement.

Heralds, Braz.
Ergocalciferol; calcium phosphate; cyanocobalamin; sodium fluoride (p.1350·1).
Vitamin and mineral supplement.

Schwarz, USA.
Ergocalciferol (p.1391·2).
Familial hypophosphataemia; gastrointestinal, liver, or biliary disease associated with malabsorption of vitamin D; hypoparathyroidism; refractory rickets.

Calciferol B12 *Medquimica, Braz.*
Ergocalciferol; vitamin B₁₂; calcium phosphate; sodium fluoride (p.1350·1).
Vitamin and mineral supplement.

Calcifluor *Crinex, Fr.*
Calcium fluoride (p.1356·1).
Dental caries prophylaxis.

Calcifolin *Ibirn, Ital.*
Calcium folinate (p.1363·1).
Antidote to folic acid antagonists; folic acid deficiency.

Calciforte *Grimberg, Fr.*
Oral liquid: Calcium gluconate (p.1188·2); calcium lactate (p.1188·2); calcium gluceptate (p.1188·1); calcium chloride (p.1188·1); yeast (Saccharomyces cerevisiae) (p.1398·1).

Powder for oral solution: Calcium gluconate (p.1188·2); calcium lactate (p.1188·2); calcium gluceptate (p.1188·1); calcium chloride (p.1188·1); calcium carbonate (p.1215·1); yeast (Saccharomyces cerevisiae) (p.1398·1).
Calcium deficiency; osteoporosis.

Calcigard *Torrent, Thai.*
Nifedipine (p.940·1).
Angina pectoris.

Calcigen D *Opfermann, Ger.*
Calcium carbonate (p.1215·1); colecalciferol (p.1391·1).
Calcium and vitamin D deficiency.

Calcigenol *Roussel, Port.*
Calcium phosphate (p.1188·3).

Calcigenol B12 *Hoechst Marion Roussel, Braz.*
Calcium phosphate; vitamin B₁₂; vitamin D; sodium fluoride (p.1350·1).
Vitamin and mineral supplement.

Calcigenol Irradiado *Hoechst Marion Roussel, Braz.*
Calcium phosphate (p.1188·3); sodium fluoride (p.1375·3).
Calcium and sodium deficiencies.

Calcigran *Nycomed, Norw.*
Oral granules: Calcium carbonate (p.1215·1); ascorbic acid (p.1389·3); colecalciferol (p.1391·1).

The symbol † denotes a preparation no longer actively marketed

Tablets: Calcium carbonate (p.1215·1); colecalciferol (p.1391·1).
Calcium supplement; osteoporosis.

Calcihep *Rhone-Poulenc Rorer, Austral.*
Heparin calcium (p.902·1).

Calcijex *Abbott, Aust.; Abbott, Austral.; Abbott, Canad.†; Abbott, Fin.; Abbott, Hong Kong; Abbott, Irl.; Abbott, Israel; Abbott, Ital.; Abbott, Mex.; Abbott, Norw.; Abbott, Singapore; Abbott, Spain; Abbott, Swed.; Abbott, Switz.; Abbott, UK; Abbott, USA.*
Calcitriol (p.1391·1).
Hyperparathyroidism; hypocalcaemia in chronic renal dialysis; osteodystrophy.

Calcilac KT *Jenapharm, Ger.*
Calcium carbonate (p.1215·1); colecalciferol (p.1391·1).
Calcium and vitamin D deficiency.

Calcilat *Eastern Pharmaceuticals, UK.*
Nifedipine (p.940·1).
Angina pectoris; hypertension; Raynaud's syndrome.

Calcilean *Organon Teknika, Canad.†*
Heparin calcium (p.902·1).
Thromboembolic disorders; thrombosis prophylaxis.

Calciless *Sam-On, Israel.*
Dibasic sodium phosphate (p.1193·2); monobasic potassium phosphate (p.1193·1).
Calcium oxalate renal calculi.

Calcilin *Laevosan, Aust.*
Calcium levulinate (p.1188·3).
Allergic and anaphylactic conditions; calcium deficiency; haemorrhage; inflammation.

Calcilin compositum *Laevosan, Aust.*
Chlorphenoxamine hydrochloride (p.412·3); calcium levulinate (p.1188·3); calcium gluconate (p.1188·2).
Allergic disorders.

Calcilos *TAD, Ger.*
Calcium carbonate (p.1215·1).
Calcium deficiency.

Calcimagon *Orion, Ger.*
Calcium carbonate (p.1215·1).
Calcium deficiency; osteoporosis.

Calcimagon-D3 *Orion, Ger.; Nycomed, Switz.*
Calcium carbonate (p.1215·1); colecalciferol (p.1391·1).
Calcium and vitamin D deficiency; osteoporosis.

Calcimar *Rhone-Poulenc Rorer, Canad.; Rhone-Poulenc Rorer, USA.*
Salcatonin (p.749·3).
Hypercalcaemia; osteoporosis; Paget's disease of bone.

Calcimax
Note.This name is used for preparations of different composition.
Carmaran, Canad.†
Calcium lactate (p.1188·2).

Wallace Mfg Chem., UK.
Calcium levulinate (p.1188·3); calcium chloride (p.1188·1); vitamins (p.1350·1).

Calcimed D₃ *Hermes, Ger.*
Calcium carbonate (p.1215·1); colecalciferol (p.1391·1).
Calcium and vitamin D deficiency.

Calcimega *Larkhall Laboratories, UK.*
Calcium with vitamins and minerals (p.1350·1).

Calci-Mix *R&D, USA.*
Calcium carbonate (p.1215·1).
Calcium deficiency; dietary supplement.

Calcimon *Byk, Port.*
Salcatonin (p.749·3).
Hypercalcaemia; osteolytic bone pain; osteoporosis; Paget's disease of bone.

Calcimonta *Byk Tosse, Ger.; Byk Gulden, Ger.*
Salcatonin (p.749·3).
Hypercalcaemia; osteolysis; osteoporosis; Paget's disease of bone; reflex sympathetic dystrophy.

Calcimore *Taro, Israel.*
Calcium carbonate (p.1215·1).
Calcium supplement; gastritis; gastrointestinal hyperacidity; heartburn; peptic ulcer.

Calcinatal *Warner-Lambert, Spain.*
Multivitamin and mineral preparation (p.1350·1).

Calcinatal-MK *Propan, S.Afr.†*
Multivitamin and mineral preparation (p.1350·1).

Calcinil *Sclavo, Ital.*
Elcatonin (p.749·2).
Hypercalcaemia; osteoporosis; Paget's disease of bone; reflex sympathetic dystrophy.

Calcio 20 Complex *Madariaga, Spain.*
Ascorbic acid (p.1389·3); calcium phosphate (p.1188·3); calcium pantothenate (p.1374·2); cyanocobalamin (p.1388·1); colecalciferol (p.1391·1); vitamin A palmitate (p.1383·2).
Calcium deficiency; osteoporosis.

Calcio Dobetin *Angelini, Ital.*
Cyanocobalamin (p.1388·1); calcium gluconate (p.1188·2); calcium gluceptate (p.1188·1).
Calcium and vitamin B₁₂ deficiency.

Calcio 20 Emulsion *Madariaga, Spain.*
Calcium phosphate (p.1188·3).
Calcium deficiency.

Calcio Faes DYC *Faes, Spain†.*
Ascorbic acid (p.1389·3); calcium carbonate (p.1215·1); calcium fluoride (p.1356·1); calcium phosphate (p.1188·3); colecalciferol (p.1391·1).
Bone and dental disorders; calcium deficiency; osteomalacia.

Calcio 20 Fuerte *Madariaga, Spain.*
Calcium phosphate (p.1188·3); colecalciferol (p.1391·1).
Calcium deficiency; osteoporosis.

Calcio Geve D y C *Reig Jofre, Spain.*
Ascorbic acid (p.1389·3); calcium carbonate (p.1215·1); calcium fluoride (p.1356·1); calcium phosphate (p.1188·3); colecalciferol (p.1391·1).
Formerly contained ascorbic acid, calcium gluceptate, calcium hypophosphite, and calcium laevulinolactogluconate.
Calcium deficiency; vitamin C and D deficiency.

Calcio Vitam D3 *Berenguer Infale, Spain†.*
Calcium hydrogen phosphate (p.1188·2); colecalciferol (p.1391·1).
Bone and dental disorders; calcium deficiency; osteomalacia.

Calcio Vitaminado *Bunker, Braz.*
Calcium phosphate; vitamin B₁₂; ergocalciferol; sodium fluoride; gastric mucosa extract (p.1350·1).
Nutritional supplement.

Calcio Vitaminado B12 *Neo Quimica, Braz.*
Calcium phosphate; calcium glycerophosphate; vitamin A; vitamin B₁₂; ergocalciferol (p.1350·1).
Calcium and vitamin supplement.

Calcioday-D *Eurodrug, Hong Kong; Eurodrug, Singapore.*
Calcium carbonate (p.1215·1); colecalciferol (p.1391·1); magnesium oxide (p.1233·2).
Calcium, magnesium, and vitamin D supplement.

Calciodie *Epifarma, Ital.*
Calcium carbonate (p.1215·1).
Calcium deficiency; calcium supplement.

Calciofix *Damor, Ital.*
L-Arginine (p.1353·3); L-lysine (p.1370·3); glycerophosphoric acid (p.1617·3).
Bone and dental disorders; tonic.

Calciomed *Lisapharma, Ital.*
Calcium carbonate (p.1215·1).
Calcium deficiency; calcium supplement.

Calciopen *Astra, Swed.†*
Phenoxymethylpenicillin potassium (p.235·1).
Bacterial infections.

Calciopiu *Lafare, Ital.*
Calcium carbonate (p.1215·1).
Calcium deficiency; calcium supplement.

Calcioral *Novartis, Port.*
Calcium carbonate (p.1215·1).

Calcioretard *Farmapros, Spain.*
Calcium ascorbate (p.1389·3); lysine hydrochloride (p.1370·3); tryptophan (p.311·3).
Bone and dental disorders; calcium deficiency; osteomalacia; rickets.

Calciosan *Provita, Ital.*
Multivitamin and mineral preparation (p.1350·1).

Calciosint *Pulitzer, Ital.*
Salcatonin (p.749·3).
Hypercalcaemia; osteoporosis; Paget's disease of bone; reflex sympathetic dystrophy.

Calcioton *San Carlo, Ital.*
Salcatonin (p.749·3).
Hypercalcaemia; osteoporosis; Paget's disease of bone; reflex sympathetic dystrophy.

Calciovit Urto *Lafare, Ital.*
Calcium oleate; ergocalciferol (p.1391·2).
Vitamin deficiency.

Calciovital Irradiado *Herald's, Braz.*
Calcium phosphate; vitamin A palmitate; ergocalciferol; cyanocobalamin (p.1350·1).
Calcium and vitamin supplement.

Calciozim *Searle, Ital.*
Vitamin and mineral preparation (p.1350·1).

Calciparin *Sanofi Winthrop, Aust.†; Sanofi Synthelabo, Ger.*
Heparin calcium (p.902·1).
Thromboembolic disorders.

Calciparina *Italfarmaco, Ital.; Sanofi Winthrop, Port.†; Sanofi Synthelabo, Spain.*
Heparin calcium (p.902·1).
Thromboembolic disorders.

Calciparine *Sanofi Synthelabo, Austral.; Sanofi Winthrop, Fr.; Sanofi Winthrop, Irl.; Choay, Israel; Mer-National, S.Afr.; Sanofi Synthelabo, Switz.; Sanofi Winthrop, UK.*
Heparin calcium (p.902·1).
Thromboembolic disorders.

Calcipen *Leo, Denm.; Leo, Norw.*
Phenoxymethylpenicillin calcium (p.235·1).
Bacterial infections.

Calciplex *Vitaplex, Austral.*
Mineral and vitamin D preparation (p.1350·1).
Calcium deficiency; osteoporosis.

Calciplus *Chemedica, Switz.*
Calcium carbonate (p.1215·1); colecalciferol (p.1391·1).
Calcium deficiency.

Calcipor *Ibirn, Ital.*
Heparin calcium (p.902·1).
Thromboembolic disorders.

Calcipot *3M, Ger.*
Effervescent tablets†: Calcium gluconate (p.1188·2).
Tablets: Calcium citrate (p.1188·1); calcium hydrogen phosphate (p.1188·2).
Calcium deficiency.

Calcipot C *Kolassa, Aust.*
Vitamin C (p.1389·3); rutoside (p.1611·2); calcium citrate (p.1188·1); calcium glycerophosphate (p.1188·2).
Calcium and vitamin C deficiency.

Calcipot D₃ *Kolassa, Aust.*
Colecalciferol (p.1391·1); calcium citrate (p.1188·1); calcium glycerophosphate (p.1188·2).
Calcium and vitamin D deficiency.

Calciprat *IPRAD, Fr.*
Calcium carbonate (p.1215·1).
Calcium deficiency; osteoporosis.

Calciprat D₃ *IPRAD, Fr.*
Calcium carbonate (p.1215·1); colecalciferol (p.1391·1).
Calcium and vitamin D deficiency; osteoporosis.

Calcipulpe *Septodont, Switz.†*
Barium sulfate (p.1032·1); calcium hydroxide (p.1588·3).
Covering for dental pulp.

Calci-Rav *Asta Medica, Israel.*
Calcium carbonate (p.1215·1).
Calcium supplement.

Calciretard *Kohler-Pharma, Ger.*
Calcium aspartate.
Hypocalcaemia.

Calcisan *Petrasch, Aust.*
Calcium hydrogen phosphate (p.1188·2); calcium carbonate (p.1215·1).
Calcium deficiency; osteoporosis.

Calcisan B + C *Petrasch, Aust.*
Calcium hydrogen phosphate (p.1188·2); calcium carbonate (p.1215·1); ascorbic acid (p.1389·3); thiamine hydrochloride (p.1975·1).
Calcium, vitamin B₁, and vitamin C deficiency; osteoporosis.

Calcisan C *Petrasch, Aust.*
Calcium hydrogen phosphate (p.1188·2); calcium carbonate (p.1215·1); ascorbic acid (p.1389·3).
Calcium and vitamin C deficiency.

Calcisan D *Petrasch, Aust.*
Calcium hydrogen phosphate (p.1188·2); calcium carbonate (p.1215·1); ergocalciferol (p.1391·2).
Calcium and vitamin D deficiency; osteoporosis.

Calcisorb *3M, Austral.; 3M, Belg.†; 3M, Israel; 3M, Neth.; 3M, NZ; 3M, S.Afr.†; 3M, UK†.*
Sodium cellulose phosphate (p.1022·3).
Hypercalcaemia; hypercalciuria; osteopetrosis; renal calculi; vitamin D intoxication.

Calcitar *Specia, Fr.†; Rhone-Poulenc Rorer, Ital.†*
Calcitonin (pork) (p.749·2).
Hypercalcaemia; osteoporosis; Paget's disease of bone.

Calcitare *Rhone-Poulenc Rorer, Austral.†; Rhone-Poulenc Rorer, Irl.†; Rhone-Poulenc Rorer, UK†.*
Calcitonin (pork) (p.749·2).
Hypercalcaemia; Paget's disease of bone.

Calcite *Riva, Canad.*
Calcium carbonate (p.1215·1).
Calcium supplement.

Calcite D *Riva, Canad.*
Calcium carbonate (p.1215·1); vitamin D (p.1391·1).
Dietary supplement.

Calcitol *Frega, Canad.†.*
Vitamin A, vitamin D, and calcium (p.1350·1).

Calcitonin *Novartis, Aust.*
Salcatonin (p.749·3).
Bone pain in malignancy; hypercalcaemia; osteoporosis; Paget's disease of bone; pancreatic disorders; reflex sympathetic dystrophy.

Calcitonina *Novartis, Ital.*
Salcatonin (p.749·3).
Hypercalcaemia; osteoporosis; Paget's disease of bone; reflex sympathetic dystrophy.

Calcitoran *Teikoku, Jpn.*
Salcatonin (p.749·3).
Osteoporosis.

Calcitran B12 *Medley, Braz.*
Cyanocobalamin; ergocalciferol; calcium phosphate; calcium glycerophosphate; sodium fluoride (p.1350·1).
Vitamin and mineral supplement.

Calcitrans *Fresenius-Praxis, Ger.†.*
Calcium gluconate (p.1188·2); calcium gluceptate (p.1188·1); calcium saccharate (p.1589·1).
Calcium deficiency.

Calcitrat *Merckle, Ger.*
Calcium citrate (p.1188·1).
Calcium deficiency; osteoporosis.

Cal-Citrate *Bio-Tech, USA.*
Calcium citrate (p.1188·1).
Calcium supplement.

Calcitridin *Opfermann, Ger.*
Calcium carbonate (p.1215·1).
Calcium deficiency; osteoporosis.

Calcitugg *Nycomed, Swed.*
Calcium carbonate (p.1215·1).
Calcium deficiency; hyperphosphataemia; osteoporosis.

Calcium 600
Note.This name is used for preparations of different composition.
Wyeth Lederle, Port.
Calcium phosphate (p.1188·3); colecalciferol (p.1391·1).

Solgar, USA.
Calcium carbonate (p.1215·1); vitamin D (p.1391·1).

Calcium 625 *Progress, Thai.*
Calcium carbonate (p.1215·1).
Calcium deficiency.

Calcium AL *Aliud, Ger.*
Calcium carbonate (p.1215·1).
Calcium supplement.

Calcium beta *Betapharm, Ger.*
Calcium carbonate (p.1215·1).
Calcium supplement; osteoporosis.

Calcium Braun *Braun, Ger.*
Calcium gluconate (p.1188·2); calcium saccharate (p.1589·1).
Calcium deficiency.

Calcium Chewable *Richlife, Hong Kong.*
Calcium; phosphorus; magnesium; vitamin D (p.1350·1).
Dietary supplement.

Calcium Clear *Nutraceuticals, UK.*
Calcium lactate (p.1188·2); magnesium carbonate (p.1232·3).
Calcium supplement.

Calcium Corbiere *Sanofi Winthrop, Fr.†.*
Calcium glucoheptogluconate (p.1188·1).
Hypocalcaemia.

Calcium Corbiere vitamine CDPP *Sanofi Winthrop, Fr.†.*
Anhydrous calcium gluceptate (p.1188·1) or calcium glucoheptogluconate with vitamins (p.1350·1).
Asthenia.

Calcium D₃ *Stada, Ger.*
Calcium carbonate (p.1215·1); colecalciferol (p.1391·1).
Osteoporosis.

Calcium D Sauter *Roche, Switz.*
Calcium hydrogen phosphate (p.1188·2); calcium gluconate (p.1188·2); calcium lactate (p.1188·2); ergocalciferol (p.1391·2); ascorbic acid (p.1389·3).
Calcium supplement; disorders of calcium and phosphorus metabolism; vitamin C and D deficiencies.

Calcium Dago *Steiner, Ger.*
Calcium carbonate (p.1215·1).
Calcium deficiency.

Calcium Docuphen *Pharmascience, Canad.†*
Docusate calcium (p.1222·3); yellow phenolphthalein (p.1244·1).
Constipation.

Calcium and Ergocalciferol Tablets *Cox, UK.*
Calcium lactate 300 mg (p.1188·2); calcium phosphate 150 mg (p.1188·3); ergocalciferol 10 μg (p.1391·2).
Each tablet contains 400 units of vitamin-D activity. They should be crushed or chewed before administration.
Distinguish from Calcium with Vitamin D Tablets (BPC 1973).

Calcium Fresenius
Note.This name is used for preparations of different composition.
Fresenius Kabi, Aust.
Calcium gluconate (p.1188·2); calcium saccharate (p.1589·1).
Hypocalcaemia; osteoporosis.

Fresenius Kabi, Ger.
Calcium gluconate (p.1188·2); calcium gluceptate (p.1188·1); calcium saccharate (p.1589·1).
Calcium deficiency.

Calcium gluconicum *Eifelfango, Ger.*
Calcium gluconate (p.1188·2); calcium levulinate (p.1188·3).
Calcium deficiency.

Calcium Heumann *Heumann, Ger.*
Calcium carbonate (p.1215·1).
Calcium deficiency.

Calcium Hexal *Hexal, Ger.*
Calcium carbonate (p.1215·1).
Calcium supplement.

Calcium 600mg *Pharmadass, UK.*
Calcium carbonate (p.1215·1); vitamins A and D (p.1350·1).

Calcium Novartis *Novartis Consumer, Aust.*
Calcium lactate gluconate (p.1188·3).
Calcium deficiency; osteoporosis.

Calcium Oyster Shell *Novopharm, Canad.*
Calcium carbonate (p.1215·1).
Calcium supplement.

Calcium Resonium *Sanofi Synthelabo, Austral.; Sanofi Synthelabo, Ger.; Sanofi Winthrop, Ger.; Sanofi Winthrop, Hong Kong; Sanofi Winthrop, Irl.; Sanofi Winthrop, Neth.†; Sanofi Winthrop, NZ; Sanofi Winthrop, UK.*
Calcium polystyrene sulfonate (p.1002·3).
Hyperkalaemia.

Calcium Rich Rolaids *Warner-Lambert, USA.*
Magnesium hydroxide (p.1233·1); calcium carbonate (p.1215·1).
Hyperacidity.

Calcium Stada *Stada, Ger.*
Calcium carbonate (p.1215·1).
Calcium deficiency; osteoporosis.

Calcium Stanley *Stanley, Canad.*
Calcium gluceptate (p.1188·1); calcium gluconate (p.1188·2).
Calcium deficiency; calcium supplement.

Calcium Truw *Truw, Ger.†.*
Calcium gluconate (p.1188·2); calcium saccharate (p.1589·1).
Calcium deficiency.

Calcium Unison *Unison, Thai.*
Calcium lactate (p.1188·2).
Calcium supplement.

Calcium Verla *Verla, Ger.*
Effervescent tablets: Calcium carbonate (p.1215·1).
Calcium deficiency; osteoporosis.
Injection: Calcium gluconate (p.1188·2); calcium saccharate (p.1589·1).
Allergic disorders; calcium deficiency; lead poisoning; tetany.
Tablets: Calcium phosphate (p.1188·3); calcium citrate (p.1188·1).
Allergic reactions; calcium deficiency; osteomalacia; osteoporosis; tetany.

Calcium Verla D *Verla, Ger.*
Calcium carbonate (p.1215·1); colecalciferol (p.1391·1).
Calcium and vitamin D₃ deficiency; osteoporosis.

Calcium Vitis *Neopharma, Ger.*
Sodium calcium edetate (p.1022·1).
Heavy-metal poisoning.

Calcium von CT *CT, Ger.*
Calcium carbonate (p.1215·1).
Calcium deficiency; osteoporosis.

Calcium-D *Roche Consumer, Neth.†.*
Calcium carbonate (p.1215·1); colecalciferol (p.1391·1).
Calcium and vitamin D deficiency.

Calcium-D-Redoxon
Roche, Hong Kong; Roche Consumer, Singapore; Roche, Thai.
Calcium; vitamin C; vitamin B₆; vitamin D (p.1350·1).
Calcium and vitamin D deficiency.

Calcium-D-Sandoz *Novartis Consumer, Ger.*
Calcium carbonate (p.1215·1); colecalciferol (p.1391·1).
Calcium and vitamin D deficiency; osteoporosis.

Calcium-dura *Merck dura, Ger.*
Calcium carbonate (p.1215·1).
Osteoporosis.

Calcium-dura Vit D₃ *Merck dura, Ger.*
Calcium phosphate (p.1188·3); colecalciferol (p.1391·1).
Calcium and vitamin D deficiency.

Calcium-EAP *Kohler-Pharma, Ger.*
Phosphorylcolamine calcium.
Multiple sclerosis.

Calcium-Rougier *Rougier, Canad.*
Calcium gluceptate (p.1188·1); calcium gluconate (p.1188·2).
Calcium supplement.

Calcium-Rutinion *Biomo, Ger.*
Rutoside (p.1611·2); calcium gluconate (p.1188·2).
Capillary disorders; epistaxis; retinopathy; skin disorders.

Calcium-Sandoz
Note.This name is used for preparations of different composition.
Novartis Consumer, Belg.; Novartis Consumer, Canad.; Novartis, Denm.; Novartis, Fin.; Novartis, Fr.; Novartis Consumer, Ger.; Novartis, Hong Kong; Novartis, Israel; Novartis Consumer, Ital.; Novartis, Mex.; Novartis Consumer, Neth.; Novartis, Norw.; Novartis, NZ; Novartis, Port.; Novartis Consumer, S.Afr.; Novartis Nutrition, Singapore; Novartis, Swed.; Novartis, Switz.; Novartis, Thai.
Effervescent tablets; powder for oral solution: Calcium lactate gluconate (p.1188·3); calcium carbonate (p.1215·1).
Bone demineralisation; calcium supplement; osteomalacia; osteoporosis; rickets; tetany.
Novartis Consumer, Belg.; Novartis, Denm.; Novartis, Fin.; Novartis, Fr.†; Novartis, Israel; Novartis Consumer, Neth.; Novartis, Norw.†; Novartis, S.Afr.; Novartis, Spain; Novartis, Swed.; Novartis, Switz.; Sandoz, UK†.
Injection: Calcium glubionate (p.1188·1).
Adjuvant in hyperkalaemia; calcium deficiency; osteomalacia; osteoporosis; poisoning with lead, fluorides, or magnesium; rickets; tetany.
Novartis, Braz.; Sandoz, Fr.†; Novartis Consumer, Ger.
Injection; syrup: Calcium gluconate (p.1188·2); calcium lactobionate (p.1188·3).
Calcium deficiency; normocalcaemic tetany; prevention of bone loss in immobilisation; rickets.
Novartis Consumer, Canad.; Novartis, Irl.; Sandoz, S.Afr.†; Alliance, UK.
Syrup: Calcium glubionate (p.1188·1); calcium lactobionate (p.1188·3).
Hypocalcaemia; osteoporosis.

Calcium-Sandoz C *Novartis, Spain.*
Ascorbic acid (p.1389·3); calcium glubionate (p.1188·1).
Calcium deficiency; vitamin C deficiency.

Calcium-Sandoz F *Novartis, Braz.*
Calcium lactate gluconate (p.1188·3); calcium carbonate (p.1215·1).
Calcium deficiency.

Calcium-Sandoz Forte *Novartis, Spain.*
Calcium carbonate (p.1215·1); calcium glubionate (p.1188·1).
Calcium deficiency; hypoparathyroidism; osteomalacia; osteoporosis; rickets.

Calcium-Sandoz Forte D *Novartis, Spain.*
Calcium gluceptate (p.1188·1); colecalciferol (p.1391·1); calcium carbonate (p.1215·1).
Deficiencies of calcium and vitamin D; osteoporosis.

Calcium-Sandoz + Vit C *Novartis, Israel.*
Calcium gluconate (p.1188·2); calcium lactate (p.1188·2); calcium carbonate (p.1215·1); vitamin C (p.1389·3).
Calcium and vitamin C supplement.

Calcium-Sandoz + Vitamina C *Novartis, Braz.*
Calcium carbonate (p.1215·1); calcium lactobionate (p.1188·3); ascorbic acid (p.1389·3).
Calcium and vitamin C supplement.

Calcium-Sorbisterit *Fresenius, Fr.†.*
Calcium polystyrene sulfonate (p.1002·3).
Hyperkalaemia related to renal insufficiency.

Calcival *Valdecasas, Mex.*
Calcium citrate (p.1188·1).
Calcium deficiency; calcium supplement; osteomalacia, rickets; osteoporosis.

Calcivit *UB Interpharm, Switz.*
Calcium hydrogen phosphate (p.1188·2); colecalciferol (p.1391·1).
Hypocalcaemia.

Calcivit D *Hexal, Ger.*
Calcium carbonate (p.1215·1); colecalciferol (p.1391·1).
Calcium and vitamin D₃ deficiency; osteoporosis.

Calcivit F *Hexal, Ger.*
Calcium carbonate (p.1215·1); sodium fluorophosphate (p.1377·2).
Osteoporosis.

calcivitase *Biosyn, Ger.*
Calcium citrate (p.1188·1); calcium gluconate (p.1188·2); calcium glycerophosphate (p.1188·2); calcium silicate (p.1189·1); colecalciferol (p.1391·1).
Calcium deficiency.

Calco
Lisapharma, Ital.; Lisapharma, Singapore; Lisapharma, Thai.
Salcatonin (p.749·3).
Hypercalcaemia; osteoporosis; Paget's disease of bone; reflex sympathetic dystrophy.

Calcort
Hoechst Marion Roussel, Braz.; Hoechst Marion Roussel, Ger.; Shire, Irl.; Hoechst Marion Roussel, Mex.; Hoechst Marion Roussel, Switz.; Shire, UK.
Deflazacort (p.1066·1).
Corticosteroid.

Cal-C-Tose *Roche, Mex.*
Multivitamin and mineral preparation (p.1350·1).

Calcufel Aqua *Hevert, Ger.*
Solidago virgaurea.
Renal calculi; urinary-tract disorders.

Calculi H *Pflüger, Ger.*
Homoeopathic preparation.

Cal-C-Vita
Roche, Aust.; Roche, Israel; Roche, Mex.; Roche, S.Afr.; Roche, Switz.
Calcium carbonate (p.1215·1); vitamins (p.1350·1).
Calcium supplement; tonic.

Cal-D3 *Cotek, Singapore.*
Calcium carbonate (p.1215·1); colecalciferol (p.1391·1).
Calcium supplement.

Cal-De *Asta Medica, Aust.; Novartis, Switz.*
Calcium carbonate (p.1215·1); colecalciferol (p.1391·1).
Vitamin D and calcium deficiency.

Caldease *Roche Consumer, Irl.*
Zinc oxide (p.1128·2); cod-liver oil (p.1357·2).
Burns; nappy rash; skin irritation; wounds.

Cal-De-Ce *Sanabo, Aust.†.*
Calcium hydrogen phosphate (p.1188·2); colecalciferol (p.1391·1); ascorbic acid (p.1389·3).
Calcium and vitamin D deficiency.

CaldeCort *Fisons, USA†.*
Hydrocortisone (p.1073·3) or hydrocortisone acetate (p.1073·3).
Skin disorders.

Calderol *Organon, USA.*
Calcifediol (p.1391·1).
Hypocalcaemia associated with renal dialysis; metabolic bone disease.

Caldesene
Note.This name is used for preparations of different composition.
Novartis Consumer, Canad.; Fisons, USA.
Ointment: Cod-liver oil (p.1357·2); zinc oxide (p.1128·2).
Skin disorders.
Novartis Consumer, Canad.; Roche Consumer, Irl.; Fisons, USA.
Topical powder: Calcium undecenoate (p.395·3).
Bromhidrosis; fungal skin infections; hyperhidrosis; minor skin irritation; nappy rash.

Caldine *Boehringer Ingelheim, Fr.*
Lacidipine (p.919·1).
Hypertension.

Caldomine-DH *Technilab, Canad.†.*
Hydrocodone tartrate (p.42·2); phenylpropanolamine hydrochloride (p.1098·1); mepyramine maleate (p.421·1); pheniramine maleate (p.422·3).
Coughs.

Caldramine *Silom, Thai.*
Calamine (p.1111·3); diphenhydramine hydrochloride (p.416·1); camphor (p.1589·3).
Skin irritation.

Cal-D-Vita *Roche, Swed.; Roche, Thai.*
Calcium (p.1187·3); colecalciferol (p.1391·1).
Calcium and vitamin D deficiency; osteomalacia; osteoporosis.

Calel-D *Rhone-Poulenc Rorer, USA.*
Calcium carbonate (p.1215·1); colecalciferol (p.1391·1).
Nutritional supplement.

Calendolon *Weleda, UK.*
Calendula (p.1589·2).
Minor wounds and abrasions.

Calendula + *Homeocan, Canad.*
Homoeopathic preparation.

Calendulene *Allergan, Fr.†.*
Calendula (p.1589·2).
Eye hygiene.

Calendumed *DHU, Ger.*
Homoeopathic preparation.

Calfate *Helfarma, Port.*
Sucralfate (p.1250·2).
Duodenitis; gastritis; gastro-oesophageal reflux; peptic ulcer.

Calfolex *Crinos, Ital.*
Calcium folinate (p.1363·1).
Antidote to folic acid antagonists; folic acid deficiency; reduction of aminopterin and methotrexate toxicity.

Calgel *Warner-Lambert, UK.*
Lignocaine [lidocaine] hydrochloride (p.1313·2); cetylpyridinium chloride (p.1138·1).
Teething pain.

Calglycine Antacid *Rugby, USA†.*
Calcium carbonate (p.1215·1); glycine (p.1365·3).
Gastrointestinal hyperacidity.

Cal-Guard *Rugby, USA†.*
Calcium carbonate (p.1215·1).

Calibral *Solvay, Port.†.*
Tenoxicam (p.87·2).
Gout; musculoskeletal, joint, and peri-articular disorders.

Calicida Indiano *Medical, Port.*
Acetic acid (p.1571·2); salicylic acid (p.1122·3); collodion.

Caliderm *Darier, Mex.*
Calcium hydroxide (p.1588·3); almond oil (p.1576·3).
Skin disorders.

Califig *Merck Consumer, UK.*
Chewable bar: Senna (p.1248·2); fig (p.1227·1); dietary fibre (p.1350·1).
Effervescent tablets: Dietary fibre supplement (p.1350·1).
Oral liquid: Senna (p.1248·2); fig (p.1227·1).
Tablets: Taraxacum (p.1669·1); peppermint oil (p.1243·3); senna (p.1248·2).
Constipation.

California Syrup of Figs *SmithKline Beecham, Irl.†.*
Senna leaf (p.1248·2).

Calimal *Sussex, UK.*
Chlorpheniramine [chlorphenamine] maleate (p.412·1).
Hypersensitivity reactions.

Calinat *Aesculapius, Ital.*
Calcium folinate (p.1363·1).
Folate deficiency; reduction of aminopterin and methotrexate toxicity.

Calinofen *Medimport, Mex.*
Paracetamol (p.71·2).
Fever; pain.

Calisvit *Menarini, Ital.*
Colecalciferol (p.1391·1); tribasic calcium phosphate (p.1188·3).
Calcium and vitamin D deficiency.

Cal-Lac *Bio-Tech, USA.*
Calcium lactate (p.1188·2).
Calcium supplement.

Callicida Brujo *Calmante Vitaminado, Spain.*
Flexible collodion; lactic acid (p.1626·2); salicylic acid (p.1122·3).
Callosities.

Callicida Brum *Brum, Spain.*
Flexible collodion; salicylic acid (p.1122·3); trichloroacetic acid (p.1674·3).
Callosities.

Callicida Cor Pik *Quimifar, Spain.*
Acetic acid (p.1571·2); flexible collodion; lactic acid (p.1626·2); castor oil; salicylic acid (p.1122·3).
Callosities.

Callicida Durcall *Llorens, Spain†.*
Acetic acid (p.1571·2); flexible collodion; lactic acid (p.1626·2); salicylic acid (p.1122·3).
Callosities.

Callicida Globodermis *Weinco, Spain.*
Salicylic acid (p.1122·3).
Callosities.

Callicida Gras *Quimifar, Spain.*
Salicylic acid (p.1122·3).
Callosities.

Callicida Rojo *Escaned, Spain.*
Acetic acid (p.1571·2); flexible collodion; benzocaine (p.1306·2); salicylic acid (p.1122·3); iodine tincture (p.1522·3).
Callosities.

Callicida Salve *Cederroth, Spain.*
Salicylic acid (p.1122·3).
Callosities.

Callimon
Note.This name is used for preparations of different composition.
Grossmann, Hong Kong.
Calcium (p.1187·3); vitamin C (p.1389·3).
Calcium and vitamin C supplement.
Grossmann, Switz.
Calcium carbonate (p.1215·1); calcium lactate (p.1188·2); ascorbic acid (p.1389·3).
Vitamin C and calcium deficiency.

Callivoro Marthand *Martinez Llenas, Spain.*
Salicylic acid (p.1122·3); benzocaine (p.1306·2).
Callosities.

Callix D *Calmante Vitaminado, Spain.*
Flexible collodion; benzocaine (p.1306·2); lactic acid (p.1626·2); salicylic acid (p.1122·3).
Callosities.

Callofin *Alcor, Spain.*
Salicylic acid (p.1122·3).
Callosities.

Callus Salve *Cress, Canad.†.*
Salicylic acid (p.1122·3).

Calma *Uno, Ital.*
Calcium carbonate (p.1215·1).
Calcium deficiency; calcium supplement.

Calmaderm *Whitehall, Fr.*
Bufexamac (p.20·3).
Pruritus.

Cal-Mag
Note.This name is used for preparations of different composition.
Seroyal, Canad.†.
Calcium carbonate (p.1215·1); magnesium oxide (p.1233·2).
Swiss Herbal, Canad.
Calcium carbonate (p.1215·1); magnesium carbonate (p.1232·3).
Quest, UK.
Calcium, magnesium, and vitamin D (p.1350·1).

Cal-Mag Citrate with Vitamin D & Zinc *Swiss Herbal, Canad.*
Calcium, magnesium, zinc, and vitamin D (p.1350·1).

Calmag D *Gerbex, Canad.*
Calcium, magnesium, and vitamin D (p.1350·1).

Cal/Mag & D *Seroyal, Canad.*
Calcium, magnesium, and vitamin D (p.1350·1).

Calmag Plus *USANA, USA.*
Calcium citrate; magnesium amino acid chelate; silicon amino acid chelate; boron amino acid chelate; vitamin D (p.1350·1).
Nutritional supplement.

Cal-Mag & Vitamin C & D *Swiss Herbal, Canad.*
Calcium and magnesium with vitamins C and D (p.1350·1).

Cal-Mag Vitamin C & Zinc *Swiss Herbal, Canad.*
Calcium, magnesium, zinc, and vitamin C (p.1350·1).

Cal-Mag with Vitamin D & Zinc *Swiss Herbal, Canad.*
Calcium, magnesium, zinc, and vitamin D (p.1350·1).

Calmag Zn *Vita Health, Singapore.*
Calcium, magnesium, and zinc (p.1350·1).
Calcium deficiency; osteoporosis.

Calman *Ativus, Braz.*
Passion flower (p.1649·1); crataegus (p.1600·2); salix (p.82·1).
Sedative.

Calmanervin *Sam-On, Israel.*
Elixir: Passion flower (p.1649·1); valerian (p.1678·3).
Tablets: Passion flower (p.1649·1); valerian (p.1678·3); thiamine hydrochloride (p.1385·1); pyridoxine hydrochloride (p.1386·3).
Anxiety; insomnia.

Calmant Martou *Sanico, Belg.†.*
Belladonna extract (p.463·1); mint oil (p.1636·2); cinnamon oil (p.1596·1); orange-peel oil; melissa oil; eugenol (p.1609·3); anethole (p.1580·1); saffron (p.1029·1).
Gastrointestinal disorders.

Calmante Creosotado *Phos-Kola, Braz.*
Eucalyptus (p.1609·2); hypophosphite; Desessartz syrup; laurana camara; tolu balsam (p.1101·3); creosote (p.1087·3).
Coughs.

Calmante Vitaminado P G *Calmante Vitaminado, Spain.*
Aspirin (p.14·2); caffeine (p.761·3); thiamine (p.1385·2).
Fever; pain.

Calmante Vitaminado PG Efervescente *Calmante Vitaminado, Spain.*
Aspirin (p.14·2); caffeine (p.761·3); thiamine mononitrate (p.1385·1); ascorbic acid (p.1389·3).
Fever; pain.

Calmante Vitaminado Rinver *Monik, Spain.*
Aspirin (p.14·2); thiamine (p.1385·2).
Fever; inflammation; pain.

Calmanticold *Calmante Vitaminado, Spain.*
Paracetamol (p.71·2).
Fever; pain.

Calmanticold Vit C *Calmante Vitaminado, Spain†.*
Ascorbic acid (p.1389·3); paracetamol (p.71·2).
Fever; pain.

Calmantina *Inexfa, Spain.*
Aspirin (p.14·2).
Fever; inflammation; pain; thromboembolism prophylaxis.

Calmapica *Calmante Vitaminado, Spain.*
Ammonia (p.1579·1).
Insect bites; stings.

Calmaril *Siam Bheasach, Thai.*
Thioridazine hydrochloride (p.708·1).
Anxiety; behaviour disorders; mania; schizophrenia.

Calmarum *Medical, Port.*
Sulfogaiacol (p.1101·1); ephedrine hydrochloride (p.1090·1); ethylmorphine (p.35·2); sodium benzoate

---

(p.1134·3); aconite (p.1572·3); thyme (p.1672·2); senega (p.1100·2).
Coughs.

Calmatel *Almirall, Spain.*
Piketoprofen (p.78·3) or piketoprofen hydrochloride (p.78·3).
Peri-articular and soft-tissue disorders.

Calmaven *Alter, Spain†.*
Diazepam (p.674·3).
Alcohol withdrawal syndrome; anxiety; epilepsy; febrile convulsions; insomnia; premedication; skeletal muscle spasm.

Calmaverine *Taphlan, Switz.*
Caroverine (p.1591·3) or caroverine hydrochloride (p.1591·3).
Smooth muscle spasm.

Calmax *Ergha, Irl.*
Alprazolam (p.654·2).
Anxiety.

Calmaxid *Lilly, Switz.*
Nizatidine (p.1238·1).
Gastric hyperacidity; gastro-oesophageal reflux; peptic ulcer.

Calmday
Will-Pharma, Belg.; Ravizza, Neth.
Nordazepam (p.696·1).
Anxiety.

Calmerphan *Doetsch, Grether, Switz.*
Dextromethorphan hydrobromide (p.1087·3).
Coughs.

Calmerphan-L *Doetsch, Grether, Switz.*
Dextromethorphan resin (p.1087·3).
Bronchitis; coughs.

Calmesine *Mepha, Switz.*
Dextromethorphan resin (p.1088·2).
Coughs.

Calmettes *Aventis, S.Afr.*
Valerian (p.1678·3).
Anxiety; nervous disorders.

Calmex
Note.This name is used for preparations of different composition.
Heralds, Braz.
Bromazepam (p.656·3).
Anxiety.

Novopharm, Canad.
Diphenhydramine hydrochloride (p.416·1).
Insomnia.

Calmine *Bouty, Ital.*
Ibuprofen (p.43·2).
Pain.

Calminex S *Schering-Plough, Braz.*
Methyl salicylate (p.55·1); zinc oxide (p.1128·2); belladonna (p.463·1); peru balsam (p.1650·2); camphor (p.1589·3).
Musculoskeletal and joint disorders.

Calmiphase *Arkomedika, Fr.*
Chamomile (p.1593·2); centella (p.1112·2).
Skin disorders.

Calmixene *Novartis, Fr.*
Pimethixene (p.423·1).
Coughs.

Calmo
Note.This name is used for preparations of different composition.
Eagle, Austral.
Mistletoe (p.1636·2); valerian (p.1678·3); vervain (p.1679·3); gentian (p.1615·3); avena (p.1583·1); passion flower (p.1649·1); skullcap (p.1664·3); tansy (p.1669·1); pulsatilla (p.1656·3).
Hypnotic; tension; tension headache.

Lab, Port.
Anemone; belladonna (p.463·1); passion flower (p.1649·1); crataegus (p.1600·2).

Calmociteno *Medley, Braz.*
Diazepam (p.674·3).
Alcohol withdrawal syndrome; anxiety; epilepsy; insomnia; premedication; sedative; skeletal muscle spasm.

Calmogel *Rhone-Poulenc Rorer, Ital.*
Isothipendyl hydrochloride (p.419·2).
Insect bites; pruritus; sunburn.

Calmogenol *Brasmedica, Braz.*
Lorazepam (p.688·3).
Alcohol withdrawal syndrome; anxiety; epilepsy; insomnia; nausea and vomiting; premedication; sedative.

Calmol *Mentholatum, USA.*
Zinc oxide (p.1128·2); bismuth subgallate (p.1213·2).
Anorectal disorders.

Calmomusc *Cardinaux, Canad.*
Methyl salicylate (p.55·1); menthol (p.1632·3); eucalyptol (p.1609·2).

Calmophytum *Holistica, Fr.*
Tilia (p.1673·2); orange buds; chamomile (p.1593·2); vervain (p.1679·3); hibiscus.
Insomnia.

Calmoplex *Teofarma, Spain.*
Codeine phosphate (p.25·2); hydroxyzine hydrochloride (p.419·1); propyphenazone (p.80·2).
Coughs; fever; pain.

Calmoroide *Warner-Lambert, UK.*
Ruscogenin (p.1660·2); vitamin A palmitate (p.1383·2).
Haemorrhoids.

Calmovarin *Faria, Braz.*
Diethylstilbestrol (p.1471·2); papaverine (p.1648·1); calcium gluconate (p.1188·2); viburnum; berberis.
Smooth muscle spasm.

Calmpose *Ranbaxy, S.Afr.*
Diazepam (p.674·3).
Alcohol withdrawal syndrome; anxiety; premedication; skeletal muscle spasm; status epilepticus.

Calms *Hylands, Canad.*
Homoeopathic preparation.

Calms Forte *Hylands, Canad.*
Homoeopathic preparation.

Calmurid
AB-Consult, Aust.; Galderma, Austral.; Galderma, Belg.; Galderma, Canad.†; Galderma, Ger.; Galderma, Irl.; Taro, Israel; Galderma, Neth.; Galderma, NZ; Bonafarma, Port.; Galderma, Switz.; Galderma, UK.
Urea (p.1127·3); lactic acid (p.1626·2).
Dry skin; hyperkeratosis.

Calmurid comp *AB-Consult, Aust.*
Urea (p.1127·3); sodium chloride (p.1196·1).
Psoriasis.

Calmurid HC
Note.This name is used for preparations of different composition.
AB-Consult, Aust.; Galderma, Canad.†; Galderma, Ger.; Galderma, Irl.; Taro, Israel; Galderma, Switz.; Galderma, UK.
Urea (p.1127·3); lactic acid (p.1626·2); hydrocortisone (p.1073·3).
Inflammatory skin disorders; keratinisation disorders.

Galderma, Neth.; Galderma, S.Afr.
Urea (p.1127·3); hydrocortisone (p.1073·3).
Skin disorders.

Calmuril
Pharmacia Upjohn, Fin.; Pharmacia Upjohn, Swed.
Urea (p.1127·3); lactic acid (p.1626·2).
Dry skin; eczema; keratinisation disorders.

Calmuril-Hydrokortison *Pharmacia Upjohn, Swed.†.*
Urea (p.1127·3); hydrocortisone (p.1073·3).
Skin disorders.

Calm-X *Republic, USA.*
Dimenhydrinate (p.415·2).
Motion sickness.

Calmydone *Technilab, Canad.*
Hydrocodone tartrate (p.42·2); etafedrine hydrochloride (p.1091·2); doxylamine succinate (p.417·1).
Coughs.

Calmylin #1 *Technilab, Canad.*
Dextromethorphan hydrobromide (p.1087·3).
Coughs.

Calmylin #2 *Technilab, Canad.*
Dextromethorphan hydrobromide (p.1087·3); pseudoephedrine hydrochloride (p.1099·2).
Formerly known as Calmylin-DM-D.
Coughs.

Calmylin #3 *Technilab, Canad.*
Dextromethorphan hydrobromide (p.1087·3); pseudoephedrine hydrochloride (p.1099·2); guaifenesin (p.1092·2).
Formerly known as Calmylin-DM-D-E.
Coughs.

Calmylin #4 *Technilab, Canad.*
Diphenhydramine hydrochloride (p.416·1); ammonium chloride (p.1085·2); dextromethorphan hydrobromide (p.1087·3).
Formerly known as Calmylin-DM.
Coughs.

Calmylin Ace *Technilab, Canad.*
Guaifenesin (p.1092·2); pheniramine maleate (p.422·3); codeine phosphate (p.25·2).
Coughs.

Calmylin with Codeine *Technilab, Canad.*
Pseudoephedrine hydrochloride (p.1099·2); codeine phosphate (p.25·2); guaifenesin (p.1092·2).
Formerly known as Calmylin Codeine D-E.
Coughs.

Calmylin Cough & Flu *Technilab, Canad.*
Dextromethorphan hydrobromide (p.1087·3); pseudoephedrine hydrochloride (p.1099·2); guaifenesin (p.1092·2); paracetamol (p.71·2).
Coughs and cold symptoms.

Calmylin Expectorant *Technilab, Canad.*
Guaifenesin (p.1092·2).
Coughs.

Calmylin Original with Codeine *Technilab, Canad.*
Diphenhydramine hydrochloride (p.416·1); ammonium chloride (p.1085·2); codeine phosphate (p.25·2).
Coughs.

Calmylin Pediatric *Technilab, Canad.*
Dextromethorphan hydrobromide (p.1087·3); pseudoephedrine hydrochloride (p.1099·2).
Coughs and cold symptoms.

Calnit *Vita Elan, Spain.*
Nimodipine (p.946·1).
Mental function impairment; neurological deficit following subarachnoid haemorrhage.

Calociclina *ISI, Ital.†.*
Tetracycline hydrochloride (p.258·3).
Bacterial infections.

Calogen
Note.This name is used for preparations of different composition.
Scientific Hospital Supplies, Austral.; Nutricia, Fin.; Scientific Hospital Supplies, Irl.; Scientific Hospital Supplies, NZ; Nutricia, NZ; SHS, Singapore; Scientific Hospital Supplies, UK.
Arachis oil (p.1581·1).
Carbohydrate malabsorption; dietary supplement; disorders of amino acid metabolism; ketogenic diet in epilepsy.

Probios, Port.; Almirall, Spain.
Salcatonin (p.749·3).
Hypercalcaemia; metastatic bone pain; osteoporosis; Paget's disease of bone.

Calomide-S *Yamanouchi, Jpn†.*
Cobamamide (p.1388·3).
Anaemias; vitamin B_{12} deficiency.

Calonat *Democal, Switz.*
Carbasalate calcium (p.23·3); ascorbic acid (p.1389·3).
Fever; pain.

Calope *Simoes, Braz.*
Phenylacetic acid; salicylic acid (p.1122·3); lactic acid (p.1626·2); thuja (p.1672·1).
Keratinisation disorders.

Caloreen
Nestle, Fr.; Clintec, Irl.†; Roussel, S.Afr.†; Nestle, UK.
Dextrin (p.1359·1).
Food for special diets.

Calox *Qualiphar, Belg.†.*
Sterculia (p.1250·2).
Formerly known as Fixobel.
Denture fixative.

Calpan *ICN, Canad.†.*
Calcium pantothenate (p.1374·1).

Calparine
Sanofi Synthelabo, Belg.; Sanofi Synthelabo, Neth.
Heparin calcium (p.902·1).
Thrombosis prophylaxis.

Calperos
Doms-Adrian, Fr.; Vifor, Switz.
Calcium carbonate (p.1215·1).
Calcium deficiency; osteoporosis.

Calperos D₃
Doms-Adrian, Fr.; Doms-Adrian, Hong Kong; Vifor, Switz.
Calcium carbonate (p.1215·1); colecalciferol (p.1391·1).
Calcium and vitamin D deficiency; osteoporosis.

Calphosan *Glenwood, USA.*
Calcium glycerophosphate (p.1188·2); calcium lactate (p.1188·2).
Calcium deficiency.

Calphron *Nephro-Tech, USA.*
Calcium acetate (p.1187·3).
Hyperphosphataemia.

Calpix *Euro-Labor, Port.*
Captopril (p.853·3).
Heart failure; hypertension.

Cal-Plus *Geriatric Pharm. Corp., USA.*
Calcium carbonate (p.1215·1).
High-potency calcium supplement.

Calpol
Glaxo Wellcome, Braz.; Glaxo Wellcome, Hong Kong; Warner-Lambert, Irl.; Glaxo Wellcome, Mex.; Glaxo Wellcome, S.Afr.; Glaxo Wellcome, Singapore; Glaxo Wellcome, Thai.; Warner-Lambert, UK.
Paracetamol (p.71·2).
Fever; pain.

Calpol Extra *Warner-Lambert, UK†.*
Paracetamol (p.71·2); codeine phosphate (p.25·2); caffeine (p.761·3).
Fever; pain.

Calporo *Eagle, Austral.*
Vitamin and mineral supplement with rose fruit, irish moss, echinacea, equisetum, lysine, and bone powder (p.1350·1).
Bone disorders; mineral supplement.

Calpred *Grossmann, Switz.*
Prednisolone acetate (p.1078·1); mepyramine maleate (p.421·1); calcium levulinate (p.1188·3).
Skin disorders.

Calprimum *Iderne, Fr.*
Calcium carbonate (p.1215·1).
Calcium deficiency; osteoporosis.

Calrub *Warner-Lambert, UK.*
Eucalyptus (p.1609·2); menthol (p.1632·3).
Respiratory-tract disorders.

Calsalettes *Torbet Laboratories, UK.*
Aloin (p.1210·2).
Constipation.

Calsan
Novartis Consumer, Canad.; Novartis, Mex.; Novartis, Switz.
Calcium carbonate (p.1215·1).
Calcium supplement; osteoporosis.

Calsein *Manuell, Mex.*
Cocarboxylase (p.1385·2).

Calshake *Fresenius, UK.*
Preparation for enteral nutrition (p.1350·1).

Calsip *Rowa, Irl.†.*
Food for special diets (p.1350·1).

Calslot *Takeda, Jpn.*
Manidipine hydrochloride (p.924·3).
Hypertension.

Calsorp *Thaipharmed, Thai.*
Calcium citrate (p.1188·1).
Calcium deficiency.

Cal-Sup
3M, Austral.; 3M, NZ; 3M, Singapore.
Calcium carbonate (p.1215·1).
Calcium deficiency; calcium supplement.

Calsyn
Rhone-Poulenc Rorer, Fr.; Rhone-Poulenc Rorer, Port.
Salcatonin (p.749·3).
Algodystrophies; hypercalcaemia; hyperphosphatasia; osteoporosis; Paget's disease of bone; prevention of bone loss in immobilisation.

Calsynar
Rhone-Poulenc Rorer, Austral.; Aventis, Belg.; Rhodia, Braz.; Rhone-Poulenc Rorer, Ger.; Rhone-Poulenc Rorer, Hong Kong; Rhone-Poulenc

Rorer, Irl.; Rhone-Poulenc Rorer, Israel; Rhone-Poulenc Rorer, Neth.†; Rhone-Poulenc Rorer, Spain; Rhone-Poulenc Rorer, UK.
Salcatonin (p.749·3) or salcatonin acetate (p.750·2).
Hypercalcaemia of malignancy; metastatic bone pain; osteoporosis; Paget's disease of bone; reflex sympathetic dystrophy.

Calsynar Lyo *Rhone-Poulenc Rorer, Ger.†.*
Salcatonin (p.749·3).
Bone pain in malignancy; hypercalcaemia; osteoporosis; Paget's disease of bone; reflex sympathetic dystrophy.

Caltab *Masa, Thai.*
Calcium carbonate (p.1215·1).
Calcium deficiency; calcium supplement.

Caltabs *Lifeplan, UK.*
Vitamin and mineral preparation (p.1350·1).

Caltheon *Chephasaar, Ger.*
Tetryzoline hydrochloride (p.1101·2).
Nasal congestion.

Caltine *Ferring, Canad.*
Salcatonin (p.749·3).
Hypercalcaemia; Paget's disease of bone.

Caltoson Balsamico *Rottapharm, Spain.*
Eucalyptol (p.1609·2); benzocaine (p.1306·2); pholcodine (p.1099·1); cherry-laurel; terpineol (p.1669·3); menthol (p.1632·3).
Respiratory-tract disorders.

Caltrate
Note.This name is used for preparations of different composition.
Whitehall, Austral.; Whitehall-Robins, Canad.; Whitehall, Fr.; Lederle, Hong Kong; Lederle, Israel; Wyeth, Mex.; Whitehall, NZ; Whitehall, S.Afr.; Whitehall, Singapore; Whitehall, Thai.; Lederle, USA.
Calcium carbonate (p.1215·1).
Calcium deficiency; calcium supplement; osteomalacia; osteoporosis.

Whitehall, Ital.; Whitehall, Port.; Whitehall, UK.
Calcium (p.1187·3); vitamin D (p.1391·1).
Calcium deficiency; osteoporosis.

Caltrate + D
Lederle, Hong Kong; Whitehall, Thai.
Calcium (p.1187·3); vitamin D (p.1391·1).
Calcium deficiency; calcium supplement; osteomalacia; osteoporosis.

Caltrate + Iron & Vitamin D
Whitehall-Robins, Canad.†; Lederle, USA.
Calcium carbonate (p.1215·1); ferrous fumarate (p.1360·1); vitamin D (p.1391·1).
Calcium and iron deficiency.

Caltrate Jr. *Lederle, USA.*
Calcium carbonate (p.1215·1).
Formerly contained calcium carbonate and vitamin D.
Calcium deficiency.

Caltrate Plus
Note.This name is used for preparations of different composition.
Whitehall, Austral.; Whitehall-Robins, Canad.
Calcium carbonate (p.1215·1); colecalciferol (p.1391·1); magnesium oxide; zinc oxide; copper oxide; manganese sulfate (p.1350·1).
Calcium deficiency; osteomalacia; osteoporosis.

Lederle, Hong Kong; Whitehall, Singapore; Whitehall, Thai.; Whitehall, UK; Lederle, USA.
Calcium (p.1187·3); colecalciferol (p.1391·1); boron; copper; magnesium; manganese; zinc (p.1350·1).
Bone disorders; calcium deficiency.

Whitehall, Port.
Calcium carbonate (p.1215·1); colecalciferol (p.1391·1); minerals.
Osteoporosis.

Caltrate + Vit D
Lederle, Israel; Whitehall, Singapore.
Calcium carbonate (p.1215·1); colecalciferol (p.1391·1).
Calcium and vitamin D deficiency.

Caltrate + Vitamin D
Whitehall, Austral.; Whitehall-Robins, Canad.; Lederle, USA.
Calcium carbonate (p.1215·1); colecalciferol (p.1391·1).
Calcium and vitamin D deficiency; calcium supplement; osteomalacia; osteoporosis.

Caltrate Vitamine D₃ *Whitehall, Fr.*
Calcium carbonate (p.1215·1); colecalciferol (p.1391·1).
Calcium and vitamin D deficiency; osteoporosis.

Caltren *Libbs, Braz.*
Nitrendipine (p.947·1).
Hypertension.

Caltro *Geneva, USA.*
Calcium with vitamin D (p.1350·1).
Calcium deficiency; dietary supplement.

Caltusine *Rudefsa, Mex.*
Carbocisteine (p.1086·3); oxolamine citrate (p.1096·2).
Coughs.

Calvakehl *Sanum-Kehlbeck, Ger.*
Homoeopathic preparation.

Calvepen *Leo, Irl.*
Phenoxymethylpenicillin calcium (p.235·1).
Bacterial infections.

Calvita *Roche Consumer, Austral.*
Calcium phosphate (p.1188·3); vitamins and iron (p.1350·1).
Calcium supplement; dietary supplement.

Calvita Osti *Roche Consumer, Austral.†.*
Calcium carbonate (p.1215·1); colecalciferol (p.1391·1).
Calcium and vitamin D deficiency; calcium and vitamin D supplement; osteomalacia; osteoporosis.

Calypsol *Gedeon Richter, Thai.*
Ketamine hydrochloride (p.1262·2).
General anaesthesia.

Calyptol *Rhone-Poulenc Rorer, Ital.; Techni-Pharma, Mon.*
Eucalyptus (p.1609·2); terpineol (p.1669·3); pine oil; thyme oil (p.1672·3); rosemary oil (p.1659·3).
Respiratory-tract congestion.

Calyptol Inhalante *Rhone-Poulenc Rorer, Spain.*
Oleum pini sylvestris; rosemary oil (p.1659·3); terpineol (p.1669·3); thyme oil (p.1672·3); eucalyptus (p.1609·2).
Respiratory-tract congestion.

CAM
Note.This name is used for preparations of different composition.
Eversil, Braz.
Theophylline calcium salicylate (p.783·2); potassium iodide (p.1522·3).
Obstructive airways disease.

Rybar, Irl.
Butetamate citrate (p.1086·2).
Formerly contained butetamate citrate and ephedrine hydrochloride.
Bronchospasm.

Cambridge Healthcare, UK.
Ephedrine hydrochloride (p.1090·1).
Formerly contained butetamate citrate and ephedrine hydrochloride.
Bronchospasm; cough.

Cama Arthritis Pain Reliever *Novartis, USA.*
Aspirin (p.14·2).
Aluminium hydroxide (p.1210·3) and magnesium oxide (p.1233·2) are included in this preparation in an attempt to limit adverse effects on the gastrointestinal mucosa.
Arthritis; pain.

Camalox *Rhone-Poulenc Rorer, Swed.*
Aluminium hydroxide (p.1210·3); magnesium hydroxide (p.1233·1); calcium carbonate (p.1215·1).
Heartburn; peptic ulcer.

Camazole *Xepa-Soul Pattinson, Singapore.*
Carbimazole (p.1521·1).
Hyperthyroidism.

Cambem *UCI, Braz.*
Cambendazole.
Strongyloidiasis.

Camboacy *Farmovy, Braz.*
Lactobacillus acidophilus (p.1626·3).
Diarrhoea; restoration of gastrointestinal flora.

Camcolit *Norgine, Belg.; Norgine, Hong Kong; Norgine, Irl.; Norgine, S.Afr.; Norgine, Singapore; Norgine, UK.*
Lithium carbonate (p.292·1).
Bipolar disorder; depression; disturbed behaviour; mania.

Camegel *Bonomelli, Ital.*
Vitamin and fibre preparation (p.1350·1).
Diarrhoea.

Cameo *Medco, USA.*
Emollient.

Camilia *Boiron, Canad.*
Homoeopathic preparation.

Camiline *Arkopharma, Fr.*
Green tea (p.1681·1).
Asthenia; slimming aid.

Camoderm
Note.This name is used for preparations of different composition.
Link, Austral.
Chamomile (p.1593·2); chamomile oil.
Nappy rash; skin irritation; sore nipples.

Norgine, Hong Kong.
Chamomile (p.1593·2); levomenol (p.1629·1).
Skin irritation.

Camomila *Catarinense, Braz.*
Aloes (p.1210·1); paregoric (p.69·3); aniseed (p.1580·2); peppermint leaf (p.1243·2); melissa (p.1632·2); chamomile (p.1593·2); centaury (p.1593·1); condurango (p.1599·1); Fuller's earth (p.1010·1); gentian (p.1615·1); absinthium (p.1571·1); quassia (p.1657·1); rhubarb (p.1248·1); bixa orellana.
Digestive disorders.

Camomilina C *Novaquimica, Braz.*
Chamomile (p.1593·2); liquorice (p.1231·2); colecalciferol; vitamin C; calcium phosphate (p.1350·1).
Nutritional supplement.

Campanyl *Temmler, Ger.*
Potassium polystyrene sulfonate (p.1020·1).
Hypercalciuria.

Campath *Berlex, USA.*
Alemtuzumab (p.506·1).
Chronic lymphocytic leukaemia.

Campel *Chiesi, Fr.*
Chromocarb diethylamine (p.1594·3).
Circulatory disorders; haemorrhoids.

Camphoderm N *Li-Il, Ger.*
Camphor (p.1589·3).
Catarrh; musculoskeletal, joint, and soft-tissue disorders.

Camphodionyl *Distri B3, Fr.*
Sulfogaiacol (p.1101·1); codeine (p.25·2).
Formerly contained sodium camsilate, sulfogaiacol, codeine, ethylmorphine hydrochloride, aconite root, Desessartz syrup, and benzoic acid.
Coughs.

Campho-Phenique *Winthrop Consumer, USA; Sterling, USA.*
Phenol (p.1152·3); camphor (p.1589·3).
Burns; cuts; herpes labialis; infections; insect bites; pain.

Campho-Phenique Antibiotic Plus Pain Reliever Ointment *Winthrop Consumer, USA†.*
Bacitracin (p.155·2); neomycin sulfate (p.228·1); polymyxin B sulfate (p.238·1); lignocaine [lidocaine] (p.1313·2).
Formerly contained diperodon hydrochloride in place of lignocaine [lidocaine].
Infection prophylaxis and pain relief in minor skin lesions.

Camphopin *Schoning-Berlin, Ger.†.*
Methyl salicylate (p.55·1); benzyl nicotinate (p.20·2); camphor (p.1589·3).
Frostbite; neuralgia; rheumatic disorders; sciatica; tendinitis.

Campho-Pneumine *Marion Merrell, Fr.*
Adult suppositories: Camphor (p.1589·3); guaiacol (p.1092·1); eucalyptol (p.1609·2); guaifenesin (p.1092·2); amylocaine hydrochloride (p.1306·1).
Suppositories child: Camphor (p.1589·3); guaiacol (p.1092·1); eucalyptol (p.1609·2); guaifenesin (p.1092·2).
Suppositories infant: Eucalyptol (p.1609·2); guaifenesin (p.1092·2).
Respiratory-tract disorders.

Camphor Linctus Compound *McGloin, Austral.*
Camphor (p.1589·3); tolu balsam (p.1101·3).
Coughs.

Camphre Compose *Valmo, Canad.*
Camphor (p.1589·3); menthol (p.1632·3); eucalyptus (p.1609·2).

Camphrice Du Canada *Homme de Fer, Fr.*
Camphor (p.1589·3).
Skin disorders.

Campral *Merck, Aust.; Alphapharm, Austral.; Merck-Belgolabo, Belg.; Lipha, Denm.; Merck, Ger.; Lipha, Irl.; Merck, Neth.; Lipha, Norw.; Merck, Port.; Merck, Singapore; Merck-Lipha, Singapore; Merck, Spain; Merck, Swed.; Lipha, Switz.; Merck, UK.*
Acamprosate calcium (p.653·3).
Alcoholism.

Campto *Aventis, Belg.; Aventis, Denm.; Rhone-Poulenc Rorer, Fin.; Rhone-Poulenc Rorer, Fr.; Rhone-Poulenc Rorer, Ger.; Rhone-Poulenc Rorer, Hong Kong; Rhone-Poulenc Rorer, Irl.; Rhone-Poulenc Rorer, Israel; Rhone-Poulenc Rorer, Ital.; Rhone-Poulenc Rorer, Neth.; Rhone-Poulenc Rorer, Norw.; Rhone-Poulenc Rorer, Port.; Aventis, S.Afr.; Rhone-Poulenc Rorer, Singapore; Pras, Spain; Rhone-Poulenc Rorer, Swed.; Rhone-Poulenc Rorer, Switz.; Rhone-Poulenc Rorer, Thai.; Rhone-Poulenc Rorer, UK.*
Irinotecan hydrochloride (p.549·1).
Colorectal cancer.

Camptosar *Pharmacia Upjohn, Austral.; Pharmacia Upjohn, Canad.; Pharmacia Upjohn, Mex.; Pharmacia Upjohn, NZ; Pharmacia Upjohn, USA.*
Irinotecan hydrochloride (p.549·1).
Colorectal cancer.

Camsilon *Cambridge, UK.*
Edrophonium chloride (p.1418·2).
Formerly known as Tensilon.
Now known as Edrophonium Chloride Ampoules.
Diagnosis of myasthenia gravis or phase-II block; reversal of competitive neuromuscular blockade.

Camyna *Nycomed, Swed.†.*
Tioxolone (p.1126·1).
Acne; seborrhoea.

Canadine *Nakorn, Thai.*
Clotrimazole (p.382·1).
Fungal skin infections.

Canadiol *Esteve, Spain.*
Itraconazole (p.387·2).
Fungal infections.

Canalba *Compu, S.Afr.*
Clotrimazole (p.382·1).
Fungal skin and vulvovaginal infections.

Canasone *Nakorn, Thai.*
Clotrimazole (p.382·1); betamethasone dipropionate (p.1063·2).
Fungal skin infections.

Canazol *Durascan, Denm.; TO-Chemicals, Thai.*
Clotrimazole (p.382·1).
Fungal skin, oropharyngeal, and vaginal infections; trichomoniasis.

Canazol-BE *TO-Chemicals, Thai.*
Clotrimazole (p.382·1); betamethasone valerate (p.1063·2).
Fungal skin infections.

Cancidas *Merck, USA.*
Caspofungin acetate (p.381·2).
Aspergillosis.

Candalba *Brauer, Austral.*
Homoeopathic preparation.

Candaspor *Be-Tabs, S.Afr.*
Clotrimazole (p.382·1).
Fungal skin and vulvovaginal infections.

Candazol *Apogepha, Ger.*
Clotrimazole (p.382·1).
Fungal infections.

Candazole *Hoe, Singapore.*
Clotrimazole (p.382·1).
Fungal skin infections.

Canderel *Searle, Mex.; Monsanto, Port.†.*
Aspartame (p.1354·3).
Sugar substitute.

Candermyl *Galderma, Austral.†.*
Emollient.

Candibene *Ratiopharm, Aust.*
Clotrimazole (p.382·1).
Fungal infections; trichomoniasis.

Candicort *Ache, Braz.*
Ketoconazole (p.389·1); betamethasone (p.1063·1).
Infected skin disorders.

Candid *Neves, Port.; Glenmark, Thai.*
Clotrimazole (p.382·1).
Fungal infections.

Candida Yeast *Homeocan, Canad.*
Homoeopathic preparation.

Candiden *Akita, UK.*
Clotrimazole (p.382·1).
Fungal infections.

Candiderm *Ache, Braz.*
Ketoconazole (p.389·1).
Fungal skin infections.

Candidine *Stallergenes, Fr.†.*
Candida albicans antigen (p.1575·3).
Diagnosis of hypersensitivity to Candida albicans; hyposensitisation to Candida albicans.

Candimon *Andromaco, Mex.*
Clotrimazole (p.382·1).
Fungal skin and vaginal infections.

Candinox *Charoen, Thai.*
Clotrimazole (p.382·1).
Fungal vaginal infections; trichomoniasis.

Candio *Hermal, Aust.; Hermal, Ger.; Boots Healthcare, Switz.†.*
Nystatin (p.392·2).
Fungal skin infections.

Candio-Hermal Plus *Hermal, Ger.*
Nystatin (p.392·2); fluprednidene acetate (p.1072·1).
Formerly known as Candio E comp N.
Inflammatory skin disorders with fungal infection.

Candiplas *Medochemie, Singapore; Medochemie, Thai.*
Miconazole nitrate (p.391·1).
Fungal and Gram-positive bacterial infections.

Candipres *Precimex, Mex.*
Amphotericin B (p.377·2).
Fungal infections.

Candistatin *Westwood-Squibb, Canad.*
Nystatin (p.392·2).
Fungal infections.

Candizol *Ache, Braz.*
Fluconazole (p.383·2).
Fungal infections.

Candizole *Aspen Consumer, S.Afr.*
Clotrimazole (p.382·1).
Fungal skin and vulvovaginal infections.

Candoral *Ache, Braz.*
Ketoconazole (p.389·1).
Fungal infections.

Candyl *Douglas, Austral.; Douglas, Thai.; TTN, Thai.*
Piroxicam (p.79·1).
Musculoskeletal and joint disorders.

Candyl-D *Douglas, NZ.*
Piroxicam (p.79·1).
Dysmenorrhoea; gout; musculoskeletal and joint disorders.

Canef *AstraZeneca, Denm.; AstraZeneca, Fin.; Astra, Mex.; Astra, Neth.; AstraZeneca, Norw.; Astra, Port.; Hassle, Swed.*
Fluvastatin sodium (p.892·1).
Hypercholesterolaemia.

Canephron N *Bionorica, Ger.; Bionorica, Hong Kong.*
Centaury (p.1593·1); lovage (p.1629·3); rosemary.
Renal calculi; urinary-tract disorders.

Canephron novo *Bionorica, Ger.*
Birch leaf (p.1585·2); java tea (p.1625·1); solidago virgaurea.
Renal calculi; urinary-tract disorders.

Canephron S *Bionorica, Ger.*
Solidago virgaurea.
Renal calculi; urinary-tract disorders.

Canesten *Bayer, Aust.; Bayer Consumer, Austral.; Bayer, Braz.; Bayer, Canad.; Bayer, Denm.; Bayer, Fin.; Bayer, Ger.; Bayer, Hong Kong; Bayer, Irl.; Bayer, Ital.; Bayer Consumer, Mex.; Bayer, Neth.; Bayer, Norw.; Bayer, NZ; Bayer, Port.; Bayer, S.Afr.; Bayer Consumer, Singapore; Bayer, Spain; Bayer, Swed.; Bayer, Thai.; Bayer Consumer, UK.*
Clotrimazole (p.382·1).
Fungal and bacterial infections; trichomoniasis.

Canesten AF *Bayer, UK.*
Bifonazole (p.381·1).
Athlete's foot.

Canesten Combi *Bayer Consumer, UK.*
Combination pack containing Canesten Cream and Canesten 1 pessary: Clotrimazole (p.382·1).
Vulvovaginal candidiasis.

Canesten HC
Bayer, Ger.; Bayer, Irl.; Bayer Consumer, Singapore; Bayer Consumer, UK.
Clotrimazole (p.382·1); hydrocortisone (p.1073·3).
Fungal skin infections with inflammation.

Canesten Oasis *Bayer Consumer, UK.*
Sodium citrate (p.1186·2).
Cystitis.

Canesten Once Daily *Bayer Consumer, Austral.*
Bifonazole (p.381·1).
Fungal skin infections.

Canestene
Bayer, Belg.; Bayer, Switz.
Clotrimazole (p.382·1).
Fungal and bacterial infections; trichomoniasis.

Canex *Alliance, S.Afr.*
Clotrimazole (p.382·1).
Fungal skin and vulvovaginal infections.

Canfomenol *Brasmedica, Braz.*
Niaouli oil (p.1640·2); camphor (p.1589·3); eucalyptol (p.1609·2); guaiacol (p.1092·1); menthol (p.1632·3); ephedrine (p.1090·1).
Respiratory-tract congestion.

Canifug *Wolff, Ger.*
Clotrimazole (p.382·1).
Fungal and bacterial infections; trichomoniasis.

Cankerol *Coradol, Ger.*
Homoeopathic preparation.

Canoderm *ACO Hud, Swed.*
Urea (p.1127·3).
Dry skin.

Canol *Jolly-Jatel, Fr.*
Cynara (p.1601·3); chimaphylla; aphloia.
Dyspepsia.

Canrenol *Prospa, Belg.*
Potassium canrenoate (p.957·1).
Cirrhosis; electrolyte disturbances; heart failure; hyperaldosteronism; hypertension; nephrotic syndrome.

Canscreen *Draxis, Canad.*
Avobenzone (p.1517·1); octinoxate (p.1517·3); oxybenzone (p.1518·1).
Sunscreen.

Canstat *Wyeth, S.Afr.*
Nystatin (p.392·2).
Candidiasis.

Cantabilin *Formenti, Ital.*
Hymecromone (p.1622·3).
Biliary-tract disorders.

Cantabiline *Merck-Belgolabo, Belg.; Lipha Sante, Fr.*
Hymecromone (p.1622·3).
Biliary-tract disorders.

Cantadrill *Pierre Fabre Sante, Fr.*
Erysimum.
Mouth and throat disorders.

Cantalene *Cooperation Pharmaceutique, Fr.*
Muramidase hydrochloride (p.1638·1); chlorhexidine acetate (p.1138·2); amethocaine [tetracaine] hydrochloride (p.1305·2).
Mouth and throat disorders.

Cantamac *Cantassium Co., UK.*
Multivitamin and mineral preparation (p.1350·1).

Cantamega *Larkhall Laboratories, UK.*
Multivitamin and mineral preparation (p.1350·1).

Cantapollen *Cantassium Co., UK.*
Dolomite; bee pollen.

Cantassium Discs *Cantassium Co., UK.*
Mineral preparation (p.1350·1).

Cantavite with FF *Cantassium Co., UK.*
Multivitamin and mineral preparation (p.1350·1).

Canthacur *Pharmascience, Canad.; Paladin, Canad.; Pharmascience, Singapore.*
Cantharidin (p.1590·3).
Molluscum contagiosum; warts.

Canthacur-PS *Paladin, Canad.*
Cantharidin (p.1590·3); podophyllum resin (p.1121·1); salicylic acid (p.1122·3).
Molluscum contagiosum; warts.

Cantharis Med Complex *Dynamit, Aust.*
Homoeopathic preparation.

Cantharone *Dormer, Canad.*
Cantharidin (p.1590·3).
Molluscum contagiosum; warts.

Cantharone Plus *Dormer, Canad.*
Cantharidin (p.1590·3); podophyllum resin (p.1121·1); salicylic acid (p.1122·3).
Warts.

Cantil
Tika, Swed.; Hoechst Marion Roussel, USA.
Mepenzolate bromide (p.470·2).
Adjunctive therapy in peptic ulcer; spasmodic disorders of the colon.

Cantipal *Loren, Mex.*
Paracetamol (p.71·2); caffeine (p.761·3); chlorpheniramine [chlorphenamine] (p.412·3); phenylephrine (p.1097·1).
Cold symptoms.

Cantopal *Larkhall Laboratories, UK.*
Calcium pantothenate (p.1374·1).

Canusal *CP Pharmaceuticals, UK.*
Heparin sodium (p.902·1).
To maintain patency of in-dwelling intravascular lines.

Caolax *Labima, Belg.†.*
Phenolphthalein (p.1244·1).
Bowel evacuation; constipation.

Caomet *Astra, Ital.*
Ubidecarenone (p.1677·1).
Cardiac disorders.

The symbol † denotes a preparation no longer actively marketed

Caosina Ern, Spain.
Calcium carbonate (p.1215·1).
Calcium supplement.

Capace
Hexal, Aust.; Amrad, Austral.; Aspen, S.Afr.
Captopril (p.853·3).
Diabetic nephropathy; heart failure; hypertension; myocardial infarction.

Capadex
Fawns & McAllan, Austral.; Pharmaco, NZ.
Dextropropoxyphene hydrochloride (p.27·1); paracetamol (p.71·2).
Pain.

Capasal
Dermal Laboratories, Irl.; Dermal, Israel; Dermal Laboratories, UK.
Salicylic acid (p.1122·3); coal tar (p.1125·1).
Scalp disorders.

Capastat
Lilly, Aust.; Lilly, Austral.; Lilly, Canad.†; Dista, Spain; Dista, UK; Dura, USA.
Capreomycin sulfate (p.159·3).
Pulmonary tuberculosis.

CAPD
Fresenius, Israel; Fresenius, Spain.
A range of electrolyte solutions with glucose (p.1184·1).
Peritoneal dialysis.

CAPD/DPCA Dicamed, Swed.
Anhydrous glucose; sodium chloride; sodium lactate; calcium chloride; magnesium chloride (p.1184·1).
Formerly known as Lockolys.
Peritoneal dialysis.

Capel Ache, Braz.
Ketoconazole (p.389·1); panthenol (p.1602·3).
Seborrhoeic dermatitis.

Capergyl Therica, Fr.
Co-dergocrine mesilate (p.1597·3).
Mental function disorders.

Capex Galderma, USA.
Fluocinolone acetonide (p.1071·1).
Formerly known as FS.
Scalp disorders.

Capginvit
Atlantic, Hong Kong; Atlantic, Thai.
Multivitamin preparation (p.1350·1).

Capibaryne Osorio de Moraes, Braz.
Vitamin B substances with minerals (p.1350·1).

Capilarema
Baldacci, Braz.; Baldacci, Port.; Zambon, Spain.
Aminaphthone (p.724·3).
Capillary disorders; haemorrhage.

Capillarema Baldacci, Ital.
Aminaphthone (p.724·3).
Capillary disorders.

Capillaron Madaus, Ger.
Homoeopathic preparation.

Capillon Gramse, Israel.
Cetrimide (p.1137·1).
Seborrhoeic dermatitis of the scalp.

Capiloton Virtus, Braz.
Jaborandi; sweet birch oil (p.55·2).
Alopecia.

Capistan Sanofi Winthrop, Fr.†.
Saw palmetto (p.1491·2).
Benign prostatic hyperplasia.

Capital with Codeine Carnrick, USA.
Paracetamol (p.71·2); codeine phosphate (p.25·2).
Pain.

Capitrol Westwood-Squibb, USA.
Chloroxine (p.214·1).
Seborrhoeic dermatitis.

Capiven Servier, Denm.
Diosmin (p.1611·1); hesperidin (p.1611·2).
Haemorrhoids; venous insufficiency.

Caplenal
Rhone-Poulenc Rorer, Hong Kong; Berk, Irl.; Berk, UK.
Allopurinol (p.397·2).
Gout; hyperuricaemia; renal calculi.

Capolax Propan, S.Afr.†.
Bisacodyl (p.1212·2).
Bowel evacuation; constipation.

Caposan Adler, Switz.
Propyphenazone (p.80·2); paracetamol (p.71·2); caffeine (p.761·3).
Fever; pain.

Caposten Chinoin, Mex.
Hydroxyprogesterone (p.1479·3).

Capota Faes, Spain†.
Cetylpyridinium chloride (p.1138·1); benzocaine (p.1306·2).
Skin and wound disinfection.

Capoten
Bristol-Myers Squibb, Austral.; Bristol-Myers Squibb, Belg.; Bristol-Myers Squibb, Braz.; Squibb, Canad.; Bristol-Myers Squibb, Denm.; Bristol-Myers Squibb, Fin.; Bristol-Myers Squibb, Hong Kong; Bristol-Myers Squibb, Irl.; Mead Johnson, Ital.; Bristol-Myers Squibb, Neth.; Bristol-Myers Squibb, Norw.; Bristol-Myers Squibb, NZ; Bristol-Myers Squibb, Port.; Bristol-Myers Squibb, S.Afr.; Bristol-Myers Squibb, Singapore; Bristol-Myers Squibb, Spain; Bristol-Myers Squibb, Swed.; Bristol-Myers Squibb, Thai.; Squibb, UK; Bristol-Myers Squibb, USA.
Captopril (p.853·3).
Diabetic nephropathy; heart failure; hypertension; myocardial infarction.

Capotena Bristol-Myers Squibb, Mex.
Captopril (p.853·3).
Diabetic nephropathy; heart failure; hypertension; myocardial infarction.

Capozid
Bristol-Myers Squibb, Denm.; Bristol-Myers Squibb, Swed.†.
Captopril (p.853·3); hydrochlorothiazide (p.907·3).
Hypertension.

Capozide
Bristol-Myers Squibb, Aust.; Bristol-Myers Squibb, Ger.; Bristol-Myers Squibb, Irl.; Bristol-Myers Squibb, Neth.; Bristol-Myers Squibb, NZ; Bristol-Myers Squibb, S.Afr.; Bristol-Myers Squibb, Switz.; Squibb, UK; Bristol-Myers Squibb, USA.
Captopril (p.853·3); hydrochlorothiazide (p.907·3).
These ingredients can be described by the British Approved Name Co-zidocapt.
Heart failure; hypertension.

Capramin Glaxo Wellcome, Aust.
Aspirin (p.14·2); carbinoxamine maleate (p.411·1); phenylephrine hydrochloride (p.1097·1); caffeine (p.761·3).
Cold and influenza symptoms.

Capricin Sisu, Canad.†.
Octanoic acid (p.1643·2).
Elimination of intestinal Candida albicans.

Caprilate Eagle, Austral.
Sodium octanoate (p.1643·2); berberis vulgaris; magnesium chloride (p.1190·3); zinc gluconate (p.1398·2); lithium chloride (p.296·2); sorbic acid (p.1157·1).
Inhibition of gastrointestinal yeast growth.

Caprilon
Note.This name is used for preparations of different composition.
Leiras, Fin.
Tranexamic acid (p.742·2).
Fibrinolysis; hereditary angioedema.

Scientific Hospital Supplies, Irl.; Cow & Gate, UK.
Medium-chain triglycerides (p.1372·1).
Formerly known as MCT(1) in the UK.
Hepatobiliary disorders; pancreatic disorders; stagnant-loop syndrome; steatorrhoea.

Caprin
Sinclair, Irl.; Sinclair, UK.
Aspirin (p.14·2).
Fever; inflammation; pain; thrombosis prophylaxis.

Caprisana Sidroga, Switz.†.
Camphor (p.1589·3); juniper oil (p.1625·2); rosemary oil (p.1659·3); turpentine oil (p.1676·3); thyme oil (p.1672·3); larch oil.
Musculoskeletal and joint pain.

Caprisset Solfran, Mex.
Multivitamin and mineral preparation (p.1350·1).

Caproamin Fides Rottapharm, Spain.
Aminocaproic acid (p.724·3).
Haemorrhage.

Caprofides Hemostatico Fides Rottapharm, Spain.
Aminocaproic acid (p.724·3); esculoside (p.1574·1); hesperidin methyl chalcone (p.1611·2); menadione (p.1395·3); creatinine sulfate.
Haemorrhage.

Caprolisin Malesci, Ital.
Aminocaproic acid (p.724·3).
Haemorrhagic disorders.

Capros Rhone-Poulenc Rorer, Ger.; Medac, Ger.
Morphine sulfate (p.56·1).
Pain.

Caprysin Leiras, Fin.
Clonidine hydrochloride (p.860·1).
Hypertension; opioid and alcohol withdrawal syndromes.

Capsamol Worwag, Ger.
Ointment: Capsicum (p.1591·1).
Musculoskeletal and joint pain.

Topical application: Camphor (p.1589·3); benzyl nicotinate (p.20·2); capsaicin (p.23·1).
Rheumatic disorders.

Capsic Pierre Fabre Sante, Fr.
Dressing: Capsicum (p.1591·1); methyl salicylate (p.55·1); camphor (p.1589·3).

Ointment: Capsaicin (p.23·1); methyl nicotinate (p.55·1).
Muscle cramp.

Capsicof Pharmacaps, Mex.
Benzonatate (p.1085·3).
Coughs.

Capsicum + Arthri-Cream Homeocan, Canad.
Homoeopathic preparation.

Capsidol
Janssen, Mex.
Capsicum oleoresin (p.1591·1).
Pain.

Vinas, Spain.
Capsaicin (p.23·1).
Muscle and joint pain.

Capsin Fleming, USA.
Capsaicin (p.23·1).
Neuralgia; pain.

Capsina Astra, Swed.
Capsaicin (p.23·1).
Postherpetic neuralgia.

Capsiplast Beiersdorf, Aust.
Capsicum (p.1591·1).
Musculoskeletal and joint disorders.

Capso RDC, Ital.
Capsicum oleoresin (p.1591·1); aloe vera (p.1110·1).
Skin disorders.

Capsoid Caps, S.Afr.
Prednisolone (p.1077·3).
Corticosteroid.

Capsolin
Note.This name is used for preparations of different composition.
Parke, Davis, Austral.
Capsicum oleoresin (p.1591·1); camphor (p.1589·3); turpentine oil (p.1676·3); cajuput oil (p.1588·1).
Joint and muscle pain.

Warner-Lambert, Ital.; Parke, Davis, Switz.†.
Capsicum oleoresin (p.1591·1); camphor (p.1589·3); turpentine oil (p.1676·3); eucalyptus oil (p.1609·2).
Musculoskeletal pain.

Capsules laxatives Nattermann Nr. 13 Piraud, Switz.†.
Senna (p.1248·2); caraway oil (p.1591·2); anise oil (p.1580·3).
Bowel evacuation; constipation.

Capsuvac Galen, UK.
Dantron (p.1221·3); docusate sodium (p.1223·1).
These ingredients can be described by the British Approved Name Co-danthrusate.
Constipation.

Capsyl Sandoz, Fr.†.
Dextromethorphan hydrobromide (p.1087·3).
Coughs.

Captagon Asta Medica, Belg.; Asta Medica, Ger.
Fenetylline hydrochloride (p.1509·3).
Hyperactivity disorders.

Captea Rhone-Poulenc Rorer, Fr.
Captopril (p.853·3); hydrochlorothiazide (p.907·3).
Hypertension.

Capti Genpharm, Israel.
Captopril (p.853·3).
Diabetic nephropathy; heart failure; hypertension; myocardial infarction.

Captimer Niddapharm, Ger.
Tiopronin (p.1025·1).
Cystinuria; heavy metal poisoning; liver disorders.

Captin Krewel, Ger.
Paracetamol (p.71·2).
Fever; pain.

Captirex Irex, Fr.
Captopril (p.853·3).
Heart failure; hypertension.

Capto CT, Ger.; ABZ, Ger.; BASF, Ger.; Eu Rho, Ger.; Isis Puren, Ger.; Lichtenstein, Ger.
Captopril (p.853·3).
Heart failure; hypertension.

Capto Comp ABZ, Ger.; BASF, Ger.; CT, Ger.; corax, Ger.; Lichtenstein, Ger.
Captopril (p.853·3); hydrochlorothiazide (p.907·3).
Hypertension.

Capto Plus Isis Puren, Ger.
Captopril (p.853·3); hydrochlorothiazide (p.907·3).
Hypertension.

capto-basan Schonenberger, Switz.
Captopril (p.853·3).
Diabetic nephropathy; heart failure; hypertension.

Captobeta Betapharm, Ger.
Captopril (p.853·3).
Heart failure; hypertension.

Captobeta Comp Betapharm, Ger.
Captopril (p.853·3); hydrochlorothiazide (p.907·3).
Hypertension.

Capto-Co Baker Norton, UK.
Captopril (p.853·3); hydrochlorothiazide (p.907·3).
These ingredients can be described by the British Approved Name Co-zidocapt.
Hypertension.

Captocomp Ebewe, Aust.†.
Verapamil hydrochloride (p.989·1); captopril (p.853·3).
Hypertension.

Captodan Pharmacodane, Denm.
Captopril (p.853·3).
Heart failure; hypertension.

Captodoc Docpharm, Ger.
Captopril (p.853·3).
Heart failure; hypertension.

Capto-dura Cor Durachemie, Ger.†.
Captopril (p.853·3).
Heart failure; hypertension.

Capto-dura M Merck dura, Ger.
Captopril (p.853·3).
Heart failure; hypertension.

Captoflux Hennig, Ger.
Captopril (p.853·3).
Heart failure; hypertension.

Captogamma Worwag, Ger.
Captopril (p.853·3).
Heart failure; hypertension.

Captogamma HCT Worwag, Ger.
Captopril (p.853·3); hydrochlorothiazide (p.907·3).
Hypertension.

Captohexal
Hexal, Austral.; Hexal, Ger.; Hexal, S.Afr.
Captopril (p.853·3).
Diabetic nephropathy; heart failure; hypertension; myocardial infarction.

Captohexal Comp Hexal, Ger.
Captopril (p.853·3); hydrochlorothiazide (p.907·3).
Hypertension.

Captol
Note.This name is used for preparations of different composition.
Durascan, Denm.
Captopril (p.853·3).
Diabetic nephropathy; heart failure; hypertension; myocardial infarction.

Pacific, NZ.
Oxprenolol hydrochloride (p.951·3).
Angina pectoris; arrhythmias; hypertension.

Captolane Rhone-Poulenc Rorer, Fr.
Captopril (p.853·3).
Diabetic nephropathy; heart failure; hypertension; myocardial infarction.

Captomax Parke-Med, S.Afr.
Captopril (p.853·3).
Heart failure; hypertension.

Captomerck Merck dura, Ger.
Captopril (p.853·3).
Heart failure; hypertension.

Captomin Medinovum, Fin.
Captopril (p.853·3).
Diabetic nephropathy; heart failure; hypertension; myocardial infarction.

Capton Diet Dexo, Switz.
Phenylpropanolamine hydrochloride (p.1098·1).
Obesity.

Captopress Bayer, Ger.†.
Captopril (p.853·3).
Heart failure; hypertension.

Captopril Comp Heumann, Ger.
Captopril (p.853·3); hydrochlorothiazide (p.907·3).
Hypertension.

Captopril Compositum Mayrhofer, Aust.
Captopril (p.853·3); hydrochlorothiazide (p.907·3).
Hypertension.

Captopril HCT Aliud, Ger.; Stada, Ger.
Captopril (p.853·3); hydrochlorothiazide (p.907·3).
Hypertension.

Captopril Plus Verla, Ger.
Captopril (p.853·3); hydrochlorothiazide (p.907·3).
Hypertension.

Captor Rowex, Irl.
Captopril (p.853·3).
Heart failure; hypertension.

Captoreal Realpharma, Ger.†.
Captopril (p.853·3).
Heart failure; hypertension.

Captoretic Hexal, S.Afr.
Captopril (p.853·3); hydrochlorothiazide (p.907·3).
Hypertension.

Captor-HCT Rowex, Irl.
Captopril (p.853·3); hydrochlorothiazide (p.907·3).
Hypertension.

Captoser Serral, Mex.
Captopril (p.853·3).
Hypertension.

Captosol Ecosol, Switz.
Captopril (p.853·3).
Diabetic nephropathy; heart failure; hypertension.

Captostad Berner, Fin.
Captopril (p.853·3).
Heart failure; hypertension.

Captral Silanes, Mex.
Captopril (p.853·3).
Heart failure; hypertension; myocardial infarction.

Captril Technilab, Canad.
Captopril (p.853·3).

Capurate Sigma, Austral.
Allopurinol (p.397·2).
Hyperuricaemia.

Capval Dreluso, Ger.
Noscapine (p.1096·1) or noscapine hydrochloride (p.1096·1).
Coughs and associated respiratory-tract disorders.

Capzasin-P
Stella, Canad.†; Thompson, USA.
Capsaicin (p.23·1).
Pain.

Carace
Du Pont, Irl.; Du Pont, UK.
Lisinopril (p.921·1).
Heart failure; hypertension; myocardial infarction.

Carace Plus
Du Pont, Irl.; Du Pont, UK.
Lisinopril (p.921·1); hydrochlorothiazide (p.907·3).
Hypertension.

Caradrin Fresenius Kabi, Aust.
Proscillaridin (p.963·3).
Cardiac disorders.

Carafate
Aventis, Austral.; Aventis, NZ; Hoechst Marion Roussel, USA.
Sucralfate (p.1250·2).
Peptic ulcer.

Caramelle alle Erbe Digestive Giuliani, Ital.
Gentian (p.1615·1); rhubarb (p.1248·1); boldo (p.1585·3).
Aid to digestion.

Caramelos Agua del Carmen Fardi, Spain.
Eucalyptol (p.1609·2); melissa (p.1632·2); menthol (p.1632·3).
Nasal congestion.

Caramelos Balsam Alcala, Spain†.
Eucalyptol (p.1609·2); oleum pini sylvestris; menthol (p.1632·3).
Throat irritation.

Caramelos Vit C *Alcala, Spain†.*
Ascorbic acid (p.1389·3).
Deficiency of vitamin C.

Carasel *Almirall, Spain.*
Ramipril (p.966·3).
Heart failure; hypertension.

Carba *ABZ, Ger.; CT, Ger.*
Carbamazepine (p.342·2).
Alcohol withdrawal syndrome; diabetic neuropathy; epilepsy; multiple sclerosis; neuralgias.

Carbabeta *Betapharm, Ger.*
Carbamazepine (p.342·2).
Alcohol withdrawal syndrome; bipolar disorder; diabetic neuropathy; epilepsy; multiple sclerosis; neuralgias.

Carbac *Syntex, Mex.*
Loracarbef (p.220·3).
Bacterial infections.

Carbacide *Fischer, Israel.*
Carbaryl (p.1429·2).
Pediculosis.

Carbactive *Cooperation Pharmaceutique, Fr.*
Activated charcoal (p.1000·2).
Gastrointestinal disorders.

Carbaflux *Hennig, Ger.*
Carbamazepine (p.342·2).
Alcohol withdrawal syndrome; bipolar disorder; diabetic neuropathy; epilepsy; multiple sclerosis; neuralgias.

Carbagamma *Worwag, Ger.*
Carbamazepine (p.342·2).
Alcohol withdrawal syndrome; diabetic neuropathy; epilepsy; multiple sclerosis; neuralgias.

Carbagen *Generics, UK.*
Carbamazepine (p.342·2).
Epilepsy.

Carbager-Plus *Streger, Mex.*
Methocarbamol (p.1329·3); ibuprofen (p.43·2).
Gout; inflammation; musculoskeletal, joint and periarticular disorders; pain.

Carbaica *Pharmafar, Ital.*
Urazamide (p.1677·2).
Liver disorders.

Carbalan *Quimica y Farmacia, Mex.*
Carbamazepine (p.342·2).
Epilepsy.

Carbalax *Pharmax, UK.*
Monobasic sodium phosphate (p.1193·2); sodium bicarbonate (p.1186·2).
Formerly known as Beogex.
Bowel evacuation; constipation.

Carbamann *Mann, Ger.*
Carbachol (p.1416·1).
Glaucoma.

Carbamid + VAS *Widmer, Ger.*
Tretinoin (p.1126·2); urea (p.1127·3).
Skin disorders.

Carbamide Creme *Widmer, Switz.*
Urea (p.1127·3); vitamin A palmitate (p.1383·2); dexpanthenol (p.1602·3).
Skin disorders.

Carbamide + VAS *Widmer, Switz.*
Tretinoin (p.1126·2); urea (p.1127·3); dexpanthenol (p.1602·3).
Skin disorders.

Carbastat
Ciba Vision, Canad.; Ciba Vision, USA.
Carbachol (p.1416·1).
Production of miosis.

Carbatil *Loren, Mex.*
Mebendazole (p.102·2).
Worm infections.

Carbatrol *Shire Richwood, USA.*
Carbamazepine (p.342·2).
Epilepsy; trigeminal neuralgia.

Carbazene *Medifive, Thai.*
Carbamazepine (p.342·2).
Epilepsy; trigeminal neuralgia.

Carbazep *Cryopharma, Mex.*
Carbamazepine (p.342·2).
Diabetic neuropathy; epilepsy; neuralgias.

Carbazina *Psicofarma, Mex.*
Carbamazepine (p.342·2).
Epilepsy; neuralgias.

Carbecin *Sanfer, Mex.*
Carbenicillin sodium (p.160·2).
Bacterial infections.

Carbellon *Torbet Laboratories, UK.*
Activated charcoal (p.1000·2); magnesium hydroxide (p.1233·1); peppermint oil (p.1243·3).
Formerly contained activated charcoal, belladonna dry extract, magnesium hydroxide, and peppermint oil.
Dyspepsia; flatulence; gastric hyperacidity.

Carbem *Lilly, Ital.†.*
Loracarbef (p.220·3).
Bacterial infections.

Carbenin *Sankyo, Jpn.*
Panipenem (p.234·3); betamipron (p.159·2).
Bacterial infections.

Carbex
Note.This name is used for preparations of different composition.
Ferring, UK.
Oral granules, sodium bicarbonate (p.1186·2); simeticone (p.1249·2); solution, anhydrous citric acid (p.1596·2).
Adjunct to contrast media for gastrointestinal radiography.

Endo, USA.
Selegiline hydrochloride (p.1177·2).
Parkinsonism.

Carbi *Gerard, Israel.*
Carbamazepine (p.342·2).
Bipolar disorder; diabetes insipidus; epilepsy; mania; trigeminal neuralgia.

Carbicalcin
Procter & Gamble, Ital.; Dreiman, Spain.
Elcatonin (p.749·2).
Hypercalcaemia; osteoporosis; Paget's disease of bone; reflex sympathetic dystrophy.

Carbilev *Aspen, S.Afr.*
Levodopa (p.1169·2); carbidopa (p.1168·2).
Parkinsonism.

Carbinib *Oftalder, Port.*
Acetazolamide (p.826·1).
Glaucoma.

Carbinoxamine Compound *Morton Grove, USA.*
Carbinoxamine maleate (p.411·1); pseudoephedrine hydrochloride (p.1099·2); dextromethorphan hydrobromide (p.1087·3).
Coughs and cold symptoms.

Carbiset *Nutripharm, USA.*
Pseudoephedrine hydrochloride (p.1099·2); carbinoxamine maleate (p.411·1).
Upper respiratory-tract symptoms.

Carbistad *Stada, Aust.*
Carbimazole (p.1521·1).
Hyperthyroidism.

Carbium
Hexal, Austral.; Hexal, Ger.
Carbamazepine (p.342·2).
Alcohol withdrawal syndrome; bipolar disorder; diabetic neuropathy; epilepsy; multiple sclerosis; neuralgias.

Carbo *Max Farma, Ital.*
Calcium carbonate (p.1215·1).
Calcium deficiency; calcium supplement.

Carbo Konigsfeld *Muller Goppingen, Ger.*
Carbo coffea (p.1681·1).
Diarrhoea.

Carbo Veg *Brauer, Austral.†.*
Homoeopathic preparation.

Ca-R-Bob *Greater Pharma, Thai.*
Activated charcoal (p.1000·2).
Abdominal distension; diarrhoea; poisoning.

Carbobel *Medgenix, Belg.*
Activated charcoal (p.1000·2); methenamine (p.223·1); magnesium citrate (p.1232·3).
Diarrhoea; dyspepsia; poisoning.

Carbocain
AstraZeneca, Denm.; AstraZeneca, Norw.; Astra, Swed.
Mepivacaine hydrochloride (p.1317·1).
Adrenaline [epinephrine] acid tartrate (p.829·2) is included in some injections as a vasoconstrictor to diminish absorption and localise the effect of the local anaesthetic.
Local anaesthesia.

Carbocaina
Note.This name is used for preparations of different composition.
Astra, Ital.
Mepivacaine hydrochloride (p.1317·1).
Adrenaline [epinephrine] acid tartrate (p.829·2) is included in some injections as a vasoconstrictor to diminish absorption and localise the effect of the local anaesthetic.
Local anaesthesia.

Bucca, Spain.
Phenol (p.1152·3); methyl salicylate (p.55·1); amethocaine [tetracaine] hydrochloride (p.1305·2).
Local anaesthesia.

Carbocaine
Astra, Austral.; Sanofi Synthelabo, Canad.; AstraZeneca, Fr.; Adcock Ingram, S.Afr.; Sanofi Winthrop, USA; Cook-Waite, USA.
Mepivacaine hydrochloride (p.1317·1).
Corbadrine (p.1599·2) is included in some injections as a vasoconstrictor to diminish absorption and localise the effect of the local anaesthetic.
Local anaesthesia.

Carbocaine with Neo-Cobefrin *Cook-Waite, USA.*
Mepivacaine hydrochloride (p.1317·1).
Corbadrine (p.1599·2) is included in this preparation as a vasoconstrictor to diminish absorption and localise the effect of the local anaesthetic.
Local anaesthesia.

Carbocal *Madariaga, Spain.*
Calcium carbonate (p.1215·1).
Hypocalcaemia; osteoporosis.

Carbocit *CT, Ital.*
Carbocisteine (p.1086·3).
Respiratory-tract disorders.

Carbo-Cort *Lagap, UK†.*
Coal tar (p.1125·1); hydrocortisone (p.1073·3).
Eczema; psoriasis.

Carbodec *Rugby, USA.*
Carbinoxamine maleate (p.411·1); pseudoephedrine hydrochloride (p.1099·2).
Allergic rhinitis; nasal congestion.

Carbodec DM *Rugby, USA.*
Pseudoephedrine hydrochloride (p.1099·2); dextromethorphan hydrobromide (p.1087·3); carbinoxamine maleate (p.411·1).
Coughs and cold symptoms.

Carbo-Dome *Lagap, UK.*
Coal tar (p.1125·1).
Psoriasis.

Carboflex *Convatec, Port.*
Activated charcoal (p.1000·2); calcium-sodium alginate (p.728·1) (p.1498·3); carmellose sodium (p.1499·3).
Ulcers; wounds.

Carbolevure
Vedim, Fr.; UCB, Switz.
Dried yeast (p.1398·1); activated charcoal (p.1000·2).
Gastrointestinal disorders.

Carbolim *Dansk-Flama, Braz.*
Lithium carbonate (p.292·1).
Bipolar disorder; depression; migraine and vascular headaches; neutropenia; schizophrenia.

Carbolit *Psicofarma, Mex.*
Lithium carbonate (p.292·1).
Bipolar disorder; psychoses.

Carbolith *ICN, Canad.*
Lithium carbonate (p.292·1).
Bipolar disorder.

Carbolithium *IFI, Ital.*
Lithium carbonate (p.292·1).
Adjunct in drug-induced leucopenia; cluster headache; psychiatric disorders.

Carbolitium *Eurofarma, Braz.*
Lithium carbonate (p.292·1).
Bipolar disorder; depression; migraine and vascular headaches; neutropenia; schizophrenia.

Carbomix
Leiras, Fin.; Pharmygiene, Fr.; Penn, Irl.; Vaillant, Ital.; Selena, Swed.; Penn, UK.
Activated charcoal (p.1000·2).
Acute poisoning; diarrhoea.

Carbondifer *Trenka Difer, Ital.*
Senna (p.1248·2); rhubarb (p.1248·1); vegetable charcoal (p.1000·3); sublimed sulfur (p.1123·3).
Formerly known as Eucarbon.
Constipation.

Carbonesia *Geymonat, Ital.*
Activated charcoal (p.1000·2); magnesium oxide (p.1233·2); calcium carbonate (p.1215·1); magnesium peroxide (p.1149·3).
Gastrointestinal disorders.

Carbonet
Smith & Nephew, Fr.; Smith & Nephew, Irl.; Smith & Nephew, UK.
Activated charcoal (p.1000·2).
Malodorous wounds.

Carboneural *Recipe, Aust.†.*
Bupivacaine hydrochloride (p.1306·3).
Local anaesthesia.

Carbonex *Aerocid, Fr.*
Magnesium hydroxide (p.1233·1).
Formerly contained sublimed sulfur and magnesium hydroxide.
Constipation.

Carbonpectate *Chew, Thai.*
Activated charcoal (p.1000·2); magnesium carbonate (p.1232·3); pectin (p.1502·3).
Diarrhoea; flatulence.

Carbophagix *Darci, Fr.*
Activated charcoal (p.1000·2); Saccharomyces cerevisiae (p.1398·1).
Gastrointestinal disorders.

Carbophos *UPSA, Fr.*
Vegetable charcoal (p.1000·3); calcium carbonate (p.1215·1); calcium phosphate (p.1188·3).
Gastrointestinal disorders.

Carboplat
Bristol-Myers Squibb, Ger.; Asofarma, Mex.
Carboplatin (p.515·1).
Malignant neoplasms.

Carbosan *Rowa, Irl.*
Carbenoxolone sodium (p.1215·3).
Aphthous stomatitis; herpes labialis; lip sores.

Carboseptol *Herbes Universelles, Canad.*
Menthol (p.1632·3); eucalyptol (p.1609·2); methyl salicylate (p.55·1); thymol (p.1158·3); zinc oxide (p.1128·2).

Carbosin
Nettopharma, Denm.; Nycomed, Fin.; Nycomed, Norw.; Asta Medica, NZ; NZ Medical & Scientific, NZ; Pharmachemie, S.Afr.; Pharmachemie, Thai.
Carboplatin (p.515·1).
Malignant neoplasms.

Carbosint *Boniscontro & Gazzone, Ital.*
Calcium carbonate (p.1215·1).
Calcium deficiency; calcium supplement.

Carbosol *Sanova, Aust.*
Carboplatin (p.515·1).
Malignant neoplasms.

Carbosorb
Pharmacia Upjohn, Austral.; Pharmacia Upjohn, NZ.
Activated charcoal (p.1000·2).
Drug overdose; poisoning.

Carbosorb S
Pharmacia Upjohn, Austral.; Pharmacia Upjohn, NZ.
Activated charcoal (p.1000·2); sorbitol (p.1377·2).
Drug overdose; poisoning.

Carbospare *Abbott, Fin.*
Food for special diets (p.1350·1).

Carbospect *Mer-National, S.Afr.†.*
Carbocisteine (p.1086·3).
Respiratory-tract disorders.

Carbostesin
Astra, Aust.; Astra, Ger.; Astra, Switz.
Bupivacaine hydrochloride (p.1306·3).
Adrenaline [epinephrine] acid tartrate (p.829·2) is included in some injections as a vasoconstrictor to diminish absorption and localise the effect of the local anaesthetic.
Local anaesthesia.

Carbosylane
Grimberg, Fr.; Trima, Israel.
Activated charcoal (p.1000·2); simeticone (p.1249·2).
Gastrointestinal disorders.

Carbosymag *Grimberg, Fr.*
Charcoal (p.1000·2); simeticone (p.1249·2); magnesium oxide (p.1233·2).
Gastrointestinal disorders.

Carbo-Syrup *Brovar, S.Afr.†.*
Carbocisteine (p.1086·3).
Respiratory-tract disorders.

Carbotec *Columbia, Mex.*
Carboplatin (p.515·1).
Malignant neoplasms.

Carboticon
Note.This name is used for preparations of different composition.
Byk, Neth.†.
Simeticone (p.1249·2).
Flatulence.

Interdelta, Switz.
Activated charcoal (p.1000·2); simeticone (p.1249·2).
Digestive disorders; flatulence.

Carbotiol *Bouty, Ital.†.*
Killed bacteria: Escherichia coli; Streptococcus ovalis; Micrococcus pyogenes var. aureus; Proteus vulgaris; vegetable charcoal (p.1000·3); kaolin (p.1229·3); sodium sulfate (p.1250·1); sodium bicarbonate (p.1186·2).
Gastrointestinal disorders.

Carbotop *Pulitzer, Ital.*
Calcium carbonate (p.1215·1).
Calcium deficiency; calcium supplement.

Carboyoghurt *SIT, Ital.*
Vegetable charcoal (p.1000·3); simeticone (p.1249·2).
Gastrointestinal disorders.

Carcinil *Abbott, Ger.†.*
Leuprorelin acetate (p.1289·2).
Prostatic cancer.

Cardace *Hoechst Marion Roussel, Fin.*
Ramipril (p.966·3).
Heart failure; hypertension; myocardial infarction.

Cardace Comp *Hoechst Marion Roussel, Fin.*
Ramipril (p.966·3); hydrochlorothiazide (p.907·3).
Hypertension.

Cardalept *Synpharma, Aust.*
Crataegus (p.1600·2); melissa (p.1632·2); rosemary.
Cardiac disorders.

Cardalin *Sintofarma, Braz.*
Nifedipine (p.940·1).
Angina pectoris; hypertension; Raynaud's syndrome.

Cardanat *Temmler, Ger.*
Etilefrine hydrochloride (p.888·1).
Hypotension.

Cardaxen *Spirig, Switz.*
Atenolol (p.841·3).
Angina pectoris; arrhythmias; hypertension; myocardial infarction.

Cardaxen plus *Spirig, Switz.*
Atenolol (p.841·3); chlortalidone (p.857·1).
Hypertension.

Cardcal *Amrad, Austral.*
Diltiazem hydrochloride (p.874·3).
Angina pectoris.

Cardec *Dermopen, Braz.*
Methyl salicylate (p.55·1); menthol (p.1632·3); camphor (p.1589·3).
Musculoskeletal and joint disorders.

Cardec DM Pediatric *Schein, USA.*
Pseudoephedrine hydrochloride (p.1099·2); dextromethorphan hydrobromide (p.1087·3); carbinoxamine maleate (p.411·1).
Coughs and cold symptoms.

Cardec-S *Barre-National, USA.*
Pseudoephedrine hydrochloride (p.1099·2); carbinoxamine maleate (p.411·1).
Upper respiratory-tract symptoms.

Cardegic
Sanofi Synthelabo, Belg.; Sanofi Synthelabo, Neth.
Lysine aspirin (p.50·3).
Thromboembolic disorders.

Cardeloc *TO-Chemicals, Thai.*
Metoprolol tartrate (p.931·2).
Angina pectoris; arrhythmias; hypertension; hyperthyroidism; myocardial infarction.

Cardem *Rhone-Poulenc Rorer, Spain.*
Celiprolol hydrochloride (p.856·1).
Angina pectoris; hypertension.

Cardene
Roche, Canad.; Yamanouchi, Irl.; Yamanouchi, Neth.; Yamanouchi, UK; Wyeth-Ayerst, USA.
Nicardipine hydrochloride (p.938·3).
Angina pectoris; hypertension.

Cardenol *TO-Chemicals, Thai.*
Propranolol hydrochloride (p.962·3).
Angina pectoris; arrhythmias; hypertension; tremor.

The symbol † denotes a preparation no longer actively marketed

1764 Preparations

Cardensiel *Lipha, Fr.*
Bisoprolol fumarate (p.850·1).
Heart failure.

Cardepine *Yamanouchi-Westmont, Thai.; Great Eastern, Thai.*
Nicardipine hydrochloride (p.938·3).
Angina pectoris; cerebrovascular disorders; heart failure; hypertension.

Cardeymin *Cantassium Co., UK.*
Magnesium orotate (p.1645·1); bromelain (p.1586·3); potassium orotate (p.1645·1).

Card-Floe II *Sisu, Canad.*
Multivitamin and mineral preparation (p.1350·1).

Cardiace *Triomed, S.Afr.*
Captopril (p.853·3).
Diabetic nephropathy; heart failure; hypertension.

Cardiacton *Byk, Aust.*
Diltiazem hydrochloride (p.874·3).
Angina pectoris; hypertension.

Cardiacum PMD *Plantamed, Ger.*
Homoeopathic preparation.

Cardiaforce *Bioforce, Switz.*
Crataegus (p.1600·2); melissa (p.1632·2); wine.
Sleep disorders; tachycardia.

Cardiagen *APS, Ger.*
Captopril (p.853·3).
Formerly contained crataegus and camphor.
Heart failure; hypertension.

Cardiagen HCT *APS, Ger.*
Captopril (p.853·3); hydrochlorothiazide (p.907·3).
Hypertension.

Cardialgine *MIP, Ger.*
Etilefrine hydrochloride (p.888·1).
Hypotension.

Cardiazidine *Monsanto, Fr.*
Trimetazidine hydrochloride (p.987·3).
Angina pectoris; vascular eye disorders; vestibular disorders.

Cardiazol-Paracodina *Knoll, Ital.*
Pentetrazol (p.1513·2); dihydrocodeine thiocyanate (p.33·3).
Coughs.

Cardibisana *Hotz, Ger.*
Crataegus (p.1600·2); cinchona bark (p.1595·3); kola (p.1681·1); convallaria (p.1599·1); cereus (p.1593·1); ephedra (p.1090·1); ginseng (p.1615·3); camphora; thiamine hydrochloride; veratrum; strophanthus; phosphor; glonoinum; ars. alb.
Cardiovascular disorders.

Cardibloc *Imperial, Singapore.*
Nicardipine hydrochloride (p.938·3).
Angina pectoris; hypertension.

Cardiblok *Xixia, S.Afr.*
Propranolol hydrochloride (p.962·3).
Angina pectoris; arrhythmias; hypertension; hyperthyroidism; phaeochromocytoma; tachycardia; tremor.

Cardicor
Merck, Denm.; Merck, Irl.; Merck, UK.
Bisoprolol fumarate (p.850·1).
Heart failure.

Cardifen *Aspen, S.Afr.*
Nifedipine (p.940·1).
Angina pectoris.

Cardil
Orion, Denm.; Orion, Singapore; Orion, Thai.
Diltiazem hydrochloride (p.874·3).
Angina pectoris; hypertension.

Cardilat *Triomed, S.Afr.*
Nifedipine (p.940·1).
Angina pectoris; hypertension.

Cardilate *Glaxo Wellcome, Ital.†.*
Note. A similar name is used for preparations of different composition (see below).
Eritrityl tetranitrate (p.886·3).
Angina pectoris.

Cardilate MR *Baker Norton, UK.*
Note. A similar name is used for preparations of different composition (see below).
Nifedipine (p.940·1).
Angina pectoris; hypertension.

Cardimax *Garec, S.Afr.†.*
Propranolol (p.963·1).
Angina pectoris; arrhythmias; hypertension; hyperthyroidism; phaeochromocytoma.

Cardimet *Errekappa, Ital.†.*
Carnitine (p.1356·1).
Carnitine deficiency; myocardial ischaemia.

Cardin *Farmoquimica, Braz.*
Methyldopa (p.927·3).
Hypertension.

Cardinit *Knoll, Mex.*
Glyceryl trinitrate (p.897·3).
Angina pectoris; heart failure.

Cardinol
Pacific, NZ; CP Pharmaceuticals, UK†.
Propranolol hydrochloride (p.962·3).
Angina pectoris; anxiety; arrhythmias; hypertension; hypertrophic obstructive cardiomyopathy; migraine; myocardial infarction; phaeochromocytoma; thyrotoxicosis; tremor.

Cardinorm *Hexal, Austral.*
Amiodarone hydrochloride (p.836·1).
Arrhythmias.

Cardinorma *Pekana, Ger.*
Homoeopathic preparation.

Cardioace *Vitabiotics, UK.*
Omega-3 fish oil; garlic; lecithin; vitamins; minerals (p.1350·1).

Cardioaspirin *Bayer, Ital.*
Aspirin (p.14·2).
Thromboembolic disorders.

Cardioaspirine *Bayer, Belg.*
Aspirin (p.14·2).
Thromboembolic disorders.

Cardiobil *Biologici Italia, Ital.*
Levocarnitine (p.1356·1).
Carnitine deficiency.

Cardiocalm *Pharmastra, Fr.*
Crataegus (p.1600·2).
Formerly contained crataegus and phenobarbital.
Insomnia; nervous disorders.

Cardiocap *Miba, Ital.*
Carbocromen hydrochloride (p.855·1).
Ischaemic heart disease.

Cardiocor *Wyeth Lederle, Fr.*
Bisoprolol fumarate (p.850·1).
Heart failure.

Cardiodisco *Juste, Spain.*
Glyceryl trinitrate (p.897·3).
Angina pectoris.

Cardiodoron
Weleda, Aust.; Weleda, Ger.
Hyoscyamus niger; onopordon acanthium; cowslip flower (p.1600·1).
Cardiac disorders; sleep disorders.

Cardiofrik *Fresenius Kabi, Aust.*
Convallaria (p.1599·1); crataegus (p.1600·2); valerian (p.1678·3).
Cardiac disorders.

Cardiogen *Vedim, Ital.*
Note. A similar name is used for preparations of different composition (see below).
Carnitine (p.1356·1).
Carnitine deficiency.

CardioGen 82 *Squibb Diagnostics, USA†.*
Note. A similar name is used for preparations of different composition (see above).
Rubidium-82 (p.1451·1).

Cardio-Green
Paesel, Ger.†; Becton Dickinson, USA.
Indocyanine green (p.1623·2).
Diagnostic aid.

Cardioguard *Clonmel, Irl.*
Folic acid (p.1361·1).
Hyperhomocysteinaemia.

Cardiol
Note. This name is used for preparations of different composition.
Roche, Port.
Carvedilol (p.855·2).
Angina pectoris; heart failure; hypertension.
Bial, Port.
Fluvastatin sodium (p.892·1).
Hypercholesterolaemia.

Cardiolan *Tosi, Ital.†.*
Metildigoxin (p.930·1).
Heart failure.

Cardiolite
Du Pont, Aust.; Du Pont, Belg.; Du Pont, Fr.; Du Pont, Spain; Du Pont, UK; Du Pont, USA.
Technetium-99m sestamibi (p.1451·1).
Diagnosis and location of myocardial infarction; diagnosis of breast cancer; diagnosis of hyperparathyroidism; diagnosis of myocardial ischaemia and ventricular dysfunction.

Cardio-Longoral *Artesan, Ger.; Cassella-med, Ger.*
Potassium aspartate (p.1195·2); magnesium aspartate (p.1190·3); crataegus (p.1600·2).
Cardiac disorders.

Cardi-Omega 3 *Thompson, USA.*
Omega-3 marine triglycerides (p.949·3).
Dietary supplement.

Cardionil *Efarmes, Spain.*
Isosorbide mononitrate (p.916·2).
Angina pectoris.

Cardio-Plantina *Plantina, Ger.*
Homoeopathic preparation.

Cardioplegia
DBL, Austral.; Faulding, Hong Kong; Bull, Singapore; Faulding, Thai.; DBL, Thai.
Magnesium chloride (p.1190·3); potassium chloride (p.1194·3); procaine hydrochloride (p.1319·1).
Induction of ischaemic cardiac arrest during heart surgery.

Cardioplegia A *Baxter, Austral.*
Sodium chloride (p.1196·1); potassium chloride (p.1194·3); magnesium chloride (p.1190·3); calcium chloride (p.1188·1).
Induction of cardiac arrest during heart surgery.

Cardioplegin N *Kohler, Ger.*
Magnesium aspartate (p.1190·3); procaine hydrochloride (p.1319·1); xylitol (p.1397·3).
Cardioplegia in open-heart surgery.

Cardiopril *Searle, Switz.*
Spirapril hydrochloride (p.973·2).
Hypertension.

Cardioprotect *BASF, Ger.*
Verapamil hydrochloride (p.989·1).
Arrhythmias; hypertension; ischaemic heart disease.

Cardioquin
Purdue Frederick, Canad.; Asta Medica, Neth.; Purdue Frederick, USA†.
Quinidine polygalacturonate (p.964·3).
Arrhythmias.

Cardioquine
Asta Medica, Fr.†; Berenguer Infale, Spain.
Quinidine polygalacturonate (p.964·3).
Arrhythmias.

Cardioreg *Rhone-Poulenc Rorer, Ital.*
β-Acetyldigoxin (p.827·3).
Heart failure.

Cardioregis *Zambon, Braz.*
Convallatoxin; nikethamide (p.1513·1).
Respiratory insufficiency.

Cardiorona *Columbia, Mex.*
Amiodarone (p.838·1).
Arrhythmias.

Cardioselect N *Dreluso, Ger.*
Homoeopathic preparation.

Cardiosolupsan *Bristol-Myers Squibb, Fr.*
Carbasalate calcium (p.23·3).
Thromboembolism prophylaxis.

Cardiostenol *Molteni, Ital.*
Morphine hydrochloride (p.56·1); atropine sulfate (p.461·1).
Adjuvant in anaesthesia; pain.

CardioTec *Squibb Diagnostics, USA†.*
Technetium-99m teboroxime (p.1451·1).
Assessment of myocardial function.

Cardioten *OFF, Ital.*
Nicardipine hydrochloride (p.938·3).
Angina pectoris; heart failure; hypertension.

Cardioton *NCSN, Ital.*
Ubidecarenone (p.1677·1).
Cardiopathy; coenzyme Q10 deficiency.

Cardiotonicum (Rowo-15) *Pharmakon, Ger.†.*
Homoeopathic preparation.
Lignocaine [lidocaine] hydrochloride (p.1313·2) is included in this preparation to alleviate the pain of injection.

Cardiovas *Knoll, Spain.*
Isosorbide mononitrate (p.916·2).
Angina pectoris; heart failure.

Cardiovasc *Rottapharm, Ital.*
Lercanidipine hydrochloride (p.920·2).
Hypertension.

Cardioxane
Chiron, Denm.; Chiron, Fr.; Chiron, Israel; Chiron, Ital.
Dexrazoxane hydrochloride (p.1006·2).
Prevention of doxorubicin cardiotoxicity.

Cardip *Francia, Ital.*
Nicardipine hydrochloride (p.938·3).
Angina pectoris; heart failure; hypertension.

Cardiphyt *Austroplant, Aust.*
Crataegus (p.1600·2).
Cardiac disorders.

Cardipin *Spirig, Switz.*
Nifedipine (p.940·1).
Angina pectoris; hypertension.

Cardiplant *Also, Ital.†; Schwabe, Switz.*
Crataegus (p.1600·2).
Cardiac disorders.

Cardipril *Liomont, Mex.*
Captopril (p.853·3).
Diabetic nephropathy; heart failure; hypertension; myocardial infarction.

Cardiprin
Reckitt & Colman, Austral.; Reckitt & Colman, Hong Kong; Reckitt Benckiser, NZ; Reckitt & Colman, Singapore; Reckitt & Colman, Thai.
Aspirin (p.14·2).
Glycine (p.1365·3) may be included in this preparation in an attempt to limit adverse effects on the gastrointestinal mucosa.
Thromboembolism prophylaxis.

Cardirene *Sanofi Synthelabo, Ital.*
Lysine aspirin (p.50·3).
Thrombosis prophylaxis.

Cardiser *Merck, Spain.*
Diltiazem hydrochloride (p.874·3).
Angina pectoris; hypertension.

Cardispan *Grossman, Mex.*
Levocarnitine (p.1356·1).
Carnitine deficiency.

Cardispare *Rolab, S.Afr.*
Propranolol hydrochloride (p.962·3).
Hypertension.

Cardium *DHA, Singapore.*
Diltiazem hydrochloride (p.874·3).
Angina pectoris; hypertension.

Cardizem
Hoechst Marion Roussel, Austral.; Boehringer de Angeli, Braz.; Hoechst Marion Roussel, Canad.; Novo Nordisk, Denm.; Pharmacia Upjohn, Fin.; Pharmacia Upjohn, Norw.; Aventis, NZ; Pharmacia Upjohn, Swed.; Hoechst Marion Roussel, USA.
Diltiazem hydrochloride (p.874·3).
Angina pectoris; arrhythmias; hypertension.

Cardol *Alphapharm, Austral.*
Sotalol hydrochloride (p.972·2).
Arrhythmias.

Cardopax *Orion, Denm.*
Isosorbide dinitrate (p.915·2).
Angina pectoris; heart failure.

Cardoral *Teva, Israel.*
Doxazosin mesilate (p.883·2).
Benign prostatic hyperplasia; hypertension.

Cardoxan *Lincoln, NZ.*
Doxazosin mesilate (p.883·2).
Benign prostatic hyperplasia; hypertension.

Cardoxin *Rafa, Israel.*
Dipyridamole (p.877·2).
Adjunct to cardiac imaging; nephrotic syndrome; pre-eclampsia; thrombosis prophylaxis.

Cardoxone *Remedica, Thai.*
Metoprolol tartrate (p.931·2).
Angina pectoris; hypertension; migraine.

Cards HCG-Urine *NZ Diagnostics, NZ.*
Pregnancy test (p.1654·3).

Carduben *Madaus, Ger.†.*
Ammi visnaga fruit (p.1579·1).
Cardiac disorders.

Cardular PP *Pfizer, Ger.*
Doxazosin mesilate (p.883·2).
Benign prostatic hyperplasia; hypertension.

Carduokatt N *Kattwiga, Ger.*
Homoeopathic preparation.

Cardura
AstraZeneca, Canad.; Pfizer, Hong Kong; Invicta, Irl.; Roerig, Ital.; Pfizer, Mex.; Pfizer, Neth.; Pfizer, S.Afr.; Pfizer, Singapore; Pfizer, Thai.; Pfizer, UK; Pfizer, USA.
Doxazosin mesilate (p.883·2).
Benign prostatic hyperplasia; hypertension.

Carduran
Pfizer, Austral.†; Pfizer, Braz.; Pfizer, Denm.; Pfizer, Norw.; Pfizer Consumer, Spain.
Doxazosin mesilate (p.883·2).
Benign prostatic hyperplasia; hypertension.

Carduus-monoplant *Weber & Weber, Ger.†.*
Silybum marianum (p.1021·3).
Liver disorders.

Cardyl *Pfizer Consumer, Spain.*
Atorvastatin calcium (p.842·3).
Hyperlipidaemias.

Care 55+ Multi *Blackmores, Austral.*
Multivitamin, mineral and ginkgo biloba preparation (p.1350·1).

Carencil *Jaba, Port.*
Captopril (p.853·3).
Heart failure; hypertension.

Carencyl *Riom, Fr.*
Multivitamin, amino-acid, and mineral preparation (p.1350·1).
Tonic.

Carentil *Almirall, Spain.*
Conjugated oestrogens (p.1467·1).
Female hypogonadism; menopausal disorders; osteoporosis.

Caress *Schering-Plough, Swed.*
Urea (p.1127·3).
Dry skin.

Carexan *Pisa, Mex.*
Itraconazole (p.387·2).
Fungal infections.

Carfenil *Chugai, Jpn†.*
Lobenzarit sodium (p.1629·2).
Rheumatoid arthritis.

Cariban *Inibsa, Spain.*
Doxylamine succinate (p.417·1); pyridoxine hydrochloride (p.1386·3).
Nausea; vomiting.

Caricef *Antibioticos, Spain.*
Cefazolin sodium (p.164·3).
Lignocaine [lidocaine] hydrochloride (p.1313·2) is included in the intramuscular injection to alleviate the pain of injection.
Bacterial infections.

Caril *Nutricia, Fr.*
Carrots, rice, dextrin-maltose, glucose, and electrolytes (p.1185·2).
Diarrhoea.

Carilax *Strallhofer, Aust.*
Senna (p.1248·2).
Bowel evacuation; constipation.

Cariomix *INTES, Ital.†.*
Xanthopterin; human placenta extract.
Corneal ulcers, burns, and wounds; herpetic keratitis.

Carisano *Bilgast, Ger.*
Garlic (p.1614·1).
Lipid disorders.

Cariso-Co *PP Lab, Thai.*
Paracetamol (p.71·2); carisoprodol (p.1327·1).
Musculoskeletal disorders.

Carisoma *Pharmax, UK.*
Carisoprodol (p.1327·1).
Skeletal muscle spasm.

Carisoma Compound *Carter Horner, Thai.*
Carisoprodol (p.1327·1); paracetamol (p.71·2).
Musculoskeletal and joint disorders.

Caritasone *Chinta, Thai.*
Carisoprodol (p.1327·1); paracetamol (p.71·2).
Musculoskeletal and joint disorders.

Carito mono
Europharm, Aust.; Hoyer, Ger.
Java tea (p.1625·1).
Urinary-tract disorders.

Carl Baders Divinal *Apotheke Heiligen Rupertus, Aust.*
Camphor and camphor spirit (p.1589·3); methyl salicylate (p.55·1); salicylic acid (p.1122·3); salol (p.82·2);

turpentine oil (p.1676·3); rosemary oil (p.1659·3); menthol (p.1632·3).
Musculoskeletal and joint disorders.

Carli *Boncour, Fr.*
Magnesium aspartate; potassium aspartate; arnica (p.1581·3).
Musculoskeletal and soft-tissue disorders.

Carloxan *Orion, Denm.*
Cyclophosphamide (p.527·3).
Malignant neoplasms.

Carlytene *Asta Medica, Fr.*
Thymoxamine [moxisylyte] hydrochloride (p.980·2).
Circulatory disorders.

Carmapine *Pharmasant, Thai.*
Carbamazepine (p.342·2).
Alcohol withdrawal syndrome; diabetic neuropathy; epilepsy; glossopharyngeal neuralgia; trigeminal neuralgia.

Carmatis *Carmaran, Canad.†*
Methyl salicylate (p.55·1); camphor (p.1589·3); menthol (p.1632·3).

Carmian *Teofarma, Ital.*
Atenolol (p.841·3); chlortalidone (p.857·1).
Hypertension.

Carmicide *Indoco, Thai.*
Sodium citrate (p.1186·2); citric acid (p.1596·2); ginger tincture (p.1227·2); aromatic cardamom tincture (p.1591·3); cinnamon tincture (p.1595·3).
Colic; flatulence.

Carmicina *Sanofi Synthelabo, Port.*
Ciprofloxacin hydrochloride (p.182·3).
Bacterial infections.

Carminagal N *Galenika, Ger.*
Cynara (p.1601·3).
Formerly contained cynara, pancreatin, and dimethicone.
Dyspepsia.

Carminative *Sanova, Aust.*
Caraway tincture (p.1591·2); coriander tincture (p.1599·2); spearmint tincture (p.1666·3).
Flatulence.

Carminative Tea *Weleda, UK.*
Fennel seed (p.1610·1); aniseed (p.1580·2); caraway seed (p.1591·2); achillea (p.1572·2); chamomile flowers (p.1593·2).
Flatulence.

Carminativo Ibys *Pharmacia Upjohn, Spain.*
Anise oil (p.1580·3); sodium bicarbonate (p.1186·2).
Aerophagia.

Carminativo Juventus *Juventus, Spain.*
Anise oil (p.1580·3); belladonna tincture (p.463·1); sodium bicarbonate (p.1186·2).
Aerophagia; meteorism; vomiting.

Carminativum Babynos
Byk, Aust.; Dentinox, Ger.
Fennel (p.1610·1); coriander (p.1599·2); chamomile (p.1593·2).
Gastrointestinal disorders.

Carminativum-Hetterich N *Galenika, Ger.*
Chamomile (p.1593·2); peppermint leaf (p.1243·2); caraway (p.1591·2); fennel (p.1610·1); dried bitter-orange peel (p.1644·2).
Gastrointestinal disorders.

Carminativum-Pascoe *Pascoe, Ger.*
Peppermint leaf (p.1243·2); chamomile (p.1593·2); caraway (p.1591·2).
Dyspepsia.

Carminetum *Galenika, Ger.*
Peppermint oil (p.1243·3).
Gastrointestinal disorders; muscle and nerve pain; respiratory-tract catarrh.

Carminex *Propan, S.Afr.*
Magnesium carbonate (p.1232·3); sodium bicarbonate (p.1186·2); sodium citrate (p.1186·2).
Constipation; hyperchlorhydria.

Carmint *Sofar, Ital.*
Peppermint oil (p.1243·3).
Gastrointestinal disorders.

Carmitol *Medinfar, Port.*
Urea (p.1127·3); panthenol (p.1602·3).
Dry skin; pruritus.

Carmol
Doak, Hong Kong; Doak, USA.
Urea (p.1127·3).
Dry skin; hyperkeratosis.

Carmol HC *Doak, USA.*
Hydrocortisone acetate (p.1073·3).
Corticosteroid.

Carmubris
Bristol-Myers Squibb, Aust.; Bristol-Myers Squibb, Ger.
Carmustine (p.516·1).
Malignant neoplasms.

Carnabol *Ache, Braz.*
Buclizine (p.411·1); caffeine (p.761·3); lysine; vitamin B substances (p.1350·1).
Reduced appetite; tonic.

Carnation
Note.This name is used for preparations of different composition.
Clintec, Canad.†
A range of preparations for enteral nutrition (p.1350·1).

Cuxson, Gerrard, Canad.; Cuxson, Gerrard, UK.
Salicylic acid (p.1122·3).
Calluses; corns; verrucas.

Carneferrol *INQ, Braz.*
Ferric ammonium citrate (p.1359·2); sodium methylarsinate (p.1666·1); tissue extracts.
Anaemias.

Carnicor *Max Farma, Ital.*
Levocarnitine (p.1356·1).
Carnitine deficiency; myocardial ischaemia.

Sigma-Tau, Spain.
Carnitine (p.1356·1).
Carnitine deficiency.

Carnigen
Hoechst Marion Roussel, Aust.; Hoechst Marion Roussel, Ger.
Oxilofrine hydrochloride (p.950·3).
Circulatory disorders; orthostatic hypotension.

Carnitene *Sigma-Tau, Ital.*
Levocarnitine (p.1356·1) or levocarnitine hydrochloride (p.1356·2).
Carnitine deficiency; myocardial ischaemia.

Carnitolo *Pharmacord, Ital.*
Carnitine hydrochloride (p.1356·2).
Carnitine deficiency.

Carnitop *Virginia, Ital.*
Carnitine (p.1356·1).
Carnitine deficiency.

Carnitor
Sigma-Tau, Canad.; Sigma-Tau, Hong Kong; Shire, UK; Sigma-Tau, USA.
Levocarnitine (p.1356·1).
Carnitine deficiency.

Carnivora VF *Carnivora, Ger.*
Dionaea muscipula.
Malignant neoplasms.

Carnizin *Bergamo, Braz.*
Buclizine (p.411·1); carnitine; lysine; vitamin B substances (p.1350·1).
Reduced appetite; tonic.

Carnotprim *Carnot, Mex.*
Metoclopramide hydrochloride (p.1235·2).
Nausea and vomiting.

Carnovis *Duncan, Ital.*
Carnitine (p.1356·1) or carnitine hydrochloride (p.1356·2).
Carnitine deficiency; myocardial ischaemia.

Carnum *FIRMA, Ital.*
Carnitine (p.1356·1).
Carnitine deficiency.

Carobel
Baxter, Austral.†; Cow & Gate, Irl.; Cow & Gate, UK.
Ceratonia (p.1500·3).
Feed thickener to control vomiting.

Carofril *Arlex, Mex.*
Paracetamol (p.71·2).
Fever; pain.

Carogil *Novartis Nutrition, Fr.*
Carrots, rice, dextrin-maltose, and electrolytes (p.1185·2).
Diarrhoea.

Caroid
Note.This name is used for preparations of different composition.
Mentholatum, Canad.†
Cascara (p.1216·1); phenolphthalein (p.1244·1); ox bile (p.1585·1).

Lepori, Port.
Capsicum (p.1591·1); cascara (p.1216·1); phenolphthalein (p.1244·1); papain (p.1647·3); bile salts (p.1585·1).

Carominthe *Lehning, Fr.*
Homoeopathic preparation.

Carotaben
Merck, Aust.; Hermal, Ger.; Boots Healthcare, Neth.; Boots Healthcare, Switz.
Betacarotene (p.1355·1).
Erythropoietic protoporphyria; photodermatoses; skin pigmentation disorders.

Carotin *Twardy, Ger.*
Betacarotene (p.1355·1); biotin (p.1355·3); calcium pantothenate (p.1374·1).
Sunburn.

Carovit *Biochimici, Ital.†*
Betacarotene with vitamin E (p.1350·1).
Nutritional supplement.

Carovit Forte *Biochimici, Ital.*
Betacarotene with vitamins E and C (p.1350·1).
Nutritional supplement.

Carovit Melanin *Biochimici, Ital.*
Amino-acid preparation with vitamins and minerals (p.1350·1).
Nutritional supplement.

Carpantin *Sanofi Synthelabo, Ital.*
Pantethine (p.952·1); carnitine chloride (p.1356·2); cyproheptadine hydrochloride (p.414·2).
Tonic.

Carpaz *Rolab, S.Afr.*
Carbamazepine (p.342·2).
Epilepsy; trigeminal neuralgia.

Carpilo *Chauvin, Fr.*
Pilocarpine nitrate (p.1422·3); carteolol hydrochloride (p.855·1).
Glaucoma; ocular hypertension.

Carpin *Novag, Mex.*
Carbamazepine (p.342·2).
Epilepsy.

Carpine *Atlantic, Thai.*
Carbamazepine (p.342·2).
Bipolar disorder; epilepsy; trigeminal neuralgia.

Carreldon *Bama, Thai.*
Diltiazem hydrochloride (p.874·3).
Angina pectoris; hypertension.

Carrier *Chiesi, Ital.*
Carnitine (p.1356·1).
Carnitine deficiency.

Carsuquin *Degorts, Mex.*
Diiodohydroxyquinoline (p.590·2).
Amoebiasis; trichomoniasis.

Carteol
Asta Medica, Belg.; Chauvin, Fr.; SIFI, Ital.
Carteolol hydrochloride (p.855·1).
Ocular hypertension; open-angle glaucoma.

Carteopil *Asta Medica, Belg.*
Pilocarpine hydrochloride (p.1422·3); carteolol hydrochloride (p.855·1).
Glaucoma; ocular hypertension.

Carter Petites Pilules *Carter-Wallace, Switz.†*
Aloin (p.1210·2); phenolphthalein (p.1244·1); liquorice (p.1231·2).
Constipation.

Carters
Note.This name is used for preparations of different composition.
Therabel, Belg.†
Aloes (p.1210·1); podophyllum resin (p.1121·1).
Constipation.

Carter-Wallace, UK†
Aloin (p.1210·2); phenolphthalein (p.1244·1).
Constipation.

Carters Little Pills *Carter Horner, Canad.*
Bisacodyl (p.1212·2).
Formerly contained aloin and phenolphthalein.
Constipation.

Carthamex *Rolmex, Canad.*
Vitamin B₆ (p.1387·1) in safflower oil.

Cartia
Note.This name is used for preparations of different composition.
SmithKline Beecham, Austral.; SmithKline Beecham, Hong Kong; SmithKline Beecham, Israel; SmithKline Beecham, NZ; Lusofarmaco, Port.
Aspirin (p.14·2).
Thrombosis prophylaxis.

Andrx, USA.
Diltiazem hydrochloride (p.874·3).
Angina pectoris; hypertension.

Cartidont *Molteni, Ital.*
Articaine hydrochloride (p.1306·1).
Adrenaline [epinephrine] acid tartrate (p.829·2) is included in this preparation as a vasoconstrictor to diminish absorption and localise the effect of the local anaesthetic.
Local anaesthesia.

Cartilag *Eagle, Austral.*
Cartilage (bovine).
Dietary supplement.

Cartivix *Jaba, Port.*
Diacerein (p.28·3).
Osteoarthritis.

Cartrax *Pfizer, Braz.*
Tioconazole (p.395·1); tinidazole (p.603·3).
Vulvovaginal infections.

Cartrol *Abbott, USA.*
Carteolol hydrochloride (p.855·1).
Hypertension.

Carudol
Note.This name is used for preparations of different composition.
Boehringer Ingelheim, Fr.†
Phenylbutazone piperazine (p.78·3).
Formerly contained phenylbutazone piperazine, methyl nicotinate, and piperazine hydrate.
Tendinitis.

Fher, Spain†
Phenylbutazone piperazine (p.78·3).
Gout; musculoskeletal and joint disorders.

Wild, Switz.†
Phenylbutazone piperazine (p.78·3); piperazine hydrate (p.106·1).
Musculoskeletal, joint, and peri-articular pain; soft-tissue disorders.

Carvasin *Wyeth Lederle, Ital.; Wyeth, NZ.*
Isosorbide dinitrate (p.915·2).
Angina pectoris; heart failure.

Carvicum *Duopharm, Ger.*
Taraxacum (p.1669·1).
Appetite loss; biliary disorders; digestive disorders; diuretic.

Carvipress *Gentili, Ital.*
Carvedilol (p.855·2).
Angina pectoris; hypertension.

Carvis *Volchem, Ital.†*
Carnitine (p.1356·1).
Tonic.

Carvit *AGIPS, Ital.*
Carnitine (p.1356·1).
Carnitine deficiency; myocardial ischaemia.

Carvomin *Wernigerode, Ger.*
Angelica (p.1580·2); cnicus benedictus (p.1597·2); peppermint leaf (p.1243·2).
Gastrointestinal disorders.

Carvomin Magentropfen mit Pomeranze
Madaus, Ger.
Bitter-orange peel (p.1644·2).
Dyspepsia.

Carylderm
Seton, Irl.; SSL, UK.
Carbaryl (p.1429·2).

Carylderm Liquid was formerly known as Derbac-C in the *UK*.
Pediculosis.

Caryolysine *Genopharm, Fr.*
Mustine [chlormethine] hydrochloride (p.561·1).
Lymphomas; mycosis fungoides; psoriasis.

Carzem *Rottapharm, Ital.*
Diltiazem hydrochloride (p.874·3).
Hypertension; ischaemic heart disease.

Carzepine *Condrugs, Thai.*
Carbamazepine (p.342·2).
Alcohol withdrawal syndrome; diabetic neuropathy; epilepsy; trigeminal neuralgia.

Carzilasa *Manuell, Mex.*
Cocarboxylase (p.1385·2).
Tonic.

Carzodelan *Gaschler, Ger.*
Pancreatin (p.1646·1).
Inflammatory disorders.

Casacol *Helsinn Birex, Irl.*
Methoxyphenamine hydrochloride (p.1094·3); guaifenesin (p.1092·2); sodium citrate (p.1186·2).
Coughs.

Casalm
Pharmacia Upjohn, Aust.; Pharmacia Upjohn, Ger.
Salcatonin (p.749·3).
Hypercalcaemia and osteolysis in malignancy; osteoporosis; Paget's disease of bone; pancreatic transplantation; reflex sympathetic dystrophy.

Casbol *Fournier SA, Spain.*
Paroxetine hydrochloride (p.302·3).
Anxiety disorders; depression; obsessive-compulsive disorder.

Cascade *Lane, UK.*
Bearberry (p.1583·3); clivers (p.1596·3); lappa root (p.1627·1).
Water retention.

Cascalax *Will-Pharma, Belg.*
Casanthranol (p.1216·1).
Constipation.

Cascapride *Merck, Ger.*
Bromopride (p.1215·1).
Gastrointestinal motility disorders; nausea; vomiting.

Cascara-Salax
Ferring, Aust.; Ferring, Ger.†; Ferring, Switz.†.
Powder for oral solution, dried magnesium sulfate (p.1191·3); tablets, cascara (p.1216·1).
Bowel evacuation.

Casec
Mead Johnson, Austral.; Mead Johnson, Israel; Mead Johnson Nutritionals, USA.
Calcium caseinate.
Protein supplement.

Casfen *Sanitas, Port.*
Infant suppositories: Aspirin (p.14·2); paracetamol (p.71·2); codeine phosphate (p.25·2).
Tablets; adult suppositories: Aspirin (p.14·2); paracetamol (p.71·2); codeine phosphate (p.25·2); caffeine (p.761·3).
Fever; pain.

Casilan *Glaxo Wellcome, Mex.*
Protein supplement (p.1350·1).

Casodex
Zeneca, Aust.; Zeneca, Belg.; AstraZeneca, Canad.; AstraZeneca, Denm.; AstraZeneca, Fin.; AstraZeneca, Fr.; Zeneca, Ger.; Zeneca, Hong Kong; Zeneca, Irl.; Zeneca, Israel; Zeneca, Ital.; Zeneca, Mex.; Zeneca, Neth.; AstraZeneca, Norw.; Zeneca, Port.; Zeneca, S.Afr.; AstraZeneca, Singapore; Zeneca, Spain; Zeneca, Swed.; Zeneca, Switz.; AstraZeneca, Thai.; AstraZeneca, UK; Zeneca, USA.
Bicalutamide (p.511·2).
Prostatic cancer.

Caspiselenio *Kin, Spain.*
Selenium sulfide (p.1123·1).
Skin disorders.

Cassadan *Dresden, Ger.; Temmler, Ger.*
Alprazolam (p.654·2).
Anxiety.

Castaderm *Lannett, USA.*
Resorcinol (p.1122·2); boric acid (p.1586·1); phenol (p.1152·3).
Fungal skin infections.

Castanha de India Composta *Infabra, Braz.*
Aesculus (p.1574·1); rutoside (p.1611·2); vitamin C (p.1389·3).
Venous insufficiency.

Castel *Syosset, USA.*
Resorcinol (p.1122·2).
Fungal skin infections.

Castellani mit Miconazol *Hollborn, Ger.*
Miconazole (p.391·1).
Fungal and bacterial skin infections.

Castilium *Hoeport, Port.*
Clobazam (p.668·1).
Anxiety.

Castindia *IMO, Ital.*
Aesculus (p.1574·1); silybum marianum (p.1021·3); hamamelis (p.1618·3).
Peripheral vascular disorders.

Castoria *Mentholatum, Canad.†*
Sennoside A and B (p.1248·3).

Castufemin N *Ardeypharm, Ger.*
Agnus castus (p.1574·2).
Mastalgia; menstrual disorders.

The symbol † denotes a preparation no longer actively marketed

Catabex
Note. This name is used for preparations of different composition.
Darci, Belg.
Dropropizine (p.1089·3).
Coughs.

Darcy, Fr.†.
Dropropizine (p.1089·3); guaifenesin (p.1092·2).
Coughs.

Catabex Expectorans Darci, Belg.
Dropropizine (p.1089·3); guaifenesin (p.1092·2).
Coughs.

Catabina Tecnifar, Port.
Dropropizine (p.1089·3).
Coughs.

Catabina Expectorante Tecnifar, Port.
Dropropizine (p.1089·3); guaifenesin (p.1092·2).
Coughs.

Cataclot Ono, Jpn†.
Ozagrel sodium (p.1645·3).
Cerebrovascular disorders.

Catacol Alcon, Fr.
Disodium inosinate phosphate.
Lens opacities.

Alcon, Switz.†.
Disodium inosinate (p.1604·3).
Eye disorders.

Cataflam
Novartis, Belg.; Novartis, Braz.; Novartis, Hong Kong; Novartis, Irl.;
Novartis, Israel; Ciba, Ital.†; Novartis, Mex.; Novartis, Neth.; No-
vartis, Norw.; Novartis, NZ; Bykomed, Port.; Novartis, S.Afr.; No-
vartis, Singapore; Novartis, Thai.; Novartis, USA.
Diclofenac (p.30·2), diclofenac diethylamine (p.30·2),
diclofenac potassium (p.30·2), diclofenac resinate
(p.31·3), or diclofenac sodium (p.30·3).
Fever; gout; inflammation; musculoskeletal, joint, and
peri-articular disorders; pain.

Catalgine Lipha Sante, Fr.
Sodium aspirin (p.16·3).
Fever; musculoskeletal and joint disorders; myocar-
dial infarction; pain.

Catalgix Rhone-Poulenc Rorer, Belg.†.
Aspirin (p.14·2).
Fever; migraine; rheumatic disorders.

Catalgix C Rhone-Poulenc Rorer, Belg.†.
Aspirin (p.14·2); ascorbic acid (p.1389·3).
Fever; migraine; rheumatic disorders.

Catalin
Takeda, Hong Kong; Takeda, Singapore; Takeda, Thai.
Pirenoxine (p.1652·2) or pirenoxine sodium
(p.1652·2).
Cataract.

Catalip Fournier, Port.
Fenofibrate (p.889·1).
Hyperlipidaemias.

Catamin Riedel-Zabinka, Braz.
Sulfur (p.1123·3); zinc oxide (p.1128·2).
Acne.

Catanac Pharmasant, Thai.
Diclofenac potassium (p.30·2).
Inflammation; pain.

Catanidin Boehringer Ingelheim, Aust.†.
Clonidine hydrochloride (p.860·1) or clonidine tosilate
(p.861·1).
Hypertension.

Catapres
Boehringer Ingelheim, Austral.; Boehringer Ingelheim, Canad.; Boe-
hringer Ingelheim, Hong Kong; Boehringer Ingelheim, Irl.; Boehringer
Ingelheim, NZ; Boehringer Ingelheim, S.Afr.; Boehringer Ingelheim,
Thai.; Boehringer Ingelheim, UK; Boehringer Ingelheim, USA.
Clonidine (p.861·1) or clonidine hydrochloride
(p.860·1).
Hypertension; menopausal flushing; migraine and vas-
cular headache.

Catapresan
Boehringer Ingelheim, Aust.; Boehringer Ingelheim, Denm.; Boehringer Ingelheim, Fin.; Boehringer Ingelheim, Ger.; Boehringer Ingelheim,
Ital.; Boehringer Ingelheim, Mex.; Boehringer Ingelheim, Neth.; Boe-
hringer Ingelheim, Norw.; Boehringer Ingelheim, Port.; Boehringer In-
gelheim, Spain; Boehringer Ingelheim, Swed.; Boehringer Ingelheim,
Switz.
Clonidine (p.861·1) or clonidine hydrochloride
(p.860·1).
Hypertension; menopausal disorders; migraine; opioid withdrawal.

Catapressan
Boehringer Ingelheim, Belg.; Boehringer Ingelheim, Fr.
Clonidine hydrochloride (p.860·1).
Hypertension.

Cataren INQ, Braz.
Diclofenac potassium (p.30·2).
Gout; inflammation; musculoskeletal, joint, and peri-
articular disorders; pain.

Cataridol Ciba Vision, Fr.
Calcium chloride (p.1188·1); magnesium chloride
(p.1190·3); sodium chloride (p.1196·1).
Formerly contained sodium iodide and calcium chlo-
ride.
Lens opacities.

Catarrh Larkhall Laboratories, UK.
Achillea (p.1572·2); vervain (p.1679·3); horehound
(p.1094·2); salvia (p.1660·3).

Catarrh Cream Weleda, UK.
Esculoside (p.1574·1); berberis fruit; prunus spinosa
fruit; bryonia alba; camphor (p.1589·3); echinacea
purp. (p.1606·2); mercurius sulph.; eucalyptus oil

(p.1609·2); peppermint oil (p.1243·3); thyme oil
(p.1672·3).
Nasal congestion.

Catarrh Mixture Potter's, UK.
Boneset (p.1586·1); blue flag (p.1624·2); lapp root
(p.1627·1); hyssop.
Catarrh.

Catarrh Pastilles
Note. This name is used for preparations of different composition.
Healthcrafts, UK.
Squill vinegar (p.1100·3); menthol (p.1632·3); pumilio
pine oil (p.1656·3); eucalyptus oil (p.1609·2).
Cough and cold symptoms.

Unichem, UK.
Menthol (p.1632·3); siberian fir oil; oleum pini sylves-
tris; creosote (p.1087·3).
Catarrh; coughs.

Catarrh Tablets Healthcrafts, UK.
Horehound (p.1094·2); squill (p.1100·3).
Catarrh; coughs.

Catarrh-eeze Peter Black, UK.
Marrubium (p.1094·2); achillea (p.1572·2); elecam-
pane (p.1089·3).
Catarrh.

Catarrh-Ex Thompson, UK.
Phenylephrine hydrochloride (p.1097·1); paracetamol
(p.71·2); caffeine (p.761·3).
Formerly contained pseudoephedrine hydrochloride
and paracetamol.
Cold symptoms.

Catarstat
Chauvin, Fr.; Chauvin Novopharma, Switz.
Pyridoxine hydrochloride (p.1386·3); amino acids.
Cataracts.

CAT-Barium (E-Z-CAT) Bracco, Switz.
Barium sulfate (p.1032·1).
Contrast medium for gastrointestinal radiography.

Catemine Tyson, USA†.
Tyrosine (p.1381·3); pyridoxal phosphate (p.1387·1).

Caterol Pharmasant, Thai.
Procaterol hydrochloride (p.770·1).
Obstructive airways disease.

Catex Cantabria, Spain.
Ciprofloxacin hydrochloride (p.182·3).
Bacterial infections.

Cathejell
Montavit, Aust.; Pfleger, Ger.; Montavit, Israel.
Diphenhydramine hydrochloride (p.416·1); chlorhexi-
dine hydrochloride (p.1138·2).
Cystoscopy; endoscopy; lubrication for catheter inser-
tion.

Cathejell with Lidocaine
Montavit, Thai.; Mediplus, UK.
Chlorhexidine hydrochloride (p.1138·2); lignocaine
[lidocaine] hydrochloride (p.1313·2).
Catheter insertion; instrument insertion.

Cathejell mit Lidocain Montavit, Aust.
Chlorhexidine hydrochloride (p.1138·2); lignocaine
[lidocaine] hydrochloride (p.1313·2).
Catheterisation; instrument insertion.

Cathejell S Pfleger, Ger.
Chlorhexidine hydrochloride (p.1138·2).
Catheterisation.

Cathejell-N Geistlich, Switz.†.
Chlorhexidine hydrochloride (p.1138·2); lignocaine
[lidocaine] hydrochloride (p.1313·2).
Catheterisation.

Catheter Preparation Pharmacia Upjohn, Austral.
Chlorhexidine gluconate (p.1138·2).
Skin disinfection before bladder catheterisation.

Catonet Nettopharm, Denm.
Captopril (p.853·3).
Heart failure; hypertension.

Catonin Magis, Ital.
Salcatonin (p.749·3).
Hypercalcaemia; osteoporosis; Paget's disease of
bone; reflex sympathetic dystrophy.

Catoprol Medley, Braz.
Captopril (p.853·3).
Heart failure; hypertension.

Catorid Boehringer Ingelheim, Belg.
Prolintane hydrochloride (p.1514·2).
Narcoleptic syndrome.

Catovit
Boehringer Ingelheim, Austral.†; Boehringer Ingelheim, S.Afr.†.
Prolintane hydrochloride (p.1514·2); multivitamins
(p.1350·1).
Tonic.

Catovit N Boehringer Ingelheim, S.Afr.
Prolintane hydrochloride (p.1514·2).
Tonic.

Catrix Donell DerMedex, USA.
Emollient and moisturiser.

Catrix Correction Donell DerMedex, USA.
SPF 15: Octinoxate (p.1517·3); methyl anthranilate;
oxybenzone (p.1518·1); titanium dioxide (p.1126·1).
Sunscreen.

Catrix Lip Donell DerMedex, USA.
SPF 15: Octinoxate (p.1517·3); oxybenzone
(p.1518·1).
Sunscreen.

Catuaba Cazi, Braz.
Erythroxylon catuaba; guarana (p.1681·1); liriosma
ovata; ginger (p.1227·2); bitter orange (p.1644·2).
Tonic.

Catuama Catarinense, Braz.
Erythroxylon catuaba; guarana (p.1681·1); liriosma
ovata; ginger (p.1227·2).

Caulophyllum Complex Dolisos, Canad.
Homoeopathic preparation.

Causat Sanofi Winthrop, Aust.†.
Procaine hydrochloride (p.1319·1); atropine sulfate
(p.461·1).
Migraine; neuralgia; neuritis.

Causat B12 N Sanofi Synthelabo, Ger.
Procaine hydrochloride (p.1319·1); atropine sulfate
(p.461·1); hydroxocobalamin hydrochloride
(p.1388·3).
Arthrosis; migraine; neuralgia; neuritis.

Causat N Sanofi Synthelabo, Ger.
Procaine hydrochloride (p.1319·1); atropine sulfate
(p.461·1).
Migraine; neuralgia; neuritis; postherpetic neuralgia;
trigeminal neuralgia.

Caustinerf forte Septodont, Switz.
Lignocaine [lidocaine] (p.1313·2); phenol (p.1152·3);
paraformaldehyde (p.1152·2).
Dental pain.

Cauterex com Gentamicina Ache, Braz.
Fibrinolysin (human) (p.890·1); dornase alfa
(p.1089·1); thiomersal (p.1158·2); gentamicin
(p.212·1).
Wounds.

Cauteridol Ederka, Mex.
Ranitidine (p.1246·3).

Cavedess Astra, Swed.†.
Deglycyrrhizinised liquorice (p.1231·2); bismuth subnitrate (p.1213·2); colloidal aluminium hydroxide
(p.1210·3); sodium bicarbonate (p.1186·2); magnesium subcarbonate (p.1232·3); fennel (p.1610·1).
Peptic ulcer.

Caved-S
Note. This name is used for preparations of different composition.
Byk, Aust.†.
Deglycyrrhizinised liquorice (p.1231·2); magnesium
carbonate (p.1232·3); aluminium hydroxide
(p.1210·3); sodium bicarbonate (p.1186·2); fennel
(p.1610·1).
Hyperacidity; peptic ulcer.

Byk, Neth.†; Pharmacia Upjohn, UK†.
Deglycyrrhizinised liquorice (p.1231·2); aluminium
hydroxide (p.1210·3); magnesium carbonate
(p.1232·3); sodium bicarbonate (p.1186·2); bismuth
subnitrate (p.1213·2).
Gastritis; gastrointestinal hyperacidity; peptic ulcer.

Casen Fleet, Spain†.
Deglycyrrhizinised liquorice (p.1231·2); colloidal aluminium hydroxide (p.1210·3); magnesium carbonate
(p.1232·3); sodium bicarbonate (p.1186·2); calamus
(p.1588·1); frangula bark (p.1227·1).
Gastrointestinal hyperacidity.

Pharmakon, Switz.†.
Deglycyrrhizinised liquorice (p.1231·2); dried aluminium hydroxide gel (p.1210·3); magnesium carbonate
(p.1232·3); sodium bicarbonate (p.1186·2); frangula
(p.1227·1); calamus (p.1588·1); fennel (p.1610·1).
Gastrointestinal disorders.

Caveril Remedica, Thai.
Verapamil hydrochloride (p.989·1).
Angina pectoris; arrhythmias; hypertension.

Caverject
Pharmacia Upjohn, Aust.; Pharmacia Upjohn, Austral.; Pharmacia
Upjohn, Belg.; Pharmacia Upjohn, Canad.; Pharmacia Upjohn,
Denm.; Pharmacia Upjohn, Fin.; Pharmacia Upjohn, Fr.; Pharmacia
Upjohn, Ger.; Pharmacia Upjohn, Hong Kong; Pharmacia Upjohn, Irl.;
Pharmacia Upjohn, Israel; Pharmacia Upjohn, Ital.; Pharmacia Up-
john, Mex.; Pharmacia Upjohn, Neth.; Pharmacia Upjohn, Norw.;
Pharmacia Upjohn, NZ; Pharmacia Upjohn, Port.; Pharmacia Upjohn,
S.Afr.; Pharmacia Upjohn, Singapore; Pharmacia Upjohn, Spain; Phar-
macia Upjohn, Swed.; Pharmacia Upjohn, Switz.; Pharmacia Upjohn,
Thai.; Pharmacia, UK; Pharmacia Upjohn, USA.
Alprostadil (p.1439·3) or alprostadil alfadex
(p.1440·1).
Erectile dysfunction.

Caviamina De Mayo, Braz.
Vitamin B substances; vitamin C; fructose (p.1350·1).

CaviD Nycomed, Denm.
Calcium carbonate (p.1215·1); colecalciferol
(p.1391·1).
Calcium and vitamin D deficiency.

Cavilon 3M, UK.
A barrier film.

Cavinton
Thieman, Ger.; Armstrong, Mex.; Biosaude, Port.; Gedeon Richter,
Singapore; Gedeon Richter, Thai.
Vinpocetine (p.1680·1).
Cerebrovascular disorders; vascular eye disoders.

Cavodine Biolab, Thai.
Povidone-iodine (p.1155·1).
Skin, burn, and wound disinfection.

Cavumox Siam Bheasach, Thai.
Amoxicillin trihydrate (p.149·2); potassium clavu-
lanate (p.187·2).
Bacterial infections.

Caye Balsam Medopharm, Ger.
Glycol salicylate (p.42·2); sodium salamidacetate
(p.81·3); benzyl nicotinate (p.20·2); capsicum
(p.1591·1); coumarin (p.1599·3).
Musculoskeletal, joint, and soft-tissue disorders.

Caziderm Cazi, Braz.
Nitrofurazone (p.231·3).
Burns; skin infections.

Cazigeran Cazi, Braz.
Vitamin B substances with magnesium and potassium
(p.1350·1).

Cazole
Malpharm, Hong Kong; Malaysia Chemist, Singapore.
Carbimazole (p.1521·1).
Hyperthyroidism.

C-1000-C Novartis, Mex.
Ascorbic acid (p.1389·3); calcium lactate gluconate
(p.1188·3).
Calcium and vitamin C supplement.

C-Calcium Streuli, Switz.
Calcium gluconate (p.1188·2); ascorbic acid
(p.1389·3); calcium saccharate (p.1589·1).
Vitamin C and calcium deficiency.

CC-Nefro Medice, Ger.
Calcium carbonate (p.1215·1).
Hyperphosphataemia.

CCNU Medac, UK.
Lomustine (p.550·2).
Malignant neoplasms.

C-Destrosio Amsa, Ital.
Ascorbic acid (p.1389·3); glucose (p.1364·2).
Vitamin C deficiency.

C-Dose Medgenix, Belg.
Ascorbic acid (p.1389·3).
Scurvy; vitamin C deficiency.

CDT
CSL, Austral.; CSL, NZ.
An adsorbed diphtheria and tetanus vaccine (p.1537·1).
Active immunisation of infants and young children.

Ceanel
Quinoderm, Irl.; Hoechst Marion Roussel, S.Afr.†; Adams, UK.
Cetrimide (p.1137·1); undecenoic acid (p.395·3);
phenethyl alcohol (p.1152·2).
Dandruff; psoriasis; seborrhoeic dermatitis.

CEA-Scan
Byk Gulden, Ital.; Mallinckrodt, Spain; Immunomedics, UK; Immuno-
medics, USA.
Technetium-99m arcitumomab (p.1451·1).
Detection of colorectal cancer.

Cebedex Chauvin, Fr.
Dexamethasone sodium phosphate (p.1067·1).
Eye disorders.

Cebedexacol Chauvin, Fr.
Chloramphenicol (p.179·1); dexamethasone sodium
phosphate (p.1067·1).
Eye infections.

Cebemyxine Chauvin, Fr.
Neomycin sulfate (p.228·1); polymyxin B sulfate
(p.238·1).
The eye ointment formerly contained neomycin sul-
fate, polymyxin B sulfate, and bacitracin zinc.
Eye infections.

Cebenicol Chauvin, Fr.
Chloramphenicol (p.179·1).
Eye infections.

Cebera Irex, Fr.
Alibendol (p.1575·2).
Dyspepsia.

Cebesine Chauvin, Fr.
Oxybuprocaine hydrochloride (p.1318·1).
Local anaesthesia.

Cebid Hauck, USA†.
Ascorbic acid (p.1389·3).
Scurvy; vitamin C deficiency.

Cebiolon Merck, Port.
Ascorbic acid (p.1389·3).
Vitamin C supplement.

Cebion
Merck, Aust.; Merck, Braz.; Merck, Ger.; Bracco, Ital.; Merck, Port.;
Merck, Spain.
Ascorbic acid (p.1389·3).
Vitamin C deficiency.

Cebion Calcio Merck, Braz.
Ascorbic acid (p.1389·3); calcium hypophosphite.
Calcium and vitamin C supplement.

Cebion Erkaltungs Merck, Ger.
Aspirin (p.14·2); ascorbic acid (p.1389·3).
Cold symptoms; fever; pain.

Cebion Glicose Merck, Braz.
Ascorbic acid (p.1389·3); glucose (p.1364·1).
Glucose and vitamin C supplement.

Cebion Multi Merck, Port.
Multivitamin and mineral preparation (p.1350·1).

Cebion N Merck, Ger.
Sodium ascorbate (p.1390·1).
Methaemoglobinaemia; vitamin C deficiency.

Cebion Plus Calcio Merck, Port.
Ascorbic acid (p.1389·3); calcium carbonate
(p.1215·1).
Nutritional supplement.

Cebion Plus Magnesio Merck, Port.
Ascorbic acid (p.1389·3); magnesium carbonate
(p.1232·3).
Nutritional supplement.

Cebion Plus Minerals Merck, Port.
Ascorbic acid and minerals (p.1350·1).
Nutritional supplement.

Cebion-Calcium N Merck, S.Afr.
Calcium carbonate (p.1215·1); ascorbic acid
(p.1389·3).
Calcium and vitamin C supplement.

Cebiopirina *Bracco, Ital.†*.
Ascorbic acid (p.1389·3); aspirin (p.14·2).
Cold symptoms; pain.

Cebran *Garant, Ital.*
Nicergoline (p.1640·2).
Cerebral and peripheral vascular disorders.

Cebrotex *Janssen-Cilag, Port.*
Glutamine.

Cebroton *Tubilux, Ital.*
Citicoline sodium (p.1596·1).
Cerebrovascular disorders; mental function impairment; parkinsonism.

Cebrotonin *Ritter, Singapore.*
Piracetam (p.1652·1).
Mental function impairment in the elderly.

Cebutid *Murat, Fr.*
Flurbiprofen (p.41·2).
Inflammation; musculoskeletal and joint disorders; pain.

Cec
Hexal, Aust.; Hexal, Ger.; Hexal, S.Afr.
Cefaclor (p.161·1).
Bacterial infections.

Cecap *Atlantic, Hong Kong.*
Vitamin C (p.1389·3).
Tonic; vitamin C deficiency.

Cecenu
Rhone-Poulenc Rorer, Belg.†; Medac, Ger.
Lomustine (p.550·2).
Malignant neoplasms.

Ceclor
Lilly, Aust.; Lilly, Austral.; Lilly, Belg.; Lilly, Braz.; Lilly, Canad.; Lilly, Hong Kong; Lilly, Israel; Lilly, Mex.; Lilly, Neth.; Lilly, NZ; Lilly, Port.; Aspen, S.Afr.; Lilly, Spain; Lilly, Switz.; Dura, USA; Lilly, USA.
Cefaclor (p.161·1).
Bacterial infections.

Ceclorbeta *Betapharm, Ger.*
Cefaclor (p.161·1).
Bacterial infections.

Cecon
Abbott, Austral.†; Abbott, Ital.; Abbott, USA.
Ascorbic acid (p.1389·3).
Scurvy; vitamin C deficiency.

Abbott, Ital.
Tablets: Sodium ascorbate (p.1390·1); ascorbic acid (p.1389·3).
Vitamin C deficiency.

Cecrisina *Janssen-Cilag, Port.*
Ascorbic acid (p.1389·3).
Vitamin C supplement.

Cedanon *Sanabo, Aust.†*
Propyphenazone (p.80·2); dihydroergotamine mesilate (p.450·3); caffeine (p.761·3).
Migraine and related vascular headache.

Cedax
Schering-Plough, Fin.; Schering-Plough, Hong Kong; Schering-Plough, Irl.; Schering-Plough, Israel; Schering-Plough, Ital.; Schering-Plough, Mex.; Schering-Plough, Neth.; Schering-Plough, S.Afr.; Schering-Plough, Singapore; Schering-Plough, Spain; Schering-Plough, Swed.; Essex, Switz.; Schering-Plough, Thai.; Schering-Plough, UK†; Schering, USA.
Ceftibuten (p.176·1).
Bacterial infections.

Cedelate *Nakorn, Thai.*
Flunarizine (p.418·2).
Migraine; vestibular disorders.

Cedilanid *Novartis, Aust.*
Injection: Deslanoside (p.867·3).
Tablets: Lanatoside C (p.919·2).
Arrhythmias; heart failure.

Cedilanide
Novartis, Braz.; Novartis, Fr.†.
Deslanoside (p.867·3).
Heart failure; supraventricular arrhythmias.

Cedine *Rowex, Irl.*
Cimetidine (p.1216·3).
Gastric hyperacidity; peptic ulcer; Zollinger-Ellison syndrome.

Cedium *Qualiphar, Belg.*
Benzalkonium chloride (p.1133·2).
Disinfection of the skin, wounds, and hands.

Cedixen *Hoechst Marion Roussel, Aust.*
Cefpirome sulfate (p.172·2).
Bacterial infections.

Cedocard
Byk, Aust.; Byk, Belg.; Paladin, Canad.; Pharmacia Upjohn, Irl.; Byk, Neth.; Pharmacia, Ital.; Pharmacia, UK.
Isosorbide dinitrate (p.915·2).
Angina pectoris; heart failure; myocardial infarction; pulmonary hypertension.

Cedol *Eurofarmaco, Ital.*
Cefamandole nafate (p.163·3).
Bacterial infections.

Cedozelim Complexo *Novaquimica, Braz.*
Vitamin B substances; fructose; vitamin C (p.1350·1).

Cedril *MC, Ital.†.*
Benzalkonium chloride (p.1133·2); benzethonium chloride (p.1134·2); didecyldimethylammonium chloride (p.1143·2).
Disinfection of ulcers, burns, and wounds.

Cedril Strumenti *MC, Ital.†.*
Benzalkonium chloride (p.1133·2); benzethonium chloride (p.1134·2); didecyldimethylammonium chloride (p.1143·2); alcohol (p.1130·3).
Instrument disinfection.

Cedrin *Schering-Plough, Braz.*
Pseudoephedrine sulfate (p.1099·3); azatadine maleate (p.409·2).
Nasal congestion.

Cedrol *Astra, Spain.*
Zolpidem tartrate (p.712·2).
Insomnia.

Cedrox *Hexal, Ger.*
Cefadroxil (p.161·2).
Bacterial infections.

Cedur
Roche, Belg.; Asta Medica, Braz.; Roche, Ger.; Roche, Switz.
Bezafibrate (p.849·1).
Hyperlipidaemias.

CeeNU
Bristol-Myers Squibb, Austral.; Bristol, Canad.; Bristol-Myers Squibb, Hong Kong; Bristol-Myers Squibb, Israel; Bristol-Myers Squibb, Mex.; Bristol-Myers Squibb, NZ; Bristol-Myers Squibb, S.Afr.†; Bristol-Myers Squibb, Singapore; Bristol-Myers Squibb, Thai.; Bristol-Myers Squibb Oncology, USA.
Lomustine (p.550·2).
Brain tumours; Hodgkin's disease.

Ceezinc *Lifeplan, UK.*
Zinc (p.1398·1); vitamin C (p.1389·3).
Tonic.

CEF-3 *Siam Bheasach, Thai.*
Ceftriaxone sodium (p.177·1).
Bacterial infections.

CEF-4 *Siam Bheasach, Thai.*
Ceftazidime (p.174·3).
Bacterial infections.

Cefa Resan *Alacan, Spain.*
Cefazolin sodium (p.164·3).
Lignocaine [lidocaine] (p.1313·2) is included in this preparation to alleviate the pain of injection.
Bacterial infections.

Cefabene *Cefak, Ger.*
Stipites dulcamarae (p.1606·2).
Eczema.

Cefabiozim *IPA, Ital.*
Cefazolin sodium (p.164·3).
Lignocaine [lidocaine] (p.1313·2) is included in this preparation to alleviate the pain of injection.
Bacterial infections.

Cefabol
Note.This name is used for preparations of different composition.
Cefak, Ger.
Boldo (p.1585·3).
Dyspepsia; gastrointestinal spasm.

Robert, Spain.
Sodium cytidine monophosphate; gamma-aminobutyric acid (p.1613·1); aminohydroxybutyric acid (p.342·2); magnesium glutamate hydrobromide (p.1631·1); trisodium uridine triphosphate; pyridoxine hydrochloride (p.1386·3).
Mental function disorders; tonic.

Cefabronchin *Cefak, Ger.*
Thyme (p.1672·2); Iceland moss; saponaria; pimpinella; eucalyptus (p.1609·2); fennel (p.1610·1); star anise.
Respiratory-tract inflammation.

Cefacene *Centrum, Spain.*
Cefazolin sodium (p.164·3).
Lignocaine [lidocaine] (p.1313·2) is included in this preparation to alleviate the pain of injection.
Bacterial infections.

Cefacet *Norgine, Fr.*
Cefalexin (p.161·3).
Bacterial infections.

Cefachol *Cefak, Ger.*
Greater celandine (p.1618·1); taraxacum (p.1669·1); silybum marianum (p.1021·3).
Biliary disorders; liver disorders.

Cefacidal
Bristol-Myers Squibb, Belg.; Bristol-Myers Squibb, Fr.; Bristol-Myers Squibb, Mex.; Bristol-Myers Squibb, Neth.; Bristol-Myers Squibb, S.Afr.; Bristol-Myers Squibb, Thai.
Cefazolin sodium (p.164·3).
Lignocaine [lidocaine] (p.1313·2) is included in the intramuscular injection to alleviate the pain of injection.
Bacterial infections.

Cefacile *Bristol-Myers Squibb, Port.*
Cefadroxil (p.161·2).
Bacterial infections.

Cefacor *Cefak, Ger.*
Scoparium (p.1661·2).
Cardiac disorders.

Cefacron *Foes, Spain†.*
Cefotaxime sodium (p.169·1).
Bacterial infections.

Cefadel *Francia, Ital.*
Cefmetazole sodium (p.167·2).
Lignocaine [lidocaine] hydrochloride (p.1313·2) is included in this preparation to alleviate the pain of injection.
Bacterial infections.

Cefadian *Cefak, Ger.†.*
Potentilla anserina.
Dysmenorrhoea.

Cefadin *Vana, Thai.*
Cefalotin sodium (p.162·3).
Bacterial infections.

Cefadol *Atlantic, Thai.*
Cefamandole nafate (p.163·3).
Bacterial infections.

Cefadolor *Cefak, Ger.*
Guaiacum wood.
Rheumatic disorders.

Cefadolor H *Cefak, Ger.*
Homoeopathic preparation.

Cefadrex *Vir, Spain.*
Cefazolin sodium (p.164·3).
Lignocaine [lidocaine] (p.1313·2) is included in the injection to alleviate the pain of injection.
Bacterial infections.

Cefadril
AGIPS, Ital.; LSP, Thai.
Cefadroxil (p.161·2).
Bacterial infections.

Cefadrox *Mer-National, S.Afr.*
Cefadroxil (p.161·2).
Bacterial infections.

Cefadyl *Apothecon, USA†.*
Cefapirin sodium (p.164·2).
Bacterial infections.

Cefadyn *Cefak, Ger.*
Ruscus aculeatus.
Chronic venous insufficiency.

Cefadysbasin *Cefak, Ger.*
Secale corn.; aesculus (p.1574·1); potentilla anserina.
Peripheral, coronary, and central circulatory disorders.

Cefagastrin *Cefak, Ger.*
Chamomile (p.1593·2); calendula (p.1589·2); peppermint leaf (p.1243·2); centaury (p.1593·1); absinthium (p.1571·1); arnica (p.1581·3); fennel (p.1610·1).
Gastrointestinal disorders.

Cefagil *Cefak, Ger.*
Homoeopathic preparation.

Cefakava *Cefak, Ger.*
Kava (p.1625·3).
Anxiety; nervousness; tension.

Cefakes *Inexfa, Spain.*
Cefazolin sodium (p.164·3).
Bacterial infections.

Cefakliman *Cefak, Ger.*
Homoeopathic preparation.

Cefakliman mono *Cefak, Ger.*
Cimicifuga (p.1595·2).
Menopausal and menstrual disorders.

Cefakliman N *Cefak, Ger.*
Homoeopathic preparation.

Cefaktivon *Cefak, Ger.*
Cerium (III)-chloride; echinacea (p.1606·2); hypericum (p.290·2); menyanthes (p.1633·1); calendula (p.1589·2).
Tonic.

Cefaktivon "novum" *Cefak, Ger.†.*
Protein-free extract of bovine blood; cerium chloride III; echinacea (p.1606·2); hypericum (p.290·2); menyanthes (p.1633·1); calendula (p.1589·2).
Adjuvant to cancer therapy; circulatory disorders.

Cefaldina *IMA, Braz.*
Isometheptene mucate (p.1624·2); dipyrone (p.34·1); caffeine (p.761·3).
Migraine.

Cefalektin *Cefak, Ger.*
Mistletoe (p.1636·2).
Adjunct to cancer therapy.

Cefalen *Byk, Thai.*
Cefalexin (p.161·3).
Bacterial infections.

Cefalexgobens *Normon, Spain.*
Cefalexin (p.161·3).
Bacterial infections.

Cefalin
Note.This name is used for preparations of different composition.
IBSA, Israel.
Cefalexin (p.161·3).
Bacterial infections.

Vana, Thai.
Cefazolin sodium (p.164·3).
Bacterial infections.

Cefaline Hauth *Homme de Fer, Fr.*
Paracetamol (p.71·2); caffeine (p.761·3).
Fever; pain.

Cefaline-Pyrazole *Homme de Fer, Fr.*
Dipyrone (p.34·1); caffeine (p.761·3).
Pain.

Cefalium *Ache, Braz.*
Paracetamol (p.71·2); dihydroergotamine mesilate (p.450·3); metoclopramide (p.1236·3); caffeine (p.761·3).
Migraine.

Cefaliv *Ache, Braz.*
Dihydroergotamine mesilate (p.450·3); dipyrone (p.34·1); caffeine (p.761·3).
Migraine.

Cefallone *Azupharma, Ger.*
Cefaclor (p.161·1).
Bacterial infections.

Cefaloject *Bristol-Myers Squibb, Fr.*
Cefapirin sodium (p.164·2).
Lignocaine [lidocaine] hydrochloride (p.1313·2) is included in the intramuscular injection to alleviate the pain of injection.
Bacterial infections.

Cefalor *Vitamed, Israel.*
Cefaclor (p.161·1).
Bacterial infections.

Cefaluffa *Cefak, Ger.*
Homoeopathic preparation.

Cefalver *Ofimex, Mex.*
Cefalexin (p.161·3).
Bacterial infections.

Cefalymphat *Cefak, Ger.*
Homoeopathic preparation.

Cefam *Magis, Ital.*
Cefamandole nafate (p.163·3).
Lignocaine [lidocaine] hydrochloride (p.1313·2) is included in this preparation to alleviate the pain of injection.
Bacterial infections.

Cefamadar *Cefak, Ger.*
Homoeopathic preparation.

Cefamar
FIRMA, Ital.; Menarini, Thai.
Cefuroxime sodium (p.178·2).
Bacterial infections.

Cefamezin
Sigma, Austral.; Hoechst Marion Roussel, Braz.; Fujisawa, Hong Kong; Teva, Israel; Pharmacia Upjohn, Ital.; Fujisawa, Jpn; Hikma, Port.†; Knoll, Spain; Fujisawa, Thai.
Cefazolin sodium (p.164·3).
Lignocaine [lidocaine] (p.1313·2) or lignocaine [lidocaine] hydrochloride (p.1313·2) may be included in the intramuscular injection to alleviate the pain of injection.
Bacterial infections.

Cefamig *Richelet, Fr.*
Chamomile (p.1593·2).
Headache.

Cefamiso *Inexfa, Spain.*
Cefalexin (p.161·3).
Bacterial infections.

Cefamox
Bristol-Myers Squibb, Braz.; Mead Johnson, Mex.; Bristol-Myers Squibb, Swed.
Cefadroxil (p.161·2).
Bacterial infections.

Cefamusel *Cruz, Spain†.*
Cefazolin sodium (p.164·3).
Lignocaine [lidocaine] (p.1313·2) is included in the intramuscular injection to alleviate the pain of injection.
Bacterial infections.

Cefanalgin *Cefak, Ger.*
Homoeopathic preparation.

Cefanephrin *Cefak, Ger.*
Solidago virgaurea; bearberry (p.1583·3).
Urinary-tract disorders.

Cefanex *Apothecon, USA.*
Cefalexin (p.161·3).
Bacterial infections.

Cefangipect *Cefak, Ger.*
Homoeopathic preparation.

Cefanorm *Cefak, Ger.*
Agnus castus (p.1574·2).
Mastalgia; menstrual disorders.

Cefaperos
Upsamedica, Belg.; Bristol-Myers Squibb, Fr.
Cefatrizine (p.164·3) or propylene glycol cefatrizine (p.164·3).
Bacterial infections.

Cefaporex *Haller, Braz.*
Cefalexin (p.161·3).
Bacterial infections.

Cefapulmon mono *Cefak, Ger.*
Hedera helix.
Bronchial catarrh.

Cefarheumin *Cefak, Ger.†.*
Homoeopathic preparation.

Cefarheumin N *Cefak, Ger.*
Pumilio pine oil (p.1656·3); rosemary oil (p.1659·3); camphor (p.1589·3).
Muscle, joint, and nerve pain; neuritis.

Cefarheumin S *Cefak, Ger.*
Homoeopathic preparation.

Cefasabal *Cefak, Ger.*
Saw palmetto (p.1491·2); solidago virgaurea; aesculus (p.1574·1).
Prostatic disorders.

Cefascillan *Cefak, Ger.*
Squill (p.1100·3); convallaria (p.1599·1).
Cardiac disorders; oedema.

Cefasedativ *Cefak, Ger.*
Valerian (p.1678·3); lupulus (p.1629·3); crataegus (p.1600·2).
Anxiety disorders; insomnia.

Cefasel
Cefak, Ger.†.
Homoeopathic preparation.

Cefak, Ger.
Sodium selenite (p.1375·2).
Selenium deficiency.

Cefasept *Cefak, Ger.*
Injection; oral drops: Homoeopathic preparation.
Tablets: Echinacea angustifolia (p.1606·2).
Infections.

Cefasept mono *Cefak, Ger.*
Echinacea purpura (p.1606·2).
Immunostimulant in respiratory-tract infections.

Cefasliymarin *Cefak, Ger.*
Silybum marianum (p.1021·3).
Liver disorders.

The symbol † denotes a preparation no longer actively marketed

Cefaspasmon N *Cefak, Ger.*
Homoeopathic preparation.

Cefasulfon N *Cefak, Ger.*
Homoeopathic preparation.

Cefatec *Cefak, Ger.*
Devil's claw root (p.26·3).
Musculoskeletal and joint disorders.

Cefatrix *Levofarma, Ital.*
Propylene glycol cefatrizine (p.164·3).
Bacterial infections.

Cefavale *Cefak, Ger.*
Lycopus europaeus.
Thyroid disorders.

Cefavora *Cefak, Ger.*
Homoeopathic preparation.

Cefawell *Cefak, Ger.*
Calendula (p.1589·2); arnica (p.1581·3).
Formerly known as Cefacutan.
Skin disorders; wounds.

Cefa-Wolff *Wolff, Ger.*
Cefaclor (p.161·1).
Bacterial infections.

Cefaxicina *CEPA, Spain†.*
Cefoxitin sodium (p.171·2).
Lignocaine [lidocaine] hydrochloride (p.1313·2) is included in the intramuscular injection to alleviate the pain of injection.
Bacterial infections.

Cefaxim *Ofimex, Mex.*
Cefotaxime (p.169·1).
Bacterial infections.

Cefaxona *Pisa, Mex.*
Ceftriaxone sodium (p.177·1).
Lignocaine [lidocaine] hydrochloride (p.1313·2) is included in the intramuscular injection to alleviate the pain of injection.
Bacterial infections.

Cefaxone *Shin Poong, Singapore.*
Ceftriaxone sodium (p.177·1).
Bacterial infections.

Cefazil *Italfarmaco, Ital.*
Cefazolin sodium (p.164·3).
Lignocaine [lidocaine] hydrochloride (p.1313·2) is included in this preparation to alleviate the pain of injection.
Bacterial infections.

Cefazillin *TP, Thai.*
Cefazolin sodium (p.164·3).
Bacterial infections.

Cefazol *General Drugs, Thai.*
Cefazolin sodium (p.164·3).
Bacterial infections.

Cefazone *Locatelli, Ital.†.*
Cefoperazone sodium (p.168·2).
Lignocaine [lidocaine] hydrochloride (p.1313·2) is included in this preparation to alleviate the pain of injection.
Bacterial infections.

Cef-Diolan *Engelhard, Ger.; Brahms, Ger.*
Cefaclor (p.161·1).
Bacterial infections.

Cefec *Tecnifar, Port.*
Cefetamet pivoxil hydrochloride (p.166·2).
Bacterial infections.

Cefedrin N *Cefak, Ger.*
Ephedra (p.1090·1); thyme (p.1672·2); ammi visnaga (p.1579·1).
Asthma; coughs.

Cefen *Pharmasant, Thai.*
Ibuprofen (p.43·2).
Fever; inflammation; musculoskeletal, joint, and soft-tissue disorders; pain.

Ceferro *Knoll, Ger.†.*
Ferrous sulfate (p.1360·3).
Iron-deficiency; iron-deficiency anaemias.

Cefexin *Unison, Thai.*
Cefalexin (p.161·3).
Bacterial infections.

Cefin *Korea United, Singapore.*
Ceftriaxone sodium (p.177·1).
Bacterial infections.

Cefine *Nakorn, Thai.*
Ceftriaxone sodium (p.177·1).
Bacterial infections.

Cefiran *Searle, Ital.†.*
Cefamandole nafate (p.163·3).
Lignocaine [lidocaine] hydrochloride (p.1313·2) is included in this preparation to alleviate the pain of injection.
Bacterial infections.

Cefirex *Irex, Fr.*
Cefradine (p.173·3).
Bacterial infections.

Cefixoral *Menarini, Ital.*
Cefixime (p.166·2).
Bacterial infections.

Cefizox
Roche, Aust.; SmithKline Beecham, Canad.; Rhone-Poulenc Rorer, Fr.; Wellcome, Irl.; Promeco, Mex.; Yamanouchi, Neth.; Hikma, Port.†; SmithKline, Spain; Fujisawa, USA.
Ceftizoxime sodium (p.176·3).
Lignocaine [lidocaine] hydrochloride (p.1313·2) may be included in the intramuscular injection to alleviate the pain of injection.
Bacterial infections.

Cefkor *Douglas, Austral.*
Cefaclor (p.161·1).
Bacterial infections.

Ceflax *Hikma, Port.†.*
Cefalexin (p.161·3).
Bacterial infections.

Ceflin *Hexal, Austral.*
Cefalexin (p.161·3).
Bacterial infections.

Cefmandol *General Drugs, Thai.*
Cefamandole (p.163·3).
Bacterial infections.

Cefmetazon
Sankyo, Hong Kong; Sankyo, Jpn; Sankyo, Thai.
Cefmetazole sodium (p.167·2).
Bacterial infections.

Cefobacter *AGIPS, Ital.*
Cefonicid sodium (p.168·1).
Lignocaine [lidocaine] hydrochloride (p.1313·2) is included in this preparation to alleviate the pain of injection.
Gram-negative bacterial infections.

Cefobid
Pfizer, Aust.; Pfizer, Braz.; Pfizer, Hong Kong; Pfizer, Singapore; Pfizer, Spain; Pfizer, Thai.; Pfizer, USA.
Cefoperazone sodium (p.168·2).
Bacterial infections.

Cefobis
Pfizer, Fr.†; Pfizer, Ger.†.
Cefoperazone sodium (p.168·2).
Bacterial infections.

Cefociclin *Francia, Ital.*
Cefoxitin sodium (p.171·2).
Lignocaine [lidocaine] hydrochloride (p.1313·2) is included in this preparation to alleviate the pain of injection.
Bacterial infections.

Cefoclin *Wayne, Mex.*
Cefotaxime (p.169·1).
Bacterial infections.

Cefodie *SmithKline Beecham, Ital.*
Cefonicid sodium (p.168·1).
Lignocaine [lidocaine] hydrochloride (p.1313·2) is included in the intramuscular injections to alleviate the pain of injection.
Bacterial infections.

Cefodime *LBS, Thai.*
Ceftazidime (p.174·3).
Bacterial infections.

Cefodox
Hoechst Marion Roussel, Irl.; Scharper, Ital.
Cefpodoxime proxetil (p.172·3).
Bacterial infections.

Cefoger *Ripari-Gero, Ital.*
Cefonicid sodium (p.168·1).
Lignocaine [lidocaine] hydrochloride (p.1313·2) is included in this preparation to alleviate the pain of injection.
Gram-negative bacterial infections.

Cefogram *Metapharma, Ital.*
Cefoperazone sodium (p.168·2).
Lignocaine [lidocaine] hydrochloride (p.1313·2) is included in this preparation to alleviate the pain of injection.
Bacterial infections.

Cefok *KBR, Ital.*
Cefonicid sodium (p.168·1).
Lignocaine [lidocaine] hydrochloride (p.1313·2) is included in this preparation to alleviate the pain of injection.
Gram-negative bacterial infections.

Cefol
Abbott, Hong Kong; Abbott, USA.
Multivitamin preparation (p.1350·1).

Cefomic *LBS, Thai.*
Cefotaxime sodium (p.169·1).
Bacterial infections.

Cefoneg *Tosi, Ital.*
Cefoperazone sodium (p.168·2).
Lignocaine [lidocaine] hydrochloride (p.1313·2) is included in the intramuscular injection to alleviate the pain of injection.
Bacterial infections.

Cefoper *Menarini, Ital.*
Cefoperazone sodium (p.168·2).
Lignocaine [lidocaine] hydrochloride (p.1313·2) is included in the intramuscular injection to alleviate the pain of injection.
Bacterial infections.

Cefoplus *Aesculapius, Ital.*
Cefonicid sodium (p.168·1).
Lignocaine [lidocaine] hydrochloride (p.1313·2) is included in this preparation to alleviate the pain of injection.
Gram-negative bacterial infections.

Cefoprim *Esseti, Ital.*
Cefuroxime sodium (p.178·2).
Lignocaine [lidocaine] hydrochloride (p.1313·2) is included in this preparation to alleviate the pain of injection.
Bacterial infections.

Ceforal
Note. This name is used for preparations of different composition.
Teva, Israel.
Cefalexin (p.161·3).
Bacterial infections.

Euro-Labor, Port.; Grunenthal, Port.
Cefadroxil (p.161·2).
Bacterial infections.

Ceforan *General Drugs, Thai.*
Cefotaxime sodium (p.169·1).
Bacterial infections.

Cefortam *Glaxo Wellcome, Port.*
Ceftazidime sodium.
Bacterial infections.

Cefosint *Crosara, Ital.†.*
Cefoperazone sodium (p.168·2).
Lignocaine [lidocaine] hydrochloride (p.1313·2) is included in this preparation to alleviate the pain of injection.
Bacterial infections.

Cefosporin *Esseti, Ital.*
Cefonicid sodium (p.168·1).
Lignocaine [lidocaine] hydrochloride (p.1313·2) is included in the intramuscular injection to alleviate the pain of injection.
Bacterial infections.

Cefossin *Cefak, Ger.*
Homoeopathic preparation.

Cefossin H *Cefak, Ger.*
Symphoricarpus; euphorbium cypariss.; gold in form of tetrachlorogold acid (p.1617·3).
Joint disorders.

Cefotan
Wyeth-Ayerst, Canad.; Zeneca, USA.
Cefotetan disodium (p.170·3).
Bacterial infections.

Cefotax *Vana, Thai.*
Cefotaxime sodium (p.169·1).
Bacterial infections.

Cefotex *Precimex, Mex.*
Cefotaxime (p.169·1).
Bacterial infections.

Cefotrizin *FIRMA, Ital.*
Propylene glycol cefatrizine (p.164·3).
Bacterial infections.

Cefovis *Ripari-Gero, Ital.*
Cefonicid sodium (p.168·1).
Lignocaine [lidocaine] hydrochloride (p.1313·2) is included in this preparation to alleviate the pain of injection.
Gram-negative bacterial infections.

Cefovit *Vitamed, Israel.*
Cefalexin (p.161·3).
Bacterial infections.

Cefoxin *Merck Sharp & Dohme, Thai.*
Cefoxitin sodium (p.171·2).
Bacterial infections.

Cefozone
Atlantic, Hong Kong; Atlantic, Singapore; Vana, Thai.
Cefoperazone sodium (p.168·2).
Bacterial infections.

Cefra *OM, Port.†.*
Cefadroxil (p.161·2).
Bacterial infections.

Cefrabiotic *Prospa, Ital.*
Cefradine (p.173·3).
Bacterial infections.

Cefraden *Merck, Mex.*
Ceftriaxone sodium (p.177·1).
Bacterial infections.

Cefradil *Merck, Mex.*
Cefotaxime sodium (p.169·1).
Bacterial infections.

Cefradur *Atral, Port.*
Cefradine (p.173·3).
Bacterial infections.

Cefril *Bristol-Myers Squibb, S.Afr.*
Cefradine (p.173·3).
Bacterial infections.

Cefrin *Julphar, UAE.*
Cefalexin (p.161·3).
Bacterial infections.

Cefrom
Hoechst Marion Roussel, Aust.; Hoechst Marion Roussel, Austral.; Aventis, Belg.; Hoechst Marion Roussel, Denm.†; Hoechst Marion Roussel, Fin.; Roussel Diamant, Fr.; Hoechst Marion Roussel, Hong Kong; Hoechst Marion Roussel, Irl.; Hoechst Marion Roussel, Mex.; Hoechst Marion Roussel, Neth.; Aventis, NZ; Aventis, S.Afr.; Hoechst Marion Roussel, Singapore; Hoechst Marion Roussel, Swed.; Hoechst Marion Roussel, Switz.†; Hoechst Marion Roussel, Thai.; Hoechst Marion Roussel, UK.
Cefpirome sulfate (p.172·2).
Bacterial infections.

Cefron *Hoechst Marion Roussel, Braz.*
Cefpirome sulfate (p.172·2).
Bacterial infections.

Cefspan
Fujisawa, Jpn; Fujisawa, Thai.
Cefixime (p.166·2).
Bacterial infections.

Ceftaran *Nakorn, Thai.*
Cefotaxime sodium (p.169·1).
Bacterial infections.

Ceftenon *Biochemie, Aust.†.*
Cefotetan disodium (p.170·3).
Bacterial infections.

Ceftim *Glaxo Allen, Ital.*
Ceftazidime (p.174·3).
Bacterial infections.

Ceftin
Glaxo Wellcome, Canad.; Glaxo Wellcome, USA.
Cefuroxime axetil (p.178·1).
Bacterial infections.

Ceftina *Galen, Mex.*
Cefalotin sodium (p.162·3).
Bacterial infections.

Ceftix *Boehringer Mannheim, Ger.†.*
Ceftizoxime sodium (p.176·3).
Bacterial infections.

Ceftrex
Columbia, Mex.; Biolab, Thai.
Ceftriaxone sodium (p.177·1).
Lignocaine [lidocaine] hydrochloride (p.1313·2) may be included in the intramuscular injection to alleviate the pain of injection.
Bacterial infections.

Ceftriphin *General Drugs, Thai.*
Ceftriaxone sodium (p.177·1).
Bacterial infections.

Cefumax *SoSe, Ital.*
Cefuroxime sodium (p.178·2).
Lignocaine [lidocaine] hydrochloride (p.1313·2) is included in this preparation to alleviate the pain of injection.
Bacterial infections.

Cefunk *Apsen, Braz.*
Mepyramine maleate (p.421·1); aspirin (p.14·2); caffeine (p.761·3); ascorbic acid (p.1389·3).
Aluminium hydroxide (p.1210·3) is included in this preparation in an attempt to limit adverse effects on the gastrointestinal mucosa.
Cold and influenza symptoms.

Cefur *Eurofarmaco, Ital.*
Cefuroxime sodium (p.178·2).
Bacterial infections.

Cefuracet *Columbia, Mex.*
Cefuroxime axetil (p.178·1).
Bacterial infections.

Cefurex *Salus, Ital.*
Cefuroxime sodium (p.178·2).
Bacterial infections.

Cefurim *General Drugs, Thai.*
Cefuroxime (p.178·1).
Bacterial infections.

Cefurin *Magis, Ital.*
Cefuroxime sodium (p.178·2).
Bacterial infections.

Cefurox-Reu *Reusch, Ger.*
Cefuroxime sodium (p.178·2).
Bacterial infections.

Cefxitin *Siam Bheasach, Thai.*
Cefoxitin sodium (p.171·2).
Bacterial infections.

Cefuzime *Julphar, UAE.*
Cefuroxime axetil (p.178·1).
Bacterial infections.

Cefzil
Bristol-Myers Squibb, Canad.; Bristol-Myers Squibb, UK; Bristol-Myers Squibb, USA.
Cefprozil (p.173·2).
Bacterial infections.

Cefzon *Fujisawa, Jpn.*
Cefdinir (p.165·2).
Bacterial infections.

Cegripe *Janssen-Cilag, Port.*
Chlorpheniramine [chlorphenamine] maleate (p.412·1); paracetamol (p.71·2); hesperidin (p.1611·2); vitamin C (p.1389·3).
Cold symptoms.

Cegrovit
Grossmann, Hong Kong; Grossmann, Switz.
Ascorbic acid (p.1389·3).
Vitamin C deficiency.

Cehafolin *Sanova, Aust.*
Calcium folinate (p.1363·1).
Enhancement of fluorouracil activity; methotrexate toxicity.

Cehapark *Sanova, Aust.†.*
Bromocriptine mesilate (p.1164·3).
Acromegaly; parkinsonism.

Cehaposid *Sanova, Aust.†.*
Etoposide (p.538·1).
Malignant neoplasms.

Cehasol *Sanova, Aust.*
Bath additive†: Eucalyptus oil (p.1609·2); camphor (p.1589·3); menthol (p.1632·3).
Cold symptoms.

Ointment: Sulfur-rich shale oil (Cehasol); vitamin F-glycerinester.
Skin disorders.

Ceklin *Klinger, Braz.*
Ascorbic acid (p.1389·3).
Vitamin C supplement.

Celamine *Pharmasant, Thai.*
Imipramine hydrochloride (p.291·1).
Depression; nocturnal enuresis; pain; panic attacks; parkinsonism.

Celance
Lilly, Braz.; Lilly, Fr.; Lilly, Hong Kong; Lilly, Irl.; Lilly, Singapore; Lilly, Thai.; Lilly, UK.
Pergolide mesilate (p.1175·1).
Parkinsonism.

Celebra *Searle, Denm.*
Celecoxib (p.24·1).
Osteoarthritis; rheumatoid arthritis.

Celebrex
Searle, Austral.; Searle, Canad.; Pfizer, Fr.; Searle, Fr.; Searle, Irl.; Searle, NZ; Searle, S.Afr.; Pfizer, Singapore; Searle, Singapore; Searle, Switz.; Searle, Thai.; Pfizer, Thai.; Pharmacia, UK; Searle, USA.
Celecoxib (p.24·1).
Adenomatous polyposis; osteoarthritis; rheumatoid arthritis.

Celectol
Rhone-Poulenc Rorer, Fr.; Pantheon, UK.
Celiprolol hydrochloride (p.856·1).
Angina pectoris; hypertension.

Celemin *Galen, Mex.*
Quinfamide.
Amoebiasis.

Celenid
Biolab, Hong Kong; Biolab, Singapore; Biolab, Thai.
Cinnarizine (p.413·1).
Cerebrovascular disorders; migraine; motion sickness; peripheral vascular disease; vestibular disorders.

Celesdepot *Schering-Plough, Port.*
Betamethasone sodium phosphate (p.1063·2); betamethasone acetate (p.1063·1).
Corticosteroid.

Celesemine *Schering-Plough, Spain.*
Betamethasone (p.1063·1); dexchlorpheniramine maleate (p.412·1).
Hypersensitivity reactions.

Celestamin *Aesca, Aust.*
Betamethasone (p.1063·1); dexchlorpheniramine maleate (p.412·1).
Hypersensitivity disorders.

Celestamine
Schering-Plough, Braz.; Schering-Plough, Fr.; Essex, Ger.; Schering-Plough, Hong Kong; Schering-Plough, Mex.; Schering-Plough, S.Afr.; Essex, Switz.
Betamethasone (p.1063·1); dexchlorpheniramine maleate (p.412·1).
Hypersensitivity reactions.

Celestamine N *Essex, Ger.*
Betamethasone (p.1063·1).
Corticosteroid.

Celestamine-F *Schering-Plough, Mex.*
Betamethasone (p.1063·1); dexchlorpheniramine maleate (p.412·1).
Hypersensitivity.

Celestan *Aesca, Aust.*
Betamethasone (p.1063·1) or betamethasone sodium phosphate (p.1063·2) and betamethasone acetate (p.1063·1).
Corticosteroid.

Celestan Depot *Essex, Ger.*
Betamethasone sodium phosphate (p.1063·2); betamethasone acetate (p.1063·1).
Corticosteroid.

Celestan solubile *Essex, Ger.*
Betamethasone sodium phosphate (p.1063·2).
Corticosteroid.

Celestan-V *Essex, Ger.*
Betamethasone valerate (p.1063·2).
Scalp disorders; skin disorders.

Celestene *Schering-Plough, Fr.*
Betamethasone (p.1063·1) or betamethasone sodium phosphate (p.1063·2).
Corticosteroid.

Celestene Chronodose *Schering-Plough, Fr.*
Betamethasone sodium phosphate (p.1063·2); betamethasone acetate (p.1063·1).
Corticosteroid.

Celestial Seasonings *Warner-Lambert, Canad.*
Menthol (p.1632·3).

Celestoderm
Schering, Canad.; Schering-Plough, Fin.; Schering-Plough, Fr.; Schering-Plough, Neth.; Schering-Plough, Norw.
Betamethasone valerate (p.1063·2).
Skin disorders.

Celestoderm cum Chinoform *Schering-Plough, Fin.*
Betamethasone valerate (p.1063·2); clioquinol (p.190·2).
Infected skin disorders.

Celestoderm cum Garamycin *Schering-Plough, Fin.*
Betamethasone valerate (p.1063·2); gentamicin sulfate (p.210·1).
Infected skin disorders.

Celestoderm Gentamicina *Schering-Plough, Spain.*
Betamethasone valerate (p.1063·2); gentamicin sulfate (p.210·1).
Infected skin disorders.

Celestoderm met Neomycine *Schering-Plough, Neth.*
Betamethasone valerate (p.1063·2); neomycin sulfate (p.228·1).
Infected skin disorders.

Celestoderm-V
Schering-Plough, Hong Kong; Schering-Plough, Israel; Schering-Plough, Ital.; Schering-Plough, Mex.; Schering-Plough, S.Afr.; Schering-Plough, Singapore; Schering-Plough, Spain; Essex, Switz.; Schering-Plough, Thai.
Betamethasone valerate (p.1063·2).
Skin disorders.

Celestoderm-V with Garamycin
Schering-Plough, Hong Kong; Schering-Plough, Israel; Schering-Plough, S.Afr.; Schering-Plough, Singapore.
Betamethasone valerate (p.1063·2); gentamicin sulfate (p.210·1).
Infected skin disorders.

Celestoderm-V with Neomycin
Schering-Plough, Hong Kong; Schering-Plough, Singapore; Schering-Plough, Thai.
Betamethasone valerate (p.1063·2); neomycin sulfate (p.228·1).
Infected skin disorders.

Celestoform *Schering-Plough, Neth.*
Betamethasone valerate (p.1063·2); clioquinol (p.190·2).
Infected skin disorders.

Celeston *Schering-Plough, Denm.*
Cream; liniment; ointment; topical solution: Betamethasone valerate (p.1063·2).
Skin disorders.

Schering-Plough, Denm.; Schering-Plough, Norw.
Injection: Betamethasone acetate (p.1063·1); betamethasone sodium phosphate (p.1063·2).
Corticosteroid.

Schering-Plough, Denm.†
Tablets: Betamethasone (p.1063·1).
Corticosteroid.

Schering-Plough, Swed.
Injection: Betamethasone sodium phosphate (p.1063·2).
Corticosteroid.

Celeston bifas *Schering-Plough, Swed.*
Betamethasone acetate (p.1063·1); betamethasone sodium phosphate (p.1063·2).
Corticosteroid.

Celeston Chronodose *Schering-Plough, Fin.*
Betamethasone acetate (p.1063·1); betamethasone sodium phosphate (p.1063·2).
Corticosteroid.

Celeston med Chinoform *Schering-Plough, Denm.*
Betamethasone valerate (p.1063·2); clioquinol (p.190·2).
Infected skin disorders.

Celeston valerat *Schering-Plough, Swed.*
Betamethasone valerate (p.1063·2).
Otitis externa; skin disorders.

Celeston valerat comp *Schering-Plough, Swed.*
Betamethasone valerate (p.1063·2); neomycin sulfate (p.228·1).
Infected skin disorders.

Celeston valerat med chinoform *Schering-Plough, Swed.*
Betamethasone valerate (p.1063·2); clioquinol (p.190·2).
Infected skin disorders; otitis externa.

Celeston valerat med gentamicin *Schering-Plough, Swed.*
Betamethasone valerate (p.1063·2); gentamicin sulfate (p.210·1).
Infected skin disorders.

Celestone
Schering-Plough, Belg.; Schering-Plough, Braz.; Schering, Canad.†; Schering-Plough, Hong Kong; Schering-Plough, Ital.; Schering-Plough, Mex.; Schering-Plough, Neth.; Schering-Plough, Port.; Schering-Plough, S.Afr.; Schering-Plough, Singapore; Schering-Plough, Spain; Essex, Switz.; Schering-Plough, Thai.; Schering, USA.
Betamethasone (p.1063·1) or betamethasone sodium phosphate (p.1063·2).
Corticosteroid.

Celestone V *Schering-Plough, Austral.*
Betamethasone valerate (p.1063·2).
Skin disorders.

Celestone Chronodose
Schering-Plough, Austral.; Schering-Plough, Belg.; Schering-Plough, Israel; Schering-Plough, Neth.; Schering-Plough, NZ; Essex, Switz.
Betamethasone sodium phosphate (p.1063·2); betamethasone acetate (p.1063·1).
Corticosteroid.

Celestone Cronodose
Schering-Plough, Ital.; Schering-Plough, Spain.
Betamethasone acetate (p.1063·1); betamethasone sodium phosphate (p.1063·2).
Corticosteroid.

Celestone M *Schering-Plough, Austral.*
Betamethasone valerate (p.1063·2).
Skin disorders.

Celestone S *Schering-Plough, Spain.*
Betamethasone (p.1063·1); sulfacetamide sodium (p.250·3).
Infected eye disorders.

Celestone Soluspan
Schering-Plough, Braz.; Schering, Canad.; Schering-Plough, Mex.; Schering-Plough, S.Afr.; Schering, USA.
Betamethasone acetate (p.1063·1); betamethasone sodium phosphate (p.1063·2).
Corticosteroid.

Celestone VG *Schering-Plough, Austral.*
Betamethasone valerate (p.1063·2); gentamicin sulfate (p.210·1).
Infected skin disorders.

Celevac *Shire, Irl.; Monmouth, UK.*
Methylcellulose (p.1502·2).
Colostomy and ileostomy management; constipation; diarrhoea; diverticular disease; obesity.

Celex *Masa, Thai.*
Cefalexin (p.161·3).
Bacterial infections.

Celexa
Lundbeck, Canad.; Forest Pharmaceuticals, USA.
Citalopram hydrobromide (p.281·2).
Depression.

Celexin
Hovid, Singapore; Vana, Thai.
Cefalexin (p.161·3).
Bacterial infections.

Ce-Limo *Asta Medica, Aust.*
Ascorbic acid (p.1389·3).
Vitamin C deficiency.

Ce-Limo plus 10 Vitamine *Asta Medica, Aust.*
Multivitamin preparation (p.1350·1).

Ce-Limo-Calcium *Asta Medica, Aust.*
Ascorbic acid (p.1389·3); calcium carbonate (p.1215·1).
Calcium and vitamin C deficiency.

Celin *Glaxo Wellcome, Hong Kong.*
Vitamin C (p.1389·3).
Vitamin C supplement.

Celipro *Lichtenstein, Ger.*
Celiprolol hydrochloride (p.856·1).
Angina pectoris; hypertension.

Celkalm *Aerocid, Fr.*
Loperamide hydrochloride (p.1231·3).
Diarrhoea.

Cellblastin *Cell Pharm, Ger.*
Vinblastine sulfate (p.577·3).
Malignant neoplasms.

CellCept
Roche, Aust.; Roche, Austral.; Roche, Belg.; Roche, Canad.; Roche, Denm.; Roche, Fin.; Roche, Fr.; Roche, Ger.; Roche, Hong Kong; Roche, Irl.; Roche, Israel; Roche, Ital.; Roche, Neth.; Roche, Norw.; Roche, NZ; Roche, Port.; Roche, S.Afr.; Roche, Singapore; Roche, Spain; Roche, Swed.; Roche, Switz.; Roche, Thai.; Roche, UK; Roche, USA.
Mycophenolate mofetil (p.561·3) or mycophenolate mofetil hydrochloride (p.562·1).
Cardiac, renal, or hepatic transplant rejection.

Cellcristin *Cell Pharm, Ger.*
Vincristine sulfate (p.578·3).
Malignant neoplasms.

Cellferon *Cell Pharm, Ger.†*
Interferon alpha-1 (p.628·1).
Hairy-cell leukaemia.

Cellidrin *Hennig, Ger.*
Allopurinol (p.397·2).
Gout; hyperuricaemia; renal calculi.

Cellidrine *Sodip, Switz.*
Allopurinol (p.397·2).
Hyperuricaemia.

cellmustin *Cell Pharm, Ger.*
Estramustine sodium phosphate (p.537·3).
Prostatic cancer.

Cellobexon *Agepha, Aust.*
Methylcellulose (p.1502·2); vitamin B₁ (p.1385·2); vitamin C (p.1389·3).
Constipation; obesity.

Celloid Compounds Magcal Plus *Blackmores, Austral.*
Dibasic sodium phosphate (p.1193·2); magnesium phosphate (p.1191·1); calcium phosphate (p.1188·3); dibasic potassium phosphate (p.1193·1); iron phosphate.

Celloid Compounds Sodical Plus *Blackmores, Austral.*
Dibasic sodium phosphate (p.1193·2); calcium phosphate (p.1188·3); iron phosphate.

Celloids CF 43 *Blackmores, Austral.*
Homoeopathic preparation.

Celloids CP 57 *Blackmores, Austral.*
Calcium phosphate (p.1188·3).

Celloids CS 36 *Blackmores, Austral.*
Calcium sulfate (p.1589·1).

Celloids IP 82 *Blackmores, Austral.*
Iron phosphate.

Celloids MP 65 *Blackmores, Austral.*
Magnesium phosphate (p.1191·1).

Celloids PC 73 *Blackmores, Austral.*
Potassium chloride (p.1194·3).

Celloids PP 85 *Blackmores, Austral.*
Potassium phosphate (p.1193·1).

Celloids PS 29 *Blackmores, Austral.*
Potassium sulfate (p.1195·1).

Celloids S 79 *Blackmores, Austral.*
Silicon dioxide (p.1503·3).

Celloids SP 96 *Blackmores, Austral.*
Dibasic sodium phosphate (p.1193·2).

Celloids SS 69 *Blackmores, Austral.*
Anhydrous sodium sulfate (p.1250·1).

Celltop *Asta Medica, Fr.*
Etoposide (p.538·1).
Malignant neoplasms.

Cellufresh
Allergan, Austral.; Allergan, Canad.; Allergan, NZ; Allergan, S.Afr.; Allergan, Singapore; Allergan, Spain; Allergan, Thai.; Allergan, USA†.
Carmellose sodium (p.1499·3).
Dry eyes; eye irritation.

Cellular Formula *General Nutrition, Canad.*
Multivitamin and trace element preparation (p.1350·1).

Cellulin Retinale *INTES, Ital.*
Retina extract.
Eye disorders.

Cellulone *Alphapharm, Austral.*
Methylcellulose (p.1502·2).
Bowel disorders; constipation; diarrhoea.

Cellulose *Grin, Mex.*
Hypromellose (p.1501·3).
Aid in ophthalmic procedures; dry eyes.

Celluson *CS, Fr.*
Bran (p.1214·2).
Dietary fibre supplement.

Celluspan *Fischer, Israel.*
Cellulose derivatives (p.1500·2); electrolytes (p.1180·1).
Aid in gonioscopy.

Celluvisc
Allergan, Austral.; Allergan, Canad.; Allergan, Denm.; Allergan, Fin.; Allergan, Fr.; Allergan, Ger.; Allergan, Hong Kong; Allergan, Ital.; Allergan, NZ; Allergan, Port.; Allergan, S.Afr.; Allergan, Singapore; Allergan, Spain; Allergan, Swed.; Allergan, Switz.; Allergan, UK; Allergan, USA.
Carmellose sodium (p.1499·3).
Dry eyes.

Celnium *Sanofi Winthrop, Fr.*
Selenium (p.1375·2) from Saccharomyces cerevisiae.
Skin and muscular disorders.

Celobar *Enila, Braz.*
Barium sulfate (p.1032·1).
Contrast medium for gastrointestinal radiography.

Celocurin *NM, Swed.*
Suxamethonium chloride (p.1340·1).
Depolarising neuromuscular blocker.

Celocurine *Pharmacia Upjohn, Fr.*
Suxamethonium iodide (p.1342·2).
Depolarising neuromuscular blocker.

Celoftal *Alcon, Ger.; Cusi, Singapore.*
Hypromellose (p.1501·3).
Aid in eye surgery.

Celol *Pacific, NZ.*
Celiprolol hydrochloride (p.856·1).
Angina pectoris; hypertension.

Celontin
Parke, Davis, Canad.; Parke, Davis, Israel; Parke, Davis, Neth.; Parke, Davis, S.Afr.†; Parke, Davis, USA.
Mesuximide (p.353·3).
Absence seizures.

Cel-U-Jec *Hauck, USA.*
Betamethasone sodium phosphate (p.1063·2).
Corticosteroid.

Celumax *Sanofi Winthrop, Braz.*
Centella (p.1112·2).
Cellulite.

Celupan *Lacer, Spain.*
Naltrexone hydrochloride (p.1016·1).
Alcoholism; opioid withdrawal.

Celvista *Lilly, Thai.*
Raloxifene hydrochloride (p.1491·1).
Osteopososis.

Cemac B12 *Larkhall Laboratories, UK.*
Vitamin B₁₂ (p.1388·1).

Cemado *Francia, Ital.*
Cefamandole nafate (p.163·3).
Lignocaine [lidocaine] hydrochloride (p.1313·2) is included in this preparation to alleviate the pain of injection.
Bacterial infections.

Cemaflavone *Therica, Fr.*
Citroflavonoids (p.1611·1); magnesium ascorbate (p.1190·3).
Circulatory disorders; haemorrhoids.

Cemalyt *Madaus, Spain.*
Triamcinolone (p.1080·1); centella (p.1112·2).
Formerly contained human placenta extract, triamcinolone acetonide, and calendula officinalis.
Bruising; skin disorders.

Cemaquin *Cimex, Hong Kong.*
Benzethonium chloride (p.1134·2); ascorbic acid (p.1389·3).
Mouth and throat infections.

Cementin
DHA, Hong Kong; DHA, Singapore.
Cimetidine (p.1216·3).
Gastro-oesophageal reflux; peptic ulcer; Zollinger-Ellison syndrome.

Cemetol *Pharmacia Upjohn, Spain†.*
Cefmetazole sodium (p.167·2).
Lignocaine [lidocaine] hydrochloride (p.1313·2) is included in the intramuscular injection to alleviate the pain of injection.
Bacterial infections.

Cemidin *Dexxon, Israel.*
Cimetidine (p.1216·3).
Gastro-oesophageal reflux; peptic ulcer; Zollinger-Ellison syndrome.

Cemidon *Alcala, Spain.*
Isoniazid (p.215·3).
Opportunistic mycobacterial infections; tuberculosis.

Cemidon B6 *Alcala, Spain.*
Isoniazid (p.215·3).
Pyridoxine hydrochloride (p.1386·3) is included in this preparation for the prophylaxis of peripheral neuropathy.
Opportunistic mycobacterial infections; tuberculosis.

Cemina *Medix, Mex.*
Ascorbic acid (p.1389·3).
Vitamin supplement.

Cemirit *Bayer, Ital.*
Aspirin (p.14·2).
Fever; inflammation; influenza symptoms; pain.

The symbol † denotes a preparation no longer actively marketed

Cenafed Century, USA.
Pseudoephedrine hydrochloride (p.1099·2).
Nasal congestion.

Cenafed Plus Century, USA.
Pseudoephedrine hydrochloride (p.1099·2); triprolidine hydrochloride (p.427·2).
Upper respiratory-tract symptoms.

Cenai The Forty-Two, Thai.
Cinnarizine (p.413·1).
Cerebrovascular disorders; migraine; motion sickness; peripheral vascular disease; vestibular disorders.

Cena-K Century, USA.
Potassium chloride (p.1194·3).
Hypokalaemia; potassium depletion.

Cenalfan Novaquimica, Braz.
Vitamins A, C, and E (p.1350·1).

Cenalfan Plus Novaquimica, Braz.
Multivitamin and mineral preparation (p.1350·1).

Cenat Madaus, Spain.
Ispaghula (p.1229·1).
Constipation; functional diarrhoeas.

Cencamet Pharmasant, Thai.
Cimetidine (p.1216·3).
Gastric hyperacidity; gastro-oesophageal reflux; peptic ulcer.

Cencopan Pharmasant, Thai.
Hyoscine butylbromide (p.468·2).
Smooth muscle spasm.

Ceneo Pensa, Spain.
Hydrocortisone butyrate (p.1073·3) or hydrocortisone propionate (p.1074·2).
Skin disorders.

Cenestin Duramed, USA.
Synthetic conjugated oestrogens, A (p.1467·1).
Menopausal disorders.

Cenilene Schering-Plough, Port.
Fluphenazine hydrochloride (p.684·3).

Cenlidac Pharmasant, Thai.
Sulindac (p.85·3).
Musculoskeletal, joint, and peri-articular disorders.

Cennlacs Westward, Canad.†.
Senna (p.1248·2); liquorice (p.1231·2).

Cenol Solvay, Belg.†.
Ascorbic acid (p.1389·3).
Dietary supplement; methaemoglobinaemia; scurvy.

Cenolate Abbott, USA.
Sodium ascorbate (p.1390·1).
Scurvy; vitamin C deficiency.

Cenpine Pharmasant, Thai.
Nicardipine hydrochloride (p.938·3).
Angina pectoris; cerebrovascular disorders; hypertension.

Centapp Pharmasant, Thai.
Brompheniramine maleate (p.410·2); phenylephrine hydrochloride (p.1097·1); phenylpropanolamine hydrochloride (p.1098·1).
Cold symptoms.

Centella Complex Peter, Ital.
Centella asiatica (p.1112·2); hamamelis (p.1618·3); aesculus (p.1574·1); pineapple.

Centella Complex C Peter, Ital.
Centella asiatica (p.1112·2); calcium phosphate (p.1188·3); vitamin C (p.1389·3); aesculus (p.1574·1); pineapple; hamamelis (p.1618·3).
Nutritional supplement.

Centellase
Hoechst Marion Roussel, Ital.; Yu Yu, Singapore.
Centella asiatica (p.1112·2).
Burns; scars; skin ulcers; venous insufficiency; wounds.

Center-Al Center, USA.
Range of allergen extracts (p.1575·3).
Hyposensitisation.

Centerfen Pharmasant, Thai.
Terfenadine (p.424·3).
Allergic rhinitis; urticaria.

Centeril H Errekappa, Ital.
Cream: Zinc oxide (p.1128·2); centella asiatica (p.1112·2); hamamelis (p.1618·3); aesculus (p.1574·1); peppermint (p.1243·2); menthol (p.1632·3).
Topical solution: Centella asiatica (p.1112·2); hamamelis (p.1618·3); aesculus (p.1574·1).
Anorectal disorders.

Centica Samjin, Singapore.
Centella asiatica (p.1112·2).
Burns; scars; skin ulcers; wounds.

Centilux Alcon Cusi, Spain.
Methylene blue [methylthioninium chloride] (p.1012·3); naphazoline hydrochloride (p.1095·1).
Eye disorders.

Centra Acid Therapex, Canad.
Aluminium hydroxide (p.1210·3); magnesium hydroxide (p.1233·1).

Centra Acid Plus Therapex, Canad.
Aluminium hydroxide (p.1210·3); magnesium hydroxide (p.1233·1); simeticone (p.1249·2).

Centracetam UCB, Port.
Piracetam (p.1652·1); vincamine (p.1680·1).

Centracol Therapex, Canad.†.
Phenylephrine hydrochloride (p.1097·1); phenylpropanolamine hydrochloride (p.1098·1); brompheniramine maleate (p.410·2).

Centracol DM Prometic, Canad.†.
Phenylpropanolamine hydrochloride (p.1098·1); pheniramine maleate (p.422·3); mepyramine maleate (p.421·1); dextromethorphan hydrobromide (p.1087·3).

Centracol Pediatrique Prometic, Canad.
Pseudoephedrine hydrochloride (p.1099·2); pheniramine maleate (p.422·3); dextromethorphan hydrobromide (p.1087·3); guaifenesin (p.1092·2).

Centralgine Amino, Switz.†.
Pethidine hydrochloride (p.75·1).
Pain; smooth muscle spasm.

Centralgol Zyma, Fr.†.
Proxibarbal (p.703·1).
Anxiety; menopausal symptoms.

Centramin Rosch & Handel, Aust.
Glycine (p.1365·3); magnesium chloride (p.1190·3); calcium chloride (p.1188·1); potassium chloride (p.1194·3).
Pruritus; tetany.

Centramina Miquel Otsuka, Spain†.
Amfetamine sulfate (p.1506·3).
Hyperactivity; narcoleptic syndrome.

Centrapryl Opus, UK†.
Selegiline hydrochloride (p.1177·2).
Parkinsonism.

Centratuss DM Therapex, Canad.†.
Dextromethorphan hydrobromide (p.1087·3).

Centratuss DM Expectorant Therapex, Canad.†.
Dextromethorphan hydrobromide (p.1087·3); guaifenesin (p.1092·2).

Centratuss DM-D Therapex, Canad.†.
Dextromethorphan hydrobromide (p.1087·3); pseudoephedrine hydrochloride (p.1099·2).

Centrax
Parke, Davis, Irl.; Parke, Davis, UK.
Prazepam (p.701·1).
Anxiety.

Centrophene Alpharma, Fr.
Trimetazidine hydrochloride (p.987·3).
Angina pectoris; vertigo; visual disorders.

Centrovite Rugby, USA.
A range of multivitamin and mineral preparations with iron and folic acid (p.1350·1).

Centrum
Note. This name is used for preparations of different composition.
Whitehall, Austral.; Whitehall, Braz.; Whitehall-Robins, Canad.; Lederle, Hong Kong; Whitehall, Irl.; Lederle, Israel; Whitehall, Port.; Whitehall, Singapore; Whitehall, Thai.; Whitehall, UK; Lederle, USA.
A range of multivitamin and mineral preparations (p.1350·1).
Poliforma, Ital.
Cytidine; uridine (p.1677·2).
Mental function impairment.

Centurion A–Z Mission Pharmacal, USA.
Iron (p.1366·3); folic acid (p.1361·1); multivitamins and minerals (p.1350·1).
Iron-deficiency anaemias.

Centyl
Leo, Denm.; Leo, Irl.; Leo, Norw.
Bendrofluazide [bendroflumethiazide] (p.844·1).
Diabetes insipidus; hypertension; oedema; renal calcium stones.

Centyl K
Leo, Irl.; Leo, UK.
Bendrofluazide [bendroflumethiazide] (p.844·1); potassium chloride (p.1194·3).
Hypertension; oedema; renal calculi.

Centyl med Kaliumklorid
Leo, Denm.; Leo, Norw.
Bendrofluazide [bendroflumethiazide] (p.844·1); potassium chloride (p.1194·3).
Diabetes insipidus; hypertension; oedema; renal calcium stones.

Ceolat
Solvay, Denm.; Solvay, Fin.; Rekawan, Ger.; Vemedia, Neth.; Solvay, Norw.; Solvay Duphar, Swed.†.
Dimethicone (p.1249·2).
Adjunct to gastroscopy and gastrointestinal radiography; flatulence.

Ceolat Compositum Lannacher, Aust.
Dimethicone (p.1410·1); metoclopramide (p.1236·3).
Gastrointestinal disorders.

Ceo-Two Beutlich, USA.
Sodium bicarbonate (p.1186·2); potassium acid tartrate (p.1244·3).
Constipation.

Ceoxil Magis, Ital.
Cefadroxil (p.161·2).
Bacterial infections.

Cepa Med Complex Dynamit, Aust.
Homoeopathic preparation.

Cepacaine
Note. This name is used for preparations of different composition.
Roche Consumer, Austral.; Roche, NZ.
Benzocaine (p.1306·2); cetylpyridinium chloride (p.1138·1).
Mouth and throat disorders.
Adcock Ingram, S.Afr.
Lozenges: Benzocaine (p.1306·2); cetylpyridinium chloride (p.1138·1).
Mouthwash: Benzocaine (p.1306·2); cinchocaine hydrochloride (p.1309·1); cetylpyridinium chloride (p.1138·1).
Mouth and throat disorders.

Cepacilina I Farmacologia, Spain.
Benzathine benzylpenicillin (p.156·2).
Bacterial infections; rheumatic fever.

Cepacilina 321, 621, or 633 CEPA, Spain†.
Benzylpenicillin sodium (p.157·2); procaine penicillin [procaine benzylpenicillin] (p.239·2); benzathine benzylpenicillin (p.156·2).
Bacterial infections; rheumatic fever.

Cepacol
Note. This name is used for preparations of different composition.
SmithKline Beecham Consumer, Canad.; Hoechst Marion Roussel, Hong Kong, NZ; Roche, NZ; Adcock Ingram, S.Afr.; Hoechst Marion Roussel, Singapore; Hoechst Marion Roussel, Thai.
Cetylpyridinium chloride (p.1138·1).
Mouth and throat disorders.
Lepetit, Ital.†.
Alkylbenzyldimethylammonium saccharinate (p.1133·3); sodium monofluorophosphate (p.1377·2); calcium hydrogen phosphate (p.1188·2).
Oral disinfection; oral hygiene.
Mer-National, S.Afr.
Linctus: Dextromethorphan hydrobromide (p.1087·3); doxylamine succinate (p.417·1); sodium citrate (p.1186·2); cetylpyridinium chloride (p.1138·1).
Coughs.

Cepacol Anaesthetic
Roche Consumer, Austral.; Roche, NZ.
Benzocaine (p.1306·2); cetylpyridinium chloride (p.1138·1).
Mouth and throat disorders.

Cepacol Anesthetic JB Williams, USA.
Benzocaine (p.1306·2); cetylpyridinium chloride (p.1138·1).
Sore throat.

Cepacol Antibacterial Roche Consumer, Austral.
Cetylpyridinium chloride (p.1138·1).
Mouth and throat disorders.

Cepacol Citrus SmithKline Beecham Consumer, Canad.
Benzocaine (p.1306·2); cetylpyridinium chloride (p.1138·1).
Formerly known as Cepacol Anesthetic.
Mouth and throat disorders.

Cepacol Cough Roche, NZ.
Dextromethorphan hydrobromide (p.1087·3); cetylpyridinium chloride (p.1138·1); benzocaine (p.1306·2); menthol (p.1632·3).
Coughs.

Cepacol Cough Discs Adcock Ingram, S.Afr.
Dextromethorphan (p.1087·3); cetylpyridinium chloride (p.1138·1); benzocaine (p.1306·2).
Coughs; sore throat.

Cepacol Cough and Sore Throat Roche Consumer, Austral.
Dextromethorphan hydrobromide (p.1087·3); cetylpyridinium chloride (p.1138·1); benzocaine (p.1306·2); menthol (p.1632·3).
Coughs; sore throat.

Cepacol with Fluoride SmithKline Beecham Consumer, Canad.
Cetylpyridinium chloride (p.1138·1); sodium fluoride (p.1375·3).

Cepacol Maximum Strength Sore Throat JB Williams, USA.
Lozenges: Benzocaine (p.1306·2); menthol (p.1632·3); cetylpyridinium chloride (p.1138·1).
Throat spray: Dyclonine hydrochloride (p.1311·3); cetylpyridinium chloride (p.1138·1).
Sore throat.

Cepacol Mint Roche Consumer, Austral.
Cetylpyridinium chloride (p.1138·1).
Mouth and throat disorders; oral hygiene.

Cepacol Mouthwash JB Williams, USA.
Cetylpyridinium chloride (p.1138·1).
Minor mouth or throat disorders.

Cepacol Regular Roche Consumer, Austral.
Cetylpyridinium chloride (p.1138·1).
Mouth and throat disorders; oral hygiene.

Cepacol Regular Strength JB Williams, USA.
Menthol (p.1632·3); cetylpyridinium chloride (p.1138·1).
Sore throat.

Cepacol Throat JB Williams, USA.
Benzyl alcohol (p.1135·2); cetylpyridinium chloride (p.1138·1).
Sore throat.

Cepacol Viractin SmithKline Beecham Consumer, Canad.
Amethocaine [tetracaine] hydrochloride (p.1305·2).

Cepacol Viractin Cold Sore Treatment JB Williams, USA.
Amethocaine [tetracaine] (p.1305·2) or amethocaine [tetracaine] hydrochloride (p.1305·2).
Topical anaesthesia.

Cepadont Agis, Israel.
Cetylpyridinium chloride (p.1138·1); chlorobutanol (p.1141·2).
Mouth disinfection.

Cepadyne Infan, Mex.
Cetylpyridinium chloride (p.1138·1).

Cepal Pharmasant, Thai.
Fenbufen (p.36·2).
Musculoskeletal and joint disorders.

Cepasium Cortunon, Canad.†.
Magnesium carbonate (p.1232·3).

Cepastat
Note. This name is used for preparations of different composition.
SmithKline Beecham Consumer, Canad.; SmithKline Beecham Consumer, USA.
Phenol (p.1152·3); menthol (p.1632·3); eucalyptus oil (p.1609·2).
Sore throat.
Hoechst Marion Roussel, Hong Kong; Hoechst Marion Roussel, Singapore.
Phenol (p.1152·3); menthol (p.1632·3).
Sore throat.

Cepastat Cherry SmithKline Beecham Consumer, USA.
Phenol (p.1152·3); menthol (p.1632·3).
Sore throat.

Cepazine Novaxo, Fr.
Cefuroxime axetil (p.178·1).
Bacterial infections.

Cepevit Darci, Fr.
Ascorbic acid (p.1389·3); hesperidin methyl chalcone (p.1611·2); hesperidin (p.1611·2); esculoside (p.1574·1).
Capillary fragility.

Cepexin Glaxo Wellcome, Aust.
Cefalexin (p.161·3).
Bacterial infections.

Cephadol
Shinyaku, Hong Kong; Shinyaku, Jpn; Shinyaku, Singapore; Shinyaku, Thai.
Difenidol hydrochloride (p.1222·1).
Dizziness; vertigo.

Cephalex CT, Ger.
Cefalexin (p.161·3).
Bacterial infections.

Cephalgan UPSA, Fr.
Carbasalate calcium (p.23·3); metoclopramide hydrochloride (p.1235·2).
Migraine.

Cephalo Infirmarius-Rovit, Ger.
Homoeopathic preparation.

Cephalobene Ratiopharm, Aust.
Cefalexin (p.161·3).
Bacterial infections.

Cephanol Riva, Canad.
Paracetamol (p.71·2).

Ceph-Biocin Orion, Ger.
Cefaclor (p.161·1).
Bacterial infections.

Cephin General Drugs, Thai.
Cefalexin (p.161·3).
Bacterial infections.

Cephoral
Merck, Ger.; Merck, Switz.
Cefixime (p.166·2).
Bacterial infections.

Cephos CT, Ital.
Cefadroxil (p.161·2).
Bacterial infections.

Cephulac
Hoechst Marion Roussel, Canad.†; Hoechst Marion Roussel, USA.
Lactulose (p.1230·1).
Hepatic encephalopathy.

Cephyl
Note. This name is used for preparations of different composition.
Boiron, Fr.
Aspirin (p.14·2); caffeine (p.761·3); belladonna; iris versicolor; nux vomica; spigelia; gelsemium.
Formerly contained aspirin, ethenzamide, caffeine hydrate, belladonna, iris versicolor, nux vomica, spigelia, and gelsemium.
Pain.
Boiron, Port.
Aspirin (p.14·2); ethenzamide (p.35·1); caffeine (p.761·3); belladonna; iris versicolor; nux vomica; spigelia; gelsemium.
Fever; pain.

Cepifran Juste, Spain.
Ceftibuten (p.176·1).
Bacterial infections.

Cepim Upsamedica, Ital.
Cefepime hydrochloride (p.165·3).
Bacterial infections.

Cepimex Mead Johnson, Ital.
Cefepime hydrochloride (p.165·3).
Bacterial infections.

Ceplac Rhone-Poulenc Rorer, UK.
Erythrosine (p.1028·2).
Disclosing agent for plaque.

Ceporacin Bioniche, Canad.
Cefalotin sodium (p.162·3).
Bacterial infections.

Ceporan Glaxo Wellcome, Mex.
Cefaloridine (p.162·2).
Bacterial infections.

Ceporex
Glaxo Wellcome, Belg.; Glaxo Wellcome, Hong Kong; Glaxo Wellcome, Irl.; Glaxo Wellcome, Ital.; Glaxo Wellcome, Mex.; Glaxo Wellcome, Port.; Glaxo Wellcome, Singapore; Glaxo Wellcome, Thai.; Glaxo Wellcome, UK.
Cefalexin (p.161·3).
Bacterial infections.

Ceporexin
Glaxo Wellcome, Braz.; Hoechst Marion Roussel, Ger.; Glaxo Wellcome, Ger.
Cefalexin (p.161·3).
Bacterial infections.

Ceporexine Glaxo Wellcome, Fr.
Cefalexin (p.161·3).
Bacterial infections.

Ceposil *Pisa, Mex.*
Potassium acetate (p.1194·3).

Cepral *Kemyos, Ital.†*
Aluminium sulfate (p.1578·2); cetylpyridinium chloride (p.1138·1).
Mouth and throat disorders.

Ceprandal *Sigma-Tau, Spain.*
Omeprazole (p.1239·1).
Gastro-oesophageal reflux; peptic ulcer; Zollinger-Ellison syndrome.

Ceprimax *Fides Rottapharm, Spain.*
Ciprofloxacin hydrochloride (p.182·3).
Bacterial infections.

Ceprin *Dolisos, Canad.*
Homoeopathic preparation.

Ceprotin *Baxter BioScience, UK.*
Protein C (p.741·2).
Thromboembolic disorders.

Ceprovit *Wider, Ger.†*
Lemon oil (p.1628·2); chamomile oil; arnica (p.1581·3).
Healing of amputations.

Ceptaz *Glaxo Wellcome, Canad.; Glaxo Wellcome, USA.*
Ceftazidime (p.174·3).
Bacterial infections.

Cepticol *Banyu, Jpn†.*
Propylene glycol cefatrizine (p.164·3).
Bacterial infections.

Cepton *Eastern Pharmaceuticals, UK.*
Chlorhexidine gluconate (p.1138·2).
Acne.

Cequinyl *SmithKline Beecham Sante, Fr.*
Paracetamol (p.71·2); pseudoephedrine hydrochloride (p.1099·2); ascorbic acid (p.1389·3).
Formerly contained paracetamol, ascorbic acid, and quinine hydrochloride.
Fever; nasal congestion; pain.

Ceradolan *Takeda, Hong Kong; Takeda, Singapore; Takeda, Thai.*
Cefotiam hydrochloride (p.171·1).
Bacterial infections.

Ceralip *Roche-Posay, Irl.*
Emollient.
Dry lips; mucous membrane damage.

Cerasorb *Curasan, Ger.*
Calcium phosphate (p.1188·3).
Artificial bone and dental enamel.

Cerat Inalterable *Roche-Posay, Fr.*
Titanium dioxide (p.1126·1); aluminium silicate (p.1211·3); white beeswax (p.1408·2); light liquid paraffin (p.1407·2).
Barrier ointment.

Cerax *Pharmasant, Thai.*
Hydroxyzine hydrochloride (p.419·1).
Hypersensitivity reactions; sedative.

Cerazette *Organon, Belg.; Organon, Fr.; Organon, Ger.; Organon, Neth.; Pharmaco, NZ; Organon, Swed.*
Desogestrel (p.1470·3).
Progestogen-only oral contraceptive.

Cerbon *Produfarma, Port.*
Pyritinol hydrochloride (p.1657·1).
Cerbrovascular disorders; mental function disorders.

Cercon *Lakeside, Mex.*
Praziquantel (p.106·3).

Cere *Kolassa, Aust.*
Ornithine aspartate (p.1374·1).
Hepatic encephalopathy.

Cerebral-Do *Grasler, Ger.*
Homoeopathic preparation.

Cerebramed *Orion, Ger.*
Amantadine hydrochloride (p.1161·2).
Drug-induced extrapyramidal disorders; influenza A; parkinsonism.

Cerebrex *Luper, Braz.*
Vitamin B substances; glutamic acid; calcium glycerophosphate; calcium phosphate (p.1350·1).
Nutritional supplement.

Cerebrino *Mandri, Spain.*
Aspirin (p.14·2); paracetamol (p.71·2); caffeine (p.761·3).
Influenza symptoms; pain.

Cerebroad *Chinta, Thai.*
Cinnarizine (p.413·1).
Cerebrovascular disorders; migraine; peripheral vascular disorders; vestibular disorders.

Cerebroforte *Azupharma, Ger.*
Piracetam (p.1652·1).
Mental function disorders.

Cerebrol
Note. This name is used for preparations of different composition.
Boehringer Ingelheim, Fr.
Diethylaminoethanol malate (p.1508·3).
Asthenia.

Actipharm, Switz.
Codeine phosphate (p.25·2); caffeine (p.761·3); paracetamol (p.71·2); propyphenazone (p.80·2).
Pain.

Cerebrol sans codeine *Actipharm, Switz.*
Caffeine (p.761·3); paracetamol (p.71·2).
Pain.

Cerebrolysin *Ebewe, Aust.; Knoll, Ger.; Ebewe, Hong Kong; Ebewe, Thai.*
Brain extract (p.1631·2).
Brain injury; epilepsy; mental function impairment; mental retardation; parkinsonism; senile dementia; stroke.

Cerebropan *ISM, Ital.*
Piracetam (p.1652·1).
Mental function impairment.

Cerebrovase *Ashbourne, UK†.*
Dipyridamole (p.877·2).
Thromboembolism prophylaxis.

Cerebroxine *Therabel, Belg.*
Vincamine (p.1680·1).
Cerebrovascular disorders.

Cerebryl *Kwizda, Aust.*
Piracetam (p.1652·1).
Cerebral disorders.

Cerebyx *Parke, Davis, Canad.; Parke, Davis, USA.*
Fosphenytoin sodium (p.349·3).
Epilepsy.

Ceredase *Genzyme, Ger.†; Genzyme, Israel; Genzyme, Ital.†; Genzyme, Jpn; Genzyme, Spain†; Genzyme, UK†; Genzyme, USA.*
Alglucerase (p.1574·3).
Gaucher disease.

Ceredopa *Ratiopharm, Aust.†.*
Levodopa (p.1169·2).
Parkinsonism.

Cereen *Rolab, S.Afr.*
Haloperidol (p.686·3).
Psychoses.

Cereginkgo *Pfluger, Ger.*
Homoeopathic preparation.

Ceregumil *Azevedos, Port.*
Preparation for enteral nutrition (p.1350·1).

Cerekinon *Tanabe, Hong Kong; Tanabe, Jpn; Tanabe, Singapore; Tanabe, Thai.*
Trimebutine maleate (p.1675·1).
Chronic gastritis; irritable bowel syndrome.

Cerella *Asche, Ger.*
Estradiol (p.1473·1).
Menopausal disorders.

Ceremin
Note. This name is used for preparations of different composition.
Madaus, Aust.
Ginkgo biloba (p.1615·2).
Cerebral and peripheral vascular disorders.

Polipharm, Thai.
Cinnarizine (p.413·1).
Cerebrovascular disorders; migraine; motion sickness; peripheral vascular disorders; vestibular disorders.

Cereon *Biogal, Israel.*
Ascorbic acid (p.1389·3).
Scurvy.

Cerepar *Mepha, Switz.*
Cinnarizine (p.413·1).
Vertigo; vestibular disorders.

Cerepar N *Merckle, Ger.*
Piracetam (p.1652·1).
Mental function impairment.

Cerestabon *Seber, Port.*
Idebenone (p.1623·1).
Cerebrovascular disorders; mental function disorders.

Ceretec *Nycomed, Austral.; Amersham, Fr.†; Sorin, Ital.; Nycomed, Spain; Nycomed Amersham, UK.*
Technetium-99m exametazime (p.1451·1).
Cerebral blood flow scintigraphy; leucocyte labelling.

Cerevon *Wellcome, Canad.†.*
Ferrous succinate (p.1360·3).
Iron-deficiency anaemia.

Cerexin *Rolab, S.Afr.†.*
Cefalexin (p.161·3).
Now known as Rolab-Cephalexin.
Bacterial infections.

Cerezyme *Genzyme, Aust.; Genzyme, Austral.; Genzyme, Denm.; Genzyme, Fr.; Genzyme, Ger.; Genzyme, Israel; Genzyme, Ital.; Genzyme, Jpn; Enzifarma, Port.; Genzyme, Spain; Genzyme, Switz.; Genzyme, UK; Genzyme, USA.*
Imiglucerase (p.1574·3).
Gaucher disease.

Cergem *Nourypharma, Ger.*
Gemeprost (p.1445·1).
Cervical dilatation.

Ceridal *Stiefel, Fin.; Rhone-Poulenc Rorer, Irl.*
A range of emollient preparations.
Dry skin and scalp disorders.

Cerina *Wyeth, Switz.*
Estradiol (p.1473·1).
Menopausal disorders; osteoporosis.

Cerivikehl *Sanum-Kehlbeck, Ger.*
Homoeopathic preparation.

Cernevit *Baxter, Aust.; Baxter, Belg.; Clintec, Fr.; Baxter, Ger.; Clintec, Irl.†; Clintec, Ital.; Clintec, Spain; Baxter, Switz.; Baxter, UK; Baxter, USA.*
A multivitamin preparation (p.1350·1).
Parenteral nutrition.

Cernilton *Strathmann, Ger.; Cernitin, Switz.†.*
Pollen extracts.
Micturation disorders; prostatitis.

Cerose DM *Wyeth-Ayerst, USA.*
Dextromethorphan hydrobromide (p.1087·3); chlorpheniramine [chlorphenamine] maleate (p.412·1); phenylephrine hydrochloride (p.1097·1).
Coughs and cold symptoms.

Cerotto Bertelli Arnikos *Kelemata, Ital.*
Capsicum oleoresin (p.1591·3).
Musculoskeletal disorders.

Cerovite *Rugby, USA.*
Multivitamin and mineral preparation with iron and folic acid (p.1350·1).

Cerox *Bouty, Ital.*
Benzalkonium chloride (p.1133·2); allantoin (p.1110·1); quaternium-14.
Skin, wound, and burn disinfection.

Ceroxmed Steril *Bouty, Ital.†.*
Benzalkonium chloride (p.1133·2).
Instrument and surface disinfection; skin, wound, and hand disinfection.

Cerson *Riemser, Ger.*
Flumetasone pivalate (p.1070·3).
Skin disorders.

Certagen *Goldline, USA.*
Oral liquid: Multivitamin and mineral preparation (p.1350·1).
Tablets: Ferrous fumarate (p.1360·1); folic acid (p.1361·1); multivitamins and minerals (p.1350·1).
Iron-deficiency anaemias.

Certagen Senior *Goldline, USA.*
Multivitamin and mineral preparation with iron and folic acid (p.1350·1).

Certain Dri *Numark, USA†.*
Aluminium chloride (p.1110·2).
Hyperhidrosis.

Certalac *Medeva, Belg.*
Lactulose (p.1230·1).
Constipation.

Certa-Vite *Major, USA.*
Multivitamin and mineral preparation (p.1350·1).

Certified Decongestant *Prodemdis, Canad.*
Xylometazoline hydrochloride (p.1102·2).

Certified Ice *Prodemdis, Canad.*
Menthol (p.1632·3).

Certified Nasal *Prodemdis, Canad.*
Sodium chloride (p.1196·1).

Certiva *North American Vaccine, USA.*
A diphtheria, tetanus, and acellular pertussis vaccine (p.1537·3).
Active immunisation.

Certobil *Metapharma, Ital.†.*
Dehydrocholic acid (p.1602·2); rhubarb (p.1248·1); cascara (p.1216·1); boldo (p.1585·3); manna (p.1233·3).
Constipation.

Certomycin *Aesca, Aust.; Essex, Ger.*
Netilmicin sulfate (p.229·3).
Bacterial infections.

Certonal *Serturner, Ger.*
Moxaverine hydrochloride (p.1638·1).
Circulatory disorders.

Certovermil *Farmedica, Braz.*
Mebendazole (p.102·2).
Worm infections.

Ceru Spray *Ghimas, Ital.*
Chamomile (p.1593·2).
Aural hygiene.

Cerubidin *Aventis, Denm.; Rhone-Poulenc Rorer, Irl.; Rhone-Poulenc Rorer, Norw.; Aventis, S.Afr.; Rhone-Poulenc Rorer, Swed.; Rhone-Poulenc Rorer, UK.*
Daunorubicin hydrochloride (p.533·1).
Leukaemias.

Cerubidine *Aventis, Belg.; Rhone-Poulenc Rorer, Canad.; Rhone-Poulenc Rorer, Fr.; Rhone-Poulenc Rorer, Israel; Rhone-Poulenc Rorer, Neth.; Aventis, NZ; Rhone-Poulenc Rorer, Switz.; Bedford, USA.*
Daunorubicin hydrochloride (p.533·1).
Malignant neoplasms.

Cerucal *Dresden, Ger.; Temmler, Ger.*
Metoclopramide hydrochloride (p.1235·2).
Gastrointestinal disorders.

Cerulisina *Bouty, Ital.*
Xylene (p.1406·3).
Ear wax removal.

Cerulyse *Chauvin, Fr.*
Xylene (p.1406·3).
Ear wax removal.

Cerumenex *Purdue Frederick, Canad.; Asta Medica, Ital.†; Aventis, S.Afr.; Mundipharma, Switz.; Purdue Frederick, USA.*
Trolamine polypeptide oleate-condensate (p.1675·2).
Ear wax removal.

Cerumenex N *Mundipharma, Ger.*
Trolamine polypeptide oleate-condensate (p.1675·2).
Ear wax removal.

Cerumenol
Note. This name is used for preparations of different composition.
Martin, Fr.
Polysorbate 80 (p.1347·3).
Ear wax removal.

Berna, Spain.
Potassium hydroxide (p.1654·1).
Ear wax removal.

Schonenberger, Switz.
Paradichlorobenzene (p.1648·3); chlorobutanol hemihydrate (p.1141·2); turpentine oil (p.1676·3); orthodichlorobenzene (p.1645·1); methoxybutyl acetate.
Ear wax removal.

Cerumin *Alcon, Braz.*
Hydroxyquinoline borate (p.1622·2); trolamine (p.1675·1).
Ear wax removal.

Cerumol
Note. This name is used for preparations of different composition.
Culver, Austral.
Paradichlorobenzene (p.1648·3); chlorobutanol (p.1141·2); orthodichlorobenzene (p.1645·1); arachis oil (p.1581·1).
Formerly contained paradichlorobenzene, chlorobutanol, turpentine oil, and arachis oil.
Ear wax removal.

Solvay, Canad.; Laboratories for Applied Biology, Irl.†.
Paradichlorobenzene (p.1648·3); chlorobutanol (p.1141·2); turpentine oil (p.1676·3).
Ear wax removal.

Laboratories for Applied Biology, Hong Kong; Pharmafrica, S.Afr.; Laboratories for Applied Biology, Singapore; Laboratories for Applied Biology, UK.
Paradichlorobenzene (p.1648·3); chlorobutanol (p.1141·2); arachis oil (p.1581·1).
The name Cerumenol has also been used for this preparation in the UK.
Ear wax removal.

Tamar, Israel.
Paradichlorobenzene (p.1648·3); chlorobutanol (p.1141·2); benzocaine (p.1306·2); turpentine oil (p.1676·3).
Ear wax removal.

Cerutil *Isis, Ger.*
Meclofenoxate hydrochloride (p.1631·3).
Cerebral circulatory disorders; mental function impairment.

Cervagem *Rhone-Poulenc Rorer, Austral.; Aventis, Denm.; Rhone-Poulenc Rorer, Fin.; Rhone-Poulenc Rorer, Hong Kong; Rhone-Poulenc Rorer, Norw.; Aventis, NZ; Rhone-Poulenc Rorer, Singapore; Rhone-Poulenc Rorer, Swed.*
Gemeprost (p.1445·1).
Cervical dilatation; termination of pregnancy.

Cervageme *Rhone-Poulenc Rorer, Fr.*
Gemeprost (p.1445·1).
Cervical dilatation prior to uterine procedures; termination of pregnancy.

Cervasta *Fournier, Ital.*
Cerivastatin sodium (p.856·1).
Hypercholesterolaemia.

Cervekanin *Romer, Mex.*
Brewers' yeast (p.1398·1).

Cervidil
Note. This name is used for preparations of different composition.
Ferring, Canad.; Forest Pharmaceuticals, USA.
Dinoprostone (p.1441·3).
Labour induction.

Serono, Ital.
Gemeprost (p.1445·1).
Cervical dilatation.

Cervilan *Hoechst Marion Roussel, Mex.*
Lomifylline; dihydroergocristine mesilate (p.1603·2).
Cerebrovascular disorders.

Cervilane *Cassenne, Fr.†; Roussel, Port.*
Lomifylline; dihydroergocristine mesilate (p.1603·2).
Cerebral circulatory disorders.

Cervinca *Basi, Port.*
Vincamine (p.1680·1).

Cerviprost *Organon, Aust.†; Nourypharma, Ger.†; Organon, Neth.†; Organon, Swed.†; Organon, Switz.†.*
Dinoprostone (p.1441·3).
Cervical dilatation; labour induction; termination of pregnancy.

Cervitec *DAB, Swed.*
Chlorhexidine acetate (p.1138·2).
Dental hygiene.

Cervoxan *Pharmafarm, Fr.; Decomed, Port.; Mabo, Spain.*
Vinburnine (p.1680·1).
Cerebrovascular disorders.

CES *ICN, Canad.*
Conjugated oestrogens (p.1467·1).
Menopausal disorders; osteoporosis.

Cesamet *Lilly, Canad.; Lilly, Irl.; Lilly, UK.*
Nabilone (p.1237·3).
Nausea and vomiting associated with cancer chemotherapy.

Cesbron *Sanofi Synthelabo, Port.*
Clenbuterol (p.763·3).

Cesol
Note. This name is used for preparations of different composition.
Merck, Ger.; Merck, Mex.
Praziquantel (p.106·3).
Cestode infections.

Cesam, Port.
Ketoconazole (p.389·1).
Pityriasis versicolor; seborrhoeic dermatitis.

Cesoline *Pharmasant, Thai.*
Hydralazine hydrochloride (p.905·3).
Hypertension.

Cesplon *Esteve, Spain.*
Captopril (p.853·3).
Diabetic nephropathy; heart failure; hypertension; myocardial infarction.

Cesplon Plus *Esteve, Spain.*
Hydrochlorothiazide (p.907·3); captopril (p.853·3).
Hypertension.

Cesra *Redel, Ger.†*
Ibuprofen (p.43·2).
Fever; gout; inflammation; musculoskeletal and joint disorders; pain.

Cesradyston *Redel, Ger.*
Hypericum (p.290·2).
Formerly contained belladonna, phenobarbital, secalia corn., gelsemium, atropine sulfate, and hamamelis.
Nervous disorders.

Cesran *Cesra, Ger.*
Hypericum (p.290·2).
Depression.

Cesrasanol *Cesra, Ger.*
Chamomile; hamamelis; calendula; arnica; achillea; centaury.
Inflammation; spasms.

Cessatosse *Regius, Braz.*
Sodium dibunate (p.1100·3); tiocol; belladonna (p.463·1); sodium benzoate (p.1134·3).
Coughs.

Cessaverm *INQ, Braz.*
Mebendazole (p.102·2).
Worm infections.

Cestox *Merck, Braz.*
Praziquantel (p.106·3).
Cestode infections; trematode infections.

Ceta *C & M, USA.*
Skin cleanser.

Ceta Plus *Seatrace, USA.*
Hydrocodone tartrate (p.42·2); paracetamol (p.71·2).
Pain.

Ceta Sulfa *Grin, Mex.*
Sulfacetamide sodium (p.250·3).
Bacterial eye infections.

Cetabon *Great Eastern, Thai.; Therapharma, Thai.*
Stanozolol (p.1491·3); vitamin B substances (p.1350·1).
Anabolic.

Cetacaine *Cetylite, USA.*
Benzocaine (p.1306·2); butyl aminobenzoate (p.1308·2); amethocaine [tetracaine] hydrochloride (p.1305·2).
Local anaesthesia.

Cetacort *Healthpoint, USA.*
Hydrocortisone (p.1073·3).
Skin disorders.

Cetafeine *Arkomedika, Fr.*
Paracetamol (p.71·2); caffeine (p.761·3).
Fever; pain.

Cetal *Parke, Davis, Aust.; Parke, Davis, Ger.; Warner-Lambert, Switz.*
Vincamine (p.1680·1).
Ménière's disease; mental function disorders; metabolic and circulatory disorders of the brain, retina, and ear.

Cetal Concentrate *Colgate Oral Care, Austral.†*
Benzalkonium chloride (p.1133·2).
Instrument and surface disinfection.

Cetal Instrument Disinfectant *Colgate Oral Care, Austral.†*
Chlorhexidine gluconate (p.1138·2); cetrimide (p.1137·1).
Disinfection of instruments, linen, and furniture.

Cetamide *Alcon, Canad.; Alcon, USA.*
Sulfacetamide sodium (p.250·3).
Eye infections.

Cetamine
Note.This name is used for preparations of different composition.
Wolfs, Belg.
Ascorbic acid (p.1389·3).
Vitamin C deficiency; vitamin C supplement.

Covan, S.Afr.
Syrup: Paracetamol (p.71·2); mepyramine maleate (p.421·1); phenylephrine hydrochloride (p.1097·1); caffeine (p.761·3).
Tablets: Quinine sulfate (p.445·1); ascorbic acid (p.1389·3); paracetamol (p.71·2); mepyramine maleate (p.421·1); phenylephrine hydrochloride (p.1097·1).
Cold and influenza symptoms.

Cetampril *Clintex, Port.*
Enalapril maleate (p.883·3).
Heart failure; hypertension.

Cetan *Pharmasant, Thai.*
Ibuprofen (p.43·2); paracetamol (p.71·2).
Musculoskeletal, joint, peri-articular, and soft-tissue disorders.

Cetanorm *Norma, UK.*
Benzalkonium chloride (p.1133·2); aldioxa (p.1109·3); chlorobutanol (p.1141·2); cetrimide (p.1137·1).

Cetaphil
Galderma, Austral.; Galderma, Braz.; Galderma, Canad.; Galderma, Hong Kong; Galderma, Mex.; Galderma, NZ; Galderma, Port.; Galderma, Singapore; Galderma, Thai.; Galderma, UK; Galderma, USA.
A range of skin cleansers and moisturisers.

Cetapon *Pharmagen, S.Afr.†*
Paracetamol (p.71·2).
Fever; pain.

Cetapred *Alcon, Belg.; Alcon, USA.*
Prednisolone acetate (p.1078·1); sulfacetamide sodium (p.250·3).
Bacterial eye infections with inflammation.

Cetapril *Dainippon, Jpn.*
Alacepril (p.833·1).
Hypertension.

Cetasil *Silom, Thai.*
Sulfacetamide sodium (p.250·3).
Bacterial eye infections.

Cetavlex
Note.This name is used for preparations of different composition.
Zeneca, Belg.
Cetrimonium bromide (p.1137·3); chlorhexidine gluconate (p.1138·2).
Disinfection of wounds, skin, and hands; skin disorders.

Bioglan, Irl.; CS, Port.; Bioglan, Singapore; Bioglan, UK.
Cetrimide (p.1137·1).
Skin disinfection.

Cetavlon
CS, Fr.; Zeneca, Neth.; Genop, S.Afr.; Zeneca, Spain.
Cetrimide (p.1137·1).
Burns; disinfection; wounds.

Cetazin *Sigmapharm, Aust.*
Sulfacetamide sodium (p.250·3).
Bacterial eye infections.

Cetebe *SmithKline Beecham, Aust.; SmithKline Beecham OTC, Ger.; SmithKline Beecham Consumer, Switz.*
Ascorbic acid (p.1389·3).
Vitamin C deficiency.

Cetildrops *Luper, Braz.*
Cetylpyridinium chloride (p.1138·1); benzocaine (p.1306·2).
Mouth and throat disorders.

Cetilsan *Sella, Ital.*
Cetylpyridinium chloride (p.1138·1).
Oral hygiene; skin and wound disinfection.

Cetimil *Lesvi, Spain.*
Nedocromil sodium (p.768·3).
Asthma.

Cetina *Infan, Mex.*
Chloramphenicol (p.179·1).
Bacterial infections.

Cetiprin
Pharmacia Upjohn, Aust.; Darrow, Braz.; Pharmacia Upjohn, Denm.; Pharmacia Upjohn, Irl.; Pharmacia Upjohn, Neth.; Pharmacia Upjohn, Norw.; Pharmacia Upjohn, NZ; Pharmacia Upjohn, Swed.; Pharmacia Upjohn, Switz.
Emepronium bromide (p.466·3) or emepronium carrageenate (p.466·3).
Bladder disorders.

Cetiprin Novum
Pharmacia Upjohn, Fin.; Pharmacia Upjohn, Hong Kong.
Emepronium carrageenate (p.466·3).
Bladder disorders.

Cetiva AE *Abbott, Braz.*
Vitamins A, C, and E (p.1350·1).

Cetoglutaran *Expanpharm, Fr.*
Calcium di-oxoglutarate.
Asthenia.

Cetona Plus *Democal, Switz.*
Aluminium acetate (p.1578·1); arnica (p.1581·3); chamomile (p.1593·2); calendula (p.1589·2); hypericum (p.290·2); comfrey (p.1598·3); dexpanthenol (p.1602·3); lignocaine [lidocaine] hydrochloride (p.1313·2).
Skin swelling.

Cetonax *Cilag, Braz.*
Ketoconazole (p.389·1).
Fungal infections.

Cetonil *Stiefel, Braz.*
Ketoconazole (p.389·1).
Fungal infections.

Cetoquina Y *Solfran, Mex.*
Fluocinolone acetonide (p.1071·1); clioquinol (p.190·2).
Infected skin disorders.

Cetornan *Chiesi, Fr.*
Ornithine oxoglurate (p.1374·1).
Nutritional supplement.

Cetovinca
Schering, Mex.; Byk Elmu, Spain.
Vincamine oxoglurate (p.1680·1).
Cerebral trauma; cerebrovascular disorders.

Cetoxil *Fustery, Mex.*
Cefuroxime axetil (p.178·1) or cefuroxime sodium (p.178·2).
Bacterial infections.

Cetoxol *Pharmacare Consumer, S.Afr.†*
Benzocaine (p.1306·2); cetylpyridinium chloride (p.1138·1).
Sore throat.

Cetozol *Cazi, Braz.*
Ketoconazole (p.389·1).
Fungal infections.

Cetraben *Sankyo, UK.*
White soft paraffin (p.1407·3); liquid paraffin (p.1407·2).
Dry skin.

Cetraben Bath Oil *Sankyo, UK.*
Light liquid paraffin (p.1407·2).
Dry skin.

Cetralon *Julphar, UAE.*
Cetirizine hydrochloride (p.411·2).
Hypersensitivity reactions.

Cetraria Salbe *Helixor, Ger.*
Iceland moss; laminaria (p.1627·1).
Skin disorders; skin ulcers.

Cetraxal *Salvat, Spain.*
Ciprofloxacin (p.182·3) or ciprofloxacin hydrochloride (p.182·3).
Bacterial infections.

Cetrazil *Virginia, Ital.*
Propylene glycol cefatrizine (p.164·3).
Bacterial infections.

Cetrexidin *Vebas, Ital.*
Chlorhexidine gluconate (p.1138·2); cetrimide (p.1137·1).
Mouth disinfection.

Cetrilan *Novaquimica, Braz.*
Cetrimide (p.1137·1); benzalkonium chloride (p.1133·2).
Skin disinfection.

Cetrin *Vitamed, Israel.*
Cetrimide (p.1137·1); chlorhexidine gluconate (p.1138·2).
Skin disinfection.

Cetrinets *Westmont, Hong Kong; Westmont, Singapore.*
Ascorbic acid (p.1389·3).
Vitamin C deficiency.

Cetrinox *Magis, Ital.*
Propylene glycol cefatrizine (p.164·3).
Bacterial infections.

Cetrisan *Gedis, Ital.*
Chlorhexidine gluconate (p.1138·2); cetrimide (p.1137·1).
Surface disinfection.

Cetrispect *Propan, S.Afr.†*
Mepyramine maleate (p.421·1); ammonium chloride (p.1085·2); sodium citrate (p.1186·2); ephedrine hydrochloride (p.1090·1).
Coughs.

Cetrizet *Sun, Thai.*
Cetirizine hydrochloride (p.411·2).
Allergic skin disorders; rhinitis.

Cetrizin *Sintofarma, Braz.*
Cetirizine hydrochloride (p.411·2).
Hypersensitivity reactions.

Cetrotide
Serono, Aust.; Serono, Austral.; Serono, Belg.; Serono, Denm.; Serono, Fin.; Serono, Fr.; Asta Medica, Ger.; Serono, Ger.; Serono, Ital.; Asta Medica, Neth.; Serono, Port.; Serono, Swed.; Serono, UK; Asta Medica, USA.
Cetrorelix acetate (p.1279·2).
Controlled ovarian stimulation.

Cetylcide II *Cetylite, USA.*
Alkyldimethylbenzylammonium chloride (p.1133·2); alkyldimethylethylbenzylammonium chloride.
Surface disinfection.

Cetylcide-G *Cetylite, USA.*
Glutaral (p.1145·2).
Instrument disinfection.

Cetylyre *Oberlin, Fr.*
Cetylpyridinium chloride (p.1138·1).
Eye disorders.

Cevalin
Lilly, Mex.; Lilly, USA†.
Ascorbic acid (p.1389·3).
Vitamin C deficiency.

Cevanil *Pharmasant, Thai.*
Pirenzepine hydrochloride (p.472·2).
Peptic ulcer.

Cevi-Bid *Geriatric Pharm. Corp., USA.*
Ascorbic acid (p.1389·3).
Vitamin C deficiency.

Cevi-Fer *Geriatric Pharm. Corp., USA.*
Ferrous fumarate (p.1360·1); folic acid (p.1361·1).
Ascorbic acid (p.1389·3) is included in this preparation to increase the absorption and availability of iron.
Iron and folic acid deficiency.

Cevirin *Esseti, Ital.*
Aciclovir (p.612·3).
Herpesvirus infections.

Ce-Vi-Sol *Mead Johnson Nutritionals, USA†.*
Ascorbic acid (p.1389·3).
Scurvy; vitamin C deficiency.

Cevi-Tabs *Ferrosan, Fin.*
Ascorbic acid (p.1389·3).
Vitamin C deficiency.

Cevitine *Warner-Lambert Consumer, Belg.†*
Ascorbic acid (p.1389·3); calcium ascorbate (p.1389·3).
Vitamin C deficiency; vitamin C supplement.

Cevitol *Lannacher, Aust.*
Ascorbic acid (p.1389·3).
Vitamin C deficiency.

Cewin *Sanofi Winthrop, Braz.*
Ascorbic acid (p.1389·3).
Vitamin C supplement.

Cezane *Laborsil, Braz.*
Acriflavinium chloride (p.1130·2); methenamine mandelate (p.223·1); methylene blue [methylthioninium chloride] (p.1012·3).
Urinary-tract infections.

Cezin *UAD, USA.*
Multivitamin and mineral preparation (p.1350·1).

Cezox *Pharmasant, Thai.*
Chlorzoxazone (p.1327·3); paracetamol (p.71·2).
Skeletal muscle pain and spasm.

C-Film
Geymonat, Ital.; Lucchini, Switz.; Arun, UK.
Nonoxinol 9 (p.1346·1).
Contraceptive.

CGT *Libbs, Braz.*
Multivitamin and mineral preparation (p.1350·1).

Chamo S *Ysatfabrik, Ger.*
Chamomile flowers (p.1593·2).
Anorectal disorders; mouth and throat inflammation; skin disorders; vaginitis; wounds.

Chamoca M *Hanosan, Ger.*
Homoeopathic preparation.

Chamomilla Comp *Weleda, Ger.*
Homoeopathic preparation.

Championyl *Sanofi Synthelabo, Ital.*
Sulpiride (p.706·1).
Dysthymia; psychoses.

Chantaline *Madaus, Spain.*
Theophylline (p.777·2).
Asthma; bronchospasm; heart failure; paroxysmal dyspnoea.

Chapstick
Note.This name is used for preparations of different composition.
Whitehall, Austral.
Padimate O (p.1518·2).

SPF 15: Padimate O (p.1518·2); oxybenzone (p.1518·1).
Dry or chapped lips; sunscreen for lips.

Whitehall, Port.†
SPF 4: Padimate (p.1518·2).
Dry or chapped lips; sunscreen.

Robins, USA.
Lip balm SPF 15: Padimate O (p.1518·2); oxybenzone (p.1518·1); titanium dioxide (p.1126·1).
Ointment SPF 15: Padimate O (p.1518·2); oxybenzone (p.1518·1).
Sunscreen.

Chapstick Lip Moisturizer *Whitehall-Robins, Canad.*
Octinoxate (p.1517·3); oxybenzone (p.1518·1).
Sunscreen.

Chapstick Medicated Lip Balm
Whitehall-Robins, Canad.; Robins, USA.
Yellow soft paraffin (p.1407·3); camphor (p.1589·3); menthol (p.1632·3); phenol (p.1152·3).

Chapstick Sun Block *Whitehall, Port.†*
SPF 15: Padimate (p.1518·2); oxybenzone (p.1518·1).
Dry or chapped lips; sunscreen.

Chapstick Sunblock *Whitehall-Robins, Canad.*
SPF 15: Padimate O (p.1518·2); oxybenzone (p.1518·1).
Sunscreen.

Charabs *Lane, UK.*
Caffeine (p.761·3); vitamin B substances (p.1350·1).
Tonic.

Charbon de Belloc *Chefaro Ardeval, Fr.*
Activated charcoal (p.1000·2).
Gastrointestinal disorders.

Charcoaid *Requa, USA.*
Activated charcoal (p.1000·2).
Emergency treatment of poisoning.

Charcoal Plus *Kramer, USA.*
Activated charcoal (p.1000·2).
Formerly contained simeticone and activated charcoal.
Flatulence.

Charcocaps
Key, Austral.; Requa, USA.
Activated charcoal (p.1000·2).
Diarrhoea; flatulence; poisoning.

Charcodote
Note.This name is used for preparations of different composition.
Pharmascience, Canad.
Activated charcoal (p.1000·2); sorbitol (p.1377·3).
Poison antidote.

Dominion, UK.
Activated charcoal (p.1000·2).
Emergency treatment of poisoning.

Charcodote Aqueous *Pharmascience, Canad.*
Activated charcoal (p.1000·2).
Poison antidote.

Charcotabs *Key, Austral.*
Activated charcoal (p.1000·2).
Diarrhoea; drug poisoning; excess gastrointestinal gas.

Chardonna-2 *Schwarz, USA.*
Belladonna (p.463·1); phenobarbital (p.355·1).
Gastrointestinal disorders.

Charlieu Anti-Poux *Mayoly-Spindler, Fr.*
Permethrin (p.1436·1); piperonyl butoxide (p.1436·2).
Lice infestation.

Charlieu Topic *Nigy, Fr.*
Urea (p.1127·3).
Dry skin disorders.

Charlieu Topicrem *Nigy, Fr.*
Urea (p.1127·3); glycerol (p.1616·3).
Dry skin disorders.

Chase Coldsorex *Stella, Canad.*
Benzoin (p.1668·3); camphor (p.1589·3); menthol (p.1632·3); myrrh (p.1639·2).

Chase Kolik Gripe Water *Stella, Canad.*
Alcohol (p.1130·3); ginger (p.1227·2); dill oil (p.1603·3); sodium bicarbonate (p.1186·2).

Chase Kolik Gripe Water Alcohol-Free *Stella, Canad.*
Fennel oil (p.1610·2); sodium bicarbonate (p.1186·2).

Chebil *Basi, Port.*
Chenodeoxycholic acid (p.1594·1).

Chefarine 4 *Chefaro, Neth.†.*
Aspirin (p.14·2); paracetamol (p.71·2).
Fever; pain.

Chefir *Drug Research, Ital.*
Cefonicid sodium (p.168·1).
Lignocaine [lidocaine] hydrochloride (p.1313·2) is included in this preparation to alleviate the pain of injection.
Bacterial infections.

Cheiranthol *Klein, Ger.*
Cheiranthus cheiri (p.2277); silybum marianum (p.1021·3); cnicus benedictus (p.1597·2); achillea (p.1572·2); hypericum (p.290·2).
Liver disorders.

Chek-Stix *Bayer, Austral.*
Positive and negative controls for tests for glucose, bilirubin, ketones, specific gravity, blood, pH, protein, urobilinogen, nitrite, and leucocytes in urine.

Chelated Bone Meal *Swiss Herbal, Canad.*
Calcium; phosphorus (p.1350·1).

Chelated Cal-Mag *GNLD, Austral.*
Calcium glycinate; magnesium glycinate; fish-liver oil.
Calcium and magnesium deficiency.

Chelated Cal-Mag plus Vitamin *Swiss Herbal, Canad.*
Calcium; magnesium; vitamin C; vitamin D (p.1350·1).

Chelated Dol Mite *Swiss Herbal, Canad.*
Calcium; magnesium (p.1350·1).

Chelated Dolomite *Jamieson, Canad.*
Calcium; magnesium (p.1350·1).

Chelated Solamins *Solgar, UK.*
Minerals as amino-acid chelates (p.1350·1).

Chelated Zinc *Richlife, Hong Kong.*
Zinc gluconate (p.1398·2); zinc proteinate (p.1398·3).
Mineral supplement.

Chelatran *SERB, Fr.*
Disodium edetate (p.1008·1).
Digitalis intoxication.

Chelidonium Compose *Boiron, Fr.*
Homoeopathic preparation.

Chelidophyt *Galenika, Ger.*
Greater celandine (p.1618·1).
Formerly contained greater celandine, achillea, peppermint leaf, and scopolia root.
Biliary and gastrointestinal spasm.

Chelintox *Braun, Switz.*
Sodium calcium edetate (p.1022·1).
Heavy-metal poisoning.

Chemacin *CT, Ital.*
Amikacin sulfate (p.148·1).
Bacterial infections.

Chemet
Janssen-Cilag, Aust.; Sanofi Winthrop, USA.
Succimer (p.1024·3).
Lead poisoning.

Chemicetina
Fournier, Ital.; Astra, Spain.
Chloramphenicol (p.179·1), chloramphenicol palmitate (p.179·2), chloramphenicol sodium succinate (p.179·2), or chloramphenicol stearate (p.181·1).
Bacterial infections.

Chemiofurin *Torlan, Spain†.*
Nitrofurantoin (p.230·3).
Urinary-tract infections.

Chemionazolo *NCSN, Ital.*
Econazole nitrate (p.382·3).
Fungal and bacterial skin and vulvovaginal infections.

Chemists Own Allergy Hayfever Sinus Relief *Hunter, Austral.*
Chlorpheniramine [chlorphenamine] maleate (p.412·1); pseudoephedrine hydrochloride (p.1099·2); paracetamol (p.71·2).
Hayfever; nasal and sinus congestion.

Chemists Own Clozole *Hunter, Austral.*
Clotrimazole (p.382·1).
Fungal skin infections; vaginal candidiasis.

Chemists Own Cold & Flu *Hunter, Austral.*
Paracetamol (p.71·2); pseudoephedrine hydrochloride (p.1099·2); codeine phosphate (p.25·2).
Cold and influenza symptoms.

Chemists Own Cold & Flu Medication for Day & Night *Hunter, Austral.*
Day tablets, Paracetamol (p.71·2); pseudoephedrine hydrochloride (p.1099·2); codeine phosphate (p.25·2); night tablets, paracetamol; pseudoephedrine hydrochloride; chlorpheniramine [chlorphenamine] maleate (p.412·1).
Cold and influenza symptoms.

Chemists Own Cold Sore *Hunter, Austral.*
Aciclovir (p.612·3).
Herpes labialis.

Chemists Own Coldeze *Hunter, Austral.*
Paracetamol (p.71·2); chlorpheniramine [chlorphenamine] maleate (p.412·1).
Cold and influenza symptoms; hayfever.

Chemists Own De Worm *Hunter, Austral.*
Mebendazole (p.102·2).
Worm infections.

Chemists Own Decongestant Nasal Spray *Hunter, Austral.*
Oxymetazoline hydrochloride (p.1096·2).
Nasal congestion.

Chemists Own Dexolix *Hunter, Austral.*
Chlorpheniramine [chlorphenamine] maleate (p.412·1); pseudoephedrine hydrochloride (p.1099·2); dextromethorphan hydrobromide (p.1087·3).
Coughs and cold symptoms.

Chemists Own Dolased *Hunter, Austral.*
Day tablets, paracetamol (p.71·2); codeine phosphate (p.25·2); night tablets, paracetamol; codeine phosphate; doxylamine succinate (p.417·1).
Pain.

Chemists Own Mucotuss *Hunter, Austral.*
Bromhexine (p.1085·3); pseudoephedrine hydrochloride (p.1099·2); guaifenesin (p.1092·2).
Coughs and cold symptoms.

Chemists Own Noesude *Hunter, Austral.*
Bromhexine hydrochloride (p.1085·3); guaifenesin (p.1092·2).
Coughs and cold symptoms.

Chemists Own Pain & Fever *Hunter, Austral.*
Paracetamol (p.71·2).
Fever; pain.

Chemists Own Pain Tablets *Hunter, Austral.*
Paracetamol (p.71·2); codeine phosphate (p.25·2).
Pain.

Chemists Own Peetalix *Hunter, Austral.*
Trimeprazine [alimemazine] tartrate (p.426·2).

Chemists Own Phescode *Hunter, Austral.*
Codeine phosphate (p.25·2); pseudoephedrine hydrochloride (p.1099·2).
Coughs and cold symptoms.

Chemists Own Sinus-Pain Relief *Hunter, Austral.*
Paracetamol (p.71·2); pseudoephedrine hydrochloride (p.1099·2).
Nasal congestion; sinusitis.

Chemists Own Ultra Sun *Hunter, Austral.*
SPF 30+: Octinoxate (p.1517·3); oxybenzone (p.1518·1); octocrilene (p.1518·1); zinc oxide (p.1128·2).
Sunscreen.

Chemists Own Zapazole *Hunter, Austral.*
Miconazole (p.391·1).
Fungal skin infections.

Chemists Own Zaymaz *Hunter, Austral.*
Chlorpheniramine [chlorphenamine] maleate (p.412·1); phenylephrine hydrochloride (p.1097·1).
Cold symptoms; hypersensitivity reactions.

Chemitrim
Biomedica, Hong Kong; Biomedica, Ital.
Co-trimoxazole (p.193·3).
Bacterial infections.

Chemoprim
Biolab, Hong Kong; Biolab, Singapore; Biolab, Thai.
Co-trimoxazole (p.193·3).
Bacterial infections.

Chemotrim *Rosemont, UK.*
Co-trimoxazole (p.193·3).
Bacterial infections.

Chemstrip 6 *Boehringer Mannheim, USA.*
Test for glucose, protein, blood, ketones, leukocytes, and pH in urine.

Chemstrip 7 *Boehringer Mannheim, USA.*
Test for glucose, protein, blood, ketones, bilirubin, leukocytes, and pH in urine.

Chemstrip 8 *Boehringer Mannheim, USA.*
Test for glucose, protein, blood, ketones, bilirubin, urobilinogen, leukocytes, and pH in urine.

Chemstrip 9 *Boehringer Mannheim, USA.*
Test for glucose, protein, blood, ketones, bilirubin, urobilinogen, nitrite, leukocytes, and pH in urine.

Chemstrip bG
Boehringer Mannheim, Canad.†; Boehringer Mannheim Diagnostics, USA.
Test for glucose in blood (p.1616·3).

Chemstrip 2 GP *Boehringer Mannheim, USA.*
Test for glucose and protein in urine.

Chemstrip K
Roche, Canad.; Boehringer Mannheim, USA.
Test for ketones in urine.

Chemstrip 2 LN *Boehringer Mannheim, USA.*
Test for nitrite and leukocytes in urine.

Chemstrip Micral *Boehringer Mannheim, USA.*
Test for albumin in urine.

Chemstrip 4 the OB *Boehringer Mannheim, USA.*
Test for glucose, protein, blood, and leukocytes in urine.

Chemstrip 10 with SG *Boehringer Mannheim, USA.*
Test for nitrite, pH, protein, glucose, ketones, urobilinogen, bilirubin, blood, leucocytes, and specific gravity in urine.

Chemstrip uG
Roche, Canad.; Boehringer Mannheim, USA.
Test for glucose in urine (p.1616·3).

Chemstrip uG 5000K *Roche, Canad.*
Test for glucose and ketones in urine.

Chemstrip uGK *Boehringer Mannheim, USA.*
Test for glucose and ketones in urine.

Chemstrip uG/K *Roche, Canad.*
Test for glucose and ketones in urine.

Chemydur *Waymade, UK.*
Isosorbide mononitrate (p.916·2).
Angina pectoris.

Chemyparin *SIT, Ital.*
Heparin sodium (p.902·1).
Eye disorders.

Chendol
CP Pharmaceuticals, Irl.†; CP Pharmaceuticals, UK†.
Chenodeoxycholic acid (p.1594·1).
Cholesterol gallstones.

Chenodex *Houde, Fr.†.*
Chenodeoxycholic acid (p.1594·1).
Cholesterol gallstones.

Chenofalk
Merck, Aust.; Codali, Belg.; Falk, Ger.; Falk, Hong Kong; Antigen, Irl.; Farmasa, Mex.; Falk, Neth.; Phardi, Switz.; Thames, UK†.
Chenodeoxycholic acid (p.1594·1).
Cholesterol gallstones.

Chephapyrin N *MIP, Ger.*
Aspirin (p.14·2); paracetamol (p.71·2); caffeine (p.761·3).
Cold symptoms; fever; pain.

Cheracap *Pharmacia Upjohn, Braz.*
Chlorpheniramine [chlorphenamine] (p.412·2); aspirin (p.14·2); caffeine (p.761·3); methoxyphenamine (p.1094·3).
Cold and influenza symptoms.

Cheracol
Note. This name is used for preparations of different composition.
Roberts, Canad.
Codeine phosphate (p.25·2); guaifenesin (p.1092·2); ammonium chloride (p.1085·2).
Coughs.

Pharmacia Upjohn, Mex.
Aspirin (p.14·2); caffeine (p.761·3); chlorpheniramine [chlorphenamine] maleate (p.412·1); methoxyphenamine hydrochloride (p.1094·3).
Cold and influenza symptoms.

Cheracol Cough *Roberts, USA.*
Codeine phosphate (p.25·2); guaifenesin (p.1092·2).
Coughs.

Cheracol D *Pharmacia Upjohn, Mex.*
Dextromethorphan hydrobromide (p.1087·3); guaifenesin (p.1092·2).
Coughs.

Cheracol D Cough *Roberts, USA.*
Dextromethorphan hydrobromide (p.1087·3); guaifenesin (p.1092·2).
Coughs.

Cheracol Nasal *Roberts, USA†.*
Oxymetazoline hydrochloride (p.1096·2).

Cheracol Plus *Lee, USA.*
Dextromethorphan hydrobromide (p.1087·3); guaifenesin (p.1092·2).
Formerly contained phenylpropanolamine hydrochloride, chlorpheniramine [chlorphenamine] maleate, and dextromethorphan hydrobromide.
Coughs and cold symptoms.

Cheracol Sore Throat *Roberts, USA.*
Phenol (p.1152·3).
Sore throat.

Cheripex *Ranbaxy, Thai.*
Diphenhydramine hydrochloride (p.416·1); sodium citrate (p.1186·2); ammonium chloride (p.1085·2); menthol (p.1632·3).
Cough and cold symptoms.

Chest Cold Relief *Brauer, Austral.*
Homoeopathic preparation.
Formerly known as Chest Cold Complex.

Chest Mixture *Potter's, UK.*
Horehound (p.1094·2); pleurisy root (p.1653·1); senega (p.1100·2); lobelia (p.1510·2); acetum scillae (p.1100·3).
Catarrh; coughs.

Chest Rub *Mentholatum, Canad.*
Camphor (p.1589·2); eucalyptus oil (p.1609·2); menthol (p.1632·3).
Formerly known as Cherry Chest Rub.

Chetotest *SPA, Ital.†.*
Test for acetone in urine.

Chew-E
Eagle, Austral.
d-Alpha tocoferil acid succinate (p.1394·1).
Vitamin E supplement.

Ranbaxy, Thai.
dl-Alpha tocoferil acetate (p.1394·1).
Vitamin E deficiency.

Chewies *Malayan, Hong Kong.*
Vitamin C (p.1389·3).
Vitamin C deficiency; vitamin C supplement.

Chiana *Bio-Diat, Ger.*
Peppermint oil (p.1243·3).
Irritable bowel syndrome.

Chibretico *Chibret, Port.*
Amiloride hydrochloride (p.835·1); hydrochlorothiazide (p.907·3).
Hypertension; oedema.

Chibro Uvelina *Merck Sharp & Dohme, Spain.*
Methylhydroxyquinoline metilsulfate (p.1635·2).
Eye irritation.

Chibro-Amuno 3 *Chibret, Ger.*
Indometacin (p.44·3).
Macular oedema following cataract surgery.

Chibro-Atropine *Merck Sharp & Dohme-Chibret, Fr.*
Atropine sulfate (p.461·1).
Eye disorders.

Chibro-Boraline *Merck Sharp & Dohme, Switz.*
Oxedrine tartrate (p.950·3); borax (p.1586·1); boric acid (p.1586·1).
Eye irritation.

Chibro-Cadron
Merck Sharp & Dohme-Chibret, Fr.; Chibret, Ger.†.
Dexamethasone sodium phosphate (p.1067·1); neomycin sulfate (p.228·1).
Eye disorders.

Chibro-Kerakain *Chibret, Ger.†.*
Proxymetacaine hydrochloride (p.1320·1).
Local anaesthesia.

Chibro-Pilocarpine *Merck Sharp & Dohme-Chibret, Fr.*
Pilocarpine nitrate (p.1422·3).
Glaucoma; reversal of mydriasis.

Chibro-Proscar *Merck Sharp & Dohme-Chibret, Fr.*
Finasteride (p.1477·2).
Benign prostatic hyperplasia.

Chibro-Timoptol *Chibret, Ger.*
Timolol maleate (p.982·1).
Glaucoma; ocular hypertension.

Chibroxin
Merck Sharp & Dohme, Braz.; Chibret, Ger.; Merck Sharp & Dohme, Hong Kong; Merck Sharp & Dohme, Israel; Merck Sharp & Dohme, Singapore; Merck Sharp & Dohme, Spain; Merck, USA.
Norfloxacin (p.232·1).
Bacterial eye infections.

Chibroxine *Merck Sharp & Dohme-Chibret, Fr.*
Norfloxacin (p.232·1).
Eye infections.

Chibroxol
Merck Sharp & Dohme, Belg.; Merck Sharp & Dohme, Neth.; Chibret, Port.; Merck Sharp & Dohme, Switz.
Norfloxacin (p.232·1).
Bacterial eye infections.

Chiclida *Torrens, Spain.*
Meclozine hydrochloride (p.420·3).
Motion sickness.

Chiggerex *Scherer, USA.*
Benzocaine (p.1306·2); camphor (p.1589·2); menthol (p.1632·3).
Skin disorders.

Chigger-Tox *Scherer, USA.*
Benzocaine (p.1306·2).
Local anaesthesia.

Chilblain Formula *Vitaplex, Austral.*
Nicotinamide (p.1372·3); acetomenaphthone (p.1395·3).
Chilblains; poor peripheral circulation.

Chilblains Ointment *Nelson, UK.*
Homoeopathic preparation.

Child Chew C *Bullivants, Austral.*
Calcium ascorbate (p.1389·3); bioflavonoids (p.1611·1).
Vitamin C supplement.

Child Formula *Avon, Canad.*
Multivitamin preparation (p.1350·1).

Children's Allerest *Ciba, USA†.*
Phenylpropanolamine hydrochloride (p.1098·1); chlorpheniramine [chlorphenamine] maleate (p.412·1).
Upper respiratory-tract symptoms.

Childrens Appetite Tonic *Bullivants, Austral.*
Lysine hydrochloride; ferric pyrophosphate; vitamin B substances (p.1350·1).
Loss of appetite; tonic.

Children's Calcium With Minerals *Cenovis, Austral.†; Vitelle, Austral.†.*
Calcium ascorbate (p.1389·3); colecalciferol (p.1391·1); ferrous fumarate (p.1360·1); folic acid (p.1361·1); zinc amino acid chelate (p.1398·3).
Dietary supplement.

Childrens Cepacol *JB Williams, USA.*
Paracetamol (p.71·2); pseudoephedrine hydrochloride (p.1099·2).
Upper respiratory-tract disorders.

Childrens Cherry Sucrets *SmithKline Beecham, Israel.*
Dyclonine hydrochloride (p.1311·3).
Sore throat.

Childrens Chesty Cough Syrup *Boots, UK.*
Guaifenesin (p.1092·2).
Formerly known as Nirolex for Children.
Coughs.

Childrens Chewable
Quest, Canad.; Quest, UK.
Multivitamin and mineral preparation (p.1350·1).

Childrens Chewable Vita-Mins *Seroyal, Canad.*
Multivitamin and mineral preparation (p.1350·1).

Childrens Chewables *Sisu, Canad.*
Multivitamin and mineral preparation (p.1350·1).

Childrens Coltalin with Vit B₁ *Fortune, Hong Kong.*
Paracetamol (p.71·2); chlorpheniramine [chlorphenamine] maleate (p.412·1); phenylephrine hydrochloride (p.1097·1); vitamin B₁ (p.1385·2).
Respiratory-tract disorders.

Childrens Diarrhoea Mixture *Unichem, UK.*
Kaolin (p.1229·3).
Diarrhoea.

Childrens Dynafed Jr *BDI, USA.*
Paracetamol (p.71·2).
Fever; pain.

The symbol † denotes a preparation no longer actively marketed

Childrens Feverhalt *Wampole, Canad.*
Paracetamol (p.71·2).
Fever; pain.

Children's Formula Cough *Pharmakon, USA.*
Dextromethorphan hydrobromide (p.1087·3); guaifenesin (p.1092·2).
Coughs.

Children's Kaopectate *Upjohn, USA.*
Attapulgite (p.1212·1).
Diarrhoea.

Childrens Mapap *Major, USA.*
Paracetamol (p.71·2).
Fever; pain.

Childrens Motion Sickness Liquid *Tanta, Canad.*
Dimenhydrinate (p.415·2).

Childrens Motrin Cold *McNeil Consumer, USA.*
Ibuprofen (p.43·2); pseudoephedrine hydrochloride (p.1099·2).
Cold and influenza symptoms.

Childrens Multi *Vitaplex, Austral.*
Multivitamin and mineral preparation with lysine hydrochloride (p.1350·1).

Children's Multivitamins *Cenovis, Austral.; Vitelle, Austral.*
Multivitamin and mineral preparation (p.1350·1).

Children's Nostril *Ciba, USA.*
Phenylephrine hydrochloride (p.1097·1).
Nasal congestion.

Childrens Nyquil *Procter & Gamble, Canad.*
Pseudoephedrine hydrochloride (p.1099·2); chlorpheniramine [chlorphenamine] maleate (p.412·1); dextromethorphan hydrobromide (p.1087·3).
Coughs and cold symptoms.

Childrens Panadol *SmithKline Beecham Consumer, Austral.*
Paracetamol (p.71·2).
Fever; pain.

Childrens Sudafed Cold & Cough *Warner-Lambert, USA.*
Pseudoephedrine hydrochloride (p.1099·2); dextromethorphan hydrobromide (p.1087·3).
Coughs and cold symptoms.

Childrens Sudafed Nasal Decongestant *Warner-Lambert, USA.*
Pseudoephedrine hydrochloride (p.1099·2).
Nasal congestion.

Children's SunKist Multivitamins Complete *Ciba, USA.*
Multivitamin and mineral preparation (p.1350·1).

Children's SunKist Multivitamins + Extra C *Ciba, USA.*
Multivitamin preparation (p.1350·1).

Children's SunKist Multivitamins + Iron *Ciba, USA.*
Multivitamin preparation with iron (p.1350·1).

Children's Tylenol Cold Multi-Symptom *McNeil Consumer, USA.*
Pseudoephedrine hydrochloride (p.1099·2); chlorpheniramine [chlorphenamine] maleate (p.412·1); paracetamol (p.71·2).
Upper respiratory-tract symptoms.

Children's Tylenol Cold Multi-Symptom Plus Cough *McNeil Consumer, USA.*
Paracetamol (p.71·2); dextromethorphan hydrobromide (p.1087·3); chlorpheniramine [chlorphenamine] maleate (p.412·1); pseudoephedrine hydrochloride (p.1099·2).
Coughs and cold symptoms.

Childrevit *Diviser Aquilea, Spain.*
Cyproheptadine hydrochloride (p.414·2); amino acids and vitamins (p.1350·1).
Tonic.

Chimar *Sanitas, Port.*
Chymotrypsin (p.1595·1); trypsin (p.1675·3).
Adjunct to antibiotics; inflammation; oedema; respiratory-tract congestion.

Chimax *Chiron, UK.*
Flutamide (p.542·3).
Prostatic cancer.

Chimodil *Yamanouchi, Ital.*
Aluminium hydroxide (p.1210·3); magnesium hydroxide (p.1233·1).
Dyspepsia associated with gastric hyperacidity.

Chimono *Lusofarmaco, Ital.*
Lomefloxacin hydrochloride (p.220·1).
Bacterial infections.

China Diarrhea L107 *Homeocan, Canad.*
Homoeopathic preparation.

China Eisenwein *Ungar, Aust.*
Ferrous citrate; tinct. cinchona comp (p.1595·3).
Iron deficiency; tonic.

China Med Complex *Dynamit, Aust.*
Homoeopathic preparation.

China-Balsam
Note. This name is used for preparations of different composition.
Sanamed, Aust.
Camphor (p.1589·3); clove oil (p.1597·1); menthol (p.1632·3).
Musculoskeletal and joint disorders; neuralgia; respiratory-tract disorders.

Bio-Diat, Ger.
Camphor (p.1589·3); clove oil (p.1597·1); eucalyptus oil (p.1609·2); Norway spruce oil; menthol (p.1632·3).
Catarrh; fatigue; headache; musculoskeletal pain; toothache.

China-Eisenwein *Mayrhofer, Aust.*
Mace flowers; gentian (p.1615·1); bitter-orange peel (p.1644·2); centaury (p.1593·1); ceratonia (p.1500·3); cinchona bark (p.1595·3); cinnamon (p.1595·3); ferrous citrate; ferrous ascorbate (p.1359·3).
Tonic.

China-Oel *Bio-Diat, Ger.*
Peppermint oil (p.1243·3).
Cold symptoms; neuromuscular pain; smooth muscle spasm.

Chinoidina *Giovanardi, Ital.*
Cinchona calisaya (p.1595·3); gentian (p.1615·1); kola (p.1681·1).
Dyspepsia.

Chinosol *Chinosolfabrik, Ger.*
Hydroxyquinoline sulfate (p.1622·2); potassium sulfate (p.1195·1).
Skin disinfection.

Chinosol S Vaseline *Chinosolfabrik, Ger.†*
Hydroxyquinoline sulfate (p.1622·2); potassium sulfate (p.1195·1).
Infective skin disorders.

Chinta *Chinta, Thai.*
Dextromethorphan hydrobromide (p.1087·3); ammonium chloride (p.1085·2); calcium pantothenate (p.1374·1); liquorice (p.1231·2).
Coughs.

Chinteina *Lafare, Ital.*
Quinidine sulfate (p.964·3).
Arrhythmias.

Chirocaine
Abbott, Neth.; Abbott, Swed.; Abbott, UK; Purdue Frederick, USA.
Levobupivacaine hydrochloride (p.1312·3).
Local anaesthesia.

Chirofossat N *Dreluso, Ger.*
Homoeopathic preparation.

Chiron Barrier Cream *Simcare, UK.*
Aluminium chlorohydrate (p.1110·2).

Chironair Odour Control Liquid *Simcare, UK.*
A deodorant for use with colostomies and ileostomies.

Chiroplexan H *Pflüger, Ger.*
Homoeopathic preparation.

Chisi *Propan, S.Afr.†.*
Turpentine oil (p.1676·3); rectified camphor oil; capsicum oleoresin (p.1591·1); methyl salicylate (p.55·1).
Musculoskeletal and joint disorders.

Chitosano *SIRC, Singapore.*
Poliglusam; hydroxycitric acid; chromium; vitamin C; guar gum; zinc sulfate; ferrous gluconate; vanadium pentoxide (p.1350·1).
Dietary aid in weight reduction.

Chlo-Amine *Hollister-Stier, USA.*
Chlorpheniramine [chlorphenamine] maleate (p.412·1).
Hypersensitivity reactions.

Chlobax *Beacons, Singapore.*
Chlordiazepoxide (p.659·2); clidinium bromide (p.465·1).
Gastrointestinal disorders.

Chloment *Denk, Hong Kong.*
Chloramphenicol (p.179·1).
Eye infections.

Chlomide *MPF, Singapore.*
Chlorpropamide (p.321·1).
Diabetes mellitus.

Chlomy-P *Sankyo, Hong Kong.*
Chloramphenicol (p.179·1); neomycin sulfate (p.228·1); prednisolone (p.1077·3).
Infected skin disorders.

Chlor *Vortech, USA†.*
Chlorpheniramine [chlorphenamine] maleate (p.412·1).
Hypersensitivity reactions.

Chlor-3 *Fleming, USA.*
Sodium chloride (p.1196·1); potassium chloride (p.1194·3); magnesium chloride (p.1190·3).
Medical condiment; table salt substitute.

Chloracil *Siam Bheasach, Thai.*
Chloramphenicol (p.179·1).
Bacterial eye or ear infections.

Chloractil *DDSA Pharmaceuticals, UK.*
Chlorpromazine hydrochloride (p.660·2).
Anxiety; intractable hiccup; premedication; psychoses; vomiting.

Chloraethyl "Dr Henning" *Henning Walldorf, Ger.*
Ethyl chloride (p.1312·1).
Local anaesthesia.

Chlorafed *Roberts, USA.*
Chlorpheniramine [chlorphenamine] maleate (p.412·1); pseudoephedrine hydrochloride (p.1099·2).
Cold symptoms.

Chloraldurat
Sanova, Aust.; Pohl, Ger.; Pohl, Neth.†; Pohl, Switz.
Chloral hydrate (p.669·3).
Insomnia; sedative.

Chloram-D *Nakornpatana, Thai.*
Chloramphenicol palmitate (p.179·2).
Bacterial infections.

Chloramex *Aspen, S.Afr.*
Chloramphenicol (p.179·1).
Eye infections.

Chloramex H *Lagamed, S.Afr.†.*
Chloramphenicol (p.179·1); hydrocortisone acetate (p.1073·3).
Inflammatory bacterial infections.

Chloraminophene *Techni-Pharma, Mon.*
Chlorambucil (p.516·3).
Glomerulonephritis; leukaemia; lymphoma.

Chlorammonic *Chiesi, Ital.*
Ammonium chloride (p.1085·2).
Alkalosis; urinary-tract disorders.

Chloramon *Streuli, Switz.*
Ammonium chloride (p.1085·2).
Bronchitis; metabolic alkalosis.

Chloramsaar N *Chephasaar, Ger.*
Chloramphenicol (p.179·1).
Bacterial infections.

Chlorasept *Baxter, UK.*
Chlorhexidine acetate (p.1138·2).
Bladder irrigation; skin disinfection.

Chloraseptic Lozenges *Procter & Gamble, Canad.*
Benzocaine (p.1306·2); menthol (p.1632·3).
Sore throat and mouth.

Chloraseptic Sore Throat Spray *Procter & Gamble, Canad.*
Phenol (p.1152·3).

Chlorasol *Seton, Israel; SSL, UK.*
Sodium hypochlorite (p.1156·2).
Skin disinfection.

Chlorate *Major, USA†.*
Chlorpheniramine [chlorphenamine] maleate (p.412·1).
Hypersensitivity reactions.

Chlorazin *Streuli, Switz.*
Chlorpromazine hydrochloride (p.660·2).
Nausea; pain; pruritus; psychoses; vertigo; vomiting.

Chlorazol *Qualiphar, Belg.*
Tosylchloramide sodium (p.1159·1).
Disinfection.

Chlorcol *Propan, S.Afr.*
Chloramphenicol (p.179·1).
Bacterial infections.

Chlordrine *Rugby, USA.*
Pseudoephedrine hydrochloride (p.1099·2); chlorpheniramine [chlorphenamine] maleate (p.412·1).
Upper respiratory-tract symptoms.

Chloresium *Rystan, USA.*
Chlorophyllin copper complex (p.1028·1).
Relief of malodour of wounds and ulcers; wound healing.

Chlorethyl *Adroka, Switz.*
Ethyl chloride (p.1312·1).
Local anaesthesia.

Chlorgest *Ranbaxy, Thai.*
Chlorpheniramine [chlorphenamine] maleate (p.412·1); phenylephrine hydrochloride (p.1097·1).
Nasal congestion.

Chlorgest-HD *Great Southern, USA†.*
Phenylephrine hydrochloride (p.1097·1); chlorpheniramine [chlorphenamine] maleate (p.412·1); hydrocodone tartrate (p.42·2).
Coughs and cold symptoms.

Chlorhexamed
Procter & Gamble, Aust.; Block, Ger.; Procter & Gamble, Switz.
Chlorhexidine gluconate (p.1138·2).
Mouth infections; oral hygiene.

Chlorhexseptic *Pharmascience, Canad.†.*
Chlorhexidine gluconate (p.1138·2).
Disinfection.

Chlorhist *Propan, S.Afr.*
Chlorpheniramine [chlorphenamine] maleate (p.412·1).
Hypersensitivity reactions.

Chlorhistan *Hua, Thai.*
Chlorpheniramine [chlorphenamine] maleate (p.412·1); phenylephrine hydrochloride (p.1097·1); paracetamol (p.71·2).
Cold symptoms; nasal congestioon.

Chlorispray *Anios, Fr.*
Chlorhexidine gluconate (p.1138·2); formaldehyde (p.1144·2); glutaral (p.1145·2); didecyldimethylammonium chloride (p.1143·2); alcohol (p.1130·3).
Surface disinfection.

Chlorleate *Silom, Thai.*
Chlorpheniramine [chlorphenamine] maleate (p.412·1).
Hypersensitivity reactions.

Chlorleate Expectorant *Silom, Thai.*
Chlorpheniramine [chlorphenamine] maleate (p.412·1); ammonium chloride (p.1085·2); sodium citrate (p.1186·2).
Coughs; nasal congestion.

Chlornicol *Genpharm, S.Afr.*
Chloramphenicol (p.179·1).
Bacterial eye infections.

Chlorochin *Streuli, Switz.*
Chloroquine phosphate (p.432·3).
Lupus erythematosus; malaria; polyarthritis.

Chlorocort *Parke, Davis, Austral.†.*
Chloramphenicol (p.179·1); hydrocortisone acetate (p.1073·3).
Eye infections.

Chlorohex
Colgate Oral Care, Austral.†; Asta Medica, Port.†; Colgate-Palmolive, UK.
Chlorhexidine gluconate (p.1138·2).
Mouth infections; oral hygiene.

Geistlich, Singapore.
Chlorhexidine (p.1138·2).
Skin and wound disinfection.

Geistlich, Switz.
Chlorhexidine gluconate (p.1138·2) and/or chlorhexidine hydrochloride (p.1138·2).
Skin and hand disinfection.

Chlorohistol *Julphar, UAE.*
Chlorpheniramine [chlorphenamine] maleate (p.412·1).
Hypersensitivity.

Chloro-Magnesion *Pautrat, Fr.*
Magnesium chloride (p.1190·3); calcium chloride (p.1188·1).
Magnesium deficiency.

Chloromycetin
Parke, Davis, Austral.; Parke, Davis, Canad.; Parke, Davis, Fin.; Goldshield, Irl.; Parke, Davis, Ital.; Warner-Lambert, Mex.; Parke, Davis, NZ; Parke, Davis, S.Afr.; Parke, Davis, Spain; Parke, Davis, Swed.; Parke, Davis, Switz.†; Forley, UK; Parke, Davis, UK†; Monarch, USA.
Chloramphenicol (p.179·1), chloramphenicol palmitate (p.179·2), chloramphenicol sodium succinate (p.179·2), or chloramphenicol succinate (p.181·1).
Bacterial eye infections.

Chloromycetin Hydrocortison *Parke, Davis, Swed.†.*
Chloramphenicol (p.179·1); hydrocortisone acetate (p.1073·3).
Eye inflammation with bacterial infection.

Chloromycetin Hydrocortisone
Parke, Davis, UK†; Parke, Davis, USA†.
Chloramphenicol (p.179·1); hydrocortisone acetate (p.1073·3).
Eye inflammation with bacterial infection.

Chloropect *Covan, S.Afr.*
Kaolin (p.1229·3); pectin (p.1502·3); bismuth subcarbonate (p.1213·1); chloroform and morphine tincture (p.56·1).
Diarrhoea.

Chloroph *Seng, Thai.*
Chloramphenicol (p.179·1).
Bacterial eye infections.

Chlorophyl liquid "Schuh" *Coradol, Ger.*
Chlorophyllin (p.1028·1); crataegus (p.1600·2).
Asthenia; deodorant.

Chlorophyll *Potter's, UK.*
Kola nut (p.1681·1); chlorophyllin (p.1028·1).
Tonic.

Chlorophyllin Salbe "Schuh" *Coradol, Ger.*
Chlorophyllin (p.1028·1); chamomilla; arnica; hamamelis (p.1618·3).
Wounds.

Chloropotassuril *Melisana, Belg.*
Potassium chloride (p.1194·3).
Potassium depletion.

Chloroptic
Allergan, Canad.†; Allergan, Irl.; Allergan, Israel; Allergan, NZ; Allergan, S.Afr.; Allergan, USA.
Chloramphenicol (p.179·1).
Bacterial eye infections.

Chlorosin *General Drugs, Thai.*
Chloramphenicol palmitate (p.179·2).
Bacterial infections.

Chlorotracin *Chew, Thai.*
Chloramphenicol (p.179·1); clioquinol (p.190·2); phthalylsulfathiazole (p.235·3).
Gastrointestinal infections.

Chlorphed-LA *Roberts, USA; Hauck, USA.*
Oxymetazoline hydrochloride (p.1096·2).
Nasal congestion.

Chlorphedrine SR *Goldline, USA.*
Pseudoephedrine hydrochloride (p.1099·2); chlorpheniramine [chlorphenamine] maleate (p.412·1).
Upper respiratory-tract symptoms.

Chlorphen *Caps, S.Afr.*
Chloramphenicol (p.179·1).
Bacterial infections.

Chlor-Pro *Schein, USA.*
Chlorpheniramine [chlorphenamine] maleate (p.412·1).
Hypersensitivity reactions.

Chlorpromanyl *Technilab, Canad.*
Chlorpromazine hydrochloride (p.660·2).
Nausea and vomiting; psychoses.

Chlorpromed *Medifive, Thai.*
Chlorpromazine hydrochloride (p.660·2).
Mania; nausea and vomiting; schizophrenia; sedation.

Chlorpyrimine
Atlantic, Hong Kong; Atlantic, Singapore; Atlantic, Thai.
Chlorpheniramine [chlorphenamine] maleate (p.412·1).
Hypersensitivity reactions.

Chlorquin
Rhone-Poulenc Rorer, Austral.; Fisons, Hong Kong.
Chloroquine phosphate (p.432·3).
Amoebic hepatitis; lupus erythematosus; malaria; rheumatoid arthritis and related collagen disease.

Chlor-Rest *Rugby, USA†.*
Phenylpropanolamine hydrochloride (p.1098·1); chlorpheniramine [chlorphenamine] maleate (p.412·1).
Upper respiratory-tract symptoms.

Chlorsig
Sigma, Austral.; Sigma, Hong Kong; Pharmaco, NZ.
Chloramphenicol (p.179·1).
Bacterial eye infections.

Chlorspan *Vortech, USA†.*
Chlorpheniramine [chlorphenamine] maleate (p.412·1).
Hypersensitivity reactions.

Chlortralim
Atlantic, Hong Kong; Atlantic, Singapore; Atlantic, Thai.
Chlortetracycline hydrochloride (p.182·1).
Bacterial eye infections.

Chlor-Trimeton
Schering-Plough, S.Afr.; Schering-Plough, USA.
Chlorpheniramine [chlorphenamine] maleate (p.412·1).
Hypersensitivity reactions.

Chlor-Trimeton Allergy Sinus *Schering-Plough, USA†.*
Phenylpropanolamine hydrochloride (p.1098·1); chlorpheniramine [chlorphenamine] maleate (p.412·1); paracetamol (p.71·2).
Upper respiratory-tract symptoms.

Chlor-Trimeton 4 Hour Relief *Schering-Plough, USA.*
Pseudoephedrine sulfate (p.1099·3); chlorpheniramine [chlorphenamine] maleate (p.412·1).
Upper respiratory-tract symptoms.

Chlor-Trimeton 12 Hour Relief *Schering-Plough, USA.*
Pseudoephedrine sulfate (p.1099·3); chlorpheniramine [chlorphenamine] maleate (p.412·1).
Upper respiratory-tract symptoms.

Chlor-Tripolon *Schering, Canad.*
Chlorpheniramine [chlorphenamine] maleate (p.412·1).
Hypersensitivity disorders; pruritus.

Chlor-Tripolon Decongestant *Schering, Canad.*
Syrup†: Chlorpheniramine [chlorphenamine] maleate (p.412·1); phenylpropanolamine hydrochloride (p.1098·1).
Tablets: Chlorpheniramine [chlorphenamine] maleate (p.412·1); pseudoephedrine sulfate (p.1099·3).
Respiratory congestion.

Chlor-Tripolon ND *Schering, Canad.*
Loratadine (p.420·1); pseudoephedrine sulfate (p.1099·3).
Upper respiratory-tract congestion.

Chlorumagene
Thepenier, Fr.†; Thepenier, Switz.
Magnesium hydroxide (p.1233·1).
Constipation.

Chlorvescent
Rhone-Poulenc Rorer, Austral.
Potassium chloride (p.1194·3); potassium bicarbonate (p.1186·1).
Potassium deficiency.

Aventis, NZ.
Potassium chloride (p.1194·3).
Potassium supplement.

Chlorzide *MPF, Singapore.*
Chlorothiazide (p.856·3).
Hypertension; oedema.

Chlorzox *Pharmasant, Thai.*
Chlorzoxazone (p.1327·3).
Skeletal muscle pain and spasm.

Chlotride
Amrad, Austral.; Merck Sharp & Dohme, Denm.; Merck Sharp & Dohme, Neth.†.
Chlorothiazide (p.856·3).
Hypertension; oedema.

Chocaton *Mirren, S.Afr.*
Multivitamin preparation (p.1350·1).

Chocovite
Torbet, Ital.†; Torbet Laboratories, UK.
Calcium gluconate (p.1188·2); ergocalciferol (p.1391·2).
Calcium and vitamin D deficiency.

Chofabol *Allen, Mex.*
Magnesium sulfate (p.1191·1); boldo (p.1585·3); cynara (p.1601·3); belladonna (p.463·1); peptone.
Biliary-tract disorders.

Chofranina *De Mayo, Braz.*
Cascara (p.1216·1); cynara (p.1601·3); carmellose (p.1499·3).
Constipation.

Choice DM
Mead Johnson, Hong Kong; Mead Johnson, Singapore; Mead Johnson Nutritionals, Thai.; Mead Johnson Nutritionals, USA.
Preparation for enteral nutrition (p.1350·1).
Abnormal glucose tolerance.

Chol 4000 *Lichtenstein, Ger.†.*
Greater celandine (p.1618·1).
Biliary and gastrointestinal spasm.

Cholac *Alra, USA.*
Lactulose (p.1230·1).
Constipation; hepatic encephalopathy.

Cholacid *Madaus, Ger.†.*
Ursodeoxycholic acid (p.1677·2).
Biliary-tract disorders.

Cholagogum F *Rhone-Poulenc Rorer, Ger.*
Turmeric (p.1029·3); greater celandine (p.1618·1).
Biliary-tract disorders.

Cholagogum N *Rhone-Poulenc Rorer, Ger.*
Greater celandine (p.1618·1); turmeric (p.1029·3); peppermint oil (p.1243·3).
Biliary disorders; gallstones.

Cholagutt *Hoeport, Port.*
Greater celandine (p.1618·1); silybum marianum (p.1021·3); peppermint leaf (p.1243·2); lavender (p.1627·2); calamus (p.1588·1); podophyllum (p.1121·1).
Biliary tract disorders.

Cholagutt-N *Albert-Roussel, Ger.; Hoechst, Ger.; Biocur, Ger.*
Greater celandine (p.1618·1); lavandula latifolia; peppermint leaf (p.1243·2).
Biliary disorders; gallstones.

Cholaktol *Medopharm, Ger.*
Peppermint oil (p.1243·3).
Gastrointestinal and biliary spasm.

Cholan-HMB *Ciba Consumer, USA†.*
Dehydrocholic acid (p.1602·2).
Biliary stasis; constipation.

Cholapret *Bionorica, Ger.*
Boldo (p.1585·3); greater celandine (p.1618·1); curcuma zanthorrhiza.
Biliary disorders; gastrointestinal disorders; liver disorders.

Chol-Arbuz N *Bittermedizin, Ger.*
Papain (p.1647·3); pancreatin (p.1646·1); turmeric (p.1029·3).
Biliary-tract disorders; liver disorders.

Cholarist *Steiner, Ger.*
Greater celandine (p.1618·1).
Smooth muscle spasm.

Cholasitrol *Lifeplan, UK.*
Sitosterol (p.970·3); vitamins; minerals (p.1350·1).
Nutritional supplement.

Cholasyn *Rolmex, Canad.*
Cascara (p.1216·1); senna (p.1248·2).
Formerly contained cascara and phenolphthalein.

Cholasyn II *Rolmex, Canad.*
Cascara (p.1216·1); senna (p.1248·2).
Biliary-tract disorders.

Choldestal *Krugmann, Ger.*
Turmeric (p.1029·3).
Dyspepsia.

Chol-Do *Grasler, Ger.*
Homoeopathic preparation.

Cholebrin *Nycomed, Swed.†.*
Iocetamic acid (p.1033·3).
Contrast medium for cholecystography.

Cholebrine
Asta Medica, Neth.; Mallinckrodt, USA†.
Iocetamic acid (p.1033·3).
Contrast medium for cholecystography.

Chole-cyl Ho-Len-Complex *Liebermann, Ger.*
Homoeopathic preparation.

Cholecysmon *SmithKline Beecham, Ger.*
Ox bile extract (p.1585·1).
Liver, bile, and pancreas disorders.

Choledyl
Parke, Davis, Canad.; Parke, Davis, Irl.; Parke, Davis, S.Afr.†; Parke, Davis, UK†; Warner Chilcott, USA.
Choline theophyllinate (p.763·3).
Obstructive airways disease.

Choledyl Expectorant *Parke, Davis, Canad.*
Choline theophyllinate (p.763·3); guaifenesin (p.1092·2).
Obstructive airways disease.

Cholegerol *Holistica, Fr.*
Soya lecithin (p.1628·1); wheat germ; shiitake; herbs (p.1350·1).
Cholesterol reduction.

Cholemin *Berk, UK†.*
Colestyramine (p.864·1).
Hyperlipidaemias.

Choleodoron
Note.This name is used for preparations of different composition.
Weleda, Aust.
Greater celandine (p.1618·1); curcuma zanthorrhiza.
Liver and gallbladder disorders.

Weleda, Fr.; Weleda, Ger.; Weleda, UK.
Homoeopathic preparation.

Cholesolvin *Cyanamid, Ital.†; Yoshitomi, Jpn†.*
Simfibrate (p.969·2).
Hyperlipidaemias.

Cholestabyl *Fournier, Ger.*
Colestipol hydrochloride (p.863·3).
Hypercholesterolaemia.

Cholesterol Support *Reese, USA.*
Sitosterol (p.970·3); zinc citrate.

Cholestin *Pharmanex, USA.*
Monascus purpureus Went.
Nutritional supplement.

Cholest-X L112 *Homeocan, Canad.*
Homoeopathic preparation.

Choletec
Squibb Diagnostics, Canad.†; Squibb Diagnostics, USA†.
Technetium-99m mebrofenin (p.1451·1).
Hepatobiliary imaging.

Cholex *Silanes, Mex.*
Menthol (p.1632·3); pinene; menthone; borneol; camphene; eucalyptol (p.1609·2).
Biliary-tract disorders.

Chol-Grandelat *Synpharma, Aust.*
Chamomile (p.1593·2); peppermint oil (p.1243·3); achillea (p.1572·2).
Gallbladder disorders.

Cholhepan N *Schuck, Ger.*
Silybum marianum (p.1021·3); greater celandine (p.1618·1); aloes (p.1210·1).
Biliary disorders; constipation.

Choliatron *Seber, Port.*
Trepibutone (p.1674·2).
Biliary-tract disorders; pancreatitis.

Cholidase *Freeda, USA.*
Vitamin B substances with vitamin E (p.1350·1).

Cholinoid *Goldline, USA.*
Vitamin B substances with vitamin C (p.1350·1); lemon bioflavonoids (p.1611·1).

Cholipin *Boehringer Ingelheim, Port.*
Fenipentol (p.1610·1); octibenzonium bromide.
Biliary-tract disorders.

Cholit-Ursan *Niddapharm, Ger.*
Ursodeoxycholic acid (p.1677·2).
Cholesterol gallstones.

Chol-Kugeletten Neu *Dolorgiet, Ger.*
Greater celandine (p.1618·1); aloes (p.1210·1).
Biliary disorders.

Chol-Less *Rafa, Israel.*
Colestyramine (p.864·1).
Atherosclerosis; hypercholesterolaemia; myocardial infarction; pruritus in partial biliary obstruction.

Cholofalk *Falk, Ger.*
Ursodeoxycholic acid (p.1677·2).
Primary biliary cirrhosis.

Cholografin
Squibb Diagnostics, Canad.†; Squibb Diagnostics, USA.
Meglumine adipiodone (p.1031·1).
Contrast medium for biliary-tract radiography.

Cholonerton *Sanova, Aust.*
Hymecromone (p.1622·3).
Liver and gallbladder disorders.

Cholosan *Spreewald, Ger.*
Raphanus sativus var nigra.
Dyspepsia.

Cholosolm Phyto *Hevert, Ger.*
Greater celandine (p.1618·1); turmeric (p.1029·3); taraxacum (p.1669·1).
Liver and bile disorders.

Cholosom SL *Hevert, Ger.*
Greater celandine (p.1618·1); curcuma zanthorrhiza; taraxacum (p.1669·1).
Liver and bile disorders.

Cholosom-Tee *Hevert, Ger.*
Caraway (p.1591·2); curcuma zanthorrhiza; taraxacum (p.1669·1); silybum marianum (p.1021·3); peppermint leaf (p.1243·2).
Biliary-tract disorders; gastrointestinal disorders.

Choloxin
Knoll, Canad.†; Boots-Flint, USA†.
Dextrothyroxine sodium (p.867·3).
Hyperlipidaemias.

Cholspasmin *Merck, Ger.*
Hymecromone (p.1622·3) or hymecromone sodium (p.1622·3).
Biliary-tract disorders.

Cholspasmin Phyto *Merck, Ger.*
Greater celandine (p.1618·1).
Biliary and gastrointestinal spasm.

Cholspasminase N *Merck, Ger.*
Pancreatin (p.1646·1).
Pancreatic disorders.

Chol-Spasmoletten *Dolorgiet, Ger.*
Hymecromone (p.1622·3).
Biliary disorders.

Cholstat
Fournier, Belg.; Fournier, Fr.†.
Cerivastatin (p.856·1) or cerivastatin sodium (p.856·1).
Hypercholesterolaemia.

Chol-Truw S *Truw, Ger.†.*
Oral drops: Homoeopathic preparation.
Tablets: Curcuma zanthorrhiza; greater celandine (p.1618·1); acetic acid (p.1571·2); absinthium (p.1571·1).
Biliary disorders.

Chomelanum
Brady, Aust.; Schur, Ger.
Choline stearate.
Burns; insect stings; skin disorders; soft-tissue disorders.

Chondrosulf *Genevrier, Fr.*
Sodium chondroitin sulfate A (p.1594·2).
Osteoarthritis.

Chooz *Schering-Plough, USA.*
Calcium carbonate (p.1215·1).
Hyperacidity.

Chophytol
Millet Roux, Braz.; Rosa-Phytopharma, Fr.; Rosa-Phytopharma, Switz.†.
Cynara (p.1601·3).
Gastrointestinal disorders; kidney disorders.

Choragon
Ferring, Ger.; Ferring, Irl.; Ferring, UK.
Chorionic gonadotrophin (p.1279·2).
Cryptorchidism; delayed puberty; female infertility; oligospermia.

Chorex *Hyrex, USA.*
Chorionic gonadotrophin (p.1279·2).
Male and female infertility; male hypogonadism; prepubertal cryptorchidism.

Chorigon *Teva, Israel.*
Chorionic gonadotrophin (p.1279·2).
Cryptorchidism; female infertility; male hypogonadism.

Choriomon
IBSA, Hong Kong; IBSA, Switz.
Chorionic gonadotrophin (p.1279·2).
Cryptorchidism; delayed puberty; female infertility; male hypogonadism.

Choron *Forest Pharmaceuticals, USA.*
Chorionic gonadotrophin (p.1279·2).
Male and female infertility; male hypogonadism; prepubertal cryptorchidism.

Chromagen *Savage, USA.*
Ferrous fumarate (p.1360·1); cyanocobalamin (p.1388·1); intrinsic factor (stomach preparation).
Ascorbic acid (p.1389·3) is included in this preparation to increase the absorption and availability of iron.
Anaemias.

Chromagen FA *Savage, USA.*
Ferrous fumarate (p.1360·1); cyanocobalamin (p.1388·1); folic acid (p.1361·1).
Ascorbic acid (p.1389·3) is included in this preparation to increase the absorption and availability of iron.
Anaemias.

Chromagen Forte *Savage, USA.*
Ferrous fumarate (p.1360·1); cyanocobalamin (p.1388·1); folic acid (p.1361·1).
Ascorbic acid (p.1389·3) is included in this preparation to increase the absorption and availability of iron.
Anaemias.

Chromagen OB *Savage, USA.*
Multivitamin and mineral preparation (p.1350·1).

Chroma-Pak *Smith & Nephew SoloPak, USA.*
Chromium trichloride (p.1357·1).
Additive for intravenous total parenteral nutrition solutions.

Chromargon *Richard, Fr.*
Hydroxyquinoline sulfate (p.1622·2); acriflavinium chloride (p.1130·2).
Skin infections.

Chrome *Eagle, Austral.*
Chromium amino acid chelate (p.1357·1).
Dietary supplement.

Chromelin Complexion Blender *Summers, USA.*
Dihydroxyacetone (p.1113·2).
Hypopigmentation; vitiligo.

Chromitope *Squibb Diagnostics, USA†.*
Chromium-51 (p.1449·2) as sodium chromate.

Chronadalate *Bayer, Fr.*
Nifedipine (p.940·1).
Angina pectoris; hypertension.

Chronexan *Asta Medica, Fr.†.*
Xipamide (p.999·2).
Hypertension; oedema.

Chronocard N *Cesra, Ger.*
Crataegus (p.1600·2).
Cardiac disorders.

Chronocorte *Streuli, Switz.*
Dexamethasone (p.1067·1); dexamethasone sodium phosphate (p.1067·1).
Corticosteroid.

Chrono-Indocid *Merck Sharp & Dohme-Chibret, Fr.*
Indometacin (p.44·3).
Musculoskeletal and joint disorders.

Chronophyllin *Byk Madaus, S.Afr.*
Theophylline (p.777·2).
Obstructive airways disease.

Chronovera *Searle, Canad.*
Verapamil hydrochloride (p.989·1).
Angina pectoris; hypertension.

Chronulac
Hoechst Marion Roussel, Canad.†; Merrell Dow, USA.
Lactulose (p.1230·1).
Constipation.

Chrysocor *Sanum-Kehlbeck, Ger.*
Placenta extracts (human).
Sexual disorders.

CHX Dental Gel *Dentsply, Ger.*
Chlorhexidine gluconate (p.1138·2).
Mouth disorders.

Chymex *Adria, USA.*
Bentiromide (p.1584·1).
Diagnosis of pancreatic insufficiency.

Chymodiactin
Knoll, Austral.; Knoll, Canad.; Knoll, Irl.†; Eight, Spain; Knoll, UK; Boots-Flint, USA.
Chymopapain (p.1594·3).
Herniated lumbar intervertebral disc.

Chymodiactine *Knoll, Fr.*
Chymopapain (p.1594·3).
Herniated lumbar intervertebral disc.

Chymol *Anglian, UK.*
Eucalyptus oil (p.1609·2); terpineol (p.1669·3); methyl salicylate (p.55·1); phenol (p.1152·3).
Bruises; chapped skin; chilblains; sprains.

Ciarbiot *Vir, Spain†.*
Ampicillin trihydrate (p.151·1).
Bacterial infections.

Ciatyl-Z *Bayer, Ger.*
Zuclopenthixol acetate (p.714·1), zuclopenthixol decanoate (p.714·1), or zuclopenthixol hydrochloride (p.714·2).
Formerly known as Sedanxol.
Psychoses.

Ciba Vision Cleaner For Sensitive Eyes *Ciba Vision, USA.*
Cleaning solution for soft contact lenses (p.1129·2).

Cibacalcin
Novartis, Aust.; Novartis, Austral.†; Novartis, Ger.; Novartis, Israel; Novartis, Ital.; Novartis, Neth.†; Novartis, Swed.
Calcitonin (human) (p.749·2).
Hypercalcaemia; osteolysis; osteoporosis; Paget's disease of bone; reflex sympathetic dystrophy.

Cibacalcina Novartis, Braz.; Novartis, Port.†; Novartis, Spain.
Calcitonin (human) (p.749·2).
Hypercalcaemia; metastatic bone pain; osteoporosis; Paget's disease of bone.

Cibacalcine Ciba-Geigy, Belg.†; Novartis, Fr.; Ciba, Switz.†.
Calcitonin (human) (p.749·2).
Hypercalcaemia; hyperphosphatasia; osteoporosis; Paget's disease of bone; prevention of bone loss in immobilisation; reflex sympathetic dystrophy.

Cibace Novartis, S.Afr.
Benazepril hydrochloride (p.843·2).
Heart failure; hypertension.

Cibacen Novartis, Aust.; Novartis, Belg.; Novartis, Denm.; Novartis, Ger.; Novartis, Irl.; Novartis, Israel; Novartis, Ital.; Novartis, Neth.; Novartis, NZ; Novartis, Spain; Novartis, Switz.
Benazepril hydrochloride (p.843·2).
Heart failure; hypertension; renal failure.

Cibacene Novartis, Fr.
Benazepril hydrochloride (p.843·2).
Hypertension.

Cibadrex Novartis, Aust.; Novartis, Denm.; Novartis, Fr.; Novartis, Ger.; Novartis, Ital.; Novartis, Neth.; Novartis, S.Afr.; Ciba-Geigy, Swed.†; Novartis, Switz.
Benazepril hydrochloride (p.843·2); hydrochlorothiazide (p.907·3).
Hypertension.

Cibaflam Ciba Vision, Ger.
Fluorometholone (p.1072·1); gentamicin sulfate (p.210·1).
Inflammatory eye infections.

Cibalena A Novartis, Braz.
Aspirin (p.14·2); paracetamol (p.71·2); caffeine (p.761·3).
Fever; pain.

Cibalgina Zyma, Ital.†; Novartis, Spain†.
Propyphenazone (p.80·2).
Formerly contained propyphenazone and allobarbital in *Ital*.
Fever; pain.

Cibalgina Compuesta Novartis, Spain†.
Codeine phosphate (p.25·2); propyphenazone (p.80·2).
Fever; pain.

Cibalgina Due Fast Novartis Consumer, Ital.
Ibuprofen (p.43·2).
Fever; influenza symptoms; pain.

Cibis Siam Bheasach, Thai.
Chlorpheniramine [chlorphenamine] maleate (p.412·1); lignocaine [lidocaine] hydrochloride (p.1313·2); hexachlorophene (p.1146·1); methyl salicylate (p.55·1); menthol (p.1632·3); camphor (p.1589·3).
Dermatitis; eczema; insect bites; pruritus; scalds; wounds.

Ciblor Inava, Fr.
Amoxicillin trihydrate (p.149·2); potassium clavulanate (p.187·2).
Bacterial infections.

Cica-Care Smith & Nephew, Fr.; Smith & Nephew Healthcare, UK.
Silicone (p.1409·3).
Hypertrophic and keloid scars.

Cicaderma Note.This name is used for preparations of different composition.
Boiron, Canad.
Homoeopathic preparation.

Boiron, Fr.†; Boiron, Port.
Calendula (p.1589·2); hypericum (p.290·2); achillea (p.1572·2); ledum palustre; pulsatilla.
Minor burns and wounds.

Cicafissan Uhlmann-Eyraud, Switz.
Casein hydrolysate; kaolin (p.1229·3); colloidal silicon dioxide (p.1503·3); bismuth subnitrate (p.1213·2); zinc oxide (p.1128·2).
Burns; skin disorders; wounds.

Cicamosa Lutsia, Fr.
Mimosa tenuiflora.
Skin disorders.

Cicatral Diviser Aquilea, Spain.
Peru balsam (p.1650·2); ergocalciferol (p.1391·2); estrone (p.1476·1); benzocaine (p.1306·2); vitamin A (p.1382·1); tyrothricin (p.267·1).
Burns; skin disorders; ulcers; wounds.

Cicatrene Note.This name is used for preparations of different composition.
Glaxo Wellcome, Braz.
Neomycin sulfate (p.228·1); bacitracin zinc (p.155·2); cysteine; glycine; threonine.
Skin infections.

Warner-Lambert, Ital.
Cream; topical powder: Neomycin sulfate (p.228·1); bacitracin zinc (p.155·2).
Topical spray: Polymixin B sulfate (p.238·1); bacitracin zinc (p.155·2).
Skin infections.

Cicatrex Glaxo Wellcome, Aust.; Glaxo Wellcome, Ger.; Warner-Lambert Consumer, Switz.
Bacitracin zinc (p.155·2); neomycin sulfate (p.228·1); cysteine; glycine; DL-threonine.
Bacterial skin infections; infected wounds and burns.

Cicatrin Glaxo Wellcome, Austral.; Glaxo Wellcome, Canad.; Glaxo Wellcome, Irl.; Wellcome, Port.; Glaxo Wellcome, S.Afr.; Wellcome, UK.
Bacitracin (p.155·2); neomycin sulfate (p.228·1); L-cysteine; glycine DL-threonine.
Bacterial skin infections; burns; wounds.

Cicatrizan Johnson & Johnson, Braz.
Neomycin sulfate (p.228·1); bacitracin zinc (p.155·2); cysteine; glycine; threonine.
Skin infections.

Cicatryl Darci, Fr.
Allantoin (p.1110·1); guaiazulene (p.1618·3); chlorocresol (p.1141·3); alpha tocoferil acetate (p.1394·1).
Superficial burns and wounds.

Cicladol Carlo Erba, Braz.; Master Pharma, Ital.
Piroxicam betadex (p.79·1).
Gout; musculoskeletal, joint, and peri-articular disorders; pain.

Ciclafast Master Pharma, Ital.
Piroxicam pivalate (p.79·3).
Musculoskeletal and joint disorders.

Ciclinalgin IMA, Braz.
Benzydamine hydrochloride (p.20·1).
Fever; inflammation; pain.

Ciclo Uniao Quimica, Braz.
Ethinylestradiol (p.1476·2); d-13-β-ethyl-17-α-ethinyl-17-beta-hydroxygon-4-en-3-one.
Combined oral contraceptive.

Ciclobiotico Atral, Port.
Capsules; oral suspension: Tetracycline hydrochloride (p.258·3).
Eye ointment; ointment: Tetracycline hydrochloride (p.258·3); prednisone (p.1079·2).
Bacterial infections.

Ciclochem Novag, Spain.
Ciclopirox olamine (p.382·1).
Fungal skin and nail infections; vulvovaginal candidiasis.

Cicloderm Trima, Israel.
Ciclopirox olamine (p.382·1).
Fungal skin infections.

Cicloderm-C Trima, Israel.
Ciclopirox olamine (p.382·1); clobetasone butyrate (p.1065·2); gentamicin sulfate (p.210·1).
Infected skin disorders.

Ciclofalina Almirall, Spain.
Piracetam (p.1652·1).
Cortical myoclonia; mental function impairment.

Cicloferon Liomont, Mex.
Aciclovir (p.612·3).
Herpesvirus infections.

Ciclolux Allergan, Ital.
Cyclopentolate hydrochloride (p.465·2).
Production of mydriasis and cycloplegia.

Ciclomestril QIF, Ital.
Ethinylestradiol (p.1476·2); levonorgestrel (p.1486·2).
Combined oral contraceptive.

Ciclople Llorens, Spain†.
Cyclopentolate hydrochloride (p.465·2).
Eye disorders; production of mydriasis.

Cicloplegicedol Oftalder, Port.
Cyclopentolate hydrochloride (p.465·2).
Production of mydriasis.

Cicloplegico Allergan-Frumtost, Braz.
Cyclopentolate hydrochloride (p.465·2).
Production of mydriasis and cycloplegia.

Cicloplejic Ciba Vision, Spain.
Cyclopentolate hydrochloride (p.465·2).
Production of mydriasis; uveitis.

Cicloplejico Alcon Cusi, Spain.
Cyclopentolate hydrochloride (p.465·2).
Production of mydriasis; uveitis.

Cicloprimogyna Schering, Braz.
White tablets, estradiol valerate (p.1473·2); red tablets, estradiol valerate; levonorgestrel (p.1486·2).
Menopausal disorders.

Ciclor Galen, Mex.
Aciclovir (p.612·3).

Ciclospasmol Yamanouchi, Ital.
Cyclandelate (p.865·2).
Vascular disorders.

Ciclotal Marcel, Mex.
Medroxyprogesterone acetate (p.1480·1).
Malignant neoplasms; progestogen-only contraceptive.

Cicloven AGIPS, Ital.
Pyricarbate (p.1656·3).
Vascular disorders.

Cicloviral Medinfar, Port.
Aciclovir (p.612·3) or aciclovir sodium (p.612·3).
Herpes simplex infections.

Ciclovular Uniao Quimica, Braz.
Estradiol enantate (p.1473·2); algestone (p.1465·1).
Injectable contraceptive.

Ciclovulon Sanval, Braz.
Ethinylestradiol (p.1476·2); norethisterone (p.1485·1).
Combined oral contraceptive.

Cicloxal Prodes, Spain†.
Cyclophosphamide (p.527·3).
Malignant neoplasms.

Cicnor Sanofi Synthelabo, Port.
Algestone acetophenide (p.1465·1); estradiol enantate (p.1473·2).

Cidalin Agis, Israel.
Mebhydrolin napadisilate (p.420·2).
Hypersensitivity reactions.

Cidegol C Hofmann & Sommer, Ger.
Chlorhexidine gluconate (p.1138·2).
Mouth and throat disorders.

Cideox Alpharma, Mex.
Oxolamine (p.1096·2).

Cidermex Medeva, Fr.
Triamcinolone acetonide (p.1080·1); neomycin sulfate (p.228·1).
Skin and eye disorders.

Cidex Johnson & Johnson Medical, Fr.; Johnson & Johnson, Ger.; Ethicon, Ital.†; Johnson & Johnson Medical, UK; Johnson & Johnson Medical, USA.
Glutaral (p.1145·2).
Instrument disinfection.

Cidilin Errekappa, Ital.
Citicoline sodium (p.1596·1).
Cerebrovascular disorders.

Cidine Note.This name is used for preparations of different composition.
Almirall, Spain.
Cinitapride acid tartrate (p.1220·1).
Gastro-oesophageal reflux; gastroparesis.

Medifive, Thai.
Cimetidine (p.1216·3).
Peptic ulcer; Zollinger-Ellison syndrome.

Cidomel Clonmel, Irl.
Indometacin (p.44·3).
Gout; musculoskeletal, joint, and peri-articular disorders.

Cidomycin Hoechst Marion Roussel, Canad.; Hoechst Marion Roussel, Irl.; Hoechst Marion Roussel, Israel; Aventis, S.Afr.; Hoechst Marion Roussel, UK.
Gentamicin sulfate (p.210·1).
Bacterial infections.

Ciella Cooperation Pharmaceutique, Fr.
Salicylic acid (p.1122·3).
Formerly contained chlorobutanol and zinc sulfate.
Eye disorders.

Ciflan Azevedos, Port.
Ciprofloxacin hydrochloride (p.182·3).
Bacterial infections.

Ciflogex Cimed, Braz.
Benzydamine hydrochloride (p.20·1).
Fever; inflammation; pain.

Ciflox Note.This name is used for preparations of different composition.
Ache, Braz.; Bayer, Fr.
Ciprofloxacin (p.182·3) or ciprofloxacin hydrochloride (p.182·3).
Bacterial infections.

Alcon, Denm.
Ciprofloxacin hydrochloride (p.182·3); hydrocortisone (p.1073·3).
Infected eye disorders.

Cifloxin Siam Bheasach, Thai.
Ciprofloxacin hydrochloride (p.182·3) or ciprofloxacin lactate (p.182·3).
Bacterial infections.

Cifolan Olan-Kemed, Thai.
Ciprofloxacin (p.182·3).
Bacterial infections.

Cifran Ranbaxy, Thai.
Ciprofloxacin hydrochloride (p.182·3) or ciprofloxacin lactate (p.182·3).
Bacterial infections.

Cifrantil Heralds, Braz.
Erythromycin (p.201·2); muramidase (p.1638·1).
Bacterial infections.

Cigamet General Drugs, Thai.
Cimetidine (p.1216·3).
Gastric hyperacidity; peptic ulcer.

Cig-Ridettes Or-Dov, Austral.
Lobeline hydrochloride (p.1510·2).
Aid to smoking withdrawal.

CIL Lichtenstein, Ger.
Fenofibrate (p.889·1).
Hyperlipidaemias.

Cilab Biolab, Thai.
Ciprofloxacin (p.182·3).
Bacterial infections.

Cilamox Sigma, Austral.
Amoxicillin trihydrate (p.149·2).
Bacterial infections.

Cildox Ciba Vision, Spain.
Doxycycline hyclate (p.200·1).
Bacterial infections; malaria.

Cilergil Cilag, Braz.
Astemizole (p.409·1).
Hypersensitivity reactions.

Cilest Janssen-Cilag, Belg.; Janssen-Cilag, Denm.; Janssen-Cilag, Fin.; Janssen-Cilag, Fr.; Janssen-Cilag, Ger.; Janssen-Cilag, Irl.; Cilag, Mex.; Janssen-Cilag, Neth.; Janssen-Cilag, Swed.; Janssen-Cilag, Switz.; Janssen-Cilag, UK.
Norgestimate (p.1486·1); ethinylestradiol (p.1476·2).
Combined oral contraceptive.

Cileste Janssen-Cilag, Aust.
Norgestimate (p.1486·1); ethinylestradiol (p.1476·2).
Combined oral contraceptive.

Cilestoderme Schering-Plough, Port.
Betamethasone valerate (p.1063·2).
Skin disorders.

Cilex Douglas, Austral.
Cefalexin (p.161·3).
Bacterial infections.

Cilfer-12-F Duphar-Interfran, Thai.
Colloidal iron (p.1366·3); vitamin B₁₂ (p.1388·1); folic acid (p.1361·1).
Anaemias.

Cilferon-A Janssen-Cilag, Ital.
Interferon alfa (p.628·1).
Malignant neoplasms; viral infections.

Ciliar Crinos, Ital.
Timonacic methyl hydrochloride (p.1673·2).
Respiratory-tract disorders associated with viscous mucus.

Cilicaine V Sigma, Austral.
Benzathine phenoxymethylpenicillin (p.157·1).
Bacterial infections.

Cilicaine Syringe Sigma, Austral.; Pharmaco, NZ.
Procaine penicillin [procaine benzylpenicillin] (p.239·2).
Bacterial infections.

Cilicaine VK Sigma, Austral.; Pharmaco, NZ.
Phenoxymethylpenicillin potassium (p.235·1).
Bacterial infections.

Cilinafosal Medical, Spain.
Ephedrine hydrochloride (p.1090·1); sulfanilamide sodium mesilate (p.256·2).
Nasal congestion and infection.

Cilinafosal DHD Estrep Medical, Spain.
Dihydrostreptomycin sulfate (p.199·2); ephedrine hydrochloride (p.1090·1); sulfanilamide sodium mesilate (p.256·2).
Nasal congestion and infection.

Cilinafosal Hidrocort Medical, Spain.
Ephedrine hydrochloride (p.1090·1); hydrocortisone acetate (p.1073·3); neomycin sulfate (p.228·1); sulfanilamide sodium mesilate (p.256·2).
Nasal congestion and infection.

Cilinafosal Neomicina Medical, Spain.
Ephedrine hydrochloride (p.1090·1); neomycin sulfate (p.228·1).
Nasal congestion and infection.

Cilinase Dovalle, Braz.
Ciclacillin (p.182·2).
Bacterial infections.

Cilinavagin Neomicina Medical, Spain.
Diethylstilbestrol dipropionate (p.1471·2); neomycin sulfate (p.228·1); sulfanilamide sodium mesilate (p.256·2); zinc sulfate (p.1398·2).
Vulvovaginal infections.

Cilipen Elofar, Braz.
Ampicillin (p.150·3).
Bacterial infections.

Cillimicina Normon, Spain.
Lincomycin hydrochloride (p.219·2).
Bacterial infections.

Cilopen VK Douglas, Austral.
Phenoxymethylpenicillin potassium (p.235·1).
Bacterial infections.

Ciloprin Janssen-Cilag, Denm.†; Janssen-Cilag, Swed.†.
Acediasulfone sodium (p.147·3); oxymethurea.
Ear infections.

Ciloprin cum Anaesthetico Janssen-Cilag, Aust.; Janssen-Cilag, Fin.
Acediasulfone (p.147·3); cinchocaine (p.1309·1); oxymethurea.
Ear disorders.

Ciloprine ca Janssen-Cilag, Switz.
Acediasulfone sodium (p.147·3); cinchocaine (p.1309·1); oxymethurea.
Otitis.

Ciloquin Ioquin, Austral.
Ciprofloxacin hydrochloride (p.182·3).
Bacterial conjunctivitis; bacterial keratitis.

Cilox Alcon, Norw.
Ciprofloxacin hydrochloride (p.182·3).
Bacterial keratitis.

Ciloxan Alcon, Aust.; Alcon, Austral.; Alcon, Belg.; Alcon, Braz.; Alcon, Canad.; Alcon, Denm.; Alcon, Fr.; Alcon, Ger.; Alcon, Hong Kong; Alcon, Israel; Alcon, Mex.; Alcon, S.Afr.; Alcon, Singapore; Alcon, Swed.; Alcon, Switz.; Alcon, Thai.; Alcon, UK; Alcon, USA.
Ciprofloxacin hydrochloride (p.182·3).
Bacterial eye infections.

Cilpen Antibioticos, Mex.
Dicloxacillin sodium (p.199·1).
Bacterial infections.

Cim Decomed, Port.
Cimetidine (p.1216·3).
Gastric hyperacidity; gastro-oesophageal reflux; gastrointestinal haemorrhage; peptic ulcer; Zollinger-Ellison syndrome.

Cimag TP, Thai.
Cimetidine (p.1216·3).
Gastric hyperacidity; peptic ulcer.

Cimagen Antigen, Irl.
Cimetidine (p.1216·3).
Gastric hyperacidity; peptic ulcer; Zollinger-Ellison syndrome.

Cimal *Alpharma, Norw.*
Cimetidine (p.1216·3).
Aspiration syndrome; gastro-oesophageal reflux; peptic ulcer; Zollinger-Ellison syndrome.

Cimascal *Belmac, Spain.*
Calcium carbonate (p.1215·1).
Calcium deficiency; osteoporosis.

Cimascal D *Belmac, Spain.*
Calcium carbonate (p.1215·1); colecalciferol (p.1391·1).
Calcium deficiency; osteoporosis.

Cime *ABZ, Ger.; Eu Rho, Ger.; Isis Puren, Ger.*
Cimetidine (p.1216·3).
Aspiration syndromes; gastro- oesophageal reflux; gastro-intestinal haemorrhage; peptic ulcer; Zollinger-Ellison syndrome.

Cimebec *Farcoral, Mex.*
Cimetidine (p.1216·3).
Peptic ulcer.

Cimebeta *Betapharm, Ger.*
Cimetidine (p.1216·3).
Aspiration syndromes; gastro-oesophageal reflux; gastrointestinal haemorrhage; peptic ulcer; Zollinger-Ellison syndrome.

Cimecodan *Pharmacodane, Denm.*
Cimetidine (p.1216·3).
Acid aspiration; gastro-oesophageal reflux; peptic ulcer; Zollinger-Ellison syndrome.

Cimehexal *Hexal, Austral.; Hexal, Ger.*
Cimetidine (p.1216·3) or cimetidine hydrochloride (p.1218·3).
Acid aspiration; gastro-oesophageal reflux; gastrointestinal haemorrhage; peptic ulcer; Zollinger-Ellison syndrome.

Cimeldine *Clonmel, Irl.*
Cimetidine (p.1216·3).
Gastric hyperacidity; peptic ulcer; Zollinger-Ellison syndrome.

Cimelin *Sanova, Aust.*
Acetylcysteine (p.1082·3).
Respiratory-tract disorders with viscous mucus.

Cimemerck *Merck, Ger.†*
Cimetidine (p.1216·3).
Acid aspiration; gastro-oesophageal reflux; gastrointestinal haemorrhage; peptic ulcer; Zollinger-Ellison syndrome.

Cimephil *Philopharm, Ger.†*
Cimetidine (p.1216·3).
Acid aspiration; gastro-oesophageal reflux; peptic ulcer; Zollinger-Ellison syndrome.

Cimet *Thiemann, Ger.*
Cimetidine (p.1216·3).
Gastro-oesophageal reflux; gastrointestinal haemorrhage; peptic ulcer; Zollinger-Ellison syndrome.

Cimeta *Jean-Marie, Hong Kong.*
Cimetidine (p.1216·3).
Dyspepsia; peptic ulcer.

Cimetag *SmithKline Beecham, Aust.; Teva, Israel; Julphar, UAE.*
Cimetidine (p.1216·3).
Acid aspiration; anaphylactoid reactions; dyspepsia; gastro-oesophageal reflux; gastrointestinal haemorrhage; pancreatic insufficiency; peptic ulcer; Zollinger-Ellison syndrome.

Cimetalgin *SmithKline Beecham, Aust.†*
Oral suspension: Cimetidine (p.1216·3); sodium alginate (p.1498·3).
Tablets: Cimetidine (p.1216·3); alginic acid (p.1498·3); sodium bicarbonate (p.1186·2).
Gastro-oesophageal reflux.

Cimetase *Liomont, Mex.*
Cimetidine (p.1216·3).
Gastro-oesophageal reflux; gastrointestinal haemorrhage; peptic ulcer; Zollinger-Ellison syndrome.

Cimetid *Nycomed, Norw.*
Cimetidine (p.1216·3).
Acid aspiration; gastro-oesophageal reflux; gastrointestinal haemorrhage; peptic ulcer; Zollinger-Ellison syndrome.

Cimetidan *Honorterapica, Braz.*
Cimetidine (p.1216·3).
Gastro-oesophageal reflux; gastrointestinal haemorrhage; peptic ulcer; Zollinger-Ellison syndrome.

Cimetil *Infabra, Braz.*
Cimetidine (p.1216·3).
Gastro-oesophageal reflux; gastrointestinal haemorrhage; peptic ulcer; Zollinger-Ellison syndrome.

Cimetimax *PMC, Austral.†*
Cimetidine (p.1216·3).
Gastro-oesophageal reflux; peptic ulcer; scleroderma oesophagus; Zollinger-Ellison syndrome.

Cimetin *Cristalia, Braz.*
Cimetidine (p.1216·3).
Acid aspiration; gastro-oesophageal reflux; gastrointestinal haemorrhage; peptic ulcer; Zollinger-Ellison syndrome.

Cimet-P *PP Lab, Thai.*
Cimetidine (p.1216·3).
Gastric hyperacidity; peptic ulcer.

Cimetrin *Cimex, Switz.†*
Erythromycin ethyl succinate (p.201·2) or erythromycin stearate (p.201·3).
Bacterial infections.

Cimex *Baldacci, Braz.; Pharmacia Upjohn, Fin.*
Cimetidine (p.1216·3).
Gastro-oesophageal reflux; gastrointestinal haemorrhage; peptic ulcer; Zollinger-Ellison syndrome.

Cimex Sirop contre la toux *Cimex, Switz.†*
Codeine phosphate (p.25·2); ephedrine hydrochloride (p.1090·1); ipecacuanha (p.1093·1); tolu balsam (p.1101·3); cherry-laurel.
Coughs.

Cimexyl *Sanova, Aust.*
Acetylcysteine (p.1082·3).
Mucolytic in asthma and bronchitis.

Cimi *Gerard, Israel.*
Cimetidine (p.1216·3).
Gastro-oesophageal reflux; peptic ulcer.

Cimicifuga comp *Steigerwald, Ger.*
Homoeopathic preparation.
Formerly known as Auroplatin.

Cimicifuga Med Complex *Dynamit, Aust.*
Homoeopathic preparation.

Cimicifuga Oligoplex *Madaus, Ger.*
Homoeopathic preparation.

Cimidine *Berlin Pharm, Thai.*
Cimetidine (p.1216·3).
Gastro-oesophageal reflux; hypersensitivity reactions; peptic ulcer; Zollinger-Ellison syndrome.

Cimifemine *Zeller, Switz.*
Cimicifuga (p.1595·2).
Menopausal disorders.

Cimipax *IPRAD, Fr.*
Cimicifuga (p.1595·2).
Insomnia; nervous disorders.

Cimisan *APS, Ger.*
Cimicifuga (p.1595·2).
Menopausal disorders.

CimLich *Lichtenstein, Ger.*
Cimetidine (p.1216·3).
Acid aspiration; gastro-oesophageal reflux; gastrointestinal haemorrhage; peptic ulcer; Zollinger-Ellison syndrome.

Cimlok *Be-Tabs, S.Afr.*
Cimetidine (p.1216·3).
Gastrointestinal hyperacidity.

Cimogal *Galen, Mex.*
Ciprofloxacin hydrochloride (p.182·3).
Bacterial infections.

Cimulcer *Biolab, Hong Kong; Biolab, Singapore; Biolab, Thai.*
Cimetidine (p.1216·3).
Gastric hyperacidity; peptic ulcer; Zollinger-Ellison syndrome.

Cinabel *Columbia, Mex.*
Clotrimazole (p.382·1).

Cinadine *Aspen, S.Afr.*
Cimetidine (p.1216·3).
Gastro-oesophageal reflux; peptic ulcer; upper gastrointestinal haemorrhage; Zollinger-Ellison syndrome.

Cinageron *Gibran, Braz.*
Cinnarizine (p.413·1).
Peripheral vascular disorders; vestibular disorders.

Cinalong *Fujirebio, Jpn.*
Cilnidipine (p.858·2).
Hypertension.

Cinaro Bilina *Semar, Spain†.*
Cynara scolymus (p.1601·3); aloes (p.1210·1).
Constipation; hepatobiliary disorders.

Cinaziere *Ashbourne, UK.*
Cinnarizine (p.413·1).

Cinazyn *Italchimici, Ital.*
Cinnarizine (p.413·1).
Vascular disorders; vestibular disorders.

Cincain *Ophtha, Denm.; Ipex, Swed.*
Cinchocaine (p.1309·1).
Eye disorders.

Cinclamina *Laborsil, Braz.*
Nikethamide (p.1513·1).
Respiratory depression.

Cincofarm *Lepori, Port.; Farma Lepori, Spain.*
Oxitriptan (p.302·2).
Depression; epilepsy; hepatic coma; myoclonus; parkinsonism; phenylketonuria; schizophrenia; sleep disorders; trigeminal neuralgia.

Cincopal *Cyanamid, Spain.*
Fenbufen (p.36·2).
Gout; musculoskeletal disorders; pain; peri-articular disorders.

Cinerine *Pharmasant, Thai.*
Cinnarizine (p.413·1).
Cerebrovascular disorders; motion sickness; peripheral vascular disorders; vestibular disorders.

Cinet *Medinfar, Port.*
Domperidone (p.1224·1).
Nausea; vomiting.

Cinetic *Teofarma, Ital.*
Thyroid (p.1526·2).
Hypothyroidism.

Cinfacromin *Cinfa, Spain.*
Merbromin (p.1150·1).
Skin disinfection.

Cinfamar *Cinfa, Spain.*
Dimenhydrinate (p.415·2).
Motion sickness; vertigo.

Cinfamar Cafeina *Cinfa, Spain.*
Caffeine (p.761·3); dimenhydrinate (p.415·2).
Motion sickness; vertigo.

Cinfatos *Cinfa, Spain.*
Dextromethorphan hydrobromide (p.1087·3).
Cough.

Cinfatos Expectorante *Cinfa, Spain.*
Dextromethorphan hydrobromide (p.1087·3); guaifenesin (p.1092·2).
Coughs and cold symptoms.

Cinifa *Nakorn, Thai.*
Rifampicin (p.243·2).
Gonorrhoea; leprosy; tuberculosis.

Cinkef-U *Faulding, Port.*
Fluorouracil (p.540·2).

Cinnabene *Ratiopharm, Aust.*
Cinnarizine (p.413·1).
Cerebral and peripheral vascular disease.

Cinnacet *Sanofi Synthelabo, Ger.*
Cinnarizine (p.413·1).
Cerebral and peripheral circulatory disorders; vestibular disorders.

Cinnageron *Streuli, Switz.*
Cinnarizine (p.413·1).
Cochlear disorders; motion sickness; vestibular disorders.

Cinnar *Atlantic, Singapore; Atlantic, Thai.*
Cinnarizine (p.413·1).
Cerebral and peripheral vascular disorders; migraine; motion sickness; vestibular disorders.

Cinnaron *Remedica, Singapore.*
Cinnarizine (p.413·1).
Motion sickness; vestibular disorders.

Cinnarplus *Gerot, Aust.*
Cinnarizine (p.413·1); etamivan (p.1509·3).
Cerebral and peripheral vascular disease.

Cinnaza *Pharmaland, Thai.*
Cinnarizine (p.413·1).
Cerebrovascular disorders; migraine; peripheral vascular disorders; vestibular disorders.

Cinnipirine *Artu, Neth.*
Cinnarizine (p.413·1).
Hypersensitivity reactions; motion sickness; vertigo; vestibular disorders.

Cinobac *Lilly, Aust.†; Lilly, Belg.†; Lilly, Ital.; Lilly, UK†; Oclassen, USA.*
Cinoxacin (p.182·2).
Urinary-tract infections.

Cinobactin *Lilly, Ger.†; Quatromed, S.Afr.; Lilly, Swed.†*
Cinoxacin (p.182·2).
Urinary-tract infections.

Cinon *Azevedos, Port.*
Cinnarizine (p.413·1).
Cerebral and peripheral vascular disorders; vestibular disorders.

Cinopal *Wyeth Lederle, Denm.†; Wyeth Lederle, Fr.†; Cyanamid, Ital.†; Wyeth, S.Afr.†; Wyeth-Ayerst, Thai.*
Fenbufen (p.36·2).
Musculoskeletal and joint disorders; pain.

Cinoxen *Ibirn, Ital.*
Cinoxacin (p.182·2).
Urinary-tract infections.

Cinquerix *SmithKline Beecham, Ital.*
A diphtheria, tetanus, pertussis, poliomyelitis, and haemophilus influenzae vaccine (p.1539·1).
Active immunisation.

Cinrizine *Medifive, Thai.*
Cinnarizine (p.413·1).
Circulatory disorders; migraine; motion sickness; vestibular disorders.

Cintilan *Medley, Braz.*
Piracetam (p.1652·1).
Alcoholism; behaviour disorders in children; cerebrovascular disorders; senile dementia; vertigo.

Cional *Nycomed, Aust.*
Aluminium formate; chamomile (p.1593·2); sage (p.1660·2); arnica (p.1581·3).
Mouth and throat disorders.

Cional S *Kreussler, Ger.†*
Aluminium formate.
Inflammatory disorders of the oropharynx.

Cipadur *Cipla-Medpro, S.Afr.*
Cefadroxil (p.161·2).
Bacterial infections.

Cipamox *Cipan, Port.*
Amoxicillin sodium (p.149·2) or amoxicillin trihydrate (p.149·2).
Bacterial infections.

Cipanfeno *Cipan, Port.*
Ketotifen fumarate (p.767·2).
Allergic conjunctivitis; allergic rhinitis; allergic skin disorders; asthma.

Cipasid *Siam Bheasach, Thai.*
Cisapride (p.1220·1).
Constipation; dyspepsia; gastro-oesophageal reflux; gastroparesis; intestinal pseudo-obstruction.

Cipex *Cipla-Medpro, S.Afr.*
Mebendazole (p.102·2).
Worm infections.

Cipflocin *Asian Pharm, Thai.*
Ciprofloxacin (p.182·3).
Bacterial infections.

Ciplox *Cipan, Port.*
Ciprofloxacin hydrochloride (p.182·3).
Bacterial infections.

Cipobacter *Rubio, Spain.*
Ciprofloxacin hydrochloride (p.182·3).
Bacterial infections.

Ciprain *Maver, Mex.*
Ciprofloxacin (p.182·3).
Bacterial infections.

Cipralan *Searle, Belg.; Bristol-Myers Squibb, Fr.*
Tablets: Cibenzoline succinate (p.857·3).
Arrhythmias.

Bristol-Myers Squibb, Fr.
Injection: Cibenzoline succinate (p.857·3); cibenzoline (p.857·2).
Arrhythmias.

Cipram *Lundbeck, Hong Kong; Lundbeck, Singapore; Lundbeck, Thai.*
Citalopram hydrobromide (p.281·2).
Depression.

Cipramil *Lundbeck, Austral.; Lundbeck, Belg.; Schering-Plough, Braz.; Lundbeck, Denm.; Lundbeck, Fin.; Lundbeck, Ger.; Lundbeck, Irl.; Lundbeck, Israel; Lundbeck, Neth.; Lundbeck, Norw.; Lundbeck, NZ; Lundbeck, S.Afr.; Lundbeck, Swed.; Lundbeck, UK.*
Citalopram hydrobromide (p.281·2) or citalopram hydrochloride (p.281·2).
Anxiety disorders; depression; obsessive-compulsive disorder; phobias.

Ciprenit Otico *Vita, Spain.*
Ciprofloxacin hydrochloride (p.182·3).
Otitis externa; otitis media.

Ciprex *Sintofarma, Braz.*
Ciprofloxacin hydrochloride (p.182·3).
Bacterial infections.

Cipride *Biolab, Thai.*
Cisapride (p.1220·1).
Anorexia nervosa; constipation; dyspepsia; gastroparesis; gastro-oesophageal reflux; intestinal pseudo-obstruction.

Cipril *Italchimici, Ital.*
Cisapride (p.1220·1).
Gastrointestinal disorders.

Cipro *Bayer, Braz.; Bayer, Canad.; Bayer, USA.*
Ciprofloxacin (p.182·3) or ciprofloxacin hydrochloride (p.182·3).
Bacterial infections.

Cipro HC *Alcon, Canad.; Bayer, USA.*
Ciprofloxacin hydrochloride (p.182·3); hydrocortisone (p.1073·3).
Infected ear disorders.

Ciprobay *Bayer, Ger.; Bayer, S.Afr.; Bayer, Singapore; Bayer, Thai.*
Ciprofloxacin (p.182·3), ciprofloxacin hydrochloride (p.182·3), or ciprofloxacin lactate (p.182·3).
Bacterial infections.

Ciprobid *Cadila, Thai.*
Ciprofloxacin (p.182·3).
Bacterial infections.

Ciprobiotic *Cryopharma, Mex.*
Ciprofloxacin hydrochloride (p.182·3).
Bacterial infections.

Ciprofin *Utopian, Thai.*
Ciprofloxacin (p.182·3).
Bacterial infections.

Ciproflox *Senosiain, Mex.*
Ciprofloxacin hydrochloride (p.182·3) or ciprofloxacin lactate (p.182·3).
Bacterial infections.

Ciprofur *Fustery, Mex.*
Ciprofloxacin hydrochloride (p.182·3).
Bacterial infections.

Ciprogen *General Drugs, Thai.*
Ciprofloxacin (p.182·3).
Bacterial infections.

Ciprogis *Agis, Israel.*
Ciprofloxacin (p.182·3).
Bacterial infections.

Ciprok *Synthelabo, Spain.*
Ciprofloxacin hydrochloride (p.182·3).
Bacterial infections.

Ciprolet *Neopharm, Thai.*
Ciprofloxacin hydrochloride (p.182·3) or ciprofloxacin lactate (p.182·3).
Bacterial infections.

Ciprolisina *AF, Mex.*
Cyproheptadine hydrochloride (p.414·2); cyanocobalamin (p.1388·1).
Tonic.

Ciprom-H *M & H, Thai.*
Ciprofloxacin lactate (p.182·3).
Bacterial infections.

Ciproquinol *Ferring, Port.*
Ciprofloxacin (p.182·3).
Bacterial infections.

Ciproser *Serral, Mex.*
Ciprofloxacin (p.182·3).
Bacterial infections.

Ciprosun Sun, Thai.
Ciprofloxacin (p.182·3).
Bacterial infections.

Ciproxin
Bayer, Aust.; Bayer, Austral.; Bayer, Denm.; Bayer, Fin.; Bayer, Hong Kong; Bayer, Irl.; Bayer, Israel; Bayer, Ital.; Bayer, Neth.; Bayer, Norw.; Bayer, NZ; Bayer, Swed.; Bayer, UK.
Ciprofloxacin (p.182·3), ciprofloxacin hydrochloride (p.182·3), or ciprofloxacin lactate (p.182·3).
Bacterial infections.

Ciproxin HC Alcon, Austral.
Ciprofloxacin hydrochloride (p.182·3); hydrocortisone (p.1073·3).
Otitis externa.

Ciproxina
Bayer, Mex.; Bayer, Port.
Ciprofloxacin hydrochloride (p.182·3) or ciprofloxacin lactate (p.182·3).
Bacterial infections.

Ciproxine
Bayer, Belg.; Bayer, Switz.
Ciprofloxacin (p.182·3), ciprofloxacin hydrochloride (p.182·3), or ciprofloxacin lactate (p.182·3).
Bacterial infections.

Ciproxin-Hydrocortison Alcon, Fin.
Ciprofloxacin hydrochloride (p.182·3); hydrocortisone (p.1073·3).
Otitis externa.

Circanetten
Note. This name is used for preparations of different composition.
Eversil, Braz.
Paraphlebon; senna (p.1248·2); sulfur (p.1123·3).
Vascular disorders.

Evers, Thai.
Potassium acid tartrate (p.1244·3); keratin; senna (p.1248·2); sulfur (p.1123·3).
Haemorrhoids; varices.

Circanol 3M, Ger.
Co-dergocrine mesilate (p.1597·3).
Adjuvant in mental function disorders; cervical disc syndrome; hypertension.

Circavite-T Circle, USA.
Multivitamin and mineral preparation with iron (p.1350·1).

Circo-Maren Krewel, Ger.
Nicergoline (p.1640·2).
Mental function disorders.

Circonyl N Medidom, Switz.†
Quinine sulfate (p.445·1).
Nocturnal leg cramps.

Circovenil Wyeth, Spain.
Buphenine hydrochloride (p.1587·3); aescin (p.1574·1); sodium polygalacturonate sulfonate.
Peripheral vascular disorders.

Circovenil Fuerte Wyeth, Spain†.
Buphenine hydrochloride (p.1587·3); aescin (p.1574·1); esculoside (p.1574·1); hesperidin (p.1611·2).
Circulatory disorders.

Circularine Lerads, Fr.
Alpha tocoferil acetate (p.1394·1); troxerutin (p.1611·2); esculoside (p.1574·1).
Peripheral vascular disorders.

Circulation Homeocan, Canad.
Homoeopathic preparation.

Circulatonic Phytomedica, Fr.
Menthol (p.1632·3); camphor (p.1589·3); cypress oil; equisetum (p.1606·3).
Circulatory disorders.

Circupon
Kolassa, Aust.; Medichemie, Switz.
Etilefrine hydrochloride (p.888·1).
Hypotension.

Circupon RR Gepepharm, Ger.
Etilefrine hydrochloride (p.888·1).
Hypotension.

Circuvit E Wernigerode, Ger.
Etilefrine hydrochloride (p.888·1).
Hypotension.

Cirflo Rhone-Poulenc Rorer, Austral.†
Oxerutins (p.1611·2); nicotinic acid (p.1372·3); bioflavonoids (p.1611·1); calcium ascorbate (p.1389·3); calcium gluconate (p.1188·2); calcium fluoride (p.1356·1); ruscus aculeatus; aesculus (p.1574·1); hamamelis (p.1618·3); pulsatilla (p.1656·3).
Circulatory disorders.

Cirkan Sinbio, Fr.
Ruscus aculeatus; ascorbic acid (p.1389·3); hesperidin methyl chalcone (p.1611·2).
Formerly contained pancreatic enzymes (expressed as chymotrypsin and trypsin activities), ruscosides, ascorbic acid, hesperidin methyl chalcone, and metescufetol sodium.
Haemorrhoids; venous insufficiency.

Cirkan a la Prednacinolone Sinbio, Fr.
Desonide (p.1066·2); lignocaine [lidocaine] hydrochloride (p.1313·2); vitamin A palmitate (p.1383·2); ruscosides; tocoferil acetate (p.1394·1); heparin sodium (p.902·1).
Anorectal disorders.

Cirkufemal Roha, Ger.
Cimicifuga (p.1595·2).
Menopausal disorders.

Cirkulin Baldrian Schulke & Mayr, Aust.
Valerian (p.1678·3).
Sedative.

Cirkuprostan Roha, Ger.†
Urtica root (p.1678·2).
Prostatic hyperplasia.

Cirkused Diafarm, Spain.
Valerian (p.1678·3).
Insomnia; nervous disorders.

Cirrus
Bios, Belg.; UCB, Fin.; UCB, Hong Kong; UCB, Singapore.
Cetirizine hydrochloride (p.411·2); pseudoephedrine hydrochloride (p.1099·2).
Nasal congestion; rhinitis.

Cirulan Novag, Mex.
Metoclopramide (p.1236·3).
Gastrointestinal motility disorders.

Cisaken Kendrick, Mex.
Cinnarizine (p.413·1).
Peripheral vascular disorders.

Cisapin LSP, Thai.
Cisapride (p.1220·1).
Constipation; dyspepsia; gastoparesis; gastro-oesophageal reflux.

Cisday BASF, Ger.
Nifedipine (p.940·1).
Angina pectoris.

Cisordinol
Lundbeck, Aust.; Lundbeck, Denm.; Lundbeck, Fin.; Lundbeck, Neth.; Lundbeck, Norw.; Dumex, Braz.; Duphar, Spain; Lundbeck, Swed.
Zuclopenthixol acetate (p.714·1), zuclopenthixol decanoate (p.714·1), or zuclopenthixol hydrochloride (p.714·2).
Psychoses.

Cisplatyl
Rhodia, Braz.; Rhone-Poulenc Rorer, Fr.; Rhone-Poulenc Rorer, Israel.
Cisplatin (p.525·1).
Malignant neoplasms.

Cispride Sintofarma, Braz.
Cisapride (p.1220·1).
Gastro-oesophageal reflux; gastroparesis.

Cistalgan Recordati, Ital.
Flavoxate hydrochloride (p.467·1); propyphenazone (p.80·2).
Spasm of the female genital tract; urinary-tract disorders.

Cistamine LBS, Thai.
Cetirizine hydrochloride (p.411·2).
Allergic conjunctivitis; allergic skin disorders; rhinitis.

Cisticid
Merck, Braz.; Merck, Mex.
Praziquantel (p.106·3).
Cestode infections; trematode infections.

Cistidil IDI, Ital.
L-Cystine (p.1359·1).
Skin disorders.

Cistobil
Bracca, Ital.; Bracco, Switz.†.
Iopanoic acid (p.1035·2).
Contrast medium for biliary-tract radiography.

Cistofuran Crosara, Ital.†
Nitrofurantoin (p.230·3).
Urinary-tract infections.

Cistomid Biotekfarma, Ital.
Pipemidic acid (p.236·1).
Urinary-tract infections.

Cistopax Zimaia, Port.†
Oxolinic acid (p.233·3).
Urinary-tract infections.

Cistus canadensis Oligoplex Madaus, Ger.
Homoeopathic preparation.

Cital Bichsel, Switz.†
Mannitol (p.924·3); sorbitol (p.1377·3).
Irrigation solution.

Citalgan Merck, Mex.
Ibuprofen (p.43·2).
Fever; inflammation; musculoskeletal, joint and peri-articular disorders; pain.

Citaloxan Faulding, Port.
Cytarabine (p.530·1).

Citanest
Note. This name is used for preparations of different composition.
Astra, Austral.; Astra, Belg.; AstraZeneca, Canad.; AstraZeneca, Fin.; Astra, Irl.; Astra, Neth.; AstraZeneca, NZ; Inibsa, Spain; Astra, Swed.; AstraZeneca, UK; Astra, USA.
Prilocaine hydrochloride (p.1318·2).
Adrenaline [epinephrine] (p.829·1) or adrenaline [epinephrine] acid tartrate (p.829·2) is included in some injections as a vasoconstrictor to diminish absorption and localise the effect of the local anaesthetic.
Local anaesthesia.

Astra, Braz.
Prilocaine hydrochloride (p.1318·2).
Felypressin (p.1283·1) is included in this preparation as a vasoconstrictor to diminish absorption and localise the effect of the local anaesthetic.
Local anaesthesia.

AstraZeneca, Fin.; AstraZeneca, Norw.
Gel: Prilocaine hydrochloride (p.1318·2); chlorhexidine gluconate (p.1138·2).
Cystitis; cystoscopy; local anaesthesia.

Citanest con Octapressin Astra, Ital.
Prilocaine hydrochloride (p.1318·2).
Felypressin (p.1283·1) is included in this preparation as a vasoconstrictor to diminish absorption and localise the effect of the local anaesthetic.
Local anaesthesia.

Citanest Dental Astra, Austral.
Prilocaine hydrochloride (p.1318·2).

Felypressin (p.1283·1) is included in this preparation as a vasoconstrictor to diminish absorption and localise the effect of the local anaesthetic.
Local anaesthesia.

Citanest Octapresin Astra, Mex.
Prilocaine hydrochloride (p.1318·2).
Felypressin (p.1283·1) is included in this preparation as a vasoconstrictor to diminish absorption and localise the effect of the local anaesthetic.
Local anaesthesia in dentistry.

Citanest Octapressin
AstraZeneca, Denm.; AstraZeneca, Fin.; AstraZeneca, Norw.; Astra-Zeneca, NZ; Astra, Port.†; Inibsa, Spain; Astra, Swed.
Prilocaine hydrochloride (p.1318·2).
Felypressin (p.1283·1) is included in this preparation as a vasoconstrictor to diminish absorption and localise the effect of the local anaesthetic.
Local anaesthesia.

Citanest with Octapressin
Astra, Irl.; AstraZeneca, UK.
Prilocaine hydrochloride (p.1318·2).
Felypressin (p.1283·1) is included in this preparation as a vasoconstrictor to diminish absorption and localise the effect of the local anaesthetic.
Local anaesthesia.

Citanest Octapressine Astra, Neth.
Prilocaine hydrochloride (p.1318·2).
Felypressin (p.1283·1) is included in this preparation as a vasoconstrictor to diminish absorption and localise the effect of the local anaesthetic.
Local anaesthesia.

Citanest Octopressin Adcock Ingram, S.Afr.†
Prilocaine (p.1318·3).
Felypressin (p.1283·1) is included in this preparation as a vasoconstrictor to diminish absorption and localise the effect of the local anaesthetic.
Local anaesthesia in dentistry.

Citavi Labocor, Port.†
Ascorbic acid (p.1389·3).
Tonic.

Citemul S Medopharm, Ger.
Mesulphen (p.1118·3).
Scabies; skin disorders.

Citicef CT, Ital.
Cefradine (p.173·3).
Bacterial infections.

Citicil CT, Ital.†
Ampicillin (p.150·3) or ampicillin sodium (p.150·3).
Bacterial infections.

Citiclor CT, Ital.
Cefaclor (p.161·1).
Bacterial infections.

Citidel Del Saz & Filippini, Ital.†
Citicoline sodium (p.1596·1).
Cerebrovascular disorders; parkinsonism.

Citidine
Atlantic, Hong Kong; Atlantic, Singapore; Atlantic, Thai.
Cimetidine (p.1216·3).
Gastro-oesophageal reflux; peptic ulcer; Zollinger-Ellison syndrome.

Citifar Lafare, Ital.
Citicoline (p.1596·1).
Cerebrovascular disorders.

Citilat CT, Ital.
Nifedipine (p.940·1).
Hypertension; ischaemic heart disease.

Citimid CT, Ital.†
Cimetidine (p.1216·3).
Gastro-oesophageal reflux; gastrointestinal haemorrhage; peptic ulcer; Zollinger-Ellison syndrome.

Citinoides Serra Pamies, Spain.
Lithium carbonate (p.292·1); sodium bicarbonate (p.1186·2).
Dyspepsia; gastrointestinal hyperacidity.

Citiolase Hoechst Marion Roussel, Ital.†
Citiolone (p.1596·2).
Liver disorders.

Citireuma CT, Ital.
Sulindac (p.85·3).
Gout; musculoskeletal, joint, and peri-articular disorders.

Citivir CT, Ital.
Aciclovir (p.612·3).
Herpesvirus infections.

Citizem CT, Ital.
Diltiazem hydrochloride (p.874·2).
Hypertension; ischaemic heart disease.

Citoburol Richter, Aust.
Calcium acetate (p.1187·3); aluminium sulfate (p.1578·2).
Bruises; inflammation.

Citocaina Cristalia, Braz.
Prilocaine hydrochloride (p.1318·2).
Felypressin (p.1283·1) is included in this preparation as a vasoconstrictor to diminish absorption and localise the effect of the local anaesthetic.
Local anaesthesia.

Citocartin Molteni, Ital.
Articaine hydrochloride (p.1306·1).
Adrenaline [epinephrine] acid tartrate (p.829·2) is included in this preparation as a vasoconstrictor to diminish absorption and localise the effect of the local anaesthetic.
Local anaesthesia in dentistry.

Citochol Strathofer, Aust.
Taraxacum (p.1669·1); achillea (p.1572·2); peppermint oil (p.1243·3).
Biliary disorders; gastrointestinal disorders.

Citodon
Durascan, Denm.; Astra, Swed.
Codeine phosphate (p.25·2); paracetamol (p.71·2).
Pain.

Citofolin Bracco, Ital.
Calcium folinate (p.1363·1).
Antidote to folic acid antagonists; folic acid deficiency; reduction of aminopterin and methotrexate toxicity.

Citofur Lusofarmaco, Ital.
Tegafur (p.573·2).
Malignant neoplasms.

Citogel Geymonat, Ital.
Sucralfate (p.1250·2).
Gastrointestinal disorders associated with hyperacidity.

Cito-Guakalin Stada, Ger.
Sodium dibunate (p.1100·3); guaifenesin (p.1092·2); thyme (p.1672·2).
Coughs and associated respiratory-tract disorders.

Citoken Kendrick, Mex.
Piroxicam (p.79·1).
Fever; inflammation; musculoskeletal and joint disorders; pain.

Citomid RU Lemery, Mex.
Vincristine sulfate (p.578·3).
Malignant neoplasms.

Citoneurin Merck, Braz.
Thiamine hydrochloride (p.1385·1); pyridoxine hydrochloride (p.1386·3); cyanocobalamin (p.1388·1).
Vitamin B deficiency; vitamin B supplement.

Citoplatino Rhone-Poulenc Rorer, Ital.
Cisplatin (p.525·1).
Malignant neoplasms.

Citosin Nettopharma, Denm.
Cisplatin (p.525·1).
Malignant neoplasms.

Citostal Bristol-Myers Squibb, Braz.
Lomustine (p.550·2).
Malignant neoplasms.

Citovirax Roche, Ital.
Ganciclovir sodium (p.623·1).
Cytomegalovirus infections.

Citra pH ValMed, USA.
Sodium citrate (p.1186·2).
Hyperacidity.

Citracal
Note. This name is used for preparations of different composition.
Mission Pharmacal, Hong Kong; Mission Pharmacal, Singapore; Mission Pharmacal, USA.
Calcium citrate (p.1188·1).
Calcium deficiency; hyperphosphataemia; osteoporosis.

Bruno, Ital.
Calcium carbonate (p.1215·1).
Calcium deficiency; calcium supplement.

Citracal + D
Mission Pharmacal, Hong Kong; Mission Pharmacal, USA.
Calcium citrate (p.1188·1); ergocalciferol (p.1391·2).
Calcium deficiency; hyperphosphataemia; osteoporosis.

Citralite Rhone-Poulenc Rorer, Austral.
Sodium bicarbonate (p.1186·2); citric acid (p.1596·2).
Urinary alkalinisation.

Citramag Bioglan, UK.
Magnesium citrate (p.1232·3).
Bowel evacuation.

Citrarginine Laphal, Fr.
Neutral arginine citrate (p.1354·1); betaine (p.1584·3); betaine hydrochloride (p.1584·3).
Liver disorders.

Citrato Espresso Gabbiani Montefarmaco, Ital.
Magnesium oxide (p.1233·2); magnesium carbonate (p.1232·3).
Gastrointestinal disorders.

Citrato Espresso S. Pellegrino Sanofi Synthelabo, Ital.
Magnesium hydroxide (p.1233·1).
Constipation.

Citravescent
Note. This name is used for preparations of different composition.
Rhone-Poulenc Rorer, Austral.
Sodium bicarbonate (p.1186·2); citric acid (p.1596·2).
Urinary alkalinisation.

Pacific, NZ.
Sodium citrotartrate.
Gastric hyperacidity; urinary alkalinisation.

Citravite Boots, NZ.
Ascorbic acid (p.1389·3).
Vitamin C supplement.

Citrazine Antigen, Irl.†
Piperazine citrate (p.105·3).
Ascariasis; enterobiasis.

Citrec Orion, Swed.
Calcium folinate (p.1363·1).
Methotrexate antagonist.

Citri Slim+Trim Bioglan, Austral.
Garcinia; chromium trichloride (p.1357·1); pectin (p.1502·3); methylcellulose (p.1502·2); magnesium amino acid chelate.
Dietary supplement; obesity.

Citrical Shire, UK†.
Calcium carbonate (p.1215·1).
Calcium deficiency.

Citrihexal *Hexal, Austral.*
Calcitriol (p.1391·1).
Hypocalcaemia; hypoparathyroidism; osteoporosis; rickets.

Citrisource *Sandoz Nutrition, Canad.†*
Preparation for enteral nutrition (p.1350·1).

Citrizan *IDI, Ital.*
Catalase (equine) (p.1592·2).
Burns; skin ulceration.

Citrizan Antibiotico *IDI, Ital.*
Catalase (equine) (p.1592·2); gentamicin sulfate (p.210·1).
Infected burns and skin ulcers.

Citrocarbonate
Note.This name is used for preparations of different composition.
Roberts, Canad.
Sodium bicarbonate (p.1186·2); sodium citrate (p.1186·2); anhydrous citric acid (p.1596·2).
Antacid; urinary alkaliniser.

Roberts, USA; Hauck, USA.
Sodium bicarbonate (p.1186·2); anhydrous sodium citrate (p.1186·2).
Hyperacidity.

Citrocholine *Therica, Fr.*
Granules for oral solution: Sodium citrate (p.1186·2); magnesium citrate (p.1232·3); choline citrate (p.1356·3).
Oral solution: Choline citrate (p.1356·3); sodium acid citrate (p.1186·2); citric acid monohydrate (p.1596·2); light magnesium carbonate (p.1232·3).
Dyspepsia.

Citrocil *I Farmacologia, Spain.*
Dihydrostreptomycin sulfate (p.199·2); sodium citrate (p.1186·2).
Gastrointestinal infections.

Citrocit *Propan, S.Afr.*
Citric acid (p.1596·2); sodium bicarbonate (p.1186·2).
Urinary alkalinisation.

Citroepatina *Roche, Ital.*
Betaine monocitrate (p.1584·3); sorbitol (p.1377·3); sodium bicarbonate (p.1186·2); anhydrous citric acid (p.1596·2).
Digestive disorders.

Citro-Flav *Goldline, USA.*
Citrus bioflavonoids complex (p.1611·1).
Capillary bleeding.

Citroflavona *Almirall, Spain.*
Ascorbic acid (p.1389·3); bioflavonoids (p.1611·1).
Capillary disorders.

Citroflavona Mag *Funk, Spain†.*
Ascorbic acid (p.1389·3); bioflavonoids (p.1611·1); hydroxyflavone.
Capillary disorders.

Citroftalmina *SIFI, Ital.*
Zinc phenolsulfonate (p.1128·3); procaine hydrochloride (p.1319·1).
Eye irritation and congestion.

Citroftalmina VC *SIFI, Ital.*
Naphazoline nitrate (p.1095·1); zinc phenolsulfonate (p.1128·3); procaine hydrochloride (p.1319·1).
Eye irritation and congestion.

Citrokehl *Sanum-Kehlbeck, Ger.*
Homoeopathic preparation.

Citrolider *Farmalider, Spain.*
Ascorbic acid (p.1389·3).
Vitamin C deficiency.

Citrolith *Beach, USA.*
Anhydrous potassium citrate (p.1186·2); anhydrous sodium citrate (p.1186·2).
Urinary alkalinising agent.

Citro-Mag *Rougier, Canad.; Rougier, Hong Kong.*
Magnesium citrate (p.1232·3).
Bowel evacuation; constipation.

Citron Chaud *Prodemdis, Canad.*
Phenylephrine hydrochloride (p.1097·1); pheniramine maleate (p.422·3); paracetamol (p.71·2); ascorbic acid (p.1389·3).
Cold and influenza symptoms; fever; pain.

Citron Chaud DM *Prodemdis, Canad.*
Phenylephrine hydrochloride (p.1097·1); pheniramine maleate (p.422·3); dextromethorphan hydrobromide (p.1087·3); ascorbic acid (p.1389·3).

Citropepsin *Byk Gulden, Ger.*
Pepsin (p.1649·3); citric acid (p.1596·2).
Gastrointestinal disorders.

Citropiperazina *Rhone-Poulenc Rorer, Ital.*
Piperazine citrate (p.105·2).
Urinary alkalinisation.

Citroplus *Medley, Braz.; Whitehall, Ital.*
Metoclopramide hydrochloride (p.1235·2).
Adjunct in gastrointestinal procedures; gastrointestinal motility disorders; nausea and vomiting.

Citrosan *Boots Healthcare, Neth.*
Paracetamol (p.71·2); ascorbic acid (p.1389·3); sodium citrate (p.1186·2).
Cold and influenza symptoms; fever; pain.

Citrosil
Note.This name is used for preparations of different composition.
Dolisos, Fr.
Thyme oil (p.1672·3); lemon oil (p.1628·2); lavender oil (p.1627·2).
House dust mite acaricide.

Manetti Roberts, Ital.
Benzalkonium chloride (p.1133·2).
Skin and wound disinfection.

Citrosil Alcolico Azzuro *Manetti Roberts, Ital.*
Benzalkonium chloride (p.1133·2); alcohol (p.1130·3); sodium nitrite (p.1023·1).
Instrument disinfection.

Citrosil Alcolico Bruno *Manetti Roberts, Ital.*
Benzalkonium chloride (p.1133·2); alcohol (p.1130·3).
Skin and wound disinfection.

Citrosil Alcolico Incolore *Manetti Roberts, Ital.*
Benzalkonium chloride (p.1133·2); alcohol (p.1130·3).
Skin and wound disinfection.

Citrosil Fazzoletto *Manetti Roberts, Ital.*
Benzalkonium chloride (p.1133·2).
Skin, wound and burns disinfection.

Citrosil Nubesan *Manetti Roberts, Ital.*
Benzalkonium chloride (p.1133·2); benzoin resin (p.1668·3).
Surface disinfection.

Citrosil Sapone *Manetti Roberts, Ital.*
Triclocarban (p.1159·2).
Skin cleansing.

Citrosil Sapoplus *Manetti Roberts, Ital.*
Benzalkonium chloride (p.1133·2).
Skin and wound disinfection.

Citrosil Spray *Manetti Roberts, Ital.*
Benzalkonium chloride (p.1133·2).
Skin and wound disinfection.

Citro-Soda *Abbott, S.Afr.*
Sodium citrate (p.1186·2); sodium bicarbonate (p.1186·2); tartaric acid (p.1669·2); citric acid (p.1596·2).
Antacid; urinary alkalinisation.

Citrosodina *Roche, Ital.*
Sodium citrate (p.1186·2).
Gastric hyperacidity.

Citrosodine *Prima, Braz.*
Citric acid (p.1596·2); sodium bicarbonate (p.1186·2); sodium citrate (p.1186·2).
Gastrointestinal hyperacidity.

Citrosteril *Fresenius, Ger.†.*
Citric acid monohydrate (p.1596·2).
Instrument disinfection.

Citrosteril Aspiratori *Sanitas, Ital.*
Orthophenylphenol (p.1152·1).
Disinfection of aspirators.

Citrosteril Deterferri *Sanitas, Ital.*
Benzalkonium chloride (p.1133·2).
Instrument disinfection.

Citrosteril Impronte *Sanitas, Ital.*
Glutaral (p.1145·2); benzalkonium chloride (p.1133·2).
Disinfection in dentistry.

Citrosteril Pronto *Sanitas, Ital.*
Benzalkonium chloride (p.1133·2); chlorhexidine (p.1138·2).
Disinfection in dentistry.

Citrosteril Sterilferri *Sanitas, Ital.*
Glutaral (p.1145·2).
Instrument disinfection.

Citrosteril Strumenti *Sanitas, Ital.*
Benzalkonium chloride (p.1133·2); alcohol (p.1130·3).
Instrument disinfection.

Citrosystem *Antipiol, Ital.*
Citronella oil (p.1596·3); basil oil; lavender oil (p.1627·2).
Insect repellent.

Citrotein
Sandoz Nutrition, Canad.†; Sandoz Nutrition, USA.
Preparation for enteral nutrition (p.1350·1).

Citrovescent *Lagamed, S.Afr.†.*
Sodium bicarbonate (p.1186·2); citric acid (p.1596·2); tartaric acid (p.1669·2).
Urinary alkalinisation.

Citrovit
Hoechst Marion Roussel, Braz.; Abello, Spain.
Ascorbic acid (p.1389·3).
Vitamin C deficiency.

Citrucel *SmithKline Beecham Consumer, USA.*
Methylcellulose (p.1502·2).
Bowel evacuation; constipation.

Citrus C with Acerola *Blackmores, Austral.*
Ascorbic acid (p.1389·3); sodium ascorbate (p.1390·1).
Vitamin C deficiency.

Citrus-flav C *Fibertone, USA.*
Citrus bioflavonoids complex (p.1611·1); vitamin C (p.1389·3); hesperidin (p.1611·2); red cherry (p.1029·1); rutoside (p.1611·2).
Capillary bleeding.

Citsav *Savio, Ital.†.*
Citicoline sodium (p.1596·1).
Cerebrovascular disorders.

Cituridina *Zambon, Ital.*
Cytidine; uridine (p.1677·2).
Hepatic encephalopathy.

Ciuk *BASF, Ger.†.*
Cimetidine (p.1216·3).
Acid aspiration; gastro-oesophageal reflux; gastrointestinal haemorrhage; peptic ulcer; Zollinger-Ellison syndrome.

Civeran *Lesvi, Spain.*
Loratadine (p.420·1).
Hypersensitivity reactions.

Civicor
Douglas, NZ; Douglas, Singapore; Douglas, Thai.; TTN, Thai.
Verapamil hydrochloride (p.989·1).
Angina pectoris; arrhythmias; hypertension.

Civigel *Ciba Vision, Fr.*
Carbomer 980 (p.1499·2).
Dry eyes.

CL tre *Nova Argentia, Ital.*
Trichloroacetic acid (p.1674·3).
Formerly known as CL 3 Bruciaporri.
Warts.

Clabin
Note.This name is used for preparations of different composition.
Chefaro, Ger.
Salicylic acid (p.1122·3).
Formerly contained salicylic acid, lactic acid, and resorcinol.
Skin disorders.

Schonenberger, Switz.
Salicylic acid (p.1122·3); lactic acid (p.1626·2); resorcinol (p.1122·2).
Calluses; corns; verrucas; warts.

Claforan
Hoechst Marion Roussel, Aust.; Hoechst Marion Roussel, Austral.; Aventis, Belg.; Hoechst Marion Roussel, Braz.; Hoechst Marion Roussel, Canad.; Aventis, Denm.; Hoechst Marion Roussel, Fin.; Roussel Diamant, Fr.; Hoechst Marion Roussel, Ger.; Hoechst Marion Roussel, Hong Kong; Hoechst Marion Roussel, Irl.; Hoechst Marion Roussel, Israel; Hoechst Marion Roussel, Ital.; Hoechst Marion Roussel, Mex.; Hoechst Marion Roussel, Neth.; Hoechst Marion Roussel, Norw.; Aventis, NZ; Aventis, S.Afr.; Hoechst Marion Roussel, Singapore; Hoechst Marion Roussel, Spain; Hoechst Marion Roussel, Swed.; Hoechst Marion Roussel, Switz.; Hoechst Marion Roussel, Thai.; Hoechst Marion Roussel, UK; Hoechst Marion Roussel, USA.
Cefotaxime sodium (p.169·1).
Lignocaine [lidocaine] hydrochloride (p.1313·2) is included in some intramuscular injections to alleviate the pain of injection.
Bacterial infections.

Claim *Apomedica, Aust.*
Curcumae oleosum extract (p.1029·3); tolynol (p.1674·1); peppermint oil (p.1243·3); eucalyptus oil (p.1609·2); camphor (p.1589·3); menthol (p.1632·3).
Gastrointestinal disorders.

Clairo Tea *Weleda, UK.*
Senna leaf (p.1248·3); peppermint leaf (p.1243·2); aniseed (p.1580·2); clove (p.1596·3).
Constipation.

Clairodermyl *BCS, Fr.†.*
Mequinol (p.1118·2).
Hyperpigmentation.

Clamarvit *Clariana, Spain.*
Ascorbic acid (p.1389·3); vitamin B substances (p.1350·1); ferrous gluconate (p.1360·1); ferrous gluceptate (p.1360·1).
Anaemias; tonic.

Clamentin *Xixia, S.Afr.*
Amoxicillin (p.149·2); clavulanic acid (p.187·2).
Bacterial infections.

Clamide *Hovid, Singapore.*
Glibenclamide (p.321·3).
Diabetes mellitus.

Clamonex *Yungjin, Singapore.*
Amoxicillin trihydrate (p.149·2); potassium clavulanate (p.187·2).
Bacterial infections.

Clamox *SmithKline Beecham, Fin.*
Amoxicillin trihydrate (p.149·2).
Bacterial infections.

Clamoxyl
Note.This name is used for preparations of different composition.
SmithKline Beecham, Aust.; SmithKline Beecham, Belg.; SmithKline Beecham, Fr.; SmithKline Beecham, Ger.; SmithKline Beecham, Neth.; Beecham, Port.; SmithKline Beecham, Spain; SmithKline Beecham, Switz.
Amoxicillin sodium (p.149·2) or amoxicillin trihydrate (p.149·2).
Bacterial infections.

SmithKline Beecham, Austral.
Amoxicillin trihydrate (p.149·2); potassium clavulanate (p.187·2).
Bacterial infections.

Clamoxyl Mucolitico *SmithKline Beecham, Spain.*
Amoxicillin trihydrate (p.149·2); bromhexine hydrochloride (p.1085·3).
Respiratory-tract infections.

Clamycin *Julphar, UAE.*
Clarithromycin (p.186·2).
Bacterial infections.

Clanzoflat *Wyeth, Spain.*
Dimethicone (p.1249·2); clebopride (p.1221·2).
Gastrointestinal disorders.

Clanzol *Wyeth, Spain†.*
Clebopride malate (p.1221·2).
Gastrointestinal disorders; nausea and vomiting.

Claradol *Nicholas, Fr.*
Paracetamol (p.71·2).
Fever; pain.

Claradol Cafeine *Nicholas, Fr.*
Paracetamol (p.71·2); caffeine (p.761·3).
Fever; pain.

Claradol Codeine *Nicholas, Fr.*
Paracetamol (p.71·2); codeine phosphate (p.25·2).
Pain.

Claragine *Nicholas, Fr.*
Aspirin (p.14·2).
Fever; pain.

Claral *Schering, Spain.*
Diflucortolone valerate (p.1069·3).
Skin disorders.

Claral Plus *Schering, Spain.*
Chlorquinaldol (p.182·1); diflucortolone valerate (p.1069·3).
Infected skin disorders.

Claramid
Zambon, Belg.; Parke, Davis, Fr.
Roxithromycin (p.247·2).
Bacterial infections.

Claratyne
Schering-Plough, Austral.; Schering-Plough, NZ.
Loratadine (p.420·1).
Allergic skin disorders; rhinitis; urticaria.

Claratyne Decongestant *Schering-Plough, NZ.*
Loratadine (p.420·1); pseudoephedrine sulfate (p.1099·3).
Upper respiratory-tract congestion.

Claraxim *Siam Bheasach, Thai.*
Cefotaxime sodium (p.169·1).
Bacterial infections.

Clarema *Damor, Ital.*
Suleparoid (p.978·2).
Thrombosis prophylaxis.

Clarens *Schiapparelli, Ital.*
Sulodexide (p.978·3).
Thrombosis prophylaxis.

Claridon *Schering-Plough, Port.*
Loratadine (p.420·1); pseudoephedrine (p.1099·2).

Claril *Alcon, Braz.*
Naphazoline hydrochloride (p.1095·1); pheniramine maleate (p.422·3).
Ocular congestion.

Clarinase
Aesca, Aust.; Schering-Plough, Austral.; Schering-Plough, Belg.; Schering-Plough, Hong Kong; Schering-Plough, Israel; Schering-Plough, Mex.; Schering-Plough, Singapore; Essex, Spain; Schering-Plough, Thai.
Loratadine (p.420·1); pseudoephedrine sulfate (p.1099·3).
Cold symptoms; rhinitis.

Clarinex *Schering-Plough, Denm.*
Loratadine (p.420·1); pseudoephedrine sulfate (p.1099·3).
Allergic rhinitis.

Claripel *Stiefel, USA.*
Hydroquinone (p.1115·1) in a sunblocking basis.
Hyperpigmented skin disorders.

Claripex AL *Sanofi Winthrop, Braz.*
Aluminium clofibrate (p.859·1).
Hyperlipidaemias.

Clarisco *Schwarz, Ital.*
Heparin sodium (p.902·1).
Vascular disorders.

Clariteyes *Schering-Plough, UK.*
Sodium cromoglicate (p.774·3).
Allergic conjunctivitis.

Claritin
Schering-Plough, Braz.; Schering, Canad.; Schering-Plough, USA.
Loratadine (p.420·1).
Allergic conjunctivitis; allergic rhinitis; hypersensitivity reactions of the skin.

Claritin Extra *Schering-Plough, Canad.*
Loratadine (p.420·1); pseudoephedrine sulfate (p.1099·3).
Upper respiratory-tract congestion.

Claritin-D *Schering-Plough, Braz.; Schering, USA.*
Loratadine (p.420·1); pseudoephedrine sulfate (p.1099·3).
Allergic rhinitis.

Claritine
Schering-Plough, Belg.; Schering-Plough, Neth.; Schering-Plough, Port.; Essex, Switz.
Loratadine (p.420·1).
Allergic rhinitis; urticaria.

Claritone *Fischer, Israel.*
Comfort solution for contact lens (p.1129·2).

Clarityn
Aesca, Aust.; Schering-Plough, Denm.; Schering-Plough, Fin.; Schering-Plough, Irl.; Schering-Plough, Ital.; Schering-Plough, Norw.; Schering-Plough, Swed.; Schering-Plough, UK.
Loratadine (p.420·1).
Allergic conjunctivitis; allergic rhinitis; pruritus; urticaria.

Clarityne
Schering-Plough, Fr.; Schering-Plough, Hong Kong; Schering-Plough, Mex.; Schering-Plough, S.Afr.; Schering-Plough, Singapore; Schering-Plough, Spain; Schering-Plough, Thai.
Loratadine (p.420·1).
Allergic conjunctivitis; allergic rhinitis; allergic skin disorders; urticaria.

Clarityne D
Schering-Plough, Mex.; Schering-Plough, S.Afr.
Loratadine (p.420·1); pseudoephedrine hydrochloride (p.1099·3) or pseudoephedrine sulfate (p.1099·2).
Upper respiratory-tract congestion.

Clarix *Cooperation Pharmaceutique, Fr.*
Erysimum; pholcodine (p.1099·1).
Formerly contained ephedrine hydrochloride, pholcodine, aconite root, belladonna, sodium camsilate, and sulfogaiacol.
Coughs.

Clarmyl *Roussel, Spain†.*
Clobazam (p.668·1).
Anxiety; insomnia.

Clarograf *Juste, Spain.*
Iopromide (p.1036·1).
Radiographic contrast medium.

Clarover Ciba Vision, Ital.
Povidone (p.1503·2).
Dry eyes.

Clarvisan
Allergan, Ital.; Hormona, Mex.; Seber, Port.; Alcon Cusi, Spain.
Pirenoxine sodium (p.1652·2).
Cataracts.

Clarvisol Allergan-Frumtost, Braz.
Pirenoxine (p.1652·2); taurine (p.1669·3).
Cataracts.

Clarvisor Alcon, Ger.
Pirenoxine sodium (p.1652·2).
Cataracts.

Clasteon Abiogen, Ital.
Disodium clodronate (p.751·2).
Hyperparathyroidism; multiple myeloma; osteolytic tumours; osteoporosis.

Clastoban Rhone-Poulenc Rorer, Fr.
Disodium clodronate (p.751·2).
Hypercalcaemia of malignancy; osteolysis of malignancy.

Claudemor
Luitpold, Braz.; Sankyo, Port.
Thromboplastin (p.742·1); benzocaine (p.1306·2); procaine (p.1319·2); zinc oxide (p.1128·2); bismuth subgallate (p.1213·2); peru balsam (p.1650·2).
Anorectal disorders.

Claudicat
Byk Gulden, Ger.; Byk, Port.
Oxpentifylline [pentoxifylline] (p.950·3).
Cerebral and peripheral vascular disorders; vascular eye disorders.

Clauparest Pekana, Ger.
Homoeopathic preparation.

Clavamel Clonmel, Irl.
Amoxicillin trihydrate (p.149·2); potassium clavulanate (p.187·2).
Bacterial infections.

Clavamox
Tyrol, Aust.; Bial, Port.
Amoxicillin sodium (p.149·2) or amoxicillin trihydrate (p.149·2); potassium clavulanate (p.187·2).
Bacterial infections.

Claventin SmithKline Beecham, Fr.
Ticarcillin sodium (p.262·3); potassium clavulanate (p.187·2).
Bacterial infections.

Clavepen
Clintex, Port.; Almirall, Spain.
Amoxicillin trihydrate (p.149·2); potassium clavulanate (p.187·2).
Bacterial infections.

Claversal
Merck, Aust.; Tramedica, Belg.; SmithKline Beecham, Ger.; Merckle, Ger.; Parke, Davis, Ital.; Byk, Port.; SmithKline, Spain.
Mesalazine (p.1234·1).
Inflammatory bowel disease.

Clavigrenin Hormosan, Ger.
Dihydroergotamine mesilate (p.450·3).
Hypotension; migraine and related vascular headaches.

Clavoxil Haller, Braz.
Amoxicillin (p.149·2); clavulanic acid (p.187·2).
Bacterial infections.

Clavucar Geymonat, Ital.
Ticarcillin sodium (p.262·3); potassium clavulanate (p.187·2).
Lignocaine [lidocaine] hydrochloride (p.1313·1) is included in the intramuscular injection to alleviate the pain of injection.
Bacterial infections.

Clavucid
Yamanouchi, Belg.; Recordati, Spain.
Amoxicillin trihydrate (p.149·2); potassium clavulanate (p.187·2).
Bacterial infections.

Clavulin
GlaxoSmithKline, Austral.; SmithKline Beecham, Braz.; SmithKline Beecham, Canad.; Fournier, Ital.; Sanfer, Mex.
Amoxicillin (p.149·2) or amoxicillin trihydrate (p.149·2); potassium clavulanate (p.187·2).
Bacterial infections.

Clavumox Pharmacia Upjohn, Spain.
Amoxicillin trihydrate (p.149·2); potassium clavulanate (p.187·2).
Bacterial infections.

Cleactor Eisai, Jpn.
Monteplase (p.936·1).
Thromboembolic disorders.

Clean & Clear Deep Cleaning Astringent
Johnson & Johnson, Canad.
Salicylic acid (p.1122·3).
Acne.

Clean & Clear Foaming Cleanser Johnson & Johnson, Canad.
Triclosan (p.1159·2).
Acne.

Clean & Clear Invisible Blemish Johnson & Johnson, Canad.
Salicylic acid (p.1122·3).
Acne.

Clean Skin Anti Acne Mentholatum, Austral.
Melaleuca oil (p.1631·3).

Clean Skin Face Wash Mentholatum, Austral.
Melaleuca oil (p.1631·3); benzalkonium chloride (p.1133·2).
Acne.

Clean-AF Floris, Israel.
Sodium chloride (p.1196·1).
Nasal congestion.

Cleancef Shin Poong, Singapore.
Cefaclor (p.161·1).
Bacterial infections.

Cleaner No 4 Fischer, Israel.
Thiomersal (p.1158·2); disodium edetate (p.1008·1)(p.1129·2).
Cleaning solution for soft contact lenses.

Clean-N-Soak
Allergan, Austral.; Allergan, Israel.
Cleaning and soaking solution for contact lens (p.1129·2).

Cleanomed Agepha, Aust.
Alcohol (p.1130·3); isopropyl alcohol (p.1149·2).
Skin disinfection.

Cleansing Herb Tablets Potter's, UK.
Senna leaves (p.1248·2); aloes (p.1210·1); cascara (p.1216·1); taraxacum (p.1669·1); fennel seed (p.1610·1).
Constipation.

Cleansing Lotion Hamilton, Austral.
Glycerol (p.1616·3); liquid paraffin (p.1407·1); chlorhexidine gluconate (p.1138·2).
Skin cleansing; skin disorders.

Cleanxate Sam Chun Dang, Singapore.
Flavoxate hydrochloride (p.467·1).
Urinary-tract disorders.

Clear Away
Schering-Plough, Austral.; Schering-Plough, Canad.†; Schering-Plough, NZ.
Salicylic acid (p.1122·3).
Warts.

Clear By Design SmithKline Beecham Consumer, USA.
Benzoyl peroxide (p.1111·1).
Acne.

Clear & Clean Persa Johnson & Johnson, Canad.
Benzoyl peroxide (p.1111·1).
Acne.

Clear Cough Be-Tabs, S.Afr.
Diphenhydramine hydrochloride (p.416·1); ammonium chloride (p.1085·2); sodium citrate (p.1186·2).
Coughs.

Clear Ear Co-Pharma, UK.
Docusate sodium (p.1223·1).
Removal of ear wax.

Clear Eyes
Abbott, Austral.; Abbott, Canad.; Abbott, NZ; Ross, USA.
Naphazoline hydrochloride (p.1095·1).
Eye irritation.

Clear Eyes ACR
Abbott, NZ; Ross, USA.
Naphazoline hydrochloride (p.1095·1); zinc sulfate (p.1398·2).
Eye irritation.

Clear Eyes CLR Ross, USA.
Sodium chloride (p.1196·1); hypromellose (p.1501·3) (p.1129·2).
Moistening drops for contact lenses.

Clear Pore
Professional Health, Canad.†; Neutrogena, Fr.
Salicylic acid (p.1122·3).
Seborrhoea.

Clear Total Lice Elimination System Care, USA.
Shampoo, pyrethrum extract (p.1436·3); piperonyl butoxide (p.1436·2); enzymic lice egg remover; comb.
Pediculosis.

Clear Tussin 30 Goldline, USA.
Guaifenesin (p.1092·2); dextromethorphan hydrobromide (p.1087·3).
Coughs.

ClearAc Hylands, Canad.
Homoeopathic preparation.

ClearAc Cleanser Hylands, Canad.
Homoeopathic preparation.

Clearamed
Procter & Gamble, Spain; Procter & Gamble, Swed.†.
Benzoyl peroxide (p.1111·1).
Acne.

Clearasil
Note. This name is used for preparations of different composition.
Procter & Gamble, Braz.
Sulfur (p.1123·3); resorcinol (p.1122·2); triclosan (p.1159·2).
Acne.

Richardson-Vicks Personal Care, USA.
Benzoyl peroxide (p.1111·1).
Acne.

Clearasil Acne Cream Procter & Gamble, Canad.
Sulfur (p.1123·3); resorcinol (p.1122·2).
Formerly contained sulfur, resorcinol, and triclosan.
Acne.

Clearasil Acne Treatment Cream Procter & Gamble, Austral.
Sulfur (p.1123·3); triclosan (p.1159·2).
Acne.

Clearasil Antibacterial Richardson-Vicks Personal Care, USA.
Triclosan (p.1159·2); glycerol (p.1616·3); titanium dioxide (p.1126·1).
Acne.

Clearasil B.P. Plus Procter & Gamble, Canad.
Benzoyl peroxide (p.1111·1).
Acne.

Clearasil Cleanser Procter & Gamble, Canad.
Salicylic acid (p.1122·3).
Acne.

Clearasil Clearstick
Procter & Gamble, Canad.; Procter & Gamble, USA.
Salicylic acid (p.1122·3).
Acne.

Clearasil Daily Face Wash
Note. This name is used for preparations of different composition.
Procter & Gamble, Austral.
Phenoxyisopropanol (p.1153·3).
Acne.

Procter & Gamble, USA.
Triclosan (p.1159·2).

Clearasil Double Clear Richardson-Vicks, USA.
Salicylic acid (p.1122·3); alcohol (p.1130·3); hamamelis (p.1618·3).
Acne.

Clearasil Double Textured Pads Procter & Gamble, USA.
Salicylic acid (p.1122·3); alcohol (p.1130·3).
Acne.

Clearasil Dual Action Pads Crookes Healthcare, UK.
Salicylic acid (p.1122·3).
Acne.

Clearasil Extra Strength Procter & Gamble, Austral.†.
Benzoyl peroxide (p.1111·1); aluminium hydroxide (p.1210·2).
Acne.

Clearasil Face Wash Procter & Gamble, Canad.
Triclosan (p.1159·2).
Formerly contained phenoxypropanol.
Acne.

Clearasil Jabon Procter & Gamble, Mex.
Triclosan (p.1159·2).
Acne.

Clearasil Max 10 Procter & Gamble (H&B Care), UK.
Benzoyl peroxide (p.1111·1).
Acne.

Clearasil Medicated Cleanser Procter & Gamble, Canad.†.
Salicylic acid (p.1122·3); alcohol (p.1130·3).
Acne.

Clearasil Medicated Face Wash Procter & Gamble (H&B Care), UK.
Phenoxypropanol (p.1153·3).
Acne.

Clearasil Medicated Foam Procter & Gamble, Austral.†.
Triclosan (p.1159·2); salicylic acid (p.1122·3).
Acne.

Clearasil Medicated Lotion Crookes Healthcare, UK.
Chlorhexidine gluconate (p.1138·2); alcohol (p.1130·3).
Acne.

Clearasil Medicated Moisturiser Procter & Gamble (H&B Care), UK.
Triclosan (p.1159·2).
Acne.

Clearasil Medicated Wipes Procter & Gamble, Austral.
Salicylic acid (p.1122·3).
Acne.

Clearasil Nightclear Procter & Gamble (H&B Care), UK.
Salicylic acid (p.1122·3).
Acne.

Clearasil Pads
Procter & Gamble, Canad.; Procter & Gamble, Mex.
Salicylic acid (p.1122·3).
Acne.

Clearasil Plus Procter & Gamble, Mex.
Benzoyl peroxide (p.1111·1).
Acne.

Clearasil Sensitive Skin Cleanser Procter & Gamble, Canad.†.
Cetrimonium bromide (p.1137·3); chlorhexidine gluconate (p.1138·2); alcohol (p.1130·3).
Acne.

Clearasil Soap Procter & Gamble (H&B Care), UK.
Triclosan (p.1159·2).
Acne.

Clearasil Treatment Cream Crookes Healthcare, UK.
Triclosan (p.1159·2); sulfur (p.1123·3).
Acne.

Clearasil Ultra
Procter & Gamble, Austral.; Procter & Gamble, Ital.†.
Benzoyl peroxide (p.1111·1).
Acne.

Clearasil Wash Antiseptico Procter & Gamble, Mex.
Triclosan (p.1159·2).
Acne.

Clearblue
Novartis Consumer, Canad.; Unipath, Fr.; Unipath, Israel; Farmades, Ital.; Warner-Lambert, NZ; Unipath, UK.
Pregnancy test (p.1654·3).

Clearblue Easy Whitehall, USA.
Pregnancy test (p.1654·3).

Clearblue One Step Warner-Lambert, Austral.
Pregnancy test (p.1654·3).

Clearex Medibrands, Israel.
Salicylic acid (p.1122·3).
Acne.

Clearex Cover Up Medibrands, Israel.
Benzoyl peroxide (p.1111·1).
Acne.

Clear-Flex Formula 13, 15, 55, 62, 91, AA, AB, AC Bieffe, Switz.†.
A range of glucose and electrolyte solutions for peritoneal dialysis (p.1184·1).

Clearly Cala-gel Tec, USA†.
Diphenhydramine hydrochloride (p.416·1); zinc acetate (p.1398·1).

Clearon Sanofi Synthelabo, Spain.
Binifibrate (p.850·1).
Hyperlipidaemias.

Clearplan
Novartis Consumer, Canad.; Unipath, Fr.; Farmades, Ital.; Warner-Lambert, NZ; Whitehall-Robins, Switz.; Unipath, UK.
Fertility test (p.1654·3).

Clearplan Easy Whitehall, USA.
Fertility test (p.1654·3).

Clearplan One Step Warner-Lambert, Austral.
Fertility test (p.1654·3).

Clearskin Acne Defense Stick Avon, Canad.
Salicylic acid (p.1122·3); alcohol (p.1130·3).
Acne.

Clearskin Cleansing Avon, Canad.
Salicylic acid (p.1122·3).
Acne.

Clearskin Medicated Cleanser Avon, Canad.
Triclosan (p.1159·2).
Acne.

Clearskin Medicated Wash Avon, Canad.
Salicylic acid (p.1122·3).
Acne.

Clearskin 2 Medicated Wash Avon, Canad.
Salicylic acid (p.1122·3).
Acne.

Clearskin Overnight Acne Treatment Avon, Canad.
Salicylic acid (p.1122·3).
Acne.

Clearskin 2 Overnight Acne Treatment Avon, Canad.
Salicylic acid (p.1122·3); alcohol (p.1130·3).
Acne.

Clearskin 2 Tinted Blemish Avon, Canad.
Sulfur (p.1123·3); resorcinol (p.1122·2).
Acne.

Clearskin 2 Triple Action Avon, Canad.
Salicylic acid (p.1122·3).
Acne.

Clearsol Coventry, UK.
Tar acids (p.1158·1).

Clear-View Colgate Oral Care, Austral.
Note. A similar name is used for preparations of different composition (see below).
Demisting solution for dental mirrors and spectacles.

Clearview HCG
Note. A similar name is used for preparations of different composition (see above).
Warner-Lambert, Austral.; Searle, Port.†; Unipath, UK; Wampole, USA.
Pregnancy test (p.1654·3).

Clebofex Quimedical, Port.
Clebopride malate (p.1221·2).
Gastrointestinal disorders; neuroses.

Cleboril Almirall, Spain.
Clebopride malate (p.1221·2).
Gastrointestinal disorders; nausea and vomiting.

Clebutec Pharmacia Upjohn, Port.
Clebopride malate (p.1221·2).
Gastrointestinal disorders.

Cledial Lipha Sante, Fr.†.
Medifoxamine (p.297·3).
Depression.

Cleensheen Florafaun, Austral.
Malathion (Maldison) (p.1434·2).
Pediculosis.

Clembroxol Ferring, Port.
Ambroxol hydrochloride (p.1084·3); clenbuterol hydrochloride (p.763·3).
Respiratory-tract disorders.

Clemental Therabel, Fr.
Tiapride hydrochloride (p.709·1).

Clements Iron Felton, Austral.
Multivitamin, mineral, and glucose preparation with iron (p.1366·3)(p.1350·1).
Iron deficiency; nutritional anaemia.

Clements Tonic Felton, Austral.
Mineral preparation with malt, honey, thiamine, and yeast (p.1350·1).
Dietary supplement.

Clemenzil ST Medopharm, Ger.
Melilotus officinalis.
Chronic venous insufficiency; haemorrhoids; thrombophlebitis.

Clemipen Biochemie, Aust.†.
Clemizole penicillin (p.188·1).
Syphilis.

Clenasma
Biomedica, Hong Kong; Biomedica, Ital.
Clenbuterol hydrochloride (p.763·3).
Obstructive airways disease.

Cleniderm Chiesi, Ital.†.
Beclometasone dipropionate (p.1061·2).
Skin disorders.

Clenil
Note.This name is used for preparations of different composition.
Farmalab, Braz.
Betamethasone dipropionate (p.1063·2).
Obstructive airways disease.

Chiesi, Hong Kong; Chiesi, Ital.; Rolab, S.Afr.; Chiesi, Singapore; Chiesi, Thai.
Beclometasone dipropionate (p.1061·2).
Obstructive airways disease.

Clenil Compositum
Note.This name is used for preparations of different composition.
Farmalab, Braz.
Betamethasone dipropionate (p.1063·2); salbutamol (p.770·3).
Obstructive airways disease.

Chiesi, Ital.; Chiesi, Singapore; Chiesi, Thai.
Beclometasone dipropionate (p.1061·2); salbutamol (p.770·3) or salbutamol sulfate (p.770·3).
Obstructive airways disease.

Clens *Alcon, USA†.*
Cleansing solution for hard contact lenses (p.1129·2).

Clen-Zym *Alcon, UK.*
Pancreatin (p.1646·1) (p.1129·2).
Soft contact lens cleanser.

Cleocin
Pharmacia Upjohn, Aust.; Kenral, Austral.; Pharmacia Upjohn, Ital.; Pharmacia Upjohn, USA.
Clindamycin hydrochloride (p.188·1) or clindamycin phosphate (p.188·2).
Bacterial infections.

Cleocin T *Pharmacia Upjohn, USA.*
Clindamycin phosphate (p.188·2).
Acne.

Cleregil *Monot, Fr.*
Deanol aceglumate (p.1507·2).
Asthenia.

Cleridium *EG, Fr.*
Dipyridamole (p.877·2).
Thromboembolism prophylaxis.

Clerz
Note.This name is used for preparations of different composition.
Ciba Vision, Austral.; Ciba Vision, Canad.
Poloxamer 407 (p.1347·1)(p.1129·2).
Lubricating, cleansing, and hydrating eye drops for use with soft contact lenses.

Alcon, USA.
Range of solutions for contact lenses (p.1129·2).

Clerz Moisturising Drops *Ciba Vision, Austral.*
Povidone (p.1503·2).
Formerly contained hyetellose and poloxamer 407.
Dry eyes.

Clesidren *FD, Ital.*
Epomediol (p.1606·3).
Liver disorders.

Cletan *Intersan, Ger.†.*
Urtica (p.1678·2).
Benign prostatic hyperplasia.

Cleveral *Aesculapius, Ital.*
Piracetam (p.1652·1).
Mental function impairment.

Clevian *Aesculapius, Ital.*
Piroxicam (p.79·1).
Musculoskeletal and joint disorders.

Clexane
Rhone-Poulenc Rorer, Austral.; Aventis, Belg.; Rhodia, Braz.; Rhone-Poulenc Rorer, Ger.; Rhone-Poulenc Rorer, Hong Kong; Rhone-Poulenc Rorer, Irl.; Rhone-Poulenc Rorer, Israel; Rhone-Poulenc Rorer, Ital.; Rhone-Poulenc Rorer, Mex.; Rhone-Poulenc Rorer, Neth.; Aventis, NZ; Aventis, S.Afr.; Rhone-Poulenc Rorer, Singapore; Rhone-Poulenc Rorer, Spain; Rhone-Poulenc Rorer, Switz.; Rhone-Poulenc Rorer, Thai.; Rhone-Poulenc Rorer, UK.
Enoxaparin sodium (p.885·1).
Deep vein thrombosis; prevention of clotting during haemodialysis; pulmonary embolism; thromboembolism prophylaxis; unstable angina.

Cliacil *Hoechst Marion Roussel, Aust.*
Phenoxymethylpenicillin potassium (p.235·1).
Bacterial infections.

Cliane *Schering, Mex.*
Estradiol (p.1473·1); norethisterone acetate (p.1485·1).
Menopausal disorders; osteoporosis.

Clifordin *Knoll, Belg.*
Doxycycline (p.200·1) or doxycycline hyclate (p.200·1).
Bacterial infections.

Climacilin *Climax, Braz.*
Benzylpenicillin sodium (p.157·2); procaine penicillin [procaine benzylpenicillin] (p.239·2); streptomycin sulfate (p.249·1).
Bacterial infections.

Climacteron *Sabex, Canad.*
Testosterone enantate benzilic acid hydrazone; estradiol dienanthate (p.1473·2); estradiol benzoate (p.1473·1).
Menopausal disorders; osteoporosis.

Climaderm
Wyeth, Braz.; Wyeth, Mex.
Estradiol (p.1473·1).
Menopausal disorders; osteoporosis.

Climagest *Novartis, UK.*
16 Tablets, estradiol valerate (p.1473·2); 12 tablets, estradiol valerate; norethisterone (p.1485·1).
Menopausal disorders.

Climara
Schering, Aust.; Schering, Austral.; Schering, Belg.; Berlex, Canad.; Schering, Denm.; Schering, Fin.; Schering, Fr.; Schering, Irl.; Schering,

Israel; Schering, Ital.; Schering, Neth.; Schering, Norw.; Schering, NZ; Schering, Port.; Schering, S.Afr.; Schering, Swed.; Schering, Switz.; Schering, Thai.; Berlex, USA.
Estradiol (p.1473·1).
Menopausal disorders; oestrogen deficiency; osteoporosis.

Climara Duo *Schering, Fin.; Schering, Port.*
4 Patches, estradiol (p.1473·1); 4 patches, estradiol; levonorgestrel (p.1486·2).
Menopausal disorders.

Climarest *LAW, Ger.*
Conjugated oestrogens (p.1467·1).
Menopausal disorders; osteoporosis.

Climaston *Solvay, Fr.*
14 Tablets, estradiol (p.1473·1); 14 tablets, estradiol; dydrogesterone (p.1472·3).
Menopausal disorders; osteoporosis.

Climatidine *Climax, Braz.*
Cimetidine (p.1216·3).
Gastro-oesophageal reflux; gastrointestinal haemorrhage; peptic ulcer; Zollinger-Ellison syndrome.

Climaval *Novartis, UK.*
Estradiol valerate (p.1473·2).
Menopausal disorders.

Climaxol *Lehning, Fr.*
Hamamelis (p.1618·3); viburnum; fragon epineux; hydrastis (p.1621·1); aesculus (p.1574·1).
Peripheral vascular disorders.

Climen
Schering, Aust.; Schering, Austral.; Schering, Belg.; Schering, Denm.; Schering, Ger.; Schering, Hong Kong; Schering, Ital.; Schering, Norw.; Schering, Port.; Schering, S.Afr.; Schering, Singapore; Schering, Switz.; Schering, Thai.
11 Tablets, estradiol valerate (p.1473·2); 10 tablets, estradiol valerate; cyproterone acetate (p.1467·3).
28-Day packs also contain 7 inert tablets.
Menopausal disorders; menstrual disorders; osteoporosis.

Schering, Spain.
Estradiol valerate (p.1473·2); cyproterone acetate (p.1467·3).
Menopausal disorders; osteoporosis.

Climene
Schering, Braz.; Schering, Fr.; Schering, Mex.
11 Tablets, estradiol valerate (p.1473·2); 10 tablets, estradiol valerate; cyproterone acetate (p.1467·3).
Menopausal disorders; osteoporosis.

Schering, Neth.
16 Tablets, estradiol valerate (p.1473·2); 12 tablets, cyproterone acetate (p.1467·3); estradiol valerate.
Menopausal disorders; osteoporosis.

Climesse *Novartis, UK.*
Estradiol valerate (p.1473·2); norethisterone (p.1485·1).
Menopausal disorders; osteoporosis.

Climopax *Wyeth, Ger.*
Conjugated oestrogens (p.1467·1); medroxyprogesterone acetate (p.1480·1).
Menopausal disorders; osteoporosis.

Climopax Cyclo *Wyeth, Ger.*
14 Tablets, conjugated oestrogens (p.1467·1); 14 tablets, conjugated oestrogens; medroxyprogesterone acetate (p.1480·1).
Menopausal disorders; osteoporosis.

Clinac
Note.This name is used for preparations of different composition.
Pacific, Hong Kong.
Clindamycin (p.189·3).
Acne.

Pacific, NZ.
Clindamycin phosphate (p.188·2).
Acne.

Oftalder, Port.
Erythromycin (p.201·2).
Acne.

Clinac BPO *Ferndale, USA.*
Benzoyl peroxide (p.1111·1).
Acne.

Clinadil *Grunenthal, Spain.*
Cinnarizine (p.413·1); dihydroergocristine mesilate (p.1603·2).
Cerebrovascular disorders.

Clinadil Compositum *Grunenthal, Spain.*
Cinnarizine (p.413·1); co-dergocrine mesilate (p.1597·3); heptaminol acephyllinate (p.765·3).
Cerebrovascular disorders.

Clinamide *Norton, S.Afr.†.*
Metoclopramide hydrochloride (p.1235·2).
Gastrointestinal disorders.

Clinasol *Gambar, Ital.†.*
Sodium tetrachloroiodite.
Infections; water purification.

Clinaten *Norton, S.Afr.†.*
Atenolol (p.841·3).
Angina pectoris; hypertension; myocardial infarction.

Clinazole *Norton, S.Afr.†.*
Metronidazole (p.594·1).
Anaerobic bacterial infections; protozoal infections.

Clinda *Lichtenstein, Ger.; Wolff, Ger.*
Clindamycin hydrochloride (p.188·1) or clindamycin palmitate hydrochloride (p.188·1).
Bacterial infections.

Clindabeta *Betapharm, Ger.*
Clindamycin hydrochloride (p.188·1).
Bacterial infections.

Clindac
Hexal, Aust.; Intramed, S.Afr.
Clindamycin (p.189·3) or clindamycin hydrochloride (p.188·1).
Bacterial infections.

Clinda-Derm *Paddock, USA.*
Clindamycin phosphate (p.188·2).
Acne.

Clindagel *Galderma, USA.*
Clindamycin phosphate (p.188·2).
Acne.

Clindahexal
Hexal, Ger.; Hexal, S.Afr.
Clindamycin hydrochloride (p.188·1) or clindamycin phosphate (p.188·2).
Bacterial infections.

Clinda-saar *Rosen, Ger.*
Clindamycin hydrochloride (p.188·1) or clindamycin phosphate (p.188·2).
Bacterial infections.

Clindastad *Stada, Ger.*
Clindamycin hydrochloride (p.188·1).
Bacterial infections.

Clindatech *Dermatech, Austral.*
Clindamycin hydrochloride (p.188·1).
Acne.

Clindazyn *Lemery, Mex.*
Clindamycin phosphate (p.188·2).
Bacterial infections.

Clindets *Stiefel, USA.*
Clindamycin phosphate (p.188·2).
Acne.

Clindex *Chelsea, USA.*
Clidinium bromide (p.465·1); chlordiazepoxide hydrochloride (p.659·2).
Gastrointestinal disorders.

Clinensol *Allergan-Frumtost, Braz.*
Miranol (p.1129·2).
Cleansing solution for contact lenses.

Clinesfar *Essex, Ger.*
Erythromycin (p.201·2); tretinoin (p.1126·2).
Acne.

Cliniben *Norton, S.Afr.†.*
Glibenclamide (p.321·3).
Diabetes mellitus.

Clinic A Retinol Vital Day *Jamieson, Canad.*
SPF20: Meradimate (p.1517·3); octinoxate (p.1517·3); octisalate (p.1518·1); oxybenzone (p.1518·1).
Sunscreen.

Clinical Program *Nutricia, Austral.*
Preparations for enteral nutrition (p.1350·1).

Clinicide *De Witt, UK†.*
Carbaryl (p.1429·2).
Pediculosis.

Cliniderm *Wild, Switz.*
Cream: Polyethylene granules (abrasive) (p.1108·3); salicylic acid (p.1122·3).
Topical solution: Triclosan (p.1159·2).
Acne; seborrhoea.

Clinifeed *Clintec, Irl.†; Nestle, UK†.*
Preparation for enteral nutrition (p.1350·1).

Cliniflam *Norton, S.Afr.†.*
Diclofenac sodium (p.30·3).
Gout; inflammation; musculoskeletal and joint disorders; pain.

Clinigel
Pharmacia Upjohn, Austral.; Pharmacia Upjohn, NZ.
Lubricating gel.

Clinimix
Clintec, Aust.; Baxter, Belg.; Clintec, Denm.; Baxter, Fin.; Baxter, Fr.; Baxter, Ger.; Clintec, Ital.; Baxter, Swed.; Baxter, UK.
A range of amino-acid and carbohydrate infusions with or without electrolytes (p.1350·1).
Parenteral nutrition.

Clinimycin *Galen, Irl.*
Oxytetracycline (p.234·1).
Bacterial infections.

Cliniretic *Norton, S.Afr.†.*
Amiloride hydrochloride (p.835·1); hydrochlorothiazide (p.907·3).
Hypertension; oedema.

Clinisorb *CliniMed, Ger.*
Activated charcoal (p.1000·2).
Formerly known as Cliniflex.
Malodorous wounds.

Clinispas *Norton, S.Afr.†.*
Baclofen (p.1322·3).
Skeletal muscle spasm or spasticity.

Clinistix
Bayer, Austral.; Miles, Canad.†; Bayer Diagnostics, Fr.; Bayer Diagnostics, Irl.; Ames, Israel; Bayer Diagnostici, Ital.; Bayer, NZ; Bayer, Port.; Bayer Diagnostics, UK; Bayer, USA.
Test for glucose in urine (p.1616·3).

Clinit *Kwizda, Aust.†.*
Ampoule 1, mofebutazone sodium (p.55·3); lignocaine [lidocaine] (p.1313·2); ampoule 2, dexamethasone (p.1067·1); cyanocobalamin (p.1388·1); lignocaine [lidocaine] (p.1313·2).
Musculoskeletal and joint disorders.

Clinit N *Hormosan, Ger.*
Sodium salamidacetate (p.81·3).
Lignocaine [lidocaine] (p.1313·2) is included in this preparation to alleviate the pain of injection.

Formerly consisted of 2 ampoules: ampoule 1, sodium salamidacetate and ampoule 2, cyanocobalamin.
Joint disorders; severe pain.

Clinitar
Shire, Irl.; Cambridge Healthcare, UK.
Coal tar (Stantar) (p.1125·1).
Dandruff; eczema; psoriasis; seborrhoeic dermatitis.

Clinitek HCG *Bayer, Austral.*
Pregnancy test (p.1654·3).

Clinitek Microalbumin *Bayer, Austral.*
Test for albumin and creatinine in urine.

Clinitest
Bayer, Austral.; Bayer, Canad.; Bayer Diagnostics, Fr.; Bayer Diagnostics, Irl.; Ames, Israel; Bayer Diagnostici, Ital.; Bayer Diagnostics, Mex.; Bayer, NZ; Bayer Diagnostics, UK; Bayer, USA.
Test for reducing substances in urine (p.1616·3).
In the UK these are described in the Drug Tariff as Copper Solution Reagent Tablets.

Clinofem *Pharmacia Upjohn, Ger.*
Medroxyprogesterone acetate (p.1480·1).
Progestogenic; test of ovarian function.

Clinofen *Norton, S.Afr.†.*
Ibuprofen (p.43·2).
Inflammation; musculoskeletal and joint disorders; pain.

Clinofug D *Wolff, Ger.*
Doxycycline hyclate (p.200·1).
Acne.

Clinofug Gel *Wolff, Ger.†.*
Erythromycin (p.201·2).
Acne.

Clinogel *Asta Medica, Fr.*
Isopropyl alcohol (p.1149·2); triclosan (p.1159·2).
Hand disinfection.

Clinolat *Norton, S.Afr.†.*
Nifedipine (p.940·1).
Angina pectoris.

Clinoleic
Baxter, Belg.; Clintec, Denm.; Baxter, Fin.; Baxter, Fr.; Baxter, Ger.; Baxter, Irl.; Baxter, Ital.; Baxter, Spain; Baxter, UK.
Olive oil (p.1643·3); soya oil (p.1378·1).
Contains egg phosphatides.
Lipid infusion for parenteral nutrition.

Clinomel
Clintec, Aust.; Baxter, Belg.; Baxter, Fin.; Baxter, Fr.; Baxter, Spain; Baxter, UK.
Amino-acid, electrolyte, glucose, and lipid (from soya oil (p.1378·1)) infusion (p.1350·1).
Contains egg phosphatides.
Parenteral nutrition.

Clinoril
Merck Sharp & Dohme, Aust.; Frosst, Austral.; Merck Sharp & Dohme, Belg.; Merck Frosst, Canad.†; Merck Sharp & Dohme, Denm.; Merck Sharp & Dohme, Hong Kong; Merck Sharp & Dohme, Irl.; Neopharmed, Ital.; Merck Sharp & Dohme, Mex.; Merck Sharp & Dohme, Neth.; Merck Sharp & Dohme, Norw.; Merck Sharp & Dohme, NZ; Merck Sharp & Dohme, S.Afr.; Merck Sharp & Dohme, Swed.; Merck Sharp & Dohme, Switz.; Merck Sharp & Dohme, Thai.; Merck Sharp & Dohme, UK; Merck, USA.
Sulindac (p.85·3).
Gout; musculoskeletal, joint, and peri-articular disorders.

Clinosyn *Norton, S.Afr.†.*
Naproxen (p.60·3).
Dysmenorrhoea; gout; musculoskeletal and joint disorders.

Clinovir *Pharmacia Upjohn, Ger.*
Medroxyprogesterone acetate (p.1480·1).
Breast cancer; endometrial cancer.

Clin-Sanorania *Lichtenstein, Ger.*
Clindamycin hydrochloride (p.188·1).
Bacterial infections.

Clinstan *Norton, S.Afr.†.*
Mefenamic acid (p.51·2).
Fever; pain.

Clinutren
Nestle, Fr.; Nestle, Ital.; Nestle, UK.
A range of preparations for enteral nutrition (p.1350·1).

Clinvit *Plants, Ital.*
Royal jelly (p.1659·3).
Nutritional supplement.

Clinwas *Wasserman, Spain.*
Clindamycin hydrochloride (p.188·1) or clindamycin phosphate (p.188·2).
Bacterial infections.

Clio-Betnovate *Glaxo Wellcome, Mex.*
Betamethasone valerate (p.1063·2); clioquinol (p.190·2).
Infected skin disorders.

Cliogan *Juste, Spain.*
Estradiol (p.1473·1).
Menopausal disorders; osteoporosis.

Clipper *Chiesi, Ital.*
Beclometasone dipropionate (p.1061·2).
Ulcerative colitis.

Clipto *Quimifar, Spain.*
Enalapril maleate (p.883·3).
Heart failure; hypertension.

Cliptol *Pierre Fabre Sante, Fr.*
Ibuprofen (p.43·2); menthol (p.1632·3).
Soft-tissue disorders.

C-Lisa *Lisapharma, Ital.*
Ascorbic acid (p.1389·3) or sodium ascorbate (p.1390·1).
Vitamin C deficiency; vitamin C supplement.

Clisemina *Juventus, Spain†.*
Doxycycline hyclate (p.200·1).
Bacterial infections.

Clisflex *Sella, Ital.*
Monobasic sodium phosphate (p.1193·2); dibasic sodium phosphate (p.1193·2).
Bowel evacuation; constipation.

Clisin *Juste, Spain.*
Estradiol valerate (p.1473·2); cyproterone acetate (p.1467·3).
Menopausal disorders; osteoporosis.

Clisma Bieffe Medital *Bieffe, Spain.*
Monobasic sodium phosphate (p.1193·2); dibasic sodium phosphate (p.1193·2).
Bowel evacuation; constipation.

Clisma Evacuante *Sofar, Ital.†.*
Monobasic sodium phosphate monohydrate (p.1193·2); dibasic sodium phosphate heptahydrate (p.1193·2).
Bowel evacuation.

Clisma Fleet *Bergamon, Ital.*
Monobasic sodium phosphate (p.1193·2); dibasic sodium phosphate (p.1193·2).
Bowel evacuation; constipation.

Clisma-Lax *Sofar, Ital.*
Monobasic sodium phosphate monohydrate (p.1193·2); hydrated dibasic sodium phosphate (p.1193·2).
Bowel evacuation; constipation.

Clivarin
Knoll, Denm.; Knoll, Fin.; Knoll, Ger.; Knoll, Norw.; Knoll, Port.; Knoll, Swed.
Reviparin sodium (p.968·3).
Thromoembolism prophylaxis.

Clivarine
Knoll, Fr.; ICN, UK.
Reviparin sodium (p.968·3).
Thromboembolism prophylaxis.

Clivoten *Italfarmaco, Ital.*
Isradipine (p.916·3).
Hypertension.

Clo Zinc *Llorens, Spain†.*
Chloramphenicol (p.179·1); naphazoline hydrochloride (p.1095·1); zinc sulfate (p.1398·2).
Eye disorders; eye infections.

Clobasone *Pharmaland, Thai.*
Clobetasol propionate (p.1065·2).
Skin disorders.

Clobegalen *Galen, Ger.*
Clobetasol propionate (p.1065·2).
Skin disorders.

Clobendian *Efarmes, Spain.*
Diltiazem hydrochloride (p.874·3).
Angina pectoris; hypertension.

Clobesol *Glaxo Wellcome, Ital.*
Clobetasol propionate (p.1065·2).
Skin disorders.

Clobeson *Dong Kook, Singapore.*
Clobetasol propionate (p.1065·2).
Skin disorders.

Clobet
Note.This name is used for preparations of different composition.
Angelini, Ital.
Clobetasone butyrate (p.1065·2).
Eye disorders.

Biolab, Thai.
Clobetasol propionate (p.1065·2).
Skin disorders.

Clobetate *Polipharm, Thai.*
Clobetasol propionate (p.1065·2).
Skin disorders.

Cloburate *Dominion, UK.*
Clobetasone butyrate (p.1065·2).
Formerly known as Eumovate Eye Drops.
Eye disorders.

Cloburate-N *Dominion, UK†.*
Clobetasone butyrate (p.1065·2); neomycin sulfate (p.228·1).
Formerly known as Eumovate-N Eye Drops.
Infected eye disorders.

Clocillin *Rolab, S.Afr.*
Cloxacillin sodium (p.192·1).
Staphylococcal infections.

Clocim *Cimex, Switz.*
Clotrimazole (p.382·1).
Fungal skin and vaginal infections.

Clocream *Roberts, USA.*
Cod-liver oil (p.1357·2); colecalciferol (p.1391·1); vitamin A palmitate (p.1383·2).
Skin disorders.

Clocreme
Pacific, Hong Kong; Pacific, NZ.
Clotrimazole (p.382·1).
Fungal infections.

Cloderm
Note.This name is used for preparations of different composition.
Dermapharm, Ger.
Clotrimazole (p.382·1).
Fungal skin infections.

Hoe, Singapore.
Clobetasol propionate (p.1065·2).
Skin disorders.

Healthpoint, USA.
Clocortolone pivalate (p.1065·3).
Skin disorders.

Clody *Chiesi, Ital.*
Disodium clodronate (p.751·2).
Hyperparathyroidism; multiple myeloma; osteolysis of malignancy; osteoporosis.

Cloel *Aesculapius, Ital.*
Cloperastine fendizoate (p.1087·2).
Coughs.

Clofec
Atlantic, Hong Kong; Vana, Thai.
Diclofenac sodium (p.30·3).
Musculoskeletal, joint, and peri-articular disorders.

Clofeme 3 Day *Hexal, Austral.*
Clotrimazole (p.382·1).
Vaginal candidiasis.

Clofen
Note.This name is used for preparations of different composition.
Alphapharm, Austral.
Baclofen (p.1322·3).
Skeletal muscle spasm or spasticity.

Julphar, UAE.
Diclofenac diethylamine (p.30·2) or diclofenac sodium (p.30·3).
Gout; inflammation; musculoskeletal, joint, peri-articular, and soft-tissue disorders; pain.

Clofenac *Hovid, Singapore.*
Diclofenac sodium (p.30·3).
Gout; musculoskeletal and joint disorders.

Clofenak *Medley, Braz.*
Diclofenac diethylamine (p.30·2) or diclofenac potassium (p.30·2).
Gout; inflammation; musculoskeletal, joint, and peri-articular disorders; pain.

Clofend *Fidia, Ital.*
Cloperastine fendizoate (p.1087·2).
Coughs.

Clofon *YF Chem, Thai.*
Diclofenac sodium (p.30·3).
Musculoskeletal, joint, and peri-articular disorders.

Clofranil *Sun, Thai.*
Clomipramine hydrochloride (p.282·1).
Depression; narcoleptic syndrome; obsessive-compulsive disorder; phobic states.

Clogar *Self-Care Products, UK.*
Cod-liver oil (p.1357·2); garlic (p.1614·1).

Clogen *UCI, Braz.*
Clotrimazole (p.382·1).
Fungal skin infections.

Clomaderm *Parke-Med, S.Afr.†.*
Clotrimazole (p.382·1).
Fungal skin infections.

Clomazem *Uniao Quimica, Braz.*
Clotrimazole (p.382·1).
Fungal skin infections.

Clomhexal
Hexal, Austral.; Hexal, Ger.
Clomifene citrate (p.1465·3).
Anovulatory infertility.

Clomid
Hoechst Marion Roussel, Aust.; Hoechst Marion Roussel, Austral.; Aventis, Belg.; Medley, Braz.; Hoechst Marion Roussel, Canad.; Marion Merrell, Fr.; Hoechst Marion Roussel, Hong Kong; Hoechst Marion Roussel, Irl.; Bruno, Ital.; Hoechst Marion Roussel, Neth.; Aventis, NZ; Mer-National, S.Afr.; Hoechst Marion Roussel, Singapore; Hoechst Marion Roussel, Switz.; Hoechst Marion Roussel, Thai.; Hoechst Marion Roussel, UK; Hoechst Marion Roussel, USA.
Clomifene citrate (p.1465·3).
Anovulatory infertility; male infertility.

Clomifen *Leiras, Fin.*
Clomifene citrate (p.1465·3).
Anovulatory infertility; male infertility.

Clomifeno *Casen Fleet, Spain.*
Clomifene citrate (p.1465·3).
Anovulatory infertility; male infertility.

Clomin
Quatromed, S.Afr.; Ranbaxy, Thai.
Dicyclomine [dicycloverine] hydrochloride (p.466·1).
Smooth muscle spasm.

Clomivid
AstraZeneca, Denm.; AstraZeneca, Norw.; Tika, Swed.
Clomifene citrate (p.1465·3).
Anovulatory infertility.

Clomycin *Roberts, USA†.*
Bacitracin (p.155·2); neomycin sulfate (p.228·1); polymyxin B sulfate (p.238·1); lignocaine [lidocaine] (p.1313·2).
Skin infections.

Clonalin *Clonmel, Irl.†.*
Diphenhydramine hydrochloride (p.416·1); sodium citrate (p.1186·2); ammonium chloride (p.1085·2); menthol (p.1632·3).
Coughs; respiratory-tract congestion.

Clonamox *Clonmel, Irl.*
Amoxicillin trihydrate (p.149·2).
Bacterial infections.

Clonamp *Clonmel, Irl.*
Ampicillin trihydrate (p.151·1).
Bacterial infections.

Clonapam *ICN, Canad.*
Clonazepam (p.347·1).
Epilepsy.

Clonazine *Clonmel, Irl.*
Chlorpromazine hydrochloride (p.660·2).
Hypothermia induction; premedication; schizophrenia; sedative; vomiting.

Clondepryl *Clonmel, Irl.*
Selegiline hydrochloride (p.1177·2).
Parkinsonism.

Clonea *Alphapharm, Austral.*
Clotrimazole (p.382·1).
Fungal skin infections.

Clonex *Teva, Israel.*
Clonazepam (p.347·1).
Epilepsy.

Clonfolic *Clonmel, Irl.*
Folic acid (p.1361·1).
Prevention of fetal neural tube defects.

Clonid-Ophtal *Winzer, Ger.*
Clonidine hydrochloride (p.860·1).
Glaucoma; ocular hypertension.

Clonilix *Clonmel, Irl.*
Indapamide (p.913·1).
Hypertension.

Clonistada *Stada, Ger.*
Clonidine hydrochloride (p.860·1).
Hypertension.

Clonix *Janssen-Cilag, Port.*
Clonixin (p.25·1).
Pain.

Clonnirit *Rafa, Israel.*
Clonidine hydrochloride (p.860·1).
Menopausal flushing; migraine and other vascular headaches.

Clonodifen *Tecnofarma, Mex.*
Diclofenac (p.30·2).
Inflammation; pain.

Clonofilin *Clonmel, Irl.*
Aminophylline (p.760·1).
Obstructive airways disease.

Clonorax *Clonmel, Irl.*
Aciclovir (p.612·3).
Herpes simplex infections of the lips and face.

Clonovate *TO-Chemicals, Thai.*
Clobetasol propionate (p.1065·2).
Skin disorders.

Clonoxifen *Clonmel, Irl.*
Tamoxifen citrate (p.571·1).
Breast cancer; endometrial cancer.

Clont *Bayer, Ger.*
Metronidazole (p.594·1).
Amoebiasis; anaerobic bacterial infections; giardiasis; trichomoniasis.

Clonteric *Clonmel, Irl.*
Aspirin (p.14·2).
Fever; inflammation; pain; thrombosis prophylaxis.

Clonuretic *Clonmel, Irl.*
Amiloride hydrochloride (p.835·1); hydrochlorothiazide (p.907·3).
Heart failure; hepatic cirrhosis; hypertension; oedema.

Clopamon *Aspen, S.Afr.*
Metoclopramide hydrochloride (p.1235·2).
Gastrointestinal disorders.

Clopan *FIRMA, Ital.*
Metoclopramide hydrochloride (p.1235·2).
Gastrointestinal disorders.

Clopine *Douglas, Austral.*
Clozapine (p.671·2).

Clopirim *Quimioterapica, Braz.*
Chloroquine phosphate (p.432·3); pyrimethamine (p.442·3).
Malaria.

Clopixol
Lundbeck, Austral.; Lundbeck, Belg.; Lundbeck, Canad.; Lundbeck, Fr.; Lundbeck, Hong Kong; Lundbeck, Irl.; Lundbeck, Israel; Lundbeck, Ital.; Organon, Mex.; Lundbeck, NZ; Lundbeck, S.Afr.; Lundbeck, Singapore; Lundbeck, Spain; Lundbeck, Switz.; Lundbeck, Thai; Lundbeck, UK.
Zuclopenthixol acetate (p.714·1), zuclopenthixol decanoate (p.714·1), or zuclopenthixol hydrochloride (p.714·2).
Psychoses.

Clopra *Quantum, USA.*
Metoclopramide hydrochloride (p.1235·2).
Nausea and vomiting.

Cloprane *Luitpold, Ital.†.*
Ronifibrate (p.969·1).
Hyperlipidaemias.

Clopress *Pacific, NZ.*
Clomipramine hydrochloride (p.282·1).
Depression; narcoleptic syndrome; nocturnal enuresis; obsessive-compulsive disorder; pain; panic attacks.

Clopsine *Psicofarma, Mex.*
Clozapine (p.671·2).
Schizophrenia.

Cloptison
Merck Sharp & Dohme, Norw.; Merck Sharp & Dohme, Switz.
Clobetasone butyrate (p.1065·2).
Eye disorders.

Cloptison-N *Merck Sharp & Dohme, Switz.†.*
Clobetasone butyrate (p.1065·2); neomycin sulfate (p.228·1).
Infected eye disorders.

CloraCEF *Ranbaxy, S.Afr.*
Cefaclor (p.161·1).
Bacterial infections.

Clorad *ACS Dobfar, Ital.*
Cefaclor (p.161·1).
Bacterial infections.

Cloradryn *Recordati, Ital.†.*
Cloprednol (p.1065·3).
Corticosteroid.

Clorafen *Merck, Mex.*
Chloramphenicol (p.179·1) or chloramphenicol palmitate (p.179·2).
Bacterial infections.

Cloramed *Medimport, Mex.*
Chloramphenicol (p.179·1).
Bacterial infections.

Cloramfen *Sclavo, Mex.*
Chloramphenicol (p.179·1).
Bacterial eye infections.

Cloramfeni *Sophia, Mex.*
Chloramphenicol (p.179·1).
Bacterial eye infections.

Cloramfenil *Pisa, Mex.*
Chloramphenicol (p.179·1).
Bacterial infections.

Cloran *Grin, Mex.*
Chloramphenicol (p.179·1).
Bacterial eye infections.

Cloran Otico *Grin, Mex.*
Chloramphenicol (p.179·1); benzocaine (p.1306·2).
Bacterial ear infections.

Clorana *Sanofi Winthrop, Braz.*
Hydrochlorothiazide (p.907·3).
Diabetes insipidus; hypertension; oedema; renal calculi.

Cloranfe *Llorens, Spain†.*
Chloramphenicol (p.179·1).
Bacterial eye infections.

Cloranfe Hemidex *Llorens, Spain.*
Boric acid (p.1586·1); chloramphenicol (p.179·1); dexamethasone phosphate (p.1067·1).
Infected eye disorders.

Cloranfenic *Ciba Vision, Spain.*
Chloramphenicol (p.179·1).
Bacterial eye infections.

Cloranfenic Zinc *Llorens, Spain.*
Chloramphenicol (p.179·1); naphazoline hydrochloride (p.1095·1); zinc sulfate (p.1398·2).
Bacterial eye infections.

Cloranpectina *Basi, Port.*
Chloramphenicol (p.179·1); phthalylsulfathiazole (p.235·3); pectin (p.1502·3).
Gastrointestinal infections.

Cloraseptic
Note.This name is used for preparations of different composition.
Legrand, Braz.
Tyrothricin (p.267·1); benzocaine (p.1306·2).
Mouth and throat disorders.

Diviser Aquilea, Spain.
Chlorhexidine gluconate (p.1138·2); chlorobutanol (p.1141·2).
Mouth and throat infections.

Cloraxene *TO-Chemicals, Thai.*
Dipotassium clorazepate (p.670·3).
Anxiety; insomnia.

Clorazin *Tecnofarma, Mex.*
Chloramphenicol (p.179·1).
Bacterial infections.

Clorcorticil *Oftalder, Port.*
Chloramphenicol (p.179·1); hydrocortisone acetate (p.1073·2).
Bacterial eye infections with inflammation.

Clordil *Diba, Mex.*
Chloramphenicol (p.179·1).
Bacterial infections.

Clordispenser *Molteni, Ital.*
Halazone (p.1145·3).
Waste disinfection.

Cloretilo Chemirosa *Ern, Spain.*
Ethyl chloride (p.1312·1).
Local anaesthesia.

Clorexan *IMS, Ital.*
Chlorhexidine gluconate (p.1138·2); isopropyl alcohol (p.1149·2).
Wound disinfection.

Clorexan Ferri *IMS, Ital.*
Chlorhexidine gluconate (p.1138·2); alcohol (p.1130·3).
Surface disinfection.

Clorexident *Warner-Lambert, Ital.†.*
Chlorhexidine gluconate (p.1138·2).
Mouth disorders; oral disinfection.

Clorexident Ortodontico *Warner-Lambert, Ital.†.*
Chlorhexidine gluconate (p.1138·2); sodium fluoride (p.1375·3).
Oral disinfection; prophylaxis of dental caries and gingivitis.

Clorfenil
Allergan-Frumtost, Braz.; Rayere, Mex.
Chloramphenicol (p.179·1).
Bacterial infections.

Clorhexitulle
Hoechst Marion Roussel, Austral.; Hoechst Marion Roussel, UK†.
Chlorhexidine acetate (p.1138·2).
Burns; infected skin disorders; skin ulcers; wounds.

Clorimet Z *Zafiro, Mex.*
Metoclopramide hydrochloride (p.1235·2).
Gastrointestinal motility disorders; nausea and vomiting.

Clorina *Lysoform, Ger.; Squibb, Spain.*
Tosylchloramide sodium (p.1159·1).
Antiseptic; skin and wound disinfection; surface disinfection; water purification.

Cloritines *Torlan, Spain.*
Halazone (p.1145·3); sodium carbonate (p.1665·1); sodium chloride (p.1196·1).
Disinfection of drinking water.

Clor-K-Zaf *Zafiro, Mex.*
Potassium chloride (p.1194·3).
Hypokalaemia; potassium supplement.

Cloroboral *Inexfa, Spain.*
Alum (p.1577·2); boric acid (p.1586·1); potassium chlorate (p.1654·1); thymol (p.1158·3); menthol (p.1632·3).
Gingivitis; mouth and throat irritation; pyorrhoea; stomatitis.

Clorocil *Oftalder, Port.*
Chloramphenicol (p.179·1).
Bacterial eye infections.

Cloromi-T *Formenti, Ital.†.*
Tosylchloramide sodium (p.1159·1).
Disinfection of minor wounds.

Clorosan *Lachifarma, Ital.*
Chlorhexidine gluconate (p.1138·2).
Disinfection of skin, wounds, and burns.

Cloro-Trimeton *Schering-Plough, Mex.*
Chlorpheniramine [chlorphenamine] maleate (p.412·1).
Hypersensitivity.

Clorpactin *Guardian, Canad.†.*
Sodium oxychlorosene (p.1152·1).
Antiseptic.

Clorpactin WCS-90 *Guardian, USA.*
Sodium oxychlorosene (p.1152·1).
Disinfection; skin infections.

Clorpamina Dopamina *Andromaco, Mex.*
Dopamine hydrochloride (p.881·3).
Heart failure; shock.

Clorpres *Bertek, USA.*
Clonidine hydrochloride (p.860·1); chlortalidone (p.857·1).
Hypertension.

Clortalil *Legrand, Braz.*
Chlortalidone (p.857·1).
Hypertension; oedema; renal calculi.

Clortanol *CT, Ital.*
Atenolol (p.841·3); chlortalidone (p.857·1).
Hypertension.

Clorxil *Rovi, Spain.*
Chlorhexidine gluconate (p.1138·2).
Disinfection of skin and wounds.

Closcript *Ranbaxy, S.Afr.*
Clotrimazole (p.382·1).
Fungal skin and vulvovaginal infections.

Closecs *Eurofarma, Braz.; Inaf, Braz.*
Loperamide (p.1232·1).
Diarrhoea.

Closina *Lilly, Austral.*
Cycloserine (p.195·3).
Tuberculosis; urinary-tract infections.

Clostedal *Silanes, Mex.*
Carbamazepine (p.342·2).
Alcohol and benzodiazepine withdrawal syndromes; bipolar disorder; diabetes insipidus; diabetic neuropathy; epilepsy; neuralgias.

Clostet *Evans, UK.*
An adsorbed tetanus vaccine (p.1565·2).
Active immunisation.

Clostilbegyt *Medphano, Ger.†; Egis, Hong Kong; Egis, Singapore.*
Clomifene citrate (p.1465·3).
Anovulatory infertility; oligospermia.

Clotam *Sanova, Aust.; Gea, Denm.; Gea, Fin.; Ecosol, Switz.; Cortecs, UK.*
Tolfenamic acid (p.88·3).
Inflammation; musculoskeletal and joint disorders; pain.

Clotan *SmithKline Beecham, Braz.*
Tolfenamic acid (p.88·3).
Musculoskeletal and joint disorders.

Clotest *Pharmacia Upjohn, Austral.†; Bripharm, Irl.*
Test for presence of *Helicobacter pylori* in gastric mucosal biopsy samples.

Cloton *Nakorn, Thai.*
Chlorpheniramine [chlorphenamine] maleate (p.412·1); ammonium chloride (p.1085·2).
Coughs; nasal congestion; rhinitis.

Clotrason *Schering-Plough, Denm.*
Betamethasone dipropionate (p.1063·2); clotrimazole (p.382·1).
Fungal skin infections.

Clotrasone *Schering-Plough, Spain; Schering-Plough, Thai.*
Betamethasone dipropionate (p.1063·2); clotrimazole (p.382·1).
Fungal skin infections.

Clotri OPT *Optimed, Ger.†.*
Clotrimazole (p.382·1).
Fungal skin infections.

Clotricin *Seng, Thai.*
Clotrimazole (p.382·1).
Fungal vaginal infections; trichomoniasis.

Clotri-Denk *Denk, Hong Kong.*
Clotrimazole (p.382·1).
Fungal and bacterial vaginal infections; fungal skin infections; trichomoniasis.

Clotriferm *Fermenta, Swed.†.*
Clotrimazole (p.382·1).
Fungal infections.

Clotrifug *Wolff, Ger.†.*
Clotrimazole (p.382·1).
Fungal and bacterial vaginal infections.

Clotrigalen *Galen, Ger.*
Clotrimazole (p.382·1).
Fungal skin infections.

Clotrimaderm *Taro, Canad.; Taro, Israel; AFT, NZ.*
Clotrimazole (p.382·1).
Fungal infections; trichomoniasis.

Clotrimix *Medley, Braz.*
Clotrimazole (p.382·1).
Fungal skin infections.

Clovate *Medeva, Spain.*
Clobetasol propionate (p.1065·2).
Skin disorders.

Clovin *Nakornpatana, Thai.*
Aciclovir (p.612·3).
Herpes simplex infections of the skin and mucous membranes.

Clovira *M & H, Thai.*
Aciclovir (p.612·3).
Herpes simplex infections of the skin and mucous membranes.

Clox *Caber, Ital.*
Ticlopidine hydrochloride (p.981·1).
Thrombosis prophylaxis.

Cloxa *Hua, Thai.; M & H, Thai.*
Cloxacillin sodium (p.192·1).
Bacterial infections.

Cloxacap *Hovid, Singapore.*
Cloxacillin sodium (p.192·1).
Bacterial infections.

Cloxalin *Siam Bheasach, Thai.*
Cloxacillin sodium (p.192·1).
Bacterial infections.

Cloxam
Note. This name is used for preparations of different composition.
Bonafarma, Port.
Cloxazolam (p.671·2).
Anxiety disorders.
Aspen, S.Afr.
Ampicillin (p.150·3); cloxacillin (p.192·1).
Bacterial infections.

Cloxan *Orion, Fin.*
Chlorprothixene hydrochloride (p.667·3).
Psychoses.

Cloxanbin *ANB, Thai.*
Cloxacillin sodium (p.192·1).
Bacterial infections.

Cloxapan *Nakornpatana, Thai.*
Cloxacillin sodium (p.192·1).
Bacterial infections.

Cloxapen *SmithKline Beecham, USA.*
Cloxacillin sodium (p.192·1).
Bacterial infections.

Cloxasian *Asian Pharm, Thai.*
Cloxacillin sodium (p.192·1).
Bacterial infections.

Cloxgen *General Drugs, Thai.*
Cloxacillin (p.192·1) or cloxacillin sodium (p.192·1).
Bacterial infections.

Cloxil
Note. This name is used for preparations of different composition.
Duopharma, Hong Kong; Ranbaxy, Thai.
Cloxacillin sodium (p.192·1).
Bacterial infections.
Ofimex, Mex.
Dicloxacillin (p.199·1).
Bacterial infections.

Cloxillin *Ibirn, Ital.*
Flucloxacillin sodium (p.207·1).
Bacterial infections.

Cloxin *Intramed, S.Afr.*
Cloxacillin sodium (p.192·1).
Staphylococcal infections.

Cloxipen *Welfer, Mex.*
Dicloxacillin (p.199·1).
Bacterial infections.

Clozan *Roerig, Belg.*
Clotiazepam (p.671·1).
Anxiety disorders.

Clozaril *Novartis, Austral.; Novartis, Canad.; Novartis, Hong Kong; Novartis, Irl.; Novartis, NZ; Novartis, Singapore; Novartis, Thai.; Novartis, UK; Novartis, USA.*
Clozapine (p.671·2).
Schizophrenia.

Clozole *Genpharm, Austral.; Jean-Marie, Hong Kong; Jean-Marie, Singapore.*
Clotrimazole (p.382·1).
Fungal skin and vaginal infections.

Clusinol *Amrad, Austral.†.*
Sulindac (p.85·3).
Musculoskeletal and joint disorders; pain with inflammation.

Clusivol *Whitehall, Braz.; Aspen Consumer, S.Afr.*
Multivitamin and mineral preparation (p.1350·1).

Clysmol *Pharmacia Upjohn, Aust.*
Monobasic sodium phosphate (p.1193·2); dibasic sodium phosphate (p.1193·2).
Bowel evacuation; constipation.

Clysodrast *Rhone-Poulenc Rorer, USA†.*
Bisacodyl tannex (p.1212·3).
Constipation.

Clyss-Go *Novag, Mex.; Prospa, Port.*
Docusate sodium (p.1223·1); sorbitol (p.1377·3).
Bowel evacuation; constipation.

C-Max *Bio-Tech, USA†.*
Vitamin C and mineral preparation (p.1350·1).

CMD *Nakorn, Thai.*
Cimetidine (p.1216·3).
Gastro-oesophageal reflux; hypersensitivity reactions; peptic ulcer; Zollinger-Ellison syndrome.

C-Mox *Columbia, S.Afr.†.*
Amoxicillin trihydrate (p.149·2).
Bacterial infections.

CMV Immunoglobulin *CSL, Austral.*
A cytomegalovirus immunoglobulin (human) (p.1536·1).
Passive immunisation.

CMV Iveegam *Immuno, Canad.†.*
A cytomegalovirus immunoglobulin (p.1536·1).
Passive immunisation.

CN-25 *Masa, Thai.*
Cinnarizine (p.413·1).
Cerebrovascular disorders; peripheral vascular disorders.

C-Naryl *Homberger, Switz.*
Ascorbic acid (p.1389·3).
Vitamin C supplement.

C'Nergil *Medinfar, Port.*
Ascorbic acid (p.1389·3).
Vitamin C deficiency.

Co Amoxin *Smaller, Spain.*
Amoxicillin trihydrate (p.149·2).
Bacterial infections.

Co Bucal *Smaller, Spain.*
Alum (p.1577·2); procaine hydrochloride (p.1319·1); salicylic acid (p.1122·3); sodium chlorate (p.1665·2); thymol (p.1158·3); cherry laurel water; peppermint oil.
Gingivitis; pyorrhoea; stomatitis.

Co Fluocin Fuerte *Smaller, Spain.*
Fluocinolone acetonide (p.1071·1).
Skin disorders.

CO₂ Granulat *Sanova, Aust.; Guerbet, Ger.*
Betaine hydrochloride (p.1584·3); sodium bicarbonate (p.1186·2); dimethicone (p.1249·2); colloidal silicon dioxide (p.1503·3).
Adjunct in double contrast radiography.

Co Hepa B12 *Smaller, Spain.*
Vitamin B substances (p.1350·1); liver extract.
Tonic; vitamin B deficiency.

Co-Acetan *Kwizda, Aust.*
Lisinopril (p.921·1); hydrochlorothiazide (p.907·3).
Hypertension.

CoActifed *Glaxo Wellcome, Canad.*
Expectorant: Triprolidine hydrochloride (p.427·2); pseudoephedrine hydrochloride (p.1099·2); guaifenesin (p.1092·2); codeine phosphate (p.25·2).
Syrup; tablets: Triprolidine hydrochloride (p.427·2); pseudoephedrine hydrochloride (p.1099·2); codeine phosphate (p.25·2).
Coughs.

Coalgan *Brothier, Fr.*
Calcium alginate (p.728·1).
Haemorrhage.

Coalip *SmithKline Beecham, Ital.*
Coenzyme A (p.1598·1).
Hypertriglyceridaemia.

Coaltar Saponine le Beuf *Gerda, Fr.*
Coal tar (p.1125·1); quillaia (p.1348·2).
Skin disorders.

Co-Amilorid *Cophar, Switz.*
Amiloride hydrochloride (p.835·1); hydrochlorothiazide (p.907·3).
Hypertension; oedema.

Co-Apap *Rugby, USA.*
Chlorpheniramine [chlorphenamine] maleate (p.412·1); dextromethorphan hydrobromide (p.1087·3); paracetamol (p.71·2); pseudoephedrine hydrochloride (p.1099·2).
Coughs and cold symptoms.

CoAprovel *Sanofi, Denm.; Bristol-Myers Squibb, Fr.; Synthelabo, Fr.; Sanofi Winthrop, Ger.; Bristol-Myers Squibb, Irl.; Sanofi Winthrop, Irl.; Sanofi Synthelabo, Ital.; Sanofi Winthrop, Neth.; Bristol-Myers Squibb, Neth.; Sanofi Winthrop, Norw.; Bristol-Myers Squibb, Norw.; Bristol-Myers Squibb, Port.; Sanofi Synthelabo, Port.; Sanofi Winthrop, Swed.; Bristol-Myers Squibb, Swed.; Sanofi Synthelabo, Spain; Sanofi Winthrop, Switz.; Bristol-Myers Squibb, Switz.; Bristol-Myers Squibb, UK; Sanofi Synthelabo, UK.*
Irbesartan (p.914·2); hydrochlorothiazide (p.907·3).
Hypertension.

Cobactin *Zambon, Braz.*
Cyproheptadine (p.414·3); cobamamide (p.1388·3).
Reduced appetite; tonic.

Cobadex *Cox, UK.*
Hydrocortisone (p.1073·3); dimeticone (p.1410·1).
Skin disorders.

Cobaforte *Scharper, Ital.*
Cobamamide (p.1388·3).
Tonic; vitamin B₁₂ deficiency.

Cobaglobal *Legrand, Braz.*
Cobamamide (p.1388·3); cyproheptadine (p.414·3).
Tonic.

Cobalatec *Caps, S.Afr.*
Cyanocobalamin (p.1388·1).
Vitamin B₁₂ deficiency.

Cobalin-H *Link, UK.*
Hydroxocobalamin (p.1388·1).
Anaemia due to B₁₂ deficiency; Leber's atrophy; tobacco amblyopia.

Cobalplex *UCI, Braz.*
Ferric ammonium citrate (p.1359·2); folic acid (p.1361·1); vitamin B₁₂; lysine hydrochloride; tryptophan; threonine; liver extract; gastric mucosa extract (p.1350·1).
Anaemias.

Cobalti *Lepori, Port.*
Ferric ammonium citrate (p.1359·2); copper sulfate (p.1358·1); manganese sulfate (p.1371·3).
Anaemias; tonic.

Cobamet *Roussel, Port.*
Mecobalamin (p.1388·3).
Anaemias.

Cobamol *Maver, Mex.*
Salbutamol (p.770·3).

Cobantril *Pfizer, Switz.*
Pyrantel embonate (p.108·1).
Nematode infections.

Cobanzyme *SERB, Fr.*
Cobamamide (p.1388·3).
Debilitated states.

Cobavital *Sintofarma, Braz.*
Cobamamide (p.1388·3); cyproheptadine hydrochloride (p.414·2).
Reduced appetite; tonic.

Cobaxid *Tecnifar, Port.*
Cobamamide (p.1388·3).
Anaemias; neuralgias; neuritis; tonic.

Co-Betaloc *Astra, Irl.; Pharmacia, UK.*
Metoprolol tartrate (p.931·2); hydrochlorothiazide (p.907·3).
Hypertension.

cobidec n *Warner-Lambert, Ger.*
Multivitamin and mineral preparation (p.1350·1).

Cobiona *Esteve, Spain.*
Oxatomide (p.422·1).
Hypersensitivity reactions.

Cobratope *Squibb Diagnostics, USA†.*
Cobalt-57 chloride (p.1449·2).

Co-Captral *Silanes, Mex.*
Captopril (p.853·2); hydrochlorothiazide (p.907·3).
Hypertension.

Co-Carnetina B12 *Sigma-Tau, Ital.*
Cobamamide (p.1388·3); carnitine (p.1356·1).
Tonic.

Coccila *Nakorn, Thai.*
Syrup: Furazolidone (p.592·1); neomycin (p.228·1); kaolin (p.1229·3).
Tablets: Diiodohydroxyquinoline (p.590·2); neomycin sulfate (p.228·1); phthalylsulfathiazole (p.235·3); light kaolin (p.1229·3); furazolidone (p.592·1).
Gastrointestinal infections.

Cocculine *Boiron, Canad.; Boiron, Fr.; Boiron, Port.*
Homoeopathic preparation.

Cocculus Oligoplex *Madaus, Ger.*
Homoeopathic preparation.

Cocillana *Orion, Fin.*
Ethylmorphine hydrochloride (p.35·2).
Coughs.

Cocillana Co *Propan, S.Afr.*
Cocillana (p.1087·2); squill (p.1100·3); menthol (p.1632·3).
Coughs.

Cocillana Compound
Note. This name is used for preparations of different composition.
Synco, Hong Kong.
Cocillana (p.1087·2); euphorbia (p.1609·3); senega (p.1100·2); squill (p.1100·3); antimony potassium tartrate (p.97·1); menthol (p.1632·3).
Coughs; respiratory-tract congestion.
Universal, Hong Kong.
Cocillana (p.1087·2); euphorbia (p.1609·3); squill (p.1100·3); senega (p.1100·2); codeine phosphate (p.25·2).
Coughs.

Cocillana-Etyfin *Pharmacia Upjohn, Swed.*
Ethylmorphine hydrochloride (p.35·2); senega (p.1100·2); cocillana (p.1087·2).
Coughs.

Co-Cillin *Docmed, S.Afr.†.*
Ampicillin trihydrate (p.151·1).
Bacterial infections.

Cocktail Reale *Sella, Ital.*
Honey (p.1366·2); pollen; ginseng (p.1615·3); royal jelly (p.1659·3); propolis (p.1655·1).
Nutritional supplement.

The symbol † denotes a preparation no longer actively marketed

Cocois *Bioglan, Hong Kong; Medeva, Irl.; Celltech, UK.*
Coal tar (p.1125·1); salicylic acid (p.1122·3); precipitated sulfur (p.1123·3).
Scalp disorders.

Cocydal *Xixia, S.Afr.*
Co-trimoxazole (p.193·3).
Bacterial infections.

Cocyntal *Boiron, Canad.*
Homoeopathic preparation.

Cod Efferalgan *Upsamedica, Spain.*
Paracetamol (p.71·2); codeine phosphate (p.25·2).
Pain.

COD N 70 *Fresenius Kabi, Ital.*
Amino-acid infusion (p.1350·1).
Parenteral nutrition.

Codabrol *Rekah, Israel.*
Paracetamol (p.71·2); codeine phosphate (p.25·2).
Coughs; fever; pain.

Cod-Acamol Forte *Teva, Israel.*
Paracetamol (p.71·2); codeine phosphate (p.25·2).
Coughs; fever; pain.

Co-Dafalgan *Upsamedica, Switz.*
Paracetamol (p.71·2); codeine phosphate (p.25·2).
Pain.

Codafen Continus
Napp, Irl.; Napp, UK.
Ibuprofen (p.43·2); codeine phosphate (p.25·2).
Inflammation; musculoskeletal, joint, and peri-articular disorders; pain.

Codalax
Napp, Irl.; Douglas, NZ; Napp, UK.
Dantron (p.1221·3); poloxamer 188 (p.1347·1).
These ingredients can be described by the British Approved Name Co-danthramer.
Constipation.

Codal-DH *Cypress, USA.*
Hydrocodone tartrate (p.42·2); phenylephrine hydrochloride (p.1097·1); mepyramine maleate (p.421·1).
Allergic rhinitis; coughs and cold symptoms.

Codal-DM *Cypress, USA.*
Dextromethorphan hydrobromide (p.1087·3); phenylephrine hydrochloride (p.1097·1); mepyramine maleate (p.421·1).
Allergic rhinitis; coughs and cold symptoms.

Codalgin
Note. This name is used for preparations of different composition.
Fawns & McAllan, Austral.
Paracetamol (p.71·2); codeine phosphate (p.25·2).
Fever; pain.

Nycomed, Norw.†
Codeine phosphate (p.25·2); phenazone (p.77·2).
Pain.

Coda-Med *Broad, UK.*
Paracetamol (p.71·2); codeine phosphate (p.25·2); caffeine citrate (p.761·3).

Codamine *Barre-National, USA†.*
Phenylpropanolamine hydrochloride (p.1098·1); hydrocodone tartrate (p.42·2).
Coughs and cold symptoms.

Codant *Antigen, Irl.*
Codeine phosphate (p.25·2).
Pain.

Codapane *Alphapharm, Austral.*
Paracetamol (p.71·2); codeine phosphate (p.25·2).
Fever; pain.

Codedrill *Pierre Fabre Sante, Fr.*
Codeine phosphate (p.25·2).
Formerly known as Pectoral Edulcor.
Coughs.

Codef *Be-Tabs, S.Afr.*
Codeine phosphate (p.25·2); mepyramine maleate (p.421·1); ephedrine hydrochloride (p.1090·1).
Coughs.

Codegest Expectorant *Great Southern, USA†.*
Phenylpropanolamine hydrochloride (p.1098·1); codeine phosphate (p.25·2); guaifenesin (p.1092·2).

Codehist DH *Geneva, USA.*
Pseudoephedrine hydrochloride (p.1099·2); chlorpheniramine [chlorphenamine] maleate (p.412·1); codeine phosphate (p.25·2).
Coughs and cold symptoms.

Codeinol *Saba, Ital.*
Codeine hydrochloride (p.25·2); ephedrine hydrochloride (p.1090·1).
Respiratory-tract symptoms with cough.

Codeisan
Note. This name is used for preparations of different composition.
Labocor, Port.†
Syrup: Codeine phosphate (p.25·2); ephedrine hydrochloride (p.1090·1); cowslip (p.1600·1); sodium benzoate (p.1134·3).
Catarrh; coughs.
Tablets: Codeine phosphate (p.25·2).
Coughs; pain.

Abello, Spain.
Codeine phosphate (p.25·2).
Coughs; diarrhoea; pain.

Codelasa *Procter & Gamble, Braz.*
Codeine (p.25·2); ephedrine hydrochloride (p.1090·1); sodium benzoate (p.1134·3); coal tar (p.1125·1); pine oil; tolu balsam (p.1101·3).
Coughs.

Codella *Napp, UK.*
Glycerol (p.1616·3); kaolin (p.1229·3); povidone-iodine (p.1155·1).
Dry skin.

Codelum *Sanova, Aust.*
Thyme (p.1672·2); codeine phosphate (p.25·2).
Coughs.

Codenfan *Bouchara, Fr.*
Codeine phosphate (p.25·2).
Pain.

Codepect *Medicap, Thai.*
Codeine phosphate (p.25·2); guaifenesin (p.1092·2); phenylpropanolamine (p.1098·1).
Cold symptoms; coughs; nasal congestion.

Codergine *Shiwa, Thai.*
Co-dergocrine mesilate (p.1597·3).
Cerebrovascular disorders; peripheral vascular disorders.

Codesan Comp *Leiras, Fin.*
Codeine phosphate (p.25·2); ephedrine hydrochloride (p.1090·1); diphenhydramine hydrochloride (p.416·1); cocillana (p.1087·2).
Coughs.

Codesan N *Leiras, Fin.*
Noscapine (p.1096·1); cocillana (p.1087·2).
Coughs.

Codesia *Asian Pharm, Thai.*
Codeine phosphate (p.25·2); guaifenesin (p.1092·2).
Coughs.

Codethyline
Hoechst Marion Roussel, Belg.†; Hoechst, Fr.†.
Ethylmorphine hydrochloride (p.35·2).
Coughs.

Codetilina-Eucaliptolo He *Teofarma, Ital.†.*
Ethylmorphine hydrochloride (p.35·2); eucalyptol (p.1609·2).
Coughs.

Codetricine *Byk, Fr.*
Tyrothricin (p.267·1).
Mouth and throat disorders.

Codetricine vitamine C *Byk, Fr.*
Tyrothricin (p.267·1); amethocaine [tetracaine] hydrochloride (p.1305·2); ascorbic acid (p.1389·3).
Mouth and throat disorders.

Codex *Zambon, Ital.*
Saccharomyces boulardii (p.1626·3).
Gastrointestinal disorders.

Cod-Guaiacol *Vitamed, Israel.*
Sulfoguaiacol (p.1101·1); codeine phosphate (p.25·2).
Coughs.

codi OPT *Optimed, Ger.*
Codeine phosphate (p.25·2).
Pain.

Codical *Sam-On, Israel.*
Codeine phosphate (p.25·2).
Coughs.

Codicaps *Thiemann, Ger.*
Codeine (p.25·2); chlorpheniramine [chlorphenamine] maleate (p.412·1).
Catarrh; coughs.

Codicaps mono *Thiemann, Ger.*
Codeine (p.25·2).
Coughs.

Codicaps N *Thiemann, Ger.*
Codeine (p.25·2).
Coughs.

Codicet *Hua, Thai.*
Codeine phosphate (p.25·2); paracetamol (p.71·2).
Pain.

Codiclear DH *Schwarz, USA.*
Hydrocodone tartrate (p.42·2); guaifenesin (p.1092·2).
Coughs.

Codicompren *Cascan, Ger.; Glaxo Wellcome, Ger.*
Codeine phosphate (p.25·2).
Coughs.

Codicontin
Asta Medica, Belg.; Mundipharma, Switz.
Dihydrocodeine tartrate (p.33·1).
Pain.

Codidol *Mundipharma, Aust.*
Dihydrocodeine tartrate (p.33·1).
Pain.

Codiforton *Sanofi Winthrop, Ger.†.*
Codeine phosphate (p.25·2).
Coughs.

Co-Dilatrend *Roche, Aust.*
Carvedilol (p.855·2); hydrochlorothiazide (p.907·3).
Hypertension.

Codimal *Schwarz, USA.*
Chlorpheniramine [chlorphenamine] maleate (p.412·1); pseudoephedrine hydrochloride (p.1099·2); paracetamol (p.71·2).
Upper respiratory-tract symptoms.

Codimal DH *Schwarz, USA.*
Hydrocodone tartrate (p.42·2); phenylephrine hydrochloride (p.1097·1); mepyramine maleate (p.421·1).
Coughs and cold symptoms.

Codimal DM *Schwarz, USA.*
Dextromethorphan hydrobromide (p.1087·3); phenylephrine hydrochloride (p.1097·1); mepyramine maleate (p.421·1).

Codimal LA *Schwarz, USA.*
Chlorpheniramine [chlorphenamine] maleate (p.412·1); pseudoephedrine hydrochloride (p.1099·2).
Cold symptoms.

Codimal PH *Schwarz, USA.*
Codeine phosphate (p.25·2); phenylephrine hydrochloride (p.1097·1); mepyramine maleate (p.421·1).
Coughs and cold symptoms.

Co-Diovan
Novartis, Aust.; Novartis, Ger.; Novartis, Irl.; Novartis, Neth.; Novartis, Port.; Novartis, S.Afr.; Novartis, Singapore; Novartis, Spain; Novartis, Switz.; Novartis, Thai.
Valsartan (p.988·3); hydrochlorothiazide (p.907·3).
Hypertension.

Co-Diovane *Novartis, Belg.*
Valsartan (p.988·3); hydrochlorothiazide (p.907·3).
Hypertension.

Codipertussin *Klinge, Aust.*
Codeine polistirex (p.26·1).
Bronchitis; coughs.

Codiphen *G.P. Laboratories, Austral.*
Codeine phosphate (p.25·2); aspirin (p.14·2).
Fever; pain.

Codipront
Pfizer, Aust.; Mack, Illert., Ger.; Mack, Hong Kong; Bracco, Ital.; Ferraz, Lynce, Port.; Mack, Singapore; Pfizer Consumer, Spain; Mack, Switz.; Mack, Thai.
Codeine (p.25·2), codeine phosphate (p.25·2), or codeine polistirex (p.26·1); phenyltoloxamine (p.423·1), phenyltoloxamine citrate (p.423·1), or phenyltoloxamine polistirex (p.423·1).
Coughs.

Codipront cum Expectorans
Note. This name is used for preparations of different composition.
Pfizer, Aust.†; Mack, Hong Kong; Mack, Switz.
Capsules: Codeine polistirex (p.26·1); phenyltoloxamine polistirex (p.423·1); guaifenesin (p.1092·2).
Coughs.
Pfizer, Aust.†; Mack, Switz.
Oral liquid: Codeine polistirex (p.26·1); phenyltoloxamine polistirex (p.423·1); guaifenesin (p.1092·2); thyme (p.1672·2).
Coughs.

Codipront mono *Mack, Illert., Ger.*
Codeine polistirex (p.26·1).
Coughs.

Codis
Reckitt & Colman, Austral.; Reckitt & Colman, Belg.; Reckitt Benckiser, Irl.; Reckitt & Colman, S.Afr.; Reckitt & Colman, Singapore; Reckitt & Colman, UK.
Aspirin (p.14·2); codeine phosphate (p.25·2).
Fever; pain.

Codisal Forte *Rafa, Israel.*
Paracetamol (p.71·2); codeine phosphate (p.25·2).
Cold symptoms; coughs; fever; pain.

Codivis *CTI, Israel.*
Codeine (p.25·2); phenyltoloxamine (p.423·1).
Coughs.

Codivite *Codilab, Port.*
Lysine hydrochloride; vitamin B substances (p.1350·1).
Tonic.

Codocalyptol *Qualiphar, Belg.†.*
Codeine (p.25·2).
Coughs.

Codoforme *Azevedos, Port.*
Codeine (p.25·2); aconite (p.1572·3); belladonna (p.463·1); trimethylamino triaminomethyl bromoform; sodium benzoate (p.1134·3); terpin (p.1101·2).
Coughs.

Codol
Note. This name is used for preparations of different composition.
Produfarma, Port.
Codeine (p.25·2); vegetable extract.

Mundipharma, Switz.
Paracetamol (p.71·2); codeine phosphate (p.25·2).
Fever; pain.

Codoliprane *Theraplix, Fr.*
Paracetamol (p.71·2); codeine phosphate (p.25·2).
Pain.

Codomill *Brunel, S.Afr.*
Mepyramine maleate (p.421·1); ephedrine hydrochloride (p.1090·1); codeine phosphate (p.25·2).
Coughs.

Codoplex *Jean-Marie, Hong Kong.*
Injection: Codeine phosphate (p.25·2); papaverine hydrochloride (p.1648·1); chlorpheniramine [chlorphenamine] maleate (p.412·1); ephedrine hydrochloride (p.1090·1).
Syrup: Codeine phosphate (p.25·2); papaverine hydrochloride (p.1648·1); guaifenesin (p.1092·2); chlorpheniramine [chlorphenamine] maleate (p.412·1).
Tablets: Codeine phosphate (p.25·2); papaverine hydrochloride (p.1648·1); chlorpheniramine [chlorphenamine] maleate (p.412·1); terpin hydrate (p.1101·2); phenolphthalein (p.1244·1); caffeine (p.761·3).
Coughs.

Codotussyl Expectorant *Whitehall, Fr.*
Oral solution: Acetylcysteine (p.1082·3).
Syrup: Carbocisteine (p.1086·3).
Respiratory-tract congestion.

Codotussyl Maux de Gorge *Whitehall, Fr.*
Lignocaine [lidocaine] hydrochloride (p.1313·3); sodium benzoate (p.1134·3); benzyl alcohol (p.1135·2).
Sore throat.

Codotussyl Toux Seche *Whitehall, Fr.*
Capsules: Dextromethorphan hydrobromide (p.1087·3).
Syrup: Pholcodine (p.1099·1).

Formerly contained pholcodine, sodium benzoate, sulfogaiacol, aconite, belladonna, cherry-laurel water, tolu syrup, and Desessartz syrup.
Coughs.

Codox *Boots, Austral.*
Aspirin (p.14·2); dihydrocodeine tartrate (p.33·1).
Coughs; fever; pain.

Codral Cold & Flu
Warner-Lambert, Austral.; Warner-Lambert, NZ.
Paracetamol (p.71·2); codeine phosphate (p.25·2); pseudoephedrine hydrochloride (p.1099·2).
Cold and influenza symptoms.

Codral Cough *Warner-Lambert, NZ.*
Dextromethorphan hydrobromide (p.1087·3); pseudoephedrine hydrochloride (p.1099·2).
Coughs.

Codral Daytime/Nightime
Warner-Lambert, Austral.; Warner-Lambert, NZ.
Day tablets, paracetamol (p.71·2); codeine phosphate (p.25·2); pseudoephedrine hydrochloride (p.1099·2); night tablets, paracetamol; codeine phosphate; triprolidine hydrochloride (p.427·2).
Cold and influenza symptoms.

Codral Dry Cough *Warner-Lambert, Austral.*
Pseudoephedrine hydrochloride (p.1099·2); codeine phosphate (p.25·2).
Coughs; nasal congestion.

Codral Expectorant *Warner-Lambert, NZ.*
Guaifenesin (p.1092·2); pseudoephedrine hydrochloride (p.1099·2).
Coughs.

Codral 4 Flu *Warner-Lambert, NZ.*
Paracetamol (p.71·2); codeine phosphate (p.25·2); pseudoephedrine hydrochloride (p.1099·2); chlorpheniramine [chlorphenamine] maleate (p.412·1).
Influenza symptoms.

Codral Forte *Glaxo Wellcome, Austral.*
Aspirin (p.14·2); codeine phosphate (p.25·2).
Coughs; pain.

Codral Linctus *Warner-Lambert, Austral.†.*
Pseudoephedrine hydrochloride (p.1099·2); codeine phosphate (p.25·2).
Cold symptoms; coughs.

Codral Pain Relief
Warner-Lambert, Austral.; Warner-Lambert, NZ.
Paracetamol (p.71·2); codeine phosphate (p.25·2).
Fever; pain.

Codrinan *Honorterapica, Braz.*
Theophylline (p.777·2).
Obstructive airways disease.

Codyl *Leo, Denm.†.*
Aspirin (p.14·2); codeine phosphate (p.25·2).
Pain.

Coedieci *Mitim, Ital.*
Ubidecarenone (p.1677·1).
Cardiopathy; coenzyme Q10 deficiency.

Co-Efferalagan *Upsamedica, Ital.*
Paracetamol (p.71·2); codeine phosphate (p.25·2).
Pain.

Coergot *Masa, Thai.*
Co-dergocrine mesilate (p.1597·3).
Cerebrovascular disorders; mental function impairment; peripheral vascular disorders; vascular headaches.

Cofasol *UCI, Braz.*
Tetramisole hydrochloride (p.108·3).
Nematode infections.

Cofed *M & H, Thai.*
Triprolidine hydrochloride (p.427·2); pseudoephedrine hydrochloride (p.1099·2).
Allergic rhinitis; cold symptoms; hayfever.

Cofena *Sanobia, Port.*
Aspirin (p.14·2); codeine phosphate (p.25·2); caffeine (p.761·3).
Fever; pain.

Cofendyl *Quatromed, S.Afr.*
Paracetamol (p.71·2); codeine phosphate (p.25·2); pseudoephedrine hydrochloride (p.1099·2).
Cold and influenza symptoms.

Coffalon *Stark, Ger.*
Paracetamol (p.71·2); salicylamide (p.82·1); caffeine (p.761·3); tiemonium iodide (p.474·2).
Pain.

Coffeemed N *Passauer, Ger.*
Caffeine (p.761·3); phenazone (p.77·2).
Influenza; migraine; neuralgia; pain.

Coffekapton *Strallhofer, Ger.*
Caffeine (p.761·3).
Fatigue; vascular headache.

Coffetylin *Bristol-Myers Squibb, Ger.*
Aspirin (p.14·2); caffeine (p.761·3).
Fever; pain.

Coffo Selt *Rosch & Handel, Aust.*
Phenazone (p.77·2); caffeine (p.761·3).
Pain.

Coff-Rest *Aspen, S.Afr.*
Triprolidine hydrochloride (p.427·2); pseudoephedrine hydrochloride (p.1099·2); dextromethorphan hydrobromide (p.1087·3).
Coughs.

Coff-Up *Propan, S.Afr.*
Pheniramine maleate (p.422·3); menthol (p.1632·3); ammonium chloride (p.1085·2); sodium citrate (p.1186·2).
Respiratory-tract congestion.

Coldil Dolisos, Canad.†
Homoeopathic preparation.

Coldistan Sigmapharm, Aust.
Eye drops; nasal drops: Diphenhydramine hydrochloride (p.416·1); naphazoline hydrochloride (p.1095·1).
Allergic eye disorders; eye irritation; rhinitis; sinusitis.

Nasal ointment: Diphenhydramine hydrochloride (p.416·1); phenylephrine hydrochloride (p.1097·1); calcium laevulinate (p.1188·3); cetylpyridinium chloride (p.1138·1); dexpanthenol (p.1602·3); sage oil (p.1660·2).
Hay fever; rhinitis; sinusitis.

Coldistop Sigmapharm, Aust.; Sigmapharm, Switz.
Vitamin A palmitate (p.1383·2); alpha tocoferil acetate (p.1394·1).
Nasal and sinus disorders.

Coldloc Fleming, USA†.
Guaifenesin (p.1092·2); phenylpropanolamine hydrochloride (p.1098·1); phenylephrine hydrochloride (p.1097·1).
Upper respiratory-tract symptoms.

Coldloc-LA Fleming, USA†.
Phenylpropanolamine hydrochloride (p.1098·1); guaifenesin (p.1092·2).
Upper respiratory-tract symptoms.

Coldophthal Sigmapharm, Aust.
Naphazoline hydrochloride (p.1095·1); mercuric oxycyanide (p.1634·3); boric acid (p.1586·1).
Conjunctivitis; eye irritation.

Coldosian Asian Pharm, Thai.
Syrup: Paracetamol (p.71·2); chlorpheniramine [chlorphenamine] maleate (p.412·1); phenylpropanolamine hydrochloride (p.1098·1).
Tablets: Paracetamol (p.71·2); chlorpheniramine [chlorphenamine] maleate (p.412·1); phenylpropanolamine hydrochloride (p.1098·1); caffeine (p.761·3).
Cold symptoms; sinusitis.

Coldrex
Note.This name is used for preparations of different composition.
SmithKline Beecham, Fin.
Aspirin (p.14·2); guaifenesin (p.1092·2); caffeine (p.761·3); ascorbic acid (p.1389·3).
Cold and influenza symptoms.

SmithKline Beecham, Irl.†; Sterling Health, UK†.
Paracetamol (p.71·2); phenylephrine hydrochloride (p.1097·1); caffeine (p.761·3); terpin hydrate (p.1101·2); ascorbic acid (p.1389·3).
Cold symptoms.

Coldrex C SmithKline Beecham Consumer, Neth.
Aspirin (p.14·2); ascorbic acid (p.1389·3).
Cold and influenza symptoms.

Coldrex Flu SmithKline Beecham, NZ.
Paracetamol (p.71·2); dextromethorphan hydrobromide (p.1087·3); chlorpheniramine [chlorphenamine] maleate (p.412·1); pseudoephedrine hydrochloride (p.1099·2).
Cold and influenza symptoms.

Coldrex Head & Chest Cold SmithKline Beecham, NZ.
Paracetamol (p.71·2); pseudoephedrine hydrochloride (p.1099·2); dextromethorphan hydrobromide (p.1087·3).
Cold and influenza symptoms.

Coldrex Head Cold SmithKline Beecham, NZ.
Paracetamol (p.71·2); pseudoephedrine hydrochloride (p.1099·2).
Sinusitis.

Coldrex Night Relief SmithKline Beecham, NZ.
Paracetamol (p.71·2); promethazine hydrochloride (p.423·2); dextromethorphan hydrobromide (p.1087·3).
Cold and influenza symptoms.

Coldrin Shinyaku, Hong Kong; Shinyaku, Singapore.
Clofedanol hydrochloride (p.1087·1).
Coughs.

Coldrine Roberts, USA; Hauck, USA.
Pseudoephedrine hydrochloride (p.1099·2); paracetamol (p.71·2).
Upper respiratory-tract symptoms.

Coldvac Byk Madaus, S.Afr.
Pneumococci; streptococci; staphylococci; *Haemophilus influenzae*(p.0·0).
Respiratory-tract disorders.

Coldvico Merck, S.Afr.†.
Paracetamol (p.71·2); ascorbic acid (p.1389·3); phenylephrine hydrochloride (p.1097·1); chlorpheniramine [chlorphenamine] maleate (p.412·1); caffeine (p.761·3).
Cold and influenza symptoms.

Coldy The Forty-Two, Thai.
Paracetamol (p.71·2); chlorpheniramine [chlorphenamine] (p.412·2) or chlorpheniramine [chlorphenamine] maleate (p.412·1); phenylpropanolamine (p.1098·1) or phenylpropanolamine hydrochloride (p.1098·1).
Allergic rhinitis; cold symptoms; hay fever; sinusitis.

Coleb Promed, Ger.; Astra, Ger.
Isosorbide mononitrate (p.916·2).
Angina pectoris; heart failure; pulmonary hypertension.

Colebrina Schering, Braz.
Iocetamic acid (p.1033·3).
Contrast medium for biliary-tract radiography.

Coledos Prospa, Braz.
Ursodeoxycholic acid (p.1677·2).
Biliary-tract disorders.

Colegraf Estedi, Spain.
Iopanoic acid (p.1035·2).
Contrast medium for biliary-tract radiography.

Colemin Biohorm, Spain.
Simvastatin (p.969·2).
Hyperlipidaemias.

Colenitral Seid, Spain†.
Glyceryl trinitrate (p.897·3).
Angina pectoris.

Colenon SIRC, Singapore.
Poliglusam; garcinia cambogia; hydroxycitric acid; chromium; vitamin C (p.1350·1).
Dietary aid.

Colepren Randall, Mex.
Hyoscine butylbromide (p.468·2); dipyrone (p.34·1).
Smooth muscle spasm.

Colerin Lab, Port.
Azintamide (p.1583·1).
Digestive insufficiency.

Colerin-F Lab, Port.
Azintamide (p.1583·1); cellulase (p.1593·1); pancreatin (p.1646·1).
Digestive insufficiency.

Colese Alphapharm, Austral.
Mebeverine hydrochloride (p.1233·3).
Irritable bowel syndrome.

Colestase Sanofi Winthrop, Braz.
Furazolidone (p.592·1); diphenoxylate hydrochloride (p.1222·2); pectin (p.1502·3); aluminium silicate (p.1211·3); magnesium hydroxide (p.1233·1).
Diarrhoea.

Colesterinex Almirall, Spain.
Pyricarbate (p.1656·3).
Hyperlipidaemias.

Colesthexal Hexal, Ger.
Colestyramine (p.864·1).
Hyperlipidaemias.

Colestid
Pharmacia Upjohn, Austral.; Pharmacia Upjohn, Belg.; Pharmacia Upjohn, Canad.; Pharmacia Upjohn, Ger.; Pharmacia Upjohn, Irl.; Pharmacia Upjohn, Israel; Pharmacia Upjohn, Mex.; Pharmacia Upjohn, Neth.; Pharmacia Upjohn, NZ; Pharmacia Upjohn, Port.; Pharmacia Upjohn, S.Afr.†; Pharmacia Upjohn, Spain; Pharmacia Upjohn, Switz.; Pharmacia, UK; Pharmacia Upjohn, USA.
Colestipol hydrochloride (p.863·3).
Hypercholesterolaemia.

Colestrol Formenti, Ital.†.
Colestyramine (p.864·1).
Hyperlipidaemias.

Colestyr CT, Ger.
Colestyramine (p.864·1).
Hyperlipidaemias.

Colex Tramedica, Neth.
Dibasic sodium phosphate (p.1193·2); monobasic sodium phosphate (p.1193·2).
Bowel evacuation; constipation.

Colfarit Bayer, Aust.†.
Aspirin (p.14·2).

Colfed-A Parmed, USA.
Pseudoephedrine hydrochloride (p.1099·2); chlorpheniramine [chlorphenamine] maleate (p.412·1).
Upper respiratory-tract symptoms.

Colfur Carter-Wallace, Mex.
Oral suspension: Colistin sulfate (p.192·3); furazolidone (p.592·1); kaolin (p.1229·3); pectin (p.1502·3).
Tablets: Colistin sulfate (p.192·3); furazolidone (p.592·1).
Gastrointestinal infections.

Colgen Bournonville, Belg.†.
Collagen (bovine, non-denatured) (p.1598·2).
Haemorrhage.

Colgout Rhone-Poulenc Rorer, Austral.; Fisons, Hong Kong.
Colchicine (p.400·1).
Gout; leukaemia; polyarthritis associated with sarcoidosis.

Coliacron Enzypharm, Neth.
Glutamine synthetase; acetylcoenzyme A kinase; oxidative phosphorylating enzymes.
Psychosomatic and neurovegetative disorders.

Colibiogen Laves, Ger.
Peptide extract from *Escherichia coli.*
Gastrointestinal disorders; hypersensitivity; musculoskeletal and joint disorders.

Colic Hylands, Canad.
Homoeopathic preparation.

Colic Relief Brauer, Austral.
Homoeopathic preparation.

Colicon Reese, USA.
Simeticone (p.1249·2).

Colicort Merck Sharp & Dohme-Chibret, Fr.
Colistimethate sodium (p.192·3); tetracycline hydrochloride (p.258·3); prednisolone sodium phosphate (p.1078·1).
Infections of the ear and nose.

Colief
Clonmel, Irl.; Forum, UK.
Tilactase (p.1673·2).
Infant colic.

Coli-Fagina S
ABC, Ital.
Lysate of *Escherichia coli; Bacillus pumilus; Morganella morgani; Alcaligenes faecalis; Shigella flexneri; Enterococcus faecalis* (p.1626·3); *Bacillus subtilis; Proteus vulgaris.*
Gastrointestinal infections; genito-urinary infections.

ABC, Port.
Lysates of *Escherichia coli; Bacillus morgani; B. faecalis alcaligenes; E. pseudodysenteriae; Bacillus subtilis; Proteus vulgaris; Enterococcus faecalis* (p.1626·3); *B. mesentericus.*
Gastrointestinal infections; genito-urinary infections.

Colifoam
Sanova, Aust.; Stafford-Miller, Austral.; Stafford-Miller Continental, Belg.†; Stafford-Miller, Denm.; Stafford-Miller, Fin.; Trommsdorff, Ger.; Stafford-Miller, Irl.; Stafford-Miller, Israel; Stafford-Miller, Ital.; Schwarz, Norw.; Stafford-Miller, NZ; Stafford-Miller, Port.; Searle, S.Afr.†; Meda, Swed.; Stafford-Miller, Switz.†; Stafford-Miller, UK.
Hydrocortisone acetate (p.1073·3).
Inflammatory bowel disease.

Colifossim Day, Ital.
Cefuroxime sodium (p.178·2).
Bacterial infections.

Colimax Qualiphar, Belg.
Ephedrine hydrochloride (p.1090·1); sodium benzoate (p.1134·3); aconite (p.1572·3); belladonna (p.463·1); thyme (p.1672·2); wild thyme; maidenhair fern.
Coughs.

Colimicina UCB, Ital.
Injection: Colistimethate sodium (p.192·3).
Tablets; oral drops: Colistin sulfate (p.192·3).
Bacterial infections.

Quimifar, Spain.
Colistin sulfate (p.192·3).
Bacterial infections.

Colimix Xepa-Soul Pattinson, Hong Kong; Xepa-Soul Pattinson, Singapore.
Dicyclomine [dicycloverine] hydrochloride (p.466·1); simeticone (p.1249·2).
Flatulence; gastrointestinal spasm; infant colic.

Colimune Rhone-Poulenc Rorer, Ger.
Sodium cromoglicate (p.774·3).
Food hypersensitivity; ulcerative colitis; ulcerative proctitis.

Colimycin Lundbeck, Denm.; Lundbeck, Norw.
Colistimethate sodium (p.192·3).
Gram-negative bacterial infections.

Colimycine Glaxo Wellcome, Belg.; Rhone-Poulenc Rorer, Fr.; Rhone-Poulenc Rorer, Neth.
Colistin sulfate (p.192·3) or colistimethate sodium (p.192·3).
Bacterial infections.

Colina Intersan, Ger.
Smectite.
Diarrhoea; gastrointestinal disorders.

Colina Spezial Intersan, Ger.
Smectite; aluminium hydroxide-magnesium carbonate gel (p.1211·2).
Diarrhoea; gastrointestinal disorders.

Colinvintol Sedar, Braz.
Adenosine (p.828·2); methionine (p.1012·2); betaine hydrochloride (p.1584·3); choline (p.1356·3); pyridoxine (p.1387·1); glucose (p.1364·1).
Liver disorders.

Coli-Om OM, Port.†.
Lysate of *Escherichia coli.*
Gastrointestinal infections; urinary-tract infections.

Coliopan Eisai, Hong Kong; Eisai, Jpn†; Eisai, Singapore.
Butropium bromide (p.464·3).
Painful gastrointestinal spasm.

Coliquifilm Allergan, Ger.; Allergan, Switz.
White soft paraffin (p.1407·3); wool alcohols (p.1410·3); light liquid paraffin (p.1407·2).
Eye disorders.

Coliracin Rafa, Israel.
Colistimethate sodium (p.192·3).
Bacterial infections.

Colircusi Gentadexa Cusi, Hong Kong.
Gentamicin sulfate (p.210·1); dexamethasone sodium phosphate (p.1067·1); tetryzoline hydrochloride (p.1101·2).
Infected eye and ear disorders.

Colircusi Iodine-Thio-Calcic Cusi, Hong Kong.
Sodium iodide (p.1522·3); potassium iodide (p.1522·3); calcium (p.1187·3); sodium thiosulfate (p.1024·2).
Cataract; fungal eye infections.

Colirio Blumen Luper, Braz.
Zinc sulfate (p.1398·2); naphazoline hydrochloride (p.1095·1).
Ocular congestion.

Colirio de Argyrol Quimioterapica, Braz.
Silver protein (p.1664·2).
Bacterial eye infections.

Colirio Helios Windson, Braz.
Zinc sulfate (p.1398·2); chlorobutanol (p.1141·2).
Eye disorders.

Colirio Legrand Legrand, Braz.
Naphazoline (p.1095·1); zinc sulfate (p.1398·2).
Ocular congestion.

Colirio Moura Brasil Hoechst Marion Roussel, Braz.
Zinc sulfate (p.1398·2); naphazoline (p.1095·1).
Ocular congestion.

Colirio Vima Dorsay, Braz.
Zinc sulfate (p.1398·2); naphazoline (p.1095·1).
Ocular congestion.

Coliriocilina Medical, Spain.
Benzylpenicillin potassium (p.157·1).
Eye infections.

Coliriocilina Adren Astr Medical, Spain.
Boric acid (p.1586·1); adrenaline [epinephrine] hydrochloride (p.829·2); naphazoline hydrochloride (p.1095·1); procaine hydrochloride (p.1319·1); zinc sulfate (p.1398·2).
Eye disorders.

Coliriocilina Espectro Medical, Spain.
Neomycin sulfate (p.228·1); oxytetracycline (p.234·1).
Bacterial eye infections.

Coliriocilina Gentam Medical, Spain.
Gentamicin sulfate (p.210·1).
Eye infections.

Coliriocilina Homatrop Medical, Spain.
Homatropine hydrobromide (p.468·1).
Production of mydriasis and cycloplegia; uveitis.

Coliriocilina Prednisona Medical, Spain.
Neomycin sulfate (p.228·1); prednisone (p.1079·2).
Eye disorders.

Colitique Lacteol du Dr Boucard, Fr.†.
Whole and lysed coliform bacteria.
Infections with coliform bacteria.

Colitofalk Codali, Belg.
Mesalazine (p.1234·1).
Inflammatory bowel disease.

Colix Prolabor, Braz.
Sodium hypochlorite (p.1156·2).
Skin, wound, instrument, and surface disinfection.

Collafilm Immuno, Fr.†.
Collagen (p.1598·2).
Ulcers; wounds.

Collaven Roche, Aust.
Centella (p.1112·2).
Chronic venous insufficiency.

Collazin Selmag, Switz.
Zinc sulfate (p.1398·2).
Zinc deficiency.

Colleofer Meda, Fin.
Iron polymaltose (p.1369·2).
Iron-deficiency anaemia.

Colli Gricar, Ital.
Benzalkonium chloride (p.1133·2); hamamelis; chamomile.
Eye disinfection; eye irritation.

Collins Elixir Collins Elixir, UK.
Ethylmorphine hydrochloride (p.35·2).
Coughs.

Collins Elixir Pastilles Collins Elixir, UK†.
Citric acid (p.1596·2); lemon oil (p.1628·2); squill vinegar (p.1100·3); glycerol (p.1616·3).
Coughs; sore throats.

Collirio Alfa Bracco, Ital.
Naphazoline nitrate (p.1095·1).
Eye irritation.

Collirio Alfa Antistaminico Bracco, Ital.
Thonzylamine hydrochloride (p.426·2); naphazoline nitrate (p.1095·1).
Conjunctival spasm.

Collirium Geymonat Geymonat, Ital.
Benzalkonium chloride (p.1133·2).
Formerly contained boric acid and agrimonia eupatoria.
Eye infections.

Collis Browne's SSL, UK.
Oral mixture: Morphine (p.56·1); peppermint oil (p.1243·3).
Coughs; diarrhoea.
Tablets: Light kaolin (p.1229·3); morphine hydrochloride (p.56·1); heavy calcium carbonate (p.1215·1).
Diarrhoea.

Collodyne Universal, S.Afr.†.
Light kaolin (p.1229·3); pectin (p.1502·3); bismuth subcarbonate (p.1213·1); chloroform and morphine tincture (p.56·1).
Diarrhoea.

Colloidine Rudefsa, Mex.
Propylhexedrine (p.1514·2).
Obesity.

Collomack
Mack, Illert., Ger.; Mack, Hong Kong; Mack, Singapore; Mack, Thai.
Salicylic acid (p.1122·3); lactic acid (p.1626·2); lauromacrogol 400 (p.1345·2).
Calluses; corns; hard skin; warts.

Collosol Amido, Fr.
Soap substitute.

Collu-Blache Chauvin Novopharma, Switz.
Chlorhexidine gluconate (p.1138·2); oxybuprocaine hydrochloride (p.1318·1).
Mouth and throat disorders.

Collubleu Medeva, Fr.
Methylene blue [methylthioninium chloride] (p.1012·3).
Bacterial mouth and throat infections.

Colludol
Aventis, Belg.; Cooperation Pharmaceutique, Fr.
Hexamidine isetionate (p.1146·2); lignocaine [lidocaine] hydrochloride (p.1313·2).
Mouth and throat disorders.

Collu-Hextril
Warner-Lambert, Fr.; Warner-Lambert Consumer, Port.
Hexetidine (p.1146·3).
Mouth and throat disorders.

Collunosol Whitehall, Fr.†.
Chlorhexidine gluconate (p.1138·2); lignocaine [lidocaine] hydrochloride (p.1313·2).
Mouth and throat disorders.

Collunosol-N Sodip, Switz.
Chlorhexidine gluconate (p.1138·2); lignocaine [lidocaine] hydrochloride (p.1313·2).
Mouth and throat disorders.

Collunovar
Note. This name is used for preparations of different composition.
Dexo, Fr.
Mouthwash; throat spray: Chlorhexidine gluconate (p.1138·2).
Formerly contained neoarsphenamine.
Pastilles: Bacitracin zinc (p.155·2); tyrothricin (p.267·1).
Formerly contained neoarsphenamine, bacitracin zinc, and amethocaine [tetracaine] hydrochloride.
Mouth and throat infections.

Actipharm, Switz.†.
Chlorhexidine gluconate (p.1138·2).
Mouth and throat disorders.

Collupressine Synthelabo, Fr.
Felypressin (p.1283·1); chlorhexidine gluconate (p.1138·2).
Mouth and throat disorders.

Collustan Oberlin, Fr.
Chlorhexidine gluconate (p.1138·2); amylocaine hydrochloride (p.1306·1); menthol.
Mouth and throat disorders.

Collylarm Vifor, Switz.
Povidone (p.1503·2); polyvinyl alcohol (p.1503·1).
Dry eyes.

Collypan Vifor, Switz.
Tetryzoline hydrochloride (p.1101·2); zinc sulfate (p.1398·2); digitalis (p.869·1); hamamelis (p.1618·3); euphrasia (p.1609·3).
Eye irritation.

Collyre Alpha Bracco, Switz.
Naphazoline nitrate (p.1095·1); camphor (p.1589·3).
Eye irritation.

Collyre Bleu
Sabex, Canad.; Leurquin, Fr.
Methylene blue [methylthioninium chloride] (p.1012·3); naphazoline hydrochloride (p.1095·1) or naphazoline nitrate (p.1095·1).
Eye disorders.

Collyre Bleu Laiter Leurquin, Switz.
Methylene blue [methylthioninium chloride] (p.1012·3); naphazoline nitrate (p.1095·1).
Eye irritation.

Collyrex SmithKline Beecham Sante, Fr.
Thiomersal (p.1158·2); phenylephrine hydrochloride (p.1097·1); pentosan polysulfate (p.953·1).
Eye disorders.

Collyria Nova Argentia, Ital.
Benzalkonium chloride (p.1133·2); guaiazulene (p.1618·3); polyvinyl alcohol (p.1503·1).
Eye hygiene; eye irritation.

Collyrium Charton, Canad.†.
Tetryzoline hydrochloride (p.1101·2); glycerol (p.1616·3).
Eye irritation.

Collyrium Fresh Wyeth-Ayerst, USA.
Tetryzoline hydrochloride (p.1101·2); glycerol (p.1616·3).
Eye irritation.

Collyrium for Fresh Eyes Bausch & Lomb, USA.
Borax (p.1586·1); boric acid (p.1586·1).
Eye irrigation.

Colme
Croma, Aust.; Ipsen, Spain.
Calcium carbimide (p.1588·2).
Alcoholism.

ColoCare Helena, USA.
Test for occult blood in faeces.

Colodium Hovid, Singapore.
Loperamide hydrochloride (p.1231·3).
Diarrhoea; ileostomy management.

Colofac
Solvay, Aust.; Solvay, Austral.; Solvay, Irl.; Solvay, NZ; Solvay, S.Afr.; Solvay, Thai.; Solvay, UK.
Mebeverine embonate (p.1234·1) or mebeverine hydrochloride (p.1233·3).
Gastrointestinal spasm; irritable bowel syndrome.

Colofiber Madaus, Belg.
Ispaghula (p.1229·1).
Colopathy; constipation.

Colofoam Norgine, Fr.
Hydrocortisone acetate (p.1073·3).
Inflammatory bowel disease.

Cololyt Spirig, Switz.
Macrogol 4000 (p.1630·3); electrolytes (p.1180·1).
Bowel evacuation.

Colomba spezial Mauermann, Ger.
Homoeopathic preparation.

Colominte Helsinn, Port.
Peppermint oil (p.1243·3).
Irritable bowel syndrome.

Colominthe Arkopharma, Fr.†.
Peppermint leaf (p.1243·2); fennel (p.1610·1); melissa (p.1632·2).
Gastrointestinal disorders.

Colomycin
Pharmax, Irl.; Pharmax, UK.
Colistin sulfate (p.192·3) or colistimethate sodium (p.192·3).
Bacterial infections.

Colonlytely Dendy, Austral.
Macrogol 3350 (p.1630·3); electrolytes (p.1180·1).
Bowel evacuation.

Colonorm Mundipharma, Aust.
Senna (p.1248·2).
Anorectal disorders; constipation.

Colonprep Dendy, Austral.
1 Sachet, macrogol 3350 (p.1630·3); electrolytes (p.1180·1) (Colonlytely); 2 sachets, sodium picosulfate (p.1249·3) (Picolax).
Bowel evacuation.

Colonsteril Orion, Fin.
Electrolytes (p.1180·1); macrogol 4000 (p.1630·3).
Bowel evacuation; constipation.

Colopeg
Roche, Belg.; Nicholas, Fr.
Electrolytes (p.1180·1); macrogol 3350 (p.1630·3) or macrogol 4000 (p.1630·3).
Bowel evacuation.

Colophos Spirig, Switz.
Monobasic sodium phosphate (p.1193·2); dibasic sodium phosphate (p.1193·2).
Bowel evacuation.

Colo-Pleon
Mayrhofer, Aust.; Henning, Ger.
Sulfasalazine (p.1251·1).
Inflammatory bowel diseases.

Colo-Prep Anmarate, S.Afr.
Monobasic sodium phosphate (p.1193·2); dibasic sodium phosphate (p.1193·2).
Bowel evacuation.

Colopriv Biotherapie, Fr.
Mebeverine hydrochloride (p.1233·3).
Gastrointestinal and biliary-tract disorders.

Colopten
Debat, Fr.†; Fournier, Ital.; Fournier SA, Spain†.
Antigenic extracts of: *Staphylococcus aureus; Escherichia coli; Klebsiella pneumoniae; Proteus vulgaris.*
Diarrhoea.

Colo-Rectal Test Roche, Canad.†.
Test for occult blood in stools.

Colosan mite Medichemie, Switz.
Sterculia (p.1250·2).
Constipation; obesity.

Colosan plus Medichemie, Switz.
Sterculia (p.1250·2); frangula (p.1227·1).
Constipation.

Coloscreen
Biolab, NZ; Helena, USA.
Test for faecal occult blood.

Colosina Lemery, Mex.
Ciclosporin (p.518·1).

Colosoft Medichemie, Switz.
Ispaghula (p.1229·1).
Constipation.

Colo-Sol Phardi, Switz.
Macrogol 3350 (p.1630·3); electrolytes (p.1180·1).
Bowel evacuation.

Colospan Hovid, Singapore.
Hyoscine butylbromide (p.468·2).
Smooth muscle spasm.

Colostrum Eagle, Austral.
Milk extract (p.1350·1).
Dietary supplement.

Colotal Agis, Israel.
Mebeverine hydrochloride (p.1233·3).
Gastrointestinal disorders.

Colovage Dynapharm, USA†.
Macrogol 3350 (p.1630·3); electrolytes (p.1180·1).
Bowel evacuation; constipation.

Coloxyl
Note. This name is used for preparations of different composition.
Fawns & McAllan, Austral.; Fawns & McAllan, NZ.
Enema; tablets: Docusate sodium (p.1223·1).
Bowel evacuation; constipation.

Fawns & McAllan, Austral.; Fawns & McAllan, NZ.
Oral drops: Poloxamer (p.1347·1).
Constipation.

Fawns & McAllan, Austral.; Fawns & McAllan, NZ.
Suppositories: Docusate sodium (p.1223·1); bisacodyl (p.1212·2).
Bowel evacuation; constipation.

Coloxyl with Senna
Fawns & McAllan, Austral.; Fawns & McAllan, NZ.
Docusate sodium (p.1223·1); sennosides (p.1248·3).
Constipation.

Colpacid Dansk-Flama, Braz.
Tyrothricin (p.267·1); nitrofurazone (p.231·3); lactic acid (p.1626·2); sodium lactate (p.1186·2).
Vulvovaginal disorders.

Colpagex N Marjan, Braz.
Neomycin (p.228·1); tyrothricin (p.267·1); nystatin (p.392·2); boric acid (p.1586·1).
Vulvovaginal infections.

Colpanist Dansk-Flama, Braz.
Metronidazole (p.594·1); nystatin (p.392·2); benzalkonium chloride (p.1133·2); urea (p.1127·3).
Vulvovaginal infections.

Colpatrin Teuto, Braz.
Metronidazole (p.594·1); nystatin (p.392·2); benzalkonium chloride (p.1133·2); urea (p.1127·3).
Vulvovaginal infections.

Colpermin
Germania, Aust.; Pharmascience, Canad.†; Tillotts, Hong Kong; Pharmacia Upjohn, Irl.; Baxter, NZ; Tillotts, NZ; Tillotts, Switz.; Tillotts, Thai.; Pharmacia, USA.
Peppermint oil (p.1243·3).
Irritable bowel syndrome.

Colphen Propan, S.Afr.
Codeine phosphate (p.25·2); chlorpheniramine [chlorphenamine] maleate (p.412·1); sodium salicylate (p.84·2); guaifenesin (p.1092·2); phenylephrine hydrochloride (p.1097·1); caffeine (p.761·3); cetylpyridinium chloride (p.1138·1).
Coughs.

Colpist MT Ativus, Braz.
Metronidazole benzoate (p.594·1); nystatin (p.392·2); benzalkonium chloride (p.1133·2).
Vulvovaginal infections.

Colpistar Farmoquimica, Braz.
Vaginal cream: Metronidazole (p.594·1); nystatin (p.392·2); benzalkonium chloride (p.1133·2); muramidase (p.1638·1).
Vaginal tablets: Metronidazole (p.594·1); nystatin (p.392·2).
Vulvovaginal infections.

Colpistatin Ache, Braz.
Metronidazole (p.594·1); nystatin (p.392·2); benzalkonium chloride (p.1133·2).
Vulvovaginal infections.

Colpogyn Angelini, Ital.
Estriol (p.1475·3).
Cervical erosion; menopausal disorders.

Colpolase De Mayo, Braz.
Topical solution: Neomycin sulfate (p.228·1); tyrothricin (p.267·1); hydroxyquinoline sulfate (p.1622·2); lactic acid (p.1626·2); menthol (p.1632·3).
Vaginal capsules: Neomycin (p.228·1); polymyxin B (p.238·3); nystatin (p.392·2); tinidazole (p.603·3).
Vulvovaginal infections.

Colpormon Lipha Sante, Fr.†.
Hydroxyestrone diacetate (p.1479·3).
Infertility caused by cervical mucus deficiency; vaginal and cervical oestrogen deficiency.

Colposeptine
Theramex, Hong Kong; Theramex, Mon.
Chlorquinaldol (p.182·1); promestriene (p.1490·3).
Leukorrhoea; vaginal atrophy.

Colpotrofin Grunenthal, Spain.
Promestriene (p.1490·3).
Vulvovaginal disorders.

Colpotrofine Byk, Braz.
Promestriene (p.1490·3).
Vulvovaginal disorders.

Colpotrophine
Theramex, Hong Kong; Theramex, Ital.; Theramex, Mon.; Sanofi Synthelabo, Port.; Theramex, Singapore; Golaz, Switz.
Promestriene (p.1490·3).
Vulvovaginal disorders.

Colpovis SIT, Ital.
Quinestradol (p.1490·3).
Vulvovaginal disorders.

Colpro
Wyeth Lederle, Belg.; Wyeth, Neth.; Akromed, S.Afr.; Wyeth, Spain; Wyeth, Switz.
Medrogestone (p.1480·1).
Benign breast disorders; endometriosis; infertility; menopausal disorders; menorrhagia; menstrual disorders.

Colpron Wyeth Lederle, Aust.
Medrogestone (p.1480·1).
Hormone replacement therapy; menorrhagia; secondary amenorrhoea.

Colprone
Wyeth-Ayerst, Canad.; Wyeth Lederle, Fr.; Wyeth-Ayerst, Hong Kong; Wyeth Lederle, Ital.; Wyeth-Ayerst, Thai.
Medrogestone (p.1480·1).
Dysfunctional uterine bleeding; endometriosis; infertility; menopausal disorders; menstrual disorders; threatened or recurrent miscarriage.

Colsanac Reprefar, Port.
Lactulose (p.1230·1).
Constipation; hepatic coma; hepatic encephalopathy.

Colser Serral, Mex.
Bezafibrate (p.849·1).
Hypercholesterolaemia.

Colsor
Note. This name is used for preparations of different composition.
Seng, Thai.
Aciclovir (p.612·3).
Herpes simplex infections of the skin and mucous membranes.

Pickles, UK.
Phenol (p.1152·3); menthol (p.1632·3); tannic acid (p.1669·1).
Herpes labialis.

Colstat
Note. This name is used for preparations of different composition.
Fournier, Port.
Cerivastatin sodium (p.856·1).
Hypercholesterolaemia.

Restan, S.Afr.
Paracetamol (p.72·1); ascorbic acid (p.1389·3); caffeine (p.761·3); phenylephrine hydrochloride

(p.1097·1); chlorpheniramine [chlorphenamine] maleate (p.412·1); atropine sulfate (p.461·1).
Cold and influenza symptoms.

Coltalin with Vit B₁ Fortune, Hong Kong.
Paracetamol (p.71·2); caffeine (p.761·3); chlorpheniramine [chlorphenamine] maleate (p.412·1); phenylephrine hydrochloride (p.1097·1); vitamin B₁ (p.1385·2).
Respiratory-tract disorders.

Coltapaste
Note. This name is used for preparations of different composition.
Smith & Nephew, Aust.
Zinc oxide (p.1128·2).
Medicated bandage.

Smith & Nephew, UK.
Zinc oxide (p.1128·2); coal tar (p.1125·1).
Medicated bandage.

Coltec Approved Prescription Services, UK†.
Mesalazine (p.1234·1).
Ulcerative colitis.

Coltramyl
Roussel Diamant, Fr.; Aventis, Port.
Thiocolchicoside (p.1330·2).
Skeletal muscle spasm.

Coltrax Hoechst Marion Roussel, Braz.
Thiocolchicoside (p.1330·2).
Painful muscle spasm.

Colubiazol Hoechst Marion Roussel, Braz.
Sulfachrysoidine (p.251·1).
Mouth infections.

Colufase Columbia, Mex.
Sodium benzoate (p.1134·3).
Hyperammonaemia.

Columina Columbia, Mex.
Cimetidine (p.1216·3).

Colutoide Honorterapica, Braz.
Prednisolone (p.1077·3); neomycin sulfate (p.228·1); bismuth sodium tartrate; procaine hydrochloride (p.1319·1).
Mouth and throat disorders.

Coly-Mycin M
Parke, Davis, Austral.; Parke, Davis, Canad.; Parke, Davis, NZ; Monarch, USA.
Colistimethate sodium (p.192·3).
Bacterial infections.

Coly-Mycin S Otic
Parke, Davis, NZ; Parke, Davis, USA.
Colistin sulfate (p.192·3); neomycin sulfate (p.228·1); hydrocortisone acetate (p.1073·3); tonzonium bromide (p.1674·1).
Bacterial ear infections.

Colyrazul Lessel, Braz.
Naphazoline hydrochloride (p.1095·1); methylene blue [methylthioninium chloride] (p.1012·3).
Ocular congestion.

CoLyte
Reed & Carnrick, Canad.; Schwarz, USA.
Macrogol 3350 (p.1630·3); electrolytes (p.1180·1).
Bowel evacuation.

Comafusin Hepar Pharmacia Upjohn, Ger.
Amino-acid, vitamin, and electrolyte infusion with xylitol (p.1350·1).
Hepatic coma.

Comagis Agis, Israel.
Bifonazole (p.381·1); fluocinonide (p.1071·2).
Infected skin disorders.

Comalose-R Rougier, Canad.
Lactulose (p.1230·1).
Hepatic encephalopathy.

Comat Milano, Thai.
Clotrimazole (p.382·1).
Fungal and bacterial vaginal infections; trichomoniasis.

Combacid Streuli, Switz.
Aluminium hydroxide-magnesium carbonate co-dried gel (p.1211·2); simeticone (p.1249·2).
Gastric hyperacidity.

Combactam
Pfizer, Aust.; Pfizer, Ger.
Sulbactam sodium (p.250·1).
Bacterial infections.

Combact-HIB Aventis, S.Afr.
An adsorbed diphtheria, tetanus, pertussis and haemophilus influenzae conjugate vaccine (p.1538·3).
Active immunisation.

Comba-Gripp Doetsch, Grether, Switz.†.
Aspirin (p.14·2); salicylamide (p.82·1); caffeine (p.761·3).
Cold symptoms.

Combantrin
Pfizer, Aust.; G.P. Laboratories, Austral.; Pfizer, Canad.; Pfizer, Fr.†; Pfizer, Hong Kong; Pfizer, Israel; Pfizer, Ital.; Pfizer, Mex.; Pfizer, NZ; Pfizer, Port.; Pfizer, S.Afr.; Pfizer, Thai.
Pyrantel embonate (p.108·1).
Worm infections.

Combantrin-1 with Mebendazole Pfizer, Austral.
Mebendazole (p.102·2).
Worm infections.

Combaren Novartis, Ger.
Diclofenac sodium (p.30·3); codeine phosphate (p.25·2).
Pain.

Combetasi ISI, Ital.
Vitamin B substances (p.1350·1).
Tonic.

The symbol † denotes a preparation no longer actively marketed

Combiamid Winzer, Ger.†
Sulfacetamide sodium (p.250·3); mafenide hydrochloride (p.221·2); naphazoline hydrochloride (p.1095·1).
Formerly contained sulfacetamide sodium, mafenide hydrochloride, naphazoline hydrochloride, and antazoline hydrochloride.
Eye infections.

Combid Glaxo Wellcome, Thai.
Lamivudine (p.635·1); zidovudine (p.645·2).
HIV infection.

Combiderm
Note.This name is used for preparations of different composition.
Convatec, Port.
Carmellose sodium (p.1499·3); pectin (p.1502·3); gelatin (p.737·2).
Ulcers; wounds.

Kalbe, Singapore.
Betamethasone dipropionate (p.1063·2); clotrimazole (p.382·1); gentamicin sulfate (p.210·1).
Infected skin disorders.

Combidol CP Pharmaceuticals, UK†.
Chenodeoxycholic acid (p.1594·1); ursodeoxycholic acid (p.1677·2).
Gallstones.

Combifusin Pharmacia Upjohn, Ger.
Amino-acid, carbohydrate, and electrolyte infusion (p.1350·1).
Parenteral nutrition.

Combilosung Agepha, Aust.
Disinfection and storage solution for contact lens (p.1129·2).

Combinovita Sedabel, Braz.
Amino-acid, vitamin, and mineral preparation (p.1350·1).
Tonic.

Combinplex Hua, Thai.
Vitamin B substances (p.1350·1).

Combion-B Merck, Thai.
Vitamin B substances (p.1350·1).

CombiPatch Rhone-Poulenc Rorer, USA.
Estradiol (p.1473·1); norethisterone acetate (p.1485·1).
Menopausal disorders.

Combiplasmal Braun, Ger.
Amino-acid, carbohydrate, and electrolyte infusion (p.1350·1).
Parenteral nutrition.

Combipres
Boehringer Ingelheim, Canad.†; Boehringer Ingelheim, USA.
Clonidine hydrochloride (p.860·1); chlortalidone (p.857·1).
Hypertension.

Combipresan
Boehringer Ingelheim, Aust.†; Boehringer Ingelheim, Ger.
Clonidine hydrochloride (p.860·1); chlortalidone (p.857·1).
Hypertension.

Combiron B 12 Ache, Braz.
Ferrous sulfate (p.1360·3); vitamin B substances (p.1350·1).
Ascorbic acid (p.1389·3) is included in this preparation to increase the absorption and availability of iron.
Anaemias.

Combisartan Menarini, Ital.
Valsartan (p.988·3); hydrochlorothiazide (p.907·3).
Hypertension.

Combistix
Bayer, Austral.†; Bayer, USA.
Test for pH, protein, and glucose in urine.

Combithyrex Biochemie, Aust.
Thyroxine [levothyroxine] sodium (p.1526·2); liothyronine sodium (p.1524·2).
Hypothyroidism.

Combitora Solvay, Spain.
Amoxicillin trihydrate (p.149·2).
Bacterial infections.

Combitorax Nezel, Spain†.
Capsules: Amoxicillin trihydrate (p.149·2); bromhexine hydrochloride (p.1085·3).
Oral suspension: Amoxicillin trihydrate (p.149·2); bromhexine (p.1085·3); guaifenesin (p.1092·2); senega (p.1100·2); liquorice (p.1231·2).
Respiratory-tract infections.

Combitrex Herals, Braz.
Tetracycline hydrochloride (p.258·3).
Bacterial infections.

Combivax SmithKline Beecham, Belg.
An adsorbed diphtheria, tetanus, and pertussis vaccine (p.1537·3).
Active immunisation.

Combivent
Boehringer Ingelheim, Aust.; Boehringer Ingelheim, Austral.; Boehringer Ingelheim, Belg.; Boehringer Ingelheim, Canad.; Boehringer Ingelheim, Denm.; Boehringer Ingelheim, Fr.; Boehringer Ingelheim, Hong Kong; Boehringer Ingelheim, Irl.; Boehringer Ingelheim, Mex.; Boehringer Ingelheim, Neth.†; Boehringer Ingelheim, NZ; Boehringer Ingelheim, Port.; Boehringer Ingelheim, S.Afr.; Boehringer Ingelheim, Singapore; Boehringer Ingelheim, Spain; Boehringer Ingelheim, Swed.; Boehringer Ingelheim, Thai.; Boehringer Ingelheim, UK; Boehringer Ingelheim, USA.
Ipratropium bromide (p.766·1); salbutamol sulfate (p.770·3).
Obstructive airways disease.

Combivir
Glaxo, Aust.; Glaxo Wellcome, Austral.; Glaxo Wellcome, Belg.; Glaxo Wellcome, Canad.; Glaxo Wellcome, Denm.; Glaxo Wellcome, Fin.; Glaxo Wellcome, Fr.; Glaxo Wellcome, Ger.; Glaxo Wellcome, Hong Kong; Glaxo Wellcome, Irl.; Glaxo Wellcome, Israel; Glaxo Wellcome, Ital.; Glaxo Wellcome, Mex.; Glaxo Wellcome, Neth.; Glaxo Wellcome, Norw.; Glaxo Wellcome, NZ; Glaxo Wellcome, Port.; Glaxo Wellcome, Singapore; Glaxo Wellcome, Spain; Glaxo Wellcome, Swed.; Glaxo Wellcome, Switz.; Glaxo Wellcome, UK; Glaxo Wellcome, USA.
Lamivudine (p.635·1); zidovudine (p.645·2).
HIV infection.

Combivite SA Druggists Self Med, S.Afr.†.
Multivitamin preparation (p.1350·1).

Combivitol Lannacher, Aust.
Multivitamin preparation (p.1350·1).

Combizym
Sankyo, Aust.; Luitpold, Belg.†; Sankyo, Fin.; Sankyo, Ger.; Sankyo, Hong Kong; Sankyo, Ital.; Will-Pharma, Neth.; Sankyo, Norw.; Sankyo, NZ; Searle, NZ; Sankyo, Port.; Selena, Swed.; Sankyo, Switz.; Sankyo, Thai.
Pancreatin (p.1646·1); enzymes from *Aspergillus oryzae*.
Cystic fibrosis; digestive disorders; pancreatic insufficiency.

Combizym Compositum
Sankyo, Aust.; Sankyo, Fin.; Sankyo, Ger.; Luitpold, Neth.†; Sankyo, NZ; Searle, NZ; Sankyo, Port.†; Selena, Swed.; Sankyo, Switz.†; Sankyo, Thai.
Pancreatin (p.1646·1); enzymes from *Aspergillus oryzae*; ox bile extract (p.1585·1).
Digestive disorders; pancreatic insufficiency.

Combudoron
Note.This name is used for preparations of different composition.
Weleda, Ger.
Arnica (p.1581·3); urtica (p.1678·2).
Burns; insect stings.

Weleda, UK.
Homoeopathic preparation.

Combur 3 Roche Diagnostics, Irl.
Test for pH, protein, and glucose in urine.

Combur 8 Roche Diagnostics, Irl.
Test for nitrite, pH, protein, glucose, ketones, urobilinogen, bilirubin, and blood in urine.

Combur 10 Roche Diagnostics, Irl.
Test for specific gravity, nitrite, pH, leucocytes, protein, glucose, ketones, urobilirubin, and blood in urine.

Combur 4 D Roche Diagnostics, Irl.
Test for protein, glucose, ketones, and blood in urine.

Combur 5 D Roche Diagnostics, Irl.
Test for pH, protein, glucose, ketones, and blood in urine.

Combur Test Roche Diagnostics, Austral.
Test for pH, protein, and glucose in urine.

Combur 7 Test Roche Diagnostics, Austral.
Test for pH, protein, glucose, bilirubin, urobilinogen, and blood in urine.

Combur 8 Test Roche Diagnostics, Austral.
Test for ketones, urobilinogen, bilirubin, blood, nitrite, pH, protein, and glucose in urine.

Combur 9 Test Roche Diagnostics, Austral.
Test for leucocytes, nitrite, pH, protein, glucose, ketones, urobilinogen, bilirubin, and blood in urine.

Combur 10 Test Roche Diagnostics, Austral.
Test for specific gravity, leucocytes, nitrite, pH, protein, glucose, ketones, urobilinogen, bilirubin, and blood in urine.

Comburic Bio-Therabel, Belg.
Allopurinol (p.397·2); benzbromarone (p.399·3).
Gout; hyperuricaemia.

Combustin Heilsalbe Combustin, Ger.
Bismuth subgallate (p.1213·2); zinc oxide (p.1128·2); benzocaine (p.1306·2).
Burns; haemorrhoids; skin disorders; skin ulceration; wounds.

Co-Mepril Kwizda, Aust.
Enalapril maleate (p.883·3); hydrochlorothiazide (p.907·3).
Hypertension.

Cometamin Yamanouchi, Jpn†.
Cycotiamine (p.1384·3).
Vitamin B₁ deficiency.

Cometon Metapharma, Ital.
Vitamin B substances (p.1350·1).
Vitamin B deficiency.

Comfeel
Note.This name is used for preparations of different composition.
Coloplast, Fr.; Coloplast, Switz.†; Coloplast, UK.
Medicated dressing: Carmellose sodium (p.1499·3).
Wounds.

Coloplast, UK.
Barrier cream.
Peristomal care.

Comfeel Plus Coloplast, UK.
Carmellose sodium (p.1499·3); calcium alginate (p.728·1).
Wounds.

Comfeel Seasorb
Note.This name is used for preparations of different composition.
Coloplast, Fr.
Calcium alginate (p.728·1); sodium alginate (p.1498·3); carmellose sodium (p.1499·3).
Bedsores; ulcers.

Coloplast, UK.
Calcium sodium alginate (p.728·1) (p.1498·3).
Exudating wounds.

Comfort Durex, Canad.
Nonoxinol 9 (p.1346·1).
Contraceptive.

Comfort Eye Drops Pilkington Barnes-Hind, USA.
Naphazoline hydrochloride (p.1095·1).
Minor eye irritation.

Comfort Tears Pilkington Barnes-Hind, USA.
Hyetellose (p.1501·1).
Dry eyes.

Comfortcare Dual Action Allergan, Canad.
Subtilisin; poloxamer (p.1129·2).
Cleanser for gas permeable contact lenses.

Comfortcare GP Pilkington Barnes-Hind, USA.
Disinfecting, wetting, and soaking solution for gas permeable contact lenses (p.1129·2).

Comfortcare GP Dual Action Allergan, Austral.†.
Subtilisin; poloxamer 338 (p.1347·1) (p.1129·2).
Cleanser for gas permeable contact lenses.

Comfortcare GP Wetting and Soaking Allergan, USA.
Wetting and soaking solution for hard gas permeable contact lenses (p.1129·2).

Comfortcare Wetting & Soaking Allergan, Canad.
Wetting and soaking solution for gas permeable contact lenses (p.1129·2).

Comfortine Dermik, USA.
Vitamin A (p.1382·1); vitamin E (p.1393·3); zinc oxide (p.1128·2); chloroxylenol (p.1142·1).
Skin disorders.

Comfrey Plus Herbal, Israel.
Comfrey (p.1598·3); allantoin (p.1110·1).
Burns; cuts; insect bites; nappy rash; soft-tissue injury.

Comfy Poliphatm, Thai.
Dextromethorphan hydrobromide (p.1087·3); chlorpheniramine [chlorphenamine] maleate (p.412·1); pseudoephedrine hydrochloride (p.1099·2); ammonium chloride (p.1085·2).
Cold symptoms; coughs; nasal congestion.

Comhist LA Procter & Gamble, USA.
Chlorpheniramine [chlorphenamine] maleate (p.412·1); phenyltoloxamine citrate (p.423·1); phenylephrine hydrochloride (p.1097·1).
Nasal congestion; rhinorrhoea.

Comilorid Mepha, Switz.
Amiloride hydrochloride (p.835·1); hydrochlorothiazide (p.907·3).
Hypertension; liver cirrhosis with ascites; oedema.

Comital L
Bayer, Port.; Bayer, Spain†.
Phenytoin (p.357·2); methylphenobarbital (p.353·3); phenobarbital (p.355·1).
Epilepsy; Sydenham's chorea.

Comixco Ashbourne, UK†.
Co-trimoxazole (p.193·3).
Bacterial infections.

Comizial Ogna, Ital.
Phenobarbital (p.355·1).
Sedative.

Comoprin British Dispensary, Thai.
Aspirin (p.14·2).
Fever; pain.

Compagel Synthelabo, Spain.
Aluminium hydroxide (p.1210·3); magnesium hydroxide (p.1233·1); magaldrate (p.1232·2).
Gastrointestinal hyperacidity.

Compagen Solfran, Mex.
Multivitamin and mineral preparation (p.1350·1).

Companion 2 Medisense, Canad.†.
Test for glucose in blood (p.1616·3).

Compazine SmithKline Beecham, USA.
Prochlorperazine (p.701·1), prochlorperazine edisilate (p.701·1), or prochlorperazine maleate (p.701·2).
Non-psychotic anxiety; psychoses; severe nausea and vomiting.

Compendium Poliforma, Ital.
Bromazepam (p.656·3).
Anxiety disorders; insomnia.

Compensal Provit, Mex.
Cyanocobalamin (p.1388·3).

Compete Mission Pharmacal, USA.
Ferrous gluconate (p.1360·1); folic acid (p.1361·1); multivitamins and minerals (p.1350·1).
Iron-deficiency anaemias.

Complamin
SmithKline Beecham, Aust.†; SmithKline Beecham, Belg.; SmithKline Beecham, Canad.; SmithKline Beecham, Ger.; Rhone-Poulenc Rorer, Ital.; SmithKline Beecham, Neth.; Tika, Swed.; Doetsch, Grether, Switz.
Xantinol nicotinate (p.999·1).
Cerebral and peripheral vascular disorders; hearing loss; hypercholesterolaemia; Ménière's disease; retinopathy.

Complamin spezial SmithKline Beecham, Ger.
Xantinol nicotinate (p.999·1).
Lipid disorders.

Complan
Boots, Hong Kong; Glaxo Wellcome, Mex.; Heinz-Wattie, NZ; Heinz, UK.
Preparation for enteral nutrition (p.1350·1).

Compleat
Novartis Nutrition, Canad.; Sandoz Nutrition, USA.
A range of preparations for enteral nutrition (p.1350·1).

Compleat Modified Novartis Nutrition, Hong Kong.
Preparation for enteral nutrition (p.1350·1).

Complegil Diepal, Fr.†.
Nutritional supplement (p.1350·1).
Convalescence.

Complejo B Carnot, Mex.
Vitamin B substances (p.1350·1).

Complenatal FF Pharmaceutical Enterprises, S.Afr.
Multivitamin and mineral preparation (p.1350·1).

Complesso B SIT, Ital.
Vitamin B substances (p.1350·1).
Formerly known as Complesso B Antitossico Jamco.
Tonic.

Complete
Allergan, Ger.†; Allergan, UK.
A range of preparations for contact lens care (p.1129·2).

Complete All-In-One Allergan, Canad.; Allergan, Israel.
A cleansing, rinsing, disinfecting and lubricating solution for soft contact lenses (p.1129·2).

Complete Comfort Plus Allergan, NZ.
Cleansing, rinsing, disinfecting, storage, and lubricating solution for contact lenses (p.1129·2).

Complete Multi Pre- and Post-Natal Wampole, Canad.
Multivitamin and mineral preparation (p.1350·1).

Complete Multi-Adult Wampole, Canad.
Multivitamin and mineral preparation (p.1350·1).

Complete Protein Remover
Allergan, Austral.; Allergan, Canad.; Allergan, Israel.
Substilisin A (p.1129·2).
Protein remover for soft contact lenses.

Complete Solution Allergan, Austral.
Cleaning, rinsing, disinfecting, storage, and lubricating solution for soft contact lenses (p.1129·2).

Compleven
Fresenius Kabi, Fin.; Fresenius Kabi, Ger.; Fresenius Kabi, Port.; Fresenius Kabi, Swed.; Fresenius Kabi, Switz.; Fresenius Kabi, UK.
Amino-acid, carbohydrate, electrolyte, and lipid (from soya oil (p.1378·1)) infusion (p.1350·1).
Contains egg phospholipid.
Parenteral nutrition.

Complevit EMS, Braz.
Buclizine (p.411·1); gamma-aminobutyric acid (p.1613·1).
Reduced appetite; tonic.

Complex 15
Schering, Canad.; Schering-Plough, USA.
Emollient and moisturiser.

Complex 75 Frega, Canad.†.
Vitamin B substances (p.1350·1).

Complex B Pharmalab, Canad.†.
Vitamin B substances (p.1350·1).

Complexan B Upsifarma, Port.
Vitamin B substances (p.1350·1).
Vitamin B deficiency.

Complexe Lehning, Fr.
A range of homoeopathic preparations.

Complexe B Compose Bio-Sante, Canad.
Vitamin B substances (p.1350·1).

Complexo B Basi, Port.
Vitamin B substances (p.1350·1).

Complidermol Medea, Spain.
Multivitamins and amino acids (p.1350·1); inositol (p.1623·3).
Skin disorders.

Complement Continus
Seton, Irl.; Mundipharma, Switz.; SSL, UK.
Pyridoxine hydrochloride (p.1386·3).
Premenstrual syndrome; vitamin B₆ deficiency.

Complutine Novartis Consumer, Spain.
Diazepam (p.674·3).
Contains pyridoxine hydrochloride.
Alcohol withdrawal syndrome; anxiety; febrile convulsions; insomnia; skeletal muscle spasm.

Comply Sherwood, USA.
Lactose-free preparation for enteral nutrition (p.1350·1).

Compocillin Abbott, NZ.
Phenoxymethylpenicillin (p.235·1).
Bacterial infections.

Compound V SSL, UK.
Salicylic acid (p.1122·3).
Verrucas.

Compound Inhalation of Menthol McGloin, Austral.
Menthol (p.1632·3); siberian fir oil; creosote (p.1087·3).
Cold symptoms.

Compound W
Whitehall-Robins, Canad.; Seton, Irl.; SSL, UK; Whitehall, USA.
Salicylic acid (p.1122·3).
Hyperkeratosis; verrucas; warts.

Compound W Plus Whitehall-Robins, Canad.
Salicylic acid (p.1122·3).
Warts.

Compoz Night-time Sleep Aid Medtech, USA.
Diphenhydramine hydrochloride (p.416·1).
Insomnia.

Compralgyl Gifrer Barbezat, Fr.
Aspirin (p.14·2); codeine phosphate (p.25·2).
Fever; pain.

Compralsol Gifrer Barbezat, Fr.
Paracetamol (p.71·2).
Fever; pain.

Comprecin Warner-Lambert, Mex.
Enoxacin (p.201·1).
Bacterial infections.

Comprimes analgesiques no 534 *Renapharm, Switz.*
Paracetamol (p.71·2).
Fever; pain.

Comprimes analgesiques "S" *Synpharma, Switz.*
Paracetamol (p.71·2); caffeine (p.761·3); propyphenazone (p.80·2).
Fever; pain.

Comprimes contre la toux *Zeller, Switz.*
Hedera helix.
Bronchial disorders with viscous mucus.

Comprimes Gynecologiques Pharmatex *Innothera, Fr.†.*
Benzalkonium chloride (p.1133·2).
Contraceptive.

Comprimes pour l'estomac *Zeller, Switz.*
Calcium carbonate (p.1215·1); magnesium trisilicate (p.1233·3).
Gastric hyperacidity.

Comprimes somniferes formule 533 *Renapharm, Switz.*
Diphenhydramine hydrochloride (p.416·1).
Insomnia.

Comprimes somniferes "S" *Synpharma, Switz.*
Diphenhydramine (p.416·1).
Agitation; insomnia; nervousness.

Compro *Paddock, USA.*
Prochlorperazine (p.701·1).
Nausea and vomiting.

Compu-Gel *Docmed, S.Afr.†.*
Aluminium hydroxide (p.1210·3); magnesium oxide (p.1233·2).
Gastric hyperacidity.

Compu-Pain *Compu, S.Afr.†.*
Paracetamol (p.71·2).
Fever; pain.

Computer Eye Drops *Bausch & Lomb, USA.*
Glycerol (p.1616·3).
Eye irritation.

Comstrong *Unison, Thai.*
Vitamin B substances (p.1350·1).

Comtan
Novartis, Aust.; Novartis, Austral.; Novartis, Belg.; Novartis, Fr.; Novartis, Ital.; Novartis, Neth.; Novartis, NZ; Novartis, Port.; Novartis, S.Afr.; Novartis, Singapore; Novartis, Spain; Novartis, Switz.; Novartis, Thai.; Novartis, USA.
Entacapone (p.1168·3).
Parkinsonism.

Comtaplex *Greater Pharma, Thai.*
Vitamin B substances (p.1350·1).

Comtess
Orion, Denm.; Orion, Fin.; Orion, Ger.; Orion, Irl.; Orion, Norw.; Orion, Swed.; Orion, UK.
Entacapone (p.1168·3).
Parkinsonism.

Comtrex *Bristol-Myers Products, USA.*
Paracetamol (p.71·2); pseudoephedrine hydrochloride (p.1099·2); chlorpheniramine [chlorphenamine] maleate (p.412·1); dextromethorphan hydrobromide (p.1087·3).
Coughs and cold symptoms.

Comtrex Allergy-Sinus *Bristol-Myers Products, USA.*
Paracetamol (p.71·2); pseudoephedrine hydrochloride (p.1099·2); chlorpheniramine [chlorphenamine] maleate (p.412·1).
Upper respiratory-tract symptoms.

Comtrex Day & Night Maximum Strength
Bristol-Myers Products, USA.
Orange caplets, dextromethorphan hydrobromide (p.1087·3); paracetamol (p.71·2); pseudoephedrine hydrochloride (p.1099·2); blue tablets, dextromethorphan hydrobromide (p.1087·3); paracetamol (p.71·2); pseudoephedrine hydrochloride (p.1099·2); chlorpheniramine [chlorphenamine] maleate (p.412·1).
Coughs and cold symptoms.

Comtrex Day & Night Multi-Symptom *Bristol-Myers Products, USA.*
Orange caplets, dextromethorphan hydrobromide (p.1087·3); paracetamol (p.71·2); pseudoephedrine hydrochloride (p.1099·2); yellow tablets, dextromethorphan hydrobromide (p.1087·3); paracetamol (p.71·2); pseudoephedrine hydrochloride (p.1099·2); chlorpheniramine [chlorphenamine] maleate (p.412·1).
Coughs and cold symptoms.

Comtrex Hot Flu Relief *Bristol-Myers Products, USA.*
Chlorpheniramine [chlorphenamine] maleate (p.412·1); dextromethorphan hydrobromide (p.1087·3); paracetamol (p.71·2); pseudoephedrine hydrochloride (p.1099·2).
Coughs and cold symptoms.

Comtrex Liqui-Gels *Bristol-Myers Products, USA†.*
Chlorpheniramine [chlorphenamine] maleate (p.412·1); dextromethorphan hydrobromide (p.1087·3); paracetamol (p.71·2); phenylpropanolamine hydrochloride (p.1098·1).
Coughs and cold symptoms.

Comvax
CSL, Austral.; Merck, USA.
A haemophilus influenzae and hepatitis B vaccine (p.1541·1).
Active immunisation in infants.

Conadyl *TO-Chemicals, Thai.*
Codeine phosphate (p.25·2); promethazine hydrochloride (p.423·1).
Coughs.

Conamic *Pharmasant, Thai.*
Mefenamic acid (p.51·2).
Inflammation; musculoskeletal and joint disorders; pain.

Conazine *Condrugs, Thai.*
Perphenazine (p.699·1).
Anxiety; nausea and vomiting.

Conazol *Liomont, Mex.*
Ketoconazole (p.389·1).
Fungal infections.

Conazole *DHA, Singapore.*
Betamethasone valerate (p.1063·2); miconazole nitrate (p.391·1); gentamicin sulfate (p.210·1).
Infected skin disorders.

Concavit *Wallace Mfg Chem., UK.*
Multivitamin preparation (p.1350·1).

Conceive *Pharmascience, Canad.†.*
Fertility test or pregnancy test (p.1654·3).

Conceive Ovulation Predictor *Quidel, USA.*
Fertility test (p.1654·3).

Conceive Pregnancy *Quidel, USA.*
Pregnancy test (p.1654·3).

Concentrated Milk of Magnesia-Cascara *Roxane, USA.*
Magnesium hydroxide (p.1233·1); cascara (p.1216·1).

Concentrin *CT, Ger.*
Aesculus (p.1574·1).
Soft-tissue disorders; venous disorders.

Conceplan M *Grunenthal, Ger.*
Ethinylestradiol (p.1476·2); norethisterone (p.1485·1).
Combined oral contraceptive.

Concept Blue *Invitech, UK.*
Pregnancy test (p.1654·3).

Concerta *Alza, USA.*
Methylphenidate hydrochloride (p.1511·3).
Attention-deficit hyperactivity disorder.

Conchae comp. *Weleda, UK.*
Conchae; oak bark (p.1643·2).
Aid to enhance calcium absorption.

Conchivit *Ghimas, Ital.†.*
Multivitamin preparation (p.1350·1).
Vitamin supplement.

Concise *BHR, UK†.*
Pregnancy test (p.1654·3).

Concor
Merck, Aust.; Merck, Ger.; Merck, Hong Kong; Merck, Israel; Bracco, Ital.; Merck, Port.; Merck, S.Afr.; Merck, Singapore; Merck, Switz.; Merck, Thai.
Bisoprolol fumarate (p.850·1).
Angina pectoris; hypertension.

Concor Plus
Merck, Aust.; Merck, Ger.; Merck, Switz.
Bisoprolol fumarate (p.850·1); hydrochlorothiazide (p.907·3).
Hypertension.

Concordin
Merck Sharp & Dohme, Denm.; Merck Sharp & Dohme, Irl.; Merck Sharp & Dohme, Swed.; Merck Sharp & Dohme, UK†.
Protriptyline hydrochloride (p.307·3).
Depression.

Condelone *Lacer, Spain†.*
Podophyllotoxin (p.1121·2).
Anogenital warts.

Condil *Protermex, Mex.; Selder, Mex.*
Podophyllum (p.1121·1).

Condiuren *Gentili, Ital.*
Enalapril maleate (p.883·3); hydrochlorothiazide (p.907·3).
Hypertension.

Condral *SPA, Ital.*
A heparinoid (p.905·2).
Osteoarthritis; pain.

Condress *Gentili, Ital.*
Collagen (p.1598·2).
Cicatrisation of wounds and skin ulcers.

Condrin-LA *Roberts, USA†; Hauck, USA†.*
Phenylpropanolamine hydrochloride (p.1098·1); chlorpheniramine [chlorphenamine] maleate (p.412·1).
Upper respiratory-tract symptoms.

Condrofer *UCB, Ital.*
Chondroitin sulfate A-iron complex (p.1357·1).
Iron deficiency; iron deficiency anaemias.

Condrosulf
Sanova, Aust.; IBSA, Switz.
Sodium chondroitin sulfate (p.1594·2).
Joint disorders.

Condrotec *Searle, UK†.*
Naproxen (p.60·3).
Misoprostol (p.1446·1) is included in this preparation in an attempt to limit adverse effects on the gastrointestinal mucosa.
Ankylosing spondylitis; osteoarthritis; rheumatoid arthritis.

Conductasa *Teofarma, Spain.*
Pyridoxine oxoglurate (p.1387·1).
Vitamin B6 deficiency.

Conducton
Klinge, Aust.; Klinge, Ger.
Carazolol (p.855·1).
Angina pectoris; arrhythmias; heart failure; hypertension; myocardial infarction.

Condyline
Hamilton, Austral.; Yamanouchi, Belg†; Canderm, Canad.; Galderma, Denm.; Galderma, Fin.; Yamanouchi, Fr.; Nycomed, Irl.; Yamanouchi, Ital.; Yamanouchi, Neth.; Galderma, Norw.; Pharmaco, NZ; Yamanouchi, Port.; Galderma, Swed.; Nycomed, Switz.; Ardern, UK.
Podophyllotoxin (p.1121·2).
Anogenital warts.

Condylox
Gerot, Aust.; Wolff, Ger.; Agis, Israel; Oclassen, USA.
Podophyllotoxin (p.1121·2).
Anogenital warts.

Conex *Forest Pharmaceuticals, USA†.*
Phenylpropanolamine hydrochloride (p.1098·1); guaifenesin (p.1092·2).
Coughs.

Conex with Codeine *Forest Pharmaceuticals, USA†.*
Phenylpropanolamine hydrochloride (p.1098·1); guaifenesin (p.1092·2); codeine phosphate (p.25·2).
Coughs.

Confetti Lassativi *Giuliani, Ital.†.*
Rhubarb (p.1248·1); cascara (p.1216·1); boldo (p.1585·3); phenolphthalein (p.1244·1).
Constipation.

Confetti Lassativi CM *Giuliani, Ital.*
Senna (p.1248·2); boldo (p.1585·3); cascara (p.1216·1).
Constipation.

Confetto *Falqui, Ital.†.*
Phenolphthalein (p.1244·1).
Constipation.

Confetto CM *Giuliani, Ital.*
Bisacodyl (p.1212·2).
Constipation.

Confetto Complex *Falqui, Ital.†.*
Phenolphthalein (p.1244·1); rhubarb (p.1248·1); boldo (p.1585·3).
Constipation.

Confiance
Helsinn, Port.; Wassen, UK.
Multivitamin and mineral preparation (p.1350·1).

Confiance Donna *Wassen, Ital.*
Multivitamin and mineral preparation (p.1350·1).
Nutritional supplement.

Confidelle *Carter Horner, Canad.*
Pregnancy test (p.1654·3).

Confidelle Progress *Bouty, Ital.*
Pregnancy test (p.1654·3).

Confidol *Medopharm, Ger.†.*
Etilefrine hydrochloride (p.888·1).
Circulatory disorders; hypotension.

Confirm *Durex, Canad.*
Pregnancy test (p.1654·3).

Confit *Procter & Gamble, Aust.*
Verapamil hydrochloride (p.989·1); triamterene (p.986·1); hydrochlorothiazide (p.907·3).
Hypertension.

Conflictan *Solvay, Fr.†.*
Oxaflozane hydrochloride (p.302·2).
Depression.

Confludin N *Bilgast, Ger.*
Homoeopathic preparation.

Confobos *Smaller, Spain.*
Famotidine (p.1225·3).
Gastro-oesophageal reflux; peptic ulcer; Zollinger-Ellison syndrome.

Conformil *Milupa, Port.*
Infant feed (p.1350·1).
Milk intolerance.

Confortid
Dumex-Alpharma, Denm.; Dumex-Alpharma, Fin.; Dumex, Ger.; Alpharma, Norw.; Dumex-Alpharma, Swed.
Indometacin (p.44·3) or indometacin sodium (p.45·1).
Gout; inflammation; musculoskeletal, joint, and periarticular disorders; pain; renal and biliary colic.

Congespirin *Bristol-Myers Squibb, USA†.*
Paracetamol (p.71·2); phenylephrine hydrochloride (p.1097·1).
Cold symptoms.

Congess *Fleming, USA†.*
Guaifenesin (p.1092·2); pseudoephedrine hydrochloride (p.1099·2).
Asthma; coughs and cold symptoms; nasal congestion.

Congest *Trianon, Canad.*
Conjugated oestrogens (p.1467·1).
Oestrogen therapy.

Congest Aid *Zee, Canad.*
Pseudoephedrine hydrochloride (p.1099·2).

Congestac *Ascher, USA.*
Pseudoephedrine hydrochloride (p.1099·2); guaifenesin (p.1092·2).
Coughs.

Congestant *Rugby, USA.*
Paracetamol (p.71·2); chlorpheniramine [chlorphenamine] maleate (p.412·1).
Upper respiratory-tract symptoms.

Congestant D *Rugby, USA†.*
Phenylpropanolamine hydrochloride (p.1098·1); chlorpheniramine [chlorphenamine] maleate (p.412·1); paracetamol (p.71·2).
Upper respiratory-tract symptoms.

Congest-Eze *Stanley, Canad.*
Pseudoephedrine hydrochloride (p.1099·2).

Congestion Relief *Schein, USA†.*
Pseudoephedrine hydrochloride (p.1099·2).
Nasal congestion.

Conidrin *Dansk-Flama, Braz.*
Naphazoline hydrochloride (p.1095·1); mepyramine (p.421·1).
Nasal congestion.

Coniel *Kyowa, Jpn.*
Benidipine hydrochloride (p.844·2).
Angina pectoris; hypertension.

Conjonctyl *Sedifa, Mon.†.*
Sodium methylsilanetriol salicylate.
Arteritis; mastalgia; osteoporosis.

Conjugen
Klinge, Aust.; Klinge, Ger.; Ridupharm, Switz.
Conjugated oestrogens (p.1467·1).
Menopausal disorders; osteoporosis.

Conjuncain-EDO *Mann, Ger.*
Oxybuprocaine hydrochloride (p.1318·1).
Local anaesthesia.

Conjunctilone *Allergan, Port.*
Neomycin sulfate (p.228·1); polymyxin B sulfate (p.238·1).
Bacterial eye infections.

Conjunctilone-S *Allergan, Port.*
Neomycin sulfate (p.228·1); polymyxin B sulfate (p.238·1); prednisolone acetate (p.1078·1).
Infected eye disorders.

Conjunctisan-A *Vitorgan, Ger.*
Homoeopathic preparation.

Conjunctisan-B *Vitorgan, Ger.*
Homoeopathic preparation.

Conjuntin *Allergan-Frumtost, Braz.*
Neomycin sulfate (p.228·1); polymyxin B sulfate (p.238·1).
Bacterial eye infections.

Conjunto Soramin Hipercalorico *Darrow, Braz.*
Amino-acid infusion (p.1350·1).
Parenteral nutrition.

Conjuvac *Stallergenes, Ital.*
An allergen extract (p.1575·3).
Hyposensitisation.

Conludag *Searle, Norw.*
Norethisterone (p.1485·1).
Progestogen-only oral contraceptive.

Conmel
Sanofi Winthrop, Braz.; Sanofi Winthrop, Mex.; Sanofi Winthrop, Port.†.
Dipyrone (p.34·1).
Fever; pain.

Connettivina
Kolassa, Aust.; Fidia, Hong Kong; Fidia, Ital.; Fidia, Thai.
Sodium hyaluronate (p.1620·1).
Burns; ulcers; varices; wounds.

Connettivina Plus *Fidia, Ital.*
Sodium hyaluronate (p.1620·1); sulfadiazine silver (p.251·3).
Burns; skin ulceration; wound.

Conotrane
Yamanouchi, Irl.; Yamanouchi, UK.
Benzalkonium chloride (p.1133·2); dimethicone (p.1410·1).
Formerly contained hydrargaphen and dimethicone in the UK.
Barrier cream.

Conova
Searle, Belg.; Searle, Denm.†.
Etynodiol diacetate (p.1477·1); ethinylestradiol (p.1476·2).
Combined oral contraceptive.

Conpec *Teral, USA†.*
Pseudoephedrine hydrochloride (p.1099·2); guaifenesin (p.1092·2).
Coughs.

Conpin *TAD, Ger.*
Isosorbide mononitrate (p.916·2).
Angina pectoris; heart failure; pulmonary hypertension.

Conprim *Condrugs, Thai.*
Co-trimoxazole (p.193·3).
Bacterial infections.

Conray
Mallinckrodt, Austral.; Mallinckrodt, Canad.; Bracco, Ital.; Mallinckrodt, UK; Mallinckrodt, USA.
Meglumine iothalamate (p.1036·2) or sodium iothalamate (p.1036·2).
Radiographic contrast medium.

Conray 30 *Mallinckrodt, Ger.*
Meglumine iothalamate (p.1036·2).
Radiographic contrast medium.

Conray 60 *Mallinckrodt, Ger.*
Meglumine iothalamate (p.1036·2).
Radiographic contrast medium.

Conray 70 *Mallinckrodt, Ger.*
Meglumine iothalamate (p.1036·2); sodium iothalamate (p.1036·2).
Radiographic contrast medium.

Conray FL *Mallinckrodt, Ger.*
Meglumine iothalamate (p.1036·2).
Contrast medium for urography.

Consept Step 1 *Allergan, Canad.*
Hydrogen peroxide (p.1147·1) (p.1129·2).
Cleansing and disinfecting solution for soft contact lenses.

Consept Step 2 *Allergan, Canad.*
Sodium thiosulfate (p.1024·2) (p.1129·2).
Wetting and soaking solution for soft contact lenses.

Consolin *Dolisos, Canad.*
Homoeopathic preparation.

The symbol † denotes a preparation no longer actively marketed

Constilac *Alra, USA.*
Lactulose (p.1230·1).
Constipation.

Constipal *Plough, Port.*
Dexbrompheniramine maleate (p.410·2); pseudoephedrine sulfate (p.1099·3).
Respiratory-tract congestion.

Constipation *Lalco, Canad.*
Frangula (p.1227·1); senna (p.1248·2).
Constipation.

Constipation L106 *Homeocan, Canad.*
Homoeopathic preparation.

Constrilia *Alcon, Fr.*
Tetryzoline hydrochloride (p.1101·2).
Eye disorders.

Constulose *Barre-National, USA.*
Lactulose (p.1230·1).
Constipation.

Consudine *Condrugs, Thai.*
Pseudoephedrine hydrochloride (p.1099·2); triprolidine hydrochloride (p.427·2).
Cold symptoms; hypersensitivity reactions; nasal congestion; rhinitis.

Consupren *Galena, Thai.; SPB, Thai.*
Ciclosporin (p.518·1).
Auto-immune disorders; graft-versus-host disease; transplant rejection.

Contac
Note. This name is used for preparations of different composition.
Sanova, Aust.†; SmithKline Beecham OTC, Ger.; SmithKline Beecham Consumer, Irl.†; SmithKline Beecham, Singapore.
Chlorpheniramine [chlorphenamine] maleate (p.412·1); phenylpropanolamine hydrochloride (p.1098·1).
Cold symptoms; hay fever; sinusitis.

SmithKline Beecham Consumer, Austral.
Atropine sulfate (p.461·1); hyoscine hydrobromide (p.468·2); hyoscyamine sulfate (p.469·3); pseudoephedrine hydrochloride (p.1099·2).
Cold symptoms.

SmithKline Beecham, Hong Kong; SmithKline Beecham, Thai.
Phenylpropanolamine hydrochloride (p.1098·1); belladonna alkaloids (p.463·1).
Cold symptoms.

SmithKline Beecham Consumer, UK.
Pseudoephedrine hydrochloride (p.1099·2).
Contac 400 formerly contained chlorpheniramine [chlorphenamine] maleate and phenylpropanolamine hydrochloride.
Cold symptoms.

Contac Allergy Formula *SmithKline Beecham Consumer, Canad.†*
Terfenadine (p.424·3).
Hypersensitivity disorders.

Contac Cold *SmithKline Beecham Consumer, Canad.†*
Chlorpheniramine [chlorphenamine] maleate (p.412·1); phenylpropanolamine hydrochloride (p.1098·1).
Formerly known as Contac C.
Respiratory congestion.

Contac Cold Nondrowsy *SmithKline Beecham Consumer, Canad.*
Pseudoephedrine hydrochloride (p.1099·2).
Formerly known as Contac C Nondrowsy.

Contac Cough Cold and Flu *SmithKline Beecham Consumer, Canad.†*
Paracetamol (p.71·2); chlorpheniramine [chlorphenamine] maleate (p.412·1); dextromethorphan hydrobromide (p.1087·3); phenylpropanolamine hydrochloride (p.1098·1).
Formerly known as Contac C Cold Care Formula.
Coughs and cold symptoms.

Contac Cough Cold and Flu Day & Night *SmithKline Beecham Consumer, Canad.*
Yellow caplets, pseudoephedrine hydrochloride (p.1099·2); dextromethorphan hydrobromide (p.1087·3); paracetamol (p.71·2); blue caplets, diphenhydramine hydrochloride (p.416·1); pseudoephedrine hydrochloride; paracetamol.
Formerly known as Contac Day & Night Cold and Flu.
Cold symptoms.

Contac Cough, Cold & Flu Nighttime *SmithKline Beecham Consumer, Canad.*
Pseudoephedrine hydrochloride (p.1099·2); diphenhydramine hydrochloride (p.416·1); paracetamol (p.71·2).
Formerly known as Contac C Nighttime.

Contac Coughcaps *SmithKline Beecham Consumer, UK†.*
Dextromethorphan hydrobromide (p.1087·3).
Coughs.

Contac Day *SmithKline Beecham Consumer, Canad.*
Pseudoephedrine hydrochloride (p.1099·2); dextromethorphan hydrobromide (p.1087·3); paracetamol (p.71·2).

Contac Day & Night Allergy Sinus *SmithKline Beecham Consumer, USA.*
Paracetamol (p.71·2); pseudoephedrine hydrochloride (p.1099·2); diphenhydramine hydrochloride (p.416·1).

Contac Day and Night Cold & Flu Caplets *SmithKline Beecham Consumer, USA.*
Pseudoephedrine hydrochloride (p.1099·2); dextromethorphan hydrobromide (p.1087·3); paracetamol (p.71·2).
Coughs and cold symptoms.

Contac Day & Night Sinus/Allergy *SmithKline Beecham Consumer, Canad.†.*
Paracetamol (p.71·2); pseudoephedrine hydrochloride (p.1099·2); diphenhydramine hydrochloride (p.416·1).
Cold symptoms; coughs.

Contac Erkaltungs-Trunk *SmithKline Beecham OTC, Ger.*
Paracetamol (p.71·2).
Fever; pain.

Contac Erkaltungs-Trunk Forte *SmithKline Beecham OTC, Ger.*
Paracetamol (p.71·2); phenylephrine hydrochloride (p.1097·1); dextromethorphan hydrobromide (p.1087·3).
Cold symptoms; influenza symptoms.

Contac H *SmithKline Beecham OTC, Ger.*
Chlorpheniramine [chlorphenamine] maleate (p.412·1); dextromethorphan hydrobromide (p.1087·3); phenylpropanolamine hydrochloride (p.1098·1).
Cold symptoms; coughs.

Contac Head & Chest Congestion *SmithKline Beecham Consumer, Canad.*
Pseudoephedrine hydrochloride (p.1099·2); guaifenesin (p.1092·2).

Contac 12 Hour *SmithKline Beecham Consumer, USA†.*
Chlorpheniramine [chlorphenamine] maleate (p.412·1); phenylpropanolamine hydrochloride (p.1098·1).
Upper respiratory-tract symptoms.

Contac 12 Hour Allergy *SmithKline Beecham Consumer, USA.*
Clemastine fumarate (p.413·2).

Contac Husten-Trunk *Fink, Ger.†.*
Ambroxol hydrochloride (p.1084·3).
Respiratory disorders associated with viscid or excessive mucus.

Contac Rhume *SmithKline Beecham Consumer, Switz.*
Chlorpheniramine [chlorphenamine] maleate (p.412·1); phenylpropanolamine hydrochloride (p.1098·1).
Cold symptoms; hay fever.

Contac Schnupfen *SmithKline Beecham, Aust.*
Chlorpheniramine [chlorphenamine] maleate (p.412·1); phenylpropanolamine hydrochloride (p.1098·1).
Allergic rhinitis; cold symptoms.

Contac Severe Cold and Flu Formula *SmithKline Beecham Consumer, USA†.*
Chlorpheniramine [chlorphenamine] maleate (p.412·1); dextromethorphan hydrobromide (p.1087·3); paracetamol (p.71·2); phenylpropanolamine hydrochloride (p.1098·1).
Coughs and cold symptoms.

Contac Severe Cold & Flu Non-Drowsy *SmithKline Beecham Consumer, USA†.*
Pseudoephedrine hydrochloride (p.1099·2); paracetamol (p.71·2); dextromethorphan hydrobromide (p.1087·3).

Contac Sinus
SmithKline Beecham Consumer, Canad.; SmithKline Beecham Consumer, USA†.
Paracetamol (p.71·2); pseudoephedrine hydrochloride (p.1099·2).
Sinus pain and congestion.

Contac Toux *SmithKline Beecham Consumer, Switz.*
Chlorpheniramine [chlorphenamine] maleate (p.412·1); phenylpropanolamine hydrochloride (p.1098·1); dextromethorphan hydrobromide (p.1087·3).
Coughs.

Contaclair *Akripan, Aust.*
Rinsing, disinfecting and storage solution for contact lens (p.1129·2).

Contact *VAAS, Ital.†.*
Chlorhexidine hydrochloride (p.1138·2).
Skin disinfection; wounds.

Contact Eyes *Abbott, Austral.*
Comfort solution for soft contact lenses (p.1129·2).

Contactol *Merck Sharp & Dohme-Chibret, Fr.†.*
Hypromellose 4000 (p.1501·3).
Contact lens and ocular prostheses; dry eye disorders.

Contafilm *Allergan, Ger.†.*
Polyvinyl alcohol (p.1503·3).
Dry eye disorders.

Contalax *3M, Fr.; Fischer, Israel.*
Bisacodyl (p.1212·2).
Bowel evacuation; constipation.

Conta-Lens Wetting *Baif, Ital.*
Benzalkonium chloride (p.1133·2); edetic acid (p.1008·3); methylcellulose (p.1502·2)(p.1129·2).
Wetting solution for hard contact lens.

Contalgin *Pharmacia Upjohn, Denm.*
Morphine sulfate (p.56·1).
Pain.

Contaren *Sintesa, Belg.*
Canrenone (p.853·3).
Hypertension; oedema.

ConTE-PAK *SoloPak, USA.*
Trace element preparation (p.1350·1).
Additive for intravenous total parenteral nutrition solutions.

Contigen *Bard, UK.*
Bovine dermal collagen (p.1598·2).
Urinary incontinence.

Contilen *Legrand, Braz.*
Chlorpheniramine [chlorphenamine] maleate (p.412·2); phenylpropanolamine (p.1098·1).
Nasal congestion.

Contimit *Lindopharm, Ger.*
Terbutaline sulfate (p.776·2).
Obstructive airways disease.

Continucor *Parke, Davis, Aust.*
Quinapril hydrochloride (p.963·3).
Heart failure; hypertension.

Contiphyllin *Lindopharm, Ger.*
Theophylline (p.777·2).
Obstructive airways disease.

Contopharma *Silhouette, Aust.*
Wetting, disinfecting, and storage solutions for contact lenses (p.1129·2).

Contra Combustiones *Vitamed, Israel.*
Aluminium acetate (p.1578·1); zinc oxide (p.1128·2); peru balsam (p.1650·2); bismuth subcarbonate (p.1213·1).
Nappy rash; skin irritation.

Contracep *Nakorn, Thai.*
Medroxyprogesterone acetate (p.1480·1).
Progestogen-only injectable contraceptive.

Contracid *Thiemann, Ger.†.*
Cimetidine (p.1216·3).
Gastro-oesophageal reflux; peptic ulcer; Zollinger-Ellison syndrome.

Contracide *Norgine, Fr.; Norgine, Ital.*
Aluminium hydroxide (p.1210·3); magnesium trisilicate (p.1233·3); dimethicone (p.1249·2).
Gastrointestinal disorders.

Contra-Coff *Universal, S.Afr.†.*
Pholcodine (p.1099·1); squill (p.1100·3).
Coughs.

Contractubex
Kolassa, Aust.; Merz, Ger.; Merz, Hong Kong; Merz, Switz.
Onion (p.1644·1); heparin (p.902·1) or heparin sodium (p.902·1); allantoin (p.1110·1).
Keloids; scars.

Contraflam *Berk, UK†.*
Mefenamic acid (p.51·2).
Inflammation; menorrhagia; pain.

Contraforte *Sanochemia, Aust.*
Propyphenazone (p.80·2); dextropropoxyphene (p.27·1); caffeine (p.761·3).
Pain.

Contralgen *Pietrasanta, Ital.*
Paracetamol (p.71·2); aspirin (p.14·2).
Cold and influenza symptoms; fever; pain.

Contralorin *Sanochemia, Aust.*
Propyphenazone (p.80·2); paracetamol (p.71·2); caffeine (p.761·3).
Fever; pain.

Contralum Ultra
Note. This name is used for preparations of different composition.
Boots Healthcare, Neth.
Enzacamene (p.1517·2); avobenzone (p.1517·1); sodium 2-phenyl-1H-benzimidazole-5-sulfonate (p.1517·2).
Photosensitive skin disorders; sunscreen.

Boots Healthcare, Switz.†.
Enzacamene (p.1517·2); avobenzone (p.1517·1); ensulizole (p.1517·2).
Sunscreen.

Contramal
Searle, Belg.; Grunenthal, Fr.; Formenti, Ital.
Tramadol hydrochloride (p.89·1).
Pain.

Contramareo *Torrens, Spain.*
Dimenhydrinate (p.415·2).
Motion sickness.

Contramutan *Rhone-Poulenc Rorer, Ger.*
Homoeopathic preparation.

Contraneural *Pfleger, Ger.*
Ibuprofen (p.43·2).
Fever; inflammation; musculoskeletal and joint disorders; pain.

Contraneural Paracetamol/Codeine *Pfleger, Ger.*
Paracetamol (p.71·2); codeine phosphate (p.25·2).
Formerly known as Contraneural Forte.
Pain.

Contrasmina *Falqui, Ital.*
Clenbuterol hydrochloride (p.763·3).
Obstructive airways disease.

Contraspasmin *Asta Medica, Ger.*
Clenbuterol hydrochloride (p.763·3).
Obstructive airways disease.

Contrasthenyl *Doms, Switz.*
Vitamin B_6 preparation with minerals (p.1350·1).
Asthenia.

Contrathion
Rhodia, Braz.; SERB, Fr.; Rhone-Poulenc Rorer, Ital.
Pralidoxime metilsulfate (p.1020·2).
Organophosphorus poisoning.

Contravert B *Sanochemia, Aust.*
Meclozine hydrochloride (p.420·3); pyridoxine hydrochloride (p.1386·3).
Motion sickness; vertigo; vomiting.

Contre-Coups de l'Abbe Perdrigeon *Pionneau, Fr.*
Aloes (p.1210·1).
Skin disorders; soft-tissue disorders.

Contre-Douleurs *Wild, Switz.*
Aspirin (p.14·2); paracetamol (p.71·2); caffeine (p.761·3).

Colloidal aluminium hydroxide (p.1210·3) is included in the tablets in an attempt to limit adverse effects on the gastrointestinal mucosa.
Fever; pain.

Contre-Douleurs C *Wild, Switz.*
Aspirin (p.14·2); paracetamol (p.71·2); caffeine (p.761·3); ascorbic acid (p.1389·3).
Cold symptoms; fever.

Contre-Douleurs P *Wild, Switz.*
Paracetamol (p.71·2).
Fever; pain.

Contrelmin *UCI, Braz.*
Tiabendazole (p.109·1); pyrvinium embonate (p.108·2).
Nematode infections.

Contrheuma *Spitzner, Ger.*
Glycol salicylate (p.42·2); benzyl nicotinate (p.20·2).
Circulatory disorders; inflammatory disorders; muscle and nerve pain; rheumatism.

Contrheuma Bad L *Spitzner, Ger.*
Salicylic acid (p.1122·3); sodium humate.
Bath additive; neuromuscular, musculoskeletal, and joint disorders.

Contrheuma V + T Bad N *Spitzner, Ger.†.*
Glycol salicylate (p.42·2); diethylamine salicylate (p.32·2); oleum pini sylvestris.
Bath additive; cold symptoms; musculoskeletal and joint disorders; neuralgia; peripheral circulatory disorders.

Contrheuma-Gel forte N *Spitzner, Ger.†.*
Bornyl salicylate (p.20·3); ethyl salicylate (p.35·1); methyl nicotinate (p.55·1).
Neuralgia; neuritis; rheumatism; sports injuries.

Contrin *Geneva, USA.*
Ferrous fumarate (p.1360·1); folic acid (p.1361·1); intrinsic factor; vitamin B_{12} substances (p.1388·1).
Vitamin C (p.1389·3) is included in this preparation to increase the absorption and availability of iron.
Anaemias.

Contrix *Codali, Belg.†.*
Meglumine iothalamate (p.1036·2).
Radiographic contrast medium.

Control
Note. This name is used for preparations of different composition.
Bio-Sante, Canad.
Cascara (p.1216·1); sennosides A and B (p.1248·3).

Bayer, Ital.
Lorazepam (p.688·3).
Convulsions; nervous disorders; sedative.

OM, Switz.†.
Mephenoxalone (p.690·3).
Anxiety; muscle tension.

Thompson, USA†.
Phenylpropanolamine hydrochloride (p.1098·1).
Obesity.

Controlip *Knoll, Mex.*
Fenofibrate (p.889·1).
Hyperlipidaemias.

Controloc
Pharma Clal, Israel; Bayer, S.Afr.; Byk Gulden, Singapore.
Pantoprazole (p.1243·1).
Gastro-oesophageal reflux; peptic ulcer.

Controlvas *Belmac, Spain.*
Enalapril maleate (p.883·3).
Heart failure; hypertension.

Contromet *Propan, S.Afr.*
Metoclopramide hydrochloride (p.1235·2).
Gastrointestinal disorders.

Contugesic *Asta Medica, Spain.*
Dihydrocodeine tartrate (p.33·1).
Pain.

Contumax *Casen Fisons, Spain.*
Sodium picosulfate (p.1249·3).
Constipation.

Contusil *Farmatre, Ital.*
Benzalkonium chloride (p.1133·2).
Skin, wound, and burn disinfection.

Contusin
Note. This name is used for preparations of different composition.
Lacer, Spain.
Diethylamine salicylate (p.32·2); camphor (p.1589·3); thymol (p.1158·3); menthol (p.1632·3); aesculus (p.1574·1).
Musculoskeletal, joint, and soft-tissue disorders.

Herbamed, Switz.
Homoeopathic preparation.

Contuss
Note. This name is used for preparations of different composition.
SmithKline Beecham, China.
Diphenhydramine hydrochloride (p.416·1); dextromethorphan hydrobromide (p.1087·3); ammonium chloride (p.1085·2); sodium citrate (p.1186·2).
Cold symptoms; coughs.

Parmed, USA†.
Phenylpropanolamine hydrochloride (p.1098·1); guaifenesin (p.1092·2); phenylephrine hydrochloride (p.1097·1).
Coughs.

Contuxin *Continentales, Mex.*
Oxolamine (p.1096·2).

Convacard *Madaus, Ger.*
Convallaria glycosides (p.1599·1).
Heart failure.

Conva-cyl Ho-Len-Complex *Liebermann, Ger.*
Homoeopathic preparation.

Convallocor Hevert, Ger.†
Homoeopathic preparation.

Convallocor-SL Hevert, Ger.
Crataegus (p.1600·2); convallaria (p.1599·1).
Cardiac disorders.

Convastabil Klein, Ger.
Convallaria (p.1599·1); crataegus (p.1600·2).
Cardiac disorders.

Convectal Vita Elan, Spain†.
Diltiazem hydrochloride (p.874·3).
Angina pectoris; hypertension; myocardial infarction.

Convertal Tecnimede, Port.
Captopril (p.853·3).

Converten Gentili, Ital.
Enalapril maleate (p.883·3).
Heart failure; hypertension; ischaemic heart disease.

Convertin Merck Sharp & Dohme, Israel.
Enalapril maleate (p.883·3).
Heart failure; hypertension.

Convulex Gerot, Aust.; Byk, Belg.; Lundbeck, Ger.; Byk, Neth.; Byk Madaus, S.Afr.; Gerot, Singapore; Gerot, Switz.; Pharmacia, UK.
Valproic acid (p.366·2) or sodium valproate (p.366·3).
Epilepsy.

Convulsofin Asta Medica, Ger.; Boehringer Mannheim, Ger.; Wernigerode, Ger.
Calcium valproate (p.368·3) or sodium valproate (p.366·3).
Epilepsy.

Cool-Mint Listerine Warner-Lambert, USA.
Thymol (p.1158·3); eucalyptol (p.1609·2); methyl salicylate (p.55·1); menthol (p.1632·3).

Cooper AR Coopervision, Canad.†.
Antazoline phosphate (p.408·3); naphazoline hydrochloride (p.1095·1).

Cooper Tears Coopervision, Canad.†.
Polyvinyl alcohol (p.1503·1).

Copal Galen, Mex.
Sulindac (p.85·3).
Gout; musculoskeletal, joint and peri-articular disorders.

Copaltra Plantes Tropicales, Fr.
Coutarea; centaury (p.1593·1).
Diabetes.

Copan Duopharma, Hong Kong.
Hyoscine butylbromide (p.468·2).
Smooth muscle spasm.

Copaxone Hoechst Marion Roussel, Austral.; Teva, Canad.; Teva, Israel; Hoechst Marion Roussel, Switz.; Aventis, UK; Teva, UK; Teva, USA.
Glatiramer acetate (p.1616·1).
Multiple sclerosis.

Cope Mentholatum, USA.
Aspirin (p.14·2); caffeine (p.761·3).
Aluminium hydroxide (p.1210·3) and magnesium hydroxide (p.1233·1) are included in this preparation in an attempt to limit adverse effects on the gastrointestinal mucosa.
Pain.

Copen Covan, S.Afr.†.
Phenoxymethylpenicillin potassium (p.235·1).
Bacterial infections.

6 Copena Ariston, Braz.
Chlorophenothiazinylscopine; vitamin B₁ (p.1385·2).
Nausea and vomiting.

Cophene No. 2 Dunhall, USA.
Pseudoephedrine hydrochloride (p.1099·2); chlorpheniramine [chlorphenamine] maleate (p.412·1).
Upper respiratory-tract symptoms.

Cophene XP Dunhall, USA.
Pseudoephedrine hydrochloride (p.1099·2); guaifenesin (p.1092·2); hydrocodone tartrate (p.42·2).
Coughs.

Cophene-B Dunhall, USA†.
Brompheniramine maleate (p.410·2).
Hypersensitivity reactions.

Cophene-X Dunhall, USA†.
Phenylephrine hydrochloride (p.1097·1); phenylpropanolamine hydrochloride (p.1098·1); pentoxyverine citrate (p.1096·3); sulfogaiacol (p.1101·1).
Coughs.

Cophenylcaine Paedpharm, Austral.
Phenylephrine hydrochloride (p.1097·1); lignocaine [lidocaine] hydrochloride (p.1313·2).
Aid in upper respiratory-tract investigations; epistaxis; preparation of nasal mucosa for surgical procedures.

Cophylac Hoechst Marion Roussel, Ger.
Expectorant: Normethadone hydrochloride (p.1095·3); oxilofrine hydrochloride (p.950·3); emetine hydrochloride (p.591·3).
Oral solution: Normethadone hydrochloride (p.1095·3); oxilofrine hydrochloride (p.950·3).
Coughs.

Copinal Vinas, Spain.
Zinc acexamate (p.1572·2).
Peptic ulcer.

Coppertone Bug & Sun Adult Schering-Plough, USA.
SPF 15: Octinoxate (p.1517·3); oxybenzone (p.1518·1); octisalate (p.1518·1); homosalate (p.1517·2).
Sunscreen.

Coppertone Bug & Sun Kids Schering-Plough, USA.
SPF 30: Octinoxate (p.1517·3); oxybenzone (p.1518·1); octocrilene (p.1518·1).
Sunscreen.

Coppertone Bug & Sunblock Schering-Plough, Canad.
SPF 15: Homosalate (p.1517·2); octinoxate (p.1517·3); octisalate (p.1518·1); oxybenzone (p.1518·1).
SPF 30: Octocrilene (p.1518·1); octinoxate (p.1517·3); oxybenzone (p.1518·1).
Insect repellent; sunscreen.

Coppertone Kids
Note. This name is used for preparations of different composition.
Schering-Plough, Canad.
SPF 15; SPF 30; SPF 40: Homosalate (p.1517·2); octinoxate (p.1517·3); octisalate (p.1518·1); oxybenzone (p.1518·1).
Sunscreen.
Schering-Plough, USA.
SPF 15: Octinoxate (p.1517·3); octisalate (p.1518·1); homosalate (p.1517·2); oxybenzone (p.1518·1).
SPF 30: Octinoxate (p.1517·3); octisalate (p.1518·1); oxybenzone (p.1518·1); octocrilene (p.1518·1).
Sunscreen.

Coppertone Lipkote Schering-Plough, Canad.†; Schering-Plough, USA.
SPF 15: Octinoxate (p.1517·3); oxybenzone (p.1518·1).
Sunscreen.

Coppertone Mist Schering-Plough, Canad.
SPF 4: Homosalate (p.1517·2); octinoxate (p.1518·1).
Sunscreen.

Coppertone Moisturizing Schering-Plough, USA.
SPF 2: Homosalate (p.1517·2).
SPF 4; SPF 6; SPF 8; SPF 15: Octinoxate (p.1517·3); oxybenzone (p.1518·1).
SPF 25; SPF 30: Octinoxate (p.1517·3); octisalate (p.1518·1); homosalate (p.1517·2); oxybenzone (p.1518·1).
SPF 45: Octinoxate (p.1517·3); octisalate (p.1518·1); octocrilene (p.1518·1); oxybenzone (p.1518·1).
Sunscreen.

Coppertone Noskote Schering-Plough, Canad.†.
SPF 15: Octinoxate (p.1517·3); octisalate (p.1518·1); oxybenzone (p.1518·1).
Sunscreen.

Coppertone Oil-Free Schering-Plough, Canad.
SPF 8; SPF 15: Octinoxate (p.1517·3); oxybenzone (p.1518·1).
SPF 30: Homosalate (p.1517·2); octinoxate (p.1517·3); octisalate (p.1518·1); oxybenzone (p.1518·1).
Sunscreen.

Coppertone Radiance Schering-Plough, Canad.
SPF 15: Homosalate (p.1517·2); octinoxate (p.1517·3); octisalate (p.1518·1); oxybenzone (p.1518·1).
Sunscreen.

Coppertone Skin Selects Schering-Plough, Canad.†.
SPF 15: Octinoxate (p.1517·3); oxybenzone (p.1518·1).
Sunscreen.

Coppertone Skin Selects Sensitive Schering-Plough, Canad.†.
SPF 15: Octinoxate (p.1517·3); titanium dioxide (p.1126·1).
Sunscreen.

Coppertone Spectra Schering-Plough, Canad.
SPF 30: Avobenzone (p.1517·1); homosalate (p.1517·2); octinoxate (p.1517·3); octisalate (p.1518·1); oxybenzone (p.1518·1).
Sunscreen.

Coppertone Sport
Note. This name is used for preparations of different composition.
Schering-Plough, Canad.; Schering-Plough, USA.
SPF 4; SPF 8; SPF 15: Octinoxate (p.1517·3); oxybenzone (p.1518·1).
Sunscreen.
Schering-Plough, Canad.; Schering-Plough, USA.
SPF 30: Octinoxate (p.1517·3); octisalate (p.1518·1); oxybenzone (p.1518·1).
Sunscreen.

Coppertone Sport Spray Schering-Plough, Canad.
SPF 15; SPF 30: Homosalate (p.1517·2); octinoxate (p.1517·3); octisalate (p.1518·1); oxybenzone (p.1518·1).
Sunscreen.

Coppertone Spray Schering-Plough, Canad.
SPF 15; SPF 30: Homosalate (p.1517·2); octinoxate (p.1517·3); octisalate (p.1518·1); oxybenzone (p.1518·1).
Sunscreen.

Coppertone Spray'n Play Schering-Plough, Canad.
SPF 30: Homosalate (p.1517·2); octinoxate (p.1517·3); octisalate (p.1518·1); oxybenzone (p.1518·1).
Sunscreen.

Coppertone Sunblock Schering-Plough, Canad.†.
SPF 45: Homosalate (p.1517·2); octinoxate (p.1517·3); octisalate (p.1518·1); oxybenzone (p.1518·1).
Sunscreen.

Coppertone Sunscreen Schering-Plough, Canad.
SPF 8: Octinoxate (p.1517·3); oxybenzone (p.1518·1).
Sunscreen.

Coppertone Sunstick Cheshire, UK.
SPF 15: Titanium dioxide (p.1126·1).
Sunscreen.

Coppertone Suntan Schering-Plough, Canad.
SPF 4: Octinoxate (p.1517·3); oxybenzone (p.1518·1).
Sunscreen.

Coppertone Supershade Cheshire, UK.
SPF 15: Oxybenzone (p.1518·1); padimate O (p.1518·2).
Sunscreen.

Coppertone Tan Magnifier Schering-Plough, USA.
SPF 2: Trolamine salicylate (p.90·1).
Gel SPF 4: Ensulizole (p.1517·2).
Lotion SPF 4: Octinoxate (p.1517·3).
Sunscreen.

Coppertone Ultrashade Cheshire, UK.
SPF 23: Octinoxate (p.1517·3); oxybenzone (p.1518·1); padimate O (p.1518·2).
Sunscreen.

Coppertone UVGuard Schering-Plough, Canad.†.
SPF 15: Avobenzone (p.1517·1); octinoxate (p.1517·3); oxybenzone (p.1518·1).
SPF 30: Avobenzone (p.1517·1); octinoxate (p.1517·3); oxybenzone (p.1518·1); octisalate (p.1518·1).
Sunscreen.

Coppertone Waterbabies Schering-Plough, Canad.; Schering-Plough, USA.
SPF 30; SPF 45: Homosalate (p.1517·2); octinoxate (p.1517·3); oxybenzone (p.1518·1); octisalate (p.1518·1).
Sunscreen.

Coppertone Waterproof Sunblock Schering-Plough, Canad.
SPF 15: Octinoxate (p.1517·3); oxybenzone (p.1518·1).
SPF 30; SPF 45: Octinoxate (p.1517·3); homosalate (p.1517·2); octisalate (p.1518·1); oxybenzone (p.1518·1).
Sunscreen.

Coptin Axcan, Canad.
Sulfadiazine (p.251·1); trimethoprim (p.264·2).
Bacterial infections of the urinary tract.

Copyrkal N Berlin-Chemie, Ger.
Propyphenazone (p.80·2); caffeine (p.761·3).
Fever; pain.

Co-Pyronil
Lilly, Thai.; Dista, USA†.
Chlorpheniramine [chlorphenamine] maleate (p.412·1); pseudoephedrine hydrochloride (p.1099·2).
Allergic rhinitis; nasal congestion.

Co-Q-10
Larkhall Laboratories, UK; Carlson, USA.
Ubidecarenone (p.1677·1).

Coquelusedal Elerte, Fr.
Niaouli (p.1640·2); grindelia (p.1618·2); gelsemium (p.1614·2).
Formerly contained niaouli oil, grindelia, gelsemium, and phenobarbital.
Coughs.

Coquelusedal Paracetamol Elerte, Fr.
Paracetamol (p.71·2); niaouli oil (p.1640·2); grindelia (p.1618·2); gelsemium (p.1614·2).
Respiratory-tract disorders.

Coquevit Brasmedica, Braz.
Sodium dibunate (p.1100·3); ephedrine (p.1090·1); vitamin C (p.1389·3).
Coughs.

CoQuinone USANA, USA.
Ubidecarenone (p.1677·1).
Nutritional supplement.

Cor Mio QIF, Braz.
Amiodarone (p.838·1).
Arrhythmias.

cor tensobon Schwarz, Ger.
Captopril (p.853·3).
Diabetic nephropathy; heart failure; hypertension.

Coraben Medic, Braz.
Ferrous sulfate (p.1360·3); folic acid (p.1361·1); vitamin B₁₂ (p.1388·3).
Succinic acid is included in this preparation to increase the absorption and availability of iron.
Anaemias.

Coracin Roberts, USA†; Hauck, USA†.
Hydrocortisone acetate (p.1073·3); neomycin sulfate (p.228·1); bacitracin zinc (p.155·2); polymyxin B sulfate (p.238·1).
Infected eye disorders.

Coracten
ICN, Hong Kong; ICN, Thai.; Celltech, UK.
Nifedipine (p.940·1).
Angina pectoris; hypertension.

Coradol Coradol, Ger.
Homoeopathic preparation.

Coradur Glaxo Wellcome, Canad.†.
Isosorbide dinitrate (p.915·2).
Angina pectoris.

Coral Drug Research, Ital.
Nifedipine (p.940·1).
Hypertension; ischaemic heart disease.

Coralen Alter, Spain.
Ranitidine hydrochloride (p.1245·2).
Acid aspiration; gastro-oesophageal reflux; gastrointestinal haemorrhage; gastrointestinal hyperacidity; peptic ulcer; Zollinger-Ellison syndrome.

Coralgesic Vesta, S.Afr.†.
Paracetamol (p.71·2); codeine phosphate (p.25·2); vitamin B substances (p.1350·1).
Fever; pain.

Coralzul Farcoral, Mex.
Furazolidone (p.592·1); homatropine (p.468·1); kaolin (p.1229·3); pectin (p.1502·3); diiodohydroxyquinoline (p.590·2).
Gastrointestinal disorders.

Coramedan Medice, Ger.
Digitoxin (p.869·2).
Arrhythmias; heart failure.

Coramil Tika, Swed.
Diltiazem hydrochloride (p.874·3).
Angina pectoris; hypertension.

Coramine Glucose Novartis Sante, Fr.
Nikethamide (p.1513·1); glucose monohydrate (p.1364·2).
Asthenia; fainting.

Corangin
Novartis, Aust.; Novartis, Ger.; Novartis, Hong Kong; Novartis, NZ.
Isosorbide mononitrate (p.916·2).
Angina pectoris; heart failure; pulmonary hypertension.

Corangin Nitrokapseln and Nitrospray Novartis, Ger.
Glyceryl trinitrate (p.897·3).
Angina pectoris; heart failure; myocardial infarction.

Corangine Novartis, Switz.
Isosorbide mononitrate (p.916·2).
Heart failure; ischaemic heart disease.

Coras Alphapharm, Austral.
Diltiazem hydrochloride (p.874·3).
Angina pectoris.

Corase Medac, Ger.
Urokinase (p.988·1).
Thromboembolic disorders.

Coraspir Armstrong, Mex.
Lysine aspirin (p.50·3).
Fever; pain; thromboembolism prophylaxis.

Corathiem Ohta, Hong Kong.
Cinnarizine (p.413·1).
Cerebrovascular disorders.

Coratol Weifa, Norw.†.
Atenolol (p.841·3).
Angina pectoris; arrhythmias; hypertension; hyperthyroidism; migraine; myocardial infarction.

Corazem Mundipharma, Aust.
Diltiazem hydrochloride (p.874·3).
Angina pectoris; heart failure; hypertension; myocardial infarction.

Corazet Mundipharma, Ger.
Diltiazem hydrochloride (p.874·3).
Angina pectoris; hypertension.

Corbar Covan, S.Afr.
Guaifenesin (p.1092·2); ephedrine hydrochloride (p.1090·1); codeine phosphate (p.25·2); chlorpheniramine [chlorphenamine] maleate (p.412·1); co. cocillana syrup (p.1087·2).
Coughs.

Corbar M Covan, S.Afr.
Carbocisteine (p.1086·3).
Respiratory-tract disorders.

Corbar S Covan, S.Afr.
Fedrilate (p.1091·3).
Coughs.

Corbeton Alphapharm, Austral.
Oxprenolol hydrochloride (p.951·3).
Angina pectoris; arrhythmias; hypertension.

Corbin Pharmaland, Thai.
Cloxacillin sodium (p.192·1).
Gram-positive bacterial infections.

Corbionax Irex, Fr.
Amiodarone hydrochloride (p.836·1).
Arrhythmias.

Corciclen Allergan-Frumtost, Braz.
Chlortetracycline hydrochloride (p.182·1); cortisone acetate (p.1065·3); bismuth loretinate.
Infected eye disorders.

Cordalin Asta Medica, Ger.
Bisoprolol fumarate (p.850·1).
Angina pectoris; hypertension.

Cordanum Asta Medica, Ger.
Talinolol (p.978·3).
Arrhythmias; hypertension; ischaemic heart disease; myocardial infarction.

Cordapur Novo APS, Ger.
Crataegus (p.1600·2).
Cardiac disorders.

Cordarene Biosintetica, Braz.
Amlodipine besilate (p.838·3).
Hypertension; ischaemic heart disease.

Cordarex Sanofi Synthelabo, Ger.
Amiodarone hydrochloride (p.836·1).
Arrhythmias.

Cordarone
Sanofi Synthelabo, Belg.; Wyeth-Ayerst, Canad.; Sanofi Winthrop, Denm.; Sanofi Winthrop, Fin.; Sanofi Winthrop, Fr.; Sanofi Winthrop, Hong Kong; Sanofi Winthrop, Irl.; Sanofi Winthrop, Mex.; Sanofi Synthelabo, Neth.; Sanofi Winthrop, Norw.; Sanofi Winthrop, NZ; Sanofi Synthelabo, Port.; Sanofi Synthelabo, Singapore; Sanofi Winthrop, Swed.; Sanofi Synthelabo, Switz.; Sanofi Synthelabo, Thai.; Wyeth-Ayerst, USA.
Amiodarone hydrochloride (p.836·1).
Arrhythmias.

Cordarone X
Sanofi Winthrop, Austral.; Sanofi Winthrop, Irl.; Sanofi Synthelabo, S.Afr.; Sanofi Winthrop, UK.
Amiodarone hydrochloride (p.836·1).
Arrhythmias.

Cordes Beta Ichthyol, Ger.
Betamethasone valerate (p.1063·2).
Skin disorders.

Cordes BPO Ichthyol, Ger.
Benzoyl peroxide (p.1111·1).
Acne.

Cordes Estriol Ichthyol, Ger.
Estriol (p.1475·3).
Vaginal disorders.

Cordes Nystatin Soft Ichthyol, Ger.
Nystatin (p.392·2).
Fungal skin infections.

Cordes VAS Ichthyol, Ger.
Tretinoin (p.1126·2).
Acne.

Cordesin Serag-Wiessner, Ger.
Potassium aspartate (p.1195·2); magnesium aspartate (p.1190·3).
Heart failure; myocardial infarction; potassium and magnesium deficiency.

Cordiax Crinos, Ital.
Celiprolol hydrochloride (p.856·1).
Angina pectoris; hypertension.

Cordicant Mundipharma, Ger.
Nifedipine (p.940·1).
Angina pectoris; hypertension.

Cordichin Knoll, Ger.
Verapamil hydrochloride (p.989·1); quinidine (p.964·2).
Arrhythmias.

Cordil Dexxon, Israel.
Isosorbide dinitrate (p.915·2).
Angina pectoris; heart failure.

Cordilan Roche, Spain.
Nifedipine (p.940·1).
Angina pectoris; hypertension; Raynaud's syndrome.

Cordilat Tecnofarma, Mex.
Nifedipine (p.940·1).
Hypertension.

Cordilox Schering, Austral.; Baker Norton, UK.
Verapamil hydrochloride (p.989·1).
Angina pectoris; arrhythmias; hypertension.

Cordiodoron Weleda, Ger.
Homoeopathic preparation.

Cordipatch Schwarz, Fr.
Glyceryl trinitrate (p.897·3).
Angina pectoris.

Cordipina IBP, Ital.
Nicardipine hydrochloride (p.938·3).
Angina pectoris; heart failure; hypertension.

Cordiplast Bayer, Spain.
Glyceryl trinitrate (p.897·3).
Angina pectoris.

Corditrine Specia, Fr.†
Glyceryl trinitrate (p.897·3).
Angina pectoris; heart failure.

Cordium
Aaciphar, Belg.†; Riom, Fr.†
Bepridil hydrochloride (p.844·3).
Angina pectoris.

Cordodopa Sanofi Synthelabo, Port.
Dopamine hydrochloride (p.881·3).
Shock.

Cordran Oclassen, USA.
Flurandrenolone [fludroxycortide] (p.1072·2).
Skin disorders.

Cordymax Pharmanex, USA.
Cordyceps sinensis mushroom mycelia.
Fatigue.

Coreg
Roche, Canad.; SmithKline Beecham, USA.
Carvedilol (p.855·2).
Heart failure; hypertension.

Coreine Germania, Aust.
Carrageenan (p.1500·1).
Constipation.

Co-Renitec
Merck Sharp & Dohme, Aust.; Merck Sharp & Dohme, Belg.; Merck Sharp & Dohme, Braz.; Merck Sharp & Dohme, Denm.; Merck Sharp & Dohme-Chibret, Fr.; Merck Sharp & Dohme, Hong Kong; Merck Sharp & Dohme, Irl.; Merck Sharp & Dohme, NZ; Merck Sharp & Dohme, S.Afr.; Merck Sharp & Dohme, Singapore; Merck Sharp & Dohme, Spain.
Enalapril maleate (p.883·3); hydrochlorothiazide (p.907·3).
Hypertension.

Co-Reniten Merck Sharp & Dohme, Switz.
Enalapril maleate (p.883·3); hydrochlorothiazide (p.907·3).
Hypertension.

Corenza C Restan, S.Afr.
Aspirin (p.14·2); ascorbic acid (p.1389·3); chlorpheniramine [chlorphenamine] maleate (p.412·1); phenylephrine hydrochloride (p.1097·1); moroxydine hydrochloride (p.636·3).
Cold and influenza symptoms.

Coreptil Sanofi Synthelabo, Ital.
Heptaminol hydrochloride (p.1619·2).
Adjunct in overdosage with neuroleptics and barbiturates; cardiac disorders.

Coretec Eisai, Jpn.
Olprinone hydrochloride (p.949·2).
Heart failure.

Corethium Johnson & Johnson Medical, UK†.
Porcine skin (p.1123·2).
Skin grafts.

Corgard
Bristol-Myers Squibb, Belg.; Bristol-Myers Squibb, Braz.; Squibb, Canad.; Sanofi Winthrop, Fr.; Bristol-Myers Squibb, Hong Kong; Bristol-Myers Squibb, Irl.†; Bristol-Myers Squibb, Ital.; Bristol-Myers Squibb, NZ; Bristol-Myers Squibb, S.Afr.; Squibb, Spain; Bristol-Myers Squibb, Switz.; Sanofi Winthrop, UK; Monarch, USA.
Nadolol (p.937·1).
Angina pectoris; arrhythmias; hypertension; hyperthyroidism; migraine.

Corgaretic
Bristol-Myers Squibb, Irl.†; Bristol-Myers Squibb, S.Afr.; Bristol-Myers Squibb, Switz.; Sanofi Winthrop, UK.
Nadolol (p.937·1); bendrofluazide [bendroflumethiazide] (p.844·1).
Hypertension.

Corguttin N plus Roland, Ger.†
Adonis vernalis (p.1573·3); convallaria (p.1599·1); crataegus (p.1600·2).
Cardiovascular disorders.

Coric Du Pont, Ger.
Lisinopril (p.921·1).
Heart failure; hypertension; myocardial infarction.

Coric Plus Du Pont, Ger.
Lisinopril (p.921·1); hydrochlorothiazide (p.907·3).
Hypertension.

Coricide le Diable Sodia, Fr.
Salicylic acid (p.1122·3).
Callosities; corns; verrucae.

Coricidil-D Plough, Port.
Paracetamol (p.71·2); chlorpheniramine [chlorphenamine] maleate (p.412·1); phenylpropanolamine hydrochloride (p.1098·1).
Cold symptoms; rhinitis; sinusitis.

Coricidin
Note.This name is used for preparations of different composition.
Schering-Plough, Ital.
Oxymetazoline hydrochloride (p.1096·2).
Allergic rhinitis; cold symptoms; sinusitis.

Schering-Plough, Spain.
Ascorbic acid (p.1389·3); caffeine (p.761·3); chlorpheniramine [chlorphenamine] maleate (p.412·1); salicylamide (p.82·1).
Fever; nasal congestion; pain.

Schering-Plough, USA.
Paracetamol (p.71·2); chlorpheniramine [chlorphenamine] maleate (p.412·1).
Upper respiratory-tract symptoms.

Coricidin Cold Schering, Canad.
Chlorpheniramine [chlorphenamine] maleate (p.412·1); aspirin (p.14·2).
Cold symptoms.

Coricidin D
Note.This name is used for preparations of different composition.
Schering, Canad.†
Long-acting tablets: Chlorpheniramine [chlorphenamine] maleate (p.412·1); phenylpropanolamine hydrochloride (p.1098·1).
Tablets: Chlorpheniramine [chlorphenamine] maleate (p.412·1); aspirin (p.14·2); phenylpropanolamine (p.1098·1).
Cold symptoms; respiratory congestion.

Schering-Plough, USA†.
Phenylpropanolamine hydrochloride (p.1098·1); chlorpheniramine [chlorphenamine] maleate (p.412·1); paracetamol (p.71·2).
Upper respiratory-tract symptoms.

Coricidin Expec Schering-Plough, Mex.
Dextromethorphan hydrobromide (p.1087·3); guaifenesin (p.1092·2); phenylpropanolamine hydrochloride (p.1098·1).
Coughs and cold symptoms.

Coricidin F Schering-Plough, Mex.
Paracetamol (p.71·2); phenylpropanolamine hydrochloride (p.1098·1); chlorpheniramine [chlorphenamine] maleate (p.412·1).
Upper respiratory-tract symptoms.

Coricidin Fuerte Schering-Plough, Spain.
Chlorpheniramine [chlorphenamine] maleate (p.412·1); phenylpropanolamine hydrochloride (p.1098·1); paracetamol (p.71·2).
Fever; nasal congestion; pain.

Coricidin Maximum Strength Sinus Headache Schering-Plough, USA†.
Phenylpropanolamine hydrochloride (p.1098·1); chlorpheniramine [chlorphenamine] maleate (p.412·1); paracetamol (p.71·2).
Upper respiratory-tract symptoms.

Coricidin Non-Drowsy Schering, Canad.†
Phenylpropanolamine hydrochloride (p.1098·1); aspirin (p.14·2).
Sinus pain and congestion.

Coricidin Pediatrico Schering-Plough, Mex.
Chlorpheniramine [chlorphenamine] maleate (p.412·1); paracetamol (p.71·2).
Fever; pain; pruritus.

Coricidin Sinus Headache Schering, Canad.†
Paracetamol (p.71·2); phenylpropanolamine hydrochloride (p.1098·1); chlorpheniramine [chlorphenamine] maleate (p.412·1).
Cold symptoms; nasal congestion; sinus headache.

Coridil Ecosol, Switz.
Diltiazem hydrochloride (p.874·3).
Hypertension; ischaemic heart disease.

Corifina Bayer, Spain.
Azelastine hydrochloride (p.409·3).
Allergic conjunctivitis; allergic rhinitis.

Corilin F Schering-Plough, Mex.
Paracetamol (p.71·2); caffeine (p.761·3); phenylephrine hydrochloride (p.1097·1); chlorpheniramine [chlorphenamine] maleate (p.412·1).
Nasal congestion.

Corilisina Pensa, Spain.
Oxymetazoline hydrochloride (p.1096·2).
Nasal congestion.

Corindocomb
Schering, Aust.†; Schering, Ger.
Mepindolol sulfate (p.926·2); hydrochlorothiazide (p.907·3).
Hypertension.

Corindolan
Schering, Aust.; Schering, Ger.
Mepindolol sulfate (p.926·2).
Angina pectoris; cardiac hyperkinetic syndrome; hypertension.

Corinfar Asta Medica, Ger.
Nifedipine (p.940·1).
Hypertension; ischaemic heart disease; Raynaud's syndrome.

Coristex-DH Technilab, Canad.
Phenylephrine hydrochloride (p.1097·1); hydrocodone tartrate (p.42·2).
Coughs.

Coristina D Schering-Plough, Braz.
Dexchlorpheniramine maleate (p.412·1); phenylephrine hydrochloride (p.1097·1); caffeine (p.761·3); aspirin (p.14·2).
Cold and influenza symptoms.

Coristina Reforcada Schering-Plough, Braz.
Dexchlorpheniramine maleate (p.412·1); phenylephrine hydrochloride (p.1097·1); caffeine (p.761·3); salicylamide (p.82·1).
Bronchodilator.

Coristine-DH Technilab, Canad.
Hydrocodone tartrate (p.42·2); phenylephrine hydrochloride (p.1097·1).
Coughs.

Coritab
Atlantic, Hong Kong; Atlantic, Singapore; Atlantic, Thai.
Paracetamol (p.71·2); phenylpropanolamine hydrochloride (p.1098·1); chlorpheniramine [chlorphenamine] maleate (p.412·1).
Cold symptoms; nasal congestion; rhinitis.

Coritussal
Mack, Hong Kong.
Dextromethorphan hydrobromide (p.1087·3); phenylephrine hydrochloride (p.1097·1); carbinoxamine maleate (p.411·1).
Coughs; rhinitis.

Mack, Singapore.
Dextromethorphan (p.1087·3); phenylephrine (p.1098·1); carbinoxamine (p.411·1).
Coughs; rhinitis.

Corium ICN, Canad.†
Chlordiazepoxide hydrochloride (p.659·2); clidinium bromide (p.465·1).
Gastrointestinal disorders with associated anxiety.

Coriver Maver, Mex.
Paracetamol (p.71·2).

Corizzina SIT, Ital.
Amethocaine [tetracaine] hydrochloride (p.1305·2); naphazoline nitrate (p.1095·1).
Nasal congestion.

cor-L 90 N Loges, Ger.
Homoeopathic preparation.

Corlan
Medeva, Irl.; Celltech, UK.
Hydrocortisone sodium succinate (p.1074·1).
Aphthous stomatitis.

Cor-loges Loges, Ger.
Squill (p.1100·3); convallaria (p.1599·1).
Cardiac disorders; oedema.

Corlopam
Segix, Ital.; Neurex, USA.
Fenoldopam mesilate (p.889·3).
Hypertension.

Cormagnesin
Asta Medica, Aust.; Worwag, Ger.
Magnesium aspartate (p.1190·3) or magnesium sulfate (p.1191·1).
Arrhythmias; eclampsia; magnesium deficiency; myocardial infarction; premature labour.

Cormax Oclassen, USA.
Clobetasol propionate (p.1065·2).
Skin disorders.

Cormelian Schering, Ital.†
Dilazep hydrochloride (p.874·3).
Cardiac disorders.

Corn Huskers Warner-Lambert, USA.
Emollient and moisturiser.

Corn Removing Liquid Scholl, Israel.
Salicylic acid (p.1122·3); camphor (p.1589·3).
Corns.

Corn Salve Cress, Canad.†
Methyl salicylate (p.55·1); salicylic acid (p.1122·3).

Cornel Almirall, Spain.
Nisoldipine (p.946·3).
Angina pectoris; hypertension.

Corneregel Mann, Ger.
Dexpanthenol (p.1602·3).
Eye disorders.

Corni Limp Sophia, Mex.
Sodium chloride (p.1196·1).

Cornina Hornhaut Beiersdorf, Ger.†
Salicylic acid (p.1122·3).
Calluses; corns.

Cornina Huhneraugen Beiersdorf, Ger.†
Salicylic acid (p.1122·3).
Corns.

Cornkil Norgine, Austral.
Benzocaine (p.1306·2); salicylic acid (p.1122·3); lactic acid (p.1626·2).
Corns.

Corocrat Biomo, Ger.
Crataegus (p.1600·2).
Heart failure.

Coroday Generics, UK.
Nifedipine (p.940·1).
Angina pectoris; hypertension.

Corodil Gea, Denm.
Enalapril maleate (p.883·3).
Heart failure; hypertension.

Corodil Comp Gea, Denm.
Enalapril maleate (p.883·3); hydrochlorothiazide (p.907·3).
Hypertension.

Corodoc S Fides, Ger.
Homoeopathic preparation.

Corodyn Schmidgall, Aust.
Crataegus tincture (p.1600·2); camphor (p.1589·3); menthol (p.1632·3).
Cardiovascular disorders.

Corogal Galen, Mex.
Nifedipine (p.940·1).
Angina pectoris; hypertension.

Coro-Lanitop Boehringer Mannheim, Aust.†
Carbocromen (p.855·1); metildigoxin (p.930·1).
Heart failure.

Corolater Vita Elan, Spain.
Diltiazem hydrochloride (p.874·3).
Angina pectoris; hypertension.

Corolin Leiras, Fin.
Simvastatin (p.969·2).
Coronary artery disease; hypercholesterolaemia.

Coronarine Negma, Fr.
Dipyridamole (p.877·2).
Thromboembolic disorders.

Coronator Roland, Ger.†
Crataegus (p.1600·2).
Heart failure.

Coronex Pacific, NZ.
Isosorbide dinitrate (p.915·2).

Coro-Nitro
3M, Ger.; Roche, UK.
Glyceryl trinitrate (p.897·3).
Angina pectoris; heart failure; myocardial infarction.

Coronorm Wolff, Ger.
Captopril (p.853·3).
Heart failure; hypertension.

Coronur Roche, Spain.
Isosorbide mononitrate (p.916·2).
Angina pectoris.

Coropres Roche, Spain.
Carvedilol (p.855·2).
Heart failure; hypertension; ischaemic heart disease.

Cororell Sanorell, Ger.
Homoeopathic preparation.

Corosan Farmacologico Milanese, Ital.
Dipyridamole (p.877·2).
Vascular disorders.

Corotal Rosch & Handel, Aust.
β-Acetyldigoxin (p.827·3).
Arrhythmias; heart failure.

Corotenol Mepha, Hong Kong.
Atenolol (p.841·3).
Angina pectoris; arrhythmias; hypertension; myocardial infarction.

Corotrend
BASF, Ger.; Rhein, Mex.; Medika, Switz.
Nifedipine (p.940·1).
Hypertension; ischaemic heart disease; Raynaud's syndrome.

Corotrop
Sanofi Winthrop, Aust.; Sanofi Synthelabo, Ger.; Sanofi Winthrop, Swed.; Sanofi Synthelabo, Spain.
Milrinone (p.934·1) or milrinone lactate (p.934·1).
Heart failure.

Corotrope
Sanofi Synthelabo, Belg.; Sanofi Winthrop, Fr.; Sanofi Synthelabo, Neth.; Sanofi Synthelabo, Spain.
Milrinone (p.934·1) or milrinone lactate (p.934·1).
Heart failure.

Coroverlan
Mayrhofer, Aust.†; Verla, Ger.
Magnesium aspartate (p.1190·3); potassium aspartate (p.1195·2); etofylline (p.765·1); crataegus (p.1600·2).
Cardiac disorders.

Corovliss Boehringer Mannheim, Ger.†
Isosorbide dinitrate (p.915·2).
Cardiac disorders.

Corpamil *Helvepharm, Switz.*
Verapamil hydrochloride (p.989·1).
Angina; arrhythmias; hypertension.

Corpea *Normon, Spain.*
Molsidomine (p.936·1).
Angina pectoris.

Corpendol *Sanofi Synthelabo, Port.*
Propranolol hydrochloride (p.962·3).
Angina pectoris; arrhythmias; essential tremor; gastrointestinal haemorrhage; hypertension; migraine; myocardial infarction; obstructive cardiomyopathy; thyrotoxicosis.

Corpotasin CL *SmithKline Beecham, Mex.*
Potassium bicarbonate (p.1186·1); potassium chloride (p.1194·3); lysine hydrochloride (p.1370·3); citric acid (p.1596·2).
Potassium and chloride supplement.

Corprilor *Rubio, Spain.*
Enalapril maleate (p.883·3).
Heart failure; hypertension.

Corque *Geneva, USA.*
Hydrocortisone (p.1073·3); clioquinol (p.190·2).
Skin disorders.

Correctol
Note.This name is used for preparations of different composition.
Schering-Plough, Canad.; Schering-Plough, Hong Kong; Schering-Plough, USA.
Bisacodyl (p.1212·2).
Formerly contained docusate sodium and phenolphthalein in the *USA*.
Constipation.

Alcon, Fr.; Alcon, Port.
Disodium inosinate (p.1604·3) or inosine monophosphate.
Visual disturbances.

Schering-Plough, Mex.
Docusate sodium (p.1223·1).

Correctol Extra Gentle *Schering-Plough, USA†.*
Docusate sodium (p.1223·1).

Correctol Stool Softener *Schering-Plough, Canad.*
Docusate sodium (p.1223·1).
Formerly contained docusate sodium and phenolphthalein.
Constipation.

Corrigast *Continental, Spain.*
Misoprostol (p.1446·1).
Peptic ulcer.

Corsalbene *Ratiopharm, Aust.*
Aspirin (p.14·2).
Migraine; myocardial infarction; thrombosis prophylaxis.

Cor-Select
Dreluso, Ger.
Ointment: Crataegus (p.1600·2); valerian (p.1678·3); camphor (p.1589·3); ol. sinapis (p.1639·1); benzyl nicotinate (p.20·2); peppermint oil (p.1243·3); melissa oil.
Cardiovascular disorders.

Dreluso, Ger.
Oral drops: Homoeopathic preparation.

Corsodyl
SmithKline Beecham, Belg.; SmithKline Beecham, Fin.; SmithKline Beecham Sante, Fr.; SmithKline Beecham OTC, Ger.; SmithKline Beecham, Hong Kong; SmithKline Beecham Consumer, Irl.; SmithKline Beecham, Israel; SmithKline Beecham, Ital.; SmithKline Beecham Consumer, Neth.; SmithKline Beecham, Norw.; Sterling, Port.; SmithKline Beecham Consumer, Swed.; SmithKline Beecham Consumer, Switz.; SmithKline Beecham Consumer, UK.
Chlorhexidine gluconate (p.1138·2).
Mouth infections; oral hygiene.

CorSotalol *Merck dura, Ger.*
Sotalol hydrochloride (p.972·2).
Arrhythmias.

Corsym *Novartis Consumer, Canad.†.*
Phenylpropanolamine polistirex (p.1098·3); chlorpheniramine [chlorphenamine] polistirex (p.412·2).
Nasal congestion.

Cortacet *Whitehall-Robins, Canad.*
Hydrocortisone acetate (p.1073·3).
Skin disorders.

Cortafriol C *Synthelabo, Spain.*
Paracetamol (p.71·2); pseudoephedrine sulfate (p.1099·3); ascorbic acid (p.1389·3).
Fever; influenza and cold symptoms; pain.

Cortafriol Complex *Synthelabo, Spain.*
Paracetamol (p.71·2); pseudoephedrine sulfate (p.1099·3); chlorpheniramine [chlorphenamine] maleate (p.412·1).
Fever; nasal congestion; pain.

CortaGel *Norstar, USA†.*
Hydrocortisone (p.1073·3).
Skin disorders.

Cortagrip *UCI, Braz.*
Dipyrone (p.34·1); sodium camsilate; guaifenesin (p.1092·2); eucalyptol (p.1609·2); niaouli oil (p.1640·2); vitamin C (p.1389·3).
Cold and influenza symptoms.

Cortagrip D *UCI, Braz.*
Dipyrone (p.34·1); chlorpheniramine [chlorphenamine] maleate (p.412·1); guaifenesin (p.1092·2); terpin hydrate (p.1101·2); sodium camsilate.
Cold and influenza symptoms.

Cortaid
Dermatech, Austral.; Carlo Erba OTC, Ital.; Pharmacia Upjohn, NZ; Pharmacia Upjohn, USA.
Hydrocortisone (p.1073·3) or hydrocortisone acetate (p.1073·3).
Skin disorders.

Cortaid with Aloe *Pharmacia Upjohn, Singapore.*
Hydrocortisone acetate (p.1073·3); aloe vera (p.1110·1).
Skin disorders.

Cortal *Organon, Swed.*
Cortisone acetate (p.1065·3).
Corticosteroid.

Cortal for Adults *SmithKline Beecham, Hong Kong.*
Aspirin (p.14·2); caffeine (p.761·3).
Fever; pain.

Cortal for Children *SmithKline Beecham, Hong Kong.*
Paracetamol (p.71·2).
Fever; pain.

Cortamed *Sabex, Canad.*
Hydrocortisone acetate (p.1073·3).
Eye disorders.

Cortamide *Ottolenghi, Ital.*
Fluocinolone acetonide (p.1071·1).
Skin disorders.

Cortancyl *Roussel Diamant, Fr.*
Prednisone (p.1079·2).
Corticosteroid.

Cortane-B Otic *Blansett, USA.*
Chloroxylenol (p.1142·1); pramocaine hydrochloride (p.1318·2); hydrocortisone (p.1073·3).

Cortanest *Piam, Ital.†.*
Hydrocortamate hydrochloride (p.1073·3); lignocaine [lidocaine] hydrochloride (p.1313·2).
Burns; skin disorders; wounds.

Cortanest Plus *Piam, Ital.*
Fluocinolone acetonide (p.1071·1); lignocaine [lidocaine] hydrochloride (p.1313·2).
Anogenital disorders; burns; skin disorders.

Cortate
Note.This name is used for preparations of different composition.
Rhone-Poulenc Rorer, Austral.
Cortisone acetate (p.1065·3).
Oral corticosteroid.

Schering, Canad.
Hydrocortisone (p.1073·3).
Skin disorders.

Cortatrigen *Goldline, USA.*
Hydrocortisone (p.1073·3); neomycin sulfate (p.228·1); polymyxin B (p.238·3).
Bacterial ear infections.

Cort-Dome *Miles, USA.*
Hydrocortisone (p.1073·3) or hydrocortisone acetate (p.1073·3).
Anorectal disorders; skin disorders.

Cortef
Pharmacia Upjohn, Austral.; Pharmacia Upjohn, Canad.; Upjohn, USA.
Hydrocortisone (p.1073·3), hydrocortisone acetate (p.1073·3), or hydrocortisone cipionate (p.1074·1).
Corticosteroid.

Cortef Feminine Itch *Upjohn, USA.*
Hydrocortisone acetate (p.1073·3).
Pruritus.

Cortegripan *Heralds, Braz.*
Dipyrone (p.34·1); guaifenesin (p.1092·2); sodium camsilate; ascorbic acid (p.1389·3); lignocaine [lidocaine] (p.1313·2).
Cold and influenza symptoms.

Cortenema
Note.This name is used for preparations of different composition.
Axcan, Canad.; Solvay, USA.
Hydrocortisone (p.1073·3).
Inflammatory bowel disease.

Casen Fleet, Spain.
Allantoin (p.1110·1); hydrocortisone hydrogen succinate (p.1074·1); homatropine methylbromide (p.468·1); zinc oxide (p.1128·2).
Anorectal disorders.

Corti Biciron N *S & K, Ger.*
Dexamethasone isonicotinate (p.1067·1); oxytetracycline hydrochloride (p.234·1).
Infected eye disorders.

Corti Jaikal *S & K, Ger.*
Hydrocortisone acetate (p.1073·3); sodium thiosulfate (p.1024·2); salicylic acid (p.1122·3).
Acne.

Corti-Arscolloid *SIT, Ital.*
Dichlorobenzyl alcohol (p.1143·2); silver protein (p.1664·2); dexamethasone sodium phosphate (p.1067·1).
Stomatitis.

Cortibiotique *Chauvin, Fr.*
Hydrocortisone acetate (p.1073·3); framycetin sulfate (p.208·2).
Infected skin disorders.

Cortic
Note.This name is used for preparations of different composition.
Sigma, Austral.
Hydrocortisone acetate (p.1073·3).
Anogenital pruritus; skin disorders.

Everett, USA.
Hydrocortisone (p.1073·3); pramocaine hydrochloride (p.1318·2); chloroxylenol (p.1142·1).
Inflammatory ear disorders.

Corticaine
Note.This name is used for preparations of different composition.
Glaxo, USA.
Rectal cream: Hydrocortisone acetate (p.1073·3); cinchocaine (p.1309·1).
Anorectal disorders.

UCB, USA.
Cream: Hydrocortisone acetate (p.1073·3).
Skin disorders.

Cortical *Caber, Ital.*
Diflucortolone valerate (p.1069·3).
Formerly contained suprarenal cortex.
Skin disorders.

Corticetine *Chauvin, Fr.; Chauvin Novopharma, Switz.*
Framycetin sulfate (p.208·2); dexamethasone sodium phosphate (p.1067·1).
Otitis.

Corticil T *Oftalder, Port.*
Oxytetracycline hydrochloride (p.234·1); hydrocortisone (p.1073·3).
Infected skin disorders.

Corti-Clyss *Braun, Switz.*
Prednisolone metasulfobenzoate sodium (p.1078·1).
Crohn's disease; ulcerative colitis.

Corticobiss *Bissendorf, Neth.†.*
Corticorelin triflutate (p.1280·2).
Diagnosis of Cushing's syndrome.

Corticoderm
Hermal, Denm.; Hermal, Norw.†; Meda, Swed.
Fluprednidene acetate (p.1072·1).
Skin disorders.

Corticotulle Lumiere
Solvay, Fr.; Hefa, Ger.
Neomycin sulfate (p.228·1); polymyxin B sulfate (p.238·1); triamcinolone acetonide (p.1080·1).
Burns; ulcers; wounds.

Corticreme
Rougier, Canad.; Rougier, Hong Kong.
Hydrocortisone acetate (p.1073·3).
Skin disorders.

Cortidene *Berna, Spain.*
Paramethasone acetate (p.1077·2).
Corticosteroid.

Cortidex *Rayere, Mex.*
Dexamethasone (p.1067·1).
Corticosteroid.

Cortidexason *Dermapharm, Ger.*
Dexamethasone (p.1067·1).
Skin and scalp disorders.

Cortidexason comp *Dermapharm, Ger.*
Dexamethasone (p.1067·1); neomycin sulfate (p.228·1).
Infected skin disorders.

Cortidro *Sofar, Ital.*
Hydrocortisone acetate (p.1073·3).
Skin disorders.

Corti-Dynexan *Kreussler, Ger.*
Prednisolone acetate (p.1078·1); lauromacrogol 400 (p.1345·2); dequalinium chloride (p.1143·1).
Inflammatory disorders of the mouth.

Cortiespec *Centrum, Spain.*
Fluocinolone acetonide (p.1071·1).
Skin disorders.

Corti-Flexiole
Mann, Ger.†; Restan, S.Afr.†.
Hydrocortisone (p.1073·3); chloramphenicol (p.179·1); vitamin A palmitate (p.1383·2).
Eye, ear, and skin disorders.

Cortifluid N *Streuli, Switz.*
Calcium pantothenate (p.1374·1); hydrocortisone acetate (p.1073·3); neomycin sulfate (p.228·1).
Infected skin disorders.

Corti-Fluoral *Schering, Ital.*
Josamycin propionate (p.217·3); diflucortolone valerate (p.1069·3).
Formerly contained chloramphenicol and diflucortolone valerate.
Mouth disorders.

Cortifoam
Reed & Carnrick, Canad.; Schwarz, USA.
Hydrocortisone acetate (p.1073·3).
Colitis; proctitis.

Cortiglanden *Disperga, Aust.*
Suprarenal cortex (p.1080·1).
Adrenocortical insufficiency; congenital adrenal hyperplasia.

Cortigripe *Zimaia, Port.*
Aspirin (p.14·2); hydrocortisone (p.1073·3).

Cortiment *Hoechst Marion Roussel, Canad.†.*
Hydrocortisone acetate (p.1073·3).
Anorectal inflammatory disorders.

Cortimycin *Medical Ophthalmics, USA.*
Eye drops: Hydrocortisone (p.1073·3); neomycin (p.228·1); polymyxin B (p.238·3).
Eye ointment: Hydrocortisone (p.1073·3); neomycin (p.228·1); bacitracin (p.155·2); polymyxin B (p.238·3).
Infected eye disorders.

Cortimycine *Drossapharm, Switz.*
Cream: Hydrocortisone acetate (p.1073·3); neomycin sulfate (p.228·1); dexpanthenol (p.1602·3).
Infected skin disorders.
Ear drops; nose drops; eye drops; eye ointment: Hydrocortisone acetate (p.1073·3); neomycin sulfate (p.228·1).
Infected inflammatory disorders.

Cortimyk *CCS, Swed.*
Miconazole nitrate (p.391·1); hydrocortisone (p.1073·3).
Fungal skin infections with inflammation.

Cortimyxin *Sabex, Canad.*
Hydrocortisone (p.1073·3); neomycin sulfate (p.228·1); polymyxin B sulfate (p.238·1).
Ear disorders.

Cort-Inal *Teofarma, Ital.*
Hydrocortisone acetate (p.1073·3); diprophylline (p.764·1).
Bronchial catarrh.

Cortine Naturelle *Roche Nicholas, Fr.†*
Suprarenal cortex (porcine) (p.1080·1).
Asthenia.

Cortinorex *Spyfarma, Spain.*
Cyanocobalamin; suprarenal cortex; glutathione; liver extract; inosine (p.1350·1).
Tonic.

Cortiphenol H *Ciba Vision, Hong Kong.*
Chloramphenicol (p.179·1); hydrocortisone acetate (p.1073·3).
Infected eye disorders.

Cortirell *Sanorell, Ger.*
Homoeopathic preparation.

Cortiron
Schering, Aust.; Schering, Ital.†.
Desoxycortone acetate (p.1066·3) or desoxycortone enantate (p.1066·3).
Adrenocortical insufficiency; hypotension.

Cortisal *Monin, Fr.*
Propylene glycol mono- and disalicylate; prednisolone (p.1077·3).
Peri-articular and soft-tissue disorders.

Cortisdin Urea *Isdin, Spain.*
Fluorometholone (p.1072·1); urea (p.1127·3).
Skin disorders.

Cortison Chemicet Topica *Astra, Spain.*
Chloramphenicol (p.179·1); hydrocortisone acetate (p.1073·3).
Infected skin disorders.

Cortison Chemicetina *Fournier, Ital.*
Chloramphenicol (p.179·1); hydrocortisone acetate (p.1073·3).
Infected eye or skin disorders.

Cortison Kemicetin *Pharmacia Upjohn, Aust.*
Chloramphenicol (p.179·1); hydrocortisone acetate (p.1073·3).
Bacterial eye infections; inflammation.

Cortison-Kemicetin *Pharmacia Upjohn, Hong Kong.*
Eye/ear drops: Chloramphenicol (p.179·1); hydrocortisone caprylate (p.1073·3).
Infected eye and ear disorders.
Ointment: Chloramphenicol (p.179·1); hydrocortisone acetate (p.1073·3).
Infected eye disorders; infected skin disorders; periodontitis.
Rectal ointment: Chloramphenicol (p.179·1); prednisolone (p.1077·3); phenylephrine hydrochloride (p.1097·1); lignocaine [lidocaine] hydrochloride (p.1313·2); tannic acid (p.1669·1); peru balsam (p.1650·2).
Anorectal disorders.

Cortisporin
Note.This name is used for preparations of different composition.
Glaxo Wellcome, Canad.; Glaxo Wellcome, Mex.; Monarch, USA.
Eye drops; ear drops: Polymyxin B sulfate (p.238·1); neomycin sulfate (p.228·1); hydrocortisone (p.1073·3).
Infected ear disorders; infected eye disorders.

Glaxo Wellcome, Canad.; Monarch, USA.
Ointment; eye ointment: Polymyxin B sulfate (p.238·1); bacitracin zinc (p.155·2); neomycin sulfate (p.228·1); hydrocortisone (p.1073·3).
Infected skin and eye disorders.

Monarch, USA.
Cream: Polymyxin B sulfate (p.238·1); neomycin sulfate (p.228·1); hydrocortisone acetate (p.1073·3).
Infected skin disorders.

Cortisporin-TC *Monarch, USA.*
Colistin sulfate (p.192·3); neomycin sulfate (p.228·1); hydrocortisone acetate (p.1073·3); tonzonium bromide (p.1674·1).
Infected ear disorders.

Cortisteron *Streuli, Switz.*
Desoxycortone acetate (p.1066·3).
Lignocaine [lidocaine] hydrochloride (p.1313·2) is included in some injections to alleviate the pain of injection.
Adrenocortical insufficiency.

Cortisumman *Winzer, Ger.*
Dexamethasone (p.1067·1).
Eye disorders.

Cortisyl *Hoechst Marion Roussel, UK.*
Cortisone acetate (p.1065·3).
Corticosteroid.

Cortivel *Ern, Spain†.*
Chloramphenicol (p.179·1); prednisolone metasulfobenzoate sodium (p.1078·1).
External ear or nasal disorders.

Cortivent *Leiras, Fin.*
Budesonide (p.1064·2).
Asthma.

Cortizone
Pfizer, Israel; Pfizer, USA.
Hydrocortisone (p.1073·3).
Skin disorders.

Cortobion *Laborsil, Braz.*
Desoxycortone (p.1066·3); ascorbic acid (p.1389·3).
Corticosteroid.

The symbol † denotes a preparation no longer actively marketed

Cortoderm
Note. This name is used for preparations of different composition.
Taro, Canad.
Hydrocortisone (p.1073·3).
Skin disorders.

Aspen, S.Afr.
Fluocinolone acetonide (p.1071·1).
Skin disorders.

Cortoftal Alcon Cusi, Spain.
Clobetasone butyrate (p.1065·2).
Inflammatory eye disorders.

Cortogen Schering-Plough, S.Afr.
Cortisone acetate (p.1065·3).
Corticosteroid.

Cortone
Merck Sharp & Dohme, Aust.; Merck Frosst, Canad.; Merck Sharp & Dohme, Ital.; Merck Sharp & Dohme, Norw.; Merck Sharp & Dohme, Swed.; Merck, USA.
Cortisone acetate (p.1065·3).
Corticosteroid.

Cortop Biologici Italia, Ital.
Hydrocortisone sodium succinate (p.1074·1).
Corticosteroid.

Cortopin Pinewood, Irl.
Hydrocortisone (p.1073·3).
Insect bites; skin disorders.

Corto-Tavegil Novartis, Ger.
Tablets: Clemastine fumarate (p.413·2); dexamethasone (p.1067·1).
Hypersensitivity reactions.
Topical gel: Clemastine fumarate (p.413·2); clocortolone pivalate (p.1065·3).
Insect stings; skin disorders; sunburn.

Cortril
Pfizer, Belg.; Pfizer, Fin.
Hydrocortisone (p.1073·3) or hydrocortisone acetate (p.1073·3).
Eye disorders; skin disorders.

Cortrophin Pinewood, UK.
Hydrocortisone (p.1073·3).
Skin disorders.

Cortrosina Akzo, Braz.
Tetracosactide (p.1298·2).
Diagnosis of adrenocortical insufficiency.

Cortrosyn
Organon, Canad.; Organon, Hong Kong; Organon, Israel; Organon, Ital.; Organon, USA.
Tetracosactide (p.1298·2) or tetracosactide hexa-acetate (p.1298·2).
Adrenocorticotrophic hormone; diagnosis of adrenocortical insufficiency.

Cortuss Pharmaland, Thai.
Dextromethorphan hydrobromide (p.1087·3).
Coughs.

Corvasal Hoechst, Fr.
Injection: Linsidomine hydrochloride (p.921·1).
Angina pectoris; cardiac investigations; coronary arterial spasm.
Tablets: Molsidomine (p.936·1).
Angina pectoris.

Corvaton
Therabel, Belg.; Hoechst Marion Roussel, Ger.; Hoechst Marion Roussel, Switz.
Molsidomine (p.936·1).
Angina pectoris; heart failure; myocardial infarction; pulmonary hypertension.

Cor-Vel Bilgast, Ger.
Camphor (p.1589·3); menthol (p.1632·3); Norway spruce oil; rosemary oil (p.1659·3).
Cardiac disorders.

Cor-Vel N Truw, Ger.†.
Oral drops: Convallaria (p.1599·1); squill (p.1100·3).
Tablets: Convallaria (p.1599·1); crataegus (p.1600·2).
Heart failure.

Corvert
Pharmacia Upjohn, Aust.; Pharmacia Upjohn, Fin.; Pharmacia Upjohn, Fr.; Pharmacia Upjohn, Ital.; Pharmacia Upjohn, Neth.; Pharmacia Upjohn, Norw.; Pharmacia Upjohn, Swed.; Pharmacia Upjohn, Switz.; Pharmacia Upjohn, USA.
Ibutilide fumarate (p.912·2).
Arrhythmias.

Corvipas Pascoe, Ger.
Homoeopathic preparation.

Corwil Zeneca, Aust.†.
Xamoterol fumarate (p.998·3).
Heart failure.

Corwin
Zeneca, Belg.†; AstraZeneca, UK†.
Xamoterol fumarate (p.998·3).
Heart failure.

Coryaid Pfizer, Hong Kong.
Salicylamide (p.82·1); caffeine (p.761·3); vitamin C (p.1389·3); chlorpheniramine [chlorphenamine] maleate (p.412·1); phenylpropanolamine hydrochloride (p.1098·1).
Cold symptoms.

Coryfin C SIT, Ital.
Menglytate (p.1094·2); ascorbic acid (p.1389·3).
Coughs; hoarseness.

Corymunun Fund a Paiva, Braz.
Corynebacterium parvum (p.527·2).
Immunostimulant.

Coryphen Rougier, Canad.
Aspirin (p.14·2).

Coryretard-C Madaus, S.Afr.†.
Carbinoxamine maleate (p.411·1); phenylephrine hydrochloride (p.1097·1).
Allergic rhinitis.

Coryx Mirren, S.Afr.
Effervescent tablets: Chlorpheniramine [chlorphenamine] maleate (p.412·1); pseudoephedrine hydrochloride (p.1099·2); aspirin (p.14·2); ascorbic acid (p.1389·3).
Syrup: Triprolidine hydrochloride (p.427·2); pseudoephedrine hydrochloride (p.1099·2); vitamin C (p.1389·3).
Cold and influenza symptoms.

Coryzalia
Boiron, Canad.; Boiron, Fr.; Boiron, Port.
Homoeopathic preparation.

Corzide
Squibb, Canad.†; Monarch, USA.
Nadolol (p.937·1); bendrofluazide [bendroflumethiazide] (p.844·1).
Hypertension.

Cosaar
Merck Sharp & Dohme, Aust.; Merck Sharp & Dohme, Switz.
Losartan potassium (p.921·3).
Heart failure; hypertension.

Cosaar Plus
Merck Sharp & Dohme, Aust.; Merck Sharp & Dohme, Switz.
Losartan potassium (p.921·3); hydrochlorothiazide (p.907·3).
Hypertension.

Cosaldon
Note. This name is used for preparations of different composition.
Hoechst Marion Roussel, Aust.; Aventis, S.Afr.
Pentifylline (p.953·1); nicotinic acid (p.1372·3).
Vascular disorders.

Hoechst Marion Roussel, Ger.
Pentifylline (p.953·1).
Cerebrovascular insufficiency; vascular eye disorders; vestibular disorders.

Cosaldon A Hoechst Marion Roussel, Ger.
Pentifylline (p.953·1); vitamin A palmitate (p.1383·2).
Vascular eye disorders; vestibular disorders.

Cosalgesic
Cox, Hong Kong; Cox, Irl.; Cox, UK.
Dextropropoxyphene hydrochloride (p.27·1); paracetamol (p.71·2).
These ingredients can be described by the British Approved Name Co-proxamol.
Pain.

Cosamin Nutramax, USA.
Glucosamine hydrochloride; sodium chondroitin sulfate; manganese ascorbate (p.1350·1).
Nutritional supplement.

Cosig Sigma, Austral.
Co-trimoxazole (p.193·3).
Bacterial infections; Pneumocystis carinii pneumonia.

Coslan Parke, Davis, Spain.
Mefenamic acid (p.51·2).
Fever; inflammation; pain.

Cosmaxil Cosmofarma, Port.†.
Atropine sulfate (p.461·1); papaverine hydrochloride (p.1648·1); ephedrine hydrochloride (p.1090·1); phenobarbital (p.355·1); theophylline (p.777·2).
Obstructive airways disease.

Cosmegen
Merck Sharp & Dohme, Aust.; Merck Sharp & Dohme, Austral.; Prodome, Braz.; Merck Frosst, Canad.; Merck Sharp & Dohme, Fin.; Merck Sharp & Dohme, Hong Kong; Merck Sharp & Dohme, Irl.; Merck Sharp & Dohme, Ital.; Merck Sharp & Dohme, Mex.; Merck Sharp & Dohme, NZ; Merck Sharp & Dohme, S.Afr.; Merck Sharp & Dohme, Swed.; Merck Sharp & Dohme, Switz.; Merck Sharp & Dohme, Thai.; Merck Sharp & Dohme, UK; Merck, USA.
Dactinomycin (p.532·2).
Malignant neoplasms.

Cosmetar-S Promedica, Fr.†.
Coal tar (Stantar) (p.1125·1).
Seborrhoeic dermatitis.

Cosmiciclina INTES, Ital.
Oxytetracycline hydrochloride (p.234·1); chloramphenicol (p.179·1); sulfacetamide sodium (p.250·3).
Bacterial infections of the eye or ear.

Cosmofer Vitaline, UK.
Iron dextran (p.1368·2).
Iron deficiency.

Coso McGloin, Austral.
Menthol (p.1632·3); camphor (p.1589·3); benzyl alcohol (p.1135·2).
Herpes labialis.

Cosopt
Merck Sharp & Dohme, Aust.; Merck Sharp & Dohme, Belg.; Merck Frosst, Canad.; Merck Sharp & Dohme, Denm.; Merck Sharp & Dohme, Fin.; Merck Sharp & Dohme-Chibret, Fr.; Chibret, Ger.; Merck Sharp & Dohme, Irl.; Merck Sharp & Dohme, Israel; Merck Sharp & Dohme, Ital.; Merck Sharp & Dohme, Mex.; Merck Sharp & Dohme, Neth.; Merck Sharp & Dohme, Norw.; Merck Sharp & Dohme, S.Afr.; Merck Sharp & Dohme, Swed.; Merck Sharp & Dohme, Switz.; Merck Sharp & Dohme, UK; Merck, USA.
Dorzolamide hydrochloride (p.883·1); timolol maleate (p.982·1).
Glaucoma; ocular hypertension.

Cospanon
Eisai, Hong Kong; Eisai, Jpn†.
Flopropione (p.1611·3).
Smooth muscle spasm.

Costi Medochemie, Thai.
Domperidone (p.1224·1).
Digestive disorders; dyspepsia; flatulence; gastrooesophageal reflux; heartburn; nausea and vomiting.

Costop Standard, Hong Kong.
Cloperastine hydrochloride (p.1087·2).
Coughs.

Cosudex Zeneca, Austral.
Bicalutamide (p.511·2).
Prostatic cancer.

Cosuric DDSA Pharmaceuticals, UK.
Allopurinol (p.397·3).
Gout; hyperuricaemia.

Cosylan
Parke, Davis, Denm.†; Warner-Lambert, Norw.; Parke, Davis, Swed.†.
Ethylmorphine hydrochloride (p.35·2); cascara (p.1216·1); menthol (p.1632·3).
Coughs; respiratory-tract irritation.

Cosyr
United American, Hong Kong; Great Eastern, Thai.; United American, Thai.
Dextromethorphan hydrobromide (p.1087·3); chlorpheniramine [chlorphenamine] maleate (p.412·1); phenylpropanolamine hydrochloride (p.1098·1); guaifenesin (p.1092·2).
Coughs.

Cotamox Asian Pharm, Thai.
Co-trimoxazole (p.193·3).
Bacterial infections.

Cotareg
Novartis, Fr.; Novartis, Ital.
Valsartan (p.988·3); hydrochlorothiazide (p.907·3).
Hypertension.

Co-Tasian Asian Pharm, Thai.
Co-trimoxazole (p.193·3).
Bacterial infections.

Cotazym
Note. This name is used for preparations of different composition.
Akzo, Braz.; Thiemann, Ger.
Pancreatin (p.1646·1).
Pancreatic enzyme deficiency.

Organon, Canad.; Pharmaco, NZ; Organon, USA.
Pancrelipase (p.1647·2).
Pancreatic enzyme deficiency.

Cotazym S Forte Organon, Austral.
Pancrelipase (p.1647·2).
Pancreatic enzyme deficiency.

Cotenol TP, Thai.
Paracetamol (p.71·2); codeine phosphate (p.25·2).
Pain.

Cotenolol Mepha, Switz.
Atenolol (p.841·3); chlortalidone (p.857·1).
Hypertension.

Cotenomel Clonmel, Irl.
Atenolol (p.841·3); chlortalidone (p.857·1).
Hypertension.

Cotet Covan, S.Afr.
Oxytetracycline hydrochloride (p.234·1).
Bacterial infections; protozoal infections.

Cothilyne Haemacure, Canad.†.
Centella (p.1112·2).
Wounds.

Cotone Emostatico Farmatre, Ital.; Iema, Ital.; Morigi, Ital.; Nova Argentia, Ital.; Olcelli, Ital.
Ferric chloride (p.1610·3).
Styptic.

Cotrane Sanofi Synthelabo, Belg.
Dimethoxanate hydrochloride (p.1089·1).
Coughs.

Cotrazol Valomed, Spain.
Guaifenesin (p.1092·2); co-trimoxazole (p.193·3).
Respiratory-tract infections.

Cotren
Biolab, Hong Kong; Biolab, Singapore; Biolab, Thai.
Clotrimazole (p.382·1).
Fungal skin and vaginal infections; trichomoniasis.

Cotribene Ratiopharm, Aust.
Co-trimoxazole (p.193·3).
Bacterial infections.

Cotridin Technilab, Canad.
Triprolidine hydrochloride (p.427·2); pseudoephedrine hydrochloride (p.1099·2); codeine phosphate (p.25·2).
Coughs.

Cotridin Expectorant Technilab, Canad.
Triprolidine hydrochloride (p.427·2); pseudoephedrine hydrochloride (p.1099·2); guaifenesin (p.1092·2); codeine phosphate (p.25·2).
Coughs.

Cotrim
Medinovum, Fin.; BASF, Ger.; Eu Rho, Ger.; Heumann, Ger.; CT, Ger.; Ratiopharm, Ger.; Holsten, Ger.; Ratiopharm, Port.; Spirig, Switz.; Lemmon, USA.
Co-trimoxazole (p.193·3).
Bacterial infections; Pneumocystis carinii pneumonia.

Cotrim E Ratiopharm, Ger.
Co-trimoxazole (p.193·3).
Bacterial infections; Pneumocystis carinii pneumonia.

Cotrim K Ratiopharm, Ger.
Co-trimoxazole (p.193·3).
Bacterial infections; Pneumocystis carinii pneumonia.

Cotrimazol Lafon, Fr.†.
Co-trimoxazole (p.193·3).
Bacterial infections; Pneumocystis carinii pneumonia; toxoplasmosis.

Cotrim-Diolan Engelhard, Ger.; Brahms, Ger.
Co-trimoxazole (p.193·3).
Bacterial infections; fungal mycetoma; paracoccidioidomycosis.

Co-Trimed Medifive, Thai.
Co-trimoxazole (p.193·3).
Bacterial infections.

Cotrimel Clonmel, Irl.
Co-trimoxazole (p.193·3).
Bacterial infections.

Cotrim-Hefa Hefa, Ger.
Co-trimoxazole (p.193·3).
Bacterial and protozoal infections.

Cotrimhexal Hexal, Ger.
Co-trimoxazole (p.193·3).
Bacterial infections.

Cotrimox-Wolff Wolff, Ger.
Co-trimoxazole (p.193·3).
Bacterial infections.

Cotrim-Puren Isis Puren, Ger.†.
Co-trimoxazole (p.193·3).
Bacterial infections; Pneumocystis carinii pneumonia.

Cotrimstada Stada, Ger.
Co-trimoxazole (p.193·3).
Bacterial infections.

Co-trim-Tablinen Sanorania, Ger.†.
Co-trimoxazole (p.193·3).
Bacterial infections; fungal mycetoma; paracoccidioidomycosis; Pneumocystis carinii pneumonia.

Cotrivan Zurich, S.Afr.†.
Co-trimoxazole (p.193·3).
Bacterial infections.

Cotron Pinewood, Irl.
Dantron (p.1221·3); poloxamer 188 (p.1347·1).
Constipation.

Co-Tuss V Rugby, USA.
Hydrocodone tartrate (p.42·2); guaifenesin (p.1092·2).
Coughs.

Cotussin TP, Thai.
Diphenhydramine hydrochloride (p.416·1); ammonium chloride (p.1085·2); sodium citrate (p.1186·2).
Coughs; nasal congestion.

Co-Tylenol Johnson & Johnson, Aust.
Paracetamol (p.71·2); carbinoxamine maleate (p.411·1); phenylephrine hydrochloride (p.1097·1).
Cold symptoms; sinusitis.

Cough & Cold Homeocan, Canad.
Homoeopathic preparation.

Cough, Cold & Allergy Relief Stanley, Canad.†.
Phenylephrine hydrochloride (p.1097·1); phenylpropanolamine hydrochloride (p.1098·1); brompheniramine maleate (p.410·2); dextromethorphan hydrobromide (p.1087·3).

Cough & Cold L52 Homeocan, Canad.
Homoeopathic preparation.

Cough Control Sucrets SmithKline Beecham, Israel.
Dextromethorphan hydrobromide (p.1087·3).
Coughs.

Cough Drops
Note. This name is used for preparations of different composition.
Zee, Canad.
Menthol (p.1632·3).

Weleda, UK.
Angelica root (p.1580·2); cinnamon (p.1595·3); clove (p.1596·3); coriander (p.1599·2); lemon oil (p.1628·2); melissa leaf (p.1632·2); nutmeg (p.1643·1); cherry-laurel water.
Coughs.

Cough Elixir Weleda, UK.
Aniseed (p.1580·2); horehound (p.1094·2); althaea root (p.1577·1); thyme (p.1672·2); drosera; ipecacuanha root; pulsatilla.
Coughs.

Cough & Flu Syrup Technilab, Canad.
Pseudoephedrine hydrochloride (p.1099·2); dextromethorphan hydrobromide (p.1087·3); guaifenesin (p.1092·2); paracetamol (p.71·2).

Cough Formula Comtrex Bristol-Myers Products, USA.
Paracetamol (p.71·2); pseudoephedrine hydrochloride (p.1099·2); guaifenesin (p.1092·2); dextromethorphan hydrobromide (p.1087·3).
Coughs and cold symptoms.

Cough L64 Homeocan, Canad.
Homoeopathic preparation.

Cough N Cold Syrup Golden Pride, Canad.; Rawleigh, Canad.
Ephedrine hydrochloride (p.1090·1); guaifenesin (p.1092·2); sodium citrate (p.1186·2).

Cough Relief Brauer, Austral.
Oral liquid: Anise oil (p.1580·3); althaea (p.1577·1); bryonia (p.1587·2); Iceland moss; echinacea (p.1606·2); chamomile (p.1593·2); thyme (p.1672·2); urtica (p.1678·2); aconitum nap.; coccus cacti; coralium rub.; drosera; ipecacuanha; kali bich.; kreosotum; spongia tosta; sticta pulm.
Coughs.

Oral spray: Homoeopathic preparation.

Cough Suppressant Syrup DM Drug Trading, Canad.
Dextromethorphan hydrobromide (p.1087·3).

Cough Syrup
Note. This name is used for preparations of different composition.
Marc-O, Canad.
Dextromethorphan hydrobromide (p.1087·3).

Stanley, Canad.†.
Pseudoephedrine hydrochloride (p.1099·2); codeine phosphate (p.25·2); guaifenesin (p.1092·2).

Technilab, Canad.
Diphenhydramine hydrochloride (p.416·1); codeine phosphate (p.25·2); ammonium chloride (p.1085·2).

Goldline, USA.
Phenylephrine hydrochloride (p.1097·1); dextromethorphan hydrobromide (p.1087·3); guaifenesin (p.1092·2).
Coughs.

Cough Syrup with Codeine Stanley, Canad.
Diphenhydramine hydrochloride (p.416·1); codeine phosphate (p.25·2); ammonium chloride (p.1085·2).
Coughs.

Cough Syrup DM Stanley, Canad.; WestCan, Canad.
Dextromethorphan hydrobromide (p.1087·3).

Cough Syrup DM Decongestant WestCan, Canad.
Dextromethorphan hydrobromide (p.1087·3); pseudoephedrine hydrochloride (p.1099·2).

Cough Syrup DM Decongestant for Children Stanley, Canad.
Dextromethorphan hydrobromide (p.1087·3); pseudoephedrine hydrochloride (p.1099·2).

Cough Syrup DM Decongestant Expectorant Stanley, Canad.
Dextromethorphan hydrobromide (p.1087·3); pseudoephedrine hydrochloride (p.1099·2); guaifenesin (p.1092·2).

Cough Syrup DM Expectorant Stanley, Canad.
Dextromethorphan hydrobromide (p.1087·3); guaifenesin (p.1092·2).

Cough Syrup DM-D-E WestCan, Canad.
Dextromethorphan hydrobromide (p.1087·3); pseudoephedrine hydrochloride (p.1099·2); guaifenesin (p.1092·2).

Cough Syrup DM-E WestCan, Canad.
Dextromethorphan hydrobromide (p.1087·3); guaifenesin (p.1092·2).

Cough Syrup Expectorant Stanley, Canad.; WestCan, Canad.
Guaifenesin (p.1092·2).

Cough Syrup with Guaifenesin & Dextromethorphan Tanta, Canad.
Dextromethorphan hydrobromide (p.1087·3); guaifenesin (p.1092·2).

Cough Syrup with Honey Hylands, Canad.
Homoeopathic preparation.

Coughcod Compu, S.Afr.
Ephedrine hydrochloride (p.1090·1); ammonium chloride (p.1085·2); sodium citrate (p.1186·2); codeine phosphate (p.25·2); mepyramine maleate (p.421·1).
Coughs.

Cough-eeze English Grains, UK†.
Ipecacuanha (p.1093·1); marrubium (p.1094·2); elecampane (p.1089·3).
Coughs.

Cough-EN Xepa-Soul Pattinson, Hong Kong; Xepa-Soul Pattinson, Singapore.
Dextromethorphan hydrobromide (p.1087·3); pseudoephedrine hydrochloride (p.1099·2); triprolidine hydrochloride (p.427·2).
Coughs; respiratory-tract congestion.

Coughlax Malaysia Chemist, Singapore.
Ammonium chloride (p.1085·2); chlorpheniramine [chlorphenamine] maleate (p.412·1); codeine phosphate (p.25·2); ephedrine hydrochloride (p.1090·1).
Coughs; respiratory-tract congestion; sneezing.

Coughmin Kyorin, Thai.
Sodium dibunate (p.1100·3); chlorpheniramine [chlorphenamine] maleate (p.412·1); dl-methylephedrine hydrochloride (p.1094·3).
Coughs.

Coughnadryl Condrugs, Thai.
Diphenhydramine hydrochloride (p.416·1); ammonium chloride (p.1085·2); sodium citrate (p.1186·2); menthol (p.1632·3).
Coughs; nasal congestion; sneezing.

Cough-X Ascher, USA.
Dextromethorphan hydrobromide (p.1087·3); benzocaine (p.1306·2).
Coughs.

Couldina Alter, Spain.
Aspirin (p.14·2); chlorpheniramine [chlorphenamine] maleate (p.412·1); phenylephrine hydrochloride (p.1097·1).
Bronchospasm; fever; nasal congestion; pain.

Couldina C Alter, Spain.
Aspirin (p.14·2); ascorbic acid (p.1389·3); chlorpheniramine [chlorphenamine] maleate (p.412·1); phenylephrine (p.1097·1).
Bronchospasm; fever; nasal congestion; pain.

Couldina Instant Alter, Spain.
Aspirin (p.14·2); chlorpheniramine [chlorphenamine] maleate (p.412·1); phenylephrine hydrochloride (p.1097·1).
Formerly contained aspirin, chlorpheniramine [chlorphenamine] maleate, and ascorbic acid.
Bronchospasm; fever; nasal congestion; pain.

Coumadin
Boots, Austral.; Du Pont, Canad.; Du Pont, Ger.; Taro, Israel; Du Pont, Ital.; Boots, NZ; Boots, S.Afr.†; Du Pont, Singapore; Du Pont, USA.
Warfarin sodium (p.992·2).
Thromboembolic disorders.

Coumadine Du Pont, Fr.
Warfarin sodium (p.992·2).
Thromboembolic disorders.

Counterpain
Bristol-Myers Squibb, Hong Kong.; Bristol-Myers Squibb, S.Afr.; Bristol-Myers Squibb, Thai.
Eugenol (p.1609·3); menthol (p.1632·3); methyl salicylate (p.55·1).
Muscle and joint pain.

Counterpain Cool Bristol-Myers Squibb, Thai.
Menthol (p.1632·3).
Muscle and joint pain.

Co-Vals Esteve, Spain.
Valsartan (p.988·3); hydrochlorothiazide (p.907·3).
Hypertension.

Covamet Covan, S.Afr.
Cyclizine hydrochloride (p.414·1).
Nausea; vestibular disorders; vomiting.

Covancaine Covan, S.Afr.
Phenazone (p.77·2); urea (p.1127·3); sulfacetamide sodium (p.250·3); benzocaine (p.1306·2).
Otitis externa; otitis media.

Covangesic Wallace, USA†.
Phenylpropanolamine hydrochloride (p.1098·1); phenylephrine hydrochloride (p.1097·1); chlorpheniramine [chlorphenamine] maleate (p.412·1); mepyramine maleate (p.421·1); paracetamol (p.71·2).
Upper respiratory-tract symptoms.

Covatine Bailly, Fr.
Captodiame hydrochloride (p.659·1).
Anxiety.

Covera Searle, USA.
Verapamil hydrochloride (p.989·1).
Angina pectoris; hypertension.

Covermark MDM, Fr.; Cupharma, Ital.
A range of covering creams.
Concealment of disfiguring skin disease.

Coversum
Servier, Aust.; Servier, Ger.; Servier, Switz.
Perindopril erbumine (p.953·2).
Heart failure; hypertension.

Coversyl
Servier, Austral.; Servier, Belg.; Servier, Canad.; Servier, Denm.; Pharmacal, Fin.; Servier, Fr.; Servier, Irl.; Servier, Ital.; Daiichi, Jpn; Sanfer, Mex.; Servier, Neth.; Servier, NZ; Servier, Port.; Servier, S.Afr.; Servier, Singapore; Servier, Spain; Servier, Thai.; Servier, UK.
Perindopril erbumine (p.953·2).
Heart failure; hypertension.

Co-Vibedoze Delta, Port.
Cobamamide (p.1388·3).
Vitamin B supplement.

Covitasa B12 Seid, Spain.
Cyproheptadine hydrochloride (p.414·2); cobamamide (p.1388·3).
Tonic.

Covite Covan, S.Afr.
Haematoporphyrin; liver extracts; caffeine; yeast (p.1350·1).
Tonic.

Covochol Covan, S.Afr.
Acetylcholine chloride (p.1415·1).
Production of miosis in eye surgery.

Covocort Covan, S.Afr.
Hydrocortisone (p.1073·3).
Corticosteroid.

Covomycin Covan, S.Afr.
Chloramphenicol (p.179·1); neomycin sulfate (p.228·1); naphazoline hydrochloride (p.1095·1).
Eye, ear, and nose infections.

Covomycin-D Covan, S.Afr.
Chloramphenicol (p.179·1); neomycin sulfate (p.228·1); dexamethasone sodium phosphate (p.1067·1).
Inflammatory eye and ear infections.

Covonia Bronchial Balsam Thornton & Ross, UK.
Dextromethorphan hydrobromide (p.1087·3); menthol (p.1632·3).
Formerly contained dextromethorphan hydrobromide, guaifenesin, menthol, and eucalyptol.
Coughs.

Covonia for Children Thornton & Ross, UK†.
Dextromethorphan hydrobromide (p.1087·3).
Coughs.

Covonia Mentholated Thornton & Ross, UK.
Menthol (p.1632·3); squill tincture (p.1100·3); liquorice (p.1231·2).
Coughs.

Covonia Night-Time Thornton & Ross, UK.
Dextromethorphan hydrobromide (p.1087·3); diphenhydramine hydrochloride (p.416·1).
Coughs.

Covosan Covan, S.Afr.
Naphazoline hydrochloride (p.1095·1); antazoline phosphate (p.408·3); sulfacetamide sodium (p.250·3).
Conjunctivitis.

Covospor Covan, S.Afr.
Clotrimazole (p.382·1).
Fungal skin and vulvovaginal infections.

Covostet Covan, S.Afr.
Amethocaine [tetracaine] hydrochloride (p.1305·2).
Local anaesthesia.

Covosulf Covan, S.Afr.
Sulfacetamide sodium (p.250·3).
Conjunctivitis.

Covotop Covan, S.Afr.
Chloramphenicol (p.179·1); benzocaine (p.1306·2).
Ear infections.

Cow & Gate Formula-S Nutricia, Hong Kong.
Infant feed (p.1350·1).
Lactose intolerance; milk protein allergy.

Cow & Gate Pepti-Junior Nutricia, Hong Kong.
Infant feed (p.1350·1).
Diarrhoea; food hypersensitivity; malabsorption syndromes; malnutrition; short-bowel syndrome.

Coxa-cyl Ho-Len-Complex Liebermann, Ger.
Homoeopathic preparation.

Coxanturenasi Teoforma, Ital.
Pyridoxine hydrochloride (p.1386·2); pyridoxal phosphate (p.1387·1).
Lignocaine [lidocaine] hydrochloride (p.1313·2) is included in the intramuscular injection to alleviate the pain of injection.
Vitamin B$_6$ and its co-enzyme deficiency.

Cozaar
Merck Sharp & Dohme, Austral.; Merck Sharp & Dohme, Belg.; Merck Sharp & Dohme, Braz.; Merck Frosst, Canad.; Merck Sharp & Dohme, Denm.; Merck Sharp & Dohme, Fin.; Merck Sharp & Dohme-Chibret, Fr.; Merck Sharp & Dohme, Hong Kong; Merck Sharp & Dohme, Irl.; Merck Sharp & Dohme, Mex.; Merck Sharp & Dohme, Neth.; Merck Sharp & Dohme, Norw.; Merck Sharp & Dohme, NZ; Merck Sharp & Dohme, Port.; Merck Sharp & Dohme, S.Afr.; Merck Sharp & Dohme, Singapore; Merck Sharp & Dohme, Spain; Merck Sharp & Dohme, Swed.; Merck Sharp & Dohme, Thai.; Merck Sharp & Dohme, UK; Merck, USA.
Losartan potassium (p.921·3).
Heart failure; hypertension.

Cozaar Comp
Merck Sharp & Dohme, Denm.; Merck Sharp & Dohme, Fin.; Merck Sharp & Dohme, Irl.; Merck Sharp & Dohme, Norw.; Merck Sharp & Dohme, S.Afr.; Merck Sharp & Dohme, Swed.; Merck Sharp & Dohme, UK.
Losartan potassium (p.921·3); hydrochlorothiazide (p.907·3).
Hypertension.

Cozaar Plus
Merck Sharp & Dohme, Belg.; Merck Sharp & Dohme, Port.; Merck Sharp & Dohme, Spain.
Losartan potassium (p.921·3); hydrochlorothiazide (p.907·3).
Hypertension.

Cozole Be-Tabs, S.Afr.
Co-trimoxazole (p.193·3).
Bacterial infections.

C-Plus Hylands, Canad.
Homoeopathic preparation.

C-Poretta Leiras, Fin.
Ascorbic acid (p.1389·3).
Dietary supplement; vitamin C deficiency.

CPS Pulver
Brady, Aust.; Gry, Ger.
Calcium polystyrene sulfonate (p.1002·3).
Hyperkalaemia.

Cracoa B Gelos, Spain.
Aluminium hydroxide (p.1210·3); calcium carbonate (p.1215·1); magnesium carbonate (p.1232·3); magnesium trisilicate (p.1233·3).
Gastrointestinal hyperacidity.

Cradocap Napp, UK.
Cetrimide (p.1137·1).
Cradle cap.

Craegium Biocur, Ger.
Crataegus (p.1600·2).
Bradycardia; heart failure.

Crafilm Francia, Ital.
Sucralfate (p.1250·2).
Gastrointestinal disorders associated with hyperacidity.

Cralonin Heel, Ger.
Homoeopathic preparation.

Cralsanic Hexal, S.Afr.†.
Sucralfate (p.1250·2).
Peptic ulcer.

Cramigen Wayne, Mex.
Amikacin (p.147·3).
Bacterial infections.

Crampex SSL, UK.
Calcium gluconate (p.1188·2); nicotinic acid (p.1372·3); ergocalciferol (p.1391·2).
Night cramps.

Crampiton Orion, Fin.
Quinine hydrochloride (p.445·1); meprobamate (p.691·1).
Muscle spasm; restless leg syndrome.

Cranberry Complex Cenovis, Austral.
Cranberry (p.1600·2); buchu (p.1587·2); bearberry (p.1583·3); ascorbic acid (p.1389·3).
Cystitis; fluid retention.

Cranio-cyl Ho-Len-Complex Liebermann, Ger.
Homoeopathic preparation.

Cranoc Astra, Ger.; Promed, Ger.
Fluvastatin sodium (p.892·1).
Hyperlipidaemias.

Crasnitin Bayer, Ital.†.
Asparaginase (p.508·3).
Leukaemia.

Crataegan Austroplant, Aust.
Crataegus (p.1600·2).
Cardiac disorders.

Crataegisan Bioforce, Switz.
Crataegus (p.1600·2).
Cardiac disorders.

Crataegitan Amino, Switz.
Crataegus (p.1600·2).
Cardiac disorders.

Crataegol LDM, Fr.
Crataegus (p.1600·2).
Insomnia; nervous disorders.

Crataegus Complex Blackmores, Austral.
Tilia platyphyllos (p.1673·2); achillea (p.1572·2); crataegus (p.1600·2); garlic (p.1614·1); ascorbic acid (p.1389·3); hesperidin (p.1611·2); rutoside (p.1611·2).
Cardiovascular disorders.

Crataegus Med Complex Dynamit, Aust.
Homoeopathic preparation.

Crataegutt
Peithner, Aust.; Schwabe, Ger.; Schwabe, Neth.†; Schwabe, Neth.; Schwabe, Spain.
Crataegus (p.1600·2).
Ischaemic heart disease.

Crataegysat F Ysatfabrik, Ger.
Crataegus (p.1600·2).
Cardiac disorders.

Crataelanat Schwabe, Ger.†.
Digoxin (p.870·1); crataegus (p.1600·2).
Heart failure.

Crataepas Pascoe, Ger.
Crataegus (p.1600·2).
Cardiac disorders.

Crataezyma Zyma, Ger.†.
Crataegus (p.1600·2).
Cardiac disorders.

Cratamed novo Redel, Ger.†.
Crataegus (p.1600·2).
Cardiac disorders.

Cratecor Bionorica, Ger.
Crataegus (p.1600·2).
Heart failure.

Cratimon Madaus, Spain.
Benzydamine aescinate.
Peri-articular disorders; soft-tissue disorders.

Craviscum mono CPF, Ger.
Crataegus (p.1600·2).
Cardiac disorders.

Cravit
Daiichi, Hong Kong; Daiichi, Jpn; Daiichi, Singapore; Daiichi, Thai.
Levofloxacin (p.219·1).
Bacterial infections.

Cravo-Espin Virtus, Braz.
Triclosan (p.1159·2); resorcinol (p.1122·2); sulfur (p.1123·3); bentonite (p.1499·2).
Acne.

Creacal Diviser Aquilea, Spain.
Calcium phosphate (p.1188·2); colecalciferol (p.1391·1).
Calcium deficiency.

Creagin Virginia, Ital.
Multivitamin and mineral preparation with creatine, ginkgo biloba and ginseng (p.1350·1).
Tonic.

Cream E45 Boots, NZ.
Emollient.
Dry skin.

Creamy Tar C & M, USA.
Coal tar (p.1125·1).
Scalp disorders.

Creanolona Bohm, Spain.
Fluocinolone acetonide (p.1071·1); neomycin (p.228·1); polymyxin B (p.238·3).
Skin infections with inflammation.

Creatile New Farma, Ital.
Creatine (p.1600·3).
Nutritional supplement.

Creatyl Volchem, Ital.
Amino-acid preparation or amino-acid and carbohydrate preparation (p.1350·1).
Nutritional supplement.

Crecil Vinas, Spain.
Cystine (p.1359·1).
Formerly known as Vitacrecil.
Cystine deficiency.

Credaxol Quimica y Farmacia, Mex.
Ranitidine (p.1246·3).
Peptic ulcer.

Crelo Blanco Yamanouchi, Ital.
Emollient.
Dry skin disorders; pharmaceutical base.

Crema Blanca Bustillos, Mex.
Hydroquinone (p.1115·1).
Skin hyperpigmentation disorders.

Crema Contracepti Lanzas Ipsen, Spain.
Benzalkonium chloride (p.1133·2).
Contraceptive.

Crema de Magnesia Cinfa, Spain.
Magnesium hydroxide (p.1233·1).
Constipation; gastrointestinal hyperacidity.

Crema Facial De Dia AHA Formula 405 Dermaclin, Mex.
SPF 15: Octinoxate (p.1517·3); oxybenzone (p.1518·1).
Sunscreen.

Crema Facial De Noche AHA Formula 405 Dermaclin, Mex.
Moisturiser.

Cremalgin Co-Pharma, UK.
Methyl nicotinate (p.55·1); glycol salicylate (p.42·2); capsicum oleoresin (p.1591·1).
Muscle and joint pain.

Crema-U Jean-Marie, Hong Kong.
Propantheline bromide (p.473·2); hyoscine methobromide (p.468·2); dicyclomine [dicycloverine] hydrochloride (p.466·1); chlorophyllin copper complex sodium (p.1028·1); methiosulfonium chloride (p.1635·1); simeticone (p.1249·2); magnesium hydrox-

ide (p.1233·1); magnesium trisilicate (p.1233·3); dried aluminium hydroxide gel (p.1210·3).
Flatulence; gastrointestinal hyperacidity; painful gastrointestinal spasm; peptic ulcer.

Creme Anti-Rides Auto-Bronzante *Clarins, Canad.*
SPF 15: Octinoxate (p.1517·3); oxybenzone (p.1518·1); titanium dioxide (p.1126·1).
Sunscreen.

Creme Auto-Bronzant *Clarins, Canad.*
SPF 15: Avobenzone (p.1517·1); enzacamene (p.1517·2); oxybenzone (p.1518·1).
Sunscreen.

Creme Autobronzante Visage *Lancome, Canad.†*
Avobenzone (p.1517·1); enzacamene (p.1517·2).
Sunscreen.

Creme de base *Glaxo Wellcome, Switz.*
Emollient.
Skin disorders.

Creme des 3 Fleurs d'Orient *Creme d'Orient, Fr.*
Cream: Hydroquinone (p.1115·1).
Ointment: Mequinol (p.1118·2).
Hyperpigmentation.

Creme Ecran Total *Lancome, Canad.*
SPF 40: Avobenzone (p.1517·1); enzacamene (p.1517·2); terephthalylidene dicamphor sulfonic acid; titanium dioxide (p.1126·1).
Sunscreen.

Creme Haute Protection *Vichy, Canad.†*
SPF 15: Avobenzone (p.1517·1); enzacamene (p.1517·2); terephthalylidene dicamphor sulfonic acid; titanium dioxide (p.1126·1).
Sunscreen.

Creme Laser Hidrante *Dermoteca, Port.*
Squalane (p.1410·2); proline (p.1374·2); urea (p.1127·3); lactic acid (p.1626·2); citric acid (p.1596·2); *dl*-alpha tocopherol (p.1394·1); ruscus aculeatus.
Dry skin; skin irritation.

Creme Protectrice *Lancome, Canad.*
SPF 15: Octinoxate (p.1517·1); enzacamene (p.1517·2); terephthalylidene dicamphor sulfonic acid; titanium dioxide (p.1126·1).
Sunscreen.

Creme Rap *Novartis Sante, Fr.*
Scoparium (p.1661·2); arnica (p.1581·3); aesculus (p.1574·1); hyoscyamus (p.470·1).
Formerly contained scoparium, arnica, aconite root, aesculus, cique, hyoscyamus, and nux vomica.
Soft-tissue disorders; venous insufficiency.

Creme Solaire Anti-Rides *Clarins, Canad.*
SPF 10: Octinoxate (p.1517·3); oxybenzone (p.1518·1); titanium dioxide (p.1126·1).
Sunscreen.

Creme Solaire Bronzage *Clarins, Canad.†*
SPF 15: Octinoxate (p.1517·3); oxybenzone (p.1518·1); titanium dioxide (p.1126·1).
Sunscreen.

Creme Solaire Bronzage Rapide *Clarins, Canad.*
SPF 10: Avobenzone (p.1517·1); octinoxate (p.1517·3); octisalate (p.1518·1); oxybenzone (p.1518·1).
Sunscreen.

Creme Solaire Bronzage Securite *Clarins, Canad.*
SPF 20: Octinoxate (p.1517·3); octisalate (p.1518·1); oxybenzone (p.1518·1); titanium dioxide (p.1126·1).
Sunscreen.

Creme Solaire Bronzage Securite Special *Clarins, Canad.*
SPF 15: Avobenzone (p.1517·1); enzacamene (p.1517·2); oxybenzone (p.1518·1).
Sunscreen.

Creme Solaire Ecran Special Visage *Clarins, Canad.*
SPF 30: Avobenzone (p.1517·1); enzacamene (p.1517·2); octinoxate (p.1517·3); oxybenzone (p.1518·1); ensulizole (p.1517·2); titanium dioxide (p.1126·1).
Sunscreen.

Creme Solaire Haute Protection *Clarins, Canad.*
Octocrilene (p.1518·1); octinoxate (p.1517·3); octisalate (p.1518·1); oxybenzone (p.1518·1); ensulizole (p.1517·2); titanium dioxide (p.1126·1).
Sunscreen.

Cremicort-H *Chefaro, Belg.*
Hydrocortisone (p.1073·3).
Skin disorders.

Cremisona *Diba, Mex.*
Fluocinolone (p.1071·1).
Skin disorders.

Cremol-P *Max Ritter, Switz.†*
Evening primrose oil (p.1613·2).
Dry skin.

Cremol-Ritter *Gebro, Switz.*
A range of skin cleansing and emollient preparations.
Skin disorders.

Cremosan *Quimica y Farmacia, Mex.*
Ketoconazole (p.389·1).
Fungal skin infections.

Cremsol *Quimifar, Spain.*
Linseed oil; calcium hydroxide (p.1588·3); benzocaine (p.1306·2); sulfathiazole (p.257·1); triamcinolone acetonide (p.1080·1); zinc oxide (p.1128·2).
Infected skin disorders.

Crenodyn *Francia, Ital.*
Cefadroxil (p.161·2).
Bacterial infections.

Creo Grippe *Marc-O, Canad.*
Camphor (p.1589·3); eucalyptol (p.1609·2); guaifenesin (p.1092·2).

Creodermol *Medical, Port.*
Creosote (p.1087·3); niaouli oil (p.1640·2); thyme oil (p.1672·3); ephedrine hydrochloride (p.1090·1).
Coughs; respiratory-tract disorders.

Creolina *Pearson, Ital.*
Cresol (p.1142·3).
Surface disinfection.

Creon
Solvay, Austral.; Solvay, Belg.; Solvay, Canad.; Solvay, Fr.; Solvay, Hong Kong; Solvay, Irl.; Solvay, Israel; Solvay, Ital.; Byk Gulden, Mex.; Solvay, Neth.; Boehringer Ingelheim, NZ; Solvay, S.Afr.; Solvay, Switz.; Solvay, UK; Solvay, USA.
Pancreatin (p.1646·1).
Pancreatic insufficiency.

Creo-Rectal *Nadeau, Canad.*
Diphenylpyraline hydrochloride (p.417·1); guaiacol carbonate (p.1092·1); camphor (p.1589·3).
Coughs.

Creo-Terpin *Lee, USA.*
Dextromethorphan hydrobromide (p.1087·3).

Crescicalcio *Prodotti, Braz.*
Calcium phosphate (p.1188·3); vitamins A, D₂, and B₁₂ (p.1350·1).
Calcium and vitamin supplement.

Crescom *Esoform, Ital.*
Sodium *o*-phenylphenol (p.1152·1).
Surface disinfection.

Cresolox *Coventry, UK.*
Tar acids (p.1158·1).

Cresophene
Note. This name is used for preparations of different composition.
Prats, Spain.
Dexamethasone (p.1067·1); hexachlorophene (p.1146·1); prajmalium bitartrate (p.957·2); parachlorophenol (p.1152·1).
Dental caries; oral disinfection.

Septodont, Switz.
Dexamethasone acetate (p.1067·1); thymol (p.1158·3); parachlorophenol (p.1152·1); camphor (p.1589·3).
Root canal infections.

Crestanon *Organon, Mex.*
Allylestrenol (p.2088·3).
Cresylate *Recsei, USA.*
m-Cresyl acetate (p.1142·3); isopropyl alcohol (p.1149·2).
Ear infection.

CRH
Ferring, Aust.; Ferring, Ger.; Ferring, Neth.
Corticorelin (p.1280·1) or corticorelin trifluoroacetate (p.1280·2).
Diagnosis of adrenal disorders.

Crilem *Lemery, Mex.*
Bromocriptine (p.1166·2).

Crimanex *Drossapharm, Switz.*
Dipyrithione (p.1113·3); undecenoic acid diethanolamide (p.396·1).
Scalp disorders.

Crinalsofex *Sofex, Port.†*
Minoxidil (p.934·2).
Alopecia androgenetica.

Criniton *Richter, Aust.; Atzinger, Ger.*
Thymol (p.1158·3); salicylic acid (p.1122·3); rosemary oil (p.1659·3).
Scalp disorders.

Crino Cordes *Ichthyol, Aust.*
Sodium bituminosulfonate (p.1115·3); sodium sulfosuccinated undecenoic acid monoethanolamide (p.396·1).
Scalp disorders.

Crino Cordes N *Ichthyol, Ger.*
Ictasol (p.1115·3).
Scalp disorders; skin disorders.

Crinohermal fem neu *Hermal, Ger.*
Fluprednidene acetate (p.1072·1); estradiol (p.1473·1).
Female hair loss.

Crino-Kaban N *Asche, Ger.*
Clocortolone pivalate (p.1065·3); salicylic acid (p.1122·3).
Scalp disorders.

Crinone *Serono, Ger.; Serono, Irl.; Sifa, Ital.; Wyeth, Mex.; Serono, Singapore; Serono, UK; Serono, USA.*
Progesterone (p.2088·3).
Female infertility; menopausal disorders; menstrual disorders.

Crinopex *Schering-Plough, Swed.†*
Pyrethrin (p.1436·3); piperonyl butoxide (p.1436·2).
Pediculosis.

Crinopex-N *Boehringer Ingelheim, Neth.†*
Pyrethrum (p.1436·3); piperonyl butoxide (p.1436·2).
Pediculosis.

Crinoren *Uriach, Spain.*
Enalapril maleate (p.883·3).
Heart failure; hypertension.

Crinoretic *Uriach, Spain.*
Enalapril maleate (p.883·3); hydrochlorothiazide (p.907·3).
Hypertension.

Crinotar *Agpharm, Switz.†*
Pyrithione zinc (p.1122·1); coal tar (p.1125·1).
Scalp disorders.

Criostat SD 2 *Grifols, Spain†.*
Factor VIII (p.734·1).
Factor VIII deficiency.

Cripar *Taurus, Ger.; Knoll, Ger.*
Dihydroergocryptine mesilate (p.1603·3).
Parkinsonism.

CRI-regen *Pekana, Ger.*
Homoeopathic preparation.

Crisinor *Rubio, Spain†.*
Auranofin (p.18·2).
Rheumatoid arthritis.

Crislaxo *Quimifar, Spain.*
Aloes (p.1210·1); aniseed (p.1580·2); cascara (p.1216·1); senna (p.1248·2); fennel (p.1610·1); rhubarb (p.1248·1); sulfur (p.1123·3); belladonna (p.463·1).
Constipation.

Crismol *Almirall, Spain.*
Fenoterol hydrobromide (p.765·1); ipratropium bromide (p.766·1).
Obstructive airways disease.

Crisolax *Italfarmaco, Ital.†*
Phenolphthalein (p.1244·1); rhubarb (p.1248·1); cascara (p.1216·1); cinchona bark (p.1595·3); frangula (p.1227·1); aloes (p.1210·1).
Constipation; gastrointestinal disorders.

Cristal
Note. This name is used for preparations of different composition.
Pfizer, Ital.†
Multivitamin preparation (p.1350·1).

Vifor, Switz.†
Glycerol (p.1616·3).
Constipation.

Cristalcrom *Cinfa, Spain.*
Chlorhexidine gluconate (p.1138·2).
Skin and wound disinfection.

Cristalmina *Salvat, Spain.*
Chlorhexidine gluconate (p.1138·2).
Skin and wound disinfection.

Cristan *Shin Poong, Singapore.*
Clotrimazole (p.382·1).
Fungal skin infections; vulvovaginal candidiasis.

Cristopal *Alcon, Fr.*
Calcium chloride (p.1188·1); sodium succinate (p.1666·2); magnesium aspartate (p.1190·3); glycine (p.1365·3).
Formerly contained calcium chloride, sodium iodide, and glycine.
Lens opacities.

Criticare HN
Mead Johnson, Austral.; Mead Johnson, Hong Kong; Mead Johnson Nutritionals, USA.
Preparation for enteral nutrition (p.1350·1).

Critichol *Angelini, Ital.*
Fenipentol hemisuccinate (p.1610·1); cascara (p.1216·1); boldo (p.1585·3); rhubarb (p.1248·1).
Constipation.

Crixivan
Merck Sharp & Dohme, Aust.; Merck Sharp & Dohme, Austral.; Merck Sharp & Dohme, Belg.; Merck Frosst, Canad.; Merck Sharp & Dohme, Denm.; Merck Sharp & Dohme, Fin.; Merck Sharp & Dohme-Chibret, Fr.; Merck Sharp & Dohme, Ger.; Merck Sharp & Dohme, Hong Kong; Merck Sharp & Dohme, Ital.; Banyu, Jpn; Merck Sharp & Dohme, Mex.; Merck Sharp & Dohme, Neth.; Merck Sharp & Dohme, Norw.; Merck Sharp & Dohme, NZ; Merck Sharp & Dohme, Port.; Merck Sharp & Dohme, S.Afr.; Merck Sharp & Dohme, Singapore; Merck Sharp & Dohme, Spain; Merck Sharp & Dohme, Swed.; Merck Sharp & Dohme, Switz.; Merck Sharp & Dohme, Thai.; Merck Sharp & Dohme, UK; Merck, USA.
Indinavir sulfate (p.625·2).
HIV infection.

Cro 50 *Investigaciones Filosoficas y Cientificas, Mex.*
Ribonuclease (p.1657·3).

Crodamols *Croda, UK.*
A range of emollient esters.

CroFab *Altana, USA.*
Crotalidae polyvalent immune fab.
Rattlesnake bites.

Croferron *Degorts, Mex.*
Ferrous fumarate (p.1360·1).
Iron-deficiency anaemia.

Croglina *Oftalder, Port.*
Sodium cromoglicate (p.774·3).
Allergic conjunctivitis.

Crolom *Dura, USA.*
Sodium cromoglicate (p.774·3).
Inflammatory disorders of the eye.

Cromabak
Thea, Fr.; Thea, Hong Kong; Pharmacia Upjohn, Singapore.
Sodium cromoglicate (p.774·3).
Allergic eye disorders.

Cromal
Mundipharma, Aust.; Cipla-Medpro, S.Afr.
Sodium cromoglicate (p.774·3).
Obstructive airways disease.

Cromantal *NCSN, Ital.†*
Disodium cromoglicate (p.774·3).
Hypersensitivity reactions.

Cro-Man-Zin *Freeda, USA.*
Chromium, manganese, and zinc preparation (p.1350·1).
Mineral supplement.

Cromaton *Menarini, Belg.†*
Liver extract; suprarenal cortex extract (p.1080·1).
Tonic.

Cromatonbic B12 *Menarini, Spain.*
Cyanocobalamin (p.1388·1).
Vitamin B12 deficiency.

Cromatonbic Ferro *Menarini, Spain.*
Ferrous lactate (p.1360·2).
Iron-deficiency anaemia.

Cromatonbic Folinico *Menarini, Spain.*
Calcium folinate (p.1363·1).
Antidote to folic acid antagonists; enhancement of fluorouracil; megaloblastic anaemia.

Cromatonferro *Menarini, Ital.*
Ferrous gluconate (p.1360·1).
Anaemias; iron deficiency.

Cromedil *Europhta, Mon.*
Sodium cromoglicate (p.774·3).
Allergic eye disorders.

Cromer Orto *Normon, Spain.*
Merbromin (p.1150·1).
Skin and wound disinfection.

Cromese *Pharmacia Upjohn, Austral.*
Sodium cromoglicate (p.774·3).
Asthma.

Cromex *Davi, Port.*
Sodium cromoglicate (p.774·3).
Allergic conjunctivitis.

Cromezin *SoSe, Ital.*
Cefazolin sodium (p.164·3).
Bacterial infections.

Cromo *Ratiopharm, Ger.; CT, Ger.; Stulln, Ger.*
Sodium cromoglicate (p.774·3).
Allergic conjunctivitis; allergic rhinitis; asthma; hypersensitivity reactions.

Cromo Asma *Aldo, Spain.*
Sodium cromoglicate (p.774·3).
Asthma; bronchospasm.

Cromo Pur *CT, Ger.*
Sodium cromoglicate (p.774·3).
Allergic rhinitis.

Cromodyn *Rappai, Switz.*
Sodium cromoglicate (p.774·3).
Allergic rhinitis.

Cromoftol *Merck Sharp & Dohme, Spain†.*
Chlorpheniramine [chlorphenamine] maleate (p.412·1); sodium cromoglicate (p.774·3).
Eye disorders.

Cromogen
Norton Waterford, Irl.; Norton, Israel; Norton, S.Afr.†; Baker Norton, UK.
Sodium cromoglicate (p.774·3).
Asthma.

Cromoglicin *Heumann, Ger.*
Sodium cromoglicate (p.774·3).
Allergic conjunctivitis; allergic rhinitis; asthma.

Cromoglin *Ratiopharm, Aust.*
Sodium cromoglicate (p.774·3).
Allergic eye disorders; obstructive airways disease; rhinitis.

Cromohexal *Hexal, Ger.; Hexal, S.Afr.*
Sodium cromoglicate (p.774·3).
Allergic conjunctivitis; allergic rhinitis; asthma.

Cromol *Betapharm, Ger.*
Sodium cromoglicate (p.774·3).
Hay fever.

Cromolerg *Allergan-Frumtost, Braz.*
Sodium cromoglicate (p.774·3).
Allergic conjunctivitis.

Cromolind *Lindopharm, Ger.*
Sodium cromoglicate (p.774·3).
Asthma.

Cromolyn
Pharmascience, Canad.; Fatol, Ger.; Orion, Ger.
Sodium cromoglicate (p.774·3).
Allergic eye disorders; allergic rhinitis; asthma.

Crom-Ophtal *Winzer, Ger.*
Sodium cromoglicate (p.774·3).
Allergic conjunctivitis; allergic rhinitis.

Cromopp *Pulmopharm, Ger.*
Sodium cromoglicate (p.774·3).
Asthma.

Cromoptic
Chauvin, Fr.; Vitamed, Israel.
Sodium cromoglicate (p.774·3).
Allergic eye disorders.

Cromosan
Note. This name is used for preparations of different composition.
Quimioterapica, Braz.
Injection: Magnesium chromate; magnesium acetate (p.1190·3).
Oral gel: Magnesium bromate; magnesium acetate (p.1190·3); magnesium oxide (p.1233·2); aluminium hydroxide (p.1210·3).
Gastrointestinal hyperacidity.

Medici, Ital.
Sodium cromoglicate (p.774·3).
Food hypersensitivity.

Cromoseptil Plus *Azevedos, Port.*
Povidone-iodine (p.1155·1).
Skin and wound disinfection.

Cromosol Ophta *Ecosol, Switz.*
Sodium cromoglicate (p.774·3).
Conjunctivitis.

Cromosol UD *Ecosol, Switz.*
Sodium cromoglicate (p.774·3).
Asthma.

Cromovisus DMG, Ital.
Calcium phosphate; bioflavonoids; yeast; vitamins (p.1350·1).
Nutritional supplement.

Cromoxin K Rius, Spain.
Carbazochrome (p.728·1); phytomenadione (p.1396·1).
Haemorrhage.

Cromozil Tubilux, Ital.
Tetryzoline hydrochloride (p.1101·2); sodium cromoglicate (p.774·3).
Conjunctivitis.

Cromunal Agis, Israel.
Sodium cromoglicate (p.774·3).
Allergic rhinitis; asthma; bronchitis.

Cronacol Biotekfarma, Ital.†
Sodium cromoglicate (p.774·3).
Food hypersensitivity.

Cronal Valdecasas, Mex.
Chlorpheniramine [chlorphenamine] (p.412·2).
Hypersensitivity.

Cronase Vitamed, Israel.
Sodium cromoglicate (p.774·3).
Allergic rhinitis.

Cronasma Orion, Ger.
Theophylline (p.777·2).
Obstructive airways disease.

Cronassial Fidia, Thai.
Gangliosides (p.1614·1).
Peripheral neuropathies; polyneuropathies.

Croneparina Vedim, Ital.
Heparin calcium (p.902·1).
Atherosclerosis; thromboembolic disorders.

Cronizat Pharmacia Upjohn, Ital.
Nizatidine (p.1238·1).
Gastro-oesophageal reflux; peptic ulcer.

Cronobe Sanus, Braz.
Vitamin B₁₂ (p.1388·1).
Anaemias; vitamin deficiency.

Cronocaps Medix, Mex.
Melatonin (p.1632·1).
Insomnia.

Cronocef Mead Johnson, Ital.
Cefprozil (p.173·2).
Bacterial infections.

Cronocol Schering-Plough, Port.
Gentamicin sulfate (p.210·1).
Bone infections.

Cronodine Alacan, Spain.
Diltiazem hydrochloride (p.874·3).
Angina pectoris; hypertension.

Cronogeron Dansk-Flama, Braz.
Cinnarizine (p.413·1).
Peripheral vascular disorders; vestibular disorders.

Cronol Solvay, Spain.
Famotidine (p.1225·3).
Gastro-oesophageal reflux; peptic ulcer; Zollinger-Ellison syndrome.

Cronomet Merck Sharp & Dohme, Braz.
Carbidopa (p.1168·2); levodopa (p.1169·2).
Parkinsonism.

Cronovera Searle, Mex.
Verapamil hydrochloride (p.989·1).
Angina pectoris; hypertension.

Cross Prep Colgate Oral Care, Austral.†
Chlorhexidine gluconate (p.1138·2); cetrimide (p.1137·1).
Surface disinfection.

Crotamitex Gepepharm, Ger.
Crotamiton (p.1112·3).
Pruritic skin disorders.

Cruex
Note. This name is used for preparations of different composition.
Novartis Consumer, Canad.†; Ciba Consumer, USA.
Aerosol; cream: Undecenoic acid (p.395·3); zinc undecenoate (p.395·3).
Bromhidrosis; fungal skin infections; hyperhidrosis; minor skin irritation; nappy rash.

Novartis Consumer, Canad.†; Rhone-Poulenc Rorer, Mex.; Ciba Consumer, USA.
Topical powder: Calcium undecenoate (p.395·3).
Bromhidrosis; fungal skin infections; hyperhidrosis; minor skin irritation; nappy rash.

Cruscasohn Antonetta, Ital.
Cereal fibre; guar gum (p.323·3); pectin (p.1502·3).
Constipation.

Crusken
Maggioni, Ital.; SmithKline Beecham, Ital.; Sterling Midy, Ital.
A range of dietary fibre supplements (p.1214·2).
Delayed gastrointestinal transit.

Cruzzy SIT, Ital.
Lotion: Pyrethrum (p.1436·3); piperonyl butoxide (p.1436·2); diethyltoluamide (p.1431·2).
Shampoo: Phenothrin (p.1436·2).
Pediculosis.

Cruzzy Antiparassitario SIT, Ital.
Pyrethrum (p.1436·3); piperonyl butoxide (p.1436·2).
Pediculosis.

Cryobutol Cryopharma, Mex.
Dobutamine (p.880·3).

Cryocriptina Cryopharma, Mex.
Bromocriptine (p.1166·2).
Hyperprolactinaemia; lactation inhibition.

Cryogesic Acorus, UK.
Ethyl chloride (p.1312·1).
Local anaesthesia; testing of regional blockade; testing of tooth vitality.

Cryometasona Cryopharma, Mex.
Dexamethasone (p.1067·1).
Corticosteroid.

Cryoperacid Cryopharma, Mex.
Loperamide hydrochloride (p.1231·3).
Diarrhoea.

Cryopina Cryopharma, Mex.
Hyoscine butylbromide (p.468·2).

Cryopril Cryopharma, Mex.
Captopril (p.853·3).
Heart failure; hypertension.

Cryosolona Cryopharma, Mex.
Methylprednisolone sodium succinate (p.1076·1).
Corticosteroid.

Cryo-Tropin Cryopharma, Mex.
Somatropin (p.1286·1).
Growth hormone deficiency; Turner's syndrome.

Cryoval Cryopharma, Mex.
Valproic acid (p.366·2).
Epilepsy.

Cryovin Cryopharma, Mex.
Ergometrine (p.1607·1).

Cryoxifeno Pizzard, Mex.
Tamoxifen (p.572·2).

Cryozol Cryopharma, Mex.
Metronidazole (p.594·1).

Cryptocur Hoechst Marion Roussel, Neth.
Gonadorelin (p.1283·3).
Cryptorchidism.

Crysanal Macarthur, Austral.
Naproxen sodium (p.61·1).
Inflammation; musculoskeletal and joint disorders; pain.

Crystacide
Medeva, Belg.; Bioglan, Ger.; Bioglan, Irl.; Bioglan, Israel; Medeva, Spain; Bioglan, UK.
Hydrogen peroxide (p.1147·1).
Skin infections.

Crystamine Dunhall, USA.
Cyanocobalamin (p.1388·1).
Schilling test; vitamin B₁₂ deficiency.

Crystapen
Bioniche, Canad.; Britannia Pharmaceuticals, Irl.; Britannia Pharmaceuticals, UK.
Benzylpenicillin sodium (p.157·2).
Bacterial infections.

Crysti 1000 Roberts, USA; Hauck, USA.
Cyanocobalamin (p.1388·1).
Schilling test; vitamin B₁₂ deficiency.

Crysticillin Apothecon, USA.
Procaine penicillin [procaine benzylpenicillin] (p.239·2).
Bacterial infections.

Crystodigin Lilly, USA.
Digitoxin (p.869·2).
Atrial flutter and fibrillation; heart failure; supraventricular tachycardia.

C-Soft Austroflex, Aust.
Rinsing and storage solution for soft contact lenses (p.1129·2).

C-Solve Syosset, USA.
Vehicle for topical preparations.

CST Pose, Thai.
Clotrimazole (p.382·1).
Fungal vaginal infections; trichomoniasis.

CT Ointment Life, Israel.
Coal tar (p.1125·1); dead sea minerals.
Psoriasis; seborrhoeic dermatitis.

CT Pommade Life, Israel.
Coal tar (p.1125·1); salicylic acid (p.1122·3); dead sea minerals.
Psoriasis of the scalp.

CT Shampoo Life, Israel.
Coal tar (p.1125·1); tar (p.1125·1); cade oil (p.1124·3); dead sea minerals.
Psoriasis; seborrhoeic dermatitis.

C-Tabs Ferrosan, Fin.
Ascorbic acid (p.1389·3).
Dietary supplement; vitamin C deficiency.

C-Tard Whitehall, Ital.
Ascorbic acid (p.1389·3).
Vitamin C deficiency.

C/T/S Hoechst Roussel, USA.
Clindamycin phosphate (p.188·2).
Acne.

Cuatroderm Schering-Plough, Spain.
Betamethasone valerate (p.1063·2); clioquinol (p.190·2); gentamicin sulfate (p.210·1); tolnaftate (p.395·2).
Infected skin disorders.

Cubitan Nutricia, Fr.
Nutritional supplement (p.1350·1).
Bedsores.

Cuerpo Amarillo Fuerte Hormona, Mex.
Progesterone (p.1488·3).

Cuidaderma Caldeira & Marques, Port.
Zinc oxide (p.1128·2); almond oil (p.1576·3); starch (p.1379·3); talc (p.1124·2).
Skin irritation.

Culat Roche, Aust.
Epoetin beta (p.731·1).
Anaemia of prematurity, chronic renal failure or malignant disease; autologous blood transfusions.

Cullens Headache Powders Cullen & Davison, UK.
Aspirin (p.14·2); caffeine (p.761·3).

Cultivo BCG Lemery, Mex.
BCG vaccine (p.1533·2).
Bladder cancer.

Culturelle LCG Nordic, UK.
Lactobacillus GG (p.1626·3).
Maintenance of healthy gastrointestinal flora.

Cunesin Recordati, Spain.
Ciprofloxacin hydrochloride (p.182·3).
Bacterial infections.

Cunil Helsinn Birex, Irl.
Ibuprofen (p.43·2).
Musculoskeletal, joint, and peri-articular disorders; pain; soft-tissue injuries.

CuNova T Leiras, Denm.
Copper-wound plastic (p.1357·3) with a silver core (p.1664·1).
Intra-uterine contraceptive device.

Cunticina Rovifarma, Spain.
Albumin tannate (p.1209·3).
Diarrhoea.

Cupanol Dermofarm, Spain.
Paracetamol (p.71·2).
Fever; pain.

Cuplaton Orion, Fin.; Orion, Singapore.
Dimethicone (p.1249·2).
Aid in gastrointestinal radiography and gastroscopy; flatulence; meteorism.

Cuplex
Trans Canaderm, Canad.; Smith & Nephew, Irl.; Smith & Nephew Healthcare, UK.
Salicylic acid (p.1122·3); lactic acid (p.1626·2).
Calluses; corns; warts.

Cupressin Takeda, Singapore.; Takeda, Thai.
Delapril hydrochloride (p.867·1).
Hypertension.

Cupridium DHU, Ger.
Homoeopathic preparation.

Cuprimine
Prodome, Braz.; Merck Frosst, Canad.; Merck Sharp & Dohme, Israel.; Merck Sharp & Dohme, Neth.†; Merck Sharp & Dohme, Norw.; Merck Sharp & Dohme, Swed.; Merck Sharp & Dohme, Thai.; Merck, USA.
Penicillamine (p.1017·1).
Cystinuria; heavy metal poisoning; rheumatoid arthritis; Wilson's disease.

Cupripen Rubio, Spain.
Penicillamine (p.1017·1).
Biliary cirrhosis; cystinuria; heavy-metal poisoning; rheumatoid arthritis; Wilson's disease.

Cuprocept CCL Cuprocept, S.Afr.
Copper-wound plastic (p.1357·3).
Intra-uterine contraceptive device.

Cuprofen SSL, UK.
Ibuprofen (p.43·2).
Cold and influenza symptoms; fever; inflammation; pain.

Cuprosodio Bier, Ital.
Cetrimide (p.1137·1); copper sulfate (p.1358·1); zinc sulfate (p.1398·2).
Personal hygiene.

Cura Arnaldi-Uscio, Ital.†
Tablets (500 mg): Aloes (p.1210·1); senna (p.1248·2); althaea (p.1577·1); liquorice (p.1231·2); ferrous sulfate (p.1360·3); vegetable charcoal (p.1000·3).
Tablets (1 g); oral powder: Melissa (p.1632·2); cascarilla; quassia (p.1657·1); senna (p.1248·2); ginger (p.1227·2); aloes (p.1210·1); althaea (p.1577·1); laurel; myrtle; bergamot oil (p.1584·2).
Constipation.

Curacit Nycomed, Norw.
Suxamethonium chloride (p.1340·1).
Depolarising neuromuscular blocker.

Curacleanse Curacel, Austral.
Cetrimide (p.1137·1); chlorhexidine gluconate (p.1138·2).
Skin and wound disinfection.

Curadent Leti, Spain.
Lignocaine [lidocaine] hydrochloride (p.1313·2).
Local anaesthesia in dentistry.

Curaderm Curacel, Austral.
Salicylic acid (p.1122·3); urea (p.1127·3); melaleuca oil (p.1631·3); linoleic acid (p.1613·2); solasodine glycosides.
UV-induced skin damage.

Curadon Tika, Swed.
Paracetamol (p.71·2).
Fever; pain.

Curafil Betamadrileno, Spain.
Chlorhexidine gluconate (p.1138·2).
Skin and wound disinfection.

Curakalos Stevia, Braz.
Salicylic acid (p.1122·3).
Keratinisation disorders.

Curam
Biochemie, Hong Kong; Biochemie, Singapore; Novartis, Thai.; Servipharm, Thai.
Amoxicillin (p.149·2); clavulanic acid (p.187·2) or potassium clavulanate (p.187·2).
Bacterial infections.

Curantyl N Berlin-Chemie, Ger.
Dipyridamole (p.877·2).
Angina pectoris; heart failure; myocardial infarction.

Curapic Leti, Spain.
Diphenhydramine hydrochloride (p.416·1); lignocaine [lidocaine] hydrochloride (p.1313·2).
Insect stings; pruritus.

Curarina Miro Palex, Spain†.
Tubocurarine chloride (p.1343·1).
Competitive neuromuscular blocker.

Curarine Taro, Israel.
Tubocurarine chloride (p.1343·1).
Competitive neuromuscular blocker.

Curash Anti-Rash Carter-Wallace, Austral.
Zinc oxide (p.1128·2).
Hyperhidrosis; nappy rash; skin irritation.

Curash Baby Wipes Carter-Wallace, Austral.
Vitamin E (p.1393·3); sorbolene.
Skin cleanser and moisturiser.

Curash Babycare Carter-Wallace, Austral.
dl-Alpha tocoferil acetate (p.1394·1); zinc oxide (p.1128·2); almond oil (p.1576·3).
Nappy rash.

Curash Medicated Carter-Wallace, Austral.
Zinc oxide (p.1128·2).
Skin irritation.

Curastain Young, USA†.
Trolamine (p.1675·1).
Reduction of dithranol-induced staining.

Curastatin Curamed, Aust.
Somatostatin acetate (p.1297·3).
Gastrointestinal haemorrhage; prevention of postoperative complications following pancreatic surgery.

Curasten Therabel, Fr.
Lysine hydrochloride (p.1370·3); calcium gluceptate (p.1188·1).
Asthenia.

Curatin Carter-Wallace, Austral.
Cream: Tolnaftate (p.395·2); chlorocresol (p.1141·3).
Powder: Tolnaftate (p.395·2).
Fungal skin infections.

Curativ QIF, Braz.
Thiomersal (p.1158·2).
Skin and wound disinfection; skin disorders.

Curatoderm
Hermal, Aust.; Boots Healthcare, Belg.; Hermal, Ger.; Hermal, Israel; Boots Healthcare, Switz.; Crookes Healthcare, UK.
Tacalcitol (p.1124·2).
Psoriasis.

Curaven Boehringer Ingelheim, Ital.
Aesculus (p.1574·1).
Peripheral vascular disorders.

Curazink Redino, Ger.
Zinc histidinate.
Zinc deficiency.

Curcumen Temmler, Ger.
Curcuma zanthorrhiza.
Dyspepsia.

Curel Bausch & Lomb, USA.
Emollient and moisturiser.

Curethyl AJC, Fr.†.
Alcohol (p.1130·3).
Alcohol withdrawal syndromes.

Curine Leti, Spain.
Benzalkonium chloride (p.1133·2); lignocaine [lidocaine] hydrochloride (p.1313·2).
Pain; pruritus.

Curlem Marcel, Mex.
Vecuronium bromide (p.1343·2).

Curocef Glaxo Wellcome, Aust.
Cefuroxime sodium (p.178·2).
Bacterial infections.

Curon-B Intramed, S.Afr.
Pancuronium bromide (p.1338·2).
Competitive neuromuscular blocker.

Curosurf
Serono, Aust.; Farmalab, Braz.; Serono, Denm.; Serono, Fin.; Serono, Fr.; Serono, Ger.; Serono, Irl.; SLE, Israel; Chiesi, Ital.; Serono, Neth.; Serono, Norw.; Serono, Port.; Serono, Spain; Serono, Swed.; Serono, Switz.; Trinity, UK; Dey, USA.
Poractant alfa (p.1656·1).
Neonatal respiratory distress syndrome.

Curoveinyl Pharmygiene, Fr.†
Aesculus (p.1574·1); hamamelis (p.1618·3); hydrastis (p.1621·1); cupressus sempervirens; scoparium (p.1661·2); nux vomica (p.1643·1).
Peripheral vascular disorders.

Curoxim Glaxo Wellcome, Ital.
Cefuroxime sodium (p.178·2).
Bacterial infections.

Curoxima Glaxo Wellcome, Spain.
Cefuroxime sodium (p.178·2).
Bacterial infections.

Curoxime Glaxo Wellcome, Port.
Cefuroxime sodium (p.178·2).
Bacterial infections.

The symbol † denotes a preparation no longer actively marketed

Curpol Warner-Lambert Consumer, Belg.
Paracetamol (p.71·2).
Fever; pain.

Cusate Pharmasant, Thai.
Docusate sodium (p.1223·1).
Constipation.

Cuscutine Geymonat, Ital.
Senna (p.1248·2); aloin (p.1210·2).
Constipation.

Cusicrom
Alcon, Hong Kong; Kener, Mex.; Alcon, Port.†; Cusi, Singapore; Alcon Cusi, Spain; Farmacusi, Spain.
Sodium cromoglicate (p.774·3).
Allergic eye disorders; allergic rhinitis; hay fever.

Cusigel Farmacusi, Spain.
Fluocinonide (p.1071·2).
Skin disorders.

Cusimolol
Alcon, Hong Kong; Alcon, Ital.; Kener, Mex.; Alcon, Port.; Alcon Cusi, Spain.
Timolol maleate (p.982·1).
Glaucoma; ocular hypertension.

Cusiter Cusi, Spain†.
Lactic acid (p.1626·2); triclocarban (p.1159·2).
Skin disinfection.

Cusiviral
Cusi, Singapore; Alcon Cusi, Spain; Britisfarma, Spain; Farmacusi, Spain.
Aciclovir (p.612·3) or aciclovir sodium (p.612·3).
Herpesvirus infections.

Custodiol
Kohler, Aust.; Kohler, Ger.
Organ perfusion solution (p.1180·1).

Customed Chefaro, Ger.†.
Bromhexine hydrochloride (p.1085·3); thymol (p.1158·3).
Coughs; respiratory-tract disorders; sinusitis.

Cutacelan Schering, Mex.
Azelaic acid (p.1110·3).
Acne.

Cutaclin ICN, Mex.
Clindamycin phosphate (p.188·2).
Acne; pyodermas.

Cutacnyl Galderma, Fr.
Benzoyl peroxide (p.1111·1).
Acne.

Cutaderm Schering-Plough, S.Afr.
Hydrocortisone (p.1073·3).
Skin disorders.

Cutanit Yamanouchi, Spain.
Fluclorolone acetonide (p.1069·3).
Skin disorders.

Cutanplast Mascia Brunelli, Ital.
Gelatin (p.737·2).
Haemostasis.

Cutanum Jenapharm, Ger.
Estradiol (p.1473·1).
Menopausal disorders.

Cutar Summers, USA.
Coal tar (p.1125·1).
Skin disorders.

Cutasept
Beiersdorf, Aust.; Bode, Ger.
Isopropyl alcohol (p.1149·2); benzalkonium chloride (p.1133·2).
Skin disinfection.

Cutemol Summers, USA.
Emollient and moisturiser.

Cutemul Medopharm, Ger.†.
Dexpanthenol (p.1602·3).
Burns; inflammatory skin disorders; wounds.

Cuterpes
Chauvin, Fr.; Chauvin, Hong Kong.
Ibacitabine (p.625·1).
Herpes simplex infections.

Cuticura DEP, USA.
Triclocarban (p.1159·2).
Skin cleanser.

Cuti-Do Grasler, Ger.
Homoeopathic preparation.

Cutifitol Llorente, Spain.
Progesterone (p.1488·3).
Hair, scalp, and skin disorders.

Cutimix Metochem, Aust.
Zinc oxide (p.1128·2); talc (p.1124·2).
Skin disorders.

Cutinova Beiersdorf, UK.
Polyurethane foam dressing.
Burns; ulcers; wounds.

Cutinova Alginate Beiersdorf, Ital.
Calcium alginate (p.728·1).
Wounds.

Cutiphile Braun, Fr.
Bismuth subgallate (p.1213·2); bismuth subnitrate (p.1213·2); zinc oxide (p.1128·2).
Skin disorders.

Cutisan Boots Healthcare, Fr.
Triclocarban (p.1159·2).
Skin disorders.

Cutisanol Millet Roux, Braz.
Magnesium silicate (p.1502·1); thymol iodide (p.1158·3); zinc oxide (p.1128·2); bismuth subgallate (p.1213·2).
Skin disorders.

cutistad
Stada, Ger.; Helvepharm, Switz.†.
Clotrimazole (p.382·1).
Fungal skin infections.

Cutivat Glaxo Wellcome, Denm.
Fluticasone propionate (p.1072·2).
Skin disorders.

Cutivate
Glaxo Wellcome, Aust.; Glaxo Wellcome, Belg.; Glaxo Wellcome, Hong Kong; Glaxo Wellcome, Israel; Glaxo Wellcome, Mex.; Glaxo Wellcome, Neth.; Glaxo Wellcome, Port.; Allen & Hanburys, S.Afr.; Glaxo Wellcome, Singapore; Glaxo Wellcome, Spain; Glaxo Wellcome, Switz.; Glaxo Wellcome, UK; Glaxo Wellcome, USA.
Fluticasone propionate (p.1072·2).
Skin disorders.

Cuvalit Schering, Ger.
Lisuride maleate (p.1174·1).
Migraine.

Cuveflam Calmante Vitaminado, Spain.
Chlorhexidine gluconate (p.1138·2).
Skin and wound disinfection.

Cuxabrain TAD, Ger.
Piracetam (p.1652·1).
Mental function disorders.

Cuxacillin TAD, Ger.†.
Amoxicillin trihydrate (p.149·2).
Bacterial infections.

Cuxafenon TAD, Ger.
Propafenone hydrochloride (p.961·3).
Arrhythmias.

Cuxaflex N TAD, Ger.†.
Ointment: Methyl salicylate (p.55·1); benzyl nicotinate (p.20·2); turpentine oil (p.1676·3).
Topical gel: Glycol salicylate (p.42·2); benzyl nicotinate (p.20·2).
Musculoskeletal, joint, and soft-tissue disorders; neuralgia.

Cuxaflex Thermo TAD, Ger.†.
Glycol salicylate (p.42·2); benzyl nicotinate (p.20·2).
Musculoskeletal, joint, and soft-tissue disorders.

Cuxanorm TAD, Ger.
Atenolol (p.841·3).
Arrhythmias; hypertension; ischaemic heart disease.

C-vimin
AstraZeneca, Fin.; Astra, Swed.
Ascorbic acid (p.1389·3).
Vitamin C deficiency.

C-Vit Novartis Consumer, Aust.
Ascorbic acid (p.1389·3).
Vitamin C deficiency.

CVP Rhone-Poulenc Rorer, Ital.†.
Bioflavonoids (p.1611·1); ascorbic acid (p.1389·3).
Gingivitis; stomatitis; vitamin C deficiency.

C-Will
Will-Pharma, Belg.; Will-Pharma, Neth.; Willpharma, Thai.
Ascorbic acid (p.1389·3).
Vitamin C deficiency.

CX Powder Adams, UK.
Chlorhexidine acetate (p.1138·2).
Skin disinfection.

Cyanide Antidote Package Lilly, USA.
Combination pack: 2 Ampoules, sodium nitrite (p.1023·1); 2 ampoules, sodium thiosulfate (p.1024·2); 12 aspirols, amyl nitrite (p.1002·1).
Cyanide poisoning.

Cyanoject Mayrand, USA.
Cyanocobalamin (p.1388·1).
Schilling test; vitamin B12 deficiency.

Cyanokit Lipha Sante, Fr.
Hydroxocobalamin (p.1388·1).
Cyanide poisoning.

Cyater Sigma-Tau, Spain.
Terfenadine (p.424·3).
Hypersensitivity reactions.

Cyclabil Schering, Fin.; Schering, Norw.; Schering, Swed.
11 Tablets, estradiol valerate (p.1473·2); 10 tablets, estradiol valerate; levonorgestrel (p.1486·2).
Menopausal disorders; menstrual disorders; osteoporosis.

Cyclacur
Schering, Aust.; Schering, Switz.
11 Tablets, estradiol valerate (p.1473·2); 10 tablets, estradiol valerate; norgestrel (p.1486·1).
Menopausal disorders; menstrual disorders.

Cycladol
Chiesi, Fr.; Wasserman, Spain.
Piroxicam betadex (p.79·1).
Gout; musculoskeletal, joint, and peri-articular disorders; pain.

Cyclafem Dolisos, Canad.
Homoeopathic preparation.

Cyclan Major, USA†.
Cyclandelate (p.865·2).
Cerebrovascular and peripheral vascular disorders.

Cycleane Monsanto, Fr.
Desogestrel (p.1470·3); ethinylestradiol (p.1476·2).
Combined oral contraceptive.

Cyclen Janssen-Ortho, Canad.
Norgestimate (p.1486·1); ethinylestradiol (p.1476·2).
28-Day packs also contain 7 inert tablets.
Combined oral contraceptive.

Cyclergine Poirier, Fr.
Cyclandelate (p.865·2).
Peripheral vascular disorders.

Cyclidox Triomed, S.Afr.
Doxycycline hyclate (p.200·1).
Bacterial infections.

Cyclimorph
Calmic, Irl.; Glaxo Wellcome, S.Afr.; CeNeS, UK.
Morphine tartrate (p.56·2); cyclizine tartrate (p.414·1).
Pain.

Cyclimycin Aspen, S.Afr.
Minocycline (p.225·3).
Bacterial infections.

Cyclinex Ross, USA.
A range of preparations for enteral nutrition including an infant feed (p.1350·1).
Gyrate atrophy; urea cycle disorder.

Cyclivex Aspen, S.Afr.
Aciclovir (p.612·3).
Herpesvirus infections.

Cyclo 3
Note. This name is used for preparations of different composition.
Pierre Fabre, Fr.; Orient, Singapore; Pierre Fabre, Singapore.
Ruscus aculeatus; melilot.
Circulatory disorders.

Pierre Fabre, Port.
Sterol heterosides from Ruscus aculeatus; hesperidin methyl chalcone (p.1611·2); ascorbic acid (p.1389·3).
Haemorrhoids; metrorrhagia; venous insufficiency.

Cyclo 3 Fort
Pierre Fabre, Fr.; Orient, Singapore; Pierre Fabre, Singapore; Pierre Fabre, Thai.
Ruscus aculeatus; hesperidin methyl chalcone (p.1611·2); vitamin C (p.1389·3).
Bleeding during oral contraceptive or intra-uterine device use; circulatory disorders; haemorrhoids.

Cyclobiol Yves Ponroy, Fr.†.
Nutritional supplement (p.1350·1).
Premenstrual syndrome.

Cycloblastin
Pharmacia Upjohn, Austral.; Pharmacia Upjohn, NZ; Pharmacia Upjohn, S.Afr.
Cyclophosphamide (p.527·3).
Auto-immune diseases; malignant neoplasms; transplant rejection.

Cycloblastine
Pharmacia Upjohn, Belg.; Pharmacia, Neth.†.
Cyclophosphamide (p.527·3).
Malignant neoplasms.

Cyclocaps
Note. This name is used for preparations of different composition.
PB, Ger.
Salbutamol sulfate (p.770·3).
Obstructive airways disease.

PB, Ger.
Beclometasone dipropionate (p.1061·2).
Respiratory-tract disorders.

Cyclo-cell Cell Pharm, Ger.
Cyclophosphamide (p.527·3).
Malignant neoplasms.

Cyclocort
Stiefel, Canad.; Fujisawa, USA.
Amcinonide (p.1061·2).
Skin disorders.

Cyclocur
Schering, Belg.; Schering, Neth.
11 Tablets, estradiol valerate (p.1473·2); 10 tablets, estradiol valerate; norgestrel (p.1486·1).
Menopausal disorders; menstrual disorders.

Cyclodox Berk, UK.
Doxycycline (p.200·1).
Bacterial infections.

Cyclofemina Carnot, Mex.
Medroxyprogesterone acetate (p.1480·1); estradiol cipionate (p.1473·2).
Injectable contraceptive.

Cyclogest
Cox, Hong Kong; Aventis, S.Afr.; Hoechst Marion Roussel, Thai.; Shire, UK.
Progesterone (p.1488·3).
Female infertility; premenstrual syndrome; puerperal depression.

Cyclogyl
Alcon, Austral.; Alcon, Canad.; Alcon, Denm.; Alcon, Neth.†; Alcon, NZ; Alcon, S.Afr.; Alcon, Singapore; Alcon, Swed.; Alcon, Switz.; Alcon, Thai.; Alcon, USA.
Cyclopentolate hydrochloride (p.465·2).
Production of mydriasis and cycloplegia.

Cyclomandol Yamanouchi, Swed.
Cyclandelate (p.865·2).
Vascular disorders.

Cyclomen Sanofi Synthelabo, Canad.
Danazol (p.1468·3).
Endometriosis; mastalgia; primary menorrhagia.

Cyclo-Menorette Wyeth, Ger.
11 Tablets, estradiol valerate (p.1473·2); estriol (p.1475·3); 10 tablets, estradiol valerate; estriol; levonorgestrel (p.1486·2).
Menopausal disorders; osteoporosis.

Cyclomin Berk, UK†.
Minocycline (p.225·3).
Bacterial infections.

Cyclomydri Thilo, Neth.†.
Cyclopentolate hydrochloride (p.465·2).
Production of mydriasis and cycloplegia.

Cyclomydril
Alcon, S.Afr.; Alcon, Singapore; Alcon, USA.
Cyclopentolate hydrochloride (p.465·2); phenylephrine hydrochloride (p.1097·1).
Production of mydriasis.

CycloOstrogynal Asche, Ger.
11 Tablets, estradiol valerate (p.1473·2); estriol (p.1475·3); 10 tablets, estradiol valerate; estriol; levonorgestrel (p.1486·2).
Menopausal disorders.

Cyclopentol Asta Medica, Belg.
Cyclopentolate hydrochloride (p.465·2).
Prevention of iridocrystalline adherences; prevention of synechiae; production of mydriasis and cycloplegia.

CycloPolar Orion, Fin.
White tablets, estradiol valerate (p.1473·2); blue tablets, estradiol valerate; medroxyprogesterone acetate (p.1480·1).
Menopausal disorders.

Cyclo-Premarin-MPA Wyeth Lederle, Aust.
Redbrown tablets, conjugated oestrogens (p.1467·1); blue tablets, conjugated oestrogens; medroxyprogesterone acetate (p.1480·1).
Menopausal disorders.

Cyclo-Premella
Wyeth Lederle, Aust.†.
14 Tablets, conjugated oestrogens (p.1467·1); 14 tablets, conjugated oestrogens; medroxyprogesterone acetate (p.1480·1).
Menopausal disorders.

Wyeth, Switz.†.
28 Tablets, conjugated oestrogens (p.1467·1); 14 tablets medroxyprogesterone acetate (p.1480·1).
Menopausal disorders; oestrogen deficiency.

Cyclo-Premella ST Wyeth, Switz.
14 Tablets, conjugated oestrogens (p.1467·1); 14 tablets, conjugated oestrogens; medroxyprogesterone acetate (p.1480·1).
Menopausal disorders; oestrogen deficiency.

Cyclo-Progynon Schering, Denm.
11 Tablets, estradiol valerate (p.1473·2); 10 tablets, estradiol valerate; levonorgestrel (p.1486·2).
Menopausal disorders; osteoporosis.

Cyclo-Progynova
Schering, Ger.; Schering, Thai.
11 Tablets, estradiol valerate (p.1473·2); 10 tablets, estradiol valerate; norgestrel (p.1486·1).
Menopausal disorders; menstrual disorders; osteoporosis.

Cyclo-Progynova 1 mg Asta Medica, UK.
11 Tablets, estradiol valerate (p.1473·2); 10 tablets, estradiol valerate; levonorgestrel (p.1486·2).
Menopausal disorders.

Cyclo-Progynova 2 mg Asta Medica, UK.
11 Tablets, estradiol valerate (p.1473·2); 10 tablets, estradiol valerate; norgestrel (p.1486·1).
Menopausal disorders.

Cyclorax Atlantic, Thai.
Aciclovir (p.612·3).
Herpes simplex infections of the skin and mucous membranes.

Cyclorel Alpharma, Fr.
Naringin sodium.
Circulatory disorders.

Cyclosa Nourypharma, Ger.
7 Tablets, ethinylestradiol (p.1476·2); 15 tablets, ethinylestradiol; desogestrel (p.1470·3).
Menstrual disorders.

Cycloserine Lilly, UK.
Cycloserine (p.195·3).
Tuberculosis; urinary-tract infections.

Cyclospasmol
Yamanouchi, Belg.; Wyeth-Ayerst, Canad.†; Yamanouchi, Fin.; Yamanouchi, Fr.; Yamanouchi, Neth.†; Yamanouchi, Port.; Wyeth-Ayerst, USA†.
Cyclandelate (p.865·2).
Peripheral and cerebral vascular disorders.

Cyclostin Pharmacia Upjohn, Ger.
Cyclophosphamide (p.527·3).
Malignant neoplasms.

Cycloteriam Roussel Diamant, Fr.†.
Triamterene (p.986·1); cyclothiazide (p.865·3).
Hypertension; oedema.

Cycloven Forte N CT, Ger.
Aesculus (p.1574·1); esculoside (p.1574·1); rutoside (p.1611·2).
Peripheral vascular disorders.

Cycloviran Sigma-Tau, Ital.
Aciclovir (p.612·3).
Herpesvirus infections.

Cycofed Cypress, USA.
Codeine phosphate (p.25·2); pseudoephedrine hydrochloride (p.1099·2); guaifenesin (p.1092·2).
Coughs.

Cycrin
Wyeth, Braz.; Wyeth, Mex.; ESI, Spain.
Medroxyprogesterone acetate (p.1480·1).
Abnormal uterine bleeding; secondary amenorrhoea.

Cydec Cypress, USA.
Carbinoxamine maleate (p.411·1); pseudoephedrine hydrochloride (p.1099·2).

Cydec DM Cypress, USA.
Carbinoxamine maleate (p.411·1); pseudoephedrine hydrochloride (p.1099·2); dextromethorphan hydrobromide (p.1087·3).

Cydoxmine-B PD, Thai.
Vitamin B1 (p.1385·2); vitamin B6 (p.1387·1); vitamin B12 (p.1388·1).
Megaloblastic anaemia; nausea and vomiting; neuritis; polyneuritis.

Cy-Gesic Cypress, USA.
Phenylephrine hydrochloride (p.1097·1); phenazone (p.77·2); benzocaine (p.1306·2).
Earache.

Cyheptine *Greater Pharma, Thai.*
Cyproheptadine (p.414·3).
Hypersensitivity reactions; pruritus; reduced appetite.

Cyklo-F *Pharmacia Upjohn, Swed.*
Tranexamic acid (p.742·2).
Menorrhagia.

Cyklokapron
Pharmacia Upjohn, Aust.; Pharmacia Upjohn, Austral.; Pharmacia Upjohn, Canad.; Pharmacia Upjohn, Denm.; Pharmacia Upjohn, Fin.; Pharmacia Upjohn, Ger.; Pharmacia Upjohn, Hong Kong; Pharmacia Upjohn, Irl.; Pharmacia Upjohn, Neth.; Pharmacia Upjohn, Norw.; Pharmacia Upjohn, NZ; Pharmacia Upjohn, S.Afr.; Pharmacia Upjohn, Singapore; Pharmacia Upjohn, Swed.; Pharmacia Upjohn, Switz.; Pharmacia, UK; Kabivitrum, USA.
Tranexamic acid (p.742·2).
Dental extraction in haemophiliacs; fibrinolysis; hereditary angioedema; menorrhagia.

Cykrina *Wyeth Lederle, Fin.; Wyeth Lederle, Swed.*
Medroxyprogesterone acetate (p.1480·1).
Endometriosis; menopausal disorders; menstrual disorders.

Cylate *Ocusoft, USA†.*
Cyclopentolate hydrochloride (p.465·2).

Cylert *Abbott, Canad.†; Abbott, Israel; Abbott, USA.*
Pemoline (p.1513·1).
Attention deficit hyperactivity disorder.

Cylex *Pharmakon, USA.*
Benzocaine (p.1306·2); cetylpyridinium chloride (p.1138·1).
Sore throat.

Cyllind *Abbott, Ger.*
Clarithromycin (p.186·2).
Bacterial infections.

Cylocide *Shinyaku, Jpn.*
Cytarabine (p.530·1).
Acute leukaemias.

Cymalon *Seton, Irl.; SSL, UK.*
Sodium citrate (p.1186·2); anhydrous citric acid (p.1596·2); sodium bicarbonate (p.1186·2); sodium carbonate (p.1665·1).
Cystitis.

Cymerin *Tokyo Tanabe, Jpn.*
Ranimustine (p.567·2).
Malignant neoplasms; polycythaemia vera; thrombocythaemia.

Cymerion *Azevedos, Port.*
Zolpidem tartrate (p.712·2).
Insomnia; sedative.

Cymevan *Roche, Fr.*
Ganciclovir (p.623·1) or ganciclovir sodium (p.623·1).
Cytomegalovirus infections.

Cymeven *Syntex, Ger.; Roche, Ger.*
Ganciclovir (p.623·1) or ganciclovir sodium (p.623·1).
Cytomegalovirus infections.

Cymevene
Roche, Aust.; Roche, Austral.; Roche, Belg.; Roche, Denm.; Roche, Fin.; Roche, Hong Kong; Roche, Irl.; Roche, Israel; Recordati, Ital.; Roche, Mex.; Roche, Neth.; Roche, Norw.; Roche, NZ; Roche, Port.; Roche, S.Afr.; Roche, Singapore; Roche, Spain; Roche, Swed.; Roche, Switz.; Roche, Thai.; Roche, UK.
Ganciclovir (p.623·1) or ganciclovir sodium (p.623·1).
Cytomegalovirus infections.

Cymex *De Witt, UK.*
Urea (p.1127·3); dimethicone (p.1410·1); cetrimide (p.1137·1); chlorocresol (p.1141·3).
Cracked lips; herpes labialis.

Cymi *Lennon, S.Afr.†.*
Cimetidine (p.1216·3).
Gastric hyperacidity; peptic ulcer; Zollinger-Ellison syndrome.

Cymine *Pharmasant, Thai.*
Dicyclomine [dicycloverine] hydrochloride (p.466·1); simeticone (p.1249·2).
Gastrointestinal colic and spasm.

Cyna Bilisan *Repha, Ger.*
Cynara (p.1601·3).
Dyspepsia.

Cynacur *Biocur, Ger.*
Cynara (p.1601·3).
Dyspepsia.

Cynafol *Kanoldt, Ger.*
Cynara (p.1601·3).
Dyspepsia.

Cynarix *Montavit, Aust.*
Cynara (p.1601·3).
Formerly contained cynara and rhubarb.
Liver and biliary disorders.

Cynarix comp *Montavit, Aust.*
Cynara (p.1601·3); salverine hydrochloride (p.1660·3).
Formerly contained cynara, rhubarb, and salverine hydrochloride.
Biliary disorders.

Cynaro Bilina *Dermofarm, Spain.*
Cynara (p.1601·3); aloes (p.1210·1).
Biliary-tract disorders; constipation.

Cynarobil *Uniao Quimica, Braz.*
Belladonna (p.463·1); boldo (p.1585·3); cynara (p.1601·3).
Liver disorders.

Cynarol *Pharmethic, Belg.*
Cynara (p.1601·3).
Biliary disorders; promotion of diuresis.

The symbol † denotes a preparation no longer actively marketed

Cynaron *Enila, Braz.*
Cynarine (p.1602·1).
Liver disorders.

Cynarzym N *Roland, Ger.*
Cynara (p.1601·3); boldo (p.1585·3); greater celandine (p.1618·1).
Digestive disorders; liver disorders.

Cynatrop *Biologia, Braz.*
Betaine hydrochloride (p.1584·3); choline (p.1356·3); liver extract.
Liver disorders.

Cyndal *Cypress, USA†.*
Codeine phosphate (p.25·2); phenylpropanolamine hydrochloride (p.1098·1); guaifenesin (p.1092·2).
Coughs; nasal and sinus congestion.

Cyndal HD *Cypress, USA.*
Hydrocodone tartrate (p.42·2); phenylephrine hydrochloride (p.1097·1); chlorpheniramine [chlorphenamine] maleate (p.412·1).

Cynomel *Enila, Braz.; Marion Merrell, Fr.; SmithKline Beecham, Mex.*
Liothyronine sodium (p.1524·2).
Hypothyroidism.

Cynovit *Julphar, UAE.*
Cyanocobalamin (p.1388·1).
Megaloblastic anaemia; vitamin B_{12} deficiency; vitamin B_{12} supplement.

Cynt
Lilly, Braz.; Lilly, Ger.; Lilly, Spain.
Moxonidine (p.936·3).
Hypertension.

Cyntex *Cypress, USA†.*
Phenylephrine hydrochloride (p.1097·1); phenylpropanolamine hydrochloride (p.1098·1); guaifenesin (p.1092·2).
Respiratory-tract congestion.

Cyomin *Forest Pharmaceuticals, USA.*
Cyanocobalamin (p.1388·1).
Schilling test; vitamin B_{12} deficiency.

Cyprid *Janssen-Cilag, Belg.*
Cisapride (p.1220·1).
Digestive disorders.

Cyprogin *Atlantic, Hong Kong; Vana, Thai.*
Cyproheptadine hydrochloride (p.414·2).
Hypersensitivity reactions; migraine; pruritus; reduced appetite.

Cypron *Generics, Israel.*
Cyproterone acetate (p.1467·3).
Androgenisation; male sexual disorders; prostatic cancer.

Cyprone *Alphapharm, Austral.*
Cyproterone acetate (p.1467·3).
Androgenisation; deviant sexual behaviour; prostatic cancer.

Cyprosian *Asian Pharm, Thai.*
Cyproheptadine hydrochloride (p.414·2).
Hypersensitivity reactions; pruritus; reduced appetite.

Cyprostat *Schering, UK.*
Cyproterone acetate (p.1467·3).
Prostatic cancer.

Cyprostol *Sanova, Aust.*
Misoprostol (p.1446·1).
Peptic ulcer.

Cyral *Gerot, Aust.*
Primidone (p.363·3).
Epilepsy.

Cyress *Yamanouchi, Neth.*
Barnidipine hydrochloride (p.843·1).
Hypertension.

Cyriamine *Pharmasant, Thai.*
Vitamin B_1 (p.1385·2); vitamin B_6 (p.1387·1); vitamin B_{12} (p.1383·3).
Vitamin B deficiency.

Cyrpon *Kolassa, Aust.*
Meprobamate (p.691·1).
Anxiety.

Cystadan *Orphan Medical, Israel.*
Betaine (p.1584·3).
Homocystinuria.

Cystadane
Orphan, Austral.; Orphan Medical, Canad.; Orphan Medical, USA.
Betaine (p.1584·3).
Homocystinuria.

Cystagon
Orphan, Austral.; Orphan, Denm.; Orphan, Fin.; Orphan, Fr.; Swedish Orphan, Swed.; Orphan, UK.
Mercaptamine bitartrate (p.1633·2).
Nephropathic cystinosis.

Cystelle Antipelliculaire *Bailleul, Fr.*
Piroctone olamine (p.1121·1).
Formerly contained soluble pyrithione.
Seborrhoeic dermatitis.

Cystelle Shampooing Cheveux Gras *Bailleul, Fr.*
Cade oil (p.1124·3); zinc gluconate (p.1398·2); pyridoxine hydrochloride (p.1386·3).
Seborrhoea.

Cystemme *Abbott, UK.*
Sodium citrate (p.1186·2).
Cystitis.

Cystex
Note.This name is used for preparations of different composition.
EMS, Braz.
Acriflavinium chloride (p.1130·2); methenamine (p.223·1); methylene blue [methylthioninium chloride] (p.1012·3); belladonna (p.463·1).
Urinary-tract infections.

Numark, USA.
Methenamine (p.223·1); sodium salicylate (p.84·2); benzoic acid (p.1134·2).
Urinary-tract infections.

Cystibosin B 48 *Bock, Ger.†.*
Homoeopathic preparation.

Cystichol *Bailleul, Fr.*
Cystine (p.1359·1); choline bitartrate (p.1356·3).
Dyspepsia.

Cysticide *Merck, Ger.; Merck, S.Afr.*
Praziquantel (p.106·3).
Neurocysticercosis.

Cystine B_6 *Bailleul, Fr.*
Cystine (p.1359·1); pyridoxine hydrochloride (p.1386·3).
Eye disorders; nail and hair disorders.

Cystinex *Sofex, Port.†.*
Gelatin; cystine; pyridoxine hydrochloride; zinc gluconate; vitamin A acetate (p.1350·1).
Skin and nail disorders.

Cystinol *Schaper & Brummer, Ger.*
Birch leaf (p.1585·2); equisetum (p.1606·3); solidago virgaurea; bearberry (p.1583·3).
Urinary-tract disorders.

Cystinol Akut *Schaper & Brummer, Ger.*
Bearberry (p.1583·3).
Urinary-tract inflammation.

Cystinol Long *Schaper & Brummer, Ger.*
Solidago virgaurea.
Renal calculi; urinary-tract disorders.

Cystiselect N *Dreluso, Ger.†.*
Homoeopathic preparation.

Cystistat *Paladin, Canad.; Dominion, UK.*
Sodium hyaluronate (p.1620·1).
Interstitial cystitis.

Cystit *Bristol-Myers Squibb, Ger.*
Nitrofurantoin (p.230·3).
Urinary-tract infections.

Cystitis Juniperus *Homeocan, Canad.*
Homoeopathic preparation.

Cystitis Relief *Thornton & Ross, UK.*
Sodium citrate (p.1186·2).
Cystitis.

Cystium Solidago *Wernigerode, Ger.*
Solidago virgaurea.
Renal calculi; urinary-tract disorders.

Cystium-wern *Wernigerode, Ger.*
Fennel oil (p.1610·2); camphor oil.
Renal calculi.

Cystit-Z *Bailleul, Fr.*
DL-Methionine (p.1012·2); zinc sulfate (p.1398·2); pyridoxine hydrochloride (p.1386·3).
Alopecia; seborrhoea.

Cysto Fink
Note.This name is used for preparations of different composition.
Kade, Ger.; SmithKline Beecham OTC, Ger.
Capsules: Rhus aromatica (p.1657·3); kava (p.1625·3); lupulus (p.1629·3); bearberry (p.1583·3); cucurbita oil.
Urinary-tract disorders.

SmithKline Beecham OTC, Ger.
Tea: Birch leaf (p.1585·2); solidago; java tea (p.1625·1); black currant (p.1389·3); bearberry (p.1583·3).
Urinary-tract disorders.

SmithKline Beecham Consumer, Switz.†.
Bearberry (p.1583·3); cucurbita oil; kava (p.1625·3); lupulus (p.1629·3); rhus aromatica (p.1657·3).
Bladder disorders.

Cystocalm *Galpharm, UK.*
Sodium citrate (p.1186·2).
Cystitis.

Cysto-Caps Chassot *Ebi, Switz.†.*
Bearberry (p.1583·3); cucurbita (p.1601·1); kava (p.1625·3); lupulus (p.1629·3); rhus aromatica (p.1657·3).
Bladder disorders.

Cysto-Conray *Mallinckrodt, Canad.; Mallinckrodt, USA.*
Meglumine iothalamate (p.1036·2).
Radiographic contrast medium.

Cysto-cyl Ho-Len-Complex *Liebermann, Ger.*
Homoeopathic preparation.

Cystofem *Sussex, UK.*
Sodium citrate (p.1186·2).
Cystitis.

Cysto-Gastreu N R18 *Reckeweg, Ger.*
Homoeopathic preparation.

Cystografin *Squibb Diagnostics, USA.*
Meglumine amidotrizoate (p.1031·2).
Radiographic contrast medium.

Cystoleve *SSL, UK.*
Sodium citrate (p.1186·2).
Cystitis.

Cysto-Myacyne N *Schur, Ger.*
Neomycin sulfate (p.228·1).
Urinary-tract infections.

Cystonorm *Esparma, Ger.*
Oxybutynin (p.471·2).
Neurogenic bladder disorders; nocturnal enuresis; urinary incontinence.

Cystopurin *Roche Consumer, Irl.; Roche Consumer, UK.*
Potassium citrate (p.1186·1).
Cystitis.

Cystosol *Unimedic, Swed.*
Sorbitol (p.1377·3).
Bladder irrigation.

Cystospaz *PolyMedica, USA.*
Hyoscyamine (p.469·3).
Urinary-tract spasm.

Cystospaz-M *PolyMedica, USA.*
Hyoscyamine sulfate (p.469·3).
Urinary-tract spasm.

Cysto-Urgenin *Hoyer, Ger.*
Cucurbita oil.
Bladder irritability.

Cystrin *Leiras, Fin.; Lorex Synthelabo, Irl.; Sanofi Synthelabo, UK.*
Oxybutynin hydrochloride (p.471·2).
Neurogenic bladder disorders; nocturnal enuresis; urinary incontinence.

Cytacon *Goldshield, Irl.; Goldshield, UK.*
Cyanocobalamin (p.1388·1).
Megaloblastic anaemia; tropical sprue; vitamin B_{12} deficiency.

Cytadren *Novartis, Austral.; Ciba, Canad.†; Novartis, NZ; Novartis, USA.*
Aminoglutethimide (p.506·3).
Breast cancer; Cushing's syndrome; prostatic cancer.

Cytagon *Pharmaland, Thai.*
Glibenclamide (p.321·3).
Diabetes mellitus.

Cytamen *DBL, Austral.; Medeva, Irl.; Celltech, UK.*
Cyanocobalamin (p.1388·1).
Anaemia due to B_{12} deficiency; Schilling test.

Cytarbel *Bellon, Fr.†.*
Cytarabine (p.530·1).
Malignant neoplasms.

Cyteal
Sinbio, Fr.; Pierre Fabre, Port.; Orient, Singapore; Pierre Fabre, Singapore.
Chlorhexidine gluconate (p.1138·2); chlorocresol (p.1141·3); hexamidine (p.1146·2) or hexamidine isetionate (p.1146·2).
Skin and vulvovaginal infections; skin and wound disinfection.

Cytelium *Ducray, Fr.*
Avena (p.1583·1); zinc oxide (p.1128·2).
Skin disorders.

Cytine *Douglas, NZ.*
Cimetidine (p.1216·3).
Gastro-oesophageal reflux; peptic ulcer; Zollinger-Ellison syndrome.

Cyto-Bifidus *Eagle, Austral.*
Lactobacillus acidophilus; L. bulgaricus; L. rhamnosus; L. casei; L. plantarum; L. salivarius; L. brevis; L. lactis (p.1626·3).
Gastrointestinal disorders.

Cytobion *Merck, Ger.*
Cyanocobalamin (p.1388·1).
Vitamin B_{12} deficiency.

CytoGam *Medimmune, USA.*
A cytomegalovirus immunoglobulin (p.1536·1).
Passive immunisation.

Cytoglobin *Bayer, Ger.*
A cytomegalovirus immunoglobulin (p.1536·1).
Passive immunisation.

Cytomel
SK-RIT, Belg.†; SmithKline Beecham, Canad.†; SmithKline Beecham, Neth.; Jones, USA.
Liothyronine sodium (p.1524·2).
Evaluation of thyroid function; hypothyroidism; non-toxic goitre.

Cytophosphan *Taro, Ger.*
Cyclophosphamide (p.527·3).
Malignant neoplasms; systemic lupus erythematosus.

Cytosar
Pharmacia Upjohn, Aust.; Pharmacia Upjohn, Belg.; Pharmacia Upjohn, Canad.; Pharmacia Upjohn, Denm.; Pharmacia Upjohn, Hong Kong; Pharmacia Upjohn, Irl.; Pharmacia Upjohn, Israel; Pharmacia Upjohn, Neth.; Pharmacia Upjohn, Norw.; Pharmacia Upjohn, Port.; Pharmacia Upjohn, S.Afr.; Pharmacia Upjohn, Singapore; Pharmacia Upjohn, Swed.; Pharmacia Upjohn, Switz.; Pharmacia, UK.
Cytarabine (p.530·1).
Leukaemias; non-Hodgkin's lymphoma.

Cytosar-U
Pharmacia Upjohn, Austral.; Pharmacia Upjohn, NZ; Pharmacia Upjohn, Thai.; Pharmacia Upjohn, USA.
Cytarabine (p.530·1).
Leukaemias; non-Hodgkin's lymphoma.

Cytosol *Cytosol, USA†.*
Electrolytes (p.1180·1).
Ocular irrigation.

Cytotec
Searle, Austral.; Searle, Belg.; Searle, Braz.; Searle, Canad.; Searle, Denm.; Searle, Fin.; Monsanto, Fr.; Heumann, Ger.; Searle, Hong Kong; Searle, Irl.; Searle, Israel; Searle, Ital.; Searle, Mex.; Searle, Neth.; Searle, Norw.; Searle, NZ; Monsanto, Port.; Searle, S.Afr.;

Searle, Singapore; Monsanto, Spain; Searle, Swed.; Searle, Switz.; Searle, Thai.; Pharmacia, UK; Searle, USA.
Misoprostol (p.1446·1).
Peptic ulcer.

Cytotect Biotest, Aust.; Biotest, Ger.; Biotest, Ital.; Biotest, Switz.
A cytomegalovirus immunoglobulin (p.1536·1).
Passive immunisation.

Cytovene Roche, Canad.; Roche, USA.
Ganciclovir (p.623·1) or ganciclovir sodium (p.623·1).
Cytomegalovirus infections.

Cytovis CTI, Israel.
Cytarabine (p.530·1).
Malignant neoplasms.

Cytoxan Bristol, Canad.; Bristol-Myers Squibb, Israel; Bristol-Myers Squibb, NZ; Bristol-Myers Squibb Oncology, USA.
Cyclophosphamide (p.527·3).
Glomerular kidney disease in children; malignant neoplasms.

Cytra-2 Cypress, USA.
Citric acid monohydrate (p.1596·2); sodium citrate (p.1186·2).
Metabolic acidosis; urinary alkalinisation.

Cytra-3 Cypress, USA.
Citric acid monohydrate (p.1596·2); potassium citrate (p.1186·1); sodium citrate (p.1186·2).
Metabolic acidosis; urinary alkalinisation.

Cytra-K Cypress, USA.
Citric acid monohydrate (p.1596·2); potassium citrate (p.1186·1).
Metabolic acidosis; urinary alkalinisation.

Cytra-LC Cypress, USA.
Citric acid monohydrate (p.1596·2); potassium citrate (p.1186·1); sodium citrate (p.1186·2).
Metabolic acidosis; urinary alkalinisation.

Cytur Test Roche Diagnostics, Austral.
Test for leucocytes in urine.

Cytuss HC Cypress, USA.
Hydrocodone tartrate (p.42·2); phenylephrine hydrochloride (p.1097·1); chlorpheniramine [chlorphenamine] maleate (p.412·1).

D-204 Gambro, Israel.
Electrolyte solution (p.1184·1).
Haemodialysis solution.

D-248 Gambro, Israel.
Electrolyte solution (p.1184·1).
Haemodialysis solution.

D-300 Gambro, Israel.
Electrolyte solution (p.1184·1).
Haemodialysis solution.

D-326 Gambro, Israel.
Electrolyte solution (p.1184·1).
Haemodialysis solution.

d Epifrin Allergan, Ger.
Dipivefrine hydrochloride (p.1604·3).
Glaucoma.

D Sucril Pierre Fabre, Fr.†.
Aspartame (p.1354·3).
Sugar substitute.

D₃ Vicotrat Heyl, Ger.
Colecalciferol (p.1391·1).
Vitamin D deficiency.

DA II Dura, USA.
Chlorpheniramine [chlorphenamine] maleate (p.412·1); phenylephrine hydrochloride (p.1097·1); hyoscine methonitrate (p.468·2).
Upper respiratory-tract symptoms.

DA Chewable Dura, USA.
Chlorpheniramine [chlorphenamine] maleate (p.412·1); phenylephrine hydrochloride (p.1097·1); hyoscine methonitrate (p.468·2).
Allergic rhinitis; cold symptoms; sinusitis.

Daben Solfran, Mex.
Mebendazole (p.102·2).
Worm infections.

Dabenzol Tecnofarma, Mex.
Albendazole (p.95·2).

Dabetil Liferpal, Mex.
Tolbutamide (p.336·3).
Diabetes mellitus.

Dabex Merck, Mex.
Metformin hydrochloride (p.332·3).
Diabetes mellitus.

Dabex G Merck, Mex.
Metformin hydrochloride (p.332·3); glibenclamide (p.321·3).
Diabetes mellitus.

Dabonal Vita, Spain.
Enalapril maleate (p.883·3).
Heart failure; hypertension.

Dabonal Plus Vita, Spain.
Hydrochlorothiazide (p.907·3); enalapril maleate (p.883·3).
Hypertension.

Dacatic Orion, Fin.
Dacarbazine (p.531·2).
Malignant neoplasms.

Dacef Aspen, S.Afr.
Cefadroxil (p.161·2).
Bacterial infections.

Daclin Pacific, NZ.
Sulindac (p.85·3).
Musculoskeletal, joint, and peri-articular disorders.

Dacoren Rhone-Poulenc Rorer, Ger.
Co-dergocrine mesilate (p.1597·3).
Hypertension; mental function disorders.

Dacortilen Meda, Swed.†.
Prednylidene (p.1079·3).
Corticosteroid.

Dacortin Merck, Spain.
Prednisone (p.1079·2).
Corticosteroid.

Dacortin H Merck, Spain.
Prednisolone (p.1077·3).
Corticosteroid.

Dacrin Merck Sharp & Dohme, Aust.; Chibret, Ger.
Hydrastinine hydrochloride; oxedrine tartrate (p.950·3).
Conjunctivitis.

Dacrine Chibret, Port.; Merck Sharp & Dohme, Switz.
Hydrastinine hydrochloride; oxedrine tartrate (p.950·3).
Conjunctivitis.

Dacriogel Alcon, Ital.
Carbomer (p.1499·2).
Dry eyes.

Dacriose Ciba Vision, USA.
Electrolytes (p.1180·1).
Eye irrigation.

Dacriosol Alcon, Denm.; Alcon, Ital.
Dextran 70 (p.729·2); hypromellose (p.1501·3).
Dry eyes.

Dacrolux Cusi, Singapore; Alcon Cusi, Spain.
Dextran 70 (p.729·2); hypromellose (p.1501·3).
Dry eyes.

Dacryne Martin, Fr.
Hydrastinine hydrochloride; oxedrine tartrate (p.950·3); chlorhexidine gluconate (p.1138·2).
Conjunctivitis; eye irritation.

Dacryoboraline Martin, Fr.
Oxedrine tartrate (p.950·3); borax (p.1586·1); boric acid (p.1586·1).
Eye irritation.

Dacryolarmes Martin, Fr.
Methylcellulose 4000 (p.1502·2).
Dry eyes; protection during eye examinations.

Dacryoseptil Martin, Fr.
Oxedrine tartrate (p.950·3); chlorhexidine gluconate (p.1138·2).
Eye disorders.

Dacryoserum Martin, Fr.
Boric acid (p.1586·1); borax (p.1586·1); sodium chloride (p.1196·1).
Minor eye disorder.

Dactil-OB
Note. This name is used for preparations of different composition.
Hoechst Marion Roussel, Braz.
Piperidolate hydrochloride (p.472·2); hesperidin (p.1611·2); ascorbic acid (p.1389·3).
Smooth muscle spasm.

Hoechst Marion Roussel, Mex.
Piperidolate hydrochloride (p.472·2).
Smooth muscle spasm.

Dacudoses Thea, Fr.
Boric acid (p.1586·1); borax (p.1586·1).
Minor eye disorders.

Dafalgan Upsamedica, Belg.; UPSA, Fr.; Upsamedica, Spain; Upsamedica, Switz.
Paracetamol (p.71·2).
Fever; pain.

Dafalgan Codeine Upsamedica, Belg.; UPSA, Fr.
Paracetamol (p.71·2); codeine phosphate (p.25·2).
Pain.

Daflon
Note. This name is used for preparations of different composition.
Servier, Aust.; Servier, Belg.; Servier, Fr.; Servier, Hong Kong; Sanfer, Mex.; Servier, Port.; Servier, Thai.
Diosmin (p.1611·1); hesperidin (p.1611·2).
Haemorrhoids; venous insufficiency.

Servier, Braz.; Servier, Spain; Servier, Switz.†.
Diosmin (p.1611·1).
Haemorrhoids; venous insufficiency.

Daflon 500 Servier, Ital.; Servier, Singapore; Servier, Spain; Servier, Switz.
Diosmin (p.1611·1); hesperidin (p.1611·2).
Haemorrhoids; venous insufficiency.

Dafloxen Liomont, Mex.
Naproxen (p.60·3) or naproxen sodium (p.61·1).
Gout; inflammation; musculoskeletal, joint and peri-articular disorders; pain.

Dafloxen F Liomont, Mex.
Naproxen sodium (p.61·1); paracetamol (p.71·2).
Fever; inflammation; pain.

Dafnegil Lepori, Port.; Poli, Switz.†.
Nifuratel (p.598·1); nystatin (p.392·2).
Balanitis; skin infections; vulvovaginal infections.

Dafnegil Neo Poli, Switz.
Ciclopirox olamine (p.382·1).
Vulvovaginal candidiasis.

Dafnegin Searle, Ital.
Ciclopirox olamine (p.382·1).
Vulvovaginal and peri-anal candidiasis.

Daforin Novaquimica, Braz.
Fluoxetine hydrochloride (p.284·2).
Depression; obsessive-compulsive disorder.

Daga Hoechst Marion Roussel, Thai.
Paracetamol (p.71·2).
Fever; pain.

Dagan Tedec Meiji, Spain.
Nicardipine hydrochloride (p.938·3).
Angina pectoris; cerebrovascular disorders; hypertension.

Dagenan Rhone-Poulenc Rorer, Canad.
Sulfapyridine (p.256·3).
Bacterial infections.

Dagra Fluor Asta Medica, Neth.†.
Sodium fluoride (p.1375·3).
Dental caries prophylaxis.

Dagracycline Asta Medica, Neth.
Doxycycline fosfatex (p.200·1).
Bacterial infections.

Dagragel Asta Medica, Port.
Bile (p.1585·1); glycerol (p.1616·3).
Bowel evacuation; constipation.

Dagramycine Asta Medica, Belg.†.
Doxycycline polyphosphate sodium (p.200·1).
Bacterial infections.

Dagravit Asta Medica, Port.
A range of vitamin preparations with or without minerals (p.1350·1).

Dagravit A Asta Medica, Belg.
Vitamin A acetate (p.1383·2).
Vitamin A deficiency.

Dagravit A Forte Asta Medica, Neth.
Vitamin A acetate (p.1383·2).
Vitamin A deficiency.

Dagravit A-E Asta Medica, Belg.
Vitamin A palmitate (p.1383·2); *dl*-alpha tocoferil acetate (p.1394·1).
Vitamin A and E deficiency.

Dagravit A-E Forte Asta Medica, Neth.
Vitamin A palmitate (p.1383·2); *dl*-alpha-tocoferil acetate (p.1394·1).
Vitamin A and E deficiency.

Dagravit B-Complex Asta Medica, Belg.; Dagra, Neth.†.
Vitamin B substances (p.1350·1).
Vitamin B deficiency.

Dagravit B-Complex Forte Asta Medica, Neth.†.
Vitamin B substances (p.1350·1); intrinsic factor.
Vitamin B deficiency.

Dagravit Becoforte Dagra, Neth.†.
Vitamin B substances (p.1350·1).
Vitamin B deficiency.

Dagravit C Asta Medica, Neth.†.
Vitamin C (p.1389·3).
Vitamin C deficiency.

Dagravit Totaal 8 Asta Medica, Neth.
Multivitamin preparation (p.1350·1).

Dagravit Total Asta Medica, Belg.†.
Multivitamin preparation with iron (p.1350·1).

Dagravit Total 8 Asta Medica, Belg.†.
Multivitamin preparation (p.1350·1).

Dagynil Asta Medica, Neth.
Conjugated oestrogens (p.1467·1).
Menopausal disorders; osteoporosis; prostatic cancer.

Dai Natha Lopes, Braz.
Tar (p.1125·1); cade oil (p.1124·3); coal tar (p.1125·1).
Seborrhoeic dermatitis.

Daiet B Humana, Ital.
Fatty-acid, lipid, and vitamin preparation (p.1350·1).
Nutritional supplement.

Dailat Pharmasant, Thai.
Serrapeptase (p.1662·1).
Inflammation; oedema.

Daily Balance Pharmavite, Canad.†.
Multivitamin preparation (p.1350·1).

Daily Conditioning Blistex, USA.
SPF 20: Octinoxate (p.1517·3); oxybenzone (p.1518·1).
Sunscreen.

Daily Fatigue Relief Herbal Concepts, UK.
Kola (p.1681·1); damiana (p.1602·1); saw palmetto (p.1491·2).
Tonic.

Daily Gold Pack Solgar, UK.
Multivitamin and mineral preparation (p.1350·1).

Daily Lip Protector Retsews, USA†.
SPF 15: Padimate O (p.1518·2); oxybenzone (p.1518·1).
Sunscreen.

Daily Menopause Relief Herbal Concepts, UK.
Tilia (p.1673·2); motherwort (p.1637·3); pulsatilla (p.1656·3); valerian (p.1678·3).
Menopausal disorders.

Daily Multi Vitaplex, Austral.
Multivitamin, mineral, and amino-acid preparation (p.1350·1).

Daily Overwork & Mental Fatigue Relief Herbal Concepts, UK.
Avena (p.1583·1); zanthoxylum (p.1682·1).
Tonic.

Daily Protection Moisturizer Kay, Canad.
SPF 15: Octinoxate (p.1517·3); oxybenzone (p.1518·1).
Sunscreen.

Daily Tension & Strain Relief Herbal Concepts, UK.
Asafetida (p.1582·3); valerian (p.1678·3); avena (p.1583·1); passion flower (p.1649·1).
Strain; tension.

Daily-Vite Rugby, USA.
Multivitamin and mineral preparation with iron and folic acid (p.1350·1).

Dairy Ease Sterling, USA.
Tilactase (p.1673·2).
Lactase insufficiency.

Dairyaid Tanta, Canad.
Tilactase (p.1673·2).
Lactase insufficiency.

Daisy Advanced Care, USA†.
Pregnancy test (p.1654·3).

Daivonex CSL, Austral.; Leo, Belg.; Schering-Plough, Braz.; Leo, Denm.; Leo, Fin.; Leo, Fr.; Leo, Ger.; Leo, Hong Kong; Leo, Israel; Formenti, Ital.; Senosiain, Mex.; Leo, Neth.; Leo, Norw.; CSL, NZ; Leo, NZ; Leo, Port.; Leo, Singapore; Farmacusi, Spain; Leo, Swed.; Leo, Switz.; Leo, Thai.
Calcipotriol (p.1112·1).
Psoriasis.

Dakar Aventis, Belg.
Lansoprazole (p.1230·3).
Gastro-oesophageal reflux; peptic ulcer; Zollinger-Ellison syndrome.

Dakin Cooperation Pharmaceutique, Fr.
Sodium hypochlorite (p.1156·2).
Skin and mucous membrane disinfection.

Dakincooper Melisana, Belg.
Sodium hypochlorite (p.1156·2).
Skin and mucous membrane disinfection.

Daktacort Janssen-Cilag, Aust.; Janssen-Cilag, Belg.; Orion, Fin.; Janssen-Cilag, Fr.†; Janssen, Hong Kong; Janssen-Cilag, Israel; Janssen, Mex.; Janssen-Cilag, Neth.; Janssen-Cilag, Norw.; Janssen-Cilag, S.Afr.; Janssen-Cilag, Singapore; Janssen-Cilag, Swed.; Janssen-Cilag, Switz.; Janssen, Thai.; Janssen-Cilag, UK.
Miconazole nitrate (p.391·1); hydrocortisone (p.1073·3).
Fungal and Gram-positive bacterial skin infections with inflammation.

Daktacort HC Johnson & Johnson MSD Consumer, UK.
Miconazole nitrate (p.391·1); hydrocortisone acetate (p.1073·3).
Infected skin disorders.

Daktagold Janssen-Cilag, Austral.
Ketoconazole (p.389·1).
Fungal skin infections.

Daktar Janssen-Cilag, Belg.; Janssen-Cilag, Ger.; Janssen-Cilag, Norw.; Janssen-Cilag, Swed.
Miconazole (p.391·1) or miconazole nitrate (p.391·1).
Fungal and Gram-positive bacterial skin infections.

Daktarin Janssen-Cilag, Aust.; Janssen-Cilag, Austral.; Janssen-Cilag, Belg.; Janssen, Braz.; Orion, Fin.; Janssen-Cilag, Fr.; Janssen, Hong Kong; Janssen-Cilag, Irl.; Janssen-Cilag, Israel; Janssen-Cilag, Ital.; Janssen, Mex.; Janssen-Cilag, Neth.; Janssen-Cilag, NZ; Janssen-Cilag, Port.; Janssen-Cilag, S.Afr.; Janssen-Cilag, Singapore; Esteve, Spain; Janssen-Cilag, Switz.; Janssen, Thai.; Janssen-Cilag, UK; Johnson & Johnson MSD Consumer, UK.
Miconazole (p.391·1) or miconazole nitrate (p.391·1).
Fungal and Gram-positive bacterial infections.

Daktarin Gold Johnson & Johnson MSD Consumer, UK.
Ketoconazole (p.389·1).
Fungal skin infections.

Daktozin Janssen-Cilag, Austral.; Janssen-Cilag, Belg.; Janssen-Cilag, NZ.
Miconazole nitrate (p.391·1); zinc oxide (p.1128·2).
Fungal skin infections.

Dalacin Pharmacia Upjohn, Aust.; Pharmacia Upjohn, Denm.; Pharmacia Upjohn, Fin.; Pharmacia Upjohn, Irl.; Pharmacia Upjohn, Norw.; Pharmacia Upjohn, NZ; Pharmacia Upjohn, Singapore; Pharmacia Upjohn, Spain; Pharmacia Upjohn, Swed.; Pharmacia Upjohn, Thai.; Pharmacia, UK.
Clindamycin hydrochloride (p.188·1), clindamycin palmitate hydrochloride (p.188·1), or clindamycin phosphate (p.188·2).
Bacterial infections.

Dalacin C Pharmacia Upjohn, Austral.; Pharmacia Upjohn, Belg.; Pharmacia Upjohn, Braz.; Pharmacia Upjohn, Canad.; Pharmacia Upjohn, Hong Kong; Pharmacia Upjohn, Irl.; Pharmacia Upjohn, Israel; Pharmacia Upjohn, Ital.; Pharmacia Upjohn, Mex.; Pharmacia Upjohn, Neth.; Pharmacia Upjohn, Port.; Pharmacia Upjohn, S.Afr.; Pharmacia Upjohn, Switz.; Pharmacia, UK.
Clindamycin hydrochloride (p.188·1), clindamycin palmitate hydrochloride (p.188·1), or clindamycin phosphate (p.188·2).
Bacterial infections.

Dalacin T Pharmacia Upjohn, Austral.; Pharmacia Upjohn, Braz.; Pharmacia Upjohn, Canad.; Pharmacia Upjohn, Hong Kong; Pharmacia Upjohn, Irl.; Pharmacia Upjohn, Ital.; Pharmacia Upjohn, Mex.; Pharmacia Upjohn, Neth.; Pharmacia Upjohn, NZ; Pharmacia Upjohn, Port.; Pharmacia Upjohn, S.Afr.; Pharmacia Upjohn, Switz.; Pharmacia, UK.
Clindamycin phosphate (p.188·2).
Acne.

Dalacin T Prewash Pharmacia Upjohn, NZ.
Triclosan (p.1159·2).
Skin cleansing.

Dalacin Topical Pharmacia Upjohn, Belg.
Clindamycin phosphate (p.188·2).
Formerly known as Dalacin T.
Acne.

Dalacin V
Pharmacia Upjohn, Austral.; Pharmacia Upjohn, Hong Kong; Pharmacia Upjohn, Mex.; Pharmacia Upjohn, NZ; Pharmacia Upjohn, Port.; Pharmacia Upjohn, Switz.
Clindamycin phosphate (p.188·2).
Bacterial vaginitis.

Dalacin Vaginal
Pharmacia Upjohn, Belg.; Pharmacia Upjohn, Canad.; Pharmacia Upjohn, Israel.
Clindamycin phosphate (p.188·2).
Bacterial vaginitis.

Dalacin VC *Pharmacia Upjohn, S.Afr.*
Clindamycin phosphate (p.188·2).
Bacterial vaginosis.

Dalacine *Pharmacia Upjohn, Fr.*
Clindamycin hydrochloride (p.188·1) or clindamycin phosphate (p.188·2).
Bacterial infections.

Dalacine T *Pharmacia Upjohn, Fr.*
Clindamycin phosphate (p.188·2).
Acne.

Dalagis T *Agis, Israel.*
Clindamycin phosphate (p.188·2).
Acne.

Dalalone *Forest Pharmaceuticals, USA.*
Dexamethasone acetate (p.1067·1).
Corticosteroid.

Dalamon *Alter, Spain.*
Capsules‡: Cobamamide (p.1388·3); pyridoxine phosphate (p.1387·1); thiamine phosphate (p.1385·2).
Injection: Cyanocobalamin (p.1388·3); dexamethasone sodium diacid phosphate (p.1067·1); pyridoxine hydrochloride (p.1386·3); thiamine hydrochloride (p.1385·1).
Lignocaine [lidocaine] hydrochloride (p.1313·2) is included in this preparation to alleviate the pain of injection.
Neuralgia; neuritis.

Dalcept *Cuprocept, S.Afr.*
Copper-wound plastic (p.1357·3).
Intra-uterine contraceptive device.

Dalcipran *Sanofi Synthelabo, Aust.*
Milnacipran hydrochloride (p.299·1).
Depression.

Dal-E *Dal-Vita, Austral.*
d-Alpha tocoferil acetate (p.1394·1).
Burns; minor wounds; skin irritation.

Dalet Med Balsam *Mauermann, Ger.*
Guaiacol (p.1092·1); methyl salicylate (p.55·1); belladonna (p.463·1); menthol (p.1632·3).
Hallux valgus; inflammation of big toe joint.

Dalfaz *Synthelabo, Spain.*
Alfuzosin hydrochloride (p.833·2).
Benign prostatic hyperplasia.

Dalgan *Astra, USA†.*
Dezocine (p.28·2).
Pain.

Dalgen *Recordati, Spain.*
Fepradinol (p.40·3) or fepradinol hydrochloride (p.40·3).
Peri-articular disorders; soft-tissue disorders.

Dalidome *Serral, Mex.*
Copper sulfate (p.1358·1); zinc sulfate (p.1398·2); camphor (p.1589·3).
Skin disorders.

Dalinar *Essex, Spain.*
Netilmicin sulfate (p.229·3).
Bacterial infections.

Dalisol *Lemery, Mex.*
Calcium folinate (p.1363·1).
Adjunct to fluorouracil therapy; antidote to folic acid antagonists; megaloblastic anaemia; reduction of methotrexate toxicity.

Dalivit
Ariston, Braz.
Vitamin B substances; vitamin C; fructose (p.1350·1).
Eastern Pharmaceuticals, UK.
Multivitamin preparation (p.1350·1).

Dallergy *Laser, USA.*
Chlorpheniramine [chlorphenamine] maleate (p.412·1); phenylephrine hydrochloride (p.1097·1); hyoscine methonitrate (p.468·2).
Upper respiratory-tract symptoms.

Dallergy-D *Laser, USA.*
Capsules: Pseudoephedrine hydrochloride (p.1099·2); chlorpheniramine [chlorphenamine] maleate (p.412·1).
Syrup: Phenylephrine hydrochloride (p.1097·1); chlorpheniramine [chlorphenamine] maleate (p.412·1).
Upper respiratory-tract symptoms.

Dallergy-JR *Laser, USA.*
Brompheniramine maleate (p.410·2); pseudoephedrine hydrochloride (p.1099·2).
Allergic rhinitis; nasal congestion.

Dalmacol *Riva, Canad.*
Hydrocodone tartrate (p.42·2); etafedrine hydrochloride (p.1091·2); sodium citrate (p.1186·2); doxylamine succinate (p.417·1).
Respiratory-tract disorders.

Dalmadorm
Roche, Braz.; ICN, Ger.; Roche, Hong Kong; Roche, Ital.; ICN, Neth.†; ICN, Port.; Pharmaco, S.Afr.; ICN, Singapore; ICN, Switz.; ICN, Thai.
Flurazepam dihydrochloride (p.685·3) or flurazepam monohydrochloride (p.685·3).
Insomnia.

Dalmane
ICN, Canad.; ICN, Irl.; ICN, UK; Roche, USA.
Flurazepam dihydrochloride (p.685·3) or flurazepam monohydrochloride (p.685·3).
Insomnia.

Dalmasin *Columbia, Mex.*
Dipyrone (p.34·1).
Fever; pain.

Dalparan *Farma Lepori, Spain.*
Zolpidem tartrate (p.712·2).
Insomnia.

Dalsy *Knoll, Spain.*
Ibuprofen (p.43·2).
Fever; musculoskeletal, joint, and peri-articular disorders; pain.

Daltroid *Lemery, Mex.*
Thyroxine [levothyroxine] sodium (p.1526·2).

Dam *Terapeutico, Ital.*
Damiana (p.1602·1); muira puama; santoreggia; kola (p.1681·1); cinnamon (p.1595·3).
Asthenia; erectile dysfunction.

Dama-Lax *Schering-Plough, Spain.*
Docusate sodium (p.1223·1).
Formerly contained docusate sodium and phenolphthalein.
Constipation.

Damason-P *Mason, USA.*
Hydrocodone tartrate (p.42·2); aspirin (p.14·2).
Pain.

Damiana and Kola Tablets *Dorwest, UK.*
Kola (p.1681·1); damiana (p.1602·1); saw palmetto (p.1491·2).
Tonic.

Damide *Benedetti, Ital.*
Indapamide (p.913·1).
Hypertension.

Damira *Wander Health Care, Switz.*
Preparation for enteral nutrition (p.1350·1).
Cow's milk intolerance.

Damosal *Salus, Mex.*
Dipyridamole (p.877·2).

Damoxicil *Byk Elmu, Spain.*
Amoxicillin trihydrate (p.149·2).
Bacterial infections.

Damoxicil Mucolitico *Byk Elmu, Spain†.*
Amoxicillin trihydrate (p.149·2); bromhexine hydrochloride (p.1085·3).
Respiratory-tract infections.

D-Amp *Dunhall, USA†.*
Ampicillin trihydrate (p.151·1).
Bacterial infections.

Dampo
Roche Consumer, Neth.
Ointment for inhalation: Camphor (p.1589·3); menthol (p.1632·3); eucalyptus oil (p.1609·2).
Cold symptoms.
Roche Nicholas, Neth.†.
Nasal spray: Oxymetazoline hydrochloride (p.1096·2).
Nasal congestion.

Dampo bij droge hoest *Roche Consumer, Neth.*
Dextromethorphan hydrobromide (p.1087·3).
Coughs.

Dampo Mucopect *Roche Consumer, Neth.†.*
Acetylcysteine (p.1082·3).
Respiratory-tract congestion.

Dampo Solvopect *Roche Consumer, Neth.*
Carbocisteine (p.1086·3).
Respiratory-tract congestion.

Danalem *Lemery, Mex.*
Danazol (p.1468·3).

Danatrol
Sanofi Synthelabo, Belg.; Sanofi Winthrop, Fr.; Sanofi Synthelabo, Ital.; Sanofi Synthelabo, Neth.; Sanofi Synthelabo, Port.; Sanofi Synthelabo, Spain; Sanofi Synthelabo, Switz.
Danazol (p.1468·3).
Benign breast disorders; endometriosis; hereditary angioedema; menorrhagia; precocious puberty.

Danazant
Antigen, Hong Kong; Antigen, Irl.
Danazol (p.1468·3).
Benign breast disorders; dysfunctional uterine bleeding; endometriosis; precocious puberty.

Dancor
Merck, Aust.; Merck, Neth.†; Merck, Port.; Merck, Spain.; Merck, Switz.
Nicorandil (p.939·2).
Angina pectoris.

Dandruff Control Pert 2 in 1 *Procter & Gamble, Austral.*
Pyrithione zinc (p.1122·1).
Dandruff.

Dandruff Treatment Shampoo *Sutton, Canad.*
Pyrithione zinc (p.1122·1).

Daneral
Hoechst Marion Roussel, Irl.; Hoechst Marion Roussel, UK†.
Pheniramine maleate (p.422·3).
Hypersensitivity reactions.

Dan-Gard
Faulding, Austral.; Stiefel, Canad.
Pyrithione zinc (p.1122·1).
Seborrhoeic dermatitis.

Danilax
Danipharm, Denm.; Danipharm, Hong Kong.
Lactulose (p.1230·1).
Constipation; hepatic encephalopathy.

Danilon
Note. This name is used for preparations of different composition.
Allergan-Frumtost, Braz.
Ibuprofen (p.43·2).
Fever; inflammation; pain.
Esteve, Spain.
Suxibuzone (p.87·2).
Musculoskeletal, joint, peri-articular, and soft-tissue disorders.

Danitin *Carnot, Mex.*
Ranitidine (p.1246·3).

Danka *Angelini, Ital.*
Levodropropizine (p.1089·3).
Coughs.

Danlax *Waymade, UK.*
Dantron (p.1221·3); poloxamer 188 (p.1347·1).
Constipation.

Danocrine
Sanofi Synthelabo, Austral.; Sanofi Winthrop, Denm.; Sanofi Winthrop, Fin.; Sanofi Winthrop, Hong Kong; Sanofi Winthrop, Israel; Sanofi Winthrop, Norw.; Sanofi Winthrop, NZ; Sanofi Winthrop, Swed.; Sanofi Winthrop, USA.
Danazol (p.1468·3).
Benign breast disease; endometriosis; hereditary angioedema; menorrhagia; precocious puberty.

Danokrin *Sanofi Winthrop, Aust.*
Danazol (p.1468·3).
Endometriosis; gynaecomastia; hereditary angioedema; precocious puberty.

Danol
Sanofi Winthrop, Irl.; Sanofi Winthrop, UK.
Danazol (p.1468·3).
Endometriosis; mastalgia; menstrual disorders; precocious puberty.

Dantamacrin
Procter & Gamble, Aust.; Procter & Gamble, Ger.; Procter & Gamble, Switz.
Dantrolene sodium (p.1328·2).
Skeletal muscle spasm; spasticity.

Dan-Tar Plus *Stiefel, Canad.*
Polytar (a blend of wood and mineral tars) (p.1124·3); pyrithione disulfide (p.1122·1).
Seborrhoeic dermatitis.

Dantrium
Pharmacia Upjohn, Austral.; Procter & Gamble, Belg.; Procter & Gamble, Canad.; Procter & Gamble, Denm.; Lipha Sante, Fr.; Procter & Gamble, Hong Kong; Procter & Gamble, Irl.; Procter & Gamble, Israel; Formenti, Ital.; Procter & Gamble, Neth.; Pharmacia Upjohn, NZ; Normal, Port.; Pharmaco, S.Afr.; Procter & Gamble, UK; Procter & Gamble, USA.
Dantrolene sodium (p.1328·2).
Malignant hyperthermia; skeletal muscle spasm; spasticity.

Danubial *Atlantis, Mex.*
Ornidazole (p.599·1).
Amoebiasis; giardiasis; trichomoniasis.

Dany *The Forty-Two, Thai.*
Domperidone (p.1224·1).
Digestive disorders; dyspepsia; nausea and vomiting.

Danzen
Allergan-Frumtost, Braz.; Takeda, Hong Kong; Takeda, Ital.; Hormona, Mex.; Takeda, Singapore; Takeda, Thai.
Serrapeptase (p.1662·1).
Inflammation; oedema; respiratory-tract congestion.

Daonil
Hoechst Marion Roussel, Aust.; Aventis, Belg.; Hoechst Marion Roussel, Braz.; Aventis, Denm.; Hoechst Marion Roussel, Fin.; Hoechst, Fr.; Hoechst Marion Roussel, Hong Kong; Hoechst Marion Roussel, Irl.; Hoechst Marion Roussel, Israel; Hoechst Marion Roussel, Ital.; Hoechst Marion Roussel, Mex.; Hoechst Marion Roussel, Neth.; Hoechst Marion Roussel, Norw.; Aventis, NZ; Hoeport, Port.; Aventis, S.Afr.; Hoechst Marion Roussel, Singapore; Hoechst Marion Roussel, Spain; Hoechst Marion Roussel, Swed.; Hoechst Marion Roussel, Switz.; Hoechst Marion Roussel, Thai.; Hoechst Marion Roussel, UK.
Glibenclamide (p.321·3).
Diabetes mellitus.

Dapa *Ferndale, USA†.*
Paracetamol (p.71·2).
Fever; pain.

Dapacin Cold *Ferndale, USA†.*
Phenylpropanolamine hydrochloride (p.1098·1); chlorpheniramine [chlorphenamine] maleate (p.412·1); paracetamol (p.71·2).
Upper respiratory-tract symptoms.

Dapamax *Parke-Med, S.Afr.*
Indapamide (p.913·1).
Hypertension; oedema.

Dapa-Tabs
Alphapharm, Austral.; Alphapharm, Hong Kong; Alphapharm, Singapore; Merck, Singapore.
Indapamide (p.913·1).
Hypertension.

Dapaz *Alter, Spain.*
Meprobamate (p.691·1).
Anxiety; insomnia; skeletal muscle spasm.

Dapotum
Sanofi Winthrop, Aust.; Bristol-Myers Squibb, Ger.; Sanofi Synthelabo, Ger.; Bristol-Myers Squibb, Switz.
Fluphenazine decanoate (p.684·3) or fluphenazine hydrochloride (p.684·3).
Psychoses.

Daprox *Nycomed, Denm.*
Naproxen (p.60·3).
Inflammation; musculoskeletal and joint disorders; pain.

Dapsoderm-X *Mex-America, Mex.*
Dapsone (p.196·1).
Bacterial mycetoma; dermatitis herpetiformis; leprosy.

Daptaral *Wyeth-Ayerst, Thai.*
Multivitamin and mineral preparation (p.1350·1).

Daptril *Xeragen, S.Afr.*
Indapamide (p.913·1).
Hypertension.

Daraclor *Glaxo Wellcome, S.Afr.†*
Pyrimethamine (p.442·3); chloroquine sulfate (p.432·3).
Malaria.

Daral *Noristan Generica, S.Afr.†*
Aminophylline (p.760·1); ephedrine hydrochloride (p.1090·1); amobarbital (p.655·2).
Asthma; bronchitis; bronchopneumonia.

Daralix *Quatromed, S.Afr.*
Promethazine hydrochloride (p.423·2).
Hypersensitivity reactions; nausea; vomiting.

Daramal *Glaxo Wellcome, S.Afr.*
Chloroquine sulfate (p.432·3).
Discoid lupus erythematosus; malaria; rheumatoid arthritis.

Daramal-Paludrine *Zeneca, S.Afr.*
Chloroquine sulfate (p.432·3); proguanil hydrochloride (p.441·3).
Malaria.

Daranide
Sigma, Austral.†; Merck Sharp & Dohme, Irl.†; Merck, USA.
Diclofenamide (p.869·1).
Glaucoma.

Daraprim
Glaxo Wellcome, Aust.; Glaxo Wellcome, Austral.; Glaxo Wellcome, Belg.; Glaxo Wellcome, Braz.; Glaxo Wellcome, Canad.; Glaxo Wellcome, Ger.; Wellcome, Irl.; Glaxo Wellcome, Israel; Glaxo Wellcome, Mex.; Glaxo Wellcome, Neth.; Glaxo Wellcome, S.Afr.; Wellcome, Spain; Glaxo Wellcome, Swed.†; Wellcome, Switz.; Glaxo Wellcome, Thai.; Glaxo Wellcome, UK; Glaxo Wellcome, USA.
Pyrimethamine (p.442·3).
Malaria; toxoplasmosis.

Dardex *Llorente Generic, Spain.*
Captopril (p.853·3).
Diabetic nephropathy; heart failure; hypertension; myocardial infarction.

Dardum
Lisapharma, Ital.; Lisapharma, Singapore.
Cefoperazone sodium (p.168·2).
Lignocaine [lidocaine] hydrochloride (p.1313·2) may be included in the intramuscular injection to alleviate the pain of injection.
Bacterial infections.

Darebon
Novartis, Aust.; Novartis, Ger.
Chlortalidone (p.857·1); reserpine (p.967·3).
Hypertension.

Daren *Delta, Singapore.*
Enalapril maleate (p.883·3).
Heart failure; hypertension.

Dari *Vita Elan, Spain.*
Nifedipine (p.940·1).
Angina pectoris; hypertension; Raynaud's syndrome.

Daricon
Pfizer, Hong Kong; Pfizer, Neth.†; Pfizer, Thai.
Oxyphencyclimine hydrochloride (p.472·1).
Irritable bowel syndrome; peptic ulcer.

Dariseb *Darier, Mex.*
Coal tar (p.1125·1); menthol (p.1632·3).
Scalp disorders.

Darkene *Bayer, Ital.*
Flunitrazepam (p.683·2).
Insomnia.

Darlin *Sandipro, Belg.*
Senna fruit (p.1248·2).
Constipation.

Darmen Salt *Ern, Spain.*
Magnesium sulfate (p.1191·1); sodium bicarbonate (p.1186·2); dibasic sodium phosphate (p.1193·2); sodium sulfate (p.1250·1).
Constipation; dyspepsia; gastric hyperacidity.

Darmol
Note. This name is used for preparations of different composition.
Schmidgall, Aust.; Iromedica, Switz.
Senna (p.1248·2).
Bowel evacuation; constipation.
Omegin, Ger.
Sodium picosulfate (p.1249·3).
Formerly contained phenolphthalein.
Constipation.

Darmol Bisacodyl *Omegin, Ger.*
Bisacodyl (p.1212·2).
Constipation.

Darmol Pico *Omegin, Ger.*
Sodium picosulfate (p.1249·3).
Constipation.

Daro *Heca, Neth.†.*
Paracetamol (p.71·2).
Fever; pain.

Daro Hoofdpijnpoeders *Heca, Neth.†.*
Paracetamol (p.71·2); propyphenazone (p.80·2); caffeine (p.761·3).
Headache.

Daro Thijm *Heca, Neth.†.*
Thyme (p.1672·2).
Coughs.

The symbol † denotes a preparation no longer actively marketed

Darob *Ebewe, Aust.; Knoll, Ger.; Knoll, Port.; Meda, Swed.†.*
Sotalol hydrochloride (p.972·2).
Arrhythmias.

Darocet *Heca, Neth.†.*
Paracetamol (p.71·2).
Fever; pain.

Darocillin *Hoechst Marion Roussel, S.Afr.†.*
Phenoxymethylpenicillin potassium (p.235·1).
Bacterial infections.

Darolan Hoestprikkeldempende *Heca, Neth.†.*
Dextromethorphan hydrobromide (p.1087·3).
Coughs.

Darolan Slijmplossende *Heca, Neth.†.*
Bromhexine hydrochloride (p.1085·3).
Respiratory-tract disorders with viscous mucus.

Daromide *Quatromed, S.Afr.*
Merbromin (p.1150·1); sulfanilamide (p.256·2); acriflavinium chloride (p.1130·2); cod-liver oil (p.1357·2); zinc oxide (p.1128·2).
Burns; skin infections; wounds.

Darosed *Hoechst Marion Roussel, S.Afr.†.*
Promethazine hydrochloride (p.423·2); codeine phosphate (p.25·2); ephedrine hydrochloride (p.1090·1).
Coughs.

Darrow-Liq *Brunel, S.Afr.*
Sodium chloride; potassium chloride; sodium citrate dihydrate; glucose (p.1185·2).
Oral rehydration therapy.

Darrowped *Pharmacare Consumer, S.Afr.†.*
Potassium chloride; sodium chloride; sodium citrate; glucose (p.1185·2).
Diarrhoea; oral rehydration therapy.

Dart *Bergamo, Braz.*
Metoclopramide (p.1236·3).
Nausea and vomiting.

Dartrox *Pisa, Mex.*
Naproxen (p.60·3).

Daruma *Wyeth Lederle, Ital.*
Idebenone (p.1623·1).
Mental and movement disturbances associated with cerebrovascular disorders.

Darvocet-N *Lilly, USA.*
Dextropropoxyphene napsilate (p.27·1); paracetamol (p.71·2).
Fever; pain.

Darvon *Lilly, Spain.; Lilly, USA.*
Dextropropoxyphene hydrochloride (p.27·1) or dextropropoxyphene napsilate (p.27·1).
Pain.

Darvon Compound *Lilly, USA.*
Dextropropoxyphene hydrochloride (p.27·1); aspirin (p.14·2); caffeine (p.761·3).
Fever; pain.

Darvon Simple *Lilly, Mex.*
Dextropropoxyphene hydrochloride (p.27·1).
Pain.

Darvon-N *Lilly, Canad.; Lilly, Mex.; Lilly, USA.*
Dextropropoxyphene napsilate (p.27·1).
Pain.

Dasc *EMS, Braz.*
Pancrelipase (p.1647·2); bile salts (p.1585·1); cellulase (p.1593·1).
Digestive disorders.

Dasen *Takeda, Jpn.*
Serrapeptase (p.1662·1).
Inflammation; respiratory-tract congestion.

Daskil *Novartis, Aust.; LPB, Ital.*
Terbinafine hydrochloride (p.394·1).
Fungal skin and nail infections.

Daskyl *Azevedos, Port.*
Terbinafine hydrochloride (p.394·1).
Fungal skin and nail infections.

Dasmetrol *Tocogino, Mex.*
Metronidazole (p.594·1).

Dasolin *Yuaquimia, Mex.*
Metronidazole (p.594·1).

Dasten *Asta Medica, Braz.*
Mazindol (p.1510·3).
Obesity.

Dastosin *Yamanouchi, Spain.*
Dimemorfan phosphate (p.1089·1).
Coughs.

Dastusin *Shiwa, Thai.*
Diphenhydramine hydrochloride (p.416·1); ammonium chloride (p.1085·2); sodium citrate (p.1186·2).
Cold symptoms; coughs.

Datolan *Faes, Spain.*
Zopiclone (p.713·1).
Insomnia.

Datril *Bristol-Myers Squibb, Mex.*
Paracetamol (p.71·2).
Fever; pain.

DaTSCAN *Nycomed Amersham, UK.*
Iodine-123 (p.1450·1) as ioflupane.
Diagnosis of parkinsonism.

Daunoblastin *Pharmacia Upjohn, Aust.; Pharmacia Upjohn, Ger.; Pharmacia Upjohn, S.Afr.*
Daunorubicin hydrochloride (p.533·1).
Leukaemias.

Daunoblastina *Pharmacia Upjohn, Braz.; Pharmacia Upjohn, Hong Kong; Pharmacia Upjohn, Ital.; Pharmacia Upjohn, Port.; Pharmacia Upjohn, Singapore; Kenfarma, Spain.*
Daunorubicin hydrochloride (p.533·1).
Malignant neoplasms.

DaunoXome *Fresenius Kabi, Aust.; Nexstar, Austral.; Nexstar, Belg.†; Nexstar, Denm.; Orphan, Fin.; Nexstar, Fr.; Nexstar, Ger.; Nexstar, Ital.; Nexstar, Neth.; Nexstar, Span; Swedish Orphan, Swed.; Fresenius Kabi, Switz.; Nexstar, UK; Nexstar, USA.*
Liposomal daunorubicin citrate (p.533·3) or liposomal daunorubicin hydrochloride (p.533·1).
HIV-related Kaposi's sarcoma.

Davedax *Bracco, Ital.*
Reboxetine mesilate (p.308·1).
Depression.

D'Aveia *Dermoteca, Port.*
A range of skin, scalp, and vaginal preparations containing avena (p.1583·1).

Daverium *Searle, Ital.*
α-Dihydroergocryptine mesilate (p.1603·3).
Age-related mental and movement disorders; headache; hyperprolactinaemia; lactation inhibition; migraine; parkinsonism.

Davicaina *Davi, Port.†.*
Metamfetamine (p.1511·1); amethocaine [tetracaine] (p.1305·2).

David Morton's Quintessential *Lifeplan, UK.*
A range of multivitamin and mineral supplements (p.1350·1).

Davilose *Davi, Port.*
Methylcellulose (p.1502·2).
Dry eyes.

Davimicina *Davi, Port.*
Bacitracin (p.155·2); hydrocortisone (p.1073·3); neomycin (p.228·1).
Infected eye disorders.

Davinefrina *Davi, Port.*
Phenylephrine (p.1097·1).

Davistar *Dansk-Flama, Braz.*
Magnesium clofibrate (p.859·1); pyricarbate (p.1656·3).
Hyperlipidaemias.

Davitamon AD *Chefaro, Neth.†.*
Vitamin A palmitate (p.1383·2); colecalciferol (p.1391·1).

Davitamon AD Fluor *Chefaro, Neth.†.*
Vitamin A palmitate (p.1383·2); colecalciferol (p.1391·1); sodium fluoride (p.1375·3).
Dental caries prophylaxis; rickets.

Davitamon E *Chefaro, Neth.†.*
dl-Alpha tocoferil acetate (p.1394·1).

Davitamon Fem *Chefaro, UK.*
A range of vitamin, mineral, and nutritional supplements (p.1350·1).

Davitamon fluor *Chefaro, Neth.†.*
Sodium fluoride (p.1375·3).
Dental caries prophylaxis.

Davixolol *Davi, Port.*
Betaxolol hydrochloride (p.848·3).
Glaucoma; ocular hypertension.

Daxon *Columbia, Mex.*
Nitazoxanide (p.598·3).
Amoebiasis; giardiasis; nematode infections.

Day Cold Comfort *Boots, UK.*
Paracetamol (p.71·2); pseudoephedrine hydrochloride (p.1099·2); pholcodine (p.1099·1).
Cold symptoms.

Day & Night *Warner-Lambert, Irl.*
15 Tablets, paracetamol (p.71·2); phenylpropanolamine hydrochloride (p.1098·1); 5 tablets, paracetamol; diphenhydramine hydrochloride (p.416·1).
Cold and influenza symptoms.

Day & Night Cold & Flu *Warner-Lambert, Austral.; Warner-Lambert, NZ.*
Day capsules, paracetamol (p.71·2); pseudoephedrine hydrochloride (p.1099·2); dextromethorphan hydrobromide (p.1087·3); night capsules, paracetamol; chlorpheniramine [chlorphenamine] maleate (p.412·1); dextromethorphan hydrobromide.
Cold and influenza symptoms.

Day Nurse
Note. This name is used for preparations of different composition.
SmithKline Beecham Consumer, Irl.
Paracetamol (p.71·2); dextromethorphan hydrobromide (p.1087·3); phenylpropanolamine hydrochloride (p.1098·1).
Cold and influenza symptoms.
GlaxoSmithKline, UK.
Paracetamol (p.71·2); pholcodine (p.1099·1); pseudoephedrine hydrochloride (p.1099·2).
Formerly contained paracetamol, dextromethorphan hydrobromide, and phenylpropanolamine hydrochloride.
Cold and influenza symptoms.

Dayalets *Abbott, Hong Kong; Abbott, USA.*
Multivitamin preparation (p.1350·1).

Dayalets + Iron *Abbott, USA.*
Multivitamin preparation with iron and folic acid (p.1350·1).

Dayalets plus Iron *Abbott, Hong Kong.*
Multivitamin preparation with iron (p.1350·1).

Dayamin *Atlantic, Thai.*
Astemizole (p.409·1).
Hypersensitivity reactions.

Dayamineral *Abbott, Spain.*
Multivitamin and mineral preparation (p.1350·1).

Daycef *Epifarma, Ital.*
Cefonicid sodium (p.168·1).
Lignocaine [lidocaine] hydrochloride (p.1313·2) is included in this preparation to alleviate the pain of injection.
Gram-negative bacterial infections.

Dayhist *The Forty-Two, Thai.*
Mebhydrolin napadisilate (p.420·2).
Hypersensitivity reactions.

Dayhist-1 *Major, USA.*
Clemastine fumarate (p.413·2).
Allergic rhinitis; urticaria.

Daypro *Searle, Canad.; Searle, USA.*
Oxaprozin (p.70·2).
Osteoarthritis; rheumatoid arthritis.

Dayquil *Procter & Gamble, Canad.*
Pseudoephedrine hydrochloride (p.1099·2); dextromethorphan hydrobromide (p.1087·3); paracetamol (p.71·2).
Cold and influenza symptoms.

Dayquil Sinus with Pain Relief *Procter & Gamble, Canad.†.*
Pseudoephedrine hydrochloride (p.1099·2); ibuprofen (p.43·2).

Days *Merck, Mex.*
Ibuprofen (p.43·2).
Fever; inflammation; pain.

Daytime Cold & Flu *Stanley, Canad.*
Pseudoephedrine hydrochloride (p.1099·2); dextromethorphan hydrobromide (p.1087·3); guaifenesin (p.1092·2); paracetamol (p.71·2).

Dayto Anase *Dayton, USA†.*
Bromelains (p.1586·3).

Dayto Himbin *Dayton, USA.*
Yohimbine hydrochloride (p.1681·3).

Dayto Sulf *Dayton, USA†.*
Sulfathiazole (p.257·1); sulfacetamide (p.250·3); sulfabenzamide (p.250·2); urea (p.1127·3).
Vaginitis due to Gardnerella vaginalis.

Daywear *Estee Lauder, Canad.*
SPF 15: Octinoxate (p.1517·3); titanium dioxide (p.1126·1).
Sunscreen.

Dazamide *Major, USA.*
Acetazolamide (p.826·1).
Epilepsy; glaucoma; oedema; symptoms associated with acute mountain sickness.

Dazen *Takeda, Fr.*
Serrapeptase (p.1662·1).
Oedema; respiratory-tract congestion.

Dazine *PP Lab, Thai.*
Thioridazine hydrochloride (p.708·1).
Anxiety; mania; schizophrenia.

Dazocan *Protein, Mex.*
Albendazole (p.95·2).

Dazol *Darrow, Braz.*
Albendazole (p.95·2).
Worm infections.

DC Softgels *Goldline, USA.*
Docusate calcium (p.1222·3).
Constipation.

DC Vin *Medicamed, Port.*
Vinpocetine (p.1680·1).
Vascular disorders.

D-Calsor *Orion, Fin.*
Calcium hydrogen phosphate (p.1188·2); colecalciferol (p.1391·1).
Calcium supplement; vitamin D deficiency.

DCCK *Fuisz, Ger.*
Co-dergocrine mesilate (p.1597·3).
Cerebral and peripheral vascular disorders; cervical disc syndrome; hypertension; migraine; shock.

D-Coate *Hua, Thai.*
Dextromethorphan hydrobromide (p.1087·3); guaifenesin (p.1092·2); terpin hydrate (p.1101·2).
Coughs.

D-Cure *SMB, Belg.*
Colecalciferol (p.1391·1).
Dietary supplement; hypoparathyroidism; pseudohypoparathyroidism; vitamin D deficiency.

DDAVP *Whitehall, Braz.; Ferring, Canad.; Ferring, Ger.; Mex-America, Mex.; Ferring, Port.; Ferring, S.Afr.; Ferring, UK; Aventis, USA.*
Desmopressin acetate (p.1281·2).
Diabetes insipidus; haemophilia; headache resulting from lumbar puncture; multiple sclerosis associated nocturia; polydipsia; polyuria; test of fibrinolytic response; test of renal concentrating capacity; von Willebrand's disease.

DDD *Austroplant, Aust.*
Lotion: Salicylic acid (p.1122·3); chlorobutanol (p.1141·2); methyl salicylate (p.55·1); thymol (p.1158·3).
Lotion, extra strong†: Salicylic acid (p.1122·3); chlorobutanol (p.1141·2); methyl salicylate (p.55·1); thymol (p.1158·3); phenol (p.1152·3).
Ointment: Salicylic acid (p.1122·3); chlorobutanol (p.1141·2); methyl salicylate (p.55·1); thymol (p.1158·3); camphor (p.1589·3).
Skin disorders.

delta pronatura, Ger.†.
Thymol (p.1158·3); salicylic acid (p.1122·3); methyl salicylate (p.55·1).
Skin disorders.

DDD, UK.
Cream: Thymol (p.1158·3); menthol (p.1632·3); methyl salicylate (p.55·1); chlorobutanol (p.1141·2); titanium dioxide (p.1126·1).
Acne; cuts; grazes.
Lotion: Thymol (p.1158·3); menthol (p.1632·3); salicylic acid (p.1122·3); chlorobutanol (p.1141·2); methyl salicylate (p.55·1).
Acne; rashes.

De Icin *Asta Medica, Belg.*
Dexamethasone sodium metasulfobenzoate (p.1067·1); neomycin sulfate (p.228·1); polymyxin B sulfate (p.238·1).
Infected eye disorders.

De Icol *Asta Medica, Belg.*
Dexamethasone sodium phosphate (p.1067·1); chloramphenicol (p.179·1).
Infected eye disorders.

de STAT *Sherman, USA.*
Range of solutions for contact lenses (p.1129·3).

De Witt's Analgesic *De Witt, UK.*
Paracetamol (p.71·2); caffeine (p.761·3).
Fever; pain.

De Witts Antacid
Note. This name is used for preparations of different composition.
Fleet, Austral.
Oral powder: Magnesium trisilicate (p.1233·3); magnesium carbonate (p.1232·3); calcium carbonate (p.1215·1); sodium bicarbonate (p.1186·2); kaolin (p.1229·3); aluminium hydroxide (p.1210·3).
Tablets†: Magnesium trisilicate (p.1233·3); magnesium carbonate (p.1232·3); calcium carbonate (p.1215·1); sodium bicarbonate (p.1186·2); aluminium hydroxide (p.1210·3).
Hyperacidity.
De Witt, UK.
Oral powder: Magnesium trisilicate (p.1233·3); light magnesium carbonate (p.1232·3); calcium carbonate (p.1215·1); sodium bicarbonate (p.1186·2); light kaolin (p.1229·3); peppermint oil (p.1243·3).
Tablets: Calcium carbonate (p.1215·1); magnesium carbonate (p.1232·3); magnesium trisilicate (p.1233·3); peppermint oil (p.1243·3).
Dyspepsia; gastric hyperacidity; heartburn.

De Witt's K & B Pills *De Witt, UK.*
Bearberry (p.1583·1); buchu (p.1587·2).
Fluid retention.

De Witt's Lozenges *De Witt, UK.*
Benzocaine (p.1306·2); cetylpyridinium chloride (p.1138·1).
Formerly contained tyrothricin, benzocaine, and cetylpyridinium chloride.
Sore throat.

De Witts New Pills *Fleet, Austral.*
Bearberry (p.1583·3); buchu (p.1587·2).
Fluid retention.

De Witts Pills *De Witt, NZ.*
Bearberry (p.1583·3); buchu (p.1587·2); caffeine (p.761·3); methylene blue [methylthioninium chloride] (p.1012·3).
Fluid retention.

Deacura *Dermapharm, Ger.*
Biotin (p.1355·3).
Biotin deficiency.

Deadyn *Boehringer Ingelheim, Ital.†.*
Pemoline (p.1513·1); levoglutamide (p.1365·2).
Tonic.

Deaftol avec lidocaine *Wild, Switz.*
Aluminium lactate (p.1578·2); lignocaine [lidocaine] hydrochloride (p.1313·2).
Mouth and throat disorders.

Dealan *Silanes, Mex.*
Coal tar (p.1125·1); clioquinol (p.190·2); allantoin (p.1110·1).
Seborrhoeic dermatitis.

Dealgic *Searle, Ital.*
Diclofenac sodium (p.30·3).
Inflammation; musculoskeletal and joint disorders; pain.

Dealyd *Rosch & Handel, Aust.*
Polyphloroglucinol phosphate (p.1121·3).
Skin disorders.

Deanxit *Lundbeck, Aust.; Lundbeck, Belg.; Lundbeck, Hong Kong; Lundbeck, Ital.; Lundbeck, Singapore; Lundbeck, Spain; Lundbeck, Switz.; Lundbeck, Thai.*
Flupentixol hydrochloride (p.684·1); melitracen hydrochloride (p.297·3).
Anxiety; depression.

Deavynfar *Remir, Mex.*
Chlorpropamide (p.321·1).
Diabetes mellitus.

Deb *Searle, Ital.*
Tetridamine maleate (p.87·3).
Cervicitis; vulvovaginitis.

Debacterol *Northern Research, USA.*
Sulfuric acid (p.1668·2); sulfonated phenols (p.1152·3).
Mouth and gum disorders.

Debax *Gebro, Aust.*
Captopril (p.853·3).
Diabetic nephropathy; heart failure; hypertension; myocardial infarction.

Debefenium *UCI, Braz.*
Bephenium hydroxynaphthoate (p.97·2).
Ancylostomiasis; ascariasis.

Debei *Eurofarma, Braz.*
Phenformin hydrochloride (p.333·2).
Diabetes mellitus.

Debeina *CPH, Port.*
Phenformin hydrochloride (p.333·2).
Diabetes mellitus.

Debekacyl *Rhone-Poulenc Rorer, Fr.†.*
Dibekacin sulfate (p.198·3).
Bacterial infections.

Debela *Brasifa, Braz.*
Dipyrone (p.34·1).
Fever; pain.

Debeone *Armstrong, Mex.*
Phenformin hydrochloride (p.333·2).
Diabetes mellitus.

Deblaston
Madaus, Aust.; Hoyer, Ger.; Byk Madaus, S.Afr.; Madaus, Switz.
Pipemidic acid (p.236·1).
Bacterial infections of the urinary tract.

Debonal *Cryopharma, Mex.*
Sodium bicarbonate (p.1186·2).
Metabolic acidosis.

Debridat
Croma, Aust.; Enila, Braz.; Parke, Davis, Fr.; Sigma-Tau, Ital.; Smith-Kline Beecham, Mex.; Parke, Davis, Port.; Parke, Davis, Singapore; Uhlmann-Eyraud, Switz.
Trimebutine (p.1675·1) or trimebutine maleate (p.1675·1).
Gastrointestinal disorders.

Debripad *Pharmacia, Neth.†.*
Dextranomer (p.1113·1).
Infected wounds.

Debrisan
Pharmacia Upjohn, Belg.; Pharmacia Upjohn, Canad.†; Pharmacia Upjohn, Fr.†; Pharmacia Upjohn, Hong Kong; Pharmacia Upjohn, Irl.; Kabi Pharmacia, Israel; Pharmacia Upjohn, Ital.; Pharmacia Upjohn, Mex.; Pharmacia Upjohn, Neth.; Pharmacia Upjohn, S.Afr.†; Pharmacia Upjohn, Swed.†; Pharmacia Upjohn, Switz.†; Pharmacia, UK; Johnson & Johnson, USA.
Dextranomer (p.1113·1).
Burns; cleansing of exudating wounds; skin ulcers.

Debrisorb
Pharmacia Upjohn, Aust.; Pharmacia Upjohn, Ger.
Dextranomer (p.1113·1).
Wounds.

Debrox
Farmila, Ital.; Marion Merrell Dow, USA.
Urea hydrogen peroxide (p.1159·3).
Ear wax removal.

Debrum *Sigma-Tau, Ital.*
Trimebutine maleate (p.1675·1); medazepam (p.690·2).
Gastrointestinal spasm with a component of anxiety.

Debrumyl
Pierre Fabre Sante, Fr.; Pierre Fabre, Port.
Deanol pidolate (p.1507·2); heptaminol hydrochloride (p.1619·2).
Mental function disorders.

Debtan *Yung Shin, Thai.*
Glibenclamide (p.321·3).
Diabetes mellitus.

Dec
Note. This name is used for preparations of different composition.
Synca, Hong Kong.
Codeine phosphate (p.25·2); ephedrine hydrochloride (p.1090·1); dexchlorpheniramine maleate (p.412·1); ammonium chloride (p.1085·2).
Coughs.

PP Lab, Thai.
Dextromethorphan hydrobromide (p.1087·3).
Coughs.

Deca
Note. This name is used for preparations of different composition.
Medinova, Switz.†.
Aluminium chloride (p.1110·2); lignocaine [lidocaine] hydrochloride (p.1313·2); cetalkonium chloride (p.1137·1); menthol (p.1632·3).
Mouth and throat disorders.

Atlantic, Thai.
Fluphenazine decanoate (p.684·3).
Schizophrenia.

Decacef *Boniscontro & Gazzone, Ital.†.*
Cefmetazole sodium (p.167·2).
Lignocaine [lidocaine] hydrochloride (p.1313·2) is included in this preparation to alleviate the pain of injection.
Bacterial infections.

Decadran *Merck Sharp & Dohme, Spain.*
Dexamethasone (p.1067·1), dexamethasone phosphate (p.1067·1), or dexamethasone sodium phosphate (p.1067·1).
Corticosteroid.

Decadran Neomicina *Merck Sharp & Dohme, Spain.*
Dexamethasone phosphate (p.1067·1); neomycin sulfate (p.228·1).
Eye or ear disorders.

Decadron
Note. This name is used for preparations of different composition.
Merck Sharp & Dohme, Austral.†; Merck Sharp & Dohme, Belg.; Prodome, Braz.; Merck Frosst, Canad.; Merck Sharp & Dohme, Denm.; Merck Sharp & Dohme, Fin.; Merck Sharp & Dohme-Chibret, Fr.; Merck Sharp & Dohme, Hong Kong; Merck Sharp & Dohme, Irl.; Merck Sharp & Dohme, Ital.; Merck Sharp & Dohme, Mex.; Merck

Sharp & Dohme, Neth.; Merck Sharp & Dohme, Norw.; Merck Sharp & Dohme, NZ; Merck Sharp & Dohme, Port.; Merck Sharp & Dohme, S.Afr.; Merck Sharp & Dohme, Swed.; Merck Sharp & Dohme, Switz.; Merck Sharp & Dohme, Thai.; Merck Sharp & Dohme, UK; Merck, USA.
Dexamethasone (p.1067·1) or dexamethasone sodium phosphate (p.1067·1).
Corticosteroid.

Merck Sharp & Dohme, Port.
Eye/ear drops: Dexamethasone sodium phosphate (p.1067·1); neomycin sulfate (p.228·1).
Infected eye and ear disorders.

Decadron avec Neomycine *Merck Sharp & Dohme, Belg.*
Dexamethasone sodium phosphate (p.1067·1); neomycin sulfate (p.228·1).
Infected eye and external ear disorders.

Decadron Con Neomicina *Merck Sharp & Dohme, Mex.*
Eye and ear drops: Dexamethasone sodium phosphate (p.1067·1); neomycin sulfate (p.228·1).
Infected eye and ear disorders.
Nasal drops: Dexamethasone sodium phosphate (p.1067·1); neomycin sulfate (p.228·1); phenylephrine hydrochloride (p.1097·1).
Rhinitis.

Decadron Con Nistatina *Merck Sharp & Dohme, Mex.*
Dexamethasone tebutate (p.1067·3); diiodohydroxyquinoline (p.590·2); nystatin (p.392·2).
Vaginitis.

Decadron cum neomycin *Merck Sharp & Dohme, Swed.*
Dexamethasone sodium phosphate (p.1067·1); neomycin sulfate (p.228·1).
Infected eye and ear disorders.

Decadron Depot *Merck Sharp & Dohme, Neth.†.*
Dexamethasone acetate (p.1067·1).
Corticosteroid.

Decadron med Neomycin *Merck Sharp & Dohme, Denm.*
Dexamethasone sodium phosphate (p.1067·1); neomycin sulfate (p.228·1).
Infected eye and ear disorders.

Decadron met neomycine *Merck Sharp & Dohme, Neth.*
Dexamethasone sodium phosphate (p.1067·1); neomycin sulfate (p.228·1).
Infected eye and ear disorders.

Decadron Nasal *Prodome, Braz.*
Dexamethasone (p.1067·1); neomycin (p.228·1); phenylephrine (p.1097·1).
Infected nasal disorders.

Decadron with Neomycin
Merck Sharp & Dohme, Hong Kong; Merck Sharp & Dohme, Thai.
Dexamethasone sodium phosphate (p.1067·1); neomycin sulfate (p.228·1).
Infected eye and ear disorders.

Decadron Oftalmico *Prodome, Braz.*
Dexamethasone (p.1067·1); neomycin sulfate (p.228·1); phenylephrine (p.1097·1).
Infected eye disorders.

Decadron Phosphat *Merck Sharp & Dohme, Ger.†.*
Dexamethasone phosphate (p.1067·1).
Corticosteroid.

Decadronal
Prodome, Braz.; Merck Sharp & Dohme, Mex.
Dexamethasone acetate (p.1067·1).
Corticosteroid.

Deca-Durabol *Organon, Swed.*
Nandrolone decanoate (p.1484·2).
Anaemia; osteoporosis.

Deca-Durabolin
Organon, Aust.; Organon, Austral.; Organon, Belg.; Akzo, Braz.; Organon, Canad.; Organon, Fin.; Organon, Ger.; Organon, Hong Kong; Organon, Irl.; Organon, Israel; Organon, Ital.; Organon, Mex.; Organon, Neth.; Organon, Norw.; Pharmaco, NZ; Organon, Port.; Donmed, S.Afr.; Organon, Singapore; Organon, Spain; Organon, Switz.; Organon, Thai.; Organon, UK; Organon, USA.
Nandrolone decanoate (p.1484·2).
Anabolic; anaemia; breast cancer; osteoporosis.

Decafar *Lafare, Ital.*
Ubidecarenone (p.1677·1).
Cardiac disorders.

Decafen *Rolab, S.Afr.†.*
Fluphenazine decanoate (p.684·3).
Psychoses.

Decagen *Goldline, USA.*
Multivitamin and mineral preparation with iron and folic acid (p.1350·1).

Decaject *Mayrand, USA.*
Dexamethasone acetate (p.1067·1) or dexamethasone sodium phosphate (p.1067·1).
Corticosteroid.

Decal *Rice Steele, Irl.*
Calcium lactate (p.1188·2); calcium gluconate (p.1188·2); calcium phosphate (p.1188·3); ergocalciferol (p.1188·2).
Calcium deficiencies; calcium supplement.

Decalcit *Neves, Port.; Geistlich, Switz.*
Ergocalciferol (p.1391·2) or colecalciferol (p.1391·1); calcium hydrogen phosphate (p.1188·2).
Calcium and vitamin D deficiency; osteomalacia; osteoporosis; rickets.

Decalogiflox *Pharmacia Upjohn, Fr.*
Lomefloxacin hydrochloride (p.220·1).
Urinary-tract infections.

Decaltrex *Ern, Spain.*
Amino-acid, vitamin, and mineral preparation (p.1350·1).

Decan *Baxter, UK.*
Electrolyte (p.1180·1) and trace element preparation (p.1350·1).
Parenteral nutrition.

Deca-Noralone *Taro, Israel.*
Nandrolone decanoate (p.1484·2).
Anabolic; breast cancer; osteoporosis; renal failure.

Decapeptyl
Ferring, Aust.; Ipsen, Belg.; Ferring, Denm.; Ferring, Fin.; Ipsen Biotech, Fr.; Ferring, Ger.; Tosse, Ger.; Ferring, Hong Kong; Ipsen, Irl.; Ferring, Israel; Ipsen, Ital.; Ferring, Neth.; Aventis, NZ; Ipsen, Port.; Adcock Ingram, S.Afr.; Ferring, Singapore; Ipsen, Spain; Ferring, Swed.; Ferring, Switz.; Ferring, Thai.; Ipsen, UK.
Triptorelin (p.1299·1), triptorelin acetate (p.1299·1), or triptorelin embonate (p.1299·1).
Breast cancer; endometriosis; female infertility; ovarian cancer; precocious puberty; prostatic cancer; uterine fibroids.

Decaprednil *Orion, Ger.*
Prednisolone (p.1077·3) or prednisolone acetate (p.1078·1).
Corticosteroid.

Decaquinon *Eisai, Thai.*
Ubidecarenone (p.1677·1).
Heart failure.

Decaris
Janssen, Hong Kong; Janssen, Mex.
Levamisole (p.101·3) or levamisole hydrochloride (p.101·2).
Nematode infections.

Decasept N *Streuli, Switz.*
Dequalinium chloride (p.1374·1); calcium pantothenate (p.1374·1); lauromacrogol 400 (p.1915·2).
Decasept formerly contained dequalinium chloride, calcium pantothenate, lauromacrogol 400, and ammonium gualenate.
Mouth and throat disorders.

Decasona *Alter, Spain.*
Beclometasone dipropionate (p.1061·2).
Asthma.

Decasone *Aspen, S.Afr.*
Dexamethasone phosphate (p.1067·1).
Corticosteroid.

Decaspray *Merck, USA.*
Dexamethasone (p.1067·1).
Skin disorders.

Decatylen
Note. This name is used for preparations of different composition.
Mepha, Hong Kong; Mepha, Singapore.
Dequalinium chloride (p.1143·1); cinchocaine hydrochloride (p.1309·1).
Mouth and throat disorders.

Protisin, Mex.
Dequalinium chloride (p.1143·1).

Decatylene *Mepha, Switz.*
Dequalinium chloride (p.1143·1).
Mouth and throat disorders.

Decatylene Neo *Mepha, Switz.*
Dequalinium chloride (p.1143·1); cinchocaine hydrochloride (p.1309·1).
Mouth and throat disorders.

Decaugh *Fortune, Hong Kong.*
Dextromethorphan hydrobromide (p.1087·3); guaifenesin (p.1092·2).
Coughs.

Decavit *Rowa, Irl.*
Multivitamin preparation (p.1350·1).

Decazate *Berk, UK†.*
Fluphenazine decanoate (p.684·3).

Decentan
Merck, Aust.; Merck, Ger.; Merck, Spain.
Perphenazine (p.699·1) or perphenazine enantate (p.699·1).
Anxiety disorders; depression; nausea; pain; psychoses; vomiting.

Decholin
Riedel-Zabinka, Braz.; Miles, USA.
Dehydrocholic acid (p.1602·2).
Biliary disorders; constipation.

Decipar *Italfarmaco, Spain.*
Enoxaparin sodium (p.885·1).
Thromboembolic disorders.

Declinax *Cambridge, UK.*
Debrisoquine sulfate (p.866·2).
Now known as Debrisoquine Tablets.
Hypertension.

Decloban *Farmacusi, Spain.*
Clobetasol propionate (p.1065·2).
Skin disorders.

Declomycin
Wyeth-Ayerst, Canad.; Lederle, USA.
Demeclocycline hydrochloride (p.198·2).
Bacterial infections; intestinal amoebiasis.

Decme *Italmex, Mex.*
Dihydroergocristine mesilate (p.1603·2).

Decocort *Hoe, Singapore.*
Miconazole nitrate (p.391·1); hydrocortisone (p.1073·3).
Fungal and Gram-positive bacterial skin infections with inflammation.

Decoderm
Hermal, Aust.; Boots Healthcare, Belg.; Hermal, Ger.; Boots Healthcare, Neth.; Boots Healthcare, Spain; Boots Healthcare, Switz.
Fluprednidene acetate (p.1072·1).
Skin disorders.

Decoderm Base *Boots Healthcare, Switz.*
Emollient.
Skin disorders.

Decoderm Basiscreme *Hermal, Ger.*
Emollient.
Skin disorders.

Decoderm bivalent *Boots Healthcare, Switz.*
Fluprednidene acetate (p.1072·1); miconazole nitrate (p.391·1).
Infected skin disorders.

Decoderm Comp
Boots Healthcare, Belg.; Hermal, Ger.
Fluprednidene acetate (p.1072·1); gentamicin sulfate (p.210·1).
Infected skin disorders.

Decoderm compositum *Hermal, Aust.*
Fluprednidene acetate (p.1072·1); gentamicin sulfate (p.210·1).
Infected skin disorders.

Decoderm tri *Hermal, Ger.*
Fluprednidene acetate (p.1072·1); miconazole nitrate (p.391·1).
Infected skin disorders.

Decoderm trivalent *Hermal, Aust.*
Fluprednidene acetate (p.1072·1); gentamicin sulfate (p.210·1); cloxiquine (p.214·1).
Infected skin disorders.

Decoderm Trivalente *Boots Healthcare, Spain.*
Fluprednidene acetate (p.1072·1); neomycin sulfate (p.228·1); cloxiquine (p.214·1).
Infected skin disorders.

Decofam Cough *DHA, Singapore.*
Ammonium chloride (p.1085·2); ephedrine hydrochloride (p.1090·1); guaifenesin (p.1092·2); menthol (p.1632·3).
Coughs.

Decofed *Barre-National, USA; Major, USA.*
Pseudoephedrine hydrochloride (p.1099·2).
Nasal congestion.

Decohistine DH *Morton Grove, USA.*
Pseudoephedrine hydrochloride (p.1099·2); chlorpheniramine [chlorphenamine] maleate (p.412·1); codeine phosphate (p.25·2).
Coughs and cold symptoms.

Decohistine Expectorant *Morton Grove, USA†.*
Guaifenesin (p.1092·2); pseudoephedrine hydrochloride (p.1099·2); codeine phosphate (p.25·2).

Decolgen
Note. This name is used for preparations of different composition.
Westmont, Hong Kong; Westmont, Singapore.
Oral liquid: Chlorpheniramine [chlorphenamine] maleate (p.412·1); paracetamol (p.71·2); phenylpropanolamine hydrochloride (p.1098·1).
Cold symptoms; upper respiratory-tract disorders.

Westmont, Singapore.
Tablets: Ascorbic acid (p.1389·3); chlorpheniramine [chlorphenamine] maleate (p.412·1); paracetamol (p.71·2); phenylpropanolamine hydrochloride (p.1098·1).
Cold symptoms; upper respiratory-tract disorders.

Great Eastern, Thai.; Westmont, Thai.
Paracetamol (p.71·2); chlorpheniramine [chlorphenamine] maleate (p.412·1).
Formerly contained phenylpropanolamine hydrochloride, paracetamol, and chlorpheniramine [chlorphenamine] maleate.
Cold symptoms; hay fever; respiratory-tract disorders; sinusitis.

Decon *Noristan Generica, S.Afr.†.*
Paracetamol (p.71·2); phenylephrine hydrochloride (p.1097·1); phenyltoloxamine citrate (p.423·1); caffeine (p.761·3); chlorpheniramine [chlorphenamine] maleate (p.412·1).
Upper respiratory-tract disorders.

Deconamine
Kenwood, Hong Kong; Kenwood, USA.
Chlorpheniramine [chlorphenamine] maleate (p.412·1); pseudoephedrine hydrochloride (p.1099·2).
Allergic rhinitis; sinusitis.

Deconamine CX *Bradley, USA.*
Guaifenesin (p.1092·2); hydrocodone tartrate (p.42·2); pseudoephedrine hydrochloride (p.1099·2).
Coughs.

Decongest
Technilab, Canad.; Technilab, Hong Kong.
Xylometazoline hydrochloride (p.1102·2).
Nasal congestion.

Decongestabs *Parmed, USA†.*
Phenylpropanolamine hydrochloride (p.1098·1); phenylephrine hydrochloride (p.1097·1); chlorpheniramine [chlorphenamine] maleate (p.412·1); phenyltoloxamine citrate (p.423·1).
Upper respiratory-tract symptoms.

Decongestant
Note. This name is used for preparations of different composition.
Moore, USA†.
Phenylpropanolamine hydrochloride (p.1098·1); phenylephrine hydrochloride (p.1097·1); chlorpheniramine [chlorphenamine] maleate (p.412·1); phenyltoloxamine citrate (p.423·1).
Upper respiratory-tract symptoms.

The symbol † denotes a preparation no longer actively marketed

Rugby, USA.
Phenylephrine hydrochloride (p.1097·1); paracetamol (p.71·2); chlorpheniramine [chlorphenamine] maleate (p.412·1).
Upper respiratory-tract symptoms.

Decongestant Antihistaminic Syrup Pharmascience, Canad.†.
Brompheniramine maleate (p.410·2); phenylephrine hydrochloride (p.1097·1); phenylpropanolamine hydrochloride (p.1098·1).
Antihistamine; decongestant.

Decongestant Expectorant Schein, USA†.
Pseudoephedrine hydrochloride (p.1099·2); guaifenesin (p.1092·2); codeine phosphate (p.25·2).
Coughs.

Decongestant Nasal Mist Prodemdis, Canad.
Oxymetazoline hydrochloride (p.1096·2).

Decongestant Nasal Spray Prodemdis, Canad.; Technilab, Canad.; Stanley, Canad.
Xylometazoline hydrochloride (p.1102·2).

Decongestant Nose Drops Prodemdis, Canad.
Xylometazoline hydrochloride (p.1102·2).

Decongestant SR Geneva, USA†.
Phenylpropanolamine hydrochloride (p.1098·1); phenylephrine hydrochloride (p.1097·1); chlorpheniramine [chlorphenamine] maleate (p.412·1); phenyltoloxamine citrate (p.423·1).
Upper respiratory-tract symptoms.

Decongestant Tablets Stanley, Canad.; Unichem, UK.
Pseudoephedrine hydrochloride (p.1099·2).

Deconhist LA Goldline, USA†.
Phenylephrine hydrochloride (p.1097·1); phenylpropanolamine hydrochloride (p.1098·1); chlorpheniramine [chlorphenamine] maleate (p.412·1); hyoscyamine sulfate (p.469·3); atropine sulfate (p.461·1); hyoscine hydrobromide (p.468·2).
Upper respiratory-tract symptoms.

Deconomed Iopharm, USA.
Pseudoephedrine hydrochloride (p.1099·2); chlorpheniramine [chlorphenamine] maleate (p.412·1).
Upper respiratory-tract disorders.

Deconsal II Medeva, USA.
Pseudoephedrine hydrochloride (p.1099·2); guaifenesin (p.1092·2).
Coughs.

Deconsal Pediatric Adams, USA.
Codeine phosphate (p.25·2); pseudoephedrine hydrochloride (p.1099·2); guaifenesin (p.1092·2).

Deconsal Sprinkle Adams, USA.
Phenylephrine hydrochloride (p.1097·1); guaifenesin (p.1092·2).
Coughs; nasal congestion.

Decontractyl
Note.This name is used for preparations of different composition.
Synthelabo, Belg.†; Robert & Carriere, Canad.†; Synthelabo, Fr.
Ointment: Mephenesin (p.1329·2); methyl nicotinate (p.55·1).
Painful muscular disorders.
Synthelabo, Fr.
Tablets: Mephenesin (p.1329·2).
Painful muscular disorders.

Decontractyl New Sanofi Synthelabo, Belg.
Ibuprofen (p.43·2).
Peri-articular and soft-tissue disorders.

Decorenone Italfarmaco, Ital.
Ubidecarenone (p.1677·1).
Cardiac disorders; co-enzyme Q deficiency.

Decorex Pisa, Mex.
Dexamethasone (p.1067·1).
Corticosteroid.

Decorin Invamed, USA†.
Pseudoephedrine hydrochloride (p.1099·2).

Decorpa Pierre Fabre, Ger.
Sterculia (p.1250·2).
Obesity.

Decortilen Merck, Ger.
Injection†: Prednylidene diethylaminoacetate hydrochloride (p.1079·3).
Tablets: Prednylidene (p.1079·3).
Corticosteroid.

Decortin Merck, Ger.
Prednisone (p.1079·2).
Oral corticosteroid.

Decortin H Merck, Ger.
Prednisolone (p.1077·3).
Oral corticosteroid.

Decos Sriprasit, Thai.
Promethazine hydrochloride (p.423·2); codeine phosphate (p.25·2).
Coughs.

Decostriol Jenapharm, Ger.
Calcitriol (p.1391·1).
Hypoparathyroidism; hypophosphataemia; pseudohypoparathyroidism; renal osteodystrophy; rickets.

Decozol Hoe, Singapore.
Miconazole nitrate (p.391·1).
Fungal skin and nail infections.

Decrelip Ferrer, Spain.
Gemfibrozil (p.896·2).
Hyperlipidaemias.

Decresco Monsanto, Spain.
Captopril (p.853·3); hydrochlorothiazide (p.907·3).
Hypertension.

Decrin Roche Consumer, Austral.†.
Aspirin (p.14·2); codeine phosphate (p.25·2).
Fever; pain.

Dectancyl Roussel Diamant, Fr.
Dexamethasone acetate (p.1067·1).
Corticosteroid.

Decubal
Dumex-Alphapharma, Fin.; Dumex, Port.; Cox, UK.
Emollient.
Dry skin disorders.

Decylenes Rugby, USA.
Undecenoic acid (p.395·3); zinc undecenoate (p.395·3).
Bromhidrosis; fungal skin infections; hyperhidrosis; minor skin irritation; nappy rash.

Dediol Rhone-Poulenc Rorer, Ital.
Alfacalcidol (p.1391·1).
Vitamin D deficiency.

Dedolor Klinge, Aust.
Diclofenac sodium (p.30·3).
Inflammation; musculoskeletal and joint disorders; pain.

Dedralen Italfarmaco, Ital.
Doxazosin mesilate (p.883·2).
Hypertension.

Dedrei Opfermann, Ger.
Colecalciferol (p.1391·1).
Osteoporosis; vitamin D deficiency.

Dedrogyl
Aventis, Belg.; Roussel Diamant, Fr.; Hoechst Marion Roussel, Ger.; Roussel, Port.
Calcifediol (p.1391·1).
Hypocalcaemia; hypoparathyroidism; osteodystrophy; osteomalacia; rickets.

Deep Cold Mentholatum, Canad.
Menthol (p.1632·3).

Deep Freeze Mentholatum, UK.
Menthol (p.1632·3); pentane.
Musculoskeletal, joint, and soft-tissue disorders.

Deep Freeze Cold Gel Mentholatum, UK.
Menthol (p.1632·3).
Musculoskeletal, joint, and peri-articular disorders.

Deep Heat Mentholatum, Austral.
Cream: Methyl salicylate (p.55·1); menthol (p.1632·3).
Topical spray: Methyl salicylate (p.55·1); ethyl salicylate (p.35·1); glycol salicylate (p.42·2); methyl nicotinate (p.55·1).
Muscular aches and pains.

Deep Heat Massage Mentholatum, UK.
Menthol (p.1632·3); methyl salicylate (p.55·1).
Musculoskeletal, joint, and soft-tissue disorders.

Deep Heat Maximum Strength Mentholatum, UK.
Menthol (p.1632·3); methyl salicylate (p.55·1).
Formerly known as Deep Heat Extra Strength.
Musculoskeletal, joint, and soft-tissue disorders.

Deep Heat Rub Mentholatum, Israel; Mentholatum, UK.
Menthol (p.1632·3); eucalyptus oil (p.1609·2); methyl salicylate (p.55·1); turpentine oil (p.1676·3).
Musculoskeletal, joint, and soft-tissue disorders.

Deep Heat Spray Mentholatum, Israel; Mentholatum, UK.
Methyl nicotinate (p.55·1); glycol salicylate (p.42·2); methyl salicylate (p.55·1); ethyl salicylate (p.35·1).
Musculoskeletal, joint, peri-articular, and soft-tissue disorders.

Deep Heating Mentholatum, Canad.
Methyl salicylate (p.55·1); menthol (p.1632·3).

Deep Heating Lotion Mentholatum, USA†.
Methyl salicylate (p.55·1); menthol (p.1632·3).
Musculoskeletal, joint, and soft-tissue pain; neuralgia.

Deep Heating Rub Mentholatum, Singapore; Mentholatum, USA†.
Methyl salicylate (p.55·1); menthol (p.1632·3).
Arthritis; musculoskeletal, joint, and soft-tissue pain; neuralgia.

Deep Heating Spray Mentholatum, Singapore.
Methyl salicylate (p.55·1); ethyl salicylate (p.35·1); glycol salicylate (p.42·2); methyl nicotinate (p.55·1).
Musculoskeletal, joint, and soft-tissue pain.

Deep Relief Mentholatum, UK.
Ibuprofen (p.43·2); menthol (p.1632·3).
Musculoskeletal, joint, and soft-tissue disorders.

Deep-Down Rub SmithKline Beecham, USA.
Methyl salicylate (p.55·1); menthol (p.1632·3); camphor (p.1589·3).
Muscle, joint, and soft-tissue pain; neuralgia.

Deetipat Ferrosan, Fin.
Colecalciferol (p.1391·1).
Vitamin D deficiency.

Defanyl Wyeth Lederle, Fr.
Amoxapine (p.279·2).
Depression.

Defatig Allergan-Frumtost, Braz.
Vitamin B substances; potassium aspartate; magnesium aspartate (p.1350·1).
Nutritional supplement.

Defaxina Smaller, Spain.
Cefalexin (p.161·3).
Bacterial infections.

DeFed Ferndale, USA.
Pseudoephedrine hydrochloride (p.1099·2).
Nasal congestion.

Defencid Duopharm, Ger.†.
Devil's claw root (p.26·3).
Musculoskeletal and joint disorders.

Defen-LA Horizon, USA.
Pseudoephedrine hydrochloride (p.1099·2); guaifenesin (p.1092·2).

Defibrase Gerot, Aust.
Batroxobin (p.726·3).
Thromboembolic disorders.

Defifical B12 Gross, Braz.
Calcium phosphate; sodium fluoride; colecalciferol; cyanocobalamin (p.1350·1).
Nutritional supplement.

Defiltran Alpharma, Fr.
Acetazolamide (p.826·1).
Soft tissue injury.

Deflam Aspen, S.Afr.
Oxaprozin (p.70·2).
Musculoskeletal and joint disorders.

Deflamat Klinge, Aust.; Sankyo, Ital.
Diclofenac sodium (p.30·3).
Gout; inflammation; musculoskeletal, joint, peri-articular, and soft-tissue disorders; pain.

Deflamm Klinge, Aust.
Diclofenac sodium (p.30·3).
Musculoskeletal pain and inflammation.

Deflamol Fumouze, Fr.
Titanium dioxide (p.1126·1); zinc oxide (p.1128·2).
Dermatitis.

Deflamon SPA, Ital.
Metronidazole (p.594·1).
Anaerobic bacterial infections; trichomoniasis.

Deflan Guidotti, Ital.
Deflazacort (p.1066·1).
Oral corticosteroid.

Deflogix Vedim, Port.
Ketoprofen lysine (p.48·1).
Inflammation; musculoskeletal, joint, and peri-articular disorders.

Deflox
Note.This name is used for preparations of different composition.
Merck, Mex.
Diclofenac potassium (p.30·2) or diclofenac resinate (p.31·3).
Inflammation; pain.
Abbott, Spain.
Terazosin hydrochloride (p.980·1).
Benign prostatic hyperplasia; hypertension.

Defluina
Note.This name is used for preparations of different composition.
Ebewe, Aust.
Raubasine (p.967·2) or raubasine hydrochloride (p.967·2); dihydroergocristine mesilate (p.1603·2); dihydroergotamine mesilate (p.450·3).
Cerebral and peripheral vascular disease.
Rhone-Poulenc Rorer, Ger.
Buflomedil hydrochloride (p.851·3).
Peripheral vascular disease.
Teofarma, Ital.
Dihydroergocristine mesilate (p.1603·2).
Vascular disorders.

Defluina N Rhone-Poulenc Rorer, Ger.
Co-dergocrine mesilate (p.1597·3).
Mental function disorders.

Defomil Nakornpatana, Thai.
Aluminium hydroxide-magnesium carbonate co-dried gel (p.1211·2); magnesium hydroxide (p.1233·1); simeticone (p.1249·2).
Flatulence; gastric hyperacidity; heartburn; peptic ulcer.

Deftan Merck, Spain.
Lofepramine hydrochloride (p.297·1).
Depression.

Defungo Siam Bheasach, Thai.
Clotrimazole (p.382·1).
Fungal skin and vaginal infections; trichomoniasis.

Defy Akorn, USA†.
Tobramycin (p.263·3).
Eye infections.

Degas Whitehall, Austral.; Invamed, USA.
Simeticone (p.1249·2).
Flatulence.

Degas Extra Whitehall, Austral.
Simeticone (p.1249·2); calcium carbonate (p.1215·1); light magnesium carbonate (p.1232·3); sodium bicarbonate (p.1186·2).
Dyspepsia; flatulence.

Degas Infant Drops Whitehall, Austral.
Simeticone (p.1249·2).
Infant colic.

Degest Akorn, USA.
Naphazoline hydrochloride (p.1095·1).
Minor eye irritation.

Degest 2 Barnes Hind, NZ.
Naphazoline hydrochloride (p.1095·1); phenazone (p.77·2).
Eye irritation.

Deglogen Sanus, Braz.
Nimesulide (p.62·3).
Fever; inflammation; pain.

Degona Prodoti, Braz.
Ampicillin (p.150·3).

Probenecid (p.401·3) is included in this preparation to reduce renal tubular excretion of the antibiotic.
Bacterial infections.

Degoran Novartis Consumer, S.Afr.
Effervescent tablets: Phenylephrine hydrochloride (p.1097·1); paracetamol (p.71·2); pheniramine maleate (p.422·3).
Formerly contained phenylpropanolamine hydrochloride, paracetamol, and pheniramine maleate.
Tablets; oral liquid: Chlorpheniramine [chlorphenamine] maleate (p.412·1); phenylpropanolamine hydrochloride (p.1098·1); dextromethorphan hydrobromide (p.1087·3); paracetamol (p.71·2).
Cold and influenza symptoms.

Degran Ranbaxy, Thai.
Ergotamine tartrate (p.452·1); caffeine (p.761·3).
Migraine and other vascular headaches.

Degranol Aspen, S.Afr.
Carbamazepine (p.342·2).
Epilepsy; trigeminal neuralgia.

Dehidrobenzperidol Roche, Spain.
Droperidol (p.682·2).
General anaesthesia; neuroleptanalgesia; premedication.

Dehistine Cypress, USA.
Chlorpheniramine [chlorphenamine] maleate (p.412·1); phenylephrine hydrochloride (p.1097·1); hyoscine methonitrate (p.468·2).
Upper respiratory-tract disorders.

Dehydral Trans Canaderm, Canad.
Methenamine (p.223·1).
Bacterial infections; hyperhidrosis.

dehydro sanol tri Sanol, Ger.
Bemetizide (p.843·2); triamterene (p.986·1).
Leg pain associated with venous insufficiency.

dehydro tri mite Sanol, Ger.
Bemetizide (p.843·2); triamterene (p.986·1).
Leg pain associated with venous insufficiency.

Dehydrobenzperidol
Janssen-Cilag, Aust.†; Janssen-Cilag, Belg.†; Janssen-Cilag, Denm.†; Orion, Fin.; Janssen-Cilag, Ger.†; Janssen, Hong Kong†; Janssen, Mex.†; Janssen-Cilag, Neth.†; Janssen-Cilag, Switz.†; Janssen, Thai.†.
Droperidol (p.682·2) or droperidol tartrate (p.682·2).
Agitation; nausea and vomiting; neuroleptanalgesia; pain; premedication.

Dehydrosin Mayrhofer, Aust.†.
Bemetizide (p.843·2); triamterene (p.986·1).
Oedema.

Deiten ABC, Ital.
Nitrendipine (p.947·1).
Hypertension.

Dekamega Omega, Spain.
Piroxicam choline (p.79·3).
Gout; musculoskeletal, joint, and peri-articular disorders; pain.

Dekamin Monico, Ital.
Amino-acid infusion (p.1350·1).
Parenteral nutrition.

Dekar 2 Pentamedical, Ital.
Benzyl benzoate (p.1428·2); quassia (p.1657·1).

Dekinet Rafa, Israel.
Biperiden hydrochloride (p.464·2) or biperiden lactate (p.464·2).
Drug-induced extrapyramidal disorders; parkinsonism.

Dekristol Jenapharm, Ger.
Colecalciferol (p.1391·1).
Hypoparathyroidism; osteomalacia; osteoporosis; pseudohypoparathyroidism; rickets; vitamin D deficiency.

Del Aqua Del-Ray, USA.
Benzoyl peroxide (p.1111·1).
Acne.

Delabarre Fumouze, Fr.
Tamarind (p.1253·2); saffron (p.1029·1).
Teething pain.

De-Lact
Nutricia, Austral.; Sharpe, NZ.
Infant feed (p.1350·1).
Lactose intolerance.

Delagil Dermapharm, Ger.
Phenol-formaldehyde-urea polycondensate sodium sulfate.
Skin disorders.

Delaket Chiesi, Ital.
Delapril (p.867·1).
Hypertension.

Delakmin Albert-Roussel, Ger.†; Hoechst, Ger.†.
(5E,7E)-9,10-Secocholesta-5,7,10(19)-triene-3β,25-diol.
Renal osteopathy.

Delapride Chiesi, Ital.
Delapril hydrochloride (p.867·1); indapamide (p.913·1).
Hypertension.

Delatestryl
Squibb, Canad.; BTG, USA.
Testosterone enantate (p.1492·2).
Breast cancer; delayed puberty (males); male hypogonadism.

Delbiase Chiesi, Ital.
Magnesium chloride (p.1190·3); magnesium bromide.
Magnesium deficiency.

Delbulasa Alpharma, Braz.
Phenylbutazone (p.78·1).
Inflammation; musculoskeletal and joint disorders.

Delcoprep *Delta, Ger.*
Macrogol 4000 (p.1630·3); electrolytes (p.1180·1).
Bowel evacuation.

Delcort *Roberts, USA†.*
Hydrocortisone (p.1073·3).
Corticosteroid.

Delecit *MDM, Ital.*
Choline alfoscerate (p.1416·2).
Mental function impairment.

Delepsine *Orion, Denm.*
Sodium valproate (p.366·3).
Epilepsy.

Delestrogen *Squibb, Canad.; Monarch, USA.*
Estradiol valerate (p.1473·2).
Breast cancer; menopausal disorders; menstrual disorders; prostatic cancer.

Delfen *Janssen-Cilag, Aust.; Janssen-Cilag, Austral.; Johnson & Johnson, Canad.; Janssen-Cilag, Irl.; Janssen-Cilag, Israel; Janssen-Cilag, Port.; Janssen-Cilag, Switz.; Janssen-Cilag, UK; Advanced Care, USA.*
Nonoxinol 9 (p.1346·1).
Contraceptive.

Delgafen *Geva, Mex.*
Fenproporex (p.1510·2).

Delgamer *Marion Merrell, Spain†.*
Diethylpropion hydrochloride (p.1508·3).
Obesity.

Delicate Skin *RCA, Ital.*
Zinc oxide (p.1128·2).
Skin irritation.

Delidose *Orion, Fr.*
Estradiol (p.1473·1).
Menopausal disorders; osteoporosis.

delimmun *Sanofi Synthelabo, Ger.*
Inosine pranobex (p.627·2).
Viral infections.

Delin *Atlantic, Hong Kong.*
Dequalinium chloride (p.1143·1).
Gingivitis; sore throat.

Delipoderm *Theramex, Mon.†; Reig Jofre, Spain.*
Promestriene (p.1490·3).
Acne; seborrhoea.

Deliproct *Schering, Fr.*
Prednisolone caproate (p.1078·1); cinchocaine hydrochloride (p.1309·1).
Formerly contained prednisolone caproate, cinchocaine hydrochloride, and clemizole undecylate.
Anorectal disorders.

Delitex N *Infectopharm, Ger.*
Lindane (p.1434·1).
Pediculosis.

Deliver *Mead Johnson, Austral.; Mead Johnson, Hong Kong; Mead Johnson, NZ.*
Preparation for enteral nutrition (p.1350·1).
Fluid or volume restriction; hypermetabolic states.

Delix *Note.This name is used for preparations of different composition.*
Hoechst Marion Roussel, Ger.
Ramipril (p.966·3).
Heart failure; hypertension.

Xepa-Soul Pattinson, Singapore.
Phenylpropanolamine hydrochloride (p.1098·1); pholcodine (p.1099·1); promethazine hydrochloride (p.423·2).
Coughs.

Delix plus *Hoechst Marion Roussel, Ger.*
Ramipril (p.966·3); hydrochlorothiazide (p.907·3).
Hypertension.

Delixi *Infectopharm, Ger.*
Permethrin (p.1436·1).
Pediculosis.

Delixir *Hamilton, Austral.*
Diphenhydramine hydrochloride (p.416·1); ammonium chloride (p.1085·2); sodium citrate (p.1186·2).
Coughs and cold symptoms.

Dellova *Poutrat, Fr.*
Bladderwrack (p.1585·2); java tea (p.1625·1).
Formerly contained ovary extracts, thyroid, digitalis purpurea, and phenolphthalein (.
Obesity.

Delmuno *Hoechst Marion Roussel, Ger.*
Felodipine (p.888·3); ramipril (p.966·3).
Hypertension.

Del-Mycin *Del-Ray, USA.*
Erythromycin (p.201·2).

Delonal *Essex, Ger.; Essex, Switz.*
Alclometasone dipropionate (p.1061·3).
Skin disorders.

Delph Sun Lotion *Fenton, UK.*
Octinoxate (p.1517·3); oxybenzone (p.1518·1); titanium dioxide (p.1126·1).
Sunscreen.

Delphi *Wyeth Lederle, Belg.; Lederle, Neth.*
Triamcinolone acetonide (p.1080·1).
Skin disorders.

Delphicort *Wyeth Lederle, Aust.; Lederle, Ger.*
Triamcinolone (p.1080·1), triamcinolone acetonide (p.1080·1), or triamcinolone diacetate (p.1080·2).
Corticosteroid.

Delphimix *Lederle, Ger.*
Triamcinolone diacetate (p.1080·2).
Musculoskeletal and joint disorders.

Delphinac *Lederle, Ger.*
Diclofenac sodium (p.30·3).
Gout; inflammation; musculoskeletal, joint, and soft-tissue disorders; pain.

Delpral *Sanofi Synthelabo, Aust.*
Tiapride hydrochloride (p.709·1).
Alcohol withdrawal syndrome; movement disorders; pain.

Delrosa *ICN, Hong Kong.*
Vitamin C (p.1389·3).
Vitamin C supplement.

Delsacid *Selvi, Ital.*
Cefonicid sodium (p.168·1).
Lignocaine [lidocaine] hydrochloride (p.1313·2) is included in this preparation to alleviate the pain of injection.
Bacterial infections.

Delsym *Novartis Consumer, Canad.; Roche Consumer, Irl.; Rhone-Poulenc Rorer, Mex.; Fisons Consumer, USA.*
Dextromethorphan (p.1087·3), dextromethorphan hydrobromide (p.1087·3), or dextromethorphan polistirex (p.1088·2).
Coughs.

Delta 80 *IDI, Ital.*
Benzoyl peroxide (p.1111·1).
Acne; skin disinfection.

Delta 80 Plus *IDI, Ital.*
Benzoyl peroxide (p.1111·1); cetylpyridinium chloride (p.1138·1).
Acne; skin disinfection.

Deltacef *Pulitzer, Ital.*
Cefuroxime sodium (p.178·2).
Bacterial infections.

Deltacid *Sintofarma, Braz.*
Deltamethrin (p.1430·3).
Scabies.

Deltacid Plus *Sintofarma, Braz.*
Deltamethrin (p.1430·3); piperonyl butoxide (p.1436·2).
Pediculosis; scabies.

Deltacillin *Lagamed, S.Afr.†.*
Phenoxymethylpenicillin potassium (p.235·1).
Bacterial infections.

Deltacina *Upsamedica, Spain.*
Neomycin sulfate (p.228·1); thiomersal (p.1158·2).
Skin infections.

Delta-Cortef *Upjohn, USA.*
Prednisolone (p.1077·3).
Corticosteroid.

Deltacortene *Lepetit, Ital.*
Prednisone (p.1079·2).
Oral corticosteroid.

Deltacortril *Pfizer, Belg.; Pfizer, Irl.; Pfizer, UK.*
Prednisolone (p.1077·3).
Corticosteroid.

Delta-D *Freeda, USA.*
Colecalciferol (p.1391·1).
Dietary supplement; vitamin D deficiency.

Delta-Diona *Reuffer, Mex.*
Prednisolone (p.1077·3).
Corticosteroid.

Deltaflogin *Delta, Braz.*
Diclofenac sodium (p.30·3).
Gout; inflammation; musculoskeletal, joint, and periarticular disorders; pain.

Delta-Hadensa *Kolassa, Aust.*
Prednisolone metasulfobenzoate sodium (p.1078·1); chlorcarvacrol; ichthammol (p.1115·2); menthol (p.1632·3); with or without chamomile oil.
Anorectal disorders.

Deltalipid *Delta, Ger.*
Soya oil (p.1378·1).
Contains egg phospholipids.
Lipid infusion for parenteral nutrition.

Deltamid *Sophia, Mex.*
Prednisolone acetate (p.1078·1); sulfacetamide sodium (p.250·3).
Eye disorders.

Deltamidrina *Tubilux, Ital.*
Prednisolone acetate (p.1078·1); atropine sulfate (p.461·1); phenylephrine hydrochloride (p.1097·1).
Inflammatory eye disorders.

Deltaren *Delta, Braz.*
Diclofenac diethylamine (p.30·2) or diclofenac potassium (p.30·2).
Gout; inflammation; musculoskeletal, joint, and periarticular disorders; pain.

Deltarhinol *Hoechst Marion Roussel, Belg.†.*
Isofluprredone acetate (p.1075·3); ephedrine hydrochloride (p.1090·1); naphazoline nitrate (p.1095·1).
Rhinitis.

Deltarhinol-Mono *Aventis, Belg.*
Naphazoline nitrate (p.1095·1).
Rhinitis.

Deltarinolo *Hoechst Marion Roussel, Ital.*
Ephedrine hydrochloride (p.1090·1); naphazoline nitrate (p.1095·1).
Nasal congestion.

Deltasiton *Faes, Spain†.*
Coal tar (p.1125·1); cloxiquine (p.214·1); gramicidin (p.213·3); neomycin sulfate (p.228·1); nystatin

(p.392·2); triamcinolone acetate (p.1080·2); keratinase (p.1626·1); titanium dioxide (p.1126·1).
Infected skin disorders.

Deltasolone *Rhone-Poulenc Rorer, Austral.†.*
Prednisolone (p.1077·3).
Corticosteroid.

Deltasone *Rhone-Poulenc Rorer, Austral.†; Pharmacia Upjohn, Canad.†; Pharmacia Upjohn, Hong Kong; Pharmacia Upjohn, NZ; Upjohn, USA.*
Prednisone (p.1079·2).
Corticosteroid.

Deltasoralen *Delta Laboratories, Irl.*
Methoxsalen (p.1118·3).
Leucoderma; psoriasis; vitiligo.

Deltastab *Waymade, UK.*
Prednisolone acetate (p.1078·1).
Corticosteroid.

Delta-Tomanol *Byk, Aust.†.*
Ramifenazone (p.80·3); phenylbutazone (p.78·1); prednisolone sodium phosphate (p.1078·1); hydroxocobalamin acetate (p.1388·3).
Cinchocaine (p.1309·1) is included in this preparation to alleviate the pain of injection.
Musculoskeletal and joint disorders; neuralgia.

Delta-Tritex *Dermol, USA.*
Triamcinolone acetonide (p.1080·1).
Skin disorders.

Deltavac *Trimen, USA.*
Sulfanilamide (p.256·2); aminoacridine hydrochloride (p.1130·2); allantoin (p.1110·1).
Vaginal infections.

Deltavagin *Biagini, Ital.*
Betamethasone (p.1063·1); tyrothricin (p.267·1); norvaline.
Formerly contained betamethasone, sulfamethoxypyridazine, tyrothricin, and norvaline.
Vaginitis.

Deltavit *Delta, Braz.*
Amino-acid, vitamin, and mineral preparation (p.1350·1).

Deltazen *Irex, Fr.*
Diltiazem hydrochloride (p.874·3).
Hypertension.

Deltison *Recip, Swed.*
Prednisone (p.1079·2).
Magnesium trisilicate (p.1233·3) and calcium hydrogen phosphate (p.1188·2) are included in this preparation in an attempt to limit adverse effects on the gastrointestinal mucosa.
Corticosteroid.

Delto-cyl Ho-Len-Complex *Liebermann, Ger.*
Homoeopathic preparation.

Delufen *Bittner, Aust.*
Homoeopathic preparation.

Delursan *Hoechst, Fr.*
Ursodeoxycholic acid (p.1677·2).
Gallstones; liver and biliary disorders.

Delvas *Berk, UK.*
Amiloride hydrochloride (p.835·1); hydrochlorothiazide (p.907·3).
These ingredients can be described by the British Approved Name Co-amilozide.
Cirrhosis with ascites; heart failure; hypertension.

Del-Vi-A *Del-Ray, USA†.*
Vitamin A (p.1382·1).
Vitamin A deficiency.

Demac *Osotspa, Thai.*
Diclofenac diethylamine (p.30·2) or diclofenac sodium (p.30·3).
Fever; inflammation; musculoskeletal, joint, periarticular, and soft-tissue disorders; pain.

Demadex *Boehringer Mannheim, Canad.†; Jouveinal, Canad.†; Roche, USA.*
Torasemide (p.985·1).
Hypertension; oedema.

Demazin *Note.This name is used for preparations of different composition.*
Schering-Plough, Austral.; Schering-Plough, NZ; Schering-Plough, S.Afr.
Delayed-release tablets; sustained-release capsules: Dexchlorpheniramine maleate (p.412·1); pseudoephedrine sulfate (p.1099·3).
Upper respiratory-tract congestion.

Schering-Plough, Austral.; Schering-Plough, NZ; Schering-Plough, S.Afr.
Syrup: Chlorpheniramine [chlorphenamine] maleate (p.412·1); phenylephrine hydrochloride (p.1097·1).
Upper respiratory-tract congestion.

Schering-Plough, Austral.
Tablets: Chlorpheniramine [chlorphenamine] maleate (p.412·1); pseudoephedrine sulfate (p.1099·3).
Upper respiratory tract congestion.

Schering-Plough, USA†.
Chlorpheniramine [chlorphenamine] maleate (p.412·1); phenylpropanolamine hydrochloride (p.1098·1).
Upper respiratory-tract symptoms.

Demazin Anti-Tussive *Schering-Plough, S.Afr.*
Chlorpheniramine [chlorphenamine] maleate (p.412·1); dextromethorphan hydrobromide (p.1087·3); phenylpropanolamine hydrochloride (p.1098·1).
Coughs.

Demazin Cold & Flu *Schering-Plough, Austral.*
Chlorpheniramine [chlorphenamine] maleate (p.412·1); pseudoephedrine sulfate (p.1099·3); paracetamol (p.71·2).
Cold and influenza symptoms; sinusitis.

Demazin Day/Night Relief *Schering-Plough, Austral.; Schering-Plough, NZ.*
Day tablets, pseudoephedrine sulfate (p.1099·3); night tablets, pseudoephedrine sulfate; dexchlorpheniramine maleate (p.412·1).
Upper respiratory-tract congestion.

Demazin Decongestant *Schering-Plough, S.Afr.*
Pseudoephedrine sulfate (p.1099·3).
Upper respiratory-tract congestion.

Demazin Expectorant *Schering-Plough, S.Afr.*
Dexchlorpheniramine maleate (p.412·1) pseudoephedrine sulfate (p.1099·3) guaifenesin (p.1092·2).
Coughs.

Demazin Non-Drowsy *Schering-Plough, NZ.*
Pseudoephedrine sulfate (p.1099·3); loratadine (p.420·1).
Upper respiratory-tract congestion.

Demazin NS *Schering-Plough, NZ.*
Loratadine (p.420·1); pseudoephedrine sulfate (p.1099·3).
Rhinitis.

Demazin Sinus *Schering-Plough, Austral.*
Pseudoephedrine sulfate (p.1099·3).
Upper respiratory-tract congestion.

Demdec *Rougier, Canad.*
Pseudoephedrine hydrochloride (p.1099·2); dextromethorphan hydrobromide (p.1087·2).
Coughs; respiratory-tract congestion.

De-menthasin *Scheurich, Ger.†.*
Dequalinium salicylate (p.1143·2); hexetidine (p.1146·3).
Mouth and throat inflammation.

Demerol *Sanofi Winthrop, Braz.; Sanofi Synthelabo, Canad.; Sanofi Winthrop, USA.*
Pethidine hydrochloride (p.75·1).
Pain.

Demetil *Farmila, Ital.*
Tetryzoline hydrochloride (p.1101·2).
Eye congestion.

Demetrin *Parke, Davis, Aust.; Godecke, Ger.; Parke, Davis, Ger.; Parke, Davis, Port.; Parke, Davis, S.Afr.; Parke, Davis, Switz.*
Prazepam (p.701·1).
Anxiety.

Demex *Berlin-Chemie, Ger.*
Propyphenazone (p.80·2).
Pain.

Demiax *Merck, Spain.*
Xipamide (p.999·2).
Hypertension; oedema.

Demi-Regroton *Rhone-Poulenc Rorer, USA.*
Chlortalidone (p.857·1); reserpine (p.967·3).
Hypertension.

Demix *Ashbourne, UK.*
Doxycycline hyclate (p.200·1).

Demo baume *Demopharm, Switz.†.*
Chlorobutanol (p.1141·2); ephedrine hydrochloride (p.1090·1); lignocaine [lidocaine] hydrochloride (p.1313·2); camphor (p.1589·3); menthol (p.1632·3); lavender oil (p.1627·2); niaouli oil (p.1640·2).
Rhinitis.

Demo elixir pectoral N *Demopharm, Switz.*
Ephedrine hydrochloride (p.1090·1); guaifenesin (p.1092·2); belladonna (p.463·1); drosera (p.1606·1); hedera helix; ipecacuanha (p.1093·1).
Demo elixir pectoral formerly contained ephedrine hydrochloride, guaifenesin, belladonna, drosera, hedera helix, ipecacuanha, and codeine phosphate.
Coughs.

Demo gouttes bronchiques *Demopharm, Switz.†.*
Thyme (p.1672·2); ground ivy (p.1618·2); liquorice (p.1231·2).
Coughs with viscous mucus.

Demo gouttes contre la toux *Demopharm, Switz.†.*
Codeine phosphate (p.25·2); ephedrine hydrochloride (p.1090·1); guaifenesin (p.1092·2); drosera (p.1606·1); hedera helix; ipecacuanha (p.1093·1); thyme oil (p.1672·3).
Coughs; respiratory-tract disorders with increased or viscous mucus.

Demo pates pectorales *Demopharm, Switz.†.*
Codeine phosphate (p.25·2); benzoic acid (p.1134·2); ipecacuanha (p.1093·1); tolu balsam (p.1101·3); drosera (p.1606·1); hedera helix; plantaginis; menthol (p.1632·3); anise oil (p.1580·3); bitter orange oil; eucalyptus oil (p.1609·2); peppermint oil (p.1243·3).
Bronchitis; coughs.

Demo pommade contre les refroidissements *Democal, Switz.*
Eucalyptus oil (p.1609·2); pine needle oil; peru balsam (p.1650·2); camphor (p.1589·3); thyme oil (p.1672·3).
Cold symptoms.

Demo pommade contre les refroidissements pour bebes *Democal, Switz.*
Eucalyptus oil (p.1609·2); pine needle oil; sage oil (p.1660·2); thyme oil (p.1672·3); juniper oil (p.1625·2); peru balsam (p.1650·2).
Respiratory-tract disorders.

Demo sirop bronchique N *Demopharm, Switz.†.*
Thyme (p.1672·2); cowslip rhizome (p.1600·1); hedera helix.
Coughs.

Demo sirop contre la toux *Demopharm, Switz.†.*
Ephedrine hydrochloride (p.1090·1); guaifenesin (p.1092·2); tolu balsam (p.1101·3); drosera (p.1606·1); ipecacuanha (p.1093·1); thyme (p.1672·2); belladonna (p.463·1); liquorice (p.1231·2).
Bronchitis; catarrh; coughs.

The symbol † denotes a preparation no longer actively marketed

Demo-Cineol *Sabex, Canad.*
Eucalyptol (p.1609·2); guaiacol (p.1092·1); camphor (p.1589·3).
Cough; rheumatic pain.

Democyl *Democal, Switz.*
Paracetamol (p.71·2).
Fever; pain.

Demodenal *Demopharm, Switz.†*
Dimenhydrinate (p.415·2).
Motion sickness.

Demodenal compositum *Demopharm, Switz.*
Dimenhydrinate (p.415·2); pyridoxine hydrochloride (p.1386·3); caffeine (p.761·3).
Motion sickness.

Demoderhin *Demopharm, Switz.†*
Diphenhydramine hydrochloride (p.416·1); mepyramine maleate (p.421·1); caffeine (p.761·3).
Nasal congestion; rhinitis.

Demodon N *Democal, Switz.*
Senna (p.1248·2).
Constipation.

Demogripal *Democal, Switz.*
Paracetamol (p.71·2).
Fever; pain.

Demogripal C *Democal, Switz.*
Paracetamol (p.71·2); ascorbic acid (p.1389·3).
Cold symptoms.

Demolaxin *Democal, Switz.*
Bisacodyl (p.1212·2).
Constipation.

Demolibral *Democal, Switz.*
Acetylcysteine (p.1082·3).
Coughs.

Demolox *Wyeth Lederle, Denm.; Cyanamid, Spain.*
Amoxapine (p.279·2).
Depression.

Demonatur Capsules contre les refroidissements *Democal, Switz.*
Brown capsules, thyme oil (p.1672·3); origanum oil; savory oil; green capsules, echinacea purpurea (p.1606·2).
Influenza symptoms.

Demonatur Dragees pour les reins et la vessie *Democal, Switz.*
Bearberry (p.1583·3); solidago virgaurea; ononis (p.1644·1); echinacea (p.1606·2); Java tea (p.1625·1).
Urinary-tract disorders.

Demonatur Gouttes pour le foie et la bile *Democal, Switz.*
Vial no 1: gentian (p.1615·1); taraxacum (p.1669·1); cynara (p.1601·3); vial no 2: silybum marianum (p.1021·3); celandine (p.1618·1); berberis.
Gastrointestinal disorders.

Demopart *Ferring, Ital.*
Demoxytocin (p.1281·1).
Induction of labour; lactation induction.

DemoPectol *Democal, Switz.*
Oral drops: Thyme (p.1672·2); hedera helix; liquorice (p.1231·2).
Syrup: Thyme (p.1672·2); cowslip root (p.1600·1); hedera helix.
Coughs.

Demoplas *Godecke, Ger.*
Phenylbutazone (p.78·1).
Lignocaine [lidocaine] hydrochloride (p.1313·2) is included in this preparation to alleviate the pain of injection.
Acute ankylosing spondylitis; rheumatism.

Demoprin nouvelle formule *Democal, Switz.*
Aspirin (p.14·2).
Fever; pain.

Demosept *Democal, Switz.*
Chlorhexidine gluconate (p.1138·2); dichlorobenzyl alcohol (p.1143·2); allantoin (p.1110·1); vitamin A (p.1382·1); colecalciferol (p.1391·1).
Skin abrasions; skin irritation.

Demostan *Demopharm, Switz.†*
Ointment: Diphenhydramine hydrochloride (p.416·1); lignocaine [lidocaine] hydrochloride (p.1313·2); menthol (p.1632·3).
Topical gel: Diphenhydramine hydrochloride (p.416·1); lignocaine [lidocaine] hydrochloride (p.1313·2).
Burns; insect bites; skin irritation.

Demostan N *Democal, Switz.*
Cream: Mepyramine maleate (p.421·1); lignocaine [lidocaine] hydrochloride (p.1313·2); calcium levulinate (p.1188·3); menthol (p.1632·3).
Topical gel and liquigel; topical spray: Mepyramine maleate (p.421·1); lignocaine [lidocaine] hydrochloride (p.1313·2); dexpanthenol (p.1602·3).
Allergic, pruritic and inflamed skin conditions.

Demosvelte N *Demopharm, Switz.†*
Agar (p.1498·3); guar gum (p.323·3); sodium alginate (p.1498·3); pectin (p.1502·3); soya (p.1378·1).
Obesity.

Demotest *Pierre Fabre, Spain.*
Budesonide (p.1064·2).
Skin disorders.

Demotherm Pommade contre le rhumatisme *Democal, Switz.*
Benzyl nicotinate (p.20·2); glycol salicylate (p.42·2).
Musculoskeletal and joint pain.

Demotussil *Demopharm, Switz.†*
Codeine phosphate (p.25·2); ephedrine hydrochloride (p.1090·1); ipecacuanha (p.1093·1); guaifenesin (p.1092·2); eucalyptol (p.1609·2).
Coughs.

Demotussol *Democal, Switz.*
Butamirate citrate (p.1086·2).
Coughs.

Demovarin *Democal, Switz.*
Heparin sodium (p.902·1).
Superficial vascular disorders.

Demoven N *Democal, Switz.*
Troxerutin (p.1611·2); aesculus (p.1574·1).
Venous insufficiency.

Demovit *Democal, Switz.*
A range of multivitamin and mineral preparations (p.1350·1).
Dietary supplementation.

Demovit C *Democal, Switz.*
Ascorbic acid (p.1389·3).
Vitamin C deficiency.

Dempol *Esoform, Ital.*
Chlorhexidine gluconate (p.1138·2).
Hand disinfection.

Demser
Merck Sharp & Dohme, Neth.†; Merck Sharp & Dohme, UK†; Merck, USA.
Metirosine (p.930·2).
Available on a named patient basis in the *UK*.
Phaeochromocytoma.

Demulcin *Ferraton, Denm.*
Codeine phosphate (p.25·2); ammonium chloride (p.1085·2).
Coughs.

Demulen
Searle, Canad.†; Searle, S.Afr.†; Searle, USA.
Etynodiol diacetate (p.1477·1); ethinylestradiol (p.1476·2).
28-Day packs also contain 7 inert tablets.
Combined oral contraceptive.

Demusin *Reig Jofre, Spain.*
Albumin tannate (p.1209·3); amylase (p.1579·3); ethylmorphine hydrochloride (p.35·2).
Diarrhoea.

Denan *Boehringer Ingelheim, Ger.*
Simvastatin (p.969·2).
Hypercholesterolaemia.

Denapril *Medinfar, Port.*
Enalapril maleate (p.883·3).
Heart failure; hypertension.

Denavir
SmithKline Beecham, Fr.; SmithKline Beecham Consumer, USA.
Penciclovir (p.638·1).
Herpes labialis.

Denaxpren *Smaller, Spain.*
Naproxen (p.60·3).
Fever; gout; musculoskeletal and joint disorders; pain.

Denazox *Remedica, Thai.*
Diltiazem hydrochloride (p.874·3).
Angina pectoris.

Dencoccult *Carter-Wallace, Austral.†*
Test for occult blood in faeces.

Dencorub *Carter-Wallace, Austral.*
Camphor (p.1589·3); menthol (p.1632·3); eucalyptus oil (p.1609·2); methyl salicylate (p.55·1).
Musculoskeletal pain.

Dencorub Arthritis *Carter-Wallace, Austral.*
Trolamine salicylate (p.90·1).
Arthritis; muscle pain.

Dencorub Arthritis Ice *Carter-Wallace, Austral.*
Menthol (p.1632·3).
Musculoskeletal pain.

Dencorub Extra Strength *Carter-Wallace, Austral.*
Methyl salicylate (p.55·1); menthol (p.1632·3).
Muscle pain.

Dencyl *SmithKline Beecham, UK†.*
Dried ferrous sulfate (p.1360·3); zinc sulfate (p.1398·2); folic acid (p.1361·1).
Prophylaxis of iron and folic acid deficiency in pregnancy.

Denerel
Medochemie, Singapore; Medochemie, Thai.
Ketotifen fumarate (p.767·2).
Allergic bronchitis; allergic rhinitis; allergic skin disorders; asthma; hay fever.

Denex
Medochemie, Singapore; Medochemie, Thai.
Metoprolol tartrate (p.931·2).
Angina pectoris; hypertension; myocardial infarction.

Deniban
Boehringer Ingelheim, Aust.†; Sanofi Synthelabo, Ital.
Amisulpride (p.655·1).
Psychoses.

Denim *Hua, Thai.*
Dimenhydrinate (p.415·2).
Motion sickness; nausea and vomiting.

Deniren *Searle, Mex.*
Amoxicillin (p.149·2).
Bacterial infections.

Denisoline *Aerocid, Fr.*
Precipitated sulfur (p.1123·3); alum (p.1577·2).
Acne.

Denkacort *Denk, Hong Kong.*
Triamcinolone acetonide (p.1080·1).
Corticosteroid.

De-Nol
Parke, Davis, Austral.; Yamanouchi, Belg.†; Gerolymatos, Hong Kong; Yamanouchi, Irl.; Agis, Israel; Yamanouchi, Ital.; Yamanouchi, Neth.; Yamanouchi, Norw.†; Pharmaco, NZ; Yamanouchi, Port.; Pharmaplan, S.Afr.; Yamanouchi, Switz.; Gerolymatos, Thai.; Yamanouchi, UK†.
Tripotassium dicitratobismuthate (p.1213·2).
Dyspepsia; gastritis; peptic ulcer.

De-Noltab
Yamanouchi, Irl.; Yamanouchi, UK.
Tripotassium dicitratobismuthate (p.1213·2).
Dyspepsia; gastritis; peptic ulcer.

Denoral
Note. This name is used for preparations of different composition.
Aventis, Belg.; Theraplix, Fr.†; Rhone-Poulenc Rorer, Hong Kong; Rhone-Poulenc Rorer, Ital.
Buzepide metiodide (p.465·1); clocinizine hydrochloride (p.413·3); phenylpropanolamine hydrochloride (p.1098·1).
Allergic rhinitis; nasal congestion; sinusitis.

Theraplix, Fr.
Syrup: Clocinizine hydrochloride (p.413·3); pholcodine (p.1099·1).
Formerly contained buzepide metiodide, clocinizine hydrochloride, and pholcodine.
Coughs.

Rhone-Poulenc Rorer, Hong Kong.
Syrup: Buzepide metiodide (p.465·1); pholcodine (p.1099·1); clocinizine hydrochloride (p.413·3).
Coughs.

Denorex
Note. This name is used for preparations of different composition.
Whitehall-Robins, Canad.; Whitehall, Irl.; Whitehall, Neth.; Whitehall, Singapore; Whitehall, UK; Whitehall, USA.
Coal tar (p.1125·1); menthol (p.1632·3).
Dandruff; psoriasis; seborrhoeic dermatitis.

Whitehall, Israel.
Coal tar (p.1125·1).
Dandruff; psoriasis; seborrhoeic dermatitis.

Denosol *Doerenkamp, Ger.*
Eucalyptol (p.1609·2); menthol (p.1632·3); camphor (p.1589·3); thymol (p.1158·3).
Colds; influenza.

Denquel *Procter & Gamble, USA.*
Potassium nitrate (p.1154·3).
Sensitive teeth.

Densical
Laphal, Fr.; Rubio, Spain.
Calcium carbonate (p.1215·1).
Calcium deficiency; osteoporosis.

Densical vitamine D₃ *Laphal, Fr.*
Calcium carbonate (p.1215·1); colecalciferol (p.1391·1).
Calcium and vitamin D deficiencies; osteoporosis.

Denson *Siam Bheasach, Thai.*
Prednisolone (p.1077·3); nitrofurazone (p.231·3).
Infected skin disorders.

Dental Ointment *Abbott, Austral.†*
Lignocaine [lidocaine] (p.1313·2); nitromersol (p.1151·2).
Denture pain; pain of dry socket and pyorrhoea.

Dentalgar *Marc-O, Canad.*
Benzocaine (p.1306·2); camphor (p.1589·3); guaiacol (p.1092·1); menthol (p.1632·3); clove oil (p.1597·1).
Toothache.

Dentalivo *IMA, Braz.*
Benzocaine (p.1306·2); cetylpyridinium chloride (p.1138·1).
Mouth disorders.

Dental-Phenjoca *Worndli, Switz.†*
Iodine (p.1522·3); camphor (p.1589·3); thymol (p.1158·3); anethole (p.1580·1); safrole; eugenol (p.1609·3); chlorobutanol (p.1141·2); phenol (p.1152·3).
Dental extraction pain.

Denta-Mint Topical Fluoride Solution *Colgate Oral Care, Austral.†*
Sodium fluoride (p.1375·3).
Fluoridation of tooth enamel.

Dentan *Ipex, Swed.*
Sodium fluoride (p.1375·3).
Dental caries prophylaxis.

Dentapaine *Reese, USA.*
Benzocaine (p.1306·2); clove oil (p.1597·1).
Toothache.

Dentaton Antisettico *Ghimas, Ital.*
Chlorhexidine gluconate (p.1138·2); benzalkonium chloride (p.1133·2).
Oral disinfection.

Dentecalcio *Melpoejo, Braz.*
Vitamin and mineral preparation (p.1350·1).

Dentese *McGloin, Austral.†*
Phenol (p.1152·3); camphor (p.1589·3); eucalyptus oil (p.1609·2); clove oil (p.1597·1).
Toothache.

Denti Gum C *Brovar, S.Afr.†*
Cetylpyridinium chloride (p.1138·1).
Mouth and throat infections.

Denti Gum CF *Brovar, S.Afr.†*
Sodium fluoride (p.1375·3); cetylpyridinium chloride (p.1138·1).
Dental caries prophylaxis; plaque removal.

Denti Gum F *Brovar, S.Afr.†*
Sodium fluoride (p.1375·3).
Dental caries prophylaxis; fluoride supplement.

Denticare *Trima, Israel.*
Sodium fluoride (p.1375·3).
Dental caries prophylaxis.

Dentigoa *Scheurich, Ger.†*
Ibuprofen (p.43·2).
Fever; pain.

Dentikrisos *Quimfar, Spain.*
Creosote (p.1087·3); benzocaine (p.1306·2); amethocaine [tetracaine] hydrochloride (p.1305·2); menthol (p.1632·3).
Toothache.

Dentin *Rekah, Israel.*
Eugenol (p.1609·3); benzocaine (p.1306·2); chlorobutanol (p.1141·2).
Toothache.

Dentinale *Montefarmaco, Ital.*
Amylocaine hydrochloride (p.1306·1); sodium benzoate (p.1134·3).
Teething pain.

Dentinox
Note. This name is used for preparations of different composition.
Byk, Aust.
Chamomile tincture (p.1593·2); myrrh tincture (p.1639·2); cetylpyridinium chloride (p.1138·1); lauromacrogol 400 (p.1345·2).
Teething pain.

DDD, Israel.
Simeticone (p.1249·2); dill oil (p.1603·3).
Infant colic.

Roche Nicholas, Neth.†
Lignocaine [lidocaine] hydrochloride (p.1313·2).
Teething pain.

DDD, Singapore.
Simeticone (p.1249·2); dill oil (p.1603·3).
Infant colic.

Dentinox, Switz.†
Chamomile (p.1593·2); lignocaine [lidocaine] hydrochloride (p.1313·2); lauromacrogol 400 (p.1345·2).
Dental pain.

Dentinox Colic Drops *DDD, UK.*
Simeticone (p.1249·2).
Colic.

Dentinox Cradle Cap
DDD, Singapore; DDD, UK.
Sodium lauril ether sulfosuccinate; sodium lauril ether sulfate (p.1496·3).
Cradle cap.

Dentinox N *Dentinox, Ger.*
Chamomile (p.1593·2); lignocaine [lidocaine] hydrochloride (p.1313·2); lauromacrogol 400 (p.1345·2).
Gingivitis.

Dentinox Teething Gel
DDD, Hong Kong; DDD, Singapore; DDD, UK.
Lignocaine [lidocaine] hydrochloride (p.1313·2); cetylpyridinium chloride (p.1138·1).
Denture irritation; sore gums; teething pain.

Dentipatch *Noven, USA.*
Lignocaine [lidocaine] (p.1313·2).
Local anaesthesia.

Dentispray
Ferraz, Lynce, Port.; Vinas, Spain.
Benzocaine (p.1306·2).
Mouth pain.

Dentogen *Anglian, UK.*
Clove oil (p.1597·1).
Toothache.

Dentohexine *Streuli, Switz.*
Chlorhexidine gluconate (p.1138·2).
Mouth and throat disorders.

Dentol Topico *Calmante Vitaminado, Spain.*
Camphor (p.1589·3); saffron (p.1029·1); clove oil (p.1597·1); cloral hydrate (p.669·3); procaine hydrochloride (p.1319·1); menthol (p.1632·3).
Toothache.

Dentolamina *Inibsa, Port.†*
Sodium perborate (p.1156·3); sodium tartrate (p.1250·2).
Mouth disorders; oral hygiene.

Dentomicin *Seid, Spain.*
Saffron (p.1029·1); tamarind (p.1253·2).
Toothache.

Dentomycin
Wyeth, Irl.; Blackwell, UK.
Minocycline hydrochloride (p.224·3).
Bacterial mouth infections.

Dentomycine *Lederle, Switz.†*
Minocycline hydrochloride (p.224·3).
Bacterial mouth infections.

Dentophar *Qualiphar, Belg.*
Amylocaine hydrochloride (p.1306·1); cloral hydrate (p.669·3); chloroform (p.1256·3); menthol (p.1632·3); thymol (p.1158·3); eugenol (p.1609·3).
Dental pain.

Dentosan Azione Intensiva *Warner-Lambert, Ital.*
Chlorhexidine gluconate (p.1138·2); peppermint oil (p.1243·3); geranium oil (p.1615·1); melissa oil; clove oil (p.1597·1); spearmint oil (p.1666·3).
Formerly known as Dentosan Pagni Collutorio.
Oral hygiene.

Dentosan Carie & Alito *Warner-Lambert, Ital.*
Sanguinaria (p.1660·3); sodium monofluorophosphate (p.1377·2).
Dental caries prophylaxis.

Dentosan Clorexidina *Warner-Lambert, Ital.*
Chlorhexidine (p.1138·2).
Gum disorders.

Dentosan Extra Fluor *Warner-Lambert, Ital.*
Sodium fluoride (p.1375·3).
Dental caries prophylaxis.

Dentosan Junior *Warner-Lambert, Ital.*
Sodium monofluorophosphate (p.1377·2); sodium fluoride (p.1375·3).
Dental caries prophylaxis.

Dentosan Mese *Warner-Lambert, Ital.*
Peppermint oil (p.1243·3); geranium oil (p.1615·1); melissa oil; clove oil (p.1597·1); spearmint oil (p.1666·3); chlorhexidine gluconate (p.1138·2).
Oral hygiene.

Dentosan Parodontale *Warner-Lambert, Ital.*
Chlorhexidine gluconate (p.1138·2).
Oral hygiene.

Dentosan Placca & Carie *Warner-Lambert, Ital.*
Chlorhexidine gluconate (p.1138·2); sodium fluoride (p.1375·3); peppermint oil (p.1243·3).
Formerly known as Dentosan Ortodontico Collutorio.
Oral hygiene.

Dentosan Sensibile *Warner-Lambert, Ital.*
Potassium nitrate (p.1154·3) sodium fluoride (p.1375·3).
Gingivitis; hypersensitive teeth.

Dentosedina *Teofarma, Ital.*
Procaine (p.1319·2); procaine hydrochloride (p.1319·1); benzocaine hydrochloride (p.1306·2); ephedrine hydrochloride (p.1090·1).
Dental pain.

Dentovax *Bouty, Ital.†.*
Inactivated cells of: *Escherichia coli; Streptococcus ovalis; Staphylococcus pyog. aur.; Proteus vulgaris;* chlorophyll (p.1028·1).
Gingivitis.

Dent's Extra Strength Toothache Gum *Dent, USA.*
Benzocaine (p.1306·2).

Dent's Lotion-Jel *Dent, USA.*
Benzocaine (p.1306·2).

Dent's Maximum Strength Toothache Drops *Dent, USA.*
Benzocaine (p.1306·2).

Dentyl pH *Grafton, UK.*
Triclosan (p.1159·2); fluoride (p.1375·3).
Oral hygiene.

Denubil *Pierre Fabre, Spain.*
Heptaminol hydrochloride (p.1619·2); deanol pidolate (p.1507·2).
Mental function disorders.

Denulcer *Ciclum, Spain.*
Ranitidine hydrochloride (p.1245·2).
Acid aspiration; gastro-oesophageal reflux; gastrointestinal haemorrhage; peptic ulcer; Zollinger-Ellison syndrome.

Denvar *Merck, Mex.; Merck, Spain.*
Cefixime (p.166·2).
Bacterial infections.

Denzo *TO-Chemicals, Thai.*
Serrapeptase (p.1662·1).
Inflammation; oedema.

Deolin *Unison, Thai.*
Drotaverine hydrochloride (p.1606·1).
Smooth muscle spasm.

Deopens *Brunel, S.Afr.*
Magnesium hydroxide (p.1233·1).
Gastro-oesophageal reflux.

Deopid *Masa, Thai.*
Gemfibrozil (p.896·2).
Hyperlipidaemias.

Depacon *Abbott, USA.*
Sodium valproate (p.366·3).
Epilepsy.

Depade *Mallinckrodt, USA.*
Naltrexone hydrochloride (p.1016·1).
Alcohol withdrawal syndrome; opioid withdrawal.

Depain Plus *Vesta, S.Afr.†.*
Paracetamol (p.71·2); codeine phosphate (p.25·2); phenobarbital (p.355·1).
Pain and associated tension.

Depakene *Abbott, Braz.; Abbott, Canad.; Kyowa, Jpn; Abbott, Mex.; Abbott, USA.*
Valproic acid (p.366·2) or sodium valproate (p.366·3).
Epilepsy.

Depakin *Sanofi Winthrop, Ital.*
Sodium valproate (p.366·3).
Epilepsy.

Depakin Chrono *Sanofi Winthrop, Ital.*
Sodium valproate (p.366·3); valproic acid (p.366·2).
Epilepsy.

Depakine *Sanofi Winthrop, Aust.; Sanofi Synthelabo, Belg.; Sanofi Winthrop, Fr.; Sanofi Synthelabo, Neth.; Sanofi Synthelabo, Port.; Sanofi Synthelabo, Spain; Sanofi Synthelabo, Switz.; Sanofi Synthelabo, Thai.*
Sodium valproate (p.366·3).
Epilepsy; febrile convulsions; infantile convulsions.

Depakine Chrono *Sanofi Winthrop, Aust.; Sanofi Winthrop, Fr.; Sanofi Synthelabo, Neth.; Sanofi Synthelabo, Port.; Sanofi Synthelabo, Switz.*
Sodium valproate (p.366·3); valproic acid (p.366·2).
Epilepsy.

Depakote *Sanofi Synthelabo, Fr.; Sanofi Synthelabo, UK; Abbott, USA.*
Valproate semisodium (p.366·3).
Bipolar disorder; epilepsy; migraine.

Depalept *CTI, Israel.*
Sodium valproate (p.366·3).
Epilepsy; porphyria.

Depalept Chrono *CTI, Israel.*
Sodium valproate (p.366·3); valproic acid (p.366·2).
Epilepsy.

Depamag *Sigma-Tau, Ital.*
Magnesium valproate (p.368·3).
Epilepsy.

Depamide
Sanofi Winthrop, Fr.; Sanofi Synthelabo, Ital.; Sanofi Synthelabo, Spain.
Valpromide (p.366·3).
Bipolar disorder; epilepsy.

depAndro *Forest Pharmaceuticals, USA†.*
Testosterone cipionate (p.1492·1).
Breast cancer; delayed puberty (males); male hypogonadism.

depAndrogyn *Forest Pharmaceuticals, USA†.*
Estradiol cipionate (p.1473·2); testosterone cipionate (p.1492·1).
Menopausal vasomotor symptoms; prevention of postpartum breast engorgement.

Depas
Fournier, Ital.; Yoshitomi, Jpn.
Etizolam (p.683·1).
Anxiety states; psychosomatic disorders; sleep disorders.

Depen
Carter Horner, Canad.; Wallace, USA.
Penicillamine (p.1017·1).
Cystinuria; rheumatoid arthritis; Wilson's disease.

Depex *Rolab, S.Afr.*
Sulpiride (p.706·1).
Now known as Rolab-Sulpiride.
Behaviour disorders; depression; peptic ulcer; psychoses; vertigo.

depGynogen *Forest Pharmaceuticals, USA.*
Estradiol cipionate (p.1473·2).
Female hypogonadism; menopausal vasomotor symptoms.

Depixol
Lundbeck, Irl.; Lundbeck, NZ; Lundbeck, UK.
Flupentixol decanoate (p.684·1) or flupentixol hydrochloride (p.684·1).
Psychoses.

depMedalone *Forest Pharmaceuticals, USA.*
Methylprednisolone acetate (p.1076·1).
Corticosteroid.

Depo Moderin *Pharmacia Upjohn, Spain.*
Methylprednisolone acetate (p.1076·1).
Corticosteroid.

Depo-Clinovir *Pharmacia Upjohn, Ger.*
Medroxyprogesterone acetate (p.1480·1).
Progestogen-only injectable contraceptive.

Depocon *Pharmacia Upjohn, Aust.*
Medroxyprogesterone acetate (p.1480·1).
Progestogen-only injectable contraceptive.

DepoCyt *Astra, USA.*
Liposomal cytarabine (p.530·1).
Lymphomatous meningitis.

Depodillar *Syntex, Neth.†.*
Paramethasone acetate (p.1077·2).
Corticosteroid.

Depogen *Hyrex, USA.*
Estradiol cipionate (p.1473·2).
Female hypogonadism; menopausal vasomotor symptoms.

Depo-Gestin *ANB, Thai.*
Medroxyprogesterone acetate (p.1480·1).
Dysfunctional uterine bleeding; endometriosis; progestogen-only injectable contraceptive.

Depoject *Mayrand, USA.*
Methylprednisolone acetate (p.1076·1).
Corticosteroid.

Depolan
Lannacher, Denm.; Nordic Drugs, Fin.; Nordic, Swed.
Morphine hydrochloride (p.56·1).
Pain.

Depolut *Taro, Israel.*
Hydroxyprogesterone caproate (p.1479·3).
Amenorrhoea; endometriosis; functional uterine bleeding; uterine cancer.

Depo-Medrate *Pharmacia Upjohn, Ger.*
Methylprednisolone acetate (p.1076·1).
Parenteral corticosteroid.

Depo-Medrol
Pharmacia Upjohn, Aust.†; Pharmacia Upjohn, Austral.; Pharmacia Upjohn, Belg.; Pharmacia Upjohn, Braz.; Pharmacia Upjohn, Canad.; Pharmacia Upjohn, Denm.; Pharmacia Upjohn, Fin.; Pharmacia Upjohn, Fr.; Pharmacia Upjohn, Hong Kong; Pharmacia Upjohn, Israel; Pharmacia Upjohn, Ital.; Pharmacia Upjohn, Mex.; Pharmacia Upjohn, Neth.; Pharmacia Upjohn, Norw.; Pharmacia Upjohn, NZ; Pharmacia Upjohn, Port.; Pharmacia Upjohn, S.Afr.; Pharmacia Upjohn, Swed.; Pharmacia Upjohn, Switz.; Pharmacia Upjohn, Thai.; Pharmacia Upjohn, USA.
Methylprednisolone acetate (p.1076·1).
Corticosteroid.

Depo-Medrol com Lidocaina *Pharmacia Upjohn, Port.*
Methylprednisolone acetate (p.1076·1); lignocaine [lidocaine] hydrochloride (p.1313·2).
Musculoskeletal, joint, and peri-articular disorders.

Depo-Medrol cum Lidocain
Pharmacia Upjohn, Fin.; Pharmacia Upjohn, Norw.
Methylprednisolone acetate (p.1076·1); lignocaine [lidocaine] hydrochloride (p.1313·2).
Musculoskeletal, joint, and peri-articular disorders.

Depo-Medrol cum Lidokain *Pharmacia Upjohn, Swed.*
Methylprednisolone acetate (p.1076·1); lignocaine [lidocaine] hydrochloride (p.1313·2).
Peri-articular disorders.

Depo-Medrol + Lidocaina *Pharmacia Upjohn, Ital.*
Methylprednisolone acetate (p.1076·1); lignocaine [lidocaine] hydrochloride (p.1313·2).
Musculoskeletal, joint, and peri-articular disorders.

Depo-Medrol with Lidocaine
Pharmacia Upjohn, Canad.; Pharmacia Upjohn, Hong Kong; Pharmacia Upjohn, Israel; Pharmacia Upjohn, NZ; Pharmacia Upjohn, S.Afr.; Pharmacia Upjohn, Switz.; Pharmacia Upjohn, Thai.
Methylprednisolone acetate (p.1076·1); lignocaine [lidocaine] hydrochloride (p.1313·2).
Musculoskeletal, joint, and peri-articular disorders.

Depo-Medrol + Lidocaine
Pharmacia Upjohn, Belg.; Pharmacia Upjohn, Neth.
Methylprednisolone acetate (p.1076·1); lignocaine [lidocaine] hydrochloride (p.1313·2).
Musculoskeletal, joint, and peri-articular disorders.

Depo-Medrol mit Lidocain *Pharmacia Upjohn, Aust.†.*
Methylprednisolone acetate (p.1076·1); lignocaine [lidocaine] hydrochloride (p.1313·2).
Musculoskeletal and joint disorders.

Depo-Medrone
Pharmacia Upjohn, Irl.; Pharmacia, UK.
Methylprednisolone acetate (p.1076·1).
Corticosteroid.

Depo-Medrone with Lidocaine
Pharmacia Upjohn, Irl.; Pharmacia, UK.
Methylprednisolone acetate (p.1076·1); lignocaine [lidocaine] hydrochloride (p.1313·2).
Musculoskeletal, joint, and peri-articular disorders.

Depo-Nisolone *Pharmacia Upjohn, Austral.*
Methylprednisolone acetate (p.1076·1).
Corticosteroid.

Deponit
Gebro, Aust.; Byk, Belg.; Schering, Braz.; Pharmacal, Fin.; Schwarz, Ger.; Schwarz, Hong Kong; Schwarz, Irl.; Schwarz, Israel; Schwarz, Ital.; Byk, Neth.; Ranbaxy, Singapore; Schwarz, Singapore; Schwarz, Switz.; Schwarz, Thai.; Schwarz, UK; Schwarz, USA.
Glyceryl trinitrate (p.897·3).
Angina pectoris; heart failure; prophylaxis of phlebitis and extravasation.

Depopred *Hyrex, USA.*
Methylprednisolone acetate (p.1076·1).
Corticosteroid.

Depo-Prodasone *Pharmacia Upjohn, Fr.*
Medroxyprogesterone acetate (p.1480·1).
Endometriosis; malignant neoplasms.

Depo-Progesta *General Drugs, Thai.*
Medroxyprogesterone acetate (p.1480·1).
Endometriosis; progestogen-only injectable contraceptive.

Depo-Progevera *Pharmacia Upjohn, Spain.*
Medroxyprogesterone acetate (p.1480·1).
Endometrial cancer; progestogen-only injectable contraceptive.

Depo-Provera
Pharmacia Upjohn, Aust.; Pharmacia Upjohn, Austral.; Pharmacia Upjohn, Belg.; Pharmacia Upjohn, Braz.; Pharmacia Upjohn, Canad.; Pharmacia Upjohn, Denm.; Pharmacia Upjohn, Fin.; Pharmacia Upjohn, Fr.; Pharmacia Upjohn, Hong Kong; Pharmacia Upjohn, Irl.; Pharmacia Upjohn, Israel; Pharmacia Upjohn, Ital.; Pharmacia Upjohn, Mex.; Pharmacia Upjohn, Neth.; Pharmacia Upjohn, Norw.; Pharmacia Upjohn, NZ; Pharmacia Upjohn, Port.; Pharmacia Upjohn, S.Afr.; Pharmacia Upjohn, Singapore; Pharmacia Upjohn, Swed.; Pharmacia Upjohn, Switz.; Pharmacia Upjohn, Thai.; Pharmacia, UK; Pharmacia Upjohn, USA.
Medroxyprogesterone acetate (p.1480·1).
Breast cancer; endometrial cancer; endometriosis; menopausal disorders; progestogen-only injectable contraceptive; renal cancer.

Depo-Ralovera *Kenral, Austral.*
Medroxyprogesterone acetate (p.1480·1).
Endometriosis; malignant neoplasms; progestogen-only injectable contraceptive.

Depostat
Schering, Aust.†; Schering, Ger.; Schering, Ital.; Schering, Spain; Schering, Switz.; Cambridge, UK.
Gestonorone caproate (p.1479·1).
Now known as Gestonorone Hexanoate Ampoules in the UK.
Benign prostatic hyperplasia; breast cancer; endometrial cancer.

Depotest *Hyrex, USA†.*
Testosterone cipionate (p.1492·1).
Breast cancer; delayed puberty (males); male hypogonadism.

Depo-Testadiol *Upjohn, USA.*
Estradiol cipionate (p.1473·2); testosterone cipionate (p.1492·1).
Menopausal vasomotor symptoms; prevention of postpartum breast engorgement.

Depotestogen *Hyrex, USA.*
Estradiol cipionate (p.1473·2); testosterone cipionate (p.1492·1).
Menopausal vasomotor symptoms; prevention of postpartum breast engorgement.

Depot-Hal
Hal, Ger.; Hal, Neth.
Allergen extracts of pollen, fungi, house dust mites and skin (p.1575·3).
Hyposensitisation.

Depot-H-Insulin *Hoechst, Ger.†.*
Neutral insulin suspension (human, highly-purified)(75% crystalline) (p.324·1).
Diabetes mellitus.

Depot-H15-Insulin *Hoechst, Ger.†.*
Neutral insulin suspension (human, highly-purified)(85% crystalline) (p.324·1).
Diabetes mellitus.

Depot-Insulin
Hoechst Marion Roussel, Aust.
Insulin injection (porcine) (p.324·1).
Diabetes mellitus.

Hoechst Marion Roussel, Ger.
Insulin injection (bovine) (p.324·1).
Diabetes mellitus.

Depot-Insulin S *Hoechst Marion Roussel, Ger.*
Insulin injection (porcine) (p.324·1).
Diabetes mellitus.

Depotrone *Propan, S.Afr.*
Testosterone cipionate (p.1492·1).
Gynaecomastia; lactation suppression; male hypogonadism; mastitis; menstrual disorders.

Depot-Thrombophob-N *Knoll, Ger.*
Heparin sodium (p.902·1).
Formerly contained heparin sodium and ephedrine hydrochloride.
Thromboembolic disorders.

Deprakine
Sanofi Winthrop, Denm.; Sanofi Winthrop, Fin.; Sanofi Winthrop, Norw.
Sodium valproate (p.366·3).
Epilepsy; manic depression.

Deprakine Depot *Sanofi Winthrop, Fin.*
Sodium valproate (p.366·3); valproic acid (p.366·2).
Bipolar disorder; epilepsy.

Deprancol *Parke, Davis, Spain.*
Dextropropoxyphene hydrochloride (p.27·1).
Pain.

Depraser *Farma Lepori, Spain†.*
Etoperidone or etoperidone hydrochloride (p.284·2).
Depression.

Deprax
Note. This name is used for preparations of different composition.
Ache, Braz.
Fluoxetine (p.288·2).
Depression; obsessive-compulsive disorder.

Farma Lepori, Spain.
Trazodone hydrochloride (p.310·1).
Depression; dyskinesias; mood disorders; premedication; tremor.

Deprece *Tecnobio, Spain.*
Almagate (p.1209·3).
Dyspepsia; gastritis; gastro-oesophageal reflux; peptic ulcer.

Deprelio *Estedi, Spain.*
Amitriptyline hydrochloride (p.273·3).
Formerly contained amitriptyline hydrochloride and perphenazine.
Bulimia nervosa; depression; nocturnal enuresis; postherpetic neuralgia.

Deprenyl
Orion, Fr.; Sanofi Winthrop, Ger.†.
Selegiline hydrochloride (p.1177·2).
Parkinsonism.

Depressan *OPW, Ger.*
Dihydralazine sulfate (p.874·2).
Hypertension.

Deprexan *Unipharm, Israel.*
Desipramine hydrochloride (p.282·3).
Depression.

Deprexin *Gedeon Richter, Singapore.*
Fluoxetine hydrochloride (p.284·2).
Depression; obsessive-compulsive disorder.

Deprilan *Biosintetica, Braz.*
Selegiline hydrochloride (p.1177·2).
Parkinsonism.

Deprilept *Lundbeck, Ger.*
Maprotiline hydrochloride (p.297·2).
Depression.

Deprimil *Merck, Port.*
Lofepramine hydrochloride (p.297·1).
Depression.

Deproic *Technilab, Canad.*
Valproic acid (p.366·2) or sodium valproate (p.366·3).
Epilepsy.

Deproist Expectorant with Codeine *Geneva, USA.*
Pseudoephedrine hydrochloride (p.1099·2); guaifenesin (p.1092·2); codeine phosphate (p.25·2).
Coughs.

Depronal
Parke, Davis, Belg.; Parke, Davis, Neth.; Warner-Lambert, Switz.
Dextropropoxyphene hydrochloride (p.27·1).
Pain.

Deproxin *Siam Bheasach, Thai.*
Fluoxetine hydrochloride (p.284·2).
Depression; obsessive-compulsive disorder.

Deptran
Note. This name is used for preparations of different composition.
Alphapharm, Austral.
Doxepin hydrochloride (p.283·3).
Depression.

Enila, Braz.
Bromazepam (p.656·3).
Anxiety; insomnia.

The symbol † denotes a preparation no longer actively marketed

Depuran Aspen Consumer, S.Afr.; Nattermann, Spain.
Senna (p.1248·2).
Constipation.

Depuran N Woelm, Ger.
Senna (p.1248·2).
Constipation.

Depuratif des Alpes Sodia, Fr.
Senna (p.1248·2); frangula bark (p.1227·1); liquorice (p.1231·2); magnesium chloride (p.1190·3).
Constipation.

Depuratif Parnel Medecine Vegetale, Fr.
Lappa (p.1627·1); viola tricolor; saponaria; fumitory (p.1612·3).
Formerly contained lappa, viola tricolor, saponaria, fumitory, sarsaparilla, and senna.
Constipation.

Depuratif Richelet Richelet, Fr.
Walnut leaves; cresson leaves; cochlearia armoracia root; cochlearia officinalis leaves; menyanthes leaves; cinnamon bark; bitter orange; gentian; tannic acid; magnesium chloride; magnesium bromide; nicotinamide (p.1350·1).
Tonic.

Depurativo IDI, Ital.
Sarsaparilla (p.1661·1); fumitory (p.1612·3); borrana; saponaria; viola; walnut leaves; clover; rhubarb (p.1248·1); senna (p.1248·2); cascara (p.1216·1); lappa (p.1627·1); chicory; dulcamara (p.1606·2); couchgrass (p.1599·3); bitter-orange (p.1644·2); gentian (p.1615·1); salix (p.82·1).
Constipation.

Depurativo Richelet Vitafarma, Spain.
Gentian (p.1615·1); potassium iodide (p.1522·3); salicylic acid (p.1122·3); tannic acid (p.1669·1); iodine (p.1522·3); cinnamon oil (p.1596·1); magnesium chloride (p.1190·3); magnesium bromide; nicotinamide (p.1372·3).
Detoxification.

Depuratum Lehning, Fr.
Birch (p.1585·2); rosemary leaf; juniper fruit (p.1625·2); rhapontic root (p.1248·1); fumitory (p.1612·3); thyme (p.1672·2).
Formerly contained ononis, birch, calamus rhizome, rosemary leaf, juniper fruit, rhapontic root, fumitory, aloes, senna, frangula bark, and thyme.
Constipation; dyspepsia.

Depurfat Herbaline, Ital.†
Rosemary; silver birch (p.1585·2); taraxacum (p.1669·1); cupressus sempervirens; juniper (p.1625·2).
Adjuvant in obesity; biliary disorders; liver disorders; venous disorders; water retention.

Depyrel Abic, Israel.
Trazodone hydrochloride (p.310·1).
Depression.

Deq Atlantic, Hong Kong; Atlantic, Singapore; Atlantic, Thai.
Dequalinium chloride (p.1143·1); tyrothricin (p.267·1).
Mouth and throat infections.

Dequacaine Boots Healthcare, Irl.; Crookes Healthcare, UK.
Benzocaine (p.1306·2); dequalinium chloride (p.1143·1).
Sore throat.

Dequa-Coff Quatromed, S.Afr.
Promethazine hydrochloride (p.423·2); codeine phosphate (p.25·2); ephedrine hydrochloride (p.1090·1).
Coughs.

Dequa/Delin Atlantic, Thai.
Dequalinium chloride (p.1143·1).
Mouth and throat disorders.

Dequadin Glaxo Wellcome, Aust.; Roberts, Canad.; Glaxo Wellcome, Hong Kong; Boots Healthcare, Irl.; Eurospital, Ital.; Boots, NZ; Aspen, S.Afr.; Inibsa, Spain; Glaxo Wellcome, Thai.; Crookes Healthcare, UK.
Dequalinium chloride (p.1143·1).
Mouth and throat infections.

Dequadin Complex Inibsa, Spain.
Lignocaine [lidocaine] hydrochloride (p.1313·2); cetylpyridinium chloride (p.1138·1); dequalinium chloride (p.1143·1).
Mouth and throat infections.

Dequadin Mouth Paint Aspen, S.Afr.
Dequalinium chloride (p.1143·1); lignocaine [lidocaine] (p.1313·2).
Mouth disorders.

Dequa-Flu Quatromed, S.Afr.
Paracetamol (p.71·2); phenylephrine hydrochloride (p.1097·1); phenyltoloxamine citrate (p.423·1); caffeine (p.761·3); chlorpheniramine [chlorphenamine] maleate (p.412·1).
Cold and influenza symptoms; rhinitis; sinusitis.

Dequafungan Provita, Aust.
Dequalinium chloride (p.1143·1); undecenoic acid (p.395·3).
Skin infections.

Dequalid Wolfs, Belg.
Dequalinium chloride (p.1143·1); lignocaine [lidocaine] hydrochloride (p.1313·2).
Mouth and throat infections.

Dequalinetten Provita, Aust.
Dequalinium chloride (p.1143·1); benzocaine (p.1306·2).
Mouth and throat disorders.

Dequalinium Wolfs, Belg.†.
Dequalinium chloride (p.1143·1); amylocaine (p.1306·1).
Mouth and throat disorders.

Dequamed Rhone-Poulenc Rorer, S.Afr.
Dequalinium chloride (p.1143·1); lignocaine [lidocaine] hydrochloride (p.1313·2).
Sore throat.

Dequasept Vitamed, Israel.
Dequalinium chloride (p.1143·1); vitamin C (p.1389·3).
Mouth and throat infections.

Dequasine Miller, USA.
Vitamin C with minerals and amino-acids (p.1350·1).

Dequavagyn Provita, Aust.
Dequalinium chloride (p.1143·1).

Dequonal Nycomed, Aust.; Kreussler, Ger.; Kreussler, Switz.
Dequalinium chloride (p.1143·1); benzalkonium chloride (p.1133·2).
Mouth and throat infections.

Dequosangola Eurospital, Ital.
Dequalinium chloride (p.1143·1).
Mouth disinfection.

Dera Ingram & Bell, Canad.†.
Zinc oxide (p.1128·2); peru balsam (p.1650·2).
Napkin rash.

Deralin Alphapharm, Austral.; Abic, Israel.
Propranolol hydrochloride (p.962·3).
Angina pectoris; arrhythmias; hypertension; hypertrophic subaortic stenosis; migraine; myocardial infarction; phaeochromocytoma; tremor.

Deratin Normon, Spain.
Chlorhexidine gluconate (p.1138·2).
Mouth and throat infections; skin and wound disinfection.

Derbac-C Seton, Irl.†.
Carbaryl (p.1429·2).
Pediculosis.

Derbac-M Seton, Irl.; Pharmaco, NZ; SSL, UK.
Malathion (p.1434·2).
Pediculosis; scabies.

Derbitan Antibiotico Normon, Spain†.
Atropine methobromide (p.460·3); streptomycin sulfate (p.249·1); phthalylsulfathiazole (p.235·3); neomycin sulfate (p.228·1).
Gastrointestinal infections.

Dercome Wolff, Ger.
Benzoyl peroxide (p.1111·1).
Acne.

Dercusan Asta Medica, Belg.
Tosylchloramide sodium (p.1159·1).
Burns; ulcers.

Dercut Pekana, Ger.
Homoeopathic preparation.

Dereme Menarini, Spain.
Beclometasone salicylate (p.1062·1).
Skin disorders.

Derifil Rystan, USA.
Chlorophyllin copper complex (p.1028·1).
Ostomy deodorant; reduction of faecal or urinary odour in incontinence.

Deril Ibirn, Ital.
Alfacalcidol (p.1391·1).
Hypoparathyroidism; osteomalacia; osteoporosis; renal osteodystrophy; rickets.

Derilate Hosban, Spain†.
Tiaprofenic acid (p.88·1).
Inflammation; musculoskeletal, joint, and peri-articular disorders; pain.

Derinase Plus Bioindustria, Ital.†.
Deoxyribonuclease (p.1089·1); bromelains (p.1586·3).
Inflammatory disorders.

Derinox Note. This name is used for preparations of different composition.
Therabel, Fr.
Prednisolone (p.1077·3); naphazoline nitrate (p.1095·1).
Formerly contained prednisolone, phenylephrine hydrochloride, and naphazoline nitrate.
Rhinopharyngitis.

Sodip, Switz.
Prednisolone (p.1077·3); phenylephrine hydrochloride (p.1097·1); naphazoline nitrate (p.1095·1).
Inflammatory and allergic disorders of upper respiratory tract.

Deripil Galderma, Spain.
Erythromycin (p.201·2).
Acne.

Derivatio H Pfluger, Ger.
Homoeopathic preparation.

Derivon Gerot, Aust.
Cream: Benzyl nicotinate (p.20·2); diethylamine salicylate (p.32·1); heparin (p.902·1).
Musculoskeletal and joint disorders; neuralgia; soft-tissue disorders.

Liniment: Benzyl nicotinate (p.20·2); camphor (p.1589·3); methyl salicylate (p.55·1).
Soft-tissue, peri-articular, musculoskeletal, and joint disorders.

Derma Care Fischer, Israel.
Salicylic acid (p.1122·3); hamamelis (p.1618·3); chamomile (p.1593·2); provitamin B_5.
Seborrhoea; skin cleansing.

Derma Keri Darier, Mex.
Urea (p.1127·3).
Hyperkeratotic skin disorders.

Derma Viva Rugby, USA.
Emollient and moisturiser.

Dermabase Paddock, USA.
Vehicle for topical preparations.

Dermabaz Sanofi Winthrop, Hong Kong.
Tretinoin (p.1126·2); erythromycin (p.201·2).
Acne.

Dermablend Sephytal, Fr.; DDC, UK.
A covering cream.
Concealment of birth marks, scars, and disfiguring skin disease.

Dermac Stiefel, Mex.
Sulfated castor oil (p.1496·2).
Seborrhoea.

Dermacalm-d Roche, Switz.
Hydrocortisone acetate (p.1073·3); dexpanthenol (p.1602·3).
Skin disorders.

Derma-Care Hermal, Israel.
Lauromacrogol 400 (p.1345·2); urea (p.1127·3).
Skin disorders.

Dermachrome Synthelabo, Fr.
Thiomersal (p.1158·2); lignocaine [lidocaine] hydrochloride (p.1313·2).
Formerly contained thiomersal, lignocaine [lidocaine] hydrochloride, and phenylephrine hydrochloride.
Burns; skin disinfection; wounds.

Dermacide CS, Fr.
Soap: Tartaric acid (p.1669·2); salicylic acid (p.1122·3); benzoic acid (p.1134·2).
Cleansing of skin.

Topical solution: Hydroxyquinoline sulfate (p.1622·2); sodium propionate (p.393·2); salicylic acid (p.1122·3); tartaric acid (p.1669·2).
Skin disinfection.

Dermacne Bio-Sante, Canad.
Benzoyl peroxide (p.1111·1).
Acne.

Dermacoat Century, USA.
Benzocaine (p.1306·2); chloroxylenol (p.1142·1); menthol (p.1632·3).
Skin disorders.

Dermacol Vitamed, Israel.
Emollient.
Dry skin.

Dermacolor Fox, UK.
A covering cream.
Concealment of birth marks, scars, and disfiguring skin disease.

Dermacombin
Taro, Israel; Taro, Thai.
Nystatin (p.392·2); neomycin (p.228·1) or neomycin sulfate (p.228·1); gramicidin (p.213·3); triamcinolone acetonide (p.1080·1).
Infected skin disorders.

Dermacort
Note. This name is used for preparations of different composition.
Medinovum, Fin.; Sankyo, UK; Solvay, USA†.
Hydrocortisone (p.1073·3).
Skin disorders.

DHA, Hong Kong.
Triamcinolone acetonide (p.1080·1).
Skin disorders.

Dermacreme Potter's, UK.
Menthol (p.1632·3); methyl salicylate (p.55·1); liquefied phenol (p.1152·3).
Antiseptic for minor skin injuries.

Dermacure Taxandria, Neth.
Miconazole nitrate (p.391·1).
Fungal skin and nail infections.

Dermacyd Sanofi Winthrop, Braz.
Lactoserum; lactic acid (p.1626·2).
Skin disorders.

Dermadex Teofarma, Ital.
Dexamethasone valerate (p.1067·3).
Skin disorders.

Dermadine Medpro, S.Afr.
Povidone-iodine (p.1155·1).
Mouth and throat disorders; skin disinfection.

Dermadrate Dermatech, Austral.
Lactic acid (p.1626·2); urea (p.1127·3); sodium pidolate (p.1123·3).
Dry skin.

Dermaflex
Note. This name is used for preparations of different composition.
Neolab, Canad.
Urea (p.1127·3).
Emollient; moisturiser.

Zila, USA†.
Lignocaine [lidocaine] (p.1313·2).

Dermaflogil NCSN, Ital.
Diflucortolone valerate (p.1069·3); kanamycin sulfate (p.218·1).
Skin disorders.

Dermaflor NCSN, Ital.
Diflorasone diacetate (p.1069·2).
Skin disorders.

Dermagor Coryne de Bruynes, Mon.
Aluminium chlorohydrate (p.1110·2).
Hyperhidrosis.

Dermagor Ecran Solar Dermoteca, Port.
Titanium dioxide (p.1126·1).
Sunscreen.

Dermagor-Antitranspirante Dermoteca, Port.
Aluminium chlorohydrate (p.1110·2).
Hyperhidrosis.

Dermagraft Smith & Nephew, UK.
Human dermal tissue (p.1123·2).
Diabetic foot ulcers.

Derm-Aid Ego, Austral.; Ego, NZ; Ego, Singapore.
Hydrocortisone (p.1073·3).
Skin disorders.

Dermaide Dermaide, USA†.
Aloe vera (p.1110·1).
Superficial burns, infections, cuts, abrasions, and irritation of the skin.

Dermal Care Bayer Diagnostici, Ital.
Urea (p.1127·3).
Dry skin and nail disorders.

Dermalar Teva, Israel.
Fluocinolone acetonide (p.1071·1).
Skin disorders.

Dermalex Sanofi Winthrop, UK†.
Hexachlorophene (p.1146·1) in an emollient base.
Prevention of bed sores; skin disinfection.

Dermalibour Ducray, Fr.
Avena (p.1583·1); zinc oxide (p.1128·2); copper sulfate (p.1358·1); zinc sulfate (p.1398·2).
Skin disorders.

Dermalife Pharmacia Upjohn, Austral.†; Pharmacia Upjohn, NZ.
Vitamin A (p.1382·1) or vitamin A palmitate (p.1383·2).
Skin disorders.

Dermalife Plus Pharmacia Upjohn, Austral.; Pharmacia Upjohn, NZ.
Calamine (p.1111·3); vitamin A (p.1382·1) or vitamin A palmitate (p.1383·2); dimethicone (p.1410·1).
Skin disorders.

Dermallerg Ratiopharm, Ger.
Hydrocortisone (p.1073·3).
Skin disorders.

Dermalo Dermal Laboratories, UK.
Liquid paraffin (p.1407·1); acetylated wool alcohols (p.1410·3).
Formerly known as Emmolate.
Dry skin.

Dermalog Bristol-Myers Squibb, Mex.
Halcinonide (p.1073·2).
Skin disorders.

Dermalog-C Bristol-Myers Squibb, Mex.
Halcinonide (p.1073·2); nystatin (p.392·2); neomycin sulfate (p.228·1).
Infected skin disorders.

derma-loges N Loges, Ger.
Peru balsam (p.1650·2); arnica (p.1581·3); hamamelis (p.1618·3); chamomile (p.1593·2); sunflower oil (p.1381·2).
Burns; haemorrhoids; skin disorders; wounds.

Dermal-Rub Hauck, USA†.
Methyl salicylate (p.55·1); camphor (p.1589·3); menthol (p.1632·3); cajuput oil (p.1588·1).
Muscle, joint, and soft-tissue pain; neuralgia.

Dermamist
Note. This name is used for preparations of different composition.
Yamanouchi, Ital.
Emollient.
Dry skin disorders.

Yamanouchi, UK.
White soft paraffin (p.1407·3).
Dry skin disorders.

Dermamycin Pfeiffer, USA.
Diphenhydramine hydrochloride (p.416·1).

Derma-Mykotral Rosen, Ger.
Miconazole nitrate (p.391·1).
Fungal infections of the skin and mucous membranes.

Dermana
Note. This name is used for preparations of different composition.
Humana, Ital.
Gamolenic acid (p.1613·1); omega-3 triglyceride (p.949·2); vitamin E (p.1393·3); vitamin A (p.1382·1).
Dry skin disorders; skin irritation.

Milte, Port.
A range of emollient and barrier preparations.

Dermanatur Sofex, Port.†.
Emollient.
Barrier preparation; dry skin.

Derman-Oil Humana, Ital.
Gamolenic acid (p.1613·1); omega-3 triglycerides (p.949·2); vitamins A (p.1382·1); vitamin E (p.1393·3).
Bath additive.

Dermaor Sam-On, Israel.
Chlorhexidine gluconate (p.1138·2); cetrimide (p.1137·1).
Skin, hand, and instrument disinfection.

Derma-Pax Recsei, USA.
Mepyramine maleate (p.421·1); chlorpheniramine [chlorphenamine] (p.412·1).
Pruritus.

Dermarell Sanorell, Ger.
Homoeopathic preparation.

Dermaren Areu, Spain.
Dichlorisone acetate (p.1069·2).
Skin disorders.

Dermarest Del, USA.
Diphenhydramine hydrochloride (p.416·1); resorcinol (p.1122·2).
Pruritus.

Dermarest Dri-Cort *Del, USA.*
Hydrocortisone acetate (p.1073·3).
Skin disorders.

Dermarest Plus *Del, USA.*
Diphenhydramine hydrochloride (p.416·1); menthol (p.1632·3).
Pruritus.

Dermase *Sanval, Braz.*
Neomycin (p.228·1); bacitracin zinc (p.155·2).
Skin infections.

Dermasept Antifungal *Pharmakon, USA.*
Tannic acid (p.1669·1); zinc chloride (p.1398·1); benzocaine (p.1306·2); methylbenzethonium chloride (p.1150·3); tolnaftate (p.395·2); undecenoic acid (p.395·3).
Fungal skin infections.

Dermasil
Note. This name is used for preparations of different composition.
Silom, Thai.
Clobetasol propionate (p.1065·2).
Skin disorders.

Chesebrough-Pond's, USA†.
Glycerol (p.1616·3); dimethicone (p.1410·1).

Derma-Smoothe/FS *Hill, USA.*
Fluocinolone acetonide (p.1071·1).
Skin disorders.

Dermasol *Olan-Kemed, Thai.*
Chloramphenicol (p.179·1); hydrocortisone acetate (p.1073·3).
Infected skin disorders.

Dermasone
Technilab, Canad.; Technilab, Hong Kong.
Clobetasol propionate (p.1065·2).
Skin and scalp disorders.

Dermaspraid *Roche Nicholas, Fr.*
Hydrocortisone acetate (p.1073·3).
Skin disorders.

Dermaspray
Roche, Aust.; Roche, Belg.; Roche Nicholas, Fr.
Chlorhexidine gluconate (p.1138·2); benzalkonium chloride (p.1133·2); benzyl alcohol (p.1135·2).
Wound and burn disinfection.

Dermaspray demangeaison *Roche Nicholas, Fr.*
Hydrocortisone (p.1073·3).
Skin disorders.

Dermatar
Note. This name is used for preparations of different composition.
Hamilton, Austral.†.
Tar (p.1125·1).
Skin inflammation and pruritus.

IDI, Ital.
Betamethasone valero-acetate (p.1063·3); salicylic acid (p.1122·3); ichthammol (p.1115·2).
Skin disorders.

Dermatech Liquid *Dermatech, Austral.*
Alcohol (p.1130·3); propylene glycol (p.1655·1).
Vehicle for topical drugs.

Dermatech Wart Treatment *Dermatech, Austral.*
Lactic acid (p.1626·2); salicylic acid (p.1122·3).
Warts.

Dermatitis Relief *Brauer, Austral.*
Homoeopathic preparation.

Dermatodoron
Weleda, Aust.; Weleda, Ger.; Weleda, UK.
Dulcamara flowers (p.1606·2); lysimachia nummularia.
Eczema.

Dermatofides *Fides, Ger.*
Homoeopathic preparation.

Dermatol *Chinosolfabrik, Ger.*
Bismuth subgallate (p.1213·2).
Burns; excoriations.

Dermatop
Hoechst Marion Roussel, Braz.; Hoechst, Ger.; Aventis, Ital.; Hoechst Marion Roussel, Thai.; Ortho Dermatological, USA.
Prednicarbate (p.1077·3).
Skin disorders.

Dermatovate *Glaxo Wellcome, Mex.*
Clobetasol propionate (p.1065·2).
Skin disorders.

Dermaval *FIRMA, Ital.*
Diflucortolone valerate (p.1069·3).

DermaVeen Acne *Dermatech, Austral.†.*
Colloidal oatmeal (p.1583·1); salicylic acid (p.1122·3).
Acne; soap-free cleanser.

DermaVeen Bath *Dermatech, Austral.*
Colloidal oatmeal (p.1583·1).
Bath additive; dry skin; pruritus.

DermaVeen Dry Skin *Dermatech, Austral.*
Colloidal oatmeal (p.1583·1).
Dry skin; pruritus; soap-free cleanser.

DermaVeen Moisturising *Dermatech, Austral.*
Colloidal oatmeal (p.1583·1); sodium pidolate (p.1123·3); white soft paraffin (p.1407·3).
Dry skin; pruritus.

DermaVeen Shower and Bath *Dermatech, Austral.*
Colloidal oatmeal (p.1583·1); sodium pidolate (p.1123·3); liquid paraffin (p.1407·1).
Dry skin; pruritus; soap-free cleanser.

DermaVite *Stiefel, USA.*
Multivitamin and mineral preparation (p.1350·1).

Dermax *Fischer, Israel.*
Triclosan (p.1159·2).
Skin disorders.

Dermazellon *Kohler, Ger.*
Silver salt of 2-aminoethyl dihydrogen phosphate.
Burns; skin infections; wounds.

Dermazin
Pharmascience, Canad.; Lek, Hong Kong; Lek, Thai.
Sulfadiazine silver (p.251·3).
Burns; infected wounds.

Dermazine *Silvestre, Braz.*
Sulfadiazine silver (p.251·3).
Bacterial skin infections; infected burns; skin ulceration.

Dermazol *Bailleul, Fr.*
Econazole nitrate (p.382·3).
Fungal skin infections.

Dermazole
Ego, Austral.; Ego, Hong Kong; Ego, NZ; Ego, Singapore.
Econazole nitrate (p.382·3).
Fungal skin infections.

Dermazon *Dinafarma, Braz.*
Dexamethasone (p.1067·1); neomycin sulfate (p.228·1).
Skin disorders.

Der-med *Permamed, Switz.*
Soap substitute.
Skin disorders.

Dermedal *Farmec, Ital.*
Tosylchloramide sodium (p.1159·1).
Disinfection of wounds and surfaces; genital hygiene.

Dermeol *Cooperation Pharmaceutique, Fr.*
Dodeclonium bromide; enoxolone (p.34·3).
Skin disorders.

Dermestril
Faulding, Austral.; Piette, Belg.; Rottapharm, Fin.; Rottapharm, Fr.; Opfermann, Ger.; Rotta, Hong Kong; LTS, Israel; Rotta, Israel; Rottapharm, Ital.; Sanofi Synthelabo, Neth.; Delta, Port.; Rottapharm, Spain; Sigma-Tau, Switz.; Strakan, UK.
Estradiol (p.1473·1).
Menopausal disorders; osteoporosis.

Dermex *Hamilton, Austral.*
Range of barrier creams.

Dermeze *Royal Childrens Hospital, Austral.*
Liquid paraffin (p.1407·1); white soft paraffin (p.1407·3).
Dry skin.

Derm-Freeze *Eagle, Austral.*
Trichlorofluoromethane (p.1199·1); dichlorodifluoromethane (p.1199·1).
Local anaesthesia; pain.

Dermic *Kinder, Braz.*
Salicylic acid (p.1122·3); sulfur (p.1123·3).
Acne.

Dermichthol *Ichthyol, Ger.*
Ictasol (p.1115·3).
Skin disorders.

Dermicin *Heralds, Braz.*
Polymyxin B sulfate (p.238·1); prednisolone (p.1077·3).
Skin disorders.

Dermicon *Bunker, Braz.*
Benzoic acid (p.1134·2); salicylic acid (p.1122·3); iodine (p.1522·3); licor de Hoffman (alcohol, solvent ether).
Fungal skin infections.

Dermi-cyl *Liebermann, Ger.*
Calcium hydroxide solution (p.1588·3).
Burns; skin disorders.

Dermi-cyl Allerg *Liebermann, Aust.*
Calcium hydroxide solution (p.1588·3).
Skin disorders.

Dermi-cyl Ho-Lens-Complex *Liebermann, Ger.*
Homoeopathic preparation.

Dermi-cyl Schrunden *Liebermann, Aust.*
Salicylic acid (p.1122·3).
Skin disorders.

Dermidex *SSL, UK.*
Lignocaine [lidocaine] (p.1313·2); alcloxa (p.1109·3); chlorobutanol (p.1141·2); cetrimide (p.1137·1).
Skin irritation.

Dermifun *Fustery, Mex.*
Miconazole nitrate (p.391·1).
Fungal skin and nail infections.

Dermil *Nettopharma, Denm.†.*
Hydrocortisone (p.1073·3).
Skin disorders.

Dermilan *Hearst, Braz.*
Nitrofurazone (p.231·3); hydrocortisone acetate (p.1073·3).
Skin disorders.

Dermilon
Caesars, Aust.; Cesra, Ger.
Zinc oxide (p.1128·2); cod-liver oil (p.1357·2).
Skin disorders.

Dermimade Bacitracina *Esfar, Port.†.*
Bacitracin (p.155·2); neomycin (p.228·1).
Skin infections.

Dermimade Cloranfenicol *Esfar, Port.*
Chloramphenicol (p.179·1).
Skin infections.

Dermimade Hidrocortisona *Esfar, Port.*
Hydrocortisone (p.1073·3).
Skin disorders.

Derminovag *Novag, Spain†.*
Hydrocortisone acetate (p.1073·3).
Skin disorders.

Dermirex *Irex, Fr.*
Minocycline (p.225·3).
Acne.

Dermirit *Medisint, Ital.*
Hydrocortisone acetate (p.1073·3).
Skin disorders.

Dermisdin *Isdin, Spain.*
Fenticlor (p.383·1); miconazole nitrate (p.391·1); salicylic acid (p.1122·3).
Formerly contained sulfur, fenticlor, miconazole nitrate, and salicylic acid.
Acne; scalp disorders; seborrhoea.

Dermisone Beclo *Zyma, Spain†.*
Beclometasone dipropionate (p.1061·2).
Skin disorders.

Dermisone Tri Antibiotic *Novartis Consumer, Spain.*
Bacitracin (p.155·2); neomycin sulfate (p.228·1); polymyxin B sulfate (p.238·1).
Skin infections.

Dermitina *Donini, Ital.*
Hamamelis (p.1618·3); sodium glutamate; fatty acids (p.1350·1).
Soap substitute.

Dermo 6 *Pharmadeveloppement, Fr.*
Pyridoxine hydrochloride (p.1386·3).
Seborrhoea.

Dermo Base Grassa *Restiva, Ital.†.*
Product basis.

Dermo Base Magra *Restiva, Ital.†.*
Product basis.

Dermo H Infantil *Novartis Consumer, Spain.*
Dimethicone (p.1410·1); benzalkonium chloride (p.1133·2); vitamin A (p.1382·1); zinc oxide (p.1128·2).
Burns; skin disorders; wounds.

Dermo Hubber *Teofarma, Spain.*
Bacitracin zinc (p.155·2); hydrocortisone acetate (p.1073·3); neomycin sulfate (p.228·1).
Infected skin disorders.

Dermo Lassar *Mex-America, Mex.*
Zinc oxide (p.1128·2).

Dermo Posterisan *Kade, Ger.*
Hydrocortisone (p.1073·3).
Skin disorders.

Dermo WAS *Montavit, Aust.*
Lecithin (p.1628·1).
Skin disorders.

Dermoangiopan *Abiogen, Ital.*
Troxerutin (p.1611·2); sulodexide (p.978·3).
Soft-tissue disorders; vascular disorders.

Dermobacter *Innotech, Fr.*
Benzalkonium chloride (p.1133·2); chlorhexidine gluconate (p.1138·2).
Bacterial skin infections.

Dermo-Bell *Mex-America, Mex.*
Araquida oil.

Dermobene *Legrand, Braz.*
Clotrimazole (p.382·1).
Fungal skin infections.

Dermobeta *Krugher, Ital.*
Fluocinolone acetonide (p.1071·1).
Skin disorders.

Dermobion *Bergamo, Braz.*
Zinc oxide (p.1128·2); boric acid (p.1586·1); dogfish-liver oil.
Barrier preparation; skin disorders.

Dermobios *Biotekfarma, Ital.†.*
Diflucortolone valerate (p.1069·3); tetracycline (p.258·3); polymyxin B sulfate (p.238·1).
Infected skin disorders.

Dermobiotico *Davi, Port.*
Neomycin sulfate (p.228·1); bacitracin (p.155·2).
Skin infections.

Dermobras *Mex-America, Mex.*
Aluminium oxide (p.1108·3); triclosan (p.1159·2).
Skin cleansing.

Dermocaine
Note. This name is used for preparations of different composition.
Ego, Austral.
Lignocaine [lidocaine] hydrochloride (p.1313·2); menthol (p.1632·3); phenoxypropanol (p.1153·3); cetrimide (p.1137·1).
Bites and stings.

Ego, NZ.
Lignocaine [lidocaine] (p.1313·2); cetrimide (p.1137·1); phenoxypropanol (p.1153·3).
Insect bites and stings; pruritus; skin irritation.

Dermocalm *Pharmadeveloppement, Fr.†.*
Vitamin A (p.1382·1); lignocaine [lidocaine] (p.1313·2); framycetin sulfate (p.208·1); hydrocortisone acetate (p.1073·3).
Burns.

Dermocica *Phytomedica, Fr.*
Arnica (p.1581·3); melaleuca oil (p.1631·3); mimosa; vervain oil.
Burns; scars; wounds.

Dermocinetic *Geymonat, Ital.*
Thyroxine [levothyroxine] sodium (p.1526·2); aescin (p.1574·1).
Cellulite; local build up of adipose tissue.

Dermocortal *Restiva, Ital.*
Hydrocortisone (p.1073·3).
Skin disorders.

Dermocrem *Ache, Braz.*
Wheat germ.
Wounds.

Dermocreme *Chauvin, Fr.†.*
Zinc oxide (p.1128·2); copper sulfate (p.1358·1).
Skin irritation.

Dermocuivre *Chauvin, Fr.*
Copper sulfate (p.1358·1); zinc oxide (p.1128·2).
Skin disorders.

Dermodex *Bristol-Myers Squibb, Braz.*
Zinc oxide (p.1128·2); nystatin (p.392·2).
Infected skin disorders.

Dermodis *Farmades, Ital.†.*
Rifaximin (p.246·3).
Bacterial skin infections.

Dermodrin *Montavit, Aust.*
Diphenhydramine hydrochloride (p.416·1).
Skin disorders.

Dermofilm *Innovatec, Singapore.*
Topical barrier preparation.

Dermofix
Azevedos, Port.; Ferrer, Spain.
Sertaconazole nitrate (p.393·3).
Fungal skin and nail infections.

Dermofug *Wolff, Ger.*
Dodecylbenzolsulfonic acid trolamine; ammonium laurilsulfate (p.1496·3).
Acne; fungal infections; seborrhoeic dermatitis.

Dermofytol *Sedar, Braz.*
Salicylic acid (p.1122·3); benzoic acid (p.1134·2); iodine (p.1522·3).
Skin infections.

Dermogaze *Ache, Braz.*
Wheat germ.
Wounds.

Dermogen *Dermopen, Braz.*
Dexamethasone sodium phosphate (p.1067·1); neomycin sulfate (p.228·1).
Skin disorders.

Dermoglos *Galderma, Braz.*
Zinc oxide (p.1128·2); cod-liver oil (p.1357·2).
Barrier preparation; skin disorders.

Dermoil *Dermofarma, Ital.*
Emollient.
Bath additive; dry skin disorders.

Dermojela *Jean-Marie, Hong Kong.*
Choline salicylate (p.24·3); benzalkonium chloride (p.1133·2); menthol (p.1632·3).
Mouth disorders.

Dermojuventus *Juventus, Spain.*
Tretinoin (p.1126·2).
Acne.

Dermol
Note. This name is used for preparations of different composition.
Pacific, NZ.
Clobetasol propionate (p.1065·2).
Skin and scalp disorders.

Dermal Laboratories, UK.
Benzalkonium chloride (p.1133·2); chlorhexidine hydrochloride (p.1138·2); liquid paraffin (p.1407·1); isopropyl myristate (p.1409·2).
Dry and pruritic skin disorders.

Dermol HC *Dermol, USA.*
Hydrocortisone (p.1073·3).

Dermolate *Schering-Plough, USA.*
Hydrocortisone (p.1073·3).
Skin disorders.

Dermolin
Note. This name is used for preparations of different composition.
Lafare, Ital.
Fluocinolone acetonide (p.1071·1).
Skin disorders.

Roberts, USA.
Methyl salicylate (p.55·1); camphor (p.1589·3); menthol (p.1632·3); mustard oil (p.1639·1).
Muscle, joint, and soft-tissue pain; neuralgia.

Dermomycin *Sigma-Tau, Ital.*
Sodium fusidate (p.208·3).
Bacterial skin infections.

Dermomycose Liquido *Reig Jofre, Spain.*
Boric acid (p.1586·1); phenol (p.1152·3); rosaniline; resorcinol (p.1122·2).
Fungal infections.

Dermomycose Talco *Reig Jofre, Spain.*
Neomycin undecylenate (p.228·1); menthol (p.1632·3).
Skin infections.

Dermophil Indien
Note. This name is used for preparations of different composition.
Dermophil Indien, Fr.; Dermophil Indien, Switz.
Peru balsam (p.1650·2); levomenol (p.1629·1); salol (p.82·2).
Emollient.

Dermophil Indien, Fr.
Lipstick: Enzacamene (p.1517·2); isopropyldibenzoylmethane (p.1517·3).
Sunscreen.

Dermophil Indien, Fr.
Maxi-stick: Enzacamene (p.1517·2); avobenzone (p.1517·1); titanium dioxide (p.1126·1).
Sunscreen.

Dermoplast
Note. This name is used for preparations of different composition.
Wyeth-Ayerst, Canad.†.
Benzocaine (p.1306·2); benzethonium chloride (p.1134·2); menthol (p.1632·3); hydroxyquinoline benzoate (p.1622·2).
Local anaesthesia.

The symbol † denotes a preparation no longer actively marketed

Mex-America, Mex.
Urea (p.1127·3).
Dry skin disorders.

Whitehall, USA.
Benzocaine (p.1306·2).
Painful conditions of the skin and perineum.

Dermoprolyn Virginia, Ital.
Aescin (p.1574·1); hamamelis (p.1618·3); ruscus aculeatus; hedera helix.
Skin disorders.

Dermoretin Sintofarma, Braz.
Tretinoin (p.1126·2).
Acne.

Dermosa Aureomicina Farmacusi, Braz.
Chlortetracycline hydrochloride (p.182·1).
Skin infections.

Dermosa Hidrocortisona Farmacusi, Spain.
Hydrocortisone acetate (p.1073·3).
Skin disorders.

Dermosed Makros, Braz.
Tyrothricin (p.267·1); salicylic acid (p.1122·3); boric acid (p.1586·1).
Skin infections.

Dermoseptic SmithKline Beecham, Spain.
Sertaconazole nitrate (p.393·3).
Fungal skin and nail infections.

Dermoskin Mex-America, Mex.
Almond oil (p.1576·3).
Moisturiser.

Dermo-Steril Ghimas, Ital.†
Triclosan (p.1159·2).
Acne.

Dermo-Sulfuryl Aerocid, Fr.
Precipitated sulfur (p.1123·3); copper sulfate (p.1358·1); zinc sulfate (p.1398·2).
Skin disorders.

Dermoswab Schwulst, S.Afr.†
Chlorhexidine (p.1138·2); isopropyl alcohol (p.1149·2).
Skin disinfection.

Dermoval
Note.This name is used for preparations of different composition.
Luper, Braz.; Tocogino, Mex.
Betamethasone (p.1063·1) or betamethasone valerate (p.1063·2).
Skin disorders.

Glaxo Wellcome, Fr.
Clobetasol propionate (p.1065·2).
Skin disorders.

Dermovan Healthpoint, USA.
Vehicle for topical preparations.

Dermovat Glaxo Wellcome, Denm.; Glaxo Wellcome, Fin.; Glaxo Wellcome, Norw.; Glaxo Wellcome, Swed.
Clobetasol propionate (p.1065·2).
Skin disorders.

Dermovate Glaxo Wellcome, Aust.; Glaxo Wellcome, Belg.; Baldassari, Braz.; Glaxo Wellcome, Canad.; Glaxo Wellcome, Hong Kong; Glaxo Wellcome, Irl.; Glaxo Wellcome, Israel; Glaxo Wellcome, Neth.; Glaxo Wellcome, NZ; Glaxo Wellcome, Port.; Allen & Hanburys, S.Afr.; Glaxo Wellcome, Singapore; Glaxo Wellcome, Switz.; Glaxo Wellcome, Thai.; Glaxo Wellcome, UK.
Clobetasol propionate (p.1065·2).
Skin and scalp disorders.

Dermovate-NN Glaxo Wellcome, Port.; Glaxo Wellcome, Switz.; Glaxo Wellcome, UK.
Clobetasol propionate (p.1065·2); neomycin sulfate (p.228·1); nystatin (p.392·2).
Skin disorders with bacterial or fungal infection.

Dermovit Kemiprogress, Ital.
Vitamin, selenium, yeast, and coenzyme Q10 (p.1350·1).
Nutritional supplement.

Dermovitamina Trenka Difer, Ital.
Cod-liver oil (p.1357·2).
Skin disorders.

Dermowas Wolff, Ger.
Soap substitute.

Dermowas N Wolff, Ger.
Dodecylbenzolsulfonic acid trolamine.
Skin disorders.

Dermowund Adler, Aust.
Acriflavinium chloride (p.1130·2); diacetylaminoazotoluene; cod-liver oil (p.1357·2); linseed oil (p.1629·1); sodium propionate (p.393·2); zinc oxide (p.1128·2).
Wounds.

Dermox Mex-America, Mex.
Methoxsalen (p.1118·3).
Psoriasis; vitiligo.

Dermoxin
Note.This name is used for preparations of different composition.
Bunker, Braz.
Fluocinolone; neomycin (p.228·1).
Skin disorders.

Glaxo Wellcome, Ger.; Cascan, Ger.
Clobetasol propionate (p.1065·2).
Skin disorders.

Dermoxinale Glaxo Wellcome, Ger.; Cascan, Ger.
Clobetasol propionate (p.1065·2).
Skin disorders.

Dermoxyl
Note.This name is used for preparations of different composition.
ICN, Canad.
Benzoyl peroxide (p.1111·1).
Acne.

RDC, Ital.
Urea hydrogen peroxide (p.1159·3).
Skin disinfection and cleansing.

Derms Uniao Quimica, Braz.
Tiabendazole (p.109·1); neomycin sulfate (p.228·1).
Skin infections.

Dermtex HC with Aloe Pfeiffer, USA.
Hydrocortisone (p.1073·3); aloe vera (p.1110·1).
Skin disorders.

Dermuspray Warner Chilcott, USA.
Trypsin (p.1675·3); peru balsam (p.1650·2); castor oil (p.1592·1).
Wounds.

Dermycose Prima, Braz.
Iodine (p.1522·3); sodium iodide (p.1522·3); salicylic acid (p.1122·3); benzoic acid (p.1134·2).
Fungal skin infections.

Deronga Heilpaste Galderma, Ger.
Natamycin (p.392·1).
Fungal skin infections.

Deroxat SmithKline Beecham, Fr.; SmithKline Beecham, Switz.
Paroxetine hydrochloride (p.302·3).
Depression; obsessive disorders; panic attacks.

Derso TCC Ache, Braz.
Triclocarban (p.1159·2).
Skin infections.

Dertrase UCB, Braz.
Carbamoylglutamic acid; inositol (p.1623·3); methionine (p.1012·2); chymotrypsin (p.1595·1); ribonucleic acid (p.1657·3); trypsin (p.1675·3); nitrofurazone (p.231·3).
Burns; skin disorders; ulcers; wounds.

Dertrin Iqfasa, Mex.
Co-trimoxazole (p.193·3).

Dervin Boniscontro & Gazzone, Ital.
Diflucortolone valerate (p.1069·3).
Skin disorders.

Derzid Unison, Thai.
Betamethasone valerate (p.1063·2).
Skin disorders.

Desacil Zambon, Braz.
Deslanoside (p.867·3).
Arrhythmias; heart failure.

Desalark Farmacologico Milanese, Ital.
Dexamethasone sodium phosphate (p.1067·1).
Eye/ear disorders.

Desalfa INTES, Ital.
Cream; ointment: Dexamethasone isonicotinate (p.1067·1); lignocaine [lidocaine] hydrochloride (p.1313·2).
Haemorrhoids; skin disorders.

Eye drops; eye ointment: Dexamethasone isonicotinate (p.1067·1); phenylephrine hydrochloride (p.1097·1); neomycin (p.228·1).
Eye disorders.

Lotion: Dexamethasone isonicotinate (p.1067·1); neomycin (p.228·1).
Formerly contained dexamethasone isonicotinate, neomycin, and nystatin.
Skin disorders.

Nasal/ear drops: Dexamethasone isonicotinate (p.1067·1); neomycin (p.228·1).
Formerly contained dexamethasone isonicotinate, neomycin, lignocaine [lidocaine] hydrochloride, phenylephrine hydrochloride, and nystatin.
Nasal and ear infections.

Desamin Same Savoma, Ital.
Naphazoline hydrochloride (p.1095·1).
Nasal congestion.

Desamix Effe Savoma, Ital.
Dexamethasone (p.1067·1); clotrimazole (p.382·1).
Infected skin disorders.

Desamix-Neomicina Savoma, Ital.
Dexamethasone (p.1067·1); neomycin sulfate (p.228·1).
Skin disorders.

Desamon Streuli, Switz.
Didecyldiammonium chloride; isopropyl alcohol (p.1149·2).
Disinfection of instruments, clothing, hands, skin, and mucous membranes.

Desanden Nycomed, Switz.
Benzoyl peroxide (p.1111·1).
Acne.

Desarell Sanorell, Ger.
Homoeopathic preparation.

Desarrol Iquinosa, Spain.
Cyproheptadine hydrochloride (p.414·2); amino acids (p.1350·1).
Tonic.

Desatura Sanofi Winthrop, Fr.†
Allopurinol (p.397·2); benzbromarone (p.399·3).
Hyperuricaemia.

Desbly Medeva, Fr.
Guaifenesin (p.1092·2); senega (p.1100·2).
Formerly contained drosera, grindelia, sodium bromide, sodium benzoate, magnesium sulfate, and wild thyme.
Respiratory-tract disorders.

Desclidium Nattermann, Ger.†
Viquidil hydrochloride (p.1680·2).
Circulatory and metabolic disorders of the brain, eyes, and inner ear.

Descon Hoechst Marion Roussel, Braz.
Chlorpheniramine [chlorphenamine] maleate (p.412·1); phenylpropanolamine hydrochloride (p.1098·1); paracetamol (p.71·2).
Nasal congestion.

Descon AP Hoechst Marion Roussel, Braz.
Chlorpheniramine [chlorphenamine] maleate (p.412·1); phenylpropanolamine hydrochloride (p.1098·1); isopropamide iodide (p.470·1).
Nasal congestion.

Descon Expectorante Hoechst Marion Roussel, Braz.
Chlorpheniramine [chlorphenamine] maleate (p.412·1); phenylpropanolamine hydrochloride (p.1098·1); guaifenesin (p.1092·2).
Respiratory-tract congestion.

Desconasal Warner-Lambert, Spain†
Xylometazoline hydrochloride (p.1102·2).
Nasal congestion.

Desconex Reig Jofre, Spain.
Loxapine hydrochloride (p.690·1) or loxapine succinate (p.690·1).
Psychoses.

Descongestan Merck, Spain.
Oxymetazoline hydrochloride (p.1096·2).
Nasal congestion.

Descutan Fresenius Kabi, Swed.
Chlorhexidine gluconate (p.1138·2).
Skin disinfection.

Desderman Schulke & Mayr, Ger.†
Alcohol (p.1130·3).
Formerly contained tetrabromocresol and alcohol.
Hand disinfection.

Desderman N Schulke & Mayr, Ger.
Orthophenylphenol (p.1152·1); alcohol (p.1130·3).
Hand disinfection.

Desec TO-Chemicals, Thai.
Omeprazole (p.1239·1).
Gastro-oesophageal reflux, Zollinger-Ellison syndrome; peptic ulcer.

Desenex
Note.This name is used for preparations of different composition.
Novartis Consumer, Canad.; Roche Consumer, Irl.; Ciba, USA.
Ointment; cream; foam; soap; spray powder; powder: Undecenoic acid (p.395·3) and/or zinc undecenoate (p.395·3).
Fungal skin infections; minor skin disorders.

Fisons, USA†.
Topical spray: Tolnaftate (p.395·2).
Fungal skin infections.

Desenfriol Schering-Plough, Spain.
Aspirin (p.14·2); caffeine (p.761·3); chlorpheniramine [chlorphenamine] maleate (p.412·1).
Fever; nasal congestion; pain.

Desenfriol C Schering-Plough, Spain.
Aspirin (p.14·2); ascorbic acid (p.1389·3); caffeine (p.761·3); chlorpheniramine [chlorphenamine] maleate (p.412·1).
Fever; nasal congestion; pain.

Desenfriol D
Note.This name is used for preparations of different composition.
Schering-Plough, Mex.
Aspirin (p.14·2); chlorpheniramine [chlorphenamine] maleate (p.412·1); phenylpropanolamine hydrochloride (p.1098·1).
Cold and influenza symptoms.

Schering-Plough, Spain.
Aspirin (p.14·2); caffeine (p.761·3); chlorpheniramine [chlorphenamine] maleate (p.412·1); phenylephrine hydrochloride (p.1097·1).
Fever; nasal congestion; pain.

Desenfriol Infantil Schering-Plough, Spain.
Aspirin (p.14·2); chlorpheniramine [chlorphenamine] maleate (p.412·1); phenylephrine hydrochloride (p.1097·1).
Fever; nasal congestion; pain.

Desenfriol-Ito Schering-Plough, Mex.
Paracetamol (p.71·2); chlorpheniramine [chlorphenamine] maleate (p.412·1); phenylpropanolamine hydrochloride (p.1098·1).
Cold and influenza symptoms.

Desensib Wiedemann, Ger.
Homoeopathic preparation.

Desensibilizante Chauvin Prima, Braz.
Sodium thiosulfate (p.1024·2); magnesium thiosulfate (p.1024·2); star anise; aniseed (p.1580·2).
Hypersensitivity reactions.

Desentol Pharmacia Upjohn, Swed.
Diphenhydramine hydrochloride (p.416·1).
Hypersensitivity reactions.

Deseril Novartis, Austral.; Novartis, Belg.; Novartis, Ger.; Novartis, Irl.; Novartis, Neth.; Novartis, S.Afr.; Novartis, Switz.; Alliance, UK.
Methysergide maleate (p.454·1).
Cluster headache; diarrhoea associated with carcinoid disease; migraine.

Deserila Novartis, Braz.
Methysergide maleate (p.454·1).
Migraine.

Desernil Novartis, Fr.
Methysergide maleate (p.454·1).
Migraine.

Deserril Sandoz, Ital.†
Methysergide maleate (p.454·1).
Migraine.

Desert Pure Calcium Cal-White, USA.
Calcium carbonate (p.1215·1); vitamin D (p.1391·1).

Desfatigan IMA, Braz.
Arginine aspartate (p.1354·1).
Nutritional supplement.

Desfatin Heralds, Braz.
Multivitamin and mineral preparation (p.1350·1).

Desferal Novartis, Aust.; Novartis, Austral.; Novartis, Belg.; Novartis, Braz.; Novartis, Canad.; Novartis, Denm.; Novartis, Fin.; Novartis, Fr.; Novartis, Ger.; Novartis, Hong Kong; Novartis, Irl.; Novartis, Israel; Novartis, Ital.; Novartis, Neth.; Novartis, Norw.; Novartis, NZ; Novartis, Port.; Novartis, S.Afr.; Novartis, Singapore; Novartis, Swed.; Novartis, Switz.; Novartis, Thai.; Novartis, UK; Novartis, USA.
Desferrioxamine mesilate (p.1003·2).
Aluminium overload; iron overload.

Desferin Padro, Spain.
Desferrioxamine mesilate (p.1003·2).
Iron overload.

Desflam Merck, Mex.
Bumadizone calcium (p.20·3).
Inflammation; peri-articular and soft-tissue disorders.

Desicort Taro, Israel.
Desoximetasone (p.1066·2).
Skin disorders.

Desidoxepin Declimed, Ger.
Doxepin hydrochloride (p.283·3).
Anxiety; depression.

Desifluvoxamin Declimed, Ger.
Fluvoxamine maleate (p.289·3).
Depression.

Desintan P Stafford-Miller, Port.
Permethrin (p.1436·1).
Pediculosis.

Desintex Richard, Fr.
Sodium thiosulfate (p.1024·2); magnesium thiosulfate (p.1024·2).
Dyspepsia; rhinitis; rhinopharyngitis.

Desintex Infantile Richard, Fr.
Sodium thiosulfate (p.1024·2); magnesium thiosulfate (p.1024·2); calcium gluconate (p.1188·2); calcium carbonate (p.1215·1).
Dyspepsia; rhinitis; rhinopharyngitis.

Desintex-Choline Richard, Fr.
Sodium thiosulfate (p.1024·2); magnesium thiosulfate (p.1024·2); choline chloride (p.1356·3).
Dyspepsia.

Desinvag Casen Fleet, Spain.
Benzalkonium chloride (p.1133·2); furazolidone (p.592·1).
Vaginal antiseptic; vulvovaginal trichomoniasis.

Desiperiden Desitin, Ger.†
Biperiden hydrochloride (p.464·2) or biperiden lactate (p.464·2).
Drug-induced extrapyramidal disorders; nicotine poisoning; parkinsonism.

Desirel Codal Synto, Thai.
Trazodone hydrochloride (p.310·1).
Anxiety; depression.

Desisulpid Desitin, Ger.
Sulpiride (p.706·1).
Depression; schizophrenia; vestibular disorders.

Desiticlopidin Desitin, Ger.
Ticlopidine hydrochloride (p.981·1).
Thromboembolic disorders.

Desitin
Note.This name is used for preparations of different composition.
Sigmapharm, Aust.; Pfizer, Canad.; Desitin, Ger.; Pfizer, Israel; Pfizer, Mex.; Leeming, USA.
Cod-liver oil (p.1357·2); zinc oxide (p.1128·2).
Nappy rash; skin disorders.

Desitin, Ger.
Topical powder: Zinc oxide (p.1128·2).
Burns; skin disorders.

Desitin Creamy Pfizer, USA.
Zinc oxide (p.1128·2); liquid paraffin (p.1407·1); white soft paraffin (p.1407·3).
Formerly known as Daily Care.
Nappy rash.

Desitin with Zinc Oxide Pfizer, USA.
Corn starch (p.1379·3); zinc oxide (p.1128·2).

Desitur Turimed, Switz.
Alcohol (p.1130·3); cetrimonium bromide (p.1137·3).
Hand disinfection.

Desketo Malesci, Ital.
Dexketoprofen trometamol (p.47·3).
Pain.

Desmanol Schulke & Mayr, Ger.
Chlorhexidine gluconate (p.1138·2); propyl alcohol (p.1155·3); isopropyl alcohol (p.1149·2).
Hand disinfection.

Desmanol G Merck, Thai.; Schulke & Mayr, Thai.
Chlorhexidine gluconate (p.1138·2).
Hand disinfection.

Desmin Grunenthal, Ger.
Ethinylestradiol (p.1476·2); desogestrel (p.1470·3).
Combined oral contraceptive.

Desmogalen Galen, Ger.
Desmopressin acetate (p.1281·2).
Diabetes insipidus; polydipsia; polyuria; test of renal concentrating capacity.

Desmoline Schering-Plough, Port.
Dithranol (p.1113·3).
Psoriasis.

Desmospray Ferring, Irl.; Ferring, Port.; Ferring, UK.
Desmopressin acetate (p.1281·2).
Diabetes insipidus; nocturia associated with multiple sclerosis; nocturnal enuresis; test of renal concentrating capacity.

Desmotabs Ferring, Irl.; Ferring, UK.
Desmopressin acetate (p.1281·2).
Diabetes insipidus; nocturnal enuresis; post-hypophysectomy polyuria or polydipsia.

Desobesi-M Asta Medica, Braz.
Fenproporex hydrochloride (p.1510·2).
Obesity.

Desocol Lampugnani, Ital.
Ursodeoxycholic acid (p.1677·2).
Biliary dyspepsia; cholesterol gallstones.

Desocort
Note.This name is used for preparations of different composition.
Galderma, Canad.
Desonide (p.1066·2).
Skin disorders.

Chauvin, Fr.
Ear drops: Dexamethasone sodium phosphate (p.1067·1).
Otitis externa.
Eye drops†: Prednisolone metasulfobenzoate sodium (p.1078·1); chlorhexidine gluconate (p.1138·2).
Eye disorders.

Desoform Lysoform, Ger.
Glyoxal (p.1145·3); formaldehyde (p.1144·2); glutaral (p.1145·2); didecyldimethylammonium chloride (p.1143·2).
Instrument disinfection.

Desogen
Note.This name is used for preparations of different composition.
Hoechst Marion Roussel, Ital.†.
Toloconium metilsulfate (p.1159·1).
Skin, burn, and wound disinfection.

Organon, USA.
21 Tablets, desogestrel (p.1470·3); ethinylestradiol (p.1476·2); 7 tablets, inert.
Combined oral contraceptive.

Desolett Organon, Swed.
Desogestrel (p.1470·3); ethinylestradiol (p.1476·2).
28-Day packs also contain 7 inert tablets.
Combined oral contraceptive.

Desomedine Chauvin, Fr.; Chauvin, Hong Kong; Chauvin, Singapore; Chauvin Novopharma, Swit.
Hexamidine isetionate (p.1146·2).
Infections of the eye or nose.

Desonol Medley, Braz.
Desonide (p.1066·2).
Skin disorders.

Desorelle Durascan, Denm.
Desogestrel (p.1470·3); ethinylestradiol (p.1476·2).
Combined oral contraceptive.

Desoren Vitamed, Israel.
Dexamethasone sodium phosphate (p.1067·1); neomycin sulfate (p.228·1); polymyxin B sulfate (p.238·1).
Ear infections.

DesOwen Galderma, Austral.; Galderma, Hong Kong; Galderma, Mex.; Galderma, NZ; Galderma, Singapore; Galderma, USA.
Desonide (p.1066·2).
Skin disorders.

Desoxil Boniscontro & Gazzone, Ital.
Ursodeoxycholic acid (p.1677·2).
Biliary disorders.

Desoxyn Abbott, USA.
Metamfetamine hydrochloride (p.1511·1).
Attention deficit hyperactivity disorder; obesity.

Despacilina Bristol-Myers Squibb, Braz.
Procaine penicillin [procaine benzylpenicillin] (p.239·2); benzylpenicillin potassium (p.157·1).
Bacterial infections.

Despamen AF, Mex.
Estradiol valerate (p.1473·2); testosterone enantate (p.1492·2).
Menopausal disorders; osteoporosis.

Desparasil Rimsa, Mex.
Piperazine hydrate (p.106·1).
Nematode infections.

Desquam Westwood-Squibb, USA.
Benzoyl peroxide (p.1111·1).
Acne.

Desquaman Hermal, Aust.; Hermal, Israel; Hermal, Port.†.
Pyrithione zinc (p.1122·1).
Scalp disorders.

De-squaman N Hermal, Ger.
Pyrithione zinc (p.1122·1).
Scalp disorders.

Desquam-X Westwood-Squibb, Canad.
Benzoyl peroxide (p.1111·1).
Acne.

Destamin Medifarma, Mex.
Histamine (p.1619·2).

deSTAT 3 Sherman, Israel; Sherman, USA.
Cleaning, disinfectant, and storage solution for gas permeable contact lenses (p.1129·2).

Destolit Aventis, Fr.†; Aventis, Port.; Norgine, UK.
Ursodeoxycholic acid (p.1677·2).
Biliary tract disorders; cholesterol gallstones.

Destrobac Rusch, Ital.; Gebro, Switz.
Povidone-iodine (p.1155·1).
Skin and wound disinfection.

Desuric Sanofi Synthelabo, Belg.; Sanofi Winthrop, Fr.; Sanfer, Mex.; Sanofi Synthelabo, Neth.; Sanofi Synthelabo, Switz.
Benzbromarone (p.399·3).
Gout; hyperuricaemia.

Desyrel Bristol, Canad.; Apothecon, USA.
Trazodone hydrochloride (p.310·1).
Depression.

DET MS Fuisz, Ger.
Dihydroergotamine mesilate (p.450·3).
Hypotension; migraine and other vascular headaches.

DET MS spezial Fuisz, Ger.
Dihydroergotamine mesilate (p.450·3).
Chronic venous insufficiency; hypotension; migraine and other vascular headaches.

Detamol PD, Thai.
Paracetamol (p.71·2).
Lignocaine [lidocaine] hydrochloride (p.1313·2) is included in this preparation to alleviate the pain of injection.
Fever; pain; post-immunisation reactions.

Detane Del, USA.
Benzocaine (p.1306·2).
Genital desensitising lubricant.

Detantol Eisai, Jpn; Eisai, Thai.
Bunazosin hydrochloride (p.852·3).
Hypertension.

Deteclo Wyeth, Irl.; Wyeth, UK.
Tetracycline hydrochloride (p.258·3); chlortetracycline hydrochloride (p.182·1); demeclocycline hydrochloride (p.198·2).
Bacterial infections.

Detemes Procter & Gamble, Aust.
Dihydroergotamine mesilate (p.450·3).
Hypotension; migraine and related vascular headaches; vascular disorders.

Detensiel Lipha Sante, Fr.
Bisoprolol fumarate (p.850·1).
Angina pectoris; hypertension.

Detensor Novartis Consumer, Switz.
Diphenhydramine hydrochloride (p.416·1); 8-chlorotheophylline.
Sleep disorders.

Detergil Manetti Roberts, Ital.
Benzalkonium chloride (p.1133·2).
Instrument disinfection; wound disinfection.

Dethamycin Vitamed, Israel.
Dexamethasone sodium phosphate (p.1067·1); neomycin sulfate (p.228·1).
Infected eye, ear, and nose disorders.

Dethaphrine Vitamed, Israel.
Dexamethasone sodium phosphate (p.1067·1); neomycin sulfate (p.228·1); phenylephrine hydrochloride (p.1097·1).
Infected eye, ear, and nose disorders.

Deticene Rhone-Poulenc Rorer, Fr.; Rhone-Poulenc Rorer, Hong Kong; Rhone-Poulenc Rorer, Israel; Rhone-Poulenc Rorer, Ital.; Rhone-Poulenc Rorer, Mex.; Rhone-Poulenc Rorer, Neth.; Rhone-Poulenc Rorer, Port.
Dacarbazine (p.531·2).
Malignant neoplasms.

Detimedac Medac, Ger.
Dacarbazine (p.531·2).
Malignant neoplasms.

Detoch PD, Thai.
Dequalinium chloride (p.1143·1); ascorbic acid (p.1389·3).
Mouth and throat infections.

Detox Reese, USA.
Red clover; liquorice; peach bark; orange grape root; stillingia; cascara; sarsaparilla; lappa root; buckthorn (p.1350·1).
Dietary supplement.

Detox Thuja Homeocan, Canad.
Homoeopathic preparation.

Detoxalgine Riom, Fr.
Glucuronamide; aspirin (p.14·2); ascorbic acid (p.1389·3).
Fever; musculoskeletal and joint disorders; pain.

Detoxergon
Note.This name is used for preparations of different composition.
Baldacci, Ital.†.
Injection: Pirglutargine (p.1652·2); pyridoxine hydrochloride (p.1386·3); taurine (p.1669·3); potassium pidolate; magnesium pidolate (p.1191·1); calcium pidolate (p.1188·3); sodium pidolate (p.1123·3).
Hyperammonaemia.

Oral powder: Pidolic acid; pirglutargine (p.1652·2); taurine (p.1669·3); pyridoxine hydrochloride (p.1386·3); sodium citrate (p.1186·2); potassium chloride (p.1194·3); magnesium chloride (p.1190·3); calcium chloride (p.1188·1).
Gastrointestinal disorders.

Baldacci, Port.
Pirglutargine (p.1652·2); taurine (p.1669·3); pyridoxine; electrolytes.
Liver disorders.

Detoxicon SIT, Ital.
Glycine (p.1365·3); acetylmethionine.
Formerly contained glucurolactone, glycine, and acetylmethionine.
Tonic.

Detraine Seid, Spain.
Hydrocortisone (p.1073·3); propanocaine hydrochloride (p.1319·3).
Insect bites and stings; pruritus; skin disorders.

Detrixin Astra, Swed.†.
Colecalciferol (p.1391·1).
Osteoporosis; vitamin D deficiency.

Detrol Pharmacia Upjohn, Canad.; Pharmacia Upjohn, USA.
Tolterodine tartrate (p.474·2).
Bladder instability.

Detrunorm Schering-Plough, UK.
Propiverine hydrochloride (p.473·3).
Bladder instability; neurogenic bladder.

Detrusitol Pharmacia Upjohn, Aust.; Pharmacia Upjohn, Belg.; Pharmacia Upjohn, Denm.; Pharmacia Upjohn, Fin.; Pharmacia Upjohn, Ger.; Pharmacia Upjohn, Hong Kong; Pharmacia Upjohn, Irl.; Pharmacia Upjohn, Israel; Pharmacia Upjohn, Ital.; Pharmacia Upjohn, Mex.; Pharmacia Upjohn, Neth.; Pharmacia Upjohn, Norw.; Pharmacia Upjohn, NZ; Pharmacia Upjohn, Port.; Pharmacia Upjohn, S.Afr.; Pharmacia Upjohn, Singapore; Pharmacia Upjohn, Spain; Pharmacia Upjohn, Swed.; Pharmacia Upjohn, Switz.; Pharmacia Upjohn, Thai.; Pharmacia, UK.
Tolterodine tartrate (p.474·2).
Bladder instability.

Dettol
Note.This name is used for preparations of different composition.
Reckitt & Colman, Austral.; Reckitt & Colman, Hong Kong; Reckitt Benckiser, Irl.; Reckitt Benckiser, NZ; Reckitt & Colman, S.Afr.; Reckitt & Colman, Singapore; Reckitt & Colman, Thai.; Reckitt & Colman, UK.
Cream: Chloroxylenol (p.1142·1); triclosan (p.1159·2).
Skin disinfection.

Reckitt & Colman, Singapore.
Medicated dressing: Ethacridine lactate (p.1130·3).
Wounds.

Reckitt & Colman, Belg.; Reckitt & Colman, Hong Kong; Reckitt Benckiser, NZ; Reckitt & Colman, S.Afr.; Reckitt & Colman, Singapore; Reckitt & Colman, Thai.; Reckitt & Colman, UK.
Topical solution: Chloroxylenol (p.1142·1).
Skin disinfection.

Reckitt & Colman, Singapore; Reckitt & Colman, UK.
Topical spray: Benzalkonium chloride (p.1133·2); lignocaine [lidocaine] hydrochloride (p.1313·2).
Insect bites and stings; minor burns; minor wounds.

Dettol Antiseptic Wash Reckitt Benckiser, UK.
Benzalkonium chloride (p.1133·2).
Wound disinfection.

Dettol Classic Reckitt & Colman, Austral.
Chloroxylenol (p.1142·1).
Bath additive; bites and stings; burns; minor abrasions; skin disorders; skin infections.

Dettol Fresh Reckitt & Colman, Austral.; Reckitt Benckiser, NZ; Reckitt & Colman, UK.
Benzalkonium chloride (p.1133·2).
Bites and stings; burns; minor abrasions; skin disorders; skin infections.

Dettol Liquid Wash Reckitt & Colman, Austral.; Reckitt & Colman, Belg.
Triclosan (p.1159·2).
Skin disinfection.

Detulin Woelm, Ger.
dl-Alpha tocoferil acetate (p.1394·1).
Vitamin E deficiency.

Deturgylone Synthelabo, Fr.
Prednisolone sodium phosphate (p.1078·1); oxymetazoline hydrochloride (p.1096·2).
Formerly contained prednazoline.
Rhinitis.

Detuss Siam Bheasach, Thai.
Syrup: Dextromethorphan hydrobromide (p.1087·3); ammonium chloride (p.1085·2); dexpanthenol (p.1602·3).
Tablets: Dextromethorphan (p.1087·3).
Coughs.

Deursil Sanofi Synthelabo, Ital.; Synthelabo, Switz.
Ursodeoxycholic acid (p.1677·2).
Biliary-tract disorders; gallstones.

Devaron Solvay, Neth.
Colecalciferol (p.1391·1).
Vitamin D deficiency.

Develin Godecke, Ger.
Dextropropoxyphene hydrochloride (p.27·1).
Pain.

Deverol Sanochemia, Aust.
Spironolactone (p.973·2).
Hyperaldosteronism; hypertension; liver cirrhosis with ascites; nephrotic syndrome; oedema.

Deverol mit Thiazid Sanochemia, Aust.
Spironolactone (p.973·2); hydrochlorothiazide (p.907·3).
Ascites; heart failure; nephrotic syndrome; oedema.

Devils Claw Plus Eagle, Austral.
Devil's claw root (p.26·3); murraya; celery (p.1592·3); hesperidin (p.1611·2).
Arthritis; rheumatism.

Devincal Almirall, Spain.
Piracetam (p.1652·1); vincamine (p.1680·1).
Cerebrovascular disorders.

Devitol Orion, Fin.
Ergocalciferol (p.1391·2).
Vitamin D deficiency.

Devitre Nycomed, Swed.
Colecalciferol (p.1391·1).
Osteoporosis; vitamin D deficiency.

Devorfungi Combe, Spain†.
Tolnaftate (p.395·2).
Fungal skin infections.

Devrom Parthenon, USA.
Bismuth subgallate (p.1213·2).
Ostomy deodorant.

Dewax Ranbaxy, Thai.
Docusate sodium (p.1223·1).
Ear wax removal.

Dex PP Lab, Thai.
Dextromethorphan hydrobromide (p.1087·3).
Coughs and cold symptoms.

Dex4 Glucose Can-Am Care, USA.
Glucose (p.1364·1).
Hypoglycaemia.

Dexa CT, Ger.; Jenapharm, Ger.; Shiwa, Thai.
Dexamethasone sodium phosphate (p.1067·1).
Corticosteroid.

Dexa Biciron Alcon, Ger.
Dexamethasone isonicotinate (p.1067·1); tramazoline hydrochloride (p.1102·1).
Allergic and inflammatory disorders of the eye.

Dexa in der Ophtiole Mann, Ger.†.
Dexamethasone sodium phosphate (p.1067·1).
Eye disorders.

Dexa Fenic Ciba Vision, Spain†.
Chloramphenicol (p.179·1); dexamethasone (p.1067·1).
Infected eye disorders.

Dexa Loscon mono Galderma, Ger.
Dexamethasone isonicotinate (p.1067·1).
Scalp disorders.

Dexa Polyspectran N Alcon, Ger.
Polymyxin B sulfate (p.238·1); neomycin sulfate (p.228·1); dexamethasone sodium phosphate (p.1067·1).
Infected eye and ear disorders.

Dexa Tavegil Novartis, Spain.
Clemastine (p.413·3); dexamethasone (p.1067·1).
Hypersensitivity reactions; inflammatory eye disorders; insect bites and stings; sunburn.

Dexa Vasoc Ciba Vision, Spain†.
Dexamethasone (p.1067·1); naphazoline hydrochloride (p.1095·1); zinc sulfate (p.1398·2).
Eye congestion; inflammatory eye disorders.

Dexa-Allvoran TAD, Ger.
Dexamethasone sodium phosphate (p.1067·1).
Corticosteroid.

Dexabene Ratiopharm, Aust.; Merckle, Ger.
Dexamethasone sodium phosphate (p.1067·1).
Corticosteroid.

Dexabion Merck, Mex.
Ampoule 1: thiamine hydrochloride (p.1385·1); pyridoxine hydrochloride (p.1386·3); cyanocobalamin (p.1388·1); ampoule 2: dexamethasone sodium phosphate (p.1067·1).
Lignocaine [lidocaine] hydrochloride (p.1313·2) is included in ampoule 2 to alleviate the pain of injection.
Inflammation; neuralgias; neuritis; peri-articular disorders.

Dexa-Brachialin N Steigerwald, Ger.
Dexamethasone sodium phosphate (p.1067·1).
Acute inflammatory rheumatic disorders.

Dexacidin Ciba Vision, USA.
Dexamethasone (p.1067·1); neomycin sulfate (p.228·1); polymyxin B sulfate (p.238·1).
Eye inflammation with bacterial infection.

Dexacin ANB, Thai.
Dexamethasone sodium phosphate (p.1067·1); neomycin sulfate (p.228·1).
Infected eye or ear disorders.

Dexacine Ciba Vision, USA.
Dexamethasone (p.1067·1); neomycin sulfate (p.228·1); polymyxin B sulfate (p.238·1).
Infected eye disorders.

Dexa-Citoneurin Merck, Braz.
Thiamine hydrochloride (p.1385·1); pyridoxine (p.1387·1); cyanocobalamin (p.1388·1); dexamethasone (p.1067·1).
Neuritis.

dexa-clinit Hormosan, Ger.
Dexamethasone sodium phosphate (p.1067·1).
Parenteral corticosteroid.

Dexacloran Dansk-Flama, Braz.
Dexamethasone (p.1067·1); diiodohydroxyquinoline (p.590·2); chloramphenicol (p.179·1).
Vulvovaginal disorders.

Dexacobal Searle, USA.
Thiamine (p.1385·2); pyridoxine hydrochloride (p.1386·3); cyanocobalamin (p.1388·1); dexamethasone (p.1067·1).
Neuritis.

Dexacort
Note.This name is used for preparations of different composition.
Gemballa, Braz.
Dexamethasone (p.1067·1); neomycin (p.228·1).
Skin disorders.

Biogal, Israel; Medeva, USA.
Dexamethasone sodium phosphate (p.1067·1).
Formerly known as Decadron in the USA.
Allergic rhinitis; nasal polyps.

Dexacortal Organon, Swed.
Dexamethasone (p.1067·1).
Corticosteroid.

Dexacortin Streuli, Switz.
Dexamethasone (p.1067·1) or dexamethasone sodium phosphate (p.1067·1).
Corticosteroid.

Dexacortin-K Streuli, Switz.
Dexamethasone (p.1067·1); lignocaine [lidocaine] hydrochloride (p.1313·2).
Joint and peri-articular disorders.

Dexacortisone ANB, Thai.
Dexamethasone sodium phosphate (p.1067·1).
Corticosteroid.

Dexacrinin Pharmagalen, Ger.†
Dexamethasone (p.1067·1); salicylic acid (p.1122·3); coal tar (p.1125·1).
Scalp disorders.

Dexadermil Legrand, Braz.
Dexamethasone (p.1067·1) or dexamethasone acetate (p.1067·1).
Skin disorders.

Dexador Ativus, Braz.
Cyanocobalamin (p.1388·1); thiamine (p.1385·2); pyridoxine (p.1387·1); dexamethasone (p.1067·1); procaine (p.1319·2).
Neuritis.

Dexadoze Teuto, Braz.
Dexamethasone (p.1067·1); thiamine hydrochloride (p.1385·1); pyridoxine (p.1387·1); cyanocobalamin (p.1388·1).
Neuritis.

Dexa-Effekton Wyeth, Ger.; LAW, Ger.
Dexamethasone sodium phosphate (p.1067·1).
Rheumatic disorders.

Dexafed Cough Mallard, USA.
Phenylephrine hydrochloride (p.1097·1); dextromethorphan hydrobromide (p.1087·3); guaifenesin (p.1092·2).
Coughs.

Dexafenicol
Allergan-Frumtost, Braz.; Ciba Vision, Spain.
Chloramphenicol (p.179·1); dexamethasone (p.1067·1).
Infected eye disorders.

Dexaflam Lichtenstein, Ger.
Dexamethasone (p.1067·1).
Corticosteroid.

Dexaflam N Lichtenstein, Ger.
Dexamethasone sodium phosphate (p.1067·1).
Musculoskeletal, joint, and peri-articular disorders.

Dexaflan Hebron, Braz.
Dexamethasone (p.1067·1).
Corticosteroid.

Dexafrin Sophia, Mex.
Dexamethasone sodium phosphate (p.1067·1); phenylephrine hydrochloride (p.1097·1).
Eye disorders.

Dexagalen Galen, Ger.
Dexamethasone (p.1067·1).
Scalp disorders.

Dexagel Mann, Ger.
Dexamethasone sodium phosphate (p.1067·1).
Eye disorders.

Dexagenta Croma, Aust.
Dexamethasone (p.1067·1) or dexamethasone sodium phosphate (p.1067·1); gentamicin sulfate (p.210·1).
Infected eye disorders.

Dexa-Gentamicin Ursapharm, Ger.
Dexamethasone (p.1067·1) or dexamethasone sodium phosphate (p.1067·1); gentamicin sulfate (p.210·1).
Infected eye disorders.

Dexagenta-POS Ursapharm, Neth.†
Dexamethasone (p.1067·1) or dexamethasone sodium phosphate (p.1067·1); gentamicin sulfate (p.210·1).
Infected eye disorders.

Dexagil Marjan, Braz.
Dexamethasone (p.1067·1); vitamin B_{12} (p.1388·1); vitamin B_1 (p.1385·2); vitamin B_6 (p.1387·1).
Neuritis.

Dexagrane Ioltech, Fr.
Dexamethasone sodium phosphate (p.1067·1); neomycin sulfate (p.228·1).
Infected eye disorders.

Dexagrin Grin, Mex.
Dexamethasone (p.1067·1) or dexamethasone phosphate (p.1067·1).
Corticosteroid.

Dexa-Helvacort Helvepharm, Switz.
Dexamethasone sodium phosphate (p.1067·1).
Corticosteroid.

Dexahexal Hexal, Ger.
Dexamethasone sodium phosphate (p.1067·1).
Corticosteroid.

Dexalgen Eurofarma, Braz.
Hydroxocobalamin (p.1388·1); dipyrone (p.34·1); dexamethasone (p.1067·1).
Neuritis.

Dexalin General Drugs, Thai.
Methyl salicylate (p.55·1); menthol (p.1632·3); cajuput oil (p.1588·1); eucalyptol (p.1609·2).
Lumbago; rheumatic conditions; sciatica.

Dexalocal
Medinova, Hong Kong; Medinova, Switz.
Dexamethasone (p.1067·1).
Skin and scalp disorders.

Dexalocal-F Medinova, Switz.
Dexamethasone (p.1067·1); framycetin sulfate (p.208·2).
Infected skin disorders.

DexAlone DexGen, USA.
Dextromethorphan hydrobromide (p.1087·3).
Coughs.

Dexaltin
Kayaku, Singapore; ANB, Thai.
Dexamethasone (p.1067·1).
Mouth ulcers.

Dexam Constric Alcon Cusi, Spain.
Chloramphenicol succinate (p.181·1); dexamethasone sodium phosphate (p.1067·1); tetryzoline hydrochloride (p.1101·2).
Eye disorders.

Dexambutol SERB, Fr.
Ethambutol hydrochloride (p.205·1).
Opportunistic mycobacterial infections; tuberculosis.

Dexambutol-INH SERB, Fr.
Ethambutol hydrochloride (p.205·1); isoniazid (p.215·3).
Opportunistic mycobacterial infections; tuberculosis.

Dexamed Medochemie, Singapore.
Dexamethasone (p.1067·1).
Corticosteroid.

Dexameth Major, USA.
Dexamethasone (p.1067·1).
Corticosteroid.

Dexamicin Grin, Mex.
Dexamethasone sodium phosphate (p.1067·1); neomycin sulfate (p.228·1).
Infected eye disorders.

Dexamin Streuli, Switz.
Dexamfetamine sulfate (p.1507·3).
Obesity.

Dexaminor Allergan-Frumtost, Braz.
Dexamethasone (p.1067·1).
Eye disorders.

Dexamol Dexxon, Israel.
Paracetamol (p.71·2).
Fever; pain.

Dexamol Cold Day Dexxon, Israel.
Paracetamol (p.71·2); guaifenesin (p.1092·2); dextromethorphan hydrobromide (p.1087·3); pseudoephedrine hydrochloride (p.1099·2).
Coughs and cold symptoms.

Dexamol Cold Night Dexxon, Israel.
Paracetamol (p.71·2); dextromethorphan hydrobromide (p.1087·3); pseudoephedrine hydrochloride (p.1099·2); chlorpheniramine [chlorphenamine] maleate (p.412·1).
Coughs and cold symptoms.

Dexamol Kid Dexxon, Israel.
Paracetamol (p.71·2).
Fever; pain.

Dexamol Plus Dexxon, Israel.
Paracetamol (p.71·2); caffeine (p.761·3).
Fever; pain.

Dexamol Sinus Day Dexxon, Israel.
Paracetamol (p.71·2); pseudoephedrine hydrochloride (p.1099·2).
Cold symptoms.

Dexamol Sinus Night Dexxon, Israel.
Paracetamol (p.71·2); pseudoephedrine hydrochloride (p.1099·2); chlorpheniramine [chlorphenamine] maleate (p.412·1).
Cold symptoms.

Dexamonozon Medice, Ger.
Dexamethasone (p.1067·1).
Oral corticosteroid.

Dexamonozon N Medice, Ger.
Lignocaine [lidocaine] hydrochloride (p.1313·2) is included in the intramuscular injection to alleviate the pain of injection.
Musculoskeletal and joint disorders.

Dexamycin Teva, Israel.
Dexamethasone sodium phosphate (p.1067·1); neomycin sulfate (p.228·1).
Infected eye disorders.

Dexamytrex
Mann, Ger.; Mann, Neth.; Lepori, Port.; Mann, Singapore; Bausch & Lomb, Thai.; Mann, Thai.
Gentamicin sulfate (p.210·1); dexamethasone (p.1067·1) or dexamethasone sodium phosphate (p.1067·1).
Infected eye disorders.

Dexa-Neuriberi Haller, Braz.
Vitamin B_1 (p.1385·2); vitamin B_6 (p.1387·1); vitamin B_{12} (p.1388·1); procaine (p.1319·2); dexamethasone (p.1067·1).
Neuritis.

Dexaneurin Uniao Quimica, Braz.
Vitamin B_{12} (p.1388·1); vitamin B_1 (p.1385·2); vitamin B_6 (p.1387·1); procaine (p.1319·2); dexamethasone (p.1067·1).
Neuritis.

Dexa-P PP Lab, Thai.
Dexamethasone (p.1067·1) or dexamethasone sodium phosphate (p.1067·1).
Corticosteroid.

Dexaphen-SA Major, USA.
Pseudoephedrine sulfate (p.1099·3); dexbrompheniramine maleate (p.410·2).
Upper respiratory-tract symptoms.

Dexa-Phlogont L Azupharma, Ger.
Prednisolone (p.1077·3); dexamethasone (p.1067·1); lignocaine [lidocaine] hydrochloride (p.1313·2).
Musculoskeletal and joint disorders.

Dexa-Polyspectran Thilo, Hong Kong.
Polymyxin B sulfate (p.238·1); neomycin sulfate (p.228·1); gramicidin (p.213·3); dexamethasone sodium phosphate (p.1067·1).
Infected eye disorders.

Dexa-POS
Ursapharm, Ger.
Dexamethasone sodium metasulfobenzoate (p.1067·1).
Allergic and inflammatory disorders of the eye.

Ursapharm, Neth.†
Dexamethasone phosphate (p.1067·1).
Inflammatory eye disorders.

Dexa-ratiopharm Ratiopharm, Ger.
Dexamethasone sodium phosphate (p.1067·1).
Corticosteroid.

Dexa-Rhinaspray
Boehringer Ingelheim, Irl.; Boehringer Ingelheim, UK†.
Tramazoline hydrochloride (p.1102·1); dexamethasone isonicotinate (p.1067·1); neomycin sulfate (p.228·1).
Allergic rhinitis.

Dexa-Rhinaspray Duo
Boehringer Ingelheim, Irl.; Boehringer Ingelheim, UK.
Tramazoline hydrochloride (p.1102·1); dexamethasone isonicotinate (p.1067·1).
Allergic rhinitis.

Dexa-Rhinospray
Note.This name is used for preparations of different composition.
Boehringer Ingelheim, Aust.†.
Tramazoline hydrochloride (p.1102·1); dexamethasone isonicotinate (p.1067·1); neomycin sulfate (p.228·1).
Rhinitis.

Boehringer Ingelheim, Belg.
Tramazoline hydrochloride (p.1102·1); dexamethasone isonicotinate (p.1067·1).
Formerly contained tramazoline hydrochloride, dexamethasone isonicotinate, and neomycin sulfate.
Rhinitis.

Dexa-Rhinospray N Boehringer Ingelheim, Ger.
Tramazoline hydrochloride (p.1102·1); dexamethasone isonicotinate (p.1067·1).
Rhinitis.

Dexasalyl
Mayrhofer, Aust.; Nourypharma, Ger.†; Medinova, Hong Kong; Medinova, Switz.
Dexamethasone (p.1067·1) or dexamethasone acetate (p.1067·1); salicylic acid (p.1122·3).
Skin and scalp disorders.

Dexasil Silom, Thai.
Dexamethasone sodium phosphate (p.1067·1); neomycin sulfate (p.228·1).
Infected eye disorders.

Dexa-sine Alcon, Ger.
Dexamethasone sodium phosphate (p.1067·1).
Eye disorders.

Dexa-Siozwo N Febena, Ger.
Dexamethasone acetate (p.1067·1); naphazoline hydrochloride (p.1095·1); peppermint oil (p.1243·3).
Catarrh; rhinitis; sinusitis.

Dexasone
ICN, Canad.; Atlantic, Hong Kong, Atlantic, Singapore; Atlantic, Thai.; Hauck, USA.
Dexamethasone (p.1067·1), dexamethasone acetate (p.1067·1), or dexamethasone sodium phosphate (p.1067·1).
Corticosteroid.

Dexasporin Moore, USA; Rugby, USA; URL, USA.
Dexamethasone (p.1067·1); neomycin sulfate (p.228·1); polymyxin B sulfate (p.238·1).
Eye inflammation with bacterial infection.

Dexatam Euromex, Mex.
Dexamethasone (p.1067·1).
Corticosteroid.

Dexatopic
Organon, Fin.; Organon, Neth.†.
Dexamethasone (p.1067·1); nandrolone decanoate (p.1484·2); chlorhexidine hydrochloride (p.1138·2).
Skin disorders.

Dexatrim
Note.This name is used for preparations of different composition.
Stella, Canad.†.
Benzocaine (p.1306·2); ferrous fumarate (p.1360·1); carmellose sodium (p.1499·3).
Obesity.

Roche, Switz.†; Thompson, USA†; Chattem, USA†.
Phenylpropanolamine hydrochloride (p.1098·1).
Obesity.

Dexatrim Plus Vitamin C Chattem, USA†.
Phenylpropanolamine hydrochloride (p.1098·1); ascorbic acid (p.1389·3).
Obesity.

Dexatrim Plus Vitamins Thompson, USA.
Caplets: Multivitamin and mineral preparation (p.1350·1).

Controlled release caplets†: Phenylpropanolamine (p.1098·1); vitamin C (p.1389·3).
Obesity.

Dexaval Tecnifar, Port.
Dexamethasone valerate (p.1067·3).
Skin disorders.

Dexaval A Tecnifar, Port.
Dexamethasone valerate (p.1067·3); chlorpheniramine [chlorphenamine] maleate (p.412·1).
Skin disorders with pruritus.

Dexaval N Tecnifar, Port.
Dexamethasone valerate (p.1067·3); neomycin sulfate (p.228·1).
Infected skin disorders.

Dexaval O Tecnifar, Port.
Dexamethasone sodium phosphate (p.1067·1); neomycin sulfate (p.228·1).
Infected eye and ear disorders.

Dexaval V Tecnifar, Port.
Dexamethasone valerate (p.1067·3); clioquinol (p.190·2).
Infected skin disorders.

Dexa-Vastrictol Allergan-Frumtost, Braz.
Dexamethasone (p.1067·1); naphazoline nitrate (p.1095·1); zinc sulfate (p.1398·2).
Infected eye disorders.

Dexavison Teuto, Braz.
Dexamethasone phosphate (p.1067·1); neomycin sulfate (p.228·1).
Infected eye disorders.

Dexchlor Schein, USA†.
Dexchlorpheniramine maleate (p.412·1).
Hypersensitivity reactions.

Dexedrine
SmithKline Beecham, Canad.; Celltech, UK; SmithKline Beecham, USA.
Dexamfetamine sulfate (p.1507·3).
Attention deficit hyperactivity disorder; narcoleptic syndrome.

Dexef Dexo, Fr.
Cefradine (p.173·3).
Bacterial infections.

Dexefrin Fischer, Israel.
Dexamethasone sodium phosphate (p.1067·1); phenylephrine (p.1097·1); neomycin sulfate (p.228·1).
Infected eye disorders.

Dexemel ML Laboratories, UK.
Icodextrin (p.1359·1).
Vehicle for peritoneal drug administration.

Dexeryl
Note.This name is used for preparations of different composition.
Pierre Fabre Sante, Fr.
Glycerol (p.1616·3); white soft paraffin (p.1407·3); liquid paraffin (p.1407·1).
Dry skin disorders.

Pascual, Hong Kong.
Dextromethorphan hydrobromide (p.1087·3); guaifenesin (p.1092·2); phenylephrine hydrochloride (p.1097·1); chlorpheniramine [chlorphenamine] maleate (p.412·1).
Respiratory-tract disorders.

DexFerrum American Regent, USA.
Iron dextran (p.1368·2).
Iron deficiency.

Dexicam OFF, Ital.
Piroxicam (p.79·1).
Gout; musculoskeletal, joint, and peri-articular disorders.

Dexicar Provit, Mex.
Dexamethasone (p.1067·1).
Corticosteroid.

Dexide
Sanofl Synthelabo, Ital.; Rottapharm, Spain.
Colextran hydrochloride (p.865·1).
Hyperlipidaemias.

Dexipan Julphar, UAE.
Dexpanthenol (p.1602·3).
Skin irritation; wounds.

Dexir
Upsamedica, Belg.; Oberlin, Fr.
Dextromethorphan hydrobromide (p.1087·3).
Coughs.

Dexiron Genpharm, Canad.
Iron dextran (p.1368·2).
Iron deficiency.

Dexit Leiras, Fin.
Dexibuprofen (p.44·1).
Fever; pain.

Dexium Sanofi Synthelabo, Ger.
Calcium dobesilate (p.1588·2).
Vascular disorders.

Dexmethsone
Rhone-Poulenc Rorer, Austral.; Fisons, Hong Kong.
Dexamethasone (p.1067·1).
Corticosteroid.

Dexnon Allen, Spain.
Thyroxine [levothyroxine] sodium (p.1526·2).
Hypothyroidism.

Dexodon Tika, Swed.
Dextropropoxyphene hydrochloride (p.27·1); paracetamol (p.71·2).
Pain.

Dexofan Nycomed, Denm.
Dextromethorphan hydrobromide (p.1087·3).
Coughs.

Dexofen *Astra, Swed.*
Dextropropoxyphene napsilate (p.27·1).
Pain.

Dexolan *Streuli, Switz.*
Dexamethasone (p.1067·1); zinc oxide (p.1128·2).
Skin disorders.

Dexoline *Ciba Vision, Ital.*
Chloramphenicol (p.179·1); dexamethasone sodium phosphate (p.1067·1); tetryzoline hydrochloride (p.1101·2).
Eye disorders.

Dexomon *Hillcross, UK.*
Diclofenac sodium (p.30·3).
Gout; inflammation; musculoskeletal, joint, peri-articular, and soft-tissue disorders; pain.

Dexon *General Drugs, Thai.*
Dexamethasone sodium phosphate (p.1067·1).
Corticosteroid.

Dexona *Jofrain, Mex.*
Dexamethasone (p.1067·1).
Corticosteroid.

Dexone *Solvay, USA†.*
Dexamethasone (p.1067·1), dexamethasone acetate (p.1067·1), or dexamethasone sodium phosphate (p.1067·1).
Corticosteroid.

Dexoph *Seng, Thai.*
Dexamethasone sodium phosphate (p.1067·1); neomycin sulfate (p.228·1).
Infected eye and ear disorders.

DexOptifen *Sping, Switz.*
Dexibuprofen (p.44·1).
Fever; inflammation; musculoskeletal, joint, and peri-articular disorders; pain.

Dex-Otic *Teva, Israel; Teva, Thai.*
Dexamethasone sodium phosphate (p.1067·1); neomycin sulfate (p.228·1); polymyxin B sulfate (p.238·1).
Infected ear disorders.

Dexpanol *Stada, Ger.*
Dexpanthenol (p.1602·3).
Wounds.

Dexpin *Greater Pharma, Thai.*
Dextromethorphan hydrobromide (p.1087·3); terpin hydrate (p.1101·2); chlorpheniramine [chlorphenamine] maleate (p.412·1).
Coughs.

Dexsal *Reckitt & Colman, Austral.*
Oral granules: Sodium citrotartrate; tartaric acid (p.1669·2); glucose; sodium bicarbonate (p.1186·2).
Dyspepsia.
Oral liquid: Calcium carbonate (p.1215·1); simeticone (p.1249·2).
Dyspepsia; flatulence.

Dexsol *Rosemont, UK.*
Dexamethasone sodium phosphate (p.1067·1).
Corticosteroid.

Dexsul *Parggon, Mex.*
Dexamethasone sodium phosphate (p.1067·1); neomycin sulfate (p.228·1); polymyxin B sulfate (p.238·1).
Infected eye disorders.

Dexthasol *Olan-Kemed, Thai.*
Dexamethasone sodium phosphate (p.1067·1).
Corticosteroid.

Dextin *Rolab, S.Afr.*
Metformin hydrochloride (p.332·3).
Diabetes mellitus.

Dextoma *Arkomedika, Fr.*
Aluminium hydroxide (p.1210·3); aluminium carbonate (p.1210·2); magnesium hydroxide (p.1233·1); magnesium carbonate (p.1232·3).
Gastrointestinal disorders.

Dexton *TP, Thai.*
Dexamethasone sodium phosphate (p.1067·1).
Corticosteroid.

Dextracin
Xepa-Soul Pattinson, Hong Kong; Xepa-Soul Pattinson, Singapore.
Dexamethasone sodium phosphate (p.1067·1); neomycin sulfate (p.228·1).
Infected eye and ear disorders.

Dextralpha *Alpha, Mex.*
Glucose (p.1364·1).
Hypoglycaemia.

Dextrarine Phenylbutazone *Synthelabo, Fr.*
Dextran sulfate (p.1603·1); phenylbutazone (p.78·1).
Tendinitis.

Dextrevit *ICN, Mex.*
Multivitamin preparation with glucose (p.1350·1).

Dextricea *Durban, Spain.*
Rice; gelatin tannate; pectin (p.1502·3); wheat germ.
Diarrhoea.

Dextro OG-T *Roche, Ger.*
Mono- and oligosaccharide mixture.
Glucose tolerance test.

Dextrocalmine *Democal, Switz.*
Dextromethorphan hydrobromide (p.1087·3).
Coughs.

Dextromine *General Drugs, Thai.*
Dextromethorphan hydrobromide (p.1087·3); chlorpheniramine [chlorphenamine] maleate (p.412·1).
Coughs.

Dextroral *General Drugs, Thai.*
Dextromethorphan hydrobromide (p.1087·3).
Coughs.

Dextrostat *Shire Richwood, USA.*
Dexamfetamine sulfate (p.1507·3).
Attention deficit hyperactivity disorder; narcoleptic syndrome.

Dextrostix
Bayer Diagnostics, Fr.†; Ames, Irl.†; Bayer, Ital.†; Bayer Diagnostics, Mex.; Bayer Diagnostics, UK†; Bayer, USA.
Test for glucose in blood (p.1616·3).

Dextrovitase *Ache, Braz.*
Vitamin B substances; ascorbic acid; glucose (p.1350·1).
Nutritional supplement.

Dexylin *General Drugs, Thai.*
Dexamethasone sodium phosphate (p.1067·1); neomycin sulfate (p.228·1).
Infected eye and ear disorders.

Dezacor *Hoechst Marion Roussel, Spain.*
Deflazacort (p.1066·1).
Corticosteroid.

Dezoral *Hoe, Singapore.*
Ketoconazole (p.389·1).
Fungal skin infections; seborrhoeic dermatitis.

DF 118
Glaxo Wellcome, Hong Kong; Galen, Irl.; Glaxo Wellcome, S.Afr.; Martindale Pharmaceuticals, UK.
Dihydrocodeine tartrate (p.33·1).
NOTE. There is no connection between Martindale, The Complete Drug Reference and Martindale Pharmaceuticals.
Pain.

D-Feda II *WE, USA.*
Pseudoephedrine hydrochloride (p.1099·2); guaifenesin (p.1092·2).

D-Fluoretten *Hoechst Marion Roussel, Ger.*
Colecalciferol (p.1391·1); sodium fluoride (p.1375·3).
Dental caries prophylaxis; rickets prophylaxis.

Dhabesol *DHA, Singapore.*
Clobetasol propionate (p.1065·2).
Skin disorders.

Dhacillin
DHA, Hong Kong; DHA, Singapore.
Ampicillin trihydrate (p.151·1).
Bacterial infections.

Dhacopan
DHA, Hong Kong; DHA, Singapore.
Hyoscine butylbromide (p.468·2).
Smooth muscle spasm.

Dhaflu *DHA, Singapore.*
Caffeine (p.761·3); chlorpheniramine [chlorphenamine] maleate (p.412·1); paracetamol (p.71·2); phenylpropanolamine hydrochloride (p.1098·1).
Cold symptoms.

Dhalumag *DHA, Singapore.*
Aluminium hydroxide (p.1210·3); magnesium trisilicate (p.1233·3).
Gastric hyperacidity; peptic ulcer.

Dhamol
DHA, Hong Kong; DHA, Singapore.
Paracetamol (p.71·2).
Fever; pain.

Dhamotil
DHA, Hong Kong; DHA, Singapore.
Diphenoxylate hydrochloride (p.1222·2).
Atropine sulfate (p.461·1) is included in this preparation to discourage abuse.
Diarrhoea.

Dhaperazine
DHA, Hong Kong; DHA, Singapore.
Prochlorperazine maleate (p.701·3).
Emotional and mental disturbances; Ménière's disease; migraine; nausea and vomiting.

Dhasedyl
DHA, Hong Kong; DHA, Singapore.
Codeine phosphate (p.25·2); ephedrine hydrochloride (p.1090·1); promethazine hydrochloride (p.423·2).
Coughs.

Dhasedyl DM *DHA, Singapore.*
Dextromethorphan hydrobromide (p.1087·3); ephedrine hydrochloride (p.1090·1); promethazine hydrochloride (p.423·2).
Coughs.

Dhasolone *DHA, Hong Kong.*
Prednisolone (p.1077·3).
Corticosteroid.

Dhatalin *DHA, Hong Kong.*
Terbutaline sulfate (p.776·2).
Asthma; bronchitis.

Dhatifen *DHA, Singapore.*
Ketotifen (p.767·2).
Asthma; hypersensitivity reactions.

Dhatrin
DHA, Hong Kong; DHA, Singapore.
Co-trimoxazole (p.193·3).
Bacterial infections.

DHC *Mundipharma, Ger.*
Dihydrocodeine tartrate (p.33·1).
Pain.

DHC Continus
Napp, Irl.; Rafa, Israel; Douglas, NZ; Napp, UK.
Dihydrocodeine tartrate (p.33·1).
Pain.

DHC Plus *Purdue Frederick, USA.*
Dihydrocodeine tartrate (p.33·1); paracetamol (p.71·2); caffeine (p.761·3).

DHE
Isis Puren, Ger.; Ratiopharm, Ger.; Novartis, USA.
Dihydroergotamine mesilate (p.450·3).
Hypotension; migraine and other vascular headaches.

DHS Sal *Person & Covey, USA†.*
Salicylic acid (p.1122·3).
Psoriasis; seborrhoeic dermatitis.

DHS Tar *Person & Covey, USA.*
Coal tar (p.1125·1).
Scalp disorders; seborrhoea.

DHS Zinc *Person & Covey, USA.*
Pyrithione zinc (p.1122·1).
Scalp disorders.

DHT *Roxane, USA.*
Dihydrotachysterol (p.1391·2).
Hypoparathyroidism; postoperative and idiopathic tetany.

Di Anatoxal *Pharmabroker, NZ.*
A diphtheria vaccine (p.1536·2).
Active immunisation.

Di Dolko *Therabel, Fr.*
Paracetamol (p.71·2); dextropropoxyphene hydrochloride (p.27·1).
Pain.

Di Retard *Llorens, Spain.*
Diclofenac sodium (p.30·3).
Dysmenorrhoea; gout; musculoskeletal, joint, and peri-articular disorders; pain; renal colic.

Di Te Anatoxal
Berna, Singapore; Berna, Thai.
An adsorbed diphtheria and tetanus vaccine (p.1537·1). Separate preparations are available for infants and young children and for older children and adults.
Active immunisation.

Di Te Per Anatoxal
Berna, Hong Kong†; Berna, Singapore†; Berna, Thai.†.
A diphtheria, tetanus, and pertussis vaccine (p.1537·1).
Active immunisation of infants and young children.

Dia-Aktivanad-N *Knoll, Ger.*
Bovine liver extract; yeast extract; caffeine (p.1350·1).
Tonic.

Diabact UBT *Diabact, Swed.*
Carbon-13 (p.1591·3) labelled urea.
Test for Helicobacter pylori infection.

Dia-BASF *BASF, Ger.*
Glibenclamide (p.321·3).
Diabetes mellitus.

Diabeedol *Sriprasit, Thai.*
Chlorpropamide (p.321·1).
Diabetes mellitus.

Diabemide *Guidotti, Ital.*
Chlorpropamide (p.321·1).
Diabetes mellitus.

Diabene *Lehning, Fr.*
Homoeopathic preparation.

Diabenol *Greater Pharma, Thai.*
Glibenclamide (p.321·3).
Diabetes mellitus.

Diabenor *IFI, Ital.*
Glisolamide (p.323·2).
Diabetes mellitus.

Diabenyl T *Chauvin ankerpharm, Ger.*
Tetryzoline hydrochloride (p.1101·2).
Eye irritation.

Diabenyl-Rhinex *Wernigerode, Ger.*
Diphenhydramine hydrochloride (p.416·1); naphazoline hydrochloride (p.1095·1).
Allergic rhinitis.

Diabeside *Chew, Thai.*
Gliclazide (p.322·2).
Diabetes mellitus.

Diabesin *TAD, Ger.*
Metformin hydrochloride (p.332·3).
Diabetes mellitus.

DiaBeta
Hoechst Marion Roussel, Canad.; Hoechst Marion Roussel, USA.
Glibenclamide (p.321·3).
Diabetes mellitus.

Diabetamide *Ashbourne, UK.*
Glibenclamide (p.321·3).
Diabetes mellitus.

Diabetan S *Schuck, Ger.*
Homoeopathic preparation.

Diabetase *Azupharma, Ger.*
Metformin hydrochloride (p.332·3).
Diabetes mellitus.

Diabetes-Gastreu N R40 *Reckeweg, Ger.*
Homoeopathic preparation.

Diabetex *Germania, Aust.*
Metformin hydrochloride (p.332·3).
Diabetes mellitus.

Diabetic Tussin *Roberts, USA.*
Dextromethorphan hydrobromide (p.1087·3); guaifenesin (p.1092·2); phenylephrine (p.1097·1).
Coughs.

Diabetic Tussin Allergy Relief *Health Care Products, USA†.*
Chlorpheniramine [chlorphenamine] maleate (p.412·1).
Upper respiratory-tract symptoms.

Diabetic Tussin DM *Roberts, USA.*
Dextromethorphan hydrobromide (p.1087·3); guaifenesin (p.1092·2).
Coughs.

Diabetic Tussin EX *Health Care Products, USA.*
Guaifenesin (p.1092·2).
Coughs.

Diabetiks *Green Turtle Bay Vitamin Co., USA.*
Vitamins; minerals; bioflavonoids; myrtillus; ginkgo biloba; green tea; pine bark; acetylcysteine; taurine; ubidecarenone; lipoic acid (p.1350·1).
Tonic.

Diabetmin *Hovid, Singapore.*
Metformin hydrochloride (p.332·3).
Diabetes mellitus.

Diabe-Tuss DM *Paddock, USA.*
Dextromethorphan hydrobromide (p.1087·3).
Coughs.

Diabex *Alphapharm, Austral.*
Metformin hydrochloride (p.332·3).
Diabetes mellitus.

Diabexan *Crosara, Ital.†.*
Chlorpropamide (p.321·1).
Diabetes mellitus.

Diabiclor *Mavi, Mex.*
Chlorpropamide (p.321·1).
Diabetes mellitus.

Diabiformine *Pfizer, Switz.*
Chlorpropamide (p.321·1); metformin hydrochloride (p.332·3).
Diabetes mellitus.

Diabines *Pfizer, Swed.†.*
Chlorpropamide (p.321·1).
Diabetes mellitus.

Diabinese
Pfizer, Austral.; Roerig, Belg.; Pfizer, Braz.; Pfizer, Canad.; Pfizer, Fr.†; Pfizer, Hong Kong; Pfizer, Irl.; Pfizer, Israel; Pfizer, Mex.; Pfizer, Norw.†; Pfizer, S.Afr.; Pfizer, Singapore; Farmasierra, Spain; Pfizer, Switz.†; Pfizer, Thai.; Pfizer, UK†; Pfizer, USA.
Chlorpropamide (p.321·1).
Diabetes insipidus; diabetes mellitus.

Diabitex *Salters, S.Afr.*
Chlorpropamide (p.321·1).
Noted FM Oct 97, but listed in MIMSSA.00.
Diabetes mellitus.

Diaborale *Pharmacia Upjohn, Ital.*
Glycyclamide (p.323·3).
Diabetes mellitus.

Diabrezide
Helsinn Birex, Irl.; Molteni, Ital.
Gliclazide (p.322·2).
Diabetes mellitus.

Diabur-5000 *Roche Diagnostics, NZ.*
Test for glucose in urine (p.1616·3).

Diabur-Test 5000
Roche Diagnostics, Austral.; Roche Diagnostics, Irl.; Roche Diagnostics, Ital.; Lakeside, Mex.; Roche Diagnostics, UK.
Test for glucose in urine (p.1616·3).

Diacard *Madaus, Ger.*
Homoeopathic preparation.

Diaceplex *Salvat, Spain.*
Diazepam (p.674·3).
Alcohol withdrawal syndrome; anxiety; febrile convulsions; insomnia; skeletal muscle spasm.

Diaceplex Simple *Salvat, Spain†.*
Diazepam (p.674·3).
Alcohol withdrawal syndrome; anxiety; epilepsy; febrile convulsions; general anaesthesia; insomnia; skeletal muscle spasm.

Dia-Chek *Searle, Austral.*
Codeine phosphate (p.25·2); aluminium hydroxide (p.1210·3).
Diarrhoea.

Diachlor *Major, USA†.*
Chlorothiazide (p.856·3).
Hypertension; oedema.

Diaclaron *Siam Bheasach, Thai.*
Gliclazide (p.322·2).
Diabetes mellitus.

Diacol *Bial, Port.*
Ethylmorphine hydrochloride (p.35·2); sodium benzoate (p.1134·3); belladonna (p.463·1); ephedrine hydrochloride (p.1090·1).
Coughs.

Dia-Colon *Piam, Ital.*
Lactulose (p.1230·1).
Gastrointestinal disorders; liver disorders.

Diacor *Dexo, Fr.*
Diltiazem hydrochloride (p.874·3).
Angina pectoris.

Di-Actane *Menarini, Fr.*
Naftidrofuryl oxalate (p.937·3).
Cerebral and peripheral vascular disorders; mental function impairment in the elderly.

Diacure
Note. This name is used for preparations of different composition.
Lehning, Fr.
Taraxacum (p.1669·1); berberis; juglans; millefolium; myrtillus (p.1639·2); centaury (p.1593·1); natrum phosphoricum.
Metabolic disorders.
Taxandria, Neth.
Loperamide hydrochloride (p.1231·3).
Diarrhoea.

Diacure Plus *Taxandria, Neth.*
Loperamide hydrochloride (p.1231·3); simeticone (p.1249·2).
Diarrhoea.

The symbol † denotes a preparation no longer actively marketed

Diadermina *Dermopen, Braz.*
Emollient.
Barrier preparation; dry skin.

Diadin M *Diadin, Ger.*
Mofebutazone (p.55·3).
Musculoskeletal, joint, and soft-tissue disorders.

Di-Adreson-F
Organon, Fin.; Organon, Hong Kong; Nourypharma, Neth.; Organon, Thai.
Prednisolone (p.1077·3) or prednisolone sodium succinate (p.1078·2).
Corticosteroid.

Dia-Eptal *Montavit, Aust.*
Glibenclamide (p.321·3).
Diabetes mellitus.

Diaformin
Alphapharm, Austral.; Alphapharm, Hong Kong.
Metformin hydrochloride (p.332·3).
Diabetes mellitus.

Diafusor
Schering-Plough, Belg.; Pierre Fabre, Fr.; Pierre Fabre, Spain.
Glyceryl trinitrate (p.897·3).
Angina pectoris.

Diagesil *Berk, UK.*
Diamorphine hydrochloride (p.28·3).
Pain.

Diaglyk *Ashbourne, UK.*
Gliclazide (p.322·2).
Diabetes mellitus.

Diagnosis *Roche Diagnostics, Ital.*
Pregnancy test (p.1654·3).

Diagnostic Skin Testing Kit *Bayer, S.Afr.†.*
Allergen extracts (p.1575·3).
Diagnostic agent.

Diagran *Bristol-Myers Squibb, Ital.*
Multivitamin preparation (p.1350·1).

Diagran Minerale *Bristol-Myers Squibb, Ital.*
Multivitamin and mineral preparation (p.1350·1).

Diagrin *Makros, Braz.*
Metoclopramide hydrochloride (p.1235·2); vitamin B₆ (p.1386·3).
Nausea and vomiting.

Diahalt *Wampole, Canad.*
Loperamide hydrochloride (p.1231·3).
Diarrhoea.

Diah-Limit *Wallis, UK.*
Loperamide hydrochloride (p.1231·3).
Diarrhoea.

Dialamine
Scientific Hospital Supplies, Austral.; SHS, Fr.; Scientific Hospital Supplies, Irl.†; Nutricia, NZ; Scientific Hospital Supplies, NZ; Scientific Hospital Supplies, UK.
Amino acid, carbohydrate, ascorbic acid, and mineral preparation (p.1350·1).
Enteral nutrition.

Dialar *Lagap, UK.*
Diazepam (p.674·3).

Dialens
Note. This name is used for preparations of different composition.
Specia, Fr.†; Chauvin Novopharma, Switz.
Dextran 60-85 (p.729·2).
Dry eyes; wetting agent for contact lenses.

Chauvin, Port.
Chlorhexidine gluconate (p.1138·2).
Contact lens care; tear deficiency.

Dialgine forte *Intermedica, Switz.*
Paracetamol (p.71·2); propyphenazone (p.80·2); caffeine (p.761·3).
Fever; pain.

Dialgirex *Irex, UK.*
Dextropropoxyphene hydrochloride (p.27·1); paracetamol (p.71·2).
Pain.

Dialibra *Dieterba, Ital.†.*
Dietary fibre supplement (p.1214·2).
Disorders of glucose and lipid metabolism.

Dialine *Teva, Israel.*
Glucose; sodium chloride; sodium lactate; calcium chloride; magnesium chloride (p.1184·1).
Peritoneal dialysis.

Dialisol *Antibioticos, Spain.*
Calcium chloride; anhydrous glucose; magnesium chloride; sodium chloride; sodium lactate (p.1184·1).
Peritoneal dialysis.

Dialoc *Masa, Thai.*
Gliclazide (p.322·2).
Diabetes mellitus.

Dialose *J&J-Merck, USA†.*
Docusate potassium (p.1223·1) or docusate sodium (p.1223·1).
Constipation; hard stools.

Dialose Plus *J&J-Merck, USA†.*
Docusate sodium (p.1223·1); yellow phenolphthalein (p.1244·1).
Constipation; hard stools.

Dialster *Esoform, Ital.*
Sodium dichloroisocyanurate (p.1156·1).
Disinfection of surfaces, water, food, and feeding bottles.

Dialudon *Novaquimica, Braz.*
Phenytoin (p.357·2); diazepam (p.674·3).
Epilepsy.

Dialume
Rhone-Poulenc Rorer, Spain; Rhone-Poulenc Rorer, USA.
Aluminium hydroxide (p.1210·3).
Hyperacidity; hyperphosphataemia.

Dialvit *Bichsel, Switz.*
Multivitamin preparation (p.1350·1).
Dietary supplement in renal failure.

Dialycare *Abbott, Ital.*
Preparation for enteral nutrition (p.1350·1).
Renal dialysis.

Dialysol Acide *Soludia, Fr.*
Sodium chloride; potassium chloride; calcium chloride; magnesium chloride; acetic acid (p.1184·1).
Haemodialysis solution.

Dialysol Bicarbonate *Soludia, Fr.*
Sodium bicarbonate; sodium chloride (p.1184·1).
Haemodialysis solution.

Dialytan H *Aguettant, Fr.*
Haemodialysis solution (p.1184·1).

Dialyte
GHP, Thai.; Gambro, USA.
Glucose; electrolytes (p.1184·1).
Peritoneal dialysis solution.

Diameb *Precimex, Mex.*
Diiodohydroxyquinoline (p.590·2).

Diamet *Weifa, Thai.*
Metformin hydrochloride (p.332·3).
Diabetes mellitus.

Diamexon *TO-Chemicals, Thai.*
Gliclazide (p.322·2).
Diabetes mellitus.

Diamicron
Servier, Aust.; Servier, Austral.; Servier, Belg.; Servier, Braz.; Servier, Canad.; Servier, Denm.; Servier, Fr.; Servier, Ger.; Servier, Hong Kong; Servier, Irl.; Servier, Ital.; Byk Gulden, Mex.; Servier, Neth.; Servier, NZ; Servier, Port.; Servier, S.Afr.; Servier, Singapore; Servier, Spain; Servier, Swed.; Servier, Thai.; Servier, UK.
Gliclazide (p.322·2).
Diabetes mellitus.

Diamin *Malaysia Chemist, Singapore.*
Metformin hydrochloride (p.332·3).
Diabetes mellitus.

Diamine TD *Major, USA†.*
Brompheniramine maleate (p.410·2).
Hypersensitivity reactions.

Diaminocillina *Fournier, Ital.*
Benzathine benzylpenicillin (p.156·2).
Bacterial infections.

Diamorf *Medeva, UK.*
Diamorphine hydrochloride (p.28·3).
Pain.

Diamoril *Chiesi, Fr.*
Benzquercin (p.1611·1).
Peripheral vascular disorders.

Diamox
Wyeth Lederle, Aust.; Lederle, Austral.; Wyeth Lederle, Belg.; Merck Sharp & Dohme, Braz.; Wyeth-Ayerst, Canad.; Wyeth Lederle, Denm.; Wyeth Lederle, Fin.; Theraplix, Fr.; Lederle, Ger.; Lederle, Hong Kong; Wyeth, Irl.; Lederle, Israel; Wyeth Lederle, Ital.; Wyeth, Mex.; Lederle, Neth.; Wyeth Lederle, Norw.; Wyeth, NZ; Wyeth, S.Afr.; Cyanamid, Spain; Wyeth Lederle, Swed.; Lederle, Switz.; Wyeth-Ayerst, Thai.; Wyeth, UK; Wyeth-Ayerst, USA.
Acetazolamide (p.826·1) or acetazolamide sodium (p.826·1).
Acute mountain sickness; epilepsy; glaucoma; heart failure; Ménière's disease; oedema; pancreatic disorders; premenstrual syndrome; respiratory insufficiency.

Diamplicil *Pharmacia Upjohn, Ital.*
Ampicillin (p.150·3); dicloxacillin (p.199·1).
Bacterial infections.

Dianben *Roche, Spain.*
Metformin hydrochloride (p.332·3).
Diabetes mellitus.

Diane
Schering, Aust.; Schering, Austral.; Schering, Belg.; Schering, Braz.; Berlex, Canad.; Schering, Denm.; Schering, Fin.; Schering, Fr.; Schering, Ger.; Schering, Hong Kong; Schering, Israel; Schering, Ital.; Schering, Mex.; Schering, Neth.; Schering, Norw.; Schering, NZ; Schering, Port.; Schering, S.Afr.; Schering, Singapore; Schering, Spain; Schering, Switz.; Schering, Thai.
Cyproterone acetate (p.1467·3); ethinylestradiol (p.1476·2).
28-Day packs also contain 7 inert tablets.
Androgen-dependent acne, seborrhoea, alopecia, and hirsutism in females; oral contraceptive in women with androgenic symptoms.

Dianeal
Baxter, Aust.; Baxter, Austral.; Baxter, Denm.; Baxter, Fin.; Baxter, Israel; Baxter, Port.†; Baxter, Spain; Baxter, Swed.; Baxter, Switz.; Baxter, UK.
Glucose; sodium chloride; sodium lactate; calcium chloride; magnesium chloride (p.1184·1).
Peritoneal dialysis.

Dianette
Schering, Irl.; Schering, UK.
Cyproterone acetate (p.1467·3); ethinylestradiol (p.1476·2).
These ingredients can be described by the British Approved Name Co-cyprindiol.
Acne and hirsutism in females.

Di-Antalvic *Hoechst, Fr.*
Dextropropoxyphene hydrochloride (p.27·1); paracetamol (p.71·2).
Pain.

Diapam
Orion, Fin.; Greater Pharma, Thai.
Diazepam (p.674·3).
Alcohol withdrawal syndromes; anxiety disorders; insomnia; muscle spasms; pain; premedication; status epilepticus.

Diapanil *Randall, Mex.*
Diazepam (p.674·3).

Diaparene Corn Starch *Personal Care, USA.*
Corn starch (p.1379·3); aloes (p.1210·1).
Nappy rash.

Diaparene Diaper Rash *Personal Care, USA.*
Zinc oxide (p.1128·2).
Nappy rash.

Diapatol *Teofarma, Ital.*
Amitriptyline hydrochloride (p.273·3); chlordiazepoxide hydrochloride (p.659·2).
Anxiety disorders; depression; insomnia.

Diaper Guard
Note. This name is used for preparations of different composition.
Del, Canad.†.
Dimethicone (p.1410·1); soft paraffin (p.1407·3); zinc oxide (p.1128·2).

Del, USA.
Dimethicone (p.1410·1); white soft paraffin (p.1407·3); vitamin A (p.1382·1); vitamin D₃ (p.1391·1); vitamin E (p.1393·3).
Nappy rash.

Diaper Rash
Note. This name is used for preparations of different composition.
Drug Trading, Canad.†.
Zinc oxide (p.1128·2).

Goldline, USA; Rugby, USA.
Zinc oxide (p.1128·2); cod-liver oil (p.1357·2).
Nappy rash.

Diaphal *Pierre Fabre, Ger.*
Frusemide [furosemide] (p.893·1); amiloride hydrochloride (p.835·1).
Ascites; hypertension; oedema.

Diapid
Sandoz, Fr.†; Novartis, USA†.
Lypressin (p.1300·1).
Diabetes insipidus.

Diapine
Atlantic, Singapore; Atlantic, Thai.
Diazepam (p.674·3).
Alcohol withdrawal syndrome; anxiety; epilepsy; skeletal muscle spasm.

Diapool *Dovalle, Braz.*
Attapulgite (p.1212·1); pectin (p.1502·3); aluminium hydroxide (p.1210·3); homatropine (p.468·1).
Diarrhoea.

Diaqua *Hauck, USA†.*
Hydrochlorothiazide (p.907·3).
Hypertension; oedema.

Diaquel *Rolab, S.Afr.*
Diazepam (p.674·3).
Now known as Rolab-Diazepam.
Alcohol withdrawal syndrome; anxiety; premedication.

Diarcalm *McGloin, Austral.*
Oral liquid: Light kaolin (p.1229·3); pectin (p.1502·3); catechu (p.1592·2); aluminium hydroxide (p.1210·3).
Tablets†: Codeine phosphate (p.25·2); attapulgite (p.1212·1); pectin (p.1502·3).
Diarrhoea; stomach pain.

Diarent *Chew, Thai.*
Loperamide hydrochloride (p.1231·3).
Diarrhoea.

Diaretyl *Cooperation Pharmaceutique, Fr.*
Loperamide hydrochloride (p.1231·3).
Diarrhoea.

Diarex *Pharmavite, Canad.*
Kaolin (p.1229·3); pectin (p.1502·3).

Diareze
Note. This name is used for preparations of different composition.
Key, Austral.
Oral suspension: Attapulgite (p.1212·1); pectin (p.1502·3); simeticone (p.1249·2).
Tablets: Attapulgite (p.1212·1); pectin (p.1502·3); aluminium hydroxide (p.1210·3).
Diarrhoea.

Boots, UK.
Loperamide hydrochloride (p.1231·3).
Diarrhoea.

Diargal *Gallia, Fr.*
Infant feed; food for special diets (p.1350·1).
Diarrhoea; lactose intolerance; sucrose intolerance.

Diarigoz *Guigoz, Fr.*
Infant feed (p.1350·1).
Diarrhoea.

Diaril *MC, Fr.*
Glutaral (p.1145·2); phenol (p.1152·3); orthophenylphenol (p.1152·1).
Formerly contained glutaral and sodium phenate.
Instrument disinfection.

Diarim *Rimsa, Mex.*
Nifuroxazide (p.230·2).

Diarlac *Urgo, Fr.*
Lactobacillus acidophilus (p.1626·3).

Diarodil *Greater Pharma, Thai.*
Loperamide hydrochloride (p.1231·3).
Diarrhoea.

Diarona *Honorterapica, Braz.*
Dipyrone (p.34·1); papaverine hydrochloride (p.1648·1).
Smooth muscle spasm.

Diaront mono *Chephasaar, Ger.*
Colistin sulfate (p.192·3).
Selective gastrointestinal tract decontamination.

Diarphen *Mepro-Pharm, UK†.*
Diphenoxylate hydrochloride (p.1222·2).
Atropine sulfate (p.461·1) is included in this preparation to discourage abuse,.
These ingredients can be described by the British Approved Name Co-phenotrope.
Diarrhoea.

Diarresec *Farmion, Braz.*
Loperamide (p.1232·1).
Diarrhoea.

Diarrest *Galen, UK.*
Codeine phosphate (p.25·2); dicyclomine [dicycloverine] hydrochloride (p.466·1); sodium chloride; potassium chloride; sodium citrate.
Diarrhoea.

Diarrest RF *Galen, Irl.*
Loperamide hydrochloride (p.1231·3); potassium chloride; sodium chloride; sodium citrate.
Diarrest formerly contained codeine phosphate, dicyclomine [dicycloverine] hydrochloride, potassium chloride, sodium chloride, and sodium citrate.
Diarrhoea.

Diarret *Geymonat, Ital.*
Nifuroxazide (p.230·2).
Acute infective diarrhoea.

Diarrex *Hylands, USA.*
Homoeopathic preparation.

Diarr-Eze *Pharmascience, Canad.*
Loperamide hydrochloride (p.1231·3).
Diarrhoea.

Diarrhea Relief *Stanley, Canad.*
Loperamide hydrochloride (p.1231·3).

Diarrheel S *Heel, Ger.†.*
Homoeopathic preparation.

Diarrhoea Complex *Brauer, Austral.†.*
Homoeopathic preparation.

Diarrhoea Relief Tablets *Brauer, Austral.*
Homoeopathic preparation.

Diarrhoesan
Vitasan, Aust.; Loges, Ger.
Apple pectin (p.1502·3); chamomile (p.1593·2).
Diarrhoea.

Diarrhoesan SC *Loges, Ger.*
Saccharomyces boulardii (p.1626·3).
Acne; diarrhoea.

Diarsed *Sanofi Winthrop, Fr.*
Diphenoxylate hydrochloride (p.1222·2).
Atropine sulfate (p.461·1) is included in this preparation to discourage abuse.
Diarrhoea.

Diarstop *Giuliani, Ital.*
Loperamide hydrochloride (p.1231·3).
Diarrhoea.

Diascan *Home Diagnostics, USA.*
Test for glucose in blood (p.1616·3).

Diascreen 3 *Marco, Austral.*
Test for glucose, protein, and pH in urine.

Diascreen 5 *Marco, Austral.*
Test for glucose, protein, ketones, pH, and blood in urine.

Diascreen 6 *Marco, Austral.*
Test for glucose, protein, ketones, pH, blood, and bilirubin in urine.

Diascreen 7 *Marco, Austral.*
Test for glucose, protein, ketones, pH, blood, bilirubin, and urobilinogen in urine.

Diascreen 8 *Marco, Austral.*
Test for glucose, protein, ketones, pH, blood, bilirubin, urobilinogen, and nitrite in urine.

Diascreen 9 *Marco, Austral.*
Test for glucose, protein, ketones, pH, blood, bilirubin, urobilinogen, nitrite, and leucocytes in urine.

Diascreen 10 *Marco, Austral.*
Test for glucose, protein, ketones, pH, blood, bilirubin, urobilinogen, nitrite, leucocytes, and specific gravity in urine.

Diascreen 40BL *Marco, Austral.*
Test for glucose, protein, blood, and leucocytes in urine.

Diascreen 1G *Marco, Austral.*
Test for glucose in urine (p.1616·3).

Diascreen 2GK *Marco, Austral.*
Test for glucose and ketones in urine.

Diascreen 2GP *Marco, Austral.*
Test for glucose and protein in urine.

Diascreen 1K *Marco, Austral.*
Test for ketones in urine.

Diascreen 4NL *Marco, Austral.*
Test for glucose, protein, nitrite, and leucocytes in urine.

Diascreen 4PH *Marco, Austral.*
Test for glucose, protein, pH, and blood in urine.

Diasectral
Aventis, Denm.; Rhone-Poulenc Rorer, Fin.
Acebutolol hydrochloride (p.825·1).
Angina pectoris; arrhythmias; hypertension; myocardial infarction.

Diasef Unison, Singapore; Unison, Thai.
Glipizide (p.322·3).
Diabetes mellitus.

Diaseptyl Ducray, Fr.
Chlorhexidine gluconate (p.1138·2).
Skin disinfection.

Diasgest Siam Bheasach, Thai.
Amylase (p.1579·3); sodium bicarbonate (p.1186·2); calcium carbonate (p.1215·1); aluminium magnesium silicate (p.1499·1); scopolia; vitamin B₁ (p.1385·2).
Dyspepsia; gastric hyperacidity; gastritis; gastrointestinal motility disorders; heartburn.

Diasorb
Note. This name is used for preparations of different composition.
Norton Healthcare, UK.
Loperamide hydrochloride (p.1231·3).
Diarrhoea.

Columbia, USA.
Activated attapulgite (p.1212·1).
Diarrhoea.

Diastabol Sanofi Winthrop, Aust.; Sanofi Winthrop, Fin.; Sanofi Winthrop, Fr.; Sanofi Synthelabo, Ger.; Sanofi Synthelabo, Port.; Sanofi Synthelabo, Spain; Sanofi Winthrop, Swed.; Sanofi Synthelabo, Switz.
Miglitol (p.333·1).
Diabetes mellitus.

Diastat Mer-National, S.Afr.†
Streptomycin (p.249·1); phthalylsulfathiazole (p.235·3); belladonna tincture (p.463·1); chloroform and morphine tincture (p.56·1); kaolin (p.1229·3); pectin (p.1502·3); tinct. card. co.
Diarrhoea.

Diastix Bayer, Austral.; Bayer, Canad.; Bayer Diagnostics, Irl.; Bayer Diagnostici, Ital.; Bayer Diagnostics, Mex.; Bayer, NZ; Bayer Diagnostics, UK; Bayer, USA.
Test for glucose in urine (p.1616·3).

Diastop Pacific, NZ.
Diphenoxylate hydrochloride (p.1222·2).
Atropine sulfate (p.461·1) is included in this preparation to discourage abuse.
Diarrhoea.

Diatelan Reuffer, Mex.
Tolbutamide (p.336·3).
Diabetes mellitus.

Diatex Medix, Mex.
Diazepam (p.674·3).
Anxiety.

Diathynil Sigma-Tau, Ital.
Biotin (p.1355·3).
Skin disorders.

Diatil Mer-National, S.Afr.
Diltiazem hydrochloride (p.874·3).
Angina pectoris; hypertension.

Diatin Ferrer, Spain.
Elcatonin (p.749·2).
Hypercalcaemia; osteoporosis; Paget's disease of bone.

Diatol
Pacific, Hong Kong; Pacific, NZ.
Tolbutamide (p.336·3).
Diabetes mellitus.

Diatolil Fardi, Spain.
Buphenine hydrochloride (p.1587·3).
Dysmenorrhoea; peripheral and cerebral circulatory disorders.

Diatracin Dista, Spain.
Vancomycin hydrochloride (p.267·2).
Bacterial infections.

Diatrum Romila, Canad.
Multivitamin and mineral preparation (p.1350·1).

Diatussin Propan, S.Afr.
Diphenhydramine hydrochloride (p.416·1); sodium citrate (p.1186·2); menthol (p.1632·3); ammonium chloride (p.1085·2); theophylline (p.777·2).
Coughs.

Diatx Pan American, USA.
Vitamin B substances and vitamin C (p.1350·1).

Diatx Fe Pan American, USA.
Vitamin B substances; vitamin C; ferrous fumarate (p.1350·1).

Diaval Valdecasas, Mex.
Tolbutamide (p.336·3).
Diabetes mellitus.

Dia-Vite R&D, Canad.
Vitamin B substances with ascorbic acid (p.1350·1).

Diawern Wernigerode, Ger.
Crataegus (p.1600·2); valerian (p.1678·3).
Heart failure.

Diaz Taro, Israel.
Diazepam (p.674·3).
Anxiety; insomnia; skeletal muscle spasm.

Diazelong Cazi, Braz.
Diazepam (p.674·3).
Alcohol withdrawal syndrome; anxiety; epilepsy; insomnia; sedative; skeletal muscle spasm.

Diazemuls Pharmacia Upjohn, Austral.; Pharmacia Upjohn, Canad.; Pharmacia Upjohn, Hong Kong; Dumex, Irl.; Pharmacia Upjohn, Ital.; CSL, NZ; Dumex, UK.
Diazepam (p.674·3).
Alcohol withdrawal syndrome; anxiety; convulsions; premedication; sedative; skeletal muscle spasm; status epilepticus; tetanus.

Diazep CT, Ger.; ABZ, Ger.
Diazepam (p.674·3).
Anxiety; premedication; skeletal muscle spasm; status epilepticus.

Diazol EMS, Braz.
Co-trimoxazole (p.193·3); calcium carbonate (p.1215·1); attapulgite (p.1212·1).
Diarrhoea.

Diazolen Degorts, Mex.
Mebendazole (p.102·2).
Worm infections.

Diazon Unison, Singapore; Unison, Thai.
Ketoconazole (p.389·1).
Fungal infections; seborrhoeic dermatitis.

Diba Manetti Roberts, Ital.
Glutaral (p.1145·2).
Instrument disinfection; surface disinfection.

Dibacilina Diba, Mex.
Ampicillin trihydrate (p.151·1).
Bacterial infections.

Dibagesic Diba, Mex.
Dextropropoxyphene (p.27·1).
Pain.

Diban Wyeth-Ayerst, Canad.
Activated attapulgite (p.1212·1); pectin (p.1502·3); prepared opium (p.69·3); hyoscyamine sulfate (p.469·3); atropine sulfate (p.461·1); hyoscine hydrobromide (p.468·2).
Diarrhoea.

Dibapec Compuesto Diba, Mex.
Furazolidone (p.592·1); kaolin (p.1229·3); pectin (p.1502·3).
Diarrhoea.

Dibaprim Diba, Mex.
Co-trimoxazole (p.193·3).
Bacterial infections.

Dibasona Diba, Mex.
Dexamethasone sodium phosphate (p.1067·1).
Corticosteroid.

Dibasul Diba, Mex.
Sulfamethoxypyridazine (p.256·1).
Bacterial infections.

Dibaterr Diba, Mex.
Tetracycline hydrochloride (p.258·3).
Bacterial infections.

Dibecon Pharmasant, Thai.
Chlorpropamide (p.321·1).
Diabetes mellitus.

Dibelet
Atlantic, Singapore; Atlantic, Thai.
Glibenclamide (p.321·3).
Diabetes mellitus.

Dibencozan Houde, Fr.†
Cobamamide (p.1388·3).
Neuralgias; neuritis.

Dibendril EMS, Braz.
Ampicillin benzathine (p.151·3); ampicillin sodium (p.150·3).
Bacterial infections.

Dibendyl Malaysia Chemist, Singapore.
Diphenhydramine hydrochloride (p.416·1); ammonium chloride (p.1085·2).
Coughs; respiratory-tract congestion; sneezing.

Dibendyl Forte CD Malaysia Chemist, Singapore.
Diphenhydramine hydrochloride (p.416·1); codeine phosphate (p.25·2); ammonium chloride (p.1085·2); sodium citrate (p.1186·2).
Coughs; respiratory-tract congestion; sneezing.

Dibent Hauck, USA.
Dicyclomine [dicycloverine] hydrochloride (p.466·1).
Functional bowel/irritable bowel syndrome.

Dibenyline SmithKline Beecham, Austral.; SmithKline Beecham, Belg.; SmithKline Beecham, Hong Kong; SmithKline Beecham, Israel; SmithKline Beecham, Neth.; SmithKline Beecham, NZ; Forley, UK.
Phenoxybenzamine hydrochloride (p.954·1).
Phaeochromocytoma; shock; urinary retention due to neurogenic bladder or beningn prostatic hyperplasia.

Dibenzyline SmithKline Beecham, USA†.
Phenoxybenzamine hydrochloride (p.954·1).
Phaeochromocytoma.

Dibenzyran Procter & Gamble, Aust.; Esparma, Ger.
Phenoxybenzamine hydrochloride (p.954·1).
Neurogenic bladder; phaeochromocytoma.

Dibertil Sandipro, Belg.
Metoclopramide hydrochloride (p.1235·2).
Adjunct in gastrointestinal examination; gastrointestinal motility disorders; nausea and vomiting.

Dibetasol Shin Poong, Singapore.
Betamethasone dipropionate (p.1063·2); betamethasone sodium phosphate (p.1063·2).
Parenteral corticosteroid.

Dibetid Arlex, Mex.
Glibenclamide (p.321·3).
Diabetes mellitus.

Dibetop Davi, Port.
Betamethasone dipropionate (p.1063·2).
Skin disorders.

Dibetop Q Davi, Port.
Betamethasone dipropionate (p.1063·2); salicylic acid (p.1122·3).
Skin disorders.

Dibilan F Byk Gulden, Mex.
Bumadizone (p.20·3).

Diblocin Astra, Ger.
Doxazosin mesilate (p.883·2).
Benign prostatic hyperplasia; hypertension.

Dibondrin Montavit, Aust.
Diphenhydramine hydrochloride (p.416·1).
Hypersensitivity disorders; prophylaxis against anaphylactic shock.

Dibro-Be Mono Dibropharm, Ger.
Potassium bromide.
Epilepsy.

Dibromol Trommsdorff, Ger.
Sodium 3,5-dibromo-4-hydroxybenzenesulfonate; bromchlorophen (p.1136·1); isopropyl alcohol (p.1149·2).
Burns; skin disinfection; wounds.

Dibroxin Tecnofarma, Mex.
Bromhexine (p.1085·3).
Respiratory-tract congestion.

Dibufen Diba, Mex.
Ibuprofen (p.43·2).
Inflammation; musculoskeletal, joint and peri-articular disorders; pain.

Dical
Note. This name is used for preparations of different composition.
Abbott, Mex.
Calcium carbonate (p.1215·1); colecalciferol (p.1391·1).
Calcium and vitamin D deficiency; calcium and vitamin D supplement.

Abbott, USA.
Calcium with vitamin D and phosphorus (p.1350·1).
Calcium deficiency; dietary supplement.

Dicalcium Abiogen, Spain.
Vitamin A palmitate (p.1383·2); colecalciferol (p.1391·1); calcium carbonate (p.1215·1).
Formerly contained vitamin A palmitate, ergocalciferol, and calcium carbonate.
Vitamin or mineral deficiency.

Dical-D Abbott, Hong Kong.
Calcium with vitamin D and phosphorus (p.1350·1).
Dietary supplement.

Dicalm Mavena, Switz.
Valerian (p.1678·3); lupulus (p.1629·3); ballota; passion flower (p.1649·1).
Anxiety; nervousness.

Dicalmir Dicofarm, Ital.
Fennel (p.1610·1); chamomile (p.1593·2); aniseed (p.1580·2); liquorice (p.1231·2); cumin; coriander (p.1599·2).
Colic; meteorism.

Dicalys 11 Dicamed, Swed.
Sodium chloride; potassium chloride; calcium chloride; magnesium chloride; sodium lactate; glucose (p.1184·1).
Haemofiltration.

Dicalys 17 Dicamed, Swed.
Sodium chloride; potassium chloride; calcium chloride; magnesium chloride; sodium lactate (p.1184·1).
Haemofiltration.

Dicap Pacific, NZ.
Loperamide hydrochloride (p.1231·3).
Diarrhoea.

Dicarbosil Bira, USA†.
Calcium carbonate (p.1215·1).
Hyperacidity.

Dicavin Quimica y Farmacia, Mex.
Difenidol (p.1222·1).
Nausea and vomiting.

Dicel Lasa, Spain†.
Fenproporex hydrochloride (p.1510·2).
Obesity.

Dicepin B6 Ipsen, Spain†.
Diazepam (p.674·3).
Contains pyridoxine hydrochloride.
Alcohol withdrawal syndrome; anxiety; febrile convulsions; insomnia; skeletal muscle spasm.

Dicetel
Solvay, Aust.; Solvay, Belg.; Byk, Braz.; Solvay, Canad.; Solvay, Fr.; Solvay, Hong Kong; Solvay, Ital.; Byk Gulden, Mex.; Solvay, Neth.†; Solvay, Port.; Solvay, Switz.; Solvay, Thai.
Pinaverium bromide (p.1651·3).
Adjunct in gastrointestinal radiography; gastrointestinal spasm.

Dichlor-Stapenor Bayer, Ger.
Dicloxacillin sodium (p.199·1).
Benzylpenicillin-resistant staphylococcal infections.

Dichlotride
Merck Sharp & Dohme, Austral.; Merck Sharp & Dohme, Belg.; Merck Sharp & Dohme, Denm.; Merck Sharp & Dohme, Neth.†; Merck Sharp & Dohme, Norw.; Merck Sharp & Dohme, Port.; Merck Sharp & Dohme, S.Afr.; Merck Sharp & Dohme, Swed.; Merck Sharp & Dohme, Thai.
Hydrochlorothiazide (p.907·3).
Hypertension; oedema; premenstrual syndrome.

Dicillin Durascan, Denm.
Dicloxacillin sodium (p.199·1).
Bacterial infections.

Dicinone
Synthelabo, Braz.; Pensa, Spain.
Etamsylate (p.732·2).
Haemorrhage.

Dicitrate Pharmascience, Singapore.
Sodium citrate (p.1186·2); citric acid monohydrate (p.1596·2).
Acid aspiration; acidosis; gout; renal calculi.

Diclac Hexal, Aust.; Hexal, Ger.; Rowex, Irl.
Diclofenac sodium (p.30·3).
Gout; inflammation; musculoskeletal and joint disorders; pain.

Diclamina Esteve, Spain.
Cinnarizine (p.413·1); heptaminol acephyllinate (p.765·3).
Vascular headache; vertigo.

Diclanil Condrugs, Thai.
Glibenclamide (p.321·3).
Diabetes mellitus.

Diclax Douglas, NZ.
Diclofenac sodium (p.30·3).
Osteoarthritis; rheumatoid arthritis.

Diclectin Duchesnay, Canad.
Doxylamine succinate (p.417·1); pyridoxine hydrochloride (p.1386·3).
Nausea and vomiting of pregnancy.

Diclex Meiji, Thai.
Dicloxacillin sodium (p.199·1).
Bacterial infections.

Diclo
Note. This name is used for preparations of different composition.
Kade, Ger.; CT, Ger.; Betapharm, Ger.; ABZ, Ger.; Eu Rho, Ger.; Sudmedica, Ger.; Ratiopharm, Ger.†; Pinewood, Irl.; Cophar, Switz.
Diclofenac sodium (p.30·3).
Gout; inflammation; musculoskeletal, joint, peri-articular, and soft-tissue disorders; pain.

FIRMA, Ital.
Dicloxacillin sodium (p.199·1).
Bacterial infections.

diclo-basan Schonenberger, Switz.
Diclofenac sodium (p.30·3).
Gout; inflammation; musculoskeletal and joint disorders; pain; soft-tissue injuries.

Diclobene Ratiopharm, Aust.
Diclofenac sodium (p.30·3).
Gout; inflammation; musculoskeletal, joint, peri-articular, and soft-tissue disorders; pain.

Diclocil
Bristol-Myers Squibb, Austral.; Bristol-Myers Squibb, Denm.; Bristol-Myers Squibb, Fin.; Bristol-Myers Squibb, Hong Kong; Bristol-Myers Squibb, Norw.; Bristol-Myers Squibb, NZ; Bristol-Myers Squibb, Port.; Bristol-Myers Squibb, Swed.; Bristol-Myers Squibb, Thai.
Dicloxacillin sodium (p.199·1).
Bacterial infections.

Diclocillin TO-Chemicals, Thai.
Dicloxacillin sodium (p.199·1).
Bacterial infections.

Diclocular Angelini, Ital.
Diclofenac sodium (p.30·3).
Adjunct in eye surgery; corneal ulcers; pain and inflammation of the eye.

Diclo-Denk Denk, Hong Kong.
Diclofenac sodium (p.30·3).
Gout; inflammation; musculoskeletal, joint, and soft-tissue disorders.

Dicloderm Forte Cruz, Spain.
Dichlorisone acetate (p.1069·2).
Skin disorders.

Diclo-Divido Isis Puren, Ger.
Diclofenac sodium (p.30·3).
Gout; inflammation; musculoskeletal, joint, and soft-tissue disorders.

Diclodoc Docpharm, Ger.
Diclofenac sodium (p.30·3).
Gout; inflammation; musculoskeletal, joint, and soft-tissue disorders.

Diclodol IPFI, Ital.
Diclofenac sodium (p.30·3).
Inflammation; muscloskeletal and joint disorders; pain.

Diclofam Aspen, S.Afr.
Diclofenac sodium (p.30·3).
Inflammation; muscloskeletal and joint disorders; pain.

Diclofan Boniscontro & Gazzone, Ital.
Diclofenac sodium (p.30·3).
Inflammation; muscloskeletal and joint disorders; pain.

Diclofen
Searle, Braz.; Jean-Marie, Hong Kong; Berlin Pharm, Thai.
Diclofenac diethylamine (p.30·2), diclofenac potassium (p.30·2), or diclofenac sodium (p.30·3).
Gout; inflammation; musculoskeletal, joint, peri-articular, and soft-tissue disorders; pain.

Diclofenbeta Betapharm, Ger.
Diclofenac sodium (p.30·3).
Gout; inflammation; musculoskeletal, joint, and soft-tissue disorders; pain.

Dicloflex Dexcel, UK.
Diclofenac sodium (p.30·3).
Gout; inflammation; musculoskeletal, joint, peri-articular, and soft-tissue disorders; pain.

Dicloftil Farmigea, Ital.
Diclofenac sodium (p.30·3).
Inflammatory eye disorders.

Diclogel Polipharm, Thai.
Diclofenac diethylamine (p.30·2).
Inflammation; pain.

Diclogrun Grunenthal, Ger.
Diclofenac sodium (p.30·3).
Inflammatory eye disorders.

Diclohexal *Hexal, Austral.; Hexal, S.Afr.*
Diclofenac sodium (p.30·3).
Gout; inflammation; musculoskeletal and joint disorders; pain.

Diclolan *Olan-Kemed, Thai.*
Diclofenac sodium (p.30·3).
Musculoskeletal, joint, and peri-articular disorders.

Diclomax *Parke, Davis, UK.*
Diclofenac sodium (p.30·3).
Inflammation; musculoskeletal, joint, peri-articular and soft-tissue disorders; pain.

Diclomel *Clonmel, Irl.*
Diclofenac sodium (p.30·3).
Gout; musculoskeletal and joint disorders; pain.

Diclomelan *Lannacher, Aust.*
Diclofenac sodium (p.30·3).
Inflammation; musculoskeletal and joint disorders; pain.

Diclomerck *Merck, Ger.†*
Diclofenac sodium (p.30·3).
Gout; inflammation; musculoskeletal and joint disorders; pain.

Diclometin *Pharmacia Upjohn, Fin.*
Diclofenac sodium (p.30·3).
Musculoskeletal and joint disorders; pain.

Diclomex *Medinovum, Fin.*
Diclofenac sodium (p.30·3).
Inflammation; musculoskeletal and joint disorders; pain.

Diclomin *Atlantis, Mex.*
Dicyclomine [dicycloverine] hydrochloride (p.466·1).
Gastrointestinal spasm and hypermotility.

Diclomol *Win-Medicare, Thai.*
Diclofenac diethylamine (p.30·2).
Inflammation; pain.

Diclon *Durascan, Denm.*
Diclofenac sodium (p.30·3).
Gout; inflammation; musculoskeletal and joint disorders; pain.

Diclophlogont *Azupharma, Ger.*
Diclofenac sodium (p.30·3).
Gout; inflammation; musculoskeletal, joint, peri-articular, and soft-tissue disorders; pain.

Dicloplast *CTI, Israel.*
Diclofenac epolamine (p.31·3).
Inflammation; musculoskeletal and joint disorders; pain.

Diclo-Puren *Isis Puren, Ger.*
Diclofenac sodium (p.30·3).
Inflammation; musculoskeletal, joint, peri-articular, and soft-tissue disorders; pain.

Dicloran *Randall, Mex.*
Diclofenac sodium (p.30·3).
Gout; inflammation; musculoskeletal and joint and peri-articular disorders; pain.

Diclorektal *Sanorania, Ger.†*
Diclofenac sodium (p.30·3).
Gout; inflammation; musculoskeletal and joint disorders.

Diclorengel *Trima, Israel.*
Diclofenac sodium (p.30·3).
Inflammation; musculoskeletal and joint disorders; pain.

Dicloreum *Wassermann, Ital.*
Diclofenac epolamine (p.31·3) or diclofenac sodium (p.30·3).
Inflammation; musculoskeletal, joint, and peri-articular disorders; pain.

Diclo-saar *Chephasaar, Ger.*
Diclofenac sodium (p.30·3).
Gout; inflammation; musculoskeletal, joint, and soft-tissue disorders; pain.

Diclosian *Asian Pharm, Thai.*
Diclofenac sodium (p.30·3).
Musculoskeletal, joint, and peri-articular disorders.

Diclosifar *Siphar, Switz.*
Diclofenac sodium (p.30·3).
Gout; inflammation; musculoskeletal and joint disorders; pain.

Dicloson *Unison, Thai.*
Dicloxacillin sodium (p.199·1).
Bacterial infections.

Diclo-Spondyril *Orion, Ger.*
Diclofenac sodium (p.30·3).
Acute; inflammation; neuralgia; neuritis; pain; rheumatic disorders; soft-tissue disorders.

Diclostad *Stada, Aust.*
Diclofenac sodium (p.30·3).
Gout; inflammation; musculoskeletal, joint, and peri-articular disorders; pain.

Diclosyl *Medicopharm, Aust.*
Diclofenac sodium (p.30·3).
Musculoskeletal, joint, peri-articular, and soft-tissue disorders; pain.

Diclo-Tablinen *Sanorania, Ger.†*
Diclofenac sodium (p.30·3).
Gout; inflammation; musculoskeletal and joint disorders.

Diclotard *Galen, UK.*
Diclofenac sodium (p.30·3).
Inflammation; musculoskeletal, joint, peri-articular, and soft-tissue disorders; pain.

Diclotec *Technilab, Canad.*
Diclofenac sodium (p.30·3).
Inflammation; pain.

Diclofenac sodium (p.30·3).
Misoprostol (p.1446·1) is included in this preparation in an attempt to limit adverse effects on the gastrointestinal mucosa.
Osteoarthritis; rheumatoid arthritis.

Diclo-Tecno *Tecnofarma, Mex.*
Dicloxacillin (p.199·1).

Diclotride *Merck Sharp & Dohme, Mex.*
Hydrochlorothiazide (p.907·3).
Hypertension; oedema.

Diclovit *Lannacher, Aust.*
Diclofenac sodium (p.30·3); thiamine hydrochloride (p.1385·1); pyridoxine hydrochloride (p.1386·3); cyanocobalamin (p.1388·1).
Gout; musculoskeletal, joint, and soft-tissue disorders; neuralgia; neuritis.

Diclovol *Arun, UK.*
Diclofenac sodium (p.30·3).
Gout; musculoskeletal, joint, peri-articular, and soft-tissue disorders; pain.

Diclowal *Ritter, Singapore.*
Diclofenac sodium (p.30·3).
Gout; musculoskeletal and joint disorders; pain.

Diclo-Wolff *Wolff, Ger.*
Diclofenac sodium (p.30·3).
Gout; inflammation; musculoskeletal, joint, and soft-tissue disorders; neuralgia; neuritis.

Diclox *PP Lab, Thai.*
Dicloxacillin sodium (p.199·1).
Bacterial infections.

Diclloxia *Asian Pharm, Thai.*
Dicloxacillin sodium (p.199·1).
Bacterial infections.

Dicloxsig *Sigma, Austral.*
Dicloxacillin sodium (p.199·1).
Gram-positive bacterial infections.

Diclozip *Ashbourne, UK.*
Diclofenac sodium (p.30·3).
Inflammation; pain.

Dicodid *Knoll, Ger.; Knoll, Switz.*
Hydrocodone hydrochloride (p.42·2) or hydrocodone tartrate (p.42·2).
Coughs; pain.

Dicodin *Asta Medica, Fr.*
Dihydrocodeine tartrate (p.33·1).
Pain.

Dicodral *Dicofarm, Ital.*
Sodium chloride; potassium chloride; sodium bicarbonate; glucose (p.1185·2).
Diarrhoea; oral rehydration therapy.

Dicofarm *Continentales, Mex.*
Pipemidic acid (p.236·1).

Dicoflor *Dicofarm, Ital.*
Food containing lactic-acid-producing organisms (p.1626·3).
Disturbances of the gastrointestinal flora.

Dicoman *Dicofarm, Ital.*
Dietary fibre supplement (p.1350·1).

Dicomin *Berlin Pharm, Thai.*
Dicyclomine [dicycloverine] hydrochloride (p.466·1).
Gastrointestinal spasm.

Diconal *Wellcome, Irl.; CeNeS, UK.*
Dipipanone hydrochloride (p.33·3); cyclizine hydrochloride (p.414·1).
Pain.

Dicopac *Nycomed Amersham, UK.*
1 capsule, cyanocobalamin (cobalt-57) (p.1449·2); 1 capsule, cyanocobalamin (cobalt-58) (p.1449·2); 1 ampoule, cyanocobalamin (p.1388·1).
Diagnosis of vitamin B₁₂ malabsorption.

Dicoplus *Almirall, Spain.*
Glucomannan (p.1616·2).
Disorders of lipid metabolism.

Dicorantil *Hoechst Marion Roussel, Braz.*
Disopyramide phosphate (p.878·2).
Arrhythmias.

Dicortal *Sigma-Tau, Ital.*
Diflucortolone valerate (p.1069·3).
Skin disorders.

Dicorten *Trima, Israel.*
Betamethasone dipropionate (p.1063·2).
Skin disorders.

Dicorvin *ICN, Spain.*
Acetylspiramycin (p.249·1).
Bacterial infections.

Dicorynan *Hoechst Marion Roussel, Spain.*
Disopyramide (p.878·2).
Arrhythmias.

Dicton *Dolorgiet, Ger.*
Codeine polistirex (p.26·1).
Coughs.

Dicynene *Delandale, Irl.; Sanofi Synthelabo, UK.*
Etamsylate (p.732·2).
Menorrhagia; periventricular haemorrhage.

Dicynone *Sanofi Synthelabo, Belg.; Synthelabo, Fr.; Synthelabo, Ital.; Sanofi Synthelabo, Singapore; OM, Switz.*
Etamsylate (p.732·2).
Haemorrhagic disorders.

Didamega *Larkhall Laboratories, UK.*
Multivitamin and mineral preparation (p.1350·1).

Didamol *Byk, Belg.†*
Dipyridamole (p.877·2).
Angina pectoris; thromboembolism prophylaxis.

Di-Delamine *Del, USA; Commerce, USA.*
Diphenhydramine hydrochloride (p.416·1); tripelennamine hydrochloride (p.427·1).
Pruritus.

Didor *Asta Medica, Port.*
Dihydrocodeine tartrate (p.33·1).
Pain.

Didralin *Medochemie, Singapore; Medochemie, Thai.*
Hydrochlorothiazide (p.907·3).
Heart failure; hypertension; oedema.

Didrex *Upjohn, USA.*
Benzfetamine hydrochloride (p.1507·1).
Obesity.

Didrica *Pensa, Spain.*
Calcium chloride; potassium chloride; sodium chloride; sodium lactate; glucose (p.1185·2).
Oral rehydration therapy.

Didrocal *Pharmacia Upjohn, Austral.; Procter & Gamble, Canad.*
White tablets, disodium etidronate (p.752·1); blue tablets, calcium carbonate (p.1215·1).
Osteoporosis.

Didrogyl *Bruno, Ital.*
Calcifediol (p.1391·1).
Hypocalcaemia; hypoparathyroidism; osteomalacia; osteoporosis; renal osteodystrophy; rickets.

Didro-Kit *Procter & Gamble, Ital.†.*
White tablets, disodium etidronate (p.752·1); blue tablets, calcium carbonate (p.1215·1).
Osteoporosis.

Didrokit *Procter & Gamble, Neth.*
Didronel tablets, disodium etidronate (p.752·1); Cacit tablets, calcium carbonate (p.1215·1).
Osteoporosis.

Didronate
Procter & Gamble, Denm.; Roche, Fin.; Procter & Gamble, Norw.; Roche, Swed.
Disodium etidronate (p.752·1).
Ectopic ossification; osteoporosis; Paget's disease of bone.

Didronate + Calcium *Procter & Gamble, Denm.; Roche, Fin.; Roche, Swed.*
14 Tablets, disodium etidronate (p.752·1) (Didronate); 76 tablets, calcium carbonate (p.1215·1).
Osteoporosis.

Didronate + Calsium *Procter & Gamble, Norw.*
14 Didronate tablets, disodium etidronate (p.752·1); 76 calcium tablets, calcium carbonate (p.1215·1).
Osteoporosis.

Didronel
Hoechst Marion Roussel, Aust.; Pharmacia Upjohn, Austral.; Procter & Gamble, Belg.; Procter & Gamble, Canad.; Knoll, Canad.; Procter & Gamble, Fr.; Procter & Gamble, Ger.; Hoechst Marion Roussel, Ger.; Procter & Gamble, Hong Kong; Procter & Gamble, Irl.; Procter & Gamble, Israel; Procter & Gamble, Ital.; Procter & Gamble, Neth.†; Pharmacia Upjohn, NZ; Normal, Port.; Boehringer Mannheim, S.Afr.†; Procter & Gamble, Switz.; Procter & Gamble, UK; Procter & Gamble, USA; MGI, USA.
Disodium etidronate (p.752·1).
Ectopic ossification; hypercalcaemia of malignancy; osteoporosis; Paget's disease of bone.

Didronel PMO
Procter & Gamble, Irl.; Procter & Gamble, UK.
Tablets, disodium etidronate (Didronel) (p.752·1); tablets, calcium carbonate (Cacit) (p.1215·1).
Osteoporosis.

Diele *Diele, Fr.†*
Food for special diets (p.1350·1).
A range of foods for patients with amino acid metabolic disorders.

Diemil *Almirall, Spain.*
Dihydroergocristine mesilate (p.1603·2); piracetam (p.1652·1).
Cerebrovascular disorders; head injury.

Dienpax *Sanofi Winthrop, Braz.*
Diazepam (p.674·3).
Alcohol withdrawal syndrome; anxiety; epilepsy; insomnia; premedication; sedative; skeletal muscle spasm; tetanus.

Dientrin *Sanofi Winthrop, Braz.*
Co-trimoxazole (p.193·3); attapulgite (p.1212·1); calcium carbonate (p.1215·1).
Diarrhoea.

Diergo *Note. This name is used for preparations of different composition.*
Novartis, Belg.
Dihydroergotamine mesilate (p.450·3).
Formerly contained dihydroergotamine mesilate and caffeine.
Migraine.

Novartis, Fr.
Dihydroergotamine mesilate (p.450·3); caffeine (p.761·3).
Migraine.

Diertina *Mundipharma, Aust.; Searle, Ital.; Sankyo, Ital.; Poli, Switz.*
Dihydroergocristine mesilate (p.1603·2).
Cerebral and peripheral vascular disorders; dopamine deficiency; hypertension.

Diertine *Yamanouchi, Spain.*
Dihydroergocristine mesilate (p.1603·2).
Cerebrovascular disorders; tinnitus; vascular eye disorders; vertigo.

Di-Ertride *Malaysia Chemist, Singapore.*
Hydrochlorothiazide (p.907·3).
Diabetes insipidus; hypertension; oedema.

Diesan *CT, Ital.*
Fluoxetine hydrochloride (p.284·2).
Bulimia nervosa; depression; obsessive-compulsive disorders.

Diesel *Neves, Port.*
Multivitamin and mineral preparation (p.1350·1).

Diespor *Biomedica, Ital.*
Cefonicid sodium (p.168·1).
Lignocaine [lidocaine] hydrochloride (p.1313·2) is included in the intramuscular preparation to alleviate the pain of injection.
Gram-negative bacterial infections.

Diestet *Searle, Mex.*
Mazindol (p.1510·3).
Obesity.

Diet Ayds *DEP, USA†.*
Benzocaine (p.1306·2).
Obesity.

Diet Sucaryl *Abbott, Ital.*
Sodium cyclamate (p.1358·3); saccharin (p.1374·3).
Sugar substitute.

Dietacil *IMA, Braz.*
Aspartame (p.1354·3).
Sugar substitute.

Dietaid *Mer-National, S.Afr.†.*
Caffeine (p.761·3); ephedrine hydrochloride (p.1090·1); phenolphthalein (p.1244·1).
Obesity.

Dietasal *Libbs, Braz.*
Sodium chloride; potassium chloride (p.1185·2).
Oral rehydration solution.

Dietene *Restan, S.Afr.*
Cathine hydrochloride (p.1507·1).
Obesity.

Dietil *Trenker, Belg.†*
Diethylpropion hydrochloride (p.1508·3).
Obesity.

Dietoman
Note. This name is used for preparations of different composition.
Schering-Plough, Braz.
Bran (p.1214·2).
Constipation; diverticular disease; irritable bowel syndrome.

Teofarma, Ital.; Armstrong, Mex.
Glucomannan (p.1616·2).
Diabetes mellitus; lipid disorders; obesity.

Dieutrim *Legere, USA†.*
Phenylpropanolamine hydrochloride (p.1098·1); benzocaine (p.1306·2); carmellose sodium (p.1499·3).
Obesity.

Dievril *FIRMA, Ital.*
Vitamin B preparation (p.1350·1).
Lignocaine [lidocaine] hydrochloride (p.1313·2) is included in the intramuscular injection to alleviate the pain of injection.
Neuralgia; neuritis.

Diezime *Recordati, Ital.*
Cefodizime sodium (p.167·3).
Lignocaine [lidocaine] hydrochloride (p.1313·2) is included in this preparation to alleviate the pain of injection.
Bacterial infections.

Dif Vitamin A Masivo *Roche, Spain.*
Vitamin A acetate (p.1383·2).
Vitamin A deficiency.

Difaterol *Aristegui, Spain.*
Bezafibrate (p.849·1).
Hyperlipidaemias.

Difedram *Mavi, Mex.*
Diphenhydramine (p.416·1).

Difelene *Nakorn, Thai.*
Diclofenac diethylamine (p.30·2) or diclofenac sodium (p.30·3).
Inflammation; musculoskeletal, joint, peri-articular, and soft-tissue disorders; pain.

Difemic *Pharmasant, Thai.*
Dicyclomine [dicycloverine] hydrochloride (p.466·1); mefenamic acid (p.51·2).
Gastrointestinal spasm.

Difen *Allergan-Frumtost, Braz.*
Pranoprofen (p.80·1).
Inflammatory eye disorders.

Difena *Standard, Hong Kong.*
Diclofenac sodium (p.30·3).
Inflammation; musculoskeletal, joint, and soft-tissue disorders.

Difenac
DHA, Hong Kong; Rolab, S.Afr.; DHA, Singapore; TP, Thai.
Diclofenac sodium (p.30·3).
Now known as Rolab-Diclofenac. sodium in S.Afr.
Gout; inflammation; musculoskeletal and joint disorders; pain.

Difene *Klinge, Irl.*
Diclofenac sodium (p.30·3).
Gout; inflammation; musculoskeletal, joint, peri-articular, and soft-tissue disorders; pain; renal colic.

Difenet *Nettopharma, Denm.*
Diclofenac sodium (p.30·3).
Gout; inflammation; musculoskeletal and joint disorders; pain.

Difenhistat *Precimex, Mex.*
Diphenhydramine (p.416·1).

Difeno *Milano, Thai.*
Diclofenac sodium (p.30·3).
Inflammation; musculoskeletal and joint disorders.

Diferin *Grossman, Mex.*
Ampicillin (p.150·3).
Bacterial infections.

Difexon *Armstrong, Mex.*
Deltamethrin (p.1430·3).
Pediculosis; scabies.

Differin
AB-Consult, Aust.; Galderma, Austral.; Galderma, Belg.; Galderma, Canad.; Galderma, Fin.; Galderma, Ger.; Galderma, Hong Kong; Galderma, Irl.; Galderma, Ital.; Galderma, Norw.; Galderma, NZ; Galderma, Port.; Galderma, S.Afr.; Galderma, Singapore; Galderma, Swed.; Galderma, Switz.; Galderma, Thai.; Galderma, UK; Galderma, USA.
Adapalene (p.1109·3).
Acne.

Differine
Galderma, Fr.; Galderma, Spain.
Adapalene (p.1109·3).
Acne.

Difflam
3M, Austral.; 3M, Hong Kong; 3M, Irl.; 3M, NZ; 3M, Singapore; 3M, Thai.; 3M, UK.
Benzydamine hydrochloride (p.20·1).
Inflammation; pain.

Difflam Anti-inflammatory Antibacterial Lozenges *3M, NZ.*
Benzydamine hydrochloride (p.20·1); cetylpyridinium chloride (p.1138·1).
Mouth and throat disorders.

Difflam Anti-inflammatory Cough Lozenges *3M, NZ.*
Benzydamine hydrochloride (p.20·1); cetylpyridinium chloride (p.1138·1); pholcodine (p.1099·1).
Coughs; mouth and throat disorders.

Difflam Anti-Inflammatory Lozenges *3M, Austral.*
Benzydamine hydrochloride (p.20·1); cetylpyridinium chloride (p.1138·1).
Mouth and throat pain.

Difflam Anti-Inflammatory Lozenges with Cough Suppressant *3M, Austral.*
Benzydamine hydrochloride (p.20·1); cetylpyridinium chloride (p.1138·1); pholcodine (p.1099·1).
Coughs; sore throat.

Difflam Anti-Inflammatory Solution *3M, Austral.*
Benzydamine hydrochloride (p.20·1).
Mouth and throat pain.

Difflam Anti-Inflammatory Throat Spray *3M, Austral.*
Benzydamine hydrochloride (p.20·1).
Mouth and throat pain.

Difflam Mouth Gel
3M, Austral.; 3M, NZ; 3M, Singapore.
Benzydamine hydrochloride (p.20·1); cetylpyridinium chloride (p.1138·1).
Formerly known as Difflam Anti-Inflammatory Antiseptic Mouth Gel in *Austral.*
Painful inflammatory mouth disorders.

Difflam-C
3M, Austral.; 3M, Hong Kong; 3M, NZ; 3M, Singapore.
Benzydamine hydrochloride (p.20·1); chlorhexidine gluconate (p.1138·2).
Mouth and throat pain.

Diffu-K *UCB, Fr.*
Potassium chloride (p.1194·3).
Hypokalaemia.

Difumal *Malesci, Ital.*
Theophylline (p.777·2).
Respiratory-tract disorders.

Diffusyl *Farmasan, Ger.*
Sodium cromoglicate (p.774·3).
Asthma.

Difilina Asmorax *Liade, Spain†.*
Diprophylline (p.764·1); ephedrine hydrochloride (p.1090·1); hydroxyzine hydrochloride (p.419·1).
Obstructive airways disease.

Difiram *Pharmasant, Thai.*
Disulfiram (p.1605·1).
Chronic alcoholism.

Difix *Chiesi, Ital.*
Calcitriol (p.1391·1).
Hypoparathyroidism; osteoporosis; pseudohypoparathyroidism; renal osteodystrophy; rickets.

Diflamil *Belmac, Spain.*
Oxyphenbutazone piperazine (p.71·1).
Gout; musculoskeletal and joint disorders.

Diflonid
Dumex-Alpharma, Denm.†; Dumex, Norw.†.
Diflunisal (p.32·2).
Musculoskeletal and joint disorders; pain.

Diflucan
Pfizer, Aust.; Pfizer, Austral.; Pfizer, Belg.; Pfizer, Canad.; Pfizer, Denm.; Pfizer, Fin.; Pfizer, Ger.; Pfizer, Hong Kong; Pfizer, Irl.; Pfizer, Israel; Roerig, Ital.; Pfizer, Mex.; Pfizer, Neth.; Pfizer, Norw.; Douglas, NZ; Roerig, Port.; Pfizer, S.Afr.; Pfizer, Singapore; Vinci, Spain; Pfizer, Swed.; Pfizer, Switz.; Pfizer, Thai.; Pfizer, UK; Pfizer, USA.
Fluconazole (p.383·2).
Fungal infections.

Difludol *Edmond Pharma, Ital.*
Diflunisal (p.32·2).
Musculoskeletal disorders; pain.

Difluid *Bioprogress, Ital.*
Dihydroergocristine mesilate (p.1603·2).
Cerebral and peripheral disorders; headache; hypertension; migraine.

Diflusal *Merck Sharp & Dohme, Belg.*
Diflunisal (p.32·2).
Pain.

Difmecor *Solvay, Ital.†.*
Fendiline hydrochloride (p.889·1).
Cardiac disorders.

Difmetre *Solvay, Ital.*
Indometacin (p.44·3); caffeine (p.761·3); prochlorperazine maleate (p.701·2).
Headache; migraine.

Difmetus Compositum *Solvay, Ital.*
Noscapine (p.1096·1); noscapine (p.1096·1); promethazine embonate (p.424·1).
Coughs.

Difnal *Ranbaxy, Singapore.*
Diclofenac sodium (p.30·3).
Inflammation; musculoskeletal, joint, peri-articular, and soft-tissue disorders; pain.

Difnan *Hikma, Port.†.*
Diclofenac (p.30·2).

Diformil *Faes, Spain.*
Formaldehyde (p.1144·2).
Mouth infections.

Diformiltricina *Faes, Spain.*
Cetrimonium bromide (p.1137·3); benzocaine (p.1306·2); formaldehyde (p.1144·2); tyrothricin (p.267·1).
Mouth and throat disorders.

Diformin *Leiras, Fin.*
Metformin hydrochloride (p.332·3).
Diabetes mellitus.

Difosfen
Rubio, Spain; Rubio, Spain.
Disodium etidronate (p.752·1).
Ectopic ossification; osteoporosis; Paget's disease of bone.

Difosfocin *Magis, Ital.*
Citicoline (p.1596·1).
Cerebrovascular disorders; parkinsonism.

Difosfonal *SPA, Ital.*
Disodium clodronate (p.751·2).
Hyperparathyroidism; multiple myeloma; osteolytic tumours; osteoporosis.

Difoxacil *Química y Farmacia, Mex.*
Norfloxacin (p.232·1).
Bacterial infections.

Dif-Per-Tet-All
Chiron, Ital.; Chiron, Thai.
An adsorbed diphtheria, tetanus, and pertussis vaccine (p.1537·3).
Active immunisation.

Difrarel
Note. This name is used for preparations of different composition.
Leurquin, Fr.
Myrtillus (p.1639·2); betacarotene (p.1355·1).
Peripheral vascular disorders.

Sigma-Tau, Ger.; Tecnifar, Port.; Sigma-Tau, Spain.
Myrtillus (p.1639·2).
Vascular disorders.

Difrarel E
Note. This name is used for preparations of different composition.
Leurquin, Fr.; Sigma-Tau, Spain.
Myrtillus (p.1639·2); vitamin E (p.1393·3).
Myopias; vascular disorders.

Leurquin, Hong Kong.
Vitamin E (p.1393·3); anthrocyanosides.
Myopias.

Difrin *Vitamed, Israel.*
Dipivefrine hydrochloride (p.1604·3).
Glaucoma.

Diftavax
Pasteur Merieux, Fr.†; Aventis, Irl.; Pasteur Merieux, Spain; Pasteur Merieux, UK.
An adsorbed diphtheria and tetanus vaccine (p.1537·3).
Active immunisation of older children and adults.

Dif-Tet-All
Chiron, Ital.; Chiron, Thai.
An adsorbed diphtheria and tetanus vaccine (p.1537·3).
Active immunisation.

Difur *Cantabria, Spain.*
Polypodium leucotomos.
Skin disorders.

Difuran *The Forty-Two, Thai.*
Furazolidone (p.592·1); kaolin (p.1229·3); pectin (p.1502·3).
Gastrointestinal infections.

Digacin *Lilly, Ger.*
Digoxin (p.870·1).
Arrhythmias; heart failure.

Digaol *Ioltech, Fr.*
Timolol maleate (p.982·1).
Glaucoma; ocular hypertension.

Digaril *Solvay, Spain.*
Fluvastatin sodium (p.892·1).
Atherosclerosis; hyperlipidaemias.

Digassim *Vitoria, Port.*
Fluoxetine hydrochloride (p.284·2).
Depression.

Digastril *Brasmedica, Braz.*
Aluminium hydroxide (p.1210·3); magnesium hydroxide (p.1233·1); kaolin (p.1229·3).
Gastrointestinal hyperacidity.

Digecap *Novaquimica, Braz.*
Bromopride (p.1215·1).
Nausea and vomiting.

Digecap-Zimatico *Novaquimica, Braz.*
Bromopride (p.1215·1); dimethicone (p.1249·2); pancreatin (p.1646·1).
Digestive disorders; nausea and vomiting.

Digedryl *Monot, Fr.*
Anhydrous sodium sulfate (p.1250·1); monobasic sodium phosphate (p.1193·2).
Dyspepsia.

Digeflash *Boehringer Ingelheim, Fr.*
Pancreas.
Dyspepsia.

Di-Gel
Plough, Port.; Schering-Plough, USA.
Aluminium hydroxide (p.1210·3); magnesium hydroxide (p.1233·1); simeticone (p.1249·2).
Dyspepsia; gastric hyperacidity.

Di-Gel Forte *Plough, Port.*
Aluminium hydroxide-magnesium carbonate co-dried gel (p.1211·2); magnesium hydroxide (p.1233·1); calcium carbonate (p.1215·1); simeticone (p.1249·2).
Dyspepsia; flatulence; gastric hyperacidity.

Digelax *Searle, Ital.*
Boldo (p.1585·3); rhubarb (p.1248·1); cascara (p.1216·1); cynara (p.1601·3); croton eleuteria; inositol (p.1623·3).
Constipation.

Digenac *Ethical Generics, UK†.*
Diclofenac sodium (p.30·3).

Digenor Plus *Rudefsa, Mex.*
Metoclopramide hydrochloride (p.1235·2); dimethicone (p.1249·2); papain (p.1647·3).
Adjunct in gastrointestinal procedures; gastrointestinal disorders.

Digepepsin *Kenwood, USA.*
Pepsin (p.1649·3); pancreatin (p.1646·1); bile salts (p.1585·1).

Digeplus *Ache, Braz.*
Metoclopramide (p.1236·3); dimethicone (p.1249·2); dehydrocholic acid (p.1602·2); cellulase (p.1593·1); pepsin (p.1649·3); pancreatin (p.1646·1).
Digestive disorders.

Digerall *Falqui, Braz.*
Alginic acid (p.1498·3); aluminium hydroxide (p.1210·3); magnesium trisilicate (p.1233·3); sodium bicarbonate (p.1186·2).
Gastrointestinal disorders.

Digerent *Polifarma, Ital.*
Trimebutine maleate (p.1675·1).
Gastrointestinal disorders.

Digerex *De Mayo, Braz.*
Bromopride (p.1215·1).
Nausea and vomiting.

Digervin *Alacan, Spain.*
Famotidine (p.1225·3).
Gastro-oesophageal reflux; peptic ulcer; Zollinger-Ellison syndrome.

Digesan *Synthelabo, Braz.*
Bromopride (p.1215·1).
Nausea and vomiting.

Di-Gesic
Dista, Austral.; Lilly, NZ.
Dextropropoxyphene hydrochloride (p.27·1) or dextropropoxyphene napsilate (p.27·1); paracetamol (p.71·2).
Pain.

Digesnorma *INQ, Braz.*
Amylase (p.1579·3); aluminium hydroxide (p.1210·3); magnesium hydroxide (p.1233·1); dimethicone (p.1249·2).
Flatulence; gastrointestinal disorders.

Digess *Axcan, Canad.†.*
Pancrelipase (p.1647·2).
Pancreatic insufficiency.

Digest
Note. This name is used for preparations of different composition.
Heralds, Braz.
Metoclopramide (p.1236·3); dimethicone (p.1249·2).
Nausea and vomiting.

Modern Health Products, UK.
Parsley (p.1648·3); centaury (p.1593·1); althaea root (p.1577·1).
Dyspepsia; flatulence.

Digestaid *Eagle, Austral.*
Betaine hydrochloride (p.1584·3); pepsin (p.1649·3); pancreatin (p.1646·1); ox bile salt (p.1585·1); bromelain (p.1586·3); papain (p.1647·3); maltase (p.1576·3); potassium chloride (p.1194·3); gentian (p.1615·1); fennel; peppermint oil (p.1243·3); chromium chelate (p.1357·1).
Gastrointestinal disorders.

Digestal *Odontofarma, Braz.*
Pancreatin (p.1646·1); ox bile (p.1585·1).
Digestive disorders.

Digestelact *Nutricia, Austral.*
Food for special diets (p.1350·1).
Lactose intolerance.

Digestif Marga *Cooperation Pharmaceutique, Fr.*
Magnesium hydroxide (p.1233·1); dried aluminium hydroxide (p.1210·3); calcium carbonate (p.1215·1).
Gastrointestinal disorders.

Digestif Rennie
Note. This name is used for preparations of different composition.
Roche, Aust.
Papain (p.1647·3); pancreatin (p.1646·1); calcium carbonate (p.1215·1); magnesium carbonate (p.1232·3).
Dyspepsia.

Roche Consumer, Irl.; Roche, S.Afr.
Calcium carbonate (p.1215·1); magnesium carbonate (p.1232·3).
Gastric hyperacidity; heartburn.

Digestif-Ara *Rafa, Israel.*
Magnesium carbonate (p.1232·3); magnesium peroxide (p.1149·3); magnesium oxide (p.1233·2); calcium carbonate (p.1215·1); kaolin (p.1229·3); peppermint oil (p.1243·3).
Calcium supplement; dyspepsia; flatulence; gastrointestinal hyperacidity.

Digestin *Chew, Thai.*
Mamylase; amylase (p.1579·3); thiamine nitrate (p.1385·1); scopolia; sodium bicarbonate (p.1186·2); calcium carbonate (p.1215·1); dried aluminium hydroxide gel (p.1210·3).
Gastrointestinal disorders.

Digestina *Uniao Quimica, Braz.*
Bromopride (p.1215·1).
Nausea and vomiting.

Digestinas Super *Geminis, Spain†.*
Aluminium glycinate (p.1210·3); aluminium hydroxide (p.1210·3).
Gastrointestinal hyperacidity.

Digestion L114 *Homeocan, Canad.*
Homoeopathic preparation.

Digestive *Dorwest, UK.*
Ginger (p.1227·2); hydrastis (p.1621·1); rhubarb (p.1248·1); valerian (p.1678·3).
Dyspepsia; heartburn.

Digestive Aid *Blackmores, Austral.*
Slippery elm (p.1665·1); fennel (p.1610·1); ginger (p.1227·2); gentian (p.1615·1); papain (p.1647·3); bromelains (p.1586·3); peppermint leaf (p.1243·2); anise oil (p.1580·3).
Digestive disorders.

Digestive Rennie *Roche Consumer, Austral.*
Calcium carbonate (p.1215·1); heavy magnesium carbonate (p.1232·3).
Dyspepsia; flatulence.

Digestivo Antonetto *Antonetto, Ital.*
Anionic resin; glycine (p.1365·3); calcium carbonate (p.1215·1).
Gastric hyperacidity.

Digestivo Giuliani *Giuliani, Ital.*
Domperidone (p.1224·1).
Dyspepsia.

Digestivo Rennie *Roche Nicholas, Spain.*
Calcium carbonate (p.1215·1); magnesium carbonate (p.1232·3); peppermint oil (p.1243·3).
Gastrointestinal hyperacidity; heartburn; meteorism.

Digestivum-Hetterich S *Galenika, Ger.*
Gentian (p.1615·1).
Gastrointestinal disorders.

Digest-Merz *Merz, Ger.*
Turmeric (p.1029·3); dimethicone (p.1249·2).
Formerly contained porcine pancreatin, Javanese turmeric, and dimethicone.
Digestive system disorders.

Digestodoron
Note. This name is used for preparations of different composition.
Weleda, Aust.
Male fern (p.102·2); polypodium leaf; scolopendrium vulgare; salix leaf (p.82·1).
Gastrointestinal disorders.

Weleda, Fr.
Homoeopathic preparation.

Weleda, UK.
Male fern (p.102·2); polypodium; scolopendrium; salix alba (p.82·1); salix purpurea (p.82·1); salix viminalis; salix vitellina.
Dyspepsia; flatulence.

Digestol *Richter, Aust.*
Gentian (p.1615·1); bitter-orange peel (p.1644·2); taraxacum (p.1669·1).
Gastrointestinal disorders.

Digestol Sanatorium *Santiveri, Spain.*
Aniseed (p.1580·2); centaurium erythraea (p.1593·1); gentian (p.1615·1); chamomile (p.1593·2); melissa (p.1632·2); peppermint (p.1243·2).
Digestive disorders; gastric hyperacidity.

Digestomen *Menarini, Belg.*
Betaine hydrochloride (p.1584·3); pepsin (p.1649·3); papain (p.1647·3); amylase (p.1579·3); pancreatin (p.1646·1); pancrelipase (p.1647·2); cellulase (p.1593·1).
Digestive disorders due to pancreatic insufficiency.

Digestomen Complex *Menarini, Spain.*
White tablets, pepsin (p.1649·3); red tablets, papain (p.1647·3); amylase (p.1579·3); green tablets, pancreatin (p.1646·1); lipase; cellulase (p.1593·1).
Digestive disorders.

Digeston *QIF, Braz.*
Bromopride (p.1215·1).
Nausea and vomiting.

Digestopan *Menarini, Ital.*
Pepsin (p.1649·3); papain (p.1647·3); amylase (p.1579·3); pancreatin (p.1646·1); pancreatic lipase; cellulase (p.1593·1).
Digestive disorders.

Digestosan *Fresenius Kabi, Aust.*
Ranitidine hydrochloride (p.1245·2).
Acid aspiration; gastro-oesophageal reflux; gastrointestinal haemorrhage; peptic ulcer; Zollinger-Ellison syndrome.

Digestovital *Puerto Galiano, Spain.*
Belladonna (p.463·1); opium (p.69·3); sodium bicarbonate (p.1186·2); sodium citrate (p.1186·2); sodium sul-

---

fate (p.1250·1); star anise; aniseed (p.1580·2) cardamom (p.1591·3).
Gastritis; gastrointestinal hyperacidity; peptic ulcer.

Digestron Lopes, Braz.
Dehydrocholic acid (p.1602·2); aesculus (p.1574·1); drimys winterii; erythroxylon catuaba; cynara (p.1601·3); cnicus benedictus (p.1597·2); sodium phosphate (p.1193·2); liver extract.
Liver disorders.

Digest-X Yucca L110 Homeocan, Canad.
Homoeopathic preparation.

Digezanol Hormona, Mex.
Albendazole (p.95·2).
Giardiasis; worm infections.

Digezyme Cantassium Co., UK.
Betaine hydrochloride (p.1584·3); ox bile (p.1585·1); pepsin (p.1649·3); pancrelipase (p.1647·3); bromelain (p.1586·3).

Digi-Aldopur Kwizda, Aust.
Spironolactone (p.973·2); β-acetyldigoxin (p.827·3).
Arrhythmias; heart failure.

Digibind Glaxo Wellcome, Austral.; Glaxo Wellcome, Canad.; Wellcome, UK; Glaxo Wellcome, USA.
Digoxin-specific antibody fragments (p.1006·3).
Digoxin or digitoxin toxicity.

Digifar Farmila, Ital.
Digitalin (p.1603·2); vitamin P (p.1611·1).
Eye disorders.

Digimed corax, Ger.
Digitoxin (p.869·2).
Heart failure.

Digimerck Merck, Aust.; Merck, Ger.
Digitoxin (p.869·2).
Arrhythmias; heart failure.

Digitaline Procter & Gamble, Belg.; Barrenne, Braz.; Welcker-Lyster, Canad.†; Procter & Gamble, Fr.; Rougier, Hong Kong.
Digitoxin (p.869·2).
Arrhythmias; heart failure.

Digitalis Antidot Boehringer Mannheim, Aust.; Roche, Belg.; Roche, Ger.; Roche, Swed.
Digoxin-specific antibody fragments (p.1006·3).
Digitalis poisoning.

Digitalis Antidote Roche, Singapore.
Digoxin-specific antibody fragments (p.1006·3).
Digitalis poisoning.

Digitalysat Scilla-Digitaloid Ysatfabrik, Ger.
Squill (p.1100·3).
Cardiac disorders.

Digitrin Astra, Norw.†; Tika, Swed.
Digitoxin (p.869·2).
Arrhythmias; heart failure.

Dignobeta Luitpold, Ger.†
Atenolol (p.841·3).
Arrhythmias; hypertension; ischaemic heart disease.

Dignobroxol Luitpold, Ger.†
Ambroxol hydrochloride (p.1084·3).
Respiratory-tract disorders associated with increased or viscous mucus.

Dignodolin Sankyo, Ger.
Flufenamic acid (p.41·1).
Musculoskeletal and joint disorders.

Dignoflex Luitpold, Ger.†
Ibuprofen (p.43·2).
Gout; inflammation; musculoskeletal and joint disorders; pain.

Dignokonstant Sankyo, Ger.
Nifedipine (p.940·1).
Angina pectoris; hypertension.

Dignometoprol Luitpold, Ger.†
Metoprolol tartrate (p.931·2).
Angina pectoris; arrhythmias; hypertension; migraine; myocardial infarction.

Dignonitrat Luitpold, Ger.†
Isosorbide dinitrate (p.915·2).
Angina pectoris; heart failure; pulmonary hypertension.

Dignoretik Sankyo, Ger.
Amiloride hydrochloride (p.835·1); hydrochlorothiazide (p.907·3).
Hypertension; oedema.

Dignotrimazol Luitpold, Ger.†
Clotrimazole (p.382·1).
Fungal skin infections.

Dignover Luitpold, Ger.†
Verapamil hydrochloride (p.989·1).
Angina pectoris; arrhythmias; hypertension.

Dignowell Luitpold, Ger.†
Phenylephrine hydrochloride (p.1097·1); a heparinoid (p.905·2).
Venous insufficiency.

Digomal Malesci, Ital.†
Digoxin (p.870·1).
Cardiac disorders.

Digophton Chauvin ankerpharm, Ger.
Digitalis (p.869·1).
Eye strain.

Digosin Chugai, Jpn.
Digoxin (p.870·1).
Arrhythmias; heart failure.

Digostada Stada, Ger.
β-Acetyldigoxin (p.827·3).
Arrhythmias; heart failure.

Digotab Asta Medica, Ger.
β-Acetyldigoxin (p.827·3).
Arrhythmias; heart failure.

Digox CT, Ger.
β-Acetyldigoxin (p.827·3).
Arrhythmias; heart failure.

Digoxin "Didier" Hormosan, Ger.
β-Acetyldigoxin (p.827·3).
Heart failure.

Digton Areu, Span.
Sulpiride (p.706·1).
Anxiety disorders; psychoses; vertigo.

Di-Hydan Synthelabo, Belg.†; Genopharm, Fr.
Phenytoin (p.357·2).
Arrhythmias; epilepsy; facial neuralgias.

Dihydergot
Note.This name is used for preparations of different composition.
Novartis, Aust.; Novartis, Austral.; Novartis, Belg.; Novartis, Braz.; Novartis, Ger.; Novartis, Neth.; Novartis, Port.; Novartis, S.Afr.; Novartis, Spain; Novartis, Switz.
Injection; oral drops; tablets: Dihydroergotamine mesilate (p.450·3).
Hypotension; migraine and other vascular headaches.
Novartis, Aust.; Novartis, Norw.†; Novartis, Switz.
Nasal spray: Dihydroergotamine mesilate (p.450·3); caffeine (p.761·3).
Migraine.

Dihydergot plus Novartis, Aust.; Novartis, Switz.
Dihydroergotamine mesilate (p.450·3); etilefrine hydrochloride (p.888·1).
Hypotension.

Dihydral Solvay, Belg.†; Solvay, Neth.
Dihydrotachysterol (p.1391·2).
Hypoparathyroidism; renal osteodystrophy; rickets.

Dihydrex Kay, USA†.
Diphenhydramine hydrochloride (p.416·1).
Motion sickness; parkinsonism.

Dihytamin Dresden, Ger.; Temmler, Ger.
Dihydroergotamine mesilate (p.450·3).
Hypotension; migraine and other vascular headaches.

Dihyzin Henning, Ger.
Dihydralazine sulfate (p.874·2).
Hypertension.

Diidergot Novartis, Ital.
Dihydroergotamine mesilate (p.450·3).
Headache; vascular disorders.

Dijex SSL, UK.
Oral liquid: Aluminium hydroxide (p.1210·3); magnesium hydroxide (p.1233·1).
These ingredients can be described by the British Approved Name Co-magaldrox.
Tablets: Aluminium hydroxide-magnesium carbonate co-dried gel (p.1211·2).
Dyspepsia.

Dikacine Continental Pharma, Belg.
Dibekacin sulfate (p.198·3).
Gram-negative bacterial infections; staphylococcal infections.

Dilabar Vita, Spain.
Captopril (p.853·3).
Diabetic nephropathy; heart failure; hypertension; myocardial infarction.

Dilabar Diu Vita, Spain.
Hydrochlorothiazide (p.907·3); captopril (p.853·3).
Hypertension.

Dilaclan CEPA, Spain.
Diltiazem hydrochloride (p.874·3).
Angina pectoris; hypertension.

Dilacor XR Watson, USA.
Diltiazem hydrochloride (p.874·3).
Angina pectoris; hypertension.

Dilacoran Knoll, Mex.
Verapamil hydrochloride (p.989·1).
Angina pectoris; arrhythmias; heart failure; hypertension; myocardial infarction.

Dilacoron Knoll, Braz.
Verapamil hydrochloride (p.989·1).
Angina pectoris; arrhythmias; hypertension; hypertrophic cardiomyopathy; migraine and other vascular headaches.

Diladel Sanofi Synthelabo, Ital.
Diltiazem hydrochloride (p.874·3).
Hypertension; ischaemic heart disease.

Dilaescol Kolassa, Aust.
Buphenine hydrochloride (p.1587·3); thiamine hydrochloride (p.1385·1); aesculus (p.1574·1).
Migraine; peripheral vascular disease; premenstrual syndrome; reflex sympathetic dystrophy.

Dilaflux Medley, Braz.
Nifedipine (p.940·1).
Angina pectoris; hypertension; Raynaud's syndrome.

Dilafurane Sanofi Synthelabo, Spain.
Benziodarone (p.400·1).
Gout; hyperuricaemia.

Dilamax Bialfar, Port.
Salmeterol xinafoate (p.773·3).
Asthma.

Dilanacin Asta Medica, Ger.
Digoxin (p.870·1).
Arrhythmias; heart failure.

Dilangio Compositum Fournier SA, Spain†.
Bencyclane acephyllinate (p.843·3); bencyclane fumarate (p.843·3).
Cardiac disorders; vascular disorders.

Dilanid Rolab, S.Afr.
Isosorbide dinitrate (p.915·2).
Angina pectoris.

Dilanorm Rhone-Poulenc Rorer, Neth.
Celiprolol hydrochloride (p.856·1).
Angina pectoris; hypertension.

Dilantin Parke, Davis, Austral.; Parke, Davis, Canad.; Parke, Davis, Fr.; Parke, Davis, Hong Kong; Parke, Davis, Israel; Parke, Davis, NZ; Parke, Davis, Singapore; Warner-Lambert, Thai.; Parke, Davis, USA.
Phenytoin (p.357·2) or phenytoin sodium (p.357·2).
Arrhythmias; epilepsy.

Dilantin with Phenobarbital Parke, Davis, Canad.†
Phenytoin sodium (p.357·2); phenobarbital (p.355·1).
Epilepsy.

Dilapres Quimifar, Spain†.
Bencyclane fumarate (p.843·3); clonidine hydrochloride (p.860·1); hydrochlorothiazide (p.907·3).
Hypertension.

Dilar Cassenne, Fr.†; Syntex, Mex.
Paramethasone acetate (p.1077·2).
Corticosteroid.

Dilarmine Syntex, Mex.
Paramethasone acetate (p.1077·2); chlorpheniramine [chlorphenamine] maleate (p.412·1).
Hypersenitivity; inflammation.

Dilarterial Llorente, Spain†.
Vincamine (p.1680·1).
Cerebral trauma; cerebrovascular disorders.

Dilatam Abic, Israel; Aspen, S.Afr.; Abic-Teva, Singapore; Abic, Thai.
Diltiazem hydrochloride (p.874·3).
Angina pectoris; hypertension.

Dilatame Sanova, Aust.†
Diltiazem hydrochloride (p.874·3).
Angina pectoris; hypertension.

Dilatol
Note.This name is used for preparations of different composition.
Kolassa, Aust.
Buphenine hydrochloride (p.1587·3).
Inhibition of labour; peripheral vascular disease; uterine relaxant; vascular headache.
Jaba, Port.
Isradipine (p.916·3).
Hypertension.

Dilatol-Chinin Kolassa, Aust.
Buphenine hydrochloride (p.1587·3); quinine sulfate (p.445·1).
Cramp.

Dilatrane Labomed, Fr.
Theophylline (p.777·2) or theophylline sodium acetate (p.783·2).
Obstructive airways disease.

Dilatrate Schwarz, USA.
Isosorbide dinitrate (p.915·2).
Angina pectoris.

Dilatrend Roche, Aust.; Roche, Austral.; Roche, Ger.; Roche, Hong Kong; Roche, Ital.; Lakeside, Mex.; Boehringer Mannheim, Norw.†; Roche, NZ; Roche, S.Afr.; Roche, Singapore; Roche, Switz.; Roche, Thai.
Carvedilol (p.855·2).
Angina pectoris; heart failure; hypertension.

Dilaudid Knoll, Austral.; Knoll, Canad.; Knoll, Ger.; Abbott, USA.
Hydromorphone hydrochloride (p.42·3).
Pain.

Dilaudid Cough Knoll, USA.
Hydromorphone hydrochloride (p.42·3); guaifenesin (p.1092·2).
Coughs.

Dilaudid-Atropin Knoll, Ger.; Knoll, Swed.; Knoll, Switz.
Hydromorphone hydrochloride (p.42·3); atropine sulfate (p.461·1).
Pain; smooth muscle spasm.

Dilbloc Roche, Port.
Carvedilol (p.855·2).
Heart failure; hypertension; ischaemic heart disease.

Dilcard Pacific, NZ.
Diltiazem hydrochloride (p.874·3).
Angina pectoris.

Dilcardia Generics, UK.
Diltiazem hydrochloride (p.874·3).
Angina pectoris; hypertension.

Dilclor Diba, Mex.
Chloramphenicol (p.179·1).
Bacterial infections.

Dilcor
Note.This name is used for preparations of different composition.
Norpharma, Denm.
Diltiazem hydrochloride (p.874·3).
Angina pectoris; hypertension.
BOI, Spain.
Nifedipine (p.940·1).
Angina pectoris; hypertension; Raynaud's syndrome.

Dilcoran Parke, Davis, Aust.†; Isis Puren, Ger.
Pentaerithrityl tetranitrate (p.952·3).
Angina pectoris.

Dilem Douglas, Hong Kong; Ist. Chim. Inter., Ital.; Douglas, Thai.; TTN, Thai.
Diltiazem hydrochloride (p.874·3).
Angina pectoris; hypertension.

Dilena Akzo, Braz.; Organon, Hong Kong; Organon, Mex.; Organon, Port.
11 Tablets, estradiol valerate (p.1473·2); 10 tablets, estradiol valerate (p.1473·2); medroxyprogesterone acetate (p.1480·1).
Menopausal disorders; osteoporosis.

Diletan Vitoria, Port.
Sumatriptan succinate (p.456·1).
Cluster headache; migraine.

Dilfar Fournier, Port.
Diltiazem hydrochloride (p.874·3).
Angina pectoris; hypertension.

Diligan
Note.This name is used for preparations of different composition.
UCB, Aust.; UCB, Port.†
Hydroxyzine (p.419·2) or hydroxyzine hydrochloride (p.419·1); meclozine (p.420·3) or meclozine hydrochloride (p.420·3); nicotinic acid (p.1372·3).
Vestibular disorders.
Rodleben, Ger.; Vedim, Ger.; UCB, Ger.
Hydroxyzine hydrochloride (p.419·1); meclozine hydrochloride (p.420·3).
Ménière's disease; vertigo.

Dilinct Restan, S.Afr.
Etofylline (p.765·1); diphenhydramine hydrochloride (p.416·1); ammonium chloride (p.1085·2); polysorbate 20 (p.1347·3).
Bronchodilator; coughs.

Diliter Pulitzer, Ital.
Diltiazem hydrochloride (p.874·3).
Angina pectoris; heart failure; hypertension.

Dilizem Berlin Pharm, Singapore; Berlin Pharm, Thai.
Diltiazem hydrochloride (p.874·3).
Angina pectoris; hypertension.

Dilmin Medinovum, Fin.
Diltiazem hydrochloride (p.874·3).
Angina pectoris; hypertension.

Diloc Tramedico, Neth.
Diltiazem hydrochloride (p.874·3).
Angina pectoris; hypertension.

Dilocaine Hauck, USA.
Lignocaine [lidocaine] hydrochloride (p.1313·2).
Local anaesthesia.

Dilomil Siam Bheasach, Thai.
Diphenoxylate hydrochloride (p.1222·2).
Atropine sulfate (p.461·1) is included in this preparation to discourage abuse.
Diarrhoea.

Dilomine Kay, USA†.
Dicyclomine [dicycloverine] hydrochloride (p.466·1).
Functional bowel/irritable bowel syndrome.

Dilor Savage, USA.
Diprophylline (p.764·1).
Obstructive airways disease.

Dilor-G Savage, USA.
Diprophylline (p.764·1); guaifenesin (p.1092·2).
Bronchospasm.

Dilosyn Sigma, Austral.
Methdilazine hydrochloride (p.421·3).
Hypersensitivity reactions; pruritus.

Dilotab Zee, Canad.†
Phenylpropanolamine hydrochloride (p.1098·1); paracetamol (p.71·2).

Dilpral Orion, Fin.
Diltiazem hydrochloride (p.874·3).
Angina pectoris; hypertension.

Dilrene Irex, Fr.
Diltiazem hydrochloride (p.874·3).
Angina pectoris; hypertension.

Dilsal TAD, Ger.
Diltiazem hydrochloride (p.874·3).
Angina pectoris; hypertension.

Dilsana Milupa, Hong Kong.
Nutritional supplement with vitamins and minerals (p.1350·1).
Pregnancy and lactation.
Milupa, Switz.†
Preparation for enteral nutrition (p.1350·1).

Dil-Sanorania Lichtenstein, Ger.
Diltiazem hydrochloride (p.874·3).
Angina pectoris; hypertension.

Dilta ABZ, Ger.
Diltiazem hydrochloride (p.874·3).
Angina pectoris; hypertension.

Diltbeta Betapharm, Ger.
Diltiazem hydrochloride (p.874·3).

Diltahexal Hexal, Austral.; Hexal, Ger.
Diltiazem hydrochloride (p.874·3).
Angina pectoris; hypertension.

Diltam Rowex, Irl.
Diltiazem hydrochloride (p.874·3).
Angina pectoris; hypertension.

Diltan Mepha, Hong Kong; Mepha, Thai.
Diltiazem hydrochloride (p.874·3).
Angina pectoris; hypertension.

Diltaretard *Betapharm, Ger.*
Diltiazem hydrochloride (p.874·3).
Angina pectoris; hypertension.

Diltec *Utopian, Thai.*
Diltiazem hydrochloride (p.874·3).
Angina pectoris; hypertension.

Dilti *CT, Ger.; BASF, Ger.*
Diltiazem hydrochloride (p.874·3).
Angina pectoris; hypertension.

Diltia *Andrx, USA.*
Diltiazem hydrochloride (p.874·3).
Angina pectoris; hypertension.

Diltiagamma *Worwag, Ger.*
Diltiazem hydrochloride (p.874·3).
Angina pectoris; hypertension.

Diltiamax *PMC, Austral.†*
Diltiazem hydrochloride (p.874·3).
Angina pectoris.

Diltiamerck *Merck, Ger.†*
Diltiazem hydrochloride (p.874·3).
Angina pectoris; hypertension.

Diltiangina *Tecnimede, Port.†*
Diltiazem hydrochloride (p.874·3).

Diltiem *Sanofi Synthelabo, Port.*
Diltiazem hydrochloride (p.874·3).
Angina pectoris; heart failure; hypertension.

Diltikard *Nycomed, Norw.*
Diltiazem hydrochloride (p.874·3).
Angina pectoris; hypertension.

Diltin *Honorterapica, Braz.*
Sodium picosulfate (p.1249·3).
Bowel evacuation; constipation.

Diltiuc *Merck dura, Ger.*
Diltiazem hydrochloride (p.874·3).
Angina pectoris; hypertension.

Diltiwas *Wasserman, Spain.*
Diltiazem hydrochloride (p.874·3).
Angina pectoris; hypertension.

Diltizem AP *Searle, Braz.*
Diltiazem hydrochloride (p.874·3).
Angina pectoris; hypertension; supraventricular arrhythmias.

Dilubrin *UCI, Braz.*
Dipyrone (p.34·1); metixene hydrochloride (p.470·2).
Fever; pain.

Dilucort *Triomed, S.Afr.*
Hydrocortisone acetate (p.1073·2).
Skin disorders.

Dilum *Tecnifar, Port.*
Isoxsuprine hydrochloride (p.1624·3).
Cerebral and peripheral vascular disorders; relaxation of the uterus.

Dilusol *Dermtek, Canad.*
Alcohol (p.1130·3); isopropyl alcohol; propylene glycol; laureth-4.
Topical vehicle.

Dilusol AHA *Dermtek, Canad.*
Alcohol (p.1130·3); glycolic acid (p.1115·1); polyquaternium 10; polysorbate 20; propylene glycol.
Topical vehicle.

Dilutol *Roche, Spain.*
Torasemide (p.985·1) or torasemide sodium (p.985·2).
Hypertension; oedema.

Dilydrin *Willvonseder, Aust.*
Buphenine hydrochloride (p.1587·3).
Dysmenorrhoea; premature labour.

Dilydrine Retard *Medichemie, Switz.*
Buphenine hydrochloride (p.1587·3).
Peripheral vascular disorders.

Dilzem *Parke, Davis, Aust.; Douglas, Austral.; Orion, Fin.; Godecke, Ger.; Douglas, Hong Kong; Elan, Irl.; Douglas, NZ; Warner-Lambert, Switz.; Pharmasant, Thai.; Elan, UK.*
Diltiazem hydrochloride (p.874·3).
Angina pectoris; arrhythmias; hypertension.

Dilzene *Sigma-Tau, Ital.*
Diltiazem hydrochloride (p.874·3).
Arrhythmias; hypertension; ischaemic heart disease.

Dilzereal *Realpharma, Ger.†*
Diltiazem hydrochloride (p.874·3).
Angina pectoris; hypertension.

Dilzicardin *Azupharma, Ger.*
Diltiazem hydrochloride (p.874·3).
Angina pectoris; hypertension.

Dima *Medochemie, Singapore.*
Nitrazepam (p.695·2).
Insomnia.

Dimac *Lilly, Aust.*
Dirithromycin (p.199·2).
Bacterial infections.

Dimacol *Wyeth, Mex.; Robins, USA.*
Guaifenesin (p.1092·2); pseudoephedrine hydrochloride (p.1099·2); dextromethorphan hydrobromide (p.1087·3).
Coughs; nasal congestion.

Dima-Fen *Stroder, Ital.†*
Fenfluramine hydrochloride (p.1510·1).
Obesity.

Dimagress *Heralds, Braz.*
Tiratricol (p.1528·3).
Lipolytic.

Dimalosio *Tipomark, Ital.*
Lactulose (p.1230·1); glucomannan (p.1616·2).
Gastrointestinal disorders.

Dim-Antos *Pharmonta, Aust.*
Propyphenazone (p.80·2).
Fever; pain.

Dimaphen *Major, USA†*
Phenylpropanolamine hydrochloride (p.1098·1); brompheniramine maleate (p.410·2).
Upper respiratory-tract symptoms.

Dimaval *Heyl, Ger.*
Unithiol (p.1025·3).
Heavy-metal poisoning.

Dimayon *Sabater, Spain†.*
Camphor (p.1589·3); eucalyptol (p.1609·2); niaouli oil (p.1640·2); oxolamine citrate (p.1096·2); paracetamol (p.71·2); choline theophyllinate (p.763·3); vitamin A (p.1382·1).
Influenza and cold symptoms.

Dimefor *Lilly, Mex.*
Metformin hydrochloride (p.332·3).
Diabetes mellitus.

Dimegan
Dexa, Fr.; Kreussler, Ger.†.
Brompheniramine maleate (p.410·2).
Allergic disorders.

Dimelor
Lilly, Canad.†; Lilly, Hong Kong; Quatromed, S.Afr.
Acetohexamide (p.320·1).
Diabetes mellitus.

Dimen *Heumann, Ger.*
Dimenhydrinate (p.415·2).
Dizziness; nausea; vomiting.

Dimenate *DHA, Hong Kong.*
Dimenhydrinate (p.415·2).
Ménière's disease; motion sickness; nausea; vomiting.

Dimenformon *Organon, Belg.*
Estradiol benzoate (p.1473·1); estradiol phenylpropionate (p.1473·2).
Menstrual disorders; oestrogen replacement therapy.

Dimeno *Milano, Thai.*
Dimenhydrinate (p.415·2).
Motion sickness; nausea and vomiting; vertigo.

Dimertest *Agen, Austral.*
Test for fibrin derivatives in plasma.

Dimetabs *Jones, USA.*
Dimenhydrinate (p.415·2).
Motion sickness.

Dimetane
Note. This name is used for preparations of different composition.
Whitehall-Robins, Canad.; Whitehall, Thai.; Robins, USA.
Brompheniramine maleate (p.410·2).
Hypersensitivity reactions.

Whitehall, Fr.
Oral liquid; syrup: Brompheniramine maleate (p.410·2); pholcodine (p.1099·1).
Formerly contained brompheniramine maleate, pholcodine, phenylephrine hydrochloride, guaifenesin, and sodium benzoate.
Coughs.

Paediatric syrup: Brompheniramine maleate (p.410·2); guaifenesin (p.1092·2); sodium benzoate (p.1134·3).
Upper respiratory-tract congestion.

Wyeth, Switz.
Codeine phosphate (p.25·2); phenylephrine hydrochloride (p.1097·1); phenylpropanolamine hydrochloride (p.1098·1); guaifenesin (p.1092·2).
Coughs and associated respiratory-tract disorders.

Dimetane DC *Robins, USA†.*
Brompheniramine maleate (p.410·2); phenylpropanolamine hydrochloride (p.1098·1); codeine phosphate (p.25·2).
Coughs.

Dimetane Decongestant *Robins, USA.*
Brompheniramine maleate (p.410·2); phenylephrine hydrochloride (p.1097·1).
Upper respiratory-tract symptoms.

Dimetane DX *Robins, USA.*
Brompheniramine maleate (p.410·2); pseudoephedrine hydrochloride (p.1099·2); dextromethorphan hydrobromide (p.1087·3).
Coughs.

Dimetane Expect *Wyeth Lederle, Fin.*
Brompheniramine maleate (p.410·2); guaifenesin (p.1092·2); phenylpropanolamine hydrochloride (p.1098·1); phenylephrine hydrochloride (p.1097·1).
Respiratory-tract disorders.

Dimetane Expect DC *Wyeth Lederle, Fin.*
Codeine phosphate (p.25·2); brompheniramine maleate (p.410·2); guaifenesin (p.1092·2); phenylpropanolamine hydrochloride (p.1098·1); phenylephrine hydrochloride (p.1097·1).
Respiratory-tract disorders.

Dimetane Expectorant
Whitehall-Robins, Canad.†; Whitehall, Thai.
Brompheniramine maleate (p.410·2); guaifenesin (p.1092·2); phenylephrine hydrochloride (p.1097·1); phenylpropanolamine hydrochloride (p.1098·1).
Upper respiratory-tract disorders.

Dimetane Expectorant C *Whitehall-Robins, Canad.†.*
Brompheniramine maleate (p.410·2); phenylephrine hydrochloride (p.1097·1); phenylpropanolamine hydrochloride (p.1098·1); guaifenesin (p.1092·2); codeine phosphate (p.25·2).
Upper respiratory-tract disorders.

Dimetane Expectorant DC
Note. This name is used for preparations of different composition.
Whitehall-Robins, Canad.†.
Brompheniramine maleate (p.410·2); hydrocodone tartrate (p.42·2); guaifenesin (p.1092·2); phenylephrine hydrochloride (p.1097·1); phenylpropanolamine hydrochloride (p.1098·1).
Upper respiratory-tract disorders.

Whitehall, Thai.
Brompheniramine maleate (p.410·2); phenylephrine hydrochloride (p.1097·1); phenylpropanolamine hydrochloride (p.1098·1); guaifenesin (p.1092·2); codeine phosphate (p.25·2).
Coughs; hypersensitivity reactions.

Dimetapp
Note. This name is used for preparations of different composition.
Whitehall, Austral.
Brompheniramine maleate (p.410·2); phenylephrine hydrochloride (p.1097·1).
Upper respiratory-tract symptoms.

Whitehall, Braz.; Whitehall-Robins, Canad.†; Robins, Hong Kong; Aspen Consumer, S.Afr.; Wyeth, Switz.; Whitehall, Thai.
Elixir; oral drops; tablets: Brompheniramine maleate (p.410·2); phenylephrine hydrochloride (p.1097·1); phenylpropanolamine hydrochloride (p.1098·1).
Upper respiratory-tract symptoms.

Robins, Hong Kong; Wyeth, Mex.; Whitehall, Thai.
Extentabs: Brompheniramine maleate (p.410·2); phenylpropanolamine hydrochloride (p.1098·1).
Upper respiratory-tract symptoms.

Whitehall-Robins, USA.
Brompheniramine maleate (p.410·2); pseudoephedrine hydrochloride (p.1099·2).
Formerly contained brompheniramine maleate and phenylpropanolamine hydrochloride.
Allergic rhinitis; nasal congestion.

Dimetapp Chewables *Whitehall-Robins, Canad.†.*
Brompheniramine maleate (p.410·2); phenylpropanolamine hydrochloride (p.1098·1).
Upper respiratory-tract disorders.

Dimetapp Clear *Whitehall-Robins, Canad.†.*
Brompheniramine maleate (p.410·2); phenylpropanolamine hydrochloride (p.1098·1).
Upper respiratory-tract symptoms.

Dimetapp Cold & Allergy Chewable *Robins, USA†.*
Brompheniramine maleate (p.410·2); phenylpropanolamine hydrochloride (p.1098·1).
Upper respiratory-tract symptoms.

Dimetapp Cold, Cough & Flu *Whitehall, Austral.*
Day & Night Liquid Capsules: Day capsules, dextromethorphan hydrobromide (p.1087·3); pseudoephedrine hydrochloride (p.1099·2); paracetamol (p.71·2); night capsules, dextromethorphan hydrobromide; pseudoephedrine hydrochloride; doxylamine succinate (p.417·1); paracetamol.
Cold and cough.

Liquid Capsules: Dextromethorphan hydrobromide (p.1087·3); pseudoephedrine hydrochloride (p.1099·2); guaifenesin (p.1092·2); paracetamol (p.71·2).
Cold and influenza symptoms; coughs.

Dimetapp Cold, Cough & Sinus *Whitehall, Austral.*
Dextromethorphan hydrobromide (p.1087·3); pseudoephedrine hydrochloride (p.1099·2); guaifenesin (p.1092·2).
Coughs; nasal congestion.

Dimetapp Cold & Fever *Whitehall-Robins, USA.*
Pseudoephedrine hydrochloride (p.1099·2); brompheniramine maleate (p.410·2); paracetamol (p.71·2).
Cold symptoms.

Dimetapp Cold & Flu
Note. This name is used for preparations of different composition.
Whitehall, Austral.
Dextromethorphan hydrobromide (p.1087·3); pseudoephedrine hydrochloride (p.1099·2); paracetamol (p.71·2).
Cold and influenza symptoms; coughs.

Robins, USA†.
Brompheniramine maleate (p.410·2); phenylpropanolamine hydrochloride (p.1098·1); paracetamol (p.71·2).
Upper respiratory-tract symptoms.

Dimetapp Cough & Cold Liqui-Gels *Whitehall-Robins, Canad.†.*
Brompheniramine maleate (p.410·2); phenylpropanolamine hydrochloride (p.1098·1); dextromethorphan hydrobromide (p.1087·3).
Coughs and cold symptoms.

Dimetapp Cough Expectorant *SA Druggists Self Med, S.Afr.†*
Guaifenesin (p.1092·2).
Coughs.

Dimetapp Decongestant *Whitehall-Robins, USA.*
Pseudoephedrine hydrochloride (p.1099·2).
Nasal congestion.

Dimetapp Decongestant Plus Cough *Whitehall-Robins, USA.*
Pseudoephedrine hydrochloride (p.1099·2); dextromethorphan hydrobromide (p.1087·3).
Coughs; nasal congestion.

Dimetapp DM
Note. This name is used for preparations of different composition.
Whitehall, Austral.
Brompheniramine maleate (p.410·2); phenylephrine hydrochloride (p.1097·1); dextromethorphan hydrobromide (p.1087·3).
Upper respiratory-tract symptoms.

Whitehall-Robins, Canad.†.
Brompheniramine maleate (p.410·2); phenylephrine hydrochloride (p.1097·1); phenylpropanolamine hydrochloride (p.1098·1); dextromethorphan hydrobromide (p.1087·3).
Cold symptoms; upper respiratory-tract disorders.

Whitehall-Robins, Canad.†.
Brompheniramine maleate (p.410·2); pseudoephedrine hydrochloride (p.1099·2); dextromethorphan hydrobromide (p.1087·3).
Formerly contained brompheniramine maleate, phenylpropanolamine hydrochloride, and dextromethorphan hydrobromide.
Coughs and cold symptoms.

Dimetapp Expectorante *Whitehall, Braz.*
Brompheniramine maleate (p.410·2); phenylephrine hydrochloride (p.1097·1); phenylpropanolamine hydrochloride (p.1098·1); guaifenesin (p.1092·2).
Nasal congestion.

Dimetapp 12 Hour Nasal *Whitehall, Austral.*
Oxymetazoline hydrochloride (p.1096·2).
Nasal congestion.

Dimetapp LA *Whitehall, Austral.†.*
Brompheniramine maleate (p.410·2); phenylephrine hydrochloride (p.1097·1); phenylpropanolamine hydrochloride (p.1098·1).
Upper respiratory tract symptoms.

Dimetapp Liqui-Gels *Whitehall-Robins, Canad.†.*
Brompheniramine maleate (p.410·2); phenylpropanolamine hydrochloride (p.1098·1).
Upper respiratory-tract disorders.

Dimetapp Nighttime Flu *Whitehall-Robins, USA.*
Pseudoephedrine hydrochloride (p.1099·2); dextromethorphan hydrobromide (p.1087·3); paracetamol (p.71·2); brompheniramine maleate (p.410·2).
Coughs and cold symptoms.

Dimetapp Non-Drowsy Flu *Whitehall-Robins, USA.*
Pseudoephedrine hydrochloride (p.1099·2); dextromethorphan hydrobromide (p.1087·3); paracetamol (p.71·2).
Coughs and cold symptoms.

Dimetapp Oral Infant Drops *Whitehall-Robins, Canad.†.*
Brompheniramine maleate (p.410·2); phenylephrine hydrochloride (p.1097·1); phenylpropanolamine hydrochloride (p.1098·1).
Cold symptoms; hypersensitivity reactions.

Dimetapp Quick Dissolve *Whitehall-Robins, Canad.†.*
Brompheniramine maleate (p.410·2); phenylpropanolamine hydrochloride (p.1098·1).
Respiratory-tract disorders.

Dimetapp Sinus
Note. This name is used for preparations of different composition.
Whitehall, Austral.
Pseudoephedrine hydrochloride (p.1099·2).
Nasal and sinus congestion.

Robins, USA.
Pseudoephedrine hydrochloride (p.1099·2); ibuprofen (p.43·2).
Nasal congestion.

Dimetapp-A Sinus *Whitehall-Robins, Canad.†.*
Phenylephrine hydrochloride (p.1097·1); phenylpropanolamine hydrochloride (p.1098·1); paracetamol (p.71·2).
Cold symptoms.

Dimetapp-C *Whitehall-Robins, Canad.†.*
Brompheniramine maleate (p.410·2); phenylpropanolamine hydrochloride (p.1098·1); phenylephrine hydrochloride (p.1097·1); codeine phosphate (p.25·2).
Cold symptoms; upper respiratory-tract disorders.

Dimethicream *Hamilton, Austral.*
Dimethicone (p.1410·1); cetrimide (p.1137·1).
Emollient barrier cream.

Dimetigal *Galen, Mex.*
Cimetidine (p.1216·3).

Dime-Time *Time-Cap, Hong Kong.*
Brompheniramine maleate (p.410·2); phenylephrine hydrochloride (p.1097·1); phenylpropanolamine hydrochloride (p.1098·1).
Upper respiratory-tract symptoms.

Dimetin-F *Farcoral, Mex.*
Dimenhydrinate (p.415·2).
Nausea and vomiting.

Dimetriose
Hoechst Marion Roussel, Austral.; Aventis, NZ; Roussel, Port.; Hoechst Marion Roussel, Singapore; Hoechst Marion Roussel, Thai.; Florizel, UK.
Gestrinone (p.1479·2).
Endometriosis.

Dimetrose
Piette, Belg.†; Hoechst Marion Roussel, Braz.; Searle, Ital.
Gestrinone (p.1479·2).
Endometriosis.

Dimex *Cazi, Braz.*
Dipyrone (p.34·1); diphenhydramine hydrochloride (p.416·1).
Fever; pain.

Dimicaps *Pharmacps, Mex.*
Dimenhydrinate (p.415·2).

Dimicin *Bergamo, Braz.*
Phthalylsulfacetamide; neomycin (p.228·1); aluminium hydroxide (p.1210·3).
Diarrhoea.

Dimicina *Codilab, Port.*
Bacitracin (p.155·2); neomycin sulfate (p.228·1).
Diarrhoea.

The symbol † denotes a preparation no longer actively marketed

Di-Mill *SIT, Ital.*
Benzalkonium chloride (p.1133·2).
Eye disinfection; eye irritation.

Diminex *Rhone-Poulenc Rorer, Mex.*
Phentermine (p.1514·1).

Diminex Antitusigeno *Vinas, Spain.*
Eucalyptol (p.1609·2); chlorcyclizine hydrochloride (p.411·3); codeine phosphate (p.25·2); guaifenesin (p.1092·2).
Respiratory-tract disorders.

Diminex Balsamico *Vinas, Spain†.*
Eucalyptol (p.1609·2); chlorcyclizine hydrochloride (p.411·3); chlorpromazine hydrochloride (p.660·2); dextromethorphan hydrobromide (p.1087·3); niaouli oil (p.1640·2); guaifenesin (p.1092·2).
Respiratory-tract disorders.

Dimiprol
Note.This name is used for preparations of different composition.
Propan, S.Afr.†.
Tablets: Paracetamol (p.71·2); codeine phosphate (p.25·2); caffeine (p.761·3); meprobamate (p.691·1).
Pain; tension.

Zurich, S.Afr.†.
Syrup: Paracetamol (p.71·2); codeine phosphate (p.25·2); promethazine hydrochloride (p.423·2).
Pain; tension.

Dimitone *Roche, Belg.; Roche, Denm.; Abic, Israel.*
Carvedilol (p.855·2).
Angina pectoris; heart failure; hypertension.

Dimodan *Hoechst Marion Roussel, Mex.*
Disopyramide (p.878·2).
Arrhythmias.

Dimophen *Nakornpatana, Thai.*
Dextromethorphan hydrobromide (p.1087·3); phenylpropanolamine hydrochloride (p.1098·1); chlorpheniramine [chlorphenamine] maleate (p.412·1); terpin hydrate (p.1101·2).
Coughs.

Dimophen DC *Nakornpatana, Thai.*
Diphenhydramine hydrochloride (p.416·1); ammonium chloride (p.1085·2); sodium citrate (p.1186·2).
Coughs.

Dimor *Nordic, Swed.*
Loperamide hydrochloride (p.1231·3).
Diarrhoea.

Dimorf *Cristalia, Braz.*
Morphine sulfate (p.56·1).
Pain.

Dimotane *Wyeth, UK.*
Brompheniramine maleate (p.410·2).
Allergic rhinitis; urticaria.

Dimotane Co *Whitehall, Irl.; Whitehall, UK.*
Brompheniramine maleate (p.410·2); codeine phosphate (p.25·2); pseudoephedrine hydrochloride (p.1099·2).
Formerly contained codeine phosphate, guaifenesin, phenylephrine hydrochloride, phenylpropanolamine hydrochloride, and brompheniramine maleate in Irl.
Coughs.

Dimotane Expectorant *Whitehall, Irl.; Whitehall, UK.*
Brompheniramine maleate (p.410·2); guaifenesin (p.1092·2); pseudoephedrine hydrochloride (p.1099·2).
Formerly contained phenylephrine hydrochloride, phenylpropanolamine hydrochloride, brompheniramine maleate, and guaifenesin.
Upper respiratory-tract disorders.

Dimotane Plus *Wyeth, UK.*
Brompheniramine maleate (p.410·2); pseudoephedrine hydrochloride (p.1099·2).
Allergic rhinitis.

Dimotapp *Whitehall, Irl.; Whitehall, UK.*
Brompheniramine maleate (p.410·2); phenylephrine hydrochloride (p.1097·1); phenylpropanolamine hydrochloride (p.1098·1).
Upper respiratory-tract disorders.

Dimotapp Expectorant *Whitehall, Fr.*
Carbocisteine (p.1086·3).
Respiratory-tract disorders.

Dina *San Carlo, Ital.*
Cimetidine (p.1216·3).
Gastrointestinal disorders associated with hyperacidity.

Dinabac *Lilly, Ital.†.*
Dirithromycin (p.199·2).
Bacterial infections.

Dinac *Douglas, Austral.; Masa, Thai.*
Diclofenac sodium (p.30·3).
Dysmenorrhoea; musculoskeletal and joint disorders; pain with inflammation.

Dinacode *Picot, Fr.*
Cream: Turpentine oil (p.1676·3); pine oil (p.1659·3); wild thyme oil; white thyme oil; niaouli oil (p.1640·2); eucalyptol (p.1609·2); quinine sulfate (p.445·1).
Respiratory congestion.

Paediatric suppositories: Potassium borotartrate (p.1653·3); sodium benzoate (p.1134·3); sodium bromide (p.1587·1); phenobarbital (p.355·1).
Paediatric syrup: Sodium benzoate (p.1134·3); grindelia (p.1618·2); wild thyme; tolu balsam (p.1101·3).

Formerly contained sodium bromide, sodium benzoate, grindelia, senega, and tolu balsam.
Coughs.

Dinacode avec codeine *Picot, Fr.*
Suppositories: Codeine (p.25·2); eucalyptol (p.1609·2).
Formerly contained codeine, belladonna, stramonium, and sodium benzoate.

Syrup; paediatric syrup: Sodium benzoate (p.1134·3); wild thyme; tolu balsam (p.1101·3); codeine (p.25·2).
Formerly contained sodium benzoate, sulfogaiacol, belladonna, grindelia, senega, tolu balsam, and codeine.
Coughs.

Dinacode N *Picot, Switz.*
Syrup: Codeine (p.25·2); sodium benzoate (p.1134·3); thyme (p.1672·2); tolu balsam (p.1101·3).
Tablets: Codeine (p.25·2); sodium benzoate (p.1134·3).
Coughs.

Dinagen *Hormona, Mex.*
Piracetam (p.1652·1).
Cerebrovascular disease.

Dinapres *Master Pharma, Ital.*
Delapril (p.867·1); indapamide (p.913·1).
Hypertension.

Dinasepte *Cosmofarma, Port.†.*
Povidone-iodine (p.1155·1).
Skin and vulvovaginal infections; skin, burn, and vaginal disinfection.

Dinate *Seatrace, USA.*
Dimenhydrinate (p.415·2).
Motion sickness.

Dinaxil *Tecnifar, Port.*
Triprolidine hydrochloride (p.427·2); pseudoephedrine hydrochloride (p.1099·2).
Allergic rhinitis; asthma; hypersensitivity; urticaria.

Dinaxin *Rayere, Mex.*
Ranitidine (p.1246·3).
Peptic ulcer.

Dinazide *TO-Chemicals, Thai.*
Triamterene (p.986·1); hydrochlorothiazide (p.907·3).
Hypertension; oedema.

Dindevan *Boots, Austral.; Goldshield, UK†.*
Phenindione (p.954·1).
Thromboembolic disorders.

Dinefec *British Dispensary, Thai.*
Diclofenac diethylamine (p.30·2).
Inflammation; musculoskeletal, joint, peri-articular, and soft-tissue disorders; pain.

Diniket *Schwarz, Ital.*
Isosorbide dinitrate (p.915·2).
Angina pectoris; heart failure.

Dinill *Allergan-Frumtost, Braz.*
Benzalkonium chloride (p.1133·2); boric acid (p.1586·1); borax (p.1586·1); hamamelis (p.1618·3); chamomile (p.1593·2).
Eye disorders.

Dinintel *Diamant, Fr.†; Diamant, Port.†; Diamant, Singapore.*
Clobenzorex hydrochloride (p.1507·2).
Obesity.

Dinisor *Parke, Davis, Spain.*
Diltiazem hydrochloride (p.874·3).
Angina pectoris; hypertension.

Dinistenile *Lepori, Port.*
Prasterone sodium sulfate (p.1488·2).
Anabolic; tonic.

Dinit *Leiras, Fin.*
Isosorbide dinitrate (p.915·2).
Angina pectoris; heart failure.

Dinneford's *SmithKline Beecham Consumer, UK†.*
Heavy magnesium carbonate (p.1232·3); citric acid monohydrate (p.1596·2); sodium bicarbonate (p.1186·2).

Dinnefords Teejel *SSL, UK.*
Choline salicylate (p.24·3).
Denture irritation; herpes labialis; mouth ulcers; teething pain.

Dinobroxol *Sankyo, Spain.*
Ambroxol hydrochloride (p.1084·3).
Respiratory-tract disorders.

Dinostral *Helvepharm, Switz.*
Oxpentifylline [pentoxifylline] (p.950·3).
Vascular disorders.

Dinoven *Sankyo, Spain.*
A heparinoid (p.905·2).
Soft-tissue disorders; varices.

Dintoina *Recordati, Ital.*
Phenytoin sodium (p.357·2).
Arrhythmias; epilepsy; trigeminal neuralgia.

Dintoinale *Recordati, Ital.*
Phenytoin sodium (p.357·2); methylphenobarbital (p.353·3).
Epilepsy.

Dinul *Tecnifar, Port.†.*
Famotidine (p.1225·3).
Gastro-oesophageal reflux; peptic ulcer; Zollinger-Ellison syndrome.

Dio *Sciencex, Fr.*
Diosmin (p.1611·1).
Capillary fragility; haemorrhoids; venous insufficiency.

Dioalgo *Bouchara, Fr.*
Dextropropoxyphene hydrochloride (p.27·1); paracetamol (p.71·2).
Pain.

Diocaine *Dioptic, Canad.*
Proxymetacaine hydrochloride (p.1320·1).
Local anaesthesia.

Diocalm *SmithKline Beecham Consumer, Irl.†.*
Morphine hydrochloride (p.56·1); attapulgite (p.1212·1); activated attapulgite.
Diarrhoea.

Diocalm Dual Action *SSL, UK.*
Morphine hydrochloride (p.56·1); attapulgite (p.1212·1).
Formerly known as Diocalm.
Diarrhoea.

Diocalm Replenish *Seton, UK†.*
Anhydrous glucose; sodium chloride; sodium citrate; potassium chloride (p.1185·2).
Formerly known as Diocalm Junior.
Diarrhoea; oral rehydration therapy.

Diocalm Ultra *SSL, UK.*
Loperamide hydrochloride (p.1231·3).
Diarrhoea.

Diocaps *Berk, UK.*
Loperamide hydrochloride (p.1231·3).
Diarrhoea.

Diocarpine *Dioptic, Canad.*
Pilocarpine hydrochloride (p.1422·3).
Cholinergic; production of miosis.

Diochloram *Dioptic, Canad.*
Chloramphenicol (p.179·1).
Bacterial eye infections.

Diocimex *Cimex, Switz.*
Doxycycline hyclate (p.200·1).
Bacterial infections.

Diocto-K *Rugby, USA†.*
Docusate potassium (p.1223·1).
Constipation.

Diocto-K Plus *Rugby, USA†.*
Docusate potassium (p.1223·1); casanthranol (p.1216·1).
Constipation.

Dioctolose Plus *Goldline, USA†.*
Docusate potassium (p.1223·1); casanthranol (p.1216·1).
Constipation.

Dioctosal *Libbs, Braz.*
Docusate sodium (p.1223·1); phenolphthalein (p.1244·1); dehydrocholic acid (p.1602·2); cascara (p.1216·1); magnesium sulfate (p.1191·1).
Constipation.

Dioctyl *Everest, Canad.; Schwarz, UK.*
Docusate sodium (p.1223·1).
Constipation.

Dioderm *Dermal Laboratories, Irl.; Dermal Laboratories, UK.*
Hydrocortisone (p.1073·3).
Dermatitis; eczema.

Diodex *Dioptic, Canad.*
Dexamethasone sodium phosphate (p.1067·1).
Corticosteroid.

Diodine *Marc-O, Canad.*
Iodine (p.1522·3); isopropyl alcohol (p.1149·2); potassium iodide (p.1522·3).
Iodine supplement.

Diodolina *Mayo, Mex.*
Diiodohydroxyquinoline (p.590·2).

Diodoquin *Glenwood, Canad.; Searle, Mex.*
Diiodohydroxyquinoline (p.590·2).
Amoebiasis.

Dioeze *Century, USA†.*
Docusate sodium (p.1223·1).
Constipation.

Diofluor *Dioptic, Canad.*
Fluorescein sodium (p.1612·1).
Aid to ophthalmic examination.

Diogent *Dioptic, Canad.*
Gentamicin sulfate (p.210·1).
Bacterial eye infections.

Diolaxil *Synthelabo, Spain.*
Sennosides A and B (p.1248·3).
Constipation.

Diolin *Chinta, Thai.*
Syrup: Streptomycin sulfate (p.249·1); furazolidone (p.592·1); kaolin (p.1229·3); pectin (p.1502·3); belladonna tincture (p.463·1); ipecacuanha tincture (p.1093·1).
Tablets: Diiodohydroxyquinoline (p.590·2); furazolidone (p.592·1); kaolin (p.1229·3); pectin (p.1502·3); atropine sulfate (p.461·1).
Gastrointestinal infections.

Diomicete *Oftalder, Port.*
Clotrimazole (p.382·1).
Fungal eye infections.

Diomycin *Dioptic, Canad.*
Erythromycin (p.201·2).
Bacterial eye infections.

Diondel *Sanofi Synthelabo, Spain†.*
Metolazone (p.930·3).
Hypertension; oedema.

Dionephrine *Dioptic, Canad.*
Phenylephrine hydrochloride (p.1097·1).

Dionosil *Glaxo Wellcome, Israel.*
Propyliodone (p.1038·2).
Radiographic contrast medium for bronchography.

Dionosil Oily *Allen & Hanburys, USA†.*
Propyliodone (p.1038·2) in arachis oil.
Radiographic contrast medium for bronchography.

Dioparine *Thea, Fr.†; Ciba Vision, Switz.*
Sodium iodoheparinate (p.1666·1).
Burns to the eye; corneal damage.

Diopentolate *Dioptic, Canad.*
Cyclopentolate hydrochloride (p.465·2).
Production of mydriasis and cycloplegia.

Diophenyl-T *Dioptic, Canad.*
Phenylephrine hydrochloride (p.1097·1); tropicamide (p.475·1).
Production of mydriasis and cycloplegia.

Diopine *Allergan, Mex.; Allergan, Neth.†; Allergan, Spain; Allergan, Switz.*
Dipivefrine hydrochloride (p.1604·3).
Glaucoma; ocular hypertension.

Diopred *Dioptic, Canad.*
Prednisolone acetate (p.1078·1).
Eye inflammation.

Diopticon *Dioptic, Canad.*
Naphazoline hydrochloride (p.1095·1).

Diopticon A *Dioptic, Canad.*
Naphazoline hydrochloride (p.1095·1); pheniramine maleate (p.422·3).

Dioptimyd *Dioptic, Canad.*
Sulfacetamide sodium (p.250·3); prednisolone acetate (p.1078·1).
Eye disorders.

Dioptrol *Dioptic, Canad.*
Neomycin sulfate (p.228·1); polymyxin B sulfate (p.238·1); dexamethasone (p.1067·1).
Eye disorders.

Dioralyte *Rhone-Poulenc Rorer, Irl.; Rhone-Poulenc Rorer, Neth.; Rhone-Poulenc Rorer, Port.; Rhone-Poulenc Rorer, UK.*
Sodium chloride; potassium chloride; sodium acid citrate; glucose (p.1185·2).
Diarrhoea; oral rehydration therapy.

Dioralyte Effervescent *Rhone-Poulenc Rorer, UK.*
Sodium chloride; sodium bicarbonate; potassium chloride; citric acid; glucose (p.1185·2).
Diarrhoea; oral rehydration therapy.

Dioralyte Relief *Rhone-Poulenc Rorer, UK.*
Rice powder; sodium citrate; sodium chloride; potassium chloride (p.1185·2).
Diarrhoea; oral rehydration therapy.

Dioralyte Rice *Rhone-Poulenc Rorer, Neth.*
Rice powder; sodium chloride; potassium chloride; sodium citrate (p.1185·2).
Diarrhoea; oral rehydration therapy.

Diosmectal *Malesci, Ital.*
Diosmectite.
Gastrointestinal disorders.

Diosmil *Theraplix, Fr.*
Diosmin (p.1611·1).
Peripheral vascular disorders.

Diosminil *Faes, Spain.*
Diosmin (p.1611·1).
Chronic venous insufficiency; haemorrhoids.

Diospor HC *Dioptic, Canad.†*
Neomycin sulfate (p.228·1); polymyxin B sulfate (p.238·1); hydrocortisone (p.1073·3).
Eye disorders.

Diosporin *Dioptic, Canad.†*
Neomycin sulfate (p.228·1); polymyxin B sulfate (p.238·1); gramicidin (p.213·3).
Bacterial eye infections.

Diostate *Roberts, USA.*
Calcium with vitamin D and phosphorus (p.1350·1).
Calcium deficiency; dietary supplement.

Diosulf *Dioptic, Canad.*
Sulfacetamide sodium (p.250·3).
Bacterial eye infections.

Diosven *CT, Ital.*
Diosmin (p.1611·1).
Peripheral vascular disorders.

Diotrope *Dioptic, Canad.*
Tropicamide (p.475·1).
Production of mydriasis and cycloplegia.

Diotroxin *Glaxo Wellcome, S.Afr.*
Thyroxine [levothyroxine] sodium (p.1526·2); liothyronine sodium (p.1524·2).
Hypothyroidism.

Dioval *Keene, USA†.*
Estradiol valerate (p.1473·2).
Female castration; female hypogonadism; menopausal vasomotor symptoms; prevention of breast engorgement; primary ovarian failure; prostatic cancer; vulval and vaginal atrophy.

Diovan *Novartis, Aust.; Novartis, Canad.; Novartis, Denm.; Novartis, Fin.; Novartis, Ger.; Novartis, Hong Kong; Novartis, Irl.; Novartis, Israel; Novartis, Mex.; Novartis, Neth.; Novartis, Norw.; Novartis, NZ; Novartis, Port.; Novartis, S.Afr.; Novartis, Singapore; Novartis, Spain; Novartis, Swed.; Novartis, Switz.; Novartis, Thai.; Novartis, UK; Novartis, USA.*
Valsartan (p.988·3).
Hypertension.

Diovan Comp
Novartis, Denm.; Novartis, Fin.; Novartis, Norw.
Valsartan (p.988·3); hydrochlorothiazide (p.907·3).
Hypertension.

Diovan HCT
Novartis, Canad.; Novartis, Mex.; Novartis, USA.
Valsartan (p.988·3); hydrochlorothiazide (p.907·3).
Hypertension.

Diovane Novartis, Belg.
Valsartan (p.988·3).
Hypertension.

Diovenor Innothera, Fr.
Diosmin (p.1611·1).
Peripheral vascular disorders.

Diovol
Note. This name is used for preparations of different composition.
Carter Horner, Canad.
Oral suspension; caplets: Aluminium hydroxide
(p.1210·3); magnesium hydroxide (p.1233·1).
Tablets: Aluminium hydroxide-magnesium carbonate
co-dried gel (p.1211·2); magnesium hydroxide
(p.1233·1).
Dyspepsia; heartburn.
Carter Horner, Thai.
Oral suspension: Aluminium hydroxide (p.1210·3);
magnesium hydroxide (p.1233·1); simeticone
(p.1249·2).
Tablets: Aluminium hydroxide-magnesium carbonate
co-dried gel (p.1211·2); magnesium hydroxide
(p.1233·1); simeticone (p.1249·2).
*Flatulence; gastric hyperacidity; gastritis; gastro-
oesophageal reflux; heartburn; peptic ulcer.*
Pharmax, UK†.
Aluminium hydroxide (p.1210·3); magnesium hydrox-
ide (p.1233·1); simeticone (p.1249·2).
Flatulence; gastrointestinal hyperacidity.

Diovol EX Carter Horner, Canad.
Aluminium hydroxide (p.1210·3); magnesium hydrox-
ide (p.1233·1).
Dyspepsia; gastro-oesophageal reflux; heartburn.

Diovol Plus
Note. This name is used for preparations of different composition.
Carter Horner, Canad.; Carter Horner, Hong Kong.
Oral suspension: Aluminium hydroxide (p.1210·3);
magnesium hydroxide (p.1233·1); simeticone
(p.1249·2).
*Dyspepsia; flatulence; gastrointestinal hyperacidity;
peptic ulcer.*
Carter Horner, Canad.; Carter Horner, Hong Kong.
Tablets: Aluminium hydroxide-magnesium carbonate
co-dried gel (p.1211·2); magnesium hydroxide
(p.1233·1); simeticone (p.1249·2).
*Dyspepsia; flatulence; gastrointestinal hyperacidity;
peptic ulcer.*

Diovol Plus AF Carter Horner, Canad.
Calcium carbonate (p.1215·1); magnesium hydroxide
(p.1233·1); simeticone (p.1249·2).
Dyspepsia; flatulence; heartburn.

Diovon Comp Novartis, Swed.
Valsartan (p.988·3); hydrochlorothiazide (p.907·3).
Hypertension.

Di-Paralene Abbott, Swed.†.
Chlorcyclizine chloride (p.411·3).
Hypersensitivity reactions.

Dipasic Atlantis, Mex.
Isoniazid aminosalicylate (p.217·2).

Dipazide Siam Bheasach, Thai.
Glipizide (p.322·3).
Diabetes mellitus.

Dipedyne Wayne, Mex.
Zidovudine (p.645·2).
HIV infection.

Dipentum
Pharmacia Upjohn, Aust.; Pharmacia Upjohn, Austral.; Pharmacia
Upjohn, Canad.; Pharmacia Upjohn, Denm.; Pharmacia Upjohn, Fin.;
Pharmacia Upjohn, Fr.; Pharmacia Upjohn, Ger.; Pharmacia Upjohn,
Hong Kong; Pharmacia Upjohn, Irl.; Sequus, Israel; Pharmacia Up-
john, Ital.; Pharmacia Upjohn, Neth.; Pharmacia Upjohn, Norw.;
Pharmacia Upjohn, NZ; Pharmacia Upjohn, S.Afr.; Pharmacia Up-
john, Swed.; Pharmacia Upjohn, Switz.; Pharmacia Upjohn, UK; Pharmacia
Upjohn, USA.
Olsalazine sodium (p.1238·3).
Ulcerative colitis.

Dipeptamin Fresenius Kabi, Ger.
L-Alanyl-L-glutamine (p.1365·2).
Parenteral nutrition.

Dipeptiven
Fresenius Kabi, Aust.; Fresenius Kabi, Denm.; Fresenius Kabi, Fin.;
Fresenius Kabi, Fr.; Fresenius Kabi, Ital.; Alpha, Mex.; Fresenius Kabi,
Port.; Fresenius Kabi, Spain; Fresenius Kabi, Swed.; Fresenius Kabi, UK.
L-Alanyl-L-glutamine (p.1365·2).
Parenteral nutrition.

Diperpen Francia, Ital.
Pipemidic acid (p.236·1).
Bacterial infections of the urinary tract.

Dipervina Farma Lepori, Spain.
Dihydroergocristine mesilate (p.1603·2); vincamine
(p.1680·1) or vincamine hydrochloride (p.1680·1).
Cerebrovascular disorders; head injury.

Diphamine Medgenix, Belg.
Diphenhydramine hydrochloride (p.416·1).
*Hypersensitivity reactions; insect stings; pruritus; sun-
burn; urticaria.*

Diphantoine Wolfs, Belg.
Phenytoin sodium (p.357·2).
Arrhythmias; epilepsy.

Diphemin Alcon, Switz.†.
Dipivefrine hydrochloride (p.1604·3).
Glaucoma.

Diphen AF Morton Grove, USA.
Diphenhydramine hydrochloride (p.416·1).

Diphen Cough Morton Grove, USA.
Diphenhydramine hydrochloride (p.416·1).
Coughs.

Diphenamill Brunel, S.Afr.
Aminophylline (p.760·1); diphenhydramine hydrochloride (p.416·1); ammonium chloride (p.1085·2); sodium citrate (p.1186·2).
Coughs.

Diphenazol Vitamed, Israel.
Diphenhydramine hydrochloride (p.416·1); naphazo-
line (p.1095·1).
Allergic conjunctivitis.

Diphenhist Rugby, USA.
Diphenhydramine hydrochloride (p.416·1).

Diphenhydramine Constrictor Asta Medica, Belg.
Diphenhydramine hydrochloride (p.416·1); naphazo-
line hydrochloride (p.1095·1).
Hypersensitivity reactions.

Diphlogen Novartis Consumer, Aust.
Aluminium sodium silicate (p.1211·3); eucalyptus oil
(p.1609·2); menthol (p.1632·3).
Formerly contained ethyl salicylate, eucalyptus oil, and
menthol.
*Musculoskeletal, joint, peri-articular, and soft-tissue
disorders.*

Diphos Procter & Gamble, Ger.
Disodium etidronate (p.752·1).
Ectopic ossification; Paget's disease of bone.

Diphuman Berna, Switz.
A diphtheria immunoglobulin (p.1536·2).
Passive immunisation.

Dipidolor
Janssen-Cilag, Aust.; Janssen-Cilag, Belg.; Janssen-Cilag, Ger.; Janssen-
Cilag, Neth.
Piritramide (p.78·3).
Pain.

Dipine Sanfer, Mex.
Dipivefrine (p.1604·3).

Dipiperon
Janssen-Cilag, Belg.; Janssen-Cilag, Denm.; Janssen-Cilag, Fr.; Janssen-
Cilag, Ger.; Janssen-Cilag, Neth.; Janssen-Cilag, Switz.
Pipamperone hydrochloride (p.700·3).
*Behaviour disorders; drug withdrawal syndromes;
psychoses.*

Dipiraxil Wayne, Mex.
Dipyrone (p.34·1).

Diplexil Tecnifar, Port.
Sodium valproate (p.366·3).
Epilepsy.

Diplogel Restiva, Ital.†.
Aluminium hydroxide (p.1210·3).
*Gastrointestinal disorders associated with hyperacidi-
ty.*

Diplovax Biovac, S.Afr.
A measles vaccine (Edmonston-Zagreb strain)
(p.1547·1).
Active immunisation.

Dipofen Arlex, Mex.
Ibuprofen (p.43·2).

Dipoquin
Ioquin, Austral.; Pacific, NZ.
Dipivefrine hydrochloride (p.1604·3).
Glaucoma.

Diposef Unison, Thai.
Dipotassium clorazepate (p.670·3).
Anxiety.

Dipot Asian Pharm, Thai.
Dipotassium clorazepate (p.670·3).
Anxiety; insomnia.

Dipres Precimex, Mex.
Dipyridamole (p.877·2).

Diprin
Alcon, Canad.†; Alcon, Swed.
Dipivefrine hydrochloride (p.1604·3).
Glaucoma.

Diprivan
Zeneca, Aust.; Zeneca, Austral.; Zeneca, Belg.; Zeneca, Braz.; Astra-
Zeneca, Canad.; AstraZeneca, Denm.; AstraZeneca, Fin.; AstraZene-
ca, Fr.; Zeneca, Ger.; Zeneca, Hong Kong; AstraZeneca, Irl.; Zeneca,
Ital.; Zeneca, Mex.; Zeneca, Neth.; Zeneca, Norw.; AstraZene-
ca, NZ; Zeneca, Port.; AstraZeneca, S.Afr.; AstraZeneca, Singapore;
Zeneca, Spain; Zeneca, Swed.; Zeneca, Thai.; AstraZeneca,
UK; Zeneca, USA.
Propofol (p.1265·3).
General anaesthesia; sedative.

Diprobase
Schering-Plough, Fr.; Schering-Plough, Irl.; Schering-Plough, Port.;
Schering-Plough, UK.
Emollient.
Dry skin conditions; topical vehicle.

Diprobath
Schering-Plough, Irl.; Schering-Plough, UK.
Light liquid paraffin (p.1407·2); isopropyl myristate
(p.1409·2).
Bath additive; dry skin; hyperkeratosis.

Diprocel
Schering-Plough, Hong Kong; Schering-Plough, Singapore.
Betamethasone dipropionate (p.1063·2).
Skin disorders.

Diproderm
Aesca, Aust.; Schering-Plough, Denm.; Schering-Plough, Fin.; Scher-
ing-Plough, Norw.; Schering-Plough, Spain; Schering-Plough, Swed.
Betamethasone dipropionate (p.1063·2).
Skin disorders.

Diprodol Sons, Mex.
Ibuprofen (p.43·2).
*Inflammation; musculoskeletal and joint disorders;
pain.*

Diprofol Taro, Israel.
Propofol (p.1265·3).
General anaesthesia; sedative.

Diproform Schering-Plough, Denm.; Schering-Plough, Ital.
Betamethasone dipropionate (p.1063·2); clioquinol
(p.190·2).
Infected skin disorders.

Diproforte Aesca, Aust.
Betamethasone dipropionate (p.1063·2).
Skin disorders.

Diprofos Schering-Plough, Port.
Betamethasone dipropionate (p.1063·2); betametha-
sone sodium phosphate (p.1063·2).
Corticosteroid.

Diprogen Schering, Canad.
Betamethasone dipropionate (p.1063·2); gentamicin
sulfate (p.210·1).
Infected skin disorders.

Diprogenta
Aesca, Aust.; Schering-Plough, Braz.; Essex, Ger.; Schering-Plough,
Hong Kong; Schering-Plough, Israel; Essex, Ital.†; Schering-Plough,
Port.; Schering-Plough, S.Afr.; Schering-Plough, Singapore; Schering-
Plough, Spain; Essex, Switz.; Schering-Plough, Thai.
Betamethasone dipropionate (p.1063·2); gentamicin
sulfate (p.210·1).
Infected skin disorders.

Diprolen Schering-Plough, Denm.; Schering-Plough, Fin.
Betamethasone dipropionate (p.1063·2).
Skin disorders.

Diprolene
Schering-Plough, Belg.; Schering-Plough, Fr.; Schering-Plough, Israel;
Essex, Switz.; Schering, USA.
Betamethasone dipropionate (p.1063·2).
Skin disorders.

Diprolene Glycol Schering, Canad.
Betamethasone dipropionate (p.1063·2).
Skin disorders.

Di-Promal Mundipharma, Aust.
Ipratropium bromide (p.766·1); salbutamol (p.770·3).
Obstructive airways disease.

Diprophos
Aesca, Aust.; Schering-Plough, Belg.; Essex, Switz.
Betamethasone dipropionate (p.1063·2); betametha-
sone sodium phosphate (p.1063·2).
Corticosteroid.

Diprosalic
Aesca, Aust.; Schering-Plough, Belg.; Schering-Plough, Braz.; Schering,
Canad.; Schering-Plough, Denm.; Schering-Plough, Fin.; Schering-
Plough, Fr.; Essex, Ger.; Schering-Plough, Hong Kong; Schering-
Plough, Irl.; Schering-Plough, Israel; Schering-Plough, Ital.; Schering-
Plough, Mex.; Schering-Plough, Neth.; Schering-Plough, Norw.; Scher-
ing-Plough, NZ; Schering-Plough, Port.; Schering-Plough, S.Afr.; Scher-
ing-Plough, Singapore; Schering-Plough, Spain; Schering-Plough,
Swed.; Essex, Switz.; Schering-Plough, Thai.; Schering-Plough, UK.
Betamethasone dipropionate (p.1063·2); salicylic acid
(p.1122·3).
Skin and scalp disorders.

Diprosept Schering-Plough, Fr.
Betamethasone dipropionate (p.1063·2); clioquinol
(p.190·2).
Infected skin disorders.

Diprosis Essex, Ger.
Betamethasone dipropionate (p.1063·2).
Skin disorders.

Diprosone
Schering-Plough, Austral.; Schering-Plough, Belg.; Schering-Plough,
Braz.; Schering, Canad.; Schering-Plough, Fr.; Essex, Ger.; Schering-
Plough, Hong Kong; Schering-Plough, Irl.; Schering-Plough, Israel;
Schering-Plough, Ital.; Schering-Plough, Mex.; Schering-Plough, Neth.;
Schering-Plough, NZ; Schering-Plough, Port.; Schering-Plough, S.Afr.;
Schering-Plough, Singapore; Essex, Switz.; Schering-Plough, Thai.;
Schering-Plough, UK; Schering, USA.
Betamethasone dipropionate (p.1063·2).
Skin and scalp disorders.

Diprosone Depot Essex, Ger.
Betamethasone dipropionate (p.1063·2); betametha-
sone sodium phosphate (p.1063·2).
Parenteral corticosteroid.

Diprosone G Schering-Plough, Mex.
Betamethasone dipropionate (p.1063·2); gentamicin
sulfate (p.210·1).
Infected skin disorders.

Diprosone Neomycine Schering-Plough, Fr.
Betamethasone dipropionate (p.1063·2); neomycin
sulfate (p.228·1).
Infected skin disorders.

Diprosone-Y Schering-Plough, Mex.
Betamethasone dipropionate (p.1063·2); clioquinol
(p.190·2).
Infected skin disorders.

Diprospan
Schering-Plough, Braz.; Schering-Plough, Denm.; Schering-Plough,

Hong Kong; Schering-Plough, Israel; Schering-Plough, Mex.; Schering-
Plough, Singapore; Schering-Plough, Thai.
Betamethasone dipropionate (p.1063·2); betametha-
sone sodium phosphate (p.1063·2).
Corticosteroid.

Diprostene Schering-Plough, Fr.
Betamethasone dipropionate (p.1063·2); betametha-
sone sodium phosphate (p.1063·2).
Corticosteroid.

Diprotop Schering-Plough, Thai.
Betamethasone dipropionate (p.1063·2).
Skin disorders.

Dipsan
Lederle, Austral.†; Wyeth, Neth.†; Lederle, S.Afr.†; Wyeth Lederle,
Swed.†.
Calcium carbimide (p.1588·2).
Alcoholism.

Dipsin CPH, Port.
Famotidine (p.1725·3).
Peptic ulcer; Zollinger-Ellison syndrome.

Dipulmin Almirall, Spain.
Salbutamol sulfate (p.770·3).
Obstructive airways disease.

Dipxapen Liferpal, Mex.
Dicloxacillin (p.199·1).
Bacterial infections.

Dipydol Valdecasas, Mex.
Dipyrone (p.34·1).
Pain.

Dipyridan Aventis, Belg.
Dipyridamole (p.877·2).
Angina pectoris; thromboembolism prophylaxis.

Dipyrin Medinovum, Fin.
Dipyridamole (p.877·2).
Heart failure; thromboembolic disorders.

Dipyrol Rolab, S.Afr.†.
Dipyridamole (p.877·2).
Thromboembolic disorders.

Dirahist Teofarma, Ital.
Triamcinolone (p.1080·1); chlorpheniramine [chlo-
rphenamine] maleate (p.412·1).
Hypersensitivity reactions.

Direct Formulary Cough Lozenges Sutton, Canad.†.
Menthol (p.1632·3).

Directim Azevedos, Port.†.
Amineptine hydrochloride (p.273·2).
Depression.

Direktan Gerot, Aust.
Sodium nicotinate.
*Decubitus ulcer; peripheral vascular disease; sports
massage.*

Dirine
Atlantic, Singapore; Atlantic, Thai.
Frusemide [furosemide] (p.893·1).
Hypertension; oedema.

Dirinol Cryopharma, Mex.
Dipyridamole (p.877·2).
Thromboembolic disorders.

Diroquine Atlantic, Thai.
Chloroquine phosphate (p.432·3).
Amoebiasis; malaria; rheumatoid arthritis.

Dirythmin AstraZeneca, UK.
Disopyramide phosphate (p.878·2).
Arrhythmias.

Dirytmin
Astra, Belg.; Astra, Neth.; Hassle, Swed.
Disopyramide phosphate (p.878·2).
Arrhythmias.

Disalcid
3M, Canad.; 3M, USA.
Salsalate (p.82·2).
Musculoskeletal and joint disorders.

Disalgil Also, Ital.
Glycol salicylate (p.42·2); camphor (p.1589·3); capsa-
icin (p.23·1).
Musculoskeletal, joint, and soft-tissue disorders.

Disalgyl Monin, Fr.
Methyl salicylate (p.55·1); capsicum oleoresin
(p.1591·1); camphor (p.1589·3).
Musculoskeletal and joint pain.

Disalpin Asta Medica, Ger.
Hydrochlorothiazide (p.907·3); reserpine (p.967·3).
Hypertension.

Disalunil Berlin-Chemie, Ger.
Hydrochlorothiazide (p.907·3).
*Diabetes insipidus; heart failure; hypertension; oede-
ma.*

Disanal Humana, Ital.†.
Gluten-free food (p.1350·1).

Disanthrol Lannett, USA†.
Docusate sodium (p.1223·1); casanthranol (p.1216·1).
Constipation.

Discase Knoll, Belg.
Chymopapain (p.1594·3).
Herniated lumbar intervertebral disc.

Dis-Cinil Complex Menarini, Ital.
Dihydroxydibutylether (p.1603·3); cascara (p.1216·1);
rhubarb (p.1248·1); boldo (p.1585·3).
Constipation.

Dis-Cinil Ilfi Menarini, Ital.†.
Dihydroxydibutylether (p.1603·3).
Constipation with digestive disorders.

Disclar *Casen Fleet, Spain†.*
Tocoferil nicotinate (p.984·3).
Hyperlipidaemias.

Disclo-Gel *Colgate Oral Care, Austral.*
Erythrosine (p.1028·2).
Disclosing agent for dental plaque.

Disclo-Plaque *Colgate Oral Care, Austral.*
Fluorescein (p.1612·1).
Disclosing agent for dental plaque.

Disclo-Tabs *Colgate Oral Care, Austral.*
Erythrosine (p.1028·2).
Disclosing agent for dental plaque.

Discmigon *Zilly, Ger.*
Hypericum oil (p.290·3); wheat-germ oil; avocado oil; birch tar oil (p.1124·3); beef hoof oil; thiamine hydrochloride (p.1385·1); formic acid (p.1612·3); garlic juice (p.1614·1); birch leaf (p.1585·2); juniper berry (p.1625·2); gentian root (p.1615·1); lupulus (p.1629·3); clove (p.1596·3); male fern leaf (p.102·3).
Joint disorders; keloid scars; rheumatism.

Disco-cyl Ho-Len-Complex *Liebermann, Ger.*
Homoeopathic preparation.

Discotrine
3M, Denm.; 3M, Fr.
Glyceryl trinitrate (p.897·3).
Angina pectoris; prevention of phlebitis and extravasation during intravenous infusion.

Discover *Carter-Wallace, UK.*
Pregnancy test (p.1654·3).

Discover Onestep *Carter-Wallace, Austral.*
Pregnancy test (p.1654·3).

Discover Onestep Ovulation Prediction *Carter-Wallace, Austral.*
Fertility test (p.1654·3).

Discromil *Pergam, Ital.*
Hydroquinone (p.1115·1).
Skin hyperpigmentation.

Discus compositum *Heel, Ger.†.*
Homoeopathic preparation.

Disdolen *Uriach, Spain.*
Fosfosal (p.42·1).
Fever; musculoskeletal, joint, peri-articular, and soft-tissue disorders; pain.

Disdolen Codeina *Uriach, Spain.*
Codeine phosphate (p.25·2); fosfosal (p.42·1).
Pain.

Disebrin *Tubilux, Ital.*
Heparin sodium (p.902·1).
Eye disorders.

Disento *Nakornpatana, Thai.*
Diiodohydroxyquinoline (p.590·2); furazolidone (p.592·1); neomycin sulfate (p.228·1); phthalylsulfathiazole (p.235·3); light kaolin (p.1229·3).
Diarrhoea; gastrointestinal infections.

Disento PF *Nakornpatana, Thai.*
Furazolidone (p.592·1); pectin (p.1502·3); light kaolin (p.1229·3).
Bacterial diarrhoea; enteritis.

Diseon *Teva, Ital.*
Alfacalcidol (p.1391·1).
Hypoparathyroidism; osteomalacia; osteoporosis; renal osteodystrophy; rickets.

Diseptil *Gedis, Ital.*
Benzalkonium chloride (p.1133·2).
Skin disinfection.

Diseptyl *Rekah, Israel.*
Co-trimoxazole (p.193·3).
Bacterial infections.

Diserinal *Pulitzer, Ital.*
Alfacalcidol (p.1391·1).
Hypoparathyroidism; osteomalacia; osteoporosis; renal osteodystrophy; rickets.

Disfil *Llorente, Spain.*
Ectylurea; phenytoin (p.357·2); phenobarbital (p.355·1); aminohydroxybutyric acid (p.342·2).
Epilepsy.

Disflatyl
Note. This name is used for preparations of different composition.
Solco, Aust.; Solco, Fin.; Solco, Hong Kong; Inibsa, Spain; Solco, Switz.; Merck, Thai.; Solco, Thai.
Simeticone (p.1249·2).
Flatulence; preparation for gastrointestinal investigations.

Solco, Hong Kong; Solco, Singapore.
Dimethicone (p.1249·2); silicon dioxide (p.1503·3).
Flatulence; preparation for gastrointestinal investigations.

Disgren *Novartis, Braz.; Poli, Ital.†; Hormonas, Mex.; Uriach, Spain.*
Triflusal (p.987·2).
Thromboembolic disorders.

Disinal *Silanes, Mex.*
Clonixin lysine (p.25·1).
Pain.

Disinclor *Tipomark, Ital.*
Tosylchloramide sodium (p.1159·1).
Disinfection of wounds and external genitals.

Disintyl *Zeta, Ital.*
Benzalkonium chloride (p.1133·2).
Disinfection of wounds, burns, and external genitals.

Disipal
3M, Austral.†; Yamanouchi, Belg.; 3M, Canad.; Yamanouchi, Denm.;

Yamanouchi, Irl.; Yamanouchi, Ital.; Yamanouchi, Norw.; Pharmaco, NZ; 3M, S.Afr.; Yamanouchi, Swed.; Yamanouchi, UK.
Orphenadrine hydrochloride (p.470·3).
Akinesia; drug-induced extrapyramidal disorders; parkinsonism; senile depression; skeletal muscle spasm; vertigo.

Diskin *Benedetti, Ital.*
Dihydroxydibutylether (p.1603·3).
Constipation with digestive disorders.

Diskinebyl *Laphal, Hong Kong.*
Dihydroxydibutylether (p.1603·3).
Biliary-tract disorders; liver disorders.

Dislax *Makros, Braz.*
Bisacodyl (p.1212·2).
Constipation.

Dismenol N *Simons, Ger.; Adroka, Switz.*
Ibuprofen (p.43·2).
Fever; inflammation; pain.

Dismenol Neu *Sanova, Aust.*
Ibuprofen (p.43·2).
Pain.

Dismozon pur *Bode, Ger.*
Magnesium monoperoxyphthalate.
Surface disinfection.

Disne Asmol *Berenguer Infale, Spain†.*
Ipratropium bromide (p.766·1).
Obstructive airways disease.

Disneumon Pernasal *Solvay, Spain.*
Phenylephrine hydrochloride (p.1097·1).
Nasal and sinus congestion.

D-Iso *Ratiopharm, Ger.*
Sodium chloride; sodium citrate; potassium chloride; glucose (p.1185·2).
Diarrhoea; oral rehydration therapy.

Disobrom *Cord, Hong Kong; Geneva, USA.*
Pseudoephedrine sulfate (p.1099·3); dexbrompheniramine maleate (p.410·2).
Upper respiratory-tract symptoms.

Disocor *Janssen-Cilag, Port.*
Carnitine (p.1356·1).

Disoderme *Plough, Port.*
Benzocaine (p.1306·2); triclosan (p.1159·2); aloe vera (p.1110·1); dl-alpha tocopherol (p.1394·1); menthol (p.1632·3); camphor (p.1589·3).
Burns; insect bites; sunburn.

Diso-Duriles *Astra, Ger.*
Disopyramide phosphate (p.878·2).
Arrhythmias.

Disofarin *Wayne, Mex.*
Disopyramide (p.878·2).

Disofrol
Schering-Plough, Braz.; Schering-Plough, Fin.; Schering-Plough, Spain; Schering-Plough, Swed.; Essex, Switz.
Pseudoephedrine sulfate (p.1099·3); dexbrompheniramine maleate (p.410·2).
Upper respiratory-tract disorders.

Disol *Siam Bheasach, Thai.*
Bromhexine hydrochloride (p.1085·3).
Respiratory-tract disorders associated with increased or viscous mucus.

Disolan *Lannett, USA†.*
Docusate sodium (p.1223·1); phenolphthalein (p.1244·1).
Constipation.

Disolan Forte *Lannett, USA†.*
Docusate sodium (p.1223·1); carmellose sodium (p.1499·3); casanthranol (p.1216·1).
Constipation.

Disomet *Orion, Fin.*
Disopyramide phosphate (p.878·2).
Arrhythmias.

Disonate *Lannett, USA†.*
Docusate sodium (p.1223·1).
Constipation.

Disonorm *Solvay, Ger.†.*
Disopyramide (p.878·2) or disopyramide phosphate (p.878·2).
Arrhythmias.

Disopam *Dexxon, Israel.*
Diazepam (p.674·3).
Alcohol withdrawal syndrome; anxiety; epilepsy; insomnia; lumbago; psychosomatic disorders; slipped disc; tremor.

Disophrol *Aesca, Aust.; Schering-Plough, USA.*
Pseudoephedrine sulfate (p.1099·3); dexbrompheniramine maleate (p.410·2).
Upper respiratory-tract symptoms.

Disoplex *Lannett, USA†.*
Docusate sodium (p.1223·1); carmellose sodium (p.1499·3).
Constipation.

Disoprivan
Zeneca, Ger.; Glaxo Wellcome, Ger.; Zeneca, Switz.
Propofol (p.1265·3).
General anaesthesia; sedative.

Disorlon *Riom, Fr.†.*
Isosorbide dinitrate (p.915·2).
Angina pectoris; heart failure.

Disotat *Isis, Ger.*
Di-isopropylammonium dichloroacetate (p.874·3) or di-isopropylammonium hydrochloride (p.874·3).
Hypertension.

Disotate *Forest Pharmaceuticals, USA†.*
Disodium edetate (p.1008·1).
Digitalis-induced cardiac arrhythmias; hypercalcaemia.

Disothiazide *Dexxon, Israel.*
Hydrochlorothiazide (p.907·3).
Hypertension; oedema.

Dispaclonidin *Ciba Vision, Ger.*
Clonidine hydrochloride (p.860·1).
Glaucoma; ocular hypertension.

Dispacromil *Ciba Vision, Ger.*
Sodium cromoglicate (p.774·3).
Allergic conjunctivitis.

Dispadex comp *Ciba Vision, Ger.*
Dexamethasone sodium phosphate (p.1067·1); neomycin sulfate (p.228·1).
Bacterial infections and inflammation of the eye.

Dispagent *Ciba Vision, Ger.*
Gentamicin sulfate (p.210·1).
Bacterial eye infections.

Dispasan *Ciba Vision, Ger.*
Sodium hyaluronate (p.1620·1).
Adjunct in ocular surgery.

Dispatenol *Ciba Vision, Ger.*
Dexpanthenol (p.1602·3); polyvinyl alcohol (p.1503·1).
Dry eyes.

Dispatetrin *Ciba Vision, Ger.†.*
Tetracycline hydrochloride (p.258·3).
Bacterial eye infections.

Dispatim
Ciba Vision, Aust.; Ciba Vision, Ger.
Timolol maleate (p.982·1).
Glaucoma; ocular hypertension.

Di-Spaz *Vortech, USA†.*
Dicyclomine [dicycloverine] hydrochloride (p.466·1).
Functional bowel/irritable bowel syndrome.

Disperbarium *Rovi, Spain.*
Barium sulfate (p.1032·1).
Contrast medium for gastrointestinal radiography.

Disperin *Orion, Fin.*
Aspirin (p.14·2).
Fever; musculoskeletal and joint disorders; pain; thromboembolism prophylaxis.

Displata *Serono, Mex.*
Carboplatin (p.515·1).

Display *Solea, Ital.*
Benzalkonium chloride (p.1133·2).
Eye disinfection; eye irritation.

Dispneitrat *IMA, Braz.*
Aminophylline (p.760·1); guaifenesin (p.1092·2).
Obstructive airways disease.

Dispon *Searle, Ital.*
Liothyronine (p.1524·3).
Cellulite; local accumulation of adipose tissue.

Dispril
Reckitt & Colman, Belg.; Reckitt & Colman, Norw.; Meda, Swed.†.
Aspirin (p.14·2).
Fever; inflammation; pain.

Disprin
Reckitt & Colman, Austral.; Reckitt & Colman, Hong Kong; Reckitt Benckiser, Irl.; Reckitt Benckiser, NZ; Reckitt Benckiser, S.Afr.; Reckitt & Colman, Singapore; Reckitt & Colman, UK.
Aspirin (p.14·2).
Fever; inflammation; pain.

Disprin CV *Reckitt & Colman, UK†.*
Aspirin (p.14·2).
Thromboembolism prophylaxis.

Disprin Direct
Reckitt & Colman, Austral.; Reckitt & Colman, UK.
Aspirin (p.14·2).
Glycine (p.1365·3) may be included in this preparation in an attempt to limit adverse effects on the gastrointestinal mucosa.
Formerly known as Solmin and Disprin Solmin in the UK.
Fever; inflammation; pain.

Disprin Extra
Reckitts, Irl.; Reckitt & Colman, UK.
Aspirin (p.14·2); paracetamol (p.71·2).
Fever; pain.

Disprin Forte *Reckitt & Colman, Austral.*
Aspirin (p.14·2); codeine phosphate (p.25·2).
Fever; inflammation; pain.

Disprol
Reckitt Benckiser, Irl.; Reckitt Benckiser, NZ; Reckitt & Colman, UK.
Paracetamol (p.71·2).
Fever; pain.

Dispromil *Diviser Aquilea, Spain.*
Famotidine (p.1225·3).
Gastro-oesophageal reflux; peptic ulcer; Zollinger-Ellison syndrome.

Disques Coricides *Seton Scholl, Fr.*
Salicylic acid (p.1122·3).
Calluses; corns.

Dissenten *SPA, Ital.*
Loperamide hydrochloride (p.1231·3).
Diarrhoea.

Dissolvurol *Dissolvurol, Mon.*
Colloidal silicon dioxide (p.1503·3).
Musculoskeletal and joint disorders.

Distaclor
Dista, Irl.; Lilly, Irl.; Lilly, Singapore; Lilly, Thai.; Dista, UK.
Cefaclor (p.161·1).
Bacterial infections.

Distalgesic
Napp, Irl.; Quatromed, S.Afr.; Lilly, Swed.; Dista, Switz.; Dista, UK.
Dextropropoxyphene hydrochloride (p.27·1) or dextropropoxyphene napsilate (p.27·1); paracetamol (p.71·2).
These ingredients can be described by the British Approved Name Co-proxamol.
Pain.

Distalgic *Lilly, Belg.*
Dextropropoxyphene hydrochloride (p.27·1); paracetamol (p.71·2).
Fever; pain.

Distamine
Lilly, Aust.†; Dista, Irl.; Lilly, Neth.†; Alliance, UK.
Penicillamine (p.1017·1).
Cystinuria; hepatitis; lead poisoning; rheumatoid arthritis; Wilson's disease.

Distaph *Alphapharm, Austral.*
Dicloxacillin sodium (p.199·1).
Gram-positive bacterial infections.

Distaquaine V-K *Dista, UK.*
Phenoxymethylpenicillin potassium (p.235·1).
Bacterial infections.

Distasil *Milana, Ital.*
Benzalkonium chloride (p.1133·2).
Skin disinfection.

Distaxid *Dista, Spain.*
Nizatidine (p.1238·1).
Gastro-oesophageal reflux; peptic ulcer.

Distensan *Esteve, Spain.*
Clotiazepam (p.671·1).
Anxiety; neuroleptanalgesia; premedication.

Disteril *Lachifarma, Ital.*
Benzalkonium chloride (p.1133·2).
Genital hygiene; skin, wound, and burn disinfection.

Distilbene *Gerda, Fr.*
Diethylstilbestrol (p.1471·2).
Prostatic cancer.

Distobram *Lilly, Port.*
Tobramycin (p.263·3).
Bacterial infections.

Distovagal *Tedec Meiji, Spain†.*
Belladonna alkaloids (p.463·1); ergotamine tartrate (p.452·1); phenobarbital (p.355·1).
Cardiovascular disorders; gastrointestinal disorders; genito-urinary disorders; menopausal disorders; premenstrual syndrome; vascular headaches.

Distraneurin
Astra, Aust.; Astra, Ger.; Astra, Switz.
Clomethiazole (p.668·2) or clomethiazole edisilate (p.668·2).
Alcohol withdrawal syndrome; insomnia; mania; pre-eclampsia and eclampsia; sedative; status epilepticus.

Distraneurine
Astra, Belg.; Astra, Neth.; Astra, Spain.
Clomethiazole (p.668·2) or clomethiazole edisilate (p.668·2).
Alcohol withdrawal syndrome; eclampsia; insomnia; sedative; status epilepticus.

Di-Su-Frone *Hua, Thai.*
Furazolidone (p.592·1); pectin (p.1502·3); kaolin (p.1229·3).
Gastrointestinal infections.

Disulone *Rhone-Poulenc Rorer, Fr.*
Dapsone (p.196·1); ferrous oxalate (p.1360·2).
Dermatitis herpetiformis; leprosy; Pneumocystis carinii pneumonia; polychondritis.

Disupril *Faria, Braz.*
Amino acids; vitamin B substances (p.1350·1).
Nutritional supplement.

Diswart *Dermatech, Austral.*
Glutaral (p.1145·2).
Common warts.

DIT1-2 *Dunhall, USA.*
Sulfanilamide (p.256·2); aminoacridine hydrochloride (p.1130·2); allantoin (p.1110·1).
Vaginal infections.

Ditanrix
SmithKline Beecham, Aust.; SmithKline Beecham, Ital.; SmithKline, Spain; SmithKline Beecham, Switz.
An adsorbed diphtheria and tetanus vaccine (p.1537·1). Separate preparations are available for infants and young children and for children and adults.
Active immunisation.

Ditaven *Merck, Aust.; Merck, Ger.*
Digitoxin (p.869·2).
Haematomas; leg oedema; peripheral vascular disease; varicose ulcers; venous insufficiency.

Ditaven comp *Merck, Aust.*
Digitoxin (p.869·2); heparin sodium (p.902·1).
Leg oedema; soft-tissue injuries; varicose ulcers; venous insufficiency.

Ditaveine *Pharmadeveloppement, Fr.*
Melilotus officinalis; red vine.
Formerly contained digitoxin and heparin sodium.
Capillary disorders.

Ditayod *Solfran, Mex.*
Phthalylsulfathiazole (p.235·3); clioquinol (p.190·2).
Amoebiasis.

DiTe Anatoxal
Berna, Hong Kong; Pharmabroker, NZ.
A diphtheria and tetanus vaccine (p.1537·1).
Active immunisation.

Ditec *Boehringer Ingelheim, Aust.; Boehringer Ingelheim, Ger.*
Fenoterol hydrobromide (p.765·1); sodium cromoglicate (p.774·3).
Obstructive airways disease.

Di-Te-Kik *Statens Serum Institut, Fin.; SSI, Swed.*
A diphtheria, tetanus, and pertussis vaccine (p.1537·3).
Active immunisation.

Di-Te-Ki-Pol *Statens Serum Institut, Denm.; Statens Serum Institut, Fin.; SSI, Swed.*
A diphtheria, tetanus, pertussis, and poliomyelitis vaccine (p.1539·1).
Active immunisation.

Ditemer *Pasteur Merieux, Belg.*
An adsorbed diphtheria and tetanus vaccine (p.1537·1).
Active immunisation.

Ditemic *SmithKline Beecham, UK†.*
Dried ferrous sulfate (p.1360·3); zinc sulfate (p.1398·2); vitamin B substances (p.1350·1); ascorbic acid (p.1389·3).

Ditenate N *Herbert, Ger.*
Theophylline (p.777·2).
Obstructive airways disease.

Ditenside *Almirall, Spain.*
Enalapril maleate (p.883·3); hydrochlorothiazide (p.907·3).
Hypertension.

Ditensor *Almirall, Spain.*
Enalapril maleate (p.883·3).
Heart failure; hypertension.

DiTePer Anatoxal *Pharmabroker, NZ.*
A diphtheria, tetanus, and pertussis vaccine (p.1537·3).
Active immunisation.

DiTePerPol Vaccin *Berna, Switz.†*
A diphtheria, tetanus, pertussis, and poliomyelitis vaccine (p.1539·1).
Active immunisation.

Di-Te-Pol *Statens Serum Institut, Denm.†*
A diphtheria, tetanus, and poliomyelitis vaccine (p.1539·1).
Active immunisation.

Diteutrin *Teuto, Braz.*
Co-trimoxazole (p.193·1); aluminium silicate (p.1211·3); magnesium hydroxide (p.1233·1).
Diarrhoea.

Dithiazid *Merck, Aust.*
Hydrochlorothiazide (p.907·3).
Hypertension; oedema.

Dithrasal *Dermatech, Austral.*
Dithranol (p.1113·3); salicylic acid (p.1122·3).
Psoriasis.

Dithrocream
Hamilton, Austral.; Dermal Laboratories, Irl.; Dermal, Israel; Dermal Laboratories, UK.
Dithranol (p.1113·3).
Psoriasis.

Ditizem *Siam Bheasach, Thai.*
Diltiazem hydrochloride (p.874·3).
Angina pectoris; hypertension.

Ditoin *Atlantic, Thai.*
Phenytoin sodium (p.357·2).
Epilepsy; migraine; trigeminal neuralgia.

Ditomed *Medifive, Thai.*
Phenytoin sodium (p.357·2).
Epilepsy.

Ditonal *Athenstaedt & Redeker, Hong Kong.*
Trichlor-dimethylethyl-salicylate; paracetamol (p.71·2).
Fever; pain.

Ditonal N *Athenstaedt, Ger.*
Paracetamol (p.71·2); caffeine (p.761·3).
Pain.

Ditopax *Schering-Plough, Mex.*
Oral suspension: Magnesium hydroxide (p.1233·1); aluminium hydroxide (p.1210·3); dimethicone (p.1249·2).
Tablets: Dimethicone (p.1249·2); aluminium hydroxide-magnesium carbonate co-dried gel (p.1211·2); magnesium hydroxide (p.1233·1).
Gastrointestinal disorders.

Ditopax-F *Schering-Plough, Mex.*
Aluminium hydroxide-magnesium carbonate co-dried gel (p.1211·2); magnesium hydroxide (p.1233·1); calcium carbonate (p.1215·3); dimethicone (p.1249·2).
Gastrointestinal disorders.

Ditran *Breves, Braz.*
Tenitramine (p.980·1).
Angina pectoris.

Ditrei *Italmex, Mex.*
Di-isopropylammonium dichloroacetate (p.874·3).
Angina pectoris; myocardial infarction; vascular disorders.

Ditrenil *Siam Bheasach, Thai.*
Nitrendipine (p.947·1).
Hypertension.

Ditrim *Orion, Fin.*
Trimethoprim (p.264·2); sulfadiazine (p.251·1).
Bacterial infections; Pneumocystis carinii pneumonia.

Ditripentat-Heyl *Heyl, Ger.*
Calcium trisodium pentetate (p.1003·1).
Poisoning with heavy or radioactive metals.

Ditropan
Sanofi Synthelabo, Aust.; Rhone-Poulenc Rorer, Austral.; Sanofi Synthelabo, Belg.; Alza, Canad.; Pharmacia Upjohn, Fr.; Synthelabo, Fr.;

Hoechst Marion Roussel, Hong Kong; Lorex, Irl.; Sanofi Synthelabo, Ital.; Aventis, NZ; Sanofi Synthelabo, Port.; Sanofi Synthelabo, S.Afr.; Synthelabo, Spain; Pharmacia Upjohn, Swed.; Pharmacia Synthelabo, Switz.; Sanofi Synthelabo, UK; Alza, USA.
Oxybutynin hydrochloride (p.471·2).
Bladder instability.

Ditropine *Asian Pharm, Thai.*
Diphenoxylate hydrochloride (p.1222·2).
Atropine sulfate (p.461·1) is included in this preparation to discourage abuse.
Diarrhoea.

Ditterolina *Fustery, Mex.*
Dicloxacillin sodium (p.199·1).
Bacterial infections.

Ditum *Nakorn, Thai.*
Dicloxacillin (p.199·1).
Bacterial infections.

Diu Rauwiplus *Lacer, Spain.*
Ajmaline (p.833·1); hydrochlorothiazide (p.907·3); methylrauhimbine; sarpagine (p.967·2); rescinnamine (p.967·3); reserpine hydrochloride (p.968·1).
Hypertension.

Diu Venostasin *Klinge, Ger.*
Tablets, triamterene (p.986·1); hydrochlorothiazide (p.907·3); controlled-release capsules, aesculus (p.1574·1).
Venous insufficiency.

Diu-Atenolol *Verla, Ger.*
Atenolol (p.841·3); chlortalidone (p.857·1).
Hypertension.

Diube *SIT, Ital.*
Atenolol (p.841·3); chlortalidone (p.857·1).
Hypertension.

Diucardin *Wyeth-Ayerst, USA.*
Hydroflumethiazide (p.911·3).
Hypertension; oedema.

Diucomb *Gebra, Aust.†; Byk, Belg.; Sanofi Synthelabo, Ger.; Schwarz, Switz.*
Bemetizide (p.843·2); triamterene (p.986·1).
Hypertension; oedema.

Diulo *Searle, Austral.†; Monsanto, Port.; Schiapparelli Searle, USA†.*
Metolazone (p.930·3).
Ascites; hypertension; oedema.

diu-melusin *Schwarz, Ger.*
Hydrochlorothiazide (p.907·3).
Hypertension; oedema.

Diumide-K Continus *Napp, Irl.; Asta Medica, UK.*
Frusemide [furosemide] (p.893·1); potassium chloride (p.1194·3).
Oedema.

Diupres *Merck, USA.*
Reserpine (p.967·3); chlorothiazide (p.856·3).
Hypertension.

Diupress *Eurofarma, Braz.*
Chlortalidone (p.857·1); amiloride hydrochloride (p.835·1).
Hypertension; oedema.

Diuprol *Protein, Mex.*
Chlortalidone (p.857·1).

Diurace *Bristol-Myers Squibb, Neth.*
Fosinopril sodium (p.892·3); hydrochlorothiazide (p.907·3).
Hypertension.

Diural
Note. This name is used for preparations of different composition.
Alpharma, Denm.; Alpharma, Norw.
Frusemide [furosemide] (p.893·1).
Forced diuresis; hypertension; oedema; renal failure.

Silanes, Mex.
Piretanide (p.956·2).
Hypertension; oedema.

Diuramid *Medphano, Ger.*
Acetazolamide (p.826·1).
Glaucoma.

Diuramin *Medinovum, Fin.*
Amiloride hydrochloride (p.835·1); hydrochlorothiazide (p.907·3).
Ascites; hypertension; oedema.

Diurana *Sanofi Winthrop, Braz.*
Frusemide [furosemide] (p.893·1); triamterene (p.986·1).
Hypertension; oedema.

Diurapid *Jenapharm, Ger.*
Frusemide [furosemide] (p.893·1) or frusemide [furosemide] sodium (p.895·1).
Oedema; oliguria.

Diuremid *Guidotti, Ital.*
Torasemide (p.985·1) or torasemide sodium (p.985·2).
Ascites; heart failure; oedema; renal failure.

Diurene *Sanofi Synthelabo, Port.*
Amiloride hydrochloride (p.835·1); hydrochlorothiazide (p.907·3).
Ascites; heart failure; hypertension.

Diuresal *Lagap, Switz.*
Frusemide [furosemide] (p.893·1).
Hypertension; oedema; renal failure.

Diurese *American Urologicals, USA.*
Trichlormethiazide (p.987·1).
Hypertension; oedema.

Diuresix *Menarini, Ital.*
Torasemide (p.985·1) or torasemide sodium (p.985·2).
Ascites; heart failure; kidney disorders; oedema.

Diuretabs *Potter's, UK.*
Buchu leaf (p.1587·2); juniper berry oil (p.1625·2); parsley piert (p.1648·3); bearberry (p.1583·3).
Fluid retention.

Diuretikum Verla *Verla, Ger.*
Triamterene (p.986·1); hydrochlorothiazide (p.907·3).
Hypertension; oedema.

Diuret-P *PP Lab, Thai.*
Hydrochlorothiazide (p.907·3).
Diuretic.

Diurex
Note. This name is used for preparations of different composition.
Honterapica, Braz.
Frusemide [furosemide] (p.893·1).
Hypercalcaemia; hypertension; oedema.

Orion, Fin.
Amiloride hydrochloride (p.835·1); hydrochlorothiazide (p.907·3).
Cirrhosis with ascites; heart failure; hypertension.

Lacer, Spain.
Xipamide (p.999·2).
Hypertension; oedema.

Diurexan
Asta Medica, Belg.; Asta Medica, Hong Kong; Asta Medica, Irl.; Asta Medica, Port.; Mer-National, S.Afr.; Asta Medica, UK.
Xipamide (p.999·2).
Hypertension; oedema.

Diurezin *Cazi, Braz.*
Hydrochlorothiazide (p.907·3).
Diabetes insipidus; hypertension; oedema; renal calculi.

Diurid *Laevosan, Aust.*
Triamterene (p.986·1); hydrochlorothiazide (p.907·3).
Heart failure; hypertension; oedema.

Diurigen *Goldline, USA.*
Chlorothiazide (p.856·3).
Hypertension; oedema.

Diuril *Merck, USA.*
Chlorothiazide (p.856·3) or chlorothiazide sodium (p.856·3).
Hypertension; oedema.

Diurin *Pacific, NZ.*
Frusemide [furosemide] (p.893·1).
Hypertension; oedema; severe renal impairment.

Diurisa *Eurofarma, Braz.*
Frusemide [furosemide] (p.893·1); amiloride hydrochloride (p.835·1).
Hypertension; oedema.

Diurix *Helvepharm, Switz.*
Frusemide [furosemide] (p.893·1).
Forced diuresis; hypertension; oedema.

Diurolan *Rayere, Mex.*
Frusemide [furosemide] (p.893·1).

Diursan *TAD, Ger.*
Hydrochlorothiazide (p.907·3); amiloride hydrochloride (p.835·1).
Hypertension; oedema.

Diutec *Garec, S.Afr.*
Amiloride hydrochloride (p.835·1); hydrochlorothiazide (p.907·3).
Hypertension; oedema.

Diutensat *Azupharma, Ger.*
Triamterene (p.986·1); hydrochlorothiazide (p.907·3).
Hypertension.

Diutensat comp *Azupharma, Ger.*
Triamterene (p.986·1); hydrochlorothiazide (p.907·3); propranolol hydrochloride (p.962·3).
Hypertension.

Diutensen-R *Wallace, USA.*
Methyclothiazide (p.927·3); reserpine (p.967·3).
Hypertension.

Diutropan *Prima, Thai.*
Oxybutynin hydrochloride (p.471·2).
Neurogenic bladder disorders.

Diuzine *I Farmacologia, Spain.*
Amiloride hydrochloride (p.835·1); hydrochlorothiazide (p.907·3).
Hypertension; oedema.

Divacuna DT *Leti, Spain.*
A diphtheria and tetanus vaccine (p.1537·1).
Formerly known as Divacuna TD.
Active immunisation of infants and young children.

Divalol W *Wernigerode, Ger.*
Curcuma zanthorrhiza; peppermint oil (p.1243·3).
Biliary disorders.

Divascan *Berlin-Chemie, Ger.*
Iprazochrome.
Diabetic retinopathy; headache; migraine.

Divegal *Sanochemia, Aust.*
Dihydroergotamine tartrate (p.450·3).
Migraine and related vascular headaches.

Divial *Merck, Spain†.*
Lorazepam pivalate (p.689·2).
Alcohol withdrawal syndrome; anxiety; chemotherapy-induced nausea and vomiting; epilepsy; insomnia.

Divical *Rottapharm, Ital.*
Calcium folinate (p.1363·1).
Folate deficiency.

Divicill *BA Farma, Port.*
Aciclovir (p.612·3).
Herpesvirus infections.

Dividol
Zambon, Braz.
Viminol para-aminobenzoate (p.415·2).
Pain.

Zambon, Ital.
Viminol hydroxybenzoate (p.90·3).
Pain.

Divigel
Orion, Denm.; Orion, Fin.; Orion, Irl.; Orion, Swed.; Orion, Switz.
Estradiol (p.1473·1).
Menopausal disorders; osteoporosis.

Divina
Organon, Austral.; Orion, Denm.; Orion, Fin.; Innothera, Fr.; Byk, Neth.; Aspen, S.Afr.; Orion, Swed.
11 Tablets, estradiol valerate (p.1473·2); 10 tablets, estradiol valerate; medroxyprogesterone acetate (p.1480·1).
Oestrogen deficiency; osteoporosis.

Divina Plus
Orion, Denm.; Orion, Swed.
16 Tablets, estradiol valerate (p.1473·2); 12 tablets, estradiol valerate; medroxyprogesterone acetate (p.1480·1).
Oestrogen deficiency; osteoporosis.

Divinal Galle *Divinal, Ger.†*
Cynara (p.1601·3).
Dyspepsia.

Divinal Gastro *Divinal, Ger.†*
Caraway (p.1591·2); peppermint leaf (p.1243·2); fennel (p.1610·1).
Dyspepsia; flatulence.

Divinal Rheuma *Divinal, Ger.†*
Camphor (p.1589·3).
Rheumatism.

Divinal Seda *Divinal, Ger.†*
Hypericum (p.290·2).
Anxiety; depression; psychovegetative states.

Divinal-Broncho-Balsam *Divinal, Ger.†*
Camphor (p.1589·3); eucalyptus oil (p.1609·2); turpentine oil (p.1676·3).
Respiratory-tract disorders.

Divinal-Hepa *Divinal, Ger.†*
Silybum marianum (p.1021·3).
Liver disorders.

Diviplus *Pharmacia Upjohn, Belg.*
16 Tablets, estradiol valerate (p.1473·2); 12 tablets, estradiol valerate; medroxyprogesterone acetate (p.1480·1).
Menopausal disorders; osteoporosis.

Divitren *Orion, Fin.*
70 Tablets, estradiol valerate (p.1473·2); 14 tablets, estradiol valerate; medroxyprogesterone acetate (p.1480·1); 7 tablets, inert.
Menopausal disorders; osteoporosis.

Diviva *Pharmacia Upjohn, Belg.*
11 Tablets, estradiol valerate (p.1473·2); 10 tablets, estradiol valerate; medroxyprogesterone acetate (p.1480·1).
Menopausal disorders; oestrogen replacement therapy.

Dixarit
Boehringer Ingelheim, Austral.†; Boehringer Ingelheim, Belg.; Boehringer Ingelheim, Canad.; Boehringer Ingelheim, Ger.; Boehringer Ingelheim, Hong Kong; Boehringer Ingelheim, Irl.; Boehringer Ingelheim, Neth.; Boehringer Ingelheim, NZ; Boehringer Ingelheim, S.Afr.; Boehringer Ingelheim, Singapore; Boehringer Ingelheim, UK.
Clonidine hydrochloride (p.860·1).
Menopausal flushing; migraine and other vascular headache.

Dixen *Maver, Mex.*
Dicloxacillin (p.199·1).
Bacterial infections.

Dixeran
Lundbeck, Aust.; Lundbeck, Belg.; Lundbeck, Switz.†.
Melitracen hydrochloride (p.297·3).
Depression.

Dixiflen *Farcoral, Mex.*
Ox bile (p.1585·1); pancreatin (p.1646·1); cellulase (p.1593·1); dimethicone (p.1249·2).
Gastrointestinal disorders.

Dixocillin *Siam Bheasach, Thai.*
Dicloxacillin sodium (p.199·1).
Gram-positive bacterial infections.

Dixonal *Medix, Mex.*
Piroxicam (p.79·1).
Gout; musculoskeletal, joint, peri-articular, and soft-tissue disorders.

Diyomex *Ofimex, Mex.*
Diiodohydroxyquinoline (p.590·2).

Diyosul *Jofrin, Mex.*
Diiodohydroxyquinoline (p.590·2).

Diyowil *Willmar, Mex.*
Diiodohydroxyquinoline (p.590·2).

Dizac *Ohmeda, USA†.*
Diazepam (p.674·3).
Anxiety; epilepsy; skeletal muscle relaxant.

Dizan *Pharmaland, Thai.*
Diazepam (p.674·3).
Anxiety; skeletal muscle spasm.

Dizepam *Masa, Thai.*
Diazepam (p.674·3).
Anxiety.

Dizmiss *JMI, USA.*
Meclozine hydrochloride (p.420·3).
Motion sickness; vertigo.

Diznil *Julphar, UAE.*
Dimenhydrinate (p.415·2).
Nausea and vomiting; vestibular disorders.

Dizolam
Atlantic, Singapore; Atlantic, Thai.
Alprazolam (p.654·2).
Anxiety; mixed anxiety depressive states.

DLPA *Cantassium Co., UK.*
DL-Phenylalanine.

DM Cough Syrup
Note.This name is used for preparations of different composition.
Prodemdis, Canad.
Diphenhydramine hydrochloride (p.416·1); dextromethorphan hydrobromide (p.1087·3); ammonium chloride (p.1085·2).
Coughs.
Technilab, Canad.; Prometic, Canad.
Dextromethorphan hydrobromide (p.1087·3).
Coughs.

DM Cough Syrup Decongestant *Prometic, Canad.*
Pseudoephedrine hydrochloride (p.1099·2); dextromethorphan hydrobromide (p.1087·3).
Coughs.

DM Cough Syrup Expectorant *Prometic, Canad.*
Dextromethorphan hydrobromide (p.1087·3); guaifenesin (p.1092·2).
Coughs.

DM Creme *Byk, Port.*
Glycol salicylate (p.42·2); menthol (p.1632·3).
Musculoskeletal, joint, peri-articular, and soft-tissue disorders; neuralgia; neuritis.

DM E Suppressant Expectorant *Drug Trading, Canad.†*
Dextromethorphan hydrobromide (p.1087·3); guaifenesin (p.1092·2).

DM Gel *Byk, Port.*
Glycol salicylate (p.42·2); menthol (p.1632·3); heparin sodium (p.902·1).
Muscular pain; neuralgia; soft-tissue injury.

DM Plus *Technilab, Canad.*
Dextromethorphan hydrobromide (p.1087·3); diphenhydramine hydrochloride (p.416·1); ammonium chloride (p.1085·2).
Formerly known as DM Syrup.
Coughs.

DM Plus Decongestant *Technilab, Canad.*
Dextromethorphan hydrobromide (p.1087·3); pseudoephedrine hydrochloride (p.1099·2).
Coughs.

DM Plus Decongestant Expectorant *Technilab, Canad.*
Dextromethorphan hydrobromide (p.1087·3); pseudoephedrine hydrochloride (p.1099·2); guaifenesin (p.1092·2).
Coughs.

DM Plus Expectorant *Technilab, Canad.*
Dextromethorphan hydrobromide (p.1087·3); guaifenesin (p.1092·2).
Coughs.

DM Sans Sucre *Trianon, Canad.*
Dextromethorphan hydrobromide (p.1087·3).
Coughs.

DM Termo *Byk, Port.*
Glycol salicylate (p.42·2); benzyl nicotinate (p.20·2).
Musculoskeletal and joint disorders; neuritis; peripheral vascular disorders.

4-DMAP
Kohler, Ger.; Kohler, Neth.
4-Dimethylaminophenol hydrochloride (p.1007·3).
Cyanide, hydrocyanic acid, nitrile, or hydrogen sulfide poisoning.

D-Med *Ortega, USA†.*
Methylprednisolone acetate (p.1076·1).
Corticosteroid.

DMG-B15 *Cantassium Co., UK.*
Calcium gluconate (p.1188·2); NN-dimethylglycine hydrochloride.

DMH *Alra, USA†.*
Dimenhydrinate (p.415·2).

DML *Person & Covey, USA.*
A range of moisturisers.

D-Mulsin *Mucos, Ger.*
Colecalciferol (p.1391·1).
Vitamin D deficiency.

D/N PR *Magis, Ital.*
Naproxen aminobutanol (p.61·3).
Gynaecological disorders.

DNCG *Mundipharma, Ger.; Stada, Ger.; Trommsdorff, Ger.; Penta, Ger.; Padia, Ger.*
Sodium cromoglicate (p.774·3).
Asthma; conjunctivitis; hypersensitivity reactions; rhinitis.

Doak-Oil *Trans Canaderm, Canad.*
Liquid paraffin; isopropyl palmitate; coal tar (p.1125·1).
Skin disorders.

Doans *Ciba Consumer, USA.*
Magnesium salicylate (p.50·3).
Fever; inflammation; pain.

Doans Backache Pills
Note.This name is used for preparations of different composition.
Novartis Consumer, Canad.
Magnesium salicylate (p.50·3).
Muscular back pain.

Eastern Pharmaceuticals, UK.
Paracetamol (p.71·2); sodium salicylate (p.84·2).
Musculoskeletal, joint, and soft-tissue pain.

Dobacen *Brandt, Switz.*
Diphenhydramine hydrochloride (p.416·1).
Insomnia.

Dobendan
Hoechst Marion Roussel, Aust.; Boots Healthcare, Ger.
Cetylpyridinium chloride (p.1138·1).
Mouth and throat disorders.

Dobesifar *Alcon, Hong Kong.*
Calcium dobesilate (p.1588·2).
Haemorrhagic eye disorders.

Dobesin *Abigo, Denm.†.*
Diethylpropion hydrochloride (p.1508·3).
Obesity.

Dobesix *Brasmedica, Braz.*
Mazindol (p.1510·3); diazepam (p.674·3).
Obesity.

Dobetin *Angelini, Ital.*
Cyanocobalamin (p.1388·1).
Tonic; vitamin B$_{12}$ deficiency.

Dobetin con Vitamina B1 *Angelini, Ital.*
Vitamin B preparation (p.1350·1).
Neuralgia; neuritis.

Dobetin Totale *Angelini, Ital.*
Vitamin B preparation (p.1350·1).
Neuralgia.

Dobica *OPW, Ger.*
Calcium dobesilate (p.1588·2).
Capillary fragility and leakage; venous insufficiency.

Dobil *Pharmaland, Thai.*
Paracetamol (p.71·2); chlorpheniramine [chlorphenamine] maleate (p.412·1); phenylpropanolamine hydrochloride (p.1098·1).
Cold symptoms; hay fever; nasal congestion; rhinitis.

Dobiron *Legrand, Braz.*
Ferrous sulfate (p.1360·3); vitamin B substances; liver extract; gastric mucosa extract (p.1350·1).
Anaemias.

Doblexan *Quimifar, Spain.*
Piroxicam (p.79·1).
Gout; musculoskeletal, joint, and peri-articular disorders; pain.

Dobren *Teofarma, Ital.*
Sulpiride (p.706·1).
Dysthymia; psychoses.

Dobriciclin *Quimifar, Spain.*
Amoxicillin trihydrate (p.149·2).
Bacterial infections.

Dobucard *Solvay, Thai.*
Dobutamine hydrochloride (p.880·2).
Heart failure.

Dobuject
Leiras, Denm.†; Leiras, Fin.; Leiras, Israel; Pisa, Mex.; Probios, Port.; Leiras, Singapore; Leiras, Swed.†; Leiras, Thai.
Dobutamine hydrochloride (p.880·2).
Heart failure; shock.

Dobupal *Almirall, Spain.*
Venlafaxine hydrochloride (p.312·2).
Depression.

Dobutam *Rafa, Israel.*
Dobutamine hydrochloride (p.880·2).
Heart failure.

Dobutina *Faulding, Port.*
Dobutamine hydrochloride (p.880·2).

Dobutrex
Lilly, Aust.; Lilly, Austral.; Lilly, Belg.; Lilly, Braz.; Lilly, Canad.; Lilly, Denm.; Lilly, Fin.; Lilly, Fr.; Lilly, Ger.; Lilly, Hong Kong; Lilly, Irl.; Lilly, Israel; Lilly, Ital.; Lilly, Mex.; Lilly, Neth.; Lilly, Norw.; Lilly, NZ; Lilly, S.Afr.; Lilly, Spain; Lilly, Swed.; Lilly, Switz.; Lilly, Thai.; Lilly, UK; Lilly, USA.
Dobutamine hydrochloride (p.880·2).
Cardiac stress testing; heart failure; shock.

Doc *SMT, Ger.*
Arnica (p.1581·3).
Musculoskeletal, joint, and soft-tissue disorders.

Docaine *M & H, Thai.*
Lignocaine [lidocaine] hydrochloride (p.1313·2).
Local anaesthesia.

Docard *Dexxon, Israel.*
Dopamine hydrochloride (p.881·3).
Shock.

Docatone *Wyeth, Spain.*
Doxapram (p.1509·2).
CNS depression; respiratory depression.

Docdol *Adcock Ingram, S.Afr.*
Paracetamol (p.71·2); codeine phosphate (p.25·2); caffeine (p.761·3).
Pain.

Docgel *Docmed, S.Afr.†.*
Dried aluminium hydroxide gel (p.1210·3); magnesium oxide (p.1233·2); simeticone (p.1249·2).
Dyspepsia; gastritis; gastro-oesophageal reflux; peptic ulcer.

Docidrazin *Zeneca, Ger.; Rhein-Pharma, Ger.*
Propranolol hydrochloride (p.962·3); hydralazine hydrochloride (p.905·3); bendrofluazide [bendroflumethiazide] (p.844·1).
Hypertension.

Dociretic *Zeneca, Ger.; Rhein-Pharma, Ger.*
Propranolol hydrochloride (p.962·3); bendrofluazide [bendroflumethiazide] (p.844·1).
Hypertension.

Dociteren *Zeneca, Ger.; Rhein-Pharma, Ger.*
Propranolol hydrochloride (p.962·3); triamterene (p.986·1); hydrochlorothiazide (p.907·3).
Hypertension.

Dociton *Zeneca, Ger.; Rhein-Pharma, Ger.*
Propranolol hydrochloride (p.962·3).
Angina pectoris; anxiety; arrhythmias; essential tremor; hypertension; hyperthyroidism; migraine; myocardial infarction.

Docline *Atlantic, Thai.*
Doxycycline (p.200·1).
Bacterial infections.

Doclis *Roche, Spain.*
Diltiazem hydrochloride (p.874·3).
Angina pectoris; hypertension.

Docostyl *Pentafarm, Spain.*
Doxycycline hyclate (p.200·1).
Bacterial infections; malaria.

Docrub *Aspen Consumer, S.Afr.*
Camphor (p.1589·3); menthol (p.1632·3); methyl salicylate (p.55·1); eucalyptus oil (p.1609·2); buchu oil (p.1587·2).
Cold symptoms; coughs; soft-tissue disorders.

Docsed *Aspen, S.Afr.*
Mepyramine maleate (p.421·1); codeine phosphate (p.25·2); pholcodine (p.1099·1); ephedrine hydrochloride (p.1090·1).
Coughs.

Doctar *Savage, USA.*
Coal tar (p.1125·1).
Scalp disorders.

Doctodermis *Medea, Spain.*
Biotin (p.1355·3); triclosan (p.1159·2).
Formerly contained biotin, methyl hydroxybenzoate, and trolamine laurilsulfate.
Skin cleansing.

Doctofril Antiinflamat *Medea, Spain.*
Phenylbutazone (p.78·1); lignocaine [lidocaine] (p.1313·2); methyl nicotinate (p.55·1); vitamin F.
Chilblains; rheumatic and muscle pain.

Doctogaster *Medea, Spain†.*
Aluminium silicate (p.1211·3); frangula bark (p.1227·1); magnesium carbonate (p.1232·3); magnesium polygalacturonate; liquorice (p.1231·2); sodium bicarbonate (p.1186·2).
Gastritis; hyperacidity; peptic ulcer.

Doctomitil *Medea, Spain.*
Eucalyptol (p.1609·2); diethylamine salicylate (p.32·2); methyl nicotinate (p.55·1).
Soft-tissue disorders.

Doctril
Martin, Fr.; Abello, Spain.
Ibuprofen lysine (p.44·1).
Fever; pain.

Doctrim *Docmed, S.Afr.†.*
Co-trimoxazole (p.193·3).
Bacterial infections.

Docucal-P *Parmed, USA†.*
Docusate calcium (p.1222·3); phenolphthalein (p.1244·1).
Constipation.

Docusoft *Taro, Israel; Reese, USA.*
Docusate sodium (p.1223·1).
Constipation.

Docusoft Plus *Reese, USA.*
Docusate sodium (p.1223·1); casanthranol (p.1216·1).
Constipation.

Docusol *Typharm, UK.*
Docusate sodium (p.1223·1).
Bowel evacuation; constipation.

Dodds *Dannorth, Canad.*
Sodium salicylate (p.84·2).
Musculoskeletal pain.

Dodecatol N *Heyl, Ger.*
Procaine hydrochloride (p.1319·1); cyanocobalamin (p.1388·1).
Inflammation; pain.

Dodecavit *SERB, Fr.*
Hydroxocobalamin acetate (p.1388·3).
Vitamin B$_{12}$ deficiency.

Dodemox *Fadim, Ital.*
Amoxicillin trihydrate (p.149·2).
Bacterial infections.

Dodepar *ABC, Port.*
Vitamin B substances (p.1350·1).
Anaemias; tonic.

Doderlein Med *Novartis Consumer, Ger.*
Lactobacillus gasseri.
Vaginal disorders.

Do-Do ChestEze *Novartis Consumer, UK.*
Theophylline (p.777·2); ephedrine hydrochloride (p.1090·1); caffeine (p.761·3).
Bronchial coughs; wheezing.

Do-Do Expectorant Linctus *Novartis Consumer, UK†.*
Guaifenesin (p.1092·2).
Coughs.

Doederlein *Novartis Consumer, Aust.*
Lactobacillus acidophilus (p.1626·3).
Vaginal candidiasis.

Dofedrin *Knoll, Mex.*
Pseudoephedrine (p.1099·2).
Upper respiratory-tract congestion.

Dofen *Knoll, Mex.*
Pseudoephedrine (p.1099·2).

Doferol *Tocogino, Mex.*
Ergocalciferol (p.1391·2).

Dogmatil
Sanofi Synthelabo, Aust.; Sanofi Synthelabo, Belg.; Synthelabo, Braz.; Sanofi Winthrop, Denm.; Synthelabo, Fr.; Sanofi Synthelabo, Ger.; Synthelabo, Hong Kong; Carnot, Mex.; Sanofi Synthelabo, Neth.; Sanofi Synthelabo, Port.; Sanofi Synthelabo, Singapore; Synthelabo, Spain; Synthelabo, Switz.
Sulpiride (p.706·1).
Depression; psychoses; psychosomatic disorders; vertigo.

Dogoxine *Rudefsa, Mex.*
Digoxin (p.870·1).

Dohyfral Vitamine AD3 *Solvay, Neth.†.*
Vitamin A (p.1382·1); colecalciferol (p.1391·1).
Vitamin A and vitamin D deficiency.

DOK *Major, USA.*
Docusate sodium (p.1223·1).
Constipation.

Doktacillin
Astra, Aust.†; AstraZeneca, Denm.; AstraZeneca, Norw.; Astra, Swed.
Ampicillin sodium (p.150·3).
Bacterial infections.

Dolac *Syntex, Mex.*
Ketorolac trometamol (p.48·2).
Pain.

Dolacet *Roberts, USA.*
Hydrocodone tartrate (p.42·2); paracetamol (p.71·2).
Pain.

Dolak *Bama, Spain.*
Isosorbide mononitrate (p.916·2).
Angina pectoris.

Dolal *Biocodex, Fr.*
Ethylmethoxy salicylate; phenylpropyl salicylate.
Musculoskeletal and joint pain.

Dolalgial *Sanofi Synthelabo, Fr.*
Clonixin lysine (p.25·1).
Pain; peri-articular disorders.

Dolamin *Sintofarma, Braz.*
Clonixin lysine (p.25·1).
Pain.

Dolan *Leiras, Fin.*
Orphenadrine citrate (p.470·3); paracetamol (p.71·2).
Skeletal muscle spasm and pain.

Dolanaest *Strathmann, Ger.*
Bupivacaine hydrochloride (p.1306·3).
Local anaesthesia; pain syndromes.

Dolanex *Lannett, USA†.*
Paracetamol (p.71·2).
Fever; pain.

Dolantin *Hoechst Marion Roussel, Ger.*
Pethidine hydrochloride (p.75·1).
Pain.

Dolantina
Hoechst Marion Roussel, Braz.; Bayer, Spain.
Pethidine hydrochloride (p.75·1).
Pain; premedication.

Dolantine *Hoechst Marion Roussel, Belg.*
Pethidine hydrochloride (p.75·1).
Pain.

Dolaren *AF, Mex.*
Cream: Diclofenac diethylamine (p.30·2).
Tablets: Diclofenac sodium (p.30·3); carisoprodol (p.1327·1).
Inflammation; musculoskeletal, joint, peri-articular and soft-tissue disorders; pain.

Dolaut *GiEnne, Ital.*
Diclofenac sodium (p.30·3).
Musculoskeletal, joint, and peri-articular disorders.

Dolcevita *Codilab, Port.*
Aspartame (p.1354·3).
Sugar substitute.

Dolcol *Dainippon, Jpn.*
Pipemidic acid (p.236·1).
Bacterial infections.

Dolcontin
Mundipharma, Fin.; Pharmacia Upjohn, Norw.; Pharmacia Upjohn, Swed.
Morphine sulfate (p.56·1).
Pain.

Dolcopin *Rottapharm, Spain.*
Magnesium trisilicate (p.1233·3); sodium bicarbonate (p.1186·2); almasilate (p.1210·1); alginic acid (p.1498·3).
Dyspepsia; gastro-oesophageal reflux.

Dolcor *Gazzoni, Ital.†.*
Aspartame (p.1354·3).
Sugar substitute.

Doldieta *Ottolenghi, Ital.†.*
Maltodextrin (p.1371·2); aspartame (p.1354·3).
Sugar substitute.

Dolefin Paracetamol *Pharmacia, Spain†.*
Paracetamol (p.71·2).
Fever; pain.

Dolemicin *Dreiman, Spain.*
Metamizole magnesium (p.34·2).
Fever; pain.

Dolene *Lederle, USA†.*
Dextropropoxyphene hydrochloride (p.27·1).
Pain.

Dolenon *Strathmann, Ger.*
Cayenne pepper (p.1591·1).
Muscle pain; nerve pain.

Dolenso *Kwizda, Aust.*
Paracetamol (p.71·2); aspirin (p.14·2).
Fever; pain.

Dolerax *Propan, S.Afr.†*
Paracetamol (p.71·2); doxylamine succinate (p.417·1); caffeine (p.761·3); codeine phosphate (p.25·2).
Pain associated with tension.

Doleron *Astra, Swed.*
Aspirin (p.14·2); dextropropoxyphene napsilate (p.27·1); phenazone (p.77·2).
Pain.

Dolestan *Whitehall-Much, Ger.*
Diphenhydramine hydrochloride (p.416·1).
Sleep disorders.

Dolestan forte comp *Whitehall-Much, Ger.*
Diphenhydramine hydrochloride (p.416·1); guaifenesin (p.1092·2).
Sleep disorders.

Dolestine *Biogal, Israel.*
Pethidine hydrochloride (p.75·1).
Pain.

Dolex
Note.This name is used for preparations of different composition.
Terramin, Aust.
Glycol salicylate (p.42·2); salicylic acid (p.1122·3); camphor (p.1589·3); turpentine oil (p.1676·3).
Rheumatic and muscle pain.

IFI, Ital.
Furprofen (p.42·1).
Pain.

Dolexaderm H *Strathmann, Ger.†*
Dulcamara (p.1606·2).
Eczema.

Dolexamed N *Strathmann, Ger.†*
Eucalyptus oil (p.1609·2); peppermint oil (p.1243·3); rosemary oil (p.1659·3).
Myalgia; neuralgia; rheumatism.

Dolflam *Rayere, Mex.*
Diclofenac sodium (p.30·3).
Gout; musculoskeletal, joint, peri-articular, and soft-tissue disorders.

Dolflash *Sanofi Winthrop, Fr.†*
Paracetamol (p.71·2).
Fever; pain.

Dolgan *Bioresearch, Mex.*
Dipyrone (p.34·1).
Fever; pain.

Dolgesic *Novag, Spain.*
Paracetamol (p.71·2).
Fever; pain.

Dolgesic Codeina *Novag, Spain.*
Codeine phosphate (p.25·2); paracetamol (p.71·2).
Pain.

Dolgit
Sanova, Aust.; Lipha Sante, Fr.; Dolorgiet, Ger.; Dolorgiet, Switz.
Ibuprofen (p.43·2).
Fever; inflammation; musculoskeletal, joint, and peri-articular disorders; pain; soft-tissue injury.

Dolgit-Diclo *Dolorgiet, Ger.*
Diclofenac sodium (p.30·3).
Gout; inflammation; musculoskeletal, joint, and soft-tissue disorders; pain.

Doli Rhume *Theraplix, Fr.*
Paracetamol (p.71·2); pseudoephedrine hydrochloride (p.1099·2).
Cold symptoms.

Dolibu *Klinge, Aust.*
Ibuprofen (p.43·2).
Fever; musculoskeletal and joint disorders; pain.

Dolical *Rekah, Israel.*
Morpholine salicylate (p.59·3).
Skeletal muscle spasm.

Dolicoccil *Dolisos, Canad.*
Homoeopathic preparation.

Dolidon *Medifa, Fr.*
Paracetamol (p.71·2); caffeine (p.761·3).
Pain.

Dolinac
Whitehall, Denm.†; Durachemie, Ger.†; Teofarma, Ital.; Whitehall, S.Afr.†
Felbinac (p.36·1) or diisopropanolamine felbinac (p.36·1).
Inflammation; pain; soft-tissue disorders.

Doline *Ferrer, Spain†.*
Benorilate (p.19·3).
Fever; musculoskeletal and joint disorders; pain.

Dolipol *Hoechst, Fr.†*
Tolbutamide (p.336·3).
Diabetes mellitus.

Doliprane *Theraplix, Fr.*
Paracetamol (p.71·2).
Fever; pain.

Dolitabs *Theraplix, Fr.*
Paracetamol (p.71·2).
Fever; pain.

Dolium *Utopian, Thai.*
Domperidone (p.1224·1).
Flatulence; nausea and vomiting.

Dolko *Therabel, Fr.*
Paracetamol (p.71·2).
Fever; pain.

Dolmatil *Delandale, Irl.; Sanofi Synthelabo, UK.*
Sulpiride (p.706·1).
Schizophrenia.

Dolmed *Leiras, Fin.*
Methadone hydrochloride (p.53·1).
Opioid dependence; pain.

Dolmen
Note.This name is used for preparations of different composition.
Sigma-Tau, Ital.
Tenoxicam (p.87·2).
Musculoskeletal disorders.

Uriach, Spain.
Aspirin (p.14·2); ascorbic acid (p.1389·3); codeine phosphate (p.25·2).
Fever; pain.

Dolmex *Ofimex, Mex.*
Aspirin (p.14·2).

Dol-Mite *Swiss Herbal, Canad.*
Calcium carbonate; magnesium carbonate (p.1350·1).

Dolmitin *Medea, Spain.*
Eucalyptol (p.1609·2); diethylamine salicylate (p.32·2).
Soft-tissue disorders.

Dolmix *Apomedica, Aust.*
Ethenzamide (p.35·1); paracetamol (p.71·2); caffeine (p.761·3).
Fever; pain.

Dolnaxen *Arlex, Mex.*
Naproxen (p.60·3).

Dolnefort *Farcoral, Mex.*
Dipyrone (p.34·1); vitamin B substances (p.1350·1).
Neuritis; pain.

Dolo Demothrex *Democal, Switz.*
Dimethyl sulfoxide (p.1402·2); benzyl nicotinate (p.20·2); glycol salicylate (p.42·2).
Musculoskeletal and joint pain.

Dolo Mobilat *Sankyo, Ger.*
Phenylephrine hydrochloride (p.1097·1); a heparinoid (p.905·2); glycol salicylate (p.42·2).
Joint, peri-articular, and soft-tissue disorders.

Dolo neos *Optimed, Ger.†*
Ibuprofen (p.43·2).
Fever; inflammation; musculoskeletal and joint disorders; pain.

Dolo Nervobion *Merck, Spain.*
Diclofenac sodium (p.30·3).
Gout; musculoskeletal, joint, and peri-articular disorders; pain; renal colic.

Dolo Target *Whitehall-Robins, Switz.*
Felbinac (p.36·1).
Musculoskeletal, joint, peri-articular, and soft-tissue injuries and disorders.

Doloana *Quimifor, Spain†.*
Aspirin (p.14·2); salicylamide (p.82·1).
Fever; pain.

Dolo-Arthrodynat *Ziethen, Ger.*
Devil's claw root (p.26·3).
Musculoskeletal and joint disorders.

Dolo-Arthrosenex *Whitehall-Robins, Switz.*
Glycol salicylate (p.42·2); heparin sodium (p.902·1); camphor (p.1589·3).
Musculoskeletal, joint, peri-articular, and soft-tissue disorders.

Dolo-Arthrosenex N *Riemser, Ger.*
Glycol salicylate (p.42·2).
Muscle, joint, and soft-tissue injuries and disorders.

Dolo-Arthrosenex sine Heparino *Whitehall-Robins, Switz.*
Glycol salicylate (p.42·2); camphor (p.1589·3); isopropyl alcohol (p.1149·2); lavender oil (p.1627·2); thyme oil (p.1672·3); Siberian fir oil.
Musculoskeletal, joint, peri-articular, and soft-tissue injuries and disorders.

Dolo-Arthrosetten H *Hotz, Ger.*
Devil's claw root (p.26·3).
Musculoskeletal and joint disorders.

Doloatrixen *Zerboni, Mex.*
Naproxen (p.60·3).

Dolobene
Ratiopharm, Aust.; Merckle, Ger.; Mepha, Hong Kong; Mepha, Switz.
Dimethyl sulfoxide (p.1402·2); heparin sodium (p.902·1); dexpanthenol (p.1602·3).
Musculoskeletal, joint, peri-articular, and soft-tissue disorders; neuralgia.

Dolobid
Merck Sharp & Dohme, Austral.; Merck Frosst, Canad.; Merck Sharp & Dohme, Hong Kong; Merck Sharp & Dohme, Irl.; Merck Sharp & Dohme, Israel; Merck Sharp & Dohme, Mex.; Merck Sharp & Dohme, Port.; Merck Sharp & Dohme, S.Afr.; Frosst, Spain; Merck Sharp & Dohme, Thai.; Merck Sharp & Dohme, UK; Merck, USA.
Diflunisal (p.32·2).
Inflammation; musculoskeletal, joint, and peri-articular disorders; pain.

Dolobis *Merck Sharp & Dohme-Chibret, Fr.*
Diflunisal (p.32·2).
Pain.

Dolocalma *Neves, Port.*
Metamizole magnesium (p.34·2).
Colic; fever; pain.

Dolocibal *Novartis, Mex.*
Ibuprofen (p.43·2); caffeine (p.761·3).
Fever; inflammation; pain.

Dolocid *Merck Sharp & Dohme, Neth.*
Diflunisal (p.32·2).
Musculoskeletal and joint disorders; pain.

Dolocod *Klinge, Aust.*
Aspirin (p.14·2); paracetamol (p.71·2); codeine phosphate (p.25·2).
Fever; pain.

Dolo-cyl *Liebermann, Ger.*
Note. A similar name is used for preparations of different composition (see below).
Arnica oil (p.1581·3); eucalyptus oil (p.1609·2); hypericum oil (p.290·3); juniper oil (p.1625·2); lavender oil (p.1627·2); pumilio pine oil (p.1656·3); rosemary oil (p.1659·3).
Musculoskeletal and joint disorders; sports injuries.

Dolocyl
Note. A similar name is used for preparations of different composition (see above).
Ciba Vision, Ital.; Novartis Consumer, Port.; Novartis, Spain†; Novartis Consumer, Switz.
Ibuprofen (p.43·2).
Fever; pain.

Dolodens *Reig Jofre, Spain.*
Codeine phosphate (p.25·2); hydroxyzine hydrochloride (p.419·1); propyphenazone (p.80·2).
Pain.

Dolodent
Note.This name is used for preparations of different composition.
OBA, Denm.
Benzocaine (p.1306·2); myrrh (p.1639·2).
Mouth pain.

Gilbert, Fr.
Amylocaine hydrochloride (p.1306·1); cloral hydrate (p.669·3).
Teething pain.

Doloderm *Theraplix, Fr.; Rhone-Poulenc Rorer, Ital.*
Methyl butetisalicylate (p.55·1).
Musculoskeletal and joint pain.

Dolo-Dismenol *Adroka, Switz.*
Ibuprofen (p.43·2).
Pain.

Dolo-Dobendan *Boots Healthcare, Ger.*
Cetylpyridinium chloride (p.1138·1); benzocaine (p.1306·2).
Mouth and throat disorders.

Dolodoc *Docpharm, Ger.*
Ibuprofen (p.43·2).
Fever; pain.

Dolofarma *Maxfarma, Spain.*
Aspirin (p.14·2); caffeine (p.761·3); paracetamol (p.71·2).
Fever; pain.

Dolofenac *Arlex, Mex.*
Diclofenac (p.30·2).

Doloflex *Byk Gulden, Ital.*
Paracetamol (p.71·2); aspirin (p.14·2).
Pain.

Dolofort *Klinge, Aust.*
Ibuprofen (p.43·2).
Pain.

Dolofur *Fustery, Mex.*
Dipyrone (p.34·1).
Fever; pain.

Dologel
Note. This name is used for preparations of different composition.
Medicamed, Port.
Capsicum (p.1591·1); eucalyptus oil (p.1609·2); methyl salicylate (p.55·1); menthol (p.1632·3).
Muscular pain.

Wander OTC, Switz.†.
Ibuprofen (p.43·2).
Musculoskeletal, joint, and soft-tissue disorders.

Dologen *Kenyaku, Thai.*
Ibuprofen (p.43·2); paracetamol (p.71·2).
Musculoskeletal, joint, peri-articular, and soft-tissue disorders.

Dologesic *Lilly, Hong Kong.*
Paracetamol (p.71·2); dextropropoxyphene napsilate (p.27·1).
Pain.

Dologex *Cinfa, Spain.*
Turpentine oil (p.1676·3); menthol (p.1632·3); camphor (p.1589·3); methyl salicylate (p.55·1).
Musculoskeletal, joint, and soft-tissue disorders.

Dologyne *Arkopharma, Fr.†.*
Artemisia vulgaris; chamomile (p.1593·2).
Pain.

Doloject *Syxyl, Ger.*
Homoeopathic preparation.

Dolokapton *Strallhofer, Aust.*
Paracetamol (p.71·2); codeine phosphate (p.25·2).
Coughs; fever; pain.

Dolokey *Inkeysa, Spain.*
Camphor (p.1589·3); lavender oil (p.1627·2); methyl salicylate (p.55·1); expressed mustard oil (p.1639·1); rosemary oil (p.1659·3); eucalyptus oil (p.1609·2); belladonna (p.463·1); capsicum (p.1591·1); menthol (p.1632·3).
Musculoskeletal and joint disorders.

Dolol *Nycomed, Denm.*
Tramadol hydrochloride (p.89·1).
Pain.

Dolomedil *Almirall, Spain.*
Codeine phosphate (p.25·2); paracetamol (p.71·2).
Pain.

Dolo-Menthoneurin
Byk, Aust.; Tosse, Ger.; Roland, Ger.; Byk Gulden, Ger.
Diethylamine salicylate (p.32·2); heparin sodium (p.902·1); menthol (p.1632·3).
Neuralgia; soft-tissue, musculoskeletal, and joint disorders.

Dolo-Menthoneurin CreSa *Tosse, Ger.†.*
Glycol salicylate (p.42·2); benzyl nicotinate (p.20·2); camphor (p.1589·3).
Muscle, joint, and peri-articular disorders.

Dolomine *Frega, Canad.*
Aspirin (p.14·2); caffeine (p.761·3).

Dolomite *Nature's Bounty, USA.*
Calcium salts (p.1187·3); magnesium salts (p.1190·3).
Dietary supplement.

Dolomo *Klinge, Aust.*
Aspirin (p.14·2); paracetamol (p.71·2); caffeine (p.761·3).
Fever; pain.

Dolomo TN *Klinge, Ger.*
White tablets, aspirin (p.14·2); paracetamol (p.71·2); caffeine (p.761·3); blue tablets, aspirin; paracetamol; codeine phosphate (p.25·2).
Pain.

Dolonerv *Gerot, Aust.*
Paracetamol (p.71·2); vitamin B substances (p.1350·1).
Pain.

Doloneuro *Merck, Ger.*
Diethylamine salicylate (p.32·2); glycol salicylate (p.42·2); methyl nicotinate (p.55·1).
Muscle, nerve, and joint pain; soft-tissue injury.

Dolo-Neurobion
Merck, Aust.; Merck, Mex.
Diclofenac sodium (p.30·3); thiamine nitrate (p.1385·1); pyridoxine hydrochloride (p.1386·3); cyanocobalamin (p.1388·1).
Musculoskeletal and joint disorders; neuralgia; neuritis; neuropathy.

Dolo-Neurobion forte *Merck, Ger.*
Vitamin B substances (p.1350·1); paracetamol (p.71·2).
Arthritis; back pain; neuralgia.

Dolo-Neurobion N
Merck, Ger.; Merck, Hong Kong.
Vitamin B substances (p.1350·1); paracetamol (p.71·2).
Joint disorders; lumbago; neuralgia; neuritis; sciatica.

Dolono *RID, USA.*
Paracetamol (p.71·2).
Fever; pain.

Dolophine *Roxane, USA.*
Methadone hydrochloride (p.53·1).
Detoxification and treatment of opioid addiction; pain.

DoloPosterine N *Kade, Ger.*
Cinchocaine hydrochloride (p.1309·1).
Anorectal disorders.

Doloproct
Schering, Denm.; Schering, Ger.; Asche, Ger.
Fluocortolone pivalate (p.1071·3); lignocaine [lidocaine] hydrochloride (p.1313·2).
Anorectal disorders.

Doloproct Comp *Schering, Denm.*
Fluocortolone pivalate (p.1071·3); lignocaine [lidocaine] hydrochloride (p.1313·2); benzyl alcohol (p.1135·2).
Formerly contained fluocortolone pivalate, lignocaine [lidocaine] hydrochloride, and chlorquinaldol.
Anorectal disorders.

Dolo-Prolixan *Siegfried, Switz.†*
Yellow tablets, azapropazone (p.19·1); dextropropoxyphene hydrochloride (p.27·1); blue tablets, azapropazone; phenprobamate (p.699·3).
Musculoskeletal, joint, and peri-articular pain.

Dolo-Puren *Isis Puren, Ger.*
Ibuprofen (p.43·2).
Fever; gout; inflammation; musculoskeletal, joint, and soft-tissue disorders; pain.

Dolopyrine *Streuli, Switz.†.*
Propyphenazone (p.80·2); atropine methobromide (p.460·3); papaverine hydrochloride (p.1648·1); diphenhydramine hydrochloride (p.416·1); codeine phosphate (p.25·2).
Pain.

Dolorac *GenDerm, USA.*
Capsaicin (p.23·1).
Pain.

Doloreduct *Azupharma, Ger.*
Paracetamol (p.71·2).
Fever; pain.

Doloren *Ratiopharm, Aust.†.*
Ibuprofen (p.43·2).
Fever; musculoskeletal and joint disorders; pain.

Dolorex *Whitehall-Robins, Switz.†.*
Glycol salicylate (p.42·2); camphor (p.1589·3); lavender oil (p.1627·2); thyme oil (p.1672·3); siberian fir oil; isopropyl alcohol (p.1149·2).
Musculoskeletal, joint, peri-articular, and soft-tissue disorders.

Dolorex Neo *Whitehall-Robins, Switz.†.*
Glycol salicylate (p.42·2); allantoin (p.1110·1).
Musculoskeletal and joint disorders; superficial circulatory disorders.

Dolorgiet *Dolorgiet, Ger.†.*
Glycol salicylate (p.42·2); benzyl nicotinate (p.20·2).
Musculoskeletal and joint disorders.

Dolor-loges *Loges, Ger.*
Homoeopathic preparation.

Dolormin Woelm, Ger.
Ibuprofen lysine (p.44·1).
Fever; pain.

Dolorol Aspen Consumer, S.Afr.
Paracetamol (p.71·2).
Fever; pain.

Dolorol Forte Aspen Consumer, S.Afr.
Paracetamol (p.71·2); codeine phosphate (p.25·2).
Fever; pain.

Dolorsan-Balsam Opfermann, Ger.
Methyl salicylate (p.55·1); menthol (p.1632·3); camphor (p.1589·3).
Catarrh; musculoskeletal and joint disorders; neuralgia; sports injuries.

Dolo-Rubriment Riemser, Ger.
Glycol salicylate (p.42·2); benzyl nicotinate (p.20·2); heparin sodium (p.902·1).
Muscle, nerve, joint, and soft-tissue disorders.

Dolosal Cristalia, Braz.; Rhone-Poulenc Rorer, Fr.
Pethidine hydrochloride (p.75·1).
Pain; premedication.

Dolosarto Biosarto, Spain.
Aspirin (p.14·2); benzydamine hydrochloride (p.20·1).
Fever; inflammation; musculoskeletal and joint disorders; pain.

Dolo-Spedifen Inpharzam, Switz.
Ibuprofen arginine (p.44·1).
Fever; pain.

Dolostop
Note. This name is used for preparations of different composition.
Bayer, Spain.
Paracetamol (p.71·2).
Fever; pain.

Zeller, Switz.
Propyphenazone (p.80·2); paracetamol (p.71·2); caffeine (p.761·3).
Fever; pain.

Dolotandex Novartis, Mex.
Naproxen sodium (p.61·3); paracetamol (p.71·2).
Fever; pain.

Dolotard Nycomed, Swed.
Dextropropoxyphene chloride (p.27·1).
Pain.

Dolotec Innothera, Fr.
Paracetamol (p.71·2).
Fever; pain.

Doloteffin Chemists Own, Austral.; Ardeypharm, Ger.
Devil's claw root (p.26·3).
Musculoskeletal and joint disorders.

DoloTendin Divinal, Ger.†.
Dexamethasone (p.1067·1); lignocaine [lidocaine] hydrochloride (p.1313·2).
Musculoskeletal, joint, and peri-articular disorders.

Dolothricin Provita, Aust.†.
Tyrothricin (p.267·1); neomycin sulfate (p.228·1); benzocaine (p.1306·2); camphor (p.1589·3); chloroxylenol (p.1142·1).
Bacterial ear infections.

Dolo-Tiaminal Silanes, Mex.
Dipyrone (p.34·1); cyanocobalamin (p.1388·1); thiamine nitrate (p.1385·1); pyridoxine hydrochloride (p.1386·3).
Neuralgia; neuritis.

Dolotor Roche, Mex.
Ketorolac trometamol (p.48·2).
Pain.

Dolotren Faes, Spain.
Diclofenac diethylamine (p.30·2) or diclofenac sodium (p.30·3).
Gout; musculoskeletal, joint, peri-articular, and soft tissue disorders; pain; renal colic.

Dolo-Veniten Whitehall-Robins, Switz.
Glycol salicylate (p.42·2); a heparinoid (p.905·2); aescin (p.1574·1).
Vascular disorders.

Dolovin Atral, Port.
Indometacin (p.44·3).
Gout; musculoskeletal and joint disorders.

DoloVisano M Kade, Ger.
Mephenesin (p.1329·2).
Cervical syndrome; lumbago; skeletal muscle spasm.

DoloVisano Salbe Kade, Ger.
Glycol salicylate (p.42·2); benzyl nicotinate (p.20·2).
Circulatory disorders of the skin; muscle, joint, and soft-tissue disorders.

Dolo-Voltaren Novartis, Spain.
Diclofenac sodium (p.30·3).
Gout; musculoskeletal, joint, and peri-articular disorders; pain; renal colic.

Doloxene Lilly, Austral.; Lilly, Denm.; Lilly, Hong Kong; Lilly, Irl.; Lilly, NZ; Quatromed, S.Afr.; Lilly, Swed.; Lilly, UK.
Dextropropoxyphene hydrochloride (p.27·1) or dextropropoxyphene napsilate (p.27·1).
Pain.

Doloxene Co Quatromed, S.Afr.
Dextropropoxyphene hydrochloride (p.27·1); aspirin (p.14·2); caffeine (p.761·3).
Pain.

Doloxene Compound Lilly, Hong Kong; Lilly, Irl.; Lilly, UK†.
Dextropropoxyphene napsilate (p.27·1); aspirin (p.14·2); caffeine (p.761·3).
Pain.

Doloxene-A Lilly, Braz.
Dextropropoxyphene napsilate (p.27·1); aspirin (p.14·2).
Pain.

Dolpocetmol Synco, Hong Kong.
Dextropropoxyphene hydrochloride (p.27·1); paracetamol (p.71·2).
Pain.

Dolprone Aventis, Belg.; Rhone-Poulenc Rorer, Switz.
Paracetamol (p.71·2).
Fever; pain.

Dolpyc
Note. This name is used for preparations of different composition.
Bournonville, Belg.†.
Capsicum oleoresin (p.1591·1); chloroform (p.1256·3).
Muscle and joint pain.

Warner-Lambert, Fr.†.
Capsicum (p.1591·1); chloroform (p.1256·3).
Pain and bruising.

Teofarma, Ital.
Capsicum oleoresin (p.1591·1).
Musculoskeletal, joint, and soft-tissue pain.

Dolsed American Urologicals, USA.
Methenamine (p.223·1); salol (p.82·2); atropine sulfate (p.461·1); hyoscyamine sulfate (p.469·3); benzoic acid (p.1134·2); methylene blue [methylthioninium chloride] (p.1012·3).
Urinary-tract infections.

Dolsinal Ferrer, Spain.
Nabumetone (p.59·3).
Osteoarthritis; rheumatoid arthritis.

Dol-Stop Warner-Lambert Consumer, Belg.†.
Paracetamol (p.71·2); codeine phosphate (p.25·2).
Fever; pain.

Doltard Nycomed, Denm.
Morphine sulfate (p.56·1).
Pain.

Dol-u-ron Neo-Farmaceutica, Port.
Paracetamol (p.71·2); codeine phosphate (p.25·2).
Pain.

Dolvan Norma, UK.
Diphenhydramine hydrochloride (p.416·1); ephedrine hydrochloride (p.1090·1); paracetamol (p.71·2); caffeine (p.761·3).
Cold and influenza symptoms; nasal congestion.

Dolver Maver, Mex.
Ibuprofen (p.43·2).
Inflammation; pain.

Dolviran Bayer, Belg.; Bayer, Port.; Bayer, Spain.
Aspirin (p.14·2); codeine phosphate (p.25·2); caffeine (p.761·3).
Fever; pain.

Dolviran N
Note. This name is used for preparations of different composition.
Hexal, Ger.
Aspirin (p.14·2); codeine phosphate (p.25·2).
Pain.

Bayer, Neth.
Aspirin (p.14·2); codeine phosphate (p.25·2); caffeine (p.761·3).
Fever; pain.

Dolviran NF Bayer, Mex.
Paracetamol (p.71·2).
Fever; pain.

Dolxen Maver, Mex.
Naproxen (p.60·3).
Inflammation; musculoskeletal and joint disorders; pain.

Dolzam Zambon, Belg.
Tramadol hydrochloride (p.89·1).
Pain.

Dolzycam Sons, Mex.
Piroxicam (p.79·1).
Gout; musculoskeletal, joint, peri-articular, and soft-tissue disorders.

Domar
Eurodrug, Hong Kong; Teofarma, Ital.; Eurodrug, Singapore; Eurodrug, Thai.
Pinazepam (p.700·2).
Alcoholism; anxiety; epilepsy; mixed anxiety depressive states; neuroses.

Domeboro Serral, Mex.; Miles, USA.
Aluminium sulfate (p.1578·2); calcium acetate (p.1187·3).
Inflammatory skin conditions.

Domenan Kissei, Jpn.
Ozagrel hydrochloride (p.1645·3).
Asthma.

Dome-Paste Miles, USA.
Zinc oxide (p.1128·2); calamine (p.1111·3); gelatin (p.737·2).
Conditions of the extremities requiring protection and support.

Domerdon Asian Pharm, Thai.
Domperidone (p.1224·1).
Delayed gastric emptying; dyspepsia; flatulence; gastro-oesophageal reflux; heartburn; nausea and vomiting.

Domes SoSe, Ital.
Nimesulide (p.62·3).
Fever; inflammation; pain.

Domex Sante Naturelle, Canad.†.
Calcium and magnesium (p.1350·1).

Domical Rhone-Poulenc Rorer, Hong Kong; Berk, Irl.†; Berk, UK†.
Amitriptyline hydrochloride (p.273·3).
Depression.

Domicetina Wiener, Mex.
Chloramphenicol (p.179·1).
Bacterial infections.

Domidone Milano, Thai.
Domperidone (p.1224·1).
Digestive disorders; dyspepsia; flatulence; gastro-oesophageal reflux; heartburn; nausea and vomiting.

Domidorm Asta Medica, Belg.†.
Prothipendyl hydrochloride (p.702·3); cyclobarbital calcium (p.674·2).
Agitation; insomnia; premedication.

Domilium LSP, Thai.
Domperidone (p.1224·1) or domperidone maleate (p.1224·1).
Delayed gastric emptying; digestive disorders; dyspepsia; nausea and vomiting.

Domin Boehringer Ingelheim, Jpn.
Talipexole hydrochloride (p.1179·1).
Parkinsonism.

Dominal Asta Medica, Aust.; Asta Medica, Belg.; Asta Medica, Ger.
Prothipendyl hydrochloride (p.702·3).
Atopic dermatitis; eclampsia; gastrointestinal spasm; postoperative vomiting; premedication; pruritus; psychiatric disorders; sedative.

Dominans Lundbeck, Ital.
Nortriptyline hydrochloride (p.301·3); fluphenazine hydrochloride (p.684·3).
Mixed anxiety depressive states.

Domnamid Lundbeck, Denm.
Estazolam (p.682·3).
Premedication; sleep disorders.

Domol Miles, USA.
Bath additive.
Lubrication of the skin; pruritus.

Dompenyl Korea United, Singapore.
Domperidone (p.1224·1).
Nausea and vomiting.

Domperamol Servier, UK.
Paracetamol (p.71·2); domperidone maleate (p.1224·1).
Migraine.

Domperdone Polipharm, Thai.
Domperidone (p.1224·1).
Digestive disorders; dyspepsia; nausea and vomiting.

Dompil Spyfarma, Spain.
Metampicillin sodium (p.222·3).
Bacterial infections.

Domutussina Proge, Ital.
Dropropizine (p.1089·3).
Coughs.

Domuvar Bioprogress, Ital.
Spores of *Bacillus subtilis*.
Gastrointestinal disorders.

Dona Rottapharm, Ital.; Opfermann, Ger.
Glucosamine sulfate (p.1616·2).
Degenerative joint disorders.

Donalg Dynacren, Ital.
Amethocaine [tetracaine] hydrochloride (p.1305·2); sulfogaiacol (p.1101·1); salicylic acid (p.1122·3); menthol (p.1632·3); sage (p.1660·2); chamomile (p.1593·2); salix (p.82·1); ginger (p.1227·2).
Dental pain.

Donamet Ravizza, Ital.
Ademetionine butanedisulfonate (p.1573·1).
Hepatic cholestasis.

Donaprox Reuffer, Mex.
Naproxen (p.60·3).

Donatiol AGIPS, Ital.
Mecysteine hydrochloride (p.1094·2); guaifenesin (p.1092·2); camphor (p.1589·3).
Respiratory-tract disorders.

Donatussin Laser, USA.
Oral drops: Chlorpheniramine [chlorphenamine] maleate (p.412·1); phenylephrine hydrochloride (p.1097·1); guaifenesin (p.1092·2).
Syrup: Chlorpheniramine [chlorphenamine] maleate (p.412·1); phenylephrine hydrochloride (p.1097·1); dextromethorphan hydrobromide (p.1087·3); guaifenesin (p.1092·2).
Coughs.

Donatussin DC Laser, USA.
Hydrocodone tartrate (p.42·2); phenylephrine hydrochloride (p.1097·1); guaifenesin (p.1092·2).
Coughs.

Doncef Pharma 2000, Fr.
Cefradine (p.173·3).
Bacterial infections.

Doneka Vita, Spain.
Lisinopril (p.921·1).
Diabetic nephropathy; heart failure; hypertension; myocardial infarction.

Doneka Plus Vita, Spain.
Lisinopril (p.921·1); hydrochlorothiazide (p.907·3).
Hypertension.

Doneurin Hexal, Ger.
Doxepin hydrochloride (p.283·3).
Anxiety; depression; withdrawal syndromes.

Dong Quai Complex Blackmores, Austral.
Angelica sinensis (p.1583·1); cimicifuga (p.1595·2); vitex agnus castus (p.1574·2); vitamins and minerals (p.1350·1).
Menopausal disorders; premenstrual syndrome; uterine cramping.

Donicer Novag, Spain†.
Amiloride hydrochloride (p.835·1); hydrochlorothiazide (p.907·3).
Hypertension; oedema.

Donix Llorens, Spain.
Lorazepam (p.688·3).
Alcohol withdrawal syndrome; anxiety disorders; chemotherapy induced nausea and vomiting; insomnia; premedication.

Donnagel
Note. This name is used for preparations of different composition.
Whitehall, Austral.
Hyoscyamine sulfate (p.469·3); atropine sulfate (p.461·1); hyoscine hydrobromide (p.468·2); kaolin (p.1229·3); pectin (p.1502·3).
Gastrointestinal disorders.

IQB, Braz.
Metronidazole (p.594·1); nystatin (p.392·3); benzalkonium chloride (p.1133·2); urea (p.1127·3).
Vulvovaginal infections.

Wyeth-Ayerst, USA.
Attapulgite (p.1212·1).
Diarrhoea.

Donnagel-PG Wyeth-Ayerst, Canad.
Capsules: Activated attapulgite (p.1212·1); pectin (p.1502·3); prepared opium (p.69·3).
Oral suspension: Kaolin (p.1229·3); pectin (p.1502·3); prepared opium (p.69·3).
Diarrhoea.

Donnalix Whitehall, Austral.
Hyoscyamine sulfate (p.469·3); atropine sulfate (p.461·1); hyoscine hydrobromide (p.468·2).
Gastrointestinal disorders.

Donnamar Marnel, USA.
Hyoscyamine sulfate (p.469·3).

Donnamor Moore, USA†.
Atropine sulfate (p.461·1); hyoscine hydrobromide (p.468·2); hyoscyamine hydrobromide (p.469·3) or hyoscyamine sulfate (p.469·3); phenobarbital (p.355·1).
Gastrointestinal disorders.

Donna-Sed Vortech, USA†.
Atropine sulfate (p.461·1); hyoscine hydrobromide (p.468·2); hyoscyamine hydrobromide (p.469·3) or hyoscyamine sulfate (p.469·3); phenobarbital (p.355·1).
Gastrointestinal disorders.

Donnatab Whitehall, Austral.
Hyoscyamine sulfate (p.469·3); atropine sulfate (p.461·1); hyoscine hydrobromide (p.468·2).
Gastrointestinal disorders.

Donnatal Wyeth-Ayerst, Canad.; Aspen, S.Afr.; Whitehall, Thai.; Robins, USA.
Hyoscyamine sulfate (p.469·3); atropine sulfate (p.461·1); hyoscine hydrobromide (p.468·2); phenobarbital (p.355·1).
Biliary-tract disorders; gastrointestinal disorders; genitourinary-tract disorders; motion sickness.

Donnazyme Robins, USA.
Pancreatin (p.1646·1).
Pancreatic insufficiency.

Donobid Merck Sharp & Dohme, Denm.; Merck Sharp & Dohme, Fin.; Merck Sharp & Dohme, Norw.; Merck Sharp & Dohme, Swed.
Diflunisal (p.32·2).
Inflammation; musculoskeletal and joint disorders; pain.

Donodol Armstrong, Mex.
Clonixin lysine (p.25·1).
Pain.

Donodol Compuesto Armstrong, Mex.
Clonixin lysine (p.25·1); hyoscine butylbromide (p.468·2).
Smooth muscle pain and spasm.

Donorest Wyeth Lederle, Port.†; Wyeth, Spain.
Fentiazac (p.40·2).
Musculoskeletal, joint, and peri-articular disorders; pain.

Donormyl Oberlin, Fr; Upsamedica, Spain.
Doxylamine succinate (p.417·1).
Insomnia.

Don't Del, USA†.
Sucrose octa-acetate (p.1668·1); isopropyl alcohol (p.1149·2).
Nail biting deterrent.

Dontisolon D Hoechst Marion Roussel, Ger.
Prednisolone (p.1077·3) or prednisolone acetate (p.1078·1).
Inflammatory disorders of the mouth.

Dontopivalone Parke, Davis, Fr.†.
Tixocortol pivalate (p.1080·1); chlorhexidine acetate (p.1138·2).
Mouth disorders.

Dontuxin Continentales, Mex.
Dextromethorphan (p.1087·3).

Donulide Wyeth Lederle, Port.
Nimesulide (p.62·3).
Fever; pain.

Donum M & H, Thai.
Domperidone (p.1224·1).
Dyspepsia; gastro-oesophageal reflux; heartburn; nausea and vomiting.

Dopacard Elan, Denm.; Ipsen, Fin.; Ipsen Biotech, Fr.†; Elan, Ger.; Elan, Irl.; NZ Medical & Scientific, NZ; Ipsen, Swed.; Galenica, Switz.; Elan, UK.
Dopexamine hydrochloride (p.882·3).
Heart failure.

Dopaflex Medphano, Ger.
Levodopa (p.1169·2).
Parkinsonism.

Dopamed
Note. This name is used for preparations of different composition.
SMP, S.Afr.†
Dopamine hydrochloride (p.881·3).
Heart failure; shock.

General Drugs, Thai.
Methyldopa (p.927·3).
Hypertension.

Dopamet Dumex-Alpharma, Denm.†; Rhone-Poulenc Rorer, Hong Kong; Berk, Irl.†; Dumex, Norw.†; Dumex, Switz.†; Berk, UK†.
Methyldopa (p.927·3).
Hypertension.

Dopamex Biolab, Thai.
Dopamine hydrochloride (p.881·3).
Acute poisoning; hypotension; shock.

Dopaminex Solvay, Hong Kong; Solvay, Thai.
Dopamine hydrochloride (p.881·3).
Hypotension; shock.

Dopar Procter & Gamble, USA.
Levodopa (p.1169·2).
Parkinsonism.

Doparid Rafa, Israel.
Tiapride hydrochloride (p.709·1).
Choreas; dyskinesias; tics; tremor.

Dopasian Asian Pharm, Thai.
Methyldopa (p.927·3).
Hypertension.

Dopegyt Thiemann, Ger.; Egis, Hong Kong; Egis, Singapore; Egis, Thai.
Methyldopa (p.927·3).
Hypertension.

Dopergin Schering, Aust.; Schering, Braz.; Schering, Ger.; Schering, Israel; Schering, Ital.; Schering, Mex.; Schering, Neth.; Schering, NZ; Schering, Spain; Schering, Switz.; Schering, Thai.
Lisuride maleate (p.1174·1).
Acromegaly; hyperprolactinaemia; infertility; lactation inhibition; mastitis; menstrual disorders; parkinsonism.

Dopergine Schering, Fr.
Lisuride maleate (p.1174·1).
Erectile dysfunction; galactorrhoea; gynaecomastia in males; infertility; menstrual disorders; parkinsonism.

Dopicar Merck Sharp & Dohme, Israel.
Carbidopa (p.1168·2); levodopa (p.1169·2).
Parkinsonism.

Dopin Pharmaland, Thai.
Dothiepin [dosulepin] hydrochloride (p.283·2).
Depression; mixed anxiety depressive states.

Dopmin Orion, Denm.; Orion, Fin.; Orion, Singapore; Orion, Thai.
Dopamine hydrochloride (p.881·3).
Heart failure; shock.

Dopo Pik Tipomark, Ital.
Triclosan (Irgasan 300) (p.1159·2); trolamine (p.1675·1); propylene glycol (p.1655·1).
Skin disinfection.

Doppelherz Energie-Tonikum N Queisser, Ger.
Vitamin B substances; honey; invert sugar; crataegus; valerian; lupulus (p.1350·1).
Tonic.

Doppelherz Ginseng Aktiv Queisser, Ger.
Ginseng; pyridoxine hydrochloride; nicotinamide; caffeine (p.1350·1).
Tonic.

Doppelherz Magenstarkung Queisser, Ger.†
Peppermint leaf (p.1243·2); absinthium (p.1571·1); silybum marianum (p.1021·3).
Gastrointestinal disorders.

Doppelherz Melissengeist Queisser, Ger.
Melissa (p.1632·2); angelica (p.1580·2); cinnamon (p.1595·3); nutmeg (p.1643·1); bitter-orange peel (p.1644·2); clove (p.1596·3); lemon peel.
Cold symptoms; insomnia; musculoskeletal and joint pain; nervous disorders.

Doppelherz Tonikum Queisser, Aust.
Crataegus (p.1600·2); melissa (p.1632·2); lupulus (p.1629·3).
Tonic.

Doppel-Spalt Compact Whitehall-Much, Ger.
Aspirin (p.14·2); caffeine (p.761·3).
Fever; inflammation; pain.

Dopram Sanova, Aust.; Wyeth-Ayerst, Austral.; Wyeth Lederle, Belg.; Wyeth-Ayerst, Canad.; Wyeth Lederle, Fin.; Robins, Hong Kong; Antigen, Irl.; Wyeth, Neth.; Wyeth Lederle, Norw.; Wyeth, NZ; Intramed, S.Afr.; Wyeth, Switz.; Anpharm, UK; Robins, USA.
Doxapram hydrochloride (p.1509·1).
Respiratory depression.

Dopress Pacific, NZ.
Dothiepin [dosulepin] hydrochloride (p.283·2).
Depression.

Doprit Farcoral, Mex.
Hydroxocobalamin (p.1388·1).

Dops
Note. This name is used for preparations of different composition.
Fuca, Fr.
Sodium bicarbonate (p.1186·2); calcium carbonate (p.1215·1); calcium phosphate (p.1188·3); magnesium hydroxide (p.1233·1); titanium dioxide (p.1126·1); magnesium carbonate (p.1232·3).
Gastric hyperacidity.

Sumitomo, Jpn.
Droxidopa (p.1168·3).
Familial amyloid polyneuropathy; parkinsonism.

Doral Wallace, USA.
Quazepam (p.703·1).
Insomnia.

Doralem Farmedica, Braz.
Aspirin (p.14·2); paracetamol (p.71·2); caffeine (p.761·3).
Aluminium hydroxide (p.1210·3) is included in this preparation in an attempt to limit adverse effects on the gastrointestinal mucosa.
Fever; pain.

Doralese SmithKline Beecham, Irl.; Bencard, UK.
Indoramin (p.914·1) or indoramin hydrochloride (p.913·3).
Benign prostatic hyperplasia.

Doralon Heralds, Braz.
Dipyrone (p.34·1); diphenhydramine (p.416·1).
Fever; pain.

Doran QIF, Braz.
Dipyrone (p.34·1).
Fever; pain.

Dorbid Prodome, Braz.
Diflunisal (p.32·2).
Gout; inflammation; musculoskeletal, joint, and peri-articular disorders; pain.

Dorcalor BA Farma, Port.
Diclofenac sodium (p.30·3).
Inflammation; musculoskeletal, joint, and peri-articular disorders; pain.

Dorcol Children's Cold Formula Novartis, USA.
Pseudoephedrine hydrochloride (p.1099·2); chlorpheniramine [chlorphenamine] maleate (p.412·1).
Cold symptoms.

Dorcol Children's Cough Syrup Novartis, USA.
Pseudoephedrine hydrochloride (p.1099·2); guaifenesin (p.1092·2); dextromethorphan hydrobromide (p.1087·3).
Coughs.

Dorcol Children's Decongestant Novartis, USA.
Pseudoephedrine hydrochloride (p.1099·2).
Nasal congestion.

Dorcol Children's Fever & Pain Reducer Novartis, USA†.
Paracetamol (p.71·2).
Fever; pain.

Dordendril Heralds, Braz.
Paracetamol (p.71·2).
Fever; pain.

Dore Immun Rentschler, Ger.
Echinacea (p.1606·2).
Immunostimulant.

Doregrippin Rentschler, Ger.
Paracetamol (p.71·2); phenylephrine hydrochloride (p.1097·1).
Cold and influenza symptoms.

Dorehydrin Procter & Gamble, Aust.
Co-dergocrine mesilate (p.1597·3).
Cervical syndrome; hypertension; mental function impairment; migraine and related vascular headache; peripheral vascular disorders.

Dorenasin Rentschler, Ger.
Xylometazoline hydrochloride (p.1102·2).
Nasal congestion.

Doreperol N Rentschler, Ger.
Hexetidine (p.1146·3).
Mouth and throat disorders; oral hygiene.

Doretrim AP Novartis, Braz.
Ibuprofen (p.43·2).
Fever; inflammation; pain.

Dorflex Hoechst Marion Roussel, Braz.
Dipyrone (p.34·1); orphenadrine citrate (p.470·3); caffeine (p.761·3).
Skeletal muscle spasm.

Dorgen Cazi, Braz.
Diclofenac sodium (p.30·3).
Gout; inflammation; musculoskeletal, joint, and peri-articular disorders; pain.

Dori Rentschler, Ger.
Benzocaine (p.1306·2); cetylpyridinium chloride (p.1138·1); tyrothricin (p.267·1).
Mouth and throat inflammation.

Doribel Luper, Braz.
Aspirin (p.14·2); caffeine (p.761·3).
Fever; pain.

Dorical Legrand, Braz.
Vitamins; sodium fluoride; calcium ferrous citrate (p.1350·1).
Nutritional supplement.

Doricin EMS, Braz.
Orphenadrine citrate (p.470·3); dipyrone (p.34·1); caffeine citrate (p.761·3).
Skeletal muscle spasm.

Dorico Sanofi Winthrop, Braz.
Paracetamol (p.71·2).
Fever; pain.

Doricum Farmila, Ital.
Fluocinolone acetonide (p.1071·1); neomycin sulfate (p.228·1).
Eye, ear, and nose disorders.

Doridamina Angelini, Ital.
Lonidamine (p.550·3).
Malignant neoplasms.

Doriflan Luper, Braz.
Diclofenac potassium (p.30·2).
Gout; inflammation; musculoskeletal, joint, and peri-articular disorders; pain.

Doril Dorsay, Braz.
Aspirin (p.14·2); caffeine (p.761·3).
Fever; pain.

Dorilax Ache, Braz.
Paracetamol (p.71·2); carisoprodol (p.1327·1); caffeine (p.761·3).
Skeletal muscle spasm.

Dorithricin Provita, Aust.
Tyrothricin (p.267·1); neomycin sulfate (p.228·1).
Mouth and throat disorders.

Dorithricin Limone Rentschler, Ger.
Tyrothricin (p.267·1); lignocaine [lidocaine] hydrochloride (p.1313·2).
Mouth and throat disorders.

Dorithricin Original Rentschler, Ger.
Tyrothricin (p.267·1); benzalkonium chloride (p.1133·2); benzocaine (p.1306·2).
Mouth and throat disorders.

Dorival Bayer, Spain.
Ibuprofen (p.43·2).
Fever; pain.

Dorixina Rhein, Mex.
Clonixin lysine (p.25·1).
Pain.

Dorken UCB, Spain.
Dipotassium clorazepate (p.670·3).
Formerly contained dipotassium clorazepate, aminohydroxybutyric acid, and pyridoxine.
Anxiety disorders; insomnia.

Dormalon Wernigerode, Ger.
Nitrazepam (p.695·2).
Sleep disorders.

Dormarex 2 Republic, USA†.
Diphenhydramine hydrochloride (p.416·1).
Insomnia; motion sickness; parkinsonism.

Dormarist Steiner, Ger.
Valerian (p.1678·3); melissa (p.1632·2).
Sleep disorders.

Dorme Hoechst Marion Roussel, S.Afr.†
Quazepam (p.703·1).
Insomnia.

Dormeasan Bioforce, Ger.
Valerian (p.1678·3); lupulus (p.1629·3).
Agitation; insomnia.

Dormeasan N Bioforce, Switz.
Lupulus (p.1629·3); valerian (p.1678·3).
Agitation; insomnia; irritability.

Dormen Labima, Belg.
Pyrithyldione (p.703·1); diphenhydramine hydrochloride (p.416·1).
Insomnia.

Dormer 211 Dormer, Canad.
Emollient.
Dry skin.

Dormex Nobel, Canad.
Diphenhydramine hydrochloride (p.416·1).
Insomnia.

Dormicum Roche, Aust.; Roche, Belg.; Roche, Denm.; Roche, Fin.; Roche, Ger.; Roche, Hong Kong; Roche, Israel; Roche, Mex.; Roche, Neth.; Roche, Norw.; Roche, Port.; Roche, S.Afr.; Roche, Singapore; Roche, Spain; Roche, Swed.; Roche, Switz.; Roche, Thai.
Midazolam (p.692·3), midazolam hydrochloride (p.692·3), or midazolam maleate (p.693·1).
General anaesthesia; insomnia; premedication; sedative.

Dormidina Pensa, Spain.
Doxylamine succinate (p.417·1).
Insomnia.

Dormi-Gastreu N R14 Reckeweg, Ger.
Homoeopathic preparation.

Dormigoa N Scheurich, Ger.†
Diphenhydramine hydrochloride (p.416·1).
Dormigoa formerly contained diphenhydramine hydrochloride and guaifenesin.
Sleep disorders.

Dormin Randob, USA.
Diphenhydramine hydrochloride (p.416·1).
Insomnia.

Dormiphen Lalco, Canad.
Diphenhydramine hydrochloride (p.416·1).
Insomnia.

Dormiplant Schwabe, Switz.†
Valerian (p.1678·3); melissa (p.1632·2).
Sleep disorders.

Dormodor ICN, Spain.
Flurazepam hydrochloride (p.685·3).
Insomnia.

Dormonid Roche, Braz.
Midazolam (p.692·3).
Adjunct in anaesthesia; premedication; sedative.

Dormonoct Aventis, Belg.; Hoechst Marion Roussel, Irl.†; Hoechst Marion Roussel, Neth.; Roussel, Port.; Aventis, S.Afr.; Hoechst Marion Roussel, UK.
Loprazolam mesilate (p.688·2).
Now marketed as Loprazolam Tablets in the UK.
Insomnia; premedication.

Dormo-Puren Isis Puren, Ger.
Nitrazepam (p.695·2).
Sleep disorders.

Dormo-Sern Serturner, Ger.
Valerian (p.1678·3); passion flower (p.1649·1).
Nervous disorders; sleep disorders.

Dormoverlan Verla, Ger.
Valerian (p.1678·3); lupulus (p.1629·3); passion flower (p.1649·1).
Agitation; insomnia.

Dormplus Pensa, Spain.
Diphenhydramine hydrochloride (p.416·1).
Insomnia.

Dormutil N Isis, Ger.
Diphenhydramine hydrochloride (p.416·1).
Sleep disorders.

Dorner Toray, Jpn.
Beraprost sodium (p.1440·3).
Thromboembolic disorders.

Dorocoff-ASS plus Hevert, Ger.†
Aspirin (p.14·2); caffeine (p.761·3).
Pain.

Dorocoff-Paracetamol Hevert, Ger.
Paracetamol (p.71·2).
Fever; pain.

Dorox M & H, Thai.
Dicloxacillin sodium (p.199·1).
Bacterial infections.

Dorpinol Heralds, Braz.
Paracetamol (p.71·2); diclofenac sodium (p.30·3); caffeine (p.761·3); carisoprodol (p.1327·1).
Skeletal muscle spasm.

Dorpiren Heralds, Braz.
Diclofenac potassium (p.30·2).
Gout; inflammation; musculoskeletal, joint, and peri-articular disorders; pain.

Dorscopena Ariston, Braz.
Dipyrone (p.34·1); chlorophenothiazinylscopine.
Skeletal muscle spasm.

Dorserol Heralds, Braz.
Carisoprodol (p.1327·1); paracetamol (p.71·2); caffeine (p.761·3).
Skeletal muscle spasm.

Dorsiflex Will-Pharma, Neth.
Mephenoxalone (p.690·3).
Muscle pain.

Dorsilon Drossapharm, Switz.†
Mephenoxalone (p.690·3); paracetamol (p.71·2).
Musculoskeletal pain.

Dorspan EMS, Braz.
Butylhyoscine (p.469·1); dipyrone (p.34·1).
Skeletal muscle spasm.

Dorveran QIF, Braz.
Belladonna (p.463·1); hyoscyamus (p.470·1); star anise; boldo (p.1585·3).
Smooth muscle spasm.

Doryl Merck, Fin.; Merck, Ger.; Merck, Switz.
Carbachol (p.1416·1).
Gastrointestinal motility disorders; urinary retention.

Doryx Faulding, Austral.; Parke, Davis, Canad.†; Gerard, Norw.; Parke, Davis, NZ; Parke-Med, S.Afr.; Faulding, Singapore; Scand Pharm, Swed.; Warner Chilcott, USA.
Doxycycline hyclate (p.200·1).
Adjunct in amoebiasis; bacterial infections.

DOS Softgel Goldline, USA.
Docusate sodium (p.1223·1).
Constipation.

Dosaflex Richwood, USA.
Senna (p.1248·2).
Constipation.

Dosalax Richwood, USA†.
Senna (p.1248·2).
Constipation.

Dosanac Siam Bheasach, Thai.
Diclofenac diethylamine (p.30·2) or diclofenac sodium (p.30·3).
Inflammation; musculoskeletal, joint, peri-articular, and soft-tissue disorders; pain.

Dosate Pharmasant, Thai.
Omeprazole (p.1239·1).
Gastro-oesophageal reflux, Zollinger-Ellison syndrome; peptic ulcer.

Dosberotec Boehringer Ingelheim, Ital.
Fenoterol hydrobromide (p.765·1).
Respiratory-tract disorders.

Doscafis Llorens, Spain.
Aspirin (p.14·2); caffeine (p.761·3); paracetamol (p.71·2).
Fever; inflammation; musculoskeletal and joint disorders; pain.

Doses-O-Son Realdyme, Fr.
Bran (p.1214·2).
Dietary fibre supplement.

Dosil Llorens, Spain.
Doxycycline hyclate (p.200·1).
Bacterial infections; malaria.

Dosil Enzimatico *Llorens, Spain.*
Doxycycline hyclate (p.200·1); chymotrypsin (p.1595·1); trypsin (p.1675·3).
Bacterial infections.

Dosiseptine *Gifrer Barbezat, Fr.*
Chlorhexidine gluconate (p.1138·2).
Wounds disinfection.

Dosoxygenee *Gifrer Barbezat, Fr.*
Hydrogen peroxide (p.1147·1).
Wound disinfection.

Dospir *Boehringer Ingelheim, Switz.*
Ipratropium bromide (p.766·1); salbutamol sulfate (p.770·3).
Obstructive airways disease.

Doss
Note.This name is used for preparations of different composition.
SmithKline Beecham, Canad.†.
Dantron (p.1221·3); docusate sodium (p.1223·1).
Constipation.
Byk Tosse, Ger.; Byk Gulden, Ger.
Alfacalcidol (p.1391·1).
Bone disorders; hypoparathyroidism.

Dossifil *Therica, Fr.†.*
Ergocalciferol (p.1391·2); calcium hypophosphite; calcium pantothenate (p.1374·1).
Vitamin D deficiency.

Dostein *Glaxo Wellcome, Mex.*
Erdosteine (p.1091·2).
Respiratory-tract congestion.

Dostil *Triomed, S.Afr.*
Paracetamol (p.71·2); codeine phosphate (p.25·2).
Fever; pain.

Dostinex *Pharmacia Upjohn, Aust.; Pharmacia Upjohn, Austral.; Pharmacia Upjohn, Belg.; Pharmacia Upjohn, Denm.; Pharmacia Upjohn, Fin.; Pharmacia Upjohn, Fr.; Pharmacia Upjohn, Ger.; Pharmacia Upjohn, Irl.; Agis, Israel; Pharmacia Upjohn, Ital.; Pharmacia Upjohn, Neth.; Pharmacia Upjohn, Norw.; Pharmacia Upjohn, NZ; Pharmacia Upjohn, Port.; Pharmacia Upjohn, S.Afr.; Pharmacia Upjohn, Singapore; Kenfarma, Spain; Pharmacia Upjohn, Swed.; Pharmacia Upjohn, Switz.; Pharmacia, UK; Pharmacia Upjohn, USA.*
Cabergoline (p.1167·3).
Hyperprolactinaemia; lactation inhibition; prolactinomas.

Dosyklin *Leiras, Fin.*
Doxycycline (p.200·1).
Bacterial infections.

Dotarem *Guerbet, Aust.; Codali, Belg.; Guerbet, Braz.; Guerbet, Denm.; Guerbet, Fin.; Guerbet, Fr.; Guerbet, Israel; Farmades, Ital.; Guerbet, Neth.†; Guerbet, Norw.; Guerbet, Port.; Guerbet, Spain; Gothia, Swed.; Guerbet, Switz.*
Meglumine gadoterate (p.1033·2).
Contrast medium for magnetic resonance imaging.

Dotest *Mentholatum, Austral.*
Pregnancy test (p.1654·3).

Dothapax *Ashbourne, UK.*
Dothiepin hydrochloride (p.283·2).

Dothep
Alphapharm, Austral.; Gerard, Irl.
Dothiepin [dosulepin] hydrochloride (p.283·2).
Depression; mixed anxiety-depressive states.

Dotur *Biochemie, Aust.*
Doxycycline hyclate (p.200·1).
Bacterial infections; protozoal infections.

Double Check *Family Planning Sales, UK.*
Nonoxinol 9 (p.1346·1).
Contraceptive.

Double-Action Toothache Kit *Dent, USA.*
Liquid, benzocaine (p.1306·2); tablets, paracetamol (p.71·2) (Maranox).

Doublebase *Dermal Laboratories, UK.*
Isopropyl myristate (p.1409·2); liquid paraffin (p.1407·1).
Dry skin; pruritus.

Doublecap *Breckenridge, USA.*
Capsaicin (p.23·1).
Musculoskeletal and joint pain.

Double-Tussin DM *Reese, USA.*
Guaifenesin (p.1092·2); dextromethorphan hydrobromide (p.1087·3).
Coughs.

Douglas Protein Plus *Douglas, NZ; Nutricia, NZ.*
Protein preparation with electrolytes (p.1350·1).
Nutritional supplement.

Doulax
Note.This name is used for preparations of different composition.
Bio-Sante, Canad.†.
Cascara (p.1216·1); phenolphthalein (p.1244·1).
Bio-Sante, Canad.
Cascara (p.1216·1); senna (p.1248·2).

Douzabox *Denk, Thai.*
Vitamin B$_1$ (p.1385·2); vitamin B$_6$ (p.1387·1); vitamin B$_{12}$ (p.1388·1).
Vitamin B deficiency.

Doval *Pharmaceutical Enterprises, S.Afr.*
Diazepam (p.674·3).
Alcohol withdrawal syndrome; anxiety; depression; premedication.

Dovate *Aspen, S.Afr.*
Clobetasol propionate (p.1065·2).
Skin disorders.

Doven *Eurofarmaco, Ital.*
Diosmin (p.1611·1).
Vascular disorders.

Doveri *Rekah, Israel.*
Opium (p.69·3); ipecacuanha (p.1093·1).
Coughs; dyspnoea.

Dovonex *Leo, Canad.; Leo, Irl.; Adcock Ingram, S.Afr.; Leo, UK; Westwood-Squibb, USA.*
Calcipotriol (p.1112·1).
Psoriasis.

Doxacor *Hexal, Ger.*
Doxazosin (p.883·2).
Hypertension.

Doxagamma *Worwag, Ger.*
Doxazosin mesilate (p.883·2).
Hypertension.

Doxakne *Hexal, Ger.*
Doxycycline (p.200·1).
Acne.

Doxal
Note.This name is used for preparations of different composition.
Novaquimica, Braz.
Pyridoxine (p.1387·1); thiamine (p.1385·2).
Vitamin supplement.
Orion, Fin.
Doxepin hydrochloride (p.283·3).
Anxiety; depression; insomnia.

Doxaloc *Unipharm, Israel.*
Doxazosin mesilate (p.883·2).
Benign prostatic hyperplasia; hypertension.

Doxam *TAD, Ger.*
Doxycycline hyclate (p.200·1); ambroxol hydrochloride (p.1084·3).
Respiratory-tract infections.

Doxa-Puren *Isis Puren, Ger.*
Doxazosin mesilate (p.883·2).
Hypertension.

Doxate-C *Richmond, Canad.†.*
Docusate calcium (p.1222·3).
Constipation.

Doxate-S *Richmond, Canad.†.*
Docusate sodium (p.1223·1).
Constipation.

Doxazomerck *Merck dura, Ger.*
Doxazosin mesilate (p.883·2).
Hypertension.

Doxergan
Aventis, Belg.; Rhone-Poulenc Rorer, Neth.†.
Oxomemazine (p.422·2).
Coughs; gastritis; hypersensitivity reactions; insomnia.

Doxi Crisol *Quimifar, Spain.*
Doxycycline hyclate (p.200·1).
Bacterial infections; malaria.

Doxi Sergo *Inexfa, Spain.*
Doxycycline hyclate (p.200·1).
Bacterial infections; malaria.

Doxibiotic *CTI, Israel.*
Doxycycline hyclate (p.200·1).
Bacterial infections; malaria.

Doxican *Azevedos, Port.*
Tenoxicam (p.87·2).
Inflammation; musculoskeletal and joint disorders.

Doxiclat *Pierre Fabre, Spain.*
Doxycycline hyclate (p.200·1).
Bacterial infections; malaria.

Doxidan
Hoechst Marion Roussel, Canad.†; Upjohn, USA.
Docusate calcium (p.1222·3); phenolphthalein (p.1244·1).
Constipation.

Doxil *Sequus, USA.*
Liposomal doxorubicin hydrochloride (p.534·3).
AIDS-related Kaposi's sarcoma.

Doxilin *MPF, Singapore.*
Doxycycline hyclate (p.200·1).
Bacterial infections.

Doximed *Medinovum, Fin.*
Doxycycline (p.200·1).
Bacterial infections.

Doximucol *Lichtenstein, Ger.*
Doxycycline hyclate (p.200·1); ambroxol hydrochloride (p.1084·3).
Bacterial infections of the respiratory tract associated with increased or viscous mucus.

Doximycin *Orion, Fin.*
Doxycycline hyclate (p.200·1).
Bacterial infections.

Doxin *Asian Pharm, Thai.*
Doxycycline hyclate (p.200·1).
Bacterial infections.

Doxina *IPFI, Ital.*
Doxycycline hyclate (p.200·1).
Bacterial infections.

Doxinate *Torlan, Spain.*
Doxycycline hyclate (p.200·1).
Bacterial infections; malaria.

Doxine
Pacific, NZ; Alphapharm, Singapore; Merck, Singapore.
Doxycycline hyclate (p.200·1).
Adjunct in amoebiasis; bacterial infections; malaria.

Doxi-Om *OM, Port.*
Calcium dobesilate (p.1588·2).
Vascular disorders.

Doxiproct
Ebewe, Aust.; OM, Port.; OM, Switz.
Calcium dobesilate (p.1588·2); lignocaine [lidocaine] hydrochloride (p.1313·2).
Anorectal disorders.

Doxiproct mit Dexamethason *Ebewe, Aust.*
Calcium dobesilate (p.1588·2); lignocaine [lidocaine] hydrochloride (p.1313·2); dexamethasone acetate (p.1067·1).
Anorectal disorders.

Doxiproct Plus
Abiogen, Ital.; OM, Switz.
Calcium dobesilate (p.1588·2); lignocaine [lidocaine] hydrochloride (p.1313·2); dexamethasone acetate (p.1067·1).
Anorectal disorders.

Doxitab *Medpro, S.Afr.*
Doxycycline hyclate (p.200·1).
Bacterial infections.

Doxiten *Zyma, Spain†.*
Doxycycline hyclate (p.200·1).
Bacterial infections.

Doxiten Bio *Teofarma, Spain.*
Doxycycline hyclate (p.200·1).
Bacterial infections; malaria.

Doxiten Enzimatico *Teofarma, Spain.*
Doxycycline hyclate (p.200·1); chymotrypsin (p.1595·1); trypsin (p.1675·3).
Bacterial infections.

Doxitin *Vitabalans, Fin.*
Doxycycline hyclate (p.200·1).
Bacterial infections.

Doxium
Ebewe, Aust.; Sanofi Synthelabo, Belg.; Allergan-Frumtost, Braz.; Ebewe, Hong Kong; Abiogen, Ital.; Knoll, Mex.; Europhta, Mon.; Esteve, Spain; OM, Switz.
Calcium dobesilate (p.1588·2).
Chronic venous insufficiency; microcirculatory disorders.

Doxivenil
OM, Port.; OM, Switz.
Calcium dobesilate (p.1588·2); dextran sulfate potassium (p.1603·1).
Inflammation; venous insufficiency.

DOXO-cell *Cell Pharm, Ger.*
Doxorubicin hydrochloride (p.534·3).
Malignant neoplasms.

Doxolem *Lemery, Mex.; Lemery, Thai.*
Doxorubicin hydrochloride (p.534·3).
Malignant neoplasms.

Doxorubin *Asta Medica, Austral.; Nettopharma, Denm.; Asta Medica, NZ.*
Doxorubicin hydrochloride (p.534·3).
Malignant neoplasms.

Doxotec *Columbia, Mex.*
Doxorubicin hydrochloride (p.534·3).
Malignant neoplasms.

Doxsig *Sigma, Austral.*
Doxycycline hyclate (p.200·1).
Adjunct in amoebiasis; bacterial infections; malaria.

Doxy
Douglas, Austral.; Elerte, Fr.; Engelhard, Ger.; CT, Ger.; BASF, Ger.; ABZ, Ger.; Brahms, Ger.; Eu Rho, Ger.; Vitamed, Israel; Douglas, NZ; Masa, Thai.; Edwards, USA.
Doxycycline (p.200·1) or doxycycline hyclate (p.200·1).
Adjunct in amoebiasis; bacterial infections; malaria.

Doxy-100 *Douglas, Thai.; TTN, Thai.*
Doxycycline (p.200·1).
Bacterial infections.

Doxy Comp *CT, Ger.*
Doxycycline hyclate (p.200·1); ambroxol hydrochloride (p.1084·3).
Respiratory-tract infections.

Doxy Komb *Engelhard, Ger.; Brahms, Ger.*
Doxycycline hyclate (p.200·1).
Bacterial infections.

Doxy Lindoxyl *Lindopharm, Ger.*
Doxycycline hyclate (p.200·1); ambroxol hydrochloride (p.1084·3).
Bacterial infections of the respiratory-tract associated with increased or viscous mucus.

Doxy M *CT, Ger.; Ratiopharm, Ger.*
Doxycycline hyclate (p.200·1).
Bacterial infections.

Doxy Plus *Stada, Ger.*
Doxycycline hyclate (p.200·1); ambroxol hydrochloride (p.1084·3).
Respiratory-tract infections.

Doxy S+K *S & K, Ger.*
Doxycycline hyclate (p.200·1).
Bacterial infections.

Doxy-basan *Schonenberger, Switz.*
Doxycycline hyclate (p.200·1).
Bacterial infections.

Doxybene *Ratiopharm, Aust.*
Doxycycline (p.200·1) or doxycycline hyclate (p.200·1).
Bacterial infections.

Doxybiocin *Orion, Ger.*
Doxycycline hyclate (p.200·1).
Bacterial infections.

Doxycap *Hovid, Singapore.*
Doxycycline hyclate (p.200·1).
Bacterial infections.

Doxychel *Rachelle, USA.*
Doxycycline hyclate (p.200·1).
Bacterial infections.

Doxcin *Riva, Canad.*
Doxycycline hyclate (p.200·1).
Bacterial infections.

Doxyclin *Pharmador, S.Afr.†.*
Doxycycline hyclate (p.200·1).
Bacterial infections.

Doxycline
Spirig, Switz.; General Drugs, Thai.
Doxycycline (p.200·1) or doxycycline hyclate (p.200·1).
Bacterial infections.

Doxycyl *Aspen, S.Afr.*
Doxycycline hyclate (p.200·1).
Bacterial infections.

Doxy-Dagra *Asta Medica, Neth.*
Doxycycline fosfatex (p.200·1).
Bacterial infections.

Doxyderm *Klinge, Aust.*
Doxycycline hyclate (p.200·1).
Acne.

Doxyderma *Dermapharm, Ger.*
Doxycycline (p.200·1).
Bacterial infections.

Doxy-Diolan *Engelhard, Ger.; Brahms, Ger.*
Doxycycline hyclate (p.200·1).
Bacterial infections.

Doxydoc *Docpharm, Ger.*
Doxycycline (p.200·1).
Bacterial infections.

Doxy-duramucal *Merck dura, Ger.*
Doxycycline hyclate (p.200·1); ambroxol hydrochloride (p.1084·3).
Bacterial infections of the respiratory-tract associated with increased or viscous mucus.

Doxydyn *Klinge, Aust.*
Doxycycline hyclate (p.200·1).
Bacterial infections.

Doxyfene *Covan, S.Afr.*
Dextropropoxyphene hydrochloride (p.27·1); paracetamol (p.71·2).
Fever; pain.

Doxyferm *Nordic, Swed.*
Doxycycline (p.200·1) or doxycycline hyclate (p.200·1).
Bacterial infections.

Doxyfim *Wolfs, Belg.*
Doxycycline hyclate (p.200·1).
Bacterial infections.

Doxygram *Pharma 2000, Fr.†.*
Doxycycline hyclate (p.200·1).
Bacterial infections.

Doxyhexal
Hexal, Aust.; Hexal, Austral.; Hexal, Ger.
Doxycycline (p.200·1) or doxycycline hyclate (p.200·1).
Adjunct in amoebiasis; bacterial infections; malaria.

Doxy-HP *Hefa, Ger.*
Doxycycline (p.200·1).
Bacterial infections.

Doxylan *Lannacher, Aust.*
Doxycycline (p.200·1) or doxycycline hyclate (p.200·1).
Bacterial infections.

Doxylar *Lagap, UK.*
Doxycycline hyclate (p.200·1).
Bacterial infections.

Doxylets
SMB, Belg.; Galephar, Fr.†; Brovar, S.Afr.†.
Doxycycline hyclate (p.200·1).
Bacterial infections.

Doxylin
Alphapharm, Austral.; Dexxon, Israel; Alpharma, Norw.; TP, Thai.
Doxycycline (p.200·1) or doxycycline hyclate (p.200·1).
Amoebiasis; bacterial infections; malaria.

Doxymerck *Merck dura, Ger.*
Doxycycline (p.200·1).
Bacterial infections.

Doxymono *Betapharm, Ger.*
Doxycycline (p.200·1).
Bacterial infections.

Doxymycin
Rhone-Poulenc Rorer, Neth.†; SA Druggists, S.Afr.†; Beacons, Singapore; Yung Shin, Thai.
Doxycycline (p.200·1) or doxycycline hyclate (p.200·1).
Bacterial infections.

Doxy-N-Tablinen *Lichtenstein, Ger.*
Doxycycline (p.200·1).
Bacterial infections.

Doxy-P
Ratiopharm, Ger.†; PP Lab, Thai.
Doxycycline hyclate (p.200·1).
Bacterial infections.

Doxypol *Beige, S.Afr.*
Dextropropoxyphene hydrochloride (p.27·1); paracetamol (p.71·2); caffeine (p.761·3).
Pain.

Doxy-Puren *Isis Puren, Ger.*
Doxycycline hyclate (p.200·1).
Bacterial infections.

Doxysol *Ecosol, Norw.; Ecosol, Switz.*
Doxycycline (p.200·1).
Bacterial infections.

Doxysolvat *Betapharm, Ger.*
Doxycycline (p.200·1); ambroxol hydrochloride (p.1084·3).
Respiratory-tract infections.

Doxystad *Stada, Aust.*
Doxycycline (p.200·1).
Bacterial infections.

Doxy-Tablinen *Sanorania, Ger.†*
Doxycycline hyclate (p.200·1).
Bacterial infections.

Doxytec *Technilab, Canad.*
Doxycycline hyclate (p.200·1).
Bacterial infections.

Doxytem *Temmler, Ger.†*
Doxycycline hyclate (p.200·1).
Bacterial infections.

Doxytrex *Helfarma, Port.*
Doxycycline hyclate (p.200·1).
Bacterial infections.

Doxytrim *Trima, Israel.*
Doxycycline hyclate (p.200·1).
Amoebiasis; bacterial infections; malaria.

Doxy-Wolff *Wolff, Ger.*
Doxycycline (p.200·1) or doxycycline hyclate (p.200·1).
Bacterial infections.

Doxy-Wolff Mucolyt *Wolff, Ger.*
Doxycycline hyclate (p.200·1); ambroxol hydrochloride (p.1084·3).
Respiratory-tract infections associated with increased or viscous mucus.

Doyle *Tanabe, Jpn†.*
Aspoxicillin (p.152·2).
Bacterial infections.

Dozbe *Profarb, Braz.*
Vitamin B_1; vitamin B_6; vitamin B_{12} (p.1350·1).
Vitamin B deficiency.

Dozebion *Baldacci, Braz.*
Vitamin B substances; iron molybdate; copper chloride; liver extract (p.1350·1).
Vitamin and mineral supplement.

Dozelin Junior *Novaquimica, Braz.*
Multivitamin and amino-acid preparation (p.1350·1).

Dozelin Lisina *Novaquimica, Braz.*
Vitamin B substances; lysine hydrochloride (p.1350·1).

Dozeneurin *Novaquimica, Braz.*
Cyanocobalamin (p.1388·1); thiamine (p.1385·2).
Vitamin B_1 and B_{12} deficiency.

Dozic *Rosemont, UK.*
Haloperidol (p.686·3).
Anxiety; intractable hiccup; motor tics; nausea and vomiting; psychoses.

Dozile
Sunspot, Austral.; Searle, NZ.
Doxylamine succinate (p.417·1).
Insomnia.

Dozol
Rice Steele, Irl.; Typharm, UK.
Paracetamol (p.71·2); diphenhydramine hydrochloride (p.416·1).
Cold and influenza symptoms; fever; pain.

DP
Note.This name is used for preparations of different composition.
Douglas, NZ.
Liquid paraffin (p.1407·1); wool fat (p.1410·3).
Dry skin; pruritus.

Douglas, Singapore.
Dimethicone (p.1410·1).
Topical barrier preparation.

dp *Scientific Hospital Supplies, UK.*
Note. A similar name is used for preparations of different composition (see above).
Low-protein food for special diets (p.1350·1).

DP Barrier Cream *Douglas, NZ.*
Dimethicone (p.1410·1).

DP HC *Douglas, NZ.*
Hydrocortisone (p.1073·3).
Skin disorders.

DP Hydrocortisone *Douglas, NZ.*
Hydrocortisone (p.1073·3).
Skin disorders.

DP Lubricating Gel *Douglas, NZ.*
Lubricating gel.

DP Warm Up *Douglas, NZ.*
Methyl salicylate (p.55·1); eucalyptus oil (p.1609·2); camphor (p.1589·3).
Muscular rub.

D-Pam *Douglas, NZ.*
Diazepam (p.674·3).
Alcohol withdrawal syndrome; anxiety; epilepsy; sedative; skeletal muscle spasm.

DPCA
Fresenius, Fr.†; Fresenius Medical, Switz.
Electrolytes; anhydrous glucose (p.1184·1).
Peritoneal dialysis.

DPE *Alcon, Canad.*
Dipivefrine hydrochloride (p.1604·3).
Glaucoma.

D-Penamine
Dista, Austral.; Dista, NZ.
Penicillamine (p.1017·1).
Cystinuria; heavy metal poisoning; rheumatoid arthritis; Wilson's disease.

DPH
Note.This name is used for preparations of different composition.
Propan, S.Afr.
Diphenhydramine hydrochloride (p.416·1); ammonium chloride (p.1085·2); sodium citrate (p.1186·2).
Coughs.

Alra, USA†.
Diphenhydramine hydrochloride (p.416·1).

DPN *Alclin, S.Afr.*
Nadide (p.1639·3).
Alcoholism; drug addiction.

DPT Merieux *Pasteur Merieux, Fr.*
An adsorbed diphtheria, tetanus, and pertussis vaccine (p.1537·3).
Active immunisation of infants and young children.

DPT-Impfstoff *Chiron Behring, Ger.†*
An adsorbed diphtheria, tetanus, and pertussis vaccine (p.1537·3).
Active immunisation of infants and young children.

DPT-Vaccinol *Procter & Gamble, Ger.†*
An adsorbed diphtheria, tetanus, and pertussis vaccine (p.1537·3).
Active immunisation of infants and young children.

Dr Caldwell Senna Laxative *Gebauer, USA†.*
Senna (p.1248·2).
Constipation.

Dr Dermi-Heal *Quality Formulations, USA.*
Allantoin (p.1110·1); zinc oxide (p.1128·2); peru balsam (p.1650·2); castor oil (p.1592·1).
Skin disorders.

Dr Ernst Richter's Abfuhrtee *Sanova, Aust.*
Senna (p.1248·2); frangula bark (p.1227·1).
Constipation.

Dr. Ernst Richter's Abfuhrtee-Filterbeutel *Hermes, Aust.*
Senna (p.1248·2); frangula (p.1227·1); calcatrippae; calendula (p.1589·2); centaurea cyanus; helianthus; rubus fruticosus; coriander (p.1599·2).
Constipation.

Dr Ernst Richter's Abfuhrtee-tassen-fertig *Sanova, Aust.*
Senna (p.1248·2); frangula bark (p.1227·1); peppermint oil (p.1243·3); liquorice (p.1231·2).
Constipation.

Dr Fischers Melissengeist *Pharmonta, Aust.†*
Nutmeg oil (p.1643·1); clove oil (p.1597·1); cinnamon oil (p.1596·1); citronella oil (p.1596·3).
Gastrointestinal disorders; musculoskeletal and joint disorders; nervous disorders.

Dr Fischer's Minzol *Pharmonta, Aust.†*
Menthae arvensis oil (p.1243·3).
Gastrointestinal disorders; headache; musculoskeletal and joint disorders; respiratory-tract disorders.

Dr Grandel Brennessel Vital Tonikum *Grandel-Synpharma, Ger.*
Urtica (p.1678·2).
Tonic.

Dr Grandel Granobil *Grandel-Synpharma, Ger.*
Usnea barbata (p.1678·2).
Bacterial infections of the mouth and throat.

Dr. Hotz Vollbad *Hotz, Ger.†*
Whey; sorbitol (p.1377·3); lactic acid (p.1626·2); alum (p.1577·2); gentian (p.1615·1); achillea (p.1572·2); crataegus (p.1600·2); olive oil (p.1643·3); arachis oil (p.1581·1); sage oil (p.1660·2); rosemary oil (p.1659·3); chamomile oil; alpha tocoferil acetate (p.1394·1).
Bath additive; skin disorders.

Dr Janssens Teebohnen *Dr Janssen, Ger.*
Aloes (p.1210·1).
Constipation.

Dr Schmidgall Halsweh *Schmidgall, Aust.*
dl-Alpha tocoferil acetate (p.1394·1); benzalkonium chloride (p.1133·2).
Mouth and throat inflammation.

Dr Scholl's Athlete's Foot *Schering-Plough, USA.*
Tolnaftate (p.395·2).
Tinea pedis.

Dr Scholl's Callus Removers *Schering-Plough, USA.*
Salicylic acid (p.1122·3).

Dr Scholl's Clear Away *Schering-Plough, USA.*
Salicylic acid (p.1122·3).
Hyperkeratosis.

Dr Scholl's Corn Removers *Schering-Plough, USA.*
Salicylic acid (p.1122·3).

Dr Scholl's Corn/Callus Remover *Schering-Plough, USA.*
Salicylic acid (p.1122·3).
Hyperkeratosis.

Dr Scholl's Cracked Heel Relief *Schering-Plough, USA.*
Lignocaine [lidocaine] (p.1313·2).

Dr Scholl's Tritin Antifungal Powder *Schering-Plough, USA†.*
Tolnaftate (p.395·2).
Tinea pedis.

Dr Scholl's Wart Remover *Schering-Plough, USA.*
Salicylic acid (p.1122·3).

Dr Wiemanns Rheumatonikum *Beethoven, Ger.*
Birch leaf (p.1585·2); salix (p.82·1); devil's claw root (p.26·3); heisteriae.
Musculoskeletal and joint disorders.

Dracodermalin *Richter, Aust.*
Camphor (p.1589·3); rosemary oil (p.1659·3); turpentine oil (p.1676·3).
Frostbite; musculoskeletal and joint disorders; respiratory-tract disorders.

Drafilyn Z *Zafiro, Mex.*
Aminophylline (p.760·1).
Obstructive airways disease.

Draganon *Roche, Ital.*
Aniracetam (p.1580·2).
Mental function disorders.

Dragee Vauban *Monot, Fr.*
Lignocaine [lidocaine] hydrochloride (p.1313·2); borax (p.1586·1).

Dragees antirhumatismales *Zeller, Switz.*
Salix (p.82·1); passion flower (p.1649·1).
Musculoskeletal and joint disorders.

Dragees aux figues avec du sene *Zeller, Switz.*
Fig (p.1227·1); senna (p.1248·2); petasites officinalis.
Constipation.

Dragees contre la toux no 536 *Renapharm, Switz.*
Butetamate citrate (p.1086·2); codeine phosphate (p.25·2); thyme (p.1672·2).
Coughs.

Dragees contre les maux de tete *Zeller, Switz.*
Salix (p.82·1); kola (p.1681·1).
Headache.

Dragees contre les maux de voyage no 537 *Renapharm, Switz.*
Dimenhydrinate (p.415·2); caffeine (p.761·3).
Motion sickness.

Dragees Fuca *Fuca, Fr.*
Frangula bark (p.1227·1); cascara (p.1216·1); bladderwrack (p.1585·2).
Constipation.

Dragees laxatives no 510 *Renapharm, Switz.†*
Aloes (p.1210·1); belladonna (p.463·1); rhubarb (p.1248·1).
Constipation.

Dragees Neunzehn *Sanova, Aust.*
Aloes (p.1210·1); frangula (p.1227·1); cascara (p.1216·1); fel sius (p.1585·1).
Constipation.

Dragees Neunzehn Senna *Sanova, Aust.*
Senna (p.1248·2).
Constipation.

Dragees pour la detente nerveuse *Zeller, Switz.*
Petasites officinalis; valerian (p.1678·3); passion flower (p.1649·1); melissa (p.1632·2).
Nervous disorders.

Dragees pour le coeur et les nerfs *Zeller, Switz.*
Crataegus (p.1600·2); passion flower (p.1649·1); lupulus (p.1629·3); valerian (p.1678·3).
Nervous disorders.

Dragees pour le sommeil nouvelle formule *Zeller, Switz.*
Valerian (p.1678·3); lupulus (p.1629·3).
Sleep disorders.

Dragees pour reins et vessie S *Synpharma, Switz.*
Java tea (p.1625·1); solidago virgaurea; ononis (p.1644·1); bearberry (p.1583·3); boldo (p.1585·3).
Urinary-tract disorders.

Dragees Vegetales Rex *Lehning, Fr.*
Frangula bark (p.1227·1); cascara (p.1216·1).
Formerly contained euonymine, bladderwrack, agar, belladonna, bile, cascara, hyoscyamus, star anise, frangula, and aloes.
Constipation.

Dragon Balm *Gerard House, UK.*
Camphor (p.1589·3); menthol (p.1632·3); turpentine oil (p.1676·3); nutmeg oil (p.1643·1); eucalyptus oil (p.1609·2); cassia oil (p.1592·1); pine oil; thymol (p.1158·3); guaiacol (p.1092·1); peru balsam (p.1650·2).
Muscular aches.

Dragosil *Daker Farmasimes, Spain†.*
Creatinolfosfate (p.1601·1) or creatinolfosfate sodium (p.1601·1).
Cardiac disorders.

Drainactil *Aerocid, Fr.*
Boldo (p.1585·3); birch leaf (p.1585·2); black currant leaf (p.1639·3).
Gastrointestinal disorders; kidney disorders.

Dralinsa *Duopharm, Ger.†*
Linseed (p.1629·1); senna leaf (p.1248·2).
Constipation.

Dramamine
Pharmacia Upjohn, Austral.; Searle, Belg.†; Pharmacia Upjohn, Fr.; Pharmacia Upjohn, Hong Kong; Pharmacia Upjohn, Irl.; Searle, Israel; Pharmacia Upjohn, Mex.; Pharmacia Upjohn, Neth.; Pharmacia Upjohn, NZ; Pharmacia Upjohn, Port.; Searle, S.Afr.†; Pharmacia Upjohn, Singapore; Searle, Switz.; Pharmacia Upjohn, Thai.; Pharmacia Upjohn, UK†; Upjohn, USA.
Dimenhydrinate (p.415·2).
Motion sickness; nausea and vomiting; vestibular disorders.

Dramamine II *Upjohn, USA.*
Meclozine hydrochloride (p.420·3).
Motion sickness.

Dramamine-compositum *Pharmacia Upjohn, Switz.*
Dimenhydrinate (p.415·2); caffeine (p.761·3).
Motion sickness.

Dramanate *Pasadena, USA.*
Dimenhydrinate (p.415·2).
Motion sickness.

Dramavit *Luper, Braz.*
Vitamin B_6 (p.1386·3); metoclopramide hydrochloride (p.1235·2).
Nausea and vomiting.

Dramigel *Drug Research, Ital.*
Amikacin sulfate (p.148·1).
Gram-negative bacterial infections.

Dramilin *Kay, USA†.*
Dimenhydrinate (p.415·2).
Motion sickness.

Dramin *Byk, Braz.*
Dimenhydrinate (p.415·2).
Hypersensitivity reactions; motion sickness; nausea and vomiting; vertigo.

Dramin B-6 *Byk, Braz.*
Dimenhydrinate (p.415·2); pyridoxine hydrochloride (p.1386·3).
Nausea and vomiting; vertigo.

Dramin B-6 DL *Byk, Braz.*
Dimenhydrinate (p.415·2); pyridoxine hydrochloride (p.1386·3); glucose (p.1364·1); fructose (p.1363·3).
Nausea and vomiting; vertigo.

Dramine *Uriach, Spain.*
Meclozine hydrochloride (p.420·3).
Motion sickness.

Drapolene
Note.This name is used for preparations of different composition.
Glaxo Wellcome, Fr.
Benzalkonium chloride (p.1133·2); cetrimonium bromide (p.1137·3).
Barrier preparation; skin disorders.

Glaxo Wellcome, Hong Kong; Wellcome, Irl.; Glaxo Wellcome, Singapore; Glaxo Wellcome, Thai.; Warner-Lambert, UK.
Benzalkonium chloride (p.1133·2); cetrimide (p.1137·1).
Minor burns and wounds; skin irritation caused by urine.

Dravyr
Drug Research, Ital.; Drug Research, Singapore.
Aciclovir (p.612·3).
Herpesvirus infections.

Draxon *Inibsa, Port.*
Flutamide (p.542·3).
Prostatic cancer.

Drazine *Pharmasant, Thai.*
Hydroxyzine hydrochloride (p.419·1).
Anxiety; hypersensitivity reactions; motion sickness.

Drazoic *Lambda, USA†.*
Benzoic acid (p.1134·2).
Fungal infections.

Dreemon *Peach, UK.*
Diphenhydramine hydrochloride (p.416·1).
Hypersensitivity reactions; insomnia.

Dreierlei *Hofmann & Sommer, Ger.*
Valerian (p.1678·3); mint oil (p.1636·2).
Digestive disorders.

Dreisacarb
Brady, Aust.; Gry, Ger.
Calcium carbonate (p.1215·1).
Calcium supplement; hyperphosphataemia.

Dreisafer *Gry, Ger.*
Ferrous sulfate (p.1360·3).
Iron deficiency.

Dreisavit *Brady, Aust.*
Multivitamin preparation (p.1350·1).

Dreisavit N
Gry, Ger.; Bichsel, Switz.
Vitamin B substances with ascorbic acid (p.1350·1).
Vitamin deficiency.

Drenian *Ern, Spain.*
Diazepam (p.674·3).
Alcohol withdrawal syndrome; anxiety; epilepsy; premedication; skeletal muscle spasticity; sleep disorders.

Dreniformio *Lilly, Braz.*
Flurandrenolone [fludroxycortide] (p.1072·2); clioquinol (p.190·2).
Skin disorders.

Drenison
Lilly, Braz.; Lilly, Canad.†; Derly, Spain†.
Flurandrenolone [fludroxycortide] (p.1072·2).
Skin disorders.

Drenison N
Lilly, Braz.; Lilly, Hong Kong.
Flurandrenolone [fludroxycortide] (p.1072·2); neomycin sulfate (p.228·1).
Infected skin disorders.

Drenison Neomicina *Derly, Spain†.*
Flurandrenolone [fludroxycortide] (p.1072·2); neomycin sulfate (p.228·1).
Infected skin disorders.

Drenoflux *Zeller, Braz.*
Diphenhydramine hydrochloride (p.416·1); ammonium chloride (p.1085·2); sodium citrate (p.1186·2); menthol (p.1632·3); sodium benzoate (p.1134·3).
Coughs; respiratory-tract congestion.

Drenol *Searle, Braz.*
Hydrochlorothiazide (p.907·3).
Diabetes insipidus; hypertension; oedema; renal calculi.

Drenomade *Esfar, Port.*
Dehydrocholic acid (p.1602·2); methionine (p.1012·2).

Drenotosse *Odontofarma, Braz.*
Diphenhydramine hydrochloride (p.416·1); ammonium chloride (p.1085·2).
Coughs.

Drenovac *Nikkho, Braz.*
Procaine penicillin [procaine benzylpenicillin] (p.239·2); benzylpenicillin potassium (p.157·1).
Bacterial infections.

Drenoxol *Vitoria, Port.*
Ambroxol hydrochloride (p.1084·3).
Respiratory-tract congestion.

Drenur *Merck, Port.†*
Fenproporex hydrochloride (p.1510·2).
Obesity.

Drenural *Grossman, Mex.*
Bumetanide (p.852·1).
Hypertension; oedema.

Dresplan *Fournier, Spain.*
Oxybutynin hydrochloride (p.471·2).
Neurogenic bladder.

Driclor *Stiefel, Austral.; Stiefel, Fr.; Stiefel, Hong Kong; Stiefel, Irl.; Stiefel, Singapore; Stiefel, UK.*
Aluminium chloride (p.1110·2).
Hyperhidrosis.

Dridase *Pharmacia Upjohn, Ger.; Byk, Neth.*
Oxybutynin hydrochloride (p.471·2).
Bladder disorders.

Dridol *Janssen-Cilag, Norw.†; Janssen-Cilag, Swed.†*
Droperidol (p.682·2).
Nausea; neuroleptanalgesia; premedication; vomiting.

Dri/Ear *Pfeiffer, USA.*
Boric acid (p.1586·1); isopropyl alcohol (p.1149·2).
Ear disorders.

Driken *Kendrick, Mex.*
Iron dextran (p.1368·2).
Iron-deficiency anaemia.

Drilix *Be-Tabs, S.Afr.*
Pseudoephedrine hydrochloride (p.1099·2).
Upper respiratory-tract congestion.

Drill
Note.This name is used for preparations of different composition.
Pierre Fabre Sante, Fr.
Chlorhexidine gluconate (p.1138·2); amethocaine [tetracaine] hydrochloride (p.1305·2).
Mouth and throat infections.

Pierre Fabre, Spain.
Chlorhexidine gluconate (p.1138·2); benzocaine (p.1306·2).
Mouth and throat infections.

Drill Expectorant *Pierre Fabre Sante, Fr.*
Carbocisteine (p.1086·3).
Respiratory-tract congestion.

Drill rhinites *Pierre Fabre Sante, Fr.*
Pseudoephedrine hydrochloride (p.1099·2).
Nasal congestion.

Drill toux seche *Pierre Fabre Sante, Fr.*
Dextromethorphan hydrobromide (p.1087·3).
Coughs.

Drimpam *Be-Tabs, S.Afr.*
Alprazolam (p.654·2).
Anxiety; mixed anxiety depressive states; panic attacks.

Drin *Wassermann, Ital.*
Aspirin (p.14·2); paracetamol (p.71·2); caffeine (p.761·3).
Fever; pain.

Driol *Bournonville, Belg.†*
Osalmid (p.1645·1).
Biliary disorders.

Drioquilen *Columbia, Mex.*
Diiodohydroxyquinoline (p.590·2).

Driptane *Fournier, Belg.; Debat, Fr.*
Oxybutynin hydrochloride (p.471·2).
Micturition disorders.

Drisdol *Sanofi Synthelabo, Canad.; Sanofi Winthrop, USA.*
Ergocalciferol (p.1391·2).
Familial hypophosphataemia; hypoparathyroidism; rickets.

Drisi-Ven *Serturner, Ger.*
Troxerutin (p.1611·2).
Vascular disorders.

Dristal Cold *Whitehall, Hong Kong.*
Chlorpheniramine [chlorphenamine] maleate (p.412·1); phenylephrine hydrochloride (p.1097·1); paracetamol (p.71·2).
Cold symptoms; upper respiratory-tract symptoms.

Dristan
Note.This name is used for preparations of different composition.
Whitehall-Robins, Canad.
Caplets; tablets: Paracetamol (p.71·2); phenylephrine hydrochloride (p.1097·1); chlorpheniramine [chlorphenamine] maleate (p.412·1).
Cold symptoms.

Capsules†: Phenylpropanolamine hydrochloride (p.1098·1); chlorpheniramine [chlorphenamine] maleate (p.412·1); aspirin (p.14·2); caffeine (p.761·3).
Cold symptoms; fever; headache; pain; upper respiratory-tract disorders.

Nasal spray: Phenylephrine hydrochloride (p.1097·1); pheniramine maleate (p.422·3).
Nasal congestion.

Whitehall-Robins, Canad.; Whitehall, Fin.; Whitehall, Irl.; Whitehall, UK.
Nasal spray: Oxymetazoline hydrochloride (p.1096·2).
Nasal congestion.

Whitehall, Irl.; Whitehall, UK.
Tablets: Aspirin (p.14·2); caffeine (p.761·3); chlorpheniramine [chlorphenamine] maleate (p.412·1); phenylephrine hydrochloride (p.1097·1).
Cold symptoms; nasal congestion.

Dristan Allergy *Whitehall, USA.*
Pseudoephedrine hydrochloride (p.1099·2); brompheniramine maleate (p.410·2).
Hypersensitivity reactions.

Dristan Cold *Whitehall, USA.*
Chlorpheniramine [chlorphenamine] maleate (p.412·1); phenylephrine hydrochloride (p.1097·1); paracetamol (p.71·2).
Formerly known as Advanced Formula Dristan.
Cold symptoms.

Dristan Cold Caplets *Whitehall, USA.*
Pseudoephedrine hydrochloride (p.1099·2); paracetamol (p.71·2).
Upper respiratory-tract symptoms.

Dristan Cold & Flu *Whitehall, USA.*
Chlorpheniramine [chlorphenamine] maleate (p.412·1); dextromethorphan hydrobromide (p.1087·3); paracetamol (p.71·2); pseudoephedrine hydrochloride (p.1099·2).
Coughs and cold symptoms.

Dristan Cold Maximum Strength *Whitehall, Hong Kong.*
Paracetamol (p.71·2); pseudoephedrine hydrochloride (p.1099·2).
Cold symptoms.

Dristan Cold Maximum Strength Multi-symptom Formula *Whitehall, USA.*
Paracetamol (p.71·2); pseudoephedrine hydrochloride (p.1099·2); brompheniramine maleate (p.410·2).
Cold symptoms; hypersensitivity reactions.

Dristan Cold Maximum Strength No Drowsiness Formula *Whitehall, USA.*
Paracetamol (p.71·2); pseudoephedrine hydrochloride (p.1099·2).
Cold symptoms.

Dristan Cold Multi-Symptom Formula *Whitehall, USA.*
Phenylephrine hydrochloride (p.1097·1); paracetamol (p.71·2); chlorpheniramine [chlorphenamine] maleate (p.412·1).
Upper respiratory-tract symptoms.

Dristan 12-hr Nasal Decongestant Spray *Whitehall, USA.*
Oxymetazoline hydrochloride (p.1096·2).
Formerly known as Dristan Long Lasting.
Nasal congestion.

Dristan Juice Mix-in *Whitehall, USA.*
Paracetamol (p.71·2); pseudoephedrine hydrochloride (p.1099·2); dextromethorphan hydrobromide (p.1087·3).
Coughs and cold symptoms.

Dristan Long Lasting *Whitehall, USA.*
Oxymetazoline hydrochloride (p.1096·2).
Nasal congestion.

Dristan N D *Whitehall-Robins, Canad.*
Pseudoephedrine hydrochloride (p.1099·2); paracetamol (p.71·2).
Formerly known as Dristan Non Drowsy.
Cold symptoms; fever; headache; pain; upper respiratory-tract disorders.

Dristan Nasal Spray *Whitehall, USA.*
Phenylephrine hydrochloride (p.1097·1); pheniramine maleate (p.422·3).
Nasal congestion.

Dristan Saline Spray *Whitehall, USA.*
Sodium chloride (p.1196·1).
Inflammation and dryness of nasal membranes.

Dristan Sinus *Whitehall-Robins, Canad.; Whitehall, USA.*
Pseudoephedrine hydrochloride (p.1099·2); ibuprofen (p.43·2).
Cold and influenza symptoms; sinusitis.

Drithocreme *Dermik, USA.*
Dithranol (p.1113·3).
Psoriasis.

Dritho-Scalp *Dermik, USA.*
Dithranol (p.1113·3).
Psoriasis.

Drivermide *Nakornpatana, Thai.*
Mebendazole (p.102·2).
Worm infections.

Drix *Pharmacal, Switz.†*
Bisacodyl (p.1212·2); frangula bark (p.1227·1); senna (p.1248·2); sodium sulfate (p.1250·1).
Constipation.

Drix Abfuhr-Dragees *Hermes, Ger.†*
Senna leaf (p.1248·2).
Constipation.

Drix N *Hermes, Ger.*
Bisacodyl (p.1212·2).
Constipation.

Drixin *Schering-Plough, Denm.*
Oxymetazoline hydrochloride (p.1096·2).
Nasal congestion.

Drixine
Schering-Plough, NZ; Schering-Plough, S.Afr.
Oxymetazoline hydrochloride (p.1096·2).
Nasal congestion.

Drixine Nasal *Schering-Plough, Austral.*
Oxymetazoline hydrochloride (p.1096·2).
Nasal congestion.

Drixomed *Iopharm, USA.*
Dexbrompheniramine maleate (p.410·2); pseudoephedrine sulfate (p.1099·3).
Respiratory-tract disorders.

Drixora *Schering-Plough, S.Afr.*
Pseudoephedrine sulfate (p.1099·3).
Upper respiratory-tract congestion.

Drixoral
Note.This name is used for preparations of different composition.
Schering, Canad.
Capsules†: Dextromethorphan hydrobromide (p.1087·3).
Coughs.
Nasal spray: Oxymetazoline hydrochloride (p.1096·2).
Upper respiratory-tract congestion.

Schering, Canad.; Schering-Plough, Hong Kong; Schering-Plough, Singapore.
Sustained release tablets: Dexbrompheniramine maleate (p.410·2); pseudoephedrine sulfate (p.1099·3).
Upper respiratory-tract congestion.

Schering-Plough, USA.
Pseudoephedrine sulfate (p.1099·3); brompheniramine maleate (p.410·2).
Upper respiratory-tract symptoms.

Drixoral Cold & Allergy *Schering-Plough, USA.*
Pseudoephedrine sulfate (p.1099·3); dexbrompheniramine maleate (p.410·2).
Upper respiratory-tract symptoms.

Drixoral Cold & Flu *Schering-Plough, USA.*
Pseudoephedrine sulfate (p.1099·3); paracetamol (p.71·2); dexbrompheniramine maleate (p.410·2).
Upper respiratory-tract symptoms.

Drixoral Cough
Schering, Canad.†; Schering-Plough, USA†.
Dextromethorphan hydrobromide (p.1087·3).
Coughs.

Drixoral Cough & Congestion *Schering-Plough, USA.*
Pseudoephedrine hydrochloride (p.1099·2); dextromethorphan hydrobromide (p.1087·3).

Drixoral Cough & Sore Throat *Schering-Plough, USA.*
Dextromethorphan hydrobromide (p.1087·3); paracetamol (p.71·2).

Drixoral Day/Night *Schering, Canad.*
Yellow tablets, pseudoephedrine sulfate (p.1099·3); white tablets, dexbrompheniramine maleate (p.410·2); pseudoephedrine sulfate.
Ear disorders; upper respiratory-tract congestion.

Drixoral ND *Schering, Canad.*
Pseudoephedrine sulfate (p.1099·3).
Ear disorders; upper respiratory-tract congestion.

Drixoral Non-Drowsy Formula *Schering, USA.*
Pseudoephedrine sulfate (p.1099·3).
Nasal congestion.

Drixoral Plus *Schering-Plough, USA.*
Pseudoephedrine sulfate (p.1099·3); paracetamol (p.71·2); dexbrompheniramine maleate (p.410·2).
Formerly known as Drixoral Allergy Sinus.
Upper respiratory-tract symptoms.

Drixtab *Schering, USA.*
Dexbrompheniramine maleate (p.410·2); pseudoephedrine sulfate (p.1099·3).
Upper respiratory-tract congestion.

Drize *Jones, USA†.*
Chlorpheniramine [chlorphenamine] maleate (p.412·1); phenylpropanolamine hydrochloride (p.1098·1).
Cold symptoms.

Droal *Vita, Spain.*
Ketorolac trometamol (p.48·2).
Pain.

Drocef *Eurofarma, Braz.*
Cefadroxil (p.161·2).
Bacterial infections.

Droclina *Vitae, Mex.*
Tetracycline (p.258·3).
Bacterial infections.

Drofaron *Democal, Switz.*
Aluminium hydroxide (p.1210·3); magnesium trisilicate (p.1233·3); dimethicone (p.1249·2).
Flatulence; gastric hyperacidity; gastritis.

Drogenil
Schering-Plough, Irl.; Essex, Ital.; Schering-Plough, Neth.; Schering-Plough, UK.
Flutamide (p.542·3).
Prostatic cancer.

Drogimed *Synpharma, Aust.*
Silver birch (p.1585·2); equisetum (p.1606·3).
Urinary-tract disorders.

Drolasona *Alter, Spain.*
Fluticasone propionate (p.1072·2).
Skin disorders.

Droleptan
Janssen-Cilag, Austral.†; Janssen-Cilag, Fr.; Janssen-Cilag, Irl.†; Janssen-Cilag, NZ†; Janssen-Cilag, UK†.
Droperidol (p.682·2).
Adjunct in neuroleptanalgesia; nausea and vomiting; premedication; psychoses.

Dromadol *Norton Healthcare, UK.*
Tramadol hydrochloride (p.89·1).
Pain.

Dromos *Sigma-Tau, Ital.*
Propionyl-L-carnitine hydrochloride.
Cardiac disorders.

Dronal *Sigma-Tau, Ital.*
Alendronate sodium (p.747·2).
Postmenopausal osteoporosis.

Dropcina *Plough, Port.*
Gramicidin (p.213·3); cetylpyridinium chloride (p.1138·1); dichlorobenzyl alcohol (p.1143·2); benzocaine (p.1306·2).
Mouth and throat disorders.

Dropgel *Ciba Vision, Ital.*
Carbomer 980 (p.1499·2).
Dry eyes.

Dropid *Progress, Thai.*
Gemfibrozil (p.896·2).
Hyperlipidaemias.

Dropilton *Bruschettini, Ital.*
Pilocarpine hydrochloride (p.1422·3).
Glaucoma.

Dropstar *Farmigea, Ital.*
Sodium hyaluronate (p.1620·1).
Dry eyes.

Droptimol *Farmigea, Ital.*
Timolol maleate (p.982·1).
Glaucoma; ocular hypertension.

Dropyal *Bruschettini, Ital.*
Sodium hyaluronate (p.1620·1); carbomer 941 (p.1499·2); glycerol (p.1616·3).
Dry eyes.

Drosera Komplex *Richter, Aust.*
Homoeopathic preparation.

Droserapect-N *Weber & Weber, Ger.*
Homoeopathic preparation.

Drosera-Weliplex *Weber & Weber, Ger.*
Homoeopathic preparation.

Drosetux
Dolisos, Canad.; Dolisos, Fr.
Homoeopathic preparation.

Drosinula N *Bioforce, Switz.*
Norway spruce buds; drosera (p.1606·1); hedera helix; pear.
Respiratory-tract disorders.

Drosithym-N *Ysatfabrik, Ger.*
Cowslip rhizome (p.1600·1); thyme (p.1672·2); drosera (p.1606·1).
Catarrh; coughs.

Drossadin *Drossapharm, Switz.*
Hexetidine (p.1146·3).
Mouth and throat disorders.

Drossanose *Drossapharm, Israel.*
Sea salt (p.1196·1).
Nasal disorders.

Drovitol *Synpharma, Aust.*
Myrrh (p.1639·2); clove (p.1596·3); tormentil (p.1674·1).
Mouth and throat disorders.

Droxaine *Whitehall, Braz.*
Aluminium hydroxide (p.1210·3); magnesium hydroxide (p.1233·1); oxetacaine (p.1317·3).
Gastrointestinal hyperacidity.

Droxaryl *Sanova, Aust.; Continental Pharma, Belg.; Sanofi Winthrop, Neth.†; Continental Pharma, Thai.*
Bufexamac (p.20·3).
Skin disorders.

Droxia *Bristol-Myers Squibb Oncology, USA.*
Hydroxyurea [hydroxycarbamide] (p.544·2).
Sickle cell anaemia.

Droxibit *Pizzard, Mex.*
Hydroxocobalamin (p.1388·1).

Droximag *PP Lab, Thai.*
Aluminium hydroxide (p.1210·3); magnesium trisilicate (p.1233·3); kaolin (p.1229·3); atropine sulfate (p.461·1).
Alkaloid poisoning; gastrointestinal infection; peptic ulcer.

Droxitop *Synpharma, Aust.*
Java tea (p.1625·1); solidago virgaurea; equisetum (p.1606·3).
Kidney and urinary-tract disorders.

Droxyl *Pharmaland, Thai.*
Aluminium hydroxide (p.1210·3); magnesium hydroxide (p.1233·1); simeticone (p.1249·2).
Gastric hyperacidity; peptic ulcer.

Drufusan N *Syxyl, Ger.*
Homoeopathic preparation.

Dry Eye Gel *Alcon, Neth.†*
Carbomer (p.1499·2).
Dry eyes.

Dry Eye Therapy *Bausch & Lomb, USA†.*
Glycerol (p.1616·3).
Dry eyes.

Dry Eyes *Bausch & Lomb, USA.*
Eye drops: Polyvinyl alcohol (p.1503·1).
Eye ointment: White soft paraffin (p.1407·3); liquid paraffin (p.1407·1); wool fat (p.1410·3).
Dry eyes.

Drylin *Merckle, Ger.*
Co-trimoxazole (p.193·3).
Bacterial infections; Pneumocystis carinii pneumonia.

Drynalken *Kendrick, Mex.*
Dopamine hydrochloride (p.881·3).
Extracorporeal circulation; hypotension; shock.

Drynalquin *Kendrick, Mex.*
Dopamine hydrochloride (p.881·3).

Dryptal
Rhone-Poulenc Rorer, Hong Kong; Berk, Irl.†; Berk, UK†.
Frusemide [furosemide] (p.893·1).
Hypertension; oedema.

Drysol *Darier, Mex.; Person & Covey, USA.*
Aluminium chloride (p.1110·2) or aluminium chlorohydrate (p.1110·2).
Hyperhidrosis.

Drytergent *C & M, USA.*
Skin cleanser.

Drytex *C & M, USA.*
Salicylic acid (p.1122·3); methylbenzethonium chloride (p.1150·3).
Acne.

DS Emulsion *Saninter, Port.*
Copper pidolate; zinc pidolate.
Seborrhoeic dermatitis; skin irritation.

D-Seb *Rydelle, Fr.; Johnson & Johnson, Ital.*
Chlorhexidine gluconate (p.1138·2).
Acne; seborrhoea.

DSMC Plus *Geneva, USA†.*
Docusate potassium (p.1223·1); casanthranol (p.1216·1).
Constipation.

D-S-S *Warner Chilcott, USA.*
Docusate sodium (p.1223·1).
Constipation.

D-S-S Plus *Warner Chilcott, USA†.*
Docusate sodium (p.1223·1); casanthranol (p.1216·1).
Constipation.

D-Stop *Ratiopharm, Ger.†.*
Loperamide hydrochloride (p.1231·3).
Diarrhoea.

DT Bis *Merieux, Fr.†.*
A diphtheria and tetanus vaccine (p.1537·1).
Active immunisation of older children and adults.

DT Coq *Pasteur Merieux, Fr.*
An adsorbed diphtheria, tetanus, and pertussis vaccine (p.1537·3).
Active immunisation.

DT Coq DTP *Pasteur Merieux, Israel.*
A diphtheria, tetanus, and pertussis vaccine (p.1537·3).
Active immunisation.

DT Polio *Pasteur Merieux, Fr.*
A diphtheria, tetanus, and poliomyelitis vaccine (p.1539·1).
Active immunisation.

DT Vax
Merieux, Fr.†; Aventis, S.Afr.; Pasteur Merieux, Thai.
An adsorbed diphtheria and tetanus vaccine (p.1537·1).
Active immunisation.

D-Tabs *Riva, Canad.†.*
Colecalciferol (p.1391·1).
Vitamin D supplement.

DTap-IPV *SSI, Swed.*
A diphtheria, tetanus, pertussis, and poliomyelitis vaccine (p.1539·1).
Active immunisation.

D-Tato *Protein, Mex.*
Benzonatate (p.1085·3).

DTCOQ/DTP *Pasteur Merieux, Braz.; Pasteur Merieux, Thai.*
An adsorbed diphtheria, tetanus, and pertussis vaccine (p.1537·3).
Active immunisation.

DT-HIB *SBL, Swed.†.*
A diphtheria, tetanus, and Haemophilus influenzae vaccine (p.1537·3).
Active immunisation.

DTIC
Bayer, Austral.; Bayer, Canad.; Rhone-Poulenc Rorer, Ger.†; Bayer, Swed.; Dome, Switz.
Dacarbazine (p.531·2) or dacarbazine citrate (p.531·3).
Malignant neoplasms.

DTIC-Dome
Bayer, Aust.; Bayer, Belg.; Bayer, Irl.; Bayer, NZ; Ebos, NZ; Bayer, S.Afr.; Bayer, Spain†; Bayer, UK; Bayer, USA.
Dacarbazine (p.531·2).
Malignant neoplasms.

DT-Impfstoff *Pasteur Merieux, Ger.; Chiron Behring, Ger.*
An adsorbed diphtheria and tetanus vaccine (p.1537·1).
Active immunisation of infants and young children.

DTP-Merieux
Aventis, S.Afr.; Pasteur Merieux, Spain.
An adsorbed diphtheria, tetanus, and pertussis vaccine (p.1537·3).
Active immunisation.

DTP-Rix *SmithKline Beecham, Ger.†.*
An adsorbed diphtheria, tetanus, and pertussis vaccine (p.1537·3).
Active immunisation.

D-Tracetten *Hoechst Marion Roussel, Ger.*
Colecalciferol (p.1391·1).
Vitamin D deficiency.

DT-reduct *Pasteur Merieux, Aust.*
An adsorbed diphtheria and tetanus vaccine (p.1537·1).
Active immunisation.

DT-Rix *SmithKline Beecham, Ger.†.*
An adsorbed diphtheria and tetanus vaccine (p.1537·1).
Active immunisation of infants and young children.

D-Tussin *Pharmco, S.Afr.†.*
Etofylline (p.765·1); diphenhydramine hydrochloride (p.416·1); ammonium chloride (p.1085·2); sodium citrate (p.1186·2).
Coughs; obstructive airways disease.

DT-Vaccinol *Procter & Gamble, Ger.†.*
An adsorbed diphtheria and tetanus vaccine (p.1537·1).
Active immunisation of infants and young children.

Duact
Glaxo Wellcome, Aust.; Glaxo Wellcome, Denm.; Glaxo Wellcome, Fin.
Acrivastine (p.408·2); pseudoephedrine hydrochloride (p.1099·2).
Allergic rhinitis.

Duadacin *Kenwood, USA†.*
Paracetamol (p.71·2); chlorpheniramine [chlorphenamine] maleate (p.412·1); phenylpropanolamine hydrochloride (p.1098·1).
Upper respiratory-tract symptoms.

Duafen *Pharmed, Aust.*
Ibuprofen (p.43·2).
Fever; pain.

Dualgan *ITF, Port.*
Etodolac (p.35·2).
Musculoskeletal, joint, and peri-articular disorders; pain.

Dualid S *Asta Medica, Braz.*
Diethylpropion hydrochloride (p.1508·3).
Obesity.

Dualizol *Degorts, Mex.*
Metronidazole (p.594·1).
Amoebiasis; giardiasis; trichomoniasis.

Dual-Lax Extra Strong *Lane, UK.*
Senna (p.1248·2); aloin (p.1210·2); cascara (p.1216·1).
Constipation.

Dual-Lax Normal Strength *Lane, UK.*
Senna (p.1248·2); cape aloes (p.1210·1); cascara (p.1216·1).
Constipation.

Duan *Pharmed, Aust.*
Aspirin (p.14·2); paracetamol (p.71·2); caffeine (p.761·3).
Fever; pain.

Duaneo *Pharmed, Aust.*
Paracetamol (p.71·2).
Fever; pain.

Duaneo mit Codein *Pharmed, Aust.*
Aspirin (p.14·2); paracetamol (p.71·2); codeine hydrochloride (p.25·2).
Pain.

Dubam *Norma, UK.*
Cream: Methyl salicylate (p.55·1); menthol (p.1632·3); eucalyptol (p.1609·2).
Topical spray: Methyl salicylate (p.55·1); ethyl salicylate (p.35·1); glycol salicylate (p.42·2); methyl nicotinate (p.55·1).
Musculoskeletal pain.

Ducase *Medecine Vegetale, Fr.†.*
Calumba (p.1589·2); quassia (p.1657·1); cascara (p.1216·1); liquorice (p.1231·2); gentian (p.1615·1); ferrous oxalate (p.1360·2).
Tonic.

Ducene *Sauter, Austral.*
Diazepam (p.674·3).
Alcohol withdrawal syndrome; anxiety disorders; skeletal muscle spasm and spasticity.

Ductopan *Neo Quimica, Braz.*
Hyoscine (p.468·2).
Smooth muscle spasm.

Duebien *PQS, Spain.*
Doxylamine succinate (p.417·1).
Insomnia.

Dueva *Menarini, Ital.*
Desogestrel (p.1470·3); ethinylestradiol (p.1476·2).
Biphasic oral contraceptive.

Dufaston *Solvay, Ital.*
Dydrogesterone (p.1472·3).
Progestogenic.

Dufine *Inibsa, Port.*
Clomifene citrate (p.1465·3).
Anovulatory infertility.

Duinum
Medochemie, Hong Kong; Medochemie, Singapore; Medochemie, Thai.
Clomifene citrate (p.1465·3).
Anovulatory infertility; oligospermia.

Dukoral
Statens Serum Institut, Denm.; SBL, Norw.; SBL, Swed.
A cholera vaccine (p.1535·2).
Active immunisation.

Dularell Classic *Sanorell, Ger.*
Homoeopathic preparation.

Dularell N *Sanorell, Ger.*
Homoeopathic preparation.

Dulax *Antigen, Irl.*
Lactulose (p.1230·1).
Constipation; hepatic encephalopathy.

Dulcagen *Goldline, USA†.*
Bisacodyl (p.1212·2).
Constipation.

Dulceril *Codilab, Port.*
Sodium cyclamate (p.1358·3); saccharin (p.1374·3).
Sugar substitute.

Dulcilarmes *Allergan, Fr.*
Povidone (p.1503·2).
Dry eyes; eye examinations.

Dulciphak *Allergan, Fr.*
Sodium monomethyltrisilanol orthohydroxybenzoate; parahydroxycinnamic acid.
Lens opacities.

Dulcivit *Abigo, Swed.*
Multivitamin preparation (p.1350·1).

Dulco Laxo *Fher, Spain.*
Bisacodyl (p.1212·2).
Constipation.

Dulcodruppels *Boehringer Ingelheim, Neth.*
Sodium picosulfate (p.1249·3).
Constipation.

Dulcolan *Boehringer Ingelheim, Mex.*
Bisacodyl (p.1212·2).
Bowel evacuation; constipation.

Dulcolax
Boehringer Ingelheim, Aust.; Boehringer Ingelheim, Belg.; Boehringer de Angeli, Braz.; Boehringer Ingelheim, Canad.; Boehringer Ingelheim, Denm.; Boehringer Ingelheim, Fr.; Boehringer Ingelheim, Ger.; Boehringer Ingelheim, Hong Kong; Boehringer Ingelheim, Irl.; Boehringer Ingelheim, Ital.; Boehringer Ingelheim, Neth.; Boehringer Ingelheim, Norw.; Boehringer Ingelheim, NZ; Boehringer Ingelheim, Port.; Boehringer Ingelheim, S.Afr.; Boehringer Ingelheim, Singapore; Boehringer Ingelheim, Swed.; Boehringer Ingelheim, Switz.; Boehringer Ingelheim, Thai.; Boehringer Ingelheim, UK; Novartis Consumer, USA.
Bisacodyl (p.1212·2).
Bowel evacuation; constipation.

Dulcolax Bowel Prep Kit *Novartis Consumer, USA†.*
Combination pack: 4 Dulcolax tablets (p.1212·2); 1 Dulcolax suppository.
Pre-operative bowel preparation.

Dulcolax Liquid
Boehringer de Angeli, Braz.; Boehringer Ingelheim, UK.
Sodium picosulfate (p.1249·3).
Bowel evacuation; constipation.

Dulcolax NP *Boehringer Ingelheim, Ger.*
Sodium picosulfate (p.1249·3).
Constipation.

Dulcolax Picosulphate *Boehringer Ingelheim, Belg.*
Sodium picosulfate (p.1249·3).
Constipation.

Dulconatur *Boehringer Ingelheim, Switz.†.*
Psyllium seed (p.1229·1).
Constipation; gastrointestinal disorders.

Dulcosol *Medifood, Ital.*
A nutritional supplement for infants (p.1350·1).

Dull-C *Freeda, USA.*
Ascorbic acid (p.1389·3).
Scurvy; vitamin C deficiency.

Dumesil *Dumex-Alpharma, Denm.†.*
Ammonium chloride (p.1085·2); diphenhydramine hydrochloride (p.416·1); menthol (p.1632·3).
Coughs; hypersensitivity reactions.

Dumex Lactose-Free *Dumex, Singapore.*
Lactose-free infant feed (p.1350·1).
Lactose intolerance.

Dumex Plus *Dumex, Singapore.*
A range of nutritional supplements (p.1350·1).

Dumicoat
Dumex-Alpharma, Denm.; Dumex-Alpharma, Fin.; Dumex, Ger.; Alpharma, Norw.; Dumex-Alpharma, Swed.; Dumex, Switz.; Dumex, UK†.
Miconazole (p.391·1).
Fungal mouth infections.

Dumirox
Pharmacia Upjohn, Ital.; Duphar, Spain.
Fluvoxamine maleate (p.389·3).
Depression; obsessive-compulsive disorder.

Dumocalcin *Dumex-Alpharma, Singapore.*
Calcium hydrogen phosphate (p.1188·2); colecalciferol (p.1391·1).
Nutritional supplement.

Dumocyclin *Dumex-Alpharma, Denm.*
Tetracycline hydrochloride (p.258·3).
Bacterial infections.

Dumolid *Dumex-Alpharma, Denm.*
Nitrazepam (p.695·2).
Epilepsy; sleep disorders.

Dumovit C *Dumex-Alpharma, Singapore.*
Ascorbic acid (p.1389·3); sodium ascorbate (p.1390·1).
Vitamin C deficiency.

Dumovital *Dumex, Port.*
Multivitamin and mineral preparation (p.1350·1).

Dumoxin
Dumex-Alpharma, Denm.†; Alpharma, Norw.; Aspen, S.Afr.; Dumex, Thai.
Doxycycline (p.200·1) or doxycycline hyclate (p.200·1).
Bacterial infections.

Dumozol *Dumex, Port.*
Metronidazole (p.594·1).
Anaerobic bacterial infections; rosacea.

Dumyrox *Solvay, Port.*
Fluvoxamine maleate (p.389·3).
Depression; obsessive-compulsive disorder.

Duna *Tedec Meiji, Spain.*
Pinazepam (p.700·2).
Anxiety.

Duo Celloids CPIP *Blackmores, Austral.*
Calcium phosphate (p.1188·3); iron phosphate.

Duo Celloids CPMP *Blackmores, Austral.*
Calcium phosphate (p.1188·3); magnesium phosphate (p.1191·1).

Duo Celloids PCCP *Blackmores, Austral.*
Potassium chloride (p.1194·3); calcium phosphate (p.1188·3).

Duo Celloids PCIP *Blackmores, Austral.*
Potassium chloride (p.1194·3); iron phosphate.

Duo Celloids PCMP *Blackmores, Austral.*
Potassium chloride (p.1194·3); magnesium phosphate (p.1191·1).

Duo Celloids PPIP *Blackmores, Austral.*
Potassium phosphate (p.1193·1); iron phosphate.

Duo Celloids PPMP *Blackmores, Austral.*
Potassium phosphate (p.1193·1); magnesium phosphate (p.1191·1).

Duo Celloids PSMP *Blackmores, Austral.*
Potassium sulfate (p.1195·1); magnesium phosphate (p.1191·1).

Duo Celloids PSPC *Blackmores, Austral.*
Potassium sulfate (p.1195·1); potassium chloride (p.1194·3).

Duo Celloids SCF *Blackmores, Austral.*
Silicon dioxide (p.1503·3); calcium fluoride.

Duo Celloids SPCF *Blackmores, Austral.*
Dibasic sodium phosphate (p.1193·2); calcium fluoride.

Duo Celloids SPCP *Blackmores, Austral.*
Dibasic sodium phosphate (p.1193·2); calcium phosphate (p.1188·3).

Duo Celloids SPIP *Blackmores, Austral.*
Dibasic sodium phosphate (p.1193·2); iron phosphate.

Duo Celloids SPMP *Blackmores, Austral.*
Dibasic sodium phosphate (p.1193·2); magnesium phosphate (p.1191·1).

Duo Celloids SPPC *Blackmores, Austral.*
Dibasic sodium phosphate (p.1193·2); potassium chloride (p.1194·3).

Duo Celloids SPPP *Blackmores, Austral.*
Dibasic sodium phosphate (p.1193·2); potassium phosphate (p.1193·1).

Duo Celloids SPPS *Blackmores, Austral.*
Dibasic sodium phosphate (p.1193·2); potassium sulfate (p.1195·1).

Duo Celloids SPS *Blackmores, Austral.*
Dibasic sodium phosphate (p.1193·2); silicon dioxide (p.1503·3).

Duo Celloids SPSS *Blackmores, Austral.*
Dibasic sodium phosphate (p.1193·2); sodium sulfate (p.1250·1).

Duo Celloids SSMP *Blackmores, Austral.*
Sodium sulfate (p.1250·1); magnesium phosphate (p.1191·1).

Duo Celloids SSPC *Blackmores, Austral.*
Sodium sulfate (p.1250·1); potassium chloride (p.1194·3).

Duo Celloids SSS *Blackmores, Austral.*
Sodium sulfate (p.1250·1); silicon dioxide (p.1503·3).

Duo Gobens *Normon, Spain.*
Doxycycline hyclate (p.200·1); chymotrypsin (p.1595·1); trypsin (p.1675·3).
Bacterial infections.

Duobact *Orion, Irl.*
Co-trimoxazole (p.193·3).
Bacterial infections.

Duobar
Scientific Hospital Supplies, Austral.; Scientific Hospital Supplies, Irl.†; Piam, Ital.; Nutricia, NZ; Scientific Hospital Supplies, NZ; Scientific Hospital Supplies, UK.
Food for special diets (p.1350·1).
Protein restriction.

Duobrus *Searle, Swed.†.*
Ibuprofen (p.43·2).
Fever; pain.

Duo-C *Geymonat, Ital.*
Ascorbic acid (p.1389·3).
Vitamin C deficiency; vitamin C supplement.

Duocal
Note. This name is used for preparations of different composition.
Scientific Hospital Supplies, Austral.; Nutricia, Fin.; SHS, Fr.; Scientific Hospital Supplies, Irl.; Piam, Ital.; Nutricia, NZ; Scientific Hospital Supplies, NZ; SHS, Singapore; Scientific Hospital Supplies, UK.
Food for special diets (p.1350·1).

Serog-Wiessner, Ger.
Glucose monohydrate (p.1364·2); xylitol (p.1397·3).
Parenteral nutrition.

Duocet *Mason, USA.*
Hydrocodone tartrate (p.42·2); paracetamol (p.71·2).
Pain.

Duocort *Orion, Fin.*
Hydrocortisone butyrate (p.1073·3); chlorhexidine gluconate (p.1138·2).
Skin disorders.

Duoctrin *Haller, Braz.*
Co-trimoxazole (p.193·3).
Bacterial infections; Pneumocystis carinii pneumonia; protozoal infections.

Duoctrin Balsamico *Haller, Braz.*
Co-trimoxazole (p.193·3); guaifenesin (p.1092·2); ammonium chloride (p.1085·2).
Bacterial infections.

Duoctrin Enterico *Haller, Braz.*
Co-trimoxazole (p.193·3); attapulgite (p.1212·1).
Diarrhoea.

Duo-CVP *Rhone-Poulenc Rorer, Canad.*
Bioflavonoids (p.1611·1); ascorbic acid (p.1389·3).
Capillary bleeding.

Duo-Cyp *Keene, USA.*
Estradiol cipionate (p.1473·2); testosterone cipionate (p.1492·1).
Menopausal vasomotor symptoms; prevention of post-partum breast engorgement.

Duo-Decadron *Prodome, Braz.*
Dexamethasone sodium phosphate (p.1067·1); dexamethasone acetate (p.1067·1).
Parenteral corticosteroid.

Duoderm
Convatec, Austral.; Bristol-Myers Squibb, Belg.†; Convatec, Fr.; Convatec, UK.
A range of hydrocolloid dressings.
Burns; ulcers; wounds.

Duodexa N *Kade, Ger.*
Dexamethasone (p.1067·1); dexamethasone sodium metasulfobenzoate (p.1067·1).
Skin disorders.

Duofer *Andreabal, Switz.*
Ferrous fumarate (p.1360·1); ferrous gluconate (p.1360·1).
Ascorbic acid (p.1389·3) is included in this preparation to increase the absorption and availability of iron.
Iron deficiency.

Duofer Fol *Andreabal, Switz.*
Ferrous fumarate (p.1360·1); ferrous gluconate (p.1360·1); folic acid (p.1361·1).
Ascorbic acid (p.1389·3) is included in this preparation to increase the absorption and availability of iron.
Iron and folic acid deficiency.

Duofilm
Note.This name is used for preparations of different composition.
Sanova, Aust.; Stiefel, Austral.; Stiefel, Canad.; Stiefel, Fr.; Stiefel, Ger.; Stiefel, Hong Kong; Stiefel, Irl.; Stiefel, Ital.; Stiefel, Mex.; Stiefel, NZ; Stiefel, Port.; Stiefel, S.Afr.; Stiefel, Singapore; Stiefel, Switz.; Stiefel, Thai.; Stiefel, UK.
Topical solution: Salicylic acid (p.1122·3); lactic acid (p.1626·2).
Warts.
Stiefel, Austral.; Stiefel, NZ; Schering-Plough, USA.
Topical gel: Salicylic acid (p.1122·3).
Calluses; corns; warts.

Duoform Novo *Mauermann, Ger.*
Ruscus aculeatus.
Haemorrhoids.

Duoforte *Stiefel, Canad.*
Salicylic acid (p.1122·3).
Warts.

Duogas
Note.This name is used for preparations of different composition.
Bracco, Ital.
Sodium bicarbonate (p.1186·2); anhydrous citric acid (p.1596·2); dimethicone (p.1249·2).
Double-contrast radiography of the oesophagus and stomach.
Bracco, Port.†
Barium sulfate (p.1032·1).

Duogastral *ISM, Ital.*
Pirenzepine hydrochloride (p.472·2).
Gastroduodenitis; peptic ulcer.

Duogink *Duopharm, Ger.*
Ginkgo biloba (p.1615·2).
Cerebrovascular disorders.

Duokapton *Strallhofer, Aust.*
Aspirin (p.14·2); paracetamol (p.71·2).
Fever; pain.

Duolax *Almirall, Spain.*
Lactulose (p.1230·1).
Constipation; hepatic encephalopathy.

Duolip
Ratiopharm, Aust.; Merckle, Ger.; Mepha, Hong Kong; Mepha, Switz.
Etofylline clofibrate (p.888·2).
Hyperlipidaemias.

Duolube *Bausch & Lomb, Canad.*
White soft paraffin (p.1407·3); liquid paraffin (p.1407·1).
Corneal dryness.

Duoluton *Schering, Hong Kong.*
Norgestrel (p.1486·1); ethinylestradiol (p.1476·2).
Endometriosis; menstrual disorders.

Duolys A *Dicamed, Swed.†*
A range of haemodialysis solutions (p.1184·1).

Duolys B *Dicamed, Swed.†*
Sodium bicarbonate; disodium edetate (p.1184·1).
Haemodialysis solution.

Duo-Medihaler *3M, USA†*
Isoprenaline hydrochloride (p.914·3); phenylephrine acid tartrate (p.1097·1).
Bronchospasm.

Duomet
Uniao Quimica, Braz.; Pacific, NZ; Propan, S.Afr.
Cimetidine (p.1216·3).
Acid aspiration; dyspepsia; gastro-oesophageal reflux; peptic ulcer; Zollinger-Ellison syndrome.

Duonalc *ICN, Canad.*
Isopropyl alcohol (p.1149·2).
Skin cleanser.

Duonalc-E *ICN, Canad.*
Alcohol (p.1130·3); isopropyl alcohol (p.1149·2).
Skin cleanser.

Duonasa *Normon, Spain.*
Amoxicillin trihydrate (p.149·2); potassium clavulanate (p.187·2).
Bacterial infections.

Duonate *URL, USA.*
Phenylephrine tannate (p.1097·3); mepyramine tannate (p.421·1).
Upper respiratory-tract disorders.

DuoNeb *Dey, USA.*
Ipratropium bromide (p.766·1); salbutamol sulfate (p.770·3).
Obstructive airways disease.

Duo-Ormogyn *Amsa, Ital.†*
Estradiol benzoate (p.1473·1); progesterone (p.1488·3).
Menstrual disorders.

Duoplant
Note.This name is used for preparations of different composition.
Stiefel, Canad.
Salicylic acid (p.1122·3); lactic acid (p.1626·2); formaldehyde (p.1144·2).
Plantar warts.
Stiefel, Mex.; Schering-Plough, USA.
Salicylic acid (p.1122·3).
Warts.

Duorol *Pharmacia Upjohn, Spain.*
Paracetamol (p.71·2).
Fever; pain.

Duo-Scabil *Agis, Israel.*
Crotamiton (p.1112·3); sulfur (p.1123·3).
Scabies.

Duospirel *Gebro, Aust.†*
Salbutamol (p.770·3); beclometasone dipropionate (p.1061·2).
Obstructive airways disease.

Duoton *TP, Thai.*
Progesterone (p.1488·3); estradiol benzoate (p.1473·1).
Menstrual disorders.

Duo-Trach Kit *Astra, USA.*
Lignocaine [lidocaine] hydrochloride (p.1313·2).
Local anaesthesia.

Duotric *Asian Pharm, Thai.*
Cimetidine (p.1216·3).
Gastric hyperacidity; peptic ulcer.

Duovax *Merck Sharp & Dohme, Belg.†*
A live measles and mumps vaccine (Enders' attenuated Edmonston strain and Jeryl Lynn B strain, respectively) (p.1548·3).
Active immunisation.

Duovent
Boehringer Ingelheim, Belg.; Boehringer de Angeli, Braz.; Boehringer Ingelheim, Canad.; Boehringer Ingelheim, Irl.; Boehringer Ingelheim, Ital.; Boehringer Ingelheim, NZ; Boehringer Ingelheim, S.Afr.; Boehringer Ingelheim, Singapore; Boehringer Ingelheim, UK.
Fenoterol hydrobromide (p.765·1); ipratropium bromide (p.766·1).
Obstructive airways disease.

Duoventrin *Schworer, Ger.*
Bismuth subnitrate (p.1213·2); linseed (p.1629·1); lactose.
Gastrointestinal disorders.

Duoventrinetten N *Schworer, Ger.*
Aluminium hydroxide-magnesium carbonate co-dried gel (p.1211·2); magnesium trisilicate (p.1233·3); magnesium hydroxide (p.1233·1).
Gastrointestinal disorders.

Duovisc
Alcon, Austral.; Alcon, Ger.; Alcon, Singapore; Alcon, Thai.
1 Syringe, sodium hyaluronate (p.1620·1) (Provisc); 1 syringe, sodium hyaluronate; sodium chondroitin sulfate (p.1594·2) (Viscoat).
Adjunct in eye surgery.

Duovitan *Asta Medica, Aust.*
Allopurinol (p.397·2); benzbromarone (p.399·3).
Gout; hyperuricaemia.

Duphalac
Solvay, Aust.; Solvay, Austral.; Solvay, Belg.; Solvay, Canad.; Solvay, Fin.; Solvay, Fr.; Solvay, Hong Kong; Solvay, Irl.; Solvay, Ital.; Solvay, Neth.; Vemedia, Neth.; Solvay, Norw.; Solvay, NZ; Solvay, Port.; Solvay, S.Afr.; Solvay, Singapore; Solvay, Spain; Solvay, Swed.; Solvay, Switz.; Solvay, Thai.; Solvay, UK; Solvay, USA.
Lactulose (p.1230·1).
Constipation; hepatic encephalopathy; salmonella enteritis.

Duphaston
Solvay, Aust.; Solvay, Austral.; Solvay, Belg.; Solvay, Fr.; Solvay, Ger.; Solvay, Hong Kong; Solvay, Irl.; Solvay, Neth.; Solvay, NZ; Solvay, Port.; Solvay, S.Afr.; Solvay, Singapore; Solvay, Spain; Solvay, Swed.; Solvay, Switz.; Solvay, Thai.; Solvay, UK.
Dydrogesterone (p.1472·3).
Dysfunctional uterine bleeding; endometriosis; female infertility; menopausal disorders; menstrual disorders; threatened or recurrent miscarriage.

Duplamin *Bruschettini, Ital.†*
Promethazine hydrochloride (p.423·2).
Skin irritation.

Duplex
Note.This name is used for preparations of different composition.
SBL, Swed.†
A diphtheria and tetanus vaccine (p.1537·1).
Active immunisation.
C & M, USA.
Skin cleanser.

Duplex T *C & M, USA.*
Coal tar (p.1125·1).
Scalp disorders.

Duplexcillina *Metapharma, Ital.*
Ampicillin (p.150·3); dicloxacillin (p.199·1).
Bacterial infections.

Duplexil *Eurofarmaco, Ital.*
Ampicillin trihydrate (p.151·1); dicloxacillin sodium (p.199·1).
Bacterial infections.

Duplicalcio *Medical, Spain†.*
Calcium levulinate (p.1188·3); vitamin B substances (p.1350·1); ergocalciferol (p.1391·2); liver extract; isoniazid (p.215·3).
Anaemias; bone and dental disorders; calcium deficiency; osteomalacia; rickets; tonic.

Duplicalcio 150 *Medical, Spain.*
Isoniazid (p.215·3); pyridoxine (p.1387·1); calcium gluconate (p.1188·2).
Tuberculosis.

Duplicalcio B12 *Medical, Spain.*
Calcium gluconate (p.1188·2); calcium levulinate (p.1188·3); cyanocobalamin (p.1388·1); isoniazid (p.215·3).
Anaemias; tonic; tuberculosis.

Duplicalcio Hidraz *Medical, Spain.*
Calcium gluconate (p.1188·2); calcium levulinate (p.1188·3); isoniazid (p.215·3).
Tonic; tuberculosis.

Duplide *Euro-Labor, Port.; Grunenthal, Port.*
Diltiazem hydrochloride (p.874·3).

Duplinal *Hexal, Aust.†.*
Dipyridamole (p.877·3); aspirin (p.14·2).
Membranous proliferative glomerulonephritis; thrombosis prophylaxis.

Duplobar *Enila, Braz.*
Barium sulfate (p.1032·1).
Contrast medium for gastrointestinal radiography.

Duplocitrin *QIF, Braz.*
Neomycin (p.228·1); bacitracin (p.155·2).
Skin infections.

Duplo-Penicillin *Teva, Israel.*
Procaine penicillin [procaine benzylpenicillin] (p.239·2); benzylpenicillin (p.157·1).
Bacterial infections.

Duplotrast *Gerot, Aust.*
Sodium bicarbonate (p.1186·2); simeticone (p.1249·2).
Adjunct in double contrast radiography.

Duplotrast Z *Gerot, Aust.*
Citric acid (p.1596·2); sodium bicarbonate (p.1186·2); simeticone (p.1249·2).
Adjunct in double contrast radiography.

Duponil *Inkeysa, Spain.*
Ammonium chloride (p.1085·2); codeine phosphate (p.25·2); diphenhydramine hydrochloride (p.416·1); ephedrine hydrochloride (p.1090·1).
Respiratory-tract disorders.

dura AL *Merck dura, Ger.*
Allopurinol (p.397·2).
Adenine-phosphoribosyl-transferase deficiency; gout; hyperuricaemia; Lesch-Nyhan syndrome.

dura AX *Durachemie, Ger.†*
Amoxicillin trihydrate (p.149·2).
Bacterial infections.

duraampicillin *Durachemie, Ger.†*
Ampicillin trihydrate (p.151·1).
Bacterial infections.

Durabezur *Durachemie, Ger.†*
Bezafibrate (p.849·1).
Hyperlipidaemias.

Durabiotic *Teva, Israel.*
Benzathine benzylpenicillin (p.156·2).
Bacterial infections.

Durabolin
Organon, Israel; Organon, USA.
Nandrolone phenylpropionate (p.1484·2).
Anabolic; breast cancer; osteoporosis.

Durabronchal *Merck dura, Ger.*
Acetylcysteine (p.1082·3).
Respiratory-tract disorders associated with increased or viscous mucus.

Duracain *Sintetica, Switz.*
Bupivacaine hydrochloride (p.1306·3).
Local anaesthesia.

Duracare
Allergan, Aust.; Allergan, Austral.; Allergan-Frumtost, Braz.; Allergan, Canad.; Allergan, Ger.†; Blairex, USA.
Disinfection and storage solution for contact lenses (p.1129·2).

duracebrol *Merck dura, Ger.*
Nicergoline (p.1640·2).
Mental function disorders.

Duracef
Bristol-Myers Squibb, Aust.; Bristol-Myers Squibb, Belg.; Bristol-Myers Squibb, Fin.; Bristol-Myers Squibb, Hong Kong; Bristol-Myers Squibb, Israel; Bristol-Myers Squibb, Mex.; Bristol-Myers Squibb, S.Afr.†; Juste, Spain; Bristol-Myers Squibb, Switz.
Cefadroxil (p.161·2).
Bacterial infections.

duracetamol *Merck dura, Ger.*
Paracetamol (p.71·2).
Fever; pain.

Duraclean
Allergan, Austral.; Allergan, Canad.
Cleansing solution for hard and gas permeable contact lenses (p.1129·2).

Duraclon *Roxane, USA.*
Clonidine hydrochloride (p.860·1).
Pain.

Duracoll *Schering-Plough, Belg.*
Gentamicin sulfate (p.210·1); collagen (bovine) (p.1598·2).
Bone infections.

duracoron *Merck dura, Ger.*
Molsidomine (p.936·1).
Angina pectoris.

Duracreme *LRC Products, UK.*
Nonoxinol 9 (p.1346·1).
Contraceptive.

duracroman *Merck dura, Ger.*
Sodium cromoglicate (p.774·3).
Allergic conjunctivitis; allergic rhinitis.

Duract *Wyeth-Ayerst, USA†.*
Bromfenac sodium (p.20·3).
Pain.

duradermal *Merck dura, Ger.*
Bufexamac (p.20·3).
Skin disorders.

duradiuret *Merck dura, Ger.*
Triamterene (p.986·1); hydrochlorothiazide (p.907·3).
Hypertension; oedema.

Duradoce *Atlantis, Mex.*
Hydroxocobalamin (p.1388·1).
Neuritis; pernicious anaemia.

Duradox *Julphar, UAE.*
Doxycycline hyclate (p.200·1).
Bacterial infections.

duradoxal *Durachemie, Ger.†*
Doxycycline (p.200·1) or doxycycline hyclate (p.200·1).
Bacterial infections.

Duradrin *Duramed, USA.*
Isometheptene mucate (p.1624·2); dichloralphenazone (p.682·1); paracetamol (p.71·2).
Migraine; tension headache.

duraerythromycin *Merck dura, Ger.*
Erythromycin stearate (p.201·3).
Bacterial infections.

durafenat *Merck dura, Ger.*
Fenofibrate (p.889·1).
Hyperlipidaemias.

Duraflor *Pharmoscience, Canad.†*
Sodium fluoride (p.1375·3).

durafungol *Merck dura, Ger.*
Clotrimazole (p.382·1).
Fungal infections; vaginal infections.

durafurid *Merck dura, Ger.*
Frusemide [furosemide] (p.893·1) or frusemide [furosemide] sodium (p.895·1).
Hypertension; oedema.

Duragel *SSL, UK.*
Nonoxinol 9 (p.1346·1).
Contraceptive.

duragentamicin *Merck dura, Ger.*
Gentamicin sulfate (p.210·1).
Bacterial infections.

Duragesic
Janssen-Ortho, Canad.; Janssen, USA.
Fentanyl (p.37·1).
Pain.

Dura-Gest *DJ, USA†.*
Phenylephrine hydrochloride (p.1097·1); phenylpropanolamine hydrochloride (p.1098·1); guaifenesin (p.1092·2).
Coughs and cold symptoms; nasal congestion.

duraglucon N *Merck dura, Ger.*
Glibenclamide (p.321·3).
Diabetes mellitus.

duraH2 *Merck dura, Ger.*
Cimetidine (p.1216·3).
Acid aspiration; gastro-oesophageal reflux; peptic ulcer; Zollinger-Ellison syndrome.

dura-Ibu *Durachemie, Ger.†*
Ibuprofen (p.43·2).
Inflammation; musculoskeletal, joint, and soft-tissue disorders; pain.

duralbuprofen *Merck dura, Ger.*
Ibuprofen (p.43·2).
Gout; inflammation; musculoskeletal, joint, and soft-tissue disorders.

durakne *Merck dura, Ger.*
Minocycline hydrochloride (p.224·3).
Acne.

Duralex *American Urologicals, USA.*
Pseudoephedrine hydrochloride (p.1099·2); chlorpheniramine [chlorphenamine] maleate (p.412·1).
Upper respiratory-tract symptoms.

Duralgin *Ethypharm, Denm.*
Morphine sulfate (p.56·1).
Pain.

duralipon *Merck dura, Ger.*
Thioctic acid (p.1671·3).
Diabetic polyneuropathy.

Duralith *Janssen-Ortho, Canad.*
Lithium carbonate (p.292·1).
Bipolar disorder.

Duralmor *Sanfer, Mex.*
Morphine sulfate (p.56·1).
Pain.

Duralone *Hauck, USA.*
Methylprednisolone acetate (p.1076·1).
Corticosteroid.

duralopid *Merck dura, Ger.*
Loperamide hydrochloride (p.1231·3).
Diarrhoea.

duralozam *Merck dura, Ger.*
Lorazepam (p.688·3).
Sleep disorders.

duraMCP *Merck dura, Ger.*
Metoclopramide hydrochloride (p.1235·2).
Gastrointestinal disorders.

duramipress *Merck dura, Ger.*
Prazosin hydrochloride (p.958·1).
Heart failure; hypertension; Raynaud's syndrome.

Duramist Plus *Pfeiffer, USA.*
Oxymetazoline hydrochloride (p.1096·2).
Nasal congestion.

duramonitat *Merck dura, Ger.*
Isosorbide mononitrate (p.916·2).
Angina pectoris; heart failure.

Duramorph *Elkins-Sinn, USA; Baxter, USA.*
Morphine sulfate (p.56·1).
Pain.

duramucal *Merck dura, Ger.*
Ambroxol hydrochloride (p.1084·3).
Respiratory-tract disorders associated with increased or viscous mucus.

Duran *Nakorn, Thai.*
Ibuprofen (p.43·2).
Fever; inflammation; musculoskeletal and joint disorders; pain.

Duranest
Astra, Aust.†; AstraZeneca, Fr.; Astra, Ger.†; Astra, USA.
Etidocaine hydrochloride (p.1312·2).
Adrenaline [epinephrine] acid tartrate (p.829·2) is included in some injections as a vasoconstrictor to diminish absorption and localise the effect of the local anaesthetic.
Local anaesthesia.

duranifin *Merck dura, Ger.*
Nifedipine (p.940·1).
Angina pectoris; hypertension; Raynaud's syndrome.

duranifin Sali *Merck dura, Ger.*
Nifedipine (p.940·1); mefruside (p.926·1).
Hypertension.

duranitrat *Merck dura, Ger.*
Isosorbide dinitrate (p.915·2).
Angina pectoris; heart failure; pulmonary hypertension.

durapaediat *Merck dura, Ger.*
Erythromycin ethyl succinate (p.201·2).
Bacterial infections.

Durapen *De Mayo, Braz.*
Ampicillin benzathine (p.151·3); ampicillin sodium (p.150·3).
Bacterial infections.

Durapen Balsamico *De Mayo, Braz.*
Ampicillin (p.150·2); guaiacol (p.1092·1); eucalyptol (p.1609·2); niaouli oil (p.1640·3).
Bacterial infections.

durapenicillin *Merck dura, Ger.*
Phenoxymethylpenicillin potassium (p.235·1).
Bacterial infections.

durapental *Merck dura, Ger.*
Oxpentifylline [pentoxifylline] (p.950·3).
Peripheral vascular disorders.

Duraphat
Austrodent, Aust.; Inpharma, Denm.; Inpharma, Fin.; Colgate-Palmolive, Ger.; Woelm, Israel; Inpharma, Norw.; Inpharma, Swed.; Colgate-Palmolive, UK.
Sodium fluoride (p.1375·3).
Dental caries prophylaxis; sensitive teeth.

duraphyllin *Merck dura, Ger.*
Theophylline (p.777·2).
Obstructive airways disease.

durapindol *Merck dura, Ger.*
Pindolol (p.955·3).
Cardiac hyperkinesis; hypertension; ischaemic heart disease.

durapirenz *Durachemie, Ger.†*
Pirenzepine hydrochloride (p.472·2).
Gastrointestinal disorders.

durapirox *Merck dura, Ger.*
Piroxicam (p.79·1).
Gout; musculoskeletal, joint, and soft-tissue disorders.

durapitrop *Merck dura, Ger.*
Piracetam (p.1652·1).
Mental function disorders.

duraprednisolon *Merck dura, Ger.; Galen, Ger.*
Prednisolone (p.1077·3) or prednisolone acetate (p.1078·1).
Corticosteroid.

durarese *Merck dura, Ger.*
Amiloride hydrochloride (p.835·1); hydrochlorothiazide (p.907·3).
Hypertension; oedema.

Durascreen
Pharmscience, Canad.
SPF 15: Octinoxate (p.1517·3); octisalate (p.1518·1); titanium dioxide (p.1126·1).
SPF 30: Octinoxate (p.1517·3); octisalate (p.1518·1); oxybenzone (p.1518·1); titanium dioxide (p.1126·1); ensulizole (p.1517·2).
Sunscreen.

Schwarz, USA.
SPF 15: Octinoxate (p.1517·3); octisalate (p.1518·1); oxybenzone (p.1518·1).

SPF 30: Octinoxate (p.1517·3); octisalate (p.1518·1); oxybenzone (p.1518·1); ensulizole (p.1517·2); titanium dioxide (p.1126·1).
Sunscreen.

durasilymarin *Merck dura, Ger.*
Silybum marianum (p.1021·3).
Liver disorders.

Durasina *SmithKline Beecham, Spain.*
Chlorpheniramine [chlorphenamine] maleate (p.412·1); phenylpropanolamine hydrochloride (p.1098·1).
Nasal congestion; sinus congestion.

durasoptin *Merck dura, Ger.*
Verapamil hydrochloride (p.989·1).
Cardiac disorders; hypertension.

duraspiron *Merck dura, Ger.*
Spironolactone (p.973·2).
Hyperaldosteronism; hypertension; liver cirrhosis with ascites; oedema.

duraspiron-comp *Merck dura, Ger.*
Spironolactone (p.973·2); frusemide [furosemide] (p.893·1).
Ascites; hyperaldosteronism; hypertension; oedema.

duratamoxifen *Durachemie, Ger.†*
Tamoxifen citrate (p.571·1).
Breast cancer.

Dura-Tap/PD *Dura, USA.*
Chlorpheniramine [chlorphenamine] maleate (p.412·1); pseudoephedrine hydrochloride (p.1099·2).
Allergic rhinitis; nasal congestion.

Duratears
Note. This name is used for preparations of different composition.
Alcon, Austral.; Alcon, Switz.†
Liquid paraffin (p.1407·1); wool fat (p.1410·3).
Dry eyes.

Alcon, Belg.; Alcon, Canad.; Alcon, Hong Kong; Alcon, Israel; Alcon, Singapore; Alcon, Thai.
White soft paraffin (p.1407·3); liquid paraffin (p.1407·1); anhydrous liquid lanolin (p.1410·3).
Dry eyes.

Alcon, Neth.†
Electrolytes (p.1180·1); hypromellose (p.1501·3); dextran 70 (p.729·2).
Dry eyes.

Alcon, NZ.
Liquid paraffin (p.1407·1); white soft paraffin (p.1407·3).
Dry eyes.

Alcon, S.Afr.
Anhydrous liquid lanolin (p.1410·3).
Dry eyes.

Duratears Free *Alcon, Neth.†*
Povidone (p.1503·2).
Dry eyes.

Duratears Naturale *Alcon, USA.*
Liquid paraffin (p.1407·1); wool fat (p.1410·3); white soft paraffin (p.1407·3).
Dry eyes.

Duratears Z *Alcon, Neth.†*
Liquid paraffin (p.1407·1); hydrous wool fat (p.1411·2); white soft paraffin (p.1407·3).
Dry eyes.

duratenol *Merck dura, Ger.*
Atenolol (p.841·3).
Angina pectoris; arrhythmias; hypertension.

duratenol comp *Merck dura, Ger.*
Atenolol (p.841·3); chlortalidone (p.857·1).
Hypertension.

Durater *Senosiain, Mex.*
Famotidine (p.1225·3).
Gastro-oesophageal reflux; peptic ulcer; Zollinger-Ellison syndrome.

Duratest *Roberts, USA†; Hauck, USA†.*
Testosterone cipionate (p.1492·1).
Breast cancer; delayed puberty (males); male hypogonadism.

Durateston *Akzo, Braz.*
Testosterone propionate (p.1492·2); testosterone phenylpropionate (p.1492·2); testosterone isocaproate (p.1492·2); testosterone caproate (p.1492·1).
Anaemia; androgenic; breast cancer; delayed puberty; male hypogonadism.

Duratestrin *Hauck, USA†.*
Estradiol cipionate (p.1473·2); testosterone cipionate (p.1492·1).
Menopausal vasomotor symptoms; prevention of postpartum breast engorgement.

Durathate *Roberts, USA†; Hauck, USA†.*
Testosterone enantate (p.1492·2).
Breast cancer; delayed puberty (males); male hypogonadism.

duratimol *Durachemie, Ger.†.*
Timolol maleate (p.982·1).
Glaucoma; ocular hypertension.

Duration
Schering-Plough, Hong Kong; Schering-Plough, USA.
Oxymetazoline hydrochloride (p.1096·2).
Nasal congestion.

Duratirs *Alcon, Ital.*
Liquid paraffin (p.1407·1).
Dry eyes.

Duratocin *Ferring, Canad.*
Carbetocin (p.1279·1).
Postpartum haemorrhage; uterine atony.

Duratuss *UCB, USA.*
Pseudoephedrine hydrochloride (p.1099·2); guaifenesin (p.1092·2).
Nasal congestion.

Duratuss DM *UCB, USA.*
Dextromethorphan hydrobromide (p.1087·3); guaifenesin (p.1092·2).
Coughs.

Duratuss G *UCB, USA.*
Guaifenesin (p.1092·2).
Respiratory-tract congestion.

Duratuss GP *UCB, USA.*
Guaifenesin (p.1092·2); pseudoephedrine hydrochloride (p.1099·2).
Coughs.

Duratuss HD *UCB, USA.*
Pseudoephedrine hydrochloride (p.1099·2); guaifenesin (p.1092·2); hydrocodone tartrate (p.42·2).
Coughs; nasal congestion.

duraultra *Ciba Vision, Ger.*
Vitamin A (p.1382·1); actinoquinol sodium (p.1573·1); naphazoline nitrate (p.1095·1).
Eye disorders.

Dura-Vent *DJ, USA†.*
Phenylpropanolamine hydrochloride (p.1098·1); guaifenesin (p.1092·2).
Respiratory-tract congestion.

Dura-Vent/A *Dura, USA†.*
Phenylpropanolamine hydrochloride (p.1098·1); chlorpheniramine [chlorphenamine] maleate (p.412·1).
Upper respiratory-tract symptoms.

Dura-Vent/DA *Dura, USA†.*
Chlorpheniramine [chlorphenamine] maleate (p.412·1); phenylephrine hydrochloride (p.1097·1); hyoscine methonitrate (p.468·2).
Upper respiratory-tract symptoms.

duravolten *Merck dura, Ger.*
Diclofenac sodium (p.30·3).
Gout; inflammation; musculoskeletal, joint, and soft-tissue disorders; pain.

durazanil *Merck dura, Ger.*
Bromazepam (p.656·3).
Anxiety disorders; insomnia.

durazepam *Merck dura, Ger.*
Oxazepam (p.697·1).
Anxiety disorders; sleep disorders.

durazidum *Merck dura, Ger.*
Magnesium hydroxide gel (p.1233·1); aluminium hydroxide gel (p.1210·3).
Gastrointestinal disorders.

Durazina *Maggioni, Ital.*
Chlorpheniramine [chlorphenamine] maleate (p.412·1); phenylpropanolamine hydrochloride (p.1098·1).
Nasal congestion.

Dura-Zok *Durascan, Denm.*
Metoprolol succinate (p.932·1).
Angina pectoris; arrhythmias; hypertension; hyperthyroidism; migraine; myocardial infarction.

Durbis
Aventis, Denm.; Hoechst Marion Roussel, Fin.; Hoechst Marion Roussel, Norw.; Hoechst Marion Roussel, Swed.
Disopyramide (p.878·2) or disopyramide phosphate (p.878·2).
Arrhythmias.

Durekal *Leo, Fin.*
Potassium chloride (p.1194·3).
Hypokalaemia.

Dur-Elix
3M, Austral.; 3M, NZ; 3M, S.Afr.
Bromhexine hydrochloride (p.1085·3).
Respiratory-tract congestion.

Dur-Elix Plus *3M, Austral.*
Bromhexine hydrochloride (p.1085·3); pseudoephedrine hydrochloride (p.1099·2).
Nasal congestion; respiratory-tract disorders associated with excess mucus.

Duremesan *Streuli, Switz.*
Suppositories: Meclozine hydrochloride (p.420·3).
Tablets: Meclozine hydrochloride (p.420·3); caffeine (p.761·3).
Nausea and vomiting.

Durex Sensilube *SSL, UK.*
Vaginal lubricant.
Formerly known as Senselle.

Duricef
Bristol, Canad.; Bristol-Myers Squibb, Singapore; Bristol-Myers Squibb, Thai.; Bristol-Myers Squibb, USA.
Cefadroxil (p.161·2).
Bacterial infections.

Duride
Alphapharm, Austral.; Pacific, NZ.
Isosorbide mononitrate (p.916·2).
Angina pectoris.

Durin *Farmasa, Mex.*
Bumetanide (p.852·1).

Durobac *Pharmaceutical Enterprises, S.Afr.*
Co-trimoxazole (p.193·3).
Bacterial infections.

Duroferon
AstraZeneca, Fin.; AstraZeneca, Norw.; Hassle, Swed.
Ferrous sulfate (p.1360·3).
Ascorbic acid (p.1389·3) may be included in this preparation to increase the absorption and availability of iron.
Iron deficiency; iron-deficiency anaemia.

Duroferon Vitamin
Astra, Denm.†; Hassle, Swed.
Multivitamin preparation with iron (p.1350·1).
Iron-deficiency anaemia of pregnancy.

Durogesic
Janssen-Cilag, Aust.; Janssen-Cilag, Austral.; Janssen-Cilag, Belg.; Janssen-Cilag, Denm.; Janssen-Cilag, Fin.; Janssen-Cilag, Fr.; Janssen-Cilag, Ger.; Janssen-Cilag, Hong Kong; Janssen-Cilag, Irl.; Janssen-Cilag, Israel; Janssen-Cilag, Ital.; Janssen-Cilag, Mex.; Janssen-Cilag, Neth.; Janssen-Cilag, Norw.; Janssen-Cilag, NZ; Janssen-Cilag, Port.; Janssen-Cilag, S.Afr.; Janssen-Cilag, Singapore; Janssen-Cilag, Spain; Janssen-Cilag, Swed.; Janssen-Cilag, Switz.; Janssen-Cilag, UK.
Fentanyl (p.37·1).
Pain.

Durolax *Boehringer Ingelheim, Austral.*
Bisacodyl (p.1212·2).
Bowel evacuation; constipation.

Durolax X-Pack *Boehringer Ingelheim, Austral.*
Combination pack: 3 Tablets, bisacodyl (p.1212·2); 1 suppository, bisacodyl; 1 sachet, citric acid (p.1596·2); heavy magnesium carbonate (p.1232·3).
Bowel evacuation.

Durolax SP *Boehringer Ingelheim, Austral.*
Sodium picosulfate (p.1249·3).
Constipation.

Duromine
3M, Austral.; 3M, Hong Kong; 3M, NZ; 3M, S.Afr.; 3M, Singapore; 3M, Thai.; 3M, UK†.
Phentermine (as an ion-exchange resin complex) (p.1514·1).
Obesity.

Duronitrin *Astra, Ital.*
Isosorbide mononitrate (p.916·2).
Cardiac disorders.

Durotan *Lilly, Ger.*
Xipamide (p.999·2); reserpine (p.967·3).
Hypertension.

Duro-Tuss
3M, Austral.; 3M, Hong Kong; 3M, NZ; 3M, Singapore.
Pholcodine (p.1099·1).
Coughs.

Duro-Tuss Cold & Allergy *3M, Austral.*
Phenylephrine hydrochloride (p.1097·1); chlorpheniramine [chlorphenamine] maleate (p.412·1).
Upper respiratory-tract congestion.

Duro-Tuss Cough Lozenges *3M, Austral.*
Pholcodine (p.1099·1); cetylpyridinium chloride (p.1138·1).
Coughs; sore throat.

Duro-Tuss Decongestant
3M, Austral.; 3M, Hong Kong; 3M, Singapore.
Pholcodine (p.1099·1); pseudoephedrine hydrochloride (p.1099·2).
Coughs; nasal congestion.

Duro-Tuss Expectorant
3M, Austral.; 3M, Hong Kong; 3M, NZ; 3M, Singapore.
Pholcodine (p.1099·1); bromhexine hydrochloride (p.1085·3).
Coughs.

Duro-Tuss Lozenges *3M, NZ.*
Pholcodine (p.1099·1); cetylpyridinium chloride (p.1138·1).
Coughs; sore throat.

Duro-Tuss Mucolytic Cough Liquid *3M, Austral.*
Bromhexine hydrochloride (p.1085·3).
Respiratory-tract congestion.

Durvitan *Seid, Spain.*
Caffeine (p.761·3).
Asthenia.

Dusil *Dumex-Alpharma, Singapore.*
Aspirin (p.14·2).
Influenza symptoms; pain.

Dusk *Seton, UK†.*
Diethyltoluamide (p.1431·2).
Insect repellent.

Merck, Aust.; Merck, Ger.
Naftidrofuryl oxalate (p.937·3).
Peripheral circulatory disorders; vascular disorders of the brain, ears, and eyes.

Duspatal
Solvay, Ger.; Solvay, Ital.; Solvay, Neth.; Solvay, Port.
Mebeverine embonate (p.1234·1) or mebeverine hydrochloride (p.1233·3).
Gastrointestinal spasm.

Duspatalin
Solvay, Belg.; Solvay, Denm.; Solvay, Fr.; Solvay, Hong Kong; Solvay, Singapore; Solvay, Spain; Solvay, Switz.
Mebeverine embonate (p.1234·1) or mebeverine hydrochloride (p.1233·3).
Enteritis; gastrointestinal spasm; irritable bowel syndrome.

Dustinex *Hal, Neth.†.*
House-dust mite extracts.
Hyposensitisation.

Dutacor *Durascan, Denm.*
Sotalol hydrochloride (p.972·2).
Arrhythmias.

Dutimelan *Hoechst Marion Roussel, Ital.†.*
10 Tablets, prednisolone acetate (p.1078·1); prednisolone (p.1077·3); 10 tablets, prednisolone; cortisone acetate (p.1065·3).
Oral corticosteroid.

Dutonin *Bristol-Myers Squibb, Aust.; Bristol-Myers Squibb, Irl.; Bristol-Myers Squibb, Neth.; Bristol-Myers, Spain; Bristol-Myers, UK.*
Nefazodone hydrochloride (p.300·3).
Depression.

Dutross *Nakorn, Thai.*
Bromhexine hydrochloride (p.1085·3).
Respiratory-tract disorders associated with increased or viscous mucus.

Duvadilan *Solvay, Austral.†; Solvay, Belg.; Solvay, Fr.; Solvay, Hong Kong; Solvay, Irl.; Solvay, Ital.†; Solvay, Neth.; Duphar, Spain†; Duphar-Interfan, Thai.*
Isoxsuprine hydrochloride (p.1624·3) or isoxsuprine resinate (p.1625·1).
Cerebral and peripheral vascular disorders; premature labour.

Duvium *Zambon, Belg.; Inpharzam, Switz.*
Benoritate (p.19·3).
Fever; musculoskeletal and joint disorders; pain.

Duvoid *Roberts, Canad.; Roberts, USA.*
Bethanechol chloride (p.1415·3).
Urinary retention.

Duxaril *Servier, Hong Kong; Servier, Singapore; Servier, Thai.*
Almitrine dimesilate (p.1506·2) or raubasine (p.967·2).
Chorioretinal ischaemia; cochleovestibular ischaemia; mental function impairment; stroke.

Duxil *Ardix, Fr.; Servier, Port.*
Almitrine (p.1506·2) or almitrine dimesilate (p.1506·2); raubasine (p.967·2).
Mental function impairment; retinal ischaemia; vestibular ischaemia.

Duxima *Ecobi, Ital.*
Cefuroxime sodium (p.178·2).
Bacterial infections.

Duxor *Servier, Spain.*
Raubasinc (p.967·2); almitrine (p.1506·2) or almitrine dimesilate (p.1506·2).
Cerebrovascular disorders; vestibular disorders.

DV *Marion Merrell Dow, USA†.*
Dienestrol (p.1471·1).
Menopausal vulval and vaginal atrophy.

D-Vi-Sol *Mead Johnson Nutritionals, Canad.*
Vitamin D (p.1391·1).
Vitamin supplement.

D-Vital *Will-Pharma, Belg.*
Calcium carbonate (p.1215·1); colecalciferol (p.1391·1).
Calcium and vitamin D deficiency; osteoporosis.

D-Worm *Triomed, S.Afr.*
Mebendazole (p.102·2).
Worm infections.

Dyazide *SmithKline Beecham, Austral.; SmithKline Beecham, Canad.; SmithKline Beecham, Hong Kong; Goldshield, Irl.; SmithKline Beecham, Mex.; SmithKline Beecham, NZ; Decomed, Port.; SmithKline Beecham, S.Afr.; SmithKline Beecham, Singapore; Doetsch, Grether, Switz.; SmithKline Beecham, Thai.; Goldshield, UK; SmithKline Beecham, USA.*
Hydrochlorothiazide (p.907·3); triamterene (p.986·1).
These ingredients can be described by the British Approved Name Co-triamterzide.
Hypertension; oedema.

Dycholium *Novartis Consumer, Canad.†.*
Dehydrocholic acid (p.1602·2).
Biliary-tract disorders.

Dycill *SmithKline Beecham, USA.*
Dicloxacillin sodium (p.199·1).
Bacterial infections.

Dyclone *Astra, USA.*
Dyclonine hydrochloride (p.1311·3).
Local anaesthesia.

Dyflex *Econo Med, USA†.*
Diprophylline (p.764·1).
Asthma; bronchospasm.

Dyflex-G *Econo Med, USA.*
Diprophylline (p.764·1); guaifenesin (p.1092·2).
Bronchospasm.

Dy-G *Cypress, USA.*
Diprophylline (p.764·1); guaifenesin (p.1092·2).
Asthma.

Dygratyl *Solvay, Denm.; Solvay, Fin.; Solvay, Swed.*
Dihydrotachysterol (p.1391·2).
Hypocalcaemia; hypoparathyroidism; osteomalacia; pseudohypoparathyroidism; renal osteodystrophy; rickets; secondary hyperparathyroidism.

Dyka-D *Covan, S.Afr.*
Chlorpheniramine [chlorphenamine] maleate (p.412·1); phenylephrine hydrochloride (p.1097·1); hyoscine methonitrate (p.468·2).
Hypersensitivity reactions; nasal congestion.

Dykatuss Co *Covan, S.Afr.*
Mepyramine maleate (p.421·1); ephedrine hydrochloride (p.1090·1); codeine phosphate (p.25·2).
Cold symptoms; coughs.

Dykatuss Expectorant *Vesta, S.Afr.†.*
Pentoxyverine citrate (p.1096·3); terpin hydrate (p.1101·2); sodium citrate (p.1186·2).
Coughs.

Dyline GG *Seatrace, USA.*
Diprophylline (p.764·1); guaifenesin (p.1092·2).
Bronchospasm.

Dylix *Lunsco, USA.*
Diprophylline (p.764·1).

Dymadon *Warner-Lambert, Austral.*
Paracetamol (p.71·2).
Fever; pain.

Dymadon Co *Warner-Lambert, Austral.*
Paracetamol (p.71·2); codeine phosphate (p.25·2).
Pain.

Dymadon Forte *Glaxo Wellcome, Austral.*
Paracetamol (p.71·2); codeine phosphate (p.25·2).
Pain.

Dymelor *Lilly, USA.*
Acetohexamide (p.320·1).
Diabetes mellitus.

Dymenate *Keene, USA.*
Dimenhydrinate (p.415·2).
Motion sickness.

Dymion *Pulitzer, Ital.†.*
Ubidecarenone (p.1677·1).
Cardiac disorders; co-enzyme Q deficiency.

Dyna Jets *Roche, S.Afr.†.*
Multivitamin preparation (p.1350·1).

Dyna-Ampcil *Salters, S.Afr.*
Ampicillin trihydrate (p.151·1).
Bacterial infections.

Dynabac *Lilly, Braz.; Pharmafarm, Fr.; Lilly, Hong Kong; Muro, USA.*
Dirithromycin (p.199·2).
Bacterial infections.

Dynablok *Dynamed, S.Afr.†.*
Propranolol hydrochloride (p.962·3).
Angina pectoris; arrhythmias; hypertension; hyperthyroidism; phaeochromocytoma; tremor.

Dynabolon *Fournier, Ital.; Theramex, Mon.†.*
Nandrolone undecylate (p.1484·2).
Anabolic; osteoporosis.

Dynacil *Schwarz, Ger.; Sanol, Ger.*
Fosinopril sodium (p.892·3).
Heart failure; hypertension.

Dynacil comp *Schwarz, Ger.; Sanol, Ger.*
Fosinopril sodium (p.892·3); hydrochlorothiazide (p.907·3).
Hypertension.

Dynacin *Medicis, USA.*
Minocycline hydrochloride (p.224·3).
Bacterial infections.

Dynacirc *Novartis, Hong Kong; Novartis, Mex.; Novartis, NZ; Novartis, S.Afr.; Novartis, Singapore; Novartis, Thai.; Novartis, USA.*
Isradipine (p.916·3).
Hypertension.

Dynacold *Thuasne, Fr.†.*
Dichlorodifluoromethane (p.1199·1); trichlorofluoromethane (p.1199·1).
Joint and muscle pain.

Dynadol *Salters, S.Afr.*
Paracetamol (p.71·2).
Fever; pain.

Dynafed Asthma Relief *BDI, USA.*
Ephedrine hydrochloride (p.1090·1); guaifenesin (p.1092·2).
Coughs.

Dynafed EX *BDI, USA.*
Paracetamol (p.71·2).
Fever; pain.

Dynafed IB *BDI, USA†.*
Ibuprofen (p.43·2).
Fever; musculoskeletal and joint disorders; pain.

Dynafed Plus *BDI, USA.*
Paracetamol (p.71·2); pseudoephedrine hydrochloride (p.1099·2).
Formerly known as Maximum Strength Dynafed.
Upper respiratory-tract symptoms.

Dynafed Pseudo *BDI, USA†.*
Pseudoephedrine hydrochloride (p.1099·2).
Nasal congestion.

Dynafemme *Diepha, Fr.*
Vitamin, mineral, and fish oil preparation (p.1350·1).
Nutritional supplement.

Dynagastrin *Salters, S.Afr.*
Dicyclomine [dicycloverine] hydrochloride (p.466·1); dried aluminium hydroxide gel (p.1210·3); light magnesium oxide (p.1233·2).
Gastric hyperacidity.

Dyna-Hex *Western Medical, USA.*
Chlorhexidine gluconate (p.1138·2).
Skin disinfection.

Dynalert *Restan, S.Afr.*
Pemoline (p.1513·1).
Fatigue.

Dynalin *Dynamed, S.Afr.†.*
Diphenhydramine hydrochloride (p.416·1); ammonium chloride (p.1085·2); sodium citrate (p.1186·2).
Coughs.

Dynametcin *Dynamed, S.Afr.†.*
Indometacin (p.44·3).
Gout; musculoskeletal and joint disorders.

Dynametron *Salters, S.Afr.*
Metronidazole (p.594·1).
Anaerobic bacterial infections; protozoal infections.

Dynamide *Salters, S.Afr.*
Metoclopramide hydrochloride (p.1235·2).
Gastrointestinal disorders.

Dynamin
Note. This name is used for preparations of different composition.
Ern, Spain.
Vitamin B substances; haematoporphyrin; amino acids; glutathione; nucleosides; procaine hydrochloride; orotic acid; magnesium molybdate; pemoline magnesium (p.1350·1).
Tonic.
Berk, UK.
Isosorbide mononitrate (p.916·2).
Angina pectoris; heart failure.

Dynamisan *Wander, Belg.†; Novartis Sante, Fr.; Mipharm, Ital.; Novartis Consumer, Port.; Novartis Consumer, Switz.*
Arginine aspartate (p.1354·1) or arginine glutamate (p.1353·3).
Tonic.

Dynamo *Key, Austral.*
Caffeine (p.761·3); glucose; thiamine hydrochloride; nicotinic acid (p.1350·1).
Drowsiness; mental fatigue.

Dynamogen *Faes, Spain.*
Arginine aspartate (p.1354·1); glutodina.
Anorexia; tonic; weight loss.

Dynamucil *Siphar, Switz.*
Acetylcysteine (p.1082·3).
Respiratory-tract disorders with viscous mucus.

Dynapam *Dynamed, S.Afr.†.*
Diazepam (p.674·3).
Alcohol withdrawal syndrome; anxiety; premedication.

Dynapayne *Salters, S.Afr.*
Syrup: Paracetamol (p.71·2); codeine phosphate (p.25·2); promethazine hydrochloride (p.423·2).
Fever; pain.
Tablets: Paracetamol (p.71·2); codeine phosphate (p.25·2); caffeine (p.761·3); meprobamate (p.691·1).
Pain and associated tension.

Dynapen
Note. This name is used for preparations of different composition.
Leo, Aust.
Sultamicillin (p.257·2) or sultamicillin tosilate (p.257·2).
Bacterial infections.
Dynamed, S.Afr.†.
Phenoxymethylpenicillin potassium (p.235·1).
Bacterial infections.
Apothecon, USA.
Dicloxacillin sodium (p.199·1).
Bacterial infections.

Dynaphlem *Dynamed, S.Afr.†.*
Carbocisteine (p.1086·3).
Respiratory-tract disorders.

Dynaphos-C *Sofar, Ital.*
Ascorbic acid (p.1389·3).
Gingivitis; stomatitis; vitamin C deficiency.

Dynaplex *Chemedica, Switz.†.*
Multivitamin and amino-acid preparation (p.1350·1).

Dynaspor *Salters, S.Afr.*
Clotrimazole (p.382·1).
Fungal infections.

Dynatra *Sintesa, Belg.; Zambon, Neth.*
Dopamine hydrochloride (p.881·3).
Hypotension; shock.

Dynavital *Monal, Fr.†.*
A range of trace element preparations (p.1350·1).

Dynazole *Salters, S.Afr.*
Co-trimoxazole (p.193·3).
Bacterial infections.

Dynef *Sigma-Tau, Ger.*
Anthocyanins from myrtillus; alpha tocoferil acetate (p.1394·1).
Eye disorders.

Dynergum *Ferring, Port.*
Citrulline malate (p.1357·2).
Tonic.

Dyneric *Henning, Ger.*
Clomifene citrate (p.1465·3).
Anovulatory infertility.

Dynese *Galen, UK.*
Magaldrate (p.1232·2).
Dyspepsia.

Dynexan
Note. This name is used for preparations of different composition.
Nycomed, Aust.; Restan, S.Afr.; Kreussler, Switz.
Amethocaine [tetracaine] hydrochloride (p.1305·2); chamomile (p.1593·2); arnica (p.1581·3); sage (p.1660·2); aluminium formate.
Mouth and throat disorders.
Kreussler, Fr.
Lignocaine [lidocaine] hydrochloride (p.1313·2).
Local anaesthesia; painful mouth lesions.

Dynexan A *Kreussler, Ger.*
Lignocaine [lidocaine] hydrochloride (p.1313·2); benzalkonium chloride (p.1133·2).
Painful inflammatory disorders of the mouth.

Dynofen *Salters, S.Afr.*
Ibuprofen (p.43·2).
Musculoskeletal and joint disorders.

Dynorm *Merck, Ger.; Roche, Ger.*
Cilazapril (p.858·1).
Hypertension.

Dynorm Plus *Merck, Ger.; Roche, Ger.*
Cilazapril (p.858·1); hydrochlorothiazide (p.907·3).
Hypertension.

Dynos *Intramed, S.Afr.*
Dopamine hydrochloride (p.881·3).
Heart failure; shock.

Dynothel *Henning, Ger.*
Dextrothyroxine sodium (p.867·3).
Hyperlipidaemias.

Dynoxytet *Salters, S.Afr.*
Oxytetracycline hydrochloride (p.234·1).
Bacterial infections.

Dyphylline-GG *Cypress, USA.*
Diprophylline (p.764·1); guaifenesin (p.1092·2).
Asthma with associated cough.

Dyprotex
Note. This name is used for preparations of different composition.
Blistex, Hong Kong.
Dimethicone (p.1410·1); zinc oxide (p.1128·2); soft paraffin (p.1407·3).
Nappy rash.
Blistex, Israel.
Zinc oxide (p.1128·2).
Nappy rash.
Blistex, USA.
Dimethicone (p.1410·1); zinc oxide (p.1128·2); cod-liver oil (p.1357·2).
Nappy rash.

Dyrenium *SmithKline Beecham, Canad.; Doetsch, Grether, Switz.†; SmithKline Beecham, USA.*
Triamterene (p.986·1).
Oedema.

Dyrenium compositum *Doetsch, Grether, Switz.*
Triamterene (p.986·1); benzthiazide (p.844·2).
Hypertension; oedema.

Dyrexan-OD *Trimen, USA†.*
Phendimetrazine tartrate (p.1513·3).
Obesity.

Dyrosol *Propan, S.Afr.*
Bismuth salicylate (p.1213·1); codeine phosphate (p.25·2); atropine sulfate (p.461·1).
Diarrhoea.

Dysalfa *Debat, Fr.*
Terazosin hydrochloride (p.980·1).
Benign prostatic hyperplasia.

Dyscornut-N *Weber & Weber, Ger.*
Homoeopathic preparation.

Dysetrin *Hua, Thai.*
Diiodohydroxyquinoline (p.590·2).
Amoebiasis.

Dyskinebyl *Zyma, Fr.†.*
Dihydroxydibutylether (p.1603·3).
Dyspepsia.

Dysman *Ashbourne, UK.*
Mefenamic acid (p.51·2).
Dysfunctional menorrhagia; fever; pain.

Dysmenalgit *Krewel, Ger.*
Naproxen (p.60·3).
Dysmenorrhoea.

Dysmenorrhoe-Gastreu R75 *Reckeweg, Ger.*
Homoeopathic preparation.

Dyspagon *Pierre Fabre Sante, Fr.*
Loperamide hydrochloride (p.1231·3).
Diarrhoea.

Dyspamet *Goldshield, Irl.; Goldshield, UK.*
Cimetidine (p.1216·3).
Gastric hyperacidity; gastro-oesophageal reflux; peptic ulcer; Zollinger-Ellison syndrome.

Dyspen *Biolab, Hong Kong; Biolab, Thai.*
Mefenamic acid (p.51·2).
Fever; pain.

Dyspne-Inhal *Augot, Fr.*
Adrenaline [epinephrine] (p.829·1).
Glottal oedema.

Dysport *Croma, Aust.; Ipsen, Belg.; Ipsen, Denm.; Ipsen, Fin.; Ipsen Biotech, Fr.; Ipsen, Ger.; Beaufour-Ipsen, Hong Kong; Ipsen, Irl.; Ipsen, Ital.; NZ Medical & Scientific, NZ; Ipsen, Spain; Ipsen, UK.*
Botulinum A toxin (p.1324·2).
Blepharospasm; foot spasticity associated with paediatric cerebral palsy; hemifacial spasm; spasmodic torticollis.

dysto-L 90 N *Loges, Ger.*
Homoeopathic preparation.

dysto-loges *Loges, Ger.*
Homoeopathic preparation.

dysto-lux *Loges, Ger.*
Hypericum (p.290·2).
Anxiety; depression.

Dystomin M *Redel, Ger.†.*
Heavy magnesium oxide (p.1233·2).
Gastric hyperacidity.

Dystonal *Pharmethic, Belg.*
Dihydroergotamine mesilate (p.450·3).
Formerly contained belladonna, ergotamine tartrate, and phenobarbital.
Migraine and other vascular headaches; orthostatic hypotension.

Dystophan *Kattwiga, Ger.*
Homoeopathic preparation.

Dystrol *Werth Lederle, Denm.†.*
Levonorgestrel (p.1486·2); ethinylestradiol (p.1476·2).
Endometriosis; menstrual disorders.

Dysurgal *Disperga, Aust.*
Atropine sulfate (p.461·1); ephedrine hydrochloride (p.1090·1); strychnine nitrate (p.1667·3).
Urinary-tract disorders.

Dysurgal N *Galenika, Ger.*
Atropine sulfate (p.461·1).
Dysurgal formerly contained atropine sulfate, ephedrine hydrochloride, and strychnine nitrate.
Dysmenorrhoea; urinary-tract disorders.

Dytac *SmithKline Beecham, Neth.; Pharmark, UK.*
Triamterene (p.986·1).
Hypertension; oedema.

Dyta-Urese *SMB, Belg.‡; SmithKline Beecham, Neth.*
Triamterene (p.986·1); epitizide (p.886·1).
Hypertension; oedema.

Dytenzide *Yamanouchi, Belg.; SmithKline Beecham, Neth.*
Triamterene (p.986·1); hydrochlorothiazide (p.907·3).
Hypertension; oedema.

Dyterene *Pharmasant, Thai.*
Hydrochlorothiazide (p.907·3); triamterene (p.986·1).
Hypertension; oedema.

Dytide *Goldshield, UK.*
Triamterene (p.986·1); benzthiazide (p.844·2).
Oedema.

Dytide H *Procter & Gamble, Aust.; Procter & Gamble, Ger.*
Triamterene (p.986·1); hydrochlorothiazide (p.907·3).
Heart failure; hypertension; oedema.

Dytuss *Lunsco, USA.*
Diphenhydramine hydrochloride (p.416·1).

Dyzole *Lincoln, NZ.*
Tinidazole (p.603·3).
Bacterial infections; protozoal infections.

D-Zol *Pacific, NZ.*
Danazol (p.1468·3).
Benign breast disease; endometriosis; hereditary angioedema; menorrhagia.

E45
Note. This name is used for preparations of different composition.
Boots, Austral.; Boots Healthcare, Irl.; Boots, S.Afr.; Crookes Healthcare, UK.
Emollient.
Dry skin disorders.

Boots, NZ.
Bath oil: Liquid paraffin (p.1407·1); dimethicone (p.1410·3).
Bath additive; dry skin; pruritus.
Wash: Liquid paraffin (p.1407·1); zinc oxide (p.1128·2).
Cleansing agent for dry skin.

E45 Itch Relief *Crookes Healthcare, UK.*
Macrogol lauril ethers (p.1345·2); urea (p.1127·3).
Pruritus; scaling skin conditions.

E Radicaps *Novaquimica, Braz.*
Vitamin E (p.1393·3).
Vitamin E supplement.

E45 Sun *Crookes Healthcare, UK.*
SPF 15; SPF 30: Titanium dioxide (p.1126·1); zinc oxide (p.1128·2).
Sunscreen.

E45 Sun Block *Crookes Healthcare, UK.*
SPF 25; SPF 50: Titanium dioxide (p.1126·1); zinc oxide (p.1128·2).
Sunscreen.

Eaca Balsamico *Nikkho, Braz.*
Aminocaproic acid (p.724·3); sodium benzoate (p.1134·3); guaifenesin (p.1092·2); ammonium chloride (p.1085·2).
Respiratory-tract congestion.

EAP-61 *Hanosan, Ger.*
Homoeopathic preparation.

Ear Clear *Key, Austral.*
Urea hydrogen peroxide (p.1159·3).
Ear wax removal.

Ear Clear for Swimmer's Ear *Key, Austral.*
Acetic acid (p.1571·2); isopropyl alcohol (p.1149·2).
Otitis externa.

Earache *Hylands, Canad.*
Homoeopathic preparation.

Earache Pain *Homeocan, Canad.*
Homoeopathic preparation.

EarCalm *Stafford-Miller, UK.*
Glacial acetic acid (p.1571·2).
Superficial ear infections.

Ear-Dry *Scherer, USA.*
Boric acid (p.1586·1); isopropyl alcohol (p.1149·2).
Ear disorders.

Earex *SSL, UK.*
Arachis oil (p.1581·1); almond oil (p.1576·3); rectified camphor oil.
Ear wax removal.

Earex Plus *SSL, UK.*
Choline salicylate (p.24·3); glycerol (p.1616·3).
Ear wax removal; earache.

Ear-Eze *Hyrex, USA.*
Hydrocortisone (p.1073·3); neomycin sulfate (p.228·1); polymyxin B (p.238·3).
Bacterial ear infections.

Early Bird
Note. This name is used for preparations of different composition.
Mentholatum, Austral.
Pyrantel embonate (p.108·1).
Enterobiasis.

Kent, UK.
Pregnancy test (p.1654·3).

EarSol *Parnell, USA.*
Alcohol (p.1130·3).
Ear disorders.

EarSol-HC *Parnell, USA.*
Hydrocortisone (p.1073·3).
Ear inflammation.

EAS *Fresenius Kabi, Switz.*
Amino-acid preparation (p.1350·1).
Nutritional supplement in renal failure.

Ease Pain Away *RMC, Canad.†*
Menthol (p.1632·3); trolamine salicylate (p.90·1).

Easistix BG *Eastern Pharmaceuticals, UK.*
Test for glucose in blood (p.1616·3).

Easistix UG *Eastern Pharmaceuticals, UK.*
Test for glucose in urine (p.1616·3).

Easprin *Lotus, USA.*
Aspirin (p.14·2).
Fever; inflammation; pain.

Easy gel *Abic, Israel.*
Benzydamine hydrochloride (p.20·1).
Musculoskeletal and joint disorders.

Easy hCG *Carter-Wallace, Austral.†*
Pregnancy test (p.1654·3).

Easy Strip *Boehringer Mannheim, Canad.†*
Test for glucose in blood (p.1616·3).

Easylax *Sam-On, Israel.*
Phenolphthalein (p.1244·1).
Constipation.

Eatan N *Desitin, Ger.*
Nitrazepam (p.695·2).
Sleep disorders.

Eau Precieuse *Warner-Lambert, Fr.*
Boric acid (p.1586·1); resorcinol (p.1122·2); salicylic acid (p.1122·3); tannic acid (p.1669·1); lysol (p.1142·3); phenol (p.1152·3); menthol (p.1632·3).
Seborrhoea.

Eau-de-vie de France avec huile de pin nain du Tirol *Luond, Switz.*
Menthol (p.1632·3); pumilio pine oil (p.1656·3).
Muscular pain and fatigue.

Eavit *Terapeutico, Ital.*
Gelatin; wheat-germ oil; carrot oil; soya lecithin; royal jelly; beeswax (p.1350·1).
Nutritional supplement.

Eavit Plus *Terapeutico, Ital.*
Gelatin; wheat-germ oil; carrot oil; lecithin; royal jelly; soya oil (p.1350·1).
Nutritional supplement.

E-Base *Barr, USA.*
Erythromycin (p.201·2).
Bacterial infections.

Ebastel *Dainippon, Jpn; Almirall, Spain.*
Ebastine (p.417·2).
Hypersensitivity reactions.

Ebefen *Ebewe, Aust.*
Tamoxifen citrate (p.571·1).
Breast cancer; endometrial cancer.

Ebenol *Strathmann, Ger.*
Hydrocortisone acetate (p.1073·3).
Burns; skin disorders.

Ebrantil *Byk, Aust.; Byk, Belg.; Byk, Braz.; Byk Gulden, Ger.; Byk Gulden, Ital.; Byk, Neth.; Byk, Port.; Byk, Switz.*
Urapidil (p.987·3), urapidil fumarate (p.988·1), or urapidil hydrochloride (p.987·3).
Hypertension; production of controlled hypotension.

Ebrocit *Robert, Spain†.*
Ebrotidine (p.1225·1).
Peptic ulcer.

Ebromin *Degorts, Mex.*
Ambroxol hydrochloride (p.1084·3).
Respiratory-tract disorders with viscous mucus.

Ebufac *DDSA Pharmaceuticals, UK.*
Ibuprofen (p.43·2).

Eburdent F *Acro, Ital.*
Miristalkonium sacchrinate (p.1151·2); sodium fluoride (p.1375·3).
Dental caries prophylaxis; oral hygiene.

Eburnal *Chiesi, Ital.*
Vinburnine phosphate (p.1680·1).
Cerebrovascular disorders.

Eburnoxin *Astra, Spain†.*
Vinburnine (p.1680·1).
Cerebrovascular disorders; retinopathies.

Eburos *Acro, Ital.*
Chlorhexidine gluconate (p.1138·2).
Oral hygiene.

EC + Complex *Seroyal, Canad.*
Vitamin preparation with zinc (p.1350·1).

Ecabil *Biologici Italia, Ital.*
Heparin calcium (p.902·1).
Thromboembolic disorders.

Ecadiu *Vita Elan, Ital.*
Hydrochlorothiazide (p.907·3); captopril (p.853·3).
Hypertension.

Ecafast *Crinos, Ital.*
Heparin calcium (p.902·1).
Thromboembolic disorders.

Ecamannan *CaDiGroup, Ital.*
Glucomannan (p.1616·2); vitamin E (p.1393·3); vitamin C (p.1389·3); betacarotene (p.1355·1).
Gastrointestinal disorders; hypercholesterolaemia; obesity.

Ecapresan *Mead Johnson, Mex.*
Captopril (p.853·3).
Hypertension.

Ecapril *Promeco, Mex.*
Captopril (p.853·3).

Ecasil *Searle, Braz.*
Aspirin (p.14·2).
Fever; inflammation; pain; thromboembolism prophylaxis.

Ecasolv *Benedetti, Ital.*
Heparin calcium (p.902·1).
Thromboembolic disorders.

Ecaten *Fustery, Mex.*
Captopril (p.853·3).
Heart failure; hypertension; myocardial infarction.

Ecazide *Bristol-Myers Squibb, Fr.; Squibb, Spain.*
Captopril (p.853·3); hydrochlorothiazide (p.907·3).
Hypertension.

Eccarvit *CaDiGroup, Ital.†*
Vitamin C; vitamin E; betacarotene (p.1350·1).
Antioxidant nutritional supplement.

Eccarvit Plus *CaDiGroup, Ital.*
Vitamin C; vitamin E; betacarotene; ginkgo biloba; chromium picolinate (p.1350·1).
Nutritional supplement.

Eccelium *Manetti Roberts, Ital.*
Econazole sulfosalicylate (p.383·1).
Fungal infections; Gram-positive bacterial superinfections.

Ecdylin *De Witt, UK.*
Diphenhydramine (p.416·1); ammonium chloride (p.1085·2).
Coughs.

Ecee Plus *Edwards, USA.*
Vitamins C and E with minerals (p.1350·1).

Echan *Biocur, Ger.*
Echinacea purpura (p.1606·2).
Respiratory- and urinary-tract infections.

Echifit *Krewel, Ger.*
Echinacea purpurea (p.1606·2).
Respiratory- and urinary-tract infections.

Echiherb *Duopharm, Ger.*
Echinacea purpurea (p.1606·2).
Respiratory- and urinary-tract infections.

Echina Pro *Planta, Canad.†*
Echinacea (p.1606·2).
Cold and influenza symptoms.

Echinacea *Potter's, UK.*
Elixir: Echinacea (p.1606·2); baptisia tinctoria; fumitory (p.1612·3).
Catarrh; immunostimulat; minor skin disorders.
Tablets: Echinacea (p.1606·2).
Immunostimulat; skin disorders.

Echinacea 4000 *Procare, Austral.*
Echinacea (p.1606·2); calcium ascorbate (p.1389·3); zinc amino acid chelate (p.1398·3).
Upper respiratory-tract symptoms.

Echinacea ACE Plus Zinc *Blackmores, Austral.*
Echinacea angustifolia (p.1606·2); vitamins (p.1350·1); zinc amino acid chelate (p.1398·3); garlic oil.
Tonic.

Echinacea ACE + Zinc *Blackmores, Austral.*
Echinacea pallida (p.1606·2); vitamins (p.1350·1); zinc (p.1398·1).
Cold and influenza symptoms.

Echinacea akut *Hevert, Ger.†*
Homoeopathic preparation.

Echinacea & Antioxidants *Vitaplex, Austral.*
Ascorbic acid (p.1389·3); d-alpha tocoferil acid succinate (p.1394·1); zinc gluconate (p.1398·2); echinacea (p.1606·2); garlic (p.1614·1).
Upper respiratory-tract disorders.

Echinacea comp
Hevert, Ger.; Steigerwald, Ger.
Homoeopathic preparation.

Echinacea Complex *Cenovis, Austral.*
Echinacea (p.1606·2); vitamins (p.1350·1); zinc amino acid chelate (p.1398·3).
Skin disorders; upper respiratory-tract infections; wounds.

Echinacea Herbal Plus Formula *Vitelle, Austral.†*
Multivitamins with echinacea and zinc amino acid chelate (p.1350·1) (p.1606·2) (p.1398·3).
Minor upper respiratory-tract disorders; skin disorders.

Echinacea L40 *Homeocan, Canad.*
Homoeopathic preparation.

Echinacea Lozenge *Blackmores, Austral.*
Echinacea purpurea (p.1606·2); sodium ascorbate (p.1390·1); eucalyptus oil (p.1609·2).
Cold and influenza symptoms.

Echinacea Med Complex *Dynamit, Aust.*
Homoeopathic preparation.

Echinacea Oligoplex *Madaus, Ger.*
Homoeopathic preparation.

Echinacea Plus *Eagle, Austral.*
Echinacea (p.1606·2); astragalus membranaceus; schizandra chinensis; tabebuia avellanedae.
Minor infections; tonic.

Echinacea Ro-Plex (Rowo-415) *Pharmakon, Ger.*
Homoeopathic preparation.

Echinacea Urtinktur *Hevert, Ger.*
Homoeopathic preparation.

Echinacea-Complex *Weber & Weber, Ger.†*
Homoeopathic preparation.

Echinacin *Madaus, Aust.; Polcopharma, Austral.; Madaus, Ger.; Madaus, Spain; Madaus, Switz.*
Echinacea purpurea (p.1606·2).
Respiratory- and urinary-tract infections; wounds.

Echinaforce *Bio-Garten, Aust.; Bioforce, Ger.; Bioforce, Switz.; Bioforce, UK.*
Echinacea purpura (p.1606·2).
Respiratory-tract infections.

EchinaMed *Bioforce, Switz.*
Echinacea (p.1606·2).
Immunostimulant.

Echinapur *Lappe, Ger.*
Echinacea purpura (p.1606·2).
Respiratory- and urinary-tract infections.

Echinarell *Sanorell, Ger.*
Homoeopathic preparation.

Echinart *Ceom, Ital.*
Homoeopathic preparation.

Echinasyx *Syxyl, Ger.*
Homoeopathic preparation.

Echine *Eagle, Austral.*
Herbal and homoeopathic antiseptic.

Echnatol *Gerot, Aust.*
Cyclizine hydrochloride (p.414·1).
Motion sickness; nausea and vomiting.

Echnatol B₆ *Gerot, Aust.*
Cyclizine hydrochloride (p.414·1); pyridoxine hydrochloride (p.1386·3).
Motion sickness; nausea and vomiting; vestibular disorders.

Echovist
Schering, Aust.; Berlex, Canad.; Schering, Denm.†; Schering, Fin.; Schering, Fr.; Schering, Ger.; Schering, Israel; Schering, Neth.; Schering, Norw.; Schering, NZ; Schering, S.Afr.; Schering, Swed.; Schering, Switz.; Schering, UK.
Galactose (p.1033·3).
Ultrasound contrast medium.

Echte Sodener Mineral-Pastillen *Twardy, Ger.*
Minerals from spring or stream (p.1180·1).
Respiratory-tract congestion.

Echtroferment-N *Weber & Weber, Ger.†*
Aniseed (p.1580·2); caraway (p.1591·2); fennel (p.1610·1); potentilla anserina.
Gastrointestinal disorders.

Echtronerval-N *Weber & Weber, Ger.†*
Homoeopathic preparation.

Echtrosept-N *Weber & Weber, Ger.†*
Homoeopathic preparation.

Echtrovit-K *Weber & Weber, Ger.†*
Procaine hydrochloride (p.1319·1); vitamins (p.1350·1); rutoside (p.1611·2).
Tonic.

Eclaran *Pierre Fabre, Fr.; Pierre Fabre, Port.*
Benzoyl peroxide (p.1111·1).
Acne.

Eclipse Lip and Face *Triangle, USA.*
SPF 15: Padimate O (p.1518·2); oxybenzone (p.1518·1).
Sunscreen.

Eclipsol *Darier, Mex.*
SPF 15; gel SPF 30: Octinoxate (p.1517·3); oxybenzone (p.1518·1).
SPF 20; SPF 27; cream SPF 30: Octinoxate (p.1517·3); avobenzone (p.1517·1).
SPF 40: Octocrilene (p.1518·1); octinoxate (p.1517·3); titanium dioxide (p.1126·1); avobenzone (p.1517·1).
SPF 50: Octocrilene (p.1518·1); octinoxate (p.1517·3); avobenzone (p.1517·1).
Sunscreen.

Eco Mi *Geymonat, Ital.*
Econazole nitrate (p.382·3).
Fungal skin or vulvovaginal infections.

Ecocain *Molteni, Ital.; Julphar, UAE.*
Lignocaine [lidocaine] hydrochloride (p.1313·2). Adrenaline [epinephrine] acid tartrate (p.829·2) is included in some injections as a vasoconstrictor to diminish absorption and localise the effect of the local anaesthetic.
Local anaesthesia.

Ecocort *Hoe, Singapore.*
Econazole nitrate (p.382·3); triamcinolone acetonide (p.1080·1).
Fungal skin infections.

Ecodergin *Farmigea, Ital.*
Econazole nitrate (p.382·3).
Vulvo-vaginal or dermatological fungal infections.

Ecoderm
Note. This name is used for preparations of different composition.
Hoe, Singapore.
Econazole nitrate (p.382·3).
Fungal skin infections.

The symbol † denotes a preparation no longer actively marketed

Chew, *Thai.*
Econazole nitrate (p.382·3); triamcinolone acetonide (p.1080·1).
Fungal skin infections.

Ecodipine *Ecosol, Switz.*
Nifedipine (p.940·1).
Hypertension; ischaemic heart disease; Raynaud's syndrome.

Ecodurex *Ecosol, Switz.*
Hydrochlorothiazide (p.907·3); amiloride hydrochloride (p.835·1).
Hypertension; oedema.

Ecoendocilli Testimonia *Istoria, Ital.†.*
Lactic-acid-producing organisms (p.1626·3); vitamins (p.1350·1).
Disturbances of the gastrointestinal flora; nutritional supplement.

Ecofenac *Ecosol, Switz.*
Diclofenac sodium (p.30·3).
Gout; inflammation; musculoskeletal, joint, and peri-articular disorders; pain.

Ecofermenti *Echo, Ital.*
Lactic-acid-producing organisms (p.1626·3); vitamins (p.1350·1).
Disturbances of the gastrointestinal flora.

Ecofibra *Echo, Ital.*
Dietary fibre supplement (p.1350·1) (p.1214·2).
Delayed gastrointestinal transit; obesity.

Ecoflorina *Ecobi, Ital.*
Lactic-acid-producing organisms (p.1626·3).
Nutritional supplement.

Ecofol *Ecobi, Ital.*
Calcium folinate (p.1363·1).
Anaemias; antidote to overdosage with folic acid antagonists; folic acid deficiency.

Ecolicin *Chauvin ankerpharm, Ger.*
Erythromycin lactobionate (p.201·3); colistimethate sodium (p.192·3).
Bacterial eye infections.

Ecomucyl *Ecosol, Switz.*
Acetylcysteine (p.1082·3).
Paracetamol overdosage; respiratory-tract disorders.

Ecomytrin *Lundbeck, Aust.†; Lundbeck, Swed.†.*
Amphomycin calcium; neomycin hydrochloride (p.228·3).
Infected skin disorders.

Ecomytrin-Hydrocortison *Lundbeck, Aust.†; Lundbeck, Swed.†.*
Amphomycin calcium; neomycin hydrochloride (p.228·3); hydrocortisone (p.1073·3).
Infected skin disorders; otitis externa.

Econ
Note.This name is used for preparations of different composition.
Orion, Denm.
Ethinylestradiol (p.1476·2); norethisterone acetate (p.1485·1).
Combined oral contraceptive.

General Drugs, Thai.
Econazole nitrate (p.382·3).
Fungal skin infections.

Econac *Goldshield, UK.*
Diclofenac sodium (p.30·3).
Gout; musculoskeletal, joint, and peri-articular disorders; pain.

Econacort *Squibb, UK.*
Econazole nitrate (p.382·3); hydrocortisone (p.1073·3).
Infected skin disorders.

Economycin *DDSA Pharmaceuticals, UK.*
Tetracycline hydrochloride (p.258·3).

Econopred *Alcon, USA.*
Prednisolone acetate (p.1078·1).
Eye disorders.

Ecopace *Goldshield, UK.*
Captopril (p.853·3).
Heart failure; hypertension; myocardial infarction.

Ecophane *Biorga, Fr.; Saninter, Port.*
Nutritional supplement (p.1350·1).
Hair and nail disorders.

Ecoprin *Sam-On, Israel.*
Aspirin (p.14·2).
Thrombosis prophylaxis.

Ecoprofen *Ecosol, Switz.*
Ibuprofen (p.43·2).
Inflammation; musculoskeletal, joint, and peri-articular disorders; pain.

Ecorex *Zambon, Ital.*
Econazole nitrate (p.382·3).
Fungal or bacterial skin or vulvovaginal infections.

Ecoro *Eu Rho, Ger.†.*
d-Alpha tocopherol (p.1393·3).
Vitamin E deficiency.

Ecosporina *Ecobi, Ital.*
Cefradine (p.173·3).
Bacterial infections.

Ecostatin *Bristol-Myers Squibb, Austral.; Westwood-Squibb, Canad.; Bristol-Myers Squibb, Irl.; Bristol-Myers Squibb, NZ; Squibb, UK.*
Econazole nitrate (p.382·3).
Fungal infections.

Ecosteril *Amsa, Ital.*
Econazole nitrate (p.382·3).
Fungal and Gram-positive skin and nail infections; vulvovaginitis.

Ecotam *Alacan, Spain.*
Econazole nitrate (p.382·3).
Fungal infections.

Ecotrin *SmithKline Beecham Consumer, Austral.†; SmithKline Beecham, Hong Kong; SmithKline Beecham, Mex.; SmithKline Beecham, NZ; SmithKline Beecham, S.Afr.; SmithKline Beecham Consumer, USA.*
Aspirin (p.14·2).
Fever; inflammation; pain; thrombosis prophylaxis.

Ecoval *Glaxo Wellcome, Ital.*
Betamethasone valerate (p.1063·2).
Skin and scalp disorders.

Ecoval con Neomicina *Glaxo Wellcome, Ital.*
Betamethasone valerate (p.1063·2); neomycin sulfate (p.228·1).
Infected skin disorders.

Ecovent *Ecosol, Switz.*
Salbutamol (p.770·3).
Obstructive airways disease.

Ecran Anti-Solaire *Clarins, Canad.*
SPF 25: Octinoxate (p.1517·3); oxybenzone (p.1518·1); ensulizole (p.1517·2); titanium dioxide (p.1126·1).
Sunscreen.

Ecran Extreme *Lutsia, Fr.*
SPF 30+: Octinoxate (p.1517·3); enzacamene (p.1517·2); ensulizole (p.1517·2); avobenzone (p.1517·1); titanium mica (p.1126·1).
Sunscreen.

Ecran Lutsia *Lutsia, Fr.*
SPF 8; SPF 10; SPF 15; SPF 25: Octinoxate (p.1517·3); enzacamene (p.1517·2); ensulizole (p.1517·2); avobenzone (p.1517·1); with or without titanium dioxide (p.1126·1).
Sunscreen.

Ecran Teinte *Lutsia, Fr.*
SPF 30+: Octinoxate (p.1517·3); enzacamene (p.1517·2); ensulizole (p.1517·2); avobenzone (p.1517·1); titanium mica (p.1126·1).
Sunscreen.

Ecran Total *Vichy, Canad.*
SPF 45: Avobenzone (p.1517·1); enzacamene (p.1517·2); terephthalylidene dicamphor sulfonic acid; titanium dioxide (p.1126·1).
Sunscreen.

Ecrans Anti-Solaires *Juvex, Fr.*
Octinoxate (p.1517·3); ensulizole (p.1517·2); avobenzone (p.1517·1).
Sunscreen.

Ecreme *Pacific, NZ.*
Econazole nitrate (p.382·3).
Fungal skin infections.

Ectaprim *Liomont, Mex.*
Co-trimoxazole (p.193·3).
Bacterial infections.

Ectinex *20th Century, Mex.*
Suxamethonium chloride (p.1340·1).
Depolarising neuromuscular blocker.

Ectodyne *Wigglesworth, UK.*
Piperazine citrate (p.105·3).
Ascariasis; enterobiasis.

Ectopal *Codal Synto, Thai.*
Danazol (p.1468·3).
Benign breast disorders; endometriosis; female infertility; gynaecomastia; hereditary angioedema; mennorhagia; precocious puberty.

Ectosone *Technilab, Canad.*
Betamethasone valerate (p.1063·2).
Skin and scalp disorders.

Ectren *Menarini, Spain.*
Quinapril hydrochloride (p.963·3).
Heart failure; hypertension.

Ectrin *EMS, Braz.*
Co-trimoxazole (p.193·3).
Bacterial infections; Pneumocystis carinii pneumonia; protozoal infections.

Ectrin Balsamico *EMS, Braz.*
Co-trimoxazole (p.193·3); guaifenesin (p.1092·2); ammonium chloride (p.1085·2).
Bacterial infections.

Ecur Test and Leucocytes *Roche Diagnostics, Austral.*
Test for protein, glucose, blood, and leucocytes in urine.

Ecural *Essex, Ger.*
Mometasone furoate (p.1077·4).
Scalp disorders; skin disorders.

Ecur-Test *Roche Diagnostics, Austral.*
Test for glucose, protein, and blood in urine.

Eczema *Homeocan, Canad.*
Homoeopathic preparation.

Eczema Cream *Hamilton, Austral.*
Coal tar (p.1125·1); silicone fluid (p.1410·1); zinc oxide (p.1128·2).
Dermatitis; eczema.

Eczema L87 *Homeocan, Canad.*
Homoeopathic preparation.

Eczema Ointment
Note.This name is used for preparations of different composition.
Stanley, Canad.†.
Bismuth subcarbonate (p.1213·1); salicylic acid (p.1122·3); zinc oxide (p.1128·2).

Potter's, UK.
Zinc oxide (p.1128·2); salicylic acid (p.1122·3); benzoic acid (p.1134·2); stellaria media.
Eczema.

Ed A-Hist *Edwards, USA.*
Phenylephrine hydrochloride (p.1097·1); chlorpheniramine [chlorphenamine] maleate (p.412·1).
Allergic rhinitis; nasal congestion.

ED Tuss HC *Edwards, USA.*
Phenylephrine hydrochloride (p.1097·1); chlorpheniramine [chlorphenamine] maleate (p.412·1); hydrocodone tartrate (p.42·2).
Coughs and cold symptoms.

Eddia *Pierre Fabre Sante, Fr.†.*
Metformin hydrochloride (p.332·3).
Diabetes mellitus.

Ede *Teofarma, Ital.†.*
Metoclopramide (p.1236·3); simeticone (p.1249·2).
Gastrointestinal disorders.

Ede 6 *Teofarma, Ital.*
Dimethicone (p.1249·2); pancreatin (p.1646·1).
Formerly contained bromelains, alpha-amylase, metoclopramide hydrochloride, dimethicone, pancreatin, and sodium dehydrocholate.
Digestive insufficiency.

Edecril *Merck Sharp & Dohme, Austral.; Merck Sharp & Dohme, NZ.*
Etacrynic acid (p.887·2).
Heart failure; hepatic cirrhosis with acites; oedema.

Edecrin *Merck Sharp & Dohme, Aust.; Merck Frosst, Canad.; Merck Sharp & Dohme, Irl.; Merck Sharp & Dohme, Ital.†; Merck Sharp & Dohme, Neth.†; Merck Sharp & Dohme, UK†; Merck, USA.*
Etacrynic acid (p.887·2) or sodium etacrynate (p.887·2).
Ascites; heart failure; oedema.

Edecrina *Merck Sharp & Dohme, Swed.*
Sodium etacrynate (p.887·2).
Oedema.

Edefen *Diba, Mex.*
Oxyphenbutazone (p.71·1).
Rheumatoid disorders.

Edemax *SIFI, Ital.*
Nimesulide (p.62·3).
Fever; inflammation; pain.

Edemox *Wasserman, Spain.*
Acetazolamide (p.826·1).
Epilepsy; glaucoma; high-altitude disorders; oedema.

Edenil *Zambon, Ital.*
Ibuprofen isobutanolammoniun (p.44·1).
Gynaecological disorders.

Edenol *Randall, Mex.*
Frusemide [furosemide] (p.893·1).
Hypertension; liver cirrhosis with acites; nephrotic syndrome; oedema.

Ederal *Esteve, Spain.*
Cinnarizine (p.413·1); calcium dobesilate (p.1588·2).
Cerebrovascular disorders; vestibular disorders.

Ederphyt *Mavena, Switz.*
Phenol undecenoate; thymol (p.1158·3); salicylic acid (p.1122·3).
Fungal foot infections.

Edex *Schwarz, Fr.; Schwarz, USA.*
Alprostadil (p.1439·3).
Erectile dysfunction.

Edhanol *Sintofarma, Braz.*
Phenobarbital (p.355·1).
Epilepsy.

Edicin *Lek, Thai.*
Vancomycin hydrochloride (p.267·2).
Staphylococcal infections.

Edifaringen *Edigen, Spain.*
Bacitracin zinc (p.155·2); benzocaine (p.1306·2); hydrocortisone acetate (p.1073·3); neomycin sulfate (p.228·1); potassium chlorate (p.1654·1).
Mouth and throat disorders.

Edigastrol *Edigen, Spain.*
Aluminium hydroxide (p.1210·3); magnesium oxide (p.1233·2).
Dyspepsia; gastrointestinal hyperacidity.

Ediluna *Vinas, Spain†.*
Ibuprofen (p.43·2).
Fever; musculoskeletal and joint disorders; pain; peri-articular disorders.

Ed-in-Sol *Edwards, USA.*
Ferrous sulfate (p.1360·3).
Iron deficiency.

Edirel *Laphal, Fr.*
Erdosteine (p.1091·2).
Respiratory-tract congestion.

Edmilla *Hanseler, Switz.*
Chamomile (p.1593·2).
Inflammatory disorders of the skin and mouth.

Ednyt *Dominion, UK.*
Enalapril maleate (p.883·3).
Heart failure; hypertension.

Edolfene *Oftalder, Port.*
Flurbiprofen sodium (p.41·2).
Ocular inflammation; prevention of intra- and postoperative miosis.

Edolglau *Oftalder, Port.*
Clonidine hydrochloride (p.860·1).
Glaucoma.

Edoltar *Oftalder, Port.*
Undecenoic acid monoethanolamide (p.396·1); coal tar (p.1125·1); salicylic acid (p.1122·3); resorcinol (p.1122·2); thymol (p.1158·3).
Skin disorders.

Edolzine *Oftalder, Port.*
Tetryzoline hydrochloride (p.1101·2).
Eye disorders.

Edoxil *Inibsa, Spain.*
Amoxicillin trihydrate (p.149·2).
Bacterial infections.

Edoxil Mucolitico *Inibsa, Spain.*
Amoxicillin trihydrate (p.149·2); bromhexine hydrochloride (p.1085·3).
Respiratory-tract infections.

EDP-Evans Dermal Powder *Boots, Austral.*
Povidone-iodine (p.1155·1).
Burns; chafing; tinea pedis; ulcers; wounds.

Edronax *Pharmacia Upjohn, Aust.; Pharmacia Upjohn, Belg.; Pharmacia Upjohn, Denm.; Pharmacia Upjohn, Fin.; Pharmacia Upjohn, Ger.; Pharmacia Upjohn, Irl.; Pharmacia Upjohn, Ital.; Pharmacia Upjohn, Mex.; Pharmacia Upjohn, Norw.; Pharmacia Upjohn, Port.; Pharmacia Upjohn, S.Afr.; Pharmacia Upjohn, Swed.; Pharmacia, UK.*
Reboxetine mesilate (p.308·1).
Depression.

E-Drops *Ranbaxy, Thai.*
dl-Alpha tocoferil acetate (p.1394·1).
Vitamin E deficiency.

ED-SPAZ *Edwards, USA.*
Hyoscyamine sulfate (p.469·3).

ED-TLC *Edwards, USA.*
Phenylephrine hydrochloride (p.1097·1); chlorpheniramine [chlorphenamine] maleate (p.412·1); hydrocodone tartrate (p.42·2).
Coughs and cold symptoms.

Eductyl *Techni-Pharma, Mon.*
Potassium acid tartrate (p.1244·3); sodium bicarbonate (p.1186·2).
Bowel evacuation; constipation.

Eduprim *F5 Profas, Spain.*
Co-trimoxazole (p.193·3).
Bacterial infections; Pneumocystis carinii pneumonia.

Eduprim Mucolitico *F5 Profas, Spain.*
Carbocisteine (p.1086·3); guaifenesin (p.1092·2); co-trimoxazole (p.193·3).
Respiratory-tract infections.

Edurid *Medipharm, Switz.*
Edoxudine (p.619·3).
Herpes simplex infections.

Edusan Fte Rectal *Casen Fleet, Spain.*
Camphor (p.1589·3); eucalyptol (p.1609·2); niaouli oil (p.1640·2); guaiacol (p.1092·1).
Respiratory-tract disorders.

Edym Sedante *Vita, Spain†.*
Diazepam (p.674·3); dimethicone (p.1249·2); metoclopramide hydrochloride (p.1235·2); pancreatin (p.1646·1).
Gastrointestinal disorders.

EES *Abbott, Austral.; Abbott, Canad.; Abbott, Hong Kong; Abbott, NZ; Abbott, Singapore; Abbott, USA.*
Erythromycin ethyl succinate (p.201·2).
Bacterial infections; intestinal amoebiasis.

Eetless *Adcock Ingram, S.Afr.*
Cathine hydrochloride (p.1507·1).
Obesity.

EFA Steri *Pharmavite, Canad.*
Sodium chloride (p.1196·1).

Efabetic *Express Care, NZ.*
Essential fatty acids; gamolenic acid; vitamin E (p.1350·1).
Dietary supplement in diabetic neuropathy.

Efacal *Efamol, Austral.; Efamol, NZ; Efamol, UK.*
Evening primrose oil (p.1613·2); fish oil (p.949·3); calcium (p.1187·3).
Calcium supplement; osteoporosis.

Efadermin *Widmer, Switz.*
Lithium succinate (p.1118·1); zinc sulfate (p.1398·2).
Seborrhoeic dermatitis.

Efagel *Mavi, Ital.*
Gamolenic acid (p.1613·1); vitamin E (p.1393·3).
Nutritional supplement.

Efalex
Note.This name is used for preparations of different composition.
Efamol, Irl.
Essential fatty acids; docosahexaenoic acid; arachidonic acid; gamolenic acid (p.1350·1).
Dietary supplement.

Novartis, UK.
Marine fatty acids (p.949·3); evening primrose oil (p.1613·2); thyme oil (p.1672·3).

Efalex Focus *Efamol, Canad.*
Evening primrose oil (p.1613·2).

Efalith *Scotia, Irl.; Scotia, NZ; Widmer, Switz.; United Drug, UK.*
Lithium succinate (p.1118·1); zinc sulfate (p.1398·2).
Seborrhoeic dermatitis.

Efamarine *Efamol, UK.*
Evening primrose oil (p.1613·2); marine fish oil (p.949·3).
Formerly known as Efamol Marine.

Efamast
Note.This name is used for preparations of different composition.
Scotia, Canad.
Gamolenic acid (p.1613·1).
Dysmenorrhoea; mastalgia.

Express Care, NZ.
Essential fatty acids; gamolenic acid (p.1613·1).
Mastalgia.

Pharmacia, UK.
Evening primrose oil (p.1613·2).
Mastalgia.

Efamax *Efamol, NZ.*
Evening primrose oil; fish oil; vitamins; minerals; herbs (p.1350·1).
Dietary supplement.

Efamol
Vitaglow, Austral.†; Efamol, Canad.; Efamol, NZ; Sidroga, Switz.; Efamol, UK.
Evening primrose oil (p.1613·2).
Nutritional supplement.

Efamol Fortify *Efamol, Canad.*
Evening primrose oil (p.1613·2); calcium carbonate (p.1215·1).

Efamol G *Covan, S.Afr.*
Gamolenic acid (p.1613·1); linoleic acid (p.1613·2).
Nutritional supplement.

Efamol Marine
Vitaglow, Austral.†; Efamol, NZ.
Evening primrose oil (p.1613·2); marine fish oil (p.949·3).
Dietary supplement to assist joint mobility.

Efamol Plus Coenzyme Q10 *Efamol, UK.*
Evening primrose oil (p.1613·2); ubidecarenone (p.1677·1).
Tonic.

Efamol PMP *Efamol, UK.*
Evening primrose oil (p.1613·2); vitamins; minerals (p.1350·1).
Premenstrual syndrome.

Efamol Safflower & Linseed *Efamol, UK.*
Evening primrose oil (p.1613·2); linseed oil (p.1629·1); safflower oil (p.1375·2).

Efanatal
Efamol, Austral.; Efamol, NZ; Efamol, UK.
Evening primrose oil; fish oil (p.1350·1).
Nutritional supplement in pregnancy and lactation.

Efaprost *Efamol, NZ.*
Fatty acids; evening primrose oil; gamolenic acid; saw palmetto; beta sitosterol (p.1350·1).
Dietary supplement; prostatic disorders.

Efargen *Teofarma, Ital.*
Cyanocobalamin (p.1388·1); folic acid (p.1361·1); nicotinamide (p.1372·3); pyridoxine hydrochloride (p.1386·3).
Vitamin deficiency.

Efasit N *Togal, Ger.†.*
Plaster: Salicylic acid (p.1122·3).
Tincture: Salicylic acid (p.1122·3); lactic acid (p.1626·2).
Calluses; corns; hard skin.

Efatime *Efamol, UK.*
Fatty acids (p.949·3); vitamin E (p.1393·3); red thyme oil.

Efavite *Efamol, UK.*
Multivitamin and mineral preparation (p.1350·1).

Efcod *Covan, S.Afr.†.*
Aminophylline (p.760·1); mepyramine maleate (p.421·1); codeine phosphate (p.25·2); ephedrine hydrochloride (p.1090·1); ipecacuanha (p.1093·1).
Coughs; obstructive airways disease.

Efcortelan *Glaxo Wellcome, UK.*
Hydrocortisone (p.1073·3).
Skin disorders.

Efcortesol *Sovereign, UK.*
Hydrocortisone sodium phosphate (p.1074·1).
Corticosteroid.

Efcospect *Covan, S.Afr.†.*
Potassium iodide (p.1522·3); ephedrine hydrochloride (p.1090·1); ipecacuanha (p.1093·1).
Respiratory-tract disorders.

Efectin *Wyeth Lederle, Aust.*
Venlafaxine hydrochloride (p.312·2).
Depression.

Efedronal *Baldassari, Braz.*
Diphenhydramine hydrochloride (p.416·1); sodium benzoate (p.1134·3); belladonna (p.463·1); lobelia (p.1510·2); guaifenesin (p.1092·2); ephedrine hydrochloride (p.1090·1).
Respiratory-tract congestion.

Efektolol *Dumex, Ger.*
Propranolol hydrochloride (p.962·3).
Angina pectoris; arrhythmias; essential tremor; hypertension; hyperthyroidism; migraine.

Efemida *Llorens, Spain†.*
Cefalexin (p.161·3).
Bacterial infections.

Efemolin *Ciba Vision, Ger.*
Fluorometholone (p.1072·1); tetryzoline hydrochloride (p.1101·2).
Allergic and inflammatory disorders of the eye.

Efemoline
Ciba Vision, Hong Kong; Ciba Vision, Ital.; Restan, S.Afr.; Ciba Vision, Singapore; Ciba Vision, Switz.; Ciba Vision, Thai.
Fluorometholone (p.1072·1); tetryzoline hydrochloride (p.1101·2).
Allergic and inflammatory disorders of the eye.

Efensol *Ipsen, Spain.*
Filicol.
Hypercholesterolaemia; pruritus associated with partial biliary obstruction.

Eferox *Hexal, Ger.*
Thyroxine [levothyroxine] sodium (p.1526·2).
Hypothyroidism.

Efexor
Wyeth Lederle, Aust.; Wyeth, Austral.; Wyeth Lederle, Belg.; Wyeth Lederle, Denm.; Wyeth Lederle, Fin.; Wyeth-Ayerst, Hong Kong; Wyeth, Irl.; Dexcel, Israel; Wyeth Lederle, Ital.; Wyeth, Mex.; Wyeth, Neth.; Wyeth Lederle, Norw.; Wyeth, NZ; Wyeth Lederle, Port.; Wyeth, S.Afr.; Wyeth, Singapore; Wyeth Lederle, Swed.; Cross, Swed.; Netpharma, Swed.; Wyeth, Switz.; Wyeth, UK.
Venlafaxine hydrochloride (p.312·2).
Depression; mixed anxiety depressive states.

Effacne
Roche-Posay, Fr.; Roche Posay, Switz.
Benzoyl peroxide (p.1111·1).
Acne.

Effagel *Roche-Posay, Fr.*
Pharmaceutical gel base.

Effective Strength Cough Formula *Barre-National, USA.*
Chlorpheniramine [chlorphenamine] maleate (p.412·1); dextromethorphan hydrobromide (p.1087·3).
Coughs and cold symptoms.

Effective Strength Cough Formula Liquid With Decongestant *Barre-National, USA.*
Dextromethorphan hydrobromide (p.1087·3); pseudoephedrine hydrochloride (p.1099·2).
Coughs and cold symptoms.

Effectsal *Shin Poong, Singapore.*
Norfloxacin (p.232·1).
Bacterial infections.

Effederm *CS, Fr.*
Tretinoin (p.1126·2).
Acne.

Effee *Propan, S.Afr.†.*
Ferrous sulfate (p.1360·3); folic acid (p.1361·1).
Iron-deficiency anaemia.

Effekton *LAW, Ger.; Wyeth, Ger.*
Diclofenac sodium (p.30·3).
Gout; inflammation; musculoskeletal, joint, and soft-tissue disorders; pain.

Efferalgan
Upsamedica, Belg.; UPSA, Fr.; Upsamedica, Ital.; Bristol-Myers Squibb, Port.; Upsamedica, Spain.
Paracetamol (p.71·2).
Fever; pain.

Efferalgan C
Upsamedica, Belg.; Upsamedica, Ital.; Upsamedica, Switz.
Paracetamol (p.71·2); ascorbic acid (p.1389·3).
Fever; pain.

Efferalgan Codeine *UPSA, Fr.*
Paracetamol (p.71·2); codeine phosphate (p.25·2).
Pain.

Efferalgan Vit C *Upsamedica, Spain.*
Paracetamol (p.71·2); ascorbic acid (p.1389·3).
Fever; pain.

Efferalgan Vitamine C *UPSA, Fr.*
Paracetamol (p.71·2); ascorbic acid (p.1389·3).
Fever; pain.

Efferbalgine *Pharmethic, Belg.*
Aspirin (p.14·2); codeine phosphate (p.25·2); ascorbic acid (p.1389·3).
Fever; pain.

Effercal
Note.This name is used for preparations of different composition.
Piam, Ital.
Calcium carbonate (p.1215·1).
Calcium deficiency; calcium supplement.
Akromed, S.Afr.†
Vitamin B₆ and mineral preparation (p.1350·1).

Effercitrate *Typharm, UK.*
Potassium citrate (p.1186·1); citric acid (p.1596·2).
Cystitis.

Effer-K *Nomax, USA.*
Potassium bicarbonate (p.1186·1); potassium citrate (p.1186·1).
Hypokalaemia; potassium depletion.

Effersol *Aspen Consumer, S.Afr.*
Sodium bicarbonate (p.1673·2); citric acid (p.1596·2).
Acidosis; urinary alkalinisation.

Effersyllium *Johnson & Johnson, Aust.*
Ispaghula (p.1229·1).
Constipation.

Effer-Syllium *J&J-Merck, USA†.*
Psyllium hydrocolloid (p.1229·1).
Anorectal disorders; constipation; irritable bowel syndrome.

Efferzyme *Bausch & Lomb, Canad.*
Subtilisin (p.1129·2).
Protein remover for soft contact lenses.

Effetre *Farmatre, Ital.*
Chlorhexidine gluconate (p.1138·2).
Disinfection of skin, wounds, burns, hands, and surgical materials; skin irritation.

Effexor
Wyeth-Ayerst, Canad.; Wyeth Lederle, Fr.; Wyeth-Ayerst, USA.
Venlafaxine hydrochloride (p.312·2).
Anxiety; depression.

Efficlean *Bausch & Lomb, Fr.†.*
Subtilisin-A(p.1129·2).
Protein remover for contact lenses.

Effico
Pharmax, Irl.
Nicotinamide; thiamine hydrochloride; caffeine (p.1350·1).
Tonic.

Efudex
ICN, Canad.; Roche, USA.
Fluorouracil (p.540·2).
Skin cancer; solar keratoses.

Pharmax, UK.
Nicotinamide; thiamine hydrochloride; caffeine; compound gentian infusion (p.1350·1).
Tonic.

Efficort *Galderma, Fr.; Galderma, Hong Kong; Galderma, Singapore.*
Hydrocortisone aceponate (p.1074·2).
Skin disorders.

Effidigest
Yves Ponroy, Fr.; Ceuta, UK.
Nutritional supplement (p.1350·1).
Gastrointestinal disorders.

Effidose *Chefaro Ardeval, Fr.†.*
A range of herbal preparations.

Effiplen *Effik, Spain.*
Buspirone hydrochloride (p.657·2).
Anxiety.

Effiprev *Effik, Fr.*
Norgestimate (p.1486·1); ethinylestradiol (p.1476·2).
Combined oral contraceptive.

Efflumidex *Allergan, Ger.*
Fluorometholone (p.1072·1).
Allergic and inflammatory disorders of the eye.

Efflumycin *Allergan, Ger.*
Fluorometholone (p.1072·1); neomycin sulfate (p.228·1).
Infected eye disorders.

Effortil
Boehringer Ingelheim, Aust.; Boehringer Ingelheim, Belg.; Boehringer Ingelheim, Fin.; Boehringer Ingelheim, Fr.; Boehringer Ingelheim, Ger.; Boehringer Ingelheim, Irl.; Boehringer Ingelheim, Mex.; Boehringer Ingelheim, Norw.; Boehringer Ingelheim, Port.; Boehringer Ingelheim, S.Afr.; Boehringer Ingelheim, Swed.; Boehringer Ingelheim, Switz.; Boehringer Ingelheim, Thai.
Etilefrine hydrochloride (p.888·1).
Hypotension.

Effortil comp *Boehringer Ingelheim, Aust.*
Etilefrine hydrochloride (p.888·1); dihydroergotamine mesilate (p.450·3).
Hypotension.

Effortil plus
Boehringer Ingelheim, Ger.; Boehringer Ingelheim, Switz.
Etilefrine hydrochloride (p.888·1); dihydroergotamine mesilate (p.450·3).
Hypotension.

Efical *Irex, Fr.*
Calcium pidolate (p.1188·3); calcium carbonate (p.1215·1).
Calcium deficiency; osteoporosis.

Efidac *Ciba, USA.*
Pseudoephedrine hydrochloride (p.1099·2).

Efidac 24-Chlorpheniramine *Ciba, USA.*
Chlorpheniramine [chlorphenamine] maleate (p.412·1).
Hypersensitivity reactions.

Efimag *Fornet, Fr.*
Magnesium pidolate (p.1191·1).
Magnesium deficiency.

Efisol S *Roland, Ger.*
Dequalinium chloride (p.1143·1).
Mouth and throat inflammation.

Eflone *Ciba Vision, USA.*
Fluorometholone acetate (p.1072·1).
Eye disorders.

Efodine *Fougera, USA.*
Povidone-iodine (p.1155·1).
Skin disinfection.

Efortil
Boehringer de Angeli, Braz.; Fher, Spain.
Etilefrine hydrochloride (p.888·1).
Hypotension.

Efrane
Abbott, Denm.; Abbott, Fin.; Abbott, Norw.; Abbott, Swed.
Enflurane (p.1258·1).
General anaesthesia.

Efrarel *Mediolanum, Ital.†.*
L-α-Glycerophosphorylethanolamine monohydrate.
Nervous disorders.

Efridol *Aesculapius, Ital.*
Nimesulide (p.62·3).
Fever; inflammation; pain.

Efrin *Fischer, Israel.*
Phenylephrine hydrochloride (p.1097·1).
Eye congestion; production of mydriasis.

Efriviral *Aesculapius, Ital.*
Aciclovir (p.612·3).
Formerly known as Efrivir.
Herpesvirus infections.

Eftab *Thornton & Ross, UK.*
Peppermint oil (p.1243·3); clove oil (p.1597·1); spearmint oil (p.1666·3); menthol (p.1632·3); thymol (p.1158·3); methyl salicylate (p.55·1).
Oral hygiene.

Eftapan
Ratiopharm, Aust.†; Merckle, Ger.
Eprazinone hydrochloride (p.1091·1).
Coughs.

Eftapan Tetra *Ratiopharm, Aust.†.*
Eprazinone hydrochloride (p.1091·1); tetracycline hydrochloride (p.258·3).
Bacterial respiratory-tract infections.

Efudex
ICN, Canad.; Roche, USA.
Fluorouracil (p.540·2).
Skin cancer; solar keratoses.

Efudix
Dermatech, Austral.; Sanico, Belg.; CSP, Fr.; ICN, Ger.; Roche, Irl.; Roche, Israel; ICN, Ital.; Roche, Mex.; ICN, Neth.†; Pacific, NZ; Pharmaco, S.Afr.; ICN, Singapore; ICN, Spain; ICN, Switz.; ICN, Thai.; ICN, UK.
Fluorouracil (p.540·2).
Anogenital warts; premalignant skin lesions; skin cancer; solar and senile keratoses.

Efurix *Roche, Braz.*
Fluorouracil (p.540·2).
Skin cancer; solar and senile keratoses.

Efxine *Pharmasant, Thai.*
Etilefrine hydrochloride (p.888·1).
Hypotension.

Egacene *Astra, Neth.*
Hyoscyamine sulfate (p.469·3).
Bradycardia; gastrointestinal spasm; hyperhidrosis.

Egarone *Formalider, Spain.*
Allantoin (p.1110·1); benzalkonium chloride (p.1133·2); muramidase hydrochloride (p.1638·1); oxymetazoline (p.1096·2).
Cold symptoms; rhinitis; sinusitis.

Egarone Oximetazolina *Alcala, Spain†.*
Oxymetazoline hydrochloride (p.1096·2).
Nasal congestion; sinus congestion.

Egazil
AstraZeneca, Denm.; AstraZeneca, Fin.; AstraZeneca, Norw.; Hassle, Swed.
Hyoscyamine sulfate (p.469·3).
Biliary colic; bladder tenesmus; hypersecretion; irritable bowel syndrome.

E/Gel *Fulton, USA†.*
Erythromycin (p.201·2).

E-Gems *Carlson, USA.*
d-Alpha tocoferil acetate (p.1394·1).
Vitamin E supplement.

Egery *Biorga, Fr.*
Erythromycin (p.201·2).
Bacterial infections.

Egibren *Chiesi, Ital.*
Selegiline hydrochloride (p.1177·2).
Psychiatric disorders.

Eglonyl *Sanofi Synthelabo, S.Afr.*
Sulpiride (p.706·1).
Depression; disturbed behaviour; peptic ulcer; psychoses; vertigo.

Ego Prickly Heat Powder *Ego, Austral.†.*
Light liquid paraffin (p.1407·2); salicylic acid (p.1122·3); zinc oxide (p.1128·2).
Prickly heat rash.

Ego Skin Cream
Ego, Austral.; Ego, Hong Kong; Ego, NZ.
Emollient.
Dry skin.

Egocappol *Ego, Austral.†.*
Salicylic acid (p.1122·3).
Cradle cap.

Egocort
Ego, Austral.; Ego, Hong Kong; Ego, NZ; Ego, Singapore.
Hydrocortisone (p.1073·3).
Skin disorders.

Egoderm
Note.This name is used for preparations of different composition.
Ego, NZ.
Cream: Allantoin (p.1110·1); ichthammol (p.1115·2).
Ointment: Dimethione (p.1410·1); zinc oxide (p.1128·2).
Skin disorders.

Ego, Singapore.
Cream: Ichthammol (p.1115·2); allantoin (p.1110·1).
Ointment: Ichthammol (p.1115·2); zinc oxide (p.1128·2).
Skin disorders.

Egoderm Cream
Note.This name is used for preparations of different composition.
Ego, Austral.
Ammoniumsulfobitol (p.1115·2).
Skin disorders.

Ego, Hong Kong.
Ichthammol (p.1115·2).
Skin disorders.

Egoderm Ointment
Note.This name is used for preparations of different composition.
Ego, Austral.
Ammoniumsulfobitol (p.1115·2); zinc oxide (p.1128·2); dimethicone (p.1410·1).
Skin disorders.

Ego, Hong Kong.
Ichthammol (p.1115·2); zinc oxide (p.1128·2).
Skin disorders.

Egogyn 30 *Schering, Ital.*
Levonorgestrel (p.1486·2); ethinylestradiol (p.1476·2).
Combined oral contraceptive.

Egomycol
Ego, Austral.; Ego, NZ.
Undecylenic alkanolamide (p.396·1); chlorhexidine gluconate (p.1138·2); salicylic acid (p.1122·3); benzoic acid (p.1134·2); resorcinol (p.1122·2).
Fungal and bacterial skin and nail infections.

Egopsoryl TA
Note.This name is used for preparations of different composition.
Ego, Austral.
Sulfur (p.1123·3); phenol (p.1152·3); menthol (p.1632·3); glycerol (p.1616·3).
Formerly contained sulfur, phenol, and coal tar.
Psoriasis.

Ego, Hong Kong.
Sulfur (p.1123·3); phenol (p.1152·3); coal tar (p.1125·1); menthol (p.1632·3).
Eczema; psoriasis.

Ego, NZ.
Allantoin (p.1110·1); sulfur (p.1123·3); menthol (p.1632·3); coal tar (p.1125·1); phenol (p.1152·3).
Psoriasis.

Ego, Singapore.
Sulfur (p.1123·3); phenol (p.1152·3); coal tar (p.1125·1).
Eczema; psoriasis.

Egozinc Pharmascience, Canad.; Pharmascience, Hong Kong.
Zinc oxide (p.1128·2) or zinc sulfate (p.1398·2).
Burns; haemorrhoids; ulcers; wounds.

Egozite Ego, Singapore.
Cream: Zinc oxide (p.1128·2); dimethicone (p.1410·1); light liquid paraffin (p.1407·2); glycerol (p.1616·3); dexpanthenol (p.1602·3).
Skin disorders.
Lotion: Dimethicone (p.1410·1).
Barrier preparation; nappy rash.

Egozite Baby Ego, NZ.
Zinc oxide (p.1128·2); dimethicone (p.1410·1); light liquid paraffin (p.1407·2).
Barrier cream; nappy rash.

Egozite Baby Cream
Note. This name is used for preparations of different composition.
Ego, Austral.
Zinc oxide (p.1128·2); dimethicone (p.1410·1); light liquid paraffin (p.1407·2); glycerol (p.1616·3); dexpanthenol (p.1602·3).
Skin disorders.

Ego, Hong Kong.
Zinc oxide (p.1128·2); dimethicone (p.1410·1); light liquid paraffin (p.1407·2); dexpanthenol (p.1602·3).
Skin disorders.

Egozite Cradle Cap Ego, Austral.; Ego, Hong Kong; Ego, NZ.
Salicylic acid (p.1122·3) in an oil basis.
Cradle cap.

Egozite Cream Ego, Austral.†
Olive oil (p.1643·3); glycerol (p.1616·3); zinc oxide (p.1128·2).
Eczema; skin irritation; vulval inflammation.

Egozite Protective Baby Ego, NZ.
Dimethicone (p.1410·1).
Barrier lotion; nappy rash.

Egozite Protective Baby Lotion Ego, Austral.
Dimethicone (p.1410·1).
Barrier preparation; nappy rash.

Ehlifena Ehlinger, Mex.
Diclofenac (p.30·2).

Ehlifung Ehlinger, Mex.
Ketoconazole (p.389·1).

Ehlindopa Ehlinger, Mex.
Methyldopa (p.927·3).

Ehliten Ehlinger, Mex.
Praziquantel (p.106·3).

Ehlixacin Ehlinger, Mex.
Ciprofloxacin (p.182·3).
Bacterial infections.

Ehrenhofer-Salbe Ehrenhofer, Aust.
Colophony (p.1598·3); lovage root (p.1629·3).
Bronchitis; skin disorders; soft-tissue, peri-articular, musculoskeletal, and joint disorders.

Ehrmann's Entschlackungstee Ehrmann, Aust.
Prunus spinosa; equisetum (p.1606·3); silver birch (p.1585·2); urtica (p.1678·2); taraxacum (p.1669·1); peppermint leaf (p.1243·2); chamomile (p.1593·2).
Urinary disorders.

Eicosapen
Nefro, Aust.; Nycomed, Ger.; Byk, Switz.
Marine fish oil (p.949·3).
Hyperlipidaemias.

Eicovis C & RF, Ital.
Omega-3 triglycerides, vitamins, and minerals (p.1350·1).
Eye disorders; nutritional supplement.

Eifelfango-Neuenahr Eifelfango, Ger.
Medicinal mud.
Gastrointestinal disorders; gout; musculoskeletal and joint disorders; neuralgia.

Einalat Bayer, Aust.†
Nifedipine (p.940·1).
Hypertension.

EinsAlpha Leo, Ger.
Alfacalcidol (p.1391·1).
Vitamin D deficiency.

Einschlafkapseln Twardy, Aust.
Valerian (p.1678·3); lupulus (p.1629·3).
Nervous disorders; sleep disorders.

Einschlaf-Kapseln biologisch Twardy, Ger.
Valerian (p.1678·3); lupulus (p.1629·3).
Nervous disorders; sleep disorders.

Eiquinon Eisai, Hong Kong.
Ubidecarenone (p.1677·1).
Heart failure.

Eisen-Diasporal Protina, Ger.
Ferrous sulfate (p.1360·3).
Iron deficiency; iron-deficiency anaemia.

Eisendragees-ratiopharm Ratiopharm, Ger.
Ferrous sulfate (p.1360·3).
Iron deficiency; iron-deficiency anaemia.

Eisen-Sandoz Novartis Consumer, Ger.
Ferrous gluconate (p.1360·1).
Iron deficiency.

EK Burger Ysatfabrik, Ger.
Homoeopathic preparation.

Ekanin Romer, Mex.
Vitamin E (p.1394·1).

Ekilid Hoechst Marion Roussel, Mex.
Sulpiride (p.706·1).
Depression; schizophrenia; vertigo.

Eksalb Kade, Ger.
Cell components and metabolic products of *Staphylococcus aureus; Enterococcus faecalis* (p.1626·3); *Pseudomonas aeruginosa; Escherichia coli;* hydrocortisone (p.1073·3).
Skin disorders.

Eksalb Simplex Kade, Ger.
Cell components and metabolic products of *Staphylococcus aureus; Enterococcus faecalis* (p.1626·3); *Pseudomonas aeruginosa; Escherichia coli.*
Skin disorders.

ektebin Hefa, Ger.
Protionamide (p.239·3).
Tuberculosis.

Ektogan Hoechst, Fr.†; Teofarma, Ital.
Zinc peroxide (p.1159·3); zinc oxide (p.1128·2); magnesium peroxide (p.1149·3).
Skin disorders; wound disinfection.

Ektoselene Robapharm, Switz.
Selenium disulfide (p.1123·1); sulfur (p.1123·3).
Scalp disorders.

Ektrofil Ecobi, Ital.
Zinc oxide (p.1128·2); aloe vera (p.1110·1).
Emollient.

Ekuba Teofarma, Ital.
Chlorhexidine gluconate (p.1138·2).
Personal hygiene.

Ekvacillin
AstraZeneca, Denm.; AstraZeneca, Fin.; AstraZeneca, Norw.; Astra, Swed.
Cloxacillin sodium (p.192·1).
Bacterial infections.

Ekzemase Azupharma, Ger.
Bufexamac (p.20·3).
Eczema; neurodermatitis.

Ekzemsalbe Agepha, Aust.
Hydrocortisone acetate (p.1073·3).
Eczema.

Ekzevowen Weber & Weber, Ger.
Acid. arsenicosum; calendula offic.; centella asiat.; lytta ves.; mahonia aquifolium; peru balsam (p.1650·2); semecarpus anacard.; viola tric.; zinc oxide (p.1128·2).
Eczema; pruritus ani; pruritus vulvae.

Elacto Novartis Consumer, Spain.
Infant feed (p.1350·1).
Eczema in infants; food-related respiratory-tract disorders.

Elacur LAW, Ger.
Propyl nicotinate (p.80·2).
Musculoskeletal and joint disorders; neuralgia.

Elacutan LAW, Ger.
Urea (p.1127·3).
Skin disorders.

Elagen Eladon, UK.
Eleutherococcus senticosis (p.1615·3).
Tonic.

ELA-Max Ferndale, USA.
Lignocaine [lidocaine] (p.1313·2).
Anorectal disorders; topical anaesthesia.

Elan Schwarz, Ital.
Isosorbide mononitrate (p.916·2).
Cardiac disorders.

Elana OTW, Ger.
Homoeopathic preparation.

Elana mono OTW, Ger.
Homoeopathic preparation.

Elantan
Note. This name is used for preparations of different composition.
Gebro, Aust.; Sanofi Synthelabo, Ger.; Schwarz, Hong Kong; Schwarz, Irl.; Knoll, Mex.; Omnimed, S.Afr.; Schwarz, Singapore; Schwarz, Switz.; Schwarz, Thai.; Schwarz, UK.
Isosorbide mononitrate (p.916·2).
Angina pectoris; heart failure; myocardial infarction.

Schering, Canad.
Isosorbide dinitrate (p.915·2).
Angina pectoris.

Elase
Parke, Davis, Austral.†; Parke, Davis, Canad.†; Parke, Davis, Fr.; Parke, Davis, Ital.; Parke, Davis, Neth.; Fujisawa, USA†.
Fibrinolysin (p.890·1); deoxyribonuclease (p.1089·1).
Cervicitis; debridement of wounds; vaginitis.

Elase-Chloromycetin
Parke, Davis, Canad.†; Fujisawa, USA†.
Fibrinolysin (p.890·1); deoxyribonuclease (p.1089·1); chloramphenicol (p.179·1).
Debridement of infected lesions.

Elastab TO-Chemicals, Thai.
Oxpentifylline [pentoxifylline] (p.950·3).
Cerebral and peripheral vascular disorders.

Elatrol Teva, Israel.
Amitriptyline hydrochloride (p.273·3).
Depression; nocturnal enuresis.

Elavil
Merck Frosst, Canad.; Merck Sharp & Dohme-Chibret, Fr.; DDSA Pharmaceuticals, UK; Zeneca, USA.
Amitriptyline hydrochloride (p.273·3).
Depression; nocturnal enuresis.

Elavil Plus Merck Frosst, Canad.
Amitriptyline hydrochloride (p.273·3); perphenazine (p.699·1).
Depression.

Elawox Riemser, Ger.
Urea hydrogen peroxide (p.1159·3).
Infected wounds.

Elazor Sigma-Tau, Ital.
Fluconazole (p.383·2).
Fungal infections.

Elbrol Pfleger, Ger.
Propranolol hydrochloride (p.962·3).
Essential tremor; hypertension; hyperthyroidism; ischaemic heart disease; migraine.

Elcarn Co-Pharma, UK.
Carnitine (p.1356·1).
Carnitine deficiency.

Elcatonin Asahi, Jpn†.
Elcatonin (p.749·2).
Hypercalcaemia; osteoporosis; Paget's disease of bone.

Elcimen Hafslund Nycomed, Aust.
Elcatonin (p.749·2).
Hypercalcaemia; osteoporosis; Paget's disease of bone; reflex sympathetic dystrophy.

Elcitonin Asahi, Jpn†.
Elcatonin (p.749·2).
Hypercalcaemia; osteoporosis; Paget's disease of bone.

Elcrit Parke, Davis, Ger.
Clozapine (p.671·2).
Schizophrenia.

Eldepryl
Reckitt & Colman, Austral.; Asta Medica, Belg.; Draxis, Canad.; Orion, Denm.; Orion, Fin.; Orion, Irl.; Asta Medica, Neth.; Orion, Norw.; Reckitt Benckiser, NZ; Reckitt Benckiser, S.Afr.; Orion, Swed.; Orion, UK; Somerset, USA.
Selegiline hydrochloride (p.1177·2).
Parkinsonism.

Eldercaps Merz, USA.
Multivitamin and mineral preparation (p.1350·1).

Elderin Lek, Hong Kong.
Etodolac (p.35·2).
Musculoskeletal, joint, and peri-articular disorders.

Eldertonic Merz, USA.
Vitamin B substances with minerals (p.1350·1).

Eldicet Solvay, Spain.
Pinaverium bromide (p.1651·3).
Gastrointestinal spasm; irritable bowel syndrome.

Eldisin Lilly, Aust.
Vindesine sulfate (p.580·1).
Malignant neoplasms.

Eldisine
Lilly, Austral.; Lilly, Belg.; Lilly, Canad.; Lilly, Fin.; Lilly, Fr.; Lilly, Ger.; Lilly, Hong Kong; Lilly, Ital.; Lilly, Neth.; Lilly, S.Afr.; Lilly, Swed.; Lilly, Switz.; Lilly, UK.
Vindesine sulfate (p.580·1).
Malignant neoplasms.

Eldopal Yamanouchi, Neth.†
Levodopa (p.1169·2).
Parkinsonism.

Eldopaque
ICN, Canad.; ICN, Hong Kong; ICN, Mex.; ICN, Singapore; ICN, USA.
Hydroquinone (p.1115·1) in a sunblocking basis.
Hyperpigmented skin conditions.

Eldoquin
ICN, Canad.; ICN, Hong Kong; ICN, Mex.; Pacific, NZ; ICN, Singapore; ICN, USA.
Hydroquinone (p.1115·1).
Hyperpigmented skin conditions.

Eldox Aspen Consumer, S.Afr.
Diphenoxylate hydrochloride (p.1222·2). Atropine sulfate (p.461·1) is included in this preparation to discourage abuse.
Diarrhoea.

Elebloc Alcon Cusi, Spain.
Carteolol hydrochloride (p.855·1).
Glaucoma; ocular hypertension.

Electopen Alter, Spain†.
Ampicillin sodium (p.150·3) or ampicillin trihydrate (p.151·1).
Bacterial infections.

Electopen Balsam Retard Alter, Spain.
Ampicillin sodium (p.150·3); ampicillin benzathine (p.151·3); niaouli oil (p.1640·2); guaifenesin (p.1092·2).
Respiratory-tract infections.

Electopen Retard Alter, Spain†.
Ampicillin sodium (p.150·3); ampicillin benzathine (p.151·3).
Bacterial infections.

Electrolade Eastern Pharmaceuticals, Irl.; Eastern Pharmaceuticals, UK.
Sodium chloride; potassium chloride; sodium bicarbonate; glucose (p.1185·2).
Diarrhoea; oral rehydration therapy.

Electrolit Pisa, Mex.
Sodium chloride; potassium chloride; calcium chloride; magnesium chloride; sodium lactate; glucose (p.1185·2).
Oral rehydration therapy.

Electrolit Pediatrico Pisa, Mex.
Glucose; sodium chloride; sodium citrate; potassium chloride (p.1185·2).
Diarrhoea; oral rehydration therapy.

Electrona Aspen Consumer, S.Afr.
Potassium chloride; sodium chloride; sodium bicarbonate; calcium lactate; sodium acid phosphate; magnesium sulfate; heavy magnesium carbonate; glucose (p.1185·2).
Diarrhoea; oral rehydration therapy.

Electropak Mirren, S.Afr.
Potassium chloride; sodium chloride; sodium bicarbonate; glucose (p.1185·2).
Diarrhoea; oral rehydration therapy.

Elegelin Sun, Singapore.
Selegiline hydrochloride (p.1177·2).
Parkinsonism.

Elemental 028
Scientific Hospital Supplies, Austral.; Nutricia, Fin.; Scientific Hospital Supplies, Irl.; Nutricia, Ital.; Nutricia, NZ; Scientific Hospital Supplies, NZ; Scientific Hospital Supplies, UK.
Preparation for enteral nutrition (p.1350·1).

Elen Yamanouchi, Jpn†.
Indeloxazine hydrochloride (p.1623·1).
Cerebrovascular disorders.

Elenol Gerda, Fr.
Lindane (p.1434·1); amylocaine hydrochloride (p.1306·1).
Scabies.

Elental Ajinomoto, Thai.
Preparation for enteral nutrition (p.1350·1).

Elentol Gerda, Fr.
Lindane (p.1434·1).
Disinfection of clothing and bedding; pediculosis.

Eleparon Luitpold, Braz.
Silymarin (p.1021·3).
Liver disorders.

Elepril Farmasa, Braz.
Selegiline (p.1178·1).
Parkinsonism.

Elequine Gilag, Mex.
Levofloxacin (p.219·1).
Bacterial infections.

Eleu-Kokk Pharmaton, Ger.; Pharmaton, Switz.
Eleutherococcus senticosis (p.1615·3).
Tonic.

Eleuphrat Essex, Austral.
Betamethasone dipropionate (p.1063·2).
Skin disorders.

Eleutheroforce Bioforce, Ger.
Eleutherococcus senticosis root (p.1615·3).
Tonic.

Eleutherokokk Arko, Ger.
Eleutherococcus senticosis root (p.1615·3).
Tonic.

Eleutherokokk-Aktiv-Kapseln SenticoMega
Twardy, Ger.†
Eleutherococcus senticosis root (p.1615·3).
Tonic.

Elevat Lagamed, S.Afr.†
Dronabinol (p.1224·3).
Anorexia with weight loss in AIDS; nausea and vomiting.

Elevit
Roche, Aust.; Roche, Switz.
Range of multivitamin or multivitamin and mineral preparations (p.1350·1).

Elevit Geriatrico Roche, Braz.
Multivitamin and mineral preparation (p.1350·1).

Elevit Pronatal Roche, Aust.
Multivitamin and mineral preparation (p.1350·1).

Elevit Vitamine B₉ Nicholas, Fr.
Multivitamin and mineral preparation (p.1350·1).

Elex Verla, Ger.
dl-Alpha tocoferil acetate (p.1394·1); magnesium oxide (p.1233·2).
Vitamin E and magnesium deficiency.

Elfanex Novartis, Aust.
Reserpine (p.967·3); dihydralazine sulfate (p.874·2); hydrochlorothiazide (p.907·3); potassium chloride (p.1194·3).
Hypertension.

Elfer Zerboni, Mex.
Ferrous sulfate (p.1360·3).

Elgadil Byk Elmu, Spain.
Urapidil hydrochloride (p.987·3).
Hypertension.

Elgam Sankyo, Spain.
Omeprazole (p.1239·1).
Gastro-oesophageal reflux; peptic ulcer; Zollinger-Ellison syndrome.

Elgydium Pierre Fabre Sante, Fr.; Chefaro, UK.
Chlorhexidine gluconate (p.1138·2).
Dental caries prophylaxis; mouth disorders.

Elibet Willmar, Mex.
Vitamin E (p.1394·1).

Elica Schering-Plough, S.Afr.; Schering-Plough, Spain.
Mometasone furoate (p.1077·2).
Skin and scalp disorders.

Elicodil Menarini, Ital.
Ranitidine bismuth citrate (p.1247·2).
Peptic ulcer.

Elidiur Bristol-Myers Squibb, Ital.
Fosinopril sodium (p.892·3); hydrochlorothiazide (p.907·3).
Hypertension.

Elimin *Cantabria, Spain.*
Sodium picosulfate (p.1249·3).
Constipation.

Elimite *Allergan, USA.*
Permethrin (p.1436·1).
Scabies.

Elimitona *Brauer, Austral.*
Homoeopathic preparation.

Elingrip *Wasserman, Spain†.*
Aspirin (p.14·2); ascorbic acid (p.1389·3); chlorpheniramine [chlorphenamine] maleate (p.412·1); kola (p.1681·1).
Cold and influenza symptoms.

Elios *Rydelle, Fr.†.*
Amino-acid, fatty-acid, and vitamin preparation (p.1350·1).
UV-induced skin damage.

Elisir Depurativo Ambrosiano *Alckamed, Ital.*
Aesculus hippocastanum (p.1574·1); hypericum perforatum (p.290·2); arnica montana (p.1581·3); knotgrass hamamelis virginiana (p.1618·3); gentiana lutea (p.1615·1).
Circulatory disorders.

Elisir Terpina *Teofarma, Ital.*
Terpin hydrate (p.1101·2); dropropizine (p.1089·3).
Coughs.

Elisor *Bristol-Myers Squibb, Fr.*
Pravastatin sodium (p.957·3).
Hypercholesterolaemia.

Elissan *Dermofarm, Spain.*
Loperamide hydrochloride (p.1231·3).
Diarrhoea.

Elitan *Medochemie, Thai.*
Metoclopramide hydrochloride (p.1235·2).
Gastrointestinal motility disorders; nausea and vomiting.

Elite *Bayer, Port.*
Test for glucose in blood (p.1616·3).
For use with Glucometer Elite.

Eliten *Bristol-Myers Squibb, Ital.*
Fosinopril sodium (p.892·3).
Heart failure; hypertension.

Elixifilin *Yamanouchi, Spain.*
Theophylline (p.777·2).
Formerly contained potassium iodide and theophylline.
Obstructive airways disease.

Elixir Bonjean *Dexo, Fr.*
Melissa (p.1632·2); bitter-orange peel (p.1644·2); aniseed (p.1580·2); cumin seed; catechu (p.1592·2); peppermint oil (p.1243·3).
Digestive disorders.

Elixir Contre La Toux Weleda *Weleda, Fr.†.*
Aniseed (p.1580·2); dulcamara (p.1606·2); drosera; althaea (p.1577·1); ipecacuanha (p.1093·1); malt (p.1371·1); white marrubium (p.1094·2); pulsatilla; thyme (p.1672·2).
Coughs.

Elixir Damiana and Saw Palmetto *Potter's, UK.*
Corn silk (p.1599·3); damiana (p.1602·1); saw palmetto (p.1491·2).
Tonic.

Elixir de Maracuja Composto *Kanda, Braz.*
Casimiroa; passion flower (p.1649·1); erythrina mulungu.
Sedative.

Elixir de Marinheiro *Phos-Kola, Braz.*
Potassium iodide (p.1522·3); cocillana (p.1087·2); sarsaparilla (p.1661·1); camphorated opium (p.69·3); anacardium occidentale.
Respiratory-tract congestion.

Elixir fortifiant *Phytomed, Switz.*
Ginkgo biloba; ginseng; calcium lactophosphate (p.1350·1).
Tonic.

Elixir Grez *Monin, Fr.*
Bitter-orange (p.1644·2); gentian (p.1615·1); cinnamon (p.1595·3); citric acid monohydrate (p.1596·2).
Digestive disorders.

Elixir Paregorico *Bergamo, Braz.; Sedar, Braz.*
Camphorated opium (p.69·3).
Diarrhoea; opioid withdrawal syndrome.

Elixir Rebleuten *Pharmacal, Switz.†.*
Aloes (p.1210·1).
Constipation.

Elixir Spark *Medecine Vegetale, Fr.*
Boldo (p.1585·3); cynara (p.1601·3).
Formerly contained cascara, senna, boldo, cynara, lupulus, bitter orange, gentian, sage, chamomile, absinthium, quassia, chicory, calumba, and centaury.
Constipation; dyspepsia.

Elixofilina *Schering, Mex.*
Theophylline (p.777·2).

Elixomin *Cenci, USA.*
Theophylline (p.777·2).
Obstructive airways disease.

Elixophyllin
Note.This name is used for preparations of different composition.
Sam-On, Israel.
Aminophylline (p.760·1).
Heart failure; obstructive airways disease.

Forest Pharmaceuticals, USA.
Theophylline (p.777·2).
Obstructive airways disease.

Elixophyllin-GG *Forest Pharmaceuticals, USA.*
Theophylline (p.777·2); guaifenesin (p.1092·2).
Obstructive airways disease.

The symbol † denotes a preparation no longer actively marketed

Elixophyllin-KI *Forest Pharmaceuticals, USA.*
Theophylline (p.777·2); potassium iodide (p.1522·3).
Tenacious mucus in asthma and bronchitis.

Elizabeth Arden Suncare *Arden, NZ.*
SPF 15: Octinoxate (p.1517·3); titanium dioxide (p.1126·1); avobenzone (p.1517·1).
Sunscreen.

Elkamol *Kendon, UK.*
Paracetamol (p.71·2).

Elkapin *Parke, Davis, Aust.†; Godecke, Ger.†; Parke, Davis, Ital.; Parke, Davis, Spain†.*
Etozolin (p.888·2).
Hypertension; oedema.

Elkin *Byk, Neth.*
Frusemide [furosemide] (p.893·1); amiloride hydrochloride (p.835·1).
Hypertension; oedema.

ELKO *Pharmacia Upjohn, Ger.*
Electrolyte infusion (p.1180·1).
Parenteral nutrition.

Ellatun *Alcon, Ger.*
Tramazoline hydrochloride (p.1102·1).
Nasal congestion.

Ell-Cranell *Galderma, Ger.*
Estradiol (p.1473·1); dexamethasone (p.1067·1); salicylic acid (p.1122·3).
Hair loss; scalp disorders.

Ell-Cranell alpha *Galderma, Ger.*
Estradiol (p.1473·1).
Alopecia androgenetica.

Elle-care *Geistlich, Switz.*
Lactic acid (p.1626·2); sodium lactate (p.1186·2); docusate sodium (p.1223·1).
Vaginal disorders.

Elleci *Lampugnani, Ital.*
Carnitine (p.1356·1).
Carnitine deficiency.

Ellence *Pharmacia Upjohn, USA.*
Epirubicin hydrochloride (p.537·1).
Breast cancer.

Elleste Duet Conti *Pharmacia, UK.*
Estradiol (p.1473·1); norethisterone acetate (p.1485·1).
Menopausal disorders; osteoporosis.

Elleste-Duet *Pharmacia, UK.*
16 Tablets, estradiol (p.1473·1); 12 tablets, estradiol; norethisterone acetate (p.1485·1).
Menopausal disorders; osteoporosis.

Elleste-Solo *Pharmacia, UK.*
Estradiol (p.1473·1).
Menopausal disorders; osteoporosis.

Ellimans *SSL, UK.*
Turpentine oil (p.1676·3); acetic acid (p.1571·2).
Musculoskeletal pain.

Elliots B *Orphan Medical, Israel.*
Electrolyte solution with glucose (p.1180·1).
Lymphocytic lymphoma; meningeal leukaemia.

Ellsurex *Galderma, Ger.*
Selenium sulfide (p.1123·1); colloidal sulfur (p.1123·3); allantoin (p.1110·1).
Scalp disorders.

Elmetacin
Sankyo, Ger.; Sankyo, NZ; Searle, NZ; Sankyo, Port.; Byk Madaus, S.Afr.†; Sankyo, Switz.; Sankyo, Thai.
Indometacin (p.44·3).
Musculoskeletal, joint, peri-articular, and soft-tissue pain and inflammation.

Elmetin *Medochemie, Thai.*
Mebendazole (p.102·2).
Worm infections.

Elmex
Note.This name is used for preparations of different composition.
Gebro, Aust.; GABA, Belg.; Orion, Fin.; Wybert, Ger.; GABA, Israel; Avantgarde, Ital.; GABA, Neth.; Dental Warehouse, S.Afr.; Inibsa, Spain; GABA, Switz.
Topical gel: Olaflur (p.1374·1); dectaflur (p.1359·1); sodium fluoride (p.1375·3).
Dental caries prophylaxis; sensitive teeth.

Gebro, Aust.; Orion, Fin.; Wybert, Ger.; GABA, Switz.
Topical solution: Olaflur (p.1374·1); dectaflur (p.1359·1).
Dental caries prophylaxis; sensitive teeth.

GABA, Fr.; GABA, Israel.
Mouthwash: Olaflur (p.1374·1); sodium fluoride (p.1375·3).
Dental caries prophylaxis.

GABA, Fr.; GABA, Israel.
Toothpaste for sensitive teeth: Olaflur (p.1374·1).
Dental caries prophylaxis.

GABA, Israel.
Toothpaste: Olaflur (p.1374·1); hetaflur.
Dental caries prophylaxis.

Inibsa, Port.
Amine fluoride.
Dental caries prophylaxis.

Elmiron *Arthropharm, Austral.; Alza, Canad.; Baker Norton, Hong Kong; Alza, USA.*
Pentosan polysulfate sodium (p.953·1).
Interstitial cystitis.

Elmogan *Lek, Hong Kong.*
Gemfibrozil (p.896·2).
Hyperlipidaemias.

Elmuten *Byk Elmu, Spain.*
Aceglutamide; acetylaspartic acid; cyanocobalamin; citrulline; inositol; thiamine nitrate; magnesium potas-

sium aspartate; pyridoxal phosphate; serine phosphate (p.1350·1).
Lignocaine [lidocaine] hydrochloride (p.1313·2) is included in this preparation to alleviate the pain of injection.
Tonic.

Elo-admix *Fresenius Kabi, Aust.*
Electrolyte infusion (p.1180·1).
Fluid and electrolyte disorders.

Eloamin *Fresenius Kabi, Aust.*
Amino-acid and electrolyte infusion (p.1350·1).
Parenteral nutrition.

Elobact *Cascan, Ger.; Glaxo Wellcome, Ger.*
Cefuroxime axetil (p.178·1).
Bacterial infections.

Elocin *Shiwa, Thai.*
Erythromycin stearate (p.201·3).
Bacterial infections.

Elocom *Schering-Plough, Belg.; Schering-Plough, Braz.; Schering, Canad.; Schering-Plough, Israel; Schering-Plough, Port.; Schering-Plough, Spain; Essex, Switz.*
Mometasone furoate (p.1077·2).
Skin disorders.

Elocon *Aesca, Aust.; Schering-Plough, Austral.; Schering-Plough, Denm.; Schering-Plough, Fin.; Schering-Plough, Irl.; Schering-Plough, Ital.; Schering-Plough, Neth.; Schering-Plough, Norw.; Schering-Plough, NZ; Schering-Plough, S.Afr.; Schering-Plough, Swed.; Schering-Plough, UK; Schering, USA.*
Mometasone furoate (p.1077·2).
Skin disorders.

Elocor *Ehlinger, Mex.*
Nifedipine (p.940·1).

Elocort *Elofar, Braz.*
Hydrocortisone (p.1073·3); nitrofurazone (p.231·3).
Skin disorders.

Eloglucose *Fresenius Kabi, Aust.*
Electrolyte infusion with glucose (p.1180·1).
Carbohydrate source; fluid and electrolyte disorders.

Elohaes *Fresenius, Belg.†; Fresenius, UK.*
Hexastarch (p.732·3) in sodium chloride.
Extracorporeal circulation; hypovolaemic shock; leucopheresis.

Elohast *Fresenius Kabi, Aust.; Fresenius Kabi, Switz.*
An etherified starch (p.732·3) in electrolytes or sodium chloride.
Hypovolaemia; shock.

Elohes *Fresenius Kabi, Fr.; Fresenius Kabi, Spain.*
An etherified starch (p.732·3) in sodium chloride.
Haemodilution; hypovolaemia; plasma exchange.

Eloisin *Alcon Cusi, Spain.*
Eledoisin trifluoroacetate (p.1606·3).
Dry eyes.

Elolipid *Fresenius Kabi, Aust.; Fresenius Kabi, Ital.*
Soya oil (p.1378·1).
Contains egg lecithin.
Lipid infusion for parenteral nutrition.

ELO-MEL *Fresenius Kabi, Aust.*
A range of electrolyte infusions with or without glucose (p.1180·1).
Carbohydrate source; fluid and electrolyte disorders.

Elomet *Schering-Plough, Hong Kong; Schering-Plough, Mex.; Schering-Plough, Singapore; Schering-Plough, Thai.*
Mometasone furoate (p.1077·2).
Skin disorders.

ELO-oral *Fresenius Kabi, Aust.*
Electrolytes (p.1180·1).
Fluid and electrolyte disorders.

Elopram *Recordati, Ital.*
Citalopram hydrobromide (p.281·2) or citalopram hydrochloride (p.281·2).
Anxiety disorders; depression.

Elorgan *Hoechst Marion Roussel, Spain.*
Oxpentifylline [pentoxifylline] (p.950·3).
Vascular disorders.

Elorheo *Fresenius Kabi, Aust.*
Dextran 40 (p.728·3) in electrolytes.
Fluid and electrolyte disorders.

Elotin *Elofar, Braz.*
Fluocinolone (p.1071·1); neomycin (p.228·1).
Ear disorders.

Elotrace *Fresenius Kabi, Aust.*
Electrolyte infusion with trace elements (p.1180·1).
Parenteral nutrition; trace element deficiency.

Elotrans *Leopold, Braz.†; Niddapharm, Ger.; Helvepharm, Switz.*
Anhydrous glucose; sodium chloride; sodium citrate; potassium chloride (p.1185·2).
Diarrhoea; oral rehydration therapy.

Eloverlan *Mayrhofer, Aust.*
Anhydrous glucose; sodium chloride; potassium chloride; sodium bicarbonate (p.1185·2).
Diarrhoea; oral rehydration therapy.

Elovol *Fresenius Kabi, Aust.*
Electrolyte infusion (p.1180·1).
Fluid and electrolyte disorders.

Eloxatin *Sanofi Synthelabo, Austral.; Sanofi Synthelabo, Belg.; Sanofi Synthelabo, Ger.; Sanofi Synthelabo, Neth.; Sanofi Synthelabo, Singapore;*

Sanofi Winthrop, Swed.; Sanofi Synthelabo, Thai.; Sanofi Winthrop, UK.
Oxaliplatin (p.563·1).
Colorectal cancer.

Eloxatine *Sanofi Winthrop, Fr.*
Oxaliplatin (p.563·1).
Colorectal cancer.

Elozell *Fresenius Kabi, Aust.*
Magnesium aspartate (p.1190·3); potassium aspartate (p.1195·2).
Cardiac disorders; digitalis toxicity; potassium and magnesium deficiency.

Elozell spezial *Fresenius Kabi, Aust.*
Potassium chloride (p.1194·3); potassium aspartate (p.1195·2); magnesium aspartate (p.1190·3).
Cardiac disorders; digitalis toxicity; potassium and magnesium deficiency.

Elozima *Elofar, Braz.*
Pancreatin (p.1646·1); dimethicone (p.1249·2).
Digestive disorders.

Elroquil N *Rodleben, Ger.*
Hydroxyzine hydrochloride (p.419·1).
Anxiety disorders; premedication; pruritus; sleep disorders.

Elspar *Prodome, Braz.; Merck Sharp & Dohme, Hong Kong; Merck, USA.*
Asparaginase (p.508·3).
Acute lymphocytic leukaemia.

Eltair *Douglas, Hong Kong; Douglas, NZ; Douglas, Singapore; Douglas, Thai.; TTN, Thai.*
Budesonide (p.1064·2).
Nasal polyps; rhinitis.

Elteans *Jaldes, Fr.*
Salmon oil (p.949·2); borage oil (p.1613·1); carrot and soya oils.
Nutritional fatty acid supplement.

Elthyrone *Knoll, Belg.*
Thyroxine [levothyroxine] sodium (p.1526·2).
Hypothyroidism.

Eltor *Hoechst Marion Roussel, Canad.*
Pseudoephedrine hydrochloride (p.1099·2).
Nasal and sinus congestion.

Eltroxin *Glaxo Wellcome, Canad.; Glaxo Wellcome, Denm.; Glaxo Wellcome, Hong Kong; Glaxo Wellcome, Israel; Glaxo Wellcome, Neth.; Glaxo Wellcome, NZ; Glaxo Wellcome, S.Afr.; Glaxo Wellcome, Singapore; Sigma-Tau, Switz.; Glaxo Wellcome, Thai.; Goldshield, UK; Roberts, USA.*
Thyroxine [levothyroxine] sodium (p.1526·2).
Hypothyroidism.

Elucent Skin Refining Day Cream *Ego, Austral.*
SPF 20: Titanium dioxide (p.1126·1); octinoxate (p.1517·3); avobenzone (p.1517·1); emollients.
Dry skin; sunscreen.

Eludril
Note.This name is used for preparations of different composition.
Inava, Fr.; Pierre Fabre, Switz.; Ceuta, UK.
Throat spray: Chlorhexidine gluconate (p.1138·2); amethocaine [tetracaine] hydrochloride (p.1305·2).
Mouth and throat disorders.

Inava, Fr.; Pierre Fabre, Port.; Orient, Singapore; Pierre Fabre, Singapore; Pierre Fabre, Spain; Pierre Fabre, Switz.; Ceuta, UK.
Mouthwash: Chlorhexidine gluconate (p.1138·2); chlorobutanol (p.1141·2).
Formerly contained chlorhexidine gluconate, chlorobutanol, and chloroform in Fr.
Mouth and throat disorders.

Elugan *Menadier, Ger.*
Simeticone (p.1249·2).
Gastrointestinal disorders.

Elugan N *Menadier, Ger.*
Simeticone (p.1249·2).
Gastrointestinal disorders.

Elugel *Pierre Fabre Sante, Fr.*
Chlorhexidine gluconate (p.1138·2).
Gum disorders; mouth hygiene.

Elum *Farmasa, Braz.*
Cloxazolam (p.671·2).
Anxiety.

Elusanes *Dolisos, Fr.*
A range of herbal preparations.

Elusanes Espino Albar *Pierre Fabre, Spain.*
Crataegus (p.1600·2).
Nervous disorders; sleep disorders.

Elutit-Calcium *Felgentrager, Ger.*
Calcium polystyrene sulfonate (p.1002·3).
Hyperkalaemia.

Elutit-Natrium *Felgentrager, Ger.*
Sodium polystyrene sulfonate (p.1023·2).
Hyperkalaemia.

Elvorine *Wyeth Lederle, Belg.; Wyeth Lederle, Fr.*
Calcium levofolinate (p.1363·1).
Adjuvant to fluorouracil therapy; drug-induced megaloblastic anaemia; folic acid deficiency; prevention of methotrexate-induced toxicity.

Elyzol *Chemomedica, Aust.; Dumex-Alpharma, Denm.; Dumex-Alpharma, Fin.; Pharmadent, Fr.; Dumex, Ger.; Dumex-Alpharma, Hong Kong; Dumex, Irl.; CTI, Israel; Cabon, Ital.; Alpharma, Mex.; Alpharma, Norw.; Dumex-Alpharma, Singapore; Dumex-Alpharma, Swed.; Dumex, Switz.; Dumex, Thai.; Dumex, UK†.*
Metronidazole (p.594·1) or metronidazole benzoate (p.594·1).
Anaerobic bacterial infections; Crohn's disease; protozoal infections; rosacea.

Elzogram Lilly, Ger.
Cefazolin sodium (p.164·3).
Bacterial infections.

Elzym Sankyo, Switz.; Sankyo, Thai.
Enzyme concentrate from *Aspergillus oryzae*; simeticone (p.1249·2); ethaverine hydrochloride (p.1608·2).
Gastrointestinal disorders with excess gas; preparation of gastrointestinal tract for radiological examination.

EM Eukal Sohan, Canad.
Eucalyptus oil (p.1609·2); menthol (p.1632·3).

Emadine Alcon, Aust.; Alcon, Belg.; Alcon, Canad.; Alcon, Denm.; Alcon, Fin.; Alcon, Fr.; Alcon, Ger.; Alcon, Irl.; Alcon, Ital.; Alcon, Port.; Alcon, Swed.; Alcon, UK; Alcon, USA.
Emedastine fumarate (p.417·3).
Allergic conjunctivitis.

Emaftol Ogna, Ital.
Policresulen.
Mouth disinfection.

Emagel Hoechst Marion Roussel, Ital.
Polygeline (p.741·1).
Plasma volume expansion.

Emagrex Dinafarma, Braz.
Bladderwrack (p.1585·2); thyroid (p.1526·2); bile salts (p.1585·1); phenolphthalein (p.1244·1).
Constipation; obesity.

Emasex A Eurim, Ger.
Bamethan sulfate (p.843·1).
Erectile dysfunction.

Emasex-N Eurim, Ger.
Bamethan sulfate (p.843·1); benzyl nicotinate (p.20·2).
Erectile dysfunction; tonic.

Emazian B12 Pfizer, Ital.
Thiamine hydrochloride (p.1385·1); riboflavin (p.1386·1); panthenol (p.1602·3); nicotinamide (p.1372·3); calcium folinate (p.1363·1); cyanocobalamin (p.1388·1).
Deficiency states; macrocytic anaemia.

EMB Fatol, Ger.; Hefa, Ger.
Ethambutol hydrochloride (p.205·1).
Tuberculosis.

Embeline E Healthpoint, USA.
Clobetasol propionate (p.1065·2).
Skin disorders.

Embial Merck, Ger.
dl-Alpha tocoferil acetate (p.1394·1).
Vitamin E deficiency.

EMB-INH Fatol, Ger.
Ethambutol hydrochloride (p.205·1); isoniazid (p.215·3).
Tuberculosis.

Emblon Berk, UK.
Tamoxifen citrate (p.571·1).
Anovulatory infertility; breast cancer.

Embol Yung Shin, Thai.
Piracetam (p.1652·1).
Alcohol withdrawal syndrome; cerebrovascular disorders; mental function impairment.

Embolex Novartis, Aust.
Certoparin sodium (p.856·2) dihydroergotamine mesilate (p.450·3).
Lignocaine [lidocaine] hydrochloride (p.1313·2) is included in this preparation to alleviate the pain of injection.
Thromboembolic disorders.

Embolex NM Novartis, Ger.
Certoparin sodium (p.856·2); dihydroergotamine mesilate (p.450·3).
Lignocaine [lidocaine] hydrochloride (p.1313·2) is included in this preparation to alleviate the pain of injection.
Thromboembolism prophylaxis.

Embrocacion Gras Quimifar, Spain.
Alcohol (p.1130·3); capsicum oleoresin (p.1591·1); methyl salicylate (p.55·1); turpentine oil (p.1676·3).
Muscle and joint pain.

Embrocation Synpharma, Aust.
Menthol (p.1632·3); peppermint oil (p.1243·3); methyl salicylate (p.55·1); eucalyptus oil (p.1609·2); rosemary oil (p.1659·3); anise oil (p.1580·3); citronella oil (p.1596·3); arnica (p.1581·3).
Musculoskeletal and joint disorders.

Embropax Taphlan, Switz.
Methyl salicylate (p.55·1); isopropyl nicotinate; capsicum (p.1591·1); camphor (p.1589·3); turpentine oil (p.1676·3); eucalyptus oil (p.1609·2); lavender oil (p.1627·2).
Peri-articular and soft-tissue disorders.

Emconcor Merck-Belgolabo, Belg.; Merck, Denm.; Merck, Fin.; Merck, Spain; Merck, Swed.
Bisoprolol fumarate (p.850·1).
Angina pectoris; heart failure; hypertension; migraine.

Emconcor Comp Merck, Fin.
Bisoprolol fumarate (p.850·1); hydrochlorothiazide (p.907·3).
Hypertension.

Emcor Merck, Irl.; Merck, Neth.; E. Merck, UK.
Bisoprolol fumarate (p.850·1).
Angina pectoris; hypertension.

Emcoretic Merck-Belgolabo, Belg.; Merck, Neth.; Merck, Spain.
Bisoprolol fumarate (p.850·1); hydrochlorothiazide (p.907·3).
Hypertension.

Emcyt Pharmacia Upjohn, Canad.; Pharmacia Upjohn, Mex.; Pharmacia Upjohn, USA.
Estramustine sodium phosphate (p.537·3).
Prostatic cancer.

Emdalen Merck, S.Afr.
Lofepramine hydrochloride (p.297·1).
Depression.

Emdar Merck, Mex.
Astemizole (p.409·1).
Hypersensitivity.

Emecheck Savage, USA†.
Phosphoric acid (p.1651·1); glucose (p.1364·1); fructose (p.1363·3).
Nausea and vomiting.

Emecort Merck, Braz.
Methylprednisolone acetate (p.1076·1); gentamicin sulfate (p.210·1).
Infected skin disorders.

Emediba Diba, Mex.
Meclozine hydrochloride (p.420·3); pyridoxine hydrochloride (p.1386·3).
Infant colic; nausea; vertigo; vomiting.

Emedrin N Streuli, Switz.
Dextromethorphan hydrobromide (p.1087·3).
Coughs.

Emedyl Montavit, Aust.
Dimenhydrinate (p.415·2).
Nausea and vomiting; vestibular disorders.

Emelis Clintec, Fr.†; Clintec, Irl.†.
High-protein semi-solid dietary supplement (p.1350·1).
Chewing or swallowing disorders.

Emeproton Cantabria, Spain.
Omeprazole (p.1239·1).
Gastro-oesophageal reflux; peptic ulcer; Zollinger-Ellison syndrome.

Emercol Pharmavite, Canad.
Benzocaine (p.1306·2); cetalkonium chloride (p.1137·1); cetylpyridinium chloride (p.1138·1).

Emercreme No 4 Pharmavite, Canad.
Cetylpyridinium chloride (p.1138·1); bacitracin (p.155·2); tyrothricin (p.267·1); diphenylpyraline hydrochloride (p.417·1); benzocaine (p.1306·2).

Emereze Plus Pharmavite, Canad.
Cetylpyridinium chloride (p.1138·1).

Emergent-Ez Healthfirst, USA.
Combination pack: 2 Ampoules, adrenaline [epinephrine] (p.829·1); 1 ampoule, aminophylline (p.760·1); 3 inhalants, ammonia (p.1579·1); 2 inhalants, amyl nitrite (p.1002·1); 2 ampoules, atropine (p.460·3); 2 ampoules, diphenhydramine hydrochloride (Benadryl) (p.416·1); tablets, glyceryl trinitrate (p.897·3); 1 vial, hydrocortisone sodium succinate (Solu-Cortef) (p.1074·1); 1 ampoule, pentazocine lactate (Talwin) (p.74·2); 1 ampoule, trimethobenzamide hydrochloride (Tigan) (p.426·3); 2 ampoules, diazepam (Valium) (p.674·3); 2 ampoules, mephentermine sulfate (Wyamine) (p.926·2).
Emergency treatment.

Emersal Medco, USA†.
Ammoniated mercury (p.1118·3); salicylic acid (p.1122·3).
Psoriasis.

Emesafene Asta Medica, Neth.
Meclozine hydrochloride (p.420·3); pyridoxine hydrochloride (p.1386·3).
Nausea; vomiting.

Emesan Lindopharm, Ger.
Diphenhydramine hydrochloride (p.416·1).
Nausea; vomiting.

Emeside Laboratories for Applied Biology, UK.
Ethosuximide (p.348·1).
Absence seizures; myoclonic seizures.

Emetal Asian Pharm, Thai.
Metoclopramide hydrochloride (p.1235·2).
Nausea and vomiting.

Emetic Elofar, Braz.
Metoclopramide (p.1236·3).
Gastrointestinal motility disorders; nausea and vomiting.

Emetrol
Note. This name is used for preparations of different composition.
Rhone-Poulenc Rorer, Austral.; Sanofi Winthrop, USA.
Fructose (p.1363·3); glucose (p.1364·2); phosphoric acid (p.1651·1).
Nausea; vomiting.
Aspen Consumer, S.Afr.
Sucrose (p.1380·3); phosphoric acid (p.1651·1).
Nausea; vomiting.

Em-eukal Soldan, Ger.
Balsam: Eucalyptus oil (p.1609·2); menthol (p.1632·3); pumilio pine oil (p.1656·3); thyme oil (p.1672·3); turpentine oil (p.1676·3); camphor (p.1589·3).
Respiratory-tract disorders.
Oral drops: Eucalyptus leaf (p.1609·2); aniseed (p.1580·2); fennel (p.1610·1); thyme (p.1672·2).
Coughs.
Oral liquid: Dextromethorphan hydrobromide (p.1087·3); menthol (p.1632·3); cetylpyridinium chloride (p.1138·1); anise oil (p.1580·3); gypsophila saponin; thymol (p.1158·3).
Catarrh; coughs.

Em-eukal forte Soldan, Ger.
Dextromethorphan hydrobromide (p.1087·3); menthol (p.1632·3); cetylpyridinium chloride (p.1138·1); euca-

lyptus oil (p.1609·2); gypsophila saponin; benzocaine (p.1306·2).
Catarrh; coughs.

Em-eukal Husten- und Brusttee Soldan, Ger.
Althaea (p.1577·1); fennel (p.1610·1); aniseed (p.1580·2); liquorice (p.1231·2); fennel oil (p.1610·2); anise oil (p.1580·3).
Coughs.

Em-eukal Mono Soldan, Ger.
Oxymetazoline hydrochloride (p.1096·2).
Rhinitis.

Emex Mirren, S.Afr.
Invert sugar (p.1366·2); phosphoric acid (p.1651·1).
Nausea.

Emfib Berk, UK†.
Gemfibrozil (p.896·2).
Hyperlipidaemias.

Emflex E. Merck, UK.
Acemetacin (p.11·2).
Inflammation; pain; rheumatoid arthritis.

Emforal Remedica, Thai.
Propranolol hydrochloride (p.962·3).
Angina pectoris; anxiety; arrhythmias; hypertension; hyperthyroidism; migraine; obstructive cardiomyopathy; tremor.

Emgecard Mayrhofer, Aust.
Magnesium aspartate hydrochloride (p.1191·3).
Magnesium deficiency.

Emgel Glaxo Wellcome, USA.
Erythromycin (p.201·2).
Acne.

Emgesan Recip, Fin.; Recip, Swed.
Magnesium hydroxide (p.1233·1).
Magnesium deficiency; renal calculi.

Emican Alter, Spain.
Salbutamol sulfate (p.770·3).
Obstructive airways disease.

Emidoxin Magis, Ital.
Cefonicid sodium (p.168·1).
Lignocaine [lidocaine] hydrochloride (p.1313·2) is included in this preparation to alleviate the pain of injection.
Gram-negative bacterial infections.

Emidrat EMS, Braz.
Sodium chloride; potassium chloride; sodium citrate; sodium phosphate; calcium lactate; magnesium citrate; citric acid; saccharin sodium; glucose (p.1185·2).
Diarrhoea; oral rehydration solution.

Emifol Solfran, Mex.
Vitamin B substances (p.1350·1).

Emiken Kener, Mex.
Domperidone (p.1224·1).

Emilace Yamanouchi, Jpn.
Nemonapride (p.695·2).
Schizophrenia.

Eminase Torrex, Austral.; Therabel, Belg.; Roberts, Canad.; SmithKline Beecham, Fr.†; Reusch, Ger.†; Roberts, Israel; SmithKline Beecham, Ital.†; Tramedico, Neth.; SmithKline Beecham, Switz.†; Monmouth, UK†; Roberts, USA.
Anistreplase (p.840·2).
Myocardial infarction.

Emistin EMS, Braz.
Clemastine fumarate (p.413·2); dexamethasone acetate (p.1067·1).
Hypersensitivity reactions.

Emitex Aspen Consumer, S.Afr.
Cyclizine hydrochloride (p.414·1).
Motion sickness; nausea; vestibular disorders; vomiting.

Emizol Lemery, Mex.
Astemizole (p.409·1).

Emko Schering-Plough, S.Afr.†; Schering, USA.
Nonoxinol 9 (p.1346·1).
Contraceptive.

Emla Astra, Aust.; Astra, Austral.; Astra, Belg.; Astra, Braz.; AstraZeneca, Canad.; AstraZeneca, Denm.; AstraZeneca, Fin.; AstraZeneca, Fr.; Astra, Ger.; Astra, Hong Kong; Astra, Irl.; Astra, Israel; Astra, Ital.; Astra, Neth.; AstraZeneca, Norw.; AstraZeneca, NZ; Astra, Port.; Astra, S.Afr.; AstraZeneca, Singapore; Astra, Spain; Astra, Swed.; Astra, Switz.; AstraZeneca, Thai.; AstraZeneca, UK; AstraZeneca, USA.
Lignocaine [lidocaine] (p.1313·2); prilocaine (p.1318·3).
Local anaesthesia.

Emlapatch AstraZeneca, Fr.
Lignocaine [lidocaine] (p.1313·2); prilocaine (p.1318·3).
Local anaesthesia.

Emmenoiasi Palmares, Ital.
Centella asiatica (p.1112·2); couch-grass (p.1599·3); lupulus (p.1629·3); melissa (p.1632·2); zinc (p.1398·1); copper (p.1357·3).
Nutritional supplement.

Emmenovis Vitoria, Port.
Estradiol benzoate (p.1473·1); progesterone (p.1488·3).
Menstrual disorders; recurrent miscarriage.

Emmetipi Sicor, Ital.†.
Methylprednisolone sodium succinate (p.1076·1).
Parenteral corticosteroid.

Emoantitossina Piam, Ital.
Calcium folinate (p.1363·1); cyanocobalamin (p.1388·1); monophosphothiamine chloride (p.1385·1); riboflavin sodium phosphate (p.1386·1);

pyridoxine hydrochloride (p.1386·3); nicotinamide (p.1372·3); panthenol (p.1602·3).
Anaemias; deficiency states.

Emoclot DI BBC, Braz.; ISI, Ital.
A factor VIII preparation (p.734·1).
Haemophilia A; von Willebrand's disease.

Emo-Cort Trans Canaderm, Canad.
Hydrocortisone (p.1073·3).
Skin disorders.

Emocrat forte Hevert, Ger.
Crataegus; rutoside sodium sulfate (p.1611·2).
Arrhythmias; ischaemic heart disease.

Emodella GABA, Switz.†.
Frangula bark (p.1227·1).
Constipation.

Emoferrina Piam, Ital.†.
Ferric sodium gluconate (p.1360·2).
Iron deficiency; iron-deficiency anaemias.

Emoflux Metapharma, Ital.
Buflomedil hydrochloride (p.851·3).
Vascular disorders.

Emoform Byk, Braz.; Warner-Lambert, Fr.†; Norgine, UK†.
Formaldehyde (p.1144·2).
Hypersensitive teeth.

Emoform nouvelle formule Wild, Switz.
Electrolytes (p.1180·1).
Oral hygiene; sensitive teeth.

Emoform-F au fluor Wild, Switz.
Electrolytes (p.1180·1); sodium monofluorophosphate (p.1377·2).
Dental caries prophylaxis; oral hygiene; sensitive teeth.

Emoklar Savio, Ital.
Heparin calcium (p.902·1).
Thromboembolic disorders.

Emol Fischer, Israel.
Bath additive.
Dry skin; skin irritation.

Emollia Gordon, USA.
Emollient and moisturiser.

Emolytar Stiefel, Ital.
Tar (p.1125·1); juniper oil (p.1625·2); coal tar (p.1125·1).
Skin disorders.

Emopads Farmalight, Port.
Aloes (p.1210·1); propylene glycol (p.1655·1); aesculus (p.1574·1); ruscus aculeatus; sage (p.1660·2); melaleuca alternifolia (p.1631·3).
Anal discomfort.

Emoplast Schiapparelli, Ital.†.
Benzalkonium chloride (p.1133·2); alum (p.1577·2).
Skin and wound disinfection.

Emopon Terapeutico, Ital.
Calcium folinate (p.1363·1); cyanocobalamin (p.1388·1); ferric ammonium citrate (p.1359·2); thiamine hydrochloride (p.1385·1); nicotinamide (p.1372·3).
Macrocytic anaemia.

Emopremarin Wyeth Lederle, Ital.
Conjugated oestrogens (p.1467·1).
Haemorrhage.

Emoren IFI, Ital.
Oxetacaine hydrochloride (p.1317·3).
Haemorrhoids.

Emorril Searle, Ital.
Hydrocortisone acetate (p.1073·3); lignocaine [lidocaine] hydrochloride (p.1313·2).
Formerly contained troxerutin, hydrocortisone acetate, nifuratel, and lignocaine [lidocaine] or lignocaine [lidocaine] hydrochloride.
Adjunct in anorectal surgery; haemorrhoids.

Emosint Sclavo, Ital.
Desmopressin acetate (p.1281·2).
Haemorrhagic disorders.

Emoton Tentan, Switz.
Agnus castus (p.1574·2).
Premenstrual disorders.

Emotonico EMS, Braz.
Ferric ammonium citrate (p.1359·2); vitamin B substances (p.1350·1).
Anaemias.

Emovat Glaxo Wellcome, Denm.; Glaxo Wellcome, Fin.; Glaxo Wellcome, Swed.
Clobetasone butyrate (p.1065·2).
Eczema.

Emovate Glaxo Wellcome, Aust.; Glaxo Wellcome, Ger.; Cascan, Ger.; Glaxo Wellcome, Neth.; Glaxo Wellcome, Port.; Medeva, Spain; Glaxo Wellcome, Switz.
Clobetasone butyrate (p.1065·2).
Skin disorders.

Emovis Boniscontro & Gazzone, Ital.
Calcium folinate (p.1363·1).
Anaemias; antidote to overdosage with folic acid antagonists; folate deficiency; reduction of aminopterin and methotrexate toxicity.

Empacod Byk Madaus, S.Afr.
Paracetamol (p.71·2); codeine phosphate (p.25·2).
Fever; pain.

Empaped Byk Madaus, S.Afr.
Paracetamol (p.71·2).
Fever; pain.

Empapol Vilardell, Spain.
Terpineol (p.1669·3); cresol (p.1142·3); pinus sylvestris resin (p.1598·3).
Mouth and throat disorders; wounds.

Emperal Orion, Denm.
Metoclopramide hydrochloride (p.1235·2).
Irritable bowel syndrome; nausea and vomiting.

Empicols Albright & Wilson, UK.
A range of sodium laurilsulfates (p.1496·3).

Empirin Wellcome, USA.
Aspirin (p.14·2).
Fever; inflammation; myocardial infarction; pain; transient ischaemic attacks.

Empirin with Codeine Wellcome, USA.
Aspirin (p.14·2); codeine phosphate (p.25·2).
Pain.

Emplatre Croix D Democal, Switz.
Cayenne pepper (p.1591·1); methyl salicylate (p.55·1); venice turpentine.
Musculoskeletal and joint pain.

Emportal Novartis Consumer, Spain.
Lactitol (p.1230·1).
Constipation; hepatic encephalopathy.

Empracet Glaxo Wellcome, Canad.
Paracetamol (p.71·2); codeine phosphate (p.25·2).
Pain.

Emprazil-A Glaxo Wellcome, S.Afr.†.
Triprolidine hydrochloride (p.427·2); pseudoephedrine hydrochloride (p.1099·2); caffeine (p.761·3); paracetamol (p.71·2).
Cold and influenza symptoms.

Empynase Kaken, Jpn†.
Pronase.
Inflammation; respiratory-tract congestion.

EMS Expectorante EMS, Braz.
Guaifenesin (p.1092·2); etafedrine hydrochloride (p.1091·2); bufylline (p.761·3); doxylamine succinate (p.417·1).
Respiratory-tract disorders.

Emser Erkaltungsgel Siemens, Ger.
Pumilio pine oil (p.1656·3); eucalyptus oil (p.1609·2); camphor (p.1589·3).
Cold symptoms.

Emser Inhalationslosung Siemens, Ger.
Natural emser salt (see Emser Salz) in isotonic solution.
Respiratory-tract disorders.

Emser Nasensalbe Hexal, Aust.
Natural emser salt; azulene (p.1583·2); nutmeg oil (p.1643·1); oleum pini sylvestris; pumilio pine oil (p.1656·3); eucalyptus oil (p.1609·2); cedar wood oil; turpentine oil (p.1676·3); camphor (p.1589·3).
Colds; hay fever.

Emser Nasensalbe N Siemens, Ger.
Natural emser salz; azulene (p.1583·2); nutmeg oil (p.1643·1); pine needle oil; pumilio pine oil (p.1656·3); eucalyptus oil (p.1609·2); cedar wood oil; camphor (p.1589·3); turpentine oil (p.1676·3).
Colds; hay fever.

Emser Nasenspray Siemens, Ger.; Hexal, Ger.
Natural emser salt (see Emser Salz) in isotonic solution.
Cold symptoms; rhinosinusitis.

Emser Pastillen Hexal, Aust.
Natural emser salt.
Respiratory-tract disorders.

Emser Pastillen mit Menthol Hexal, Aust.
Natural emser salt; menthol (p.1632·3); peppermint oil (p.1243·3); eucalyptus oil (p.1609·2).
Respiratory-tract disorders.

Emser Pastillen mit Mentholfrische Siemens, Ger.
Natural emser salt (see Emser Salz); menthol (p.1632·3).
Formerly known as Emser Pastillen mit Menthol N.
Throat disorders.

Emser Pastillen ohne Menthol Siemens, Ger.
Natural emser salt (see Emser Salz).
Throat disorders.

Emser Pastillen zuckerfrei Siemens, Ger.
Natural emser salt (see Emser Salz).
Mouth and throat disorders.

Emser Salz Siemens, Ger.
Natural emser salt (containing lithium, sodium, potassium, magnesium, calcium, manganese, ferrous, ferric, fluoride, chloride, bromide, iodide, nitrite, sulfate, bicarbonate, and carbonate ions).
Dyspepsia; respiratory-tract disorders.

Emser Sole Siemens, Ger.†.
Cations: sodium, potassium; anions: chloride, sulfate, bicarbonate.
Respiratory-tract disorders.

Emsilat Siemens, Ger.†.
Eucalyptus oil (p.1609·2); pine needle oil.
Cold symptoms.

Emsogen
Scientific Hospital Supplies, Austral.; Scientific Hospital Supplies, Irl.; Nutricia, NZ; Scientific Hospital Supplies, NZ.
Preparation for enteral nutrition (p.1350·1).

Emsyn Compu, S.Afr.
Erythromycin estolate (p.201·2).
Bacterial infections.

Emtec-30 Technilab, Canad.
Paracetamol (p.71·2); codeine phosphate (p.25·2).
Cold symptoms; pain; upper respiratory-tract disorders.

Emthexat
Nycomed, Fin.; Nycomed, Norw.; Nycomed, Swed.
Methotrexate (p.553·2).
Malignant neoplasms; psoriasis; rheumatoid arthritis.

Emthexate
Nettopharma, Denm.; Pharmachemie, Israel; Asta Medica, NZ; Pharmachemie, S.Afr.; Pharmachemie, Singapore; Pras, Spain; Pharmachemie, Thai.
Methotrexate (p.553·2) or methotrexate sodium (p.553·2).
Malignant neoplasms; psoriasis; rheumatoid arthritis.

Emuclens Ovelle, Irl.
Cleanser in an emollient base.
Water-free cleansing.

Emucream Ovelle, Irl.
Emollient.
Dry skin.

Emu-K Pharmacia Upjohn, S.Afr.†.
Erythromycin estolate (p.201·2).
Bacterial infections.

Emulave
Rydelle, Fr.; Ovelle, Irl.; Johnson & Johnson, Ital.; Dermoteca, Port.†.
Avena (p.1583·1).
Soap substitute.

Emulax
Note.This name is used for preparations of different composition.
Hassle, Swed.
Cascara (p.1216·1); docusate sodium (p.1223·1).
Constipation.

British Dispensary, Thai.
Oral liquid: Liquid paraffin (p.1407·1); phenolphthalein (p.1244·1); carmellose sodium (p.1499·3).
Tablets: Bisacodyl (p.1212·2).
Constipation.

Emuliquen Laxante Lainco, Spain.
Sodium picosulfate (p.1249·3); paraffin (p.1407·1).
Formerly contained phenolphthalein and paraffin.
Constipation.

Emuliquen Simple Lainco, Spain.
Paraffin (p.1407·1).
Constipation.

Emulsan Leiras, Swed.†.
Fractionated soya oil (p.1378·1).
Contains fractionated egg lecithin.
Lipid infusion for parenteral nutrition.

Emulsao Scott SmithKline Beecham, Braz.
Cod-liver oil; soya oil; vitamin A; vitamin D; electrolytes (p.1350·1).
Nutritional supplement.

Emulsiderm
Dermal Laboratories, Irl.; Dermal, Israel; Dermal Laboratories, UK.
Isopropyl myristate (p.1409·2); liquid paraffin (p.1407·1); benzalkonium chloride (p.1133·2).
Dry skin conditions.

E-Mulsin Mucos, Ger.
Alpha tocoferil acetate (p.1394·1).
Vitamin E deficiency.

Emulsoil Paddock, USA.
Castor oil (p.1592·1).
Constipation.

Emu-V
Pharmacia Upjohn, Austral.; Pharmacia Upjohn, S.Afr.†.
Erythromycin (p.201·2).
Bacterial infections.

Emuvin Pharmacia Upjohn, Aust.†.
Erythromycin (p.201·2).
Bacterial infections.

E-Mycin
Alphapharm, Austral.; Alphapharm, Canad.†; Pharmacia Upjohn, Hong Kong; Pharmacia Upjohn, Israel; Pacific, NZ; Docmed, S.Afr.†; Pharmacia Upjohn, Singapore; Knoll, USA.
Erythromycin (p.201·2), erythromycin estolate (p.201·2), or erythromycin ethyl succinate (p.201·2).
Bacterial infections.

En Ravizza, Ital.
Delorazepam (p.674·2).
Anxiety disorders; sleep disorders.

Enacard Approved Prescription Services, UK.
Enalapril maleate (p.883·3).
Heart failure; hypertension.

Enada Health & Diet Food Co., UK.
Nadide (p.1639·3).
Chronic fatigue syndrome.

Enadil United Nordic, Denm.
Enalapril maleate (p.883·3).
Heart failure; hypertension.

enadura Merck dura, Ger.
Enalapril maleate (p.883·3).
Heart failure; hypertension.

Enahexal Hexal, Ger.
Enalapril maleate (p.883·3).
Heart failure; hypertension.

Enaladil Rhein, Mex.
Enalapril maleate (p.883·3).
Heart failure; hypertension.

Enalagamma Worwag, Ger.
Enalapril (p.883·3).
Heart failure; hypertension.

Enaloc Leiras, Fin.
Enalapril maleate (p.883·3).
Heart failure; hypertension.

Enaloc Comp Leiras, Fin.
Enalapril maleate (p.883·3); hydrochlorothiazide (p.907·3).
Hypertension.

Enam Neopharm, Thai.
Enalapril maleate (p.883·3).
Heart failure; hypertension.

Enanton
Orion, Denm.; Orion, Fin.; Orion, Norw.; Orion, Swed.
Leuprorelin acetate (p.1289·2).
Endometriosis; prostatic cancer; uterine leiomyomas.

Enantone
Takeda, Aust.; Takeda, Fr.; Takeda, Ger.; Takeda, Hong Kong; Takeda, Ital.; Takeda, Thai.
Leuprorelin acetate (p.1289·2).
Breast cancer; endometriosis; precocious puberty; prostatic cancer; uterine fibroids.

Enantone-Gyn Takeda, Ger.
Leuprorelin acetate (p.1289·2).
Breast cancer; endometriosis.

Enantyum
Menarini, Ital.; Menarini, Spain.
Dexketoprofen trometamol (p.47·3).
Pain.

Enap Rowex, Irl.
Enalapril maleate (p.883·3).
Heart failure; hypertension.

Enapren Merck Sharp & Dohme, Ital.
Enalapril maleate (p.883·3).
Heart failure; hypertension; ischaemic heart disease.

Enapril Sintofarma, Braz.
Enalapril maleate (p.883·3).
Heart failure; hypertension.

Enaril
Biolab, Singapore; Biolab, Thai.
Enalapril maleate (p.883·3).
Heart failure; hypertension.

Enatia Pentafarma, Port.
Enalapril maleate (p.883·3); hydrochlorothiazide (p.907·3).
Hypertension.

Enatus Medisint, Ital.
Iceland moss; plantago; althaea; aesculus; thyme; melissa; drosera; papaver.
Tonic.

Enbrel
Wyeth, UK; Immunex, USA.
Etanercept (p.1608·1).
Rheumatoid arthritis.

Encare
Stella, Canad.†; Thompson, USA.
Nonoxinol 9 (p.1346·1).
Contraceptive.

Encaskin Creme Farmalight, Port.
Salnacedin.
Acne.

Encaskin Detergente Farmalight, Port.
Salnacedin.
Skin wash.

Encebrin Lilly, Hong Kong.
Multivitamin and mineral preparation (p.1350·1).

Encefabol
Merck, Braz.; Bracco, Ital.
Pyritinol (p.1657·1) or pyritinol hydrochloride (p.1657·1).
Cerebrovascular disorders; impaired mental function.

Encegam Centeon, Ger.†; Chiron Behring, Ger.†.
A tick-borne encephalitis immunoglobulin (p.1539·3).
Passive immunisation.

Encelin Crosara, Ital.†.
Citicoline sodium (p.1596·1).
Cerebrovascular disorders; parkinsonism.

Encephabol
Merck, Aust.; Lipha Sante, Fr.; Merck, Ger.; Merck, Hong Kong; Merck, Mex.; Merck, S.Afr.; Merck, Singapore; Merck, Thai.
Pyritinol (p.1657·1) or pyritinol hydrochloride (p.1657·1).
Cerebrovascular disorders; impaired mental function.

Encepur
Chiron Behring, Aust.; Chiron Behring, Fin.; Chiron Behring, Ger.; Meda, Swed.
An inactivated tick-borne encephalitis vaccine (p.1539·3).
Separate preparations are available for infants and children and for older children and adults.
Active immunisation.

Encetrop Dumex, Ger.
Piracetam (p.1652·1).
Mental function disorders.

Encialina Bucca, Spain.
Aconite (p.1572·3); arnica (p.1581·3); ipecacuanha (p.1093·1); chamomile (p.1593·2); rhatany (p.1657·3); iodine (p.1522·3).
Mouth inflammation; pyorrhoea.

Encorate Sun, Singapore.
Sodium valproate (p.366·3).
Epilepsy.

Encypalmed Trima, Israel.
Pancreatin (p.1646·1); ox bile (p.1585·1); rhubarb (p.1248·1); frangula bark (p.1227·1); sodium bicarbonate (p.1186·2).
Dyspepsia; gastro-enteritis; meteorism.

End Lice Thompson, USA.
Pyrethrins; piperonyl butoxide (p.1436·2).
Pediculosis.

Endacil Sydenham, Mex.
Indometacin (p.44·3).

Endafed UAD, USA.
Pseudoephedrine hydrochloride (p.1099·2); brompheniramine maleate (p.410·2).
Allergic rhinitis; nasal congestion.

Endagen-HD Abana, USA.
Phenylephrine hydrochloride (p.1097·1); chlorpheniramine [chlorphenamine] maleate (p.412·1); hydrocodone tartrate (p.42·2).
Coughs and cold symptoms.

Endak
Madaus, Aust.†; Madaus, Ger.
Carteolol hydrochloride (p.855·1).
Angina pectoris; arrhythmias; hypertension; myocardial infarction.

Endal UAD, USA.
Phenylephrine hydrochloride (p.1097·1); guaifenesin (p.1092·2).
Coughs.

Endal Expectorant UAD, USA†.
Phenylpropanolamine hydrochloride (p.1098·1); guaifenesin (p.1092·2); codeine phosphate (p.25·2).
Coughs.

Endalbumin Alfa Biotech, Ital.†.
Albumin (p.724·1).
Hypoalbuminaemia.

Endal-HD Forest Pharmaceuticals, USA.
Chlorpheniramine [chlorphenamine] maleate (p.412·1); phenylephrine hydrochloride (p.1097·1); hydrocodone tartrate (p.42·2).
Coughs and cold symptoms.

Endal-HD Plus UAD, USA.
Chlorpheniramine [chlorphenamine] maleate (p.412·1); phenylephrine hydrochloride (p.1097·1); hydrocodone tartrate (p.42·2).
Coughs and cold symptoms.

Endantadine Endo, Canad.
Amantadine hydrochloride (p.1161·2).
Influenza A; parkinsonism.

Endcol SA Druggists Self Med, S.Afr.†.
Paracetamol (p.71·2); ascorbic acid (p.1389·3); phenylephrine hydrochloride (p.1097·1); chlorpheniramine [chlorphenamine] maleate (p.412·1); caffeine (p.761·3).
Cold symptoms.

Endcol Cold & Flu Aspen Consumer, S.Afr.
Paracetamol (p.71·2); vitamin C (p.1389·3); phenylephrine hydrochloride (p.1097·1); chlorpheniramine [chlorphenamine] maleate (p.412·1); caffeine (p.761·3).
Cold and influenza symptoms.

Endcol Cough Linctus SA Druggists Self Med, S.Afr.†.
Triprolidine hydrochloride (p.427·2); pseudoephedrine hydrochloride (p.1099·2); codeine phosphate (p.25·2).
Coughs.

Endcol Decongestant SA Druggists Self Med, S.Afr.†.
Triprolidine hydrochloride (p.427·2); pseudoephedrine hydrochloride (p.1099·2).
Cold symptoms.

En-De-Kay Manx, UK.
Sodium fluoride (p.1375·3).
Dental caries prophylaxis.

Endep
Alphapharm, Austral.; Rolab, S.Afr.
Amitriptyline hydrochloride (p.273·1).
Now known as Rolab-Amitriptyline HCl in S.Afr.
Depression; nocturnal enuresis.

Endermyl Galderma, Canad.
Emollient.
Dry skin.

Endiaron Medphano, Ger.
Loperamide hydrochloride (p.1231·3).
Diarrhoea.

Endium Dexo, Fr.
Diosmin (p.1611·1).
Haemorrhoids; peripheral vascular disorders.

Endobil Gerot, Aust.†; Merck, Irl.
Meglumine iodoxamate (p.1034·3).
Contrast medium for cholecystography and cholangiography.

Endobulin
Immuno, Aust.; Baxter, Denm.; Baxter, Fin.; Baxter, Fr.; Immuno, Ger.; Immuno, Israel; Immuno, Ital.; Adcock-Ingram Critical Care, S.Afr.; Baxter, Spain; Baxter, Swed.; Baxter, Switz.; Immuno, UK†.
A normal immunoglobulin (p.1551·3).
Hypogammaglobulinaemia; idiopathic thrombocytopenic purpura; immunodeficiency disorders; Kawasaki disease; passive immunisation.

Endocal Pisa, Mex.
Salcatonin (p.749·3).

Endocet Endo, Canad.
Oxycodone hydrochloride (p.70·2); paracetamol (p.71·2).
Fever; pain.

Endocodone Endo, USA.
Oxycodone hydrochloride (p.70·2).
Pain.

Endocris Cristalia, Braz.
Sodium laurilsulfate (p.1496·3).
Dental disorders.

Endodan Endo, USA.
Oxycodone hydrochloride (p.70·2); aspirin (p.14·2).
Fever; inflammation; pain.

Endofalk Falk, Ger.
Macrogol 3350 (p.1630·3); electrolytes (p.1180·1).
Bowel cleansing for endoscopy.

The symbol † denotes a preparation no longer actively marketed

Endofolin Marjan, Braz.
Folic acid (p.1361·1).
Anaemias; folic acid deficiency.

Endogest Siam Bheasach, Thai.
Amylase (p.1579·3); vitamin B₁ (p.1385·2); scopolia; sodium bicarbonate (p.1186·2); calcium carbonate (p.1215·1).
Dyspepsia; gastric hyperacidity; gastritis; gastrointestinal motility disorders; heartburn.

Endol Cruz, Spain†.
Tiadenol (p.980·1).
Hyperlipidaemias.

Endolipid Darrow, Braz.
Lipid emulsion (p.1350·1).
Parenteral nutrition.

Endolipide Braun, Fr.
Soya oil (p.1378·1).
Contains egg lecithin.
Lipid infusion for parenteral nutrition.

Endolor Keene, USA.
Paracetamol (p.71·2); caffeine (p.761·3); butalbital (p.658·3).
Pain.

Endomethasone Septodont, Switz.†
Powder, hydrocortisone acetate (p.1073·3); thymol iodide (p.1158·3); barium sulfate (p.1032·1); liquid, eugenol (p.1609·3); peppermint oil (p.1243·3); anise oil (p.1580·3).
Root canal sealant.

Endomethazone Austrodent, Aust.
Dexamethasone (p.1067·1); hydrocortisone acetate (p.1073·3).
Root canal filling.

Endone Boots, Austral.
Oxycodone hydrochloride (p.70·2).
Pain.

Endoneutralio Crosara, Ital.†
Sodium citrate (p.1186·2); potassium citrate (p.1186·1).
Gastric hyperacidity.

Endopancrine 40 Organon, Fr.†
Insulin injection (crystalline) (porcine, highly purified) (p.324·1).
Diabetes mellitus.

Endopancrine 100 Organon, Fr.†
Insulin zinc suspension (porcine, highly purified) (p.324·1).
Diabetes mellitus.

Endopancrine Protamine Organon, Fr.†
Isophane insulin injection (crystalline) (porcine, highly purified) (p.324·1).
Diabetes mellitus.

Endopancrine Zinc Protamine Organon, Fr.†
A protamine zinc insulin suspension (porcine, highly purified) (p.324·1).
Diabetes mellitus.

Endo-Paractol Temmler, Ger.
Simeticone (p.1249·2).
Adjuvant for endoscopy and double contrast radiography.

Endophleban Rentschler, Ger.†
Dihydroergotamine mesilate (p.450·3).
Chronic venous insufficiency; hypotension; migraine and related vascular headache.

Endoprost Italfarmaco, Ital.
Iloprost trometamol (p.1445·2).
Buerger's disease.

Endorem Guerbet, Aust.; Codali, Belg.; Guerbet, Denm.; Guerbet, Fin.; Guerbet, Fr.; Guerbet, Ger.; Farmades, Ital.; Guerbet, Neth.†; Guerbet, Norw.; Guerbet, Port.; Guerbert, Spain; Gothia, Swed.; Guerbet, Switz.
Ferumoxides (p.1032·3).
Contrast medium for magnetic resonance imaging of the liver.

Endorphenyl Tyson, USA†.
Phenylalanine (p.1374·2).

Endosalil Elofar, Braz.
Aspirin (p.14·2).
Fever; inflammation; pain; thromboembolism prophylaxis.

Endosgel Solco, Aust.; Farco, Ger.; Almed, Switz.†
Chlorhexidine gluconate (p.1138·2); sodium lactate (p.1186·2).
Aid to endoscopy and catheterisation.

Endosporine Peters, Fr.
Glutaral (p.1145·2).
Instrument disinfection.

Endospray Axcan, Canad.
Benzocaine (p.1306·2); amethocaine [tetracaine] hydrochloride (p.1305·2).
Local anaesthesia.

Endotelon Sanofi Winthrop, Fr.
Grape seeds.
Lymphoedema; peripheral vascular disorders.

Endoxan Asta Medica, Aust.; Asta Medica, Austral.; Asta Medica, Belg.; Asta Medica, Fr.; Asta Medica, Ger.; Asta Medica, Hong Kong; Asta Medica, Ital.; Asta Medica, Mex.; Asta Medica, NZ; Baxter, NZ; Asta Medica, Port.; Aventis, S.Afr.; Asta Medica, Singapore; Asta Medica, Switz.
Cyclophosphamide (p.527·3).
Auto-immune disorders; malignant neoplasms.

Endoxana Asta Medica, Thai.; Asta Medica, UK.
Cyclophosphamide (p.527·3).
Malignant neoplasms.

Endrate Abbott, USA.
Disodium edetate (p.1008·1).
Digitalis-induced cardiac arrhythmias; hypercalcaemia.

Endrine
Wyeth Lederle, Aust.; Christiaens, Belg.
Ephedrine (p.1090·1); camphor (p.1589·3); menthol (p.1632·3); eucalyptol (p.1609·2).
Cold symptoms.

Endrine Doux Christiaens, Belg.
Ephedrine (p.1090·1); camphor (p.1589·3); eucalyptol (p.1609·2).
Cold symptoms.

Endrine mild Wyeth Lederle, Aust.
Ephedrine (p.1090·1); camphor (p.1589·3); eucalyptol (p.1609·2).
Catarrh; rhinitis.

Endronax Sintofarma, Braz.
Alendronate sodium (p.747·2).
Bone metastases; hypercalcaemia; osteoporosis; Paget's disease of bone.

Enduron Abbott, Austral.†; Abbott, Hong Kong; Abbott, USA.
Methyclothiazide (p.927·3).
Hypertension; oedema.

Enduronil Abbott, Ital.
Methyclothiazide (p.927·3); deserpidine (p.867·2).
Hypertension.

Enduronyl Abbott, Hong Kong; Abbott, USA.
Methyclothiazide (p.927·3); deserpidine (p.867·2).
Hypertension.

Enduxan Abbott, Braz.
Cyclophosphamide (p.527·3).
Malignant neoplasms.

Enecat Lafayette, USA†.
Barium sulfate (p.1032·1).
Contrast medium for gastrointestinal radiography.

Enelbin-Paste N Cassella-med, Ger.
Zinc oxide (p.1128·2); salicylic acid (p.1122·3); aluminium silicate (p.1211·3).
Inflammation.

Enelbin-Salbe N Cassella-med, Ger.
Heparin sodium (p.902·1); salicylic acid (p.1122·3).
Muscle, joint, and soft-tissue disorders.

Enelbin-Venen Salbe Cassella-med, Ger.†
Heparin sodium (p.902·1).
Soft-tissue injury; superficial vascular disorders.

Enelfa
Sanova, Aust.; Dolorgiet, Ger.
Paracetamol (p.71·2).
Fever; pain.

Enema Casen Casen Fleet, Spain.
Dibasic sodium phosphate (p.1193·2); monobasic sodium phosphate (p.1193·2).
Bowel evacuation.

Enemac Eurospital, Ital.
Monobasic sodium phosphate (p.1193·2); dibasic sodium phosphate (p.1193·2).
Bowel evacuation; constipation.

Enemol Pharmascience, Canad.
Dibasic sodium phosphate (p.1193·2); monobasic sodium phosphate (p.1193·2).
Laxative.

Ener-B Nature's Bounty, USA†.
Vitamin B₁₂ (p.1388·1).
Dietary supplement.

Enercal Plus Wyeth, Singapore.
Lactose-free nutritional supplement (p.1350·1).

Enercomplex Provita, Ital.
Mineral preparation with vitamin C, carnitine, creatine, and ginseng (p.1350·1).
Tonic.

Ener-E Wassen, Ital.
Vitamin E (p.1393·3); ubidecarenone (p.1677·1).
Nutritional supplement.

Ener-G General Dietary, UK.
Gluten-free bread, flour bran, and pasta (p.1350·1).
Gluten-sensitive enteropathies.

Energeia Sanitalia, Ital.
Ginseng; ginkgo biloba; eleuterococcus; minerals (p.1350·1).
Nutritional supplement.

Energen Volchem, Ital.
Glucose (p.1364·1) or maltodextrin (p.1371·2).
Energy loss; hypoglycaemia.

Energex Fort Frega, Canad.†.
Multivitamin and mineral preparation (p.1350·1).

Energil C Legrand, Braz.
Ascorbic acid (p.1389·3).
Vitamin C supplement.

Energisan Ache, Braz.
Vitamin B substances; fructose; succinic dinitrile (p.1350·1).
Tonic.

Energitum SmithKline Beecham Sante, Fr.†
Arginine glutamate (p.1353·3).
Tonic.

Energivit
Note.This name is used for preparations of different composition.
Scientific Hospital Supplies, Austral.; Scientific Hospital Supplies, UK.
Nutritional supplement for infants and children (p.1350·1).

Ache, Braz.
Piracetam (p.1652·1); fructose; vitamin B substances; ascorbic acid; tocopherol acetate (p.1350·1).
Alcoholism; behaviour disorders in children; cerebrovascular disorders; senile dementia; vertigo.

Energona Maurer, Ger.
Norfenefrine hydrochloride (p.949·1).
Hypotension.

Energoplex Libbs, Braz.
Vitamins; fructose; arginine (p.1350·1).
Nutritional supplement.

Energy Alfa Dolisos, Canad.
Homoeopathic preparation.

Energyn-T DHA, Singapore.
Multivitamin and mineral preparation (p.1350·1).

Enerjets Chilton, USA.
Caffeine (p.761·3).
Fatigue.

Ener-Mix Also, Ital.
Multivitamin and mineral preparation (p.1350·1).

Enertonic Bifarma, Ital.
Eleutherococcus senticosis (p.1615·3); ginkgo biloba (p.1615·2); guarana (p.1681·1); echinacea (p.1606·2).
Dietary supplement.

Enervit
EMS, Braz.; Also, Ital.
A range of nutritional supplements (p.1350·1).

Enervon-C
United American, Hong Kong; United American, Singapore; Great Eastern, Thai.; United American, Thai.
Vitamin B substances and vitamin C (p.1350·1).

United American, Singapore.
Syrup: Multivitamin preparation (p.1350·1).

Enervon-C Plus United American, Hong Kong.
Multivitamin preparation (p.1350·1).

Enfalac AR
Mead Johnson, Canad.; Mead Johnson Nutritionals, Canad.; Mead Johnson, NZ.
Infant feed (p.1350·1).
Gastro-oesophageal reflux.

Enfalac HA Mead Johnson, Port.
Infant feed (p.1350·1).
Milk intolerance.

Enfalac Lactofree Mead Johnson Nutritionals, Canad.
Lactose-free infant feed (p.1350·1).
Formerly known as Enfalac Lactose Free.
Lactose intolerance.

Enfalac Lytren Mead Johnson Nutritionals, Canad.
Glucose; potassium citrate; sodium chloride; sodium citrate; citric acid (p.1185·2).
Diarrhoea.

Enfalac Nutramigen Mead Johnson Nutritionals, Canad.
Gluten-free, lactose-free casein hydrolysate preparation for special diets (p.1350·1).
Galactosaemia; protein sensitivity.

Enfalac Pregestimil Mead Johnson Nutritionals, Canad.
Infant feed (p.1350·1).
Malabsorption syndromes.

Enfalac Prosobee Soy Mead Johnson Nutritionals, Canad.
Soy based infant feed (p.1350·1).
Hypersensitivity to cow's milk.

Enfamil AR
Mead Johnson, Hong Kong; Mead Johnson, Irl.; Mead Johnson, Port.; Mead Johnson Nutritionals, UK.
Infant feed (p.1350·1).
Gastro-oesophageal reflux.

Enfamil Lactofree Mead Johnson, Irl.
Infant feed (p.1350·1).
Lactose intolerance.

Enfamil Natalins Rx Mead Johnson Nutritionals, USA.
Multivitamin and mineral preparation (p.1350·1).
Formerly known as Natalins Rx.

Enfran Pisa, Mex.
Enflurane (p.1258·1).
General anaesthesia.

Engerix-B
SmithKline Beecham, Aust.; SmithKline Beecham, Austral.; SmithKline Beecham, Belg.; SmithKline Beecham, Braz.; SmithKline Beecham, Canad.; SmithKline Beecham, Denm.; SmithKline Beecham, Fin.; SmithKline Beecham, Fr.; SmithKline Beecham, Ger.; SSW, Ger.; SmithKline Beecham, Hong Kong; SmithKline Beecham, Irl.; SmithKline Beecham, Israel; SmithKline Beecham, Ital.; SmithKline Beecham, Mex.; SmithKline Beecham, Neth.; SmithKline Beecham, Norw.; SmithKline Beecham, NZ; Smith Kline & French, Port.; SmithKline Beecham, S.Afr.; SmithKline Beecham, Singapore; SmithKline, Spain; SmithKline Beecham, Swed.; SmithKline Beecham, Switz.; SmithKline Beecham, Thai.; SmithKline Beecham, UK; SmithKline Beecham, USA.
A hepatitis B vaccine (recombinant DNA) (p.1542·2).
Active immunisation.

Engov Newlab, Braz.
Aspirin (p.14·2); caffeine (p.761·3); mepyramine (p.421·1).
Aluminium hydroxide (p.1210·3) is included in this preparation in an attempt to limit adverse effects on the gastrointestinal mucosa.
Fever; pain.

Engystol Heel, Ger.
Homoeopathic preparation.

Engystol N Heel, Ger.; Heel, S.Afr.
Homoeopathic preparation.

Enhancin Ranbaxy, Singapore.
Amoxicillin (p.149·2); potassium clavulanate (p.187·2).
Bacterial infections.

Eni Grossman, Mex.
Ciprofloxacin hydrochloride (p.182·3).
Bacterial infections.

Enicul Apomedica, Aust.
Magnesium trisilicate (p.1233·3); algeldrate (p.1210·3); ammonium glycyrrhizinate (p.1085·2).
Gastrointestinal disorders.

Enirant Gepepharm, Ger.
Co-dergocrine mesilate (p.1597·3).
Cerebral circulatory disorders; hypertension.

Enison Lilly, Spain.
Vindesine sulfate (p.580·1).
Malignant neoplasms.

Enjomin Codilab, Port.
Dimenhydrinate (p.415·2).
Motion sickness; nausea; vomiting.

Enjoy Heralds, Braz.
Aspirin (p.14·2); mepyramine (p.421·1).
Aluminium hydroxide (p.1210·3) is included in this preparation in an attempt to limit adverse effects on the gastrointestinal mucosa.
Fever; pain.

Enlirane Zeneca, Mex.
Enflurane (p.1258·1).
General anaesthesia.

Enlive Abbott, Austral.; Abbott, Irl.; Abbott, Ital.; Abbott Nutrition, UK.
A range of products for enteral nutrition (p.1350·1).

Enlon AstraZeneca, Canad.; Baxter, USA.
Edrophonium chloride (p.1418·2).
Differential diagnosis of myasthenia gravis; reversal of competitive neuromuscular blockade.

Enlon-Plus Baxter, USA.
Edrophonium chloride (p.1418·2).
Atropine sulfate (p.461·1) is included in this preparation to protect against the muscarinic actions.
Curare antagonist; reversal of competitive neuromuscular blockade.

Eno
Note.This name is used for preparations of different composition.
Reckitt & Colman, Austral.; SmithKline Beecham, Ital.†; SmithKline Beecham Consumer, UK.
Citric acid (p.1596·2); sodium bicarbonate (p.1186·2); anhydrous sodium carbonate (p.1665·1).
Dyspepsia; flatulence; nausea.

SmithKline Beecham Consumer, Canad.
Sodium citrate (p.1186·2).
Dyspepsia.

SmithKline Beecham, Israel.
Sodium bicarbonate (p.1186·2); tartaric acid (p.1669·2); citric acid (p.1596·2).
Dyspepsia; flatulence.

Sterling, Port.
Citric acid (p.1596·2); sodium carbonate (p.1665·1).

Enofosforina Vigor Serra Pamies, Spain.
Calcium lactophosphate; magnesium glycerophosphate; kola; pyridoxine; sodium glycerophosphate; potassium glycerophosphate; nicotinamide; glycerol (p.1350·1).
Tonic.

Enomdan Pharmacia Upjohn, Swed.
Multivitamin preparation (p.1350·1).

Enomine Major, USA†.
Phenylpropanolamine hydrochloride (p.1098·1); guaifenesin (p.1092·2); phenylephrine hydrochloride (p.1097·1).
Coughs.

Enoton Pensa, Spain.
Cyproheptadine aspartate (p.414·3); mecobalamin (p.1388·3).
Anorexia; tonic; weight loss.

Enovid Searle, USA†.
Noretynodrel (p.1486·1); mestranol (p.1482·1).
Endometriosis; hypermenorrhoea; production of cyclical withdrawal bleeding.

Enoxen C & RF, Ital.
Enoxacin (p.201·1).
Bacterial infections.

Enoxin Faulding, Austral.
Enoxacin (p.201·1).
Bacterial infections.

Enoxor Sinbio, Fr.; Pierre Fabre, Fr.
Enoxacin (p.201·1).
Bacterial infections.

Enpott Ranbaxy, Thai.
Potassium chloride (p.1194·3).
Hypokalaemia.

Enpovax HDC CSL, Austral.
An inactivated poliomyelitis vaccine (p.1558·2).
Active immunisation.

Enpresse Duramed, USA.
Levonorgestrel (p.1486·2); ethinylestradiol (p.1476·2).
Triphasic oral contraceptive.

Enprin Galpharm, UK.
Aspirin (p.14·2).
Thrombosis prophylaxis.

Enrich
Abbott, Fr.; Abbott, Fr.; Abbott, Irl.; Abbott, Ital.; Abbott, Switz.; Abbott Nutrition, UK.
Preparation for enteral nutrition (p.1350·1).

Ensinger Schiller-Quelle Heilwasser Ensinger, Ger.
Electrolytes (p.1180·1); silicic acid; boric acid (p.1586·1); carbon dioxide (p.1198·2).
Gastrointestinal disorders; urinary-tract infections.

Ensini Nutricia, Fin.
Preparation for enteral nutrition (p.1350·1).

Ensure
Abbott, Austral.; Abbott, Braz.; Abbott, Fin.; Abbott, Hong Kong; Abbott, Irl.; Abbott, Israel; Abbott, Ital.; Abbott, NZ; Abbott, Singapore; Abbott, Switz.; Abbott, Thai.; Abbott Nutrition, UK; Ross, USA.
A range of preparations for enteral nutrition (p.1350·1).

Ensure Plus
Abbott, Hong Kong; Abbott, Irl.; Abbott, Ital.; Abbott, Singapore; Abbott, Switz.; Abbott Nutrition, UK.
High calorie preparation for enteral nutrition (p.1350·1).

ENT
Note.This name is used for preparations of different composition.
Iomed, Hong Kong; Ion, USA†.
Phenylpropanolamine hydrochloride (p.1098·1); brompheniramine maleate (p.410·2).
Nasal congestion; sinusitis.

Covan, S.Afr.
Phenylephrine hydrochloride (p.1097·1); naphazoline nitrate (p.1095·1).
Nasal congestion.

Entacyl Roberts, Canad.
Piperazine adipate (p.105·3).
Ascariasis; enterobiasis.

Entalgic Salters, S.Afr.
Paracetamol (p.71·2).
Fever; pain.

Entamizole Sovereign, UK.
Diloxanide furoate (p.590·3); metronidazole (p.594·1).
Amoebiasis.

Entecet Sorin-Maxim, Fr.
Hordeum sativum germ; enzymes derived from aspergillus including amylase and protease; lipase derived from rhizopus.
Dyspepsia.

Entera Rowa, Irl.†
Preparation for enteral nutrition (p.1350·1).
Formerly known as Fresium High Energy.

Enteral 400 Scientific Hospital Supplies, UK.
Preparation for enteral nutrition (p.1350·1).

Enterasin Crinos, Ital.
Mesalazine (p.1234·1).
Crohn's disease; ulcerative colitis.

Entercal Luper, Braz.
Co-trimoxazole (p.193·3); attapulgite (p.1212·1).
Diarrhoea.

Enterex Pisa, Mex.
Preparation for enteral nutrition (p.1350·1).

Entermid Nakornpatana, Thai.
Loperamide hydrochloride (p.1231·3).
Diarrhoea.

Entero Heractrin Heralds, Braz.
Co-trimoxazole (p.193·3); calcium carbonate (p.1215·1).
Diarrhoea.

Enterobacticel Armstrong, Mex.
Co-trimoxazole (p.193·3).

Enterobene Ratiopharm, Aust.
Loperamide hydrochloride (p.1231·3).
Diarrhoea.

Enterobion Makros, Braz.
Furazolidone (p.592·1); homatropine (p.468·1); pectin (p.1502·3).
Diarrhoea.

Enterocare Phytocare, Austral.
Ispaghula (p.1229·1); plum; black currant (p.1389·3); slippery elm (p.1665·1); Lactobacillus acidophilus (p.1626·3); pectin (p.1502·3); sterculia (p.1250·2).
Constipation.

Enterocler Heralds, Braz.
Neomycin (p.228·1); attapulgite (p.1212·1); pectin (p.1502·3); electroytes (p.1180·1).
Diarrhoea.

Enterodina Luper, Braz.
Neomycin (p.228·1); sulfadiazine (p.251·1); phthalylsulfathiazole (p.235·3); pectin (p.1502·3).
Diarrhoea.

Entero-Diyod Serral, Mex.
Diiodohydroxyquinoline (p.590·2).
Amoebiasis; giardiasis; shigellosis; trichomoniasis.

Enterodrip Diepal, Fr.†
Preparation for enteral nutrition (p.1350·1).

Enterodyne Adcock Ingram, S.Afr.
Bismuth carbonate (p.1213·1); calcium carbonate (p.1215·1); chloroform and morphine tincture (p.56·1); aromatic ammonia liquid (p.1579·1); nutmeg oil (p.1643·1); clove oil (p.1597·1); cardamom tincture (p.1591·3); catechu tincture (p.1592·3); conc. cinnamon water; cinnamon oil (p.1596·1).
Gastrointestinal disorders.

Enteroftal Windson, Braz.
Neomycin (p.228·1); sulfaguanidine (p.253·2); phthalylsulfathiazole (p.235·3); ceratonia (p.1500·3).
Diarrhoea.

Enterogermina Sanofi Synthelabo, Ital.
Spores of Bacillus subtilis.
Gastrointestinal disorders.

Enterogil Diepal, Fr.†
Preparation for enteral nutrition (p.1350·1).

Enterol Merck, Port.
Saccharomyces boulardii (p.1626·3).
Gastrointestinal disorders.

Enterolyte Propan, S.Afr.
Kaolin (p.1229·3); pectin (p.1502·3); sodium lactate; potassium chloride; sodium chloride (p.1185·2).
Diarrhoea.

Enteromicina
Note.This name is used for preparations of different composition.
Gross, Braz.
Streptomycin sulfate (p.249·1); phthalylsulfathiazole (p.235·3); menadione (p.1395·3).
Diarrhoea.

Produfarma, Port.
Neomycin sulfate (p.228·1).

Enteromix Bioprogress, Ital.
Piromidic acid (p.237·1).
Bacterial infections of the gastrointestinal tract.

Enteromucilage Bayer, Fr.†
Sterculia (p.1250·2).
Constipation.

Enterone Heralds, Braz.
Co-trimoxazole (p.193·3).
Bacterial infections; Pneumocystis carinii pneumonia; protozoal infections.

Enteronorm Apsen, Braz.
Loperamide hydrochloride (p.1231·3).
Diarrhoea.

Enteropathyl Monot, Fr.
Sulfaguanidine (p.253·2).

Enteropen Cazi, Braz.
Attapulgite (p.1212·1); pectin (p.1502·3); homatropine (p.468·1).
Diarrhoea.

Enteroplant Schwabe, Ger.; Spitzner, Ger.
Peppermint oil (p.1243·3); caraway oil (p.1591·2).
Dyspepsia.

Enteropride
Cilag, Braz.; Cilag, Mex.
Cisapride (p.1220·1).
Gastro-oesophageal reflux; gastrointestinal motility disorders.

Enterosan Monmouth, UK†.
Light kaolin (p.1229·3); morphine hydrochloride (p.56·1); belladonna (p.463·1).
Diarrhoea.

Enterosilicona Estedi, Spain.
Dimethicone (p.1249·2).
Flatulence; infant colic; meteorism.

Enterostop Teofarma, Ital.
Bacitracin (p.155·2); neomycin sulfate (p.228·1).
Gastrointestinal infections.

Entero-Teknosal Taco, Ger.
Colloidal silicon dioxide (p.1503·3).
Diarrhoea.

Enterotonus Breves, Braz.
Physostigmine (p.1421·3); atropine (p.460·3); cascara (p.1216·1).
Constipation.

Enterovaccino ISI (Antitifico) ISI, Ital.
A killed oral typhoid vaccine (p.1566·3).
Active immunisation.

Enterovaccino Nuovo ISM ISM, Ital.†.
A killed oral typhoid vaccine (p.1566·3).
Active immunisation.

Enterozol Dinafarma, Braz.
Neomycin sulfate (p.228·1); sulfadiazine (p.251·1).
Diarrhoea.

Entertainer's Secret KLI, USA.
Aloe vera (p.1110·1); carmellose sodium (p.1499·3); glycerol (p.1616·3).
Formerly known as Moi-Stir 10.
Throat discomfort.

Entex
Note.This name is used for preparations of different composition.
Purdue Frederick, Canad.†.
Phenylpropanolamine hydrochloride (p.1098·1); guaifenesin (p.1092·2).
Upper respiratory-tract congestion.

Andrx, USA.
Phenylephrine hydrochloride (p.1097·1); guaifenesin (p.1092·2).
Formerly contained phenylephrine hydrochloride, phenylpropanolamine hydrochloride, and guaifenesin.
Coughs and cold symptoms; nasal congestion.

Entex HC Andrx, USA.
Hydrocodone tartrate (p.42·2); phenylephrine hydrochloride (p.1097·1); guaifenesin (p.1092·2).
Coughs.

Entex LA Andrx, USA.
Phenylephrine hydrochloride (p.1097·1); guaifenesin (p.1092·2).
Formerly contained phenylpropanolamine hydrochloride and guaifenesin.
Respiratory-tract congestion.

Entex PSE Dura, USA.
Pseudoephedrine hydrochloride (p.1099·2); guaifenesin (p.1092·2).
Coughs; nasal congestion.

Entir
Unison, Singapore.; Unison, Thai.
Aciclovir (p.612·3).
Herpesvirus infections.

Entocord
Astra, S.Afr.; Astra, Spain.
Budesonide (p.1064·2).
Crohn's disease; ulcerative colitis.

Entocort
Astra, Aust.; Astra, Austral.; AstraZeneca, Canad.; AstraZeneca, Denm.; AstraZeneca, Fin.; AstraZeneca, Fr.; Astra, Ger.; Astra, Hong Kong; Astra, Irl.; Abic, Israel; Astra, Neth.; AstraZeneca, Norw.; AstraZeneca, NZ; AstraZeneca, Singapore; Tika, Swed.; Astra, Switz.; AstraZeneca, UK; AstraZeneca, USA.
Budesonide (p.1064·2).
Inflammatory bowel disease.

Entodiba Diba, Mex.
Diiodohydroxyquinoline (p.590·2).
Amoebiasis.

Entom Dynacren, Ital.
Diethyltoluamide (p.1431·2); piperonyl butoxide (p.1436·2); pyrethrum (p.1436·3).
Insect repellent.

Entom Nature Dynacren, Ital.
Geranium oil (p.1615·1).
Insect repellent.

Entonox BOC, UK.
Nitrous oxide (p.1264·3); oxygen (p.1199·3).
Obstructive airways disease; pain.

Entoplus Diba, Mex.
Albendazole (p.95·2).
Worm infections.

Entosorbine-N Roche Consumer, Neth.
Albumin tannate (p.1209·3).
Diarrhoea.

Entox-P Wyeth-Ayerst, Thai.
Activated attapulgite (p.1212·1).
Diarrhoea.

Entrarin Asian Pharm, Thai.
Aspirin (p.14·2).
Fever; inflammation; pain.

Entrin Acidophilus Murdock, USA†.
Lactobacillus rhamnosus (p.1626·3); Lactobacillus acidophilus (p.1626·3).

Entrin Bifidus Murdock, USA†.
Bifidobacterium longum; Bifidobacterium breve; Lactobacillus rhamnosus; Lactobacillus acidophilus (p.1626·3).

Entrition Clintec, USA.
A range of lactose-free preparations for enteral nutrition (p.1350·1).

Entrobar Lafayette, USA.
Barium sulfate (p.1032·1).
Contrast medium for gastrointestinal radiography.

Entrocalm Galpharm, UK.
Capsules: Loperamide hydrochloride (p.1231·3).
Tablets: Kaolin (p.1229·3).
Diarrhoea.

Entrocalm Replace Galpharm, UK.
Glucose monohydrate; sodium chloride; potassium chloride; sodium citrate; citric acid (p.1185·2).
Oral rehydration therapy.

Entrodyn Ravensberg, Ger.
Phenylephrine (p.1097·1); caffeine (p.761·3).
Hypotension.

Entrophen Johnson & Johnson, Canad.
Aspirin (p.14·2).
Fever; musculoskeletal and joint disorders; myocardial infarction; pain; transient ischaemic attacks.

Entrotabs Monmouth, UK.
Aluminium hydroxide (p.1210·3); attapulgite (p.1212·1); pectin (p.1502·3).
Diarrhoea; dyspepsia.

Entrydil Orion, Irl.
Diltiazem hydrochloride (p.874·3).
Angina pectoris; hypertension.

Entschlackender Abfuhrtee Smetana, Aust.
Senna (p.1248·2); equisetum (p.1606·3); sambucus (p.1660·3); calcatrippae flowers.
Constipation.

Entschlackungstee Sanova, Aust.
Silver birch (p.1585·2); taraxacum (p.1669·1); prunus spinosa; rose fruit (p.1389·3).
Herbal preparation.

Entumin Novartis, Ital.
Clotiapine (p.671·1).
Anxiety disorders; psychoses.

Entumine Novartis, Switz.
Clotiapine (p.671·1).
Alcohol withdrawal syndrome; anxiety disorders; hyperactivity; psychoses; sleep disorders.

Enturen Cida Vision, Israel.
Sulfinpyrazone (p.402·2).
Thromboembolic disorders.

Entuss Expectorant Roberts, USA; Hauck, USA.
Oral liquid: Hydrocodone tartrate (p.42·2); sulfogaiacol (p.1101·1).
Tablets: Hydrocodone tartrate (p.42·2); guaifenesin (p.1092·2).
Coughs.

Entuss-D Roberts, USA.
Liquid: Hydrocodone tartrate (p.42·2); pseudoephedrine hydrochloride (p.1099·2).

Tablets: Hydrocodone tartrate (p.42·2); pseudoephedrine hydrochloride (p.1099·2); guaifenesin (p.1092·2).
Coughs.

Entuss-D Jr Roberts, USA.
Hydrocodone tartrate (p.42·2); pseudoephedrine hydrochloride (p.1099·2); guaifenesin (p.1092·2).
Coughs.

Entzundungstropfen Cosmochema, Ger.
Homoeopathic preparation.

Enuclen N Alcon, Ger.
Tyloxapol (p.1349·3).
Cleansing and lubrication of eye prostheses.

Enuclene
Alcon, Canad.; Alcon, NZ; Alcon, USA.
Tyloxapol (p.1349·3).
Lubrication, cleaning, and wetting of artificial eyes.

Enulose Barre-National, USA.
Lactulose (p.1230·1).
Hepatic encephalopathy.

EnurAid Hylands, Canad.
Homoeopathic preparation.

Enuretine Le Marchand, Fr.†
Isopropamide iodide (p.470·1); vitamin E (p.1393·3); thiamine (p.1385·2); ephedrine hydrochloride (p.1090·1); phenobarbital (p.355·1).
Urinary incontinence.

Enuroplant DHU, Ger.
Homoeopathic preparation.

Enveloppements ECR ECR, Switz.†.
Hay flowers; chamomile (p.1593·2); achillea (p.1572·2); linseed (p.1629·1); equisetum (p.1606·3).
Cold symptoms.

Enviro-Stress Vitaline, USA.
Vitamin B substances with vitamin C and minerals (p.1350·1).

Enxak Luitpold, Braz.
Ergotamine tartrate (p.452·1).
Migraine and other vascular headaches.

Enzace Sigma, Austral.
Captopril (p.853·3).
Diabetic nephropathy; heart failure; hypertension; myocardial infarction.

Enziagil Magenplus Serturner, Ger.
Gentian (p.1615·1).
Digestive system disorders.

Enzicoba Farmasa, Braz.
Cobamamide (p.1388·3).
Reduced appetite; tonic.

Enzipan Ravizza, Ital.
Pancreatin (p.1646·1).
Pancreatic disorders.

Enziprid Brasmedica, Braz.
Bromopride (p.1215·1); lipase; amylase (p.1579·3).
Digestive-system disorders; nausea and vomiting.

Enzivital Farmasa, Braz.
Cobamamide; carnitine; lysine; vitamin B substances (p.1350·1).
Tonic.

Enzone UAD, USA.
Hydrocortisone acetate (p.1073·3); pramocaine (p.1318·2).

Enzyflat Solvay, Aust.
Pancreatin (p.1646·1); dimethicone (p.1249·2).
Flatulence; meteorism; preparation for gastrointestinal radiography and ultrasound.

Enzymatic Cleaner Alcon, USA.
Pancreatin (p.1646·1) (p.1129·2).
Cleansing solution for soft contact lenses.

Enzyme
Note.This name is used for preparations of different composition.
GNLD, USA.
Pancreatin (p.1646·1); pepsin (p.1649·3); ox bile (p.1585·1); papain (p.1647·3); amylase (p.1579·3).
Digestive disorders.

Nature's Bounty, USA.
Amylase (p.1579·3); cellulase (p.1593·1); lipase; protease.
Gastrointestinal disorders.

Enzyme Digest Quest, UK.
Betaine hydrochloride (p.1584·3); papain (p.1647·3); bromelain (p.1586·3); amylase (p.1579·3).

Enzymet Ranbaxy, Thai.
Pancreatin (p.1646·1); simeticone (p.1249·2).
Digestive system disorders; flatulence.

Enzym-Harongan Schwabe, Ger.
Harongae; curcuma zanthorrhiza; pancreas.
Digestive system disorders.

Enzym-Lefax Asche, Ger.
Pancreatin (p.1646·1); simeticone (p.1249·2).
Digestive system disorders.

Enzym-Wied Wiedemann, Ger.
Pancreatin (p.1646·1); bromelains (p.1586·3); papain (p.1647·3); triacylglycerollipase; amylase (p.1579·3); trypsin (p.1675·3); chymotrypsin (p.1595·1); rutoside (p.1611·2).
Arteriosclerosis; soft-tissue injury; thrombosis; venous inflammation.

Enzynorm
Ebewe, Aust.; Knoll, Ger.; Hoechst Marion Roussel, S.Afr.†.
Stomach extract.
Gastrointestinal disorders.

The symbol † denotes a preparation no longer actively marketed

Enzynorm forte Knoll, Ger.
Gastric mucous membrane extract; amino acids (p.1350·1).
Gastrointestinal disorders.

Enzyplex
Westmont, Hong Kong; Westmont, Singapore; Great Eastern, Thai.; Westmont, Thai.
Rizolipase; amylase (p.1579·3); protease; deoxycholic acid; simeticone (p.1249·2); vitamin B substances (p.1350·1).
Digestive system disorders with execess gas.

Eogran Synpharma, Aust.
Chamomile (p.1593·2); peppermint leaf (p.1243·2); tormentil (p.1674·1).
Diarrhoea.

Eoline Pfizer, Belg.
Hydrocortisone (p.1073·3); nystatin (p.392·2); oxytet-racycline calcium (p.234·1).
Infected skin disorders.

Eolus Sigma-Tau, Ital.
Eformoterol [formoterol] fumarate (p.764·2).
Obstructive airways disease.

E.P. Pharmax, UK.
Paracetamol (p.71·2); caffeine (p.761·3); codeine phosphate (p.25·2).
Pain.

Epabetina OFF, Ital.
Betaine glucuronate (p.1584·3); trigonelline.
Liver disorders.

Epa-Bon Sifarma, Ital.†
Cyclobutyrol sodium (p.1601·2).
Biliary disorders.

Epacaps Byk Roland, Switz.
Marine fish oil (p.949·3).
Hyperlipidaemias; nutritional supplement.

Epacrosil Uniao Quimica, Braz.
Adenosine (p.828·2); methionine (p.1012·2); betaine hydrochloride (p.1584·3); choline citrate (p.1356·3); vitamin B₆ (p.1386·3).
Liver disorders.

Epadel Mochida, Jpn.
Ethyl icosapentate.
Arteriosclerosis obliterans; hyperlipidaemias.

Epaderm SSL, UK.
Yellow soft paraffin (p.1407·3); emulsifying wax (p.1409·1); liquid paraffin (p.1407·1).
Dry skin.

Epagogo Kopkins, Braz.
Boldo (p.1585·3); rhubarb (p.1248·1); cynara (p.1601·3); cascara (p.1216·1).
Liver disorders.

Epailis DHN, Fr.
Nutritional supplement (p.1350·1).
Regurgitation.

Epalat EPS OFF, Ital.
Lactulose (p.1230·1).
Liver disorders.

Epalfen Zambon, Ital.
Lactulose (p.1230·1).
Bacterial gastrointestinal infections; constipation; digestive disorders; hepatic encephalopathy.

Epamin Parke, Davis, Mex.
Phenytoin (p.357·2) or phenytoin sodium (p.357·2).
Epilepsy.

Epanutin
Parke, Davis, Aust.; Parke, Davis, Belg.; Parke, Davis, Ger.; Parke, Davis, Irl.; Parke, Davis, Israel; Parke, Davis, Neth.; Parke, Davis, S.Afr.; Parke, Davis, Spain; Parke, Davis, Swed.; Parke, Davis, Switz.; Parke, Davis, UK.
Phenytoin (p.357·2) or phenytoin sodium (p.357·2).
Arrhythmias; epilepsy; seizures associated with neuro-surgery or head injury; trigeminal neuralgia.

Epaplex 40 Uno, Ital.
Ferric sodium gluconate (p.1360·2).
Sideropenic anaemia.

Epaq
Note.This name is used for preparations of different composition.
Kolassa, Aust.; Arrow, Austral.; 3M, Ger.
Salbutamol sulfate (p.770·3).
Obstructive airways disease.

3M, Mex.
Metronidazole (p.594·1).
Bacterial vaginosis.

Eparema Byk, Braz.; SIT, Ital.
Cascara (p.1216·1); boldo (p.1585·3); rhubarb (p.1248·1).
Constipation.

Eparema-Levul SIT, Ital.
Cascara (p.1216·1); boldo (p.1585·3); rhubarb (p.1248·1); fructose (p.1363·3).
Constipation.

Eparex Newlab, Braz.
Adenosine (p.828·2); methionine (p.1012·2); betaine hydrochloride (p.1584·3).
Liver disorders.

Epargriseovit
Pharmacia Upjohn, Hong Kong; Pharmacia Upjohn, Ital.
Cyanocobalamin (p.1388·1); folic acid (p.1361·1); nicotinamide (p.1372·3); ascorbic acid (p.1389·3).
Anaemias; peripheral neuropathies; tonic.

Eparical Rhone-Poulenc Rorer, Ital.
Heparin calcium (p.902·1).
Thromboembolic disorders.

Eparinlider Pharmaland, Ital.
Heparin calcium (p.902·1).
Thromboembolic disorders.

Eparinovis INTES, Ital.
Heparin sodium (p.902·1).
Eye disorders.

Eparmefolin Bracco, Ital.
Cyanocobalamin (p.1388·1); calcium folinate (p.1363·1).
Anaemias; deficiency states.

Eparsil Pulitzer, Ital.†
Silymarin (p.1021·3).
Liver disorders.

Epativan B6 Honorterapica, Braz.
Adenosine (p.828·2); methionine (p.1012·2); choline (p.1356·3); betaine hydrochloride (p.1584·3); vitamin B₆ (p.1386·3).
Liver disorders.

Epatovis Dorsay, Braz.
Cynara (p.1601·3); cascara (p.1216·1); persea americana; rhubarb (p.1248·1); boldo (p.1585·3).
Liver disorders.

Epatoxil Tosi, Ital.
Cogalactoisomerase sodium (p.1598·1).
Liver disorders.

Epa-Treis Ecobi, Ital.
Calcium oxoglurate; choline orotate (p.1645·1).
Liver disorders.

Epaxal
Berna, Belg.; Berna, Canad.; Berna, Denm.; Berna, Fin.; Niddapharm, Ger.; Berna, Hong Kong; Berna, Ital.; Berna, Norw.; Pharmabroker, NZ; Cortec, Swed.; Berna, Switz.
An inactivated hepatitis A vaccine (p.1541·2).
Active immunisation.

EP&C Essence Potter's, UK.
Bayberry bark (p.1583·3); hemlock spruce; sambucus (p.1660·3); peppermint oil (p.1243·3).
Formerly called Elder Flowers with Peppermint and Composition Essence.
Colds; sore throat.

Epelin Ache, Braz.
Phenytoin sodium (p.357·2).
Epilepsy; trigeminal neuralgia.

Ephed 20th 20th Century, Mex.
Ephedrine (p.1090·1).

Ephedroides Richelet, Fr.
Pseudoephedrine hydrochloride (p.1099·2).
Nasal congestion.

Ephedyl Synco, Hong Kong.
Promethazine hydrochloride (p.423·2); codeine phosphate (p.25·2); ephedrine hydrochloride (p.1090·1).
Coughs and cold symptoms; rhinitis.

Ephepect Bolder, Ger.
Ephedrine hydrochloride (p.1090·1); ammonium chloride (p.1085·2); thyme (p.1672·2); cowslip rhizome (p.1600·1); anise oil (p.1580·3); fennel oil (p.1610·2); peppermint oil (p.1243·3); eucalyptus oil (p.1609·2).
Bronchitis; catarrh.

Ephepect-Blocker-Pastillen N Bolder, Ger.
Sodium dibunate (p.1100·3); dequalinium chloride (p.1143·1).
Coughs and associated respiratory-tract disorders.

Ephex Teral, USA†.
Guaifenesin (p.1092·2); ephedrine hydrochloride (p.1090·1).

Ephydion Theratech, Fr.
Syrup: Ethylmorphine hydrochloride (p.35·2); sulfogaiacol (p.1101·1); grindelia (p.1618·2).
Formerly contained ephedrine hydrochloride, ethylmorphine hydrochloride, sulfogaiacol, belladonna, grindelia, and drosera.
Tablets; oral drops: Ethylmorphine hydrochloride (p.35·2); sodium benzoate (p.1134·3); grindelia (p.1618·2).
Formerly contained ephedrine hydrochloride, ethylmorphine hydrochloride, sodium benzoate, belladonna, grindelia, and drosera.
Coughs.

Ephydrol CS, Fr.
Cream: Fioravanti; lavender oil (p.1627·2); bergamot oil (p.1584·2); lemon oil (p.1628·2); camphor (p.1589·3); menthol (p.1632·3); salicyl alcohol; formaldehyde solution (p.1144·2).
Topical solution (with brush or aeosol spray): Fioravanti; camphor (p.1589·3); menthol (p.1632·3); salicyl alcohol; bergamot oil (p.1584·2); lemon oil (p.1628·2); lavender oil (p.1627·2); formaldehyde solution (p.1144·2); plantain (p.1652·3).
Topical spray: Sanicula; fioravanti; camphor (p.1589·3); lavender oil (p.1627·2); bergamot oil (p.1584·2); lemon oil (p.1628·2); menthol (p.1632·3); salicyl alcohol; formaldehyde solution (p.1144·2).
Hyperhidrosis.

Ephynal
Roche, Aust.; Roche, Belg.; Roche, Braz.; Roche, Fr.; Roche Nicholas, Ger.; Roche Consumer, Irl.; Roche, Israel; Roche, Ital.; Roche, Mex.; Roche, Port.; Roche, S.Afr.; Roche Nicholas, Spain; Roche, Swed.†; Roche, Switz.; Roche Consumer, UK.
Alpha tocoferil acetate (p.1394·1).
Vitamin E deficiency.

Epi EZ Allerex, Canad.†
Adrenaline [epinephrine] (p.829·1).
Anaphylactic shock.

Epi-Aberel Janssen-Cilag, Ger.†
Tretinoin (p.1126·2).
Acne.

Epianal Will-Pharma, Neth.
Sodium oleate (p.1497·1); oxypolyethoxydodecanum; chlorocarvacrol.
Haemorrhoids.

Epi-C Lafayette, USA.
Barium sulfate (p.1032·1).
Contrast medium for gastrointestinal radiography.

Epicef Lisapharma, Ital.
Cefonicid sodium (p.168·1).
Lignocaine [lidocaine] hydrochloride (p.1313·2) is included in the intramuscular preparation to alleviate the pain of injection.
Gram-negative bacterial infections.

Epiclodina Pisa, Mex.
Clonidine (p.861·1).
Pain.

Epicordin
Note.This name is used for preparations of different composition.
Solvay, Aust.
Isosorbide mononitrate (p.916·2).
Angina pectoris; heart failure; pulmonary hypertension.

Solvay, Ger.
Captopril (p.853·3).
Heart failure; hypertension.

Epicrin Gebro, Switz.
Vitamin A; biotin; dexpanthenol; zinc amino acid chelate; millet extract; cystine; wheat-germ oil (p.1350·1).
Hair and nail disorders.

Epidermil Kinder, Braz.
Betamethasone (p.1063·1).
Skin disorders.

Epidex Kinder, Braz.
Desonide (p.1066·2).
Skin disorders.

Epidosin Solvay, Ger.†
Valethamate bromide (p.475·3).
Smooth muscle spasms.

Epiestrol
Helsinn Birex, Irl.; Roerig, Ital.; Rottapharm, Switz.
Estradiol (p.1473·1).
Menopausal disorders; osteoporosis.

Epifoam
Stafford-Miller, Israel; Schwarz, USA.
Hydrocortisone acetate (p.1073·3); pramocaine hydrochloride (p.1318·2).
Skin disorders.

Epifrin
Allergan, Canad.; Allergan, S.Afr.†; Allergan, USA.
Adrenaline [epinephrine] hydrochloride (p.829·2).
Open-angle glaucoma.

Epiglu ICN, UK.
Ethyl 2-cyanocrylate (p.1601·2); polymethylmethacrylate (p.1635·2).
Skin wounds.

Epiject Abbott, Canad.
Sodium valproate (p.366·3).
Epilepsy.

Epikur Agepha, Aust.
Meprobamate (p.691·1).
Anxiety; sleep disturbances.

Epilan Gerot, Aust.
Mephenytoin (p.353·2).
Epilepsy.

Epilan-D Gerot, Aust.
Phenytoin (p.357·2).
Epilepsy.

Epilantin Otsuka, Spain.
Phenytoin (p.357·2); phenobarbital (p.355·1).
Epilepsy.

Epilantine Streuli, Switz.
Phenytoin sodium (p.357·2).
Epilepsy.

Epilem Lemery, Mex.
Epirubicin hydrochloride (p.537·1).
Malignant neoplasms.

Epilim
Reckitt & Colman, Austral.; Sanofi Winthrop, Hong Kong; Sanofi Winthrop, Irl.; Reckitt Benckiser, NZ; Sanofi Synthelabo, S.Afr.; Sanofi Synthelabo, Singapore; Sanofi Winthrop, UK.
Sodium valproate (p.366·3).
Epilepsy.

Epilim Chrono
Sanofi Winthrop, Irl.; Sanofi Synthelabo, UK.
Sodium valproate (p.366·3); valproic acid (p.366·2).
Epilepsy.

E-Pilo
Ciba Vision, Canad.†; Ciba Vision, USA.
Adrenaline [epinephrine] acid tartrate (p.829·2); pilocarpine hydrochloride (p.1422·3).
Glaucoma; raised intra-ocular pressure.

Epi-Lyt
Stiefel, Canad.†; Stiefel, USA.
Glycerol (p.1616·3); lactic acid (p.1626·2).
Dry skin.

Epimaz Norton, UK.
Carbamazepine (p.342·2).

Epi-Monistat Janssen-Cilag, Ger.†
Miconazole nitrate (p.391·1).
Fungal infections.

Epinal Alcon, USA.
Adrenaline [epinephrine] borate complex (p.831·1).
Open-angle glaucoma.

Epipen Nycomed, Norw.
Phenytoin (p.357·2) or phenytoin sodium (p.357·2).
Arrhythmias; epilepsy.

Epione Schering-Plough, Port.
Betamethasone valerate (p.1063·2); gentamicin sulfate (p.210·1).
Infected skin disorders.

Epipak Espe, Ger.
Aluminium chlorohydrate (p.1110·2); polyethylene-imine hydrochloride.
Mouth disorders.

Epipen
Epipharm, Aust.; CSL, Austral.; ALK, Belg.; Allerex, Canad.; ALK, Denm.; ALK, Fin.; Center, Israel; ALK Norw.; CSL, NZ; Merck, S.Afr.; ALK, Swed.; Trimedal, Switz.; ALK, UK; Dey, USA.
Adrenaline [epinephrine] (p.829·1) or adrenaline [epinephrine] hydrochloride (p.829·2).
Anaphylaxis.

Epi-Pevaryl Janssen-Cilag, Ger.
Econazole nitrate (p.382·3).
Fungal skin and nail infections.

Epi-Pevaryl Heilpaste Janssen-Cilag, Ger.
Econazole nitrate (p.382·3); zinc oxide (p.1128·2).
Fungal skin infections.

Epi-Pevaryl Pv Janssen-Cilag, Ger.
Econazole (p.383·1).
Pityriasis versicolor.

Epipevisone Janssen-Cilag, Ger.
Econazole nitrate (p.382·3); triamcinolone acetonide (p.1080·1).
Fungal skin infections.

Epiphane Biorga, Fr.
Gelatin (p.737·2).
Fragile nails and hair.

Epiphane 7 Saninter, Port.
Gelatin (p.737·2).
Fragile hair and nails.

Epiphysan Disperga, Aust.
Bovine pineal gland extract (p.1631·2).
Hypersexuality; psychoses.

Epipropane Medgenix, Belg.
Phenobarbital magnesium (p.356·2); amfetamine sulfate (p.1506·3).
Agitation; epilepsy; hypertension.

Episcorit Sanum-Kehlbeck, Ger.
Echinacea purpura (p.1606·2).
Respiratory- and urinary-tract infections.

Episec Odan, Canad.
Liquid paraffin (p.1407·1); propylene glycol (p.1655·1); trolamine stearate.

Episoft LED, Fr.
Moisturiser.
Dry skin disorders.

Episol Schering-Plough, Port.
SPF 15: Padimate O (p.1518·2); oxybenzone (p.1518·1).
Sunscreen.

Epistaxol Medical, Spain.
Adrenaline [epinephrine] (p.829·1); phenazone (p.77·2); naphazoline hydrochloride (p.1095·1); rutoside (p.1611·2).
Epistaxis; mucous membrane haemorrhage.

Epitelizante Ciba Vision, Spain.
Amino acids (p.1350·1); chloramphenicol (p.179·1); vitamin A palmitate (p.1383·2).
Corneal damage.

Epitezan Allergan-Frumtost, Braz.
Vitamin A (p.1382·1); chloramphenicol (p.179·1); amino acids.
Eye infections.

Epitheliale Ducray, Fr.
Avena (p.1583·1); vitamins A and E (p.1350·1).
Skin disorders.

Epitol Lemmon, USA.
Carbamazepine (p.342·2).
Epilepsy; trigeminal neuralgia.

Epitomax Janssen-Cilag, Fr.
Topiramate (p.365·2).
Epilepsy.

Epitopic Gerda, Fr.
Difluprednate (p.1069·3).
Skin disorders.

Epival
Abbott, Canad.; Abbott, Mex.
Valproate semisodium (p.366·3).
Epilepsy; mania; migraine.

Epivir
Glaxo, Aust.; Glaxo Wellcome, Belg.; Glaxo Wellcome, Denm.; Glaxo Wellcome, Fin.; Glaxo Wellcome, Fr.; Glaxo Wellcome, Ger.; Glaxo Wellcome, Israel; Glaxo Wellcome, Ital.; Glaxo Jpn; Glaxo Wellcome, Neth.; Glaxo Wellcome, Norw.; Glaxo Wellcome, Port.; Glaxo Wellcome, Singapore; Glaxo Wellcome, Spain; Glaxo Wellcome, Swed.; Glaxo Wellcome, Thai.; Glaxo Wellcome, UK; Glaxo Wellcome, USA.
Lamivudine (p.635·1).
HIV infection.

Epixian UCB, Spain†.
Cocarboxylase (p.1385·2); magnesium phosphate (p.1191·1); magnesium succinate; pyridoxal phosphate (p.1387·1); chymotrypsin (p.1595·1); trypsin (p.1675·3).
Renal calculi.

Epizon Mepha, Hong Kong.
Rectocaps for children: Paracetamol (p.71·2); propyphenazone (p.80·2); guaifenesin (p.1092·2).
Rectocaps for infants: Paracetamol (p.71·2); propyphenazone (p.80·2); guaifenesin (p.1092·2); valerian (p.1678·3); passion flower (p.1649·1).
Fever; pain.

Eplonat *Infirmarius-Rovit, Ger.*
d-Alpha tocopherol (p.1393·3).
Vitamin E deficiency.

E.P.O. & E *Quest, UK.*
Evening primrose oil (p.1613·2); vitamin E.

Epo + Maxepa + Vitamin E Herbal Plus Formula 8 *Vitelle, Austral.†.*
d-Alpha tocopherol (p.1393·3); evening primrose oil (p.1613·2); marine fish oil (p.949·3).
Nutritional supplement.

EPOC *Evening Primrose Oil Co., UK†.*
Evening primrose oil (p.1613·2).

EPOC Marine *Evening Primrose Oil Co., UK†.*
Evening primrose oil (p.1613·2); marine fish oil (p.949·3).

Epocelin
Orion, Fin.; Fujisawa, Jpn; CEPA, Spain†; Fujisawa, Thai.
Ceftizoxime sodium (p.176·3).
Lignocaine [lidocaine] (p.1313·2) or lignocaine [lidocaine] hydrochloride (p.1313·2) may be included in the intramuscular injection to alleviate the pain of injection.
Bacterial infections.

Epocler
Note.This name is used for preparations of different composition.
Whitehall, Braz.
Adenosine (p.828·2); methionine (p.1012·2); choline (p.1356·3); betaine hydrochloride (p.1584·3); vitamin B₆ (p.1386·3).
Liver disorders.

Whitehall, Ital.
Hydroquinone (p.1115·1).
Skin hyperpigmentation.

Epogam
Searle, Austral.†; Strathmann, Ger.; Searle, Irl.; Whitehall, Ital.; Pharmacia, UK.
Evening primrose oil (p.1613·2).
Eczema.

Scotia, Denm.; Scotia, NZ; Covan, S.Afr.; Leti, Spain.
Gamolenic acid (p.1613·1).
Eczema.

Epogen *Amgen, USA.*
Epoetin alfa (p.731·1).
Anaemia in cancer patients on chemotherapy; anaemia in zidovudine-treated HIV-infected patients; anaemia of chronic renal failure.

Epogin *Chugai, Jpn.*
Epoetin beta (p.731·1).
Anaemia in renal dialysis patients; autologous blood transfusion.

Epomax *Cryopharma, Mex.*
Epoetin alfa (p.731·1).
Anaemias.

Epopa *Vitalia, UK.*
Safflower oil (p.1375·1); salmon oil (p.949·2); evening primrose oil (p.1613·2); borage oil (p.1613·1); nicotinic acid (p.1372·3).

Epopen *Pensa, Spain.*
Epoetin alfa (p.731·1).
Anaemia of chronic renal failure; autologous blood transfusions; cisplatin-induced anaemia.

Eposerin *Pharmacia Upjohn, Ital.*
Ceftizoxime sodium (p.176·3).
Lignocaine [lidocaine] hydrochloride (p.1313·2) is included in the intramuscular injection to alleviate the pain of injection.
Bacterial infections.

Eposid *Nettopharma, Denm.*
Etoposide (p.538·1).
Malignant neoplasms.

Eposin
Nycomed, Norw.; Pharmachemie, S.Afr.; Tedec Meiji, Spain; Nycomed, Swed.
Etoposide (p.538·1).
Malignant neoplasms.

Epotin *Julphar, UAE.*
Epoetin (p.730·2).
Anaemias; autologous blood transfusions.

Epoxide *PP Lab, Thai.*
Chlordiazepoxide hydrochloride (p.659·2).
Anxiety.

Epoxitin *Janssen-Cilag, Ital.*
Epoetin alfa (p.731·1).
Anaemias; autologous blood transfusions.

Eppy
Allergan, Fr.†; Chauvin, Irl.; Visufarma, Ital.†; Smith & Nephew, S.Afr.†; Abigo, Swed.; Chauvin, UK.
Adrenaline [epinephrine] (p.829·1).
Open-angle glaucoma.

Eppy/N *Pilkington Barnes-Hind, USA†.*
Adrenaline [epinephrine] borate complex (p.831·1).
Open-angle glaucoma.

Eppystabil *Pharmacia Upjohn, Aust.†.*
Adrenaline [epinephrine] (p.829·1).
Open-angle glaucoma.

Epresat *Salus, Fr.*
Multivitamin preparation with plant extracts and yeast (p.1350·1).
Tonic.

Eprex
Janssen-Cilag, Austral.; Janssen-Cilag, Belg.; Janssen-Ortho, Canad.; Janssen-Cilag, Denm.; Janssen-Cilag, Fr.; Cilag, Hong Kong; Janssen-Cilag, Irl.; Janssen-Cilag, Israel; Janssen-Cilag, Ital.; Cilag, Mex.; Janssen-Cilag, Neth.; Janssen-Cilag, Norw.; Janssen-Cilag, NZ; Janssen-Cilag, S.Afr.; Janssen-Cilag, Singapore; Janssen-

Cilag, Spain; Janssen-Cilag, Swed.; Janssen-Cilag, Switz.; Janssen, Thai.; Janssen-Cilag, UK.
Epoetin alfa (p.731·1).
Anaemias; autologous blood transfusions.

Eprofil *Columbia, Mex.*
Tiabendazole (p.109·1).

Epromate *Major, USA†.*
Aspirin (p.14·2); meprobamate (p.691·1).
Pain.

Epsicaprom *Bial, Port.*
Aminocaproic acid (p.724·3).

Epsitron *Remedica, Thai.*
Captopril (p.853·3).
Heart failure; hypertension.

Epsoclar *Biologici Italia, Ital.*
Heparin sodium (p.902·1).
Thromboembolic disorders.

ept Stick Test *Warner-Lambert, USA.*
Pregnancy test (p.1654·3).

Eptadone *Zambon, Ital.*
Methadone hydrochloride (p.53·1).
Opioid withdrawal; pain.

Eptico *Watsons, Canad.*
Camphor (p.1589·3); zinc oxide (p.1128·2).

Epulor *Vistapharm, USA.*
Preparation for enteral nutrition (p.1350·1).

Epuram *Pharmafarm, Fr.*
Citrulline (p.1357·2); arginine hydrochloride (p.1353·3); ornithine hydrochloride (p.1374·1).
Liver disorders.

Equagesic
Note.This name is used for preparations of different composition.
Wyeth-Ayerst, Canad.†; Akromed, S.Afr.†; Wyeth, UK.
Aspirin (p.14·2); meprobamate (p.691·1); ethoheptazine citrate (p.35·1).
Musculoskeletal pain.

Wyeth-Ayerst, USA.
Aspirin (p.14·2); meprobamate (p.691·1).
Musculoskeletal pain.

Equal
Nutrasweet, NZ; Searle, Thai.
Aspartame (p.1354·3).
Sugar substitute.

Equalactin *Numark, USA.*
Polycarbophil calcium (p.1244·2).
Constipation; diarrhoea.

Equanil
Wyeth, Austral.†; Wyeth-Ayerst, Canad.; Sanofi Winthrop, Fr.; Aspen, S.Afr.; Wyeth, UK†; Wyeth-Ayerst, USA.
Meprobamate (p.691·1).
Alcohol withdrawal sydrome; anxiety; premedication; sedative; skeletal muscle spasm.

Equanox *Linde, UK.*
Nitrous oxide (p.1264·3); oxygen (p.1199·3).

Equasym *Celltech, UK.*
Methylphenidate hydrochloride (p.1511·3).
Attention-deficit hyperactivity disorder.

Equazine M *Rugby, USA†.*
Aspirin (p.14·2); meprobamate (p.691·1).
Pain.

Equiday *Algol, Fin.*
d-Alpha tocopherol (p.1393·3).
Vitamin E deficiency.

Equiday E *Solvay, Ger.†.*
d-Alpha tocopherol (p.1393·3).
Vitamin E deficiency.

Equiderm *Galderma, Mex.*
Emollient; moisturiser.

Equidral *Scherer, Ital.†.*
Maltodextrin; electrolytes (p.1180·1).
Electrolyte depletion in hyperhidrosis.

Equilet *Mission Pharmacal, USA.*
Calcium carbonate (p.1215·1).
Hyperacidity.

Equilibrin *Rhone-Poulenc Rorer, Ger.*
Amitriptylinoxide (p.278·1).
Depression.

Equilibrium *SFD, Port.*
A range of emollients, moisturisers, and shampoos.

Equilibrium Creme Anti-transpirante *SFD, Port.*
Aluminium chlorohydrate (p.1110·2); centella (p.1112·2); aloe vera (p.1110·1).
Hyperhidrosis.

Equilid
Hoechst Marion Roussel, Braz.; Bruno, Ital.
Sulpiride (p.706·1).
Adjuvant in gastric ulcer; depression; nausea and vomiting; nervous disorders; psychoses.

Equilium *Fumouze, Fr.*
Tiapride (p.709·1).
Aggressive states; agitation; choreiform movements; pAIN.

Equilon *Chefaro, UK.*
Mebeverine hydrochloride (p.1233·3).
Irritable bowel syndrome.

Equilon Herbal *Chefaro, UK.*
Peppermint oil (p.1243·3).
Irritable bowel syndrome.

Equin
Aldo-Union, Hong Kong; Aldo, Spain.
Conjugated oestrogens (p.1467·1).
Dysfunctional uterine haemorrhage; lactation inhibition; menopausal disorders; osteoporosis.

Equinorm *Aspen, S.Afr.*
Clomipramine hydrochloride (p.282·1).
Depression; narcoleptic syndrome.

Equipax *Parke, Davis, Spain.*
Gabapentin (p.350·2).
Epilepsy.

Equipur *Medipharma, Ger.†.*
Vincamine (p.1680·1).
Ménière's disease; mental function disorders; metabolic and circulatory disorders of the brain, retina, and inner ear.

Equisil *Klein, Ger.*
Equisetum (p.1606·3); plantago lanceolata; castanea vulgaris; cowslip rhizome (p.1600·1); verbascum flowers; thyme (p.1672·2); ephedrine hydrochloride (p.1090·1); colloidal silicon dioxide (p.1503·3).
Coughs and associated respiratory-tract disorders.

Equitam
Note.This name is used for preparations of different composition.
Eurofarma, Braz.
Ginkgo biloba (p.1615·2).
Cerebrovascular disorders.

Biotherapie, Fr.
Lorazepam (p.688·3).
Alcohol withdrawal syndrome; anxiety.

Equiton *Bruschettini, Ital.*
Timolol maleate (p.982·1); pilocarpine hydrochloride (p.1422·3).
Glaucoma; ocular hypertension.

ER Cream *Curacel, Austral.*
Coal tar (p.1125·1); zinc oxide (p.1128·2); allantoin (p.1110·1).
Skin disorders.

Era *Abbott, NZ.*
Erythromycin lactobionate (p.201·3) or erythromycin stearate (p.201·3).
Bacterial infections.

Eracillin *Chew, Thai.*
Ampicillin trihydrate (p.151·1).
Bacterial infections.

Eracine *Sanofi Winthrop, Fr.*
Acrosoxacin [rosoxacin] (p.147·3).
Bacterial infections.

Eradacil
Sanofi Winthrop, Braz.; Sanofi Synthelabo, Port.
Acrosoxacin [rosoxacin] (p.147·3).
Gonorrhoea.

Eralga *Chew, Thai.*
Hyoscine butylbromide (p.468·2).
Smooth muscle spasm.

Eramox *Nycomed, Aust.*
Amoxicillin trihydrate (p.149·2).
Bacterial infections.

Eramycin *Wesley, USA.*
Erythromycin stearate (p.201·3).
Bacterial infections.

Erantin *Boehringer Mannheim, Spain†.*
Epoetin beta (p.731·1).
Anaemia of chronic renal failure; cisplatin-induced anaemia.

Eranz *Wyeth, Mex.*
Donepezil hydrochloride (p.1417·2).
Alzheimer's disease.

Erasis *Orion, Fin.*
Erythromycin acistrate (p.201·2).
Bacterial infections.

Erasol *McGloin, Austral.*
Phenazone (p.77·2).
Ear ache.

Erathrom *Asian Pharm, Thai.*
Erythromycin estolate (p.201·2) or erythromycin stearate (p.201·3).
Bacterial infections.

Eraverm *Gemballa, Braz.*
Mebendazole (p.102·2).
Worm infections.

Erbazid *Pharmacia Upjohn, Mex.*
Isoniazid (p.215·3).

Ercaf *Geneva, USA.*
Ergotamine tartrate (p.452·1); caffeine (p.761·3).
Migraine and related vascular headache.

Ercal *Syntex, Mex.*
Fluocinolone acetonide (p.1071·1); bismuth subgallate (p.1213·2); lignocaine [lidocaine] hydrochloride (p.1313·2).
Anorectal disorders.

Ercar *Almirall, Spain.*
Carboplatin (p.515·1).
Bladder cancer; head and neck cancer; ovarian cancer; small-cell lung cancer.

Ercefuryl
Sanofi Synthelabo, Belg.; Synthelabo, Fr.; Synthelabo, Hong Kong; Lu-itpold, Fr.; Sanofi Synthelabo, Singapore; Sanofi Synthelabo, Thai.
Nifuroxazide (p.230·2).
Gastrointestinal infections.

Erceryl *Sanofi Synthelabo, Fr.*
Nifuroxazide (p.230·2).
Diarrhoea.

Ercestop *Sanofi Synthelabo, Fr.*
Loperamide hydrochloride (p.1231·3).
Formerly known as Delalande Diarrhee.
Diarrhoea.

Ercestopyl *Sanofi Synthelabo, Belg.*
Loperamide hydrochloride (p.1231·3).
Diarrhoea.

Ercevit *Synthelabo, Fr.†.*
Rutoside (p.1611·2); rutoside propylsulfonate sodium.
Peripheral vascular disorders.

Erco-Fer *Orion, Swed.*
Ferrous fumarate (p.1360·1).
Iron deficiency; iron-deficiency anaemia.

Erco-Fer vitamin *Orion, Swed.†.*
Multivitamin preparation with ferrous fumarate (p.1360·1)(p.1350·1).
Iron deficiency; iron-deficiency anaemia.

Ercolax *Ercopharm, Switz.†.*
Bisacodyl (p.1212·2).
Bowel evacuation; constipation.

Ercoquin
Ercopharm, Denm.†; Nycomed, Norw.
Hydroxychloroquine sulfate (p.437·2).
Lupus erythematosus; malaria; photosensitivity; rheumatoid arthritis; Sjögren's syndrome.

Ercorax Roll-on *Ercopharm, Switz.†.*
Propantheline bromide (p.473·2).
Hyperhidrosis.

Ercoril *Ercopharm, Denm.†.*
Propantheline bromide (p.473·2).
Gastrointestinal spasm; hyperhidrosis.

Ercotina *Orion, Fin.*
Propantheline bromide (p.473·2).
Gastrointestinal disorders.

Erdopect *Pharmacal, Fin.*
Erdosteine (p.1091·2).
Respiratory-tract disorders.

Erdotin *Edmond Pharma, Ital.*
Erdosteine (p.1091·2).
Respiratory-tract congestion.

Erecnos *Fournier, UK†.*
Thymoxamine [moxisylyte] hydrochloride (p.980·2).
Erectile dysfunction.

Eremfat *Fatol, Aust.; Fatol, Ger.*
Rifampicin (p.243·2) or rifampicin sodium (p.245·3).
Brucellosis; leprosy; meningococcal meningitis prophylaxis; staphylococcal infections; tuberculosis.

Eres N *Muller Goppingen, Ger.*
Verbascum flowers.
Bronchial catarrh.

Erevan *Fournier, Ital.*
A heparinoid (p.905·2).
Thrombosis prophylaxis; vascular disorders.

Erfolgan *Roche, Austral.*
Ibopamine hydrochloride (p.912·1).
Heart failure.

Erg XXI *Farmorcore, Port.†.*
Nicergoline (p.1640·2).
Cerebral and peripheral vascular disorders; hypertension.

Ergamisol
Janssen-Cilag, Austral.; Janssen-Cilag, Belg.; Janssen-Ortho, Canad.; Janssen-Cilag, Ger.; Janssen-Cilag, Israel; Janssen-Cilag, Ital.†; Janssen-Cilag, Neth.; Janssen-Cilag, S.Afr.; Janssen, USA.
Levamisole hydrochloride (p.101·2).
Adjunct to fluorouracil in colon cancer.

Ergate *Propan-Vernleigh, S.Afr.†.*
Ergotamine tartrate (p.452·1).
Migraine.

Ergenyl
Sanofi Synthelabo, Ger.; Sanofi Winthrop, Swed.
Sodium valproate (p.366·3).
Epilepsy.

Ergenyl Chrono *Sanofi Synthelabo, Ger.*
Sodium valproate (p.366·3); valproic acid (p.366·2).
Epilepsy.

Ergix *Monot, Fr.*
Capsules: Dextromethorphan hydrobromide (p.1087·3).
Coughs.
Lozenges: Tyrothricin (p.267·1); lignocaine [lidocaine] hydrochloride (p.1313·2).
Sore throat.
Syrup: Carbocisteine (p.1086·3).
Respiratory-tract congestion.
Tablets: Ibuprofen (p.43·2).
Fever; pain.

ergo sanol spezial N *Sanol, Ger.*
Ergotamine tartrate (p.452·1).
Migraine and other vascular headache.

ergobel *Hormosan, Ger.*
Nicergoline (p.1640·2).
Mental function disorders.

Ergocaf *Galen, Mex.*
Ergotamine tartrate (p.452·1); caffeine (p.761·3).
Migraine.

Ergocalm
Note.This name is used for preparations of different composition.
Mayrhofer, Aust.
Lorazepam (p.688·3).
Anxiety disorders; premedication; sleep disorders.

Wyeth, Ger.
Lormetazepam (p.689·3).
Premedication; sleep disorders.

Ergocris *Magis, Ital.*
Dihydroergocristine mesilate (p.1603·2).
Cerebral and peripheral vascular disorders; dopaminergic deficiency; headache; hypertension; migraine.

The symbol † denotes a preparation no longer actively marketed

Ergodavur Belmac, Spain.
Dihydroergocristine mesilate (p.1603·2).
Cerebrovascular disorders; vascular eye disorders; vestibular disorders.

Ergodesit Desitin, Ger.
Co-dergocrine mesilate (p.1597·3).
Hypertension; mental function disorders.

Ergodilat Diviser Aquilea, Spain.
Co-dergocrine mesilate (p.1597·3).
Cerebrovascular disorders; circulatory disorders.

Ergodose Murat, Fr.
Co-dergocrine mesilate (p.1597·3).
Mental function impairment in the elderly.

Ergodryl
Parke, Davis, Austral.; Parke, Davis, Canad.; Parke, Davis, NZ.
Ergotamine tartrate (p.452·1); caffeine citrate (p.761·3); diphenhydramine hydrochloride (p.416·1).
Migraine and other vascular headaches.

Ergodryl Mono Parke, Davis, Austral.
Ergotamine tartrate (p.452·1).
Migraine and other vascular headaches.

Ergofar Continentales, Mex.
Ergometrine (p.1607·1).

Ergoffin Dresden, Ger.; Temmler, Ger.
Ergotamine tartrate (p.452·1); caffeine (p.761·3).
Headache; migraine.

Ergofit Bonomelli, Ital.†
Vitamin C (p.1389·3).
Nutritional supplement.

Ergo-Fort Odontofarma, Braz.
Amino acids; vitamin B substances (p.1350·1).

Ergohepat B12 IMA, Braz.
Acetylmethionine; choline (p.1356·3); vitamine B₁₂ (p.1388·1).
Liver disorders.

Ergohydrine Streuli, Switz.
Co-dergocrine mesilate (p.1597·3).
Cerebrovascular disorders.

Ergokapton Strallhofer, Aust.
Ergotamine tartrate (p.452·1).
Migraine and related vascular headaches.

Ergokoffin OBA, Denm.
Ergotamine tartrate (p.452·1); caffeine (p.761·3).
Migraine.

Ergo-Kranit Krewel, Ger.
Ergotamine tartrate (p.452·1); propyphenazone (p.80·2); paracetamol (p.71·2).
Headache; migraine.

Ergo-Kranit mono Krewel, Ger.
Ergotamine tartrate (p.452·1).
Migraine and other vascular headaches.

Ergolefrin Gepepharm, Ger.
Dihydroergotamine mesilate (p.450·3); etilefrine hydrochloride (p.888·1).
Hypotension.

Ergolin Boniscontro & Gazzone, Ital.
Nicergoline (p.1640·2).
Cerebrovascular disorders.

Ergo-Lonarid PD Boehringer Ingelheim, Ger.
Dihydroergotamine tartrate (p.450·3); paracetamol (p.71·2).
Headache; migraine.

Ergomar
Rhone-Poulenc Rorer, Canad.; Lotus, USA.
Ergotamine tartrate (p.452·1).
Migraine and related vascular headache.

Ergomed Kwizda, Aust.
Co-dergocrine mesilate (p.1597·3).
Cerebral insufficiency; hypertension; migraine and related vascular headache.

Ergomemor QIF, Braz.
Glutamic acid; calcium glycerophosphate; calcium; thiamine (p.1350·1).
Dietary supplement.

Ergomimet Klinge, Ger.
Dihydroergotamine mesilate (p.450·3).
Hypotension; migraine and other vascular headaches; vascular disorders.

Ergomimet plus Klinge, Ger.
Dihydroergotamine mesilate (p.450·3); etilefrine hydrochloride (p.888·1).
Hypotension.

Ergont
Sigmapharm, Aust.; Desitin, Ger.
Dihydroergotamine mesilate (p.450·3).
Hypotension; migraine and related vascular headache; vascular disorders.

Ergoplex Kwizda, Aust.†
Co-dergocrine mesilate (p.1597·3).
Cerebral insufficiency; hypertension; migraine and related vascular headache.

ergoplus Hormosan, Ger.
Co-dergocrine mesilate (p.1597·3).
Cervical disc syndrome; hypertension; mental function disorders.

Ergoram Bonomelli, Ital.†
Amino-acid preparation (p.1350·1).
Nutritional supplement.

Ergosanol a la cafeine Schwarz, Switz.
Suppositories: Ergotamine tartrate (p.452·1); ethenzamide (p.35·1); caffeine (p.761·3); caffeine citrate (p.761·3).

Tablets: Ergotamine tartrate (p.452·1); ethenzamide (p.35·1); caffeine (p.761·3).
Cluster headache; migraine and related vascular headache.

Ergosanol special Schwarz, Switz.†
Ergotamine tartrate (p.452·1); phenyltoloxamine citrate (p.423·1); ethenzamide (p.35·1); caffeine (p.761·3).
Cluster headache; migraine and related vascular headache.

Ergosanol special a la cafeine Schwarz, Switz.
Ergotamine tartrate (p.452·1); ethenzamide (p.35·1); caffeine (p.761·3); caffeine citrate (p.761·3); phenyltoloxamine citrate (p.423·1).
Cluster headache; migraine and other vascular headaches.

Ergosia Asian Pharm, Thai.
Ergotamine tartrate (p.452·1).
Migraine.

ergotam CT, Ger.
Dihydroergotamine mesilate (p.450·3).
Hypotension; migraine and other vascular headaches; vascular disorders.

Ergotan Salf, Ital.
Ergotamine tartrate (p.452·1).
Migraine and related vascular headache.

Ergotonine Streuli, Switz.
Dihydroergotamine mesilate (p.450·3).
Fatigue; hypotension; migraine.

Ergotop Kwizda, Aust.
Nicergoline (p.1640·2).
Peripheral and cerebral vascular disorders.

ergotox CT, Ger.
Co-dergocrine mesilate (p.1597·3).
Hypertension; mental function disorders.

Ergotrate
Lilly, Braz.; Lilly, Canad.†; Lilly, Mex.; Lilly, S.Afr.†; Bedford, USA.
Ergometrine maleate (p.1607·1).
Postpartum or postabortal haemorrhage.

Ergotyl Lek, Thai.
Methylergometrine maleate (p.1635·1).
Management of third stage of labour; postpartum haemorrhage; postpartum uterine atony.

Ergovasan Klinge, Aust.
Dihydroergotamine mesilate (p.450·3).
Circulatory disorders; hypotension; migraine and related vascular headaches.

Ergovis Bonomelli, Ital.
A range of nutritional supplements (p.1350·1).

Ergybiol Nutergia, Fr.
Mineral preparation (p.1350·1).

Ergymag Nutergia, Fr.
Vitamin B and mineral preparation (p.1350·1).

Ergyphilus Nutergia, Fr.
Lactobacillus species, fibre, and mineral preparation (p.1350·1).
Maintenance of normal gastrointestinal flora.

Eriber Berman, Mex.
Erythromycin (p.201·2).
Bacterial infections.

Eribiotic Teuto, Braz.
Erythromycin stearate (p.201·3).
Bacterial infections.

Eribus Welfer, Mex.
Erythromycin (p.201·2).
Bacterial infections.

Ericin Chew, Thai.
Erythromycin stearate (p.201·3).
Bacterial infections.

Ericosol Ecosol, Switz.
Erythromycin stearate (p.201·3).
Bacterial infections.

Eridamin Brasmedica, Braz.
Benzydamine hydrochloride (p.20·1).
Fever; inflammation; pain.

Eridan SIT, Ital.†
Diazepam (p.674·3).
Adjuvant in epilepsy; anxiety disorders.

Eridosis Stiefel, Spain.
Erythromycin (p.201·2).
Acne.

Eriflogin Asta Medica, Braz.
Erythromycin estolate (p.201·2).
Bacterial infections.

Erifoscin I Farmacologia, Spain.
Erythromycin estolate (p.201·2); fosfomycin calcium (p.208·2).
Bacterial infections.

Eril
Note. This name is used for preparations of different composition.
Savio, Ital.
Piperacillin sodium (p.236·1).
Lignocaine [lidocaine] hydrochloride (p.1313·2) is included in this preparation to alleviate the pain of injection.
Bacterial infections.

Asahi, Jpn.
Fasudil hydrochloride (p.888·2).
Cerebral vasospasm following subarachnoid haemorrhage.

Erimicina Medifarma, Mex.
Erythromycin (p.201·2).
Bacterial infections.

Erimin Sumitomo, Jpn†.
Nimetazepam (p.695·2).
Insomnia.

Erimit TP, Thai.
Erythromycin estolate (p.201·2) or erythromycin stearate (p.201·3).
Bacterial infections.

Erimycin Siam Bheasach, Thai.
Erythromycin ethyl succinate (p.201·2) or erythromycin stearate (p.201·3).
Bacterial infections.

Erios Mepha, Switz.
Erythromycin ethyl succinate (p.201·2) or erythromycin stearate (p.201·3).
Bacterial infections.

Erispan Sumitomo, Jpn†.
Fludiazepam (p.683·2).
Autonomic imbalance; psychosomatic disorders.

Erisuspen Medifarma, Mex.
Erythromycin (p.201·2).
Bacterial infections.

Eritina Sanitas, Port.
Erythromycin propionate (p.201·3).
Bacterial infections.

Eritolat Marcel, Mex.
Erythromycin (p.201·2).
Bacterial infections.

Eritos Searle, Braz.
Dropropizine (p.1089·3).
Coughs.

Eritrerba Pharmacia Upjohn, Mex.
Erythromycin (p.201·2).
Bacterial infections.

Eritrex Ache, Braz.
Erythromycin estolate (p.201·2).
Bacterial infections.

Eritrex A Ache, Braz.
Erythromycin estolate (p.201·2); oxolamine (p.1096·2).
Bacterial skin infections.

Eritrocina
Abbott, Ital.; Abbott, Port.
Erythromycin ethyl succinate (p.201·2) or erythromycin lactobionate (p.201·3).
Bacterial infections.

Eritrocist Edmond Pharma, Ital.
Erythromycin stinoprate (p.203·3).
Bacterial infections.

Eritrofar Elofar, Braz.
Erythromycin estolate (p.201·2).
Bacterial infections.

Eritrofarmin Rayere, Mex.
Erythromycin (p.201·2).
Bacterial infections.

Eritrogen Boehringer Mannheim, Ital.†.
Epoetin beta (p.731·1).
Anaemia associated with renal impairment; autologous blood transfusion.

Eritrogobens Normon, Spain.
Erythromycin ethyl succinate (p.201·2).
Bacterial infections.

Eritrolat Liferpal, Mex.
Erythromycin (p.201·2).
Bacterial infections.

Eritromicina Sanofi Synthelabo, Port.
Erythromycin lactobionate (p.201·3).
Bacterial infections.

Eritroquim Quimica y Farmacia, Mex.
Erythromycin (p.201·2).
Bacterial infections.

Eritrosima Quirnioterapica, Braz.
Erythromycin estolate (p.201·2); muramidase hydrochloride (p.1638·1).
Bacterial infections.

Eritrosol Solfran, Mex.
Erythromycin (p.201·2).
Bacterial infections.

Eritroveinte Madariaga, Spain.
Erythromycin estolate (p.201·2).
Bacterial infections.

Eritrovier Tecnofarma, Mex.
Erythromycin ethyl succinate (p.201·2) or erythromycin stearate (p.201·3).
Bacterial infections.

Eritrovit B12 Lisapharma, Ital.
Cyanocobalamin (p.1388·1).
Anaemia; neuritis.

Eritrowel Welfer, Mex.
Erythromycin (p.201·2).
Bacterial infections.

Erjean Erjean, Fr.
Sodium chloride (p.1196·1).
Fluid and electrolyte disorders.

Erkaltungsbad Agepha, Aust.
Eucalyptus oil (p.1609·2); pumilio pine oil (p.1656·3); menthol (p.1632·3).
Catarrh.

Erkaltungsbalsam
Note. This name is used for preparations of different composition.
Agepha, Aust.
Peppermint oil (p.1243·3); camphor (p.1589·3); menthol (p.1632·3).
Catarrh.

Genericon, Aust.
Menthol (p.1632·3); camphor (p.1589·3); methyl salicylate (p.55·1).
Cold symptoms; musculoskeletal and joint disorders.

Sanofi Winthrop, Aust.
Eucalyptus oil (p.1609·2); pumilio pine oil (p.1656·3); oleum pini sylvestris; camphor (p.1589·3); menthol (p.1632·3).
Cold symptoms.

Erkaltungsbalsam forte Salbe Twardy, Ger.
Camphor (p.1589·3); menthol (p.1632·3); clove oil (p.1597·1).
Bronchitis; cold symptoms; coughs.

Erkaltungsbalsam-ratiopharm E Salbe Ratiopharm, Ger.
Eucalyptus oil (p.1609·2); camphor (p.1589·3); turpentine oil (p.1676·3).
Cold symptoms.

Erkaltungstee
Note. This name is used for preparations of different composition.
Sanova, Aust.
Thyme leaf (p.1672·2); althaea (p.1577·1); verbascum flowers; drosera (p.1606·1); plantago lanceolata leaf.
Mouth and throat disorders; respiratory-tract disorders.

Sanova, Aust.†
Thyme leaf (p.1672·2); althaea (p.1577·1); verbascum flowers; plantago lanceolata leaf.
Mouth and throat disorders; respiratory-tract disorders.

Erladexone Malaysia Chemist, Singapore.
Dexamethasone (p.1067·1).
Corticosteroid.

Erliten Malaysia Chemist, Singapore.
Ketotifen fumarate (p.767·2).
Allergic bronchitis; allergic conjunctivitis; allergic rhinitis; allergic skin disorders; asthma; hay fever.

Erlivin Malaysia Chemist, Singapore.
Griseofulvin (p.386·2).
Fungal skin, hair, and nail infections.

Erlmetin Malaysia Chemist, Singapore.
Cimetidine (p.1216·3).
Acid aspiration; adjunct in pancreatic insufficiency; gastro-oesophageal reflux; peptic ulcer; Zollinger-Ellison syndrome.

Erloric Malaysia Chemist, Singapore.
Allopurinol (p.397·2).
Gout; hyperuricaemia; renal calculi.

Erlotyl Malaysia Chemist, Singapore.
Diphenoxylate hydrochloride (p.1222·2).
Atropine sulfate (p.461·1) is included in this preparation to discourage abuse.
Diarrhoea.

Erlvirax Malaysia Chemist, Singapore.
Aciclovir (p.612·3).
Herpesvirus infections.

Ermsech Heumann, Ger.
Calcium lactate (p.1188·2); echinacea (p.1606·2).
Hypersensitivity disorders; increase of immune capacity.

Ermycin Remedica, Singapore.
Erythromycin stearate (p.201·3).
Bacterial infections.

Ermysin Orion, Fin.
Erythromycin (p.201·2) or erythromycin ethyl succinate (p.201·2).
Bacterial infections.

Ernodasa Ern, Spain.
Streptodornase (p.1667·2); streptokinase (p.975·3).
Inflammation; soft-tissue damage; ulcers.

ERO Scherer, USA.
Urea hydrogen peroxide (p.1159·3).
Ear wax removal.

Ero Test Heralds, Braz.
Conjugated oestrogens (p.1467·1); methyltestosterone (p.1482·3); vitamin C (p.1389·3).
Erectile dysfunction.

Erocap Douglas, Austral.†
Fluoxetine hydrochloride (p.284·2).
Depression.

Erole Forte Orion, Fin.
d-Alpha tocopherol; selenium yeast (p.1350·1).
Dietary supplement.

Erole-C Orion, Fin.
Capsules, d-alpha tocopherol; selenium yeast; tablets, ascorbic acid (p.1350·1).
Dietary supplement.

Eromel Aspen, S.Afr.
Erythromycin stearate (p.201·3).
Bacterial infections.

Eromel-S Lagamed, S.Afr.†
Erythromycin ethyl succinate (p.201·2).
Bacterial infections.

Eromycin
Dista, NZ; Julphar, UAE.
Erythromycin (p.201·2), erythromycin estolate (p.201·2), erythromycin ethyl succinate (p.201·2), or erythromycin stearate (p.201·3).
Bacterial infections.

Erotab Hovid, Singapore.
Erythromycin estolate (p.201·2).
Bacterial infections.

Eroxade Osoth, Thai.
Roxithromycin (p.247·2).
Bacterial infections.

Erpalfa *INTES, Ital.*
Cytarabine (p.530·1).
Viral keratitis.

Erpecalm *Prisfar, Port.*
Thyme oil (p.1672·3); oregao oil; sweet marjoram oil; lavender (p.1627·2); lemon; chamomile (p.1593·2); thuja (p.1672·1); lappa (p.1627·1); plantain (p.1652·3).
Herpes labialis.

Erremox *RKG, Ital.*
Amoxicillin trihydrate (p.149·2).
Bacterial infections.

Errevit Combi *Erredici, Ital.†*
Vitamin E; betacarotene; selenium (p.1350·1).
Nutritional supplement.

Errevit Forte Gamma *Erredici, Ital.*
Betacarotene; vitamin E; selenium; gamolenic acid (p.1613·1).
Nutritional supplement.

Erthiol *American de Mexico, Mex.*
Merbromin (p.1150·1).

Ervevax
SmithKline Beecham, Aust.; SmithKline Beecham, Austral.; SmithKline Beecham, Belg.; SmithKline Beecham, Ger.; Dresden, Ger.; SmithKline Beecham, Irl.; SmithKline Beecham, Israel; SmithKline Beecham, Mex.; SmithKline Beecham, NZ; SmithKline Beecham, Switz.; SmithKline Beecham, Thai.; SmithKline Beecham, UK.
A rubella vaccine (Wistar RA 27/3 strain) (p.1562·3).
Active immunisation.

Ervin *Nokorn, Thai.*
Thiamphenicol (p.261·3).
Bacterial infections.

Erwinase
Ipsen, Austral.; Ipsen, Fin.; Ipsen, Ger.; NZ Medical & Scientific, NZ; Ipsen, Swed.; Beaufour-Ipsen, Thai.; Ipsen, UK.
Crisantaspase (asparaginase) (p.508·3).
Acute lymphocytic leukaemia.

Ery *Bouchara, Fr.; Bouchara, Switz.†*
Erythromycin ethyl succinate (p.201·2) or erythromycin propionate (p.201·3).
Bacterial infections.

Eryacne
Galderma, Austral.; Galderma, Fr.; Galderma, Hong Kong; Galderma, Ital.; Galderma, Neth.; Galderma, NZ; Galderma, Singapore; Galderma, Thai.; Galderma, UK.
Erythromycin (p.201·2).
Acne.

Eryacnen *Galderma, Braz.; Galderma, Mex.*
Erythromycin (p.201·2).
Acne.

Eryaknen *AB-Consult, Aust.; Galderma, Ger.; Galderma, Switz.*
Erythromycin (p.201·2).
Acne.

Eryase *Ducray, Fr.*
Avena (p.1583·1); zinc oxide (p.1128·2); copper sulfate (p.1358·1).
Nappy rash.

Erybesan *Biochemie, Aust.†*
Erythromycin ethyl succinate (p.201·2) or erythromycin stearate (p.201·3).
Bacterial infections.

Erybeta *Betapharm, Ger.*
Erythromycin ethyl succinate (p.201·2) or erythromycin stearate (p.201·3).
Bacterial infections.

Erybid *Abbott, Canad.*
Erythromycin (p.201·2).
Bacterial infections.

Eryc
Faulding, Austral.; Parke, Davis, Canad.; Faulding, Hong Kong; Taro, Israel; Parke, Davis, Neth.; Parke, Davis, NZ; Faulding, Port.; Warner Chilcott, USA.
Erythromycin (p.201·2) or erythromycin lactobionate (p.201·3).
Bacterial infections.

Erycen *Berk, UK†.*
Erythromycin (p.201·2).
Bacterial infections.

Erycette
Janssen-Cilag, S.Afr.; Ortho Dermatological, USA.
Erythromycin (p.201·2).
Acne.

Erycin *Nycomed, Denm.; Atlantic, Thai.*
Erythromycin (p.201·2), erythromycin ethyl succinate (p.201·2), or erythromycin stearate (p.201·3).
Bacterial infections.

Erycinum *Schering, Aust.†; CytoChemia, Ger.*
Erythromycin (p.201·2), erythromycin lactobionate (p.201·3), or erythromycin stearate (p.201·3).
Bacterial infections.

Erycocci *Pharmafarm, Fr.†*
Erythromycin ethyl succinate (p.201·2).
Bacterial infections.

Erycytol *Lannacher, Aust.*
Hydroxocobalamin (p.1388·1).
Herpes zoster infections; liver disorders; macrocytic anaemias; neuralgia; neuritis; tobacco amblyopia; vitamin B₁₂ deficiency.

Eryderm
Abbott, Belg.; Abbott, Israel; Abbott, Mex.; Abbott, Neth.; Abbott, S.Afr.; Abbott, Singapore; Abbott, Switz.; Abbott, USA.
Erythromycin (p.201·2).
Acne.

Erydermec *Hexal, Ger.*
Erythromycin (p.201·2).
Acne.

Ery-Diolan *Engelhard, Ger.; Brahms, Ger.*
Erythromycin ethyl succinate (p.201·2) or erythromycin stearate (p.201·3).
Bacterial infections.

Eryfer *Cassella-med, Ger.*
Ferrous sulfate (p.1360·3).
Iron deficiency; iron-deficiency anaemias.

Eryfer comp *Cassella-med, Ger.*
Ferrous sulfate (p.1360·3); cyanocobalamin (p.1388·1); folic acid (p.1361·1).
Iron and vitamin deficiency.

Eryfluid *Pierre Fabre, Fr.; Pierre Fabre, Port.*
Erythromycin (p.201·2).
Acne.

Erygel *Allergan, USA.*
Erythromycin (p.201·2).
Acne; skin infections.

Eryhexal *Hexal, Aust.; Hexal, Austral.; Hexal, Ger.*
Erythromycin (p.201·2), erythromycin ethyl succinate (p.201·2), or erythromycin stearate (p.201·3).
Bacterial infections.

Erylar *Arlex, Thai.*
Erythromycin (p.201·2).
Bacterial infections.

Erylik *Biorga, Fr.*
Erythromycin (p.201·2); tretinoin (p.1126·2).
Acne.

Erymax
Elan, Irl.; Parke-Med, S.Afr.†; Elan, UK; Allergan, USA.
Erythromycin (p.201·2).
Bacterial infections.

Ery-Max
AstraZeneca, Norw.; I Farmacologia, Spain; Astra, Swed.
Erythromycin (p.201·2), erythromycin ethyl succinate (p.201·2), or erythromycin lactobionate (p.201·3).
Bacterial infections.

Ery-Maxin *Astra, Aust.†.*
Erythromycin (p.201·2) or erythromycin ethyl succinate (p.201·2).
Bacterial infections.

Erymin *Milano, Thai.; Elan, UK†.*
Erythromycin estolate (p.201·2) or erythromycin ethyl succinate (p.201·2).
Bacterial infections.

Erymin S *Parke-Med, S.Afr.†.*
Erythromycin estolate (p.201·2).
Bacterial infections.

Erymycin *Triomed, S.Afr.*
Erythromycin estolate (p.201·2) or erythromycin stearate (p.201·3).
Bacterial infections.

Eryped
Abbott, Hong Kong; Abbott, Singapore.
Erythromycin ethyl succinate (p.201·2).
Bacterial infections.

Ery-Ped *Abbott, USA.*
Erythromycin ethyl succinate (p.201·2).
Bacterial infections.

Eryplast *Lutsia, Fr.*
Barrier cream.
Nappy rash.

Erypo
Janssen-Cilag, Aust.; Janssen-Cilag, Fr.
Epoetin alfa (p.731·1).
Anaemias; autologous blood transfusion.

Ery-Reu *Reusch, Ger.†.*
Erythromycin lactobionate (p.201·3).
Bacterial infections.

Erysec *Lindopharm, Ger.*
Erythromycin stinoprate (p.203·3).
Bacterial infections.

Erysidoron 1 *Weleda, UK.*
Homoeopathic preparation.

Erysidoron 2 *Weleda, UK.*
Birch (p.1585·2); sulphur.
Boils; tonsillitis.

Erysidoron Nr 1 *Weleda, Aust.*
Homoeopathic preparation.

Erysidoron Nr 2 *Weleda, Aust.*
Homoeopathic preparation.

Erysil *Silom, Thai.*
Erythromycin estolate (p.201·2).
Bacterial infections.

Erysol
Stiefel, Canad.; Xepa-Soul Pattinson, Hong Kong; Xepa-Soul Pattinson, Singapore.
Erythromycin (p.201·2) or erythromycin ethyl succinate (p.201·2).
Bacterial infections.

Erysolvan *Fresenius Kabi, Aust.*
Erythromycin stinoprate (p.203·3).
Bacterial infections.

Eryson *Beacons, Singapore.*
Erythromycin (p.201·2) or erythromycin ethyl succinate (p.201·2).
Bacterial infections.

Erystat *Medpro, S.Afr.†.*
Erythromycin estolate (p.201·2).
Bacterial infections.

Erystrat *Orion, Denm.*
Erythromycin acistrate (p.201·2).
Bacterial infections.

Erytab *Abbott, Israel.*
Erythromycin (p.201·2).
Bacterial infections.

Ery-Tab
Abbott, Thai.; Abbott, USA.
Erythromycin (p.201·2).
Bacterial infections.

Erytab-S *Xepa-Soul Pattinson, Singapore.*
Erythromycin stearate (p.201·3).
Bacterial infections.

Eryteal *Pierre Fabre Sante, Fr.*
Cod-liver oil (p.1357·2); halibut-liver oil (p.1366·1); zinc oxide (p.1128·2); cetrimonium bromide (p.1137·3).
Burns; nappy rash.

Erythra-Derm *Paddock, USA.*
Erythromycin (p.201·2).
Formerly known as ETS-2%.
Acne.

Erythro *CT, Ger.*
Erythromycin ethyl succinate (p.201·2) or erythromycin stearate (p.201·3).
Bacterial infections.

Erythro Ethyl *DHA, Hong Kong.*
Erythromycin ethyl succinate (p.201·2).
Bacterial infections.

Erythrocin
Abbott, Aust.; Abbott, Austral.; Abbott, Canad.; Abbott, Ger.; Abbott, Hong Kong; Abbott, Irl.; Abbott, Israel; Abbott, S.Afr.; Abbott, Singapore; Abbott, Thai.; Abbott, UK; Abbott, USA.
Erythromycin (p.201·2), erythromycin ethyl succinate (p.201·2), erythromycin lactobionate (p.201·3), or erythromycin stearate (p.201·3).
Bacterial infections.

Erythrocin Neo *Abbott, Ger.*
Erythromycin stearate (p.201·3).
Bacterial infections.

Erythrocine
Abbott, Belg.; Abbott, Fr.; Abbott, Neth.; Abbott, Switz.
Erythromycin ethyl succinate (p.201·2), erythromycin lactobionate (p.201·3), or erythromycin stearate (p.201·3).
Bacterial infections.

Erythroderm *Agis, Israel.*
Erythromycin (p.201·2).
Acne.

Erythroforte *Abbott, Belg.*
Erythromycin ethyl succinate (p.201·2).
Bacterial infections.

Erythrogel *Biorga, Fr.*
Erythromycin (p.201·2).
Acne.

Erythrogenat *Azupharma, Ger.*
Erythromycin ethyl succinate (p.201·2) or erythromycin stearate (p.201·3).
Bacterial infections.

Erythrogram *Pharma 2000, Fr.*
Erythromycin ethyl succinate (p.201·2).
Bacterial infections.

Erythro-Hefa *Hefa, Ger.*
Erythromycin stearate (p.201·3).
Bacterial infections.

Erythrol *Vitamed, Israel.*
Erythromycin ethyl succinate (p.201·2).
Bacterial infections.

Erythromid
Abbott, Canad.; Abbott, Irl.†; Abbott, S.Afr.†; Abbott, UK.
Erythromycin (p.201·2).
Bacterial infections.

Erythroped
Abbott, Irl.; Abbott, Israel; Abbott, S.Afr.; Abbott, UK.
Erythromycin ethyl succinate (p.201·2).
Bacterial infections.

Erythro-Teva *Teva, Israel.*
Erythromycin (p.201·2), erythromycin ethyl succinate (p.201·2), or erythromycin stearate (p.201·3).
Bacterial infections.

Erytop *Stada, Ger.*
Erythromycin (p.201·2).
Acne.

Erytran *Spirig, Switz.*
Erythromycin stearate (p.201·3).
Bacterial infections.

Erytrociclin *Lisapharma, Ital.*
Erythromycin stearate (p.201·3).
Bacterial infections.

Eryval *Smetana, Aust.*
Absinthium (p.1571·1); centaury (p.1593·1); hypericum (p.290·2); peppermint leaf (p.1243·2); valerian (p.1678·3).
Gastrointestinal disorders.

Eryzole *Alra, USA.*
Erythromycin ethyl succinate (p.201·2); acetyl sulfafurazole (p.253·1).
Otitis media.

ES Bronchial Mixture *Torbet Laboratories, UK.*
Squill (p.1100·3); ipecacuanha tincture (p.1093·1); senega (p.1100·2); ammonium bicarbonate (p.1085·1).
Coughs.

Esacinone *Lisapharma, Ital.*
Fluocinolone acetonide (p.1071·2).
Skin disorders.

Esafosfina
Biomedica, Hong Kong; Biomedica, Ital.; Biomedica, Thai.
Sodium fructose-1,6-diphosphate.
Hypophosphataemia; ischaemia of lower limbs; myocardial infarction; regional ischaemia; shock.

Esafosfina Glutammica *Biomedica, Hong Kong.*
Calcium fructose-1,6-diphosphate; vitamin B substances (p.1350·1); levoglutamide (p.1365·2).
Metabolic disorders.

Esaglut *Biomedica, Ital.*
Levoglutamide (p.1365·2); dicalcium fructose-1,6-diphosphate; thiamine nitrate (p.1385·1); pyridoxine hydrochloride (p.1386·3); calcium pantothenate (p.1374·1).
Asthenia; mental function impairment; tonic.

Esametone *Lisapharma, Ital.*
Methylprednisolone (p.1076·1).
Oral corticosteroid.

Esapent *Pharmacia Upjohn, Ital.*
Omega-3 triglycerides (p.949·2).
Hypertriglyceridaemia.

Esarondil *Terapeutico, Ital.*
Methacycline hydrochloride (p.222·3).
Bacterial infections.

Esavir *Boniscontro & Gazzone, Ital.*
Aciclovir (p.612·3).
Herpesvirus infections.

Esbelcaps *Medix, Mex.*
Fenproporex hydrochloride (p.1510·2); diazepam (p.674·3).
Obesity.

Esbelt *Virtus, Braz.*
Thyroid (p.1526·2); bladderwrack (p.1585·2); bile salts (p.1585·1); phenolphthalein (p.1244·1).
Obesity.

Esbeltex *Medix, Mex.*
Glucomannan (p.1616·2).
Hyperglycaemia; hyperlipidaemias; obesity.

Esbeltrat *Luper, Braz.*
Thyroid (p.1526·2); bladderwrack (p.1585·2); phenolphthalein (p.1244·1).

Esbericard
Europharm, Aust.; Asta Medica, Switz.†.
Crataegus (p.1600·2).
Cardiac disorders.

Esbericard novo *Schaper & Brummer, Ger.*
Crataegus (p.1600·2).
Cardiac disorders.

Esbericum
Europharm, Aust.; Schaper & Brummer, Ger.
Hypericum (p.290·2).
Anxiety; depression.

Esberigal N *Schaper & Brummer, Ger.†*
Cnicus benedictus (p.1597·2); silybum marianum (p.1021·3); greater celandine (p.1618·1); chamomile (p.1593·2).
Biliary disorders.

Esberitop *Zeller, Switz.*
Thuja (p.1672·1); echinacea (p.1606·2); baptisia tinctoria; vitamin C (p.1389·3).
Cold symptoms.

Esberitox mono *Schaper & Brummer, Ger.*
Echinacea purpurea (p.1606·2).
Respiratory-tract infections.

Esberitox N
Schaper & Brummer, Ger.; Asta Medica, Switz.†.
Thuja (p.1672·1); baptisia tinctoria; echinacea purpurea et pallida (p.1606·2).
Respiratory-tract infections; tonic.

Esberiven
Note.This name is used for preparations of different composition.
Knoll, Fr.
Melilot; heparin sodium (p.902·1).
Peripheral vascular disorders.

Iquinosa, Spain.
Melilot; troxerutin (p.1611·2).
Peripheral vascular disorders.

Esberiven Forte *Knoll, Fr.*
Melilot; rutoside (p.1611·2).
Peripheral vascular disorders.

Esberizym N *Schaper & Brummer, Ger.†.*
Porcine pancreatin (p.1646·1); bromelains (p.1586·3); dimethicone (p.1249·2).
Digestive system disorders.

Escabin *Virtus, Braz.*
Lindane (p.1434·1).
Pediculosis; scabies.

Escacin *Reuffer, Mex.*
Benzyl benzoate (p.1428·2).

Escalgin sans codeine *Streuli, Switz.†.*
Salicylamide (p.82·1); propyphenazone (p.80·2); caffeine (p.761·3).
Fever; pain.

Escandine
Strallhofer, Aust.; Zambon, Braz.; Pharmazam, Spain.
Ibopamine hydrochloride (p.912·1).
Heart failure.

Escapin-N *Streger, Mex.*
Hyoscine butylbromide (p.468·2); paracetamol (p.71·2).
Smooth muscle pain and spasm.

Escarbicida *Stafford, Mex.*
Lindane (p.1434·1).

Escarine *Rivadis, Fr.*
Barrier preparation.

The symbol † denotes a preparation no longer actively marketed

Escarol *Muller Goppingen, Ger.*
Asarabacca (p.1582·3).
Respiratory-tract disorders.

Escatitona *Madaus, Aust.†.*
Homoeopathic preparation.

Escinogel *Doms-Adrian, Fr.*
Bamethan sulfate (p.843·1); aescin (p.1574·1).
Formerly contained bamethan sulfate, buphenine hydrochloride, and aescin.
Peripheral vascular disorders.

Esclama *Pharmacia Upjohn, Ger.*
Nimorazole (p.598·3).
Protozoal infections.

Esclebin *Wasserman, Spain.*
Norfloxacin (p.232·1).
Bacterial infections.

Esclerobion *Merck, Port.*
Vitamin A acetate (p.1383·2); pyridoxine hydrochloride (p.1386·3); dl-alpha tocoferil acetate (p.1394·1).
Atherosclerosis; vascular disorders.

Esclerovitan *Merck, Braz.*
Vitamins A, B₆, and E (p.1350·1).

Esclerovitan A O *Merck, Mex.*
Multivitamin and mineral preparation (p.1350·1).

Esclim *Women First, USA.*
Estradiol (p.1473·1).
Menopausal disorders; osteoporosis.

Escogripp sans codeine *Streuli, Switz.*
Propyphenazone (p.80·2); salicylamide (p.82·1); caffeine (p.761·3); ascorbic acid (p.1389·3); mepyramine maleate (p.421·1).
Cold and influenza symptoms.

Escophylline *Streuli, Switz.*
Aminophylline (p.760·1).
Obstructive airways disease.

Escoprim *Streuli, Switz.*
Co-trimoxazole (p.193·3).
Bacterial infections.

Escor *E. Merck, Denm.†; Pharmacal, Fin.; Trommsdorff, Ger.; Merck, Hong Kong.*
Nilvadipine (p.946·1).
Hypertension.

Escoretic *Streuli, Switz.*
Amiloride hydrochloride (p.835·1); hydrochlorothiazide (p.907·3).
Hypertension; oedema.

Escotussin *Streuli, Switz.*
Dihydrocodeine thiocyanate (p.33·3); belladonna (p.463·1); drosera (p.1606·1); guaifenesin (p.1092·2).
Coughs.

Escouflaire *Denolin, Belg.†.*
Belladonna leaf (p.463·1); stramonium leaf (p.474·1); hyoscyamus leaf (p.470·1); peppermint leaf (p.1243·2); potassium nitrate (p.1154·3).
Respiratory disorders.

Escumycin *Orion, Denm.*
Erythromycin (p.201·2) or erythromycin ethyl succinate (p.201·2).
Bacterial infections.

ESE *Abbott, Port.*
Erythromycin ethyl succinate (p.201·2).
Bacterial infections.

Esedril *Lipha, Ital.†.*
Naftidrofuryl oxalate (p.937·3).
Cerebral and peripheral vascular disorders.

Eselin *Ravizza, Ital.*
Etamsylate (p.732·2).
Haemorrhage; vascular disorders.

Esgic *Forest Pharmaceuticals, USA.*
Butalbital (p.658·3); paracetamol (p.71·2); caffeine (p.761·3).
Tension headache.

Esgic-Plus *Forest Pharmaceuticals, USA.*
Butalbital (p.658·3); paracetamol (p.71·2); caffeine (p.761·3).
Tension headache.

Esidrex *Novartis, Aust.; Ciba-Geigy, Belg.†; Novartis, Fr.; Novartis, Ital.; Novartis, Neth.; Novartis, Norw.†; Novartis, Spain; Novartis, Swed.; Novartis, Switz.*
Hydrochlorothiazide (p.907·3).
Diabetes insipidus; heart failure; hypercalciuria; hypertension; oedema.

Esidrix *Novartis, Ger.; Ciba, USA.*
Hydrochlorothiazide (p.907·3).
Hypertension; oedema.

Esilgan *Takeda, Ital.*
Estazolam (p.682·3).
Insomnia.

Esimil *Novartis, Ger.; Ciba, USA.*
Guanethidine monosulfate (p.901·1); hydrochlorothiazide (p.907·3).
Hypertension.

Esiteren *Novartis, Ger.*
Hydrochlorothiazide (p.907·3); triamterene (p.986·1).
Hypertension; oedema.

Eskacef *Julphar, UAE.*
Cefradine (p.173·3).
Bacterial infections.

Eskaflam *SmithKline Beecham, Mex.*
Nimesulide (p.62·3).
Fever; inflammation; pain; peri-articular and soft-tissue disorders.

Eskalith *SmithKline Beecham, USA.*
Lithium carbonate (p.292·1).
Bipolar disorder.

Eskamel *Dermatech, Austral.; Goldshield, UK.*
Resorcinol (p.1122·2); precipitated sulfur (p.1123·3).
Acne.

Eskapar *SmithKline Beecham, Mex.*
Nifuroxazide (p.230·2).
Diarrhoea.

Eskazine *SmithKline Beecham, Spain.*
Trifluoperazine hydrochloride (p.710·3).
Anxiety; psychoses.

Eskazole *SmithKline Beecham, Aust.; SmithKline Beecham, Austral.; SmithKline Beecham, Fr.; SmithKline Beecham, Ger.; SmithKline Beecham, Israel; Armstrong, Mex.; SmithKline Beecham, Neth.; SmithKline, Spain; SmithKline Beecham, UK†.*
Albendazole (p.95·2).
Cestode infections; giardiasis; intestinal nematode infections.

Eskim *Prospa, Ital.†.*
Omega-3 triglycerides (p.949·2).
Hypertriglyceridaemia.

Eskornade *Pharmaco, S.Afr.; Goldshield, UK.*
Phenylpropanolamine hydrochloride (p.1098·1); diphenylpyraline hydrochloride (p.417·1).
Formerly contained isopropamide, phenylpropanolamine hydrochloride, and diphenylpyraline hydrochloride in S.Afr.
Nasal and sinus congestion.

Esmacen *Smaller, Spain.*
Astemizole (p.409·1).
Hypersensitivity reactions.

Esmalorid *Merck, Ger.*
Trichlormethiazide (p.987·1); amiloride hydrochloride (p.835·1).
Hypertension; oedema.

Esmeron *Organon Teknika, Aust.; Organon Teknika, Austral.; Organon Teknika, Belg.; Organon Teknika, Denm.; Organon Teknika, Fin.; Organon Teknika, Fr.; Organon Teknika, Ger.; Organon Teknika, Hong Kong; Organon Teknika, Irl.; Organon Teknika, Israel; Organon Teknika, Ital.; Organon Teknika, Neth.; Organon Teknika, Norw.; Pharmaco, NZ; Organon, Port.; Sanofi Synthelabo, S.Afr.; Organon, Singapore; Organon Teknika, Spain; Organon Teknika, Swed.; Organon, Thai.; Organon, UK.*
Rocuronium bromide (p.1339·2).
Competitive neuromuscular blocker.

Eso Cem *Esoform, Ital.*
Glutaral (p.1145·2).
Instrument disinfection.

Eso Deterferri *Esoform, Ital.*
Benzalkonium chloride (p.1133·2).
Instrument disinfection.

Eso Din *Esoform, Ital.*
Glutaral (p.1145·2); phenol (p.1152·3).
Instrument disinfection.

Eso Ferri *Esoform, Ital.*
Benzalkonium chloride (p.1133·2).
Instrument disinfection.

Eso Ferri Alcolico *Esoform, Ital.*
Benzalkonium chloride (p.1133·2); alcohol (p.1130·3).
Instrument disinfection.

Eso Ferri Alcolico Plus *Esoform, Ital.*
Benzalkonium chloride (p.1133·2); isopropyl alcohol (p.1149·2).
Instrument disinfection.

Eso Ferri Plus *Esoform, Ital.*
Chlorhexidine gluconate (p.1138·2); isopropyl alcohol (p.1149·2).
Instrument disinfection and storage.

Eso HI, HP, and HPI *Esoform, Ital.*
Glutaral (p.1145·2).
Instrument disinfection.

Eso S 80 *Esoform, Ital.*
Benzalkonium chloride (p.1133·2); chlorhexidine gluconate (p.1138·2).
Instrument disinfection.

Esoalcolico Incolore *Esoform, Ital.*
Benzalkonium chloride (p.1133·2); alcohol (p.1130·3).
Skin, hand, and wound disinfection.

Esofenol 60 *Esoform, Ital.*
Sodium o-phenylphenol (p.1152·1).
Waste disinfection.

Esofenol Ferri *Esoform, Ital.*
Orthobenzyl parachlorophenol (p.1152·1); orthophenylphenol (p.1152·1).
Instrument disinfection.

Esofex *Leiras, Fin.*
Ranitidine hydrochloride (p.1245·2).
Dyspepsia; heartburn; peptic ulcer.

Esoform 92 *Esoform, Ital.*
Benzalkonium chloride (p.1133·2); glutaral (p.1145·2); alkylphenoxypolyglycol ether.
Surface disinfection.

Esoform Alcolico *Esoform, Ital.*
Benzalkonium chloride (p.1133·2); methyl salicylate; camphor; thyme oil; alcohol (p.1130·3); acetone; chloroform.
Skin disinfection.

Esoform Deterferri *Esoform, Ital.†.*
Benzalkonium chloride (p.1133·2).
Instrument disinfection.

Esoform Ferri *Esoform, Ital.†.*
Benzalkonium chloride (p.1133·2); sodium nitrite (p.1023·1); methylene blue [methylthioninium chloride].
Instrument disinfection.

Esoform Ferri Alcolico *Esoform, Ital.†.*
Benzalkonium chloride (p.1133·2); alcohol (p.1130·3); sodium nitrite (p.1023·1); acetone; chloroform.
Instrument disinfection.

Esoform Jod 20 and 50 *Esoform, Ital.*
Iodine (p.1522·3); potassium iodide (p.1522·3); alcohol; chloroform; isopropyl alcohol.
Skin and hand disinfection.

Esoform Jod 25 *Esoform, Ital.*
Alkylphenoxypolyglycol-iodine-ether complex.
Room and surface disinfection.

Esoform Jod 35 and 75 *Esoform, Ital.*
Povidone-iodine (p.1155·1).
Skin, wound, and hand disinfection.

Esoform Mani *Esoform, Ital.*
Chlorhexidine gluconate (p.1138·2); isopropyl alcohol; chloroform; alcohol.
Skin and hand disinfection.

Esoform Maniferri *Esoform, Ital.†.*
Chlorhexidine gluconate (p.1138·2); isopropyl alcohol (p.1149·2).
Skin, hand, and instrument disinfection.

Esoform 7 mc *Esoform, Ital.*
Paraformaldehyde (p.1152·2); hydrogen peroxide (40-45 volume) (p.1147·1).
Surface and room disinfection.

Esoform 70 mc *Esoform, Ital.*
Paraformaldehyde (p.1152·2); hydrogen peroxide (40-45 volume) (p.1147·1).
Room disinfection.

Eso-Jod 100 500 *Esoform, Ital.*
Povidone-iodine (p.1155·1).
Wound disinfection.

Esol *Leiras, Fin.*
d-Alpha tocopherol (p.1393·3).
Vitamin E deficiency.

Esolut *Angelini, Ital.*
Progesterone (p.1488·3).
Luteal insufficiency.

E-Solve *Syosset, USA.*
Vehicle for topical preparations.

Esosan *Esoform, Ital.*
Benzalkonium chloride (p.1133·2).
Skin and surface disinfection.

Esosan Pronto *Esoform, Ital.*
Chlorhexidine gluconate (p.1138·2); benzalkonium chloride (p.1133·2).
Disinfection.

Esoterica
Note. This name is used for preparations of different composition.
Medicis, Canad.
Hydroquinone (p.1115·1); oxybenzone (p.1518·1); padimate O (p.1518·2).
Skin pigmentation disorders.

Lenthéric, UK†.
Hydroquinone (p.1115·1).

Esoterica Facial and Sunscreen *Medicis, USA.*
Hydroquinone (p.1115·1); padimate O (p.1518·2); oxybenzone (p.1518·1).
Hyperpigmentation.

Esoterica Regular *Medicis, Canad.*
Hydroquinone (p.1115·1).
Skin pigmentation disorders.

Esoterica Sensitive Skin and Regular *Medicis, USA.*
Hydroquinone (p.1115·1).
Hyperpigmentation.

Esoterica Unscented *Medicis, Canad.*
Hydroquinone (p.1115·1).
Skin pigmentation disorders.

Esotran *Almirall, Spain.*
Estradiol (p.1473·1).
Menopausal disorders; osteoporosis.

Esoxid *Esoform, Ital.*
Glutaral (p.1145·2).
Instrument disinfection.

Espabion *Degorts, Mex.*
Trimebutine (p.1675·1).
Gastrointestinal motility disorders.

espa-butyl *Esparma, Ger.†.*
Hyoscine butylbromide (p.468·2).
Smooth muscle spasm.

Espacil *ICN, Mex.*
Hyoscine butylbromide (p.468·2).
Smooth muscle spasm.

Espacil Compuesto *ICN, Mex.*
Hyoscine butylbromide (p.468·2); clonixin lysine (p.25·1).
Smooth muscle pain and spasm.

espa-dorm *Esparma, Ger.*
Zopiclone (p.713·1).
Sleep disorders.

espa-formin *Esparma, Ger.*
Metformin hydrochloride (p.332·3).
Diabetes mellitus.

espa-lepsin *Esparma, Ger.*
Carbamazepine (p.342·2).
Alcohol withdrawal syndrome; diabetic neuropathy; epilepsy; multiple sclerosis; neuralgias.

espa-lipon *Esparma, Ger.*
Thioctic acid (p.1671·3) or ethylenediamine thioctate (p.1671·3).
Diabetic polyneuropathy.

espa-moxin *Esparma, Ger.*
Amoxicillin trihydrate (p.149·2).
Bacterial infections.

Espar *Greater Pharma, Thai.*
Aspartame (p.1354·3).
Sugar substitute.

Esparil *Esparma, Ger.†.*
Captopril (p.853·3).
Heart failure; hypertension.

Esparon *Orion, Ger.*
Alprazolam (p.654·2).
Anxiety.

Espasantral *Carnot, Mex.*
Hyoscine methobromide (p.468·2).

Espasmacid *Gemballa, Braz.*
Aluminium hydroxide (p.1210·3); magnesium hydroxide (p.1233·1); dimethicone (p.1249·2).
Flatulence; gastrointestinal hyperacidity.

Espasmalgon *Dovalle, Braz.*
Papaverine hydrochloride (p.1648·1); phenobarbital (p.355·1); homatropine methylbromide (p.468·1); phenazone (p.77·2); hyoscyamus (p.470·1).
Smooth muscle spasm.

Espasmo Canulasa *Novartis, Spain†.*
Cellulase (p.1593·1); dimethicone (p.1249·2); glutamic acid hydrochloride (p.1365·2); metixene hydrochloride (p.470·2); pancreatin (p.1646·1); pepsin (p.1649·3); dehydrocholic acid (p.1602·2).
Digestive system insufficiency; meteorism.

Espasmo Canulase *Novartis, Port.*
Cellulase (p.1593·1); dimethicone (p.1249·2); glutamic acid hydrochloride (p.1365·2); metixene hydrochloride (p.470·2); pancreatin (p.1646·1); pepsin (p.1649·3); sodium dehydrocholate (p.1602·2).

Espasmo Cibalgina *Novartis, Mex.*
Drofenine hydrochloride (p.466·3); propyphenazone (p.80·2).
Smooth muscle pain and spasm.

Espasmo Colic *Makros, Braz.*
Homatropine methylbromide (p.468·1); dimethicone (p.1249·2).
Smooth muscle spasm.

Espasmo Digestomen *Menarini, Spain.*
Amylase (p.1579·3); methionine phenylbutyrate; nicotinic acid (p.1372·3); papain (p.1647·3); pepsin (p.1649·3); flopropione (p.1611·3); betaine hydrochloride (p.1584·3); pancreatin (p.1646·1); lipase; bile extract (p.1585·1); cellulase (p.1593·1); hemicellulase (p.1593·1).
Biliary-tract disorders; digestive system insufficiency; dyspepsia; meteorism.

Espasmo Luftal *Bristol-Myers Squibb, Braz.*
Homatropine methylbromide (p.468·1); dimethicone (p.1249·2).
Smooth muscle spasm.

Espasmo Novozyme *Novartis, Braz.*
Metixene hydrochloride (p.470·2); dimethicone (p.1249·2); cellulase (p.1593·1); pepsin (p.1649·3); glutamic acid hydrochloride (p.1365·2); pancreatin (p.1646·1); sodium dehydrocholate (p.1602·2).
Digestive-system disorders.

Espasmo Silidron *Enila, Braz.*
Dimethicone (p.1249·2); camylofin (p.1590·1).
Smooth muscle spasm.

Espasmobel *Opofarm, Braz.*
Dipyrone (p.34·1); adiphenine hydrochloride; papaverine (p.1648·1); homatropine (p.468·1).
Smooth muscle spasm.

Espasmocron *Delta, Braz.*
Atropine (p.460·3); papaverine (p.1648·1); thiamine (p.1385·2); phenazone (p.77·2).
Smooth muscle spasm.

Espasmodid Composto *Uniao Quimica, Braz.*
Hyoscine butylbromide (p.468·2); dipyrone (p.34·1).
Smooth muscle spasm.

Espasmolex *Bergamo, Braz.*
Papaverine hydrochloride (p.1648·1); belladonna (p.463·1); star anise; hyoscyamus (p.470·1); boldo (p.1585·3).
Smooth muscle spasm.

Espasmosan *Leofarma, Braz.*
Belladonna (p.463·1); papaverine hydrochloride (p.1648·1).
Smooth muscle spasm.

Espasmosan Composto *Leofarma, Braz.*
Belladonna (p.463·1); papaverine hydrochloride (p.1648·1); dipyrone (p.34·1).
Smooth muscle spasm.

Espaven *ICN, Mex.*
Dimethicone (p.1249·2); calcium pantothenate (p.1374·1).
Gastrointestinal disorders.

Espaven Alcalino *ICN, Mex.*
Aluminium hydroxide (p.1210·3); magnesium hydroxide (p.1233·1); dimethicone (p.1249·2).
Gastrointestinal hyperacidity.

Espaven Enzimatico *ICN, Mex.*
Pancreatin (p.1646·1); dimethicone (p.1249·2); ox bile (p.1585·1); Aspergillus niger cellulase (p.1593·1).
Gastrointestinal disorders.

Espaven MD *ICN, Mex.*
Metoclopramide hydrochloride (p.1235·2); dimethicone (p.1249·2).
Gastrointestinal disorders.

Espaven Pediatrico *ICN, Mex.*
Dimethicone (p.1249·2).
Gastrointestinal disorders.

Especies Calmantes *Bergamo, Braz.*
Passion flower (p.1649·1); erythrina mulungu; melissa (p.1632·2).
Sedative.

Espectral *Centrum, Spain.*
Ampicillin trihydrate (p.151·1); muramidase hydrochloride (p.1638·1).
Bacterial infections.

Espectral Balsamico *Centrum, Spain.*
Ampicillin trihydrate (p.151·1); guaifenesin (p.1092·2); muramidase hydrochloride (p.1638·1).
Respiratory-tract infections.

Espectrin *Glaxo Wellcome, Braz.*
Co-trimoxazole (p.193·3).
Bacterial infections; Pneumocystis carinii pneumonia; protozoal infections.

Espectrosira *Clariana, Spain.*
Ampicillin sodium (p.150·3); ampicillin benzathine (p.151·3); bromhexine hydrochloride (p.1085·3); guaifenesin (p.1092·2).
Lignocaine (lidocaine) hydrochloride (p.1313·3) is included in this preparation to alleviate the pain of injection.
Respiratory-tract infections.

Espeden *Vita, Spain.*
Norfloxacin (p.232·1).
Bacterial infections.

Esperal *Sanofi Winthrop, Fr.*
Disulfiram (p.1605·1).
Chronic alcoholism.

Esperson *Hoechst Marion Roussel, Braz.; Hoechst Marion Roussel, Hong Kong; Hoechst Marion Roussel, Thai.*
Desoximetasone (p.1066·2).
Skin disorders.

Esperson N *Hoechst Marion Roussel, Braz.*
Desoximetasone (p.1066·2); neomycin sulfate (p.228·1).
Infected skin disorders.

Espesil *Orion, Fin.*
Acebutolol hydrochloride (p.825·1).
Angina pectoris; arrhythmias; hypertension; myocardial infarction.

Espidifen *Zambon, Spain.*
Ibuprofen arginine (p.44·1).
Fever; musculoskeletal, joint, and peri-articular disorders; pain.

Espiran *ICT, Ital.†*
Fenspiride hydrochloride (p.765·3).
Respiratory-tract disorders.

Espiride *Aspen, S.Afr.*
Sulpiride (p.706·1).
Behaviour disorders; depression; peptic ulcer; psychoses; vertigo.

Espledol *Fher, Spain.*
Acemetacin (p.11·2).
Musculoskeletal and joint disorders; peri-articular disorders.

Espo *Kirin, Jpn.*
Epoetin alfa (p.731·1).
Anaemia; autologous blood transfusion.

Espongostan *Byk Leo, Spain†.*
Gelatin (p.737·2).
Mucous membrane haemorrhage.

Espotabs *Combe, Canad.†; Combe, USA†.*
Yellow phenolphthalein (p.1244·1).
Constipation.

Esprenit *Hennig, Ger.*
Ibuprofen (p.43·2) or ibuprofen sodium (p.44·1).
Fever; inflammation; musculoskeletal, joint, and soft-tissue disorders; pain.

Esprit *Bayer, Austral.*
Test for glucose in blood (p.1616·3).

Esprit Sensor *Bayer Diagnostics, Irl.*
Test for glucose in blood.
For use with Esprit Glucometer.

Espritin *Petrasch, Aust.*
Lactic acid (p.1626·2).
Psoriasis.

Espumisan *Berlin-Chemie, Ger.*
Simeticone (p.1249·2).
Defoaming agent in radiography and endoscopy of the gastrointestinal tract.

Esquinon *Sankyo, Jpn†.*
Carboquone (p.516·1).
Malignant neoplasms.

Esracain *Rafa, Israel.*
Lignocaine (lidocaine) hydrochloride (p.1313·2).
Arrhythmias; local anaesthesia.

Esradin *Sigma-Tau, Ital.*
Isradipine (p.916·3).
Hypertension.

Essamin *Torre, Ital.*
Amino-acid preparation (p.1350·1).
Renal failure.

Essaven
Note. This name is used for preparations of different composition.
Rhone-Poulenc Rorer, Ger.; Rhone-Poulenc Rorer, Ital.; Aventis, S.Afr.
Topical gel: Aescin (p.1574·1); heparin sodium (p.902·1); essential phospholipids.
Soft-tissue trauma; vascular disorders.

Rhone-Poulenc Rorer, Hong Kong; Aventis, S.Afr.; Rhone-Poulenc Rorer, Thai.
Capsules: Aescin (p.1574·1); rutoside (p.1611·2); essential phospholipids.
Vascular disorders.

Rhone-Poulenc Rorer, Ital.
Capsules: Aescin (p.1574·1); phosphatidyl choline (p.1651·1).
Formerly contained aescin, rutoside, and phosphatidylcholine.
Venous insufficiency.

Essaven 60 000 *Rhone-Poulenc Rorer, Ger.*
Heparin sodium (p.902·1).
Soft-tissue disorders; superficial vascular disorders.

Essaven Mono *Nattermann, Ger.†.*
Aesculus (p.1574·1).
Chronic venous insufficiency.

Essaven N *Rhone-Poulenc Rorer, Ger.*
Aesculus (p.1574·1); trimethylhesperidin chalcone (p.1611·2).
Soft-tissue disorders; vascular disorders.

Essaven Sport *Rhone-Poulenc Rorer, Ger.*
Glycol salicylate (p.42·2); arnica tincture (p.1581·3).
Sports injuries.

Essaven Tri-Complex *Rhone-Poulenc Rorer, Ger.*
Heparin sodium (p.902·1); allantoin (p.1110·1); dexpanthenol (p.1602·3).
Soft-tissue disorders; superficial vascular disorders.

Essaven ultra *Rhone-Poulenc Rorer, Ger.*
Aesculus (p.1574·1); trimethylhesperidin chalcone (p.1611·2); essential phospholipids.
Soft-tissue injury; vascular disorders.

Essavenon *Nattermann, Spain.*
Aescin (p.1574·1); phospholipids; heparin sodium (p.902·1).
Peripheral vascular disorders; soft-tissue disorders.

Essen *Abbott, Braz.*
Metoclopramide hydrochloride (p.1235·2); dimethicone (p.1249·2); dehydrocholic acid (p.1602·2); cellulase (p.1593·1); pepsin (p.1649·3); lipase; amylase (p.1579·3); pancreatin (p.1646·1).
Digestive-system disorders.

Essen Enzimatico *Scharper, Ital.*
Pepsin (p.1649·3); amylase (p.1579·3); lipase; trypsin (p.1675·3); chymotrypsin (p.1595·1); cellulase (p.1593·1).
Dyspepsia.

Essence Algerienne *Toulade, Fr.*
Eucalyptol (p.1609·2); menthol (p.1632·3); guaiacol (p.1092·1).
Upper respiratory-tract congestion.

Essential B *General Nutrition, Canad.*
Vitamin B substances (p.1350·1).

Essential Balance *Pharmavite, Canad.*
Multivitamin and mineral preparation (p.1350·1).

Essential ProPlus *Nutrisoy, USA.*
Preparation for enteral nutrition (p.1350·1).

Essentiale
Note. This name is used for preparations of different composition.
Gerot, Aust.; Rhone-Poulenc Rorer, Hong Kong; Aventis, S.Afr.; Rhone-Poulenc Rorer, Thai.
Essential phospholipids; vitamins (p.1350·1).
Liver disorders.

Rhone-Poulenc Rorer, Ital.
Phosphatidyl choline (p.1651·1).
Liver disorders.

Essentiale N *Rhone-Poulenc Rorer, Ger.*
Essential phospholipids.
Gallstones; liver disorders; psoriasis; radiation trauma.

Essentielle Aminosauren *Fresenius Kabi, Ger.*
Amino-acid preparation (p.1350·1).
Dietary supplement in renal failure.

Essex
Schering-Plough, Denm.; Essex, Ger.; Essex, Switz.
Emollient.
Skin disorders.

Schering-Plough, Fin.
A range of vehicles for topical preparations.

Essigsaure Tonerde-Salbe *Michallik, Ger.*
Aluminium acetotartrate (p.1578·2).
Soft-tissue disorders.

Essitol *Athenstaedt, Ger.*
Aluminium acetotartrate (p.1578·2).
Insect stings; soft-tissue injury.

EST *Rosch & Handel, Aust.*
Alum (p.1577·2); calcium acetate (p.1187·3); calcium carbonate (p.1215·1).
Bruises; insect bites; sprains; swelling.

Establix *BA Farma, Port.†.*
Buspirone hydrochloride (p.657·2).
Anxiety; insomnia.

Estac *Gross, Braz.*
Metoclopramide hydrochloride (p.1235·2); pyridoxine hydrochloride (p.1386·3).
Nausea and vomiting.

Estafan *Herals, Braz.*
Arginine; vitamin C (p.1350·1).
Nutritional supplement.

Estafiloide *IQB, Braz.*
A staphylococcal vaccine (toxoid) (p.1565·1).
Active immunisation.

Estalis
Novartis, Fin.; Novartis, Swed.
Estradiol (p.1473·1); norethisterone acetate (p.1485·1).
Menopausal disorders; osteoporosis.

Estalis Continuous *Novartis, Austral.*
Estradiol (p.1473·1); norethisterone acetate (p.1485·1).
Menopausal disorders; osteoporosis.

Estalis Sekvens
Novartis, Fin.; Novartis, Swed.
4 Patches, estradiol (p.1473·1); 4 patches, estradiol; norethisterone acetate (p.1485·1).
Menopausal disorders; osteoporosis.

Estalis Sequi
Novartis, Austral.; Novartis, Port.
4 Patches, estradiol (p.1473·1); 4 patches, estradiol; norethisterone acetate (p.1485·1).
Menopausal disorders; osteoporosis.

Estandron *Organon, Aust.†.*
Estradiol benzoate (p.1473·1); estradiol phenylpropionate (p.1473·2); testosterone propionate (p.1492·2); testosterone phenylpropionate (p.1492·2); testosterone isocaproate (p.1492·2).
Menopausal disorders.

Estandron P *Akzo, Braz.*
Estradiol benzoate (p.1473·1); estradiol phenylpropionate (p.1473·2); testosterone propionate (p.1492·2); testosterone phenylpropionate (p.1492·2); testosterone isocaproate (p.1492·2).
Menopausal disorders.

Estar
Westwood-Squibb, Canad.; Westwood-Squibb, USA.
Coal tar (p.1125·1).
Psoriasis.

Estecina
APS, Port.; Normon, Spain.
Ciprofloxacin (p.182·3), ciprofloxacin hydrochloride (p.182·3), or ciprofloxacin lactate (p.182·3).
Bacterial infections.

Esteclin *Lakeside, Mex.*
Erdosteine (p.1091·2).
Respiratory-tract disorders with viscous mucus.

Esteclin Bac *Lakeside, Mex.*
Amoxicillin trihydrate (p.149·2); erdosteine (p.1091·2).
Respiratory-tract infections.

Esten *Rhone Poulenc Rorer, Austral.†.*
Vitamins and minerals (p.1350·1); arizona garlic (p.1614·1); lecithin (p.1628·1); cimicifuga (p.1595·2); viburnum opulus; passion flower (p.1649·1); smilax (p.1661·1).
Menopausal disorders.

Esteprim *Solfran, Mex.*
Co-trimoxazole (p.193·3).
Bacterial infections.

Ester Aces *Sisu, Canad.*
Betacarotene, selenium, vitamin C, and vitamin E (p.1350·1).

Ester C EVC *Sisu, Canad.*
Vitamins A, B, and C with zinc (p.1350·1).

Esterasine *Baxter, Fr.*
Complement C1 esterase inhibitor (p.1599·1).
Hereditary angioedema.

Esterbiol *Inexfa, Spain.*
Pyricarbate (p.1656·3).
Hypercholesterolaemia.

Ester-C
Note. This name is used for preparations of different composition.
Quest, Canad.; Sisu, Canad.; Stanley, Canad.
Calcium ascorbate (p.1389·3).

Solgar, UK.
Vitamin C with bioflavonoids (p.1350·1).

Ester-C Plus *Solgar, USA.*
Vitamin C (p.1389·3); citrus bioflavonoids complex (p.1611·1); red cherry (p.1029·1); rose hips (p.1389·3); rutoside (p.1611·2); calcium (p.1187·3).
Capillary bleeding.

Ester-C Plus Multi-Mineral *Solgar, USA.*
Vitamin C (p.1389·3); citrus bioflavonoids complex (p.1611·1); red cherry (p.1029·1); rose hips (p.1389·3); rutoside (p.1611·2); calcium; magnesium; potassium; zinc (p.1180·1).
Capillary bleeding.

Estericlean *Braun, Spain.*
Sodium chloride (p.1196·1).
Fluid and electrolyte replacement; hypovolaemia.

Esterofundina *Braun, Fr.*
Electrolyte infusion with or without glucose (p.1180·1).
Fluid and electrolyte disorders.

Esterol *Laborest, Ital.*
Rice oil; vitamin E; oleic acid; linoleic acid; linolenic acid; gamma-orizanol (p.1350·1).
Nutritional supplement.

Esterol Plus *Laborest, Ital.*
Rice oil; tocotrienol; vitamin E; gamma-orizanol (p.1350·1).
Nutritional supplement.

Esteromicin *Universales, Mex.*
Erythromycin (p.201·2).
Bacterial infections.

Estigyn *Glaxo Wellcome, Austral.†.*
Ethinylestradiol (p.1476·2).
Amenorrhoea; menopausal disorders.

Estilsona *Astra, Spain.*
Prednisolone steaglate (p.1078·2).
Corticosteroid.

Estima *Effik, Fr.*
Progesterone (p.1488·3).

Estimulocel *Synthelabo, Spain†.*
Procodazole ethyl ester (p.1655·1).
Immunotherapy.

Estinyl *Schering, Canad.†; Schering-Plough, S.Afr.; Schering, USA.*
Ethinylestradiol (p.1476·2).
Breast cancer; female hypogonadism; menopausal disorders; prostatic cancer.

Estivan *Aventis, Belg.*
Ebastine (p.417·2).
Allergic conjunctivitis; allergic rhinitis; urticaria.

Estivin *Alcon, USA†.*
Naphazoline hydrochloride (p.1095·1); hypromellose (p.1501·3).
Minor eye irritation.

Esto *Angelini, Ital.*
Alfoscerate olamine.
Anxiety disorders.

Estomagel *Neo Quimica, Braz.*
Aluminium hydroxide (p.1210·3); magnesium trisilicate (p.1233·3).
Gastrointestinal hyperacidity.

Estomaplus *QIF, Braz.*
Metoclopramide (p.1236·3).
Gastrointestinal motility disorders; nausea and vomiting.

Estomazil *Dorsay, Braz.*
Sodium carbonate (p.1665·1); sodium bicarbonate (p.1186·2); citric acid (p.1596·2).
Gastrointestinal hyperacidity.

Estomil *Merck, Spain.*
Lansoprazole (p.1230·3).
Gastro-oesophageal reflux; peptic ulcer.

Estomycin *Columbia, S.Afr.†.*
Erythromycin estolate (p.201·2).
Bacterial infections.

Estovyn-T *Grossman, Mex.*
Tinidazole (p.603·3).

Estrabeta *Betapharm, Ger.*
Estradiol (p.1473·1).
Menopausal disorders; osteoporosis.

Estrace
Roberts, Canad.; Bristol-Myers Squibb, USA.
Estradiol (p.1473·1).
Breast cancer; female castration; female hypogonadism; menopausal vasomotor symptoms; osteoporosis; primary ovarian failure; prostatic cancer; vulval and vaginal atrophy.

Estracomb
Novartis, Aust.; Novartis, Braz.; Novartis, Canad.; Novartis, Denm.; Novartis, Fin.; Novartis, Ger.; Novartis, Hong Kong; Novartis, Ital.; Byk Gulden, Mex.; Novartis, Neth.; Novartis, Norw.; Novartis, Port.; Novartis, Singapore; Novartis, Spain; Novartis, Swed.; Novartis, Switz.
4 Patches, estradiol (p.1473·1) (Estraderm); 4 patches, estradiol; norethisterone acetate (p.1485·1) (Estragest).
Menopausal disorders; oestrogen deficiency; osteoporosis.

Estracombi
Novartis, Austral.; Novartis, Belg.; Novartis, Irl.; Novartis, S.Afr.; Novartis, UK.
4 Patches, estradiol (p.1473·1) (Estraderm TTS); 4 patches, estradiol; norethisterone acetate (p.1485·1) (Estragest TTS).
Menopausal disorders; osteoporosis.

Estracyt
Pharmacia Upjohn, Aust.; Pharmacia Upjohn, Austral.†; Pharmacia Upjohn, Belg.; Pharmacia Upjohn, Denm.; Pharmacia Upjohn, Fin.; Pharmacia Upjohn, Fr.; Pharmacia Upjohn, Ger.; Pharmacia Upjohn, Hong Kong; Pharmacia Upjohn, Israel; Pharmacia Upjohn, Ital.; Shinyaku, Jpn; Pharmacia Upjohn, Neth.; Pharmacia Upjohn, Norw.; Pharmacia Upjohn, Port.; Pharmacia Upjohn, S.Afr.; Pharmacia Upjohn, Singapore; Pharmacia Upjohn, Spain; Pharmacia Upjohn, Swed.; Pharmacia Upjohn, Switz.; Pharmacia, UK.
Estramustine meglumine phosphate, estramustine phosphate (p.537·3), or estramustine sodium phosphate (p.537·3).
Prostatic cancer.

Estraderm
Novartis, Aust.; Novartis, Austral.; Novartis, Belg.; Novartis, Braz.; Novartis, Canad.; Novartis, Denm.; Novartis, Fin.; Novartis, Fr.; Novartis, Ger.; Novartis, Hong Kong; Novartis, Israel; Novartis, Ital.; Byk Gulden, Mex.; Novartis, Neth.; Novartis, Norw.; Novartis, NZ; Novartis, Port.; Novartis, S.Afr.; Novartis, Singapore; Novartis, Spain; Novartis, Swed.; Novartis, Switz.; Novartis, UK; Novartis, USA.
Estradiol (p.1473·1).
Menopausal disorders; oestrogen deficiency; osteoporosis.

Estradurin
Pharmacia Upjohn, Aust.; Pharmacia Upjohn, Denm.; Pharmacia Upjohn, Fin.; Pharmacia Upjohn, Ger.; Pharmacia Upjohn, Neth.; Pharmacia Upjohn, Norw.; Pharmacia Upjohn, Spain†; Pharmacia Upjohn, Swed.; Pharmacia Upjohn, Switz.; Pharmacia Upjohn, UK†.
Polyestradiol phosphate (p.1488·1).
Mepivacaine hydrochloride (p.1317·1) is included in this preparation to alleviate the pain of injection.
Amenorrhoea; breast cancer; menopausal disorders; prostatic cancer.

Estradurine *Pharmacia Upjohn, Belg.*
Polyestradiol phosphate (p.1488·1).
Mepivacaine hydrochloride (p.1317·1) is included in this preparation to alleviate the pain of injection.
Prostatic cancer.

Estrafemol *Henning, Ger.*
12 Capsules, estradiol valerate (p.1473·2); 14 capsules, estradiol valerate; medroxyprogesterone acetate (p.1480·1).
Menopausal disorders.

The symbol † denotes a preparation no longer actively marketed

Estragest *Ciba-Geigy, Aust.; Novartis, Ger.; Novartis, Switz.*
Estradiol (p.1473·1); norethisterone acetate (p.1485·1).
Menopausal disorders; osteoporosis.

Estra-L *Pasadena, USA†.*
Estradiol valerate (p.1473·2).
Female castration; female hypogonadism; menopausal vasomotor symptoms; prevention of breast engorgement; primary ovarian failure; prostatic cancer; vulval and vaginal atrophy.

Estramon *Hexal, Aust.; Hexal, Ger.; Rowex, Irl.; Ecosol, Switz.*
Estradiol (p.1473·1).
Menopausal disorders; osteoporosis.

Estrapak
Note. This name is used for preparations of different composition.
Novartis, Austral.
8 Patches, estradiol (p.1473·1) (Estraderm); 14 tablets, medroxyprogesterone acetate (p.1480·1) (Provera).
Menopausal disorders; osteoporosis.

Novartis, Irl.; Novartis, Mex.; Novartis, NZ; Novartis, UK.
Transdermal patches, estradiol (p.1473·1) (Estraderm); tablets, norethisterone acetate (p.1485·1).
Menopausal disorders; osteoporosis.

Estratab *Solvay, USA.*
Esterified oestrogens (p.1473·1).
Breast cancer; menopausal vasomotor symptoms; oestrogen deficiency; osteoporosis; prostatic cancer; vulval and vaginal atrophy.

Estratest *Solvay, USA.*
Esterified oestrogens (p.1473·1); methyltestosterone (p.1482·3).
Menopausal disorders.

Estrefen *Solfran, Mex.*
Dihydrostreptomycin (p.199·2); sulfadiazine (p.251·1).
Diarrhoea.

Estregur *Tegur, Mex.*
Chlorotrianisene (p.1465·3).

Estreptoenterol *Juste, Spain.*
Dihydrostreptomycin sulfate (p.199·2); phthalylsulfathiazole (p.235·3); pectin (p.1502·3).
Gastrointestinal infections.

Estreva *Theramex, Hong Kong; Theramex, Mon.*
Estradiol (p.1473·1).
Oestrogen deficiency.

Estrex *Lake, USA.*
Homoeopathic preparation.

Estriagel *Medicamed, Port.*
Collagen (p.1598·2); cerais oil; placenta filatol.
Firming cream.

Estrifam *Novo Nordisk, Ger.*
Estradiol (p.1473·1).
Menopausal disorders; oestrogen deficiency; osteoporisis.

Estring *Pharmacia Upjohn, Aust.†; Pharmacia Upjohn, Austral.; Pharmacia Upjohn, Canad.; Pharmacia Upjohn, Denm.; Pharmacia Upjohn, Fin.; Pharmacia Upjohn, Ger.; Pharmacia Upjohn, Neth.; Pharmacia Upjohn, Norw.; Pharmacia Upjohn, NZ; Pharmacia Upjohn, S.Afr.; Pharmacia Upjohn, Switz.; Pharmacia, UK; Pharmacia Upjohn, USA.*
Estradiol (p.1473·1).
Postmenopausal atrophy of the vagina or lower urinary-tract.

Estrocare *Pharmanex, USA.*
Cordyceps sinensis; cimicifuga (p.1595·2).
Menopausal disorders.

Estroclim *Sigma-Tau, Ital.*
Estradiol (p.1473·1).
Menopausal disorders; osteoporosis.

Estro-Cyp *Keene, USA†.*
Estradiol cipionate (p.1473·2).
Female hypogonadism; menopausal vasomotor symptoms.

Estrofem *Novo Nordisk, Aust.; Novo Nordisk, Austral.; Novo Nordisk, Belg.; Novo Nordisk, Denm.; Novo Nordisk, Fin.; Rhone-Poulenc Rorer, Fr.; Novo Nordisk, Hong Kong; Novo Nordisk, Irl.; Novo Nordisk, Israel; Novo Nordisk, Neth.; Novo Nordisk, NZ; Novo Nordisk, Port.; Novo Nordisk, S.Afr.; Novo Nordisk, Singapore; Novo Nordisk, Thai.*
Estradiol (p.1473·1).
Formerly contained estradiol and estriol in *Fr.* and *S.Afr.*
Menopausal disorders; oestrogen deficiency; osteoporosis.

Estrofem N *Novo Nordisk, Switz.*
Estradiol (p.1473·1).
Estrofem formerly contained estradiol and estriol.
Oestrogen deficiency.

Estrogel *Asta Medica, Aust.; Schering, Canad.; Leiras, Denm.; Leiras, Fin.*
Estradiol (p.1473·1).
Menopausal disorders; osteoporosis.

Estronar *Sanitas, Port.*
Estradiol (p.1473·1).
Menopausal disorders; prostatic cancer.

Estronorm *Jenapharm, Ger.*
Estradiol (p.1473·1).
Menopausal disorders; osteoporosis.

Estro-Pause *Adcock Ingram, S.Afr.*
Estradiol valerate (p.1473·2).
Menopausal disorders.

Estrostep *Parke, Davis, USA.*
Norethisterone acetate (p.1485·1); ethinylestradiol (p.1476·2).
Triphasic oral contraceptive.

Estrostep Fe *Parke, Davis, USA.*
21 Tablets, norethisterone acetate (p.1485·1); ethinylestradiol (p.1476·2); 7 tablets, ferrous fumarate (p.1360·1).
Triphasic oral contraceptive.

Estroxyn *Pharmacia Upjohn, Austral.*
Tamoxifen citrate (p.571·1).
Breast cancer.

Estulic *Novartis, Belg.; Novartis, Fr.; Novartis, Ger.; Asta Medica, Neth.*
Guanfacine hydrochloride (p.901·3).
Hypertension.

Esucos *UCB, Aust.; UCB, Belg.; UCB, Denm.; UCB, Fin.; SIT, Ital.; UCB, Norw.; UCB, Swed.*
Dixyrazine (p.682·1).
Alcohol withdrawal syndrome; anxiety; depression; nausea; neuroleptanalgesia; premedication; psychiatric disorders; vomiting.

Eta Biocortilen *SIFI, Ital.*
Dexamethasone sodium phosphate (p.1067·1); neomycin sulfate (p.228·1).
Formerly contained dexamethasone sodium phosphate, neomycin sulfate, and gramicidin.
Infected eye disorders.

Eta Biocortilen VC *SIFI, Ital.*
Dexamethasone sodium phosphate (p.1067·1); neomycin sulfate (p.228·1); gramicidin (p.213·3); tetryzoline hydrochloride (p.1101·2).
Infected eye disorders.

Eta Cortilen *SIFI, Ital.†.*
Dexamethasone sodium phosphate (p.1067·1).
Eye disorders.

Etabus *Columbia, Mex.*
Disulfiram (p.1605·1).

Etalontin *Parke, Davis, Aust.†.*
Ethinylestradiol (p.1476·2); norethisterone acetate (p.1485·1).
Combined oral contraceptive.

Etalpha *Leo, Aust.; Leo, Denm.; Leo, Fin.; Leo, Neth.; Leo, Norw.; Farmacusi, Spain; Leo, Swed.*
Alfacalcidol (p.1391·1).
Hypoparathyroidism; osteomalacia; osteoporosis; renal osteodystrophy; rickets; vitamin D deficiency.

Etamucin *Sanova, Aust.*
Sodium hyaluronate (p.1620·1).
Adjunct in ophthalmic surgery.

Etanicozid B6 *Piam, Ital.*
Ethambutol hydrochloride (p.205·1); isoniazid (p.215·3).
Pyridoxine hydrochloride (p.1386·3) is included in this preparation for the prophylaxis of peripheral neuropathy.
Tuberculosis.

Etapiam *Piam, Ital.*
Ethambutol hydrochloride (p.205·1).
Tuberculosis.

Etaretin *Etapharm, Aust.*
Retinal phosphatides; sodium bicarbonate (p.1186·2).
Eye disorders.

Etaverol *Dinafarma, Braz.*
Homatropine (p.468·1); belladonna (p.463·1).
Smooth muscle spam.

Etaxene *Wassermann, Ital.*
Somatostatin acetate (p.1297·3).
Gastrointestinal haemorrhage.

ETDR *SIFI, Ital.*
Vitamin C; vitamin E; rutoside; sambucus (p.1350·1).
Nutritional supplement.

Eterciclina *Uniao Quimica, Braz.*
Guaifenesin (p.1092·2); potassium iodide (p.1522·3).
Respiratory-tract congestion.

Etermol *Quimpe, Spain.*
Aconite (p.1572·3); calcium lactophosphate; ephedrine hydrochloride (p.1090·1); beech; lemon; sulfogaiacol (p.1101·1).
Upper-respiratory-tract disorders.

Etermol Antitusivo *Quimpe, Spain.*
Benzydamine hydrochloride (p.20·1); dextromethorphan hydrobromide (p.1087·3); guaifenesin (p.1092·2); sodium benzoate (p.1134·3).
Coughs.

Ethamolin *DBL, Austral.†; Glaxo Wellcome, Braz.; Reed & Carnrick, Canad.†; Questcor, USA.*
Monoethanolamine oleate (p.1636·3).
Haemorrhoids; oesophageal varices; varicose veins.

Ethatyl *Aventis, S.Afr.*
Ethionamide (p.206·1).
Tuberculosis.

Ethbutol *Pharmasant, Thai.*
Ethambutol hydrochloride (p.205·1).
Tuberculosis.

Etheophyl *Lindopharm, Ger.†.*
Theophylline (p.777·2).
Obstructive airways disease.

Ethibloc *Johnson & Johnson, Switz.†.*
Sodium amidotrizoate (p.1031·2).
Packing of pancreatic duct following partial pancreatic resection; pre-operative vascular embolisation for renal tumours.

Ethibloc Okkklusions-Emulsion *Ethicon, Ger.*
Sodium amidotrizoate (p.1031·2).
Packing the residual pancreatic duct after partial resection of the pancreas; pre-operative vascular embolisation for renal tumours.

Ethical Nutrients 45+ *Health World, Austral.*
Multivitamin and mineral supplement (p.1350·1).

Ethical Nutrients Antioxidant Fish Oil Garlic Plus *Health World, Austral.*
Fish oil (p.949·3); garlic oil; betacarotene; folic acid; vitamin B$_{12}$; vitamin B$_6$; vitamin E (p.1350·1).
Peripheral vascular disorders.

Ethical Nutrients Bioflavonoids Plus *Health World, Austral.*
Ascorbic acid (p.1389·3); bioflavonoids (p.1611·1).
Cold and influenza symptoms; peripheral vascular disorders.

Ethical Nutrients HRT Support *Health World, Austral.*
Multivitamin and mineral preparation (p.1350·1).

Ethical Nutrients Inner Health Powder *Health World, Austral.*
Lactobacillus acidophilus (p.1626·3).
Maintenance of normal gastrointestinal flora.

Ethical Nutrients Iron Plus *Health World, Austral.*
Iron amino-acid chelate; vitamin B substances; calcium ascorbate; calcium succinate (p.1350·1).
Iron supplement.

Ethical Nutrients Maxepa *Health World, Austral.*
Omega-3 marine triglycerides (p.949·3).
Premenstrual disorder; psoriasis.

Ethical Nutrients Maxi Bifidus *Health World, Austral.*
Bifidobacterium bifidum (p.1626·3).
Maintence of normal gastrointestinal flora.

Ethical Nutrients Maxi Dophilus *Health World, Austral.*
Lactobacillus acidophilus (p.1626·3).
Maintenance of normal gastrointestinal flora.

Ethical Nutrients Super Multi *Health World, Austral.*
Vitamins; minerals; bladderwrack; vanadium; molybdenum (p.1350·1).

Ethical Nutrients Womens Multi *Health World, Austral.*
Vitamins; minerals; taraxacum (p.1350·1).

Ethicholine *Baxter, NZ; DBL, NZ; Bull, Singapore.*
Suxamethonium chloride (p.1340·1).
Depolarising neuromuscular blocker.

Ethimil *Dexcel, UK.*
Verapamil hydrochloride (p.989·1).
Angina pectoris; hypertension.

Ethimycin *Noristan Generica, S.Afr.†.*
Erythromycin stearate (p.201·3).
Bacterial infections.

Ethiodol *Savage, USA.*
Iodised oil (p.1034·1).
Contrast medium for hysterosalpingography and lymphography.

Ethipam *Noristan Generica, S.Afr.†.*
Diazepam (p.674·3).
Alcohol withdrawal syndrome; anxiety; premedication.

Ethipramine *Aspen, S.Afr.*
Imipramine hydrochloride (p.291·1).
Alcohol withdrawal syndrome; behaviour disorders; depression; parkinsonism.

Ethipurinol *Noristan Generica, S.Afr.†.*
Allopurinol (p.397·2).
Gout; hyperuricaemia.

Ethmozine *Monmouth, Irl.; Monmouth, UK†; Roberts, USA.*
Moracizine hydrochloride (p.936·1).
Ventricular arrhythmias.

Ethrane *Abbott, Aust.; Abbott, Austral.; Abbott, Belg.†; AstraZeneca, Canad.; Abbott, Ger.; Abbott, Hong Kong; Abbott, Irl.; Abbott, Israel; Abbott, Mex.; Abbott, Neth.; Abbott, S.Afr.; Abbott, Switz.; Baxter, USA.*
Enflurane (p.1258·1).
Anaesthesia and analgesia in obstetrics; general anaesthesia.

Ethyol *Schering-Plough, Austral.; Schering-Plough, Belg.; Lilly, Canad.; US Bioscience, Denm.; Schering-Plough, Fin.; Schering-Plough, Fr.; Essex, Ger.; Schering-Plough, Hong Kong; Bioscience, Israel; Schering-Plough, Ital.; Schering-Plough, Mex.; Schering-Plough, Neth.; Schering-Plough, NZ; Schering-Plough, Port.; Schering-Plough, S.Afr.; Schering-Plough, Singapore; Schering-Plough, Spain; Schering-Plough, Swed.; Essex, Switz.; Schering-Plough, Thai.; Schering-Plough, UK; Alza, USA; US Bioscience, USA.*
Amifostine (p.1001·3).
Radiation-associated xerostomia; reduction of nephrotoxicity due to cisplatin; reduction of neutropenia due to cyclophosphamide and cisplatin therapy for ovarian cancer.

Etiaxil *Interdelta, Switz.*
Aluminium chloride (p.1110·2).
Hyperhidrosis.

Etibi *Gerot, Aust.; ICN, Canad.; Zoja, Hong Kong; Formenti, Ital.†.*
Ethambutol hydrochloride (p.205·1).
Tuberculosis.

Etibi-INH *Formenti, Ital.†.*
Ethambutol hydrochloride (p.205·1); isoniazid (p.215·3).
Tuberculosis.

Etidron *Abiogen, Ital.*
Disodium etidronate (p.752·1).
Paget's disease of bone.

Etifollin *Nycomed, Norw.*
Ethinylestradiol (p.1476·2).
Menopausal disorders; prostatic cancer.

etil *CT, Ger.*
Etilefrine hydrochloride (p.888·1).
Hypotension.

Etiltox *AFOM, Ital.*
Disulfiram (p.1605·1).
Alcoholism.

Etimonis *Ecosol, Switz.†.*
Isosorbide mononitrate (p.916·2).
Heart failure; ischaemic heart disease.

Etioven *Cassenne, Fr.*
Naftazone (p.739·2).
Peripheral vascular disorders.

Eti-Puren *Isis Puren, Ger.*
Etilefrine hydrochloride (p.888·1).
Hypotension.

Etizem *Neo-Farmaceutica, Port.*
Diltiazem hydrochloride (p.874·3).
Angina pectoris; hypertension.

Etmoren *Evers, Ger.†.*
Silver birch (p.1585·2); java tea (p.1625·1); solidago virgaurea.
Diuretic.

ETO CS *Pharmacia Upjohn, Ger.*
Etoposide (p.538·1).
Malignant neoplasms.

Etocin *Malaysia Chemist, Singapore.*
Erythromycin ethyl succinate (p.201·2) or erythromycin stearate (p.201·3).
Bacterial infections.

Etocoderm *Richter, Aust.*
Alpha tocopherol (p.1394·1).
Skin disorders.

Etocovit *Richter, Aust.*
d-Alpha-tocopherol (p.1393·3).
Vitamin E deficiency.

Etofen *Ecosol, Switz.*
Etofenamate (p.35·3).
Musculoskeletal, joint, and soft-tissue disorders.

Eto-Gry *Gry, Ger.*
Etoposide (p.538·1).
Malignant neoplasms.

Etomedac *Medac, Ger.*
Etoposide (p.538·1).
Malignant neoplasms.

Etomine *Novartis, S.Afr.*
Clotiapine (p.671·1).
Agitation; anxiety; depression; psychoses.

Etono *Chefaro, Fin.*
Tripelennamine hydrochloride (p.427·1).
Insect stings and bites.

Etonox *Charoen, Thai.*
Etodolac (p.35·2).
Musculoskeletal and joint disorders; pain.

Etopan *Taro, Israel.*
Etodolac (p.35·2).
Osteoarthritis; pain; rheumatoid arthritis.

Etopofos *Bristol-Myers Squibb, Denm.; Bristol-Myers Squibb, Fin.; Bristol-Myers Squibb, Norw.; Bristol-Myers Squibb, Swed.*
Etoposide phosphate (p.538·3).
Malignant neoplasms.

Etopophos *Bristol-Myers Squibb, Austral.; Bristol-Myers Squibb, Belg.; Bristol-Myers Squibb, Fr.; Bristol-Myers Squibb, Ger.; Bristol-Myers Squibb, Irl.; Bristol-Myers Squibb, Israel; Bristol-Myers Squibb, NZ; Bristol-Myers Squibb, S.Afr.; Bristol-Myers Squibb, Switz.; Bristol-Myers Squibb, UK; Bristol-Myers Squibb Oncology, USA.*
Etoposide phosphate (p.538·3).
Malignant neoplasms.

Etopos *Lemery, Mex.*
Etoposide (p.538·1).
Malignant neoplasms.

Etoxisclerol *Bama, Spain.*
Lauromacrogol 400 (p.1345·2).
Varices.

Etrafon *Schering, Canad.; Schering-Plough, S.Afr.; Schering, USA.*
Perphenazine (p.699·1); amitriptyline hydrochloride (p.273·3).
Mixed anxiety depressive states.

Etramon *Janssen-Cilag, Spain†.*
Econazole nitrate (p.382·3).
Fungal infections.

Etrane *Abbott, Braz.*
Enflurane (p.1258·1).
General anaesthesia.

Etrat
Note. This name is used for preparations of different composition.
Klinge, Aust.; Novartis Consumer, Port.†.
Heparin sodium (p.902·1); menthol (p.1632·3); glycol salicylate (p.42·2).
Musculoskeletal and joint disorders; soft-tissue injury.

Gemballa, Braz.
A heparinoid (p.905·2); glycol salicylate (p.42·2); benzyl nicotinate (p.20·2).
Soft-tissue injury.

Etrat Sportgel *Klinge, Ger.*
Heparin sodium (p.902·1); menthol (p.1632·3); glycol salicylate (p.42·2).
Sports injuries.

Etrat Sportsalbe MPS *Klinge, Ger.*
A heparinoid (p.905·2).
Soft-tissue injury; superficial vascular disorders.

Etro *Inexfa, Spain.*
Ampicillin sodium (p.150·3); ampicillin benzathine (p.151·3).
Lignocaine [lidocaine] hydrochloride (p.1313·2) is included in this preparation to alleviate the pain of injection.
Bacterial infections.

Etro Balsamico *Inexfa, Spain.*
Ampicillin sodium (p.150·3); ampicillin benzathine (p.151·3); eucalyptol (p.1609·2); niaouli oil (p.1640·2); guaifenesin (p.1092·2).
Lignocaine [lidocaine] hydrochloride (p.1313·2) is included in this preparation to alleviate the pain of injection.
Respiratory-tract infections.

Etumina *Novartis, Spain.*
Clotiapine (p.671·1).
Anxiety; insomnia; psychoses.

Etumine *Novartis, Belg.*
Clotiapine (p.671·1).
Agitation; alcohol withdrawal syndrome; anxiety; psychoses.

Etumin/Entumin *Novartis, Israel.*
Clotiapine (p.671·1).
Alcohol withdrawal syndrome; anxiety; bipolar disorder; schizophrenia.

Etyzem *Caber, Ital.*
Diltiazem hydrochloride (p.874·3).
Angina pectoris; heart failure; hypertension.

Eubetal *SIFI, Ital.*
Betamethasone sodium phosphate (p.1063·2); antazoline phosphate (p.408·3).
Eye disorders.

Eubetal Antibiotico *SIFI, Ital.*
Eye drops: Betamethasone sodium phosphate (p.1063·2); rolitetracycline (p.247·1); chloramphenicol (p.179·1); colistimethate sodium (p.192·3).
Eye disorders.
Eye ointment: Betamethasone sodium phosphate (p.1063·2); tetracycline (p.258·3); chloramphenicol (p.179·1); colistimethate sodium (p.192·3).
Eye disorders.

Eubine *Chiesi, Fr.*
Oxycodone hydrochloride (p.70·2).
Pain.

Eubiol *Chephasaar, Ger.*
Arginine aspartate (p.1354·1).
Liver disorders.

Eubiolac *Verla, Ger.*
Calcium lactate (p.1188·2).
Vaginal disorders.

Eubispasme Codethyline *Promedica, Fr.†.*
Opium (p.69·3); ethylmorphine (p.35·2); camphoric acid; anisohydrocinnamol hydrochloride.
Coughs.

Euboral *Reig Jofre, Spain.*
Naphazoline hydrochloride (p.1095·1); borax (p.1586·1).
Eye irritation.

Eubos *Hobein, Hong Kong.*
Skin cleanser.

Eubucal *Sanopharm, Switz.*
Chlorhexidine gluconate (p.1138·2); myrrh (p.1639·2); chamomile (p.1593·2); arnica (p.1581·3); rhatany (p.1657·3); menthol (p.1632·3).
Mouth disorders.

Eucabal *Esparma, Ger.†.*
Plantago lanceolata; thyme (p.1672·2).
Catarrh.

Eucabal-Balsam S *Esparma, Ger.*
Eucalyptus oil (p.1609·2); oleum pini sylvestris.
Respiratory-tract disorders.

Eucafluid N *Steigerwald, Ger.*
Eucalyptus oil (p.1609·2); oleum pini sylvestris; peppermint oil (p.1243·3); rosemary oil (p.1659·3).
Musculoskeletal and joint disorders; neuralgia.

Eucalcic *Byk, Fr.*
Calcium carbonate (p.1215·1).
Renal osteodystrophy.

Eucaliptina *Restiva, Ital.†.*
Eucalyptol (p.1609·2); guaiacol (p.1092·1).
Respiratory disorders.

Eucalipto Composto *Dynacren, Ital.*
Eucalyptus oil (p.1609·2); camphor (p.1589·3); levomenthol (p.1632·3); thymol (p.1158·3).
Nasal congestion.

Eucaliptol *Neo Quimica, Braz.*
Dipyrone (p.34·1); guaifenesin (p.1092·2); eucalyptol (p.1609·2); sodium camisalate; ascorbic acid (p.1389·3).
Lignocaine [lidocaine] hydrochloride (p.1313·2) is included in this preparation to alleviate the pain of injection.
Cold and influenza symptoms.

Eucaliptol Composto
Note.This name is used for preparations of different composition.
Bunker, Braz.
Dipyrone (p.34·1); eucalyptol (p.1609·2); guaifenesin (p.1092·2).
Cold and influenza symptoms.

INQ, Braz.
Dipyrone (p.34·1); guaifenesin (p.1092·2); eucalyptol (p.1609·2); terpineol (p.1669·3); ascorbic acid (p.1389·3); chlorpheniramine [chlorphenamine] maleate (p.412·1).
Cold and influenza symptoms.

Eucalyptamint *Ciba, USA.*
Menthol (p.1632·3); eucalyptus oil (p.1609·2).

Eucalyptine
Note.This name is used for preparations of different composition.
Millet Roux, Braz.
Camphor (p.1589·3); eucalyptol (p.1609·2); phenol (p.1152·3); guaiacol (p.1092·1).
Respiratory-tract congestion.

Martin, Fr.
Adult suppositories: Eucalyptol (p.1609·2); guaifenesin (p.1092·2); camphor (p.1589·3).
Formerly contained eucalyptol, guaiacol, phenol, camphor, and codeine phosphate.
Infant suppositories: Eucalyptol (p.1609·2); guaifenesin (p.1092·2).
Coughs.

Eucalyptine Le Brun
Note.This name is used for preparations of different composition.
Medgenix, Belg.
Capsules: Eucalyptol (p.1609·2); codeine (p.25·2).
Formerly contained eucalyptol, guaiacol, phenol, codeine, camphor, and bromoform.
Coughs.
Suppositories for adults and children: Codeine phosphate (p.25·2); eucalyptol (p.1609·2).
Formerly contained camphor, phenol, eucalyptol, and guaiacol.
Coughs.
Suppositories for infants: Codeine phosphate (p.25·2); eucalyptol (p.1609·2).
Formerly contained camphor, eucalyptol, and guaiacol.
Respiratory disorders.
Syrup: Codeine (p.25·2); eucalyptol (p.1609·2).
Formerly contained sulfogaiacol, sodium phenolsulfonate, sodium camisalate, codeine, belladonna, aconite, bromoform, and eucalyptol.
Coughs.

Martin, Fr.
Capsules†: Eucalyptol (p.1609·2); guaiacol (p.1092·1); phenol (p.1152·3); camphor (p.1589·3); bromoform (p.1587·1); codeine (p.25·2).
Coughs.
Neonatal suppositories: Eucalyptol (p.1609·2); sulfogaiacol (p.1101·1).
Formerly contained eucalyptol, sulfogaiacol, and sodium camisalate.
Respiratory-tract disorders.
Syrup: Eucalyptol (p.1609·2); codeine (p.25·2).
Formerly contained eucalyptus oil, sodium phenolsulfonate, sodium camisalate, sulfogaiacol, bromoform, codeine, belladonna, and aconite.
Coughs.

Eucalyptine Pholcodine *Martin, Fr.*
Eucalyptol (p.1609·2); pholcodine (p.1099·1).
Formerly contained eucalyptol, guaiacol, phenol, camphor, and pholcodine.
Coughs.

Eucalyptine Pholcodine Le Brun *Medgenix, Belg.*
Suppositories for adults and children: Eucalyptol (p.1609·2); camphor (p.1589·3); phenol (p.1152·3); guaiacol (p.1092·1); pholcodine (p.1099·1).
Suppositories for infants: Eucalyptol (p.1609·2); camphor (p.1589·3); guaiacol (p.1092·1); pholcodine (p.1099·1).
Syrup: Sulfogaiacol (p.1101·1); sodium camisalate; sodium phenolsulfonate; pholcodine (p.1099·1); belladonna (p.463·1); aconite (p.1572·3); eucalyptol (p.1609·2).
Formerly contained eucalyptol, sodium camisalate, sodium phenolsulfonate, pholcodine, belladonna, aconite, bromoform, and eucalyptol.
Respiratory disorders.

Eucalyptospirine *Rovifarma, Spain.*
Aspirin (p.14·2); eucalyptol (p.1609·2); guaiacol (p.1092·1).
Formerly ocntained aspirin, amylocaine hydrochloride, eucalyptol, ethylmorphine, guaiacol, and sodium camsilate.
Influenza and cold symptoms.

Eucalyptospirine Lact *Rovi, Spain†.*
Aspirin (p.14·2); amylocaine hydrochloride (p.1306·1); eucalyptol (p.1609·2); guaiacol (p.1092·1); sodium camsilate.
Influenza and cold symptoms.

Eucalyptrol L *Medapharm, Ger.†.*
Eucalyptus oil (p.1609·2).
Cold symptoms.

Eucament *Catinense, Braz.*
Benzocaine (p.1306·2); camphor (p.1589·3); cetylpyridinium chloride (p.1138·1); tyrothricin (p.267·1).
Mouth and throat disorders.

Eucamenth *Planta, Canad.†.*
Camphor oil; eucalyptus oil (p.1609·2); menthol (p.1632·3).
Coughs; nasal and sinus congestion.

Eucar *Salus, Ital.*
Levocarnitine hydrochloride (p.1356·2).
Carnitine deficiency.

Eucarbon
Note.This name is used for preparations of different composition.
Trenka, Aust.; Trenker, Belg.
Senna (p.1248·2); rhubarb (p.1248·1); vegetable charcoal (p.1000·3); sulfur (p.1123·3); peppermint oil (p.1243·3); fennel oil (p.1610·2).
Constipation; dyspepsia; flatulence.
Trenka, Israel.
Senna (p.1248·2); rhubarb (p.1248·1); vegetable charcoal (p.1000·3); sulfur (p.1123·3).
Constipation; meteorism.
Trenka, Switz.†.
Senna (p.1248·2); rhubarb (p.1248·1); vegetable charcoal (p.1000·3); peppermint oil (p.1243·3); fennel oil (p.1610·2).
Constipation; flatulence.

Eucardic
Roche, Irl.; Roche, Neth.; Boehringer Mannheim, Swed.†; Roche, UK.
Carvedilol (p.855·2).
Formerly known as Dilatrend in *Neth.*
Angina pectoris; heart failure; hypertension.

Eucardina *Italmex, Mex.*
Tripsepar.
Thromboembolic disorders.

Eucardion *Dompe Biotec, Ital.†.*
Dexrazoxane hydrochloride (p.1006·2).
Prevention of doxorubicin cardiotoxicity.

Eucarnil *Pulitzer, Ital.*
Levocarnitine (p.1356·1).
Carnitine deficiency; myocardial ischaemia.

Eucebral-N *Sudmedica, Ger.†.*
Etofylline (p.765·1); cyclandelate (p.865·2).
Cerebral and peripheral vascular disorders.

Eucerin
Note.This name is used for preparations of different composition.
Beiersdorf, Austral.; Smith & Nephew, Canad.†; Beiersdorf, Irl.; Beiersdorf, Thai.; Beiersdorf, UK; Beiersdorf, USA.
A range of skin cleansing and emollient preparations.
Beiersdorf, USA.
SPF 25: Octinoxate (p.1517·3); octisalate (p.1518·1); titanium dioxide (p.1126·1); zinc oxide (p.1128·2).
Dry skin; sunscreen.

Eucerin Dry Skin Care Daily Facial *Beiersdorf, USA.*
SPF 20: Octinoxate (p.1517·3); titanium dioxide (p.1126·1); ensulizole (p.1517·2); octisalate (p.1518·1).
Sunscreen.

Eucerin Omega Fettsauren Olbad *Beiersdorf, Ger.*
Soya oil (p.1378·1).
Bath additive; dry skin.

Eucerin Pele com tendencia para o acne *Beiersdorf, Port.*
A range of cleansing and moisturising preparations.
Acne.

Eucerin Pele com tendencia para o acne creme anti-borbulhas *Beiersdorf, Port.*
Zinc oxide (p.1128·2); panthenol (p.1602·3).
Acne.

Eucerin Pele Seca *Beiersdorf, Port.*
Urea (p.1127·3).
Dry skin.

Eucerin Pele Sensivel *Beiersdorf, Port.*
A range of soap substitutes and moisturisers.

Eucerin Plus *Beiersdorf, USA.*
SPF 15: Octinoxate (p.1517·3); oxybenzone (p.1518·1); octisalate (p.1518·1).
Dry skin; sunscreen.

Eucerin Salbe *Beiersdorf, Ger.*
Urea (p.1127·3).
Dry skin.

Euceta
Novartis Consumer, Aust.; Sandoz, Ital.†; Wander, Neth.†; Novartis Consumer, Switz.
Aluminium acetotartrate (p.1578·2).
Skin disorders.

Euceta avec camomille et arnica *Novartis Consumer, Switz.*
Aluminium acetotartrate (p.1578·2); chamomile (p.1593·2); arnica (p.1581·3).
Skin disorders.

Euceta mit Kamille *Novartis Consumer, Aust.*
Aluminium acetotartrate (p.1578·2); chamomile (p.1593·2).
Skin disorders.

Euceta Pic *Novartis Consumer, Switz.*
Aluminium acetotartrate (p.1578·2); mepyramine maleate (p.421·1); lignocaine [lidocaine] hydrochloride (p.1313·2).
Insect bites.

Euchessina *Antonetta, Ital.†; Antonetto, Switz.*
Phenolphthalein (p.1244·1).
Constipation.

Euchessina CM *Antonetto, Ital.*
Sodium picosulfate (p.1249·3).
Constipation.

Euci *Falqui, Ital.†.*
Paracetamol (p.71·2); ascorbic acid (p.1389·3); pseudoephedrine hydrochloride (p.1099·2); dextromethorphan hydrobromide (p.1087·3).
Cold symptoms.

Eucid *Greater Pharma, Thai.*
Omeprazole (p.1239·1).
Gastro-oesophageal reflux, Zollinger-Ellison syndrome; peptic ulcer.

Eucil *Farmasa, Braz.*
Metoclopramide (p.1236·3).
Gastrointestinal motility disorders; nausea and vomiting.

Eucillin *Petrasch, Aust.*
Bacitracin (p.155·2); dequalinium chloride (p.1143·1); diphenylpyraline hydrochloride (p.417·1).
Infected skin disorders.

Euclorina *SmithKline Beecham, Ital.*
Tosylchloramide sodium (p.1591·1).
Skin, wound, and genital disinfection.

Eucol *Augot, Fr.*
Arginine oxoglurate (p.1354·1).
Hepatic encephalopathy; tonic.

Eucoprost *Frosst, Spain.*
Finasteride (p.1477·2).
Benign prostatic hyperplasia.

Eucorten *Trima, Israel.*
Clobetasone butyrate (p.1065·2).
Skin disorders.

Eudal-SR *UAD, USA.*
Pseudoephedrine hydrochloride (p.1099·2); guaifenesin (p.1092·2).
Coughs.

Eudemine *Celltech, UK; Goldshield, UK.*
Diazoxide (p.868·1).
Hypertensive crises; hypoglycaemia.

Eudent con Glysan *Bioprogress, Ital.*
Glysan (enoxolone (p.34·3); sanguinaria (p.1660·3)); sodium monofluorophosphate (p.1377·2) or sodium fluoride (p.1375·3).
Gum disorders; oral hygiene.

Euderm *Xepa-Soul Pattinson, Hong Kong.*
Urea (p.1127·3).
Dry skin disorders.

Eudermal Pasta *Pentaderm, Ital.*
Barrier cream.

Eudermal Sapone Allo Zolfo pH 5 *Pentaderm, Ital.*
Sulfur (p.1123·3).
Skin cleansing.

Eudermico *Novogaleno, Ital.*
Urea (p.1127·3); lactic acid (p.1626·2).
Dry skin disorders.

Eudextran *Bieffe, Ital.*
Dextran 40 (p.728·3) in sodium chloride or glucose.
Plasma volume expansion; thromboembolic disorders.

Eudigestio *Ogna, Ital.*
Pancreatin (p.1646·1); pepsin (p.1649·3).
Dyspepsia.

Eudigox *Astra, Ital.*
Digoxin (p.870·1).
Arrhythmias; heart failure.

Eudolene *Savio, Ital.*
Nimesulide (p.62·3).
Fever; inflammation; pain.

Eudorlin *Berlin-Chemie, Ger.*
Propyphenazone (p.80·2); paracetamol (p.71·2); caffeine (p.761·3).
Pain.

Eudur *Recipe, Aust.†; Astra, Ger.†.*
Terbutaline sulfate (p.776·2); theophylline (p.777·2).
Obstructive airways disease.

Eudyna *Ebewe, Aust.; BASF, Ger.; Knoll, Hong Kong; Knoll, Mex.; Knoll, Singapore.*
Tretinoin (p.1126·2).
Acne.

Eufans *Sigma-Tau, Ital.*
Amtolmetin guacil (p.14·1).
Musculoskeletal and joint disorders; pain.

Eufenil *Pharmacaps, Mex.*
Ibuprofen (p.43·2).

Eufermen *Luitpold, Braz.*
Enzymes from *Aspergillus oryzae*; ethaverine hydrochloride (p.1608·2); dimethicone (p.1249·2).
Digestive-system disorders.

Eufibron *Berlin-Chemie, Ger.*
Propyphenazone (p.80·2).
Fever; pain.

Eufilin *Byk, Braz.*
Aminophylline (p.760·1).
Neonatal apnoea; obstructive airways disease.

Eufilina *Byk, Port.; Byk Elmu, Spain.*
Theophylline (p.777·2).
Formerly contained aminophylline in Spain.
Obstructive airways disease.

Eufimenth N mild *Lichtenstein, Ger.†.*
Eucalyptus oil (p.1609·2); Norway spruce oil.
Respiratory-tract disorders.

Eufimenth-Balsam N *Lichtenstein, Ger.*
Eucalyptus oil (p.1609·2); Norway spruce oil; menthol (p.1632·3).
Respiratory-tract disorders.

Euflat *Sanova, Aust.†.*
Pancreatin (p.1646·1); papaverine hydrochloride (p.1648·1); angelica (p.1580·2); aloes (p.1210·1); fel tauri (p.1585·1); carbo coffea (p.1681·1).
Gastrointestinal disorders.

Euflat I *Stegropharm, Ger.*
Dimethicone (p.1249·2); caraway oil (p.1591·2); fennel oil (p.1610·2).
Digestive system disorders.

Euflat-E *Sudmedica, Ger.*
Pancreatin (p.1646·1).
Digestive system disorders.

Euflex *Schering, Canad.*
Flutamide (p.542·3).
Prostatic cancer.

Euflux-N *Sudmedica, Ger.*
Pumilio pine oil (p.1656·3); camphor (p.1589·3).
Cardiac disorders; respiratory disorders.

Eufor *Farmasa, Braz.*
Fluoxetine (p.288·2).
Depression; obsessive-compulsive disorder.

Eufusin *Clarmed, Ital.*
Succinylated gelatin (p.737·2).
Hypovolaemia.

Eugalac
Chepharin, Aust.†; Topfer, Ger.
Lactulose (p.1230·1).
Constipation; hepatic encephalopathy; salmonella infections.

Eugalan Topfer forte *Topfer, Ger.*
Bifidum bacteria; albumin; lactose (p.1370·2); lactulose (p.1230·1); minerals.
Cirrhosis; gastrointestinal disorders.

Eugalan Topfer forte LC *Topfer, Ger.*
Bifidobacteria; lactulose (p.1230·1); albumin; lactose (p.1370·2); galactose; minerals.
Constipation; hepatic encephalopathy.

Eugerminal *Medix, Mex.*
Vitamin E (p.1394·1).
Vitamin E supplement.

Eugiron *Denolin, Belg.*
Clove flower (p.1596·3); althaea root and leaf (p.1577·1); raspberry leaf (p.1657·2); tilia flower (p.1673·2); eucalyptus leaf (p.1609·2); aniseed fruit (p.1580·2); fennel fruit (p.1610·1).
Mouth and throat disorders.

Euglamin *Medinovum, Fin.*
Glibenclamide (p.321·3).
Diabetes mellitus.

Euglucan *Roche, Fr.*
Glibenclamide (p.321·3).
Diabetes mellitus.

Euglucon
Roche, Aust.; Hoechst Marion Roussel, Aust.; Boehringer Mannheim, Austral.†; Roche, Belg.; Asta Medica, Braz.; Pharmascience, Canad.; Roche, Denm.; Roche, Fin.; Roche, Hong Kong; Roche, Ital.; Boehringer Mannheim, Jpn†; Lakeside, Mex.; Boehringer Mannheim, Neth.†; Roche, Norw.; Roche, Port.; Roche, S.Afr.; Roche, Singapore; Roche, Spain; Roche, Swed.; Roche, Switz.; Roche, Thai.; Hoechst Marion Roussel, UK.
Glibenclamide (p.321·3).
Diabetes mellitus.

Euglucon N *Roche, Ger.; Hoechst Marion Roussel, Ger.*
Glibenclamide (p.321·3).
Diabetes mellitus.

Eugrippine *Synthelabo, Belg.†*
Diphenhydramine hydrochloride (p.416·1); caffeine (p.761·3); quinine sulfate (p.445·1); ascorbic acid (p.1389·3).
Fever associated with influenza.

Eugune *Palmares, Ital.*
Magnesium; bioflavonoids; proline oxide; lupulus; hydroxyapatite (p.1350·1).
Menopausal disorders.

Eugynon
Schering, Hong Kong; Schering, Ital.; Schering, Norw.; Schering, Spain†.
Norgestrel (p.1486·1); ethinylestradiol (p.1476·2).
Combined oral contraceptive; menstrual disorders.

Eugynon 30 *Schering, UK.*
Levonorgestrel (p.1486·2); ethinylestradiol (p.1476·2).
Combined oral contraceptive.

Eugynon 250 *Schering, Thai.*
Levonorgestrel (p.1486·2); ethinylestradiol (p.1476·2).
28-Day packs also contain 7 inert tablets.
Combined oral contraceptive.

Euhypnos
Sigma, Austral.; Pharmacia Upjohn, Belg.; Pharmacia Upjohn, Irl.; Pharmaco, NZ; Pharmacia, S.Afr.†; Pharmacia Upjohn, Thai.; Farmitalia Carlo Erba, UK.
Temazepam (p.707·2).
Insomnia; premedication.

Euipnos *Pharmacia Upjohn, Ital.*
Temazepam (p.707·2).
Insomnia.

Euka *Pharmonta, Aust.*
Fennel (p.1610·1); aniseed (p.1580·2); rosemary; eucalyptus (p.1609·2); lavender flowers (p.1627·2); laurel leaves; camphor (p.1589·3); peppermint oil (p.1243·3); spearmint oil (p.1666·3).
Gastrointestinal disorders.

Eukalisan forte *Steigerwald, Ger.*
Cyanocobalamin (p.1388·1); nicotinamide (p.1372·3); rutoside sodium sulfate (p.1611·2).
Lignocaine [lidocaine] hydrochloride (p.1313·2) is included in this preparation to alleviate the pain of injection.
Liver disorders.

Eukalisan N *Steigerwald, Ger.*
Cyanocobalamin (p.1388·1); nicotinamide (p.1372·3); rutoside sodium sulfate (p.1611·2).
Procaine hydrochloride (p.1319·1) is included in this preparation to alleviate the pain of injection.
Liver disorders; neuralgia; peripheral vascular disorders; tonic.

Eukamillat *Biocur, Ger.*
Chamomile (p.1593·2).
Gastrointestinal, anogenital, dental, respiratory-tract, and skin disorders.

Eukavan *Duopharm, Ger.*
Kava (p.1625·3).
Anxiety disorders.

Euky Bear Cough Syrup *Felton, Austral.*
Chlorpheniramine [chlorphenamine] (p.412·2); dextromethorphan (p.1087·3); sodium citrate (p.1186·2).
Coughs and cold symptoms.

Euky Bear Eu-Clear Inhalant *Felton, Austral.*
Eucalyptus oil (p.1609·2); menthol (p.1632·3).
Cold symptoms; respiratory-tract congestion.

Euky Bear Nasex *Felton, Austral.†*
Oxymetazoline hydrochloride (p.1096·2); eucalyptol (p.1609·2); menthol (p.1632·3).
Nasal congestion.

Euky Bearub *Felton, Austral.*
Eucalyptus oil (p.1609·2); eucalyptol (p.1609·2); menthol (p.1632·3); camphor (p.1589·3); rosemary oil (p.1659·3).
Cold and influenza symptoms; insect bites; muscular aches and pains; nasal congestion.

Eulactol *Eulactol, S.Afr.*
Urea (p.1127·3).
Dry skin.

Eulatin N *Lichtwer, Ger.*
Lignocaine [lidocaine] (p.1313·2); bismuth subgallate (p.1213·2).
Anorectal disorders.

Eulatin NN *Lichtwer, Ger.*
Hamamelis (p.1618·3); bismuth subgallate (p.1213·2); benzocaine (p.1306·2).
Anorectal disorders.

Eulexin
Schering-Plough, Austral.; Schering-Plough, Belg.; Schering-Plough, Braz.; Schering-Plough, Denm.; Schering-Plough, Fin.; Schering-Plough, Israel; Schering-Plough, Ital.; Schering-Plough, Mex.; Schering-Plough, Neth.; Schering-Plough, Norw.; Schering-Plough, NZ; Schering-Plough, Port.; Schering-Plough, S.Afr.; Schering-Plough, Spain; Schering-Plough, Swed.; Schering, USA.
Flutamide (p.542·3).
Prostatic cancer.

Eulexine *Schering-Plough, Fr.*
Flutamide (p.542·3).
Prostatic cancer.

Eulip *SIT, Ital.†.*
Tiadenol (p.980·3).
Hyperlipidaemias.

Eulitop
Roche, Belg.; Roche, Spain.
Bezafibrate (p.849·1).
Hyperlipidaemias.

Eulyptan *Labima, Belg.*
Codeine (p.25·2).
Coughs.

Eu-Med
Note.This name is used for preparations of different composition.
Novartis Consumer, Aust.
Paracetamol (p.71·2); caffeine (p.761·3); propyphenazone (p.80·2).
Formerly contained salacetamide, caffeine, propyphenazone, and phenazone.
Fever; pain.

Zyma, Ger.†.
Phenazone (p.77·2).
Fever; pain.

Eumetinex *Lakeside, Mex.*
Amoxicillin trihydrate (p.149·2); clavulanic acid (p.187·2).
Bacterial infections.

Euminz *Lichtwer, Ger.*
Peppermint oil (p.1243·3).
Neuralgia; tension-type headache.

Eumol *Arlex, Mex.*
Oxolamine (p.1096·2).

Eumotol *Byk, Braz.*
Bumadizone calcium (p.20·3).
Gout; musculoskeletal and joint disorders.

Eumovate
Glaxo Wellcome, Belg.; Glaxo Wellcome, Braz.; Glaxo Wellcome, Canad.; Glaxo Wellcome, Hong Kong; Glaxo Wellcome, Irl.; Glaxo Wellcome, Israel; Glaxo Wellcome, Ital.; Glaxo Wellcome, NZ; Allen & Hanburys, S.Afr.; Glaxo Wellcome, Singapore; Glaxo Wellcome, Thai.; Glaxo Wellcome, UK.
Clobetasone butyrate (p.1065·2).
Skin disorders.

Eunasin *Bracco, Ital.†.*
Metizoline hydrochloride (p.1094·3).
Upper respiratory-tract disorders.

Eunerpan *Knoll, Ger.*
Melperone hydrochloride (p.690·3).
Psychiatric disorders; sleep disorders.

Eunova *SmithKline Beecham OTC, Ger.*
Multivitamin and mineral preparation (p.1350·1).

Eupantol *Byk, Fr.*
Pantoprazole sodium (p.1243·2).
Gastro-oesophageal reflux; peptic ulcer.

Eupatal *Madaus, Ger.*
Thyme (p.1672·2); star anise oil.
Cold symptoms.

Eupatol *Donini, Ital.*
Cascara (p.1216·1); boldo (p.1585·3); rhubarb (p.1248·1).
Constipation.

Eupatorium Oligoplex *Madaus, Ger.*
Homoeopathic preparation.

Eupeclanic *Uriach, Spain.*
Amoxicillin trihydrate (p.149·2); potassium clavulanate (p.187·2).
Bacterial infections.

Eupen *Uriach, Spain.*
Amoxicillin trihydrate (p.149·2).
Bacterial infections.

Eupen Bronquial *Uriach, Spain.*
Amoxicillin trihydrate (p.149·2); brovanexine hydrochloride (p.1086·1).
Respiratory-tract infections.

Eupeptina *Diviser Aquilea, Spain.*
Dibasic sodium phosphate (p.1193·2); magnesium carbonate (p.1232·3); magnesium phosphate (p.1191·1); magnesium oxide (p.1233·2); pepsin carbonate.
Constipation; dyspepsia.

Euphidra G2 Radical *Zeta, Ital.*
Multivitamin and mineral preparation (p.1350·1).
Nutritional supplement.

Euphon
Note.This name is used for preparations of different composition.
ACP, Belg.
Codeine (p.25·2); aconite (p.1572·3); sodium formate (p.1612·3); erysimin; elecampane (p.1089·3).
Throat disorders.

Mayoly-Spindler, Fr.
Oral solution†: Codeine (p.25·2); aconite (p.1572·3); sodium formate (p.1612·3); erysimin.
Coughs.
Pastilles: Erysimin.
Sore throat.
Syrup; capsules: Erysimin; codeine (p.25·2).
Coughs.

Mayoly-Spindler, Singapore.
Erysimin.
Catarrh; cough; throat disorders.

Euphon N *Mayoly-Spindler, Switz.; Uhlmann-Eyraud, Switz.*
Codeine (p.25·2); tolu balsam (p.1101·3).
Coughs and associated respiratory-tract disorders.

Euphorbia Complex *Blackmores, Austral.*
Passion flower (p.1649·1); thyme (p.1672·2); grindelia (p.1618·2); euphorbia (p.1609·3); vitamins (p.1350·1).
Asthma; bronchitis; catarrh.

Euphorbium Compositum S *Heel, S.Afr.*
Homoeopathic preparation.

Euphorbium compositum-Nasentropfen S *Heel, Ger.*
Homoeopathic preparation.

Euphyllin
Byk, Aust.; Byk, Belg.; Meda, Fin.; Byk Gulden, Ger.†; Byk, Neth.; Byk Gulden, Norw.†; Byk Madaus, S.Afr.; Byk, Switz.
Aminophylline (p.760·1) or theophylline (p.777·2).
Obstructive airways disease.

Euphyllina *Byk Gulden, Ital.*
Aminophylline (p.760·1) or theophylline (p.777·2).
Obstructive airways disease.

Euphyllin-Calcium *Byk, Aust.†.*
Aminophylline (p.760·1); calcium gluconate (p.1188·2).

Euphylline *Byk, Fr.*
Theophylline (p.777·2).
Obstructive airways disease.

Euphylong
Byk Gulden, Ger.; Byk Gulden, Hong Kong; Byk, Neth.; Swedish Orphan, Swed.; Byk, Switz.†.
Theophylline (p.777·2).
Obstructive airways disease.

Euphytose *Nicholas, Fr.*
Crataegus (p.1600·2); passion flower (p.1649·1); guarana (p.1681·1); kola (p.1681·1); valerian (p.1678·3); ballota.
Nervous disorders.

Eupneron *E Pharma, Fr.*
Eprozinol hydrochloride (p.1091·2).
Obstructive airways disease.

Eupnol *Rottapharm, Spain.*
Benzethonium chloride (p.1134·2); eucalyptol (p.1609·2); cherry-laurel; procaine hydrochloride (p.1319·1); terpineol (p.1669·3); menthol (p.1632·3).
Mouth and throat inflammation.

Eupond *Sudmedica, Ger.†.*
Theobromine (p.777·2); dehydrocholic acid (p.1602·3); ox bile (p.1585·1); atropine sulfate (p.461·1); aloes (p.1210·1); frangula bark (p.1227·1); cichorium; ononis (p.1644·1); parsley (p.1648·3); birch leaf (p.1585·2).
Heart conditions; obesity.

Eupond-F *Sudmedica, Ger.†.*
Frangula bark (p.1227·1).
Constipation.

Eupragin *Alcon, Ger.*
Erythromycin estolate (p.201·2).
Bacterial eye infections.

Eupres *Searle, Ital.*
Atenolol (p.841·3); chlortalidone (p.857·1).
Hypertension.

Eupressin *Biosintetica, Braz.*
Enalapril maleate (p.883·3).
Heart failure; hypertension.

Eupressin H *Biosintetica, Braz.*
Enalapril maleate (p.883·3); hydrochlorothiazide (p.907·3).
Hypertension.

Eupressyl *Byk, Fr.*
Urapidil (p.987·3) or urapidil hydrochloride (p.987·3).
Hypertension.

Euproctol *Sanophorm, Switz.†*
Ointment: Resorcinol (p.1122·2); ephedrine hydrochloride (p.1090·1); lignocaine [lidocaine] hydrochloride (p.1313·2); menthol (p.1632·3).
Suppositories: Sozoiodol zinc (p.1157·2); resorcinol (p.1122·2); zinc oxide (p.1128·2).
Anorectal disorders.

Euprotin *Almirall, Spain.*
Lenograstim (p.738·1).
Mobilisation of autologous peripheral blood progenitor cells; reduction of neutropenia associated with cancer chemotherapy.

Euradal *Lacer, Spain.*
Bisoprolol fumarate (p.850·1).
Angina pectoris; hypertension.

Euralben *Reuffer, Mex.*
Albendazole (p.95·2).

Eurax
Novartis Consumer, Aust.; Novartis Consumer, Austral.; Novartis Consumer, Belg.; Novartis Consumer, Canad.; Novartis Sante, Fr.; Novartis, Hong Kong; Novartis Consumer, Irl.; Novartis, Israel; Novartis Consumer, Ital.; Novartis, Mex.; Novartis, Norw.; Novartis, NZ; Novartis Consumer, Port.; Novartis, S.Afr.; Novartis Nutrition, Singapore; Novartis Consumer, Switz.; Novartis Consumer, UK; Westwood-Squibb, USA.
Crotamiton (p.1112·3).
Pediculosis; pruritus; scabies.

Eurax-Hydrocortisone
Novartis Consumer, Irl.; Novartis Consumer, UK.
Crotamiton (p.1112·3); hydrocortisone (p.1073·3).
Pruritic skin disorders.

Euraxil
Gepepharm, Ger.; Padro, Spain.
Crotamiton (p.1112·3).
Pediculosis; pruritus; scabies.

Euraxil Hidrocort *Padro, Spain.*
Crotamiton (p.1112·3); hydrocortisone (p.1073·3).
Skin disorders.

Eureceptor *Zambon, Ital.*
Cimetidine (p.1216·3).
Gastrointestinal disorders.

Eurelix *Hoechst, Fr.*
Piretanide (p.956·2).
Hypertension.

Eurex *Sanofi Synthelabo, Ger.*
Prazosin hydrochloride (p.958·1).
Heart failure; hypertension.

Eurhyton *Adima, Switz.†.*
Crataegus (p.1600·2).
Cardiac disorders.

Eurifam *Euromex, Mex.*
Rifampicin (p.243·2).

Euritmin *Rhein, Mex.*
Verapamil (p.991·1).

Eurixor
Richter, Aust.; Biosyn, Ger.
Mistletoe (p.1636·2).
Joint disorders; malignant neoplasms.

Eurobiol
Parke, Davis, Fr.; Interdelta, Switz.†.
Pancreas extract.
Digestive disorders; pancreatic insufficiency.

Eurocal D *Procter & Gamble, Ital.*
Calcium carbonate (p.1215·1); colecalciferol (p.1391·1).
Calcium and vitamin D deficiency; osteoporosis.

Eurodin *Takeda, Jpn.*
Estazolam (p.682·3).
Insomnia; premedication.

Euroflash *Lifescan, Port.*
Test for glucose in blood (p.1616·3).

Eurogel *Cielle, Ital.*
Royal jelly (p.1659·3); dried yeast (p.1398·1); wheat germ.
Nutritional supplement.

Eurolat *Euromex, Mex.*
Ketoconazole (p.389·1).

Eurolol *Euromex, Mex.*
Metoprolol (p.932·1).

Euronac *Europhta, Mon.*
Acetylcysteine (p.1082·3).
Eye ulceration.

Europranolol *Euromex, Mex.*
Propranolol (p.963·1).

Europrazosin *Euromex, Mex.*
Prazosin (p.958·1).

Eurosan *Mepha, Switz.*
Clotrimazole (p.382·1).
Fungal skin and nail infections.

Euroxi *Copernico, Ital.*
Piroxicam (p.79·1).
Musculoskeletal, joint, and peri-articular disorders.

Eusaprim
Glaxo Wellcome, Aust.; Glaxo Wellcome, Belg.; Glaxo Wellcome, Fr.; Glaxo Wellcome, Ital.; Glaxo Wellcome, Neth.; Glaxo Wellcome, Swed.; Wellcome, Switz.†.
Co-trimoxazole (p.193·3).
Bacterial infections; Pneumocystis carinii pneumonia; toxoplasmosis.

Eusedon mono *Krewel, Ger.*
Promethazine hydrochloride (p.423·2).
Hypersensitivity reactions; nervous disorders; sleep disorders.

Euskin *Sankyo, Spain.*
Erythromycin (p.201·2).
Acne.

Eusovit *Strathmann, Ger.*
dl-Alpha tocoferil acetate (p.1394·1).
Vitamin E deficiency.

Euspirax *Asche, Ger.*
Choline theophyllinate (p.763·3).
Obstructive airways disease.

Eutalgic *Pierre Fabre Sante, Fr.*
Menthol (p.1632·3); methyl salicylate (p.55·1); camphor (p.1589·3).
Soft-tissue injury.

Euthyral *Lipha Sante, Fr.*
Liothyronine sodium (p.1524·2); thyroxine [levothyroxine] sodium (p.1526·2).
Hypothyroidism.

Euthyrox
Merck, Aust.; Merck-Belgolabo, Belg.; Merck, Ger.; Merck, Neth.; Merck, Singapore.
Thyroxine [levothyroxine] sodium (p.1526·2).
Goitre; hypothyroidism; thyroid cancer.

Eutirox
Bracco, Ital.; Merck, Mex.
Thyroxine [levothyroxine] sodium (p.1526·2).
Hypothyroidism.

Eutrodin *GD, Ital.*
Zinc oxide (p.1128·2); titanium dioxide (p.1126·1).
Barrier cream.

Eutrofic *Dermoteca, Port.*
A range of moisturisers.

Eutrofic Forte Gel Despigmentante *Dermoteca, Port.*
Glycolic acid (p.1115·1); hydroquinone (p.1115·1).
Hyperpigmentation; keratoses.

Eutys-Kili *Farmila, Ital.*
Vitamin B₆; chromium; citrin; kelp; kola (p.1350·1).
Nutritional supplement.

Euvaderm *Parke, Davis, Ger.†*
Cream: Betamethasone benzoate (p.1063·1).
Ointment: Betamethasone benzoate (p.1063·1); salicylic acid (p.1122·3).
Skin disorders.

Euvaderm N *Parke, Davis, Ger.†*
Betamethasone benzoate (p.1063·1); salicylic acid (p.1122·3).
Skin disorders.

Euvalon *Hotz, Ger.†*
Crataegus (p.1600·2); valerian (p.1678·3).
Cardiac disorders.

Euvanol *Monot, Fr.†*
Geranium oil (p.1615·1); niaouli oil (p.1640·2); camphor (p.1589·3); benzalkonium bromide (p.1133·1).
Rhinopharyngeal infections.

Euvax-B *LG Chem, Thai.*
A hepatitis B vaccine (recombinant DNA) (p.1542·2).
Active immunisation.

Euvegal Entspannungs- und Einschlafdragees *Spitzner, Ger.*
Valerian (p.1678·3); melissa (p.1632·2).
Nervous disorders; sleep disorders.

Euvegal forte *Spitzner, Ger.†*
Valerian (p.1678·3); melissa (p.1632·2).
Insomnia; nervous disorders.

Euvegal N *Spitzner, Ger.*
Valerian (p.1678·3); melissa (p.1632·2); passion flower (p.1649·1).
Neurosedative.

Euvifor *Vedim, Port.*
Piracetam (p.1652·1); co-dergocrine mesilate (p.1597·3).
Cerebrovascular disorders; mental function disorders; vestibular disorders.

Euvitan *Baer, Ger.*
Caffeine and sodium benzoate (p.763·1); rutoside sodium sulfate (p.1611·2); tinct. amara; angelica (p.1580·2); calluna vulgaris; juglans regia; valerian (p.1678·3).
Dystonias; reduced appetite.

Euviterin *Sudmedica, Ger.†*
Caffeine (p.761·3); nucleoside-nucleotide; melissa (p.1632·2); lavender flower (p.1627·2).
Hypotension.

Euvitol *Bracco, Ital.*
Vitamin A palmitate (p.1383·2).
Skin disorders.

Euzymina Lisina I *Menarini, Spain.*
Lysine hydrochloride (p.1370·3); nicotinic acid (p.1372·3); pepsin (p.1649·3); citrus aurantium; lactic acid (p.1626·2).
Digestive enzyme deficiency.

Euzymina Lisina II *Menarini, Spain.*
Lysine hydrochloride (p.1370·3); nicotinic acid (p.1372·3); pepsin (p.1649·3); citrus aurantium.
Digestive disorders.

Evacode *Norton, UK.*
Codeine phosphate (p.25·2).

Evac-Q-Kit *Adria, USA†.*
Combination pack: Evac-Q-Mag; Evac-Q-Tabs, 2 tablets; Evac-Q-Sert, 2 suppositories.
Colon preparation prior to radiology.

Evac-Q-Kwik
Note.This name is used for preparations of different composition.
Pharmacia Upjohn, Canad.†.

Combination preparation: Solution, magnesium citrate (p.1232·3); tablets, phenolphthalein (p.1244·1); suppository, bisacodyl (p.1212·2).
Colonic evacuation.

Savage, USA.

Combination pack: Evac-Q-Mag; Evac-Q-Tabs, 2 tablets; Evac-Q-Kwik Suppositories, 1 suppository.
Bowel evacuation.

Evac-Q-Kwik Suppository *Savage, USA.*
Bisacodyl (p.1212·2).

Evac-Q-Mag *Savage, USA.*
Magnesium citrate (p.1232·3).

Evac-Q-Sert *Adria, USA†.*
Potassium acid tartrate (p.1244·3); sodium bicarbonate (p.1186·2).

Evac-Q-Tabs *Savage, USA.*
Bisacodyl (p.1212·2).
Formerly contained phenolphthalein.

Evacuante *Bohm, Spain; Lainco, Spain.*
Macrogol (p.1630·1); electrolytes (p.1180·1).
Bowel evacuation.

Evac-U-Gen *Walker Pharmacal, USA†.*
Yellow phenolphthalein (p.1244·1).
Constipation.

Evac-U-Lax *Hauck, USA†.*
Phenolphthalein (p.1244·1).
Constipation.

Evacuol *Almirall, Spain.*
Sodium picosulfate (p.1249·3).
Constipation.

Evadene *Wyeth Lederle, Ital.*
Butriptyline hydrochloride (p.281·2).
Depression.

Evadermin *Gambar, Ital.*
Povidone-iodine (p.1155·1).
Genital hygiene.

Evadol *Degorts, Mex.*
Diclofenac (p.30·2).
Inflammation; pain.

Evagrip *Mavda, Spain.*
An influenza vaccine (p.1544·3).
Active immunisation.

Evalgan *Pharmacia Upjohn, Aust.*
Dimeticone (p.1410·2); zinc oxide (p.1128·2).
Skin disorders.

Evalin *Queisser, Ger.*
Cimicifuga (p.1595·2).
Menopausal disorders.

Evalose *Copley, USA†.*
Lactulose (p.1230·1).

Evana *Pharmaton, Switz.*
Agnus castus (p.1574·2).
Premenstrual syndrome.

Evanor *Wyeth, Braz.*
Levonorgestrel (p.1486·2); ethinylestradiol (p.1476·2).
Combined oral contraceptive.

Evanor-D *Wyeth Lederle, Ital.*
Levonorgestrel (p.1486·2); ethinylestradiol (p.1476·2).
Combined oral contraceptive.

Evans Blue Dye *New World Trading Corporation, USA†.*
Aid for plasma volume measurement.

Evaphol *Norton, UK.*
Pholcodine (p.1099·1).

Evaplan *Roche Diagnostics, Austral.*
Fertility test (p.1654·3).

Evasen Crema *Evapharm, Ital.*
Vitamin E (p.1393·3).
Cracked nipples.

Evasen Dischetti *Evapharm, Ital.*
Potassium sorbate (p.1157·1); glycerol (p.1616·3).
Cracked nipples.

Evasidol *Wyeth Lederle, Aust.*
Butriptyline hydrochloride (p.281·2).
Anxiety; depression.

Evasprin *Euro-Labor, Port.; Grunenthal, Port.*
Lysine aspirin (p.50·3).
Fever; pain.

Evastel *Rhone-Poulenc Rorer, Mex.*
Ebastine (p.417·2).
Hypersensitivity.

Evatest One Step *Roche Diagnostics, Austral.*
Pregnancy test (p.1654·3).

Evazol
Petrasch, Aust.; Ravensberg, Ger.
Dequalinium chloride (p.1143·1).
Infected wounds; skin infections.

EVC *Sisu, Canad.*
Vitamin and mineral preparation (p.1350·1).

Eve *Grunenthal, Aust.*
Ethinylestradiol (p.1476·2); norethisterone (p.1485·2).
Combined oral contraceptive.

Evening Gold *Larkhall Laboratories, UK.*
Evening primrose oil (p.1613·2).

Evercid *Boniscontro & Gazzone, Ital.*
Flucloxacillin sodium (p.207·1).
Bacterial infections.

Ever-fit Cardio *Prisfar, Port.*
Multivitamin and mineral preparation (p.1350·1).

Ever-Fit Plus *Prisfar, Port.*
Vitamin and mineral preparation (p.1350·1).

Evergin *Eversil, Braz.*
Metamizole magnesium (p.34·2).
Fever; pain.

Everon *Weleda, Aust.*
Pepsin (p.1649·3); lemon juice; menthol (p.1632·3).
Colds.

Everone *Hyrex, USA†.*
Testosterone enantate (p.1492·2).
Breast cancer; delayed puberty (males); male hypogonadism.

Eversun *Pfizer, NZ.*
SPF 30+: Avobenzone (p.1517·1); octinoxate (p.1517·3); oxybenzone (p.1518·1).
Sunscreen.

E-Vicotrat *Heyl, Ger.*
Alpha tocoferil acetate (p.1394·1).
Vitamin E deficiency.

E-Vicotrat + Magnesium *Heyl, Ger.*
dl-Alpha tocoferil acetate (p.1394·1); magnesium oxide (p.1233·2).
Vitamin E and magnesium deficiency.

E-vidon *Abigo, Swed.*
d-Alpha tocoferil acetate (p.1394·1).
Vitamin E deficiency.

Eviepar *Eversil, Braz.*
Adenosine (p.828·2); methionine (p.1012·2); betaine (p.1584·3); choline citrate (p.1356·3); pyridoxine hydrochloride (p.1386·3).
Liver disorders.

Eviletten N *Evers, Ger.†*
Modified keratin.
Haemorrhoids; varicose veins.

E-vimin *Astra, Swed.*
dl-Alpha-tocoferil acetate (p.1394·1).
Vitamin E deficiency.

Evina *Rodisma, Ger.*
d-Alpha tocopherol with ascorbic acid (p.1350·1).
Vitamin E and C deficiency.

Evion
Merck, Ger.; Bracco, Ital.
dl-Alpha tocoferil acetate (p.1394·1).
Vitamin E deficiency.

Eviprostat
Note.This name is used for preparations of different composition.
Eversil, Braz.
Manganese amino acid chelate; populus tremula (p.1653·2); pulsatilla (p.1656·3); salicylic acid (p.1122·3); kaolin (p.1229·3).
Urinary-tract disorders.

Evers, Hong Kong.
Wheat-germ oil; manganese chloride (p.1371·3); chimaphila umbellata; populus tremulula (p.1653·2); pulsatilla (p.1656·3); equisetum (p.1606·3); sodium taurocholate.
Benign prostatic hyperplasia.

Shinyaku, Singapore.
Wheat-germ oil; chimaphila umbellata; populus tremula (p.1653·2); pulsatilla (p.1656·3); equisetum (p.1606·3); choleinic sodium; manganese chloride (p.1371·3).
Benign prostatic hyperplasia.

Interdelta, Switz.†.
Wheat-germ oil; chimaphila umbellata; populus tremula (p.1653·2); pulsatilla (p.1656·3); equisetum (p.1606·3).
Prostatic disorders.

Eviprostat N *Evers, Ger.*
Chimaphila umbellata; populus tremula (p.1653·2); pulsatilla (p.1656·3); equisetum (p.1606·3).
Prostatic hyperplasia.

Eviprostat-S *Evers, Ger.*
Saw palmetto (p.1491·2).
Micturition disorders associated with benign prostatic hyperplasia.

Evisco Mistel Urtinktur *Evisco, Ger.*
Homoeopathic preparation.

Evisco Misteltropfen N *Evisco, Ger.*
Homoeopathic preparation.

Evista
Note. A similar name is used for preparations of different composition (see below).
Lilly, Aust.; Lilly, Austral.; Lilly, Belg.; Lilly, Canad.; Lilly, Denm.; Lilly, Fin.; Lilly, Fr.; Lilly, Ger.; Lilly, Irl.; Lilly, Israel; Lilly, Ital.; Lilly, Mex.; Lilly, Neth.; Lilly, Norw.; Lilly, NZ; Lilly, Port.; Lilly, S.Afr.; Lilly, Singapore; Lilly, Spain; Lilly, Swed.; Lilly, UK; Lilly, USA.
Raloxifene hydrochloride (p.1491·1).
Osteoporosis.

E-Vista *Seatrace, USA†.*
Note. A similar name is used for preparations of different composition (see above).
Hydroxyzine hydrochloride (p.419·1).
Anxiety; hypersensitivity reactions.

Evit
Europharm, Aust.; Chefaro, Ger.; Mavena, Switz.
d-Alpha tocopherol (p.1393·3) or alpha tocoferil acetate (p.1394·1).
Vitamin E deficiency.

Evitas *Heralds, Braz.*
Algestone acetophenide (p.1465·1); estradiol enantate (p.1473·2).
Injectable contraceptive.

Evitex *Alcon, Ital.*
Vitamin A (p.1382·1); tocoferil nicotinate (p.984·3).
Vitamin A and E deficiency.

Evitex A E Fuerte *Alcon Cusi, Spain.*
Vitamin A palmitate (p.1383·2); tocoferil nicotinate (p.984·3).
Deficiency of vitamins A and E; eye disorders; infertility; recurrent miscarriage; skin disorders.

Evitina *CT, Ital.*
dl-Alpha tocoferil acetate (p.1394·1).

Evitocor *Apogepha, Ger.*
Atenolol (p.841·3).
Angina pectoris; arrhythmias; cardiovascular disorders; hypertension.

Evitocor plus *Apogepha, Ger.†*
Atenolol (p.841·3); chlortalidone (p.857·1).
Hypertension.

Evitol
Lannacher, Aust.; Teva, Israel.
Alpha tocoferil acetate (p.1394·1).
Vitamin E deficiency; vitamin E supplement.

E-Vitum *Lipha, Ital.*
d-Alpha tocoferil acetate (p.1394·1).
Haemolytic anaemia; intermittent claudication; vitamin E deficiency.

Evo-Conti *Janssen-Cilag, Denm.*
Estradiol (p.1473·1); norethisterone acetate (p.1485·1).
Menopausal disorders.

Evolis *Solvay, Fr.*
Betahistine hydrochloride (p.1584·2).
Vestibular disorders.

Evopad *Janssen-Cilag, Spain.*
Estradiol (p.1473·1).
Menopausal disorders; osteoporosis.

Evoprim *Bioceuticals, UK.*
Evening primrose oil (p.1613·2).

Evorel
Janssen-Cilag, Denm.; Janssen-Cilag, Fin.; Janssen-Cilag, Ger.; Janssen-Cilag, Irl.; Janssen-Cilag, Israel; Janssen-Cilag, Norw.; Janssen-Cilag, S.Afr.; Janssen-Cilag, Swed.; Janssen-Cilag, UK.
Estradiol (p.1473·1).
Menopausal disorders; oestrogen deficiency; osteoporosis.

Evorel Conti
Janssen-Cilag, Fin.; Janssen-Cilag, Irl.; Janssen-Cilag, S.Afr.; Janssen-Cilag, UK.
Estradiol (p.1473·1); norethisterone acetate (p.1485·1).
Menopausal disorders; osteoporosis.

Evorel Micronor *Janssen-Cilag, Swed.*
Patches, estradiol (p.1473·1); tablets, norethisterone (p.1485·1).
Oestrogen deficiency; osteoporosis.

Evorel Pak *Janssen-Cilag, UK.*
Transdermal patches, estradiol (p.1473·1); tablets, norethisterone (p.1485·1).
Menopausal disorders; osteoporosis.

Evorel Sequi
Janssen-Cilag, Fin.; Janssen-Cilag, UK.
4 Patches, estradiol (Evorel) (p.1473·1); 4 patches, estradiol; norethisterone acetate (Evorel Conti) (p.1485·1).
Menopausal disorders; osteoporosis.

Evo-Sequi *Janssen-Cilag, Denm.*
Patch I, estradiol (p.1473·1); patch II, estradiol; norethisterone acetate (p.1485·1).
Menopausal disorders.

Evoxac *Daiichi, USA.*
Cevimeline hydrochloride (p.1416·2).
Dry mouth associated with Sjögren's syndrome.

Evril *Boehringer de Angeli, Braz.*
Flurbiprofen (p.41·2).
Dysmenorrhoea; musculoskeletal, joint, and peri-articular disorders.

Ewadyl *Masa, Thai.*
Diphenhydramine hydrochloride (p.416·1); ammonium chloride (p.1085·2); sodium citrate (p.1186·2).
Cold symtoms; coughs; hypersensivity disorders of the respiratory tract.

Exacor *Monsanto, Fr.*
Cibenzoline succinate (p.857·3).
Arrhythmias.

Exact *Premier, USA.*
Benzoyl peroxide (p.1111·1).
Acne.

Exactech *Medisense, UK.*
Test for glucose in blood (p.1616·3).

Exacyl
Bournonville, Belg.†; Sanofi Winthrop, Fr.
Tranexamic acid (p.742·2).
Haemorrhagic disorders.

Ex'ail
Solvay, Belg.†; Warner-Lambert, Fr.
Garlic (p.1614·1); rutoside (p.1611·2); copper chlorophyll (p.1028·1).
Circulatory disorders.

Exalamin *Pharmacos, Mex.*
Oxolamine (p.1096·2).
Coughs.

Exalgin *Sons, Mex.*
Dipyrone (p.34·1).
Fever; pain.

The symbol † denotes a preparation no longer actively marketed

Exalver Maver, Mex.
Paracetamol (p.71·2); pseudoephedrine hydrochloride (p.1099·2); dextromethorphan hydrobromide (p.1087·3).
Coughs; nasal congestion.

Examicyn Pharmacos, Mex.
Erythromycin (p.201·2).
Bacterial infections.

Exangina N Muller Goppingen, Ger.
Homoeopathic preparation.

Exasul Pharmacos, Mex.
Sulfamethoxypyridazine (p.256·1).
Bacterial infections.

Exatech
Medisense, Austral.; Medica, NZ.
Test for glucose in blood (p.1616·3).

Exaverm Pharmacos, Mex.
Mebendazole (p.102·2).
Worm infections.

Exbenzol Sons, Mex.
Mebendazole (p.102·2).
Worm infections.

Excaugh Fortune, Hong Kong.
Guaifenesin (p.1092·2).
Coughs.

Excedrin
Note.This name is used for preparations of different composition.
Bristol-Myers Squibb, Canad.
Paracetamol (p.71·2); caffeine (p.761·3).
Fever; pain.

Bristol-Myers Squibb, USA.
Aspirin (p.14·2); paracetamol (p.71·2); caffeine (p.761·3).
Pain.

Excedrin Migraine Bristol-Myers Squibb, USA.
Paracetamol (p.71·2); aspirin (p.14·2); caffeine (p.761·3).
Migraine.

Excedrin PM Bristol-Myers Squibb, USA.
Paracetamol (p.71·2); diphenhydramine citrate (p.416·1) or diphenhydramine hydrochloride (p.416·1).
Pain associated with sleeplessness.

Excegran Dainippon, Jpn.
Zonisamide (p.371·2).
Epilepsy.

Excel ET Selfcare, Austral.
Test for glucose in blood (p.1616·3).

Excelcur MFI Maeil, Hong Kong.
Preparation for enteral nutrition (p.1350·1).
Gastro-enteritis.

Excelsior Grisi, Mex.
Tolnaftate (p.395·2).
Fungal skin infections.

Excillin Propan, S.Afr.
Ampicillin trihydrate (p.151·1).
Bacterial infections.

Excipial
Mayrhofer, Aust.†; Spirig, Switz.
Emollient.
Skin disorders.

Excipial U
Mayrhofer, Aust.†; Spirig, Switz.
Urea (p.1127·3).
Skin disorders.

Excita Schmid, USA†.
Nonoxinol 9 (p.1346·1).
Contraceptive.

Exdol Lioh, Canad.
Paracetamol (p.71·2); caffeine citrate (p.761·3); codeine phosphate (p.25·2).
Fever; pain.

Executive B Cenovis, Austral.; Vitelle, Austral.
Vitamins and minerals (p.1350·1); valerian (p.1678·3); passion flower (p.1649·1).
Stress; vitamin and mineral deficiencies.

Exelderm
Bioglan, Irl.; Schwarz, Ital.†; Syntex, Mex.; Bioglan, UK; Westwood-Squibb, USA.
Sulconazole nitrate (p.393·3).
Fungal skin infections.

Exelmin UCI, Braz.
Cambendazole; mebendazole (p.102·2).
Worm infections.

Exelon
Novartis, Aust.; Novartis, Austral.; Novartis, Belg.; Novartis, Canad.; Novartis, Denm.; Novartis, Fin.; Novartis, Ger.; Knoll, Ger.; Novartis, Hong Kong; Novartis, Irl.; Novartis, Israel; Novartis, Ital.; Novartis, Mex.; Novartis, Neth.; Novartis, Norw.; Novartis, NZ; Novartis, Port.; Novartis, S.Afr.; Novartis, Singapore; Novartis, Spain; Novartis, Swed.; Novartis, Switz.; Novartis, Thai.; Novartis, UK; Novartis, USA.
Rivastigmine hydrogen tartrate (p.1424·3).
Alzheimer's disease.

Exeu Biocur, Ger.
Eucalyptus oil (p.1609·2).
Cold symptoms.

Exgest LA Carnrick, USA†.
Phenylpropanolamine hydrochloride (p.1098·1); guaifenesin (p.1092·2).
Respiratory-tract congestion.

Exhirud
Sanofi Winthrop, Aust.; Sanofi Synthelabo, Ger.
Leech extract (p.905·3).
Soft-tissue disorders; vascular disorders.

Ex-Histine WE, USA.
Phenylephrine (p.1097·1); chlorpheniramine [chlorphenamine] (p.412·2); hyoscine (p.468·2).
Upper respiratory-tract disorders.

Exidine Baxter, USA.
Chlorhexidine gluconate (p.1138·2).
Skin disinfection.

Exil Esoform, Ital.
Cetylpyridinium chloride (p.1138·1).
Genital hygiene.

Exipan Agis, Israel.
Piroxicam (p.79·1).
Inflammation; pain.

Exirel
Byk, Aust.; 3M, UK†.
Pirbuterol acetate (p.769·3) or pirbuterol hydrochloride (p.769·3).
Obstructive airways disease.

Exit Farmasa, Braz.
Cinnarizine (p.413·1); piracetam (p.1652·1).
Cerebral and peripheral vascular disorders; impaired mental function.

Exitop
Asta Medica, Aust.; Asta Medica, Fin.; Asta Medica, Ger.; Asta Medica, Swed.
Etoposide (p.538·1).
Malignant neoplasms.

Ex-Lax
Novartis Consumer, Canad.; Novartis Consumer, UK; Novartis Consumer, USA.
Senna (p.1248·2).
Formerly contained phenolphthalein.
Constipation.

Ex-Lax Extra Gentle Pills Novartis, USA†.
Docusate sodium (p.1223·1); phenolphthalein (p.1244·1).
Constipation.

Ex-Lax Gentle Nature Novartis, USA†.
Calcium sennoside A (p.1248·3); calcium sennoside B (p.1248·3).
Constipation.

Ex-Lax Light Sandoz, Canad.†.
Yellow phenolphthalein (p.1244·1); docusate sodium (p.1223·1).
Constipation.

Ex-Lax Stool Softener
Novartis Consumer, Canad.; Novartis Consumer, USA.
Docusate sodium (p.1223·1).
Constipation.

Exlutena Organon, Swed.
Lynestrenol (p.1480·1).
Progestogen-only oral contraceptive.

Exluton
Organon, Belg.†; Organon, Fin.; Organon, Fr.; Organon, Mex.; Organon, Neth.†; Organon, Port.; Donmed, S.Afr.†; Organon, Thai.
Lynestrenol (p.1480·1).
Progestogen-only oral contraceptive.

Exlutona
Organon, Denm.; Organon, Ger.; Organon, Norw.; Organon, Switz.
Lynestrenol (p.1480·1).
Progestogen-only oral contraceptive.

Exmykehl Sanum-Kehlbeck, Ger.
Homoeopathic preparation.

Exna Robins, USA.
Benzthiazide (p.844·2).
Hypertension; oedema.

Exneural BASF, Ger.
Ibuprofen (p.43·2).
Fever; inflammation; musculoskeletal, joint, and soft-tissue disorders; pain.

Exocaine Del, USA; Commerce, USA.
Methyl salicylate (p.55·1).
Muscle and joint pain.

Exocin
Allergan, Denm.; Allergan, Fin.; Allergan, Irl.; Allergan, Ital.; Allergan, Port.; Allergan, S.Afr.; Allergan, Spain; Allergan, UK.
Ofloxacin (p.232·3).
Bacterial eye infections.

Exocine Allergan, Fr.
Ofloxacin (p.232·3).
Bacterial eye infections.

Exodalina Sons, Mex.
Dipyrone (p.34·1).
Pain.

Exoderil
Novartis, Aust.; Rentschler, Ger.; Biochemie, Hong Kong; Biochemie, Singapore.
Naftifine hydrochloride (p.392·1).
Fungal skin and nail infections.

Exoderil Zinkpaste Sanabo, Aust.†.
Naftifine hydrochloride (p.392·1); zinc oxide (p.1128·2).
Fungal skin infections.

Exofat Sunspot, Austral.
Poliglusam; oligofructose; ascorbic acid (p.1389·3).
Obesity.

Exofur Sons, Mex.
Furazolidone (p.592·1).
Diarrhoea.

Exolise Arkopharma, Fr.
Green tea (p.1681·1).
Obesity.

Exolit
Medochemie, Singapore; Medochemie, Thai.
Bromhexine hydrochloride (p.1085·3).
Respiratory-tract disorders associated with increased or viscous mucus.

Exolyt Abigo, Swed.
Chlorcyclizine hydrochloride (p.411·3); guaifenesin (p.1092·2); ammonium chloride (p.1085·2).
Coughs.

Exomega Ducray, Fr.
Avena (p.1583·1); omega-6 fatty acids (p.1613·1).
Skin disorders.

Exomuc Bouchara, Fr.
Acetylcysteine (p.1082·3).
Respiratory-tract congestion.

Exorex
Cybermed, Aust.; Pharmax, UK.
Coal tar (p.1125·1).
Eczema; psoriasis.

Exormin Health Care, Hong Kong.
Ginkgo biloba (p.1615·2).
Cerebral disorders; peripheral vascular disorders; tinnitis; vertigo.

Exorvit Sons, Mex.
Cyanocobalamin (p.1388·1).

Exorvit VM Sons, Mex.
Vitamin and mineral preparation (p.1350·1).

Exoseptoplix Diepha, Fr.
Chlorhexidine gluconate (p.1138·2).
Formerly contained sulfanilamide.
Bacterial skin infections.

Exosurf
Glaxo Wellcome, Aust.; Glaxo Wellcome, Austral.; Glaxo Wellcome, Belg.; Glaxo Wellcome, Braz.; Glaxo Wellcome, Canad.; Glaxo Wellcome, Denm.†; Glaxo Wellcome, Fin.; Glaxo Wellcome, Ger.; Glaxo Wellcome, Hong Kong; Wellcome, Irl.; Glaxo Wellcome, Israel; Glaxo Wellcome, Ital.; Glaxo Wellcome, Mex.; Glaxo Wellcome, Neth.; Glaxo Wellcome, S.Afr.; Glaxo Wellcome, Singapore; Wellcome, Spain; Glaxo Wellcome, Swed.; Wellcome, Switz.; Glaxo Wellcome, Thai.; Wellcome, UK; Glaxo Wellcome, USA.
Colfosceril palmitate (p.1656·1).
Neonatal respiratory distress syndrome.

Ex-Ova Fustery, Mex.
Estreptoprogestageno.

Expafusin
Fresenius Kabi, Aust.; Pharmacia Upjohn, Ger.; Fresenius Kabi, Spain.
An etherified starch (p.732·3) with electrolytes.
Plasma volume expansion.

Expahes
Fresenius Kabi, Aust.; Fresenius Kabi, Switz.
Hetastarch (p.732·3).
Haemodilution; hypovolaemia.

Expal Sons, Mex.
Pipenzolate (p.472·2).
Gastrointestinal disorders.

Expandox Expanpharm, Fr.
Paracetamol (p.71·2).
Formerly known as Expandol.
Fever; pain.

Expanfen Expanpharm, Fr.
Ibuprofen (p.43·2).
Fever; pain.

Expec Legrand, Braz.
Oxomemazine (p.422·2); potassium iodide (p.1522·3); sodium benzoate (p.1134·3); guaifenesin (p.1092·2); ipecacuanha (p.1093·1).
Respiratory-tract congestion.

Expectal N Bayer, Ger.†.
Thyme (p.1672·2).
Catarrh; coughs.

Expectal-Balsam Kolassa, Aust.
Pumilio pine oil (p.1656·3); camphor (p.1589·3); eucalyptus oil (p.1609·2); nutmeg oil (p.1643·1); thyme oil (p.1672·3); benzyl nicotinate (p.20·2).
Respiratory-tract disorders.

Expectalin Parke-Med, S.Afr.
Diphenhydramine hydrochloride (p.416·1); ammonium chloride (p.1085·2).
Coughs.

Expectalin with codeine Parke-Med, S.Afr.
Diphenhydramine hydrochloride (p.416·1); ammonium chloride (p.1085·2); codeine phosphate (p.25·2).
Coughs.

Expectal-Tropfen Kolassa, Aust.
Codeine (p.25·2); thyme extract (p.1672·2); orange extract; anise oil (p.1580·3).
Respiratory-tract disorders.

Expectamin Legrand, Braz.
Dexchlorpheniramine (p.412·2); pseudoephedrine (p.1099·2).
Respiratory-tract disorders.

Expectco Covan, S.Afr.†
Pseudoephedrine hydrochloride (p.1099·2); mepyramine maleate (p.421·1); ipecacuanha (p.1093·1).
Coughs.

Expectil Bunker, Braz.
Diphenhydramine hydrochloride (p.416·1); ammonium chloride (p.1085·2); sulfogaiacol (p.1101·1); sodium citrate (p.1186·2).
Respiratory-tract congestion.

Expectocilin Balsamico EMS, Braz.
Ampicillin sodium (p.150·3); ampicillin benzathine (p.151·3); guaifenesin (p.1092·2).
Bacterial infections.

Expectofar Esfar, Port.
Codeine (p.25·2); ephedrine (p.1090·1); mepiraxamine; vitamin C (p.1389·3).

Expectolu Bergamo, Braz.
Potassium iodide (p.1522·3); lobelia (p.1510·2); hyoscyamus (p.470·1).
Respiratory-tract congestion.

Expectomel Cazi, Braz.
Rorippa nasturtium aquaticum; aconite (p.1572·3); ipecacuanha (p.1093·1); senega (p.1100·2); tolu balsam (p.1101·3); honey (p.1366·2).
Respiratory-tract congestion.

Expectoran Codein Grossmann, Switz.
Codeine phosphate (p.25·2); thyme (p.1672·2); senega (p.1100·2); quillaia (p.1348·2).
Adjuvant in bronchitis; coughs.

Expectorant Cough Formula Tanta, Canad.
Guaifenesin (p.1092·2).

Expectorant Cough Syrup Technilab, Canad.
Guaifenesin (p.1092·2).

Expectorant Syrup Marc-O, Canad.
Guaifenesin (p.1092·2).

Expectotussin "C" Adcock Ingram, S.Afr.
Mepyramine maleate (p.421·1); ammonium chloride (p.1085·2); sodium citrate (p.1186·2); phenylephrine hydrochloride (p.1097·1); ascorbic acid (p.1389·3).
Coughs.

Expectovac Nikkho, Braz.
Procaine penicillin [procaine benzylpenicillin] (p.239·2); benzylpenicillin potassium (p.157·1); aminocaproic acid (p.724·3); bacterial antigens.
Bacterial infections.

Expectuss EMS, Braz.
Ambroxol hydrochloride (p.1084·3).
Respiratory-tract congestion.

Expectussin Dinafarma, Braz.
Noscapine (p.1096·1); mepyramine maleate (p.421·1).
Coughs.

Expectysat N Ysatfabrik, Ger.
Cowslip root (p.1600·1); thyme (p.1672·2).
Cold symptoms.

Expeflen Diba, Mex.
Ambroxol hydrochloride (p.1084·3).
Respiratory-tract disorders.

Expicin Sons, Mex.
Ampicillin (p.150·3).
Bacterial infections.

Expigen
Note.This name is used for preparations of different composition.
Sanova, Aust.
Polysorbate 20 (p.1347·3); ammonium chloride (p.1085·2); sodium benzoate (p.1134·3); anise oil (p.1580·3); niaouli oil (p.1640·2); thyme oil (p.1672·3); menglytate (p.1094·2).
Coughs; respiratory congestion.

Pharmacia Upjohn, Fin.; Pharmacia Upjohn, Norw.; Adcock Ingram, S.Afr.
Polysorbate 20 (p.1347·3); ammonium chloride (p.1085·2).
Coughs.

Expiran British Dispensary, Thai.
Chlorpheniramine [chlorphenamine] maleate (p.412·1); ammonium chloride (p.1085·2); sulfogaiacol (p.1101·1).
Coughs.

Expit PB, Ger.
Ambroxol hydrochloride (p.1084·3).
Respiratory-tract disorders associated with increased or viscous mucus.

Exposis Osler, Fr.
SPF 20; SPF 30: Octinoxate (p.1517·3); titanium dioxide (p.1126·1); avobenzone (p.1517·1).
Sunscreen.

Exprep Mundipharma, Fin.
Senna (p.1248·2).
Bowel evacuation.

Expros Orion, Fin.
Tamsulosin hydrochloride (p.978·3).
Benign prostatic hyperplasia.

Expulin
Shire, Irl.
Pholcodine (p.1099·1); pseudoephedrine hydrochloride (p.1099·2); chlorpheniramine [chlorphenamine] maleate (p.412·1).
Coughs; respiratory-tract congestion.

Shire, UK.
Pholcodine (p.1099·1); pseudoephedrine hydrochloride (p.1099·2); chlorpheniramine [chlorphenamine] maleate (p.412·1).
Coughs.

Expulin Chesty Cough Monmouth, UK.
Guaifenesin (p.1092·2).
Coughs.

Expulin Childrens Cough
Monmouth, Irl.; Monmouth, UK.
Pholcodine (p.1099·1); chlorpheniramine [chlorphenamine] maleate (p.412·1).
Coughs.

Expulin Decongestant Monmouth, UK.
Ephedrine hydrochloride (p.1090·1); chlorpheniramine [chlorphenamine] maleate (p.412·1).
Nasal congestion.

Expulin Dry Cough
Monmouth, Irl.; Monmouth, UK.
Pholcodine (p.1099·1).
Coughs.

Exputex Shire, Irl.
Carbocisteine (p.1086·3).
Respiratory-tract disorders with excessive or viscous mucus.

exrheudon OPT *Optimed, Ger.*
Ointment: Glycol salicylate (p.42·2); benzyl nicotinate (p.20·2).
Frostbite; inflammatory disorders; soft-tissue, nerve, and joint disorders; sports injuries.
Tablets: Phenylbutazone (p.78·1).
Acute ankylosing spondylitis; gout; rheumatism.

Exrhinin *Wernigerode, Ger.*
Tetryzoline hydrochloride (p.1101·2).
Nasal congestion.

Exsel *Allergan, USA.*
Selenium sulfide (p.1123·1).
Dandruff; pityriasis versicolor; seborrhoeic dermatitis.

Extencilline *Rhone-Poulenc Rorer, Fr.*
Benzathine benzylpenicillin (p.156·2).
Bacterial infections.

Extendryl *Fleming, USA.*
Phenylephrine hydrochloride (p.1097·1); hyoscine methonitrate (p.468·2); chlorpheniramine [chlorphenamine] maleate (p.412·1).
Allergic rhinitis; respiratory congestion; urticaria and angioedema.

Exteny *Iqfasa, Mex.*
Mebendazole (p.102·2).

Exterol *Dermal Laboratories, Irl.; Dermal, Israel; Dermal Laboratories, UK.*
Urea hydrogen peroxide (p.1159·3).
Ear wax removal.

Extin *Opfermann, Ger.*
Adipic acid (p.1573·3); ammonium chloride (p.1085·2).
Urinary-tract infections.

Extiser Q *Serral, Mex.*
Praziquantel (p.106·3).
Cysticercosis.

Extovyl *Dexo, Fr.*
Betahistine mesilate (p.1584·3).
Vertigo.

Extra Action Cough *Rugby, USA.*
Dextromethorphan hydrobromide (p.1087·3); guaifenesin (p.1092·2).
Coughs.

Extra Once A Day *Quest, Canad.*
Multivitamin, mineral, and trace element preparation (p.1350·1).

Extra Strength Acetaminophen with Codeine *WestCan, Canad.*
Paracetamol (p.71·2); caffeine (p.761·3); codeine phosphate (p.25·2).
Fever; pain.

Extra Strength Alenic Alka *Rugby, USA.*
Aluminium hydroxide (p.1210·3); magnesium carbonate (p.1232·3).
Hyperacidity.

Extra Strength Alka-Seltzer Effervescent Tablets *Bayer, USA.*
Sodium bicarbonate (p.1186·2); citric acid (p.1596·2); aspirin (p.14·2).
Hyperacidity.

Extra Strength Allergy Sinus *Stanley, Canad.; WestCan, Canad.*
Pseudoephedrine hydrochloride (p.1099·2); chlorpheniramine [chlorphenamine] maleate (p.412·1); paracetamol (p.71·2).

Extra Strength Analgesic *Prodemdis, Canad.*
Methyl salicylate (p.55·1); camphor (p.1589·3); menthol (p.1632·3); eucalyptus oil (p.1609·2).

Extra Strength Bayer Plus *Sterling Health, USA.*
Aspirin (p.14·2).
Calcium carbonate (p.1215·1), magnesium carbonate (p.1232·3), and magnesium oxide (p.1233·2) are included in this preparation in an attempt to limit adverse effects on the gastrointestinal mucosa.

Extra Strength Biotin Forte *Vitaline, USA†.*
Multivitamin preparation (p.1350·1).

Extra Strength Cold Medication Daytime Relief *Stanley, Canad.; WestCan, Canad.*
Pseudoephedrine hydrochloride (p.1099·2); dextromethorphan hydrobromide (p.1087·3); paracetamol (p.71·2).

Extra Strength Cold Medication Nightime *Stanley, Canad.*
Pseudoephedrine hydrochloride (p.1099·2); chlorpheniramine [chlorphenamine] maleate (p.412·1); dextromethorphan hydrobromide (p.1087·3); paracetamol (p.71·2).

Extra Strength Cold Medication Nighttime Relief *WestCan, Canad.*
Pseudoephedrine hydrochloride (p.1099·2); chlorpheniramine [chlorphenamine] maleate (p.412·1); dextromethorphan hydrobromide (p.1087·3); paracetamol (p.71·2).

Extra Strength Doans PM *Ciba, USA.*
Magnesium salicylate (p.50·3); diphenhydramine hydrochloride (p.416·1).

Extra Strength Genaton *Goldline, USA.*
Aluminium hydroxide (p.1210·3); magnesium carbonate (p.1232·3).
Hyperacidity.

Extra Strength Maalox Antacid/Anti-Gas *Novartis Consumer, USA.*
Aluminium hydroxide (p.1210·3); magnesium hydroxide (p.1233·1); simeticone (p.1249·2).
Hyperacidity.

Extra Strength Mintox Plus *Major, USA.*
Simeticone (p.1249·2).

Extra Strength Pyrroxate *Roberts, USA†.*
Phenylpropanolamine hydrochloride (p.1098·1); chlorpheniramine [chlorphenamine] maleate (p.412·1); paracetamol (p.71·2).
Upper respiratory-tract symptoms.

Extra Strength Sinus and Congestion Relief *WestCan, Canad.*
Pseudoephedrine hydrochloride (p.1099·2); paracetamol (p.71·2).

Extra Strength Sinus Medication *Stanley, Canad.*
Pseudoephedrine hydrochloride (p.1099·2); paracetamol (p.71·2).

Extra Strength Tylenol Headache Plus *McNeil Consumer, USA†.*
Paracetamol (p.71·2); calcium carbonate (p.1215·1).
Gastrointestinal pain associated with hyperacidity.

Extra Strength Tylenol PM *McNeil Consumer, USA.*
Diphenhydramine hydrochloride (p.416·1); paracetamol (p.71·2).
Insomnia.

Extra Strength Vicks Cough Drops *Procter & Gamble, USA.*
Menthol (p.1632·3).

Extra Strong Formula 12 *Hilarys, Canad.*
Aloes (p.1210·1); bisacodyl (p.1212·2); cascara (p.1216·1); frangula (p.1227·1); rhubarb (p.1248·1); senna (p.1248·2).
Constipation.

Extracort *Galderma, Ger.*
Triamcinolone acetonide (p.1080·1).
Skin disorders.

Extracort Rhin sine *Alcon, Ger.*
Triamcinolone acetonide (p.1080·1); phenylephrine hydrochloride (p.1097·1).
Allergic nasal disorders.

Extracort Tinktur N *Galderma, Ger.*
Triamcinolone acetonide (p.1080·1); salicylic acid (p.1122·3).
Skin disorders.

Extrafer *SoSe, Ital.*
Ferric sodium gluconate (p.1360·2).
Anaemias.

Extralife Arthri-Care *Felton, Austral.*
Turmeric (p.1029·3); ginger (p.1227·2); feverfew (p.453·3); devil's claw root (p.26·3); lecithin (p.1628·1).
Musculoskeletal and joint disorders.

Extralife Extra-Brite *Felton, Austral.*
Ginkgo biloba (p.1615·2); ginseng (p.1615·3); lecithin (p.1628·1).
Alzheimer's disease; mental function disorders.

Extralife Eye-Care *Felton, Austral.*
Myrtillus (p.1639·2); ginkgo biloba (p.1615·2); big marigold; riboflavin (p.1386·1); zinc gluconate (p.1398·2).
Eye disorders.

Extralife Flow-Care *Felton, Austral.*
Saw palmetto (p.1491·2); urtica (p.1678·2); pyridoxine hydrochloride (p.1386·3); zinc gluconate (p.1398·2).
Benign prostatic hyperplasia; micturition disorders in men.

Extralife Fluid-Care *Felton, Austral.*
Taraxacum (p.1669·1); equisetum (p.1606·3); parsley (p.1648·3); bearberry (p.1583·3); solidago virgaurea; pyridoxine hydrochloride (p.1386·3).
Fluid retention.

Extralife Leg-Care *Felton, Austral.*
Aesculus (p.1574·1); ruscus aculeatus; centella (p.1112·2); ginkgo biloba (p.1615·2); myrtillus (p.1639·2); hesperidin (p.1611·2); rutoside (p.1611·2); ascorbic acid (p.1389·3).
Varicose veins.

Extralife Liva-Care *Felton, Austral.*
Silybum marianum (p.1021·3); greater celandine (p.1618·1); cynara (p.1601·3); turmeric (p.1029·3); astragalus; taraxacum (p.1669·1); lecithin (p.1628·1).
Acne; gastrointestinal disorders; halitosis; hyperlipidaemias; hypersensitivity disorders; hypoglycaemia; menopausal disorders; migraine; obesity; premenstrual syndrome.

Extralife Meno-Care *Felton, Austral.*
Soya bean (p.1378·1); cimicifuga (p.1595·2); chaste tree; dong quai; calcium phosphate (p.1188·3).
Menopausal disorders; osteoporosis.

Extralife Migrai-Care *Felton, Austral.*
Feverfew (p.453·3); salix (p.82·1); magnesium phosphate (p.1191·1).
Migraine and other headaches.

Extralife PMS-Care *Felton, Austral.*
Salix (p.82·1); chaste tree; cimicifuga (p.1595·2); viburnum opulus; bearberry (p.1583·3); pyridoxine hydrochloride (p.1386·3); ferrous fumarate (p.1360·1).
Premenstrual syndrome.

Extralife Sleep-Care *Felton, Austral.*
Valerian (p.1678·3); passion flower (p.1649·1); gentian (p.1615·1); lupulus (p.1629·3); magnesium phosphate (p.1191·1); calcium phosphate (p.1188·3).
Nervous disorders; sleep disorders.

Extralife Uri-Care *Felton, Austral.*
Cranberry (p.1600·2); bearberry (p.1583·3); buchu (p.1587·2); pyridoxine hydrochloride (p.1386·3); ascorbic acid (p.1389·3); potassium sulfate (p.1195·1).
Cystitis.

Extranase *Rottapharm, Fr.*
Bromelains (p.1586·3).
Post-traumatic and postoperative oedema.

Extraneal *Baxter, Denm.; Baxter, Fin.; Baxter, Spain; Baxter, Swed.; Baxter, Switz.*
Icodextrin; sodium chloride; sodium lactate; calcium chloride; magnesium chloride (p.1184·1).
Peritoneal dialysis.

Extraplus *Pierre Fabre, Spain.*
Ketoprofen (p.47·3).
Musculoskeletal, joint disorders, peri-articular, and soft-tissue disorders.

Extrato Hepatico Composto
Note. This name is used for preparations of different composition.

Delta, Braz.
Methionine (p.1012·2); choline (p.1356·3); liver extract.
Liver disorders.

Herals, Braz.
Methionine (p.1012·2); choline (p.1356·3); pyridoxine hydrochloride (p.1386·3).
Liver disorders.

Extravite *Vitalia, UK.*
Multivitamin and mineral preparation (p.1350·1).

Extravits *Lifeplan, UK.*
Multivitamin and mineral preparation (p.1350·1).

Extur *Normon, Spain.*
Indapamide (p.913·1).
Hypertension; oedema.

Exuracid *Rosch & Handel, Aust.*
Tisopurine (p.403·2).
Gout; hyperuricaemia; urinary calculi.

Exzem Oil *Pharmadass, UK.*
Vitamin E oil (p.1393·3); evening primrose oil (p.1613·2); castor oil (p.1592·1); olive oil (p.1643·3); safflower oil (p.1375·1); grapeseed oil; chamomile oil.

Eye Dew *Crookes Healthcare, UK.*
Hamamelis (p.1618·3); naphazoline hydrochloride (p.1095·1).
Formerly known as Optrex Eye Dew.
Eye irritation.

Eye Drops *Rivex, Canad.; Zee, Canad.; Reese, USA.*
Tetryzoline hydrochloride (p.1101·2).
Eye irritation.

Eye Drops Extra *Ocusoft, USA.*
Phenylephrine hydrochloride (p.1097·1).

Eye Eze *Pharmavite, Canad.*
Boric acid (p.1586·1); borax (p.1586·1).

Eye Formula Euphr *Homeocan, Canad.*
Homoeopathic preparation.

Eye Health Herbal Plus Formula 4 *Vitelle, Austral.*
Euphrasia (p.1609·3); ginkgo biloba (p.1615·2); betacarotene (p.1355·1); d-alpha tocoferil acid succinate (p.1394·1); ascorbic acid (p.1389·3); rutoside (p.1611·2); hesperidin (p.1611·2).
Eye strain.

Eye Mo *SmithKline Beecham, Hong Kong; SmithKline Beecham, Singapore; Sterling, Thai.*
Boric acid (p.1586·1); borax (p.1586·1).
Eye irritation.

Eye Mo 36 *SmithKline Beecham, Hong Kong.*
Boric acid (p.1586·1); tetryzoline hydrochloride (p.1101·2).
Eye irritation.

Eye Mo Moist *SmithKline Beecham, Singapore.*
Hypromellose (p.1501·3).
Dry eyes.

Eye Scrub *Ciba Vision, USA.*
Eyelid cleanser.

Eye Wash *Rivex, Canad.*
Boric acid (p.1586·1).

Eyedex *Siam Bheasach, Thai.*
Dexamethasone sodium phosphate (p.1067·1); neomycin sulfate (p.228·1).
Infected eye and ear disorders.

Eyelube *Sabex, Canad.*
Hypromellose (p.1501·3).
Dry eyes.

Eye-Lube-A *Optopics, USA.*
Glycerol (p.1616·3).
Dry eyes.

Eye-Sed *Scherer, USA.*
Zinc sulfate (p.1398·2).
Minor eye irritation.

Eyesine *Akorn, USA.*
Tetryzoline hydrochloride (p.1101·2).
Minor eye irritation.

Eyestil *Ophtapharma, Canad.*
Sodium hyaluronate (p.1620·1).
Dry eyes.

Eye-Stream *Alcon, Austral.; Alcon, Canad.; Alcon, Hong Kong; Alcon, NZ; Alcon, Singapore; Alcon Cusi, Spain; Alcon, USA.*
Electrolytes (p.1180·1).
Eye irrigation.

Eye-vit *Pharmadass, UK.*
Multivitamin, mineral, and trace element preparation (p.1350·1).

Eyevite *Allergan, Austral.; Allergan, NZ.*
Vitamin and mineral preparation (p.1350·1).
Eye disorders.

Eyewash *Rivex, Canad.; Zee, Canad.*
Electrolyte solution (p.1180·1).
Eye irrigation.

Eye-Zine *Ocumed, USA.*
Tetryzoline hydrochloride (p.1101·2).
Eye irritation.

EZ Detect
Marco, Austral.; Biomerica, USA.
Test for occult blood in faeces or urine.

E-Z-Cat *Therapex, Canad.†; E-Z-EM, Port.; E-Z-EM, UK.*
Barium sulfate (p.1032·1).
Contrast medium for computerised axial tomography of the gastrointestinal tract.

E-Z-Gas II
Note. This name is used for preparations of different composition.

Therapex, Canad.
Sodium bicarbonate (p.1186·2); tartaric acid (p.1669·2); simeticone (p.1249·2).
Production of CO_2 in double contrast radiography of the gastrointestinal tract.

Bracco, Switz.
Sodium bicarbonate (p.1186·2); citric acid (p.1596·2); simeticone (p.1249·2).
Production of CO_2 in double contrast radiography of the gastrointestinal tract.

Ez-HBT *Metabolic Solutions, USA.*
Carbon-13 (p.1591·3) labelled urea (Helicosol); test meal (Ensure).
Diagnosis of Helicobacter pylori infection.

E-Z-HD *E-Z-EM, Israel; E-Z-EM, Port.; E-Z-EM, UK.*
Barium sulfate (p.1032·1).
Contrast medium for gastrointestinal radiography.

Ezon-T *Unison, Thai.*
Ointment: Tolnaftate (p.395·2).
Topical solution: Tolnaftate (p.395·2); triacetin (p.395·3).
Fungal skin infections.

Ezosina *Fournier, Ital.*
Terazosin hydrochloride (p.980·1).
Hypertension.

E-Z-Paque *E-Z-EM, Belg.; E-Z-EM, UK.*
Barium sulfate (p.1032·1).
Contrast medium for gastrointestinal radiography.

I + I-F *Dunhall, USA.*
Hydrocortisone (p.1073·3); clioquinol (p.190·2); pramocaine (p.1318·2).
Skin disorders.

F080 *Baxter, Ital.*
Amino-acid infusion for parenteral nutrition (p.1350·1).
Liver disorders.

F 99 Sulgan N *Divapharma, Ger.†.*
Hamamelis (p.1618·3).
Anorectal disorders.

FAB *Medical Research, Austral.*
Iron and vitamin B substances (p.1350·1).

FAB Co *Medical Research, Austral.*
Iron, vitamin B substances, and vitamin C (p.1350·1).

FAB Tri-Cal *Medical Research, Austral.*
Calcium hydrogen phosphate (p.1188·2); calcium carbonate (p.1215·1); calcium gluconate (p.1188·2); zinc oxide (p.1128·2); magnesium oxide (p.1233·2); colecalciferol (p.1391·1).
Nutritional supplement.

Fabahistin *Bayer, Austral.†; Bayer, S.Afr.†.*
Mebhydrolin napadisilate (p.420·2).
Hypersensitivity reactions.

Fabasma *Propan, S.Afr.†.*
Amobarbital (p.655·2); ephedrine hydrochloride (p.1090·1); aminophylline (p.760·1).
Asthma.

Fabrazyme *Genzyme, UK.*
Agalsidase beta (p.1574·2).
Fabry disease.

Fabrol *Ciba-Geigy, Swed.†.*
Acetylcysteine (p.1082·3).
Bronchitis.

Fabroven *Pierre Fabre, Spain.*
Capsules: Ascorbic acid (p.1389·3); hesperidin methyl chalcone (p.1611·2); ruscus aculeatus.
Cream: Dextran sulfate (p.1603·1); melilotus; ruscus aculeatus.
Peripheral vascular disorders.

Fabubac *Brunel, S.Afr.*
Co-trimoxazole (p.193·3).
Bacterial infections.

Face Foundation *Avon, Canad.†.*
SPF 15: Octinoxate (p.1517·3); titanium dioxide (p.1126·1).
Sunscreen.

Face Zone *Clinique, Canad.*
SPF 30: Homosalate (p.1517·2); octinoxate (p.1517·3); octisalate (p.1518·1); oxybenzone (p.1518·1).
Sunscreen.

Faces Only *Schering-Plough, USA.*
SPF 6; SPF 15: Octinoxate (p.1517·3); oxybenzone (p.1518·1).
Sunscreen.

Facicam *Senosiain, Mex.*
Piroxicam (p.79·1).
Gout; musculoskeletal, joint, peri-articular and soft-tissue disorders.

The symbol † denotes a preparation no longer actively marketed

Facilit *Fides Rottapharm, Spain.*
Allopurinol (p.397·2); benzbromarone (p.399·3).
Gout; hyperuricaemia.

Facogen *NBF-Lanes, Ital.*
Lipid, protein, carbohydrate, multivitamin, and trace-element preparation (p.1350·1).
Nutritional supplement.

Facort *Biolab, Thai.*
Triamcinolone acetonide (p.1080·1).
Skin disorders.

Facovit *Teofarma, Ital.*
Testosterone propionate (p.1492·2); rubidium iodide (p.1660·1); potassium iodide (p.1522·3); riboflavin (p.1386·1).
Cataract.

Fact Plus *Medisense, Canad.; Advanced Care, USA.*
Pregnancy test (p.1654·3).

Factor AF2 *Biosyn, Ger.*
Liver and spleen extract.
Supportive tumour therapy.

Factrel *Wyeth-Ayerst, Canad.; Wyeth-Ayerst, USA.*
Gonadorelin hydrochloride (p.1284·2).
Diagnostic evaluation of anterior pituitary function.

Fa-Cyl *Medley, Braz.*
Tinidazole (p.603·3).
Anaerobic bacterial infections; protozoal infections.

Fa-Cyl M *Medley, Braz.*
Tinidazole (p.603·3); miconazole (p.391·1).
Vulvovaginal infections.

FAD Ophthalmic Soln *Santen, Hong Kong.*
Flavine adenine dinucleotide disodium.
Blepharitis; keratitis.

Fadiamone *CS, Fr.*
Phyto-oestrogens; centella (p.1112·2).
Formerly contained estrone, estradiol, testosterone propionate, pregnenolone acetate, and allantoin.
Skin ageing.

Fadig *Dansk-Flama, Braz.*
Amino acids and vitamin B substances (p.1350·1).

Fadine *Biolab, Thai.*
Famotidine (p.1225·3).
Gastro-oesophageal reflux; peptic ulcer; Zollinger-Ellison syndrome.

Fadol *Lemery, Mex.*
Hydrocortisone (p.1073·3).
Corticosteroid.

Faexojodan *Kanoldt, Ger.†*
Saccharomyces cerevisiae (non-fermentable) (p.1398·1).
Skin disorders.

Fagastril *Quimfar, Spain.*
Famotidine (p.1225·3).
Gastro-oesophageal reflux; peptic ulcer; Zollinger-Ellison syndrome.

Fagizol *Continentales, Mex.*
Metronidazole (p.594·1).

Fagolipo *Libbs, Braz.*
Mazindol (p.1510·3).
Obesity.

Fagorutin Buchweizen *SmithKline Beecham OTC, Ger.*
Tablets: Fagopyrum esculentum; troxerutin (p.1611·2).
Peripheral vascular disorders.

Tea: Fagopyrum esculentum.
Capillary disorders; peripheral vascular disorders.

Fagorutin Roßkastanien-Balsam F *SmithKline Beecham OTC, Ger.*
Aesculus (p.1574·1); arnica (p.1581·3); rutoside sodium sulfate (p.1611·2); menthol (p.1632·3); rosemary oil (p.1659·3).
Superficial vascular disorders.

Fagorutin Ruscus *SmithKline Beecham OTC, Ger.*
Ruscus aculeatus.
Chronic venous insufficiency; haemorrhoids.

Fagus *Knoll, Spain.*
Ranitidine hydrochloride (p.1245·2).
Acid aspiration; gastro-oesophageal reflux; gastrointestinal haemorrhage; peptic ulcer; Zollinger-Ellison syndrome.

Fagusan *Spreewald, Ger.*
Guaifenesin (p.1092·2).
Coughs and related respiratory-tract disorders.

Faktu
Meda, Fin.; Tosse, Ger.; Byk Gulden, Ger.; Roland, Ger.; Byk Gulden, Hong Kong; Byk, Port.; Byk Gulden, Singapore; Byk, Switz.; Byk Gulden, Thai.
Policresulen; cinchocaine hydrochloride (p.1309·1).
Anorectal disorders.

Faktu akut *Byk Gulden, Ger.; Roland, Ger.*
Bufexamac (p.20·3); bismuth subgallate (p.1213·2); titanium dioxide (p.1126·1); lignocaine [lidocaine] hydrochloride (p.1313·2).
Anorectal disorders.

Falcol *Farma Lepori, Spain.*
Aceclofenac (p.11·1).
Musculoskeletal, joint, and peri-articular disorders; pain.

Falexol *Protein, Mex.*
Cefalexin (p.161·3).
Bacterial infections.

Falicard *Asta Medica, Ger.*
Verapamil hydrochloride (p.989·1).
Arrhythmias; hypertension; ischaemic heart disease.

Falimint *Berlin-Chemie, Ger.*
Acetylaminopropoxybenzene.
Mouth and throat disorders.

Falithrom *Hexal, Ger.*
Phenprocoumon (p.954·3).
Thromboembolism prophylaxis.

Falitonsin *Asta Medica, Ger.*
Atenolol (p.841·3).
Arrhythmias; hypertension; ischaemic heart disease.

Falkamin
Note.This name is used for preparations of different composition.
Falk; Ger.; Knoll, Ital.
Leucine (p.1370·3); valine (p.1381·3); isoleucine (p.1370·1).
Nutritional supplement in liver disorders.

Falk, Hong Kong; Falk, Singapore.
Amino-acid preparation (p.1350·1).
Nutritional supplement in liver disorders.

Falmonox *Sanofi Winthrop, Braz.*
Teclozan (p.603·2).
Intestinal amoebiasis.

Falqui *Unipharma, Switz.†*
Phenolphthalein (p.1244·1); liquid paraffin (p.1407·1); agar (p.1498·3); prune (p.1245·1).
Constipation.

Falquigut *Falqui, Ital.*
Sodium picosulfate (p.1249·3).
Constipation.

Falquilax *Falqui, Ital.*
Senna (p.1248·2).
Constipation.

Faltium *Almirall, Spain.*
Veralipride (p.711·2).
Menopausal disorders.

Falvin *Theramex, Ital.*
Fenticonazole nitrate (p.383·2).
Dermatological and gynaecological fungal infections.

Famcod *Salters, S.Afr.*
Paracetamol (p.71·4); codeine phosphate (p.25·2).
Pain.

Famel
Note.This name is used for preparations of different composition.
Boots, Ital.
Lactocreosote (p.1087·3); calcium lactophosphate; ephedrine hydrochloride (p.1090·1).
Bronchial catarrh.

Boots Healthcare, Neth.
Creosote (p.1087·3); ephedrine hydrochloride (p.1090·1).
Coughs.

Boots Healthcare, Switz.
Lactocreosote (p.1087·3); calcium lactophosphate; codeine (p.25·2); drosera (p.1606·1); grindelia (p.1618·2).
Bronchitis; coughs; sore throat.

Famel Broomhexine *Boots Healthcare, Neth.*
Bromhexine hydrochloride (p.1085·3).
Coughs.

Famel Catarrh & Throat Pastilles *Seton, UK†.*
Creosote (p.1087·3); cinnamon leaf oil; lemon oil (p.1628·2); menthol (p.1632·3).
Coughs; sore throat.

Famel cum Codein *Brady, Aust.*
Lactocreosote (p.1087·3); calcium lactophosphate; codeine hydrochloride (p.25·2).
Asthma; bronchitis; catarrh; cold symptoms.

Famel cum Ephedrin *Brady, Aust.*
Lactocreosote (p.1087·3); calcium lactophosphate; ephedrine hydrochloride (p.1090·1).
Asthma; bronchitis; catarrh; cold symptoms.

Famel Expectorant *SSL, UK.*
Guaifenesin (p.1092·2).
Coughs.

Famel Linctus *Seton, UK†.*
Pholcodine (p.1099·1).
Coughs.

Famel Original *SSL, UK.*
Creosote (p.1087·3); codeine phosphate (p.25·2).
Coughs.

Famethacin *Be-Tabs, S.Afr.*
Indometacin (p.44·3).
Gout; musculoskeletal and joint disorders.

Family Medicated First Aid Treatment *Tender, Canad.*
Benzalkonium chloride (p.1133·2); lignocaine [lidocaine] hydrochloride (p.1313·2).

Family Medicated Sunburn Relief *Tender, Canad.†.*
Lignocaine [lidocaine] (p.1313·2).

Fam-Lax *Torbet Laboratories, UK.*
Yellow phenolphthalein (p.1244·1); rhubarb (p.1248·1).
Constipation.

Fam-Lax Senna *Torbet Laboratories, UK.*
Turkey rhubarb (p.1248·1); senna leaf (p.1248·2); carrageenan (p.1500·1).
Constipation.

Famo *CTI, Israel.*
Famotidine (p.1225·3).
Gastro-oesophageal reflux; peptic ulcer; Zollinger-Ellison syndrome.

Famoc
Berlin Pharm, Singapore; Berlin Pharm, Thai.
Famotidine (p.1225·3).
Gastro-oesophageal reflux; peptic ulcer; Zollinger-Ellison syndrome.

Famocid
Sun, Singapore; Sun, Thai.
Famotidine (p.1225·3).
Peptic ulcer; Zollinger-Ellison syndrome.

Famodil *Sigma-Tau, Ital.*
Famotidine (p.1225·3).
Gastrointestinal disorders.

Famodine
Farmasa, Braz.; Duopharma, Hong Kong.
Famotidine (p.1225·3).
Acid aspiration; gastro-oesophageal reflux; peptic ulcer; Zollinger-Ellison syndrome.

Famonox *Charoen, Thai.*
Famotidine (p.1225·3).
Peptic ulcer; Zollinger-Ellison syndrome.

Famopsin
Remedica, Hong Kong; Remedica, Singapore; Remedica, Thai.
Famotidine (p.1225·3).
Dyspepsia; gastric hyperacidity; heartburn; peptic ulcer; Zollinger-Ellison syndrome.

Famoset *Sintofarma, Braz.*
Famotidine (p.1225·3).
Acid aspiration; gastro-oesophageal reflux; peptic ulcer; Zollinger-Ellison syndrome.

Famotal *Alphama, Norw.*
Famotidine (p.1225·3).
Gastro-oesophageal reflux; peptic ulcer; Zollinger-Ellison syndrome.

Famotec *Julphar, UAE.*
Famotidine (p.1225·3).
Gastro-oesophageal reflux; peptic ulcer; Zollinger-Ellison syndrome.

Famotin
DHA, Singapore; LSP, Thai.
Famotidine (p.1225·3).
Gastro-oesophageal reflux; peptic ulcer; Zollinger-Ellison syndrome.

Famox
Ache, Braz.; Pacific, Hong Kong; Pacific, NZ; Alphapharm, Singapore; Merck, Singapore.
Famotidine (p.1225·3).
Acid aspiration; gastro-oesophageal reflux; peptic ulcer; Zollinger-Ellison syndrome.

Famoxal *Silanes, Mex.*
Famotidine (p.1225·3).
Acid aspiration; gastro-oesophageal reflux; peptic ulcer; Zollinger-Ellison syndrome.

Fampin *Wayne, Mex.*
Rifampicin (p.243·2).

Famstim *Genpharm, S.Afr.*
Ammonium bicarbonate (p.1085·1); aromatic ammonium spirit (p.1579·1); spirit of ether (p.1403·2).
Coughs.

Famtuss *Genpharm, S.Afr.*
Diphenhydramine hydrochloride (p.416·1); ammonium chloride (p.1085·2); sodium citrate (p.1186·2); menthol (p.1632·3).
Coughs.

Famucaps *Brunel, S.Afr.*
Phenylephrine hydrochloride (p.1097·1); chlorpheniramine [chlorphenamine] maleate (p.412·1); ascorbic acid (p.1389·3); caffeine (p.761·3); paracetamol (p.71·2); atropine sulfate (p.461·1).
Upper respiratory-tract disorders.

Famulcer *Inkeysa, Spain.*
Famotidine (p.1225·3).
Gastro-oesophageal reflux; peptic ulcer; Zollinger-Ellison syndrome.

Famvir
SmithKline Beecham, Aust.; SmithKline Beecham, Austral.; SmithKline Beecham, Belg.; SmithKline Beecham, Canad.; SmithKline Beecham, Denm.; SmithKline Beecham, Fin.; SmithKline Beecham, Ger.; SmithKline Beecham, Hong Kong; Novartis, Irl.; SmithKline Beecham, Israel; SmithKline Beecham, Neth.; SmithKline Beecham, NZ; SmithKline Beecham, Spain; SmithKline Beecham, Swed.; SmithKline Beecham, Switz.; SmithKline Beecham, Thai.; Novartis, UK; SmithKline Beecham, USA.
Famciclovir (p.620·3) or penciclovir (p.638·1).
Herpesvirus infections.

Fanalgic *Mitchell, UK.*
Paracetamol (p.71·2).
Fever; pain.

Fanalgin *Weifa, Norw.*
Phenazone (p.77·2); caffeine (p.761·3).
Fever; pain.

Fanasil *Roche, Ital.†.*
Sulfadoxine (p.252·3).
Bacterial infections.

Fanaxal *Esteve, Spain.*
Alfentanil hydrochloride (p.11·3).
General anaesthesia.

Fanciadazol *Novag, Mex.*
Mebendazole (p.102·2).
Worm infections.

Fandall *Maver, Mex.*
Dipyrone (p.34·1).
Fever; pain.

Fangopress *Geistlich, Switz.†.*
Compress.
Musculoskeletal and joint disorders.

Fango-Rubriment *Riemser, Ger.*
Medicinal mud; sulfur (p.1123·3).
Musculoskeletal and joint disorders.

Fangotherm
Eifelfango, Ger.; Eifelfango, Switz.†.
Medicinal mud.
Gastrointestinal, liver, and kidney disorders; gout; musculoskeletal and joint disorders; neuralgia.

Fanhdi
Grifols, Ger.; Grifols, Ital.; Grifols, Spain; Grifols, UK.
A factor VIII preparation (p.734·1).
Haemophilia A.

Fanosin *Abello, Spain.*
Famotidine (p.1225·3).
Gastro-oesophageal reflux; peptic ulcer; Zollinger-Ellison syndrome.

Fanox *Lesvi, Spain.*
Famotidine (p.1225·3).
Gastro-oesophageal reflux; peptic ulcer; Zollinger-Ellison syndrome.

Fansia *Eurodrug, Thai.*
Phenylpropanolamine hydrochloride (p.1098·1).
Obesity.

Fansidar
Roche, Aust.†; Roche, Austral.; Roche, Belg.†; Roche, Braz.; Roche, Canad.; Roche, Denm.; Roche, Fr.; Roche, Irl.; Roche, Israel; Roche, Neth.†; Roche, S.Afr.; Roche, Swed.†; Roche, Switz.; Roche, UK; Roche, USA.
Sulfadoxine (p.252·3); pyrimethamine (p.442·3).
Malaria; Pneumocystis carinii pneumonia; toxoplasmosis.

Fansidol *NCSN, Ital.*
Nimesulide (p.62·3).
Fever; inflammation; pain.

Fansimef *Roche, Switz.*
Mefloquine hydrochloride (p.438·2); sulfadoxine (p.252·3); pyrimethamine (p.442·3).
Malaria.

Fantomalt
Nutricia, Fin.; Nutricia, Ital.; Nutricia, Port.
Maltodextrin (p.1371·2).
Preparation for enteral nutrition.

Fantrodol *Farmaco, Mex.*
Ambroxol (p.1084·3).
Respiratory-tract disorders.

Farakil *Chew, Thai.*
Prednisolone (p.1077·3); neomycin (p.228·1).
Infected skin disorders.

Faraxen *Randall, Mex.*
Naproxen (p.60·3).

Farbee with Vitamin C *Major, USA.*
Vitamin B substances with vitamin C (p.1350·1).

Farco-Oxicyanid-Tupfer *Farco, Ger.*
Mercuric oxycyanide (p.1634·3).
Disinfection of skin and mucous membranes.

Farco-Tril *Farco, Ger.*
Oxytetracycline calcium (p.234·1); polymyxin B sulfate (p.238·1); hydrocortisone (p.1073·3).
Genito-urinary-tract disorders.

Farco-Uromycin *Farco, Ger.*
Neomycin sulfate (p.228·1); lignocaine [lidocaine] hydrochloride (p.1313·2).
Urinary-tract infections.

Fardixon *Farcoral, Mex.*
Nalidixic acid (p.227·1).
Urinary-tract infections.

Fardolpin *Farcoral, Mex.*
Dipyrone (p.34·1).
Fever; pain.

Farecef *Lafare, Ital.*
Cefoperazone sodium (p.168·2).
Bacterial infections.

Faremicin *Lafare, Ital.*
Fosfomycin calcium (p.208·2).
Bacterial infections.

Faremid *Lafare, Ital.*
Pipemidic acid (p.236·1).
Bacterial infections.

Fareston
Orion, Aust.; Schering-Plough, Austral.; Asta Medica, Belg.; Ercopharm, Denm.†; Orion, Fin.; Orion, Fr.; Asta Medica, Ger.; Orion, Irl.; Schering-Plough, Ital.; Schering-Plough, Mex.; Asta Medica, Neth.†; Schering-Plough, NZ; Schering-Plough, Port.; Schering-Plough, S.Afr.; Schering-Plough, Spain; Orion, Swed.; Orion, Switz.; Schering-Plough, Thai.; Orion, UK; Schering-Plough, USA.
Toremifene citrate (p.576·1).
Breast cancer.

Faretrizin *Lafare, Ital.*
Propylene glycol cefatrizine (p.164·3).
Bacterial infections.

Fargan *Carlo Erba OTC, Ital.*
Promethazine (p.423·2).
Skin irritation.

Farganesse *Pharmacia Upjohn, Ital.*
Promethazine hydrochloride (p.423·2).
Hypersensitivity reactions; premedication.

Fargestium *Cazi, Braz.*
Rhubarb (p.1248·1); aniseed (p.1580·2); melissa (p.1632·2); clove (p.1596·3); quassia (p.1657·1); pichurim; gentian (p.1615·1); nux vomica (p.1643·1).
Digestive-system disorders.

Fargo *Elexsam, Austral.†.*
Lignocaine [lidocaine] (p.1313·2).
Bites and stings; muscle pain; pain; pruritus; skin irritation.

Farial *Riemser, Ger.*
Indanazoline hydrochloride (p.1092·3).
Colds.

Farin Gola *Montefarmaco, Ital.*
Cetylpyridinium chloride (p.1138·1).
Mouth and throat disinfection.

Faringesic *Diafarm, Spain.*
Chlorhexidine hydrochloride (p.1138·2); benzocaine (p.1306·2).
Mouth and throat disorders.

Faringina *SIT, Ital.*
Dequalinium chloride (p.1143·1).
Mouth disinfection.

Faringotricina *SIT, Ital.*
Tyrothricin (p.267·1).
Stomatitis.

Farlac *Farmasa, Braz.*
Lactulose (p.1230·1).
Constipation; hepatic encephalopathy.

Farlin *Continentales, Mex.*
Dipyrone (p.34·1).

Farlutal
Pharmacia Upjohn, Aust.; Pharmacia, Austral.†; Pharmacia Upjohn, Belg.; Carlo Erba, Braz.; Pharmacia Upjohn, Fin.; Pharmacia Upjohn, Fr.; Pharmacia Upjohn, Ger.; Pharmacia Upjohn, Hong Kong; Carlo Erba OTC, Ital.; Pharmacia Upjohn, Mex.; Pharmacia Upjohn, Neth.; Pharmacia Upjohn, Norw.; Pharmacia Upjohn, NZ; Pharmacia Upjohn, S.Afr.; Pharmacia Upjohn, Singapore; Kenfarma, Spain; Pharmacia Upjohn, Swed.; Pharmacia Upjohn, Switz.; Pharmacia Upjohn, Thai.; Pharmacia, UK.
Medroxyprogesterone acetate (p.1480·1).
Malignant neoplasms; metrorrhagia; secondary amenorrhoea.

Farmabroxol *Farmasan, Ger.†*
Ambroxol hydrochloride (p.1084·3).
Respiratory disorders associated with viscid or excessive mucus.

Farmacetamol *Docmed, S.Afr.†*
Paracetamol (p.71·2).
Fever; pain.

Farmacola *Roche Nicholas, Spain.*
Ginseng (p.1615·3); multivitamins and minerals (p.1350·1); caffeine (p.761·3).
Tonic.

Farmacrom *Alcon Cusi, Spain.*
Sodium cromoglicate (p.774·3).
Allergic rhinitis; hay fever.

Farmadiuril *Farmacusi, Spain.*
Bumetanide (p.852·1).
Oedema, hypertension.

Farmaflebon *Farmasa, Mex.*
Hydroxypolyethoxydodecanol (p.1345·2).
Oesophageal varices; telangiectasis.

Farmagripine *Pensa, Spain.*
Chlorpheniramine [chlorphenamine] maleate (p.412·1); phenylpropanolamine hydrochloride (p.1098·1); paracetamol (p.71·2).
Fever; influenza and cold symptoms; pain.

Farmalcohol *Cinfa, Spain.*
Alcohol (p.1130·3); cetylpyridinium chloride (p.1138·1).
Disinfection.

Farmaproina *I Farmacologia, Spain.*
Procaine penicillin [procaine benzylpenicillin] (p.239·2).
Bacterial infections.

Farmeban *Farmasa, Mex.*
Diiodohydroxyquinoline (p.590·2); dimethicone (p.1249·2).
Amoebiasis.

Farmiblastina *Kenfarma, Spain.*
Doxorubicin hydrochloride (p.534·3).
Malignant neoplasms.

Farmicam *Continentales, Mex.*
Piroxicam (p.79·1).

Farmicetina P7 *Darrow, Braz.*
Chloramphenicol (p.179·1).
Bacterial infections.

Farmidal S *Continentales, Mex.*
Astemizole (p.409·1).

Farmin *Farcoral, Mex.*
Diazepam (p.674·3).

Farmistin *Pharmacia Upjohn, Ger.*
Vincristine sulfate (p.578·3).
Malignant neoplasms.

Farmitrexat *Pharmacia Upjohn, Ger.*
Methotrexate sodium (p.553·2).
Malignant neoplasms; psoriasis.

Farmorubicin
Pharmacia Upjohn, Aust.; Pharmacia Upjohn, Denm.; Pharmacia Upjohn, Fin.; Pharmacia Upjohn, Ger.; Farmitalia, Israel; Pharmacia Upjohn, Mex.; Pharmacia Upjohn, Norw.; Pharmacia Upjohn, S.Afr.; Pharmacia Upjohn, Swed.; Pharmacia Upjohn, Switz.; Pharmacia Upjohn, Thai.
Epirubicin hydrochloride (p.537·1).
Malignant neoplasms.

Farmorubicina
Pharmacia Upjohn, Braz.; Pharmacia Upjohn, Ital.; Pharmacia Upjohn, Port.; Kenfarma, Spain.
Epirubicin hydrochloride (p.537·1).
Malignant neoplasms.

Farmorubicine
Pharmacia Upjohn, Belg.; Pharmacia Upjohn, Fr.; Pharmacia Upjohn, Neth.
Epirubicin hydrochloride (p.537·1).
Malignant neoplasms.

Farmospasmina *Giuliani, Ital.*
Papaverine hydrochloride (p.1648·1); belladonna (p.463·1).
Gastrointestinal spasm.

Farmotal *Pharmacia Upjohn, Ital.*
Thiopental sodium (p.1269·1).
General anaesthesia.

Farmotex *Liomont, Mex.*
Famotidine (p.1225·3).
Peptic ulcers.

Farnerate *Kuraray, Jpn.*
Prednisolone farnesil.
Skin disorders.

Farnezone *Taiho, Jpn.*
Prednisolone farnesil.
Skin disorders.

Farnitin *Lafare, Ital.*
Carnitine (p.1356·1).
Carnitine deficiency; myocardial ischaemia.

Farnitran *Fariberica, Port.*
Nitrendipine (p.947·1).
Hypertension.

Farom *Suntory, Jpn.*
Faropenem sodium (p.206·3).
Bacterial infections.

Faros *Lichtwer, Ger.; Medichemie Bioline, Switz.*
Crataegus (p.1600·2).
Cardiac disorders.

Farpectol *Farcoral, Mex.*
Kaolin (p.1229·3); pectin (p.1502·3).
Gastrointestinal disorders.

Farpik *Farcoral, Mex.*
Paracetamol (p.71·2).
Fever; pain.

Farpresse *Fariberica, Port.*
Lisinopril (p.921·1).
Heart failure; hypertension.

Fartoxol *Farcoral, Mex.*
Oxolamine citrate (p.1096·2).
Coughs.

Fartricon *Farcoral, Mex.*
Metronidazole (p.594·1).
Amoebiasis; giardiasis; trichomoniasis.

Farvicett *Farmec, Ital.*
Chlorhexidine gluconate (p.1138·2); cetrimide (p.1137·1).
Skin, wound, burn, and mucous membrane disinfection.

Farviran *Farmigea, Ital.*
Inosine pranobex (p.627·2).
Viral gynaecological infections.

Farxen *Farcoral, Mex.*
Naproxen (p.60·3); paracetamol (p.71·2).
Fever; pain.

Fasax *BASF, Ger.*
Piroxicam (p.79·1).
Gout; musculoskeletal, joint, and soft-tissue disorders.

Fase *Schwarz, Ital.†*
Aprotinin (p.725·3).
Oedema; pancreatic disorders; prevention of post-surgical adhesions; pulmonary embolism; shock.

Fasidine *Siam Medicare, Thai.*
Famotidine (p.1225·3).
Peptic ulcer; Zollinger-Ellison syndrome.

Fasigin *Pfizer, Ital.*
Tinidazole (p.603·3).
Trichomoniasis.

Fasigin N *Pfizer, Ital.*
Tinidazole (p.603·3); nystatin (p.392·2).
Vulvovaginal trichomoniasis and candidiasis.

Fasigyn
Pfizer, Aust.†; Pfizer, Austral.; Pfizer, Belg.; Pfizer, Braz.; Pfizer, Hong Kong; Pfizer, Israel; Pfizer, Mex.; Pfizer, Neth.; Roerig, Port.; Pfizer, S.Afr.; Pfizer, Singapore.; Pfizer, Swed.; Pfizer, Thai.; Pfizer, UK.
Tinidazole (p.603·3).
Anaerobic bacterial infections; protozoal infections.

Fasigyn VT *Pfizer, Mex.*
Tinidazole (p.603·3); tioconazole (p.395·1).
Vaginal fungal and bacterial infections.

Fasigyne
Pfizer, Fr.†; Pfizer, Switz.
Tinidazole (p.603·3).
Anaerobic bacterial infections; protozoal infections.

Fasolan *Cilag, Mex.*
Flunarizine hydrochloride (p.418·1).
Cerebral and peripheral vascular disorders; migraine; vertigo.

Faspic *Zambon, Ital.; Robapharm, Spain†; Inpharzam, Switz.*
Ibuprofen (p.43·2).
Fever; gout; musculoskeletal, joint, and peri-articular disorders; pain.

Fast Powder *Medochemie, Singapore.*
Bacitracin zinc (p.155·2); neomycin sulfate (p.228·1).
Bacterial skin infections.

Fast-Acting Mylanta *J&J-Merck, USA.*
Oral liquid: Aluminium hydroxide (p.1210·3); magnesium hydroxide (p.1233·1); simeticone (p.1249·2).
Flatulence; hyperacidity.
Tablets: Calcium carbonate (p.1215·1); magnesium hydroxide (p.1233·1).
Hyperacidity.

Fastenyl *Sarget, Fr.*
Arginine aspartate (p.1354·1); vitamin C (p.1389·3).
Tonic.

Fastin *SmithKline Beecham, Canad.†; SmithKline Beecham, USA†.*
Phentermine hydrochloride (p.1514·1).
Obesity.

Fastium *Sanus, Braz.*
Diethylpropion hydrochloride (p.1508·3); diazepam (p.674·3).
Obesity.

Fastjekt *Allergopharma, Ger.; Bracco, Ital.*
Adrenaline [epinephrine] (p.829·1) or adrenaline [epinephrine] hydrochloride (p.829·2).
Anaphylactic shock.

Fastum
Menarini, Belg.; Menarini, Hong Kong; Menarini, Irl.; Menarini, Ital.; Sanitas, Port.; Restan, S.Afr.; Menarini, Singapore; Guidotti, Spain; Menarini, Switz.; Menarini, Thai.
Ketoprofen (p.47·3).
Gout; inflammation; musculoskeletal, joint, peri-articular, and soft-tissue disorders; pain; thrombophlebitis.

Fasturtec *Sanofi Synthelabo, UK.*
Rasburicase (p.403·3).
Hyperuricaemia.

Fasupond *Eu Rho, Ger.*
Phenylpropanolamine hydrochloride (p.1098·1).
Obesity.

Fate Low Protein *Fate, UK.*
A range of low-protein foods for special diets (p.1350·1).

Father John's Medicine Plus *Oakhurst, USA.*
Phenylephrine hydrochloride (p.1097·1); dextromethorphan hydrobromide (p.1087·3); chlorpheniramine [chlorphenamine] maleate (p.412·1); ammonium chloride (p.1085·2); guaifenesin (p.1092·2).
Coughs.

Fatidin *Cipan, Port.*
Famotidine (p.1225·3).
Peptic ulcer; Zollinger-Ellison syndrome.

Fatigue *Homeocan, Canad.*
Homoeopathic preparation.

Fatigue L5 *Homeocan, Canad.*
Homoeopathic preparation.

Fat-Solv *Cantassium Co., UK.*
Inositol (p.1623·3); choline bitartrate (p.1356·3); methionine (p.1012·2); betaine hydrochloride (p.1584·3); alfalfa (p.1574·3); kelp (p.1625·3); glutamic acid hydrochloride (p.1365·2); vitamin B$_6$ (p.1386·3).

Faulcris *Faulding, Port.*
Vincristine sulfate (p.578·3).

Faulcurium *Faulding, Port.*
Atracurium besilate (p.1333·1).
Competitive neuromuscular blocker.

Fauldetic *Faulding, Port.*
Dacarbazine (p.531·2).

Fauldexato *Faulding, Port.*
Methotrexate (p.553·2).

Fauldoxo *Faulding, Port.*
Doxorubicin hydrochloride (p.534·3).

Faulplatin *Faulding, Port.*
Cisplatin (p.525·1).

Faulviral *Faulding, Port.*
Aciclovir (p.612·3).

Faustan *Dresden, Ger.; Temmler, Ger.*
Diazepam (p.674·3).
Anxiety disorders; premedication; skeletal muscle spasm; sleep disorders; status epilepticus.

Fave di Fuca *Arnold, Ital.*
Bladderwrack (p.1585·2); cascara (p.1216·1); frangula (p.1227·1).
Constipation.

Faverin
Arrow, Austral.; Solvay, Hong Kong; Solvay, Irl.; Solvay, Singapore; Solvay, Thai.; Solvay, UK.
Fluvoxamine maleate (p.289·3).
Depression; obsessive-compulsive disorder.

Favistan
Biochemie, Aust.; Temmler, Ger.
Metimazole [thiamazole] (p.1525·1).
Hyperthyroidism.

Favorex *TAD, Ger.*
Sotalol hydrochloride (p.972·2).
Arrhythmias.

Favoxil *Agis, Israel.*
Fluvoxamine maleate (p.289·3).
Depression; obsessive-compulsive disorder.

Fawodin *Wayne, Mex.*
Famotidine (p.1225·3).

Fazol *Rhone-Poulenc Rorer, Fr.*
Isoconazole nitrate (p.387·2).
Fungal skin infections.

Fazol G *Rhone-Poulenc Rorer, Fr.*
Isoconazole nitrate (p.387·2).
Vaginal candidiasis.

Fazolin *Siam Bheasach, Thai.*
Cefazolin (p.164·3).
Bacterial infections.

Fazoplex *Inkeysa, Spain.*
Cefazolin sodium (p.164·3).
Bacterial infections.

FBC *Ranbaxy, Thai.*
Ferrous fumarate (p.1360·1); vitamins; calcim phosphate (p.1350·1).
Anaemias.

Fe^{50} *UCB, USA.*
Dried ferrous sulfate (p.1360·3).
Iron-deficiency anaemia.

Febichol *Medphano, Ger.*
Fenipentol (p.1610·1).
Biliary disorders.

Febracyl *Vifor, Switz.*
Propyphenazone (p.80·2); paracetamol (p.71·2).
Fever; pain.

Febralgin *Boehringer de Angeli, Braz.*
Dipyrone (p.34·1).
Fever; pain.

Febranine *Roche Nicholas, Spain.*
Paracetamol (p.71·2).
Fever; pain.

Febrax *Syntex, Mex.*
Naproxen sodium (p.61·1); paracetamol (p.71·2).
Fever; pain.

Febrectal
Note.This name is used for preparations of different composition.
Almirall, Spain.
Paracetamol (p.71·2).
Formerly known as Febrectal Simple.
Fever; pain.

Funk, Spain†.
Mucopolysaccharidases; paracetamol (p.71·2); oleum pini sylvestris.
Fever; pain.

Febrectol *Irex, Fr.*
Adult suppositories: Paracetamol (p.71·2); pine needle oil.
Dispersible tablets; tablets: Paracetamol (p.71·2).
Paediatric and infant suppositories: Paracetamol (p.71·2); pine needle oil.
Formerly contained paracetamol, pine needle oil, and phenobarbital.
Fever; pain.

Febricol
Xepa-Soul Pattinson, Hong Kong; Xepa-Soul Pattinson, Singapore.
Chlorpheniramine [chlorphenamine] maleate (p.412·1); paracetamol (p.71·2); phenylpropanolamine hydrochloride (p.1098·1).
Cold symptoms.

Febridol *Genpharm, Austral.*
Paracetamol (p.71·2).
Fever; pain.

Febrim *Rimsa, Mex.*
Paracetamol (p.71·2).
Fever; pain.

Febrinal *Singer, Switz.*
Paracetamol (p.71·2); dextromethorphan hydrobromide (p.1087·3); phenylephrine hydrochloride (p.1097·1).
Cold and influenza symptoms.

Febro-cyl Ho-Len-Complex *Liebermann, Ger.*
Homoeopathic preparation.

Febronyl *Rhone-Poulenc Rorer, Mex.*
Paracetamol (p.71·2).
Fever; pain.

Febs *Boots, Singapore.*
Paracetamol (p.71·2); ascorbic acid (p.1389·3); caffeine (p.761·3); phenylephrine hydrochloride (p.1097·1).
Cold and influenza symptoms; fever; pain; sinus congestion.

Febupen *EMS, Braz.*
Oxyphenbutazone (p.71·1); paracetamol (p.71·2).
Fever; inflammation; pain.

Fecol *Nakornpatana, Thai.*
Syrup: Paracetamol (p.71·2); salicylamide (p.82·1); chlorpheniramine [chlorphenamine] maleate (p.412·1); phenylephrine hydrochloride (p.1097·1).
Tablets: Paracetamol (p.71·2); chlorpheniramine [chlorphenamine] maleate (p.412·1); phenylephrine hydrochloride (p.1097·1).
Cold symptoms; nasal congestion.

Fectri *Parggon, Mex.*
Co-trimoxazole (p.193·3).
Bacterial infections.

Fectrim *DDSA Pharmaceuticals, UK.*
Co-trimoxazole (p.193·3).

Fedac
DHA, Hong Kong; DHA, Singapore.
Pseudoephedrine hydrochloride (p.1099·2); triprolidine hydrochloride (p.427·2).
Allergic rhinitis; cold symptoms; sinusitis; upper respiratory-tract congestion.

Fedac Compound
DHA, Hong Kong; DHA, Singapore.
Codeine phosphate (p.25·2); pseudoephedrine hydrochloride (p.1099·2); triprolidine hydrochloride (p.427·2).
Coughs; nasal congestion.

Fedahist *Schwarz, USA.*
Pseudoephedrine hydrochloride (p.1099·2); chlorpheniramine [chlorphenamine] maleate (p.412·1).
Cold symptoms; fever; other upper respiratory tract allergies; sinusitis.

Fedahist Expectorant *Schwarz, USA†.*
Guaifenesin (p.1092·2); pseudoephedrine hydrochloride (p.1099·2).
Coughs and cold symptoms.

Fedip
Gebro, Aust.; Gebro, Switz.†.
Nifedipine (p.940·1).
Angina pectoris; hypertension; Raynaud's syndrome.

Fedra *Schering, Ital.*
Gestodene (p.1479·1); ethinylestradiol (p.1476·2).
Combined oral contraceptive.

Feel Perfecte *L'Oreal, Canad.*
SPF 15: Octinoxate (p.1517·3).
Sunscreen.

Feen-A-Mint
Schering-Plough, Canad.; Schering-Plough, USA.
Bisacodyl (p.1212·2).
Formerly contained phenolphthalein.
Constipation.

Feen-a-mint Pills *Schering-Plough, USA†.*
Docusate sodium (p.1223·1); phenolphthalein
(p.1244·1).
Constipation.

Fefol
Pfizer, Austral.; Medeva, Irl.; Xixia, S.Afr.; ICN, Singapore; Celltech, UK.
Dried ferrous sulfate (p.1360·3); folic acid (p.1361·1).
Iron and folic acid deficiency in pregnancy.

Fefol Z *Medeva, UK†.*
Dried ferrous sulfate (p.1360·3); zinc sulfate
(p.1398·2); folic acid (p.1361·1).
Iron and folic acid deficiency in pregnancy.

Fefol-Vit *Xixia, S.Afr.*
Dried ferrous sulfate (p.1360·3); folic acid (p.1361·1);
vitamin B and C substances (p.1350·1).
Iron, folic acid, and vitamin deficiency in pregnancy.

FegaCoren *Vitorgan, Ger.*
Protein extracts from hepar, pancreas, thymus, lien,
cor, ren, aorta, gland. suprarenal., mucosa intest., amnion, testes, gland. thyreoidea, diencephalon.
Cardiovascular and liver disorders.

FegaCoren N *Vitorgan, Ger.*
Protein extracts from hepar, pancreas, thymus, lien,
cor, ren, aorta, gland. suprarenal., mucosa intest., amnion, testes, gland. thyreoidea, diencephalon; metenolone acetate; prednisolone acetate; liothyronine
hydrochloride; deslanoside; alpha-tocoferil acetate; cyanocobalamin; pyridoxine hydrochloride.
Cardiovascular and liver disorders.

Fegatex *Vifor, Switz.†.*
Vegetable extracts.
Digestive disorders.

Fegenor *Leurquin, Fr.*
Fenofibrate (p.889·1).
Hyperlipidaemias.

Feiba
Baxter, Belg.; Immuno, Braz.; Baxter, Canad.; Baxter, Denm.; Baxter, Fin.; Baxter, Fr.; Immuno, Ital.; Baxter, Swed.; Baxter, Switz.; Hyland Immuno, UK; Immuno, USA.
A factor VIII inhibitor bypassing fraction (p.734·3).
Haemorrhagic disorders.

Feiba S-TIM 4
Immuno, Aust.; Immuno, Fr.
A factor VIII inhibitor bypassing fraction (p.734·3).
Haemorrhagic disorders.

Feiba TIM 4
Immuno, Hong Kong; Immuno, Israel; Adcock-Ingram Critical Care, S.Afr.; Baxter, Spain.
A factor VIII inhibitor bypassing fraction (p.734·3).
Haemophilia.

Felbatol *Wallace, USA.*
Felbamate (p.349·1).
Epilepsy.

Felcam *Asian Pharm, Thai.*
Piroxicam (p.79·1).
Gout; musculoskeletal and joint disorders.

Felden
Pfizer, Aust.; Pfizer, Denm.; Pfizer, Fin.; Mack, Illert., Ger.; Pfizer, Ger.; Pfizer, Norw.; Pfizer, Swed.; Pfizer, Switz.
Piroxicam (p.79·1).
*Gout; inflammation; musculoskeletal, joint, peri-artic-
ular, and soft-tissue disorders; pain.*

Feldene
Pfizer, Austral.; Pfizer, Belg.; Pfizer, Braz.; Pfizer, Canad.; Pfizer, Fr.; Pfizer, Hong Kong; Pfizer, Irl.; Pfizer, Israel; Pfizer, Ital.; Pfizer, Mex.; Pfizer, Neth.; Pfizer, NZ; Pfizer, Port.; Pfizer, S.Afr.; Pfizer, Singapore; Nefax, Spain; Pfizer Consumer, Spain; Pfizer, Thai.; Pfizer, UK; Pfizer, USA.
Piroxicam (p.79·1).
*Gout; inflammation; musculoskeletal, joint, peri-artic-
ular, and soft-tissue disorders; pain.*

Feldexican *INQ, Braz.*
Piroxicam (p.79·1).
*Gout; musculoskeletal, joint, peri-articular, and soft-
tissue disorders; pain.*

Feldox *Farmion, Braz.*
Piroxicam (p.79·1).
*Gout; musculoskeletal, joint, peri-articular, and soft-
tissue disorders; pain.*

Felexin
Remedica, Hong Kong; Remedica, Singapore; Remedica, Thai.
Cefalexin (p.161·3).
Bacterial infections.

Feliberal *Silanes, Mex.*
Enalapril maleate (p.883·3).
*Angina pectoris; heart failure; hypertension; myocar-
dial infarction.*

Felicium
Stada, Aust.; Opus, UK.
Fluoxetine hydrochloride (p.284·2).
*Bulimia nervosa; depression; obsessive-compulsive
disorder.*

Felidon neu *Sanova, Aust.*
Absinthium (p.1571·1); achillea (p.1572·2); taraxacum
(p.1669·1).
Hepatobiliary disorders.

Felis
Biocur, Ger.; Ecosol, Switz.
Hypericum (p.290·2).
Anxiety; depression.

Felison *Bayer, Ital.*
Flurazepam monohydrochloride (p.685·3).
Insomnia.

Felix *Apotheke Heiligen Josef, Aust.*
Hamamelis (p.1618·3); panthenol (p.1602·3); zinc ox-
ide (p.1128·2).
Haemorrhoids; pruritus ani.

Felixene *Wasserman, Spain.*
Ciprofloxacin hydrochloride (p.182·3).
Bacterial infections.

Feller *Makros, Braz.*
Mebendazole (p.102·2).
Worm infections.

Fellesan
Recip, Fin.; Recip, Swed.†.
Cholic acid; dehydrocholic acid (p.1602·2).
Biliary-tract disorders; gallstones.

Felnan *EMS, Braz.*
Piroxicam (p.79·1).
*Gout; musculoskeletal, joint, peri-articular, and soft-
tissue disorders; pain.*

Feloday *Novartis, Ital.*
Felodipine (p.888·3).
Angina pectoris; hypertension.

Felodur *PMC, Austral.*
Felodipine (p.888·3).
Hypertension.

Felrox *Seng, Thai.*
Piroxicam (p.79·1).
*Gout; musculoskeletal, joint, peri-articular, and soft-
tissue disorders.*

Felsol Neo *Roland, Ger.*
Phenazone (p.77·2); nikethamide calcium thiocyanate
(p.1513·1); ephedrine hydrochloride (p.1090·1).
Asthma; bronchitis; dyspnoea; emphysema; silicosis.

Fem-I *BDI, USA.*
Paracetamol (p.71·2); pamabrom (p.952·1).
Pain.

Fem 7
Merck, Ger.; Merck, Mex.; Merck, Neth.; Merck, Singapore.
Estradiol (p.1473·1).
Menopausal disorders; osteoporosis.

Femafen *Nicholas, UK†.*
Ibuprofen (p.43·2).

Femanest
Durascan, Denm.; Tika, Swed.
Estradiol (p.1473·1).
Menopausal disorders; osteoporosis.

Femanor
Durascan, Denm.; Tika, Swed.
Estradiol (p.1473·1); norethisterone acetate (p.1485·1).
Menopausal disorders; osteoporosis.

Femapak *Solvay, UK.*
Combination pack: Patches, estradiol (p.1473·1) (Fematrix); tablets, dydrogesterone (p.1472·3) (Duphaston).
Menopausal disorders; osteoporosis.

Femapirin *Chefaro, Neth.†.*
Ibuprofen (p.43·2).
Dysmenorrhoea.

Femaplus spezial Dr Hagedorn *Naturarzneimittel,
Ger.*
Homoeopathic preparation.

Femaprin *Chefaro, Spain.*
Ibuprofen (p.43·2).
*Fever; musculoskeletal, joint, and peri-articular disor-
ders; pain.*

Femar
Novartis, Denm.; Novartis, Fin.; Novartis, Norw.; Novartis, Swed.
Letrozole (p.550·1).
Breast cancer.

Femara
*Novartis, Aust.; Novartis, Austral.; Novartis, Belg.; Novartis, Canad.; Novartis, Fin.; Novartis, Ger.; Novartis, Hong Kong; Novartis, Irl.; No-
vartis, Israel; Novartis, Ital.; Novartis, Neth.; Novartis, NZ; Novartis, Port.; Novartis, S.Afr.; Novartis, Singapore; Novartis, Spain; Novartis, Switz.; Novartis, Thai.; Novartis, UK; Novartis, USA.*
Letrozole (p.550·1).
Breast cancer.

Femasekvens
Durascan, Denm.; Tika, Swed.
16 Tablets, estradiol (p.1473·1); 12 tablets, estradiol;
norethisterone acetate (p.1485·1).
Menopausal disorders; osteoporosis.

Fematab *Solvay, Irl.*
Estradiol (p.1473·1).
Menopausal disorders.

Fematrix
Solvay, Irl.; Solvay, UK.
Estradiol (p.1473·1).
Menopausal disorders; osteoporosis.

Femavit *Pharmacia Upjohn, Ger.*
21 Tablets, conjugated oestrogens (p.1467·1); 7 tablets,
inert.
Menopausal disorders; osteoporosis.

FemCal *Freeda, USA.*
Calcium carbonate (p.1215·1); colecalciferol
(p.1391·1); vitamin B; minerals (p.1350·1).

Femcet *Russ, USA†.*
Paracetamol (p.71·2); caffeine (p.761·3); butalbital
(p.658·3).
Pain.

Femease *Robinson, UK.*
Self-heating adhesive pad.
Dysmenorrhoea.

Femepen *Nycomed, Norw.*
Phenoxymethylpenicillin potassium (p.235·1).
Bacterial infections.

Femerital *Asta Medica, Neth.†.*
Ambucetamide (p.1578·3); paracetamol (p.71·2); caf-
feine hydrate (p.761·3).
Dysmenorrhoea.

Femeron *Johnson & Johnson MSD Consumer, UK†.*
Miconazole nitrate (p.391·1).
Vaginal candidiasis.

Fem-Etts *Roberts, USA†.*
Paracetamol (p.71·2); pamabrom (p.952·1).
Pain.

Femex *Roche, Neth.*
Naproxen sodium (p.61·1).
*Fever; inflammation; musculoskeletal and joint disor-
ders; pain.*

femhrt *Parke, Davis, USA.*
Ethinylestradiol (p.1476·2); norethisterone acetate
(p.1485·1).
Menopausal disorders; osteoporosis.

Femicine *Lake, USA†.*
Pulsatilla; mercurius vivus; sulfur.
Vaginal irritation.

Femicur N *Schaper & Brummer, Ger.*
Agnus castus (p.1574·2).
Mastalgia; menstrual disorders.

Femi-cyl Ho-Len-Complex *Liebermann, Ger.*
Homoeopathic preparation.

Femidine *AVP, UK.*
Povidone-iodine (p.1155·1).
Vaginal disorders.

Femidol *Merck, Spain.*
Ibuprofen (p.43·2).
Fever; pain.

Femigel *Scientific, S.Afr.*
Estradiol (p.1473·1).
Menopausal disorders.

Femigoa *Wyeth, Ger.; Lederle, Ger.*
Levonorgestrel (p.1486·2); ethinylestradiol (p.1476·2).
Combined oral contraceptive.

Femikliman uno *Biocur, Ger.*
Cimicifuga (p.1595·2).
Menopausal disorders.

Femilar *Schering, Fin.*
Cyproterone acetate (p.1467·3); estradiol valerate
(p.1473·2).
Biphasic oral contraceptive.

Femilax *G & W, USA†.*
Docusate sodium (p.1223·1); phenolphthalein
(p.1244·1).
Constipation.

Femilla N *Steigerwald, Ger.*
Cimicifuga (p.1595·2).
Dysmenorrhoea.

Feminalin *Farma Lepori, Spain.*
Ibuprofen (p.43·2).
Fever; pain.

Feminax
Roche Consumer, Irl.; Roche Consumer, UK.
Paracetamol (p.71·2); codeine phosphate (p.25·2); caf-
feine (p.761·3); hyoscine hydrobromide (p.468·2).
Dysmenorrhoea.

Femin-Do *Grasler, Ger.*
Homoeopathic preparation.

Feminease *Parnell, USA.*
Vaginal moisturising and lubricating cream with eriodictyon (p.1091·2).

Feminesse *Anglian, UK.*
Sorbic acid; glycerol; liquid paraffin; polycarbophil.
Vaginal odour.

Feminex *Sante Naturelle, Canad.*
Multivitamin and mineral preparation (p.1350·1).

Feminine Herbal Complex *GNLD, Austral.*
Wild yam root; red sage (p.1660·2); hypericum
(p.290·2); vitex agnus castus (p.1574·2); alchemilla
vulgaris (p.1648·3); angelica sinensis; skullcap
(p.1664·3); ginger (p.1227·2); taraxacum (p.1669·1);
liquorice (p.1231·2).
Menstrual disorders.

Feminique
Note. This name is used for preparations of different composition.
QHP, USA.
Sodium benzoate (p.1134·3); sorbic acid (p.1157·1);
lactic acid (p.1626·2); octoxinol 9 (p.1346·3).
Vaginal disorders.

QHP, USA.
Vinegar (p.1571·2).
Vaginal disorders.

Feminique with Iron and Calcium *Stanley, Canad.†.*
Multivitamin preparation with calcium and iron
(p.1350·1).

Feminon A *Cesra, Ger.*
Agnus castus (p.1574·2).
Mastalgia; menstrual disorders.

Feminon C *Cesra, Ger.*
Cimicifuga (p.1595·2).

Feminon N *Cesra, Ger.*
Homoeopathic preparation.

Feminova *Merck-Belgolabo, Belg.*
Estradiol (p.1473·1).
Menopausal disorders; osteoporosis.

Femiplexe *Lehning, Fr.†.*
Copper gluconate (p.1357·3); zinc gluconate
(p.1398·2).
Menopausal disorders; menstrual disorders.

Femipres *Schwarz, Ital.*
Moexipril hydrochloride (p.935·3).
Hypertension.

Femipres Plus *Schwarz, Ital.*
Moexipril hydrochloride (p.935·3); hydrochlorothi-
azide (p.907·3).
Hypertension.

Femiron *Menley & James, USA.*
Ferrous fumarate (p.1360·1).
Iron-deficiency anaemias.

Femiron Multi-Vitamins and Iron *Menley & James,
USA.*
Multivitamin preparation with iron and folic acid
(p.1350·1).

Femisana *Hotz, Ger.*
Agnus castus (p.1574·2); greater celandine (p.1618·3);
cimicifuga (p.1595·2); phosphorus.
Gynaecological disorders.

Femisana H *Hotz, Ger.*
Homoeopathic preparation.

Femit *Mitim, Ital.*
Ferritin (p.1359·3).
Iron deficiency; iron-deficiency anaemias.

Femizol-M *Lake, USA.*
Miconazole nitrate (p.391·1).
Fungal vaginal infections.

Fem-Mono
Generics, Denm.; Scand Pharm, Swed.
Isosorbide mononitrate (p.916·2).
Angina pectoris.

Femodeen *Schering, Neth.*
Ethinylestradiol (p.1476·2); gestodene (p.1479·1).
Combined oral contraceptive.

Femoden *Schering, Fin.*
Ethinylestradiol (p.1476·2); gestodene (p.1479·1).
Combined oral contraceptive.

Femoden ED *Schering, Austral.*
21 Tablets, ethinylestradiol (p.1476·2); gestodene
(p.1479·1); 7 tablets, inert.
Combined oral contraceptive.

Femodene
*Schering, Belg.; Schering, Irl.; Schering, NZ; Schering, S.Afr.; Schering,
UK.*
Ethinylestradiol (p.1476·2); gestodene (p.1479·1).
28-Day packs also contain 7 inert tablets.
Combined oral contraceptive.

Femodette *Schering, UK.*
Ethinylestradiol (p.1476·2); gestodene (p.1479·1).
Combined oral contraceptive.

Femogex *Germiphene, Canad.†.*
Estradiol valerate (p.1473·2).
Oestrogenic.

Femoston
*Solvay, Aust.; Solvay, Austral.; Solvay, Belg.; Solvay, Fin.; Solvay, Ger.;
Solvay, Hong Kong; Solvay, Irl.; Solvay, Ital.; Solvay, Neth.; Solvay,
Port.; Solvay, Singapore; Solvay, Switz.; Solvay, UK.*
14 Tablets, estradiol (p.1473·1); 14 tablets, estradiol;
dydrogesterone (p.1472·3).
Menopausal disorders; osteoporosis.

Femoston Conti
Solvay, Irl.; Solvay, Switz.; Solvay, UK.
Estradiol (p.1473·1); dydrogesterone (p.1472·3).
Menopausal disorders; osteoporosis.

Femoston mono *Solvay, Ger.*
Estradiol (p.1473·1).
Menopausal disorders; osteoporosis.

Femovan *Schering, Ger.*
Ethinylestradiol (p.1476·2); gestodene (p.1479·1).
Combined oral contraceptive.

FemPatch *Parke, Davis, USA.*
Estradiol (p.1473·1).
Menopausal disorders; oestrogen deficiency.

Femplan-MA *Antigen, Irl.*
Estradiol (p.1473·1); medroxyprogesterone acetate
(p.1480·1).
Menopausal disorders; osteoporosis.

Fempress
Isis, Ger.; Schwarz, Switz.
Moexipril hydrochloride (p.935·3).
Hypertension.

Fempress Plus *Isis, Ger.*
Moexipril hydrochloride (p.935·3); hydrochlorothi-
azide (p.907·3).
Hypertension.

Femranette mikro *LAW, Ger.*
Ethinylestradiol (p.1476·2); levonorgestrel (p.1486·2).
Combined oral contraceptive.

Femsept *Lipha Sante, Fr.*
Estradiol (p.1473·1).
Menopausal disorders.

FemSeven
Merck, Aust.; Merck, Denm.; Merck, Fin.; Bracco, Ital.; Merck, Swed.; Merck, Switz.; E. Merck, UK.
Estradiol (p.1473·1).
Menopausal disorders; osteoporosis.

Femstal *Syntex, Mex.*
Butoconazole nitrate (p.381·2).
Vulvovaginal candidiasis.

Femstat *Bayer Consumer, USA.*
Butoconazole nitrate (p.381·2).
Vulvovaginal candidiasis.

Femtran
3M, Austral.; 3M, NZ.
Estradiol (p.1473·1).
Menopausal disorders; osteoporosis.

Femulen
Searle, Austral.; Searle, NZ; Searle, S.Afr.†; Pharmacia, UK.
Etynodiol diacetate (p.1477·1).
Progestogen-only oral contraceptive.

Fenac
Alphapharm, Austral.; LBS, Thai.
Diclofenac diethylamine (p.30·2) or diclofenac sodium (p.30·3).
Inflammation; musculoskeletal, joint, peri-articular, and soft-tissue disorders.

Fenadol *Proge, Ital.*
Diclofenac sodium (p.30·3).
Inflammation; musculoskeletal and joint disorders; pain.

Fenaflan *Teuto, Braz.*
Diclofenac (p.30·2).
Gout; inflammation; musculoskeletal, joint, and peri-articular disorders; pain.

Fenalgin *Geminis, Spain†.*
Caffeine (p.761·3); paracetamol (p.71·2); propyphenazone (p.80·2).
Pain.

Fenam *Solvay, Ital.†.*
Isoxsuprine resinate (polistirex) (p.1625·1).
Cerebrovascular disorders.

Fenamic *Siam Bheasach, Thai.*
Mefenamic acid (p.51·2).
Pain.

Fenamide *Farmigea, Ital.*
Diclofenamide (p.869·1).
Glaucoma.

Fenamin *Aspen, S.Afr.*
Mefenamic acid (p.51·2).
Dysmenorrhoea; musculoskeletal, joint, and soft-tissue disorders.

Fenamine *Fawns & McAllan, Austral.*
Pheniramine maleate (p.422·3).
Hypersensitivity reactions; motion sickness; vestibular disorders.

Fenamon
Medochemie, Singapore; Medochemie, Thai.
Nifedipine (p.940·1).
Angina pectoris; hypertension.

Fenantoin *NM, Swed.*
Phenytoin (p.357·2).
Epilepsy.

Fenaren
Mundipharma, Aust.; Uniao Quimica, Braz.
Diclofenac diethylamine (p.30·2) or diclofenac sodium (p.30·3).
Gout; inflammation; musculoskeletal, joint, and peri-articular disorders; pain; renal and biliary colic.

Fenasil *Sintofarma, Braz.*
Terfenadine (p.424·3).
Hypersensitivity reactions.

Fenason *Unison, Thai.*
Terfenadine (p.424·3).
Hypersensitivity reactions.

Fenasten *Sintofarma, Braz.*
Cinasteride.
Malignant neoplasms.

Fenazil *Sella, Ital.*
Promethazine hydrochloride (p.423·2).
Hypersensitivity reactions.

Fenazol *Hokuriku, Jpn†.*
Ufenamate (p.90·2).
Skin disorders.

Fenbid *Goldshield, UK.*
Ibuprofen (p.43·2).
Inflammation; pain.

Fenburil *De Mayo, Braz.*
Diclofenac (p.30·2).
Gout; inflammation; musculoskeletal, joint, and peri-articular disorders; pain.

Fenchelsaft N *Chauvin ankerpharm, Ger.*
Fennel oil (p.1610·2).
Catarrh.

Fendazol *Lepori, Port.†.*
Ditazole (p.880·1).
Thromboembolic disorders.

Fendin *Ranbaxy, S.Afr.*
Terfenadine (p.424·3).
Hypersensitivity reactions.

Fenemal
Nycomed, Denm.; Nycomed, Norw.; NM, Swed.
Phenobarbital (p.355·1).
Epilepsy; pre-eclampsia; withdrawal syndromes.

Fenergan
Rhodia, Braz.; Vitoria, Port.
Promethazine hydrochloride (p.423·2).
Adjunct to analgesia and anaesthesia; hypersensitivity reactions; insomnia; nausea and vomiting; sedative.

Fenergan Creme *Rhodia, Braz.*
Promethazine (p.423·2).
Cutaneous hypersensitivity reactions.

Fenergan Expectorante
Rhodia, Braz.; Rhone-Poulenc Rorer, Spain.
Promethazine hydrochloride (p.423·2); sulfogaiacol (p.1101·1); ipecacuanha (p.1093·1).
Upper-respiratory-tract disorders.

Fenergan Topico *Rhone-Poulenc Rorer, Spain.*
Promethazine (p.423·2).
Cutaneous hypersensitivity reactions.

Fenesin *DJ, USA.*
Guaifenesin (p.1092·2).
Coughs.

Fenesin DM *Dura, USA.*
Dextromethorphan hydrobromide (p.1087·3); guaifenesin (p.1092·2).
Coughs.

Fenfedrin *Xepa-Soul Pattinson, Hong Kong.*
Chlorpheniramine [chlorphenamine] maleate (p.412·1); pseudoephedrine hydrochloride (p.1099·2).
Allergic rhinitis; nasal congestion.

Fengam *Pharmasant, Thai.*
Tiaprofenic acid (p.88·1).
Gout; inflammation; musculoskeletal, joint, and soft-tissue disorders; pain.

Feniben *Zerboni, Mex.*
Phenylbutazone (p.78·1).

Fenicol
Rolab, S.Afr.; Pharmasant, Thai.
Chloramphenicol! (p.179·1).
Bacterial infections.

Fenidantoin S *Byk Gulden, Mex.*
Phenytoin sodium (p.357·2).
Epilepsy.

Fenidex *Allergan-Frumtost, Braz.*
Dexamethasone (p.1067·1); chloramphenicol (p.179·1).
Infected eye disorders.

Fenidina *Boniscontro & Gazzone, Ital.*
Nifedipine (p.940·1).
Angina pectoris; hypertension.

Feniken *Kener, Mex.*
Nifedipine (p.940·1).

Fenil-Livre *Mead Johnson, Port.*
Preparation for enteral nutrition (p.1350·1).
Phenylketonuria.

Fenil-V *Vitoria, Port.*
Diclofenac sodium (p.30·3).
Musculoskeletal, joint, and soft-tissue disorders; neuralgia; neuritis.

Fenint *Pharmacia Upjohn, Ger.*
Thioctic acid (p.1671·3).
Diabetic polyneuropathy.

Fenipencil *Marcel, Mex.*
Ampicillin (p.150·3).
Bacterial infections.

Fenisal *Sofar, Ital.*
Nimesulide (p.62·3).
Inflammation; musculoskeletal and joint disorders; pain.

Fenisec *Hoechst Marion Roussel, Mex.*
Fenproporex (p.1510·2).

Fenisol *Reuffer, Mex.*
Chloramphenicol (p.179·1).
Bacterial infections.

Fenistil
Note.This name is used for preparations of different composition.
Novartis Consumer, Aust.; Novartis Consumer, Belg.; Novartis, Israel; Zyma, Ital.; Novartis Consumer, Neth.; Novartis, Norw.; Novartis Consumer, Port.; Novartis Consumer, Spain; Novartis Consumer, Switz.; Novartis, Thai.
Dimetindene maleate (p.415·3).
Hypersensitivity reactions; pruritic skin disorders.

Novartis Consumer, Ger.
Capsules; tablets; injection; syrup; oral drops; topical gel: Dimetindene maleate (p.415·3).
Hypersensitivity reactions; pruritic skin disorders.
Cream: Tripelennamine hydrochloride (p.427·1).
Pruritic skin disorders.
Ointment: Hydrocortisone acetate (p.1073·3).
Skin disorders.

Fenitron *Psicofarma, Mex.*
Phenytoin sodium (p.357·2).
Epilepsy.

Fenizolan
Grunenthal, Aust.; Nourypharma, Ger.
Fenticonazole nitrate (p.383·2).
Genital candidiasis; vulvovaginal Gram-positive bacterial infections.

Fenizzard *Pizzard, Mex.*
Chloramphenicol (p.179·1).
Bacterial eye infections.

Fennings Children's Powders *Anglian, UK.*
Paracetamol (p.71·2).
Fever; pain.

Fennings Little Healers *Anglian, UK.*
Ipecacuanha (p.1093·1).
Coughs.

Fenobeta *Betapharm, Ger.*
Fenofibrate (p.889·1).
Hyperlipidaemias.

Fenocris *Cristalia, Braz.*
Phenobarbital (p.355·1).
Anxiety; epilepsy; hyperbilirubinaemia; insomnia; premedication; sedation.

Fenocriz *Fustery, Mex.*
Phenobarbital (p.355·1).

Fenogal *SMB, Belg.*
Fenofibrate (p.889·1).
Hyperlipidaemias.

Fenogel *Basi, Port.*
Etofenamate (p.35·3).

Fenoket *Opus, UK.*
Ketoprofen (p.47·3).
Gout; musculoskeletal, joint, and peri-articular disorders; pain.

Fenolip
Note.This name is used for preparations of different composition.
Lannacher, Aust.
Fenofibrate (p.889·1).
Hyperlipidaemias.

Lepori, Port.
Sodium cromoglicate (p.774·3).
Allergic rhinitis; conjunctivitis.

Fenomel *Clonmel, Irl.*
Flurbiprofen (p.41·2).
Musculoskeletal and joint disorders.

Fenopron
Lilly, Hong Kong; Dista, Irl.; Quatromed, S.Afr.; Novex Pharma, UK.
Fenoprofen calcium (p.36·3).
Fever; gout; musculoskeletal and joint disorders; pain.

Fenoptic *Allergan, Port.*
Chloramphenicol (p.179·1).
Bacterial eye infections.

Fenospen *Pharmacia Upjohn, Ital.*
Phenoxymethylpenicillin (p.235·1).
Bacterial infections.

Fenotricin *Dinafarma, Braz.*
Cetylpyridinium chloride (p.1138·1); benzocaine (p.1306·2).
Mouth and throat disorders.

Fenox
Note.This name is used for preparations of different composition.
Boots Healthcare, Irl.†; Boots, S.Afr.†.
Nasal drops: Phenylephrine hydrochloride (p.1097·1); naphazoline nitrate (p.1095·1).
Nasal congestion; sinusitis.

Boots, S.Afr.†; SSL, UK.
Nasal spray: Phenylephrine hydrochloride (p.1097·1).
Nasal congestion; sinusitis.

Fenoxcillin *Novo Nordisk, Denm.†.*
Phenoxymethylpenicillin potassium (p.235·1).
Bacterial infections.

Fenoxypen *Novo Nordisk, Switz.†.*
Phenoxymethylpenicillin potassium (p.235·1).
Bacterial infections.

Fensaid *Amrad, Austral.†.*
Piroxicam (p.79·1).
Ankylosing spondylitis; osteoarthritis; rheumatoid arthritis.

Fensel *Pharmacia Upjohn, Spain.*
Felodipine (p.888·3).
Angina pectoris; hypertension.

Fensol *Rolab, S.Afr.†.*
Fenoterol hydrobromide (p.765·1).
Obstructive airways disease.

Fenspin *Basi, Port.*
Fenspiride hydrochloride (p.765·3).

Fenspir *Ibirn, Ital.*
Fenspiride hydrochloride (p.765·3).
Respiratory-tract disorders.

Fensum *Merckle, Ger.*
Paracetamol (p.71·2).
Fever; pain.

Fentalim *Angelini, Ital.*
Alfentanil hydrochloride (p.11·3).
General anaesthesia; neuroleptanalgesia.

Fentamox *Opus, UK†.*
Tamoxifen citrate (p.571·1).
Anovulatory infertility; breast cancer.

Fentanest
Pharmacia Upjohn, Ital.; Janssen, Mex.; Roche, Spain.
Fentanyl (p.37·1) or fentanyl citrate (p.37·1).
Analgesia during anaesthesia; premedication.

Fentatienil *Angelini, Ital.*
Sufentanil citrate (p.84·3).
General anaesthesia; neuroleptanalgesia.

Fentazin
Goldshield, Irl.†; Forley, UK.
Perphenazine (p.699·1).
Anxiety; nausea; psychoses; vomiting.

Fentiderm *Zyma, Ital.*
Fenticonazole nitrate (p.383·2).
Fungal skin and anogenital infections.

Fentigyn *Novartis, Ital.*
Fenticonazole nitrate (p.383·2).
Fungal vulvovaginal infections.

Fentrinol *Fresenius Kabi, Aust.*
Amidefrine mesilate (p.1085·1).
Rhinitis.

Fenugrene *Aerocid, Fr.*
Fenugreek (p.1610·3).
Appetite stimulant.

Fenulin *Gerard House, UK.*
Fenugreek (p.1610·3); slippery elm (p.1665·1); hydrastis (p.1621·1).
Gastrointestinal disorders.

Fenuril
Pharmacia Upjohn, Fin.; Pharmacia Upjohn, Swed.
Urea (p.1127·3).
Dry skin.

Fenuril-Hydrokortison *Pharmacia Upjohn, Swed.*
Urea (p.1127·3); hydrocortisone (p.1073·3).
Eczema.

Fenwal ACD *Baxter, Denm.†.*
Citric acid monohydrate (p.1596·2); anhydrous glucose (p.1364·1); sodium citrate (p.1186·2).
Anticoagulant for blood transfusions.

Feocyte *Dunhall, USA.*
Iron (p.1366·3); liver extracts; folic acid (p.1361·1); vitamin B substances (p.1350·1); copper.
Vitamin C (p.1389·3) is included in this preparation to increase the absorption and availability of iron.
Iron-deficiency anaemias.

Feosol *SmithKline Beecham Consumer, USA.*
Ferrous sulfate (as dried or hydrate) (p.1360·3).
Iron deficiency; iron-deficiency anaemia.

Feospan
ICN, Hong Kong; Medeva, Irl.; Celltech, UK.
Dried ferrous sulfate (p.1360·3).
Iron deficiency; iron-deficiency anaemia.

Feostat *Forest Pharmaceuticals, USA.*
Ferrous fumarate (p.1360·1).
Iron-deficiency anaemia.

Feparil *Madaus, Spain.*
Tablets: Aescin (p.1574·1).
Oedema; peripheral vascular disorders.
Topical gel: Diethylamine salicylate (p.32·2); aescin (p.1574·1); sodium aescin polysulfate (p.1574·1).
Peripheral vascular disorders.

Feprapax *Ashbourne, UK.*
Lofepramine hydrochloride (p.297·1).
Depression.

Fepron
Lilly, Ital.; Lilly, Neth.†.
Fenoprofen calcium (p.36·3).
Inflammation; musculoskeletal, joint, and peri-articular disorders.

Fer UCB *UCB, Fr.*
Ferrous chloride (p.1359·3).
Anaemias.

Feraken *Kendrick, Mex.*
Moclobemide (p.299·3).
Depression.

Ferancee *J&J-Merck, USA†.*
Ferrous fumarate (p.1360·1).
Ascorbic acid (p.1389·3) is included in this preparation to increase the absorption and availability of iron.
Iron-deficiency anaemias.

Feraplex *Lambda, UK†.*
Vitamin B substance and iron (p.1350·1).

Feratab *Upsher-Smith, USA.*
Ferrous sulfate (p.1360·3).
Iron-deficiency anaemias.

Fercayl *Pharmacobel, Belg.*
Iron dextran (p.1368·2).
Iron-deficiency anaemia.

Ferdek *Ranbaxy, Thai.*
Ferrous fumarate (p.1360·1).
Iron-deficiency anaemia.

Ferfolic SV *Durbin, UK.*
Ferrous gluconate (p.1360·1); folic acid (p.1361·1).
Iron and folic acid deficiency; neural tube defect prophylaxis.

Fer-gen-sol *Goldline, USA.*
Ferrous sulfate (p.1360·3).
Iron deficiency anaemia.

Fergon
Sanofi Synthelabo, Austral.; Sanofi Winthrop, Irl.; ICN, NZ; Winthrop Consumer, USA.
Ferrous gluconate (p.1360·1).
Iron deficiency; iron-deficiency anaemia.

Feridex *Advanced Magnetics, Israel; Eiken, Jpn; Berlex, USA.*
Ferumoxides (p.1032·3).
Contrast medium for magnetic resonance imaging of the liver.

Ferifer *Streger, Mex.*
Ferrous sulfate (p.1360·3).
Iron-deficiency anaemia.

Fer-In-Sol
Bristol-Myers Squibb, Braz.; Mead Johnson Nutritionals, Canad.; Mead Johnson, Hong Kong; Bristol-Myers Squibb, Irl.; Mead Johnson, Ital.; Mead Johnson, Mex.; Mead Johnson Nutritionals, Thai.; Mead Johnson Nutritionals, USA.
Ferrous sulfate (p.1360·3).
Iron-deficiency anaemias.

Fer-Iron *Rugby, USA.*
Ferrous sulfate (p.1360·3).
Iron-deficiency anaemias.

Ferlactis *AGIPS, Ital.*
Streptococcus lactis.
Gastrointestinal disorders.

Ferlasin Martin, Spain†.
Multivitamin, mineral, and amino-acid preparation (p.1350·1).
Tonic.

Ferlatum Lifepharma, Ital.
Iron succinyl-protein complex (p.1369·3).
Anaemias; iron deficiency.

Ferlis B12 Iodo Suma, Braz.
Ferrous citrate; copper; vitamin B substances (p.1350·1).
Iron deficiency; iron-deficiency anaemia.

Ferlixir Aspen, S.Afr.
Multivitamin and mineral preparation (p.1350·1).

Ferlixit Rhone-Poulenc Rorer, Ital.
Ferric sodium gluconate (p.1360·2).
Anaemias; iron deficiency.

Fermalac Rougier, Canad.
Lactobacillus acidophilus (p.1626·3); *Lactobacillus bulgaricus* (p.1626·3); *Streptococcus lactis.*
Diarrhoea.

Fermalac Vaginal Rougier, Canad.
Lactobacillus acidophilus (p.1626·3); *Lactobacillus bulgaricus* (p.1626·3); *Streptococcus lactis.*
Adjunct in treatment of vaginal infections.

Fermasian Asian Pharm, Thai.
Ferrous fumarate (p.1360·1).
Iron-deficiency anaemia.

Fermate Kenyaku, Thai.
Ferrous fumarate (p.1360·1).
Iron-deficiency anaemia.

Fermathron Biomet, Austral.; Biomet Merck, UK.
Sodium hyaluronate (p.1620·1).
Osteoarthritis of the knee.

Fermentmycin Intramed, S.Afr.
Gentamicin sulfate (p.210·1).
Bacterial infections.

Fermento duodenal Sanol, Ger.; Schwarz, Switz.
Pancreatin (p.1646·1); dimethicone (p.1249·2).
Digestive disorders.

Fermentol Carter Horner, Canad.
Pepsin (p.1649·3).
Dyspepsia without hyperacidity; oral vehicle.

Fermenturto-Lio Teknofarma, Ital.
Lactobacillus bulgaricus (p.1626·3); *Lactobacillus casei.*
Gastrointestinal disorders.

Fermetone Composto Lepori, Port.
Bile extract (p.1585·1); dimethicone (p.1249·2); hemicellulose (p.1500·2); pancreatin (p.1646·1).
Digestive disorders.

Fernadin Liferpal, Mex.
Ferrous fumarate (p.1360·1).

Fernore Knoll, Belg.
Ferrous gluconate (p.1360·1).
Iron-deficiency anaemia.

Ferocyl Hudson, USA†.
Ferrous fumarate (p.1360·1).
Docusate sodium (p.1223·1) is included in this preparation to reduce the constipating effects of iron.
Iron-deficiency anaemias.

Ferodan Odan, Canad.
Ferrous sulfate (p.1360·3).
Anaemias.

Fero-Folic
Abbott, S.Afr.; Abbott, Switz.; Abbott, USA.
Ferrous sulfate (p.1360·3); folic acid (p.1361·1).
Sodium ascorbate (p.1390·1) is included in this preparation to increase the absorption and availability of iron.
Folic acid deficiency; iron deficiency.

Feroglobin Vitabiotics, Hong Kong.
Iron, vitamin B, and mineral preparation (p.1350·1).
Anaemias.

Vitabiotics, UK.
Capsules: Vitamin B substances; folic acid; iron; copper; zinc (p.1350·1).
Oral liquid: Vitamin B substances; vitamin C; minerals; honey; malt; lysine (p.1350·1).

Fero-Grad
Abbott, Belg.; Abbott, Canad.; Abbott, S.Afr.; Abbott, USA.
Ferrous sulfate (p.1360·3).
Sodium ascorbate (p.1390·1) is included in this preparation to increase the absorption and availability of iron.
Iron deficiency; iron-deficiency anaemia.

Fero-Grad vitamine C Abbott, Fr.
Ferrous sulfate (p.1360·3).
Ascorbic acid (p.1389·3) is included in this preparation to increase the absorption and availability of iron.
Anaemias.

Fero-Gradumet
Abbott, Belg.; Abbott, Neth.; Abbott, Spain; Abbott, USA†.
Ferrous sulfate (p.1360·3).
Iron deficiency; iron-deficiency anaemia.

Feron Toray, Jpn.
Interferon beta (p.632·2).
Hepatitis; malignant neoplasms.

Ferosof Banner, Hong Kong.
Ferrous fumarate (p.1360·1).
Docusate sodium (p.1223·1) is included in this preparation to reduce the constipating effects of iron.
Iron-deficiency anaemia.

Ferospace Hudson, USA†.
Ferrous sulfate (p.1360·3).
Iron-deficiency anaemia.

Ferotrinsic Rugby, USA.
Ferrous fumarate (p.1360·1); folic acid (p.1361·1); intrinsic factor; vitamin B_{12} substances (p.1388·1).
Vitamin C (p.1389·3) is included in this preparation to increase the absorption and availability of iron.
Anaemias.

Ferplex Italfarmaco, Ital.; Italfarmaco, Spain.
Iron succinyl-protein complex (p.1369·3).
Iron-deficiency anaemia.

Ferplus-B Chew, Thai.
Ferrous fumarate (p.1360·1); vitamins; minerals (p.1350·1).
Iron-deficiency anaemia; vitamin deficiency.

Ferquifa B_{12} Merck, Port.†.
Ferrous citrate; copper sulfate; liver extract; folic acid; cyanocobalamin (p.1350·1).
Anaemias.

Ferralet Mission Pharmacal, USA†.
Ferrous gluconate (p.1360·1).
Iron-deficiency anaemia.

Ferralet Plus Mission Pharmacal, USA.
Ferrous gluconate (p.1360·1); folic acid (p.1361·1); vitamin B_{12} substances (p.1388·1).
Vitamin C (p.1389·3) is included in this preparation to increase the absorption and availability of iron.
Iron-deficiency anaemias.

Ferralyn Lannett, USA†.
Dried ferrous sulfate (p.1360·3).
Iron-deficiency anaemias.

Ferranina Byk Gulden, Mex.
Iron polymaltose (p.1369·2).
Iron deficiency; iron-deficiency anaemia.

Ferranina Fol Byk Gulden, Mex.
Iron polymaltose (p.1369·2); folic acid (p.1361·1).
Iron-deficiency anaemias.

Ferrascorbin Streuli, Switz.
Oral drops: Ferrous chloride (p.1359·3).
Ascorbic acid (p.1389·3) is included in this preparation to increase the absorption and availability of iron.
Tablets: Ferrous chloride (p.1359·3); ferrous gluconate (p.1360·1).
Ascorbic acid (p.1389·3) is included in this preparation to increase the absorption and availability of iron.
Iron deficiency; iron-deficiency anaemia.

Ferra-TD Goldline, USA†.
Dried ferrous sulfate (p.1360·3).
Iron-deficiency anaemias.

Ferrematos Boniscontro & Gazzone, Ital.†.
Ferrous gluconate (p.1360·1).
Iron deficiency; iron-deficiency anaemias.

Ferremon Medici, Ital.
Iron succinyl-protein complex (p.1369·3).
Anaemias; iron deficiency.

Ferretab
Lannacher, Aust.; Ridupharm, Switz.
Ferrous fumarate (p.1360·1).
Ascorbic acid (p.1389·3) may be included in this preparation to increase the absorption and availability of iron.
Iron-deficiency anaemia.

Ferretab comp Lannacher, Aust.
Ferrous fumarate (p.1360·1); sodium folate (p.1361·3).
Iron and folic acid deficiency.

Ferretts Pharmics, USA†.
Ferrous fumarate (p.1360·1).

Ferrex Breckenridge, USA.
Polysaccharide-iron complex (p.1374·3).
Iron-deficiency anaemia.

Ferrex Forte Breckenridge, USA.
Polysaccharide-iron complex (p.1374·3); folic acid (p.1361·1); cyanocobalamin (p.1388·1).
Iron-deficiency anaemia.

Ferrex PC Breckenridge, USA.
Multivitamin and mineral preparation with polysaccharide-iron complex (p.1374·3) (p.1350·1).
Nutritional supplement.

Ferricure Trenker, Belg.
Polysaccharide-iron complex (p.1374·3).
Iron-deficiency anaemia.

Ferri-Emina Lafare, Ital.
Ferric sodium gluconate (p.1360·2).
Anaemias; iron deficiency.

Ferrifol Sanico, Belg.
Ferrous succinate (p.1360·3); folic acid (p.1361·1).
Iron and folic acid deficiencies; megaloblastic anaemia.

Ferrifol-3 CTI, Israel.
Iron polymaltose (p.1369·2); folic acid (p.1361·1).
Anaemias.

Ferrifol B12 Sanico, Belg.
Ferric ammonium citrate (p.1359·2); folic acid (p.1361·1); vitamin B_{12} (p.1388·1).
Anaemias; growth disorders.

Ferrimed Byk Madaus, S.Afr.
Capsules: Iron polymaltose (p.1369·2); folic acid (p.1361·1).
Injection; syrup: Iron polymaltose (p.1369·2).
Iron-deficiency anaemias.

Ferrimed DS Byk Madaus, S.Afr.
Iron polymaltose (p.1369·2).
Iron-deficiency anaemias.

Ferrin Ativus, Braz.
Ferrous fumarate (p.1360·1) or ferrous gluconate (p.1360·1).
Iron deficiency; iron-deficiency anaemia.

Ferripel-3 CTI, Israel.
Iron polymaltose (p.1369·2).
Iron-deficiency anaemia.

Ferriprox Chiesi, Fr.; Chiesi, Ital.; Orphan, UK.
Deferiprone (p.1003·1).
Iron overload.

Ferriseltz
Bracco, Ital.; Rovi, Spain.
Ferric ammonium citrate (p.1359·2).
Contrast medium for magnetic resonance imaging.

Ferriseptil Gedis, Ital.
Glutaral (p.1145·2).
Disinfection.

Ferritamin Abigo, Swed.
Multivitamin preparation with iron and caffeine (p.1350·1).

Ferritin Complex ABC, Ital.
Ferric sodium gluconate (p.1360·2); calcium folinate (p.1363·3).
Anaemias.

Ferritin Oti ABC, Ital.
Ferric sodium gluconate (p.1360·2).
Anaemias; iron deficiency.

Ferrivenin Laevosan, Aust.†.
Iron sucrose (p.1370·1).
Hypochromic anaemias.

Ferrlecit
Rhone-Poulenc Rorer, Ger.; Rhone-Poulenc Rorer, Israel; Schein, USA.
Ferric sodium gluconate (p.1360·2).
Iron deficiency; iron-deficiency anaemias.

Ferrlecit 2 Nattermann, Ger.
Ferrous succinate (p.1360·3).
Iron deficiency; iron-deficiency anaemias.

Ferro
AstraZeneca, Denm.; Sam-On, Israel.
Ferrous gluconate (p.1360·1) or ferrous sulfate (p.1360·3).
Iron-deficiency anaemia.

Ferro-12 Wassen, Ital.
Ferrous fumarate (p.1360·1).
Vitamin C (p.1389·3) is included in this preparation to increase the absorption and availability of iron.
Iron supplement.

Ferro 66 Byk Gulden, Ger.†.
Ferrous chloride (p.1359·3).
Iron deficiency; iron-deficiency anaemias.

Ferro Complex Pharmafar, Ital.
Sodium feredetate (p.1375·3).
Anaemias.

Ferro Drops L Aspen, S.Afr.
Ferrous lactate (p.1360·2).
Iron-deficiency anaemias.

Ferro Folico Abbott, Mex.
Ferrous sulfate (p.1360·3); folic acid (p.1361·1).
Ascorbic acid (p.1389·3) is included in this preparation to increase the absorption and availability of iron.
Iron and folic acid deficiency.

Ferro sanol Sanol, Ger.
Ferrous glycine sulfate (p.1360·2).
Iron deficiency; iron-deficiency anaemia.

Ferro sanol comp Sanol, Ger.
Ferrous glycine sulfate (p.1360·3); folic acid (p.1361·1); cyanocobalamin (p.1388·1).
Iron and vitamin B deficiency; iron-deficiency anaemias.

Ferro sanol duodenal Sanol, Ger.; Schwarz, Ger.
Ferrous glycine sulfate (p.1360·2).
Iron deficiency; iron-deficiency anaemias.

Ferro sanol gyn Sanol, Ger.; Schwarz, Ger.
Ferrous glycine sulfate (p.1360·3); folic acid (p.1361·1).
Iron and folic acid deficiency.

Ferro Semar Sanofi Synthelabo, Spain.
Ferrous ascorbate (p.1359·3).
Iron-deficiency anaemia.

Ferro-Agepha Agepha, Aust.
Ferrous gluconate (p.1360·1).
Iron-deficiency anaemia.

Ferroben Teuto, Braz.
Oral solution: Ferric ammonium citrate (p.1359·2); vitamin B substances; copper sulfate (p.1350·1).
Tablets: Ferrous sulfate (p.1360·3); vitamin B substances (p.1350·1).
Iron deficiency; iron-deficiency anaemia.

Ferro-Be-Sian Asian Pharm, Thai.
Ferrous gluconate (p.1360·1); vitamins (p.1350·1).
Iron-deficiency anaemia.

Ferrobet Montavit, Aust.
Ferrous fumarate (p.1360·1).
Iron-deficiency anaemia.

Ferrocal Rekah, Israel.
Calcium ferrous citrate.
Iron-deficiency anaemia.

Ferrocap F Consolidated Chemicals, Irl.
Ferrous fumarate (p.1360·1); folic acid (p.1361·1).
Anaemia during pregnancy.

Ferro-C-Calcium Hotz, Ger.
Ferrous gluconate (p.1360·1); calcium gluconate (p.1188·2); ascorbic acid (p.1389·3).
Iron deficiency, especially with elevated calcium and vitamin C requirements.

Ferrocel Medifarma, Mex.
Iron dextran (p.1368·2).

Ferrocitol Delta, Braz.
Iron (p.1366·3); copper; vitamin B substances (p.1350·1).
Iron deficiency; iron-deficiency anaemia.

Ferrocomplex Farmalab, Braz.
Ferrous sulfate (p.1360·3); aluminium hydroxide (p.1210·3); magnesium hydroxide (p.1233·1); thiamine.
Ascorbic acid (p.1389·3) is included in this preparation to increase the absorption and availability of iron.
Iron deficiency; iron-deficiency anaemia.

Ferrocontin Continus Asta Medica, UK†.
Ferrous glycine sulfate (p.1360·2).
Iron-deficiency anaemia.

Ferrocontin Folic Continus Asta Medica, UK†.
Ferrous glycine sulfate (p.1360·2); folic acid (p.1361·1).
Iron and folic acid deficiency in pregnancy.

Ferrocur CIC, Spain.
Iron succinyl-protein complex (p.1369·3).
Iron-deficiency anaemia.

Ferrocutid Labocor, Port.†.
Ferrous glycine sulfate (p.1360·2).
Iron deficiency; iron-deficiency anaemia.

Ferrocyte
Eisai, Singapore; Eisai, Thai.
Ferrous sodium citrate.
Iron-deficiency anaemia.

Ferro-Dok Major, USA.
Ferrous fumarate (p.1360·1).
Docusate sodium (p.1223·1) is included in this preparation to reduce the constipating effects of iron.
Iron-deficiency anaemia.

Ferro-Folgamma Worwag, Ger.
Ferrous sulfate (p.1360·3); folic acid (p.1361·1); cyanocobalamin (p.1388·1).
Iron and vitamin deficiency.

Ferrofolin Farmades, Ital.
Iron succinyl-protein complex (p.1369·3); calcium folinate (p.1363·1).
Anaemias; folic acid deficiency; iron deficiency.

Ferrofolin Simplex Farmades, Ital.†.
Iron succinyl-protein complex (p.1369·3).
Anaemias; iron deficiency.

Ferro-Folsan
Solvay, Ger.; Solvay, Port.
Ferrous sulfate (p.1360·3); folic acid (p.1361·1).
Iron and folic acid deficiency.

Ferrofran Faria, Braz.
Ferrous sulfate (p.1360·3); aluminium hydroxide (p.1210·3); magnesium hydroxide (p.1233·1); thiamine.
Ascorbic acid (p.1389·3) is included in this preparation to increase the absorption and availability of iron.
Iron deficiency; iron-deficiency anaemia.

Ferrogamma Worwag, Ger.
Ferrous sulfate (p.1360·3).
Iron deficiency.

Ferrograd
Abbott, Irl.; Abbott, Ital.; Abbott, UK.
Ferrous sulfate (p.1360·3).
Iron-deficiency anaemia.

Ferrograd C
Abbott, Aust.; Abbott, Austral.; Abbott, Irl.; Abbott, Ital.; Abbott, NZ; Abbott, UK.
Ferrous sulfate (p.1360·3).
Sodium ascorbate (p.1390·1) is included in this preparation to increase the absorption and availability of iron.
Iron-deficiency anaemia.

Ferrograd Fol Abbott, Aust.
Ferrous sulfate (p.1360·3); folic acid (p.1361·1).
Iron and folic acid deficiency.

Ferrograd Folic
Abbott, Irl.; Abbott, Israel; Abbott, Ital.; Abbott, NZ; Abbott, UK.
Ferrous sulfate (p.1360·3); folic acid (p.1361·1).
Ascorbic acid (p.1389·3) may be included in this preparation to increase the absorption and availability of iron.
Iron and folic acid deficiency in pregnancy.

Ferrograd Folico Abbott, Port.
Ferrous sulfate (p.1360·3); folic acid (p.1361·1).
Iron and folic acid deficiency in pregnancy.

Ferro-Gradumet
Abbott, Aust.; Abbott, Austral.; Abbott, Israel; Abbott, NZ; Abbott, Port.; Abbott, Switz.
Ferrous sulfate (p.1360·3).
Iron deficiency; iron-deficiency anaemia.

Ferroin Pisa, Braz.
Iron dextran (p.1368·2).
Anaemias.

FERROinfant N Rubiepharm, Ger.
Ferrous sulfate (p.1360·3).
Iron deficiency; iron-deficiency anaemias.

FERROinfant Neu Rubiepharm, Ger.
Iron sucrose (p.1370·1).
Iron deficiency; iron-deficiency anaemias.

Ferrokapsul Strathmann, Ger.
Ferrous fumarate (p.1360·1).
Iron deficiency; iron-deficiency anaemia.

Ferroklinge *Ariston, Braz.*
Ferrous sulfate (p.1360·3).
Succinic acid is included in this preparation to increase the absorption and availability of iron.
Iron deficiency; iron-deficiency anaemia.

Ferrol *Chemil, Ital.†*
Chondroitin sulfate-iron complex (p.1357·1).
Iron deficiency; iron-deficiency anaemias.

Ferromar *Marnel, USA†.*
Ferrous fumarate (p.1360·1).
Ascorbic acid (p.1389·3) is included in this preparation to increase the absorption and availability of iron.

Ferromax *Weifa, Norw.*
Ferrous sulfate (p.1360·3).
Iron deficiency; iron-deficiency anaemia.

Ferromex *Dumex-Alpharma, Singapore.*
Ferrous sulfate (p.1360·3); copper sulfate (p.1358·1); manganese sulfate (p.1371·3).
Iron-deficiency anaemia.

Ferromia *Eisai, Jpn.*
Ferrous sodium citrate.
Iron-deficiency anaemia.

Ferromina *Provita, Ital.*
Ferrous gluconate; vitamin C; magnesium stearate; folic acid; vitamin B$_{12}$ (p.1350·1).
Nutritional supplement.

Ferromyn *Astra, Denm.†.*
Ferrous succinate (p.1360·3).
Succinic acid is included in this preparation to increase the absorption and availability of iron.
Iron deficiency.

Ferromyn S *Hassle, Swed.*
Ferrous succinate (p.1360·3).
Iron deficiency; iron-deficiency anaemia.

Ferroplex *Honorterapica, Braz.*
Ferrous sulfate (p.1360·3); cyanocobalamin (p.1388·1); folic acid (p.1361·1).
Ascorbic acid (p.1389·3) is included in this preparation to increase the absorption and availability of iron.
Iron deficiency; iron-deficiency anaemia.

Ferroplex-frangula *ERA, Denm.*
Iron salts (p.1366·3); frangula bark (p.1227·1).
Iron deficiency.

Ferroprotina
AF, Mex.; Faes, Spain.
Ferritin (p.1359·3).
Iron-deficiency anaemia.

Ferro-Retard *Nycomed, Norw.*
Ferrous sulfate (p.1360·3).
Iron deficiency; iron-deficiency anaemia.

Ferrosanol duodenal *Schwarz, Switz.*
Ferrous glycine sulfate (p.1360·2).
Iron deficiency; iron-deficiency anaemia.

Ferro-Sequels *Lederle, USA†.*
Ferrous fumarate (p.1360·1).
Docusate sodium (p.1223·1) is included in this preparation to reduce the constipating effects of iron.
Iron deficiency; iron deficiency anaemias.

Ferrosprint *Searle, Ital.*
Ferric sodium gluconate (p.1360·2).
Anaemias.

Ferrostrane *Parke, Davis, Fr.*
Sodium feredetate (p.1375·2).
Anaemias.

Ferrotab *Antigen, Irl.*
Dried ferrous sulfate (p.1360·3); copper sulfate (p.1358·1); manganese sulfate (p.1371·3).
Iron-deficiency anaemia.

Ferrotemp *Medix, Mex.*
Ferrous fumarate (p.1360·1); thiamine hydrochloride (p.1385·1).
Iron-deficiency anaemia.

Ferro-Terapina *Degorts, Mex.*
Ferrous fumarate (p.1360·1).
Iron-deficiency anaemia.

Ferrotonico B12 *Neo Quimica, Braz.*
Ferric ammonium citrate (p.1359·2); lysine hydrochloride; vitamin B$_6$; vitamin B$_{12}$; tryptophan; acetylmethionine; fraction G (p.1350·1).
Anaemias.

Ferrotrat *Medley, Braz.*
Ferrous sulfate (p.1360·3); folic acid (p.1361·1); vitamin B$_{12}$ (p.1388·1).
Iron deficiency; iron-deficiency anaemia.

Ferrotrat B12 *Medley, Braz.*
Ferric ammonium citrate (p.1359·2); vitamin B$_{12}$; liver extract; stomach extract; carnitine hydrochloride; lysine; sodium glycerophosphate; manganese sulfate; copper sulfate (p.1350·1).
Anaemias.

Ferro-Tre *Mediolanum, Ital.*
Iron acetyltransferrin.
Formerly contained ferritin and folic acid.
Iron-deficiency anaemias.

Ferrotron *VAAS, Ital.*
Amino-acid preparation with vitamins and minerals (p.1350·1).
Nutritional supplement.

Ferroven *Geymonat, Ital.†.*
Iron sucrose (p.1370·1).
Anaemias.

Ferrovin-Chinaeisenwein *Pharmonta, Aust.*
Ferric ammonium citrate (p.1359·2); manganese hypophosphite; cinchona bark (p.1595·3); citrus aurantium.
Anaemias; iron deficiency; tonic.

Ferrovin-Eisenelixier *Pharmonta, Aust.*
Iron sucrose (p.1370·1); aromatic tincture; bitter orange tincture (p.1644·2).
Iron deficiency; tonic.

Ferrum *Hausmann, Irl.*
Iron polymaltose (p.1369·2).
Iron-deficiency anaemia.

Ferrum Fol *Ferraz, Lynce, Port.*
Iron polymaltose (p.1369·2); folic acid (p.1361·1).
Iron and folic acid deficiency.

Ferrum H *Sigma, Austral.; Pharmaco, NZ.*
Iron polymaltose (p.1369·2).
Iron-deficiency anaemias.

Ferrum Hausmann
Richter, Aust.; Bio-Therabel, Belg.; Yamanouchi, Ger.; Vifor, Hong Kong; Geymonat, Ital.; Ferraz, Lynce, Port.; Vifor, Singapore; Vifor International, Switz.
Ferrous fumarate (p.1360·1), iron dextran (p.1368·2), or iron polymaltose (p.1369·2).
Iron deficiency; iron-deficiency anaemia.

Ferrum phosphoricum comp *Weleda, Ger.*
Homoeopathic preparation.

Ferrum Verla *Verla, Ger.*
Ferrous gluconate (p.1360·1).
Iron deficiency.

Ferrum-Quarz *Weleda, Aust.*
Ferrous sulfate (p.1360·3); quartz.
Migraine and related vascular headaches; tonic.

Fersaday *Goldshield, UK.*
Ferrous fumarate (p.1360·1).
Iron deficiency.

Fersamal *Forley, UK.*
Ferrous fumarate (p.1360·1).
Iron deficiency.

Fertibion *Tegur, Mex.*
Arginine (p.1353·3).

Fertilan *Codal Synto, Hong Kong.*
Clomifene citrate (p.1465·3).
Anovulatory infertility.

Fertiline *Organon, Fr.†.*
Urofollitropin (p.1299·3).
Female infertility.

Fertility Score *FertiPro, Irl.*
Test for male fertility (p.1654·3).

Fertinex *Serono, USA.*
Urofollitropin (p.1299·3).
Female infertility.

Fertinic *Desbergers, Canad.*
Ferrous gluconate (p.1360·1).
Iron-deficiency anaemias.

Fertinorm
Serono, Aust.†; Serono, Canad.; Serono, Ger.; Serono, Swed.†.
Urofollitropin (p.1299·3).
Anovulatory infertility.

Fertiral *Hoechst Marion Roussel, UK†.*
Gonadorelin (p.1283·3).
Amenorrhoea; male and female infertility.

Fertodur *Schering, Braz.; Schering, Mex.*
Cyclofenil (p.1467·2).
Anovulatory infertility.

Fertomcidina-U *Theriaca, Ital.*
Magnesium glycerophosphate (p.1191·1); salicylic acid (p.1122·3); sodium iodide (p.1522·3); ammonium bromide (p.1587·1).
Disinfection.

Fertomid *Cipla-Medpro, S.Afr.*
Clomifene citrate (p.1465·3).
Anovulatory infertility.

Ferumat *Continental Pharma, Belg.; Searle, Neth.†.*
Ferrous fumarate (p.1360·1).
Iron deficiency; iron-deficiency anaemias.

Ferval *Valdecasas, Mex.*
Ferrous fumarate (p.1360·1).
Iron-deficiency anaemia.

Fervex *Oberlin, Fr.*
Pheniramine maleate (p.422·3); paracetamol (p.71·2); ascorbic acid (p.1389·3).
Upper respiratory-tract disorders.

Fervex Rhume *Oberlin, Fr.†.*
Paracetamol (p.71·2); phenylpropanolamine hydrochloride (p.1098·1).
Cold symptoms.

Fervical *Garant, Ital.*
Calcium carbonate (p.1215·1).
Calcium deficiency; calcium supplement.

Ferxal *Silanes, Mex.*
Iron succinyl-protein complex (p.1369·3).
Iron-deficiency anaemia.

Ferybar *Pinewood, Irl.*
Liver extract; vitamin B substances; minerals (p.1350·1).
Vitamin and mineral supplement.

Fesofor *Xixia, S.Afr.†.*
Ferrous sulfate (p.1360·3).
Iron-deficiency anaemias.

Fesovit *Evans Medical, Irl.*
Dried ferrous sulfate (p.1360·3); vitamin B and C substances (p.1350·1).
Iron deficiency.

Fesovit Z *Medeva, UK†.*
Ferrous sulfate (p.1360·3); zinc sulfate (p.1398·2); vitamin B and C substances (p.1350·1).
Iron deficiency.

Fess *Paedpharm, Austral.*
Sodium chloride (p.1196·1).
Nasal congestion; sinusitis.

Festal *Hoechst Marion Roussel, Aust.†.*
Pancreatic lipase; pancreatic amylase (p.1579·3); pancreatic protease; hemicellulase (p.1593·1); ox bile (p.1585·1).
Digestive system disorders.

Festal N *Hoechst Marion Roussel, Ital.†.*
Pancreatin (p.1646·1).
Digestive system disorders.

Fe-Tinic *Ethex, USA.*
Polysaccharide-iron complex (p.1374·3).
Iron-deficiency anaemia.

Fe-Tinic Forte *Ethex, USA.*
Polysaccharide-iron complex (p.1374·3); folic acid (p.1361·1); vitamin B$_{12}$ (p.1388·1).
Iron-deficiency anaemia.

Feto-Longoral *Artesan, Ger.; Cassella-med, Ger.*
Multivitamin and mineral preparation (p.1350·1).

Fetrin *Lunsco, USA.*
Ferrous fumarate (p.1360·1); cyanocobalamin (p.1388·1); intrinsic factor.
Ascorbic acid (p.1389·3) is included in this preparation to increase the absorption and availability of iron.

Fetrival *Probios, Port.*
Iron succinyl-protein complex (p.1369·3).
Iron deficiency; iron-deficiency anaemia.

Feuille de Saule *Gilbert, Fr.*
Salicylic acid (p.1122·3).
Callus; corns; verrucas.

Fevamol *Aspen Consumer, S.Afr.*
Paracetamol (p.71·2).
Fever; pain.

Fevarin
Solvay, Denm.; Solvay, Fin.; Solvay, Ger.; Solvay, Ital.; Solvay, Neth.; Solvay, Norw.; Solvay, Swed.
Fluvoxamine maleate (p.289·3).
Depression; obsessive-compulsive disorder.

Fever & Inflammation Relief *Brauer, Austral.*
Homoeopathic preparation.

Feverall *Upsher-Smith, USA.*
Paracetamol (p.71·2).
Fever; pain.

Fevital Simplex *Prospa, Ital.*
Ferric sodium gluconate (p.1360·2).
Iron deficiency; iron-deficiency anaemias.

Fexicam *Technilab, Canad.*
Piroxicam (p.79·1).
Fever; inflammation; pain.

Fexin *Compu, S.Afr.*
Cefalexin (p.161·3).
Bacterial infections.

Fezona *Diba, Mex.*
Phenylbutazone (p.78·1).
Musculoskeletal and joint disorders; pain.

FGF Tabs *Abbott, Austral.*
Dried ferrous sulfate (p.1360·3); folic acid (p.1361·1).
Iron and folate deficiency; iron-deficiency anaemia; megaloblastic anaemia.

Fhbc *Baxter, Ital.*
Amino-acid infusion (p.1350·1).
Parenteral nutrition.

Fiacin *Biosarto, Spain.*
Indometacin (p.44·3); prednisone (p.1079·2).
Musculoskeletal and joint disorders; peri-articular disorders.

Fialetta Odontalgica Dr Knapp *Montefarmaco, Ital.*
Benzocaine (p.1306·2); chlorobutanol (p.1141·2); clove oil (p.1597·1); colophony (p.1598·3).
Toothache.

Fiberall *Ciba Consumer, USA.*
Chewable tablets†: Polycarbophil calcium (p.1244·2).
Constipation; diarrhoea; stool softener in haemorrhoids.
Oral powder; wafers: Psyllium hydrophilic mucilloid (p.1229·1).
Constipation; stool softener in haemorrhoids.

Fibercon
Lederle, Israel; Wyeth, Mex.; Lederle, USA.
Polycarbophil calcium (p.1244·2).
Bowel disorders; constipation.

Fiberform
Solvay, Neth.; Boehringer Ingelheim, Swed.
Wheat germ.
Constipation.

Fiberform Mix *Boehringer Ingelheim, Swed.*
Wheat germ.
Constipation.

Fiberlan *Galagen, USA.*
Lactose-free, gluten-free preparation for enteral nutrition (p.1350·1).

Fiber-Lax *Rugby, USA.*
Polycarbophil calcium (p.1244·2).
Constipation; diarrhoea.

FiberNorm *G & W, USA.*
Polycarbophil calcium (p.1244·2).
Constipation.

Fibersource *Novartis Nutrition, Singapore.*
Preparation for enteral nutrition with fibre (p.1350·1).

Fibertabletter *Kabi, Swed.†.*
Oat fibre (p.1214·2).
Dietary supplement.

Fibion *Asta Medica, Switz.*
Soya bran (p.1214·2).
Constipation.

Fiblaferon *Biosyn, Ger.*
Interferon beta (human) (p.632·2).
Viral infections.

Fiboran
Christiaens, Belg.; Nycomed, Fr.; Nycomed, Spain.
Aprindine hydrochloride (p.841·1).
Arrhythmias.

Fibra Light *Farmalight, Port.*
Fibre; guar gum (p.323·3).
Dietary fibre supplement.

Fibra Line *Investigacion, Mex.*
A range of dietary fibre supplements (p.1350·1).
Gastrointestinal disorders; obesity.

Fibracol *Johnson & Johnson Medical, UK.*
Collagen alginate (p.1598·2).
Wounds.

Fibrad *Ross, USA†.*
Dietary fibre preparation (p.1350·1).

Fibraflex
Nycomed, Ger.†.
Topical emulsion: Diethylamine salicylate (p.32·2); turpentine oil (p.1676·3); benzyl nicotinate (p.20·2).
Musculoskeletal and joint disorders; sports injuries.
Orion, Ger.
Ointment: Heparin sodium (p.902·1); glycol salicylate (p.42·2); benzyl nicotinate (p.20·2).
Musculoskeletal, joint, and nerve disorders; sports injuries.
Tablets: Ibuprofen (p.43·2).
Fever; musculoskeletal, joint, and soft-tissue disorders; pain.
Topical gel: Heparin sodium (p.902·1); glycol salicylate (p.42·2); menthol (p.1632·3).
Musculoskeletal and joint disorders; sports injuries.

Fibraflex-W-Creme N *Dorsch, Ger.†; Orion, Ger.†.*
Glycol salicylate (p.42·2); benzyl nicotinate (p.20·2).
Formerly contained heparin, glycol salicylate, and benzyl nicotinate.
Neuralgia; rheumatism.

Fibraguar *Fardi, Spain.*
Guar gum (p.323·3).
Diabetes mellitus.

Fibralime *Bio2, Fr.*
Nutritional supplement (p.1350·1).
Obesity.

Fibramucil *Procter & Gamble, Spain.*
Ispaghula (p.1229·1).
Constipation.

Fibrasan *Errekappa, Ital.*
Cellulose (p.1500·2).
Gastrointestinal disorders.

Fibrase
Note. This name is used for preparations of different composition.
Teoforma, Ital.
Pentosan polysulfate sodium (p.953·1).
Peripheral vascular disorders; soft-tissue disorders; thrombosis prophylaxis.
Warner-Lambert, Mex.
Chloramphenicol (p.179·1); fibrinolysin (bovine) (p.890·1); dornase alfa (p.1089·1).
Infected burns, ulcers, and wounds.

Fibrase com Clorafenicol *Ache, Braz.*
Fibrinolysin (human) (p.890·1); dornase alfa (p.1089·1); chloramphenicol (p.179·1).
Skin infections.

Fibrase SA *Warner-Lambert, Mex.*
Fibrinolysin (bovine) (p.890·1); dornase alfa (p.1089·1).
Burns; ulcers; wounds.

Fibrax *Whitehall-Robins, Canad.†.*
Grain and citrus fibre.
Constipation.

Fibre Dophilus *Pharmadass, UK.*
Acidophilus; bifidophilus.

Fibre Plus *Pharmadass, UK.*
Ispaghula (p.1229·1).
Formerly known as Fibrelax.

Fibrepur *Hoechst Marion Roussel, Canad.†.*
Ispaghula (p.1229·1).
Constipation.

Fibresource *Novartis Nutrition, Hong Kong.*
Preparation for enteral nutrition (p.1350·1).

Fibre-Vit *Vitalia, UK.*
Multivitamin, mineral, and fibre preparation (p.1350·1).

Fibrex Hot Drink *Berlin-Chemie, Ger.*
Aspirin (p.14·2); ascorbic acid (p.1389·3).
Fever; inflammation; pain.

Fibrex Tabletten *Berlin-Chemie, Ger.*
Aspirin (p.14·2); paracetamol (p.71·2).
Fever; pain.

Fibrezym *Bene, Ger.*
Pentosan polysulfate sodium (p.953·1).
Thromboembolism prophylaxis.

Fibrinol *Baldacci, Braz.*
Fibrin (bovine) (p.735·3).
Haemorrhage.

The symbol † denotes a preparation no longer actively marketed

Fibrinomer *ISI, Ital.†*
Fibrinogen (p.736·1).
Haemorrhagic disorders; hypofibrinogenaemia.

Fibrit *Neo-Farmaceutica, Port.†*
Anistreplase (p.840·2).
Myocardial infarction.

Fibrocid *Lacer, Spain.*
Pentosan polysulfate sodium (p.953·1).
Hyperlipidaemias; thromboembolic disorders.

Fibrocide *Neo-Farmaceutica, Port.†*
Pentosan polysulfate sodium (p.953·1).
Hyperlipidaemias; thromboembolic disorders.

Fibrocit *CT, Ital.*
Gemfibrozil (p.896·2).
Hyperlipidaemias.

Fibrocol *Zambon, Braz.*
Bran (p.1214·2).
Constipation; diverticulitis; irritable bowel syndrome; nutritional supplement.

Fibroderm *Torlan, Spain.*
Acedoben potassium (p.1571·2).
Skin disorders.

Fibrogammin
Centeon, Aust.; Centeon, Ger.
A factor XIII preparation (p.735·3).
Factor XIII deficiency; haemorrhagic disorders.

Fibrogammin P
Centeon, Israel; Aventis Behring, UK.
A factor XIII preparation (p.735·3).
Factor XIII deficiency.

Fibrolan
Parke, Davis, Aust.; Parke, Davis, Ger.; Parke, Davis, Switz.
Fibrinolysin (bovine) (p.890·1); deoxyribonuclease (p.1089·1).
Wounds.

Fibrolax *Giuliani, Ital.*
Ispaghula (p.1229·1).
Constipation.

Fibrolax Complex *Giuliani, Ital.*
Ispaghula (p.1229·1); senna (p.1248·2).
Constipation.

Fibromucil *Collins, Mex.*
Ispaghula (p.1229·1).
Constipation; hypercholesterolamia.

Fibronevrina *Ceccarelli, Ital.*
Thiamine hydrochloride (p.1385·1); cyanocobalamin (p.1388·1).
Formerly contained d-isopropylammonium dichloroacetate, thiamine, and cyanocobalamin.
Peripheral neuralgia and neuritis.

Fibroral *Novartis Nutrition, Fr.*
Preparation for enteral nutrition (p.1350·1).

Fibros *Boniscontro & Gazzone, Ital.*
Gemfibrozil (p.896·2).
Hyperlipidaemias.

Fibrosine
Note. This name is used for preparations of different composition.
Whitehall, Irl.†; Whitehall, Port.
Maltodextrin (p.1371·2).
Constipation.

Whitehall, Singapore; Whitehall, Thai.
Dietary fibre preparation (p.1350·1).

Fibro-Vein
Australasian Medical, Austral.; STD, Irl.; Mac, Ital.; NZ Medical & Scientific, NZ.
Sodium tetradecyl sulfate (p.1497·2).
Varicose veins.

Fibrovein *Intramed, S.Afr.*
Sodium tetradecyl sulfate (p.1497·2).
Varicose veins.

Fibro-Vein *STD Pharmaceutical Products, UK.*
Sodium tetradecyl sulfate (p.1497·2).
Formerly known as STD Injection.
Varicose veins.

Fibrovit *Provita, Ital.*
Glucomannan (p.1616·2); pectin; inulin; guar; garcinia cambogia (p.1214·2).
Dietary fibre supplement.

Fibroxyn *Aspen, S.Afr.*
Naproxen (p.60·3).
Inflammation; musculoskeletal and joint disorders; pain.

Fibsol *Arrow, Austral.*
Lisinopril (p.921·1).
Heart failure; hypertension; myocardial infarction.

Fibyrax
Rhone-Poulenc Rorer, Austral.; Whitehall-Robins, Canad.†
Grain and citrus fibres (p.1214·2).
Constipation; dietary fibre supplement.

Fichtensirup N *Jukunda, Ger.*
Spruce needles; thyme (p.1672·2); sage (p.1660·2); liquorice (p.1231·2); thyme oil (p.1672·3); sage oil (p.1660·2).
Respiratory-tract disorders; tonic.

Ficortril
Pfizer, Ger.; Pfizer, Swed.
Hydrocortisone (p.1073·3) or hydrocortisone acetate (p.1073·3).
Anogenital pruritus; eczema; inflammatory eye disorders.

Fideine *Bergamo, Braz.*
Phenolphthalein (p.1244·1); rhubarb (p.1248·1); cascara (p.1216·1); gentian (p.1615·1); papain (p.1647·3).
Constipation.

Fidium *Fides Rottapharm, Spain.*
Betahistine hydrochloride (p.1584·2).
Vertigo.

Fienamina *Recordati, Ital.*
Chlorpheniramine [chlorphenamine] maleate (p.412·1); ephedrine hydrochloride (p.1090·1).
Hypersensitivity reactions.

Fiery Jack *Pickles, UK.*
Cream: Glycol salicylate (p.42·2); diethylamine salicylate (p.32·2); capsicum oleoresin (p.1591·1); methyl nicotinate (p.55·1).
Ointment: Capsicum oleoresin (p.1591·1).
Musculoskeletal and joint disorders; pain.

Figadobil *Dorsay, Braz.*
Adenosine (p.828·2); methionine (p.1012·2); betaine hydrochloride (p.1584·3); choline citrate (p.1356·3); pyridoxine hydrochloride (p.1386·3).
Liver disorders.

Figadosan *La-Sante, Braz.*
Cynara (p.1601·3); cascara (p.1216·1); boldo (p.1585·3); rhubarb (p.1248·1); persea americana.
Liver disorders.

Figatil *Catarinense, Braz.*
Cynara (p.1601·3); boldo (p.1585·3); ox bile (p.1585·1).
Liver disorders.

Figen *ERA, Denm.*
Senna (p.1248·2); fig (p.1227·1).
Constipation.

Figsen *Carter-Wallace, Austral.†*
Phenolphthalein (p.1244·1).
Constipation.

FIII Hc *Baxter, Ital.*
Amino-acid infusion (p.1350·1).
Parenteral nutrition.

Filair *3M, UK.*
Beclometasone dipropionate (p.1061·2).
Obstructive airways disease.

Filcrin *Serono, Mex.*
Vincristine (p.579·3).

Filena
Organon, Aust.; Organon, Ital.
11 White tablets, estradiol valerate (p.1473·2); 10 blue tablets, estradiol valerate; medroxyprogesterone acetate (p.1480·1).
Menopausal disorders; osteoporosis.

Filesna *Serono, Mex.*
Mesna (p.1011·3).

Filibon
Wyeth, Mex.; Wyeth, S.Afr.
Multivitamin and mineral preparation (p.1350·1).
Supplement for pregnant or lactating women.

Filinasma *Searle, Braz.*
Theophylline (p.777·2); ephedrine hydrochloride (p.1090·1); phenobarbital (p.355·1); homatropine (p.468·1).
Respiratory-tract disorders.

Filivir *Serono, Mex.*
Aciclovir (p.612·3).

Filmagene *Confar, Port.*
Barrier cream.

Filmcel *Allergan-Frumtost, Braz.*
Hypromellose (p.1501·3).
Dry eyes.

Filmogen Same *Savoma, Ital.*
Barrier cream.

Filogargan *Heralds, Braz.*
Tyrothricin (p.267·1); benzocaine (p.1306·2); cetylpyridinium chloride (p.1138·1).
Mouth and throat disorders.

Filogaster *Climax, Braz.*
Amylase (p.1579·3); papain (p.1647·3); pepsin (p.1649·3); homocysteine thiolactone; pancreatin (p.1646·1); sodium dehydrocholate (p.1602·2); vitamin B substances (p.1350·1); magnesium chloride.
Digestive-system disorders.

Filokloral *Sabater, Spain.*
Cefazolin sodium (p.164·3).
Lignocaine [lidocaine] hydrochloride (p.1313·2) is included in this preparation to alleviate the pain of injection.
Bacterial infections.

Filotempo *Asta Medica, Port.*
Aminophylline (p.760·1).
Asthma.

Filter Oil Free *Dermoteca, Port.*
SPF 16: Neoheliopan E; zinc oxide (p.1128·2).
SPF 30: Neoheliopan E; zinc oxide (p.1128·2); titanium dioxide (p.1126·1); ferric oxide (p.1028·2).
Sunscreen.

Filter OTC *Dermoteca, Port.*
Topical emulsion SPF 15; SPF 20: Amiloxate (p.1516·3); zinc oxide (p.1128·2); titanium dioxide (p.1126·1).
Topical spray SPF 15: Amiloxate (p.1516·3); zinc oxide (p.1128·2).
SPF 40: Amiloxate (p.1516·3); padimate (p.1518·2); enzacamene (p.1517·2); zinc oxide (p.1128·2).
Sunscreen.

Filtrax *Ipso, Ital.*
Pipemidic acid (p.236·1).
Bacterial urinary-tract infections.

Fin-A *Ehlinger, Mex.*
Ketotifen (p.767·2).

Finac *C & M, USA.*
Sulfur (p.1123·3); methylbenzethonium chloride (p.1150·3).
Acne.

Finalgon
Boehringer Ingelheim, Aust.; Boehringer Ingelheim, Austral.; Boehringer Ingelheim, Canad.; Thomae, Ger.; Boehringer Ingelheim, NZ; Boehringer Ingelheim, Port.; Fher, Spain.
Nonivamide (p.63·1); nicoboxil (p.62·2).
Musculoskeletal, joint, peri-articular, and soft-tissue disorders; peripheral vascular disorders.

Finalgon N Schmerzpflaster *Thomae, Ger.†*
Cayenne pepper (p.1591·1); methyl salicylate (p.55·1).
Musculoskeletal and joint disorders; sprains.

Finamicina *Fustery, Mex.*
Rifampicin (p.243·2).
Tuberculosis.

Finan *Solfran, Mex.*
Multivitamin and mineral preparation (p.1350·1).

Finastid *Neopharmed, Ital.*
Finasteride (p.1477·2).
Benign prostatic hyperplasia.

Finatux *Jaba, Port.*
Carbocisteine (p.1086·3).
Respiratory-tract congestion.

Fincoid *Orion, Switz.†*
Copper-wound polyethylene (p.1357·3).
Intra-uterine contraceptive device.

Findol *Senosiain, Mex.*
Ketorolac trometamol (p.48·2).
Pain.

Findol N *Mundipharma, Ger.*
Tilidate hydrochloride (p.88·2).
Naloxone hydrochloride (p.1014·3) is included in this preparation to discourage abuse.
Pain.

Findor *Sibras, Braz.*
Aspirin (p.14·2); caffeine (p.761·3).
Fever; pain.

Finedal *Llorente, Spain.*
Clobenzorex hydrochloride (p.1507·2).
Obesity.

Fineural N *Molimin, Ger.*
Aspirin (p.14·2); paracetamol (p.71·2); caffeine (p.761·3).
Cold symptoms; fever; neuralgia; pain.

Finevin *Berlex, USA.*
Azelaic acid (p.1110·3).
Acne.

Finfo *Osotspa, Thai.*
Piroxicam (p.79·1).
Fever; inflammation; musculoskeletal and joint disorders; pain.

Finidol *Novartis, Fr.*
Aspirin (p.14·2); caffeine (p.761·3).
Colloidal aluminium hydroxide (p.1210·3) is included in this preparation in an attempt to limit adverse effects on the gastrointestinal mucosa.
Fever; pain.

Finigas *Apsen, Braz.*
Dimethicone (p.1249·2).
Flatulence.

Finil *Coradol, Ger.*
Homoeopathic preparation.

Finimal
Roche, Belg.†; Roche Consumer, Neth.
Paracetamol (p.71·2); caffeine (p.761·3).
Fever; pain.

Finipect *Roche Nicholas, Neth.†*
Noscapine (p.1096·1).
Coughs.

Finiweh *Dentinox, Ger.*
Paracetamol (p.71·2).
Fever; pain.

Finlepsin *Asta Medica, Ger.*
Carbamazepine (p.342·2).
Alcohol withdrawal syndrome; epilepsy; neurogenic pain; psychoses.

Finn *Boehringer de Angeli, Braz.*
Aspartame (p.1354·3).
Sugar substitute.

Finnferon-Alpha *Veripalvelu, Fin.*
Interferon alfa (p.628·1).
Malignant neoplasms.

Finprob *Farcoral, Mex.*
Pipenzolate (p.472·2); dimethicone (p.1249·2).
Gastrointestinal disorders.

Finrexin *Leiras, Fin.*
Aspirin (p.14·2); caffeine (p.761·3); ascorbic acid (p.1389·3).
Fever; pain.

Fiorgen PF *Goldline, USA†.*
Aspirin (p.14·2); caffeine (p.761·3); butalbital (p.658·3).
Pain.

Fioricet *Novartis, USA.*
Butalbital (p.658·3); paracetamol (p.71·2); caffeine (p.761·3).
Tension headache.

Fioricet with Codeine *Novartis, USA.*
Codeine phosphate (p.25·2); butalbital (p.658·3); paracetamol (p.71·2); caffeine (p.761·3).
Tension headache.

Fiorinal
Note. This name is used for preparations of different composition.
Novartis, Austral.
Codeine phosphate (p.25·2); doxylamine succinate (p.417·1); paracetamol (p.71·2).
Pain.

Novartis, Canad.; Novartis, USA.
Aspirin (p.14·2); butalbital (p.658·3); caffeine (p.761·3).
Pain; vascular or tension headaches.

Novartis, Canad.
Aspirin (p.14·2); caffeine (p.761·3); paracetamol (p.71·2).
Pain.

Fiorinal C *Novartis, Canad.*
Butalbital (p.658·3); caffeine (p.761·3); aspirin (p.14·2); codeine phosphate (p.25·2).
Anxiety; pain; tension.

Fiorinal Codeina *Novartis, Spain.*
Aspirin (p.14·2); caffeine (p.761·3); codeine phosphate (p.25·2); paracetamol (p.71·2).
Pain.

Fiorinal with Codeine *Novartis, USA.*
Aspirin (p.14·2); butalbital (p.658·3); caffeine (p.761·3); codeine phosphate (p.25·2).
Tension headache.

Fiormil *Inpharzam, Switz.*
Enterococcus faecium (p.1626·3).
Restoration of normal gastrointestinal flora.

Fiorpap *Geneva, USA†.*
Butalbital (p.658·3); paracetamol (p.71·2); caffeine (p.761·3).
Pain.

Fiortal *Geneva, USA†.*
Aspirin (p.14·2); caffeine (p.761·3); butalbital (p.658·3).
Pain.

Fiortal with Codeine *Geneva, USA.*
Aspirin (p.14·2); caffeine (p.761·3); butalbital (p.658·3); codeine (p.25·2).
Pain.

FiProFLAX *Arkopharma, UK.*
Flax oil; fibre; protein; carbohydrate; lignans (p.1350·1).
Dietary supplement.

Firac *Grossman, Mex.*
Clonixin lysine (p.25·1).
Pain.

Firac Plus *Grossman, Mex.*
Clonixin lysine (p.25·1); pargeverine hydrochloride.
Smooth muscle pain and spasm.

Firin *Hoyer, Ger.*
Norfloxacin (p.232·1).
Bacterial infections.

Firmacef *FIRMA, Ital.*
Cefazolin sodium (p.164·3).
Lignocaine [lidocaine] hydrochloride (p.1313·2) is included in the intramuscular injection to alleviate the pain of injection.
Bacterial infections.

Firmacort *FIRMA, Ital.*
Methylprednisolone (p.1076·1) or methylprednisolone sodium succinate (p.1076·1).
Corticosteroid.

Firmavit *FIRMA, Ital.*
Cobamamide (p.1388·3); pyridoxal phosphate (p.1387·1); thiamine diphosphate (p.1385·2).
Neuritis.

Fironetta *Schering, Denm.*
21 Tablets, ethinylestradiol (p.1476·2); levonorgestrel (p.1486·2); 7 tablets, inert.
Triphasic oral contraceptive.

First Choice *Polymer Technology, USA.*
Test for glucose in blood (p.1616·3).

First Response
Carter-Wallace, Austral.†; Carter Horner, Canad.; Carter-Wallace, UK; Carter-Wallace, USA.
Fertility test or pregnancy test (p.1654·3).

Fisamox *Rhone-Poulenc Rorer, Austral.*
Amoxicillin sodium (p.149·2).
Bacterial infections.

Fish Factor *Farmila, Ital.*
Omega-3 marine triglycerides (p.949·3).
Arteriosclerosis; disorders of lipid metabolism.

Fishaphos *Felton, Austral.*
Omega-3 marine triglycerides (p.949·3).
Dietary supplement.

Fisherman's Friend *Lofthouse of Fleetwood, Canad.*
Menthol (p.1632·3).
Coughs; sore throat.

Fisherman's Friend Original *Lofthouse of Fleetwood, Canad.*
Menthol (p.1632·3); eucalyptus oil (p.1609·2).
Cold symptoms.

Fisher's Phospherine *Felton, Austral.*
Vitamins and minerals; alstonia constricta; quassia; valerian (p.1350·1).
Tonic.

Fishogar *Self-Care Products, UK.*
Fish oil; garlic (p.1614·1).

Fisifax *Septa, Spain.*
Nicergoline (p.1640·2).
Cerebral and peripheral vascular disorders; vascular headache.

Fisiobil *Salvat, Spain.*
Dimecrotic acid, magnesium salt.
Hepatobiliary disorders.

Fisiodar *Abiogen, Ital.*
Diacerein (p.28·3).
Osteoarthritis.

Fisiofer
Eurofarma, Braz.; Molteni, Ital.
Ferric sodium gluconate (p.1360·2) or iron succinyl-protein complex (p.1369·3).
Iron deficiency; iron-deficiency anaemias.

Fisiogastrol *Salvat, Spain.*
Cisapride (p.1220·1).
Gastro-oesophageal reflux; gastroparesis.

Fisiologica *Farmasur, Spain; Fardi, Spain.*
Sodium chloride (p.1196·1).
Nasal congestion.

Fisiologico
Labormedica, Braz.
Sodium chloride (p.1196·1).
Fluid and electrolyte depletion.

Betamadrileno, Spain; Neusc, Spain; Orrava, Spain; Calmante Vitaminado, Spain.
Sodium chloride (p.1196·1).
Nasal congestion.

Fisiologico Bieffe M *Baxter, Spain.*
Sodium chloride (p.1196·1).
Fluid and electrolyte depletion; hypovolaemia.

Fisiologico Braun *Braun, Spain.*
Sodium chloride (p.1196·1).
Fluid and electrolyte depletion; hypovolaemia.

Fisiologico Farmacelsia *Farmacelsia, Spain.*
Sodium chloride (p.1196·1).
Fluid and electrolyte disorders.

Fisiologico Mein *Fresenius Kabi, Spain.*
Sodium chloride (p.1196·1).
Fluid and electrolyte depletion; hypovolaemia.

Fisiologico Vitulia *Ern, Spain.*
Sodium chloride (p.1196·1).
Fluid and electrolyte depletion; hypovolaemia.

Fisohex *SmithKline Beecham, Braz.*
Triclosan (p.1159·2).
Skin disinfection.

Fisopred *Rhone-Poulenc Rorer, Mex.*
Prednisolone sodium phosphate (p.1078·1).
Corticosteroid.

Fissan *Uhlmann-Eyraud, Switz.*
Casein hydrolysate; colloidal silicon dioxide (p.1503·3); polysilic acid fluoride; bismuth subnitrate (p.1213·2); kaolin (p.1229·3); silica clay (p.1503·3); titanium dioxide (p.1126·1); zinc oxide (p.1128·2).
Skin irritation.

Fissan-Silberpuder *Salitine, Ger.*
Methenamine silver nitrate compound.
Umbilical cord care; wounds.

Fissan-Zinkschuttelmixtur *Salitine, Ger.*
Zinc oxide (p.1128·2).
Skin disorders.

Fitacnol *Arkopharma, Fr.*
Lappa (p.1627·1); pensee sauvage; ortie dioique.
Acne.

Fitaxal *Phygiene, Fr.†.*
Lactulose (p.1230·1).
Constipation.

Fitocrem *Andromaco, Spain†.*
Paraffin; wheat germ; phenoxyethanol.
Burns; ulcers; wounds.

Fitocreme *Fariberica, Port.*
Wheat germ; phenoxyethanol.
Burns; ulcers; wounds.

Fitodorf Alghe Marine *Fitodorfarma, Ital.*
Quercia marine extract; frangula (p.1227·1); rhubarb (p.1248·1).
Constipation; dietary supplement.

Fitodorf Rabarbaro *Fitodorfarma, Ital.*
Boldo (p.1585·3); rhubarb (p.1248·1).
Digestive disorders; reduced intestinal motility.

Fitoestimulina *Grossman, Mex.*
Wheat germ; phenoxyethanol (p.1153·3).
Burns; ulcers; vaginal lesions; wounds.

Fitolax *IMA, Braz.*
Senna (p.1248·2); cassia pulp (p.1216·2); tamarind (p.1253·2); coriander (p.1599·2).
Constipation.

Fitolinea *Pharbenia, Ital.*
Bladderwrack (p.1585·2); senna (p.1248·2).
Constipation; obesity.

Fitosonno *Pharbenia, Ital.*
Eschscholtzia californica; passion flower (p.1649·1); valerian (p.1678·3).
Insomnia.

Fitostimoline *Damor, Ital.*
Cream; medicated dressing; pessaries; vaginal wash: Wheat germ; phenoxyethanol (p.1153·3).
Burns; skin disorders; vaginal disorders; vascular disorders; wounds.
Injection: Wheat germ.
Burns; skin disorders; vascular disorders; wounds.

Fitostress *Pharbenia, Ital.*
Ginseng (p.1615·3); kola (p.1681·1).
Tonic.

Fitosvelt *Arkochim, Spain.*
Black currant (p.1389·3); tea (p.1681·1).
Diuretic.

Fitton *Teva, Israel.*
Fenetylline (p.1509·3).
CNS stimulant.

Fittydent *Hoeveler, Aust.*
Eucalyptus oil (p.1609·2); sage oil (p.1660·2); clove oil (p.1597·1).
Mouth and throat inflammation; toothache.

Fitzecalm *Julphar, UAE.*
Carbamazepine (p.342·2).
Bipolar disorder; epilepsy.

Fivasa *Norgine, Fr.*
Mesalazine (p.1234·1).
Inflammatory bowel disease.

Fiverocil *Serono, Mex.*
Fluorouracil (p.540·2).

Fivoflu *Dabur, Thai.*
Fluorouracil (p.540·2).
Malignant neoplasms.

Fixateur phospho-calcique *Bichsel, Switz.*
Calcium carbonate (p.1215·1).
Hyperphosphataemia.

Fixca *Lesvi, Spain.*
Ondansetron hydrochloride (p.1241·3).
Nausea and vomiting.

Fixical *Pharmascience, Fr.*
Calcium carbonate (p.1215·1).
Calcium deficiency; osteoporosis.

Fixical Vitamine D₃ *Pharmascience, Fr.*
Calcium carbonate (p.1215·1); colecalciferol (p.1391·1).
Calcium and vitamin D deficiency; osteoporosis.

Fixim *Yamanouchi, Neth.*
Cefixime (p.166·2).
Bacterial infections.

Fixime *Merck, S.Afr.*
Cefixime (p.166·2).
Bacterial infections.

Fixoten *Cryopharma, Mex.*
Oxpentifylline [pentoxifylline] (p.950·3).
Vascular disorders.

Fizz *Stanley, Canad.†.*
Multivitamin preparation (p.1350·1).

Flacar *Schwabe, Ger.*
Betaine dihydrogen citrate (p.1584·3); sorbitol (p.1377·3).
Liver disorders.

Flagenase *Liomont, Mex.*
Metronidazole (p.594·1) or metronidazole benzoate (p.594·1).
Anaerobic bacterial infections; protozoal infections.

Flagenase 400 *Liomont, Mex.*
Metronidazole (p.594·1) or metronidazole benzoate (p.594·1); diiodohydroxyquinoline (p.590·2).
Amoebiasis.

Flagentyl
Rhone-Poulenc Rorer, Fr.; Vitoria, Port.
Secnidazole (p.602·1).
Protozoal infections.

Flaginazol *Vitae, Mex.*
Metronidazole (p.594·1).
Amoebiasis; giardiasis; trichomoniasis.

Flagyl
Rhone-Poulenc Rorer, Aust.; Rhone-Poulenc Rorer, Austral.; Aventis, Belg.; Rhodia, Braz.; Rhone-Poulenc Rorer, Canad.; Baxter, Canad.; Aventis, Denm.; Rhone-Poulenc Rorer, Fin.; Rhone-Poulenc Rorer, Fr.; Rhone-Poulenc Rorer, Ger.; Rhone-Poulenc Rorer, Hong Kong; Rhone-Poulenc Rorer, Irl.; Rhone-Poulenc Rorer, Israel; Pharmacia Upjohn, Ital.; Rhone-Poulenc Rorer, Mex.; Rhone-Poulenc Rorer, Neth.; Rhone-Poulenc Rorer, Norw.; Aventis, NZ; Vitoria, Port.; Aventis, S.Afr.; Rhone-Poulenc Rorer, Singapore; Rhone-Poulenc Rorer, Spain; Rhone-Poulenc Rorer, Swed.; Rhone-Poulenc Rorer, Switz.; Rhone-Poulenc Rorer, Thai.; Hawgreen, UK; Rhone-Poulenc Rorer, UK; SCS, USA; Searle, USA.
Metronidazole (p.594·1), metronidazole benzoate (p.594·1), or metronidazole hydrochloride (p.594·1).
Anaerobic bacterial infections; Crohn's disease; protozoal infections; rosacea.

Flagyl Comp *Rhone-Poulenc Rorer, Fin.*
Metronidazole (p.594·1); nystatin (p.392·2).
Bacterial vaginosis; vaginal trichomoniasis.

Flagyl Compak
Rhone-Poulenc Rorer, Irl.; Hawgreen, UK.
Combination preparation: Tablets, metronidazole (p.594·1); *pessaries,* nystatin (p.392·2).
Vaginitis.

Flagyl Nistatina *Rhodia, Braz.*
Metronidazole (p.594·1); nystatin (p.392·2).
Vulvovaginal candidiasis and trichomoniasis.

Flagystatin
Rhone-Poulenc Rorer, Canad.; Rhone-Poulenc Rorer, Singapore.
Metronidazole (p.594·1); nystatin (p.392·2).
Vaginal trichomoniasis and candidiasis.

Flagystatin V *Rhone-Poulenc Rorer, Mex.*
Metronidazole (p.594·1); nystatin (p.392·2).
Vaginal trichomoniasis and candidiasis.

Flamadene *Heralds, Braz.*
Piroxicam (p.79·1).
Dysmenorrhoea; gout; musculoskeletal, joint, and peri-articular disorders.

Flamanan *Legrand, Braz.*
Paracetamol (p.71·2); oxyphenbutazone (p.71·1).
Fever; inflammation; pain.

Flamarene *Sanus, Braz.*
Piroxicam (p.79·1).
Dysmenorrhoea; gout; musculoskeletal, joint, and peri-articular disorders.

Flamaret *Xixia, S.Afr.*
Indometacin (p.44·3).
Dysmenorrhoea; gout; musculoskeletal and joint disorders.

Flamatak *Cox, UK.*
Diclofenac sodium (p.30·3).
Gout; inflammation; musculoskeletal, joint, peri-articular, and soft-tissue disorders; pain.

Flamatrol
Teva, Hong Kong; Berk, UK.
Piroxicam (p.79·1).
Inflammation; musculoskeletal and joint disorders; pain.

Flamazine
Smith & Nephew, Canad.; Smith & Nephew, Denm.; Smith & Nephew, Fin.; Smith & Nephew, Hong Kong; Smith & Nephew, Irl.; Smith & Nephew, Norw.; Solvay, Port.; Smith & Nephew, S.Afr.; Smith & Nephew, Singapore; Smith & Nephew, Thai.; Smith & Nephew Healthcare, UK.
Sulfadiazine silver (p.251·3).
Infected wounds and burns.

Flamazine C *Smith & Nephew, Canad.*
Sulfadiazine silver (p.251·3); chlorhexidine gluconate (p.1138·2).
Burns; ulcers; wounds.

Flamecid *Propan, S.Afr.†.*
Indometacin (p.44·3).
Gout; musculoskeletal and joint disorders.

Flameril
Novartis, NZ; Normal, Port.
Diclofenac (p.30·2), diclofenac diethylamine (p.30·2), or diclofenac sodium (p.30·3).
Gout; inflammation; musculoskeletal and joint disorders; pain.

Flamic *Siam Bheasach, Thai.*
Piroxicam (p.79·1).
Gout; musculoskeletal, joint, peri-articular, and soft-tissue disorders.

Flamicina *Fustery, Mex.*
Ampicillin (p.150·3), ampicillin sodium (p.150·3), or ampicillin trihydrate (p.151·1).
Bacterial infections.

Flamilon *OM, Switz.†.*
Suxibuzone (p.87·3).
Inflammation.

Flaminase *Formenti, Ital.*
Promelase (p.1655·1).
Respiratory-tract disorders.

Flamirex *Irex, Fr.*
Tiaprofenic acid (p.88·1).
Musculoskeletal and joint disorders.

Flammacerium
Solvay, Belg.; Solvay, Fr.; Solvay, Israel; Solvay, Neth.; Solvay, UK.
Sulfadiazine silver (p.251·3); cerous nitrate (p.1112·3).
Available on a named patient basis in the UK.
Infected burns.

Flammazine
Solvay, Aust.; Solvay, Belg.; Solvay, Fr.; Solvay, Ger.; Solvay, Neth.; Solvay, Spain; Solvay, Switz.
Sulfadiazine silver (p.251·3).
Burns; infected skin disorders; infected wounds.

Flamon *Mepha, Switz.*
Verapamil hydrochloride (p.989·1).
Arrhythmias; hypertension; ischaemic heart disease.

Flamostat *Honorterapica, Braz.*
Piroxicam (p.79·1).
Dysmenorrhoea; gout; musculoskeletal, joint, and peri-articular disorders.

Flamrase *Berk, UK.*
Diclofenac sodium (p.30·3).
Musculoskeletal, joint, peri-articular, and soft-tissue disorders; pain.

Flanamox *Wolff, Ger.*
Amoxicillin trihydrate (p.149·2); flucloxacillin sodium (p.207·1).
Bacterial infections.

Flanaren *Teuto, Braz.*
Diclofenac sodium (p.30·3).
Gout; inflammation; musculoskeletal, joint, and peri-articular disorders; pain.

Flanax
Hoechst Marion Roussel, Braz.; Syntex, Mex.
Naproxen sodium (p.61·1).
Fever; gout; inflammation; pain.

Flanders Buttocks *Flanders, USA.*
Zinc oxide (p.1128·2); peru balsam (p.1650·2).
Nappy rash.

Flanid *Pierre Fabre, Fr.*
Tiaprofenic acid (p.88·1).

Flanil
Biolab, Singapore; Biolab, Thai.
Methyl salicylate (p.55·1); menthol (p.1632·3); eugenol (p.1609·3).
Insect bites; muscle pain; pruritus.

Flanoquin *Liomont, Mex.*
Diiodohydroxyquinoline (p.590·2).

Flantadin *Lepetit, Ital.*
Deflazacort (p.1066·1).
Oral corticosteroid.

Flar *ISM, Mex.*
Streptococcus lactis; *Lactobacillus acidophilus* (p.1626·3); nicotinamide (p.1372·3).
Gastrointestinal disorders.

Flarex
Alcon, Aust.; Alcon, Austral.; Alcon, Canad.; Alcon, Israel; Alcon, Ital.;

Alcon, Mex.; Alcon, Neth.†; Pacific, NZ; Alcon, Switz.; Alcon, Thai.; Alcon, USA.
Fluorometholone acetate (p.1072·1).
Inflammatory eye disorders.

Flaspas *Daito, Jpn.*
Aranidipine (p.841·2).
Hypertension.

Flatoril *Almirall, Spain.*
Clebopride malate (p.1221·2); simeticone (p.1249·2).
Dyspepsia; gastro-oesophageal reflux; hiatus hernia.

Flatulence Gastulence *Greater Pharma, Thai.*
Cascara (p.1216·1); capsicum (p.1591·1); amylase (p.1579·3); ginger (p.1227·2); nux vomica (p.1643·1); asafetida (p.1582·3).
Constipation; flatulence.

Flatulex
Note.This name is used for preparations of different composition.
Globopharm, Switz.
Chewable tablets: Simeticone (p.1249·2); caraway oil (p.1591·2); fennel oil (p.1610·2); peppermint oil (p.1243·3).
Oral drops: Simeticone (p.1249·2).
Adjunct prior to gastrointestinal examination; flatulence.
Dayton, USA.
Oral drops: Simeticone (p.1249·2).
Tablets: Simeticone (p.1249·2); activated charcoal (p.1000·2).
Flatulence.

Flavamed Halstabletten *Berlin-Chemie, Ger.*
Benzocaine (p.1306·2).
Sore throat.

Flavan *Pharmafarm, Fr.*
Leucocianidol (p.1611·2).
Peripheral vascular disorders.

Flavangin *Streuli, Switz.*
Ethacridine lactate (p.1130·3); cetylpyridinium chloride (p.1138·1); lignocaine [lidocaine] hydrochloride (p.1313·2); menthol (p.1632·3).
Mouth and throat disorders.

Flavettes
CCM, Hong Kong; CCM, Singapore.
Vitamin C (p.1389·3).
Vitamin C deficiency.

Flaviastase *Iphym, Fr.*
Enzymes derived from Aspergillus.
Digestive disorders.

Flavinol *Chew, Thai.*
Euflavine (p.1130·3); thymol (p.1158·3).
Burns; wounds.

Flavion *Terapeutico, Ital.*
Aesculus; centella; lemon; bearberry (p.1350·1).
Nutritional supplement.

Flavis *Pulitzer, Ital.*
Piracetam (p.1652·1).
Mental function impairment.

Flavogin *Baif, Ital.*
Ginkgo biloba; bioflavonoids; dog rose; myrtillus; vitamin C (p.1350·1).
Tonic.

Flavon *General Drugs, Thai.*
Flavonoids (p.1611·1).
Haemorrhoids; vascular insufficiency.

Flavone 500 *Ecobi, Ital.*
Ascorbic acid (p.1389·3); hesperidin (p.1611·2).

Flavonex *Ross, USA.*
Preparation for enteral nutrition (p.1350·1).

Flavonoid C *Vitaglow, Austral.†.*
Calcium ascorbate (p.1389·3); bioflavonoids (p.1611·1); hesperidin (p.1611·2); rutoside (p.1611·2).
Cold symptoms; hypersensitivity reactions; peripheral vascular disorders; vitamin C deficiency.

Flavonoid Complex *Neo-Life, Austral.†.*
Cranberry; kale; green tea; red beetroot; mixed berry; oregon grape; grape; orange extract; lemon extract; grapefruit (p.1611·1).
Flavonoid supplement.

Flavons
Note.This name is used for preparations of different composition.
Eagle, Austral.
Ascorbic acid (p.1389·3); sodium ascorbate (p.1390·1); calcium ascorbate (p.1389·3); hesperidin (p.1611·2); bioflavonoids (p.1611·1); rutoside (p.1611·2); rose fruit (p.1389·3); boneset (p.1586·1); echinacea (p.1606·2); achillea (p.1572·2).
Minor wounds; tonic.

Freeda, USA.
Citrus bioflavonoids complex (p.1611·1); hesperidin (p.1611·2).
Capillary bleeding.

Flavoquine *Roussel Diamant, Fr.*
Amodiaquine hydrochloride (p.430·3).
Malaria.

Flavorcee *Hudson, USA†.*
Ascorbic acid (p.1389·3).
Scurvy; vitamin C deficiency.

Flavorin *TO-Chemicals, Thai.*
Flavoxate hydrochloride (p.467·1).
Urinary-tract disorders.

Flavorola C *Lifeplan, UK.*
Vitamin C (p.1389·3); bioflavonoids (p.1611·1).
Nutritional supplement.

Flavovenyl *Plan, Switz.*
Capsules; oral drops: Bioflavonoids (p.1611·1); hesperidin methyl chalcone (p.1611·2); esculoside (p.1574·1).

Ointment: Bioflavonoids (p.1611·1); hesperidin methyl chalcone (p.1611·2); esculoside (p.1574·1); menthol (p.1632·3).
Peripheral vascular disorders.

Flavo-Zinc *Solgar, UK.*
Zinc gluconate (p.1398·2); zinc citrate.
Dietary supplement.

Flaxedil
Rhone-Poulenc Rorer, Austral.†; Rhodia, Braz.; Rhone-Poulenc Rorer, Canad.†; Rhone-Poulenc Rorer, Neth.†; Concord, UK.
Gallamine triethiodide (p.1337·1).
Competitive neuromuscular blocker.

Flebeside *Jorba, Spain.*
Carbazochrome (p.728·1); troxerutin (p.1611·2).
Vascular disorders.

Flebil *Molteni, Ital.*
Troxerutin (p.1611·2).
Peripheral vascular disorders.

Flebo Stop *Inexfa, Spain.*
Bromelains (p.1586·3); esculoside (p.1574·1); etofylline (p.765·1); hydrochlorothiazide (p.907·3).
Oedema; vascular disorders.

Flebobag Fisio *Grifols, Spain.*
Sodium chloride infusion (p.1196·1).
Fluid and electrolyte depletion; hypovolaemia.

Flebobag Glucosal *Grifols, Spain.*
Sodium chloride infusion (p.1196·1) with glucose (p.1364·2).
Fluid and electrolyte depletion; hypovolaemia.

Flebocortid
Hoechst Marion Roussel, Braz.; Lepetit, Ital.; Cilag, Mex.
Hydrocortisone sodium succinate (p.1074·1).
Corticosteroid.

Flebogamma
Grifols, Ger.; Grifols, Ital.; Grifols, Spain; Grifols, UK.
A normal immunoglobulin (p.1551·3).
Formerly known as Alphaglobin in the *UK.*
Hypogammaglobulinaemia; idiopathic thrombocytopenic purpura; passive immunisation.

Fleboplast Fisio *Grifols, Spain.*
Sodium chloride infusion (p.1196·1).
Fluid and electrolyte depletion; hypovolaemia.

Fleboplast Glucosal *Grifols, Spain.*
Sodium chloride infusion (p.1196·1) with glucose (p.1364·2).
Fluid and electrolyte depletion; hypovolaemia.

Fleboplast Plurisal *Grifols, Spain.*
Electrolyte infusion (p.1180·1) with sodium lactate (p.1186·2).
Fluid and electrolyte depletion; hypovolaemia.

Fleboside *Pharmafar, Ital.*
Troxerutin (p.1611·2); carbazochrome (p.728·1).
Capillary fragility; haemorrhoids; varicose ulcers.

Flebosmil *Socopharm, Fr.*
Diosmin (p.1611·1).
Peripheral vascular disorders.

Flebostasin
Sankyo, Ital.
Aesculus (p.1574·1).
Chronic venous insufficiency.

Sankyo, Spain.
Aescin (p.1574·1).
Oedema; peripheral vascular disorders.

Fleboton *Sanofi Winthrop, Port.†*
Hidrosmin (p.1611·2).
Oedema; vascular disorders.

Flebozin *Depofarma, Ital.*
Melilot; aesculus; centella (p.1350·1).
Nutritional supplement.

Flebs *Pierre Fabre, Ital.*
Heparin (p.902·1); a heparinoid (p.905·2).
Haemorrhoids; phlebitis; soft-tissue injury; thrombophlebitis.

Flecaine *3M, Fr.*
Flecainide acetate (p.890·1).
Arrhythmias.

Flecatab *Alphapharm, Austral.*
Flecainide acetate (p.890·1).
Arrhythmias.

Flectadol *Sanofi Synthelabo, Ital.*
Lysine aspirin (p.50·3).
Cold symptoms; fever; musculoskeletal and joint disorders; pain.

Flector
Genevrier, Fr.; IBSA, Hong Kong; IBSA, Ital.; IBSA, Switz.
Diclofenac epolamine (p.31·3) or diclofenac sodium (p.30·3).
Inflammation; musculoskeletal, joint, peri-articular, and soft-tissue disorders; pain.

Fleet
De Witt, Denm.; De Witt, Irl.; Pisa, Mex.
Monobasic sodium phosphate (p.1193·2); dibasic sodium phosphate (p.1193·2).
Bowel evacuation; constipation.

Fleet Babylax
Fleet, Singapore; Fleet, USA.
Glycerol (p.1616·3).
Constipation in children.

Fleet Bagenema *Fleet, USA.*
Liquid castile soap (p.1496·2).

Fleet Bisacodyl *Fleet, USA.*
Bisacodyl (p.1212·2).
Bowel evacuation; constipation.

Fleet Enema
Wolfs, Belg.; Whitehall, Braz.; Johnson & Johnson, Canad.; Fleet-De-witt, Hong Kong; Dexxon, Israel; Fleet, Singapore; Fleet, USA.
Dibasic sodium phosphate (p.1193·2); monobasic sodium phosphate (p.1193·2).
Bowel evacuation; constipation.

Fleet Enema Mineral Oil *Johnson & Johnson, Canad.*
Liquid paraffin (p.1407·1).
Bowel evacuation; constipation.

Fleet Klysma *Fleet, Neth.†*
Monobasic sodium phosphate (p.1193·2).
Bowel evacuation.

Fleet Laxative
Fleet, Austral.; Fleet, USA.
Bisacodyl (p.1212·2).
Bowel evacuation; constipation.

Fleet Medicated Pads *Fleet, USA.*
Hamamelis water (p.1618·3); alcohol; glycerol.
Anorectal disorders.

Fleet Micro *Ferring, Swed.*
Sodium citrate (p.1186·2); sodium lauril sulfoacetate (p.1496·3).
Constipation.

Fleet Micro-Enema
Note. This name is used for preparations of different composition.
Fleet, Austral.
Sodium citrate (p.1186·2); sodium lauril sulfoacetate (p.1496·3); sorbitol (p.1377·3).
Bowel evacuation; constipation.

Fleet-Dewitt, Hong Kong; Baxter, NZ; Fleet, NZ; De Witt, UK†.
Sodium citrate (p.1186·2); sodium lauril sulfoacetate (p.1496·3).
Bowel evacuation; constipation.

Fleet Pain Relief *Fleet, USA.*
Pramocaine hydrochloride (p.1318·2).
Anorectal disorders.

Fleet Phosphate Enema *Baxter, NZ; Fleet, NZ.*
Monobasic sodium phosphate (p.1193·2); dibasic sodium phosphate (p.1193·2).
Bowel evacuation; constipation.

Fleet Phospho-Soda
De Witt, Aust.; Fleet, Austral.; Wolfs, Belg.; Johnson & Johnson, Canad.; Ferring, Fr.; Ferring, Ger.; Fleet-Dewitt, Hong Kong; Fleet, Singapore; De Witt, UK; Fleet, USA.
Monobasic sodium phosphate (p.1193·2); dibasic sodium phosphate (p.1193·2).
Bowel evacuation; constipation.

Fleet Prep Kit No. 1 *Fleet, USA.*
Combination pack: Fleet Phospho-Soda; Fleet Bisacodyl Tablets (p.1212·2), 4 tablets; Fleet Bisacodyl Suppositories, 1 suppository.
Bowel evacuation.

Fleet Prep Kit No. 2 *Fleet, USA.*
Combination pack: Fleet Phospho-Soda; Fleet Bisacodyl Tablets (p.1212·2), 4 tablets; Fleet Bagenema, 1 enema.
Bowel evacuation.

Fleet Prep Kit No. 3 *Fleet, USA.*
Combination pack: Fleet Phospho-Soda; Fleet Bisacodyl Tablets (p.1212·2), 4 tablets; Fleet Bisacodyl Enema.
Bowel evacuation.

Fleet Prep Kit No. 4 *Fleet, USA†.*
Combination pack: Fleet Magnesium Citrate (p.1232·3); Fleet Bisacodyl Tablets (p.1212·2), 4 tablets; Fleet Bisacodyl Suppositories, 1 suppository.
Bowel evacuation.

Fleet Prep Kit No. 5 *Fleet, USA†.*
Combination pack: Fleet Magnesium Citrate (p.1232·3); Fleet Bisacodyl Tablets (p.1212·2), 4 tablets; Fleet Bagenema, 1 enema.
Bowel evacuation.

Fleet Prep Kit No. 6 *Fleet, USA†.*
Combination pack: Fleet Magnesium Citrate (p.1232·3); Fleet Bisacodyl Tablets (p.1212·2), 4 tablets; Fleet Bisacodyl Enema.
Bowel evacuation.

Fleet Ready-to-Use
Fleet, Austral.; De Witt, UK.
Monobasic sodium phosphate (p.1193·2); dibasic sodium phosphate (p.1193·2).
Bowel evacuation; constipation.

Flemex
Note. This name is used for preparations of different composition.
Precimex, Mex.
Hydrocortisone (p.1073·3).
Corticosteroid.

Parke, Davis, S.Afr.
Carbocisteine (p.1086·3).
Respiratory-tract disorders.

Flemeze *Parke-Med, S.Afr.*
Orciprenaline sulfate (p.769·1); bromhexine hydrochloride (p.1085·3).
Coughs.

Flemgo *Alliance, S.Afr.*
Carbocisteine (p.1086·3).
Respiratory-tract disorders.

Flemina *Precimex, Mex.*
Dopamine (p.881·3).

Flemizyme *Pascual, Hong Kong.*
Muramidase hydrochloride (p.1638·1).
Haemorrhage; sinusitis.

Flemlite *Aspen Consumer, S.Afr.*
Carbocisteine (p.1086·3).
Respiratory-tract disorders.

Flemoxin
Yamanouchi, Belg.; Yamanouchi, Denm.; Yamanouchi, Fin.; Ya-

manouchi, Neth.; Yamanouchi, Port.; Yamanouchi, Swed.†; Yamanouchi, Switz.
Amoxicillin (p.149·2), amoxicillin sodium (p.149·2), or amoxicillin trihydrate (p.149·2).
Bacterial infections.

Flemoxine *Yamanouchi, Fr.*
Amoxicillin trihydrate (p.149·2).
Bacterial infections.

Flemoxon *Merck, Mex.*
Amoxicillin trihydrate (p.149·2).
Bacterial infections.

Flemun *Intermuti, Ger.*
Sitosterol (p.970·3).
Rheumatic disorders.

Flenalgin *Kanda, Braz.*
Metixene hydrochloride (p.470·2); dipyrone (p.34·1).
Smooth muscle spasm.

Flenid *Merckle, Ger.*
Sodium cromoglicate (p.774·3).
Hypersensitivity reactions.

Flenin *Schuck, Ger.*
Homoeopathic preparation.

Flenverme *Hipolabor, Braz.*
Mebendazole (p.102·2); tiabendazole (p.109·1).
Worm infections.

Flerudin *Janssen-Cilag, Spain.*
Flunarizine hydrochloride (p.418·1).
Migraine; vertigo.

Fletanol *Sante Naturelle, Canad.*
Vitamin A and vitamin D (p.1350·1).

Fletchers Arachis Oil Retention Enema *Pharmax, UK.*
Arachis oil (p.1581·1).
Constipation.

Fletchers Castoria *Mentholatum, USA.*
Senna (p.1248·2).
Constipation.

Fletchers Childrens Laxative *Mentholatum, USA†.*
Yellow phenolphthalein (p.1244·1).
Constipation.

Fletchers Enemette
Pharmax, Irl.; Pharmax, UK.
Docusate sodium (p.1223·1).
Bowel evacuation; constipation.

Fletchers Phosphate Enema
Pharmax, Irl.; Pharmax, UK.
Monobasic sodium phosphate (p.1193·2); dibasic sodium phosphate (p.1193·2).
Bowel evacuation; constipation.

Fletchers Sore Mouth Medicine *Nasmark, Canad.*
Alum (p.1577·2); potassium chlorate (p.1654·1).
Canker sores; denture irritation; herpes labialis.

Flexafen *Diba, Mex.*
Ibuprofen (p.43·2).
Inflammation; musculoskeletal, joint, and peri-articular disorders; pain.

Flexagen *Aspen, S.Afr.*
Diclofenac sodium (p.30·3).
Inflammation; musculoskeletal and joint disorders; pain.

Flexagil *Diviser Aquilea, Spain.*
Carisoprodol (p.1327·1); propyphenazone (p.80·2).
Musculoskeletal spasms.

Flex-All *Chattem, Canad.*
Topical gel: Menthol (p.1632·3).
Muscle and joint pain.
Topical stick: Menthol (p.1632·3); methyl salicylate (p.55·1).
Musculoskeletal, joint, peri-articular, and soft-tissue disorders.

Flex-all 454 *Chattem, USA.*
Menthol (p.1632·3); methyl salicylate (p.55·1).
Musculoskeletal pain and stiffness.

Flexaphen *Trimen, USA.*
Chlorzoxazone (p.1327·3); paracetamol (p.71·2).
Musculoskeletal pain.

Flexar *Sanitas, Port.*
Piroxicam (p.79·1).
Gout; musculoskeletal, joint, and peri-articular disorders; pain.

Flexase *TAD, Ger.*
Piroxicam (p.79·1).
Gout; musculoskeletal, joint, and soft-tissue disorders.

Flex-Care
Alcon, Braz.; Alcon, USA.
Range of solutions for contact lenses (p.1129·2).

Flexdor *Bunker, Braz.*
Orphenadrine citrate (p.470·3); dipyrone (p.34·1); caffeine (p.761·3).
Skeletal muscle spasm.

Flexen
Note. This name is used for preparations of different composition.
Italfarmaco, Ital.
Ketoprofen (p.47·3) or ketoprofen sodium (p.48·1).
Gout; musculoskeletal, joint, peri-articular, and soft-tissue disorders.

Rayere, Mex.
Naproxen (p.60·3).
Inflammation; musculoskeletal and joint disorders.

Flexeril
Merck Frosst, Canad.; Merck, USA.
Cyclobenzaprine hydrochloride (p.1328·1).
Skeletal muscle spasm.

Flexfree *Whitehall, Belg.†*
Felbinac (p.36·1).
Soft-tissue, peri-articular, and joint pain and inflammation.

Flexiban
Neopharmed, Ital.; Frosst, Port.
Cyclobenzaprine hydrochloride (p.1328·1).
Skeletal muscle spasm.

Flexidin *Mundipharma, Aust.*
Indometacin (p.44·3).
Gout; inflammation; musculoskeletal, joint, and peri-articular disorders; oedema; pain.

Flexidol *Almirall, Spain.*
Fepradinol hydrochloride (p.40·3).
Peri-articular disorders; soft-tissue disorders.

Flexidone *Poli, Ital.†*
Carisoprodol (p.1327·1); propyphenazone (p.80·2).
Musculoskeletal and joint disorders.

flexi-loges *Loges, Ger.*
Devil's claw root (p.26·3).
Musculoskeletal and joint disorders.

Flexin
Note. This name is used for preparations of different composition.
Taro, Israel.
Orphenadrine citrate (p.470·3).
Skeletal muscle spasm.

Douglas, Thai.; TTN, Thai.
Naproxen (p.60·3).
Dysmenorrhoea; gout; musculoskeletal, joint, and peri-articular disorders.

Flexin Continus *Napp, Irl.; Napp, UK.*
Indometacin (p.44·3).
Gout; inflammation; musculoskeletal, joint, and peri-articular disorders; pain.

Flexirox *Asta Medica, Fr.*
Piroxicam (p.79·1).
Musculoskeletal, joint, and peri-articular disorders.

Flexital
Sun, Singapore; Sun, Thai.
Oxpentifylline [pentoxifylline] (p.950·3).
Cerebral, ocular, and peripheral vascular disorders.

Flexium *Aventis, Belg.*
Etofenamate (p.35·3).
Lumbar spondylosis; peri-articular disorders; soft-tissue injury.

Flexocutan N *Orion, Ger.*
Flufenamic acid (p.41·1); glycol salicylate (p.42·2); benzyl nicotinate (p.20·2).
Bruising; muscle and joint disorders; neuralgia.

Flexogyne *Biogyne, Fr.*
Benzalkonium chloride (p.1133·2).
Contraceptive.

Flexoject *Mayrand, USA.*
Orphenadrine citrate (p.470·3).
Musculoskeletal pain.

Flexon *Keene, USA.*
Orphenadrine citrate (p.470·3).
Musculoskeletal pain.

Flexotard *Pharmacia, UK.*
Diclofenac sodium (p.30·3).
Gout; inflammation; musculoskeletal, joint, peri-articular, and soft-tissue disorders; pain.

Flextra *Poly, USA.*
Paracetamol (p.71·2); phenyltoloxamine citrate (p.423·1).
Pain.

Flexurat
Note. This name is used for preparations of different composition.
Nycomed, Aust.
Suprarenal cortex (p.1080·1); pentosan polysulfate sodium (p.953·1).
Peri-articular, and soft-tissue disorders.

Truw, Ger.†
Bovine suprarenal cortex (p.1080·1); diethylamine salamidacetate (p.81·3); pentosan polysulfate sodium (p.953·1).
Joint and soft tissue disorders.

Flicum *Esteve, Spain.*
Flubendazole (p.99·2).
Ascariasis; enterobiasis; hookworm infections; trichuriasis.

Flindix *Vitoria, Port.*
Isosorbide dinitrate (p.915·2).
Angina pectoris; heart failure; myocardial infarction.

flint *Togal, Ger.*
Poly(butylmethacrylate, methylmethacrylate) (p.1635·2).
Wounds.

Flintstones
Bayer, Canad.; Bayer, Singapore; Miles Consumer Healthcare, USA.
Multivitamins or multivitamins and minerals (p.1350·1).

Flivas *Asahi, Jpn.*
Naftopidil (p.938·1).

Flixonase
Glaxo Wellcome, Aust.; Glaxo Wellcome, Belg.; Glaxo Wellcome, Denm.; Glaxo Wellcome, Fin.; Glaxo Wellcome, Fr.; Glaxo Wellcome, Hong Kong; Allen & Hanburys, Irl.; Glaxo Wellcome, Israel; Glaxo Wellcome, Ital.; Glaxo Wellcome, Mex.; Glaxo Wellcome, Neth.; Glaxo Wellcome, NZ; Glaxo Wellcome, S.Afr.; Glaxo Wellcome, Singapore; Glaxo Wellcome, Spain; Glaxo Wellcome, Thai.; Allen & Hanburys, UK.
Fluticasone propionate (p.1072·2).
Allergic rhinitis; nasal polyps.

Flixotaide *Glaxo Wellcome, Port.*
Fluticasone propionate (p.1072·2).
Asthma.

Flixotide
Glaxo Wellcome, Aust.; Glaxo Wellcome, Austral.; Glaxo Wellcome, Belg.; Glaxo Wellcome, Denm.; Glaxo Wellcome, Fin.; Glaxo Wellcome, Fr.; Glaxo Wellcome, Hong Kong; Allen & Hanburys, Irl.; Glaxo Wellcome, Israel; Glaxo Wellcome, Ital.; Glaxo Wellcome, Mex.; Glaxo Wellcome, Neth.; Glaxo Wellcome, NZ; Glaxo Wellcome, S.Afr.; Glaxo Wellcome, Singapore; Glaxo Wellcome, Spain; Glaxo Wellcome, Thai.; Allen & Hanburys, UK.
Fluticasone propionate (p.1072·2).
Asthma.

Flobacin *Sigma-Tau, Ital.*
Ofloxacin (p.232·3).
Bacterial infections.

Flociprin *Ibi, Ital.*
Ciprofloxacin hydrochloride (p.182·3) or ciprofloxacin lactate (p.182·3).
Bacterial infections.

Flo-Coat *Lafayette, USA.*
Barium sulfate (p.1032·1).
Contrast medium for gastrointestinal radiography.

Flocofil *Serono, Mex.*
Mercaptopurine (p.552·2).

Flocur *Pharmacia Upjohn, Mex.*
Tolfenamic acid (p.88·3).

Flodermol *Juventus, Spain.*
Fluocinolone acetonide (p.1071·1); gramicidin (p.213·3); neomycin sulfate (p.228·1).
Infected skin disorders.

Flodil *AstraZeneca, Fr.*
Felodipine (p.888·3).
Angina pectoris; hypertension.

Flodol *Uno, Ital.*
Piroxicam (p.79·1).
Musculoskeletal, joint, and peri-articular disorders.

Flogan *Merck, Braz.*
Diclofenac potassium (p.30·2).
Gout; inflammation; musculoskeletal, joint, and peri-articular disorders; pain.

Flogecyl *Wild, Switz.*
Aescin beta (p.1574·1); carrageenan (p.1500·1).
Mouth disorders.

Flogen *Fustery, Mex.*
Naproxen sodium (p.61·1).
Inflammation; pain.

Flogencyl *Expanpharm, Fr.*
Aescin (p.1574·1).
Mouth ulcers.

Flogene
Note. This name is used for preparations of different composition.
Ache, Braz.
Piroxicam betadex (p.79·1).
Dysmenorrhoea; gout; musculoskeletal, joint, and peri-articular disorders.

Polifarma, Ital.
Fentiazac (p.40·2) or fentiazac calcium (p.40·2).
Fever; inflammation; pain.

Flogiftalmina *Davi, Port.*
Phenylephrine hydrochloride (p.1097·1); prednisolone metasulfobenzoate sodium (p.1078·1).
Eye disorders.

Floginax *Teofarma, Ital.*
Naproxen (p.60·3).
Musculoskeletal and joint disorders; pain.

Flogi-Ped *Stiefel, Braz.*
Benzydamine hydrochloride (p.20·1).
Fever; inflammation; pain.

Flogiren *Sanval, Braz.*
Diclofenac (p.30·2).
Gout; inflammation; musculoskeletal, joint, and peri-articular disorders; pain.

Flogo Rosa *Asta Medica, Braz.*
Benzydamine hydrochloride (p.20·1).
Vaginal irritation.

Flogobene *Upsamedica, Ital.*
Piroxicam (p.79·1).
Musculoskeletal and joint disorders.

Flogocan *Quimedical, Port.*
Piroxicam (p.79·1).
Gout; musculoskeletal, joint, and peri-articular disorders; pain.

Flogocid
Note. This name is used for preparations of different composition.
Continental Pharma, Belg.
Bufexamac (p.20·3); neomycin sulfate (p.228·1); nystatin (p.392·2).
Infected skin disorders.

Continental Pharma, Switz.
Bufexamac (p.20·3).
Skin disorders.

Flogocid NN *Continental Pharma, Switz.†.*
Bufexamac (p.20·3); nystatin (p.392·2); neomycin sulfate (p.228·1).
Infected skin disorders.

Flogofenac *Ecobi, Ital.*
Diclofenac diethylamine (p.30·2) or diclofenac sodium (p.30·3).
Musculoskeletal, joint, and soft-tissue disorders.

Flogogin *Tosi, Ital.†.*
Tablets; injection; suppositories: Naproxen sodium (p.61·1).

Lignocaine [lidocaine] hydrochloride (p.1313·2) and lignocaine [lidocaine] (p.1313·2) are included in the intramuscular injection to alleviate the pain of injection.
Musculoskeletal and joint disorders; pain.

Topical gel: Naproxen sodium (p.61·1); a heparinoid (p.905·2).
Inflammation; musculoskeletal and joint disorders; pain.

Flogoken *Kener, Mex.*
Diclofenac (p.30·2).

Flogoprofen *Wasserman, Spain.*
Etofenamate (p.35·3).
Pain; peri-articular disorders.

Flogoral
Asta Medica, Braz.; Lepori, Port.
Benzydamine hydrochloride (p.20·1).
Mouth and throat disorders.

Flogosan *Liomont, Mex.*
Piroxicam (p.79·1).
Inflammation; musculoskeletal and joint disorders; pain.

Flogoter *Estedi, Spain.*
Indometacin (p.44·3).
Gout; inflammation; musculoskeletal and joint disorders; pain; peri-articular disorders.

Flogotisol
Zambon, Braz.; Zambon, Ital.
Thiamphenicol sodium glycinate isophthalolate (p.262·1).
Lignocaine [lidocaine] (p.1313·2) may be included in the injection to alleviate the pain of injection.
Bacterial infections.

Flogoxen *Medley, Braz.*
Piroxicam (p.79·1).
Dysmenorrhoea; gout; musculoskeletal, joint, and peri-articular disorders.

Flogozen *Valeas, Ital.*
Imidazole salicylate (p.44·3).
Fever; otorhinolaryngeal inflammation.

Flolan
Glaxo Wellcome, Aust.; Glaxo Wellcome, Belg.; Glaxo Wellcome, Canad.; Glaxo Wellcome, Denm.; Glaxo Wellcome, Fr.; Wellcome, Irl.; Glaxo Wellcome, Ital.; Glaxo Wellcome, Neth.; Wellcome, Spain; Wellcome, UK; Glaxo Wellcome, USA.
Epoprostenol sodium (p.1443·3).
Pulmonary hypertension; thrombosis prophylaxis during renal dialysis.

Flolid *CT, Ital.*
Nimesulide (p.62·3).
Fever; inflammation; pain.

Flomax
Note. This name is used for preparations of different composition.
CSL, Austral.; Boehringer Ingelheim, Canad.; Pharmaplan, S.Afr.; Yamanouchi, UK; Boehringer Ingelheim, USA.
Tamsulosin hydrochloride (p.978·3).
Benign prostatic hyperplasia.

Chiesi, Ital.
Morniflumate (p.56·1).
Fever; inflammation; pain.

Flomed *Pulitzer, Ital.*
Buflomedil hydrochloride (p.851·3).
Cerebral and peripheral vascular disorders.

Flomox *Shionogi, Jpn.*
Cefcapene pivoxil hydrochloride (p.165·2).
Bacterial infections.

Flonase *Glaxo Wellcome, Canad.; Glaxo Wellcome, USA.*
Fluticasone propionate (p.1072·2).
Allergic rhinitis.

Flopen *CSL, Austral.*
Flucloxacillin magnesium (p.207·1) or flucloxacillin sodium (p.207·1).
Gram-positive coccal infections.

florabio Mann-Feigen-Sirup mit Senna *Florabio, Ger.*
Fig (p.1227·1); cassia; manna (p.1233·3).
Constipation.

florabio naturreiner Heilpflanzensaft *Florabio, Ger.*
A range of plant extracts.

Floradix *Salus, Fr.*
Nutritional supplement with iron (p.1350·1).

Floradix Krauterblut *Salushaus, Ger.*
Urtica; couch-grass; thall. rhodophyceae; crataegus; centaury; rose fruit; dried yeast; ferrous gluconate; vitamins.
Tonic.

Floradix Krauterblut-S-Saft *Salushaus, Ger.*
Thall. macrocystis pyrifera; urtica; couch-grass; achillea; fennel; rad. dauc. carot.; wheat-germ; dried bitter-orange peel; angelica; equisetum; juniper; ferrous gluconate; vitamins; rose fruit.
Tonic.

Floradix Maskam *Duopharm, Ger.†.*
Frangula bark (p.1227·1); rhubarb (p.1248·1); senna (p.1248·2); fennel (p.1610·1).
Constipation.

Floradix Multipretten *Salushaus, Ger.*
Caraway (p.1591·2); caraway oil (p.1591·2); fennel (p.1610·1); fennel oil (p.1610·2); anise oil (p.1580·3); coriander (p.1599·2); coriander oil (p.1599·2); peppermint leaf (p.1243·2); peppermint oil (p.1243·3); absinthium (p.1571·1); achillea (p.1572·3); imperatoria root; bromelains (p.1586·3); enzymes from *Aspergillus oryzae.*
Gastrointestinal disorders.

Floralac *Fresenius Kabi, Aust.*
Lactulose (p.1230·1).
Constipation; hepatic encephalopathy.

Floralax *Flora, Canad.†.*
Ispaghula (p.1229·1).

Floralaxative *Lalco, Canad.†.*
Buckthorn (p.1215·1); senna (p.1248·2).

Floran Effervescent *McGloin, Austral.†.*
Sodium fluoride (p.1375·3).
Dental caries prophylaxis.

Floraquin
Note. This name is used for preparations of different composition.
Searle, Austral.†; Searle, Thai.
Diiodohydroxyquinoline (p.590·2); boric acid (p.1586·1); phosphoric acid (p.1651·1).
Vaginal infections.

Searle, S.Afr.†.
Diiodohydroxyquinoline (p.590·2).
Vaginal infections.

Florate *Alcon, Braz.*
Fluorometholone acetate (p.1072·1).
Eye disorders.

Floratil
Merck, Braz.; Merck, Mex.
Lysate of *Saccharomyces boulardii* (p.1626·3).
Diarrhoea; restoration of gastrointestinal flora.

Florbiox *Crinos, Ital.*
Multivitamin and mineral preparation with *Lactobacillus acidophilus* (p.1350·1)(p.1626·3).
Maintenance of gastrointestinal flora.

Floregin *Abbott, Braz.*
Muramidase hydrochloride (p.1638·1); nimorazole (p.598·3).
Vulvovaginal infections.

Floregin Composto *Abbott, Braz.*
Nimorazole (p.598·3); clotrimazole (p.382·1); muramidase (p.1638·1).
Vulvovaginal infections.

Florelax *Sanofi Synthelabo, Ital.*
Dried yeast (p.1398·1); lactic-acid-producing organisms (p.1626·3); chamomile (p.1593·2); angelica (p.1580·2); valerian (p.1678·3); peppermint leaf (p.1243·2); caraway (p.1591·2); vitamin B substances (p.1350·1).
Gastrointestinal disorders.

Florelax Stomaco *Sanofi Synthelabo, Ital.*
Pineapple stem; rice starch; dog rose; green tea (p.1350·1).
Gastrointestinal disorders.

Florerbe Lassativa *Bonomelli, Ital.*
Senna (p.1248·2); boldo (p.1585·3); cynara (p.1601·3); aniseed (p.1580·2); liquorice (p.1231·2).
Constipation.

Floresse *Roche Consumer, UK.*
Borage oil (p.1613·1) with or without vitamins.

Florgynal *Lyocentre, Fr.*
Estriol (p.1475·3); progesterone (p.1488·3); *Lactobacillus casei* var. *Rhamnosus* (p.1626·3).

Floriabene *Cefak, Ger.*
Ethyl linoleate.
Skin disorders.

Florical *Mericon, USA.*
Calcium carbonate (p.1215·1); sodium fluoride (p.1375·3).
Dietary supplement.

Florida Sunburn Relief *Pharmacel, USA†.*
Benzyl alcohol (p.1135·2); phenol (p.1152·3); camphor (p.1589·3); menthol (p.1632·3).

Floridine *DHN, Fr.*
Preparation for enteral nutrition (p.1350·1).

Florigien *Schering, Ital.*
Nonoxinol 9 (p.1346·1); phenoxyethanol (p.1153·3); sodium laurilsulfate (p.1496·3); thymol (p.1158·3).
Vaginal infections.

Florilax
Note. This name is used for preparations of different composition.
Floris, Israel.
Senna (p.1248·2).
Constipation.

Confar, Port.
Glucomannan (p.1616·2).
Constipation; hyperlipidaemias; obesity.

Florinef
Bristol-Myers Squibb, Austral.; Roberts, Canad.; Bristol-Myers Squibb, Denm.; Bristol-Myers Squibb, Fin.; Bristol-Myers Squibb, Hong Kong; Bristol-Myers Squibb, Irl.; Bristol-Myers Squibb, Neth.; Bristol-Myers Squibb, Norw.; Bristol-Myers Squibb, NZ; Bristol-Myers Squibb, S.Afr.; Bristol-Myers Squibb, Singapore; Bristol-Myers Squibb, Swed.; Bristol-Myers Squibb, Switz.; Bristol-Myers Squibb, Thai.; Squibb, UK; Monarch, USA.
Fludrocortisone acetate (p.1070·1).
Adrenocortical insufficiency; congenital adrenal hyperplasia.

Florinefe *Bristol-Myers Squibb, Braz.*
Fludrocortisone acetate (p.1070·1).
Adrenocortical insufficiency; congenital adrenal hyperplasia; orthostatic hypotension.

Florisan N *Boehringer Ingelheim, Ger.†.*
Bisacodyl (p.1212·2).
Constipation.

Florisene *Lamberts Healthcare, UK.*
Ferrous glycine sulfate; vitamin C; vitamin B$_{12}$; lysine (p.1350·1).
Hair loss in women.

Florissamol *Andrae, Aust.*
Urtica (p.1678·2); camphor (p.1589·3).
Chillblains; muscle and joint pain; scalp disorders; soft-tissue disorders.

Florlax *Cazi, Braz.*
Senna (p.1248·2); tamarind (p.1253·2); coriander (p.1599·2); cassia pulp (p.1216·2).
Constipation.

Florocycline *SmithKline Beecham, Fr.†.*
Tetracycline hydrochloride (p.258·3).
Bacterial infections.

Florone
Pharmacia Upjohn, Canad.†; Galderma, Ger.; Dermik, USA.
Diflorasone diacetate (p.1069·2).
Skin disorders.

Floropryl *Merck Sharp & Dohme, USA†.*
Dyflos (p.1417·3).
Open-angle glaucoma; strabismus.

Florvite *Everett, USA.*
A range of vitamin and fluoride (p.1375·3) preparations with or without minerals (p.1350·1).
Dental caries prophylaxis; dietary supplement.

Flosa *Merckle, Ger.*
Ispaghula (p.1229·1).
Constipation; stool softener.

Flosine *Bittermedizin, Ger.*
Ispaghula (p.1229·1).
Constipation; stool softener.

Flossac *Caber, Ital.*
Norfloxacin (p.232·1).
Bacterial urinary-tract infections.

Flotiran *Schering-Plough, Port.*
Betamethasone dipropionate (p.1063·2); clotrimazole (p.382·1).
Infected skin disorders.

Flotrin *Abbott, Ger.; Kanoldt, Ger.*
Terazosin hydrochloride (p.980·1).
Benign prostatic hyperplasia.

Flovent *Glaxo Wellcome, Canad.; Glaxo Wellcome, USA.*
Fluticasone propionate (p.1072·2).
Asthma.

Flowmega *Lifeplan, UK.*
Omega-3 marine triglycerides (p.949·3).

Floxacin
Merck Sharp & Dohme, Braz.; Medix, Mex.
Norfloxacin (p.232·1).
Bacterial infections.

Floxacipron *BA Farma, Port.†.*
Ciprofloxacin (p.182·3).
Bacterial infections.

Floxakin *Kener, Mex.*
Ciprofloxacin (p.182·3).
Bacterial infections.

Floxal
Riel, Aust.; Mann, Ger.; Chauvin Novopharma, Switz.
Ofloxacin (p.232·3).
Bacterial eye infections.

Floxalin *Salus, Ital.*
Naproxen sodium (p.61·1).
Musculoskeletal and joint disorders; pain.

Floxapen
SmithKline Beecham, Aust.; SmithKline Beecham, Austral.; SmithKline Beecham, Belg.; SmithKline Beecham, Irl.; SmithKline Beecham, Mex.; SmithKline Beecham, Neth.; SmithKline Beecham, NZ; Beecham, Port.; SmithKline Beecham, S.Afr.; SmithKline Beecham, Switz.; SmithKline Beecham, UK.
Flucloxacillin magnesium (p.207·1) or flucloxacillin sodium (p.207·1).
Bacterial infections.

Floxedol *Oftalder, Port.*
Ofloxacin (p.232·3).
Bacterial eye infections.

Floxenor *Pose, Thai.*
Norfloxacin (p.232·1).
Bacterial infections.

Floxil
Note. This name is used for preparations of different composition.
Dumex-Alpharma, Hong Kong.
Menthol (p.1632·3); tartaric acid (p.1669·2).
Sore throat.

Janssen, Mex.
Ofloxacin (p.232·3).
Bacterial infections.

Tecnimede, Port.
Flucloxacillin sodium (p.207·1).
Bacterial infections.

Dumex-Alpharma, Singapore.
Dichlorobenzyl alcohol (p.1143·2); amylmetacresol (p.1133·2); menthol (p.1632·3).
Sore throat.

Floxin
Note. This name is used for preparations of different composition.
Janssen-Ortho, Canad.; Ortho McNeil, USA; Daiichi, USA.
Ofloxacin (p.232·3).
Bacterial infections.

Sriprasit, Thai.
Flunarizine hydrochloride (p.418·1).
Cerebral and peripheral vascular disorders.

Floxinol *Millet Roux, Braz.*
Norfloxacin (p.232·1).
Bacterial infections.

The symbol † denotes a preparation no longer actively marketed

Floxstat *Cilag, Braz.; Cilag, Mex.*
Ofloxacin (p.232·3).
Bacterial infections.

Floxyfral *Solvay, Aust.; Solvay, Belg.; Solvay, Fr.; Solvay, Switz.*
Fluvoxamine maleate (p.289·3).
Depression; obsessive-compulsive disorder.

Flu-21 *Uno, Ital.*
Fluocinonide (p.1071·2).
Skin disorders.

Flu, Cold & Cough Medicine *Major, USA.*
Chlorpheniramine [chlorphenamine] maleate (p.412·1); dextromethorphan hydrobromide (p.1087·3); paracetamol (p.71·2); pseudoephedrine hydrochloride (p.1099·2).
Coughs and cold symptoms.

Flu & Fever Relief *Brauer, Austral.*
Homoeopathic preparation.

Flu Oph *Seng, Thai.*
Fluorometholone (p.1072·1).
Inflammatory eye disorders.

Fluad *Chiron, Ital.*
An influenza vaccine (p.1544·3).
Active immunisation.

Fluagel *EMS, Braz.*
Aluminium hydroxide (p.1210·3).
Gastrointestinal hyperacidity.

Flu-Amp *Generics, UK.*
Ampicillin trihydrate (p.151·1); flucloxacillin sodium (p.207·1).
These ingredients can be described by the British Approved Name Co-fluampicil.
Bacterial infections.

Fluanxol
Lundbeck, Aust.; Lundbeck, Austral.; Lundbeck, Belg.; Lundbeck, Canad.; Lundbeck, Denm.; Lundbeck, Fin.; Lundbeck, Fr.; Bayer, Ger.; Lundbeck, Hong Kong; Lundbeck, Irl.; Lundbeck, Israel; Organon, Mex.; Lundbeck, Neth.; Lundbeck, Norw.; Dumex, Port.; Lundbeck, S.Afr.; Lundbeck, Singapore; Lundbeck, Swed.; Lundbeck, Switz.; Lundbeck, Thai.; Lundbeck, UK.
Flupentixol (p.684·2), flupentixol decanoate (p.684·1), or flupentixol hydrochloride (p.684·1).
Alcohol withdrawal syndrome; anxiety; depression; psychoses.

Fluarix
SmithKline Beecham, Aust.; SmithKline Beecham, Austral.; SmithKline Beecham, Denm.; SmithKline Beecham, Fin.; SmithKline Beecham, Fr.; SmithKline Beecham, Hong Kong; SmithKline Beecham, Irl.; SmithKline Beecham, Ital.; SmithKline Beecham, Mex.; SmithKline Beecham, Neth.; SmithKline Beecham, Norw.; SmithKline Beecham, NZ; Smith Kline & French, Port.†; SmithKline Beecham, Spain; SmithKline Beecham, Swed.; SmithKline Beecham, Switz.; SmithKline Beecham, UK.
An inactivated influenza vaccine (split virion) (p.1544·3).
Active immunisation.

Fluaton *Tubilux, Ital.*
Fluorometholone (p.1072·1).
Inflammatory eye disorders.

Flubason
Hoechst Marion Roussel, Ital.; Hoechst Marion Roussel, Spain.
Desoximetasone (p.1066·2).
Skin disorders.

Flubenil *Formenti, Ital.†.*
Ibuprofen guaiacol (p.44·1).
Cold symptoms; fever; pain.

Flubilar *Byk, Fr.*
Sodium methylcamphorate.
Constipation; digestive disorders.

Flubiotic NF *Pharmazam, Spain.*
Amoxicillin trihydrate (p.149·2).
Flubiotic formerly contained acetylcysteine and amoxicillin trihydrate.
Bacterial infections.

Fluciderm *Shiwa, Thai.*
Fluocinolone acetonide (p.1071·1).
Skin disorders.

Fluciderm-N *Shiwa, Thai.*
Fluocinolone acetonide (p.1071·1); neomycin sulfate (p.228·1).
Infected skin disorders.

Flucil
Note. This name is used for preparations of different composition.
Rhone-Poulenc Rorer, Austral.
Flucloxacillin sodium (p.207·1).
Gram-positive coccal infections.

Masa, Thai.
Acetylcysteine (p.1082·3).
Respiratory-tract disorders associated with increased or viscous mucus.

Flucillin
Pinewood, Irl.; Rolab, S.Afr.
Flucloxacillin sodium (p.207·1).
Now known as Rolab-Flucloxacillin in S.Afr.
Bacterial infections.

Flucin *Wayne, Mex.*
Fluocinolone (p.1071·1).
Skin disorders.

Flucinal *Nobel, Ital.*
Flucloxacillin sodium (p.207·1).
Bacterial infections.

Flucinar *Medphano, Ger.*
Fluocinolone acetonide (p.1071·1).
Skin disorders.

Flucinome *Essex, Switz.*
Flutamide (p.542·3).
Prostatic cancer.

Fluclomix *Ashbourne, UK.*
Flucloxacillin sodium (p.207·1).
Bacterial infections.

Fluclon *Clonmel, Irl.†.*
Flucloxacillin sodium (p.207·1).
Gram-positive bacterial infections.

Flucloxil *Duopharma, Hong Kong.*
Flucloxacillin (p.207·1).
Bacterial infections.

Flucloxin
Douglas, NZ; Rivopharm, Switz.†.
Flucloxacillin sodium (p.207·1).
Gram-positive bacterial infections.

Fluclox-Reu *Reusch, Ger.*
Flucloxacillin sodium (p.207·1).
Bacterial infections.

Flucol *Apotex, S.Afr.†; Garec, S.Afr.†.*
Paracetamol (p.71·2); codeine phosphate (p.25·2); caffeine (p.761·3); mepyramine maleate (p.421·1); phenylephrine hydrochloride (p.1097·1).
Cold and influenza symptoms; sinusitis.

Flucon
Alcon, Aust.; Alcon, Belg.; Alcon, Fr.; Alcon, Hong Kong; Alcon, NZ; Alcon, S.Afr.; Alcon, Thai.
Fluorometholone (p.1072·1).
Inflammatory eye disorders.

Fluconal *Libbs, Braz.*
Fluconazole (p.383·2).
Fungal infections.

Flu-Cortanest *Piam, Ital.*
Diflucortolone valerate (p.1069·3).
Burns; insect stings; skin disorders.

Flucozole *Siam Bheasach, Thai.*
Fluconazole (p.383·2).
Fungal infections.

Fluctin *Lilly, Ger.*
Fluoxetine hydrochloride (p.284·2).
Bulimia nervosa; depression; obsessive-compulsive disorder.

Fluctine
Lilly, Aust.; Lilly, Switz.
Fluoxetine hydrochloride (p.284·2).
Bulimia nervosa; depression; obsessive-compulsive disorder.

Flucur *Shigaken, Singapore.*
Chlorpheniramine [chlorphenamine] maleate (p.412·1); naphazoline hydrochloride (p.1095·1).
Cold symptoms; rhinitis; sinusitis.

Fludactil *Aspen Consumer, S.Afr.*
Triprolidine hydrochloride (p.427·2); pseudoephedrine hydrochloride (p.1099·2).
Cold and influenza symptoms.

Fludactil Co *Aspen Consumer, S.Afr.*
Triprolidine hydrochloride (p.427·2); pseudoephedrine hydrochloride (p.1099·2); codeine phosphate (p.25·2).
Coughs.

Fludactil Expectorant *Aspen Consumer, S.Afr.*
Triprolidine hydrochloride (p.427·2); pseudoephedrine hydrochloride (p.1099·2); guaifenesin (p.1092·2).
Coughs.

Fludan *Biolab, Thai.*
Flunarizine (p.418·2).
Cerebrovascular disorders; migraine.

Fludan Codeina *Ipsen, Spain.*
Codeine phosphate (p.25·2).
Coughs; diarrhoea; pain.

Fludapamide *Spirig, Switz.*
Indapamide (p.913·1).
Hypertension.

Fludara
Schering, Aust.; Schering, Austral.; Schering, Belg.; Berlex, Canad.; Schering, Denm.; Schering, Fin.; Schering, Fr.; Medac, Ger.; Schering, Ger.; Schering, Israel; Schering, Ital.; Schering, Mex.; Schering, Neth.; Schering, Norw.; Schering, NZ; Schering, Port.; Schering, S.Afr.; Schering, Singapore; Schering, Swed.; Schering, Switz.; Schering, Thai.; Schering, UK; Berlex, USA.
Fludarabine phosphate (p.539·3) or fludarabine phosphate sodium (p.540·1).
Chronic lymphocytic leukaemia.

Fludarene *Merck Sharp & Dohme, Ital.*
Chromocarb diethylamine (p.1594·3).
Capillary fragility.

Fludecate
Unipharm, Israel; Intramed, S.Afr.
Fluphenazine decanoate (p.684·3).
Psychoses.

Fluden *Rekah, Israel.*
Sodium fluoride (p.1375·3).
Dental caries prophylaxis.

Fludent
Alpharma, Fin.; Dumex-Alpharma, Swed.
Sodium fluoride (p.1375·3).
Dental caries prophylaxis.

Fludestrin *Bristol-Myers Squibb, Ger.*
Testolactone (p.574·2).
Breast cancer.

Fludeten
Alter, Spain; Alter, Spain.
Paracetamol (p.71·2); codeine phosphate (p.25·2).
Pain.

Fludex
Servier, Aust.; Servier, Belg.; Servier, Denm.; Eutherapie, Fr.; Servier, Neth.; Servier, Port.; Servier, Switz.
Indapamide (p.913·1).
Hypertension.

Fludilat
Akzo, Braz.; Thiemann, Ger.; Organon, Hong Kong; Organon, Port.; Organon, Switz.†; Organon, Thai.
Bencyclane fumarate (p.843·3).
Vascular disorders.

Fluditec *Innotech, Fr.*
Carbocisteine (p.1086·3).
Respiratory-tract congestion.

Fludren *Diafarm, Spain.*
Dextromethorphan hydrobromide (p.1087·3); ephedrine hydrochloride (p.1090·1); chlorpheniramine [chlorphenamine] maleate (p.412·1).
Coughs.

Fludronef *Iquinosa, Spain.*
Fludrocortisone acetate (p.1070·1); gramicidin (p.213·3); neomycin sulfate (p.228·1).
Eye disorders; infected skin disorders.

Fluend
Note. This name is used for preparations of different composition.
Herbaline, Ital.†.
Silver birch (p.1585·2); salix (p.82·1); thyme (p.1672·1); tilia (p.1673·2); cynara (p.1601·3); rose fruit (p.1389·3); citrus aurantium.
Cold and influenza symptoms.

Genpharm, S.Afr.†.
Diphenhydramine hydrochloride (p.416·1); paracetamol (p.71·2); phenylephrine hydrochloride (p.1097·1); ascorbic acid (p.1389·3).
Cold symptoms.

Fluental *Hoechst Marion Roussel, Ital.*
Sobrerol (p.1100·3); paracetamol (p.71·2).
Respiratory-tract disorders.

Fluenzen *Ecupharma, Ital.*
Imidazole salicylate (p.44·3).
Fever; otorhinolaryngeal inflammation.

Flufenan *Cristalia, Braz.*
Fluphenazine (p.684·3).
Psychoses.

Fluforte *Allergan, Mex.*
Fluorometholone (p.1072·1).

Flugen *Ciba Vision, Spain.*
Fluorometholone (p.1072·1); gentamicin sulfate (p.210·1).
Ocular inflammation following cataract surgery.

Flugeral *Italfarmaco, Ital.*
Flunarizine hydrochloride (p.418·1).
Migraine; vertigo.

Flui-Amoxicillin *Zambon, Ger.*
Amoxicillin trihydrate (p.149·2).
Bacterial infections.

Fluibil *Zambon, Braz.*
Chenodeoxycholic acid (p.1594·1).
Cholesterol gallstones.

Fluibron
Farmalab, Braz.; Chiesi, Ital.; Chiesi, Singapore; Chiesi, Switz.
Ambroxol hydrochloride (p.1084·3).
Respiratory-tract disorders associated with increased or viscous mucus.

Fluid Loss
Note. This name is used for preparations of different composition.
Vitaglow, Austral.
Celery (p.1592·3); juniper (p.1625·2); bearberry (p.1583·3); parsley (p.1648·3); potassium chloride (p.1194·3).
Fluid retention.

Vitaplex, Austral.
Celery (p.1592·3); buchu (p.1587·2); taraxacum (p.1669·1); bearberry (p.1583·3).
Fluid retention.

Fluidasa
Knoll, Mex.; Knoll, Spain.
Mepifylline (p.421·1).
Obstructive airways disease.

Fluide Hydratant Matifiant *Vichy, Canad.†.*
SPF 13: Octinoxate (p.1517·3); ensulizole (p.1517·2).
Sunscreen.

Fluide Hydratant Quotidien *L'Oreal, Canad.*
SPF 15: Octinoxate (p.1517·3); ensulizole (p.1517·2).
Sunscreen.

Fluide Multi-Confort *Clarins, Canad.*
SPF 15: Octinoxate (p.1517·3); oxybenzone (p.1518·1); titanium dioxide (p.1126·1).
Sunscreen.

Fluide Multi-Regenerant Lift Jour *Clarins, Canad.*
SPF 15: Octinoxate (p.1517·3); oxybenzone (p.1518·1).
Sunscreen.

Fluide Protecteur Jeunesse des Mains *Clarins, Canad.*
SPF 15: Avobenzone (p.1517·1); octinoxate (p.1517·3); octisalate (p.1518·1); oxybenzone (p.1518·1).
Sunscreen.

Fluidema *Baldacci, Port.*
Indapamide (p.913·1).
Hypertension.

Fluiden *Lagos, Ital.*
Fenspiride hydrochloride (p.765·3).
Respiratory-tract disorders.

Fluidex *O'Connor, USA†.*
Buchu (p.1587·2); couch-grass (p.1599·3); corn silk (p.1599·3); hydrangea (p.1621·1).
Oedema.

Fluidex with Pamabrom *O'Connor, USA†.*
Pamabrom (p.952·1).
Oedema associated with premenstrual syndrome.

Fluidin
Note. This name is used for preparations of different composition.
Ativus, Braz.
Ambroxol (p.1084·3).
Respiratory-tract congestion.

Lasa, Spain†.
Guaifenesin (p.1092·2).
Coughs.

Fluidin Adulto *Merck, Port.*
Codeine (p.25·2); guaifenesin (p.1092·2); sodium benzoate (p.1134·3); ammonium acetate (p.1085·1); ephedrine hydrochloride (p.1090·1); caffeine (p.761·3); sodium iodide (p.1522·3); ipecacuanha (p.1093·1).
Coughs and other respiratory-tract disorders.

Fluidin Antiasmatico *Merck, Port.*
Aminophylline (p.760·1); potassium iodide (p.1522·3); ephedrine hydrochloride (p.1090·1); phenobarbital (p.355·1); sodium benzoate (p.1134·3); senega (p.1100·2); ipecacuanha (p.1093·1); belladonna (p.463·1); thyme (p.1672·2).
Asthma.

Fluidin Infantil *Merck, Port.*
Guaifenesin (p.1092·2); sodium benzoate (p.1134·3); ammonium acetate (p.1085·1); cowslip (p.1600·1); senega (p.1100·2); pine oil; drosera (p.1606·1); belladonna (p.463·1).
Coughs and other respiratory-tract disorders.

Fluidin Mucolitico NF *Ipsen, Spain.*
Carbocisteine (p.1086·3).
Fluidin Mucolitico formerly contained butetamate citrate, carbocisteine, diprophylline, and guaifenesin.
Respiratory-tract disorders.

Fluidin Nocturno *Merck, Port.†.*
Codeine (p.25·2); ethylmorphine hydrochloride (p.35·2); terpin hydrate (p.1101·2); homatropine methylbromide (p.468·1); phenobarbital (p.355·1); eucalyptol (p.1609·2).
Coughs.

Flui-DNCG *Zambon, Ger.*
Sodium cromoglicate (p.774·3).
Asthma.

Fluidox *Baldacci, Port.*
Ambroxol hydrochloride (p.1084·3).
Respiratory tract disorders.

Fluifort *Dompe, Ital.*
Carbocisteine lysine (p.1086·3).
Respiratory disorders associated with excessive or viscous mucus.

Fluilast *Boniscontro & Gazzone, Ital.*
Ticlopidine hydrochloride (p.981·1).
Thrombosis prophylaxis.

Fluimucil
Strallhofer, Aust.; Zambon, Braz.; Zambon, Fr.; Zambon, Ger.; Inpharzam, Hong Kong; Zambon, Ital.; Zambon, Neth.; Zambon, Port.; Zambon, Singapore; Zambon, Spain; Inpharzam, Switz.; Sermmitr, Thai.; Zambon, Thai.
Acetylcysteine (p.1082·3).
Poisoning with paracetamol, acrylonitrile, methacrynitrile, or methyl bromide; respiratory-tract disorders associated with increased or viscous mucus; urotoxicity caused by ifosfamide and cyclophosphamide.

Fluimucil Antibiotic
Note. This name is used for preparations of different composition.
Zambon, Belg.
Thiamphenicol glycine acetylcysteinate (p.262·1).
Bacterial infections of the respiratory tract associated with increased or viscous mucus.

Zambon, Fr.
Thiamphenicol acetylcysteinate (p.262·1).
Respiratory-tract infections.

Sermmitr, Thai.; Zambon, Thai.
Thiamphenicol (p.261·3); acetylcysteine (p.1082·3).
Respiratory-tract infections associated with increased or viscous mucus.

Fluimucil Antibiotico
Zambon, Ital.; Zambon, Spain.
Thiamphenicol glycine acetylcysteinate (p.262·1).
Respiratory-tract infections.

Fluimucil Biotic *Zambon, Braz.*
Acetylcysteine (p.1082·3); thiamphenicol (p.261·3).
Respiratory-tract infections.

Fluimucil Solucao Nasal *Zambon, Braz.*
Acetylcysteine (p.1082·3); benzalkonium chloride (p.1133·2); sodium chloride (p.1196·1).
Nasal congestion.

Flu-Imune *Lederle-Praxis, USA†.*
An influenza vaccine (p.1544·3).

Fluinol *Almirall, Spain.*
Fluticasone propionate (p.1072·2).
Nasal polyps; rhinitis.

Fluisedal *Elerte, Fr.*
Meglumine benzoate; polysorbate 20 (p.1347·3); promethazine hydrochloride (p.423·2).
Respiratory-tract congestion.

Fluisedal sans promethazine *Elerte, Fr.*
Meglumine benzoate; polysorbate 20 (p.1347·3).
Respiratory-tract congestion.

Flui-Theophylline *Zambon, Ger.†.*
Theophylline (p.777·2).
Obstructive airways disease.

Fluiven *Herbaline, Ital.†.*
Achillea (p.1572·2); centella (p.1112·2); hamamelis (p.1618·3); myrtillus (p.1639·2).
Peripheral vascular disorders.

Fluixol *Nutrifar, Ital.*
Ambroxol hydrochloride (p.1084·3).
Respiratory-tract disorders.

Fluken *Kendrick, Mex.*
Flutamide (p.542·3).
Prostatic cancer.

Flukenol *Kendrick, Mex.*
Fluconazole (p.383·2).
Fungal infections.

Flukezol *Kener, Mex.*
Fluconazole (p.383·2).
Fungal infections.

Flukit *Julphar, UAE.*
Syrup: Paracetamol (p.71·2); pseudoephedrine hydrochloride (p.1099·2); chlorpheniramine [chlorphenamine] maleate (p.412·1).
Cold and influenza symptoms.
Tablets: Paracetamol (p.71·2); salicylamide (p.82·1); promethazine hydrochloride (p.423·2); phenylephrine hydrochloride (p.1097·1).
Cold and influenza symptoms; rhinitis.

Flulem *Lemery, Mex.*
Flutamide (p.542·3).
Prostatic cancer.

Flulium
Note.This name is used for preparations of different composition.
Pharmasant, Thai.
Dipotassium clorazepate (p.670·3).
Anxiety; depression; dystonias.
Utopian, Thai.
Flunarizine (p.418·2).
Cerebrovascular disorders.

Flumach *Mayoly-Spindler, Fr.*
Spironolactone (p.973·2).
Hyperaldosteronism; hypertension; myasthenia gravis; oedema.

Flumadine *Forest, Israel; Forest Pharmaceuticals, USA.*
Rimantadine hydrochloride (p.640·1).
Influenza A.

Flumarin *Shionogi, Jpn.*
Flomoxef sodium (p.206·3).
Bacterial infections.

Flumark *Dainippon, Jpn.*
Enoxacin (p.201·1).
Bacterial infections.

Flumasalen *TO-Chemicals, Thai.*
Flumetasone pivalate (p.1070·3); salicylic acid (p.1122·3).
Skin disorders.

Flumed *Medifive, Thai.*
Fluoxetine (p.288·2).
Depression; obsessive-compulsive disorder.

Flumetol *Farmila, Ital.*
Fluorometholone (p.1072·1); tetryzoline hydrochloride (p.1101·2).
Inflammatory eye disorders.

Flumetol Antibiotico *Farmila, Ital.*
Fluorometholone (p.1072·1); tetracycline (p.258·3).
Infected eye disorders.

Flumetol Semplice *Farmila, Ital.*
Fluorometholone (p.1072·1).
Inflammatory eye disorders.

Flumex *Allergan-Frumtost, Braz.*
Fluorometholone (p.1072·1).
Eye disorders.

Flumex-N *Allergan-Frumtost, Braz.*
Neomycin sulfate (p.228·1); fluorometholone (p.1072·1).
Infected eye disorders.

Flumid *Hexal, Ger.*
Flutamide (p.542·3).
Prostatic cancer.

Flumox *Rolab, S.Afr.*
Amoxicillin (p.149·2); flucloxacillin (p.207·1).
Bacterial infections.

Flumural *SPA, Ital.†.*
Flumequine (p.207·3).
Urinary-tract infections.

Flunagen *Gentili, Ital.*
Flunarizine hydrochloride (p.418·1).
Migraine; vertigo.

Flunarin *Asta Medica, Braz.*
Flunarizine hydrochloride (p.418·1).
Hemiplegia; migraine and other vascular headaches; subarachnoid haemorrhage.

Flunarium *Greater Pharma, Thai.*
Flunarizine hydrochloride (p.418·1).
Cerebrovascular disorders; migraine; motion sickness; vertigo.

Flunase *Teva, Israel.*
Flunisolide (p.1070·3).
Rhinitis.

Flunavert *Hennig, Ger.*
Flunarizine hydrochloride (p.418·1).
Migraine; vertigo.

Flunaza *Pharmaland, Thai.*
Flunarizine (p.418·2).
Cerebrovascular disorders.

Flunazine *Shiwa, Thai.*
Flunarizine (p.418·2).
Cerebral and peripheral vascular disorders; vestibular disorders.

Flunazol *Sintofarma, Braz.*
Fluconazole (p.383·2).
Fungal infections.

Fluneurin *Hexal, Ger.*
Fluoxetine hydrochloride (p.284·2).
Depression.

Flunidor *Chibret, Port.†.*
Diflunisal (p.32·2).
Inflammation; pain.

Fluniget *Merck Sharp & Dohme, Aust.; Merck Sharp & Dohme, Ger.†.*
Diflunisal (p.32·2).
Musculoskeletal and joint disorders; pain.

Flunimerck *Merck dura, Ger.*
Flunitrazepam (p.683·2).
Insomnia.

Fluninoc *Hexal, Ger.*
Flunitrazepam (p.683·2).
Insomnia.

Flunipam
Alpharma, Denm.; Alpharma, Norw.
Flunitrazepam (p.683·2).
Insomnia; premedication.

Flunir *Oberlin, Fr.*
Niflumic acid (p.62·3).
Sprains.

Flunitec *Boehringer de Angeli, Braz.; Boehringer Ingelheim, Denm.†; Boehringer Ingelheim, Norw.*
Flunisolide (p.1070·3).
Asthma; nasal congestion.

Flunolone *Atlantic, Hong Kong; Atlantic, Singapore.*
Fluocinolone acetonide (p.1071·1); neomycin sulfate (p.228·1).
Infected skin disorders.

Flunolone-V *Atlantic, Hong Kong; Atlantic, Singapore.*
Fluocinolone acetonide (p.1071·1).
Skin disorders.

Flunox *Roche, Ital.*
Flurazepam monohydrochloride (p.685·3).
Insomnia.

Fluo Fenic *Ciba Vision, Spain.*
Chloramphenicol (p.179·1); fluocinolone acetonide (p.1071·1).
Infected eye disorders.

Fluo Grin *Grin, Mex.*
Fluocinolone acetonide (p.1071·1); neomycin sulfate (p.228·1).
Infected eye disorders.

Fluo Vasoc *Ciba Vision, Spain.*
Fluocinolone acetonide (p.1071·1); naphazoline hydrochloride (p.1095·1); neomycin sulfate (p.228·1); zinc sulfate (p.1398·2).
Infected eye disorders.

Fluocal com Pectina *Breves, Braz.*
Neomycin sulfate (p.228·1); dihydrostreptomycin sulfate (p.199·2); pectin (p.1502·3); apple juice; attapulgite (p.1212·1); calcium lactate (p.1188·2).
Diarrhoea.

Fluo-calc *Searle, Switz.*
Sodium monofluorophosphate (p.1377·2); calcium carbonate (p.1215·1).
Osteoporosis.

Fluocalcic *Asta Medica, Aust.; Yamanouchi, Belg.; Yamanouchi, Fr.†.*
Sodium monofluorophosphate (p.1377·2); calcium carbonate (p.1215·1).
Osteoporosis.

Fluocaril *Asta Medica, Braz.*
Sodium fluoride (p.1375·3).
Dental caries prophylaxis.

Fluocaril Bi-Fluore *Synthelabo, Fr.; Goupil, Fr.*
Sodium monofluorophosphate (p.1377·2); sodium fluoride (p.1375·3).
Dental caries prophylaxis.

Fluocid Forte *Inkeysa, Spain.*
Fluocinolone acetonide (p.1071·1).
Skin disorders.

Fluocim *Cimex, Switz.*
Fluoxetine hydrochloride (p.284·2).
Bulimia; depression.

Fluoclox *Ranbaxy, Singapore.*
Flucloxacillin sodium (p.207·1).
Bacterial infections.

Fluocortan *Centrum, Spain.*
Fluocinolone acetonide (p.1071·1).
Skin disorders.

Fluodel *QIF, Braz.*
Sodium fluoride (p.1375·3).
Dental caries prophylaxis.

Fluodent *Scherer, Ital.†.*
Sodium fluoride (p.1375·3).
Dietary-fluoride deficiency.

Fluoderm *Taro, Canad.; Lennon, S.Afr.†.*
Fluocinolone acetonide (p.1071·1).
Skin disorders.

Fluodermo Fuerte *Septa, Spain.*
Fluocinolone acetonide (p.1071·1).
Skin disorders.

Fluodonil *Biologici Italia, Ital.†.*
Diflunisal (p.32·2).
Musculoskeletal and joint disorders; pain.

Fluodont *Gebro, Aust.*
Sodium fluoride (p.1375·3).
Dental caries prophylaxis.

Fluodontyl *Synthelabo, Fr.; Synthelabo, Spain.*
Sodium fluoride (p.1375·3).
Formerly contained sodium fluoride and formaldehyde in *Fr.*.
Dental caries prophylaxis.

Fluodrazin F *Breves, Braz.*
Isoniazid (p.215·3); ascorbic acid (p.1389·3).
Tuberculosis.

Fluo-Fenicol *Allergan-Frumtost, Braz.*
Fluocinolone acetonide (p.1071·1); chloramphenicol (p.179·1).
Infected eye disorders.

Fluoftal *Agepha, Aust.*
Fluorescein sodium (p.1612·1).
Diagnosis of corneal disorders.

Fluogel *Dentoria, Fr.*
Sodium fluoride (p.1375·3); ammonium difluoride (p.1376·2).
Dental caries prophylaxis following radiotherapy.

Fluogen *Parkedale, USA†.*
An influenza vaccine (p.1544·3).
Active immunisation.

Fluogum *Synthelabo, Fr.*
Sodium fluoride (p.1375·3).
Dental caries prophylaxis.

Fluohexal *Hexal, Austral.*
Fluoxetine hydrochloride (p.284·2).
Depression; obsessive-compulsive disorder.

Fluomicetina *Formenti, Ital.†.*
Fluocinolone acetonide (p.1071·1); kanamycin sulfate (p.218·1).
Anogenital pruritus; skin disorders.

Fluomix Same *Savoma, Ital.*
Fluocinolone acetonide (p.1071·1).
Skin disorders.

Fluomycin N *Nourypharma, Ger.*
Dequalinium chloride (p.1143·1).
Vaginal infections.

Fluon *Rabi & Solabo, Fr.*
Metesculetol sodium (p.1635·1); hamamelis (p.1618·3); aesculus (p.1574·1); viburnum.
Haemorrhoids; oedema; peripheral vascular disorders.

Fluonex *ICN, USA†.*
Fluocinonide (p.1071·2).
Skin disorders.

Fluonid *Allergan, USA.*
Fluocinolone acetonide (p.1071·1).
Skin disorders.

Fluonid-N *Biolab, Thai.*
Fluocinolone acetonide (p.1071·1); neomycin sulfate (p.228·1).
Infected skin disorders.

Fluonilid *Ascot, Austral.†.*
Loflucarban (p.390·3).
Skin infections.

Fluonolone *Vana, Thai.*
Fluocinolone acetonide (p.1071·1); neomycin sulfate (p.228·1).
Infected skin disorders.

Fluonolone-V *Vana, Thai.*
Fluocinolone acetonide (p.1071·1).
Skin disorders.

Fluopate *Laphal, Fr.*
Sodium fluoride (p.1375·3); calcium fluoride (p.1356·1).
Dental caries prophylaxis.

Fluoplexe *Lehning, Fr.*
Sodium fluoride (p.1375·3).
Peri-articular disorders.

Fluor *Or-Dov, Austral.; Crinex, Fr.; Lacer, Spain; Kin, Spain.*
Sodium fluoride (p.1375·3).
Dental caries prophylaxis.

Fluor Microsol *Herbaxt, Fr.*
Sodium fluoride (p.1375·3).
Peri-articular disorders.

Fluoracaine *Dioptic, Canad.; Akorn, USA.*
Fluorescein sodium (p.1612·1); proxymetacaine hydrochloride (p.1320·1).
Aid to eye examination; local anaesthesia.

Fluor-A-Day *Pharmascience, Canad.; Dental Health Products, UK.*
Sodium fluoride (p.1375·3).
Dental caries prophylaxis.

Fluoralfa *INTES, Ital.*
Fluorescein sodium (p.1612·1).
Diagnosis of eye disorders.

Fluordent *Warner-Lambert, Ital.†.*
Sodium fluoride (p.1375·3).
Dental caries prophylaxis.

Fluorescite
Alcon, Austral.; Alcon, Canad.; Alcon, Hong Kong; Alcon, NZ; Alcon, S.Afr.; Alcon, Singapore; Alcon, Thai.; Alcon, USA.
Fluorescein sodium (p.1612·1).
Aid to eye examination.

Fluorets
Smith & Nephew, Austral.; Ophtpharma, Canad.; Dioptic, Canad.; Chauvin, Hong Kong; Chauvin, Irl.; Smith & Nephew, NZ; Smith & Nephew, S.Afr.; Chauvin, Singapore; Chauvin, UK; Akorn, USA.
Fluorescein sodium (p.1612·1).
Aid to eye examination.

Fluorette
Fertin, Denm.; Fertin, Norw.; Meda, Swed.
Sodium fluoride (p.1375·3).
Dental caries prophylaxis.

Fluoretten *Hoechst Marion Roussel, Ger.*
Sodium fluoride (p.1375·3).
Dental caries prophylaxis.

Fluorex *Crinex, Fr.*
Sodium fluoride (p.1375·3).
Dental caries prophylaxis.

Fluorex Plus *Gerot, Aust.*
Tetracycline hydrochloride (p.258·3); dequalinium chloride (p.1143·1); prednisone (p.1079·2).
Colpitis.

Fluorhinose *Monot, Fr.*
Benzododecinium bromide (p.1135·1); sodium chloride (p.1196·1).

Fluoridrops *WestCan, Canad.*
Sodium fluoride (p.1375·3).
Fluoride supplement.

Fluorigard *Colgate-Palmolive, Ital.; Colgate-Palmolive, UK; Colgate-Palmolive, USA.*
Sodium fluoride (p.1375·3).
Dental caries prophylaxis.

Fluorigard Gel-Kam *Colgate-Palmolive, UK.*
Stannous fluoride (p.1379·3).
Dental caries prophylaxis.

Fluorigard Ortho *Asta Medica, Port.†.*
Sodium fluoride (p.1375·3).
Dental caries prophylaxis.

Fluoril *Novartis, Ger.*
Sodium monofluorophosphate (p.1377·2); calcium lactate gluconate (p.1188·3); calcium carbonate (p.1215·1).
Osteoporosis.

Fluorilette *Leiras, Fin.*
Sodium fluoride (p.1375·3).
Dental caries prophylaxis.

Fluori-Methane *Gebauer, USA.*
Dichlorodifluoromethane (p.1199·1); trichlorofluoromethane (p.1199·2).
Local anaesthesia.

Fluorin *Sanofi Synthelabo, Ital.*
Sodium fluoride (p.1375·3).
Fluoride supplement.

Fluor-In *Sanofi Synthelabo, Port.*
Sodium fluoride (p.1375·3).
Dental caries prophylaxis.

Fluorinse *Oral-B, Canad.; Oral-B, USA.*
Sodium fluoride (p.1375·3).
Dental caries prophylaxis.

Fluor-I-Strip *Bausch & Lomb, USA.*
Fluorescein sodium (p.1612·1).
Aid to eye examination.

Fluor-I-Strip AT *Bausch & Lomb, Canad.†.*
Fluorescein sodium (p.1612·1).
Aid to eye examination.

Fluoritab *Fluoritab, USA.*
Sodium fluoride (p.1375·3).
Dental caries prophylaxis.

Fluoritabs *WestCan, Canad.*
Sodium fluoride (p.1375·3).

Fluornatrium *Odontomed, Braz.*
Sodium fluoride (p.1375·3).
Dental caries prophylaxis.

Fluorobioptal *Farmila, Ital.*
Dexamethasone (p.1067·1); chloramphenicol (p.179·1).
Formerly contained dexamethasone, chloramphenicol, nitrofurazone, and phenylephrine hydrochloride.
Inflammatory eye disorders.

Fluorocaine *Medical Ophthalmics, USA.*
Fluorescein sodium (p.1612·1); proxymetacaine hydrochloride (p.1320·1).

Fluorocalciforte *Serozym, Fr.†.*
Calcium chloride (p.1188·1); calcium gluceptate (p.1188·1); calcium gluconate (p.1188·2); calcium lactate (p.1188·2); calcium carbonate (p.1215·1); sodium monofluorophosphate (p.1377·2); yeast (p.1398·1).
Osteoporosis.

Fluorocare *Colgate Oral Care, Austral.*
Sodium monofluorophosphate (p.1377·2).
Dental caries prophylaxis; sensitive teeth.

Fluorogum *Schwulst, S.Afr.†.*
Sodium fluoride (p.1375·3).
Fluoride supplement.

Fluor-Op *Ciba Vision, USA.*
Fluorometholone (p.1072·1).
Inflammatory eye disorders.

Fluoroplex
Allergan, Austral.; Allergan, Canad.†; Allergan, USA.
Fluorouracil (p.540·2).
Solar keratoses.

Fluoropos *Ursapharm, Ger.*
Fluorometholone (p.1072·1).
Inflammatory eye disorders.

Fluororinil *Farmila, Ital.*
Betamethasone (p.1063·1); chlorpheniramine [chlorphenamine] maleate (p.412·1).
Rhinitis.

Fluoros *Jenapharm, Ger.*
Sodium fluoride (p.1375·3).
Osteoporosis.

Fluorosol *WestCan, Canad.*
Sodium fluoride (p.1375·3).

Fluorox *Medical Ophthalmics, USA.*
Fluorescein sodium (p.1612·1); oxybuprocaine (p.1318·1).

Fluorthyrin *Agepha, Aust.*
Fluorotyrosine (p.1522·3).
Hyperthyroidism.

Fluortop *GABA, Switz.*
Sodium fluoride (p.1375·3).
Dental caries prophylaxis.

Fluorvas *Llorens, Spain.*
Fluorometholone (p.1072·1); tetryzoline hydrochloride (p.1101·2).
Eye disorders.

Fluor-Vigantoletten *Merck, Ger.*
Colecalciferol (p.1391·1); sodium fluoride (p.1375·3).
Dental caries prophylaxis; vitamin D deficiency.

Fluorvitin *IPFI, Ital.*
Sodium fluoride (p.1375·3).
Dental caries prophylaxis.

Fluoselgine *Teofarma, Fr.*
Domiphen bromide (p.1143·3); sodium fluoride (p.1375·3).
Dental hygiene; gingivitis.

Fluosept *Inava, Fr.†*
Ammonium difluoride (p.1376·2); benzyl salicylate.
Dental caries prophylaxis.

Fluotest *Alcon Cusi, Spain†.*
Fluorescein sodium (p.1612·1); oxybuprocaine hydrochloride (p.1318·1).
Aid to eye examination.

Fluothane *Zeneca, Aust.; Zeneca, Austral.; Zeneca, Belg.; Zeneca, Braz.; Astra-Zeneca, Fr.; Zeneca, Ger.; Zeneca, Hong Kong; Zeneca, Irl.; Zeneca, Israel; Zeneca, Ital.; Zeneca, Mex.; Zeneca, Neth.; Zeneca, Norw.†; AstraZeneca, NZ; Zeneca, Port.; Zeneca, S.Afr.; Zeneca, Spain; Zeneca, Swed.; Zeneca, Switz.; AstraZeneca, Thai.; AstraZeneca, UK†; Wyeth-Ayerst, USA.*
Halothane (p.1259·3).
General anaesthesia.

Fluotic *Hoechst Marion Roussel, Canad.*
Sodium fluoride (p.1375·3).
Otospongiosis.

Fluotrat *Searle, Braz.*
Xylitol (p.1397·3); sodium fluoride (p.1375·3).
Dental caries prophylaxis.

Fluo-Vaso *Allergan-Frumtost, Braz.*
Fluocinolone acetonide (p.1071·1); naphazoline hydrochloride (p.1095·1); neomycin (p.228·1); zinc sulfate (p.1398·2).
Infected eye disorders.

Fluovitef *Teofarma, Ital.*
Fluocinolone acetonide (p.1071·1).
Skin disorders.

Fluox *Pacific, NZ.*
Fluoxetine hydrochloride (p.284·2).
Depression.

Fluoxac *Psicofarma, Mex.*
Fluoxetine hydrochloride (p.284·2).
Depression.

Fluoxemerck *Merck dura, Ger.*
Fluoxetine hydrochloride (p.284·2).
Depression.

Fluoxeren *Menarini, Ital.*
Fluoxetine hydrochloride (p.284·2).
Bulimia nervosa; depression; obsessive-compulsive disorder.

Fluoxibene *Ratiopharm, Aust.*
Fluoxetine hydrochloride (p.284·2).
Bulimia nervosa; depression; obsessive-compulsive disorder.

Fluoxifar *Siphar, Switz.*
Fluoxetine hydrochloride (p.284·2).
Depression.

Flu-Oxinate *Pasadena, USA.*
Fluorescein sodium (p.1612·1); oxybuprocaine hydrochloride (p.1318·1).

Fluoxine *TO-Chemicals, Thai.*
Fluoxetine (p.288·2).
Depression.

Fluox-Puren *Isis Puren, Ger.*
Fluoxetine hydrochloride (p.284·2).
Depression.

Flupam *Tika, Swed.†*
Flunitrazepam (p.683·2).
Premedication; sleep disorders.

Flupar *Orion, Fin.*
An inactivated influenza vaccine (p.1544·3).
Active immunisation.

Flupazine *Psicofarma, Mex.*
Trifluoperazine hydrochloride (p.710·3).
Nausea and vomiting; psychoses.

Flupress *Drug Research, Ital.*
Buflomedil pyridoxal phosphate compound (p.852·1).
Cerebral and peripheral vascular disorders.

Fluprim Tosse *Roche, Ital.†.*
Dextromethorphan hydrobromide (p.1087·3).
Coughs.

Flura *Kirkman, USA.*
Sodium fluoride (p.1375·3).
Dental caries prophylaxis.

Flurablastin *Pharmacia Upjohn, Denm.; Pharmacia Upjohn, Fin.; Pharmacia Upjohn, Norw.; Pharmacia Upjohn, Swed.*
Fluorouracil (p.540·2) or fluorouracil sodium (p.541·2).
Malignant neoplasms.

Fluracedyl *Pharmachemie, Israel; Nycomed, Norw.; Nycomed, Swed.*
Fluorouracil (p.540·2) or fluorouracil sodium (p.541·2).
Malignant neoplasms.

Flurate *Bausch & Lomb, USA.*
Fluorescein sodium (p.1612·1); oxybuprocaine hydrochloride (p.1318·1).
Local anaesthesia.

Flurekain *Croma, Aust.*
Oxybuprocaine hydrochloride (p.1318·1); fluorescein sodium (p.1612·1).
Local anaesthesia.

Fluress *Allergan, Austral.; Allergan, Canad.; Barnes Hind, NZ; Abigo, Swed.; Akorn, USA.*
Fluorescein sodium (p.1612·1); oxybuprocaine hydrochloride (p.1318·1).
Aid to eye examination; local anaesthesia.

Flurets *Oral-B, Austral.*
Sodium fluoride (p.1375·3).
Prevention of tooth decay.

Fluricin *Seng, Thai.*
Flunarizine hydrochloride (p.418·1).
Cerebral and peripheral vascular disorders; vestibular disorders.

Flurinol *Promeco, Mex.*
Epinastine hydrochloride (p.417·3).
Hypersensitivity.

Flurizic *Pharmacia Upjohn, Ital.*
Flurithromycin ethyl succinate (p.207·3).
Bacterial infections.

Fluroblastin *Pharmacia Upjohn, Ger.; Pharmacia Upjohn, S.Afr.*
Fluorouracil (p.540·2).
Malignant neoplasms.

Fluroblastine *Pharmacia Upjohn, Belg.*
Fluorouracil sodium (p.541·2).
Malignant neoplasms.

Fluro-Ethyl *Gebauer, USA.*
Ethyl chloride (p.1312·1); cryofluorane (p.1199·1).
Topical anaesthesia.

Flurofen *Knoll, Denm.*
Flurbiprofen (p.41·2).
Inflammation; musculoskeletal and joint disorders.

Flurolon *Allergan, Denm.*
Fluorometholone (p.1072·1).
Inflammatory eye disorders.

Flurop *Davi, Port.*
Fluorometholone (p.1072·1).
Eye disorders.

Flurosyn *Rugby, USA.*
Fluocinolone acetonide (p.1071·1).
Skin disorders.

Flurox
Note. This name is used for preparations of different composition.
Lemery, Mex.
Fluorouracil (p.540·2).
Malignant neoplasms.

Ocusoft, USA.
Fluorescein sodium (p.1612·1); oxybuprocaine hydrochloride (p.1318·1).

Flurozin *Remedica, Thai.*
Flurbiprofen (p.41·2).
Musculoskeletal and joint disorders.

Flurpax *Hoechst Marion Roussel, Spain.*
Flunarizine hydrochloride (p.418·1).
Migraine; vertigo.

Flusan *Novag, Mex.*
Tolbutamide (p.336·3).
Diabetes mellitus.

Fluscand *Enapharm, Swed.*
Flunitrazepam (p.683·2).
Premedication; sleep disorders.

Flusemide *UCB, Spain.*
Nicardipine hydrochloride (p.938·3).
Angina pectoris; cerebral vasospasm; hypertension.

Fluserin *Novaquimica, Braz.*
Flunitrazepam (p.683·2).
Adjunct in general anaesthesia; insomnia; premedication.

Flushield
Wyeth, Mex.; Wyeth-Ayerst, USA.
An inactivated influenza vaccine (split virion) (p.1544·3).
Active immunisation.

Flusin *Aspen Consumer, S.Afr.*
Chlorpheniramine [chlorphenamine] maleate (p.412·1); ephedrine hydrochloride (p.1090·1); paracetamol (p.71·2); caffeine (p.761·3).
Cold and influenza symptoms.

Flusin C *Aspen Consumer, S.Afr.*
Chlorpheniramine [chlorphenamine] maleate (p.412·1); pseudoephedrine hydrochloride (p.1099·2); vitamin C (p.1389·3).
Cold and influenza symptoms.

Flusin DM *Aspen Consumer, S.Afr.*
Chlorpheniramine [chlorphenamine] maleate (p.412·1); pseudoephedrine hydrochloride (p.1099·2); dextromethorphan hydrobromide (p.1087·3); ascorbic acid (p.1389·3).
Coughs; upper respiratory-tract congestion.

Flusin S *Aspen Consumer, S.Afr.*
Chlorpheniramine [chlorphenamine] maleate (p.412·1); paracetamol (p.71·2); pseudoephedrine hydrochloride (p.1099·2); vitamin C (p.1389·3).
Cold and influenza symptoms.

Flusol *Ecosol, Switz.*
Fluoxetine hydrochloride (p.284·2).
Bulimia; depression.

Flusonal *Almirall, Spain.*
Fluticasone propionate (p.1072·2).
Asthma.

Fluspi *Hexal, Ger.*
Fluspirilene (p.686·1).
Schizophrenia.

Fluspiral *Menarini, Ital.*
Fluticasone propionate (p.1072·2).
Obstructive airways disease.

Flusporan *Menarini, Spain.*
Flutrimazole (p.386·1).
Fungal skin infections.

Fluss 40 *Scharper, Ital.*
Frusemide [furosemide] (p.893·1); triamterene (p.986·1).
Ascites; hyperaldosteronism; hypertension; oedema.

Flussorex *Lampugnani, Ital.*
Citicoline sodium (p.1596·1).
Cerebrovascular disorders; mental function disorders; parkinsonism.

Flu-Stat *Be-Tabs, S.Afr.*
Capsules: Paracetamol (p.71·2); ascorbic acid (p.1389·3); phenylephrine hydrochloride (p.1097·1); chlorpheniramine [chlorphenamine] maleate (p.412·1); caffeine (p.761·3).
Syrup: Paracetamol (p.71·2); phenylpropanolamine hydrochloride (p.1098·1); dextromethorphan hydrobromide (p.1087·3).
Cold and influenza symptoms.

Fluta *ABZ, Ger.*
Flutamide (p.542·3).
Prostatic cancer.

Flutabene *Ratiopharm, Aust.*
Flutamide (p.542·3).
Prostatic cancer.

Flutacan *Leiras, Denm.; Ferring, Swed.*
Flutamide (p.542·3).
Prostatic cancer.

Fluta-cell *Cell Pharm, Ger.*
Flutamide (p.542·3).
Prostatic cancer.

Fluta-Gry *Gry, Ger.*
Flutamide (p.542·3).
Prostatic cancer.

Flutaide *Glaxo Wellcome, Port.*
Fluticasone propionate (p.1072·2).
Rhinitis.

Flutamex *Sanofi Synthelabo, Ger.*
Flutamide (p.542·3).
Prostatic cancer.

Flutamin
Alphapharm, Austral.; Pacific, NZ.
Flutamide (p.542·3).
Prostatic cancer.

Flutan
Medochemie, Hong Kong; Medochemie, Thai.
Flutamide (p.542·3).
Prostatic cancer.

Flutaplex *Abbott, Belg.; Nettopharma, Denm.*
Flutamide (p.542·3).
Prostatic cancer.

Flutenal *Recordati, Spain.*
Flupamesone (p.1080·2).
Skin disorders.

Flutenal Gentamicina *Recordati, Spain.*
Flupamesone (p.1080·2); gentamicin sulfate (p.210·1).
Infected skin disorders.

Flutenal Sali *Recordati, Spain.*
Flupamesone (p.1080·2); salicylic acid (p.1122·3).
Skin disorders.

Flutex
Note. This name is used for preparations of different composition.
Aspen Consumer, S.Afr.
Capsules: Ascorbic acid (p.1389·3); salicylamide (p.82·1); paracetamol (p.71·2); caffeine (p.761·3); phenylephrine hydrochloride (p.1097·1); chlorpheniramine [chlorphenamine] maleate (p.412·1).
Syrup: Paracetamol (p.71·2); phenylephrine hydrochloride (p.1097·1).
Cold and influenza symptoms.

Syosset, USA.
Triamcinolone acetonide (p.1080·1).
Skin disorders.

Flutex Cough Linctus *Aspen Consumer, S.Afr.*
Diphenhydramine hydrochloride (p.416·1); codeine phosphate (p.25·2); ammonium chloride (p.1085·2).
Coughs.

Flutide
Glaxo Wellcome, Ger.; Glaxo Wellcome, Norw.; Glaxo Wellcome, Swed.
Fluticasone propionate (p.1072·2).
Allergic rhinitis; asthma; nasal polyps.

Flutin
Orion, Denm.; Julphar, UAE.
Fluoxetine hydrochloride (p.284·2).
Bulimia nervosa; depression; obsessive-compulsive disorder.

Flutinase *Glaxo Wellcome, Switz.*
Fluticasone propionate (p.1072·2).
Nasal polyps; rhinitis.

Flutine
Teva, Israel; Pharmasant, Thai.
Fluoxetine hydrochloride (p.284·2).
Depression; obsessive-compulsive disorder.

Flutivate *Glaxo Wellcome, Ger.; Cascan, Ger.; Glaxo Wellcome, Norw.; Glaxo Wellcome, Swed.*
Fluticasone propionate (p.1072·2).
Skin disorders.

Flutol *Douglas, NZ.*
Flutamide (p.542·3).

Flutox *Pharmazam, Spain.*
Cloperastine fendizoate (p.1087·2) or cloperastine hydrochloride (p.1087·2).
Coughs.

Flutraz *Tika, Norw.†*
Flunitrazepam (p.683·2).
Insomnia.

Fluvaccin *SBL, Swed.†.*
An influenza vaccine (p.1544·3).
Active immunisation.

Fluvaleas *Valeas, Ital.*
Isopropamide iodide (p.470·1); paracetamol (p.71·2); diphenhydramine hydrochloride (p.416·1); caffeine (p.761·3).
Fever; inflammation; pain.

Fluvax
CSL, Austral.; CSL, NZ.
An inactivated influenza vaccine (split virion) (p.1544·3).
Active immunisation.

Fluvean *Formenti, Ital.*
Fluocinolone acetonide (p.1071·1).
Skin disorders.

Fluvermal
Janssen-Cilag, Fr.; Janssen-Cilag, Port.
Flubendazole (p.99·2).
Veterinary names include Flubenol.
Intestinal nematode infections.

Fluvert *Medley, Braz.*
Flunarizine hydrochloride (p.418·1).
Hemiplegia; migraine and other vascular headaches; subarachnoid haemorrhage.

Fluvic *Pierre Fabre Sante, Fr.*
Carbocisteine (p.1086·3).
Respiratory-tract congestion.

Fluviral
Note. This name is used for preparations of different composition.
Virtus, Braz.
Mepyramine maleate (p.421·1); caffeine (p.761·3); phenylpropanolamine hydrochloride (p.1098·1); dipyrone (p.34·1).
Cold and influenza symptoms.

Biochem, Canad.
An inactivated influenza vaccine (whole and split virion) (p.1544·3).
Active immunisation.

Fluvirin
Ebos, Austral.; Medeva, Belg.; Medeva, Fin.; Medeva, Irl.; Evans Medical, Israel; Farmarekord, Ital.†; Medeva, Norw.; Helsinn, Port.; Medpro, S.Afr.; SBL, Swed.; Evans, UK; Medeva, USA.
An inactivated influenza vaccine (surface antigen) (p.1544·3).
Active immunisation.

Fluvirine *Medeva, Fr.*
An influenza vaccine (p.1544·3).
Active immunisation.

Fluvium *Rekah, Israel.*
Sodium fluoride (p.1375·3).
Osteoporosis.

Fluvoxadura *Merck dura, Ger.*
Fluvoxamine maleate (p.289·3).
Depression; obsessive-compulsive disorder.

Flux
Note. This name is used for preparations of different composition.
Hexal, Aust.
Fluoxetine hydrochloride (p.284·2).
Bulimia nervosa; depression; obsessive-compulsive disorder.

Alpharma, Norw.
Sodium fluoride (p.1375·3).
Dental caries prophylaxis.

Fluxal *Pfizer Consumer, Spain.*
Lysine aspirin (p.50·3); calcium ascorbate (p.1389·3); chlorpheniramine [chlorphenamine] maleate (p.412·1); phenylephrine hydrochloride (p.1097·1).
Influenza and cold symptoms.

Fluxantin *Gea, Denm.; Gea, Fin.*
Fluoxetine hydrochloride (p.284·2).
Bulimia; depression.

Fluxapril *Wyeth Lederle, Aust.; Lederle, Ger.†*
Flucloxacillin sodium (p.207·1); piperacillin sodium (p.236·1).
Bacterial infections.

Fluxarten *SmithKline Beecham, Ital.*
Flunarizine hydrochloride (p.418·1).
Migraine; vertigo.

Fluxedan *AF, Mex.*
Bromhexine hydrochloride (p.1085·3); oxeladin citrate (p.1096·1).
Respiratory-tract disorders with viscous mucus.

Fluxema *Zimaia, Port.†*
Bencyclane fumarate (p.843·3).

Fluxene *Eurofarma, Braz.*
Fluoxetine hydrochloride (p.284·2).
Depression; obsessive-compulsive disorder.

Fluxet *Krewel, Ger.*
Fluoxetine hydrochloride (p.284·2).
Depression.

Fluxetil *Unison, Thai.*
Fluoxetine (p.288·2).
Depression; obsessive-complusive disorder.

Fluxetin *Atlantic, Singapore; Atlantic, Thai.*
Fluoxetine hydrochloride (p.284·2).
Depression.

Fluxine *Rudefsa, Mex.*
Aesculus (p.1574·1).

Fluxocor *Cibran, Braz.*
Dipyridamole (p.877·2).
Adjunct in myocardial imaging; ischaemic heart disease; thromboembolism prophylaxis.

Fluxoten *Herbaline, Ital.†*
Melissa (p.1632·2); centaury (p.1593·1); calendula (p.1589·2); artemisia vulgaris; saffron (p.1029·1).
Menstrual disorders.

Fluxum *Wassermann, Ital.*
Parnaparin sodium (p.952·2).
Thrombosis prophylaxis; vascular disorders.

Fluzac *LBS, Thai.*
Fluoxetine hydrochloride (p.284·2).
Depression; obsessive-compulsive disorder.

Fluzal *Julphar, UAE.*
Carbinoxamine maleate (p.411·1); phenylpropanolamine hydrochloride (p.1098·1).
Upper respiratory-tract disorders.

Fluzine *PP Lab, Thai.*
Fluphenazine hydrochloride (p.684·3).
Anxiety; schizophrenia.

Fluzone *Connaught, Canad.; Pasteur Merieux, Irl.; Connaught, Norw.†; Meda, Swed.†; Pasteur Merieux, UK; Pasteur Merieux, USA.*
An inactivated influenza vaccine (split virion) (p.1544·3).
Active immunisation.

Flynoken A *Kendrick, Mex.*
Calcium folinate (p.1363·1).
Antidote to folic acid antagonists; megaloblastic anaemia; reduction of methotrexate toxicity.

FML
Allergan, Austral.; Allergan, Belg.; Allergan, Canad.; Allergan, Hong Kong; Allergan, Irl.; Allergan, Israel; Allergan, Mex.; Allergan, NZ; Allergan, S.Afr.; Allergan, Singapore; Allergan, Spain; Allergan, Switz.; Allergan, Thai.; Allergan, USA.
Fluorometholone (p.1072·1).
Inflammatory eye disorders.

FML Liquifilm *Allergan, Fin.; Allergan, Neth.†; Allergan, Port.; Allergan, UK.*
Fluorometholone (p.1072·1).
Inflammatory eye disorders.

FML Neo
Allergan, Israel; Allergan, Port.; Allergan, S.Afr.; Allergan, Spain; Allergan, Switz.; Allergan, Thai.
Fluorometholone (p.1072·1); neomycin sulfate (p.228·1).
Inflammatory eye infections.

FML Neo Liquifilm *Allergan, UK†.*
Fluorometholone (p.1072·1); neomycin sulfate (p.228·1).
Inflammatory eye infections.

FML-S *Allergan, USA.*
Fluorometholone (p.1072·1); sulfacetamide sodium (p.250·3).
Inflammatory eye infections.

FMP *Nakorn, Thai.*
21 Tablets, norgestrel (p.1486·1); ethinylestradiol (p.1476·2); 7 tablets, inert.
Combined oral contraceptive.

FNZ *Pose, Thai.*
Flunarizine hydrochloride (p.418·1).
Cerebrovascular disorders.

Foamicon *Invamed, USA.*
Aluminium hydroxide (p.1210·3); magnesium trisilicate (p.1233·3); sodium bicarbonate (p.1186·2); alginic acid (p.1498·3).
Hyperacidity.

Foban *Hoe, Singapore.*
Fusidic acid (p.208·3).
Staphylococcal skin infections; streptococcal skin infections.

Fobidon *Biomedica, Ital.*
Domperidone (p.1224·1).
Gastric discomfort; nausea; vomiting.

Focalin *Novartis, USA.*
d-Methylphenidate hydrochloride (p.1512·2).
Attention deficit hyperactivity disorder.

Focus Care All-in-One *Ciba Vision, Austral.; Ciba Vision, NZ.*
Cleansing, rinsing, disinfecting, and storage solution for soft contact lenses (p.1129·2).

Focus Care One Step *Ciba Vision, Austral.; Ciba Vision, NZ.*
Hydrogen peroxide (p.1147·1) (p.1129·2).
Disinfection, neutralisation, and storage of contact lenses.

Focusan *Lundbeck, Aust.†*
Tolnaftate (p.395·2); cetylpyridinium chloride (p.1138·1).
Fungal skin infections.

Fohn- und Wettertropfen N *Biomedica, Ger.*
Homoeopathic preparation.

Fohnetten N *Ziethen, Ger.*
Benzyl mandelate; caffeine (p.761·3); paracetamol (p.71·2).
Migraine; pain.

Foille
Note. This name is used for preparations of different composition.
Blistex, Canad.†.
Benzocaine (p.1306·2); benzyl alcohol (p.1135·2).
Burns; insect bites; wounds.
Sanofi Synthelabo, Ital.
Benzocaine (p.1306·2); benzyl alcohol (p.1135·2); chloroxylenol (p.1142·1).
Formerly contained benzocaine, benzyl alcohol, hydroxyquinoline, and colloidal sulfur.
Burns; skin irritation; wounds.
Blistex, USA.
Benzocaine (p.1306·2); chloroxylenol (p.1142·1).
Local anaesthesia.

Foille Insetti *Sanofi Synthelabo, Ital.*
Hydrocortisone (p.1073·3).
Insect stings; skin irritation.

Foille Sole *Sanofi Synthelabo, Ital.*
Benzocaine (p.1306·2); benzyl alcohol (p.1135·2); chloroxylenol (p.1142·1).
Formerly known as Foille Plus.
Skin irritation; wounds.

Foipan *Ono, Jpn.*
Camostat mesilate (p.1589·3).
Gastro-oesophageal reflux; pancreatitis.

Fokalepsin *Lundbeck, Ger.*
Carbamazepine (p.342·2).
Diabetic neuropathy; epilepsy; neuralgias.

Fol Sang B12 *IQB, Braz.*
Cyanocobalamin (p.1388·1); hydroxocobalamin (p.1388·1); thiamine (p.1385·2); liver extract.
Megaloblastic anaemia.

Folacin
Note. This name is used for preparations of different composition.
Ativus, Braz.
Oral drops; oral solution: Folic acid (p.1361·1); ascorbic acid (p.1389·3).
Folic acid deficiency; megaloblastic anaemia.
Ativus, Braz.; Pharmacia Upjohn, Swed.
Tablets: Folic acid (p.1361·1).
Folic acid deficiency; megaloblastic anaemia.

Folacin 12 *Quest, Canad.*
Vitamin B12 (p.1388·1); folic acid (p.1361·1).

Folarell *Sanorell, Ger.*
Folic acid (p.1361·1).
Antidote to treatment with folic acid antagonists; folate deficiency; megaloblastic anaemia.

Folaren *Ist. Chim. Inter., Ital.*
Calcium folinate (p.1363·1).
Antidote to folic acid antagonists; folate deficiency; reduction of aminopterin and methotrexate toxicity.

Fol-Asmedic *Dyckerhoff, Ger.*
Folic acid (p.1361·1).
Folic acid deficiency; megaloblastic anaemia.

Folatine *Lifeplan, UK.*
Folic acid (p.1361·1).
Nutritional supplement.

Folavit *Wolfs, Belg.*
Folic acid (p.1361·1).
Anaemias; prevention of neural tube defects in pregnancy.

Folaxin *Zambon, Spain.*
Calcium folinate (p.1363·1).
Adjunct to fluorouracil therapy; antidote to folic acid antagonists; reduction of methotrexate toxicity.

Folcane *Rhone-Poulenc Rorer, Mex.*
Folinic acid (p.1363·1).

Folcodex *Sanico, Belg.*
Pholcodine (p.1099·1); ephedrine hydrochloride (p.1090·1); belladonna (p.463·1); aconite (p.1572·3); sulfogaiacol (p.1101·1); ipecacuanha (p.1093·1); tolu balsam (p.1101·3).
Bronchopulmonary disorders.

Folcofen *Alliance, S.Afr.*
Diphenhydramine hydrochloride (p.416·1); pholcodine (p.1099·1); guaifenesin (p.1092·2).
Coughs.

Folcress *Grisi, Mex.*
Minoxidil (p.934·2).
Alopecia androgenetica.

Foldan *Searle, Braz.*
Tiabendazole (p.109·1).
Nematode infections.

Folderm *Kinder, Braz.*
Tiabendazole (p.109·1).
Nematode infections.

Folepar B12 *Lisapharma, Ital.*
Folic acid (p.1361·1); nicotinamide (p.1372·3); thiamine hydrochloride (p.1385·1); cyanocobalamin (p.1388·1).
Deficiency states; macrocytic anaemia.

Folergot-DF *Marnel, USA.*
Phenobarbital (p.355·1); ergotamine tartrate (p.452·1); belladonna (p.463·1).
Gastrointestinal disorders.

Folex
Note. This name is used for preparations of different composition.
Qualiphar, Belg.
Pholcodine (p.1099·1); ephedrine hydrochloride (p.1090·1); sodium citrate (p.1186·2).
Bronchitis; coughs; laryngitis.
Rybar, Irl.; Pharmateam, Israel; Pharmateam, UK.
Ferrous fumarate (p.1360·1); folic acid (p.1361·1).
Iron and folic acid deficiency in pregnancy.
Adria, USA†.
Methotrexate sodium (p.553·2).
Malignant neoplasms.

Folgamma *Worwag, Ger.*
Cyanocobalamin (p.1388·1); folic acid (p.1361·1).
Vitamin B12 and folic acid deficiency.

Folgamma Mono *Worwag, Ger.*
Folic acid (p.1361·1).
Folic acid deficiency.

Folgard *Upsher-Smith, USA.*
Folic acid; cyanocobalamin; pyridoxine hydrochloride; riboflavin (p.1350·1).
Dietary supplement.

Foliamin
Takeda, Hong Kong; Takeda, Thai.
Folic acid (p.1361·1).
Anaemias.

Foliben *FIRMA, Ital.*
Calcium folinate (p.1363·1).
Antidote to folic acid antagonists; folate deficiency; reduction of aminopterin and methotrexate toxicity.

Folic Acid Plus *Cenovis, Austral.; Vitelle, Austral.*
Vitamin and mineral preparation with iron and folic acid (p.1350·1).

Folic Plus *Peter Black, UK.*
Folic acid (p.1361·1); calcium (p.1187·3); vitamin D (p.1391·1).

Folicare *Rosemont, UK.*
Folic acid (p.1361·1).

FOLI-cell *Cell Pharm, Ger.*
Calcium folinate (p.1363·1).
Antidote to treatment with folic acid antagonists; folate deficiency.

Folicil *Bial, Port.*
Folic acid (p.1361·1).
Folic acid deficiency.

Folicombin *Jenapharm, Ger.*
Ammonium iron sulfate; folic acid (p.1361·1).
Iron and folate deficiency.

Folicum *Julphar, UAE.*
Folic acid (p.1361·1).
Folate deficiency.

Folidan *Almirall, Spain.*
Calcium folinate (p.1363·1).
Adjunct to fluorouracil therapy; megaloblastic anaemia; methotrexate poisoning.

Folidar *Italfarmaco, Ital.*
Calcium folinate (p.1363·1).
Folate deficiency; reduction of aminopterin and methotrexate toxicity.

Folifer *Bial, Port.*
Ferrous sulfate (p.1360·3); folic acid (p.1361·1).
Iron and folic acid deficiency.

Foliferron *Wyeth, Spain.*
Folic acid (p.1361·1); ferrous fumarate (p.1360·1).
Iron and folic acid deficiency.

Foligan
Henning, Ger.; Synthelabo, Switz.†.
Allopurinol (p.397·2).
Gout; hyperuricaemia; renal calculi.

Foliglobin *Pharmaceutical Enterprises, S.Afr.*
Ferrous sulfate (p.1360·3); folic acid (p.1361·1); vitamin B12 (p.1388·1).
Ascorbic acid (p.1389·3) is included in this preparation to increase the absorption and availability of iron.
Anaemias; iron deficiency.

Folina *Schwarz, Ital.*
Folic acid (p.1361·1) or sodium folate (p.1361·3).
Folate deficiency.

Folinac *Bioprogress, Ital.*
Calcium folinate (p.1363·1).
Antidote to overdosage with folic acid antagonists; folate deficiency; reduction of aminopterin and methotrexate toxicity.

Folinemic Ferro *FIRMA, Ital.*
Iron succinyl-protein complex (p.1369·3).
Iron deficiency; iron-deficiency anaemias.

Folingrav *Anmol, Ital.*
Folic acid (p.1361·1).
Folic acid supplement.

Folinoral *Therabel, Fr.*
Calcium folinate (p.1363·1).
Drug-induced megaloblastic anaemia; methotrexate toxicity.

Folinvit *Garant, Ital.*
Calcium folinate (p.1363·1).
Anaemias; folate deficiency; reduction of aminopterin and methotrexate toxicity.

Foliplus *Sanofi Synthelabo, Ital.*
Calcium folinate (p.1363·1).
Anaemias; folate deficiency; reduction of aminopterin and methotrexate toxicity.

Foli-Rivo *Rivopharm, Switz.*
Folic acid (p.1361·1).
Megaloblastic anaemias.

Folitab *Rhone-Poulenc Rorer, Mex.*
Folic acid (p.1361·1).

Folitabs *Abello, Spain.*
Finasteride (p.1477·2).
Alopecia androgenetica.

Folivit *Siam Bheasach, Thai.*
Folic acid (p.1361·1).
Anaemias.

Folix *Caber, Ital.†.*
Calcium folinate (p.1363·1).
Antidote to overdosage with folic acid antagonists; folate deficiency; reduction of aminopterin and methotrexate toxicity.

Follegon *Organon, Neth.*
Urofollitropin (p.1299·3).
Male and female infertility.

Follimin *Wyeth Lederle, Norw.; Wyeth Lederle, Swed.*
Levonorgestrel (p.1486·2); ethinylestradiol (p.1476·2).
28-Day packs also contain 7 inert tablets.
Combined oral contraceptive.

Follinett *Wyeth Lederle, Swed.*
Levonorgestrel (p.1486·2); ethinylestradiol (p.1476·2).
Combined oral contraceptive.

Follistim *Organon, USA.*
Follitropin beta (p.1283·1).
Female infertility.

Follistrel *Wyeth Lederle, Swed.*
Levonorgestrel (p.1486·2).
Progestogen-only oral contraceptive.

Follitrin *Fustery, Mex.*
Urofollitropin (p.1299·3).
Female infertility.

Folsan
Solvay, Aust.; Solvay, Ger.
Folic acid (p.1361·1).
Folic acid deficiency.

Folsana *Hotz, Ger.†.*
Ferrous gluconate (p.1360·1); folic acid (p.1361·1).
Formerly known as Ferro-Folsan.
Iron-deficiency anaemia.

Foltene *Crinos, Hong Kong.*
Tricosaccaride.
Alopecia.

FOLTX *Pan American, USA.*
Folic acid (p.1361·1); cyanocobalamin (p.1388·1); pyridoxine hydrochloride (p.1386·3).
Homocysteinaemia; homocystinuria; nutritional supplement.

Folverlan *Verla, Ger.*
Folic acid (p.1361·1).
Antidote to treatment with folic acid antagonists; folic acid deficiency; megaloblastic anaemia.

Folvite
Wyeth-Ayerst, Canad.†; Wyeth Lederle, Fin.; Lederle, Switz.; Lederle, USA.
Folic acid (p.1361·1) or sodium folate (p.1361·3).
Folate deficiency; megaloblastic anaemia.

Fomac *Berk, UK†.*
Mebeverine hydrochloride (p.1233·3).
Colonic spasm; irritable bowel syndrome.

Fomagrippin N *Michallik, Ger.*
Propyphenazone (p.80·2); ephedrine hydrochloride (p.1090·1); ascorbic acid (p.1389·3).
Cold symptoms.

Fomene *Almirall, Spain.*
Tetridamine maleate (p.87·3).
Vaginitis.

Fomentil *SIT, Ital.*
Eucalyptus oil (p.1609·2); menthol (p.1632·3); thyme oil (p.1672·3); peru balsam (p.1650·2); benzoin (p.1668·3).
Laryngitis; respiratory congestion; rhinitis; sore throat.

Fomos *Luitpold, Ger.†.*
Terfenadine (p.424·3).
Hypersensitivity reactions.

Fon Wan Eleuthero *Giuliani, Ital.*
Honey (p.1366·2); eleutherococcus senticosis (p.1615·3).
Nervous tension.

Fon Wan Ginsenergy *Giuliani, Ital.*
Honey (p.1366·2); royal jelly (p.1659·3); ginseng (p.1615·3).
Nutritional supplement.

Fon Wan Pocket Energy *Giuliani, Ital.†.*
Ginseng (p.1615·3); honey (p.1366·2).
Nutritional supplement.

The symbol † denotes a preparation no longer actively marketed

Fon Wan Pollen Giuliani, Ital.
Pollen; honey (p.1366·2); royal jelly (p.1659·3); ginseng (p.1615·3).
Nutritional supplement.

Foncitril Lafon, Fr.
Citric acid monohydrate (p.1596·2); monobasic potassium citrate; monosodium citrate.
Formerly contained trimethylphloroglucinol, citric acid monohydrate, monobasic potassium citrate, and monosodium citrate.
Metabolic acidosis; urinary alkalinisation.

Fondril Procter & Gamble, Ger.
Bisoprolol fumarate (p.850·1).
Angina pectoris; hypertension.

Fondril-5 HCT Procter & Gamble, Ger.
Bisoprolol fumarate (p.850·1); hydrochlorothiazide (p.907·3).
Hypertension.

Fondur Durascan, Denm.
Fluoxetine hydrochloride (p.284·2).
Bulimia nervosa; depression.

Fonergin Hoechst Marion Roussel, Braz.
Prednisolone (p.1077·3); framycetin sulfate (p.208·2); gramicidin (p.213·3); amylocaine (p.1306·1); procaine (p.1319·2).
Mouth disorders.

Fongamil Biorga, Fr.; Juste, Spain.
Omoconazole nitrate (p.393·1).
Fungal infections.

Fongarex Piette, Belg.; Besins-Iscovesco, Fr.
Omoconazole nitrate (p.393·1).
Fungal skin and vulvovaginal infections.

Fongeryl SERB, Fr.
Econazole nitrate (p.382·3).
Formerly contained laurcetium bromide and lemoxinol.
Fungal skin infections.

Fongitar Stiefel, Austral.; Stiefel, Hong Kong; Stiefel, Ital.†; Stiefel, NZ; Stiefel, Port.; Stiefel, Singapore; Stiefel, Thai.
Pyrithione zinc (p.1122·1); tar (p.1125·1); cade oil (p.1124·3); coal tar (p.1125·1).
Scalp disorders.

Fonicef Errekappa, Ital.
Cefonicid sodium (p.168·1).
Lignocaine [lidocaine] hydrochloride (p.1313·2) is included in this preparation to alleviate the pain of injection.
Bacterial infections.

Fonisal Salus, Ital.
Cefonicid sodium (p.168·1).
Lignocaine [lidocaine] hydrochloride (p.1313·2) is included in this preparation to alleviate the pain of injection.
Gram-negative bacterial infections.

Fonlipol Lafon, Fr.
Tiadenol (p.980·3).
Hyperlipidaemias.

Fonofos Pulitzer, Ital.†
Fosfomycin calcium (p.208·2).
Bacterial infections.

Fontego Polifarma, Ital.
Bumetanide (p.852·1).
Oedema.

Fontex Lilly, Denm.; Lilly, Fin.; Lilly, Norw.; Lilly, Swed.
Fluoxetine hydrochloride (p.284·2).
Bulimia; depression; obsessive-compulsive disorder.

Fonx Yamanouchi, Fr.
Oxiconazole nitrate (p.393·1).
Fungal skin infections.

Fonzac Gemelli, Denm.
Fluoxetine hydrochloride (p.284·2).
Bulimia nervosa; depression.

Fonzylane Lafon, Fr.; Lafon, Hong Kong.
Buflomedil hydrochloride (p.851·3).
Cerebral and peripheral vascular disorders.

Foot Zeta Zeta, Ital.
Undecenoic acid (p.395·3); usnic acid (p.1678·2).
Fungal skin disorders.

For Liver Tosi, Ital.†
Injection: Uridine (p.1677·2); inosine (p.1623·3); guanosine; cytidine; cyanocobalamin (p.1388·3); riboflavin sodium phosphate (p.1386·1); pyridoxine hydrochloride (p.1386·3); nicotinamide (p.1372·3); calcium folinate (p.1363·1).
Oral liquid: Uridine (p.1677·2); inosine (p.1623·3); guanosine; cytidine; cyanocobalamin (p.1388·3); thiamine hydrochloride (p.1385·1); riboflavin sodium phosphate (p.1386·1); pyridoxine hydrochloride (p.1386·3); nicotinamide (p.1372·3); calcium folinate (p.1363·1).
Anaemias; liver disorders.

For Men Jamieson, Canad.
Multivitamin and mineral preparation (p.1350·1).

For Peripheral Circulation Herbal Plus Formula 5 Vitelle, Austral.
Ginkgo biloba (p.1615·2); crataegus (p.1600·2); zanthoxylum (p.1682·1); capsicum (p.1591·1); rutoside (p.1611·2); hesperidin (p.1611·2).
Peripheral vascular disorders.

For the Post-Menopausal Years Jamieson, Canad.
Multivitamin and mineral preparation (p.1350·1).

For Women Active Woman Formula Blackmores, Austral.
Eleutherococcus senticosis; damiana; avena; centella; minerals; vitamin C (p.1350·1).
Dietary supplement.

For Women Multi Plus EPO Blackmores, Austral.
Evening primrose oil (p.1613·2); vitamins; minerals; choline bitartrate; bioflavonoids; rutoside (p.1350·1).
Dietary supplement.

Foradil Novartis, Aust.; Novartis, Belg.; Novartis, Canad.; Novartis, Denm.; Novartis, Fin.; Novartis, Fr.; Novartis, Ger.; Novartis, Hong Kong; Novartis, Irl.; Novartis, Israel; Novartis, Ital.; Novartis, Mex.; Novartis, Neth.; Novartis, Norw.; Novartis, NZ; Novartis, Port.; Novartis, S.Afr.; Novartis, Singapore; Novartis, Spain; Novartis, Swed.; Novartis, Switz.; Novartis, UK; Novartis, USA.
Eformoterol [formoterol] fumarate (p.764·2).
Obstructive airways disease.

Foradile Novartis, Austral.
Eformoterol [formoterol] fumarate (p.764·2).
Asthma.

Foral Grossmann, Switz.
Codeine phosphate (p.25·2); ephedrine hydrochloride (p.1090·1); sodium benzoate (p.1134·3); hedera helix; senega (p.1100·2); liquorice (p.1231·2); star anise oil.
Coughs.

Forane Abbott, Aust.; Abbott, Braz.; AstraZeneca, Canad.; Abbott, Hong Kong; Abbott, Irl.; Abbott, Israel; Abbott, Ital.; Abbott, Mex.; Abbott, NZ; Abbott, S.Afr.; Abbott, Singapore; Abbott, Spain; Abbott, Thai.; Baxter, USA.
Isoflurane (p.1261·1).
General anaesthesia.

Forapin Pfizer, Aust.†
Note.This name is used for preparations of different composition.
Pfizer, Aust.†
Liniment: Apis mellifera (p.1581·1); benzyl nicotinate (p.20·2); bornyl salicylate (p.20·3); camphor (p.1589·3); methyl nicotinate (p.55·1).
Frostbite; musculoskeletal, joint, and peri-articular disorders; neuralgias.
Pfizer, Aust.†; Mack, Belg.†; Mack, Switz.
Ointment: Apis mellifera (p.1581·1); benzyl nicotinate (p.20·2); bornyl salicylate (p.20·3); nonivamide (p.63·1).
Frostbite; musculoskeletal, joint, and peri-articular disorders; neuralgias; sports injuries.

Forapin E Mack, Illert., Ger.
Liniment: Bee venom (p.1581·1); bornyl salicylate (p.20·3); methyl nicotinate (p.55·1).
Ointment: Bee venom (p.1581·1); benzyl nicotinate (p.20·2); bornyl salicylate (p.20·3).
Cold damage; musculoskeletal and joint disorders; sports injuries.

Forcaltonin Unigene, UK.
Salcatonin (p.749·3).
Hypercalcaemia of malignancy; Paget's disease of bone.

Forcapil Arkopharma, Fr.
Calcium pantothenate (p.1374·1); biotin (p.1355·3); pyridoxine (p.1387·1); zinc pidolate; cystine (p.1359·1); methionine (p.1012·2).
Hair and nail tonic.

Forcemil Normon, Spain.
Multivitamin and mineral preparation with ginseng (p.1350·1).

Forceval
Unigene, Irl.; Unigreg, UK.
Multivitamin and mineral preparation (p.1350·1).

Forceval Protein
Unigreg, Irl.; Unigreg, UK.
Preparation for enteral nutrition (p.1350·1).
Hypoproteinaemia; malabsorption states; nutritional supplement.

Forcicline Tocogino, Mex.
Tetracycline (p.258·3).
Bacterial infections.

Forcil Continentales, Mex.
Ferrous sulfate (p.1360·3).

Ford Fibre Vitelle, Austral.
Ispaghula (p.1229·1).
Constipation; digestive disorders.

Ford Pills Faulding, Austral.
Aloin (p.1210·2); phenolphthalein (p.1244·1).
Constipation.

Fordiuran Farmacusi, Spain.
Bumetanide (p.852·1).
Hypertension; oedema.

Fordtran Hanseler, Switz.; Streuli, Switz.
Macrogol 4000 (p.1630·3) with electrolytes.
Bowel evacuation.

Forehead-C Lina, UK.
Aloe vera (p.1110·1).
Fever.

Forene
Abbott, Belg.; Abbott, Denm.; Abbott, Fin.; Abbott, Ger.; Abbott, Neth.; Abbott, Norw.; Abbott, Swed.; Abbott, Switz.
Isoflurane (p.1261·1).
General anaesthesia.

Foresight Cantassium Co., UK.
Multivitamin preparation (p.1350·1).

Foresight Iron Formula Cantassium Co., UK.
Ferrous gluconate (p.1360·1); copper gluconate (p.1357·3).

Forexin Pharmaland, Thai.
Ciprofloxacin (p.182·3).
Bacterial infections.

Forgenac Formenti, Ital.
Diclofenac sodium (p.30·3).
Inflammation; musculoskeletal and joint disorders; oedema.

Foric Sam-On, Israel.
Ferrous fumarate (p.1360·1); folic acid (p.1361·1).
Anaemias; folic acid supplement.

Forilin Novo Nordisk, Denm.
Roxithromycin (p.247·2).
Bacterial infections.

Forlax Beaufour, Fr.; Intersan, Ger.; Beaufour-Ipsen, Hong Kong; Beaufour-Ipsen, Thai.
Macrogol 4000 (p.1630·3).
Constipation.

Formadon Gordon, USA.
Formaldehyde (p.1144·2).
Hyperhidrosis.

Formalyde Pedinol, USA.
Formaldehyde (p.1144·2).
Drying agent in surgical removal of warts; hyperhidrosis and offensive odour of the feet.

Formance Abbott, Hong Kong; Abbott, Irl.; Abbott, Mex.; Abbott, Thai.
Nutritional supplement (p.1350·1).

Formasan Sanum-Kehlbeck, Ger.
Homoeopathic preparation.

Formedico Uragme, Ital.
Zinc chloride (p.1398·1); alcohol (p.1130·3); sodium monofluorophosphate (p.1377·2).
Mouth disorders.

Formicain DHU, Ger.
Homoeopathic preparation.

Formicare Bath Hamilton, Austral.†
Tar (p.1125·1).
Inflammation; pruritus; skin irritation.

Formicare Shower Hamilton, Austral.†
Tar (p.1125·1).
Inflammation; pruritus; skin irritation.

Formicare Skin Gel Hamilton, Austral.†
Tar (p.1125·1).
Inflammation; pruritus; skin irritation.

Formicare Skin Relief Hamilton, Austral.†
Menthol (p.1632·3); cetrimide (p.1137·1); dimethicone (p.1410·1); tar (p.1125·1).
Dermatitis; dry skin; eczema.

Formicare Skin Wash Hamilton, Austral.†
Tar (p.1125·1).
Dermatitis; dry skin; eczema; soap substitute.

Formidium DHU, Ger.
Homoeopathic preparation.

Formin Pharmaland, Thai.
Metformin hydrochloride (p.332·3).
Diabetes mellitus.

Formisoton Staufen, Ger.
Homoeopathic preparation.

Formistin Lusofarmaco, Ital.
Cetirizine hydrochloride (p.411·2).
Hypersensitivity reactions.

Formitonicum Simoes, Braz.
Chinaria officinalis; sterculia (p.1250·2); gentian (p.1615·1); iodine (p.1522·3); cinnamon (p.1595·3).

Formitrol Novartis Consumer, Ital.
Dextromethorphan hydrobromide (p.1087·3).
Coughs.

Formocarbine SmithKline Beecham Sante, Fr.
Activated charcoal (p.1000·2).
Gastrointestinal disorders.

Formo-Cresol Mitis Colgate Oral Care, Austral.
Formaldehyde (p.1144·2); cresol (p.1142·3).
Endodontics.

Formoftil Farmigea, Ital.
Formocortal (p.1073·2).
Inflammatory eye disorders.

Formomicin Farmigea, Ital.
Formocortal (p.1073·2); gentamicin sulfate (p.210·1).
Infected inflammatory eye disorders.

Formula 2 Nutrifarma, Mex.
Preparation for enteral nutrition (p.1350·1).

Formula III Sisu, Canad.†
Multivitamin and mineral preparation (p.1350·1).

Formula IV GNLD, Austral.
Nutritional supplement with vitamins and minerals (p.1350·1).

Formula 28 QIF, Braz.
Vitamin, mineral, and enzyme preparation (p.1350·1).

Formula 44 Procter & Gamble, Canad.
Dextromethorphan hydrobromide (p.1087·3).
Coughs.

Formula 405 Doak, USA.
Skin cleanser.

Formula B Plus Major, USA.
Ferrous fumarate (p.1360·1); folic acid (p.1361·1); multivitamins and minerals (p.1350·1).
Iron-deficiency anaemias.

Formula CDC Seroyal, Canad.
Vitamin C, manganese, and zinc (p.1350·1).

Formula CI Seroyal, Canad.†
Chromium proteinate (p.1357·1); inositol nicotinate (p.914·1).

Formula 44D Procter & Gamble, Canad.
Dextromethorphan hydrobromide (p.1087·3); pseudoephedrine hydrochloride (p.1099·2).
Coughs and cold symptoms.

Formula E Procter & Gamble, Mex.
Guaifenesin (p.1092·2).

Formula 44E Procter & Gamble, Canad.
Dextromethorphan hydrobromide (p.1087·3); guaifenesin (p.1092·2).
Coughs.

Formula EM Major, USA.
Glucose (p.1364·1); fructose (p.1363·3); phosphoric acid (p.1651·1).
Nausea and vomiting.

Formula Forte Senior Hall, Canad.
Multivitamin and mineral preparation (p.1350·1).

Formula Gly Seroyal, Canad.
Multivitamin and mineral preparation (p.1350·1).

Formula Gyn Seroyal, Canad.
Vitamin B₆ (p.1387·1); magnesium proteinate (p.1190·3).

Formula 44M Procter & Gamble, Canad.
Dextromethorphan hydrobromide (p.1087·3); pseudoephedrine hydrochloride (p.1099·2); chlorpheniramine [chlorphenamine] maleate (p.412·1); paracetamol (p.71·2).
Coughs and cold symptoms.

Formula 44M Pediatric Procter & Gamble, Canad.
Dextromethorphan hydrobromide (p.1087·3); pseudoephedrine hydrochloride (p.1099·2); chlorpheniramine [chlorphenamine] maleate (p.412·1).
Cold symptoms.

Formula O General Nutrition, Canad.
Multivitamin preparation with zinc (p.1350·1).

Formula OSG Seroyal, Canad.
Vitamins A, C, and D, and minerals (p.1350·1).

Formula OSX Seroyal, Canad.
Mineral preparation (p.1350·1).

Formula S Procter & Gamble, Mex.
Dextromethorphan (p.1087·3).

Formula 33 SE Nutrition Care, Austral.
Vitamins; minerals; selenium; bladderwrack; echinacea purpurea; hydrastis (p.1350·1).
Dietary supplement.

Formula Three Vitaglow, Austral.†
Pyridoxine hydrochloride (p.1386·3); magnesium oxide (p.1233·2); zinc amino acid chelate (p.1398·3).
Nutritional supplement.

Formula Three Triple Strength Vitaglow, Austral.†
Pyridoxine hydrochloride (p.1386·3); magnesium oxide (p.1233·2); zinc amino acid chelate (p.1398·3); manganese amino acid chelate.
Nutritional supplement.

Formula VM Solgar, USA.
A range of vitamin preparations (p.1350·1).

Formula VM-75 Solgar, UK.
Multivitamin and mineral preparation (p.1350·1).

Formulaexpec Procter & Gamble, Spain.
Guaifenesin (p.1092·2).
Coughs.

Formula-S Nutricia, Singapore.
Lactose-free, soya-based infant feed (p.1350·1).

Formulatus Procter & Gamble, Spain.
Dextromethorphan hydrobromide (p.1087·3).
Coughs.

Formule de l'Abbe Chaupitre Arkopharma, Fr.
A range of homoeopathic preparations.

Formule 115 DM Frega, Canad.†
Pseudoephedrine hydrochloride (p.1099·2); chlorpheniramine [chlorphenamine] maleate (p.412·1); dextromethorphan hydrobromide (p.1087·3).

Formule No 203 Profil Pharmalab, Canad.†
Multivitamin and mineral preparation (p.1350·1).

Formule No 204 Profil Pharmalab, Canad.†
Vitamin C, iron, and potassium (p.1350·1).

Formule W Whitehall, Neth.
Salicylic acid (p.1122·3).
Corns; warts.

Formulex ICN, Canad.
Dicyclomine [dicycloverine] hydrochloride (p.466·1).
Antispasmodic.

Formulix Ortho, UK.
Paracetamol (p.71·2); codeine phosphate (p.25·2).
These ingredients can be described by the British Approved Name Co-codamol.
Pain.

Forpyn Rolab, S.Afr.
Paracetamol (p.71·2); codeine phosphate (p.25·2); caffeine (p.761·3); doxylamine succinate (p.417·1).
Pain and associated tension.

Forsalil UCI, Braz.
Cetylpyridinium chloride (p.1138·1); borax (p.1586·1); benzocaine (p.1306·2); phenosalyl; menthol (p.1632·3); eucalyptus oil (p.1609·2); mallow.
Mouth and throat disorders.

Forta Ross, USA.
A range of preparations for enteral nutrition (p.1350·1).

Forta B Continental Pharma, Belg.
Hydroxocobalamin acetate (p.1388·3).
Megaloblastic anaemia; neuralgia; vitamin B₁₂ deficiency.

Fortacet *Interdelta, Switz.*
Aluminium acetotartrate (p.1578·2); chamomile (p.1593·2); arnica (p.1581·3).
Insect bites; skin irritation; soft-tissue injuries.

Fortacil *Manuell, Mex.*
Amino-acid and mineral preparation (p.1350·1).
Anaemia; tonic.

Fortagesic *Sanofi Winthrop, Irl.*
Pentazocine hydrochloride (p.74·2); paracetamol (p.71·2).
Musculoskeletal pain.

Fortakehl *Sanum-Kehlbeck, Ger.*
Homoeopathic preparation.

Fortal
Note. This name is used for preparations of different composition.
Sanofi Synthelabo, Belg.; Sanofi Winthrop, Fr.
Pentazocine (p.74·2).
Pain.

Prisfar, Port.
Calcium and magnesium preparation (p.1350·1).
Nutritional supplement.

Fortalgesic *Sanofi Winthrop, Swed.†; Sanofi Synthelabo, Switz.*
Pentazocine (p.74·2), pentazocine hydrochloride (p.74·2), or pentazocine lactate (p.74·2).
Neuroleptanalgesia; pain; premedication.

Fortalgex GH *Laborsil, Braz.*
Multivitamin and mineral preparation (p.1350·1).

Fortalidon P *Novartis Consumer, Switz.*
Paracetamol (p.71·2).
Fever; pain.

Fortalis *Interdelta, Switz.*
Methyl salicylate (p.55·1); salicylic acid (p.1122·3); formic acid (p.1612·3); camphor (p.1589·3).
Musculoskeletal and joint pain.

Fortam *Glaxo Wellcome, Spain; Glaxo Wellcome, Switz.*
Ceftazidime (p.174·3).
Bacterial infections.

Fortamines 10 *Rougier, Canad.*
Multivitamin preparation (p.1350·1).

Fortamol *Merck, Denm.*
Codeine phosphate (p.25·2); paracetamol (p.71·2).
Pain.

Fortaneurin *Continental Pharma, Belg.*
Vitamin B substances (p.1350·1).
Megaloblastic anaemia; neuralgia; polyneuritis; vitamin B_1 and/or B_{12} deficiency.

Fortasec *Esteve, Spain.*
Loperamide hydrochloride (p.1231·3).
Diarrhoea.

Fortasept *Wander, Aust.†*
Oxybuprocaine hydrochloride (p.1318·1).

Fortaz *Glaxo Wellcome, Braz.; Glaxo Wellcome, Canad.; Glaxo Wellcome, USA.*
Ceftazidime (p.174·3).
Bacterial infections.

Fortecortin *Merck, Aust.; Merck, Ger.; Merck, Spain; Merck, Switz.*
Dexamethasone (p.1067·1), dexamethasone phosphate (p.1067·1), or dexamethasone sodium phosphate (p.1067·1).
Corticosteroid.

Fortefog *Agropharm, UK.*
Cypermethrin (Fortemethrin) (p.1430·3); piperonyl butoxide (p.1436·2); bioallethrin (p.1428·3); N-octylbicycloheptene dicarboximide.
Insecticide and repellent.

Fortel *Biomerica, USA.*
Fertility test or pregnancy test (p.1654·3).

Fortel One Step *Marco, Austral.*
Pregnancy test (p.1654·3).

Forten *Farmalab, Braz.*
Amino-acid preparation with hydroxocobalamin (p.1350·1).
Nutritional supplement.

Fortenac *Interdelta, Switz.*
Diclofenac sodium (p.30·3).
Musculoskeletal, joint, and peri-articular disorders.

Fortepen *Biochemie, Aust.†*
Procaine penicillin [procaine benzylpenicillin] (p.239·2); benzylpenicillin sodium (p.157·1).
Bacterial infections.

Fortespan *SmithKline Beecham, UK†.*
Ferrous sulfate (p.1360·3); folic acid (p.1361·1).
Iron and folic acid deficiency in pregnancy.

Fortevital *Tentan, Switz.*
Multivitamin and mineral preparation with caffeine, ginseng, and gingko biloba (p.1350·1).
Tonic.

Fortfen *Compu, S.Afr.*
Diclofenac sodium (p.30·3).
Gout; inflammation; musculoskeletal and joint disorders; pain.

Forthane *Abbott, Austral.*
Isoflurane (p.1261·1).
General anaesthesia.

Fortical *Rubio, Spain.*
Calcium carbonate (p.1215·1).
Hypocalcaemia; osteoporosis.

Forticine *Wolfs, Belg.*
Nutritional supplement (p.1350·1).

Forticol *Medinfar, Port.*
Deanol acetoglutamate (p.1507·2); heptaminol hydrochloride (p.1619·2).
Mental function disorders.

Forticreme *Nutricia, Fr.; Nutricia, Irl.; Nutricia, Port.; Nutricia Clinical, UK.*
Preparation for enteral nutrition (p.1350·1).

Forticrin *Panzera, Ital.*
Vitamin B substances (p.1350·1); vitamin E (p.1393·3); achillea (p.1572·2); ginkgo biloba (p.1615·2); ginseng (p.1615·3).
Hair loss.

Fortifier *United American, Hong Kong.*
Ferrous fumarate (p.1360·1); vitamin B substances; liver (p.1350·1).
Anaemias.

Fortifresh *Nutricia, Fin.; Nutricia, Fr.†; Nutricia, Irl.; Nutricia, Ital.; Nutricia, Port.†.*
Preparation for enteral nutrition (p.1350·1).

Fortijuice *Nutricia, Austral.; Nutricia, Irl.; Douglas, NZ; Nutricia, Singapore; Nutricia Clinical, UK.*
Preparation for enteral nutrition (p.1350·1).

Fortimel *Nutricia, Fin.; Nutricia, Fr.; Nutricia, Irl.; Nutricia, Ital.; Douglas, NZ; Nutricia, NZ; Nutricia, Port.; Nutricia Clinical, UK.*
High protein nutritional supplement (p.1350·1).

Fortimicin *Kyowa, Jpn.*
Astromicin sulfate (p.152·3).
Bacterial infections.

Fortinic *Lambda, USA†.*
Vitamin B substances and iron (p.1350·1).

Fortipine *Goldshield, UK.*
Nifedipine (p.940·1).
Angina pectoris; hypertension; Raynaud's syndrome.

Fortiplex *Sante Naturelle, Canad.*
Vitamin B_{12} (p.1388·1); ferrous fumarate (p.1360·1).

Fortipudding *Nutricia, Fr.†; Nutricia, Irl.†; Nutricia, Ital.; Nutricia, Port.†; Nutricia Clinical, UK.*
Nutritional supplement (p.1350·1).

Fortisip *Nutricia, Austral.; Nutricia, Irl.; Nutricia, Ital.; Baxter, NZ; Nutricia, NZ; Nutricia, Singapore; Nutricia Clinical, UK.*
A range of preparations for enteral nutrition (p.1350·1).

Fortistress *Sante Naturelle, Canad.*
Vitamin B substances and vitamin C (p.1350·1).

Fortolin *Fortune, Hong Kong.*
Paracetamol (p.71·2).
Fever; pain.

Fortonal *Medic, Braz.*
Iron (p.1366·3); calcium glycerophosphate; sodium glycerophosphate.
Iron deficiency; iron-deficiency anaemia.

Fortovase *Roche, Aust.; Roche, Austral.; Roche, Belg.; Roche, Canad.; Roche, Denm.; Roche, Fin.; Roche, Fr.; Roche, Ger.; Roche, Ital.; Roche, Neth.; Roche, NZ; Roche, Port.; Roche, S.Afr.; Roche, Spain; Roche, Swed.; Roche, Switz.; Roche, Thai.; Roche, UK; Roche, USA.*
Saquinavir (p.641·1).
HIV infection.

Fortplex *Cazi, Braz.*
Multivitamin and mineral preparation (p.1350·1).

Fortradol *Bayer, Ital.*
Tramadol hydrochloride (p.89·1).
Pain.

Fortral *Sanofi Winthrop, Aust.†; Sanofi Synthelabo, Austral.; Sanofi Winthrop, Denm.; Sanofi Synthelabo, Fr.; Sanofi Winthrop, Irl.; Sanofi Synthelabo, Neth.; Sanofi Winthrop, NZ; Sterwin, UK.*
Pentazocine (p.74·2), pentazocine hydrochloride (p.74·2), or pentazocine lactate (p.74·2).
Pain.

Fortralin *Sanofi Winthrop, Norw.*
Pentazocine (p.74·2), pentazocine hydrochloride (p.74·2), or pentazocine lactate (p.74·2).
Pain.

Fortrans *Beaufour, Fr.; Beaufour-Ipsen, Hong Kong; Beaufour-Ipsen, Singapore; Emerging Pharma, Rus.*
Macrogol 4000 (p.1630·3); anhydrous sodium sulfate; sodium bicarbonate; sodium chloride; potassium chloride (p.1180·1).
Bowel evacuation.

Fortravel *Asta Medica, Aust.*
Cyclizine hydrochloride (p.414·1).
Motion sickness.

Fortum *Glaxo Wellcome, Aust.; Glaxo Wellcome, Austral.; Glaxo Wellcome, Denm.; Glaxo Wellcome, Fr.; Cascan, Ger.; Glaxo Wellcome, Ger.; Glaxo Wellcome, Hong Kong; Glaxo Wellcome, Irl.; Glaxo Wellcome, Israel; Glaxo Wellcome, Mex.; Glaxo Wellcome, Neth.; Glaxo Wellcome, Norw.; Glaxo Wellcome, NZ; Glaxo Wellcome, S.Afr.; Glaxo Wellcome, Singapore; Glaxo Wellcome, Swed.; Glaxo Wellcome, Thai.; Glaxo Wellcome, UK.*
Ceftazidime (p.174·3).
Bacterial infections.

Fortumset *Glaxo Wellcome, Fr.*
Ceftazidime (p.174·3).
Bacterial infections.

Fortwin *Ranbaxy, Thai.*
Pentazocine lactate (p.74·2).
Pain.

Fortyplan *Lifeplan, UK.*
Vitamin, mineral, and nutritional preparation (p.1350·1).

Fortzaar *Merck Sharp & Dohme, Denm.; Merck Sharp & Dohme-Chibret, Fr.*
Losartan potassium (p.921·3); hydrochlorothiazide (p.907·3).
Hypertension.

Forverm *Elofar, Braz.*
Mebendazole (p.102·2); tiabendazole (p.109·1).
Worm infections.

Forvital *Whitehall, Fr.*
Multivitamin and iron preparation (p.1350·1).

Forzid *Atlantic, Thai.*
Ceftazidime (p.174·3).
Bacterial infections.

Fosalan *Merck Sharp & Dohme, Israel.*
Alendronate sodium (p.747·2).
Osteoporosis.

Fosamax *Merck Sharp & Dohme, Aust.; Merck Sharp & Dohme, Austral.; Merck Sharp & Dohme, Belg.; Merck Sharp & Dohme, Braz.; Merck Frosst, Canad.; Merck Sharp & Dohme, Denm.; Merck Sharp & Dohme-Chibret, Fr.; Merck Sharp & Dohme, Fin.; Merck Sharp & Dohme, Ger.; Merck Sharp & Dohme, Hong Kong; Merck Sharp & Dohme, Irl.; Merck Sharp & Dohme, Ital.; Merck Sharp & Dohme, Mex.; Merck Sharp & Dohme, Neth.; Merck Sharp & Dohme, Norw.; Merck Sharp & Dohme, NZ; Merck Sharp & Dohme, Port.; Merck Sharp & Dohme, S.Afr.; Merck Sharp & Dohme, Singapore; Merck Sharp & Dohme, Spain; Merck Sharp & Dohme, Swed.; Merck Sharp & Dohme, Switz.; Merck Sharp & Dohme, Thai.; Merck Sharp & Dohme, UK; Merck, USA.*
Alendronate sodium (p.747·2).
Osteoporosis; Paget's disease of bone.

Foscan *Scotia, UK.*
Temoporfin (p.573·3).
Photodynamic therapy of head and neck cancers.

Foscavir *Astra, Aust.; Astra, Austral.; Astra, Belg.; AstraZeneca, Fin.; AstraZeneca, Fr.; Astra, Ger.; Astra, Hong Kong; Astra, Israel; Astra, Ital.; Astra, Jpn; Astra, Neth.; AstraZeneca, Norw.; Astra, Port.; Astra, Spain; Astra, Swed.; Astra, Switz.; AstraZeneca, Thai.; AstraZeneca, UK; Astra, USA.*
Foscarnet sodium (p.621·2).
Cytomegalovirus retinitis; herpes simplex infections.

Foscovir *AstraZeneca, Denm.*
Foscarnet sodium (p.621·2).
Cytomegalovirus infections; herpes simplex infections.

Fosfalugel *Yamanouchi, Ital.*
Aluminium phosphate (p.1211·3).
Gastric hyperacidity.

Fosfalumina *Schering-Plough, Spain†.*
Aluminium phosphate (p.1211·3).
Gastrointestinal hyperacidity; phosphate deficiency.

Fosfarsile Forte *Fitobucaneve, Ital.*
Oral liquid: Royal jelly (p.1659·3); propolis (p.1655·1); selenium (p.1375·2); ginseng (p.1615·3).
Tablets: Glucose (p.1364·1); royal jelly (p.1659·3); ginseng (p.1615·3).
Nutritional supplement.

Fosfarsile Yunior *Fitobucaneve, Ital.*
Royal jelly (p.1659·3); vitamins (p.1350·1); phosphorus proteinate (p.1350·1); cod-liver oil (p.1357·2).
Nutritional supplement.

Fosfaseron *Serono, Mex.*
Cyclophosphamide (p.527·3).

Fosfatan *Farmavy, Braz.*
Vitamin B_1; magnesium glycerophosphate; calcium glycerophosphate; sodium glycerophosphate; guarana; kola; cinchona bark; nux vomica (p.1350·1).

Fosfo Plus *FAMA, Ital.*
Levoglutamide (p.1365·2); DL-phosphoserine; cyanocobalamin (p.1388·1).
Tonic.

Fosfo-Astenil *Sanofi Synthelabo, Port.*
Sodium hydroxybenzylphosphinate; phosphoric acid; manganese chloride; calcium glycerophosphate; magnesium glycerophosphate; potassium glycerophosphate; sodium glycerophosphate; totamine; thiamine hydrochloride (p.1350·1).
Tonic.

Fosfocaps *Novaquimica, Braz.*
Amino-acid, vitamin, and mineral preparation (p.1350·1).

Fosfocil *Senosiain, Mex.*
Fosfomycin calcium (p.208·2) or fosfomycin disodium (p.208·2).
Lignocaine [lidocaine] hydrochloride (p.1313·2) is included in the intramuscular injection to alleviate the pain of injection.
Bacterial infections.

Fosfocin *Infectopharm, Ger.; Crinos, Ital.; Boehringer Mannheim, Switz.†.*
Fosfomycin calcium (p.208·2) or fosfomycin disodium (p.208·2).
Bacterial infections.

Fosfocina *I Farmacologia, Spain.*
Fosfomycin calcium (p.208·2) or fosfomycin disodium (p.208·2).
Lignocaine [lidocaine] hydrochloride (p.1313·2) is included in the intramuscular injection to alleviate the pain of injection.
Bacterial infections.

Fosfocine *Sanofi Winthrop, Fr.*
Fosfomycin sodium (p.208·2).
Bacterial infections.

Fosfocrisolo *Zambon, Ital.*
Sodium aurotiosulfate (p.84·1).
Rheumatoid arthritis.

Fosfoglutina B6 *Baldacci, Port.*
Calcium pyrrolidonecarboxylate; levoglutamide; tetraethylamonium phosphate; pyridoxine (p.1350·1).
Mental function impairment.

Fosfoguaaiacol *Ogna, Ital.*
Guaiacol (p.1092·1); eucalyptus (p.1609·2).
Respiratory congestion.

Fosfor *Consolidated Chemicals, Irl.; Cortecs, UK.*
Phosphorylcolamine.
Tonic.

Fosforal *Fournier, Ital.†.*
Fosfomycin calcium (p.208·2).
Bacterial infections.

Fosforil Calcium *SPA, Ital.†.*
Calcium glucose-1-phosphate; pyridoxine hydrochloride (p.1386·3); ergocalciferol (p.1391·2).
Calcium and vitamin deficiency.

Fosforilasi *Polifarma, Ital.*
Cocarboxylase (p.1385·2); riboflavin sodium phosphate (p.1386·1); pyridoxal phosphate (p.1387·1); nicotinamide (p.1372·3).
Lignocaine [lidocaine] hydrochloride (p.1313·2) is included in this preparation to alleviate the pain of injection.
Neuritis; toxicosis.

Fosforina *Francia, Ital.*
Vitamin B substances; vitamin E (p.1350·1).
Nutritional supplement.

Fosfosoda *Casen Fleet, Spain.*
Monobasic sodium phosphate (p.1193·2); dibasic sodium phosphate (p.1193·2).
Bowel evacuation.

Fosfo-Soda Fleet *Bergamon, Ital.*
Monobasic sodium phosphate (p.1193·2); dibasic sodium phosphate (p.1193·2).
Constipation.

Fosfosol *Virtus, Braz.*
Kola; guarana; nux vomica; sodium glycerophosphate; glutamic acid; phosphoric acid (p.1350·1).

Fosfoutipi Vitaminico *Terapeutico, Ital.*
Uridine triphosphate (p.1677·2); cyanocobalamin (p.1388·1); thiamine hydrochloride (p.1385·1).
Peripheral neuropathies.

Fosfree *Mission Pharmacal, USA.*
Multivitamin preparation with iron and calcium (p.1350·1).
Calcium supplement; nocturnal leg cramping.

Fosgluten Reforzado *Alter, Spain.*
Calcium magnesium phytate; vitamin B substances; glutamine (p.1350·1).
Tonic.

Fosgluten Super Reforcado *Alter, Port.*
Levoglutamide; calcium glycerophosphate; vitamin B substances (p.1350·1).

Fosicomb *Bristol-Myers Squibb, Aust.*
Fosinopril sodium (p.892·3); hydrochlorothiazide (p.907·3).
Hypertension.

Fosicombi *Menarini, Ital.*
Fosinopril sodium (p.892·3); hydrochlorothiazide (p.907·3).
Hypertension.

Fosicomp *Bristol-Myers Squibb, Switz.*
Fosinopril sodium (p.892·3); hydrochlorothiazide (p.907·3).
Hypertension.

Foside *Solvay, Belg.*
Fosinopril sodium (p.892·3); hydrochlorothiazide (p.907·3).
Hypertension.

Fosinil *Solvay, Belg.; Squibb, Spain.*
Fosinopril sodium (p.892·3).
Heart failure; hypertension.

Fosinorm *Bristol-Myers Squibb, Ger.*
Fosinopril sodium (p.892·3).
Heart failure; hypertension.

Fosinorm comp *Bristol-Myers Squibb, Ger.*
Fosinopril sodium (p.892·3); hydrochlorothiazide (p.907·3).
Hypertension.

Fosipres *Menarini, Ital.*
Fosinopril sodium (p.892·3).
Heart failure; hypertension.

Fositen *Bristol-Myers Squibb, Port.; Bristol-Myers Squibb, Switz.*
Fosinopril sodium (p.892·3).
Heart failure; hypertension.

Fositens *Bristol-Myers Squibb, Aust.; Squibb, Ital.*
Fosinopril sodium (p.892·3).
Heart failure; hypertension.

Fositens Plus *Squibb, Spain.*
Fosinopril sodium (p.892·3); hydrochlorothiazide (p.907·3).
Hypertension.

Fosmicin *Meiji, Thai.*
Fosfomycin sodium (p.208·2).
Bacterial infections.

Fosmicin-S *Meiji, Jpn.*
Fosfomycin sodium (p.208·2).
Bacterial infections.

The symbol † denotes a preparation no longer actively marketed

Fossyol Merckle, Ger.
Metronidazole (p.594·1).
Trichomoniasis.

Fostex Westwood, USA.
Benzoyl peroxide (p.1111·1).
Acne.

Fostex Acne Medication Cleansing Bristol-Myers Products, USA.
Salicylic acid (p.1122·3).
Acne; hyperkeratosis.

Fostex Medicated Westwood-Squibb, USA.
Salicylic acid (p.1122·3); sulfur (p.1123·3).
Acne.

Fostex Medicated Cleansing Bristol-Myers Squibb, Canad.
Salicylic acid (p.1122·3).
Acne; oily skin.

Fostimon IBSA, Ital.; IBSA, Switz.
Urofollitropin (p.1299·3).
Female infertility.

Fostril Westwood, USA.
Sulfur (p.1123·3); zinc oxide (p.1128·2).
Acne.

Fosvital IMA, Braz.
Vitamin B substances; amino acids; minerals (p.1350·1).
Tonic.

Fotax M & H, Thai.
Cefotaxime sodium (p.169·1).
Bacterial infections.

Fotexina Pisa, Mex.
Cefotaxime sodium (p.169·1).
Lignocaine [lidocaine] (p.1313·2) is included in the intramuscular injection to alleviate the pain of injection.
Bacterial infections.

Fotil Santen, Denm.; Santen, Fin.; Ciba Vision, Ger.; Santen, Norw.; Santen, Swed.; Ciba Vision, Switz.; Santen, Thai.
Pilocarpine hydrochloride (p.1422·3); timolol maleate (p.982·1).
Glaucoma; ocular hypertension.

Fotofil INTES, Ital.
Sodium aminobenzoate; actinoquinol (p.1573·1); naphazoline nitrate (p.1095·1); borax (p.1586·1).
Blepharitis; conjunctivitis; corneal damage.

Fotoprotectores Isdin, Port.
SPF 15; SPF 20; SPF 25; SPF 50: A range of sunscreen preparations.

Fototar ICN, USA.
Coal tar (p.1125·1).
Psoriasis; seborrhoeic dermatitis.

Fotrec DHA Visufarma, Ital.
Docosahexaenoic acid (p.949·2); omega-3 triglycerides (p.949·2).
Nutritional supplement.

Four-Ton Body Spring, Ital.
Guarana (p.1681·1); damiana (p.1602·1); ginseng (p.1615·3); royal jelly (p.1659·3).
Nutritional supplement.

Fovysat Ysatfabrik, Ger.
Crataegus (p.1600·2); ginger (p.1227·2).
Dystonias; neuroses.

Fowlers Novartis Consumer, Canad.
Attapulgite (p.1212·1).

Foxil Ibirn, Ital.
Cefadroxil (p.161·2).
Bacterial infections.

Foximin Euro-Pharma, Ital.
Fosfomycin calcium (p.208·2).
Bacterial infections.

Foxin Pharmaland, Thai.
Norfloxacin (p.232·1).
Bacterial infections.

Foxinon M & H, Thai.
Norfloxacin (p.232·1).
Bacterial infections.

Foy Lepetit, Ital.; Ono, Jpn.
Gabexate mesilate (p.1613·1).
Disseminated intravascular coagulation; pancreatitis.

Foziretic Lipha Sante, Fr.
Fosinopril sodium (p.892·3); hydrochlorothiazide (p.907·3).
Hypertension.

Fozitec Lipha Sante, Fr.
Fosinopril sodium (p.892·3).
Heart failure; hypertension.

Fractal Sinbio, Fr.
Fluvastatin sodium (p.892·1).
Hypercholesterolaemia.

Frademicina Rhodia, Braz.
Lincomycin (p.219·3).
Bacterial infections.

Fradicilina Reig Jofre, Spain†
Procaine penicillin [procaine benzylpenicillin] (p.239·2).
Bacterial infections.

Fradilen Chibret, Port.
Chromocarb diethylamine (p.1594·3).
Capillary fragility.

Frador Fenton, UK.
Menthol (p.1632·3); chlorobutanol (p.1141·2); storax (p.1667·2); benzoin (p.1668·3).
Mouth ulcers.

Fragador Weleda, UK.
Cochlearia offic.; conchae; fragaria vesca fruit; glycogen; lovage (p.1629·3); mel; natrium carb.; pimpinella anisum fruit; sage leaves (p.1660·2); wheat germ; urtica leaves (p.1678·2); ferrum phos.
Stress.

Fragmin Pharmacia Upjohn, Aust.; Pharmacia Upjohn, Austral.; Pharmacia Upjohn, Belg.; Pharmacia Upjohn, Canad.; Pharmacia Upjohn, Denm.; Pharmacia Upjohn, Fin.; Pharmacia Upjohn, Ger.; Pharmacia Upjohn, Hong Kong; Kabi Pharmacia, Israel; Pharmacia Upjohn, Ital.; Pharmacia Upjohn, Neth.; Pharmacia Upjohn, Norw.; Pharmacia Upjohn, NZ; Pharmacia Upjohn, Port.; Pharmacia Upjohn, S.Afr.; Pharmacia Upjohn, Singapore; Pharmacia Upjohn, Spain; Pharmacia Upjohn, Swed.; Pharmacia Upjohn, Switz.; Pharmacia, UK; Pharmacia Upjohn, USA.
Dalteparin sodium (p.865·3).
Prevention of clotting during haemodialysis or haemofiltration; thromboembolic disorders; unstable angina.

Fragmine Pharmacia Upjohn, Fr.
Dalteparin sodium (p.865·3).
Prevention of clotting during haemodialysis; thromboembolic disorders.

Fragonal Phygiene, Fr.†
Ruscus aculeatus; esculoside (p.1574·1).
Circulatory disorders; haemorrhoids.

Frakidex Chauvin, Fr.; Chauvin, Port.; Chauvin Novopharma, Switz.
Dexamethasone phosphate (p.1067·1) or dexamethasone sodium phosphate (p.1067·1); framycetin sulfate (p.208·2).
Infected eye disorders.

Frakitacine Chauvin Novopharma, Switz.
Framycetin sulfate (p.208·2).
Bacterial eye infections.

Framecef Levofarma, Ital.
Cefonicid sodium (p.168·1).
Lignocaine [lidocaine] hydrochloride (p.1313·2) is included in this preparation to alleviate the pain of injection.
Gram-negative bacterial infections.

Framil Francia, Ital.†
Bicarnitine chloride (p.1356·2).
Anorexia; dyspepsia.

Framin SIFRA, Ital.†
Amino-acid infusion (p.1350·1).
Parenteral nutrition.

Framybiotal Martin, Fr.†
Framycetin sulfate (p.208·2).
Rhinopharyngeal infections.

Framyxone Theratech, Fr.
Dexamethasone sodium phosphate (p.1067·1); framycetin sulfate (p.208·2); polymyxin B sulfate (p.238·1).
Formerly known as Dexapolyfra.
Ear and nose infections.

Francital Francia, Ital.
Fosfomycin calcium (p.208·2).
Bacterial infections.

Frangulina Bruschettini, Ital.
Frangula (p.1227·1); boldo (p.1585·3).
Constipation.

Franol
Note.This name is used for preparations of different composition.
Sanofi Winthrop, Braz.; Sanofi Winthrop, Irl.; Sanofi Winthrop, UK.
Ephedrine hydrochloride (p.1090·1) or ephedrine sulfate (p.1090·2); theophylline (p.777·2).
Formerly contained phenobarbital, ephedrine hydrochloride, and theophylline in the UK.
Obstructive airways disease.

Sanofi Synthelabo, Thai.
Theophylline (p.777·2).
Obstructive airways disease.

Franol Expectorant Sanofi Winthrop, Irl.
Theophylline hydrate (p.777·2); guaifenesin (p.1092·2).
Formerly contained ephedrine, theophylline hydrate, and guaifenesin.
Obstructive airways disease.

Franol Plus Sanofi Winthrop, UK.
Ephedrine sulfate (p.1090·2); theophylline (p.777·2).
Formerly contained phenobarbital, thenyldiamine hydrochloride, ephedrine sulfate, and theophylline.
Obstructive airways disease.

Franolyn Expectorant Johnson & Johnson MSD Consumer, UK.
Ephedrine (p.1090·1); guaifenesin (p.1092·2); theophylline (p.777·2).
Formerly known as Strong Franolyn.
Coughs.

Franolyn Sedative Johnson & Johnson MSD Consumer, UK.
Dextromethorphan hydrobromide (p.1087·3).
Formerly known as Soothing Franolyn.
Coughs.

Franzbranns Hilarys, Canad.
Menthol (p.1632·3); alcohol (p.1130·3); eucalyptus oil (p.1609·2); salol (p.82·2).

Franzbranntwein Klosterfrau, Ger.†
Menthol (p.1632·3); camphor (p.1589·3); alcohol (p.1130·3).
Muscle and joint pain; soft-tissue disorders.

Franzbranntwein mit Fichtennadelol Hetterich, Ger.
Camphor (p.1589·3); alcohol (p.1130·3); Norway spruce oil.
Muscle and joint pain; soft-tissue disorders.

Fraurs Francia, Ital.
Ursodeoxycholic acid (p.1677·2).
Biliary disorders; gallstones.

Fraxidol Edmond Pharma, Ital.
Tramadol hydrochloride (p.89·1).
Pain.

Fraxiforte Sanofi Synthelabo, Switz.
Nadroparin calcium (p.937·2).
Deep-vein thrombosis.

Fraxiparin Sanofi Winthrop, Aust.; Sanofi Synthelabo, Ger.
Nadroparin calcium (p.937·2).
Thromboembolic disorders.

Fraxiparina Sanofi Winthrop, Braz.; Sanofi Synthelabo, Ital.; Sanofi Synthelabo, Port.; Sanofi Synthelabo, Spain.
Nadroparin calcium (p.937·2).
Prevention of clotting during haemodialysis; thromboembolic disorders.

Fraxiparine Sanofi Synthelabo, Austral.; Sanofi Synthelabo, Belg.; Sanofi Synthelabo, Canad.; Sanofi Winthrop, Denm.†; Sanofi Winthrop, Fin.; Sanofi Synthelabo, Fr.; Sanofi Winthrop, Hong Kong; Sanofi Winthrop, Mex.; Sanofi Synthelabo, Neth.; Sanofi Winthrop, Norw.; Sanofi Winthrop, NZ; Sanofi Synthelabo, Singapore; Sanofi Winthrop, Swed.; Sanofi Synthelabo, Switz.; Sanofi Synthelabo, Thai.
Nadroparin calcium (p.937·2).
Prevention of clotting during haemodialysis; thromboembolic disorders.

Fraxodi Sanofi Winthrop, Fr.; Sanofi Synthelabo, Neth.
Nadroparin calcium (p.937·2).
Thromboembolic disorders.

Frazim Francia, Ital.
Pirenzepine hydrochloride (p.472·2).
Peptic ulcer.

Frazoline Bouchara, Fr.
Framycetin sulfate (p.208·2); naphazoline nitrate (p.1095·1); amylocaine hydrochloride (p.1306·1).
Nasal infection and congestion.

FreAmine Braun McGaw, Hong Kong; Baxter, Ital.; McGaw, NZ; Pharmacia Upjohn, Spain; Fresenius, UK†; McGaw, USA.
A range of amino-acid infusions with or without electrolytes (p.1350·1).
Parenteral nutrition.

Fre-bre Self-Care Products, UK.
Parsley seed (p.1648·3); peppermint oil (p.1243·3); spearmint oil (p.1666·3).

Fredcina Bunker, Braz.
Lincomycin (p.219·3).
Bacterial infections.

Free & Clear Pharmaceutical Specialties, USA.
Skin cleanser.

Freedavite Freeda, USA.
Multivitamin and mineral preparation with iron (p.1350·1).

Freedox Pharmacia Upjohn, Aust.; Pharmacia Upjohn, Austral.; Pharmacia Upjohn, Belg.; Pharmacia Upjohn, Denm.†; Pharmacia Upjohn, Fin.; Pharmacia Upjohn, Norw.; Pharmacia Upjohn, S.Afr.; Pharmacia Upjohn, Swed.; Pharmacia Upjohn, Switz.
Tirilazad mesilate (p.983·1).
Subarachnoid haemorrhage.

Freezone Medtech, Canad.; Whitehall, Irl.; Whitehall, UK†; Whitehall, USA.
Salicylic acid (p.1122·3).
Corn and callus removal.

Freimax Caldeira & Marques, Port.
Methyl salicylate (p.55·1); turpentine oil (p.1676·3); camphor (p.1589·3); thymol (p.1158·3); pine oil.
Inflammation; musculoskeletal and joint disorders.

Freka-cid Niddapharm, Ger.
Povidone-iodine (p.1155·1).
Burns; skin disinfection; wounds.

Freka-Clyss Fresenius Kabi, Switz.
Dibasic sodium phosphate (p.1193·2); monobasic sodium phosphate (p.1193·2).
Bowel evacuation; constipation.

Frekaderm Fresenius, Fr.†; Fresenius Kabi, Ger.; Fresenius Kabi, Switz.
Alcohol (p.1130·3); benzalkonium chloride (p.1133·2); orthophenylphenol (p.1152·1); clorophene (p.1142·3).
Skin disinfection.

Freka-Drainjet Fresenius Kabi, Ger.
Sodium chloride (p.1196·1).
Irrigation fluid.

Freka-Drainjet Purisole Fresenius Kabi, Ger.
Sorbitol (p.1377·3); mannitol (p.924·3).
Bladder irrigation.

Freka-Nol Fresenius Kabi, Ger.
Alcohol (p.1130·3); glyoxal (p.1145·3); didecyldimethylammonium chloride (p.1143·2).
Surface and instrument disinfection.

Freka-Sept 80 Fresenius Kabi, Ger.
Alcohol (p.1130·3); orthophenylphenol (p.1152·1); clorophene (p.1142·3); benzalkonium chloride (p.1133·2).
Hand disinfection.

Freka-Steril Fresenius Kabi, Ger.
Propyl alcohol (p.1155·3); isopropyl alcohol (p.1149·2).
Hand disinfection; skin disinfection.

FrekaVit Fresenius Kabi, Ger.
Multivitamin infusion (p.1350·1).
Parenteral nutrition.

Fremet Recordati, Spain.
Cimetidine (p.1216·3).
Acid aspiration; gastro-oesophageal reflux; gastrointestinal haemorrhage; gastrointestinal hyperacidity; peptic ulcer; short-bowel syndrome; Zollinger-Ellison syndrome.

Frenactil Janssen-Cilag, Belg.; Janssen-Cilag, Neth.
Benperidol (p.656·2).
Agitation; delirium; hallucinations; nausea and vomiting; sexually deviant behaviour.

Frenadol Abello, Spain.
Paracetamol (p.71·2); chlorpheniramine [chlorphenamine] maleate (p.412·1); dextromethorphan hydrobromide (p.1087·3).
Coughs; fever; influenza and cold symptoms; pain.

Frenadol Complex Abello, Spain.
Ascorbic acid (p.1389·3); caffeine citrate (p.761·3); chlorpheniramine [chlorphenamine] maleate (p.412·1); dextromethorphan hydrobromide (p.1087·3); paracetamol (p.71·2).
Cold and influenza symptoms; coughs; fever; pain.

Frenadol PS Abello, Spain.
Paracetamol (p.71·2); pseudoephedrine hydrochloride (p.1099·2); dextromethorphan hydrobromide (p.1087·3); chlorpheniramine [chlorphenamine] maleate (p.412·1).
Cold and influenza symptoms; coughs; fever; pain.

Frenal Searle, Ital.; Sigma-Tau, Spain.
Sodium cromoglicate (p.774·3).
Asthma; bronchospasm.

Frenal Compositum Sigma-Tau, Spain.
Sodium cromoglicate (p.774·3); isoprenaline sulfate (p.914·3).
Allergic bronchitis; asthma.

Frenal Rinologico Searle, Ital.
Sodium cromoglicate (p.774·3).
Allergic rhinitis.

Frenaseltz Abello, Spain.
Paracetamol (p.71·2); chlorpheniramine [chlorphenamine] maleate (p.412·1); phenylpropanolamine hydrochloride (p.1098·1).
Cold and influenza symptoms.

Frendox Errekappa, Ital.
Bioflavonoids; vitamin E (p.1350·1).
Nutritional supplement.

frenopect Hefa, Ger.
Ambroxol hydrochloride (p.1084·3).
Respiratory-tract disorders associated with increased or viscous mucus.

Frenotosse Cimed, Braz.
Bromoform (p.1587·1); tolu balsam (p.1101·3); sodium benzoate (p.1134·3).
Coughs.

Frenotossil Infabra, Braz.
Potassium iodide (p.1522·3); sulfogaiacol (p.1101·1); tolu balsam (p.1101·3).
Respiratory-tract congeston.

Frenovex Hearst, Braz.
Rutoside (p.1611·2); menadione (p.1395·3); ascorbic acid (p.1389·3).
Haemorrhagic disorders.

Frerichs Maldifassi Pharbenia, Ital.
Aloes (p.1210·1); rhubarb (p.1248·1); calamus (p.1588·1); gentian (p.1615·1).
Constipation.

Fresco Rekah, Israel.
Calcium carbonate (p.1215·1); magnesium carbonate (p.1232·3); magnesium trisilicate (p.1233·3).
Gastrointestinal hyperacidity; peptic ulcer.

Fresenius OPD Rowa, Irl.†
Preparation for enteral nutrition (p.1350·1).
Inflammatory bowel disease.

Fresenizol Alpha, Mex.
Metronidazole (p.594·1).
Anaerobic bacterial infections.

FreshBurst Listerine Warner-Lambert, USA.
Thymol (p.1158·3); eucalyptol (p.1609·2); methyl salicylate (p.55·1); menthol (p.1632·3).
Mouth disorders.

Fresofol Alpha, Mex.
Propofol (p.1265·3).
General anaesthesia.

Fresubin Fresenius, Fin.; Rowa, Irl.†; Fresenius Kabi, Ital.; Alpha, Mex.; Fresenius Kabi, Port.; Fresenius Kabi, Switz.; Fresenius, Thai.; Fresenius, UK.
A range of preparations for enteral nutrition (p.1350·1).

Freudal Ifusa, Mex.
Diazepam (p.674·3).

Frialgina Prodes, Spain†
Aspirin (p.14·2); ascorbic acid (p.1389·3); caffeine (p.761·3).
Fever; pain.

Friax Zeller, Port.†
Cetrimide (p.1137·1); benzyl alcohol (p.1135·3); eucalyptus oil (p.1609·2).
Chilblains.

Friccex Bergamo, Braz.
Methacholine; thymol (p.1158·3); menthol (p.1632·3); methyl salicylate (p.55·1); camphor (p.1589·3).
Musculoskeletal and joint disorders.

Friction Rub Mathieu, Canad.
Isopropyl alcohol (p.1149·2).

Frigol Brady, Aust.
Xantinol nicotinate (p.999·1).
Cerebral and peripheral vascular disorders.

Frigoplasma Kropf, Switz.
Aluminium acetotartrate (p.1578·2); chamomile (p.1593·2); hamamelis (p.1618·3); camphor (p.1589·3); cajuput oil (p.1588·1); rosemary oil (p.1659·3); thyme oil (p.1672·3).
Phlebitis; soft-tissue and peri-articular disorders.

Friliver Bracco, Ital.
Amino-acid preparations (p.1350·1).
Hepatic failure; tonic.

Frinova Rhone-Poulenc Rorer, Spain.
Promethazine (p.423·2).
Hypersensitivity reactions; motion sickness; nausea and vomiting.

Friosmin N Michallik, Ger.
Bismuth subgallate (p.1213·2); emplastrum lithargyri.
Burns; wounds.

Frisium Hoechst Marion Roussel, Aust.; Hoechst Marion Roussel, Austral.; Aventis, Belg.; Hoechst Marion Roussel, Braz.; Hoechst Marion Roussel, Canad.; Aventis, Denm.; Hoechst Marion Roussel, Fin.; Hoechst Marion Roussel, Ger.; Hoechst Marion Roussel, Hong Kong; Hoechst Marion Roussel, Irl.; Hoechst Marion Roussel, Israel; Aventis, Ital.; Hoechst Marion Roussel, Mex.; Hoechst Marion Roussel, Neth.; Aventis, NZ; Hoechst Marion Roussel, Singapore; Hoechst Marion Roussel, Thai.; Hoechst Marion Roussel, UK.
Clobazam (p.668·1).
Anxiety; epilepsy; insomnia.

Frisogrow Friesland, Singapore.
Nutritional supplement (p.1350·1).

Frisolac BA Farma, Port.
Ketoconazole (p.389·1).
Fungal infections.

Frisolona Allergan, Port.
Prednisolone acetate (p.1078·1).
Eye disorders.

Frisomum Friesland, Hong Kong; Friesland, Singapore.
Preparation for enteral nutrition (p.1350·1).
Pregnancy and lactation.

Frisosoy Friesland, Hong Kong; Friesland, Singapore.
Infant feed (p.1350·1).
Cow's milk protein allergy; lactose intolerance.

Frisovom Friesland, Hong Kong; Friesland, Singapore.
Infant feed (p.1350·1).
Colic; constipation; vomiting.

Fristamin FIRMA, Ital.
Loratadine (p.420·1).
Allergic rhinitis; hypersensitivity reactions.

Frivent Dompe, Ital.
Theophylline (p.777·2).
Asthma; bronchospasm.

Frixodon Brasmedica, Braz.
Methacholine hydrochloride (p.1419·3); thymol (p.1158·3); menthol (p.1632·3); methyl salicylate (p.55·1).
Musculoskeletal and joint disorders.

Frixopel EMS, Braz.
Turpentine oil (p.1676·3); methyl salicylate (p.55·1); camphor (p.1589·3); menthol (p.1632·3).
Musculoskeletal and joint disorders.

Froben Ebewe, Aust.; Knoll, Belg.; Knoll, Canad.; Kanoldt, Ger.; Boots, Hong Kong; Knoll, Irl.; GNR, Ital.; Promeco, Mex.; Knoll, Neth.; Knoll, NZ; Knoll, Port.; Knoll, S.Afr.; Knoll, Singapore; Cantabria, Spain; Knoll, Switz.; Knoll, UK.
Flurbiprofen (p.41·2).
Musculoskeletal, joint, peri-articular, and soft-tissue disorders; pain.

Froidir Orion, Fin.
Clozapine (p.671·2).
Schizophrenia.

Frone Serono, Braz.; Serono, Ital.†; Serono, Spain.
Interferon beta (p.632·2).
Anogenital warts; malignant neoplasms; viral infections.

Frontal Pharmacia Upjohn, Braz.; Solvay, Ital.
Alprazolam (p.654·2).
Anxiety disorders; insomnia; panic disorders; tremor.

Froop Ashbourne, UK.
Frusemide [furosemide] (p.893·1).
Oedema; oliguria.

Froop Co Ashbourne, UK.
Frusemide [furosemide] (p.893·1); amiloride hydrochloride (p.835·1).
These ingredients can be described by the British Approved Name Co-amilofruse.
Ascites with cirrhosis; oedema.

Frosinor Novartis, Spain.
Paroxetine hydrochloride (p.302·3).
Anxiety disorders; depression.

Frost Cream Weleda, UK.
Abrotanum; arnica (p.1581·3); peru balsam (p.1650·2); rosemary oil (p.1659·3); stibium metallicum.
Chilblains.

Frostsalbe Weleda, Aust.
Homoeopathic preparation.

Frova Elan, USA.
Frovatriptan (p.454·1).
Migraine.

Froxal Galen, Mex.
Cefuroxime sodium (p.178·2).
Bacterial infections.

Frubiase Calcium Boehringer Ingelheim, Ger.
Calcium carbonate (p.1215·1).
Calcium deficiency; osteoporosis.

Frubiase Calcium forte 500 Boehringer Ingelheim, Ger.
Calcium gluconate (p.1188·2); calcium lactate (p.1188·2); ergocalciferol (p.1391·2).
Osteomalacia; osteoporosis.

Frubiase Calcium T Boehringer Ingelheim, Ger.
Calcium gluconate (p.1188·2); calcium lactate (p.1188·2).
Calcium deficiency.

Frubienzym Boehringer Ingelheim, Ger.
Muramidase (p.1638·1); cetylpyridinium chloride (p.1138·1).
Mouth and throat disorders.

Frubilurgyl Boehringer Ingelheim, Ger.
Chlorhexidine gluconate (p.1138·2).
Mouth and throat disorders.

Frubiose Calcium Wild, Switz.†.
Calcium gluconate (p.1188·2); calcium lactate (p.1188·2); ergocalciferol (p.1391·2); phosphoric acid (p.1651·1).
Calcium deficiency.

Frubiose Vitamine D Boehringer Ingelheim, Fr.
Ergocalciferol (p.1391·2); calcium gluconate (p.1188·2); calcium lactate (p.1188·2).
Formerly known as Frubiose Calcique.
Hypocalcaemia; osteomalacia; rickets; vitamin D and calcium deficiency.

Frubizin Boehringer Ingelheim, Ger.
Cetylpyridinium chloride (p.1138·1).
Mouth and throat disorders.

Frubizin Forte Boehringer Ingelheim, Ger.
Cetylpyridinium chloride (p.1138·1); benzocaine (p.1306·2).
Mouth and throat disorders.

Frucalde Euro-Labor, Port.
Ergocalciferol (p.1391·2); calcium gluconate (p.1188·2); calcium lactate (p.1188·2).
Hypocalcaemia; osteomalacia; osteoporosis.

Fru-Co Norton Waterford, Irl.; Baker Norton, UK.
Frusemide [furosemide] (p.893·1); amiloride hydrochloride (p.835·1).
These ingredients can be described by the British Approved Name Co-amilofruse.
Ascites; nephrotic syndrome; oedema.

Fructal Bieffe, Ital.
Fructose (p.1363·3).

Fructan Searle, Ital.
Fructose (p.1363·3).
Sugar substitute.

Fructines Pharmethic, Belg.; DB, Fr.
Sodium picosulfate (p.1249·3).
Constipation.

Fructines nouvelle formule DB, Switz.
Sodium picosulfate (p.1249·3).
Constipation.

Fructofin Also, Ital.
Fructose (p.1363·3).
Sugar substitute.

Fructogenase Luper, Braz.
Fructose; vitamins (p.1350·1).
Vitamin supplement.

Fructopiran Monico, Ital.
Fructose (p.1363·3).

Fructosil Volchem, Ital.
Fructose (p.1363·3).
Supplementation of glycogen reserves.

Frudemisan Bioquimico, Mex.
Frusemide [furosemide] (p.893·1).

Frugelletten Bregenzer, Aust.
Fig (p.1227·1); senna (p.1248·2); tamarind (p.1253·2).
Constipation.

Fruhjahrs-Elixier ohne Alkohol Ehrmann, Aust.
Urtica (p.1678·2); silver birch (p.1585·2); taraxacum (p.1669·1).
Diuretic.

Fruit of the Earth Moisturizing Aloe Fruit of the Earth, Canad.
SPF 8; SPF 15: Octinoxate (p.1517·3); oxybenzone (p.1518·1).
SPF 30; SPF 45: Octinoxate (p.1517·3); octocrilene (p.1518·1); octisalate (p.1518·1); oxybenzone (p.1518·1); titanium dioxide (p.1126·1).
Sunscreen.

Fruit of the Earth Moisturizing Aloe Baby Fruit of the Earth, Canad.
SPF 45: Octinoxate (p.1517·3); octocrilene (p.1518·1); octisalate (p.1518·1); oxybenzone (p.1518·1); titanium dioxide (p.1126·1).
Sunscreen.

Fruit of the Earth Moisturizing Aloe Kids Fruit of the Earth, Canad.
Topical liquid SPF 30: Octinoxate (p.1517·3); octocrilene (p.1518·1); octisalate (p.1518·1); oxybenzone (p.1518·1); titanium dioxide (p.1126·1).
Topical spray SPF 30: Octinoxate (p.1517·3); octocrilene (p.1518·1); octisalate (p.1518·1); DEA-methoxycinnamate.
Sunscreen.

Fruit of the Earth Moisturizing Aloe Sport Fruit of the Earth, Canad.
SPF 8; SPF 15: Octinoxate (p.1517·3); oxybenzone (p.1518·1).
SPF 30: Octinoxate (p.1517·3); octisalate (p.1518·1); oxybenzone (p.1518·1).
Sunscreen.

Fruitatives Rogers, Canad.
Bisacodyl (p.1212·2); docusate sodium (p.1223·1); prune (p.1245·1).

Fruity Chews Goldline, USA.
A range of vitamin preparations (p.1350·1).

Frumax Ashbourne, UK†.
Frusemide [furosemide] (p.893·1).
Oedema.

Frumeron Remedica, Hong Kong; Remedica, Thai.
Indapamide (p.913·1).
Hypertension.

Frumil Rhone-Poulenc Rorer, Hong Kong; Rhone-Poulenc Rorer, Irl.; Aventis, NZ; Rhone-Poulenc Rorer, Switz.; Helios, UK.
Frusemide [furosemide] (p.893·1); amiloride hydrochloride (p.835·1).
These ingredients can be described by the British Approved Name Co-amilofruse.
Ascites; heart failure; oedema.

Frusamil Aventis, Belg.; Aventis, Denm.
Frusemide [furosemide] (p.893·1); amiloride hydrochloride (p.835·1).
Hypertension; oedema.

Frusehexal Hexal, Austral.
Frusemide [furosemide] (p.893·1).
Hypertension; oedema.

Frusemek Berk, UK.
Frusemide [furosemide] (p.893·1); amiloride hydrochloride (p.835·1).
These ingredients can be described by the British Approved Name Co-amilofruse.
Ascites; fluid retention; heart failure.

Frusene Rhone-Poulenc Rorer, Irl.†; Orion, UK.
Frusemide [furosemide] (p.893·1); triamterene (p.986·1).
Ascites; heart failure; oedema.

Frusid Douglas, Austral.; Douglas, Hong Kong; Douglas, NZ; Douglas, Singapore; Douglas, Thai.; TTN, Thai.; DDSA Pharmaceuticals, UK.
Frusemide [furosemide] (p.893·1).
Ascites; hypertension; oedema.

Frusol Rosemont, UK.
Frusemide [furosemide] (p.893·1).
Hypertension; oedema.

Frutalax QIF, Braz.
Senna (p.1248·2); cassia pulp (p.1216·2); tamarind (p.1253·2); coriander (p.1599·2).
Constipation.

Frutarine Farmalab, Braz.
Senna (p.1248·2); cassia pulp (p.1216·2); tamarind (p.1253·2); liquorice (p.1231·2).
Constipation.

Frutin Prisfar, Port.
Natural dolomite.
Gastric hyperacidity.

Frutoplex Marjan, Braz.
Adenosine; fructose; betaine hydrochloride; methionine; choline citrate; vitamin B_6; vitamin B_2; nicotinamide (p.1350·1).
Vitamin supplement.

Frutovena Farmalab, Braz.
Vitamin B substances; vitamin C (p.1350·1); coriander (p.1599·2).
Vitamin supplement.

Frutovitam Cristalia, Braz.
Multivitamin preparation (p.1350·1).

Fruttocal Sigma-Tau, Ital.
Ergocalciferol (p.1391·2); calcium ascorbate (p.1389·2); calcium gluconate (p.1188·2); inosine (p.1623·3).
Dental caries prophylaxis; osteoporosis; rickets.

Fruver Bonomelli, Ital.
Multivitamin preparation (p.1350·1).

Fruxucre Etajesa, Fr.†.
Fructose (p.1363·3).
Sugar substitute.

FSME-Bulin Immuno, Aust.; Baxter-Hyland, Ger.; Baxter, Switz.
A tick-borne encephalitis immunoglobulin (p.1539·3).
Passive immunisation.

FSME-Immun Immuno, Aust.; Immuno, Belg.†; Immuno, Ger.; Baxter, Switz.
A tick-borne encephalitis vaccine (p.1539·3).
Active immunisation.

Ftoral Abic, Hong Kong; Abic, Israel.
Tegafur (p.573·2).
Malignant neoplasms.

Ftoralon Sanova, Aust.†.
Tegafur (p.573·2).
Malignant neoplasms.

Ftorocort Gedeon Richter, Thai.
Triamcinolone acetonide (p.1080·1).
Skin disorders.

Fuca Cassella-med, Switz.†.
Frangula bark (p.1227·1); cascara (p.1216·1).
Constipation.

Fucafibres Fuca, Fr.†.
Fruit and cereal fibres (p.1350·1); lactitol (p.1230·1).
Gastrointestinal disorders.

Fucibet Farmacusi, Spain; Leo, UK.
Betamethasone valerate (p.1063·2); fusidic acid (p.208·3).
Infected skin disorders.

Fucicort Leo, Belg.; Leo, Denm.; Leo, Fin.; Leo, Ger.; Leo, Hong Kong; Leo, Israel; Senosiain, Mex.; Bomac, NZ; Leo, Port.; Leo, Singapore; Leo, Switz.; Leo, Thai.
Fusidic acid (p.208·3); betamethasone valerate (p.1063·2).
Infected skin disorders.

Fucidin Leo, Aust.; CSL, Austral.; Leo, Belg.; Leo, Canad.; Leo, Denm.; Leo, Fin.; Leo, Hong Kong; Leo, Irl.; Leo, Israel; Senosiain, Mex.; Leo, Neth.; Leo, Norw.; CSL, NZ; Adcock Ingram, S.Afr.; Leo, Singapore; Leo, Swed.; Leo, Thai.; Leo, UK.
Fusidic acid (p.208·3) or sodium fusidate (p.208·3).
Gram-positive bacterial infections.

Fucidin H Leo, Canad.; Leo, Irl.; Discotrade, Israel; Adcock Ingram, S.Afr.; Leo, Singapore; Leo, Switz.; Leo, UK.
Fusidic acid (p.208·3) or sodium fusidate (p.208·3); hydrocortisone acetate (p.1073·3).
Infected skin disorders.

Fucidin Hydrocortisone Leo, Belg.
Fusidic acid (p.208·3); hydrocortisone acetate (p.1073·3).
Infected skin disorders.

Fucidine Leo, Fr.; Boehringer Ingelheim, Ger.; Leo, Ger.; Leo, Port.; Farmacusi, Spain; Leo, Switz.
Fusidic acid (p.208·3) or sodium fusidate (p.208·3).
Bacterial infections.

Fucidine H Leo, Port.; Farmacusi, Spain.
Fusidic acid (p.208·3); hydrocortisone acetate (p.1073·3).
Infected skin disorders.

Fucidine plus Boehringer Ingelheim, Ger.
Sodium fusidate (p.208·3); hydrocortisone butyrate (p.1073·3).
Infected skin disorders.

Fucidin-Hydrocortison Leo, Denm.; Leo, Fin.; Leo, Norw.; Leo, Swed.
Fusidic acid (p.208·3); hydrocortisone (p.1073·3) or hydrocortisone acetate (p.1073·3).
Infected skin disorders.

Fucithalmic Leo, Aust.; Leo, Belg.; Leo, Denm.; Leo, Fin.; Leo, Fr.; Thomae, Ger.; Alcon, Ger.; Leo, Hong Kong; Leo, Irl.; Leo, Israel; Formenti, Ital.; Leo, Neth.; Leo, Norw.; CSL, NZ; Leo, NZ; Leo, Port.; Adcock Ingram, S.Afr.; Leo, Singapore; Alcon Cusi, Spain; Leo, Swed.; Leo, Switz.; Leo, Thai.; Leo, UK.
Fusidic acid (p.208·3).
Bacterial eye infections.

Fuclode Bioprogress, Ital.
Cefaclor (p.161·1).
Bacterial infections.

Fucus Homeocan, Canad.
Homoeopathic preparation.

Fucus Composto Simoes, Braz.
Pokeroot (p.1653·1); bladderwrack (p.1585·2); calotropis gigantea.

Fudimun Kanoldt, Ger.†.
Echinacea purpura (p.1606·2).
Respiratory- and urinary-tract infections.

Fudirine PP Lab, Thai.
Frusemide [furosemide] (p.893·1).
Hypertension; oedema.

FUDR Roche, Singapore; Roche, USA.
Floxuridine (p.539·2).
Gastrointestinal adenocarcinoma metastatic to the liver.

Fugacar Janssen, Thai.
Mebendazole (p.102·2).
Worm infections.

Fugaten Lysoform, Ger.
Alcohol (p.1130·3).
Surface disinfection.

Fugerel Aesca, Aust.; Schering-Plough, Austral.; Essex, Ger.; Schering-Plough, Hong Kong; Schering-Plough, Singapore; Schering-Plough, Thai.
Flutamide (p.542·3).
Prostatic cancer.

Fugisept Lysoform, Ger.
Didecyldimethylammonium chloride (p.1143·2); glyoxal (p.1145·3).
Fungal and bacterial skin infections.

Fulcin Zeneca, Austral.; Zeneca, Braz.; AstraZeneca, Denm.; AstraZeneca, Fin.; Zeneca, Hong Kong; Zeneca, Irl.; SIT, Ital.; Zeneca, Mex.; ICI, Neth.†; AstraZeneca, Norw.; Zeneca, Port.; Zeneca, S.Afr.; Astra-Zeneca, Singapore; Zeneca, Spain; Zeneca, Swed.; Zeneca, Switz.; AstraZeneca, Thai.; AstraZeneca, UK†.
Griseofulvin (p.386·2).
Fungal skin, hair, and nail infections.

Fulcin S Zeneca, Aust.
Griseofulvin (microfine) (p.386·2).
Fungal infections.

The symbol † denotes a preparation no longer actively marketed

Fulcine AstraZeneca, Fr.†
Griseofulvin (p.386·2).
Fungal infections.

Fulcro Fournier, Ital.
Fenofibrate (p.889·1).
Hyperlipidaemias.

Fulgium Teofarma, Spain.
Benzydamine salicylate (p.20·1).
Peri-articular and soft-tissue disorders.

Ful-Glo Allergan, Austral.; Barnes Hind, NZ; Akorn, USA.
Fluorescein sodium (p.1612·1).
Aid to eye examination.

Fulgram ABC, Ital.
Norfloxacin (p.232·1).
Urinary-tract infections.

Full Marks SSL, UK.
Phenothrin (p.1436·2).
Pediculosis.

Full Service Sunblock Clinique, Canad.
SPF 15; SPF 20: Octinoxate (p.1517·3); octisalate (p.1518·1); oxybenzone (p.1518·1).
Sunscreen.

Full-Fort Kopkins, Braz.
Ptychopetalum uncinatum; erythroxylon catuaba.
Tonic.

Fullvita Multivitaminas e Minerais Farmalight, Port.
Multivitamin and mineral preparation (p.1350·1).

Fulvicin Schering, Canad.; Schering, USA.
Griseofulvin (p.386·2).
Fungal infections of the skin, hair, and nails.

Fulvina Schering-Plough, Mex.
Griseofulvin (p.386·2).
Fungal infections.

Fumaderm Fumedica, Ger.; Hermal, Ger.
Dimethyl fumarate; calcium monoethyl fumarate (p.1114·3); magnesium monoethyl fumarate (p.1114·3); zinc monoethyl fumarate (p.1114·3).
Psoriasis.

Fumafer Sanofi Winthrop, Fr.
Ferrous fumarate (p.1360·1).
Anaemias.

Fumasorb Milance, USA†.
Ferrous fumarate (p.1360·1).
Iron-deficiency anaemias.

Fumatinic Laser, USA.
Ferrous fumarate (p.1360·1); cyanocobalamin (p.1388·1).
Ascorbic acid (p.1389·3) is included in this preparation to increase the absorption and availability of iron.
Iron-deficiency anaemias.

Fumerin Laser, USA†.
Ferrous fumarate (p.1360·1).
Iron-deficiency anaemias.

Funa LBS, Thai.
Fluconazole (p.383·2).
Fungal infections.

Funcenal Farma Lepori, Spain.
Flutrimazole (p.386·1).
Fungal skin infections.

Funchicorea Melpoejo, Braz.
Cichorium intybus; rhubarb (p.1248·1); fennel (p.1610·1).
Gastrointestinal spasm.

Funcort Nakorn, Thai.
Miconazole nitrate (p.391·1).
Fungal skin and nail infections.

Fundamin Biomedis, Hong Kong; Biomedis, Singapore.
Vitamin B substances (p.1350·1).
Nausea and vomiting; neuritis; tonic.

Fundamin-E Biomedis, Hong Kong; Biomedis, Singapore; Biomedis, Thai.; Great Eastern, Thai.
Vitamin B substances; vitamin E (p.1350·1).

Funduscein Ciba Vision, Canad.†; Iolab, USA.
Fluorescein sodium (p.1612·1).
Aid to eye examination.

Fungamizol Ofimex, Mex.
Ketoconazole (p.389·1).
Fungal infections.

Funganiline Squibb, Spain.
Amphotericin B (p.377·2).
Oropharyngeal candidiasis.

Fungarest Janssen-Cilag, Spain.
Ketoconazole (p.389·1).
Fungal infections.

Fungata Pfizer, Aust.; Mack, Illert., Ger.
Fluconazole (p.383·2).
Vaginal candidiasis.

Fungazol Ofimex, Mex.; Biolab, Thai.
Ketoconazole (p.389·1).
Fungal infections.

Fungederm Nucare, UK.
Clotrimazole (p.382·1).
Fungal skin infections.

Fungex Streuli, Switz.
Ointment: Undecenoic acid (p.395·3); zinc undecenoate (p.395·3).

Topical powder: Undecenoic acid (p.395·3); zinc undecenoate (p.395·3); aluminium acetotartrate (p.1578·2); calcium lactate (p.1188·2).
Fungal skin infections.

Fungibacid Asche, Ger.†
Tioconazole (p.395·1).
Fungal infections.

Fungicide Torrent, Thai.
Ketoconazole (p.389·1).
Fungal infections.

Fungiderm Note.This name is used for preparations of different composition.
Nycomed, Aust.
Bifonazole (p.381·1).
Fungal skin and nail infections.

Terra-Bio, Ger.; Greater Pharma, Thai.
Clotrimazole (p.382·1).
Fungal skin and vaginal infections; trichomoniasis.

Janssen-Cilag, Ital.†.
Miconazole nitrate (p.391·1).
Fungal infections.

Fungiderm-B Greater Pharma, Thai.
Clotrimazole (p.382·1); betamethasone (p.1063·1).
Fungal skin infections.

Fungidermo Cinfa, Spain.
Clotrimazole (p.382·1).
Fungal skin infections.

Fungidexan Hermal, Ger.
Clotrimazole (p.382·1); urea (p.1127·3).
Fungal skin infections.

Fungifos Combustin, Ger.
Tolciclate (p.395·2).
Fungal skin infections.

Fungilin Bristol-Myers Squibb, Austral.; Bristol-Myers Squibb, Denm.; Bristol-Myers Squibb, Hong Kong; Bristol-Myers Squibb, Israel; Bristol-Myers Squibb, Ital.; Bristol-Myers Squibb, NZ; Squibb, UK.
Amphotericin B (p.377·2).
Candidiasis.

Fungi-M Nakornpatana, Thai.
Miconazole nitrate (p.391·1).
Fungal skin, nail, and hair infections.

Fungimax Neo Quimica, Braz.
Metronidazole (p.594·1); nystatin (p.392·2).
Vulvovaginal infections.

Fungimon Trima, Israel.
Zinc undecenoate (p.395·3); undecenoic acid (p.395·3); aluminium chlorohydrate (p.1110·2).
Fungal skin infections.

Fungi-Nail Kramer, USA.
Resorcinol (p.1122·2); salicylic acid (p.1122·3); chloroxylenol (p.1142·1); benzocaine (p.1306·2); isopropyl alcohol (p.1149·2).
Fungal and bacterial skin infections; fungal nail infections.

Funginox Charoen, Thai.
Ketoconazole (p.389·1).
Fungal infections.

Fungiquim Quimica y Farmacia, Mex.
Miconazole (p.391·1).
Fungal infections.

Fungireduct Azupharma, Ger.
Nystatin (p.392·2).
Candidiasis.

Fungisan Galderma, Ger.
Omoconazole nitrate (p.393·1).
Fungal skin infections.

Fungisdin Isdin, Spain.
Miconazole (p.391·1) or miconazole nitrate (p.391·1).
Candidiasis; fungal skin infections.

Fungisil Silom, Thai.
Miconazole nitrate (p.391·1).
Fungal infections of the skin, nails, and mucous membranes.

Fungisil-T Silom, Thai.
Miconazole nitrate (p.391·1); triamcinolone acetonide (p.1080·1).
Fungal infections of the skin, nails, and mucous membranes.

Fungistat Cilag, Mex.
Terconazole (p.395·1).
Vulvovaginal candidiasis.

Fungisten Weifa, Norw.
Clotrimazole (p.382·1).
Fungal infections.

Fungizid Ratiopharm, Ger.; Ratiopharm, Hong Kong; Douglas, NZ.
Clotrimazole (p.382·1).
Fungal infections.

Fungizon Bristol-Myers Squibb, Braz.
Amphotericin B (p.377·2).
Fungal infections.

Fungizona Squibb, Spain.
Amphotericin B (p.377·2).
Fungal infections.

Fungizone Bristol-Myers Squibb, Austral.; Bristol-Myers Squibb, Belg.; Squibb, Canad.; Bristol-Myers Squibb, Fin.; Bristol-Myers Squibb, Fr.; Bristol-Myers Squibb, Hong Kong; Bristol-Myers Squibb, Irl.; Bristol-Myers Squibb, Israel; Bristol-Myers Squibb, Ital.; Bristol-Myers Squibb, Neth.; Bristol-Myers Squibb, Norw.; Bristol-Myers Squibb, NZ; Bristol-Myers Squibb, S.Afr.; Bristol-Myers Squibb, Singapore; Bristol-Myers Squibb, Swed.; Bristol-Myers Squibb, Switz.; Bristol-Myers Squibb, Thai.; Squibb, UK; Bristol-Myers Squibb Oncology, USA.
Amphotericin B (p.377·2).
Fungal infections; leishmaniasis.

Fungo Note.This name is used for preparations of different composition.
Ego, Austral.
Balm: Miconazole nitrate (p.391·1); bufexamac (p.20·3).
Fungal skin infections.

Cream; vaginal cream; topical powder: Miconazole nitrate (p.391·1).
Fungal skin and vaginal infections.

Topical solution: Miconazole (p.391·1).
Fungal skin and nail infections.

Ego, Hong Kong; Ego, NZ; Ego, Singapore.
Miconazole nitrate (p.391·1).
Fungal and bacterial skin infections.

Fungo Hubber ICN, Spain.
Ketoconazole (p.389·1).
Fungal infections.

Fungocort Douglas, NZ.
Miconazole nitrate (p.391·1); hydrocortisone (p.1073·3).
Infected skin disorders.

Fungoid Pedinol, USA.
Topical solution†: Clotrimazole (p.382·1).
Fungal infections.

Topical tincture: Miconazole nitrate (p.391·1).
Fungal nail infections.

Fungoid AF Pedinol, USA†.
Undecenoic acid (p.395·3).
Fungal skin infections.

Fungoid HC Pedinol, USA.
Miconazole nitrate (p.391·1); hydrocortisone (p.1073·3).
Bacterial and fungal skin infections.

Fungol Hoechst Marion Roussel, Braz.
Iodine (p.1522·3); potassium iodide (p.1522·3); salicylic acid (p.1122·3); boric acid (p.1586·1); magenta (p.1149·3).
Fungal skin infections.

Fungoral Janssen-Cilag, Aust.; Farmion, Braz.; Cilag, Mex.; Janssen-Cilag, Norw.; Janssen-Cilag, Swed.
Ketoconazole (p.389·1).
Fungal infections; seborrhoeic dermatitis.

Fungotox Mepha, Switz.
Clotrimazole (p.382·1).
Fungal skin and vaginal infections.

Fungowas Wasserman, Spain.
Ciclopirox olamine (p.382·1).
Cutaneous, mucosal and nail fungal infections.

Fungur M Hexal, Ger.
Miconazole nitrate (p.391·1).
Fungal skin and vaginal infections.

Fungusol Roche Nicholas, Spain.
Boric acid (p.1586·1); chlorocresol (p.1141·3); zinc oxide (p.1128·2).
Fungal skin infections; intertrigo.

Funida Nakornpatana, Thai.
Tinidazole (p.603·3).
Amoebiasis; anaerobic bacterial infections; giardiasis; trichomoniasis.

Furabid Procter & Gamble, Neth.
Nitrofurantoin (p.230·3).
Urinary-tract infections.

Furacin Schering-Plough, Braz.; Formenti, Ital.†; Rhein, Mex.; SmithKline Beecham, S.Afr.; Seid, Spain; Procter & Gamble, USA; Roberts, USA.
Nitrofurazone (p.231·3).
Burns; skin disinfection; ulcers; wounds.

Furacine Norgine, Belg.; Norgine, Neth.
Nitrofurazone (p.231·3).
Infected wounds and burns; infection prophylaxis for skin grafts.

Furacin-Sol Bioglan, Ger.
Nitrofurazone (p.231·3).
Skin disorders; wounds.

Furadantin Roche, Aust.; Pharmacia Upjohn, Austral.; Procter & Gamble, Ger.; Procter & Gamble, Irl.; Formenti, Ital.; Recip, Norw.; Pharmacia Upjohn, NZ; SmithKline Beecham, S.Afr.; Recip, Swed.; Procter & Gamble, UK; Dura, USA.
Nitrofurantoin (p.230·3).
Urinary-tract infections.

Furadantina Boehringer Ingelheim, Mex.; Normal, Port.†.
Nitrofurantoin (p.230·3).
Urinary-tract infections.

Furadantine Procter & Gamble, Belg.; Lipha Sante, Fr.; Procter & Gamble, Switz.
Nitrofurantoin (p.230·3).
Urinary-tract infections.

Furadantine MC Procter & Gamble, Neth.
Nitrofurantoin (macrocrystalline) (p.230·3).
Urinary-tract infections.

Furadoine Lipha Sante, Fr.
Nitrofurantoin (p.230·3).
Cystitis.

Furamid Knoll, Switz.
Diloxanide furoate (p.590·3).
Amoebiasis.

Furamide Knoll, Irl.†; Sovereign, UK†.
Diloxanide furoate (p.590·3).
Amoebiasis.

Furanthril Medphano, Ger.
Frusemide [furosemide] (p.893·1) or frusemide [furosemide] sodium (p.895·1).
Forced diuresis; hypertension; oedema; oliguria.

Furantoina Uriach, Spain.
Nitrofurantoin (p.230·3).
Urinary-tract infections.

Furanton Randall, Mex.
Nitrofurantoin (p.230·3); methenamine mandelate (p.223·1).
Urinary-tract infections.

Furanvit SIFI, Ital.
Nitrofurazone (p.231·3); pyridoxine hydrochloride (p.1386·3).
Bacterial eye infections.

Furasept Beige, S.Afr.
Nitrofurazone (p.231·3).
Burns; skin infections; ulcers; wounds.

Furasian Asian Pharm, Thai.
Syrup: Furazolidone (p.592·1); kaolin (p.1229·3); pectin (p.1502·3).

Tablets: Furazolidone (p.592·1).
Diarrhoea; enteritis.

Furazolin De Mayo, Braz.
Furazolidone (p.592·1); phthalylsulfathiazole (p.235·3); pectin (p.1502·3).
Diarrhoea.

Furazolon Heralds, Braz.
Hydrocortisone (p.1073·3); nitrofurazone (p.231·3).
Infected skin disorders.

Furedan Scharper, Ital.
Nitrofurantoin (p.230·3).
Urinary-tract infections.

Furese Durascan, Denm.
Frusemide [furosemide] (p.893·1).
Hypertension; oedema.

Furesis Orion, Fin.
Frusemide [furosemide] (p.893·1).
Hypertension; oedema; renal failure.

Furesis comp Orion, Fin.; Orion, Swed.
Frusemide [furosemide] (p.893·1); triamterene (p.986·1).
Hypertension; oedema.

Furetic Siam Bheasach, Thai.
Frusemide [furosemide] (p.893·1).
Ascites; barbiturate poisoning; eclampsia; oedema.

Furex Aspen, S.Afr.
Nitrofurazone (p.231·3).
Burns; skin infections; ulcers; wounds.

Furide Polipharm, Thai.
Frusemide [furosemide] (p.893·1).
Ascites; hypertension; oedema.

Furil OFF, Ital.
Nitrofurantoin (p.230·3).
Urinary-tract infections.

Furion Chew, Thai.
Furazolidone (p.592·1).
Diarrhoea; enteritis.

Furix Nycomed, Denm.; Nycomed, Norw.; Nycomed, Swed.
Frusemide [furosemide] (p.893·1).
Forced diuresis; hypertension; oedema; renal failure.

Furmidal Sydenham, Mex.
Frusemide [furosemide] (p.893·1).

Furo CT, Ger.; ABZ, Ger.; Ratiopharm, Ger.
Frusemide [furosemide] (p.893·1) or frusemide [furosemide] sodium (p.895·1).
Forced diuresis; heart failure; hypertension; oedema; oliguria.

Furo-Aldopur Kwizda, Aust.; Hormosan, Ger.
Frusemide [furosemide] (p.893·1); spironolactone (p.973·2).
Ascites; oedema.

Furobactina Dexter, Spain.
Nitrofurantoin (p.230·3).
Urinary-tract infections.

furo-basan Schonenberger, Switz.
Frusemide [furosemide] (p.893·1).
Hypertension; oedema.

Furo-BASF BASF, Ger.
Frusemide [furosemide] (p.893·1).
Ascites; hypertension; oedema; oliguria.

Furobeta Betapharm, Ger.
Frusemide [furosemide] (p.893·1).
Ascites; hypertension; oedema; oliguria.

Furocloran AF, Mex.
Chloramphenicol (p.179·1).
Bacterial infections.

Furodermal Streuli, Switz.
Camphor (p.1589·3); ichthammol (p.1115·2); bismuth oxyiodogallate (p.1214·1); thymol (p.1158·3).
Skin infections.

Furodermil Vifor, Switz.†
Ichthammol (p.1115·2); salicylic acid (p.1122·3); bismuth hydroxyquinoline (p.1214·1); peru balsam (p.1650·2).
Skin disorders.

Furodrix Streuli, Switz.
Frusemide [furosemide] sodium (p.895·1).
Heart failure; hypertension; oedema; oliguria in pregnancy; renal failure.

Furohexal Hexal, Aust.
Frusemide [furosemide] (p.893·1).
Hypertension; oedema.

Furoic Searle, Ital.
Calcium mefolinate (p.1363·2).
Antidote in overdosage with folic acid antagonists; folate deficiency; reduction of aminopterin and methotrexate toxicity.

Furolacton Lannacher, Aust.
Spironolactone (p.973·2); frusemide [furosemide] (p.893·1).
Oedema.

Furomed Wolff, Ger.
Frusemide [furosemide] (p.893·1).
Hypertension; oedema; oliguria.

Furomil Euromex, Mex.
Frusemide [furosemide] (p.893·1).

Furomin Medinovum, Fin.
Frusemide [furosemide] (p.893·1).
Hypertension; oedema.

Furon Ratiopharm, Aust.
Frusemide [furosemide] (p.893·1) or frusemide [furosemide] sodium (p.895·1).
Forced diuresis; hypercalcaemic crises; hypertension; oedema; renal failure.

Furonet Nettopharma, Denm.†
Frusemide [furosemide] (p.893·1).
Hypertension; oedema.

Furonex Zerboni, Mex.
Frusemide [furosemide] (p.893·1).

Furopectin PP Lab, Thai.
Furazolidone (p.592·1); kaolin (p.1229·3); pectin (p.1502·3).
Bacterial diarrhoea; enteritis.

Furo-Puren Isis Puren, Ger.
Frusemide [furosemide] (p.893·1).
Ascites; heart failure; hypertension; oedema.

Furorese Hexal, Ger.
Frusemide [furosemide] (p.893·1) or frusemide [furosemide] sodium (p.895·1).
Ascites; forced diuresis; hypertension; oedema; oliguria.

Furorese Comp Hexal, Ger.
Frusemide [furosemide] (p.893·1); spironolactone (p.973·2).
Ascites; oedema.

Furosal TAD, Ger.
Frusemide [furosemide] (p.893·1).
Ascites; hypertension; oedema; oliguria.

Furosan Fustery, Mex.
Frusemide [furosemide] (p.893·1).

Furoscand Enapharm, Swed.†
Frusemide [furosemide] (p.893·1).
Hypertension; oedema.

Furosemid comp Upsamedica, Switz.†
Frusemide [furosemide] (p.893·1); spironolactone (p.973·2).
Ascites; oedema.

Furosemida Composta Heralds, Braz.
Frusemide [furosemide] (p.893·1); potassium chloride (p.1194·3).
Hypertension; oedema.

Furosifar Siphar, Switz.
Frusemide [furosemide] (p.893·1).
Hypertension; oedema; renal failure.

Furospir Mepha, Switz.
Frusemide [furosemide] (p.893·1); spironolactone (p.973·2).
Oedema.

Furo-Spirobene Ratiopharm, Aust.
Frusemide [furosemide] (p.893·1); spironolactone (p.973·2).
Aldosteronism; oedema.

Furostad Stada, Aust.
Frusemide [furosemide] (p.893·1).
Hypertension; oedema.

Furoter Protein, Mex.
Frusemide [furosemide] (p.893·1).

Furotricina Finderm, Ital.
Tyrothricin (p.267·1); nitrofurazone (p.231·3).
Gynaecological infections.

Furotyrol Tyrol, Aust.
Frusemide [furosemide] (p.893·1).
Hypertension; oedema.

Furovite Vitamed, Israel.
Frusemide [furosemide] (p.893·1).
Hypertension; oedema.

Furoxime Siam Bheasach, Thai.
Cefuroxime axetil (p.178·1) or cefuroxime sodium (p.178·2).
Bacterial infections.

Furoxona Boehringer Ingelheim, Mex.
Furazolidone (p.592·1).
Gastrointestinal infections.

Furoxone Formenti, Ital.†; Xixia, S.Afr.†; Roberts, USA.
Furazolidone (p.592·1).
Gastrointestinal infections.

Fursemida Biochimico, Braz.; Legrand, Braz.
Frusemide [furosemide] (p.893·1).
Hypercalcaemia; hypertension; oedema.

Fursol Ecosol, Switz.
Frusemide [furosemide] (p.893·1).
Hypertension; oedema.

Furtulon Roche, Jpn.
Doxifluridine (p.534·2).
Malignant neoplasms.

Furunkulosin Merckle, Ger.
Yeast (p.1398·1).
Furunculosis.

Fusalar Fustery, Mex.
Fluocinolone (p.1071·1).
Skin disorders.

Fusaloyos Danval, Spain.
Fusafungine (p.208·3).
Upper respiratory-tract infections and inflammation.

Fusanidazol Universales, Mex.
Metronidazole (p.594·1).

Fusid
Note. This name is used for preparations of different composition.
Gry, Ger.; Teva, Israel; ICN, Neth.†.
Frusemide [furosemide] (p.893·1) or frusemide [furosemide] sodium (p.895·1).
Forced diuresis; heart failure; hypertension; oedema; oliguria.

Chew, Thai.
Fusidic acid (p.208·3).
Bacterial skin infections.

Fustaren Fustery, Mex.
Diclofenac sodium (p.30·3).
Inflammation; musculoskeletal and joint disorders; pain.

Fustermicina Fustery, Mex.
Gentamicin (p.212·1).
Bacterial infections.

Fustermid Fustery, Mex.
Pipemidic acid (p.236·1).

Fustermizol Fustery, Mex.
Astemizole (p.409·1).
Hypersensitivity.

Futasole Julphar, UAE.
Fusidic acid (p.208·3).
Bacterial skin infections.

Futasone Julphar, UAE.
Fusidic acid (p.208·3); betamethasone valerate (p.1063·2).
Infected skin disorders.

Futraful Otsuka, Hong Kong; Taiho, Jpn†.
Tegafur (p.573·2).
Malignant neoplasms.

Futroken Kener, Mex.
Nitrofurantoin (p.230·3).

Futura Marano, Ital.
Aspartame (p.1354·3).
Sugar substitute.

Futuran Madaus, Ger.
Hypericum (p.290·2).
Depression.

Future E L'Oreal, Canad.
SPF 15: Avobenzone (p.1517·1); octocrilene (p.1518·1).
Sunscreen.

Fuxen Fustery, Mex.
Naproxen (p.60·3).
Gout; inflammation; musculoskeletal, joint, and peri-articular disorders; pain.

Fuxol Columbia, Mex.
Furazolidone (p.592·1).
Gastrointestinal infections.

Fuzoltec Tecnofarma, Mex.
Itraconazole (p.387·2).
Fungal infections.

Fuzotyl Rayere, Mex.
Furazolidone (p.592·1); homatropine (p.468·1); kaolin (p.1229·3); pectin (p.1502·3).
Gastrointestinal disorders.

FX Passage
Hestag, Aust.; Worwag, Ger.
Magnesium sulfate (p.1191·1).
Constipation; stool softener.

Fybogel
Reckitt & Colman, Austral.; Reckitt & Colman, Belg.; Reckitt & Colman, Hong Kong; Reckitt Benckiser, Irl.; Schering-Plough, Mex.; Reckitt Benckiser, S.Afr.; Reckitt & Colman, Singapore; Reckitt & Colman, Spain†; Reckitt & Colman, Thai.; Reckitt & Colman, UK.
Ispaghula (p.1229·1).
Constipation; dietary fibre supplement.

Fybogel Mebeverine
Reckitt Benckiser, Irl.; Reckitt & Colman, Singapore; Reckitt & Colman, UK.
Ispaghula (p.1229·1); mebeverine hydrochloride (p.1233·3).
Formerly known as Colven in Irl. and UK.
Gastrointestinal disorders.

Fybozest Reckitt & Colman, UK.
Ispaghula (p.1229·1).
Hypercholesterolaemia.

Fymnal Farmasa, Braz.
Ibuprofen (p.43·2); fenoterol (p.765·2).
Fever; inflammation; pain.

Fynnon Calcium Aspirin Seton, UK†.
Aspirin (p.14·2).
Calcium carbonate (p.1215·1) is included in this preparation in an attempt to limit adverse effects on the gastrointestinal mucosa.
Fever; pain.

Fynnon Salt SSL, UK.
Sodium sulfate (p.1250·1).
Constipation.

Fysioquens
Aaciphar, Belg.†; Nourypharma, Neth.
7 Tablets, ethinylestradiol (p.1476·2); 15 tablets, ethinylestradiol; lynestrenol (p.1480·1).
Sequential-type oral contraceptive.

Fytosid Dabur, Thai.
Etoposide (p.538·1).
Malignant neoplasms.

G-204 Teva, Israel.
Electrolyte solution (p.1184·1).
Haemodialysis.

G-248 Teva, Israel.
Electrolyte solution (p.1184·1).
Haemodialysis.

G Tril Vinas, Spain†.
Febarbamate (p.683·2).
Alcohol withdrawal syndrome; insomnia; tremor.

Gaba Nikkho, Braz.
Gamma-aminobutyric acid (p.1613·1); papaverine hydrochloride (p.1648·1); nicotinic acid (p.1372·3); calcium pantothenate (p.1374·1).
Impaired mental function.

Gabacet Synthelabo, Fr.
Piracetam (p.1652·1).
Cerebrovascular disorders; vertigo.

Gaballon Nikkho, Braz.
Gamma-aminobutyric acid; lysine hydrochloride; vitamin B_1; vitamin B_2; calcium pantothenate (p.1350·1).
Nutritional supplement.

Gabax Nikkho, Braz.
Gamma-aminobutyric acid (p.1613·1); pyridoxine hydrochloride (p.1386·3).
Impaired mental function.

Gabbromicina Pharmacia Upjohn, Hong Kong.
Paromomycin sulfate (p.599·2).
Amoebiasis; bacterial infections.

Gabbroral Pharmacia Upjohn, Belg.; Pharmacia Upjohn, Ital.
Paromomycin sulfate (p.599·2).
Amoebiasis; bacterial intestinal infections; giardiasis.

Gabil Tecnifar, Port.†
Barbetonium iodide; idanpramine; chlordiazepoxide (p.659·2).
Gastrointestinal motility disorders.

Gabisedil Seber, Port.
Amino-hydroxybutyric acid (p.342·2); valerian (p.1678·3); passion flower (p.1649·1); chamomile (p.1593·2); crataegus (p.1600·2).
Anxiety; excitability; infantile convulsions; insomnia.

Gabitran Solfran, Mex.
Multivitamin preparation (p.1350·1).

Gabitril
Sanofi Winthrop, Aust.; Sanofi Synthelabo, Austral.; Sanofi Synthelabo, Belg.; Sanofi Winthrop, Denm.; Sanofi Winthrop, Fin.; Sanofi Winthrop, Fr.; Sanofi Synthelabo, Ger.; Novo Nordisk, Irl.; Sanofi Synthelabo, Ital.; Sanofi Synthelabo, Port.; Sanofi Synthelabo, Spain; Sanofi Synthelabo, Switz.; Sanofi Winthrop, UK; Abbott, USA.
Tiagabine hydrochloride (p.365·1).
Epilepsy.

Gabomade Esfar, Port.
4-Amino-3-hydroxybutyric acid (p.342·2).
Convulsions; headache; mental function disorders; nocturnal enuresis.

Gabormon Nikkho, Braz.
Gamma-aminobutyric acid (p.1613·1); methyltestosterone (p.1482·3).
Androgen deficiency; breast cancer (females); delayed growth; delayed puberty (males).

Gabrene Synthelabo, Fr.†
Progabide (p.364·2).
Epilepsy.

Gabrilen Kreussler, Ger.
Ketoprofen (p.47·3).
Inflammation; musculoskeletal, joint, peri-articular, and soft-tissue disorders; pain.

Gabunat Strathmann, Ger.
Biotin (p.1355·3).
Biotin deficiency.

Gacida Hoechst Marion Roussel, Thai.
Magnesium trisilicate (p.1233·3); dried aluminium hydroxide gel (p.1210·3).
Gastric hyperacidity; gastritis; heartburn; peptic ulcer.

Gadovist Schering, Switz.
Gadobutrol.
Contrast medium for magnetic resonance imaging.

Gaduol Climax, Braz.
Vitamin A palmitate (p.1383·2); ergocalciferol (p.1391·2).
Vitamin supplement.

Gaiarsol Monin, Fr.
Methylarsinic acid; guaiacol (p.1092·1); aconite root (p.1572·3); codeine (p.25·2); tolu balsam (p.1101·3).
Coughs.

Galacordin Biomo, Ger.
Potassium aspartate (p.1195·2); magnesium aspartate (p.1190·3).
Potassium and magnesium deficiency.

Galactogil Gallia, Fr.
Galega; calcium phosphate (p.1188·2); malt extract (p.1371·1).
Lactation insufficiency.

Galactomin
Scientific Hospital Supplies, Irl.; Piam, Ital.; Cow & Gate, UK.
Food for special diets (p.1350·1).
Lactose, glucose, or galactose intolerance.

Galactoquin Mundipharma, Aust.†
Quinidine polygalacturonate (p.964·3).
Arrhythmias.

Galake Galen, UK.
Dihydrocodeine tartrate (p.33·1); paracetamol (p.71·2).
These ingredients can be described by the British Approved Name Co-dydramol.
Pain.

Galama Pharmonta, Aust.
Silver birch (p.1585·2).
Kidney disorders.

Galamila Mavena, Switz.
Dexpanthenol (p.1602·3); chlorhexidine gluconate (p.1138·2) or chlorhexidine hydrochloride (p.1138·2).
Nipple care during breastfeeding.

Galanol GLX Lifeplan, UK.
Evening primrose oil (p.1613·2).
Nutritional supplement.

Galanol Gold Lifeplan, UK.
Evening primrose oil (p.1613·2); borage oil (p.1613·1).
Nutritional supplement.

Galantase
Tokyo Tanabe, Jpn; Hoechst Marion Roussel, S.Afr.†
Tilactase (p.1673·2).
Lactose intolerance.

Galcdexan Grin, Mex.
Aluminium hydroxide (p.1210·3).

Galcodine Galen, UK.
Codeine phosphate (p.25·2).
Dry coughs.

Galecin Galen, Mex.
Clindamycin phosphate (p.188·2).
Bacterial infections.

Galedol Galen, Mex.
Diclofenac sodium (p.30·3).
Gout; musculoskeletal, joint, peri-articular and soft-tissue disorders; pain.

Galenamet Galen, Irl.; Galen, UK.
Cimetidine (p.1216·3).
Gastric hyperacidity; peptic ulcer; Zollinger-Ellison syndrome.

Galenamox Galen, Irl.; Galen, UK.
Amoxicillin trihydrate (p.149·2).
Bacterial infections.

Galenat Kamill N Hetterich, Ger.
Chamomile (p.1593·2).
Gastrointestinal disorders; inflammatory disorders of skin and mucous membranes.

Galenavowen-N Weber & Weber, Ger.†.
Homoeopathic preparation.

Galenpamil Galen, Mex.
Verapamil (p.991·1).
Angina pectoris.

Galenphol Galen, UK.
Pholcodine (p.1099·1).
Formerly known as Galphol.
Coughs.

Galentromicina Galen, Mex.
Erythromycin (p.201·2).
Bacterial infections.

Galfer Galen, Irl.; Galen, UK.
Ferrous fumarate (p.1360·1).
Iron-deficiency anaemia.

Galfer FA Galen, Irl.; Galen, UK.
Ferrous fumarate (p.1360·1); folic acid (p.1361·1).
Iron and folic acid deficiency in pregnancy.

Galfloxin Galen, UK.
Flucloxacillin sodium (p.207·1).
Bacterial infections.

Galidrin Galen, Mex.
Ranitidine hydrochloride (p.1245·2).
Gastro-oesophageal reflux; peptic ulcer; Zollinger-Ellison syndrome.

Galirene Alpharma, Fr.
Calcium bromide (p.1587·1); calcium lactate (p.1188·2).
Insomnia; nervous disorders.

Galium Complex Blackmores, Austral.
Clivers (p.1596·3); echinacea angustifolia (p.1606·2); calendula (p.1589·2); baptisia tinctoria; vitamins (p.1350·1); zinc amino acid chelate (p.1398·3).
Tonic.

Galivert Luhr-Lehrs, Ger.
Homoeopathic preparation.

Galleb S Hoyer, Ger.†
Taraxacum (p.1669·1).
Biliary-tract disorders; dyspepsia.

Galle-Donau Sanova, Aust.
Tolynol nicotinate (p.1674·1); α-naphthylacetic acid (p.1639·3).
Biliary-tract disorders.

Gallemolan forte Cesra, Ger.
Greater celandine (p.1618·1); absinthium (p.1571·1); taraxacum (p.1669·1).
Biliary-tract disorders; dyspepsia.

The symbol † denotes a preparation no longer actively marketed

Gallemolan G Cesra, Ger.
Absinthium (p.1571·1); boldo leaves (p.1585·3); chamomile flowers (p.1593·2); greater celandine (p.1618·1); taraxacum (p.1669·1).
Biliary-tract disorders; dyspepsia.

Gallen- und Lebertee Smetana, Aust.
Agrimony herb (p.1574·3); marrubium vulgare (p.1094·2); peppermint leaf (p.1243·2); achillea (p.1572·2); taraxacum (p.1669·1).
Biliary-tract disorders.

Gallenja OTW, Ger.
Homoeopathic preparation.

Gallenperlen Agepha, Aust.
Phenylpropanol (p.1650·3).
Biliary-tract disorders.

Gallesyn Wenig, Aust.
Oral drops: Frangula (p.1227·1); herba teucrii; peppermint oil (p.1243·3).
Tablets: Frangula (p.1227·1); herba teucrii; menthol (p.1632·3).
Biliary-tract disorders.

Gallesyn neu Wenig, Aust.
Oral drops: Cynara (p.1601·3); taraxacum (p.1669·1); peppermint leaf (p.1243·2).
Tablets: Cynara (p.1601·3); taraxacum (p.1669·1); menthol (p.1632·3).
Biliary-tract disorders.

Gallexier
Note.This name is used for preparations of different composition.
Salus, Fr.
Cynara (p.1601·3).
Gastrointestinal and liver disorders.

Salushaus, Ger.
Oral liquid: Cynara (p.1601·3); taraxacum (p.1669·1); curcuma zanthorrhiza; silybum marianum (p.1021·3); cnicus benedictus (p.1597·2); menyanthes (p.1633·1); achillea (p.1572·2); gentian (p.1615·1); absinthium (p.1571·1); calamus (p.1588·1); chamomile (p.1593·2); fennel (p.1610·1); fructose (p.1363·3).
Digestive system disorders.
Tablets: Curcuma zanthorrhiza; cynara (p.1601·3); silybum marianum (p.1021·3); taraxacum (p.1669·1); chamomile (p.1593·2); peppermint leaf (p.1243·2).
Biliary disorders.

Gallia HA Gallia, Fr.
Infant feed (p.1350·1).
Milk-protein intolerance.

Gallia Lactofidus Gallia, Fr.
Infant feed (p.1350·1).
Gastrointestinal disorders.

Gallia Soja Gallia, Fr.
Infant feed (p.1350·1).
Diarrhoea; gluten intolerance; milk-intolerance.

Galliagene Gallia, Fr.
Infant feed (p.1350·1).
Diarrhoea; malabsorption syndromes; milk-protein intolerance.

Gallith Evers, Ger.
Hedera helix.
Cholesterol gallstones.

Gallo Merz Kolassa, Aust.
Dehydrocholic acid (p.1602·2); pancreatin (p.1646·1); cellulase (p.1593·1); dimethicone (p.1249·2); turmeric (p.1029·3).
Biliary-tract and pancreatic disorders.

Gallo Merz N Merz, Ger.
Dimethicone (p.1249·2); turmeric (p.1029·3).
Biliary-tract disorders.

Gallo Merz Spasmo Merz, Ger.
Hymecromone (p.1622·3).
Biliary-tract spasm.

Gallobeta Betapharm, Ger.
Gallopamil hydrochloride (p.896·3).
Angina pectoris; arrhythmias; hypertension.

Gallogen Torii, Hong Kong.
Tocamphyl.
Biliary-tract disorders; liver disorders.

Gallogran Synpharma, Aust.
Taraxacum (p.1669·1); achillea (p.1572·2); absinthium (p.1571·1).
Biliary- and gastrointestinal tract disorders.

Gallopas Pascoe, Ger.
Greater celandine (p.1618·1).
Gastrointestinal and biliary-tract spasm.

Galloselect Dreluso, Ger.
Homoeopathic preparation.

Galloselect M Dreluso, Ger.
Greater celandine (p.1618·1); taraxacum (p.1669·1); silybum marianum (p.1021·3); cynara (p.1601·3); chamomile (p.1593·2); peppermint oil (p.1243·3); caraway oil (p.1591·2).
Biliary-tract disorders.

Galloway's Cough Syrup Pfizer Consumer, UK.
Ipecacuanha liquid extract (p.1093·1); squill vinegar (p.1100·3).
Coughs.

Galmarin Lifeplan, UK.
Evening primrose oil (p.1613·2); borage oil (p.1613·1); omega-3 marine triglycerides (p.949·3).
Nutritional supplement.

Galmax Max Farma, Ital.
Sodium succinate ursodeoxycholate (p.1677·3).
Biliary disorders; gallstones.

Galotam Normon, Spain†.
Ampicillin sodium (p.150·3); sulbactam sodium (p.250·1).
Bacterial infections.

Galpamol Galpharm, UK.
Paracetamol (p.71·2).
Pain.

Galpharm Flu Relief Galpharm, UK.
Paracetamol (p.71·2); phenylephrine hydrochloride (p.1097·1).
Cold and influenza symptoms.

Galprofen Galpharm, UK.
Ibuprofen (p.43·2).
Fever; pain.

Galpseud Galen, Irl.†; Galen, UK.
Pseudoephedrine hydrochloride (p.1099·2).
Respiratory-tract congestion.

Galpseud Plus Galen, UK.
Pseudoephedrine hydrochloride (p.1099·2); chlorpheniramine [chlorphenamine] maleate (p.412·1).
Allergic rhinitis.

Galusan Almirall, Spain.
Pipemidic acid (p.236·1).
Urinary-tract infections.

Gama Venina Centeon, Braz.
A normal immunoglobulin (p.1551·3).
Agammaglobulinaemia; chronic demyelinated polyneuropathy; hypogammaglobulinaemia; idiopathic thrombocytopenic purpura; Kawasaki disease; lymphocytic leukaemia; passive immunisation.

Gamactrin Delta, Braz.
Sulfamethoxazole (p.254·1); trimethoprim (p.264·2).
Bacterial infections; Pneumocystis carinii pneumonia; protozoal infections.

Gamalat Novaquimica, Braz.
Dimethicone (p.1249·2); aluminium hydroxide (p.1210·3); magnesium hydroxide (p.1233·1).
Flatulence; gastrointestinal hyperacidity.

Gamalate B6 Novag, Spain.
Gamma-aminobutyric acid (p.1613·1); aminohydroxybutyric acid (p.342·2); magnesium glutamate hydrobromide (p.1631·1); pyridoxine (p.1387·1).
Mental function impairment; senility.

Gamanil Merck, Irl.; E. Merck, UK.
Lofepramine hydrochloride (p.297·1).
Depression.

Gamatol LED, Fr.
Borage oil (p.1613·1).

Gamavate Julphar, UAE.
Clobetasol propionate (p.1065·2).
Skin disorders.

Gambex Aspen Consumer, S.Afr.
Lindane (p.1434·1).
Pediculosis.

Gambrolys Gambro, Swed.†.
Sodium chloride; sodium hydroxide; potassium chloride; magnesium chloride; calcium chloride; acetic acid (p.1184·1).
Haemodialysis solution.

Gambrosol
Gambro, Denm.; Gambro, Fin.; Gambro, Spain; Gambro, Swed.; Bichsel, Switz.
Glucose; sodium chloride; sodium lactate; calcium chloride; magnesium chloride (p.1184·1).
Peritoneal dialysis.

Gamibetal
Dansk-Flama, Braz.; SIT, Ital.; Italmex, Mex.; Seber, Port.
Aminohydroxybutyric acid (p.342·2).
Behaviour disorders; epilepsy; infantile convulsions.

Gamibetal Complex
Dansk-Flama, Braz.; SIT, Ital.
Aminohydroxybutyric acid (p.342·2); phenobarbital (p.355·1); phenytoin (p.357·2) or phenytoin sodium (p.357·2).
Epilepsy.

Gamibetal Compositum Seber, Port.
Aminohydroxybutyric acid (p.342·2); diazepam (p.674·3).
Epilepsy.

Gamibetal Plus SIT, Ital.
Aminohydroxybutyric acid (p.342·2); diazepam (p.674·3).
Epilepsy.

Gamikal Galen, Mex.
Amikacin sulfate (p.148·1).
Bacterial infections.

Gamimune N
Bayer, Canad.; Bayer Biological, Hong Kong; Bayer, Israel; Cutter, UK†; Bayer, USA.
A normal immunoglobulin (p.1551·3).
Agammaglobulinaemia; hypogammaglobulinaemia; idiopathic thrombocytopenic purpura; immunodeficiency; passive immunisation.

Gamma Anti D Grifols, Spain.
An anti-D immunoglobulin (p.1532·1).
Prevention of rhesus sensitisation.

Gamma Antihep B Grifols, Spain.
A hepatitis B immunoglobulin (p.1542·1).
Passive immunisation.

Gamma Antitenos Grifols, Spain.
A tetanus immunoglobulin (p.1565·1).
Passive immunisation.

Gamma Antitetanos Grifols, Spain.
A tetanus immunoglobulin (p.1565·1).
Passive immunisation.

Gamma EPA Quest, UK.
Concentrated fish oil (p.949·3).

Gamma Glob Anti Rh ICN, Spain†.
An anti-D immunoglobulin (p.1532·1).
Prevention of rhesus sensitisation.

Gamma Glob Antihep B Alonga, Spain†.
A hepatitis B immunoglobulin (p.1542·1).
Passive immunisation.

Gamma Marine Quest, UK.
Evening primrose oil (p.1613·2); borage oil (p.1613·1); fish oil (p.949·3).
Nutritional supplement.

Gamma Oil
Quest, Canad.; Quest, UK.
Evening primrose oil (p.1613·2).
Nutritional supplement.

Gamma Oil Marine Quest, Canad.
Gamolenic acid (p.1613·1); linoleic acid (p.1613·2); vitamins (p.1350·1).

Gammabulin
Immuno, Austral.†; Immuno, Ger.†; Immuno, Hong Kong; Immuno, Irl.; Immuno, Ital.; Immuno, Swed.†; Hyland Immuno, UK.
A normal immunoglobulin (p.1551·3).
Agammaglobulinaemia; hypogammaglobulinaemia; passive immunisation.

Gammabulin A Immuno, Ger.†.
A hepatitis A immunoglobulin (p.1541·2).
Passive immunisation.

Gammacur Biocur, Ger.
Evening primrose oil (p.1613·2).
Eczema.

Gammadin OFF, Ital.
Povidone-iodine (p.1155·1).
Skin and mucous membrane disinfection.

Gammagard
Baxter, Aust.; Baxter, Belg.; Baxter, Canad.; Baxter, Denm.; Baxter, Fin.; Baxter, Fr.; Baxter-Hyland, Ger.; Baxter-Hyland, Hong Kong; Baxter, Israel; Baxter, Ital.; Baxter, Singapore; Baxter, Spain; Baxter, Swed.; Baxter, Switz.; Baxter, UK; Baxter, USA.
A normal immunoglobulin (p.1551·3).
Auto-immune disorders; B-cell chronic lymphocytic leukaemia; Guillain-Barré syndrome; hypogammaglobulinaemia; idiopathic thrombocytopenic purpura; Kawasaki disease; passive immunisation.

Gammaglob Grifols, Spain.
A normal immunoglobulin (p.1551·3).
Passive immunisation.

Gammaglob Anti D Grifols, Spain.
An anti-D immunoglobulin (p.1532·1).
Prevention of rhesus sensitisation.

Gammaglob Antihep B P CE Centeon, Spain.
A hepatitis B immunoglobulin (p.1542·1).
Passive immunisation.

Gammaglob Antite ICN, Spain; Centeon, Spain.
A tetanus immunoglobulin (p.1565·1).
Passive immunisation.

Gammaglobulin
Pharmacia Upjohn, Denm.; Pharmacia Upjohn, Norw.
A normal immunoglobulin (p.1551·3).
Hypogammaglobulinaemia; passive immunisation.

Gammaglobulin SPR Veripalvelu, Fin.
A normal immunoglobulin (p.1551·3).
Hypogammaglobulinaemia; passive immunisation.

Gammakine Dompe Biotec, Ital.
Interferon gamma-1b (p.634·1).
Chronic granulomatous disease.

Gammalon
Daiichi, Hong Kong; Daiichi, Thai.
Gamma-aminobutyric acid (p.1613·1).
Cerebrovascular disorders; hypertension; mental function impairment.

Gamma-Men Nuovo ISM, Ital.†.
An anti-D immunoglobulin (p.1532·1).
Prevention of rhesus sensitisation.

Gammamida Complex Laproquifar, Spain†.
Cyanocobalamin (p.1388·1); glutamic acid (p.1365·2); pyridoxine (p.1387·1); thiamine (p.1385·2).
Alcoholism; muscular dystrophies; nausea and vomiting in pregnancy; vitamin B deficiency.

Gammanorm
Pharmacia Upjohn, Denm.; Pharmacia Upjohn, Norw.; Pharmacia Upjohn, Swed.
A normal immunoglobulin (p.1551·3).
Hypogammaglobulinaemia.

Gamma-OH SERB, Fr.
Sodium oxybate (p.1268·2).
General anaesthesia.

GammaOil Premium Quest, UK.
Evening primrose oil (p.1613·2).

Gammaplus Fidia, Ital.
Omega-3 triglycerides (p.949·2); omega-6 triglycerides.
Nutritional supplement.

Gammar Nikkho, Braz.
Gamma-aminobutyric acid (p.1613·1).
Impaired mental function.

Gammariza Toyo, Hong Kong.
Oryzanol (p.1645·1).
Autonomic nervous-system disorders; menopausal disorders.

Gammar-P Centeon, USA.
A normal immunoglobulin (p.1551·3).
Immunoglobulin deficiency; passive immunisation.

Gammatet Propan, S.Afr.†.
Tetracycline hydrochloride (p.258·3).
Bacterial infections.

Gamma-Tet P Centeon, Ital.
A tetanus immunoglobulin (p.1565·1).
Passive immunisation.

Gammatetanos Lab Francais du Fractionnement, Fr.
A tetanus immunoglobulin (p.1565·1).
Passive immunisation.

Gamma-Venin
Centeon, Aust.; Centeon, Ger.; Behringwerke, Israel; Centeon, Spain.
A normal immunoglobulin (p.1551·3).
Hypogammaglobulinaemia; passive immunisation.

Gamma-Venin P Centeon, Ital.
A normal immunoglobulin (p.1551·3).
Bacterial infections.

Gammavit Sessa, Ital.
Borage oil (p.1613·1).
Nutritional supplement.

Gammonativ
Pharmacia Upjohn, Aust.†; Pharmacia Upjohn, Denm.; Pharmacia Upjohn, Ger.; Pharmacia Upjohn, Norw.; Pharmacia Upjohn, Swed.
A normal immunoglobulin (p.1551·3).
Hypogammaglobulinaemia; idiopathic thrombocytopenic purpura.

Gamonil
Merck, Ger.; Merck, Switz.
Lofepramine hydrochloride (p.297·1).
Depression.

Gamophen
Johnson & Johnson, Austral.; Johnson & Johnson Medical, UK.
Triclosan (p.1159·2).
Acne; soap substitute.

Gamulin Rh Armour, USA†.
An anti-D immunoglobulin (p.1532·1).
Prevention of rhesus sensitisation.

Ganaton Hokuriku, Jpn.
Itopride hydrochloride (p.1229·2).
Gastrointestinal symptoms of chronic gastritis.

Ganavit Pharmaton, Switz.
Guarana (p.1681·1); caffeine (p.761·3); vitamins; minerals (p.1350·1).
Tonic.

Ganda
Chauvin, Irl.; Smith & Nephew, S.Afr.†; Chauvin, UK.
Guanethidine monosulfate (p.901·1); adrenaline [epinephrine] (p.829·1).
Glaucoma.

Gandhour Dermoteca, Port.
A range of soap substitutes and moisturisers.

Gandin Polipharm, Thai.
Mefenamic acid (p.51·2).
Pain.

Ganidin NR Cypress, USA.
Guaifenesin (p.1092·2).

Ganite Fujisawa, USA†.
Gallium nitrate (p.753·1).
Hypercalcaemia of malignancy.

Gani-Tuss NR Cypress, USA.
Guaifenesin (p.1092·2); codeine phosphate (p.25·2).
Coughs.

Gani-Tuss-DM NR Cypress, USA.
Guaifenesin (p.1092·2); dextromethorphan hydrobromide (p.1087·3).
Coughs.

Ganor Boehringer Ingelheim, Ger.
Famotidine (p.1225·3).
Peptic ulcer; Zollinger-Ellison syndrome.

Gantanol Roche, USA†.
Sulfamethoxazole (p.254·1).
Adjunct in falciparum malaria; bacterial infections.

Gantrim Geymonat, Ital.
Co-trimoxazole (p.193·3).
Bacterial infections; Pneumocystis carinii pneumonia.

Gantrimex Geymonat, Ital.
Oxolamine citrate (p.1096·2) or oxolamine phosphate (p.1096·2).
Respiratory-tract disorders.

Gantrisin Roche, USA.
Acetyl sulfafurazole (p.253·1) or sulfafurazole diolamine (p.253·1).
Bacterial eye infections; urinary-tract infections.

Gaopathyl Monot, Fr.
Aluminium hydroxide (p.1210·3); magnesium hydroxide (p.1233·1).
Antacid.

Gaoptol Europhta, Mon.
Timolol maleate (p.982·1).
Glaucoma; ocular hypertension.

Gaosedal Codeine Monot, Fr.
Paracetamol (p.71·2); codeine phosphate (p.25·2).

Garacol Schering-Plough, Neth.
Gentamicin sulfate (p.210·1).
Bacterial infections.

Garacoll Schering-Plough, Mex.
Gentamicin sulfate (p.210·1).
Bacterial infections.

Garalen Galen, Mex.
Gentamicin (p.212·1).
Bacterial infections.

Garalone Schering-Plough, Port.
Gentamicin sulfate (p.210·1).
Bacterial infections.

Garamicina
Schering-Plough, Braz.; Schering-Plough, Mex.
Gentamicin sulfate (p.210·1).
Bacterial infections.

Garamicina V *Schering-Plough, Mex.*
Gentamicin sulfate (p.210·1); betamethasone valerate (p.1063·2).
Infected skin disorders.

Garamycin
Schering-Plough, Austral.†; Schering, Canad.; Schering-Plough, Denm.; Schering-Plough, Hong Kong; Schering-Plough, Israel; Schering-Plough, Neth.; Schering-Plough, Norw.; Schering-Plough, S.Afr.; Schering-Plough, Singapore; Schering-Plough, Swed.; Essex, Switz.; Schering-Plough, Thai.; Schering-Plough, UK; Schering, USA.
Gentamicin sulfate (p.210·1).
Bacterial infections.

Garanil *Zambon, Spain.*
Captopril (p.853·3).
Diabetic nephropathy; heart failure; hypertension; myocardial infarction.

Garasone
Schering-Plough, Belg.; Schering-Plough, Braz.; Schering, Canad.; Schering-Plough, Hong Kong; Schering-Plough, Mex.; Schering-Plough, S.Afr.; Schering-Plough, Singapore.
Gentamicin sulfate (p.210·1); betamethasone sodium phosphate (p.1063·2).
External ear disorders; inflammatory eye infections.

Garatec *Technilab, Canad.*
Gentamicin sulfate (p.210·1).
Bacterial infections.

Gardenal
Aventis, Belg.; Rhodia, Braz.; Rhone-Poulenc Rorer, Fr.; Rhone-Poulenc Rorer, Hong Kong; Aventis, NZ; Aventis, S.Afr.; Rhone-Poulenc Rorer, Spain; Rhone-Poulenc Rorer, Thai.; Concord, UK.
Phenobarbital (p.355·1) or phenobarbital sodium (p.355·1).
Epilepsy; febrile convulsions; insomnia; sedative.

Gardenale *Rhone-Poulenc Rorer, Ital.*
Phenobarbital (p.355·1) or phenobarbital sodium (p.355·1).
Epilepsy; insomnia; sedative.

GA-301-Redskin 301 *Madaus, Ger.†.*
Histamine hydrochloride (p.1619·1); clove oil (p.1597·1); juniper oil (p.1625·2).
Migraine; musculoskeletal and joint disorders; neuritis; respiratory-tract disorders.

Garfield
Whitehall-Robins, Canad.; Menley & James, USA.
A range of multivitamin preparations with or without minerals (p.1851·1).

Gargarisma *ankerpharm, Ger.†.*
Aluminium chloride (p.1110·2); potassium chlorate (p.1654·1).
Mouth and throat inflammation.

Gargarisma zum Gurgeln *Krewel, Ger.*
Aluminium chloride (p.1110·2).
Mouth infections.

Gargarol *Boiron, Canad.*
Homoeopathic preparation.

Gargaron *Sam-On, Israel.*
Cetylpyridinium chloride (p.1138·1).
Mouth and throat infectons.

Gargilon *Vemedia, Neth.*
Dequalinium chloride (p.1143·1).
Sore throat.

Gargocetil *Bunker, Braz.*
Cetylpyridinium chloride (p.1138·1).
Mouth and throat disorders.

Gargol *Rekah, Israel.*
Boric acid (p.1586·1); thymol (p.1158·3); menthol (p.1632·3); terpineol (p.1669·3); eucalyptol (p.1609·2); methyl salicylate (p.55·1); chloroxylenol (p.1142·1).
Mouth and throat disorders.

Gargosedans *INQ, Braz.*
Tyrothricin (p.267·1); neomycin sulfate (p.228·1); sulfadiazine (p.251·1); benzocaine (p.1306·2); chlorophyll (p.1028·1).
Mouth and throat disorders.

Gargotrat *Bergamo, Braz.*
Cetylpyridinium chloride (p.1138·1); allantoin (p.1110·1); benzocaine (p.1306·2); chlorophyll (p.1028·1); peppermint leaf (p.1243·2); eucalyptol (p.1609·2).
Mouth and throat disorders.

Garlic Allium Complex *GNLD, Austral.*
Garlic (p.1614·1); onion (p.1644·1); chive; leek; rosemary.
Upper respiratory-tract congestion.

Garlic, Horseradish, A & C Capsules *Vitaplex, Austral.*
Garlic oil; horseradish (p.1620·1); ascorbic acid (p.1389·3); vitamin A palmitate (p.1383·2).
Excess body fluids; excess mucus formation.

Garlic and Horseradish + C Complex *Cenovis, Austral.; Vitelle, Austral.*
Horseradish (p.1620·1); garlic (p.1614·1); sodium ascorbate (p.1390·1); ascorbic acid (p.1389·3); fenugreek (p.1610·3); althaea (p.1577·1).
Upper respiratory-tract symptoms.

Garlimega *Cantassium Co., UK.*
Garlic (p.1614·1).

Garlix *Blackmores, Austral.*
Garlic (p.1614·1).
Cold and influenza symptoms.

Garlodex *Modern Health Products, UK.*
Althaea root (p.1577·1); parsley (p.1648·3); garlic oil.
Catarrh; colds.

Garmastan
Austroplant, Aust.; Protina, Ger.
Guaiazulene (p.1618·3).
Mastitis prophylaxis.

Garoin *Rhone-Poulenc Rorer, S.Afr.†.*
Phenytoin sodium (p.357·2); phenobarbital sodium (p.355·1).
Epilepsy.

Garonsept *Sam-On, Israel.*
Benzalkonium chloride (p.1133·2); menthol (p.1632·3); thymol (p.1158·3); lemon oil (p.1628·2).
Mouth and throat infections.

Gartech *Eagle, Austral.*
Astragalus; echinacea pallida (p.1606·2); garlic (p.1614·1); berberis vulgaris; paraformaldehyde (p.1152·2); garlic oil; anise oil (p.1580·3); thymol (p.1158·3); savory oil.
Cold and influenza symptoms.

Gartricin *Cantabria, Spain.*
Benzocaine (p.1306·2).
Mouth and throat disorders.

Garydol *Cinfa, Spain.*
Chlorhexidine gluconate (p.1138·2); benzocaine (p.1306·2).
Sore throat.

Garze Disinfettanti alla Pomata Betadine
Asta Medica, Ital.
Povidone-iodine (p.1155·1).
Medicated dressing.

Gas Ban *Roberts, USA.*
Calcium carbonate (p.1215·1); simeticone (p.1249·2).
Flatulence.

Gas Ban DS *Roberts, USA.*
Aluminium hydroxide (p.1210·3); magnesium hydroxide (p.1233·1); simeticone (p.1249·2).
Flatulence.

Gas Permeable Daily Cleaner *Allergan, Austral.†.*
Cleansing solution for hard and gas permeable contact lenses (p.1129·2).

Gas Relief *Rugby, USA.*
Simeticone (p.1249·2).
Flatulence.

Gasam *Sriprasit, Thai.*
Tiaprofenic acid (p.88·1).
Gout; musculoskeletal, joint, and soft-tissue disorders.

Gasbrand-Antitoxin *Chiron Behring, Ger.*
A gas-gangrene antitoxin (p.1540·1).
Gas gangrene.

Gascop *Valdecasas, Mex.*
Albendazole (p.95·2).
Worm infections.

Gasec *Mepha, Port.*
Omeprazole (p.1239·1).
Gastro-oesophageal reflux; peptic ulcer; Zollinger-Ellison syndrome.

Gaslon N *Shinyaku, Jpn.*
Irsogladine maleate (p.1228·3).
Gastric ulcer.

Gasmol *Hilarys, Canad.†.*
Magnesium carbonate (p.1232·3); magnesium hydroxide (p.1233·1); magnesium trisilicate (p.1233·3); calcium carbonate (p.1215·1); rhubarb (p.1248·1).

Gasmotin *Dainippon, Jpn.*
Mosapride citrate (p.1237·3).
Gastritis.

Gaspiren *Sanus, Braz.*
Omeprazole (p.1239·1).
Gastro-oesophageal reflux; gastrointestinal hyperacidity; peptic ulcer.

Gastab *Greater Pharma, Thai.*
Sodium bicarbonate (p.1186·2); cataria.
Flatulence.

Gasteel
Note. This name is used for preparations of different composition.
Shinfuso, Hong Kong.
Dimethicone (p.1249·2).
Flatulence.

Shinfuso, Thai.
Simeticone (p.1249·2); dried aluminium hydroxide gel (p.1210·3).
Flatulence; preparation for gastrointestinal examinations.

Gaster
Note. This name is used for preparations of different composition.
SoSe, Ital.
Sodium cromoglicate (p.774·3).
Food hypersensitivity; proctitis; ulcerative colitis.

Yamanouchi, Jpn.
Famotidine (p.1225·3).
Gastro-oesophageal reflux; gastrointestinal haemorrhage; peptic ulcer; premedication; Zollinger-Ellison syndrome.

Gastidine *Vida, Hong Kong.*
Cimetidine (p.1216·3).
Peptic ulcer.

Gastopride *Solvay, Port.†.*
Famotidine (p.1225·3).
Peptic ulcer; Zollinger-Ellison syndrome.

Gastracol *Streuli, Switz.*
Aluminium hydroxide (p.1210·3).
Gastric hyperacidity.

Gastral *Novag, Spain†.*
Sucralfate (p.1250·2).
Gastrointestinal haemorrhage; peptic ulcer.

Gastralgin *De Angeli, Ital.*
Roxatidine acetate hydrochloride (p.1248·1).
Gastrointestinal disorders associated with hyperacidity.

Gastralgine *UPSA, Fr.†.*
Aluminium hydroxide (p.1210·3); aluminium glycinate (p.1210·3); magnesium trisilicate (p.1233·3); simeticone (p.1249·2).
Gastrointestinal disorders.

Gastralon N *Cesra, Ger.*
Chamomile (p.1593·2); gentian (p.1615·1); absinthium (p.1571·1).
Gastrointestinal disorders.

Gastralsan
Note. This name is used for preparations of different composition.
Dolisos, Ger.
Homoeopathic preparation.

Dolisos, Fr.†.
Cynara (p.1601·3); boldo (p.1585·3); fumitory (p.1612·3).
Biliary-tract disorders.

Gastran
Note. This name is used for preparations of different composition.
Johnson & Johnson, Braz.
Dimethicone (p.1249·2); aluminium hydroxide (p.1210·3); magnesium hydroxide (p.1233·1).
Flatulence; gastrointestinal hyperacidity.

Delta, Singapore.
Ranitidine (p.1246·3).
Gastro-oesophageal reflux; peptic ulcer.

Gastrarctin N *Serum-Werk Bernburg, Ger.*
Colloidal silver (p.1664·2); chamomile flowers (p.1593·2); peppermint leaf (p.1243·2).
Gastrointestinal disorders.

Gastrax *Asche, Ger.*
Nizatidine (p.1238·3).
Peptic ulcer.

Gastrec *Tecnofarma, Mex.*
Ranitidine (p.1246·3).

Gastregan *Synpharma, Aust.*
Chamomile flower (p.1593·2); melissa leaf (p.1632·2); peppermint leaf (p.1243·2).
Gastrointestinal pain and inflammation.

Gastrex
Note. This name is used for preparations of different composition.
Simoes, Braz.
Aluminium hydroxide (p.1210·3); magnesium hydroxide (p.1233·1); calcium carbonate (p.1215·1).
Gastrointestinal hyperacidity.

Boehringer Ingelheim, Fr.
Aluminium histidinate; magnesium hydroxide (p.1233·1).
Gastrointestinal disorders.

Gastribien *Cinfa, Spain.*
Aluminium hydroxide (p.1210·3); magnesium trisilicate (p.1233·3).
Dyspepsia; peptic ulcer.

Gastricalm *OJG, Belg.*
Magaldrate (p.1232·2).
Gastrointestinal disorders associated with hyperacidity.

Gastricard N *Ysatfabrik, Ger.*
Oral drops: Gentian (p.1615·1); ginger oil; crataegus (p.1600·2); fennel oil (p.1610·2); peppermint oil (p.1243·3); caraway oil (p.1591·2); coriander oil (p.1599·2).

Tablets: Crataegus (p.1600·2); peppermint oil (p.1243·3); caraway oil (p.1591·2); fennel oil (p.1610·2); coriander oil (p.1599·2); dimethicone (p.1249·2).

Gastrointestinal disorders.

Gastricholan-L *Sudmedica, Ger.*
Chamomile flowers (p.1593·2); peppermint leaf (p.1243·2); fennel (p.1610·1).
Gastrointestinal disorders.

Gastricin *Odontofarma, Braz.*
Dicyclomine [dicycloverine] hydrochloride (p.466·1); aluminium hydroxide (p.1210·3); magnesium hydroxide (p.1233·1); simeticone (p.1249·2).
Flatulence; gastrointestinal hyperacidity.

Gastricur *Heumann, Ger.*
Pirenzepine hydrochloride (p.472·2).
Dyspepsia; gastritis; peptic ulcer.

Gastricure *Bio-Familia, Switz.*
Ceratonia (p.1500·3); marine algae; magnesium trisilicate (p.1233·3).
Bloating; gastric hyperacidity; gastric irritation.

Gastridin *Merck Sharp & Dohme, Ital.*
Famotidine (p.1225·3).
Gastrointestinal disorders.

Gastridina *Medibial, Port.*
Ranitidine hydrochloride (p.1245·2).
Acid aspiration; dyspepsia; gastro-oesophageal reflux; peptic ulcer; Zollinger-Ellison syndrome.

Gastrifam *Helsinn, Port.*
Famotidine (p.1225·3).
Dyspepsia; gastro-oesophageal reflux; peptic ulcer; Zollinger-Ellison syndrome.

Gastrifom *Tanta, Canad.*
Aluminium hydroxide (p.1210·3); alginic acid (p.1498·3).
Gastrointestinal disorders.

gastri-L 90 N *Loges, Ger.*
Homoeopathic preparation.

Gastrilax *Saunier-Daguin, Fr.†.*
Anhydrous sodium sulfate (p.1250·1); dibasic sodium phosphate (p.1193·2); citric acid monohydrate (p.1596·2).
Gastrointestinal disorders.

Gastrils *Ernest Jackson, UK†.*
Aluminium hydroxide-magnesium carbonate co-dried gel (p.1211·2).
Dyspepsia.

Gastrimagal *Azupharma, Ger.†.*
Magaldrate (p.1232·2).
Gastrointestinal disorders associated with hyperacidity.

Gastrimut *Normon, Spain.*
Omeprazole (p.1239·1).
Gastro-oesophageal reflux; peptic ulcer; Zollinger-Ellison syndrome.

Gastrimuto *Medibial, Port.*
Ranitidine bismuth citrate (p.1247·2).
Peptic ulcer.

Gastrin-Do *Grasler, Ger.*
Homoeopathic preparation.

Gastrinol *Frega, Canad.*
Magnesium hydroxide (p.1233·1); aluminium hydroxide-magnesium carbonate co-dried gel (p.1211·2); simeticone (p.1249·2).

Gastrion *Vita, Spain.*
Famotidine (p.1225·3).
Gastro-oesophageal reflux; peptic ulcer; Zollinger-Ellison syndrome.

Gastri-P *Sanorania, Ger.†.*
Pirenzepine hydrochloride (p.472·2).
Gastrointestinal disorders.

Gastripan
Note. This name is used for preparations of different composition.
Ratiopharm, Aust.†.
Aluminium glycinate (p.1210·3); almasilate (p.1210·1); liquorice (p.1231·2); ethaverine hydrochloride (p.1608·2).
Gastrointestinal disorders.

Merckle, Ger.
Magaldrate (p.1232·2).
Gastric hyperacidity; heartburn; peptic ulcer.

Gastriselect *Dreluso, Ger.*
Homoeopathic preparation.

Gastritol *Klein, Ger.*
Potentilla anserina; absinthium (p.1571·1); cnicus benedictus (p.1597·2); liquorice (p.1231·2); angelica (p.1580·2); chamomile (p.1593·2); hypericum (p.290·2).
Gastrointestinal disorders.

Gastrium *Ache, Braz.*
Omeprazole (p.1239·1).
Gastro-oesophageal reflux; gastrointestinal hyperacidity; peptic ulcer.

Gastri-Vyr *Cazi, Braz.*
Calcium carbonate (p.1215·1); aluminium hydroxide (p.1210·3).
Gastrointestinal hyperacidity.

Gastro *Unipharm, Israel.*
Famotidine (p.1225·3).
Gastrointestinal hyperacidity; heartburn; peptic ulcer; Zollinger-Ellison syndrome.

Gastro Gobens *Normon, Spain.*
Aluminium hydroxide (p.1210·3); dimethicone (p.1249·2); levoglutamide (p.1365·2); metoclopramide hydrochloride (p.1235·2).
Dyspepsia; gastritis; meteorism; nausea; oesophagitis; peptic ulcer.

Gastro H2 *Lesvi, Spain.*
Cimetidine (p.1216·3).
Acid aspiration; gastro-oesophageal reflux; gastrointestinal haemorrhage; gastrointestinal hyperacidity; peptic ulcer; short-bowel syndrome; Zollinger-Ellison syndrome.

Gastroalgine *Novag, Spain.*
Aluminium hydroxide (p.1210·3); dimethicone (p.1249·2); enoxolone aluminium (p.1225·2); magnesium hydroxide (p.1233·1).
Gastrointestinal hyperacidity; meteorism; peptic ulcer.

Gastrobario *Bial, Port.*
Barium sulfate (p.1032·1).
Radiographic contrast medium.

Gastrobid Continus
Napp, Irl.; Napp, UK.
Metoclopramide hydrochloride (p.1235·2).
Gastrointestinal disorders; nausea and vomiting.

Gastrobitan *Gea, Norw.†.*
Cimetidine (p.1216·3).
Aspiration syndrome; gastro-oesophageal reflux; peptic ulcer; Zollinger-Ellison syndrome.

Gastrobon *Byk Madaus, S.Afr.†.*
Magaldrate (p.1232·2).
Dyspepsia; gastritis; gastro-oesophageal reflux disease; peptic ulcer.

Gastrobrom *Fawns & McAllan, Austral.†.*
Powdered milk; glucose; magnesium trisilicate (p.1233·3); magnesium hydroxide (p.1233·1); magnesium carbonate (p.1232·3); calcium carbonate (p.1215·1).
Dyspepsia.

Gastrobul
Codali, Belg.; Guerbet, Fr.
Betaine hydrochloride (p.1584·3); sodium bicarbonate (p.1186·2); dimethicone (p.1249·2).
Gas production for double-contrast radiography.

Gastrocalm *Bio-Sante, Canad.*
Aluminium hydroxide-magnesium carbonate co-dried gel (p.1211·2); simeticone (p.1249·2).

Gastrocaps A *Riemser, Ger.*
Aluminium hydroxide (p.1210·3).
Gastrointestinal disorders associated with hyperacidity; hyperphosphaturia.

Gastroccult *SmithKline Diagnostics, USA.*
Test for occult blood in gastric contents.

Gastrocolon *Pharmagen, S.Afr.†.*
Metoclopramide hydrochloride (p.1235·2).
Gastrointestinal disorders.

Gastrocote
Stanley, Canad.†; SA Druggists, S.Afr.†; SSL, UK.
Alginic acid (p.1498·3) or sodium alginate (p.1498·3); aluminium hydroxide (p.1210·3); magnesium trisilicate (p.1233·3); sodium bicarbonate (p.1186·2).
Gastro-oesophageal reflux; heartburn; hiatus hernia.

Gastrocrom *Medeva, USA.*
Sodium cromoglicate (p.774·3).
Mastocytosis.

Gastrocure *Taxandria, Neth.*
Domperidone maleate (p.1224·1).
Gastrointestinal disorders.

Gastrocynesine
Boiron, Fr.; Boiron, Port.
Homoeopathic preparation.

Gastrodenol *Yamanouchi, Spain.*
Tripotassium dicitratobismuthate (p.1213·2).
Gastritis; peptic ulcer.

Gastrodin *Shiwa, Thai.*
Cimetidine (p.1216·3).
Gastric hyperacidity; peptic ulcer; Zollinger-Ellison syndrome.

Gastrodina *Degorts, Mex.*
Cimetidine (p.1216·3).
Peptic ulcer.

Gastrodine *Apsen, Braz.*
Cimetidine (p.1216·3).
Acid aspiration; gastro-oesophageal reflux; gastrointestinal haemorrhage; peptic ulcer; Zollinger-Ellison syndrome.

Gastrodomina
Almirall, Hong Kong; Almirall, Spain.
Famotidine (p.1225·3).
Gastro-oesophageal reflux; peptic ulcer; Zollinger-Ellison syndrome.

Gastrodyn *Leiras, Fin.*
Glycopyrronium bromide (p.467·2).
Premedication; protection against muscarininc effects of anticholinesterases used to reverse neuromuscular blockade.

Gastrodyn comp *Leiras, Fin.*
Glycopyrronium bromide (p.467·2); diazepam (p.674·3).
Gastrointestinal disorders.

Gastrofilm *Will-Pharma, Belg.*
Algeldrate (p.1210·3); magnesium carbonate (p.1232·3); calcium carbonate (p.1215·1); magnesium trisilicate (p.1233·3); bismuth subnitrate (p.1213·2); belladonna (p.463·1).
Dyspepsia; gastric hyperacidity.

Gastroflat *Bunker, Braz.*
Dimethicone (p.1249·2).
Flatulence.

Gastroflux *Ashbourne, UK.*
Metoclopramide hydrochloride (p.1235·2).
Gastrointestinal disorders.

Gastrofrenal
Searle, Ital.; Sigma-Tau, Spain†.
Sodium cromoglicate (p.774·3).
Food hypersensitivity; inflammatory bowel disease.

Gastrofusine *Braun, Switz.*
Electrolyte infusion with glucose (p.1180·1).
Fluid and electrolyte disorders.

Gastrogard-R *Nutricia, Austral.*
Antirotavirus hyperimmune bovine colostrum (p.1535·1).
Diarrhoea due to rotavirus.

Gastrogel
Note.This name is used for preparations of different composition.
Fawns & McAllan, Austral.; Sigma, Hong Kong.
Oral liquid: Aluminium hydroxide (p.1210·3); magnesium hydroxide (p.1233·1); magnesium trisilicate (p.1233·3).
Gastrointestinal hyperacidity.

Fawns & McAllan, Austral.; Sigma, Hong Kong; Fawns & McAllan, NZ.
Tablets: Aluminium hydroxide (p.1210·3); magnesium hydroxide (p.1233·1); magnesium trisilicate (p.1233·3); simeticone (p.1249·2).
Gastrointestinal hyperacidity.

Medquimica, Braz.
Aluminium hydroxide (p.1210·3); magnesium hydroxide (p.1233·1); dimethicone (p.1249·2).
Flatulence; gastrointestinal hyperacidity.

Giuliani, Ital.; Synthelabo, Switz.
Sucralfate (p.1250·2).
Gastrointestinal disorders.

Gastrogenol *Profarb, Braz.*
Guarana (p.1681·1); kola (p.1681·1); cinchona bark (p.1595·3).

Gastroglutal *Tedec Meiji, Spain.*
Magnesium oxide (p.1233·2); levoglutamide (p.1365·2); aluminium glycinate (p.1210·3).
Gastrointestinal hyperacidity.

Gastrografin
Schering, Aust.; Squibb Diagnostics, Canad.†; Schering, Fin.; Schering, Ger.; Schering, Ital.; Schering, Neth.; Schering, Norw.; Schering, NZ;

Schering, S.Afr.; Schering, Spain; Schering, Swed.; Schering, Switz.; Schering, UK; Squibb Diagnostics, USA.
Meglumine amidotrizoate (p.1031·2); sodium amidotrizoate (p.1031·2).
Contrast medium for gastrointestinal radiography; meconium ileus.

Gastrografina *Schering, Port.*
Meglumine amidotrizoate (p.1031·2); sodium amidotrizoate (p.1031·2).
Contrast medium for gastrointestinal radiography.

Gastrografine *Schering, Fr.*
Meglumine amidotrizoate (p.1031·2); sodium amidotrizoate (p.1031·2).
Contrast medium for gastrointestinal radiography.

Gastrol
Note.This name is used for preparations of different composition.
Luper, Braz.
Aluminium hydroxide (p.1210·3); magnesium hydroxide (p.1233·1); calcium carbonate (p.1215·1).
Gastrointestinal hyperacidity.

Salus, Ital.
Pirenzepine hydrochloride (p.472·2).
Gastroduodenitis; peptic ulcer.

Gastrol S *Fides, Ger.*
Gentian (p.1615·1); chamomile (p.1593·2); melissa (p.1632·2); caraway (p.1591·2); fennel (p.1610·1); coriander (p.1599·2); sweet basil; absinthium (p.1571·1); hypericum (p.290·2); cinchona bark (p.1595·3); juniper (p.1625·2); calamus (p.1588·1); turmeric (p.1029·3).
Gastrointestinal disorders.

Gastrolav *Vitoria, Port.*
Ranitidine hydrochloride (p.1245·2).
Dyspepsia; gastro-oesophageal reflux; peptic ulcer; Zollinger-Ellison syndrome.

Gastrolem *Lemery, Mex.*
Cimetidine (p.1216·3).

Gastroloc *Stern, Ger.†.*
Omeprazole (p.1239·1).
Gastro-oesophageal reflux; peptic ulcer; Zollinger-Ellison syndrome.

Gastroluft
Fuji, Swed.†; Nycomed, Switz.†.
Sodium bicarbonate (p.1186·2); tartaric acid (p.1669·2); dimethicone (p.1249·2).
Adjunct in gastrointestinal double-contrast radiography.

Gastrolux *Goldham, Ger.*
Sodium amidotrizoate (p.1031·2); meglumine amidotrizoate (p.1031·2) or lysine amidotrizoate (p.1032·1).
Contrast medium for gastrointestinal radiography.

Gastrolyte
Rhone-Poulenc Rorer, Austral.; Rhone-Poulenc Rorer, Canad.; Aventis, NZ.
Sodium chloride; potassium chloride; sodium acid citrate; glucose (p.1185·2).
Diarrhoea; oral rehydration therapy.

Gastrolyte-R
Rhone-Poulenc Rorer, Austral.; Rhone-Poulenc Rorer, Hong Kong.
Rice powder; sodium chloride; sodium citrate; potassium chloride (p.1185·2).
Diarrhoea; oral rehydration therapy.

Gastrom *Tanabe, Jpn.*
Ecabet sodium (p.1225·2).
Gastric ulcer; gastritis.

Gastromag *Windson, Braz.*
Dicyclomine [dicycloverine] hydrochloride (p.466·1); aluminium hydroxide (p.1210·3); magnesium hydroxide (p.1233·1); simeticone (p.1249·2).
Flatulence; gastrointestinal hyperacidity.

Gastromax *Pfizer, UK†.*
Metoclopramide hydrochloride (p.1235·2).
Gastrointestinal disorders; nausea and vomiting.

Gastromet *Bayer, Ital.†.*
Cimetidine (p.1216·3) or cimetidine hydrochloride (p.1218·3).
Gastrointestinal disorders.

Gastromiro
Gerot, Aust.; E. Merck, Irl.; Bracco, Israel; Bracco, Ital.; Bracco, Port.; Merck, UK.
Iopamidol (p.1035·2).
Contrast medium for gastrointestinal radiography.

Gastromol *Byk Elmu, Spain.*
Magaldrate (p.1232·2).
Dyspepsia; gastro-oesophageal reflux; gastrointestinal hyperacidity.

Gastron *Aspen, S.Afr.*
Loperamide hydrochloride (p.1231·3).
Colostomies; diarrhoea; ileostomies.

Gastronerton
Sanova, Aust.; Dolorgiet, Ger.
Metoclopramide (p.1236·3) or metoclopramide hydrochloride (p.1235·2).
Gastrointestinal disorders.

Gastronol *Bioforce, Switz.*
Homoeopathic preparation.

Gastronorm *Janssen-Cilag, Ital.*
Domperidone (p.1224·1).
Dyspepsia; nausea.

Gastro-Pasc *Pascoe, Ger.*
Homoeopathic preparation.

Gastropax *Lehning, Fr.*
Kaolin (p.1229·3); calcium carbonate (p.1215·1); magnesium trisilicate (p.1233·3); magnesium carbonate (p.1232·3); calcium phosphate (p.1188·3); sodium bicarbonate (p.1186·2); magnesium hydroxide (p.1233·1).

Formerly contained belladonna, star anise, kaolin, calcium carbonate, magnesium trisilicate, magnesium carbonate, vegetable charcoal, thyme, calcium phosphate, liquorice, sodium bicarbonate, sodium sulfate, and magnesium hydroxide.

Gastropeache Susp *Italfarmaco, Spain.*
Aluminium hydroxide (p.1210·3); magnesium hydroxide (p.1233·1).
Dyspepsia; gastrointestinal hyperacidity.

Gastropect *Aspen, S.Afr.*
Kaolin (p.1229·3); pectin (p.1502·3).
Diarrhoea.

Gastropen *I Farmacologia, Spain.*
Famotidine (p.1225·3).
Gastro-oesophageal reflux; peptic ulcer; Zollinger-Ellison syndrome.

Gastro-Pepsin *Ceccarelli, Ital.*
Pepsin (p.1649·3); gastric mucosa; hydrochloric acid (p.1621·2); lactic acid (p.1626·2); bitter orange.
Formerly contained pepsin, gastric mucosa, hydrochloric acid, lactic acid, nux vomica, kola, gentian, condurango, cascarilla, and bitter orange.
Dyspepsia; hypoacidity.

Gastropin *Boehringer Ingelheim, Mex.*
Pirenzepine hydrochloride (p.472·2).

Gastropiren *AGIPS, Ital.*
Pirenzepine hydrochloride (p.472·2).
Gastrointestinal disorders.

Gastroplant *DHU, Ger.*
Homoeopathic preparation.

Gastroplex *Codilab, Port.†.*
Bismuth carbonate (p.1213·1); calcium carbonate (p.1215·1); magnesium carbonate (p.1232·3); sodium bicarbonate (p.1186·2); aluminium silicate (p.1211·3).
Gastrointestinal disorders.

Gastroplus *QIF, Braz.*
Magnesium hydroxide (p.1233·1); aluminium hydroxide (p.1210·3); dimethicone (p.1249·2).
Flatulence; gastrointestinal hyperacidity.

Gastroprotect *LAW, Ger.; Wyeth, Ger.*
Cimetidine (p.1216·3).
Aspiration syndrome; gastro-oesophageal reflux; gastrointestinal haemorrhage; peptic ulcer; Zollinger-Ellison syndrome.

Gastropulgit *Spitzner, Ger.*
Attapulgite (p.1212·1); aluminium hydroxide-magnesium carbonate co-dried gel (p.1211·2).
Gastrointestinal disorders.

Gastropulgite
Ipsen, Belg.†; Beaufour, Fr.; Beaufour, Switz.
Attapulgite (p.1212·1); aluminium hydroxide-magnesium carbonate co-dried gel (p.1211·2).
Gastrointestinal disorders.

Gastrosan
Note.This name is used for preparations of different composition.
Inkeysa, Spain.
Aluminium hydroxide (p.1210·3); magnesium hydroxide (p.1233·1).
Dyspepsia; gastrointestinal hyperacidity.

Bioforce, Switz.
Achillea (p.1572·2); taraxacum (p.1669·1); melissa (p.1632·2); gentian (p.1615·1); cnicus benedictus (p.1597·2); angelica (p.1580·2); centaury (p.1593·1).
Digestive disorders.

Gastrosecur *Duopharm, Ger.*
Chirata; gentian (p.1615·1); ginger (p.1227·2); cinnamon (p.1595·3); dried bitter-orange peel (p.1644·2); caraway (p.1591·2).
Gastrointestinal disorders.

Gastrosed
Note.This name is used for preparations of different composition.
Amsa, Ital.
Pirenzepine hydrochloride (p.472·2).
Gastritis; peptic ulcer.

Roberts, USA.
Hyoscyamine sulfate (p.469·3).

Gastrosedyl *Monin, Fr.†.*
Belladonna (p.463·1); hyoscyamus (p.470·1).
Gastrointestinal and biliary-tract disorders.

Gastrosil
Sanova, Aust.; Heumann, Ger.; Heumann, Switz.
Metoclopramide (p.1236·3) or metoclopramide hydrochloride (p.1235·2).
Adjunct in gastrointestinal examination; gastrointestinal disorders.

Gastrosine *Boiron, Canad.*
Homoeopathic preparation.

Gastrostad *Stada, Ger.†.*
Magaldrate (p.1232·2).
Gastrointestinal disorders associated with hyperacidity.

Gastro-Stop *Rhone-Poulenc Rorer, Austral.*
Note. A similar name is used for preparations of different composition (see below).
Loperamide hydrochloride (p.1231·3).
Diarrhoea.

Gastrostop *Biomedica, Ital.†.*
Note. A similar name is used for preparations of different composition (see above).
Aluminium glycinate (p.1210·3); magnesium hydroxide (p.1233·1).
Hyperchlorhydria.

Gastrotat *Noristan Generica, S.Afr.†.*
Metoclopramide hydrochloride (p.1235·2).
Gastrointestinal disorders.

Gastrotest *Sanochemia, Aust.*
2 White tablets, caffeine and sodium benzoate (p.763·1); 3 yellow tablets, phenazopyridine (p.78·1).
Test for gastric acid production.

Gastro-Timelets
Sanova, Aust.; Temmler, Denm.; Temmler, Ger.; Asta Medica, Switz.†.
Metoclopramide hydrochloride (p.1235·2).
Gastrointestinal disorders.

Gastrotranquil *Azupharma, Ger.*
Metoclopramide hydrochloride (p.1235·2).
Gastrointestinal disorders.

Gastrovegetalin *Verla, Ger.*
Melissa (p.1632·2).
Gastrointestinal disorders; sleep disorders.

Gastrovison *Schering, Ital.†.*
Sodium bicarbonate (p.1186·2); citric acid (p.1596·2); simeticone (p.1249·2); silicon dioxide (p.1503·3).
Gas production for double-contrast radiography.

Gastrozepin
Boehringer Ingelheim, Aust.; Boehringer Ingelheim, Ger.; Boehringer Ingelheim, Ital.; Boehringer Ingelheim, S.Afr.
Pirenzepine hydrochloride (p.472·2).
Duodenitis; gastritis; gastrointestinal haemorrhage; peptic ulcer; Zollinger-Ellison syndrome.

Gastrozepina *Boehringer Ingelheim, Port.*
Pirenzepine hydrochloride (p.472·2).

Gastrozepine *Boehringer Ingelheim, Switz.†.*
Pirenzepine hydrochloride (p.472·2).
Gastroduodenitis; peptic ulcer.

Gastrulcer *Fariberica, Port.*
Ranitidine hydrochloride (p.1245·2).
Gastro-oesophageal reflux; gastrointestinal haemorrhage; peptic ulcer; Zollinger-Ellison syndrome.

Gastyl *ANB, Thai.*
Simeticone (p.1249·2).
Excess gastrointestinal gas.

Gasulsol *Herbes Universelles, Canad.*
Aluminium hydroxide (p.1210·3); magnesium trisilicate (p.1233·3).

Gasva *Gerbex, Canad.†.*
Aluminium hydroxide (p.1210·3); magnesium trisilicate (p.1233·3).

Gas-X
Novartis Consumer, Canad.; General Drugs, Thai.; Novartis, USA.
Simeticone (p.1249·2).
Flatulence.

Gasyran *Loren, Mex.*
Ranitidine (p.1246·3).
Peptic ulcer.

Gaszym *Ranbaxy, Thai.*
Simeticone (p.1249·2); pancreatin (p.1646·1).
Digestive system disorders; flatulence.

Gat Globulina Antitimocitaria *Butantan, Braz.*
An antilymphocyte immunoglobulin (p.508·2).

Gatinar
Novartis, Spain†; Novartis Consumer, Switz.
Lactulose (p.1230·1).
Constipation; hepatic encephalopathy; salmonella enteritis.

Gaviscon
Note.This name is used for preparations of different composition.
Reckitt & Colman, Austral.; Novartis Consumer, Belg.; SmithKline Beecham, Fr.; Reckitt Benckiser, Irl.; Novartis Consumer, Ital.; Novartis Consumer, Neth.; Reckitt & Colman, S.Afr.; Reckitt & Colman, Singapore; Reckitt & Colman, UK.
Oral suspension: Sodium alginate (p.1498·3); calcium carbonate (p.1215·1); sodium bicarbonate (p.1186·2).
Gastro-oesophageal reflux; heartburn.

Reckitt & Colman, Austral.; Novartis Consumer, Belg.; Reckitt & Colman, Hong Kong; Reckitt Benckiser, Irl.; Novartis Consumer, Ital.; Reckitt Benckiser, NZ; Helsinn, Port.†; Reckitt & Colman, S.Afr.; Reckitt & Colman, Singapore; Reckitt & Colman, UK; SmithKline Beecham Consumer, USA.
Oral powder; tablets: Alginic acid (p.1498·3); aluminium hydroxide (p.1210·3); magnesium trisilicate (p.1233·3); sodium bicarbonate (p.1186·2).
Gastro-oesophageal reflux; heartburn.

SmithKline Beecham Consumer, Canad.
Alginic acid (p.1498·3) or sodium alginate (p.1498·3); aluminium hydroxide (p.1210·3).
Formerly known as Gaviscon Heartburn Relief.
Gastro-oesophageal reflux; heartburn.

Ferring, Denm.; Ferring, Fin.; Ferring, Israel; Ferring, Norw.; Ferring, Swed.; Novartis Consumer, Switz.
Oral suspension: Sodium alginate (p.1498·3); aluminium hydroxide (p.1210·3); sodium bicarbonate (p.1186·2); calcium carbonate (p.1215·1).
Abdominal distension; gastric hyperacidity; gastro-oesophageal reflux; heartburn.

Ferring, Denm.; Ferring, Fin.; Novartis Consumer, Ger.; Ferring, Israel; Ferring, Norw.; Ferring, Swed.; Novartis Consumer, Switz.
Tablets: Alginic acid (p.1498·3); sodium bicarbonate (p.1186·2); aluminium hydroxide (p.1210·3).
Abdominal distension; gastric hyperacidity; gastro-oesophageal reflux; heartburn.

SmithKline Beecham, Fr.
Tablets: Alginic acid (p.1498·3); sodium alginate (p.1498·3); dried colloidal aluminium hydroxide (p.1210·3); sodium bicarbonate (p.1186·2); magnesium trisilicate (p.1233·3).
Gastro-oesophageal reflux.

Novartis Consumer, Ger.
Oral suspension: Sodium alginate (p.1498·3); potassium bicarbonate (p.1186·2); calcium carbonate (p.1215·1).

Formerly contained sodium alginate, sodium bicarbonate, aluminium hydroxide, and calcium carbonate.
Gastro-oesophageal reflux; heartburn.

Reckitt & Colman, Hong Kong.
Oral liquid: Sodium alginate (p.1498·3); sodium bicarbonate (p.1186·2).
Flatulence; gastro-oesophageal reflux; heartburn.

Novartis Consumer, Neth.
Tablets: Alginic acid (p.1498·3); algeldrate (p.1210·3); sodium bicarbonate (p.1186·2); calcium carbonate (p.1215·1); magnesium trisilicate (p.1233·3).
Gastro-oesophageal reflux.

Reckitt Benckiser, NZ.
Infant oral powder: Magnesium alginate (p.1499·1); sodium alginate (p.1498·3).
Gastro-oesophageal reflux.

Reckitt Benckiser, NZ.
Oral liquid: Sodium alginate (p.1498·3); calcium carbonate (p.1215·1); potassium bicarbonate (p.1186·1) or sodium bicarbonate (p.1186·2).
Gastro-oesophageal reflux.

Reckitt Benckiser, S.Afr.
Oral liquid (peppermint): Sodium alginate (p.1498·3).
Gastrointestinal disorders.

Novartis Consumer, Spain.
Alginic acid (p.1498·3); sodium bicarbonate (p.1186·2).
Gastro-oesophageal reflux.

SmithKline Beecham Consumer, USA.
Oral liquid: Aluminium hydroxide (p.1210·3); magnesium carbonate (p.1232·3); sodium alginate (p.1498·3).
Dyspepsia.

Gaviscon Acid SmithKline Beecham Consumer, Canad.†
Magnesium hydroxide (p.1233·1); calcium carbonate (p.1215·1).

Gaviscon Advance
Reckitt Benckiser, Irl.; Reckitt & Colman, UK.
Sodium alginate (p.1498·3); potassium bicarbonate (p.1186·1).
Dyspepsia; gastro-oesophageal reflux; heartburn.

Gaviscon Extra Strength SmithKline Beecham Consumer, USA.
Aluminium hydroxide (p.1210·3); magnesium carbonate (p.1232·3).
Dyspepsia.

Gaviscon Extra Strength Relief Formula
SmithKline Beecham Consumer, USA.
Aluminium hydroxide (p.1210·3); magnesium carbonate (p.1232·3); simeticone (p.1249·2).
Hyperacidity.

Gaviscon Heartburn Relief SmithKline Beecham Consumer, Canad.
Alginic acid (p.1498·3); magnesium carbonate (p.1232·3).
Formerly known as Gaviscon Heartburn Relief Aluminium-Free.
Gastro-oesophageal reflux; heartburn.

Gaviscon Infant
Note.This name is used for preparations of different composition.
Reckitt Benckiser, Irl.
Alginic acid (p.1498·3); magnesium alginate (p.1499·1); aluminium hydroxide (p.1210·3).
Gastro-oesophageal reflux.

Reckitt & Colman, UK.
Magnesium alginate (p.1499·1); sodium alginate (p.1498·3).
Formerly known as Infant Gaviscon and contained aluminium hydroxide, magnesium alginate, and sodium alginate.
NOTE. In view of its high sodium content this preparation should not be used in premature infants or in situations where excess water-loss is likely, such as fever or high room-temperature; some sources have recommended that it should be avoided altogether in children less than 6 months of age.
Gastro-oesophageal reflux.

Gaviz Searle, Braz.
Oral liquid: Aluminium hydroxide (p.1210·3); magnesium carbonate (p.1232·3).
Tablets: Aluminium hydroxide (p.1210·3); magnesium trisilicate (p.1233·3).
Gastrointestinal hyperacidity.

Gaz Away Swiss Herbal, Canad.
α-galactosidase.

GB Tablets Potter's, UK.
Leptandra virginica; euonymus (p.1225·3); kava root (p.1625·3); lappa root (p.1627·1).
Formerly known as Gall Bladder Tablets.
Abdominal discomfort; gall bladder disorders.

GBN
Malpharm, Hong Kong; Malaysia Chemist, Singapore.
Glibenclamide (p.321·3).
Diabetes mellitus.

GE Thai Otsuka, Thai.
Carbohydrate, electrolyte, and trace element infusion (p.1350·1).
Parenteral nutrition.

Geangin
Gea, Denm.; Gea, Norw.†
Verapamil hydrochloride (p.989·1).
Angina pectoris; arrhythmias; hypertension; myocardial infarction.

Geasalol Gea, Denm.
Methenamine hippurate (p.223·1).
Urinary-tract infections.

Geavir
Gea, Denm.; Gea, Fin.; Gea, Norw.; Gea, Swed.
Aciclovir (p.612·3) or aciclovir sodium (p.612·3).
Herpesvirus infections.

Gebauer "114" Spray Gebauer, USA†.
Cryofluorane (p.1199·1).
Topical anaesthetic.

Gee-Gee Jones, USA.
Guaifenesin (p.1092·2).
Coughs.

Geepenil Orion, Fin.
Benzylpenicillin sodium (p.157·2).
Bacterial infections.

Gefanil Sumitomo, Jpn†.
Gefarnate (p.1227·2).
Gastritis; peptic ulcer.

Geffer Roche, Ital.
Metoclopramide hydrochloride (p.1235·2); dimethicone (p.1249·2); potassium citrate (p.1186·1); citric acid (p.1596·2); tartaric acid (p.1669·2); sodium bicarbonate (p.1186·2).
Gastrointestinal disorders associated with hyperacidity.

Gegorvit Fher, Ital.
Multivitamin preparation with ginseng (p.1350·1).
Nutritional supplement.

Gehwol Fungizid Gerlach, Ger.
Cream: Undecenoic acid monoethanolamide (p.396·1); chloroxylenol (p.1142·1); 3,4,5,6-tetrabromo-o-cresol (p.1158·1).
Topical liquid: Undecenoic acid monoethanolamide (p.396·1); chloroxylenol (p.1142·1); 3,4,5,6-tetrabromo-o-cresol (p.1158·1); copper-trolamine complex.
Topical powder: Bromosalicylic acid (p.1122·3); undecenoic acid monoethanolamide (p.396·1); chloroxylenol (p.1142·1); 3,4,5,6-tetrabromo-o-cresol (p.1158·1).
Fungal infections.

Gehwol Huhneraugen Tinktur Gerlach, Ger.
Salicylic acid (p.1122·3); glacial acetic acid (p.1571·2).
Calluses; corns.

Gehwol Huhneraugenpflaster Gerlach, Ger.
Salicylic acid (p.1122·3); lactic acid (p.1626·2).
Calluses; corns.

Gehwol Nagelpilz Gerlach, Ger.
Zinc chloride (p.1398·1); bromosalicylic acid (p.1122·3); salicylic acid (p.1122·3); undecenoic acid monoethanolamide (p.396·1).
Fungal nail infections.

Gehwol Schalpaste Gerlach, Ger.
Salicylic acid (p.1122·3).
Calluses; corns.

Gel 4000 Bruschettini, Ital.
Hypromellose (p.1501·3).
Aid in ophthalmic procedures.

Gel a la consoude Phytomed, Switz.
Comfrey (p.1598·3); calendula (p.1589·2); hypericum (p.290·2); echinacea (p.1606·2); mint (p.1666·3).
Soft-tissue injuries.

Gel a l'Acetotartrate d'Alumine Defresne Synthelabo, Fr.
Hesperidin methyl chalcone (p.1611·2); aluminium acetotartrate (p.1578·2).
Formerly contained methylcitrine and aluminium acetotartrate.
Soft-tissue injury; venous insufficiency.

Gel Creme Protector Vichy, Canad.
SPF 15: Avobenzone (p.1517·1); enzacamene (p.1517·2); terephthalylidene dicamphor sulfonic acid; titanium dioxide (p.1126·1).
Sunscreen.

Gel de Calamine Therica, Fr.
Calamine (p.1111·3); zinc oxide (p.1128·2).
Skin disorders.

Gel Kam
Asta Medica, Port.†; Scherer, USA.
Stannous fluoride (p.1379·3).
Dental caries prophylaxis.

Gel Solaire Bronzage Clarins, Canad.†
SPF 3: Ensulizole (p.1517·2).
Sunscreen.

Gel Solaire Bronzage Securite Clarins, Canad.
SPF 15: Octocrilene (p.1518·1); octinoxate (p.1517·3); octisalate (p.1518·1) oxybenzone (p.1518·1).
Sunscreen.

Gel Solaire Bronzage Securite Special Sport
Clarins, Canad.
SPF 15: Avobenzone (p.1517·1); octinoxate (p.1517·3); octisalate (p.1518·1); oxybenzone (p.1518·1).
Sunscreen.

Gelacet
Hermal, Aust.; Boots Healthcare, Switz.
Vitamin A acetate (p.1383·2); L-cystine (p.1359·1); gelatin (p.737·2).
Hair and nail disorders.

Gelacet N Hermal, Ger.
Vitamin A acetate (p.1383·2); cystine (p.1359·1); gelatin (p.737·2).
Hair and nail disorders.

Gelafundin
Braun, Ger.; Braun, Hong Kong; Braun, Thai.
Gelatin polysuccinate (p.737·2) with electrolytes.
Extracorporeal circulation; haemodilution; hypotension; hypovolaemia.

Gelafundina Braun, Port.
Modified gelatin (p.737·2) with electrolytes.
Extracorporeal circulation; hypovolaemia.

Gelafusal-N in Ringeracetat Serum-Werk Bernburg, Ger.
Gelatin polysuccinate (p.737·2) in electrolytes.
Hypovolaemia; thrombosis prophylaxis.

Gelamel Morado, Ital.
Royal jelly (p.1659·3).
Nutritional supplement.

Gelan Plus Chinoin, Mex.
Aluminium hydroxide (p.1210·3); magnesium hydroxide (p.1233·1); dimethicone (p.1249·2).
Flatulence; gastrointestinal hyperacidity.

Gelaspon Chauvin ankerpharm, Ger.
Gelatin (p.737·2).
Haemorrhage; haemostatic.

Gelastypt Hoechst Marion Roussel, Ger.
Gelatin (p.737·2).
Wounds.

Gelcen Centrum, Spain.
Capsaicin (p.23·1).
Muscle and joint pain.

Gelclair Sinclair, UK.
Povidone (p.1503·2); sodium hyaluronate (p.1620·1); enoxolone (p.34·3).
Painful mouth lesions.

Gelcosal Quinoderm, UK†.
Coal tar (p.1125·1); tar (p.1125·1); salicylic acid (p.1122·3).
Dermatitis; psoriasis.

Gelcotar
Note.This name is used for preparations of different composition.
Quinoderm, Hong Kong; Quinoderm, Irl.; Quinoderm, UK†.
Shampoo: Coal tar (p.1125·1); cade oil (p.1124·3).
Dandruff; psoriasis of the scalp; seborrhoeic dermatitis.

Quinoderm, Irl.; Quinoderm, UK†.
Topical gel: Coal tar (p.1125·1); tar (p.1125·1).
Dermatitis; psoriasis.

Geldene Pfizer, Fr.
Piroxicam (p.79·1).
Soft-tissue disorders; tendinitis.

Gelenkja OTW, Ger.
Homoeopathic preparation.

Gelestra Abiogen, Ital.
Estradiol (p.1473·1).
Menopausal disorders.

Gelfilm
Pharmacia Upjohn, Austral.; Pharmacia Upjohn, Canad.; Pharmacia Upjohn, Hong Kong; Pharmacia Upjohn, Neth.; Pharmacia Upjohn, NZ; Upjohn, USA.
Gelatin (p.737·2).
Haemostatic.

Gelflex Bunker, Braz.
Turpentine oil (p.1676·3); methyl salicylate (p.55·1); camphor (p.1589·3); mustard oil (p.1639·1); rosemary oil (p.1659·3); lavender oil (p.1627·2); menthol (p.1632·3).
Musculoskeletal and joint disorders.

Gelfoam
Pharmacia Upjohn, Austral.; Pharmacia Upjohn, Belg.; Pharmacia Upjohn, Canad.; Pharmacia Upjohn, Hong Kong; Pharmacia Upjohn, Israel; Pharmacia Upjohn, Neth.; Pharmacia Upjohn, NZ; Pharmacia Upjohn, Singapore; Pharmacia Upjohn, Switz.†; Upjohn, USA.
Gelatin (p.737·2).
Haemostatic.

Gelhist Econolab, USA.
Phenylephrine tannate (p.1097·3); chlorpheniramine [chlorphenamine] tannate (p.412·2); mepyramine tannate (p.421·1).
Nasal congestion; rhinitis.

Gelicain Curasan, Ger.
Lignocaine [lidocaine] hydrochloride (p.1313·2).
Local anaesthesia.

Gelictar Nigy, Fr.
Ichthammol (p.1115·2).
Seborrhoeic dermatitis.

Gelictar Fort Nigy, Fr.
Ichthammol (p.1115·2); salicylic acid (p.1122·3); resorcinol (p.1122·2).
Keratinisation disorders; seborrhoeic dermatitis.

Gelidina Yamanouchi, Spain.
Fluocinolone acetonide (p.1071·1).
Skin disorders.

Gelifundol
Biotest, Aust.; Biotest, Ger.; Biotest, Hong Kong; Mednostica, S.Afr.; Biotest, Switz.†; Biotest, Thai.
Oxypolygelatin (p.739·2).
Hypovolaemia; resuspension of concentrated erythrocytes.

Gelimag British Dispensary, Thai.
Magnesium trisilicate (p.1233·3); aluminium hydroxide (p.1210·3).
Gastric hyperacidity; peptic ulcer.

Geliofil Effik, Fr.
Lactic acid (p.1626·2); glycogen.
Vaginal disorders.

Geliperm
Yamanouchi, Ger.; Geistlich, Switz.†; Geistlich, UK.
Hydrogel dressing.
Burns; ulcers; wounds.

Gelisyn Syntex, Mex.
Fluocinonide (p.1071·2).
Skin disorders.

Gel-Larmes Thea, Fr.
Carbomer 934 P (p.1499·2).
Dry eyes.

Gelmax EMS, Braz.
Aluminium hydroxide (p.1210·3); calcium carbonate (p.1215·1); magnesium hydroxide (p.1233·1).
Gastrointestinal hyperacidity.

Geloalumin Gelos, Spain.
Aluminium hydroxide (p.1210·3); dimethicone (p.1249·2); magnesium hydroxide (p.1233·1).
Gastrointestinal hyperacidity and flatulence.

Gelocast Beiersdorf, Ital.
Zinc oxide (p.1128·2).
Medicated dressing.

Gelocatil Gelos, Spain.
Paracetamol (p.71·2).
Fever; pain.

Gelocatil Codeina Gelos, Spain.
Paracetamol (p.71·2); codeine (p.25·2).
Pain.

Gelodiet DHN, Fr.
Gelatin (p.737·2); sucrose (p.1380·3).
Dehydration.

Gelodrin Pohl, Ger.
Sodium cromoglicate (p.774·3).
Allergic conjunctivitis; allergic rhinitis.

Gelodrox Gelos, Spain.
Dried aluminium hydroxide (p.1210·3); calcium carbonate (p.1215·1); magnesium carbonate (p.1232·3); magnesium trisilicate (p.1233·3).
Gastrointestinal hyperacidity.

Gelodual Gelos, Spain.
Dried aluminium hydroxide (p.1210·3); magnesium hydroxide (p.1233·1); magnesium trisilicate (p.1233·3).
Gastrointestinal hyperacidity.

Gelofalk Falk, Ger.†
Smectite; aluminium magnesium gel (p.1210·3); magnesium hydroxide (p.1233·1).
Gastrointestinal disorders.

Geloflex Braun, UK.
Succinylated gelatin (p.737·2) in sodium chloride.
Hypovolaemia.

Gelofrix Delta, Braz.
Turpentine oil (p.1676·3); mustard oil (p.1639·1); rosemary oil (p.1659·3); lavender oil (p.1627·2); methyl salicylate (p.55·1); camphor (p.1589·3); menthol (p.1632·3).
Musculoskeletal and joint disorders.

Gelofusin Braun, Aust.
Gelatin (p.737·2) with electrolytes.
Haemodilution; hypovolaemia.

Gelofusine
Braun, Austral.; Braun, Belg.; Braun, Fin.; Braun, Fr.; Braun, Hong Kong; Braun Omnimed, S.Afr.; Braun, Singapore; Braun, Thai.; Braun, UK.
Succinylated gelatin (p.737·2) in sodium chloride.
Extracorporeal circulation; plasma volume expansion.

Gelogastrine Monot, Fr.†.
Agar (p.1498·3); gelatin (p.737·2); kaolin (p.1229·3).
Gastrointestinal disorders.

Gelogel Stevia, Braz.
Methyl salicylate (p.55·1); camphor (p.1589·3); menthol (p.1632·3); turpentine oil (p.1676·3).
Musculoskeletal and joint disorders.

Gelol Dorsay, Braz.
Methyl salicylate (p.55·1); camphor (p.1589·3); menthol (p.1632·3); turpentine oil (p.1676·3); mustard oil (p.1639·1); rosemary oil (p.1659·3); lavender oil (p.1627·2).
Musculoskeletal and joint disorders.

Gelomyrtol
Sanova, Aust.; Pohl, Ger.; Pohl, Hong Kong.
Myrtol.
Bronchitis; sinusitis.

Gelonasal Pohl, Ger.
Xylometazoline hydrochloride (p.1102·2).
Nasal congestion.

Gelonevral Teuto, Braz.
Turpentine oil (p.1676·3); methyl salicylate (p.55·1); camphor (p.1589·3); mustard oil (p.1639·1); rosemary oil (p.1659·3); lavender oil (p.1627·2).
Musculoskeletal and joint disorders.

Gelonic Dermoteca, Port.†
Amino-acid and mineral preparation (p.1350·1).
Hair and nail disorders.

Gelonic Forte Dermoteca, Port.
Amino-acid, vitamin and mineral preparation (p.1350·1).
Hair and nail disorders.

Gelonida
Note.This name is used for preparations of different composition.
Lundbeck, Denm.
Aspirin (p.14·2); codeine phosphate (p.25·2).
Pain.

Godecke, Ger.
Paracetamol (p.71·2); codeine phosphate (p.25·2).
Pain.

Gelonida NA Godecke, Ger.
Oral liquid: Sodium salicylate (p.84·2); paracetamol (p.71·2); codeine phosphate (p.25·2).
Cold symptoms; fever; neuralgia; neuritis; pain.
Suppositories: Aspirin (p.14·2); paracetamol (p.71·2); codeine phosphate (p.25·2).
Coughs and cold symptoms; pain.

The symbol † denotes a preparation no longer actively marketed

Gelopectose Gallia, Fr.
Pectin (p.1502·3); microcrystalline cellulose (p.1500·2); hydrated colloidal silicon dioxide (p.1503·3).
Regurgitation in infants.

Geloplasma
Pasteur Merieux, Belg.†; Rhone-Poulenc Rorer, Neth.†; Rhone-Poulenc Rorer, Spain.
Gelatin (p.737·2) with electrolytes.
Blood-volume expansion.

Gelostretch Beiersdorf, Ital.
Zinc oxide (p.1128·2).
Medicated dressing.

Gelotricar Gelos, Spain.
Calcium carbonate (p.1215·1); magnesium carbonate (p.1232·3); sodium bicarbonate (p.1186·2).
Gastrointestinal hyperacidity; peptic ulcer.

Gelotrisin Gelos, Spain.
Aluminium hydroxide (p.1210·3); magnesium trisilicate (p.1233·3).
Dyspepsia; gastrointestinal hyperacidity.

Gelovit Almirall, Spain†.
Androstanolone (p.1465·2).
Atrophic vaginitis; gynaecomastia; male hypogonadism and androgen deficiency.

Gelox Beaufour, Fr.
Montmorillonite; aluminium hydroxide (p.1210·3); magnesium hydroxide (p.1233·1).
Gastrointestinal disorders.

Gelparine Streuli, Switz.
Heparin sodium (p.902·1).
Soft-tissue injury; superficial inflammation and thrombosis.

Gel-Phan Pierre Fabre, Fr.
Gelatin (p.737·2).
Fragile hair or nails.

Gelpirin Alra, USA†.
Paracetamol (p.71·2); aspirin (p.14·2); caffeine (p.1116·3).

Gelpirin-CCF Alra, USA†.
Paracetamol (p.71·2); guaifenesin (p.1092·2); phenylpropanolamine hydrochloride (p.1098·1); chlorpheniramine [chlorphenamine] maleate (p.412·1).
Coughs and cold symptoms.

Gelplex Fresenius Kabi, Ital.
Polygeline (p.741·1) with electrolytes.
Plasma volume expansion.

Gelsemium Oligoplex Madaus, Ger.
Homoeopathic preparation.

Gelsica Resinag, Switz.
Aluminium chlorohydrate (p.1110·2).
Wounds.

Geltears
Smith & Nephew, Austral.; Chauvin, Irl.; Chauvin, UK.
Carbomer 940 (p.1499·2).
Dry eyes.

Gel-Tin Young, USA.
Stannous fluoride (p.1379·3).
Dental caries prophylaxis.

Gelucystine Parke, Davis, Fr.
Cystine (p.1359·1).
Fragile nails and hair.

Gelufene Cooperation Pharmaceutique, Fr.
Ibuprofen (p.43·2).
Fever; pain.

Gelum Medicopharm, Aust.†
Potassium iron phosphate-citrate complex.

Gelumag Synco, Hong Kong.
Magnesium trisilicate (p.1233·3); aluminium hydroxide (p.1210·3).
Gastrointestinal hyperacidity; peptic ulcer.

Gelumaline Solvay, Fr.
Belladonna (p.463·1); codeine (p.25·2); caffeine (p.761·3); paracetamol (p.71·2).
Fever; pain.

Gelumen Medpro, S.Afr.
Dicyclomine [dicycloverine] hydrochloride (p.466·1); dried aluminium hydroxide gel (p.1210·3); light magnesium oxide (p.1233·2).
Gastric hyperacidity.

Gelum-Gel Dreluso, Ger.
Potassium-iron (III)-citrate-phosphate complex-polycitric acid glycerol ester.
Inflammatory disorders; soft-tissue injuries.

Gelumina Sanitas, Port.
Oral liquid: Aluminium hydroxide (p.1210·3).
Tablets: Aluminium hydroxide (p.1210·3); calcium carbonate (p.1215·1).
Gastrointestinal disorders.

Gelum-Supp Dreluso, Ger.
Potassium-iron (III)-citrate-phosphate complex; benzocaine (p.1306·2).
Anorectal disorders.

Gelum-Tropfen Dreluso, Ger.
Potassium-iron(III)-citrate-phosphate complex(p.0·0); lactic acid (p.1626·2).
Liver disorders; oxygen deficiency; sclerosis.

Geluprane Theraplix, Fr.
Paracetamol (p.71·2).
Fever; pain.

Gelusil
Note. This name is used for preparations of different composition.
Parke, Davis, Aust.; Warner-Lambert, Ger.; Warner-Lambert Consumer, Switz.
Almasilate (p.1210·1).
Gastrointestinal disorders.

Parke, Davis, Austral.; Parke, Davis, USA.
Aluminium hydroxide (p.1210·3); magnesium hydroxide (p.1233·1); simeticone (p.1249·2).
Gastrointestinal hyperacidity.

Warner-Lambert Consumer, Belg.; Warner-Lambert, Fr.; Warner-Lambert, Hong Kong; Warner-Lambert, Neth.†; Parke, Davis, S.Afr.; Parke, Davis, Singapore; Warner-Lambert, Thai.; Parke, Davis, UK†.
Aluminium hydroxide (p.1210·3); magnesium trisilicate (p.1233·3).
Gastrointestinal hyperacidity.

Warner-Lambert, Canad.
Aluminium hydroxide (p.1210·3); magnesium hydroxide (p.1233·1).
Gastrointestinal hyperacidity.

Warner-Lambert Consumer, Port.
Aluminium hydroxide (p.1210·3); calcium phosphate (p.1188·3); magnesium trisilicate (p.1233·3).
Formerly contained aluminium hydroxide, magnesium hydroxide, and magnesium trisilicate.
Gastrointestinal disorders.

Gelusil M Ache, Braz.
Aluminium hydroxide (p.1210·3); magnesium hydroxide (p.1233·1); dimethicone (p.1249·2).
Flatulence; gastrointestinal hyperacidity.

Gelusil MPS Warner-Lambert, Thai.
Aluminium hydroxide (p.1210·3); magnesium hydroxide (p.1233·1); simeticone (p.1249·2).
Flatulence; gastric hyperacidity; peptic ulcer.

Gelusil Plus
Warner-Lambert, Hong Kong; Parke, Davis, Singapore.
Aluminium hydroxide (p.1210·3); magnesium hydroxide (p.1233·1); simeticone (p.1249·2).
Dyspepsia; flatulence; gastric hyperacidity; gastritis; peptic ulcer.

Gelusil S Parke, Davis, S.Afr.
Aluminium hydroxide (p.1210·3); magnesium hydroxide (p.1233·1); simeticone (p.1249·2).
Bloating; gastric hyperacidity; peptic ulcer.

Gelusil Simethicone Warner-Lambert Consumer, Belg.
Aluminium hydroxide (p.1210·3); magnesium hydroxide (p.1233·1); simeticone (p.1249·2).
Flatulence; gastrointestinal disorders associated with hyperacidity.

Gelusil-Lac
Warner-Lambert, Ger.; Warner-Lambert Consumer, Switz.
Almasilate (p.1210·1); milk powder.
Gastrointestinal disorders.

Gely Ipsen, Spain.
Glycerol (p.1616·3).
Barrier preparation; lubricant.

Gem Nycomed, Norw.
Sodium chloride; potassium chloride; sodium citrate; glucose (p.1185·2).
Diarrhoea; oral rehydration therapy.

Gemalt Pharmavite, Canad.
Multivitamin preparation with iron (p.1350·1).

Gemcor Upsher-Smith, USA†.
Gemfibrozil (p.896·2).

Gemfibril Siam Bheasach, Thai.
Gemfibrozil (p.896·2).
Hyperlipidaemias.

Gemfibromax PMC, Austral.†.
Gemfibrozil (p.896·2).
Hyperlipidaemias.

Gemhexal Hexal, Austral.
Gemfibrozil (p.896·2).
Hyperlipidaemias.

Gemicina Gastroenterologicos, Mex.
Neomycin (p.228·1).

Gemini Restan, S.Afr.
Antazoline hydrochloride (p.408·3); tetryzoline hydrochloride (p.1101·2).
Eye irritation; inflammatory eye disorders.

Gemizol Pacific, NZ.
Gemfibrozil (p.896·2).
Hyperlipidaemias.

Gemlipid FIRMA, Ital.
Gemfibrozil (p.896·2).
Hyperlipidaemias.

Gemnpid CCPC, Hong Kong.
Gemfibrozil (p.896·2).
Hyperlipidaemias.

Gemvites Pharmavite, Canad.
Multivitamin preparation (p.1350·1).

Gemzar
Lilly, Aust.; Lilly, Austral.; Lilly, Belg.; Lilly, Canad.; Lilly, Denm.; Lilly, Fin.; Lilly, Fr.; Lilly, Ger.; Lilly, Hong Kong; Lilly, Israel; Lilly, Ital.; Lilly, Mex.; Lilly, Neth.; Lilly, Norw.; Lilly, NZ; Lilly, Port.; Lilly, S.Afr.; Lilly, Singapore; Lilly, Spain; Lilly, Swed.; Lilly, Switz.; Lilly, Thai.; Lilly, UK; Lilly, USA.
Gemcitabine hydrochloride (p.543·3).
Bladder cancer; non-small cell lung cancer; pancreatic cancer.

Gemzil Pharmasant, Thai.
Captopril (p.853·3).
Heart failure; hypertension.

Gen H-B-Vax
Pasteur Merieux, Aust.; Chiron Behring, Ger.; Pasteur Merieux, Ger.; Pro Vaccine, Switz.
A hepatitis B vaccine (recombinant DNA) (p.1542·0). Separate preparations are available for children, adults, and adult dialysis patients.
Active immunisation.

Genabid Goldline, USA†.
Papaverine hydrochloride (p.1648·1).
Cerebral and peripheral ischaemia; smooth muscle spasm.

Genac
Note. This name is used for preparations of different composition.
Genevrier, Fr.
Acetylcysteine (p.1082·3).
Corneal ulceration.

Goldline, USA.
Pseudoephedrine hydrochloride (p.1099·2); triprolidine hydrochloride (p.427·2).
Upper respiratory-tract symptoms.

Genacol Goldline, USA.
Chlorpheniramine [chlorphenamine] maleate (p.412·1); dextromethorphan hydrobromide (p.1087·3); paracetamol (p.71·2); pseudoephedrine hydrochloride (p.1099·2).
Coughs and cold symptoms.

Genagesic Goldline, USA†.
Dextropropoxyphene hydrochloride (p.27·1); paracetamol (p.71·2).
Pain.

Genahist Goldline, USA.
Diphenhydramine hydrochloride (p.416·1).
Insomnia; motion sickness; parkinsonism.

Genalfa INTES, Ital.
Gentamicin sulfate (p.210·1); naphazoline nitrate (p.1095·1).
Eye infections.

Genalgen Farmaco, Mex.
Naproxen (p.60·3).
Inflammation; musculoskeletal and joint disorders; pain.

Genalin Great Eastern, Thai.; Therapharma, Thai.
Multivitamin and mineral preparation (p.1350·1).

Gen-Allerate Goldline, USA†.
Chlorpheniramine [chlorphenamine] maleate (p.412·1).

Genamin Goldline, USA†.
Phenylpropanolamine hydrochloride (p.1098·1); chlorpheniramine [chlorphenamine] maleate (p.412·1).
Upper respiratory-tract symptoms.

Genapap Goldline, USA.
Paracetamol (p.71·2).
Fever; pain.

Genaphed Goldline, USA.
Pseudoephedrine hydrochloride (p.1099·2).
Nasal congestion.

Genaprost Gentili, Ital.
Finasteride (p.1477·2).
Benign prostatic hyperplasia.

Genasal Goldline, USA.
Oxymetazoline hydrochloride (p.1096·2).
Nasal congestion.

Genasoft Plus Softgels Goldline, USA.
Docusate sodium (p.1223·1); casanthranol (p.1216·1).
Constipation.

Genaspor Goldline, USA.
Tolnaftate (p.395·2).
Fungal skin infections.

Genaton Goldline, USA.
Oral liquid: Aluminium hydroxide (p.1210·3); magnesium carbonate (p.1232·3).
Tablets: Aluminium hydroxide (p.1210·3); magnesium trisilicate (p.1233·3); sodium bicarbonate (p.1186·2); alginic acid (p.1498·3).
Hyperacidity.

Genatrop INTES, Ital.
Gentamicin sulfate (p.210·1); atropine sulfate (p.461·1).
Bacterial eye infections.

Genatropine Amido, Fr.
Atropine oxide hydrochloride (p.462·1).
Biliary tract disorders; gastrointestinal disorders.

Genatuss Goldline, USA.
Guaifenesin (p.1092·2).
Coughs.

Genatuss DM Goldline, USA.
Dextromethorphan hydrobromide (p.1087·3); guaifenesin (p.1092·2).
Coughs.

Genavit General Drugs, Thai.
Vitamin B₁ (p.1385·2); vitamin B₆ (p.1387·1); vitamin B₁₂ (p.1388·1).
Anaemia; beri-beri; nausea and vomiting; vitamin B deficiency.

Gen-Beclo Genpharm, Canad.
Beclometasone dipropionate (p.1061·2).
Corticosteroid.

Gen-bee with C Goldline, USA.
Vitamin B substances with vitamin C (p.1350·1).

Gencalc Goldline, USA.
Calcium carbonate (p.1215·1).
Calcium deficiency; dietary supplement.

Gencardia Genus, UK.
Aspirin (p.14·2).

Gencefal Llorente, Spain.
Cefazolin sodium (p.164·3).
Bacterial infections.

GenCept 10/11 Gencon, USA†.
Norethisterone (p.1485·1); ethinylestradiol (p.1476·2).
Biphasic oral contraceptive.

GenCept 0.5/35 and 1/35 Gencon, USA†.
Norethisterone (p.1485·1); ethinylestradiol (p.1476·2).
28-Day packs also contain 7 inert tablets.
Combined oral contraceptive.

Gencifrice Baume Ire Dents Synthelabo, Fr.
Casein hydrolysate.
Teething pain.

Gencin Curasan, Ger.; Rolab, S.Afr.
Gentamicin sulfate (p.210·1).
Now known as Rolab-Gentamicin in S.Afr.
Bacterial infections.

Gencolax General Drugs, Thai.
Bisacodyl (p.1212·2).
Bowel evacuation; constipation.

Gencold Goldline, USA†.
Phenylpropanolamine hydrochloride (p.1098·1); chlorpheniramine [chlorphenamine] maleate (p.412·1).
Upper respiratory-tract symptoms.

Gencydo
Weleda, Aust.; Weleda, Ger.; Weleda, UK.
Citrus limonum; cydonia.
Hypersensitivity reactions.

Gendazel General Drugs, Thai.
Albendazole (p.95·2).
Worm infections.

Gendecon
Note. This name is used for preparations of different composition.
General Drugs, Thai.
Phenylpropanolamine hydrochloride (p.1098·1); paracetamol (p.71·2); chlorpheniramine [chlorphenamine] maleate (p.412·1).
Fever; muscle pain; nasal congestion; rhinitis.

Goldline, USA.
Phenylephrine hydrochloride (p.1097·1); paracetamol (p.71·2); chlorpheniramine [chlorphenamine] maleate (p.412·1).
Upper respiratory-tract symptoms.

Genebs Goldline, USA.
Paracetamol (p.71·2).
Fever; pain.

Genemicin Diba, Mex.
Gentamicin (p.212·1).
Bacterial infections.

Generaid
Scientific Hospital Supplies, Austral.; Scientific Hospital Supplies, Irl.†; Nutricia, NZ; Scientific Hospital Supplies, NZ; Scientific Hospital Supplies, UK.
Amino-acid and protein preparation (p.1350·1).
Chronic liver disease; porto-hepatic encephalopathy.

Genercin General Drugs, Thai.
Chloramphenicol (p.179·1).
Bacterial infections.

Generet Goldline, USA.
Ferrous sulfate (p.1360·3); vitamin B substances with vitamin C (p.1350·1).
Iron-deficiency anaemias.

Genergin General Drugs, Thai.
Dipyrone (p.34·1).
Fever; pain.

Generix-T Goldline, USA.
Multivitamin and mineral preparation with iron (p.1350·1).

Generlog General Drugs, Thai.
Triamcinolone acetonide (p.1080·1).
Oral lesions.

Generman Byk Gulden, Ital.
Multivitamin preparation with calcium glycerophosphate and sodium fluoride (p.1350·1).
Bone and dental weakness.

Genesa Gensia, Swed.†; Gensia, USA.
Arbutamine hydrochloride (p.841·2).
Pharmacological stress testing in heart disease.

Geneserine Amido, Fr.
Eseridine salicylate (p.1419·1).
Dyspepsia.

Genesis Wassen, UK.
Multivitamin and mineral preparation (p.1350·1).

Genevis D2 Rudefsa, Mex.
Vitamin D (p.1391·2).
Vitamin D deficiency.

Genexal Mediforma, Mex.
Gentamicin (p.212·1).
Bacterial infections.

Geneye AC Allergy Goldline, USA†.
Tetryzoline hydrochloride (p.1101·2); zinc sulfate (p.1398·2).
Eye irritation.

Geneye Extra Goldline, USA.
Tetryzoline hydrochloride (p.1101·2).
Eye irritation.

Gen-Formula Thai Otsuka, Thai.
Preparation for enteral nutrition (p.1350·1).

Gengigel
Knoll, Port.; Professional Dental, UK.
Hyaluronic acid (p.1620·1) or sodium hyaluronate (p.1620·1).
Mouth disorders.

Gengivario Farmatre, Ital.; Iema, Ital.; AFOM, Ital.
Myrrh (p.1639·2); rhatany root (p.1657·3).
Astringent.

Gengivarium Kemyos, Ital.†.
Benzocaine (p.1306·2).
Mouth disorders.

Gen-Glybe Genpharm, Canad.
Glibenclamide (p.321·3).
Diabetes mellitus.

Gengraf *Abbott, USA.*
Ciclosporin (p.518·1).
Psoriasis; rheumatoid arthritis; transplant rejection.

GenHevac B *Pasteur Vaccins, Fr.*
A hepatitis B vaccine (recombinant DNA) (p.1542·2).
Active immunisation.

Genin *General Drugs, Thai.*
Quinine sulfate (p.445·1).
Malaria.

Genisol
Fisons, Irl.; Teofarma, Ital.
Coal tar (p.1125·1); sodium sulfosuccinated undecenoic acid monoethanolamide (p.396·1).
Seborrhoeic dermatitis.

Genite *Goldline, USA.*
Pseudoephedrine hydrochloride (p.1099·2); dextromethorphan hydrobromide (p.1087·3); doxylamine succinate (p.417·1); paracetamol (p.71·2).
Coughs and cold symptoms.

Genitopen *IQB, Braz.*
Ampicillin benzathine (p.151·3); ampicillin sodium (p.150·3); antigens from *Neisseria, Escherichia, Streptococcus, Staphylococcus, Proteus,* and *Pseudomonas.*
Bacterial infections.

Gen-K *Goldline, USA.*
Potassium chloride (p.1194·3).
Hypokalaemia; potassium depletion.

Genkova *Sons, Mex.*
Gentamicin sulfate (p.210·1).
Bacterial infections.

Gen-Lac *Genpharm, Canad.*
Lactulose (p.1230·1).
Constipation.

Genlip *Warner-Lambert, Ital.*
Gemfibrozil (p.896·2).
Hyperlipidaemias.

Gen-Medroxy *Genpharm, Canad.*
Medroxyprogesterone acetate (p.1480·1).

Genocin *General Drugs, Thai.*
Chloroquine phosphate (p.432·3).
Amoebiasis; malaria.

Genogris *Vita, Spain.*
Piracetam (p.1652·1).
Cerebrovascular disorders; cortical myoclonia; mental function impairment.

Genola *CCD, Fr.*
Hexylresorcinol (p.1146·3); benzododecinium bromide (p.1135·1); allantoin (p.1110·1); boric acid (p.1586·1).
Spermicide.

Genoptic
Allergan, Austral.; Allergan, Hong Kong; Allergan, NZ; Allergan, S.Afr.; Allergan, Singapore; Allergan, USA.
Gentamicin sulfate (p.210·1).
Bacterial eye infections.

Genora 0.5/35 and 1/35 *Rugby, USA†.*
Ethinylestradiol (p.1476·2); norethisterone (p.1485·1).
28-Day packs also contain 7 inert tablets.
Combined oral contraceptive.

Genora 1/50 *Rugby, USA†.*
Mestranol (p.1482·1); norethisterone (p.1485·1).
28-Day packs also contain 7 inert tablets.
Combined oral contraceptive.

Genoral *Kenral, Austral.*
Estropipate (p.1476·1).
Menopausal disorders; oestrogen deficiency.

Genoscopamine *Amido, Fr.†*
Hyoscine oxide hydrobromide (p.469·1).
Parkinsonism.

Genotonorm
Pharmacia Upjohn, Belg.; Pharmacia Upjohn, Fr.; Pharmacia Upjohn, Spain.
Somatropin (p.1286·1).
Growth hormone deficiency; Turner's syndrome.

Genotropin
Pharmacia Upjohn, Aust.; Pharmacia Upjohn, Austral.; Pharmacia Upjohn, Braz.; Pharmacia Upjohn, Denm.; Pharmacia Upjohn, Fin.; Pharmacia Upjohn, Ger.; Pharmacia Upjohn, Hong Kong; Pharmacia Upjohn, Irl.; Pharmacia Upjohn, Israel; Pharmacia Upjohn, Ital.; Pharmacia Upjohn, Mex.; Pharmacia Upjohn, Neth.; Pharmacia Upjohn, Norw.; Pharmacia Upjohn, NZ; Pharmacia Upjohn, Port.; Pharmacia Upjohn, S.Afr.; Pharmacia Upjohn, Singapore; Pharmacia Upjohn, Swed.; Pharmacia Upjohn, Switz.; Pharmacia, UK; Pharmacia Upjohn, USA.
Somatropin (p.1286·1).
Growth disorders in renal failure; growth hormone deficiency; Prader-Willi syndrome; Turner's syndrome.

Genox
Alphapharm, Austral.; Pacific, NZ.
Tamoxifen citrate (p.571·1).
Breast cancer; endometrial cancer.

Genoxal
Sanfer, Mex.; Pras, Spain.
Cyclophosphamide (p.527·3).
Auto-immune disorders; malignant neoplasms; transplant rejection.

Genoxal Trofosfamida *Pras, Spain.*
Trofosfamide (p.577·1).
Malignant neoplasms.

Genoxen
Antigen, Hong Kong; Antigen, Irl.†
Naproxen (p.60·3).
Gout; musculoskeletal, joint, peri-articular, and soft-tissue disorders.

Genozil *Pulitzer, Ital.*
Gemfibrozil (p.896·2).
Hyperlipidaemias.

Genpril *Goldline, USA.*
Ibuprofen (p.43·2).
Fever; osteoarthritis; pain; rheumatoid arthritis.

Genprin *Goldline, USA.*
Aspirin (p.14·2).
Fever; inflammation; myocardial infarction; pain; transient ischaemic attacks.

Genquin *Seng, Thai.*
Gentamicin sulfate (p.210·1); bacitracin (p.155·2); clioquinol (p.190·2); glycine; threonine; cystine.
Infected skin disorders.

Genrex *Rayere, Mex.*
Gentamicin sulfate (p.210·1).
Bacterial infections.

Genrex-B *Rayere, Mex.*
Gentamicin sulfate (p.210·1); betamethasone (p.1063·1).
Infected skin disorders.

Gensan *Goldline, USA†.*
Aspirin (p.14·2); caffeine (p.761·3).

Gensil *General Drugs, Thai.*
Metoclopramide (p.1236·3).
Nausea and vomiting.

Gensumycin
Aventis, Denm.; Hoechst Marion Roussel, Fin.; Hoechst Marion Roussel, Norw.; Hoechst Marion Roussel, Swed.
Gentamicin sulfate (p.210·1).
Bacterial infections.

Genta
CT, Ger.; Grin, Mex.; M & H, Thai.; Shiwa, Thai.
Gentamicin sulfate (p.210·1).
Bacterial infections.

Genta Gobens *Normon, Spain.*
Gentamicin sulfate (p.210·1).
Bacterial infections.

Gentabac *Infan, Mex.*
Gentamicin (p.212·1).
Bacterial infections.

Gentabilles *Schering-Plough, Fr.†*
Gentamicin sulfate (p.210·1).
Bacterial infections.

Gentac *Samakeephaesaj, Thai.*
Gentamicin sulfate (p.210·1).
Bacterial infections.

Gentacarnot *Carnot, Mex.*
Gentamicin (p.212·1).
Bacterial infections.

Gentacidin
Ciba Vision, Canad.†; Ciba Vision, USA.
Gentamicin sulfate (p.210·1).
Bacterial eye infections.

Gentacin
Carter-Wallace, Mex.; Olan-Kemed, Thai.
Gentamicin sulfate (p.210·1).
Bacterial infections.

Gentacoll
Schering-Plough, Denm.; Schering-Plough, Fin.
Gentamicin sulfate (p.210·1).
Bone infection.

Gentacort
Note. This name is used for preparations of different composition.
Allergan-Frumtost, Braz.
Gentamicin sulfate (p.210·1); betamethasone (p.1063·1).
Infected eye disorders.

Ciba Vision, Ital.
Gentamicin sulfate (p.210·1); fluorometholone (p.1072·1).
Infected eye disorders.

Gentadexa
Alcon, Port.; Alcon Cusi, Spain.
Gentamicin sulfate (p.210·1); dexamethasone sodium phosphate (p.1067·1); tetryzoline hydrochloride (p.1101·2).
External ear infections; eye infections with inflammation.

GentaGobens *APS, Port.*
Gentamicin sulfate (p.210·1).
Bacterial infections.

Gentak *Akorn, USA.*
Gentamicin sulfate (p.210·1).
Bacterial infections.

Gental
General Drugs, Thai.; Julphar, UAE.
Gentamicin sulfate (p.210·1).
Bacterial infections.

Gental-F *General Drugs, Thai.*
Gentamicin sulfate (p.210·1); fluocinolone acetonide (p.1071·1).
Infected skin disorders.

Gentalline *Schering-Plough, Fr.*
Gentamicin sulfate (p.210·1).
Bacterial infections.

Gentalodina *Rhone-Poulenc Rorer, Spain†.*
Gentamicin sulfate (p.210·1).
Bacterial infections.

Gentalyn *Schering-Plough, Ital.*
Gentamicin sulfate (p.210·1).
Bacterial infections.

Gentalyn Beta *Schering-Plough, Ital.*
Gentamicin sulfate (p.210·1); betamethasone valerate (p.1063·2).
Infected skin disorders.

Gentamedical *Medical, Ital.*
Gentamicin sulfate (p.210·1).
Bacterial infections.

Gentamen *Fournier, Ital.*
Gentamicin sulfate (p.210·1).
Bacterial infections.

Gentamival *Rovi, Spain.*
Gentamicin sulfate (p.210·1).
Bacterial infections.

Gentamytrex
Tramedica, Belg.; Mann, Ger.; Mann, Neth.; Mann, Singapore.
Gentamicin sulfate (p.210·1).
Bacterial eye infections.

Gentanacin *Loren, Mex.*
Gentamicin (p.212·1).
Bacterial infections.

Genta-Oph *Seng, Thai.*
Gentamicin sulfate (p.210·1).
Bacterial infections.

Gentapat *Parggon, Mex.*
Gentamicin (p.212·1).
Bacterial infections.

Gentaplus *Abbott, Braz.*
Gentamicin sulfate (p.210·1).
Bacterial infections.

Gentarim *Rimsa, Mex.*
Gentamicin sulfate (p.210·1).
Bacterial infections.

Gentasol *Ocusoft, USA.*
Gentamicin sulfate (p.210·1).
Bacterial infections.

Gentasone *Schering-Plough, Fr.*
Gentamicin sulfate (p.210·1); betamethasone sodium phosphate (p.1063·2).
Bacterial eye infections with inflammation.

Gentatrim *Trima, Israel.*
Gentamicin sulfate (p.210·1).
Bacterial skin infections.

Gentavasor *Alcon Cusi, Spain.*
Gentamicin sulfate (p.210·1); tetryzoline hydrochloride (p.1101·2).
Eye disorders.

Gentavivant *Vivant, Mex.*
Gentamicin (p.212·1).
Bacterial infections.

Gentax *Agepha, Aust.*
Gentamicin sulfate (p.210·1).
Bacterial eye infections.

Gentaxil *Haller, Mex.*
Gentamicin (p.212·1).
Bacterial infections.

Gentazaf Z *Zafira, Mex.*
Gentamicin sulfate (p.210·1).
Bacterial infections.

Genteal
Ciba Vision, Austral.; Novartis Ophthalmics, Canad.; Ciba Vision, NZ; Ciba Vision, USA.
Hypromellose (p.1501·3).
Dry eyes; eye irritation.

Ciba Vision, Ital.
Hypromellose (p.1501·3) (p.1129·2).
Wetting solution for contact lenses.

Gentialoquin *Collins, Mex.*
Gentamicin (p.212·1).
Bacterial infections.

Gentibioptal *Farmila, Ital.*
Gentamicin sulfate (p.210·1).
Bacterial eye infections.

Genticin
Roche, Irl.; Roche, UK.
Gentamicin sulfate (p.210·1).
Bacterial infections.

Genticina *Pharmacia Upjohn, Spain.*
Gentamicin sulfate (p.210·1).
Bacterial infections.

Genticol *SIFI, Ital.*
Gentamicin sulfate (p.210·1).
Eye infections.

Gentipress *Gentili, Ital.*
Enalapril maleate (p.883·3); hydrochlorothiazide (p.907·3).
Hypertension.

Gentisone HC
Roche, Irl.; Roche, UK.
Gentamicin sulfate (p.210·1); hydrocortisone acetate (p.1073·3).
Bacterial ear infections.

Gentlax *Blair, USA†.*
Senna (p.1248·2).
Constipation.

Gentlax S *Blair, USA†.*
Docusate sodium (p.1223·1); senna (p.1248·2).
Constipation.

Gentle C with Bioflavonoids *Cenovis, Austral.*
Calcium ascorbate (p.1389·3); lemon bioflavonoids (p.1611·1); rutoside (p.1611·2); hesperidin (p.1611·2).
Capillary disorders; cold and influenza symptoms; wounds.

Gentlees *Delamac, Austral.*
Hamamelis water (p.1618·3); glycerol; cetylpyridinium chloride (p.1138·1).
Anogenital wounds; anorectal disorders; napppy rash; nipple care.

Gent-L-Tip *Chester, Canad.*
Monobasic sodium phosphate (p.1193·2); dibasic sodium phosphate (p.1193·2).
Bowel evacuation.

Gentocil *Oftalder, Port.*
Gentamicin sulfate (p.210·1).
Bacterial infections.

Gentomil *Biologici Italia, Ital.*
Gentamicin sulfate (p.210·1).
Bacterial infections.

Gent-Ophtal *Winzer, Ger.*
Gentamicin sulfate (p.210·1).
Bacterial eye infections.

Gentos
Note. This name is used for preparations of different composition.
Bittner, Aust.
Homoeopathic preparation.

Llorente, Spain.
Clofedanol hydrochloride (p.1087·1).
Coughs.

Gentralay *Plevifarma, Spain†.*
Gentamicin sulfate (p.210·1).
Bacterial infections.

Gentran 40
Baxter, Canad.; Baxter, UK; Baxter, USA.
Dextran 40 (p.728·3) in glucose or sodium chloride.
Extracorporeal circulation; plasma volume expansion; thromboembolism prophylaxis.

Gentran 70
Baxter, Canad.; Baxter, UK; Baxter, USA.
Dextran 70 (p.729·2) in glucose or sodium chloride.
Plasma volume expansion.

Gentran 75 *Baxter, USA†.*
Dextran 75 (p.730·1) in sodium chloride.
Plasma volume expansion.

Gentrisone *Shin Poong, Singapore.*
Betamethasone dipropionate (p.1063·2); clotrimazole (p.382·1); gentamicin sulfate (p.210·1).
Infected skin disorders.

Gentus *Gentili, Ital.†*
Dimemorfan phosphate (p.1089·1).
Coughs.

Gentussiin *General Drugs, Thai.*
Guaifenesin (p.1092·2); dextromethorphan hydrobromide (p.1087·3).
Coughs.

Genu-cyl Ho-Len-Complex *Liebermann, Ger.*
Homoeopathic preparation.

Genuine Australian Eucalyptus Drops *Felton, Austral.*
Eucalyptus oil (p.1609·2); menthol (p.1632·3); lemon oil (p.1628·2).
Cough; nasal congestion; sore throat.

Genurat *Soria Natural, Spain.*
Bearberry (p.1583·3); betula alba (p.1585·2); oleum pini sylvestris; calluna vulgaris.
Urinary-tract infections.

Genurin
Recordati, Hong Kong; Recordati, Ital.; Recordati, Singapore.
Flavoxate hydrochloride (p.467·1).
Genito-urinary tract disorders.

Genurin-S *Hoechst Marion Roussel, Braz.*
Flavoxate hydrochloride (p.467·1).
Urinary-tract spasm.

Genuxal *Asta Medica, Braz.*
Cyclophosphamide (p.527·3).
Malignant neoplasms.

Gen-Xene *Alra, USA.*
Dipotassium clorazepate (p.670·3).
Alcohol withdrawal syndrome; anxiety; epilepsy.

Geocillin *Pfizer, USA.*
Carindacillin sodium (p.160·3).
Bacterial infections.

Geodon *Pfizer, USA.*
Ziprasidone hydrochloride (p.712·1).
Schizophrenia.

Geo-magnit *Biomo, Ger.*
Magnesium glutamate; dibasic magnesium phosphate.
Magnesium deficiency.

Geomicina *Atral, Port.*
Oxytetracycline hydrochloride (p.234·1).
Bacterial infections.

Geomycine *Schering-Plough, Belg.*
Gentamicin sulfate (p.210·1).
Bacterial infections.

Geopen
Note. This name is used for preparations of different composition.
Pfizer, Hong Kong.
Carindacillin sodium (p.160·3).
Bacterial infections of the urinary tract.

Pfizer, Ital.†; Pfizer, Spain†.
Carbenicillin sodium (p.160·2).
Bacterial infections.

Geophagol *Sanval, Braz.*
Mebendazole (p.102·2).
Worm infections.

Georkacina *Ehlinger, Mex.*
Amikacin (p.147·3).
Bacterial infections.

Geracin *Reuffer, Mex.*
Gentamicin (p.212·1).
Bacterial infections.

Geralen *Gerot, Aust.*
5-Methoxypsoralen (p.1120·3).
Psoriasis.

Geram *Vedim, Fr.*
Piracetam (p.1652·1).
Cerebrovascular disorders; improvement of mental function in the elderly; vertigo.

The symbol † denotes a preparation no longer actively marketed

Geramet Gerard, Irl.
Cimetidine (p.1216·3).
Gastric hyperacidity; gastro-oesophageal reflux; peptic ulcer; Zollinger-Ellison syndrome.

Geramox Gerard, Irl.
Amoxicillin (p.149·2) or amoxicillin trihydrate (p.149·2).
Infections.

Gerard 99 Gerard House, UK.
Lupulus (p.1629·3); passion flower (p.1649·1); valerian (p.1678·3).
Irritability; tenseness.

Gerard House Buchu Compound Peter Black, UK.
Taraxacum (p.1669·1); buchu (p.1587·2); bearberry (p.1583·3); clivers (p.1596·3).
Fluid retention.

Gerard House Cranesbill Peter Black, UK.
Geranium maculatum.
Diarrhoea.

Gerard House Curzon Peter Black, UK.
Damiana (p.1602·1).
Tonic.

Gerard House Gladlax Peter Black, UK.
Aloes (p.1210·1); fennel (p.1610·1); valerian (p.1678·3); cnicus benedictus (p.1597·2).
Constipation.

Gerard House Golden Seal Compound Peter Black, UK.
Althaea root (p.1577·1); hydrastis (p.1621·1); geranium maculatum; taraxacum (p.1669·1).
Gastrointestinal disorders.

Gerard House Helonias Compound Peter Black, UK.
Helonias (p.1619·1); parsley (p.1648·3); cimicifuga (p.1595·2); raspberry leaf (p.1657·2).
Fluid retention.

Gerard House Ligvites Peter Black, UK.
Guaiacum (p.1618·2); cimicifuga (p.1595·2); white willow bark (p.82·1); sarsaparilla (p.1661·1); poplar bark (p.1653·2).
Musculoskeletal and joint disorders.

Gerard House Motherwort Compound Peter Black, UK.
Passion flower (p.1649·1); motherwort (p.1637·3); tilia flower (p.1673·2).
Stresses and strains.

Gerard House Reumalex Peter Black, UK.
Guaiacum resin (p.1618·2); cimicifuga (p.1595·2); salix (p.82·1); sarsaparilla (p.1661·1); poplar bark (p.1653·2).
Musculoskeletal and joint disorders.

Gerard House Serenity Peter Black, UK.
Lupulus (p.1629·3); passion flower (p.1649·1); valerian (p.1678·3).
Irritability; stress.

Gerard House Somnus Peter Black, UK.
Valerian (p.1678·3); lupulus (p.1629·3); wild lettuce (p.1680·3).
Insomnia.

Gerard House Valerian Compound Peter Black, UK.
Lupulus (p.1629·3); passion flower (p.1649·1); valerian (p.1678·3); wild lettuce (p.1680·3); Jamaica dogwood (p.1625·1); skullcap (p.1664·3).
Insomnia; restlessness.

Gerard House Waterlex Peter Black, UK.
Taraxacum (p.1669·1); equisetum (p.1606·3); bearberry (p.1583·3).
Water retention.

Geratam Bios, Belg.
Piracetam (p.1652·1).
Mental function impairment.

Geratar UCB, S.Afr.
Inositol nicotinate (p.914·1); multivitamins (p.1350·1); meclozine (p.420·3); hydroxyzine hydrochloride (p.419·1).
Vascular disorders; vertigo.

Geravim Major, USA.
Vitamin B substances with minerals (p.1350·1).

Geravitine Dinafarma, Braz.
Erythroxylon catuaba; liriosma ovata; vitamin E; vitamin B substances (p.1350·1); yohimbine hydrochloride (p.1681·3).

Gerax Gerard, Irl.
Alprazolam (p.654·2).
Alcohol withdrawal syndrome; anxiety disorders; depression; mixed anxiety-depressive states; panic attacks; phobias.

Gerbin ICN, Spain.
Aceclofenac (p.11·1).
Gout; inflammation; musculoskeletal, joint, peri-articular, and soft-tissue disorders; pain.

Gercid forte Henkel, Ger.
Didecyldimethylammonium chloride (p.1143·2); isopropyl alcohol (p.1149·2).
Disinfection.

Geref
Serono, Aust.; Serono, Canad.†; Serono, Fin.; Serono, Hong Kong; Serono, Irl.; Serono, Israel; Serono, Ital.; Serono, Mex.; Serono, Norw.; Serono, Port.; Serono, S.Afr.; Serono, Spain; Serono, Swed.†; Serono, Switz.; Serono, Thai.; Serono, UK; Serono, USA.
Sermorelin (p.1297·2) or sermorelin acetate (p.1297·1).
Test for growth hormone secretion.

Gerelax Gerard, Irl.
Lactulose (p.1230·1).
Constipation; hepatic encephalopathy.

Geriaforce
Note.This name is used for preparations of different composition.
Bioforce, Ger.
Homoeopathic preparation.

Bioforce, Switz.
Ginkgo biloba (p.1615·2).
Atherosclerosis.

Gerial B12 Allen, Mex.
Amino-acids and vitamin B substances with iron (p.1350·1).

Gerialong Heralds, Braz.
Multivitamin, amino-acid, and mineral preparation (p.1350·1).

Geriaplasma Ardeypharm, Ger.
Bovine heart extract; bovine liver extract; bovine spleen extract.
Tonic.

Geriaton Ache, Braz.
Multivitamin and mineral preparation with ginseng (p.1350·1).

Geriatric Stanley, Canad.; Herbes Universelles, Canad.
Multivitamin and mineral preparation (p.1350·1).

Geriatric Pharmaton
Boehringer Ingelheim, Aust.†
Deanol tartrate; ginseng; vitamins; minerals; rutoside (p.1350·1).
Tonic.

Pharmaton, Israel.
Multivitamin and mineral preparation with ginseng (p.1350·1).
Tonic; vitamin and mineral deficiency.

Pharmaton, Thai.
Deanol tartrate; vitamins; minerals; rutoside; linoleic acid; linolenic acid (p.1350·1).
Tonic.

Geriatric Pharmaton-neu Boehringer Ingelheim, Aust.
Ginseng; vitamins; minerals; lecithin (p.1350·1).

Geriatrie-Mulsin Mucos, Ger.
Multivitamin preparation (p.1350·1).

Geriavit Pharmaton, Switz.
Ginseng; deanol bitartrate; multivitamins; minerals; rutoside; lecithin (p.1350·1).
Tonic.

Geriavite Sintofarma, Braz.
Multivitamins with ginseng, inositol, and rutoside (p.1350·1).

Gericaps Pharmadass, UK.
Multivitamin and mineral preparation (p.1350·1).

Gericarb Gerard, Irl.
Carbamazepine (p.342·2).
Alcohol withdrawal syndrome; epilepsy; pain.

Gericin Seid, Spain.
Nitrendipine (p.947·1).
Angina pectoris; hypertension; Raynaud's syndrome.

Gericomplex Boehringer Ingelheim, S.Afr.
Multivitamins; minerals; dimethylaminoethanol bitartrate; ginseng (p.1350·1).
Tonic.

Geridium Goldline, USA†.
Phenazopyridine hydrochloride (p.77·3).
Irritation of the lower urinary tract.

Geriflox Gerard, Irl.
Flucloxacillin sodium (p.207·1).
Gram-positive bacterial infections.

Gerigoa Sanova, Aust.
Procaine resinate; procaine hydrochloride; buphenine resinate; haematoporphyrin; orotic acid; vitamins (p.1350·1).
Tonic.

Geri-Kan H3 Kanda, Braz.
Etofylline (p.765·1); procaine hydrochloride (p.1319·1); potassium aspartate; magnesium aspartate; adenosine; linoleic acid; linolenic acid; choline bitartrate; methionine; biotin; vitamin E acetate; vitamin A; vitamin C; vitamin B substances; folic acid; inositol (p.1350·1).
Tonic.

Gerimal Rugby, USA.
Co-dergocrine mesilate (p.1597·3).
Senile dementia.

Gerimax
Note.This name is used for preparations of different composition.
Dansk, Fr.
Ginseng (p.1615·3).
Tonic.

Vitalia, UK†.
Multivitamin and mineral preparation with ginseng (p.1350·1).

Gerimax adultes Richelet, Fr.
Multivitamin and mineral preparation with ginseng (p.1350·1).

Gerimax enfants Richelet, Fr.
Multivitamin and mineral preparation (p.1350·1).

Gerimax Junior Dansk, Israel.
Multivitamin and mineral preparation (p.1350·1).

Gerimax NF Dansk, Israel.
Multivitamin and mineral preparation with ginseng (p.1350·1).

Gerimed Fielding, USA.
Multivitamin and mineral preparation (p.1350·1).
Osteoporosis.

Gerinap Gerard, Irl.
Naproxen (p.60·3).
Gout; musculoskeletal and joint disorders.

Geriot Goldline, USA.
Ferrous fumarate (p.1360·1); folic acid (p.1361·1); multivitamins and minerals (p.1350·1).
Iron-deficiency anaemias.

Geripan Heralds, Braz.
Guarana (p.1681·1); erythroxylon catuaba; liriosma ovata; ginger (p.1227·2).
Nutritional supplement.

Geriplex Parke, Davis, USA†.
Multivitamin and mineral preparation (p.1350·1).

Geri-Plus Herbes Universelles, Canad.
Betacarotene, selenium, vitamin C, and vitamin E (p.1350·1).

Geriso Asta Medica, Port.
Linoleic acid (p.1613·2); vitamin A; vitamin E; pyridoxine; lecithin (p.1350·1).
Atherosclerosis; hypercholesterolaemia; vascular disorders.

Geritol
SmithKline Beecham Consumer, Canad.; SmithKline Beecham Consumer, USA.
Ferric ammonium citrate (p.1359·2); vitamin B substances with methionine (p.1350·1).
Iron-deficiency anaemias.

Geritol Complete SmithKline Beecham Consumer, USA.
Iron (p.1366·3); folic acid (p.1361·1); multivitamins and minerals (p.1350·1).
Iron-deficiency anaemias.

Geritol Extend SmithKline Beecham Consumer, USA.
Multivitamin and mineral preparation with iron and folic acid (p.1350·1).

Geriton Gerbex, Canad.
Vitamin B substances, calcium, and iron (p.1350·1).

Geritonic Geriatric Pharm. Corp., USA.
Ferric ammonium citrate (p.1359·2); liver fraction; vitamin B substances and minerals (p.1350·1).
Iron-deficiency anaemias.

Gerivent Gerard, Irl.
Salbutamol (p.770·3).
Obstructive airways disease.

Gerivit
Note.This name is used for preparations of different composition.
Sanoreform, Ger.†
Ginseng (p.1615·3).
Tonic.

Westmont, Hong Kong.
Methyltestosterone (p.1482·3); ethinylestradiol (p.1476·2); vitamins; minerals; amino acids (p.1350·1).
Geriatric nutritional supplement.

Gerivite Goldline, USA.
Multivitamin and mineral preparation (p.1350·1).

Gerivites Rugby, USA.
Ferrous sulfate (p.1360·3); vitamin B substances with vitamin C (p.1350·1).
Iron-deficiency anaemias.

Germanin Bayer, Ger.
Suramin (p.602·2).
Onchocerciasis; trypanosomiasis.

Germentin Gerard, Irl.
Amoxicillin trihydrate (p.149·2); potassium clavulanate (p.187·2).
Bacterial infections.

Germex SA Druggists Self Med, S.Afr.†
Nitrofurazone (p.231·3).
Bacterial infections; burns; wounds.

Germicidin IMS, Ital.
Benzalkonium chloride (p.1133·2).
Surface and instrument disinfection.

Germisdin Antiseptico Isdin, Port.
Antiseptic cleanser for skin and hair.

Germisdin Higiene Intima Isdin, Port.
Preparation for vaginal hygiene.

Germolene
Note.This name is used for preparations of different composition.
SmithKline Beecham Consumer, Irl.; Bayer, UK.
Ointment: Zinc oxide (p.1128·2); methyl salicylate (p.55·1); octafonium chloride (p.1151·3); phenol (p.1152·3).
Skin disinfection.

Bayer, UK.
Cream: Chlorhexidine gluconate (p.1138·2); phenol (p.1152·3).
Skin disinfection.

SmithKline Beecham Consumer, UK.
Topical spray: Triclosan (p.1159·2); dichlorophen (p.98·1).
Skin disinfection.

SmithKline Beecham Consumer, UK.
Topical wipes: Benzalkonium chloride (p.1133·2); chlorhexidine gluconate (p.1138·2).
Skin disinfection.

Germolene First Aid SmithKline Beecham Consumer, Irl.
Chlorhexidine gluconate (p.1138·2); phenol (p.1152·3).
Skin disinfections.

Germoloids Bayer, UK.
Cream; ointment; suppositories: Lignocaine [lidocaine] hydrochloride (p.1313·2); zinc oxide (p.1128·2).

Topical wipes: Chlorhexidine gluconate (p.1138·2); benzalkonium chloride (p.1133·2); menthol (p.1632·3).
Haemorrhoids.

Germose Besins-Iscovesco, Fr.
Sodium benzoate (p.1134·3); sulfogaiacol (p.1101·1); grindelia (p.1618·2); crataegus (p.1600·2); peppermint (p.1243·2); thyme (p.1672·2).
Respiratory-tract congestion.

Germozero Carlo Erba OTC, Ital.
Tosylchloramide sodium (p.1159·1).
Skin disinfection.

Germozero Hospital Carlo Erba OTC, Ital.†
Chlorhexidine gluconate (p.1138·2); cetrimide (p.1137·1).
Disinfection of wounds, external genitalia, surfaces, and instruments.

Germozero Plus Carlo Erba OTC, Ital.
Benzalkonium chloride (p.1133·2); orthophenylphenol (p.1152·1).
Wounds disinfection.

Gernebcin Lilly, Ger.
Tobramycin sulfate (p.263·3).
Bacterial infections.

Gernel Gerbex, Canad.
Cresol (p.1142·3); zinc oxide (p.1128·2).

Gero H3 Sedabel, Braz.
Multivitamins, amino acids, and minerals with erythroxylon catuaba and adenosine (p.1350·1).

Gero H3 Aslan Chefaro, Ger.
Procaine hydrochloride (p.1319·1); benzoic acid; potassium disulfite; sodium phosphate (p.1350·1).

Geroaslan H3 Sanova, Aust.
Procaine hydrochloride (p.1319·1).
Tonic.

Geroderm
Note.This name is used for preparations of different composition.
Avantgarde, Ital.
Triclosan (p.1159·2).
Skin cleansing.

Maxwell, S.Afr.†
Soap substitute.

Geroderm Zolfo Avantgarde, Ital.
Sulfur (p.1123·3); lactic acid (p.1626·2); triclosan (p.1159·2).
Skin cleansing in acne.

Gerodorm Gerot, Aust.
Cinolazepam (p.667·3).
Sleep disorders.

Geroforte IMA, Braz.
Multivitamins with guarana and erythroxylon catuaba (p.1350·1).

Gerogelat Metochem, Aust.
Vitamin A palmitate (p.1383·2); tocoferil acetate (p.1394·1).
Hearing loss; mucous membrane disorders; tinnitus; vitamin A and E deficiency.

Gerolin CT, Ital.
Citicoline sodium (p.1596·1).
Cerebrovascular disorders; parkinsonism.

Gerontamin Heilit, Ger.
Gelatin (p.737·2); cystine (p.1359·1).
Joint disorders.

Gerontex Marjan, Braz.
Multivitamin, amino-acid, and mineral preparation (p.1350·1).

Gerontin Pharmonta, Aust.
Procaine hydrochloride (p.1319·1); caffeine (p.761·3).
Tonic.

Gerosenil Delta, Braz.
Methyltestosterone (p.1482·3); alpha tocoferil acetate (p.1394·1); yohimbine (p.1681·3); caffeine (p.761·3); ephedrine (p.1090·1).
Erectile dysfunction.

Geroten Gerard, Irl.
Captopril (p.853·3).
Heart failure; hypertension.

Geroton Forte Bradley, USA†.
Multivitamin and mineral preparation (p.1350·1).

Gerotrex H3 Bunker, Braz.
Multivitamin, amino-acid, and mineral preparation (p.1350·1).

Gerovital H3
Sanova, Aust.; Sicomed, Hong Kong.
Procaine hydrochloride (p.1319·1).
Tonic.

Geroxalen
Galderma, Denm.; Sanofi Synthelabo, Neth.; Galderma, Norw.
Methoxsalen (p.1118·3).
Mycosis fungoides; psoriasis.

Geroxicam Gerard, Irl.
Piroxicam (p.79·1).
Dysmenorrhoea; gout; musculoskeletal and joint disorders.

Gerozac Gerard, Irl.
Fluoxetine hydrochloride (p.284·2).
Depression.

Gertac Gerard, Irl.
Ranitidine hydrochloride (p.1245·2).
Gastro-oesophageal reflux; peptic ulcer; Zollinger-Ellison syndrome.

Gerviton Andreabal, Switz.†
Multivitamin and mineral preparation (p.1350·1).

GES 45
Milupa, Fr.
Glucose; sucrose; potassium citrate; sodium bicarbonate; sodium chloride (p.1185·2).
Diarrhoea; oral rehydration therapy.

Milupa, Hong Kong; **Milupa,** Singapore.
Glucose; potassium chloride; sodium bicarbonate; sodium chloride (p.1185·2).
Diarrhoea; oral rehydration therapy.

Milupa, Switz.
Oral rehydration solution (p.1185·2).
Diarrhoea; gastro-enteritis.

Gesamtnahrlosung Fresenius Kabi, Aust.
A range of amino-acid, glucose, and lipid (from soya oil (p.1378·1)) infusions (p.1350·1).
Contains egg lecithin.
Parenteral nutrition.

Gesidine Lilly, Port.
Vindesine sulfate (p.580·1).

Gesiprox Kalbe, Singapore.
Naproxen sodium (p.61·1).
Gout; musculoskeletal and joint disorders; pain.

Gestadinona Schering, Braz.
Hydroxyprogesterone caproate (p.1479·3); estradiol valerate (p.1473·2).
Endometriosis; menopausal disorders; menstrual disorders.

Gestaferron Arlex, Mex.
Ferrous fumarate (p.1360·1).

Gestafortin Merck, Ger.
Chlormadinone acetate (p.1465·3).
Endometriosis; menstrual disorders.

Gestakadin Kade, Ger.
Norethisterone acetate (p.1485·1).
Menopausal disorders; menstrual disorders.

Gestamater Cyanamid, Spain.
Multivitamin and mineral preparation (p.1350·1).

Gestamestrol N Hermal, Ger.
Chlormadinone acetate (p.1465·3); mestranol (p.1482·1).
Androgen-dependent alopecia, acne, and seborrhoea; hirsutism.

Gestamine Nadeau, Canad.
Multivitamin preparation with calcium and iron (p.1350·1).

Gestanon
Organon, Aust.†; Organon, Mex.
Allylestrenol (p.1465·2).
Threatened miscarriage.

GestaPolar Orion, Ger.
Medroxyprogesterone acetate (p.1480·1).

Gestapuran
Leo, Fin.; Leo, Swed.
Medroxyprogesterone acetate (p.1480·1).
Endometriosis; menopausal disorders; menstrual disorders.

Gestarelle IPRAD, Fr.
Multivitamin and mineral preparation (p.1350·1).

Gesterol Germiphene, Canad.†
Progesterone (p.1488·3).
Progestogenic.

Gestid Ranbaxy, Singapore.
Oral suspension: Aluminium hydroxide (p.1210·3); magnesium hydroxide (p.1233·1); simeticone (p.1249·2).
Tablets: Aluminium hydroxide (p.1210·3); magnesium trisilicate (p.1233·3); magnesium hydroxide (p.1233·1); simeticone (p.1249·2).
Flatulence; gastric hyperacidity; gastritis; gastro-oesophageal reflux; peptic ulcer.

Gestiferrol Wolfs, Belg.
Ferrous fumarate (p.1360·1); folic acid (p.1361·1).
Anaemias; dietary supplement during pregnancy.

Gestinol Libbs, Braz.
Gestodene (p.1479·1); ethinylestradiol (p.1476·2).
Combined oral contraceptive.

Gestone
Ferring, Israel; NZ Medical & Scientific, NZ; Paines & Byrne, Thai.; Ferring, UK.
Progesterone (p.1488·3).
Adjunct in infertility disorders; dysfunctional uterine bleeding; threatened or recurrent miscarriage.

Gestoral Novartis, Fr.
Medroxyprogesterone acetate (p.1480·1).
Menopausal disorders.

Gets-It Oakhurst, USA.
Salicylic acid (p.1122·3); zinc chloride (p.1398·1).
Hyperkeratosis.

Gevatran Lipha Sante, Fr.
Naftidrofuryl oxalate (p.937·3).
Peripheral and cerebral vascular disorders.

Gevilon
Parke, Davis, Aust.; Orion, Fin.; Parke, Davis, Ger.; Warner-Lambert, Switz.
Gemfibrozil (p.896·2).
Hyperlipidaemias.

Gevirol Gerbex, Canad.
Multivitamin and mineral preparation (p.1350·1).

Gevrabon Lederle, USA.
Vitamin B substances with minerals (p.1350·1).

Gevral
Whitehall, Braz.; Cyanamid, Ital.†; Whitehall, S.Afr.; Lederle, UK†; Lederle, USA.
Multivitamin and mineral preparation (p.1350·1).

Gevral Instant Protein
Whitehall, Irl.; Whitehall-Robins, Switz.
Multivitamin, mineral, and protein preparation (p.1350·1).
Tonic.

Gevral Protein
Lederle, UK†; Lederle, USA.
Multivitamin, mineral, and protein preparation (p.1350·1).

Gevral Proteina Cyanamid, Spain.
Protein, vitamin, and mineral preparation (p.1350·1).
Nutritional supplement.

Gevral T Lederle, USA.
Ferrous fumarate (p.1360·1); folic acid (p.1361·1); multivitamins and minerals (p.1350·1).
Iron-deficiency anaemias.

Gevral Tablets Whitehall, Irl.
Multivitamin and mineral preparation (p.1350·1).

Gevramycin Schering-Plough, Spain.
Gentamicin sulfate (p.210·1).
Bacterial infections.

Gevramycin Topica Schering-Plough, Spain.
Gentamicin sulfate (p.210·1).
Bacterial skin infections; ulcers.

Gewacalm Nycomed, Aust.
Diazepam (p.674·3).
Anxiety disorders; eclampsia; neuroses; panic attacks; phobias; premedication; skeletal muscle spasm; sleep disorders; status epilepticus.

Gewacyclin Nycomed, Aust.
Doxycycline hyclate (p.200·1).
Bacterial infections.

Gewadal Nycomed, Aust.
Paracetamol (p.71·2); propyphenazone (p.80·2); caffeine (p.761·3).
Fever; pain.

Gewadilat Bayer, Aust.†.
Nifedipine (p.940·1).
Angina pectoris; hypertension; Raynaud's syndrome.

Gewaglucon Nycomed, Aust.
Glibenclamide (p.321·3).
Diabetes mellitus.

Gewapurol Nycomed, Aust.
Allopurinol (p.397·2).
Gout; hyperuricaemia; renal calculi.

Gewazem Nycomed, Aust.
Diltiazem hydrochloride (p.874·3).
Angina pectoris.

Gewodin Gewo, Ger.
Famprofazone (p.36·1); paracetamol (p.71·2); propyphenazone (p.80·2); caffeine (p.761·3).
Pain.

Gewodine Geistlich, Switz.
Paracetamol (p.71·2); caffeine (p.761·3); propyphenazone (p.80·2).
Fever; pain.

Gewusst wie Beruhigungs Metochem, Aust.†.
Valerian (p.1678·3).
Anxiety disorders.

Geyderm Geymonat, Ital.
Benzalkonium chloride (p.1133·2).
Disinfection of mucous membranes, wounds, burns, surfaces, and instruments.

Geyderm Sepsi Geymonat, Ital.
Cetylpyridinium chloride (p.1138·1).
Disinfection of wounds and burns.

Geyfritz Geymonat, Ital.
Aspirin (p.14·2); caffeine (p.761·3).
Glycine (p.1365·3) is included in this preparation in an attempt to limit adverse effects on the gastrointestinal mucosa.
Cold symptoms; pain.

Gezon Laborsil, Braz.
Diclofenac potassium (p.30·2).
Gout; inflammation; musculoskeletal, joint, and periarticular disorders; pain.

G-Farlutal Pharmacia Upjohn, Ger.
Medroxyprogesterone acetate (p.1480·1).
Menstrual disorders; test of ovarian function.

G-Fen General Drugs, Thai.
Ibuprofen (p.43·2).
Fever; inflammation; pain.

GFN/DM Cypress, USA.
Guaifenesin (p.1092·2); dextromethorphan hydrobromide (p.1087·3).
Coughs.

GFN/PSE Cypress, USA.
Guaifenesin (p.1092·2); pseudoephedrine hydrochloride (p.1099·2).
Respiratory-tract disorders associated with increased or viscous mucus.

GG-Cen Schwarz, USA†.
Guaifenesin (p.1092·2).
Coughs.

GHRH
Ferring, Belg.; Ferring, Ital.; Sanofi Synthelabo, Neth.; Ferring, Neth.; Ferring, UK.
Somatorelin acetate (p.1297·2).
Diagnosis of growth hormone deficiency.

GI
Note. This name is used for preparations of different composition.
Sankyo, Hong Kong.
Taka-diastase (p.1579·3); lipase; aluminium magnesium silicate (p.1499·1); hydrotalcite (p.1228·1); sodium bicarbonate (p.1186·2); calcium carbonate (p.1215·1); scopolia; cinnamon (p.1595·3); fennel (p.1610·1); ginger (p.1227·2); menthol (p.1632·3); liquorice (p.1231·2); clove (p.1596·3); phellodendron.
Gastrointestinal disorders.

Provit, Mex.
Gentamicin sulfate (p.210·1).
Bacterial infections.

Giarlam UCI, Braz.
Furazolidone (p.592·1).
Cholera; diarrhoea; giardiasis.

Gibicef Metapharma, Ital.
Cefuroxime sodium (p.178·2).
Bacterial infections.

Gibifer Metapharma, Ital.
Ferric sodium gluconate (p.1360·2).
Iron-deficiency anaemias.

Gibiflu Metapharma, Ital.
Flunisolide (p.1070·3).
Rhinitis.

Gibinap Metapharma, Ital.
Naproxen sodium (p.61·1).
Lignocaine [lidocaine] hydrochloride (p.1313·2) is included in the intramuscular injection to alleviate the pain of injection.
Musculoskeletal and joint disorders; pain.

Gibixen Metapharma, Ital.
Naproxen (p.60·3).
Musculoskeletal and joint disorders; pain.

Gichtex Gerot, Aust.
Allopurinol (p.397·2).
Gout; hyperuricaemia; renal calculi.

Gichtex plus Gerot, Aust.
Allopurinol (p.397·2); benzbromarone (p.399·3).
Gout; hyperuricaemia.

Giflorex Errekappa, Ital.
Lactobacillus casei var *rhamnosus* (p.1626·3); maltodextrin (p.1371·2); fructose (p.1363·3).
Maintenance of gastrointestinal flora.

Gigasept Schulke & Mayr, Ger.
Succinic dialdehyde (p.1145·1); dimethoxytetrahydrofuran; formaldehyde (p.1144·2).
Instrument disinfection.

Gigasept AF Schulke & Mayr, Ger.
Didecyldimethylammonium chloride (p.1143·2); phenoxypropanol (p.1153·3); aminoalkylglycine.
Instrument disinfection.

Gigasept FF Schulke & Mayr, Ger.
Succinic dialdehyde (p.1145·1); dimethoxytetrahydrofuran.
Instrument disinfection.

Gigasept Med Schulke & Mayr, Ger.
Didecyldimethylammonium chloride (p.1143·2); phenoxypropanol (p.1153·3); aminoalkylglycine.
Instrument disinfection.

Gilemal Enzypharm, Aust.
Glibenclamide (p.321·3).
Diabetes mellitus.

Gilex Rekah, Israel.
Doxepin hydrochloride (p.283·3).
Depression; mixed anxiety depressive states.

Gillazyme Sandoz OTC, Switz.†.
Pancreatin (p.1646·1); dehydrocholic acid (p.1602·2); dimethicone (p.1249·2).
Digestive-system disorders.

Gillazyme plus Sandoz OTC, Switz.†.
Pancreatin (p.1646·1); dehydrocholic acid (p.1602·2); dimethicone (p.1249·2); metixene hydrochloride (p.470·2).
Digestive-system disorders.

Gilt Lacoer, Ger.
Clotrimazole (p.382·1).
Fungal skin infections.

Gilucor Solvay, Ger.
Sotalol hydrochloride (p.972·2).
Arrhythmias.

Giludop
Solvay, Denm.; Solvay, Swed.
Dopamine hydrochloride (p.881·3).
Shock.

Gilurytmal
Solvay, Aust.; Solvay, Ger.; Lacer, Spain.
Ajmaline (p.833·1).
Arrhythmias.

Gilustenon Solvay, Ger.†.
Glyceryl trinitrate (p.897·3).
Angina pectoris; heart failure.

Gimalxina Collins, Mex.
Amoxicillin trihydrate (p.149·2).
Bacterial infections.

Ginatren LPB, Ital.†.
A trichomonal vaccine containing *Lactobacillus acidophilus* (p.1566·2).
Vaginitis.

Gincaps Medix, Mex.
Ginseng (p.1615·3).

Gincoben Ipsen, Port.
Ginkgo biloba (p.1615·2).
Cerebral and peripheral vascular disorders; vestibular disorders.

Gincola Biocontrolfarm, Ital.†.
Ginseng (p.1615·3); kola (p.1681·1).

Gincosan Pharmaton, Switz.
Ginkgo biloba (p.1615·2); ginseng (p.1615·3).
Mental function impairment.

Gine Canesten Bayer, Spain.
Clotrimazole (p.382·1).
Balanitis; vulvovaginal candidiasis.

Gine Heyden Squibb, Spain.
Amphotericin B (p.377·2); tetracycline hydrochloride (p.258·3).
Vulvovaginal infections.

Gine Zalain Robert, Spain.
Sertaconazole nitrate (p.393·3).
Vulvovaginal candidiasis.

Gineburno Dovalle, Braz.
Estrone (p.1476·1); aminophenazone (p.13·3); viburnum prunifolium.
Dysmenorrhoea.

Ginecofuran Crosara, Ital.†.
Nifuroxime (p.392·2); furazolidone (p.592·1).
Vaginitis.

Ginecoside Darrow, Braz.
Injection: Progesterone (p.1488·3); estradiol (p.1473·1).
Tablets: Normethandrone; methyloestradiol.
Menopausal disorders.

Ginecrin Abbott, Spain.
Leuprorelin acetate (p.1289·2).
Endometriosis; prostatic cancer; uterine fibroma.

Ginedak Akzo, Braz.
Miconazole nitrate (p.391·1).
Vulvovaginal candidiasis.

Ginedermofix Ferrer, Spain.
Sertaconazole nitrate (p.393·3).
Vulvovaginal candidiasis.

Ginedisc
Schering, Braz.; Schering, Mex.
Estradiol (p.1473·1).
Menopausal disorders; osteoporosis.

Gineflor Mitim, Ital.
Ibuprofen isobutanolammonium (p.44·1).
Gynaecological disorders.

Ginejuvent Juventus, Spain.
Benzalkonium chloride (p.1133·2); calcium lactate (p.1188·2); lactic acid (p.1626·2); chamomile (p.1593·2).
Vulvovaginal candidiasis; vulvovaginal trichomoniasis.

Ginenorm Aesculapius, Ital.
Ibuprofen isobutanolammonium (p.44·1).
Gynaecological inflammatory disorders.

Ginesal Farmigea, Ital.
Benzydamine hydrochloride (p.20·1).
Gynaecological disorders; vaginal hygiene.

Ginestatin Akzo, Braz.
Metronidazole (p.594·1); benzalkonium chloride (p.1133·2).
Vulvovaginal infections.

Ginetris Pharmacia Upjohn, Hong Kong.
Chloramphenicol (p.179·1); myralact; cloponone.
Vaginal disorders.

Ginexin-F SK, Singapore.
Ginkgo biloba (p.1615·2).
Organic brain disorders; peripheral vascular disorders; tinnitus; vertigo.

Gingicain D Hoechst Marion Roussel, Ger.
Amethocaine [tetracaine] (p.1305·2); benzalkonium chloride (p.1133·2).
Local anaesthesia; skin disinfection.

Gingiloba Biocur, Ger.
Ginkgo biloba (p.1615·2).
Dizziness; mental function disorders; peripheral vascular disorders; tinnitus.

Gingilone
Note. This name is used for preparations of different composition.
Allergan-Frumtost, Braz.
Hydrocortisone acetate (p.1073·3); neomycin sulfate (p.228·1); troxerutin (p.1611·2); ascorbic acid (p.1389·3).
Mouth disorders.

Teofarma, Spain.
Ascorbic acid (p.1389·3); cortisone acetate (p.1065·3); neomycin sulfate (p.228·1); rutoside (p.1611·2).
Bleeding gums; mouth ulcers; stomatitis.

Gingi-Pak Gingi-Pak, Switz.†.
A range of threads and tampons impregnated with adrenaline [epinephrine] hydrochloride (p.829·2).
Dental haemorrhage.

Gingisan Teva, Israel.
Mouthwash: Chamomile (p.1593·2); eucalyptus (p.1609·2); liquorice (p.1231·2).
Ointment: Chamomile (p.1593·2); eucalyptus (p.1609·2); liquorice (p.1231·2); benzocaine (p.1306·2).
Mouth disorders.

Gingium Hexal, Ger.
Ginkgo biloba (p.1615·2).
Dizziness; intermittent claudication; mental function disorders; tinnitus.

Gingivitol N Hennig, Ger.
Hydrastis (p.1621·1).
Inflammatory disorders of the mouth.

Gingo A Eagle, Austral.
Ginkgo biloba (p.1615·2); crataegus (p.1600·2); eleutherococcus senticosis (p.1615·3); liquorice (p.1231·2); choline bitartrate (p.1356·3); cayenne (p.1591·1); nicotinic acid (p.1372·3); potassium phosphate (p.1193·1).

Gingobeta Betapharm, Ger.
Ginkgo biloba (p.1615·2).
Dizziness; headache; mental function disorders; peripheral vascular disorders; tinnitus.

Gingopret Bionorica, Ger.
Ginkgo biloba (p.1615·2).
Headache; mental function disorders; peripheral vascular disorders; tinnitus; vertigo.

The symbol † denotes a preparation no longer actively marketed

Gingosol *Ecosol, Switz.*
Ginkgo biloba (p.1615·2).
Mental function impairment.

Gingviton *Sam Chun Dang, Singapore.*
Multivitamin and mineral preparation with ginseng and lecithin (p.1350·1).

Ginkapran *Yungjin, Singapore.*
Ginkgo biloba (p.1615·2).
Cerebral disorders; peripheral vascular disorders.

Ginkgo ACE *Vitaglow, Austral.†.*
Ginkgo biloba (p.1615·2); betacarotene (p.1355·1); ascorbic acid (p.1389·3); alpha tocoferil succinate (p.1394·2); zinc amino acid chelate (p.1398·3); cysteine hydrochloride (p.1358·3); bioflavonoids (p.1611·1); choline bitartrate (p.1356·3); inositol (p.1623·3); calcium phosphate (p.1188·3).
Free radical scavenger.

Ginkgo biloba comp *Hevert, Ger.*
Homoeopathic preparation.

Ginkgo Biloba Plus *Eagle, Austral.*
Ginkgo biloba (p.1615·2); crataegus (p.1600·2); eleutherococcus senticosis (p.1615·3); ginseng (p.1615·3).
Peripheral circulatory disorders; tinnitus.

Ginkgo Complex *Blackmores, Austral.*
Ginkgo biloba (p.1615·2); crataegus (p.1600·2); ginseng (p.1615·3); d-alpha tocoferil acid succinate (p.1394·1).
Cerebral and peripheral vascular disorders.

Ginkgo Plus *Biohorma, Ital.*
Hamamelis (p.1618·3); aesculus (p.1574·1); ginkgo biloba (p.1615·2); cupressus sempervirens.
Peripheral vascular disorders.

Ginkgo Plus Herbal Plus Formula 10 *Vitelle, Austral.*
Ginkgo biloba (p.1615·2); ginger (p.1227·2); potassium phosphate (p.1193·1); magnesium oxide (p.1233·2).
Peripheral vascular disorders.

Ginkgobakehl *Sanum-Kehlbeck, Ger.*
Homoeopathic preparation.

Ginkgoforce *Weber & Weber, Ger.†*
Homoeopathic preparation.

Ginkgorell *Sanorell, Ger.*
Homoeopathic preparation.

Ginkoba
Fher, Ital.; Pharmaton, Switz.
Ginkgo biloba (p.1615·2).
Mental function disorders.

Ginkobil *Ratiopharm, Ger.*
Ginkgo biloba (p.1615·2).
Headache; mental function disorders; peripheral vascular disorders; tinnitus; vertigo.

Ginkodilat *Azupharma, Ger.*
Ginkgo biloba (p.1615·2).
Headache; mental function disorders; peripheral vascular disorders; tinnitus; vertigo.

Ginkoftal *Tubilux, Ital.*
Bioflavonoids (p.1611·1); ginkgo biloba (p.1615·2).
Eye disorders; nutritional supplement.

Ginkogink *URPAC, Fr.*
Ginkgo biloba (p.1615·2).
Mental function impairment in the elderly; peripheral and cerebral vascular disorders; vertigo.

Ginkopur *Isis Puren, Ger.*
Ginkgo biloba (p.1615·2).
Dizziness; headache; mental function disorders; peripheral vascular disorders; tinnitus.

Ginkor *Beaufour, Fr.*
Ginkgo biloba (p.1615·2); troxerutin (p.1611·2).
Peripheral vascular disorders.

Ginkor Fort
Beaufour, Fr.; Beaufour-Ipsen, Hong Kong; Beaufour-Ipsen, Thai.
Ginkgo biloba (p.1615·2); heptaminol (p.1619·2) or heptaminol hydrochloride (p.1619·2); troxerutin (p.1611·2).
Haemorrhoids; venous insufficiency.

Ginkor Procto *Beaufour, Fr.†*
Ginkgo biloba (p.1615·2); butyl aminobenzoate (p.1308·2).
Haemorrhoids.

Ginkosen *Tai Guk, Singapore.*
Ginkgo biloba (p.1615·2).
Circulatory disorders.

Ginkovital *Pharmadass, UK.*
Ginkgo biloba (p.1615·2).

Gino Clotrimix *Medley, Braz.*
Clotrimazole (p.382·1).
Vulvovaginal candidiasis.

Gino Loprox *Hoechst Marion Roussel, Braz.*
Ciclopirox olamine (p.382·1).
Vulvovaginal candidiasis.

Gino Pletil *Searle, Braz.*
Tinidazole (p.603·3); miconazole nitrate (p.391·1).
Vulvovaginal infections.

Gino Tralen *Pfizer, Braz.*
Tioconazole (p.395·1).
Vulvovaginal candidiasis.

Gino-Canesten *Bayer, Port.*
Clotrimazole (p.382·1).

Ginocap *Biocontrolfarm, Ital.†.*
Bearberry (p.1583·3).

Gino-Cauterex *Ache, Braz.*
Fibrinolysin (human) (p.890·1); dornase alfa (p.1089·1); chloramphenicol (p.179·1).
Vulvovaginal infections.

Ginoday *Biocontrolfarm, Ital.†*
Birch (p.1585·2); alga clorella.

Ginoden *Schering, Ital.*
Gestodene (p.1479·1); ethinylestradiol (p.1476·2).
Combined oral contraceptive.

Gino-Fibrase *Ache, Braz.*
Fibrinolysin (human) (p.890·1); dornase alfa (p.1089·1); chloramphenicol (p.179·1).
Vulvovaginal infections.

Ginolax *Biocontrolfarm, Ital.†.*
Psyllium seed (p.1229·1); frangula (p.1227·1).

Gino-Lotremine *Schering-Plough, Port.*
Clotrimazole (p.382·1).

Ginomains *Gandhour, Fr.*
Emollient.
Dry skin disorders.

Ginometrim *Nikkho, Braz.*
Tinidazole (p.603·3); nystatin (p.392·2); gentamicin (p.212·1); benzalkonium chloride (p.1133·2).
Vulvovaginal infections.

Ginomineral *Biocontrolfarm, Ital.†.*
Mineral preparation (p.1350·1).
Nutritional supplement.

Ginomizol *Tocogino, Mex.*
Astemizole (p.409·1).

Ginopil *Biocontrolfarm, Ital.†.*
Pilosella.

Ginosutin *Akzo, Braz.*
Tinidazole (p.603·3).
Vulvovaginal infections.

Ginosutin M *Akzo, Braz.*
Tinidazole (p.603·3); miconazole (p.391·1).
Vulvovaginal infections.

Gino-Travogen *Schering, Port.*
Isoconazole nitrate (p.387·2).
Vulvovaginal infections.

Gino-Trosyd *Pfizer, Port.*
Tioconazole (p.395·1).
Fungal vaginal infections.

Ginoven *Biocontrolfarm, Ital.†.*
Aesculus (p.1574·1).

Ginoxil *RDC, Ital.*
Urea hydrogen peroxide (p.1159·3).
Vaginal disorders; vaginal hygiene.

Ginoxil Ecoschiuma *RDC, Ital.*
Hamamelis (p.1618·3); aloe vera (p.1110·1); allantoin (p.1110·1).
Personal hygiene.

Ginroy *Medisculab, Ger.†*
Ginseng (p.1615·3).
Tonic.

Ginsana
Boehringer Ingelheim, Aust.; Boehringer de Angeli, Braz.; Quest, Canad.; Boehringer Ingelheim, Fr.; Pharmaton, Ger.; Fher, Ital.; Boehringer Ingelheim, Port.; Boehringer Ingelheim, S.Afr.; Pharmaton, Singapore; Fher, Spain; GPL, Switz.; Pharmaton, Thai.
Ginseng (p.1615·3).
Tonic.

Ginsatonic *Arkopharma, Fr.†.*
Ginseng (p.1615·3).
Tonic.

Ginseng Med Complex *Dynamit, Aust.*
Homoeopathic preparation.

Ginseng-Complex "Schuh" *Coradol, Ger.*
Panax ginseng (p.1615·3); chlorophyllin (p.1028·1); crataegus (p.1600·2).
Tonic.

Ginsroy *Schumit, Thai.*
Ginseng (p.1615·3).
Tonic.

Ginurovac *Nikkho, Braz.*
Procaine penicillin [procaine benzylpenicillin] (p.239·2); benzylpenicillin potassium (p.157·1); aminocaproic acid (p.724·3); antigens from *Neisseria gonorrhoea, Escherichia coli, Staphylococcus aureus, Streptococcus pyogenes, Proteus vulgaris,* and *Pseudomonas aeruginosa.*
Bacterial infections.

Ginvapast
Note. This name is used for preparations of different composition.
Ogna, Ital.
Calcium gluconate (p.1188·2); procaine hydrochloride (p.1319·1); cetylpyridinium chloride (p.1138·1).
Gum disorders; skin ulcers.
Wild, Switz.
Calcium gluconate (p.1188·2); procaine hydrochloride (p.1319·1); vitamins A and D (p.1350·1).
Gum disorders.

Ginzing *Vitaglow, Austral.*
Ginseng (p.1615·3).
Tonic.

Ginzing E *Vitaglow, Austral.*
Ginseng (p.1615·3); d-alpha tocopherol (p.1393·3).
Tonic.

Ginzing G *Vitaglow, Austral.*
Ginseng (p.1615·3); ginkgo biloba (p.1615·2).
Tonic.

Girha "Schuh" *Coradol, Ger.*
Homoeopathic preparation.

Girheulit H *Pfluger, Ger.*
Homoeopathic preparation.

Giroflox *Tecnimede, Port.*
Ciprofloxacin (p.182·3).
Bacterial infections.

Gi-Sen *Giuliani, Ital.*
Ginseng (p.1615·3).

Gittalun *Boehringer Ingelheim, Ger.*
Doxylamine succinate (p.417·1).
Sleep disorders.

Gityl *Krewel, Ger.*
Bromazepam (p.656·3).
Anxiety; sleep disorders.

Givalex
Norgine, Belg.; Norgine, Fr.; Norgine, Ger.
Hexetidine (p.1146·3); choline salicylate (p.24·3); chlorobutanol (p.1141·2).
Mouth and throat disorders.

Givitol
Galen, Irl.; Galen, UK.
Ferrous fumarate (p.1360·1); folic acid (p.1361·1); vitamin B and C substances (p.1350·1).
Iron and folic acid deficiency in pregnancy.

GLA-130 *Shaklee, Canad.*
Borage oil (p.1613·1); safflower oil (p.1375·1).

Glaan *Neo-Farmaceutica, Port.†*
Emollient.
Skin disorders.

Gladem
Boehringer Ingelheim, Aust.; Boehringer Ingelheim, Ger.; Boehringer Ingelheim, Switz.
Sertraline hydrochloride (p.308·3).
Depression; obsessive-compulsive disorder.

Gladiaton *Sedar, Braz.*
Ferric ammonium citrate (p.1359·2); phosphoric acid; dibasic sodium phosphate; melissa; vitamin B substances; vitamin C (p.1350·1).
Iron deficiency; iron-deficiency anaemia.

Gladixol *Kolassa, Aust.*
β-Acetyldigoxin (p.827·3); potassium aspartate (p.1195·2); magnesium aspartate (p.1190·3).
Arrhythmias; heart failure.

Gladixol N *corax, Ger.*
β-Acetyldigoxin (p.827·3).
Heart failure.

Glakay *Eisai, Jpn.*
Menatetrenone (p.1396·3).
Osteoporosis.

Glamidolo
Angelini, Italgeni; Angelini, Ital.
Dapiprazole hydrochloride (p.1602·2).
Glaucoma; reversal of mydriasis.

Glamin
Pharmacia Upjohn, Ger.; Pharmacia Upjohn, Irl.; Fresenius Kabi, Ital.; Pharmacia Upjohn, Neth.; Fresenius Kabi, Port.; Fresenius Kabi, Spain; Fresenius Kabi, Switz.; Fresenius, UK.
Amino-acid infusion (p.1350·1).
Parenteral nutrition.

Glandicin *Degorts, Mex.*
Piroxicam (p.79·1).
Inflammation; pain.

Glandol *Boots Healthcare, Switz.*
Borage oil (p.1613·1).
Dietary supplement.

Glandosane
Stada, Aust.; Cell Pharm, Ger.; Fresenius, Israel; Fresenius Kabi, Port.; Helvepharm, Switz.; Fresenius, Thai.; Fresenius, UK; Kenwood, USA†.
Carmellose sodium (p.1499·3); sorbitol (p.1377·3); electrolytes (p.1180·1).
Dry mouth.

Glandulae-F-Gastreu R20 *Reckeweg, Ger.*
Homoeopathic preparation.

Glandulae-M-Gastreu R19 *Reckeweg, Ger.*
Homoeopathic preparation.

Glanil *Janssen, Swed.†*
Cinnarizine (p.413·1).
Motion sickness.

GLA-Plus Vitamin E *Shaklee, Canad.*
Essential fatty acids with vitamin E (p.1350·1).
Nutritional supplement.

Glaucadrine
Merck Sharp & Dohme-Chibret, Fr.; Merck Sharp & Dohme, Switz.†.
Aceclidine hydrochloride (p.1415·1); adrenaline [epinephrine] (p.829·1).
Glaucoma.

Glaucocare
Bournonville, Belg.†; Bournonville, Neth.†.
Aceclidine (p.1415·1) or aceclidine hydrochloride (p.1415·1).
Glaucoma; raised intra-ocular pressure.

Glaucocarpine *Taro, Israel.*
Pilocarpine hydrochloride (p.1422·3).
Glaucoma.

Glaucofrin
Bournonville, Belg.†; Bournonville, Neth.†.
Aceclidine (p.1415·1) or aceclidine hydrochloride (p.1415·1); adrenaline [epinephrine] (p.829·1).
Glaucoma; raised intra-ocular pressure.

Glaucol
Note. This name is used for preparations of different composition.
Croma, Aust.
Diclofenamide (p.869·1).
Glaucoma.
Norton, UK.
Timolol maleate (p.982·1).
Ocular hypertension.

Glaucon *USA.*
Adrenaline [epinephrine] hydrochloride (p.829·2).
Open-angle glaucoma.

Glauconex
Alcon, Aust.; Bournonville, Belg.†; Alcon, Ger.; Thilo, Neth.†.
Befunolol hydrochloride (p.843·2).
Glaucoma; ocular hypertension.

Glauconide *Llorens, Spain.*
Diclofenamide (p.869·1).
Glaucoma.

Glauco-Oph *Seng, Thai.*
Timolol maleate (p.982·1).
Glaucoma; ocular hypertension.

Glaucosan *Hexal, S.Afr.*
Timolol maleate (p.982·1).
Raised intra-ocular pressure.

Glaucostat
Merck Sharp & Dohme-Chibret, Fr.; Chibret, Port.; Merck Sharp & Dohme, Spain; Merck Sharp & Dohme, Switz.
Aceclidine hydrochloride (p.1415·1).
Glaucoma; ocular hypertension.

Glauco-Stulln *Stulln, Ger.*
Pindolol (p.955·3).
Glaucoma.

Glaucotat *Chibret, Ger.*
Aceclidine hydrochloride (p.1415·1).
Glaucoma.

Glaucothil
Alcon, Aust.; Alcon, Ger.
Dipivefrine hydrochloride (p.1604·3).
Glaucoma.

GlaucTabs *Akorn, USA.*
Methazolamide (p.927·1).
Glaucoma.

Glaudrops *Alcon Cusi, Spain.*
Dipivefrine hydrochloride (p.1604·3).
Glaucoma; ocular hypertension.

Glaufrin *Allergan, Swed.†.*
Adrenaline [epinephrine] hydrochloride (p.829·2).
Open-angle glaucoma.

Glauko Biciron *S & K, Ger.*
Pilocarpine hydrochloride (p.1422·3); phenylephrine hydrochloride (p.1097·1).
Glaucoma.

Glaumid *SIFI, Ital.*
Diclofenamide (p.869·1).
Glaucoma.

Glaunorm *Farmigea, Ital.*
Aceclidine hydrochloride (p.1415·1).
Glaucoma.

Glau-opt *Trinity, UK.*
Timolol maleate (p.982·1).
Glaucoma; ocular hypertension.

Glaupax
Orion, Denm.; Ciba Vision, Ger.; Orion, Irl.; Ciba Vision, Neth.; Orion, Norw.; Orion, Swed.†; Ciba Vision, Switz.; Ercopharm, Thai.
Acetazolamide (p.826·1).
Epilepsy; glaucoma; oedema.

Glautarakt *Pekana, Ger.*
Homoeopathic preparation.

Glautimol *Alcon, Braz.*
Timolol (p.982·2).
Glaucoma; ocular hypertension.

Glavamin
Fresenius Kabi, Aust.; Fresenius Kabi, Denm.; Fresenius Kabi, Fin.; Fresenius Kabi, Norw.; Fresenius Kabi, Swed.
Amino-acid infusion (p.1350·1).
Parenteral nutrition.

Glaxal Base *Roberts, Canad.*
Moisturiser.
Dermatological base.

Glazidim
Glaxo Wellcome, Belg.; Glaxo Wellcome, Fin.; Glaxo Wellcome, Ital.
Ceftazidime (p.174·3).
Bacterial infections.

Gleevec *Novartis, USA.*
Imatinib mesylate (p.547·1).
Chronic myeloid leukaemia.

Gleitgelen *Wolff, Ger.*
Liquid paraffin (p.1407·1); medium-chain triglycerides (p.1372·1).
Vaginal dryness.

Gleitmittel *Bichsel, Switz.*
Chlorhexidine gluconate (p.1138·2); macrogol (p.1630·3).
Lubrication before catheterisation or endoscopy.

Gliadel
Rhone-Poulenc Rorer, Canad.; Rhone-Poulenc Rorer, Fr.; Guilford, Israel; Aventis, NZ; Aventis, Port.; Rhone-Poulenc Rorer, Singapore; Rhone-Poulenc Rorer, USA.
Carmustine (p.516·1).
Glioblastoma multiforme.

Glianimon *Bayer, Ger.*
Benperidol (p.656·2).
Psychoses.

Gliatilin *Italfarmaco, Ital.*
Choline alfoscerate (p.1416·2).
Mental function impairment.

Glib *ABZ, Ger.*
Glibenclamide (p.321·3).
Diabetes mellitus.

gli-basan *Schonenberger, Switz.*
Glibenclamide (p.321·3).
Diabetes mellitus.

Glibemid *MPF, Singapore.*
Glibenclamide (p.321·3).
Diabetes mellitus.

Gliben
CT, Ger.; Lichtenstein, Ger.; Abiogen, Ital.; Pacific, NZ; Biolab, Thai.
Glibenclamide (p.321·3).
Diabetes mellitus.

Gliben F Abiogen, Ital.
Glibenclamide (p.321·3); phenformin hydrochloride (p.333·2).
Diabetes mellitus.

Gliben-Azu Azupharma, Ger.
Glibenclamide (p.321·3).
Diabetes mellitus.

Glibenbeta Betapharm, Ger.
Glibenclamide (p.321·3).
Diabetes mellitus.

Glibendoc Docpharm, Ger.
Glibenclamide (p.321·3).
Diabetes mellitus.

Glibenese
Pfizer, Aust.; Roerig, Belg.; Pfizer, Denm.; Pfizer, Fin.; Pfizer, Fr.; Pfizer, Ger.†; Pfizer, Irl.; Pfizer, Neth.; Pfizer Consumer, Spain; Pfizer, Swed.†; Mack, Switz.; Pfizer, UK.
Glipizide (p.322·3).
Diabetes mellitus.

Glibenhexal Hexal, Ger.
Glibenclamide (p.321·3).
Diabetes mellitus.

Glibenil Cryopharma, Mex.
Glibenclamide (p.321·3).
Diabetes mellitus.

Gliben-Puren N Isis Puren, Ger.
Glibenclamide (p.321·3).
Diabetes mellitus.

Glibesifar Siphar, Switz.
Glibenclamide (p.321·3).
Diabetes mellitus.

Glibesyn
Medochemie, Singapore; Medochemie, Thai.
Glibenclamide (p.321·3).
Diabetes mellitus.

Glibetic
Teva, Israel; The Forty-Two, Thai.
Glibenclamide (p.321·3).
Diabetes mellitus.

Glibic Progress, Thai.
Glibenclamide (p.321·3).
Diabetes mellitus.

Glibomet Guidotti, Ital.
Glibenclamide (p.321·3); metformin hydrochloride (p.332·3).
Diabetes mellitus.

Gliboral
Guidotti, Hong Kong; Guidotti, Ital.
Glibenclamide (p.321·3).
Diabetes mellitus.

Glib-ratiopharm Ratiopharm, Ger.
Glibenclamide (p.321·3).
Diabetes mellitus.

Glicacil Bioprogress, Ital.†
Sodium cromoglicate (p.774·3).
Asthma; chronic intestinal inflammatory disease; food hypersensitivity.

Glicamin Lafare, Ital.
A heparinoid (p.905·2).
Thrombosis prophylaxis.

Glicermina Bescansa, Spain†.
Stearic acid; glycerol.
Skin disorders.

Glicerolax Dynacren, Ital.
Glycerol (p.1616·2); mallow.
Constipation.

Glicerotens Llorens, Spain.
Glycerol (p.1616·3).
Glaucoma; ocular hypertension; ocular surgery.

Glicero-Valerovit Teofarma, Ital.
Sodium glycerophosphate (p.1617·3); valerian (p.1678·3).
Lignocaine [lidocaine] hydrochloride (p.1313·2) is included in the intramuscular injection to alleviate the pain of injection.
Hyperexcitability; tonic.

Glicinal Ogera, Switz.
Sodium cromoglicate (p.774·3).
Asthma.

Glico Test Callegari, Ital.†
Test for glucose in blood (p.1616·3).

Glico Urine B Callegari, Ital.†
Test for glucose in urine (p.1616·3).

Glicobase Formenti, Ital.
Acarbose (p.319·2).
Diabetes mellitus.

Glicoderm Mex-America, Mex.
Glycolic acid (p.1115·1).
Skin disorders.

Glicodin Novaquimica, Braz.
Potassium iodide (p.1522·3); ammonium chloride (p.1085·2); hyoscyamus (p.470·1).
Respiratory-tract congestion.

Glico-Fita Lilly, Braz.
Test for glucose in urine (p.1616·3).

Gliconorm Abiogen, Ital.
Glibenclamide (p.321·3); metformin hydrochloride (p.332·3).
Diabetes mellitus.

Glicosado Labormedica, Braz.
Glucose infusion (p.1364·1).
Parenteral nutrition.

Glicoxem Precimex, Mex.
Glibenclamide (p.321·3).
Diabetes mellitus.

Glicron Siam Medicare, Thai.
Gliclazide (p.322·2).
Diabetes mellitus.

Glidiab CCPC, Hong Kong.
Glipizide (p.322·3).
Diabetes mellitus.

Glifage Merck, Braz.
Metformin (p.332·3).
Diabetes mellitus.

Glifarcal Farcoral, Mex.
Glibenclamide (p.321·3).
Diabetes mellitus.

Gliformin Guidotti, Ital.
Glibenclamide (p.321·3); phenformin hydrochloride (p.333·2).
Diabetes mellitus.

Glimbal CSC, Aust.
Clocortolone pivalate (p.1065·3).
Skin disorders.

Glimel
Alphapharm, Austral.; Alphapharm, Hong Kong.
Glibenclamide (p.321·3).
Diabetes mellitus.

Glimicron Hovid, Singapore.
Gliclazide (p.322·2).
Diabetes mellitus.

Glimide Beacons, Singapore.
Glibenclamide (p.321·3).
Diabetes mellitus.

Glimidstada Stada, Ger.
Glibenclamide (p.321·3).
Diabetes mellitus.

Glimiton Bristol-Myers Squibb, Braz.
Mineral preparation with vitamin B substances (p.1350·1).

Glineon Dovalle, Braz.
Mineral preparation with vitamin B substances and sorbitol (p.1350·1).

Glinor Medinovum, Fin.
Sodium cromoglicate (p.774·3).
Allergic conjunctivitis; allergic rhinitis.

Glinorboral Silanes, Mex.
Glibenclamide (p.321·3); phenformin.
Diabetes mellitus.

Glios Pharmacia Upjohn, Ital.†.
Serine alfoscerate.
Cerebrovascular disorders; mental function impairment.

Glioten Armstrong, Mex.
Enalapril maleate (p.883·3).
Heart failure; hypertension.

Glipep Faulding, Port.
Vancomycin (p.269·1).

Glipid Pacific, NZ.
Glipizide (p.322·3).
Diabetes mellitus.

Glipiscand Scand Pharm, Swed.
Glipizide (p.322·3).
Diabetes mellitus.

Gliplex Farmasa, Braz.
Vitamin B substances with glucose (p.1350·1).

Glipressina Ferring, Ital.
Terlipressin acetate (p.1298·1).
Haemorrhage from oesophageal varices.

Gliptide Crinos, Ital.
Sulglicotide (p.1253·2).
Gastrointestinal disorders; peptic ulcer.

Glisuret Pisa, Mex.
Glycine (p.1365·3).

Glitisol
Zambon, Braz.; Zambon, Ital.
Thiamphenicol (p.261·3) or thiamphenicol glycinate hydrochloride (p.262·1).
Bacterial infections.

Glivec Novartis, UK.
Imatinib mesilate (p.547·1).
Chronic myeloid leukaemia.

Globenicol Yamanouchi, Neth.
Chloramphenicol (p.179·1).
Bacterial eye infections.

Globentyl Nycomed, Norw.
Aspirin (p.14·2).
Fever; pain; rheumatic disorders.

Globocef
Roche, Aust.†; Roche, Braz.; Roche, Ger.; Roche, Hong Kong; Roche, Ital.; Roche, Mex.; Roche, Port.; Roche, Switz.
Cefetamet pivoxil hydrochloride (p.166·2).
Bacterial infections.

Globoid Nycomed, Norw.
Aspirin (p.14·2).
Fever; pain; rheumatic disorders.

Globuce Sigma-Tau, Spain.
Ciprofloxacin hydrochloride (p.182·3).
Bacterial infections.

Globuli Jacoby, Aust.
Homoeopathic preparation.

Globulina Lloren Anti RH Llorente, Spain.
An anti-D immunoglobulin (p.1532·1).
Prevention of rhesus sensitivity.

Globuman
Note. This name is used for preparations of different composition.
Kwizda, Aust.†.
A hepatitis A immunoglobulin (p.1541·2).
Passive immunisation.

Berna, Belg.†; Berna, Hong Kong; Berna, Ital.; Berna, Port.; Byk Madaus, S.Afr.; Berna, Spain; Berna, Switz.; Berna, Thai.
A normal immunoglobulin (p.1551·3).
Idiopathic thrombocytopenic purpura; immune deficiency; passive immunisation.

Globuman Hepatite A
Berna, Belg.†; Berna, Port.†; Berna, Switz.†.
A hepatitis A immunoglobulin (p.1541·2).
Passive immunisation.

Globuman Hepatitis A
Berna, Hong Kong†; Byk Madaus, S.Afr.; Berna, Thai.†.
A hepatitis A immunoglobulin (p.1541·2).
Passive immunisation.

Globuman iv CMV Berna, Switz.
A cytomegalovirus immunoglobulin (p.1536·1).
Passive immunisation.

Globuren Dompe Biotec, Ital.
Epoetin alfa (p.731·1).
Anaemias; autologous blood transfusions.

Gloceda Medgenix, Belg.
Erysimin; aconite (p.1572·3); belladonna (p.463·1); euphorbia (p.1609·3); drosera (p.1606·1); cherry-laurel; codeine phosphate (p.25·2).
Coughs.

Glofil Cypros, USA.
Iodine-125 (p.1450·1) as sodium iothalamate.
Evaluation of glomerular filtration rate.

Glogama Antihepatitis B Evans, Spain†.
A hepatitis B immunoglobulin (p.1542·1).
Passive immunisation.

Glonoin Coradol, Ger.
Herbal and homoeopathic preparation.

Glononinum Hevert, Ger.†.
Homoeopathic preparation.

Gloquat C Rhone Poulenc Chemicals, UK.
Alkylaryltrimethylammonium chloride.
Disinfection.

Glossderm Columbia, Mex.
Cod-liver oil (p.1357·2); benzalkonium chloride (p.1133·2); zinc oxide (p.1128·2); allantoin (p.1110·1).
Napkin rash.

Glossithiase Jolly-Jatel, Fr.
Thenoate monoethanolamine (p.261·3); muramidase hydrochloride (p.1638·1).
Infections of the mouth and throat.

Glossware & Brush Clinique, Canad.
SPF 8: Octinoxate (p.1517·3).
Sunscreen.

Glotil Brasifa, Braz.
Sodium dibunate (p.1100·3); phenethylamine citrate; homatropine methylbromide (p.468·1).
Coughs.

Glotone Vita, Spain.
Cyproheptadine hydrochloride (p.414·2); embryo extract; gastric mucosa extract; muscle extract.
Tonic.

Glottyl
Note. This name is used for preparations of different composition.
Asta Medica, Belg.
Codeine phosphate (p.25·2).
Formerly contained aconite, codeine phosphate, cherry-laurel, belladonna, drosera, erysimin, and euphorbia.
Coughs.

Marion Merrell, Fr.
Amylocaine hydrochloride (p.1306·1); erysimum; grindelia (p.1618·2).
Sore throat.

Glovan Teva, Israel.
Nonoxinol 9 (p.1346·1); ricinoleic acid (p.1658·1).
Contraceptive.

Gluben Dexcel, Israel.
Glibenclamide (p.321·3).
Diabetes mellitus.

Gluborid
Sanochemia, Aust.; Grunenthal, Ger.; Grunenthal, Switz.
Glibornuride (p.322·2).
Diabetes mellitus.

GlucaGen
Novo Nordisk, Aust.; Novo Nordisk, Austral.; Novo Nordisk, Belg.; Novo Nordisk, Denm.; Novo Nordisk, Fin.; Novo Nordisk, Fr.; Novo Nordisk, Ger.; Novo Nordisk, Hong Kong; Novo Nordisk, Irl.; Novo Nordisk, Israel; Novo Nordisk, Ital.; Novo Nordisk, NZ; Novo Nordisk, Port.; Novo Nordisk, S.Afr.; Novo Nordisk, Switz.; Novo Nordisk, Thai.; Novo Nordisk, UK.
Glucagon hydrochloride (p.1010·2).
Aid in gastrointestinal examination; beta-blocker poisoning; hypoglycaemia.

Glucagon
Lilly, Mex.; Lilly, UK.
Glucagon (p.1010·1) or glucagon hydrochloride (p.1010·2).
Aid in gastrointestinal radiography; hypoglycaemia.

Glucal Galen, Mex.
Glibenclamide (p.321·3).
Diabetes mellitus.

Glucal B12 Dansk-Flama, Braz.
Calcium, fluoride, phosphoric acid, and lysine (p.1350·1).
Nutritional supplement.

Glucalcium Renaudin, Fr.
Calcium gluconate (p.1188·2); calcium glucepate (p.1188·1).
Hypocalcaemia.

Glucamet Opus, UK.
Metformin hydrochloride (p.332·3).
Diabetes mellitus.

Glucantim Rhone-Poulenc Rorer, Ital.
Meglumine antimonate (p.587·2).
Leishmaniasis.

Glucantime
Rhodia, Braz.; Rhone-Poulenc Rorer, Fr.; Rhone-Poulenc Rorer, Spain.
Meglumine antimonate (p.587·2).
Leishmaniasis.

Glucerna
Abbott, Austral.; Abbott, Canad.; Abbott, Fin.; Abbott, Hong Kong; Abbott, Irl.; Ross, Israel; Abbott, Ital.; Abbott, NZ; Abbott, Singapore; Abbott, Thai.; Ross, USA.
Preparation for enteral nutrition (p.1350·1).
Glucose intolerance.

Glucidoral Servier, Fr.
Carbutamide (p.321·1).
Diabetes mellitus.

Glucinan Lipha Sante, Fr.
Metformin chlorophenoxyacetate (p.332·3).
Diabetes mellitus.

Glucobay
Bayer, Aust.; Bayer, Austral.; Bayer, Belg.; Bayer, Braz.; Bayer, Denm.; Bayer, Fin.; Bayer, Ger.; Bayer, Hong Kong; Bayer, Irl.; Bayer, Ital.; Bayer, Mex.; Bayer, Neth.; Bayer, Norw.; Bayer, NZ; Bayer, Port.; Bayer, S.Afr.; Bayer, Singapore; Bayer, Spain; Bayer, Swed.; Bayer, Switz.; Bayer, Thai.; Bayer, UK.
Acarbose (p.319·2).
Diabetes mellitus.

Glucobene Ratiopharm, Aust.
Glibenclamide (p.321·3).
Diabetes mellitus.

Glucobon Biomo, Ger.
Metformin hydrochloride (p.332·3).
Diabetes mellitus.

Gluco-Calcium
Note. This name is used for preparations of different composition.
Lilly, Hong Kong.
Calcium (p.1187·3).
Alkalosis; hypocalcaemia; parathyroid deficiency; vitamin D deficiency.

Lilly, Thai.
Calcium (p.1187·3); glucose (p.1364·1).
Hypocalcaemia.

Glucocalcium Streuli, Switz.
Calcium gluconate (p.1188·2); calcium sucrate.
Hypocalcaemia; poisoning.

Glucocard NZ Medical & Scientific, NZ.
Test for glucose in blood (p.1616·3).

Glucochaux Darci, Belg.†.
Calcium gluconate (p.1188·2); calcium hydrogen phosphate (p.1188·2).
Calcium deficiency; calcium supplement.

Glucodex Rougier, Canad.
Glucose (p.1364·2).
Oral glucose tolerance test.

Glucodin Boots Healthcare, Irl.†.
Glucose (p.1364·2); vitamin C (p.1389·3).

Glucoferro Guidotti, Ital.
Ferrous gluconate (p.1360·1).
Iron deficiency; iron-deficiency anaemias.

Glucofilm
Bayer, Austral.; Miles, Canad.†; Bayer Diagnostics, Fr.†; Bayer Diagnostici, Ital.; Bayer, NZ; Bayer, USA.
Test for glucose in blood (p.1616·3).

Glucoformin Biobras, Braz.
Metformin hydrochloride (p.332·3).
Diabetes mellitus.

Glucohexal Hexal, Austral.
Metformin hydrochloride (p.332·3).
Diabetes mellitus.

Glucolon Sabater, Spain.
Glibenclamide (p.321·3).
Diabetes mellitus.

Glucolyte Thai Otsuka, Thai.
Electrolyte infusion with glucose (p.1180·1).
Carbohydrate source; fluid and electrolyte disorders.

Glucoman Volchem, Ital.
Dietary fibre supplement containing glucomannan (p.1616·2), galactomannan, and minerals (p.1350·1).
Disorders of carbohydrate and lipid metabolism; gastrointestinal disorders; obesity.

Glucomen Menarini, Irl.
Test for glucose in blood (p.1616·3).

Glucomet
Douglas, Austral.; Douglas, NZ; Hua, Thai.
Metformin hydrochloride (p.332·3).
Diabetes mellitus.

Glucometer
Bayer, Austral.; Bayer Diagnostici, Ital.; Bayer, NZ.
Test for glucose in blood (p.1616·3).
For use with Glucometer Elite blood glucose meter.

Glucometer Esprit Bayer, NZ.
Test for glucose in blood (p.1616·3).
For use with Glucometer Esprit blood glucose meter.

The symbol † denotes a preparation no longer actively marketed

Glucomide Lipha, Ital.
Metformin hydrochloride (p.332·3); glibenclamide (p.321·3).
Diabetes mellitus.

Glucomin Dexcel, Israel.
Metformin hydrochloride (p.332·3).
Diabetes mellitus.

Glucomore Hayes, Israel.
Glucose polymers (p.1350·1).
High-calorie supplement.

Gluconil Utopian, Thai.
Glibenclamide (p.321·3).
Diabetes mellitus.

Gluconorm
Note. This name is used for preparations of different composition.
Novo Nordisk, Canad.
Repaglinide (p.334·1).
Diabetes mellitus.

Wolff, Ger.
Glibenclamide (p.321·3).
Diabetes mellitus.

Glucophage
Merck, Aust.; 3M, Austral.; Merck-Belgolabo, Belg.; Hoechst Marion Roussel, Canad.; Lipha, Denm.; Merck, Fin.; Lipha Sante, Fr.; Lipha, Hong Kong; Lipha, Irl.; Abic, Israel; Lipha, Ital.; Lakeside, Mex.; Merck, Neth.; Lipha, Norw.; Pacific, NZ; Merck, Port.; Mer-National, S.Afr.; Merck, Singapore; Merck-Lipha, Singapore; Boehringer Mannheim, Spain†; Merck, Swed.; Lipha, Switz.; Merck, Thai.; Merck, UK; Bristol-Myers Squibb, USA.
Metformin hydrochloride (p.332·3).
Diabetes mellitus.

Glucophage S Merck, Ger.
Metformin hydrochloride (p.332·3).
Diabetes mellitus.

Glucoplasmal
Braun, Aust.; Braun, Ger.; Braun, Spain.
Amino-acid, glucose, and electrolyte infusion (p.1350·1).
Parenteral nutrition.

Glucoplex Geistlich, UK†.
Carbohydrate, electrolyte, and trace element infusion (p.1350·1).
Parenteral nutrition.

Glucoplurisalina Fresenius Kabi, Spain.
Electrolyte infusion with glucose (p.1180·1).
Fluid and electrolyte depletion.

Glucopolielectrol Baxter, Spain.
Electrolyte infusion with glucose (p.1350·1).
Fluid and electrolyte depletion.

Glucopotasica Braun, Spain†; Mein, Spain†.
Potassium chloride infusion (p.1194·3) with glucose (p.1364·2).
Fluid and electrolyte depletion.

Glucopotasico Bieffe, Spain; Ern, Spain.
Potassium chloride infusion (p.1194·3) with glucose (p.1364·2).
Fluid and electrolyte depletion.

Glucor Bayer, Fr.
Acarbose (p.319·2).
Diabetes mellitus.

Glucoremed Lichtenstein, Ger.
Glibenclamide (p.321·3).
Diabetes mellitus.

Gluco-Rite Agis, Israel.
Glipizide (p.322·3).
Diabetes mellitus.

Glucosada Grifols, Port.
Glucose (p.1364·2).
Carbohydrate souce; fluid depletion.

Glucosado Braun, Port.
Glucose (p.1364·2).
Carbohydrate source; fluid depletion.

Glucosalin Baxter, Switz.; Bioren, Switz.
Anhydrous glucose (p.1364·1); sodium chloride (p.1196·1).
Carbohydrate source; fluid and electrolyte disorders.

Glucosalina Braun, Spain; Grifols, Spain; Instituto Farmacologico, Spain; Fresenius Kabi, Spain.
Sodium chloride infusion (p.1196·1) with glucose (p.1364·2).
Fluid and electrolyte depletion.

Glucosalina Modific Mein, Spain†.
Sodium chloride (p.1196·1) and sodium lactate (p.1186·2) infusion with glucose (p.1364·2).
Fluid and electrolyte depletion.

Glucosalino Bieffe, Spain; Ern, Spain; Braun, Spain; Baxter, Spain.
Sodium chloride (p.1196·1) infusion with glucose (p.1364·2).
Fluid and electrolyte depletion.

Glucosan
Note. This name is used for preparations of different composition.
Laevosan, Aust.†.
Anhydrous glucose (p.1364·1).
Carbohydrate source; fluid depletion.

Ortho, Ital.
Test for glucose in blood (p.1616·3).

Glucoseral Streuli, Switz.
Electrolyte infusion with glucose (p.1180·1).
Fluid and electrolyte disorders; parenteral nutrition.

Glucosmon Byk Elmu, Spain.
Glucose (p.1364·2).
Carbohydrate source; hypoglycaemia.

Glucosteril
Orion, Fin.; Fresenius Kabi, Ger.; Fresenius Kabi, Port.
Glucose (p.1364·2) with or without sodium chloride.
Carbohydrate source; fluid depletion.

Glucostix
Bayer, Austral.; Bayer, Canad.†; Bayer Diagnostics, Fr.†; Bayer Diagnostics, Irl.; Bayer Diagnostici, Ital.; Bayer Diagnostics, Mex.; Bayer, NZ; Bayer, Port.; Bayer Diagnostics, UK; Bayer, USA.
Test for glucose in blood (p.1616·3).

Glucostrip Biodiagnostics, Austral.
Test for glucose in blood (p.1616·3).

Glucosulfa Lipha, Ital.
Metformin (p.332·3); tolbutamide (p.336·3).
Diabetes mellitus.

Gluco-Tablinen Sanorania, Ger.†
Glibenclamide (p.321·3).
Diabetes mellitus.

Glucotard Boehringer Mannheim, Ger.†
Guar gum (p.323·3).
Diabetes mellitus.

Glucotide
Bayer Diagnostics, Fr.; Bayer Diagnostics, Irl.; Bayer Diagnostics, Mex.; Bayer Diagnostics, UK.
Test for glucose in blood (p.1616·3).

Glucotouch Lifescan, Port.
Test for glucose in blood (p.1616·3).

Glucotrend
Roche Diagnostics, Austral.; Roche Diagnostics, Irl.
Test for glucose in blood (p.1616·3).

Glucotrol
Pfizer, Hong Kong; Pfizer, USA.
Glipizide (p.322·3).
Diabetes mellitus.

Glucovance Bristol-Myers Squibb, USA.
Glibenclamide (p.321·3); metformin hydrochloride (p.332·3).
Diabetes mellitus.

Glucoven Chinoin, Mex.
Note. A similar name is used for preparations of different composition (see below).
Glibenclamide (p.321·3).
Diabetes mellitus.

Glucoven infant Fresenius Kabi, Ger.
Note. A similar name is used for preparations of different composition (see above).
Carbohydrate and electrolyte infusion (p.1350·1).
Formerly known as Glucovenos pad.
Parenteral nutrition.

Glucozide
Unison, Singapore; Unison, Thai.
Gliclazide (p.322·2).
Diabetes mellitus.

Glufer-C Nakornpatana, Thai.
Ferrous gluconate (p.1360·1); manganese sulfate; copper sulfate (p.1350·1).
Ascorbic acid (p.1389·3) is included in this preparation to increase the absorption and availability of iron.
Iron-deficiency anaemia.

Glufor CTI, Israel.
Metformin hydrochloride (p.332·3).
Diabetes mellitus.

Gluformin Condrugs, Thai.
Metformin hydrochloride (p.332·3).
Diabetes mellitus.

Glukacel Braun, Norw.
Electrolyte infusion with glucose (p.1180·1).
Carbohydrate source; fluid and electrolyte disorders.

Gluketurtest Roche Diagnostics, Ital.
Test for glucose and ketone bodies in urine.

Gluko Savio, Ital.†.
Glutathione sodium (p.1010·3).
Alcohol and drug poisoning; radiation trauma.

Glukolyt Kohler, Ger.
Carbohydrate and electrolyte infusion (p.1350·1).
Carbohydrate source; fluid depletion.

Glukoreduct Sanofi Synthelabo, Ger.
Glibenclamide (p.321·3).
Diabetes mellitus.

Glukos-El Braun, Swed.
Carbohydrate and electrolyte infusion (p.1350·1).
Parenteral nutrition.

Glukovital Wolff, Ger.
Glibenclamide (p.321·3).
Diabetes mellitus.

Glukurtest Roche Diagnostics, Ital.
Test for glucose in urine (p.1616·3).

Glumal
Kyowa, Jpn; Knoll, Spain†.
Aceglutamide aluminium (p.1209·2).
Peptic ulcer.

Glumida Pensa, Spain.
Acarbose (p.319·2).
Diabetes mellitus.

Gluparin Locatelli, Ital.†.
A heparinoid (p.905·2).
Hyperlipidaemias; peripheral vascular disorders; thrombosis prophylaxis.

Glu-Phos SPA, Ital.
Disodium glucose-1-phosphate.
Glucose deficiency.

Glupital Lilly, Mex.
Glipizide (p.322·3).
Diabetes mellitus.

Glurenor
Guidotti, Ital.; Boehringer Ingelheim, Port.; Yamanouchi, Spain; Menarini, Thai.
Gliquidone (p.323·1).
Diabetes mellitus.

Glurenorm
Boehringer Ingelheim, Aust.; Menarini, Belg.; Yamanouchi, Ger.; Sanofi Winthrop, UK.
Gliquidone (p.323·1).
Diabetes mellitus.

Glustress Pond's, Thai.
Metformin hydrochloride (p.332·3).
Diabetes mellitus.

Gluta Complex UCB, Ital.
Cobamamide (p.1388·3); amino acids (p.1350·1).
Tonic.

Glutabeina A Allergan-Frumtost, Braz.
Glutamic acid; vitamin A acetate; thiamine; pyridoxine (p.1350·1).
Nutritional supplement.

Glutabeina E Allergan-Frumtost, Braz.
Glutamic acid; tocoferil acetate; thiamine; pyridoxine (p.1350·1).
Nutritional supplement.

Glutacerebro AFOM, Ital.
Levoglutamide (p.1365·2).
Mental function impairment.

Glutacid Nycomed, Norw.
Glutamic acid (p.1365·2).
Achlorhydria; hypochlorhydria.

Glutaferro Medix, Spain.
Ferrous glutamate or ferrous glycine sulfate (p.1360·2).
Ascorbic acid (p.1389·3) is included in the capsules to increase absorption and availability of iron and docusate sodium (p.1223·1) is included to reduce the constipating effects of iron.
Anaemias.

Glutafin
Nutricia, Irl.; Nutricia, Ital.; Nutricia, NZ; Nutricia Dietary, UK.
A range of gluten-free foods (p.1350·1).
Gluten sensitivity.

Glutamag Vitamine Euform, Fr.
Magnesium glutamate; riboflavin sodium phosphate (p.1386·1); nicotinamide (p.1372·3).
Tonic.

Glutamed Boehringer Mannheim, Ital.†
Glutathione sodium (p.1010·3).
Alcohol and drug poisoning; protection against toxicity induced by cytotoxic chemotherapy; radiation trauma.

Glutamin Verla, Ger.
Glutamic acid (p.1365·2).
Tonic.

Glutamin Fosforo SIT, Ital.
Levoglutamide (p.1365·2); DL-phosphoserine; cyanocobalamin (p.1388·1).
Mental function impairment.

Glutanil Bioprogress, Ital.
Reduced glutathione sodium (p.1010·3).
Alcohol and drug poisoning; radiation trauma.

Glutarall Colgate Oral Care, Austral.†.
Glutaral (p.1145·2).
Disinfection.

Glutarex Ross, USA.
A range of lysine- and tryptophan-free preparations for enteral nutrition including an infant feed (p.1350·1).
Glutaric aciduria type I.

Glutargin Terapeutico, Ital.
Arginine glutamate (p.1353·3); arginine aspartate (p.1354·1).
Liver disorders.

Glutarin Pharmaland, Thai.
Glutaral (p.1145·2).
Instrument disinfection.

Glutarol
Dermal Laboratories, Irl.; Vifor, Switz.†; Dermal Laboratories, UK.
Glutaral (p.1145·2).
Warts.

Glutarsin E Berlin-Chemie, Ger.
Glutamic acid (p.1365·2); arginine hydrochloride (p.1353·3); potassium hydroxide (p.1654·1); sodium hydroxide (p.1665·3).
Hyperammonaemia.

Glutasan San Carlo, Ital.
Glutathione sodium (p.1010·3).
Alcohol and drug poisoning; radiation trauma.

Glutaven Teofarma, Ital.
Levoglutamide (p.1365·2).
Mental function impairment.

Gluthion CT, Ital.
Reduced glutathione sodium (p.1010·3).
Alcohol and drug poisoning; radiation trauma.

Gluti-Agil mono Serturner, Ger.
Glutamic acid (p.1365·2).
Mental function disorders.

Glutisal Ravensberg, Ger.
Salicylamide (p.82·1); ethenzamide (p.35·1).
Fever; gout; neuralgia; pain.

Glutofac
Kenwood, Hong Kong.
Multivitamin and mineral preparation (p.1350·1).

Kenwood, USA.
A range of vitamin preparations (p.1350·1).

Glutose Paddock, USA.
Glucose (p.1364·2).
Hypoglycaemia.

Glutoxil Rottapharm, Ital.
Glutathione sodium (p.1010·3).
Alcohol and drug poisoning; radiation trauma.

Glutril
ICN, Aust.; CSP, Fr.; ICN, Ger.; ICN, Switz.
Glibornuride (p.322·2).
Diabetes mellitus.

Gluzo Pharmasant, Thai.
Glibenclamide (p.321·3).
Diabetes mellitus.

Gluzolyte Pharmasant, Thai.
Metformin hydrochloride (p.332·3).
Diabetes mellitus.

Gly Derm Super Sunblock ICN, Canad.
Meradimate (p.1517·3); octinoxate (p.1517·3); octisalate (p.1518·1); titanium dioxide (p.1126·1).
Sunscreen.

Glyade Alphapharm, Austral.
Gliclazide (p.322·2).
Diabetes mellitus.

Glyate Geneva, USA.
Guaifenesin (p.1092·2).
Coughs.

Glyben Rolab, S.Afr.
Glibenclamide (p.321·3).
Diabetes mellitus.

Glycemin Siam Bheasach, Thai.
Chlorpropamide (p.321·1).
Diabetes mellitus.

Glycemirex Irex, Fr.
Gliclazide (p.322·2).
Diabetes mellitus.

Glyceol
Chugai, Hong Kong; Chugai, Jpn; Chugai, Thai.
Glycerol (p.1616·3) with fructose and sodium chloride.
Cerebral oedema; raised intracranial pressure.

Glycerosteril
Fresenius Kabi, Ger.; Fresenius, Thai.
Glycerol (p.1616·3) with glucose and sodium chloride.
Cerebral oedema.

Glycerotone Ciba Vision, Fr.
Glycerol (p.1616·3).
Ocular hypertension; raised intracranial pressure.

Glyceryl-T Rugby, USA.
Theophylline (p.777·2); guaifenesin (p.1092·2).
Bronchospasm.

Glycifer Nycomed, Denm.
Ferrous glycine sulfate (p.1360·2).
Iron deficiency.

Glycilax Engelhard, Ger.
Glycerol (p.1616·3).
Constipation.

Glycirenan Disperga, Aust.
Adrenaline [epinephrine] hydrochloride (p.829·2).
Bronchospasm.

Glycobal Nadeau, Canad.
Multivitamin and mineral preparation (p.1350·1).

Glycocortison Ciba Vision, Ger.
Hydrocortisone acetate (p.1073·3).
Eye disorders.

Glycocortisone H Ciba Vision, Switz.
Hydrocortisone acetate (p.1073·3) in glucose.
Corneal disorders.

Glycofed Pal-Pak, USA.
Pseudoephedrine hydrochloride (p.1099·2); guaifenesin (p.1092·2).
Coughs.

glycolande N Sanofi Synthelabo, Ger.
Glibenclamide (p.321·3).
Diabetes mellitus.

Glycomin Aspen, S.Afr.
Glibenclamide (p.321·3).
Diabetes mellitus.

Glycon
Note. This name is used for preparations of different composition.
Farmalab, Braz.
Potassium iodide (p.1522·3); ammonium benzoate; tolu balsam (p.1101·3).
Respiratory-tract congestion.

ICN, Canad.
Metformin hydrochloride (p.332·3).
Diabetes mellitus.

Siam Bheasach, Thai.
Gliclazide (p.322·2).
Diabetes mellitus.

Glyconon DDSA Pharmaceuticals, UK.
Tolbutamide (p.336·3).
Diabetes mellitus.

Glycophos
Fresenius Kabi, Aust.; Fresenius Kabi, Fin.; Pharmacia, Neth.†; Fresenius Kabi, Port.; Fresenius Kabi, Swed.; Fresenius Kabi, Switz.
Sodium glycerophosphate (p.1617·3).
Phosphate supplement for parenteral nutrition.

Glycoplex Vitaplex, Austral.
Vitamins, minerals, and amino acids (p.1350·1); liquorice (p.1231·2); taraxacum (p.1669·1).
Dietary supplement.

Glycoprep
Pharmatel, Austral.; Pharmatel, NZ.
Macrogol 3350 (p.1630·3); electrolytes (p.1180·1).
Bowel evacuation; constipation.

Glycoprep-C *Pharmatel, Austral.*
Macrogol 3350 (p.1630·3); electrolytes (p.1180·1); ascorbic acid (p.1389·3).
Bowel evacuation; constipation.

Gly-Coramin *Novartis Consumer, Switz.*
Nikethamide (p.1513·1); glucose and other reduced sugars (p.1364·1).
Tonic.

Glycoran *Shinyaku, Singapore.*
Metformin hydrochloride (p.332·3).
Diabetes mellitus.

Glycostigmin *Leiras, Fin.*
Neostigmine metilsulfate (p.1420·1).
Glycopyrronium bromide (p.467·2) is included in this preparation to protect against muscarinic actions.
Reversal of competitive neuromuscular blockade.

Glyco-Thymoline *Labomed, Fr.*
Sodium benzoate (p.1134·3); sodium bicarbonate (p.1186·2); borax (p.1586·1); sodium salicylate (p.84·2); thymol (p.1158·3); eucalyptol (p.1609·2); oleum pini sylvestris; menthol (p.1632·3); glycerol (p.1616·3).
Mouth disorders.

Glycotuss *Pal-Pak, USA.*
Guaifenesin (p.1092·2).
Coughs.

Glycotuss-dM *Pal-Pak, USA.*
Dextromethorphan hydrobromide (p.1087·3); guaifenesin (p.1092·2).
Coughs.

Glycovit *Alifarma, Ital.*
Amino-acid, multivitamin, and mineral preparation (p.1350·1).
Nutritional supplement.

Glycron *Aspen, S.Afr.*
Gliclazide (p.322·2).
Diabetes mellitus.

Glycylpressin *Ferring, Aust.; Ferring, Ger.*
Terlipressin acetate (p.1298·1).
Haemorrhagic gastritis; variceal haemorrhage.

Glycyron *Minophagen, Jpn†.*
Ammonium glycyrrhizinate (p.1085·2).
Liver disorders; skin disorders; stomatitis.

Glycyrrhiza Complex *Blackmores, Austral.*
Liquorice (p.1231·2); avena (p.1583·1); rose fruit (p.1389·3); vitamins (p.1350·1); ginseng (p.1615·3).
Tonic.

Glyderm
ICN, Hong Kong; ICN, Singapore.
Esterified glycolic acid (p.1115·1).
Dry skin disorders.

Glygen *General Drugs, Thai.*
Glipizide (p.322·3).
Diabetes mellitus.

Glymax *LPN, Fr.*
Metformin hydrochloride (p.332·3).
Diabetes mellitus.

Glymese *DDSA Pharmaceuticals, UK.*
Chlorpropamide (p.321·1).
Diabetes mellitus.

Glynase
Julphar, UAE; Pharmacia Upjohn, USA.
Glibenclamide (p.321·3).
Diabetes mellitus.

Glyoktyl *Medic, Denm.*
Docusate sodium (p.1223·1); glycerol (p.1616·3).
Bowel evacuation; constipation.

Gly-Oxide *SmithKline Beecham Consumer, USA.*
Urea hydrogen peroxide (p.1159·3).
Oral hygiene; oral inflammation.

Glyphyllin *Rekah, Israel.*
Theophylline sodium glycinate (p.783·2).
Obstructive airways disease.

Glypolix *Stroder, Ital.†.*
Dexfenfluramine hydrochloride (p.1508·3).
Obesity.

Glypressin
Ferring, Belg.; Ferring, Denm.; Ferring, Fin.; Ferring, Hong Kong; Ferring, Irl.; Ferring, Neth.; Ferring, Singapore; Ferring, Spain; Ferring, Thai.; Ferring, UK.
Terlipressin (p.1298·1) or terlipressin acetate (p.1298·1).
Variceal haemorrhage.

Glypressine
Ferring, Fr.; Ferring, Switz.
Terlipressin acetate (p.1298·1).
Variceal haemorrhage.

Gly-Rectal *Valmo, Canad.*
Glycerol (p.1616·3).

Glyrol *Iolab, USA†.*
Glycerol (p.1616·3).
Glaucoma; raised intra-ocular pressure before ophthalmic surgery.

Glysan *LAW, Ger.; Wyeth, Ger.*
Magaldrate (p.1232·2).
Gastric hyperacidity; heartburn; peptic ulcer.

Glysennid *Novartis Consumer, Canad.*
Sennosides (p.1248·3).
Constipation.

Glyset *Bayer, USA.*
Miglitol (p.333·1).
Diabetes mellitus.

Glytrin
Bioglan, Denm.; Bioglan, Hong Kong; Sanofi Winthrop, Irl.; Tramedi-

co, Neth.; Bioglan, Singapore; Bioglan, Swed.; Bioglan, Thai.; Sanofi Synthelabo, UK.
Glyceryl trinitrate (p.897·3).
Angina pectoris.

Glytuss *Mayrand, USA.*
Guaifenesin (p.1092·2).
Coughs.

Glyvenol
Novartis, Aust.; Novartis, Belg.; Novartis, Braz.; Novartis, Hong Kong; Novartis, Mex.; Novartis, Switz.; Novartis, Thai.
Tribenoside (p.1674·2).
Haemorrhoids; venous insufficiency.

Glyzide *Julphar, UAE.*
Gliclazide (p.322·2).
Diabetes mellitus.

G-Myticin *Pedinol, USA.*
Gentamicin sulfate (p.210·1).
Bacterial infections.

GNC *General Nutrition, Canad.*
Range of vitamin and mineral preparations (p.1350·1).

Go Kit *Pharmatel, Austral.*
3 Tablets, bisacodyl (p.1212·2); 1 sachet, magnesium citrate (p.1232·3).
Bowel evacuation.

Go Kit Plus *Pharmatel, Austral.*
3 Tablets, bisacodyl (p.1212·2); 1 suppository, bisacodyl (p.1212·2); 1 sachet, magnesium citrate (p.1232·3).
Bowel evacuation.

Goanna Analgesic Ice *Herron, Austral.*
Glycol salicylate (p.42·2); menthol (p.1632·3).
Musculoskeletal and joint pain.

Goanna Arthritis Cream *Herron, Austral.*
Trolamine salicylate (p.90·1).
Musculoskeletal and joint pain.

Goanna Bite-Eze *Herron, Austral.*
Eucalyptus (p.1609·2); citronella; peppermint flower (p.1243·2).
Bites; cold and influenza symptoms; skin disorders.

Goanna Heat Cream *Herron, Austral.*
Methyl salicylate (p.55·1); menthol (p.1632·3); camphor (p.1589·3); eucalyptus oil (p.1609·2); pumilio pine oil (p.1656·3); turpentine oil (p.1676·3); peppermint oil (p.1243·3); cajuput oil (p.1588·1); capsicum oleoresin (p.1591·1).
Musculoskeletal, joint, and soft-tissue pain.

Goanna Liniment *Herron, Austral.*
Methyl salicylate (p.55·1); turpentine oil (p.1676·3); eucalyptus oil (p.1609·2); camphor (p.1589·3); peppermint oil (p.1243·3); pumilio pine oil (p.1656·3); menthol (p.1632·3).
Musculoskeletal and joint pain.

Goanna Salve *Herron, Austral.*
Eucalyptus oil (p.1609·2); pumilio pine oil (p.1656·3); peppermint oil (p.1243·3); camphor (p.1589·3); methyl salicylate (p.55·1); menthol (p.1632·3); turpentine oil (p.1676·3).
Musculoskeletal and joint pain.

Gobanal *Normon, Spain.*
Diazepam (p.674·3).
Contains pyridoxine hydrochloride.
Alcohol withdrawal syndrome; anxiety; febrile convulsions; insomnia; skeletal muscle spasm.

Gobemicina *Normon, Spain.*
Ampicillin trihydrate (p.151·1) or ampicillin sodium (p.150·3).
Bacterial infections.

Gobemicina Retard *Normon, Spain.*
Ampicillin sodium (p.150·3); ampicillin benzathine (p.151·3).
Lignocaine [lidocaine] hydrochloride (p.1313·2) is included in this preparation to alleviate the pain of injection.
Bacterial infections.

Gobens Trim *Normon, Spain.*
Co-trimoxazole (p.193·3).
Bacterial infections; Pneumocystis carinii pneumonia.

Gobrosan *Protein, Mex.*
Ibuprofen (p.43·2).

Gocce Antonetto *Antonetto, Ital.†.*
Sodium picosulfate (p.1249·3).
Constipation.

Gocce Lassative Aicardi *SIT, Ital.*
Sodium picosulfate (p.1249·3).
Constipation.

Goccemed *Iodosan, Ital.*
Iodine (p.1522·3).
Oral hygiene.

Godabion B6 *Merck, Spain.*
Pyridoxine hydrochloride (p.1386·3).
Vitamin B6 deficiency.

Godal *Merck, Spain.*
Bisoprolol fumarate (p.850·3).
Angina pectoris; hypertension.

Godamed *Pfleger, Ger.*
Aspirin (p.14·2).
Glycine (p.1365·3) is included in Godamed 500 in an attempt to limit adverse effects on the gastrointestinal mucosa.
Fever; pain; thromboembolic disorders.

Goddards White Oil Embrocation *LRC Products, UK.*
Turpentine oil (p.1676·3); dilute acetic acid (p.1571·3); dilute ammonia solution (p.1579·1).
Muscular aches and pains.

Go-Evac *Copley, USA†.*
Macrogol 3350 (p.1630·3); electrolytes (p.1180·1).
Bowel evacuation.

Gofreely *Promedical, Ital.*
Macrogol 3350 (p.1630·3); electrolytes (p.1180·1).
Bowel evacuation.

Golac *Elofar, Braz.*
Potassium citrate; sodium chloride; sodium citrate; calcium lactate; magnesium citrate; glucose (p.1185·2).
Diarrhoea; oral rehydration therapy.

Golacetin *Vaillant, Ital.*
Cetylpyridinium chloride (p.1138·1).
Oral disinfection.

Goladin *Sofar, Ital.*
Dequalinium chloride (p.1143·3).
Oral disinfection.

Golamed *Iodosan, Ital.*
Cicliomenol.
Mouth and throat disinfection.

Golamed Due *Iodosan, Ital.*
Cicliomenol; hexylresorcinol (p.1146·3).
Mouth and throat disinfection; sore throat.

Golamed Oral *Iodosan, Ital.*
Iodinated glycerol (p.1092·3); domiphen bromide (p.1143·3).
Oropharyngeal disinfection.

Golamixin *Fournier, Ital.*
Tyrothricin (p.267·1); cetrimonium bromide (p.1137·3); benzocaine (p.1306·2).
Bacterial stomatitis.

Golan *Mavi, Mex.*
Frusemide [furosemide] (p.893·1).

Golapiol *Antipiol, Ital.*
Propolis (p.1655·1).

Golasan *Dynacren, Ital.*
Chlorhexidine gluconate (p.1138·2) or chlorhexidine hydrochloride (p.1138·2).
Mouth and throat disinfection; oral hygiene.

Golasept *Zeta, Ital.*
Povidone-iodine (p.1155·1).
Oral disinfection.

Golasol *Gambar, Ital.*
Chlorhexidine gluconate (p.1138·2).
Mouth and throat disinfection; oral hygiene.

Golaval *Carlo Erba OTC, Ital.*
Cetrimonium tosilate (p.1137·3).
Mouth and throat disinfection.

Gold-50 *Schering-Plough, Austral.*
Aurothioglucose (p.18·3).
Rheumatoid arthritis.

Gold Alka-Seltzer *Bayer, USA.*
Sodium bicarbonate (p.1186·2); citric acid (p.1596·2); potassium bicarbonate (p.1186·1).
Hyperacidity.

Gold Bond *Chattem, Canad.†.*
Menthol (p.1632·3); zinc oxide (p.1128·2).
Pruritus.

Gold Cross Antihistamine Elixir *Biotech, Austral.*
Promethazine hydrochloride (p.423·2).
Hypersensitivity reactions; insomnia; motion sickness.

Goldcare *Vitabiotics, UK.*
Multivitamin and mineral preparation with ginkgo biloba and bioflavonoids (p.1350·1).

Golden Eye Drops *Typharm, UK.*
Propamidine isetionate (p.1155·3).
Eye infections.

Golden Eye Ointment
Note. This name is used for preparations of different composition.
Sigma, Austral.
Yellow mercuric oxide (p.1633·3).
Bacterial eye infections.

Typharm, UK.
Dibrompropamidine isetionate (p.1143·1).
Eye infections.

Golden Star *Duopharm, Ger.*
Vitamin A palmitate (p.1383·2); riboflavin sodium phosphate (p.1386·1).
Eye disorders.

Goldgeist *Gerlach, Ger.*
Pyrethrum (p.1436·3); piperonyl butoxide (p.1436·2).
Pediculosis.

Goldgesic *Ranbaxy, S.Afr.*
Paracetamol (p.71·2); codeine phosphate (p.25·2); promethazine hydrochloride (p.423·2).
Fever; pain.

Goldgestant *Searle, S.Afr.†.*
Chlorpheniramine [chlorphenamine] maleate (p.412·1); phenylpropanolamine hydrochloride (p.1098·1); phenylephrine hydrochloride (p.1097·1).
Cold symptoms.

Gold-Komplex *Steigerwald, Ger.*
Homoeopathic preparation.

Goldtropfen N *DHU, Ger.*
Homoeopathic preparation.

Goldtropfen S *DHU, Ger.*
Homoeopathic preparation.

Goldtropfen-Hetterich *Galenika, Ger.*
Crataegus (p.1600·2); valerian (p.1678·3); convallaria (p.1599·1); scoparium (p.1661·2); camphor (p.1589·3); gold chloride.
Cardiac disorders.

GoLytely
Stafford-Miller, Austral.; Baxter, Canad.; Stafford-Miller, NZ; Kloster, S.Afr.; Braintree, USA.
Macrogol 3350 (p.1630·3); electrolytes (p.1180·1).
Bowel evacuation.

Gomec *General Drugs, Thai.*
Omeprazole (p.1239·1).
Gastro-oesophageal reflux, Zollinger-Ellison syndrome; peptic ulcer.

Gomenol *Gomenol, Fr.*
Niaouli oil (p.1640·2).
Respiratory-tract disorders.

Gomenoleo *Gomenol, Fr.*
Niaouli oil (p.1640·2).
Burns; infections; instrument lubrication; ulcers; wounds.

Gomenol-Syner-Penicilline *Gomenol, Fr.†.*
Benzylpenicillin sodium (p.157·2); niaouli oil (p.1640·2).
Bacterial infections.

Gonadotraphon LH *Paines & Byrne, Irl.; Ferring, UK†.*
Chorionic gonadotrophin (p.1279·2).
Anovulatory infertility; delayed puberty, cryptorchidism, and oligospermia in the male.

Gonadotropyl C *Hoechst Marion Roussel, Mex.*
Chorionic gonadotrophin (p.1279·2).
Cryptorchidism; delayed puberty; hypogonadism; male and female infertility.

Gonak *Akorn, USA.*
Hypromellose (p.1501·3).
Gonioscopic examination.

Gonakor *Sanfer, Mex.*
Chorionic gonadotrophin (p.1279·2); hydroxocobalamin (p.1388·3).
Erectile dysfunction; hypogonadism; oligospermia.

Gonal-F
Serono, Aust.; Serono, Austral.; Serono, Canad.; Serono, Denm.; Serono, Fin.; Serono, Fr.; Serono, Ger.; Serono, Hong Kong; Serono, Irl.; Serono, Israel; Serono, Ital.; Serono, Mex.; Serono, Neth.; Serono, Norw.; Serono, NZ; Serono, Port.; Serono, Singapore; Serono, Spain; Serono, Swed.; Serono, Switz.; Serono, Thai.; Serono, UK; Serono, USA.
Follitropin alfa (p.1283·1).
Male and female infertility; stimulation of ovulation.

Gonaplex *Carter-Wallace, Mex.*
Chorionic gonadotrophin (p.1279·2).

Gonasi HP *Amsa, Ital.*
Chorionic gonadotrophin (p.1279·2).
Formerly known as Gonadotrafon LH.
Amenorrhoea; cryptorchidism; hypogonadism; infertility; threatened or recurrent miscarriage.

Gonasone *Fustery, Mex.*
Chorionic gonadotrophin (p.1279·2).
Cryptorchidism; female infertility; hypogonadism and delayed puberty in the male; recurrent miscarriage.

Gonic *Hauck, USA.*
Chorionic gonadotrophin (p.1279·2).
Male and female infertility; male hypogonadism; prepubertal cryptorchidism.

Gonioscopic *Alcon, USA.*
Hyetellose (p.1501·1).
Gonioscopic examination.

Goniosoft *Ocusoft, USA.*
Hypromellose (p.1501·3).

Goniosol *Ciba Vision, USA.*
Hypromellose (p.1501·3).
Gonioscopic examination.

Gonne Balm *Lane, UK.*
Camphor (p.1589·3); menthol (p.1632·3); eucalyptus oil (p.1609·2); methyl salicylate (p.55·1); turpentine oil (p.1676·3).
Joint and muscular pain.

Gonocilin *Uniao Quimica, Braz.*
Ampicillin (p.150·3).
Probenecid (p.401·3) is included in this preparation to reduce renal tubular excretion of the antibiotic.
Bacterial infections.

Gonoform *Ratiopharm, Aust.*
Amoxicillin trihydrate (p.149·2).
Bacterial infections.

Gonol *Neo Quimica, Braz.*
Ampicillin (p.150·3).
Probenecid (p.401·3) is included in this preparation to reduce renal tubular excretion of the antibiotic.
Bacterial infections.

Gonorcin *General Drugs, Thai.*
Norfloxacin (p.232·1).
Bacterial infections.

Gonorrels *Gilton, Braz.*
Ampicillin (p.150·3).
Probenecid (p.401·3) is included in this preparation to reduce renal tubular excretion of the antibiotic.
Bacterial infections.

Goodnight *Aventis, NZ.*
Promethazine hydrochloride (p.423·2).
Insomnia.

Goodnight Formula *Vitaplex, Austral.*
Valerian (p.1678·3); chamomile (p.1593·2); passion flower (p.1649·1); skullcap (p.1664·3); vitamin B substances (p.1350·1); zinc sulfate (p.1398·2).
Insomnia.

Goodypops *Health Imports, UK.*
Echinacea (p.1606·2); vitamin C (p.1389·3); pectin (p.1502·3).
Sore throat.

The symbol † denotes a preparation no longer actively marketed

Goody's Headache Powders *Goodys, USA.*
Aspirin (p.14·2); paracetamol (p.71·2); caffeine (p.761·3).

Go-Pain *PD Pharm, S.Afr.*
Syrup: Paracetamol (p.71·2); codeine phosphate (p.25·2); promethazine hydrochloride (p.423·2).
Fever; pain.
Tablets: Paracetamol (p.71·2); codeine phosphate (p.25·2); caffeine (p.761·3); meprobamate (p.691·1).
Pain with tension.

Gopten
Knoll, Austral.; Knoll, Braz.; Knoll, Denm.; Knoll, Fin.; Knoll, Fr.; Knoll, Ger.; Knoll, Irl.; Knoll, Ital.; Knoll, Mex.; Knoll, Neth.; Knoll, Norw.; Knoll, NZ; Knoll, Port.; Knoll, S.Afr.; Knoll, Spain; Knoll, Swed.; Knoll, Switz.; Knoll, UK.
Trandolapril (p.985·2).
Hypertension; left ventricular dysfunction following myocardial infarction.

Gordobalm *Gordon, USA.*
Methyl salicylate (p.55·1); menthol (p.1632·3); camphor (p.1589·3).
Muscle, joint, and soft-tissue pain; neuralgia.

Gordochom *Gordon, USA.*
Undecenoic acid (p.395·3); chloroxylenol (p.1142·1).
Fungal skin infections.

Gordofilm *Gordon, USA.*
Salicylic acid (p.1122·3).
Verrucas.

Gordogesic *Gordon, USA.*
Methyl salicylate (p.55·1).
Muscle, joint, and soft-tissue pain; neuralgia.

Gorgonium *Drossapharm, Switz.*
Heparin (p.902·1); allantoin (p.1110·1); dexpanthenol (p.1602·3); collagen (p.1598·2).
Scars.

Gormel *Gordon, USA.*
Urea (p.1127·3).
Dry skin; hyperkeratosis.

Gota Cebrina *Irisfarma, Spain.*
Multivitamin preparation (p.1350·1).

Gotas Binelli *Sanofi Winthrop, Braz.*
Fedrilate (p.1091·3).
Coughs.

Gotas Digestivas *Bunker, Braz.; Dakota, Braz.*
Chamomile (p.1593·2); gentian (p.1615·1); nux vomica (p.1643·1); boldo (p.1585·3).
Liver disorders.

Gotas Hepaticas *Ariston, Braz.*
Cascara (p.1216·1); rhubarb (p.1248·1); boldo (p.1585·3); cynara (p.1601·3); belladonna (p.463·1).
Liver disorders.

Gotas Nican *Prima, Braz.*
Belladonna (p.463·1); grindelia (p.1618·2); aconite (p.1572·3); bromoform (p.1587·1); sodium dibunate (p.1100·3); passion flower (p.1649·1); sodium benzoate (p.1134·3).
Coughs.

Gotas Ototilan *Prodotti, Braz.*
Fluocinolone (p.1071·1); neomycin (p.228·1); lignocaine [lidocaine] (p.1313·2).
Infected ear disorders.

Gotas Zimaia *Zimaia, Port.*
Ephedrine (p.1090·1); ethylmorphine (p.35·2).
Coughs.

Gothaplast Capsicum-Warmepflaster *Gothaplast, Ger.*
Nonivamide (p.63·1).
Musculoskeletal and joint disorders.

Gotil-AD *Laborsil, Braz.*
Vitamin A (p.1382·1); vitamin D (p.1391·1).
Vitamin supplement.

Gouttes aux Essences *Dolisos, Fr.*
Peppermint oil (p.1243·3); clove oil (p.1597·1); thyme oil (p.1672·3); cinnamon oil (p.1596·1); lavender oil (p.1627·2).
Respiratory-tract disorders.

Gouttes contre la toux "S" *Synpharma, Switz.*
Codeine phosphate (p.25·2); aromatic tincture; hyoscyamus (p.470·1); ipecacuanha (p.1093·1); drosera (p.1606·1); plantago lanceolata.
Coughs.

Gouttes Dentaires *Valmo, Canad.*
Benzocaine (p.1306·2); camphor (p.1589·3); guaiacol (p.1092·1); menthol (p.1632·3); clove oil (p.1597·1).

Gouttes homeopathiques contre le rhume des foins *Phytomed, Switz.†; Herbamed, Switz.*
Homoeopathic preparation.

Gouttes nasales *Spirig, Switz.*
Phenylephrine (p.1097·1).
Nasal congestion; rhinitis; sinusitis.

Gouttes nasales N *Spirig, Switz.*
Naphazoline nitrate (p.1095·1); phenylephrine (p.1097·1).
Nasal congestion; rhinitis; sinusitis.

Gouttes pour le coeur et les nerfs Concentrees *Zeller, Switz.*
Crataegus (p.1600·2); passion flower (p.1649·1).
Cardiac disorders; nervous disorders.

Gouttes pour Mal d'Orreilles *Valmo, Canad.*
Benzocaine (p.1306·2); camphor (p.1589·3); chlorobutanol (p.1141·2).

Goxil *Pharmacia Upjohn, USA.*
Azithromycin (p.153·1).
Bacterial infections.

Gozid *General Drugs, Thai.*
Gemfibrozil (p.896·2).
Hyperlipidaemias.

G/P *Cypress, USA.*
Guaifenesin (p.1092·2); pseudoephedrine hydrochloride (p.1099·2).
Respiratory-tract congestion.

GP-500 *Marnel, USA.*
Pseudoephedrine hydrochloride (p.1099·2); guaifenesin (p.1092·2).
Coughs.

Gracial
Organon, Aust.; Organon, Belg.; Organon, Denm.; Organon, Fin.; Organon, Hong Kong; Organon, Ital.; Organon, Neth.; Organon, Port.; Organon, Switz.
Desogestrel (p.1470·3); ethinylestradiol (p.1476·2).
Biphasic oral contraceptive.

Gradient *Polifarma, Ital.*
Flunarizine hydrochloride (p.418·1).
Migraine; vertigo.

Gradin Del D Andreu *Roche Nicholas, Spain.*
Benzalkonium chloride (p.1133·2); benzocaine (p.1306·2); tyrothricin (p.267·1).
Mouth and throat disorders.

Gradulon *Ebewe, Aust.†*
Digoxin (p.870·1); verapamil hydrochloride (p.989·1).
Arrhythmias; heart failure; myocardial infarction.

Grafco batonnets de bois *Salzmann, Switz.*
Silver nitrate (p.1664·2); potassium nitrate (p.1154·3).
Granulation tissue; verrucas.

Grageniil *Reig Jofre, Spain.*
Codeine phosphate (p.25·2); diphenhydramine hydrochloride (p.416·1); ephedrine hydrochloride (p.1090·1).
Cough; respiratory-tract disorders.

Grains de Vals
Note.This name is used for preparations of different composition.
Qualiphar, Belg.
Aloes (p.1210·1); belladonna (p.463·1); cascara (p.1216·1); frangula bark (p.1227·1); intestinal mucosa extract; ox bile extract (p.1585·1); phenolphthalein (p.1244·1).
Constipation.
Nogues, Fr.; Nogues, Switz.
Boldo (p.1585·3); cascara (p.1216·1); senna (p.1248·2).
Formerly contained aloes, belladonna, cascara, frangula bark, and ox bile extract in Fr.
Constipation.

Gral *Boniscontro & Gazzone, Ital.†*
Dihydroergocristine mesilate (p.1603·2).
Cerebrovascular disorders; dopaminergic deficiency; headache; hypertension; migraine; peripheral vascular disorders.

Gramal *Probiomed, Mex.*
Molgramostim (p.738·3).
Reduction of neutropenia associated with cytotoxic therapy or bone marrow transplants.

Gramaxin *Roche, Israel.; Boehringer Mannheim, Ger.†*
Cefazolin sodium (p.164·3).
Lignocaine [lidocaine] hydrochloride (p.1313·2) may be included in the intramuscular preparation to alleviate the pain of injection.
Bacterial infections.

Gramcal *Sandoz, Canad.†*
Calcium lactate gluconate (p.1188·3); calcium carbonate (p.1215·1).
Calcium supplement; osteoporosis.

Gramcilina *Medley, Braz.*
Ampicillin (p.150·3).
Bacterial infections.

Gramidil *EG, Fr.*
Amoxicillin trihydrate (p.149·2).
Bacterial infections.

Graminflor *Adroka, Switz.*
Hay flower.
Musculoskeletal and joint disorders.

Gramipan *Mayoly-Spindler, Switz.*
Dequalinium chloride (p.1143·1); ascorbic acid (p.1389·3).
Mouth and throat infections.

Gramixina *Merck, Port.*
Polymyxin B sulfate (p.238·1); gramicidin (p.213·3); chlorpheniramine [chlorphenamine] maleate (p.412·1); naphazoline hydrochloride (p.1095·1); procaine hydrochloride (p.1319·1).
Bacterial infections.

Grammicin *Siam Bheasach, Thai.*
Gentamicin sulfate (p.210·1).
Bacterial infections.

Grammixin *Siam Bheasach, Thai.*
Gentamicin sulfate (p.210·1).
Bacterial skin infections.

Gramoce A *Vir, Spain.*
Ascorbic acid (p.1389·3); vitamin A (p.1382·1).
Deficiency of vitamins A and C.

Gramplus *Chiesi, Ital.*
Clofoctol (p.192·1).
Bacterial infections.

Gram-Val *Polifarma, Ital.*
Doxycycline hyclate (p.200·1).
Bacterial infections.

Gran *Kirin, Jpn.*
Filgrastim (p.736·1).
Neutropenia.

Granamon *Norgine, Ger.*
Sterculia (p.1250·2).
Constipation.

Grandaxin
EGIS, Hung.; Egis, Thai.
Tofisopam (p.709·3).
Alcohol withdrawal syndrome; anxiety; menopausal disorders.

Graneodin *Bristol-Myers Squibb, Irl.; Squibb, UK.*
Neomycin sulfate (p.228·1); gramicidin (p.213·3).
Bacterial infections of the skin and ear.

Graneodine *Bristol-Myers Squibb, Belg.†*
Neomycin sulfate (p.228·1); gramicidin (p.213·3).
Skin infections.

Grani di Vals *Geymonat, Ital.*
Cascara (p.1216·1); aloes (p.1210·1); aloin (p.1210·2).
Constipation.

Granions *Granions, Mon.*
A range of mineral supplements (p.1350·1).

Granobil *Synpharma, Aust.*
Fennel (p.1610·1); cowslip root (p.1600·1); thyme leaf (p.1672·2).
Catarrh; coughs.

Granocol *Schering, Austral.; Schering, NZ.*
Sterculia (p.1250·2); frangula bark (p.1227·1).
Constipation.

Granocyte
Rhone-Poulenc Rorer, Aust.; Amrad, Austral.; Aventis, Belg.; Chugai, Denm.; Rhone-Poulenc Rorer, Fin.; Rhone-Poulenc Rorer, Fr.; Rhone-Poulenc Rorer, Ger.; Aventis, Irl.; Rhone-Poulenc Rorer, Israel; Rhone-Poulenc Rorer, Ital.; Rhone-Poulenc Rorer, Neth.; Chugai, Norw.; Amrad, NZ; Rhone-Poulenc Rorer, Port.; Aventis, S.Afr.; Rhone-Poulenc Rorer, Singapore; Rhone-Poulenc Rorer, Spain; Rhone-Poulenc Rorer, Swed.; Rhone-Poulenc Rorer, Switz.; Chugai, Thai.; Chugai, UK.
Lenograstim (p.738·1).
Mobilisation of autologous peripheral blood progenitor cells; reduction of neutropenia associated with cytotoxic therapy or bone marrow transplantation.

Granoleina *SIFI, Ital.*
dl-Alpha tocoferil acetate (p.1394·1); linoleic acid (p.1613·2); vitamin A palmitate (p.1383·2); ergocalciferol (p.1391·2).
Vitamin deficiencies.

Granon *Nycomed, Denm.*
Acetylcysteine (p.1082·3).
Respiratory-tract congestion.

Granoton *Grandel-Synpharma, Ger.*
Tocopherol; tritici sativi e embryo; ethanol.
Tonic.

Grans Remedy *Grans Remedy, NZ.*
Zinc oxide (p.1128·2); zinc undecenoate (p.395·3); alum (p.1577·2); talc (p.1124·2).
Foot odour.

Granudoxy *Pierre Fabre, Fr.*
Doxycycline (p.200·1).
Bacterial infections.

Granufink Kurbiskern *SmithKline Beecham OTC, Ger.*
Cucurbita (p.1601·1).
Urinary-tract disorders.

Granufink Kurbiskern N *SmithKline Beecham OTC, Ger.*
Cucurbita (p.1601·1); cucurbita oil.
Urinary-tract disorders.

Granuflex *Convatec, Israel; Bristol-Myers Squibb, S.Afr.; Convatec, UK.*
Hydrocolloid dressing.
Burns; skin ulcers; wounds.

Granugel
Note.This name is used for preparations of different composition.
Convatec, Israel.
Hydrocolloid gel.
Skin ulcers; wounds.
Bristol-Myers Squibb, S.Afr.
Pectin (p.1502·3); carmellose sodium (p.1499·3).
Wounds.

Granugen *Knoll, Austral.*
Paraffin oil (p.1407·1); zinc oxide (p.1128·2); titanium dioxide (p.1126·1); paraffin viscous; ethyl vanillin; soft paraffin.
Minor wounds and ulcers.

Granuderm *Copley, USA.*
Trypsin (p.1675·3); peru balsam (p.1650·2); castor oil (p.1592·1).
Wounds.

Granules Boripharm *Dolisos, Fr.*
A range of homoeopathic preparations.
Formerly known as Granules Boribel.

Granulex *Bertek, USA.*
Trypsin (p.1675·3); peru balsam (p.1650·2); castor oil (p.1592·1).
Wound dressing.

Granulokine *Roche, Braz.; Roche, Ital.; Pensa, Spain.*
Filgrastim (p.736·1).
Mobilisation of autologous peripheral blood progenitor cells; neutropenia.

GranuMed *Rugby, USA.*
Trypsin (p.1675·3); peru balsam (p.1650·2); castor oil (p.1592·1).
Wounds.

Gran-Verm *Brasmedica, Braz.*
Mebendazole (p.102·2).
Worm infections.

Granvit *Plants, Ital.*
Royal jelly (p.1659·3) with wheat-germ oil, carrot oil, and soya lecithin (p.1350·1).
Nutritional supplement.

Grasmin *Almirall, Spain†.*
Fenproporex resinate (p.1510·1).
Obesity.

Graten *Pisa, Mex.*
Morphine sulfate (p.56·1).
Pain.

Gratusminal
Note.This name is used for preparations of different composition.
Zambon, Braz.
Phenobarbital diethylamine (p.356·2); deslanoside (p.867·3).
Cardiac disorders.
Almirall, Spain.
Phenobarbital diethylamine (p.356·2).
Agitation; convulsive disorders; depression; insomnia; smooth muscle spasm.

Gravergol *Carter Horner, Canad.; Carter Horner, Hong Kong.*
Ergotamine tartrate (p.452·1); caffeine (p.761·3); dimenhydrinate (p.415·2).
Migraine and other vascular headaches.

Gravibinan *Schering, Aust.; Schering, Ger.*
Hydroxyprogesterone caproate (p.1479·3); estradiol valerate (p.1473·2).
Threatened or recurrent miscarriage.

Gravibinon *Schering, Aust.; Schering, Ger.*
Hydroxyprogesterone caproate (p.1479·3); estradiol valerate (p.1473·2).
Threatened or recurrent miscarriage.

Gravidex
Note.This name is used for preparations of different composition.
Provita, Ital.
Multivitamin and mineral preparation (p.1350·1).
Almirall, Spain†.
Dinoprostone (p.1441·3).
Hydatidiform mole; labour induction; termination of pregnancy.

Gravidinona *Schering, Mex.*
Hydroxyprogesterone caproate (p.1479·3); estradiol valerate (p.1473·2).
Recurrent miscarriage.

Gravigard *SPA, Ital.†*
Copper-wound plastic (p.1357·3).
Intra-uterine contraceptive device.

Gravigen *Byk Gulden, Ital.*
Multivitamin and mineral preparation (p.1350·1).

Gravindex *Ortho, Israel.*
Pregnancy test (p.1654·3).

Gravistat *Jenapharm, Ger.*
Ethinylestradiol (p.1476·2); levonorgestrel (p.1486·2).
Combined oral contraceptive; menstrual disorders.

Gravitamon *Chefaro, Neth.†*
Multivitamin and mineral preparation (p.1350·1).

Gravol *Carter Horner, Canad.; Carter Horner, Hong Kong; Carter Horner, Thai.*
Dimenhydrinate (p.415·2).
Nausea; vomiting.

Greatbloc *Creative Brands, Austral.*
SPF 15; SPF 30+: Padimate O (p.1518·2); oxybenzone (p.1518·1); avobenzone (p.1517·1).
Sunscreen.

Greater-Gloxa *Greater Pharma, Thai.*
Cloxacillin sodium (p.192·1).
Bacterial infections.

Greatofen *Greater Pharma, Thai.*
Ibuprofen (p.43·2).
Musculoskeletal and joint disorders.

Green Antiseptic Mouthwash & Gargle *Lee-Adams, Canad.*
Alcohol (p.1130·3); cetylpyridinium chloride (p.1138·1).

Greenosan *Bang & Tegner, Denm.†*
Multivitamin and mineral preparation (p.1350·1).

Grefen *Doetsch, Grether, Switz.*
Ibuprofen (p.43·2).
Fever; inflammation; musculoskeletal and joint disorders; pain.

Gregoderm *Unigreg, UK.*
Neomycin sulfate (p.228·1); polymyxin B sulfate (p.238·1); hydrocortisone (p.1073·3); nystatin (p.392·2).
Infected skin disorders.

Greosin *Allen, Spain.*
Griseofulvin (p.386·2).
Fungal skin and nail infections.

Grexin *Pharmasant, Thai.*
Digoxin (p.870·1).
Arrhythmias; heart failure.

Gricin
Dresden, Ger.†; LAW, Ger.
Griseofulvin (p.386·2).
Fungal infections of the skin, hair, or nails.

Grietalgen *Diviser Aquilea, Spain.*
Peru balsam (p.1650·2); bismuth subnitrate (p.1213·2); ergocalciferol (p.1391·2); estrone (p.1476·1); benzocaine (p.1306·2); vitamin A (p.1382·1).
Cracked nipples; mastitis.

Grietalgen Hidrocort *Diviser Aquilea, Spain.*
Bismuth subnitrate (p.1213·2); colecalciferol (p.1391·1); estrone (p.1476·1); benzocaine (p.1306·2);

vitamin A (p.1382·1); hydrocortisone glycyrrhetinate (p.1074·2); neomycin sulfate (p.228·1).
Burns; cracked nipples; mastitis; skin disorders; wounds.

Grifed *Syntex, Mex.*
Naproxen sodium (p.61·1); pseudoephedrine hydrochloride (p.1099·2).
Cold and influenza symptoms.

Grifulin *Teva, Israel.*
Griseofulvin (p.386·2).
Fungal skin infections.

Grifulvin *General Drugs, Thai.*
Griseofulvin (p.386·2).
Fungal skin, hair, and nail infections.

Grifulvin V *Ortho Dermatological, USA.*
Griseofulvin (microsize) (p.386·2).
Fungal skin, hair, and nail infections.

Gripakin *Fournier SA, Spain‡.*
Chlorpheniramine [chlorphenamine] maleate (p.412·1); paracetamol (p.71·2).
Cold symptoms; nasal congestion.

Gripalgine *Pharmetic, Belg.†.*
Aspirin (p.14·2); codeine phosphate (p.25·2); ascorbic acid (p.1389·3).
Fever; pain.

Gripavac *Pasteur Merieux, Spain.*
An influenza vaccine (p.1544·3).
Active immunisation.

Gripcaps C *Infabra, Braz.*
Phenylephrine (p.1097·1); paracetamol (p.71·2); ascorbic acid (p.1389·3).
Cold and influenza symptoms.

Gripefago C *Baldassari, Braz.*
Dipyrone (p.34·1); sodium camsilate; guaifenesin (p.1092·2); eucalyptol (p.1609·2); niaouli oil (p.1640·2); ascorbic acid (p.1389·3); mepyramine maleate (p.421·1).
Lignocaine [lidocaine] hydrochloride (p.1313·2) is included in this preparation to alleviate the pain of injection.
Cold and influenza symptoms.

Gripefin *Faria, Braz.*
Carbasalate calcium (p.23·3); phenylpropanolamine hydrochloride (p.1098·1); pheniramine maleate (p.422·3); mepyramine maleate (p.421·1).
Cold and influenza symptoms.

Gripen *EMS, Braz.*
Dimetindene (p.415·3); rutoside (p.1611·2); ascorbic acid (p.1389·3); phenylephrine (p.1097·1); paracetamol (p.71·2).
Cold and influenza symptoms.

Gripenil *Windson, Braz.*
Phenylephrine (p.1097·1); carbinoxamine (p.411·1).
Nasal congestion.

Gripeonil *Faria, Braz.*
Paracetamol (p.71·2).
Fever; pain.

Gripetral *Atral, Port.*
Aspirin (p.14·2); ascorbic acid (p.1389·3); caffeine (p.761·3).
Cold and influenza symptoms.

Gripex *Lambda, USA†.*
Guaifenesin (p.1092·2); dextromethorphan hydrobromide (p.1087·3); phenylephrine hydrochloride (p.1097·1).
Coughs.

Gripidor *Medical, Port.*
Aspirin (p.14·2); paracetamol (p.71·2).
Fever; pain.

Gripin C *Medquimica, Braz.*
Salicylamide (p.82·1); chlorpheniramine [chlorphenamine] (p.412·2); caffeine (p.761·3); vitamin C (p.1389·3).
Cold and influenza symptoms.

Gripion *Makros, Braz.*
Diphenhydramine hydrochloride (p.416·1); dipyrone (p.34·1); ascorbic acid (p.1389·3).
Cold and influenza symptoms.

Gripionex *Delta, Braz.*
Paracetamol (p.71·2); caffeine (p.761·3); phenylephrine hydrochloride (p.1097·1); tripelennamine maleate (p.427·2).
Cold and influenza symptoms.

Gripol C *Delta, Braz.*
Dipyrone (p.34·1); mepyramine maleate (p.421·1); caffeine (p.761·3); ascorbic acid (p.1389·3).
Cold and influenza symptoms.

Gripol C Capuride *INQ, Braz.*
Dipyrone (p.34·1); guaifenesin (p.1092·2); sodium camsilate; eucalyptol (p.1609·2).
Cold and influenza symptoms.

Gripol Composto *INQ, Braz.*
Dipyrone (p.34·1); mepyramine maleate (p.421·1); caffeine (p.761·3); ascorbic acid (p.1389·3).
Cold and influenza symptoms.

Gripomatine *QIF, Braz.*
Dipyrone (p.34·1); sodium camsilate; guaifenesin (p.1092·2); eucalyptol (p.1609·2); niaouli oil (p.1640·2); vitamin C (p.1389·3).
Cold and influenza symptoms.

Griponal *Merck, Port.*
Paracetamol (p.71·2); phenylephrine hydrochloride (p.1097·1); chlorpheniramine [chlorphenamine] maleate (p.412·1).
Cold and influenza symptoms.

Griponia *Bunker, Braz.*
Dipyrone (p.34·1); sodium camsilate; guaifenesin (p.1092·2); eucalyptol (p.1609·2); niaouli oil (p.1640·2); ascorbic acid (p.1389·3).
Cold and influenza symptoms.

Grippal *Bayer, Spain.*
Aspirin (p.14·2); chlorpheniramine [chlorphenamine] maleate (p.412·1); phenylpropanolamine (p.1098·1).
Influenza and cold symptoms; nasal congestion.

Grippalgine N *DP-Medica, Switz.*
Paracetamol (p.71·2); salicylamide (p.82·1); caffeine (p.761·3).
Cold and influenza symptoms.

Grippalin & C *Multi-Pro, Canad.*
Chlorpheniramine [chlorphenamine] maleate (p.412·1); paracetamol (p.71·2); ascorbic acid (p.1389·3).
Cold and influenza symptoms.

Grippefloran *Bioflora, Aust.*
Salix purpurea (p.82·1); tilia flower (p.1673·2); vitamin C (p.1389·3).
Cold symptoms.

Grippe-Gastreu R6 *Reckeweg, Ger.*
Homoeopathic preparation.

Grippetee Dr Zeidler *Apotheke Erzengel Michael, Aust.*
Tilia flower (p.1673·2); sambucus flower (p.1660·3); rose fruit (p.1389·3); thyme leaf (p.1672·2); drosera (p.1606·1).
Cold symptoms.

Grippetee EF-EM-ES *Smetana, Aust.*
Sambucus flower (p.1660·3); tilia flower (p.1673·2); plantago lanceolata.
Cold symptoms.

Gripp-Heel *Heel, Ger.; Heel, S.Afr.*
Homoeopathic preparation.

Grippin-Merz *Merz, Ger.†.*
Amantadine sulfate (p.1161·2).
Influenza A.

Grippinon *Nycomed, Aust.*
Aspirin (p.14·2); ascorbic acid (p.1389·3).
Cold symptoms.

Grippogran *Synpharma, Aust.*
Sambucus flower (p.1660·3); tilia flower (p.1673·2); centaury (p.1593·1).
Cold symptoms.

Grippon *Adcock Ingram, S.Afr.*
Capsules: Paracetamol (p.71·2); caffeine (p.761·3); ascorbic acid (p.1389·3); phenylephrine hydrochloride (p.1097·1); chlorpheniramine [chlorphenamine] maleate (p.412·1).
Cold and influenza symptoms.
Propan, S.Afr.; Adcock Ingram, S.Afr.
Syrup: Paracetamol (p.71·2); chlorpheniramine [chlorphenamine] maleate (p.412·1); ephedrine (p.1090·1).
Cold and influenza symptoms.

Grippostad C *Note. This name is used for preparations of different composition.*
Stada, Ger.
Paracetamol (p.71·2); ascorbic acid (p.1389·3); caffeine (p.761·3); chlorpheniramine [chlorphenamine] maleate (p.412·1).
Cold symptoms; influenza.
Medika, Switz.
Paracetamol (p.71·2); ascorbic acid (p.1389·3).
Cold symptoms.

Grippostad Gute Nacht-Saft *Stada, Ger.*
Dextromethorphan hydrobromide (p.1087·3); paracetamol (p.71·2).
Cold and influenza symptoms.

Grippostad Heissgetrank *Stada, Ger.*
Paracetamol (p.71·2).
Cold symptoms; pain.

Gripps *Pascoe, Ger.*
Homoeopathic preparation.

Gripsay *Delta, Braz.*
Dipyrone (p.34·1); sodium camsilate; guaifenesin (p.1092·2); eucalyptol (p.1609·2); niaouli oil (p.1640·2); lignocaine [lidocaine] hydrochloride (p.1313·2); mepyramine maleate (p.421·1); ascorbic acid (p.1389·3).
Cold and influenza symptoms.

Griptol *Brasmedica, Braz.*
Aspirin (p.14·2); caffeine (p.761·3); vitamin C (p.1389·3).
Fever; pain.

Grisactin *Wyeth-Ayerst, USA.*
Griseofulvin (p.386·2).
Fungal skin infections.

Grise *Cesam, Port.*
Emollient.
Skin disorders.

Grisefuline *Sanofi Winthrop, Fr.*
Griseofulvin (p.386·2).
Fungal infections.

Griseo *CT, Ger.*
Griseofulvin (p.386·2).
Fungal skin infections.

Griseoful *Ofimex, Mex.*
Griseofulvin (p.386·2).
Fungal infections.

Griseomed *Sanochemia, Aust.*
Griseofulvin (p.386·2).
Superficial fungal infections.

Griseostatin *Schering-Plough, Austral.; Schering-Plough, Hong Kong.*
Griseofulvin (p.386·2).
Fungal infections of the skin, hair, and nails.

Grisetin *Note. This name is used for preparations of different composition.*
Merck, Port.†.
Vitamin B$_{12}$; vitamin B$_1$ (p.1350·1).
Tonic.
Ipsen, Spain.
Flutamide (p.542·3).
Prostatic cancer.

Grisflavin *Asian Pharm, Thai.*
Griseofulvin (p.386·2).
Fungal skin, hair, and nail infections.

Grisol *Gebro, Switz.*
Griseofulvin (p.386·2).
Tinea pedis.

Grisomicon *Sanitas, Port.*
Griseofulvin (p.386·2).
Fungal infections.

Grisovin *Glaxo Wellcome, Aust.; Sigma, Austral.; Glaxo Wellcome, Hong Kong; Glaxo Wellcome, Mex.; Glaxo Wellcome, NZ; Glaxo Wellcome, Port.; Glaxo Wellcome, S.Afr.†; Glaxo Wellcome, Thai.; Glaxo Wellcome, UK.*
Griseofulvin (p.386·2).
Fungal infections of the skin, hair, and nails.

Grisovin FP *Roberts, Canad.†.*
Griseofulvin (p.386·2).
Fungal skin infections.

Grisovina FP *Teofarma, Ital.*
Griseofulvin (p.386·2).
Fungal skin and nail infections.

Gris-PEG *Allergan, USA.*
Griseofulvin (ultramicrosize) (p.386·2).
Fungal skin, hair, and nail infections.

Grivin *Atlantic, Singapore; Atlantic, Thai.*
Griseofulvin (p.386·2).
Fungal infections.

Grodurex *Grossmann, Switz.*
Hydrochlorothiazide (p.907·3); amiloride hydrochloride (p.835·1).
Hypertension; oedema.

Grofenac *Grossmann, Hong Kong; Grossmann, Switz.*
Diclofenac sodium (p.30·3).
Gout; inflammation; musculoskeletal, joint, and periarticular disorders; pain.

Gromazol *Grossmann, Switz.*
Clotrimazole (p.382·1).
Fungal foot infections.

Groprim *Grossmann, Switz.*
Co-trimoxazole (p.193·3).
Bacterial infections; blastomycosis; Pneumocystis carinii pneumonia.

Grotanat *Schulke & Mayr, Ger.*
Chlorocresol (p.1141·3); clorophene (p.1142·3); orthophenylphenol (p.1152·1).
Instrument disinfection.

Grovixim *Torlan, Spain.*
Carnitine chloride; cobamamide; cocarboxylase.
Tonic.

Gruncef *Grunenthal, Ger.*
Cefadroxil (p.161·2).
Bacterial infections.

Grune Salbe "Schmidt" N *Wider, Ger.†.*
Urea (p.1127·3); silver (p.1664·1); magnesium chloride (p.1190·3).
Ulcers; wounds.

Grunicina *Lakeside, Mex.*
Amoxicillin trihydrate (p.149·2).
Bacterial infections.

Grunlicht Dreierlei Tropfen *Lichtenheldt, Ger.*
Peppermint oil (p.1243·3); valerian (p.1678·3).
Dizziness; nausea; nervous disorders.

Grunlicht Hingfong Essenz *Lichtenheldt, Ger.*
Peppermint oil (p.1243·3); anise oil (p.1580·3); cassia oil (p.1592·1); fennel oil (p.1610·2); rosemary oil (p.1659·3); thyme oil (p.1672·3); menthol (p.1632·3); camphor (p.1589·3); peppermint leaf (p.1243·2); bay leaf; arnica (p.1581·3); tilia (p.1673·2); chamomile (p.1593·2); aniseed (p.1580·2); fennel (p.1610·1); calamus (p.1588·1); valerian (p.1678·3).
Cold symptoms; nausea; nervous disorders; neuralgias; rheumatic disorders.

Grunlicht Magenbalsam Tropfen *Lichtenheldt, Ger.*
Anise oil (p.1580·3); fennel oil (p.1610·2); caraway oil (p.1591·2).
Dyspepsia; gastrointestinal spasm; meteorism.

Gruntin Tropfen *Grunenthal, Ger.*
Tilidate hydrochloride (p.88·2).
Naloxone hydrochloride (p.1014·3) is included in this preparation to discourage abuse.
Pain.

G.Test *Sabiluc, Fr.*
Pregnancy test (p.1654·3).

Guafen *Agepha, Aust.*
Guaifenesin (p.1092·2).
Catarrh; coughs.

Guaiacalcium Complex *SIT, Ital.*
Dropropizine (p.1089·3); sulfogaiacol (p.1101·1).
Formerly contained dropropizine, sodium benzoate, calcium gluceptate, sulfogaiacol, and ephedrine hydrochloride.
Coughs.

Guaiaspir *Lampugnani, Ital.*
Guacetisal (p.1092·1).
Respiratory-tract disorders.

Guaifed *Muro, USA.*
Pseudoephedrine hydrochloride (p.1099·2); guaifenesin (p.1092·2).
Coughs; nasal congestion.

Guaifed-PD *Muro, USA.*
Pseudoephedrine hydrochloride (p.1099·2); guaifenesin (p.1092·2).
Coughs; nasal congestion.

Guaifenesin AC *Morton Grove, USA†.*
Codeine phosphate (p.25·2); guaifenesin (p.1092·2).

Guaifenesin DAC *Cypress, USA.*
Codeine phosphate (p.25·2); pseudoephedrine hydrochloride (p.1099·2); guaifenesin (p.1092·2).
Coughs and associated respiratory-tract disorders.

Guaifenex DM *Silarx, USA.*
Guaifenesin (p.1092·2); dextromethorphan hydrobromide (p.1087·3).
Coughs.

Guaifenex *Ethex, USA†.*
Guaifenesin (p.1092·2); phenylpropanolamine hydrochloride (p.1098·1); phenylephrine hydrochloride (p.1097·1).
Coughs.

Guaifenex DM *Ethex, USA.*
Guaifenesin (p.1092·2); dextromethorphan hydrobromide (p.1087·3).
Coughs.

Guaifenex G *Ethex, USA.*
Guaifenesin (p.1092·2).
Coughs.

Guaifenex LA *Ethex, USA.*
Guaifenesin (p.1092·2).
Coughs.

Guaifenex PPA *Ethex, USA†.*
Guaifenesin (p.1092·2); phenylpropanolamine hydrochloride (p.1098·1).
Coughs.

Guaifenex PSE *Ethex, Hong Kong; Ethex, USA.*
Guaifenesin (p.1092·2); pseudoephedrine hydrochloride (p.1099·2).
Coughs; nasal congestion.

Guaifenex Rx *Ethex, USA.*
AM tablets, guaifenesin (p.1092·2); pseudoephedrine hydrochloride (p.1099·2); PM tablets, guaifenesin.
Coughs.

Guaifenex Rx DM *Ethex, USA.*
AM tablets, guaifenesin (p.1092·2); pseudoephedrine hydrochloride (p.1099·2); PM tablets, guaifenesin; dextromethorphan hydrobromide (p.1087·3).
Coughs.

Guaimax-D *Schwarz, USA.*
Guaifenesin (p.1092·2); pseudoephedrine hydrochloride (p.1099·2).
Coughs.

Guaipax *Eon, USA†.*
Guaifenesin (p.1092·2); phenylpropanolamine hydrochloride (p.1098·1).
Coughs.

Guaitab *Muro, USA.*
Guaifenesin (p.1092·2); pseudoephedrine hydrochloride (p.1099·2).
Coughs; nasal congestion.

Guaivent *Ethex, USA.*
Guaifenesin (p.1092·2); pseudoephedrine hydrochloride (p.1099·2).
Coughs.

Guai-Vent/PSE *Dura, USA.*
Guaifenesin (p.1092·2); pseudoephedrine hydrochloride (p.1099·2).
Coughs.

Guajabronc *Molteni, Ital.†.*
Guacetisal (p.1092·1).
Respiratory-tract disorders.

Guanor *Rosemont, UK.*
Diphenhydramine hydrochloride (p.416·1); ammonium chloride (p.1085·2); sodium citrate (p.1186·2); menthol (p.1632·3).
Coughs.

Guar Verlan *Verla, Ger.*
Guar gum (p.323·3).
Diabetes mellitus; hyperlipidaemias.

Guarasex *Heralds, Braz.*
Vitamin preparation with guarana and erythroxylon catuaba (p.1350·1).

Guarem *Orion, Fin.; Shire, Hong Kong; Rybar, Irl.; Orion, Israel; Shire, UK.*
Guar gum (p.323·3).
Diabetes mellitus; hyperlipidaemias.

Guastil *Uriach, Spain.*
Sulpiride (p.706·1).
Anxiety; psychoses; vertigo.

Guaxan *Roche, Spain.*
Nimesulide (p.62·3).
Fever; inflammation; pain.

Gubamine *Gubler, Switz.†.*
Paracetamol (p.71·2); caffeine (p.761·3); propyphenazone (p.80·2).
Fever; pain.

Guep'Away *Clement, Fr.*
(N-Butyl-N-acetyl)-3-ethylaminopropionate; Frepylate.
Insect repellent.

The symbol † denotes a preparation no longer actively marketed

Guethural *Elerte, Fr.*
Lozenges†; oral granules†: Guethol carbonate (p.1092·3).
Tablets: Guaietolin (p.1092·1).
Respiratory-tract congestion.

Gufen N *Steigerwald, Ger.*
Guaifenesin (p.1092·2).
Respiratory-tract disorders.

Gugecin *Lilly, Mex.*
Cinoxacin (p.182·2).
Urinary-tract infections.

GuiaCough CF *Schein, USA†.*
Phenylpropanolamine hydrochloride (p.1098·1); dextromethorphan hydrobromide (p.1087·3); guaifenesin (p.1092·2).
Coughs.

GuiaCough PE *Schein, USA†.*
Pseudoephedrine hydrochloride (p.1099·2); guaifenesin (p.1092·2).
Coughs.

Guiatex *Rugby, USA†.*
Phenylephrine hydrochloride (p.1097·1); phenylpropanolamine hydrochloride (p.1098·1); guaifenesin (p.1092·2).
Coughs.

Guiatex LA *Rugby, USA†.*
Phenylpropanolamine hydrochloride (p.1098·1); guaifenesin (p.1092·2).
Coughs.

Guiatex PSE *Rugby, USA.*
Pseudoephedrine hydrochloride (p.1099·2); guaifenesin (p.1092·2).
Coughs.

Guiatuss *Goldline, USA.*
Guaifenesin (p.1092·2).
Coughs; respiratory-tract congestion.

Guiatuss CF *Barre-National, USA†.*
Phenylpropanolamine hydrochloride (p.1098·1); dextromethorphan hydrobromide (p.1087·3); guaifenesin (p.1092·2).
Coughs.

Guiatuss PE *Barre-National, USA.*
Pseudoephedrine hydrochloride (p.1099·2); guaifenesin (p.1092·2).
Coughs.

Guiatussin with Codeine Expectorant *Rugby, USA.*
Codeine phosphate (p.25·2); guaifenesin (p.1092·2).
Coughs.

Guiatussin DAC *Rugby, USA.*
Pseudoephedrine hydrochloride (p.1099·2); guaifenesin (p.1092·2); codeine phosphate (p.25·2).
Coughs.

Guiatussin with Dextromethorphan *Rugby, USA.*
Dextromethorphan hydrobromide (p.1087·3); guaifenesin (p.1092·2).
Coughs.

Guigoz Hypoallergenique *Guigoz, Fr.*
Infant feed (p.1350·1).
Milk-protein allergy.

Gumbaral *Asta Medica, Ger.*
Ademetionine tosilate bis(sulfate) (p.1573·1).
Degenerative joint disorders.

Gumbix *Solvay, Aust.; Solvay, Ger.*
Aminomethylbenzoic acid (p.725·2).
Haemorrhage.

Gum-Ese *McGloin, Austral.*
Lignocaine [lidocaine] hydrochloride (p.1313·2); benzalkonium chloride (p.1133·2).
Mouth ulcers.

Gumilk *Gallia, Fr.*
Ceratonia (p.1500·3); maltodextrin (p.1371·2).
Regurgitation in infants.

Gunevax
Chiron, Ital.; Chiron, Thai.
A rubella vaccine (Wistar RA 27/3 strain) (p.1562·3).
Active immunisation.

Gupisone *Julphar, UAE.*
Prednisolone (p.1077·3).
Corticosteroid.

Gurfix *Novartis Consumer, Aust.*
Hexetidine (p.1146·3).
Mouth and throat inflammation.

Gurgellosung Chauvin *Chauvin ankerpharm, Ger.*
Chlorhexidine gluconate (p.1138·2).
Mouth and throat disorders.

Gurgellosung-ratiopharm *Ratiopharm, Ger.*
Dequalinium chloride (p.1143·1).
Mouth and throat infections.

Guronamin *Chugai, Jpn†.*
Glucuronamide.
Eclampsia; hyperbilirubinaemia; skin disorders; vomiting of pregnancy.

Guronsan
Note.This name is used for preparations of different composition.
Exel, Belg.; Riom, Fr.; Jaba, Port.
Glucuronamide; ascorbic acid (p.1389·3); caffeine (p.761·3).
Asthenia.

Chugai, Hong Kong.
Injection: Glucuronic acid (p.1350·1).
Oral liquid: Vitamin B$_2$; vitamin B$_1$; glucuronolactone; vitamin B$_6$ (p.1350·1).

Tablets: Glucuronolactone; glucuronamide; vitamin C; thiamine disulfide (p.1350·1).
Tonic.

Chugai, Jpn†.
Glucurolactone or sodium glucuronate.
Eclampsia; hyperbilirubinaemia; skin disorders; vomiting of pregnancy.

Gustase *Geriatric Pharm. Corp., USA.*
Standardised amylolytic enzyme (Gerilase) (p.1579·3); standardised proteolytic enzyme (Geriprotase); standardised cellulolytic enzyme (Gericellulase) (p.1593·1).
Gastrointestinal disorders.

Gustase Plus *Geriatric Pharm. Corp., USA.*
Phenobarbital (p.355·1); homatropine methylbromide (p.468·1); standardised amylolytic enzyme (Gerilase) (p.1579·3); standardised proteolytic enzyme (Geriprotase); standardised cellulolytic enzyme (Gericellulase) (p.1593·1).
Gastrointestinal disorders.

Gutalax *Fher, Spain.*
Sodium picosulfate (p.1249·3).
Constipation.

Gutnacht *Salushaus, Ger.*
Oral liquid: Valerian (p.1678·3); hypericum (p.290·2); rosemary; melissa (p.1632·2); chamomile (p.1593·2); peppermint leaf (p.1243·2).
Tablets: Valerian (p.1678·3); passion flower (p.1649·1); lupulus (p.1629·3); hypericum (p.290·2); melissa (p.1632·2); rhiz. jatamansi.
Insomnia; nervous disorders.

Gutron
Nycomed, Aust.; Nycomed, Fr.; Nycomed, Ger.; Nycomed, Hong Kong; Nycomed, Israel; Lusofarmaco, Ital.; Sanofi Winthrop, Mex.; Douglas, NZ; Lab, Port.; Nycomed, Switz.; Hafslund Nycomed, Thai.
Midodrine hydrochloride (p.933·3).
Ejaculation disorders; hypotension; urinary incontinence.

Guttacor *Galenika, Ger.*
Convallaria (p.1599·1); crataegus (p.1600·2); valerian (p.1678·3).
Cardiac disorders.

Guttacor-Balsam N *Galenika, Ger.*
Rosemary oil (p.1659·3); camphor (p.1589·3).
Cardiovascular disorders.

Guttae 20 Hustentropfen N *Palmicol, Ger.†.*
Thyme (p.1672·3); wild thyme; primrose flower (p.1600·1).
Catarrh; coughs.

Guttalax
Boehringer Ingelheim, Aust.; Wolfs, Belg.; Boehringer de Angeli, Braz.; Boehringer Ingelheim, Ital.; Boehringer Ingelheim, Port.; Byk, Switz.
Sodium picosulfate (p.1249·3).
Bowel evacuation; constipation; stool softener.

Guttaplast *Beiersdorf, Ger.*
Salicylic acid (p.1122·3).
Hyperkeratosis.

G-well *Goldline, USA.*
Lindane (p.1434·1).
Pediculosis; scabies.

GX *Pharmacia Upjohn, Ger.; Braun, Ger.; Delta, Ger.; Serum-Werk Bernburg, Ger.*
Carbohydrate infusion (p.1350·1).
Parenteral nutrition.

GX E *Pharmacia Upjohn, Ger.; Braun, Ger.*
Carbohydrate and electrolyte infusion (p.1350·1).
Parenteral nutrition.

Gyalme *Effik, Fr.*
Sodium laurilsulfate (p.1496·3).
Genito-urinary cleansing.

Gydrelle *IPRAD, Fr.*
Estriol (p.1475·3).
Menopausal disorders.

Gynaemine *Sriprasit, Thai.*
Ergotamine tartrate (p.452·1); ergometrine maleate (p.1607·1).
Oxytocic.

Gynamon *Jenapharm, Ger.*
Orange tablets, estradiol (p.1473·1); grey tablets, estradiol; norethisterone acetate (p.1485·1).
Menopausal disorders; osteoporosis.

Gynasan *Bastian, Ger.*
Estriol (p.1475·3).
Menopausal disorders; oestrogenic.

Gynaseptol *Bravir, Braz.*
Hydroxyquinoline sulfate (p.1622·2); boric acid (p.1586·1).
Vulvovaginal infections.

Gynasol *Wild, Switz.†.*
Tartaric acid (p.1669·2); aluminium lactate (p.1578·2); aluminium sulfate (p.1578·2); anhydrous glucose (p.1364·1); sodium bicarbonate (p.1186·2).
Vaginal disorders.

Gynatren *Strathmann, Ger.*
A trichomonal vaccine (p.1566·2).

Gynatrol *Wyeth Lederle, Denm.*
Ethinylestradiol (p.1476·2); levonorgestrel (p.1486·2).
Combined oral contraceptive.

Gynax-N *Ativus, Braz.*
Dexamethasone (p.1067·1); nystatin (p.392·2); neomycin sulfate (p.228·1); tyrothricin (p.267·1); sodium propionate (p.393·2); boric acid (p.1586·1).
Vulvovaginal disorders.

Gynazole *Ther-Rx, USA.*
Butoconazole nitrate (p.381·2).
Vulvovaginal candidiasis.

Gynebo *Chew, Thai.*
Clotrimazole (p.382·1).
Trichomoniasis; vaginal fungal infections.

Gynecort *Combe, USA.*
Hydrocortisone acetate (p.1073·3).
Skin disorders.

Gynecure *Pfizer, Canad.*
Tioconazole (p.395·1).
Vulvovaginal candidiasis.

Gynefix
Besins-Iscovesco, Fr.; Contrel, UK.
Copper-wound polypropylene thread (p.1357·3).
Intra-uterine contraceptive device.

Gynegella P *Guieu, Ital.*
Salicaria; α-ketoglutaric acid.
Vaginal douche.

Gynelle 375 *CCD, Fr.*
Copper-wound polyethylene (p.1357·3).
Intra-uterine contraceptive device.

Gyne-Lotremin
Schering-Plough, Hong Kong; Schering-Plough, Singapore.
Clotrimazole (p.382·1).
Vaginitis; vulvovaginal candidiasis.

Gyne-Lotrimin
Schering-Plough, Austral.; Schering-Plough, USA.
Clotrimazole (p.382·1).
Vulvovaginal candidiasis.

Gyne-Moistrin
Schering-Plough, Canad.; Schering-Plough, USA†.
Polyglyceryl methacrylate; propylene glycol (p.1655·1).
Vaginal dryness.

Gynera
Schering, Braz.; Schering, Denm.; Schering, Hong Kong; Schering, Israel; Schering, Port.; Schering, Singapore; Schering, Switz.; Schering, Thai.
Gestodene (p.1479·1); ethinylestradiol (p.1476·2). 28-Day packs also contain 7 inert tablets.
Combined oral contraceptive.

Gynergen Comp *Novartis, Denm.*
Bellafolin; butalbital (p.658·3); caffeine (p.761·3); ergotamine tartrate (p.452·1).
Migraine.

Gynergene *Novartis, Braz.*
Ergotamine tartrate (p.452·1).
Migraine and other vascular headaches.

Gynergene Cafeine *Novartis, Fr.*
Ergotamine tartrate (p.452·1); caffeine (p.761·3).
Migraine.

Gynescal *CCD, Fr.†.*
Paraformaldehyde (p.1152·2); salicylic acid (p.1122·3); benzoic acid (p.1134·2); borax (p.1586·1); sodium bicarbonate (p.1186·2).
Topical antiseptic.

Gynestin *Kenyaku, Thai.*
Clotrimazole (p.382·1); urea (p.1127·3).
Trichomoniasis.

Gynestrel *Recordati, Ital.*
Naproxen sodium (p.61·1).
Gynaecological disorders.

Gyne-Sulf *G & W, USA†.*
Sulfathiazole (p.257·1); sulfacetamide (p.250·3); sulfabenzamide (p.250·2).
Vaginitis due to Gardnerella vaginalis.

Gyne-T
Janssen-Ortho, Canad.; Janssen-Cilag, Denm.†; Janssen-Cilag, Fr.; Janssen-Cilag, Ger.†; Ortho, Hong Kong; Ortho, Israel; Janssen-Cilag, Neth.†; Janssen-Cilag, UK.
Copper-wound plastic (p.1357·3).
Intra-uterine contraceptive device.

Gynezol *Parke-Davis, S.Afr.†.*
Clotrimazole (p.382·1).
Vaginal fungal infections.

Gyn-Hydralin *Nicholas, Fr.*
Glycine (p.1365·3).
Pruritus.

Gynintim Film *Piette, Belg.*
Nonoxinol 9 (p.1346·1).
Contraceptive.

Gynipral
Nycomed, Aust.; Nycomed, Switz.
Hexoprenaline sulfate (p.766·1).
Premature labour.

Gyno Icaden *Schering, Braz.*
Isoconazole nitrate (p.387·2).
Vulvovaginal candidiasis.

Gyno Iruxol *Knoll, Braz.*
Chloramphenicol (p.179·1); collagenase (p.1598·2).
Vulvovaginal infections.

Gyno Oceral *Asta Medica, Aust.*
Oxiconazole nitrate (p.393·1).
Fungal and Gram-positive vaginal infections.

Gyno-Canesten
Bayer, Ger.; Bayer, Ital.
Clotrimazole (p.382·1).
Balanitis; fungal vulvovaginal infections.

Gyno-Canestene
Bayer, Belg.; Bayer, Neth.
Clotrimazole (p.382·1).
Fungal vaginal infections.

Gynocastus *Zilly, Ger.*
Vitex agnus castus (p.1574·2).
Mastalgia; menstrual disorders.

Gynoco *TO-Chemicals, Thai.*
Nystatin (p.392·2); diiodohydroxyquinoline (p.590·2); benzalkonium chloride (p.1133·2).
Trichomoniasis; vaginal fungal infections.

Gyno-Daktar *Janssen-Cilag, Ger.*
Miconazole nitrate (p.391·1).
Balanitis; fungal vaginal infections.

Gyno-Daktarin
Janssen-Cilag, Aust.; Janssen-Cilag, Austral.†; Janssen, Belg.; Janssen, Braz.; Orion, Fin.; Janssen-Cilag, Fr.; Janssen, Hong Kong; Janssen-Cilag, Irl.; Janssen-Cilag, Israel; Janssen, Mex.; Janssen-Cilag, Neth.; Janssen-Cilag, NZ; Janssen-Cilag, Port.; Janssen-Cilag, S.Afr.; Janssen-Cilag, UK.
Miconazole nitrate (p.391·1).
Vulvovaginal candidiasis with Gram-positive superinfection.

Gynodian Depot
Schering, Aust.; Schering, Ger.; Schering, Ital.; Schering, Spain; Schering, Switz.
Estradiol valerate (p.1473·2); prasterone enantate (p.1488·2).
Menopausal disorders.

Gynodiol *Fielding, USA.*
Estradiol (p.1473·1).
Breast cancer; menopausal disorders; oestrogen deficiency; osteoporosis; prostatic cancer.

Gynoflor
Pharmacia Upjohn, Aust.; Prospa, Belg.; Nourypharma, Ger.; Medinova, Switz.
Lactobacillus acidophilus (p.1626·3); estriol (p.1475·3).
Restoration of vaginal flora; vaginal disorders.

Gyno-Flor E *Medinova, Hong Kong.*
Lactobacillus acidophilus (p.1626·3); estriol (p.1475·3).
Resoration of vaginal flora; vaginal disorders.

Gynofug *Wolff, Ger.*
Ibuprofen (p.43·2).
Inflammation; pain.

Gyno-Fungistat *Cilag, Braz.*
Terconazole (p.395·1).
Vulvovaginal candidiasis.

Gyno-Fungix *Janssen, Braz.*
Terconazole (p.395·1).
Vulvovaginal candidiasis.

Gynokadin *Kade, Ger.; Besins, Ger.*
Estradiol (p.1473·1) or estradiol valerate (p.1473·2).
Menopausal disorders; osteoporosis.

Gynol *Advanced Care, USA.*
Nonoxinol 9 (p.1346·1).
Contraceptive.

Gynol II
Janssen-Cilag, Irl.; Janssen-Cilag, UK.
Nonoxinol 9 (p.1346·1).
Contraceptive.

Gyno-Liderman *Jacoby, Aust.*
Oxiconazole nitrate (p.393·1).
Fungal and Gram-positive vaginal infections.

Gyno-Monistat *Janssen-Cilag, Ger.†.*
Miconazole nitrate (p.391·1).
Balanitis; fungal vaginal infections.

Gyno-Mycel *Sanus, Braz.*
Isoconazole nitrate (p.387·2).
Vaginal candidiasis.

Gyno-Myfungar
Rhein, Mex.; Klinge, Switz.
Oxiconazole nitrate (p.393·1).
Fungal and Gram-positive vulvovaginal infections.

Gynomyk
Will-Pharma, Belg.; Cassenne, Fr.; Will-Pharma, Neth.
Butoconazole nitrate (p.381·2).
Fungal vulvovaginal infections.

Gyno-Mykotral *Rosen, Ger.*
Miconazole nitrate (p.391·1).
Fungal genital infections.

Gyno-Neuralgin *Pfleger, Ger.*
Ibuprofen (p.43·2).
Dysmenorrhoea.

Gyno-Pevaryl
Janssen-Cilag, Aust.; Janssen-Cilag, Belg.; Janssen-Cilag, Fr.; Janssen-Cilag, Ger.; Cilag, Hong Kong; Janssen-Cilag, Irl.; Janssen-Cilag, Israel; ICN, NZ; Janssen-Cilag, Port.; Roche, S.Afr.; Janssen-Cilag, Singapore; Pensa, Spain; Janssen-Cilag, Switz.; Janssen-Cilag, UK.
Econazole nitrate (p.382·3).
Fungal balanitis; fungal vulvovaginal infections.

Gynoplix Theraplix *Vaillant, Ital.†.*
Acetarsol (p.587·2).
Vaginal dryness.

Gynospasmine *Synthelabo, Fr.†.*
Paracetamol (p.71·2).
Fever; pain.

Gynospor *Aspen, S.Afr.*
Miconazole nitrate (p.391·1).
Vaginal fungal infections.

Gynosyl *Homberger, Switz.*
Homoeopathic preparation.

Gyno-Tardyferon *Robapharm, Switz.*
Ferrous sulfate (p.1360·3); folic acid (p.1361·1).
Iron and folic acid deficiency; iron-deficiency anaemia.

Gyno-Terazol
Janssen-Cilag, Belg.; Janssen-Cilag, Neth.; Janssen-Cilag, Switz.
Terconazole (p.395·1).
Fungal genital infections.

Gyno-Travogen *Schering, Aust.; Schering, Belg †; Schering, Hong Kong; Schering, Israel; Schering, NZ; Schering, Singapore; Schering, Switz.*
Isoconazole nitrate (p.387·2).
Fungal and Gram-positive vaginal infections.

Gyno-Trimaze *Aspen Consumer, S.Afr.*
Clotrimazole (p.382·1).
Fungal vaginal infections.

Gyno-Trosyd *Pfizer, Aust.†; Pfizer, Fin.; Pfizer, Fr.†; Pfizer, Hong Kong; Pfizer, NZ; Pfizer, S.Afr.; Pfizer, Singapore; Pfizer, Switz.*
Tioconazole (p.395·1).
Fungal vaginal infections; vaginal trichomoniasis.

Gynovin *Schering, Aust.; Schering, Mex.; Schering, Spain.*
Ethinylestradiol (p.1476·2); gestodene (p.1479·1).
Combined oral contraceptive.

Gynovite Plus *Optimox, USA.*
Multivitamin and mineral preparation with iron and folic acid (p.1350·1).

GynPolar *Orion, Ger.*
Estradiol (p.1473·1).
Menopausal disorders.

Gyrablock *Medochemie, Singapore; Medochemie, Thai.*
Norfloxacin (p.232·1).
Bacterial infections.

Gyramid *Parke, Davis, Aust.†*
Enoxacin (p.201·1).
Bacterial infections.

Gyrol *Brasmedica, Braz.*
Tyrothricin (p.267·1); thymol (p.1158·3); boric acid (p.1586·1).
Vulvovaginal infections.

Gy-Sol *Provit, Mex.*
Gentamicin sulfate (p.210·1).
Bacterial infections.

H1 *Esoform, Ital.*
Glutaral (p.1145·2).
Instrument disinfection.

H 2 Blocker *Ratiopharm, Ger.*
Cimetidine (p.1216·3) or cimetidine hydrochloride (p.1218·3).
Aspiration syndromes; gastro-oesophageal reflux; gastrointestinal haemorrhage; hypersensitivity reactions; peptic ulcer; Zollinger-Ellison syndrome.

H Tussan *Inibsa, Spain.*
Anise oil (p.1580·3); hedera helix; thyme oil (p.1672·3).
Coughs.

Habekacin *Meiji, Jpn†.*
Arbekacin sulfate (p.152·2).
Staphylococcal infections.

Habitrol *Novartis Consumer, Canad.; Novartis Consumer, USA.*
Nicotine (p.1640·3).
Aid to smoking withdrawal.

Habstal-Cor N *Steierl, Ger.*
Homoeopathic preparation.

Habstal-Nerv N *Steierl, Ger.*
Passion flower (p.1649·1); valerian root (p.1678·3).
Insomnia; nervous disorders.

Habstal-Pulm N *Steierl, Ger.*
Homoeopathic preparation.

HAC *Zeneca, Belg.*
Cetrimonium bromide (p.1137·3); chlorhexidine gluconate (p.1138·2).
Burns; disinfection of skin, instruments, textiles, and surfaces; wounds.

Hacdil-S *Zeneca, Belg.*
Cetrimonium bromide (p.1137·3); chlorhexidine gluconate (p.1138·2).
Disinfection of wounds and instruments.

Hachemina Fuerte *Medea, Spain.*
Aminobenzoic acid (p.1516·3).
Alopecia; leucopenia; skin disorders.

Hacks *Ernest Jackson, UK.*
Menthol (p.1632·3); eucalyptus oil (p.1609·2); vitamin C (p.1389·3).
Cold symptoms; coughs.

Hacks Blackcurrant *Ernest Jackson, UK.*
Menthol (p.1632·3); vitamin C (p.1389·3).
Cold symptoms; coughs.

Hactos *Hubert, UK.*
Capsicum (p.1591·1); peppermint oil (p.1243·3); anise oil (p.1580·3); clove oil (p.1597·1).
Catarrh; cold symptoms; coughs.

Hadarax *Greater Pharma, Thai.*
Hydroxyzine hydrochloride (p.419·1).
Pruritus.

Hadensa
Note. This name is used for preparations of different composition.
Kolassa, Aust.; Leiras, Fin.; Ferrer, Spain.
Ointment: Chlorocarvacrol; ichthammol (p.1115·2); menthol (p.1632·3).
Anorectal disorders.

Kolassa, Aust.; Leiras, Fin.
Suppositories: Chlorocarvacrol; ichthammol (p.1115·2); menthol (p.1632·3); chamomile oil.
Anorectal disorders.

Hadiel *Piam, Ital.*
Bezafibrate (p.849·1).
Hyperlipidaemias.

H-Adiftal *ISM, Ital.*
An adsorbed diphtheria vaccine (p.1536·2).
Active immunisation.

H-Adiftetal *ISM, Ital.*
An adsorbed diphtheria and tetanus vaccine (p.1537·1).
Active immunisation.

Haelan *Dista, Irl.; Novex Pharma, UK.*
Flurandrenolone [fludroxycortide] (p.1072·2).
Skin disorders.

Haemaccel
Hoechst Marion Roussel, Aust.; Hoechst Marion Roussel, Austral.; Aventis, Belg.; Hoechst Marion Roussel, Braz.; Aventis, Denm.; Hoechst Marion Roussel, Fin.; Hoechst, Fr.; Hoechst Marion Roussel, Ger.; Hoechst Marion Roussel, Hong Kong; Hoechst Marion Roussel, Irl.; Hoechst Marion Roussel, Israel; Hoechst Marion Roussel, Mex.; Behring, Neth.; Hoechst Marion Roussel, Norw.; Aventis, NZ; Hoechst Marion Roussel, Port.; Aventis, S.Afr.; Hoechst Marion Roussel, Singapore; Hoechst Marion Roussel, Swed.; Hoechst Marion Roussel, Switz.; Hoechst Marion Roussel, Thai.; Hoechst Marion Roussel, UK.
Polygeline (p.741·1) with electrolytes.
Extra-corporeal circulation; organ perfusion; plasma exchange; plasma volume expansion.

Haemanal *Sigmapharm, Aust.*
Hydrastinine hydrochloride; chlorocarvacrol; zinc oxide (p.1128·2); tannic acid (p.1669·1); menthol (p.1632·3).
Anorectal disorders.

Haemate
Centeon, Denm.; Centeon, Ger.; Centeon, Ital.; Aventis, Neth.; Centeon, Spain; Centeon, Swed.
A factor VIII preparation (p.734·1).
Haemorrhagic disorders.

Haemate HS *Centeon, Switz.*
A factor VIII preparation (p.734·1).
Haemorrhagic disorders.

Haemate P
Centeon, Israel; Centeon, UK.
A factor VIII preparation (p.734·1).
Haemorrhagic disorders.

Haematicum Glausch *Terramin, Aust.*
Iron; manganese (p.1350·1).
Tonic.

Haemiton *Asta Medica, Ger.*
Clonidine hydrochloride (p.860·1).
Hypertension.

Haemiton compositum *Asta Medica, Ger.*
Clonidine hydrochloride (p.860·1); triamterene (p.986·1); hydrochlorothiazide (p.907·3).
Hypertension.

Haemo Duoform *Mauermann, Ger.*
Hamamelis leaves (p.1618·3).
Haemorrhoids.

Haemocomplettan
Centeon, Aust.; Centeon, Ger.; Centeon, Switz.
Fibrinogen (p.736·1).
Haemorrhagic disorders; hypofibrinogenaemia.

Haemocomplettan P *Centeon, UK.*
Fibrinogen (p.736·1).
Fibrinogen disorders.

Haemocortin *Streuli, Switz.*
Ointment: Hydrocortisone acetate (p.1073·3); bismuth oxychloride (p.1214·1); lignocaine [lidocaine] hydrochloride (p.1313·2); zinc oxide (p.1128·2).
Suppositories: Hydrocortisone acetate (p.1073·3); bismuth oxychloride (p.1214·1); lignocaine [lidocaine] hydrochloride (p.1313·2); zinc oxide (p.1128·2); ethacridine lactate (p.1130·3); menthol (p.1632·3); adrenaline [epinephrine] hydrochloride (p.829·2); hamamelis (p.1618·3); peru balsam (p.1650·2).
Anorectal disorders.

Haemoctin SDH
Biotest, Ger.; Boehringer Ingelheim, Port.; Biotest, Singapore.
A factor VIII preparation (p.734·1).
Haemorrhagic disorders.

Haemodyn *Klinge, Aust.*
Oxpentifylline [pentoxifylline] (p.950·3).
Peripheral vascular disorders.

Haemo-Exhirud *Sanofi Synthelabo, Ger.*
Leech extract (p.905·3); allantoin (p.1110·1); lauromacrogol 400 (p.1345·2).
Anorectal disorders; urogenital venous disorders.

Haemo-Exhirud Bufexamac Zapfchen *Sanofi Synthelabo, Ger.*
Bufexamac (p.20·3); bismuth subgallate (p.1213·2); titanium dioxide (p.1126·1); lignocaine [lidocaine] hydrochloride (p.1313·2).
Haemorrhoids.

Haemofusin *Pharmacia Upjohn, Ger.*
Pentastarch (p.732·3) in sodium chloride.
Plasma volume expansion.

Haemoglukotest 20-800 *Roche Diagnostics, Ital.*
Test for glucose in blood (p.1616·3).

Haemo-Glukotest 20-800 *Lakeside, Mex.*
Test for glucose in blood (p.1616·3).

Haemolan *Streuli, Switz.*
Ointment: Lignocaine [lidocaine] hydrochloride (p.1313·2); bismuth oxychloride (p.1214·1); zinc oxide (p.1128·2); menthol (p.1632·3); peru balsam (p.1650·2).
Suppositories: Lignocaine [lidocaine] hydrochloride (p.1313·2); bismuth oxychloride (p.1214·1); zinc oxide (p.1128·2); menthol (p.1632·3); peru balsam (p.1650·2); ethacridine lactate (p.1130·3); ephedrine hydrochloride (p.1090·1); hamamelis (p.1618·3).
Anorectal disorders.

Haemomac *CT, Ger.†*
Bufexamac (p.20·3); lignocaine [lidocaine] hydrochloride (p.1313·2); bismuth subgallate (p.1213·2); titanium dioxide (p.1126·1).
Haemorrhoids.

Haemonase P *SA Druggists Self Med, S.Afr.†*
Bromelains (p.1586·3); dl-alpha tocoferil acetate (p.1394·1).
Anorectal disorders; inflammation; oedema.

Haemopressin *Curatis, Ger.*
Terlipressin acetate (p.1298·1).
Variceal haemorrhage.

Haemoproct *Julphar, UAE.*
Tribenoside (p.1674·2); lignocaine [lidocaine] (p.1313·2) or lignocaine [lidocaine] hydrochloride (p.1313·2).
Haemorrhoids.

Haemoprotect *Betapharm, Ger.*
Ferrous sulfate (p.1360·3).
Iron deficiency; iron-deficiency anaemia.

Haemo-Red Formula *Eagle, Austral.*
Multivitamin and mineral preparation with yellow dock and urtica (p.1350·1).

Haemorrhoid Cream *Nelson, UK.*
Homoeopathic preparation.

Haemosol *Eisai, Hong Kong.*
Alpha tocoferil calcium succinate; phytomenadione (p.1396·1); rutoside (p.1611·2); muramidase hydrochloride (p.1638·1); pluronic F-68.
Anorectal disorders.

Haemosolvate *NBI, S.Afr.*
Factor VIII (p.734·1).
Factor VIII deficiency.

Haemosolvex *NBI, S.Afr.*
Factor IX (p.735·1).
Coagulation disorders.

Haemovex 4 *Hospamed, Swed.*
Sodium chloride; potassium chloride; calcium chloride; magnesium chloride; sodium lactate; glucose (p.1184·1).
Haemofiltration.

Haemovex 8 *Hospamed, Swed.*
Sodium chloride; calcium chloride; magnesium chloride; sodium lactate; glucose (p.1184·1).
Haemofiltration.

Haemovital *Pharmadass, UK.*
Vitamin, mineral, and nutritional preparation (p.1350·1).

Haenal *Strathmann, Ger.†*
Quinisocaine hydrochloride (p.1320·2).
Anorectal disorders; insect stings.

HAES *Fresenius Kabi, Aust.*
Pentastarch (p.732·3) in sodium chloride.
Haemodilution; plasma volume expansion; shock.

HAES Esteril *Fresenius Kabi, Spain.*
Pentastarch (p.732·3).
Plasma volume expansion.

HAES-Rheopond *Serag-Wiessner, Ger.*
Pentastarch (p.732·3) in sodium chloride.
Hypovolaemia; shock.

HAES-steril
Fresenius, Belg.†; Fresenius Kabi, Denm.; Meda, Fin.; Fresenius Kabi, Ger.; Fresenius, Israel; Fresenius Kabi, Ital.; Alpha, Mex.; Fresenius Kabi, Norw.; Fresenius Kabi, Port.; Fresenius Kabi, S.Afr.; Fresenius Kabi, Singapore; Fresenius Kabi, Swed.; Fresenius Kabi, Switz.; Fresenius, Thai.; Fresenius, UK.
Pentastarch (p.732·3) in sodium chloride.
Haemodilution; plasma volume expansion; shock.

Hafif *Biogal, Israel.*
Carbaryl (p.1429·2).
Pediculosis.

Haimabig *ISI, Ital.*
A hepatitis B immunoglobulin (p.1542·1).
Passive immunisation.

Haimacig *ISI, Ital.*
A cytomegalovirus immunoglobulin (p.1536·1).
Passive immunisation.

Haima-D *ISI, Ital.*
An anti-D immunoglobulin (p.1532·1).
Prevention of rhesus sensitisation.

Haimaferone *ISI, Ital.*
Interferon alfa (p.628·1).
Malignant neoplasms; viral infections.

Haimalbumin *Nuovo ISM, Ital.*
Albumin (p.724·1).
Hypoalbuminaemia.

Haima-Parot *ISI, Ital.*
A mumps immunoglobulin (p.1551·1).
Passive immunisation.

Haimapertus *ISI, Ital.*
A pertussis immunoglobulin (p.1555·3).
Passive immunisation.

Haimarab *ISI, Ital.*
A rabies immunoglobulin (p.1560·2).
Passive immunisation.

Haimaserum *ISI, Ital.†*
Plasma protein fraction (p.740·2).
Hypoproteinaemia; hypovolaemia.

Haima-Tetanus *ISI, Ital.*
A tetanus immunoglobulin (p.1565·1).
Passive immunisation.

Haimaven *ISI, Ital.*
A normal immunoglobulin (p.1551·3).
Idiopathic thrombocytopenic purpura; immunodeficiency; passive immunisation.

Haimazig *Nuovo ISM, Ital.*
A varicella-zoster immunoglobulin (p.1567·3).
Passive immunisation.

Haiprex *3M, Denm.*
Methenamine hippurate (p.223·1).
Urinary-tract infections.

4 Hair *Marlyn, USA.*
Multivitamin, mineral, and amino-acid preparation (p.1350·1).

Hair Booster *Nature's Bounty, USA.*
Vitamin B substances with minerals, iron, and folic acid (p.1350·1).

Hair Nutrition *Contassium Co., UK.*
Multivitamin and mineral preparation (p.1350·1).

Hair & Scalp *ICN, Canad.; ICN, Hong Kong.*
Pyrithione zinc (p.1122·1).
Scalp irritation; seborrhoeic dermatitis.

Hair and Skin Formula *Vitaplex, Austral.*
Calcium pantothenate (p.1374·1); inositol (p.1623·3); aminobenzoic acid (p.1516·3); ascorbic acid (p.1389·3); dl-alpha tocoferil acetate (p.1394·1).
Multivitamin preparation.

Hairgaine *Agis, Israel.*
Minoxidil (p.934·2).
Alopecia androgenetica.

Hairscience *Ego, Singapore.*
Miconazole nitrate (p.391·1); salicylic acid (p.1122·3).
Dandruff; seborrhoeic dermatitis.

Hair-vit *Pharmadass, UK.*
Multivitamin, mineral, and trace element preparation (p.1350·1).

Halamid *Asta Medica, Ger.*
Nedocromil sodium (p.768·3).
Obstructive airways disease.

Halbmond *Whitehall-Much, Ger.*
Diphenhydramine hydrochloride (p.416·1).
Sleep disorders.

Halciderm
Note. This name is used for preparations of different composition.
Bristol-Myers Squibb, Austral.; Bristol-Myers Squibb, Ital.; Squibb, Neth.†; Squibb, UK.
Cream; ointment: Halcinonide (p.1073·2).
Skin disorders.

Bristol-Myers Squibb, Ital.
Tincture: Halcinonide (p.1073·2); salicylic acid (p.1122·3).
Formerly contained halcinonide, benzoxonium chloride, and salicylic acid.
Skin disorders.

Halciderm Combi *Bristol-Myers Squibb, Ital.*
Halcinonide (p.1073·2); neomycin sulfate (p.228·1).
Formerly contained halcinonide, neomycin sulfate, and nystatin.
Infected skin disorders.

Halcion
Pharmacia Upjohn, Aust.; Pharmacia Upjohn, Austral.; Pharmacia Upjohn, Belg.; Pharmacia Upjohn, Canad.; Pharmacia Upjohn, Denm.; Pharmacia Upjohn, Fin.; Pharmacia Upjohn, Ger.; Pharmacia Upjohn, Hong Kong; Pharmacia Upjohn, Irl.; Pharmacia Upjohn, Israel; Pharmacia Upjohn, Ital.; Pharmacia Upjohn, Mex.; Pharmacia Upjohn, Neth.; Pharmacia Upjohn, NZ; Pharmacia Upjohn, Port.; Pharmacia Upjohn, S.Afr.; Pharmacia Upjohn, Spain; Pharmacia Upjohn, Swed.; Pharmacia Upjohn, Switz.; Pharmacia Upjohn, Thai.; Pharmacia Upjohn, USA.
Triazolam (p.709·3).
Insomnia.

Haldid *Janssen-Cilag, Denm.*
Fentanyl citrate (p.37·1).
Analgesia in anaesthesia.

Haldol
Janssen-Cilag, Aust.; Janssen-Cilag, Austral.; Janssen-Cilag, Belg.; Janssen, Braz.; Janssen-Ortho, Canad.; Janssen-Cilag, Fr.; Janssen-Cilag, Ger.; Janssen, Hong Kong; Janssen-Cilag, Irl.; Janssen-Cilag, Israel; Janssen-Cilag, Ital.; Janssen, Mex.; Janssen-Cilag, Neth.; Janssen-Cilag, Norw.; Janssen-Cilag, NZ; Janssen-Cilag, Swed.; Janssen-Cilag, Switz.; Janssen, Thai.; Janssen-Cilag, UK; Ortho McNeil, USA.
Haloperidol (p.686·3), haloperidol decanoate (p.686·3), or haloperidol lactate (p.687·2).
Alcohol withdrawal syndrome; anxiety; behaviour disorders in children; bipolar disorder; intractable hiccup; movement disorders; nausea and vomiting; psychoses; psychosomatic disorders; stuttering; tics; Tourette syndrome.

Halenol *Halsey, USA.*
Paracetamol (p.71·2).
Fever; pain.

Haley's M-O *Sterling Health, USA.*
Magnesium hydroxide (p.1233·1); liquid paraffin (p.1407·1).
Constipation.

Half Betadur CR *Monmouth, UK.*
Propranolol hydrochloride (p.962·3).

Half Beta-Prograne *Tillomed, UK.*
Propranolol hydrochloride (p.962·3).
Angina pectoris; anxiety; essential tremor; hyperthyroidism; migraine; prophylaxis of gastrointestinal bleeding.

Half Inderal
Zeneca, Irl.; AstraZeneca, UK.
Propranolol hydrochloride (p.962·3).
Angina pectoris; anxiety; essential tremor; hypertension; hyperthyroidism; migraine; variceal haemorrhage.

Half Securon *Knoll, UK.*
Verapamil hydrochloride (p.989·1).
Angina pectoris; hypertension; myocardial infarction.

Half Sinemet
Du Pont, Irl.; Du Pont, UK.
Carbidopa (p.1168·2); levodopa (p.1169·2).
These ingredients can be described by the British Approved Name Co-careldopa.
Parkinsonism.

Halfan
SmithKline Beecham, Aust.†; SmithKline Beecham, Belg.; SmithKline Beecham, Fr.; SmithKline Beecham, Ger.; SmithKline Beecham, Neth.; Smith Kline & French, Port.; SmithKline Beecham, S.Afr.; SmithKline, Spain; SmithKline Beecham, Switz.; SmithKline Beecham, UK†; SmithKline Beecham, USA.
Halofantrine hydrochloride (p.436·2).
Malaria.

Halfprin *Kramer, USA.*
Aspirin (p.14·2).
Myocardial infarction.

Haliborange
Eurospital, Ital.; Boots, NZ; Inibsa, Spain; Seven Seas, UK.
Vitamins A, C, and D (p.1350·1).

Haliborange Calcium Plus Vitamin D *Seven Seas, UK.*
Calcium (p.1187·3); vitamin D (p.1391·1).

Haliborange Halibonbons *Seven Seas, UK.*
Vitamin C (p.1389·3).

Haliborange High Strength Vitamin C *Seven Seas, UK.*
Vitamin C with or without vitamin E and bioflavonoids (p.1350·1).

Haliborange Multivitamins *Seven Seas, UK.*
Multivitamins with or without calcium and iron (p.1350·1).

Halibut
Note.This name is used for preparations of different composition.
Andramaco, Port.
Halibut oil (p.1366·1); zinc oxide (p.1128·2).
Anorectal disorders; skin disorders; vulvovaginal disorders.

Novartis Consumer, Spain.
Benzethonium chloride (p.1134·2); vitamin A (p.1382·1); zinc oxide (p.1128·2).
Burns; cracked nipples; skin irritation; ulcers; wounds.

Adroka, Switz.
Halibut-liver oil (p.1366·1).
Tonic; vitamin A and D deficiency.

Halibut Hidrocortisona *Novartis Consumer, Spain.*
Hydrocortisone acetate (p.1073·3); vitamin A (p.1382·1); zinc oxide (p.1128·2); benzethonium chloride (p.1134·2).
Insect bites; skin disorders.

Halicar *DHU, Ger.*
Homoeopathic preparation.

Halitol *Reig Jofre, Spain.*
Amoxicillin trihydrate (p.149·2).
Respiratory-tract infections.

Halitol Mucolitico *Reig Jofre, Spain.*
Amoxicillin trihydrate (p.149·2); guaifenesin (p.1092·2).
Formerly known as Amoxyvinco Mucolitico.
Respiratory-tract infections.

Halitran *Roche Nicholas, Neth.†.*
Vitamin A (p.1382·1); colecalciferol (p.1391·1).
Vitamin A and D deficiency.

Halivite *Whitehall, Fr.*
Cod-liver oil (p.1357·2); zinc oxide (p.1128·2).
Skin disorders.

Halivol *Warner-Lambert, Austral.†.*
Vitamin A (p.1382·1); ergocalciferol (p.1391·1).
Vitamin A and D deficiency.

Halloo-Wach N *Roland, Ger.*
Caffeine (p.761·3); glucose monohydrate.
Fatigue.

Halls
Adams, Canad.; Adams Confectionery, UK.
Eucalyptus oil (p.1609·2); menthol (p.1632·3).
Cold symptoms; nasal congestion; sore throat.

Hall's Sugar Free Mentho-Lyptus *Warner-Lambert, USA.*
Menthol (p.1632·3); eucalyptus oil (p.1609·2).
Sore throats.

Halls Zinc Defense *Warner-Lambert, USA.*
Zinc acetate (p.1398·1).
Zinc supplement.

Halls-Plus Maximum Strength *Warner-Lambert, USA.*
Menthol (p.1632·3).

Halofed *Halsey, USA.*
Pseudoephedrine hydrochloride (p.1099·2).
Nasal congestion.

Halog
Bristol-Myers Squibb, Aust.; Bristol-Myers Squibb, Braz.; Westwood-Squibb, Canad.; Bristol-Myers Squibb, Fr.†; Bristol-Myers Squibb, Ger.; Bristol-Myers Squibb, Hong Kong; Bristol-Myers Squibb, Norw.; Squibb, Spain; Westwood-Squibb, USA.
Halcinonide (p.1073·2).
Skin disorders.

Halog Neomycine *Bristol-Myers Squibb, Fr.†.*
Halcinonide (p.1073·2); neomycin sulfate (p.228·1).
Infected skin disorders.

Halog Tri *Bristol-Myers Squibb, Ger.*
Halcinonide (p.1073·2); neomycin sulfate (p.228·1); nystatin (p.392·2).
Infected skin disorders.

Halogedol *Fardi, Spain.*
Camphor (p.1589·3); methyl salicylate (p.55·1).
Muscle and joint pain.

Halomed *Medifive, Thai.*
Haloperidol (p.686·3).
Alcohol withdrawal syndrome; anxiety; psychomotor agitation.

Halomycetin *Kwizda, Aust.*
Chloramphenicol (p.179·1).
Bacterial eye infections.

Haloneural *Hexal, Ger.*
Haloperidol (p.686·3).
Psychoses.

Halo-P *PP Lab, Thai.*
Haloperidol (p.686·3).
Anxiety; psychomotor agitation.

Haloper
CT, Ger.; CTI, Israel.
Haloperidol (p.686·3).
Extrapyramidal disorders; pain; psychoses; vomiting.

Haloperil *Psicofarma, Mex.*
Haloperidol (p.686·3).
Psychoses.

Halopol *General Drugs, Thai.*
Haloperidol (p.686·3).
Alcohol withdrawal syndrome; anxiety; behaviour disorders in children; psychomotor agitation.

Hal-oral *Hal, Ger.*
Allergen extracts of pollen, fungi, house dust mites and skin (p.1575·3).
Hyposensitisation.

Haloral *Hal, Neth.†.*
Allergen extracts (p.1575·3).
Hyposensitisation.

Halotestin
Pharmacia Upjohn, Austral.; Pharmacia Upjohn, Canad.; Pharmacia Upjohn, Fr.†; Pharmacia Upjohn, Hong Kong; Pharmacia Upjohn, Israel; Pharmacia Upjohn, Ital.; Pharmacia Upjohn, Neth.; Pharmacia Upjohn, Norw.†; Pharmacia Upjohn, S.Afr.; Pharmacia Upjohn, Singapore; Upjohn, Swed.†; Pharmacia Upjohn, Thai.; Upjohn, USA.
Fluoxymesterone (p.1478·2).
Breast cancer; delayed puberty; male hypogonadism; osteoporosis; postpartum mastalgia.

Halotex *Westwood, USA.*
Haloprogin (p.387·1).
Fungal skin infections.

Halotussin *Halsey, USA.*
Guaifenesin (p.1092·2).
Coughs.

Halotussin-DM *Halsey, USA.*
Dextromethorphan hydrobromide (p.1087·3); guaifenesin (p.1092·2).
Coughs.

Halset *Novartis Consumer, Aust.*
Cetylpyridinium chloride (p.1138·1).
Mouth and throat inflammation.

Haltran *Roberts, USA.*
Ibuprofen (p.43·2).
Fever; osteoarthritis; pain; rheumatoid arthritis.

Halycitrol
Tamar, Israel; Laboratories for Applied Biology, UK.
Vitamin A and D substances (p.1350·1).

Hamadin *Schwabe, Ger.; Spitzner, Ger.*
Saccharomyces boulardii (p.1626·3).
Acne; diarrhoea.

Hamamelis Complex *Blackmores, Austral.*
Hamamelis (p.1618·3); stone root (p.1667·1); plantain seed (p.1652·3); rhubarb (p.1248·1); ascorbic acid (p.1389·3); rutoside (p.1611·2); hesperidin (p.1611·2).
Haemorrhoids.

Hamamelis Compose *Boiron, Fr.*
Homoeopathic preparation.

Hamamilla *Pharmasette, Ital.*
Benzalkonium chloride (p.1133·2); hamamelis (p.1618·3); chamomile (p.1593·2); hypromellose (p.1501·3).
Eye disinfection; eye irritation.

Hamasana *Robugen, Ger.*
Hamamelis (p.1618·3).
Burns; haemorrhoids; skin disorders; varicose veins; wounds.

Hamatopan *Wolff, Ger.*
Ferrous sulfate (p.1360·3).
Iron deficiency; iron-deficiency anaemias.

Hamatopan F *Wolff, Ger.*
Dried ferrous sulfate (p.1360·3); folic acid (p.1361·1).
Iron deficiency; iron-deficiency anaemia.

Hametum
Peithner, Aust.; Spitzner, Ger.; Schwabe, Ger.; Schwabe, Switz.†; TTN, Thai.; Willmar, Thai.
Hamamelis (p.1618·3).
Bleeding gums; epistaxis; haemorrhoids; skin disorders.

Hametum-N
Note.This name is used for preparations of different composition.
Spitzner, Ger.; Schwabe, Ger.
Hamamelis (p.1618·3); aesculus (p.1574·1).
Anorectal disorders; haemorrhoids.

Schwabe, Switz.†.
Hamamelis (p.1618·3).
Haemorrhoids.

HAMFL *Fresenius, Aust.*
A range of electrolyte infusions with or without glucose (p.1184·1).
Haemofiltration.

Hamilton Dry Skin *Hamilton, Austral.*
Bath oil: Light liquid paraffin (p.1407·2).
Bath additive; dry skin; eczema; psoriasis.
Cream: Urea (p.1127·3).
Dry skin.
Lotion: Liquid paraffin (p.1407·1); glycerol (p.1616·3).
Dry skin.
Wash: Soap substitute.
Dry skin.

Hamilton Lip Balm *Hamilton, Austral.*
Octinoxate (p.1517·3); avobenzone (p.1517·1).
Dry chapped lips; sunscreen.

Hamilton Sensitive Broad Spectrum Milk
Hamilton, Austral.
SPF 15: Octinoxate (p.1517·3); titanium dioxide (p.1126·1).
SPF 30+: Octinoxate (p.1517·3); titanium dioxide (p.1126·1); zinc oxide (p.1128·2).
Sunscreen.

Hamilton Skin Repair
Hamilton, Austral.; Hamilton, Hong Kong.
Dimethicone (p.1410·1); cetrimide (p.1137·1).
Dermatitis; dry skin.

Hamilton Solastick Broad Spectrum *Hamilton, Austral.*
SPF 15: Octinoxate (p.1517·3); avobenzone (p.1517·1).
SPF 30+: Octinoxate (p.1517·3); avobenzone (p.1517·1); oxybenzone (p.1518·1); titanium dioxide (p.1126·1).
Sunscreen.

Hamilton Sportblock Broad Spectrum Milk
Hamilton, Austral.
SPF 30+: Octinoxate (p.1517·3); enzacamene (p.1517·2); avobenzone (p.1517·1); titanium dioxide (p.1126·1).
Sunscreen.

Hamilton Sunscreen *Hamilton, NZ.*
Octinoxate (p.1517·3); octisalate (p.1518·1); avobenzone (p.1517·1).
Sunscreen.

Hamilton Sunscreen Clear *Hamilton, NZ.*
Octinoxate (p.1517·3); oxybenzone (p.1518·1); avobenzone (p.1517·1).
Sunscreen.

Hamilton Sunscreen Clear Lotion Broad Spectrum *Hamilton, Austral.*
SPF 15; SPF 30+: Octinoxate (p.1517·3); oxybenzone (p.1518·1); avobenzone (p.1517·1).
Sunscreen.

Hamilton Sunscreen Cream Broad Spectrum *Hamilton, Austral.*
SPF 15: Octinoxate (p.1517·3); octisalate (p.1518·1); avobenzone (p.1517·1).
SPF 30+: Octinoxate (p.1517·3); enzacamene (p.1517·2); avobenzone (p.1517·1); titanium dioxide (p.1126·1).
Sunscreen.

Hamilton Sunscreen 4 Hour *Hamilton, Austral.†.*
Octinoxate (p.1517·3); oxybenzone (p.1518·1); padimate O (p.1518·2); titanium dioxide (p.1126·1).
Sunscreen.

Hamilton Sunscreen Kidscreen, Low Allergy, Sunsport Sunstick *Hamilton, NZ.*
Octinoxate (p.1517·3); titanium dioxide (p.1126·1).
Sunscreen.

Hamilton Sunscreen Low Allergy *Hamilton, Austral.†.*
Octinoxate (p.1517·3); titanium dioxide (p.1126·1).
Sunscreen.

Hamilton Sunscreen Milk Broad Spectrum
Hamilton, Austral.
SPF 15: Octinoxate (p.1517·3); avobenzone (p.1517·1); enzacamene (p.1517·2).
SPF 30+: Octinoxate (p.1517·3); enzacamene (p.1517·2); avobenzone (p.1517·1); titanium dioxide (p.1126·1).
Sunscreen.

Hamilton Sunscreen Quadblock *Hamilton, NZ.*
Cream SPF 40: Octinoxate (p.1517·3); oxybenzone (p.1518·1); padimate O (p.1518·2); titanium dioxide (p.1126·1).
Stick: Octinoxate (p.1517·3); enzacamene (p.1517·2); avobenzone (p.1517·1).
Sunscreen.

Hamilton Sunscreen Quadblock, Water Resistant *Hamilton, NZ.*
Milk (lotion): Octinoxate (p.1517·3); enzacamene (p.1517·2); titanium dioxide (p.1126·1).
Sunscreen.

Hamilton Sunscreen Sunsport *Hamilton, NZ.*
Lotion: Octinoxate (p.1517·3); enzacamene (p.1517·2); avobenzone (p.1517·1).
Sunscreen.

Hamilton Superblock Broad Spectrum Milk
Hamilton, Austral.
SPF 30+: Octinoxate (p.1517·3); enzacamene (p.1517·2); avobenzone (p.1517·1); titanium dioxide (p.1126·1).
Sunscreen.

Hamilton Toddler Broad Spectrum Milk *Hamilton, Austral.*
SPF 30+: Octinoxate (p.1517·3); enzacamene (p.1517·2); avobenzone (p.1517·1); titanium dioxide (p.1126·1).
Sunscreen.

Hamilton Watersport Broad Spectrum Milk
Hamilton, Austral.
SPF 30+: Octinoxate (p.1517·3); enzacamene (p.1517·2); titanium dioxide (p.1126·1).
Sunscreen.

Hamoagil plus *Chefaro, Ger.*
Bufexamac (p.20·3); lignocaine [lidocaine] hydrochloride (p.1313·2); bismuth dihydroxide-(3,4,5-trihydroxybenzoate) or bismuth subgallate (p.1213·2); titanium dioxide (p.1126·1).
Haemorrhoids.

Hamo-Europuran N *Scheurich, Ger.†.*
Lauromacrogol 400 (p.1345·2).
Anorectal disorders.

Hamofiltrasol *Alte Kreis, Aust.*
Anhydrous glucose; electrolytes (p.1184·1).
Haemofiltration solution.

Hamo-ratiopharm *Ratiopharm, Ger.*
Ointment: Butoxycaine hydrochloride (p.1308·2); zinc oxide (p.1128·2); chamomile (p.1593·2).
Suppositories: Bismuth subgallate (p.1213·2); zinc oxide (p.1128·2); chamomile (p.1593·2).
Anal fissure; haemorrhoids.

Hamorrhoidal-Zapfchen *Weleda, Aust.*
Antimony.
Anorectal disorders.

Hamos N *Dr Janssen, Ger.*
Menthol (p.1632·3); aesculus (p.1574·1).
Haemorrhoids.

Hamos-Tropfen-S *Dr Janssen, Ger.*
Aesculus (p.1574·1).
Vascular disorders.

Hamovannad *Bastian, Ger.*
Inositol nicotinate (p.914·1).
Haemorrhoids; peripheral vascular disorders.

Hamo-Vibolex *Chephasaar, Ger.*
Cyanocobalamin (p.1388·1).
Hyperchromic anaemia.

Hand Cream with Sunscreen *Kay, Canad.*
SPF 4: Octinoxate (p.1517·3).
Sunscreen.

Handexin *Rusch, Ital.*
Chlorhexidine gluconate (p.1138·2); aminoxide.
Hand disinfection.

Hanotoxin N *Hanosan, Ger.*
Homoeopathic preparation.

Hanp *Suntory, Jpn.*
Carperitide (p.855·1).
Heart failure.

Hansamed Spray *Beiersdorf, Ger.*
Chlorhexidine gluconate (p.1138·2).
Wound disinfection.

Hansaplast Herbal Heat Plaster *Beiersdorf, UK.*
Capsicum (p.1591·1); arnica (p.1581·3).
Musculoskeletal and joint pain.

Hansaplast Hornhaut-Pflaster *Beiersdorf, Ger.*
Salicylic acid (p.1122·3).
Keratinisation disorders.

Hansaplast Huhneraugen-Pflaster *Beiersdorf, Ger.*
Salicylic acid (p.1122·3).
Corns.

Hansaplast Spruhpflaster *Beiersdorf, Ger.*
Methacrylate copolymer (p.1635·2).
Wounds.

Happinose *Dendron, UK.*
Menthol (p.1632·3).
Nasal congestion.

Haricon *Condrugs, Thai.*
Haloperidol (p.686·3).
Alcohol withdrawal syndrome; anxiety; psychomotor agitation.

Haridol *Atlantic, Thai.*
Haloperidol (p.686·3) or haloperidol decanoate (p.686·3).
Anxiety; behaviour disorders in children; nausea and vomiting; psychoses; psychosomatic disorders.

Harmogen
Pharmacia Upjohn, Irl.; Pharmacia, UK.
Estropipate (p.1476·1).
Menopausal disorders; osteoporosis.

Harmomed *Kwizda, Aust.*
Dothiepin [dosulepin] hydrochloride (p.283·2); diazepam (p.674·3).
Depression.

Harmonet
Wyeth Lederle, Belg.; Wyeth Lederle, Denm.; Wyeth Lederle, Fin.; Wyeth Lederle, Fr.; Wyeth-Ayerst, Hong Kong; Wyeth Lederle, Israel; Wyeth Lederle, Ital.; Wyeth, Neth.; Wyeth Lederle, Port.; Wyeth, Spain; Wyeth, Switz.
Gestodene (p.1479·1); ethinylestradiol (p.1476·2).
Combined oral contraceptive.

Harmonette *Wyeth Lederle, Aust.*
Gestodene (p.1479·1); ethinylestradiol (p.1476·2).
Combined oral contraceptive.

Harmosin *Hormosan, Ger.*
Melperone hydrochloride (p.690·3).
Psychiatric disorders; sleep disorders.

Harnal
Yamanouchi, Jpn; Yamanouchi, Thai.
Tamsulosin hydrochloride (p.978·3).
Benign prostatic hyperplasia.

Harnosal *TAD, Ger.†.*
Sulfaethidole; sulfamethizole (p.253·3).
Urinary-tract infections.

Harnsauretropfen F Syxyl, Ger.
Homoeopathic preparation.

Harnsauretropfen N Syxyl, Ger.†
Homoeopathic preparation.

Harntee 400 TAD, Ger.
Birch leaf (p.1585·2); calendula (p.1589·2); equisetum (p.1606·3); fennel (p.1610·1); couch-grass (p.1599·3); juniper (p.1625·2); liquorice (p.1231·2); ononis (p.1644·1); java tea (p.1625·1); phaseolus vulgaris; solidago virgaurea; bearberry (p.1583·3).
Urinary-tract infections.

Harntee 450 Bad Heilbrunner, Ger.
Birch leaf (p.1585·2); java tea (p.1625·1); solidago virgaurea.
Urinary-tract disorders.

Harntee STADA Stada, Ger.
Bearberry (p.1583·3); birch leaf (p.1585·2); fructus phaseoli; solidago virgaurea; java tea (p.1625·1); equisetum (p.1606·3).
Urinary-tract disorders.

Harntee-Steiner Steiner, Ger.
Silver birch (p.1585·2); java tea (p.1625·1); solidago virgaurea.
Urinary-tract disorders.

Harntreibender Tee Sanova, Aust.
Urtica (p.1678·2); silver birch (p.1585·2); taraxacum (p.1669·1); prunus spinosa; ononis (p.1644·1).
Diuretic.

Harongan Schwabe, Ger.
Haronga.
Dyspepsia.

Harpadol Arkopharma, Fr.
Devil's claw root (p.26·3).
Joint pain.

Harpagin Merz, Ger.
Benzbromarone (p.399·3); allopurinol (p.397·2).
Hyperuricaemia.

Harpagocid Phytomedica, Fr.
Devil's claw root (p.26·3).
Musculoskeletal and joint disorders.

Harpagofito Orto Norman, Spain.
Devil's claw root (p.26·3).
Rheumatic and joint pain.

Harpagoforte Asmedic Dyckerhoff, Ger.
Devil's claw root (p.26·3).
Gastrointestinal disorders; musculoskeletal and joint disorders.

HarpagoMega Twardy, Ger.
Devil's claw root (p.26·3).
Degenerative joint disorders; dyspepsia.

Harpagophytum Complex Blackmores, Austral.
Salix alba (p.82·1); cimicifuga racemosa (p.1595·2); devil's claw root (p.26·3); bryonia alba (p.1587·2); vitamins and minerals (p.1350·1); hesperidin (p.1611·2); rutoside (p.1611·2).
Musculoskeletal and joint disorders.

Hartiosen Inkeysa, Spain.
Devil's claw root (p.26·3).
Rheumatic and joint pain.

Hartmannsche Enzypharm, Aust.
Electrolyte infusion (p.1180·1).
Fluid and electrolyte disorders.

Hartsorb Siam Bheasach, Thai.
Isosorbide dinitrate (p.915·2).
Angina pectoris.

Harzer Hustenelixier Wernigerode, Ger.
Plantago lanceolata.
Catarrh; mouth and throat inflammation.

Harzer Hustenloser Wernigerode, Ger.
Thyme (p.1672·3); cowslip root (p.1600·1).
Cold symptoms.

Harzol Europharm, Aust.; Hoyer, Ger.
Sitosterol (p.970·3).
Benign prostatic hyperplasia.

HA-Tabletten N Boehringer Ingelheim, Ger.
Aspirin (p.14·2); paracetamol (p.71·2); caffeine (p.761·3).
Cold symptoms; fever; neuralgia; pain; rheumatism.

H-Atetal ISM, Ital.
An adsorbed tetanus vaccine (p.1565·2).
Active immunisation.

Hautfunktionstropfen S Cosmochema, Ger.
Homoeopathic preparation.

Hautplus N Dr Hagedorn Naturarzneimittel, Ger.
Homoeopathic preparation.

Haut-Vital N Twardy, Ger.
Vitamins (p.1350·1); calcium lactate (p.1188·2); Saccharomyces cerevisiae (p.1398·1); lecithin (p.1628·1).
Hair, skin, and nail disorders.

Havlane Roussel Diamant, Fr.
Loprazolam mesilate (p.688·2).
Insomnia.

Havrix
SmithKline Beecham, Aust.; SmithKline Beecham, Austral.; SmithKline Beecham, Belg.; SmithKline Beecham, Canad.; SmithKline Beecham, Denm.; SmithKline Beecham, Fin.; SmithKline Beecham, Fr.; SmithKline Beecham, Ger.; SSW, Ger.; SmithKline Beecham, Hong Kong; SmithKline Beecham, Israel; SmithKline Beecham, Ital.; SmithKline Beecham, Mex.; SmithKline Beecham, Neth.; SmithKline Beecham, Norw.; SmithKline Beecham, NZ; SmithKline & French, Port.; SmithKline Beecham, S.Afr.; SmithKline Beecham, Singapore; SmithKline Beecham, Spain; SmithKline Beecham,

Swed.; SmithKline Beecham, Switz.; SmithKline Beecham, Thai.; SmithKline Beecham, UK; SmithKline Beecham, USA.
An adsorbed inactivated hepatitis A vaccine (HM 175 strain) (p.1541·2).
Separate preparations are available for children and adults.
Active immunisation.

Hawaiian Tropic
Note. This name is used for preparations of different composition.
Tanning Research, Canad.
SPF 10: Meradimate (p.1517·3); octinoxate (p.1517·3); oxybenzone (p.1518·1).
SPF 30; SPF 45: Octinoxate (p.1517·3); octisalate (p.1518·1); titanium dioxide (p.1126·1).
Sunscreen.

Tanning Research, USA.
SPF 8+; SPF 10+: Octinoxate (p.1517·3); oxybenzone (p.1518·1); meradimate (p.1517·3).
Gel SPF 15+: Octinoxate (p.1517·3); octocrilene (p.1518·1); oxybenzone (p.1518·1); meradimate (p.1517·3).
Lotion SPF 15+: Octinoxate (p.1517·3); oxybenzone (p.1518·1); meradimate (p.1517·3).
SPF 30+: Octinoxate (p.1517·3); meradimate (p.1517·3); oxybenzone (p.1518·1); octisalate (p.1518·1); homosalate (p.1517·2).
SPF 45+: Octinoxate (p.1517·3); octocrilene (p.1518·1); oxybenzone (p.1518·1); octisalate (p.1518·1); titanium dioxide (p.1126·1).
SPF 45+: Octinoxate (p.1517·3); oxybenzone (p.1518·1); octisalate (p.1518·1); titanium dioxide (p.1126·1); meradimate (p.1517·3).
Sunscreen.

Hawaiian Tropic Baby Faces
Note. This name is used for preparations of different composition.
Tanning Research, Canad.
SPF 35; SPF 50: Octinoxate (p.1517·3); octisalate (p.1518·1); titanium dioxide (p.1126·1).
Sunscreen.

Tanning Research, USA.
SPF 20: Octinoxate (p.1517·3); octocrilene (p.1518·1); oxybenzone (p.1518·1); meradimate (p.1517·3).
SPF 35; SPF 50: Octinoxate (p.1517·3); octocrilene (p.1518·1); oxybenzone (p.1518·1); octisalate (p.1518·1); titanium dioxide (p.1126·1).
Sunscreen.

Hawaiian Tropic Bioshield Tanning Research, Canad.
SPF 15: Octinoxate (p.1517·3); octisalate (p.1518·1); oxybenzone (p.1518·1).
SPF 30: Octinoxate (p.1517·3); octocrilene (p.1518·1); octisalate (p.1518·1); titanium dioxide (p.1126·1).
Sunscreen.

Hawaiian Tropic Cool Aloe with I.C.E. Tanning Research, Canad.
Lignocaine [lidocaine] (p.1313·2); menthol (p.1632·3); aloe vera (p.1110·1).

Hawaiian Tropic Dark Tanning
Note. This name is used for preparations of different composition.
Tanning Research, Canad.
Lotion SPF 4: Octinoxate (p.1517·3); octisalate (p.1518·1).
Formerly contained octinoxate and meradimate.
Oil SPF 4: Octinoxate (p.1517·3); padimate O (p.1518·2).
Sunscreen.

Tanning Research, USA.
Gel SPF 2; gel SPF 4: Ensulizole (p.1517·2).
Oil SPF 2; oil SPF 4: Octinoxate (p.1517·3); padimate O (p.1518·2).
Sunscreen.

Hawaiian Tropic Herbal Tanning Research, Canad.
SPF 4: Octinoxate (p.1517·3); oxybenzone (p.1518·1).
SPF 2; SPF 15: Ensulizole (p.1517·2); sulisobenzone (p.1518·3).
Sunscreen.

Hawaiian Tropic Just For Kids
Note. This name is used for preparations of different composition.
Tanning Research, Canad.
SPF 30: Octinoxate (p.1517·3); octisalate (p.1518·1); titanium dioxide (p.1126·1).
Sunscreen.

Tanning Research, USA.
SPF 30: Octinoxate (p.1517·3); oxybenzone (p.1518·1); octisalate (p.1518·1); homosalate (p.1517·2).
SPF 45: Octinoxate (p.1517·3); oxybenzone (p.1518·1); octisalate (p.1518·1); octocrilene (p.1518·1); titanium dioxide (p.1126·1).
Sunscreen.

Hawaiian Tropic Lipbalm Tanning Research, Canad.†
SPF 45: Octinoxate (p.1517·3); meradimate (p.1517·3); octisalate (p.1518·1); oxybenzone (p.1518·1); titanium dioxide (p.1126·1).
Sunscreen.

Hawaiian Tropic Protective Tanning Tanning Research, USA.
SPF 6: Titanium dioxide (p.1126·1).
Sunscreen.

Hawaiian Tropic Protective Tanning Dry Tanning Research, USA.
Gel SPF 6: Ensulizole (p.1517·2); sulisobenzone (p.1518·3).
Oil SPF 6: Octinoxate (p.1517·3); homosalate (p.1517·2); meradimate (p.1517·3).
Sunscreen.

Hawaiian Tropic Self Tanning Sunblock Tanning Research, USA.
Octinoxate (p.1517·3); oxybenzone (p.1518·1).
Sunscreen.

Hawaiian Tropic Sport
Note. This name is used for preparations of different composition.
Tanning Research, Canad.
SPF 8: Octinoxate (p.1517·3); octocrilene (p.1518·1); oxybenzone (p.1518·1).
SPF 15; SPF 30: Octinoxate (p.1517·3); octisalate (p.1518·1); titanium dioxide (p.1126·1).
Tanning Research, USA.
SPF 15: Octinoxate (p.1517·3); octocrilene (p.1518·1); oxybenzone (p.1518·1).
SPF 30: Octinoxate (p.1517·3); octocrilene (p.1518·1); oxybenzone (p.1518·1); octisalate (p.1518·1); titanium dioxide (p.1126·1).
Sunscreen.

Hawaiian Tropic Sport Sunblock Tanning Research, Canad.
SPF 30: Octinoxate (p.1517·3); octocrilene (p.1518·1); octisalate (p.1518·1); oxybenzone (p.1518·1); titanium dioxide (p.1126·1).
Sunscreen.

Hawaiian Tropic Total Sport Tanning Research, Canad.
SPF 20: Octinoxate (p.1517·3); octisalate (p.1518·1); oxybenzone (p.1518·1).
Sunscreen.

Hawkmide LBS, Thai.
Frusemide [furosemide] (p.893·1).
Hypertension; oedema.

Hawkperan LBS, Thai.
Metoclopramide (p.1236·3).
Gastrointestinal motility disorders; nausea and vomiting.

Hay Fever
Homeocan, Canad.; Hylands, Canad.
Homoeopathic preparation.

Hay Fever Relief Brauer, Austral.
Homoeopathic preparation.

Hay Fever & Sinus Relief Herbal Concepts, UK.
Echinacea (p.1606·2); sambucus (p.1660·3); garlic (p.1614·1).
Catarrh; hayfever; sinus congestion.

Hayclear Novartis, NZ.
Budesonide (p.1064·2).
Allergic rhinitis.

Hay-Crom
Norton Waterford, Irl.; Norton, S.Afr.†; Norton Healthcare, UK.
Sodium cromoglicate (p.774·3).
Formerly known as Eye-Crom in the UK.
Allergic conjunctivitis.

Hayfebrol Scot-Tussin, USA.
Pseudoephedrine hydrochloride (p.1099·2); chlorpheniramine [chlorphenamine] maleate (p.412·1).
Upper respiratory-tract symptoms.

Hayfever Eye Drops Dominion, UK.
Sodium cromoglicate (p.774·3).
Ocular symptoms of hayfever.

Hayfever Relief Thornton & Ross, UK.
Beclometasone dipropionate (p.1061·2).
Allergic rhinitis.

Hayfever & Sinus Relief Herbal Concepts, UK.
Echinacea (p.1606·2); sambucus (p.1660·3); garlic (p.1614·1).
Catarrh; hayfever; sinus congestion.

Haymine Pharmax, UK.
Chlorpheniramine [chlorphenamine] maleate (p.412·1); ephedrine hydrochloride (p.1090·1).
Hypersensitivity reactions.

H-BIG Abbott, USA†.
A hepatitis B immunoglobulin (p.1542·1).
Passive immunisation.

H-B-Vax
Pasteur Merieux, Denm.; Pasteur Merieux, Swed.
A hepatitis B vaccine (recombinant DNA) (p.1542·2).
Active immunisation.

H-B-Vax II
CSL, Austral.; Pasteur Merieux, Belg.; Merck Sharp & Dohme, Hong Kong; Aventis, Irl.; Merck Sharp & Dohme, Mex.; Merck Sharp & Dohme, NZ; Merck Sharp & Dohme, S.Afr.; Merck Sharp & Dohme, Singapore; Merck Sharp & Dohme, Thai.; Pasteur Merieux, UK.
A hepatitis B vaccine (recombinant DNA) (p.1542·2).
Active immunisation.

HB-Vax-DNA
Pasteur Merieux, Fr.; Pasteur Merieux, Neth.
An adsorbed hepatitis B vaccine (recombinant DNA) (p.1542·2).
Active immunisation.

HBvaxPRO Aventis, UK.
A hepatitis B vaccine (recombinant) (p.1542·2).
Active immunisation.

Hc45
Boots Healthcare, Irl.; Crookes Healthcare, UK.
Hydrocortisone acetate (p.1073·3).
Dermatitis; eczema; insect bites.

HC Derma-Pax Recsei, USA.
Hydrocortisone acetate (p.1073·3); mepyramine maleate (p.421·1); chlorpheniramine [chlorphenamine] maleate (p.412·1).
Skin disorders.

HCT Hexal, Ger.; CT, Ger.
Hydrochlorothiazide (p.907·3).
Heart failure; hypertension; oedema.

HCT-ISIS Isis Puren, Ger.
Hydrochlorothiazide (p.907·3).
Heart failure; hypertension; oedema.

HD Braun, Braz.
Electrolytes with or without glucose (p.1184·1).
Dialysis solution.

HD 85 Lafayette, USA.
Barium sulfate (p.1032·1).
Contrast medium for gastrointestinal radiography.

HD 200 Plus Lafayette, USA.
Barium sulfate (p.1032·1).
Contrast medium for gastrointestinal radiography.

Head Cold Relief Brauer, Austral.
Homoeopathic preparation.

Head & Shoulders
Procter & Gamble, Canad.; Procter & Gamble, USA.
Pyrithione zinc (p.1122·1).
Seborrhoeic dermatitis.

Head & Shoulders Intensive Treatment Procter & Gamble, USA.
Selenium sulfide (p.1123·1).
Dandruff; seborrhoeic dermatitis.

Headache Complex Brauer, Austral.
Homoeopathic preparation.

Headache & Migraine Homeocan, Canad.
Homoeopathic preparation.

Headache Relief Brauer, Austral.
Homoeopathic preparation.

Headache Tablets Romilo, Canad.
Aspirin (p.14·2).

Headmaster Seton, Irl.
Phenothrin (p.1436·2).
Pediculosis.

Headrin Extra Strength Reese, USA.
Aspirin (p.14·2); paracetamol (p.71·2); caffeine (p.761·3).

Heads Shampoo Hamilton, Hong Kong.
Econazole nitrate (p.382·3).
Scalp irritation; seborrhoeic dermatitis.

Headway
Pacific, Hong Kong; Pacific, NZ.
Minoxidil (p.934·2).
Alopecia androgenetica.

Heafusine Braun, Fr.
Pentastarch (p.732·3).
Haemodilution; shock.

Heal Aid Plus Reese, USA.
Resorcinol (p.1122·2); phenol (p.1152·3).

Healing Ointment Nelson, UK.
Homoeopathic preparation.

Healon
Pharmacia Upjohn, Austral.; Pharmacia Upjohn, Belg.; Pharmacia Upjohn, Canad.; Pharmacia Upjohn, Fin.; Pharmacia Upjohn, Fr.†; Pharmacia Upjohn, Ger.; Pharmacia Upjohn, Hong Kong; Pharmacia Upjohn, Israel; Pharmacia Upjohn, Ital.†; Pharmacia, Neth.†; Pharmacia Upjohn, Norw.†; Pharmacia Upjohn, NZ; Pharmacia Upjohn, S.Afr.; Pharmacia Upjohn, Singapore; Pharmacia Upjohn, Swed.†; Pharmacia Upjohn, Switz.; Pharmacia Upjohn, Thai.; Pharmacia Upjohn, USA.
Sodium hyaluronate (p.1620·1).
Adjunct in eye surgery.

Healon Yellow
Pharmacia Upjohn, Ital.†; Pharmacia, Swed.†; Kabi Pharmacia, USA.
Sodium hyaluronate (p.1620·1); fluorescein sodium (p.1612·1).
Adjunct in eye surgery.

Healonid
Pharmacia Upjohn, Aust.; Pharmacia Upjohn, Irl.; Pharmacia, UK.
Sodium hyaluronate (p.1620·1).
Adjunct in eye surgery.

Healonid Yellow Pharmacia Upjohn, Aust.†
Sodium hyaluronate (p.1620·1); fluorescein sodium (p.1612·1).
Adjunct in eye surgery.

HealthAid Boldo-Plus Pharmadass, UK.
Boldo (p.1585·3); taraxacum (p.1669·1); bladderwrack (p.1585·2); clivers (p.1596·3); bearberry (p.1583·3); juniper oil (p.1625·2); vitamin B₆ (p.1386·3).
Formerly known as HealthAid AquaFall.
Water retention.

HealthAid FemmeVit PMS Formula Pharmadass, UK.
Multivitamin and mineral preparation (p.1350·1).

Healtheries Musseltone Health Imports, UK.
Green-lipped mussel (p.1618·2).
Musculoskeletal and joint disorders.

Healtheries Musseltone & Glucosamine Health Imports, UK.
Green-lipped mussel (p.1618·2); glucosamine (p.1616·2).
Musculoskeletal and joint disorders.

Healthy Feet Pickles, UK.
Undecenoic acid (p.395·3); dibrompropamidine isetionate (p.1143·1).
Fungal skin infections.

Heartburn & Indigestion Liquid Unichem, UK.
Sodium alginate (p.1498·3).
Dyspepsia; heartburn.

Heartburn Relief Stanley, Canad.
Aluminium hydroxide (p.1210·3); alginic acid (p.1498·3).

Heartline BDI, USA†.
Aspirin (p.14·2).
Myocardial infarction.

Heat Cream *General Drugs, Thai.*
Methyl salicylate (p.55·1); menthol (p.1632·3); eugenol (p.1609·3).
Muscle pain; sprains.

Heat Rub *Stanley, Canad.*
Methyl salicylate (p.55·1); camphor (p.1589·3); menthol (p.1632·3); eucalyptus oil (p.1609·2).
Muscle, joint, and soft-tissue pain; neuralgia.

Heath & Heather Becalm *Peter Black, UK.*
Valerian (p.1678·3); lupulus (p.1629·3); passion flower (p.1649·1).
Stress.

Heath & Heather Inner Fresh Tablets *Peter Black, UK.*
Frangula bark (p.1227·1).
Constipation.

Heath & Heather Quiet Night *Peter Black, UK.*
Valerian (p.1678·3); lupulus (p.1629·3); passion flower (p.1649·1).
Insomnia.

Heath & Heather Skin Tablets *Peter Black, UK.*
Lappa root (p.1627·1); wild pansy.
Eczema; skin blemishes.

Heath & Heather Water Relief Tablets *Peter Black, UK.*
Bladderwrack (p.1585·2); clivers (p.1596·3); ground ivy (p.1618·2); lappa (p.1627·1).
Water retention.

Heb *Pilkington Barnes-Hind, USA†.*
Vehicle for topical preparations.

Hebagam IM *NBI, S.Afr.*
Hepatitis B immunoglobulin (p.1542·1).
Passive immunisation.

Heberbiovac HB *Fustery, Mex.*
A hepatitis B vaccine (recombinant DNA) (p.1542·2).
Active immunisation.

Hebrin *Searle, Braz.*
Iodine (p.1522·3); cade oil (p.1124·3); salicylic acid (p.1122·3).
Fungal skin infections.

Hebucol *Chiesi, Fr.†.*
Cyclobutyrol sodium (p.1601·2).
Dyspepsia.

HEC
Note. This name is used for preparations of different composition.
Chauvin, Fr.; Chauvin, Singapore.
Tannin (p.1669·1); hamamelis (p.1618·3); phenazone (p.77·2).
Haemorrhoids; nose bleeds; wounds.

Chauvin Novopharma, Switz.
Tannin (p.1669·1); pectin (p.1502·3); peru balsam (p.1650·2); hamamelis (p.1618·3).
Mucous membrane disorders of the nose.

Hectonona *Milo, Spain.*
Dried aluminium hydroxide (p.1210·3); magnesium carbonate (p.1232·3); sodium bicarbonate (p.1186·2); tartaric acid (p.1669·2).
Dyspepsia.

Hectorol *Bone Care, USA.*
Doxercalciferol (p.1391·2).
Hyperparathyroidism.

Hedazol *Alpha, Mex.*
Mebendazole (p.102·2).

Hedelix *Krewel, Ger.*
Hedera helix.
Respiratory-tract disorders.

Hederix
Note. This name is used for preparations of different composition.
Saba, Ital.
Codeine hydrobromide (p.26·1); hedera helix.
Coughs.

Plan, Switz.
Noscapine hydrochloride (p.1096·1); hedera; senega (p.1100·2); helenium (p.1089·3); orris; marrubium (p.1094·2).
Coughs.

Hedex
SmithKline Beecham Consumer, Irl.; SmithKline Beecham Consumer, Neth.†; SmithKline Beecham, Spain; SmithKline Beecham Consumer, UK.
Paracetamol (p.71·2).
Fever; pain.

Hedex Extra *SmithKline Beecham Consumer, UK.*
Paracetamol (p.71·2); caffeine (p.761·3).
Fever; pain.

Hedex Headcold *Sterling Health, UK†.*
Oral powder: Paracetamol (p.71·2); phenylephrine (p.1097·1); ascorbic acid (p.1389·3).
Tablets: Paracetamol (p.71·2); phenylephrine (p.1097·1); ascorbic acid (p.1389·3); caffeine (p.761·3).

Hedex Ibuprofen *SmithKline Beecham Consumer, UK.*
Ibuprofen (p.43·2).
Cold and influenza symptoms; fever; pain.

Hedonin *Gerot, Aust.*
Phenylpropanol (p.1650·3); moxaverine hydrochloride (p.1638·1).
Biliary-tract disorders; gastrointestinal disorders.

Heelbalm *Co-Pharma, UK.*
Allantoin (p.1110·1); peppermint oil (p.1243·3); urea (p.1127·3); moisturisers.
Dry, cracked skin on the heels and soles of the feet.

Heemex *Lane, UK.*
Hamamelis (p.1618·3); compound benzoin tincture; zinc oxide (p.1128·2).
Haemorrhoids.

Heer-More *Eagle, Austral.*
Homoeopathic preparation.

Heet
Medtech, Canad.; Whitehall, USA.
Methyl salicylate (p.55·1); camphor (p.1589·3); capsaicin (p.23·1).
Muscle, joint, and soft-tissue pain; neuralgia.

hefasolon *Hefa, Ger.*
Prednisolone (p.1077·3) or prednisolone sodium phosphate (p.1078·1).
Corticosteroid.

Hegor *Procter & Gamble, Aust.*
Shampoo.
Scalp and hair disorders.

Hegor Antipoux *Incomex, Mon.*
d-Phenothrin (p.1436·2).
Pediculosis.

Hegrimarin *Strathmann, Ger.†.*
Silybum marianum (p.1021·3).
Liver disorders.

Heilit *Heilit, Ger.*
Camphor (p.1589·3); methyl salicylate (p.55·1); benzyl nicotinate (p.20·2).
Musculoskeletal and joint disorders.

Heilit Rheuma-Olbad *Heilit, Ger.*
Camphor (p.1589·3); menthol (p.1632·3); methyl salicylate (p.55·1).
Bath additive; musculoskeletal and joint disorders.

Heitrin *Abbott, Ger.*
Terazosin hydrochloride (p.980·1).
Hypertension.

Hekbilin Kapseln *Strathmann, Ger.†.*
Cynara (p.1601·3).
Dyspepsia.

Heksavit *Leiras, Fin.*
Pyridoxine hydrochloride (p.1386·3).
Vitamin B$_6$ deficiency.

Helago-oel N *Helago, Ger.*
Chamomile (p.1593·2); sage (p.1660·2).
Mouth and throat inflammation.

Helarium *Bionorica, Ger.*
Hypericum (p.290·2).
Depression; nervous disorders.

Helastop *Hamilton, Austral.*
Propolis (p.1655·1).
Herpes labialis.

Helberina *Galen, Mex.*
Heparin (p.902·1).

Helcon *Polipharm, Thai.*
Co-dergocrine mesilate (p.1597·3).
Mental function disorders.

Helfergin *Lundbeck, Ger.*
Meclofenoxate hydrochloride (p.1631·3).
Cerebral insufficiency; cerebrovascular disorders.

Helianthus comp *Plantina, Ger.*
Homoeopathic preparation.

Heliclar *Abbott, Belg.*
Clarithromycin (p.186·2).
Helicobacter pylori-associated peptic ulcer.

Heliclear *Wyeth, UK.*
Capsules, lansoprazole (Zoton) (p.1230·3); tablets, clarithromycin (Klaricid) (p.186·2); capsules, amoxicillin (p.149·2).
Helicobacter pylori-associated duodenal ulcer.

Helicocin *Biochemie, Aust.†.*
Oval tablet, amoxicillin trihydrate (p.149·2); round tablet, metronidazole (p.594·1).
Helicobacter pylori infection.

Helicosec *AstraZeneca, NZ.*
Capsules, omeprazole (p.1239·1); capsules, amoxicillin trihydrate (p.149·2); tablets, metronidazole (p.594·1).
Helicobacter pylori-associated peptic ulcer.

Helidac *Pharmacia Upjohn, Austral.*
Chewable tablets, tripotassium dicitratobismuthate (p.1213·2); tablets, metronidazole (p.594·1); capsules, tetracycline hydrochloride (p.258·3).
Peptic ulcer.

Procter & Gamble, USA.
Combination pack: Pink tablets, bismuth salicylate (p.1213·1); white tablets, metronidazole (p.594·1); orange/white capsules, tetracycline hydrochloride (p.258·3).
Duodenal ulcer.

Helifenicol *Ariston, Braz.*
Dextromethorphan hydrobromide (p.1087·3); helicin.
Coughs.

HeliMet *Wyeth, UK.*
Capsules, lansoprazole (Zoton) (p.1230·3); tablets, clarithromycin (Klaricid) (p.186·2); tablets, metronidazole (p.594·1).
Peptic ulcer.

Helimox *Essex, Ital.†.*
Amoxicillin (p.149·2).
Bacterial infections.

Helioban *Galderma, Mex.*
SPF 15: Octinoxate (p.1517·3); titanium dioxide (p.1126·1).
Sunscreen.

Heliobloc *Galderma, Fr.*
SPF 25: Titanium dioxide (p.1126·1); avobenzone (p.1517·1); terephthalylidene dicamphor sulfonic acid.
Sunscreen.

Heliobloc Fort *Galderma, Fr.*
SPF 60: Titanium dioxide (p.1126·1); avobenzone (p.1517·1); terephthalylidene dicamphor sulfonic acid; enzacamene (p.1517·2).
Sunscreen.

Helioblock
Note. This name is used for preparations of different composition.
Galderma, Mex.
SPF 25UVB/15UVA; SPF 60UVB/15UVA: Terephthalylidene dicamphor sulfonic acid; avobenzone (p.1517·1); enzacamene (p.1517·2); titanium dioxide (p.1126·1).
Sunscreen.

Galderma, Singapore.
SPF 25; SPF 60: Terephthalylidene dicamphor sulfonic acid; avobenzone (p.1517·1); enzacamene (p.1517·2); titanium dioxide (p.1126·1).
Sunscreen.

Galderma, Thai.
SPF 25; SPF 60: Eusolex 6300; avobenzone (p.1517·1); mexoryl SX; titanium dioxide (p.1126·1).
Sunscreen.

Heliopar *Orion, Fin.*
Chloroquine phosphate (p.432·3).
Amoebiasis; light-sensitive skin disorders; lupus erythematosus; malaria; musculoskeletal and joint disorders.

Helipak A *Orion, Fin.*
Enteric-coated capsules, lansoprazole (Lanzo) (p.1230·3); tablets, amoxicillin (Amorion) (p.149·2); tablets, metronidazole (Trikozol) (p.594·1).
Peptic ulcer.

Helipak K *Orion, Fin.*
Enteric-coated capsules, lansoprazole (Lanzo) (p.1230·3); tablets, clarithromycin (Zeclar) (p.186·2); tablets, amoxicillin (Amorion) (p.149·2).
Peptic ulcer.

Helipak T *Orion, Fin.*
Enteric-coated capsules, lansoprazole (Lanzo) (p.1230·3); tablets, tetracycline (Oricyclin) (p.258·3); tablets, metronidazole (Trikozol) (p.594·1).
Peptic ulcer.

Heliplant *Kanoldt, Ger.†.*
Silybum marianum (p.1021·3).
Liver disorders.

Helipur *Braun, Ger.; Braun, Ital.*
Chlorocresol (p.1141·3); clorophene (p.1142·3); orthophenylphenol (p.1152·1).
Surface and instrument disinfection.

Helipur H plus *Braun, Ger.*
Glyoxal (p.1145·3); glutaral (p.1145·2).
Instrument disinfection.

Helipur H plus N *Braun, Ger.*
Glutaral (p.1145·2); isopropyl alcohol (p.1149·2); ethylhexanal.
Instrument disinfection.

Helirad *Allen, Aust.*
Ranitidine bismuth citrate (p.1247·2).
Peptic ulcer.

Helis *Bifarma, Ital.*
Benzalkonium chloride (p.1133·2).
Eye disinfection.

Heli-Sal *Strallhofer, Aust.*
Note. A similar name is used for preparations of different composition (see below).
Crataegus (p.1600·2); mistletoe (p.1636·2); garlic (p.1614·1).
Cardiovascular disorders.

Helisal
Note. A similar name is used for preparations of different composition (see above).
Cortecs, Irl.; Cortecs, USA.
Test for *Helicobacter pylori* infection.

Helistat *Marion Merrell Dow, USA†.*
Absorbable collagen sponge (p.1598·2).
Haemostatic.

Heliton *Columbia, Mex.*
Nitazoxanide (p.598·3); tripotassium dicitratobismuthate (p.1213·2).
Peptic ulcer.

Helix I *Braun, Ital.*
Sodium o-phenylphenol (p.1152·1).
Instrument disinfection.

Helixate
Bayer, Aust.; Bayer, Denm.; Centeon, Fin.; Centeon, Fr.; Centeon, Ger.; Centeon, Ital.; Bayer, Neth.; Centeon, Spain; Centeon, Swed.; Centeon, Switz.; Centeon, UK; Centeon, USA.
A factor VIII preparation (recombinant) (p.734·1).
Haemophilia A.

Helixor
Germania, Aust.; Helixor, Ger.
Mistletoe (p.1636·2) from fir trees, pine trees, or apple trees.
Malignant neoplasms.

Helmex *Pfizer, Ger.*
Pyrantel embonate (p.108·1).
Worm infections.

Helmiben *Searle, Braz.*
Mebendazole (p.102·2); tiabendazole (p.109·1).
Worm infections.

Helmidrax *Haller, Braz.*
Mebendazole (p.102·2); tiabendazole (p.109·1).
Worm infections.

Helmifar *Farcoral, Mex.*
Piperazine citrate (p.105·3).
Worm infections.

Helmine *Glaxo Wellcome, Spain.*
Ondansetron hydrochloride (p.1241·3).
Nausea and vomiting.

Helmintal *Sanus, Braz.*
Albendazole (p.95·2).
Giardiasis; worm infections.

Helmintox *Innotech, Fr.*
Pyrantel embonate (p.108·1).
Intestinal nematode infections.

Helminzole *Randall, Mex.*
Mebendazole (p.102·2).

Helmi-Ped *Stiefel, Braz.*
Mebendazole (p.102·2); tiabendazole (p.109·1).
Worm infections.

Helmisons *Sons, Mex.*
Albendazole (p.95·2).
Worm infections.

Helmizil *Heralds, Braz.*
Mebendazole (p.102·2).
Worm infections.

Helo-acid *Rosch & Handel, Aust.*
Citric acid (p.1596·2); tartaric acid (p.1669·2); lactic acid (p.1626·2); pepsin (p.1649·3).
Digestive disorders.

Helol *Italfarmaco, Spain†.*
Tripotassium dicitratobismuthate (p.1213·2).
Gastritis; peptic ulcer.

Helopanflat
Rosch & Handel, Aust.; Knoll, Port.; Knoll, Switz.
Pancreatin (p.1646·1); simeticone (p.1249·2).
Gastrointestinal disorders; preparation for gastrointestinal radiography.

Helopanflat N *BASF, Ger.*
Porcine pancreatin (p.1646·1); simeticone (p.1249·2).
Digestive system disorders.

Helopanzym *Rosch & Handel, Aust.*
Pepsin (p.1649·3); pancreatin (p.1646·1); porcine bile (p.1585·1).
Digestive system disorders.

Helopyrin *Rosch & Handel, Aust.*
Ethenzamide (p.35·1); ascorbic acid (p.1389·3); flavonoids (p.1611·1); rutoside (p.1611·2); ephedrine hydrochloride (p.1090·1).
Cold symptoms.

Helpin *Berlin-Chemie, Ger.*
Brivudine (p.616·2).
Herpes and varicella infections.

Helvamox *Helvepharm, Switz.*
Amoxicillin trihydrate (p.149·2).
Bacterial infections.

Helvecin *Helvepharm, Switz.*
Indometacin (p.44·3).
Gout; musculoskeletal, joint, and peri-articular disorders.

Helvedoclyn *Helvepharm, Switz.*
Doxycycline hyclate (p.200·1).
Bacterial infections.

Helvedstensstifter *Braun, Denm.*
Silver nitrate (p.1664·2).
Hyperkeratosis.

Helvegeron *Helvepharm, Switz.*
Amino-acid, multivitamin and mineral preparation with ginseng and lecithin (p.1350·1).
Tonic.

Helvemycin *Helvepharm, Switz.†.*
Erythromycin ethyl succinate (p.201·2) or erythromycin stearate (p.201·3).
Bacterial infections.

Helveprim *Helvepharm, Switz.*
Co-trimoxazole (p.193·3).
Bacterial infections; blastomycosis; malaria; Pneumocystis carinii pneumonia.

Helver Sal *Bauxili, Spain.*
Aspirin (p.14·2).
Fever; musculoskeletal, joint, and peri-articular disorders; pain; thromboembolism prophylaxis.

Hem Anth *Llorens, Spain.*
Chlorpheniramine [chlorphenamine] maleate (p.412·1); dexamethasone phosphate (p.1067·1).
Eye disorders.

Hem Fe *Wakefield, USA.*
Ferrous fumarate (p.1360·1); vitamin B$_{12}$ (p.1388·1); desiccated gastric substance.
Ascorbic acid (p.1389·3) is included in this preparation to increase the absorption and availability of iron.
Docusate sodium (p.1223·1) is included in this preparation to reduce the constipating effects of iron.
Iron deficiency anaemias.

Hemabate
Pharmacia Upjohn, Hong Kong; Pharmacia, UK; Upjohn, USA.
Carboprost trometamol (p.1441·1).
Postpartum haemorrhage; termination of pregnancy.

Hema-Chek
Bayer Diagnostics, UK; Bayer, USA.
Test for blood in faeces.

Hema-Combistix
Bayer, Austral.; Bayer Diagnostics, Irl.; Bayer Diagnostics, UK; Bayer, USA†.
Test for pH, protein, glucose, and blood in urine.

Hemagene Tailleur *Elerte, Fr.*
Ibuprofen (p.43·2).
Formerly contained aspirin, phenacetin, menthol, and methyl nonyl ketone.
Fever; pain.

Hemapep SA Druggists Self Med, S.Afr.†.
Potassium chloride; sodium chloride; calcium carbonate; glucose (p.1185·2).
Oral rehydration therapy.

Hemarate Biomedis, Thai.; Great Eastern, Thai.
Ferrous fumarate (p.1360·1); vitamins.
Iron-deficiency anaemia.

Hemarexin Technilab, Canad.
Multivitamins; minerals; kola (p.1350·1).
Tonic.

Hemaspan Sanofi Winthrop, USA.
Ferrous fumarate (p.1360·1).
Vitamin C (p.1389·3) is included in this preparation to increase the absorption and availability of iron. Docusate sodium (p.1223·1) is included in this preparation to reduce the constipating effects of iron.
Iron-deficiency anaemias.

Hemastix
Bayer, Austral.; Bayer Diagnostics, Fr.; Bayer Diagnostics, Irl.; Bayer Diagnostics, Ital.; Bayer, NZ; Bayer Diagnostics, UK; Bayer, USA.
Test for blood in urine.

Hematest
Bayer, Austral.; Bayer, Canad.†; Bayer, USA.
Test for blood in faeces.

Hematiase B12 Gross, Braz.
Liver extract; gastric mucosa extract; ferric ammonium citrate (p.1359·2); cyanocobalamin (p.1388·1).
Anaemias; iron-deficiency.

Hematinic Solgar, UK.
Liver (desiccated); vitamin B_{12} (p.1388·1); iron (p.1366·3); calcium ascorbate (p.1389·3); folic acid (p.1361·1).
Dietary supplement.

Hematon Dexa, Fr.†.
Arginine aspartate; cobalt gluconate; manganese gluconate (p.1350·1).
Tonic.

Hematone Thuna, Canad.†.
Vitamin B substances, vitamin C, and iron (p.1350·1).

Hemax Bio Sidus, Thai.
Epoetin alfa (p.731·1).
Anaemias.

Hemax-Eritron Biosintetica, Braz.
Epoetin alfa (p.731·1).
Anaemias.

Hemcort HC
Technilab, Canad.; Technilab, Hong Kong.
Hydrocortisone acetate (p.1073·3); zinc sulfate (p.1398·2).
Anorectal disorders.

Hemedonine Creme d'Orient, Fr.
Haematoporphyrin (p.1618·3).
Tonic.

Hemeran
Note. This name is used for preparations of different composition.
Novartis Consumer, Aust.; Novartis Consumer, Belg.; Novartis Consumer, Port.; Novartis Consumer, Switz.
A heparinoid (p.905·2).
Haematomas; thrombophlebitis; venous insufficiency.

Novartis Consumer, Ger.
Heparin sodium (p.902·1).
Skin trauma; soft-tissue injury.

Hemerven Interdelta, Switz.
Diosmin (p.1611·1).
Peripheral vascular disorders.

HemeSelect SmithKline Diagnostics, USA.
Test for occult blood in faeces.

Hemestal Silanes, Mex.
Hemezol.
Anaerobic bacterial infections; protozoal infections.

Hemetiken Kener, Mex.
Difenidol (p.1222·1).

Hemicraneal Knoll, Spain.
Caffeine (p.761·3); ergotamine tartrate (p.452·1); paracetamol (p.71·2).
Headache; migraine.

Hemi-Daonil
Hoechst, Fr.; Hoechst Marion Roussel, Neth.
Glibenclamide (p.321·3).
Diabetes mellitus.

Hemigoxine Nativelle Procter & Gamble, Fr.
Digoxin (p.870·1).
Arrhythmias; heart failure.

Hemineurin
Astra, Austral.; AstraZeneca, NZ.
Clomethiazole (p.668·2) or clomethiazole edisilate (p.668·2).
Alcohol withdrawal syndrome; disturbed behaviour and sleep disorders in the elderly; insomnia; pre-eclampsia and eclampsia; sedative; status epilepticus.

Heminevrin
AstraZeneca, Denm.; AstraZeneca, Fin.; Astra, Hong Kong; Astra, Irl.; AstraZeneca, Norw.; Astra, S.Afr.; Astra, Swed.; AstraZeneca, UK.
Clomethiazole (p.668·2) or clomethiazole edisilate (p.668·2).
Alcohol withdrawal syndrome; behaviour disorders in the elderly; eclampsia; insomnia; pre-eclamptic toxaemia; psychomotor agitation; sedative; status epilepticus.

Hemipralon URPAC, Fr.
Propranolol hydrochloride (p.962·3).
Cardiovascular disorders; migraine.

Hemo Rekah, Israel.
Ointment: Bismuth subgallate (p.1213·2); benzocaine (p.1306·2); zinc oxide (p.1128·2); chloroxylenol (p.1142·1); zinc sulfate (p.1398·2).

Suppositories: Bismuth subgallate (p.1213·2); benzocaine (p.1306·2); zinc oxide (p.1128·2); peru balsam (p.1650·2).
Anorectal disorders.

Hemo 141 Esteve, Spain.
Etamsylate (p.732·2).
Haemorrhage.

Hemoaenus Simoes, Braz.
Rutoside (p.1611·2); hamamelis (p.1618·3); aesculus (p.1574·1); polygonum acre.
Haemorrhoids.

Hemoal Combe, Spain.
Ephedrine (p.1090·1); benzocaine (p.1306·2).
Anorectal disorders.

Hemobion Merck, Mex.
Ferrous sulfate (p.1360·3).
Iron-deficiency anaemia.

Hemocalcin Vinas, Spain.
Disodium clodronate (p.751·2).
Hypercalcaemia of malignancy; osteolytic bone metastases.

Hemocane
Note. This name is used for preparations of different composition.
Key, Austral.
Lignocaine [lidocaine] (p.1313·2) or lignocaine [lidocaine] hydrochloride (p.1313·2); allantoin (p.1110·1); hamamelis (p.1618·3); zinc oxide (p.1128·2); chlorhexidine acetate (p.1138·2).
Anal pruritus; haemorrhoids.

Eastern Pharmaceuticals, UK.
Lignocaine [lidocaine] hydrochloride (p.1313·2); zinc oxide (p.1128·2); bismuth oxide (p.1213·1); benzoic acid (p.1134·2); cinnamic acid (p.1142·2).
Haemorrhoids.

Hemoccult
Prevention et Biologie, Fr.; SmithKline Diagnostics, USA.
A range of tests for occult blood in faeces.

Hemoce Hoechst Marion Roussel, Spain.
Polygeline (p.741·1).
Perfusion fluid for extracorporeal circulation; plasma volume expansion; shock.

Hemoclar Sanofi Winthrop, Fr.
Pentosan polysulfate (p.953·1).
Soft-tissue disorders; superficial vascular disorders.

Hemocromo Francia, Ital.
Ferric sodium gluconate (p.1360·2).
Iron-deficiency anaemia.

Hemocyte US Pharmaceutical, USA.
Injection: Ferrous gluconate (p.1360·1); vitamin B substances (p.1350·1).
Procaine hydrochloride (p.1319·1) is included in this preparation to alleviate the pain of injection.
Tablets: Ferrous fumarate (p.1360·1).
Iron-deficiency anaemias.

Hemocyte Plus US Pharmaceutical, USA.
Ferrous fumarate (p.1360·1); folic acid (p.1361·1); sodium ascorbate (p.1390·1); vitamin B substances and minerals (p.1350·1).
Iron-deficiency anaemias.

Hemocyte-F US Pharmaceutical, USA.
Elixir: Polysaccharide-iron complex (p.1374·3); folic acid (p.1361·1); vitamin B_{12} (p.1388·1).
Anaemias.
Tablets: Ferrous fumarate (p.1360·1); folic acid (p.1361·1).
Iron-deficiency anaemias.

Hemocyte-V US Pharmaceutical, USA.
Ferrous gluconate (p.1360·1); vitamin B substances (p.1350·1).
Iron-deficiency anaemias.

Hemo-Cyto-Serum Hua, Thai.
Monosodium glutamate (p.1372·2); strychnine sulfate (p.1667·3); iron (p.1366·3).
Anaemias; tonic.

Hemodex Pharmacia Upjohn, Fr.
Dextran 60 (p.729·2) with electrolytes.
Blood volume expansion.

Hemodren Compuesto Llorens, Spain.
Bismuth subgallate (p.1213·2); aesculus (p.1574·1); hamamelis (p.1618·3); hydrocortisone acetate (p.1073·3); ruscogenin (p.1660·2); tyrothricin (p.267·1); amylocaine hydrochloride (p.1306·1); benzocaine (p.1306·2).
Anorectal disorders.

Hemodren Simple Llorens, Spain†.
Ruscogenin (p.1660·2).
Anorectal disorders.

Hemofactor HT Grifols, Spain.
Factor IX (p.735·1); factor X; prothrombin; factor VII (p.733·3).
Clotting-factor deficiencies; haemorrhage.

Hemofer
Note. This name is used for preparations of different composition.
Profarb, Braz.
Iron (p.1366·3); intrinsic factor; liver extract; vitamins (p.1350·1).
Iron deficiency; iron-deficiency anaemias.

Willmar, Mex.
Ferrous sulfate (p.1360·3).

Hemofibrine Spugna Ogna, Ital.†.
Fibrin (p.735·3).
Absorbable haemostatic for dental use.

Hemofil Baxter-Hyland, Ger.
A factor VIII preparation (p.734·1).
Factor VIII deficiency.

Hemofil HT Baxter, UK.
A factor VIII preparation (p.734·1).
Haemophilia A.

Hemofil M
Baxter, Fr.†; Baxter-Hyland, Hong Kong; Baxter, Ital.; Baxter, Port.†; Baxter, Singapore; Baxter, Spain; Baxter, Swed.; Baxter, UK; Baxter, USA.
A factor VIII preparation (monoclonal) (p.734·1).
Haemorrhagic disorders.

Hemofiltracion E2 and E3 Baxter, Spain.
Sodium chloride; potassium chloride; calcium chloride; magnesium chloride; sodium lactate; glucose (p.1184·1).
Haemofiltration solution.

Hemofiltracion E4 and E5 Baxter, Spain.
Sodium chloride; potassium chloride; calcium chloride; magnesium chloride; sodium lactate (p.1184·1).
Haemofiltration solution.

Hemofiltracion HF 01 Fresenius, Spain.
Sodium chloride; calcium chloride; magnesium chloride; sodium lactate; glucose (p.1184·1).
Haemofiltration solution.

Hemofiltracion HF 02 Fresenius, Spain.
Sodium chloride; calcium chloride; magnesium chloride; sodium acetate (p.1184·1).
Haemofiltration solution.

Hemofiltracion HF 11 and HF 23 Fresenius, Spain.
Sodium chloride; potassium chloride; calcium chloride; magnesium chloride; sodium lactate; glucose (p.1184·1).
Haemofiltration solution.

Hemofiltrasol Gambro, Swed.
Anhydrous glucose; electrolytes (p.1184·1).
Haemofiltration.

Hemofiltrationslosning 401 Baxter, Swed.
Anhydrous glucose; sodium chloride; sodium lactate; calcium chloride; magnesium chloride; potassium chloride (p.1184·1).
Haemofiltration.

Hemofissural Baldacci, Port.
Zinc oxide (p.1128·2); titanium dioxide (p.1126·1); hamamelis (p.1618·3); amethocaine [tetracaine] hydrochloride (p.1305·2).
Anorectal disorders.

Hemofluss Fonten, Ital.
Heparin calcium (p.902·1).
Thromboembolic disorders.

Hemogenin Hoechst Marion Roussel, Braz.
Oxymetholone (p.1487·3).
Anaemias; growth retardation; hereditory angioedema.

Hemogrin Al Grin, Mex.
Homatropine (p.468·1).

Hemohes
Braun, Fin.; Braun, Ger.; Braun, Norw.; Braun, Singapore; Braun, Swed.; Braun, Switz.; Braun Melsungen, UK.
Pentastarch (p.732·3) in sodium chloride or electrolytes.
Extracorporeal perfusion; haemodilution; plasma volume expansion.

Hemo-Ice Key, Israel.
Freezable solution in plastic applicator.
Haemorrhoids.

Hemolax Hua, Thai.
Ferrous fumarate (p.1360·1); vitamin B_1 (p.1385·2); vitamin B_6 (p.1387·1); vitamin B_{12} (p.1388·1); cascara (p.1216·1).
Beri-beri; constipation; iron-deficiency anaemia; vitamin B_{12} deficiency.

Hemoleven Lab Francais du Fractionnement, Fr.
A factor XI preparation.
Factor XI deficiency.

Hemoluol Warner-Lambert, Fr.†.
Aesculus (p.1574·1); shepherd's purse (p.1662·3); cupressus sempervirens.
Peripheral vascular disorders.

Hemonet Diafarm, Spain.
Amethocaine [tetracaine] hydrochloride (p.1305·2).
Haemorrhoids.

Hemorhin Hua, Thai.
Docusate sodium (p.1223·1); spermaceti.
Haemorrhoids.

Hemoid For Women Thompson, USA.
Cream: White soft paraffin (p.1407·3); liquid paraffin (p.1407·1); pramocaine hydrochloride (p.1318·2); phenylephrine hydrochloride (p.1097·1); aloe vera (p.1110·1).
Lotion: Liquid paraffin (p.1407·1); yellow soft paraffin (p.1407·3); glycerol (p.1616·3).
Suppositories: Zinc oxide (p.1128·2); phenylephrine hydrochloride (p.1097·1).
Anorectal disorders.

Hemorrane Byk Elmu, Spain.
Hydrocortisone acetate (p.1073·3).
Formerly contained aesculus, benzocaine, hydrocortisone acetate, and prednisone.
Haemorrhoids.

Hemorrhoid Ointment Stanley, Canad.
Pramocaine hydrochloride (p.1318·2); zinc sulfate (p.1398·2).
Haemorrhoids.

Hemorrogel Arkopharma, Fr.
Capsules†: Aesculus (p.1574·1).
Haemorrhoids; peripheral vascular disorders.
Rectal gel: Pilewort (p.1651·3); aesculus (p.1574·1); calendula (p.1589·2).
Haemorrhoids.

Hemorroidex Medic, Braz.
Rutoside (p.1611·2); hamamelis (p.1618·3); aesculus (p.1574·1).
Haemorrhoids.

Hemorrol QIF, Braz.
Rutoside (p.1611·2); aesculus (p.1574·1); hamamelis (p.1618·3).
Venous insufficiency.

Hemosan Sanval, Braz.
Hamamelis (p.1618·3); polygonum acre; aesculus (p.1574·1).
Venous insufficiency.

Hemosedan Centrapharm, Belg.
Prednisolone (p.1077·3); hexachlorophene (p.1146·1); cinchocaine hydrochloride (p.1309·1); belladonna (p.463·1).
Haemorrhoids.

Hemoset A Pharmalink, Swed.
Sodium chloride; potassium chloride; magnesium chloride; calcium chloride (p.1184·1).
Haemodialysis.

Hemoset A glucos Pharmalink, Swed.
Sodium chloride; potassium chloride; magnesium chloride; calcium chloride; anhydrous glucose (p.1184·1).
Haemodialysis.

Hemosin-K Hormonas, Mex.
Carbazochrome sodium sulfonate (p.728·1); vitamin K (p.1395·3).
Haemorrhage.

Hemosol B0 Gambro, Swed.
Sodium chloride; calcium chloride; magnesium chloride; lactic acid or sodium lactate; sodium bicarbonate (p.1184·1).
Haemofiltration.

Hemosol Bicar Hospal, Denm.
Calcium chloride; magnesium chloride; sodium chloride; sodium bicarbonate; sodium lactate (p.1184·1).
Haemodialysis; haemofiltration.

Hemo-Somaton Desbergers, Canad.
Combination preparation: Oral solution, bovine plasma; tablets, multivitamins and minerals (p.1350·1).
Tonic.

Hemo-Somaton with Vitamin C Desbergers, Canad.
Combination preparation: Oral solution, bovine plasma; tablets multivitamins and minerals (p.1350·1).
Tonic.

Hemostatico Antisep Asen Asens, Spain†.
Benzalkonium chloride (p.1133·2); phenazone (p.77·2); hamamelis water (p.1618·3).
Epistaxis; wounds.

Hemotene Astra, USA.
Absorbable collagen (p.1598·2).
Haemostatic.

Hemototal Euro-Labor, Port.
Ferrous gluconate (p.1360·1).
Iron deficiency; iron-deficiency anaemia.

Hemovas Robert, Spain.
Oxpentifylline [pentoxifylline] (p.950·3).
Vascular disorders.

Hemovasal Manetti Roberts, Ital.
Suleparoid (p.978·2).
Soft-tissue disorders; superficial vascular disorders; thrombosis prophylaxis.

Hemovirtu's Virtus, Braz.
Aesculus (p.1574·1); hamamelis (p.1618·3); polygonum.
Haemorrhoids.

Hemovirtu's Pomada Virtus, Braz.
Davila rugosa; belladonna (p.463·1).
Haemorrhoids.

Hem-Prep G & W, USA.
Shark-liver oil; phenylmercuric nitrate (p.1154·1); bismuth subgallate (p.1213·2); zinc oxide (p.1128·2); benzocaine (p.1306·2).
Anorectal disorders.

Hemril Upsher-Smith, USA.
Bismuth subgallate (p.1213·2); bismuth resorcinol compound (p.1214·1); benzyl benzoate (p.1428·2); peru balsam (p.1650·2); zinc oxide (p.1128·2).

Hemril-HC Upsher-Smith, USA.
Hydrocortisone acetate (p.1073·3).

Henexal Pisa, Mex.
Frusemide [furosemide] (p.893·1).

Henofin Ehlinger, Mex.
Astemizole (p.409·1).

Hepa Kolassa, Aust.
Ornithine aspartate (p.1374·1).
Hyperammonaemia associated with liver disorders.

Hepa Factor Sigma-Tau, Spain†.
Folic acid (p.1361·1); cobamamide (p.1388·3).
Folic acid deficiency; liver disorders.

Hepabene Ratiopharm, Aust.
Fumitory (p.1612·3); silybum marianum (p.1021·3).
Biliary-tract disorders.

Hepabionta Merck, S.Afr.
Vitamin B substances (p.1350·1); orotic acid (p.1645·1); folic acid (p.1361·1).
Liver disorders.

Hepabuzone Spirig, Switz.
Heparin sodium (p.902·1); phenylbutazone (p.78·1).
Musculoskeletal, joint, peri-articular, and soft-tissue disorders; peripheral vascular disorders; thrombophlebitis.

The symbol † denotes a preparation no longer actively marketed

Hepacal *Benedetti, Ital.*
Heparin calcium (p.902·1).
Thromboembolic disorders.

Hepacalmina *Prisfar, Port.*
Bioflavonoids (p.1611·1).
Liver disorders.

Hepacap *Medicap, Thai.*
Essential phospholipids and multivitamins (p.1350·1).
Liver disorders.

Hepaccine-B *Biovac, S.Afr.*
A hepatitis B vaccine (p.1542·2).
Active immunisation.

Hepacholine Sorbitol *Synthelabo, Fr.*
Choline citrate (p.1356·3); sorbitol (p.1377·3).
Constipation; dyspepsia.

Hepacitol *Andromaco, Spain.*
Arginine timonacicate (p.1354·1).
Liver disorders.

Hepaclem *Clement Thionville, Fr.*
Cynara (p.1601·3); boldo (p.1585·3); kinkeliba (p.1626·1); curcuma zanthorrhiza.
Digestive-system disorders; renal disorders.

Hepacoban B12 *Bohm, Spain.*
Vitamin B substances (p.1350·1); liver extract.
Tonic; vitamin B deficiency.

Hepacomplet B12 1000 *Reig Jofre, Spain†.*
Vitamin B substances (p.1350·1); liver; adenine hydrochloride (p.1573·2).
Anaemias; tonic.

Hepacomplet B12 Triple *Reig Jofre, Spain.*
Vitamin B substances (p.1350·1); liver; amino acids.
Anaemias; tonic.

Hepadial *Biocodex, Fr.*
Dimecrotic acid, magnesium salt.
Dyspepsia.

Hepadif *Reig Jofre, Spain.*
Oral solution: Carnitine orotate (p.1645·1); carnitine (p.1356·1); vitamin B substances (p.1350·1); liver extract.
Tablets: Carnitine orotate (p.1645·1); vitamin B substances (p.1350·1); liver extract; sorbitol (p.1377·3); adenine hydrochloride (p.1573·2).
Acetonaemia; hepatitis.

Hepadigest *Uriach, Spain†.*
Cyclobutyrol calcium (p.1601·2); metoclopramide hydrochloride (p.1235·2); procaine (p.1319·2); tiopronin (p.1025·1).
Dyspepsia; hepatobiliary disorders.

Hepadoddi *Merck, Port.*
Magnesium dimecrotate.
Biliary-tract disorders.

Hepaduran V *OTW, Ger.*
Silybum marianum (p.1021·3).
Liver disorders.

Hepa-Factor *Max Farma, Ital.*
Folinic acid (p.1363·1); hydroxocobalamin (p.1388·1).
Hyperchromic anaemia; liver disorders.

Hepaflex *Baxter, Fin.*
Heparin sodium (p.902·1).
Thrombosis prophylaxis.

Hepagallin N *Pfluger, Ger.*
Cynara (p.1601·3).
Dyspepsia.

Hepa-Gastreu R7 *Reckeweg, Ger.*
Homoeopathic preparation.

Hepa-Gel *Lichtenstein, Ger.*
Heparin sodium (p.902·1).
Skin trauma; swelling.

HepaGel *Spirig, Switz.*
Heparin sodium (p.902·1).
Peripheral vascular disorders; soft-tissue disorders.

Hepagrisevit Forte-N *Pharmacia Upjohn, Ger.*
Injection: Cyanocobalamin (p.1388·1); folic acid (p.1361·1); nicotinamide (p.1372·3).
Lignocaine [lidocaine] hydrochloride (p.1313·2) is included in this preparation to alleviate the pain of injection.
Tablets: Cyanocobalamin (p.1388·1); folic acid (p.1361·1); pyridoxine hydrochloride (p.1386·3).
Liver disorders.

Hepagrume *EG, Fr.*
Arginine (p.1353·3); betaine (p.1584·3); choline dihydrogen citrate (p.1356·3); inositol (p.1623·3); sorbitol (p.1377·3).
Constipation; dyspepsia.

Hepal *Rigers, Mex.*
Liver extract.

hepa-L 90 N *Loges, Ger.*
Homoeopathic preparation.

Hepalac *Berlin Pharm, Thai.*
Lactulose (p.1230·1).
Constipation; hepatic encephalopathy.

Hepalean *Organon Teknika, Canad.*
Heparin sodium (p.902·1).
Thromboembolic disorders; thrombosis prophylaxis.

Hepalean-Lok *Organon Teknika, Canad.*
Heparin sodium (p.902·1).
To maintain patency of intravenous injection devices.

Hepalin *Bergamo, Braz.*
Adenosine (p.828·2); methionine (p.1012·2); betaine hydrochloride (p.1584·3); choline (p.1356·3); pyridoxine (p.1387·1); sorbitol (p.1377·3).
Liver disorders.

Hepalipon N *Rhenomed, Ger.†*
Methionine (p.1012·2); choline hydrogen tartrate (p.1356·3); inositol (p.1623·3).
Liver disorders.

Hepa-loges N *Loges, Ger.*
Silybum marianum (p.1021·3).
Liver disorders.

Hepa-Merz
Merz, Ger.; Merz, Hong Kong.
Ornithine aspartate (p.1374·1).
Liver disorders.

Hepa-Merz KT *Merz, Ger.*
Ornithine aspartate (p.1374·1).
Liver disorders.

Hepa-Merz Lact *Merz, Ger.*
Lactulose (p.1230·1).
Constipation; liver disorders; salmonella enteritis.

Hepa-Merz Sil *Merz, Ger.*
Silybum marianum (p.1021·3).
Liver disorders.

Hepamig *Welcker-Lyster, Canad.*
Tilia (p.1673·2).
Biliary-tract disorders.

Hepanephrol
Laphal, Fr.; Knoll, Port.
Cynara (p.1601·3).
Formerly contained cynara and hesperidin in *Fr.*
Dyspepsia; fluid retention.

Hepanisan *Heralds, Braz.*
Carnitine (p.1356·1); liver extract; vitamin B₂; vitamin B₆; vitamin B₁₂ (p.1350·1).
Liver disorders.

Hepanutrin
JP, Braz.; Geistlich, UK.
Amino-acid infusion (p.1350·1).
Parenteral nutrition.

Hepaplus *Hexal, Ger.*
Heparin sodium (p.902·1).
Soft-tissue injury; superficial vascular disorders.

Hepa-POS *Ursapharm, Ger.†*
Cynara (p.1601·3).
Dyspepsia.

Hepar 10% *Pharmacia Upjohn, Ger.*
Amino-acid preparation (p.1350·1).
Liver disorders.

Hepar H *Pfluger, Ger.*
Homoeopathic preparation.

Hepar 202 N *Staufen, Ger.*
Homoeopathic preparation.

Hepar Pasc Mono *Koch, Aust.*
Silybum marianum (p.1021·3).
Liver disorders.

Hepar SL *Serturner, Ger.*
Cynara (p.1601·3).
Dyspepsia.

Heparano N *Pfluger, Ger.*
Silybum marianum (p.1021·3).
Liver disorders.

Heparegen *Drossapharm, Switz.*
Timonacic (p.1673·2).
Liver disorders.

Heparexine *Murat, Fr.*
Fosforylcholine magnesium (p.1612·3).
Constipation; dyspepsia.

Hepargitol *Elerte, Fr.*
Arginine hydrochloride (p.1353·3); sorbitol (p.1377·3); anhydrous sodium sulfate (p.1250·1); sodium phosphate (p.1193·2); citric acid (p.1596·2).
Constipation; dyspepsia.

Heparin Comp *CT, Ger.*
Heparin sodium (p.902·1); arnica (p.1581·3); aesculus (p.1574·1).
Soft-tissue injury; superficial vascular disorders.

Heparinol *Streuli, Switz.*
Heparin sodium (p.902·1); thymol.
Haematomas; thrombophlebitis; ulcers; varicose veins.

Heparos *Desbergers, Canad.*
Cyanocobalamin (p.1388·1); ferric ammonium citrate (p.1359·2).
Iron-deficiency anaemias.

Hepar-Pasc *Pascoe, Ger.*
Silybum marianum (p.1021·3).
Liver disorders.

Hepar-Pasc duo *Pascoe, Ger.*
Silybum marianum (p.1021·3); methionine (p.1012·2).
Liver disorders.

Hepar-Pasc N *Pascoe, Ger.†*
Methionine (p.1012·2); greater celandine (p.1618·1); silybum marianum (p.1021·3).
Liver disorders.

Hepar-POS *Ursapharm, Ger.*
Cynara (p.1601·3).
Dyspepsia.

Heparstad *Stada, Ger.*
Cynara (p.1601·3).
Biliary-tract disorders.

Heparsyx *Syxyl, Ger.*
Silybum marianum (p.1021·3).
Liver disorders.

Heparth *20th Century, Mex.*
Heparin sodium (p.902·1).

Hepa-S
Lichtwer, Aust.; Medichemie Bioline, Switz.
Cynara (p.1601·3).
Digestive disorders.

Hepa-Salbe *Lichtenstein, Ger.*
Heparin sodium (p.902·1).
Inflammation; swelling.

Hepasedan *Delta, Braz.*
Vitamin B₁₂ (p.1388·1); methionine (p.1012·2); betaine tartrate (p.1584·3); choline tartrate (p.1356·3); liver extract; gastric mucosa extract; cynara (p.1601·3).
Liver disorders.

Hepasil Composto *Edmond Pharma, Ital.*
Fencibutirol sodium (p.1610·2); rhubarb (p.1248·1); frangula (p.1227·1); cascara (p.1216·1); boldo (p.1585·3).
Constipation.

Hepasol *G.P. Laboratories, Austral.*
Vitamin and mineral preparation with liver extract (p.1350·1).
Tonic.

Hepatamine
Braun McGaw, Hong Kong; McGaw, NZ; McGaw, USA.
Amino-acid infusion (p.1350·1).
Parenteral nutrition in hepatic encephalopathy.

Scientific Hospital Supplies, Israel; SHS, Singapore.
Amino-acid preparation (p.1350·1).
Nutritional supplement in liver disorders.

Hepatect
Biotest, Aust.; Biotest, Ger.; Biotest, Hong Kong; Intra Pharma, Irl.; Biotest, Israel; Biotest, Ital.; Boehringer Ingelheim, Port.; Biotest, Switz.
A hepatitis B immunoglobulin (p.1542·1).
Passive immunisation.

Hepathromb *LAW, Ger.; Brenner-Efeka, Ger.*
Heparin sodium (p.902·1).
Inflammation; swelling.

Hepathrombin *Godecke, Ger.*
Heparin sodium (p.902·1).
Skin trauma; soft-tissue disorders; vascular disorders.

Hepathrombine *Lyron, Switz.*
Heparin sodium (p.902·1); allantoin (p.1110·1); dexpanthenol (p.1602·3).
Scars; soft-tissue injury; venous insufficiency.

Hepatic-Aid *McGaw, NZ.*
Food for special diets (p.1350·1).
Liver disease.

Hepatic-Aid II *McGaw, USA.*
Preparation for enteral nutrition (p.1350·1).
Liver disease.

Hepaticum novo *Pascoe, Ger.*
Curcuma zanthorrhiza; peppermint leaf (p.1243·2); absinthium (p.1571·1).
Biliary disorders.

Hepaticum-Lac-Medice *Medice, Ger.*
Lactulose (p.1230·1).
Constipation; liver disorders; salmonella enteritis.

Hepaticum-Medice H *Medice, Ger.*
Cinchona bark (p.1595·3); silybum marianum (p.1021·3); greater celandine (p.1618·1); gentian (p.1615·1); turmeric (p.1029·3).
Adjunct in skin disorders; biliary disorders; gastrointestinal disorders.

Hepatimed N *Medice, Ger.†*
Greater celandine (p.1618·1); hydrastis (p.1621·1); silybum marianum (p.1021·3).
Acne; biliary disorders; constipation.

Hepato Fardi *Fardi, Spain.*
Choline orotate (p.1645·1); almond milk.
Liver disorders.

Hepatobyl *Breves, Braz.*
Dehydrocholic acid (p.1602·2); ox bile (p.1585·1); boldo (p.1585·3); belladonna (p.463·1).
Liver disorders.

Hepatocler *Heralds, Braz.*
Methionine (p.1012·2); choline chloride (p.1356·3); betaine hydrochloride (p.1584·3); thiamine nitrate; pyridoxine hydrochloride; riboflavin (p.1350·1).
Liver disorders.

Hepatodoron
Weleda, Aust.; Weleda, Ger.†
Fragaria vesca; vitis vinifera.
Constipation; eczema; liver disorders.

Hepato-Drainol *Boiron, Port.†*
Homoeopathic preparation.

Hepatofalk
Note. This name is used for preparations of different composition.
Falk, Ger.
Choline orotate (p.1645·1); adenosine (p.828·2); cyanocobalamin (p.1388·1); hydroxocobalamin acetate (p.1388·3).
Lignocaine [lidocaine] hydrochloride (p.1313·2) is included in the intramuscular injection to alleviate the pain of injection.
Liver disorders.
Falk, Hong Kong.
Injection: Choline orotate (p.1645·1); adenosine (p.828·2); vitamin B₁₂ (p.1388·1).
Lignocaine [lidocaine] (p.1313·2) is included in this preparation to alleviate the pain of injection.
Tablets: Choline orotate (p.1645·1); cysteine hydrochloride (p.1358·3); vitamin B substances (p.1350·1); folic acid (p.1361·1); ox bile (p.1585·1); greater celandine (p.1618·1); curcuma zanthorrhiza; cynara (p.1601·3); taraxacum (p.1669·1); frangula (p.1227·1); rhubarb (p.1248·1).
Liver disorders.

Hepatofalk Neu *Falk, Ger.*
Choline orotate (p.1645·1); cysteine hydrochloride (p.1358·3); vitamins (p.1350·1); ox bile (p.1585·1); ammi visnaga (p.1579·1); absinthium (p.1571·1); boldo (p.1585·3); greater celandine (p.1618·1); curcuma zanthorrhiza; cynara (p.1601·3); taraxacum (p.1669·1).
Liver and biliary-tract disorders.

Hepatofalk Planta
Falk, Hong Kong.
Silymarin (p.1021·3); turmeric (p.1029·3); greater celandine (p.1618·1).
Liver disorders.
Falk, Singapore.
Silybum marianum (p.1021·3); curcuma zanthorrhiza; greater celandine (p.1618·1).
Colic; dyspepsia; liver disorders.

Hepatofalk Planta N *Falk, Ger.*
Silybum marianum (p.1021·3); curcuma zanthorrhiza.
Liver disorders.

Hepato-Flux *Prodotti, Braz.*
Belladonna (p.463·1); boldo (p.1585·3); cascara (p.1216·1); colato; nicotinamide (p.1372·3).
Liver disorders.

Hepatogenol *Profarb, Braz.*
Inositol (p.1623·3); acetylmethionine; vitamin B₁₂ (p.1350·1).
Liver disorders.

Hepatoregius *Dovalle, Braz.*
Pepsin (p.1649·3); pancreatin (p.1646·1); boldo (p.1585·3); cynara (p.1601·3).
Digestive-system disorders.

Hepatorell *Sanorell, Ger.*
Silybum marianum (p.1021·3).
Liver disorders.

Hepatos
Note. This name is used for preparations of different composition.
Hevert, Ger.
Silybum marianum (p.1021·3).
Liver disorders.
Teofarma, Ital.
Cascara (p.1216·1); boldo (p.1585·3).
Constipation.

Hepatos B12 *Teofarma, Ital.*
Cascara sagrada (p.1216·1); boldo (p.1585·3); inositol (p.1623·3); cyanocobalamin (p.1388·1).
Constipation.

Hepatotris *Medic, Braz.*
Methionine (p.1012·2); vitamin B₁₂ (p.1388·1); choline (p.1356·3).
Liver disorders.

Hepatoum *Hepatoum, Fr.*
Oral liquid: Pulsatilla (p.1656·3); turmeric (p.1029·3); peppermint oil (p.1243·3); alverine citrate (p.1211·3).
Formerly contained pulsatilla, turmeric, and peppermint oil.
Gastrointestinal disorders.
Tablets: Pepsin (p.1649·3); pancreatin (p.1646·1); amylase (p.1579·3).
Formerly known as Tridigestine Hepatoum.
Dyspepsia.

Hepatoxane *Esplanade, Fr.†*
Tocamphyl.
Dyspepsia.

Hepatyrix *SmithKline Beecham, UK.*
A hepatitis A and typhoid vaccine (p.1544·2).
Active immunisation.

Hepavax-Gene *Korea Green Cross, Thai.*
A hepatitis B vaccine (recombinant DNA) (p.1542·2).
Active immunisation.

Hepa-Vibolex *MIP, Ger.*
Ornithine aspartate (p.1374·1).
Hepatic encephalopathy.

Hepavirmo *Cazi, Braz.*
Solanum paniculatum; cynara (p.1601·3); boldo (p.1585·3); cascara (p.1216·1); belladonna (p.463·1); liver extract; vitamin B₁₂; magnesium sulfate; nicotinamide (p.1350·1).
Liver disorders.

Hepavit
Note. This name is used for preparations of different composition.
Fresenius Kabi, Braz.
Hydroxocobalamin acetate (p.1388·3).
Anaemias; neurologic disorders.
General Drugs, Thai.
Liver extract.
Anaemias.

Hepavite *Covan, S.Afr.*
Choline bitartrate (p.1356·3); inositol (p.1623·3); methionine (p.1012·2); vitamin B substances; bioflavonoids; magnesium sulfate; zinc sulfate; potassium chloride (p.1350·1).
Hepatic disorders.

Hepavitose *Climax, Braz.*
Ferric ammonium citrate (p.1359·2); vitamin B substances; manganese hypophosphite; copper chloride (p.1350·1).
Iron deficiency; iron-deficiency anaemias.

Hepax *UPSA, Fr.*
Cynara (p.1601·3); kinkeliba (p.1626·1); boldo (p.1585·3); rosemary.
Digestive disorders.

Hep-Flush *Leo, UK.*
Heparin sodium (p.902·1).
Now known as Heparin Sodium ampoules.
To maintain patency of in-dwelling intravenous lines.

Hepflush *American Pharmaceutical, USA.*
Heparin sodium (p.902·1).
To maintain patency of indwelling intravenous catheters.

Hep-Forte *Marlyn, USA.*
Multivitamin, amino-acid, and mineral preparation (p.1350·1).

Heplant *Spitzner, Ger.*
Silybum marianum (p.1021·3).
Liver disorders.

HeplexAmine *Fresenius, UK†.*
Amino-acid infusion (p.1350·1).
Parenteral nutrition.

Hep-Lock *Elkins-Sinn, USA.*
Heparin sodium (p.902·1).
To maintain patency of in-dwelling intravenous lines.

Heplok
Leo, Irl.; Leo, UK.
Heparin sodium (p.902·1).
Now known as Heparin Sodium ampoules in the UK.
To maintain patency of in-dwelling intravenous lines.

Hepofilina *INQ, Braz.*
Adenosine (p.828·2); betaine hydrochloride (p.1584·3); choline (p.1356·3).
Liver disorders.

Heprecomb *Berna, Switz.*
A hepatitis B vaccine (recombinant DNA) (p.1542·2).
Active immunisation.

Hep-Rinse *Leo, Irl.*
Heparin sodium (p.902·1).
To maintain patency of intravenous lines.

Hepro *Casen Fleet, Spain.*
Allantoin (p.1110·1); aminoacridine hydrochloride (p.1130·2); hydrocortisone hydrogen succinate (p.1074·1); lignocaine [lidocaine] hydrochloride (p.1313·2).
Anorectal disorders.

Hepsal
CP Pharmaceuticals, Irl.; CP Pharmaceuticals, UK.
Heparin sodium (p.902·1).
To maintain patency of in-dwelling intravenous lines.

Heptadon *Ebewe, Aust.*
Methadone hydrochloride (p.53·1).
Pain.

Heptalac *Copley, USA†.*
Lactulose (p.1230·1).

Hept-A-Myl
Synthelabo, Belg.‡; Synthelabo, Fr.
Heptaminol (p.1619·2) or heptaminol hydrochloride (p.1619·2).
Hypotension.

Heptan *Aguettant, Fr.*
Minerals and trace element preparation (p.1350·1).
Parenteral nutrition.

Heptovir *Glaxo Wellcome, Canad.*
Lamivudine (p.635·1).
Hepatitis B.

Heptylon *Delalande, Port.*
Heptaminol hydrochloride (p.1619·2).
Alcohol withdrawal syndrome; hypotension; neuromuscular and nervous disorders.

Hepuman
Berna, Belg.†; Berna, Hong Kong; Berna, Spain; Berna, Switz.; Berna, Thai.
A hepatitis B immunoglobulin (p.1542·1).
Passive immunisation.

Hepuman B *Berna, Ital.*
A hepatitis B immunoglobulin (p.1542·1).
Passive immunisation.

Heracillin
AstraZeneca, Denm.; Astra, Swed.
Flucloxacillin magnesium (p.207·1) or flucloxacillin sodium (p.207·1).
Bacterial infections.

Heracline *Technilab, Canad.*
Adrenal cortex extract (p.1080·1); testis extract (p.1492·1); liver extract.
Tonic.

Heractrin *Heralds, Braz.*
Co-trimoxazole (p.193·3); guaifenesin (p.1092·2); ammonium chloride (p.1085·2).
Bacterial infections.

Heralvent *Luhr-Lehrs, Ger.*
Homoeopathic preparation.

Herb and Honey Cough Elixir *Weleda, UK.*
Honey (p.1366·2); althaea (p.1577·1); Iceland moss; marrubium (p.1094·2); pimpinella anisum; sambucus (p.1660·3); thyme (p.1672·2).
Coughs.

Herbadon *Mavena, Ger.*
Devil's claw root (p.26·3).
Musculoskeletal and joint disorders.

Herbagola *Gricar, Ital.*
Cetylpyridinium chloride (p.1138·1).
Oral disinfection.

Herbagyn *Mavena, Ger.*
Cimicifuga (p.1595·2).
Menopausal disorders.

Herbal Anxiety Formula *Faulding, Austral.*
Passion flower (p.1649·1); chamomile (p.1593·2).
Anxiety; nervous tension.

Herbal Arthritis Formula *Faulding, Austral.*
Ginkgo biloba (p.1615·2); devil's claw root (p.26·3).
Arthritis; rheumatism.

Herbal Booster *Pharmadass, UK.*
Kola (p.1681·1); bissy nut (p.1681·1); echinacea (p.1606·2); spirulina (p.1667·1); yellow dock (p.1681·3); ginger (p.1227·2); liquorice (p.1231·2).

Herbal Capillary Care *Faulding, Austral.*
Ginkgo biloba (p.1615·2); aesculus (p.1574·1).
Nocturnal leg cramps; tinnitus; tired legs and feet.

Herbal Cleanse *Vitaplex, Austral.*
Aloes (p.1210·1); taraxacum (p.1669·1); ispaghula (p.1229·1); yellow dock (p.1681·3); sarsaparilla (p.1661·1); lappa (p.1627·1); clivers (p.1596·3); hydrastis (p.1621·1); slippery elm (p.1665·1); echinacea purpurea (p.1606·2); ginger (p.1227·2); silybum marianum (p.1021·3).
Constipation; liver disorders.

Herbal Cold & Flu Relief *Faulding, Austral.*
Echinacea angustifolia (p.1606·2); liquorice (p.1231·2); garlic (p.1614·1).
Catarrh; cold and influenza symptoms.

Herbal Cold Relief *Jamieson, Canad.*
Ephedra (p.1090·1); eucalyptus oil (p.1609·2); grindelia (p.1618·2).

Herbal Cough Expectorant *Jamieson, Canad.*
Elm bark (p.1665·1); eucalyptus oil (p.1609·2); honey (p.1366·2); anise oil (p.1580·3); camphor oil; white pine.

Herbal Digestive Formula *Faulding, Austral.*
Liquorice (p.1231·2); turmeric (p.1029·3); ginger (p.1227·2).
Dyspepsia; flatulence.

Herbal Diuretic Formula *Faulding, Austral.*
Taraxacum (p.1669·1); bearberry (p.1583·3).
Fluid retention.

Herbal Expectorant *Jamieson, Canad.*
Aclenophora; apricot; asparagus officinalis; citrus reticulata; ginger; liquorice; mulberry; ophiopogon japonicus; schizandra; skullcap.

Herbal Eye Care Formula *Faulding, Austral.*
Myrtillus (p.1639·2).
Eye disorders.

Herbal Headache Relief *Faulding, Austral.*
Feverfew (p.453·3).
Headache.

Herbal Indigestion Naturtabs *Cantassium Co., UK.*
Skullcap (p.1664·3); valerian (p.1678·3); fennel (p.1610·1); myrrh (p.1639·2); papain (p.1647·3); capsicum oleoresin (p.1591·1).

Herbal Laxative
Note. This name is used for preparations of different composition.
Vitaplex, Austral.‡.
Senna (p.1248·2); ispaghula (p.1229·1); liquorice (p.1231·2).
Constipation.

Quest, Canad.
Cascara (p.1216·1); rhubarb (p.1248·1).

Shaklee, Canad.
Senna (p.1248·2).
Formerly contained senna, buckthorn, and leptandra virginica.
Constipation.

Swiss Herbal, Canad.
Senna leaves (p.1248·2); cascara (p.1216·1); rhubarb root (p.1248·1); gentian root (p.1615·1); liquorice root (p.1231·2); juniper berries (p.1625·2); buchu leaves (p.1587·2); peppermint oil (p.1243·3).
Constipation.

Nature's Bounty, USA†.
Senna (p.1248·2); cascara (p.1216·1).
Constipation.

Herbal Liver Formula *Faulding, Austral.*
Silybum marianum (p.1021·3).
Digestive disorders; liver disorders.

Herbal Nerve *Swiss Herbal, Canad.*
Valerian root (p.1678·3); skullcap (p.1664·3); gentian root (p.1615·1); liquorice (p.1231·2).

Herbal Pain Relief *Cantassium Co., UK.*
Salix bark (p.82·1); passion flower (p.1649·1); valerian (p.1678·3).
Pain.

Herbal PMS Formula *Faulding, Austral.*
Myrtillus (p.1639·2); liquorice (p.1231·2); cimicifuga (p.1595·2).
Menstrual disorders.

Herbal Premens *Swisshealth, UK.*
Agnus castus (p.1574·2).
Premenstrual syndrome.

Herbal Sleep Aid *Wampole, Canad.*
Lupulus (p.1629·3); passion flower (p.1649·1); valerian (p.1678·3).
Sleep disorders.

Herbal Sleep Formula *Faulding, Austral.*
Valerian (p.1678·3).
Insomnia.

Herbal Stress Relief *Faulding, Austral.*
Ginseng (p.1615·3).
Stress.

Herbal Throat *Jamieson, Canad.*
Camphor (p.1589·3); elm bark (p.1665·1); marrubium (p.1094·2); menthol (p.1632·3); parsley (p.1648·3); thyme (p.1672·2).

Herb-a-Lax *Blooms, Austral.*
Senna (p.1248·2); frangula bark (p.1227·1); ispaghula (p.1229·1); dill seed; liquorice (p.1231·2).
Constipation.

Herbalax *Sante Naturelle, Canad.*
Cascara (p.1216·1); frangula (p.1227·1); rhubarb (p.1248·1); senna (p.1248·2); bile salts (p.1585·1).

Herbalax Forte *Sante Naturelle, Canad.†.*
Cascara (p.1216·1); phenolphthalein (p.1244·1); bile salts (p.1585·1); capsicum oleoresin (p.1591·1); papain (p.1647·3).

Herbaneurin *Mavena, Ger.*
Hypericum (p.290·2).
Depression.

Herbatar *Erredici, Ital.*
Cream: Pine oil; birch oil (p.1124·3); castor oil (p.1592·1); chamomile (p.1593·2); allantoin (p.1110·1).
Skin disorders.
Scalp application: Pine oil; birch oil (p.1124·3); cedar oil.
Seborrhoeic dermatitis.

Herbatar Plus *Erredici, Ital.*
Ammonium lactate (p.1110·3); tar (p.1125·1); allantoin (p.1110·1).
Hyperkeratosis.

Herbatorment *Herbapharm, Ger.†.*
Tormentil (p.1674·1).
Diarrhoea.

Herbavit *Erredici, Ital.*
Biotin (p.1355·3); a heparinoid (p.905·2); arnica (p.1581·3); urtica (p.1678·2); polyglycopolyamine; dexpanthenol (p.1602·3); menthol (p.1632·3).
Prevention of hair loss.

Herbe *Recordati, Ital.*
Benzalkonium chloride (p.1133·2); hamamelis (p.1618·3).
Eye disinfection.

Herbelax *Sanochemia, Aust.*
Calcium sennoside A (p.1248·3); calcium sennoside B (p.1248·3); bran (p.1214·2); fig (p.1227·1).
Bowel evacuation; constipation; stool softener.

Herbelix *Lane, UK.*
Lobelia (p.1510·2); tolu solution; sodium bicarbonate (p.1186·2).
Nasal congestion.

Herbesan *Warner-Lambert, Fr.*
Senna (p.1248·2); aniseed (p.1580·2); peppermint leaf (p.1243·2); couch-grass (p.1599·3).
Constipation.

Herbesan Instantane *Warner-Lambert, Fr.*
Sennosides B (p.1248·3).
Constipation.

Herbesser
Tanabe, Hong Kong; Tanabe, Jpn; Delta, Port.; Tanabe, Singapore; Tanabe, Thai.
Diltiazem hydrochloride (p.874·3).
Angina pectoris; arrhythmias; hypertension.

Herb-Fibe *Shaklee, Canad.*
Fibre.
Constipation.

Herbheal Ointment *Potter's, UK.*
Colophony (p.1598·3); starch (p.1379·3); sublimed sulfur (p.1123·3); zinc oxide (p.1128·2); althaea root (p.1577·1); stellaria media.
Skin irritation.

Herbogesic *Seroyal, Canad.*
Magnesium salicylate (p.50·3).

Herbolax *Seroyal, Canad.*
Cascara (p.1216·1); rhubarb (p.1248·1); senna (p.1248·2); liquorice (p.1231·2).

Herbopyrine *Herbes Universelles, Canad.*
Aspirin (p.14·2); caffeine citrate (p.761·3).

Herborex *Rolmex, Canad.*
Cascara (p.1216·1); yellow dock (p.1681·3).

Herbulax *Peter Black, UK.*
Frangula bark (p.1227·1); taraxacum (p.1669·1).
Constipation.

Herceptin
Roche, Austral.; Roche, Fr.; Roche, Irl.; Roche, Singapore; Roche, Switz.; Roche, UK; Genentech, USA.
Trastuzumab (p.576·1).
Breast cancer.

Herden *Remedica, Thai.*
Oxpentifylline [pentoxifylline] (p.950·3).
Peripheral vascular disorders.

Herisan *Rougier, Canad.*
Zinc oxide (p.1128·2).
Superficial skin irritations.

Herklin *Armstrong, Mex.*
Lotion: Lindane (p.1434·1); lignocaine [lidocaine] (p.1313·2).
Shampoo: Lindane (p.1434·1).
Pediculosis; scabies.

Hermal *Merck-Clevenot, Fr.†.*
Pyrithione zinc (p.1122·1).
Seborrhoeic dermatitis.

Hermalind *Hermal, Ger.*
Dexpanthenol (p.1602·3); chlorhexidine gluconate (p.1138·2).
Burns; wounds.

Hermasept *Merck, Aust.†.*
Dexpanthenol (p.1602·3); chlorhexidine gluconate (p.1138·2).
Burns; infected wounds.

Hermes ASS *Hermes, Ger.*
Aspirin (p.14·2).
Fever; pain.

Hermes ASS plus *Hermes, Ger.†.*
Aspirin (p.14·2); caffeine (p.761·3).
Pain.

Hermes Cevitt *Hermes, Ger.*
Ascorbic acid (p.1389·3).
Vitamin C deficiency.

Hermes Cevitt + Calcium *Hermes, Ger.†.*
Ascorbic acid (p.1389·3); calcium carbonate (p.1215·1).
Vitamin C and calcium deficiency.

Hermes Drix Abfuhr-Tee *Hermes, Ger.†.*
Senna (p.1248·2).
Constipation.

Hermixsofex *Sofex, Port.†.*
Aciclovir (p.612·3).
Herpes simplex infections.

Hermocil *Ofalder, Port.*
Aciclovir (p.612·3).

Hermolepsin *Orion, Swed.*
Carbamazepine (p.342·2).
Alcohol withdrawal syndrome; epilepsy; trigeminal neuralgia.

Hernia-Tee *Steierl, Ger.†.*
Bearberry (p.1583·3); herniaria (p.1619·2); equisetum (p.1606·3).
Urinary-tract disorders.

Hernidisc *Eagle, Austral.*
Homoeopathic preparation.

Herniol *Steierl, Ger.*
Bearberry (p.1583·3); herniaria (p.1619·2).
Urinary-tract disorders.

Heroid *Chew, Thai.*
Diosmin (p.1611·1); hesperidin (p.1611·2).
Haemorrhoids; phlebitis; varicose veins; venous insufficiency.

Herpecin-L *Chattem, USA.*
Allantoin (p.1110·1); padimate O (p.1518·2).
Oral lesions.

Herpen *Sumitomo, Jpn†.*
Ampicillin sodium (p.150·3).
Bacterial infections.

Herpenon *Polipharm, Thai.*
Aciclovir (p.612·3).
Herpes simplex infections of the skin and mucous membranes.

Herpes Soothing Cream *Homeocan, Canad.*
Homoeopathic preparation.

Herpesan
Rowa, Hong Kong; Rowa, Singapore.
Carbenoxolone sodium (p.1215·3).
Orofacial lesions.

Herpes-Gel *Master Pharma, Ital.†.*
Ibacitabine (p.625·1).
Herpesvirus infections.

Herpesine *Nikkho, Braz.*
Idoxuridine (p.625·1); thiomersal (p.1158·2).
Herpesvirus skin infections.

Herpesnil *Sofar, Ital.*
Aciclovir (p.612·3).
Herpesvirus infections.

Herpetad
TAD, Ger.; Boehringer Ingelheim, UK.
Aciclovir (p.612·3).
Herpes simplex infections.

Herpetrol *Alva, USA.*
Multivitamin preparation with zinc and lysine (p.1350·1).

Herpex
Note. This name is used for preparations of different composition.
Germania, Aust.†.
Bacillus subtilis.
Herpes zoster infection.

Searle, Braz.
Tromantadine hydrochloride (p.642·3).
Viral skin infections.

Herphonal *Dresden, Ger.; Temmler, Ger.*
Trimipramine maleate (p.311·2).
Depression; pain.

Herpid *Yamanouchi, UK.*
Idoxuridine (p.625·1) in dimethyl sulfoxide.
Herpesvirus skin infections.

Herpidu
Ciba Vision, Hong Kong; Ciba Vision, Thai.
Idoxuridine (p.625·1).
Herpes simplex infections of the eye.

Herpilem *Lemery, Mex.*
Aciclovir (p.612·3).
Herpesvirus infections.

Herplex
Allergan, Canad.; Allergan, Hong Kong; Allergan, USA†.
Idoxuridine (p.625·1).
Herpes simplex keratitis.

Herplex Liquifilm *Allergan, Austral.†.*
Idoxuridine (p.625·1).
Herpes simplex infections of the eye.

Herplex-D
Allergan, Austral.; Allergan, S.Afr.†.
Idoxuridine (p.625·1).
Herpes simplex skin infections.

Herpofug *Berner, Fin.*
Aciclovir (p.612·3).
Herpesvirus infections.

Herpolips *Berner, Fin.*
Aciclovir (p.612·3).
Herpes labialis.

Herposicc *Nycomed, Aust.*
Benzocaine (p.1306·2); sulfur (p.1123·3); zinc oxide (p.1128·2); talc (p.1124·2); phenol (p.1152·3).
Herpes labialis.

Herpotern *Rentschler, Ger.†*
Aciclovir sodium (p.612·3).
Herpes and varicella virus infections.

Herpoviric *Azupharma, Ger.†*
Aciclovir (p.612·3).
Herpesvirus infections.

Herron Baby Teething Gel *Herron, Austral.*
Choline salicylate (p.24·3).
Sore gums; teething pain.

Herten *Vir, Spain.*
Enalapril maleate (p.883·3).
Heart failure; hypertension.

Herviros
Hermal, Aust.; Hermal, Ger.; Hermal, Hong Kong.
Amethocaine [tetracaine] hydrochloride (p.1305·2); aminoquinuride hydrochloride (p.1133·1).
Infected mouth disorders.

Herz- und Kreislauftonikum Bioflora *Bioflora, Aust.*
Crataegus (p.1600·2); mistletoe (p.1636·2); melissa (p.1632·2); rosemary; lavender flower (p.1627·2).
Cardiovascular disorders.

HerzASS *Ratiopharm, Ger.*
Aspirin (p.14·2).
Thrombosis prophylaxis.

Herz-Punkt Starkungstonikum mit Ginseng N *Herzpunkt, Ger.*
Ginseng (p.1615·3).
Tonic.

Herz-Punkt Vitaltonikum N *Herzpunkt, Ger.*
Crataegus; melissa; ferrous gluconate (p.1350·1).
Tonic.

Herz-Starkung N *Jukunda, Ger.*
Crataegus (p.1600·2); lycopus virg.; cactus; kalmia latifolia; camphora.
Cardiac disorders.

Herztropfen CM *Cosmochema, Ger.*
Homoeopathic preparation.

Herz-Tropfen Eu Rho *Eu Rho, Ger.*
Crataegus (p.1600·2).
Cardiac disorders.

Herztropfen Truw Gold *Truw, Ger.†*
Homoeopathic preparation.

Hespan *Geistlich, UK; Du Pont, USA.*
Hetastarch (p.732·3) in sodium chloride.
Extracorporeal circulation; leucopheresis; plasma volume expansion.

Hespander *Kyorin, Jpn; Kyorin, Thai.*
Hetastarch (p.732·3) in glucose with electrolytes.
Haemodiluent; plasma volume expansion.

Hespercorbin *Fides Rottapharm, Spain.*
Glucosamine sulfate (p.1616·2).
Arthrosis.

Hesteril *Fresenius Kabi, Fr.*
Pentastarch (p.732·3).
Haemodilution; plasma volume expansion.

Heteroid *Chew, Thai.*
Diosmin (p.1611·1).
Haemorrhoids; phlebitis; varicose veins; venous insufficiency.

Hetrazan
Lederle, Austral.†; Wyeth-Ayerst, Canad.†; Lederle, UK.
Diethylcarbamazine citrate (p.98·1).
Worm infections.

Hetrogalen *Galenika, Ger.*
Hedera helix.
Catarrh.

Heumann Abfurhtee Solubilax N *Sanofi Synthelabo, Ger.*
Senna (p.1248·2); frangula bark (p.1227·1).
Constipation.

Heumann Beruhigungstee Tenerval N *Sanofi Synthelabo, Ger.*
Valerian root (p.1678·3); melissa (p.1632·2); valerian oil.
Nervous disorders; sleep disorders.

Heumann Blasen- und Nierentee Solubitrat N *Sanofi Synthelabo, Ger.*
Java tea (p.1625·1); solidago virgaurea; birch leaf (p.1585·2); fennel oil (p.1610·2).
Urinary-tract disorders.

Heumann Bronchialtee Solubifix N *Sanofi Synthelabo, Ger.*
Althaea (p.1577·1); liquorice (p.1231·2); cowslip root (p.1600·1); anise oil (p.1580·3); thyme oil (p.1672·3).
Respiratory-tract disorders.

Heumann Hustenstiller *Sanova, Aust.†*
Drosera (p.1606·1); thyme (p.1672·2).
Coughs and cold symptoms.

Heumann Leber- und Gallentee Solu-Hepar NT *Sanofi Synthelabo, Ger.*
Boldo (p.1585·3); greater celandine (p.1618·1); silybum marianum (p.1021·3); peppermint oil (p.1243·3).
Biliary-tract disorders; liver disorders.

Heumann Magentee Solu-Vetan Novo *Sanofi Synthelabo, Ger.*
Liquorice root (p.1231·2); peppermint leaf (p.1243·2); peppermint oil (p.1243·3).
Gastrointestinal disorders.

Heumann's Bronchial *Sanova, Aust.†*
Thyme (p.1672·2).
Catarrh; coughs.

Heumann's Bronchialtee *Sanova, Aust.*
Althaea (p.1577·1); liquorice (p.1231·2); cowslip root (p.1600·1); anise oil (p.1580·3); thyme oil (p.1672·3).
Bronchitis; catarrh; coughs.

Heuschnupfenmittel *DHU, Ger.*
Homoeopathic preparation.

Heusin *Hotz, Ger.*
Aesculus (p.1574·1); mistletoe (p.1636·2); crataegus (p.1600·2); hamamelis (p.1618·3); arnica (p.1581·3); silybum marianum (p.1021·3).
Peripheral vascular disorders.

Hevac B
Pfizer, Aust.†; Pasteur Merieux, Braz.
A hepatitis B vaccine (recombinant) (p.1542·2).
Active immunisation.

Hevert Enzym Novo *Hevert, Ger.†*
Dimethicone (p.1249·2); pancreatin (p.1646·1); trypsin (p.1675·3).
Hevert Enzym formerly contained thiamine hydrochloride, cholesterol, dimethicone, fel tauri, folic acid, pancreatin, papain, riboflavin, and trypsin.
Digestive system disorders.

Hevert-Aktivon Mono *Hevert, Ger.†*
Ginseng (p.1615·3).
Tonic.

Hevert-Blasen- und Nieren- Tee *Hevert, Ger.*
Java tea (p.1625·1); bearberry (p.1583·3); birch leaf (p.1585·2); equisetum (p.1606·3); ononis (p.1644·1); couch-grass (p.1599·3); tilia (p.1673·2); centaurea cyanus.
Urinary-tract disorders.

Hevert-Card forte *Hevert, Ger.†*
Herbal and homoeopathic preparation.

Hevert-Carmin symbio *Hevert, Ger.*
Vegetable charcoal (p.1000·3); aniseed (p.1580·2); caraway (p.1591·2); anise oil (p.1580·3); caraway oil (p.1591·2); fennel oil (p.1610·2); peppermint oil (p.1243·3).
Gastrointestinal disorders.

Hevert-Dorm *Hevert, Ger.*
Diphenhydramine hydrochloride (p.416·1).
Sleep disorders.

Hevert-Entwasserungs-Tee *Hevert, Ger.†*
Pterocarpus santalinus; rosemary; juniper (p.1625·2); asparagus; lovage (p.1629·3); ononis (p.1644·1); taraxacum (p.1669·1); rose fruit (p.1389·3); calendula (p.1589·2); squill (p.1100·3); birch leaf (p.1585·2); buchu (p.1587·2); centaurea cyanus.
Cystitis; oedema; renal calculi.

Hevert-Erkaltungs-Tee *Hevert, Ger.†*
Sambucus (p.1660·3); thyme (p.1672·2); salix bark (p.82·1).
Cold symptoms.

Hevert-Gall S *Hevert, Ger.*
Greater celandine (p.1618·1); cnicus benedictus (p.1597·2); chamomile (p.1593·2); taraxacum (p.1669·1); caraway oil (p.1591·2); peppermint oil (p.1243·3); boldo (p.1585·3); calamus (p.1588·1); silybum marianum (p.1021·3); turmeric (p.1029·3).
Biliary disorders; duodenal disorders; liver disorders.

Hevert-Gicht-Rheuma-Tee comp *Hevert, Ger.†*
Salix (p.82·1); sambucus (p.1660·3); birch leaf (p.1585·2); juniper (p.1625·2); achillea (p.1572·2); liquorice (p.1231·2); ononis (p.1644·1).
Rheumatic disorders.

Hevertigon *Hevert, Ger.*
Homoeopathic preparation.

Hevert-Mag *Hevert, Ger.*
Magaldrate (p.1232·2).
Gastric hyperacidity; heartburn; peptic ulcer.

Hevert-Magen-Galle-Leber-Tee *Hevert, Ger.†*
Calendula (p.1589·2); fennel (p.1610·1); absinthium (p.1571·1); centaurea (p.1593·1); greater celandine (p.1618·1); mylabris cichorii; achillea (p.1572·2); thyme (p.1672·2); calamus (p.1588·1).
Digestive system disorders.

Hevert-Migrane *Hevert, Ger.*
Homoeopathic preparation.

Hevert-Nerv plus Eisen *Hevert, Ger.†*
Minerals; kola; ginseng; iron phosphate; lecithin (p.1350·1).
Tonic.

Hevert-Nier II *Hevert, Ger.†*
Hevert-Nier II injection: Homoeopathic preparation.

Hevertnier Complex *Hevert, Ger.†*
Homoeopathic preparation.

Hevertnier spasmo *Hevert, Ger.†*
Homoeopathic preparation.

Hevertolax duo *Hevert, Ger.*
Frangula bark (p.1227·1); senna (p.1248·2).
Constipation.

Hevertolax Phyto *Hevert, Ger.†*
Senna fruit (p.1248·2).
Constipation.

Hevertopect *Hevert, Ger.*
Anise oil (p.1580·3); eucalyptus oil (p.1609·2); fennel oil (p.1610·2); peppermint oil (p.1243·3); pumilio pine oil (p.1656·3); turpentine oil (p.1676·3); ammi visnaga (p.1579·1); ephedrine hydrochloride (p.1090·1); eucalyptus (p.1609·2); thyme (p.1672·2); verbascum.
Respiratory-tract disorders.

Hevertotox *Hevert, Ger.*
Homoeopathic preparation.

Hevertoval mono *Hevert, Ger.*
Homoeopathic preparation.

Hevertozym *Hevert, Ger.*
Pancreatin (p.1646·1).
Pancreatic insufficiency.

Hevert-Vitan N *Hevert, Ger.*
Multivitamin and mineral preparation (p.1350·1).
Calcium and vitamin deficiency.

Hewallergia *Hevert, Ger.*
Homoeopathic preparation.

Heweberberol-Tee *Hevert, Ger.*
Birch leaf (p.1585·2); solidago virgaurea; ononis (p.1644·1); java tea (p.1625·1); pterocarpus santalinus; liquorice root (p.1231·2).
Urinary-tract disorders.

Hewechol Artischockendragees *Hevert, Ger.*
Cynara (p.1601·3).
Dyspepsia.

Hewedolor *Hevert, Ger.*
Rhus toxicodendron (p.1657·3); capsicum (p.1591·1); methyl salicylate (p.55·1).
Neuromuscular disorders; scars.

Hewedolor forte *Hevert, Ger.*
Sodium salamidacetate (p.81·3).
Nerve pain.

Hewedolor neuro *Hevert, Ger.*
Thiamine hydrochloride (p.1385·1); pyridoxine hydrochloride (p.1386·3); lignocaine [lidocaine] hydrochloride (p.1313·2).
Nerve pain.

Hewedolor plus Coffein *Hevert, Ger.†*
Procaine hydrochloride (p.1319·1); caffeine (p.761·3).
Nerve pain.

Hewedolor Procain *Hevert, Ger.*
Procaine hydrochloride (p.1319·1).
Pain.

Hewedormir *Hevert, Ger.*
Valerian (p.1678·3).
Nervousness; sleep disorders.

Hewedormir forte *Hevert, Ger.*
Doxylamine succinate (p.417·1).
Anxiety; hypersensitivity reactions; sleep disorders.

Heweformica *Hevert, Ger.†*
Homoeopathic preparation.

Hewegingko *Hevert, Ger.*
Homoeopathic preparation.

Hewekliman *Hevert, Ger.*
Homoeopathic preparation.

Hewekzem novo *Hevert, Ger.*
Panthenol (p.1602·3); vitamin A palmitate (p.1383·2); alpha tocoferil acetate (p.1394·1); chamomile oil; echinacea; sarsaparilla.
Skin disorders.

Hewelymphon N *Hevert, Ger.*
Homoeopathic preparation.

Hewenephron duo *Hevert, Ger.*
Solidago virgaurea; echinacea (p.1606·2).
Renal calculi.

Heweneural *Hevert, Ger.*
Lignocaine [lidocaine] hydrochloride (p.1313·2).
Migraine; nervous system disorders.

Hewepsychon duo *Hevert, Ger.*
Kava (p.1625·3); hypericum (p.290·2).
Depression; dystonias; hypertension; menopausal disorders; migraine; nocturnal enuresis; tonic.

Hewepsychon uno *Hevert, Ger.*
Homoeopathic preparation.

Hewerheum *Hevert, Ger.†*
Homoeopathic preparation.

Hewesabal comp *Hevert, Ger.*
Homoeopathic preparation.

Hewesabal mono *Hevert, Ger.*
Homoeopathic preparation.

Heweselen *Hevert, Ger.*
Homoeopathic preparation.

Hewethyreon *Hevert, Ger.*
Homoeopathic preparation.

Hewetraumen *Hevert, Ger.*
Homoeopathic preparation.

Heweurat *Hevert, Ger.†*
Homoeopathic preparation.

Heweven P 3 *Hevert, Ger.*
Hamamelis (p.1618·3); aesculus (p.1574·1); aescin (p.1574·1).
Vascular disorders.

Heweven P 7 *Hevert, Ger.†*
Hamamelis (p.1618·3); aesculus (p.1574·1); aescin; aesculin; echinacea.
Vascular disorders.

Hewletts *Kestrel, UK.*
Zinc oxide (p.1128·2); hydrous wool fat (p.1411·2); arachis oil (p.1581·1); white soft paraffin (p.1407·3).
Dry skin.

Hexa-Blok *Hexal, S.Afr.*
Atenolol (p.841·3).
Angina pectoris; hypertension.

Hexabiotin *Durascan, Denm.*
Erythromycin ethyl succinate (p.201·2) or erythromycin stearate (p.201·3).
Bacterial infections.

Hexabrix
Sanova, Aust.†; Mallinckrodt, Austral.; Codali, Belg.; Guerbet, Braz.;
Mallinckrodt, Canad.; Guerbet, Denm.; Guerbet, Fin.; Guerbet, Fr.; Guerbet, Ger.; Guerbet, Israel; Guerbet, Ital.; Guerbet, Neth.†; Guerbet, Norw.; Aventis, NZ; Guerbet, Port.; Guerbet, Spain; Gothia, Swed.; Guerbet, Switz.; May & Baker, UK; Mallinckrodt, USA.
Meglumine ioxaglate (p.1037·1); sodium ioxaglate (p.1037·1).
Radiographic contrast medium.

Hexacillin *Garec, S.Afr.†*
Ampicillin trihydrate (p.151·1).
Bacterial infections.

Hexacortone *Spirig, Switz.*
Prednisolone acetate (p.1078·1).
Skin disorders.

Hexacroman *Durascan, Denm.*
Sodium cromoglicate (p.774·3).
Allergic conjunctivitis.

Hexadilat *Durascan, Denm.*
Nifedipine (p.940·1).
Angina pectoris; hypertension; Raynaud's syndrome.

Hexadreps *Diepha, Fr.†*
Biclotymol (p.1136·1).
Mouth and throat infections.

Hexadrol
Organon Teknika, Canad.; Organon, USA.
Dexamethasone (p.1067·1) or dexamethasone sodium phosphate (p.1067·1).
Corticosteroid.

Hexafen *EMS, Braz.*
Deltamethrin (p.1430·3).
Scabies.

Hexafene *Vifor, Switz.†*
Inositol nicotinate (p.914·1); buclizine hydrochloride (p.411·1); hydroxyzine hydrochloride (p.419·1).
Vertigo.

Hexafluid *Diepha, Fr.†*
Carbocisteine (p.1086·3).
Respiratory-tract congestion.

Hexagastron *Durascan, Denm.*
Sucralfate (p.1250·2).
Gastro-oesophageal reflux; peptic ulcer.

Hexaglucon *Durascan, Denm.*
Glibenclamide (p.321·3).
Diabetes mellitus.

Hexakapron *Teva, Israel.*
Tranexamic acid (p.742·2).
Haemorrhage.

Hexalacton *Durascan, Denm.*
Spironolactone (p.973·2).
Ascites; hyperaldosteronism; oedema.

Hexalen
DBL, Austral.; Lilly, Canad.; US Bio, Israel; US Bioscience, Norw.; Swedish Orphan, Swed.; Ipsen, UK; MGI, USA.
Altretamine (p.506·2).
Ovarian cancer.

Hexalense *Ioltech, Fr.*
Aminocaproic acid (p.724·3).
Inflammatory eye disorders.

Hexalid *Durascan, Denm.*
Diazepam (p.674·3).
Alcohol withdrawal syndrome; anxiety; spasticity.

Hexalyse *Doms-Adrian, Fr.; Doms-Adrian, Hong Kong.*
Biclotymol (p.1136·1); muramidase hydrochloride (p.1638·1); enoxolone (p.34·3).
Formerly contained biclotymol, dequalinium chloride, muramidase, papain, and enoxolone in *Fr.*
Mouth and throat disorders.

Hexamet *Hexal, S.Afr.*
Cimetidine (p.1216·3).
Gastro-oesophageal reflux; peptic ulcer; Zollinger-Ellison syndrome.

Hexamon *Beiersdorf-Lilly, Ger.; Gastropharm, Ger.*
Hexylresorcinol (p.1146·3); lauromacrogol 400 (p.1345·2).
Anorectal disorders.

Hexamycin *Durascan, Denm.*
Gentamicin sulfate (p.210·1).
Bacterial infections.

Hexanicit *Promed, Ger.; Astra, Swed.*
Inositol nicotinate (p.914·1).
Hyperlipidaemias; peripheral and central circulatory disorders.

Hexanios G+R *Anios, Fr.*
Polihexanide (p.1154·2); didecyldimethylammonium chloride (p.1143·2).
Instrument disinfection.

Hexanitrat *Hexal, Aust.*
Isosorbide dinitrate (p.915·2).
Angina pectoris; heart failure; myocardial infarction; pulmonary hypertension.

Hexanium *Fides Rottapharm, Spain†.*
Emepronium bromide (p.466·3).
Urinary-tract disorders.

Hexanurat *Durascan, Denm.*
Allopurinol (p.397·2).
Gout.

Hexaphane *Biorga, Fr.; Saninter, Port.*
Gelatin; cystine; zinc gluconate; vitamin B substances (p.1350·1).
Fragile hair and nails.

Hexaphenyl *Ingram & Bell, Canad.†*
Hexachlorophene sodium (p.1146·2).
Disinfection.

Hexapindol *Durascan, Denm.; Tika, Norw.†; Tika, Swed.†.*
Pindolol (p.955·3).
Angina pectoris; arrhythmias; hypertension; myocardial infarction.

Hexapneumine
Note.This name is used for preparations of different composition.
Doms-Adrian, Fr.
Adult suppositories; paediatric suppositories: Biclotymol (p.1136·1); eucalyptol (p.1609·2); pholcodine (p.1099·1).
Formerly contained biclotymol, eucalyptol, pholcodine, and paracetamol.
Coughs.

Adult syrup; paediatric syrup: Biclotymol (p.1136·1); chlorpheniramine [chlorphenamine] maleate (p.412·1); pholcodine (p.1099·1).
Formerly contained biclotymol, chlorpheniramine [chlorphenamine] maleate, guaifenesin, and pholcodine.
Coughs.

Infant suppositories: Biclotymol (p.1136·1); eucalyptol (p.1609·2).
Formerly contained biclotymol, eucalyptol, and paracetamol.
Respiratory-tract disorders.

Infant syrup: Biclotymol (p.1136·1); chlorpheniramine [chlorphenamine] maleate (p.412·1); tolu balsam (p.1101·3).
Formerly contained biclotymol, chlorpheniramine [chlorphenamine] maleate, guaifenesin, paracetamol, and tolu balsam.
Coughs.

Tablets: Biclotymol (p.1136·1); chlorpheniramine [chlorphenamine] maleate (p.412·1); phenylephrine hydrochloride (p.1097·1).
Nasal congestion.

Doms-Adrian, Hong Kong.
Adult syrup; paediatric syrup: Biclotymol (p.1136·1); chlorpheniramine [chlorphenamine] maleate (p.412·1); guaifenesin (p.1092·2); pholcodine (p.1099·1).
Coughs.

Infant syrup: Biclotymol (p.1136·1); chlorpheniramine [chlorphenamine] maleate (p.412·1); guaifenesin (p.1092·2); paracetamol (p.71·2); tolu balsam (p.1101·3).
Coughs; fever.

Tablets: Biclotymol (p.1136·1); chlorpheniramine [chlorphenamine] maleate (p.412·1); phenylephrine hydrochloride (p.1097·1).
Nasal congestion.

Hexapress *Durascan, Denm.*
Prazosin hydrochloride (p.958·1).
Heart failure; hypertension; Raynaud's syndrome.

Hexaquart L *Braun, Ger.*
Didecyldimethylammonium chloride (p.1143·2); benzalkonium chloride (p.1133·2).
Surface disinfection.

Hexaquart plus *Braun, Ger.*
Didecyldimethylammonium chloride (p.1143·2); lauryldipropylene triamine; biguanidinium acetate.
Surface and instrument disinfection.

Hexaquart S *Braun, Ger.*
Didecyldimethylammonium chloride (p.1143·2); benzalkonium chloride (p.1133·2).
Fungal skin infection prophylaxis; surface disinfection.

Hexaquine *Gomenol, Fr.*
Quinine benzoate (p.447·1); thiamine hydrochloride (p.1385·1); niaouli oil (p.1640·2).
Muscle cramps.

Hexaretic *Hexal, S.Afr.*
Amiloride (p.835·3); hydrochlorothiazide (p.907·3).
Hypertension; oedema.

Hexarone *Hexal, S.Afr.*
Amiodarone hydrochloride (p.836·1).
Arrhythmias.

Hexaseptine *Gifrer Barbezat, Fr.*
Hexamidine isetionate (p.1146·2).
Bacterial skin infections; skin and mucous membrane disinfection.

Hexasoptin *Durascan, Denm.*
Verapamil hydrochloride (p.989·1).
Angina pectoris; arrhythmias; hypertension; myocardial infarction.

Hexaspray *Doms-Adrian, Fr.; Doms-Adrian, Hong Kong.*
Biclotymol (p.1136·1).
Mouth and throat disorders.

Hexastat *Bellon, Fr.†; Rhone-Poulenc Rorer, Hong Kong; Rhone-Poulenc Rorer, Ital.†; Rhone-Poulenc Rorer, Neth.†; Rhone-Poulenc Rorer, Norw.†.*
Altretamine (p.506·2).
Malignant neoplasms.

Hexatin *Agepha, Aust.*
Hexetidine (p.1146·3).
Mouth and throat inflammation.

Hexatrione *Wyeth Lederle, Fr.*
Triamcinolone hexacetonide (p.1080·2).
Musculoskeletal and joint disorders.

Hexavitamin *Upsher-Smith, USA.*
Multivitamin preparation (p.1350·1).

Hexavitamins *Novopharm, Canad.*
Multivitamin preparation (p.1350·1).

Hexene *Osoth, Thai.*
Chlorhexidine gluconate (p.1138·2).
Skin disinfection.

Hexide *Milano, Thai.*
Chlorhexidine gluconate (p.1138·2).
Antiseptic lubricant for vaginal examination.

Hexidin
Note.This name is used for preparations of different composition.
Genericon, Aust.; Nycomed, Norw.†.
Chlorhexidine gluconate (p.1138·2).
Mouth infections; oral hygiene.

Allergan, Austral.†; Fischer, Israel.
Chlorhexidine gluconate (p.1138·2); thiomersal (p.1158·2)(p.1129·2).
Disinfecting solution for soft contact lenses.

Hexifluor *Warner-Lambert, Port.*
Hexetidine (p.1146·3).

Hexigel *Warner-Lambert Consumer, Switz.†.*
Hexetidine (p.1146·3).
Mouth disorders.

Hexilium *Pharmasant, Thai.*
Flunarizine (p.418·2).
Cerebral and peripheral vascular disorders; vestibular disorders.

Hexinawas *Wasserman, Spain†.*
Altretamine (p.506·2).
Lung cancer; ovarian cancer.

Hexit *Odan, Canad.*
Lindane (p.1434·1).
Pediculosis; scabies.

Hexobion *Merck, Ger.*
Pyridoxine hydrochloride (p.1386·3).
Vitamin B deficiency.

Hexogen *Antigen, Irl.*
Inositol nicotinate (p.914·1).
Peripheral and cerebral vascular disorders.

Hexo-Imotryl *Cassenne, Fr.†.*
Benzydamine hydrochloride (p.20·1); hexamidine isetionate (p.1146·2).
Mouth and throat disorders.

Hexokain *Nycomed, Denm.*
Benzocaine (p.1306·2); chlorhexidine hydrochloride (p.1138·2).
Mouth disorders; oral hygiene.

Hexol *Sigma, Austral.; Sigma, Hong Kong; Pharmaland, Thai.*
Chlorhexidine gluconate (p.1138·2).
Skin disinfection.

Hexoll *Asta Medica, Neth.†.*
Acetic acid (p.1571·2); citric acid (p.1596·2).
Pediculosis.

Hexomedin *Rhone-Poulenc Rorer, Spain.*
Hexamidine isetionate (p.1146·2).
Burns; skin infections; wounds.

Hexomedin N *Rhone-Poulenc Rorer, Ger.*
Hexamidine isetionate (p.1146·2).
Acne; paronychia.

Hexomedine
Note.This name is used for preparations of different composition.
Aventis, Belg.; Theraplix, Fr.; Rhone-Poulenc Rorer, Neth.†; Rhone-Poulenc Rorer, Switz.†.
Topical solution; topical gel: Hexamidine isetionate (p.1146·2).
Skin disinfection; skin disorders.

Rhodia, Braz.; Theraplix, Fr.
Throat spray: Hexamidine isetionate (p.1146·2); amethocaine [tetracaine] (p.1305·2) or amethocaine [tetracaine] hydrochloride (p.1305·2).
Infections of the mouth and throat.

Hexopal *Sanofi Winthrop, Irl.; Sanofi Winthrop, UK.*
Inositol nicotinate (p.914·1).
Intermittent claudication; Raynaud's syndrome.

Hexoral *Parke, Davis, Aust.; Warner-Lambert, Ger.*
Hexetidine (p.1146·3).
Mouth and throat disorders.

Hexoraletten N *Warner-Lambert, Ger.*
Chlorhexidine hydrochloride (p.1138·2); benzocaine (p.1306·2).
Mouth and throat disorders.

Hextril *Warner-Lambert Consumer, Belg.; Warner-Lambert, Fr.; Warner-Lambert, Neth.; Warner-Lambert Consumer, Port.; Warner-Lambert Consumer, Switz.*
Hexetidine (p.1146·3).
Mouth and throat disorders.

Hextriletten *Warner-Lambert Consumer, Switz.*
Cetylpyridinium chloride (p.1138·1); 2,4-dichlorobenzyl alcohol (p.1143·2); lignocaine [lidocaine] hydrochloride (p.1313·2).
Sore throat.

HF *Fresenius Medical, Switz.*
A range of electrolyte infusions with or without glucose (p.1184·1).
Haemofiltration.

HF-BIC35+HF-EL010 *Dicamed, Swed.*
Sodium chloride; sodium bicarbonate; calcium chloride; magnesium chloride; glucose (p.1184·1).
Haemofiltration.

HF-BIC35+HF-EL210 *Dicamed, Swed.*
Sodium chloride; sodium bicarbonate; calcium chloride; magnesium chloride; potassium chloride; glucose (p.1184·1).
Haemofiltration.

Hi Potency B Compound *Swiss Herbal, Canad.*
Vitamin B substances (p.1350·1).

Hi Potency Cal *Swiss Herbal, Canad.*
Calcium carbonate (p.1215·1).

Hi Potency Multi-Mineral *Swiss Herbal, Canad.*
Mineral and trace element preparation (p.1350·1).

Hi Potency Stress B with C *Lee-Adams, Canad.*
Vitamin B substances; vitamin C (p.1350·1).

Hialid *Santen, Hong Kong.*
Sodium hyaluronate (p.1620·1).
Keratoconjunctival epithelial damage.

HIB Merieux *Pasteur Merieux, Ger.*
A haemophilus influenzae conjugate vaccine (diphtheria toxoid conjugate) (p.1540·2).
Active immunisation.

HIB-DPT *Pasteur Merieux, Ger.*
A diphtheria, tetanus, pertussis and haemophilus influenzae vaccine (p.1538·3).
Active immunisation.

HIB-DT *Pasteur Merieux, Ger.*
A diphtheria, tetanus, and haemophilus influenzae vaccine (p.1537·3).
Active immunisation.

Hiberix *SmithKline Beecham, Austral.; SmithKline Beecham, Belg.; SmithKline Beecham, Fin.; SmithKline Beecham, Irl.; SmithKline Beecham, Ital.; SmithKline Beecham, Singapore; SmithKline Beecham, Spain; SmithKline Beecham, Switz.; SmithKline Beecham, Thai.*
A haemophilus influenzae conjugate vaccine (tetanus toxoid conjugate) (p.1540·2).
Active immunisation.

Hibernal *Rhone-Poulenc Rorer, Swed.*
Chlorpromazine embonate (p.660·2) or chlorpromazine hydrochloride (p.660·2).
Adjunct to analgesia; psychoses.

HIBest *Pasteur Vaccins, Fr.*
A haemophilus influenzae conjugate vaccine (tetanus protein conjugate) (p.1540·2).
Active immunisation.

Hibicet *Zeneca, Austral.; Zeneca, Irl.; Zeneca, Ital.; AstraZeneca, NZ; Zeneca, S.Afr.; AstraZeneca, Thai.; SSL, UK.*
Chlorhexidine gluconate (p.1138·2); cetrimide (p.1137·1).
Formerly known as Savlon Hospital Concentrate in the UK.
Disinfection.

Hibicet concentraat *Zeneca, Neth.*
Chlorhexidine gluconate (p.1138·2); cetrimide (p.1137·1).
Formerly known as Savlon.
Disinfection.

Hibicet Hospital Concentrate
Zeneca, Hong Kong; AstraZeneca, Singapore.
Chlorhexidine gluconate (p.1138·2); cetrimide (p.1137·1).
Disinfection.

Hibicet verdunning *Zeneca, Neth.*
Chlorhexidine gluconate (p.1138·2); cetrimide (p.1137·1).
Formerly known as Savlodil.
Disinfection.

Hibiclens *Zeneca, Austral.; AstraZeneca, NZ; Zeneca, USA.*
Chlorhexidine gluconate (p.1138·2).
Skin disinfection.

Hibicol *Zeneca, Austral.*
Chlorhexidine gluconate (p.1138·2); isopropyl alcohol (p.1149·2).
Hand disinfection.

Hibident *SmithKline Beecham, Aust.; SmithKline Beecham Consumer, Belg.†; SmithKline Beecham, Neth.†.*
Chlorhexidine gluconate (p.1138·2).
Mouth infections; oral hygiene.

Hibidil *Zeneca, Belg.; AstraZeneca, Canad.; AstraZeneca, Fr.; Zeneca, S.Afr.; Zeneca, Switz.*
Chlorhexidine gluconate (p.1138·2).
Skin, mucous membrane, wound, and instrument disinfection.

Hibigel *SmithKline Beecham, Neth.†.*
Chlorhexidine gluconate (p.1138·2).
Mouth infections.

Hibiguard *Zeneca, Belg.*
Chlorhexidine gluconate (p.1138·2).
Disinfection of hands and skin.

Hibimax *Zeneca, Spain.*
Chlorhexidine gluconate (p.1138·2).
Burns; instrument disinfection; skin disinfection; skin disorders; wounds.

Hibiscrub *Zeneca, Belg.; AstraZeneca, Fin.; AstraZeneca, Fr.; Zeneca, Hong Kong; Zeneca, Irl.; Zeneca, Ital.; Zeneca, Mex.; Zeneca, Neth.; AstraZeneca, Norw.; Zeneca, Port.; Zeneca, S.Afr.; AstraZeneca, Singapore; Zeneca, Spain; Zeneca, Swed.; Zeneca, Switz.; AstraZeneca, Thai.; SSL, UK.*
Chlorhexidine gluconate (p.1138·2).
Skin disinfection.

Hibisol *Zeneca, Hong Kong; Zeneca, Irl.; Zeneca, Neth.; AstraZeneca, Singapore; SSL, UK.*
Chlorhexidine gluconate (p.1138·2); isopropyl alcohol (p.1149·2).
Skin disinfection.

Hibisprint *AstraZeneca, Fr.*
Chlorhexidine gluconate (p.1138·2).
Skin disinfection.

Hibistat *Zeneca, USA.*
Chlorhexidine gluconate (p.1138·2).
Skin disinfection.

Hibital *Zeneca, Switz.*
Chlorhexidine gluconate (p.1138·2); isopropyl alcohol (p.1149·2).
Skin and hand disinfection.

Hibitane
Note.This name is used for preparations of different composition.
Zeneca, Austral.; Zeneca, Belg.; Zeneca, Braz.; AstraZeneca, Canad.; Bioglan, Denm.; AstraZeneca, Fr.; Zeneca, Hong Kong; Zeneca, Irl.; Zeneca, Neth.; Bioglan, Norw.; AstraZeneca, NZ; CS, Port.; Genop, S.Afr.; AstraZeneca, Singapore; Bioglan, Singapore; Bioglan, Swed.; Zeneca, Switz.; AstraZeneca, Thai.; Bioglan, UK.
Chlorhexidine gluconate (p.1138·2) or chlorhexidine hydrochloride (p.1138·2).
Disinfection; gynaecological and obstetric lubricant and disinfectant.

Zeneca, Austral.
Tincture: Chlorhexidine gluconate (p.1138·2); isopropyl alcohol (p.1149·2).
Skin disinfection.

SmithKline Beecham Consumer, Belg.
Pastilles: Chlorhexidine hydrochloride (p.1138·2); lignocaine [lidocaine] hydrochloride (p.1313·2).
Formerly contained chlorhexidine hydrochloride and benzocaine.
Mouth and throat disorders.

Sterling, Port.; SmithKline Beecham, Spain.
Pastilles: Chlorhexidine hydrochloride (p.1138·2); benzocaine (p.1306·2).
Mouth and throat disorders.

Hibizene *Zeneca, Ital.*
Cetrimide (p.1137·1); chlorhexidine gluconate (p.1138·2).
Disinfection of burns, wounds, and external genitalia.

Hibon *Tokyo Tanabe, Hong Kong.*
Riboflavin tetrabutyrate (p.1386·2).
Vitamin B_2 deficiency.

Hibor *Rovi, Spain.*
Bemiparin sodium.
Thromboembolism prophylaxis.

HibTITER *Wyeth Lederle, Aust.; Lederle, Austral.; Wyeth Lederle, Belg.; Wyeth, Braz.; Wyeth-Ayerst, Canad.†; Wyeth Lederle, Denm.; Wyeth Lederle, Fin.; Lederle, Ger.; Lederle Irl.; Lederle, Israel; Wyeth Lederle, Ital.; Wyeth, Mex.; Wyeth, NZ; Wyeth Lederle, Port.; Wyeth, S.Afr.; Wyeth, Singapore; Cyanamid, Spain; Wyeth Lederle, Swed.; Lederle, Switz.; Wyeth, UK; Lederle, USA.*
A haemophilus influenzae conjugate vaccine (diphtheria CRM₁₉₇ protein conjugate) (p.1540·2).
Active immunisation.

HIB-Vaccinol *Procter & Gamble, Ger.†.*
A haemophilus influenzae conjugate vaccine (diphtheria toxoid conjugate) (p.1540·2).
Active immunisation.

Hi-Cal VM *NCI, USA†.*
Supplemental nutrition bar for immunocompromised individuals (p.1350·1).

Hicarlex *Ferrer, Spain.*
Fosinopril sodium (p.892·3).
Heart failure; hypertension.

Hicee *Takeda, Thai.*
Ascorbic acid (p.1389·3).
Vitamin C deficiency.

Hicin *Douglas, Austral.†.*
Indometacin (p.44·3).
Gout; inflammation; musculoskeletal, joint, peri-articular, and soft-tissue disorders; oedema; pain.

Hicomp *GHP, Thai.*
Vitamin B substances with glucose (p.1350·1).
Nutritional supplement.

Hiconcil *Bristol-Myers Squibb, Belg.; Bristol-Myers Squibb, Braz.; UPSA, Fr.; Bristol-Myers Squibb, Israel.*
Amoxicillin trihydrate (p.149·2).
Bacterial infections.

Hiconcil-NS *Bristol-Myers Squibb, S.Afr.†.*
Amoxicillin trihydrate (p.149·2); nystatin (p.392·2).
Bacterial infections; candidiasis.

Hi-Cor *C & M, USA.*
Hydrocortisone (p.1073·3).
Skin disorders.

Hicoseen *Piraud, Switz.†.*
Butamirate citrate (p.1086·2); dextromethorphan (p.1087·3); guaifenesin (p.1092·2).
Bronchitis; coughs.

Hicoton *Medika, Ger.*
Ferric saccharose complex (p.1370·1); calcium glycerophosphate (p.1188·2); rhus toxicodendron (p.1657·3); lupulus (p.1629·3); cinchona bark (p.1595·3); lecithin (p.1628·1); camphor monobromide.
Urinary-tract disorders.

Hidalone *Schering-Plough, Port.*
Hydrocortisone (p.1073·3).
Skin disorders.

Hidantal *Hoechst Marion Roussel, Braz.*
Phenytoin (p.357·2).
Arrhythmias; epilepsy; neuralgia; skeletal muscle spasm.

Hidantil *Ofimex, Mex.*
Phenytoin sodium (p.357·2).

Hidantina *Vitoria, Port.*
Phenytoin sodium (p.357·2).
Epilepsy; neuralgia.

Hidantina Composta *Vitoria, Port.*
Phenytoin sodium (p.357·2); phenobarbital (p.355·1).
Epilepsy.

The symbol † denotes a preparation no longer actively marketed

Hidantoina Rudefsa, Mex.
Phenytoin sodium (p.357·2).
Epilepsy.

Hiderm Baypharm, Austral.†.
Clotrimazole (p.382·1).
Fungal skin and vulvovaginal infections.

Hidil
Berlin Pharm, Singapore; Berlin Pharm, Thai.
Gemfibrozil (p.896·2).
Hyperlipidaemias.

Hidine PD, Thai.
Chlorhexidine gluconate (p.1138·2).
Disinfection.

Hidonac Zambon, Ital.
Acetylcysteine (p.1082·3).
Paracetamol poisoning.

Hidra Rydelle, Fr.†.
Amino-acid, fatty-acid, vitamin, and mineral preparation (p.1350·1).
Skin disorders.

Hidrabene Legrand, Braz.
Sodium chloride; potassium chloride; sodium phosphate; sodium citrate; potassium citrate; magnesium citrate; calcium lactate; homatropine methylbromide (p.1185·2).
Oral rehydration therapy.

Hidrafil Stiefel, Mex.
SPF 14: Oxybenzone (p.1518·1); octinoxate (p.1517·3).
Sunscreen.

Hidrafix Byk, Braz.
Sodium citrate; sodium chloride; potassium chloride; glucose (p.1185·2).
Oral rehydration therapy.

Hidrafix 90 Byk, Braz.
Potassium citrate; sodium citrate; sodium chloride; glucose (p.1185·2).
Oral rehydration therapy.

Hidralma Wasserman, Spain†.
Hydrotalcite (p.1228·1).
Hyperacidity.

Hidramox Carter-Wallace, Mex.
Amoxicillin trihydrate (p.149·2).
Bacterial infections.

Hidramox-M Carter-Wallace, Mex.
Amoxicillin trihydrate (p.149·2); bromhexine hydrochloride (p.1085·3).
Respiratory-tract infections.

Hidrasal Medifarma, Mex.
Frusemide [furosemide] (p.893·1).

Hidrasix Serral, Mex.
Isoniazid (p.215·3).

Hidratante Isdin, Port.
Polyglycerylmethacrylate; glycerol (p.1616·3); carbomer (p.1499·2).
Vaginal lubricant.

Hidratoderme Sofex, Port.†.
Urea (p.1127·3); allantoin (p.1110·1).
Skin disorders.

Hidratoil Free Dermoteca, Port.
A range of moisturisers and skin cleansers.

Hidrazida Zimaia, Port.
Isoniazid (p.215·3).
Tuberculosis.

Hidrion Gross, Mex.
Frusemide [furosemide] (p.893·1); potassium chloride (p.1194·3).
Hypertension; oedema.

Hidroaltesona Alter, Spain.
Hydrocortisone (p.1073·3).
Corticosteroid.

Hidroazer Zerboni, Mex.
Ketotifen (p.767·2).

Hidroc Cloranf Ciba Vision, Spain.
Chloramphenicol (p.179·1); hydrocortisone acetate (p.1073·3).
Eye disorders.

Hidroc Neomic Ciba Vision, Spain.
Hydrocortisone acetate (p.1073·3); neomycin sulfate (p.228·1).
Eye disorders.

Hidrociclina Grossman, Mex.
Benzylpenicillin (p.157·1).
Bacterial infections.

Hidrocil Oftalder, Port.
Hypromellose (p.1501·3).
Dry eyes.

Hidrocin Asta Medica, Braz.
Dexamethasone (p.1067·2); neomycin (p.228·1); naphazoline (p.1095·1).
Infected nasal disorders.

Hidrocorete Legrand, Braz.
Clioquinol (p.190·2); hydrocortisone (p.1073·3).
Skin disorders.

Hidroferol Faes, Spain.
Calcifediol (p.1391·1).
Hypoparathyroidism; hypophosphataemia; osteodystrophy; osteomalacia; rickets.

Hidro-Lact Cesam, Port.
A range of moisturisers and soap substitutes.

Hidrolyte QIF, Braz.
Sodium chloride; acetylmethionine (p.1185·2).
Oral rehydration therapy.

Hidrona Fustery, Mex.
Chlortalidone (p.857·1).
Hypertension; oedema.

Hidropolicin Grin, Mex.
Polymyxin B sulfate (p.238·1); neomycin sulfate (p.228·1); hydrocortisone acetate (p.1073·3).
Infected eye disorders.

Hidropolivit Menarini, Spain.
Multivitamin preparation (p.1350·1).

Hidropolivit Mineral Menarini, Spain.
Multivitamins and minerals (p.1350·1); orotic acid; hesperidin.
Tonic.

Hidroquin Mex-America, Mex.
Hydroquinone (p.1115·1).
Skin hyperpigmentation.

Hidroral JP, Braz.
Sodium chloride; potassium chloride; sodium lactate; glucose (p.1185·2).
Oral rehydration therapy.

Hidrosaluretil Alcala, Spain.
Hydrochlorothiazide (p.907·3).
Diabetes insipidus; hypertension; oedema; renal calculi.

Hidrosol Pacific, NZ.
Aluminium chloride (p.1110·2).
Hyperhidrosis.

Hidrowil Willmar, Mex.
Hydroxocobalamin (p.1388·1).

Hidroxil B12 B6 B1 Almirall, Spain.
Hydroxocobalamin (p.1388·1); pyridoxine hydrochloride (p.1386·3); thiamine hydrochloride (p.1385·1).
Vitamin B deficiency.

Hidroxogel Delta, Braz.
Aluminium hydroxide (p.1210·3); magnesium hydroxide (p.1233·1); dimethicone (p.1249·2).
Flatulence; gastrointestinal hyperacidity.

Hierco Ern, Spain.
Ferritin (p.1359·3).
Iron-deficiency anaemia.

Hi-Fluor Alphapharm, Austral.†.
Sodium fluoride (p.1375·3).
Bone pain in multiple myeloma; osteoporosis; Paget's disease of bone.

Higado Potenciado Medic Medical, Spain†.
Vitamin B substances (p.1350·1); glutathione (p.1010·3); liver extract; procaine ascorbate (p.1319·2).
Tonic; vitamin B deficiency.

High Potency Cal-Mag Plus Quest, Canad.
Calcium; magnesium; zinc; vitamin C; vitamin D (p.1350·1).

High Potency Lightening Serum Ocean Health, Singapore.
Lactic acid (p.1626·2); hydroquinone (p.1115·1); kojic acid; liquorice (p.1231·2).
Skin hyperpigmentation.

High Potency N-Vites Nion, USA.
Vitamin B substances with vitamin C (p.1350·1).

Higienex Sanval, Braz.
Tyrothricin (p.267·1); thymol (p.1158·3); hydroxyquinoline sulfate (p.1622·2); menthol (p.1632·3); chlorophyll (p.1028·1); sodium bicarbonate (p.1186·2); alum (p.1577·2); lactic acid (p.1626·2).
Vulvovaginal infections.

Higigripe CPH, Port.
Aspirin (p.14·2); caffeine (p.761·3); ascorbic acid (p.1389·3).

Higroton
Novartis, Braz.; Novartis, Mex.
Chlortalidone (p.857·1).
Ascites; heart failure; hypertension; oedema; renal calculi.

Higroton Reserpina Novartis, Braz.
Chlortalidone (p.857·1); reserpine (p.967·3).
Hypertension.

Higrotona Novartis, Spain.
Chlortalidone (p.857·1).
Diabetes insipidus; hypertension; oedema.

Higrotona Reserpina Novartis, Spain.
Chlortalidone (p.857·1); reserpine (p.967·3).
Hypertension.

Higroton-Res Novartis, Mex.
Chlortalidone (p.857·1); reserpine (p.967·3).
Hypertension.

Hijuven
Eisai, Hong Kong; Eisai, Thai.
dl-Alpha tocoferil nicotinate (p.984·3).
Cerebral and peripheral vascular disorders; hyperlipidaemias.

Hill's Balsam Chesty Cough Boehringer Ingelheim, UK.
Guaifenesin (p.1092·2).
Coughs.

Hill's Balsam Chesty Cough for Children Boehringer Ingelheim, UK.
Citric acid (p.1596·2); ipecacuanha (p.1093·1).
Coughs.

Hill's Balsam Chesty Cough Pastilles Boehringer Ingelheim, UK.
Compound benzoin tincture; peppermint oil (p.1243·3); ipecacuanha (p.1093·1); menthol (p.1632·3).
Cough and cold symptoms.

Hill's Balsam Dry Cough Boehringer Ingelheim, UK.
Pholcodine (p.1099·1).
Coughs.

Hill's Balsam Extra Strong Boehringer Ingelheim, UK.
Compound benzoin tincture; peppermint oil (p.1243·3); ipecacuanha (p.1093·1); menthol (p.1632·3).
Coughs and cold symptoms.

Hill's Balsam Nasal Congestion Pastilles Boehringer Ingelheim, UK.
Eucalyptus oil (p.1609·2); menthol (p.1632·3).
Nasal congestion.

Hima-Pasta nouvelle formule Mundipharma, Switz.
Zinc sulfate (p.1398·2); zinc oxide (p.1128·2).
Herpes labialis.

Himega
Sigma, Austral.; Sigma, Hong Kong.
Eicosapentaenoic acid (p.949·3); docosahexaenoic acid (p.949·2).
Dietary supplement.

Himus Grossman, Mex.
Thymomodulin (p.1672·3).

Hingfong-Essenz Hofmanns Tropfen Hofmann & Sommer, Ger.
Valerian (p.1678·3); peppermint oil (p.1243·3); rosemary oil (p.1659·3); fennel oil (p.1610·2); anise oil (p.1580·3); camphor (p.1589·3).
Headache; nausea; pain; psychosomatic disorders.

H-Insulin Hoechst, Ger.†.
Insulin injection (human, highly purified) (p.324·1).
Diabetes mellitus.

Hiosinotil Loren, Mex.
Hyoscine butylbromide (p.468·2).

Hioxyl
Croma, Aust.; Quinoderm, Irl.; Adams, UK.
Hydrogen peroxide (p.1147·1).
Skin infections; skin ulcers; wounds.

Hipeksal Leiras, Fin.
Methenamine hippurate (p.223·1).
Urinary-tract infections.

Hiperbiotico Atral, Port.
Ampicillin sodium (p.150·3) or ampicillin trihydrate (p.151·1).
Bacterial infections.

Hiperbiotico Retard Atral, Port.
Ampicillin sodium (p.150·3); ampicillin benzathine (p.151·3).
Bacterial infections.

Hipercol Helfarma, Port.
Citicoline (p.1596·1).
Cerebrovascular disorders.

Hiperdipina Pentafarma, Port.
Nitrendipine (p.947·1).

Hiperico Diviser Aquilea, Spain.
Hypericum (p.290·2).
Sleep disorders; tonic.

Hiperikan Farmasa, Mex.
Hypericum (p.290·2).
Depression.

Hiperlex Ferrer, Spain.
Fosinopril sodium (p.892·3).
Heart failure; hypertension.

Hiperlex Plus Ferrer, Spain.
Fosinopril sodium (p.892·3); hydrochlorothiazide (p.907·3).
Hypertension.

Hipersex Medical, Port.
Testis; pituitary; fitine; zinc phosphate; strychnine sulfate; adonis vernalis; boldo (p.1350·1).
Tonic.

Hipertenol Sanofi Synthelabo, Port.
Nitrendipine (p.947·1).

Hipertex Rayere, Mex.
Captopril (p.853·3).
Hypertension.

Hipertil Normal, Port.
Captopril (p.853·3).

Hiperton Grin, Mex.
Sodium chloride (p.1196·1).
Corneal oedema.

Hipoartel Ipsen, Braz.
Enalapril maleate (p.883·3).
Heart failure; hypertension.

Hipoartel Plus Ipsen, Spain.
Enalapril maleate (p.883·3); hydrochlorothiazide (p.907·3).
Hypertension.

Hipocatril Cibran, Braz.
Captopril (p.853·3).
Heart failure; hypertension.

Hipocol Valdecasas, Mex.
Nicotinic acid (p.1372·3).
Hypercholesterolaemia; pellagra.

Hipoderme Teuto, Braz.
Vitamin A (p.1382·1); colecalciferol (p.1391·1); boric acid (p.1586·1); zinc oxide (p.1128·2).
Barrier preparation.

Hipodermon Neo Quimica, Braz.
Vitamin A (p.1382·1); vitamin D (p.1391·1); boric acid (p.1586·1); zinc oxide (p.1128·2).
Barrier preparation; emollient.

Hipodex Bunker, Braz.
Vitamin A (p.1382·1); vitamin D (p.1391·1); neomycin (p.228·1); benzethonium chloride (p.1134·2).
Barrier preparation; infected skin disorders.

Hipodor Lepori, Port.
Hexyl nicotinate (p.42·2); methyl salicylate (p.55·1).
Musculoskeletal and joint disorders; neuritis; soft-tissue disorders.

Hipofagin S Byk, Braz.
Diethylpropion hydrochloride (p.1508·3).
Obesity.

Hipoglos Procter & Gamble, Braz.
Vitamin A palmitate (p.1383·2); ergocalciferol (p.1391·2); boric acid (p.1586·1); zinc oxide (p.1128·2); hydrocortisone (p.1073·3); aluminium magnesium silicate (p.1499·1).
Barrier preparation; emollient.

Hipoglos com Hidrocortisona Procter & Gamble, Braz.
Hydrocortisone (p.1073·3); vitamin A (p.1382·1); vitamin D (p.1391·1); zinc oxide (p.1128·2); boric acid (p.1586·1); aluminium magnesium silicate (p.1499·1).
Skin disorders.

Hipoglos Oftalmico Procter & Gamble, Braz.
Vitamin A palmitate (p.1383·2); ergocalciferol (p.1391·2); chloramphenicol (p.179·1); hydrocortisone (p.1073·3).
Infected eye disorders.

Hipoglos Plus Andromaco, Mex.
Vitamin A (p.1382·1); zinc oxide (p.1128·2); allantoin (p.1110·1); boric acid (p.1586·1).
Skin disorders.

Hipokinon Psicofarma, Mex.
Benzhexol [trihexyphenidyl] hydrochloride (p.463·3).
Extrapyramidal disorders; parkinsonism.

Hiposan Sanval, Braz.
Zinc oxide (p.1128·2); cod-liver oil (p.1357·2).
Barrier preparation; skin disorders.

Hiposcler Basi, Port.
Clofibrate nicotinyl alcohol.

Hiposul Mex-America, Mex.
Sodium thiosulfate (p.1024·2).

Hipotensil Medinfar, Port.
Captopril (p.853·3).
Heart failure; hypertension.

Hipotest Marlop, USA.
Multivitamin and mineral preparation with iron (p.1350·1).

Hipotosse Inibsa, Port.
Ambroxol hydrochloride (p.1084·3).
Respiratory-tract congestion.

Hi-Po-Vites Hudson, USA.
Multivitamin and mineral preparation with iron and folic acid (p.1350·1).

Hippophan Weleda, Fr.
Sea buckthorn.
Tonic.

Hippramine 3M, S.Afr.
Methenamine hippurate (p.223·1).
Urinary-tract infections.

Hippuran Orion, Swed.†.
Methenamine hippurate (p.223·1).
Urinary-tract infections.

Hipputope Squibb Diagnostics, USA†.
Iodine-131 (p.1450·1) as sodium iodohippurate.

Hipranol Zurich, S.Afr.†.
Propranolol hydrochloride (p.962·3).
Angina pectoris; arrhythmias; hypertension.

Hiprex
Sanova, Aust.; 3M, Austral.; 3M, Belg.; 3M, Canad.†; 3M, Fin.; 3M, Irl.; 3M, Israel; 3M, Norw.; 3M, NZ; 3M, Swed.; 3M, UK; Hoechst Marion Roussel, USA.
Methenamine hippurate (p.223·1).
Urinary-tract infections.

Hipten
Note. This name is used for preparations of different composition.
Ofimex, Mex.
Methyldopa (p.927·3).

Farmorcore, Port.†.
Enalapril maleate (p.883·3).

Hirtonin Takeda, Jpn.
Protirelin tartrate (p.1296·1).
Prolonged disturbance of consciousness; spinocerebellar degeneration.

Hirucreme Nicholas, Fr.
Hirudin (p.905·3).
Peripheral vascular disorders.

Hirudex Pharmafar, Ital.
Leech extract (p.905·3); esculoside (p.1574·1).
Bruises; inflammation; oedema; phlebitis; varices.

Hirudoid
Sankyo, Aust.; Sankyo, Austral.; Sankyo, Belg.; Luitpold, Braz.; Sankyo, Denm.; Sankyo, Fin.; Sankyo, Ger.; Sankyo, Hong Kong; Sankyo, Ital.; Sankyo, Neth.; Sankyo, NZ; Searle, NZ; Sankyo, Port.; Sankyo, Singapore; Sankyo, Spain; Selena, Swed.†; Sankyo, Switz.; Sankyo, Thai.; Sankyo, UK.
A heparinoid (p.905·2).
Soft-tissue injury; thrombophlebitis; venous insufficiency; wounds.

Hiscifed Greater Pharma, Thai.
Pseudoephedrine hydrochloride (p.1099·2); triprolidine hydrochloride (p.1129·1).
Cold symptoms; hypersensitivity reactions; nasal congestion; rhinitis.

Hiscolgen Greater Pharma, Thai.
Paracetamol (p.71·2); phenylpropanolamine hydrochloride (p.1098·1); chlorpheniramine [chlorphenamine] maleate (p.412·1).
Cold symptoms; hay fever; nasal congestion.

Hisfedin *Wolff, Ger.*
Terfenadine (p.424·3).
Hypersensitivity reactions.

Hismacon *Condrugs, Thai.*
Astemizole (p.409·1).
Allergic conjunctivitis; allergic rhinitis; allergic skin disorders.

Hismadrin *Janssen-Cilag, Aust.*
Astemizole (p.409·1); pseudoephedrine hydrochloride (p.1099·2).
Hypersensitivity reactions.

Hismanal
Janssen-Cilag, Aust.†; Janssen-Cilag, Austral.†; Janssen-Cilag, Belg.†; Janssen, Braz.†; McNeil Consumer, Canad.†; Janssen-Cilag, Denm.†; Janssen-Cilag, Fr.†; Janssen-Cilag, Ger.†; Janssen-Cilag, Irl.†; Janssen-Cilag, Israel†; Janssen-Cilag, Ital.†; Janssen, Mex.†; Janssen-Cilag, Neth.†; Janssen-Cilag, Port.†; Janssen-Cilag, S.Afr.†; Janssen-Cilag, Spain†; Janssen-Cilag, Switz.†; Janssen-Cilag, UK†; Janssen, USA†.
Astemizole (p.409·1).
Allergic conjunctivitis; allergic rhinitis; urticaria.

Hismanal-D *Janssen-Cilag, S.Afr.†*
Pseudoephedrine hydrochloride (p.1099·2); astemizole (p.409·1).
Hypersensitivity reactions.

Hismizol *TO-Chemicals, Thai.*
Astemizole (p.409·1).
Allergic rhinitis; allergic skin disorders.

Hisno *Milano, Thai.*
Astemizole (p.409·1).
Hypersensitivity reactions.

Hisnot *Farmasa, Braz.*
Astemizole (p.409·1).
Hypersenxitivity reactions.

Hisocel *Fresenius, Braz.*
Gelatin (p.737·2) in electrolytes.
Plasma volume expansion.

Hisof *Banner, Hong Kong.*
Docusate sodium (p.1223·1).
Constipation; stool softener.

Hisoplex com Glicose *Fresenius, Braz.*
Electrolyte infusion with glucose (p.1180·1).
Plasma volume expansion.

Hispamicina Retard *Inkeysa, Spain.*
Ampicillin sodium (p.150·3); ampicillin benzathine (p.151·3).
Bacterial infections.

Hisprin *Shiwa, Thai.*
Paracetamol (p.71·2); chlorpheniramine [chlorphenamine] maleate (p.412·1); phenylpropanolamine (p.1098·1).
Cold symptoms.

Histabloc *Medley, Braz.*
Astemizole (p.409·1).
Hypersensitivity reactions.

Histac *Ranbaxy, Thai.*
Ranitidine (p.1246·3).
Gastro-oesophageal reflux; peptic ulcer; Zollinger-Ellison syndrome.

Histacon *Quatromed, S.Afr.*
Paracetamol (p.71·2); phenylephrine hydrochloride (p.1097·1); chlorpheniramine [chlorphenamine] maleate (p.412·1); caffeine (p.761·3).
Allergic rhinitis; cold symptoms.

Histacyl Compositum *Streuli, Switz.*
Diphenhydramine hydrochloride (p.416·1); mepyramine maleate (p.421·1).
Hypersensitivity reactions.

Histacylettes *Streuli, Switz.*
Diphenhydramine hydrochloride (p.416·1); mepyramine hydrochloride (p.421·1); caffeine (p.761·3).
Hypersensitivity reactions.

Histadane *Cibran, Braz.*
Terfenadine (p.424·3).
Hypersensitivity reactions.

Histade *Breckenridge, USA†.*
Phenylpropanolamine hydrochloride (p.1098·1); chlorpheniramine [chlorphenamine] maleate (p.412·1).
Cold symptoms; rhinitis.

Histadestal *Bioimmun, Ger.*
A normal immunoglobulin (p.1551·3); histamine hydrochloride (p.1619·2).
Hypersensitivity reactions.

Histadex *Vitamed, Israel.*
Dexchlorpheniramine maleate (p.412·1); pseudoephedrine hydrochloride (p.1099·2).
Respiratory-tract congestion.

Histafed *Trima, Israel.*
Triprolidine hydrochloride (p.427·2); pseudoephedrine hydrochloride (p.1099·2).
Respiratory-tract congestion.

Histafed Comp *Trima, Israel.*
Triprolidine hydrochloride (p.427·2); pseudoephedrine hydrochloride (p.1099·2); codeine phosphate (p.25·2).
Coughs; upper respiratory-tract infections.

Histafed Expectorant *Trima, Israel.*
Triprolidine hydrochloride (p.427·2); pseudoephedrine hydrochloride (p.1099·2); guaifenesin (p.1092·2).
Coughs.

Histafen
Note. This name is used for preparations of different composition.
Xepa-Soul Pattinson, Hong Kong; Berk, UK.
Terfenadine (p.424·3).
Allergic rhinitis; allergic skin reactions.

Douglas, NZ.
Chlorpheniramine [chlorphenamine] maleate (p.412·1).
Hypersensitivity reactions.

Histafilin *Estedi, Spain.*
Theophylline (p.777·2).
Heart failure; obstructive airways disease; paroxysmal dyspnoea.

Histagesic Modified *Jones, USA.*
Phenylephrine hydrochloride (p.1097·1); paracetamol (p.71·2); chlorpheniramine [chlorphenamine] maleate (p.412·1).
Upper respiratory-tract symptoms.

Histaglobin
Germania, Aust.; Mirren, S.Afr.; Promedica, Thai.
A normal immunoglobulin (p.1551·3); histamine hydrochloride (p.1619·2).
Hypersensitivity reactions.

Histajodol N *Kattwiga, Ger.*
Nonivamide (p.63·1); salicylic acid (p.1122·3); rosemary oil (p.1659·3).
Circulatory disorders; neuralgia; rheumatism; sciatica.

Histak *Ranbaxy, S.Afr.*
Ranitidine hydrochloride (p.1245·2).
Acid aspiration; gastro-oesophageal reflux; peptic ulcer; Zollinger-Ellison syndrome.

Histalerg *Dermopen, Braz.*
Fluocinolone acetonide (p.1071·1); neomycin (p.228·1).
Infected skin disorders.

Histalerg Profen *Dermopen, Braz.*
Pheniramine maleate (p.422·3).
Hypersensitivity reactions.

Histalet *Numark, USA.*
Pseudoephedrine hydrochloride (p.1099·2); chlorpheniramine [chlorphenamine] maleate (p.412·1).
Upper respiratory-tract symptoms.

Histalet X *Numark, USA.*
Pseudoephedrine hydrochloride (p.1099·2); guaifenesin (p.1092·2).
Coughs.

Histalet Forte *Numark, USA†.*
Phenylpropanolamine hydrochloride (p.1098·1); phenylephrine hydrochloride (p.1097·1); chlorpheniramine [chlorphenamine] maleate (p.412·1); mepyramine maleate (p.421·1).
Upper respiratory-tract symptoms.

Histalgane *Spirig, Switz.*
Nonivamide (p.63·1); benzyl nicotinate (p.20·2); glycol salicylate (p.42·2); dimethyl sulfoxide (p.1402·2).
Musculoskeletal, joint, and peri-articular pain.

Histalgane mite *Spirig, Switz.*
Glycol salicylate (p.42·2); dimethyl sulfoxide (p.1402·2).
Musculoskeletal, joint, and peri-articular pain.

Histalino *Arlex, Mex.*
Astemizole (p.409·1).

Histalix
Note. This name is used for preparations of different composition.
Roche, S.Afr.
Diphenhydramine hydrochloride (p.416·1); codeine phosphate (p.25·2).
Coughs; nasal congestion.

Wallace Mfg Chem., UK.
Diphenhydramine hydrochloride (p.416·1); ammonium chloride (p.1085·2); sodium citrate (p.1186·2); menthol (p.1632·3).
Coughs.

Histalix-C *Roche, S.Afr.†.*
Dextromethorphan hydrobromide (p.1087·3); paracetamol (p.71·2); pseudoephedrine hydrochloride (p.1099·2); ascorbic acid (p.1389·3).
Cold symptoms.

Histaloc *Julphar, UAE.*
Promethazine hydrochloride (p.423·2).
Hypersensitivity; motion sickness.

Histalon *ICN, Canad.*
Chlorpheniramine [chlorphenamine] maleate (p.412·1).

Histamed
Note. This name is used for preparations of different composition.
Covan, S.Afr.
Lotion: Diphenhydramine hydrochloride (p.416·1); calamine (p.1111·3); camphor (p.1589·3); benzocaine (p.1306·2).
Skin disorders.

Propan, Braz.
Elixir: Chlorpheniramine [chlorphenamine] maleate (p.412·1).
Hypersensitivity reactions.

Propan-Vernleigh, S.Afr.†
Cream: Mepyramine maleate (p.421·1).
Skin disorders.

Histamed Compound *Propan, S.Afr.*
Chlorpheniramine [chlorphenamine] maleate (p.412·1); ascorbic acid (p.1389·3); salicylamide (p.82·1); paracetamol (p.71·2); caffeine (p.761·3); phenylephrine hydrochloride (p.1097·1).
Cold symptoms.

Histamen *Polifarma, Ital.†*
Astemizole (p.409·1).
Allergic conjunctivitis; rhinitis; urticaria.

Histamin *Heralds, Braz.; Neo Quimica, Braz.*
Dexchlorpheniramine (p.412·2).
Hypersensitivity reactions.

Histaminos *Lesvi, Spain.*
Astemizole (p.409·1).
Hypersensitivity reactions.

Histan *Siam Bheasach, Thai.*
Hydroxyzine hydrochloride (p.419·1).
Anxiety; hypersensitivity reactions.

Histantil *Pharmascience, Canad.*
Promethazine hydrochloride (p.423·2).
Antihistamine.

Histaoph *Seng, Thai.*
Antazoline hydrochloride (p.408·3); tetryzoline hydrochloride (p.1101·2).
Allergic eye disorders; conjunctivitis.

Histaser *Serral, Mex.*
Astemizole (p.409·1).
Hypersensitivity.

Histatab Plus *Century, USA.*
Phenylephrine hydrochloride (p.1097·1); chlorpheniramine [chlorphenamine] maleate (p.412·1).
Upper respiratory-tract symptoms.

Histatapp *Pharmasant, Thai.*
Chlorpheniramine [chlorphenamine] maleate (p.412·1).
Hypersensitivity reactions.

Histaterfen *Azupharma, Ger.†*
Terfenadine (p.424·3).
Hypersensitivity reactions.

Histatex *Medix, Mex.*
Pheniramine (p.422·3).
Hypersensitivity.

Hista-Vadrin *Scherer, USA†.*
Phenylpropanolamine hydrochloride (p.1098·1); phenylephrine hydrochloride (p.1097·1); chlorpheniramine [chlorphenamine] maleate (p.412·1).
Upper respiratory-tract symptoms.

Hista-Vent DA *Ethex, USA.*
Chlorpheniramine [chlorphenamine] maleate (p.412·1); phenylephrine hydrochloride (p.1097·1); hyoscine methonitrate (p.468·2).
Upper respiratory-tract symptoms.

Histaverin *Estedi, Spain.*
Codeine phosphate (p.25·2).
Cough; diarrhoea; pain.

Histaxin *Asta Medica, Aust.*
Diphenhydramine hydrochloride (p.416·1).
Dermatologic hypersensitivity reactions.

Histazine *Trima, Israel.*
Cetirizine (p.411·3).
Hypersensitivity reactions.

Histema *Unison, Thai.*
Astemizole (p.409·1).
Allergic conjunctivtis; allergic rhinitis; allergic skin disorders.

Histenol Cold *Zee, Canad.*
Pseudoephedrine hydrochloride (p.1099·2); dextromethorphan hydrobromide (p.1087·3); paracetamol (p.71·2).

Histergan *Norma, UK.*
Diphenhydramine hydrochloride (p.416·1).
Hypersensitivity reactions.

Histerone *Roberts, USA†; Hauck, USA†.*
Testosterone (p.1492·1).
Androgen replacement therapy; delayed puberty.

Histex *CTEX, USA.*
Pseudoephedrine hydrochloride (p.1099·2); chlorpheniramine [chlorphenamine] maleate (p.412·1).
Upper respiratory-tract symptoms.

Histex CT *CTEX, USA.*
Carbinoxamine maleate (p.411·1).
Hypersensitivity reactions.

Histex HC *CTEX, USA.*
Pseudoephedrine hydrochloride (p.1099·2); hydrocodone tartrate (p.42·2); carbinoxamine hydrochloride (p.411·1) or carbinoxamine maleate (p.411·1).
Coughs; respiratory-tract congestion; rhinitis.

Histex PD *CTEX, USA.*
Carbinoxamine (p.411·1).
Allergic rhinitis.

Histex SR *CTEX, USA.*
Paracetamol (p.71·2); phenylephrine (p.1097·1); chlorpheniramine [chlorphenamine] (p.412·2).
Allergic rhinitis; cold symptoms; sinusitis.

Histiacil *Columbia, Mex.*
Dextromethorphan hydrobromide (p.1087·3); ambroxol hydrochloride (p.1084·3).
Respiratory-tract disorders.

Histilos *UCB, Swed.*
Nicotinic acid (p.1372·3); meclozine hydrochloride (p.420·3); hydroxyzine hydrochloride (p.419·1).
Ménière's disease.

Histin *Kenyaku, Thai.*
Carbinoxamine maleate (p.411·1).
Allergic rhinitis; allergic skin disorders.

Histine DM *Ethex, USA†.*
Phenylpropanolamine hydrochloride (p.1098·1); brompheniramine maleate (p.410·2); dextromethorphan hydrobromide (p.1087·3).
Coughs.

Histiness *Biomedica, Ger.*
Homoeopathic preparation.

Histinex D *Ethex, USA.*
Hydrocodone tartrate (p.42·2); pseudoephedrine hydrochloride (p.1099·2).
Coughs and cold symptoms.

Histinex DM *Ethex, USA†.*
Dextromethorphan hydrobromide (p.1087·3); phenylpropanolamine hydrochloride (p.1098·1); brompheniramine maleate (p.410·2).
Coughs and cold symptoms.

Histinex HC *Ethex, USA.*
Hydrocodone tartrate (p.42·2); phenylephrine hydrochloride (p.1097·1); chlorpheniramine [chlorphenamine] maleate (p.412·1).
Coughs.

Histinex PV *Ethex, USA.*
Hydrocodone tartrate (p.42·2); pseudoephedrine hydrochloride (p.1099·2); chlorpheniramine [chlorphenamine] maleate (p.412·1).
Cough and cold symptoms.

Histoacryl *Braun, UK.*
Enbucrilate (p.1601·2).
Tissue adhesive for closure of minor wounds.

Histodil *Gedeon Richter, Thai.*
Cimetidine hydrochloride (p.1218·3).
Gastro-oesophageal reflux; gastrointestinal haemorrhage; peptic ulcer; Zollinger-Ellison syndrome.

Histodor *Aspen, S.Afr.*
Cream: Mepyramine maleate (p.421·1); diphenhydramine hydrochloride (p.416·1).
Insect bites; skin disorders.

Tablets: Mepyramine maleate (p.421·1); promethazine hydrochloride (p.423·2); caffeine (p.761·3).
Hypersensitivity reactions.

Histodor Expectorant *Aspen Consumer, S.Afr.*
Diphenhydramine hydrochloride (p.416·1); ammonium chloride (p.1085·2); sodium citrate (p.1186·2).
Coughs.

Histodryl *Biolab, Thai.*
Diphenhydramine hydrochloride (p.416·1); ammonium chloride (p.1085·2); sodium citrate (p.1186·2); menthol (p.1632·3).
Cold symptoms; coughs.

Histo-Fluine P *Richard, Fr.*
Aesculus (p.1574·1); hamamelis (p.1618·3); shepherd's purse (p.1662·3); pulsatilla (p.1656·3); esculoside (p.1574·1).
Peripheral vascular disorders.

Histofreezer
Hamilton, Austral.; Braun, Fr.
Dimethyl ether (p.1199·1); propane (p.1200·3).
Warts.

Histol *Julphar, UAE.*
Pheniramine maleate (p.422·3).
Hypersensitivity.

Histolyn-CYL *ALK, USA.*
Histoplasmin (p.1619·3).
Diagnostic test.

Histophtal *Metochem, Aust.†*
Naphazoline hydrochloride (p.1095·1); antazoline hydrochloride (p.408·3).
Eye disorders.

Histor-D *Roberts, USA.*
Phenylephrine hydrochloride (p.1097·1); chlorpheniramine [chlorphenamine] maleate (p.412·1).
Upper respiratory-tract symptoms.

Histor-D Timecelles *Roberts, USA.*
Chlorpheniramine [chlorphenamine] maleate (p.412·1); phenylephrine hydrochloride (p.1097·1); hyoscine methonitrate (p.468·2).
Upper respiratory-tract symptoms.

Histosal *Ferndale, USA†.*
Phenylpropanolamine hydrochloride (p.1098·1); paracetamol (p.71·2); caffeine (p.761·3); mepyramine maleate (p.421·1).
Upper respiratory-tract symptoms.

Histussin D *Sanofi Winthrop, USA.*
Hydrocodone tartrate (p.42·2); pseudoephedrine hydrochloride (p.1099·2).
Coughs; respiratory-tract congestion.

Histussin HC *Sanofi Winthrop, USA.*
Chlorpheniramine [chlorphenamine] maleate (p.412·1); phenylephrine hydrochloride (p.1097·1); hydrocodone tartrate (p.42·2).
Coughs and cold symptoms.

Hitocobamin *Hishiyama, Thai.*
Mecobalamin (p.1388·3).
Peripheral neuropathy.

Hitrechol *Evers, Hong Kong.*
Hedera helix.
Gallstones.

Hi-Vegi-Lip *Freeda, USA.*
Pancreatin (p.1646·1); pancrelipase (p.1647·2).
Deficiency of digestive enzymes.

Hivensteril *Orion, Fin.*
Mineral preparation for infusion (p.1350·1).

Hivernum *Arkopharma, Fr.*
Homoeopathic preparation.
Formerly known as Formule de l' Abbe Chaupitre no 5.

Hives *Hylands, Canad.*
Homoeopathic preparation.

Hivid
Roche, Aust.; Roche, Austral.; Roche, Belg.; Roche, Braz.; Roche, Canad.; Roche, Denm.; Roche, Fin.; Roche, Fr.; Roche, Ger.; Roche, Hong Kong; Roche, Irl.; Roche, Israel; Roche, Ital.; Roche, Jpn; Roche, Mex.; Roche, Neth.; Roche, Norw.; Roche, NZ; Roche, Port.; Roche, S.Afr.; Roche, Singapore; Roche, Spain; Roche, Swed.; Roche, Switz.; Roche, Thai.; Roche, UK; Roche, USA.
Zalcitabine (p.644·1).
HIV infection.

Hivita *Mega Vitamin, Austral.*
A range of multivitamin and mineral preparations (p.1350·1).

Hivita Childvita *Mega Vitamin, Austral.*
Multivitamin and mineral preparation with enzymes (p.1350·1).

Hivita Liquivita *Mega Vitamin, Austral.*
Multivitamin and mineral preparation with plant extracts (p.1350·1).

Hi-Z *Otsuka, Jpn†.*
Oryzanol (p.1645·1).
Head and neck injury; hyperlipidaemia; irritable bowel syndrome; menopausal disorders.

Hizaar *Merck Sharp & Dohme, Ital.*
Losartan potassium (p.921·3); hydrochlorothiazide (p.907·3).
Hypertension.

Hizin *Ranbaxy, Thai.*
Hydroxyzine hydrochloride (p.419·1).
Hypersensitivity reactions.

Hjertealbyl *Leo, Denm.†.*
Aspirin (p.14·2).
Ischaemic heart disease; myocardial infarction.

Hjertemagnyl *Nycomed, Denm.*
Aspirin (p.14·2).
Ischaemic heart disease; myocardial infarction.

HMG *Farma Lepori, Spain.*
Menotrophin (p.1288·2).
Female infertility; male infertility.

HMG Massone *Fustery, Mex.*
Menotrophin (p.1288·2).
Male and female infertility.

H-Mide *LBS, Thai.*
Frusemide [furosemide] (p.893·1).
Hypertension; oedema.

HMS
Allergan, S.Afr.†; Allergan, Switz.; Allergan, USA.
Medrysone (p.1075·3).
Inflammatory eye disorders.

HMS Liquifilm
Allergan, Austral.; Allergan, Neth.†.
Medrysone (p.1075·3).
Inflammatory eye disorders.

HN 25
Milupa, Fr.; Milupa, Hong Kong; Milupa, Irl.; Milupa, Singapore.
Food for special diets (p.1350·1).
Gastro-enteritis in infants and children.

Milupa, Port.; Milupa, Switz.
Preparation for enteral nutrition (p.1350·1).
Gastrointestinal disorders.

HN RL *Milupa, Fr.*
Lactose-free infant feed (p.1350·1).
Diarrhoea.

Hocimin *Durascan, Denm.*
Cimetidine (p.1216·3).
Acid aspiration; gastro-oesophageal reflux; peptic ulcer; Zollinger-Ellison syndrome.

Hocura-Spondylose novo *Pascoe, Ger.*
Hypericum (p.290·2); camphor (p.1589·3).
Nerve and muscle pain.

Hodernal *Rottapharm, Spain.*
Liquid paraffin (p.1407·1).
Constipation.

Hoecutin Olbad *Hoernecke, Ger.†.*
Soya oil (p.1378·1).
Bath additive; dry skin; pruritus.

Hoecutin Olbad F *Hoernecke, Ger.†.*
Arachis oil (p.1581·1); light liquid paraffin (p.1407·2).
Bath additive; dry skin; pruritus.

Hoemarin Derma *Hoernecke, Ger.*
Ichthammol (p.1115·2); sage oil (p.1660·2).
Bath additive; eczema.

Hoemarin Rheuma *Hoernecke, Ger.†.*
Methyl salicylate (p.55·1); turpentine oil (p.1676·3); eucalyptus oil (p.1609·2).
Bath additive; circulatory disorders; musculoskeletal and joint disorders; neuralgia.

Hoepixin Bad N *Hoernecke, Ger.*
Coal tar (p.1125·1).
Bath additive; pruritic skin disorders.

Hoepixin N *Hoernecke, Ger.*
Coal tar (p.1125·1); thyme oil (p.1672·3).
Bath additive; eczema; psoriasis.

Hoevenol *Hoernecke, Ger.*
Capsules: Aesculus (p.1574·1).
Soft-tissue injury; venous insufficiency.
Topical emulsion†: Methyl salicylate (p.55·1); aesculus (p.1574·1).
Haemorrhoids; peripheral vascular disorders; venous insufficiency.

Hoevenol A *Hoernecke, Ger.†.*
Topical application: Arnica (p.1581·3).
Venous insufficiency.
Topical gel: Arnica (p.1581·3); aesculus (p.1574·1).
Circulatory disorders; phlebitis; venous insufficiency.

Hofcomant *Merck, Aust.*
Amantadine sulfate (p.1161·2).
Drug-induced extrapyramidal disorders; herpes zoster; parkinsonism.

Hofels White Willow and Burdock *Seven Seas, UK.*
Salix (p.82·1); lappa (p.1627·1); southern prickly ash (p.1682·1); bearberry (p.1583·3); poplar bark (p.1653·2).
Musculoskeletal and joint pain.

Hoffmannstropfen *Hofmann & Sommer, Ger.*
Ether; alcohol.
Tonic.

Hoggar N *Stada, Ger.*
Doxylamine succinate (p.417·1).
Sleep disorders.

Hokunalin *Hokuriku, Jpn.*
Tulobuterol (p.785·2).
Obstructive airways disease.

Hold DM *Ascher, USA.*
Dextromethorphan hydrobromide (p.1087·3).
Coughs.

Holfungin *Hollborn, Ger.*
Clotrimazole (p.382·1).
Fungal and bacterial skin infections.

Hollihesive *Sigma, Austral.†.*
Skin barrier dressing.

Hollister Karaya Paste *Sigma, Austral.†.*
Sterculia (p.1250·2).
Barrier paste.

Hollister Skin Gel *Sigma, Austral.†.*
Barrier gel.

Holofusine *Braun, Switz.*
Electrolyte infusion with or without glucose (p.1180·1).
Fluid and electrolyte disorders.

Holopon *Byk Gulden, Hong Kong.*
Hyoscine methobromide (p.468·2).
Gastritis; motion sickness; peptic ulcer; smooth muscle spasm.

Holoxan
Asta Medica, Aust.; Asta Medica, Austral.; Asta Medica, Belg.; Asta, Denm.; Asta Medica, Fin.; Asta Medica, Fr.; Asta Medica, Ger.; Asta Medica, Hong Kong; Asta Medica, Ital.; Sanfer, Mex.; Asta Medica, Neth.; Asta Medica, Norw.; Asta Medica, NZ; NZ Medical & Scientific, NZ; Asta Medica, Port.; Aventis, S.Afr.; Asta Medica, Singapore; Asta Medica, Swed.; Asta Medica, Switz.; Asta Medica, Thai.
Ifosfamide (p.546·1).
Malignant neoplasms.

Holoxane *Asta Medica, Braz.*
Ifosfamide (p.546·1).
Malignant neoplasms.

Holsten aktiv *Holsten, Ger.†.*
Ethyl chloride (p.1312·1).
Local anaesthesia.

Homasedin *Medifarma, Mex.*
Homatropine (p.468·1).

Homatrocil *Oftalder, Port.*
Homatropine hydrobromide (p.468·1).
Production of mydriasis and cycloplegia.

Homatrop *Llorens, Spain.*
Homatropine hydrobromide (p.468·1).
Production of mydriasis and cycloplegia; uveitis.

Homatropil *Rhone-Poulenc Rorer, Mex.*
Homatropine (p.468·1).

Homeocoksinum *Homeocan, Canad.*
Homoeopathic preparation.

Homeodent
Boiron, Canad.; Boiron, Port.
Homoeopathic preparation.

Homeodose
Dolisos, Canad.; Dolisos, Fr.
A range of homoeopathic preparations.

Homeogene
Boiron, Canad.; Boiron, Fr.; Boiron, Port.
A range of homoeopathic preparations.

Homeoplasmine
Note.This name is used for preparations of different composition.
Boiron, Fr.
Calendula (p.1589·2); pokeroot (p.1653·1); bryonia (p.1587·2); Siam benzoin (p.1662·3); boric acid (p.1586·1).
Skin irritation.

Boiron, Port.
Homoeopathic preparation.

Homeovox
Boiron, Canad.; Boiron, Port.
Homoeopathic preparation.

Hominex *Ross, USA.*
A range of methionine-free preparations for enteral nutrition including an infant feed (p.1350·1).
Vitamin B₆-nonresponsive homocystinuria or hypermethioninaemia.

Homo *Grin, Mex.*
Homatropine (p.468·1).
Production of mydriasis.

Homoclomin
Eisai, Hong Kong; Eisai, Jpn; Eisai, Thai.
Homochlorcyclizine hydrochloride (p.418·3).
Allergic rhinitis; pruritus; urticaria.

Homoderma *Brauer, Austral.*
Homoeopathic preparation.

Honey Lemon Cough Lozenges *Sutton, Canad.*
Menthol (p.1632·3).

Honey & Molasses *Lane, UK.*
Ipecacuanha liquid extract (p.1093·1); marrubium (p.1094·2); squill vinegar (p.1100·3); capsicum (p.1591·1); peppermint oil (p.1243·3); tolu solution; honey (p.1366·2); molasses; glycerol (p.1616·3); liquorice (p.1231·2); anise oil (p.1580·3).
Coughs.

Honeyflu *Home, Ital.*
Paracetamol (p.71·2); dextromethorphan hydrobromide (p.1087·3).
Cough; fever.

Hongosan *Medea, Spain.*
Acedoben (p.1571·3); aluminium chlorohydrate (p.1110·2); cetrimonium bromide (p.1137·3); dexamethasone (p.1067·1); salicylic acid (p.1122·3).
Fungal skin infections.

Hongoseril *Isdin, Spain.*
Itraconazole (p.387·2).
Fungal infections.

Honsa *M & H, Thai.*
Hydroxyzine hydrochloride (p.419·1).
Anxiety; pruritus.

Honvan
Asta Medica, Aust.; Asta Medica, Austral.; Asta Medica, Belg.; Abbott, Braz.; Asta Medica, Ger.; Asta Medica, Hong Kong; Sanfer, Mex.; Asta Medica, Neth.; Asta Medica, Norw.†; Asta Medica, NZ; NZ Medical & Scientific, NZ; Asta Medica, Port.; Noristan, S.Afr.†; Asta Medica, Singapore; Pras, Spain; Asta Medica, Swed.†; Asta Medica, Switz.; Asta Medica, Thai.
Fosfestrol (p.1478·3) or fosfestrol sodium (p.1478·3).
Prostatic cancer.

Honvol *Carter Horner, Canad.*
Fosfestrol sodium (p.1478·3).
Prostatic cancer.

Honzil *Arlex, Mex.*
Ketoconazole (p.389·1).

Hopacem *Hommel, Ger.*
Mianserin hydrochloride (p.298·1).
Depression.

Hordenol *Aerocid, Fr.†.*
Hordenine sulfate; caffeine (p.761·3).
Diarrhoea.

Horehound and Aniseed Cough Mixture *Potter's, UK.*
Pleurisy root (p.1653·1); elecampane (p.1089·3); horehound (p.1094·3); skunk cabbage (p.1664·3); lobelia (p.1510·2).
Coughs.

Hormo Hepatico *Iodo Suma, Braz.*
Adenosine (p.828·2); methionine (p.1012·2); betaine hydrochloride (p.1584·3); choline (p.1356·3); inositol (p.1623·3); pyridoxine (p.1387·1); liver extract; sorbitol (p.1377·3).
Liver disorders.

Hormocervix *Millet Roux, Braz.*
Hydroxyestrone diacetate (p.1479·3).
Vulvovaginal disorders.

Hormodausse *Technilab, Canad.*
Vitamin B substances; iron; liver extract; beef serum (p.1350·1).

Hormodausse plus Calcium and Vitamin D *Charton, Canad.†.*
Multivitamin and mineral preparation (p.1350·1).

Hormoginase *Sanval, Braz.*
Estradiol benzoate (p.1473·1); progesterone (p.1488·3); ergocalciferol (p.1391·2).
Menopausal disorders.

Hormolax *Hormona, Mex.*
Ispaghula (p.1229·1).
Constipation.

Hormone Multicap *Scherer, Thai.*
Methyltestosterone (p.1482·3); ethinylestradiol (p.1476·2); vitamins; rutoside; inositol; methionine; choline bitartrate (p.1350·1).
Nutritional supplement.

Hormonin
Shire, Hong Kong; Shire, UK.
Estriol (p.1475·3); estradiol (p.1473·1); estrone (p.1476·1).
Menopausal disorders; osteoporosis.

Horon *Scherer, Thai.*
Methyltestosterone (p.1482·3); ethinylestradiol (p.1476·2); vitamins; minerals; inositol; methionine; choline bitartrate (p.1350·1).
Nutritional supplement.

Horse Radish and Garlic Tablets *Vitaglow, Austral.*
Horseradish (p.1620·1); garlic (p.1614·1); ascorbic acid (p.1389·3); zinc sulfate (p.1398·2).
Catarrh; coughs; hayfever; sinusitis; upper respiratory-tract congestion.

Horton *Warner-Lambert Consumer, Belg.†.*
Bisacodyl (p.1212·2).
Bowel evacuation; constipation.

Horvilan N *Schoning-Berlin, Ger.†.*
Turmeric (p.1029·3); peppermint oil (p.1243·3); greater celandine (p.1618·1).
Biliary-tract disorders.

Hosboral *Hoechst Marion Roussel, Spain.*
Amoxicillin trihydrate (p.149·2).
Bacterial infections.

Hosboral Bronquial *Roussel, Spain.*
Amoxicillin trihydrate (p.149·2); bromhexine hydrochloride (p.1085·3).
Respiratory-tract infections.

Hospidermin *Lysoform, Ger.*
Alcohol (p.1130·3); potassium thiocyanate; 5-chloro-2-hydroxybenzoic acid.
Skin disinfection.

Hospisept *Lysoform, Ger.*
Propyl alcohol (p.1155·3); alcohol (p.1130·3).
Hand disinfection; skin disinfection.

Hostacyclin
Hoechst Marion Roussel, Aust.; Hoechst, Ger.†.
Tetracycline hydrochloride (p.258·3).
Amoebiasis; bacterial infections.

Hostacycline
Hoechst Marion Roussel, Belg.†; Hoechst Marion Roussel, Irl.†; Quatromed, S.Afr.
Tetracycline hydrochloride (p.258·3).
Bacterial infections.

Hostid *Fournier, Ger.*
Urtica root (p.1678·2).
Micturition disorders associated with prostatic cancer.

Hostop *Nettopharma, Denm.†.*
Acetylcysteine (p.1082·3).
Respiratory-tract congestion.

Hot Coldrex *SmithKline Beecham Consumer, Neth.*
Paracetamol (p.71·2); ascorbic acid (p.1389·3).
Cold and influenza symptoms.

Hot Lemon *Prodemdis, Canad.*
Phenylephrine hydrochloride (p.1097·1); pheniramine maleate (p.422·3); paracetamol (p.71·2); ascorbic acid (p.1389·3).

Hot Lemon Relief *Apotex, Canad.*
Phenylephrine hydrochloride (p.1097·1); pheniramine maleate (p.422·3); paracetamol (p.71·2); ascorbic acid (p.1389·3).

Hot Thermo *Merck dura, Ger.*
Glycol salicylate (p.42·2); benzyl nicotinate (p.20·2).
Musculoskeletal, joint, and soft-tissue disorders; superficial vascular disorders.

Hotemin *Egis, Hong Kong.*
Piroxicam (p.79·1).
Gout; musculoskeletal and joint disorders.

12 Hour Antihistamine Nasal Decongestant *URL, USA.*
Pseudoephedrine sulfate (p.1099·3); dexbrompheniramine maleate (p.410·2).
Upper respiratory-tract symptoms.

8-Hour Bayer Timed-Release *Glenbrook, USA†.*
Aspirin (p.14·2).
Fever; inflammation; myocardial infarction; pain; transient ischaemic attacks.

12 Hour Cold
Note.This name is used for preparations of different composition.
Goldline, USA.
Pseudoephedrine sulfate (p.1099·3); dexbrompheniramine maleate (p.410·2).
Upper respiratory-tract symptoms.

Hudson, USA†.
Phenylpropanolamine hydrochloride (p.1098·1); chlorpheniramine [chlorphenamine] maleate (p.412·1).
Upper respiratory-tract symptoms.

12 Hour Sinarest *Ciba Consumer, USA†.*
Oxymetazoline hydrochloride (p.1096·2).
Nasal congestion.

Hova
Novartis Consumer, Aust.; Gebro, Switz.
Valerian (p.1678·3); lupulus (p.1629·3).
Anxiety disorders; sleep disorders.

Hovaletten N *Zyma, Ger.†.*
Lupulus (p.1629·3); valerian (p.1678·3).
Nervous disorders; sleep disorders.

H₂Oxyl *Stiefel, Canad.†.*
Benzoyl peroxide (p.1111·1).
Acne.

H-Peran *LBS, Thai.*
Metoclopramide (p.1236·3).
Gastrointestinal motility disorders; nausea and vomiting.

Hp-Pac *Abbott, Canad.*
Capsules, lanzoprazole (Prevacid) (p.1230·3); tablets, clarithromycin (Biaxin) (p.186·2); capsules, amoxicillin trihydrate (p.149·2).
Helicobacter pylori-associated peptic ulcer.

H-R Lubricating Jelly *Wallace, USA.*
Vaginal lubricant.

HRF
Wyeth-Ayerst, Austral.; Wyeth Lederle, Belg.; Wyeth, Braz.; Monmouth, Irl.; Sigma-Tau, Neth.; Wyeth, NZ; Akromed, S.Afr.†; Intrapharm, UK.
Gonadorelin (p.1283·3) or gonadorelin hydrochloride (p.1284·2).
Anovulatory infertility; sterility or delayed puberty due to hypogonadotrophic hypogonadism; test of hypothalamic function.

HRI Calm Life *Jessup, UK.*
Jamaica dogwood (p.1625·1); lupulus (p.1629·3); skullcap (p.1664·3); chamomile (p.1593·2); valerian (p.1678·3).
Irritability; restlessness.

HRI Clear Complexion *Jessup, UK.*
Sarsaparilla (p.1661·1); iris versicolor (p.1624·2); lappa (p.1627·1).
Skin disorders.

HRI Golden Seal Digestive *Jessup, UK.*
Ginger (p.1227·2); myrrh (p.1639·2); hydrastis (p.1621·1); rhubarb (p.1248·1); valerian (p.1678·3).
Dyspepsia; flatulence.

HRI Night *Jessup, UK.*
Valerian (p.1678·3); passion flower (p.1649·1); wild lettuce (p.1680·3); vervain (p.1679·3); lupulus (p.1629·3).
Insomnia.

HRI Water Balance *Jessup, UK.*
Taraxacum (p.1669·1); buchu (p.1587·2); parsley piert (p.1648·3); bearberry (p.1583·3).
Water retention.

H-Sal *Zambon, Braz.*
Homatropine (p.468·1); sodium; potassium; calcium; vitamin B₂; nicotinamide; glucose (p.1185·2).
Gastrointestinal spasm; oral rehydration therapy.

HT903 *Optimal, Hong Kong.*
Melatonin (p.1632·1).
Jet lag; melatonin deficiency.

H-Tab *Pharmaland, Thai.*
Haloperidol (p.686·3).
Hypomania; mania; psychoses.

H-Tronin *Hoechst Marion Roussel, Ger.*
Insulin injection (human) (p.324·1).
Diabetes mellitus.

H-Tuss-D *Cypress, USA.*
Hydrocodone tartrate (p.42·2); pseudoephedrine hydrochloride (p.1099·2).
Coughs.

Huberdilat *ICN, Spain.*
Cetiedil (p.856·3).
Peripheral vascular disorders.

Huberdoxina *ICN, Spain.*
Ciprofloxacin hydrochloride (p.182·3) or ciprofloxacin lactate (p.182·3).
Bacterial infections.

Hubergrip *ICN, Spain.*
Suppositories: Caffeine (p.1116·3); calcium pantothenate (p.1374·1); citiolone (p.1596·2); chlorpheniramine [chlorphenamine] maleate (p.412·1); paracetamol (p.71·2); vitamin A (p.1382·1).
Tablets: Caffeine (p.1116·3); chlorpheniramine [chlorphenamine] maleate (p.412·1); propyphenazone (p.80·2); salicylamide (p.82·1).
Influenza and cold symptoms.

Huberlitren *ICN, Spain†.*
Calcium lactate; citric acid; magnesium sulfate; potassium chloride; sodium citrate; sodium chloride; tribasic sodium phosphate; glucose (p.1185·2).
Oral rehydration therapy.

Hubermizol *ICN, Spain.*
Astemizole (p.409·1).
Hypersensitivity reactions.

Huberplex *Teofarma, Spain.*
Chlordiazepoxide hydrochloride (p.659·2).
Alcohol withdrawal syndrome; anxiety; insomnia; skeletal muscle spasm.

Huile analgesique "Polar-Bar" *Panax, Switz.*
Mint oil (p.1636·2); camphor (p.1589·3); menthol (p.1632·3); eucalyptus oil (p.1609·2); methyl salicylate (p.55·1); thymol (p.1158·3).
Headache.

Huile de Bain Therapeutique *Atlas, Canad.*
Wool fat (p.1410·3); liquid paraffin (p.1407·1).

Huile de Haarlem *Lefevre, Fr.†*
Sulfur (p.1123·3); linseed oil (p.1629·1); turpentine oil (p.1676·3).
Arthritic disorders; respiratory-tract disorders.

Huile de millepertuis A. Vogel (huile de St. Jean) *Bioforce, Switz.*
Hypericum (p.290·2); sunflower oil (p.1381·2).
Superficial wounds.

Huile Gomenolee *Gomenol, Fr.*
Niaouli oil (p.1640·2).
Nasal infections.

Huile Po-Ho A. Vogel *Bioforce, Switz.*
Peppermint oil (p.1243·3); eucalyptus oil (p.1609·2); juniper oil (p.1625·2); caraway oil (p.1591·2); fennel oil (p.1610·2).
Cold symptoms; headache; muscular tension.

Huile Solaire Bronzage *Clarins, Canad.†*
SPF 3: Octinoxate (p.1517·3); oxybenzone (p.1518·1).
Sunscreen.

Humacart 3/7 *Lilly, Jpn.*
A mixture of insulin injection (human, prb) and isophane insulin injection (human, prb) (p.324·1).
Diabetes mellitus.

Humaject 10/90, 20/80, 30/70, 40/60, 50/50 *Lilly, Neth.*
Mixtures of insulin injection (human) and isophane insulin injection (human) respectively in the proportions indicated (p.324·1).
Diabetes mellitus.

Humaject 20/80, 30/70, 40/60, 50/50 *Lilly, Belg.*
Mixtures of insulin injection (human) and isophane insulin injection (human) respectively in the proportions indicated (p.324·1).
Diabetes mellitus.

Humaject I *Lilly, UK.*
Injection device containing Humulin I (p.324·1).
Diabetes mellitus.

Humaject M1, M2, M3, M4, M5 *Lilly, UK.*
Injection device containing Humulin M1, M2, M3, M4, and M5 respectively (p.324·1).
Diabetes mellitus.

Humaject NPH
Lilly, Belg.; Lilly, Neth.
Isophane insulin injection (human) (p.324·1).
Diabetes mellitus.

Humaject Regular
Lilly, Belg.; Lilly, Neth.
Insulin injection (human) (p.324·1).
Diabetes mellitus.

Humaject S *Lilly, UK.*
Injection device containing Humulin S (p.324·1).
Diabetes mellitus.

Humal *Rosch & Handel, Aust.*
Humic acid; salicylic acid (p.1122·3).
Rheumatism.

Humalog
Lilly, Aust.; Lilly, Austral.; Lilly, Belg.; Lilly, Canad.; Lilly, Denm.; Lilly, Fin.; Lilly, Fr.; Lilly, Ger.; Lilly, Hong Kong; Lilly, Irl.; Lilly, Israel; Lilly, Ital.; Lilly, Mex.; Lilly, Neth.; Lilly, Norw.; Lilly, NZ; Lilly, Port.; Lilly, S.Afr.; Lilly, Singapore; Lilly, Spain; Lilly, Swed.; Lilly, Switz.; Lilly, Thai.; Lilly, UK; Lilly, USA.
Insulin lispro (p.324·1).
Diabetes mellitus.

Humalog Mix 25
Lilly, Aust.; Lilly, Neth.; Lilly, Norw.
Mixture of insulin lispro 25% and isophane insulin lispro 75% (p.324·1).
Diabetes mellitus.

Humalog Mix 25 and 50
Lilly, Aust.; Lilly, Denm.; Lilly, Fin.; Lilly, Fr.; Lilly, Irl.; Lilly, UK.
A mixture of insulin lispro 25% or 50% and isophane insulin lispro 75% or 50%, respectively (p.324·1).
Diabetes mellitus.

Humalog Mix 75/25 and 50/50 *Lilly, USA.*
Mixtures of isophane insulin lispro 75% and 50% and insulin lispro 25% and 50% respectively (p.324·1).
Diabetes mellitus.

Human Actraphane *Novo Nordisk, UK†.*
Mixture of neutral insulin injection (human, pyr) 30% and isophane insulin injection (human, pyr) 70% (p.324·1).
Diabetes mellitus.

Human Actrapid *Novo Nordisk, UK.*
Neutral insulin injection (human, pyr) (p.324·1).
Diabetes mellitus.

Human Initard 50/50 *Novo Nordisk, UK†; Wellcome, UK†.*
Mixture of neutral insulin injection (human, emp, highly purified) 50% and isophane insulin injection (human, emp, highly purified) 50% (p.324·1).
Diabetes mellitus.

Human Insulatard *Novo Nordisk, UK.*
Isophane insulin injection (human, pyr, highly purified) (p.324·1).
Formerly known as Human Protaphane.
Diabetes mellitus.

Human Mixtard 10, 20, 30, 40, and 50 *Novo Nordisk, UK.*
Mixture of neutral insulin injection (human, pyr, highly purified) 10, 20, 30, 40, or 50% and isophane insulin injection (human, pyr, highly purified) 90, 80, 70, 60, or 50% respectively (p.324·1).
Human Mixtard 30 ge was formerly known as Human Actraphane 30/70 and contained human insulin (emp).
Diabetes mellitus.

Human Monotard *Novo Nordisk, UK.*
Insulin zinc suspension (amorphous 30%, crystalline 70%) (human, pyr) (p.324·1).
Diabetes mellitus.

Human Ultratard *Novo Nordisk, UK.*
Insulin zinc suspension (crystalline) (human, pyr) (p.324·1).
Diabetes mellitus.

Human Velosulin *Novo Nordisk, UK.*
Neutral insulin injection (human, emp, highly purified) (p.324·1).
Diabetes mellitus.

Humana AR *Humana, Ital.*
Infant feed (p.1350·1).
Gastro-oesophageal reflux; regurgitation.

Humana Disanal *Humana, Ital.*
Food for special diets (p.1350·1).
Gastrointestinal disorders.

Humana HA *Humana, Ital.*
Infant feed (p.1350·1).
Food intolerance.

Humana Sinelac *Humana, Ital.*
Infant feed (p.1350·1).
Formerly known as Humana SL.
Milk intolerance.

Humanalbin *Centeon, Ger.*
Albumin (p.724·1).
Hypovolaemia.

Humanilusin *Cryopharma, Mex.*
Human insulin (p.324·1).
Diabetes mellitus.

Humaplus 10/90, 20/80, 30/70, 40/60, 50/50 *Lilly, Spain.*
Mixtures of insulin injection (human) and isophane insulin injection (human) respectively in the proportions indicated (p.324·1).
Diabetes mellitus.

Humaplus NPH *Lilly, Spain.*
Isophane insulin injection (human) (p.324·1).
Diabetes mellitus.

Humaplus Regular *Lilly, Spain.*
Insulin injection (human) (p.324·1).
Diabetes mellitus.

Humate-P *Centeon, USA.*
A factor VIII preparation (p.734·1).
Haemophilia A.

Humatin
Parke, Davis, Aust.; Parke, Davis, Canad.; Parke, Davis, Ger.; Parke, Davis, Ital.; Parke, Davis, Spain; Parke, Davis, Switz.; Parke, Davis, USA.
Paromomycin sulfate (p.599·2).
Bacterial enteritis; hepatic encephalopathy and coma; intestinal amoebiasis; preoperative intestinal sterilisation; taeniasis.

Humatrope
Lilly, Aust.; Lilly, Austral.; Lilly, Belg.; Lilly, Braz.; Lilly, Canad.; Lilly, Denm.; Lilly, Fin.; Lilly, Ger.; Lilly, Hong Kong; Lilly, Ital.; Lilly, Mex.;

Lilly, Neth.; Lilly, Norw.; Lilly, Port.; Lilly, S.Afr.; Lilly, Singapore; Lilly, Spain; Lilly, Swed.; Lilly, Switz.; Lilly, UK; Lilly, USA.
Somatropin (p.1286·1).
Growth disorders in renal failure; growth hormone deficiency; Turner's syndrome.

Humatro-Pen *Aza, Austral.*
Somatropin (p.1286·1).
Growth hormone deficiency.

Humavent *WE, USA.*
Guaifenesin (p.1092·2).

Humectante *Alcon Cusi, Spain.*
Methylcellulose (p.1502·2); sodium chloride (p.1196·1).
Dry eyes in contact lens wearers.

Humectol *Virtus, Braz.*
Bisacodyl (p.1212·2); docusate (p.1222·3).
Constipation.

Humedia *APS, Ger.*
Glibenclamide (p.321·3).
Diabetes mellitus.

Humegon
Organon, Aust.; Organon, Austral.; Organon, Belg.; Akzo, Braz.; Organon, Canad.; Organon, Fr.†; Organon, Ger.; Organon, Hong Kong; Organon, Irl.; Organon, Israel; Organon, Ital.; Organon, Mex.; Organon, Neth.†; Organon, Norw.†; Organon, Port.†; Donmed, S.Afr.; Organon, Singapore; Organon, Swed.†; Organon, Switz.; Organon, Thai.; Organon, UK†; Organon, USA.
Menotrophin (p.1288·2).
Male and female infertility.

Humektan *Orion, Fin.*
Moisturiser; vehicle for topical drugs.

Humex
Note.This name is used for preparations of different composition.
Fournier, Belg.; Fournier SA, Spain†.
Dextromethorphan hydrobromide (p.1087·3).
Coughs.

Urgo, Fr.
Adult syrup: Pholcodine (p.1099·1).
Formerly contained ethylmorphine hydrochloride, squill, ipecacuanha, and belladonna.
Coughs.
Capsules: Carbinoxamine maleate (p.411·1); phenylpropanolamine hydrochloride (p.1098·1); paracetamol (p.71·2).
Upper respiratory-tract disorders.
Lozenges: Ethylmorphine hydrochloride (p.35·1); ipecacuanha (p.1093·1); belladonna (p.463·1).
Coughs.
Nasal solution: Benzalkonium chloride (p.1133·2).
Formerly contained benzododecinium bromide.
Nasal infections.
Paediatric syrup: Pholcodine (p.1099·1).
Formerly contained pholcodine, sodium benzoate, drosera, belladonna, and tolu balsam.
Coughs.
Pastilles: Biclotymol (p.1136·1).
Sore throat.
Throat spray: Benzalkonium chloride (p.1133·2); lignocaine [lidocaine] hydrochloride (p.1313·2).
Mouth and throat disorders.

Humex Expectorant *Urgo, Fr.*
Lozenges: Acetylcysteine (p.1082·3).
Syrup: Carbocisteine (p.1086·3).
Respiratory-tract congestion.

Humex Kinaldine *Urgo, Fr.*
Dequalinium chloride (p.1143·1); ascorbic acid (p.1389·3).
Mouth and throat disorders.

Humex Rhume *Urgo, Fr.*
Tablets (daytime), paracetamol (p.71·2); pseudoephedrine hydrochloride (p.1099·2); capsules (evening), paracetamol; chlorpheniramine [chlorphenamine] maleate (p.412·1).
Cold symptoms.

Humibid *Medeva, USA.*
Guaifenesin (p.1092·2).
Coughs.

Humibid DM *Adams, USA.*
Dextromethorphan hydrobromide (p.1087·3); guaifenesin (p.1092·2).
Coughs.

Humiderm *Convatec, UK†.*
Sodium pidolate (p.1123·3).
Dry skin disorders.

Huminsulin *Lilly, Ger.*
Insulin injection (human, prb) (p.324·1).
Diabetes mellitus.

Huminsulin Basal
Lilly, Aust.; Lilly, Ger.; Lilly, Switz.
Isophane insulin injection (human, prb) (p.324·1).
Diabetes mellitus.

Huminsulin Long
Lilly, Aust.; Lilly, Ger.†; Lilly, Switz.
Insulin zinc suspension (crystalline 70%, amorphous 30%) (human, prb) (p.324·1).
Diabetes mellitus.

Huminsulin Normal
Lilly, Aust.; Lilly, Ger.; Lilly, Switz.
Insulin injection (human, prb) (p.324·1).
Diabetes mellitus.

Huminsulin Profil I, II, III, and IV
Lilly, Aust.; Lilly, Ger.; Lilly, Switz.
Mixtures of insulin injection (human, prb) 10%, 20%, 30%, and 40% and isophane insulin injection (human, prb) 90%, 80%, 70%, and 60% respectively (p.324·1).
Diabetes mellitus.

Huminsulin Ultralong
Lilly, Aust.; Lilly, Ger.†; Lilly, Switz.
Insulin zinc suspension (crystalline) (human, prb) (p.324·1).
Diabetes mellitus.

HuMist Nasal Mist *Scherer, USA.*
Sodium chloride (p.1196·1).
Nasal irritation.

Humoferon *Sigma-Tau, Ital.*
Interferon alfa-n1 (p.628·1).
Chronic hepatitis; leukaemias.

Humopin N *Schoning-Berlin, Ger.†*
Salicylic acid (p.1122·3).
Bath additive; musculoskeletal and joint disorders.

Humorsol *Merck, USA.*
Demecarium bromide (p.1416·3).
Open-angle glaucoma; strabismus.

Humoryl *Synthelabo, Fr.*
Toloxatone (p.309·2).
Depression.

Humoxal
Note.This name is used for preparations of different composition.
Freda, Port.†
Phenylephrine hydrochloride (p.1097·1).
Nasal congestion.

Fournier SA, Spain†.
Oxymetazoline hydrochloride (p.1096·2).
Nasal congestion; sinus congestion.

Humulin 10/90, 20/80, 30/70, 40/60, and 50/50
Lilly, Austral.; Lilly, Canad.; Lilly, Ital.; Lilly, S.Afr.; Lilly, Singapore.
Mixtures of insulin injection (human) and isophane insulin injection (human) respectively in the proportions indicated (p.324·1).
Diabetes mellitus.

Humulin 70/30, 80/20, and 90/10
Lilly, Braz.; Lilly, Hong Kong; Lilly, Israel; Lilly, Mex.; Lilly, NZ; Lilly, Thai.; Lilly, USA.
Mixtures of isophane insulin injection (human) and insulin injection (human) (p.324·1) respectively in the proportions indicated.
Diabetes mellitus.

Humulin I
Lilly, Irl.; Lilly, Ital.; Lilly, UK.
Isophane insulin injection (human, prb) (p.324·1).
Diabetes mellitus.

Humulin L
Lilly, Austral.; Lilly, Canad.; Lilly, Hong Kong; Lilly, Ital.; Lilly, Mex.; Lilly, NZ; Lilly, S.Afr.; Lilly, Singapore; Lilly, USA.
Insulin zinc suspension (human) (p.324·1).
Diabetes mellitus.

Humulin Lenta
Lilly, Braz.; Lilly, Port.
Insulin zinc suspension (30% amorphous, crystalline 70%) (human) (p.324·1).
Diabetes mellitus.

Humulin Lente
Lilly, Irl.; Lilly, UK.
Insulin zinc suspension (30% amorphous, 70% crystalline) (human, prb) (p.324·1).
Diabetes mellitus.

Humulin M1, M2, M3, M4, M5
Lilly, Irl.; Lilly, Port.; Lilly, UK.
Mixtures of insulin injection (human) 10%, 20%, 30%, 40%, and 50% and isophane insulin injection (human) 90%, 80%. 70%, 60%, and 50%, respectively (p.324·1).
Diabetes mellitus.

Humulin Mix 30/70
Lilly, Denm.; Lilly, Fin.; Lilly, Norw.; Lilly, Swed.
A mixture of insulin injection (human) 30% and isophane insulin injection (human) 70% (p.324·1).
Diabetes mellitus.

Humulin N
Lilly, Canad.; Lilly, Hong Kong; Lilly, Israel; Lilly, Mex.; Lilly, NZ; Lilly, S.Afr.; Lilly, Singapore; Lilly, Thai.; Lilly, USA.
Isophane insulin injection (human) (p.324·1).
Diabetes mellitus.

Humulin NPH
Lilly, Austral.; Lilly, Braz.; Lilly, Denm.; Lilly, Fin.; Lilly, Norw.; Lilly, Port.; Lilly, Swed.
Isophane insulin injection (human) (p.324·1).
Diabetes mellitus.

Humulin R
Lilly, Austral.; Lilly, Canad.; Lilly, Hong Kong; Lilly, Israel; Lilly, Ital.; Lilly, Mex.; Lilly, NZ; Lilly, S.Afr.; Lilly, Singapore; Lilly, Thai.; Lilly, USA.
Insulin injection (human) (p.324·1).
Diabetes mellitus.

Humulin Regular
Lilly, Braz.; Lilly, Denm.; Lilly, Fin.; Lilly, Norw.; Lilly, Port.; Lilly, Swed.
Insulin injection (human) (p.324·1).
Diabetes mellitus.

Humulin S
Lilly, Irl.; Lilly, UK.
Insulin injection (human, prb) (p.324·1).
Diabetes mellitus.

Humulin U
Lilly, Canad.; Lilly, Israel; Lilly, Mex.; Lilly, NZ; Lilly, S.Afr.†.
Insulin zinc suspension (crystalline) (human) (p.324·1).
Diabetes mellitus.

Humulin U Ultralente *Lilly, USA.*
Insulin zinc suspension, extended (human, crb) (p.324·1).
Diabetes mellitus.

Humulin UL *Lilly, Austral.*
Insulin zinc suspension (crystalline) (human, prb) (p.324·1).
Diabetes mellitus.

Humulin Ultralenta *Lilly, Port.*
Insulin zinc suspension (crystalline) (human) (p.324·1).
Diabetes mellitus.

Humulin Zn
Lilly, Irl.; Lilly, UK.
Insulin zinc suspension (crystalline) (human, prb) (p.324·1).
Diabetes mellitus.

Humulina 10:90, 20:80, 30:70, 40:60, 50:50 *Lilly, Spain.*
Mixture of insulin injection (human, prb) and isophane insulin injection (human, prb) (p.324·1) respectively in the proportions indicated.
Diabetes mellitus.

Humulina Lenta *Lilly, Spain.*
Insulin zinc suspension (human) (p.324·1).
Diabetes mellitus.

Humulina NPH *Lilly, Spain.*
Isophane insulin injection (human, prb) (p.324·1).
Diabetes mellitus.

Humulina Regular *Lilly, Spain.*
Insulin injection (human, prb) (p.324·1).
Diabetes mellitus.

Humulina Ultralenta *Lilly, Spain.*
Insulin zinc suspension (crystalline 70%, amorphous 30%) (human) (p.324·1).
Diabetes mellitus.

Humuline 10/90, 20/80, 30/70, 40/60, 50/50
Lilly, Belg.; Lilly, Neth.
Mixtures of insulin injection (human) and isophane insulin injection (human) respectively in the proportions indicated (p.324·1).
Diabetes mellitus.

Humuline Long *Lilly, Belg.*
Insulin suspension (human, biosynthetic) (p.324·1).
Diabetes mellitus.

Humuline NPH
Lilly, Belg.; Lilly, Neth.
Isophane insulin injection (human) (p.324·1).
Diabetes mellitus.

Humuline Regular
Lilly, Belg.; Lilly, Neth.
Neutral insulin injection (human) (p.324·1).
Diabetes mellitus.

Humuline Ultralong *Lilly, Belg.*
Insulin suspension (human, biosynthetic) (p.324·1).
Diabetes mellitus.

Humuline Zink *Lilly, Neth.†*
Insulin zinc suspension (crystalline, human) (p.324·1).
Diabetes mellitus.

Humutard
Lilly, Fin.; Lilly, Swed.†
Insulin zinc suspension (human) (amorphous 30%, crystalline 70%) (p.324·1).
Diabetes mellitus.

Humutard Ultra
Lilly, Denm.; Lilly, Fin.
Insulin zinc suspension (crystalline) (human)(p.324·1).
Diabetes mellitus.

Hurricaine
Clarben, Spain; Beutlich, USA.
Benzocaine (p.1306·2).
Local anaesthesia.

Hustagil Erkaltungsbalsam *Dentinox, Ger.*
Thyme oil (p.1672·3); oleum pini sylvestris; eucalyptus oil (p.1609·2); clove oil (p.1597·1).
Coughs and associated respiratory-tract disorders.

Hustagil Inhalationsol *Dentinox, Ger.*
Thyme oil (p.1672·3); eucalyptus oil (p.1609·2); pumilio pine oil (p.1656·3); pine needle oil; clove oil (p.1597·1).
Coughs and associated respiratory-tract disorders.

Hustagil Thymian-Hustensaft *Dentinox, Ger.*
Thyme (p.1672·2).
Coughs and associated respiratory-tract disorders.

Hustagil Thymiantropfen *Dentinox, Ger.*
Thyme (p.1672·2).
Coughs and associated respiratory-tract disorders.

Hustazol *Yoshitomi, Jpn†.*
Cloperastine fendizoate (p.1087·2) or cloperastine hydrochloride (p.1087·2).
Coughs.

Hustazol-C *Takeda, Thai.*
Cloperastine hydrochloride (p.1087·2); sulfogaiacol (p.1101·1); dl-methylephedrine hydrochloride (p.1094·3).
Coughs.

Husten ACC *Hexal, Aust.*
Acetylcysteine (p.1082·3).
Respiratory-tract disorders with viscous secretions.

Husten- und Fieber-Saft *Ratiopharm, Ger.*
Paracetamol (p.71·2); dextromethorphan hydrobromide (p.1087·3).
Coughs; fever.

Hustensaft Weleda *Weleda, Aust.*
Herbal and homoeopathic preparation.

Hustensaft-Dr Schmidgall *Schmidgall, Aust.*
Plantago lanceolata; thyme (p.1672·2); cowslip (p.1600·1).
Catarrh; coughs and cold symptoms.

Hustenstiller *Ratiopharm, Ger.*
Dextromethorphan hydrobromide (p.1087·3).
Coughs.

Hustenstiller N *Palmicol, Ger.†*
Menthol (p.1632·3); benzocaine (p.1306·2).
Catarrh; coughs.

Hustentabs *Ratiopharm, Ger.*
Bromhexine hydrochloride (p.1085·3).
Respiratory-tract disorders associated with increased or viscous mucus.

Husties *Eu Rho, Ger.*
Thyme (p.1672·2).
Catarrh; coughs.

HVM *Scherer, Singapore.*
Multivitamin and mineral preparation (p.1350·1).

Hya-ject *Hexal, Ger.*
Sodium hyaluronate (p.1620·1).
Joint disorders.

Hyalart
Bayer, Ger.; SPA, Ital.
Sodium hyaluronate (p.1620·1).
Musculoskeletal and joint disorders.

Hyalase
Rhone-Poulenc Rorer, Austral.; CP, Israel; Artex, NZ; Xixia, S.Afr.; CP Pharmaceuticals, UK.
Hyaluronidase (p.1620·3).
Enhance absorption of intramuscular and subcutaneous injections; extravasation; haematoma; hypodermoclysis; oedema.

Hyalein *Santen, Jpn.*
Sodium hyaluronate (p.1620·1).
Keratoconjunctival disorders.

Hyalgan
Kolassa, Aust.; Nycomed, Denm.; Nycomed, Fin.; Fournier, Fr.†; Fidia, Hong Kong; Shire, Irl.; Fidia, Ital.; Nycomed, Swed.; Shire, UK; Sanofi Winthrop, USA.
Sodium hyaluronate (p.1620·1).
Osteoarthritis of the knee.

Hyalistil *SIFI, Ital.*
Sodium hyaluronate (p.1620·1).
Dry eyes.

Hyalofill
Convatec, Fr.; Convatec, UK.
Hyaff (p.1620·1).
Ulcers; wounds.

Hyalogran *Convatec, Fr.*
Sodium alginate (p.1498·3); Hyaff (p.1620·1).
Ulcers; wounds.

Hyalozima *Apsen, Braz.*
Hyaluronidase (p.1620·3).
Enhancement of absorption of intramuscular and subcutaneous injections; reduction of extravasation.

Hyanit N *Strathmann, Ger.†*
Urea (p.1127·3).
Skin disorders.

Hya-Ophtal *Winzer, Ger.*
Sodium hyaluronate (p.1620·1).
Aid in eye surgery.

Hyason *Organon, Neth.*
Hyaluronidase (p.1620·3).
Adjunct to local anaesthesia of the eye.

Hyate:C
Porton, Israel; Speywood, Switz.; Ipsen, UK; Speywood, USA.
A porcine factor VIII:C preparation (p.734·1).
Haemophilia in patients with antibodies to human factor VIII.

Hy-Bio *Solgar, UK.*
Vitamin C with bioflavonoids (p.1350·1).

Hybloc *Pacific, NZ.*
Labetalol hydrochloride (p.918·1).
Hypertension.

Hybolin *Hyrex, USA.*
Nandrolone phenylpropionate (p.1484·2) or nandrolone decanoate (p.1484·2).
Anaemia in renal disease; breast cancer.

Hybutyl *Pharmaland, Thai.*
Hyoscine butylbromide (p.468·2).
Smooth muscle spasm.

Hycal
SmithKline Beecham, Irl.; SmithKline Beecham Drinks, UK†.
Glucose syrup solids (p.1364·2).
Food for special diets.

Hycamtin
SmithKline Beecham, Aust.; SmithKline Beecham, Austral.; SmithKline Beecham, Belg.; SmithKline Beecham, Canad.; SmithKline Beecham, Denm.; SmithKline Beecham, Fin.; SmithKline Beecham, Fr.; SmithKline Beecham, Ger.; SmithKline Beecham, Hong Kong; SmithKline Beecham, Irl.; SmithKline Beecham, Israel; SmithKline Beecham, Ital.; SmithKline Beecham, Neth.; SmithKline Beecham, Norw.; Beecham, Port.; SmithKline Beecham, S.Afr.; SmithKline Beecham, Singapore; SmithKline Beecham, Spain; SmithKline Beecham, Swed.; SmithKline Beecham, Switz.; SmithKline Beecham, Thai.; Merck, UK; SmithKline Beecham, USA.
Topotecan hydrochloride (p.575·3).
Ovarian cancer; small-cell lung cancer.

Hyceral *Condrugs, Thai.*
Co-dergocrine mesilate (p.1597·3).
Mental function impairment; peripheral vascular disorders.

Hycocin *Rekah, Israel.*
Hydrocortisone acetate (p.1073·3); neomycin sulfate (p.228·1).
Infected eye, ear, and nose disorders.

HycoClear Tuss *Ethex, USA.*
Hydrocodone tartrate (p.42·2); guaifenesin (p.1092·2).
Coughs.

Hycodan
Note.This name is used for preparations of different composition.
Du Pont, Canad.
Hydrocodone tartrate (p.42·2).
Coughs.
Endo, USA.
Hydrocodone tartrate (p.42·2); homatropine methylbromide (p.468·1).
Coughs.

Hycomine
Note.This name is used for preparations of different composition.
Boots, Austral.†
Hydrocodone tartrate (p.42·2); homatropine methylbromide (p.468·1); mepyramine maleate (p.421·1); phenylephrine hydrochloride (p.1097·1); ammonium chloride (p.1085·2).
Coughs.
Du Pont, Canad.
Hydrocodone tartrate (p.42·2); mepyramine maleate (p.421·1); phenylephrine hydrochloride (p.1097·1); ammonium chloride (p.1085·2).
Coughs; upper respiratory-tract congestion.
Endo, USA†.
Hydrocodone tartrate (p.42·2); phenylpropanolamine hydrochloride (p.1098·1).
Coughs and cold symptoms.

Hycomine Compound *Endo, USA.*
Hydrocodone tartrate (p.42·2); chlorpheniramine [chlorphenamine] maleate (p.412·1); phenylephrine hydrochloride (p.1097·1); paracetamol (p.71·2); caffeine (p.761·3).
Coughs and cold symptoms.

Hycomycin *Teva, Israel.*
Hydrocortisone acetate (p.1073·3); neomycin sulfate (p.228·1).
Infected eye, ear, nose, and skin disorders.

Hyco-Pap *Lunsco, USA†.*
Hydrocodone tartrate (p.42·2); paracetamol (p.71·2).

Hycor *Sigma, Austral.*
Hydrocortisone (p.1073·3) or hydrocortisone acetate (p.1073·3).
Inflammatory eye disorders.

Hycort
ICN, Canad.; Everett, USA.
Hydrocortisone (p.1073·3).
Inflammatory bowel diseases; skin disorders.

Hycotuss *Endo, USA.*
Hydrocodone tartrate (p.42·2); guaifenesin (p.1092·2).
Coughs.

Hydac
Aventis, Denm.; Hoechst Marion Roussel, Fin.; Hoechst Marion Roussel, Swed.
Felodipine (p.888·3).
Hypertension.

Hydal *Mundipharma, Aust.*
Hydromorphone hydrochloride (p.42·3).
Pain.

Hydantin *Orion, Fin.*
Phenytoin (p.357·2).
Epilepsy.

Hydeltrasol *Merck Sharp & Dohme, USA.*
Prednisolone sodium phosphate (p.1078·1).
Corticosteroid.

Hydeltra-TBA *Merck Sharp & Dohme, USA†.*
Prednisolone tebutate (p.1078·2).
Acute gouty arthritis; acute nonspecific tenosynovitis; bursitis; cystic tumours; epicondylitis; post-traumatic osteoarthritis; rheumatoid arthritis; synovitis of osteoarthritis.

Hydergin
Novartis, Aust.; Novartis, Fin.; Novartis, Ger.; Novartis, Swed.
Co-dergocrine mesilate (p.1597·3).
Cerebral and peripheral vascular disorders; cervical syndrome; hypertensive crises; mental function impairment; migraine and other vascular headaches; shock.

Hydergina
Novartis, Ital.; Novartis, Mex.; Novartis, Spain.
Co-dergocrine mesilate (p.1597·3).
Cerebral and peripheral vascular disorders; hypertension; mental function disorders; migraine and other vascular headache.

Hydergine
Novartis, Belg.; Novartis, Braz.; Novartis, Canad.; Novartis, Fr.; Novartis, Hong Kong; Novartis, Irl.; Novartis, Israel; Novartis, Neth.; Novartis, Port.; Novartis, Singapore; Novartis, Switz.; Novartis, Thai.; Novartis, UK; Novartis, USA.
Co-dergocrine mesilate (p.1597·3).
Cerebral and peripheral vascular disorders; mental function impairment; migraine and other vascular headache.

Hyderm *Taro, Canad.*
Hydrocortisone acetate (p.1073·3).
Skin disorders.

Hydiphen *Dresden, Ger.*
Clomipramine hydrochloride (p.282·1).
Depression; nocturnal enuresis; pain; psychoses; sleep disorders.

Hydoftal *Agepha, Aust.*
Hydrocortisone (p.1073·3); hydrocortisone acetate (p.1073·3); neomycin sulfate (p.228·1).
Inflammatory eye disorders.

Hydol *Napp, Irl.*
Dihydrocodeine tartrate (p.33·1).
Pain.

Hydopa *Alphapharm, Austral.*
Methyldopa (p.927·3).
Hypertension.

Hydra Perfecte *L'Oreal, Canad.*
SPF 10: Octinoxate (p.1517·3).
Sunscreen.

Hydrabak
Note.This name is used for preparations of different composition.
Transphyto, Fr.
Wetting solution for contact lenses (p.1129·2).
Farmila, Ital.
Sodium chloride (p.1196·1) (p.1129·2).
Adjunct to use of contact lenses.

Hydracillin *SmithKline Beecham, Ger.†*
Procaine penicillin [procaine benzylpenicillin] (p.239·2); benzylpenicillin sodium (p.157·2).
Lignocaine [lidocaine] hydrochloride (p.1313·2) is included in this preparation to alleviate the pain of injection.
Bacterial infections.

Hydracort *Galderma, Fr.*
Hydrocortisone (p.1073·3).
Skin disorders.

Hydraderm *Sigma, Austral.*
Moisturiser.

Hydragel *Nicholas, Fr.*
Vaginal lubricant.

Hydralin *Nicholas, Fr.*
Powder for topical solution: Sodium perborate (p.1156·3); borax (p.1586·1); sodium bicarbonate (p.1186·2); sodium carbonate anhydrous (p.1665·1).
Soap: Borax (p.1586·1).
Skin cleansing.

Hydralyte *River Foods, Austral.*
Oral rehydration solution (p.1185·2).
Diarrhoea; oral rehydration therapy.

Hydramox *Caber, Ital.*
Amoxicillin trihydrate (p.149·2).
Bacterial infections.

Hydramyn *Lu Chem, USA†.*
Diphenhydramine hydrochloride (p.416·1).
Coughs.

Hydran
Note.This name is used for preparations of different composition.
Orion, Fin.
Vehicle for topical preparations.
Teva, Israel.
Sodium chloride; anhydrous trisodium citrate; potassium chloride; glucose (p.1185·2).
Diarrhoea; oral rehydration therapy.

Hydranorme *Roche-Posay, Irl.*
Emollient.
Dry skin; psoriasis.

Hydrap-ES *Parmed, USA.*
Hydrochlorothiazide (p.907·3); reserpine (p.967·3); hydralazine hydrochloride (p.905·3).
Hypertension.

Hydraplus *SFD, Port.*
Emollient.
Dry skin.

Hydrapres *Rubio, Spain.*
Hydralazine hydrochloride (p.905·3).
Heart failure; hypertension.

Hydrares *Pharmasant, Thai.*
Reserpine (p.967·3); hydralazine hydrochloride (p.905·3); hydrochlorothiazide (p.907·3).
Hypertension.

Hydrasense *Schering, Canad.*
Isotonic desalinated sea water.
Nasal congestion; nasal dryness.

Hydrasorb *Knoll, Canad.†*
Polyurethane foam dressing.
Wounds.

Hydrastis Complex *Blackmores, Austral.*
Liquorice (p.1231·2); althaea (p.1577·1); chamomile (p.1593·2); hydrastis (p.1621·1); vitamin A acetate (p.1383·2).
Gastrointestinal disorders.

Hydrastis Salbe *Steigerwald, Ger.*
Homoeopathic preparation.

Hydrate *Hyrex, USA.*
Dimenhydrinate (p.415·2).
Motion sickness.

Hydra-zide *Par, USA.*
Hydralazine hydrochloride (p.905·3); hydrochlorothiazide (p.907·3).

Hydrea
Bristol-Myers Squibb, Austral.; Bristol-Myers Squibb, Belg.; Bristol-Myers Squibb, Braz.; Squibb, Canad.; Bristol-Myers Squibb, Fin.; Bristol-Myers Squibb, Fr.; Bristol-Myers Squibb, Hong Kong; Bristol-Myers Squibb, Irl.; Bristol-Myers Squibb, Israel; Bristol-Myers Squibb, NZ; Bristol-Myers Squibb, Neth.; Bristol-Myers Squibb, NZ; Bristol-Myers Squibb, S.Afr.; Bristol-Myers Squibb, Singapore; Bristol-Myers Squibb, Spain; Bristol-Myers Squibb, Swed.; Bristol-Myers Squibb, Thai.; Squibb, UK; Bristol-Myers Squibb Oncology, USA.
Hydroxyurea [hydroxycarbamide] (p.544·2).
Malignant neoplasms.

Hydrene *Alphapharm, Austral.*
Triamterene (p.986·1); hydrochlorothiazide (p.907·3).
Hypertension; oedema.

Hydrenox *Knoll, UK†.*
Hydroflumethiazide (p.911·3).
Hypertension; oedema.

Hydrex
Note.This name is used for preparations of different composition.
Orion, Fin.
Hydrochlorothiazide (p.907·3).
Diabetes insipidus; hypertension; oedema.

Adams, Hong Kong; Unitech, Irl.; Adams, Thai.; Adams, UK.
Chlorhexidine gluconate (p.1138·2).
Skin disinfection.

Rolab, S.Afr.
Frusemide [furosemide] (p.893·1).
Now known as Rolab-Furosemide.
Oedema.

Hydrigoz Guigoz, Fr.
Maltodextrin; sucrose; sodium chloride; citric acid; potassium citrate (p.1185·2).
Diarrhoea; oral dehydration.

Hydrine TO-Chemicals, Thai.
Co-dergocrine mesilate (p.1597·3).
Cerebrovascular disorders; mental function impairment.

Hydrisalic Pedinol, USA.
Salicylic acid (p.1122·3).
Hyperkeratotic skin.

Hydrisea Pedinol, USA.
Emollient and moisturiser.

Hydrisinol Pedinol, USA.
Emollient and moisturiser.

Hydro Cobex Pasadena, USA.
Hydroxocobalamin (p.1388·1).
Schilling test; vitamin B₁₂ deficiency.

Hydro Cordes Ichthyol, Ger.
Allantoin (p.1110·1); dexpanthenol (p.1602·3); ethyl linoleate.
Skin disorders.

Hydro PC Cypress, USA.
Hydrocodone tartrate (p.42·2); phenylephrine hydrochloride (p.1097·1); chlorpheniramine [chlorphenamine] maleate (p.412·1).
Coughs; upper respiratory-tract congestion.

Hydro-Adreson Organon, Neth.; Organon, Singapore; Organon, Thai.
Hydrocortisone sodium succinate (p.1074·1).
Corticosteroid.

Hydroagisten Agis, Israel.
Hydrocortisone acetate (p.1073·3); clotrimazole (p.382·1).
Infected skin disorders.

Hydrocal Bioglan, Irl.; Bioglan, UK†.
Hydrocortisone acetate (p.1073·3); calamine (p.1111·3).
Skin disorders.

Hydrocare Allergan, Austral.†; Allergan-Frumtost, Braz.; Allergan, Ger.†; Allergan, Ital.
Range of solutions for contact lenses (p.1129·2).

Hydrocare Cleaning/Soaking Allergan, Israel.
Solution for cleaning, soaking, and disinfecting soft contact lenses (p.1129·2).

Hydrocare Enzymatic Protein Remover Allergan, Austral.
Papain (p.1647·3) (p.1129·2).
Cleanser for soft and gas permeable contact lenses.

Hydrocare Fizzy Allergan, Port.
Solution for contact lenses (p.1129·2).

Hydrocare Fizzy Protein Remover Allergan, NZ.
Papain (p.1647·3) (p.1129·2).
Protein removal from soft and gas-permeable contact lenses.

Hydrocare Preserved Saline Allergan, NZ.
Sodium chloride (p.1196·1) (p.1129·2).

Hydrocare Protein Remover Allergan, Canad.
Papain (p.1647·3)(p.1129·2).
Protein remover for soft contact lenses.

Allergan, Israel.
Enzymatic protein remover for soft contact lenses (p.1129·2).

Hydro-Cebral Ratiopharm, Ger.
Co-dergocrine mesilate (p.1597·3).
Mental function disorders.

Hydrocet Carnrick, USA.
Hydrocodone tartrate (p.42·2); paracetamol (p.71·2).
Pain.

Hydro-Chlor Vortech, USA†.
Hydrochlorothiazide (p.907·3).
Hypertension; oedema.

Hydrocil Instant Numark, USA.
Psyllium hydrophilic mucilloid (p.1229·1).
Constipation.

Hydroclonazone Chiesi, Fr.
Tosylchloramide sodium (p.1159·1).
Water purification.

Hydrocobamine Byk, Neth.
Hydroxocobalamin (p.1388·1).
Megaloblastic anaemia; vitamin B₁₂ deficiency.

Hydrocodeinon Streuli, Switz.
Dihydrocodeine hydrochloride (p.33·3).
Coughs.

Hydrocodone CP Morton Grove, USA.
Hydrocodone tartrate (p.42·2); phenylephrine hydrochloride (p.1097·1); chlorpheniramine [chlorphenamine] maleate (p.412·1).
Upper respiratory-tract symptoms.

Hydrocodone GF Morton Grove, USA.
Hydrocodone tartrate (p.42·2); guaifenesin (p.1092·2).
Upper respiratory-tract symptoms.

Hydrocodone HD Morton Grove, USA.
Hydrocodone tartrate (p.42·2); phenylephrine hydrochloride (p.1097·1); chlorpheniramine [chlorphenamine] maleate (p.412·1).
Upper respiratory-tract symptoms.

Hydrocodone PA Morton Grove, USA†.
Hydrocodone tartrate (p.42·2); phenylpropanolamine hydrochloride (p.1098·1).
Upper respiratory-tract symptoms.

Hydrocoll Hartmann, Fr.
Carmellose sodium (p.1499·3); pectin (p.1502·3); gelatin (p.737·2).
Burns; ulcers; wounds.

Hydrocomp Lichtenstein, Ger.
Amiloride hydrochloride (p.835·1); hydrochlorothiazide (p.907·3).
Hypertension; oedema.

Hydrocort
CT, Ger.
Hydrocortisone acetate (p.1073·3).
Skin disorders.

Abic, Israel.
Hydrocortisone sodium succinate (p.1074·1).
Corticosteroid.

Hydrocort Mild CT, Ger.†
Hydrocortisone (p.1073·3).
Skin disorders.

Hydrocortancyl Roussel Diamant, Fr.
Prednisolone (p.1077·3) or prednisolone acetate (p.1078·1).
Corticosteroid.

Hydrocortimycin Kolassa, Aust.
Hydrocortisone acetate (p.1073·3); neomycin sulfate (p.228·1).
Inflammatory eye disorders.

Hydrocortisone comp Streuli, Switz.
Hydrocortisone acetate (p.1073·3); zinc stearate (p.1497·3).
Skin disorders.

Hydrocortistab Waymade, UK.
Hydrocortisone acetate (p.1073·3).
Corticosteroid.

Hydrocortisyl Hoechst Marion Roussel, Irl.; Hoechst Marion Roussel, UK†.
Hydrocortisone (p.1073·3).
Skin disorders.

Hydrocortone Merck Sharp & Dohme, Aust.; Merck Sharp & Dohme, Irl.; Merck Sharp & Dohme, Port.; Merck Sharp & Dohme, Switz.; Merck Sharp & Dohme, UK; Merck, USA.
Hydrocortisone (p.1073·3), hydrocortisone acetate (p.1073·3), or hydrocortisone sodium phosphate (p.1074·1).
Corticosteroid.

Hydrocream Paddock, USA.
Vehicle for topical preparations.

Hydro-Crysti-12 Roberts, USA; Hauck, USA.
Hydroxocobalamin (p.1388·1).
Schilling test; vitamin B₁₂ deficiency.

Hydrocutan Dermapharm, Ger.
Hydrocortisone (p.1073·3) or hydrocortisone acetate (p.1073·3).
Skin disorders.

Hydrocutan mild Dermapharm, Ger.
Hydrocortisone (p.1073·3).
Skin disorders.

Hydroderm
Note. This name is used for preparations of different composition.
Aesca, Aust.
Hydrocortisone (p.1073·3).
Skin disorders.

Pacific, NZ.
Dewaxed oil-soluble lanolin fraction (p.1410·3); liquid paraffin (p.1407·1).
Dry skin disorders; pruritus.

Hydroderm HC Karrer, Ger.
Hydrocortisone (p.1073·3).
Skin disorders.

Hydrodermed Karrer, Ger.
Erythromycin (p.201·2).
Acne.

Hydrodexan
Procter & Gamble, Aust.; Hermal, Ger.
Hydrocortisone (p.1073·3); urea (p.1127·3).
Skin and scalp disorders.

HydroDiuril
Merck Frosst, Canad.†; Merck, USA.
Hydrochlorothiazide (p.907·3).
Hypertension; oedema.

Hydrofluoric Acid Antidote Malaysia Chemist, Singapore.
Calcium gluconate (p.1188·2).
Hydrofluoric acid burns.

Hydroform Dermacare, Austral.
Hydrocortisone (p.1073·3); clioquinol (p.190·2).
Inflammatory skin disorders.

Hydrogalen Galen, Ger.
Hydrocortisone (p.1073·3).
Skin disorders.

Hydrogesic Edwards, USA.
Hydrocodone tartrate (p.42·2); paracetamol (p.71·2).
Pain.

Hydroheal Algin Faulding, Austral.
Calcium alginate (p.728·1).
Burns; ulcers; wounds.

Hydroheal Colloid Faulding, Austral.
Hydrocolloid dressing.
Burns; ulcers; wounds.

Hydroheal Gel Faulding, Austral.
Hydrogel dressing.
Burns; ulcers; wounds.

Hydrol Janssen-Cilag, S.Afr.
Potassium chloride; sodium chloride; sodium citrate; glucose (p.1185·2).
Oral rehydration therapy.

Hydrolac Milk Industries, Israel.
Protein hydrolysate (p.1350·1).
Nutritional supplement.

Hydro-Less Aspen, S.Afr.
Indapamide (p.913·1).
Hypertension.

Hydrolid Helvepharm, Switz.
Amiloride hydrochloride (p.835·1); hydrochlorothiazide (p.907·3).
Hypertension; oedema.

Hydro-long Lichtenstein, Ger.
Chlortalidone (p.857·1).
Diabetes insipidus; hypertension; oedema.

Hydrolotion Spirig, Singapore.
Emollient and moisturiser.

Hydromal Hauck, USA†.
Hydrochlorothiazide (p.907·3).
Hypertension; oedema.

Hydromedin Merck Sharp & Dohme, Ger.
Etacrynic acid (p.887·2) or sodium etacrynate (p.887·2).
Ascites; oedema.

Hydromet
Note. This name is used for preparations of different composition.
Prodome, Braz.; Merck Sharp & Dohme, Irl.†; Merck Sharp & Dohme, Neth.†; Merck Sharp & Dohme, Swed.†
Hydrochlorothiazide (p.907·3); methyldopa (p.927·3).
Hypertension.

Barre-National, USA.
Hydrocodone tartrate (p.42·2); homatropine methylbromide (p.468·1).
Coughs.

Hydromol
Note. This name is used for preparations of different composition.
Quinoderm, Hong Kong; Quinoderm, Irl.; Adams, UK.
Emollient: Light liquid paraffin (p.1407·2); isopropyl myristate (p.1409·2).
Dry skin conditions.

Quinoderm, Irl.
Cream: Sodium pidolate (p.1123·3); arachis oil (p.1581·1); isopropyl myristate (p.1409·2); liquid paraffin (p.1407·1); sodium lactate (p.1186·2).
Dry skin.

Adams, UK.
Cream: Isopropyl myristate (p.1409·2); liquid paraffin (p.1407·1); sodium pidolate (p.1123·3); sodium lactate (p.1186·2).
Dry skin conditions.

Hydromorph Purdue Frederick, Canad.
Hydromorphone hydrochloride (p.42·3).
Pain.

Hydromox Lederle, USA.
Quinethazone (p.964·2).
Hypertension; oedema.

Hydromycin PP Lab, Thai.
Tetracycline hydrochloride (p.258·3).
Bacterial infections.

Hydron KGS Cypress, USA.
Hydrocodone tartrate (p.42·2); sulfogaiacol (p.1101·1).
Coughs.

Hydronet Nettopharma, Denm.†
Amiloride hydrochloride (p.835·1); hydrochlorothiazide (p.907·3).
Hypertension; oedema.

Hy-Drop Fidia, Ital.
Sodium hyaluronate (p.1620·1).
Dry eyes.

Hydropane Halsey, USA.
Hydrocodone tartrate (p.42·2); homatropine methylbromide (p.468·1).
Coughs.

Hydropel C & M, USA.
Topical barrier preparation.

Hydrophed Rugby, USA.
Theophylline (p.777·2); ephedrine sulfate (p.1090·2); hydroxyzine hydrochloride (p.419·1).
Bronchospasm.

Hydrophene DH Morton Grove, USA†.
Hydrocodone tartrate (p.42·2); phenylephrine hydrochloride (p.1097·1); mepyramine maleate (p.421·1).
Coughs.

Hydrophil Omega, Canad.
Urea (p.1127·3); white soft paraffin (p.1407·3).
Dry skin.

Hydrophilic Rugby, USA.
Vehicle for topical preparations.

Hydroplus Eurofarma, Braz.
Oral rehydration solution (p.1185·2).

Hydropres Merck Sharp & Dohme, Canad.†; Merck, USA.
Hydrochlorothiazide (p.907·3); reserpine (p.967·3).
Hypertension.

Hydro-rapid Lichtenstein, Ger.
Frusemide [furosemide] (p.893·1).
Hypertension; oedema; oliguria.

Hydros G Chaix et du Marais, Fr.
Glucose, sodium chloride, and potassium chloride infusion (p.1180·1).
Carbohydrate source; fluid and electrolyte disorders.

HydroSaluric Merck Sharp & Dohme, Irl.; Merck Sharp & Dohme, UK†.
Hydrochlorothiazide (p.907·3).
Hypertension; oedema.

Hydro-Serp Rugby, USA.
Hydrochlorothiazide (p.907·3); reserpine (p.967·3).
Hypertension.

Hydroserpine Rugby, USA.
Hydrochlorothiazide (p.907·3); reserpine (p.967·3).
Hypertension.

Hydrosil
Xepa-Soul Pattinson, Hong Kong; Xepa-Soul Pattinson, Singapore.
Aluminium hydroxide (p.1210·3); magnesium hydroxide (p.1233·1); simeticone (p.1249·2).
Dyspepsia; flatulence; gastric hyperacidity; gastro-oesophageal reflux; peptic ulcer.

HydroSkin Rugby, USA.
Hydrocortisone (p.1073·3).
Skin disorders.

Hydrosol Polyvitamin BON Doms-Adrian, Hong Kong.
Multivitamin preparation (p.1350·1).

Hydrosol Polyvitamine Roche, Fr.
Multivitamin preparation (p.1350·1).

Hydrosol Polyvitamine BON Doms-Adrian, Fr.
Multivitamin preparation (p.1350·1).

Hydrosone Technilab, Canad.
Hydrocortisone (p.1073·3).

HydroStat IR Richwood, USA†.
Hydromorphone hydrochloride (p.42·3).
Pain.

HydroTex Syosset, USA.
Hydrocortisone (p.1073·3).
Skin disorders.

Hydrotricine Rhone-Poulenc Rorer, Ital.; Vitoria, Port.
Tyrothricin (p.267·1).
Bacterial stomatitis.

Hydrotrix Kolassa, Aust.; Trommsdorff, Ger.; Medice, Ger.; Medice, Switz.
Frusemide [furosemide] (p.893·1); triamterene (p.986·1).
Heart failure; hypertension; oedema.

Hydro-Tussin DM Ethex, USA.
Guaifenesin (p.1092·2); dextromethorphan hydrobromide (p.1087·3).
Coughs and cold symptoms.

Hydro-Tussin HD Ethex, USA.
Guaifenesin (p.1092·2); hydrocodone tartrate (p.42·2); pseudoephedrine hydrochloride (p.1099·2).
Coughs and cold symptoms.

Hydroxin Shiwa, Thai.
Hydroxyzine hydrochloride (p.419·1).
Anxiety; hypersensitivity reactions.

Hydroxium Knoll, Neth.†
Co-dergocrine mesilate (p.1597·3).
Alzheimer's disease.

Hydroxo Merck-Belgolabo, Belg.†
Hydroxocobalamin (p.1388·1).
Nerve pain.

Hydroxy-Cal Sisu, Canad.
Vitamin C and minerals (p.1350·1).

Hydro-Z Mayrand, USA†.
Hydrochlorothiazide (p.907·3).
Hypertension; oedema.

Hydrozide
Note. This name is used for preparations of different composition.
Douglas, Austral.†; Douglas, Hong Kong; Douglas, NZ.
Hydrochlorothiazide (p.907·3); amiloride hydrochloride (p.835·1).
Hepatic cirrhosis with ascites; hypertension; oedema.

Atlantic, Hong Kong; Atlantic, Singapore; Atlantic, Thai.; Williams, USA†.
Hydrochlorothiazide (p.907·3).
Hypertension; oedema.

Hydrozole Dermacare, Austral.
Hydrocortisone (p.1073·3); clotrimazole (p.382·1).
Skin disorders.

Hyfac Saninter, Port.
Pyrithione zinc (p.1122·1); piroctone olamine (p.1121·1); vitamin E.
Acne.

Hyfac AHA Saninter, Port.
Piroctone olamine (p.1121·1); glycolic acid (p.1115·1); malic acid (p.1631·1).
Acne.

Hy-GAG Curasan, Ger.
Sodium hyaluronate (p.1620·1).
Degenerative joint disorders.

Hygeol Wampole, Canad.
Sodium hypochlorite (p.1156·2).
Disinfection; wound cleansing.

Hygienist Bayer, USA.
Chlorocresol (preventol CMK) (p.1141·3); clorophene (preventol BP) (p.1142·3); orthophenylphenol (preventol extra) (p.1152·1).
Surface disinfection.

Hygienist Pavimenti e Piastrelle Bayer, Ital.
Benzalkonium chloride (p.1133·2).
Surface disinfection.

The symbol † denotes a preparation no longer actively marketed

Hygine In Geymonat, Ital.†.
Lactobacillus acidophilus (p.1626·3).
Disturbances of vaginal flora.

Hygiodermil Vifor, Switz.
Bornyl salicylate (p.20·3); neroli oil (p.1640·1); lavender oil (p.1627·2); menthol (p.1632·3).
Skin disorders.

Hygroton
Novartis, Aust.; Novartis, Austral.; Novartis, Belg.; Geigy, Canad.†; Novartis, Denm.; Novartis, Fr.†; Novartis, Ger.; Novartis, Hong Kong; Novartis, Israel; Novartis, Norw.†; Novartis, NZ; Novartis, Port.; Novartis, S.Afr.; Ciba-Geigy, Swed.†; Novartis, Switz.; Alliance, UK; Rhone-Poulenc Rorer, USA.
Chlortalidone (p.857·1).
Diabetes insipidus; heart failure; hypertension; oedema.

Hygroton-Reserpine
Novartis, S.Afr.; Novartis, Switz.
Chlortalidone (p.857·1); reserpine (p.967·3).
Hypertension.

Hykaten Zeneca, Neth.†.
Atenolol (p.841·3); hydrochlorothiazide (p.907·3); amiloride hydrochloride (p.835·1).
Hypertension.

Hylaform Collagen, Ger.
Sodium hyaluronate (p.1620·1).
Skin disorders.

Hylak Ratiopharm, Aust.
Metabolic products of lactic-acid producing organisms (p.1626·3); lactic acid (p.1626·2); amino acids.
Gastrointestinal disorders; liver disorders; skin disorders.

Hylak forte Ratiopharm, Aust.
Metabolic products of lactic-acid producing organisms (p.1626·3); metabolic products of Gram-positive and Gram-negative intestinal flora; lactic acid (p.1626·2); amino acids.
Gastrointestinal disorders; liver disorders; skin disorders.

Hylak forte N Merckle, Ger.
Metabolic products of: Lactobacillus helveticus (p.1626·3); Escherichia coli; Lactobacillus acidophilus (p.1626·3).
Gastrointestinal disorders.

Hylak N Merckle, Ger.
Metabolic products of Lactobacillus helveticus (p.1626·3).
Gastrointestinal disorders.

Hylakombun Ratiopharm, Aust.
Phthalylsulfathiazole (p.235·3); ethaverine hydrochloride (p.1608·2); ox bile (p.1585·1); metabolic products of Escherichia coli; Enterococcus faecalis (p.1626·3); Lactobacillus acidophilus (p.1626·3).
Bacterial infections of the gastrointestinal tract.

Hylands Hylands, Canad.
A range of homoeopathic preparations.

Hylase Dessau, Ger.
Hyaluronidase (p.1620·3).
Adjunct in ocular surgery; adjuvant to increase absorption and dispersion of drugs; inflammation; prevention of episiotomy.

Hylashield I-Med, Canad.†.
Hylan A (p.1620·1).
Eye disorders.

Hylidone Major, USA†.
Chlortalidone (p.857·1).
Hypertension; oedema.

Hylo-Comod Ursapharm, Ger.
Sodium hyaluronate (p.1620·1).
Dry eyes.

Hylorel Medeva, USA.
Guanadrel sulfate (p.900·3).
Hypertension.

Hylutin Hyrex, USA.
Hydroxyprogesterone caproate (p.1479·3).
Abnormal uterine bleeding; amenorrhoea; metrorrhagia.

Hymecel Ciba Vision, Ger.†.
Hypromellose (p.1501·3).
Adjunct in intra-ocular surgery; moistening of artificial lenses.

Hymed Medifive, Thai.
Co-dergocrine mesilate (p.1597·3).
Cerebrovascular disorders; mental function impairment.

Hyomide Beacons, Singapore.
Hyoscine butylbromide (p.468·2).
Smooth muscle spasm.

Hyoscal N Steierl, Ger.
Scopolia carniolica root.
Smooth muscle spasm.

Hyosophen Rugby, USA.
Atropine sulfate (p.461·1); hyoscine hydrobromide (p.468·2); hyoscyamine hydrobromide (p.469·3) or hyoscyamine sulfate (p.469·3); phenobarbital (p.355·1).
Gastrointestinal disorders.

Hyospasmol Aspen, S.Afr.
Hyoscine butylbromide (p.468·2).
Gastrointestinal spasm.

Hyostan Pharmaland, Thai.
Hyoscine butylbromide (p.468·2).
Gastro-duodenitis; nausea and vomiting; peptic ulcer; smooth muscle spasm.

Hyozin Samakeephaesaj, Thai.
Hyoscine butylbromide (p.468·2).
Nausea and vomiting; peptic ulcer; smooth muscle spasm.

Hypace Xeragen, S.Afr.
Enalapril maleate (p.883·3).
Heart failure; hypertension.

Hypadil Kowa, Jpn.
Nipradilol (p.946·3).
Glaucoma; ocular hypertension.

Hypam Pacific, NZ.
Triazolam (p.709·3).
Insomnia.

Hypaque
Sanofi Winthrop, Braz.; Nycomed Amersham, Canad.; Sanofi Winthrop, Irl.†; Intrapharm, UK; Nycomed, USA.
Meglumine amidotrizoate (p.1031·2) or sodium amidotrizoate (p.1031·2).
Radiographic contrast medium.

Hypaque-M
Sanofi Winthrop, Braz.; Nycomed Amersham, Canad.
Meglumine amidotrizoate (p.1031·2); sodium amidotrizoate (p.1031·2).
Radiographic contrast medium.

Hypaque-M, Hypaque-76 Nycomed, USA.
Meglumine amidotrizoate (p.1031·2); sodium amidotrizoate (p.1031·2).
Radiographic contrast medium.

Hypen Shinyaku, Jpn.
Etodolac (p.35·2).
Musculoskeletal and joint disorders; pain.

Hyperab
Bayer, Canad.†; Cutter, Israel.
A rabies immunoglobulin (p.1560·2).
Passive immunisation.

Hyperamine
Braun, Fr.; Braun, UK.
Amino-acid infusion (p.1350·1).
Parenteral nutrition.

Hypercal
Note.This name is used for preparations of different composition.
Novartis Nutrition, Fr.
Nutritional supplement (p.1350·1).

Nelson, UK.
Homoeopathic preparation.

Hypercalcio Luper, Braz.
Calcium, vitamin D, vitamin B_{12}, and fluoride supplement (p.1350·1).

Hypercard Hotz, Ger.
Olive leaves; mistletoe (p.1636·3); ginseng (p.1615·3); convallaria (p.1599·1); rauwolfia; silicea; sumbul. moschat.; conium.
Cardiovascular disorders.

Hypercidin Electramed, Irl.
Sodium hypochlorite (p.1156·2).
Surface disinfection.

Hyperdine Masa, Thai.
Clopamide (p.863·1); dihydroergocristine mesilate (p.1603·2); reserpine (p.967·3).
Hypertension.

Hyperesa Dolorgiet, Ger.
Valerian (p.1678·3); hypericum (p.290·2).
Insomnia; nervous disorders.

Hyperforat Klein, Ger.
Hypericum (p.290·2).
Depression; migraine; nocturnal enuresis; stuttering.

Hyperforat-forte Klein, Ger.
Hypericum (p.290·2); rauwolfia vomitoria (p.967·2).
Depression; excitation; irritability.

HyperHep Bayer, Canad.†.
A hepatitis B immunoglobulin (p.1542·1).
Passive immunisation.

Hyperhes Fresenius Kabi, Aust.
An etherified starch (p.732·3) in sodium chloride.
Plasma volume expansion; shock.

Hypericaps Duopharm, Ger.
Hypericum (p.290·2).
Anxiety.

Hyperiforce Bioforce, Switz.
Hypericum (p.290·2).
Sleep disorders; tension.

Hyperiforce comp Bioforce, Switz.
Hypericum (p.290·2); melissa (p.1632·2); lupulus (p.1629·3).
Exhaustion; irritability; sleep disorders.

Hyperiforte Blackmores, Austral.
Hypericum (p.290·2).
Anxiety; depression; nervous disorders.

Hyperilex Medice, Ger.
Pemoline (p.1513·1).
Behaviour disorders in children.

HyperiMed Bioforce, Switz.
Hypericum (p.290·2).
Sleep disorders; tension.

Hyperimerck Merck dura, Ger.
Hypericum (p.290·2).
Anxiety; depression.

Hyperiplant Schwabe, Switz.
Hypericum (p.290·2).
Depression; insomnia; tension.

Hyperium
Biopharma, Fr.; Servier, Port.
Rilmenidine phosphate (p.968·3).
Hypertension.

Hyperlipen
Sanofi Synthelabo, Belg.; Sanofi Synthelabo, Switz.
Ciprofibrate (p.858·3).
Hyperlipidaemias.

Hyperlite Pharmacia Upjohn, Spain.
Electrolyte infusion (p.1180·1).
Fluid and electrolyte depletion.

Hyperlyte McGaw, USA.
A range of electrolyte preparations (p.1180·1).
Fluid and electrolyte disorders.

Hypermol Pacific, NZ.
Timolol maleate (p.982·1).
Angina pectoris; arrhythmias; hypertension; migraine; myocardial infarction.

Hypernol DHA, Hong Kong.
Atenolol (p.841·3).
Angina pectoris; arrhythmias; hypertension.

Hyperphen S.Afr.
Hydralazine hydrochloride (p.905·3).
Hypertension.

Hyperpur Isis Puren, Ger.
Hypericum (p.290·2).
Depression.

Hyperretic Pharmasant, Thai.
Amiloride hydrochloride (p.835·1); hydrochlorothiazide (p.907·3).
Hepatic cirrhosis with ascites; hypertension; oedema.

Hyperstat
Schering-Plough, Belg.; Schering, Canad.; Schering-Plough, Fr.†; Schering-Plough, Ital.; Schering-Plough, Mex.; Schering-Plough, Neth.; Schering-Plough, S.Afr.; Schering-Plough, Spain; Schering-Plough, Swed.; Essex, Switz.; Schering, USA.
Diazoxide (p.868·1).
Hypertension; hypoglycaemia.

Hyper-Tet Bayer, Canad.†.
A tetanus immunoglobulin (p.1565·1).
Passive immunisation.

Hypertonalum Essex, Ger.
Diazoxide (p.868·1).
Hypertension.

Hypertorr Henning, Ger.
Triamterene (p.986·1); hydrochlorothiazide (p.907·3).
Heart failure; hypertension; oedema.

Hyperval Novartis Consumer, Switz.
Hypericum (p.290·2).
Anxiety; insomnia; tension.

Hypery Pond's, Thai.
Reserpine (p.967·3); hydralazine hydrochloride (p.905·3); hydrochlorothiazide (p.907·3).
Hypertension.

Hyphed Cypress, USA.
Hydrocodone tartrate (p.42·2); pseudoephedrine hydrochloride (p.1099·2); chlorpheniramine [chlorphenamine] maleate (p.412·1).
Coughs.

Hy-Phen Ascher, USA.
Hydrocodone tartrate (p.42·2); paracetamol (p.71·2).
Coughs.

Hypnasmine Elerte, Fr.
Butobarbital (p.659·1); theophylline (p.777·2).
Formerly contained caffeine, butobarbital, and theophylline.
Respiratory-tract disorders.

Hypnodorm
Alphapharm, Austral.; Teva, Israel.
Flunitrazepam (p.683·2).
General anaesthesia; insomnia; premedication.

Hypnol Cristalia, Braz.
Pentobarbital (p.698·2).
Cerebrovascular disorders; epilepsy; premedication.

Hypnomidate
Janssen-Cilag, Aust.; Janssen-Cilag, Belg.; Janssen, Braz.; Janssen-Cilag, Fr.; Janssen-Cilag, Ger.; Janssen, Mex.; Janssen-Cilag, Neth.; Janssen-Cilag, S.Afr.; Janssen-Cilag, Spain; Janssen-Cilag, Switz.†; Janssen-Cilag, UK.
Etomidate (p.1259·2).
General anaesthesia.

Hypnor Rolab, S.Afr.
Flunitrazepam (p.683·2).
Now known as Rolab-Flunitrazepam.
Insomnia.

Hypnorex Sanofi Synthelabo, Ger.
Lithium carbonate (p.292·1).
Bipolar disorder; depression; mania.

Hypnovel
Roche, Austral.; Roche, Fr.; Roche, Irl.; Roche, NZ; Roche, UK.
Midazolam hydrochloride (p.692·3) or midazolam maleate (p.693·1).
Induction of anaesthesia; insomnia; premedication; sedative.

Hypo Tears Ciba Vision, Spain.
Polyvinyl alcohol (p.1503·1).
Dry eyes.

Hypoca Yamanouchi, Jpn.
Barnidipine hydrochloride (p.843·1).
Hypertension.

Hypocaina Hypofarma, Braz.
Lignocaine [lidocaine] hydrochloride (p.1313·2).
Local anaesthesia.

Hypochylin
Recip, Fin.; Recip, Swed.
Glutamic acid hydrochloride (p.1365·2).
Hypochylia.

Hypodyn Novartis, Aust.
Dihydroergotamine mesilate (p.450·3); etilefrine hydrochloride (p.888·1).
Hypotension.

Hypoguard Priory, Irl.
Test for glucose in blood (p.1616·3).

Hypoguard GA Hypoguard, UK.
Test for glucose in blood (p.1616·3).

Hypol Felton, Austral.
Capsules: Cod-liver oil (p.1357·2).
Arthritis; cardiovascular disorders; cold and influenza symptoms; dietary supplement; inflammatory disorders.
Oral emulsion: Cod-liver oil (p.1357·2); soya oil (p.1378·1); calcium hypophosphite; sodium hypophosphite.
Arthritis; cardiovascular disorders; cold and influenza symptoms; dietary supplement; inflammatory disorders.
Tablets: Vitamin A; colecalciferol; vitamin C; calcium dihydrogen phosphate (p.1350·1).
Vitamin and calcium supplement.

Hypolac Neo Abello, Ital.
Infant feed (p.1350·1).
Food intolerance.

Hypolar Retard Lagap, UK.
Nifedipine (p.940·1).
Angina pectoris; hypertension.

Hypomide Aspen, S.Afr.
Chlorpropamide (p.321·1).
Diabetes mellitus.

Hyposedon N Harras-Curarina, Ger.
Kava (p.1625·3); passion flower (p.1649·1).
Agitation; sleep disorders.

Hypostamin Novartis Consumer, Aust.
Tritoqualine (p.427·3).
Hypersensitivity reactions.

Hypostamine Chiesi, Fr.
Tritoqualine (p.427·3).
Hypersensitivity reactions.

Hypotears
Note.This name is used for preparations of different composition.
Ciba Vision, Canad.; Ciba Vision, Israel; Ciba Vision, Singapore.
Eye drops: Polyvinyl alcohol (p.1503·1).
Dry eyes.

Ciba Vision, Hong Kong; Ciba Vision, Ital.; Ciba Vision, Switz.; Novartis Ophthalmics, UK; Ciba Vision, USA.
Eye drops: Polyvinyl alcohol (p.1503·1); macrogol 400 (p.1630·3) or macrogol 8000 (p.1630·3).
Dry eyes.

Ciba Vision, Canad.; Ciba Vision, Israel; Ciba Vision, USA.
Eye ointment: White soft paraffin (p.1407·3); light liquid paraffin (p.1407·2).
Dry eyes.

Restan, S.Afr.
Povidone (p.1503·2).
Contact lens lubricant; dry eyes.

Hypotears PF Ciba Vision, Israel.
Polyvinyl alcohol (p.1503·1); macrogol 400 (p.1630·3).
Dry eyes.

Hypotears Plus
Ciba Vision, Hong Kong; Ciba Vision, Thai.
Povidone (p.1503·2).
Dry eyes.

Hypoten Covan, S.Afr.
Sodium nitroprusside (p.971·1).
Hypertension.

Hypotens Dexxon, Israel.
Prazosin hydrochloride (p.958·1).
Benign prostatic hyperplasia; hypertension.

Hy-Po-Tone Aspen, S.Afr.
Methyldopa (p.927·3).
Hypertension.

Hypotonie-Gastreu R44 Tropfen Reckeweg, Ger.
Homoeopathic preparation.

Hypovase
Invicta, Irl.; Pfizer, UK.
Prazosin hydrochloride (p.958·1).
Benign prostatic hyperplasia; heart failure; hypertension; Raynaud's syndrome.

Hypren Astra, Aust.
Ramipril (p.966·3).
Heart failure; hypertension; myocardial infarction.

Hypren plus Astra, Aust.
Ramipril (p.966·3); hydrochlorothiazide (p.907·3).
Hypertension.

Hyprenan
Astra, Denm.†; Astra, Norw.†; Hassle, Swed.†.
Prenalterol hydrochloride (p.959·2).
Hypotension; reversal of beta blockade; shock.

HypRho-D Bayer, Canad.†.
An anti-D immunoglobulin (p.1532·1).
Prevention of rhesus sensitisation.

Hyprim Italchimici, Ital.†.
Brodimoprim (p.159·3).
Otorhinolaryngeal disorders; respiratory-tract infections.

Hyprogest Keene, USA†.
Hydroxyprogesterone caproate (p.1479·3).
Abnormal uterine bleeding; amenorrhoea; metrorrhagia.

Hyprosia Asian Pharm, Thai.
Etilefrine (p.888·1).
Hypotension.

Hyprosin Pacific, NZ.
Prazosin hydrochloride (p.958·1).
Benign prostatic hyperplasia; heart failure; hypertension; Raynaud's disease.

Hypurin 30/70 *CP Pharmaceuticals, UK.*
Mixture of neutral insulin injection (porcine, highly purified) 30% and isophane insulin injection (porcine, highly purified) 70% (p.324·1).
Diabetes mellitus.

Hypurin Isophane
Rhone-Poulenc Rorer, Austral.; CP Pharmaceuticals, UK.
Isophane insulin injection (bovine or porcine, highly purified) (p.324·1).
Diabetes mellitus.

Hypurin Lente *CP Pharmaceuticals, UK.*
Insulin zinc suspension (30% amorphous, 70% crystalline) (bovine, highly purified) (p.324·1).
Diabetes mellitus.

Hypurin Neutral
Rhone-Poulenc Rorer, Austral.; CP Pharmaceuticals, UK.
Neutral insulin injection (bovine or porcine, highly purified) (p.324·1).
Diabetes mellitus.

Hypurin Protamine Zinc *CP Pharmaceuticals, UK.*
Protamine zinc insulin injection (bovine, highly purified) (p.324·1).
Diabetes mellitus.

Hyrexin *Hyrex, USA.*
Diphenhydramine hydrochloride (p.416·1).
Motion sickness; parkinsonism.

Hyrin *Merckle, Ger.*
Metoclopramide (p.1236·3).
Gastrointestinal disorders.

Hyrvalan *Monot, Fr.†.*
Paracetamol (p.71·2); ascorbic acid (p.1389·3); chlorpheniramine [chlorphenamine] maleate (p.412·1).
Upper respiratory-tract disorders.

Hyseke *Saninter, Port.*
Sodium pidolate (p.1123·3); zinc pidolate; enoxolone (p.34·3).
Dry skin.

Hyskon
Dermatech, Austral.; Pharmacia Upjohn, Canad.†; Reusch, Ger.†; Medisan, Swed.†; Pharmacia, UK; Pharmacia, USA.
Dextran 70 (p.729·2) in glucose.
Aid to hysteroscopy.

Hysone
Note. This name is used for preparations of different composition.
Alphapharm, Austral.
Hydrocortisone (p.1073·3).
Corticosteroid.

Roberts, USA.
Clioquinol (p.190·2); hydrocortisone (p.1073·3).
Inflammatory skin disorders.

Hysopan *Denk, Hong Kong.*
Hyoscine butylbromide (p.468·2).
Smooth muscle spasm.

Hytacand *AstraZeneca, Fr.*
Candesartan cilexetil (p.853·2); hydrochlorothiazide (p.907·3).
Hypertension.

Hytakerol
Sanofi Synthelabo, Canad.; Sanofi Winthrop, USA.
Dihydrotachysterol (p.1391·2).
Hypoparathyroidism; postoperative and idiopathic tetany.

Hyteneze *Opus, UK†.*
Captopril (p.853·3).
Heart failure; hypertension.

Hytic *Seng, Thai.*
Hyoscine butylbromide (p.468·2).
Smooth muscle spasm.

Hytinic *Hyrex, USA.*
Capsules: Polysaccharide-iron complex (p.1374·3).
Injection: Ferrous gluconate (p.1360·1); vitamin B substances (p.1350·1).
Procaine hydrochloride (p.1319·1) is included in this preparation to alleviate the pain of injection.
Iron-deficiency anaemias.

Hytisone
Atlantic, Hong Kong; Atlantic, Thai.
Hydrocortisone (p.1073·3) or hydrocortisone acetate (p.1073·3).
Inflammatory skin disorders.

Hytone *Dermik, USA.*
Hydrocortisone (p.1073·3).
Skin disorders.

Hytrast
Guerbet, Braz.; Guerbet, Fr.†; Byk Gulden, Ger.†.
Iopydol (p.1036·2); iopydone (p.1036·2).
Contrast medium for upper respiratory-tract radiography.

Hytrin
Abbott, Austral.; Abbott, Belg.; Abbott, Braz.; Abbott, Canad.; Abbott, Hong Kong; Abbott, Irl.; Abbott, Israel; Abbott, Mex.; Abbott, Neth.; Abbott, NZ; Abbott, Port.; Abbott, S.Afr.; Abbott, Singapore; Abbott, Thai.; Abbott, UK; Abbott, USA; Wellcome, USA.
Terazosin hydrochloride (p.980·1).
Benign prostatic hyperplasia; hypertension.

Hytrin BPH *Abbott, Switz.*
Terazosin hydrochloride (p.980·1).
Benign prostatic hyperplasia.

Hytrine *Abbott, Fr.*
Terazosin hydrochloride (p.980·1).
Benign prostatic hyperplasia.

Hytrinex *Astra, Swed.*
Terazosin hydrochloride (p.980·1).
Benign prostatic hyperplasia; hypertension.

Hytuss *Hyrex, USA.*
Guaifenesin (p.1092·2).
Coughs.

Hyzaar
Merck Frosst, Canad.; Merck Sharp & Dohme-Chibret, Fr.; Merck Sharp & Dohme, Hong Kong; Merck Sharp & Dohme, Neth.; Merck Sharp & Dohme, Singapore; Merck Sharp & Dohme, Thai.; Merck, USA.
Losartan potassium (p.921·3); hydrochlorothiazide (p.907·3).
Hypertension.

Hyzine *Hyrex, USA†.*
Hydroxyzine hydrochloride (p.419·1).
Anxiety; hypersensitivity reactions.

Hyzum N *Merckle, Ger.*
Arnica (p.1581·3).
Inflammation; muscle and joint pain; soft-tissue injury.

Ial
Fidia, Hong Kong; Fidia, Ital.; Trans Bussan, Switz.; Fidia, Thai.
Sodium hyaluronate (p.1620·1).
Adjunct in ocular surgery.

Ialugen *IBSA, Switz.*
Sodium hyaluronate (p.1620·1).
Burns; wounds.

Ialugen Plus *IBSA, Switz.*
Sodium hyaluronate (p.1620·1); sulfadiazine silver (p.251·3).
Infected wounds and burns.

Ialum *Fidia, Ital.*
Sodium hyaluronate (p.1620·1).
Adjunct in eye surgery.

Ialurex *Fidia, Ital.*
Sodium hyaluronate (p.1620·1).
Dry eyes.

Iamin Hydrating Gel *Procyte, USA.*
Prezatide copper acetate (p.1121·3).
Burns; ulcers; wounds.

Iba-Cide *Ingram & Bell, Canad.†.*
Chloroxylenol (p.1142·1); terpineol (p.1669·3); isopropyl alcohol (p.1149·2).
Antiseptic.

Ibaril
Aventis, Denm.; Hoechst Marion Roussel, Fin.; Bipharma, Neth.; Hoechst Marion Roussel, Norw.; Hoechst Marion Roussel, Swed.
Desoximetasone (p.1066·2).
Skin disorders.

Ibaril med salicylsyra *Hoechst Marion Roussel, Swed.*
Desoximetasone (p.1066·2); salicylic acid (p.1122·3).
Skin disorders.

Ibaril med salicylsyre
Aventis, Denm.; Hoechst Marion Roussel, Norw.
Desoximetasone (p.1066·2); salicylic acid (p.1122·3).
Skin disorders.

Ibenon *Diviser Aquilea, Spain.*
Ibuprofen (p.43·2).
Fever; pain.

Ibercal *BOI, Spain.*
Calcium pidolate (p.1188·3).
Hypocalcaemia; osteoporosis.

Iberet
Abbott, Canad.; Abbott, Hong Kong; Abbott, Mex.; Abbott, S.Afr.; Abbott, Singapore; Abbott, Spain†; Abbott, Thai.; Abbott, USA.
Ferrous sulfate (p.1360·3); vitamin B substances (p.1350·1).
Sodium ascorbate (p.1390·1) or ascorbic acid (p.1389·3) is included in this preparation to increase the absorption and availability of iron.
Iron-deficiency anaemias.

Iberet-Folic
Abbott, Hong Kong; Abbott, Singapore; Abbott, USA.
Ferrous sulfate (p.1360·3); folic acid (p.1361·1); vitamin B substances (p.1350·1).
Sodium ascorbate (p.1390·1) is included in this preparation to increase the absorption and availability of iron.
Folic acid deficiency; iron-deficiency anaemias.

Iberin Folico *Abbott, Braz.*
Ferrous sulfate (p.1360·3); folic acid (p.1361·1).
Ascorbic acid (p.1389·3) is included in this preparation to increase the absorption and availability of iron.
Iron deficiency; iron-deficiency anaemia.

Iberogast
Steigerwald, Ger.
Iberis amara; chamomile (p.1593·2); peppermint leaf (p.1243·2); greater celandine (p.1618·1); silybum marianum (p.1021·3); melissa (p.1632·2); caraway (p.1591·2); liquorice (p.1231·2); angelica (p.1580·2).
Gastrointestinal disorders.

Steigerwald, Switz.
Iberis amara; angelica (p.1580·2); silybum marianum (p.1021·3); cuminum cyminum; chamomile (p.1593·2); greater celandine (p.1618·1); liquorice (p.1231·2); melissa (p.1632·2); peppermint leaf (p.1243·2).
Gastrointestinal disorders.

Iberol
Abbott, Braz.; Abbott, Mex.
Ferrous sulfate (p.1360·3); vitamin B substances (p.1350·1).
Ascorbic acid (p.1389·3) is included in this preparation to increase the absorption and availability of iron.
Iron-deficiency anaemia; vitamin B deficiency.

Ibexone *Sandipro, Belg.*
Co-dergocrine mesilate (p.1597·3).
Mental function impairment.

Ibiamox
Fisons, Austral.†; Ibi, Ital.; Douglas, NZ; IBI, Thai.
Amoxicillin (p.149·2), amoxicillin sodium (p.149·2), or amoxicillin trihydrate (p.149·2).
Bactrial infections.

Ibifon *Ampharco, USA†.*
Ibuprofen (p.43·2).

Ibilex
Alphapharm, Austral.; IBI, Thai.
Cefalexin (p.161·3) or cefalexin sodium (p.162·2).
Bacterial infections.

Ibimicyn *Ibi, Ital.*
Note. A similar name is used for preparations of different composition (see below).
Ampicillin sodium (p.150·3).
Bacterial infections.

Ibimycin *IBI, Thai.*
Note. A similar name is used for preparations of different composition (see above).
Doxycycline (p.200·1).
Bacterial infections.

Ibis *Pharmaland, Thai.*
Ketotifen fumarate (p.767·2).
Asthma; hypersensitivity reactions.

Ibopain *Docmed, S.Afr.†.*
Ibuprofen (p.43·2).
Musculoskeletal and joint disorders.

Ibrofen *TO-Chemicals, Thai.*
Ibuprofen (p.43·2).
Musculoskeletal and joint disorders.

Ibrufhalal *Halal, UK.*
Ibuprofen (p.43·2).
Inflammation; pain.

IBS Relief *Thornton & Ross, UK.*
Mebeverine hydrochloride (p.1233·3).
Irritable bowel syndrome.

Ibu
ABZ, Ger.; Eu Rho, Ger.; Kade, Ger.; Pose, Thai.; Boots, USA.
Ibuprofen (p.43·2).
Fever; gout; inflammation; musculoskeletal, joint, and soft-tissue disorders; pain.

Ibu-4, -6, -8 *Truxton, USA.*
Ibuprofen (p.43·2).

Ibualgic *EG, Fr.*
Ibuprofen (p.43·2).
Pain.

Ibubest *CT, Ger.†.*
Ibuprofen (p.43·2).
Fever; pain.

Ibubeta *Betapharm, Ger.*
Ibuprofen (p.43·2).
Fever; gout; inflammation; musculoskeletal, joint, and soft-tissue disorders; pain.

Ibudol *Sanova, Aust.*
Ibuprofen (p.43·2).
Fever; inflammation; musculoskeletal and joint disorders; pain.

Ibudolor *Stada, Ger.*
Ibuprofen (p.43·2).
Fever; pain.

Ibudros *Manetti Roberts, Ital.*
Ibuproxam (p.44·3).
Musculoskeletal, joint, peri-articular, and soft-tissue disorders; phlebitis; superficial thrombophlebitis.

Ibufac
Unison, Thai.; DDSA Pharmaceuticals, UK.
Ibuprofen (p.43·2).
Fever; musculoskeletal and joint disorders; pain.

Ibufarm *Noristan, S.Afr.†.*
Ibuprofen (p.43·2).
Musculoskeletal and joint disorders.

Ibufem *Galpharm, UK.*
Ibuprofen (p.43·2).
Dysmenorrhoea.

Ibufen
Dexxon, Israel; Beacons, Singapore; Siam Bheasach, Thai.
Ibuprofen (p.43·2).
Musculoskeletal and joint disorders; pain.

Ibufen-L *Amino, Switz.*
Suppositories: Ibuprofen lysine (p.44·1); lignocaine [lidocaine] hydrochloride (p.1313·2).
Tablets: Ibuprofen lysine (p.44·1).
Gout; musculoskeletal, joint, and peri-articular disorders.

Ibuflam *Lichtenstein, Ger.*
Ibuprofen (p.43·2).
Fever; gout; inflammation; musculoskeletal, joint, and soft-tissue disorders; pain.

Ibuflex *Rayere, Mex.*
Ibuprofen (p.43·2).
Inflammation; pain.

Ibufug *Wolff, Ger.*
Ibuprofen (p.43·2).
Gout; inflammation; musculoskeletal and joint disorders; pain.

Ibugan *Hoechst Marion Roussel, Thai.*
Ibuprofen (p.43·2).
Musculoskeletal and joint disorders; pain.

Ibugel
Mayrhofer, Aust.†; Dermal Laboratories, Irl.; Medinova, Switz.†; Dermal Laboratories, UK.
Ibuprofen (p.43·2).
Musculoskeletal, joint, peri-articular, and soft-tissue disorders.

Ibuhexal *Hexal, Ger.*
Ibuprofen (p.43·2) or ibuprofen sodium (p.44·1).
Fever; gout; inflammation; musculoskeletal, joint, and soft-tissue disorders; pain.

Ibulan *Olan-Kemed, Thai.*
Ibuprofen (p.43·2).
Fever; inflammation; musculoskeletal and joint disorders; pain.

Ibular *Lagap, UK.*
Ibuprofen (p.43·2).
Inflammation; pain.

Ibuleve
Dermal, Israel; Searle, S.Afr.; Dendron, UK.
Ibuprofen (p.43·2).
Musculoskeletal, joint, and soft-tissue disorders.

Ibuloid *Reddy, Singapore.*
Ibuprofen (p.43·2).
Musculoskeletal and joint disorders; pain.

Ibumax *Vitabalans, Fin.*
Ibuprofen (p.43·2).
Fever; gout; musculoskeletal and joint disorders; pain.

Ibumed
Pharmethic, Belg.; SmithKline Beecham, S.Afr.; Helvepharm, Switz.†.
Ibuprofen (p.43·2).
Fever; pain.

Ibumerck *Merck dura, Ger.*
Ibuprofen (p.43·2).
Fever; gout; inflammation; musculoskeletal, joint, and soft-tissue disorders; pain.

Ibumetin
Nycomed, Aust.; Nycomed, Denm.; United Nordic, Denm.; Nycomed, Fin.; Nycomed, Norw.; Nycomed, Swed.
Ibuprofen (p.43·2).
Fever; gout; inflammation; musculoskeletal and joint disorders; pain.

Ibumousse *Dermal Laboratories, UK.*
Ibuprofen (p.43·2).
Musculoskeletal and joint pain; neuralgia.

Ibunet *Nettopharma, Denm.†.*
Ibuprofen (p.43·2).
Gout; musculoskeletal and joint disorders; pain.

Ibupax *Alter, Port.*
Ibuprofen (p.43·2).
Fever; gout; musculoskeletal, joint, peri-articular, and soft-tissue disorders; pain.

Ibuphlogont *Azupharma, Ger.*
Ibuprofen (p.43·2).
Gout; inflammation; musculoskeletal, joint, and soft-tissue disorders; pain.

Ibupril *Liomont, Mex.*
Ibuprofen (p.43·2).
Inflammation; pain.

Ibuprin *Thompson, USA†.*
Ibuprofen (p.43·2).
Fever; osteoarthritis; pain; rheumatoid arthritis.

Ibuprof *CT, Ger.*
Ibuprofen (p.43·2) or ibuprofen lysine (p.44·1).
Gout; inflammation; musculoskeletal, joint, and soft-tissue disorders; pain.

Ibuprohm *Ohm, USA†.*
Ibuprofen (p.43·2).
Fever; osteoarthritis; pain; rheumatoid arthritis.

Ibupron *Ratiopharm, Aust.†.*
Ibuprofen (p.43·2).
Fever; inflammation; musculoskeletal and joint disorders; pain.

Ibu-ratiopharm *Ratiopharm, Ger.*
Ibuprofen (p.43·2).
Fever; gout; inflammation; musculoskeletal, joint, and soft-tissue disorders; pain.

Iburem *Sanova, Aust.†.*
Ibuprofen (p.43·2).
Pain.

Iburen *Hua, Thai.*
Ibuprofen (p.43·2).
Gout; musculoskeletal and joint disorders.

Ibureumin *Durascan, Denm.*
Ibuprofen (p.43·2).
Gout; musculoskeletal and joint disorders; pain.

Ibusal *Orion, Fin.*
Ibuprofen (p.43·2).
Fever; musculoskeletal and joint disorders; pain.

Ibuscent *Vita Elan, Spain.*
Ibuprofen (p.43·2).
Fever; pain.

Ibusifar *Siphar, Switz.*
Ibuprofen (p.43·2).
Fever; inflammation; pain.

Ibu-Slow *Bio-Therabel, Belg.*
Ibuprofen (p.43·2).
Musculoskeletal, joint, and peri-articular disorders.

Ibuslow *Eurodrug, Hong Kong.*
Ibuprofen (p.43·2).
Dysmenorrhoea; fever; musculoskeletal, joint, peri-articular, and soft-tissue disorders.

Ibuspray *Dermal Laboratories, UK.*
Ibuprofen (p.43·2).
Musculoskeletal, joint, and soft-tissue disorders; neuralgia.

Ibustrin
Pharmacia Upjohn, Aust.; Pharmacia Upjohn, Ital.; Pharmacia Upjohn, Mex.; Pharmacia Upjohn, Port.; Pharmacia Upjohn, Thai.
Indobufen (p.913·2) or indobufen sodium (p.913·2).
Thromboembolic disorders; thrombosis prophylaxis.

Ibu-Tab *Alra, USA.*
Ibuprofen (p.43·2).
Fever; osteoarthritis; pain; rheumatoid arthritis.

Ibutad *TAD, Ger.*
Ibuprofen (p.43·2) or ibuprofen sodium (p.44·1).
Gout; inflammation; musculoskeletal, joint, and soft-tissue disorders; pain.

Ibutop *Sanova, Aust.; Chefaro, Belg.; Dolorgiet, Denm.; Chefaro Ardeval, Fr.; Chefaro, Ger.*
Ibuprofen (p.43·2).
Inflammation; musculoskeletal, joint, peri-articular, and soft-tissue disorders; pain; sports injuries.

Ibutop Cuprofen *SSL, UK.*
Ibuprofen (p.43·2).
Musculoskeletal, joint, and soft-tissue disorders.

Ibutop Ralgex *SSL, UK.*
Ibuprofen (p.43·2).
Inflammation; musculoskeletal pain.

Ibu-Vivimed *Mann, Ger.†*
Ibuprofen (p.43·2).
Fever; pain.

Ibux *Weifa, Norw.*
Ibuprofen (p.43·2).
Fever; musculoskeletal and joint disorders; pain.

Ibuxin *Medinovum, Fin.*
Ibuprofen (p.43·2).
Fever; gout; musculoskeletal and joint disorders; pain.

IC Green *Akorn, USA.*
Indocyanine green (p.1623·2).
Ophthalmic angiography.

Icaden *Schering, Braz.; Schering, Mex.*
Isoconazole (p.387·1) or isoconazole nitrate (p.387·2).
Fungal and Gram-positive vulvovaginal infections; fungal skin infections.

Icaps *Alcon, Canad.; Ciba Vision, USA.*
Multivitamin and mineral preparation (p.1350·1).

Icar *Hawthorn, USA.*
Carbonyl iron (p.1366·3).
Iron deficiency; iron supplement.

Icavex *Asta Medica, Fr.*
Thymoxamine [moxisylyte] hydrochloride (p.980·2).
Erectile dysfunction.

Icaz *Novartis, Ital.*
Isradipine (p.916·3).
Hypertension.

Ice Cool Stress & Tension Relief *Amirose, UK.*
Menthol (p.1632·3).
Headache; tension.

Ice Gel *Mentholatum, Austral.; Hyde, Canad.*
Menthol (p.1632·3).
Muscular aches and pains.

Ice Gel Therapy *Sutton, Canad.*
Menthol (p.1632·3).

Ice Lipbalm *Mentholatum, Canad.*
SPF 12: Padimate O (p.1518·2).
Sunscreen.

Ice Therapy *Stella, Canad.†*
Menthol (p.1632·3).
Muscle pain.

Icespray *Rhone-Poulenc Rorer, Spain.*
Menthol (p.1632·3).
Insect bites; pruritus; sprains.

Ic-Gel *Germiphene, Canad.*
Chlorhexidine gluconate (p.1138·2); isopropyl alcohol (p.1149·2).

ICG-Pulsion *Pulsion, Ger.; Pulsion, Israel.*
Indocyanine green (p.1623·2).
Diagnostic agent.

Ichthalgan *Ichthyol, Ger.*
Heparin sodium (p.902·1); ictasol (p.1115·3).
Muscle, joint, and peri-articular disorders; neuritis.

Ichthalgan forte *Ichthyol, Aust.*
Heparin sodium (p.902·1); ictasol (p.1115·3).
Musculoskeletal, joint, and peri-articular disorders.

Ichtho-Bad *Ichthyol, Aust.; Ichthyol, Ger.; Ichthyol, Switz.*
Ichthammol (p.1115·2).
Bath additive; hyperhidrosis; musculoskeletal and joint disorders; neuralgia; pelvic disorders; skin disorders; superficial circulatory disorders; wounds.

Ichtho-Bellol *Ichthyol, Aust.; Ichthyol, Ger.*
Ictasol (p.1115·3); atropine sulfate (p.461·1).
Pelvic disorders.

Ichtho-Bellol compositum S *Ichthyol, Ger.*
Ictasol (p.1115·3); atropine sulfate (p.461·1); propyphenazone (p.80·2).
Pelvic disorders.

Ichtho-Cadmin *Ichthyol, Aust.*
Ictasol (p.1115·3); cadmium sulfide (p.1588·1).
Scalp disorders.

Ichtho-Cortin *Ichthyol, Aust.*
Hydrocortisone (p.1073·3) or hydrocortisone acetate (p.1073·3); ictasol (p.1115·3).
Skin disorders.

Ichthocortin *Ichthyol, Ger.*
Hydrocortisone (p.1073·3) or hydrocortisone acetate (p.1073·3); ictasol (p.1115·3).
Skin disorders.

Ichthoderm *Ichthyol, Ger.*
Ictasol (p.1115·3).
Scalp disorders.

Ichth-Oestren *Ichthyol, Aust.*
Estradiol benzoate (p.1473·1); light ammonium bituminosulfonate (p.1115·2); urea (p.1127·3); lactose (p.1370·2).
Vaginal disorders.

Ichtholan *Ichthyol, Aust.; Ichthyol, Ger.; Ichthyol, Switz.*
Ichthammol (p.1115·2).
Inflammatory skin disorders; musculoskeletal, joint, and peri-articular disorders; thrombophlebitis.

Ichtholan spezial *Ichthyol, Ger.*
Ichthammol (p.1115·2).
Musculoskeletal and joint disorders.

Ichtholan T *Ichthyol, Ger.*
Ictasol (p.1115·3).
Skin disorders.

Ichthopaste *Smith & Nephew, Ital.; Smith & Nephew, UK.*
Ichthammol (p.1115·2); zinc oxide (p.1128·2).
Medicated bandage.

Ichthoseptal *Ichthyol, Ger.*
Chloramphenicol (p.179·1); ictasol (p.1115·3).
Infected skin disorders.

Ichthosin *Ichthyol, Ger.*
Ictasol (p.1115·3).
Skin disorders.

Ichthraletten *Ichthyol, Aust.; Ichthyol, Ger.; Ichthyol, Switz.†*
Sodium bituminosulfonate (p.1115·3).
Mastitis; skin disorders.

Ichthyol Hochviskose Flussigkeit *Ichthyol, Ger.*
Ichthammol (p.1115·2).
Skin disorders.

Ichtopur *Ichthyol, Aust.*
Ichthammol (p.1115·2).
Urogenital disorders.

Icht-Oral *Ichthyol, Ger.†*
Minocycline hydrochloride (p.224·3).
Bacterial infections.

Ichtyosoft *LED, Fr.*
Cream: Ictasol (p.1115·3); ammonium lactate (p.1110·3).
Formerly contained ictasol, ammonium lactate, and gamolenic acid.
Skin disorders.
Shampoo: Ictasol (p.1115·3); ammonium lactate (p.1110·3); salicylic acid (p.1122·3).
Scalp disorders.

Icodial *Baxter, Spain.*
Icodextrin (p.1359·1).
Peritoneal dialysis.

Icol *Alcon Cusi, Spain.*
Chloramphenicol (p.179·1) or chloramphenicol succinate (p.181·1); dexamethasone sodium phosphate (p.1067·1).
Infected eye disorders.

Icolamida *Alcon Cusi, Spain.*
Chloramphenicol (p.179·1); sulfacetamide sodium (p.250·3).
Eye infections.

Ictage 6 *Nuova ICT, Ital.*
Gamolenic acid (p.1613·1).
Skin disorders.

Ictan *Synthelabo, Spain.*
Clotrimazole (p.382·1).
Fungal skin infections.

Icthaband *Seton Scholl, Austral.; SSL, UK.*
Ichthammol (p.1115·2); zinc oxide (p.1128·2).
Eczema; leg ulcers; medicated bandage.

Ictholin *Hilarys, Austral.†*
Ichthammol (p.1115·2); phenol (p.1152·3).

Ictiomen *Casen Fleet, Spain.*
Ichthammol (p.1115·2); talc (p.1124·2); menthol (p.1632·3).
Skin disorders.

Ictom 3 *ICT, Ital.*
Omega-3 triglycerides (p.949·2); vitamin E (p.1393·3).
Dry skin; psoriasis.

Ictotest *Bayer, Austral.; Bayer Diagnostics, Irl.; Ames, Israel; Bayer Diagnostici, Ital.; Bayer Diagnostics, UK; Bayer, USA.*
Test for bilirubin in urine.

Icy Hot *Chattem, Singapore; Chattem, USA.*
Methyl salicylate (p.55·1); menthol (p.1632·3).
Muscle, joint, and soft-tissue pain; neuralgia.

Id Sedin *Nikkho, Braz.*
Gamma-aminobutyric acid (p.1613·1); reserpine (p.967·3).
Cerebral disorders.

Ida *The Forty-Two, Thai.*
Bromhexine hydrochloride (p.1085·3).
Respiratory-tract disorders associated with increased or viscous mucus.

Ida-D *The Forty-Two, Thai.*
Bromhexine hydrochloride (p.1085·3); dextromethorphan hydrobromide (p.1087·3).
Respiratory-tract disorders associated with increased or viscous mucus.

Idalon *Hoechst Marion Roussel, Neth.*
Floctafenine (p.40·3).
Pain.

Idalprem *Novartis Consumer, Spain.*
Lorazepam (p.688·3).
Alcohol withdrawal syndrome; anxiety; insomnia; nausea and vomiting.

Idamycin *Pharmacia Upjohn, Canad.; Pharmacia Upjohn, Mex.; Pharmacia Upjohn, USA.*
Idarubicin hydrochloride (p.545·2).
Leukaemias.

Idaptan *Danval, Spain.*
Trimetazidine hydrochloride (p.987·3).
Angina pectoris; neurosensorial ischaemia.

Idarac *Hoechst Marion Roussel, Belg.†; Hoechst Marion Roussel, Braz.; Sanofi Synthelabo, Canad.; Roussel Diamant, Fr.; Hoechst Marion Roussel, Ital.†; Hoechst Marion Roussel, Ital.†; Roussel, Spain; Hoechst Marion Roussel, Thai.*
Floctafenine (p.40·3).
Pain.

Idasal Nebulizador *Warner-Lambert, Spain.*
Oxymetazoline hydrochloride (p.1096·2).
Nasal congestion.

Idazole *Chew, Thai.*
Tinidazole (p.603·3).
Amoebiasis; bacterial mouth infections; giardiasis; trichomoniasis.

Idc *Pharmaland, Thai.*
Indometacin (p.44·3).
Gout; musculoskeletal and joint disorders.

Idealid *AF, Mex.*
Lidamidine (p.1231·2).
Diarrhoea; irritable bowel syndrome.

Idecortex *Pentafarma, Port.*
Idebenone (p.1623·1).

Ideolaxyl *SmithKline Beecham Sante, Fr.*
Aloes (p.1210·1); senna (p.1248·2).
Formerly contained aloes, frangula bark, hyoscyamus, and senna.
Constipation.

Ideolider *IPFI, Ital.*
Acetylaspartic acid; citrulline (p.1357·2).
Memory impairment.

Ideos *Ferring, Fin.; Innothera, Fr.; Henning, Ger.; Helsinn Birex, Irl.; Segix, Ital.; Innothera, Norw.; Helsinn, Port.; Vita, Spain; Ferring, Swed.*
Calcium carbonate (p.1215·1); colecalciferol (p.1391·1).
Calcium and vitamin D deficiency; osteoporosis.

Iderpes *Pierre Fabre, Switz.*
Idoxuridine (p.625·1).

Idina *Grin, Mex.*
Idoxuridine (p.625·1).
Herpes simplex infections.

IDM Solution *Rougier, Canad.†*
Guaifenesin (p.1092·2); potassium iodide (p.1522·3); ephedrine hydrochloride (p.1090·1); mepyramine maleate (p.421·1).
Cold symptoms.

Ido A 50 *Byk Leo, Spain.*
Vitamin A palmitate (p.1383·2).
Vitamin A deficiency.

Ido-C *Abigo, Swed.*
Ascorbic acid (p.1389·3).
Some tablets also contain sodium ascorbate.
Vitamin C deficiency.

I-Doc *Mentholatum, UK.*
Hamamelis (p.1618·3).
Sore eyes.

Idocyklin *Roerig, Swed.†*
Doxycycline (p.200·1) or doxycycline hyclate (p.200·1).
Bacterial infections.

Ido-E *Pharmacia Upjohn, Fin.; Pharmacia Upjohn, Norw.; Pharmacia Upjohn, Swed.*
d-Alpha tocoferil acetate (p.1394·1).
Vitamin E deficiency.

Idom *Kanoldt, Ger.†*
Dothiepin [dosulepin] hydrochloride (p.283·2).
Depression.

Idomed *Rowex, Irl.†*
Indometacin (p.44·3).
Gout; musculoskeletal, joint, and peri-articular disorders; pain.

Idopamil *Therabel, Belg.*
Ibopamine hydrochloride (p.912·1).
Heart failure.

Idotrim *Abigo, Swed.*
Trimethoprim (p.264·2).
Urinary-tract infections.

Idotyl *Ferrosan, Denm.*
Aspirin (p.14·2).
Fever; inflammation; musculoskeletal and joint disorders; pain.

IDR *Asta Medica, Port.†*
Fentiazac (p.40·2).
Inflammation; pain.

Idracemi *Farmigea, Ital.*
Eye drops: Hydrocortisone sodium phosphate (p.1074·1).
Eye ointment: Hydrocortisone hydrogen succinate (p.1074·1); neomycin sulfate (p.228·1); chloramphenicol (p.179·1).
Eye disorders.

Idracemi Eparina *Farmigea, Ital.*
Hydrocortisone sodium phosphate (p.1074·1); heparin sodium (p.902·1).
Eye disorders.

Idratante Samil *Sandoz, Ital.†*
Emollient.

Idril sine *Winzer, Ger.*
Actinoquinol sodium (p.1573·1); naphazoline nitrate (p.1095·1).
Eye disorders.

Idro P2 *Sanofi Synthelabo, Ital.*
Sulmarin sodium; ascorbic acid (p.1389·3).
Capillary disorders; haemorrhage.

Idro-C *Restiva, Ital.†*
Ascorbic acid (p.1389·3).

Idrocet *Lusofarmaco, Ital.*
Hydrocortisone acetate (p.1073·3); neomycin sulfate (p.228·1).
Inflammatory eye and ear disorders.

Idrocol *Lafon, Fr.*
Poloxamer 188 (p.1347·1).
Constipation.

Idrolac *Aesculapius, Ital.*
Lactulose (p.1230·1).
Hepatic encephalopathy and cirrhosis.

Idrolattone *Formenti, Ital.*
Spironolactone (p.973·2).
Hyperaldosteronism; hypertension; oedema.

Idrolone *Sanofi Synthelabo, Ital.*
Fenquizone potassium (p.890·1).
Hypertension; oedema.

Idroneomicil *Searle, Ital.*
Neomycin sulfate (p.228·1); hydrocortisone acetate (p.1073·3); naphazoline nitrate (p.1095·1).
Infection and inflammation of the eye, nose, and ear.

Idropan B *Lisapharma, Ital.*
Vitamin B substances (p.1350·1); calcium folinate (p.1363·1).
Deficiency states; megaloblastic anaemia.

Idroplurivit *Menarini, Ital.*
Multivitamin preparation (p.1350·1).

Idropulmina *ISI, Ital.*
Guaifenesin (p.1092·2).
Coughs; respiratory-tract disorders.

Idroquark *Polifarma, Ital.*
Ramipril (p.966·3); hydrochlorothiazide (p.907·3).
Hypertension.

Idroskin *Mavi, Ital.*
Collagen (p.1598·2).
Dry skin.

Idrovel *Savoma, Ital.*
Emollient.

Idrum *FIRMA, Ital.*
Electrolytes (p.1180·1); carmellose sodium (p.1499·3).
Dry mouth.

Iducher *Farmigea, Ital.*
Idoxuridine (p.625·1).
Herpesvirus infections of the eye.

Iducol *SIFI, Ital.*
Idoxuridine (p.625·1); colistimethate sodium (p.192·3); rolitetracycline (p.247·1) or tetracycline (p.258·3); xanthopterin.
Herpesvirus infections of the eye.

Iducutit *Pharmagalen, Ger.†*
Idoxuridine (p.625·1) in dimethyl sulfoxide.
Herpes simplex and zoster infections.

Idulamine *Schering-Plough, Mex.*
Azatadine maleate (p.409·2).
Allergic skin reactions; rhinitis.

Idulanex *Schering-Plough, Mex.*
Azatadine maleate (p.409·2); pseudoephedrine sulfate (p.1099·3).
Allergic rhinitis.

Iduridin *Geymonat, Ital.†; Ferring, Norw.†; Ferring, UK†.*
Idoxuridine (p.625·1) in dimethyl sulfoxide.
Herpesvirus skin infections.

Idustatin *Sanofi Synthelabo, Ital.*
Ointment (1.5%)†: Idoxuridine (p.625·1); neomycin sulfate (p.228·1); cod-liver oil (p.1357·2).
Ointment (3%); topical solution: Idoxuridine (p.625·1).
Herpes simplex infections of the skin and mucous membranes.

Iduviran *Chauvin, Fr.*
Idoxuridine (p.625·1).
Herpes simplex eye infections.

Iecatec *Tedec Meiji, Spain.*
Enalapril maleate (p.883·3).
Heart failure; hypertension.

Ietepar *Rottapharm, Ital.*
Betaine glucuronate (p.1584·3); diolamine glucuronate (p.1604·1); nicotinamide ascorbate.
Liver disorders; poisoning.

Ifa Dex *Investigacion, Mex.*
Fenproporex (p.1510·2).
Obesity.

Ifa Diety *Investigacion, Mex.*
Fenproporex hydrochloride (p.1510·2).
Obesity.

Ifa Norex *Investigacion, Mex.*
Diethylpropion hydrochloride (p.1508·3).
Obesity.

Ifa Reduccing S *Investigacion, Mex.*
Phentermine hydrochloride (p.1514·1).
Obesity.

Ifecin *Hormona, Mex.*
Ampicillin (p.150·3).
Bacterial infections.

Ifemed *Medifive, Thai.*
Piroxicam (p.79·1).
Gout; musculoskeletal and joint disorders.

Ifenec *Italfarmaco, Ital.*
Econazole (p.383·1) or econazole nitrate (p.382·3).
Fungal infections; Gram-positive bacterial infections.

Ifersol *Investigacion, Mex.*
Ferrous sulfate (p.1360·3).

Ifex
Bristol, Canad.; Bristol-Myers Squibb Oncology, USA.
Ifosfamide (p.546·1).
Malignant neoplasms.

Ifiral *Unique, Thai.*
Sodium cromoglicate (p.774·3).
Allergic rhinitis; hay fever.

IFO-cell *Cell Pharm, Ger.*
Ifosfamide (p.546·1).
Malignant neoplasms.

Ifolem *Lemery, Mex.*
Ifosfamide (p.546·1).
Malignant neoplasms.

Ifomida *Asoforma, Mex.*
Ifosfamide (p.546·1).
Malignant neoplasms.

Ifoxan
Teva, Israel; Sanfer, Mex.
Ifosfamide (p.546·1).
Malignant neoplasms.

Ifumelus *Ifusa, Mex.*
Tolbutamide (p.336·3).
Diabetes mellitus.

Ifutemp *Ifusa, Mex.*
Paracetamol (p.71·2).
Fever; pain.

IG Gamma *Sclavo, Israel.*
A normal immunoglobulin (p.1551·3).
Hypogammaglobulinaemia; passive immunisation.

Ig Tetano *Sclavo, Israel.*
A tetanus immunoglobulin (p.1565·1).
Passive immunisation.

Ig Vena N *Biagini, Ital.*
A normal immunoglobulin (p.1551·3).
Hypogammaglobulinaemia; idiopathic thrombocytopenic purpura; passive immunisation.

Igabulin *Human, Aust.†*
Immunoglobulin A (p.1552·2).
Prevention of necrotising enterocolitis in babies.

Igantet *Grifols, Ital.*
A tetanus immunoglobulin (p.1565·1).
Passive immunisation.

IgeE *Grands Espaces, Fr.*
Black currant (p.1389·3); raspberry (p.1028·3).
Cold symptoms.

Igitur-antirheumatische *Apomedica, Aust.*
Diethylamine salicylate (p.32·2); salicylic acid (p.1122·3); benzyl nicotinate (p.20·2); camphor (p.1589·3).
Musculoskeletal, joint, and peri-articular disorders.

I-Glo *Aspen, S.Afr.*
Phenylephrine hydrochloride (p.1097·1).
Eye irritation.

IgRho *Sclavo, Israel.*
An anti-D immunoglobulin (p.1532·1).
Prevention of rhesus sensitisation.

Igril *Wellcome, Spain.*
Caffeine hydrate (p.761·3); cyclizine hydrochloride (p.414·1); ergotamine tartrate (p.452·1).
Headache; migraine.

Igroseles *Schwarz, Ital.*
Atenolol (p.841·3); chlortalidone (p.857·1).
Hypertension.

Igroton *Novartis, Ital.*
Chlortalidone (p.857·1).
Hypertension; oedema.

Igroton-Lopresor *Novartis, Ital.*
Chlortalidone (p.857·1); metoprolol tartrate (p.931·2).
Hypertension.

Igroton-Reserpina *Novartis, Ital.*
Chlortalidone (p.857·1); reserpine (p.967·3).
Hypertension.

Iguassina *Zambon, Braz.*
Triamterene (p.986·1); hydrochlorothiazide (p.907·3).
Hypertension; oedema.

Iiyalgon *Bioiberica, Spain.*
Hyaluronic acid (p.1620·1).
Osteoarthritis.

Ikaclomin *Teva, Israel.*
Clomifene citrate (p.1465·3).
Anovulatory infertility; oligospermia.

Ikacor *Teva, Israel.*
Verapamil hydrochloride (p.989·1).
Angina pectoris; arrhythmias; hypertension.

Ikapress *Teva, Israel.*
Verapamil hydrochloride (p.989·1).
Angina pectoris; hypertension.

Ikaran
Exel, Belg.†; Pierre Fabre, Fr.; Formenti, Ital.; Robapharm, Switz.
Dihydroergotamine mesilate (p.450·3).
Hypotension; migraine and vascular headache; venous insufficiency.

Ikatin *Pisa, Mex.*
Gentamicin sulfate (p.210·1).
Bacterial infections.

Ikeriane *Ducray, Fr.*
Guanidine glycolate.
Dry skin disorders.

Ikestatina *Crinos, Ital.*
Somatostatin acetate (p.1297·3).
Diabetic ketoacidosis; gastrointestinal haemorrhage; gastrointestinal radiography; prevention of complications following pancreatic surgery.

Iketoncid *Iketon, Ital.*
Glutaral (p.1145·2); cetrimide (p.1137·1).
Instrument disinfection.

Ikorel
Rhone-Poulenc Rorer, Austral.; Rhone-Poulenc Rorer, Fr.; Rhone-Poulenc Rorer, Irl.; Rhone-Poulenc Rorer, Neth.; Aventis, NZ; Rhone-Poulenc Rorer, UK.
Nicorandil (p.939·2).
Angina pectoris.

Iktorivil *Roche, Swed.*
Clonazepam (p.347·1).
Epilepsy.

Ilagane *Daker Farmasimes, Spain†.*
Naproxen (p.60·3).
Musculoskeletal, joint, and peri-articular disorders.

Ila-med m *Paesel, Ger.*
Pipenzolate bromide (p.472·2).
Gastrointestinal disorders.

Ildamen
Asta Medica, Aust.; Asta Medica, Ger.; Asta Medica, Hong Kong; Asta Medica, Port.
Oxyfedrine hydrochloride (p.952·1).
Angina pectoris; arrhythmias; heart failure; myocardial infarction.

Ildor *Esteve, Spain†.*
Nedocromil sodium (p.768·3).
Obstructive airways disease.

Iletin Lente *Lilly, Canad.*
Insulin zinc suspension (bovine and porcine) (p.324·1).
Diabetes mellitus.

Iletin NPH *Lilly, Canad.*
Isophane insulin injection (bovine and porcine) (p.324·1).
Diabetes mellitus.

Iletin II Pork Lente *Lilly, Canad.*
Insulin zinc suspension (porcine) (p.324·1).
Diabetes mellitus.

Iletin II Pork NPH *Lilly, Canad.*
Isophane insulin injection (porcine) (p.324·1).
Diabetes mellitus.

Iletin II Pork Regular *Lilly, Canad.*
Neutral insulin injection (porcine) (p.324·1).
Diabetes mellitus.

Iletin Regular *Lilly, Canad.*
Neutral insulin injection (bovine and porcine) (p.324·1).
Diabetes mellitus.

Iliadin
Merck, Denm.; Merck, Hong Kong; Merck, Mex.; Merck, Norw.; Merck, S.Afr.; Merck, Singapore; Merck, Swed.; Merck, Thai.
Oxymetazoline hydrochloride (p.1096·2).
Nasal congestion; otitis media; rhinitis; sinusitis.

Ilio-Funkton *Robugen, Ger.*
Dimethicone (p.1249·2).
Reduction of gastrointestinal gas.

Ilja Rogoff *Roche Nicholas, Ger.*
Garlic (p.1614·1); mistletoe (p.1636·2); crataegus (p.1600·2); sophora japonica; lupulus (p.1629·3).
Vascular disorders.

Ilja Rogoff Forte *Roche Nicholas, Ger.*
Garlic (p.1614·1).
Vascular disorders.

Illings Bozner Maycur-Tee *Esplanade, Aust.*
Senna (p.1248·2); magnesium sulfate (p.1191·1); chamomile (p.1593·2); fennel (p.1610·1).

Iloban *Merck, Braz.*
Cyanocobalamin (p.1388·1); ferrous fumarate (p.1360·1); folic acid (p.1361·1).
Ascorbic acid (p.1389·3) is included in this preparation to increase the absorption and availability of iron.
Anaemias; iron deficiency.

Ilocin *Haller, Braz.*
Erythromycin (p.201·2).
Bacterial infections.

Ilocit *Juste, Spain.*
Iloprost trometamol (p.1445·2).
Thromboangitis obliterans.

Ilomedin
Schering, Aust.; Schering, Denm.; Schering, Fin.; Schering, Ger.; Schering, Israel; Schering, Ital.†; Schering, Norw.; Schering, NZ; Schering, Port.; Schering, Spain; Schering, Swed.; Schering, Switz.
Iloprost trometamol (p.1445·2).
Peripheral vascular disorders; thromboangitis obliterans.

Ilomedine
Schering, Fr.; Schering, Neth.
Iloprost trometamol (p.1445·2).
Peripheral ischaemia; thromboangiitis obliterans.

Ilon Abszess
Caesaro, Aust.†; Cesra, Ger.
Turpentine; turpentine oil (p.1676·3).
Infected skin disorders.

Ilopan *Savage, USA.*
Dexpanthenol (p.1602·3).
Intestinal atony; paralytic ileus.

Ilopan-Choline *Savage, USA.*
Dexpanthenol (p.1602·3); choline bitartrate (p.1356·3).
Flatulence.

Ilosone
Lilly, Aust.; Lilly, Austral.; Lilly, Braz.; Lilly, Canad.; Lilly, Hong Kong; Dista, Irl.; Lilly, Ital.†; Lilly, Mex.; Aspen, S.Afr.; Lilly, Thai.; Lilly, UK†; Dista, USA.
Erythromycin (p.201·2) or erythromycin estolate (p.201·2).
Bacterial infections.

Ilotrex *Uniao Quimica, Braz.*
Erythromycin stearate (p.201·3).
Bacterial infections.

Ilotycin
Lilly, Canad.†; Lilly, S.Afr.; Lilly, Switz.†; Dista, USA.
Erythromycin (p.201·2) or erythromycin gluceptate (p.201·3).
Bacterial infections.

Ilozyme *Adria, USA.*
Pancrelipase (p.1647·2).
Pancreatic enzyme deficiency.

Ilsatec
Boehringer de Angeli, Braz.; Boehringer Ingelheim, Mex.
Lansoprazole (p.1230·3).
Gastro-oesophageal reflux; peptic ulcer; Zollinger-Ellison syndrome.

Ilube
Alcon, Irl.; Alcon, UK.
Acetylcysteine (p.1082·3); hypromellose (p.1501·3).
Dry eye syndromes.

Ilvico
Note.This name is used for preparations of different composition.
Merck, Irl.
Brompheniramine maleate (p.410·2); calcium ascorbate (p.1389·3); paracetamol (p.71·2); caffeine hydrate (p.761·3).
Cold and influenza symptoms.

Merck, S.Afr.
Syrup: Brompheniramine maleate (p.410·2); sodium ascorbate (p.1390·1); methylephedrine hydrochloride (p.1094·3); phenazone (p.77·2); sodium salicylate (p.84·2); codeine phosphate (p.25·2).
Tablets: Brompheniramine maleate (p.410·2); calcium ascorbate (p.1389·3); propyphenazone (p.80·2); salicylamide (p.82·1); quinine hydrochloride (p.445·1); caffeine (p.761·3).
Allergic rhinitis; cold and influenza symptoms; sinusitis.

Merck, Switz.
Brompheniramine maleate (p.410·2); caffeine (p.761·3); paracetamol (p.71·2).
Fever; nasal congestion; pain.

Ilvico grippal *Merck, Ger.*
Ibuprofen (p.43·2).
Fever; pain.

Ilvico mit Vitamin C *Merck, Aust.*
Paracetamol (p.71·2); ascorbic acid (p.1389·3).
Fever; pain.

Ilvico N
Merck, Ger.†; Merck, Port.
Brompheniramine maleate (p.410·2); calcium ascorbate (p.1389·3); caffeine (p.761·3); paracetamol (p.71·2).
Cold symptoms; fever; pain.

Ilvispect *Merck, S.Afr.*
Carbocisteine (p.1086·3).
Respiratory-tract disorders.

I-L-X *Kenwood, USA.*
A range of preparations containing iron (p.1366·3), liver extracts, and vitamin B substances (p.1350·1).
Vitamin C (p.1389·3) is included in some preparations to increase the absorption and availability of iron.
Iron-deficiency anaemias.

I-L-X B₁₂ *Kenwood, USA.*
Iron preparation with multivitamins (p.1350·1).

Imacillin
AstraZeneca, Denm.; AstraZeneca, Norw.; Astra, Swed.
Amoxicillin (p.149·2) or amoxicillin trihydrate (p.149·2).
Bacterial infections.

Imacol *Marcel, Mex.*
Tetracycline (p.258·3).
Bacterial infections.

Imacort *Spirig, Switz.*
Clotrimazole (p.382·1); hexamidine isetionate (p.1146·2); prednisolone acetate (p.1078·1).
Infected skin disorders.

Imadrax *Durascan, Denm.*
Amoxicillin trihydrate (p.149·2).
Bacterial infections.

Imagopaque
Nycomed, Aust.; Nycomed, Fin.; Nycomed, Ger.; Nycomed, Ital.; Nycomed Imaging, Norw.†; Nycomed, Spain; Nycomed, Switz.
Iopentol (p.1035·3).
Radiographic contrast medium.

Imanance *Lancome, Canad.*
SPF 15: Octinoxate (p.1517·3); titanium dioxide (p.1126·1).
Sunscreen.

Imap
Janssen-Cilag, Belg.; Janssen-Ortho, Canad.†; Janssen-Cilag, Ger.; Abic, Israel; Janssen-Cilag, Neth.; Janssen-Cilag, Norw.†; Janssen-Cilag, Switz.†
Fluspirilene (p.686·1).
Anxiety; psychoses.

Imaplus *MVM, Fr.†*
Vegetable oils (p.1350·1).
Gastrointestinal disorders; hypercholesterolaemia.

Imazin *Napp, UK.*
Aspirin (p.14·2); isosorbide mononitrate (p.916·2).
Angina pectoris; myocardial infarction.

Imazol
Note.This name is used for preparations of different composition.
Karrer, Ger.; Spirig, Switz.
Cream: Clotrimazole (p.382·1); hexamidine isetionate (p.1146·2).
Fungal skin infections.

Karrer, Ger.
Paste: Clotrimazole (p.382·1); phenethyl alcohol (p.1152·2).
Fungal skin infections.

Spirig, Switz.
Paste: Clotrimazole (p.382·1).
Skin disorders.

Imazol comp *Karrer, Ger.*
Clotrimazole (p.382·1); hexamidine isetionate (p.1146·2); prednisolone acetate (p.1078·1).
Fungal skin infections.

Imbak *Mucos, Ger.*
Acidophilus-milk powder (p.1626·3); yeast (p.1398·1); juniper (p.1625·2); ginger (p.1227·2).
Gastrointestinal disorders.

Imbrilon
Rhone-Poulenc Rorer, Hong Kong; Berk, Irl.†; Berk, UK†.
Indometacin (p.44·3).
Gout; inflammation; musculoskeletal, joint, and peri-articular disorders; pain.

Imbun
Ratiopharm, Aust.; Merckle, Ger.
Ibuprofen (p.43·2) or ibuprofen lysine (p.44·1).
Fever; gout; inflammation; musculoskeletal, joint, and soft-tissue disorders; pain.

IMD *Malaysia Chemist, Singapore.*
Loperamide hydrochloride (p.1231·3).
Diarrhoea.

Imdex *CCM, Singapore.*
Isosorbide mononitrate (p.916·2).
Angina pectoris.

Imdur
Astra, Aust.; Astra, Austral.; AstraZeneca, Canad.; AstraZeneca, Denm.; AstraZeneca, Fin.; Astra, Hong Kong; Astra, Irl.; Astra, Mex.; AstraZeneca, Norw.; AstraZeneca, NZ; Astra, Port.; Astra, S.Afr.; AstraZeneca, Singapore; Hassle, Swed.; Astra, Switz.; AstraZeneca, Thai.; AstraZeneca, UK; Key, USA.
Isosorbide mononitrate (p.916·2).
Angina pectoris.

Imegul *Arkopharma, Fr.*
Cascara (p.1216·1); ispaghula (p.1229·1).
Constipation.

Imepas *Marcel, Mex.*
Diazepam (p.674·3).

Imeron *Byk Gulden, Ger.*
Iomeprol (p.1035·1).
Radiographic contrast medium.

Imeson *Taurus, Ger.*
Nitrazepam (p.695·2).
Sleep disorders.

Imet *FIRMA, Ital.*
Indometacin (p.44·3).
Musculoskeletal and joint disorders.

Imex *Merz, Ger.*
Tetracycline hydrochloride (p.258·3).
Acne.

Imexim *Cimex, Switz.†*
Co-trimoxazole (p.193·3).
Bacterial infections.

Imferon
Rhone-Poulenc Rorer, Mex.; Llorente, Spain.
Iron dextran (p.1368·2).
Iron-deficiency anaemia.

Imidazyl *Recordati, Ital.*
Naphazoline nitrate (p.1095·1).
Conjunctivitis.

Imidazyl Antistaminico *Recordati, Ital.*
Naphazoline nitrate (p.1095·1); thonzylamine hydrochloride (p.426·2).
Conjunctivitis.

Imidin K *Wernigerode, Ger.*
Xylometazoline hydrochloride (p.1102·2).
Nasal congestion; rhinitis.

Imidin N *Wernigerode, Ger.*
Xylometazoline hydrochloride (p.1102·2).
Nasal congestion; rhinitis.

Imigran
Glaxo Wellcome, Aust.; Glaxo Wellcome, Austral.; Glaxo Wellcome, Braz.; Glaxo Wellcome, Denm.; Glaxo Wellcome, Fin.; Glaxo Wellcome, Ger.; Cascan, Ger.; Glaxo Wellcome, Hong Kong; Glaxo Wellcome, Irl.; Glaxo Wellcome, Israel; Glaxo Wellcome, Mex.; Glaxo Wellcome, Neth.; Glaxo Wellcome, Norw.; Glaxo Wellcome, NZ; Glaxo Wellcome, Port.; Glaxo Wellcome, S.Afr.; Glaxo Wellcome, Singapore; Glaxo Wellcome, Spain; Glaxo Wellcome, Swed.; Glaxo Wellcome, Switz.; Glaxo Wellcome, Thai.; Glaxo Wellcome, UK.
Sumatriptan (p.457·2), sumatriptan hemisulfate (p.457·2), or sumatriptan succinate (p.456·1).
Cluster headache; migraine.

The symbol † denotes a preparation no longer actively marketed

Imigrane *Glaxo Wellcome, Fr.*
Sumatriptan (p.457·2) or sumatriptan succinate (p.456·1).
Migraine; vascular facial pain.

Imiject *Glaxo Wellcome, Fr.*
Sumatriptan succinate (p.456·1).
Vascular facial pain.

Imilgamma *Worwag, Ger.*
Benfotiamine (p.1384·3).
Formerly known as Benfogamma.
Vitamin B₁ deficiency.

Iminase *Madaus, Spain.*
Anistreplase (p.840·2).
Myocardial infarction.

Imipem *Neopharmed, Ital.*
Imipenem (p.214·1); cilastatin sodium (p.182·2).
Lignocaine [lidocaine] (p.1313·2) is included in the intramuscular injection to alleviate the pain of injection.
Bacterial infections.

Imitrex *Glaxo Wellcome, Belg.; Glaxo Wellcome, Canad.; Glaxo Wellcome, Israel; Glaxo Wellcome, USA.*
Sumatriptan (p.457·2), sumatriptan hemisulfate (p.457·2), or sumatriptan succinate (p.456·1).
Cluster headache; migraine.

Imizol *Farmigea, Ital.†*
Naphazoline nitrate (p.1095·1).
Eye irritation.

Immignost *Richter, Aust.†; GN, Ger.†*
Tetanus toxoid; diphtheria toxoid; Streptococcal group C antigen; tuberculin (p.1675·3); Candida albicans antigen; Trichophyton mentagrophytes antigen; proteus mirabilis antigen.
Assessment of cell-mediated immunity.

Immubron *Bruschettini, Ital.*
Lysates of: Staphylococcus aureus; Streptococcus pyogenes; Streptococcus viridans; Klebsiella pneumoniae; Klebsiella ozaenae; Haemophilus influenzae; Moraxella catarrhalis; strains of Streptococcus pneumoniae.
Respiratory-tract infections.

ImmuCyst *Pasteur Merieux, Aust.; Rhone-Poulenc Rorer, Austral.; Pasteur Merieux, Belg.; Connaught, Canad.; Pasteur Merieux, Fr.; CytoChemia, Ger.†; Pasteur Merieux, Hong Kong; Connaught, Israel; Wassermann, Ital.; Aventis, NZ; Inibsa, Port.; Pasteur Merieux, Singapore; Inibsa, Spain; Sanofi Synthelabo, Switz.; Pasteur Merieux, Thai.; Pasteur Merieux, UK.*
A BCG vaccine (p.1533·2).
Bladder cancer.

Immucytal *Pierre Fabre, Ital.*
Ribosomal fractions of Klebsiella pneumoniae; Streptococcus pneumoniae; Streptococcus pyogenes; Haemophilus influenzae; membrane fraction of Klebsiella pneumoniae.
Bronchial infections; otorhinolaryngeal infections.

Immudynal *Ardeypharm, Ger.*
Homoeopathic preparation.

Immugrip *Pierre Fabre, Fr.*
An inactivated influenza vaccine (p.1544·3).
Active immunisation.

Immukin *Boehringer Ingelheim, Hong Kong; Boehringer Ingelheim, Irl.; Boehringer Ingelheim, UK.*
Interferon gamma-1b (rbe) (p.634·1).
Infections in chronic granulomatous disease.

Immukine *Boehringer Ingelheim, Belg.; Boehringer Ingelheim, Neth.*
Interferon gamma-1b (p.634·1).
Infections in chronic granulomatous disease.

Immulem *Lemery, Mex.*
Ciclosporin (p.518·1).
Transplant rejection.

Immunace *Vitabiotics, UK.*
Multivitamin, mineral, and bioflavonoid preparation (p.1350·1).

Immun-Aid *Pisa, Mex.; McGaw, NZ; McGaw, USA.*
Preparation for enteral nutrition (p.1350·1).
Immunosuppression.

Immunate *Osterreichisches Institut, Aust.; Baxter, Swed.*
A factor VIII preparation (p.734·1).
Haemorrhagic disorders.

Immunate STIM *Immuno, Ger.; Immuno, Ital.*
A factor VIII preparation (p.734·1).
Haemorrhagic disorders.

Immunate STIM plus *Baxter, Switz.*
A factor VIII preparation (p.734·1).
Haemorrhagic disorders.

Immunex CRP *Wampole, USA.*
Test for C-reactive protein in serum.

Immunine *Osterreichisches Institut, Aust.; Baxter, Canad.; Baxter, Denm.; Baxter, Spain; Baxter, Swed.*
A factor IX preparation (p.735·1).
Haemorrhagic disorders.

Immunine STIM *Immuno, Ger.; Immuno, Ital.*
A factor IX preparation (p.735·1).
Haemorrhagic disorders.

Immunine STIM plus *Baxter, Switz.*
A factor IX preparation (p.735·1).
Haemorrhagic disorders.

Immunja *OTW, Ger.*
Homoeopathic preparation.

Immunocal *Immunotec, USA.*
Preparation for enteral nutrition (p.1350·1).

Immunoendocig *Nuovo ISM, Ital.*
A cytomegalovirus immunoglobulin (p.1536·1).
Passive immunisation.

Immunoendozig *ISI, Ital.*
A varicella-zoster immunoglobulin (p.1567·3).
Passive immunisation.

ImmunoHBs *ISI, Ital.*
A hepatitis B immunoglobulin (p.1542·1).
Passive immunisation.

Immunokine *Oxo, Thai.*
Tetrachlorodecaoxide (p.1670·1).
Post-radiation-therapy syndromes.

Immunomega *Larkhall Laboratories, UK.*
Multivitamin and mineral preparation (p.1350·1).

Immunomorb *ISI, Ital.*
A measles immunoglobulin (p.1547·3).
Passive immunisation.

Immunoparot *ISI, Ital.*
A mumps immunoglobulin (p.1551·1).
Passive immunisation.

Immunopertox *ISI, Ital.*
A pertussis immunoglobulin (p.1555·3).
Passive immunisation.

Immunopret *Bionorica, Ger.*
Echinacea purpurea (p.1606·2).
Respiratory- and urinary-tract infections.

Immunoprin *Ashbourne, UK.*
Azathioprine (p.509·3).
Inflammatory disorders; organ transplants.

Immunorho *ISI, Ital.*
An anti-D immunoglobulin (p.1532·1).
Prevention of rhesus sensitisation.

Immunoros *ISI, Ital.*
A rubella immunoglobulin (p.1562·2).
Passive immunisation.

Immunotetan *ISI, Ital.*
A tetanus immunoglobulin (p.1565·1).
Passive immunisation.

Immunovac *Artu, Neth.*
Allergen extracts (p.1575·3).
Hyposensitisation.

Immunozig *ISI, Ital.*
A varicella-zoster immunoglobulin (p.1567·3).
Passive immunisation.

Immunozima *Salus, Ital.†*
Muramidase hydrochloride (p.1638·1).
Viral infections.

Immutone *Pharmadass, UK.*
Shark-liver oil.

Imoclone *Orion, Denm.*
Zopiclone (p.713·1).
Insomnia.

Imocur
Note.This name is used for preparations of different composition.
Pharmacia Upjohn, Fin.
Loperamide hydrochloride (p.1231·3).
Diarrhoea; ileostomy management.
Zambon, Fr.
Bacterial fractions of Haemophilus influenzae; Streptococcus pneumoniae; Klebsiella ozaenae; Klebsiella pneumoniae; Staphylococcus aureus; Streptococcus viridans; Streptococcus pyogenes; Moraxella catarrhalis.
Prevention of upper respiratory-tract infection.

Imodium *Janssen-Cilag, Aust.; Janssen-Cilag, Austral.; Janssen-Cilag, Belg.; McNeil Consumer, Canad.; Janssen-Ortho, Canad.; Janssen-Cilag, Denm.; Orion, Fin.; Janssen-Cilag, Fr.; Janssen Cilag, Ger.; Woelm, Ger.; Janssen, Hong Kong; Janssen-Cilag, Irl.; Janssen-Cilag, Israel; Janssen-Cilag, Ital.; Janssen-Cilag, Mex.; Janssen-Cilag, Neth.; Janssen-Cilag, Norw.; Janssen-Cilag, NZ; Janssen-Cilag, Port.; Janssen-Cilag, S.Afr.; Janssen-Cilag, Singapore; Abello, Spain; Janssen-Cilag, Swed.; Janssen-Cilag, Switz.; Janssen, Thai.; Janssen-Cilag, UK; Johnson MSD Consumer, UK; McNeil Consumer, USA; Janssen, USA.*
Loperamide hydrochloride (p.1231·3).
Diarrhoea; ileostomy management.

Imodium Advanced *Janssen-Cilag, Austral.; McNeil Consumer, Canad.; Janssen-Cilag, NZ; McNeil Consumer, USA.*
Loperamide hydrochloride (p.1231·3); simeticone (p.1249·2).
Diarrhoea; excess gastrointestinal gas.

Imodium Plus *Woelm, Ger.; Janssen-Cilag, S.Afr.; Abello, Spain; Janssen-Cilag, Switz.; Johnson & Johnson MSD Consumer, UK.*
Loperamide hydrochloride (p.1231·3); simeticone (p.1249·2).
Diarrhoea; excess gastrointestinal gas.

Imogam *CSL, Austral.; Connaught, Canad.*
A rabies immunoglobulin (p.1560·2).
Passive immunisation.

Imogam Rabia *Rhone-Poulenc Rorer, Spain†.*
A rabies immunoglobulin (p.1560·2).
Passive immunisation.

Imogam Rabies *Pasteur Merieux, Israel; Pasteur Merieux, USA.*
A rabies immunoglobulin (p.1560·2).
Passive immunisation.

Imogam Rage *Pasteur Merieux, Fr.*
A rabies immunoglobulin (p.1560·2).
Passive immunisation.

Imogam Tetano *Pasteur Merieux, Ital.*
A tetanus immunoglobulin (p.1565·1).
Passive immunisation.

Imosec *Janssen, Braz.; Abello, Spain.*
Loperamide hydrochloride (p.1231·3).
Diarrhoea.

Imossel *Martin, Fr.*
Loperamide hydrochloride (p.1231·3).
Diarrhoea.

Imosselduo *Martin, Fr.; Martin-Johnson & Johnson, Fr.*
Loperamide hydrochloride (p.1231·3); simeticone (p.1249·2).
Diarrhoea; flatulence.

Imovane *Rhone-Poulenc Rorer, Aust.; Rhone-Poulenc Rorer, Austral.; Aventis, Belg.; Rhodia, Braz.; Rhone-Poulenc Rorer, Canad.; Aventis, Denm.; Rhone-Poulenc Rorer, Fin.; Rhone-Poulenc Rorer, Fr.; Rhone-Poulenc Rorer, Hong Kong; Rhone-Poulenc Rorer, Israel; Rhone-Poulenc Rorer, Ital.; Rhone-Poulenc Rorer, Mex.; Rhone-Poulenc Rorer, Neth.; Rhone-Poulenc Rorer, Norw.; Aventis, NZ; Aventis, S.Afr.; Rhone-Poulenc Rorer, Singapore; Rhone-Poulenc Rorer, Swed.; Rhone-Poulenc Rorer, Switz.*
Zopiclone (p.713·1).
Sleep disorders.

Imovax *Pasteur Merieux, Braz.; Merieux, Fr.†*
A mumps vaccine (Urabe Am 9 strain) (p.1551·1).
Active immunisation.

Imovax BCG *Pasteur Merieux, Ital.*
A BCG vaccine (p.1533·2).
Active immunisation.

Imovax Colera *Pasteur Merieux, Ital.†*
A cholera vaccine (p.1535·2).
Active immunisation.

Imovax DT *Pasteur Merieux, Ital.*
A diphtheria and tetanus vaccine (p.1537·1).
Active immunisation.

Imovax DTP *Pasteur Merieux, Ital.†*
A diphtheria, tetanus, and pertussis vaccine (p.1537·3).
Active immunisation.

Imovax Meningo A & C *Aventis, S.Afr.*
A meningococcal vaccine (p.1550·1).
Active immunisation.

Imovax Mumps *Pasteur Merieux, Hong Kong.*
A mumps vaccine (live attenuated Urabe Am 9 strain) (p.1551·1).
Active immunisation.

Imovax Polio *Pasteur Merieux, Belg.; Meda, Fin.; Pasteur Merieux, Fr.; Pasteur Merieux, Hong Kong; Pasteur Merieux, Israel; Pasteur Merieux, Ital.; Pasteur Merieux, Norw.; Pasteur Merieux, Singapore; Pasteur Merieux, Swed.*
An inactivated poliomyelitis vaccine (p.1558·2).
Active immunisation.

Imovax Rabbia *Pasteur Merieux, Ital.*
A rabies vaccine (p.1560·2).
Active immunisation.

Imovax Rabies *Connaught, Canad.; Pasteur Merieux, USA.*
A rabies vaccine (human diploid cell) (p.1560·2).
Active immunisation.

Imovax Tetano *Pasteur Merieux, Ital.*
A tetanus vaccine (p.1565·2).
Active immunisation.

Imozop *Durascan, Denm.*
Zopiclone (p.713·1).
Insomnia.

Impact *Novartis, Fin.; Novartis Nutrition, Hong Kong; Novartis Consumer, Ital.; Novartis Consumer, Port.; Novartis Nutrition, Singapore; Novartis Consumer, UK; Novartis Nutrition, USA.*
Preparation for enteral nutrition (p.1350·1).

Impalud *Sanus, Braz.*
Quinine sulfate (p.445·1).
Babesiosis; leg cramps; malaria.

Impelium *TO-Chemicals, Thai.*
Loperamide hydrochloride (p.1231·3).
Diarrhoea.

Impetex *Roche, Ital.*
Diflucortolone valerate (p.1069·3); chlorquinaldol (p.182·1).
Infected skin disorders.

Implanon *Organon, Austral.; Organon, Denm.; Organon, Fin.; Organon, Fr.; Nourypharma, Ger.; Organon, Neth.; Organon, Swed.; Organon, UK.*
Etonogestrel (p.1477·1).
Progestogen-only implantable contraceptive.

Implementor *Pentafarma, Port.†*
Pirlindole hydrochloride (p.307·3).

Impletol *Bayer, Ger.*
Procaine hydrochloride (p.1319·1); caffeine (p.761·3).
Nervous system disorders.

Impore *Unison, Thai.*
Loperamide hydrochloride (p.1231·3).
Diarrhoea.

Importal *Novartis Consumer, Aust.; Novartis Consumer, Belg.; Novartis, Denm.; Novartis, Fin.; Novartis Sante, Fr.; Novartis Consumer, Ger.; Novartis, Israel; Novartis Consumer, Neth.; Novartis, Norw.; Novartis, NZ; Novartis Consumer, Port.; Novartis Consumer, S.Afr.†; Novartis, Swed.; Novartis Consumer, Switz.; Novartis, Thai.*
Lactitol (p.1230·1).
Constipation; hepatic encephalopathy.

Imposit N *Madaus, Ger.*
Cetylpyridinium chloride (p.1138·1); benzocaine (p.1306·2).
Mouth and throat disorders.

Impregon *Fleming, USA.*
Tetrachlorosalicylanilide.
Napkin disinfection.

Impresso *Isis Puren, Ger.*
Oxprenolol hydrochloride (p.951·3); hydralazine hydrochloride (p.905·3); chlortalidone (p.857·1).
Hypertension.

Impril *ICN, Canad.†*
Imipramine hydrochloride (p.291·1).
Depression.

Impromen *Janssen-Cilag, Belg.; Janssen-Cilag, Ger.; Formenti, Ital.; Janssen-Cilag, Neth.; Janssen, Thai.*
Bromperidol (p.657·1), bromperidol decanoate (p.657·1), or bromperidol lactate (p.657·1).
Psychoses.

Improntal *Fides Rottapharm, Spain.*
Piroxicam (p.79·1).
Gout; musculoskeletal, joint, peri-articular, and soft-tissue disorders; pain.

Improved Analgesic *Rugby, USA.*
Methyl salicylate (p.55·1); menthol (p.1632·3).
Muscle, joint, and soft-tissue pain; neuralgia.

Improved Once A Day *UK.*
Multivitamin and mineral preparation (p.1350·1).

Improved Versal *Clay Park, Hong Kong.*
Zinc oxide (p.1128·2); calamine (p.1111·3).
Anorectal disorders.

Improvera *Pharmacia, UK.*
28 Tablets, estropipate (p.1476·1); 12 tablets, medroxyprogesterone acetate (p.1480·1).
Menopausal disorders; osteoporosis.

Improvil *Monsanto, Austral.*
21 Tablets, norethisterone (p.1485·1); ethinylestradiol (p.1476·2); 7 tablets, inert.
Triphasic oral contraceptive.

Imp-Tab *Alra, USA†.*
Imipramine hydrochloride (p.291·1).

Impugan *Dumex-Alpharma, Denm.†; Dumex-Alpharma, Swed.; Dumex, Switz.; Dumex, Thai.*
Frusemide [furosemide] (p.893·1).
Ascites; hypertension; nephrotic syndrome; oedema; renal insufficiency.

Imtack *Astra, Irl.†; AstraZeneca, UK†.*
Isosorbide dinitrate (p.915·2).
Angina pectoris.

Imtrate *Douglas, Austral.; Douglas, NZ.*
Isosorbide mononitrate (p.916·2).
Angina pectoris.

Imuderm *Goldshield, UK.*
Cream: White soft paraffin (p.1407·3); fractionated coconut oil (p.1372·1); glycerol (p.1616·3).
Hand & face wash; shower gel: Soap substitute.
Oil: Light liquid paraffin (p.1407·2); almond oil (p.1576·3).
Dry skin disorders.

Imudon *Solvay, Fr.*
Lysates of Lactobacillus acidophilus (p.1626·3); Lactobacillus helveticus (p.1626·3); Lactobacillus lactis (p.1626·3); Lactobacillus fermentum (p.1626·3); Streptococcus pyogenes; Enterococcus faecium (p.1626·3); Enterococcus faecalis (p.1626·3); Streptococcus sanguis; Staphylococcus aureus; Klebsiella pneumoniae; Corynebacterium pseudodiphtheriticum; Fusiformis fusiformis; Candida albicans.
Mouth disorders.

Imufor *Boehringer Ingelheim, Aust.*
Interferon gamma-1b (p.634·1).
Infections in chronic granulomatous disease.

Imugins *Schumit, Thai.*
Ginseng (p.1615·3); multivitamins and minerals (p.1350·1).
Tonic.

Imukin *Boehringer Ingelheim, Aust.; Boehringer Ingelheim, Austral.; Boehringer Ingelheim, Denm.; Boehringer Ingelheim, Fin.; Boehringer Ingelheim, Ger.; Boehringer Ingelheim, Ital.; Boehringer Ingelheim, Norw.; Boehringer Ingelheim, NZ; Boehringer Ingelheim, Port.; Boehringer Ingelheim, Spain; Boehringer Ingelheim, Swed.; Boehringer Ingelheim, Thai.*
Interferon gamma-1b (rbe) (p.634·1).
Infections in chronic granulomatous disease.

Imuneprim *IQB, Braz.*
Co-trimoxazole (p.193·3).
Bacterial infections; Pneumocystis carinii pneumonia; protozoal infections.

Imunoferon *Fariberica, Port.*
Glicofosfopeptical (p.1616·2).
Immunodeficiency.

Imunovir *Rivex, Canad.; Newport, Irl.; NZ Medical & Scientific, NZ; Ardern, UK.*
Inosine pranobex (p.627·2).
Viral infections.

Imuprel *Adcock Ingram, S.Afr.*
Isoprenaline hydrochloride (p.914·3).
Bronchospasm; heart block; shock.

Imuprin *Pharmacia Upjohn, Fin.*
Azathioprine (p.509·3).
Auto-immune disorders; lupus erythematosus; rheumatoid arthritis; transplant rejection.

Imuran *Glaxo Wellcome, Austral.; Glaxo Wellcome, Belg.; Glaxo Wellcome, Braz.; Glaxo Wellcome, Canad.; Glaxo Wellcome, Hong Kong; Wellcome, Irl.; Glaxo Wellcome, Israel; Glaxo Wellcome, Mex.; Glaxo Wellcome, Neth.; Glaxo Wellcome, NZ; Glaxo Wellcome, Port.; Glaxo Wellcome, S.Afr.; Glaxo Wellcome, Singapore; Glaxo Wellcome, Thai.; Glaxo Wellcome, UK; Faro, USA.*
Azathioprine (p.509·3) or azathioprine sodium (p.510·2).
Auto-immune disorders; transplant rejection.

Imurek *Glaxo Wellcome, Aust.; Glaxo Wellcome, Ger.; Wellcome, Switz.*
Azathioprine (p.509·3) or azathioprine sodium (p.510·2).
Auto-immune disorders; transplant rejection.

Imurel *Glaxo Wellcome, Denm.; Glaxo Wellcome, Fin.; Glaxo Wellcome, Fr.; Glaxo Wellcome, Norw.; Medeva, Spain; Glaxo Wellcome, Swed.*
Azathioprine (p.509·3).
Auto-immune disorders; transplant rejection.

Imuvac *Solvay, Spain.*
An influenza vaccine (p.1544·3).
Active immunisation.

Imuvit
Kunzle, Switz.; Rueckert, Thai.
Ginseng (p.1615·3); multivitamins and minerals (p.1350·1).
Tonic.

In A Wink
Note. This name is used for preparations of different composition.
Ciba Vision, Austral.
Naphazoline nitrate (p.1095·1); zinc sulfate (p.1398·2).
Conjunctivitis; eye irritation.

Ciba Vision, Canad.
A range of solutions for contact lenses (p.1129·2).

Ciba Vision, NZ.
Povidone (p.1503·2).
Dry eyes.

In A Wink Allergy *Ciba Vision, Austral.*
Antazoline hydrochloride (p.408·3); tetryzoline hydrochloride (p.1101·2).
Allergic conjunctivitis; hay fever.

In A Wink Moisturing *Ciba Vision, Austral.*
Povidone (p.1503·2).
Dry eyes.

Inabrin
Pharmacia Upjohn, Belg.†; Pharmacia Upjohn, Port.†.
Ibuprofen (p.43·2).
Fever; pain.

Inac *Recon, Singapore.*
Diclofenac sodium (p.30·3).
Gout; musculoskeletal, joint, peri-articular, and soft-tissue disorders.

Inacid *Merck Sharp & Dohme, Spain.*
Indometacin (p.44·3) or indometacin sodium (p.45·1).
Gout; inflammation; musculoskeletal, joint, peri-articular, and soft-tissue disorders; pain; patent ductus arteriosus.

Inacol *Medifarma, Mex.*
Tetracycline (p.258·3).
Bacterial infections.

Inadine
Johnson & Johnson, Ger.; Johnson & Johnson, Irl.; Ethicon, Ital.; Johnson & Johnson, Swed.†; Johnson & Johnson Medical, UK.
Povidone-iodine (p.1155·1).
Burns; skin ulcers; wounds.

Inalacor *Faes, Spain.*
Fluticasone propionate (p.1072·2).
Asthma.

Inalador Vick *Procter & Gamble, Braz.*
Menthol (p.1632·3); camphor (p.1589·3); methyl salicylate (p.55·1); siberian fir oil.
Respiratory-tract congestion.

Inalar *Montefarmaco, Ital.*
Xylometazoline hydrochloride (p.1102·2); domiphen bromide (p.1143·3).
Nasal congestion.

Inalgon Neu *Fresenius Kabi, Aust.*
Dipyrone (p.34·1).
Fever; pain.

Inalintra *Diviser Aquilea, Spain.*
Oxymetazoline hydrochloride (p.1096·2).
Nasal congestion.

Inalobel *Sedabel, Braz.*
Ephedrine (p.1090·1); eucalyptol (p.1609·2); menthol (p.1632·3); niaouli oil (p.1640·2); tolu balsam (p.1101·3); sumatra benzoin (p.1668·3).
Respiratory-tract congestion.

Inalpin *Qualiphar, Belg.*
Codeine phosphate (p.25·2); guaifenesin (p.1092·2).
Formerly contained codeine phosphate, bromoform, sulfogaiacol, sodium camsilate, guaiacol, and aconite.
Coughs.

Inamide *Gerard, Irl.*
Indapamide (p.913·1).
Hypertension.

Inapsin *Janssen-Cilag, S.Afr.†.*
Droperidol (p.682·2).
Neuroleptanalgesia; premedication.

Inapsine
Janssen-Ortho, Canad.†; Janssen, USA†.
Droperidol (p.682·2).
Nausea and vomiting in surgical and diagnostic procedures; neuroleptanalgesia; premedication.

Inarub *Frega, Canad.†.*
Methyl salicylate (p.55·1); menthol (p.1632·3); eucalyptol (p.1609·2).

Inaspir *Almirall, Spain.*
Salmeterol xinafoate (p.773·3).
Obstructive airways disease.

Inatrex Balsamico *Eurofarma, Braz.*
Dipyrone (p.34·1); niaouli oil (p.1640·2); eucalyptol (p.1609·2); guaifenesin (p.1092·2); sodium camsilate; diphenhydramine hydrochloride (p.416·1).
Cold and influenza symptoms.

Inca's Gold *Larkhall Laboratories, UK.*
Jojoba oil.

Incidal
Bayer, Hong Kong; Bayer, Ital.†; Bayer, Neth.†; Bayer, Thai.
Mebhydrolin napadisilate (p.420·2).
Hypersensitivity reactions.

Incidin *Henkel, Ger.*
Isopropyl alcohol (p.1149·2); propyl alcohol (p.1155·3).
Equipment disinfection.

Incidin Extra *Henkel, Ger.*
Benzalkonium chloride (p.1133·2); oligo(di(iminoimidocarbonyl)iminohexamethylene) (p.1152·1); orthophenylphenol (p.1152·1).
Surface disinfection.

Incidin extra N *Henkel, Ger.*
Glucoprotamine; benzalkonium chloride (p.1133·2).
Surface disinfection.

Incidin M Spray Extra *Henkel, Ger.*
Tributyltin benzoate; isopropyl alcohol (p.1149·2).
Skin disinfection.

Incidin perfekt *Henkel, Ger.*
Formaldehyde (p.1144·2); glyoxal (p.1145·3); glutaral (p.1145·2); benzalkonium chloride (p.1133·2); oligo(di(iminoimidocarbonyl)iminohexamethylene).
Surface disinfection.

Incidin Plus *Henkel, Ger.*
Glucoprotamine.
Surface disinfection.

Incidin Spezial
Note. This name is used for preparations of different composition.
Henkel, Ger.
Formaldehyde (p.1144·2); glyoxal (p.1145·3); glutaral (p.1145·2); alcohol (p.1130·3).
Surface disinfection.

Henkel, Ital.
Alcohol (p.1130·3); glyoxal (p.1145·3); glutaral (p.1145·2); benzalkonium chloride (p.1133·2).
Surface disinfection.

Incidine *Parogerm, Fr.*
Glutaral (p.1145·2); formaldehyde (p.1144·2); glyoxal (p.1145·3).
Surface and instrument disinfection.

Incidur *Henkel, Ger.*
Glutaral (p.1145·2); glyoxal (p.1145·3).
Surface disinfection.

Incidur Spray *Henkel, Ger.*
Glutaral (p.1145·2); benzalkonium chloride (p.1133·2); 5-bromo-5-nitro-1,3-dioxacyclohexane; alcohol (p.1130·3); propyl alcohol (p.1155·3).
Surface disinfection.

Inconturina *OTW, Ger.*
Solidago virgaurea; clove (p.1596·3).
Urinary-tract disorders.

Incremin
Note. This name is used for preparations of different composition.
Cyanamid, Ital.†; Wyeth, Mex.
Lysine hydrochloride; vitamin B substances (p.1350·1).
Nutritional supplement.

Wyeth Lederle, Port.
Lysine (p.1370·3).

Incremin Con Hierro *Wyeth, Mex.*
Ferric pyrophosphate (p.1359·3); vitamin B substances; lysine hydrochloride (p.1350·1).
Iron-deficiency anaemia.

Incremin Iron *Whitehall, Austral.*
Ferric pyrophosphate (p.1359·3); vitamin B substances (p.1350·1); lysine hydrochloride.
Dietary supplement.

Incremin with Iron
Whitehall, NZ.
Iron; vitamin B substances; lysine hydrochloride (p.1350·1).
Dietary supplement.

Lederle, USA†.
Ferric pyrophosphate (p.1359·3); vitamin B substances; L-lysine (p.1350·1).
Iron-deficiency anaemias.

Incremin with Vitamin C *Whitehall, Austral.*
Vitamin B substances; lysine hydrochloride; vitamin C (p.1350·1).
Dietary supplement.

Incutin *Andreabal, Switz.*
Benzyl nicotinate (p.20·2); glycol salicylate (p.42·2); methyl salicylate (p.55·1); camphor (p.1589·3); capsicum (p.1591·1); pine oil; rosemary oil (p.1659·3).
Musculoskeletal, joint, peri-articular, and soft-tissue pain and inflammation.

Indaco *Ciba Vision, Ital.*
Naphazoline nitrate (p.1095·1); zinc sulfate (p.1398·2).
Eye irritation.

Indaflex *Lampugnani, Ital.*
Indapamide (p.913·1).
Hypertension.

Indahexal *Hexal, Austral.*
Indapamide (p.913·1).
Hypertension.

Indalgin *Orion, Fin.*
Indometacin (p.44·3); ethylmorphine hydrochloride (p.35·2).
Pain.

Indalix *Triomed, S.Afr.*
Indapamide (p.913·1).
Hypertension.

Indamol *Rhone-Poulenc Rorer, Ital.*
Indapamide (p.913·1).
Hypertension.

Indanorm *Julphar, UAE.*
Indapamide (p.913·1).
Hypertension.

Indarzona-N *Streger, Mex.*
Dexamethasone (p.1067·1).
Corticosteroid.

Inderal
Zeneca, Aust.; Zeneca, Austral.; Zeneca, Belg.; Zeneca, Braz.; Wyeth-Ayerst, Canad.; AstraZeneca, Denm.; AstraZeneca, Fin.; Zeneca, Hong Kong; Zeneca, Irl.; Zeneca, Israel; Zeneca, Ital.; Zeneca, Neth.; AstraZeneca, Norw.; Zeneca, Port.; Zeneca, S.Afr.; AstraZeneca, Singapore; Zeneca, Swed.; Zeneca, Switz.; AstraZeneca, Thai.; AstraZeneca, UK; Wyeth-Ayerst, USA.
Propranolol hydrochloride (p.962·3).
Angina pectoris; anxiety; arrhythmias; essential tremor; hypertension; hyperthyroidism; hypertrophic obstructive cardiomyopathy; migraine; myocardial infarction; phaeochromocytoma; variceal haemorrhage.

Inderal comp *Zeneca, Aust.*
Propranolol hydrochloride (p.962·3); triamterene (p.986·1); hydrochlorothiazide (p.907·3).
Hypertension.

Inderalici *Zeneca, Mex.*
Propranolol hydrochloride (p.962·3).
Angina pectoris; anxiety; arrhythmias; essential tremor; glaucoma; hypertension; hyperthyroidism; migraine; myocardial infarction; obstructive cardiomyopathy; phaeochromocytoma; variceal haemorrhage.

Inderetic
Zeneca, Aust.; Zeneca, Belg.; Zeneca, Irl.; Zeneca, Neth.; S.Afr.; Zeneca, Switz.; AstraZeneca, UK.
Propranolol hydrochloride (p.962·3); bendrofluazide [bendroflumethiazide] (p.844·1).
Hypertension.

Inderex *AstraZeneca, UK.*
Propranolol hydrochloride (p.962·3); bendrofluazide [bendroflumethiazide] (p.844·1).
Hypertension.

Inderide
Wyeth-Ayerst, Canad.; Wyeth-Ayerst, USA.
Propranolol hydrochloride (p.962·3); hydrochlorothiazide (p.907·3).
Hypertension.

Inderm
Sankyo, Belg.; Dermapharm, Ger.; Sankyo, Neth.; Sankyo, Switz.
Erythromycin (p.201·2).
Acne.

Indermil *Davis & Geck, UK.*
Enbucrilate (p.1601·2).
Wound closure.

Indian Brandee *Anglian, UK.*
Capsicum (p.1591·1); compound cardamom tincture (p.1591·3).
Dyspepsia; flatulence.

Indianische Frauenwurzel Kapseln *NAM, Ger.*
Cimicifuga (p.1595·2).
Menopausal disorders.

Indiaral *Gifrer Barbezat, Fr.*
Loperamide hydrochloride (p.1231·3).
Diarrhoea.

Indicatest *Polidis, Fr.*
Pregnancy test (p.1654·3).

Indigestion *Hylands, Canad.*
Homoeopathic preparation.

Indigestion Complex *Brauer, Austral.†.*
Homoeopathic preparation.

Indigestion and Flatulence *Cantassium Co., UK.*
Capsicum oleoresin (p.1591·1); valerian (p.1678·3); fennel (p.1610·1); myrrh (p.1639·2); papain (p.1647·3).

Indigestion and Flatulence Tablets *Healthcrafts, UK.*
Peppermint oil (p.1243·3); fennel oil (p.1610·2); capsicum oleoresin (p.1591·1).
Dyspepsia; flatulence.

Indigestion Mixture *Potter's, UK.*
Meadowsweet (p.1631·2); gentian (p.1615·1); euonymus (p.1225·3).
Dyspepsia; flatulence; heartburn.

Indigestion Relief
Note. This name is used for preparations of different composition.
Galpharm, UK.
Ranitidine (p.1246·3).
Dyspepsia; heartburn.

Herbal Concepts, UK.
Leptandra virginica; capsicum (p.1591·1); fringetree bark; ginger (p.1227·2).
Colic; dyspepsia; nausea.

Indigestion Relief Liquid *Boots, UK.*
Simeticone (p.1249·2); aluminium hydroxide (p.1210·3); magnesium hydroxide (p.1233·1).
Formerly known as Double Action Indigestion Mixture.
Dyspepsia.

Indigestion Relief Tablets *Boots, UK.*
Simeticone (p.1249·2); dried aluminium hydroxide gel (p.1210·3); magnesium hydroxide (p.1233·1).
Formerly known as Double Action Indigestion Tablets.
Dyspepsia.

Indigestion Tablets *Brauer, Austral.*
Homoeopathic preparation.

Indivina *Orion, UK.*
Estradiol valerate (p.1473·2); medroxyprogesterone acetate (p.1480·1).
Menopausal disorders; osteoporosis.

Indo
Agepha, Aust.; CT, Ger.
Indometacin (p.44·3).
Gout; inflammation; musculoskeletal, joint, and soft-tissue disorders; oedema; pain.

Indo Framan *Inexfa, Spain.*
Indometacin (p.44·3).
Gout; musculoskeletal, joint, and peri-articular disorders; pain.

Indo Top *Ratiopharm, Ger.*
Indometacin (p.44·3).
Inflammation; musculoskeletal, joint, and soft-tissue disorders; pain.

Indobene *Ratiopharm, Aust.*
Indometacin (p.44·3).
Aluminium glycinate (p.1210·3) is included in this preparation in an attempt to limit adverse effects on the gastrointestinal mucosa.
Formerly known as Gaurit.
Gout; inflammation; musculoskeletal, joint, peri-articular, and soft-tissue disorders; pain.

Indobiotic *Chauvin, Fr.*
Indometacin (p.44·3); gentamicin sulfate (p.210·1).
Inflammation and bacterial infections after cataract surgery.

Indobloc *Asta Medica, Ger.*
Propranolol hydrochloride (p.962·3).
Anxiety; arrhythmias; essential tremor; hypertension; hyperthyroidism; migraine; myocardial infarction.

Indoblok *Parke-Med, S.Afr.†.*
Propranolol hydrochloride (p.962·3).
Angina pectoris; anxiety; arrhythmias; hypertension; phaeochromocytoma.

Indocaf *Reig Jofre, Spain; Tedec Meiji, Spain.*
Indometacin (p.44·3).
Aluminium hydroxide (p.1210·3) is included in the capsules in an attempt to limit adverse effects on the gastrointestinal mucosa.
Gout; inflammation; musculoskeletal, joint, peri-articular, and soft-tissue disorders; pain.

Indocarsil *Solfran, Mex.*
Indometacin (p.44·3).
Musculoskeletal and joint disorders.

Indochron *Inwood, USA†.*
Indometacin (p.44·3).
Acute gouty arthritis; ankylosing spondylitis; bursitis; osteoarthritis; rheumatoid arthritis; tendinitis.

Indocid
Merck Sharp & Dohme, Aust.; Merck Sharp & Dohme, Austral.; Merck Sharp & Dohme, Belg.; Prodome, Braz.; Merck Frosst, Canad.; Merck Sharp & Dohme, Denm.; Merck Sharp & Dohme, Fin.; Merck Sharp & Dohme-Chibret, Fr.; Merck Sharp & Dohme, Hong Kong; Merck Sharp & Dohme, Irl.; Merck Sharp & Dohme, Ital.; Merck Sharp & Dohme, Mex.; Merck Sharp & Dohme, Neth.; Merck Sharp & Dohme, Norw.; Merck Sharp & Dohme, NZ; Merck Sharp & Dohme, Port.; Merck Sharp & Dohme, S.Afr.; Merck Sharp & Dohme, Switz.; Merck Sharp & Dohme, Thai.; Merck Sharp & Dohme, UK.
Indometacin (p.44·3) or indometacin sodium (p.45·1).
Closure of patent ductus arteriosus in premature neonates; fever; gout; inflammation; musculoskeletal, joint and peri-articular disorders; pain; prevention of oedema and miosis during cataract extraction.

Indocid Colirio *Merck Sharp & Dohme, Braz.*
Indometacin (p.44·3).
Prevention of miosis and inflammation during ocular surgery.

Indocid PDA
Merck Sharp & Dohme, Austral.; Merck Frosst, Canad.; Merck Sharp & Dohme, Hong Kong; Merck Sharp & Dohme, Irl.; Merck Sharp & Dohme, Neth.; Merck Sharp & Dohme, NZ; Merck Sharp & Dohme, UK.
Indometacin sodium (p.45·1).
Closure of patent ductus arteriosus.

Indocin
Merck Sharp & Dohme, USA.
Injection: Indometacin sodium (p.45·1).
Closure of patent ductus arteriosus.

Merck, USA; Forte, USA.
Capsules; oral suspension; suppositories; sustained-release capsules: Indometacin (p.44·3).
Acute gouty arthritis; ankylosing spondylitis; bursitis; osteoarthritis; rheumatoid arthritis; tendinitis.

Indocollirio *SIFI, Ital.*
Indometacin (p.44·3).
Prevention of miosis and inflammation during cataract surgery.

Indocollyre
Germania, Aust.; Ophtapharma, Canad.†; Chauvin, Fr.; Chauvin, Hong Kong; Chauvin, Port.; Chauvin, Singapore; Chauvin, Thai.
Indometacin (p.44·3).
Ocular inflammation following eye surgery; postoperative eye pain; prevention of intra-operative miosis.

Indocontin Mundipharma, Ger.
Indometacin (p.44·3).
Inflammation; musculoskeletal, joint, and soft-tissue disorders; pain.

Indoflam
Compu, S.Afr.†; Recon, Singapore.
Indometacin (p.44·3).
Gout; musculoskeletal and joint disorders; pain.

Indoflex Laser, S.Afr.†
Indometacin (p.44·3).
Gout; inflammation; musculoskeletal and joint disorders; pain.

Indoftol Merck Sharp & Dohme, Spain.
Indometacin (p.44·3).
Postoperatve ocular inflammation.

Indohexal Hexal, Aust.
Indometacin (p.44·3).
Gout; inflammation; musculoskeletal, joint, and peri-articular disorders; oedema; pain.

Indolar SR Lagap, UK.
Indometacin (p.44·3).
Inflammation; musculoskeletal, joint, and peri-articular disorders; pain.

Indolgina Uriach, Spain.
Indometacin (p.44·3).
Gout; inflammation; musculoskeletal, joint, and peri-articular disorders; pain.

Indolin Virginia, Ital.
Indapamide (p.913·1).
Hypertension.

Indom Collirio INTES, Ital.
Indometacin (p.44·3).
Prevention of miosis and inflammation during cataract surgery.

Indoman Berman, Mex.
Indometacin (p.44·3).

Indomax Ashbourne, UK.
Indometacin (p.44·3).
Gout; inflammation; musculoskeletal and joint disorders; pain.

Indomed
Amrad, Austral.†; Merck Sharp & Dohme, Israel; Noristan, S.Afr.†; Greater Pharma, Thai.
Indometacin (p.44·3).
Gout; inflammation; musculoskeletal, joint, and peri-articular disorders; oedema; pain.

Indomee Merck Sharp & Dohme, Swed.
Indometacin (p.44·3).
Gout; musculoskeletal, joint and peri-articular disorders.

Indomelan Lannacher, Aust.
Indometacin (p.44·3).
Gout; inflammation; musculoskeletal, joint, and peri-articular disorders; oedema; pain.

Indo-Mepha Mepha, Switz.
Indometacin (p.44·3).
Musculoskeletal, joint, peri-articular, and soft-tissue pain and inflammation.

Indomet Heumann, Ger.
Indometacin (p.44·3).
Gout; inflammation; musculoskeletal, joint, and soft-tissue disorders; pain.

Indometacinum-mp Medphano, Ger.
Indometacin (p.44·3).
Gout; inflammation; musculoskeletal, joint, and soft-tissue disorders; pain.

Indometin Orion, Fin.
Indometacin (p.44·3).
Fever; gout; inflammation; musculoskeletal and joint disorders; pain.

Indomet-ratiopharm Ratiopharm, Ger.
Indometacin (p.44·3).
Gout; inflammation; musculoskeletal, joint, peri-articular, and soft-tissue disorders; pain.

Indomet-ratiopharm m Ratiopharm, Ger.
Indometacin (p.44·3).
Aluminium glycinate (p.1210·3) is included in this preparation in an attempt to limit adverse effects on the gastrointestinal mucosa.
Gout; inflammation; musculoskeletal, joint, and soft-tissue disorders; pain.

Indomisal Riemser, Ger.
Indometacin (p.44·3).
Gout; inflammation; musculoskeletal, joint, and soft-tissue disorders; pain.

Indomod
Pharmacia Upjohn, Irl.†; Pharmacia, UK.
Indometacin (p.44·3).
Gout; musculoskeletal, joint, and peri-articular disorders.

Indonet Nettopharma, Denm.†
Indometacin (p.44·3).
Dysmenorrhoea; gout; musculoskeletal and joint disorders.

Indonilo Sigma-Tau, Spain.
Indometacin (p.44·3).
Gout; inflammation; musculoskeletal, joint, and peri-articular disorders; pain.

Indo-paed Hexal, Ger.
Indometacin (p.44·3).
Gout; inflammation; musculoskeletal, joint, peri-articular, and soft-tissue disorders; pain.

Indo-Phlogont Azupharma, Ger.
Indometacin (p.44·3).
Gout; inflammation; musculoskeletal, joint, and soft-tissue disorders; pain.

Indophtal Chauvin Novopharma, Switz.
Indometacin (p.44·3).
Eye disorders.

Indoptic
Merck Sharp & Dohme, Israel; Merck Sharp & Dohme, Switz.
Indometacin (p.44·3).
Prevention of oedema after cataract surgery.

Indoptol
Merck Sharp & Dohme, Aust.; Sigma, Austral.; Merck Sharp & Dohme, Belg.; Merck Sharp & Dohme, Neth.
Indometacin (p.44·3).
Inhibition of intra-operative miosis; prevention of cystoid macular oedema after cataract surgery.

Indorektal Sanorania, Ger.†
Indometacin (p.44·3).
Gout; inflammation; musculoskeletal and joint disorders; pain.

Indosan Sanfer, Mex.
Indometacin (p.44·3).

Indospray Rhone-Poulenc Rorer, Austral.
Indometacin (p.44·3).
Musculoskeletal, joint, peri-articular, and soft-tissue disorders.

Indo-Tablinen Sanorania, Ger.†
Indometacin (p.44·3).
Gout; inflammation; musculoskeletal and joint disorders; pain.

Indotal Pharmagen, S.Afr.†
Indometacin (p.44·3).
Gout; inflammation; musculoskeletal and joint disorders; pain.

Indotard
CTI, Israel; Galen, UK†.
Indometacin (p.44·3).
Inflammation; musculoskeletal, joint, and peri-articular disorders; pain.

Indotec Technilab, Canad.
Indometacin (p.44·3).
Gout; musculoskeletal and joint disorders; ovarian hyperstimulation syndrome; pain; renal calculi; renal colic.

Indotrin Liferpal, Mex.
Indometacin (p.44·3).
Musculoskeletal and joint disorders.

Indovis CTI, Israel.
Indometacin (p.44·3).
Gout; musculoskeletal and joint disorders.

Indoxen Sigma-Tau, Ital.
Indometacin (p.44·3).
Musculoskeletal disorders.

Inductal 20th Century, Mex.
Thiopental sodium (p.1269·1).

Inductol 20th Century, Mex.
Propanidid (p.1265·3).

Indulfan Henkel, Ital.
Glyoxal (p.1145·3); benzalkonium chloride (p.1133·2).
Surface disinfection.

Indulfan plus Henkel, Ger.†
Formaldehyde (p.1144·2); glyoxal (p.1145·3); glutaral (p.1145·2); benzalkonium chloride (p.1133·2).
Surface disinfection.

Indurgan Solvay, Spain.
Omeprazole (p.1239·1).
Gastro-oesophageal reflux; peptic ulcer; Zollinger-Ellison syndrome.

Indusil Recordati, Ital.
Cobamamide (p.1388·3).
Vitamin B_{12} deficiency.

Indusil T Diamant, Fr.†
Cobamamide (p.1388·3).
Tonic.

Inesfay Mavi, Mex.
Cimetidine (p.1216·3).

Inexbron Inexfa, Spain.
Amoxicillin trihydrate (p.149·2).
Bacterial infections.

Inexbron Mucolitico Inexfa, Spain.
Amoxicillin trihydrate (p.149·2); bromhexine hydrochloride (p.1085·3).
Respiratory-tract infections.

Inexfal Inexfa, Spain.
Cytidine; muramidase hydrochloride (p.1638·1); uridine (p.1677·2).
Liver disorders.

Infacol
Warner-Lambert, Austral.; Rosken, Hong Kong; Pharmax, Irl.; Warner-Lambert, NZ; Rosken, Singapore; Pharmax, UK.
Simeticone (p.1249·2).
Colic; flatulence; meteorism.

Infa-C-Vit Pisa, Mex.
Vitamin C (p.1389·3).

Infaderm Goldshield, UK.
Light liquid paraffin (p.1407·3); almond oil (p.1576·3).
Dry skin disorders.

Infadrops Goldshield, UK.
Paracetamol (p.71·2).

Infafren Simple Pisa, Mex.
Homatropine (p.468·1).

Infalgina Pisa, Mex.
Paracetamol (p.71·2).
Fever; pain.

Infalyte Mead Johnson Nutritionals, USA.
Electrolytes and rice syrup solids (p.1185·2).
Formerly known as Ricelyte.
Oral rehydration therapy.

Infanolyte GHP, Thai.
Calcium chloride; glucose; magnesium chloride; potassium chloride; sodium chloride; sodium citrate (p.1185·2).
Diarrhoea; oral rehydration therapy.

Infanrix
SmithKline Beecham, Aust.; SmithKline Beecham, Austral.; SmithKline Beecham, Belg.; SmithKline Beecham, Fin.; SmithKline Beecham, Ger.; SmithKline Beecham, Irl.; SmithKline Beecham, Israel; SmithKline Beecham, Ital.; SmithKline Beecham, Mex.; SmithKline Beecham, Norw.; SmithKline Beecham, NZ; SmithKline Beecham, Port.; SmithKline Beecham, Singapore; SmithKline Beecham, Spain; SBL, Swed.; SmithKline Beecham, Thai.; SmithKline Beecham, UK; SmithKline Beecham, USA.
A diphtheria, tetanus, and acellular pertussis vaccine (p.1537·3).
Active immunisation.

Infanrix DTPa SmithKline Beecham, Switz.
A diphtheria, tetanus, and pertussis vaccine (p.1537·3).
Active immunisation.

Infanrix DTPa-HepB SmithKline Beecham, Switz.
A diphtheria, tetanus, pertussis, and hepatitis B vaccine (p.1538·3).
Active immunisation.

Infanrix DTPa-Hib SmithKline Beecham, Switz.
A diphtheria, tetanus, pertussis, and haemophilus influenzae vaccine (p.1538·3).
Active immunisation.

Infanrix DTPa-IPV+Hib SmithKline Beecham, Switz.
A diphtheria, tetanus, pertussis, poliomyelitis, and haemophilus influenzae vaccine (p.1539·1).
Active immunisation.

Infanrix HepB
SmithKline Beecham, Austral.; SmithKline Beecham, Fin.; SmithKline Beecham, Ital.; SmithKline Beecham, NZ; SmithKline Beecham, Spain; SBL, Swed.
A diphtheria, tetanus, pertussis, and hepatitis B vaccine (p.1538·3).
Active immunisation.

Infanrix Hib SmithKline Beecham, Spain.
A diphtheria, tetanus, pertussis, and haemophilus influenzae vaccine (p.1538·3).
Active immunisation.

Infanrix + Hib
SmithKline Beecham, Aust.; SmithKline Beecham, Belg.; SmithKline Beecham, Ger.
A diphtheria, tetanus, acellular pertussis, and haemophilus influenzae vaccine (p.1538·3).
Active immunisation.

Infanrix IPV + Hib SmithKline Beecham, Belg.
A diphtheria, tetanus, pertussis, poliomyelitis, and haemophilus influenzae vaccine (p.1539·1).
Active immunisation.

Infanrix Polio SmithKline Beecham, Fr.
A diphtheria, tetanus, pertussis, and poliomyelitis vaccine (p.1539·1).
Active immunisation.

Infanrix Polio-Hib
SmithKline Beecham, Fr.; SmithKline Beecham, Israel.
A diphtheria, tetanus, pertussis, poliomyelitis, and haemophilus influenzae vaccine (p.1539·1).
Active immunisation.

Infanrix Polio+Hib SmithKline Beecham, Fin.
A diphtheria, tetanus, pertussis, poliomelitis, and haemophilus influenzae vaccine (p.1539·1).
Active immunisation.

Infanrix-Hib
SmithKline Beecham, Austral.; SmithKline Beecham, UK.
A diphtheria, tetanus, acellular pertussis, and haemophilus influenzae vaccine (p.1538·3).
Active immunisation.

Infanrix-IPV+Hib
SmithKline Beecham, Aust.; SmithKline Beecham, Ger.; SmithKline Beecham, Singapore.
A diphtheria, tetanus, acellular pertussis, poliomyelitis, and haemophilus influenzae vaccine (p.1539·1).
Active immunisation.

Infanrix-Polio+Hib SBL, Swed.
A diphtheria, tetanus, pertussis, poliomyelitis, and haemophilus influenzae vaccine (p.1539·1).
Active immunisation.

Infant Calm Brauer, Austral.
Passion flower (p.1649·1); aconitum nap; belladonna; chamomilla.
Insomnia; irritability or restlessness in children.

Infant Gaviscon Reckitt Benckiser, S.Afr.
Alginic acid (p.1498·3); magnesium trisilicate (p.1233·3); dried aluminium hydroxide gel (p.1210·3); sodium bicarbonate (p.1186·2).
Gastro-oesophageal reflux.

Infant Multiple Vitamin Stanley, Canad.
Vitamins A, C, and D (p.1350·1).

Infant Tonic Brauer, Austral.
Angelica (p.1580·2); ascorbic acid (p.1389·3); kola (p.1681·1); hypericum (p.290·2); ginseng (p.1615·3); urtica (p.1678·2); aurum mur.; calc. phos.; ferrum met.; ferrum phos.; kali phos.; mag. phos.; phosphoricum acidum.
Tonic.

Infantol Carter Horner, Canad.
Multivitamin preparation (p.1350·1).
Dietary supplement.

Infants Tylenol Cold Decongestant & Fever Reducer McNeil Consumer, USA.
Paracetamol (p.71·2); pseudoephedrine hydrochloride (p.1099·2).
Congestion; fever; pain.

Infantussin N Palmicol, Ger.†
Anise oil (p.1580·3); fennel oil (p.1610·2); thyme (p.1672·2); althaea (p.1577·1).
Coughs and cold symptoms.

Infapain Alliance, S.Afr.
Paracetamol (p.71·2); codeine phosphate (p.25·2).
Fever; pain.

Infapain Forte Alliance, S.Afr.
Paracetamol (p.71·2); codeine phosphate (p.25·2); promethazine hydrochloride (p.423·2).
Fever; pain.

Infasoy
Wyeth Health, Austral.; Cow & Gate, Irl.; Wyeth, NZ; Cow & Gate, UK.
Infant feed (p.1350·1).
Formerly known as Nutrilon Soya in the UK.
Cow's milk intolerance; galactosaemia; lactose intolerance.

Infasurf Forest Pharmaceuticals, USA.
Calfactant (p.1656·1).
Neonatal respiratory distress syndrome.

Infa-Tardyferon Germania, Aust.
Ferrous sulfate (p.1360·3).
Iron deficiency; iron-deficiency anaemia.

Infatrini Nutricia Clinical, UK.
Preparation for enteral nutrition in infants (p.1350·1).

Infazinc Atlas, Canad.
Zinc oxide (p.1128·2).

Infecteracin INQ, Braz.
Co-trimoxazole (p.193·3).
Bacterial infections; Pneumocystis carinii pneumonia; protozoal infections.

InfectoBicillin Infectopharm, Ger.
Benzathine phenoxymethylpenicillin (p.157·1).
Bacterial infections.

InfectoBicillin H Infectopharm, Ger.
Azidocillin sodium (p.153·1).
Bacterial infections.

InfectoCef Infectopharm, Ger.
Cefaclor (p.161·1).
Bacterial infections.

InfectoCillin Infectopharm, Ger.
Phenoxymethylpenicillin potassium (p.235·1).
Bacterial infections.

InfectoDyspept Infectopharm, Ger.
Carrot; rice; sodium chloride; sodium citrate; potassium citrate; citric acid (p.1185·2).
Diarrhoea; oral rehydration.

Infectoflam
Ciba Vision, Hong Kong; Ciba Vision, Singapore; Ciba Vision, Switz.; Ciba Vision, Thai.
Fluorometholone (p.1072·1); gentamicin sulfate (p.210·1).
Bacterial eye infections; inflammatory eye disorders.

InfectoFlu Infectopharm, Ger.
Amantadine hydrochloride (p.1161·2).
Formerly known as Infectogripp.
Influenza A.

InfectoFos Infectopharm, Ger.
Fosfomycin sodium (p.208·2).
Bacterial infections.

InfectoKrupp Infectopharm, Ger.
Adrenaline [epinephrine] (p.829·1).
Obstructive airways disease.

InfectoMox Infectopharm, Ger.
Amoxicillin (p.149·2).
Bacterial infections.

InfectoMycin Infectopharm, Ger.
Erythromycin estolate (p.201·2).
Bacterial infections.

InfectoPedicul Infectopharm, Ger.
Permethrin (p.1436·1).
Pediculosis.

InfectoSoor Infectopharm, Ger.
Ointment: Miconazole nitrate (p.391·1); zinc oxide (p.1128·2).
Napkin rash.
Oral gel: Miconazole (p.391·1).
Mouth and throat candidiasis.

Infectoss Heralds, Braz.
Erythromycin (p.201·2).
Bacterial infections.

InfectoTop Infectopharm, Ger.
Lodoxamide trometamol (p.768·1).
Allergic conjunctivitis.

InfectoTrimet Infectopharm, Ger.
Trimethoprim (p.264·2).
Urinary-tract infections.

Infectracina Apsen, Braz.
Neomycin (p.228·1); bacitracin (p.155·2).
Bacterial skin infections.

Infectrin
Note. This name is used for preparations of different composition.
Boehringer de Angeli, Braz.
Co-trimoxazole (p.193·3).
Bacterial infections; Pneumocystis carinii pneumonia; protozoal infections.

Searle, Ital.†
Ampicillin (p.150·3); flucloxacillin (p.207·1).
Bacterial infections.

Infectrin Balsamico *Boehringer de Angeli, Braz.*
Co-trimoxazole (p.193·3); guaifenesin (p.1092·2); ammonium chloride (p.1085·2).
Bacterial infections.

INFeD *Schein, USA.*
Iron dextran (p.1368·2).
Iron deficiency.

Infekt-Komplex Ho-Fu-Complex *Liebermann, Ger.*
Homoeopathic preparation.

Inferax *Yamanouchi, Ger.*
Interferon alfacon-1 (p.630·1).
Hepatitis B and C.

Infergen
Amgen, Canad.; Yamanouchi, Ital.; Yamanouchi, Neth.; Amgen, USA.
Interferon alfacon-1 (p.630·1).
Hepatitis C.

Inferil *Pharmarecord, Ital.*
Ferric sodium gluconate (p.1360·2).
Iron-deficiency anaemias.

Infesol *Berlin-Chemie, Ger.*
Amino-acid, electrolyte, and xylitol infusion (p.1350·1).
Protein and fluid deficiency.

Infestat *Opus, UK†.*
Nystatin (p.392·2).
Gastrointestinal candidiasis.

Infex
Note.This name is used for preparations of different composition.
Elofar, Braz.
Tetracycline (p.258·3).
Bacterial infections.

Merz, Ger.
Amantadine sulfate (p.1161·2).
Influenza A.

Infibran
Expanpharm, Fr.; Sanitas, Port.
Wheat bran (p.1214·2).
Constipation.

Infi-China *Infirmarius-Rovit, Ger.*
Homoeopathic preparation.

Infidyston *Infirmarius-Rovit, Ger.*
Homoeopathic preparation.

Infi-Echinacea *Infirmarius-Rovit, Ger.*
Homoeopathic preparation.

Infifer *Infirmarius-Rovit, Ger.*
Homoeopathic preparation.

Infihepan *Infirmarius-Rovit, Ger.*
Homoeopathic preparation.

Infi-Lymphect *Infirmarius-Rovit, Ger.*
Homoeopathic preparation.

Infiossan N *Infirmarius-Rovit, Ger.*
Homoeopathic preparation.

Infi-Symphytum *Infirmarius-Rovit, Ger.*
Homoeopathic preparation.

Infi-tract N *Infirmarius-Rovit, Ger.*
Scopolia carniolica; curcuma zanthorrhiza; greater celandine (p.1618·1); gentian (p.1615·1); angelica (p.1580·2); manna (p.1233·3); saffron (p.1029·1); zedoary; myrrh (p.1639·2); ascorbic acid (p.1389·3).
Biliary disorders; digestive disorders; gastrointestinal spasm.

Infla-Ban *Triomed, S.Afr.*
Diclofenac sodium (p.30·3).
Gout; inflammation; musculoskeletal and joint disorders.

Inflaced *Biotherapie, Fr.*
Piroxicam (p.79·1).
Musculoskeletal, joint, and peri-articular disorders.

Infladerm *Cazi, Braz.*
Nitrofurazone (p.231·3); hydrocortisone acetate (p.1073·3).
Infected skin disorders.

Infladoren *QIF, Braz.*
Diclofenac (p.30·2).
Gout; inflammation; musculoskeletal, joint, and peri-articular disorders; pain.

Inflam *Lichtenstein, Ger.*
Capsules; slow-release capsules; topical spray: Indometacin (p.44·3).
Gout; inflammation; musculoskeletal, joint, and soft-tissue disorders; pain.
Ointment: Indometacin (p.44·3); lauromacrogol 400 (p.1345·2).
Inflammation; musculoskeletal, joint, and soft-tissue disorders; pain.

Inflamac *Spirig, Switz.*
Diclofenac sodium (p.30·3).
Fever; gout; inflammation; musculoskeletal, joint, and peri-articular disorders; pain.

Inflamase
Ciba Vision, Canad.; Ciba Vision, USA.
Prednisolone sodium phosphate (p.1078·1).
Inflammatory eye disorders.

Inflamate *TO-Chemicals, Thai.*
Indometacin (p.44·3).
Gout; musculoskeletal and joint disorders; rheumatic fever.

Inflamene *Farmalab, Braz.*
Piroxicam (p.79·1).
Dysmenorrhoea; gout; musculoskeletal, joint, and peri-articular disorders.

Inflammide
Boehringer Ingelheim, S.Afr.; Boehringer Ingelheim, Singapore; Boehringer Ingelheim, Thai.
Budesonide (p.1064·2).
Asthma.

Inflanac
Biolab, Hong Kong; Biolab, Singapore; Biolab, Thai.
Diclofenac sodium (p.30·3).
Musculoskeletal, joint, and peri-articular disorders.

Inflanan *Marjan, Braz.*
Piroxicam (p.79·1).
Dysmenorrhoea; gout; musculoskeletal, joint, and peri-articular disorders.

Inflanefran *Allergan, Ger.*
Prednisolone acetate (p.1078·1).
Eye disorders.

Inflanegent *Allergan, Ger.*
Prednisolone acetate (p.1078·1); gentamicin sulfate (p.210·1).
Infected eye disorders.

Inflanox *Farmoquimica, Braz.*
Piroxicam (p.79·1).
Dysmenorrhoea; gout; musculoskeletal, joint, and peri-articular disorders.

Inflaren *Cibran, Braz.*
Diclofenac sodium (p.30·3).
Gout; inflammation; musculoskeletal, joint, and peri-articular disorders; pain.

Inflax *Ativus, Braz.*
Piroxicam (p.79·1).
Dysmenorrhoea; gout; musculoskeletal, joint, and peri-articular disorders.

Inflazone *Aspen, S.Afr.*
Phenylbutazone (p.78·1).
Ankylosing spondylitis.

Inflexal
Kwizda, Aust.; Berna, Hong Kong†; Berna, Ital.; Berna, Port.†; Byk Madaus, S.Afr.; Berna, Singapore; Berna, Spain; Berna, Switz.
An influenza vaccine (p.1544·3).
Active immunisation.

Inflexal S *Niddapharm, Ger.*
An influenza vaccine (p.1544·3).
Active immunisation.

Infloran
Kwizda, Aust.; Berna, Hong Kong; Berna, Ital.; Vieira, Port.; Berna, Spain; Berna, Switz.; Berna, Thai.
Bifidobacterium bifidum (p.1626·3) or Bifidobacterium infantis; Lactobacillus acidophilus (p.1626·3).
Constipation; digestive disorders in infants on an artificial diet; enterocolitis; restoration of intestinal flora.

Infloxa *Alpharma, Mex.*
Ciprofloxacin (p.182·3).
Bacterial infections.

Influaforce *Bioforce, Switz.*
Homoeopathic preparation.

Influamin *Serum-Werk Bernburg, Ger.*
Amino-acid, electrolyte, and xylitol infusion (p.1350·1).
Parenteral nutrition.

Influbene *Ratiopharm, Aust.*
Paracetamol (p.71·2); etilefrine hydrochloride (p.888·1); butetamate citrate (p.1086·2); chlorpheniramine [chlorphenamine] maleate (p.412·1).
Cold and influenza symptoms.

Influbene C *Mepha, Switz.*
Paracetamol (p.71·2); ascorbic acid (p.1389·3).
Fever; pain.

Influbene N *Mepha, Switz.*
Paracetamol (p.71·2).
Fever; pain.

Infludo
Weleda, Aust.; Weleda, Fr.; Weleda, Ger.; Weleda, UK.
Homoeopathic preparation.

Influex *Steigerwald, Ger.*
Homoeopathic preparation.

Influpiol C *Antipiol, Ital.*
Vitamin C; propolis; salix (p.1350·1).

Influpozzi *IVP, Ital.*
An influenza vaccine (p.1544·3).
Active immunisation.

Influrem *Edmond Pharma, Ital.*
Propyphenazone (p.80·2); caffeine (p.761·3); paracetamol (p.71·2).
Cold symptoms; pain.

Influsplit *Valda, Ital.*
An inactivated influenza vaccine (p.1544·3).
Active immunisation.

Influsplit SSW *SmithKline Beecham, Ger.*
An influenza vaccine (p.1544·3).
Active immunisation.

Influtruw *Bilgast, Ger.*
Homoeopathic preparation.

Influtux *Antipiol, Ital.*
Hedera; propolis; dog rose; echinacea (p.1350·1).

Influvac
Solvay, Aust.; Solvay, Belg.; Solvay, Denm.; Solvay, Fin.; Solvay, Fr.; Solvay, Ger.; Solvay, Irl.; Solvay, Israel; Solvay, Neth.; Solvay, Port.; Solvay, S.Afr.; Solvay, Swed.; Solvay, Switz.; Solvay, UK.
An inactivated influenza vaccine (surface antigen) (p.1544·3).
Active immunisation.

Influvac S *Solvay, Ital.*
An influenza vaccine (p.1544·3).
Active immunisation.

Influvidon *Sanochemia, Aust.*
Salicylamide (p.82·1); caffeine (p.761·3); propyphenazone (p.80·2); hesperidin phosphate (p.1611·2); calcium ascorbate (p.1389·3); piprin hydrate (p.423·1).
Cold and influenza symptoms.

Influvirus *Nuovo ISM, Ital.*
An influenza vaccine (p.1544·3).
Active immunisation.

Influvit
Note.This name is used for preparations of different composition.
DHU, Ger.
Homoeopathic preparation.

Recordati, Ital.
Paracetamol (p.71·2); ascorbic acid (p.1389·3); propyphenazone (p.80·2).
Fever; pain.

Inf-Oph *Seng, Thai.*
Prednisolone acetate (p.1078·1).
Conjunctivitis.

Infosan *Nycomed Imaging, Norw.†.*
Albumin (p.724·1).
Contrast medium for echocardiography.

Infoson *Nycomed, Swed.†.*
Albumin (p.724·1).
Contrast medium for echocardiography.

Infraline *Rolmex, Canad.†.*
Methyl salicylate (p.55·1); menthol (p.1632·3); eucalyptol (p.1609·2).

Inframin *Fresenius Kabi, Ital.*
Amino-acid infusion (p.1350·1).
Parenteral nutrition in renal failure.

Infrarub
Note.This name is used for preparations of different composition.
Whitehall, Braz.
Methyl nicotinate (p.55·1); capsaicin (p.23·1); histamine hydrochloride (p.1619·2); glycol salicylate (p.42·2).
Musculoskeletal and joint disorders.

Whitehall, USA.
Methyl salicylate (p.55·1); menthol (p.1632·3).
Muscle, joint, and soft-tissue pain; neuralgia.

Infree *Eisai, Jpn.*
Indometacin farnesil (p.46·1).
Musculoskeletal, joint, and peri-articular disorders.

Infrotto Ultra *Cassella-med, Ger.*
Glycol salicylate (p.42·2); nonivamide (p.63·1).
Muscular and neuromuscular disorders; rheumatic disorders.

Infufer *Sabex, Canad.*
Iron dextran (p.1368·2).
Iron deficiency.

Infukoll HES *Serum-Werk Bernburg, Ger.; Schwarz, Ger.*
Hetastarch (p.732·3) in sodium chloride.
Hypovolaemia.

Infukoll M 40 *Serum-Werk Bernburg, Ger.*
Dextran 40 (p.728·3) in sodium chloride.
Hypovolaemia; thrombosis prophylaxis.

Infumal *Serum-Werk Bernburg, Ger.*
Arginine (p.1353·3); malic acid (p.1631·1); sodium hydroxide (p.1665·3).
Hyperammonaemia.

Infumix *Orion, Fin.*
A range of amino-acid, carbohydrate, lipid, and electrolyte infusions (p.1350·1).
Parenteral nutrition.

Infumorph *Elkins-Sinn, USA.*
Morphine sulfate (p.56·1).
Pain.

Ingastri *Ipsen, Spain.*
Famotidine (p.1225·3).
Gastro-oesophageal reflux; peptic ulcer; Zollinger-Ellison syndrome.

Ingelan
Germania, Aust.; Boehringer Ingelheim, Ger.
Topical gel: Isoprenaline sulfate (p.914·3).
Skin disorders.

Germania, Aust.; Boehringer Ingelheim, Ger.
Topical powder: Isoprenaline sulfate (p.914·3); salicylic acid (p.1122·3).
Skin disorders.

Ingro *Farmacologico Milanese, Ital.†.*
Sulfogaiacol (p.1101·1); dextromethorphan hydrobromide (p.1087·3); eucalyptus (p.1609·2).
Coughs.

Ingrown Toe Nail Salve *Cress, Canad.†.*
Boric acid (p.1586·1); camphor (p.1589·3); salicylic acid (p.1122·3).

Inhacort *Boehringer Ingelheim, Ger.*
Flunisolide (p.1070·3).
Asthma.

Inhalador *Fournier SA, Spain†.*
Camphor (p.1589·3); methyl salicylate (p.55·1); oleum pini sylvestris; sassafras oil (p.1661·1); menthol (p.1632·3).
Nasal congestion.

Inhalene *Sanofi Synthelabo, Belg.*
Menthol (p.1632·3); eucalyptol (p.1609·2).
Cold symptoms; laryngitis; sinusitis.

Inhepar *Pisa, Mex.*
Heparin sodium (p.902·1).

Inhibac *Pharmaland, Thai.*
Chlorhexidine gluconate (p.1138·2); cetrimide (p.1137·1).
Disinfection.

Inhibace
Note.This name is used for preparations of different composition.
Roche, Aust.; Bayer, Austral.†; Roche, Belg.; Roche, Canad.; Roche, Hong Kong; Syntex, Mex.; Roche, NZ; Roche, S.Afr.; Roche, Singapore; Roche, Spain; Roche, Swed.; Roche, Switz.; Roche, Thai.
Cilazapril (p.858·1).
Heart failure; hypertension.

Bristol-Myers Squibb, Israel.
Captopril (p.853·3).
Diabetic nephropathy; heart failure; hypertension; myocardial infarction.

Inhibace comp *Roche, Swed.*
Cilazapril (p.858·1); hydrochlorothiazide (p.907·3).
Hypertension.

Inhibace Plus
Roche, Aust.; Roche, Canad.; Roche, NZ; Roche, S.Afr.; Roche, Spain; Roche, Switz.
Cilazapril (p.858·1); hydrochlorothiazide (p.907·3).
Hypertension.

Inhibin *Asta Medica, Neth.*
Hydroquinine hydrobromide (p.1622·1).
Nocturnal muscle cramps.

Inhibitron *Liomont, Mex.*
Omeprazole (p.1239·1).
Acid aspiration; gastro-oesophageal reflux; peptic ulcer; Zollinger-Ellison syndrome.

Inhibostamin *Novartis Consumer, Ger.*
Tritoqualine (p.427·3).
Minor allergic disorders; pruritus.

Inhiston *Biomedica, Ital.*
Pheniramine maleate (p.422·3).
Hypersensitivity reactions.

Inibace *Roche, Ital.; Roche, Port.*
Cilazapril (p.858·1).
Heart failure; hypertension.

Inibace Plus *Roche, Ital.; Roche, Port.*
Cilazapril (p.858·1); hydrochlorothiazide (p.907·3).
Hypertension.

Inibex S *Medley, Braz.*
Diethylpropion (p.1508·3).
Obesity.

Inibina *Apsen, Braz.*
Isoxsuprine hydrochloride (p.1624·3).
Cerebral and peripheral vascular disorders; dysmenorrhoea; premature labour.

Inimur *Taurus, Ger.*
Nifuratel (p.598·1).
Fungal infections; trichomoniasis.

Inipomp *Synthelabo, Fr.*
Pantoprazole sodium (p.1243·2).
Gastro-oesophageal reflux; peptic ulcer.

Iniprol *Bournonville, Belg.†.*
Aprotinin (p.725·3).
Fatty emboli; haemorrhage; shock.

Inistolin Antitusivo Ped *Warner-Lambert, Spain.*
Dextromethorphan hydrobromide (p.1087·3); pseudoephedrine hydrochloride (p.1099·2).
Coughs; nasal congestion.

Inistolin Expectoran Ped *Warner-Lambert, Spain.*
Pseudoephedrine hydrochloride (p.1099·2); guaifenesin (p.1092·2).
Respiratory-tract congestion.

Iniston *Warner-Lambert, Spain.*
Pseudoephedrine hydrochloride (p.1099·2); triprolidine hydrochloride (p.427·2).
Cold symptoms; nasal congestion.

Iniston Antitusivo *Warner-Lambert, Spain.*
Dextromethorphan hydrobromide (p.1087·3); pseudoephedrine hydrochloride (p.1099·2); triprolidine hydrochloride (p.427·2).
Coughs; nasal congestion.

Iniston Expectorante *Warner-Lambert, Spain.*
Guaifenesin (p.1092·2); pseudoephedrine hydrochloride (p.1099·2); triprolidine hydrochloride (p.427·2).
Coughs; nasal congestion.

Initard 50/50 *Novo Nordisk, UK†; Wellcome, UK†.*
Mixture of neutral insulin injection (porcine, highly purified) 50% and isophane insulin injection (porcine, highly purified) 50% (p.324·1).
Diabetes mellitus.

Initiss *Pharmacia Upjohn, Ital.*
Cilazapril (p.858·1).
Hypertension.

Initiss Plus *Pharmacia Upjohn, Ital.*
Cilazapril (p.858·1); hydrochlorothiazide (p.907·3).
Hypertension.

Injectio Lymphatica N EKF *Biomedica, Ger.*
Homoeopathic preparation.

Inkamil *Ipsen, Spain.*
Ciprofloxacin hydrochloride (p.182·3).
Bacterial infections.

Inmunobalt *Rudefsa, Mex.*
Oral solution: A lysate of Streptococcus pneumoniae; Klebsiella pneumoniae; Klebsiella ozaenae; Streptococcus viridans; Streptococcus pyogenes; Staphylococcus aureus; Neiserria catarrhalis; Haemophilus influenzae.

Tablets: A lysate of Streptococcus pneumoniae; Klebsiella pneumoniae(p.0·0); Streptococcus haemolyticus; Staphylococcus aureus; Neiserria catarrhalis; Haemophilus influenzae.

Respiratory-tract infections.

Inmunoferon *Andromaco, Mex.; Cantabria, Spain.*
Glicofosfopeptical (p.1616·2).
Immunotherapy.

Inmunol *Andromaco, Mex.*
Glicofosfopeptical (p.1616·2).
Immunostimulant.

Inmupen *Llorente, Spain.*
Amoxicillin trihydrate (p.149·2); potassium clavulanate (p.187·2).
Bacterial infections.

Innerfresh Pro *Murdock, USA†.*
Chlorophyllin copper complex (p.1028·1).

Innersource *Quest, Canad.*
Multivitamin and mineral preparation (p.1350·1).

Inno Rheuma *Naturland, Aust.*
Cream: Camphor (p.1589·3); menthol (p.1632·3); rosemary oil (p.1659·3).
Oil: Lavender oil (p.1627·2); menthol (p.1632·3); rosemary oil (p.1659·3).
Musculoskeletal and joint disorders; nerve pain.

Innobrand *Lab Francais du Fractionnement, Fr.*
A complex of factor VIII and von Willebrand's factor (p.734·1).
Von Willebrand's disease.

InnoGel Plus *Hogil, USA.*
Pyrethrins; piperonyl butoxide (p.1436·2).

Innohep
Leo, Belg.; Leo, Canad.; Leo, Denm.; Leo, Fin.; Leo, Fr.; Braun, Ger.; Leo, Ger.; Leo, Irl.; Formenti, Ital.†; Leo, Neth.; Leo, Norw.; CSL, NZ; Leo, Port.; Leo, Singapore; Farmacusi, Spain; Leo, Swed.; Leo, UK; Du Pont, USA.
Tinzaparin sodium (p.982·3).
Thromboembolic disorders.

Innomel *Clonmel, Irl.*
Enalapril maleate (p.883·3).
Heart failure; hypertension.

Innovace *Merck Sharp & Dohme, Irl.; Merck Sharp & Dohme, UK.*
Enalapril maleate (p.883·3).
Heart failure; hypertension; ischaemic heart disease.

Innovar *Janssen, USA†.*
Fentanyl citrate (p.37·1); droperidol (p.682·2).
Anaesthesia; neuroleptanalgesia; premedication.

Innozide *Merck Sharp & Dohme, Irl.; Merck Sharp & Dohme, UK.*
Enalapril maleate (p.883·3); hydrochlorothiazide (p.907·3).
Hypertension.

Inobesin *Windson, Braz.*
Fenproporex hydrochloride (p.1510·2).
Obesity.

Inocar *Solvay, Spain.*
Cilazapril (p.858·1).
Heart failure; hypertension.

Inocar Plus *Solvay, Spain.*
Cilazapril (p.858·1); hydrochlorothiazide (p.907·3).
Hypertension.

Inocor
Sanofi Winthrop, Belg.†; Sanofi Winthrop, Braz.; Sanofi Winthrop, Canad.†; Sanofi Winthrop, Fr.†; Sanofi Winthrop, Israel; Sanofi Synthelabo, Ital.; Sanofi Synthelabo, Port.; Sanofi Winthrop, Swed.; Sanofi Winthrop, USA.
Amrinone (p.839·2) or amrinone lactate (p.839·2).
Heart failure.

Inofer *AJC, Fr.*
Ferrous succinate (p.1360·3).
Succinic acid is included in this preparation to increase the absorption and availability of iron.
Anaemia.

Inoflox *Biomedis, Singapore.*
Ofloxacin (p.232·3).
Bacterial infections.

Inolaxine *Debat, Fr.; Dales, Hong Kong; Fournier, Switz.*
Sterculia (p.1250·2).
Constipation; inflammatory bowel disease.

Inolaxol *Selena, Swed.*
Sterculia (p.1250·2).
Adjunct in treatment of diarrhoea; constipation.

Inolin *Tanabe, Jpn.*
Tretoquinol hydrochloride (p.785·2).
Obstructive airways disease.

INOmax *INO Therapeutics, USA.*
Nitric oxide (p.947·2).
Neonatal respiratory distress syndrome.

Inongan *Fumouze, Fr.*
Menthol (p.1632·3); methyl salicylate (p.55·1); camphor (p.1589·3); eucalyptus oil (p.1609·2).
Formerly contained salicylic acid, menthol, methyl salicylate, camphor, isobornyl acetate, and eucalyptus oil.
Muscle pain.

Inopamil *Astra, Ital.; Zambon, Neth.*
Ibopamine hydrochloride (p.912·1).
Heart failure.

Inopin *Siam Bheasach, Thai.*
Dopamine hydrochloride (p.881·3).
Shock.

Inosital *Toyo, Hong Kong.*
Inositol (p.1623·3).
Peripheral vascular disorders.

Inotop *Torrex, Aust.*
Dobutamine hydrochloride (p.880·2).
Heart failure; shock.

Inotrex *Lilly, Port.*
Dobutamine hydrochloride (p.880·2).

Inotropisa *Pisa, Mex.*
Dopamine hydrochloride (p.881·3).
Cardiac surgery; hypovolaemia; shock.

Inotyol
Note.This name is used for preparations of different composition.
Brady, Aust.; Hoechst Marion Roussel, Ital.
Ointment: Ichthammol (p.1115·2); hamamelis (p.1618·3); zinc oxide (p.1128·2); titanium dioxide (p.1126·1).
Burns; skin disorders; wounds.

Fournier, Belg.; Debat, Denm.; Debat, Norw.; Selena, Swed.
Ointment: Ichthammol (p.1115·2); zinc oxide (p.1128·2); titanium dioxide (p.1126·1).
Formerly contained ichthammol, hamamelis, zinc oxide, titanium dioxide, borax in *Belg.*
Skin disorders; superficial wounds and burns.

Debat, Fr.; Urgo, Israel.
Ointment: Ichthammol (p.1115·2); hamamelis (p.1618·3); zinc oxide (p.1128·2); titanium dioxide (p.1126·1); siam benzoin (p.1662·3).
Burns; skin disorders; wounds.

Brady, Aust.
Topical powder: Ichthammol (p.1115·2); hamamelis (p.1618·3); zinc oxide (p.1128·2); calcium carbonate (p.1215·1).
Skin disorders.

Hoechst Marion Roussel, Ital.†.
Topical powder: Ichthammol (p.1115·2); zinc oxide (p.1128·2); hamamelis (p.1618·3).
Skin irritation.

Inoval *Janssen, Braz.†.*
Fentanyl citrate (p.37·1); droperidol (p.682·2).
Neuroleptanalgesia.

Inovan *Kyowa, Jpn.*
Dopamine hydrochloride (p.881·3).
Anuria; oliguria; shock.

Inovapar *Zerboni, Mex.*
Bromocriptine (p.1166·2).

Inoven *Johnson & Johnson MSD Consumer, UK.*
Ibuprofen (p.43·2).
Fever; inflammation; pain.

Inpanol *DHA, Hong Kong; DHA, Singapore.*
Propranolol hydrochloride (p.962·3).
Angina pectoris; arrhythmias; hypertension; hyperthyroidism; myocardial infarction.

Insacial *Byk Gulden, Mex.*
Cathine resinate (p.1507·1).

Insadol *Sanofi Winthrop, Braz.; Expanpharm, Fr.; Expanpharm, Switz.*
Maize (p.1599·3).
Dental disorders.

Insect Ecran *Osler, Fr.*
Paediatric spray: Ethohexadiol (p.1432·3).
Insect repellent.
Solution: Permethrin (p.1436·1).
Insect repellent for clothing and bedding.
Spray: Diethyltoluamide (p.1431·2).
Insect repellent.

Insensye *Merck Sharp & Dohme, Austral.*
Norfloxacin (p.232·1).
Bacterial infections.

Inside *Antula, Swed.*
Ranitidine hydrochloride (p.1245·2).
Gastro-oesophageal reflux.

Insidon *Novartis, Aust.; Ciba-Geigy, Belg†; Ciba-Geigy, Fr.†; Novartis, Ger.; Novartis, Irl.; Ciba, Ital.†; Novartis, Neth.†; Novartis, Switz.*
Opipramol hydrochloride (p.302·2).
Anxiety; depression; sleep disorders.

Insig *Sigma, Austral.*
Indapamide (p.913·1).
Hypertension.

Insogen *Byk Gulden, Mex.*
Chlorpropamide (p.321·1).
Diabetes mellitus.

Insogen Plus *Byk Gulden, Mex.*
Metformin hydrochloride (p.332·3); chlorpropamide (p.321·1).
Diabetes mellitus.

Insom *Lennon, S.Afr.†.*
Flunitrazepam (p.683·2).
Insomnia.

Insoma *Pacific, NZ.*
Nitrazepam (p.695·2).
Insomnia.

Insomin *Orion, Fin.*
Nitrazepam (p.695·2).
Epilepsy; insomnia.

Insomnal *Rougier, Canad.*
Diphenhydramine hydrochloride (p.416·1).
Insomnia.

Insomn-Eze *Rhone-Poulenc Rorer, Austral.*
Promethazine hydrochloride (p.423·2).
Insomnia.

Insomnia *Homeocan, Canad.*
Homoeopathic preparation.

Insomnia Passiflora *Homeocan, Canad.*
Homoeopathic preparation.

Inspirol Halsschmerztabletten *Hotz, Ger.*
Tyrothricin (p.267·1); benzocaine (p.1306·2); dequalinium chloride (p.1143·1).
Mouth and throat infections.

Inspirol Heilpflanzenol *Hotz, Ger.*
Peppermint oil (p.1243·3).
Cold symptoms; gastrointestinal disorders.

Inspirol Mundwasser konzentrat *Hotz, Ger.†.*
Menthol (p.1632·3); eucalyptus oil (p.1609·2); peppermint oil (p.1243·3); pumilio pine oil (p.1656·3).
Mouth and throat disorders.

Inspirol P *Hotz, Ger.*
Myrrh (p.1639·2).
Mouth and throat inflammation.

Inspiryl *Astra, Mex.; AstraZeneca, Norw.; Draco, Swed.*
Salbutamol sulfate (p.770·3).
Obstructive airways disease.

Instacare *Ciba Vision, Austral.; Ciba Vision, NZ.*
Cleansing and disinfecting solutions for soft contact lenses (p.1129·2).

Instacyl *Streuli, Switz.*
Aspirin (p.14·2); ascorbic acid (p.1389·3).
Cold symptoms.

Insta-Glucose *Dermatech, Austral.*
Glucose (p.1364·1).
Hypoglycaemia.

Instant Rub *Lioh, Canad.*
Methyl salicylate (p.55·1); menthol (p.1632·3).

Instantine *Bayer, Canad.*
Aspirin (p.14·2); caffeine (p.761·3).
Fever; headache; pain.

Instat *Johnson & Johnson, Aust.; Ethicon, Ital.†; Johnson & Johnson, Switz.†; Johnson & Johnson Medical, UK; Johnson & Johnson Medical, USA†.*
Collagen (bovine) (p.1598·2).
Haemorrhage.

Instenon *Nycomed, Aust.; Nycomed, Hong Kong; Hafslund Nycomed, Thai.*
Hexobendine hydrochloride (p.905·3); etofylline (p.765·3); etamivan (p.1509·3).
Cerebrovascular disorders.

Instillagel *Solco, Aust.; Farco, Denm.; Farco, Ger.; Farco, Hong Kong; Farco, Irl.; Farco, Israel; Selena, Swed.; Almed, Switz.†; CliniMed, UK.*
Lignocaine [lidocaine] hydrochloride (p.1313·2); chlorhexidine gluconate (p.1138·2).
Catheterisation; cystoscopy; endoscopy.

Instrunet *Inibsa, Port.*
A range of solutions for skin and instrument disinfection.

Instru-Safe *Eagle, Austral.*
Silicone (p.1409·3).
Instrument lubrication.

Instruzyme *Peters, Fr.*
Mixed quaternary ammonium salts; polihexanide (p.1154·2).
Instrument disinfection.

Insulatard *Novo Nordisk, Denm.; Novo Nordisk, Irl.; Novo Nordisk, Neth.; Novo Nordisk, Norw.; Novo Nordisk, Port.; Novo Nordisk, Swed.; Novo Nordisk, Thai.*
Isophane insulin injection (recombinant human monocomponent) (p.324·1).
Formerly known as Human Insulatard in *Irl.*
Diabetes mellitus.

Insulatard HM *Novo Nordisk, Belg.; Novo Nordisk, Neth.; Novo Nordisk, Singapore; Novo Nordisk, Switz.*
Isophane insulin injection (human, monocomponent) (p.324·1).
Formerly known as Protaphan HM in *Switz.*
Diabetes mellitus.

Insulatard Human *Novo Nordisk, Ger.*
Isophane insulin injection (human) (p.324·1).
Diabetes mellitus.

Insulatard MC *Novo Nordisk, Ger.; Novo Nordisk, Switz.*
Isophane insulin injection (porcine, highly purified) (p.324·1).
Diabetes mellitus.

Insulatard NPH *Novo Nordisk, Spain.*
Isophane insulin injection (human) (p.324·1).
Diabetes mellitus.

Insulex *Pisa, Mex.*
Insulin (p.324·1).
Diabetes mellitus.

Insulin 2 *Novo Nordisk, Austral.†.*
Acid insulin injection (bovine) (p.324·1).
Diabetes mellitus.

Insulin Basal *Hoechst Marion Roussel, Norw.*
Isophane insulin injection (human, emp) (p.324·1).
Diabetes mellitus.

Insulin Infusat *Hoechst Marion Roussel, Norw.*
Insulin injection (human, emp) (p.324·1).
Diabetes mellitus.

Insulin Komb 25/75 *Hoechst Marion Roussel, Norw.*
Mixture of insulin injection (human, emp) and isophane insulin injection (human, emp) (p.324·1).
Diabetes mellitus.

Insulin Lente MC *Novo Nordisk, Fin.*
Insulin zinc suspension (porcine/bovine) (amorphous 34%, crystalline 66%) (p.324·1).
Diabetes mellitus.

Insulin Lyhyt *Orion, Fin.*
Insulin injection (human) (p.324·1).
Diabetes mellitus.

Insulin Pitka *Orion, Fin.*
Isophane insulin injection (human) (p.324·1).
Diabetes mellitus.

Insulin Rapid *Hoechst Marion Roussel, Norw.*
Insulin injection (human, emp) (p.324·1).
Diabetes mellitus.

Insulin Reaction *Sherwood, USA.*
Glucose (p.1364·2).
Hypoglycaemia.

Insulin S *Berlin-Chemie, Ger.*
Insulin injection (pork) (p.324·1).
Diabetes mellitus.

Insulin SNC *Berlin-Chemie, Ger.*
Insulin injection (porcine) (p.324·1).
Diabetes mellitus.

Insuline Semi Tardum *Organon, Fr.†.*
Insulin zinc suspension (amorphous) (porcine, highly purified) (p.324·1).
Diabetes mellitus.

Insuline Tardum MX *Organon, Fr.†.*
Mixture of insulin zinc suspension (amorphous) (porcine, highly purified) 30% and insulin zinc suspension (crystalline) (bovine, highly purified) 70% (p.324·1).
Diabetes mellitus.

Insuline Ultra Tardum *Organon, Fr.†.*
Insulin zinc suspension (crystalline) (bovine, highly purified) (p.324·1).
Diabetes mellitus.

Insuman Basal
Hoechst Marion Roussel, Aust.; Hoechst Marion Roussel, Fin.; Hoechst, Fr.; Hoechst Marion Roussel, Ger.; Aventis, Irl.; Hoechst Marion Roussel, Neth.; Hoechst Marion Roussel, Swed.; Hoechst Marion Roussel, Switz.; Aventis, UK.
Isophane insulin injection (human) (p.324·1).
Diabetes mellitus.

Insuman Comb 15, 25, and 50
Hoechst Marion Roussel, Aust.; Hoechst Marion Roussel, Fin.; Hoechst, Fr.; Hoechst Marion Roussel, Ger.; Aventis, Irl.; Hoechst Marion Roussel, Neth.; Hoechst Marion Roussel, Swed.; Hoechst Marion Roussel, Switz.; Aventis, UK.
Mixtures of soluble insulin injection (human) 15%, 25%, and 50% and isophane insulin injection (human) 85%, 75%, and 50% respectively (p.324·1).
Diabetes mellitus.

Insuman Infusat
Hoechst Marion Roussel, Aust.; Hoechst Marion Roussel, Fin.; Hoechst, Fr.; Hoechst Marion Roussel, Swed.; Hoechst Marion Roussel, Switz.
Soluble insulin injection (human) (p.324·1).
Diabetes mellitus.

Insuman Intermediaire 25/75 *Hoechst, Fr.†.*
Mixture of insulin injection (human, emp, highly purified) 25% and isophane insulin injection (human, emp, highly purified) 75% (p.324·1).
Diabetes mellitus.

Insuman Intermediaire 100% *Hoechst, Fr.†.*
Isophane insulin injection (human, emp, highly purified) (p.324·1).
Diabetes mellitus.

Insuman komb Typ 15, Typ 25, and Typ 50
Hoechst Marion Roussel, Aust.
Mixtures of soluble insulin injection (human) 15%, 25%, and 50% and isophane insulin injection (human) 85%, 75%, and 50% respectively (p.324·1).
Diabetes mellitus.

Insuman Rapid
Hoechst Marion Roussel, Aust.; Hoechst Marion Roussel, Fin.; Hoechst, Fr.; Hoechst Marion Roussel, Ger.; Aventis, Irl.; Hoechst Marion Roussel, Neth.; Hoechst Marion Roussel, Swed.; Hoechst Marion Roussel, Switz.; Aventis, UK.
Neutral insulin injection (human) (p.324·1).
Diabetes mellitus.

Insup *Smaller, Spain.*
Enalapril maleate (p.883·3).
Heart failure; hypertension.

Insuvac *Sanus, Braz.*
Extracts of bacterial antigens and allergens (p.1575·3).
Hyposensitisation.

Insuven *Almirall, Spain.*
Diosmin (p.1611·1).
Haemorrhoids; vascular disorders.

Intacglobin *Grossman, Mex.*
Immunoglobulin G (p.1551·3).

Intal
Sanova, Aust.; Rhone-Poulenc Rorer, Austral.; Fisons, Braz.; Rhone-Poulenc Rorer, Canad.; Rhone-Poulenc Rorer, Ger.; Rhone-Poulenc Rorer, Hong Kong; Rhone-Poulenc Rorer, Irl.; Rhone-Poulenc Rorer, Mex.; Aventis, NZ; Rhone-Poulenc Rorer, Port.; Rhone-Poulenc Rorer, Singapore; Rhone-Poulenc Rorer, Spain; Rhone-Poulenc Rorer, Thai.; Rhone-Poulenc Rorer, UK; Rhone-Poulenc Rorer, USA.
Sodium cromoglicate (p.774·3).
Allergic rhinitis; asthma; bronchitis.

Intapan *Duopharma, Hong Kong.*
Nalbuphine hydrochloride (p.60·1).
Adjunct in general anaesthesia; pain.

Intard *Julphar, UAE.*
Diphenoxylate hydrochloride (p.1222·2).
Atropine sulfate (p.461·1) is included in this preparation to discourage abuse.
Diarrhoea.

Inteflora *Restan, S.Afr.*
Saccharomyces boulardii (p.1626·3).
Gastrointestinal disorders.

Integrilin
Key, Canad.; Schering-Plough, Denm.; Schering-Plough, Fin.; Schering-Plough, Fr.; Essex, Ger.; Schering-Plough, Irl.; Schering-Plough, Israel; Schering-Plough, Ital.; Schering-Plough, Neth.; Schering-Plough, Port.;

Intensain Hoechst, Ger.†
Carbocromen hydrochloride (p.855·1).
Cardiac disorders.

Intensol Roxane, USA†.
Metoclopramide hydrochloride (p.1235·2).
Gastrointestinal disorders.

Inter IF Sanus, Braz.
Interferon alfa (p.628·1).
Viral skin infections.

Interacton Enzypharm, Neth.†
Amine oxidase; glutaminase; allyl sulfide.
Asthma; bronchitis; hypersensitivity reactions; pertussis; sinusitis; skin disorders.

Interberin Wyeth Lederle, Aust.†
Sargramostim (p.741·3).
Neutropenia after bone marrow transplantation.

Interceed Johnson & Johnson Medical, Fr.†; Johnson & Johnson, Ger.†; Johnson & Johnson Medical, UK.
Oxidised cellulose (p.728·1).
Postoperative adhesions.

Interceed (TC7) Johnson & Johnson Medical, USA†.
Oxidised cellulose (p.728·1).
Gynaecological surgery.

Intercron Laphal, Fr.
Sodium cromoglicate (p.774·3).
Food hypersensitivity.

Intercyton Medeva, Fr.; Sanofi Synthelabo, Spain.
Flavodate sodium (p.1611·1).
Circulatory disorders.

Interderm Interpharma, Spain.
Gentamicin sulfate (p.210·1); nystatin (p.392·2); triamcinolone acetonide (p.1080·1).
Infected skin disorders.

Interferon Alfanative Bionative, Swed.
Interferon alfa (leucocyte) (p.628·1).
Chronic myeloid leukaemia; hairy-cell leukaemia.

Intestinol Rosch & Handel, Aust.
Pancreatin (p.1646·1); sodium cholate; duodenum extract; charcoal (p.1000·2).
Gastrointestinal disorders.

Intetrix Ipsen, Belg.†; Beaufour, Fr.
Tiliquinol (p.603·3); tiliquinol laurilsulfate (p.603·3); tilbroquinol (p.603·2).
Infective diarrhoea; intestinal amoebiasis.

Intetrix P Beaufour, Fr.†
Tilbroquinol (p.603·2).
Formerly contained tilbroquinol and furoylbromomethyloxine.
Infective diarrhoea.

Inthacine The Forty-Two, Thai.
Indometacin (p.44·3).
Gout; musculoskeletal and joint disorders.

Intim ICIM, Ital.
Hamamelis (p.1618·3); levomenol (p.1629·1).
Personal hygiene.

Intracef Aspen, S.Afr.
Cefuroxime sodium (p.178·2).
Bacterial infections.

Intradermi Fluid N Eberth, Ger.
Dihydroxymethylrutin; aesculus (p.1574·1); benzyl nicotinate (p.20·3).
Bath additive; circulatory disorders; musculoskeletal and joint disorders; neuromuscular disorders and trauma.

Intradermi N Eberth, Ger.
Ointment: Bovine ovarian extract (p.1487·2); bovine testicular extract (p.1492·1); bovine adrenal extract.
Musculoskeletal disorders; peripheral circulatory disorders.
Oral drops: Troxerutin (p.1611·2); aesculus (p.1574·1); scoparium (p.1661·2).
Brachialgia paraesthetica; circulatory disorders.

Intradermo Cort Ant Fung Cederroth, Spain.
Fluocinolone acetonide (p.1071·1); gramicidin (p.213·3); neomycin sulfate (p.228·1); nystatin (p.392·2).
Infected skin disorders.

Intrafat Nihon, Jpn.
Soya oil (p.1378·1).
Contains egg lecithin.
Lipid infusion for parenteral nutrition.

Intrafer Geymonat, Ital.
Iron polymaltose (p.1369·2).
Iron deficiency; iron-deficiency anaemia.

Intrafusin Fresenius Kabi, Aust.; Pharmacia Upjohn, Ger.; Fresenius Kabi, Switz.; Fresenius, UK.
Amino-acid infusion with or without electrolytes (p.1350·1).

Intrafusin E Pharmacia Upjohn, Ger.
Amino-acid and electrolyte infusion (p.1350·1).
Parenteral nutrition.

Intragam Serotherapeutiscihes, Aust.; CSL, Austral.; CSL, NZ; NBI, S.Afr.
A normal immunoglobulin (p.1551·3).
Idiopathic thrombocytopenic purpura; immunodeficiency; passive immunisation.

Intraglobin Biotest, Aust.; Intra Pharma, Irl.; Biotest, Ital.; Biotest, Thai.
A normal immunoglobulin (p.1551·3).
Agammaglobulinaemia; hypogammaglobulinaemia; idiopathic thrombocytopenic purpura; Kawasaki syndrome; passive immunisation; Wiskott-Aldrich syndrome.

Intraglobin F Biotest, Ger.; Biotest, Hong Kong; Mednostica, S.Afr.; Biotest, Singapore; Biotest, Switz.
A normal immunoglobulin (p.1551·3).
Hypogammaglobulinaemia; idiopathic thrombocytopenic purpura; immunodeficiency disorders; Kawasaki syndrome; passive immunisation.

Intrait de Marron D'Inde P Aerocid, Fr.
Aesculus (p.1574·1); metesculetol sodium (p.1635·1).
Haemorrhoids.

Intralgin 3M, S.Afr.†; 3M, UK.
Benzocaine (p.1306·2); salicylamide (p.82·1).
Inflammation; muscle pain.

Intralgis Urgo, Fr.
Ibuprofen (p.43·2).
Fever; musculoskeletal, joint, peri-articular, and soft-tissue disorders; pain.

Intralipid Fresenius Kabi, Aust.; Baxter, Austral.; Pharmacia Upjohn, Belg.†; Baxter, Canad.; Fresenius Kabi, Denm.; Fresenius Kabi, Fin.; Pharmacia Upjohn, Hong Kong; Pharmacia Upjohn, Irl.; Pharmacia Upjohn, Israel; Fresenius Kabi, Ital.; Pharmacia Upjohn, Neth.; Fresenius Kabi, Norw.; Baxter, NZ; Kabi Pharmacia, NZ; Fresenius Kabi, Port.; Fresenius Kabi, S.Afr.; Fresenius Kabi, Singapore; Fresenius Kabi, Swed.; Fresenius Kabi, Switz.; Pharmacia Upjohn, Thai.; Fresenius, UK; Clintec, USA.
Soya oil (p.1378·1).
Contains egg phospholipids.
Lipid infusion for parenteral nutrition.

Intralipide Fresenius Kabi, Fr.
Soya oil (p.1378·1).
Contains egg lecithin.
Lipid infusion for parenteral nutrition.

Intralipos Green Cross Guangzhou, Singapore.
Purified soya oil (p.1378·1).
Contains egg lecithin.
Lipid infusion for parenteral nutrition.

Intramin Pharmacia Upjohn, Ger.
Amino-acid, carbohydrate, and electrolyte infusion (p.1350·1).
Parenteral nutrition.

Intramin G Fresenius Kabi, Aust.
Amino-acid, electrolyte, and glucose infusion (p.1350·1).
Parenteral nutrition.

Intrasil BASF, Ger.
Sulpiride (p.706·1).
Depression; dizziness; Ménière's disease; schizophrenia.

Intrasite
Note. This name is used for preparations of different composition.
Smith & Nephew, Austral.; Smith & Nephew, S.Afr.
Crilanomer (p.1112·3).
Wounds.

Smith & Nephew, Fr.
Carmellose sodium (p.1499·3); propylene glycol (p.1655·1).
Formerly contained crilanomer.
Leg ulcers.

Smith & Nephew, Irl.
Hydrogel starch copolymer.
Wounds.

Smith & Nephew, UK.
Carmellose (p.1499·3).
Formerly known as Scherisorb. Formerly contained hydrogel starch copolymer.
Wound dressing.

Intrasol Wondli, Switz.†.
Thymol iodide (p.1158·3).
Oral hygiene.

Intrastigmina Lusofarmaco, Ital.
Neostigmine metilsulfate (p.1420·1).
Abdominal distension; post-operative intestinal atony; urinary retention.

Intraval Aventis, NZ.
Thiopental sodium (p.1269·1).
General anaesthesia.

Intraval Sodium Rhone-Poulenc Rorer, Hong Kong; Rhone-Poulenc Rorer, Irl.; Rhone-Poulenc Rorer, S.Afr.†; Rhone-Poulenc Rorer, Thai.; Rhone-Poulenc Rorer, UK†.
Thiopental sodium (p.1269·1).
Convulsive states; general anaesthesia; raised intracranial pressure in neurosurgery.

Intra-Vite B Group plus Ascorbic Acid Roche, Austral.
Vitamin B substances with vitamin C (p.1350·1).

Intrazig ISI, Ital.
A varicella-zoster immunoglobulin (p.1567·3).
Passive immunisation.

Intrazolina Torlan, Spain.
Cefazolin sodium (p.164·3).
Lignocaine [lidocaine] hydrochloride (p.1313·2) is included in this preparation to alleviate the pain of injection.
Bacterial infections.

Intricon Great Eastern, Thai.; United American, Thai.
Ferrous fumarate (p.1360·1); vitamin B substances; liver (p.1350·1).
Anaemias.

Intrimun Biotest, Ger.
A normal immunoglobulin (p.1551·3).
Immune deficiency.

Introlan Galagen, USA.
Lactose-free, gluten-free preparation for enteral nutrition (p.1350·1).

Introlite Abbott, Irl.; Abbott, UK; Ross, USA.
Preparation for enteral nutrition (p.1350·1).

Intron A Aesca, Austral.; Schering-Plough, Austral.; Schering-Plough, Belg.; Schering-Plough, Braz.; Schering, Canad.; Essex, Ger.; Schering-Plough, Hong Kong; Schering-Plough, Israel; Schering-Plough, Ital.; Schering-Plough, Mex.; Schering-Plough, Neth.; Schering-Plough, NZ; Schering-Plough, Port.; Schering-Plough, S.Afr.; Schering-Plough, Singapore; Schering-Plough, Spain; Essex, Swed.; Schering, USA.
Interferon alfa-2b (rbe) (p.628·1).
Anogenital warts; hepatitis B; hepatitis C; malignant neoplasms.

Intron A/Rebetol Essex, Switz.
Capsules, ribavirin (Rebetol) (p.639·1); injection, interferon alfa-2b (p.628·1).
Hepatitis C.

Introna Schering-Plough, Denm.; Schering-Plough, Fin.; Schering-Plough, Fr.; Schering-Plough, Irl.; Schering-Plough, Norw.; Schering-Plough, Swed.; Schering-Plough, Thai.; Schering-Plough, UK.
Interferon alfa-2b (rbe) (p.628·1).
Formerly known as Intron A in Irl. and UK.
Anogenital warts; hepatitis; malignant neoplasms.

Intropin Du Pont, Canad.; Du Pont, Hong Kong; Du Pont, Irl.†; Sanofi Synthelabo, S.Afr.; Du Pont, Singapore; Meda, Swed.; Du Pont, USA.
Dopamine hydrochloride (p.881·3).
Shock.

Inulac Coryphama, Ital.
Lactic-acid-producing organisms (p.1626·3).
Maintenance of normal gastrointestinal flora.

Inutest Fresenius Kabi, Aust.; Kemiflor, Swed.†; Laevosan, Switz.†.
Polyfructosan (p.1624·2).
Determination of glomerular filtration rate.

Invenol Hoechst Marion Roussel, Aust.†
Carbutamide (p.321·1).
Diabetes mellitus.

Inversine Layton, USA.
Mecamylamine hydrochloride (p.925·3).
Hypertension.

Invertos Pharmacia Upjohn, Norw.†
Anhydrous glucose (p.1364·1); fructose (p.1363·3).
Carbohydrate source.

Invigan Almi, Spain.
Famotidine (p.1225·3).
Gastro-oesophageal reflux; peptic ulcer; Zollinger-Ellison syndrome.

Invirase Roche, Aust.; Roche, Austral.; Roche, Belg.; Roche, Canad.; Roche, Denm.; Roche, Fin.; Roche, Fr.; Roche, Ger.; Roche, Hong Kong; Roche, Irl.; Roche, Israel; Roche, Ital.; Roche, Jpn; Roche, Mex.; Roche, Neth.; Roche, Norw.; Roche, NZ; Roche, Port.†; Roche, S.Afr.; Roche, Singapore; Roche, Spain; Roche, Swed.; Roche, Switz.; Roche, Thai.; Roche, UK; Roche, USA.
Saquinavir (p.641·1) or saquinavir mesilate (p.641·1).
HIV infection.

Invoigin Chew, Thai.
Dipyrone (p.34·1).
Fever; pain.

Invoril Ranbaxy, Singapore; Ranbaxy, Thai.
Enalapril maleate (p.883·3).
Heart failure; hypertension.

Inyesprin Grunenthal, Spain.
Lysine aspirin (p.50·3).
Fever; musculoskeletal, joint, and peri-articular disorders; pain; thromboembolism prophylaxis.

Inza
Note. This name is used for preparations of different composition.
Alphapharm, Austral.; Alphapharm, Hong Kong; Alphapharm, Singapore; Merck, Singapore.
Naproxen (p.60·3).
Inflammation; musculoskeletal and joint disorders; pain.

Aspen, S.Afr.
Ibuprofen (p.43·2).
Gout; musculoskeletal and joint disorders.

Inzelloval Kohler-Pharma, Ger.
Mineral preparation (p.1350·1).

Inzitan Roche, Spain.
Cyanocobalamin (p.1388·1); dexamethasone (p.1067·1); thiamine hydrochloride (p.1385·1).
Lignocaine [lidocaine] hydrochloride (p.1313·2) is included in this preparation to alleviate the pain of injection.
Musculoskeletal and joint disorders.

Inzolen Kohler, Ger.
A range of electrolyte (p.1180·1) and trace element (p.1350·1) infusions.
Electrolyte disorders; metabolic disorders.

Iobid DM Iomed, USA.
Guaifenesin (p.1092·2); dextromethorphan hydrobromide (p.1087·3).
Coughs.

Iocare Ciba Vision, Ital.
Electrolytes (p.1180·1).
Eye irrigation.

Iocare Balanced Salt Solution Ciba Vision, UK; Ciba Vision, USA.
Electrolytes (p.1180·1).
Eye irrigation.

Iocare BSS Ciba Vision, Ger.
Electrolytes (p.1180·1).
Eye irrigation.

Iocon Healthpoint, USA.
Coal tar (p.1125·1).
Scalp disorders.

Iodal Iomed, USA.
Hydrocodone tartrate (p.42·2); phenylephrine hydrochloride (p.1097·1); chlorpheniramine [chlorphenamine] maleate (p.412·1).
Upper respiratory-tract symptoms.

Iodax Rekah, Israel.
Iodine (p.1522·3); potassium iodide (p.1522·3).
Disinfection of minor cuts and bruises.

Iode Valmo, Canad.; Atlas, Canad.
Iodine (p.1522·3); potassium iodide (p.1522·3).

Iodepol Ache, Braz.
Potassium iodide (p.1522·3); guaifenesin (p.1092·2).
Respiratory-tract congestion.

Iodermol Heralds, Braz.
Iodine (p.1522·3); salicylic acid (p.1122·3); benzoic acid (p.1134·2).
Fungal skin infections.

Iodesin EMS, Braz.
Oxomemazine hydrochloride (p.422·2); potassium iodide (p.1522·3); sodium benzoate (p.1134·3); guaifenesin (p.1092·2); ipecacuanha (p.1093·1).
Respiratory-tract congestion.

Iodetal Sanval, Braz.
Sulfogaiacol (p.1101·1); potassium iodide (p.1522·3); tolu balsam (p.1101·3).
Respiratory-tract congestion.

Iodeto de Potassio Composto Delta, Braz.
Potassium iodide (p.1522·3); guaifenesin (p.1092·2); carbinoxamine (p.411·1).
Respiratory-tract congestion.

Iodeto de Potassium Composto Farmedica, Braz.
Potassium iodide (p.1522·3); oxomemazine (p.422·2).
Respiratory-tract congestion.

Iodex
Note. This name is used for preparations of different composition.
Qualiphar, Belg.†
Iodine (p.1522·3).
Superficial wounds.

Lee, USA.
Povidone-iodine (p.1155·1).
Skin disinfection.

Iodex Buccal Qualiphar, Belg.
Povidone-iodine (p.1155·1).
Mouth and throat infections.

Iodex Dermique Qualiphar, Belg.
Povidone-iodine (p.1155·1).
Disinfection of skin and instruments; infected skin disorders.

Iodex with Methyl Salicylate Medtech, USA.
Iodine (p.1522·3); methyl salicylate (p.55·1).
Muscle, joint, and soft-tissue pain; neuralgia.

Iodiflor Floris, Israel.
Povidone-iodine (p.1155·1).
Skin disinfection.

Iodina Montplet, Spain.
Povidone-iodine (p.1155·1).
Skin, wound, and burn disinfection.

Iodisis Prisfar, Port.
Iodine (p.1522·3).
Mouth and throat infections and inflammation.

Iodobec Farmedica, Braz.
Potassium iodide (p.1522·3); guaifenesin (p.1092·2); sodium benzoate (p.1134·3); oxomemazine (p.422·2); ipecacuanha (p.1093·1).
Respiratory-tract congestion.

Iodocid Bergamon, Ital.
Povidone-iodine (p.1155·1).
Skin disinfection.

Iodoflex Smith & Nephew, Irl.; Smith & Nephew Healthcare, UK.
Cadexomer-iodine (p.1136·3).
Leg ulcers; wounds.

Iodopen American Pharmaceutical, USA.
Sodium iodide (p.1522·3).
Additive for intravenous total parenteral nutrition solutions.

Iodosan Collutorio SmithKline Beecham, Ital.
Iodine (p.1522·3).
Oral hygiene.

Iodosorb Lannacher, Aust.; Smith & Nephew, Canad.; Smith & Nephew, Denm.; Smith & Nephew, Fin.; Strathmann, Ger.; Valeas, Ital.; Almirall, Spain; Smith & Nephew, Swed.; Perstorp, Switz.; Smith & Nephew Healthcare, UK.
Cadexomer-iodine (p.1136·3).
Infected wounds and ulcers.

Iodosteril IMS, Ital.
Povidone-iodine (p.1155·1).
Skin disinfection.

Iodoten Pierrel, Ital.
Povidone-iodine (p.1155·1).
Wound disinfection.

Iodotope Squibb Diagnostics, USA.
Iodine-131 (p.1450·1) as sodium iodide.
Hyperthyroidism; thyroid cancer.

The symbol † denotes a preparation no longer actively marketed

Iodo-Vit *Vitamed, Israel.*
Povidone-iodine (p.1155·1).
Skin and wound disinfection.

Iofed *Iomed, USA.*
Brompheniramine maleate (p.410·2); pseudoephedrine hydrochloride (p.1099·2).
Upper respiratory-tract symptoms.

Iofoscal *Virtus, Braz.*
Guarana (p.1681·1); kola (p.1681·1); minerals (p.1350·1).
Nutritional supplement.

Iohist D *Iomed, USA†.*
Phenylpropanolamine hydrochloride (p.1098·1); phenyltoloxamine citrate (p.423·1); mepyramine maleate (p.421·1); pheniramine maleate (p.422·3).
Respiratory-tract disorders.

Iohist DM *Iomed, USA†.*
Dextromethorphan hydrobromide (p.1087·3); phenyl-propanolamine hydrochloride (p.1098·1); brompheniramine maleate (p.410·2).
Upper respiratory-tract symptoms.

Ioimbina Composta
Note.This name is used for preparations of different composition.
Delta, Braz.
Yohimbine hydrochloride (p.1681·3); vitamin B substances; inositol (p.1350·1).
Tonic.

Neo Quimica, Braz.
Methyltestosterone (p.1482·3); yohimbine hydrochloride (p.1681·3); vitamin E (p.1393·3); caffeine (p.761·3); ephedrine (p.1090·1).
Erectile dysfunction.

Ioiro *Regional Health, NZ.*
Ioidol.
Radiographic contrast medium.

Iolin NPH *Biobras, Braz.*
Isophane insulin injection (bovine and porcine, highly purified) (p.324·1).
Diabetes mellitus.

Iolin Regular *Biobras, Braz.*
Insulin injection (bovine and porcine, highly purified) (p.324·1).
Diabetes mellitus.

Iomeron
Gerot, Aust.; HCP, Austral.; Byk, Belg.; Bracco, Denm.; Astra Tech, Fin.; Byk, Fr.; Bracco, Israel; Bracco, Ital.; Eisai, Jpn; Byk, Neth.; Astra Tech, Norw.; Regional Health, NZ; Bracco, Port.; Rovi, Spain; Astra Tech, Swed.; Bracco, Switz.; Merck, UK.
Iomeprol (p.1035·1).
Radiographic contrast medium.

Ionamin
Medeva, Belg.†; Rhone-Poulenc Rorer, Canad.; Rhone-Poulenc Rorer, Irl.†; Rhone-Poulenc Rorer, Mex.; Searle, Singapore; Cambridge Healthcare, UK†; Medeva, USA.
Phentermine (as an ion-exchange resin complex) (p.1514·1).
Obesity.

Ionamine *Medeva, Switz.*
Phentermine (as an ion-exchange resin complex) (p.1514·1).
Obesity.

Ionarthrol *Picot, Fr.*
Copper gluconate (p.1357·3).
Formerly contained manganese sulfate, magnesium sulfate, calcium chloride, nickel chloride, ferrous sulfate, and sodium sulfate.
Joint disorders; viral infections.

Ionax Astringent *Healthpoint, USA.*
Salicylic acid (p.1122·3); allantoin (p.1110·1).
Acne.

Ionax Foam *Healthpoint, USA.*
Skin cleanser.

Ionax Scrub
Note.This name is used for preparations of different composition.
Galderma, Austral.; Galderma, Fr.; Galderma, Irl.; Galderma, Singapore; Galderma, Thai.; Galderma, UK; Healthpoint, USA.
Polyethylene granules (abrasive) (p.1108·3).
Acne; oily skin conditions.

Galderma, Braz.
Benzalkonium chloride (p.1133·2).
Skin cleanser.

Ionax T
Galderma, Fr.†; Galderma, Port.†.
Coal tar (p.1125·1); salicylic acid (p.1122·3).
Seborrhoeic dermatitis.

Ionil
Galderma, Braz.; Galderma, Canad.†; Galderma, Mex.; Healthpoint, USA.
Salicylic acid (p.1122·3).
Seborrhoeic dermatitis.

Ionil P *Galderma, Braz.*
Piroctone olamine (p.1121·1); salicylic acid (p.1122·3).
Scalp disorders.

Ionil Plus
Galderma, Braz.; Galderma, Mex.; Healthpoint, USA.
Salicylic acid (p.1122·3).
Scalp psoriasis; seborrhoeic dermatitis.

Ionil Rinse *Galderma, Braz.*
Hydrolised collagen proteins (p.1598·1).
Dry brittle hair.

Ionil Scalp Cleanser *Galderma, Austral.*
Salicylic acid (p.1122·3).
Scalp disorders.

Ionil-T
Note.This name is used for preparations of different composition.
Galderma, Austral.; Galderma, Braz.; Galderma, Hong Kong; Galder-ma, Irl.; Galderma, Ital.†; Galderma, Mex.; Galderma, NZ; Galderma, Singapore; Galderma, Thai.; Galderma, UK; Healthpoint, USA.
Coal tar (p.1125·1); salicylic acid (p.1122·3).
Scalp disorders.

Galderma, Canad.†.
Coal tar (p.1125·1).
Scalp disorders.

Ionil-T Plus
Note.This name is used for preparations of different composition.
Galderma, Austral.; Galderma, Canad.†; Galderma, Mex.; Health-point, USA.
Coal tar (Owentar II) (p.1125·1).
Scalp disorders.

Galderma, Braz.
Salicylic acid (p.1122·3).
Scalp psoriasis; seborrhoeic dermatitis.

Ionimag *Byk, Fr.*
Magnesium lactate (p.1191·1).
Magnesium deficiency.

Ionitan *Aguettant, Fr.*
Electrolyte infusion (p.1180·1).
Parenteral nutrition.

Ionosteril *Fresenius Kabi, Port.*
Electrolyte infusion with or without glucose (p.1180·1).
Plasma substitute.

Ionyl *Pharmadeveloppement, Fr.*
Phosphoric acid (p.1651·1); sodium glycerophosphate (p.1617·3); magnesium glycerophosphate (p.1191·1); manganese glycerophosphate (p.1617·3).
Tonic.

Iopamiro
Astra Tech, Denm.; Astra Tech, Fin.; Bracco, Israel; Bracco, Ital.; Da-gra, Neth.†; Astra Tech, Norw.; Bracco, Port.; Rovi, Spain; Astra Tech, Swed.; Bracco, Switz.
Iopamidol (p.1035·2).
Radiographic contrast medium.

Iopamiron
Schering, Braz.; Schering, Fr.
Iopamidol (p.1035·2).
Radiographic contrast medium.

Iophen *Rugby, USA.*
Iodinated glycerol (p.1092·3).
Coughs.

Iopidine
Alcon, Aust.; Alcon, Austral.; Alcon, Belg.; Alcon, Canad.; Alcon, Denm.; Alcon, Fin.; Alcon, Fr.; Alcon, Ger.; Alcon, Hong Kong; Alcon, Irl.; Alcon, Israel; Alcon, Ital.; Alcon, Jpn; Alcon, Mex.; Alcon, Norw.; Alcon, NZ; Alcon, Port.; Alcon, S.Afr.; Alcon, Singapore; Alcon, Swed.; Alcon, Switz.; Alcon, UK; Alcon, USA.
Apraclonidine hydrochloride (p.840·3).
Control of intra-ocular pressure following eye surgery; glaucoma.

Iopimax *Alcon Cusi, Spain.*
Apraclonidine hydrochloride (p.840·3).
Glaucoma; prevention of ocular hypertension in laser surgery.

Iosal II *Iomed, USA.*
Pseudoephedrine (p.1099·2); guaifenesin (p.1092·2).
Coughs.

Iosalide *Yamanouchi, Ital.*
Josamycin (p.217·3) or josamycin propionate (p.217·3).
Bacterial infections.

Iosopan *Goldline, USA.*
Magaldrate (p.1232·2).
Hyperacidity.

Iosopan Plus *Goldline, USA.*
Magaldrate (p.1232·2); simeticone (p.1249·2).
Hyperacidity.

Iotrovist *Schering, Port.†.*
Iotrolan (p.1036·3).
Radiographic contrast medium.

Iotussin HC *Iomed, USA.*
Hydrocodone tartrate (p.42·2); phenylephrine hydrochloride (p.1097·1); chlorpheniramine [chlorphenamine] maleate (p.412·1).
Upper respiratory-tract symptoms.

Ipacef *IPA, Ital.*
Cefuroxime sodium (p.178·2).
Bacterial infections.

Ipacid *IPA, Ital.*
Cefonicid sodium (p.168·1).
Lignocaine [lidocaine] hydrochloride (p.1313·2) is included in this preparation to alleviate the pain of injection.
Bacterial infections.

Ipagastril *IPA, Ital.*
Sucralfate (p.1250·2).
Gastritis; gastro-oesophageal reflux; peptic ulcer.

Ipalat *Pfleger, Ger.*
Ointment: Pumilio pine oil (p.1656·3); eucalyptus oil (p.1609·2).
Pastilles: Cowslip root (p.1600·1).
Syrup†: Cowslip root (p.1600·1); thyme (p.1672·2).
Respiratory-tract disorders.

Ipamicina *IPA, Ital.*
Fosfomycin calcium (p.208·2).
Bacterial infections.

Ipamix *Gentili, Ital.*
Indapamide (p.913·1).
Hypertension.

Iparen *NCSN, Ital.*
Suleparoid (p.978·2).
Thrombosis prophylaxis.

Ipatox *IPA, Ital.*
Glutathione sodium (p.1010·3).
Alcohol and drug poisoning; radiation trauma.

Ipatrizina *IPA, Ital.*
Propylene glycol cefatrizine (p.164·3).
Bacterial infections.

Ipaviran *NCSN, Ital.*
Aciclovir (p.612·3).
Herpesvirus infections.

Ipavit *IPA, Ital.*
Vitamin B substances with calcium folinate (p.1350·1)(p.1363·1).

Ipazone *IPA, Ital.*
Cefoperazone sodium (p.168·2).
Bacterial infections.

Ipcamox *Nat Druggists, S.Afr.*
Amoxicillin trihydrate (p.149·2).
Bacterial infections.

Ipeca
Note.This name is used for preparations of different composition.
Orion, Fin.
Ipecacuanha (p.1093·1).
Poisoning.

Amino, Switz.
Emetine hydrochloride (p.591·3); ethylmorphine hydrochloride (p.35·2); ephedrine hydrochloride (p.1090·1); codeine phosphate (p.25·2); cherry-laurel water; tolu balsam (p.1101·3).
Respiratory-tract disorders.

Ipecol *Iodo Suma, Braz.*
Sodium dibunate (p.1100·3); ipecacuanha (p.1093·1); sodium benzoate (p.1134·3).
Respiratory-tract congestion.

Ipercortis *AGIPS, Ital.*
Triamcinolone (p.1080·1).
Corticosteroid.

Iperiton *Lampugnani, Ital.*
Mutivitamin and mineral preparation with hypericum and dog rose (p.1350·1).
Nutritional supplement.

Iperix *Palmares, Ital.*
Inositol; vitamin B₆; hypericum (p.1350·1).
Nutritional supplement.

Iperplasin *CSC, Aust.*
Mepartricin (p.390·3).
Benign prostatic hyperplasia.

Iperten *Chiesi, Ital.*
Manidipine hydrochloride (p.924·3).
Hypertension.

Ipertrofan *SPA, Ital.*
Mepartricin (p.390·3).
Benign prostatic hyperplasia.

Ipervital *IDI, Ital.*
Nutritional supplement (p.1350·1).

Ipesandrine *Novartis Consumer, Port.*
Dextromethorphan hydrobromide (p.1087·3); ephedrine hydrochloride (p.1090·1).
Coughs.

Ipesil *Antigen, Irl.*
Ipecacuanha (p.1093·1); squill (p.1100·3).
Coughs.

Ipetitrin *Agepha, Aust.*
Ipecacuanha (p.1093·1).
Bronchitis; coughs.

Ipnovel *Roche, Ital.*
Midazolam (p.692·3).
General anaesthesia; premedication; sedative.

Ipoazotal *SIT, Ital.*
Arginine hydrochloride (p.1353·3); ornithine hydrochloride (p.1374·1); citrulline (p.1357·2).
Hyperammonaemia.

Ipoazotal Complex *SIT, Ital.*
Arginine hydrochloride (p.1353·3); ornithine hydrochloride (p.1374·1); citrulline (p.1357·2); acetyl aspartate; aceglumic acid; calcium oxoglurate.
Hyperammonaemia.

Ipocalcin *Salus, Ital.*
Salcatonin (p.749·3).
Hypercalcaemia; osteoporosis; Paget's disease of bone; reflex sympathetic dystrophy.

Ipocol *Lagap, Switz.*
Divistyramine (p.880·2).
Biliary-tract disorders; hypercholesterolaemia.

Ipocromo *Ripari-Gero, Ital.*
Ferric sodium gluconate (p.1360·2).
Iron-deficiency anaemias.

Ipogen *Gentili, Ital.†.*
Dihydralazine tartrate (p.874·2); chlorothiazide (p.856·3).
Hypertension.

Ipoglusan *Bioquimico, Mex.*
Tolbutamide (p.336·3).
Diabetes mellitus.

Ipol
CSL, Austral.; CSL, NZ; Pasteur Merieux, USA.
An inactivated poliomyelitis vaccine (p.1558·2).
Active immunisation.

Ipolab *Finmedical, Ital.*
Labetalol hydrochloride (p.918·1).
Hypertension.

Ipolipid
Medochemie, Hong Kong; Medochemie, Singapore; Medochemie, Thai.
Gemfibrozil (p.896·2).
Hyperlipidaemias.

Iposeb *Rydelle, Fr.†.*
Amino-acid, vitamin, and mineral preparation (p.1350·1).
Seborrhoea.

Ippi Verde *Henkel, Ital.*
Triclosan (Irgasan DP 300) (p.1159·2).
Skin and hand disinfection.

Ipradol
Nycomed, Aust.; Nycomed, Hong Kong; Aspen, S.Afr.; Lacer, Spain†; Hafslund Nycomed, Thai.
Hexoprenaline (p.766·1), hexoprenaline hydrochloride (p.766·1), or hexoprenaline sulfate (p.766·1).
Obstructive airways disease; prevention of uterine contractions.

Iprafen *Chiesi, Ital.*
Fenoterol hydrobromide (p.765·1); ipratropium bromide (p.766·1).
Obstructive airways disease.

Ipral
Bristol-Myers Squibb, Irl.; Squibb, UK†.
Trimethoprim (p.264·2).
Urinary- and respiratory-tract infections.

Ipratrin *Alphapharm, Austral.*
Ipratropium bromide (p.766·1).
Obstructive airways disease.

Ipravent *Pharmacia, Austral.*
Ipratropium bromide (p.766·1).
Obstructive airways disease.

Ipren *Nycomed, Denm.; Pharmacia Upjohn, Swed.*
Ibuprofen (p.43·2).
Fever; inflammation; musculoskeletal and joint disorders; pain.

Iproben *Mepha, Switz.*
Ibuprofen (p.43·2).
Fever; pain.

Iprogel *Mepha, Switz.*
Ibuprofen (p.43·2).
Musculoskeletal, joint, peri-articular and soft-tissue pain and inflammation.

Iprosten *Takeda, Ital.*
Ipriflavone (p.753·3).
Osteoporosis.

Ipsatol *Orion, Fin.*
Biperiden hydrochloride (p.464·2) or biperiden lactate (p.464·2).
Drug-induced extrapyramidal disorders; parkinsonism; trigeminal neuralgia.

Ipsatol Cough Formula Liquid for Children and Adults *Kenwood, USA†.*
Guaifenesin (p.1092·2); dextromethorphan hydrobromide (p.1087·3); phenylpropanolamine hydrochloride (p.1098·1).
Coughs.

Ipser Europe *Pasteur Vaccins, Fr.†.*
A snake venom antiserum (*Vipera ammodytes, V. aspis, and V. berus*) (p.1563·3).
Viper bites.

Ipsilon *Nikkho, Braz.*
Aminocaproic acid (p.724·3).
Haemorrhage.

Ipsovir *Ipso, Ital.*
Aciclovir (p.612·3).
Herpesvirus infections.

Ipstyl
Ipsen, Ital.; Ipsen, Norw.
Lanreotide (p.1289·2).
Acromegaly; carcinoid tumours.

IPV Merieux *Pasteur Merieux, Ger.*
An inactivated poliomyelitis vaccine (type 1, 2, and 3) (p.1558·2).
Active immunisation.

Ipvent *Cipla-Medpro, S.Afr.*
Ipratropium bromide (p.766·1).
Obstructive airways disease.

IPV-Virelon *Chiron Behring, Ger.*
An inactivated poliomyelitis vaccine (type I, II, and III) (p.1558·2).
Active immunisation.

Iqfacilina *Iqfasa, Mex.*
Ampicillin (p.150·3).
Bacterial infections.

Iqfadina *Iqfasa, Mex.*
Ranitidine (p.1246·3).

Irban *Pharmabest, Israel.*
Irbesartan (p.914·2).
Hypertension.

Ircon *Kenwood, USA.*
Iron carbonyl.
Formerly contained ferrous fumarate.
Iron-deficiency anaemias.

Ircon-FA *Kenwood, USA.*
Iron carbonyl; folic acid (p.1361·1).
Formerly contained ferrous fumarate and folic acid.
Iron-deficiency anaemias.

Irenat
Kolassa, Aust.; Bayer, Ger.
Sodium perchlorate (p.1526·1).
Adjunct in radionuclide brain scanning; hyperthyroidism.

Irene *Pharmaland, Thai.*
Astemizole (p.409·1).
Allergic conjunctivitis; allergic rhinitis; urticaria.

Irfen *Mepha, Switz.*
Ibuprofen (p.43·2).
Musculoskeletal and joint disorders; pain.

Irgaman *Rusch, Ital.*
Triclosan (Irgasan DP 300) (p.1159·2).
Skin disinfection.

Irgamid
Ciba Vision, Denm.; Ciba Vision, Fin.; Ciba Vision, Neth.; Ciba Vision, Switz.
Sulfadicramide (p.252·1).
Bacterial eye infections.

Iricil *Cantabria, Spain.*
Lisinopril (p.921·1).
Diabetic nephropathy; heart failure; hypertension; myocardial infarction.

Iridina Due *Montefarmaco, Ital.*
Naphazoline hydrochloride (p.1095·1).
Eye irritation.

Iridina Light *Montefarmaco, Ital.*
Benzalkonium chloride (p.1133·2).
Eye disinfection; eye irritation.

Iridus *Hoechst Marion Roussel, Mex.*
Naftidrofuryl.

Iridux *Hoechst Marion Roussel, Braz.*
Naftidrofuryl.
Vascular disorders.

Irigate *Optopics, USA†.*
Sodium chloride (p.1196·1).
Eye irrigation.

Iris Med Complex *Dynamit, Aust.*
Homoeopathic preparation.

Iri-Sol *Ocumed, USA.*
Eye irrigation.

Iristamina *Montefarmaco, Ital.*
Thonzylamine hydrochloride (p.426·2); naphazoline nitrate (p.1095·1).
Conjunctivitis; eye irritation.

Irocombivit *Schmidgall, Aust.*
Multivitamin preparation (p.1350·1).

Irocopar cC *Schmidgall, Aust.*
Carbasalate calcium (p.23·3); paracetamol (p.71·2); codeine phosphate (p.25·2).
Pain.

Irocophan *Schmidgall, Aust.*
Carbasalate calcium (p.23·3); paracetamol (p.71·2); caffeine (p.761·3).
Fever; pain.

Irocovit C *Schmidgall, Aust.†.*
Vitamin C (p.1389·3).
Vitamin C deficiency.

Iromin *Schmidgall, Aust.*
Carbasalate calcium (p.23·3).
Cold symptoms; fever; pain.

Iromin Chinin C *Schmidgall, Aust.*
Carbasalate calcium (p.23·3); quinine hydrochloride (p.445·1); calcium ascorbate (p.1389·3).
Cold symptoms; fever; pain.

Iromin-G *Mission Pharmacal, USA.*
Ferrous gluconate (p.1360·1); folic acid (p.1361·1); multivitamins and minerals (p.1350·1).
Iron-deficiency anaemias.

Iron Complex *Jamieson, Canad.*
Multivitamin and mineral preparation (p.1350·1).

Iron Compound *Blackmores, Austral.*
Sodium sulfate (p.1250·1); ferrous phosphate; potassium chloride (p.1194·3).
Iron deficiency.

Iron Jelloids *Seton, UK†.*
Ferrous fumarate (p.1360·1); vitamin B substances (p.1350·1).
Iron deficiency.

Iron Plus
Cenovis, Austral.; Vitelle, Austral.
Multivitamin preparation with iron (p.1350·1).
Tonic; vitamin and iron supplement.

Swiss Herbal, Canad.
Multivitamin and mineral preparation (p.1350·1).

Ironax *Caber, Ital.†.*
Ferrous gluconate (p.1360·1).
Iron deficiency; iron-deficiency anaemia.

Ironorm *Wallace Mfg Chem., UK.*
Capsules: Dried ferrous sulfate (p.1360·3); folic acid (p.1361·1); vitamin B substances; vitamin C (p.1350·1).
Elixir: Ferric ammonium citrate (p.1359·2); vitamin B substances; minerals (p.1350·1).
Oral drops: Ferrous sulfate (p.1360·3).
Iron deficiency.

Irontona *Brauer, Austral.*
Angelica (p.1580·2); ascorbic acid (p.1389·3); kola (p.1681·1); ferrous sulfate (p.1360·3); hypericum (p.290·2); ginseng (p.1615·3); urtica (p.1678·2); aurum muriaticum; calcarea phosphorica; ferrum metallicum; ferrum phosphoricum; kali phosphoricum; magnesia phosphorica; phosphoric acid.
Tonic.

Irospan *Fielding, USA.*
Ferrous sulfate (p.1360·3).
Ascorbic acid (p.1389·3) is included in this preparation to increase the absorption and availability of iron.
Iron-deficiency anaemias.

Iroviton-Irocombivit *Schmidgall, Aust.*
Multivitamin preparation with hesperidin (p.1350·1).

Irriclens
Convatec, Fr.; Convatec, UK.
Sodium chloride (p.1196·1).
Wound cleansing and irrigation.

Irritos *Faes, Spain.*
Phenylpropanolamine hydrochloride (p.1098·1); dextromethorphan hydrobromide (p.1087·3).
Coughs; nasal congestion.

Irritren
Byk, Aust.; Tosse, Ger.†; Byk Gulden, Hong Kong.
Lonazolac calcium (p.50·2).
Inflammation; musculoskeletal, joint, peri-articular, and soft-tissue disorders; pain.

Irrodan
Biomedica, Hong Kong; Biomedica, Ital.; Biomedica, Thai.
Buflomedil hydrochloride (p.851·3).
Cerebral and peripheral vascular disorders.

IRS 19 *Solvay, Fr.*
Lysates of *Streptococcus pneumoniae; Streptococcus group G; Streptococcus pyogenes; Staphylococcus aureus; Acinetobacter calcoaceticus; Neisseria subflava; Klebsiella pneumoniae; Moraxella catarrhalis; Haemophilus influenzae; Streptococcus dysgalactiae; Enterococcus faecium; Enterococcus faecalis* (p.1626·3).
Respiratory-tract disorders.

Hefa, Ger.
Lysate of: *Streptococcus pneumoniae; Streptococcus pyogenes; Enterococcus faecalis* (p.1626·3)*; Staphylococcus aureus; Moraxella catarrhalis; Neisseria flava; Neisseria perflava; Haemophilus influenzae; Klebsiella pneumoniae; Gaffkya tetragena; Moraxella.*
Respiratory-tract infections.

Irtan
Rhone-Poulenc Rorer, Ger.; Rhone-Poulenc Rorer, Mex.
Nedocromil sodium (p.768·3).
Allergic conjunctivitis; allergic rhinitis; keratoconjunctivitis.

Irtonin *Takeda, Ital.*
Protirelin tartrate (p.1296·1).
Mental function disorders.

Irudil *Roche, Aust.*
Hirudin (p.905·3).
Peripheral vascular disorders.

Iruxol
Knoll, Braz.; Knoll, Fin.; Knoll, Ger.; Knoll, Ital.
Collagenase (p.1598·2); chloramphenicol (p.179·1).
Burns; skin ulcers and wounds.

Iruxol Mono
Knoll, Fin.; Knoll, Hong Kong; Knoll, Irl.; Knoll, S.Afr.; Knoll, Spain; Knoll, Switz.
Collagenase (p.1598·2); proteases.
Ulcers; wounds.

Iruxol Neo *Knoll, Spain.*
Collagenase (p.1598·2); neomycin sulfate (p.228·1).
Burns; ulcers; wounds.

Iruxolum mono *Ebewe, Aust.*
Enzymes from *Clostridium histolyticum.*
Necrotic ulcers; wounds.

IS 5 Mono *Ratiopharm, Ger.*
Isosorbide mononitrate (p.916·2).
Angina pectoris; heart failure; myocardial infarction; pulmonary hypertension.

Isacilin *Eurofarma, Braz.*
Benzylpenicillin potassium (p.157·1).
Procaine (p.1319·2) is included in this preparation to alleviate the pain of injection.
Bacterial infections.

Isadol *Pisa, Mex.*
Zidovudine (p.645·2).
HIV infection.

Isairon *Pfizer, Ital.*
Chondroitin sulfate–iron complex (p.1357·2).
Iron deficiency; iron-deficiency anaemias.

Isavir *Pisa, Mex.*
Aciclovir sodium (p.612·3).
Cytomegalovirus infections; herpesvirus infections.

Isaxion *Ferring, Port.*
Ticlopidine hydrochloride (p.981·1).
Thrombo-embolism prophylaxis.

Iscador
Weleda, Aust.; Weleda, Ger.
Mistletoe (p.1636·2) from apple trees, pine trees or oak trees.
Neoplasms.

Ischelium *Polifarma, Ital.*
Co-dergocrine mesilate (p.1597·3).
Cerebral and peripheral vascular disorders; hypertension.

Ischelium Papaverina *Polifarma, Ital.†.*
Co-dergocrine mesilate (p.1597·3); papaverine hydrochloride (p.1648·1).
Cerebral and peripheral vascular disorders; hypertension.

Ischemol *Rhone-Poulenc Rorer, Mex.*
Tetryzoline hydrochloride (p.1101·2).

Ischemol A *Formila, Ital.*
Tetryzoline hydrochloride (p.1101·2); chlorpheniramine [chlorphenamine] maleate (p.412·1).
Eye disorders.

Isclofen *Isis, UK.*
Diclofenac sodium (p.30·3).
Musculoskeletal and joint disorders.

Iscover
Bristol-Myers Squibb, Austral.; Bristol-Myers Squibb, Ger.; Bristol-My-

ers Squibb, Port.; Bristol-Myers, Spain; Bristol-Myers Squibb, Switz.; Bristol-Myers Squibb, UK.
Clopidogrel bisulfate (p.863·1).
Atherosclerosis.

Isdinex *Isdin, Spain.*
Benzethonium chloride (p.1134·2); diphenhydramine hydrochloride (p.416·1).
Pruritus.

Isdinium *Isdin, Spain.*
Hydrocortisone butyrate (p.1073·3) or hydrocortisone propionate (p.1074·2).
Skin disorders.

Isdol *Isdin, Spain.*
Ibuprofen (p.43·2).
Fever; pain.

I-Sense *Akorn, USA.*
Multivitamin preparation (p.1350·1).

Isepacin
Schering-Plough, Ital.; Schering-Plough, Mex.; Schering-Plough, Port.
Isepamicin sulfate (p.215·2).
Bacterial infections.

Isepacine *Schering-Plough, Belg.*
Isepamicin sulfate (p.215·2).
Bacterial infections.

Isepalline *Schering-Plough, Fr.*
Isepamicin sulfate (p.215·2).
Bacterial infections.

Isephca S *Iso, Ger.*
Thyme (p.1672·2).
Coughs.

Isib *Ashbourne, UK.*
Isosorbide mononitrate (p.916·2).
Angina pectoris.

Isi-Calcin *ISI, Ital.†.*
Elcatonin (p.749·2).
Hypercalcaemia; osteoporosis; Paget's disease of bone; reflex sympathetic dystrophy.

Isicom *Desitin, Ger.*
Carbidopa (p.1168·2); levodopa (p.1169·2).
Parkinsonism.

Isiferone *ISI, Ital.*
Interferon alfa (p.628·1).
Malignant neoplasms; viral infections.

Isiflu Zonale *ISI, Ital.*
An influenza vaccine (p.1544·3).
Active immunisation.

ISI-F/2/ST *ISI, Ital.*
Amino acids (p.1350·1).
Nutritional supplement in renal insufficiency.

Isilung *Exel, Belg.*
Eprazinone hydrochloride (p.1091·1).
Respiratory-tract disorders.

Isimoxin *ISI, Ital.*
Amoxicillin (p.149·2).
Bacterial infections.

Isisfen *Isis, UK.*
Ibuprofen (p.43·2).
Inflammation; pain.

Isitab *Agepha, Aust.*
Disinfection tablets for soft contact lenses (p.1129·2).

Isiven *ISI, Ital.*
A normal immunoglobulin (p.1551·3).
Hypogammaglobulinaemia; idiopathic thrombocytopenic purpura; passive immunisation.

Iskaemyl *Astra, Denm.†.*
Aspirin (p.14·2).
Ischaemic heart disease; thrombosis prophylaxis.

Iskedyl
Pierre Fabre, Fr.; Pierre Fabre, Spain.
Dihydroergocristine mesilate (p.1603·2); raubasine (p.967·2).
Cerebral and peripheral vascular disorders; head injury; mental function disorders of the elderly.

Iskemil *Ache, Braz.*
Dihydroergocristine mesilate (p.1603·2).
Impaired mental function.

Isketam *Ache, Braz.*
Piracetam (p.1652·1); dihydroergocristine mesilate (p.1603·2).
Impaired mental function.

Iskevert *Medley, Braz.*
Dihydroergocristine mesilate (p.1603·2).
Impaired mental function.

Isla-Mint
Sanova, Aust.; Engelhard, Ger.; Engelhard, Hong Kong.
Iceland moss.
Catarrh; coughs; sore throat.

Islamint *Ceuta, UK.*
Iceland moss.
Dry throat; respiratory-tract congestion.

Isla-Moos
Engelhard, Ger.; Engelhard, Hong Kong.
Iceland moss.
Catarrh; coughs; sore throat.

Ismelin
Novartis, Aust.; Novartis, Austral.; Novartis, Mex.; Novartis, NZ; Novartis, S.Afr.; Ciba Vision, Switz.†; Sovereign, UK; Ciba, USA.
Guanethidine monosulfate (p.901·1).
Hypertension; reflex sympathetic dystrophy.

Ismeline *Ciba Vision, Fr.†.*
Guanethidine sulfate (p.901·1).
Eye disorders.

Ismexin *Medinovum, Fin.*
Isosorbide mononitrate (p.916·2).
Angina pectoris; heart failure.

Ismipur *ISM, Ital.*
Mercaptopurine (p.552·2).
Acute leukaemia.

Ismo
Wyeth-Ayerst, Canad.; Ercopharm, Denm.†; Roche, Ger.; Roche, Hong Kong; Boehringer Mannheim, Israel; Roche, Ital.; Boehringer Mannheim, Neth.†; Roche, Norw.; Roche, NZ; Roche, Port.; Roche, S.Afr.; Roche, Singapore; Roche, Swed.; Roche, Switz.; Roche, Thai.; Roche, UK; Wyeth-Ayerst, USA.
Isosorbide mononitrate (p.916·2).
Angina pectoris; heart failure; myocardial infarction; pulmonary hypertension.

Ismotic *Alcon, USA.*
Isosorbide (p.915·2).
Raised intra-ocular pressure.

Ismox *Roche, Fin.*
Isosorbide mononitrate (p.916·2).
Angina pectoris; heart failure.

Iso *Lacer, Spain.*
Isosorbide dinitrate (p.915·2).
Angina pectoris; heart failure.

Iso Mack
Pfizer, Aust.; Mack, Denm.; Mack, Illert., Ger.; Mack, Hong Kong; Mack, Singapore; Mack, Switz.; Mack, Thai.
Isosorbide dinitrate (p.915·2).
Angina pectoris; heart failure; myocardial infarction; pulmonary hypertension; pulmonary oedema.

Iso Triraupin *Roche, Hong Kong.*
Butizide (p.853·1); reserpine (p.967·3); rescinnamine (p.967·3); raubasine (p.967·2); potassium chloride (p.1194·3).
Hypertension.

ISO-Augentropfen C *Iso, Ger.*
Homoeopathic preparation.

Iso-B *Tyson, USA.*
Multivitamin preparation (p.1350·1).

Isobac *Carnot, Mex.*
Co-trimoxazole (p.193·3).
Bacterial infections.

Isobar *Chiesi, Fr.*
Methyclothiazide (p.927·3); triamterene (p.986·1).
Hypertension.

Iso-Betadine *Asta Medica, Belg.*
Povidone-iodine (p.1155·1).
Burns; disinfection of the skin and mucous membranes; mouth and throat infections; skin infections; ulcers; vulvovaginal infections; wounds.

Isobib *Korea United, Singapore.*
Isosorbide dinitrate (p.915·2).
Angina pectoris; heart failure.

Isobinate *General Drugs, Thai.*
Isosorbide dinitrate (p.915·2).
Angina pectoris.

Isobranch *Bieffe, Ital.*
L-Isoleucine (p.1370·1); L-leucine (p.1370·3); L-valine (p.1381·3).
Hepatic encephalopathy; post-trauma disorders.

Isocaine *Novocol, USA.*
Mepivacaine hydrochloride (p.1317·1).
Corbadrine (p.1599·2) is included in some injections as a vasoconstrictor to diminish absorption and localise the effect of the local anaesthetic.
Local anaesthesia.

Isocal
Mead Johnson, Austral.; Mead Johnson Nutritionals, Canad.; Mead Johnson, Hong Kong; Mead Johnson, Israel; Mead Johnson, NZ; Mead Johnson, Singapore; Mead Johnson Nutritionals, Thai.; Mead Johnson Nutritionals, USA.
A range of preparations for enteral nutrition (p.1350·1).

Isocard
Note. A similar name is used for preparations of different composition (see below).
Sintesa, Belg.†; Schwarz, Fr.; Eastern Pharmaceuticals, UK.
Isosorbide dinitrate (p.915·2).
Angina pectoris.

Iso-Card *Triomed, S.Afr.†.*
Note. A similar name is used for preparations of different composition (see above).
Verapamil hydrochloride (p.989·1).
Angina pectoris; arrhythmias; hypertension.

Isocardide *Sam-On, Israel.*
Isosorbide dinitrate (p.915·2).
Angina pectoris.

Isocef *Recordati, Ital.*
Ceftibuten (p.176·1).
Bacterial infections.

IsoCell *Antonetto, Ital.*
Multivitamin and mineral preparation with plant extracts (p.1350·1).

Isocet *Rugby, USA†.*
Paracetamol (p.71·2); caffeine (p.761·3); butalbital (p.658·3).

Isochinol
Schwarzhaupt, Ger.; Democal, Switz.
Quinisocaine hydrochloride (p.1320·2).
Burns; haemorrhoids; skin disorders; wounds.

Isocillin *Hoechst Marion Roussel, Ger.*
Phenoxymethylpenicillin potassium (p.235·1).
Bacterial infections.

Isoclar *Boniscontro & Gazzone, Ital.*
Heparin sodium (p.902·1).
Thromboembolic disorders.

Isoclor Ciba, USA.
Chlorpheniramine [chlorphenamine] maleate (p.412·1); pseudoephedrine hydrochloride (p.1099·2).
Cold symptoms.

Isoclor Expectorant Fisons, USA.
Codeine phosphate (p.25·2); pseudoephedrine hydrochloride (p.1099·2); guaifenesin (p.1092·2).
Coughs.

Isocolan
Giuliani, Ital.; Synthelabo, Switz.
Macrogol 4000 (p.1630·3); electrolytes (p.1180·1).
Colonic lavage; constipation.

Isocom Nutripharm, USA.
Isometheptene mucate (p.1624·2); dichloralphenazone (p.682·1); paracetamol (p.71·2).
Tension and vascular headaches.

Isocord Asta Medica, Braz.
Isosorbide dinitrate (p.915·2).
Angina pectoris.

Isocort Pharma Clal, Israel.
Isoconazole nitrate (p.387·2); diflucortolone valerate (p.1069·3).
Fungal skin infections.

Isoday Tillotts, Switz.†
Isosorbide dinitrate (p.915·2).
Heart failure; ischaemic heart disease; myocardial infarction.

Isoderm Alkapharm, Singapore.
Skin cleanser.

Isodex Braun, Braz.
Dextran 40 (p.728·3) in electrolytes.
Plasma volume expansion.

Isodine
Faulding, Austral.; Meiji, Jpn†; Boehringer Ingelheim, Mex.; Sidefarma, Port.; Meiji, Thai.
Povidone-iodine (p.1155·1).
Mouth and throat infections; skin, mucous membrane, and instrument disinfection; vaginitis.

Isodinit Hexal, Ger.
Isosorbide dinitrate (p.915·2).
Angina pectoris; heart failure; pulmonary hypertension.

Isodiur Italfarmaco, Spain.
Torasemide (p.985·1) or torasemide sodium (p.985·2).
Hypertension; oedema.

Isodol Magis, Ital.
Nimesulide (p.62·3).
Fever; inflammation; pain.

Isodril Monot, Fr.†
Chlorhexidine gluconate (p.1138·2); phenylephrine hydrochloride (p.1097·1).
Eye disorders.

Isodrink Volchem, Ital.
Isotonic rehydration solution (p.1350·1).

Isodur
Durascan, Denm.; Tika, Swed.; Galen, UK.
Isosorbide mononitrate (p.916·2).
Angina pectoris.

Iso-Eremfat Fatol, Ger.
Rifampicin (p.243·2); isoniazid (p.215·3).
Tuberculosis.

Isoess Bieffe, Ital.
Amino-acid infusion (p.1350·1).
Parenteral nutrition in renal failure.

Isoetam Ferrer, Spain†.
Ethambutol (p.205·3); isoniazid (p.215·3).
Pyridoxine hydrochloride (p.1386·3) is included in this preparation for the prophylaxis of peripheral neuropathy.
Tuberculosis.

Isoflurane Abbott, UK.
Isoflurane (p.1261·1).
Formerly available as Forane.
General anaesthesia.

Isofor Rhone-Poulenc Rorer, S.Afr.†
Isoflurane (p.1261·1).
General anaesthesia.

Isofort Bieffe, Ital.
Amino-acid infusion (p.1350·1).
Parenteral nutrition.

Isofra Bouchara, Fr.
Framycetin sulfate (p.208·2).
Bacterial nose and throat infections.

Isoftal Agepha, Aust.
Naphazoline hydrochloride (p.1095·1).
Conjunctivitis.

Isogaine Clarben, Spain.
Mepivacaine hydrochloride (p.1317·1).
Local anaesthesia.

Isogel
Glaxo Wellcome, NZ; Charwell, Singapore; Pfizer Consumer, UK.
Ispaghula (p.1229·1).
Colostomy control; constipation; diarrhoea; irritable bowel syndrome.

Isogen
Note.This name is used for preparations of different composition.
Wyeth, Austral.†
Isosorbide dinitrate (p.915·2).
Heart failure; ischaemic heart disease.

Pharma Clal, Israel.
Isoconazole nitrate (p.387·2).
Fungal skin infections.

Isoginkgo Merck dura, Ger.
Ginkgo biloba (p.1615·2).
Cerebral circulatory disorders.

Isoglaucon
Agepha, Aust.; Alcon, Ger.; Alcon, Ital.; Alcon Cusi, Spain.
Clonidine hydrochloride (p.860·1).
Glaucoma.

Isogrow Bieffe, Ital.
Amino-acid infusion (p.1350·1).
Parenteral nutrition in neonates.

Isogutt Winzer, Ger.
Monobasic sodium phosphate (p.1193·2); dibasic sodium phosphate (p.1193·2).
Ocular burns.

Isogutt akut Winzer, Ger.
Sodium chloride (p.1196·1).
Eye injuries and burns.

Isogyn Crosara, Ital.
Isoconazole nitrate (p.387·2).
Fungal vulvovaginal infections.

Isohes
Fresenius Kabi, Aust.; Fresenius Kabi, Switz.
Pentastarch (p.732·3).
Haemodilution; plasma volume expansion.

Isohexal Hexal, Austral.
Isotretinoin (p.1115·3).
Acne.

Isoket
Gebro, Aust.; Schwarz, Ger.; Sanol, Ger.; Schwarz, Hong Kong; Schwarz, Irl.; Schwarz, Israel; Knoll, Mex.; Neo-Farmaceutica, Port.; Omnimed, S.Afr.; Ranbaxy, Singapore; Schwarz, Singapore; Schwarz, Switz.; Schwarz, Thai.; Schwarz, UK.
Isosorbide dinitrate (p.915·2).
Angina pectoris; coronary spasm; heart failure; pulmonary hypertension.

Isolan Galagen, USA.
Lactose-free, gluten-free preparation for enteral nutrition (p.1350·1).

Isoliv Bieffe, Ital.
An amino-acid infusion (p.1350·1).
Parenteral nutrition in liver disease.

Isollyl Improved Rugby, USA†.
Aspirin (p.14·2); caffeine (p.761·3); butalbital (p.658·3).
Pain.

Isolyt CT, Ger.†.
Glucose monohydrate; sodium chloride; sodium citrate; potassium chloride (p.1185·2).
Diarrhoea; oral rehydration therapy.

Isolyte
Braun McGaw, Hong Kong; McGaw, NZ; McGaw, USA.
A range of electrolyte infusions with or without glucose (p.1180·1).
Fluid and electrolyte disorders.

Isolyte P 45 E 90 Darrow, Braz.
Sodium lactate; potassium chloride; sodium chloride; calcium chloride; magnesium chloride (p.1185·2).
Oral rehydration therapy.

Isomel Clonmel, Irl.
Isosorbide mononitrate (p.916·2).
Angina pectoris; heart failure.

Isomeride
Servier, Ital.†; Servier, Neth.†.
Dexfenfluramine hydrochloride (p.1508·3).
Obesity.

Isomet M & H, Thai.
Methyldopa (p.927·3).
Hypertension.

Isomide Monmouth, UK.
Disopyramide (p.878·2) or disopyramide phosphate (p.878·2).
Arrhythmias.

Isomil
Abbott, Austral.; Abbott, Braz.; Abbott, Canad.; Abbott, Fin.; Abbott, Hong Kong; Abbott, Israel; Abbott, Ital.; Abbott, Mex.; Abbott, NZ; Abbott, Singapore; Abbott, Thai.; Abbott Nutrition, UK; Ross, USA.
Lactose-free soy protein infant feed (p.1350·1).
Galactosaemia; lactose intolerance; milk intolerance.

Isomil DF Ross, USA.
Lactose-free soy protein infant feed (p.1350·1).
Diarrhoea.

Isomil SF Ross, USA.
Lactose-free, sucrose-free soy protein infant feed (p.1350·1).
Milk intolerance; sucrose intolerance.

Isomol Schwarz, Ger.; Sanol, Ger.
Macrogol 3350 (p.1630·3); electrolytes (p.1180·1).
Constipation.

Isomonat Roche, Aust.
Isosorbide mononitrate (p.916·2).
Heart failure; ischaemic heart disease; pulmonary hypertension.

Isomonit
Hexal, Austral.; United Nordic, Denm.; Hexal, Ger.; Rowex, Irl.
Isosorbide mononitrate (p.916·2).
Angina pectoris; heart failure; pulmonary hypertension.

Isomonoreal Realpharma, Ger.†
Isosorbide mononitrate (p.916·2).
Angina pectoris; heart failure; myocardial infarction; pulmonary hypertension.

Isomyrtine Schwarz, Fr.
Pholcodine (p.1099·1); isomyrtol.
Formerly contained oxytetracycline, isomyrtol, terpineol, and pholcodine.
Coughs.

Isonefrine Tubilux, Ital.
Phenylephrine hydrochloride (p.1097·1).
Production of mydriasis.

Isonitril Rubio, Spain.
Isosorbide mononitrate (p.916·2).
Angina pectoris.

Isopamil General Drugs, Thai.
Verapamil hydrochloride (p.989·1).
Angina pectoris; arrhythmias; hypertension; myocardial infarction.

Isopap Geneva, USA; Marsam, USA.
Isometheptene mucate (p.1624·2); dichloralphenazone (p.682·1); paracetamol (p.71·2).
Tension and vascular headaches.

Isopaque
Nycomed, Belg.†; Nycomed Imaging, Denm.†.
Calcium metrizoate (p.1037·3); magnesium metrizoate (p.1037·3); meglumine metrizoate (p.1037·3); sodium metrizoate (p.1037·3).
Radiographic contrast medium for cystography.

Isopaque Amin Nycomed, Swed.†.
Calcium metrizoate (p.1037·3); meglumine metrizoate (p.1037·3).
Radiographic contrast medium.

Isopaque Cysto
Nycomed Imaging, Norw.†; Nycomed, Swed.†; Nycomed Amersham, UK.
Calcium metrizoate (p.1037·3); magnesium metrizoate (p.1037·3); meglumine metrizoate (p.1037·3); sodium metrizoate (p.1037·3).
Radiographic contrast medium.

Isopen Siam Bheasach, Thai.
Isosorbide mononitrate (p.916·2).
Angina pectoris; heart failure; myocardial infarction.

Isophyl Ego, Austral.†.
Salicylic acid (p.1122·3).
Miliaria rubra; pruritus.

Isophyllen Laevosan, Aust.
Diprophylline (p.764·1).
Cardiovascular disorders; Cheyne Stokes respiration; oedema.

Isoplasmal G Braun, Spain.
Amino-acid, carbohydrate, and electrolyte infusion (p.1350·1).
Parenteral nutrition.

Isopredon Albert-Roussel, Aust.†.
Fluprednisolone (p.1072·2).
Corticosteroid.

Isoprinosina Synthelabo, Ital.†.
Inosine pranobex (p.627·2).
Viral infections.

Isoprinosine
Sanofi Synthelabo, Belg.; Synthelabo, Fr.; Degab, Ger.; Newport, Irl.; Hoechst Marion Roussel, Mex.
Inosine pranobex (p.627·2).
Viral infections.

Isoprochin P Merckle, Ger.
Propyphenazone (p.80·2).
Fever; pain.

Isoprodian
Croma, Aust.; Fatol, Ger.
Isoniazid (p.215·3); protionamide (p.239·3); dapsone (p.196·1).
Mycobacterial infections including leprosy.

Isopront Ferraz, Lynce, Port.
Isosorbide dinitrate (p.915·2).
Angina pectoris; heart failure; myocardial infarction; pulmonary oedema.

Isoptin
Ebewe, Aust.; Knoll, Austral.; Knoll, Canad.; Knoll, Denm.; Knoll, Fin.; Knoll, Ger.; Knoll, Hong Kong; Knoll, Irl.; Knoll, Ital.; Knoll, Neth.; Knoll, Norw.; Knoll, NZ; Knoll, Port.; Knoll, S.Afr.; Knoll, Singapore; Knoll, Swed.; Knoll, Switz.; Knoll, Thai.; Abbott, USA.
Verapamil hydrochloride (p.989·1).
Angina pectoris; arrhythmias; coronary spasm; heart failure; hypertension; hypertrophic cardiomyopathy; myocardial infarction.

Isoptin plus Knoll, Ger.
Verapamil hydrochloride (p.989·1); hydrochlorothiazide (p.907·3).
Hypertension.

Isoptine
Knoll, Belg.; Knoll, Fr.
Verapamil hydrochloride (p.989·1).
Angina pectoris; arrhythmias; hypertension; myocardial infarction.

Isopto Alkaline
Alcon, Fin.; Alcon, Irl.; Alcon, UK; Alcon, USA†.
Hypromellose (p.1501·3).
Dry eyes.

Isopto B 12 Alcon Cusi, Spain.
Cyanocobalamin (p.1388·1).
Corneal damage.

Isopto Biotic Alcon, Swed.
Polymyxin B sulfate (p.238·1); neomycin sulfate (p.228·1); phenylephrine hydrochloride (p.1097·1).
Bacterial eye infections.

Isopto Carpina Alcon Cusi, Spain.
Pilocarpine hydrochloride (p.1422·3).
Glaucoma; ocular hypertension; reversal of mydriasis.

Isopto Carpine
Alcon, Austral.; Alcon, Belg.; Alcon, Braz.; Alcon, Canad.; Alcon, Fin.; Alcon, Hong Kong; Alcon, Israel; Alcon, Ital.; Alcon, Norw.; Alcon, NZ; Alcon, S.Afr.; Alcon, Switz.†; Alcon, Thai.; Alcon, UK†; Alcon, USA.
Pilocarpine hydrochloride (p.1422·3).
Glaucoma; ocular hypertension; reversal of mydriasis.

Isopto Cetamide
Alcon, Belg.; Alcon, USA.
Sulfacetamide sodium (p.250·3).
Eye infections.

Isopto Cetapred
Alcon, Belg.; Alcon, Braz.; Alcon, USA.
Prednisolone acetate (p.1078·1); sulfacetamide sodium (p.250·3).
Infected eye disorders.

Isopto Dex Alcon, Ger.
Dexamethasone (p.1067·1).
Eye disorders.

Isopto Fenicol
Alcon, Hong Kong; Alcon, NZ; Alcon, Singapore; Alcon Cusi, Spain; Alcon, Swed.
Chloramphenicol (p.179·1).
Bacterial eye infections.

Isopto Flucon
Alcon, Ger.; Alcon Cusi, Spain.
Fluorometholone (p.1072·1).
Eye disorders.

Isopto Fluid Alcon, Ger.
Hypromellose (p.1501·3).
Dry eyes.

Isopto Frin
Alcon, Austral.; Sanofi Synthelabo, Belg.; Alcon, Irl.; Alcon, NZ; Alcon, Singapore; Alcon, UK; Alcon, USA†.
Phenylephrine hydrochloride (p.1097·1).
Eye fatigue; eye irritation; wetting agent for hard contact lenses.

Isopto Karbakolin Alcon, Swed.
Carbachol (p.1416·1).
Glaucoma.

Isopto Max Alcon, Ger.
Dexamethasone (p.1067·1); neomycin sulfate (p.228·1); polymyxin B sulfate (p.238·1).
Infected eye disorders.

Isopto Maxidex
Alcon, Norw.; Alcon, Swed.
Dexamethasone (p.1067·1).
Inflammatory eye disorders.

Isopto Naturale Alcon, Ger.
Dextran 70 (p.729·2); hypromellose (p.1501·3).
Dry eyes.

Isopto Pilomin Alcon, Ger.
Pilocarpine hydrochloride (p.1422·3); physostigmine salicylate (p.1421·3).
Glaucoma.

Isopto Plain
Alcon, Fin.; Alcon, Irl.; Alcon, Swed.; Alcon, UK; Alcon, USA.
Hypromellose (p.1501·3).
Dry eyes.

Isopto Tears
Alcon, Austral.; Alcon, Belg.; Alcon, Canad.; Alcon, Hong Kong; Alcon, NZ; Alcon, Singapore; Alcon, Switz.; Alcon, Thai.; Alcon, USA.
Hypromellose (p.1501·3).
Dry eyes.

Isopuramin Bieffe, Ital.
A range of amino-acid infusions (p.1350·1).
Parenteral nutrition.

Iso-Puren Isis Puren, Ger.
Isosorbide dinitrate (p.915·2).
Heart failure; ischaemic heart disease.

Isoram Bieffe, Ital.
L-Arginine (p.1353·3); L-isoleucine (p.1370·1); L-leucine (p.1370·3); L-valine (p.1381·3).
Hepatic encephalopathy; post-trauma disorders.

Isorbid Wyeth, Mex.
Isosorbide dinitrate (p.915·2).
Angina pectoris; heart failure.

Isordil
Wyeth-Ayerst, Austral.; Wyeth Lederle, Belg.; Wyeth, Braz.; Wyeth-Ayerst, Canad.; Wyeth-Ayerst, Hong Kong; Shire, Irl.; Wyeth, Neth.; Aspen, S.Afr.; Wyeth, Singapore; Wyeth-Ayerst, Thai.; Monmouth, UK; Wyeth-Ayerst, USA.
Isosorbide dinitrate (p.915·2).
Angina pectoris; heart failure; myocardial infarction.

Isorel Novipharm, Aust.
Mistletoe (p.1636·2) from fir trees, apple trees or pine trees.
Malignant neoplasms.

Isorem
Remedica, Hong Kong; Remedica, Thai.
Isosorbide dinitrate (p.915·2).
Angina pectoris; heart failure.

Isoren Bieffe, Ital.
Amino-acid infusion (p.1350·1).
Parenteral nutrition in renal failure.

Isoritmon Basi, Port.
Chloroprocainamide.
Arrhythmias.

Isorythm Lipha Sante, Fr.
Disopyramide (p.878·2) or disopyramide phosphate (p.878·2).
Arrhythmias.

Isosal Sanochemia, Aust.
Cream: Salicylamide (p.82·1).

Topical fluid: Salicylamide (p.82·1); camphor (p.1589·3).
Musculoskeletal, joint, and peri-articular disorders; neuralgia; soft-tissue injury.

Isoselect Bieffe, Ital.
Amino-acid infusion (p.1350·1).
Hepatic encephalopathy; parenteral nutrition.

Isosource *Novartis Nutrition, Canad.; Novartis Nutrition, Hong Kong; Novartis Nutrition, Singapore; Sandoz Nutrition, USA.*
A range of preparations for enteral nutrition (p.1350·1).

Isostad *Stada, Aust.*
Isosorbide dinitrate (p.915·2).
Angina pectoris; heart failure; hypertension; myocardial infarction.

Isostenase *Azupharma, Ger.*
Isosorbide dinitrate (p.915·2).
Angina pectoris; heart failure; myocardial infarction; pulmonary hypertension.

Isosteril *Fresenius Kabi, Switz.*
Electrolyte infusion with glucose (p.1180·1).
Fluid and electrolyte disorders.

Isotamine *ICN, Canad.*
Isoniazid (p.215·3).
Tuberculosis.

Isotard
Note. This name is used for preparations of different composition.
CTI, Israel.
Isosorbide dinitrate (p.915·2).
Angina pectoris.

Strakan, UK.
Isosorbide mononitrate (p.916·2).
Angina pectoris.

Isotard MC *Novo Nordisk, Austral.*
Note. A similar name is used for preparations of different composition (see above).
Isophane insulin injection (bovine, monocomponent) (p.324·1).
Diabetes mellitus.

Isotein HN *Sandoz Nutrition, USA.*
Lactose-free, gluten-free preparation for enteral nutrition (p.1350·1).

Isoten *Wyeth Lederle, Belg.*
Bisoprolol fumarate (p.850·1).
Angina pectoris; cardiac hyperkinetic syndrome; hypertension.

Isotol *Diaco, Ital.*
Mannitol (p.924·3).
Raised intra-ocular pressure; raised intracranial pressure.

Isotone Kochsalz *Braun, Ger.; Pharmacia Upjohn, Ger.*
Sodium chloride (p.1196·1).
Fluid and electrolyte disorders.

Isotrate
Note. This name is used for preparations of different composition.
Bioglan, Hong Kong; Helsinn Birex, Irl.; Bioglan, Irl.; Bioglan, Singapore; Bioglan, UK.
Isosorbide mononitrate (p.916·2).
Angina pectoris.

Berlin Pharm, Thai.; Hauck, USA†.
Isosorbide dinitrate (p.915·2).
Angina pectoris.

Isotrex *Sanova, Aust.; Stiefel, Austral.; Stiefel, Canad.; Stiefel, Denm.; Stiefel, Fr.; Stiefel, Ger.; Stiefel, Hong Kong; Stiefel, Israel; Stiefel, Ital.; Stiefel, Mex.; Stiefel, NZ; Stiefel, Port.; Stiefel, S.Afr.; Stiefel, Singapore; Stiefel, Spain; Stiefel, Thai.; Stiefel, UK.*
Isotretinoin (p.1115·3).
Acne.

Isotrex Eritromicina *Stiefel, Spain.*
Isotretinoin (p.1115·3); erythromycin (p.201·2).
Acne.

Isotrexin *Stiefel, Ger.; Stiefel, Irl.; Stiefel, Ital.; Stiefel, Port.; Stiefel, UK.*
Isotretinoin (p.1115·3); erythromycin (p.201·2).
Acne.

Isotrim *Ghimas, Ital.†.*
Co-trimoxazole (p.193·3).
Bacterial infections.

Iso-Triraupin *Roche, Thai.*
Butizide (p.853·1); reserpine (p.967·3); rescinnamine (p.967·3); raubasine (p.967·2).
Hypertension.

Isovir *Sanofi Synthelabo, Port.*
Inosine pranobex (p.627·2).
Viral infections.

Isovist *Schering, Aust.; Schering, Denm.; Schering, Fin.; Schering, Ger.; Schering, Ital.†; Schering, Neth.; Schering, Norw.†; Schering, NZ; Schering, S.Afr.; Schering, Swed.†; Schering, Switz.; Schering, UK.*
Iotrolan (p.1036·3).
Radiographic contrast medium.

Isovorin *Wyeth Lederle, Aust.; Wyeth Lederle, Denm.; Wyeth Lederle, Fin.; Lederle, Neth.; Wyeth Lederle, Norw.; Wyeth, S.Afr.; Cyanamid, Spain; Wyeth Lederle, Swed.; Lederle, Switz.†; Wyeth, UK.*
Calcium levofolinate (p.1363·1).
Adjunct to fluorouracil therapy for colorectal cancer; antidote to folic acid antagonists; reduction of high-dose methotrexate toxicity.

Isovue *HCP, Austral.; Squibb Diagnostics, Canad.†; Squibb Diagnostics, USA.*
Iopamidol (p.1035·2).
Radiographic contrast medium.

Isox *Senosiain, Mex.*
Itraconazole (p.387·2).
Fungal infections.

Isoxan *NHS, Fr.*
Multivitamin and mineral preparation (p.1350·1).

I-Soyalac *Nutricia-Luma Lindar, USA.*
Corn- and lactose-free soy protein infant feed (p.1350·1).

Isozid *Fatol, Ger.*
Isoniazid (p.215·3).
Tuberculosis.

Isozid comp N *Fatol, Ger.*
Isoniazid (p.215·3).
Pyridoxine hydrochloride (p.1386·3) is included in this preparation for the prophylaxis of peripheral neuropathy.
Formerly known as Isozid-compositum.
Tuberculosis.

Isozid-H *Gebro, Aust.*
Hexetidine (p.1146·3).
Skin disinfection.

Ispagel *Richmond Pharmaceuticals, UK.*
Ispaghula (p.1229·1).

Ispenoral *Rosen, Ger.*
Phenoxymethylpenicillin potassium (p.235·1).
Bacterial infections.

Isquebral *Iquinosa, Spain.*
Dihydroergocristine mesilate (p.1603·2); raubasine (p.967·2).
Cerebral and peripheral vascular disorders; head injury.

Issium *Lifepharma, Ital.*
Flunarizine hydrochloride (p.418·1).
Migraine; vertigo.

Istamyl *Monot, Fr.†.*
Isothipendyl hydrochloride (p.419·2).
Hypersensitivity reactions.

Isteropac *Bracco, Switz.*
Iodamide (p.1034·1).
Contrast medium for hysterosalpingography.

Isteropac ER *Bracco, Ital.*
Meglumine iodamide (p.1034·1).
Contrast medium for hysterosalpingography.

Istin *Pfizer, Irl.; Pfizer, UK.*
Amlodipine besilate (p.838·3).
Angina pectoris; hypertension.

Istivac *Aventis, Port.*
An inactivated influenza vaccine (p.1544·3).
Active immunisation.

Istix *Sons, Mex.*
Tetracycline (p.258·3).
Bacterial infections.

Istopar *Disperga, Aust.*
Mineral preparation with liver extract and thiamine hydrochloride (p.1350·1).
Iron-deficiency anaemia; tonic.

Istopril *Condad Synto, Thai.*
Enalapril maleate (p.883·3).
Heart failure; hypertension.

Isudrine *Boehringer Ingelheim, Fr.*
Aluminium phosphate (p.1211·3); magnesium oxide (p.1233·2).
Gastrointestinal disorders.

Isugran *Synpharma, Aust.*
Mistletoe (p.1636·2).
Circulatory disorders.

Isuhuman Basal *Hoechst Marion Roussel, Neth.†; Hoeport, Port.; Hoechst Marion Roussel, Swed.†.*
Isophane insulin injection (human) (p.324·1).
Diabetes mellitus.

Isuhuman Comb 25/75, 50/50 *Hoechst Marion Roussel, Swed.†.*
Mixtures of insulin injection (human, emp) and isophane insulin injection (human, emp) respectively in the proportions indicated (p.324·1).
Diabetes mellitus.

Isuhuman Comb 15, Comb 25, Comb 50 *Hoechst Marion Roussel, Neth.†; Hoeport, Port.*
Mixtures of isophane insulin injection (human) 85%, 75% and 50% and neutral insulin injection (human) 15%, 25% and 50% respectively (p.324·1).
Diabetes mellitus.

Isuhuman Infusat *Hoechst Marion Roussel, Neth.; Hoechst Marion Roussel, Swed.†.*
Insulin injection (human) (p.324·1).
Diabetes mellitus.

Isuhuman Rapid *Hoechst Marion Roussel, Neth.†; Hoeport, Port.; Hoechst Marion Roussel, Swed.†.*
Insulin injection (human) (p.324·1).
Diabetes mellitus.

Isuprel *Abbott, Austral.; Abbott, Belg.; Sanofi Synthelabo, Canad.; Abbott, Fr.; Sanofi Winthrop, Israel; Abbott, NZ; Abbott, Singapore; Abbott, Thai.; Sanofi Winthrop, USA.*
Isoprenaline hydrochloride (p.914·3).
Bronchospasm in anaesthesia; heart block; heart failure; pulmonary hypertension in anaesthesia; shock; Stokes-Adams syndrome.

Itagil *Dumex, Port.*
Buspirone hydrochloride (p.657·2).
Anxiety.

Italdermol *Italmex, Mex.*
Wheat germ; phenoxyethanol (p.1153·3).
Burns; cervicitis; skin irritation; ulcers; vulvovaginitis; wounds.

Italmicin *Italmex, Mex.*
Chloramphenicol (p.179·1).
Bacterial infections.

Italnik *Italmex, Mex.*
Ciprofloxacin (p.182·3).
Bacterial infections.

Italprid *Teofarma, Ital.*
Tiapride hydrochloride (p.709·1).
Alcohol withdrawal syndrome; behaviour disorders; gastrointestinal motility disorders; headache; movement disorders.

Ital-Ultra *Italmex, Mex.*
Ambroxol hydrochloride (p.1084·3).
Respiratory-tract congestion.

Italviron *Italmex, Mex.*
Asparagine; acetylglutamine; pyridoxine; phosphorylserine (p.1350·1).
Memory disorders.

Itax Antipoux *Pierre Fabre, Fr.†.*
Topical spray: Phenothrin (p.1436·2); tetramethrin (p.1437·3); piperonyl butoxide (p.1436·2).
Pediculosis.

Pierre Fabre Sante, Fr.
Shampoo: Phenothrin (p.1436·2).
Pediculosis.

Itax Preventif *Pierre Fabre, Fr.†.*
Repellent 3535.
Head lice repellent.

ITC *Asta Medica, Belg.†.*
Sodium iodide (p.1522·3); potassium iodide (p.1522·3); calcium chloride (p.1188·1); sodium thiosulfate (p.1024·2).
Cataracts.

Itch-X *Ascher, USA.*
Pramocaine hydrochloride (p.1318·2); benzyl alcohol (p.1135·2).
Local anaesthesia.

Item Antipoux *Gandhour, Fr.*
Lotion; shampoo: Phenothrin (p.1436·2).
Pediculosis.

Topical spray: Diethyltoluamide (p.1431·2).
Head lice repellent.

Iteor *Pierre Fabre Sante, Fr.†.*
A range of vitamin and mineral preparations (p.1350·1).

Itinerol B₆ *Vifor, Switz.*
Meclozine hydrochloride (p.420·3); pyridoxine hydrochloride (p.1386·3); caffeine (p.761·3).
Nausea; vomiting.

Itorex *Chong Kun Dang, Ital.*
Cefuroxime sodium (p.178·2).
Bacterial infections.

Itranax *Cilag, Braz.; Cilag, Mex.*
Itraconazole (p.387·2).
Fungal infections.

Itrin *Abbott, Ital.*
Terazosin hydrochloride (p.980·1).
Hypertension.

Itrop *Boehringer Ingelheim, Aust.; Boehringer Ingelheim, Ger.*
Ipratropium bromide (p.766·1).
Arrhythmias.

Iuvacor *Inverni della Beffa, Ital.*
Ubidecarenone (p.1677·1).
Cardiac disorders; co-enzyme Q₁₀ deficiency.

Ivacin *Wyeth Lederle, Denm.; Wyeth Lederle, Swed.*
Piperacillin sodium (p.236·1).
Bacterial infections.

Ivadal *Sanofi Synthelabo, Aust.; Grunenthal, Fr.†; Vita, Ital.†.*
Zolpidem tartrate (p.712·2).
Insomnia.

I-Valex *Ross, USA.*
A range of leucine-free preparations for enteral nutrition including an infant feed (p.1350·1).
Leucine catabolism disorders.

Ivamix *Fresenius Kabi, Norw.*
Amino-acid and lipid (from soya oil (p.1378·1)) infusion (p.1350·1).
Parenteral nutrition.

Ivarest *Blistex, USA.*
Calamine (p.1111·3); diphenhydramine hydrochloride (p.416·1).
Formerly contained calamine and benzocaine.
Minor skin irritation.

Iveegam *Baxter, Canad.; Immuno, USA.*
A normal immunoglobulin (p.1551·3).
Hypogammaglobulinaemia; Kawasaki syndrome; passive immunisation.

Ivel *Knoll, Mex.*
Lupulus (p.1629·3); valerian (p.1678·3).
Anxiety; insomnia.

Ivel Schlaf *Kanoldt, Ger.*
Lupulus (p.1629·3); valerian (p.1678·3).
Restlessness; sleep disorders.

Ivelip *Baxter, Belg.; Baxter, Fr.; Clintec, Israel; Clintec, Ital.; Baxter, Spain; Baxter, UK.*
Soya oil (p.1378·1).
Contains egg lecithin.
Lipid infusion for parenteral nutrition.

Ivemix *Clintec, Fr.†.*
Amino-acid, lipid (from soya oil (p.1378·1)), and glucose infusion (p.1350·1).
Contains egg lecithin.
Parenteral nutrition.

Ivepaque *Nycomed, Fr.*
Iopentol (p.1035·3).
Radiographic contrast medium.

Ivofol *Juste, Spain.*
Propofol (p.1265·3).
General anaesthesia; sedative.

Ivracain *Sintetica, Switz.*
Chloroprocaine hydrochloride (p.1308·3).
Local anaesthesia.

Ivy Block *Enviroderm, USA.*
Bentoquatam (p.1111·1).
Prophylaxis against poison ivy, oak-, or sumac-induced contact dermatitis.

Ivy Dry *Ivy Corp, USA.*
Zinc acetate (p.1398·1).
Minor skin irritation.

Ivy-Chex *JMI, USA.*
Polyvinylpyrrolidone vinylacetate copolymers; methyl salicylate (p.55·1).
Minor skin irritation.

Ivy-Rid *Roberts, USA.*
Polyvinylpyrrolidone vinylacetate copolymers.
Minor skin irritation.

Iwamet *Masa, Thai.*
Cimetidine (p.1216·3).
Gastro-oesophageal reflux; hypersensitivity reactions; peptic ulcer; Zollinger-Ellison syndrome.

Iwazin *Masa, Thai.*
Tyrothricin (p.267·1); benzethonium chloride (p.1134·2); benzocaine (p.1306·2).
Mouth and throat infections.

Ixel *Pierre Fabre, Aust.; Pierre Fabre, Fr.; Pierre Fabre, Israel; Pierre Fabre, Port.*
Milnacipran hydrochloride (p.299·1).
Depression.

Ixoten *Asta Medica, Aust.; Asta Medica, Ger.*
Trofosfamide (p.577·1).
Malignant neoplasms.

Iyafin *Nakorn, Thai.*
Junior syrup: Dextromethorphan hydrobromide (p.1087·3); pseudoephedrine hydrochloride (p.1099·2); chlorpheniramine [chlorphenamine] maleate (p.412·1); guaifenesin (p.1092·2); sodium citrate (p.1186·2).

Syrup: Dextromethorphan hydrobromide (p.1087·3); pseudoephedrine hydrochloride (p.1099·2); chlorpheniramine [chlorphenamine] maleate (p.412·1); guaifenesin (p.1092·2); ammonium chloride (p.1085·2); sodium citrate (p.1186·2).

Tablets: Dextromethorphan hydrobromide (p.1087·3); phenylpropanolamine hydrochloride (p.1098·1); chlorpheniramine [chlorphenamine] maleate (p.412·1); guaifenesin (p.1092·2).
Coughs.

Izacef *Intramed, S.Afr.*
Cefazolin sodium (p.164·3).
Bacterial infections.

Izadima *Pisa, Mex.*
Ceftazidime (p.174·3).
Bacterial infections.

Izo *Pond's, Thai.*
Isosorbide dinitrate (p.915·2).
Angina pectoris.

Jaa Pyral *Jaapharm, Canad.*
Pyrantel embonate (p.108·1).

Jaaps Health Salt *Askit, UK.*
Sodium bicarbonate (p.1186·2); tartaric acid (p.1669·2); sodium potassium tartrate (p.1250·1).
Constipation; dyspepsia; heartburn.

Jaba B₁₂ *Jaba, Port.*
Cobamamide (p.1388·3).
Anaemias; liver disorders; neuralgia; neuritis.

Jabasulide *Jaba, Port.*
Nimesulide (p.62·3).
Fever; inflammation; pain.

Jabon Antiseptico Asens *Asens, Spain†.*
Hexachlorophene (p.1146·1).
Skin disinfection.

Jack and Jill Children's Formula *Buckley, Canad.*
Dextromethorphan hydrobromide (p.1087·3); chlorpheniramine maleate (p.412·1).
Formerly known as Jack and Jill Children's DM Formula Cough Liquid.
Cold symptoms; coughs.

Jack and Jill Cough Syrup *Buckley, Canad.*
Guaifenesin (p.1092·2); mepyramine maleate (p.421·1).
Cold symptoms; coughs.

Jack & Jill Rub *Buckley, Canad.*
Camphor (p.1589·3); menthol (p.1632·3); eucalyptol (p.1609·2).
Cold symptoms.

Jackson's All Fours *Anglian, UK.*
Guaifenesin (p.1092·2).
Coughs.

Jackson's Bronchial Balsam *Anglian, UK.*
Guaifenesin (p.1092·2).
Coughs.

Jackson's Febrifuge *Anglian, UK.*
Sodium salicylate (p.84·2).
Cold and influenza symptoms; musculoskeletal, joint, and soft-tissue disorders.

The symbol † denotes a preparation no longer actively marketed

Jackson's Lemon Linctus *Anglian, UK.*
Glycerol (p.1616·3); honey (p.1366·2).
Coughs; sore throat.

Jackson's Troublesome Coughs *Anglian, UK.*
Ipecacuanha (p.1093·1); glycerol (p.1616·3); honey (p.1366·2).
Coughs.

Jacutin
Hermal, Aust.; Hermal, Ger.; Boots Healthcare, Switz.; Boots, Thai.; Hermal, Thai.
Lindane (p.1434·1).
Pediculosis; scabies.

Jacutin N *Hermal, Ger.*
Bioallethrin (p.1428·3); piperonyl butoxide (p.1436·2).
Pediculosis.

Jadelle *Leiras, Fin.*
Levonorgestrel (p.1486·2).
Progestogen-only contraceptive implant.

Jadit *Hoechst Marion Roussel, Braz.*
Buclosamide (p.381·1); salicylic acid (p.1122·3).
Fungal skin infections.

Jaikal *S & K, Ger.*
Sodium thiosulfate (p.1024·2); salicylic acid (p.1122·3); resorcinol (p.1122·2).
Acne.

Jaikin N *Galderma, Ger.*
Dimethicone (p.1410·1).
Acne.

Jakava *Queisser, Ger.*
Kava (p.1625·3).
Agitation; anxiety.

Jalapa comp *Pfluger, Ger.*
Homoeopathic preparation.

Jalovis *Coli, Ital.†.*
Hyaluronidase (p.1620·3); chlorhexidine hydrochloride (p.1138·2).
Bruising; chilblains; haemorrhoids; skin ulceration; wounds.

Jaluran *Pfizer, Ital.*
Hyaluronidase (p.1620·3).
Facilitates subcutaneous absorption of drugs.

Jamaican Sarsaparilla *Potter's, UK.*
Sarsaparilla root (p.1661·1); capsicum (p.1591·1); liquorice (p.1231·2); peppermint oil (p.1243·3).
Skin disorders.

Jamylene *Expanpharm, Fr.*
Docusate sodium (p.1223·1).
Constipation.

Janacin *Biolab, Thai.*
Norfloxacin (p.232·1).
Bacterial infections.

Janimine *Abbott, USA†.*
Imipramine hydrochloride (p.291·1).
Depression; nocturnal enuresis.

Japan Freeze-Dried Tuberculin *Vaccina, S.Afr.*
Tuberculin purified protein derivative (p.1675·3).
Tuberculosis test.

Japanol *Liebermann, Ger.*
Mint oil (p.1636·2).
Cold symptoms; dyspepsia; myalgia.

Japomin *Bano, Aust.*
Peppermint oil (p.1243·3).
Catarrh; gastrointestinal disorders; headache.

Jarabe Manceau *Alcor, Spain.*
Senna (p.1248·2); coriander (p.1599·2); pyrus malus.
Constipation.

Jarabe Manzanas Siken *Diafarm, Spain.*
Senna (p.1248·2); coriander (p.1599·2); prune (p.1245·1); frangula (p.1227·1); fennel (p.1610·1).
Constipation.

Jardin *Rolab, S.Afr.*
Dothiepin [dosulepin] hydrochloride (p.283·2).
Depression.

Jarsin *Kwizda, Aust.; Lichtwer, Ger.; Medichemie Bioline, Switz.*
Hypericum (p.290·2).
Agitation; anxiety; depression; insomnia; tension.

Jasicholin N *Bolder, Ger.*
Butinoline phosphate (p.1587·3); dimethicone (p.1249·2).
Gastrointestinal disorders.

Jasimenth CN *Bolder, Ger.*
Dequalinium chloride (p.1143·1); ascorbic acid (p.1389·3).
Mouth and throat disorders.

Jatroneural
Procter & Gamble, Aust.; Procter & Gamble, Ger.†.
Trifluoperazine hydrochloride (p.710·3).
Anxiety disorders.

Jatropur *Procter & Gamble, Ger.†.*
Triamterene (p.986·1).
Oedema.

Jatrosom N *Esparma, Ger.*
Tranylcypromine sulfate (p.309·3).
Depression.

Jatrox *Procter & Gamble, Ger.†.*
Bismuth salicylate (p.1213·1).
Gastritis; peptic ulcer; traveller's diarrhoea.

Jecobiase *Pionneau, Fr.*
Sodium sulfate (p.1250·1); sodium citrate (p.1186·2); sodium bicarbonate (p.1186·2); magnesium chloride (p.1190·3).
Gastrointestinal disorders.

Jecopeptol *Alpharma, Fr.*
Aluminium hydroxide (p.1210·3); calcium carbonate (p.1215·1); magnesium hydroxide (p.1233·1); sodium bicarbonate (p.1186·2); boldo (p.1585·3); kinkeliba (p.1626·1); euonymus (p.1225·3).
Digestive disorders.

Jectofer
Astra, Aust.; AstraZeneca, Canad.; AstraZeneca, Denm.; Astra, Ger.; Astra, Irl.; Astra, Neth.; AstraZeneca, Norw.; Astra, Swed.; Astra-Zeneca, UK.
Iron sorbitol (p.1369·2).
Iron deficiency; iron-deficiency anaemia.

Jedipin
Jenapharm, Ger.; Jenapharm, Thai.
Nifedipine (p.940·1).
Angina pectoris; hypertension; myocardial infarction; Raynaud's syndrome.

Jekovit *Orion, Fin.*
Ergocalciferol (p.1391·2).
Vitamin D deficiency.

Jellin *Grunenthal, Ger.*
Fluocinolone acetonide (p.1071·1).
Skin disorders.

Jellin polyvalent *Grunenthal, Ger.*
Fluocinolone acetonide (p.1071·1); neomycin sulfate (p.228·1); nystatin (p.392·2).
Infected skin disorders.

Jellin-Neomycin *Grunenthal, Ger.*
Fluocinolone acetonide (p.1071·1); neomycin sulfate (p.228·1).
Infected skin disorders.

Jellisoft *Grunenthal, Ger.*
Fluocinolone acetonide (p.1071·1).
Skin disorders.

Jellisoft-Neomycin *Grunenthal, Ger.*
Fluocinolone acetonide (p.1071·1); neomycin sulfate (p.228·1).
Infected skin disorders.

Jelonet
Smith & Nephew, Austral.; Smith & Nephew, Fr.; Smith & Nephew, Ital.; Smith & Nephew, S.Afr.; Smith & Nephew, UK.
Soft paraffin (p.1407·3).
Wound dressing.

Jemalt 13+13 *Wander Health Care, Switz.*
Multivitamin and mineral preparation (p.1350·1).

Jemizym *Jean-Marie, Hong Kong.*
Muramidase hydrochloride (p.1638·1).
Haemorrhage; respiratory-tract disorders.

Jenabroxol *Jenapharm, Ger.†.*
Ambroxol hydrochloride (p.1084·3).
Respiratory disorders associated with viscous or excessive mucus.

Jenabroxol comp *Jenapharm, Ger.*
Doxycycline hyclate (p.200·1); ambroxol hydrochloride (p.1084·3).
Respiratory-tract infections.

Jenacard *Jenapharm, Ger.*
Isosorbide dinitrate (p.915·2).
Angina pectoris; heart failure; pulmonary hypertension.

Jenacillin A *Jenapharm, Ger.*
Benzylpenicillin (p.157·2); procaine penicillin [procaine benzylpenicillin] (p.239·2).
Bacterial infections.

Jenacillin O *Jenapharm, Ger.*
Procaine penicillin [procaine benzylpenicillin] (p.239·2).
Bacterial infections.

Jenacillin V *Jenapharm, Ger.*
Phenoxymethylpenicillin potassium (p.235·1).
Bacterial infections.

Jenacyclin *Jenapharm, Ger.*
Doxycycline (p.200·1).
Bacterial infections.

Jenacysteine *Jenapharm, Ger.†.*
Acetylcysteine (p.1082·3).
Respiratory disorders associated with viscous or excessive mucus.

Jenafenac *Jenapharm, Ger.*
Diclofenac sodium (p.30·3).
Inflammation; musculoskeletal, joint, and soft-tissue disorders.

Jenamazol *Jenapharm, Ger.*
Clotrimazole (p.382·1).
Corynebacterium infections; fungal infections.

Jenametidin *Jenapharm, Ger.†.*
Cimetidine (p.1216·3).
Aspiration syndrome; gastro-oesophageal reflux; peptic ulcer; Zollinger-Ellison syndrome.

Jenamicin *Hauck, USA†.*
Gentamicin sulfate (p.210·1).
Bacterial infections.

Jenamoxazol *Jenapharm, Ger.†.*
Co-trimoxazole (p.193·3).
Bacterial infections.

Jenampin *Jenapharm, Ger.†.*
Ampicillin trihydrate (p.151·1).
Bacterial infections.

Jenapamil *Jenapharm, Ger.*
Verapamil hydrochloride (p.989·1).
Angina pectoris; hypertension; tachycardia.

Jenapirox *Jenapharm, Ger.*
Piroxicam (p.79·1).
Musculoskeletal and joint disorders.

Jenaprofen *Jenapharm, Ger.*
Ibuprofen (p.64·2).
Fever; gout; inflammation; musculoskeletal, joint, and soft-tissue disorders; pain.

Jenapurinol *Jenapharm, Ger.*
Allopurinol (p.397·2).
Gout; hyperuricaemia; renal calculi.

Jenaspiron *Jenapharm, Ger.*
Spironolactone (p.973·2).
Ascites; hyperaldosteronism; oedema.

Jenatacin *Jenapharm, Ger.†.*
Indometacin (p.44·3).
Gout; musculoskeletal, joint, and soft-tissue disorders; pain.

Jenatenol *Jenapharm, Ger.*
Atenolol (p.841·3).
Arrhythmias; hypertension; ischaemic heart disease.

Jenateren comp *Jenapharm, Ger.*
Triamterene (p.986·1); hydrochlorothiazide (p.907·3).
Heart failure; hypertension; oedema.

Jenest *Organon, USA.*
21 Tablets, norethisterone (p.1485·1); ethinylestradiol (p.1476·2); 7 tablets, inert.
Biphasic oral contraceptive.

Jenoxifen *Jenapharm, Ger.*
Tamoxifen citrate (p.571·1).
Breast cancer.

Jephagynon *Jenapharm, Ger.*
Estradiol benzoate (p.1473·1); progesterone (p.1488·3).
Amenorrhoea.

Jephoxin *Jenapharm, Ger.*
Amoxicillin trihydrate (p.149·2).
Bacterial infections.

Jeprolol *Jenapharm, Ger.*
Metoprolol tartrate (p.931·2).
Arrhythmias; hypertension; migraine; myocardial infarction.

Jeridin *Berk, UK†.*
Isosorbide dinitrate (p.915·2).
Angina pectoris; heart failure.

Jestryl *Chauvin ankerpharm, Ger.*
Carbachol (p.1416·1).
Glaucoma; production of miosis.

Jetepar
Rotta, Hong Kong; Rotta, Singapore.
Betaine glucuronate (p.1584·3); diolamine glucuronate (p.1604·1); nicotinamide ascorbate.
Biliary-tract disorders; liver disorders.

Jets *Freeda, USA.*
Multivitamin preparation with lysine (p.1350·1).

JE-Vaccine *Kaketsuken, Thai.*
An inactivated Japanese encephalitis vaccine, Beijing strain (p.1539·2).
Active immunisation.

JE-Vax
CSL, Austral.; Connaught, Canad.; Pasteur Merieux, USA.
A Japanese encephalitis vaccine (p.1539·2).
Active immunisation.

Jevity
Abbott, Austral.; Abbott, Braz.; Abbott, Canad.; Abbott, Hong Kong; Abbott, Irl.; Ross, Israel; Abbott, NZ; Abbott, Singapore; Abbott, Thai.; Abbott Nutrition, UK; Ross, USA.
Preparation for enteral nutrition (p.1350·1).

Jezil *Alphapharm, Austral.*
Gemfibrozil (p.896·2).
Hyperlipidaemias.

JHP Rodler Tropfen *Woelm, Ger.*
Mint oil (p.1636·2).
Cold symptoms; gastrointestinal disorders; headache.

Jiffy Corn Plasters *Brovar, S.Afr.†.*
Salicylic acid (p.1122·3).
Calluses; corns; warts.

Jiffy Toothache Drops *Block, Canad.*
Benzocaine (p.1306·2); eugenol (p.1609·3).
Toothache.

Jinda *Lichtwer, Ger.*
Cimicifuga (p.1595·2).
Menopausal disorders.

Jodetten *Henning, Ger.*
Potassium iodide (p.1522·3).
Iodine-deficiency disorders.

Jodid *Merck, Ger.; Ratiopharm, Ger.; Verla, Ger.*
Potassium iodide (p.1522·3).
Iodine-deficiency disorders.

Jodieci *Esoform, Ital.*
Povidone-iodine (p.1155·1); alcohol (p.1130·3).
Infected skin disorders; disinfection of skin and superficial wounds.

Jodix *Orion, Fin.*
Potassium iodide (p.1522·3).
Protection of the thyroid from radio-iodine.

Jodlauge, Tolzer *Jodquellen, Ger.*
Anions: chloride, bromide, iodide, bicarbonate; cations: sodium, magnesium, potassium, calcium.
Circulatory disorders.

jodminerase *GN, Ger.†.*
Potassium iodide (p.1522·3).
Iodine-deficiency disorders.

Jodobac
Note. This name is used for preparations of different composition.
Bode, Germ.
Povidone-iodine (p.1155·1).
Catheter care; disinfection of the skin, mucous membranes, and hands; wounds.

Beiersdorf, Switz.
Propyl alcohol (p.1155·3); povidone-iodine (p.1155·1).
Skin and wound disinfection.

Jodo-Calcio-Vitaminico *Bruschettini, Ital.*
Sodium iodide (p.1522·3); potassium iodide (p.1522·3); rubidium iodide (p.1660·1); calcium gluconate (p.1188·2); ascorbic acid (p.1389·3).
Eye disorders.

Jodocur *Farmacologico Milanese, Ital.*
Povidone-iodine (p.1155·1).
Disinfection of skin, wounds, and burns; mouth and throat infections; vaginal hygiene.

Jodoform *Lohmann, Ger.*
Iodoform (p.1149·1).
Wounds.

Jodogard *Gedis, Ital.*
Povidone-iodine (p.1155·1).
Skin and hand disinfection.

Jodonorm *Biochemie, Aust.*
Sodium iodide (p.1522·3).
Iodine-deficiency goitre.

Jodoplex *Streuli, Switz.*
Povidone-iodine (p.1155·1).
Burns; infected skin disorders; skin, hand, and mucous-membrane disinfection; ulcers; wounds.

Jodosan *Superfos Biosector, Norw.*
Iodine (p.1522·3).
Formerly known as Idu-Phor.
Disinfection of skin and wounds.

Jodthyrox
Merck, Aust.; Merck, Ger.
Thyroxine [levothyroxine] sodium (p.1526·2); potassium iodide (p.1522·3).
Goitre; iodine deficiency.

Joggers *Solgar, UK.*
Multivitamin and mineral preparation with bee pollen and ginseng (p.1350·1).

Joghurt Milkitten *Apotheke Roten Krebs, Aust.†.*
Yogurt; lactose (p.1370·2); senna (p.1248·2); fruit paste (plums and figs); wheat germ oil.
Constipation.

John Plunketts Protective Day Cream *Sunspot, Austral.*
SPF 25: Elastin; collagen (p.1598·2); vitamin A (p.1382·1); Dermasome SOD; Dermasome E; Megasol Complex; oxybenzone (p.1518·1); octinoxate (p.1517·3).
Emollient; sunscreen.

John Plunketts Super Wrinkle Cream *Sunspot, Austral.*
Active soluble elastin; active soluble collagen (p.1598·2).
Dry skin; wrinkles.

John Plunketts Vita-Pore *Sunspot, Austral.*
Soluble bio-sulfur CLR (p.1123·3); vitamin B; hamamelis (p.1618·3).
Oily skin.

Johnson & Johnson Burn Cream *Johnson & Johnson, Canad.*
Benzocaine (p.1306·2).

Johnson's Antiseptic Powder *Pharmedica, S.Afr.†.*
Benzethonium chloride (p.1134·2).
Skin disorders.

Johnsons Baby *Johnson & Johnson, Canad.*
SPF 15: Meradimate (p.1517·3); octinoxate (p.1517·3); titanium dioxide (p.1126·1).
Sunscreen.

Johnson's Baby Clear *Johnson & Johnson, Thai.*
Ethyl butylacetylaminopropionate.
Insect repellent.

Johnson's Baby Nappy Rash Ointment *Pharmedica, S.Afr.†.*
Zinc oxide (p.1128·2).
Napkin rash.

Johnson's Baby Prickly Heat Powder *Johnson & Johnson, Thai.*
Eucalyptus oil (p.1609·2); zinc oxide (p.1128·2); chloroxylenol (p.1142·1).
Heat rash.

Johnson's Baby Sunblock *Johnson & Johnson, USA.*
SPF 15: Zinc oxide (p.1128·2); titanium dioxide (p.1126·1).
SPF 30: Oxybenzone (p.1518·1); octinoxate (p.1517·3) octisalate (p.1518·1); titanium dioxide (p.1126·1).
Sunscreen.

Johnsons Baby Sunblock Broad Spectrum
Johnson & Johnson, Austral.†.
SPF15+: Octinoxate (p.1517·3); oxybenzone (p.1518·1); octisalate (p.1518·1); avobenzone (p.1517·1).
Sunscreen.

Johnsons Clean & Clear Daily Facial Moisturiser *Johnson & Johnson, Austral.*
SPF 15: Salicylic acid (p.1122·3); octinoxate (p.1517·3); enzacamene (p.1517·2); avobenzone (p.1517·1).
Moisturiser; sunscreen.

Johnsons Clean & Clear Facial Cleansing Bar *Johnson & Johnson, Austral.*
Triclosan (p.1159·2).
Acne; soap substitute.

Johnsons Clean & Clear Foaming Facial Wash *Johnson & Johnson, Austral.*
Triclosan (p.1159·2).
Acne; soap substitute.

Johnsons Clean & Clear Invisible Blemish Treatment *Johnson & Johnson, Austral.*
Salicylic acid (p.1122·3); alcohol (p.1130·3).
Acne.

Johnsons Clean & Clear Oil Controlling Toner *Johnson & Johnson, Austral.*
Salicylic acid (p.1122·3); alcohol (p.1130·3).
Acne.

Johnsons Clean & Clear Skin Balancing Moisturiser *Johnson & Johnson, Austral.*
Salicylic acid (p.1122·3).
Acne.

Johnson's Diaper Rash *Johnson & Johnson, Canad.*
Zinc oxide (p.1128·2).
Nappy rash.

Johnson's Medicated *Johnson & Johnson, Canad.*
Zinc oxide (p.1128·2).
Nappy rash.

Johnson's Penaten Crema Disinfettante *Johnson & Johnson, Ital.*
Cetylpyridinium chloride (p.1138·1).
Nappy rash.

Joint & Muscle Complex *Brauer, Austral.†*
Homoeopathic preparation.

Joint & Muscle Oral Spray and Tablets *Brauer, Austral.†*
Homoeopathic preparation.

Joint & Muscle Relief Cream *Brauer, Austral.*
Arnica (p.1581·3); bellis perennis; bryonia (p.1587·2); hypericum (p.290·2); kalmia latifolia; ledum palustre; rue (p.1660·1); ranunculus bulbosus; toxicodendron radicans; belladonna; camphora; symphytum.
Musculoskeletal, joint, peri-articular, and soft-tissue disorders.

Jointace *Vitabiotics, UK.*
Glucosamine; omega-3 fish oil; cod-liver oil; vitamins; trace elements (p.1350·1).
Nutritional supplement.

Jomax *Hexal, Ger.*
Bufexamac (p.20·3).
Skin disorders.

Jomethid *Cox, UK.*
Ketoprofen (p.47·3).
Gout; musculoskeletal, joint, and peri-articular disorders; pain.

Jonctum *Marion Merrell, Fr.*
Oxaceprol (p.1645·2).
Burns; rheumatic disorders.

Jonil T *Galderma, Switz.†*
Coal tar (p.1125·1); salicylic acid (p.1122·3); benzalkonium chloride (p.1133·2).
Scalp disorders.

Jonosteril *Fresenius Kabi, Ger.*
A range of electrolyte infusions with or without carbohydrate (p.1180·1).
Fluid and electrolyte disorders.

Jopamiro *Gerot, Aust.*
Iopamidol (p.1035·2).
Radiographic contrast medium.

Jopinol *Bernhauer, Aust.†.*
Iodine (p.1522·3); pumilio pine oil (p.1656·3).
Catarrh.

Jorkil *Bohm, Spain†.*
Silicone (p.1249·2); metoclopramide hydrochloride (p.1235·2); levoglutamide (p.1365·2); aluminium glycinate (p.1210·3); mannitol (p.924·3).
Dyspepsia; meteorism.

Josacine *Rhone-Poulenc Rorer, Fr.; Yamanouchi, Switz.*
Josamycin (p.217·3) or josamycin propionate (p.217·3).
Bacterial infections.

Josalid *Biochemie, Aust.*
Josamycin (p.217·3).
Bacterial infections; toxoplasmosis.

Josamina *Novag, Spain.*
Josamycin (p.217·3) or josamycin propionate (p.217·3).
Bacterial infections.

Josamy *Yamanouchi, Jpn.*
Josamycin propionate (p.217·3).
Bacterial infections.

Josaxin *UCB, Ital.; Yamanouchi, Spain.*
Josamycin (p.217·3) or josamycin propionate (p.217·3).
Bacterial infections.

Josir *Boehringer Ingelheim, Fr.*
Tamsulosin hydrochloride (p.978·3).
Benign prostatic hyperplasia.

Jossalind *Hexal, Ger.†.*
Sodium hyaluronate (p.1620·1).
Ulcers; wounds.

Jour Apres Jour *Lactel, Fr.*
Nutritional supplement (p.1350·1).

Jouvence *Carmaran, Canad.†.*
Hydroquinone (p.1115·1).

Jouvence de l'Abbe Soury *Chefaro Ardeval, Fr.*
Oral solution; tablets: Hamamelis (p.1618·3); calamus (p.1588·1); piscidia (p.1625·1); viburnum.
Peripheral vascular disorders.

Topical gel: Hamamelis (p.1618·3); viburnum.
Peripheral vascular disorders; venous insufficiency.

Joy-Rides *Stafford-Miller, UK.*
Hyoscine hydrobromide (p.468·2).
Motion sickness.

Jsoskleran *Iso, Ger.*
Homoeopathic preparation.

Jsostoma S *Iso, Ger.*
Homoeopathic preparation.

Juaflor *Terapia, Mex.*
Metronidazole benzoate (p.594·1).

JuBronchan C *Jukunda, Ger.*
Homoeopathic preparation.

JuCholan S *Jukunda, Ger.†.*
Silybum marianum (p.1021·3); hypericum (p.290·2); taraxacum (p.1669·1); peppermint leaf (p.1243·2); cheldionium (p.1618·1).
Liver and biliary-tract disorders.

JuCor *Jukunda, Ger.*
Homoeopathic preparation.

JuCurba N *Strathmann, Ger.†.*
Devil's claw root (p.26·3).
Musculoskeletal and joint disorders.

JuCystan S *Jukunda, Ger.*
Homoeopathic preparation.

JuDorm *Jukunda, Ger.*
Lupulus (p.1629·3); melissa (p.1632·2); valerian (p.1678·3); hypericum (p.290·2).
Insomnia; stress.

JuGrippan *Jukunda, Ger.†.*
Echinacea (p.1606·2); centaury (p.1593·1); chamomile (p.1593·2); calendula (p.1589·2); hamamelis; achillea; ysop; arnica; bryonia; aconit; belladonna; ferrum phos.; kalium chloratum; silicea; ammonium carb.
Cold symptoms.

JuGrippan S *Jukunda, Ger.*
Homoeopathic preparation.

JuHepan *Jukunda, Ger.*
Homoeopathic preparation.

Jukunda Melissen-Krautergeist Tropfen *Jukunda, Ger.*
Melissa; ginger; rosemary oil; lavender oil; pimentol; cinnamon oil; clove oil (p.1350·1).
Tonic.

Jukunda Rotol *Jukunda, Ger.*
Hypericum (p.290·2).
Gastrointestinal disorders; nervous disorders; wounds.

Julab *Biolab, Thai.*
Selegiline hydrochloride (p.1177·2).
Parkinsonism.

JuLax S *Jukunda, Ger.†.*
Senna (p.1248·2).
Constipation.

Julmentin *Julphar, UAE.*
Amoxicillin sodium (p.149·2) or amoxicillin trihydrate (p.149·2); potassium clavulanate (p.187·2).
Bacterial infections.

Julphamox *Julphar, UAE.*
Amoxicillin trihydrate (p.149·2).
Bacterial infections.

JuMenstran *Jukunda, Ger.*
Homoeopathic preparation.

Jumex *Sanofi Winthrop, Aust.; Sanofi Winthrop, Hong Kong; Dexxon, Israel; Chiesi, Ital.; Novartis, Port.; Sanofi Synthelabo, Singapore; Sanofi Synthelabo, Thai.*
Selegiline hydrochloride (p.1177·2).
Parkinsonism.

Jumexal *Sanofi Synthelabo, Switz.*
Selegiline hydrochloride (p.1177·2).
Parkinsonism.

Jumexil *Farmalab, Braz.*
Selegiline hydrochloride (p.1177·2).
Parkinsonism.

Junamac *Cantassium Co., UK.*
Multivitamin and mineral preparation (p.1350·1).

Junce *Inibsa, Spain†.*
Ascorbic acid (p.1389·3).
Adjunct in treatment of iron supplementation; vitamin C deficiency.

JuNeuron S *Jukunda, Ger.†.*
Scopaminum hydrobromic.; avena sativa; valerian (p.1678·3); passion flower (p.1649·1); lupulus (p.1629·3); hypericum (p.290·2); melissa (p.1632·2).
Insomnia; nervousness.

Jungborn *Taro, Israel.*
Oral granules: Senna (p.1248·2).

Teabags: Senna (p.1248·2); tilia (p.1673·2); caraway (p.1591·2); aniseed (p.1558·2); fennel (p.1610·1); bearberry (p.1583·3); chamomile (p.1593·2); peppermint leaf (p.1243·2).
Constipation.

Jungle Formula Insect Repellent *Chefaro, UK.*
Diethyltoluamide (p.1431·2).

Jungle Formula Insect Repellent Plus U.V. Sunscreens *Chefaro, UK.*
Padimate O (p.1518·2); oxybenzone (p.1518·1); diethyltoluamide (p.1431·2).

Jungle Formula Sting Relief Cream *Chefaro, UK.*
Hydrocortisone (p.1073·3).
Insect bites and stings.

Junifen
Boots Healthcare, Belg.; Boots, Thai.; Crookes Healthcare, UK†.
Ibuprofen (p.43·2).
Fever; inflammation; pain.

Junik *Klinge, Ger.*
Beclometasone dipropionate (p.1061·2).
Asthma.

Junior Ideal Quota *Cantassium Co., UK.*
Multivitamin and mineral preparation (p.1350·1).

Junior Kao-C *Seton, UK†.*
Calcium carbonate (p.1215·1); light kaolin (p.1229·3).
Diarrhoea.

Junior Strength Cold DM *WestCan, Canad.*
Pseudoephedrine hydrochloride (p.1099·2); chlorpheniramine [chlorphenamine] maleate (p.412·1); dextromethorphan hydrobromide (p.1087·3); paracetamol (p.71·2).

Junior Time C *Vitaplex, Austral.*
Vitamin C substances (p.1350·1).

Juniormen *Retrain, Spain.*
Nicametate; ginseng; pyritinol hydrochloride; rutoside; vitamins (p.1350·1); deanol acid tartrate.
Tonic.

Juniorvit *Pharmadass, UK.*
Multivitamin and mineral preparation (p.1350·1).

Juniperus-Komplex-Injektopas *Pascoe, Ger.†.*
Homoeopathic preparation.

Junisana *Hotz, Ger.*
Althaea (p.1577·1); thyme (p.1672·2); guaiacum; liquorice (p.1231·2); iron(III)-sucrose-complex; juniper (p.1625·2); calcium lactate (p.1188·2).
Bronchitis; catarrh; coughs.

Junivite *Boots, Thai.*
Multivitamin preparation (p.1350·1).

Juno Junipah *Torbet Laboratories, UK.*
Oral powders: Sodium sulfate (p.1250·1); sodium phosphate (p.1193·2); sodium bicarbonate (p.1186·2); juniper oil (p.1625·2).

Tablets: Sodium sulfate (p.1250·1); sodium phosphate (p.1193·2); phenolphthalein (p.1244·1); juniper oil (p.1625·2).
Constipation.

JuPhlebon S *Jukunda, Ger.†.*
Melilotus; scoparium (p.1661·2); aesculus (p.1574·1); hamamelis; cuprum aceticum.
Venous insufficiency.

Jusline 70/30 *Julphar, UAE.*
Insulin injection (human) (p.324·1).
Diabetes mellitus.

Jusline N *Julphar, UAE.*
Insulin injection (human) (p.324·1).
Diabetes mellitus.

Jusline R *Julphar, UAE.*
Insulin injection (human) (p.324·1).
Diabetes mellitus.

Jusprin *Julphar, UAE.*
Aspirin (p.14·2).
Fever; inflammation; pain; thromboembolism prophylaxis.

Just One Per Day *Reese, USA†.*
Phenylpropanolamine hydrochloride (p.1098·1).

Justar *Intersan, Ger.*
Cicletanine hydrochloride (p.857·3).
Hypertension.

Justebarin *Juste, Spain.*
Barium sulfate (p.1032·1).
Contrast medium for gastrointestinal radiography.

Justegas *Juste, Spain.*
Citric acid (p.1596·2); sodium bicarbonate (p.1186·2).
Gastrointestinal hyperacidity.

Justelax *Juste, Spain.*
Sennosides A and B (p.1248·3).
Bowel evacuation.

Justogen mono *Wernigerode, Ger.*
Taraxacum (p.1669·1).
Biliary-tract disorders; dyspepsia; reduced appetite.

Justor *Chiesi, Fr.*
Cilazapril (p.858·1).
Heart failure; hypertension.

Jutussin N R8 *Reckeweg, Ger.*
Homoeopathic preparation.

Jutussin neo *Koch, Aust.*
Plantago lanceolata; thyme (p.1672·2); verbascum.
Coughs.

Juvela
Note. This name is used for preparations of different composition.
Scientific Hospital Supplies, Irl.; Scientific Hospital Supplies, UK.
Food for special diets (p.1350·1).
Gluten-sensitive enteropathies.

Eisai, Jpn; Eisai, Singapore.
dl-Alpha tocoferil acetate (p.1394·1) or tocoferil nicotinate (p.984·3).
Arteriosclerosis; cerebrovascular disorders; hyperlipidaemia; hypertension.

Juvental *Hennig, Ger.*
Atenolol (p.841·3).
Cardiovascular disorders.

Juvepirine *Asta Medica, Fr.†.*
Aspirin (p.14·2).
Glycine (p.1365·3) is included in this preparation in an attempt to limit adverse effects on the gastrointestinal mucosa.
Fever; musculoskeletal and joint disorders; pain.

JuViton *Jukunda, Ger.*
Crataegus (p.1600·2); rosemary; hypericum (p.290·2); primrose flower (p.1600·1); ginger (p.1227·2); primula veris; kola; cactus; kalmia; lilium tigrinum; ambra; aurum colloidale; lycopus virg.
Cardiovascular disorders.

Juwoment Sport *Serum-Werk Bernburg, Ger.*
Heparin sodium (p.902·1).
Soft-tissue injury.

K-10 *SmithKline Beecham, Canad.*
Potassium chloride (p.1194·3).
Potassium depletion.

K-50 *ICN, Mex.*
Menadione sodium bisulfite (p.1395·3).
Haemorrhagic disorders.

K + 8 *Alra, USA.*
Potassium chloride (p.1194·3).
Hypokalaemia; potassium depletion.

K + 10 *Alra, USA.*
Potassium chloride (p.1194·3).
Hypokalaemia; potassium depletion.

K + Care *Alra, USA.*
Potassium bicarbonate (p.1186·1).
Hypokalaemia; potassium depletion.

K 1000 T *Hanosan, Ger.*
Homoeopathic preparation.

K Thrombin *Fawns & McAllan, Austral.*
Menadione sodium bisulfite (p.1395·3).
Prothrombin deficiency.

Kabala *IMA, Braz.*
Coal tar (p.1125·1); jaborandi.
Keratinisation disorders; seborrhoeic dermatitis.

Kaban *Asche, Ger.*
Clocortolone pivalate (p.1065·3); clocortolone caproate (p.1065·3).
Burns; skin disorders.

Kabanimat *Asche, Ger.*
Clocortolone pivalate (p.1065·3); clocortolone caproate (p.1065·3).
Burns; skin disorders.

Kabiglobulin *Pharmacia, UK.*
A normal immunoglobulin (p.1551·3).
Agammaglobulinaemia; hypogammaglobulinaemia; passive immunisation.

Kabikinase
Pharmacia Upjohn, Aust.; Pharmacia Upjohn, Austral.; Pharmacia Upjohn, Belg.; Carlo Erba, Braz.; Pharmacia Upjohn, Canad.; Pharmacia Upjohn, Denm.; Pharmacia Upjohn, Fin.; Pharmacia Upjohn, Fr.; Pharmacia Upjohn, Ger.; Pharmacia Upjohn, Hong Kong; Pharmacia Upjohn, Irl.; Pharmacia Upjohn, Israel; Pharmacia Upjohn, Mex.; Pharmacia Upjohn, Neth.; Pharmacia Upjohn, Norw.; Pharmacia Upjohn, NZ; Pharmacia Upjohn, Port.†; Pharmacia Upjohn, S.Afr.; Pharmacia Upjohn, Singapore; Pharmacia Upjohn, Spain; Pharmacia Upjohn, Swed.†; Pharmacia Upjohn, Switz.; Pharmacia Upjohn, Thai.; Pharmacia, UK†; Kabi Pharmacia, USA†.
Streptokinase (p.975·3).
Thromboembolic disorders.

KabiMix
Fresenius Kabi, Aust.; Fresenius Kabi, Denm.; Fresenius Kabi, Fr.; Pharmacia Upjohn, Ital.; Pharmacia Upjohn, Neth.; Fresenius Kabi, Norw.; Fresenius Kabi, Port.; Fresenius Kabi, Spain; Fresenius Kabi, Swed.; Fresenius, UK.
Amino-acid, carbohydrate, and lipid (from soya oil (p.1378·1)) infusion with or without electrolytes (p.1350·1).
Contains egg lecithin.
Parenteral nutrition.

KabiMix Basal *Fresenius Kabi, Fin.*
Amino-acid, glucose, lipid (from soya oil (p.1378·1)), and electrolyte infusion (p.1350·1).
Contains egg phospholipids.
Parenteral nutrition.

Kabiven
Fresenius Kabi, Fin.; Fresenius Kabi, Port.; Fresenius Kabi, Swed.
Amino-acid, carbohydrate, lipid (from soya oil (p.1378·1)), and electrolyte infusion (p.1350·1).
Parenteral nutrition.

KA-Cilone *SM, Thai.*
Triamcinolone acetonide (p.1080·1); kanamycin sulfate (p.218·1).
Infected skin disorders.

Kacinth *Intramed, S.Afr.*
Amikacin sulfate (p.148·1).
Bacterial infections.

Kadalex *Diaco, Ital.*
Potassium chloride (p.1194·3).
Hypokalaemia.

KadeFungin *Kade, Ger.*
Clotrimazole (p.382·1).
Fungal and bacterial infections of the vagina.

Kadian *Knoll, Canad.; Faulding, USA.*
Morphine sulfate (p.56·1).
Pain.

Kadiur *GiEnne, Ital.*
Potassium canrenoate (p.957·1); butizide (p.853·1).
Hyperaldosteronism.

Kadol *Teofarma, Ital.*
Phenylbutazone (p.78·1).
Musculoskeletal and soft-tissue disorders; skin irritation.

Kadolax *Hua, Thai.*
Bisacodyl (p.1212·2).
Constipation.

Kaergona Hidrosoluble *Ern, Spain.*
Menadione (p.1395·3).
Hypoprothrombinaemia.

Kafa *Democal, Switz.*
Propyphenazone (p.80·2); paracetamol (p.71·2); caffeine (p.761·3).
Pain.

Kainever *Seber, Port.*
Estazolam (p.682·3).
Insomnia.

Kajel Alacan, Spain.
Hypericum (p.290·2).
Sleep disorders; tonic.

Kajos
AstraZeneca, Norw.; Hassle, Swed.
Potassium citrate (p.1186·1).
Potassium supplement.

Kal Sept Elofar, Braz.
Kaolin (p.1229·3); pectin (p.1502·3); aluminium hydroxide (p.1210·3).
Diarrhoea.

Kala Freeda, USA.
Lactobacillus acidophilus (p.1626·3).
Dietary supplement.

Kalaf Sam-On, Israel.
Xylometazoline hydrochloride (p.1102·2).
Nasal congestion.

Kalbeten Sam-On, Israel.
Bismuth salicylate (p.1213·1).
Abdominal cramps; diarrhoea; dyspepsia; flatulence; nausea.

Kalci-300 Be-Tabs, S.Afr.
Calcium gluconate (p.1188·2).
Calcium supplement.

Kalcidon
Verman, Fin.; Abigo, Swed.
Calcium carbonate (p.1215·1).
Calcium deficiency; hyperphosphataemia; osteoporosis.

Kalcipos
Recip, Fin.; Recip, Swed.
Calcium carbonate (p.1215·1).
Calcium deficiency; hyperphosphataemia; osteoporosis.

Kalcipos-D
Recip, Fin.; Recip, Swed.
Calcium carbonate (p.1215·1); colecalciferol (p.1391·1).
Calcium and vitamin D deficiencies; osteoporosis.

Kalcitena ACO, Swed.
Calcium carbonate (p.1215·1).
Calcium deficiency; hyperphosphataemia; osteoporosis.

Kaleorid
Leo, Denm.; Leo, Fr.; Leo, Norw.; Leo, Swed.
Potassium chloride (p.1194·3).
Hypokalaemia; potassium supplement.

Kaletra
Abbott, UK; Abbott, USA.
Lopinavir (p.636·2); ritonavir (p.640·2).
HIV infection.

Kalgaron Rafa, Israel.
Tyrothricin (p.267·1); benzocaine (p.1306·2).
Mouth and throat disorders.

Kalgut Tanabe, Jpn.
Denopamine (p.867·1).
Heart failure.

Kali Mag Vitaplex, Austral.
Potassium amino acid chelate; magnesium amino acid chelate.
Potassium and magnesium supplement.

Kalicet Hoechst Marion Roussel, Ital.
Fexofenadine hydrochloride (p.417·3).
Allergic rhinitis; urticaria.

Kalicitrine Promedica, Fr.†.
Choline citrate (p.1356·3); potassium citrate (p.1186·1).
Dyspepsia.

Kaliglutol Streuli, Switz.
Potassium chloride (p.1194·3).
Hypokalaemia.

Kaliklora Jod med Queisser, Ger.†.
Potassium iodide (p.1522·3).
Iodine deficiency.

Kalimate Nikken, Jpn.
Calcium polystyrene sulfonate (p.1002·3).
Hyperkalaemia.

Kalinor Knoll, Ger.
Potassium citrate (p.1186·1); potassium bicarbonate (p.1186·1).
Potassium deficiency, particularly in association with metabolic acidosis.

Kalinorm
Nycomed, Denm.†; Nycomed, Fin.; Nycomed, Norw.
Potassium chloride (p.1194·3).
Hypokalaemia; potassium supplement.

Kalinor-retard P Knoll, Ger.
Potassium chloride (p.1194·3).
Potassium deficiency.

Kaliolite Merck, Mex.
Potassium chloride (p.1194·3).
Hypokalaemia.

Kalioral Fresenius Kabi, Aust.
Anhydrous potassium citrate (p.1186·1); potassium bicarbonate (p.1186·1); citric acid (p.1596·2).
Oedema; potassium deficiency.

Kalisol Orion, Fin.
Potassium chloride (p.1194·3).
Hypokalaemia.

Kalisteril Orion, Fin.
Potassium chloride (p.1194·3).
Potassium supplement.

Kalisyl Solvay, Aust.†.
Diethylamine salicylate (p.32·2); myrtecaine (p.1317·3).
Inflammation; pain.

Kalitabs Leo, Swed.
Potassium chloride (p.1194·3).
Potassium deficiency; potassium supplement.

Kalitrans Niddapharm, Ger.
Potassium bicarbonate (p.1186·1).
Potassium deficiency.

Kalitrans retard Fresenius, Ger.†.
Potassium chloride (p.1194·3).
Potassium deficiency.

Kalium
Apogepha, Ger.
Potassium adipate.
Potassium deficiency.

Vifor, Hong Kong.
Potassium chloride (p.1194·3).
Potassium deficiency.

Kalium Duretter
AstraZeneca, Fin.; Hassle, Swed.
Potassium chloride (p.1194·3).
Potassium deficiency; potassium supplement.

Kalium Durettes
Astra, Belg.; Astra, Neth.
Potassium chloride (p.1194·3).
Hypokalaemia; potassium supplement.

Kalium Durules
Astra, Canad.†; AstraZeneca, Singapore.
Potassium chloride (p.1194·3).
Hypokalaemia.

Kalium Retard Nycomed, Swed.
Potassium chloride (p.1194·3).
Hypokalaemia; potassium supplement.

Kalium-Can Ratiopharm, Ger.
Potassium canrenoate (p.957·1).
Ascites; hyperaldosteronism; oedema.

Kalium-Duriles Astra, Ger.
Potassium chloride (p.1194·3).
Potassium deficiency.

Kalium-Magnesium Apogepha, Ger.
Potassium adipate; magnesium adipate.
Potassium and magnesium deficiency.

Kalium-Magnesium-Asparaginat Berlin-Chemie, Ger.
Potassium hydroxide (p.1654·1); magnesium oxide (p.1233·2); DL-aspartic acid; xylitol (p.1397·3).
Cardiac disorders.

Kalius Fermenti, Ital.†.
Trimebutine maleate (p.1675·1).
Gastrointestinal disorders.

Kalkurenal Goldrute Muller Goppingen, Ger.
Solidago virgaurea.
Renal calculi.

Kalloplast Newlab, Braz.
Salicylic acid (p.1122·3); zinc chloride (p.1398·1).
Keratinisation disorders.

Kalma
Note.This name is used for preparations of different composition.
Fresenius Kabi, Aust.; Niddapharm, Ger.
Tryptophan (p.311·3).
Depression; sleep disorders.

Alphapharm, Austral.
Alprazolam (p.654·2).
Anxiety; panic disorders.

Schering-Plough, Spain.
Ibuprofen (p.43·2).
Fever; pain.

Kalm-B Cantassium Co., UK.
Multivitamin and mineral preparation (p.1350·1).

Kalmocaps Medix, Mex.
Chlordiazepoxide (p.659·2).

Kalms Lane, UK.
Lupulus (p.1629·3); valerian (p.1678·3); gentian (p.1615·1).
Menopausal disorders; sleep disorders; stresses and strains.

Kaloplasmal Braun, Ger.†.
Glucose monohydrate (p.1364·2); xylitol (p.1397·3).
Parenteral nutrition.

Kaloplasmal E Braun, Ger.†.
Electrolyte infusion with glucose and xylitol (p.1180·1).
Parenteral nutrition.

Kalostop QIF, Braz.
Salicylic acid (p.1122·3); lactic acid (p.1626·2); acetic acid (p.1571·2).
Keratinisation disorders.

Kalovowen-N Weber & Weber, Ger.†.
Homoeopathic preparation.

Kalpress Zeneca, Spain.
Valsartan (p.988·3).
Hypertension.

Kalpress Plus Zeneca, Spain.
Valsartan (p.988·3); hydrochlorothiazide (p.907·3).
Hypertension.

Kalsimin Byk Elmu, Spain.
Salcatonin (p.749·3).
Hypercalcaemia; metastatic bone pain; osteoporosis; Paget's disease of bone.

Kalspare Dominion, UK.
Chlortalidone (p.857·1); triamterene (p.986·1).
Ascites; hypertension; oedema.

Kalten
Zeneca, Belg.; Zeneca, Spain; Zeneca, Switz.; AstraZeneca, UK.
Atenolol (p.841·3); amiloride hydrochloride (p.835·1); hydrochlorothiazide (p.907·3).
Hypertension.

Kaltocarb
Note.This name is used for preparations of different composition.
Faulding, Austral.†; Convatec, UK†.
Calcium alginate (p.728·1); activated charcoal (p.1000·2).
Discharging, purulent and contaminated wounds.

Convatec, Israel.
Calcium alginate (p.728·1); sodium alginate (p.1498·3); activated charcoal (p.1000·2).
Malodorous wounds.

Kaltostat
Note.This name is used for preparations of different composition.
Convatec, Austral.; Convatec, UK; Calgon Vestal, USA†.
Calcium alginate (p.728·1).
Haemostatic wound dressing.

Convatec, Irl.; Convatec, Israel; Convatec, Ital.; Bristol-Myers Squibb, S.Afr.
Calcium alginate (p.728·1); sodium alginate (p.1498·3).
Haemostatic wound dressing.

Convatec, Port.
Calcium sodium alginate (p.1498·3) (p.728·1).
Haemostatic wound dressing.

Kaluril
Note.This name is used for preparations of different composition.
Alphapharm, Austral.
Amiloride hydrochloride (p.835·1).
Hypertension; oedema.

Merck Sharp & Dohme, Israel.
Amiloride hydrochloride (p.835·1); hydrochlorothiazide (p.907·3).
Hypertension; oedema.

Kalyamon B12 Cilag, Braz.
Minerals; vitamin B$_{12}$; vitamin D$_3$ (p.1350·1).

Kalymin Dresden, Ger.; Temmler, Ger.
Pyridostigmine bromide (p.1423·3).
Antimuscarinic toxicity; myasthenia gravis; reversal of competitive neuromuscular blockade; smooth muscle atony.

Kalzonorm Merck, Aust.
Calcium carbonate (p.1215·1).
Hypocalcaemia; increased calcium requirements; osteoporosis.

Kamacaine Kamada, Israel.
Bupivacaine hydrochloride (p.1306·3).
Local anaesthesia.

Kamfeine Wolfs, Belg.
Sodium camsilate; ephedrine hydrochloride (p.1090·1); lobelia (p.1510·2); sodium benzoate (p.1134·3).
Convalescence after influenza; dyspnoea.

Kamidex Dexcel, Israel.
Loperamide hydrochloride (p.1231·3).
Diarrhoea.

Kamil Blue Fischer, Israel.
Liquid soap: Azulene (p.1583·2); chamomile (p.1593·2).
Skin cleansing; skin disorders.
Lotion: Azulene (p.1583·2); glycerol (p.1616·3); silicone (p.1409·3); panthenol (p.1602·3).
Barrier preparation; skin disorders.
Ointment: Chamomile (p.1593·2); panthenol (p.1602·3); wool fat (p.1410·3); white soft paraffin (p.1407·3); silicone (p.1409·3); zinc oxide (p.1128·2).
Barrier preparation; skin disorders.
Topical oil: Azulene (p.1583·2).
Barrier preparation; skin disorders.

Kamillan plus Wernigerode, Ger.
Chamomile (p.1593·2); achillea (p.1572·2).
Burns; gastrointestinal disorders; inflammation of mucous membranes; wounds.

Kamillan supra Wernigerode, Ger.
Chamomile (p.1593·2).
Gastrointestinal disorders; inflammation and infections of the skin and mucous membranes; respiratory-tract disorders.

Kamillat Hexal, Aust.
Chamomile (p.1593·2).
Mouth, throat, and anorectal disorders; respiratory-tract disorders; skin disorders.

Kamille N Spitzner, Ger.
Chamomile (p.1593·2).
Gastrointestinal disorders; inflammation of skin and mucous membranes; upper respiratory-tract inflammation.

Kamillen
Wernigerode, Aust.; Robugen, Ger.
Chamomile flowers (p.1593·2).
Mouth, throat, gastrointestinal and anorectal disorders; skin disorders.

Kamillen-Bad Mediapharm, Switz.
Chamomile flowers (p.1593·2).
Skin disorders.

Kamillenbad Intradermi Eberth, Ger.
Chamomile oil.
Anogenital disorders; bath additive; skin and mucous membrane disorders.

Kamillen-Bad N Ritsert Ritsert, Ger.
Chamomile oil.
Anorectal disorders; bath additive; inflammation of skin and mucous membranes.

Kamillen-Bad-Robugen Robugen, Ger.
Chamomile (p.1593·2).
Anogenital disorders; bath additive; skin and mucous membrane disorders; wounds.

Kamillencreme N Ratiopharm, Ger.
Chamomile (p.1593·2).
Skin disorders; wounds.

Kamillenextract Steierl, Ger.
Chamomile (p.1593·2).
Anogenital disorders; gastrointestinal disorders; respiratory-tract disorders; skin and mucous membrane disorders.

Kamillin Robugen, Ger.
Chamomile (p.1593·2).
Gastrointestinal disorders; skin and mucous membrane disorders.

Kamillobad Asta Medica, Ger.†.
Chamomile (p.1593·2); chamomile oil.
Bath additive; inflammation of skin and mucous membranes.

Kamilloderm Serum-Werk Bernburg, Ger.
Chamomile (p.1593·2).
Burns; skin irritation; wounds.

Kamillofluid Amino, Switz.
Chamomile (p.1593·2).
Mouth and throat disorders; skin disorders.

Kamillomed Kottas-Heldenberg, Aust.
Chamomile (p.1593·2).
Gastrointestinal disorders; skin and mucous membrane inflammation.

Kamillosan
Note.This name is used for preparations of different composition.
Asta Medica, Aust.
Chamomile oil.
Anal disorders; gastrointestinal disorders; mouth and throat disorders; respiratory-tract disorders; skin disorders; vulvovaginal disorders.

Asta Medica, Belg.; Asta Medica, Ger.; Goldshield, Irl.; Sanfer, Mex.; Dagra, Neth.†; Norgine, NZ; CSL, NZ; Norgine, S.Afr.†; Asta Medica, Spain; Goldshield, UK.
Chamomile (p.1593·2).
Burns; gastrointestinal disorders; inflammation of mucous membranes; skin disorders; wounds.

Asta Medica, Hong Kong; Asta Medica, Thai.
Chamazulene; levomenol (p.1629·1).
Burns; minor cuts and abrasions; skin irritation.

Asta Medica, Switz.
Buccal spray: Chamomile (p.1593·2); peppermint oil (p.1243·3); anise oil (p.1580·3).
Mouth and throat disorders.
Liquid; cream; ointment; topical powder: Chamomile (p.1593·2).
Mouth and throat disorders; skin disorders.
Topical gel†: Vitamin A (p.1382·1); chlorhexidine gluconate (p.1138·2); chamomile (p.1593·2).
Skin disorders.

Kamillosan Mundspray Asta Medica, Ger.
Chamomile (p.1593·2); peppermint oil (p.1243·3); anise oil (p.1580·3).
Mouth and throat disorders.

Kamillosan-M Asta Medica, Thai.
Chamomile (p.1593·2); chamazulene; essential oil.
Mouth and throat disorders.

Kamiloderm Mex-America, Mex.
Chamomile (p.1593·2); vitamin A (p.1382·1).
Skin disorders.

Kamilotract Tamar, Israel.
Chamomile (p.1593·2); sage (p.1660·2).
Mucous membrane inflammation.

Kamiltract Baby Vitamed, Israel.
Chamomile (p.1593·2); sage (p.1660·2); calamine (p.1111·3); zinc oxide (p.1128·2).
Burns; insect bites; skin disorders; sore nipples; wounds.

Kamistad
Stada, Ger.; Stada, Hong Kong; Stada, Singapore; Stada, Thai.
Lignocaine [lidocaine] hydrochloride (p.1313·2); thymol (p.1158·3); chamomile (p.1593·2).
Inflammatory disorders of the mouth.

Kamol Whitehall, Fr.
Capsicum oleoresin (p.1591·1); menthol (p.1632·3); eucalyptus oil (p.1609·2); camphor (p.1589·3); methyl salicylate (p.55·1).
Formerly contained capsicum oleoresin, menthol, eucalyptus oil, camphor, chloroform, and methyl salicylate.
Soft-tissue disorders.

Kamoxin Chew, Thai.
Amoxicillin trihydrate (p.149·2).
Bacterial infections.

KamRho-D Kamada, Israel.
An anti-D immunoglobulin (p.1532·1).
Prevention of rhesus sensitisation.

Kamu Jay Jamieson, Canad.
Ascorbic acid (p.1389·3).
Vitamin supplement.

Kamu Jay Multi Complex Jamieson, Canad.†.
Vitamin and mineral preparation (p.1350·1).

Kamycine Bristol-Myers Squibb, Fr.†.
Kanamycin sulfate (p.218·1).
Bacterial infections.

Kanacolirio Medical, Spain.
Kanamycin sulfate (p.218·1).
Bacterial eye infections.

Kanacyl Oftalder, Port.
Bekanamycin sulfate (p.156·1).
Bacterial eye infections.

Kanafosal Medical, Spain.
Ephedrine hydrochloride (p.1090·1); kanamycin sulfate (p.218·1); naphazoline hydrochloride (p.1095·1); procaine hydrochloride (p.1319·1); sulfanilamide sodium mesilate (p.256·2).
Nasal congestion and infection.

Kanafosal Predni *Medical, Spain.*
Ephedrine hydrochloride (p.1090·1); kanamycin sulfate (p.218·1); naphazoline hydrochloride (p.1095·1); prednisone (p.1079·2); procaine hydrochloride (p.1319·1); sulfanilamide sodium mesilate (p.256·2).
Nasal congestion and infection.

Kanakion *Roche, Braz.; Roche, Port.*
Phytomenadione (p.1396·1).
Haemorrhagic disorders; vitamin K deficiency.

Kanamytrex *Alcon, Ger.*
Kanamycin sulfate (p.218·1).
Bacterial eye infections.

Kanapat *Parggon, Mex.*
Kanamycin (p.218·2).
Bacterial infections.

Kanapomada *Medical, Spain.*
Kanamycin sulfate (p.218·1); prednisolone (p.1077·3); trypsin (p.1675·3); urea (p.1127·3); lignocaine [lidocaine] (p.1313·2).
Infected skin disorders.

Kana-Stulln *Stulln, Ger.*
Kanamycin sulfate (p.218·1).
Eye infections.

Kanavit *Medphano, Ger.*
Phytomenadione (p.1396·1).
Vitamin K deficiency.

Kanazima *Kinder, Braz.*
Erythromycin (p.201·2).
Bacterial infections.

Kanazone *SIT, Ital.*
Dexamethasone phosphate (p.1067·1); kanamycin sulfate (p.218·1); phenylephrine hydrochloride (p.1097·1).
Eye, nose, and ear disorders.

Kanbine *Rovi, Spain.*
Amikacin sulfate (p.148·1).
Bacterial infections.

Kancin *Atlantic, Thai.*
Kanamycin sulfate (p.218·1).
Bacterial infections.

Kancin-L *Atlantic, Singapore.*
Kanamycin sulfate (p.218·1).
Bacterial infections.

Kanendomycin *Meiji, Jpn†.*
Bekanamycin sulfate (p.156·1).
Bacterial infections.

Kanendos *Fournier, Ital.†.*
Bekanamycin sulfate (p.156·1).
Adjuvant in hyperammonaemia; intestinal infections.

Kanescin *Torlan, Spain.*
Kanamycin sulfate (p.218·1).
Bacterial infections.

Kaneuron *SERB, Fr.*
Phenobarbital (p.355·1).
Formerly contained phenobarbital, caffeine, crataegus, and passion flower.
Epilepsy.

Kangen *General Drugs, Thai.*
Kanamycin acid sulfate (p.218·1).
Bacterial infections.

Kanibel *Willmar, Mex.*
Kanamycin (p.218·2).
Bacterial infections.

Kanin *LBS, Thai.*
Hyoscine butylbromide (p.468·2).
Gastro-duodenitis; nausea and vomiting; peptic ulcer; smooth muscle spasm.

Kank-A
Note. This name is used for preparations of different composition.
Blistex, Canad.
Benzocaine (p.1306·2); cetylpyridinium chloride (p.1138·1).
Canker sores; mouth irritation.
Blistex, Israel.
Benzocaine (p.1306·2); cetylpyridinium chloride (p.1138·1); siam benzoin (p.1662·3).
Mouth irritation.
Blistex, USA.
Benzocaine (p.1306·2); compound benzoin tincture.
Mouth disorders.

Kan-Mycin *Olan-Kemed, Thai.*
Kanamycin sulfate (p.218·1).
Bacterial infections.

Kannasyn *Sanofi Winthrop, Irl.†; Sanofi Winthrop, UK†.*
Kanamycin acid sulfate (p.218·1).
Bacterial infections.

Kanolone *LBS, Thai.*
Triamcinolone acetonide (p.1080·1).
Musculoskeletal and joint disorders; skin disorders.

Kan-Ophtal *Winzer, Ger.*
Kanamycin sulfate (p.218·1).
Bacterial eye infections.

Kanrenol *GNR, Ital.*
Potassium canrenoate (p.957·1).
Hyperaldosteronism; hypertension.

Kantrex *Bristol-Myers, Spain; Apothecon, USA.*
Kanamycin sulfate (p.218·1).
Bacterial infections.

Kantrexil *Opus, S.Afr.*
Kanamycin sulfate (p.218·1); dimevamide (p.466·2); pectin (p.1502·3); bismuth subcarbonate (p.1213·1); activated attapulgite (p.1212·1).
Gastro-enteritis.

Kao *Covan, S.Afr.*
Kaolin (p.1229·3); pectin (p.1502·3).
Formerly contained kaolin, bismuth subcarbonate, and dicyclomine [dicycloverine] hydrochloride.
Diarrhoea.

Kao Lectrolyte *Pharmacia Upjohn, USA†.*
Oral rehydration solution (p.1185·2).
Diarrhoea; vomiting.

Kaobrol *SmithKline Beecham Sante, Fr.*
Magnesium carbonate (p.1232·3); calcium carbonate (p.1215·1); heavy kaolin (p.1229·3).
Gastrointestinal disorders.

Kaochlor *Pharmacia Upjohn, Canad.; Adria, USA.*
Potassium chloride (p.1194·3).
Hypokalaemia; potassium depletion.

Kaodene *Waymade, UK.*
Codeine phosphate (p.25·2); light kaolin (p.1229·3).
Diarrhoea.

Kaodene Non-Narcotic *Pfeiffer, USA.*
Kaolin (p.1229·3); pectin (p.1502·3); bismuth salicylate (p.1213·1).
Diarrhoea.

Kaologeais *Chiesi, Fr.*
Magnesium oxide (p.1233·2); meprobamate (p.691·1); magnesium sulfate (p.1191·1); kaolin (p.1229·3); sterculia (p.1250·2).
Gastrointestinal disorders.

Kaomagma
Note. This name is used for preparations of different composition.
Whitehall, Austral.
Kaolin (p.1229·3); aluminium hydroxide (p.1210·3).
Diarrhoea.
Whitehall, Braz.
Kaolin (p.1229·3); aluminium hydroxide (p.1210·3); pectin (p.1502·3).
Diarrhoea.

Kaomagma with Pectin *Whitehall, Austral.*
Kaolin (p.1229·3); aluminium hydroxide (p.1210·3); pectin (p.1502·3).
Diarrhoea.

Kaomuth *Bailly, Fr.*
Kaolin (p.1229·3); magnesium hydroxide (p.1233·1).
Gastrointestinal disorders.

Kaomycin *Armstrong, Mex.*
Neomycin sulfate (p.228·1); kaolin (p.1229·3); pectin (p.1502·3).
Gastro-enteritis.

Kaon *Pharmacia Upjohn, Canad.; Savage, USA.*
Potassium gluconate (p.1194·3).
Hypokalaemia; potassium depletion.

Kaon-Cl *Savage, USA.*
Potassium chloride (p.1194·3).
Hypokalaemia; potassium depletion.

Kaoneo *Covan, S.Afr.†.*
Kaolin (p.1229·3); pectin (p.1502·3); dicyclomine [dicycloverine] hydrochloride (p.466·1); neomycin sulfate (p.228·1).
Diarrhoea.

Kao-Paverin *Reese, USA.*
Capsules: Loperamide hydrochloride (p.1231·3).
Oral liquid: Kaolin (p.1229·3); pectin (p.1502·3); bismuth salicylate (p.1213·1).

Kaopectal *Silom, Thai.*
Kaolin (p.1229·3); pectin (p.1502·3).
Diarrhoea; dysentery; food poisoning.

Kaopectal-N *Silom, Thai.*
Neomycin sulfate (p.228·1); kaolin (p.1229·3); pectin (p.1502·3).
Diarrhoea; dysentery; enterocolitis.

Kaopectate *Pharmacia Upjohn, Austral.; Pharmacia Upjohn, Belg.; Pharmacia Upjohn, Braz.; Johnson & Johnson, Canad.; Pharmacia Upjohn, Irl.; Pharmacia Upjohn, Mex.; Pharmacia Upjohn, Switz.; Pharmacia Upjohn, Thai.; Pharmacia Upjohn, UK†.*
Kaolin (p.1229·3); pectin (p.1502·3).

Kaopectate II *Upjohn, USA.*
Loperamide hydrochloride (p.1231·3).
Diarrhoea.

Kaopectate Advanced Formula *Upjohn, USA.*
Attapulgite (p.1212·1).
Diarrhoea.

Kaopectate Maximum Strength *Upjohn, USA.*
Attapulgite (p.1212·1).
Diarrhoea.

Kaopectin *Dinafarma, Braz.; Vitamed, Israel; Adcock Ingram, S.Afr.*
Kaolin (p.1229·3); pectin (p.1502·3).
Diarrhoea.

Kaoprompt-H *Pharmacia Upjohn, Ger.*
Kaolin (p.1229·3); pectin (p.1502·3).
Diarrhoea.

Kao-Pront *Lachifarma, Ital.†.*
Kaolin (p.1229·3).
Diarrhoea.

Kao-Spen *Century, USA.*
Kaolin (p.1229·3); pectin (p.1502·3).
Diarrhoea.

Kaostatex *Aspen, S.Afr.*
Light kaolin (p.1229·3); pectin (p.1502·3); sodium lactate; potassium chloride; sodium chloride (p.1185·2).
Diarrhoea.

Kaotalil *Tocogino, Mex.*
Phthalylsulfathiazole (p.235·3).

Kapake *Galen, Israel; Galen, UK.*
Paracetamol (p.71·2); codeine phosphate (p.25·2).
These ingredients can be described by the British Approved Name Co-codamol.
Pain.

Kapanol *Glaxo Wellcome, Aust.; Glaxo Wellcome, Austral.; Glaxo Wellcome, Belg.; Glaxo Wellcome, Denm.†; Glaxo Wellcome, Fr.; Glaxo Wellcome, Ger.; Glaxo Wellcome, Israel; Glaxo Wellcome, Mex.; Glaxo Wellcome, Neth.; Glaxo Wellcome, Norw.†; Glaxo Wellcome, NZ; Glaxo Wellcome, Switz.*
Morphine sulfate (p.56·1).
Pain.

Kapectin Forte *Taro, Israel.*
Kaolin (p.1229·3); pectin (p.1502·3).
Diarrhoea.

Kaplon *Approved Prescription Services, UK.*
Captopril (p.853·3).
Heart failure; hypertension.

Kapodin *Eformes, Spain†.*
Minoxidil (p.934·2).
Alopecia.

Kaptin *Julphar, UAE.*
Light kaolin (p.1229·3); pectin (p.1502·3).
Gastrointestinal disorders.

Kaptin II *Julphar, UAE.*
Activated attapulgite (p.1212·1).
Diarrhoea.

Kaput *Maxfarma, Spain†.*
Povidone-iodine (p.1155·1).
Skin and instrument disinfection; skin disorders.

Karacil *ICN, Canad.†.*
Ispaghula (p.1229·1).

Karaya Bismuth *Sanofi Synthelabo, Ger.*
Bismuth subnitrate (p.1213·2); sterculia (p.1250·2).
Diarrhoea; inflammatory bowel disease.

Karayal *Chiesi, Fr.*
Magnesium oxide (p.1233·2); magnesium sulfate (p.1191·1); kaolin (p.1229·3); sterculia (p.1250·2).
Gastrointestinal disorders.

Karbasal *CCS, Swed.*
Urea (p.1127·3).
Dry skin.

Karbolytt *Fresenius Kabi, Denm.; Fresenius Kabi, Norw.*
Electrolyte infusion with glucose (p.1180·1).
Carbohydrate source; fluid and electrolyte disorders.

Karbons *Eagle, Austral.*
Activated charcoal (p.1000·2).
Digestive system disorders.

Kardegic *Synthelabo, Fr.; Synthelabo, Switz.*
Lysine aspirin (p.50·3).
Thrombosis prophylaxis.

Karden *Novartis, Aust.*
Nicardipine hydrochloride (p.938·3).
Angina pectoris; hypertension.

Kardiamed *Medice, Ger.*
β-Acetyldigoxin (p.827·3).
Arrhythmias; heart failure.

Kardil *Orion, Norw.†.*
Diltiazem hydrochloride (p.874·3).
Angina pectoris.

Kardion *Lemery, Mex.*
Dobutamine (p.880·3).

Kardioplex *SAD, Denm.*
Electrolytes (p.1180·1); procaine hydrochloride (p.1319·1).
Cardioplegia in open heart surgery.

Kardopal *Orion, Fin.*
Levodopa (p.1169·2); carbidopa (p.1168·2).
Parkinsonism.

Karelyne *Urgo, Fr.*
Sweet almond oil peroxide (p.1576·3).
Anorectal disorders.

Karex *Wolff, Ger.*
Erythromycin stinoprate (p.203·3).
Bacterial infections.

Karicare AR *Nutricia, Austral.; Karicare, NZ.*
Infant feed (p.1350·1).
Gastro-oesophageal reflux.

Karicare Baby Bath Oil *Karicare, NZ.*
Hydrous wool fat (p.1410·3); light liquid paraffin (p.1407·2).
Dry skin; pruritus.

Karicare Barrier Cream *Karicare, NZ.*
Dimethicone (p.1410·1); cetrimide (p.1137·1).
Nappy rash; skin irritation.

Karicare Breast Care *Karicare, NZ.*
Glycerol (p.1616·3); light liquid paraffin (p.1407·2).
Nipple care during pregnancy and lactation.

Karicare Food Thickener *Nutricia, Austral.; Karicare, NZ.*
Pregelatinised maize starch (p.1379·3).
Dysphagia; gastro-oesophageal reflux in infants.

Karicare Goat Milk *Nutricia, Austral.*
Infant feed (p.1350·1).
Cow's milk intolerance.

Karicare Mother and Baby *Karicare, NZ.*
Hydrous wool fat (p.1410·3); light liquid paraffin (p.1407·2).
Dry skin.

Karicare Nutrilon *Nutricia, Austral.†.*
Infant feed (p.1350·1).
Cow's milk, lactose, and disaccharide intolerance; galactosaemia.

Karicare Ointment *Karicare, NZ.*
Zinc oxide (p.1128·2); glycerol (p.1616·3).
Nappy rash; skin irritation.

Karicare Soya *Nutricia, Austral.*
Infant feed (p.1350·1).
Cow's milk or lactose intolerance.

Karidina *Kerifarm, Spain.*
Cefazolin sodium (p.164·3).
Bacterial infections.

Karidium *Lorvic, Canad.; Lorvic, USA.*
Sodium fluoride (p.1375·3).
Dental caries prophylaxis.

Karigel *Lorvic, USA.*
Sodium fluoride (p.1375·3).
Dental caries prophylaxis.

Karigel-N *Lorvic, USA.*
Sodium fluoride (p.1375·3).
Dental caries prophylaxis.

Karil *Novartis, Ger.*
Salcatonin acetate (p.750·2).
Hypercalcaemia; osteolysis; osteoporosis; Paget's disease of bone; sympathetic pain syndromes.

Karilexina *Reig Jofre, Spain.*
Cefalexin (p.161·3).
Bacterial infections.

Karin
Note. This name is used for preparations of different composition.
Gilton, Braz.
Levonorgestrel (p.1486·2); ethinylestradiol (p.1476·2).
Combined oral contraceptive.
Unipharm, Israel.
Clarithromycin (p.186·2).
Bacterial infections.

Karison *Dermapharm, Ger.*
Clobetasol propionate (p.1065·2).
Skin disorders.

Karotena ACO *Kabi, Swed.†.*
Betacarotene (p.1355·1).

Karoyan S *Daiichi, Hong Kong.*
Carpronium chloride; pantothenyl ethyl ether; tocoferil acetate (p.1394·1); salicylic acid (p.1122·3); diphenhydramine hydrochloride (p.416·1); asunaron; menthol (p.1632·3).
Alopecia; dandruff.

Karrer *Lisapharma, Ital.*
Carnitine (p.1356·1).
Carnitine deficiency; myocardial ischaemia.

Karvea *Sanofi Synthelabo, Austral.; Bristol-Myers Squibb, Ger.; Bristol-Myers Squibb, Ital.; Bristol-Myers, Spain.*
Irbesartan (p.914·2).
Hypertension.

Karvezide *Sanofi Synthelabo, Austral.; Bristol-Myers Squibb, Ger.; Bristol-Myers Squibb, Ital.; Bristol-Myers, Spain.*
Irbesartan (p.914·2); hydrochlorothiazide (p.907·3).
Hypertension.

Karvisin *Synpharma, Aust.*
Fennel (p.1610·1); chamomile (p.1593·2); caraway (p.1591·2).
Gastrointestinal disorders.

Karvol
Note. This name is used for preparations of different composition.
Boots, Austral.
Menthol (p.1632·3); oleum pini sylvestris; pumilio pine oil (p.1656·3); terpineol (p.1669·3).
Nasal congestion.
Boots Healthcare, Irl.; Crookes Laboratories, UK.
Chlorobutanol (p.1141·2); menthol (p.1632·3); oleum pini sylvestris; pumilio pine oil (p.1656·3); terpineol (p.1669·3); thymol (p.1158·3).
Respiratory-tract congestion.
Boots, Israel.
Menthol (p.1632·3); cinnamon oil (p.1596·1); terpineol (p.1669·3); chlorobutanol (p.1141·2); oleum pini sylvestris; thymol (p.1158·3); pumilio pine oil (p.1656·3).
Cold symptoms.
Boots, NZ.
Menthol (p.1632·3); pine oil; cinnamon oil (p.1596·1).
Nasal congestion.
Boots, S.Afr.; Boots, Singapore.
Chlorobutanol (p.1141·2); menthol (p.1632·3); cinnamon oil (p.1596·1); pine oil; terpineol (p.1669·3); thymol (p.1158·3).
Upper respiratory-tract congestion.

Kary Uni *Santen, Hong Kong.*
Pirenoxine (p.1652·2).
Cataract.

Kas-Bah *Potter's, UK.*
Buchu (p.1587·2); clivers (p.1596·3); couch-grass (p.1599·3); equisetum (p.1606·3); bearberry (p.1583·3); senna (p.1248·2).
Urinary and bladder discomfort.

Kaskadil *Lab Francais du Fractionnement, Fr.*
A factor IX preparation (p.735·1).
Haemorrhagic disorders.

Kasmal *Silanes, Mex.*
Ketotifen fumarate (p.767·2).
Asthma; bronchitis; rhinitis.

The symbol † denotes a preparation no longer actively marketed

Kasof J&J-Merck, USA†.
Docusate potassium (p.1223·1).
Anorectal disorders; severe constipation.

Katabios SIT, Ital.
Multivitamin preparation (p.1350·1).

Katadolon
Asta Medica, Braz.; Asta Medica, Ger.
Flupirtine maleate (p.41·1).
Pain.

Katagrip Lepori, Port.
Ethenzamide (p.35·1); paracetamol (p.71·2).
Cold symptoms.

Katalem Lemery, Mex.
Ranitidine (p.1246·3).
Peptic ulcer.

Katapekt Vitabalans, Fin.
Codeine phosphate (p.25·2); guaifenesin (p.1092·2); ammonium chloride (p.1085·2); thyme (p.1672·2).
Coughs.

Katar Berna, Ital.†.
Streptococcus pneumoniae; Staphylococcus aureus; Staphylococcus albus; Streptococcus; Klebsiella pneumoniae; Moraxella catarrhalis; Haemophilus influenzae; Corynebacterium pseudodiphtheriae.
Respiratory-tract congestion.

Katasma Bruschettini, Ital.
Diprophylline (p.764·1).
Obstructive airways disease.

Kataval Farmigea, Ital.
Triamcinolone acetonide (p.1080·1); neomycin sulfate (p.228·1).
Anorectal disorders; otitis externa; skin disorders.

Katifen General Drugs, Thai.
Ketotifen (p.767·2).
Asthma; hypersensitivity reactions.

Kation Searle, Ital.†.
Potassium citrate (p.1186·1).
Hypokalaemia.

Kationen Fresenius Kabi, Aust.
A trace element preparation (p.1350·1).
Parenteral nutrition.

Katoderm Deverge, Ital.
Emollient.
Formerly contained collagen and silver.
Skin irritation.

Katogel Deverge, Ital.
Emollient.
Dry skin; skin irritation.

Katomed Deverge, Ital.
Silver (p.1664·1).
Burns; skin ulcers; wounds.

Katopril Delta, Singapore.
Captopril (p.853·3).
Heart failure; hypertension.

Katosilver Deverge, Ital.
Silver sucralfate.
Prevention of decubitus ulcers; skin irritation.

Katovit Fher, Spain.
Prolintane hydrochloride (p.1514·2); vitamins.
Tonic.

Katoxyn Deverge, Ital.
Silver (p.1664·1); benzoyl peroxide (p.1111·1); kaolin (p.1229·3); calcium gluconate (p.1188·2).
Disinfection of wounds and burns.

Katrim Kanda, Braz.
Co-trimoxazole (p.193·3).
Bacterial infections; Pneumocystis carinii pneumonia; protozoal infections.

Katrim Balsamico Kanda, Braz.
Co-trimoxazole (p.193·3); guaifenesin (p.1092·2); ammonium chloride (p.1085·2).
Bacterial infections.

Katrum Smaller, Spain.
Capsaicin (p.23·1).
Muscle and joint pain.

Katsin M & H, Thai.
Ketoconazole (p.389·1).
Fungal infections; seborrhoeic dermatitis.

Kattwilact Kattwiga, Ger.
Lactulose (p.1230·1).
Constipation; hepatic encephalopathy; salmonella enteritis.

Kattwilon N Kattwiga, Ger.
Isoprenaline sulfate (p.914·3).
Allergic rashes; midge bites; pruritus; vaccination pocks; varicella.

Katulcin-R Kattwiga, Ger.
Bismuth salicylate (p.1213·1).
Gastritis; peptic ulcer.

Katulcin-Rupha Kattwiga, Ger.†.
Bismuth subnitrate (p.1213·2); bismuth salicylate (p.1213·1).
Gastritis; hyperchlorhydria; peptic ulcer.

Kavacur Biocur, Ger.
Kava (p.1625·3).
Anxiety disorders.

Kavaform Novartis Consumer, Aust.
Capsules: Kawain (p.1625·3); magnesium orotate (p.1645·1); vitis vinifera rubra.
Oral suspension: Kawain (p.1625·3); magnesium orotate (p.1645·1).
Tonic.

Kavaform N Klinge, Ger.
Kawain (p.1625·3).
Mental function disorders; psychiatric disorders.

Kavain Harras Plus Harras-Curarina, Ger.
Kawain (p.1625·3); kava (p.1625·3).
Anxiety disorders.

Kava-Phyton Merckle, Ger.
Kava (p.1625·3).
Anxiety disorders.

Kavasedon
Harras-Curarina, Ger.; Mavena, Switz.
Kava (p.1625·3).
Anxiety disorders.

Kavasol Ecosol, Switz.
Kava (p.1625·3).
Anxiety disorders; insomnia.

Kavatino Bionorica, Ger.
Kava (p.1625·3).
Anxiety disorders.

Kavavit Novartis, Aust.
Kawain (p.1625·3); vitamins (p.1350·1).
Tonic.

Kavepenin
AstraZeneca, Norw.; Astra, Swed.
Phenoxymethylpenicillin potassium (p.235·1).
Bacterial infections.

Kaveri Lichtwer, Ger.
Ginkgo biloba leaf (p.1615·2).
Cerebral and peripheral circulatory disorders.

Kavipen Maver, Mex.
Phenoxymethylpenicillin potassium (p.235·1).
Bacterial infections.

Kavitol Lannacher, Aust.
Menadione sodium bisulfite (p.1395·3).
Haemorrhage; overdosage with coumarin anticoagulants.

Kavosan Oral-B, Ital.
Sodium perborate (p.1156·3).
Formerly known as Oral-B Kavosan.
Oral hygiene.

Kavosporal comp Muller Goppingen, Ger.
Kava (p.1625·3); valerian (p.1678·3).
Anxiety disorders.

Kavosporal forte Muller Goppingen, Ger.
Kava (p.1625·3).
Anxiety disorders.

Kawaform Klinge, Switz.
Kawain (p.1625·3); magnesium orotate (p.1645·1); vitis vinifera.
Insomnia; tension; tonic.

Kay Ciel Forest Pharmaceuticals, USA.
Potassium chloride (p.1194·3).
Hypokalaemia; potassium depletion.

Kay-Cee-L
Geistlich, Irl.; Geistlich, UK.
Potassium chloride (p.1194·3).
Hypokalaemia; potassium depletion.

Kayexalate
Sanofi Synthelabo, Canad.; Sanofi Winthrop, Fr.; Sanofi Winthrop, Israel; Sanofi Synthelabo, Ital.; Sanofi Synthelabo, Thai.; Sanofi Winthrop, USA.
Sodium polystyrene sulfonate (p.1023·2).
Hyperkalaemia.

Kayexalate Calcium Sanofi Synthelabo, Belg.
Calcium polystyrene sulfonate (p.1002·3).
Hyperkalaemia.

Kayexalate Sodium Sanofi Synthelabo, Belg.
Sodium polystyrene sulfonate (p.1023·2).
Hyperkalaemia.

Kaylixir Lannett, USA†.
Potassium gluconate (p.1194·3).
Hypokalaemia; potassium depletion.

Kaytwo Eisai, Jpn.
Menatetrenone (p.1396·3).
Vitamin K deficiency.

Kaz McGloin, Austral.†.
Menthol (p.1632·3).
Inhalation.

Kazak Knoll, Austral.
Cerivastatin sodium (p.856·1).
Hypercholesterolaemia.

Kazinal Asian Pharm, Thai.
Ketoconazole (p.389·1).
Fungal infections.

K-Biofen Alpha, Mex.
Chloramphenicol (p.179·1).
Bacterial infections.

K-C Century, USA.
Kaolin (p.1229·3); pectin (p.1502·3); bismuth subcarbonate (p.1213·1).
Diarrhoea.

K-Cil TP, Thai.
Cloxacillin sodium (p.192·1).
Bacterial infections.

KCl-retard
Novartis Consumer, Aust.; Zyma, Ger.
Potassium chloride (p.1194·3).
Hypokalaemia.

Kdiron Julphar, UAE.
Ferrous sulfate (p.1360·3).
Iron deficiency anaemia.

K-Dur
Key, Canad.; Schering-Plough, Mex.; Key, USA.
Potassium chloride (p.1194·3).
Hypokalaemia.

Keal EG, Fr.
Sucralfate (p.1250·2).
Peptic ulcer.

Kedacillin Hormona, Mex.
Sulbenicillin sodium (p.250·2).
Mepivacaine hydrochloride (p.1317·1) is included in this preparation to alleviate the pain of injection.
Bacterial infections.

Kedacillina Bracco, Ital.†.
Sulbenicillin sodium (p.250·2).
Lignocaine [lidocaine] hydrochloride (p.1313·2) is included in this preparation to alleviate the pain of injection.
Bacterial infections.

Keduril
Rhodia, Braz.; Rhone-Poulenc Rorer, Mex.
Ketoprofen (p.47·3) or ketoprofen sodium (p.48·1).
Gout; musculoskeletal, joint, and peri-articular disorders; pain.

Keefloxin Helfarma, Port.
Ciprofloxacin hydrochloride (p.182·3).
Bacterial infections.

Keep Alert Reese, USA.
Caffeine (p.761·3).

Keep Clear Anti-Dandruff Shampoo Avon, Canad.
Pyrithione zinc (p.1122·1).

Kefaclor LSP, Thai.
Cefaclor (p.161·1).
Bacterial infections.

Kefadim
Lilly, Belg.; Lilly, Braz.; Lilly, Thai.; Lilly, UK.
Ceftazidime (p.174·3).
Bacterial infections.

Kefadol
Lilly, Irl.; Dista, UK.
Cefamandole nafate (p.163·3).
Bacterial infections.

Kefalex Medinovum, Fin.
Cefalexin (p.161·3).
Bacterial infections.

Kefamin Lilly, Spain.
Ceftazidime (p.174·3).
Bacterial infections.

Kefandol Lilly, Fr.
Cefamandole formate sodium (p.163·3).
Bacterial infections.

Kefazim Lilly, Aust.
Ceftazidime (p.174·3).
Bacterial infections.

Kefazin Vitamed, Israel.
Cefazolin sodium (p.164·3).
Bacterial infections.

Kefazol Lilly, Braz.
Cefazolin sodium (p.164·3).
Bacterial infections.

Kefazon Esseti, Ital.
Cefoperazone sodium (p.168·2).
Lignocaine [lidocaine] hydrochloride (p.1313·2) is included in this preparation to alleviate the pain of injection.
Bacterial infections.

Kefen Pacific, NZ.
Ketoprofen (p.47·3).
Gout; musculoskeletal, joint, and peri-articular disorders; pain.

Kefentech JE IL, Singapore.
Ketoprofen (p.47·3).
Inflammation; musculoskeletal, joint, and peri-articular disorders; pain.

Kefexin
Orion, Fin.; Orion, Irl.
Cefalexin (p.161·3).
Bacterial infections.

Keflex
Lilly, Aust.; Lilly, Austral.; Lilly, Braz.; Lilly, Canad.; Lilly, Denm.; Lilly, Hong Kong; Lilly, Irl.; Lilly, Israel; Lilly, Mex.; Lilly, Norw.; Lilly, NZ; Lilly, Port.; Aspen, S.Afr.; Lilly, Swed.; Lilly, Switz.†; Lilly, Thai.; Lilly, UK; Dista, USA.
Cephalexin (p.161·3).
Bacterial infections.

Keflin
Lilly, Aust.; Lilly, Braz.; Lilly, Canad.; Lilly, Denm.; Lilly, Fin.; Lilly, Fr.†; Lilly, Israel; Lilly, Ital.; Lilly, Mex.; Lilly, Neth.; Lilly, Norw.; Lilly, NZ; Aspen, S.Afr.; Lilly, Swed.†; Lilly, Thai.
Cefalotin sodium (p.162·3).
Bacterial infections.

Keflin Neutral Lilly, Austral.
Cefalotin sodium (p.162·3).
Bacterial infections.

Keflor Alphapharm, Austral.
Cefaclor (p.161·1).
Bacterial infections.

Kefloridina Lilly, Spain.
Cefalexin (p.161·3).
Bacterial infections.

Kefloridina Mucolitico Lilly, Spain.
Bromhexine hydrochloride (p.1085·3); cefalexin (p.161·3).
Respiratory-tract infections.

Kefol Lilly, Spain.
Cefazolin sodium (p.164·3).
Bacterial infections.

Kefolor
Lilly, Fin.; Lilly, Swed.†.
Cefaclor (p.161·1).
Bacterial infections.

Keforal
Lilly, Belg.; Lilly, Fr.; Lilly, Ital.; Lilly, Neth.
Cefalexin (p.161·3).
Bacterial infections.

Kefox CT, Ital.
Cefuroxime sodium (p.178·2).
Bacterial infections.

Kefoxina CT, Ital.
Propylene glycol cefatrizine (p.164·3).
Bacterial infections.

Kefspor Asta Medica, Ger.
Cefaclor (p.161·1).
Bacterial infections.

Keftab DJ, USA.
Cefalexin hydrochloride (p.162·1).
Bacterial infections.

Keftid
Galen, Irl.; Galen, UK.
Cefaclor (p.161·1).
Bacterial infections.

Kefurim Vitamed, Israel.
Cefuroxime sodium (p.178·2).
Bacterial infections.

Kefurion Orion, Fin.
Cefuroxime sodium (p.178·2).
Bacterial infections.

Kefurox
Lilly, Belg.; Lilly, Canad.; Lilly, USA.
Cefuroxime sodium (p.178·2).
Bacterial infections.

Kefzim Lilly, S.Afr.
Ceftazidime (p.174·3).
Bacterial infections.

Kefzol
Lilly, Aust.; Lilly, Austral.; Lilly, Belg.; Lilly, Canad.; Lilly, Fr.†; Lilly, Israel; Lilly, Neth.; Lilly, NZ; Lilly, S.Afr.; Lilly, Switz.; Lilly, Thai.; Lilly, UK; Lilly, USA.
Cefazolin sodium (p.164·3).
Lignocaine [lidocaine] hydrochloride (p.1313·2) may be included in the solvent for intramuscular injection to alleviate the pain of injection.
Bacterial infections.

Keimax Essex, Ger.
Ceftibuten (p.176·1).
Bacterial infections.

Keimicina Boehringer Mannheim, Ital.†.
Kanamycin sulfate (p.218·1).
Genito-urinary bacterial infections.

Kela TO-Chemicals, Thai.
Triamcinolone acetonide (p.1080·1).
Skin disorders.

Kelaplus TO-Chemicals, Thai.
Miconazole nitrate (p.391·1); triamcinolone acetonide (p.1080·1).
Fungal skin infections.

Kelatin
Yamanouchi, Belg.; Yamanouchi, Neth.
Penicillamine (p.1017·1).
Cystinuria; heavy-metal poisoning; rheumatoid arthritis; Wilson's disease.

Kelatine Yamanouchi, Port.
Penicillamine (p.1017·1).
Heavy-metal poisoning; rheumatoid arthritis.

Kelavitam Iodo Suma, Braz.
Buclizine (p.411·1); carnitine; vitamin B substances; gamma-aminobutyric acid (p.1350·1).
Reduced appetite; tonic.

Kelbium Faes, Spain.
Cefpodoxime proxetil (p.172·3).
Bacterial infections.

Kelefusin Pisa, Mex.
Potassium chloride (p.1194·3).

Kelfiprim
Pharmacia Upjohn, Ital.; Pharmacia Upjohn, Mex.; Pharmacia Upjohn, Thai.
Trimethoprim (p.264·2); sulfametopyrazine (p.256·1).
Bacterial infections; Pneumocystis carinii pneumonia.

Kelfizina
Pharmacia Upjohn, Belg.†; Pharmacia Upjohn, Ital.
Sulfametopyrazine (p.256·1).
Bacterial infections; toxoplasmosis.

Kelfizine W
Pharmacia Upjohn, Irl.; Pharmacia, UK.
Sulfametopyrazine (p.256·1).
Bacterial infections.

Keli-med Permamed, Switz.
Garlic (p.1614·1); hyoscyamus (p.470·1); allantoin (p.1110·1); heparin sodium (p.902·1); avobenzone (p.1517·1); enzacamene (p.1517·2).
Scars.

Kelnac
Sankyo, Jpn; Sankyo, Thai.
Plaunotol (p.1244·2).
Gastritis; peptic ulcer.

Kelocyanor
3M, Austral.†; SERB, Fr.; Lipha, Irl.; Restan, S.Afr.†; Cambridge, UK.
Dicobalt edetate (p.1006·3).
Cyanide poisoning.

Kelofibrase Azupharma, Ger.
Urea (p.1127·3); heparin sodium (p.902·1); camphor (p.1589·3).
Keloids; scars.

Kelosal Ipsen, Spain.
Cisapride (p.1220·1).
Gastro-oesophageal reflux; gastroparesis.

Kelosoft *Chemomedica, Aust.; Geistlich, Switz.*
Hyoscyamus oil (p.470·1).
Nasal disorders; scars.

Kelp Plus 3 *Larkhall Laboratories, UK.*
Kelp (p.1625·3); vitamin B$_6$ (p.1386·3); soya lecithin (p.1628·1); cider vinegar.

Kelsef *Alpharma, Fr.*
Cefradine (p.173·3).
Bacterial infections.

Kelsopen *Faes, Spain†.*
Amoxicillin trihydrate (p.149·2); potassium clavulanate (p.187·2).
Bacterial infections.

Keltican N *Trommsdorff, Ger.*
Trisodium uridine triphosphate; disodium uridine diphosphate; disodium uridine phosphate; disodium cytidine phosphate.
Lignocaine [lidocaine] hydrochloride (p.1313·2) is included in the injection to alleviate the pain of injection.
Neuralgia; neuritis; neuropathy.

Keltrol *Kelco International, UK.*
Xanthan gum (p.1504·3).
Pharmaceutical suspending agent.

Kelual *Ducray, Fr.*
Keluamid (p.1118·1).
Seborrhoeic dermatitis.

Kelual Zinc *Ducray, Fr.*
Keluamid (p.1118·1); zinc sulfate (p.1398·2).
Seborrhoeic dermatitis.

Kemadren *Wellcome, Spain.*
Procyclidine hydrochloride (p.473·1).
Drug-induced extrapyramidal disorders; parkinsonism.

Kemadrin *Glaxo Wellcome, Aust.; Glaxo Wellcome, Austral.; Glaxo Wellcome, Belg.; Glaxo Wellcome, Canad.; Glaxo Wellcome, Denm.; Wellcome, Irl.; Glaxo Wellcome, Israel; Glaxo Wellcome, Ital.; Glaxo Wellcome, Neth.; Glaxo Wellcome, NZ; Glaxo Wellcome, Swed.†; Wellcome, Switz.; Wellcome, UK; Glaxo Wellcome, USA.*
Procyclidine hydrochloride (p.473·1).
Drug-induced extrapyramidal disorders; parkinsonism.

Kemeol *Interdelta, Switz.*
Ephedrine (p.1090·1); neroli oil (p.1640·1); eucalyptus oil (p.1609·2).
Nasal congestion.

Kemerhine *Interdelta, Switz.*
Ephedrine hydrochloride (p.1090·1); neroli oil (p.1640·1); eucalyptus oil (p.1609·2).
Nasal congestion.

Kemerhinose *Interdelta, Switz.*
Sodium chloride (p.1196·1); benzododecinium bromide (p.1135·1).
Nasal congestion.

Kemicetin *Pharmacia Upjohn, Aust.*
Chloramphenicol (p.179·1).
Bacterial infections.

Kemicetina *Pharmacia Upjohn, Belg.*
Chloramphenicol (p.179·1).
Bacterial infections.

Kemicetine *Pharmacia Upjohn, Hong Kong; Pharmacia Upjohn, Singapore; Pharmacia Upjohn, Thai.; Pharmacia, UK.*
Chloramphenicol (p.179·1) or chloramphenicol sodium succinate (p.179·2).
Bacterial infections.

Kemocarb *Dabur, Thai.*
Carboplatin (p.515·1).
Malignant neoplasms.

Kemodyn *Esseti, Ital.*
Citicoline sodium (p.1596·1).
Cerebrovascular disorders; parkinsonism.

Kemoplat *Dabur, Thai.*
Cisplatin (p.525·1).
Malignant neoplasms.

Kemphor *Salusif, Port.*
Zinc chloride (p.1398·1); sumatra benzoin (p.1668·3); guathesia oil; menthol (p.1632·3).
Mouth disorders.

Kempi *Pharmacia Upjohn, Spain.*
Spectinomycin hydrochloride (p.248·2).
Gonorrhoea.

Kemsol *Carter Horner, Canad.*
Dimethyl sulfoxide (p.1402·2).
Scleroderma.

Kemzid *Unison, Singapore; Unison, Thai.*
Triamcinolone acetonide (p.1080·1).
Skin disorders.

Kenacomb *Bristol-Myers Squibb, Austral.; Westwood-Squibb, Canad.; Bristol-Myers Squibb, Hong Kong; Bristol-Myers Squibb, Irl.; Bristol-Myers Squibb, Israel; Bristol-Myers Squibb, Mex.; Bristol-Myers Squibb, NZ; Bristol-Myers Squibb, Port.; Bristol-Myers Squibb, S.Afr.; Bristol-Myers Squibb, Singapore; Bristol-Myers Squibb, Thai.*
Triamcinolone acetonide (p.1080·1); neomycin sulfate (p.228·1); gramicidin (p.213·3); nystatin (p.392·2).
Infected skin disorders; otitis externa.

Kenacombin *Bristol-Myers Squibb, Swed.†*
Triamcinolone acetonide (p.1080·1); neomycin sulfate (p.228·1); gramicidin (p.213·3); nystatin (p.392·2).
Infected skin disorders.

Kenacombin Novum *Bristol-Myers Squibb, Swed.*
Triamcinolone acetonide (p.1080·1); nystatin (p.392·2).
Fungal skin infections.

Kenacort *Bristol-Myers Squibb, Belg.; Bristol-Myers Squibb, Fin.; UPSA, Fr.; Bristol-Myers Squibb, Mex.; Squibb, Neth.†; Bristol-Myers Squibb, Swed.†; Bristol-Myers Squibb, Switz.; Bristol-Myers Squibb, Thai.; Apothecon, USA†.*
Triamcinolone (p.1080·1) or triamcinolone acetonide (p.1080·1).
Corticosteroid.

Kenacort Solubile *Bristol-Myers Squibb, Belg.*
Triamcinolone acetonide dipotassium phosphate (p.1080·2).
Corticosteroid.

Kenacort-A
Note.This name is used for preparations of different composition.
Bristol-Myers Squibb, Austral.; Bristol-Myers Squibb, Belg.; Bristol-Myers Squibb, Hong Kong; Bristol-Myers Squibb, Ital.; Bristol-Myers Squibb, Neth.; Bristol-Myers Squibb, NZ.
Triamcinolone acetonide (p.1080·1).
Corticosteroid.

Bristol-Myers Squibb, Switz.
Injection; oral paste: Triamcinolone acetonide (p.1080·1).
Corticosteroid.

Tincture: Triamcinolone acetonide (p.1080·1); salicylic acid (p.1122·3).
Skin disorders.

Kenacort-A Solubile *Bristol-Myers Squibb, Switz.*
Triamcinolone acetonide dipotassium phosphate (p.1080·2).
Corticosteroid.

Kenacort-T *Bristol-Myers Squibb, Norw.; Bristol-Myers Squibb, Swed.*
Triamcinolone acetonide (p.1080·1).
Corticosteroid.

Kenacort-T comp *Bristol-Myers Squibb, Fin.; Bristol-Myers Squibb, Norw.; Bristol-Myers Squibb, Swed.*
Triamcinolone acetonide (p.1080·1); salicylic acid (p.1122·3).
Otitis externa; skin disorders.

Kenacutan *Bristol-Myers Squibb, Denm.; Bristol-Myers Squibb, Norw.; Bristol-Myers Squibb, Swed.*
Triamcinolone acetonide (p.1080·1); halquinol (p.214·1).
Infected skin disorders.

Kenaject *Mayrand, USA.*
Triamcinolone acetonide (p.1080·1).
Corticosteroid.

Kenalcol *Bristol-Myers Squibb, Fr.*
Triamcinolone acetonide (p.1080·1); salicylic acid (p.1122·3); benzalkonium chloride (p.1133·2).
Skin disorders.

Kenalin *Kendrick, Mex.*
Sulindac (p.85·3).
Gout; musculoskeletal, joint, and peri-articular disorders.

Kenalog
Note.This name is used for preparations of different composition.
Westwood-Squibb, Canad.; Bristol-Myers Squibb, Denm.; Bristol-Myers Squibb, Ger.; Bristol-Myers Squibb, Irl.; Bristol-Myers Squibb, Israel; Squibb, UK; Westwood-Squibb, USA.
Triamcinolone acetonide (p.1080·1).
Corticosteroid.

Bristol-Myers Squibb, Neth.
Triamcinolone acetonide (p.1080·1); salicylic acid (p.1122·3).
Keratinisation disorders; psoriasis.

Kenalog Comp *Bristol-Myers Squibb, Denm.*
Triamcinolone acetonide (p.1080·1); gramicidin (p.213·3); neomycin sulfate (p.228·1).
Infected skin disorders.

Kenalog Comp med Mycostatin *Bristol-Myers Squibb, Denm.*
Triamcinolone acetonide (p.1080·1); gramicidin (p.213·3); neomycin sulfate (p.228·1); nystatin (p.392·2).
Infected skin disorders.

Kenalog Dental *Bristol-Myers Squibb, Mex.*
Triamcinolone (p.1080·1).

Kenalog med Salicylsyre *Bristol-Myers Squibb, Denm.*
Triamcinolone acetonide (p.1080·1); salicylic acid (p.1122·3).
Skin disorders.

Kenalog in Orabase *Bristol-Myers Squibb, Austral.; Westwood-Squibb, Canad.; Bristol-Myers Squibb, Hong Kong; Bristol-Myers Squibb, Israel; Bristol-Myers Squibb, NZ; Bristol-Myers Squibb, S.Afr.; Bristol-Myers Squibb, Singapore; Squibb, Spain; Bristol-Myers Squibb, Thai.; Apothecon, USA.*
Triamcinolone acetonide (p.1080·1).
Oral lesions.

Kenalone *Bristol-Myers Squibb, Austral.*
Triamcinolone acetonide (p.1080·1).
Skin disorders.

Kenalyn *Silom, Thai.*
Ketoconazole (p.389·1).
Fungal scalp infections.

Kenapril *Kener, Mex.*
Captopril (p.853·3).

Kenaprol *Kener, Mex.*
Metoprolol tartrate (p.931·2).

Kenaprox *Kener, Mex.*
Naproxen (p.60·3).

Kenazol
Note.This name is used for preparations of different composition.
Kendrick, Mex.
Etoposide (p.538·1).

Pharmasant, Thai.
Ketoconazole (p.389·1).
Fungal infections.

Kenazole *Greater Pharma, Thai.*
Ketoconazole (p.389·1).
Fungal infections.

Kenciclen *Kener, Mex.*
Doxycycline (p.200·1).
Bacterial infections.

Kendazol *Kener, Mex.*
Danazol (p.1468·3).

Kendural *Abbott, Switz.*
Ferrous sulfate (p.1360·3).
Sodium ascorbate (p.1390·1) is included in this preparation to increase the absorption and availability of iron.
Iron deficiency; iron-deficiency anaemia.

Kendural C *Abbott, Ger.*
Ferrous sulfate (p.1360·3).
Ascorbic acid (p.1389·3) is included in this preparation to increase the absorption and availability of iron.
Iron deficiency; iron-deficiency anaemias.

Kendural-Fol-500 *Abbott, Ger.*
Ferrous sulfate (p.1360·3); folic acid (p.1361·1).
Ascorbic acid (p.1389·3) is included in this preparation to increase the absorption and availability of iron.
Iron and folic acid deficiency; iron-deficiency anaemias.

Kendural-Plus *Abbott, Ger.*
Ferrous sulfate (p.1360·3); vitamins.
Iron deficiency.

Kenefen *Pharmasant, Thai.*
Ketotifen fumarate (p.767·2).
Asthma; bronchitis; hypersensitivity reactions.

Kenergon *Magistra, Switz.*
Lignocaine [lidocaine] (p.1313·2).
Premature ejaculation.

Kenesil *Ipsen, Spain.*
Nimodipine (p.946·1).
Mental function impairment; neurological deficit following subarachnoid haemorrhage.

Kenhancer *Emerging Pharma, Singapore; Sang-A Pharm, Singapore.*
Ketoprofen (p.47·3).
Musculoskeletal, joint, peri-articular, and soft-tissue disorders.

Keno *TO-Chemicals, Thai.*
Triamcinolone acetonide (p.1080·1).
Oral lesions.

Kenoid *Bristol-Myers Squibb, NZ.*
Triamcinolone acetonide (p.1080·1); lignocaine [lidocaine] hydrochloride (p.1313·2); nystatin (p.392·2).
Anorectal disorders; skin disorders.

Kenoket *Kendrick, Mex.*
Clonazepam (p.347·1).
Epilepsy.

Kenolan *Kendrick, Mex.*
Captopril (p.853·3).
Heart failure; hypertension.

Kenona *Kener, Mex.*
Propafenone (p.962·2).

Kenonel *Marnel, USA.*
Triamcinolone acetonide (p.1080·1).
Skin disorders.

Kenopril *Kendrick, Mex.*
Enalapril maleate (p.883·3).
Hypertension.

Kenoral *General Drugs, Thai.*
Ketoconazole (p.389·1).
Fungal infections.

Kenspa *Kenyaku, Thai.*
Chlordiazepoxide (p.659·2); clidinium bromide (p.465·1).
Gastrointestinal disorders; smooth muscle spasm.

Kentadin *Kendrick, Mex.*
Oxpentifylline [pentoxifylline] (p.950·3).
Vascular disorders.

Kentamol *Norton, UK.*
Salbutamol (p.770·3).
Asthma.

Kentosanil *Kener, Mex.*
Oxolamine citrate (p.1096·2).

Kenwood Therapeutic Liquid *Kenwood, USA.*
Multivitamin and mineral preparation (p.1350·1).

Kenya-Mox *Kenyaku, Thai.*
Amoxicillin trihydrate (p.149·2).
Bacterial infections.

Kenzen *Takeda, Fr.*
Candesartan cilexetil (p.853·2).
Hypertension.

Kenzoflex *Collins, Mex.*
Ciprofloxacin hydrochloride (p.182·3).
Bacterial infections.

Kephalodoron *Weleda, Aust.*
Ferrous sulfate (p.1360·3); silicon dioxide (p.1503·3).
Migraine; nervous disorders; vasomotor headache.

Kepinol *Pfleger, Ger.*
Co-trimoxazole (p.193·3).
Bacterial infections; Pneumocystis carinii pneumonia.

Keppra *UCB, Irl.; UCB, UK; UCB, USA.*
Levetiracetam (p.353·1).
Epilepsy.

Keppur *Drossapharm, Switz.*
Cream: Heparin sodium (p.902·1); comfrey (p.1598·3); hypericum oil (p.290·3); calendula oil (p.1589·2).
Topical gel: Heparin sodium (p.902·1); comfrey (p.1598·3).
Musculoskeletal, joint, peri-articular, and soft-tissue disorders; peripheral vascular disorders.

Keprodol *Ratiopharm, Aust.*
Ketoprofen (p.47·3).
Inflammation; musculoskeletal and joint disorders; pain.

Kepsidol *Kener, Mex.*
Haloperidol (p.686·3).

Kerafilm *Pierre Fabre Sante, Fr.*
Salicylic acid (p.1122·3); lactic acid (p.1626·2).
Formerly contained salicylic acid, lactic acid, iodine, and butyl aminobenzoate.
Calluses; corns; verrucae.

Keral
Menarini, Irl.; Menarini, UK.
Dexketoprofen trometamol (p.47·3).
Pain.

Keralac Plus *LED, Fr.*
Ammonium lactate (p.1110·3); salicylic acid (p.1122·3); zinc gluconate (p.1398·2).
Acne.

Keraliss 14 *LED, Fr.*
Ammonium lactate (p.1110·3); zinc gluconate (p.1398·2).
Acne.

Keralyt *Westwood-Squibb, Canad.; Westwood-Squibb, USA.*
Salicylic acid (p.1122·3).
Hyperkeratosis.

Keranon *Pentamedical, Ital.*
Salicylic acid (p.1122·3).
Keratinisation disorders.

Kerapil *LED, Fr.*
Ammonium lactate (p.1110·3).
Skin disorders.

Kerasal *Spirig, Switz.*
Salicylic acid (p.1122·3); urea (p.1127·3).
Skin disorders.

Keratisdin *Isdin, Spain.*
Lactic acid (p.1626·2).
Skin disorders.

Kerato Biciron *N S & K, Ger.*
Calcium pantothenate (p.1374·1).
Corneal injury.

Keratocynesine *Boiron, Canad.*
Homoeopathic preparation.

Keratolip *Ogna, Ital.*
Betacarotene (p.1355·1); propolis (p.1655·1).
Emollient for lips.

Keratosane *Biorga, Fr.*
Urea (p.1127·3); pentosan polysulfate (p.953·1).
Skin disorders.

Keratosis *Widmer, Aust.*
Urea (p.1127·3); dexpanthenol (p.1602·3).
Hyperkeratotic skin disorders.

Keratosis forte *Widmer, Aust.*
Urea (p.1127·3); dexpanthenol (p.1602·3); tretinoin (p.1126·2).
Skin disorders.

Keratospor *Agis, Israel.*
Bifonazole (p.381·1); urea (p.1127·3).
Fungal nail infections.

Keratotal *Collagen, Ital.*
Ammonium lactate (p.1110·3).
Dry skin; scalp disorders.

Keratyl
Chauvin, Fr.; Chauvin ankerpharm, Ger.; Chauvin Novopharma, Switz.; Chauvin, Thai.
Nandrolone sodium sulfate (p.1484·2).
Eye disorders.

Keri
Bristol-Myers Squibb, Hong Kong; Westwood, Singapore; Bristol-Myers Squibb, UK; Westwood, USA.
Emollient and moisturiser.
Dry skin.

Keri Lotion *Bristol-Myers Squibb, Canad.*
SPF 15: Octinoxate (p.1517·3); octisalate (p.1518·1); oxybenzone (p.1518·1).
Sunscreen.

Keri Silky Smooth *Bristol-Myers, Austral.*
Emollient.
Dry skin disorders; pruritus; skin irritation.

Keri Soap *Bristol-Myers Squibb, Canad.*
Emollient.

Kerledex *Searle, USA†.*
Betaxolol hydrochloride (p.848·3); chlortalidone (p.857·1).
Hypertension.

Kerlocal *Pierre Fabre, Fr.*
Tretinoin (p.1126·2).
Keratinisation disorders.

Kerlon
Lorex, Denm.; Leiras Synthelabo, Fin.; Sanofi Synthelabo, Ital.; Sanofi Synthelabo, Neth.; Searle, Neth.; Synthelabo, Switz.
Betaxolol hydrochloride (p.848·3).
Angina pectoris; hypertension.

Kerlone
Sanofi Synthelabo, Belg.; Synthelabo, Fr.; Sanofi Synthelabo, Ger.;

The symbol † denotes a preparation no longer actively marketed

Synthelabo, Hong Kong; Synthelabo, Israel; Sanofi Synthelabo, Singapore; Sanofi Synthelabo, Thai.; Sanofi Synthelabo, UK; Searle, USA.
Betaxolol hydrochloride (p.848·3).
Angina pectoris; hypertension.

Kernit *CT, Ital.*
Carnitine (p.1356·1).
Carnitine deficiency; myocardial ischaemia.

Kernosan Elixir *Kern, Switz.*
Aniseed (p.1580·2); horseradish (p.1620·1); calamus (p.1588·1); fennel (p.1610·1); hedera helix; imperatoria root; Iceland moss; pimpinella root; plantain seed (p.1652·3); oak bark (p.1643·2); cowslip root (p.1600·1); liquorice (p.1231·2).
Bronchitis; catarrh; coughs.

Kernosan Heidelberger Poudre *Kern, Switz.*
Absinthium (p.1571·1); aniseed (p.1580·2); caraway (p.1591·2); fennel (p.1610·1); juniper (p.1625·2); achillea (p.1572·2); pimpinella root.
Digestive system disorders.

Kernosan Huile de Massage *Kern, Switz.†*
Plum oil; camphor (p.1589·3); methyl salicylate (p.55·1); eucalyptus oil (p.1609·2); lavender oil (p.1627·2); mint oil (p.1636·2); rosemary oil (p.1659·3); sage oil (p.1660·2); thyme oil (p.1672·3); turpentine oil (p.1676·3); hyoscyamus oil (p.470·1).
Musculoskeletal, joint, and peri-articular pain.

Keroderm *Turimed, Switz.*
Linoleic acid ethyl ester; triclosan (p.1159·3); cholesterol; cod-liver oil (p.1357·2); zinc oxide (p.1128·2); titanium dioxide (p.1126·1).
Eczema; inflammation; minor skin lesions.

Kerodex
Miba, Ital.; Whitehall, USA.
Barrier cream.

Keromask *Network Health & Beauty, UK.*
A covering cream.
Concealment of birth marks, scars, and disfiguring skin disease.

Kertyol *Ducray, Fr.*
Salicylic acid (p.1122·3).
Dandruff.

Kesint *Copernico, Ital.*
Cefuroxime sodium (p.178·2).
Bacterial infections.

Kessar
Pharmacia Upjohn, Aust.; Pharmacia Upjohn, Austral.; Pharmacia Upjohn, Fr.; Pharmacia Upjohn, Ger.; Pharmacia Upjohn, Ital.; Pharmacia Upjohn, Mex.; Pharmacia Upjohn, S.Afr.; Pharmacia Upjohn, Switz.
Tamoxifen citrate (p.571·1).
Breast cancer; endometrial cancer.

Kest *Torbet Laboratories, UK.*
Magnesium sulfate (p.1191·1); phenolphthalein (p.1244·1).
Constipation.

Kestine
Aventis, Denm.; Rhone-Poulenc Rorer, Fin.; Rhone-Poulenc Rorer, Hong Kong; Rhone-Poulenc Rorer, Israel; Rhone-Poulenc Rorer, Neth.; Rhone-Poulenc Rorer, Norw.; Aventis, S.Afr.; Rhone-Poulenc Rorer, Singapore; Rhone-Poulenc Rorer, Swed.
Ebastine (p.417·2).
Allergic conjunctivitis; allergic rhinitis; pruritus; urticaria.

Kestomatine *Sanofi Synthelabo, Belg.*
Algeldrate (p.1210·3); simeticone (p.1249·2).
Gastrointestinal disorders.

Kestomatine Baby *Sanofi Synthelabo, Belg.*
Simeticone (p.1249·2); ceratonia (p.1500·3).
Abdominal distension; flatulence; vomiting.

Kestomatine Bebe *Synthelabo, Switz.*
Dimethicone (p.1249·2); carob fruit and seed (p.1500·3).
Gastrointestinal disorders.

Kestomicol *Farmaco, Mex.*
Ketoconazole (p.389·1).
Fungal infections.

Kestrone *Hyrex, USA.*
Estrone (p.1476·1).
Abnormal uterine bleeding; breast cancer; female castration; female hypogonadism; menopausal vulval and vaginal atrophy; primary ovarian failure; prostatic cancer.

Ketalar
Parke, Davis, Aust.; Parke, Davis, Austral.; Parke, Davis, Belg.; Ache, Braz.; Parke, Davis, Canad.; Parke, Davis, Denm.; Parke, Davis, Fin.; Parke, Davis, Fr.; Parke, Davis, Hong Kong; Parke, Davis, Ital.; Parke, Davis, Israel; Parke, Davis, Ital.; Parke, Davis, Neth.; Warner-Lambert, Norw.; Parke, Davis, NZ; Parke, Davis, S.Afr.†; Parke, Davis, Swed.; Parke, Davis, Switz.; Warner-Lambert, Thai.; Parke, Davis, UK; Monarch, USA.
Ketamine hydrochloride (p.1262·2).
General anaesthesia.

Ketalgesic *Max Farma, Ital.*
Ketoprofen (p.47·3).
Pain.

Ketalgine *Amino, Switz.*
Methadone hydrochloride (p.53·1).
Pain.

Ketalin *Galen, Mex.*
Ketamine hydrochloride (p.1262·2).
General anaesthesia.

Ketanest
Parke, Davis, Aust.; Parke, Davis, Fin.; Parke, Davis, Ger.; Parke, Davis, Neth.
Ketamine hydrochloride (p.1262·2).
Aid in intubation; general anaesthesia; regional anaesthesia; status asthmaticus.

Ketanine *Korea United, Singapore.*
Captopril (p.853·3).
Heart failure; hypertension.

Ketartrium *Esseti, Ital.*
Ketoprofen (p.47·3).
Gout; inflammation; musculoskeletal, joint, and peri-articular disorders; phlebitis; superficial thrombophlebitis.

Ketas *Kyorin, Jpn.*
Ibudilast (p.766·1).
Asthma; cerebrovascular disorders.

Ketasma *Lesvi, Spain.*
Ketotifen fumarate (p.767·2).
Allergic rhinitis; asthma.

Ketazol *Shiwa, Thai.*
Ketoconazole (p.389·1).
Fungal infections.

Ketazon
Note.This name is used for preparations of different composition.
Gerot, Aust.; Medphano, Ger.
Kebuzone (p.47·2) or kebuzone sodium (p.47·3).
Trimecaine (p.1321·3) is included in the injection to alleviate the pain of injection.
Gout; inflammation; musculoskeletal and joint disorders; neuralgia; neuritis; pain; thrombophlebitis.

Siam Bheasach, Thai.
Ketoconazole (p.389·1).
Fungal infections.

Ketek *Aventis, UK.*
Telithromycin (p.258·2).
Bacterial infections of the respiratory tract.

Keten *Siam Bheasach, Thai.*
Ketotifen (p.767·2).
Asthma; hypersensitivity reactions.

Ketensin *Pharmacia Upjohn, Neth.*
Ketanserin tartrate (p.917·2).
Hypertension.

Ketesse
Lusofarmaco, Ital.; Sanitas, Port.; Tecefarma, Spain.
Dexketoprofen trometamol (p.47·3).
Pain.

Ketifen *Biolab, Thai.*
Ketotifen fumarate (p.767·2).
Asthma; bronchitis; hypersensitivity reactions.

Ketil *Tillomed, UK.*
Ketoprofen (p.47·3).
Dysmenorrhoea; musculoskeletal, joint, and peri-articular disorders.

Ketina *Pisa, Mex.*
Ketamine (p.1262·3).

Keto
Note.This name is used for preparations of different composition.
Vitabalans, Fin.
Ketoprofen (p.47·3).
Fever; gout; inflammation; musculoskeletal and joint disorders; pain.

Masa, Thai.
Ketotifen fumarate (p.767·2).
Asthma; hypersensitivity reactions.

Ketocid *Trinity, UK.*
Ketoprofen (p.47·3).
Gout; musculoskeletal, joint, and peri-articular disorders; pain.

Ketocine *Progress, Thai.*
Ketoconazole (p.389·1).
Fungal infections.

Ketocon *Cibran, Braz.*
Ketoconazole (p.389·1).
Fungal infections.

Ketoderm *Janssen-Cilag, Fr.*
Ketoconazole (p.389·1).
Fungal skin infections.

Keto-Diabur Test *Roche Diagnostics, Irl.*
Test for glucose and ketones in urine.

Keto-Diabur Test 5000
Roche Diagnostics, Austral.; Roche Diagnostics, Fr.; Lakeside, Mex.; Roche Diagnostics, NZ; Roche Diagnostics, UK.
Test for glucose and ketones in urine.

Ketodiaburtest 5000 *Roche Diagnostics, Ital.*
Test for glucose and ketones in urine.

Keto-Diastix
Bayer, Austral.; Bayer, Canad.; Bayer Diagnostics, Fr.; Bayer Diagnostics, Irl.; Bayer Diagnostici, Ital.; Bayer Diagnostics, Mex.; Bayer, NZ; Bayer Diagnostics, UK; Bayer, USA.
Test for glucose and ketones in urine.

Ketodiastix *Bayer, Port.*
Test for glucose and ketones in urine.

Ketodol *Wassermann, Ital.*
Ketoprofen (p.47·3).
Sucralfate (p.1250·2) is included in this preparation in an attempt to limit adverse effects on the gastrointestinal mucosa.
Pain.

Ketodur
Searle, Denm.; Searle, Norw.; Searle, Swed.
Ketobemidone hydrochloride (p.47·3).
Pain.

Ketof *Hexal, Ger.*
Ketotifen fumarate (p.767·2).
Hypersensitivity reactions.

Ketofar *Farcoral, Mex.*
Ketoconazole (p.389·1).
Fungal infections.

Ketofen
Note.This name is used for preparations of different composition.
Pharmacia Upjohn, Fin.; Del Saz & Filippini, Ital.†.
Ketoprofen (p.47·3) or ketoprofen lysine (p.48·1).
Fever; gout; inflammation; musculoskeletal and joint disorders; pain.

Asian Pharm, Thai.
Ketotifen fumarate (p.767·2).
Asthma; hypersensitivity reactions.

Ketofene *Alter, Port.*
Ketoprofen (p.47·3).

Ketoflam *Parke-Med, S.Afr.*
Ketoprofen (p.47·3).
Gout; musculoskeletal, joint, and peri-articular disorders; pain.

Ketogan *Searle, Denm.; Searle, Norw.; Searle, Swed.*
Ketobemidone hydrochloride (p.47·3); 3-dimethylamino-1,1-diphenylbuten-(1)hydrochloride.
Pain.

Ketogan Novum *Searle, Swed.*
Ketobemidone hydrochloride (p.47·3).
Adjunct in regional anaesthesia; pain.

Ketoisdin *Isdin, Spain.*
Ketoconazole (p.389·1).
Fungal infections.

Ketolan *Olan-Kemed, Thai.*
Ketoconazole (p.389·1).
Fungal infections.

Ketolar *Parke, Davis, Spain.*
Ketamine hydrochloride (p.1262·2).
General anaesthesia.

Ketolist *Thiemann, Ger.*
Ketoprofen (p.47·3).
Gout; musculoskeletal, joint, and soft-tissue disorders.

Ketomed *Medifive, Thai.*
Ketoconazole (p.389·1).
Fungal infections.

Ketomex *Medinovum, Fin.*
Ketoprofen (p.47·3).
Fever; gout; inflammation; musculoskeletal and joint disorders; pain.

Ketomizol *Reuffer, Mex.*
Ketoconazole (p.389·1).
Fungal infections.

Ketonal *Agis, Israel.*
Ketoprofen (p.47·3).
Musculoskeletal and joint disorders; pain.

Ketonan *Marjan, Braz.*
Ketoconazole (p.389·1).
Fungal infections.

Ketonazole *Polipharm, Thai.*
Ketoconazole (p.389·1).
Fungal infections.

Ketone *Wayne, Mex.*
Ketoconazole (p.389·1).
Fungal infections.

Ketonex *Abbott, Austral.; Ross, USA.*
Isoleucine, leucine, and valine free preparation for enteral nutrition (p.1350·1).
Maple syrup urine disease.

Ketoplus *Benedetti, Ital.*
Ketoprofen (p.47·3).
Gout; inflammation; musculoskeletal, joint, peri-articular, and soft-tissue disorders; pain; phlebitis.

Ketorax *Searle, Norw.*
Ketobemidone hydrochloride (p.47·3).
Pain.

Ketorin *Orion, Fin.*
Ketoprofen (p.47·3).
Fever; gout; inflammation; musculoskeletal and joint disorders; pain.

Ketosil *Silom, Thai.*
Ketoconazole (p.389·1).
Fungal infections.

Ketosolan *Spyfarma, Spain.*
Ketoprofen (p.47·3).
Gout; musculoskeletal, joint, and peri-articular disorders; pain.

Ketosteril
Fresenius Kabi, Aust.; Fresenius Kabi, Fr.; Fresenius Kabi, Ger.; Alpha, Mex.; Fresenius Kabi, Port.; Fresenius Kabi, Singapore; Fresenius Kabi, Switz.; Fresenius Kabi, Thai.
Amino-acid preparation (p.1350·1).
Nutritional supplement in renal failure.

Ketostix
Bayer, Austral.; Bayer, Canad.; Bayer Diagnostics, Irl.; Bayer Diagnostici, Ital.; Bayer, NZ; Bayer Diagnostics, UK; Bayer, USA.
Test for ketones in urine, plasma, and serum.

Ketotab *Nakorn, Thai.*
Ketotifen fumarate (p.767·2).
Asthma; hypersensitivity reactions.

Ketotard *Galen, UK.*
Ketoprofen (p.47·3).
Dysmenorrhoea; gout; musculoskeletal, joint, and peri-articular pain; sciatica.

Ketotop *Pacific, Singapore.*
Ketoprofen (p.47·3).
Musculoskeletal, joint, peri-articular, and soft-tissue disorders.

Ketovail *Approved Prescription Services, UK†.*
Ketoprofen (p.47·3).
Inflammation; musculoskeletal and joint disorders; pain.

Ketovite *Paines & Byrne, Irl.*
Oral liquid: Vitamin A, choline chloride, vitamin D, and cyanocobalamin (p.1350·1).
Dietary supplement.

Paines & Byrne, Irl.; Paines & Byrne, NZ; Paines & Byrne, UK.
Tablets: Multivitamin preparation (p.1350·1).
Dietary supplement.

Ketozip *Ashbourne, UK.*
Ketoprofen (p.47·3).
Dysmenorrhoea; gout; musculoskeletal, joint, and peri-articular disorders; sciatica.

Ketozole *DHA, Singapore.*
Ketoconazole (p.389·1).
Fungal infections.

Ketrax *Zeneca, Irl.; IDIS, UK.*
Levamisole hydrochloride (p.101·2).
Worm infections.

Ketrel
Biorga, Fr.; Saninter, Port.
Tretinoin (p.1126·2).
Acne; keratinisation disorders.

Ketrizin *Esseti, Ital.*
Propylene glycol cefatrizine (p.164·3).
Bacterial infections.

Ketum *Menarini, Fr.*
Ketoprofen (p.47·3).
Musculoskeletal, joint, and soft-tissue disorders.

Ketur-Test
Roche Diagnostics, Irl.; Roche Diagnostics, Ital.; Roche Diagnostics, NZ; Roche Diagnostics, UK.
Test for ketones in urine.
Formerly known as BM-Test Ketur in Irl.

Kevatril *Bristol-Myers Squibb, Ger.; SmithKline Beecham, Ger.*
Granisetron hydrochloride (p.1227·3).
Nausea and vomiting associated with cytotoxic chemotherapy or radiotherapy.

Kevis *Pfizer Consumer, Ital.*
Pyrithione magnesium (p.1122·1); iceland moss.
Seborrhoeic dermatitis.

Kevopril *Rhone-Poulenc Rorer, Aust.*
Quinupramine (p.308·1).
Depression.

Kexelate *Adcock Ingram, S.Afr.*
Sodium polystyrene sulfonate (p.1023·2).
Hyperkalaemia.

Kexidil *Kener, Mex.*
Benzhexol [trihexyphenidyl] hydrochloride (p.463·3).

Key-Plex *Hyrex, USA.*
Vitamin B substances and vitamin C (p.1350·1).
Parenteral nutrition.

Key-Pred *Hyrex, USA.*
Prednisolone acetate (p.1078·1).
Corticosteroid.

Key-Pred-SP *Hyrex, USA.*
Prednisolone sodium phosphate (p.1078·1).
Corticosteroid.

Kezepin *Wayne, Mex.*
Carbamazepine (p.342·2).

Kezer *Zerboni, Mex.*
Ketoprofen (p.47·3).

K-Flebo *Sclavo, Ital.*
Potassium aspartate (p.1195·2).
Hyperammonaemia; hypokalaemia.

K-Fosfosteril *Orion, Fin.*
Dibasic potassium phosphate (p.1193·1).
Potassium deficiency.

K-G Elixir *Geneva, USA.*
Potassium gluconate (p.1194·3).
Hypokalaemia; potassium depletion.

KH3
Schwarzhaupt, Aust.; Schwarzhaupt, Hong Kong; Neo-Farmaceutica, Port.†; Torbet Laboratories, UK.
Procaine hydrochloride (p.1319·1); haematoporphyrin (p.1618·3).
Tonic.

Schwarzhaupt, Ger.; Bamford, NZ; Schwarzhaupt, Thai.
Procaine hydrochloride (p.1319·1); haematoporphyrin (p.1618·3); magnesium carbonate; magnesium phosphate; potassium chloride; sodium phosphate.
Tonic.

KH3 Powel *Kenfarma, Spain.*
Procaine hydrochloride (p.1319·1); haematoporphyrin (p.1618·3).
Tonic.

Khellangan N *Ardeypharm, Ger.*
Ammi visnaga fruit (p.1579·1).
Cardiac disorders; obstructive airways disease.

Kiatrium *Gross, Braz.*
Diazepam (p.674·3).
Alcohol withdrawal syndrome; anxiety; epilepsy; insomnia; premedication; sedative; skeletal muscle spasm.

Kid Kare Childrens Cough/Cold *Rugby, USA.*
Chlorpheniramine [chlorphenamine] maleate (p.412·1); dextromethorphan hydrobromide (p.1087·3); pseudoephedrine hydrochloride (p.1099·2).
Coughs and cold symptoms.

Kid Kare Pediatric Nasal Decongestant *Rugby, USA.*
Pseudoephedrine hydrochloride (p.1099·2).
Nasal congestion.

Kiddi
Pharmaton, Israel.
Lysine hydrochloride; multivitamins and minerals (p.1350·1).
Nutritional supplement.

Pharmaton, Switz.
Multivitamin and mineral preparation (p.1350·1).
Formerly known as Kiddi Nouvelle formule.

Kiddi Pharmaton
Boehringer Ingelheim, Hong Kong; Boehringer Ingelheim, Irl.; Pharmaton, Singapore; Pharmaton, Thai.
Multivitamin and mineral preparation with lysine (p.1350·1).
Tonic.

Kiddicrom *Boehringer Ingelheim, S.Afr.†*
Sodium cromoglicate (p.774·3).
Asthma.

Kiddie Vite *Covan, S.Afr.*
Ferrous gluconate (p.1360·1); vitamin B₁ (p.1385·2).
Iron-deficiency anaemia.

Kiddiekof *Covan, S.Afr.*
Codeine phosphate (p.25·2); mepyramine maleate (p.421·1); ephedrine hydrochloride (p.1090·1).
Coughs.

Kiddy Chews *Schein, USA†.*
A range of vitamin preparations (p.1350·1).

Kiddyflu *Caps, S.Afr.*
Paracetamol (p.71·2); dextromethorphan hydrobromide (p.1087·3); phenylephrine hydrochloride (p.1097·1); chlorpheniramine [chlorphenamine] maleate (p.412·1).
Cold and influenza symptoms.

Kiditard *Dagra, Neth.†*
Quinidine bisulfate (p.964·2).
Arrhythmias.

Kidmin *Otsuka, Jpn; Thai Otsuka, Thai.*
Amino-acid infusion (p.1350·1).
Parenteral nutrition in renal failure.

Kidrolase
Rhone-Poulenc Rorer, Canad.; Rhone-Poulenc Rorer, Fr.; Rhone-Poulenc Rorer, Israel.
Asparaginase (p.508·3).
Malignant neoplasms.

Kidscreen *Hamilton, Austral.†*
Octinoxate (p.1517·3); titanium dioxide (p.1126·1).
Sunscreen.

KIE *Laser, USA.*
Ephedrine hydrochloride (p.1090·1); potassium iodide (p.1522·3).
Coughs.

KI-Expectorante *Cimed, Braz.*
Oxomemazine hydrochloride (p.422·2); potassium iodide (p.1522·3); guaifenesin (p.1092·2); sodium benzoate (p.1134·3); ipecacuanha (p.1093·1).
Respiratory-tract congestion.

Kiflone *Berk, UK†.*
Cefalexin (p.161·3).
Bacterial infections.

Kilios *Pharmacia Upjohn, Ital.*
Aspirin (p.14·2).
Fever; pain.

Kilkof *Bell, UK.*
Cetylpyridinium chloride (p.1138·1); benzoin tincture (p.1668·3); ipecacuanha tincture (p.1093·1); capsicum tincture (p.1591·1).
Cold symptoms; coughs; sore throat.

Killgrip *Sedabel, Braz.*
Dipyrone (p.34·1); sodium camsilate; guaifenesin (p.1092·2); eucalyptol (p.1609·2); niaouli oil (p.1640·2); lignocaine [lidocaine] hydrochloride (p.1313·2); ascorbic acid (p.1389·3); mepyramine maleate (p.421·1).
Cold and influenza symptoms.

Killpan *Labitec, Spain.*
Camphor (p.1589·3); arnica (p.1581·3); capsicum (p.1591·1); aesculus (p.1574·3); scrophularia aquatica; menthol (p.1632·3); rosemary; turpentine oil (p.1676·3).
Rheumatic and muscle pain.

Kilmicen *Pharmacia Upjohn, Mex.*
Tolciclate (p.395·2).
Fungal skin infections.

Kimafan *Duopharma, Hong Kong.*
Captopril (p.853·3).
Diabetic nephropathy; heart failure; hypertension; myocardial infarction.

Kiminto *Rhone-Poulenc Rorer, UK.*
Peppermint oil (p.1243·3).

Kin Soff *Kanion, Israel.*
Pyrethrum (p.1436·3); piperonyl butoxide (p.1436·2).
Pediculosis.

Kincare *Moraz, UK.*
Parsley (p.1648·3); garlic (p.1614·1).
Pediculosis.

Kinciclina *Kin, Spain.*
Tetracycline megallate (p.260·3).
Bacterial infections.

Kindelmin *Kinder, Braz.*
Mebendazole (p.102·2).
Worm infections.

Kinder Em-eukal Hustensaft *Soldan, Ger.*
Thyme (p.1672·2); cowslip root (p.1600·1).
Catarrh; respiratory-tract congestion.

Kinder Erkaltungsbalsam
Note. This name is used for preparations of different composition.
Generican, Aust.
Menthol (p.1632·3); camphor (p.1589·3); eucalyptus oil (p.1609·2).
Catarrh; cold symptoms.

Ratiopharm, Aust.
Camphor (p.1589·3); turpentine oil (p.1676·3); eucalyptus oil (p.1609·2).
Cold symptoms.

Kinder Finimal *Roche Consumer, Neth.*
Paracetamol (p.71·2).
Fever; pain.

Kinder Luuf *Apomedica, Aust.*
Camphor (p.1589·3); menthol (p.1632·3); eucalyptus oil (p.1609·2); turpentine oil (p.1676·3); thymol (p.1158·3).
Catarrh; coughs and cold symptoms.

Kindercal *Mead Johnson Nutritionals, USA.*
Preparation for enteral nutrition (p.1350·1).

Kindergen *Scientific Hospital Supplies, UK.*
Preparation for enteral nutrition (p.1350·1).

Kindergen Prod
Scientific Hospital Supplies, Irl.†; Nutricia, NZ; Scientific Hospital Supplies, NZ.
Preparation for enteral nutrition (p.1350·1).
Peritoneal dialysis in renal failure.

Kindivite *Wyeth Health, Austral.†.*
Vitamins and minerals with fat, protein and carbohydrate (p.1350·1).

Kinedak *Ono, Jpn.*
Epalrestat (p.321·3).
Diabetic neuropathy.

Kinerase
ICN, Singapore; ICN, USA.
N⁶-furfuryladenine.
Photodamaged skin; skin hyperpigmentation.

Kineret *Amgen, USA.*
Anakinra (p.1624·1).
Rheumatoid arthritis.

Kinestase *Liomont, Mex.*
Cisapride (p.1220·1).
Dyspepsia; gastro-oesophageal reflux; gastroparesis; impaired gastric motility.

Kinet *Solvay, Spain.*
Cisapride (p.1220·1).
Gastro-oesophageal reflux; gastroparesis.

Kinevac *Bracco, Canad.; Bracco, USA.*
Sincalide (p.1664·3).
Diagnosis of biliary-tract and pancreatic disorders.

Kinidin
Note. This name is used for preparations of different composition.
Astra, Austral.; Durascan, Denm.; AstraZeneca, Fin.; Astra, Hong Kong; Astra, Irl.; Astra, Norw.†; AstraZeneca, NZ; Hassle, Swed.; Astra, Switz.; AstraZeneca, Thai.; AstraZeneca, UK.
Quinidine bisulfate (p.964·2).
Arrhythmias.

Nycomed, Denm.
Quinidine sulfate (p.964·2).
Arrhythmias.

Kinidine *Astra, Neth.*
Quinidine bisulfate (p.964·2).
Arrhythmias.

Kinidine Durettes *Astra, Belg.*
Quinidine bisulfate (p.964·2).
Arrhythmias.

Kiniduron *Orion, Fin.*
Quinidine bisulfate (p.964·2).
Arrhythmias.

Kinin *Nycomed, Denm.; NM, Swed.*
Quinine hydrochloride (p.445·1).
Malaria; myotonia; night cramps.

Kinline *Siam Bheasach, Thai.*
Selegiline hydrochloride (p.1177·2).
Parkinsonism.

Kinogen *Geymonat, Ital.*
Tyrothricin (p.267·1); hydrocortisone sodium succinate (p.1074·1).
Vulvovaginal infections.

Kinolymphat *PGM, Ger.*
Homoeopathic preparation.

Kinot *Farex, Canad.*
Camphor (p.1589·3); expressed mustard oil (p.1639·1).

Kinson *Alphapharm, Austral.*
Levodopa (p.1169·2); carbidopa (p.1168·2).
Parkinsonism.

Kintavit *Synthelabo, Switz.*
Multivitamin and mineral preparation with ginseng (p.1350·1).

Kinupril *Rhone-Poulenc Rorer, Fr.†.*
Quinupramine (p.308·1).
Depression.

Kinurea H *Fuca, Fr.*
Quinine and urea hydrochloride (p.1657·1).
Anorectal disorders.

Kionex *Paddock, USA.*
Sodium polystyrene sulfonate (p.1023·2).
Hyperkalaemia.

Kir Richter *Lepetit, Ital.†.*
Aprotinin (p.725·3).
Antidote to thrombolytics; haemorrhage; shock.

Kira
Kwizda, Aust.; Lichtwer, Ger.; Lichtwer, UK.
Hypericum (p.290·2).
Depression.

kirim *Hormosan, Ger.*
Bromocriptine mesilate (p.1164·3).
Parkinsonism.

kirim gyn *Taurus, Ger.*
Bromocriptine mesilate (p.1164·3).
Hyperprolactinaemia; lactation inhibition.

Kirin *Medochemie, Hong Kong.*
Spectinomycin hydrochloride (p.248·2).
Gonorrhoea.

Kiro Rub *Prodemdis, Canad.*
Methyl salicylate (p.55·1); camphor (p.1589·3); menthol (p.1632·3); eucalyptus oil (p.1609·2).

Kisitan *Lambda, USA†.*
Oral liquid: Phenylephrine tannate (p.1097·3); chlorpheniramine [chlorphenamine] tannate (p.412·2); mepyramine tannate (p.421·1).
Tablets: Phenylephrine tannate (p.1097·3); chlorpheniramine [chlorphenamine] tannate (p.412·2).

Kisitex *Lambda, USA†.*
Phenylephrine hydrochloride (p.1097·1); phenylpropanolamine (p.1098·1); guaifenesin (p.1092·2).
Coughs.

Kisolv *Ecupharma, Ital.*
Urokinase (p.988·1).
Thromboembolic disorders.

Kitapen *Dansk-Flama, Braz.*
Benzathine benzylpenicillin (p.156·2); bacterial antigens.
Bacterial infections.

Kitnos
Carlo Erba, Braz.; Pharmacia Upjohn, Mex.
Etofamide (p.592·1).
Amoebiasis.

Kiton *Pulitzer, Ital.*
Isosorbide mononitrate (p.916·2).
Cardiac stenosis; ischaemic heart disease.

kivat *Hormosan, Ger.*
Fluspirilene (p.686·1).
Anxiety disorders.

Klacid
Abbott, Aust.; Abbott, Austral.; Abbott, Denm.; Abbott, Fin.; Abbott, Ger.; Abbott, Hong Kong; Abbott, Irl.; Abbott, Israel; Abbott, Ital.; Abbott, Neth.; Abbott, Norw.; Abbott, NZ; Abbott, Port.; Abbott, S.Afr.; Abbott, Singapore; Abbott, Spain; Abbott, Swed.; Abbott, Switz.; Abbott, Thai.
Clarithromycin (p.186·2) or clarithromycin lactobionate (p.187·1).
Bacterial infections.

Klacid HP 7
Abbott, Austral.; Abbott, NZ.
Capsules, omeprazole (Losec) (p.1239·1); capsules, amoxicillin trihydrate (Amoxil) (p.149·2); tablets, clarithromycin (Klacid) (p.186·2).
Helicobacter pylori-associated peptic ulcer.

Klaciped *Abbott, Switz.*
Clarithromycin (p.186·2).
Bacterial infections.

Klamacin *Hua, Thai.*
Clotrimazole (p.382·1).
Trichomoniasis.

Klaricid
Abbott, Braz.; Abbott, Mex.; Abbott, UK.
Clarithromycin (p.186·2) or clarithromycin lactobionate (p.187·1).
Bacterial infections.

Klariderm *Clariana, Spain.*
Fluocinonide (p.1071·2).
Skin disorders.

Klarivitina *Clariana, Spain.*
Cyproheptadine hydrochloride (p.414·2).
Allergic rhinitis; reduced appetite; urticaria.

Klaron *Dermik, USA.*
Sulfacetamide sodium (p.250·3).
Acne.

KLB6 *Nature's Bounty, USA.*
Pyridoxine hydrochloride (p.1386·3); soya lecithin (p.1628·1); kelp (p.1625·3); cider vinegar.

Klean-Prep
Norgine, Aust.; Norgine, Belg.; Rivex, Canad.; Norgine, Denm.; Sabora, Fin.; Norgine, Fr.; Norgine, Ger.; Norgine, Hong Kong; Helsinn Birex, Irl.; Norgine, Neth.; Norgine, Norw.; CSL, NZ; Norgine, NZ; Helsinn, Port.; Norgine, S.Afr.; Norgine, Singapore; Biolac, Swed.; Norgine, Switz.; Norgine, UK.
Macrogol 3350 (p.1630·3); electrolytes (p.1180·1).
Bowel evacuation.

K-Lease *Adria, USA.*
Potassium chloride (p.1194·3).
Potassium deficiency.

Kleen-Handz *American Medical, USA.*
Alcohol (p.1130·3).
Hand disinfection.

Kleenocid *Agepha, Aust.*
Chlorhexidine acetate (p.1138·2).
Skin disinfection.

Kleenosept *Agepha, Aust.*
Hexetidine (p.1146·3).
Skin disinfection.

Kleer *Modern Health Products, UK.*
Echinacea (p.1606·2); urtica (p.1678·2); lappa root (p.1627·1).
Skin disorders.

Kleer Cream *Lane, UK.*
Hamamelis (p.1618·3); eucalyptus oil (p.1609·2); methyl salicylate (p.55·1); camphor (p.1589·3); ti-tree oil (p.1631·3); zinc oxide (p.1128·2).
Formerly known as Soothene.
Minor skin disorders.

Klerist-D *Nutripharm, USA.*
Pseudoephedrine hydrochloride (p.1099·2); chlorpheniramine [chlorphenamine] maleate (p.412·1).
Upper respiratory-tract symptoms.

Klexane
Aventis, Denm.; Rhone-Poulenc Rorer, Fin.; Rhone-Poulenc Rorer, Norw.; Rhone-Poulenc Rorer, Swed.
Enoxaparin sodium (p.885·1).
Thromboembolic disorders.

KLGH 3 *Faria, Braz.*
Procaine hydrochloride (p.1319·1); magnesium aspartate; potassium aspartate; calcium fluoride; calcium phosphate; ferrous sulfate; zinc oxide; magnesium sulfate; sodium molybdate; adenosine; etofylline; linoleic acid; gamolenic acid; tartaric acid (p.1350·1).
Tonic.

Kliacef *Fonten, Ital.*
Cefaclor (p.161·1).
Bacterial infections.

Klifem *Pekana, Ger.*
Homoeopathic preparation.

Klimadynon
Bionorica, Ger.; Bionorica, Hong Kong; Bionorica, Singapore.
Cimicifuga (p.1595·2).
Menopausal disorders.

Klimaktoplant *Omida, Switz.*
Homoeopathic preparation.

Klimaktoplant H *DHU, Ger.*
Homoeopathic preparation.

Klimaktosin *Meckel, Ger.*
Homoeopathic preparation.

Klimalet *Organon, Denm.*
11 Tablets, estradiol valerate (p.1473·2); 10 tablets, estradiol valerate; medroxyprogesterone acetate (p.1480·1).
Menopausal disorders; osteoporosis.

Klimapur *Kwizda, Aust.*
Estradiol (p.1473·1).
Menopausal disorders; osteoporosis.

Klimasyx *Syxyl, Ger.*
Homoeopathic preparation.

Klimax-Gastreu N R10 *Reckeweg, Ger.*
Homoeopathic preparation.

Klimaxil *Leo, Denm.*
12 Tablets, estradiol (p.1473·1); 10 tablets, estradiol; medroxyprogesterone acetate (p.1480·1).
Menopausal disorders; osteoporosis.

Klimicin *Lek, Thai.*
Clindamycin hydrochloride (p.188·1) or clindamycin phosphate (p.188·2).
Bacterial infections.

Klimofol *Ivamed, Ger.*
Propofol (p.1265·3).
General anaesthesia.

Klimonorm
Jenapharm, Ger.; Jenapharm, Hong Kong; Jenapharm, Thai.
9 Tablets, estradiol valerate (p.1473·2); 12 tablets, estradiol valerate; levonorgestrel (p.1486·2).
Menopausal disorders; osteoporosis.

Klinna *Greater Pharma, Thai.*
Clindamycin phosphate (p.188·2).
Acne.

Klinoc *Wyeth Lederle, Aust.*
Minocycline hydrochloride (p.224·3).
Acne.

Klinomycin *Lederle, Ger.*
Minocycline hydrochloride (p.224·3).
Bacterial infections.

Klinotab *Wyeth Lederle, Belg.*
Minocycline hydrochloride (p.224·3).
Bacterial infections.

Klinoxid *Lederle, Ger.*
Benzoyl peroxide (p.1111·1).
Acne.

Kliofem *Novo Nordisk, UK.*
Estradiol (p.1473·1); norethisterone acetate (p.1485·1).
Oestrogen deficiency; postmenopausal osteoporosis.

Kliogest
Novo Nordisk, Aust.; Novo Nordisk, Austral.; Novo Nordisk, Belg.; Novo Nordisk, Denm.; Novo Nordisk, Fin.; Rhone-Poulenc Rorer, Fr.; Novo Nordisk, Hong Kong; Novo Nordisk, Irl.; Novo Nordisk, Israel; Novo Nordisk, Ital.; Novo Nordisk, Mex.; Novo Nordisk, NZ; Novo Nordisk, Port.; Novo Nordisk, S.Afr.; Novo Nordisk, Singapore; Novo Nordisk, Swed.; Novo Nordisk, Thai.
Estradiol (p.1473·1); norethisterone acetate (p.1485·1).
Formerly contained estradiol, estriol, and norethisterone acetate in *Fr.* and *Irl.*
Menopausal disorders; osteoporosis.

Kliogest N
Novo Nordisk, Ger.; Novo Nordisk, Switz.
Estradiol (p.1473·1); norethisterone acetate (p.1485·1).
Formerly contained estradiol, estriol, and norethisterone acetate in *Switz.*
Menopausal disorders.

Klion *Gedeon Richter, Thai.*
Metronidazole (p.594·1).
Anaerobic bacterial infections.

The symbol † denotes a preparation no longer actively marketed

Kliovance
Novo Nordisk, Austral.; Novo Nordisk, NZ; Novo Nordisk, UK.
Estradiol (p.1473·1); norethisterone acetate (p.1485·1).
Menopausal disorders; osteoporosis.

Klipal *Robapharm, Fr.*
Paracetamol (p.71·2); codeine phosphate (p.25·2).
Pain.

Klismacort *Bene, Ger.*
Prednisolone (p.1077·3).
Rectal corticosteroid.

Klistier *Fresenius Kabi, Ger.*
Dibasic sodium phosphate (p.1193·2); monobasic sodium phosphate (p.1193·2).
Bowel evacuation; constipation.

Klizin *Honorterapica, Braz.*
Buclizine (p.411·1); vitamin B substances (p.1350·1).
Reduced appetite; tonic.

KLN *Roche Consumer, UK.*
Kaolin (p.1229·3); pectin (p.1502·3); sodium citrate (p.1186·2); peppermint oil (p.1243·3).
Diarrhoea.

Kloclor *Adcock Ingram, S.Afr.†*
Cefaclor (p.161·1).
Bacterial infections.

Klodin *Savio, Ital.*
Ticlopidine hydrochloride (p.981·1).
Thrombosis prophylaxis.

Klonopin *Roche, USA.*
Clonazepam (p.347·1).
Epilepsy; panic attacks.

Klont *Medochemie, Thai.*
Metronidazole (p.594·1).
Amoebiasis; anaerobic bacterial infections; giardiasis; trichomoniasis.

Klopoxid *Nycomed, Denm.*
Chlordiazepoxide (p.659·2).
Alcohol withdrawal syndrome; anxiety.

K-Lor *Abbott, Canad.; Abbott, USA.*
Potassium chloride (p.1194·3).
Hypokalaemia; potassium depletion.

Kloraetyl *Apodan, Denm.*
Ethyl chloride (p.1312·1).
Local anaesthesia.

Klor-Con *Upsher-Smith, USA.*
Potassium chloride (p.1194·3).
Hypokalaemia.

Klor-Con/EF *Upsher-Smith, USA.*
Potassium bicarbonate (p.1186·1); potassium citrate (p.1186·1).
Hypokalaemia.

Klor-De *Medentech, Israel.*
Sodium dichloroisocyanurate (p.1156·1).
Surface and instrument disinfection.

Kloref *Knoll, S.Afr.; Cox, UK.*
Betaine hydrochloride (p.1584·3); potassium bicarbonate (p.1186·1); potassium chloride (p.1194·3); potassium benzoate (p.1195·2).
Hypokalaemia; potassium depletion.

Kloref-S *Cox, UK†.*
Betaine hydrochloride (p.1584·3); potassium bicarbonate (p.1186·1); potassium chloride (p.1194·3).
Hypokalaemia; potassium depletion.

Klorhexol *Leiras, Fin.*
Chlorhexidine gluconate (p.1138·1).
Hand and skin disinfection.

Klor-Kleen *Medentech, Irl.†*
Sodium dichloroisocyanurate (p.1156·1); sodium dodecylbenzenesulfonate.
Surface disinfection.

Klorokin *Zerboni, Mex.*
Chloroquine (p.432·2).

Klorproman *Orion, Fin.*
Chlorpromazine hydrochloride (p.660·2).
Alcohol withdrawal syndrome; nausea and vomiting; pain; psychoses; sedative.

Klorsept
Medentech, Irl.†; Medentech, Israel.
Sodium dichloroisocyanurate (p.1156·1).
Skin and wound disinfection; surface disinfection.

Klorvess *Novartis, USA.*
Effervescent tablets: Potassium chloride (p.1194·3); potassium bicarbonate (p.1186·1); lysine hydrochloride (p.1370·3).
Oral effervescent granules: Potassium chloride (p.1194·3); potassium bicarbonate (p.1186·1); potassium citrate (p.1186·1); lysine hydrochloride (p.1370·3).
Oral liquid: Potassium chloride (p.1194·3).
Hypokalaemic-hypochloraemic alkalosis; potassium depletion.

Klosterfrau Aktiv V *Klosterfrau, Ger.*
Garlic; hypericum; vitamin A; alpha tocoferil acetate (p.1350·1).
Tonic.

Klosterfrau Franzbranntwein *Klosterfrau, Ger.*
Menthol (p.1632·3); camphor (p.1589·3); alcohol (p.1130·3).
Musculoskeletal, joint, and soft-tissue disorders.

Klosterfrau Franzbranntwein Latschenkiefer *Klosterfrau, Ger.*
Topical gel: Camphor (p.1589·3); pumilio pine oil (p.1656·3).

Topical lotion: Camphor (p.1589·3); alcohol (p.1130·3).
Musculoskeletal, joint, and soft-tissue disorders.

Klosterfrau Melissengeist *Klosterfrau, Ger.*
Melissa; elecampane; angelica; ginger; clove; gentian; fruct. piperis nigri; galanga; nutmeg; dried bitter-orange peel; cinnamon bark; senna; cardamom; alcohol.
Tonic.

Klotricid *Pharmacia Upjohn, Fin.*
Clotrimazole (p.382·1).
Fungal skin infections.

Klotriptyl *Orion, Fin.*
Amitriptyline hydrochloride (p.273·3).
Depression; insomnia.

Klotrix *Apothecon, USA.*
Potassium chloride (p.1194·3).
Hypokalaemia; potassium depletion.

Klyndaken *Kendrick, Mex.*
Clindamycin phosphate (p.188·2).
Bacterial infections.

Klysma Salinisch
Pharmacia Upjohn, Aust.†; Pharmacia Upjohn, Ger.
Monobasic sodium phosphate (p.1193·2); dibasic sodium phosphate (p.1193·2).
Bowel evacuation.

Klysma Sorbit *Pharmacia Upjohn, Ger.*
Sorbitol (p.1377·3); potassium sorbate (p.1157·1).
Bowel evacuation; constipation.

K-Lyte
Note. This name is used for preparations of different composition.
Roberts, Canad.
Potassium citrate (p.1186·1).
Potassium depletion.

Apothecon, USA.
Potassium bicarbonate (p.1186·1).
Potassium deficiency.

K-Lyte DS *Apothecon, USA.*
Potassium bicarbonate (p.1186·1); potassium citrate (p.1186·1).
Potassium deficiency.

K-Lyte/Cl
Note. This name is used for preparations of different composition.
Roberts, Canad.
Potassium chloride (p.1194·3).
Potassium depletion.

Apothecon, USA.
Effervescent powder: Potassium chloride (p.1194·3).
Effervescent tablets: Potassium chloride (p.1194·3); potassium bicarbonate (p.1186·1).
Potassium deficiency.

Klyx
Ferring, Denm.; Ferring, Fin.; Ferring, Norw.; Ferring, Swed.
Docusate sodium (p.1223·1); sorbitol (p.1377·3).
Bowel evacuation; constipation.

Klyx Magnum *Ferring, Switz.*
Docusate sodium (p.1223·1); dried magnesium sulfate (p.1191·3); urea (p.1127·3).
Bowel evacuation; constipation.

KMA *Berlin-Chemie, Ger.*
Potassium hydroxide (p.1654·1); magnesium oxide (p.1233·2).
Cardiac disorders.

K-Mag *Vitaglow, Austral.*
Potassium aspartate (p.1195·2); magnesium aspartate (p.1190·3).
Potassium and magnesium supplement.

K-Med *Riva, Canad.†*
Potassium chloride (p.1194·3); magnesium gluconate (p.1190·3).
Potassium supplement.

KMG Plus *Seroyal, Canad.*
Vitamin B₆ with magnesium and potassium (p.1350·1).

KMH *M & H, Thai.*
Kanamycin sulfate (p.218·1).
Bacterial infections.

K-MIC *Hassle, Swed.†*
Potassium chloride (p.1194·3).
Hypokalaemia; potassium supplement.

K-Mizol *Arlex, Mex.*
Miconazole (p.391·1) or miconazole nitrate (p.391·1).

Kneipp Abfuhr Herbagran *Kneipp, Ger.*
Ispaghula (p.1229·1).
Constipation.

Kneipp Abfuhr Tee N *Kneipp, Ger.*
Senna (p.1248·2).
Constipation.

Kneipp Baldrian *Kneipp, Ger.*
Valerian (p.1678·3).
Anxiety disorders; sleep disorders.

Kneipp Baldrian + Hopfen *Kneipp, Ger.*
Valerian (p.1678·3); lupulus (p.1629·3).
Anxiety; sleep disorders.

Kneipp Baldrian Pflanzensaft Nerventrost *Kneipp, Ger.*
Valerian (p.1678·3).
Nervousness; sleep disorders.

Kneipp Balsamo *Fher, Spain.*
Camphor (p.1589·3); peru balsam (p.1650·2); eucalyptol (p.1609·2); oleum pini sylvestris; thymol (p.1158·3); menthol (p.1632·3).
Upper-respiratory-tract disorders.

Kneipp Beruhigungs-Bad spezial *Kneipp, Ger.*
Citronella (p.1596·3).
Anxiety; bath additive; tension.

Kneipp Birkenblatter Pflanzensaft *Kneipp, Ger.*
Birch leaf (p.1585·2).
Urinary-tract disorders.

Kneipp Blasen- und Nieren-Tee *Kneipp, Ger.*
Equisetum (p.1606·3); solidago virgaurea; birch leaf (p.1585·2); ononis (p.1644·1).
Urinary-tract disorders.

Kneipp Brennesselkraut Pflanzensaft Kneippianum *Kneipp, Ger.*
Urtica (p.1678·2).
Rheumatic disorders; urinary-tract disorders.

Kneipp Brunnenkresse-Pflanzensaft *Kneipp, Ger.†*
Nasturtium.
Diuretic.

Kneipp Calcium compositum N *Kneipp, Ger.*
Multivitamin and mineral preparation (p.1350·1).
Calcium deficiency.

Kneipp Drei-Pflanzen-Dragees N *Kneipp, Ger.*
Combination pack: Tablets, Crataegus (p.1600·2); tablets, garlic (p.1614·1); tablets, mistletoe (p.1636·2).
Arteriosclerosis.

Kneipp Entschlackungs-Tee *Kneipp, Ger.*
Juniper (p.1625·2); peppermint leaf (p.1243·2); birch leaf (p.1585·2).
Diuretic.

Kneipp Entwasserungstee *Kneipp, Aust.*
Juniper (p.1625·2); peppermint leaf (p.1243·2); silver birch leaf (p.1585·2).
Diuretic.

Kneipp Erkaltungs-Bad *Kneipp, Ger.*
Thyme oil (p.1672·3).
Bath additive; cold symptoms.

Kneipp Erkaltungsbad Spezial *Kneipp, Ger.*
Eucalyptus oil (p.1609·2); camphor (p.1589·3).
Bath additive; catarrh.

Kneipp Erkaltungs-Balsam N *Kneipp, Ger.*
Eucalyptus oil (p.1609·2); siberian fir oil; rosemary oil (p.1659·3); pumilio pine oil (p.1656·3); thyme oil (p.1672·3); turpentine oil (p.1676·3).
Coughs and associated respiratory-tract disorders.

Kneipp Erkaltungs-Tee *Kneipp, Ger.*
Tilia (p.1673·2); sambucus (p.1660·3); thyme (p.1672·2).
Cold symptoms.

Kneipp Fichtennadel Franzbranntwein *Kneipp, Ger.*
Menthol (p.1632·3); alcohol (p.1130·3).
Musculoskeletal, joint, and soft-tissue disorders; peripheral circulatory disorders.

Kneipp Flatulo *Kneipp, Ger.*
Fennel (p.1610·1); caraway (p.1591·2); peppermint leaf (p.1243·2); gentian (p.1615·1).
Flatulence; meteorism.

Kneipp Galle- und Leber-Tee *Kneipp, Aust.*
Peppermint leaf (p.1243·2); turmeric (p.1029·2); taraxacum (p.1669·1).
Gallbladder and liver disorders.

Kneipp Galle- und Leber-Tee N *Kneipp, Ger.*
Peppermint leaf (p.1243·2); turmeric (p.1029·2); taraxacum (p.1669·1).
Biliary and liver disorders; herbal tea.

Kneipp Ginsenetten *Kneipp, Ger.†*
Ginseng (p.1615·3).
Tonic.

Kneipp Grippe-Tee *Kneipp, Aust.*
Tilia (p.1673·2); salix purpurea (p.82·1); plantago lanceolata; thyme (p.1672·2); chamomile (p.1593·2).
Cold symptoms.

Kneipp Herz- und Kreislauf-Tee *Kneipp, Ger.*
Rosemary; crataegus (p.1600·2); motherwort (p.1637·3); hypericum (p.290·2); Paraguay tea.
Cardiovascular disorders.

Kneipp Herz- und Kreislauf-Unterstutzungs-Tee *Kneipp, Aust.*
Rosemary leaf; crataegus (p.1600·2); maté leaf (p.1681·1).
Cardiovascular disorders.

Kneipp Herzsalbe Unguentum Cardiacum Kneipp *Kneipp, Ger.*
Rosemary oil (p.1659·3); camphor (p.1589·3); menthol (p.1632·3).
Cardiac disorders.

Kneipp Heupack Herbatherm N *Kneipp, Ger.*
Cut grasses and flowers.
Biliary-tract, kidney, and bladder disorders; rheumatic and arthritic disorders.

Kneipp Husten- und Bronchial-Tee
Kneipp, Aust.; Kneipp, Ger.
Fennel (p.1610·1); cowslip flowers and calyx (p.1600·1); thyme (p.1672·2); plantago lanceolata.
Bronchitis; catarrh; coughs.

Kneipp Hustensaft Spitzwegerich *Kneipp, Ger.*
Plantago lanceolata.
Catarrh.

Kneipp Knoblauch Dragees N *Kneipp, Ger.*
Garlic (p.1614·1).
Arteriosclerosis.

Kneipp Knoblauch-Pflanzensaft *Kneipp, Ger.*
Garlic (p.1614·1).
Arteriosclerosis; digestive system disorders; hypertension.

Kneipp Krauter Hustensaft N Kneipp Tannolsaft *Kneipp, Ger.*
Norway spruce oil; pumilio pine oil (p.1656·3); cowslip flower (p.1600·1); thyme (p.1672·2).
Coughs and associated respiratory-tract disorders.

Kneipp Krauter Taschenkur Nerven und Schlaf N *Kneipp, Ger.*
Combination pack: Tablets, valerian (p.1678·3); tablets, hypericum (p.290·2); tablets, melissa leaves (p.1632·2); citronella oil (p.1596·3); lemon grass oil (p.1628·2).
Nervous disorders.

Kneipp Kreislauf-Bad Rosmarin-Aquasan *Kneipp, Ger.†*
Camphor (p.1589·3); rosemary oil (p.1659·3).
Bath additive; circulatory disorders.

Kneipp Latschenkiefer Franzbranntwein *Kneipp, Ger.†*
Camphor (p.1589·3); oleum pini sylvestris; alcohol (p.1130·3).
Musculoskeletal and joint disorders; peripheral vascular disorders; soft-tissue disorders.

Kneipp Lowenzahn-Pflanzensaft *Kneipp, Ger.*
Taraxacum (p.1669·1).
Gall bladder and liver disorders.

Kneipp Magen-Tee *Kneipp, Ger.*
Aniseed (p.1580·2); fennel (p.1610·1); caraway (p.1591·2).
Gastrointestinal disorders.

Kneipp Melisse Pflanzensaft *Kneipp, Ger.*
Melissa (p.1632·2).
Nervous disorders.

Kneipp Milch-Molke-Bad *Kneipp, Ger.†*
Skimmed milk; whey; lactic acid (p.1626·2).
Bath additive; burns; skin disorders.

Kneipp Minzol Trost Tropfen *Kneipp, Ger.*
Mint oil (p.1636·2).
Cold symptoms; gastrointestinal disorders; myalgia; neuralgia.

Kneipp Mistel-Pflanzensaft *Kneipp, Ger.*
Mistletoe (p.1636·2).
Circulatory disorders.

Kneipp Nerven- und Schlaf-Tee *Kneipp, Aust.*
Melissa (p.1632·2); valerian (p.1678·3); citrus sinensis.
Nervous disorders; sleep disorders.

Kneipp Nerven- und Schlaf-Tee N *Kneipp, Ger.*
Melissa (p.1632·2); valerian (p.1678·3); sweet orange peel.
Nervous disorders.

Kneipp Neurodermatitis-Bad *Kneipp, Ger.†*
Soya oil (p.1378·1).
Bath additive; dry skin; pruritus.

Kneipp Nieren- und Blasen-Tee *Kneipp, Aust.*
Silver birch (p.1585·2); equisetum (p.1606·3); solidago virgaurea; ononis (p.1644·1); peppermint leaf (p.1243·2); calendula (p.1589·2).
Urinary-tract disorders.

Kneipp Petersilie N *Kneipp, Ger.*
Parsley (p.1648·3).
Diuretic.

Kneipp Pflanzen-Dragees Brennessel *Kneipp, Ger.*
Urtica (p.1678·2).
Urinary-tract disorders.

Kneipp Pflanzen-Dragees Mistel *Kneipp, Ger.*
Mistletoe (p.1636·2).
Circulatory disorders.

Kneipp Pflanzen-Dragees Weissdorn *Kneipp, Ger.*
Crataegus leaves, flowers, and fruit (p.1600·2).
Cardiac disorders.

Kneipp Rettich-Pflanzensaft *Kneipp, Ger.†*
Raphanus.
Gall bladder and liver disorders.

Kneipp Rheuma Salbe *Kneipp, Ger.*
Cayenne pepper (p.1591·1).
Musculoskeletal and joint disorders; neuralgia; sciatica.

Kneipp Rheuma Stoffwechsel-Bad Heublumen-Aquasan *Kneipp, Ger.*
Coumarin (p.1599·3); peppermint oil (p.1243·2); caraway oil (p.1591·2); sage oil (p.1660·2); thyme oil (p.1672·3).
Bath additive; tonic bath.

Kneipp Rheuma Tee N *Kneipp, Ger.†*
Dulcamara stalk (p.1606·2); salix bark (p.82·1); sambucus leaf (p.1660·3); juniper berry (p.1625·2); red sandalwood.
Rheumatic disorders.

Kneipp Rheuma-Bad *Kneipp, Ger.*
Juniper oil (p.1625·2); sweet birch oil (p.55·2).
Bath additive; rheumatism and spinal disorders.

Kneipp Rosmarin-Pflanzensaft *Kneipp, Ger.†*
Rosemary leaf.
Circulatory disorders.

Kneipp Schafgarbe-Pflanzensaft Frauentost N *Kneipp, Ger.†*
Achillea (p.1572·2).
Anorexia; digestive system disorders.

Kneipp Spitzwegerich-Pflanzensaft Hustentrost *Kneipp, Ger.*
Plantago lanceolata.
Catarrh; mouth and throat disorders.

Kneipp Stoffwechsel-Unterstutzungs-Tee *Kneipp, Aust.*
Prunus spinosa; taraxacum (p.1669·1); peppermint leaf (p.1243·2); lovage (p.1629·3); hibiscus.
Stimulation of metabolic activity.

Kneipp Tonikum-Bad Fichtennadel-Aquasan *Kneipp, Ger.†.*
Norway spruce oil; eucalyptus oil (p.1609·2); turpentine oil (p.1676·3).
Bath additive; tonic bath.

Kneipp Verdauungs-Tee *Kneipp, Aust.*
Prunus spinosa; chamomile (p.1593·2); fennel (p.1610·1); centaury (p.1593·1).
Gastrointestinal disorders.

Kneipp Verdauungs-Tee N *Kneipp, Ger.*
Chamomile (p.1593·2); fennel (p.1610·1); centaury (p.1593·1).
Gastrointestinal disorders.

Kneipp Wacholderbeer-Pflanzensaft *Kneipp, Ger.†.*
Juniper (p.1625·2).
Diuretic; gastrointestinal disorders.

Kneipp Weissdorn-Pflanzensaft Sebastianeum *Kneipp, Ger.*
Crataegus (p.1600·2).
Cardiac disorders.

Kneipp Weissdorn-Tee *Kneipp, Ger.*
Crataegus (p.1600·2).
Cardiac disorders.

Kneipp Woerisettes *Roche, Switz.†.*
Aloes (p.1210·1); plant extracts.
Constipation.

Kneipp Worisetten S *Kneipp, Ger.*
Senna (p.1248·2).
Constipation.

Kneipp Zinnkraut-Pflanzensaft *Kneipp, Ger.*
Equisetum (p.1606·3).
Urinary-tract disorders.

Kneipplax N *Kneipp, Ger.†.*
Ispaghula (p.1229·1); senna (p.1248·2).
Constipation.

Knoblauch-Vital *Bioflora, Aust.*
Garlic; vitamin E (p.1350·1).
Tonic.

Knochenzement *Synthes, Aust.*
Methylmethacrylate/polymethylmethacrylate (p.1635·2).
Bone cement in orthopaedic surgery.

K-Norm *Fisons, USA.*
Potassium chloride (p.1194·3).
Hypokalaemia; potassium depletion.

Koate *Kolassa, Aust.†.*
A factor VIII preparation (p.734·1).
Factor VIII deficiency.

Koate-DVI *Bayer, USA.*
A factor VIII preparation (p.734·1).
Haemorrhagic disorders.

Koate-HP
Bayer, Canad.†; Bayer Biological, Hong Kong; Bayer, Israel; Probifasa, Mex.; Bayer, Singapore; Bayer, USA†.
A factor VIII preparation (p.734·1).
Haemophilia A.

Koate-HS *Sclavo, Ital.†.*
A factor VIII preparation (p.734·1).
Haemorrhagic disorders.

Kochsalz mit Glucose *Braun, Ger.*
Sodium chloride (p.1196·1); glucose (p.1364·1).
Fluid and electrolyte disorders.

Kodamid *Nycomed, Denm.*
Codeine phosphate (p.25·2); caffeine (p.761·3); propyphenazone (p.80·2); salicylamide (p.82·1).
Magnesium hydroxide (p.1233·1) is included in this preparation in an attempt to limit adverse effects on the gastrointestinal mucosa.
Pain.

Kodan Tinktur Forte *Schulke & Mayr, Ger.*
Isopropyl alcohol (p.1149·2); propyl alcohol (p.1155·3); orthophenylphenol (p.1152·1).
Skin disinfection.

Kodapon *Pharmagen, S.Afr.†.*
Paracetamol (p.71·2); codeine phosphate (p.25·2).
Fever; pain.

Kodimagnyl *Nycomed, Denm.*
Aspirin (p.14·2); codeine phosphate (p.25·2).
Magnesium hydroxide (p.1233·1) is included in some dosage forms in an attempt to limit adverse effects on the gastrointestinal mucosa.
Pain.

Kodipar *Nycomed, Denm.*
Codeine phosphate (p.25·2); paracetamol (p.71·2).
Pain.

Kof-Eze *Roberts, USA.*
Menthol (p.1632·3).
Coughs; sore throats.

Koffazon *Recip, Swed.*
Caffeine (p.761·3); phenazone (p.77·2).
Pain.

Koffex *Rougier, Canad.*
Dextromethorphan hydrobromide (p.1087·3).

Koffex DM *Rougier, Canad.*
Dextromethorphan hydrobromide (p.1087·3).
Coughs.

Koffex DM-D *Rougier, Canad.*
Dextromethorphan hydrobromide (p.1087·3); pseudoephedrine hydrochloride (p.1099·2).
Coughs.

Koffex DM-D-E *Rougier, Canad.*
Dextromethorphan hydrobromide (p.1087·3); pseudoephedrine hydrochloride (p.1099·2); guaifenesin (p.1092·2).
Coughs; respiratory-tract congestion.

Koffex DM-E *Rougier, Canad.*
Dextromethorphan hydrobromide (p.1087·3); guaifenesin (p.1092·2).
Coughs.

Koffex Expectorant *Rougier, Canad.*
Guaifenesin (p.1092·2).

Koffisal *Nycomed, Denm.*
Caffeine (p.761·3); phenazone salicylate (p.77·2); salicylamide (p.82·1).
Pain.

Kofron *Guidotti, Spain.*
Clarithromycin (p.186·2).
Bacterial infections.

Kogenate
Bayer, Aust.; Bayer, Austral.; Bayer, Belg.; Bayer, Canad.; Bayer, Denm.; Bayer, Fr.; Bayer, Ger.; Bayer, Irl.; Bayer, Ital.; Bayer, Neth.; Bayer, Norw.; Bayer, NZ; Bayer, Port.; Bayer, Spain; Bayer, Swed.; Bayer, Switz.; Bayer, UK; Bayer, USA.
A factor VIII preparation (recombinant) (p.734·1).
Haemorrhagic disorders.

Kohle-Compretten *Merck, Ger.*
Activated charcoal (p.1000·2).
Acute poisoning; diarrhoea.

Kohle-Hevert *Hevert, Ger.*
Activated charcoal (p.1000·2).
Acute poisoning; diarrhoea.

Kohlensaurebad Bastian *Bastian, Ger.*
Sodium bicarbonate (p.1186·2).
Bath additive; cardiac and circulatory disorders.

Kohle-Pulvis *Kohler, Ger.*
Activated charcoal (p.1000·2).
Acute poisoning; diarrhoea.

Kohle-Tabletten *Boxo, Ger.*
Activated charcoal (p.1000·2).
Acute poisoning; diarrhoea.

Kohrsolin *Bode, Ger.*
Glutaral (p.1145·2); 1,6-dihydroxy-2,5-dioxahexan; polymethylolurea derivative.
Surface and instrument disinfection.

Kohrsolin FF *Bode, Ger.*
Glutaral (p.1145·2); benzalkonium chloride (p.1133·2); didecyldimethylammonium chloride (p.1143·2).
Surface disinfection.

Kohrsolin iD *Bode, Ger.*
Glutaral (p.1145·2); 1,6-dihydroxy-2,5-dioxahexan; polymethylolurea derivative.
Instrument disinfection.

Kola Astier *URPAC, Fr.*
Kola (p.1681·1); caffeine (p.761·3).
Asthenia.

Kola Fosfatada Soel *Regius, Braz.*
Kola (p.1681·1); nux vomica (p.1643·1); sodium glycerophosphate; calcium glycerophosphate (p.1350·1).
Tonic.

Kola-Dallmann *Dallmann, Ger.†.*
Kola (p.1681·1); caffeine (p.761·3).
Fatigue.

Kola-Dallmann mit Lecithin *Dallmann, Ger.†.*
Kola (p.1681·1); caffeine (p.761·3); egg lecithin (p.1628·1).
Fatigue.

Koladex *Laboratories for Applied Biology, UK.*
Caffeine (p.761·3); kola nut (p.1681·1).
Tonic.

Kolampept *Teuto, Braz.*
Aluminium hydroxide (p.1210·3); magnesium hydroxide (p.1233·1); dimethicone (p.1249·2).
Flatulence; gastrointestinal hyperacidity.

Kolanticon
Peckforton, Irl.; Peckforton, UK.
Aluminium hydroxide (p.1210·3); dicyclomine [dicycloverine] hydrochloride (p.466·1); light magnesium oxide (p.1233·2); simeticone (p.1249·2).
Dyspepsia; gastritis; gastro-oesophageal reflux; peptic ulcer.

Kolantyl
Note.This name is used for preparations of different composition.
Medley, Braz.
Dicyclomine [dicycloverine] hydrochloride (p.466·1); aluminium hydroxide (p.1210·3); magnesium hydroxide (p.1233·1); methylcellulose (p.1502·2); magnesium trisilicate (p.1233·3).
Gastrointestinal hyperacidity.

Adcock Ingram, S.Afr.
Oral gel: Dicyclomine [dicycloverine] hydrochloride (p.466·1); aluminium hydroxide (p.1210·3); magnesium oxide (p.1233·2); methylcellulose (p.1502·2).
Wafers: Dicyclomine [dicycloverine] hydrochloride (p.466·1); aluminium hydroxide (p.1210·3); magnesium hydroxide (p.1233·1); methylcellulose (p.1502·2); magnesium trisilicate (p.1233·3).
Gastrointestinal disorders.

Kolantyl DMP *Medley, Braz.*
Aluminium hydroxide (p.1210·3); magnesium hydroxide (p.1233·1); methylcellulose (p.1502·2); dimethicone (p.1249·2).
Flatulence; gastrointestinal hyperacidity.

Kolemed *Rosch & Handel, Aust.*
Activated charcoal (p.1000·2).
Diarrhoea; flatulence.

Kolephrin *Pfeiffer, USA.*
Pseudoephedrine hydrochloride (p.1099·2); paracetamol (p.71·2); chlorpheniramine [chlorphenamine] maleate (p.412·1).
Upper respiratory-tract symptoms.

Kolephrin GG/DM *Pfeiffer, USA.*
Dextromethorphan hydrobromide (p.1087·3); guaifenesin (p.1092·2).
Coughs.

Kolephrin/DM *Pfeiffer, USA.*
Chlorpheniramine [chlorphenamine] maleate (p.412·1); dextromethorphan hydrobromide (p.1087·3); paracetamol (p.71·2); pseudoephedrine hydrochloride (p.1099·2).
Coughs and cold symptoms.

Kolestop *Omni, UK.*
Sitosterol (p.970·3); beta sitostanol.
Nutritional supplement to reduce serum cholesterol.

Kollaps-Gastreu N R67 *Reckeweg, Ger.*
Homoeopathic preparation.

Kollateral *Ursapharm, Ger.*
Moxaverine hydrochloride (p.1638·1).
Coronary disorders; peripheral and cerebral circulatory disorders.

Kollateral A + E *Ursapharm, Ger.*
Moxaverine hydrochloride (p.1638·1); vitamin A acetate (p.1383·2); alpha tocoferil acetate (p.1394·1).
Cerebral, coronary, and ocular vascular disorders.

Kolsuspension *Abigo, Swed.*
Activated charcoal (p.1000·2).
Diarrhoea; poisoning.

Kolton bronchiale Erkaltungssaft *Promonta, Ger.†.*
Thyme (p.1672·2).
Bronchitis; catarrh; coughs.

Kolton grippale N *Byk Gulden, Ger.*
Piprinhydrinate (p.423·1); paracetamol (p.71·2); ethenzamide (p.35·1).
Cold and influenza symptoms.

Kolyum *Fisons, USA.*
Potassium gluconate (p.1194·3); potassium citrate (p.1186·1).
Hypokalaemia; potassium depletion.

Kombetin
Boehringer Mannheim, Ger.†; Roche, Ital.
Strophanthin-K (p.978·2).
Cardiac disorders.

Komb-H-Insulin *Hoechst, Ger.†.*
Mixture of insulin injection (human) 50% and isophane insulin (human) 50% (p.324·1).
Diabetes mellitus.

Kombicrom *Fisons, Denm.*
Sodium cromoglicate (p.774·3); xylometazoline hydrochloride (p.1102·2).
Allergic rhinitis.

Kombinax *Bracco, Ital.*
Sulfadiazine (p.251·1); trimethoprim (p.264·2).
Bacterial infections.

Komb-Insulin
Hoechst Marion Roussel, Aust.
Insulin injection (porcine) (p.324·1).
Diabetes mellitus.

Hoechst Marion Roussel, Ger.
Insulin (chromatographically purified, bovine), comprising a mixture of Insulin and Depot-Insulin (Hoechst, Ger.) (p.324·1).
Diabetes mellitus.

Komb-Insulin S *Hoechst Marion Roussel, Ger.*
Insulin (chromatographically purified, porcine), comprising a mixture of Insulin S and Depot-Insulin S (Hoechst, Ger.) (p.324·1).
Diabetes mellitus.

Kombistrat *UCB, Swed.†.*
Hydroxyzine hydrochloride (p.419·1); oxyphencyclimine hydrochloride (p.472·1).
Gastrointestinal disorders.

Kombi-Stulln *Stulln, Ger.*
Polymyxin B sulfate (p.238·1); neomycin sulfate (p.228·1); gramicidin (p.213·3).
Eye infections.

Kompensan
Pfizer, Ger.; Pfizer, Port.; Pfizer, Switz.
Dihydroxyaluminum sodium carbonate (p.1222·1).
Gastrointestinal disorders associated with hyperacidity.

Kompensan-S
Pfizer, Ger.; Pfizer, Port.; Pfizer, Switz.
Dihydroxyaluminum sodium carbonate (p.1222·1); dimethicone (p.1249·2).
Gastrointestinal disorders.

Kona *M & H, Thai.*
Dextromethorphan hydrobromide (p.1087·3); diphenhydramine hydrochloride (p.416·1); pseudoephedrine hydrochloride (p.1099·2).
Cold symptoms; coughs; nasal congestion.

Konaderm *ICN, Mex.*
Ketoconazole (p.389·1).
Fungal skin infections.

Konakion
Roche, Aust.; Roche, Austral.; Roche, Belg.; Roche, Denm.; Roche, Fin.; Roche, Ger.; Roche, Hong Kong; Roche, Irl.; Roche, Israel; Roche, Ital.; Roche, Mex.; Roche, Neth.; Roche, NZ; Roche, S.Afr.; Roche, Singapore; Roche, Spain; Roche, Swed.; Roche, Switz.; Roche, Thai.; Roche, UK; Roche, USA†.
Phytomenadione (p.1396·1).
Anticoagulant antidote; haemorrhagic disease of the newborn; hypoprothrombinaemia; salicylate poisoning; vitamin K deficiency.

Konakion Novum *Roche, Norw.*
Phytomenadione (p.1396·1).
Haemorrhage in neonates; hypoprothrombinaemia; warfarin overdose.

Konazil *Sintofarma, Braz.*
Ketoconazole (p.389·1).
Fungal infections.

Konazol *PP Lab, Thai.*
Ketoconazole (p.389·1).
Fungal infections.

Kondon's Nasal *Kondon, USA.*
Ephedrine (p.1090·1).
Nasal congestion.

Kondremul *Fisons, USA.*
Liquid paraffin (p.1407·1).
Constipation.

Kondremul with Phenolphthalein *Fisons, USA†.*
Liquid paraffin (p.1407·1); phenolphthalein (p.1244·1).
Constipation.

Konjax *Murat, Fr.†.*
Glucomannan (p.1616·2).
Obesity.

Konjunktival *Thilo, Hong Kong.*
Naphazoline hydrochloride (p.1095·1); pheniramine maleate (p.422·3).
Conjunctivitis.

Konjunktival Thilo *Alcon, Ger.*
Naphazoline hydrochloride (p.1095·1); pheniramine maleate (p.422·3).
Eye disorders.

Konlax
Shinyaku, Hong Kong; Shinyaku, Thai.
Pridinol mesilate (p.1330·1).
Skeletal muscle spasm.

Konor *Italzama, Ital.*
Tar (p.1125·1).
Seborrhoeic dermatitis.

Konorderm *Italzama, Ital.*
Inositol, vitamin PP, vitamin E, betacarotene, selenium, L-cystine (p.1350·1).
Antioxidant nutritional supplement.

Konovid *TO-Chemicals, Thai.*
Ofloxacin (p.232·3).
Bacterial infections.

Konstitutin *CytoChemia, Ger.*
Eleutherococcus senticosis (p.1615·3).
Tonic.

Konsyl
Glaxo Wellcome, Mex.; Pacific, NZ; Mepha, Switz.; Eastern Pharmaceuticals, UK; Konsyl, USA.
Ispaghula (p.1229·1).
Constipation; diarrhoea; irritable bowel syndrome.

Konsyl Fiber *Konsyl, USA†.*
Polycarbophil calcium (p.1244·2).

Konsyl-D *Konsyl, USA.*
Psyllium hydrophilic mucilloid (p.1229·1).
Constipation.

Kontagripp Mono *Azupharma, Ger.*
Ibuprofen (p.43·2).
Fever; pain.

Kontakto Derm Lotio *Combe, Ger.*
Benzocaine (p.1306·2); benzyl benzoate (p.1428·2).
Eczema; pruritus.

Kontal *Leiras, Fin.*
Niclosamide (p.104·2).
Worm infections.

Kontexin
Pharmacia Upjohn, Aust.†; Pharmacia Upjohn, Switz.
Phenylpropanolamine hydrochloride (p.1098·1).
Urinary incontinence.

Konyne *Cutter, Israel.*
A factor IX preparation (p.735·1).
Haemophilia B.

Konyne 80
Bayer Biological, Hong Kong; Probifasa, Mex.; Bayer, USA†.
Factor IX complex (p.735·1).
Haemophilia B; haemorrhagic disorders.

Kop Alerge Vacina *Kopkins, Braz.*
An oral anticatarrh vaccine.
Active immunisation.

Kop Hepar *Kopkins, Braz.*
Solanum paniculatum; boldo (p.1585·3); cynara (p.1601·3).
Liver disorders.

Kopen *Athlone, Irl.*
Phenoxymethylpenicillin (p.235·1).
Gram-positive bacterial infections.

Kophane Cough and Cold Formula *Pfeiffer, USA†.*
Phenylpropanolamine hydrochloride (p.1098·1); chlorpheniramine [chlorphenamine] maleate (p.412·1); dextromethorphan hydrobromide (p.1087·3).
Coughs and cold symptoms.

Korandil *Remedica, Thai.*
Enalapril maleate (p.883·3).
Heart failure; hypertension.

Koreberon *Asta Medica, Ger.*
Sodium fluoride (p.1375·3).
Osteoporosis.

Korec *Sanofi Winthrop, Fr.*
Quinapril hydrochloride (p.963·3).
Heart failure; hypertension.

Koretic *Sanofi Winthrop, Fr.*
Quinapril hydrochloride (p.963·3); hydrochlorothiazide (p.907·3).
Hypertension.

The symbol † denotes a preparation no longer actively marketed

Koro M & H, Thai.
Chloramphenicol (p.179·1).
Bacterial eye infections.

Korodin
Note.This name is used for preparations of different composition.
Robugen, Ger.
Camphor (p.1589·3); crataegus (p.1600·2).
Cardiac disorders; circulatory disorders.

Medipharm, Switz.†.
Chamomile (p.1593·2); crataegus (p.1600·2).
Cardiac disorders.

Koromex QHP, USA.
Vaginal cream: Octoxinol (p.1346·3).
Vaginal jelly; vaginal gel; condom: Nonoxinol 9 (p.1346·1).
Contraceptive.

Korseng Self-Care Products, UK.
Ginseng (p.1615·3).

Korsolex AF Bode, Ger.
Laurylpropylenediamine; dodecylbispropylenetriamine.
Instrument disinfection.

Korsolex basic Bode, Ger.
Glutaral (p.1145·2); dihydroxydioxahexane.
Instrument disinfection.

Korsolex FF Bode, Ger.†.
Glutaral (p.1145·2); succindialdehyde; polyoxyethylene cocosamine.
Instrument disinfection.

Korsolex-Endo-Disinfectant Bode, Ger.
Glutaral (p.1145·2).
Disinfection of endoscopes.

Korticoid Cophar, Switz.
Fluocinonide (p.1071·2).
Skin disorders.

Korticoid polyvalent Cophar, Switz.
Fluocinonide (p.1071·2); gramicidin (p.213·3); neomycin sulfate (p.228·1); nystatin (p.392·2).
Infected skin disorders.

Kortikoid-ratiopharm Ratiopharm, Ger.
Triamcinolone acetonide (p.1080·1).
Burns; skin disorders.

Korynase Kyorin, Thai.
Promelase (p.1655·1).
Inflammation; oedema.

Korzen Korean Drug, Singapore.
Serrapeptase (p.1662·1).
Inflammation; respiratory-tract congestion.

Kos Crinos, Ital.†.
Ibuprofen pyridoxine (p.44·1).
Musculoskeletal and joint disorders; pain.

Kovilen Mediolanum, Ital.
Nedocromil sodium (p.768·3).
Ocular hypersensitivity reactions.

Kovinal Mediolanum, Ital.
Nedocromil sodium (p.768·3).
Allergic rhinitis.

Kovitonic Freeda, USA.
Ferric pyrophosphate (p.1359·3); folic acid (p.1361·1); vitamin B substances with L-lysine (p.1350·1).
Iron-deficiency anaemias.

KP PP Lab, Thai.
Phytomenadione (p.1396·1).
Haemorrhagic disorders.

K-Pek Rugby, USA.
Attapulgite (p.1212·1).
Diarrhoea.

K-Phen Kay, USA†.
Promethazine hydrochloride (p.423·2).
Hypersensitivity reactions; motion sickness; nausea; postoperative pain (adjunct); sedative; vomiting.

K-Phos MF Beach, USA.
Monobasic potassium phosphate (p.1193·1); monobasic sodium phosphate (p.1193·2).
Urinary acidification.

K-Phos Neutral Beach, USA.
Dibasic sodium phosphate (p.1193·2); monobasic potassium phosphate (p.1193·1); monobasic sodium phosphate (p.1193·2).
Phosphorus supplement.

K-Phos No.2 Beach, USA.
Monobasic potassium phosphate (p.1193·1); monobasic sodium phosphate (p.1193·2).
Urinary acidification.

K-Phos Original Beach, USA.
Monobasic potassium phosphate (p.1193·1).
Urinary acidification.

KPN Freeda, USA.
Multivitamin and mineral preparation with iron and folic acid (p.1350·1).

K-Profen Medix, Mex.
Ketoprofen (p.47·3).
Musculoskeletal, joint, and peri-articular disorders.

Kraftol Profarb, Braz.
Vitamin and mineral preparation (p.1350·1).

Krama Miba, Ital.
Barrier cream.

Kratalgin Kwizda, Aust.
Ibuprofen (p.43·2).
Pain.

Kratium Medochemie, Hong Kong.
Diazepam (p.674·3).
Anxiety; skeletal muscle spasm; sleep disorders.

Kratofin Kwizda, Aust.†.
Paracetamol (p.71·2); aluminium aspirin (p.13·3); caffeine (p.761·3).
Fever; pain.

Kratofin simplex Kwizda, Aust.
Paracetamol (p.71·2).
Fever; pain.

Krauter Hustensaft Apomedica, Aust.
Thyme (p.1672·2); ononis (p.1644·1); cowslip root (p.1600·1); liquorice (p.1231·2); castanea vulgaris; sambucus (p.1660·3).
Catarrh; coughs.

Krauterdoktor Beruhigungstropfen Kollerics, Aust.
Lupulus (p.1629·3); melissa (p.1632·2); orange flower.
Anxiety; nervous disorders.

Krauterdoktor Entschlackungs-Elixier Kollerics, Aust.
Taraxacum (p.1669·1); viola tricolor; manna (p.1233·3); bitter-orange peel (p.1644·2); rose fruit (p.1389·3).
Tonic.

Krauterdoktor Entspannungs- und Einschlaftropfen Kollerics, Aust.
Valerian (p.1678·3); lupulus (p.1629·3); melissa (p.1632·2).
Anxiety disorders; sleep disorders.

Krauterdoktor Entwasserungs-Elixier Kollerics, Aust.
Silver birch (p.1585·2); equisetum (p.1606·3); urtica (p.1678·2).
Urinary-tract disorders.

Krauterdoktor Erkaltungstropfen Kollerics, Aust.
Sambucus (p.1660·3); tilia (p.1673·2); centaury (p.1593·1).
Cold symptoms.

Krauterdoktor Gallentreibende Tropfen Kollerics, Aust.
Taraxacum (p.1669·1); achillea (p.1572·2); absinthium (p.1571·1).
Biliary-tract disorders.

Krauterdoktor Harnstein- und Nierengriesstropfen Kollerics, Aust.
Ononis (p.1644·1); taraxacum (p.1669·1); centaury (p.1593·1).
Urinary-tract disorders.

Krauterdoktor Hustentropfen Kollerics, Aust.
Fennel (p.1610·1); cowslip root (p.1600·1); thyme (p.1672·2).
Catarrh; coughs.

Krauterdoktor Krampf- und Reizhustensirup Kollerics, Aust.
Aniseed (p.1580·2); drosera (p.1606·1); thyme (p.1672·2).
Coughs.

Krauterdoktor Magen-Darmtropfen Kollerics, Aust.
Valerian (p.1678·3); caraway (p.1591·2); melissa (p.1632·2).
Gastrointestinal disorders.

Krauterdoktor Nerven-Tonikum Kollerics, Aust.
Valerian (p.1678·3); lupulus (p.1629·3); melissa (p.1632·2).
Anxiety; nervousness; sleep disorders.

Krauterdoktor Rosmarin-Wein Kollerics, Aust.
Rosemary; melissa (p.1632·2).
Circulatory disorders.

Krauterdoktor Verdauungsfordernde Tropfen Kollerics, Aust.
Angelica (p.1580·2); centaury (p.1593·1); absinthium (p.1571·1).
Gastrointestinal disorders.

Krautergeist S Jukunda, Ger.†.
Melissa; sloe; ginger; melissa oil; rosemary oil; lavender oil; capsicum oil; cinnamon oil; clove oil (p.1350·1).
Tonic.

Krauterhaus Mag Kottas Babytee Kottas-Heldenberg, Aust.
Chamomile (p.1593·2); mallow leaf; melissa (p.1632·2); caraway (p.1591·2); fennel (p.1610·1).
Gastrointestinal disorders.

Krauterhaus Mag Kottas Blasentee Kottas-Heldenberg, Aust.
Silver birch (p.1585·2); java tea (p.1625·1); herniaria (p.1619·2); couch-grass (p.1599·3); ononis (p.1644·1); peppermint leaf (p.1243·2).
Urinary-tract disorders.

Krauterhaus Mag Kottas Blutreinigungstee Kottas-Heldenberg, Aust.†.
Peppermint leaf (p.1243·2); urtica (p.1678·2); viola tricolor; taraxacum (p.1669·1); achillea (p.1572·2); calendula (p.1589·2).
Tonic.

Krauterhaus Mag Kottas Entschlackungstee Kottas-Heldenberg, Aust.
Silver birch (p.1585·2); peppermint leaf (p.1243·2); taraxacum (p.1669·1); urtica (p.1678·2); ononis (p.1644·1); chamomile (p.1593·2).
Diuretic.

Krauterhaus Mag Kottas Entwasserungstee Kottas-Heldenberg, Aust.
Equisetum (p.1606·3); parsley root (p.1648·3); couch-grass (p.1599·3); solidago virgaurea; urtica (p.1678·2); peppermint leaf (p.1243·2); calendula (p.1589·2).
Urinary-tract disorders.

Krauterhaus Mag Kottas Fruhjahrs- und Herbstkurtee Kottas-Heldenberg, Aust.
Peppermint leaf (p.1243·2); equisetum (p.1606·3); achillea (p.1572·2); urtica (p.1678·2); viola tricolor; calendula (p.1589·2); mallow flower.
Tonic.

Krauterhaus Mag Kottas Gallen- und Lebertee Kottas-Heldenberg, Aust.
Mallow leaf; peppermint leaf (p.1243·2); menyanthes (p.1633·1); agrimony (p.1574·3); taraxacum (p.1669·1); calendula (p.1589·2).
Biliary-tract disorders.

Krauterhaus Mag Kottas Grippetee Kottas-Heldenberg, Aust.
Sambucus (p.1660·3); tilia (p.1673·2); plantago lanceolata; rose fruit (p.1389·3).
Cold symptoms.

Krauterhaus Mag Kottas Husten- und Bronchialtee Kottas-Heldenberg, Aust.
Verbascum flower; althaea (p.1577·1); plantago lanceolata; thyme (p.1672·2); mallow flower.
Catarrh; coughs; sore throat.

Krauterhaus Mag Kottas Magen- und Darmtee Kottas-Heldenberg, Aust.
Chamomile (p.1593·2); mallow leaf; melissa (p.1632·2); peppermint leaf (p.1243·2); achillea (p.1572·2); calendula (p.1589·2).
Gastrointestinal disorders.

Krauterhaus Mag Kottas milder Abfuhrtee Kottas-Heldenberg, Aust.
Prunus spinosa; fennel (p.1610·1); mallow leaf; peppermint leaf (p.1243·2); rose fruit (p.1389·3).
Constipation.

Krauterhaus Mag Kottas Nerven- und Schlaftee Kottas-Heldenberg, Aust.
Citrus aurantium; melissa (p.1632·2); peppermint leaf (p.1243·2); valerian (p.1678·3); lupulus (p.1629·3); calendula (p.1589·2).
Anxiety disorders; sleep disorders.

Krauterhaus Mag Kottas Nierentee Kottas-Heldenberg, Aust.
Java tea (p.1625·1); equisetum (p.1606·3); herniaria (p.1619·2); ononis (p.1644·1); rose fruit (p.1389·3); peppermint leaf (p.1243·2).
Urinary-tract disorders.

Krauterhaus Mag Kottas Tee fur die Verdauung Kottas-Heldenberg, Aust.
Mallow leaf; peppermint leaf (p.1243·2); caraway (p.1591·2); absinthium (p.1571·1); bitter-orange peel (p.1644·2); calendula (p.1589·2).
Gastrointestinal disorders.

Krauterhaus Mag Kottas Tee gegen Blahungen Kottas-Heldenberg, Aust.
Mallow leaf; peppermint leaf (p.1243·2); caraway (p.1591·2); fennel (p.1610·1); achillea (p.1572·2); calendula (p.1589·2).
Flatulence.

Krauterhaus Mag Kottas Tee gegen Durchfall Kottas-Heldenberg, Aust.
Erwachsene Tee: Tormentil (p.1674·1); chamomile (p.1593·2); mallow leaf; myrtillus (p.1639·2); bitter-orange peel (p.1644·2); mallow flower.
Kinder Tee: Chamomile (p.1593·2); mallow leaf; myrtillus (p.1639·2); rubus fruticosus; aniseed (p.1580·2).
Diarrhoea.

Krauterhaus Mag Kottas Wechseltee Kottas-Heldenberg, Aust.
Melissa (p.1632·2); peppermint leaf (p.1243·2); achillea (p.1572·2); sage (p.1660·2); valerian (p.1678·3); chamomile (p.1593·2); calendula (p.1589·2).
Menopausal disorders.

Krauterlax A Dolorgiet, Ger.
Aloes (p.1210·1).
Constipation.

Krauterlax-S Henk, Ger.†.
Sennoside (p.1248·3).
Constipation.

Krautertee Nr I Neuners, Aust.
Valerian (p.1678·3); lupulus (p.1629·3); melissa (p.1632·2); lavender flower (p.1627·2); chamomile (p.1593·2).
Nervous disorders.

Krautertee Nr 2 Neuners, Aust.
Silver birch (p.1585·2); lovage root (p.1629·3); solidago virgaurea; couch-grass (p.1599·3); prunus spinosa; sambucus (p.1660·3); calendula (p.1589·2).
Urinary tract disorders.

Krautertee Nr 3 Neuners, Aust.
Bearberry (p.1583·3); parsley (p.1648·3); veronica; solidago virgaurea; equisetum (p.1606·3); rosemary.
Urinary tract disorders.

Krautertee Nr 4 Neuners, Aust.
Equisetum (p.1606·3); juniper (p.1625·2); solidago virgaurea; parsley (p.1648·3); rose fruit (p.1389·3); peppermint leaf (p.1243·2).
Urinary tract disorders.

Krautertee Nr 7 Neuners, Aust.
Althaea (p.1577·1); plantago lanceolata; thyme (p.1672·2); aniseed (p.1580·2); marrubium vulgare (p.1094·2).
Catarrh; coughs.

Krautertee Nr 8 Neuners, Aust.
Urtica (p.1678·2); sage (p.1660·2); fennel (p.1610·1); peppermint leaf (p.1243·2); chamomile (p.1593·2).
Gastrointestinal disorders.

Krautertee Nr 9 Neuners, Aust.
Centaury (p.1593·1); menyanthes (p.1633·1); valerian (p.1678·3); melissa (p.1632·2); chamomile (p.1593·2); fennel (p.1610·1).
Gastrointestinal disorders.

Krautertee Nr 10 Neuners, Aust.
Tilia (p.1673·2); thyme (p.1672·2); sage (p.1660·2); sambucus (p.1660·3); aniseed (p.1580·2); fennel (p.1610·1).
Cold and influenza symptoms.

Krautertee Nr 11 Neuners, Aust.
Althaea (p.1577·1); plantago lanceolata; aniseed (p.1580·2); fennel (p.1610·1); galeopsis ochroleuca.
Upper respiratory-tract disorders.

Krautertee Nr 12 Neuners, Aust.
Prunus spinosa; linaria vulgaris; fennel (p.1610·1); caraway (p.1591·2); centaury (p.1593·1); peppermint leaf (p.1243·2).
Gastrointestinal disorders.

Krautertee Nr 16 Neuners, Aust.
Sage (p.1660·2); orange flowers; achillea (p.1572·2); melissa (p.1632·2); lupulus (p.1629·3); calendula (p.1589·2).
Menopausal disorders.

Krautertee Nr 17 Neuners, Aust.
Taraxacum (p.1669·1); turmeric (p.1029·3); centaury (p.1593·1); absinthium (p.1571·1); chamomile (p.1593·2); caraway (p.1591·2).
Liver and biliary disorders.

Krautertee Nr 18 Neuners, Aust.
Juniper (p.1625·2); parsley (p.1648·3); ononis (p.1644·1).
Urinary tract disorders.

Krautertee Nr 19 Neuners, Aust.
Silver birch (p.1585·2); urtica (p.1678·2); juniper (p.1625·2); lovage root (p.1629·3); viola tricoloris.
Diuresis.

Krautertee Nr 20 Neuners, Aust.
Crataegus (p.1600·2); taraxacum (p.1669·1); gentian (p.1615·1); centaury (p.1593·1); mistletoe (p.1636·2); rosemary.
Cardiovascular disorders.

Krautertee Nr 25 Neuners, Aust.
Parsley (p.1648·3); silver birch (p.1585·2); ononis (p.1644·1); taraxacum (p.1669·1); rubus fruticosus; rose fruit (p.1389·3).
Tonic.

Krautertee Nr 28 Neuners, Aust.
Marrubium vulgare (p.1094·2); agrimony herb (p.1574·3); absinthium (p.1571·1); cichorium intybus; angelica (p.1580·2); peppermint leaf (p.1243·2).
Biliary disorders.

Krautertee Nr 29 Neuners, Aust.
Silver birch (p.1585·2); taraxacum (p.1669·1); juniper (p.1625·2); rosemary; flos bellidis.
Diuresis.

Krautertee Nr 30 Neuners, Aust.
Juniper (p.1625·2); ononis (p.1644·1); silver birch (p.1585·2); rosemary; absinthium (p.1571·1); herba majoranae.
Diuresis.

Krautertee Nr 31 Neuners, Aust.
Bearberry (p.1583·3); java tea (p.1625·1); lovage root (p.1629·3).
Diuresis.

Krautertee Nr 32 Neuners, Aust.
Mistletoe (p.1636·2); crataegus (p.1600·2); equisetum (p.1606·3); prunus spinosa.
Circulatory and metabolic disorders.

Krautertee Nr 44 Neuners, Aust.
Crataegus (p.1600·2); juglans leaf; achillea (p.1572·2); linaria vulgaris; angelica (p.1580·2); calendula flower (p.1589·2).
Circulatory disorders; gastrointestinal disorders.

Krautertee Nr 107 Neuners, Aust.
Angelica (p.1580·2); sage (p.1660·2); caraway (p.1591·2); peppermint leaf (p.1243·2); aniseed (p.1580·2); sweet basil.
Gastrointestinal disorders.

Krautertee Nr 124 Neuners, Aust.
Valerian (p.1678·3); achillea (p.1572·2); chamomile (p.1593·2); plantago lanceolata; peppermint leaf (p.1243·2).
Labour.

Krautertee Nr 126 Neuners, Aust.
Caraway (p.1591·2); aniseed (p.1580·2); fennel (p.1610·1); parsley (p.1648·3); thyme (p.1672·2).
Breast feeding.

Krautertee Nr 141 Neuners, Aust.
Lupulus (p.1629·3); valerian (p.1678·3); melissa (p.1632·2); lavender flower (p.1627·2); peppermint leaf (p.1243·2).
Nervous disorders.

Krautertee Nr 201 Neuners, Aust.
Melissa (p.1632·2); lavender flower (p.1627·2); lupulus (p.1629·3); peppermint leaf (p.1243·2); orange flower.
Nervous disorders.

Krautertee Nr 204 Neuners, Aust.
Silver birch (p.1585·2); ononis (p.1644·1); solidago virgaurea; bearberry (p.1583·3); peppermint leaf (p.1243·2).
Urinary tract disorders.

Krautertee Nr 207 Neuners, Aust.
Galeopsis ochroleuca; wild thyme; rose fruit (p.1389·3); calendula (p.1589·2).
Catarrh; coughs.

Krautertee Nr 209 Neuners, Aust.
Chamomile (p.1593·2); peppermint leaf (p.1243·2); melissa (p.1632·2); orange flower.
Gastrointestinal disorders.

Krautertee Nr 210 *Neuners, Aust.*
Tilia (p.1673·2); sambucus (p.1660·3); peppermint leaf (p.1243·2); bitter-orange peel (p.1644·2).
Cold symptoms.

Krautertee Nr 211 *Neuners, Aust.*
Thyme (p.1672·2); drosera (p.1606·1); aniseed (p.1580·2); verbascum flowers.
Catarrh; coughs.

Krautertee Nr 217 *Neuners, Aust.*
Chamomile (p.1593·2); fennel (p.1610·1); caraway (p.1591·2); peppermint leaf (p.1243·2); bitter-orange peel (p.1644·2).
Gastrointestinal disorders.

Krautertee Nr 311 *Neuners, Aust.*
Peppermint leaf (p.1243·2); thyme (p.1672·2); chamomile (p.1593·2); sage (p.1660·2).
Catarrh; coughs.

Krebsilasi *Wyeth Lederle, Ital.*
Pancrelipase (p.1647·2).
Cystic fibrosis; malabsorption syndromes.

Kredex
Roche, Belg.; Roche, Fr.; SmithKline Beecham, Ital.†; Roche, Norw.; Lusofarmaco, Port.†; Roche, Spain; Roche, Swed.
Carvedilol (p.855·2).
Angina pectoris; heart failure; hypertension.

Kreislauf Katovit *Boehringer Ingelheim, Ger.*
Etilefrine hydrochloride (p.888·1).
Hypotension.

Kreislaufja *OTW, Ger.*
Homoeopathic preparation.

Kreislauftropen *APS, Ger.*
Crataegus (p.1600·2); camphor (p.1589·3).
Formerly known as Cardiagen.
Cardiovascular disorders.

Kremil-S *Great Eastern, Thai.; Therapharma, Thai.*
Aluminium hydroxide-magnesium carbonate co-dried gel (p.1211·2); simeticone (p.1249·2); dicyclomine [dicycloverine] hydrochloride (p.466·1).
Gastrointestinal disorders.

Krenosin
Sanofi Winthrop, Fr.; Sanofi Synthelabo, Ital.
Adenosine (p.828·2).
Diagnosis of arrhythmias; paroxysmal supraventricular tachycardia.

Krenosine *Sanofi Synthelabo, Switz.*
Adenosine (p.828·2).
Supraventricular tachycardia.

Kreon
Solvay, Aust.; Solvay, Ger.; Solvay, Port.; Solvay, Spain.
Pancreatin (p.1646·1).
Pancreatic insufficiency.

Kresse *Pharmacia Upjohn, Spain†.*
Minoxidil (p.934·2).
Alopecia.

Kreuzlinger Klosterliniment *Luond, Switz.*
Salicylic acid (p.1122·3); camphor (p.1589·3); plant extracts.
Musculoskeletal, joint, and soft-tissue disorders.

Kriptiser *Serral, Mex.*
Bromocriptine (p.1166·2).

Kripton *Alphapharm, Austral.*
Bromocriptine mesilate (p.1164·3).
Acromegaly; hyperprolactinaemia; lactation inhibition; parkinsonism.

Krisovin *Beacons, Singapore.*
Griseofulvin (p.386·2).
Fungal skin, hair, and nail infections.

Kristalose *Bertek, USA.*
Lactulose (p.1230·1).
Constipation.

Kronofed-A *Ferndale, USA.*
Pseudoephedrine hydrochloride (p.1099·2); chlorpheniramine [chlorphenamine] maleate (p.412·1).
Respiratory-tract congestion.

Krophan N *Repha, Ger.*
Bladderwrack (p.1585·2); potassium iodide (p.1522·3); thyreoidinum.
Iodine-deficiency disorders.

Krucef *Krugher, Ital.*
Cefonicid sodium (p.168·1).
Lignocaine [lidocaine] hydrochloride (p.1313·2) is included in this preparation to alleviate the pain of injection.
Gram-negative bacterial infections.

Kruschels *Pharmethic, Belg.†.*
Dried magnesium sulfate (p.1191·3); sodium chloride (p.1196·1); anhydrous sodium sulfate (p.1250·1); potassium sulfate (p.1195·1); potassium chloride (p.1194·3).
Constipation.

Kruses Fluid Magnesia *Felton, Austral.*
Magnesium bicarbonate.
Gastrointestinal hyperacidity.

Kryobulin *Immuno, Braz.*
A factor VIII preparation (p.734·1).
Haemorrhagic disorders.

Kryobulin s-TIM 3 *Immuno, Aust.†.*
A factor VIII preparation (p.734·1).
Factor VIII deficiency.

Kryobulin TIM 3 *Immuno, Spain†.*
A factor VIII preparation (p.734·1).
Factor VIII deficiency.

Kryobulin TIM 3-I *Immuno, Ital.†.*
A factor VIII preparation (p.734·1).
Haemorrhagic disorders.

Kryobuline S-TIM 3 *Immuno, Switz.†.*
A factor VIII preparation (p.734·1).
Haemophilia A; von Willebrand's disease.

Kryptocur
Hoechst Marion Roussel, Aust.; Hoechst Marion Roussel, Belg.†; Hoechst Marion Roussel, Ger.; Hoechst Marion Roussel, Ital.; Hoechst Marion Roussel, Switz.
Gonadorelin (p.1283·3).
Cryptorchidism.

KSR
Alphapharm, Austral.; Alphapharm, Hong Kong; Pacific, NZ; Alphapharm, Singapore; Merck, Singapore.
Potassium chloride (p.1194·3).
Hypokalaemia.

K-Tab *Abbott, USA.*
Potassium chloride (p.1194·3).
Hypokalaemia; potassium depletion.

K-Thrombin *Fawns & McAllan, NZ.*
Menadione sodium bisulfite (p.1395·3).
Menorrhagia; post-extraction haemorrhage; prothrombin deficiency; urticaria.

Kudrox Double Strength *Schwarz, USA†.*
Aluminium hydroxide (p.1210·3); magnesium hydroxide (p.1233·1); simeticone (p.1249·2).
Hyperacidity.

Kuhlprednon *Gerot, Aust.*
Prednisolone (p.1077·3).
Skin disorders.

Kupa *M & H, Thai.*
Bromhexine hydrochloride (p.1085·3); guaifenesin (p.1092·2).
Respiratory-tract disorders associated with increased or viscous mucus.

Kuracid *Gea, Denm.*
Ranitidine hydrochloride (p.1245·2).
Acid aspiration; gastro-oesophageal reflux; peptic ulcer; Zollinger-Ellison syndrome.

Kurgan
APS, Port.; Normon, Spain.
Cefazolin sodium (p.164·3).
Lignocaine [lidocaine] hydrochloride (p.1313·2) may be included in the intramuscular injection to alleviate the pain of injection.
Bacterial infections.

Kuson *Labitec, Spain.*
Potassium hydroxide (p.1654·1).
Verrucas; warts.

Kutapressin *Schwarz, USA.*
Liver-derivative complex.
Skin disorders.

Kutesan Crema *Plurisystem, Ital.*
Emollient.

Kutrase *Schwarz, USA.*
Lipase; amylase (p.1579·3); protease.
Formerly contained lipase, amylase, protease, cellulase, hyoscyamine sulfate, and phenyltoloxamine citrate.
Functional dyspepsia devoid of organic pathology (nervous dyspepsia).

Ku-Zyme *Schwarz, USA.*
Lipase; amylase (p.1579·3); protease.
Functional dyspepsia due to enzyme deficiency or imbalance.

Ku-Zyme HP *Schwarz, USA.*
Pancrelipase (p.1647·2).
Pancreatic insufficiency.

Kvilla *Pharmacia Upjohn, Fin.*
Quillaia (p.1348·2); ammonium chloride (p.1085·2).
Coughs.

Kwai
Kwizda, Aust.; Lederle, Austral.†; Lichtwer, Ger.; Solvay, Ital.; Lichtwer, Switz.; Lichtwer, UK.
Garlic (p.1614·1).
Arteriosclerosis; cold and influenza symptoms.

Kwan Loong Oil *DHA, Canad.*
Methyl salicylate (p.55·1); menthol (p.1632·3); eucalyptus oil (p.1609·2).

Kwelcof *Ascher, USA.*
Hydrocodone tartrate (p.42·2); guaifenesin (p.1092·2).

Kwellada *Reed & Carnrick, Canad.†.*
Lindane (p.1434·1).
Pediculosis; scabies.

Kwellada-P *Reed & Carnrick, Canad.*
Permethrin (p.1436·1).
Pediculosis; scabies.

Kwells
Roche Consumer, Austral.; Roche Consumer, Irl.; Roche Consumer, UK.
Hyoscine hydrobromide (p.468·2).
Motion sickness.

Kwikprep *Dendy, Austral.*
Monobasic sodium phosphate (p.1193·2); dibasic sodium phosphate (p.1193·2).
Bowel evacuation; constipation.

K-Y
Johnson & Johnson Medical, Fr.; Johnson & Johnson, Israel; Ethicon, Ital.; Johnson & Johnson, NZ; Johnson & Johnson, Switz.†; Johnson & Johnson, UK; Johnson & Johnson, USA.
Lubricating gel.
Aid in ultrasound scanning; lubrication of mucous membranes and instruments.

K-Y Personal Lubricant *Johnson & Johnson, Canad.*
Nonoxinol 9 (p.1346·1).
Contraceptive; vaginal lubricant.

Kyaugutt *Krewel, Ger.*
Crataegus (p.1600·2).
Heart failure.

Kybernin *Centeon, Switz.*
An antithrombin III preparation (p.725·2).
Antithrombin III deficiency.

Kybernin P
Centeon, Aust.; Centeon, Ger.; Centeon, Ital.; Centeon, Spain; Centeon, UK†.
Antithrombin III (p.725·2).
Antithrombin III deficiency; disseminated intravascular coagulation.

Kyolarte *Kyorin, Thai.*
Electrolyte infusion with glucose (p.1180·1).
Fluid and electrolyte disorders.

Kyolic *Quest, UK.*
Garlic (p.1614·1).

Kyolic Formula 103 *Quest, Canad.*
Calcium ascorbate (p.1389·3).
Dietary supplement.

Kyolic Formula 105 *Quest, Canad.*
Betacarotene, selenium, vitamin C, and vitamin E (p.1350·1).
Bacterial infections.

Kytril
SmithKline Beecham, Aust.; SmithKline Beecham, Belg.; SmithKline Beecham, Braz.; SmithKline Beecham, Denm.; SmithKline Beecham, Fin.; SmithKline Beecham, Fr.; SmithKline Beecham, Hong Kong; Roche, Irl.; SmithKline Beecham, Israel; SmithKline Beecham, Ital.; SmithKline Beecham, Mex.; SmithKline Beecham, Neth.; SmithKline Beecham, Norw.; Smith Kline & French, Port.; SmithKline Beecham, S.Afr.; SmithKline Beecham, Singapore; SmithKline, Spain; SmithKline Beecham, Swed.; SmithKline Beecham, Thai.; Roche, UK; SmithKline Beecham, USA.
Granisetron hydrochloride (p.1227·3).
Nausea and vomiting.

Kytta *Merck, Ger.*
Glycol salicylate (p.42·2).
Inflammation; pain; superficial vascular disorders.

Kytta Baume *Whitehall-Robins, Switz.†.*
Comfrey (p.1598·3); methyl nicotinate (p.55·1).
Musculoskeletal pain.

Kytta Pommade *Whitehall-Robins, Switz.†.*
Comfrey (p.1598·3); pine-needle oil; lavender oil (p.1267·2).
Musculoskeletal pain; soft-tissue injury; wounds.

Kytta-Balsam f *Merck, Ger.*
Comfrey (p.1598·3); methyl nicotinate (p.55·1).
Local circulatory disorders; musculoskeletal, joint, and soft-tissue disorders.

Kytta-Cor *Merck, Ger.*
Crataegus (p.1600·2).
Cardiac disorders.

Kytta-Femin *Merck, Ger.*
Agnus castus (p.1574·2).
Mastalgia; menstrual disorders.

Kytta-Kava *Merck, Ger.*
Kava (p.1625·3).
Anxiety disorders.

Kytta-Kliman *Merck, Ger.*
Cimicifuga (p.1595·2).
Menopausal disorders.

Kytta-Modal *Merck, Ger.*
Hypericum (p.290·2).
Depression.

Kytta-Plasma f *Merck, Ger.*
Comfrey (p.1598·3).
Soft-tissue disorders.

Kytta-Rheumabad N *Merck, Ger.*
Noble fir oil; norway spruce oil.
Bath additive; rheumatism.

Kytta-Salbe f *Merck, Ger.*
Comfrey (p.1598·3).
Soft-tissue disorders.

Kytta-Sedativ f *Merck, Ger.*
Valerian (p.1678·3); lupulus (p.1629·3); passion flower (p.1649·1).
Agitation; sleep disorders.

Kytta-Thermopack Moor-Fangoparaffin *Merck, Ger.*
Peat; medicinal mud.
Hemiplegia; musculoskeletal, joint, and soft-tissue disorders; myelitis.

Kyypakkaus *Orion, Fin.*
Hydrocortisone (p.1073·3).
Bee and wasp stings; snake bites.

L 25 *Lehning, Fr.*
Homoeopathic preparation.

L 28 *Lehning, Fr.*
Homoeopathic preparation.

L 52 *Lehning, Fr.*
Homoeopathic preparation.

L 72 *Lehning, Fr.*
Homoeopathic preparation.

L 114 *Lehning, Fr.*
Homoeopathic preparation.

LA-12 *Hyrex, USA.*
Hydroxocobalamin (p.1388·1).
Schilling test; vitamin B₁₂ deficiency.

LA Morph *Pharmacia Upjohn, NZ.*
Morphine sulfate (p.56·1).
Pain.

Lab/A *Tosi, Ital.*
Lactobacillus (p.1626·3).
Vulvovaginal candidiasis.

Labdiazina *Lab, Port.*
Sulfadiazine (p.251·1).
Bacterial infections.

Label *Asta Medica, Braz.*
Ranitidine hydrochloride (p.1245·2).
Acid aspiration; gastro-oesophageal reflux; gastrointestinal haemorrhage; peptic ulcer; Zollinger-Ellison syndrome.

Labello Active *Beiersdorf, Canad.*
SPF 15: Octinoxate (p.1517·3); oxybenzone (p.1518·1).
Sunscreen.

Labello UV *Beiersdorf, Canad.*
SPF 30: Octocrilene (p.1518·1); octinoxate (p.1517·3); oxybenzone (p.1518·1); titanium dioxide (p.1126·1).
Sunscreen.

Labfcilina *Faria, Braz.*
Ampicillin trihydrate (p.151·1); bromelains (p.1586·3).
Bacterial infections.

Labileno *Faes, Spain.*
Lamotrigine (p.351·2).
Epilepsy.

Labiosan *Henselwerk, Ger.*
Zinc oxide (p.1128·2).
Lip disorders.

Labisan *Schutz, Aust.*
Phenol (p.1152·3); zinc oxide (p.1128·2); precipitated sulfur (p.1123·3).
Fever blisters.

Labiton *Laboratories for Applied Biology, UK.*
Thiamine (p.1385·2); caffeine (p.761·3); kola nuts (p.1681·1); alcohol.
Tonic.

Labitrix *Bioquimico, Mex.*
Metronidazole (p.594·1).

Labmist *Laboratories for Applied Biology, UK.*
Sodium chloride (p.1196·1).
Nasal dryness.

Labocaina *Combe, Ital.*
Benzocaine (p.1306·2); resorcinol (p.1122·2); chlorothymol (p.1142·1).
Pruritus.

Labocane *Combe, Ger.*
Benzocaine (p.1306·2); benzyl cinnamate; benzyl benzoate (p.1428·2).
Eczema; pruritus.

Labopal *Beecham, Spain.*
Benazepril hydrochloride (p.843·2).
Heart failure; hypertension; renal failure.

Labosept
Laboratories for Applied Biology, Irl.†; Laboratories for Applied Biology, UK.
Dequalinium chloride (p.1143·1).
Mouth and throat infections.

Labrocol *Lagap, UK.*
Labetalol hydrochloride (p.918·1).
Angina pectoris; hypertension.

Labstix
Bayer, Austral.†; Bayer, Canad.†; Bayer Diagnostics, Irl.; Bayer Diagnostici, Ital.; Bayer Diagnostics, UK; Bayer, USA.
Test for pH, protein, glucose, ketones, and blood in urine.

Labstix SG
Bayer, Canad.†; Bayer Diagnostics, UK.
Test for pH, protein, glucose, ketones, blood, and specific gravity in urine.

Laburide *Wolfs, Belg.*
Pheneturide (p.354·3).
Epilepsy.

Labycarbol *Arlex, Mex.*
Methocarbamol (p.1329·3).

Labydon *Arlex, Mex.*
Nalidixic acid (p.227·1).

Labymetacyn *Arlex, Mex.*
Indometacin (p.44·3).

Labypurol *Arlex, Mex.*
Allopurinol (p.397·2).

Labysal *Arlex, Mex.*
Aspirin (p.14·2).

Lac 4 n *Parke, Davis, Ger.†.*
Almasilate (p.1210·1).
Gastrointestinal disorders.

Lacalut *Pietrasanta, Ital.*
Aluminium lactate (p.1578·2); aluminium fluoride (p.1376·2); aluminium hydroxide (p.1210·3); silicon dioxide (p.1503·3).
Gum disorders; oral hygiene; sensitive teeth.

Lacbon *Sankyo, Thai.*
Lactobacillus spp. (p.1626·3).
Constipation; restoration of intestinal flora.

Laccoderme a l'huile de cade *Pierre Fabre, Fr.*
Rectified cade oil (p.1124·3); hyoscyamus oil (p.470·1); salicylic acid (p.1122·3).
Psoriatic skin disorders.

Lacdigest *Grogg, Switz.*
Tilactase (p.1673·2).
Lactase deficiency.

Lac-Dol *Douglas, Austral.*
Lactulose (p.1230·1).
Constipation; hepatic encephalopathy.

Laceran Beiersdorf, Ger.†; Beiersdorf, Port.†.
Urea (p.1127·3).
Dry skin disorders.

Lacerdermol Lacer, Spain.
Biotin (p.1355·3); calcium pantothenate (p.1374·1); vitamin A (p.1382·1).
Blepharitis; fragile nails; glossitis; skin disorders.

Lacerdermol Complex Lacer, Spain.
Vitamin B substances (p.1350·1); vitamin A (p.1382·1).
Seborrhoeic blepharitis; skin disorders.

Lacermucin Lacer, Spain.
Tyloxapol (p.1349·3).
Respiratory-tract disorders.

Lacerol Lacer, Spain.
Diltiazem hydrochloride (p.874·3).
Angina pectoris; hypertension.

Lachemistol Wiedemann, Ger.
Homoeopathic preparation.

Lac-Hydrin Westwood-Squibb, Canad.; Bristol-Myers Squibb, Mex.; Bristol-Myers Squibb, NZ; Westwood-Squibb, USA.
Ammonium lactate (p.1110·3).
Formerly contained lactic acid in Canad.
Dry skin disorders; pruritus.

Lachydrin Westwood, Singapore.
Lactic acid (p.1626·2).
Dry skin.

Laciken Kendrick, Mex.
Aciclovir (p.612·3).
Viral infections.

Lacimen Menarini, Spain.
Lacidipine (p.919·1).
Hypertension.

Lacin Vana, Thai.
Clindamycin hydrochloride (p.188·1).
Bacterial infections.

Lacipil Glaxo Wellcome, Braz.; Glaxo Wellcome, Hong Kong; Glaxo Wellcome, Ital.; Glaxo Wellcome, Mex.; Glaxo Wellcome, Port.; Glaxo Wellcome, Singapore; Glaxo Wellcome, Spain.
Lacidipine (p.919·1).
Hypertension.

Lacirex Guidotti, Ital.
Lacidipine (p.919·1).
Hypertension.

Lacoerdin-N Weber & Weber, Ger.
Convallaria (p.1599·1); potassium aspartate (p.1195·2); magnesium aspartate (p.1190·3); magnesium phosphate trihydrate (p.1191·1); magnesium sulfate (p.1191·1); crataegus (p.1600·2).
Cardiovascular disorders.

Lacomannan CaDiGroup, Ital.
Glucomannan (p.1616·2); lactulose (p.1230·1).
Obesity.

Lac-Oph Seng, Thai.
Hypromellose (p.1501·3) (p.1129·2).
Dry eyes; wetting solution for contact lenses.

Lacophtal Winzer, Ger.
Povidone (p.1503·2).
Dry eye disorders.

Lacovin Galderma, Spain.
Minoxidil (p.934·2).
Alopecia androgenetica.

Lacribase Tubilux, Ital.
Benzalkonium chloride (p.1133·2).
Eye disinfection.

Lacrifluid Europhta, Mon.
Carbomer 940 (p.1499·2).
Dry eyes.

Lacrigel
Note. This name is used for preparations of different composition.
Winzer, Ger.
Hyetellose (p.1501·1).
Dry eyes.

Farmigea, Ital.; Europhta, Mon.
Carbomer 940 (p.1499·2).
Dry eyes.

Lacri-Gel Medical Ophthalmics, USA.
Note. A similar name is used for preparations of different composition (see above).
Soft paraffin (p.1407·3); liquid paraffin (p.1407·1); wool fat (p.1410·3).
Dry eyes.

Lacril
Note. This name is used for preparations of different composition.
Allergan-Frumtost, Braz.; Allergan, Denm.
Polyvinyl alcohol (p.1503·1).
Dry eyes.

Allergan, Canad.; Allergan, USA.
Hypromellose (p.1501·3).
Formerly contained methylcellulose in Canad.
Dry eyes.

Lacri-Lube
Note. This name is used for preparations of different composition.
Allergan, Austral.; Allergan, Canad.; Allergan, Irl.; Allergan, UK; Allergan, USA.
White soft paraffin (p.1407·3); liquid paraffin (p.1407·1); wool alcohol (p.1410·3) or wool fat (p.1410·3).
Dry eyes.

Allergan, Israel.
White soft paraffin (p.1407·3); liquid paraffin (p.1407·1).
Dry eyes.

Lacrilube
Note. This name is used for preparations of different composition.
Allergan, Ital.; Allergan, NZ; Allergan, S.Afr.; Allergan, Singapore.
White soft paraffin (p.1407·3); liquid paraffin (p.1407·1); wool alcohols (p.1410·3).
Dry eyes.

Allergan, Spain.
Soft paraffin (p.1407·3).
Dry eyes.

Lacrilux Tubilux, Ital.
Polyvinyl alcohol (p.1503·1).
Dry eyes.

Lacrima Alcon, Braz.
Dextran; hypromellose (p.1501·3); benzalkonium chloride (p.1133·2).
Dry eyes.

Lacrima Plus Alcon, Braz.
Dextran; hypromellose (p.1501·3); polyquad.
Dry eyes.

Lacrimal Allergan, Ger.
Polyvinyl alcohol (p.1503·1).
Dry eyes.

Lacrimal OK Allergan, Ger.
Polyvinyl alcohol (p.1503·1); povidone (p.1503·2).
Dry eyes.

Lacrimalfa INTES, Ital.
Sodium chloride; sodium bicarbonate; sodium acid phosphate; magnesium sulfate.
Dry eyes.

Lacrimart Baif, Ital.
Methylcellulose (p.1502·2).
Dry eyes; eye disinfection.

Lacrime Ogna, Ital.
Elixir: Oleum pini sylvestris; storax (p.1667·2); eucalyptol (p.1609·2).
Pastilles: Oleum pini sylvestris; storax (p.1667·2); eucalyptol (p.1609·2); menthol (p.1632·3).
Bronchial catarrh; coughs; sore throat.

Lacrimill Ottolenghi, Ital.
Hypromellose (p.1501·3).
Dry eyes; eye disinfection; eye irritation.

Lacrimol Fischer, Israel.
Eye drops: Povidone (p.1503·2).
Eye ointment: White soft paraffin (p.1407·3); liquid paraffin (p.1407·1); wool fat (p.1410·3).
Dry eyes.

Lacrinorm Ophtapharma, Canad.; Chauvin, Fr.; Farmigea, Ital.; Chauvin Novopharma, Switz.
Carbomer 940 (p.1499·2).
Dry eyes.

Lacrisert Sigma, Austral.; Merck Frosst, Canad.; Merck Sharp & Dohme, Denm.†; Merck Sharp & Dohme, Fin.; Merck Sharp & Dohme-Chibret, Fr.; Merck Sharp & Dohme, Neth.; Merck Sharp & Dohme, Norw.; Merck Sharp & Dohme, S.Afr.; Merck Sharp & Dohme, Swed.; Merck, USA.
Hyprolose (p.1501·2).
Dry eyes.

Lacrisic
Note. This name is used for preparations of different composition.
Agepha, Aust.†.
Carbomer (p.1499·2).
Dry eyes.

Alcon, Ger.
Hypromellose (p.1501·3); povidone (p.1503·2); glycerol (p.1616·3).
Dry eyes.

Lacrisifi
SIFI, Ital.; SIFI, Singapore.
Hypromellose (p.1501·3).
Dry eyes; eye irritation.

Lacrisol Bruschettini, Ital.
Hypromellose (p.1501·3).
Dry eyes; eye disinfection.

Lacri-Stulln Stulln, Ger.
Povidone (p.1503·2).
Dry eyes.

Lacri-Tears Medical Ophthalmics, USA.
Hypromellose (p.1501·3); dextran (p.729·2).
Dry eyes.

Lacromycin Fischer, Israel.
Gentamicin sulfate (p.210·1).
Eye infections.

Lacrypos Alcon, Fr.
Sodium chondroitin sulfate (p.1594·2).
Eye disorders.

Lacrystat Asta Medica, Belg.
Hypromellose (p.1501·3); dextran 70 (p.729·2).
Dry eyes.

Lacrytube Asta Medica, Belg.
Liquid paraffin (p.1407·1); white soft paraffin (p.1407·3); wool fat (p.1410·3).
Corneal protection in comatose or anaesthetised patients; keratoconjunctivitis sicca.

Lacryvisc Alcon, Fr.; Alcon, Hong Kong; Alcon, Port.; Alcon, Singapore; Alcon Cusi, Spain; Alcon, Swed.; Alcon, Switz.; Alcon, Thai.
Carbomer (p.1499·2).
Dry eyes.

Lacson Aspen, S.Afr.
Lactulose (p.1230·1).
Constipation; hepatic encephalopathy.

Lactacyd SmithKline Beecham Sante, Fr.; Sanofi Winthrop, Hong Kong; Sterling, Port.; Sanofi Synthelabo, Singapore; Sanofi Synthelabo, Thai.
Milk serum; lactic acid (p.1626·2).
Skin disorders; vulvovaginal disorders.

Lactacyd Antibatterico SmithKline Beecham, Ital.
Triclosan (p.1159·2).
Skin disinfection.

Lactacyd Derma SmithKline Beecham, Ital.
Milk serum; lactic acid (p.1626·2).
Acne; soap substitute.

Lactacyd Intimo SmithKline Beecham, Ital.
Milk serum; lactic acid (p.1626·2).
Genital hygiene.

Lactagel Creme d'Orient, Fr.
Ammonium lactate (p.1110·3).
Skin disorders.

Lacta-Gynecogel Medgenix, Belg.
Lactic acid (p.1626·2).
Vulvovaginal infections.

Lactaid Sunrise, Austral.; McNeil Consumer, Canad.; Clonmel, Irl.†; Iketon, Ital.†; Myplan, UK†; McNeil Consumer, USA.
Tilactase (p.1673·2) (derived from Kluyveromyces lactis or Aspergillus oryzae).
Lactose intolerance.

Lactal Kabi, Swed.†.
Lactic acid (p.1626·2); glycogen.
Bacterial vaginosis.

Lactar Creme d'Orient, Fr.
Ammonium lactate (p.1110·3); cade oil (p.1124·3).
Seborrhoeic dermatitis.

Lact-Easy Sunrise, Austral.
Tilactase (p.1673·2).
Lactose intolerance.

Lactel Lactel, Fr.
Nutritional supplement (p.1350·1).
Lactose intolerance.

Lacteol Menarini, Belg.; Lacteol du Dr Boucard, Fr.; Lacteol, Hong Kong; Bruschettini, Ital.; Biosaude, Port.; Lacteol, Singapore; Ramon Sala, Spain; Lacteol, Switz.; Lacteol, Thai.; Morrow, Thai.
Lactobacillus acidophilus (p.1626·3).
Colopathy; diarrhoea; enterocolitis.

Lacteol Fort Carnot, Mex.
Lactobacillus acidophilus (Boucardii) (p.1626·3).
Diarrhoea; restoration of gastrointestinal flora.

Lactess Protein, Mex.
Bromocriptine (p.1166·2).

Lacticare
Note. This name is used for preparations of different composition.
Stiefel, Austral.†; Stiefel, Canad.; Stiefel, Fr.; Stiefel, Hong Kong; Stiefel, Irl.; Stiefel, Mex.; Stiefel, Singapore; Stiefel, Thai.; Stiefel, UK.
Lactic acid (p.1626·2); sodium pidolate (p.1123·3).
Dry skin disorders.

Stiefel, USA.
Lactic acid (p.1626·2); liquid paraffin (p.1407·1).
Emollient and moisturiser.

Lacticare-HC Stiefel, Mex.; Stiefel, USA.
Hydrocortisone (p.1073·3).
Skin disorders.

Lactidorm Galactopharm, Ger.
Lupulus (p.1629·3).
Anxiety; insomnia.

Lactifero Bergamo, Braz.
Urtica (p.1678·2); gentian (p.1615·1); calcium phosphate; sodium glycerophosphate; citric acid; lactic acid (p.1350·1).

Lactinex Becton Dickinson, USA.
Lactobacillus acidophilus (p.1626·3); Lactobacillus bulgaricus (p.1626·3).
Dietary supplement.

Lactinol Pedinol, USA.
Lactic acid (p.1626·2).
Dry skin.

Lactinol-E Pedinol, USA.
Lactic acid (p.1626·2); vitamin E (p.1393·3).
Dry skin.

Lactipan Byk, Braz.; Ibi, Ital.
Lactobacillus bulgaricus (p.1626·3); Lactobacillus acidophilus (p.1626·3); Streptococcus lactis.
Diarrhoea; maintenance of normal gastrointestinal flora.

Lactisan Galactopharm, Ger.
Sour milk whey concentrate (p.1626·2).
Gynaecological disorders; skin disinfection.

Lactisol Galactopharm, Ger.
Lactic acid (p.1626·2).
Gastrointestinal disorders; skin disorders; wounds.

Lactisona Stiefel, Port.; Stiefel, Spain.
Hydrocortisone (p.1073·3).
Skin disorders.

Lactisporin Medisint, Ital.
Lactic-acid-producing organisms (p.1626·3); dried yeast (p.1398·1).
Restoration of normal gastrointestinal flora.

Lactivis Fitobucaneve, Ital.
Capsules: Vitamins (p.1350·1); Lactobacillus acidophilus (p.1626·3); dried yeast (p.1398·1); dried yogurt.
Powder for oral liquid: Vitamins (p.1350·1); lactic-acid-producing organisms (p.1626·3).
Nutritional supplement.

Lacto Calamine
Note. This name is used for preparations of different composition.
CSL, NZ.
Calamine (p.1111·3); hamamelis (p.1618·3).
Insect bites; sunburn.

Boots, S.Afr.†; Schering-Plough, UK.
Lotion: Calamine (p.1111·3); zinc oxide (p.1128·2); hamamelis (p.1618·3); phenol (p.1152·3).
Skin irritation; sunburn.

Schering-Plough, UK.
Cream: Calamine (p.1111·3); zinc oxide (p.1128·2); hamamelis (p.1618·3).
Dry skin; sunburn.

Lacto Pregomine Milupa, Fr.
Infant feed (p.1350·1).
Cow's milk intolerance.

Lacto Vagin UCI, Braz.
Tyrothricin (p.267·1); hydroxyquinoline (p.1622·2); tannic acid (p.1669·1); lactic acid (p.1626·2); acetic acid (p.1571·2); camphor (p.1589·3).
Vulvovaginal disorders.

Lactobac Nutrition Care, Austral.
Lactobacillus acidophilus (p.1626·3); Bifidobacterium bifidum (p.1626·3).
Dietary supplement.

Lactocal-F Laser, USA.
Multivitamin and mineral preparation with iron and folic acid (p.1350·1).
Supplement for pregnant or lactating women.

Lactocol Ogna, Ital.
Guaiacol (p.1092·1); lactic acid (p.1626·2); calcium phosphate (p.1188·3); calcium lactate (p.1188·2); codeine hydrochloride (p.25·2); aconite (p.1572·3).
Coughs.

Lactocol Expectorante Alcala, Spain†.
Guaifenesin (p.1092·2).
Coughs.

Lactocur Biocur, Ger.
Lactulose (p.1230·1).
Constipation; hepatic encephalopathy; salmonella enteritis.

Lactofalk Falk, Ger.
Lactulose (p.1230·1).
Constipation; liver disorders; salmonella enteritis.

Lactoferment Novartis Consumer, Switz.
Lactobacillus acidophilus (p.1626·3).
Gastrointestinal disorders.

Lactoferrina Wasserman, Spain.
Iron succinyl-protein complex (p.1369·3).
Iron deficiency anaemia.

Lactofilus Llorente, Spain.
Lactobacillus acidophilus (p.1626·3).
Restoration of the gastrointestinal flora.

Lactofree Mead Johnson Nutritionals, USA.
Lactose-free infant feed (p.1350·1).

Lactoger Schwarz, Ital.
Lactulose (p.1230·1).
Gastrointestinal infections; hepatic encephalopathy.

Lactogermine Humana, Ital.
Lactic-acid-producing organisms (p.1626·3); vitamins (p.1350·1).
Nutritional supplement.

Lacto-Gin Precifarma, Braz.
Tyrothricin (p.267·1); hydroxyquinoline (p.1622·2); acetic acid (p.1571·2); lactic acid (p.1626·2); tannic acid (p.1669·1); camphor (p.1589·3).
Vulvovaginal disorders.

Lactolas Virginia, Ital.
Lactulose (p.1230·1); inulin (p.1624·1); rhubarb (p.1248·1); frangula (p.1227·1); senna (p.1248·2); vitamin B substances (p.1350·1).
Gastrointestinal disorders.

Lactolavol Rosch & Handel, Aust.
Calcium lactate (p.1188·2); tartaric acid (p.1669·2); atropine sulfate (p.461·1).
Vaginal disorders.

Lactolife Fitolife, Ital.
Dried yeast (p.1398·1); lactic-acid-producing organisms (p.1626·3).
Gastrointestinal disorders; nutritional supplement.

Lactoliofil Belmac, Spain.
Lactobacillus acidophilus (p.1626·3).
Restoration of the gastrointestinal flora.

Lactonico Dermoteca, Port.
Ammonium lactate (p.1110·3); squalane (p.1410·2); levomenol (p.1629·1); vitamin E.
Barrier preparation; dry skin disorders.

Lactonorm Geymonat, Ital.
Lactobacillus acidophilus (p.1626·3).
Disturbances in vaginal flora.

Lactophilus Organon, Fin.
Lactobacillus rhamnosus (p.1626·3).
Restoration of gastrointestinal flora.

Lacto-Purga Newlab, Braz.
Phenolphthalein (p.1244·1); lactose (p.1370·2).
Constipation.

Lactopurum Pfluger, Ger.
Homoeopathic preparation.

Lactored Fides, Spain†.
Tilactase (p.1673·2); lipase; silicone (p.1249·2).
Milk intolerance.

Lactosec Aspen, S.Afr.
Pyridoxine hydrochloride (p.1386·3).
Vitamin deficiency.

Lactovit *Herbaline, Ital.†.*
Dried yeast (p.1398·1); myrtillus (p.1639·2); *Lactobacillus acidophilus* (p.1626·3).
Nutritional supplement.

Lactrase *Rivex, Canad.; Schwarz, USA.*
Tilactase (p.1673·2).
Lactase insufficiency; lactose intolerance.

Lactucol *Distifarma, Port.*
Sodium benzoate (p.1134·3); bromoform (p.1587·1); ephedrine hydrochloride (p.1090·1); cherry-laurel water; balsamic syrup; maidenhair; peca; aconite (p.1572·3); belladonna (p.463·1); drosera (p.1606·1); grindelia (p.1618·2); lobelia (p.1510·2).
Coughs.

Lactuflor *MIP, Ger.*
Lactulose (p.1230·1).
Constipation; liver disorders; salmonella enteritis.

Lactugal *Intrapharm, UK.*
Lactulose (p.1230·1).
Constipation; hepatic encephalopathy.

Lactulax *Rougier, Canad.; Senosiain, Mex.*
Lactulose (p.1230·1).
Constipation; hepatic encephalopathy.

Lactulona *Luitpold, Braz.*
Lactulose (p.1230·1).
Constipation; hepatic encephalopathy.

Lactuverlan *Verla, Ger.*
Lactulose (p.1230·1).
Constipation; liver disorders; salmonella enteritis.

Lactyl *Ibirn, Ital.*
Lactulose (p.1230·1).
Cirrhosis; hepatic encephalopathy.

Ladazol *Mer-National, S.Afr.*
Danazol (p.1468·3).
Endometriosis; hereditary angioedema; mastalgia.

Ladip *Duncan, Ital.*
Lacidipine (p.919·1).
Hypertension.

Ladocort *LBS, Thai.*
Miconazole nitrate (p.391·1); hydrocortisone (p.1073·3).
Infected skin disorders.

Ladogal *Sanofi Winthrop, Braz.; Sanofi Winthrop, Mex.; Sanofi Synthelabo, Singapore; Sanofi Synthelabo, Thai.*
Danazol (p.1468·3).
Benign breast disorders; endometriosis; gynaecomastia; hereditary angioedema; mennorhagia; precocious puberty.

Ladropen *Berk, Irl.†; Berk, UK†.*
Flucloxacillin (p.207·1) or flucloxacillin sodium (p.207·1).
Bacterial infections.

Lady-35 *Masa, Thai.*
Cyproterone acetate (p.1467·3); ethinylestradiol (p.1476·2).
Oral contraceptive in women with androgenic symptoms.

Ladymega *Cantassium Co., UK.*
Multivitamin and mineral preparation (p.1350·1).

Ladytone *Vitabiotics, UK.*
Multivitamin and mineral preparation (p.1350·1).

Ladyvital *Pharmadass, UK.*
Multivitamin, mineral, and nutritional preparation (p.1350·1).

Laevadosin *Fresenius Kabi, Aust.*
Buccal tablets: Adenosine (p.828·2); guanosine; adenosine phosphate disodium (p.1573·3); disodium cytidine phosphate; guanosine monophosphate, disodium salt; disodium uridine monophosphate.
Injection: Adenosine triphosphate, disodium salt (p.1573·3); adenosine phosphate disodium (p.1573·3); guanosine monophosphate, disodium salt; adenosine (p.828·2); inosine (p.1623·3); guanosine; uridine (p.1677·2).
Myopathies; peripheral, cerebral, and coronary vascular disorders.

Laev-Amin *Laevosan, Aust.*
Amino-acid infusion (p.1350·1).
Parenteral nutrition.

Laevilac S *Fresenius Kabi, Ger.*
Lactulose (p.1230·1).
Constipation; liver disorders; salmonella enteritis.

Laevodex *Laevosan, Aust.*
Dextran 40 (p.728·3) or dextran 60 (p.729·2) in sodium chloride infusion.
Plasma volume expansion; thrombosis prophylaxis.

Laevofusin Isoton *Fresenius Kabi, Aust.*
Electrolyte infusion (p.1180·1).
Fluid and electrolyte disorders.

Laevofusin-Starter *Laevosan, Aust.*
Sodium, chloride, lactate, and acetate infusion (p.1180·1).
Fluid and electrolyte disorders.

Laevolac *Fresenius Kabi, Aust.; Roche, Ital.; Douglas, NZ; Ferraz, Lynce, Port.; Byk Madaus, S.Afr.†; Medichemie Bioline, Switz.*
Lactulose (p.1230·1).
Constipation; disturbances of gastrointestinal flora; hepatic encephalopathy.

Laevoral *Fresenius Kabi, Aust.*
Fructose (p.1363·3).
Carbohydrate source; gastrointestinal disorders; glucose substitute; liver disorders.

Laevosan *Laevosan, Aust.; Roche, Ital.*
Fructose (p.1363·3).
Asthenia; cardiac disorders; diabetes; liver disorders; poisoning.

Laevostrophan *Fresenius Kabi, Aust.*
Strophanthin-K (p.978·2).
Angina; arrhythmias; heart failure.

Laevostrophan compositum *Laevosan, Aust.*
Strophanthin-K (p.978·2); diprophylline (p.764·1).
Heart failure.

Laevovit D₃ *Fresenius Kabi, Aust.*
Colecalciferol (p.1391·1).
Osteomalacia; rickets; vitamin D supplementation.

Lafarin *Lafare, Ital.*
Cefalexin (p.161·3).
Bacterial infections.

Lafena *Cinfa, Spain.*
Aspirin (p.14·2).
Fever; inflammation; pain.

Lafol *Wyeth, Ger.*
Folic acid (p.1361·1).
Folic acid supplement.

Lafurex *Lafare, Ital.*
Cefuroxime sodium (p.178·2).
Bacterial infections.

Lagarmicin *Bohm, Spain.*
Erythromycin stearate (p.201·3).
Bacterial infections.

Lagatrim *Lagap, Switz.*
Co-trimoxazole (p.193·3).
Bacterial infections; Pneumocystis carinii pneumonia.

Lagenbach *Mex-America, Mex.*
Senna (p.1248·2).
Constipation.

Lagin *Epifarma, Ital.*
Benzydamine hydrochloride (p.20·1).
Gynaecological disorders; mouth and throat disorders.

Lagrifilm Plus *Allergan, Mex.*
Polyvinyl alcohol (p.1503·1); povidone (p.1503·2).
Dry eyes.

Lagun *Pharmacal, Fin.*
Dextromethorphan hydrobromide (p.1087·3).
Coughs.

Lagylan *Alpha, Mex.*
Metronidazole (p.594·1).

Laidor *Esseti, Ital.*
Nimesulide (p.62·3).
Fever; inflammation; pain.

Laif *Steigerwald, Ger.*
Hypericum (p.290·2).
Depression.

Laiken *Farmasa, Mex.*
Kava extract (p.1625·3).
Anxiety.

Lait Auto-Bronzant *Clarins, Canad.*
SPF 6: Octinoxate (p.1517·3); avobenzone (p.1517·1).
Formerly contained octinoxate, oxybenzone, and titanium dioxide.
Sunscreen.

Lait Bronzage *Clarins, Canad.*
SPF 6; SPF 10: Octinoxate (p.1517·3); oxybenzone (p.1518·1); titanium dioxide (p.1126·1).
SPF 19: Octinoxate (p.1517·3); oxybenzone (p.1518·1); ensulizole (p.1517·2); titanium dioxide (p.1126·1).
Sunscreen.

Lait Ecran Total *Vichy, Canad.*
SPF 25; SPF 30: Avobenzone (p.1517·1); octocrilene (p.1518·1); terephthalylidene dicamphor sulfonic acid; titanium dioxide (p.1126·1).
Sunscreen.

Lait Hydratant Bronzage *Vichy, Canad.†.*
SPF 8: Avobenzone (p.1517·1); enzacamene (p.1517·2); terephthalylidene dicamphor sulfonic acid; titanium dioxide (p.1126·1).
Sunscreen.

Lait Protecteur *Lancome, Canad.; Vichy, Canad.*
SPF 8; SPF 15: Avobenzone (p.1517·1); octocrilene (p.1518·1); terephthalylidene dicamphor sulfonic acid; titanium dioxide (p.1126·1).
Formerly contained avobenzone, enzacamene, terephthalylidene dicamphor sulfonic acid, and titanium dioxide.
Sunscreen.

Lait Solaire Ecran Total *Lancome, Canad.*
SPF 25: Avobenzone (p.1517·1); enzacamene (p.1517·2); terephthalylidene dicamphor sulfonic acid; titanium dioxide (p.1126·1).
Sunscreen.

Lait Solaire Haute Protection *Lancome, Canad.*
SPF 15: Avobenzone (p.1517·1); enzacamene (p.1517·2); octocrilene (p.1518·1); terephthalylidene dicamphor sulfonic acid; titanium dioxide (p.1126·1).
Sunscreen.

Laitan *Schwabe, Ger.; Spitzner, Ger.; Schwabe, Switz.*
Kava (p.1625·3).
Anxiety disorders; sleep disorders.

Lake *Faes, Spain.*
Ranitidine hydrochloride (p.1245·2).
Acid aspiration; gastro-oesophageal reflux; gastrointestinal haemorrhage; peptic ulcer; short-bowel syndrome; Zollinger-Ellison syndrome.

Lakriment Neu *Dolorgiet, Ger.*
Liquorice (p.1231·2).
Catarrh.

Laktipex *Selena, Swed.*
Lactulose (p.1230·1).
Constipation; hepatic encephalopathy.

Lalax *Orion, Fin.*
Lactitol (p.1230·1).
Constipation; hepatic encephalopathy.

Lamaline *Solvay, Fr.*
Paracetamol (p.71·2); opium (p.69·3); caffeine (p.761·3).
Formerly contained paracetamol, belladonna, opium, and caffeine.
Pain.

Lambda *Isdin, Port.*
Cream: Triclosan (p.1159·2); aluminium hydroxide (p.1210·3).
Roll-on: Aluminium chlorohydrate (p.1110·2).
Hyperhidrosis.

Lamblit *Novag, Mex.*
Metronidazole (p.594·1).
Amoebiasis; giardiasis; trichomoniasis.

Lambutol *Atlantic, Hong Kong; Atlantic, Thai.*
Ethambutol hydrochloride (p.205·1).
Tuberculosis.

Lamicitin *Glaxo Wellcome, S.Afr.*
Lamotrigine (p.351·2).
Epilepsy.

Lamictal *Glaxo Wellcome, Aust.; Glaxo Wellcome, Austral.; Glaxo Wellcome, Belg.; Glaxo Wellcome, Braz.; Glaxo Wellcome, Canad.; Glaxo Wellcome, Denm.; Glaxo Wellcome, Fin.; Glaxo Wellcome, Fr.; Glaxo Wellcome, Ger.; Desitin, Ger.; Glaxo Wellcome, Hong Kong; Glaxo Wellcome, Irl.; Glaxo Wellcome, Israel; Glaxo Wellcome, Ital.; Glaxo Wellcome, Mex.; Glaxo Wellcome, Neth.; Glaxo Wellcome, Norw.; Glaxo Wellcome, NZ; Glaxo Wellcome, Port.; Glaxo Wellcome, Singapore; Wellcome, Spain; Glaxo Wellcome, Swed.; Glaxo Wellcome, Thai.; Wellcome, UK; Glaxo Wellcome, USA.*
Lamotrigine (p.351·2).
Epilepsy.

Lamisil *Novartis, Aust.; Novartis, Austral.; Novartis Consumer, Austral.; Novartis, Belg.; Novartis, Braz.; Novartis, Canad.; Novartis, Denm.; Novartis, Fin.; Novartis, Fr.; Novartis, Ger.; Novartis, Hong Kong; Novartis, Irl.; Novartis, Israel; Novartis, Ital.; Novartis, Mex.; Novartis, Neth.; Novartis, Norw.; Novartis, NZ; Novartis, Port.; Novartis, S.Afr.; Novartis, Singapore; Novartis, Spain; Novartis, Swed.; Novartis, Switz.; Novartis, Thai.; Novartis, UK; Novartis, USA.*
Terbinafine (p.394·3) or terbinafine hydrochloride (p.394·1).
Fungal skin and nail infections.

Lamnotyl *Farmasur, Spain.*
Boric acid (p.1586·1); hamamelis (p.1618·3); ichthammol (p.1115·2); zinc oxide (p.1128·2).
Burns; grazes; skin disorders.

Lamoryl *Leo, Norw.†; Lovens, Swed.†.*
Griseofulvin (p.386·2).
Fungal infections.

Lampicin *Lakeside, Mex.*
Ampicillin (p.150·3), ampicillin sodium (p.150·3), or ampicillin trihydrate (p.151·1).
Bacterial infections.

Lampit *Bayer, Ger.†.*
Nifurtimox (p.598·2).
Trypanosomiasis.

Lampocef *Lampugnani, Ital.*
Cefonicid sodium (p.168·1).
Lignocaine [lidocaine] hydrochloride (p.1313·2) is included in this preparation to alleviate the pain of injection.
Gram-negative bacterial infections.

Lampocillina *Salus, Ital.*
Ampicillin sodium (p.150·3).
Bacterial infections.

Lampoflex *Lampugnani, Ital.*
Piroxicam (p.79·1).
Musculoskeletal, joint, and peri-articular disorders.

Lampomandol *AGIPS, Ital.*
Cefamandole nafate (p.163·3).
Lignocaine [lidocaine] hydrochloride (p.1313·2) is included in this preparation to alleviate the pain of injection.
Bacterial infections.

Lampren *Ciba-Geigy, Jpn; Novartis, Neth.; Padro, Spain.*
Clofazimine (p.191·1).
Leprosy.

Lamprene *Novartis, Austral.; Novartis, Fr.; Novartis, Hong Kong; Novartis, Irl.†; Novartis, NZ; Novartis, S.Afr.; Novartis, Switz.; Alliance, UK; Geigy, USA.*
Clofazimine (p.191·1).
Leprosy.

Lamra *Merckle, Ger.*
Diazepam (p.674·3).
Anxiety.

Lamuran *Roche, Aust.; SIT, Ital.*
Raubasine (p.967·2).
Peripheral and cerebral vascular disorders.

Lanabiotic
Note.This name is used for preparations of different composition.
Combe, Canad.†.
Bacitracin (p.155·2); polymyxin B sulfate (p.238·1).
Wounds.
Combe, USA.
Polymyxin B sulfate (p.238·1); neomycin sulfate (p.228·1); bacitracin (p.155·2); lignocaine [lidocaine] (p.1313·2).
Bacterial skin infections.

Lanacane
Note.This name is used for preparations of different composition.
Combe, Israel; Combe, Spain; Combe, UK; Combe, USA.
Benzocaine (p.1306·2).
Skin irritation.
Formula, NZ.
Benzocaine (p.1306·2); resorcinol (p.1122·2).
Skin irritation.

Lanacane Medicated Cream *Combe, Canad.*
Benzocaine (p.1306·2); resorcinol (p.1122·2).
Skin disorders.

Lanacane Medicated Powder *Combe, UK.*
Menthol (p.1632·3); zinc oxide (p.1128·2).
Skin irritation.

Lanacine *Lannacher, Aust.*
Clindamycin hydrochloride (p.188·1) or clindamycin phosphate (p.188·2).
Bacterial infections.

Lanacordin *Wellcome, Spain.*
Digoxin (p.870·1).
Arrhythmias; heart failure.

Lanacort *Combe, Canad.†; Combe, Israel; Combe, Ital.; Combe, UK; Combe, USA.*
Hydrocortisone acetate (p.1073·3).
Skin disorders.

Lanacrist *Tika, Swed.*
Digoxin (p.870·1).
Arrhythmias; heart failure.

Lanaphilic
Note.This name is used for preparations of different composition.
Medco, USA.
Urea (p.1127·3).
Dry skin; hyperkeratosis.
Medco, USA.
Vehicle for topical preparations.

Lanate *Douglas, NZ.*
Ammonium lactate (p.1110·3).
Dry skin disorders.

Lanatilin *Nycomed, Aust.*
α-Acetyldigoxin (p.827·3).
Heart failure.

Lanatin *Nycomed, Denm.*
Lisinopril (p.921·1).
Heart failure; hypertension.

Lancome-Creme Gelee *Lancome, Canad.*
SPF 8: Enzacamene (p.1517·2); octinoxate (p.1517·3); terephthalylidene dicamphor sulfonic acid; titanium dioxide (p.1126·1).
Sunscreen.

Lancome-Creme Solaire *Lancome, Canad.*
SPF 15: Avobenzone (p.1517·1); enzacamene (p.1517·2); terephthalylidene dicamphor sulfonic acid; titanium dioxide (p.1126·1).
Sunscreen.

Lander Dandruff Control *Lander, Canad.*
Pyrithione zinc (p.1122·1).
Dandruff.

Lanexat *Roche, Braz.; Roche, Denm.; Roche, Fin.; Roche, Mex.; Roche, Swed.*
Flumazenil (p.1008·3).
Benzodiazepine overdosage; reversal of benzodiazepine-induced sedation.

Lanfast *Julphar, UAE.*
Lansoprazole (p.1230·3).
Formerly known as Lanso.
Gastro-oesophageal reflux; peptic ulcer; Zollinger-Ellison syndrome.

Langoran *Marion Merrell, Fr.*
Isosorbide dinitrate (p.915·2).
Angina pectoris; heart failure.

Laniazid *Lannett, USA.*
Isoniazid (p.215·3).
Tuberculosis.

Lanicor *Roche, Aust.; Roche, Ger.*
Digoxin (p.870·1).
Heart failure; tachycardia.

Lanirapid *Boehringer Mannheim, Jpn†; Roche, Spain.*
Metildigoxin (p.930·3).
Heart failure; tachycardia.

Lanitop *Roche, Aust.; Roche, Belg.; Asta Medica, Braz.; Roche, Ger.; Roche, Hong Kong; Boehringer Mannheim, Ital.; Roche, Port.; Roche, Switz.*
Metildigoxin (p.930·1).
Arrhythmias; heart failure.

Lanoc *Lannacher, Aust.*
Metoprolol tartrate (p.931·2).
Angina pectoris; arrhythmias; hypertension; migraine; myocardial infarction.

Lanofene *Augot, Fr.†.*
Zinc oxide (p.1128·2).
Eczema; nappy rash.

The symbol † denotes a preparation no longer actively marketed

Lanohex *Rougier, Canad.; Rougier, Hong Kong.*
Phenoxyethanol (p.1153·3).
Scalp disorders; skin cleansing.

Lanol *Nakornpatana, Thai.*
Calamine (p.1111·3); zinc oxide (p.1128·2); phenol (p.1152·3); camphor (p.1589·3); menthol (p.1632·3).
Skin disorders.

Lanolelle *Warner-Lambert, Canad.†.*
Hydrous wool fat (p.1411·2).
Dry skin.

Lanolor *Squibb, USA.*
Emollient and moisturiser.

Lanophyllin *Lannett, USA†.*
Theophylline (p.777·2).
Asthma; bronchospasm.

Lanorinal *Lannett, USA†.*
Aspirin (p.14·2); caffeine (p.761·3); butalbital (p.658·3).
Pain.

Lanoxicaps *Glaxo Wellcome, USA.*
Digoxin (p.870·1).
Atrial fibrillation; heart failure.

Lanoxin
Glaxo Wellcome, Austral.; Glaxo Wellcome, Belg.; Glaxo Wellcome, Braz.; Glaxo Wellcome, Canad.; Glaxo Wellcome, Hong Kong; Wellcome, Irl.; Glaxo Wellcome, Israel; Glaxo Wellcome, Ital.; Glaxo Wellcome, Mex.; Glaxo Wellcome, Neth.; Glaxo Wellcome, Norw.; Glaxo Wellcome, NZ; Wellcome, Port.; Glaxo Wellcome, S.Afr.; Glaxo Wellcome, Singapore; Glaxo Wellcome, Swed.; Wellcome, Switz.; Glaxo Wellcome, Thai.; Glaxo Wellcome, UK; Glaxo Wellcome, USA.
Digoxin (p.870·1).
Heart failure; supraventricular arrhythmias.

Lansinoh *Meriana, Austral.*
Wool fat (p.1410·3).
Burns; dry, damaged skin; minor cuts.

Lansox *Takeda, Ital.*
Lansoprazole (p.1230·3).
Gastro-oesophageal reflux; peptic ulcer; Zollinger-Ellison syndrome.

Lansoyl *Warner-Lambert, Belg.; Axcan, Canad.; Warner-Lambert, Fr.; Parke, Davis, Switz.*
Liquid paraffin (p.1407·1).
Constipation.

Lantanon *Organon, Ital.; Donmed, S.Afr.; Organon, Spain.*
Mianserin hydrochloride (p.298·1).
Depression.

Lantarel *Lederle, Ger.*
Methotrexate sodium (p.553·2).
Psoriasis vulgaris; psoriatic arthritis; rheumatoid arthritis.

Lantigen B
COB, Belg†; Bruschettini, Ital.; Seber, Port.; Bruschettini, Switz.†.
Antigenic extracts from *Streptococcus pneumoniae; Streptococcus pyogenes; Moraxella catarrhalis; Staphylococcus aureus; Klebsiella pneumoniae; Haemophilus influenzae.*
Respiratory-tract disorders.

Lantogent *Bio Terapico Ralay, Spain.*
Gentamicin sulfate (p.210·1).
Bacterial infections.

Lantus *Aventis Pharma, USA.*
Insulin glargine (p.324·1).
Diabetes mellitus.

Lanuretic *Lannacher, Aust.*
Hydrochlorothiazide (p.907·3); amiloride hydrochloride (p.835·1).
Hypertension; oedema.

Lanvis
Glaxo Wellcome, Austral.; Glaxo Wellcome, Belg.; Glaxo Wellcome, Braz.; Glaxo Wellcome, Canad.; Glaxo Wellcome, Hong Kong; Wellcome, Irl.; Glaxo Wellcome, Israel; Glaxo Wellcome, Neth.; Glaxo Wellcome, NZ; Glaxo Wellcome, Swed.; Wellcome, Switz.; Glaxo Wellcome, Thai.; Glaxo Wellcome, UK.
Tioguanine (p.575·1).
Leukaemias.

Lanzo
Wyeth Lederle, Denm.; Wyeth Lederle, Fin.; Orion, Fin.; Wyeth Lederle, Norw.; Wyeth Lederle, Swed.
Lansoprazole (p.1230·3).
Gastro-oesophageal reflux; peptic ulcer; Zollinger-Ellison syndrome.

Lanzor *Hoechst, Fr.; Hoechst Marion Roussel, Ger.; Aventis, S.Afr.*
Lansoprazole (p.1230·3).
Formerly known as Lanazor in *S.Afr.*
Gastro-oesophageal reflux; gastrointestinal hyperacidity; peptic ulcer; Zollinger-Ellison syndrome.

Lao-Dal *Synthelabo, Fr.†.*
Camphor (p.1589·3); menthol (p.1632·3); lignocaine [lidocaine] hydrochloride (p.1313·2); chloroform (p.1256·3); methyl salicylate (p.55·1); turpentine oil (p.1676·3); glycol salicylate (p.42·2).
Soft-tissue disorders.

Lapices Epiderm Metadier *Prats, Spain.*
Dithranol (p.1113·3); salicylic acid (p.1122·3).
Skin disorders.

Lapidar *Swiss Herbal, Canad.*
Cascara (p.1216·1); frangula (p.1227·1); senna (p.1248·2).

Lapidar 10 *Kunzle, Switz.*
Capsules†: Frangula bark (p.1227·1); cascara (p.1216·1); senna (p.1248·2).

Tablets: Frangula bark (p.1227·1); senna (p.1248·2); liquorice (p.1231·2).
Constipation.

Lapidar 14 *Kunzle, Switz.†.*
Frangula bark (p.1227·1); senna (p.1248·2); marian thistle (p.1021·3).
Constipation.

Lapidar 10 plus *Kunzle, Switz.†.*
Frangula bark (p.1227·1); senna (p.1248·2); mint oil (p.1636·2); fennel oil (p.1610·2).
Constipation.

Lapril *Pharmasant, Thai.*
Enalapril maleate (p.883·3).
Heart failure; hypertension.

Laprilen *Baldacci, Port.*
Enalapril maleate (p.883·3); hydrochlorothiazide (p.907·3).
Hypertension.

Laracit *Lemery, Mex.*
Cytarabine (p.530·1).
Leukaemias; lymphomas.

Laractone *Lagap, UK.*
Spironolactone (p.973·2).
Ascites; heart failure; hyperaldosteronism; oedema.

Larafen *Lagap, UK.*
Ketoprofen (p.47·3).
Musculoskeletal and joint disorders; pain.

Laraflex *Lagap, UK.*
Naproxen (p.60·3).
Gout; inflammation; musculoskeletal disorders; pain.

Larapam *Lagap, UK.*
Piroxicam (p.79·1).
Gout; inflammation; musculoskeletal disorders; pain.

Laratrim *Lagap, UK.*
Co-trimoxazole (p.193·3).
Bacterial infections.

Larch Resin comp. *Weleda, UK.*
Ananassa fruit; lavender oil (p.1627·2); larch resin.
Sore eyes.

Largactil
Rhone-Poulenc Rorer, Aust.; Rhone-Poulenc Rorer, Austral.; Rhone-Poulenc Rorer, Belg.†; Rhone-Poulenc Rorer, Canad.; Aventis, Denm.; Rhone-Poulenc Rorer, Fr.; Rhone-Poulenc Rorer, Hong Kong; Rhone-Poulenc Rorer, Irl.; Rhone-Poulenc Rorer, Ital.; Rhone-Poulenc Rorer, Mex.; Rhone-Poulenc Rorer, Neth.; Rhone-Poulenc Rorer, Norw.; Aventis, NZ; Vitoria, Port.; Aventis, S.Afr.; Rhone-Poulenc Rorer, Spain; Rhone-Poulenc Rorer, Switz.†; Hawgreen, UK.
Chlorpromazine (p.660·2), chlorpromazine embonate (p.660·2), or chlorpromazine hydrochloride (p.660·2).
Alcohol or opioid withdrawal syndrome; anxiety; autism; eclampsia; induction of hypothermia; intractable hiccup; nausea and vomiting; pain; premedication; psychoses; sedative.

Largal ultra *Septodont, Switz.†.*
Edetate sodium; cetrimonium bromide (p.1137·3).
Adjunct in dental surgery.

Largatrex
*Note.*This name is used for preparations of different composition.
Vitoria, Port.
Chlorpromazine hydrochloride (p.660·2).

Rhone-Poulenc Rorer, Spain.
Chlorpromazine (p.660·2); heptaminol (p.1619·2); benzhexol [trihexyphenidyl] (p.464·1).
Aggression; anxiety; psychoses.

Largitor *Italfarmaco, Spain.*
Myrtillus (p.1639·2).
Vascular disorders.

Largon
*Note.*This name is used for preparations of different composition.
Klinge, Aust.
Kawain (p.1625·3).
Nervous disorders.

Wyeth-Ayerst, USA†.
Propiomazine hydrochloride (p.424·3).
Sedative.

Lariam
Roche, Aust.; Roche, Austral.; Roche, Belg.; Roche, Canad.; Roche, Denm.; Roche, Fin.; Roche, Fr.; Roche, Ger.; Roche, Hong Kong; Roche, Irl.; Roche, Israel; Roche, Ital.; Roche, Neth.; Roche, Norw.; Roche, NZ; Roche, S.Afr.; Roche, Singapore; Roche, Swed.; Roche, Switz.; Roche, UK; Roche, USA.
Mefloquine hydrochloride (p.438·2).
Malaria.

Laridal *Elfar, Spain.*
Astemizole (p.409·1).
Hypersensitivity reactions.

Larifikehl *Sanum-Kehlbeck, Ger.*
Homoeopathic preparation.

Larilon *Bioprogress, Ital.*
Chlorhexidine gluconate (p.1138·2); benzododecinium chloride (p.1135·2).
Disinfection of wounds and burns.

Larimicina *Novaquimica, Braz.*
Diphenhydramine hydrochloride (p.416·1); ammonium chloride (p.1085·2); sodium citrate (p.1186·2).
Coughs.

Laringex *Cazi, Braz.*
Tyrothricin (p.267·1); cetrimonium; vitamin C (p.1389·3); lignocaine [lidocaine] (p.1313·2).
Mouth and throat disorders.

Larintil *Brasmedica, Braz.*
Tyrothricin (p.267·1); neomycin sulfate (p.228·1); benzocaine (p.1306·2).
Mouth and throat disorders.

Larmabak *Thea, Fr.; Thea, Hong Kong; Pharmacia Upjohn, Singapore.*
Sodium chloride (p.1196·1).
Dry eyes.

Larmes Artificielles *Ciba Vision, Fr.*
Sodium chloride (p.1196·1).
Dry eyes.

Larodopa *Roche, S.Afr.†; Cambridge, UK; Roche, USA.*
Levodopa (p.1169·2).
Now known as Levodopa Tablets in the *UK.*
Parkinsonism.

Laroferon *Roche, Fr.*
Interferon alfa-2a (p.628·1).
Hepatitis C.

Laroscorbine *Roche Nicholas, Fr.*
Ascorbic acid (p.1389·3).
Vitamin C deficiency.

Laroxyl *Roche, Fr.; Roche, Ital.*
Amitriptyline hydrochloride (p.273·3).
Depression; nocturnal enuresis; pain.

LarvE *SMTL, UK.*
Sterile larvae of *Lucilia sericata* (p.1118·2).
Infected or necrotic wounds.

Larvitan *Cimed, Braz.*
Amino-acid, vitamin, and mineral preparation (p.1350·1).

Larydol *Dolisos, Canad.*
Homoeopathic preparation.

Larylin Heissgetrank gegen Schmerzen und Fieber *Bayer, Ger.†.*
Paracetamol (p.71·2).
Fever; pain.

Larylin Husten-Heissgetrank *Bayer, Ger.†.*
Ambroxol hydrochloride (p.1084·3).
Respiratory disorders associated with viscid or excessive mucus.

Larylin Husten-Loser Pastillen *Merck, Ger.*
Ambroxol hydrochloride (p.1084·3).
Respiratory disorders associated with viscid or excessive mucus.

Larylin Husten-Loser Saft *Merck, Ger.*
Ambroxol hydrochloride (p.1084·3).
Respiratory disorders associated with viscid or excessive mucus.

Larylin Hustensirup N *Bayer, Ger.†.*
Dropropizine (p.1089·3).
Catarrh; coughs.

Larylin Husten-Stiller *Merck, Ger.*
Dropropizine (p.1089·3).
Coughs.

Larylin NAC Husten-Loser *Merck, Ger.*
Acetylcysteine (p.1082·3).
Respiratory-tract disorders associated with viscid or excessive mucus.

Larylin Nasenspray N *Bayer, Ger.†.*
Oxymetazoline hydrochloride (p.1096·2).
A similar preparation formerly contained naphazoline nitrate and pheniramine maleate.
Colds; middle ear inflammation; nasal congestion.

Laryngarsol *Sanofi Synthelabo, Belg.*
Ascorbic acid (p.1389·3); sodium ascorbate (p.1390·1); dequalinium chloride (p.1143·1).
Mouth and throat disorders.

Laryng-O-Jet *Medeva, UK.*
Lignocaine [lidocaine] hydrochloride (p.1313·2).
Local anaesthesia.

Laryngomedin N *Rhone-Poulenc Rorer, Ger.*
Hexamidine isetionate (p.1146·2).
Mouth and throat disorders.

Laryngsan N *Opfermann, Ger.*
Camphor (p.1589·3); caffeine and sodium benzoate (p.763·1); ammonia solution (p.1579·1); peppermint oil (p.1243·3).
Cold and influenza symptoms; laryngitis; pharyngitis.

Lasa Antiasmatico *Lasa, Spain†.*
Aminophylline (p.760·1); potassium iodide (p.1522·3).
Obstructive airways disease.

Lasa Con Codeina *Ipsen, Spain.*
Chlorpheniramine [chlorphenamine] maleate (p.412·1); codeine phosphate (p.25·2); pseudoephedrine hydrochloride (p.1099·2).
Coughs; nasal congestion.

Lasain *Inibsa, Spain.*
Metamizole magnesium (p.34·2).
Fever; pain.

Lasalar-Y *Alpharma, Mex.*
Fluocinolone acetonide (p.1071·1); clioquinol (p.190·2).
Skin disorders.

Lasalar-Y Simple *Alpharma, Mex.*
Clioquinol (p.190·2).
Skin disorders.

Lasar *Biocur, Ger.*
dl-Alpha tocoferil acetate (p.1394·1); magnesium oxide (p.1233·2).
Vitamin E or magnesium deficiency.

Laser *Tosi, Ital.*
Naproxen (p.60·3).
Gout; musculoskeletal and joint disorders; neuralgia.

Laser Slim 'n Trim *Laser, S.Afr.†.*
Cathine hydrochloride (p.1507·1).
Obesity.

Laservis *Chemedica, Ger.; Chemedica, Switz.*
Sodium hyaluronate (p.1620·1).
Adjunct in ocular procedures.

Lasikal *Hoechst Marion Roussel, Irl.†; Borg, UK.*
Frusemide [furosemide] (p.893·1); potassium chloride (p.1194·3).
Oedema.

Lasilacton *Hoechst Marion Roussel, Aust.; Hoechst Marion Roussel, Mex.*
Frusemide [furosemide] (p.893·1); spironolactone (p.973·2).
Ascites; hyperaldosteronism; oedema.

Lasilactona *Hoechst Marion Roussel, Braz.*
Frusemide [furosemide] (p.893·1); spironolactone (p.973·2).
Hypertension; oedema.

Lasilactone *Hoechst Marion Roussel, Switz.; Borg, UK.*
Frusemide [furosemide] (p.893·1); spironolactone (p.973·2).
Hypertension; oedema.

Lasiletten *Hoechst Marion Roussel, Neth.*
Frusemide [furosemide] (p.893·1).
Hypertension; oedema.

Lasilix *Hoechst, Fr.*
Frusemide [furosemide] (p.893·1).
Hypertension; oedema.

Lasitace *Hoechst Marion Roussel, Aust.*
Frusemide [furosemide] (p.893·1); ramipril (p.966·3).
Heart failure; hypertension.

Lasitone *Hoechst Marion Roussel, Ital.*
Frusemide [furosemide] (p.893·1); spironolactone (p.973·2).
Oedema.

Lasix
Hoechst Marion Roussel, Aust.; Hoechst Marion Roussel, Austral.; Aventis, Belg.; Hoechst Marion Roussel, Braz.; Hoechst Marion Roussel, Canad.; Aventis, Denm.; Hoechst Marion Roussel, Fin.; Hoechst Marion Roussel, Fr.; Hoechst Marion Roussel, Hong Kong; Hoechst Marion Roussel, Irl.; Hoechst Marion Roussel, Israel; Hoechst Marion Roussel, Ital.; Hoechst Marion Roussel, Mex.; Hoechst Marion Roussel, Neth.; Aventis, NZ; Hoeport, Port.; Aventis, S.Afr.; Hoechst Marion Roussel, Singapore; Hoechst Marion Roussel, Swed.; Hoechst Marion Roussel, Switz.; Hoechst Marion Roussel, Thai.; Borg, UK; Hoechst Marion Roussel, USA.
Frusemide [furosemide] (p.893·1) or frusemide [furosemide] sodium (p.895·1).
Forced diuresis; heart failure; hypertension; nephrotic syndrome; oedema; renal failure.

Lasix + K *Borg, UK†.*
White tablets, frusemide [furosemide] (p.893·1); yellow tablets, potassium chloride (p.1194·3).
Oedema.

Lasma
Pharmax, Irl.; Pharmax, UK†.
Theophylline (p.777·2).
Obstructive airways disease.

Lasonil
*Note.*This name is used for preparations of different composition.
Bayer, Aust.; Bayer, Ital.; Bayer, Neth.; Bayer, Port.; Bayer Consumer, UK.
A heparinoid (p.905·2).
Formerly contained a heparinoid and hyaluronidase.
Soft-tissue injury.

Bayer, Austral.; Bayer, Belg.; Bayer, Fr.†; Bayer, Israel; Bayer, NZ; Bayer, Spain.
A heparinoid (p.905·2); hyaluronidase (p.1620·3).
Soft-tissue injury; thrombophlebitis; varicose ulcers.

Lasonil H *Bayer, Ital.*
A heparinoid (p.905·2); hyaluronidase (p.1620·3); vitamin A palmitate (p.1383·2); calcium pantothenate (p.1374·1); menthol (p.1632·3).
Anorectal disorders.

Lasonil N *Bayer, Ger.*
A heparinoid (p.905·2).
Lasonil formerly contained a heparinoid and hyaluronidase.
Soft-tissue injury; superficial venous disorders.

Lasoproct *Bayer, Ital.†.*
A heparinoid (p.905·2); hyaluronidase (p.1620·3); vitamin A palmitate (p.1383·2); calcium pantothenate (p.1374·1); dexamethasone (p.1067·1); amethocaine [tetracaine] hydrochloride (p.1305·2); menthol (p.1632·3).
Anorectal disorders.

Lasoreuma *Bayer, Ital.†.*
A heparinoid (p.905·2); glycol salicylate (p.42·2); benzyl nicotinate (p.20·2).
Inflammation; pain.

Lasoride *Hoechst Marion Roussel, Irl.; Borg, UK.*
Frusemide [furosemide] (p.893·1); amiloride hydrochloride (p.835·1).
These ingredients can be described by the British Approved Name Co-amilofruse.
Oedema.

Lasoven *Bayer, Ital.*
A heparinoid (p.905·2).
Peripheral vascular disorders; soft-tissue disorders.

Laspar *Intramed, S.Afr.*
Asparaginase (p.508·3).
Lymphoblastic leukaemias.

Lassadermil *Oftalder, Port.*
Zinc oxide (p.1128·2).

Lassarmex *Precimex, Mex.*
Zinc oxide (p.1128·2).

Lassatina ISI, Ital.
Senna (p.1248·2); cascara (p.1216·1); rhubarb (p.1248·1); liquorice (p.1231·2); belladonna (p.463·1); nux vomica (p.1643·1); aniseed (p.1580·2).
Constipation.

Lassifar Lafare, Ital.
Lactulose (p.1230·1).
Hepatic encephalopathy.

Lasten/Barn Ferrosan, Fin.
Multivitamin preparation with manganese (p.1350·1).

Lastet
Pharmacia Upjohn, Ital.; Kayaku, Jpn†; Sanfer, Mex.; Probios, Port.; Pras, Spain.
Etoposide (p.538·1).
Malignant neoplasms.

Lasticom Asta Medica, Aust.
Azelastine hydrochloride (p.409·3).
Asthma; bronchitis.

Lastin
AstraZeneca, Fin.; Tika, Swed.
Azelastine hydrochloride (p.409·3).
Allergic conjunctivitis; allergic rhinitis.

Lastrim Chew, Thai.
Co-trimoxazole (p.193·3).
Bacterial infections.

Latensin Sanum-Kehlbeck, Ger.
Bacillus cereus.
Immunotherapy.

Latesil Solvay, Port.
Flufenamic acid (p.41·1); diethylamine salicylate (p.32·2); myrtecaine (p.1317·3).
Musculoskeletal, joint, peri-articular, and soft-tissue disorders.

Latesyl Medicopharm, Aust.
Diethylamine salicylate (p.32·2); myrtecaine (p.1317·3).
Musculoskeletal and joint disorders; neuralgia.

Laticort Medphano, Ger.
Hydrocortisone butyrate (p.1073·3).
Skin disorders.

Latimit Medphano, Ger.†
Hydrocortisone acetate (p.1073·3).
Skin disorders.

Latocef Del Saz & Filippini, Ital.†
Propylene glycol cefatrizine (p.164·3).
Bacterial infections.

Latonid Abbott, Swed.
Meloxicam (p.51·3).
Osteoarthritis.

Latotryd Atlantis, Mex.
Erythromycin (p.201·2).
Bacterial infections.

Lattulac Sofar, Ital.
Lactulose (p.1230·1).
Cirrhosis; hepatic encephalopathy.

Latycin
Biochemie, Aust.†; Boucher & Muir, Austral.; Biochemie, Singapore.
Tetracycline hydrochloride (p.258·3).
Bacterial eye infections.

Laubeel Desitin, Ger.
Lorazepam (p.688·3).
Anxiety disorders.

Laudamonium Henkel, Ger.
Benzalkonium chloride (p.1133·2).
Skin and surface disinfection.

Laudefen Wayne, Mex.
Difenidol (p.1222·1).

Laur Sons, Mex.
Tetracycline (p.258·3).
Bacterial infections.

Lauricin Sons, Mex.
Erythromycin estolate (p.201·2) or erythromycin stearate (p.201·3).
Bacterial infections.

Laurimic Effik, Spain.
Fenticonazole nitrate (p.383·2).
Fungal skin and nail infections; vulvovaginal candidiasis.

Laurimicina Mavi, Mex.
Erythromycin stearate (p.201·3).
Bacterial infections.

Lauritran Chinoin, Mex.
Erythromycin estolate (p.201·2).
Bacterial infections.

Lauroderme Baldacci, Port.
Salicylic acid (p.1122·3); zinc oxide (p.1128·2).
Skin inflammation and irritation.

Lauromentol Lepori, Port.
Menthol (p.1632·3); methyl salicylate (p.55·1); salicylic acid (p.1122·3); laurel oil; turpentine oil (p.1676·3).
Musculoskeletal, joint, peri-articular, and soft-tissue disorders.

Lauromicina Lafare, Ital.
Ointment: Fluocinolone acetonide (p.1071·1); erythromycin stearate (p.201·3).
Infected skin disorders.
Tablets: Laurilsulfate salt of erythromycin stearate (p.201·3).
Bacterial infections.

Lavaflac Antibioticos, Spain.
Sodium chloride (p.1196·1).
Fluid and electrolyte disorders.

Lavagin Mayrhofer, Aust.
Lactic acid (p.1626·2); sodium lactate (p.1186·2).
Vaginal disorders.

Lavanda Sofar Sofar, Ital.
Anhydrous citric acid (p.1596·2); sodium citrate (p.1186·2); alum (p.1577·2); phenol (p.1152·3).
Vaginal disinfection.

Lavasept Fresenius Kabi, Switz.
Polihexanide (p.1154·2).
Bone and soft-tissue infections; wounds.

Lavement au Phosphate Norgine, Belg.
Monobasic sodium phosphate (p.1193·2); dibasic sodium phosphate (p.1193·2).
Bowel evacuation.

Laveran Brasmedica, Braz.
Cimetidine (p.1216·3).
Gastro-oesophageal reflux; gstro-intestinal haemorrhage; peptic ulcer; Zollinger-Ellison syndrome.

Lavichthol Ichthyol, Aust.
Ictasol (p.1115·3).
Skin disorders.

Lavisa Lesvi, Spain.
Fluconazole (p.383·2).
Fungal infections.

Lavolen Lacer, Spain.
Trisodium polysaccharide sulfate; a nonoxinol (p.1346·1).
Contraceptive.

Lavolho Regius, Braz.
Boric acid (p.1586·1); chlorobutanol (p.1141·2).
Eye disorders.

Lax Pills G & W, USA†.
Yellow phenolphthalein (p.1244·1).

Laxa Nobel, Canad.†.
Aloin (p.1210·2); cascara (p.1216·1); phenolphthalein (p.1244·1); bile salts (p.1585·1).

Laxabon
AstraZeneca, Norw.; Tika, Swed.
Macrogol 3350 (p.1630·3); electrolytes (p.1180·1).
Bowel evacuation.

Laxaco Jamieson, Canad.
Cascara sagrada (p.1216·1); senna (p.1248·2).
Constipation.

Laxadin Teva, Israel.
Bisacodyl (p.1212·2).
Constipation.

Laxadoron Weleda, UK.
Caraway (p.1591·2); clove (p.1596·3); centaury (p.1593·1); peppermint leaf (p.1243·2); achillea (p.1572·2); senna leaf (p.1248·2); aniseed (p.1580·2); nectar hoyae carnosae.
Constipation.

Laxagel Everest, Canad.
Capsules: Docusate sodium (p.1223·1).
Constipation.
Oral powder: Ispaghula (p.1229·1).
Constipation.

Laxagetten CT, Ger.
Bisacodyl (p.1212·2).
Constipation.

Laxal Julphar, UAE.
Senna (p.1248·2).
Bowel evacuation; constipation.

Laxalpin Kwizda, Aust.
Senna (p.1248·2); frangula bark (p.1227·1); fennel (p.1610·1); chamomile (p.1593·2); guaiacum wood; liquorice (p.1231·2); sambucus (p.1660·3); adiantum capillus veneris; sodium potassium tartrate (p.1250·1).
Constipation.

Laxamalt
Bouchara, Fr.; Bouchara, Switz.
Liquid paraffin (p.1407·1).
Constipation.

Laxamucil Orion, Fin.
Ispaghula (p.1229·1).
Constipation.

Laxan
Note. This name is used for preparations of different composition.
QIF, Braz.
Senna (p.1248·2); tamarind (p.1253·2); cassia pulp (p.1216·2).
Constipation.

Chew, Thai.
Methocarbamol (p.1329·3).
Musculoskeletal pain.

Laxanin N Schwarzhaupt, Ger.
Bisacodyl (p.1212·2).
Constipation.

Laxans Schulke & Mayr, Aust.
Ispaghula (p.1229·1).

Laxans-ratiopharm Ratiopharm, Ger.
Bisacodyl (p.1212·2).
Bowel evacuation; constipation.

Laxante Bescansa Bescansa, Spain.
Carrageenan mucilage (p.1500·1); phenolphthalein (p.1244·1).
Formerly contained calcium carbonate, carrageenan mucilage, and phenolphthalein.

Laxante Bescansa Aloico Bescansa, Spain.
Aloin (p.1210·2); belladonna (p.463·1); phenolphthalein (p.1244·1); rhubarb (p.1248·1).
Constipation.

Laxante Derly Derly, Spain.
Cascara (p.1216·1); senna (p.1248·2).
Constipation.

Laxante Olan Puerto Galiano, Spain.
Senna (p.1248·2).
Formerly contained ipomoea, phenolphthalein, sodium bicarbonate, and tartaric acid.
Constipation.

Laxante Salud Boots Healthcare, Spain.
Senna (p.1248·2).
Formerly contained aloes and phenolphthalein.
Constipation.

Laxante Sanatorium Santiveri, Spain.
Aloes (p.1210·1); aniseed (p.1580·2); sulfur (p.1123·3); senna (p.1248·2); chamomile (p.1593·2).
Constipation.

Laxarine Farmion, Braz.
Senna (p.1248·2); cassia pulp (p.1216·2); tamarind (p.1253·2); coriander (p.1599·2); liquorice (p.1231·2).
Constipation.

Laxarol Therapex, Canad.†.
Phenolphthalein (p.1244·1); liquid paraffin (p.1407·1).

Laxaron Monot, Fr.
Lactulose (p.1230·1).
Constipation.

Laxasan
Note. This name is used for preparations of different composition.
Dolisos, Canad.
Homoeopathic preparation.

Dolisos, Fr.†.
Senna (p.1248·2); tamarind (p.1253·2).
Constipation.

Gebro, Switz.
Sodium picosulfate (p.1249·3); fennel oil (p.1610·2); peppermint oil (p.1243·3).
Constipation.

Laxative
Note. This name is used for preparations of different composition.
Lalco, Canad.
Aloes (p.1210·1); cascara sagrada (p.1216·1); bile salts (p.1585·1).
Constipation.

Trima, Israel.
Aloin (p.1210·2); phenolphthalein (p.1244·1); belladonna (p.463·1).
Constipation.

Laxative Comp Teva, Israel.
Aloin (p.1210·2); phenolphthalein (p.1244·1); aloes (p.1210·1); ipecacuanha (p.1093·1); belladonna (p.463·1).
Constipation.

Laxative Pills
Note. This name is used for preparations of different composition.
Stanley, Canad.
Sennosides (p.1248·3).
Formerly contained phenolphthalein.

Rugby, USA†.
Yellow phenolphthalein (p.1244·1).
Constipation.

Laxative & Stool Softener Rugby, USA.
Docusate sodium (p.1223·1); casanthranol (p.1216·1).
Constipation.

Laxative Tablets Herbal Concepts, UK.
Aloes (p.1210·1); cascara (p.1216·1); senna (p.1248·2); valerian (p.1678·3).
Constipation.

Laxativum Nouvelle Formule Giuliani, Switz.†.
Cascara (p.1216·1); boldo (p.1585·3); senna (p.1248·2).
Constipation.

Laxavit Wolfs, Belg.
Docusate sodium (p.1223·1); glycerol (p.1616·3).
Constipation.

Laxbene
Note. This name is used for preparations of different composition.
Ratiopharm, Aust.; Merckle, Ger.
Suppositories: Bisacodyl (p.1212·2).
Bowel evacuation; constipation.

Ratiopharm, Aust.
Tablets: Bisacodyl (p.1212·2); dimethicone (p.1249·2).
Bowel evacuation; constipation.

Laxbene N Merckle, Ger.
Bisacodyl (p.1212·2).
Constipation.

Laxcodyl Pharmasant, Thai.
Bisacodyl (p.1212·2).
Constipation.

Laxen Farmasa, Mex.
Ispaghula (p.1229·1).

Laxen Busto Salvat, Spain.
Phenolphthalein (p.1244·1).
Constipation.

Laxette Medpro, S.Afr.
Lactulose (p.1230·1).
Constipation; hepatic encephalopathy.

Laxettes Mentholatum, Austral.
Chocolate: Phenolphthalein (p.1244·1).
Tablets: Calcium sennoside A (p.1248·3); calcium sennoside B (p.1248·3).
Constipation.

Laxicaps Propan-Vernleigh, S.Afr.†.
Phenolphthalein (p.1244·1); ferrous sulfate (p.1360·3).
Constipation.

Laxicaps P Propan, S.Afr.
Phenolphthalein (p.1244·1).
Constipation.

Laxikal Forte Teva, Israel.
Senna (p.1248·2).
Constipation.

Laxilose Technilab, Canad.
Lactulose (p.1230·1).
Constipation.

Laxiplant cum Senna Wander OTC, Switz.†.
Ispaghula (p.1229·1); senna (p.1248·2).
Constipation.

Laxiplant Soft
Schwabe, Ger.; Schwabe, Switz.
Ispaghula (p.1229·1).
Constipation; diarrhoea.

Laxisoft Sanofi Synthelabo, Spain.
Ispaghula (p.1229·1).
Constipation.

Laxo Vian Alcala, Spain†.
Atropine sulfate (p.461·1); hyoscyamus (p.470·3); cascara (p.1216·1); phenolphthalein (p.1244·1); podophyllum (p.1121·1); sodium bicarbonate.
Constipation.

Laxoberal
Boehringer Ingelheim, Denm.; Boehringer Ingelheim, Ger.; Boehringer Ingelheim, Irl.; Boehringer Ingelheim, Swed.; Boehringer Ingelheim Self Medication, UK.
Sodium picosulfate (p.1249·3).
Bowel evacuation; constipation.

Laxoberal Bisa Boehringer Ingelheim, Ger.
Bisacodyl (p.1212·2).
Constipation.

Laxoberon
Boehringer Ingelheim, Belg.; Boehringer Ingelheim, Fin.; Boehringer Ingelheim, Mex.; Boehringer Ingelheim, Neth.†; Boehringer Ingelheim, Switz.
Sodium picosulfate (p.1249·3).
Bowel evacuation; constipation.

Laxocodyl Julphar, UAE.
Bisacodyl (p.1212·2).
Bowel evacuation; constipation.

Laxol Enila, Braz.
Castor oil (p.1592·1); peppermint oil (p.1243·3).
Constipation.

Laxolen Basi, Port.
Cascara (p.1216·1).
Constipation.

Laxolind Metochem, Aust.†.
Senna (p.1248·2); frangula (p.1227·1); chamomile (p.1593·2).
Bowel regulation.

Laxolyne Julphar, UAE.
Glycerol (p.1616·3).
Constipation.

Laxomild Renapharm, Switz.†.
Calcium sennoside A (p.1248·3); calcium sennoside B (p.1248·3).
Constipation.

Laxomundin Mundipharma, Ger.†.
Lactulose (p.1230·1).
Constipation.

Laxonol Madaus, Spain.
Sodium picosulfate (p.1249·3).
Constipation.

Laxopol
Pohl, Ger.; Pohl, Israel.
Castor oil (p.1592·1).
Constipation.

Laxose
Pinewood, Irl.; Berk, UK†.
Lactulose (p.1230·1).
Constipation; hepatic encephalopathy.

Laxtam Merck, Braz.
Senna (p.1248·2); cassia pulp (p.1216·2); tamarind (p.1253·2); coriander (p.1599·2); liquorice (p.1231·2).
Constipation.

Laxucil Novopharm, Canad.
Ispaghula (p.1229·1).

Laxvital Maxfarma, Spain.
Carmellose (p.1499·3); docusate sodium (p.1223·1); casanthranol (p.1216·1).
Constipation.

Laxyl Solfran, Mex.
Diazepam (p.674·3).

Laxysat Burger Ysatfabrik, Ger.
Bisacodyl (p.1212·2).
Constipation.

Laxysat mono Ysatfabrik, Ger.†.
Buckthorn (p.1215·1).
Constipation.

Lazercreme Pedinol, USA.
Vitamin E (p.1393·3); vitamin A (p.1382·1).
Minor skin irritation.

Lazerformaldehyde Pedinol, USA.
Formaldehyde (p.1144·2).
Bromhidrosis (feet); hyperhidrosis; warts.

LazerSporin-C Pedinol, USA.
Neomycin sulfate (p.228·1); polymyxin B sulfate (p.238·1); hydrocortisone (p.1073·3).
Bacterial ear infections.

LBC-LAX Murdock, USA†.
Cascara (p.1216·1).

LC-65
Allergan, Austral.; Allergan, Israel; Allergan, NZ; Allergan, Port.; Allergan, USA.
Range of solutions for contact lenses (p.1129·2).

The symbol † denotes a preparation no longer actively marketed

L-Carn *Sigma-Tau, Ger.*
Carnitine (p.1356·1).
Carnitine deficiency.

L-Cimexyl *Cimex, Switz.*
Acetylcysteine (p.1082·3).
Respiratory-tract disorders.

L-Combur-5-Test *Roche Diagnostics, Austral.*
Test for pH, protein, glucose, ketones, and blood in urine.

Le 100 B *Pharmalab, Canad.†*
Cascara (p.1216·1); phenolphthalein (p.1244·1).

Le 500 D *Pharmalab, Canad.*
Cascara (p.1216·1).

Le Face Protection *Creative Brands, Austral.*
SPF 15+: Octinoxate (p.1517·3); avobenzone (p.1517·1).
Sunscreen.

Le Fibre *Or-Dov, Austral.*
Wheat fibre.
Dietary fibre supplement; obesity.

Le Stick a Levres *Duchesnay, Canad.*
Cinoxate (p.1517·1); allantoin (p.1110·1); vitamin A palmitate (p.1383·2).
Sunscreen.

Le Tan Broad Spectrum *Creative Brands, Austral.*
SPF15+: Octinoxate (p.1517·3); avobenzone (p.1517·1).
Sunscreen.

Le Tan Fast Extra Dark *Creative Brands, Austral.*
Dihydroxyacetone (p.1113·2).
Artificial suntan.

Le Tan Fast Plus *Creative Brands, Austral.*
SPF 15: Octinoxate (p.1517·3); avobenzone (p.1517·1); dihydroxyacetone (p.1113·2).
Artificial suntan; sunscreen.

Le Tan Fast Self Tan *Creative Brands, Austral.*
Dihydroxyacetone (p.1113·2).
Artificial suntan.

Le Tan Gel *Creative Brands, Austral.*
SPF 8: Octinoxate (p.1517·3); benzophenone (p.1517·1).
SPF 15: Octinoxate (p.1517·3); benzophenone (p.1517·1); avobenzone (p.1517·1).
Sunscreen.

Le Tan Natural *Creative Brands, Austral.*
SPF 15: Titanium dioxide (p.1126·1); zinc oxide (p.1128·2).
Sunscreen.

Le Tan Roll On Lotion *Creative Brands, Austral.*
SPF 15: Octinoxate (p.1517·3); avobenzone (p.1517·1).
Sunscreen.

Le Tan Sensitive *Creative Brands, Austral.*
SPF 30+: Octinoxate (p.1517·3); amiloxate (p.1516·3); octisalate (p.1518·1); zinc oxide (p.1128·2).
Sunscreen.

Le Tan Sport Dry Lotion *Creative Brands, Austral.*
SPF 15: Octinoxate (p.1517·3); oxybenzone (p.1518·1); avobenzone (p.1517·1).
Sunscreen.

Le Tan Sport & Surf *Creative Brands, Austral.*
SPF 30+: Octinoxate (p.1517·3); amiloxate (p.1516·3); octisalate (p.1518·1); zinc oxide (p.1128·2).
Sunscreen.

Le Tan Sunblock Stick *Creative Brands, Austral.*
SPF 15: Octinoxate (p.1517·3); avobenzone (p.1517·1).
Sunscreen.

Le Tan Sunscreen Lotion *Creative Brands, Austral.*
SPF4; SPF8: Octinoxate (p.1517·3).
SPF15: Octinoxate (p.1517·3); avobenzone (p.1517·1).
SPF 30+: Octinoxate (p.1517·3); enzacamene (p.1517·2); avobenzone (p.1517·1).
Sunscreen.

Le Tan Sunscreen Lotion Broad Spectrum
Creative Brands, Austral.
SPF 15+: Octinoxate (p.1517·3); avobenzone (p.1517·1).
Sunscreen.

Le Tan Ultimate *Creative Brands, Austral.*
SPF 8: Octinoxate (p.1517·3); benzophenone (p.1517·1).
SPF 15+: Octinoxate (p.1517·3); avobenzone (p.1517·1); benzophenone (p.1517·1).
Sunscreen.

Le Thermogene *Tradiphar, Fr.*
Capsicum oleoresin (p.1591·1); glycol salicylate (p.42·2).
Musculoskeletal and peri-articular pain; respiratory-tract congestion.

Le Trim-BM *Or-Dov, Austral.*
Benzocaine (p.1306·2); methylcellulose (p.1502·2); ferrous gluconate; vitamins (p.1350·1).
Obesity.

Lealgin *Janssen-Cilag, Swed.†*
Phenoperidine hydrochloride (p.78·1).
Adjunct in neuroleptanalgesia; pain in surgical procedures; respiratory depressant in intensive care.

Leanor *Aspen Consumer, S.Afr.*
Cathine hydrochloride (p.1507·1).
Obesity.

Leaton fur Erwachsene *Pharmacia Upjohn, Aust.*
Multivitamins (p.1350·1) with caffeine (p.761·3).
Tonic.

Leaton fur Kinder *Pharmacia Upjohn, Aust.*
Multivitamins (p.1350·1).
Tonic.

Lebensenergie-Kapseln *Twardy, Ger.*
Eleutherococcus (p.1615·3).
Tonic.

Leber- und Galletee *Sanova, Aust.*
Absinthium (p.1571·1); calamus (p.1588·1); angelica (p.1580·2); peppermint leaf (p.1243·2); bitter-orange leaf.
Liver and biliary disorders.

Leberetic *Ern, Spain.*
Potassium sulfate (p.1195·1); sodium bicarbonate (p.1186·2); sodium sulfate (p.1250·1).
Liver disorders.

Leber-Galle-Tropfen 83 *Bio-Diat, Ger.*
Sage (p.1660·2); absinthium (p.1571·1); gentian (p.1615·1); fennel (p.1610·1); centaury (p.1593·1); elecampane (p.1089·3); anise oil (p.1580·3); peppermint oil (p.1243·3); calamus oil; lavender oil (p.1627·2).
Biliary disorders; dyspepsia.

Leber-Galletropfen S *Cosmochema, Ger.*
Homoeopathic preparation.

Leberinfusion *Fresenius Kabi, Aust.*
Arginine (p.1353·3); malic acid (p.1631·1); sodium hydroxide (p.1665·3); potassium hydroxide (p.1654·1).
Liver disorders.

Lebersal *Ern, Spain.*
Magnesium sulfate (p.1191·1); sodium bicarbonate (p.1186·2); dibasic sodium phosphate (p.1193·2); sodium sulfate (p.1250·1).
Gastrointestinal disorders; hepatic insufficiency.

Lebic *Isis Puren, Ger.*
Baclofen (p.1322·3).
Skeletal muscle spasm or spasticity.

Lebopride *Spyfarma, Spain.*
Sulpiride (p.706·1).
Anxiety disorders; psychoses; vertigo.

Lebriton N *Zeppenfeldt, Ger.*
Homoeopathic preparation.

Lebrocetin *Liferpal, Mex.*
Chloramphenicol (p.179·1).
Bacterial infections.

Lecia *Caldeira & Marques, Port.*
Ortho-oxybenzoic acid; lactic acid (p.1626·2); phenol (p.1152·3); glacial acetic acid (p.1571·2); turpentine oil (p.1676·3).
Corns; verrucas.

Lecibral *Solvay, Spain.*
Nicardipine hydrochloride (p.938·3).
Angina pectoris; cerebrovascular disorders; hypertension.

Lecicarbon
Note.This name is used for preparations of different composition.
Brady, Aust.
Sodium bicarbonate (p.1186·2); potassium acid tartrate (p.1244·3).
Constipation.

Athenstaedt, Ger.; Athenstaedt, Switz.
Sodium bicarbonate (p.1186·2); monobasic sodium phosphate (p.1193·2).
Bowel evacuation; constipation.

Leciderm *Darier, Mex.*
Lecithin (p.1628·1).
Dry skin disorders.

Lecikur *Agepha, Aust.*
Lecithin (p.1628·1); caffeine (p.761·3).
Tonic.

Lecinova *Novartis Consumer, Ital.*
Nutritional supplement containing phospholipids and vitamins (p.1350·1).

Leciplus *Novartis Consumer, Ital.*
Nutritional supplement containing phospholipids and vitamins (p.1350·1).

Lecitone *Yves Ponroy, Fr.*
A range of nutritional supplements containing phospholipids (p.1350·1).
Tonic.

Lecival *Agepha, Aust.*
Oral solution: Lecithin (p.1628·1); caffeine (p.761·3).
Tablets: Lecithin (p.1628·1); vitamin E acetate (p.1394·1).
Tonic.

Leclor A *Provit, Mex.*
Chloramphenicol (p.179·1).
Bacterial infections.

Lecrolyn *Santen, Denm.; Santen, Fin.; Santen, Norw.; Santen, Swed.; Santen, Thai.*
Sodium cromoglicate (p.774·3).
Allergic conjunctivitis; allergic rhinitis.

Lectil *Bouchara, Fr.*
Betahistine hydrochloride (p.1584·2).
Vertigo.

Lectopam *Roche, Canad.*
Bromazepam (p.656·3).
Anxiety.

Ledclair *Sinclair, Irl.; Durbin, UK.*
Sodium calcium edetate (p.1022·1).
Heavy metal poisoning.

Ledercillin VK
Wyeth-Ayerst, Canad.†; Lederle, USA†.
Phenoxymethylpenicillin potassium (p.235·1).
Bacterial infections.

Ledercort
Wyeth Lederle, Belg.; Wyeth Lederle, Ital.; Lederle, Neth.; Wyeth, S.Afr.; Cyanamid, Spain; Lederle, Switz.; Lederle, UK.
Triamcinolone (p.1080·1), triamcinolone acetonide (p.1080·1), or triamcinolone diacetate (p.1080·2).
Corticosteroid.

Lederderm *Lederle, Ger.*
Minocycline hydrochloride (p.224·3).
Bacterial infections.

Lederfen
Wyeth Lederle, Aust.; Lederle, Irl.; Lederle, Israel; Wyeth, UK.
Fenbufen (p.36·2).
Musculoskeletal and joint disorders.

Lederfolat *Lederle, Ger.*
Calcium folinate (p.1363·1).
Folate deficiency.

Lederfolin
Wyeth Lederle, Ital.; Cyanamid, Spain; Lederle, UK.
Calcium folinate (p.1363·1).
Drug-induced folic acid deficiency; megaloblastic anaemia; methotrexate overdose; potentiation of fluorouracil activity.

Lederfoline
Wyeth Lederle, Fr.; Wyeth Lederle, Port.
Calcium folinate (p.1363·1).
Drug-induced megaloblastic anaemia; folic acid deficiency; prevention of methotrexate toxicity.

Lederlind *Lederle, Ger.*
Nystatin (p.392·2).
Fungal infections of the skin and mucous membranes.

Lederlon *Lederle, Ger.*
Triamcinolone hexacetonide (p.1080·2).
Parenteral corticosteroid.

Ledermicina *Cyanamid, Ital.†*
Demeclocycline hydrochloride (p.198·2).
Bacterial infections.

Ledermix
Note.This name is used for preparations of different composition.
Wyeth Lederle, Aust.; Wyeth, Irl.; Wyeth, S.Afr.; Lederle, Switz.; Lederle, UK.
Paste, triamcinolone acetonide (p.1080·1); demeclocycline calcium (p.198·2); cement, triamcinolone acetonide; demeclocycline hydrochloride (p.198·2); solution, eugenol (p.1609·3).
Bacterial infection and inflammatory disorders in dentistry.

Wyeth Lederle, Denm.
Paste, triamcinolone acetonide (p.1080·1); demeclocycline calcium (p.198·2); cement, triamcinolone acetonide; demeclocycline calcium; hardener N, macrogol 400 (p.1630·3); hardener S, eugenol (p.1609·3).
Bacterial infection and inflammatory disorders in dentistry.

Lederle, Israel.
Triamcinolone acetonide (p.1080·1); demeclocycline calcium (p.198·2).
Bacterial infection and inflammatory disorders in dentistry.

Ledermycin
Wyeth Lederle, Aust.; Lederle, Austral.; Wyeth Lederle, Belg.†; Wyeth, Irl.; Lederle, Neth.; Lederle, NZ; Lederle, S.Afr.†; Wyeth, UK.
Demeclocycline hydrochloride (p.198·2).
Amoebiasis; bacterial infections; hyponatraemia.

Lederpaediat *Lederle, Ger.†*
Erythromycin ethyl succinate (p.201·2).
Bacterial infections.

Lederpax *Wyeth, Mex.; Cyanamid, Spain.*
Erythromycin (p.201·2).
Acne.

Lederplatin
Teva, Denm.; Wyeth Lederle, Swed.†
Cisplatin (p.525·1).
Malignant neoplasms.

Lederscon *Lederle, Hong Kong.*
Aluminium hydroxide (p.1210·3); magnesium hydroxide (p.1233·1); mannitol (p.924·3); simeticone (p.1249·2).
Flatulence; meteorism.

Lederspan
Wyeth Lederle, Aust.†; Wyeth Lederle, Belg.†; Wyeth Lederle, Denm.†; Wyeth Lederle, Fin.†; Wyeth, Irl.†; Lederle, Neth.†; Wyeth Lederle, Norw.†; Wyeth, S.Afr.; Wyeth Lederle, Swed.†; Wyeth, UK†.
Triamcinolone hexacetonide (p.1080·2).
Corticosteroid.

Ledertam *Wyeth Lederle, Ital.; Wyeth Lederle, Swed.†*
Tamoxifen citrate (p.571·1).
Breast cancer.

Ledertepa *Wyeth Lederle, Belg.; Lederle, Neth.*
Thiotepa (p.574·3).
Malignant neoplasms.

Ledertrexate
Lederle, Austral.; Wyeth Lederle, Belg.; Wyeth Lederle, Fr.; Wyeth, Mex.; Lederle, Neth.; Wyeth Lederle, NZ.
Methotrexate (p.553·2) or methotrexate sodium (p.553·2).
Malignant neoplasms; mycosis fungoides; psoriasis; rheumatoid arthritis.

Ledervorin
Wyeth Lederle, Belg.; Lederle, Neth.
Calcium folinate (p.1363·1).
Adjunct to fluorouracil in colorectal cancer; adjunct to high-dose methotrexate therapy; overdosage with folic acid antagonists.

Ledoren *Boniscontro & Gazzone, Ital.*
Nimesulide (p.62·3).
Fever; inflammation; pain.

Ledovit C *Bama, Spain.*
Ascorbic acid (p.1389·3).
Adjunct in treatment of iron supplementation; vitamin C deficiency.

Ledox *Weifa, Norw.*
Naproxen (p.60·3).
Gout; musculoskeletal and joint disorders; pain.

Ledoxid Acne *Lederle, Switz.†*
Benzoyl peroxide (p.1111·1).
Acne.

Ledoxina *Lemery, Mex.*
Cyclophosphamide (p.527·3).
Malignant neoplasms.

Ledum Med Complex *Dynamit, Aust.*
Homoeopathic preparation.

Lefax
Asche, Ger.; Pharmacia Upjohn, Switz.
Simeticone (p.1249·2).
Anti-foaming agent in radiography of the gastrointestinal tract; detergent intoxication; gastrointestinal disorders associated with excess gas.

Lefaxin *Lannacher, Aust.*
Simeticone (p.1249·2).
Flatulence.

Lefcar *Glaxo Wellcome, Ital.*
Carnitine (p.1356·1) or carnitine hydrochloride (p.1356·2).
Carnitine deficiency; myocardial ischaemia.

Leferdivin *Hotz, Ger.*
Vitamin B substances; lecithin; ferrous citrate; glutamic acid (p.1350·1).
Tonic.

Lefrine *Grin, Mex.*
Phenylephrine hydrochloride (p.1097·1).
Nasal congestion.

Leftose
Shinyaku, Jpn; Shinyaku, Singapore; Shinyaku, Thai.
Muramidase hydrochloride (p.1638·1).
Haemmorhage; infections; inflammation.

Leg Cramps with Quinine *Hylands, Canad.*
Homoeopathic preparation.

Legalon
Madaus, Aust.; Madaus, Fr.; Madaus, Ger.
Silybum marianum (p.1021·3).
Liver disorders.

Madaus, Belg.; Madaus, Hong Kong; Ibi, Ital.; Byk Gulden, Mex.; Neo-Farmaceutica, Port.; Byk Madaus, S.Afr.; Madaus, Spain; Madaus, Switz.; Madaus, Thai.
Silymarin (p.1021·3).
Liver disorders.

Legalon SIL *Madaus, Ger.; Madaus, Switz.*
Disodium silibinin dihemisuccinate (p.1021·3).
Mushroom poisoning.

Madaus, Spain.
Silibinin dihydrogensuccinate.
Mushroom poisoning.

Legapas *Ebi, Switz.†*
Cascara (p.1216·1).
Constipation.

Legapas comp *Pascoe, Ger.†*
Cascara (p.1216·1); silybum marianum (p.1021·3); greater celandine (p.1618·1); taraxacum (p.1669·1).
Formerly known as Legapas N.
Liver disorders.

Legapas mono *Pascoe, Ger.*
Cascara (p.1216·1).
Constipation.

Legatrin PM *Columbia, USA.*
Paracetamol (p.71·2); diphenhydramine hydrochloride (p.416·1).
Insomnia.

Legatrin Rub *Columbia, USA.*
Menthol (p.1632·3); benzocaine (p.1306·2).

Legedern
Schering-Plough, Denm.; Schering-Plough, Fin.; Schering-Plough, Ital.; Schering-Plough, Norw.
Alclometasone dipropionate (p.1061·1).
Skin disorders.

Legendal *Zambon, Neth.; Inpharzam, Switz.*
Lactulose (p.1230·1).
Constipation; hepatic encephalopathy.

Legil *Millet Roux, Braz.*
Tenoxicam (p.87·2).
Musculoskeletal, joint, and peri-articular disorders.

Legofer
Asta Medica, Ital.; ITF, Port.
Iron succinyl-protein complex (p.1369·3).
Iron deficiency; iron-deficiency anaemia.

Lehydan *Abigo, Swed.*
Phenytoin (p.357·2).
Epilepsy.

Leiba *Uniao Quimica, Braz.*
Lactobacillus acidophilus (p.1626·3).
Diarrhoea; restoration of intestinal flora.

Leicester Retard *Polifarma, Ital.*
Isosorbide mononitrate (p.916·2).
Angina pectoris.

Leiguar *Labatec, Switz.*
Guar gum (p.323·3).
Diabetes mellitus; hyperlipidaemias.

Leioderm *LAW, Ger.*
Hydroxyquinoline sulfate (p.1622·2).
Impetigo.

Leioderm P *LAW, Ger.*
Hydroxyquinoline sulfate (p.1622·2); prednisolone (p.1077·3).
Infected skin disorders.

Leios *Wyeth, Ger.*
Levonorgestrel (p.1486·2); ethinylestradiol (p.1476·2).
Combined oral contraceptive.

Leite de Magnesia *Sterling, Port.*
Magnesium hydroxide (p.1233·1).

Leite de Magnesia de Phillips *SmithKline Beecham, Braz.*
Magnesium hydroxide (p.1233·1).
Constipation.

Leite de Magnesia Honfar *Honorterapica, Braz.*
Magnesium hydroxide (p.1233·1).
Constipation.

Lejguar *Meta Fackler, Ger.*
Guar gum (p.323·3).
Diabetes mellitus; hyperlipidaemias.

Lektinol *Madaus, Ger.*
Mistletoe (p.1636·2).
Malignant neoplasms.

Lelong Contusions *SmithKline Beecham Sante, Fr.†.*
Arnica (p.1581·3); tamus communis.
Soft-tissue disorders.

Lelong Irritations *SmithKline Beecham Sante, Fr.†.*
Enoxolone (p.34·3); propanocaine hydrochloride (p.1319·3).
Inflammatory and pruritic skin disorders.

Lema C *Ern, Spain.*
Ascorbic acid (p.1389·3); borax (p.1586·1).
Halitosis; mouth and throat inflammation; pyorrhoea.

Lemazol *Petrasch, Aust.*
Ascorbic acid (p.1389·3); potassium orotate (p.1645·1); inositol (p.1623·3); sorbitol (p.1377·3).
Liver disorders.

Lemblastine *Lemery, Mex.*
Vinblastine sulfate (p.577·3).
Malignant neoplasms.

Lemdopa *Lemery, Mex.*
Levodopa (p.1169·2); carbidopa (p.1168·2).
Parkinsonism.

L-Emental *Nutrition Medical, Israel.*
A range of preparations for enteral nutrition (p.1350·1).

Lemgrip *Reckitt & Colman, Belg.*
Paracetamol (p.71·2).
Fever; pain.

Lemivit *Kemiprogress, Ital.*
Vitamins (p.1350·1); lecithin (p.1628·1).
Fatigue.

Lemlax *Co-Pharma, UK.*
Lactulose (p.1230·1).
Constipation.

Lemocin
Note. This name is used for preparations of different composition.
Novartis Consumer, Aust.; Novartis Consumer, Belg.
Tyrothricin (p.267·1); cetrimide (p.1137·1); lignocaine [lidocaine] (p.1313·2).
Mouth and throat disorders.

Novartis Consumer, Ger.; Novartis Consumer, Switz.
Tyrothricin (p.267·1); cetrimonium bromide (p.1137·3); lignocaine [lidocaine] (p.1313·2) or lignocaine [lidocaine] hydrochloride (p.1313·2).
Mouth and throat disorders.

Lemocin CX *Novartis Consumer, Ger.*
Chlorhexidine gluconate (p.1138·2).
Mouth and throat disorders.

Lemocin Flexibels *Novartis Consumer, Ger.*
Benzoxonium chloride (p.1135·2); lignocaine [lidocaine] hydrochloride (p.1313·2).
Mouth and throat disorders.

Lemon Time *Buckley, Canad.*
Paracetamol (p.71·2); phenylphrine hydrochloride (p.1097·1); mepyramine maleate (p.421·1); ascorbic acid (p.1389·3).
Cold symptoms.

Lemonvit *Molteni, Ital.*
Ascorbic acid (p.1389·3).
Vitamin C deficiency.

Lemophar *Alpharma, Mex.*
Hyoscine butylbromide (p.468·2).

Lem-Plus *Adcock Ingram, UK.*
Capsules: Paracetamol (p.71·2); caffeine (p.761·3); phenylephrine (p.1097·1).

Oral powder: Paracetamol (p.71·2); ascorbic acid (p.1389·3).
Cold symptoms.

Lemsip
Note. This name is used for preparations of different composition.
Reckitt & Colman, Austral.; Meda, Swed.†.
Paracetamol (p.71·2).
Cold and influenza symptoms.

Reckitt & Colman, Hong Kong; Reckitts, Irl.
Paracetamol (p.71·2); sodium citrate (p.1186·2); ascorbic acid (p.1389·3).
Cold and influenza symptoms.

Reckitt & Colman, S.Afr.†.
Paracetamol (p.71·2); phenylephrine hydrochloride (p.1097·1); sodium citrate (p.1186·2).
Cold and influenza symptoms.

Lemsip Chesty Cough
Reckitt Benckiser, Austral.; Reckitt Benckiser, NZ.
Guaifenesin (p.1092·2).
Coughs.

Lemsip Childrens Six+ Cold & Flu Relief
Reckitt & Colman, UK.
Paracetamol (p.71·2); phenylephrine hydrochloride (p.1097·1).
Cold and influenza symptoms.

Lemsip Cold & Flu Breathe Easy *Reckitt & Colman, UK.*
Paracetamol (p.71·2); phenylephrine hydrochloride (p.1097·1); ascorbic acid (p.1389·3).
Cold and influenza symptoms.

Lemsip Cold & Flu Combined Relief *Reckitt & Colman, UK.*
Paracetamol (p.71·2); phenylephrine hydrochloride (p.1097·1); caffeine (p.761·3).
Cold and influenza symptoms.

Lemsip Cold & Flu Headcold *Reckitt Benckiser, NZ.*
Paracetamol (p.71·2); menthol (p.1632·3).
Cold and influenza symptoms.

Lemsip Cold & Flu Max Strength *Reckitt & Colman, UK.*
Paracetamol (p.71·2); phenylephrine hydrochloride (p.1097·1); ascorbic acid (p.1389·3).
Cold and influenza symptoms.

Lemsip Cold & Flu Max Strength Capsules *Reckitt & Colman, UK.*
Paracetamol (p.71·2); phenylephrine hydrochloride (p.1097·1); caffeine (p.761·3).
Cold and influenza symptoms.

Lemsip Cold & Flu Original *Reckitt & Colman, UK.*
Paracetamol (p.71·2); ascorbic acid (p.1389·3); phenylephrine hydrochloride (p.1097·1).
Cold and influenza symptoms.

Lemsip Cold & Flu Original, Cold & Flu Max *Reckitt Benckiser, NZ.*
Paracetamol (p.71·2).
Cold and influenza symptoms.

Lemsip Cough & Cold Chesty Cough *Reckitt & Colman, UK.*
Guaifenesin (p.1092·2).
Coughs.

Lemsip Cough & Cold Dry Cough *Reckitt & Colman, UK.*
Honey (p.1366·2); terpeneless lemon oil (p.1628·2); glycerol (p.1616·3); citric acid (p.1596·2).
Coughs; sore throat.

Lemsip Flu *Reckitt & Colman, Austral.*
Paracetamol (p.71·2); pseudoephedrine hydrochloride (p.1099·2); dextromethorphan hydrobromide (p.1087·3); chlorpheniramine [chlorphenamine] maleate (p.412·1).
Cold and influenza symptoms; coughs.

Lemsip Flu Strength
Note. This name is used for preparations of different composition.
Reckitt & Colman, Hong Kong; Reckitt Benckiser, NZ.
Paracetamol (p.71·2); pseudoephedrine hydrochloride (p.1099·2); ascorbic acid (p.1389·3).
Cold and influenza symptoms.

Reckitt & Colman, UK†.
Paracetamol (p.71·2); phenylephrine (p.1097·1); ascorbic acid (p.1389·3).
Cold and influenza symptoms.

Lemsip Headcold *Reckitt Benckiser, Austral.*
Paracetamol (p.71·2).
Fever; pain.

Lemsip Lozenges *Reckitt & Colman, Austral.*
Cetylpyridinium chloride (p.1138·1).
Sore throat.

Lemsip Max *Reckitt Benckiser, Austral.*
Paracetamol (p.71·2).
Fever; pain.

Lemsip Night Time *Reckitt & Colman, UK†.*
Dextromethorphan hydrobromide (p.1087·3); chlorpheniramine [chlorphenamine] maleate (p.412·1); phenylpropanolamine hydrochloride (p.1098·1); paracetamol (p.71·2).
Influenza symptoms.

Lemsip Non-Decongestant *Reckitt Benckiser, UK.*
Paracetamol (p.71·2); ascorbic acid (p.1389·3).
Cold and influenza symptoms.

Lemsip Pharmacy Power+ *Reckitt & Colman, UK.*
Paracetamol (p.71·2); pseudoephedrine hydrochloride (p.1099·2); ascorbic acid (p.1389·3).
Cold and influenza symptoms.

Lemsip Pharmacy Powercaps *Reckitt & Colman, UK.*
Ibuprofen (p.43·2); pseudoephedrine hydrochloride (p.1099·2).
Cold and influenza symptoms.

Lemsip with Phenylephrine *Reckitts, Irl.*
Paracetamol (p.71·2); phenylephrine hydrochloride (p.1097·1); ascorbic acid (p.1389·3).
Cold and influenza symptoms.

Lemsip Power + *Reckitt & Colman, UK†.*
Ibuprofen (p.43·2); pseudoephedrine hydrochloride (p.1099·2).
Cold and flu symptoms.

Lemsip Sore Throat *Reckitt & Colman, UK.*
Hexylresorcinol (p.1146·3).
Sore throat.

Lemsip Throat Lozenges *Reckitt Benckiser, NZ.*
Cetylpyridinium chloride (p.1138·1).
Sore throat.

Lemsip Vapo-Patches *Reckitt Benckiser, UK.*
Camphor (p.1589·3); eucalyptus oil (p.1609·2).
Respiratory-tract congestion.

Lemtosid *Lemery, Mex.*
Benzonatate (p.1085·3).
Coughs.

Lemuval *Bayer, Aust.*
A heparinoid (p.905·2); hyaluronidase (p.1620·3); vitamin A palmitate (p.1383·2); calcium pantothenate (p.1374·1); menthol (p.1632·3).
Anorectal disorders.

Lemyflox *Lemery, Mex.*
Ciprofloxacin (p.182·3).
Bacterial infections.

Len V.K. *Aspen, S.Afr.*
Phenoxymethylpenicillin potassium (p.235·1).
Bacterial infections.

Lenactin *Roche, NZ.*
Dextromethorphan hydrobromide (p.1087·3); cetylpyridinium chloride (p.1138·1); benzocaine (p.1306·2); menthol (p.1632·3).
Coughs.

Lenadol *Lennon, S.Afr.†.*
Paracetamol (p.71·2); codeine phosphate (p.25·2); diphenhydramine hydrochloride (p.416·1); caffeine (p.761·3).
Fever; pain and associated tension.

Lenamet *Aspen, S.Afr.*
Cimetidine (p.1216·3).
Gastric hypersecretion; peptic ulcer.

Lenapain *Aspen Consumer, S.Afr.*
Doxylamine succinate (p.417·1); codeine phosphate (p.25·2); caffeine (p.761·3); paracetamol (p.71·2).
Pain and associated tension.

Lenasone *Aspen, S.Afr.*
Betamethasone sodium phosphate (p.1063·2).
Corticosteroid.

Lenazine *Aspen, S.Afr.*
Promethazine hydrochloride (p.423·2).
Hypersensitivity reactions.

Lenazine Forte *Aspen, S.Afr.*
Promethazine hydrochloride (p.423·2); codeine phosphate (p.25·2); ephedrine hydrochloride (p.1090·1).
Coughs.

Len-B Co *SA Druggists Self Med, S.Afr.†.*
Vitamin B substances (p.1350·1).

Lendianon *QIF, Braz.*
Lindane (p.1434·1).
Pediculosis; scabies.

Lendorm
Boehringer Ingelheim, Aust.; Roche, Denm.
Brotizolam (p.657·2).
Insomnia.

Lendormin
Boehringer Ingelheim, Belg.; Boehringer Ingelheim, Ger.; Boehringer Ingelheim, Ital.; Boehringer Ingelheim, Jpn†; Boehringer Ingelheim, Neth.; Boehringer Ingelheim, Port.; Boehringer Ingelheim, S.Afr.
Brotizolam (p.657·2).
Insomnia.

Lendormine *Boehringer Ingelheim, Switz.*
Brotizolam (p.657·2).
Sleep disorders.

Lenen *Schering, Ger.; Scherax, Ger.*
Fluocortin butyl (p.1071·3).
Rhinitis.

Leniartril *San Carlo, Ital.*
Naproxen (p.60·3).
Musculoskeletal and joint disorders; neuritis.

Lenicalm *Dolisos, Fr.; Dolisos, Ital.*
Asperula odorata; crataegus (p.1600·2); tilia (p.1673·2).
Insomnia; nervous disorders.

Lenicet *Athenstaedt, Ger.*
Aluminium diacetate hydroxide; aluminium hydroxide (p.1210·3).
Skin disorders.

Lenident *Zeta, Ital.*
Procaine hydrochloride (p.1319·1).
Local anaesthesia.

Lenidermyl *Oberlin, Fr.†.*
Palmitoyl collagen acid (p.1598·2).
Skin disorders.

Lenide-T *Aspen Consumer, S.Afr.*
Loperamide hydrochloride (p.1231·3).
Diarrhoea; ostomy management.

Lenidolor *Menarini, Ital.*
Meclenamic acid (p.51·1) or meclofenamate sodium (p.51·1).
Musculoskeletal and joint disorders; pain.

Lenidor *Simoes, Braz.*
Thymol (p.1158·3); methyl salicylate (p.55·1); menthol (p.1632·3); camphor (p.1589·3).
Musculoskeletal and joint disorders.

Lenil *Zeta, Ital.*
Chlorhexidine hydrochloride (p.1138·2).
Disinfection of wounds and burns.

Leniline *Erredici, Ital.*
Vitamin E; vitamin C; ginkgo biloba; melilotus; bioflavonoids (p.1350·1).
Nutritional supplement.

Lenipasta *Novogaleno, Ital.*
Zinc oxide (p.1128·2); rice starch (p.1379·3); enoxolone (p.34·3).
Skin irritation; wounds.

Lenirit *Bonomelli, Ital.*
Hydrocortisone acetate (p.1073·3).
Skin disorders.

Lenirose *Novogaleno, Ital.*
Sulfur (p.1123·3); titanium dioxide (p.1126·1); panthenol (p.1602·3); rusco; calendula (p.1589·2); oryzanol (p.1645·1); enoxolone (p.34·3).
Rosacea; seborrhoeic dermatitis; skin irritation.

Lenisolone *Aspen, S.Afr.*
Prednisolone (p.1077·3).
Corticosteroid.

Lenitin *Teva, Israel.*
Bromazepam (p.656·3).
Anxiety; premedication; sedative.

Lenitral
Besins-Iscovesco, Fr.; Besins, Hong Kong; Besins-Iscovesco, Singapore.
Glyceryl trinitrate (p.897·3).
Angina pectoris; heart failure; hypotension.

Lenium
SmithKline Beecham, Irl.; Johnson & Johnson MSD Consumer, UK†.
Selenium sulfide (p.1123·1).
Dandruff; scalp seborrhoea.

Lenixil *Europital, Ital.†.*
Chlorhexidine gluconate (p.1138·2).
Disinfection of minor wounds and burns.

Lennacol *Lennon, S.Afr.†.*
Chloramphenicol (p.179·1).
Bacterial infections.

Lennamine *Lennon, S.Afr.†.*
Diphenhydramine hydrochloride (p.416·1); ammonium chloride (p.1085·2); sodium citrate (p.1186·2); menthol (p.1632·3).
Coughs; nasal congestion.

Lenocef *Aspen, S.Afr.*
Cefalexin (p.161·3).
Bacterial infections.

Lenocin *General Drugs, Thai.*
Tetracycline hydrochloride (p.258·3).
Bacterial infections.

Lenolax *Aspen Consumer, S.Afr.*
Dibasic sodium phosphate (p.1193·2); monobasic sodium phosphate (p.1193·2).
Bowel evacuation; constipation.

Lenoltec No 1, No 2, or No 3 *Technilab, Canad.*
Paracetamol (p.71·2); caffeine (p.761·3); codeine phosphate (p.25·2).
Formerly known as Lenoltec with Codeine No 1, No 2, or No 3.
Cold symptoms; pain.

Lenoltec No 4 *Technilab, Canad.*
Paracetamol (p.71·2); codeine phosphate (p.25·2).
Formerly known as Lenoltec with Codeine No 4.
Pain.

Lenoprel *Intramed, S.Afr.†.*
Isoprenaline hydrochloride (p.914·3).
Bronchospasm; shock.

Lenovate *Aspen, S.Afr.*
Betamethasone valerate (p.1063·2).
Corticosteroid.

Lenovor *Serono, Mex.*
Folinic acid (p.1363·1).

Lenoxin *Glaxo Wellcome, Ger.*
Digoxin (p.870·1).
Heart failure; tachycardia.

Lenpryl *Galen, Mex.*
Captopril (p.853·3).
Heart failure; hypertension.

Lens Fresh
Allergan, Aust.†; Allergan, Ger.†; Allergan, USA†.
Range of solutions for contact lenses (p.1129·2).

Lens Lubricant *Bausch & Lomb, USA.*
Wetting solution for hard contact lenses (p.1129·2).

Lens Plus
Allergan, Austral.; Allergan, NZ; Allergan, USA.
Range of solutions for contact lenses (p.1129·2).

Lens Plus Buffered Saline Solution *Allergan, Canad.*
Buffered sodium chloride (p.1196·1) (p.1129·2).
Rinsing solution for contact lenses.

Lens Plus Rewetting Drops *Allergan, Canad.†.*
Wetting solution for soft contact lenses (p.1129·2).

Lens Tears *Agepha, Aust.*
Wetting solution for contact lenses (p.1129·2).

Lens Wet *Agepha, Aust.*
Wetting solution for contact lenses (p.1129·2).

Lensan A *Ciba Vision, Aust.*
Hydrogen peroxide (p.1147·1) (p.1129·2).
Disinfecting solution for contact lenses.

Lensan B *Ciba Vision, Aust.*
Catalase (p.1592·2) (p.1129·2).
Neutralising solution for contact lenses.

Lensept
Ciba Vision, Aust.; Ciba Vision, USA†.
Hydrogen peroxide (p.1147·1) (p.1129·2).
Disinfecting solution for soft contact lenses.

Lensrins NT *Ciba Vision, Aust.*
Storage and rinsing solution for soft contact lenses (p.1129·2).

Lentard MC *Novo Nordisk, UK†.*
Insulin zinc suspension (amorphous porcine 30%, crystalline bovine 70%, monocomponent) (p.324·1).
Diabetes mellitus.

The symbol † denotes a preparation no longer actively marketed

Lentare Novartis, S.Afr.
Formestane (p.543·1).
Breast cancer.

Lentaron
Novartis, Aust.; Ciba-Geigy, Belg.†; Ciba, Canad.†; Novartis, Denm.; Novartis, Fr.; Novartis, Ger.; Novartis, Hong Kong; Novartis, Irl.; Novartis, Israel; Novartis, Ital.; Novartis, Neth.; Novartis, Port.; Novartis, Spain; Novartis, Switz.; Novartis, UK†.
Formestane (p.543·1).
Breast cancer.

Lente
Novo Nordisk, Ger.
Insulin zinc suspension (porcine with bovine, monocomponent) (p.324·1).
Diabetes mellitus.

Novo Nordisk, USA.
Insulin zinc suspension (bovine or porcine) (p.324·1).
Diabetes mellitus.

Lente Iletin I Lilly, USA†.
Insulin zinc suspension (bovine and porcine) (p.324·1).
Diabetes mellitus.

Lente Iletin II Lilly, USA.
Insulin zinc suspension (porcine) (p.324·1).
Diabetes mellitus.

Lente L Novo Nordisk, USA†.
Insulin zinc suspension (porcine) (p.324·1).
Diabetes mellitus.

Lente MC
Novo Nordisk, Aust.
Insulin zinc suspension (p.324·1).
Diabetes mellitus.

Novo Nordisk, Austral.†; Novo Nordisk, Belg.; Novo Nordisk, Fr.†; Novo Nordisk, Spain; Novo Nordisk, Switz.
Insulin zinc suspension (amorphous porcine 30%, crystalline bovine 70%, monocomponent) (p.324·1).
Diabetes mellitus.

Lentizol
Parke, Davis, Irl.; Parke, Davis, UK.
Amitriptyline hydrochloride (p.273·3).
Depression.

Lento C Eurofarma, Braz.
Ascorbic acid (p.1389·3).
Vitamin C deficiency; vitamin C supplement.

Lentocilin-S Atral, Port.
Benzathine benzylpenicillin (p.156·2).
Rheumatic fever; syphilis.

Lentogesic Mer-National, S.Afr.
Capsules: Dextropropoxyphene hydrochloride (p.27·1); paracetamol (p.71·2); pemoline (p.1513·1); levoglutamide (p.1365·2).
Pain.

Syrup: Paracetamol (p.71·2); codeine phosphate (p.25·2); promethazine hydrochloride (p.423·2).
Fever; pain.

Lentogest Amsa, Ital.
Hydroxyprogesterone caproate (p.1479·3).
Infertility; menstrual and menopausal disorders; threatened or recurrent miscarriage.

Lento-Kalium Roche, Ital.
Potassium chloride (p.1194·3).
Hypokalaemia.

Lentolith Mer-National, S.Afr.
Lithium carbonate (p.292·1).
Bipolar disorder; depression.

Lentopenil Grossman, Mex.
Benzathine benzylpenicillin (p.156·2).
Bacterial infections.

Lentoquine Almirall, Spain.
Hydroquinidine hydrochloride (p.912·1).
Arrhythmias.

Lentorem Remir, Mex.
Hydroxocobalamin (p.1388·1).

Lentorsil Italfarmaco, Ital.
Ursodeoxycholic acid (p.1677·2).
Biliary disorders; cholesterol gallstones.

Leo-400 Charoen, Thai.
Albendazole (p.95·2).
Worm infections.

Leo-Doce Solfran, Mex.
Hydroxocobalamin (p.1388·1).

Leonal Byk Leo, Spain.
Ibuprofen (p.43·2).
Fever; pain.

Leopin Quest, Canad.
Vitamin B substances (p.1350·1).
Dietary supplement.

Leotrim Leofarma, Braz.
Co-trimoxazole (p.193·3).
Bacterial infections; Pneumocystis carinii pneumonia; protozoal infections.

Leparan Italfarmaco, Ital.
Suleparoid (p.978·2).
Thrombosis prophylaxis.

Lepheton Pharmacia Upjohn, Swed.
Ethylmorphine hydrochloride (p.35·2); ephedrine hydrochloride (p.1090·1).
Bronchitis; coughs.

Lepicortinolo Decomed, Port.
Prednisolone (p.1077·3) or prednisolone hydrogen succinate (p.1078·1).
Corticosteroid.

Lepinal Desitin, Ger.
Phenobarbital (p.355·1).
Epilepsy.

Lepinaletten Desitin, Ger.
Phenobarbital (p.355·1).
Epilepsy.

Lepobron Lepori, Port.
Theophylline (p.777·2).
Obstructive airways disease.

Leponex
Novartis, Aust.; Novartis, Belg.; Novartis, Braz.; Novartis, Denm.; Novartis, Fin.; Novartis, Fr.; Novartis, Ger.; Novartis, Israel; Novartis, Ital.; Novartis, Mex.; Novartis, Neth.; Novartis, Norw.; Novartis, Port.; Novartis, S.Afr.; Novartis, Spain; Novartis, Swed.; Novartis, Switz.
Clozapine (p.671·2).
Parkinsonism; schizophrenia.

Leptanal
Janssen-Cilag, Norw.; Janssen-Cilag, Swed.
Fentanyl citrate (p.37·1).
Adjunct in neuroleptanalgesia; pain.

Lepticur Roussel Diamant, Fr.
Tropatepine hydrochloride (p.474·3).
Extrapyramidal disorders; parkinsonism.

Leptilan
Novartis, Denm.; Novartis, Ger.; Du Pont, Ger.; Novartis, Mex.
Sodium valproate (p.366·3).
Epilepsy.

Leptilanil Novartis, Aust.
Sodium valproate (p.366·3).
Epilepsy; febrile convulsions.

Leptofen Pharmacia Upjohn, Ital.
Fentanyl (p.37·1); droperidol (p.682·2).
Neuroleptanalgesia; premedication.

Leptoprol Mavi, Mex.
Metoprolol (p.932·1).

Leptopsique Psicofarma, Mex.
Perphenazine (p.699·1).
Anxiety disorders; nausea and vomiting; pain; psychoses.

Lercadip
Zeneca, Ital.; Biohorm, Spain.
Lercanidipine hydrochloride (p.920·2).
Hypertension.

Lercan Pierre Fabre, Fr.
Lercanidipine hydrochloride (p.920·2).
Hypertension.

Lerdip Byk, Neth.
Lercanidipine hydrochloride (p.920·2).
Hypertension.

Lergigan Recip, Swed.
Promethazine hydrochloride (p.423·2).
Alcoholism; anxiety; croup; hypersensitivity reactions; nausea; premedication; sedative; sleep disorders; tension; vertigo.

Lergigan comp Recip, Swed.
Promethazine hydrochloride (p.423·2); caffeine (p.761·3); ephedrine sulfate (p.1090·2).
Alcoholism; anxiety; croup; hypersensitivity reactions; nausea; premedication; sedative; sleep disorders; tension; vertigo.

Lergocil Juste, Spain.
Azatadine maleate (p.409·2).
Hypersensitivity reactions.

Lerin Allergan-Frumtost, Braz.
Naphazoline hydrochloride (p.1095·1); zinc phenolsulfonate (p.1128·3); berberine sulfate (p.1584·2).
Ocular congestion.

Leritine Merck Frosst, Canad.
Anileridine hydrochloride (p.14·1) or anileridine phosphate (p.14·2).
Adjunct in general anaesthesia; anxiety; pain.

Lerivon
Organon, Austral.; Organon, Belg.
Mianserin hydrochloride (p.298·1).
Depression.

Lertamine Lilly, Mex.
Loratadine (p.420·1).
Allergic rhinitis; urticaria.

Lertamine-D Lilly, Mex.
Loratadine (p.420·1); pseudoephedrine sulfate (p.1099·3).
Allergic rhinitis; nasal congestion.

Lertus Gunther, Braz.
Fluconazole (p.383·2).
Fungal infections.

Lervipan Emilio, Spain.
Pivampicillin (p.237·2).
Bacterial infections.

Lerzam Pharmazam, Spain.
Lercanidipine hydrochloride (p.920·2).
Hypertension.

Les Yeux 1 Bilosa, Aust.
Hydrogen peroxide (p.1147·1) (p.1129·2).
Disinfecting solution for gas-permeable contact lenses.

Les Yeux 2 Bilosa, Aust.
Catalase (p.1592·2) (p.1129·2).
Neutralising solution for gas-permeable contact lenses.

Lescol
Novartis, Aust.; Novartis, Austral.; Novartis, Belg.; Novartis, Braz.; Novartis, Canad.; Novartis, Denm.; Novartis, Fr.; Novartis, Ger.; Novartis, Hong Kong; Novartis, Irl.; Novartis, Israel; Novartis, Ital.; Novartis, Mex.; Novartis, Neth.; Novartis, Norw.; Novartis, NZ; Novartis, Port.; Novartis, Swed.; Novartis, Switz.; Novartis, Thai.; Novartis, UK; Novartis, USA.
Fluvastatin sodium (p.892·1).
Atherosclerosis; hypercholesterolaemia.

Leshcutan Teva, Israel.
Paromomycin; methylbenzethonium chloride (p.1150·3).
Cutaneous leishmaniasis.

Lesil Farmatrading, Port.
Tolu balsam (p.1101·3); sulfogaiacol (p.1101·1); pine oil.
Coughs.

Lespenefril
Produfarma, Port.; Nattermann, Spain.
Lespedeza capitata.
Diuretic.

Lespenephryl
UCB, Aust.; Darci, Fr.
Lespedeza capitata.
Diuresis.

Lessmusec Brunel, S.Afr.
Carbocisteine (p.1086·3).
Respiratory-tract disorders.

Lesspain Be-Tabs, S.Afr.†.
Paracetamol (p.71·2); codeine phosphate (p.25·2); promethazine hydrochloride (p.423·2).
Fever; pain.

Lesterol
Hoechst Marion Roussel, Braz.; Hoechst Marion Roussel, Mex.
Probucol (p.959·2).
Hyperlipidaemias.

Lestid
Pharmacia Upjohn, Denm.; Pharmacia Upjohn, Fin.; Pharmacia Upjohn, Norw.; Pharmacia Upjohn, Swed.
Colestipol hydrochloride (p.863·3).
Hyperlipidaemias.

Letequatro Upsifarma, Port.
Thyroxine [levothyroxine] sodium (p.1526·2).
Hypothyroidism.

Lethyl Aspen, S.Afr.
Phenobarbital (p.355·1).
Anxiety; insomnia; migraine.

Letigen Nycomed, Denm.
Caffeine (p.761·3); ephedrine hydrochloride (p.1090·1).
Obesity.

Letofort Salus, Ital.
Letosteine (p.1094·1).
Respiratory-tract disorders associated with increased or viscous mucus.

Letoprol Mavi, Mex.
Metoprolol (p.932·1).

Letter Rhone-Poulenc Rorer, Port.
Thyroxine [levothyroxine] sodium (p.1526·2).
Hypothyroidism.

Letus Unison, Thai.
Co-trimoxazole (p.193·3).
Bacterial infections.

Leuco-4 Pharmascience, Fr.
Adenine (p.1573·2).
Asthenia.

Leuco Hubber
Rhone-Poulenc Rorer, Port.†; Teofarma, Spain.
Hydrocortisone acetate (p.1073·3); neomycin sulfate (p.228·1).
Vulvovaginal inflammatory disorders.

Leucobasal
Germania, Aust.; Biabasal, Switz.
Mequinol (p.1118·2).
Hyperpigmentation.

Leucocida Simoes, Braz.
Hydroxyquinoline sulfate (p.1622·2); borax (p.1586·1); cetrimonium bromide (p.1137·3); alum (p.1577·2).
Vulvovaginal disorders.

Leucodin Synthelabo, Braz.
Mequinol (p.1118·2).
Vitiligo.

Leucodinine B Chiesi, Fr.
Mequinol (p.1118·2).
Hyperpigmentation.

Leucogen Ache, Braz.
Thymomodulin (p.1672·3).
Diabetes mellitus; immunodeficiencies; malignant neoplasms; rheumatoid arthritis; skin disorders.

Leucomax
Aesca, Aust.; Novartis, Aust.; Novartis, Belg.; Novartis, Braz.; Novartis, Denm.; Schering-Plough, Denm.; Schering-Plough, Fin.; Novartis, Fin.; Schering-Plough, Fin.; Novartis, Ger.; Essex, Ger.; Novartis, Hong Kong; Schering-Plough, Hong Kong; Novartis, Irl.; Novartis, Israel; Novartis, Ital.; Schering-Plough, Mex.; Novartis, Mex.; Novartis, Neth.; Schering-Plough, Norw.; Novartis, NZ; Novartis, Port.; Novartis, S.Afr.; Schering-Plough, Singapore; Schering-Plough, Singapore; Novartis, Spain; Schering-Plough, Swed.; Novartis, Swed.; Essex, Switz.; Novartis, Switz.; Schering-Plough, Thai.; Schering-Plough, Thai.; Novartis, UK.
Molgramostim (p.738·3).
Aplastic anaemia; myelodysplastic syndromes; neutropenia induced by antineoplastic agents, bone marrow transplantation, or ganciclovir.

Leucorsan Zilliken, Ital.†.
Vaginal capsules: Benzydamine hydrochloride (p.20·1); hydroxyquinoline sulfate (p.1622·2); hydroxyquinoline benzoate (p.1622·2).

Vaginal douche: Benzydamine hydrochloride (p.20·1); hydroxyquinoline sulfate (p.1622·2); hydroxyquinoline benzoate (p.1622·2); cetrimonium tosilate (p.1137·3).
Vaginal and cervical inflammation.

Leucotrofina
Note.This name is used for preparations of different composition.
Pharmacia Upjohn, Aust.†.
Bovine thymus extract.
Leucopenia.

Pierre Fabre, Ital.†; Pharmacia Upjohn, Mex.
Thymomodulin (p.1672·3).
Hypersensitivity; infections; leucopenia.

Leukase Merck, Aust.
Framycetin sulfate (p.208·2); trypsin (p.1675·3).
Burns; infective skin disorders.

Leukase N SmithKline Beecham, Ger.
Topical gel: Framycetin sulfate (p.208·2); lignocaine [lidocaine] hydrochloride (p.1313·2).

Topical powder; ointment: Framycetin sulfate (p.208·2).
Infected skin disorders; infected wounds.

Leukase-Kegel Merck, Aust.
Framycetin sulfate (p.208·2); trypsin (p.1675·3); lignocaine [lidocaine] hydrochloride (p.1313·2).
Infective skin and mouth disorders.

Leukeran
Glaxo Wellcome, Aust.; Glaxo Wellcome, Austral.; Glaxo Wellcome, Belg.; Glaxo Wellcome, Braz.; Glaxo Wellcome, Canad.; Glaxo Wellcome, Denm.; Glaxo Wellcome, Fin.; Glaxo Wellcome, Fr.; Glaxo Wellcome, Ger.; Glaxo Wellcome, Hong Kong; Wellcome, Irl.; Glaxo Wellcome, Israel; Glaxo Wellcome, Ital.; Glaxo Wellcome, Mex.; Glaxo Wellcome, Neth.; Glaxo Wellcome, Norw.; Glaxo Wellcome, NZ; Wellcome, Port.; Glaxo Wellcome, S.Afr.; Glaxo Wellcome, Singapore; Wellcome, Spain; Glaxo Wellcome, Switz.; Glaxo Wellcome, Thai.; Glaxo Wellcome, UK; Glaxo Wellcome, USA.
Chlorambucil (p.516·3).
Malignant neoplasms.

Leukichtan Ichthyol, Aust.
Ictasol (p.1115·3); cod-liver oil (p.1357·2).
Burns; skin disorders; wounds.

Leukichtan N Ichthyol, Ger.†.
Ictasol (p.1115·3).
Ulcers; wounds.

Leukine Immunex, USA.
Sargramostim (p.741·3).
Mobilisation of autologous peripheral blood progenitor cells; neutropenia.

Leuko Fungex Antifungal Beiersdorf, Austral.
Miconazole (p.391·1).
Fungal skin infections.

leukominerase Biosyn, Ger.
Lithium carbonate (p.292·1).
Bipolar disorder; depression; mania.

Leukona-Eukalpin-Bad Atzinger, Ger.
Norway spruce oil; eucalyptus oil (p.1609·2).
Bath additive; respiratory-tract disorders.

Leukona-Jod-Bad
Richter, Aust.; Atzinger, Ger.
Iodine (p.1522·3).
Arteriosclerosis; bath additive; iodine-deficiency goitre; neuralgia; spinal disorders.

Leukona-Kreislauf-Bad Atzinger, Ger.
Rosemary oil (p.1659·3); camphor (p.1589·3); eucalyptus oil (p.1609·2).
Bath additive; circulatory disorders.

Leukona-Mintol Atzinger, Ger.†.
Peppermint oil (p.1243·3).
Gastrointestinal disorders; respiratory-tract disorders.

Leukona-Rheuma-Bad Richter, Aust.
Pumilio pine oil (p.1656·3); turpentine oil (p.1676·3); methyl salicylate (p.55·1).
Formerly contained pumilio pine oil, camphor, thyme oil, turpentine oil, and methyl salicylate.
Musculoskeletal and joint disorders; prostatitis; skin disorders.

Leukona-Rheuma-Bad N Atzinger, Ger.
Methyl salicylate (p.55·1); turpentine oil (p.1676·3); Norway spruce oil.
Bath additive; rheumatic disorders.

Leukona-Rheumasalbe Atzinger, Ger.
Camphor (p.1589·3); turpentine oil (p.1676·3); rosemary oil (p.1659·3).
Cold symptoms; frostbite; rheumatism; soft-tissue injury.

Leukona-Sedativ-Bad Atzinger, Ger.
Cloral hydrate (p.669·2); lupulus (p.1629·3); valerian (p.1678·3).
Bath additive; nervous disorders; sleep disorders; spasmophilia.

Leukona-Sedativ-Bad sine Chloralhydrat Atzinger, Ger.
Valerian (p.1678·3); lupulus (p.1629·3).
Bath additive; nervous disorders; sleep disorders.

Leukona-Stoffwechsel-Bad Atzinger, Ger.
Juniper oil (p.1625·2).
Allergic skin disorders; bath additive; metabolic disorders.

Leukona-Sulfomoor-Bad Richter, Aust.
Sulfurated potash (p.1124·1); colloidal sulfur (p.1123·3); sodium humate; peat.
Musculoskeletal and joint disorders.

Leukona-Sulfomoor-Bad N Atzinger, Ger.
Sulfurated potash (p.1124·1); peat; sodium humate.
Bath additive; musculoskeletal and joint disorders; skin disorders.

Leukona-Wundsalbe Atzinger, Ger.
Cod-liver oil (p.1357·2); hamamelis water (p.1618·3); allantoin (p.1110·1).
Skin ulcers; wounds.

LeukoNorm *CytoChemia, Ger.*
Leucocytes (p.738·2).
Immunological disorders.

LeukoScan *Byk Gulden, Ital.*
Technetium-99m (p.1451·1) sulesomab.
Bone scanning in osteomyelitis.

Leunase
Rhone-Poulenc Rorer, Austral.; Kyowa, Hong Kong; Kyowa, Jpn; San-fer, Mex.; Aventis, NZ; Kyowa, Singapore; Kyowa, Thai.
Asparaginase (p.508·3).
Acute leukaemias; malignant lymphomas.

Leuplin *Takeda, Jpn.*
Leuprorelin acetate (p.1289·2).
Breast cancer; endometriosis; precocious puberty; prostatic cancer; uterine myoma.

Leustat *Janssen-Cilag, UK.*
Cladribine (p.527·1).
Chronic lymphocytic leukaemia; hairy-cell leukaemia.

Leustatin
Janssen-Cilag, Aust.; Janssen-Cilag, Austral.; Cilag, Braz.; Janssen-Ortho, Canad.; Janssen-Cilag, Denm.; Janssen-Cilag, Fin.; Janssen-Cilag, Ger.; Cilag, Hong Kong; Janssen-Cilag, Ital.; Janssen-Cilag, Neth.; Janssen-Cilag, Norw.; Janssen-Cilag, NZ; Janssen-Cilag, S.Afr.; Janssen-Cilag, Spain; Janssen-Cilag, Swed.; Janssen-Cilag, Switz.; Janssen, Thai.; Ortho Biotech, USA.
Cladribine (p.527·1).
Chronic lymphocytic leukaemia; hairy-cell leukaemia.

Leustatine *Janssen-Cilag, Fr.*
Cladribine (p.527·1).
Hairy-cell leukaemia.

Leutrol *Abbott, Ital.*
Meloxicam (p.51·3).
Ankylosing spondylitis; osteoarthritis; rheumatoid arthritis.

Levadin *Wiener, Mex.*
Yeast (p.1398·1).

Levadol *IPFI, Ital.*
Paracetamol (p.71·2).
Fever; pain.

Levaknel *Crinos, Ital.†*
Zinc oxide (p.1128·2); chlorhexidine (p.1138·2); triclosan (Irgasan DP 300) (p.1159·2).
Seborrhoea.

Levaliver *Byk Elmu, Spain.*
Aceglutamide (p.1571·2); amino acids (p.1350·1); betaine hydrochloride (p.1584·3); cyclobutyrol sodium (p.1601·2); pyridoxal phosphate (p.1387·1); sorbitol (p.1377·3).
Liver disorders.

Levall *CTEX, USA.*
Phenylephrine hydrochloride (p.1097·1); hydrocodone tartrate (p.42·2); guaifenesin (p.1092·2).
Coughs.

Levamin *Pisa, Mex.*
An amino-acid preparation with or without electrolytes (p.1350·1).
Parenteral nutrition.

Levanxol
Strallhofer, Aust.; Pharmacia Upjohn, Belg.; Pharmacia, S.Afr.†
Temazepam (p.707·2).
Anxiety disorders; sleep disorders.

Levaquin
Janssen-Ortho, Canad.; Ortho McNeil, USA.
Levofloxacin (p.219·1).
Bacterial infections.

Levate *ICN, Canad.†*
Amitriptyline hydrochloride (p.273·3).
Depression.

Levatol *Schwarz, USA.*
Penbutolol sulfate (p.952·2).
Hypertension.

Levaxin *Nycomed, Swed.*
Thyroxine [levothyroxine] sodium (p.1526·2).
Hypothyroidism; thyroid cancer.

Levbid *Schwarz, USA.*
Hyoscyamine sulfate (p.469·3).
Biliary and renal colic; gastrointestinal disorders; parkinsonism; rhinitis; urinary-tract disorders.

Levicor *Bioindustria, Ital.†*
Metaraminol tartrate (p.926·3).
Hypotension.

Leviden *Toho, Hong Kong.*
Liver hydrolysate.
Liver disorders.

Levifusa *Ifusa, Mex.*
Yeast (p.1398·1).

Levium *Hexal, Ger.*
Methotrimeprazine [levomepromazine] maleate (p.692·1).
Pain; psychoses.

Levlen
Schering, Aust.; Berlex, USA.
Levonorgestrel (p.1486·2); ethinylestradiol (p.1476·2).
28-Day packs also contain 7 inert tablets.
Combined oral contraceptive.

Levlen ED
Schering, Austral.; Schering, NZ.
21 Tablets, Levonorgestrel (p.1486·2); ethinylestradiol (p.1476·2); 7 tablets, inert.
Combined oral contraceptive.

Levlite *Berlex, USA.*
Levonorgestrel (p.1486·2); ethinylestradiol (p.1476·2).
28-Day packs also contain 7 inert tablets.
Combined oral contraceptive.

Levobren *GiEnne, Ital.*
Levosulpiride (p.706·2).
Gastrointestinal disorders; headache; migraine; vertigo.

Levocarb *Sanus, Braz.*
Levodopa (p.1169·2); carbidopa (p.1168·2).
Parkinsonism.

Levocarb-GRY *Teva, Ger.*
Carbidopa (p.1168·2); levodopa (p.1169·2).
Parkinsonism.

Levocarnil *Sigma-Tau, Fr.*
Carnitine (p.1356·1).
Carnitine deficiency.

Levocarvit *Mitim, Ital.*
Levocarnitine (p.1356·1).
Carnitine deficiency; myocardial ischaemia.

Levocina *Cryopharma, Mex.*
Methotrimeprazine [levomepromazine] maleate (p.692·1).
Psychoses.

Levodex *Dexxon, Israel.*
Diltiazem hydrochloride (p.874·3).
Angina pectoris.

Levodexan *Grin, Mex.*
Dexamethasone sodium phosphate (p.1067·1); chloramphenicol (p.179·1).
Infected eye disorders.

Levodopa comp B *Stada, Ger.*
Levodopa (p.1169·2); benserazide hydrochloride (p.1164·2).
Drug-induced extrapyramidal disorders; parkinsonism.

Levodopa comp C *Stada, Ger.*
Levodopa (p.1169·2); carbidopa (p.1168·2).
Parkinsonism.

Levo-Dromoran *ICN, USA.*
Levorphanol tartrate (p.50·1).
Pain.

Levofenil *Grin, Mex.*
Dexamethasone sodium phosphate (p.1067·1); chloramphenicol (p.179·1); phenylephrine hydrochloride (p.1097·1).
Inflammatory eye infections.

Levofolene *Farmades, Ital.*
Calcium levofolinate (p.1363·1).
Antidote to folic acid antagonists; folate deficiency anaemia.

Levoglusalino Vitulia *Ern, Spain†.*
Electrolyte infusion with fructose (p.1180·1).
Carbohydrate source; fluid and electrolyte depletion.

Levograf *Juste, Spain.*
Galactose (p.1033·3).
Ultrasound contrast medium.

Levolac *Leiras, Fin.; Fresenius Kabi, Norw.*
Lactulose (p.1230·1).
Constipation; hepatic encephalopathy.

Levomed *Medochemie, Thai.*
Levodopa (p.1169·2); carbidopa (p.1168·2).
Parkinsonism.

Levomet *Chiesi, Ital.*
Levodopa methyl hydrochloride (p.1172·3).
Parkinsonism.

Levomycetin *Chew, Thai.*
Chloramphenicol (p.179·1).
Bacterial infections.

Levonelle *Schering, UK.*
Levonorgestrel (p.1486·2).
Postcoital oral contraceptive.

Levonova
Leiras, Denm.; Leiras, Norw.; Leiras, Swed.
Levonorgestrel (p.1486·2).
Menorrhagia; progestogen-only oral contraceptive.

Leiras, Fin.
Levonorgestrel (p.1486·2).
Menstrual disorders; progestogen-releasing intra-uterine contraceptive device.

Levopar *Hexal, Ger.*
Levodopa (p.1169·2); benserazide (p.1164·2).
Drug-induced extrapyramidal disorders; parkinsonism.

Levopar Plus *Teva, Israel.*
Levodopa (p.1169·2); benserazide hydrochloride (p.1164·2).
Parkinsonism.

Levophed
Abbott, Austral.; Abbott, Belg.; Sanofi Synthelabo, Canad.; Abbott, Hong Kong; Abbott, Irl.; Sanofi Winthrop, Israel; Abbott, NZ; Abbott, Singapore; Abbott, UK; Abbott, USA.
Noradrenaline [norepinephrine] acid tartrate (p.948·2).
Now known as Noradrenaline (Norepinephrine) 1:1000 in the *UK*.
Cardiac arrest; hypotensive states.

Levophta
Chauvin, Fr.; Ciba Vision, Ger.; Winzer, Ger.
Levocabastine hydrochloride (p.419·3).
Allergic conjunctivitis.

Levoplus *Montefarmaco, Ital.*
Dietary fibre (p.1214·2); lactulose (p.1230·1); lactitol (p.1230·1); mannitol (p.924·3).

Levopraid *Ravizza, Ital.*
Levosulpiride (p.706·2).
Gastrointestinal disorders; headache; psychiatric disorders; vertigo.

Levoprome *Lederle, USA.*
Methotrimeprazine [levomepromazine] hydrochloride (p.691·3).
Pain; premedication.

Levopront
Mack, Singapore; Mack, Thai.
Levodropropizine (p.1089·3).
Coughs.

Levoptin *Archifar, Thai.*
Chloramphenicol (p.179·1); prednisolone sodium phosphate (p.1078·1); naphazoline hydrochloride (p.1095·1).
Eye disorders.

Levora *Watson, USA.*
Levonorgestrel (p.1486·2); ethinylestradiol (p.1476·2).
28-Day packs also contain 7 inert tablets.
Combined oral contraceptive.

Levordiol *Novaquimica, Braz.*
Levonorgestrel (p.1486·2); ethinylestradiol (p.1476·2); vitamin B₆.
Triphasic oral contraceptive.

Levorin *Wyeth Lederle, Aust.*
Calcium levofolinate (p.1363·1).
Enhancement of fluorouracil activity; methotrexate toxicity.

Levostab *Formenti, Ital.*
Levocabastine hydrochloride (p.419·3).
Allergic conjunctivitis; allergic rhinitis.

Levo-T
Pharmascience, Canad.†; Lederle, USA.
Thyroxine [levothyroxine] sodium (p.1526·2).
Hypothyroidism; TSH suppression.

Levotec *Technilab, Canad.*
Thyroxine [levothyroxine] sodium (p.1526·2).
Hypothyroidism.

Levothroid
Rhone-Poulenc Rorer, Spain; Forest Laboratories, USA.
Thyroxine [levothyroxine] sodium (p.1526·2).
Hypercholesterolaemia; hypothyroidism; TSH suppression.

Levothym *Lundbeck, Ger.*
Oxitriptan (p.302·2).
Depression; neurological disorders; sleep disorders.

Levothyrox *Lipha Sante, Fr.*
Thyroxine [levothyroxine] sodium (p.1526·2).
Hypothyroidism.

Levotiroxina *Farmedica, Braz.*
Thyroxine [levothyroxine] sodium (p.1526·2); liothyronine sodium (p.1524·2).
Hypothyroidism.

Levotonine *Panpharma, Fr.*
Oxitriptan (p.302·2).
Myoclonus.

Levotuss
Janssen-Cilag, Belg.; Dompe, Ital.; Almirall, Spain.
Levodropropizine (p.1089·3).
Coughs.

Levovist
Schering, Aust.; Berlex, Canad.; Schering, Denm.; Schering, Fin.; Schering, Fr.; Schering, Ger.; Schering, Israel; Schering, Ital.; Schering, Neth.; Schering, Norw.; Schering, NZ; Schering, Port.; Schering, Spain; Schering, Swed.; Schering, Switz.; Schering, UK.
Galactose (p.1033·3).
Ultrasound contrast medium.

Levoxacin *Glaxo Wellcome, Ital.*
Levofloxacin (p.219·1).
Bacterial infections.

Levoxyl *Jones, USA.*
Thyroxine [levothyroxine] sodium (p.1526·2).
Formerly known as Levoxine.
Hypothyroidism; TSH suppression.

Levozin *Orion, Fr.*
Methotrimeprazine [levomepromazine] maleate (p.692·1) or methotrimeprazine [levomepromazine] embonate (p.692·1).
Agitation; insomnia; pain; psychoses.

Levozine *Cristalia, Braz.*
Methotrimeprazine [levomepromazine] (p.691·3).
Adjunct in general anaesthesia; pain in obstetrics; premedication; psychoses.

Levsin
Rivex, Canad.; Schwarz, USA.
Hyoscyamine sulfate (p.469·3).
Adjunct to hypotonic duodenography; biliary and renal colic; gastrointestinal disorders; improvement of radiological visibility of the kidneys; parkinsonism; partial heart block associated with vagal activity; premedication; rhinitis.

Levsin with Phenobarbitone *Schwarz, USA.*
Phenobarbital (p.355·1); hyoscyamine sulfate (p.469·3).
Gastrointestinal disorders.

Levsinex *Schwarz, USA.*
Hyoscyamine sulfate (p.469·3).
Biliary and renal colic; gastrointestinal disorders; parkinsonism; rhinitis; urinary-tract disorders.

Levudin *GD, Ital.*
Yeast (p.1398·1); betacarotene (p.1355·1).

Levugen *Travenol, UK.*
Fructose (p.1363·3).

Levulan Kerastick *DUSA, USA.*
Aminolevulinic acid hydrochloride (p.507·2).
Actinic keratoses.

Levulosado *Bieffe, Spain; Braun, Spain; Ern, Spain.*
Fructose (p.1363·3).
Fluid and electrolyte disorders; liver disorders.

Levulosalino Isot *Braun, Spain.*
Sodium chloride (p.1196·1); fructose (p.1363·3).
Carbohydrate source; fluid and electrolyte disorders.

Levuplex *Apsen, Braz.*
Multivitamin preparation with fructose (p.1350·1).

Levupotasico *Ern, Spain†.*
Fructose (p.1363·3); potassium chloride (p.1194·3).
Hypokalaemia.

Levurinetten *Novartis Consumer, Aust.*
Dried yeast (p.1398·1); vitamin B substances (p.1350·1).
Skin disorders.

Levurinetten N *Zyma, Ger.†*
Dried yeast (p.1398·1).
Appetite loss; skin disorders.

Levusalino *Ern, Spain.*
Fructose (p.1363·3); sodium chloride (p.1196·1).
Carbohydrate source; fluid and electrolyte disorders.

Lexat *Eagle, Austral.*
Bile salts (p.1585·1); pancreatin (p.1646·1); boldo (p.1585·3); greater celandine (p.1618·1); aloes (p.1210·1); agar (p.1498·3); sanguinaria (p.1660·3).
Constipation; digestive system disorders.

Lexatin *Roche, Austral.*
Bromazepam (p.656·3).
Anxiety.

Lexemin *Unison, Thai.*
Fenofibrate (p.889·1).
Hyperlipidaemias.

Lexfor *Nakorn, Thai.*
Norfloxacin (p.232·1).
Bacterial infections.

Lexibiotico *Llano, Spain.*
Cefalexin (p.161·3).
Bacterial infections.

Lexiflox *Duopharma, Hong Kong.*
Norfloxacin (p.232·1).
Bacterial infections.

Lexil *Roche, Ital.*
Bromazepam (p.656·3); propantheline bromide (p.473·2).
Gastrointestinal disorders.

Lexilium *Remedica, Hong Kong.*
Bromazepam (p.656·3).
Anxiety.

Lexincef *Serra Pamies, Spain.*
Cefalexin (p.161·3).
Bacterial infections.

Lexinor
AstraZeneca, Fin.; Astra, Hong Kong; AstraZeneca, Singapore; Astra, Swed.; AstraZeneca, Thai.
Norfloxacin (p.232·1).
Bacterial infections.

Lexobene *Merckle, Ger.*
Diclofenac sodium (p.30·3).
Lignocaine [lidocaine] hydrochloride (p.1313·2) is included in this preparation to alleviate the pain of injection.
Gout; inflammation; musculoskeletal, joint, and soft-tissue disorders; neuralgia; neuritis; pain.

Lexomil *Roche, Fr.*
Bromazepam (p.656·3).
Alcohol withdrawal syndrome; anxiety.

Lexostad *Stada, Ger.*
Bromazepam (p.656·3).
Anxiety disorders; insomnia.

Lexotan
Roche, Austral.; Roche, Belg.; Roche, Braz.; Roche, Denm.; Roche, Hong Kong; Roche, Irl.; Roche, Ital.; Roche, Mex.; Roche, Port.; Roche, S.Afr.; Roche, Singapore; Roche, Thai.; Roche, UK.
Bromazepam (p.656·3).
Anxiety; insomnia; psychosomatic disorders.

Lexotanil
Roche, Aust.; Roche, Ger.; Roche, Neth.; Roche, Switz.
Bromazepam (p.656·3).
Anxiety disorders; insomnia; psychosomatic symptoms.

Lexpec *Rosemont, UK.*
Folic acid (p.1361·1).
Anaemias.

Lexpec with Iron *Rosemont, UK.*
Ferric ammonium citrate (p.1359·2); folic acid (p.1361·1).
Iron and folic acid deficiency.

Lexpec with Iron-M *Rosemont, UK.*
Ferric ammonium citrate (p.1359·2); folic acid (p.1361·1).
Iron and folic acid deficiency.

Lexxel *Astra, USA.*
Enalapril maleate (p.883·3); felodipine (p.888·3).
Hypertension.

Leza *Bioclon, Mex.*
Yeast (p.1398·1).
Modification of gastrointestinal flora.

Lezidim *Lemery, Mex.*
Ceftazidime (p.174·3).
Bacterial infections.

L-Gel *Medical Industries, Austral.*
Lubricating gel.

LH Predict *Aptus, NZ.*
Fertility test (p.1654·3).

Li 450 *Ziethen, Ger.*
Lithium carbonate (p.292·1).
Bipolar disorders; depression; mania.

Liatriz Solfran, Mex.
Meclozine (p.420·3); pyridoxine (p.1387·1).
Nausea and vomiting.

Libenar SmithKline Beecham, Ital.; Sterling Health, Spain†.
Sodium chloride (p.1196·1).
Nasal dryness; nasal hygiene.

Liberal Asian Pharm, Thai.
Flunarizine hydrochloride (p.418·1).
Cerebrovascular disorders; vestibular disorders.

Liberalgium Diviser Aquilea, Spain.
Diclofenac sodium (p.30·3).
Gout; inflammation; musculoskeletal, joint, and peri-articular disorders; pain; renal colic.

Liberan AF, Mex.
Simeticone (p.1249·2).
Flatulence.

Liberanas OTC, Spain.
Sodium chloride (p.1196·1).
Nasal congestion.

Liberbil Ferrer, Spain†.
Cyclobutyrol sodium (p.1601·2); theophylline dehydrocholinate; metoclopramide hydrochloride (p.1235·2).
Hepatobiliary disorders.

Liberen Lisapharma, Ital.
Dextropropoxyphene hydrochloride (p.27·1).
Pain; renal and hepatic colic.

Liberol Galactina, Switz.†.
Camphor (p.1589·3); methyl salicylate (p.55·1); guaiacol (p.1092·1); mustard spirit (p.1639·1); pumilio pine oil (p.1656·3); thyme oil (p.1672·3); eucalyptus oil (p.1609·2); turpentine oil (p.1676·3); hyoscyamus oil (p.470·1).
Chilblains; cold symptoms; muscle and joint pain.

Liberol Baby N Mavena, Switz.
Eucalyptus oil (p.1609·2); pumilio pine oil (p.1656·3); anise oil (p.1580·3); juniper oil (p.1625·2).
Cold symptoms.

Liberol Bain Mavena, Switz.
Thyme oil (p.1672·3); pumilio pine oil (p.1656·3); eucalyptus oil (p.1609·2); rosemary oil (p.1659·3); lavender oil (p.1627·2); niaouli oil (p.1640·2).
Coughs and cold symptoms.

Liberol Dragees contre la toux Mavena, Switz.
Thyme (p.1672·2); hedera helix.
Coughs.

Liberol N Mavena, Switz.
Camphor (p.1589·3); pumilio pine oil (p.1656·3); thyme oil (p.1672·3); eucalyptus oil (p.1609·2).
Cold symptoms.

Liberol Pastilles contre la toux Mavena, Switz.
Thyme (p.1672·2); senega root (p.1100·2).
Coughs.

Liberol Sirop contre la toux Mavena, Switz.
Thyme (p.1672·2); hedera helix; senega root (p.1100·2); liquorice (p.1231·2).
Coughs.

Libertrim AF, Mex.
Trimebutine (p.1675·1).
Gastrointestinal motility disorders; irritable bowel syndrome.

Libetist Opus, UK.
Salbutamol sulfate (p.770·3).
Asthma; bronchitis; emphysema.

Libexin Mucolitico Chiesi, Ital.
Prenoxdiazine hibenzate (p.1099·2); carbocisteine (p.1086·3).
Coughs.

Libexine Labatec, Switz.
Prenoxdiazine hibenzate (p.1099·2) or prenoxdiazine hydrochloride (p.1099·2).
Coughs.

Libexine Compositum Labatec, Switz.
Prenoxdiazine hydrochloride (p.1099·2); guaifenesin (p.1092·2); terpin hydrate (p.1101·2).
Coughs.

Libidomega Cantassium Co., UK.
Amino-acid, vitamin, and mineral preparation (p.1350·1).

Liblan Yung Shin, Thai.
Chlordiazepoxide (p.659·2); clidinium bromide (p.465·1).
Dysmenorrhoea; gastric hyperacidity; gastroduodenitis; gastrointestinal motility disorders; irritable or spastic colon; peptic ulcer; ureteric spasm and dyskinesia.

Librax Roche, Aust.†; Roche, Belg.†; ICN, Canad.; Medilink, Fin.; CSP, Fr.; Roche, Hong Kong; Roche, Israel; ICN, Ital.; ICN, Port.; Pharmaco, S.Afr.; ICN, Singapore; Roche, Swed.†; ICN, Switz.; ICN, Thai.; Roche, USA.
Chlordiazepoxide (p.659·2) or chlordiazepoxide hydrochloride (p.659·2); clidinium bromide (p.465·1).
Biliary dyskinesia; dysmenorrhoea; dyspepsia; irritable colon; nocturnal enuresis; peptic ulcer; smooth muscle spasm; ureteric spasm.

Libritabs Roche Products, USA.
Chlordiazepoxide (p.659·2).
Anxiety.

Librium ICN, Ger.; ICN, Hong Kong; ICN, Irl.; ICN, Ital.; Roche, Neth.†; Pharmaco, S.Afr.; ICN, UK; ICN, USA.
Chlordiazepoxide (p.659·2) or chlordiazepoxide hydrochloride (p.659·2).
Alcohol withdrawal syndrome; anxiety; insomnia; premedication; skeletal muscle spasm.

Librofem Eastern Pharmaceuticals, UK.
Ibuprofen (p.43·2).
Pain.

Libronchin Byk, Neth.
Acetylcysteine (p.1082·3).
Respiratory-tract disorders with increased or viscous mucus.

Libronchin Prikkelhoest Byk, Neth.
Noscapine hydrochloride (p.1096·1).
Coughs.

Licab Torrent, Thai.
Lithium carbonate (p.292·1).
Bipolar disorder; depression; mania.

Licain Curasan, Ger.
Lignocaine [lidocaine] hydrochloride (p.1313·2).
Local anaesthesia.

Licarb Abic, Thai.
Lithium carbonate (p.292·1).
Bipolar disorder; depression; mania.

Licarbium Rekah, Israel.
Lithium carbonate (p.292·1).
Bipolar disorder.

Licarpin Allergan, Swed.†.
Pilocarpine nitrate (p.1422·3).
Glaucoma.

Lice Rid Florafaun, Austral.
Malathion (Maldison) (p.1434·2).
Pediculosis.

Licide Reese, USA.
Pyrethrum (p.1436·3); piperonyl butoxide (p.1436·2).
Pediculosis.

Liconar Biolab, Thai.
Miconazole nitrate (p.391·1).
Fungal and Gram-positive bacterial skin infections.

Licoplex DS Keene, USA†.
Ferrous gluconate (p.1360·1); vitamin B substances (p.1350·1).
Procaine hydrochloride (p.1319·1) is included in this preparation to alleviate the pain of injection.
Iron-deficiency anaemias.

Licor Amoniacal Asens, Spain†.
Alcohol (p.1130·3); ammonia (p.1579·1); ammonium carbonate (p.1085·1).
Exhaustion; nausea; shock.

Licor de Cacau Virtus, Braz.
Piperazine (p.105·3); citric acid (p.1596·2); theobroma (p.1671·3); cinnamon (p.1595·3); cascara (p.1216·1).
Intestinal nematode infections.

Licor de Tayuya Dansk-Flama, Braz.
Sarsaparilla (p.1661·1); tayuya; ceratonia (p.1500·3).

Licrease Laphal, Fr.
Pancreatin (p.1646·1).
Pancreatic insufficiency.

Lidaltrin Lacer, Spain.
Quinapril hydrochloride (p.963·3).
Heart failure; hypertension.

Lidaltrin Diu Lacer, Spain.
Quinapril hydrochloride (p.963·3); hydrochlorothiazide (p.907·3).
Hypertension.

Lida-Mantle-HC Miles, USA.
Hydrocortisone acetate (p.1073·3); lignocaine [lidocaine] (p.1313·2).
Skin disorders.

Lidaprim Note.This name is used for preparations of different composition.
Hafslund Nycomed, Aust.; Nycomed, Hong Kong; Lisapharma, Ital.; Hafslund Nycomed, Thai.
Sulfametrole (p.256·2); trimethoprim (p.264·2).
Bacterial infections.

Hormona, Mex.
Co-trimoxazole (p.193·3).
Bacterial infections.

Lidazon Democal, Switz.
Cetylpyridinium chloride (p.1138·1); dichlorobenzyl alcohol (p.1143·2); lignocaine [lidocaine] (p.1313·2) or lignocaine [lidocaine] hydrochloride (p.1313·2).
Lidazon lozenges formerly contained cetylpyridinium chloride, dichlorobenzyl alcohol, lignocaine [lidocaine], and chlorquinaldol.
Mouth and throat disorders.

Lid-Care Ciba Vision, Austral.; Ciba Vision, NZ; Novartis Ophthalmics, UK.
Eyelid cleanser.

Lidemol Medicis, Canad.
Fluocinonide (p.1071·2).
Skin disorders.

Lidene Cooperation Pharmaceutique, Fr.
Doxylamine succinate (p.417·1).
Insomnia.

Lident Adrenalina Warner-Lambert, Ital.
Lignocaine [lidocaine] hydrochloride (p.1313·2).
Adrenaline [epinephrine] acid tartrate (p.829·2) is included in this preparation as a vasoconstrictor to diminish absorption and localise the effect of the local anaesthetic.
Local anaesthesia in dentistry.

Lident Andrenor Warner-Lambert, Ital.
Lignocaine [lidocaine] hydrochloride (p.1313·2).
Adrenaline [epinephrine] acid tartrate (p.829·2) and noradrenaline [norepinephrine] acid tartrate (p.948·2) are included in this preparation as vasoconstrictors to diminish absorption and localise the effect of the local anaesthetic.
Local anaesthesia in dentistry.

Liderflex Farmalider, Spain.
Camphor (p.1589·3); methyl salicylate (p.55·1); menthol (p.1632·3).
Muscular and joint pain.

Liderman Jacoby, Aust.
Oxiconazole nitrate (p.393·1).
Fungal skin infections.

Liderplus Farmalider, Spain.
Paracetamol (p.71·2); pseudoephedrine sulfate (p.1099·3); chlorpheniramine [chlorphenamine] maleate (p.412·1).
Cold and influenza symptoms; respiratory-tract congestion.

Lidesthesin Ritsert, Ger.
Lignocaine [lidocaine] hydrochloride (p.1313·2).
Local anaesthesia.

Lidex Yamanouchi, Belg.; Medicis, Canad.; Medicis, USA.
Fluocinonide (p.1071·2).
Skin disorders.

Lidifen Berk, UK.
Ibuprofen (p.43·2).
Fever; inflammation; musculoskeletal and joint disorders; pain.

Lidinal Fustery, Mex.
Nalidixic acid (p.227·1).

Lidixin Ofimex, Mex.
Nalidixic acid (p.227·1).

Lido Tea Trima, Israel.
Senna (p.1248·2); caraway (p.1591·2); liquorice (p.1231·2); chamomile (p.1593·2); peppermint leaf (p.1243·2).
Constipation.

Lidobama Complex Bama, Spain†.
Cellulase (p.1593·1); cyclobutyrol (p.1601·2); dimethicone (p.1249·2); lignocaine [lidocaine] hydrochloride (p.1313·2); pancreatin (p.1646·1).
Digestive-system disorders.

Lidocard Orion, Fin.
Lignocaine [lidocaine] hydrochloride (p.1313·2).
Arrhythmias.

Lidocation Weimer, Thai.
Lignocaine [lidocaine] hydrochloride (p.1313·2).
Adrenaline [epinephrine] (p.829·1) is included in this preparation as a vasoconstrictor to diminish absorption and localise the effect of the local anaesthetic.
Local anaesthesia.

Lidocaton Weimer, Ger.†; Weimer, Switz.†; Weimer, Thai.
Lignocaine [lidocaine] hydrochloride (p.1313·2).
Adrenaline [epinephrine] (p.829·1) is included in this preparation as a vasoconstrictor to diminish absorption and localise the effect of the local anaesthetic.
Local anaesthesia.

Lidocord Apsen, Braz.
Lignocaine [lidocaine] hydrochloride (p.1313·2).
Arrhythmias.

Lidocorit Gebro, Aust.
Lignocaine [lidocaine] hydrochloride (p.1313·2).
Arrhythmias.

Lidodan Odan, Canad.
Lignocaine [lidocaine] (p.1313·2) or lignocaine [lidocaine] hydrochloride (p.1313·2).
Local anaesthesia.

Lidoderm Endo, USA.
Lignocaine [lidocaine] (p.1313·2).
Postherpetic neuralgia.

Lidohex Bichsel, Switz.†.
Lignocaine [lidocaine] hydrochloride (p.1313·2); chlorhexidine gluconate (p.1138·2).
Catheterisation; endoscopy.

Lido-Hyal Ogna, Ital.; Wild, Switz.
Hyaluronidase (p.1620·3); lignocaine [lidocaine] hydrochloride (p.1313·2).
Local anaesthesia; prophylaxis of soft-tissue disorders.

Lidoject Hexal, Ger.; Mayrand, USA.
Lignocaine [lidocaine] hydrochloride (p.1313·2).
Local anaesthesia.

Lidomyxin Sabex, Canad.
Polymyxin B sulfate (p.238·1); lignocaine [lidocaine] hydrochloride (p.1313·2).
Ear infections, pain, and pruritus.

Lidonostrum Nostrum, Port.
Lignocaine [lidocaine] hydrochloride (p.1313·2).
Local anaesthesia.

LidoPen Meridian, Israel; Survival Technology, USA.
Lignocaine [lidocaine] hydrochloride (p.1313·2).
Arrhythmias.

LidoPosterine Kade, Ger.
Lignocaine [lidocaine] (p.1313·2).
Anorectal disorders.

Lidosen Senese, Ital.
Lignocaine [lidocaine] hydrochloride (p.1313·2).
Local anaesthesia.

Lidosporin Note.This name is used for preparations of different composition.
Glaxo Wellcome, Braz.
Polymyxin B sulfate (p.238·1); lignocaine [lidocaine] (p.1313·2).
Ear infections.

Warner-Lambert, Canad.
Cream: Polymyxin B sulfate (p.238·1); gramicidin (p.213·3); lignocaine [lidocaine] hydrochloride (p.1313·2).
Skin disorders.
Ear drops: Polymyxin B sulfate (p.238·1); lignocaine [lidocaine] hydrochloride (p.1313·2).
Ear infections.

Lidox Major, USA†.
Chlordiazepoxide hydrochloride (p.659·2); clidinium bromide (p.465·1).
Irritable bowel syndrome; peptic ulcer (adjunct).

Lidoxin Unison, Thai.
Cloxacillin sodium (p.192·1).
Bacterial infections.

Lid-Pack Ciba Vision, Canad.
Polymyxin B sulfate (p.238·1); bacitracin zinc (p.155·2).

Lidrian Clarmed, Ital.
Lignocaine [lidocaine] hydrochloride (p.1313·2).
Local anaesthesia.

Lidrone Serra Pamies, Spain.
Phenylephrine hydrochloride (p.1097·1); naphazoline nitrate (p.1095·1); prednisolone (p.1077·3); cetrimide (p.1137·1).
Cold symptoms; rhinitis; sinusitis.

Lievistar Skills, Ital.
Dried yeast (p.1398·1); cynara (p.1601·3).
Nutritional supplement.

Lievitosohn Antonetto, Ital.
Saccharomyces cerevisiae (p.1398·1); vitamin B substances (p.1350·1).
Restoration of normal gastrointestinal flora.

Lievitovit Novartis Consumer, Ital.
Dried yeast (p.1398·1); vitamin B substances (p.1350·1).
Restoration of normal gastrointestinal flora.

Lievitovit 300 Gazzoni, Ital.†.
Dried yeast (p.1398·1).

Lifaton B12 Sabater, Spain.
Cyanocobalamin (p.1388·1).
Vitamin B12 deficiency.

Life Brand Baby Sunblock and Kids Sunblock Tanning Research, Canad.
SPF 30: Octinoxate (p.1517·3); octisalate (p.1518·1); titanium dioxide (p.1126·1).
Sunscreen.

Life Brand Cough Lozenges Sutton, Canad.†.
Menthol (p.1632·3).

Life Brand Natural Source Tanning Research, Canad.†.
SPF 25: Titanium dioxide (p.1126·1).
Sunscreen.

Life Brand Sport Sunblock Tanning Research, Canad.
SPF 15; SPF 30: Octinoxate (p.1517·3); octisalate (p.1518·1); oxybenzone (p.1518·1).
Sunscreen.

Life Brand Sunblock Tanning Research, Canad.
SPF 15: Octinoxate (p.1517·3); oxybenzone (p.1518·1).
SPF 30: Octinoxate (p.1517·3); homosalate (p.1517·2); octisalate (p.1518·1); oxybenzone (p.1518·1).
Formerly contained octinoxate, avobenzone, and homosalate.
Sunscreen.

Life Drops Potter's, UK.
Capsicum (p.1591·1); sambucus (p.1660·3); peppermint oil (p.1243·3).
Cold symptoms; sore throat.

Lifechange Circulation Aid Cenovis, Austral.
Fish oil (p.949·3); dl-alpha tocoferil acetate (p.1394·1); ginkgo biloba (p.1615·2); crataegus (p.1600·2).
Peripheral circulatory disorders; wounds.

Lifechange Menopause Formula Cenovis, Austral.
Soya bean (p.1378·1); red clover (p.1657·2).
Menopausal disorders.

Lifechange Mens Complex with Saw Palmetto Cenovis, Austral.
Zinc amino acid chelate (p.1398·3); cucurbita (p.1601·1); saw palmetto (p.1491·2).
Tonic.

Lifechange Multi Plus Antioxidant Cenovis, Austral.
Vitamins and minerals (p.1350·1); vitis vinifera; ginkgo biloba (p.1615·2).
Peripheral circulatory disorders; vitamin and mineral deficiencies.

Lifedrops Lifeplan, UK.
Sambucus (p.1660·3); peppermint (p.1243·2).
Coughs and cold symptoms; flatulence.

Lifenac Liferpal, Mex.
Diclofenac sodium (p.30·3).
Musculoskeletal, joint, and peri-articular disorders.

Liferxina Liferpal, Mex.
Ciprofloxacin (p.182·3).
Bacterial infections.

Lifestyles Ansell, Canad.
Nonoxinol 9 (p.1346·1).
Contraceptive.

Lifesystem Herbal Formula 1 Arthritic Aid Cenovis, Austral.
Celery (p.1592·3); juniper (p.1625·2); devil's claw root (p.26·3); salix (p.82·1).
Arthritic and rheumatic pain.

Lifesystem Herbal Formula 7 Liver Tonic Cenovis, Austral.
Silybum marianum (p.1021·3); taraxacum (p.1669·1); cynara (p.1601·3); garlic (p.1614·1).
Digestive disorders; liver tonic.

Lifesystem Herbal Formula 6 For Peripheral Circulation Cenovis, Austral.
Ginkgo biloba (p.1615·2); crataegus (p.1600·2); zanthoxylum (p.1682·1); capsicum (p.1591·4); rutoside (p.1611·2); hesperidin (p.1611·2).
Peripheral circulatory disorders.

Lifesystem Herbal Formula 12 Willowbark Cenovis, Austral.†.
Skullcap (p.1664·3); devil's claw root (p.26·3); salix (p.82·1).
Headache.

Lifesystem Herbal Formula 4 Women's Formula Cenovis, Austral.
Angelica (p.1580·2); cimicifuga (p.1595·2); blue cohosh (p.1585·3); pulsatilla (p.1656·3); agnus castus (p.1574·2).
Menstrual disorders.

Lifesystem Herbal Plus Formula 8 Echinacea Cenovis, Austral.†.
Echinacea (p.1606·2); d-alpha tocoferil acid succinate (p.1394·1); betacarotene (p.1355·1); ascorbic acid (p.1389·3); sodium ascorbate (p.1390·1); zinc amino acid chelate (p.1398·3).
Minor upper respiratory-tract disorders; skin disorders; wounds.

Lifesystem Herbal Plus Formula 5 Eye Relief Cenovis, Austral.
Euphrasia officinalis (p.1609·3); ginkgo biloba (p.1615·2); betacarotene (p.1355·1); d-alpha tocoferil acid succinate (p.1394·1); ascorbic acid (p.1389·3); rutoside (p.1611·2); hesperidin (p.1611·2).
Eye strain; tired eyes.

Lifesystem Herbal Plus Formula 9 Fatty Acids And Vitamin E Cenovis, Austral.†.
d-Alpha tocopherol (p.1393·3); evening primrose oil (p.1613·2); omega-3 marine triglycerides (p.949·3).
Dietary supplement.

Lifesystem Herbal Plus Formula 11 Ginkgo Cenovis, Austral.
Ginkgo biloba (p.1615·2); ginger (p.1227·2); dibasic potassium phosphate (p.1193·1); magnesium oxide (p.1233·2).
Peripheral circulatory disorders; tonic.

Lifesystem Herbal Plus Formula 3 Male Formula Cenovis, Austral.
Eleutherococcus senticosis; equisetum; sarsaparilla; liquorice; damiana; zinc amino acid chelate; betacarotene; pyridoxine hydrochloride; d-alpha tocoferil acid succinate; magnesium oxide (p.1350·1).
Tonic.

Lifesystem Herbal Plus Formula 2 Valerian Cenovis, Austral.
Valerian (p.1678·3); passion flower (p.1649·1); dibasic potassium phosphate (p.1193·1); magnesium oxide (p.1233·2).
Nervous tension; sleep disorders.

Lifesystem Mineral Plus Formula 10 Osteoporosis Cenovis, Austral.†.
Calcium carbonate (p.1215·1); colecalciferol (p.1391·4).
Calcium deficiency; osteoporosis.

Lifo-Scrub Braun, Switz.
Chlorhexidine gluconate (p.1138·2).
Skin and hand disinfection.

Lifril Casen Fleet, Spain†.
Pirlindole (p.307·3).
Depression.

Lifurom Lilly, S.Afr.
Cefuroxime sodium (p.178·2).
Bacterial infections.

Lifurox Lilly, Denm.†; Lilly, Fin.; Lilly, Norw.; Lilly, Spain; Lilly, Swed.†.
Cefuroxime sodium (p.178·2).
Bacterial infections.

Liga Jacobs, UK.
Gluten-free food for special diets (p.1350·1).

Lightening Crinos, Ital.
Glycolic acid (p.1115·1); phytic acid (p.1023·1).
Hyperpigmentation disorders.

Lightning Cough Remedy Potter's, UK.
Liquorice (p.1231·2); anise oil (p.1580·3).
Coughs.

Lignospan Dentsply, Austral.; Septodont, Switz.
Lignocaine [lidocaine] hydrochloride (p.1313·2).
Adrenaline [epinephrine] acid tartrate (p.829·1) is included in this preparation as a vasoconstrictor to diminish absorption and localise the effect of the local anaesthetic.
Local anaesthesia.

Lignospan Special Dental Warehouse, S.Afr.
Lignocaine (p.1313·2).
Adrenaline [epinephrine] (p.829·1) is included in this preparation as a vasoconstrictor to diminish absorption and localise the effect of the local anaesthetic.
Local anaesthesia.

Lignosporin Glaxo Wellcome, Singapore.
Polymyxin B sulfate (p.238·1); lignocaine [lidocaine] hydrochloride (p.1313·2).
Ear infections.

Lignostab-A AstraZeneca, UK.
Lignocaine [lidocaine] hydrochloride (p.1313·2).

Adrenaline [epinephrine] (p.829·1) is included in this preparation as a vasoconstrictor to diminish absorption and localise the effect of the local anaesthetic.
Local anaesthesia.

Li-iL Rheuma-Bad Li-il, Ger.
Glycol salicylate (p.42·2); methyl salicylate (p.55·1).
Bath additive; musculoskeletal, joint, and soft-tissue disorders.

Likacin Lisapharm, Israel; Lisapharma, Ital.
Amikacin (p.147·3) or amikacin sulfate (p.148·1).
Bacterial infections.

Likenil Vedim, Spain.
Lisinopril (p.921·1).
Diabetic nephropathy; heart failure; hypertension; myocardial infarction.

Likuden M Hoechst Marion Roussel, Ger.
Griseofulvin (microfine) (p.386·2).
Fungal infections.

Lilacillin Takeda, Jpn.
Sulbenicillin sodium (p.250·2).
Mepivacaine hydrochloride (p.1317·1) is included in the intramuscular injection to alleviate the pain of injection.
Bacterial infections.

Li-Liquid Rosemont, UK.
Lithium citrate (p.292·1).
Depression; mania; psychoses.

Lilium Med Complex Dynamit, Aust.
Homoeopathic preparation.

Lillypen Profil 10, 20, 30, and 40 Lilly, Fr.
Mixtures of insulin injection (human, prb) 10%, 20%, 30%, and 40% and isophane insulin injection (human, prb) 90%, 80%, 70%, and 60% respectively (p.324·1).
Diabetes mellitus.

Lillypen Protamine Isophane Lilly, Fr.
Isophane insulin injection (human, prb) (p.324·1).
Diabetes mellitus.

Lillypen Rapide Lilly, Fr.
Insulin injection (human, prb) (p.324·1).
Diabetes mellitus.

Liman Solvay, Aust.; Solvay, Ger.†.
Tenoxicam (p.87·2).
Gout; musculoskeletal and joint disorders.

Limao Bravo
Note. This name is used for preparations of different composition.
Catarinense, Braz.
Siparuna guyanensis; aconite (p.1572·3); grindelia (p.1618·2); senega (p.1100·2); sodium benzoate (p.1134·3).
Respiratory-tract congestion.

Farmedica, Braz.
Siparuna guyanensis; sodium benzoate (p.1134·3); aconite (p.1572·3); bromoform (p.1587·1); grindelia (p.1618·2); menthol (p.1632·3).
Coughs.

Herald's, Braz.
Siparuna guyanensis; rorippa nasturtium aquaticum; mikania; fig (p.1227·1).
Respiratory-tract congestion.

Legrand, Braz.
Siparuna guyanensis; bromoform (p.1587·1); althaea (p.1577·1); aconite (p.1572·3); sodium benzoate (p.1134·3); guaifenesin (p.1092·2).
Coughs.

Limao Bravo com Vitamina C Cazi, Braz.
Cetylpyridinium chloride (p.1138·1); vitamin C (p.1389·3); siparuna guyanensis.
Mouth and throat disorders.

Limbao Kanoldt, Ger.
Kava (p.1625·3).
Anxiety disorders.

Limbatril ICN, Ger.
Amitriptyline hydrochloride (p.273·3); chlordiazepoxide (p.659·2).
Dystonias; non-psychotic mental disorders.

Limbial Chiesi, Ital.
Oxazepam (p.697·1).
Anxiety; insomnia; nervous disorders.

Limbitrol ICN, Aust.; Roche, Belg.†; Roche, Braz.; Medilink, Fin.; ICN, Neth.†; Pharmaco, S.Afr.; ICN, Switz.; ICN, USA.
Amitriptyline hydrochloride (p.273·3); chlordiazepoxide (p.659·2).
Mixed anxiety depressive states.

Limbitryl ICN, Ital.
Amitriptyline hydrochloride (p.273·3); chlordiazepoxide (p.659·2).
Mixed anxiety depressive states.

Limclair Sinclair, Irl.; Durbin, UK.
Trisodium edetate (p.1008·1).
Calcareous corneal opacities; digitalis-induced arrhythmias; hypercalcaemia; parathyroidism.

Limed Medifive, Thai.
Lithium carbonate (p.292·1).
Bipolar disorder.

Limethason Green Cross, Hong Kong; Yoshitomi, Jpn; Yoshitomi, Singapore.
Dexamethasone palmitate (p.1067·3).
Rheumatoid arthritis.

Limican Sanofi Synthelabo, Ital.
Alizapride hydrochloride (p.1209·3).
Nausea and vomiting.

Limifen Janssen-Cilag, Spain.
Alfentanil hydrochloride (p.11·3).
General anaesthesia.

Liminate Modern Health Products, UK.
Turkey rhubarb (p.1248·1); senna leaf (p.1248·2); chondrus (p.1500·1).
Constipation.

Limit-X UB Interpharm, Switz.
Cathine hydrochloride (p.1507·1).
Obesity.

Limonal Falqui, Ital.
Light magnesium carbonate (p.1232·3); anhydrous citric acid (p.1596·2).
Constipation.

Limone CliniMed, UK.
A deodorant spray for stoma care.

Limovan Rhone-Poulenc Rorer, Spain.
Zopiclone (p.713·1).
Insomnia.

Limoxin Liferpal, Mex.
Amoxicillin (p.149·2).
Bacterial infections.

Limpele Conjugado Dovalle, Braz.
Econazole (p.383·1).
Fungal skin infections.

Limpidex Sigma-Tau, Ital.
Lansoprazole (p.1230·3).
Gastro-oesophageal reflux; peptic ulcer; Zollinger-Ellison syndrome.

Limptar Hoechst Marion Roussel, Aust.; Cassella-med, Ger.; Hoechst Marion Roussel, Switz.†.
Quinine sulfate (p.445·1); aminophylline (p.760·1).
Cramp.

Limptar N Cassella-med, Ger.
Quinine sulfate (p.445·1).
Night cramp.

Linadin Sedabel, Braz.
Attapulgite (p.1212·1); pectin (p.1502·3); homatropine (p.468·1).
Diarrhoea.

Linamin Plus Seber, Port.
Fursultiamine (p.1384·3); cyanocobalamin (p.1388·3) or hydroxocobalamin (p.1388·1); pyridoxine hydrochloride (p.1386·3).
Mepivacaine hydrochloride (p.1317·1) is included in the intramuscular injection to alleviate the pain of injection.
Neuralgia; neuritis; neuropathy; rheumatoid arthritis.

Linapen Welfer, Mex.
Ampicillin (p.150·3).
Bacterial infections.

Linaris RAN, Ger.†.
Co-trimoxazole (p.193·3).
Bacterial infections.

Linatil Gea, Fin.
Enalapril maleate (p.883·3).
Heart failure; hypertension.

Linatil Comp Gea, Fin.
Enalapril maleate (p.883·3); hydrochlorothiazide (p.907·3).
Hypertension.

Linazine Asian Pharm, Thai.
Cinnarizine (p.413·1).
Cerebrovascular disorders; migraine; motion sickness; peripheral vascular disorders; vestibular disorders.

Lincaina Braun, Port.
Lignocaine [lidocaine] hydrochloride (p.1313·2).
Adrenaline [epinephrine] hydrochloride (p.829·2) is included in some injections as a vasoconstrictor to diminish absorption and localise the effect of the local anaesthetic.
Local anaesthesia.

Lincil Almirall, Spain.
Nicardipine hydrochloride (p.938·3).
Angina pectoris; cerebrovascular disorders; hypertension.

Linco General Drugs, Thai.
Lincomycin (p.219·3).
Gram-positive bacterial infections.

Lincocin Pharmacia Upjohn, Austral.; Pharmacia Upjohn, Belg.; Pharmacia Upjohn, Canad.; Pharmacia Upjohn, Hong Kong; Pharmacia Upjohn, Ital.; Pharmacia Upjohn, Mex.; Pharmacia Upjohn, Neth.; Pharmacia Upjohn, S.Afr.; Pharmacia Upjohn, Singapore; Pharmacia Upjohn, Spain; Pharmacia Upjohn, Swed.†; Pharmacia Upjohn, Switz.; Pharmacia Upjohn, Thai.; Upjohn, USA.
Lincomycin hydrochloride (p.219·2).
Bacterial infections.

Lincocina Pharmacia Upjohn, Port.
Lincomycin hydrochloride (p.219·2).
Bacterial infections.

Lincocine Pharmacia Upjohn, Fr.
Lincomycin hydrochloride (p.219·2).
Bacterial infections.

Lincogin Samakeephaesaj, Thai.
Lincomycin hydrochloride (p.219·2).
Gram-positive bacterial infections.

Lincolan Olan-Kemed, Thai.
Lincomycin (p.219·2).

Lincomy Nakorn, Thai.
Lincomycin hydrochloride (p.219·2).
Gram-positive bacterial infections.

Linco-Plus Cibran, Braz.
Lincomycin hydrochloride (p.219·2).
Bacterial infections.

Lincorex Hyrex, USA.
Lincomycin hydrochloride (p.219·2).
Bacterial infections.

Linctifed Glaxo Wellcome, S.Afr.
Triprolidine hydrochloride (p.427·2); pseudoephedrine hydrochloride (p.1099·2); codeine phosphate (p.25·2); guaifenesin (p.1092·2).
Coughs.

Linctodyl Pharmaceutical Enterprises, S.Afr.
Dextromethorphan hydrobromide (p.1087·3); ephedrine hydrochloride (p.1090·1); ammonium chloride (p.1085·2).
Coughs.

Linctosan Aspen, S.Afr.
Diphenhydramine hydrochloride (p.416·1); ammonium chloride (p.1085·2); sodium citrate (p.1186·2); menthol (p.1632·3).
Coughs.

Linctus Tussi Infans Propan, S.Afr.
Ipecacuanha (p.1093·1); squill (p.1100·3); tolu (p.1101·3).
Coughs.

Lindanoxil Dakota, Braz.
Ointment; topical liquid: Lindane (p.1434·1).
Pediculosis; scabies.

Soap: Lindane (p.1434·1); hexachlorophene (p.1146·1).
Skin disinfection.

Lindemil Knoll, Spain.
Alum (p.1577·2); benzalkonium chloride (p.1133·2).
Vaginal antiseptic; vulvovaginal trichomoniasis (adjuvant).

Lindigoa S Brenner-Efeka, Ger.; LAW, Ger.; Riemser, Ger.
Aesculus (p.1574·1); troxerutin (p.1611·2).
Vascular disorders.

Lindilane Grunenthal, Fr.
Paracetamol (p.71·2); codeine phosphate (p.25·2).
Pain.

Lindofluid N Lindopharm, Ger.
Bornyl acetate (p.1586·3); α-pinene; arnica (p.1581·3); melissa (p.1632·2).
Muscle, joint, and nerve pain.

Lindormin Boehringer Ingelheim, Mex.
Brotizolam (p.657·2).
Insomnia.

Lindotab Lindopharm, Ger.†.
Tiaprofenic acid (p.88·1).
Inflammation; musculoskeletal, joint, and soft-tissue disorders.

Lindoxyl Lindopharm, Ger.
Ambroxol hydrochloride (p.1084·3).
Respiratory-tract disorders associated with increased or viscous mucus.

Linea Valeas, Ital.†.
Diethylpropion hydrochloride (p.1508·3).
Obesity.

Linea F Angelini, Ital.
Benzalkonium chloride (p.1133·2); benzydamine hydrochloride (p.20·1).
Disinfection of wounds and burns.

Lineafarm Wyeth, Spain†.
Nonoxinol 9 (p.1346·1).
Contraceptive.

Linervidol Interdelta, Switz.
Paracetamol (p.71·2); pyridoxine hydrochloride (p.1386·3); promethazine hydrochloride (p.423·2).
Agitation; fever; pain.

Linfocilin Climax, Braz.
Benzylpenicillin potassium (p.157·1); procaine penicillin [procaine benzylpenicillin] (p.239·2).
Bacterial infections.

Linfogex Climax, Braz.
Vitamin B substances (p.1350·1).
Vitamin B deficiency.

Linfoglobulina Rhone-Poulenc Rorer, Spain.
Antilymphocyte immunoglobulin (horse) (p.508·2).
Organ transplant rejection.

Linfolysin Nuovo ISM, Ital.
Chlorambucil (p.516·3).
Chronic lymphoid leukaemia; Hodgkin's disease; lymphoma.

Lingo Siam Bheasach, Thai.
Lincomycin hydrochloride (p.219·2).
Gram-positive bacterial infections.

Lingraine Sanofi Winthrop, Irl.; Sanofi Synthelabo, UK†.
Ergotamine tartrate (p.452·1).
Migraine and other vascular headaches.

Lini-Bombe Thepenier, Fr.†.
Veratrol; menthol (p.1632·3); cloral hydrate (p.669·3); salicylic acid (p.1122·3).
Formerly contained veratrol, menthol, cloral hydrate, and phenazone gentisate.
Musculoskeletal and joint disorders.

Liniment Balm Greenridge, Austral.
Sweet birch oil (p.55·2); menthol (p.1632·3).
Musculoskeletal, joint, and soft-tissue pain.

Linimento de Sloan Warner-Lambert Consumer, Port.
Turpentine oil (p.1676·3); capsicum oil; pine oil; camphor oil; methyl salicylate (p.55·1).
Musculoskeletal pain.

The symbol † denotes a preparation no longer actively marketed

Linimento Klari *Clariana, Spain.*
Camphor (p.1589·3); capsicum (p.1591·1); amyl salicylate (p.14·1); rosemary oil (p.1659·3); sassafras oil
(p.1661·1); turpentine oil (p.1676·3).
Rheumatic and muscle pain.

Linimento Naion *Puerto Galiano, Spain.*
Camphor (p.1589·3); alcohol (p.1130·3); salicylic acid
(p.1122·3); turpentine; menthol (p.1632·3); soft soap
(p.1496·1); capsicum (p.1591·1); methyl salicylate
(p.55·1); rosemary; lavender (p.1627·2).
Rheumatic and muscle pain.

Linimento Sloan *Warner-Lambert, Spain.*
Ammonia (p.1579·1); capsicum (p.1591·1); methyl
salicylate (p.55·1); oleum pini sylvestris; sassafras; turpentine oil (p.1676·3); camphor (p.1589·3).
Rheumatic and muscle pain.

Liniplant *Spitzner, Ger.*
Eucalyptus oil (p.1609·2); cajuput oil (p.1588·1).
Upper respiratory-tract disorders.

Linisol *Braun, Belg.*
Lignocaine [lidocaine] hydrochloride (p.1313·2).
Local anaesthesia.

Linitul *Bama, Spain.*
Peru balsam (p.1650·2); castor oil.
Burns; wounds.

Linitul Antibiotico *Bama, Spain.*
Acexamic acid (p.1572·2); bacitracin (p.155·2); neomycin sulfate (p.228·1); polymyxin B sulfate
(p.238·1).
Burns; infected skin disorders; ulcers; wounds.

Link
Note. This name is used for preparations of different composition.
Alpharma, Denm.; Alpharma, Fin.; Alpharma, Norw.; Dumex-Alphar-
ma, Swed.
Aluminium hydroxide-magnesium carbonate co-dried
gel (p.1211·2).
*Dyspepsia; gastric hyperacidity; gastritis; heartburn;
peptic ulcer.*

Savio, Ital.
Citicoline sodium (p.1596·1).
Cerebrovascular disorders.

Linmycin *Vana, Thai.*
Lincomycin hydrochloride (p.219·2).
Gram-positive bacterial infections.

Linobion-Globuli *Linobion, Aust.*
Fatty acids; cod-liver oil (p.1357·2); thymol
(p.1158·3).
Vaginal disorders.

Linobion-Heilsalbe *Linobion, Aust.*
Fatty acids.
Skin disorders.

Linobion-Kapseln *Linobion, Aust.*
Fatty acids.
Skin disorders.

Linobion-Salbenstift *Linobion, Aust.*
Fatty acids; thymol (p.1158·3).
Skin disorders.

Linobion-Sulfonamid *Linobion, Aust.*
Fatty acids; sulfathiazole (p.257·1).
Infected skin disorders.

Linobion-Zinksalbe *Linobion, Aust.*
Fatty acids; zinc oxide (p.1128·2).
Skin disorders.

Linoforce *Bioforce, Switz.*
Linseed (p.1629·1); senna (p.1248·2); frangula bark
(p.1227·1).
Constipation.

Linola
Wolff, Ger.; Cimex, Switz.
Linoleic acid (p.1613·2); 9,11-octadecadienoic acid.
Skin disorders.

Linola gamma *Wolff, Ger.*
Evening primrose oil (p.1613·2).
Skin disorders.

Linola gras *Cimex, Switz.*
Linoleic acid (p.1613·2); 9,11-octadecadienoic acid;
betacarotene (p.1355·1); colecalciferol (p.1391·1); tocoferil acetate (p.1394·1).
Skin disorders.

Linola mi-gras *Cimex, Switz.*
Linoleic acid (p.1613·2); 9,11-octadecadienoic acid.
Skin disorders.

Linoladiol
Note. This name is used for preparations of different composition.
Montavit, Aust.
Estradiol (p.1473·1).
Vaginal disorders.

Cimex, Switz.
Estradiol (p.1473·1); linoleic acid (p.1613·2); 9,11-oc-
tadecadienoic acid.
Vulvovaginal disorders.

Linoladiol N *Wolff, Ger.*
Estradiol (p.1473·1).
*Oestrogen deficiency; skin disorders; vaginal disor-
ders.*

Linoladiol-H N *Wolff, Ger.*
Estradiol (p.1473·1); prednisolone (p.1077·3).
Acne; ulcus cruris; vaginal disorders.

Linola-Fett *Montavit, Aust.*
Fatty acids, betacarotene, colecalciferol-cholesterin,
vitamin E (p.1350·1).
Skin disorders.

Linola-Fett 2000 *Wolff, Ger.*
Linoleic acid (p.1613·2).
Skin disorders.

Linola-Fett N *Wolff, Ger.*
Linoleic acid (p.1613·2); 9,11-octadecadienoic acid.
Skin disorders.

Linola-Fett-N Olbad *Wolff, Ger.*
Bath additive; emollient.

Linola-H N *Wolff, Ger.*
Prednisolone (p.1077·3).
Skin disorders.

Linola-H-compositum N *Wolff, Ger.*
Prednisolone (p.1077·3); neomycin sulfate (p.228·1).
Burns; infected skin disorders; skin ulcers.

Linola-H-Fett N *Wolff, Ger.*
Prednisolone (p.1077·3).
Skin disorders.

Linola-sept *Wolff, Ger.*
Clioquinol (p.190·2).
Infected skin disorders.

Linotar
Linotar, Austral.; MZ, S.Afr.
Coal tar (p.1125·1).
Skin and scalp disorders.

Linsal *Sigma, Austral.*
Methyl salicylate (p.55·1).
Rubefacient and topical analgesic.

L-Insulin *Berlin-Chemie, Ger.*
Neutral insulin suspension (porcine) (p.324·1).
Diabetes mellitus.

L-Insulin SNC *Berlin-Chemie, Ger.*
Neutral insulin suspension (porcine) (p.324·1).
Diabetes mellitus.

Linusit Creola *Fink, Ger.†*
Linseed (p.1629·1).
Gastrointestinal disorders.

Linusit Darmaktiv Leinsamen *Fink, Ger.†*
Linseed (p.1629·1).
Gastrointestinal disorders.

Linusit Gold *Drogenhansa, Aust.*
Linseed (p.1629·1).
Gastrointestinal disorders.

Linvite *Linton, S.Afr.†*
Multivitamin and mineral preparation (p.1350·1).

Liocarpina *SIFI, Ital.*
Pilocarpine hydrochloride (p.1422·3).
Glaucoma; ocular hypertension.

Liofindol *ICN, Mex.*
Mazindol (p.1510·3).

Liogynon *Schering, Aust.*
Levonorgestrel (p.1486·2); ethinylestradiol (p.1476·2).
Triphasic oral contraceptive.

Lio-Levedura *Vitoria, Port.†*
Saccharomyces cerevisiae (p.1398·1).

Liometacen
Gerot, Aust.; Chiesi, Ital.; Chiesi, Thai.
Meglumine indometacin (p.46·1).
*Gout; musculoskeletal and joint disorders; pain; renal
and biliary colic; thrombophlebitis.*

Lio-Morbillo *Nuovo ISM, Ital.*
A measles vaccine (Schwarz strain) (p.1547·1).
Active immunisation.

Lion Cleansing Herbs *Potter's, UK.*
Buckthorn (p.1215·1); psyllium seed (p.1229·1); senna
(p.1248·2); sambucus (p.1660·3); fennel (p.1610·1);
maté (p.1681·1).
Constipation.

Lioresal
Novartis, Aust.; Novartis, Austral.; Novartis, Belg.; Novartis, Braz.;
Novartis, Canad.; Novartis, Denm.; Novartis, Fin.; Novartis, Fr.; No-
vartis, Ger.; Du Pont, Ger.; Novartis, Hong Kong; Novartis, Irl.; No-
vartis, Israel; Novartis, Ital.; Novartis, Neth.; Novartis, Norw.;
Novartis, NZ; Novartis, Port.; Novartis, S.Afr.; Novartis, Singapore;
Novartis, Spain; Novartis, Swed.; Novartis, Switz.; Novartis, Thai.;
Novartis, UK; Geigy, USA.
Baclofen (p.1322·3).
Skeletal muscle spasm or spasticity.

Liosiero *Nuovo ISM, Ital.*
A botulism antitoxin (types A, B, and E) (p.1534·3).
Botulism.

Liotec *Technilab, Canad.*
Baclofen (p.1322·3).

Lioton
Menarini, Hong Kong; Sanofi Synthelabo, Ital.; Menarini, Switz.
Heparin sodium (p.902·1).
Peripheral vascular disorders; soft-tissue disorders.

Liotropina *SIFI, Ital.†*
Atropine sulfate (p.461·1).
Eye disorders.

Liozim *Farmanova, Ital.*
Fructose (p.1363·3); acacia honey (p.1366·2); lactic-
acid-producing organisms (p.1626·3).
Nutritional supplement.

Lip Block Sunscreen *Norwood, Canad.*
SPF 15: Octinoxate (p.1517·3); oxybenzone
(p.1518·1); titanium dioxide (p.1126·1).
Sunscreen.

Lip Medex
Note. This name is used for preparations of different composition.
Blistex, Canad.
Camphor (p.1589·3); phenol (p.1152·3); menthol
(p.1632·3).
Dry, cracked lips; herpes labialis.

Blistex, USA.
Camphor (p.1589·3); phenol (p.1152·3).
Oral lesions.

Lip Tone *Blistex, USA.*
SPF 15: Octinoxate (p.1517·3); meradimate
(p.1517·3).
Sunscreen.

Lipactin
Novartis Consumer, Canad.; Widmer, Ger.; Widmer, Switz.
Heparin sodium (p.902·1); zinc sulfate (p.1398·2).
*Herpes simplex infections of the lips and orofacial ar-
ea.*

Lipanon *Allergan-Frumtost, Braz.*
Fenofibrate (p.889·1).
Hyperlipidaemias.

Lipanor
Sanofi Winthrop, Fr.; CTI, Israel; Sanofi Synthelabo, Port.
Ciprofibrate (p.858·3).
Hyperlipidaemias.

Lipanthyl
Fournier, Belg.; Fournier, Fr.; Fournier, Ger.; Formenti, Ital.; Fournier,
Port.; Fournier, Singapore; Fournier, Switz.; Fournier, Thai.
Fenofibrate (p.889·1).
Hyperlipidaemias.

Lipantil
Fournier, Irl.; Fournier, UK.
Fenofibrate (p.889·1).
Hyperlipidaemias.

Liparison *Novartis, Spain.*
Fenofibrate (p.889·1).
Hyperlipidaemias.

Liparol *Ashbourne, UK.*
Bezafibrate (p.849·1).
Hyperlipidaemias.

Lipaten *Merck, S.Afr.*
Clofibrate (p.859·1); nicotinyl alcohol tartrate
(p.939·3).
Hyperlipidaemias.

Lipavlon *Zeneca, Fr.†*
Clofibrate (p.859·1).
Hyperlipidaemias.

Lipaxan *Italfarmaco, Ital.*
Fluvastatin sodium (p.892·1).
Hypercholesterolaemia.

Lipazil *Douglas, Austral.*
Gemfibrozil (p.896·2).
Hyperlipdaemias.

Lipazym *Bittermedizin, Ger.*
Pancreatin (p.1646·1).
Pancreatic insufficiency.

Lipbalm with Sunscreen *Hyde, Canad.*
Padimate O (p.1518·2).
Sunscreen.

Lipcor
Note. This name is used for preparations of different composition.
Nycomed, Aust.
Fenofibrate (p.889·1).
Hyperlipidaemias.

Carlo Erba, Braz.
Eicosapentaenoic acid (p.949·3); docosahexaenoic
acid (p.949·2).
Hyperlipidaemias; nutritional supplement.

Lipemol *Squibb, Spain.*
Pravastatin sodium (p.957·3).
Hyperlipidaemias.

Lipex *Amrad, Austral.*
Simvastatin (p.969·2).
Hyperlipidaemias.

Lip-Eze *SmithKline Beecham Consumer, Austral.*
SPF 15+: Octinoxate (p.1517·3); avobenzone
(p.1517·1).
Dry, cracked, and chapped lips; sunscreen.

Lipidal *Pharmabest, Israel.*
Pravastatin sodium (p.957·3).
Hypercholesterolaemia.

Lipidavit *Rodisma, Ger.*
Garlic (p.1614·1); alpha tocoferil acetate (p.1394·1);
lecithin (p.1628·1).
Hyperlipidaemias.

Lipidax *UCB, Ital.*
Fenofibrate (p.889·1).
Hyperlipidaemias.

Lipidem *Braun, Switz.*
Soya oil (p.1378·1).
Contains egg lecithin.
Lipid infusion for parenteral nutrition.

Lipiderm *Chauvin, Fr.*
Moisturiser.
Dry skin disorders.

Lipidil
Fournier, Canad.; Fournier, Ger.; Schering-Plough, Mex.
Fenofibrate (p.889·1).
Hyperlipidaemias.

Lipidys *Medifive, Thai.*
Gemfibrozil (p.896·2).
Hyperlipidaemias.

Lipikar *Roche-Posay, Irl.*
Emollient.
Dry skin; psoriasis.

Lipilim *Atlantic, Hong Kong.*
Clofibrate (p.859·1).
Hyperlipidaemias.

Lipiodol
Sanova, Aust.†; Mallinckrodt, Austral.; Codali, Belg.; Guerbet, Braz.;
Guerbet, Denm.; Guerbet, Fr.; Guerbet, Ger.; Guerbet, Israel; Guer-
bet, Ital.; Guerbet, Neth.†; Guerbet, Norw.; Aventis, NZ; Guerbet,
Port.; May & Baker, UK.
Iodised oil (p.1034·1).
Radiographic contrast medium.

Lipirex *Irex, Fr.*
Fenofibrate (p.889·1).
Hyperlipidaemias.

Lipiscor *Sanum-Kehlbeck, Ger.*
Marine fish oil (p.949·3).
Hyperlipidaemias.

Lipison *Unison, Thai.*
Gemfibrozil (p.896·2).
Hyperlipidaemias.

Lipisorb
Mead Johnson, Austral.; Mead Johnson Nutritionals, Canad.†; Mead
Johnson Nutritionals, Thai.; Mead Johnson Nutritionals, USA.
Food for special diets (p.1350·1).
Fat malabsorption.

Lipitor
Parke, Davis, Austral.; Parke, Davis, Belg.; Parke, Davis, Canad.;
Parke, Davis, Fin.; Pfizer, Fin.; Parke, Davis, Hong Kong; Parke, Davis,
Irl.; Parke, Davis, Israel; Warner-Lambert, Ital.; Parke, Davis, Mex.;
Parke, Davis, Neth.; Pfizer, Norw.; Parke, Davis, NZ; Parke, Davis,
S.Afr.; Parke, Davis, Singapore; Pfizer, Singapore; Parke, Davis, Swed.;
Pfizer, Swed.; Warner-Lambert, Thai.; Parke, Davis, UK; Parke, Davis,
USA; Pfizer, USA.
Atorvastatin calcium (p.842·3).
Hypercholesterolaemia.

Lipitrol *Julphar, UAE.*
Bezafibrate (p.849·1).
Hyperlipidaemias.

Lipivas *Merck Sharp & Dohme, Denm.†*
Lovastatin (p.922·3).
Hypercholesterolaemia.

Liplat *Esteve, Spain.*
Pravastatin sodium (p.957·3).
Hyperlipidaemias.

Liple *Yoshitomi, Jpn.*
Alprostadil (p.1439·3).
*Maintenance of patent ductus arteriosus; mesenteric
arterial portography; peripheral vascular disorders;
skin ulcers.*

Lipmagik *Reese, USA.*
Benzocaine (p.1306·2); phenol (p.1152·3); alcohol
(p.1130·3).

Lipo Cordes *Ichthyol, Ger.*
Allantoin (p.1110·1); dexpanthenol (p.1602·3); ethyl
linoleate.
Skin disorders.

Lipo Sol *Widmer, Switz.*
Triclosan (p.1159·2).
Acne; seborrhoea.

Lipoabsorver *Neves, Port.*
Poliglusam; vitamin C.
Hypercholesterolaemia; slimming aid.

Lipobalsamo *Teofarma, Ital.*
Eucalyptol (p.1609·2); guaiacol (p.1092·1).
Respiratory-tract disorders.

Lipobase
Yamanouchi, Irl.; Yamanouchi, NZ; Yamanouchi, UK.
Emollient.
Skin disorders; vehicle for Locoid Lipocream.

Lipobay
Bayer, Aust.†; Bayer, Austral.†; Bayer, Belg†; Bayer, Denm.†; Bayer,
Fin.†; Bayer, Ger.†; Bayer, Irl.†; Bayer, Ital.†; Bayer, Neth.†; Bayer,
Norw.†; Bayer, Port.†; Bayer, Singapore†; Bayer, Spain†; Bayer,
Swed.†; Bayer, Switz.†; Bayer, Thai.†; Bayer, UK†.
Cerivastatin sodium (p.856·1).
Hypercholesterolaemia.

Lipocal *Mex-America, Mex.*
Calcium hydroxide (p.1588·3).

Lipochol
Note. This name is used for preparations of different composition.
Takeda, Hong Kong.
Orotic acid (p.1645·1); thioctic acid amide (p.1671·3);
turmeric (p.1029·3); methionine (p.1012·2); vitamin B
substances; vitamin C (p.1350·1); inositol (p.1623·3).
Liver disorders.

Takeda, Ital.
Orotic acid (p.1645·1); thioctic acid amide (p.1671·3);
methionine (p.1012·2); vitamin B substances; vitamin
C (p.1350·1); inositol (p.1623·3).
Liver disorders.

Lipocin *Kener, Mex.*
Bezafibrate (p.849·1).

Lipoclar *Crinos, Ital.*
Fenofibrate (p.889·1).
Hyperlipidaemias.

Lipoclin
Kwizda, Aust.†; Sumitomo, Jpn.
Clinofibrate (p.859·1).
Hyperlipidaemias.

Lipocol *Merz, Ger.*
Colestyramine (p.864·1).
Hypercholesterolaemia.

Lipodel *Synthelabo, Ital.†*
Pantethine (p.952·1).
Lipid disorders.

Lipoenergy *Farma Energy, Ital.*
Choline; inositol; methionine; carnitine; vitamin B$_6$
(p.1350·1).
Nutritional supplement.

Lipofacton *Akzo, Braz.*
Clofibrate (p.859·1); nicotinyl alcohol tartrate
(p.939·3).
Hyperlipidaemias.

Lipofen *Vitoria, Port.†.*
Fenofibrate (p.889·1).
Hyperlipidaemias.

Lipofene *Teofarma, Ital.*
Fenofibrate (p.889·1).
Hyperlipidaemias.

Lipoflavonoid *Numark, USA.*
Multivitamin preparation with lemon bioflavonoids (p.1611·1)(p.1350·1).

Lipofor *Remedica, Singapore.*
Gemfibrozil (p.896·2).
Hyperlipidaemias.

Lipofren *Abella, Spain.*
Lovastatin (p.922·3).
Atherosclerosis; hypercholesterolaemia.

Lipofundin
Braun, Aust.; Braun, Denm.†; Braun, UK.
Soya oil (p.1378·1).
Lipid infusion for parenteral nutrition.

Lipofundin MCT
Braun, Ger.; Braun, Ital.; Braun, Switz.
Soya oil (p.1378·1); medium-chain triglycerides (p.1372·1).
Contains egg phospholipids.
Lipid infusion for parenteral nutrition.

Lipofundin MCT/LCT
Braun, Hong Kong; Braun, Israel; Omnimed, S.Afr.; Braun, Singapore; Braun, Thai.; Braun, UK.
Soya oil (p.1378·1); medium-chain triglycerides (p.1372·1).
Contains egg lecithin.
Lipid infusion for parenteral nutrition.

Lipofundin mit MCT *Braun, Aust.*
Soya oil (p.1378·1); medium-chain triglycerides (p.1372·1).
Contains egg phospholipid.
Lipid infusion for parenteral nutrition.

Lipofundin N *Braun, Ger.*
Soya oil (p.1378·1).
Contains egg phospholipid.
Lipid infusion for parenteral nutrition.

Lipofundin S
Braun, Braz.; Braun, Irl.†; Braun, Ital.; Braun, Thai.
Soya oil (p.1378·1).
Lipid infusion for parenteral nutrition.

Lipofundina MCT/LCT
Braun, Port.; Braun, Spain.
Soya oil (p.1378·1); medium-chain triglycerides (p.1372·1).
Contains egg lecithin.
Lipid infusion for parenteral nutrition.

Lipogen
Note.This name is used for preparations of different composition.
Ibirn, USA.
Gemfibrozil (p.896·2).
Hyperlipidaemias.

Goldline, USA.
Vitamin B substances (p.1350·1).
It may also contain vitamin C.

Lipogis *Agis, Israel.*
Cerivastatin sodium (p.856·1).
Hypercholesterolaemia.

Lipograsil *Uriach, Spain.*
Cynara (p.1601·3); cascara (p.1216·1); phenol-phthalein (p.1244·1); bladderwrack (p.1585·2).
Formerly contained cynara, cascara, phenolphthalein, bladderwrack, caffeine citrate, thyroid extract, magnesium chloride, and sodium bicarbonate.
Obesity.

Lipoicin
Takeda, Hong Kong; Takeda, Thai.
Thioctic acid (p.1671·3).
Liver disorders.

Lipoite *Helfarma, Port.*
Gemfibrozil (p.896·2).
Hyperlipidaemias.

Lipolan *Orion, Fin.*
Emollient.
Dry skin disorders.

Lipolest *Ardern, UK.*
Ispaghula (p.1229·1); guar gum (p.323·3).
Hypercholesterolaemia.

Lipoleum *SFD, Port.*
Emollient.
Barrier preparation; skin disorders.

Lipolotion *Spirig, Singapore.*
Emollient and moisturiser.
Dry skin disorders.

Lipomax *Makros, Braz.*
Fenproporex hydrochloride (p.1510·2).
Obesity.

Lipomega *Nutri-Well, Hong Kong.*
Omega-3 marine triglycerides (p.949·3).
Hypercholesterolaemia.

Lipo-Merz
Kolassa, Aust.; Merz, Ger.; Merz, Hong Kong; Medinfar, Port.; Merz, Singapore; Merz, Switz.
Etofibrate (p.888·2).
Hyperlipidaemias.

Lipomul *Roberts, USA.*
High calorie preparation containing maize oil for enteral nutrition (p.1350·1)(p.1371·2).

Liponet *UCB, Spain.*
Pantethine (p.952·1).
Hyperlipidaemias.

Liponol *Rugby, USA.*
Vitamin B substances with methionine (p.1350·1).

Liponorm *Gentili, Ital.*
Simvastatin (p.969·2).
Coronary arteriosclerosis; hypercholesterolaemia; ischaemic heart disease.

Lipopharm N *Pharmasan, Ger.*
Soya phospholipid (p.1378·1).
Hypercholesterolaemia.

Liporon *General Drugs, Thai.*
Choline bitartrate (p.1356·3); inositol (p.1623·3); methionine (p.1012·2); vitamin B substances (p.1350·1).
Liver disorders.

Liposcler *CEPA, Spain.*
Lovastatin (p.922·3).
Atherosclerosis; hypercholesterolaemia.

Liposic *Mann, Ger.*
Carbomer (p.1499·2).
Dry eyes.

Liposit *Merz, Ger.†.*
Sitosterol (p.970·3).
Hyperlipidaemias.

Liposom *Fidia, Ital.*
Hypothalamic phospholipids (p.1631·2).
Neuroendocrine disorders.

Liposperse *Summit, Port.†.*
Vegetable lipids.
Adjunct in cholecystography.

Lipostabil
Note.This name is used for preparations of different composition.
Rhone-Poulenc Rorer, Ger.
Essential phospholipids.
Lipid disorders.

Rhone-Poulenc Rorer, Hong Kong.
Essential phospholipids; vitamins (p.1350·1); theophylline (p.777·2).
Hyperlipidaemias; thromboembolic disorders; vascular disorders.

Rhone-Poulenc Rorer, Ital.
Phosphatidyl choline (p.1651·1).
Fat emboli; hyperlipidaemias.

Aventis, S.Afr.
Capsules: Essential phospholipids; multivitamins (p.1350·1); theophylline (p.777·2).
Injection: Essential phospholipids; multivitamins (p.1350·1); adenosine phosphate (p.1573·3).
Atherosclerosis; diabetic angiopathies; hyperlipidaemias; thromboembolism prophylaxis.

Lipostat
Note.This name is used for preparations of different composition.
Bristol-Myers Squibb, Irl.; Bristol-Myers Squibb, Israel; Bristol-Myers Squibb, NZ; Bristol-Myers Squibb, UK.
Pravastatin sodium (p.957·3).
Atherosclerosis; hypercholesterolaemia; myocardial infarction; stroke prophylaxis.

Del Saz & Filippini, Ital.†.
A heparinoid (p.905·2).
Thrombosis prophylaxis.

Liposterol *Vita, Spain.*
Cerivastatin sodium (p.856·1).
Hypercholesterolaemia.

Lipostop *Francia, Ital.†.*
A heparinoid (p.905·2).
Thrombosis prophylaxis.

Liposyn
Abbott, Denm.; Abbott, Fin.; Abbott, Israel; Abbott, Ital.; Abbott, Mex.; Abbott, Swed.
Safflower oil (p.1375·1); soya oil (p.1378·1).
Contains egg phosphatides.
Lipid infusion for parenteral nutrition.

Liposyn II *Abbott, USA.*
Safflower oil (p.1375·1); soya oil (p.1378·1).
Contains egg phospholipids.
Lipid infusion for parenteral nutrition.

Liposyn III *Abbott, USA.*
Soya oil (p.1378·1).
Contains egg phospholipids.
Lipid infusion for parenteral nutrition.

Lipotalon *Merckle, Ger.*
Dexamethasone palmitate (p.1067·3).
Rheumatic disorders.

Lipoton *Basi, Port.*
Choline; inositol; methionine (p.1350·1).

Lipotrend Cholesterol *Roche Diagnostics, Ital.*
Test for cholesterol in blood.

Lipotriad *Numark, USA.*
Multivitamin and mineral preparation (p.1350·1).

Lipotropic Factors *Solgar, USA.*
Choline bitartrate (p.1356·3); inositol (p.1623·3); methionine (p.1012·2).
Dietary supplement.

Lipoven *Fresenius Kabi, Fr.*
Soya oil (p.1378·1).
Contains egg lecithin.
Lipid infusion for parenteral nutrition.

Lipovenoes
Fresenius, Belg.†; Alpha, Mex.; Fresenius Kabi, Port.; Fresenius Kabi, S.Afr.
Soya oil (p.1378·1).
Contains egg lecithin.
Lipid infusion for parenteral nutrition.

Lipovenos
Fresenius Kabi, Aust.; Fresenius, Braz.; Fresenius Kabi, Denm.; Fresenius Kabi, Ger.; SIFRA, Ital.; Fresenius Kabi, Norw.; Fresenius Kabi,
Spain; Fresenius Kabi, Swed.; Fresenius Kabi, Switz.; Fresenius, Thai.; Fresenius, UK†.
Fractionated soya oil (p.1378·1).
Contains egg lecithin.
Lipid infusion for parenteral nutrition.

Lipovenos MCT *Fresenius Kabi, Ger.*
Soya oil (p.1378·1); medium-chain triglycerides (p.1372·1).
Contains egg phospholipid.
Lipid infusion for parenteral nutrition.

Lipovit *Brunel, S.Afr.*
Multivitamin preparation (p.1350·1).

Lipovitan *Medphano, Ger.*
Choline bitartrate (p.1356·3); dexpanthenol (p.1602·3); myo-inositol (p.1623·3); methionine (p.1012·2); vitamin B substances (p.1350·1); alpha tocoferil acetate (p.1394·1).
Liver disorders.

Lipovitasi-Or *Atlantis, Mex.*
Carnitine orotate (p.1385·1); thiamine nitrate (p.1385·1); DL-methionine (p.1012·2).
Liver disorders.

Lipox *TAD, Ger.*
Bezafibrate (p.849·1).
Hyperlipidaemias.

Lipozid *Searle, Ital.*
Gemfibrozil (p.896·2).
Hyperlipidaemias.

Lipozil *M & H, Thai.*
Gemfibrozil (p.896·2).
Hyperlipidaemias.

Lipraken *Kener, Mex.*
Enalapril (p.883·3).

Lipram *Global, USA.*
Pancrelipase (p.1647·2).
Pancreatic insufficiency.

Liprevil *Schwarz, Ger.; Sanol, Ger.*
Pravastatin sodium (p.957·3).
Hyperlipidaemias.

Lipril *Merck, Port.*
Lisinopril (p.921·1).
Heart failure; hypertension.

Liprocil *Nestle, Fr.*
Medium-chain triglycerides (p.1372·1); vitamins (p.1350·1).
Nutritional supplement.

Lip-Sed
Note.This name is used for preparations of different composition.
Parke, Davis, Austral.
Medicated stick: Octinoxate (p.1517·3); oxybenzone (p.1518·1); avobenzone (p.1517·1).
Chapped, cracked, or blistered lips; sunscreen.

Warner-Lambert, Austral.†.
Topical gel: Padimate O (p.1518·2).
Dry, cracked, or chapped lips; sunscreen.

Lipshield Lipbalm *Mentholatum, Canad.*
SPF 21: Padimate O (p.1518·2); octinoxate (p.1517·3); oxybenzone (p.1518·1).
Sunscreen.

Lipsin
Nycomed, Aust.; Caber, Ital.; Aventis, S.Afr.
Fenofibrate (p.889·1).
Hyperlipidaemias.

Lipur *Parke, Davis, Fr.*
Gemfibrozil (p.896·2).
Hyperlipidaemias.

Lipus *BA Farma, Port.*
Lovastatin (p.922·3).
Hypercholesterolaemia.

Liqiprin *SmithKline Beecham, Israel.*
Paracetamol (p.71·2).
Fever; pain.

Liquemin
Roche, Aust.; Roche, Ital.
Heparin (p.902·1) or heparin sodium (p.902·1).
Thromboembolic disorders.

Liquemin N *Roche, Ger.*
Heparin sodium (p.902·1).
Thromboembolic disorders.

Liquemine
Roche, Belg.; Roche, Braz.; Roche, Switz.
Heparin sodium (p.902·1).
Hyperlipidaemias; thromboembolic disorders.

Liqfruta Cough Medicine *LRC Products, UK†.*
Ipecacuanha (p.1093·1); menthol (p.1632·3); glucose (p.1364·1).
Coughs.

Liqfruta Garlic Cough Medicine *Pfizer Consumer, UK.*
Garlic oil; guaifenesin (p.1092·2).
Coughs.

Liquibid *Capellon, USA.*
Guaifenesin (p.1092·2).

Liquibid-D *Capellon, USA.*
Guaifenesin (p.1092·2); phenylephrine hydrochloride (p.1097·1).
Upper respiratory-tract symptoms.

Liquicard *Duopharm, Ger.†.*
Crataegus (p.1600·2).
Circulatory disorders; heart failure.

Liqui-Char
Oxford Pharmaceuticals, UK; Jones, USA.
Activated charcoal (p.1000·2).
Emergency treatment of poisoning.

Liquid Antacid *Pennex, Israel.*
Magnesium hydroxide (p.1233·1); aluminium hydroxide (p.1210·3).
Gastrointestinal hyperacidity; heartburn.

Liquid Antacid Plus Simethicon *Pennex, Israel.*
Magnesium hydroxide (p.1233·1); aluminium hydroxide (p.1210·3); simeticone (p.1249·2).
Flatulence; gastrointestinal hyperacidity; heartburn.

Liquid B Complex *Jamieson, Canad.†.*
Vitamin B substances (p.1350·1).

Liquid Pred *Muro, USA.*
Prednisone (p.1079·2).
Corticosteroid.

Liquid Soap Pre-Op *Pharmacia Upjohn, Austral.*
Triclosan (p.1159·2).
Skin cleansing.

Liquidepur *Woelm, Ger.*
Senna (p.1248·2).
Constipation.

Liquidorm N *Hanosan, Ger.*
Homoeopathic preparation.

Liqui-Doss *Ferndale, USA.*
Liquid paraffin (p.1407·1).
Constipation.

Liquifer
Note.This name is used for preparations of different composition.
Abbott, Aust.; Abbott, Ital.; Abbott, Switz.
Ferrous polystyrene sulfonate.
Ascorbic acid (p.1389·3) or sodium ascorbate (p.1390·1) is included in this preparation to increase the absorption and availability of iron.
Iron-deficiency anaemias.

Abbott, Neth.
Ferrous sulfate (p.1360·3).
Iron-deficiency anaemia.

Liquifilm
Allergan, Aust.; Allergan, Austral.; Allergan, Belg.; Allergan, Canad.; Allergan, Fin.; Allergan, Fr.†; Allergan, Ger.; Allergan, Hong Kong; Allergan, Irl.; Allergan, Neth.†; Allergan, NZ; Allergan, Port.; Allergan, Switz.; Allergan, USA.
Polyvinyl alcohol (p.1503·1) (p.1129·2).
Dry eyes; wetting and lubricating solution for contact lenses.

Liquifilm Lagrimas *Allergan, Spain.*
Polyvinyl alcohol (p.1503·1).
Dry eyes.

Liquifilm Tears
Allergan, Israel; Allergan, S.Afr.; Allergan, Singapore; Allergan, Thai.; Allergan, UK.
Polyvinyl alcohol (p.1503·1) (p.1129·2).
Dry eyes; lubricant for hard contact lenses.

Liquifilm Wetting
Allergan, Israel; Allergan, Spain.
Wetting solution for hard contact lenses (p.1129·2).

Liquifresh *Allergan, Spain.*
Polyvinyl alcohol (p.1503·1); povidone (p.1503·2) (p.1129·2).
Contact lens discomfort; dry eyes.

Liquigen
Scientific Hospital Supplies, Austral.; Nutricia, Fin.; SHS, Fr.; Scientific Hospital Supplies, Irl.; Nutricia, NZ; Scientific Hospital Supplies, NZ; SHS, Singapore; Scientific Hospital Supplies, UK.
Medium-chain triglycerides (p.1372·1).
Food for special diets.

Liquigesic Co *Paedpharm, Austral.*
Paracetamol (p.71·2); codeine phosphate (p.25·2).
Pain.

Liqui-Histine DM *Liquipharm, USA†.*
Dextromethorphan hydrobromide (p.1087·1); phenylpropanolamine hydrochloride (p.1098·1); brompheniramine maleate (p.410·2).
Upper respiratory-tract symptoms.

Liquimat *Healthpoint, USA.*
Sulfur (p.1123·3).
Acne; oily skin.

Liquipake *Lafayette, USA.*
Barium sulfate (p.1032·1).
Contrast medium for gastrointestinal radiography.

Liquipom Dexa Antib *Iquinosa, Spain.*
Dexamethasone sodium phosphate (p.1067·1); neomycin sulfate (p.228·1); polymyxin B sulfate (p.238·1).
Infected eye and ear disorders.

Liquipom Dexa Const *Iquinosa, Spain.*
Dexamethasone sodium phosphate (p.1067·1); phenylephrine hydrochloride (p.1097·1).
Eye disorders.

Liquipom Dexamida *Iquinosa, Spain.*
Dexamethasone sodium phosphate (p.1067·1); phenylephrine hydrochloride (p.1097·1); sulfacetamide sodium (p.250·3).
Infected eye disorders.

Liquipom Medrisone *Iquinosa, Spain.*
Medrysone (p.1075·3).
Eye disorders.

Liquiprin *Menley & James, USA.*
Paracetamol (p.71·2).
Fever; pain.

Liquirit N *Loges, Ger.*
Algeldrate (p.1210·3); magnesium carbonate (p.1232·3); liquorice (p.1231·2).
Gastrointestinal disorders.

Liquisorbon MCT *Nutricia, Irl.†.*
Gluten-free, fructose-free, low-lactose food for special diets (p.1350·1).

Liroken Kendrick, Mex.
Diclofenac sodium (p.30·3).
Gout; musculoskeletal and joint disorders.

Lis Lisapharma, Ital.
Lactulose (p.1230·1).
Constipation; disturbances of the gastrointestinal flora; hepatic cirrhosis; hepatic encephalopthy.

Lisa Lisapharma, Ital.
Cefonicid sodium (p.168·1).
Lignocaine [lidocaine] hydrochloride (p.1313·2) is included in the intramuscular injection to alleviate the pain of injection.
Bacterial infections.

Lisacef Lisapharma, Ital.
Cefradine (p.173·3).
Lignocaine [lidocaine] hydrochloride (p.1313·2) is included in the intramuscular injection to alleviate the pain of injection.
Bacterial infections.

Lisador Farmasa, Braz.
Dipyrone (p.34·1); promethazine (p.423·2); adiphenine.
Smooth muscle spasm.

Lisaglucon Farmasa, Braz.
Glibenclamide (p.321·3).
Diabetes mellitus.

Lisal Pharmacia, Swed.†
Sodium chloride (p.1196·1).
Contact lens care; eye wash.

Lisanirc Lisapharma, Ital.
Nicardipine hydrochloride (p.938·3).
Angina pectoris; heart failure; hypertension.

Lisapres Libbs, Braz.
Guanabenz acetate (p.900·2).
Hypertension.

Lisaspin Euro-Labor, Port.; Grunenthal, Port.
Lysine aspirin (p.50·3).
Fever; pain.

Lisbak Savio, Ital.
A *Bacillus subtilis* preparation.
Gastrointestinal disorders.

Lisedema Climax, Braz.
Piroxicam (p.79·1).
Dysmenorrhoea; gout; musculoskeletal, joint, and peri-articular disorders.

Lisenteral Lisapharma, Ital.
Lysates of various *Escherichia coli* strains and other coliform bacteria.
Colibacilliary gastrointestinal and genito-urinary infections.

Liserdol
Wyeth, Ger.; Pharmacia Upjohn, Hong Kong; Pharmacia Upjohn, Ital.; Pharmacia Upjohn, S.Afr.†; Pharmacia Upjohn, Singapore; Wyeth, Switz.
Metergoline (p.1175·1).
Gastric motility disorders; lactation inhibition; menstrual disorders; migraine.

Lisigamma Worwag, Ger.
Lisinopril (p.921·1).
Heart failure; hypertension.

Lisigon Ofimex, Mex.
Danazol (p.1468·3).

Lisihexal Hexal, Ger.
Lisinopril (p.921·1).
Heart failure; hypertension; myocardial infarction.

Lisil KBR, Ital.
Carbocisteine (p.1086·3).
Respiratory-tract disorders associated with increased or viscous mucus.

Lisin Sorb Nikkho, Braz.
Lysine (p.1370·3); vitamin B substances (p.1350·1).
Tonic.

Lisino Essex, Ger.
Loratadine (p.420·1).
Hypersensitivity reactions.

Lisinvitan Quimioterapica, Braz.
Buclizine (p.411·1); lysine; tryptophan; vitamin B₆; vitamin B₁₂ (p.1350·1).
Reduced appetite; tonic.

Lisiofer Garant, Ital.
Ferric sodium gluconate (p.1360·2).
Anaemia.

Lisipril Orion, Fin.
Lisinopril (p.921·1).
Heart failure; hypertension; myocardial infarction.

Lisipril Comp Orion, Fin.
Lisinopril (p.921·1); hydrochlorothiazide (p.907·3).
Hypertension.

Liskantin Desitin, Ger.
Primidone (p.363·3).
Epilepsy.

Liskonum SmithKline Beecham, UK.
Lithium carbonate (p.292·1).
Bipolar disorder; mania.

Lismol Lesvi, Spain.
Colestyramine (p.864·1).
Hyperlipidaemias.

Lisodren Bristol-Myers Squibb, Braz.
Mitotane (p.559·2).
Adrenal cortex cancer; Cushing's syndrome.

Lisodur Alphapharm, Austral.
Lisinopril (p.921·1).
Heart failure; hypertension.

Lisodura Merck dura, Ger.
Lisinopril (p.921·1).
Heart failure; hypertension; myocardial infarction.

Lisofenicol IMA, Braz.
Chloramphenicol (p.179·1); muramidase hydrochloride (p.1638·1); hydroxyquinoline sulfate (p.1622·2); boric acid (p.1586·1); glucose (p.1364·1).
Vulvovaginal disorders.

Lisoflu Sanofi Synthelabo, Ital.
Paracetamol(p.71·2); ascorbic acid (p.1389·3); pseudoephedrine hydrochloride (p.1099·2); dextromethorphan hydrobromide (p.1087·3).
Cold symptoms.

Lisolac Tecnimede, Port.
Tilactase (p.1673·2).
Digestive disorders.

Lisomalen Varos, Braz.
Magnesium oxide (p.1233·2); vitamin B₆ (p.1386·3).
Renal calculi.

Lisomucil Sanofi Synthelabo, Ital.
Carbocisteine (p.1086·3).
Respiratory-tract disorders.

Lisomucil Gola Sanofi Synthelabo, Ital.
Dequalinium chloride (p.1143·1); enoxolone (p.34·3).
Mouth and throat disorders.

Lisomucin Cipan, Port.
Bromhexine hydrochloride (p.1085·3).
Coughs.

Lisopride Sanofi Synthelabo, Port.
Sulpiride (p.706·1).

Lisopulm Esseti, Ital.
Ambroxol hydrochloride (p.1084·3).
Respiratory-tract disorders.

Lisoquinol IMA, Braz.
Muramidase hydrochloride (p.1638·1); furazolidone (p.592·1); hydroxyquinoline sulfate (p.1622·2); boric acid (p.1586·1).
Vulvovaginal disorders.

Lisorane Zeneca, Mex.
Isoflurane (p.1261·1).
General anaesthesia.

Lisotox Synthelabo, Braz.
Acetylmethionine; choline citrate (p.1356·3); cyanocobalamin (p.1388·1).
Liver disorders.

Lisotrex Profarb, Braz.
Erythromycin (p.201·2).
Bacterial infections.

Lispril Siam Bheasach, Thai.
Lisinopril (p.921·1).
Hypertension.

Listerfluor Parke, Davis, S.Afr.
Sodium fluoride (p.1375·3).
Dental caries prophylaxis.

Listerine
Note.This name is used for preparations of different composition.
Warner-Lambert, Canad.
Eucalyptol (p.1609·2); thymol (p.1158·3); menthol (p.1632·3).
Dental plaque prophylaxis; oral hygiene.

Warner-Lambert, Irl.†; Warner-Lambert, Port.; Warner-Lambert, USA.
Eucalyptol (p.1609·2); menthol (p.1632·3); methyl salicylate (p.55·1); thymol (p.1158·3).
Dental plaque prophylaxis; oral hygiene.

Warner-Lambert, NZ.
Benzoic acid (p.1134·2); eucalyptol (p.1609·2); thymol (p.1158·3).
Oral hygiene.

Listerine Antiseptic Mouthwash Warner-Lambert, UK.
Eucalyptol (p.1609·2); menthol (p.1632·3); methyl salicylate (p.55·1); thymol (p.1158·3).
Oral hygiene.

Listermint Warner-Lambert, UK.
Cetylpyridinium chloride (p.1138·1); zinc chloride (p.1398·1).
Oral hygiene.

Listermint Arctic Mint Mouthwash Warner-Wellcome, USA.
Glycerol (p.1616·3).

Listermint with Fluoride
Warner-Lambert, Irl.†; Warner-Lambert, UK.
Sodium fluoride (p.1375·3); cetylpyridinium chloride (p.1138·1).
Dental plaque prophylaxis; oral hygiene.

Listran Uriach, Spain.
Nabumetone (p.59·3).
Osteoarthritis; rheumatoid arthritis.

Lisvifar Farcoral, Mex.
Multivitamin preparation (p.1350·1).

Lit-300 Hua, Thai.
Lithium carbonate (p.292·1).
Bipolar disorder.

Litalgin Leiras, Fin.
Dipyrone (p.34·1); pitofenone hydrochloride (p.1652·3).
Gastrointestinal, biliary, and renal colic.

Litalir
Bristol-Myers Squibb, Ger.; Bristol-Myers Squibb, Switz.
Hydroxyurea [hydroxycarbamide] (p.544·2).
Malignant neoplasms.

Litarek Ipsen, Braz.
Gemfibrozil (p.896·2).
Hyperlipidaemias.

Litarex
Dumex-Alpharma, Denm.; Astra, Norw.†; Astra, Swed.†; Dumex, Switz.; Dumex, UK†.
Lithium citrate (p.292·1).
Bipolar disorder; mania.

Lithane Pfizer, Canad.
Lithium carbonate (p.292·1).
Bipolar disorder.

Litheum Valdecasas, Mex.
Lithium carbonate (p.292·1).
Bipolar disorder.

Lithiabyl Plantes et Medecines, Fr.†
Berberis vulgaris; urtica (p.1678·2); taraxacum (p.1669·1).
Formerly contained berberis and methenamine.
Digestive disorders.

Lithiagel Cochon, Fr.†
Basic aluminium carbonate (p.1210·2).
Diagnosis of hyperparathyroidism; hyperphosphataemia.

Lithias-cyl N Ho-Len-Complex Liebermann, Ger.
Homoeopathic preparation.

Lithicarb
Rhone-Poulenc Rorer, Austral.; Fisons, Hong Kong; Pacific, Hong Kong; Pacific, NZ.
Lithium carbonate (p.292·1).
Bipolar disorder; depression; mania.

Lithiofor
Vifor, Hong Kong; Vifor, Switz.
Lithium sulfate (p.296·2).
Bipolar disorders; depression.

Lithionit
AstraZeneca, Norw.; Astra, Swed.
Lithium sulfate (p.296·2).
Bipolar disorder; mania.

Lithiumeel Peithner, Aust.
Homoeopathic preparation.

Lithizine Technilab, Canad.†
Lithium carbonate (p.292·1).
Bipolar disorder.

Lithobid Solvay, USA.
Lithium carbonate (p.292·1).
Bipolar disorder.

Lithofalk
Merck, Aust.; Falk, Ger.; Phardi, Switz.; Thames, UK†.
Chenodeoxycholic acid (p.1594·1); ursodeoxycholic acid (p.1677·2).
Adjunct to lithotripsy; gallstones.

Lithonate
Approved Prescription Services, UK; Solvay, USA†.
Lithium carbonate (p.292·1).
Bipolar disorder; depression; mania.

Lithostat Mission Pharmacal, USA.
Acetohydroxamic acid (p.1571·3).
Adjunct in urinary-tract infection with urea-splitting organisms.

Lithosun Sun, Singapore.
Lithium carbonate (p.292·1).
Bipolar disorder.

Lithotabs Solvay, USA†.
Lithium carbonate (p.292·1).
Bipolar disorder; mania.

Lithurex Phonix, Ger.
Pyridoxine hydrochloride; magnesium citrate (p.1232·3); citric acid (p.1596·2); sodium citrate (p.1186·2); potassium citrate (p.1186·1).
Urinary-tract disorders.

Litiax Novag, Spain.
Quercus infectoria (p.1613·1).
Renal calculi.

Litican
Sanofi Synthelabo, Belg.; Lorex Synthelabo, Neth.†
Alizapride hydrochloride (p.1209·3).
Nausea; vomiting.

Litiocar Biosintetica, Braz.
Lithium carbonate (p.292·1).
Bipolar disorder; depression; migraine and other vascular headaches; neutropenia; schizophrenia.

Lito Orion, Fin.
Lithium carbonate (p.292·1).
Bipolar disorder.

Litobile Poli, Ital.†
Magnesium trihydrate salt of chenodeoxycholic (p.1594·1) and ursodeoxycholic acids (p.1677·2).
Biliary dyspepsia; gallstones.

Litoff Caber, Ital.
Ursodeoxycholic acid (p.1677·2).
Biliary-tract disorders.

Litosmil Evans, Fr.†
Diosmin (p.1611·1).
Peripheral vascular disorders.

Litoxol Centrapharm, Fr.
Sulfaguanidine (p.253·2); aluminium salicylate.
Infective diarrhoea.

Litrison
Note.This name is used for preparations of different composition.
Klinger, Braz.
Cynara (p.1601·3); solanum paniculatum; boldo (p.1585·3); choline bitartrate (p.1356·3); magnesium sulfate (p.1191·2).
Liver disorders.

Roche, Ital.
Alpha tocoferil acetate; vitamin B substances (p.1350·1).
Formerly contained choline bitartrate, DL-methionine, and vitamin B substances.

Litursol Crinos, Ital.
Ursodeoxycholic acid (p.1677·2).
Biliary-tract disorders.

Liv 52 Ebi, Switz.
Capparis spinosa; cichorium intybus; solanum nigrum; cassia occidentalis; terminalia arjuna; achillea millefolium; tamarix gallica; ferrum bhasma.
Gastrointestinal disorders; tonic.

Livadex Restan, S.Afr.
Vitamin B substances; liver extracts; caffeine (p.1350·1).
Tonic.

Livaid Lagamed, S.Afr.†
Vitamin B substances; liver extracts (p.1350·1).
Tonic.

Livamine Bioceuticals, UK.
Multivitamin and mineral preparation (p.1350·1).

Liv-Detox Blackmores, Austral.
DL-Methionine (p.1012·2); choline bitartrate (p.1356·3); inositol (p.1623·3); levoglutamide (p.1365·2); pyridoxine hydrochloride (p.1386·3); riboflavin (p.1386·1); sodium sulfate (p.1250·1).
Liver disorders.

Liver Tonic Capsules Vitaglow, Austral.
Silybum marianum (p.1021·3).
Dyspepsia; stress.

Liver Tonic Herbal Formula 6 Vitelle, Austral.
Silybum marianum (p.1021·3); taraxacum (p.1669·1); cynara (p.1601·3); garlic (p.1614·1).
Digestive disorders; liver tonic.

Liverall Sankyo, Hong Kong.
Di-isopropylammonium dichloroacetate (p.874·3); calcium gluconate (p.1188·2).
Liver disorders.

Liverasi Francia, Ital.
Cogalactoisomerase sodium (p.1598·1).
Liver disorders.

Livercrom Byk Elmu, Spain.
Arginine timonacicate (p.1354·1).
Liver disorders.

Liverguard Pharmadass, UK†.
Capparis spinosa; achorium intybus; solanum nigrum; cassia occidentalis; terminalia arjuna; achillea (p.1572·2); tamarix gallica; mandur bhasma.

Livial
Organon, Austral.; Organon, Belg.; Akzo, Braz.; Organon, Denm.; Organon, Fin.; Organon, Hong Kong; Organon, Irl.; Organon, Ital.; Organon, Mex.; Organon, Neth.; Organon, Norw.; Pharmaco, NZ; Organon, Port.; Organon, Singapore; Organon, Swed.; Organon, Switz.; Organon, Thai.; Organon, UK.
Tibolone (p.1495·1).
Menopausal disorders; osteoporosis.

Liviane Compuesto Knoll, Spain†.
Aescin (p.1574·1); thiocolchicoside (p.1330·2).
Musculoskeletal lesions; peripheral vascular disorders.

Liviel Organon, Aust.
Tibolone (p.1495·1).
Menopausal disorders; osteoporosis.

Liviella Organon, Ger.; Nourypharma, Ger.
Tibolone (p.1495·1).
Menopausal disorders.

Livifem Donmed, S.Afr.
Tibolone (p.1495·1).
Menopausal disorders; osteoporosis.

Liviton Restan, S.Afr.
Vitamins; minerals; caffeine; liver extracts (p.1350·1).
Tonic.

Livitrinsic-f Goldline, USA.
Ferrous fumarate (p.1360·1); folic acid (p.1361·1); intrinsic factor; vitamin B₁₂ substances (p.1388·1).
Vitamin C (p.1389·3) is included in this preparation to increase the absorption and availability of iron.
Anaemias.

Livocab
Janssen-Cilag, Ger.; Taxandria, Neth.; Janssen-Cilag, Spain.
Levocabastine hydrochloride (p.419·3).
Allergic conjunctivitis; allergic rhinitis.

Livostin
Janssen-Cilag, Aust.; Janssen-Cilag, Austral.; Janssen-Cilag, Belg.; Janssen-Ortho, Canad.; Janssen-Cilag, Denm.; Janssen-Cilag, Fin.; Janssen-Cilag, Israel; Janssen-Cilag, Ital.; Shinyaku, Jpn; Janssen, Mex.; Janssen-Cilag, Norw.; Janssen-Cilag, NZ; Janssen-Cilag, S.Afr.; Janssen-Cilag, Swed.; Janssen-Cilag, Switz.; Ciba Vision, Thai.; Janssen, Thai.; Novartis Ophthalmics, UK; Ciba Vision, USA.
Levocabastine hydrochloride (p.419·3).
Allergic conjunctivitis; allergic rhinitis.

Lixacol Schering-Plough, Spain.
Mesalazine (p.1234·1).
Ulcerative colitis.

Lixidol Roche, Ital.
Ketorolac trometamol (p.48·2).
Pain.

Lixir Abigo, Swed.
Multivitamins (p.1350·1); caffeine.

Lixogan Tocogino, Mex.
Naproxen (p.60·3).

Lizipaina Upsamedica, Spain.
Bacitracin (p.155·2); muramidase (p.1638·1); papain (p.1647·3).
Mouth and throat inflammation.

Lizovag Novag, Mex.
Ketoconazole (p.389·1).
Fungal infections.

LKV-Drops Freeda, USA†.
Multivitamin preparation (p.1350·1).

Llorentecaina Noradrenal *Llorente, Spain.*
Lignocaine [lidocaine] hydrochloride (p.1313·2).
Noradrenaline [norepinephrine] acid tartrate (p.948·2)
is included in this preparation as a vasoconstrictor to
diminish absorption and localise the effect of the local
anaesthetic.
Local anaesthesia.

Lloyd's Cream *SSL, UK.*
Diethylamine salicylate (p.32·2).
Muscular pain.

LM6 *AF, Mex.*
Paracetamol (p.71·2); mepyramine maleate (p.421·1);
phenylephrine hydrochloride (p.1097·1); caffeine
(p.761·3).
Cold symptoms.

Lobac *Seatrace, USA.*
Salicylamide (p.82·1); phenyltoloxamine (p.423·1);
paracetamol (p.71·2).
Musculoskeletal pain.

Lobacin *TO-Chemicals, Thai.*
Neomycin sulfate (p.228·1); bacitracin (p.155·2); amy-
locaine hydrochloride (p.1306·1).
Mouth and throat disorders.

Lobak *Zurich, S.Afr.†.*
Chlormezanone (p.660·1); paracetamol (p.71·2).
Pain; skeletal muscle spasm.

Lobamine-Cysteine
Pierre Fabre, Fr.; Actipharm, Switz.†.
Methionine (p.1012·2); cysteine hydrochloride
(p.1358·3).
Hair and nail disorders.

Lobana *Ulmer, USA.*
Soap-free skin cleanser.

Lobana Body *Ulmer, USA.*
Emollient and moisturiser.

Lobana Derm-Aide *Ulmer, USA.*
Vitamin A (p.1382·1); vitamin D (p.1391·1); vitamin E
(p.1393·3).
Skin disorders.

Lobana Peri-Garde *Ulmer, USA.*
Vitamin A (p.1382·1); vitamin D (p.1391·1); vitamin E
(p.1382·1); chloroxylenol (p.1142·1).
Skin disorders.

Lobelia Composta *Simoes, Braz.*
Grindelia (p.1618·2); lobelia (p.1510·2); mephitis pu-
torius.
Coughs.

Lobelia Compound *Gerard House, UK.*
Lobelia (p.1510·2); gum ammoniacum; squill
(p.1100·3).
Cough and cold symptoms.

Lobelia Med Complex *Dynamit, Aust.*
Homoeopathic preparation.

Lobione *Aventis, Belg.*
Betahistine mesilate (p.1584·3).
Vertigo.

Lobivon *Menarini, Ital.; Menarini, Spain.*
Nebivolol hydrochloride (p.938·2).
Hypertension.

Lobu *Ohara, Jpn.*
Loxoprofen sodium (p.50·2).
Inflammation; pain.

Locabase *Pierre Fabre, Fr.*
Basis for topical preparations.

Locabiosol
Servier, Aust.; Servier, Ger.; Servier, Port.
Fusafungine (p.208·3).
Upper respiratory-tract infections and inflammation.

Locabiotal
*Servier, Belg.; Servier, Braz.; Therval, Fr.; Servier, Hong Kong; Servier,
Irl.; Stroder, Ital.; AF, Mex.; Servier, S.Afr.; Servier, Switz.; Servier, UK.*
Fusafungine (p.208·3).
Upper respiratory-tract infection and inflammation.

Locacid
Pierre Fabre, Fr.; Pierre Fabre, Israel; Pierre Fabre, Port.
Tretinoin (p.1126·2).
Acne; psoriasis.

Locacorten
Note. This name is used for preparations of different composition.
*Ciba, Canad.†; Novartis, Ger.; Novartis, Israel; Novartis, Neth.; No-
vartis, Switz.*
Flumetasone pivalate (p.1070·3).
Skin disorders.

Novartis, Israel.
Cream; ointment: Flumetasone pivalate (p.1070·3); ne-
omycin sulfate (p.228·1).
Skin disorders.

Locacorten med Salicylsyre *Novartis, Denm.*
Flumetasone pivalate (p.1070·3); salicylic acid
(p.1122·3).
Skin disorders.

Locacorten mit Neomycin *Novartis, Aust.*
Flumetasone pivalate (p.1070·3); neomycin sulfate
(p.228·1).
Infected skin disorders.

Locacorten Tar
*Novartis, Aust.; Novartis, Hong Kong; Novartis, Israel; Ciba-Geigy,
S.Afr.†; Max Ritter, Switz.†.*
Flumetasone pivalate (p.1070·3); coal tar (p.1125·1);
salicylic acid (p.1122·3).
Skin disorders.

Locacorten Triclosan *Max Ritter, Switz.†.*
Flumetasone pivalate (p.1070·3); triclosan (p.1159·2).
Infected skin disorders.

Locacorten Vioform
*Novartis, Aust.; Novartis, Austral.; Novartis, Canad.; Novartis,
Denm.; Novartis, Fin.; Novartis, Ger.; Novartis, Neth.; Novartis,
Norw.; Novartis, S.Afr.; Novartis, Swed.*
Flumetasone pivalate (p.1070·3); clioquinol (p.190·2).
External ear disorders; infected skin disorders.

Locacortene *Novartis Consumer, Belg.*
Flumetasone pivalate (p.1070·3).
Skin disorders.

Locacortene Tar *Novartis Consumer, Belg.*
Flumetasone pivalate (p.1070·3); coal tar (p.1125·1);
salicylic acid (p.1122·3).
Skin disorders.

Locacortene Vioforme *Novartis Consumer, Belg.*
Flumetasone pivalate (p.1070·3); clioquinol (p.190·2).
External ear disorders; skin disorders.

Localin *Fischer, Israel.*
Oxybuprocaine hydrochloride (p.1318·1).
Local anaesthesia.

Localone
Pierre Fabre, Fr.; Pierre Fabre, Port.
Triamcinolone acetonide (p.1080·1); salicylic acid
(p.1122·3).
Skin disorders.

Localyn *Recordati, Ital.*
Ear drops: Fluocinolone acetonide (p.1071·1); neomy-
cin sulfate (p.228·1).
Formerly contained fluocinolone acetonide, neomycin
sulfate, polymyxin B sulfate, and ketocaine hydrochlo-
ride.
Ear disorders.
Lotion; ointment; topical solution: Fluocinolone aceto-
nide (p.1071·1).
Skin disorders.
Nasal spray: Fluocinolone acetonide (p.1071·1); clon-
azoline hydrochloride (p.1087·1).
Nasal inflammation and hypersensitivity.

Localyn SV *Recordati, Ital.*
Fluocinolone acetonide (p.1071·1).
Nasal inflammation and hypersensitivity.

Localyn-Neomicina *Recordati, Ital.*
Fluocinolone acetonide (p.1071·1); neomycin sulfate
(p.228·1).
Infected skin disorders.

Locao Mancha Branca *Stevia, Braz.*
Benzoic acid (p.1134·2); iodine (p.1522·3); licor de
Hoffman (alcohol, solvent ether).
Fungal skin disorders.

Locapred
Pierre Fabre, Fr.; Pierre Fabre, Port.; Pierre Fabre, Switz.
Desonide (p.1066·2).
Skin disorders.

Locasalen
*Novartis, Aust.; Novartis Consumer, Belg.; Novartis, Canad.†; No-
vartis, Ger.; Novartis, Hong Kong; Novartis, Israel; Novartis, Neth.;
Novartis, Norw.†; Novartis, Singapore; Ciba-Geigy, Swed.†; Novartis,
Switz.; Novartis, Thai.*
Flumetasone pivalate (p.1070·3); salicylic acid
(p.1122·3).
Skin disorders.

Locaseptil-Neo *Drossapharm, Switz.*
Prednisolone acetate (p.1078·1); cinchocaine
(p.1309·1).
Nasal and buccal lesions.

Locasil *Locatelli, Ital.†.*
Silymarin (p.1021·3).
Liver disorders.

Locasol
Nutricia, Austral.; Baxter, NZ; Nutricia, NZ; Cow & Gate, UK.
Low-calcium milk substitute (p.1350·1).
Calcium intolerance.

Locasol New Formula *Scientific Hospital Supplies, Irl.*
Low-calcium food for special diets (p.1350·1).

Locasyn *Roche, Denm.*
Flunisolide (p.1070·3).
Rhinitis.

Locatop
Pierre Fabre, Fr.; Pierre Fabre, Switz.
Desonide (p.1066·2).
Skin disorders.

Loceptin *Nycomed, Swed.†.*
Morphine sulfate (p.56·1).
Pain.

Loceryl
*AB-Consult, Aust.; Galderma, Austral.; Galderma, Belg.; Roche,
Braz.; Galderma, Denm.; Galderma, Fin.; Galderma, Fr.; Galderma,
Ger.; Roche, Hong Kong; Galderma, Israel; Galderma, Ital.; Galderma,
Norw.; Galderma, NZ; Galderma, S.Afr.; Galderma, Singapore; Gal-
derma, Swed.; Galderma, Switz.; Galderma, UK.*
Amorolfine hydrochloride (p.377·1).
Fungal skin and nail infections.

Locetar
Galderma, Port.; Galderma, Spain.
Amorolfine hydrochloride (p.377·1).
Fungal nail infections.

Lochol *Novartis, Jpn.*
Fluvastatin sodium (p.892·1).
Hyperlipidaemias.

Locholes *TO-Chemicals, Thai.*
Gemfibrozil (p.896·2).
Hyperlipidaemias.

Locholest *Warner Chilcott, USA.*
Colestyramine (p.864·1).
*Hypercholesterolaemia; pruritus associated with bil-
iary obstruction.*

Locilan *Monsanto, Austral.*
Norethisterone (p.1485·1).
Progestogen-only contraceptive.

**Locion Corporal Suavizante AHA Formula
405** *Dermaclin, Mex.*
SPF 15: Octinoxate (p.1517·3); oxybenzone
(p.1518·1).
Skin disorders; sunscreen.

Locion Limpiadora AHA Formula 405 *Derma-
clin, Mex.*
Soap substitute.
Acne; xerosis.

Lockets *Mars, UK.*
Menthol (p.1632·3); eucalyptol (p.1609·2); honey
(p.1366·2); glycerol (p.1616·3).
Nasal congestion; sore throat.

Lockets Medicated Linctus *Thornton & Ross, UK.*
Ipecacuanha (p.1093·1); honey (p.1366·2); glucose
(p.1364·1); glycerol (p.1616·3); menthol (p.1632·3).
Coughs; sore throats.

Locko *General Drugs, Thai.*
Dextromethorphan hydrobromide (p.1087·3); chlorpheniramine [chlorphenamine] maleate (p.412·1);
phenylpropanolamine hydrochloride (p.1098·1); paracetamol (p.71·2).
Cold and influenza symptoms.

Lockolys
Fresenius, Denm.; Fresenius Medical, Fin.
Range of solutions containing glucose; sodium chlo-
ride; sodium lactate; calcium chloride; magnesium
chloride (p.1184·1).
Peritoneal dialysis.

Locobase
Yamanouchi, Fin.; Yamanouchi, Ital.; Yamanouchi, Switz.
Emollient; vehicle for topical preparations.

Locoid
*Yamanouchi, Belg.; Yamanouchi, Denm.; Yamanouchi, Fin.; Ya-
manouchi, Fr.; Yamanouchi, Irl.; Sanofi Winthrop, Mex.; Yamanouchi,
Neth.; Yamanouchi, Norw.; Pharmaco, NZ; Yamanouchi, Port.; Phar-
maplan, S.Afr.; Yamanouchi, Swed.; Yamanouchi, Switz.; Ya-
manouchi, UK; Ferndale, USA.*
Hydrocortisone butyrate (p.1073·3).
Skin disorders.

Locoid C
*Yamanouchi, Irl.; Pharmaco, NZ; Yamanouchi, Port.; 3M, S.Afr.†; Ya-
manouchi, UK.*
Hydrocortisone butyrate (p.1073·3); chlorquinaldol
(p.182·1).
Skin disorders with bacterial or fungal infection.

Locoid Crelo *Yamanouchi, Swed.*
Hydrocortisone butyrate (p.1073·3).
Eczema; otitis externa; psoriasis.

Locoide N *Yamanouchi, Fr.*
Hydrocortisone butyrate (p.1073·3); neomycin sulfate
(p.228·1).
Infected skin disorders.

Locoidol
Yamanouchi, Denm.; Yamanouchi, Fin.; Yamanouchi, Norw.
Hydrocortisone butyrate (p.1073·3); chlorquinaldol
(p.182·1).
Infected skin disorders.

Locoidon
CSC, Aust.; Yamanouchi, Ital.
Hydrocortisone butyrate (p.1073·3).
Skin disorders.

LOCOL *Novartis, Ger.*
Fluvastatin sodium (p.892·1).
Hyperlipidaemias.

Locomin *UCB, Switz.*
Aceclofenac (p.11·1).
Musculoskeletal and joint disorders.

Locomucil *Pharmazam, Spain.*
Acetylcysteine (p.1082·3).
Respiratory-tract disorders.

Locorten *Novartis, Ital.*
Cream; ointment: Flumetasone pivalate (p.1070·3); ne-
omycin sulfate (p.228·1).
Otitis externa; skin disorders.
Ear drops; oral drops: Flumetasone pivalate
(p.1070·3); clioquinol (p.190·2).
Gingivitis; oral inflammatory lesions; otitis.
Lotion: Flumetasone pivalate (p.1070·3).
Otitis externa; skin disorders.

Locorten Neomicina *Novartis, Braz.*
Flumetasone pivalate (p.1070·3); neomycin sulfate
(p.228·1).

Locorten Tar *Zyma, Ital.†.*
Flumetasone pivalate (p.1070·3); salicylic acid
(p.1122·3); coal tar (p.1125·1).
Skin disorders.

Locorten Vioform
Novartis, NZ; Novartis Consumer, UK.
Flumetasone pivalate (p.1070·3); clioquinol (p.190·2).
*Inflammatory disorders of the ear with bacterial or fun-
gal infection; otorrhoea.*

Locorten Vioformio
Novartis, Braz.; Novartis, Ital.; Novartis Consumer, Port.
Flumetasone pivalate (p.1070·3); clioquinol (p.190·2).
Infected skin disorders.

Locortene *Novartis, Spain.*
Flumetasone pivalate (p.1070·3).
Skin disorders.

Locortene Vioformo *Novartis, Spain.*
Clioquinol (p.190·2); flumetasone pivalate (p.1070·3).
Infected skin disorders.

Lodales *Sanofi Winthrop, Fr.*
Simvastatin (p.969·2).
Hypercholesterolaemia.

Lodema *Hamilton, Austral.†.*
Coumarin (p.1599·3).
*Lymphoedema and elephantitis associated with filaria-
sis; oedema.*

Loderix *EGIS, Hung.*
Setastine hydrochloride (p.424·3).
Hypersensitivity reactions.

Loderm *Vinas, Spain.*
Erythromycin (p.201·2) or erythromycin laurilsulfate.
Acne.

Loderm Retinoico *Vinas, Spain.*
Erythromycin laurilsulfate; tretinoin (p.1126·2).
Acne.

Lodiar *Ashbourne, UK†.*
Loperamide hydrochloride (p.1231·3).
Diarrhoea.

Lodiarid *Clement, Fr.*
Loperamide hydrochloride (p.1231·3).
Diarrhoea.

Lodimol *Kener, Mex.*
Dipyridamole (p.877·2).

Lodine
*Sanofi Winthrop, Aust.; Fornet, Fr.; Wyeth-Ayerst, Hong Kong; Wyeth
Lederle, Ital.; Wyeth, Mex.; Wyeth Lederle, Port.; Sigma-Tau, Switz.;
Shire, UK; Wyeth-Ayerst, USA.*
Etodolac (p.35·2).
*Gout; inflammation; musculoskeletal and joint disor-
ders; pain.*

Lodis *Eugal, Ital.†.*
Loperamide hydrochloride (p.1231·3).
Diarrhoea.

Lodixal *Knoll, Belg.*
Verapamil hydrochloride (p.989·1).
Hypertension.

Lodopin *Fujisawa, Jpn.*
Zotepine (p.713·3).
Schizophrenia.

Lodosyn *Merck, USA.*
Carbidopa (p.1168·2).
Parkinsonism.

Lodoz *Lipha Sante, Fr.*
Bisoprolol fumarate (p.850·1); hydrochlorothiazide
(p.907·3).
Hypertension.

Lodrane *ECR, USA.*
Pseudoephedrine hydrochloride (p.1099·2); bromphe-
niramine maleate (p.410·2).
Allergic rhinitis; nasal congestion.

Lodrane Allergy *ECR, USA.*
Brompheniramine maleate (p.410·2).

Lodronat *Roche, Aust.*
Disodium clodronate (p.751·2).
*Hypercalcaemia of malignancy; osteolysis of malig-
nancy.*

Loesfer *Searle, Switz.*
Ferrous gluconate (p.1360·1).
Ascorbic acid (p.1389·3) is included in this preparation
to increase the absorption and availability of iron.
Iron deficiency; iron-deficiency anaemia.

Loesfer + acide folique *Searle, Switz.†.*
Ferrous gluconate (p.1360·1); folic acid (p.1361·1).
Ascorbic acid (p.1389·3) is included in this preparation
to increase the absorption and availability of iron.
*Folic acid deficiency; iron deficiency; iron-deficiency
anaemia.*

Loestrin
Parke, Davis, UK; Parke, Davis, USA.
Norethisterone acetate (p.1485·1); ethinylestradiol
(p.1476·2).
Combined oral contraceptive.

Loestrin 1.5/30 *Parke, Davis, Canad.*
Norethisterone acetate (p.1485·1); ethinylestradiol
(p.1476·2).
Combined oral contraceptive.

Loestrin Fe *Parke, Davis, USA.*
21 Tablets, norethisterone acetate (p.1485·1); ethinylestradiol (p.1476·2); 7 tablets, ferrous fumarate
(p.1360·1).
Combined oral contraceptive.

Loette
Wyeth-Ayerst, Austral.; Wyeth Lederle, Ital.; Wyeth, NZ.
Levonorgestrel (p.1486·2); ethinylestradiol (p.1476·2).
28-Day packs also contain 7 inert tablets.
Combined oral contraceptive.

Lofenac *Chew, Thai.*
Diclofenac diethylamine (p.30·2).
Musculoskeletal, joint, and peri-articular disorders.

Lofenalac
*Mead Johnson, Austral.; Bristol-Myers Squibb, Belg.†; Mead Johnson
Nutritionals, Canad.; Bristol-Myers Squibb, Fr.; Mead Johnson Nu-
tritionals, Israel; Mead Johnson, Ital.; Mead Johnson, NZ; Mead
Johnson, Port.; Mead Johnson Nutritionals, Thai.; Mead Johnson Nu-
tritionals, UK†; Mead Johnson Nutritionals, USA.*
Food for special diets (p.1350·1).
Phenylketonuria.

Lofenoxal *Monsanto, Austral.*
Diphenoxylate hydrochloride (p.1222·2).
Atropine sulfate (p.461·1) is included in this prepara-
tion to discourage abuse.
Diarrhoea.

Lofensaid *Opus, UK.*
Diclofenac sodium (p.30·3).
*Inflammation; musculoskeletal, joint, and peri-articu-
lar disorders; pain.*

Lofoxin Locatelli, Ital.†.
Fosfomycin calcium (p.208·2).
Bacterial infections.

Loftan Cascan, Ger.; Glaxo Wellcome, Ger.
Salbutamol sulfate (p.770·3).
Obstructive airways disease.

Lofton Abbott, Spain.
Buflomedil hydrochloride (p.851·3).
Peripheral vascular disorders.

Loftyl
Abbott, Aust.; Abbott, Belg.; Abbott, Fr.; Abbott, Ital.; Abbott, Mex.;
Abbott, Neth.; Abbott, Port.; Abbott, S.Afr.; Abbott, Switz.
Buflomedil hydrochloride (p.851·3).
Cerebral and peripheral vascular disorders.

Logacron Inexfa, Spain.
Merbromin (p.1150·1).
Wound disinfection.

Logan Ist. Chim. Inter., Ital.
Citicoline sodium (p.1596·1).
Arteriosclerosis; cerebral vascular disorders; parkinsonism.

Logastric Bio-Therabel, Belg.
Omeprazole (p.1239·1).
Gastro-oesophageal reflux; peptic ulcer; Zollinger-Ellison syndrome.

Logat Libbs, Braz.
Ranitidine hydrochloride (p.1245·2).
Acid aspiration; gastro-oesophageal reflux; gastrointestinal haemorrhage; peptic ulcer; Zollinger-Ellison syndrome.

Logecine Genopharm, Fr.
Erythromycin (p.201·2).
Bacterial infections.

Logen Goldline, USA.
Diphenoxylate hydrochloride (p.1222·2).
Atropine sulfate (p.461·1) is included in this preparation to discourage abuse.
Diarrhoea.

Logesic Carter-Wallace, Mex.
Diclofenac sodium (p.30·3).
Gout; inflammation; musculoskeletal, joint, and soft-tissue disorders; pain.

Logicin Chest Rub Sigma, Austral.
Menthol (p.1632·3); camphor (p.1589·3); eucalyptus oil (p.1609·2); thymol (p.1158·3); clove oil (p.1597·1); cedar wood oil; turpentine oil (p.1676·3).
Nasal congestion.

Logicin Cough & Cold Sigma, Austral.
Codeine phosphate (p.25·2); paracetamol (p.71·2); pseudoephedrine hydrochloride (p.1099·2).
Cold and influenza symptoms.

Logicin Cough Mixture for Congested Chesty Coughs
Sigma, Austral.; Sigma, Hong Kong.
Guaifenesin (p.1092·2); pseudoephedrine hydrochloride (p.1099·2).
Coughs; nasal congestion.

Logicin Cough Mixture for Dry Coughs
Sigma, Austral.; Sigma, Hong Kong.
Dextromethorphan hydrobromide (p.1087·3); pseudoephedrine hydrochloride (p.1099·2).
Coughs; nasal congestion.

Logicin Cough Suppressant Sigma, Austral.
Pholcodine (p.1099·1).
Coughs.

Logicin Expectorant Sigma, Austral.
Bromhexine bromide; guaifenesin (p.1092·2).
Coughs and cold symptoms.

Logicin Flu Strength Sigma, Austral.
Dextromethorphan hydrobromide (p.1087·3); pseudoephedrine hydrochloride (p.1099·2); paracetamol (p.71·2).
Cold and influenza symptoms.

Logicin Flu Strength Day & Night Sigma, Austral.
Daytime tablets, paracetamol (p.71·2); pseudoephedrine hydrochloride (p.1099·2); dextromethorphan hydrobromide (p.1087·3); night-time tablets, paracetamol; pseudoephedrine hydrochloride; chlorpheniramine [chlorphenamine] maleate (p.412·1).
Cold and influenza symptoms.

Logicin Hay Fever Sigma, Austral.
Paracetamol (p.71·2); pseudoephedrine hydrochloride (p.1099·2); chlorpheniramine [chlorphenamine] maleate (p.412·1).
Hay fever.

Logicin Junior Childrens Cough Mixture
Sigma, Austral.; Sigma, Hong Kong.
Dextromethorphan hydrobromide (p.1087·3); pseudoephedrine hydrochloride (p.1099·2).
Coughs; nasal congestion.

Logicin Rapid Relief Sigma, Austral.
Lozenges: Lignocaine [lidocaine] hydrochloride (p.1313·2); benzydamine hydrochloride (p.20·1); dichlorobenzyl alcohol (p.1143·2).
Sore throat.
Nasal spray: Oxymetazoline hydrochloride (p.1096·2).
Nasal congestion.

Logicin Sinus Sigma, Austral.
Pseudoephedrine hydrochloride (p.1099·2).
Upper respiratory-tract congestion.

Logiflox Pharmacia Upjohn, Fr.
Lomefloxacin hydrochloride (p.220·1).
Cystitis in women.

Logimat Astra, Belg.
Felodipine (p.888·3); metoprolol succinate (p.932·1).
Hypertension.

Logimax
Astra, Aust.; AstraZeneca, Denm.; AstraZeneca, Fin.; AstraZeneca, Fr.; Astra, Mex.; Astra, Norw.†; Astra, Spain; Hassle, Swed.; Astra, Switz.
Felodipine (p.888·3); metoprolol succinate (p.932·1).
Hypertension.

Astra, Hong Kong.
Felodipine (p.888·3); metoprolol tartrate (p.931·2).
Hypertension.

Logiparin Novo Nordisk, Aust.; Novo Nordisk, S.Afr.†.
Tinzaparin sodium (p.982·3).
Thromboembolic disorders.

Logirene Pharmacia Upjohn, Fr.
Frusemide [furosemide] (p.893·1); amiloride hydrochloride (p.835·1).
Heart failure.

Logoderm
Schering-Plough, Austral.; Schering-Plough, Mex.; Schering-Plough, NZ.
Alclometasone dipropionate (p.1061·1).
Skin disorders.

Logomed Allergie-Tabletten Logomed, Ger.†.
Terfenadine (p.424·3).
Hypersensitivity reactions.

Logomed Beruhigungs-Tabletten Logomed, Ger.†.
Diphenhydramine hydrochloride (p.416·1).
Sleep disorders.

Logomed Desinfektions-Salbe Logomed, Ger.†.
Povidone-iodine (p.1155·1).
Infected skin disorders; skin ulceration; wounds.

Logomed Durchfall-Kapseln Logomed, Ger.†.
Loperamide hydrochloride (p.1231·3).
Diarrhoea.

Logomed Ekzem-Salbe Logomed, Ger.†.
Bufexamac (p.20·3).
Eczema; neurodermatitis.

Logomed Erkaltungs-Balsam Logomed, Ger.†.
Camphor (p.1589·3); eucalyptus oil (p.1609·2); oleum pini sylvestris; turpentine oil (p.1676·3).
Upper respiratory-tract disorders.

Logomed Galle-Dragees Logomed, Ger.†.
Hymecromone (p.1622·3).
Biliary disorders.

Logomed Hamorrhoiden Logomed, Ger.†.
Bufexamac (p.20·3); lignocaine [lidocaine] hydrochloride (p.1313·2); bismuth subgallate (p.1213·2); titanium dioxide (p.1126·1).
Haemorrhoids.

Logomed Hautpilz-Salbe Logomed, Ger.†.
Clotrimazole (p.382·1).
Fungal skin infections.

Logomed Herz Logomed, Ger.†.
Crataegus (p.1600·2).
Cardiac disorders.

Logomed Heuschnupfen-Spray Logomed, Ger.†.
Sodium cromoglicate (p.774·3).
Allergic rhinitis.

Logomed Husten Logomed, Ger.†.
Ambroxol hydrochloride (p.1084·3).
Respiratory disorders associated with viscid or excessive mucus.

Logomed Juckreiz Logomed, Ger.†.
Gel: Diphenhydramine hydrochloride (p.416·1).
Allergic skin disorders; insect stings; pruritus; sunburn.

Logomed Kreislauf-Tabletten Logomed, Ger.†.
Etilefrine hydrochloride (p.888·1).
Hypotension.

Logomed Leber-Kapseln Logomed, Ger.†.
Silybum marianum (p.1021·3).
Liver disorders.

Logomed Magen Logomed, Ger.†.
Magaldrate (p.1232·2).
Gastric hyperacidity; peptic ulcer.

Logomed Nasen-Tropfen Logomed, Ger.†.
Xylometazoline hydrochloride (p.1102·2).
Nasal congestion.

Logomed Neuro-Aktiv-Tabletten Logomed, Ger.†.
Pyritinol hydrochloride (p.1657·1).
Cerebrovascular disorders; mental function disorders.

Logomed Prostata-Kapseln Logomed, Ger.†.
Urtica (p.1678·2).
Micturition disorders associated with prostatic cancer.

Logomed Reise-Tabletten Logomed, Ger.†.
Dimenhydrinate (p.415·2).
Motion sickness; nausea and vomiting; vertigo.

Logomed Schmerz Logomed, Ger.†.
Ibuprofen (p.43·2).
Fever; pain.

Logomed Schmerz- /Fieber Logomed, Ger.†.
Paracetamol (p.71·2).
Fever; pain.

Logomed Sport-Gel Logomed, Ger.†.
Heparin sodium (p.902·1).
Soft-tissue injury.

Logomed Venen-Salbe Logomed, Ger.†.
Heparin sodium (p.902·1).
Soft-tissue injury.

Logopharm Immun Logomed, Ger.†.
Echinacea purpura (p.1606·2).
Respiratory- and urinary-tract infections.

Logradin Juste, Spain.
Loratadine (p.420·1); pseudoephedrine sulfate (p.1099·3).
Allergic rhinitis.

Logroton Recipe, Aust.†; Novartis, Belg.; Novartis, Fr.; Novartis, Neth.†; Novartis, Switz.
Metoprolol tartrate (p.931·2); chlortalidone (p.857·1).
Hypertension.

Logryx Wyeth Lederle, Fr.
Minocycline hydrochloride (p.224·3).
Bacterial infections.

Logynon Schering, Irl.; Schering, Israel; Schering, UK.
Levonorgestrel (p.1486·2); ethinylestradiol (p.1476·2).
28-Day packs also contain 7 inert tablets.
Triphasic oral contraceptive.

Logynon ED Schering, Austral.; Schering, S.Afr.
21 Tablets, levonorgestrel (p.1486·2); ethinylestradiol (p.1476·2); 7 tablets, inert.
Menstrual disorders; triphasic oral contraceptive.

Loitin Vita, Spain.
Fluconazole (p.383·2).
Fungal infections.

Lokalicid Dermapharm, Ger.
Clotrimazole (p.382·1).
Fungal skin infections.

Lokalison-antimikrobiell Creme N Dermapharm, Ger.
Dexamethasone (p.1067·1); neomycin sulfate (p.228·1); nystatin (p.392·2).
Infected skin disorders.

Lokilan Roche, Norw.
Flunisolide (p.1070·3).
Rhinitis.

Lokilan Nasal Roche, Swed.†.
Flunisolide (p.1070·3).
Allergic rhinitis.

Lomabronchin N Lomapharm, Ger.
Homoeopathic preparation.

Lomacin Novartis, Mex.
Lomefloxacin hydrochloride (p.220·1).
Bacterial eye infections.

Lomaherpan Madaus, Aust.; Lomapharm, Ger.
Melissa (p.1632·2).
Superficial herpesvirus infections.

Lomahypericum Lomapharm, Ger.; Lomapharm, Singapore.
Hypericum (p.290·2).
Formerly known as Lophakomp-Hypericum in Ger.
Psychiatric disorders.

Lomarheumin N Lomapharm, Ger.
Homoeopathic preparation.

Lomarin Geymonat, Ital.
Dimenhydrinate (p.415·2).
Nausea; vertigo; vomiting.

Lomasatin M Lomapharm, Ger.
Myrrh (p.1639·2).
Mouth and throat inflammation.

Lomatol Lomapharm, Ger.
Oral drops: Peppermint leaf (p.1243·2); fennel (p.1610·1); caraway (p.1591·2); absinthium (p.1571·1).
Tablets: Absinthium (p.1571·1); caraway (p.1591·2); peppermint leaf (p.1243·2); caraway oil (p.1591·2); peppermint oil (p.1243·3).
Gastrointestinal disorders.

Lomatuell H Lohmann, Ital.
White soft paraffin (p.1407·3).
Wound dressing.

Lomax Julphar, UAE.
Lomefloxacin hydrochloride (p.220·1).
Bacterial infections.

Lomazell forte N Lomapharm, Ger.
Benzyl nicotinate (p.20·2); nonivamide (p.63·1); bovine placental extract.
Circulatory disorders of the skin.

Lombriareu Areu, Spain.
Pyrantel embonate (p.108·1).
Worm infections.

Lombrimade Esfar, Port.†.
Piperazine (p.105·3).

Lomeflon Senju, Jpn†.
Lomefloxacin hydrochloride (p.220·1).
Bacterial eye and ear infections.

Lomexin Grunenthal, Aust.; Effik, Fr.; S & K, Ger.; Recordati, Ital.; Aspen, S.Afr.; Recordati, Spain; Akita, UK.
Fenticonazole nitrate (p.383·2).
Fungal skin and nail infections; vulvovaginal candidiasis.

Lomide
Note. This name is used for preparations of different composition.
Alcon, Austral.; Alcon, NZ.
Lodoxamide trometamol (p.768·1).
Conjunctivitis.
Siam Bheasach, Thai.
Loperamide hydrochloride (p.1231·3).
Diarrhoea.

Lomine Riva, Canad.
Dicyclomine [dicycloverine] hydrochloride (p.466·1).
Smooth muscle spasm.

Lomir
Novartis, Aust.; Novartis, Belg.; Novartis, Braz.; Novartis, Denm.; Novartis, Fin.; Novartis, Ger.; Novartis, Ital.; Novartis, Neth.; Novartis, Norw.; Novartis, Port.; Mizar, Spain; Novartis, Swed.; Novartis, Switz.
Isradipine (p.916·3).
Hypertension.

Lomont Rosemont, UK.
Lofepramine hydrochloride (p.297·1).
Depression.

Lomotil Searle, Austral.; Searle, Braz.; Searle, Canad.; Searle, Hong Kong; Goldshield, Irl.; Searle, Mex.; Searle, NZ; Monsanto, Port.†; Searle, S.Afr.; Searle, Singapore; Searle, Thai.; Goldshield, UK; Searle, USA.
Diphenoxylate hydrochloride (p.1222·2).
Atropine sulfate (p.461·1) is included in this preparation to discourage abuse.
These ingredients can be described by the British Approved Name Co-phenotrope.
Diarrhoea; ostomy management.

Lomper Esteve, Spain.
Mebendazole (p.102·2).
Worm infections.

Lomudal
Aventis, Belg.; Fisons, Denm.; Rhone-Poulenc Rorer, Fin.; Rhone-Poulenc Rorer, Fr.; Fisons, Israel; Rhone-Poulenc Rorer, Ital.; Rhone-Poulenc Rorer, Neth.; Fisons, Norw.; Aventis, S.Afr.; Rhone-Poulenc Rorer, Swed.; Rhone-Poulenc Rorer, Switz.
Sodium cromoglicate (p.774·3).
Allergic conjunctivitis; allergic rhinitis; asthma; bronchial hypersensitivity; food hypersensitivity; inflammatory bowel disease.

Lomupren Rhone-Poulenc Rorer, Ger.
Sodium cromoglicate (p.774·3).
Allergic rhinitis.

Lomupren compositum Rhone-Poulenc Rorer, Ger.
Sodium cromoglicate (p.774·3); xylometazoline hydrochloride (p.1102·2).
Allergic rhinitis.

Lomusol
Sigmapharm, Aust.; Aventis, Belg.; Rhone-Poulenc Rorer, Fr.; Rhone-Poulenc Rorer, Neth.; Rhone-Poulenc Rorer, Switz.
Sodium cromoglicate (p.774·3).
Allergic conjunctivitis; allergic rhinitis.

Lomusol comp Sigmapharm, Aust.†.
Sodium cromoglicate (p.774·3); xylometazoline hydrochloride (p.1102·2).
Allergic rhinitis.

Lomusol plus Xylometazoline Aventis, Belg.
Sodium cromoglicate (p.774·3); xylometazoline hydrochloride (p.1102·2).
Allergic rhinitis; nasal congestion.

Lomusol-X Rhone-Poulenc Rorer, Switz.
Sodium cromoglicate (p.774·3); xylometazoline hydrochloride (p.1102·2).
Allergic rhinitis; nasal congestion.

Lomuspray Rhone-Poulenc Rorer, Ital.
Sodium cromoglicate (p.774·3).
Asthma.

Lomy Masa, Thai.
Loperamide hydrochloride (p.1231·3).
Diarrhoea.

Lonactene Ferring, UK.
Carbetocin (p.1279·1).
Postpartum haemorrhage; postpartum uterine atony.

Lonalac Mead Johnson Nutritionals, USA.
Preparation for enteral nutrition (p.1350·1).

Lonarid Boehringer Ingelheim, Ger.; Boehringer Ingelheim, Ital.
Paracetamol (p.71·2); codeine phosphate (p.25·2).
Pain.

Lonarid Mono Boehringer Ingelheim, Belg.
Paracetamol (p.71·2).
Fever; pain.

Lonarid N Boehringer Ingelheim, Belg.
Paracetamol (p.71·2); caffeine (p.761·2); codeine phosphate (p.25·2).
Pain.

Lonavar CSL, Austral.
Oxandrolone (p.1487·2).
Anabolic.

London Drugs Dark Tanning Tanning Research, Canad.†.
SPF 4: Meradimate (p.1517·3); octinoxate (p.1517·3).
Sunscreen.

London Drugs Kids Sunblock Tanning Research, Canad.
SPF 30: Octinoxate (p.1517·3); homosalate (p.1517·2); octisalate (p.1518·1); oxybenzone (p.1518·1).
Formerly known as London Drugs Baby Sunblock.
Sunscreen.

London Drugs Sport Tanning Research, Canad.
SPF 15†: Octinoxate (p.1517·3); oxybenzone (p.1518·1).
SPF 30: Octinoxate (p.1517·3); octisalate (p.1518·1); oxybenzone (p.1518·1).
Sunscreen.

London Drugs Sunblock Tanning Research, Canad.
SPF 15: Octinoxate (p.1517·3); oxybenzone (p.1518·1).
SPF 30: Octinoxate (p.1517·3); homosalate (p.1517·2); octisalate (p.1518·1); oxybenzone (p.1518·1).
Sunscreen.

London Drugs Sunscreen Tanning Research, Canad.†.
SPF 8: Octinoxate (p.1517·3); oxybenzone (p.1518·1).
Sunscreen.

Longachin *Teofarma, Ital.*
Quinidine arabogalactane sulfate (p.966·1).
Arrhythmias.

Longacilin *Sanus, Braz.*
Benzathine benzylpenicillin (p.156·2).
Bacterial infections.

Longacor *Procter & Gamble, Fr.†; Rovi, Spain; Elaiapharm, Switz.*
Quinidine arabogalactane sulfate (p.966·1).
Arrhythmias.

Longalgic *Evans, Fr.†*
Benorilate (p.19·3).
Pain.

Longastatina *Italfarmaco, Ital.*
Octreotide (p.1292·1).
Acromegaly; diarrhoea associated with immunodeficiency; malignant neoplasms; pancreatic disorders.

Longasteril 40 *Fresenius Kabi, Ger.*
Dextran 40 (p.728·3) in glucose or sodium chloride.
Plasma volume expansion; thrombosis prophylaxis; vascular disorders.

Longasteril 70 *Fresenius Kabi, Ger.*
Dextran 70 (p.729·2) with electrolytes.
Plasma volume expansion; thrombosis prophylaxis.

Longatren *Bayer, Aust.*
Azidocillin sodium (p.153·1).
Bacterial infections.

Longazem *De Salute, Ital.*
Diltiazem hydrochloride (p.874·3).
Hypertension; ischaemic heart disease.

Longevit E *QIF, Braz.*
Caffeine (p.761·3); vitamin E; vitamin B substances (p.1350·1); erythroxylon catuaba.

Longevital *Sanitalia, Ital.*
Pollen; royal jelly (p.1659·3).
Nutritional supplement.

Longifene *Bios, Belg.; UCB, Hong Kong; Covan, S.Afr.; UCB, Singapore; UCB, Switz.†*
Buclizine hydrochloride (p.411·1).
Appetite loss; hypersensitivity reactions; motion sickness; nausea and vomiting.

Longivol *Medical, Spain.*
Embryo extract; methyltestosterone; vitamins (p.1350·1); caffeine; calcium magnesium phytate; ethinylestradiol.
Tonic.

Longtussin *Klinge, Aust.†*
Day capsules, etamiphylline hydrochloride (p.765·1); guaifenesin (p.1092·2); night capsules, codeine (p.25·2); chlorphenoxamine hydrochloride (p.412·3).
Bronchitis; cough.

Longum *Pharmacia Upjohn, Belg.; Pharmacia Upjohn, Ger.*
Sulfametopyrazine (p.256·1).
Bacterial infections; malaria; toxoplasmosis.

Loniten *Pharmacia Upjohn, Aust.; Pharmacia Upjohn, Austral.; Pharmacia Upjohn, Braz.; Pharmacia Upjohn, Canad.; Pharmacia Upjohn, Hong Kong; Pharmacia Upjohn, Irl.; Pharmacia Upjohn, Ital.; Pharmacia Upjohn, NZ; Pharmacia Upjohn, Port.; Pharmacia Upjohn, S.Afr.; Pharmacia Upjohn, Singapore; Pharmacia Upjohn, Spain; Pharmacia Upjohn, Switz.; Pharmacia Upjohn, Thai.; Pharmacia Upjohn, UK; Upjohn, USA.*
Minoxidil (p.934·2).
Alopecia androgenetica; hypertension.

Lonnoten *Pharmacia Upjohn, Belg.; Pharmacia Upjohn, Neth.*
Minoxidil (p.934·2).
Hypertension.

Lonol
Note. This name is used for preparations of different composition.
Boehringer Ingelheim, Mex.
Benzydamine hydrochloride (p.20·1).
Musculoskeletal, joint and peri-articular disorders.

Aspen, S.Afr.
Allopurinol (p.397·2).
Gout; hyperuricaemia.

Lonol Sport *Boehringer Ingelheim, Mex.*
Benzydamine hydrochloride (p.20·1); methyl salicylate (p.55·1); menthol (p.1632·3).
Musculoskeletal, joint, peri-articular and soft-tissue disorders.

Lonolox *Pharmacia Upjohn, Ger.*
Minoxidil (p.934·2).
Hypertension.

Lonoten *Pharmacia Upjohn, Fr.*
Minoxidil (p.934·2).
Hypertension.

Lonox *Geneva, USA.*
Diphenoxylate hydrochloride (p.1222·2).
Atropine sulfate (p.461·1) is included in this preparation to discourage abuse.
Diarrhoea.

Lonseren *Rhone-Poulenc Rorer, Spain.*
Pipotiazine palmitate (p.700·3).
Anxiety; psychoses.

Loortan *Therabel, Belg.*
Losartan potassium (p.921·3).
Hypertension.

Loortan Plus *Therabel, Belg.*
Losartan potassium (p.921·3); hydrochlorothiazide (p.907·3).
Hypertension.

Lo/Ovral *Wyeth-Ayerst, USA.*
Norgestrel (p.1486·1); ethinylestradiol (p.1476·2).

28-Day packs also contain 7 inert tablets.
Combined oral contraceptive.

Lopalind *Lindopharm, Ger.*
Loperamide hydrochloride (p.1231·3).
Diarrhoea.

Lopamine *Shiwa, Thai.*
Loperamide hydrochloride (p.1231·3).
Diarrhoea.

Lo-P-Caps *ST, Thai.*
Calcium acetate (p.1187·3).
Hyperphosphataemia.

Lop-Dia *Philopharm, Ger.*
Loperamide hydrochloride (p.1231·3).
Diarrhoea.

Lopedium *Hexal, Ger.; Hexal, S.Afr.*
Loperamide hydrochloride (p.1231·3).
Diarrhoea.

Lopela *Pharmasant, Thai.*
Loperamide hydrochloride (p.1231·3).
Diarrhoea.

Lopelin *Fumouze, Fr.†*
Loperamide hydrochloride (p.1231·3).
Diarrhoea.

Lopemid *Gentili, Ital.*
Loperamide hydrochloride (p.1231·3).
Diarrhoea; ileostomy management.

Loperacap *ICN, Canad.*
Loperamide hydrochloride (p.1231·3).

LoperaGen *Goldshield, UK.*
Loperamide hydrochloride (p.1231·3).
Diarrhoea.

Loperamerck *Merck, Ger.†*
Loperamide hydrochloride (p.1231·3).
Diarrhoea.

Loperan *Wasserman, Spain.*
Loperamide hydrochloride (p.1231·3).
Diarrhoea.

Loperastat *Be-Tabs, S.Afr.*
Loperamide hydrochloride (p.1231·3).
Diarrhoea; ostomy management.

Loperax *Xepa-Soul Pattinson, Hong Kong.*
Loperamide hydrochloride (p.1231·3).
Diarrhoea.

Lopercin *Polipharm, Thai.*
Loperamide hydrochloride (p.1231·3).
Diarrhoea.

Loperdium *General Drugs, Thai.*
Loperamide hydrochloride (p.1231·3).
Diarrhoea.

Loperhoe *Betapharm, Ger.*
Loperamide hydrochloride (p.1231·3).
Diarrhoea.

Loperia *Great Eastern, Thai.; Therapharma, Thai.*
Loperamide hydrochloride (p.1231·3).
Diarrhoea.

Loperid *Vitamed, Israel.*
Loperamide hydrochloride (p.1231·3).
Diarrhoea.

Loperium *Remedica, Hong Kong; Pharbita, Israel.*
Loperamide hydrochloride (p.1231·3).
Diarrhoea.

Loperkey *Inkeysa, Spain.*
Loperamide hydrochloride (p.1231·3).
Diarrhoea.

Lopermide *Atlantic, Hong Kong; Vana, Thai.*
Loperamide hydrochloride (p.1231·3).
Diarrhoea.

Loperol *Rolab, S.Afr.*
Loperamide hydrochloride (p.1231·3).
Now known as Rolab-Loperamide HCl.
Diarrhoea.

Loperyl *SmithKline Beecham, Ital.†*
Loperamide hydrochloride (p.1231·3).
Diarrhoea.

Lopetrans *Fresenius-Praxis, Ger.†*
Loperamide hydrochloride (p.1231·3).
Diarrhoea.

Lopex *Leiras, Fin.*
Loperamide hydrochloride (p.1231·3).
Diarrhoea; ileostomy management.

Lophakomp-B1 *Lomapharm, Ger.*
Thiamine hydrochloride (p.1385·1).
Vitamin B_1 deficiency.

Lophakomp-B6 *Lomapharm, Ger.*
Pyridoxine hydrochloride (p.1386·3).
Vitamin B_6 deficiency.

Lophakomp-B 12 *Lomapharm, Ger.*
Cyanocobalamin (p.1388·1).
Vitamin B_{12} deficiency.

Lophakomp-B 12 Depot *Lomapharm, Ger.*
Hydroxocobalamin acetate (p.1388·3).
Vitamin B_{12} deficiency.

Lophakomp-Echinacea H *Lomapharm, Ger.*
Homoeopathic preparation.

Lophakomp-Hamamelis H *Lomapharm, Ger.*
Homoeopathic preparation.

Lophakomp-Procain N *Lomapharm, Ger.*
Procaine hydrochloride (p.1319·1).
Nervous system disorders.

Lopid *Parke, Davis, Austral.; Parke, Davis, Belg.†; Ache, Braz.; Parke, Davis, Canad.; Parke, Davis, Denm.; Parke, Davis, Fin.; Parke, Davis, Hong Kong; Parke, Davis, Irl.; Parke, Davis, Ital.; Parke, Davis, Mex.; Parke, Davis, Neth.; Parke, Davis, NZ; Parke, Davis, Port.; Parke, Davis, S.Afr.; Parke, Davis, Singapore; Parke, Davis, Spain; Parke, Davis, Swed.; Warner-Lambert, Thai.; Parke, Davis, UK; Parke, Davis, USA.*
Gemfibrozil (p.896·2).
Hyperlipidaemias.

Lopimed *Ecosol, Switz.*
Loperamide hydrochloride (p.1231·3).
Diarrhoea.

Lopiretic *Bristol-Myers Squibb, Port.*
Captopril (p.853·3); hydrochlorothiazide (p.907·3).
Hypertension.

Lopirin *Bristol-Myers Squibb, Aust.; Bristol-Myers Squibb, Ger.; Bristol-Myers Squibb, Switz.*
Captopril (p.853·3).
Formerly known as Lopirin Cor in Ger.
Diabetic nephropathy; heart failure; hypertension; myocardial infarction.

Lopitrex *Bristol-Myers Squibb, Hong Kong.*
Cefapirin sodium (p.164·2).
Bacterial infections.

Loporic *M & H, Thai.*
Allopurinol (p.397·2).
Gout; hyperuricaemia; renal calculi; uric acid nephropathy.

Lopranol LA *Opus, UK.*
Propranolol hydrochloride (p.962·3).
Angina pectoris; hypertension.

Lopresor *Astra, Aust.; Novartis, Austral.; Novartis, Belg.; Novartis, Canad.; Novartis, Ger.; Novartis, Irl.; Novartis, Israel; Novartis, Ital.; Novartis, Mex.; Novartis, Neth.; Novartis, NZ; Novartis, Port.; Novartis, S.Afr.; Padro, Spain; Novartis, Switz.; Novartis, UK.*
Metoprolol fumarate (p.932·1) or metoprolol tartrate (p.931·2).
Angina pectoris; arrhythmias; hypertension; hyperthyroidism; migraine; myocardial infarction.

Lopress *Siam Bheasach, Thai.*
Prazosin hydrochloride (p.958·1).
Hypertension.

Lopressor *Novartis, Braz.; Novartis, Fr.; Novartis, USA.*
Metoprolol tartrate (p.931·2).
Angina pectoris; arrhythmias; hypertension; migraine; myocardial infarction.

Lopressor HCT *Novartis, USA.*
Metoprolol tartrate (p.931·2); hydrochlorothiazide (p.907·3).
Hypertension.

Lopril *Orion, Fin.; Bristol-Myers Squibb, Fr.*
Captopril (p.853·3).
Diabetic nephropathy; heart failure; hypertension; myocardial infarction.

Lopril D *Bristol-Myers Squibb, Braz.*
Captopril (p.853·3); hydrochlorothiazide (p.907·3).
Heart failure; hypertension.

Loprofin *SHS, Fr.; Scientific Hospital Supplies, Irl.; Nutricia, Ital.; Nutricia, NZ; Scientific Hospital Supplies, UK.*
A range of gluten-free, low protein foods for special diets (p.1350·1).
Phenylketonuria; protein restriction.

Loprox *Hoechst Marion Roussel, Braz.; Hoechst Marion Roussel, Canad.; Hoechst Marion Roussel, Mex.; Bipharma, Neth.; Hoechst Marion Roussel, Thai.; Hoechst Marion Roussel, USA.*
Ciclopirox (p.382·1) or ciclopirox olamine (p.382·1).
Fungal skin and nail infections.

Loptomit *Bournonville, Neth.†*
Timolol maleate (p.982·1).
Glaucoma; raised intra-ocular pressure.

Lora *Atlantic, Thai.; PP Lab, Thai.*
Lorazepam (p.688·3).
Anxiety; insomnia.

Lorabenz *Norton Healthcare, Denm.*
Lorazepam (p.688·3).
Anxiety.

Lorabid *Lilly, Aust.; Lilly, Hong Kong; Lilly, Mex.; Lilly, S.Afr.; Lilly, Swed.; Monarch, USA.*
Loracarbef (p.220·3).
Bacterial infections.

Loradur *Pharmacia Upjohn, Aust.*
Amiloride hydrochloride (p.835·1); hydrochlorothiazide (p.907·3).
Ascites; hypertension; oedema.

Lorafem *Zambon, Ger.*
Loracarbef (p.220·3).
Bacterial infections.

Loraga *Parke, Davis, Fin.; Parke, Davis, Swed.*
Lactulose (p.1230·1).
Constipation; hepatic encephalopathy.

Loramed *Medifive, Thai.*
Lorazepam (p.688·3).
Anxiety; insomnia.

Loramet *Wyeth Lederle, Belg.; Wyeth-Ayerst, Hong Kong; Wyeth, Irl.; Wyeth, Neth.; Aspen, S.Afr.; Wyeth, Singapore; Wyeth, Spain; Wyeth, Switz.; Wyeth-Ayerst, Thai.*
Lormetazepam (p.689·3).
Insomnia; sedative.

Loranil *Libbs, Braz.*
Loratadine (p.420·1).
Hypersensitivity reactions.

Loranox *Charoen, Thai.*
Loratadine (p.420·1).
Allergic rhinitis; allergic skin disorders.

Lorans *Schwarz, Ital.; Medochemie, Singapore.*
Lorazepam (p.688·3).
Anxiety; insomnia.

Lorapam *Pacific, NZ; Siam Bheasach, Thai.*
Lorazepam (p.688·3).
Anxiety; premedication.

Lorasifar *Siphar, Switz.*
Lorazepam (p.688·3).
Anxiety; sedative; sleep disorders.

Lorastine *Schering-Plough, Israel.*
Loratadine (p.420·1).
Allergic rhinitis; urticaria.

Lorastyne *Schering-Plough, Austral.*
Loratadine (p.420·1).
Allergic rhinitis; dermatological hypersensitivity reactions; urticaria.

Loratin *Julphar, UAE.*
Loratadine (p.420·1).
Allergic conjunctivitis; allergic rhinitis; pruritus; urticaria.

Loratyn *Aesca, Aust.*
Loratadine (p.420·1).
Allergic rhinitis; urticaria.

Loratyne *Schering-Plough, S.Afr.*
Loratadine (p.420·1).
Allergic rhinitis; urticaria.

Lorax
Note. This name is used for preparations of different composition.
Lilly, Aust.; Lilly, Neth.
Loracarbef (p.220·3).
Bacterial infections.

Wyeth, Braz.
Lorazepam (p.688·3).
Alcohol withdrawal syndrome; anxiety; epilepsy; insomnia; nausea and vomiting; premedication.

Lorazene *Berlin Pharm, Thai.*
Lorazepam (p.688·3).
Anxiety; epilepsy; muscle relaxation.

Lorazep *Asian Pharm, Thai.*
Lorazepam (p.688·3).
Anxiety.

Lorcet 10/650 *Forest Pharmaceuticals, USA.*
Hydrocodone tartrate (p.42·2); paracetamol (p.71·2).
Pain.

Lorcet Plus *Forest Pharmaceuticals, USA.*
Hydrocodone tartrate (p.42·2); paracetamol (p.71·2).
Pain.

Lorcet-HD *Forest Pharmaceuticals, USA.*
Hydrocodone tartrate (p.42·2); paracetamol (p.71·2).
Pain.

Lorenin *Wyeth Lederle, Port.*
Lorazepam (p.688·3).

Lorenzo's Oil *Scientific Hospital Supplies, UK.*
Glycerol trioleate; glycerol trierucate (p.1629·2).
Adrenoleucodystrophy.

Loretam *Wyeth, Ger.*
Lormetazepam (p.689·3).
Insomnia; premedication.

Loretic *Xixia, S.Afr.†*
Triamterene (p.986·1); hydrochlorothiazide (p.907·3).
Hypertension; oedema.

Lorexen *Loren, Mex.*
Naproxen (p.60·3).
Fever; inflammation; pain.

Loricin *Sigma-Tau, Ital.*
Sulbactam sodium (p.250·1); ampicillin sodium (p.150·3).
Lignocaine [lidocaine] hydrochloride (p.1313·2) is included in the intramuscular injection to alleviate the pain of injection.
Bacterial infections.

Loridem *Sandipro, Belg.*
Lorazepam (p.688·3).
Anxiety; insomnia; premedication.

Lorien *Aspen, S.Afr.*
Fluoxetine hydrochloride (p.284·2).
Bulimia nervosa; depression.

Lorinden T *Medphano, Ger.*
Flumetasone pivalate (p.1070·3); coal tar (p.1125·1); salicylic acid (p.1122·3).
Skin disorders.

Lorityne *LSP, Thai.*
Loratadine (p.420·1).
Allergic rhinitis; allergic skin disorders.

Lorium *Ache, Braz.*
Lorazepam (p.688·3).
Alcohol withdrawal syndrome; anxiety; epilepsy; insomnia; nausea and vomiting; premedication.

Lorivan *Remedica, Hong Kong; Dexxon, Israel.*
Lorazepam (p.688·3).
Anxiety; insomnia; premedication.

Lornazol *Loren, Mex.*
Ketoconazole (p.389·1).
Fungal infections.

The symbol † denotes a preparation no longer actively marketed

Loron *Ercopharm, Denm.†; Boehringer Mannheim, Irl.; Roche, UK.*
Disodium clodronate (p.751·2).
Hypercalcaemia of malignancy; tumour-induced osteolysis and bone pain.

Lorophyn *Columbia, Mex.*
Nonoxinol 9 (p.1346·1).
Contraception.

Loroxide *Dermik, Canad.†; Dermik, USA.*
Benzoyl peroxide (p.1111·1).
Acne.

Lorpa *Beacons, Singapore.*
Loperamide (p.1232·1).
Diarrhoea.

Lorsedal *Prospa, Port.*
Lorazepam (p.688·3).

Lorsedin *Siam Bheasach, Thai.*
Loratadine (p.420·1).
Allergic conjunctivitis; allergic rhinitis; allergic skin disorders.

Lortaan *Merck Sharp & Dohme, Ital.; Medinfar, Port.*
Losartan potassium (p.921·3).
Hypertension.

Lortaan Plus *Medinfar, Port.*
Losartan potassium (p.921·3); hydrochlorothiazide (p.907·3).
Hypertension.

Lortab *UCB, USA.*
Hydrocodone tartrate (p.42·2); paracetamol (p.71·2).
Pain.

Lortab ASA *UCB, USA.*
Hydrocodone tartrate (p.42·2); aspirin (p.14·2).
Pain.

Lortadine *Olan-Kemed, Thai.*
Loratadine (p.420·1).
Allergic rhinitis; allergic skin disorders.

Lorvas *Torrent, Thai.*
Indapamide (p.913·1).
Hypertension.

Lorzaar *MSD Chibropharm, Ger.*
Losartan potassium (p.921·3).
Heart failure; hypertension.

Lorzaar plus *MSD Chibropharm, Ger.*
Losartan potassium (p.921·3); hydrochlorothiazide (p.907·3).
Hypertension.

Lorzem *Douglas, NZ.*
Lorazepam (p.688·3).
Anxiety.

Losalen *Novartis, Braz.; Novartis, Ital.; Novartis Consumer, Port.; Novartis, Spain.*
Flumetasone pivalate (p.1070·3); salicylic acid (p.1122·3).
Skin disorders.

Losan Fe *Hexal, Ger.†.*
Ferrous gluconate (p.1360·1).
Iron deficiency.

Losapan *Duopharm, Ger.*
Cynara (p.1601·3).
Dyspepsia.

Losaprex *Sigma-Tau, Ital.*
Losartan potassium (p.921·3).
Hypertension.

Losazid *Sigma-Tau, Ital.*
Losartan potassium (p.921·3); hydrochlorothiazide (p.907·3).
Hypertension.

Loscalcon *Lilly, Ger.*
Calcium carbonate (p.1215·1).
Calcium deficiency.

Loscon *Galderma, Ger.*
Tioxolone (p.1126·1); benzoxonium chloride (p.1135·2).
Scalp disorders.

Losec *Astra, Aust.; Astra, Austral.; Astra, Belg.; Astra, Braz.; AstraZeneca, Canad.; AstraZeneca, Denm.; AstraZeneca, Fin.; Astra, Hong Kong; Astra, Irl.; Abic, Israel; Schering-Plough, Ital.; Astra, Mex.; Astra, Neth.; AstraZeneca, Norw.; AstraZeneca, NZ; Astra, Port.; Astra, S.Afr.; AstraZeneca, Singapore; Astra, Spain; Hassle, Swed.; AstraZeneca, Thai.; AstraZeneca, UK.*
Omeprazole (p.1239·1), omeprazole magnesium (p.1239·1), or omeprazole sodium (p.1239·1).
Acid aspiration; gastro-oesophageal reflux; peptic ulcer; Zollinger-Ellison syndrome.

Losec 1-2-3 A *AstraZeneca, Canad.*
Omeprazole magnesium (p.1239·1); amoxicillin (p.149·2); clarithromycin (p.186·2).
Helicobacter pylori-associated peptic ulcer.

Losec Heliara *AstraZeneca, Fin.*
Tablets I, metronidazole (p.594·1); tablets II, omeprazole magnesium (Losec) (p.1239·1); tablets III, amoxicillin trihydrate (p.149·2).
Helicobacter pylori-associated peptic ulcer.

Losec Helicopak *AstraZeneca, Austral.*
Tablets, omeprazole magnesium (Losec) (p.1239·1); capsules, amoxicillin trihydrate (Amoxil) (p.149·2); tablets, metronidazole (Flagyl) (p.594·1).
Peptic ulcer associated with Helicobacter pylori infection.

Losec Hp7 *AstraZeneca, Austral.*
Tablets, omeprazole magnesium (Losec) (p.1239·1); capsules, amoxicillin trihydrate (Amoxil) (p.149·2); tablets, clarithromycin (Klacid) (p.186·2).
Helicobacter pylori-associated peptic ulcer.

AstraZeneca, NZ.
Capsules, omeprazole (p.1239·1); capsules, amoxicillin trihydrate (p.149·2); tablets, clarithromycin (p.186·2).
Helicobacter pylori-associated peptic ulcer.

Losec 1-2-3 M *AstraZeneca, Canad.*
Omeprazole magnesium (p.1239·1); metronidazole (p.594·1); clarithromycin (p.186·2).
Helicobacter pylori-associated peptic ulcer.

Losec 20 Triple *Astra, S.Afr.*
Capsules, omeprazole (Losec) (p.1239·1); tablets, clarithromycin (Klacid) (p.186·2); capsules, amoxicillin (Moxan) (p.149·2).
Peptic ulcer associated with Helicobacter pylori infection.

Losferon *Besins-Iscovesco, Fr.†.*
Ferrous gluconate (p.1360·1).
Iron deficiency anaemia.

Losferron *Asta Medica, Aust.; Prospa, Belg.; Lilly, Ger.; SPA, Ital.; Will-Pharma, Neth.; Prospa, Port.*
Ferrous gluconate (p.1360·1).
Ascorbic acid (p.1389·3) may be included in this preparation to increase the absorption and availability of iron.
Iron-deficiency anaemia.

Losferron-Fol *Asta Medica, Aust.*
Ferrous gluconate (p.1360·1); folic acid (p.1361·1).
Ascorbic acid (p.1389·3) is included in this preparation to increase the absorption and availability of iron.
Iron and folic acid deficiency anaemias.

Losnesium *Lilly, Ger.*
Magnesium carbonate (p.1232·3); magnesium oxide (p.1233·2).
Magnesium deficiency.

Lostatin *Reddy, Singapore.*
Lovastatin (p.922·3).
Hypercholesterolaemia.

Lotagen *Byk, Belg.†.*
Metacresolsulfonic acid-formaldehyde (p.738·3).
Gynaecological disorders.

Lotem *Adcock Ingram, S.Afr.*
Ibuprofen (p.43·2); paracetamol (p.71·2).
Fever; pain.

Lotemax *Bausch & Lomb, USA.*
Loteprednol etabonate (p.1075·3).
Eye disorders.

Lo-Ten *Pacific, Hong Kong; Pacific, NZ.*
Atenolol (p.841·3).
Angina pectoris; arrhythmias; hypertension; myocardial infarction.

Lotensin *Novartis, Braz.; Novartis, Canad.; Novartis, Mex.; Novartis, USA.*
Benazepril hydrochloride (p.843·2).
Heart failure; hypertension; renal failure.

Lotensin HCT *Novartis, USA.*
Benazepril hydrochloride (p.843·2); hydrochlorothiazide (p.907·3).
Hypertension.

Lotharin *Berk, UK.*
Diphenoxylate hydrochloride (p.1222·2).
Atropine sulfate (p.461·1) is included in this preparation to discourage abuse.
The ingredients in this preparation can be described by the British Approved Name Co-phenotrope.
Diarrhoea.

Lotil *Fenton, UK.*
Emollient.
Dry skin.

Lotio decapans *Widmer, Switz.*
Resorcinol (p.1122·2); salicylic acid (p.1122·3).
Scalp disorders.

Lotio Zinc *Sam-On, Israel.*
Zinc oxide (p.1128·2).
Skin irritation.

Lotion Ecran Solaire Extreme *Prodemdis, Canad.*
SPF 30: Avobenzone (p.1517·1); octinoxate (p.1517·3); oxybenzone (p.1518·1); titanium dioxide (p.1126·1).
Sunscreen.

Lotion pour Feux Sauvages
Note. This name is used for preparations of different composition.
Atlas, Canad.
Camphor (p.1589·3); zinc salicylate.

Sabex, Canad.
Benzoin (p.1668·3); camphor (p.1589·3); menthol (p.1632·3); myrrh (p.1639·2).

Valmo, Canad.
Benzoin (p.1668·3); camphor (p.1589·3); menthol (p.1632·3).

Lotocreme *Abbott, S.Afr.†.*
Hexachlorophene (p.1146·1).
Skin disorders.

Lotrel *Novartis, USA.*
Amlodipine besilate (p.838·3); benazepril hydrochloride (p.843·2).
Hypertension.

Lotremin *Schering-Plough, Hong Kong; Schering-Plough, Singapore.*
Clotrimazole (p.382·1).
Fungal skin infections.

Lotremine *Schering-Plough, Port.*
Clotrimazole (p.382·1).

Lotricomb *Essex, Ger.; Schering-Plough, NZ.*
Betamethasone dipropionate (p.1063·2); clotrimazole (p.382·1).
Skin disorders with fungal infection.

Lotriderm *Schering-Plough, Belg.; Schering, Canad.; Dominion, Irl.; Schering-Plough, S.Afr.; Dominion, UK†.*
Betamethasone dipropionate (p.1063·2); clotrimazole (p.382·1).
Fungal skin infections.

Lotrimin *Schering-Plough, Mex.; Schering, USA.*
Clotrimazole (p.382·1).
Fungal skin infections.

Lotrimin AF
Note. This name is used for preparations of different composition.
Schering-Plough, Mex.
Miconazole nitrate (p.391·1).
Fungal skin infections.

Schering-Plough, USA.
Cream; lotion; topical solution: Clotrimazole (p.382·1).
Powder; spray: Miconazole nitrate (p.391·1).
Fungal skin infections.

Lotrisone *Schering, USA.*
Betamethasone dipropionate (p.1063·2); clotrimazole (p.382·1).
Fungal skin infections.

Lotronex *Glaxo Wellcome, USA†.*
Alosetron hydrochloride (p.1210·2).
Irritable bowel syndrome.

Lotusix *Torlan, Spain†.*
Phenylephrine hydrochloride (p.1097·1); guaifenesin (p.1092·2); co-trimoxazole (p.193·3).
Respiratory-tract infections.

Lotussin *Searle, S.Afr.*
Diphenhydramine hydrochloride (p.416·1); dextromethorphan hydrobromide (p.1087·3); ephedrine hydrochloride (p.1090·1); guaifenesin (p.1092·2).
Coughs.

Lotussin Expectorant *Searle, S.Afr.*
Diphenhydramine (p.416·1); aminophylline (p.760·1); ammonium chloride (p.1085·2).
Coughs.

Lo-Uric *Rolab, S.Afr.*
Allopurinol (p.397·2).
Gout; hyperuricaemia.

Lovacol *Orion, Fin.*
Lovastatin (p.922·3).
Hyperlipidaemias.

Lovalip *Merck Sharp & Dohme, Israel.*
Lovastatin (p.922·3).
Hypercholesterolaemia.

Lovamine *MVM, Fr.*
Nutritional supplement (p.1350·1).

Lovan *Alphapharm, Austral.; Lilly, NZ.*
Fluoxetine hydrochloride (p.284·2).
Bulimia; depression; obsessive-compulsive disorder; premenstrual dysphoric disorder.

Lovelle *Organon, Austral.*
Desogestrel (p.1470·3); ethinylestradiol (p.1476·2).
Combined oral contraceptive.

Lovenox *Gerot, Aust.; Rhone-Poulenc Rorer, Canad.; Rhone-Poulenc Rorer, Fr.; Rhone-Poulenc Rorer, Port.; Roche, Switz.; Rhone-Poulenc Rorer, USA.*
Enoxaparin sodium (p.885·1).
Thromboembolic disorders.

Loveral *Rayere, Mex.*
Albendazole (p.95·2).
Worm infections.

Lovina *Hexal, Ger.*
Desogestrel (p.1470·3); ethinylestradiol (p.1476·2).
Combined oral contraceptive.

Lovir *Douglas, Austral.; Douglas, NZ; Ranbaxy, Singapore.*
Aciclovir (p.612·3).
Herpesvirus infections.

Lovire *Ranbaxy, S.Afr.*
Aciclovir (p.612·3).
Herpesvirus infections.

Loviscol *Wyeth, Mex.*
Carbocisteine (p.1086·3).

Lovrak *Julphar, UAE.*
Aciclovir (p.612·3).
Herpes simplex skin infections; varicella-zoster skin infections.

Low Liquemine *Roche, Switz.†.*
Dalteparin sodium (p.873·3).
Anticoagulant during haemodialysis or haemofiltration; thromboembolic disorders.

Lowadina *Wayne, Mex.*
Loratadine (p.420·1).

Lowasa *Central, Irl.*
Aspirin (p.14·2).
Thromboembolism prophylaxis.

Lowe-Komplex *Infirmarius-Rovit, Ger.*
A range of homoeopathic preparations.

Lowgan *Yamanouchi, Jpn†.*
Amosulalol hydrochloride (p.839·1).
Hypertension.

Lowila Cake
Note. This name is used for preparations of different composition.
Bristol-Myers Squibb, Hong Kong.
Sodium lauril sulfoacetate (p.1496·3).
Soap substitute.

Westwood-Squibb, USA.
Skin cleanser.

Lowpre *Ehlinger, Mex.*
Captopril (p.853·3).

Lowsium Plus *Rugby, USA.*
Magaldrate (p.1232·2); simeticone (p.1249·2).
Hyperacidity.

Loxapac *Wyeth Lederle, Belg.†; Wyeth-Ayerst, Canad.; Wyeth Lederle, Denm.; Wyeth Lederle, Fr.; Wyeth, Irl.; Wyeth, NZ; Wyeth, UK.*
Loxapine (p.690·1), loxapine hydrochloride (p.690·1), or loxapine succinate (p.690·1).
Psychoses.

Loxavit *Vitamed, Israel.*
Cloxacillin sodium (p.192·1).
Bacterial infections.

Loxazol *Glaxo Wellcome, Neth.; Warner-Lambert, Neth.; Warner-Lambert Consumer, Switz.*
Permethrin (p.1436·1).
Pediculosis; scabies.

Loxen *Novartis, Fr.*
Nicardipine hydrochloride (p.938·3).
Hypertension.

Loxin *Mann, Ger.*
Azelastine hydrochloride (p.409·3).
Allergic conjunctivitis.

Loxina *Neves, Port.*
Lomefloxacin hydrochloride (p.220·1).
Bacterial infections.

Loxitane *Watson, USA.*
Loxapine hydrochloride (p.690·1) or loxapine succinate (p.690·1).
Psychoses.

Loxonin *Sankyo, Jpn; Sankyo, Thai.*
Loxoprofen sodium (p.50·2).
Inflammation; musculoskeletal, joint, and peri-articular disorders; pain.

Lozide *Servier, Canad.*
Indapamide (p.913·1).
Hypertension.

Lozione Same AS *Savoma, Ital.†.*
Methionine (p.1012·2); zinc sulfate (p.1398·2); pyridoxine (p.1387·1).
Seborrhoea.

Lozione Vittoria *Ottolenghi, Ital.*
Benzalkonium chloride (p.1133·2).
Skin cleansing.

Lozol *Rhone-Poulenc Rorer, USA.*
Indapamide (p.913·1).
Heart failure; hypertension.

LP Mix *Braun, Fr.*
Amino-acid and lipid infusion (p.1350·1).
Parenteral nutrition.

L-Polamidon *Hoechst Marion Roussel, Ger.*
Levomethadone hydrochloride (p.50·1).
Pain.

LP-Truw mono *Truw, Ger.†.*
Sitosterol (p.970·3).
Hyperlipidaemias.

LPV *CSL, Austral.*
Phenoxymethylpenicillin potassium (p.235·1).
Bacterial infections.

LSP *Seroyal, Canad.*
Calcium aspartate; magnesium aspartate (p.1190·3).

Luan *Molteni, Ital.*
Lignocaine [lidocaine] hydrochloride (p.1313·2).
Local anaesthesia.

Luase *Sankyo, Spain.*
Diclofenac sodium (p.30·3).
Gout; inflammation; musculoskeletal, joint, and peri-articular disorders; pain; renal colic.

Lubafax *Douglas, Austral.*
Lubricant for skin or for medical instruments.

Lubalix *Drossapharm, Switz.*
Cloxazolam (p.671·2).
Anxiety disorders; insomnia.

Lubarol *Biovital, Austral.*
Nonoxinol 9 (p.1346·1).
Contraceptive.

Lubentyl *Synthelabo, Fr.*
Liquid paraffin (p.1407·1).
Constipation.

Lubentyl a la Magnesie *Synthelabo, Fr.*
Liquid paraffin (p.1407·1); magnesium hydroxide (p.1233·1).
Constipation.

Lubex *Permamed, Switz.*
Sodium sulfosuccinated undecenoic acid monoethanolamide (p.396·1).
Skin disorders.

Lubexyl *Permamed, Switz.*
Benzoyl peroxide (p.1111·1).
Acne.

Lubo *Synthelabo, Switz.*
Guar mucilage (p.323·3).
Lubricant.

Lubogliss *Streuli, Switz.†.*
Lignocaine [lidocaine] hydrochloride (p.1313·2).
Catheterisation; endoscopy.

Luborant
Note. This name is used for preparations of different composition.
Antigen, Irl.; Antigen, UK.
Electrolytes (p.1180·1); carmellose sodium (p.1499·3); sorbitol (p.1377·3).
Saliva substitute.

Antigen, NZ; Baxter, NZ.
Electrolytes (p.1180·1); sodium fluoride (p.1375·3).
Saliva substitute.

LubraSol *Pharmaceutical Specialties, USA.*
Emollient.

Lubricans *Vitamed, Israel.*
Emollient.
Dry skin.

Lubricating Gel *Lake, USA†.*
Vaginal lubricant.

Lubricating Jelly *Lake, USA†.*
Vaginal lubricant.

Lubriderm
Note. This name is used for preparations of different composition.
Warner-Lambert, Canad.
Wool fat (p.1410·3); liquid paraffin (p.1407·1).
Skin disorders.

Warner-Lambert, USA.
Emollient and moisturiser.

Lubriderm AHA *Warner-Lambert, Canad.*
Lactic acid (p.1626·2).

Lubriderm Daily UV
Warner-Lambert, Canad.; Warner-Lambert, USA.
SPF 15: Octinoxate (p.1517·3); octisalate (p.1518·1); oxybenzone (p.1518·1).
Formerly contained avobenzone, octinoxate, and ensulizole in *Canad.*
Sunscreen.

Lubrifilm
Cusi, Singapore; Alcon Cusi, Spain.
Soft paraffin (p.1407·3); liquid paraffin (p.1407·1); wool fat (p.1410·3).
Dry eyes; eye irritation.

Lubrigel *Rudefsa, Mex.*
Carbomers (p.1499·2).

Lubrik *Grin, Mex.*
Polyvinyl alcohol (p.1503·1).
Dry eyes.

Lubrilax *Normon, Spain.*
Sodium picosulfate (p.1249·3).
Constipation.

Lubrilent *SIFI, Ital.†.*
Wetting solution for hard contact lenses (p.1129·2).

Lubrilin *Grin, Mex.*
White soft paraffin (p.1407·3).

Lubrin
Note. This name is used for preparations of different composition.
Upsher Smith, Israel.
Macrogols (p.1630·1); glycerol (p.1616·3); polysorbate 80 (p.1347·3); macrogol stearate; neobee m-5.
Vaginal lubricant.

Kenwood, USA.
Tricaprylin; glycerol (p.1616·3); laureth 23 (p.1345·2).
Vaginal lubricant.

Lubrirhin *Alcon, Ger.*
Bromhexine (p.1085·3).
Rhinitis.

Lubri-Tears *Alcon, UK.*
Liquid paraffin (p.1407·1); white soft paraffin (p.1407·3); wool fat (p.1410·3).
Eye lubrication and protection.

LubriTears *Bausch & Lomb, USA.*
Eye drops: Hypromellose (p.1501·3); dextran 70 (p.729·2).
Eye ointment: White soft paraffin (p.1407·3); liquid paraffin (p.1407·1); wool fat (p.1410·3).
Dry eyes.

Lucenfal *Farma Lepori, Spain.*
Nicardipine hydrochloride (p.938·3).
Angina pectoris; cerebrovascular disorders; hypertension.

Lucibran *Bracco, Ital.†.*
Alfoscerate olamine.
Anxiety; confusion.

Lucidril
Kolassa, Aust.; Lipha Sante, Fr.
Meclofenoxate hydrochloride (p.1631·3).
Mental function disorders.

Lucilium *Ecosol, Switz.*
Hypericum (p.290·2).
Insomnia; tension.

Lucisan *Pfizer Consumer, Ital.*
Naphazoline nitrate (p.1095·1).
Eye irritation.

Luco-Oph *Seng, Thai.*
Sulfamethizole (p.253·3).
Eye and ear infections.

Lucopenin *Durascan, Denm.†.*
Meticillin sodium (p.223·3).
Staphylococcal infections.

Lucosil *Lundbeck, Aust.†; Rosco, Denm.; Rosco, Norw.*
Sulfamethizole (p.253·3).
Bacterial infections.

Lucostine *Lundbeck, Swed.†.*
Lomustine (p.550·2).
Malignant neoplasms.

Lucretin *Abbott, Braz.*
Boric acid (p.1586·1); salicylic acid (p.1122·3); ammonium alum.
Vulvovaginal disorders.

Lucrin
Abbott, Austral.; Abbott, Belg.; Abbott, Fr.; Abbott, Hong Kong; Takeda, Israel; Abbott, Israel; Abbott, Mex.; Abbott, Neth.; Abbott, NZ; Abbott, Port.; Abbott, S.Afr.; Abbott, Singapore; Abbott, Switz.
Leuprorelin (p.1289·3) or leuprorelin acetate (p.1289·2).
Endometriosis; precocious puberty; prostatic cancer; uterine fibroids.

Luctor *Sanofi Synthelabo, Ger.*
Naftidrofuryl oxalate (p.937·3).
Peripheral vascular disorders.

Ludilat *Organon, Aust.†.*
Bencyclane fumarate (p.843·3).
Peripheral and cerebral vascular disorders.

Ludiomil
Novartis, Aust.; Novartis, Belg.; Novartis, Braz.; Novartis, Canad.; Novartis, Denm.; Novartis, Fin.; Novartis, Ger.; Du Pont, Ger.; Novartis, Hong Kong; Novartis, Israel; Novartis, Ital.; Novartis, Mex.; Novartis, Neth.; Novartis, NZ; Novartis, Port.; Novartis, S.Afr.; Novartis, Singapore; Novartis, Spain; Novartis, Swed.; Novartis, Switz.; Novartis, Thai.; Novartis, UK; Novartis, USA†.
Maprotiline hydrochloride (p.297·2) or maprotiline mesilate (p.297·3).
Depression.

Luffa comp-Heel Nasentropfen *Heel, Ger.*
Homoeopathic preparation.

Luffa compositum *Heel, Ger.*
Homoeopathic preparation.

Luffa comp.-Tropfen-Pascoe N *Pascoe, Ger.†.*
Homoeopathic preparation.

Luffa Med Complex *Dynamit, Aust.*
Homoeopathic preparation.

Luffa Nasentropfen *DHU, Ger.*
Homoeopathic preparation.

luffa-loges *Loges, Ger.*
Homoeopathic preparation.

Luforan *Serono, Spain.*
Gonadorelin (p.1283·3).
Hypothalamic-pituitary dysfunction.

Luftgaz *Gilton, Braz.*
Dimethicone (p.1249·2); calcium pantothenate (p.1374·1).
Flatulence.

Lufyllin *Wallace, USA.*
Diprophylline (p.764·1).
Asthma; reversible bronchospasm.

Lufyllin-EPG *Wallace, USA.*
Diprophylline (p.764·1); ephedrine hydrochloride (p.1090·1); guaifenesin (p.1092·2); phenobarbital (p.355·1).
Bronchospasm.

Lufyllin-GG *Wallace, USA.*
Diprophylline (p.764·1); guaifenesin (p.1092·2).
Asthma; reversible bronchospasm.

Lugesteron *Leiras, Fin.*
Progesterone (p.1488·3).
Female infertility; menstrual and menopausal disorders; progesterone deficiency.

Luiflex
Sankyo, Aust.; Sankyo, Belg.
Indometacin (p.44·3).
Musculoskeletal and joint disorders; soft-tissue injury.

Luitase *Sankyo, Ital.*
Pancrelipase (p.1647·2).
Cystic fibrosis; malabsorption.

Luivac
Sankyo, Ger.; Byk Gulden, Mex.
Lysates of *Staphylococcus aureus*; *Streptococcus mitis*; *Streptococcus pyogenes*; *Streptococcus pneumoniae*; *Klebsiella pneumoniae*; *Moraxella catarrhalis*; *Haemophilus influenzae*(p.0·0).
Respiratory-tract infections.

Luizym
Note. This name is used for preparations of different composition.
Luitpold, Ger.†.
Enzyme extract from *Aspergillus oryzae*.
Digestive system disorders.

Luitpold, Ital.†.
Protease; cellulase (p.1593·1); amylase (p.1579·3).
Digestive disorders.

Sankyo, Port.†.
Amylase (p.1579·3); protease.

Lukadin *San Carlo, Ital.*
Amikacin sulfate (p.148·1).
Gram-negative bacterial infections.

Lukasm *Sigma-Tau, Ital.*
Montelukast sodium (p.768·1).
Asthma.

Lumbago-Gastreu R11 *Reckeweg, Ger.*
Homoeopathic preparation.

Lumbalgine *Cooperation Pharmaceutique, Fr.*
Glycol salicylate (p.42·2); menthol (p.1632·3); camphor (p.1589·3); turpentine oil (p.1676·3); benzyl nicotinate (p.20·2).
Muscular disorders.

Lumbaxol Para *Aldo, Spain†.*
Chlormezanone (p.660·1); paracetamol (p.71·2).
Dysmenorrhoea; neuralgias; peri-articular disorders; premenstrual syndrome.

Lumbinon *Lichtenstein, Ger.*
Glycol salicylate (p.42·2).
Migraine; musculoskeletal, joint, and soft-tissue disorders; neuralgia.

Lumbriquil *Regius, Braz.*
Piperazine (p.105·3); prune (p.1245·1).
Intestinal nematode infections.

Lumiactiv *Vichy, Canad.*
Avobenzone (p.1517·1); octocrilene (p.1518·1); terephthalylidene dicamphor sulfonic acid.
Sunscreen.

Lumifurex *Irex, Fr.*
Nifuroxazide (p.230·2).
Diarrhoea.

Lumigan *Allergan, USA.*
Bimatoprost (p.1440·3).
Glaucoma; ocular hypertension.

Lumin *Alphapharm, Austral.*
Mianserin hydrochloride (p.298·1).
Depression.

Luminal
Desitin, Ger.; Sanofi Winthrop, Israel; Bayer, Port.; Bayer, Spain; Merck, Switz.; Sanofi Winthrop, USA.
Phenobarbital (p.355·1) or phenobarbital sodium (p.355·1).
Adjunct in the treatment of poisoning; epilepsy; insomnia; sedative.

Luminale *Bracco, Ital.*
Phenobarbital (p.355·1) or phenobarbital sodium (p.355·1).
Barbiturate withdrawal; epilepsy; sedative.

Luminaletas
Bayer, Port.; Bayer, Spain.
Phenobarbital (p.355·1).
Anxiety; convulsive disorders; depression; insomnia; smooth muscle spasm.

Luminalette *Bracco, Ital.*
Phenobarbital (p.355·1).
Barbiturate withdrawal; epilepsy; sedative.

Luminaletten *Desitin, Ger.*
Phenobarbital (p.355·1).
Epilepsy.

Luminovag *Novag, Mex.*
Ketoconazole (p.389·1).
Amoebiasis.

Lumirelax *Alpharma, Fr.*
Methocarbamol (p.1329·3).
Musculoskeletal and joint disorders.

Lumirem
Sanova, Aust.†; Guerbet, Denm.; Guerbet, Fin.; Guerbet, Fr.; Guerbet, Ger.; Guerbet, Ital.; Guerbet, Neth.†; Gothia, Swed.; Guerbet, Switz.†.
Ferumoxsil (p.1032·3).
Contrast medium for magnetic resonance imaging of the gastrointestinal tract.

Lumitens *Solvay, Fr.*
Xipamide (p.999·2).
Hypertension; oedema.

Lunadon *Singer, Switz.*
Tolazoline hydrochloride (p.984·3); drofenine hydrochloride (p.466·3); diphenhydramine hydrochloride (p.416·1).
Nervous disorders; sleep disorders.

Lundiran *Vir, Spain.*
Naproxen (p.60·3).
Fever; gout; musculoskeletal and joint disorders; pain.

Lunelax
AstraZeneca, Norw.; Tika, Swed.
Ispaghula (p.1229·1).
Adjunct in treatment of diarrhoea; bowel evacuation; constipation.

Lunelax comp *Tika, Swed.†.*
Ispaghula (p.1229·1); sennosides (p.1248·3).
Constipation.

Lunelle *Pharmacia Upjohn, USA.*
Medroxyprogesterone acetate (p.1480·1); estradiol cipionate (p.1473·2).
Injectable contraceptive.

Lunerin
AstraZeneca, Fin.; Tika, Swed.†.
Brompheniramine maleate (p.410·2); phenylpropanolamine hydrochloride (p.1098·1).
Rhinitis.

Lunibron-A *Valeas, Ital.*
Flunisolide (p.1070·3).
Hypersensitivity disorders of the respiratory tract.

Lunis *Valeas, Ital.*
Flunisolide (p.1070·3).
Rhinitis.

Lupectrim *Luper, Braz.*
Co-trimoxazole (p.193·3).
Bacterial infections; Pneumocystis carinii pneumonia; protozoal infections.

Lupectrim Balsamico *Luper, Braz.*
Co-trimoxazole (p.193·3); guaifenesin (p.1092·2); ammonium chloride (p.1085·2).
Bacterial infections.

Lu-Peracina *Reuffer, Mex.*
Piperazine (p.105·3).

Lupercaina *Luper, Braz.*
Yohimbine hydrochloride (p.1681·3); vitamin B substances; vitamin E (p.1350·1); ptychopetalum uncinatum; erythroxylon catuaba.
Erectile dysfunction.

Luperzol *Quimica y Farmacia, Mex.*
Ketoconazole (p.389·1).

Lupidon *Seid, Spain.*
Calcium pantothenate (p.1374·1); dimethicone (p.1249·2); magnesium polygalacturonate.
Flatulence.

Lupidon G *Bruschettini, Hong Kong; Bruschettini, Ital.*
A herpes simplex type 2 vaccine (p.1544·3).
Active immunisation.

Lupidon H *Bruschettini, Ital.*
A herpes simplex type 1 vaccine (p.1544·3).
Active immunisation.

Lupidon H+G *Boots Healthcare, Switz.*
Lupidon H, a herpes simplex vaccine (type I); Lupidon G, a herpes simplex vaccine (type II) (p.1544·3).
Herpes simplex infections.

Lupovalin *Selz, Spain.*
Diphenhydramine hydrochloride (p.416·1).
Insomnia.

Lupron *Abbott, Braz.; Abbott, Canad.; TAP, USA.*
Leuprorelin acetate (p.1289·2).
Endometriosis; fibroids; precocious puberty; prostatic cancer.

Lurdex *Liferpal, Mex.*
Albendazole (p.95·2).
Worm infections.

Luret *Sanofi Synthelabo, Ger.*
Azosemide (p.843·1).
Oedema.

Luride *Colgate-Palmolive, USA.*
Sodium fluoride (p.1375·3).
Dental caries prophylaxis.

Lurline PMS *Fielding, USA.*
Paracetamol (p.71·2); pamabrom (p.952·1); pyridoxine (p.1387·1).
Premenstrual syndrome.

Lurselle
Hoechst Marion Roussel, Austral.; Hoechst, Ger.†; Hoechst Marion Roussel, Hong Kong; Mer-National, S.Afr.; Hoechst Marion Roussel, Thai.
Probucol (p.959·2).
Hypercholesterolaemia.

Lusap *Interdelta, Switz.*
Malathion (p.1434·2).
Pediculosis.

Lustra *Medicis, USA.*
Hydroquinone (p.1115·1).
Hyperpigmentation.

Lustral
Invicta, Irl.; Pfizer, Israel; Pfizer, UK.
Sertraline hydrochloride (p.308·3).
Depression; mixed anxiety depressive states; obsessive-compulsive disorder.

Lustys Herbalene *Lane, UK.*
Senna leaf (p.1248·2); frangula bark (p.1227·1); sambucus (p.1660·3); fennel (p.1610·1).
Constipation.

Lutenil *Byk, Braz.*
Nomegestrol acetate (p.1484·3).
Menstrual disorders.

Lutenyl
Theramex, Hong Kong; Theramex, Ital.; Theramex, Mon.; Sanofi Synthelabo, Port.
Nomegestrol acetate (p.1484·3).
Endometriosis; menopausal disorders; menstrual disorders.

Luteran *Solymes, Fr.*
Chlormadinone acetate (p.1465·3).
Endometriosis; fibromas; menstrual disorders.

Lutestral *Cassenne, Fr.†.*
Chlormadinone acetate (p.1465·3); ethinylestradiol (p.1476·2).
Menstrual disorders.

Lutionex *Roussel, Fr.†.*
Demegestone (p.1470·3).
Endometriosis; fibromas; menstrual disorders.

Lutoginestryl F *Hoechst Marion Roussel, Mex.*
Progesterone (p.1488·3); estradiol benzoate (p.1473·1).
Menstrual disorders.

Lutometrodiol *Monsanto, Fr.†.*
Etynodiol diacetate (p.1477·1).
Endometriosis; fibromas; mastopathy; menstrual disorders; progestogen-only oral contraceptive.

Lutopolar *Orion, Fin.*
Medroxyprogesterone acetate (p.1480·1).
Dysfunctional uterine bleeding; endometriosis; malignant neoplasms; menstrual disorders.

Lutoral
Note. This name is used for preparations of different composition.
Sanofi Winthrop, Ital.†.
Medroxyprogesterone acetate (p.1480·1).
Menstrual disorders; premature labour; prostatic hyperplasia; threatened abortion.

Searle, Mex.
Chlormadinone acetate (p.1465·3).
Menstrual disorders; uterine cancer; uterine fibroids.

Lutoral E *Searle, Mex.*
Chlormadinone acetate (p.1465·3); mestranol (p.1482·1).
Endometriosis; menstrual disorders.

Lutrax *Alcon, Mex.*
Azapentacene.

Lutrelef
Sigmapharm, Aust.; Ferring, Fr.; Ferring, Ger.; Ferring, Israel; Ferring, Ital.; Ferring, Neth.; Ferring, Swed.; Ferring, Switz.
Gonadorelin acetate (p.1284·2).
Delayed puberty; male and female infertility.

Lutrepulse
Ferring, Canad.; Ferring, USA†.
Gonadorelin acetate (p.1284·2).
Infertility.

Luuf Balsam *Apomedica, Aust.*
Camphor (p.1589·3); menthol (p.1632·3); eucalyptus oil (p.1609·2); turpentine oil (p.1676·3); pumilio pine oil (p.1656·3); oleum pini sylvestris; thymol (p.1158·3).
Respiratory-tract disorders.

Luuf-Erkaltungssol *Apomedica, Aust.*
Oleum pini sylvestris; eucalyptus oil (p.1609·2); pumilio pine oil (p.1656·3).
Respiratory-tract disorders.

Luuf-Heilpflanzenol *Apomedica, Aust.*
Eucalyptus oil (p.1609·2); peppermint oil (p.1243·3); cajuput oil (p.1588·1).
Digestive disorders; flatulence; migraine; pain; respiratory-tract disorders; soft-tissue injury.

Luuf-Hustentee *Apomedica, Aust.*
Thyme (p.1672·2); guaifenesin (p.1092·2); menthol (p.1632·3); camphor (p.1589·3); fennel oil (p.1610·2); anise oil (p.1580·3); eucalyptus oil (p.1609·2); thyme oil (p.1672·3).
Coughs and cold symptoms.

Luuf-Nasenspray *Apomedica, Aust.*
Naphazoline hydrochloride (p.1095·1); diphenhydramine hydrochloride (p.416·1).
Colds; hay fever; sinusitis.

Luva Invisivel *Dermoteca, Port.†.*
Barrier preparation.

Luvased
Wyeth Lederle, Aust.; Biocur, Ger.
Valerian (p.1678·3); lupulus (p.1629·3).
Anxiety disorders; sleep disorders.

Luvased-Tropfen N *Biocur, Ger.*
Valerian (p.1678·3); lupulus (p.1629·3); melissa (p.1632·2); passion flower (p.1649·1).
Nervous disorders; sleep disorders.

Luvatren *Janssen-Cilag, Switz.†.*
Moperone hydrochloride (p.695·1).
Alcohol withdrawal syndrome; epilepsy; psychoses.

Luveris *Serono, UK.*
Lutropin alfa (p.1290·2).
Female infertility.

Luvion *GiEnne, Ital.*
Canrenone (p.853·3) or potassium canrenoate (p.957·1).
Hyperaldosteronism; hypertension.

Luvos Heilerde *Luvos, Ger.†.*
Natural loess.
Gastrointestinal disorders; skin disorders.

Luvox
Solvay, Austral.; Solvay, Canad.; Pharmacia Upjohn, Mex.; Solvay, S.Afr.; Solvay, USA.
Fluvoxamine maleate (p.289·3).
Depression; obsessive-compulsive disorder.

Luxazone *Allergan, Ital.*
Dexamethasone (p.1067·1).
Eye disorders.

Luxazone Eparina *Tubilux, Ital.*
Dexamethasone (p.1067·1); heparin sodium (p.902·1).
Eye disorders.

Luxiq *Connetics, USA.*
Betamethasone valerate (p.1063·2).
Skin disorders.

Luxivia *Norman, Canad.*
SPF 15: Octinoxate (p.1517·3); titanium dioxide (p.1126·1).
Sunscreen.

Luxivia Ultra *Norman, Canad.*
SPF 15: Octinoxate (p.1517·3); oxybenzone (p.1518·1).
Sunscreen.

Luxoben *Asta Medica, Ital.†.*
Tiapride hydrochloride (p.709·1).
Anxiety; dyskinesia.

Luxofort *Solfran, Mex.*
Vitamin B substances (p.1350·1).

Luxomicina *Tubilux, Ital.*
Micronomicin sulfate (p.224·3).
Eye infections.

Luzone *Sigma-Tau, Spain.*
Sulodexide (p.978·3).
Atherosclerosis; hyperlipidaemias; thromboembolic disorders.

Lyasin *MC, Ital.†.*
Chlorhexidine gluconate (p.1138·2).
Hand disinfection.

Lyban *Rhone-Poulenc Rorer, Austral.†.*
Pyrethrins; piperonyl butoxide (p.1436·1).
Pediculosis.

Lybovit *Frankin, Hong Kong.*
Cyproheptadine (p.414·3); vitamins; lysine (p.1350·1).
Appetite loss; vitamin supplement.

Lycamed *UCB, Ital.†.*
Lysine calcium citrate hydrochloride.
Calcium supplement.

Lycia Luminique *Artsana, Ital.*
Benzalkonium chloride (p.1133·2); hamamelis (p.1618·3); chamomile (p.1593·2).
Eye disinfection; eye irritation.

Lyclear
Warner-Lambert, Austral.; Warner-Lambert, Irl.; Glaxo Wellcome, Irl.; Glaxo Wellcome, Israel; Glaxo Wellcome, NZ; Glaxo Wellcome, S.Afr.; Kestrel, UK.
Permethrin (p.1436·1).
Pediculosis; scabies.

Lycoaktin *Steigerwald, Ger.*
Injection: Homoeopathic preparation.

Lycoaktin M *Steigerwald, Ger.*
Lycopus virginicus.
Hyperthyroidism with nervous disorders.

Lycovowen-N *Weber & Weber, Ger.†.*
Homoeopathic preparation.

Lyderm
Note.This name is used for preparations of different composition.
Taro, Canad.
Fluocinonide (p.1071·2).
Skin disorders.

PSM, NZ.
Permethrin (p.1436·1).
Scabies.

Lydonide *Technilab, Canad.*
Fluocinonide (p.1071·2).
Skin disorders.

Lygal E Creme *Taurus, Ger.*
Betamethasone benzoate (p.1063·1).
Skin disorders.

Lygal E Tinktur *Taurus, Ger.*
Betamethasone benzoate (p.1063·1); salicylic acid (p.1122·3).
Skin disorders.

Lygal Kopfsalbe N *Taurus, Ger.*
Salicylic acid (p.1122·3).
Scalp disorders.

Lygal Kopftinktur *Taurus, Ger.*
Prednisolone (p.1077·3); salicylic acid (p.1122·3); dexpanthenol (p.1602·3).
Scalp disorders.

Lygal Wundsalbe *Taurus, Ger.*
Wheat-germ oil.
Burns; wounds.

Lyman *Drossapharm, Switz.*
Heparin sodium (p.902·1); allantoin (p.1110·1); dexpanthenol (p.1602·3); lavender oil (p.1627·2).
Peripheral vascular disorders; soft-tissue disorders.

LYMErix
SmithKline Beecham, Canad.; SmithKline Beecham, USA.
A lyme disease vaccine (recombinant) (p.1546·2).
Active immunisation.

Lymetel *Almirall, Spain.*
Fluvastatin sodium (p.892·1).
Atherosclerosis; hypercholesterolaemia.

Lymphaden *Hevert, Ger.*
Homoeopathic preparation.

Lymphaden N *Hevert, Ger.*
Homoeopathic preparation.

Lymphazurin *US Surgical, USA.*
Sulphan blue (p.1668·2).
Adjunct to lymphography.

Lymphdiaral *Pascoe, Ger.*
Homoeopathic preparation.

Lymphex *Drossapharm, Switz.†.*
Coumarin (p.1599·3).
Lymphoedema.

Lymphoglobulin *Imtix, Ger.*
An antilymphocyte immunoglobulin (horse) (p.508·2).
Aplastic anaemia; organ transplantation.

Lymphoglobuline
Imtix, Belg.; Imtix, Fr.; Pasteur Merieux, Hong Kong; Pasteur Merieux, Israel; Imtix, Ital.; Imtix, Neth.; Aventis, S.Afr.; Imtix, Switz.; Pasteur Merieux, Thai.
An antilymphocyte immunoglobulin (horse) (p.508·2).
Formerly known as Lymfoglobuline in Neth.
Aplastic anaemia; graft-versus-host disease; transplant rejection.

Lymphomyosot
Heel, Ger.; Heel, S.Afr.
Homoeopathic preparation.

Lymphozil *Cesra, Ger.*
Echinacea pallida (p.1606·2); calc. carbonic.; lachesis.
Tonic.

Lymphtropfen S *Cosmochema, Ger.*
Homoeopathic preparation.

Lyndak *Eurofarmaco, Ital.*
Sulindac (p.85·3).
Gout; musculoskeletal and joint disorders; neuritis; soft-tissue injury.

Lyndiol
Organon, Aust.; Organon, Belg.†; Organon, Denm.†; Organon, Ger.†; Organon, Hong Kong; Organon, Swed.†; Organon, Thai.
Lynestrenol (p.1480·1); ethinylestradiol (p.1476·2).
Combined oral contraceptive.

Lyndiolett *Organon, Swed.*
Lynestrenol (p.1480·1); ethinylestradiol (p.1476·2).
Combined oral contraceptive.

Lynoral *Organon, Neth.*
Ethinylestradiol (p.1476·2).
Breast cancer; menstrual disorders; oestrogen deficiency; postcoital contraceptive; prostatic cancer.

Lyn-ratiopharm *Ratiopharm, Ger.*
Lynestrenol (p.1480·1); ethinylestradiol (p.1476·2).
Combined oral contraceptive; menstrual disorders.

Lyn-ratiopharm-Sequenz *Ratiopharm, Ger.*
7 Capsules, ethinylestradiol (p.1476·2); 15 capsules, lynestrenol (p.1480·1); ethinylestradiol.
Sequential-type oral contraceptive.

Lyobalsam *Truw, Ger.†.*
Camphor (p.1589·3); eucalyptus oil (p.1609·2).
Respiratory-tract disorders.

Lyo-Bifidus *Alpharma, Fr.*
Bifidobacterium bifidus (Bacillus bifidus) (p.1626·3).
Diarrhoea.

Lyofoam *SSL, UK.*
Polyurethane foam dressing.
Ulcers; wounds.

Lyofoam C *SSL, UK.*
Activated charcoal (p.1000·2).
Malodorous wounds.

Lyogen *Lundbeck, Ger.*
Fluphenazine decanoate (p.684·3) or fluphenazine hydrochloride (p.684·3).
Psychoses.

Lyorodin *Rodleben, Ger.; UCB, Ger.*
Fluphenazine decanoate (p.684·3) or fluphenazine hydrochloride (p.684·3).
Psychoses.

Lyostypt
Braun Surgical, Switz.†; Davis & Geck, UK.
Collagen (p.1598·2).
Haemorrhage.

Lyovac Cosmegen
Merck Sharp & Dohme, Belg.; Merck Sharp & Dohme, Ger.; Merck Sharp & Dohme, Neth.
Dactinomycin (p.532·2).
Malignant neoplasms.

Lyphocin
Fujisawa, Hong Kong; American Pharmaceutical, USA.
Vancomycin hydrochloride (p.267·2).
Bacterial infections.

Lypholyte *American Pharmaceutical, USA.*
A range of electrolyte preparations (p.1180·1).
Fluid and electrolyte disorders.

Lyprinex *Life Plus, UK.*
Green-lipped mussel lipid extract (p.1618·2).
Formerly known as Lyprinol.

Lypsyl Cold Sore Gel *Novartis Consumer, UK.*
Lignocaine [lidocaine] hydrochloride (p.1313·2); zinc sulfate (p.1398·2); cetrimide (p.1137·1).
Herpes labialis.

Lyptocodine *Monot, Fr.†.*
Adult and paediatric syrup: Pholcodine (p.1099·1); codeine camsilate (p.26·1); eucalyptol (p.1609·2); sulfogaiacol (p.1101·1); magnesium sulfate (p.1191·1).
Infant syrup: Calcium bromide (p.1587·1); guaifenesin (p.1092·2); mannitol (p.924·3); syrup diacode.
Coughs.

Lysalgo *SIT, Ital.*
Mefenamic acid (p.51·2).
Inflammation; pain.

Lysantin *Gea, Denm.*
Orphenadrine hydrochloride (p.470·3).
Drug-induced extrapyramidal disorders; parkinsonism.

Lysanxia
Parke, Davis, Belg.; Parke, Davis, Fr.
Prazepam (p.701·1).
Alcohol withdrawal syndrome; anxiety.

Lysbex *Provita, Aust.*
Bibenzonium bromide (p.1085·3).
Coughs.

Lysedem *Knoll, Fr.†.*
Coumarin (p.1599·3).
Post-mastectomy lymphoedema.

Lysedil *Vifor, Switz.*
Promethazine hydrochloride (p.423·2); belladonna (p.463·1).
Coughs; gastrointestinal disorders; hypersensitivity reactions; sedative.

Lysedil compositum *Vifor, Switz.*
Promethazine hydrochloride (p.423·2); belladonna (p.463·1); paracetamol (p.71·2).
Coughs; fever; gastrointestinal disorders; hypersensitivity reactions; pain; sedative.

Lyseen
Hommel, Ger.†; Novartis Consumer, Ital.
Pridinol mesilate (p.1330·1).
Skeletal muscle spasm.

Lyseen New *Therabel, Belg.†.*
Chlormezanone (p.660·1).
Formerly contained pridinol mesilate.
Skeletal muscle spasm.

Lysetol V *Schulke & Mayr, Ger.*
Formaldehyde (p.1144·2); glutaral (p.1145·2); didecyldimethylammonium chloride (p.1143·2).
Formerly contained formaldehyde, glutaral, and ethylhexanal.
Instrument disinfection.

Lysetol FF *Schulke & Mayr, Ger.*
Glutaral (p.1145·2); ethylhexanal.
Instrument disinfection.

Lysetol Med *Schulke & Mayr, Ger.*
Cocospropylendiaminguaniacetat; phenoxypropanol (p.1153·3); benzalkonium chloride (p.1133·2).
Instrument disinfection.

Lysinotol *Asta Medica, Spain.*
Lysine aspirin (p.50·3).
Fever; musculoskeletal, joint, and peri-articular disorders; pain; thromboembolism prophylaxis.

Lysivit B12 a l'inositol *Sarget, Fr.†.*
Lysine hydrochloride; inositol; cyanocobalamin (p.1350·1).
Tonic.

Lyso-6
Darci, Fr.; UCB, Switz.
Muramidase hydrochloride (p.1638·1); pyridoxine hydrochloride (p.1386·3).
Mouth and throat disorders.

Lysocalm *Darci, Fr.*
Muramidase hydrochloride (p.1638·1); menthol (p.1632·3).
Mouth and throat infections.

Lysocline *Parke, Davis, Fr.*
Methacycline hydrochloride (p.222·3).
Formerly contained methacycline hydrochloride and muramidase hydrochloride.
Bacterial infections.

Lysodren
Bristol, Canad.; Bristol-Myers Squibb Oncology, USA.
Mitotane (p.559·2).
Adrenal cortical cancer.

Lysodrop *Asta Medica, Belg.*
Acetylcysteine (p.1082·3).
Dry eyes.

Lysofon *Lafon, Fr.*
Lozenges: Chlorhexidine acetate (p.1138·2); amethocaine [tetracaine] hydrochloride (p.1305·2).
Formerly contained tricarbaurinium and amethocaine [tetracaine] hydrochloride.
Mouth and throat pain.

Throat spray: Chlorhexidine gluconate (p.1138·2).
Formerly contained tricarbaurinium.
Mouth and throat disorders.

Lysoform *Lysoform, Ger.*
Formaldehyde (p.1144·2).
Hyperhidrosis; skin disorders; surface and linen disinfection.

Lysoform Killavon *Lysoform, Ger.*
Benzalkonium chloride (p.1133·2).
Disinfection of skin, mucous membranes, and surfaces; skin disorders.

Lysoformin *Lysoform, Ger.*
Formaldehyde (p.1144·2); glutaral (p.1145·2).
Surface disinfection.

Lysoformin 3000 *Lysoform, Ger.*
Glyoxal (p.1145·3); glutaral (p.1145·2); didecyldimethylammonium chloride (p.1143·2).
Disinfection of instruments and surfaces.

Lysoformin spezial *Lysoform, Ger.*
Guanidine derivative; didecyldimethylammonium chloride (p.1143·2).
Disinfection of surfaces.

Lysokana *Zambon, Spain†.*
Kanamycin sulfate (p.218·1); muramidase hydrochloride (p.1638·1); bacitracin (p.1647·3).
Mouth and throat inflammation.

Lysomucil *Zambon, Belg.*
Acetylcysteine (p.1082·3).
Paracetamol overdose; respiratory-tract disorders associated with viscous mucus.

Lysopaine
Boehringer Ingelheim, Fr.
Muramidase hydrochloride (p.1638·1); papaya sap; bacitracin (p.155·2).
Mouth and throat infections.

Boehringer Ingelheim, Switz.
Muramidase hydrochloride (p.1638·1); papain (p.1647·3); bacitracin (p.155·2).
Mouth and throat disorders.

Lysoprin *Rafa, Israel.*
Lysine aspirin (p.50·3).
Glycine (p.1365·3) is included in this preparation in an attempt to limit adverse effects on the gastrointestinal mucosa.
Fever; pain.

Lysovir *Alliance, UK.*
Amantadine hydrochloride (p.1161·2).
Influenza A.

Lysox *Menarini, Belg.*
Acetylcysteine (p.1082·3).
Respiratory-tract disorders associated with viscous secretions.

Lyspafen *Janssen-Cilag, Switz.†.*
Difenoxin hydrochloride (p.1222·1).
Atropine sulfate (p.461·1) is included in this preparation to discourage abuse.
Diarrhoea.

Lyssavac N
Berna, Hong Kong; Berna, Ital.; Berna, Switz.; Berna, Thai.
A rabies vaccine (p.1560·2).
Active immunisation.

Lyssuman *Berna, Spain†.*
A rabies immunoglobulin (p.1560·2).
Passive immunisation.

Lysthenon
Nycomed, Aust.; Nycomed, Ger.; Nycomed, Switz.
Suxamethonium chloride (p.1340·1).
Depolarising neuromuscular blocker.

Lystin
Biolab, Hong Kong; Biolab, Thai.
Nystatin (p.392·2).
Fungal infections.

Lysuron *Roche, Switz.*
Allopurinol (p.397·2).
Gout; hyperuricaemia; renal calculi.

Lyteca *Zurich, S.Afr.†*
Paracetamol (p.71·2).
Pain.

Lyteers *Fischer, Israel.*
Sodium chloride (p.1196·1); potassium chloride (p.1194·3).
Dry eyes.

Lyteprep *Therapex, Canad.*
Electrolyte solution (p.1180·1).
Gastrointestinal lavage.

Lytos
Boehringer Mannheim, Aust.†; Roche, Fr.
Disodium clodronate (p.751·2).
Malignant hypercalcaemia; malignant osteolysis; Paget's disease of bone.

Lytren
Mead Johnson Nutritionals, Canad.
Glucose; potassium citrate; sodium chloride; sodium citrate; citric acid (p.1185·2).
Diarrhoea; oral rehydration therapy.

Mead Johnson, Fr.
Maltodextrin; glucose; potassium citrate; sodium chloride; citric acid; sodium citrate; calcium gluconate; magnesium phosphate (p.1185·2).
Diarrhoea; oral rehydration therapy.

Lytren RHS *Mead Johnson Nutritionals, Canad.*
Citric acid; potassium citrate; sodium chloride; sodium citrate (p.1185·2).

Lyzyme *Shin Poong, Singapore.*
Muramidase hydrochloride (p.1638·1).
Haemorrhage; respiratory-tract congestion; sinusitis.

M & M *Malam, UK.*
Cod-liver oil (p.1357·2); purified honey (p.1366·2).

Ma Ma Sustagen *Mead Johnson, Hong Kong.*
Preparation for enteral nutrition (p.1350·1).
Pregnancy and lactation.

Maagersan *Cermak, Aust.†*
Vitamin A (p.1382·1); colecalciferol (p.1391·1).
Vitamin A and D deficiency.

Maalox
Gerot, Aust.; Aventis, Belg.; Novartis Consumer, Canad.; Theraplix, Fr.; Rhone-Poulenc Rorer, Ger.; Rhone-Poulenc Rorer, Hong Kong; Rhone-Poulenc Rorer, Irl.; Rhone-Poulenc Rorer, Israel; Rhone-Poulenc Rorer, Ital.; Rhone-Poulenc Rorer, Neth.; Aventis, S.Afr.; Rhone-Poulenc Rorer, Spain; Rhone-Poulenc Rorer, UK; Novartis Consumer, USA.
Algeldrate or aluminium hydroxide (p.1210·3); magnesium hydroxide (p.1233·1).
These ingredients can be described by the British Approved Name Co-magaldrox.
Gastrointestinal hyperacidity.

Maalox Antacid *Rhone-Poulenc Rorer, USA.*
Calcium carbonate (p.1215·1).
Hyperacidity.

Maalox Anti-Diarrheal *Rhone-Poulenc Rorer, USA†.*
Loperamide hydrochloride (p.1231·3).
Diarrhoea.

Maalox Anti-Gas *Rhone-Poulenc Rorer, USA.*
Simeticone (p.1249·2).
Flatulence.

Maalox Anti-Gas Extra Strength *Novartis, USA.*
Aluminium hydroxide (p.1210·3); magnesium hydroxide (p.1233·1); simeticone (p.1249·2).
Antacid; flatulence.

Maalox Ballonnements *Theraplix, Fr.*
Aluminium hydroxide (p.1210·3); magnesium hydroxide (p.1233·1); simeticone (p.1249·2).
Flatulence; gastric hyperacidity.

Maalox Daily Fiber *Rhone-Poulenc Rorer, USA†.*
Psyllium hydrophilic mucilloid (p.1229·1).

Maalox GRF *Novartis Consumer, Canad.†*
Simeticone (p.1249·2).
Dyspepsia; flatulence.

Maalox H₂ Acid Controller *Novartis Consumer, Canad.*
Famotidine (p.1225·3).

Maalox Heartburn Relief *Rhone-Poulenc Rorer, USA.*
Aluminium hydroxide-magnesium carbonate co-dried gel (p.1211·2); magnesium carbonate (p.1232·3).
Hyperacidity.

Maalox HRF *Novartis Consumer, Canad.*
Calcium carbonate (p.1215·1); sodium alginate (p.1498·3); magnesium carbonate (p.1232·3).
Formerly contained aluminium hydroxide-magnesium carbonate co-dried gel, magnesium alginate, and magnesium carbonate.
Dyspepsia; gastro-oesophageal reflux; heartburn.

Maalox Plus
Rhodia, Braz.; Novartis Consumer, Canad.; Rhone-Poulenc Rorer, Hong Kong; Rhone-Poulenc Rorer, Irl.; Rhone-Poulenc Rorer, Israel; Rhone-Poulenc Rorer, Ital.; Rhone-Poulenc Rorer, Neth.; Rhone-Poulenc Rorer, Port.; Aventis, S.Afr.; Rhone-Poulenc Rorer, UK; Rhone-Poulenc Rorer, USA†.
Aluminium hydroxide (p.1210·3); magnesium hydroxide (p.1233·1); simeticone (p.1249·2).
Dyspepsia; flatulence; gastrointestinal hyperacidity; heartburn.

Maalox Quick Dissolve
Novartis Consumer, Canad.; Novartis, USA.
Calcium carbonate (p.1215·1).
Antacid.

The symbol † denotes a preparation no longer actively marketed

Maalox TC
Rhodia, Braz.; Novartis Consumer, Canad.; Rhone-Poulenc Rorer, Ital.; Rhone-Poulenc Rorer, UK.
Aluminium hydroxide (p.1210·3); magnesium hydroxide (p.1233·1).
Formerly known as Maalox Concentrate. These ingredients can be described by the British Approved Name Co-magaldrox.
Gastrointestinal hyperacidity; peptic ulcer.

Maaloxan
Rhone-Poulenc Rorer, Ger.; Piraud, Switz.†.
Aluminium hydroxide (p.1210·3); magnesium hydroxide (p.1233·1).
Gastrointestinal disorders associated with gastric hyperacidity.

Maaloxan Ca *Rhone-Poulenc Rorer, Switz.*
Aluminium hydroxide (p.1210·3); magnesium hydroxide (p.1233·1); calcium carbonate (p.1215·1).
Formerly known as Camalox.
Gastric hyperacidity.

Mab *Whitehall, Fr.*
Magnesium carbonate (p.1232·3); calcium carbonate (p.1215·1); sodium bicarbonate (p.1186·2).
Gastrointestinal disorders.

MabCampath *Schering, UK.*
Alemtuzumab (p.506·1).
Chronic lymphocytic leukaemia.

Mabicrol *Promeco, Mex.*
Clarithromycin (p.186·2).
Bacterial infections.

Mabogastrol *Merck, Spain.*
Aluminium hydroxide (p.1210·3); magnesium carbonate (p.1232·3); sodium bicarbonate (p.1186·2).
Formerly contained anethole, aluminium hydroxide, magnesium carbonate, and sodium bicarbonate.
Dyspepsia.

Mabosil *Mabo, Spain†.*
Magnesium trisilicate (p.1233·3).
Gastrointestinal hyperacidity.

Maboterpen
Note. This name is used for preparations of different composition.
Mabo, Spain†.
Suppositories: Camphor (p.1589·3); eucalyptol (p.1609·2); dextromethorphan (p.1087·3); niaouli oil (p.1640·2); guaiacol (p.1092·1).
Respiratory-tract disorders.

Tedec Meiji, Spain†.
Syrup: Tolu balsam (p.1101·3); diphenhydramine hydrochloride (p.416·1); ephedrine hydrochloride (p.1090·1); niaouli oil (p.1640·2); oleum pini sylvestris; sodium benzoate (p.1134·3); bitter orange; sulfogaiacol (p.1101·1).
Upper-respiratory-tract disorders.

Mabron
Medochemie, Hong Kong; Medochemie, Singapore; Medochemie, Thai.
Tramadol hydrochloride (p.89·1).
Pain.

Mabthera
Roche, Aust.; Roche, Austral.; Roche, Belg.; Roche, Denm.; Roche, Fin.; Roche, Fr.; Roche, Ger.; Roche, Israel; Roche, Ital.; Roche, Mex.; Roche, Neth.; Roche, Norw.; Roche, NZ; Roche, Port.; Roche, S.Afr.; Roche, Singapore; Roche, Spain; Roche, Swed.; Roche, Switz.; Roche, Thai.; Roche, UK.
Rituximab (p.567·3).
Follicular lymphoma.

Mac *Ernest Jackson, UK.*
Amylmetacresol (p.1133·2); menthol (p.1632·3).
Sore throat.

Mac Dual Action *Ernest Jackson, UK.*
Hexylresorcinol (p.1146·3).
Formerly known as Mac Extra.
Sore throat.

Mac Sugar Free *Ernest Jackson, UK.*
Dequalinium chloride (p.1143·1).
Mouth and throat infections.

Macaine *Adcock Ingram, S.Afr.*
Bupivacaine hydrochloride (p.1306·3).
Adrenaline [epinephrine] (p.829·1) is included in some injections as a vasoconstrictor to diminish absorption and localise the effect of the local anaesthetic.
Local anaesthesia.

Macalvit
Note. This name is used for preparations of different composition.
Novartis Consumer, Aust.; Novartis, Swed.
Calcium gluconate (p.1188·3); calcium carbonate (p.1215·1); ascorbic acid (p.1389·3).
Calcium and vitamin C deficiency.

Novartis Consumer, Ger.
Ascorbic acid (p.1389·3); calcium lactate gluconate (p.1188·3); calcium phosphinate.
Cold and influenza symptoms; tonic.

Novartis, Spain†.
Multivitamin and mineral preparation (p.1350·1).

Mach-2 *Tocogino, Mex.*
Dipyrone (p.34·1).

Machlor *Eagle, Austral.*
Magnesium chloride (p.1190·3); magnesium oxide (p.1233·2); magnesium amino acid chelate.
Magnesium supplement.

Machto *Nakornpatana, Thai.*
Oral gel: Aluminium hydroxide-magnesium carbonate co-dried gel (p.1211·2); magnesium hydroxide (p.1233·1); simeticone (p.1249·2).

Tablets: Aluminium hydroxide (p.1210·3); magnesium trisilicate (p.1233·3); magnesium hydroxide (p.1233·1); peppermint oil (p.1243·3).
Flatulence; gastric hyperacidity; heartburn; peptic ulcer.

Mack Pen *Pfizer, Aust.†*
Phenoxymethylpenicillin potassium (p.235·1).
Bacterial infections.

Mackenzies Menthoids *BML, Austral.†.*
Phenolphthalein (p.1244·1); potassium nitrate (p.1154·3); methylene blue [methylthioninium chloride] (p.1012·3).
Backache; rheumatic pain.

Mackenzies Smelling Salts *Cox, UK.*
Ammonia (p.1579·1); eucalyptus oil (p.1609·2).
Catarrh; colds.

Macladin *Guidotti, Ital.*
Clarithromycin (p.186·2).
Bacterial infections.

Maclar
Abbott, Aust.; Abbott, Belg.; Abbott, Port.
Clarithromycin (p.186·2).
Opportunistic mycobacterial infections.

Maclean Indigestion Tablets *SmithKline Beecham Consumer, UK.*
Calcium carbonate (p.1215·1); light magnesium carbonate (p.1232·3); aluminium hydroxide (p.1210·3).
Gastrointestinal disorders.

Macleans Mouthguard *SmithKline Beecham Consumer, UK.*
Cetylpyridinium chloride (p.1138·1); sodium fluoride (p.1375·3).
Oral hygiene.

Macleans Sensitive *SmithKline Beecham Consumer, Austral.*
Sodium fluoride (p.1375·3); strontium acetate.
Dental caries prophylaxis; pain associated with sensitive teeth.

Macmiror
Sanova, Aust.; Poli, Hong Kong; Searle, Ital.; Italmex, Mex.; Farma Lepori, Spain†; Poli, Switz.†.
Nifuratel (p.598·1).
Gastrointestinal amoebiasis; genito-urinary tract infections.

Macmiror Complex
Poli, Hong Kong; Searle, Ital.
Nifuratel (p.598·1); nystatin (p.392·2).
Vulvovaginal infections.

Macmiror Complex V *Italmex, Mex.*
Nifuratel (p.598·1); nystatin (p.392·2).
Vulvovaginal infections.

Macodin *Parggon, Mex.*
Dipyrone (p.34·1).
Fever; pain.

Macosil *Vifor, Switz.*
Aluminium hydroxide (p.1210·3); magnesium hydroxide (p.1233·1); simeticone (p.1249·2).
Gastrointestinal disorders.

Macro Antioxidant *Whitehall, Austral.*
Vitamin and mineral preparation (p.1350·1).
Dietary supplement.

Macro Anti-Stress *Whitehall, Austral.*
Vitamin B substances, ascorbic acid, and valerian (p.1678·3)(p.1350·1).
Dietary supplement; stress.

Macro B *Whitehall, Austral.*
Vitamin B substances and ascorbic acid (p.1350·1).
Dietary supplement.

Macro C *Whitehall, Austral.*
Ascorbic acid (p.1389·3); calcium ascorbate (p.1389·3); citrus bioflavonoids (p.1611·1); rutoside (p.1611·2); hesperidin (p.1611·2).
Vitamin C supplement.

Macro C + Garlic with Zinc *Whitehall, Austral.†.*
Ascorbic acid (p.1389·3); calcium ascorbate (p.1389·3); zinc (p.1998·1); garlic (p.1614·1).
Cold and influenza symptoms; zinc and vitamin C deficiencies.

Macro E *Whitehall, Austral.*
d-Alpha tocopherol (p.1393·3).
Vitamin E deficiency; vitamin E supplement.

Macro Garlic *Whitehall, Austral.*
Odourless Arizona garlic (p.1614·1).
Cold and influenza symptoms.

Macro Go *Whitehall, Austral.†.*
Vitamin B substances with ascorbic acid (p.1350·1).
Dietary supplement.

Macro M *Whitehall, Austral.*
Multivitamin and mineral preparation (p.1350·1).
Dietary supplement.

Macro Maxepa *Whitehall, Austral.*
Eicosapentaenoic acid (p.949·3); docosahexaenoic acid (p.949·2); d-alpha tocoferil acetate.
Omega-3 fatty acid supplement.

Macro Natural Vitamin E Cream *Whitehall, Austral.*
d-Alpha tocoferil acetate (p.1394·1); vitamin A palmitate (p.1383·2); panthenol (p.1602·3); allantoin (p.1110·1); avocado oil.
Dry skin; minor skin disorders.

Macro PMT *Whitehall, Austral.†.*
Vitamins B and C and mineral preparation (p.1350·1).
Dietary supplement.

Macro Sports Supplement *Whitehall, Austral.†.*
Multivitamin, mineral, electrolyte and nutritional supplement preparation (p.1350·1).

Macrobid
Alza, Canad.; Procter & Gamble, Irl.; Procter & Gamble, UK; Procter & Gamble, USA.
Nitrofurantoin (p.230·3).
Urinary-tract infections.

Macrocilin *Ofimex, Mex.*
Tetracycline (p.258·3).

Macrodantin
Pharmacia Upjohn, Austral.; Alza, Canad.; Goldshield, Irl.; Procter & Gamble, Israel; Geymonat, Ital.; SmithKline Beecham, S.Afr.; Procter & Gamble, UK; Procter & Gamble, USA.
Nitrofurantoin (macrocrystalline) (p.230·3).
Urinary-tract infections.

Macrodantina *Schering-Plough, Braz.; Boehringer Ingelheim, Mex.*
Nitrofurantoin (p.230·3).
Urinary-tract infections.

Macrodex
Torrex, Aust.; Pharmacia Upjohn, Austral.†; Pharmacia Upjohn, Canad.†; Pharmalink, Denm.; Pharmalink, Ger.; Pharmacia Upjohn, Israel; Pisa, Mex.; Pharmacia Upjohn, Norw.; Pharmacia Upjohn, S.Afr.; Pharmacia Upjohn, Spain; Pharmalink, Swed.; Braun, Switz.; Pharmacia, UK; Pharmacia, USA.
Dextran 60 (p.729·2) or dextran 70 (p.729·2) in glucose or sodium chloride.
Plasma volume expansion; thromboembolism prophylaxis.

Macrodexin *Braun, Braz.*
Dextran in glucose.
Plasma volume expansion.

Macrodoxine *Lagamed, S.Afr.†*
Vitamin B substances with vitamin C (p.1350·1).

Macrofurin *Mavi, Mex.*
Nitrofurantoin (p.230·3).

Macrolate *Pharmagen, S.Afr.†*
Erythromycin estolate (p.201·2).
Bacterial infections.

Macrolax *Carlo Erba OTC, Ital.*
Docusate sodium (p.1223·1); sorbitol (p.1377·3).
Constipation.

Macrolin
Note. This name is used for preparations of different composition.
Haller, Braz.
Lincomycin (p.219·3).
Bacterial infections.

Chiron, Fr.
Aldesleukin (p.547·3).
HIV infection.

Macro-P *Promefarm, Ital.*
Macrogol 4000 (p.1630·3); electrolytes (p.1180·1).
Bowel evacuation.

Macropen
Note. This name is used for preparations of different composition.
Sanitas, Port.
Cefatrizine (p.164·3).
Bacterial infections.

Xixia, S.Afr.
Amoxicillin (p.149·2); flucloxacillin (p.207·1).
Bacterial infections.

Macroral *Malesci, Ital.*
Midecamycin acetate (p.224·3).
Bacterial infections.

Macrosil *Faes, Spain.*
Roxithromycin (p.247·2).
Bacterial infections.

Macrotec *Squibb Diagnostics, USA†.*
Technetium-99m (p.1451·1) labelled albumin.

Macroten *Bergamo, Braz.*
Phenolphthalein (p.1244·1); bladderwrack (p.1585·2); thyroid (p.1526·2); bile salts (p.1585·1).
Constipation.

Mactam *Coli, Ital.†.*
Latamoxef disodium (p.218·2).
Gram-negative bacterial infections.

Madar *Ravizza, Ital.*
Nordazepam (p.696·1).
Sleep disorders.

Made B12 *Esfar, Port.*
Vitamin B₁₂ (p.1388·1).

Madecassol
Roche, Aust.; Roche, Belg.; Nicholas, Fr.; Sanofi Winthrop, Mex.; Laroche Navarron, Neth.†; Serdex, Port.; Syntex, Switz.†.
Centella (p.1112·2).
Burns; cellulite; keloids; ulcers; venous insufficiency; wounds.

Madecassol C *Sanofi Winthrop, Mex.*
Centella (p.1112·2); metronidazole (p.594·1); nitrofurazone (p.231·3).
Bacterial vaginosis; trichomoniasis.

Madecassol Neomycine Hydrocortisone *Nicholas, Fr.*
Centella (p.1112·2); neomycin sulfate (p.228·1); hydrocortisone acetate (p.1073·3).
Skin disorders; wounds.

Madecassol Tulgras *Nicholas, Fr.*
Centella (p.1112·2).
Ulcers; wounds.

Maderan *Nycomed, Switz.†.*
Sulfametrole (p.256·2); trimethoprim (p.264·3).
Bacterial infections.

Maderil *Medifarma, Neth.*
Oxyphenbutazone (p.71·1).

Madicure *Taxandria, Neth.*
Mebendazole (p.102·2).
Enterobiasis.

Madiplot *Takeda, Thai.*
Manidipine hydrochloride (p.924·3).
Hypertension.

Madiprazole *Pharmadica, Thai.*
Omeprazole (p.1239·1).
Gastro-oesophageal reflux; peptic ulcer; Zollinger-Ellison syndrome.

Madol *Masa, Thai.*
Tramadol hydrochloride (p.89·1).
Pain.

Madola *Pharmaland, Thai.*
Tramadol hydrochloride (p.89·1).
Pain.

Madomine *Atlantic, Singapore.*
Sulfadoxine (p.252·3); pyrimethamine (p.442·3).
Malaria.

Madonna *Biolab, Thai.*
Levonorgestrel (p.1486·2).
Postcoital oral contraceptive.

Madopar
Roche, Aust.; Roche, Austral.; Roche, Denm.; Roche, Fin.; Roche, Ger.; Roche, Hong Kong; Roche, Irl.; Roche, Ital.; Roche, Mex.; Roche, Neth.; Roche, Norw.; Roche, NZ; Roche, Port.; Roche, S.Afr.; Roche, Singapore; Roche, Spain; Roche, Switz.; Roche, Thai.; Roche, UK.
Levodopa (p.1169·2); benserazide hydrochloride (p.1164·2).
These ingredients can be described by the British Approved Name Co-beneldopa.
Parkinsonism.

Madopark *Roche, Swed.*
Levodopa (p.1169·2); benserazide hydrochloride (p.1164·2).
Parkinsonism.

Madurase *Tecnobio, Spain†.*
Clebopride malate (p.1221·2).
Adjunct in gastrointestinal radiography and intubation; gastro-oesophageal reflux; gastroparesis; nausea and vomiting.

Mafen *Osotspa, Thai.*
Ibuprofen (p.43·2).
Fever; inflammation; pain.

Mafena *Maver, Mex.*
Diclofenac (p.30·2).
Inflammation.

Maflurell *Sanorell, Ger.*
Homoeopathic preparation.

Maformin *Pharmadica, Thai.*
Metformin hydrochloride (p.332·3).
Diabetes mellitus.

Mafu *Bayer, Ital.*
Tetramethrin (p.1437·3); piperonyl butoxide (p.1436·2).
Insecticide.

Mag-200 *Optimox, USA.*
Magnesium oxide (p.1233·2).
Magnesium deficiency.

Mag 2
Charton, Canad.†; Theraplix, Fr.; Sanofi Synthelabo, Ital.; Casen Fisons, Spain†; Rhone-Poulenc Rorer, Switz.
Magnesium carbonate (p.1232·3) or magnesium pidolate (p.1191·1).
Eclampsia; magnesium deficiency; muscular cramp; nervous disorders.

Mag 50 *Vitaplex, Austral.*
Magnesium amino acid chelate.
Magnesium supplement.

Mag 77 *Osotspa, Thai.*
Aluminium hydroxide (p.1210·3); magnesium hydroxide (p.1233·1); simeticone (p.1249·2).
Flatulence; gastric hyperacidity; gastritis; gastro-oesophageal reflux; peptic ulcer.

Mag Cit Prep *Medefield, Austral.*
Magnesium citrate (p.1232·3).
Bowel evacuation.

Mag Doskar's Leber-Galletonikum *Doskar, Aust.*
Cynara (p.1601·3); taraxacum (p.1669·1); peppermint leaf (p.1243·2).
Liver and biliary-tract disorders.

Mag Doskar's Magentonikum *Doskar, Aust.*
Chamomile (p.1593·2); peppermint leaf (p.1243·2); melissa (p.1632·2).
Gastrointestinal disorders.

Mag Doskar's Nerventonikum *Doskar, Aust.*
Valerian (p.1678·3); lupulus (p.1629·3); melissa (p.1632·2); chamomile (p.1593·2).
Nervous disorders.

Mag Doskar's Nieren- und Blasentonikum *Doskar, Aust.*
Urtica (p.1678·2); equisetum (p.1606·3); silver birch (p.1585·2).
Renal and bladder disorders.

Mag Kottas Baby-Tee *Kottas-Heldenberg, Aust.*
Chamomile (p.1593·2); mallow leaves; spearmint (p.1666·3); caraway (p.1591·2); fennel (p.1610·1).
Gastrointestinal disorders.

Mag Kottas Beruhigungstee *Kottas-Heldenberg, Aust.*
Tea: Melissa (p.1632·2); spearmint (p.1666·3); valerian (p.1678·3); flos aurantii; mallow leaves; rose fruit (p.1389·3); mallow flowers.
Tea bags: Melissa (p.1632·2); spearmint (p.1666·3); valerian (p.1678·3); flos aurantii; mallow leaves; rose fruit (p.1389·3).
Nervous disorders.

Mag Kottas Blahungs-Verdauungstee *Kottas-Heldenberg, Aust.*
Tea: Mallow leaves; peppermint leaf (p.1243·2); caraway (p.1591·2); fennel (p.1610·1); centaury (p.1593·1); calendula (p.1589·2).
Tea bags: Mallow leaves; peppermint leaf (p.1243·2); caraway (p.1591·2); fennel (p.1610·1); centaury (p.1593·1).
Gastrointestinal disorders.

Mag Kottas Entschlackungstee *Kottas-Heldenberg, Aust.*
Tea: Silver birch (p.1585·2); peppermint leaf (p.1243·2); urtica (p.1678·2); violae tricoloris; taraxacum (p.1669·1); calendula (p.1589·2).
Tea bags: Silver birch (p.1585·2); peppermint leaf (p.1243·2); urtica (p.1678·2); violae tricoloris; taraxacum (p.1669·1).
Tonic.

Mag Kottas Entwasserungstee *Kottas-Heldenberg, Aust.*
Tea: Java tea (p.1625·1); equisetum (p.1606·3); herniaria (p.1619·2); taraxacum (p.1669·1); peppermint leaf (p.1243·2); calendula (p.1589·2).
Tea bags: Java tea (p.1625·1); equisetum (p.1606·3); herniaria (p.1619·2); taraxacum (p.1669·1); peppermint leaf (p.1243·2).
Renal and bladder disorders.

Mag Kottas Grippe-Tee *Kottas-Heldenberg, Aust.*
Tea: Sambucus (p.1660·3); tilia (p.1673·2); plantago lanceolata; rose fruit (p.1389·3).
Tea bags: Sambucus (p.1660·3); tilia (p.1673·2); plantago lanceolata; orris; rose fruit (p.1389·3).
Cold symptoms.

Mag Kottas Herz- und Kreislauftee *Kottas-Heldenberg, Aust.*
Flos aurantii; crataegus (p.1600·2); maté leaves (p.1681·1); peppermint leaf (p.1243·2); rosemary.
Cardiovascular disorders.

Mag Kottas Husten-Bronchialtee *Kottas-Heldenberg, Aust.*
Tea: Althaea leaves and root (p.1577·1); plantago lanceolata; thyme (p.1672·2); aniseed (p.1580·2); verbascum flowers.
Tea bags: Plantago lanceolata; thyme (p.1672·2); aniseed (p.1580·2); althaea root (p.1577·1); iceland moss.
Catarrh; cough.

Mag Kottas Krauterexpress-Nerven-Schlaf-Tee *Kottas-Heldenberg, Aust.*
Lupulus (p.1629·3); flos aurantii; melissa (p.1632·2); peppermint leaf (p.1243·2); valerian (p.1678·3).
Nervous disorders.

Mag Kottas Leber-Gallentee *Kottas-Heldenberg, Aust.*
Tea: Mallow leaves; peppermint leaf (p.1243·2); menyanthes (p.1633·1); cnicus benedictus (p.1597·2); taraxacum (p.1669·1); calendula (p.1589·2).
Tea bags: Chamomile (p.1593·2); peppermint leaf (p.1243·2); menyanthes (p.1633·1); herba teucrii; taraxacum (p.1669·1).
Biliary disorders.

Mag Kottas Magen-Darmtee *Kottas-Heldenberg, Aust.*
Tea: Mallow leaves; melissa (p.1632·2); peppermint leaf (p.1243·2); chamomile (p.1593·2); calamus (p.1588·1); calendula (p.1589·2).
Tea bags: Chamomile (p.1593·2); mallow leaves; peppermint leaf (p.1243·2); centaury (p.1593·1); calamus (p.1588·1); fennel (p.1610·1).
Gastrointestinal disorders.

Mag Kottas Nerven-Beruhigungstee *Kottas-Heldenberg, Aust.*
Melissa (p.1632·2); peppermint leaf (p.1243·2); valerian (p.1678·3); flos aurantii; mistletoe (p.1636·2); calendula (p.1589·2).
Nervous disorders.

Mag Kottas Nieren-Blasentee *Kottas-Heldenberg, Aust.*
Tea: Peppermint leaf (p.1243·2); java tea (p.1625·1); equisetum (p.1606·3); herniaria (p.1619·2); bearberry (p.1583·3); calendula (p.1589·2).
Tea bags: Peppermint leaf (p.1243·2); java tea (p.1625·1); equisetum (p.1606·3); herniaria (p.1619·2); ononis (p.1644·1).
Renal and bladder disorders.

Mag Kottas Schlaftee *Kottas-Heldenberg, Aust.*
Lupulus (p.1629·3); flos aurantii; melissa (p.1632·2); peppermint leaf (p.1243·2); valerian (p.1678·3).
Nervous disorders.

Mag Kottas Tee fur stillende Mutter *Kottas-Heldenberg, Aust.*
Tea: Melissa (p.1632·2); mallow leaves; peppermint leaf (p.1243·2); caraway (p.1591·2); fennel (p.1610·1); calendula (p.1589·2).
Tea bags: Melissa (p.1632·2); mallow leaves; peppermint leaf (p.1243·2); caraway (p.1591·2); fennel (p.1610·1).
Gastrointestinal disorders during lactation.

Mag Kottas Wechseltee *Kottas-Heldenberg, Aust.*
Tea: Melissa (p.1632·2); peppermint leaf (p.1243·2); chamomile (p.1593·2); potentilla anserina; valerian (p.1678·3).
Tea bags: Melissa (p.1632·2); peppermint leaf (p.1243·2); chamomile (p.1593·2); achillea (p.1572·2); valerian (p.1678·3).
Menopausal disorders.

Magagel *Genpharm, S.Afr.†.*
Aluminium oxide (p.1108·3); magnesium trisilicate (p.1233·3).
Gastro-oesophageal reflux; peptic ulcer.

Magalan *Invamed, USA†.*
Aluminium hydroxide (p.1210·3); magnesium hydroxide (p.1233·1); simeticone (p.1249·2).

Magalba *Salters, S.Afr.†.*
Magnesium sulfate (p.1191·1); magnesium carbonate (p.1232·3).
Constipation.

Magalox Plus *Invamed, USA†.*
Aluminium hydroxide (p.1210·3); magnesium hydroxide (p.1233·1); simeticone (p.1249·2).

Magalphil *Philopharm, Ger.†.*
Magaldrate (p.1232·2).
Gastrointestinal disorders associated with hyperacidity.

Magan *Savage, USA.*
Magnesium salicylate (p.50·3).
Fever; osteoarthritis; pain; rheumatoid arthritis.

Magasan *Gastropharm, Ger.†.*
Magaldrate (p.1232·2).
Gastric hyperacidity.

Magastron *Hexal, Ger.*
Magaldrate (p.1232·2).
Gastric hyperacidity; peptic ulcer.

Mag-Cal Mega *Freeda, USA.*
Magnesium (p.1190·3); calcium (p.1187·3).
Dietary supplement.

Magcal Plus *Blackmores, Austral.†.*
Magnesium phosphate (p.1191·1); calcium phosphate (p.1188·3); dibasic potassium phosphate (p.1193·1); iron phosphate; dibasic sodium phosphate (p.1193·2).

Mag-Carb *R&D, USA.*
Magnesium carbonate (p.1232·3).
Nutritional supplement.

Magcol *Pharmasant, Thai.*
Aluminium hydroxide (p.1210·3); magnesium hydroxide (p.1233·1); simeticone (p.1249·2).
Flatulence; gastric hyperacidity; peptic ulcer.

Magel *Vitamed, Israel.*
Aluminium hydroxide (p.1210·3); magnesium hydroxide (p.1233·1).
Gastritis; gastrointestinal hyperacidity; peptic ulcer.

Magen-Darmtropfen S *Cosmochema, Ger.*
Homoeopathic preparation.

Magenpulver Hafter *Streuli, Switz.*
Bismuth subnitrate (p.1213·2); calcium carbonate (p.1215·1); magnesium peroxide (p.1149·3).
Gastric hyperacidity.

Magentabletten Hafter *Streuli, Switz.*
Bismuth subnitrate (p.1213·2); calcium carbonate (p.1215·1); magnesium carbonate (p.1232·3).
Gastric hyperacidity.

Magentee
Note.This name is used for preparations of different composition.
Sanova, Aust.
Chamomile (p.1593·2); peppermint leaf (p.1243·2); caraway (p.1591·2); valerian (p.1678·3).
Gastrointestinal disorders.
Weleda, Aust.
Angelica (p.1580·2); gentian (p.1615·3); menyanthes (p.1633·1); caraway (p.1591·2); parsley (p.1648·3); achillea (p.1572·2).
Gastrointestinal disorders.
Bad Heilbrunner, Ger.
Chamomile (p.1593·2); fennel (p.1610·1); peppermint leaf (p.1243·2).
Dyspepsia; flatulence.

Magentee EF-EM-ES *Smetana, Aust.*
Absinthium (p.1571·1); centaury (p.1593·1); taraxacum (p.1669·1); skin powder; cort. aurantii dulc; hypericum (p.290·2).
Gastrointestinal disorders.

Magen-Tee Stada N *Stada, Ger.†.*
Chamomile (p.1593·2); peppermint leaf (p.1243·2); achillea (p.1572·2).
Gastrointestinal disorders.

Magentropen N Legastol *Twardy, Aust.*
Peppermint leaf (p.1243·2); cynara (p.1601·3); taraxacum (p.1669·1).
Gastrointestinal and biliary-tract disorders.

Magesto
Takeda, Hong Kong; Takeda, Thai.
Mamylase; amylase (p.1579·3); vitamin B₁; scopolia; sodium bicarbonate (p.1186·2); calcium carbonate (p.1215·1); cinnamon oil (p.1596·1); clove oil (p.1597·1); fennel oil (p.1610·2); ginger oil; orange peel oil (p.1644·1); menthol (p.1632·3); aluminium hydroxide gel (p.1210·3).
Gastrointestinal tract disorders.

Mag-G *Cypress, USA.*
Magnesium gluconate (p.1190·3).
Dietary supplement.

Magic Mix *Taranis, Fr.*
Maize starch (p.1379·3).
Dietary aid; gastro-oesophageal reflux in infants.

Magicul *Alphapharm, Austral.*
Cimetidine (p.1216·3).
Gastro-oesophageal reflux; peptic ulcer; Zollinger-Ellison syndrome.

Magion *Ern, Spain.*
Magaldrate (p.1232·2).
Dyspepsia; gastro-oesophageal reflux; gastrointestinal hyperacidity.

Magisbile *Magis, Ital.*
Fencibutirol (p.1610·1); boldo (p.1585·3); rhubarb (p.1248·1); cascara (p.1216·1); sorbitol (p.1377·3).
Constipation; dyspepsia; haemorrhoids.

Magium *Hexal, Ger.*
Magnesium aspartate (p.1190·3) or magnesium oxide (p.1233·2).
Magnesium deficiency.

Magium E *Hexal, Ger.*
dl-Alpha tocoferil acetate (p.1394·1); magnesium oxide (p.1233·2).
Vitamin E and magnesium deficiency.

Magium K *Hexal, Ger.*
Potassium aspartate (p.1195·2); magnesium aspartate (p.1190·3).
Potassium and magnesium deficiency.

Maglid *Aventis, Belg.*
Aluminium hydroxide (p.1210·3); magnesium hydroxide (p.1233·1).
Gastrointestinal disorders associated with hyperacidity.

Maglucate *Pharmascience, Canad.*
Magnesium gluconate (p.1190·3).
Hypomagnesaemia.

Magluphen *Tyrol, Aust.*
Diclofenac sodium (p.30·3).
Gout; inflammation; musculoskeletal and joint disorders; pain; renal and biliary colic.

Maglut *Magis, Ital.*
Glutathione (p.1010·3).
Alcohol and drug poisoning; radiation trauma.

Magmed *Lichtenstein, Ger.†.*
Magaldrate (p.1232·2).
Gastric hyperacidity; peptic ulcer.

Magmin *Vitaglow, Austral.*
Magnesium aspartate (p.1190·3).
Magnesium deficiency; magnesium supplement.

Mag-Min *Selmag, Switz.*
Magnesium aspartate (p.1190·3).
Magnesium deficiency; magnesium supplement.

Magnacal *Sherwood, USA.*
Lactose-free preparation for enteral nutrition (p.1350·1).

Magnalox *Schein, USA†.*
Aluminium hydroxide (p.1210·3); magnesium hydroxide (p.1233·1).
Hyperacidity.

Magnalum *Protein, Mex.*
Aluminium hydroxide (p.1210·3).

Magnapen *CP Pharmaceuticals, UK.*
Capsules: Ampicillin trihydrate (p.151·1); flucloxacillin sodium (p.207·1).
Injection: Ampicillin sodium (p.150·3); flucloxacillin sodium (p.207·1).
Syrup: Ampicillin trihydrate (p.151·1); flucloxacillin magnesium (p.207·1).
These ingredients can be described by the British Approved Name Co-fluampicil.
Bacterial infections.

Magnaprin *Rugby, USA.*
Aspirin (p.14·2).
Aluminium hydroxide (p.1210·3), calcium carbonate (p.1215·1), and magnesium hydroxide (p.1233·1) are included in this preparation in an attempt to limit adverse effects on the gastrointestinal mucosa.
Fever; inflammation; myocardial infarction; pain; transient ischaemic attacks.

Magnaspart *Rosen, Ger.*
Magnesium aspartate (p.1190·3).
Magnesium deficiency.

Magnatex *Propan, S.Afr.†.*
Ibuprofen (p.43·2).
Musculoskeletal and joint disorders.

Magnatol *Sterling Health, UK†.*
Potassium bicarbonate (p.1186·1); alexitol sodium (p.1209·3); magnesium carbonate (p.1232·3).
Gastro-oesophageal reflux.

Magne-B₆ *Sanofi Winthrop, Fr.*
Oral solution: Magnesium lactate (p.1191·1); magnesium pidolate (p.1191·1); pyridoxine hydrochloride (p.1386·3).
Tablets: Magnesium lactate (p.1191·1); pyridoxine hydrochloride (p.1386·3).
Magnesium deficiency.

MagneBind *Nephro-Tech, USA.*
Magnesium carbonate (p.1232·3); calcium carbonate (p.1215·1).
Dietary phosphate binder.

Magnecyl *Pharmacia Upjohn, Swed.*
Aspirin (p.14·2).
Fever; inflammation; pain.

Magnecyl-koffein *Pharmacia Upjohn, Swed.*
Aspirin (p.14·2); caffeine (p.761·3).
Fever; inflammation; pain.

Magnefusin *Pisa, Mex.*
Magnesium sulfate (p.1191·1).

Magnerot A *Worwag, Ger.*
Magnesium aspartate (p.1190·3).
Magnesium deficiency.

magnerot Classic *Worwag, Ger.*
Magnesium orotate (p.1645·1).
Magnesium deficiency.

Magnerot N Worwag, Ger.†.
Magnesium phosphate (p.1191·1); magnesium citrate (p.1232·3).
Magnesium deficiency.

Magnesia
Nycomed, Denm.; Cinfa, Spain.
Magnesium hydroxide (p.1233·1).
Constipation; gastritis; gastro-oesphageal reflux; peptic ulcer.

Magnesia Bisurada Whitehall, Braz.
Magnesium carbonate (p.1232·3); bismuth subcarbonate (p.1213·1); calcium carbonate (p.1215·1); sodium bicarbonate (p.1186·2).
Gastrointestinal hyperacidity.

Magnesia Bisurata Wyeth Lederle, Ital.†.
Magnesium carbonate (p.1232·3); sodium bicarbonate (p.1186·2); kaolin (p.1229·3).
Gastrointestinal disorders associated with hyperacidity.

Magnesia Bisurata Aromatic Wyeth Lederle, Ital.
Magnesium carbonate (p.1232·3); sodium bicarbonate (p.1186·2); calcium carbonate (p.1215·1).
Gastrointestinal hyperacidity.

Magnesia Bisurata Aromatic Plus Wyeth Lederle, Ital.
Oxetacaine (p.1317·3); aluminium hydroxide (p.1210·3); magnesium carbonate (p.1232·3) or magnesium oxide (p.1233·2).
Gastrointestinal disorders associated with hyperacidity.

Magnesia Effervescente Sella Sella, Ital.
Magnesium hydroxide (p.1233·1); tartaric acid (p.1669·2); sodium bicarbonate (p.1186·2).
Constipation; gastrointestinal hyperacidity.

Magnesia Fluida Virtus, Braz.
Magnesium hydroxide (p.1233·1).
Gastrointestinal hyperacidity.

Magnesia S Pellegrino
Saprochi, Israel; Sanofi Synthelabo, Ital.; Saprochi, Switz.
Magnesium hydroxide (p.1233·1).
Constipation; gastrointestinal hyperacidity.

Magnesia san Pellegrino Seid, Spain.
Magnesium hydroxide (p.1233·1).
Constipation; dyspepsia.

Magnesia Volta Edmond Pharma, Ital.
Magnesium hydroxide (p.1233·1).
Constipation; gastrointestinal hyperacidity.

Magnesiamaito Orion, Fin.
Magnesium hydroxide (p.1233·1).
Gastrointestinal disorders.

Magnesie Plus Whitehall, Belg.†.
Magnesium carbonate (p.1232·3); sodium bicarbonate (p.1186·2); calcium carbonate (p.1215·1).
Gastrointestinal disorders associated with hyperacidity.

Magnesie S Pellegrino Centrapharm, Fr.
Magnesium hydroxide (p.1233·1).
Constipation.

Magnesioboi BOI, Spain.
Magnesium lactate (p.1191·1).
Magnesium depletion.

Magnesiocard
Verla, Ger.; Tecnimede, Port.; Verla, Switz.
Magnesium aspartate hydrochloride (p.1191·3).
Magnesium deficiency; magnesium supplement.

Magnesiomix Provita, Ital.
Multivitamin preparation with magnesium (p.1350·1).

Magnesit Byk Madaus, S.Afr.
Magnesium l-aspartate hydrochloride (p.1191·3).
Hypomagnesaemia.

Magnesium Biomed Verla, Switz.
Effervescent tablets; granules for oral liquid: Magnesium aspartate (p.1190·3).
Tablets: Magnesium glutamate; magnesium citrate (p.1232·3).
Magnesium deficiency; magnesium supplement.

Magnesium Complexe Golaz, Switz.
Magnesium chloride (p.1190·3); magnesium glutamate; magnesium glycerophosphate (p.1191·1); magnesium orotate (p.1645·1); magnesium aspartate (p.1190·3).
Magnesium deficiency; magnesium supplement.

Magnesium compositum OPW, Ger.
Magnesium adipate; magnesium nicotinate.
Circulatory disorders.

Magnesium Diasporal
Austroplant, Aust.; Protina, Ger.; Protina, Switz.
Magnesium citrate (p.1232·3), magnesium levulinate (p.1191·3), magnesium oxide (p.1233·2), or magnesium sulfate (p.1191·1).
Magnesium deficiency.

Magnesium Glycocolle Lafarge SERP, Mon.
Magnesium lactate (p.1191·1); glycine (p.1365·3).
Magnesium deficiency.

Magnesium Plus Cenovis, Austral.; Vitelle, Austral.
Magnesium orotate (p.1645·1); magnesium oxide (p.1233·2); magnesium amino acid chelate; monobasic potassium phosphate (p.1193·2); calcium hydrogen phosphate (p.1188·2).
Mineral supplement.

Magnesium Pyre Salvat, Spain.
Magnesium bromide; magnesium chloride (p.1190·3); magnesium fluoride; magnesium iodide.
Magnesium depletion.

Magnesium Tonil APS, Ger.
Capsules: Heavy magnesium oxide (p.1233·2); *dl*-alpha tocoferil acetate (p.1394·1).
Magnesium or vitamin E deficiency.
Injection: Magnesium sulfate (p.1191·1).
Magnesium deficiency.

Magnesium Tonil N APS, Ger.
Magnesium citrate (p.1232·3).
Magnesium deficiency.

Magnesium Tonil Vitamin E Richter, Aust.
Magnesium oxide (p.1233·2); *dl*-alpha tocoferil acetate (p.1394·1).
Vitamin E and magnesium deficiency.

Magnesium Vital Golaz, Switz.
Magnesium aspartate (p.1190·3).
Magnesium deficiency; magnesium supplement.

Magnesium-Eufidol Medopharm, Ger.†.
Potassium aspartate (p.1195·2); magnesium aspartate (p.1190·3).
Cardiac disorders; magnesium or potassium deficiency.

Magnesium-OK
Wassen, Ital.; Helsinn, Port.; Wassen, UK.
Magnesium; vitamins; minerals (p.1350·1).
Nutritional supplement.

Magnesium-Plus-Hevert Hevert, Ger.
Magnesium oxide (p.1233·2); *d*-alpha tocopherol (p.1393·3).
Magnesium or vitamin E deficiency.

Magnesona Vitoria, Port.
Magnesium pidolate (p.1191·1).
Magnesium deficiency.

Magnesorot Worwag, Ger.
Magnesium orotate (p.1645·1).
Magnesium deficiency.

Magnespasmil Euro-Labor, Port.; Grunenthal, Port.
Magnesium lactate (p.1191·1).
Magnesium deficiency.

Magnespasmyl
Meuse, Belg.; Cooperation Pharmaceutique, Fr.; Sanofi Synthelabo, Switz.
Magnesium lactate (p.1191·1).
Magnesium deficiency; magnesium supplement.

Magnesplus Chemedica, Switz.
Magnesium carbonate (p.1232·3); vitamin B_6 (p.1386·3).
Magnesium deficiency.

Magnetrans forte Niddapharm, Ger.
Magnesium oxide (p.1233·2).
Magnesium deficiency.

Magnevist
Schering, Aust.; Schering, Belg.; Berlex, Canad.; Schering, Denm.; Schering, Fin.; Schering, Fr.; Schering, Ger.; Schering, Ital.; Schering, Neth.; Schering, Norw.; Schering, NZ; Schering, Port.; Schering, Spain; Schering, Swed.; Schering, Switz.; Schering, UK; Berlex, USA.
Meglumine gadopentetate (p.1033·1).
Contrast medium for magnetic resonance imaging.

Magnevistan Schering, Braz.
Meglumine gadopentetate (p.1033·1).
Contrast medium for magnetic resonance imaging.

Magnezie Lifeplan, UK.
Vitamin and mineral preparation (p.1350·1).

Magnezyme Reckitt & Colman, Belg.
Magnesium carbonate (p.1232·3).
Fatigue.

Magnidol-Plus Streger, Mex.
Paracetamol (p.71·2).
Fever; pain.

Magnil Sons, Mex.
Dipyrone (p.34·1).
Pain.

Magnofit
Asta Medica, Aust.
Chewable tablets: Magnesium citrate (p.1232·3); magnesium carbonate (p.1232·3).
Magnesium deficiency.
Effervescent tablets: Magnesium oxide (p.1233·2).
Magnesium deficiency.
Asta Medica, Ital.
Magnesium carbonate (p.1232·3).
Magnesium deficiency.

Magnogene
Note. This name is used for preparations of different composition.
Novartis Sante, Fr.; Interdelta, Switz.
Magnesium chloride (p.1190·3).
Magnesium deficiency; magnesium supplement.
Diviser Aquilea, Spain.
Magnesium bromide; magnesium chloride (p.1190·3); magnesium fluoride; magnesium iodide.
Magnesium depletion.

Magnograf Juste, Spain.
Meglumine gadopentetate (p.1033·1).
Contrast medium for gastrointestinal radiography; contrast medium for magnetic resonance imaging.

Magnol Atlantis, Mex.
Dipyrone (p.34·1).
Fever; pain.

Magnolax Wampole, Canad.
Magnesium hydroxide (p.1233·1); liquid paraffin (p.1407·1).
Constipation.

Magnolex Sante Naturelle, Canad.
Magnesium chloride (p.1190·3) or magnesium gluceptate (p.1190·3).

Magnonorm Genericon, Aust.
Magnesium oxide (p.1233·2).
Magnesium deficiency.

Magnoplasm Faulding, Austral.
Glycerol (p.1616·3); magnesium sulfate (p.1191·1).
Poultice for abscesses, boils, and carbuncles.

Magnopyrol
Abbott, Braz.; Rhein, Mex.
Metamizole magnesium (p.34·2).
Fever; pain.

Magnoral Medinfar, Port.
Magnesium chloride (p.1190·3).
Magnesium deficiency.

Magnorbin Merck, Ger.†.
Magnesium ascorbate (p.1190·3).
Magnesium deficiency.

Magnorell Sanorell, Ger.
Magnesium citrate (p.1232·3).
Magnesium deficiency.

Magnorol Rolmex, Canad.
Magnesium gluceptate (p.1190·3).

Magnoscorbol Roche Nicholas, Fr.†.
Magnesium chloride (p.1190·3); ascorbic acid (p.1389·3).
Anxiety attacks; magnesium deficiency.

Magnosol
Sarget, Fr.; Asta Medica, Ital.
Magnesium carbonate (p.1232·3); magnesium oxide (p.1233·2).
Magnesium deficiency.

Magnosolv Asta Medica, Aust.
Precipitated magnesium carbonate (p.1232·3); magnesium oxide (p.1233·2).
Magnesium deficiency.

Magnostase Neo Quimica, Braz.
Furazolidone (p.592·1); diphenoxylate hydrochloride (p.1222·2); attapulgite (p.1212·1); pectin (p.1502·3).
Diarrhoea.

Magnox Lennod, USA.
Aluminium hydroxide (p.1210·3); magnesium hydroxide (p.1233·1).
Hyperacidity.

Magnurol Esteve, Spain.
Terazosin hydrochloride (p.980·1).
Benign prostatic hyperplasia; hypertension.

Magnyl Nycomed, Denm.
Aspirin (p.14·2).
Magnesium hydroxide (p.1233·1) is included in this preparation in an attempt to limit adverse effects on the gastrointestinal mucosa.
Fever; inflammation; ischaemic heart disease; pain; thromboembolism prophylaxis.

Magocean Proceane, Fr.
Magnesium oxide (p.1233·2).
Magnesium supplement.

Magonate Fleming, USA.
Magnesium gluconate (p.1190·3).
Dietary supplement.

Magopsor Strathmann, Ger.†.
Dexamethasone (p.1067·3); allantoin (p.1110·1); vitamin A palmitate (p.1383·2); alpha tocoferil acetate (p.1394·1).
Skin disorders.

Magoral ST, Thai.
Magnesium oxide (p.1233·2).
Gastric hyperacidity; magnesium deficiency.

Mag-Oro Eagle, Austral.
Magnesium orotate (p.1645·1); magnesium aspartate (p.1190·3); magnesium amino acid chelate; potassium aspartate (p.1195·2); pyridoxine hydrochloride (p.1386·3).
Magnesium, potassium, and vitamin B_6 supplement.

Mag-Ox Blaine, USA.
Magnesium oxide (p.1233·2).
Hyperacidity; magnesium deficiency.

Magrilan
Medochemie, Hong Kong; Medochemie, Singapore; Medochemie, Thai.
Fluoxetine hydrochloride (p.284·2).
Depression; mixed anxiety depressive states.

Magrinex Heralds, Braz.
Mazindol (p.1510·3).
Obesity.

Magroton Sanval, Braz.
Phenolphthalein (p.1244·1); thyroid (p.1526·2); bladderwrack (p.1585·2); bile salts (p.1585·1).
Constipation; obesity.

Magsal US Pharmaceutical, USA.
Magnesium salicylate (p.50·3); phenyltoloxamine citrate (p.423·1).
Pain.

Magsil Fortune, Hong Kong.
Aluminium hydroxide (p.1210·3); magnesium hydroxide (p.1233·1); dimethicone (p.1249·2).
Gastrointestinal hyperacidity; meteorism.

Magsons Sons, Mex.
Dipyrone (p.34·1).
Fever; pain.

Mag-SR Cypress, USA.
Magnesium chloride (p.1190·3).
Magnesium supplement.

Mag-Tab SR Niche, USA.
Magnesium lactate (p.1191·1).
Magnesium deficiency.

Magtrate Mission Pharmacal, USA.
Magnesium gluconate (p.1190·3).
Dietary supplement.

Magtrom Trommsdorff, Ger.†.
Magnesium aspartate (p.1190·3).
Magnesium deficiency.

Magvital
Panderma, Aust.; Vifor, Switz.†.
Magnesium hydrogen aspartate (p.1190·3); or magnesium sulfate (p.1191·1).
Eclampsia; magnesium deficiency; premature labour.

Mahiou Vectem, Spain.
Phenolphthalein (p.1244·1); vitamin F.
Chilblains; haematomas; haemorrhoids; insect bites and stings; varices.

Mainnox Charoen, Thai.
Mefenamic acid (p.51·2); dicyclomine [dicycloverine] hydrochloride (p.466·1).
Smooth muscle spasm.

Maintain Schmid, Israel.
Benzocaine (p.1306·2).
Local anaesthesia.

Maiorad
Rotta, Ital.; Delta, Port.; Rotta, Thai.
Tiropramide hydrochloride (p.1673·3).
Smooth muscle spasm.

Majeptil
Aventis, Belg.; Rhone-Poulenc Rorer, Canad.; Rhone-Poulenc Rorer, Fr.; Rhone-Poulenc Rorer, Mex.; Rhone-Poulenc Rorer, Spain.
Thioproperazine mesilate (p.708·1).
Anxiety; psychoses.

Majocarmin-Tee Hevert, Ger.
Aniseed (p.1580·2); fennel (p.1610·1); caraway (p.1591·2); chamomile (p.1593·2); peppermint leaf (p.1243·2).
Gastrointestinal disorders.

Majolat Klinge, Aust.
Nifedipine (p.940·1).
Angina pectoris; hypertension.

Major-Con Major, USA.
Simeticone (p.1249·2).
Flatulence.

Major-gesic Major, USA.
Phenyltoloxamine citrate (p.423·1); paracetamol (p.71·2).
Upper respiratory-tract symptoms.

Majorpen Ipso, Ital.
Amoxicillin trihydrate (p.149·2).
Bacterial infections.

Makatussin
Note. This name is used for preparations of different composition.
Gebro, Aust.†.
Camphor (p.1589·3); menthol (p.1632·3); cypress oil; eucalyptus oil (p.1609·2); pumilio pine oil (p.1656·3); oleum pini sylvestris; turpentine oil (p.1676·3); thyme oil (p.1672·3); peppermint oil (p.1243·3).
Respiratory-tract disorders.

Gebro, Switz.
Ointment: Camphor (p.1589·3); menthol (p.1632·3); cypress oil; eucalyptus oil (p.1609·2); pumilio pine oil (p.1656·3); oleum pini sylvestris; turpentine oil (p.1676·3); thyme oil (p.1672·3).
Respiratory-tract disorders.

Oral drops: Drosera (p.1606·1); liquorice (p.1231·2); pimpinella; senega root (p.1100·2); thyme (p.1672·2); anise oil (p.1580·3); eucalyptus oil (p.1609·2); camphor (p.1589·3); menthol (p.1632·3).
Catarrh; coughs.

Syrup: Drosera (p.1606·1); liquorice (p.1231·2); senega root (p.1100·2); thyme (p.1672·2).
Bronchitis.

Makatussin Balsam mit Menthol Roland, Ger.
Eucalyptus oil (p.1609·2); menthol (p.1632·3); thyme oil (p.1672·3).
Bronchitis; catarrh.

Makatussin forte Gebro, Switz.
Dihydrocodeine hydrochloride (p.33·3); drosera (p.1606·1); liquorice (p.1231·2); pimpinella; senega root (p.1100·2); thyme (p.1672·2); anise oil (p.1580·3); eucalyptus oil (p.1609·2); camphor (p.1589·3); menthol (p.1632·3).
Bronchitis; coughs.

Makatussin Saft Roland, Ger.
Thyme (p.1672·2).
Bronchitis; catarrh.

Makatussin Saft Drosera Roland, Ger.
Drosera (p.1606·1).
Coughs.

Makatussin Tropfen Roland, Ger.
Thyme (p.1672·2); star anise oil.
Bronchitis; catarrh.

Makatussin Tropfen Drosera Roland, Ger.
Drosera (p.1606·1).
Coughs.

Makatussin Tropfen forte Roland, Ger.
Dihydrocodeine hydrochloride (p.33·3); drosera (p.1606·1).
Coughs.

Makrocilin Makros, Braz.
Ampicillin (p.150·3).
Bacterial infections.

Malafene Knoll, Belg.
Ibuprofen (p.43·2).
Fever; inflammation; pain.

Malandil Bohm, Spain.
Carnitine hydrochloride (p.1356·2); cobamamide (p.1388·3); lysine hydrochloride (p.1370·3).
Anaemias; tonic.

The symbol † denotes a preparation no longer actively marketed

Malarex *Dumex-Alpharma, Denm.*
Chloroquine phosphate (p.432·3).
Amoebiasis; lupus erythematosus; malaria; photosensitivity; rheumatoid arthritis.

Malarone *Glaxo Wellcome, Aust.; Glaxo Wellcome, Austral.; Glaxo Wellcome, Belg.; Glaxo Wellcome, Canad.; Glaxo Wellcome, Denm.; Glaxo Wellcome, Fr.; Glaxo Wellcome, Ger.; Cascan, Ger.; Glaxo Wellcome, Singapore; Glaxo Wellcome, Swed.; Glaxo Wellcome, Switz.; Glaxo Wellcome, UK; Glaxo Wellcome, USA.*
Atovaquone (p.588·3); proguanil hydrochloride (p.441·3).
Malaria.

Malatal *Hauck, USA†.*
Atropine sulfate (p.461·1); hyoscine hydrobromide (p.468·2); hyoscyamine hydrobromide (p.469·3) or hyoscyamine sulfate (p.469·3); phenobarbital (p.355·1).
Gastrointestinal disorders.

Malaviron *Wallace Mfg Chem., UK.*
Chloroquine phosphate (p.432·3).
Malaria.

Male Formula Herbal Plus Formula 2 *Vitelle, Austral.*
Eleutherococcus senticosis; equisetum; sarsaparilla; liquorice; damiana; zinc amino acid chelate; betacarotene; pyridoxine hydrochloride; d-alpha tocoferil acid succinate; magnesium oxide (p.1350·1).
Tonic.

Malexin *BASF, Ger.*
Naproxen (p.60·3).
Gout; inflammation; musculoskeletal, joint, and soft-tissue disorders; pain.

Malfin *Nettopharma, Denm.†.*
Morphine sulfate (p.56·1).
Pain.

Maliasin *Ebewe, Aust.; Knoll, Braz.; BASF, Ger.; Ravizza, Ital.; Knoll, Switz.*
Barbexaclone (p.342·2).
Epilepsy.

Malimed *Ecosol, Switz.*
Cimetidine (p.1216·3).
Gastric hyperacidity; gastro-oesophageal reflux; gastrointestinal haemorrhage; peptic ulcer; Zollinger-Ellison syndrome.

Malinert *Strathmann, Ger.†.*
Aspirin (p.14·2); paracetamol (p.71·2).
Inflammation; pain.

Malipuran *Heumann, Ger.*
Bufexamac (p.20·3).
Skin disorders.

Malival *Silanes, Mex.*
Indometacin (p.44·3).
Gout; musculoskeletal, joint and peri-articular disorders.

Malival Compuesto *Silanes, Mex.*
Methocarbamol (p.1329·3); indometacin (p.44·3).
Musculoskeletal, joint and peri-articular disorders; skeletal muscle spasm.

Malix *Lagap, UK.*
Glibenclamide (p.321·3).
Diabetes mellitus.

Mallamint *Roberts, USA.*
Calcium carbonate (p.1215·1).
Hyperacidity.

Mallazine *Roberts, USA; Hauck, USA.*
Tetryzoline hydrochloride (p.1101·2).
Minor eye irritation.

Mallebrin *Krewel, Ger.*
Hexaurea aluminium chloride.
Formerly known as Mallebrinetten.
Mouth and throat disorders.

Mallebrin Konzentrat *Krewel, Ger.*
Aluminium chloride (p.1110·2).
Mouth and throat inflammation.

Mallisol *Hauck, USA†.*
Povidone-iodine (p.1155·1).
Skin disinfection.

Mallorol *Novartis, Swed.*
Thioridazine (p.708·1) or thioridazine hydrochloride (p.708·1).
Alcohol withdrawal syndrome; pain; psychoses.

Malocide *Rhone-Poulenc Rorer, Fr.*
Pyrimethamine (p.442·3).
Toxoplasmosis.

Malocin *M & H, Thai.*
Erythromycin stearate (p.201·3).
Bacterial infections.

Malogen Aqueous *Germiphene, Canad.†.*
Testosterone (p.1492·1).
Androgenic.

Malogen in Oil *Germiphene, Canad.†.*
Testosterone propionate (p.1492·2).
Androgenic.

Malogex *Germiphene, Canad.†.*
Testosterone enantate (p.1492·2).
Androgenic.

Maloprim *Glaxo Wellcome, Austral.†; Wellcome, Irl.; Glaxo Wellcome, S.Afr.; Wellcome, UK.*
Pyrimethamine (p.442·3); dapsone (p.196·1).
Malaria.

Maltlevol *Carter Horner, Canad.*
Multivitamin preparation (p.1350·1) with ferric ammonium citrate (p.1359·2).
Food supplement; iron-deficiency anaemia.

Maltlevol-M *Carter Horner, Canad.*
Multivitamin and mineral preparation (p.1350·1).

Maltofer *Meda, Fin.; Therabel, Fr.; Vifor International, Switz.*
Iron polymaltose (p.1369·2).
Formerly known as Fer Lucien in *Fr.*
Iron deficiency; iron-deficiency anaemias.

Maltofer Fol *Vifor International, Switz.*
Iron polymaltose (p.1369·2); folic acid (p.1361·1).
Iron and folic acid deficiency.

Maltogen *Nestle, Austral.*
Infant feed supplement (p.1350·1).
Anorexia; constipation.

Malton E *Serturner, Ger.*
d-Alpha tocopherol (p.1393·3).
Vitamin E deficiency.

Maltovis *Volchem, Ital.*
Maltodextrin (p.1371·2).
Carbohydrate source.

Maltsupex *Wallace, USA.*
Malt extract (p.1371·1).
Constipation.

Maltyl *Merckle, Ger.*
Dequalinium chloride (p.1143·1).
Mouth and throat disorders.

Maludil *Durascan, Denm.*
Maprotiline hydrochloride (p.297·2).
Depression.

Malugel *Charoen, Thai.*
Calcium carbonate (p.1215·1); simeticone (p.1249·2).
Flatulence; gastric hyperacidity; heartburn; peptic ulcer.

Malva Composta *Windson, Braz.*
Mallow; benzocaine (p.1306·2); menthol (p.1632·3).
Mouth and throat disorders.

Malvatricin *Daudt, Braz.*
Sodium fluoride (p.1375·3); tyrothricin (p.267·1).
Dental caries prophylaxis.

Malvedrin *Adroka, Switz.*
Ointment: Mallow leaves; vitamin A (p.1382·1); vitamin D (p.1391·1); chamomile oil; hypericum oil (p.290·3); linseed oil (p.1629·1).
Skin irritation; superficial wounds.

Topical liquid: Mallow leaves.
Mouth and throat disorders; superficial wounds.

Malveol *Magistra, Switz.*
Althaea leaves (p.1577·1); mallow leaves; salicylic acid (p.1122·3); mint oil (p.1636·2).
Mouth and throat disorders.

Malvitona *Leo, Fin.; Leo, Swed.*
Vitamin B substances (p.1350·1); caffeine (p.761·3).
Tonic.

Malvodon *IMA, Braz.*
Mallow; poppy (p.1099·2).
Mouth disorders.

Malvol *Hearst, Braz.*
Cetylpyridinium chloride (p.1138·1); benzocaine (p.1306·2); phenosalyl; menthol (p.1632·3); mallow; eucalyptus oil (p.1609·2).
Mouth and throat disorders.

Malvona *Prima, Braz.*
Phenosalyl; menthol (p.1632·3); benzocaine (p.1306·2); mallow; cetylpyridinium chloride (p.1138·1).
Mouth and throat disorders.

Malvosulfam *Hearst, Braz.*
Sulfanilamide (p.256·2); phenosalyl; salol (p.82·2); procaine hydrochloride (p.1319·1); myrrh (p.1639·2); mallow; peppermint oil (p.1243·3).
Mouth and throat disorders.

Mamellin *Fresenius Kabi, Aust.*
Vitamin F; peru balsam (p.1650·2); alpha tocoferil acetate (p.1394·1).
Skin damage.

Mammol *Abbott, USA.*
Bismuth subnitrate (p.1213·2); castor oil (p.1592·1); peru balsam (p.1650·2).
Nipple care.

Man Formula *Avon, Canad.*
Multivitamin and mineral preparation (p.1350·1).

Manceau *SmithKline Beecham Consumer, Belg.†.*
Senna (p.1248·2); mali comm. syrup.
Constipation.

Mancef *Lafare, Ital.*
Cefamandole nafate (p.163·3).
Lignocaine [lidocaine] hydrochloride (p.1313·2) is included in this preparation to alleviate the pain of injection.
Bacterial infections.

Mandal 425 *Golaz, Switz.*
Hypericum (p.290·2).
Insomnia; nervous disorders.

Mandanol *Pharmachem, UK.*
Paracetamol (p.71·2).
Fever; pain.

Mandarine *Boiron, Canad.*
Homoeopathic preparation.

Mandelamine *Parke, Davis, Canad.; Parke, Davis, Ger.†; Aspen, S.Afr.; Warner-Lambert, Switz.†; Warner Chilcott, USA.*
Methenamine mandelate (p.223·1).
Urinary-tract infections.

Mandelan *Sydenham, Mex.*
Methenamine (p.223·1).

Mandelip *Dermoteca, Port.*
Mandelic acid (p.221·2) with sunscreens.
Chapped lips.

Mandelo-katt *Kattwiga, Ger.*
Homoeopathic preparation.

Mandepiril *Tegur, Mex.*
Methenamine (p.223·1).

Mandocarbine *Monal, Fr.†.*
Activated charcoal (p.1000·2).
Formerly contained vegetable charcoal, magnesium hydroxide, and calcium mandelate.
Gastrointestinal disorders.

Mandokef *Lilly, Aust.; Lilly, Ger.; Lilly, Ital.; Lilly, Port.; Aspen, S.Afr.; Lilly, Spain; Lilly, Switz.*
Cefamandole nafate (p.163·3).
Lignocaine [lidocaine] hydrochloride (p.1313·2) may be included in the intramuscular injection to alleviate the pain of injection.
Bacterial infections.

Mandol *Lilly, Austral.; Lilly, Belg.; Lilly, Canad.†; Lilly, Hong Kong; Lilly, Neth.; Lilly, NZ; Lilly, Thai.; Lilly, USA.*
Cefamandole nafate (p.163·3).
Bacterial infections.

Mandolgin *Durascan, Denm.*
Tramadol hydrochloride (p.89·1).
Pain.

Mandolsan *San Carlo, Ital.*
Cefamandole nafate (p.163·3).
Lignocaine [lidocaine] hydrochloride (p.1313·2) is included in the intramuscular injection to alleviate the pain of injection.
Bacterial infections.

Mandragora comp *Weleda, Ger.*
Homoeopathic preparation.

Mandragora Med Complex *Dynamit, Aust.*
Homoeopathic preparation.

Mandrogripp *Dolorgiet, Ger.†.*
Paracetamol (p.71·2).
Fever; pain.

Mandrolax *Dolorgiet, Ger.†.*
Bisacodyl (p.1212·2).
Constipation.

Mandrolax Lactu *Dolorgiet, Ger.†.*
Lactulose (p.1230·1).
Constipation; hepatic encephalopathy; salmonella enteritis.

Mandrolax Pico *Dolorgiet, Ger.†.*
Sodium picosulfate (p.1249·3).
Constipation.

Mandros Diarstop *Dolorgiet, Ger.†.*
Loperamide hydrochloride (p.1231·3).
Diarrhoea.

Mandros Reise *Dolorgiet, Ger.†.*
Dimenhydrinate (p.415·2).
Motion sickness; nausea; vertigo; vomiting.

Maneon *Poli, Ital.†.*
Amineptine hydrochloride (p.273·2).
Depression.

Manerix *Roche, Canad.; Roche, Irl.; Roche, Spain; Roche, UK.*
Moclobemide (p.299·3).
Depression.

Manevac *Galen, UK.*
Ispaghula (p.1229·1); senna fruit (p.1248·2).
A similar product was formerly marketed in the *UK* under the name Agiolax.
Bowel evacuation; constipation.

Mangaplexe *Lehning, Fr.*
Manganese gluconate (p.1371·3).
Hypersensitivity.

Manibee Complejo *Rhone-Poulenc Rorer, Mex.*
Vitamin B substances (p.1350·1).

Manibee-C *Rhone-Poulenc Rorer, Mex.*
Vitamin B substances; vitamin C (p.1350·1).

Manic *Medifive, Thai.*
Mefenamic acid (p.51·2).
Pain.

Manicol *Martin, Fr.†.*
Mannitol (p.924·3).
Bowel evacuation; constipation; dyspepsia.

Manidon *Knoll, Spain.*
Verapamil hydrochloride (p.989·1).
Angina pectoris; arrhythmias; hypertension; myocardial infarction.

Manimon *Asta Medica, Ger.*
Propranolol hydrochloride (p.962·3); triamterene (p.986·1); hydrochlorothiazide (p.907·3).
Hypertension.

Maninil *Berlin-Chemie, Ger.*
Glibenclamide (p.321·3).
Diabetes mellitus.

Maniprex *Wolfs, Belg.*
Lithium carbonate (p.292·1).
Bipolar disorder; depression.

Maniton *Kyorin, Thai.*
Mannitol (p.924·3).
Anuria; oliguria; raised intracranial pressure.

Mannex *Bioceuticals, UK.*
Multivitamin and mineral preparation (p.1350·1).

Mannistol *Bieffe, Ital.*
Mannitol (p.924·3).
Cranial and ocular hypertension.

Mannite *Saprochi, Switz.*
Mannitol (p.924·3).
Constipation.

Mannit-Losung *Serag-Wiessner, Ger.*
Mannitol (p.924·3).
Forced diuresis; oedema; renal failure.

Manoderm *Propan, S.Afr.†.*
Clioquinol (p.190·2); hydrocortisone (p.1073·3).
Skin disorders.

Manorfen *Manor, UK.*
Ibuprofen (p.43·2).

Mansal *Vita, Spain.*
Cimetidine (p.1216·3).
Acid aspiration; gastro-oesophageal reflux; gastrointestinal haemorrhage; gastrointestinal hyperacidity; peptic ulcer; Zollinger-Ellison syndrome.

Mansil *Pfizer, Ger.*
Oxamniquine (p.105·1).
Schistosomiasis.

Mantadan *Boehringer Ingelheim, Ital.*
Amantadine hydrochloride (p.1161·2).
Influenza A; mental function impairment; parkinsonism.

Mantadil *Wellcome, USA†.*
Chlorcyclizine hydrochloride (p.411·3); hydrocortisone acetate (p.1073·3).

Mantadix *Du Pont, Belg.†; Du Pont, Fr.*
Amantadine hydrochloride (p.1161·2).
Influenza A; parkinsonism.

Mantai *Tecnimede, Port.*
Minoxidil (p.934·2).

Mantidan *Boehringer de Angeli, Braz.*
Amantadine hydrochloride (p.1161·2).
Drug-induced extrapyramidal disorders; fatigue associated with multiple sclerosis; influenza A; parkinsonism.

Manusept
Note.This name is used for preparations of different composition.
Bode, Ger.; Beiersdorf, Switz.
Orthophenylphenol (p.1152·1).
Hand disinfection.

SSL, UK.
Triclosan (p.1159·2); isopropyl alcohol (p.1149·2).
Skin disinfection.

Manusept HD *Bode, Ger.*
Alcohol (p.1130·3).
Hand disinfection.

Maolate *Upjohn, USA.*
Chlorphenesin carbamate (p.1327·2).
Musculoskeletal pain.

Maoni *Lichtwer, Ger.*
Kava (p.1625·3).
Nervous disorders.

MAOtil *Hormosan, Ger.*
Selegiline (p.1178·1).
Parkinsonism.

Maox *Manne, USA.*
Magnesium oxide (p.1233·2).
Hyperacidity.

Mapap *Major, USA.*
Paracetamol (p.71·2).
Fever; pain.

Mapap Cold Formula *Major, USA.*
Paracetamol (p.71·2); chlorpheniramine [chlorphenamine] maleate (p.412·1); pseudoephedrine hydrochloride (p.1099·2); dextromethorphan hydrobromide (p.1087·3).

Mapezine *Siam Bheasach, Thai.*
Carbamazepine (p.342·1).
Epilepsy; trigeminal neuralgia.

Maple Melts *Green Turtle Bay Vitamin Co., USA.*
Vitamin and mineral preparation (p.1350·1).
Tonic.

Mapluxin *Novartis, Mex.*
Digoxin (p.870·1).
Heart failure; paroxysmal supraventricular tachycardia.

Mapox *Niddapharm, Ger.*
Aciclovir (p.612·3).
Herpesvirus infections.

Mapro-GRY *Gry, Ger.†.*
Maprotiline hydrochloride (p.297·2).
Depression.

Maprolu *Hexal, Ger.*
Maprotiline hydrochloride (p.297·2).
Depression.

Mapurit *Sanum-Kehlbeck, Ger.*
dl-Alpha tocoferil acetate (p.1394·1); magnesium oxide (p.1233·2).
Magnesium or vitamin E deficiency.

Maquil *Pharmaton, Ger.†.*
Cynara (p.1601·3).
Dyspepsia.

Maqui-Libre *Lancome, Canad.*
SPF 15: Octinoxate (p.1517·3).
Sunscreen.

Mar *Masa, Thai.*
Dried aluminium hydroxide gel (p.1210·3); magnesium hydroxide (p.1233·1); simeticone (p.1249·2).
Flatulence; gastric hyperacidity; peptic ulcer.

mar plus *Stada, Ger.*
Dexpanthenol (p.1602·3); sodium chloride (p.1196·1).
Nasal congestion.

Maracugina Composta *Virtus, Braz.*
Passion flower (p.1649·1); erythrina mulungu; crataegus (p.1600·2).
Sedative.

Marament Balsam W *Wider, Ger.†*
Camphor (p.1589·3); methyl salicylate (p.55·1); benzyl nicotinate (p.20·2).
Neuralgia; rheumatism; sciatica; sprains.

Marament-N *Amino, Switz.*
Camphor (p.1589·3); methyl salicylate (p.55·1); benzyl nicotinate (p.20·2); oleum pini sylvestris.
Musculoskeletal, joint, and soft-tissue disorders.

Maranon H *Henkel, Ger.*
Sodium hypochlorite (p.1156·2).
Instrument disinfection.

Maranox *Dent, USA.*
Paracetamol (p.71·2).
Fever; pain.

Marax
Note.This name is used for preparations of different composition.
Pfizer, Braz.
Hydroxyzine hydrochloride (p.419·1); ephedrine sulfate (p.1090·2); theophylline (p.777·2).
Bronchospastic disorders.

Asche, Ger.
Magaldrate (p.1232·2).
Gastrointestinal hyperacidity; peptic ulcer.

Pfizer, USA.
Ephedrine sulfate (p.1090·2); theophylline (p.777·2); hydroxyzine hydrochloride (p.419·1).
Bronchospasm.

Marben *Medifarma, Mex.*
Mebendazole (p.102·2).

Marblen *Fleming, USA.*
Calcium carbonate (p.1215·1); magnesium carbonate (p.1232·3).
Hyperacidity.

Marcain
Astra, Austral.; AstraZeneca, Denm.; AstraZeneca, Fin.; Astra, Irl.; AstraZeneca, Norw.; AstraZeneca, NZ; AstraZeneca, Singapore; Astra, Swed.; AstraZeneca, UK.
Bupivacaine hydrochloride (p.1306·3).
Adrenaline [epinephrine] (p.829·1) or adrenaline [epinephrine] acid tartrate (p.829·2) is included in some injections as a vasoconstrictor to diminish absorption and localise the effect of the local anaesthetic.
Local anaesthesia.

Marcain with Fentanyl
Astra, Austral.; AstraZeneca, NZ.
Bupivacaine hydrochloride (p.1306·3); fentanyl citrate (p.37·1).
Epidural analgesia.

Marcain with Pethidine
Astra, Austral.; AstraZeneca, NZ.
Bupivacaine hydrochloride (p.1306·3); pethidine hydrochloride (p.75·1).
Epidural analgesia.

Marcaina
Astra, Braz.; Astra, Ital.; Astra, Port.†.
Bupivacaine hydrochloride (p.1306·3).
Adrenaline [epinephrine] acid tartrate (p.829·2) is included in some injections as a vasoconstrictor to diminish absorption and localise the effect of the local anaesthetic.
Local anaesthesia.

Marcaine
Astra, Belg.; Sanofi Synthelabo, Canad.; AstraZeneca, Fr.; Astra, Hong Kong; Astra, Israel; Astra, Neth.; AstraZeneca, Thai.; Sanofi Winthrop, USA.
Bupivacaine hydrochloride (p.1306·3).
Adrenaline [epinephrine] (p.829·1) or adrenaline [epinephrine] acid tartrate (p.829·2) is included in some injections as a vasoconstrictor to diminish absorption and localise the effect of the local anaesthetic.
Analgesia; local anaesthesia.

Marcelle Multi-Defense *Professional Health, Canad.*
SPF 15: Meradimate (p.1517·3); octinoxate (p.1517·3); ensulizole (p.1517·2).
Sunscreen.

Marcelle Protective Block *Professional Health, Canad.*
SPF 15: Titanium dioxide (p.1126·1).
SPF 25: Titanium dioxide (p.1126·1); zinc oxide (p.1128·2).
Sunscreen.

Marcelle Sunblock *Professional Health, Canad.*
SPF 8: Octinoxate (p.1517·3); oxybenzone (p.1518·1).
SPF 15; SPF 20: Octinoxate (p.1517·3); octisalate (p.1518·1); oxybenzone (p.1518·1).
Sunscreen.

Marcen *Pharmacia Upjohn, Spain.*
Ketazolam (p.688·2).
Anxiety; insomnia; skeletal muscle spasm.

Marcillin *Marnel, USA.*
Ampicillin trihydrate (p.151·1).

Marco Rub Camphorated *Marc-O, Canad.*
Camphor (p.1589·3); menthol (p.1632·3); eucalyptol (p.1609·2).

Marcocid *Willvonseder, Aust.*
Propyl alcohol (p.1155·3); isopropyl alcohol (p.1149·2).
Skin disinfection.

Marcof *Marnel, USA.*
Hydrocodone tartrate (p.42·2); sulfogaiacol (p.1101·1).
Coughs.

Marcoumar
Roche, Aust.; Roche, Belg.; Roche, Braz.; Roche, Denm.; Roche, Neth.; Roche, Switz.
Phenprocoumon (p.954·3).
Thromboembolic disorders.

Marcumar *Roche, Ger.*
Phenprocoumon (p.954·3).
Thromboembolic disorders.

marcuphen *CT, Ger.*
Phenprocoumon (p.954·3).
Thromboembolic disorders.

Marduk *S & K, Ger.*
Benzoyl peroxide (p.1111·1).
Acne.

Mareen *Krewel, Ger.*
Doxepin hydrochloride (p.283·3).
Anxiety disorders; depression; sleep disorders; withdrawal syndromes.

Marespin *Abiogen, Ital.*
Sulfamazone sodium (p.253·3).
Respiratory-tract infections.

Marevan
Boots, Austral.; Bio-Therabel, Belg.; Glaxo Wellcome, Braz.; Nycomed, Denm.; Orion, Fin.; Nycomed, Norw.; Glaxo Wellcome, NZ; Goldshield, UK.
Warfarin sodium (p.992·2).
Thromboembolic disorders.

Marevit *Pensa, Spain.*
Meclozine hydrochloride (p.420·3).
Motion sickness.

Marezine *Himmel, USA.*
Cyclizine hydrochloride (p.414·1).
Motion sickness.

Margesic *Marnel, USA.*
Butalbital (p.658·3); paracetamol (p.71·2); caffeine (p.761·3).
Tension headache.

Margesic H *Marnel, USA.*
Hydrocodone tartrate (p.42·2); paracetamol (p.71·2).
Pain.

Marianon *Klein, Ger.*
Silybum marianum (p.1021·3); greater celandine (p.1618·1); achillea (p.1572·2); absinthium (p.1571·1); hypericum (p.290·2).
Biliary disorders.

Mariazeller *Apotheke Gnadenmutter, Aust.*
Cinnamon (p.1595·3); cinchona bark (p.1595·3); dried bitter-orange peel (p.1644·2); clove (p.1596·3); flos aurantii; chamomile (p.1593·2); folium aurantium; melissa (p.1632·2); menyanthes (p.1633·1); cardamom fruit (p.1591·3); fructus aurantii immat; coriander (p.1599·2); absinthium (p.1571·1); cnicus benedictus (p.1597·2); centaury (p.1593·1); achillea moschata; achillea (p.1572·2); guaiacum wood; juniper (p.1625·2); galanga; gentian (p.1615·1); ginger (p.1227·2); nutmeg (p.1643·1).
Gastrointestinal disorders.

Marienbader Pillen N *Riemser, Ger.*
Bisacodyl (p.1212·2).
Constipation.

Mariendistel Curarina *Harras-Curarina, Ger.*
Silybum marianum (p.1021·3).
Liver disorders.

Maril
Atlantic, Singapore; Atlantic, Thai.
Metoclopramide hydrochloride (p.1235·2).
Gastrointestinal motility disorders; nausea and vomiting.

Marine Lipid Concentrate *Vitaline, USA.*
Omega-3 marine triglycerides with vitamin E (p.949·3).
Dietary supplement.

Marinepa *Lifeplan, UK.*
Omega-3 marine triglycerides (p.949·3).
Nutritional supplement.

Marinol
Sanofi Synthelabo, Canad.; Roxane, USA.
Dronabinol (p.1224·3).
Appetite stimulant; nausea and vomiting associated with cancer chemotherapy.

Pharmaceveloppement, Fr.
Iodine (p.1522·3); marine algae; calcium dihydrogen phosphate (p.1588·2); tannic acid (p.1669·1); phosphoric acid (p.1651·1); sea water.
Tonic.

Mariston *Codal Synto, Thai.*
Gemfibrozil (p.896·2).
Hyperlipidaemias.

Markalakt
Koch, Aust.; Pascoe, Ger.
Chamomile (p.1593·2).
Allergic disorders; gastrointestinal disorders; skin disorders.

Marks-Losung *Serag-Wiessner, Ger.*
Electrolyte infusion with glucose (p.1180·1).
Fluid and electrolyte disorders.

Marlidan *Vinas, Spain†.*
Liver extract.
Tonic.

Marlin Salt System *Marlin, USA.*
Sodium chloride (p.1196·1)(p.1129·2).
Rinsing and storage solution for soft contact lenses.

Marlyn Formula 50 *Marlyn, USA.*
Amino acids; pyridoxine hydrochloride (p.1386·3).
Nail disorders; postnatal hair-loss.

Marly-Skin *Sandoz, Ital.†.*
Barrier preparation.

Marmine *Vortech, USA†.*
Dimenhydrinate (p.415·2).
Motion sickness.

Marnal *Vortech, USA†.*
Aspirin (p.14·2); caffeine (p.761·3); butalbital (p.658·3).
Pain.

Marnatal-F *Marnel, USA.*
Multivitamin and mineral preparation with iron and folic acid (p.1350·1).

Marolderm *Dermapharm, Ger.†.*
Dexpanthenol (p.1602·3).
Burns; skin ulceration; sunburn; wounds.

Maronil *Unipharm, Israel.*
Clomipramine hydrochloride (p.282·1).
Depression; obsessive-compulsive disorder.

Marovilina *Atlantis, Mex.*
Ampicillin trihydrate (p.151·1).
Bacterial infections.

Marplan
Medilink, Denm.; Cambridge, UK; Roche, USA.
Isocarboxazid (p.292·1).
Now known as Isocarboxazid Tablets in the UK.
Depression.

Marpres *Marnel, USA.*
Hydrochlorothiazide (p.907·3); reserpine (p.967·3); hydralazine hydrochloride (p.905·3).
Hypertension.

Marrubene Codethyline *Lemoine, Fr.†*
Elecampane (p.1089·3); marrubium (p.1094·2); terpin (p.1101·2); sodium benzoate (p.1134·3); ethylmorphine hydrochloride (p.35·2).
Respiratory-tract congestion.

Marsil *Crosara, Ital.†.*
Silybum marianum (p.1021·3).
Liver disorders.

Marsilid *Laphal, Fr.*
Iproniazid phosphate (p.291·3).
Depression.

Marsonil *Makros, Braz.*
Ephedrine hydrochloride (p.1090·1); homatropine methylbromide (p.468·1).
Obstructive airways disease.

Marten-Tab *Marnel, USA.*
Butalbital (p.658·3); paracetamol (p.71·2).
Tension headache.

Marthritic *Marnel, USA.*
Salsalate (p.82·2).

Martigene *Ciba Vision, Fr.*
Phenylephrine hydrochloride (p.1097·1); brompheniramine maleate (p.410·2).
Allergic conjunctivitis.

Martimil *Synthelabo, Spain.*
Nortriptyline hydrochloride (p.301·3).
Depression.

Martindale Methadone Mixture DTF *Martindale Pharmaceuticals, UK.*
Methadone hydrochloride (p.53·1).
It contains hydroxybenzoate esters as preservatives.
NOTE. There is no connection between Martindale, The Complete Drug Reference and Martindale Pharmaceuticals.
Opioid withdrawal.

Martos-10 *Otsuka, Jpn†.*
Maltose (p.1371·2).
Carbohydrate source; diabetes mellitus.

Marvelon
Organon, Aust.; Organon, Austral.; Organon, Belg.; Organon, Canad.; Organon, Denm.; Organon, Fin.; Organon, Ger.; Organon, Hong Kong; Organon, Mex.; Organon, Neth.; Organon, Norw.; Pharmaco, NZ; Organon, Port.; Donmed, S.Afr.; Organon, Singapore; Organon, Switz.; Organon, Thai.; Organon, UK.
Desogestrel (p.1470·3); ethinylestradiol (p.1476·2).
28-Day packs also contain 7 inert tablets.
Combined oral contraceptive.

Marviol *Organon, Irl.*
Desogestrel (p.1470·3); ethinylestradiol (p.1476·2).
Combined oral contraceptive.

Marzine
Glaxo Wellcome, Aust.†; Glaxo Wellcome, Canad.†; Warner-Lambert, Denm.; Warner-Lambert, Fin.; Glaxo Wellcome, Fin.; Glaxo Wellcome, Hong Kong; Warner-Lambert, Norw.; Warner-Lambert, NZ; Glaxo Wellcome, Singapore; Glaxo Wellcome, Swed.; Warner-Lambert Consumer, Switz.
Cyclizine hydrochloride (p.414·1) or cyclizine lactate (p.414·1).
Motion sickness; nausea and vomiting; vestibular disorders.

Masa Balm
Note.This name is used for preparations of different composition.
British Dispensary, Thai.
Methyl salicylate (p.55·1); menthol (p.1632·3); camphor (p.1589·3); eucalyptus oil (p.1609·2).
Musculoskeletal and joint pain.

Masa, Thai.
Methyl salicylate (p.55·1); menthol (p.1632·3); eugenol (p.1609·3).
Musculoskeletal and joint pain; sprains; strains.

Masaga *Nakornpatana, Thai.*
Methyl salicylate (p.55·1); menthol (p.1632·3); camphor (p.1589·3); eucalyptus oil (p.1609·2); clove oil (p.1597·1).
Musculoskeletal pain; neuralgia; sciatica.

Masagil *Calmante Vitaminado, Spain.*
Liniment: Camphor (p.1589·3); ammonia (p.1579·1); methyl salicylate (p.55·1); rosemary oil (p.1659·3); turpentine oil (p.1676·3).

Topical Spray: Camphor (p.1589·3); methyl salicylate (p.55·1); turpentine oil (p.1676·3); menthol (p.1632·3).
Rheumatic and muscle pain.

Masarax *Masa, Thai.*
Hydroxyzine hydrochloride (p.419·1).
Hypersensitivity reactions; sedative.

Masaren *Masa, Thai.*
Diclofenac diethylamine (p.30·2).
Musculoskeletal, joint, and peri-articular disorders.

Masarol *Masa, Thai.*
Ketoconazole (p.389·1).
Fungal infections.

Masawarm *Masa, Thai.*
Albendazole (p.95·2).
Worm infections.

Masaworm-I *Masa, Thai.*
Mebendazole (p.102·2).
Worm infections.

Masculine Herbal Complex *GNLD, Austral.*
Saw palmetto; avena; celery; damiana; achillea; hypericum; skullcap; astragalus; chillies.
Tonic.

Masdil *Esteve, Spain.*
Diltiazem hydrochloride (p.874·3).
Angina pectoris; arrhythmias; hypertension.

Masern-Impfstoff Merieux *Pasteur Merieux, Ger.*
A live measles vaccine (attenuated Schwarz strain) (p.1547·1).
Active immunisation.

Masern-Lebend-Impfstoff *Chiron Behring, Ger.†.*
A live measles vaccine (more attenuated Enders strain) (p.1547·1).
Active immunisation.

Masern-Vaccinol *Procter & Gamble, Ger.†.*
A live measles vaccine (attenuated Schwarz strain) (p.1547·1).
Active immunisation.

Masern-Virus-Impfstoff *Chiron Behring, Ger.†.*
A live measles vaccine (more attenuated Enders strain) (p.1547·1).
Active immunisation.

Masferol *Quimica y Farmacia, Mex.*
Paracetamol (p.71·2).
Fever; pain.

Masflex *Abbott, Mex.*
Meloxicam (p.51·3).
Gout; inflammation; musculoskeletal, joint, and peri-articular disorders; pain.

Masigel K *Boehringer Ingelheim, Ger.†.*
Dimagnesium aluminium trisilicate.
Gastrointestinal disorders.

Maskam Krauter-Tee *Duopharm, Ger.†.*
Senna (p.1248·2).
Constipation; exogenous obesity.

Masnoderm *Dominion, UK†.*
Clotrimazole (p.382·1).
Fungal skin infections.

Masor *Formenti, Ital.†.*
Stepronin lysine (p.1101·1).
Respiratory-tract disorders.

Massage Balm Arnica *Weleda, UK.*
Arnica flower oil; birch leaf oil (p.55·2); lavender oil (p.1627·2); rosemary oil (p.1659·3).
Rheumatic and muscular pain.

Massage Balm Calendula *Weleda, UK.*
Calendula (p.1589·2); betula alba (p.1585·2); lavender oil (p.1627·2).
Muscle tension.

Massageol *Neo Quimica, Braz.*
Camphor (p.1589·3); turpentine oil (p.1676·3); menthol (p.1632·3); methyl salicylate (p.55·1); chlorophyll (p.1028·1).
Musculoskeletal and joint disorders.

Massagim *Vitoria, Port.*
Diethylamine salicylate (p.32·2).

Masse
Note.This name is used for preparations of different composition.
Janssen-Cilag, Austral.†; Janssen-Cilag, Irl.; Janssen-Cilag, UK†; Advanced Care, USA.
Emollient and moisturiser.
Nipple care.

Janssen-Cilag, S.Afr.
Allantoin (p.1110·1); aminoacridine (p.1130·3).
Napkin rash; nipple care.

Massengill *SmithKline Beecham Consumer, USA.*
Concentrated solution: Lactic acid (p.1626·2); sodium lactate (p.1186·2); sodium bicarbonate (p.1186·2); alcohol (p.1130·3); octoxinol 9 (p.1346·3).
Powder: Ammonium alum; phenol (p.1152·3); methyl salicylate (p.55·1); eucalyptus oil (p.1609·2); menthol (p.1632·3); thymol (p.1158·3); sodium chloride (p.1196·1).
Vaginal disorders.

Massengill Disposable
Note.This name is used for preparations of different composition.
SmithKline Beecham Consumer, USA.
Vinegar (p.1571·2).
Vaginal disorders.

SmithKline Beecham Consumer, USA.
Alcohol (p.1130·3); lactic acid (p.1626·2); sodium lactate (p.1186·2); octoxinol 9 (p.1346·3); propylene glycol (p.1655·1); cetylpyridinium chloride (p.1138·1); diazolidinyl urea.
Vaginal disorders.

The symbol † denotes a preparation no longer actively marketed

Massengill Feminine Cleansing Wash *SmithKline Beecham Consumer, USA.*
Vaginal cleanser.

Massengill Medicated
Note.This name is used for preparations of different composition.
SmithKline Beecham Consumer, Canad.†; SmithKline Beecham, Israel.
Povidone-iodine (p.1155·1).
Vaginal irritation.

SmithKline Beecham Consumer, USA.
Soft cloth towelette: Hydrocortisone (p.1073·3).
Corticosteroid.

Vaginal douche: Povidone-iodine (p.1155·1).
Vaginal disorders.

Massorax *RTA, Switz.*
Methyl salicylate (p.55·1); isopropyl nicotinate; capsicum (p.1591·1); camphor (p.1589·3); turpentine oil (p.1676·3); eucalyptus oil (p.1609·2); lavender oil (p.1627·2).
Musculoskeletal, joint, and soft-tissue disorders.

Massubal *Dermopen, Braz.*
Methyl salicylate (p.55·1); turpentine oil (p.1676·3); guaiacol (p.1092·1).
Musculoskeletal and joint disorders.

Mastia *Inexfa, Spain.*
Aspirin (p.14·2); caffeine (p.761·3).
Contains thiamine.
Fever; pain.

Mastical *Byk Elmu, Spain.*
Calcium carbonate (p.1215·1).
Hypocalcaemia; osteoporosis.

Mastika *Goldshield, UK.*
Mastic gum (p.1631·2).
Peptic ulcer.

Mastiol *Reig Jofre, Spain.*
Chlorhexidine acetate (p.1138·2); benzocaine (p.1306·2); vitamin A (p.1382·1).
Mastitis.

Mastodanatrol *Sanofi Synthelabo, Port.*
Danazol (p.1468·3).
Benign breast disorders.

Mastodynon
Bionorica, Ger.; Bionorica, Thai.
Homoeopathic preparation.

Mastu S
Stada, Ger.; Stada, Hong Kong.
Bufexamac (p.20·3); bismuth subgallate (p.1213·2); titanium dioxide (p.1126·1); lignocaine [lidocaine] hydrochloride (p.1313·2).
Anorectal disorders.

Maswin *Masa, Thai.*
Piroxicam (p.79·1).
Gout; musculoskeletal and joint disorders.

Matcine
Atlantic, Singapore; Atlantic, Thai.
Chlorpromazine hydrochloride (p.660·2).
Affective disorders; controlled hypotension; hypothermia induction; nausea and vomiting; premedication; schizophrenia; sedative.

Matergam *Centeon, Braz.*
An anti-D immunoglobulin (p.1532·1).
Prevention of rhesus sensitisation.

Materna
Wyeth, Braz.; Wyeth-Ayerst, Canad.; Wyeth-Ayerst, Israel; Wyeth, Mex.; Lederle, USA.
Multivitamin and mineral preparation (p.1350·1).
Dietary supplement during pregnancy and lactation.

Materna Nova *Lederle, Switz.*
Multivitamin and mineral preparation (p.1350·1).

Materna Tsimchit *Maabarot, Israel.*
Infant feed (p.1350·1).
Milk intolerance.

Maternity One *Swiss Herbal, Canad.*
Multivitamin and mineral preparation (p.1350·1).

Mathieu Cough Syrup *Mathieu, Canad.*
Ammonium chloride (p.1085·2); potassium iodide (p.1522·3).

Mathoine *Wolfs, Belg.*
Phenytoin (p.357·2); methylphenobarbital (p.353·3).
Epilepsy.

Matiga *Pierre Fabre, Fr.†.*
Arachis oil (p.1581·1); menthol (p.1632·3).
Musculoskeletal, joint, peri-articular, and soft-tissue disorders.

Matmille *Ritsert, Ger.*
Bath additive: Chamomile (p.1593·2); chamomile oil.
Skin and mucous-membrane disorders.

Ointment; oral liquid: Chamomile (p.1593·2).
Gastrointestinal disorders; skin and mucous-membrane disorders.

Mato *Hevert, Ger.*
Homoeopathic preparation.

Matrabec *Warner-Lambert, Spain.*
Multivitamin and mineral preparation (p.1350·1).

Matricaria Vitam AED *Dansk-Flama, Braz.*
Chamomile (p.1593·2); vitamin A; vitamin D; calcium phosphate; calcium carbonate; pepsin (p.1350·1).

Matrifolin *Orion, Fin.*
Vitamin B substances with ferrous fumarate (p.1360·1) (p.1350·1).
Iron-deficiency anaemia; vitamin supplement.

Matrix *Wyeth Lederle, Ital.*
A heparinoid (p.905·2).
Osteoarthritis.

Matulane *Roche, USA.*
Procarbazine hydrochloride (p.566·2).
Malignant neoplasms.

Mature Balance *Pharmavite, Canad.*
Multivitamin and mineral preparation (p.1350·1).

Maveral *Farmades, Ital.*
Fluvoxamine maleate (p.289·3).
Depression; obsessive-compulsive disorder.

Mavid *Abbott, Ger.*
Clarithromycin (p.186·2).
Mycobacterial infections.

Mavigen Sebo *Mavi, Ital.*
Cystine (p.1359·1).
Seborrhoea.

Mavik
Knoll, Canad.; Abbott, USA.
Trandolapril (p.985·2).
Heart failure following myocardial infarction; hypertension.

Mavipiu *Mavi, Ital.*
Calamine (p.1111·3); zinc oxide (p.1128·2); oryzanol (p.1645·1).
Barrier preparation; nappy rash.

Max *Unison, Thai.*
Ambroxol hydrochloride (p.1084·3).
Respiratory-tract disorders associated with increased or viscous mucus.

Maxadol *Restan, S.Afr.*
Capsules: Paracetamol (p.71·2); codeine phosphate (p.25·2).

Syrup: Paracetamol (p.71·2); codeine phosphate (p.25·2); promethazine hydrochloride (p.423·2).
Fever; pain.

Maxadol Forte *Restan, S.Afr.*
Paracetamol (p.71·2); codeine phosphate (p.25·2); caffeine (p.761·3); meprobamate (p.691·1).
Pain.

Maxadol-P *Restan, S.Afr.*
Paracetamol (p.71·2).
Fever; pain.

Maxair
3M, Canad.†; Jouveinal, Canad.†; 3M, Fr.; 3M, Switz.; 3M, USA.
Pirbuterol acetate (p.769·3).
Obstructive airways disease.

Maxalt
Merck Sharp & Dohme, Austral.; Merck Sharp & Dohme, Belg.; Merck Frosst, Canad.; Merck Sharp & Dohme, Denm.; Merck Sharp & Dohme, Fin.; Merck Sharp & Dohme, Ger.; Merck Sharp & Dohme, Ital.; Merck Sharp & Dohme, Mex.; Merck Sharp & Dohme, Neth.; Merck Sharp & Dohme, Norw.; Merck Sharp & Dohme, NZ; Merck Sharp & Dohme, Port.; Merck Sharp & Dohme, S.Afr.; Merck Sharp & Dohme, Spain; Merck Sharp & Dohme, Swed.; Merck Sharp & Dohme, UK; Merck, USA.
Rizatriptan benzoate (p.455·2).
Migraine.

Maxamaid MSUD
SHS, Fr.; Scientific Hospital Supplies, UK.
Leucine-, isoleucine-, and valine-free food (p.1350·1).
Maple syrup urine disease.

Maxamaid RVHB
Nutricia, NZ; Scientific Hospital Supplies, NZ; Scientific Hospital Supplies, UK.
Methionine-free food (p.1350·1).
Homocystinuria; hypermethioninaemia.

Maxamaid XLEU *SHS, Fr.*
Food for special diets (p.1350·1).
Isovaleric acidaemia.

Maxamaid XLYS, Low Try *SHS, Fr.*
Food for special diets (p.1350·1).
Glutaric aciduria.

Maxamaid XLYS, TRY *Scientific Hospital Supplies, UK.*
Lysine- and tryptophan-free food (p.1350·1).
Glutaric aciduria.

Maxamaid XMET *SHS, Fr.*
Food for special diets (p.1350·1).
Homocystinuria.

Maxamaid XMET, Cys *SHS, Fr.*
Food for special diets (p.1350·1).
Sulfite oxidase deficiency.

Maxamaid XMET, THRE, VAL, ISOLEU *Scientific Hospital Supplies, UK.*
Methionine-, threonine-, valine-free, and low isoleucine food (p.1350·1).
Methylmalonic acidaemia; propionic acidaemia.

Maxamaid XMTVI *SHS, Fr.*
Food for special diets (p.1350·1).
Methylmalonic or propionic acidaemia.

Maxamaid XP
SHS, Fr.; Scientific Hospital Supplies, Israel; Medifood, Ital.; Nutricia, NZ; Scientific Hospital Supplies, NZ; Scientific Hospital Supplies, UK.
Food for special diets (p.1350·1).
Phenylketonuria.

Maxamaid XPHEN, TYR *Scientific Hospital Supplies, UK.*
Phenylalanine- and tyrosine-free food (p.1350·1).
Tyrosinaemia.

Maxamaid XPTM *SHS, Fr.*
Food for special diets (p.1350·1).
Tyrosinaemia.

Maxamum MSUD
SHS, Fr.; Nutricia, NZ; Scientific Hospital Supplies, NZ.
Food for special diets (p.1350·1).
Maple syrup urine disease.

Maxamum XLYS, Try *SHS, Fr.*
Food for special diets (p.1350·1).
Glutaric aciduria.

Maxamum XMET *SHS, Fr.*
Food for special diets (p.1350·1).
Homocystinuria.

Maxamum XMTVI *SHS, Fr.*
Food for special diets (p.1350·1).
Methylmalonic or propionic acidaemia.

Maxamum XP
SHS, Fr.; Scientific Hospital Supplies, Israel; Medifood, Ital.; Scientific Hospital Supplies, NZ; Scientific Hospital Supplies, UK.
Food for special diets (p.1350·1).
Phenylketonuria.

Maxamum XPhen, Tyr
Scientific Hospital Supplies, Austral.; SHS, Fr.
Food for special diets (p.1350·1).
Tyrosinaemia.

Maxaquin
Searle, Braz.; Searle, Hong Kong; Searle, Israel; Searle, Ital.; Searle, Mex.; Monsanto, Port.; Aspen, S.Afr.; Searle, Switz.; Searle, Thai.; Unimed, USA.
Lomefloxacin hydrochloride (p.220·1).
Bacterial infections.

Maxcef
Bristol-Myers Squibb, Braz.; Bristol-Myers Squibb, Israel.
Cefepime (p.165·3) or cefepime hydrochloride (p.165·3).
Bacterial infections.

Maxcil *Triomed, S.Afr.*
Amoxicillin trihydrate (p.149·2).
Bacterial infections.

Maxenal *McNeil Consumer, Canad.*
Pseudoephedrine hydrochloride (p.1099·2).
Nasal congestion.

Maxepa
Cenovis, Austral.; Vitelle, Austral.; Pierre Fabre, Fr.; Scherer, Hong Kong; Novartis Consumer, Ital.; Seven Seas, UK; Solgar, USA.
Omega-3 marine triglycerides (p.949·3).
Dietary supplement; lipid disorders.

Maxepa & EPO *Vitaplex, Austral.*
Marine fish oil (p.949·3); evening primrose oil (p.1613·2).
Dietary supplement.

Maxepa Plus *Vitaglow, Austral.*
Marine fish oil (p.949·3); magnesium phosphate (p.1191·1).
Psoriasis; rheumatoid arthritis.

Maxeran *Hoechst Marion Roussel, Canad.*
Metoclopramide hydrochloride (p.1235·2).
Adjunct in gastrointestinal radiography; delayed gastric emptying; facilitation of small bowel intubation; postoperative vomiting.

Maxi-6 *Desbergers, Canad.*
Multivitamin preparation (p.1350·1).

Maxi-10 *Desbergers, Canad.*
Multivitamin preparation (p.1350·1).

Maxi-B
Sanofi Synthelabo, Belg.; Sanofi Winthrop, Neth.†.
Vitamin B substances (p.1350·1).
Neurological or rheumatic pain.

Maxibol *Hoechst Marion Roussel, Mex.*
Cobamamide (p.1388·3).

Maxicaine *Sanofi Synthelabo, Fr.*
Parethoxycaine hydrochloride (p.1318·2).
Throat disorders.

Maxi-calc *Searle, Switz.*
Calcium carbonate (p.1215·1).
Calcium deficiency; calcium supplement.

Maxi-Calsor *Orion, Fin.*
Calcium carbonate (p.1215·1).
Calcium deficiency; calcium supplement.

Maxicilina *Pharmacia Upjohn, Mex.*
Ampicillin sodium (p.150·3); ampicillin benzathine (p.151·3).
Bacterial infections.

Maxicrom
Alcon, Braz.; Alcon, Mex.
Sodium cromoglicate (p.774·3).
Allergic conjunctivitis.

Maxid *Fonten, Ital.*
Cefonicid sodium (p.168·1).
Lignocaine [lidocaine] hydrochloride (p.1313·2) is included in this preparation to alleviate the pain of injection.
Gram-negative bacterial infections.

Maxidex
Alcon, Austral.; Alcon, Belg.; Alcon, Braz.; Alcon, Canad.; Alcon, Denm.; Alcon, Fr.; Alcon, Ger.; Alcon, Hong Kong; Alcon, Israel; Alcon, Neth.†; Alcon, NZ; Alcon, S.Afr.; Alcon, Singapore; Alcon Cusi, Spain; Alcon, Switz.; Alcon, UK; Alcon, USA.
Dexamethasone (p.1067·1) or dexamethasone sodium phosphate (p.1067·1).
Inflammatory external ear disorders; inflammatory eye disorders.

Maxidon *Astra, Swed.*
Morphine sulfate (p.56·1).
Pain.

Maxidone *Watson, USA.*
Hydrocodone tartrate (p.42·2); paracetamol (p.71·2).
Pain.

Maxidrol *Alcon, Fr.*
Dexamethasone (p.1067·1); neomycin sulfate (p.228·1); polymyxin B sulfate (p.238·1).
Infected eye disorders.

Maxifed *MCR, USA.*
Guaifenesin (p.1092·2); pseudoephedrine hydrochloride (p.1099·2).
Nasal Congestion.

Maxifed DM *MCR, USA.*
Guaifenesin (p.1092·2); pseudoephedrine hydrochloride (p.1099·2); dextromethorphan hydrobromide (p.1087·3).
Coughs; nasal congestion.

Maxifed G *MCR, USA.*
Guaifenesin (p.1092·2); pseudoephedrine hydrochloride (p.1099·2).
Coughs; nasal Congestion.

Maxiflor *Allergan, USA.*
Diflorasone diacetate (p.1069·2).
Skin disorders.

Maxijul
Note.This name is used for preparations of different composition.
Scientific Hospital Supplies, Austral.; Scientific Hospital Supplies, Israel.
Maltodextrin (p.1371·2).
Carbohydrate food supplement.

SHS, Fr.; Scientific Hospital Supplies, Irl.; Scientific Hospital Supplies, UK.
Food for special diets (p.1350·1).

Maxi-Kalz *Asta Medica, Aust.*
Calcium monocitrate (p.1188·1); calcium dicitrate (p.1188·1).
Calcium supplementation.

Maxi-Kalz Vit D3 *Asta Medica, Aust.*
Calcium carbonate (p.1215·1); colecalciferol (p.1391·1).
Osteoporosis.

Maxilase
Sanofi Winthrop, Fr.; Sanofi Synthelabo, Port.; Sanofi Winthrop, Spain†.
Amylase (p.1579·3).
Oedema; upper respiratory-tract congestion.

Maxilase-Bacitracine *Sanofi Winthrop, Fr.*
Alpha-amylase (p.1579·3); bacitracin (p.155·2).
Bacterial infections of the mouth and throat.

Maxilube *Mission Pharmacal, USA.*
Dimethicone (p.1410·1); glycerol (p.1616·3); carbomer 934 (p.1499·2); trolamine (p.1675·1); sodium laurilsulfate (p.1496·3).
Vaginal lubricant.

Maximet SR *Opus, UK.*
Indometacin (p.44·3).
Inflammation; musculoskeletal, joint, and peri-articular disorders; pain.

Maximum Blue Label *Vitaline, USA.*
Multivitamin and mineral preparation (p.1350·1).

Maximum Green Label *Vitaline, USA.*
Multivitamin and mineral preparation (p.1350·1).

Maximum Once A Day *Quest, Canad.*
Multivitamin and mineral preparation (p.1350·1).

Maximum Red Label *Vitaline, USA.*
Multivitamin and mineral preparation with iron and folic acid (p.1350·1).

Maximum Relief Ex-Lax *Novartis Consumer, USA.*
Senna (p.1248·2).
Formerly contained phenolphthalein.
Constipation.

Maximum Strength Allergy Drops *Bausch & Lomb, USA.*
Naphazoline hydrochloride (p.1095·1); hypromellose (p.1501·3).
Minor eye irritation.

Maximum Strength Anbesol *Whitehall, USA.*
Benzocaine (p.1306·2); alcohol (p.1130·3).
Local anaesthesia.

Maximum Strength Aqua-Ban *Thompson, USA.*
Pamabrom (p.952·1).
Premenstrual water retention.

Maximum Strength Arthriten *Alva, USA†.*
Paracetamol (p.71·2); magnesium salicylate (p.50·3); caffeine (p.761·3).

Maximum Strength Dermarest Dricort *Del, USA†.*
Hydrocortisone acetate (p.1073·3).

Maximum Strength Desenex Antifungal *Ciba, USA.*
Miconazole nitrate (p.391·1).

Maximum Strength Dristan Cold *Whitehall, USA.*
Paracetamol (p.71·2); pseudoephedrine hydrochloride (p.1099·2); brompheniramine maleate (p.410·2).
Cold symptoms; nasal congestion.

Maximum Strength Flexall 454 *Chattem, USA.*
Menthol (p.1632·3); aloe vera (p.1110·1); eucalyptus oil (p.1609·2); methyl salicylate (p.55·1); thyme oil (p.1672·3).
Musculoskeletal disorders; pain.

Maximum Strength KeriCort-10 *Bristol-Myers Squibb, USA†.*
Hydrocortisone (p.1073·3).

Maximum Strength Nasal Decongestant *Taro, USA†.*
Oxymetazoline hydrochloride (p.1096·2).
Nasal congestion.

Maximum Strength Ornex *Menley & James, USA.*
Pseudoephedrine hydrochloride (p.1099·2); paracetamol (p.71·2).
Upper respiratory-tract symptoms.

Maximum Strength Sine-Aid *McNeil Consumer, USA.*
Pseudoephedrine hydrochloride (p.1099·2); paracetamol (p.71·2).
Upper respiratory-tract symptoms.

Maximum Strength Sinutab Without Drowsiness *Warner-Lambert, USA.*
Pseudoephedrine hydrochloride (p.1099·2); paracetamol (p.71·2).
Upper respiratory-tract symptoms.

Maximum Strength Sleepinal *Thompson, USA.*
Diphenhydramine hydrochloride (p.416·1).
Insomnia.

Maximum Strength Sudogest Sinus *Major, USA.*
Paracetamol (p.71·2); pseudoephedrine hydrochloride (p.1099·2).
Upper respiratory-tract congestion.

Maximum Strength TheraFlu Non-Drowsy *Novartis, USA.*
Paracetamol (p.71·2); dextromethorphan hydrobromide (p.1087·3); pseudoephedrine hydrochloride (p.1099·2).
Coughs and cold symptoms.

Maximum Strength Tylenol Allergy Sinus *McNeil Consumer, USA.*
Pseudoephedrine hydrochloride (p.1099·2); chlorpheniramine [chlorphenamine] maleate (p.412·1); paracetamol (p.71·2).
Upper respiratory-tract symptoms.

Maximum Strength Tylenol Allergy Sinus NightTime *McNeil Consumer, USA.*
Pseudoephedrine hydrochloride (p.1099·2); diphenhydramine hydrochloride (p.416·1); paracetamol (p.71·2).
Upper respiratory-tract symptoms.

Maximum Strength Tylenol Sinus *McNeil Consumer, USA.*
Pseudoephedrine hydrochloride (p.1099·2); paracetamol (p.71·2).
Upper respiratory-tract symptoms.

Maximum Strength Unisom SleepGels *Pfizer Consumer, USA.*
Diphenhydramine hydrochloride (p.416·1).
Insomnia.

Maxipime
Bristol-Myers Squibb, Aust.; Bristol-Myers Squibb, Austral.; Bristol-Myers Squibb, Belg.; Bristol-Myers Squibb, Canad.; Bristol-Myers Squibb, Denm.; Bristol-Myers Squibb, Fin.; Bristol-Myers Squibb, Ger.; Bristol-Myers Squibb, Hong Kong; Bristol-Myers Squibb, Irl.; Bristol-Myers Squibb, Ital.; Bristol-Myers Squibb, Mex.; Bristol-Myers Squibb, Neth.; Bristol-Myers Squibb, NZ; Bristol-Myers Squibb, Port.; Bristol-Myers Squibb, S.Afr.; Bristol-Myers Squibb, Singapore; Bristol-Myers, Spain; Bristol-Myers Squibb, Swed.; Bristol-Myers Squibb, Switz.; Bristol-Myers Squibb, Thai.; Bristol-Myers Squibb, USA.
Cefepime hydrochloride (p.165·3).
Bacterial infections.

Maxipro HBV
Scientific Hospital Supplies, Irl.†; Scientific Hospital Supplies, UK.
Food for special diets (p.1350·1).
Hypoproteinaemia.

Maxisorb
Scientific Hospital Supplies, Irl.; Scientific Hospital Supplies, UK.
Food for special diets (p.1350·1).

Maxisporin *Yamanouchi, Neth.*
Cefradine (p.173·3).
Bacterial infections.

Maxitone *Brunel, S.Afr.*
Haematoporphyrin; cyanocobalamin; caffeine; rose hip; yeast (p.1350·1).
Tonic.

Maxitrol
Alcon, Belg.; Alcon, Braz.; Alcon, Canad.; Alcon, Fin.; Alcon, Hong Kong; Alcon, Irl.; Alcon, Israel; Alcon, Mex.; Alcon, Neth.†; Alcon, Norw.; Alcon, NZ; Alcon, S.Afr.; Alcon, Singapore; Alcon Cusí, Spain; Alcon, Switz.; Alcon, Thai.; Alcon, UK; Alcon, USA.
Dexamethasone (p.1067·1); neomycin sulfate (p.228·1); polymyxin B sulfate (p.238·1).
Inflammatory eye infections.

Maxius *OM, Port.*
Tibezonium iodide (p.1673·1).
Mouth and throat disorders.

Maxivate *Westwood-Squibb, USA.*
Betamethasone dipropionate (p.1063·2).
Skin disorders.

Maxivent *Norton, UK.*
Salbutamol (p.770·3).
Asthma; bronchospasm.

Maxivision *Medical Ophthalmics, USA.*
Vitamin, mineral, and nutrient preparation (p.1350·1).

Maxivit *Pfizer, Switz.*
Multivitamin and mineral preparation (p.1350·1).

Maxi-Vite *Goldline, USA.*
Multivitamin, mineral, and amino-acid preparation (p.1350·1).

Maxolon
SmithKline Beecham, Austral.; ICN, Hong Kong; Shire, Irl.; ICN, NZ; Pharmaco, S.Afr.; ICN, Singapore; Monmouth, UK; SmithKline Beecham, USA.
Metoclopramide hydrochloride (p.1235·2).
Aid in gastrointestinal investigations; gastrointestinal disorders; migraine; nausea and vomiting.

Maxomat *Sanofi Winthrop, Fr.*
Somatropin (p.1286·1).
Growth-hormone deficiency; Turner's syndrome.

Maxor *Alphapharm, Austral.*
Omeprazole (p.1239·1).
Gastro-oesophageal reflux; peptic ulcer; Zollinger-Ellison syndrome.

Maxoral *Armstrong, Mex.*
Tibezonium iodide (p.1673·1).
Mouth and throat disorders.

Maxovite *Tyson, USA.*
Multivitamin and mineral preparation (p.1350·1).
Premenstrual syndrome.

Max-Pax *Sanus, Braz.*
Lorazepam (p.688·3).
Alcohol withdrawal syndrome; anxiety; epilepsy; insomnia; nausea and vomiting; premedication.

Maxsoten *Wyeth Lederle, Belg.*
Bisoprolol fumarate (p.850·1); hydrochlorothiazide (p.907·3).
Hypertension.

Maxtrex *Pharmacia, UK.*
Methotrexate (p.553·2).
Malignant neoplasms; psoriasis.

Maxtrim *Bristol-Myers Squibb, Mex.*
Co-trimoxazole (p.193·3).
Bacterial infections; Pneumocystis carinii pneumonia.

Maxum Multi-vite *Seroyal, Canad.*
Multivitamin and mineral preparation (p.1350·1).

Maxzide
Wyeth Lederle, Belg.; Bertek, USA.
Triamterene (p.986·1); hydrochlorothiazide (p.907·3).
Hypertension; oedema.

Maycor
Parke, Davis, Ger.; Godecke, Ger.; Parke, Davis, Spain†.
Isosorbide dinitrate (p.915·2).
Angina pectoris; heart failure; myocardial infarction; peripheral vascular disorders; pulmonary hypertension.

May-Cur-Tee *Gersthofer, Aust.*
Frangula bark (p.1227·1); senna (p.1248·2); fennel (p.1610·1); chamomile (p.1593·2); magnesium sulfate (p.1191·1).
Bowel evacuation; constipation.

Maydil *Parke, Davis, Aust.†.*
Isosorbide dinitrate (p.915·2).
Angina pectoris; heart failure; myocardial infarction.

Mayfit akut *Mayrhofer, Aust.†.*
Methyl salicylate (p.55·1); camphor (p.1589·3); menthol (p.1632·3).
Musculoskeletal and joint disorders.

Mayfit chronisch *Mayrhofer, Aust.†.*
Methyl salicylate (p.55·1); capsicum (p.1591·1); turpentine oil (p.1676·3).
Musculoskeletal and joint disorders.

Mayfung *Mayrhofer, Aust.*
Bath additive: Disodium sulfosuccinated undecenoic acid monoethanolamide (p.396·1).
Topical solution: Undecenoic acid monoethanolamide (p.396·1).
Fungal infections.

Maygace *Bristol-Myers, Spain.*
Megestrol acetate (p.1481·2).
AIDS-associated cachexia; breast cancer; endometrial cancer.

Maynar *Novag, Spain.*
Aciclovir (p.612·3) or aciclovir sodium (p.612·3).
Herpesvirus infections.

Mayogel *Propan, S.Afr.*
Aluminium hydroxide (p.1210·3); magnesium oxide (p.1233·2).
Gastrointestinal disorders.

Mayopirina *Mayo, Mex.*
Dipyrone (p.34·1).

May-Vita *Merz, USA.*
Vitamin B substances with minerals (p.1350·1).

Mazanor *Wyeth-Ayerst, USA†.*
Mazindol (p.1510·3).
Obesity.

Mazon Medicated Cream *Nasmark, Canad.*
Coal tar (p.1125·1); resorcinol (p.1122·2); salicylic acid (p.1122·3).
Skin disorders.

Mazon Medicated Shampoo *Nasmark, Canad.*
Coal tar (p.1125·1); salicylic acid (p.1122·3); sulfur (p.1123·3).
Scalp disorders.

Mazon Medicated Soap *Nasmark, Canad.*
Coal tar (p.1125·1).
Skin disorders.

MB-Combi *Ciba-Geigy, S.Afr.†.*
30 capsules, clofazimine (p.191·1); 2 capsules, rifampicin (p.243·2); 28 tablets, dapsone (p.196·1).
Leprosy.

M-beta *Betapharm, Ger.*
Morphine sulfate (p.56·1).
Pain.

MB-Tab *Alra, USA†.*
Meprobamate (p.691·1).

M-Caps *Pal-Pak, USA.*
Methionine (p.1012·2).
Odour, dermatitis, and ulceration in incontinent adults.

MCP *CT, Ger.; Hexal, Ger.; Aliud, Ger.; Betapharm, Ger.; Isis Puren, Ger.; Ratiopharm, Ger.; Stada, Ger.*
Metoclopramide (p.1236·3) or metoclopramide hydrochloride (p.1235·2).
Gastrointestinal disorders.

MCR *Rafa, Israel.*
Note. A similar name is used for preparations of different composition (see below).
Morphine sulfate (p.56·1).
Pain.

MCR-50 *Pharmacia, UK.*
Note. A similar name is used for preparations of different composition (see above).
Isosorbide mononitrate (p.916·2).
Angina pectoris.

MCT
Mead Johnson, Israel; Medifood, Ital.; Mead Johnson, Singapore; Mead Johnson Nutritionals, USA.
Medium-chain triglycerides (p.1372·1).
Adjunct in the management of disorders of fat absorption and transport.

MCT Duocal
Scientific Hospital Supplies, Irl.; Scientific Hospital Supplies, UK.
Protein-, lactose-, gluten-, fructose-, and sucrose-free food for special diets (p.1350·1).
Fat malabsorption.

MCT Oil
Mead Johnson, Austral.; Scientific Hospital Supplies, Austral.; Mead Johnson Nutritionals, Canad.; Nutricia, Port.; Mead Johnson Nutritionals, Thai.; Mead Johnson Nutritionals, UK; Cow & Gate, UK.
Medium-chain triglycerides (p.1372·1).
Disorders of fat digestion and absorption; ketogenic diets.

MCT Oljymoduli *Nutricia, Fin.*
Medium-chain triglycerides (p.1372·1).
Fat malabsorption.

MCT Pepdite
Scientific Hospital Supplies, Irl.; Scientific Hospital Supplies, UK.
Infant feed (p.1350·1).
Disorders of fat absorption; protein intolerance.

mct Psycho Dragees N *Eurim, Ger.†.*
Hypericum (p.290·2).
Anxiety disorders; depression.

M-D *Milano, Thai.*
Diphenhydramine hydrochloride (p.416·1); calamine (p.1111·3).
Contact dermatitis; urticaria.

MD-60 *Mallinckrodt, Austral.*
Meglumine amidotrizoate (p.1031·2); sodium amidotrizoate (p.1031·2).
Radiographic contrast medium.

MD-76
Mallinckrodt, Austral.; Mallinckrodt, Canad.; Mallinckrodt, USA.
Meglumine amidotrizoate (p.1031·2); sodium amidotrizoate (p.1031·2).
Radiographic contrast medium.

MD Complejo *Liferpal, Mex.*
Vitamin B substances (p.1350·1).

MD-Gastroview
Mallinckrodt, Austral.; Mallinckrodt, USA.
Meglumine amidotrizoate (p.1031·2); sodium amidotrizoate (p.1031·2).
Contrast medium for gastrointestinal radiography.

Mdiltiwas *Wasserman, Spain.*
Diltiazem hydrochloride (p.874·3).
Angina pectoris; hypertension.

M-Dolor
Ethypharm, Aust.; Hexal, Ger.
Morphine sulfate (p.56·1).
Pain.

MDP-Squibb *Squibb Diagnostics, USA†.*
Technetium-99m medronate (p.1451·1).

MDR Fitness Tabs *MDR, USA.*
Multivitamin and mineral preparation (p.1350·1).

Mealin *Pharmasant, Thai.*
Mianserin hydrochloride (p.298·1).
Depression.

Measlegam *NBI, S.Afr.†.*
Measles immunoglobulin (p.1547·1).
Passive immunisation.

Meaverin *Rhone-Poulenc Rorer, Ger.*
Injection: Mepivacaine hydrochloride (p.1317·1).
Local anaesthesia.
Topical gel: Mepivacaine hydrochloride (p.1317·1); lauromacrogol 400 (p.1345·2).
Catheterisation; intubation; local anaesthesia.

Meaverin "A" mit Adrenalin *Rhone-Poulenc Rorer, Ger.†.*
Mepivacaine hydrochloride (p.1317·1).
Adrenaline [epinephrine] acid tartrate (p.829·2) is included in this preparation as a vasoconstrictor to diminish absorption and localise the effect of the local anaesthetic.
Local anaesthesia.

Meaverin hyperbar *Rhone-Poulenc Rorer, Ger.*
Mepivacaine hydrochloride (p.1317·1).
Local anaesthesia.

Meaverin "N" mit Noradrenaline *Rhone-Poulenc Rorer, Ger.†.*
Mepivacaine hydrochloride (p.1317·1).
Noradrenaline [norepinephrine] acid tartrate (p.948·2) is include in this preparation as a vasoconstrictor to diminish absorption and localise the effect of the local anaesthetic.
Local anaesthesia.

Meba *Polipharm, Thai.*
Mebendazole (p.102·2).
Worm infections.

Meban *Kener, Mex.*
Mebendazole (p.102·2).

Mebandozer *Zerboni, Mex.*
Mebendazole (p.102·2).

Mebaral *Sanofi Winthrop, USA.*
Methylphenobarbital (p.353·3).
Anxiety; epilepsy.

Mebaxin *Milano, Thai.*
Methocarbamol (p.1329·3).
Musculoskeletal pain.

Mebeciclol *Sanofi Winthrop, Mex.*
Mebendazole (p.102·2); tinidazole (p.603·3).
Nematode infections; protozoal infections.

Mebelmin *Jofrain, Mex.*
Mebendazole (p.102·2).

Mebemerck *Merck dura, Ger.*
Mebeverine hydrochloride (p.1233·3).
Irritable bowel syndrome.

Meben *UCI, Braz.; General Drugs, Thai.*
Mebendazole (p.102·2).
Worm infections.

Mebendan *Tedec Meiji, Spain.*
Mebendazole (p.102·2).
Worm infections.

Mebenda-P *PP Lab, Thai.*
Mebendazole (p.102·2).
Worm infections.

Mebendazotil *Iodo Suma, Braz.*
Mebendazole (p.102·2).
Worm infections.

Mebendil *Uniao Quimica, Braz.*
Mebendazole (p.102·2).
Worm infections.

Mebenix *Honorterapica, Braz.*
Albendazole (p.95·2).
Worm infections.

Mebenlax *British Dispensary, Thai.*
Mebendazole (p.102·2).
Worm infections.

Mebentiasis *Keton, Mex.*
Mebendazole (p.102·2).

Mebentine *Vitae, Mex.*
Mebendazole (p.102·2).
Worm infections.

Mebetin *Sam Chun Dang, Singapore.*
Mebeverine hydrochloride (p.1233·3).
Gastrointestinal spasm; irritable bowel syndrome.

Mebo
Mebo, Thai.; Julphar, UAE.
Sitosterol (p.970·3).
Burns; haemorrhoids; ulcers; wounds.

Mebocaina *Novartis Consumer, Port.*
Tyrothricin (p.267·1); cetylpyridinium chloride (p.1138·1); oxybuprocaine hydrochloride (p.1318·1).
Mouth and throat disorders.

Mebonat *Roche, Spain.*
Disodium clodronate (p.751·2).
Hypercalcaemia of malignancy; osteolytic bone metastases.

Mebran *Willmar, Mex.*
Dextromethorphan (p.1087·3).

Mebron
Nikkho, Braz.; Daiichi, Jpn.
Epirizole (p.35·1).
Fever; inflammation; pain.

Mebucaine *Novartis Consumer, Switz.*
Cetylpyridinium chloride (p.1138·1); oxybuprocaine hydrochloride (p.1318·1); tyrothricin (p.267·1).
Mouth and throat disorders.

Mebutan *SmithKline Beecham, Neth.*
Nabumetone (p.59·3).
Osteoarthritis; rheumatoid arthritis.

Mebzol *Julphar, UAE.*
Mebendazole (p.102·2).
Worm infections.

Mecain *Curasan, Ger.*
Mepivacaine hydrochloride (p.1317·1).
Local anaesthesia.

Mecca *Mentholatum, Canad.*
Camphor (p.1589·3); phenol (p.1152·3); zinc oxide (p.1128·2).

Mecholyl *Gordon, USA.*
Methacholine chloride (p.1419·3).
Iontophoresis.

Mechovit *Streuli, Switz.*
DL-methionine (p.1012·2); vitamins (p.1350·1).
Liver disorders.

Meclan *Ortho Dermatological, USA.*
Meclocycline sulfosalicylate (p.222·1).
Acne.

Meclifar *Farcoral, Mex.*
Meclozine (p.420·3); vitamin B₆ (p.1387·1).
Nausea and vomiting; vertigo.

Mecloderm *Istoria, Ital.*
Meclocycline sulfosalicylate (p.222·1).
Bacterial skin infections.

Mecloderm Antiacne *Istoria, Ital.*
Meclocycline sulfosalicylate (p.222·1).
Acne; seborrhoeic dermatitis.

Mecloderm F *Istoria, Ital.*
Meclocycline sulfosalicylate (p.222·1); fluocinolone acetonide (p.1071·1).
Infected skin disorders.

Mecloderm Ovuli *Istoria, Ital.*
Meclocycline sulfosalicylate (p.222·1).
Vulvovaginal and cervical infections.

Mecloderm Polvere Aspersoria *Istoria, Ital.*
Meclocycline sulfosalicylate (p.222·1).
Bacterial skin infections.

Meclodol *Parke, Davis, Ital.*
Meclofenamate sodium (p.51·1).
Musculoskeletal and joint disorders; pain.

Meclomen
Parke, Davis, Aust.; Parke, Davis, Hong Kong; Parke-Med, S.Afr.†; Parke, Davis, Spain.
Meclofenamate sodium (p.51·1).
Inflammation; menorrhagia; musculoskeletal, joint, and peri-articular disorders; pain.

Meclomid *Randall, Ital.*
Metoclopramide hydrochloride (p.1235·2).
Gastrointestinal motility disorders; nausea and vomiting.

Meclon *Farmigea, Ital.*
Clotrimazole (p.382·1); metronidazole (p.594·1).
Vulvovaginal and cervical infections.

Meclosorb *S & K, USA.*
Meclocycline sulfosalicylate (p.222·1).
Bacterial skin infections.

Meclutin *ABC, Ital.*
Meclocycline sulfosalicylate (p.222·1); fluocinolone acetonide (p.1071·1).
Infected skin disorders.

Meclutin Semplice *ABC, Ital.*
Meclocycline sulfosalicylate (p.222·1).
Bacterial skin infections.

Mecoten *Promeco, Mex.*
Dipyrone (p.34·1).
Pain.

Mectizan
Merck Sharp & Dohme-Chibret, Fr.; Merck, USA.
Ivermectin (p.99·3).
Veterinary names include: Eqvalan; Ivomec; Oramec.
Lymphatic filariasis; onchocerciasis.

Meda *Circle, USA.*
Paracetamol (p.71·2).
Fever; pain.

Medacaps N *Palmicol, Ger.†*
Deanol hydrogen tartrate (p.1507·1).
Medacaps formerly contained inositol nicotinate, deanol hydrogen tartrate, crataegus, procaine hydrochloride, haematoporphyrin, hesperidin, and alpha tocoferil acetate.
Tonic.

Medacote *Dal-Med, USA†.*
Mepyramine maleate (p.421·1); dimethicone (p.1410·1); zinc oxide (p.1128·2); menthol (p.1632·3); camphor (p.1589·3).
Pruritus.

Med-Actigen *Medical Supply, Thai.*
Triprolidine hydrochloride (p.427·2); pseudoephedrine hydrochloride (p.1099·2).
Cold symptoms; hay fever; rhinitis; upper respiratory-tract congestion.

Medalgin *Medical Supply, Thai.*
Dipyrone (p.34·1).
Pain.

Medalginan *Medinfar, Port.*
Benzyl nicotinate (p.20·2); capsicum (p.1591·1); camphor (p.1589·3); diethylamine salicylate (p.32·2).
Musculoskeletal and joint disorders; neuritis.

Medamet *Caps, S.Afr.*
Metronidazole (p.594·1).
Anaerobic bacterial infections; protozoal infections.

Medamol Co *Medical Supply, Thai.*
Paracetamol (p.71·2); chlorpheniramine [chlorphenamine] maleate (p.412·1); phenylpropanolamine hydrochloride (p.1098·1).
Cold and influenza symptoms; hay fever; sinusitis.

Medamor *Merck Sharp & Dohme, Fin.*
Amiloride hydrochloride (p.835·1).
Hypertension; liver cirrhosis with ascites; oedema.

Med-Anspasmic *Medical Supply, Thai.*
Mefenamic acid (p.51·2); dicyclomine [dicycloverine] hydrochloride (p.466·1).
Smooth muscle spasm.

Medapur *Rentschler, Ger.*
Diphenhydramine hydrochloride (p.416·1).
Pruritus; skin irritation.

Medaren *Medical Supply, Thai.*
Diclofenac sodium (p.30·3).
Musculoskeletal, joint, and peri-articular disorders; pain.

Medaspor *Medpro, S.Afr.*
Clotrimazole (p.382·1).
Fungal infections.

Medazine *Medpro, S.Afr.*
Cyclizine hydrochloride (p.414·1).
Motion sickness; nausea and vomiting; vestibular disorders.

Medazole *Asian Pharm, Thai.*
Mebendazole (p.102·2).
Worm infections.

Medazyl *M & H, Thai.*
Metronidazole (p.594·1).
Anaerobic bacterial infections.

Med-Broncodil *Medical Supply, Thai.*
Terbutaline sulfate (p.776·2).
Obstructive airways disease.

Med-Broncodil Expectorant *Medical Supply, Thai.*
Terbutaline sulfate (p.776·2); guaifenesin (p.1092·2).
Obstructive airways disease.

Med-Circuron *Medical Supply, Thai.*
Cinnarizine (p.413·1).
Cerebrovascular disorders; migraine; motion sickness; peripheral vascular disorders; vestibular disorders.

Medebar
Medefield, Austral.; Medefield, NZ.
Barium sulfate (p.1032·1).
Contrast medium for gastrointestinal radiography.

Medebiotin *Medea, Spain.*
Biotin sodium (p.1355·3).
Biotin deficiency.

Medecitral *Medea, Spain.*
Belladonna alkaloids (p.463·1); sodium bromide (p.1587·1); sodium citrate (p.1186·2).
Vomiting.

Medefizz
Medefield, Austral.; Medefield, NZ.
Potassium bicarbonate; citric acid.
Adjunct in gastrointestinal radiography.

Medefoam *NZ.*
Simeticone (p.1249·2).
Adjunct in gastrointestinal radiography.

Medefoam-2 *Medefield, Austral.*
Simeticone (p.1249·2).
Antifoaming agent for barium radiography.

Medemycin *Meiji, Jpn.*
Midecamycin (p.224·3).
Bacterial infections.

Medenorex *Medea, Spain.*
Cyproheptadine hydrochloride (p.414·2); amino acids and vitamins (p.1350·1).
Tonic.

Medent-DM *Stewart Jackson, USA.*
Guaifenesin (p.1092·2); pseudoephedrine hydrochloride (p.1099·2); dextromethorphan hydrobromide (p.1087·3).
Coughs.

Mede-Prep
Medefield, Austral.; Medefield, NZ.
Mannitol (p.924·3).
Bowel evacuation.

Mederebro *Medea, Spain.*
Cyanocobalamin (p.1388·1); thiamine (p.1385·2); pyridoxine hydrochloride (p.1386·3).
Formerly contained cynocobalamin, cerebral medullary neuropeptides, and thiamine nitrate.
Neurological disorders.

Mederebro Compuesto *Medea, Spain†.*
Cyanocobalamin (p.1388·1); cerebral medullary neuropeptides; pyridoxine hydrochloride (p.1386·3); phosphoserine; thiamine nitrate (p.1385·1); levoglutamide (p.1365·2).
Neurological disorders.

Mederma *Merz, USA.*
Onion (p.1644·1).
Scars.

Mederreumol *Medea, Spain.*
Indometacin (p.44·3).
Gout; inflammation; musculoskeletal, joint, and peri-articular disorders; pain.

Medescan *Medefield, Austral.*
Barium sulfate (p.1032·1).
Radiographic contrast medium.

Medeserpine Co *Medical Supply, Thai.*
Reserpine (p.967·3); hydrochlorothiazide (p.907·3).
Hypertension.

Medesup *Medea, Spain†.*
Bisacodyl (p.1212·2).
Bowel evacuation; constipation.

Medeton *TP, Thai.*
Medroxyprogesterone acetate (p.1480·1).
Endometriosis; progestogen-only injectable contraceptive.

Medevac
Medefield, Austral.; Medefield, NZ.
Arachis oil (p.1581·1); sorbitol (p.1377·3).
Gallbladder evacuant for oral cholecystography.

Med-Gastramet *Medical Supply, Thai.*
Cimetidine (p.1216·3).
Gastric hyperacidity; gastro-oesophageal reflux; peptic ulcer.

Med-Glionil *Medical Supply, Thai.*
Glibenclamide (p.321·3).
Diabetes mellitus.

Med-Guaiphan *Medical Supply, Thai.*
Dextromethorphan hydrobromide (p.1087·3); guaifenesin (p.1092·2); terpin hydrate (p.1101·2).
Coughs.

Medi Creme *Warner-Lambert, Austral.*
Chlorhexidine acetate (p.1138·2); cetrimide (p.1137·1); hexamidine isetionate (p.1146·2); allantoin (p.1110·1); lignocaine [lidocaine] (p.1313·2).
Abrasions; cuts; insect bites and stings; minor burns; skin irritation.

Medi Pulv *Warner-Lambert, Austral.*
Hexamidine isetionate (p.1146·2); chlorhexidine hydrochloride (p.1138·2); allantoin (p.1110·1).
Cuts; minor burns and scalds.

Mediabet *Medice, Ger.*
Metformin hydrochloride (p.332·3).
Diabetes mellitus.

Medialipide
Braun, Belg.; Braun, Fr.
Soya oil (p.1378·1); medium-chain triglycerides (p.1372·1).
Contains egg lecithin.
Lipid infusion for parenteral nutrition.

Medianox *Grossmann, Switz.*
Cloral hydrate (p.669·3).
Nervousness; sleep disorders.

Medianut *Braun, Fr.*
Amino-acid and lipid infusion (p.1350·1).
Parenteral nutrition.

Mediatensyl *Debat, Fr.*
Urapidil (p.987·3).
Hypertension.

Mediator
Biopharma, Fr.; Servier, Port.
Benfluorex hydrochloride (p.844·2).
Adjunct in asymptomatic diabetes; hyperlipidaemias.

Mediaven
Will-Pharma, Belg.; Drossapharm, Switz.
Naftazone (p.739·2).
Diabetic retinopathy; venous insufficiency.

Mediaxal
Servier, Hong Kong; Servier, Ital.; Servier, Singapore; Servier, Switz.†.
Benfluorex hydrochloride (p.844·2).
Diabetes mellitus; hyperlipidaemias.

Medibronc *Monot, Fr.†.*
Carbocisteine (p.1086·3).
Respiratory-tract congestion.

Medica *Qualiphar, Belg.*
Chlorhexidine gluconate (p.1138·2); lignocaine [lidocaine] hydrochloride (p.1313·2).
Throat disorders.

Medicaid *Eastern Pharmaceuticals, UK.*
Cetrimide (p.1137·1).
Minor cuts and burns; nappy rash; skin irritation.

Medicaina *Cristalia, Braz.*
Lignocaine [lidocaine] (p.1313·2); prilocaine (p.1318·3).
Local anaesthesia.

Medical Pic *Artsana, Ital.*
Chlorhexidine gluconate (p.1138·2); parahydroxybenzoate phenoxyethanol.
Wound and burn disinfection.

Medicament Sinus *Prodemdis, Canad.*
Pseudoephedrine hydrochloride (p.1099·2); paracetamol (p.71·2).

Medicap *Xepa-Soul Pattinson, Hong Kong.*
Mefenamic acid (p.51·2).
Pain; soft-tissue injury.

Medicated Analgesic Cream *Prodemdis, Canad.*
Methyl salicylate (p.55·1); camphor (p.1589·3); menthol (p.1632·3); eucalyptus oil (p.1609·2).

Medicated Chest Rub *Hyde, Canad.*
Camphor (p.1589·3); eucalyptus oil (p.1609·2); menthol (p.1632·3).

Medicated Extract of Rosemary *Potter's, UK.*
Geranium oil (p.1615·1); rosemary oil (p.1659·3); methyl salicylate (p.55·1); bay oil (p.1583·3).
Scalp disorders.

Medichrom *Qualiphar, Belg.*
Merbromin (p.1150·1).
Disinfection of minor wounds.

Medicillin *Medinovum, Fin.*
Phenoxymethylpenicillin potassium (p.235·1).
Bacterial infections.

Medicinal Gargle *Weleda, UK.*
Rhatany (p.1657·3); myrrh (p.1639·2); clove oil (p.1597·1); eucalyptus oil (p.1609·2); geranium oil (p.1615·1); lavender oil (p.1627·2); peppermint oil (p.1243·2); sage oil (p.1660·2); aesculus; argentum nitricum; calcium fluoricum; magnesium sulfuricum.
Mouth and throat disorders.

Mediclear *Boots, UK.*
Benzoyl peroxide (p.1111·1).
Acne.

Medicoal *Concord, UK.*
Activated charcoal (p.1000·2).
Acute poisoning; drug overdosage.

Medicod *Propan, S.Afr.†.*
Paracetamol (p.71·2); codeine phosphate (p.25·2); caffeine (p.761·3).
Pain.

Medicone *Dickinson, USA.*
Yeast extract (p.1398·1); shark-liver oil.

Medicone Derma *Medicone, USA.*
Benzocaine (p.1306·2); zinc oxide (p.1128·2); hydroxyquinoline sulfate (p.1622·2); ichthammol (p.1115·2); menthol (p.1632·3).
Skin disorders.

Medicone Dressing *Medicone, USA†.*
Benzocaine (p.1306·2); zinc oxide (p.1128·2); hydroxyquinoline sulfate (p.1622·2); cod-liver oil (p.1357·2); menthol (p.1632·3).
Skin disorders.

Medicone Rectal *Medicone, USA.*
Ointment: Benzocaine (p.1306·2); hydroxyquinoline sulfate (p.1622·2); zinc oxide (p.1128·2); menthol (p.1632·3); castor oil (p.1592·1); peru balsam (p.1650·2).
Suppositories: Benzocaine (p.1306·2); hydroxyquinoline sulfate (p.1622·2); zinc oxide (p.1128·2); menthol (p.1632·3); peru balsam (p.1650·2).
Anorectal disorders.

Mediconet *Medicone, USA†.*
Hamamelis (p.1618·3).
Perianal cleansing.

Medicreme
Rosken, Hong Kong.
Chlorhexidine acetate (p.1138·2); cetrimide (p.1137·1); hexamidine isetionate (p.1146·2); lignocaine [lidocaine] (p.1313·2); allantoin (p.1110·1).
Burns; cuts and abrasions; skin irritation.

Warner-Lambert, NZ.
Chlorhexidine acetate (p.1138·2); cetrimide (p.1137·1); hexamidine isetionate (p.1146·2); lignocaine [lidocaine] (p.1313·2).
Burns; wounds.

Medicyclomine *Brunel, S.Afr.*
Dicyclomine [dicycloverine] hydrochloride (p.466·1).
Gastrointestinal spasm; urinary-tract spasm.

Medi-Dan *Mahdeen, Canad.*
Coal tar (p.1125·1); benzalkonium chloride (p.1133·2); salicylic acid (p.1122·3).

Medident *Medibrands, Israel.*
Chlorhexidine gluconate (p.1138·2).
Mouth disinfection.

Medifed *Medpro, S.Afr.*
Triprolidine hydrochloride (p.427·2); pseudoephedrine hydrochloride (p.1099·2); dextromethorphan hydrobromide (p.1087·3).
Coughs.

Medifen *Grisi, Mex.*
Ibuprofen (p.43·2).

Medifer *Medimport, Mex.*
Ferrous fumarate (p.1360·1).
Iron-deficiency anaemia.

Mediflex *Crown, S.Afr.*
Indometacin (p.44·3).
Musculoskeletal and joint disorders.

Mediflor Tisane Antirhumatismale No 2
Monot, Fr.†.
Birch (p.1585·2); ash; meadowsweet (p.1631·2); strawberry plant; parietaria; couch-grass (p.1599·3); asparagus; juniper (p.1625·2); bearberry (p.1583·3); black currant (p.1389·3); tilia (p.1673·2); frangula bark (p.1227·1).
Muscular pain; rheumatic pain.

Mediflor Tisane Calmante Troubles du Sommeil No 14 *Monot, Fr.†.*
Passion flower (p.1649·1); bitter orange (p.1644·2); crataegus (p.1600·2); melissa (p.1632·2); tilia (p.1673·2); valerian (p.1678·3).
Insomnia; nervous disorders.

Mediflor Tisane Circulation du Sang No 12
Monot, Fr.†.
Aesculus (p.1574·1); red vine; hyssop; valerian (p.1678·3); hamamelis (p.1618·3); cypress nut; mistletoe (p.1636·2); willow leaf (p.82·1); melissa (p.1632·2); crataegus (p.1600·2); frangula bark (p.1227·1).
Peripheral vascular disorders.

Mediflor Tisane Contre la Constipation Passagere No 7 *Monot, Fr.†.*
Senna (p.1248·2); ash; fennel (p.1610·1); liquorice (p.1231·2); rosemary.
Formerly known as Mediflor Tisane Laxative.
Constipation.

Mediflor Tisane Digestive No 3 *Monot, Fr.†.*
Aniseed (p.1580·2); mint (p.1666·3); angelica (p.1580·2); lavender (p.1627·2); orange leaf; rosemary; elecampane (p.1089·3); fennel (p.1610·1); coriander (p.1599·2); hyssop.
Digestive disorders.

Mediflor Tisane Hepatique No 5 *Monot, Fr.†.*
Boldo (p.1585·3); kinkeliba (p.1626·1); elecampane root (p.1089·3); rosemary; liquorice (p.1231·2); berberis; mercury herb; mallow leaves; senna leaves (p.1248·2).
Digestive disorders; liver disorders.

Mediflor Tisane No 4 Diuretique *Monot, Fr.*
Asparagus; fennel (p.1610·1); couch-grass (p.1599·3); bearberry (p.1583·3); ash; meadowsweet (p.1631·2); strawberry root; althaea leaf (p.1577·1); liquorice (p.1231·2).
Diuresis; renal calculi.

Mediflor Tisane Pectorale d'Alsace *Monot, Fr.*
Mallow; althaea flowers (p.1577·1); poppy (p.1099·2); coltsfoot flowers and leaves (p.1087·2); verbascum flowers and leaves; gnaphalium dioicum; althaea herb and root (p.1577·1); calendula (p.1589·2); wild thyme; ground ivy (p.1618·2); liquorice (p.1231·2); melissa (p.1632·2); meadowsweet (p.1631·2); couch-grass (p.1599·3).
Respiratory-tract disorders.

Medi-Flu *Parke, Davis, USA†.*
Chlorpheniramine [chlorphenamine] maleate (p.412·1); dextromethorphan hydrobromide (p.1087·3); paracetamol (p.71·2); pseudoephedrine hydrochloride (p.1099·2).
Coughs and cold symptoms.

Medifolin *Medinfar, Port.*
Calcium folinate (p.1363·1).
Drug-induced folic acid deficiency; folate deficiency; megaloblastic anaemia.

Medifon *Medinfar, Port.*
Tyrothricin (p.267·1); benzocaine (p.1306·2); dequalinium chloride (p.1143·1); vitamin C (p.1389·3); menthol (p.1632·3).
Mouth and throat disorders.

Medigel
Note. This name is used for preparations of different composition.
Medice, Ger.
Bamethan sulfate (p.843·1); ephedrine sulfate (p.1090·2); lauromacrogol 400 (p.1345·2).
Soft-tissue injury; venous insufficiency.

Medifood, Ital.
Nutritional supplement (p.1350·1).
Vomiting.

Propan, S.Afr.; Mer-National, S.Afr.
Dicyclomine [dicycloverine] hydrochloride (p.466·1); aluminium hydroxide gel (p.1210·3); magnesium ox-

ide (p.1233·2); simeticone (p.1249·2); sodium laurilsulfate (p.1496·3); methylcellulose (p.1502·2).
Formerly contained dicyclomine [dicycloverine] hydrochloride, aluminium hydroxide gel, magnesium oxide, and simeticone.
Gastrointestinal disorders.

Medigesic *US Pharmaceutical, USA.*
Butalbital (p.658·3); paracetamol (p.71·2); caffeine (p.761·3).
Tension headache.

Medihaler-Epi
3M, Austral.†; 3M, S.Afr.†; 3M, Switz.†; 3M, UK†.
Adrenaline [epinephrine] acid tartrate (p.829·2).
Anaphylaxis; bronchospasm.

Medihaler-Ergotamine *3M, UK†.*
Ergotamine tartrate (p.452·1).
Migraine.

Medihaler-Iso
Sanova, Aust.†; 3M, Belg.†; 3M, Neth.†; 3M, Port.†; 3M, S.Afr.†; 3M, UK†; 3M, USA.
Isoprenaline sulfate (p.914·3).
Bronchospasm.

Medijel
Key, Austral.; DDD, Hong Kong; DDD, Israel; DDD, Singapore; DDD, UK.
Lignocaine [lidocaine] hydrochloride (p.1313·2); aminoacridine hydrochloride (p.1130·2).
Mouth ulcers; sore gums.

Medikasma *Propan, S.Afr.†.*
Amobarbital (p.655·2); ephedrine hydrochloride (p.1090·1); aminophylline (p.760·1).
Asthma.

Medi-Keel A *Restan, S.Afr.*
Lozenges: Cetylpyridinium chloride (p.1138·1); benzocaine (p.1306·2).
Sore throat.
Throat spray: Phenol (p.1152·3).
Mouth and throat infections.

Mediker *SIT, Ital.*
Phenothrin (p.1436·2).
Pediculosis.

Medikol *Selena, Swed.*
Activated charcoal (p.1000·2).
Diarrhoea; poisoning.

Medi-Kord *Medirel, Switz.†.*
Adrenaline [epinephrine] hydrochloride (p.829·2); zinc phenolsulfonate octahydrate (p.1128·3).
Adjunct in dental procedures.

Medil *Crosara, Ital.†.*
Buflomedil hydrochloride (p.851·3).
Cerebral and peripheral vascular disorders.

Medilan *Westbrook, UK.*
Wool fat (p.1410·3).

Medilar *Fidia, Ital.*
Multivitamin and mineral preparation with gamolenic acid (p.1350·1).
Nutritional supplement.

Medilax *Mission Pharmacal, USA†.*
Phenolphthalein (p.1244·1).
Constipation.

Medilet *Medice, Ger.*
Lactulose (p.1230·1).
Constipation; hepatic encephalopathy; salmonella enteritis.

Medilium *Medifive, Thai.*
Flunarizine (p.418·2).
Cerebrovascular disorders; migraine.

Medilyn *Medpro, S.Afr.*
Diphenhydramine hydrochloride (p.416·1); ammonium chloride (p.1085·2); sodium citrate (p.1186·2).
Coughs.

Medimegen *Medical Supply, Thai.*
Brompheniramine maleate (p.410·2); phenylephrine hydrochloride (p.1097·1); phenylpropanolamine hydrochloride (p.1098·1).
Hypersensitivity reactions; nasal congestion.

Medinait *Procter & Gamble, Spain†.*
Dextromethorphan hydrobromide (p.1087·3); doxylamine succinate (p.417·1); ephedrine sulfate (p.1090·2); paracetamol (p.71·2).
Cold and influenza symptoms.

Medinat Esten *Bioglan, Austral.*
Vitamins; minerals (p.1350·1); equisetum (p.1606·3); eleutherococcus senticosis (p.1615·3); damiana (p.1602·1); cimicifuga (p.1595·2); angelica (p.1580·2).
Menopausal disorders.

Medinat PMT-Eze *Bioglan, Austral.*
Pyridoxine hydrochloride (p.1386·3); cyanocobalamin (p.1388·1); ferrous fumarate (p.1360·1); buchu (p.1587·2); bearberry (p.1583·3); parsley (p.1648·3); juniper oil (p.1625·2); evening primrose oil (p.1613·2).
Premenstrual syndrome.

Medinex *Whitehall, UK†.*
Diphenhydramine hydrochloride (p.416·1).
Insomnia.

Medinol *SSL, UK.*
Paracetamol (p.71·2).
Formerly known as Cupanol.
Fever; pain.

Mediocin *Medical Supply, Thai.*
Diiodohydroxyquinoline (p.590·2); furazolidone (p.592·1); phthalylsulfathiazole (p.235·3).
Diarrhoea; dysentery; food poisoning.

Mediolax *Medice, Ger.*
Bisacodyl (p.1212·2).
Constipation.

Medipain *Medi-Plex, USA†.*
Hydrocodone tartrate (p.42·2); paracetamol (p.71·2).

Medipam *Medinovum, Fin.*
Diazepam (p.674·3).
Anxiety disorders; insomnia; neuroses; pain; premedication; psychosomatic disorders; skeletal muscle spasm.

Medipax *Tecnifar, Port.*
Dipotassium clorazepate (p.670·3).
Anxiety.

Medipe *Sam-On, Israel.*
Chlorhexidine gluconate (p.1138·2).
Mouth disinfection.

Medipekt *Orion, Fin.*
Bromhexine hydrochloride (p.1085·3).
Respiratory-tract congestion.

Medipina *Medinfar, Port.†.*
Nifedipine (p.940·1).
Angina pectoris; hypertension.

Medipirol *Medimport, Mex.*
Metamizole magnesium (p.34·2).
Pain.

Mediplant *Roche, Aust.*
Ointment: Menthol (p.1632·3); camphor (p.1589·3); eucalyptus oil (p.1609·2).
Pastilles: Menthol (p.1632·3); eucalyptus oil (p.1609·2).
Respiratory-tract disorders.

Mediplant Inhalations *Roche, Aust.*
Menthol (p.1632·3); camphor (p.1589·3); eucalyptus oil (p.1609·2).
Respiratory-tract disorders.

Mediplant Krauter *Roche, Aust.*
Althaea (p.1577·1); thyme (p.1672·2); ammonium chloride (p.1085·2).
Respiratory-tract disorders.

Mediplast *Beiersdorf, USA.*
Salicylic acid (p.1122·3).
Hyperkeratosis.

Mediplex *US Pharmaceutical, USA.*
Multivitamin and mineral preparation (p.1350·1).

Mediplus *Angelini, Ital.*
Benzalkonium chloride (p.1133·2); benzydamine hydrochloride (p.20·1).
Disinfection of skin, wounds, and burns.

Medipo *Mediolanum, Ital.*
Simvastatin (p.969·2).
Coronary arteriosclerosis; hypercholesterolaemia; ischaemic heart disease.

Medipramine *Propan, S.Afr.†.*
Imipramine hydrochloride (p.291·1).
Depression; nocturnal enuresis.

Medi-Prep *SSL, UK.*
Cetrimide (p.1137·1).
Skin disinfection.

Medipulv
Rosken, Hong Kong; Warner-Lambert, NZ.
Chlorhexidine hydrochloride (p.1138·2); hexamidine isetionate (p.1146·2); allantoin (p.1110·1).
Burns; wounds.

Medi-Quik
Note. This name is used for preparations of different composition.
Mentholatum, Canad.†.
Aerosol: Benzalkonium chloride (p.1133·2); camphor (p.1589·3); lignocaine [lidocaine] (p.1313·2).
Mentholatum, Canad.; Mentholatum, USA.
Topical spray: Lignocaine [lidocaine] (p.1313·2); benzalkonium chloride (p.1133·2).
Skin disorders.

Medised *SSL, UK.*
Paracetamol (p.71·2); promethazine hydrochloride (p.423·2).
Fever; pain.

Medised Infant *SSL, UK.*
Diphenhydramine hydrochloride (p.416·1); paracetamol (p.71·2).
Cold symptoms.

Medisense *Abbott, Irl.*
Test for glucose and ketones in blood (p.1616·3).

Medisense G2 *Medisense, UK.*
Test for glucose in blood (p.1616·3).

Medismon *Medice, Ger.*
Erythromycin stinoprate (p.203·3).
Bacterial infections.

Medi-Sol *Mykal, UK.*
Adhesive remover.

Medisport Athlete's Foot *Medisport, UK.*
Clotrimazole (p.382·1).
Tinea pedis.

Medi-Swab *SSL, UK.*
Isopropyl alcohol (p.1149·2).
Pre-injection swab.

Medi-Swab H *SSL, UK.*
Isopropyl alcohol (p.1149·2); chlorhexidine acetate (p.1138·2).
Pre-injection swab.

Meditapp *Medifive, Thai.*
Brompheniramine maleate (p.410·2); phenylephrine hydrochloride (p.1097·1); phenylpropanolamine hydrochloride (p.1098·1).
Coughs; hypersensitivity reactions.

Meditapp Expectorant *Medifive, Thai.*
Guaifenesin (p.1092·2); brompheniramine maleate (p.410·2); phenylephrine hydrochloride (p.1097·1); phenylephrine hydrochloride (p.1098·1).
Coughs; hypersensitivity reactions.

Meditar *Yamanouchi, Ital.*
Coal tar (Stantar) (p.1125·1).
Seborrhoeic dermatitis of the scalp.

Medi-Test Combi 2 *BHR, UK.*
Test for glucose and protein in urine.

Medi-Test Combi 5 *Dutec, Austral.*
Test for glucose, blood, ascorbic acid, protein, and pH in urine.

Medi-Test Combi 7 *Dutec, Austral.*
Test for glucose, blood, ketones, ascorbic acid, nitrite, protein, and pH in urine.

Medi-Test Combi 9
Dutec, Austral.; BHR, UK.
Test for glucose, ascorbic acid, ketones, blood, protein, nitrite, pH, bilirubin, and urobilinogen in urine.

Medi-Test Combi 3A *Dutec, Austral.*
Test for glucose, protein, pH, and ascorbic acid in urine.

Medi-Test Combi 4A *Dutec, Austral.*
Test for nitrite, blood, protein, pH, and ascorbic acid in urine.

Medi-Test Combi 6A *Dutec, Austral.*
Test for blood, bilirubin, protein, ketones, ascorbic acid, glucose, and pH in urine.

Medi-Test Combi 5N *Dutec, Austral.*
Test for pH, glucose, blood, ascorbic acid, protein, and nitrite in urine.

Medi-Test Glucose
Dutec, Austral.; BHR, UK.
Test for glucose in urine (p.1616·3).

Medi-Test Glucose 2 *Dutec, Austral.*
Test for glucose and ascorbic acid in urine.

Medi-Test Glucose 3 *Dutec, Austral.*
Test for glucose, ketones, and ascorbic acid in urine.

Medi-Test Glycaemie C *BHR, UK.*
Test for glucose in blood (p.1616·3).

Medi-Test Keton *Dutec, Austral.*
Test for ketones in urine.

Medi-Test Nitrit *Dutec, Austral.*
Test for nitrite in urine.

Medi-Test Protein 2 *Dutec, Austral.*
Test for protein and pH in urine.

Medi-Test Urbi *Dutec, Austral.*
Test for urobilinogen and bilirubin in urine.

Medi-Tissue *SSL, UK.*
Alcohol (p.1130·3); benzalkonium chloride (p.1133·2).
Skin and instrument disinfection.

Meditonsin H *Medice, Ger.*
Homoeopathic preparation.

Medituss *Crown, S.Afr.*
Mepyramine maleate (p.421·1); ammonium chloride (p.1085·2); sodium citrate (p.1186·2); cetrimide (p.1137·1); menthol (p.1632·3); ephedrine hydrochloride (p.1090·1).
Respiratory-tract congestion.

Mediuresix *Medical Supply, Thai.*
Frusemide [furosemide] (p.893·1).
Ascites; oedema.

Mediveine *Elerte, Fr.*
Diosmin (p.1611·1).
Haemorrhoids; peripheral vascular disorders.

Medivitan N *Medice, Ger.*
Hydroxocobalamin (p.1388·1); sodium folate (p.1361·3); pyridoxine hydrochloride (p.1386·3).
Lignocaine [lidocaine] hydrochloride (p.1313·2) is included in this preparation to alleviate the pain of injection.
Alcoholism; anaemias; cachexia; peripheral neuropathies; vitamin deficiency.

Medivitan N Neuro *Medice, Ger.*
Thiamine hydrochloride (p.1385·1); pyridoxine hydrochloride (p.1386·3).
Neuralgia; neuritis; polyneuropathies.

Medi-Wipe *SSL, UK.*
Chlorhexidine gluconate (p.1138·2); alcohol (p.1130·3).
Hard surface disinfection.

Medixin *Pierrel, Ital.†.*
Co-trimoxazole (p.193·3).
Bacterial infections.

Medizinalbad *Synpharma, Aust.*
Camphor (p.1589·3); anise oil (p.1580·3); eucalyptus oil (p.1609·2); methyl salicylate (p.55·1); niaouli oil (p.1640·2); citronella oil (p.1596·3); peppermint oil (p.1243·3); rosemary oil (p.1659·3); thyme oil (p.1672·3).
Musculoskeletal and joint disorders.

Medizol
Note. This name is used for preparations of different composition.
Medinovum, Fin.
Miconazole nitrate (p.391·1).
Fungal skin infections.
Medimport, Mex.
Metronidazole (p.594·1).
Trichomoniasis.

Medizyme *Utopian, Thai.*
Serrapeptase (p.1662·1).
Inflammation; respiratory-tract congestion.

Med-Kafuzone *Medical Supply, Thai.*
Furazolidone (p.592·1); kaolin (p.1229·3); pectin (p.1502·3).
Bacterial gastro-enteritis; diarrhoea; dysentery.

Medkofen *Medifive, Thai.*
Ketotifen fumarate (p.767·2).
Asthma; hypersensitivity reactions.

Med-Mucolo *Medical Supply, Thai.*
Bromhexine hydrochloride (p.1085·3); sulfogaiacol (p.1101·1).
Respiratory-tract disorders associated with increased or viscous mucus.

Med-Myolax *Medical Supply, Thai.*
Orphenadrine citrate (p.812·1); paracetamol (p.71·2).
Musculoskeletal and joint pain; neuralgia.

Mednil *Pharmaland, Thai.*
Mefenamic acid (p.51·2).
Pain.

Medobeta *Medochemie, Singapore.*
Betamethasone (p.1063·1).
Skin disorders.

Medobiotin
Apotheke Roten Krebs, Aust.; Medopharm, Ger.
Biotin (p.1355·3).
Biotin deficiency; hair and nail disorders.

Medocalcum *Medochemie, Singapore.*
Chlordiazepoxide (p.659·2); clidinium bromide (p.465·1).
Gastrointestinal disorders; nocturnal enuresis; smooth muscle spasm.

Medocarnitin *Medosan, Ital.*
Carnitine (p.1356·1).
Carnitine deficiency.

Medocef *Medochemie, Singapore; Medochemie, Thai.*
Cefoperazone sodium (p.168·2).
Bacterial infections.

Medociprin *Medochemie, Thai.*
Ciprofloxacin (p.182·3).
Bacterial infections.

Medoclazide *Medochemie, Singapore.*
Gliclazide (p.322·2).
Diabetes mellitus.

Medocodene *Schwarz, UK.*
Paracetamol (p.71·2); codeine phosphate (p.25·2).
These ingredients can be described by the British Approved Name Co-codamol.
Fever; pain.

Medocriptine *Medochemie, Hong Kong.*
Bromocriptine mesilate (p.1164·3).
Acromegaly; benign breast disorders; hyperprolactinaemia; hypogonadism; infertility; lactation inhibition; menstrual disorders; parkinsonism.

Medocycline *Medochemie, Hong Kong.*
Tetracycline hydrochloride (p.258·3).
Bacterial infections.

Medodermone
Medochemie, Hong Kong; Medochemie, Singapore; Medochemie, Thai.
Clobetasol propionate (p.1065·2).
Skin disorders.

Medofulvin *Medochemie, Singapore.*
Griseofulvin (p.386·2).
Fungal infections.

Medolexin *Medochemie, Hong Kong.*
Cefalexin (p.161·3).
Bacterial infections.

Medolin
Medochemie, Singapore; Medochemie, Thai.
Salbutamol sulfate (p.770·3).
Obstructive airways disease.

Medomet *DDSA Pharmaceuticals, UK.*
Methyldopa (p.927·3).

Medomycin
Medochemie, Hong Kong; Medochemie, Singapore; Medochemie, Thai.
Doxycycline hyclate (p.200·1).
Bacterial infections.

Medopa
Note. This name is used for preparations of different composition.
Medinfar, Port.
Dopamine hydrochloride (p.881·3).
Shock.
Atlantic, Thai.
Methyldopa (p.927·3).
Hypertension.

Medopal *Fustery, Mex.*
Methyldopa (p.927·3).

Medopam *Schwulst, S.Afr.†.*
Oxazepam (p.697·1).
Alcohol withdrawal syndrome; anxiety.

Medopate *Atlantic, Thai.*
Methyldopa (p.927·3).
Hypertension.

Medophyll *Li-il, Ger.*
Thymol (p.1158·3).
Skin ulceration; superficial skin disorders; wounds.

Medopren *Malesci, Ital.*
Methyldopa (p.927·3).
Hypertension.

Medoric *Medifive, Thai.*
Allopurinol (p.397·2).
Gout; hyperuricaemia.

The symbol † denotes a preparation no longer actively marketed

Medostatin *Medochemie, Hong Kong.*
Lovastatin (p.922·3).
Atherosclerosis; hypercholesterolaemia.

Medotar *Medca, USA.*
Coal tar (p.1125·1); zinc oxide (p.1128·2).
Skin disorders.

Medotifen *Medical Supply, Thai.*
Ketotifen fumarate (p.767·2).
Asthma; hypersensitivity reactions.

Medovent *Medochemie, Thai.*
Ambroxol hydrochloride (p.1084·3).
Respiratory-tract disorders associated with increased or viscous mucus.

Medovir
Medochemie, Singapore; Medochemie, Thai.
Aciclovir (p.612·3).
Herpesvirus infections.

Medoxim *Medici, Ital.*
Cefuroxime sodium (p.178·2).
Bacterial infections.

Medoxin *Milano, Thai.*
Doxycycline hyclate (p.200·1).
Bacterial infections.

Medozem *Medochemie, Thai.*
Diltiazem hydrochloride (p.874·3).
Angina pectoris; hypertension.

Medozide *Malesci, Ital.*
Methyldopa (p.927·3); hydrochlorothiazide (p.907·3).
Hypertension.

Medozine *Medochemie, Thai.*
Cinnarizine (p.413·1).
Cerebrovascular disorders; migraine; peripheral vascular disorders.

Medphlem *Medpro, S.Afr.†*
Carbocisteine (p.1086·3).
Respiratory-tract disorders.

Med-Phylline *Medical Supply, Thai.*
Theophylline (p.777·2).
Obstructive airways disease.

Medpramol *Schwulst, S.Afr.†*
Paracetamol (p.71·2).
Fever; pain.

Medralone *Keene, USA.*
Methylprednisolone acetate (p.1076·1).
Corticosteroid.

Medramil *Farmigea, Ital.†*
Medrysone (p.1075·3); tetryzoline hydrochloride (p.1101·2); pheniramine maleate (p.422·3).
Eye disorders.

Medramine retard *Mepha, Switz.†*
Dimenhydrinate (p.415·2); pyridoxine hydrochloride (p.1386·3).
Nausea; vomiting.

Medramine-B₆ Rectocaps *Mepha, Switz.†*
Dimenhydrinate (p.415·2); pyridoxine hydrochloride (p.1386·3); caffeine (p.761·3).
Nausea; vomiting.

Medrate *Pharmacia Upjohn, Ger.*
Methylprednisolone (p.1076·1) or methylprednisolone sodium succinate (p.1076·1).
Corticosteroid.

Medricol *Alcon Cusi, Spain.*
Chloramphenicol (p.179·1); medroxyprogesterone acetate (p.1480·1).
Eye disorders.

Medrisocil *Oftalder, Port.*
Medrysone (p.1075·3).
Eye disorders.

Medrivas
Alcon, Port.†; Alcon Cusi, Spain.
Medroxyprogesterone acetate (p.1480·1); tetryzoline hydrochloride (p.1101·2).
Eye disorders.

Medrivas Antib *Alcon Cusi, Spain.*
Chloramphenicol succinate (p.181·1); medroxyprogesterone acetate (p.1480·1); tetryzoline hydrochloride (p.1101·2).
Infected eye disorders.

Medrivas Antibiotico *Alcon, Port.*
Chloramphenicol (p.179·1); medroxyprogesterone acetate (p.1480·1); tetryzoline hydrochloride (p.1101·2).
Eye disorders.

Medrol
Pharmacia Upjohn, Austral.; Pharmacia Upjohn, Belg.; Pharmacia Upjohn, Canad.; Pharmacia Upjohn, Denm.; Pharmacia Upjohn, Fin.; Pharmacia Upjohn, Fr.; Pharmacia Upjohn, Hong Kong; Pharmacia Upjohn, Israel; Pharmacia Upjohn, Ital.; Upjohn, Neth.†; Pharmacia Upjohn, Norw.; Pharmacia Upjohn, NZ; Pharmacia Upjohn, Port.; Pharmacia Upjohn, S.Afr.; Pharmacia Upjohn, Swed.; Pharmacia Upjohn, Switz.; Pharmacia Upjohn, USA.
Methylprednisolone (p.1076·1).
Corticosteroid.

Medrol Acne Lotion *Pharmacia Upjohn, Canad.*
Methylprednisolone acetate (p.1076·1); aluminium chlorohydrate complex (p.1110·2); sulfur (p.1123·3).
Acne; seborrhoeic dermatitis.

Medrol Lozione Antiacne *Pharmacia Upjohn, Ital.*
Methylprednisolone acetate (p.1076·1); aluminium chlorohydrate (p.1110·2); colloidal sulfur (p.1123·3).
Acne.

Medrol Veriderm *Pharmacia Upjohn, Canad.*
Methylprednisolone acetate (p.1076·1).
Formerly called Medrol Topical.
Skin disorders.

Medrone
Pharmacia Upjohn, Irl.; Pharmacia, UK.
Methylprednisolone (p.1076·1).
Corticosteroid.

MED-Rx *Iomed, USA.*
Blue tablets, pseudoephedrine hydrochloride (p.1099·2); guaifenesin (p.1092·2); white tablets, guaifenesin.
Upper respiratory-tract symptoms.

MED-Rx DM *Iopharm, USA.*
Blue tablets, pseudoephedrine hydrochloride (p.1099·2); guaifenesin (p.1092·2); green tablets, guaifenesin; dextromethorphan hydrobromide (p.1087·3).
Upper respiratory-tract symptoms.

Medsara *Asofarma, Mex.*
Cytarabine (p.530·1).
Malignant neoplasms.

Medsatrexate *Asofarma, Mex.*
Methotrexate (p.553·2).
Malignant neoplasms.

Medsavorina *Asofarma, Mex.*
Folinic acid (p.1363·1) or calcium folinate (p.1363·1).
Megaloblastic anaemia; reduction of methotrexate toxicity.

Med-Spastic *Medical Supply, Thai.*
Oxyphencyclimine hydrochloride (p.472·1).
Gastrointestinal disorders; genito-urinary disorders.

Med-Sultrim *Medical Supply, Thai.*
Co-trimoxazole (p.193·3).
Bacterial infections.

Med-Tricocide *Medical Supply, Thai.*
Metronidazole (p.594·1).
Trichomoniasis.

Med-Tussin *Medical Supply, Thai.*
Diphenhydramine hydrochloride (p.416·1); ammonium chloride (p.1085·2); sodium citrate (p.1186·2).
Coughs.

Medusit *Grunenthal, Port.*
Sodium fluoride (p.1375·3).
Osteoporosis.

Med-Xyzarax *Medical Supply, Thai.*
Hydroxyzine hydrochloride (p.419·1).
Allergic skin disorders; anxiety.

Medyn *Medice, Ger.*
Pyridoxine hydrochloride (p.1386·3); folic acid (p.1361·1); cyanocobalamin (p.1388·1).
Prevention of elevated homocysteine concentration.

ME-F *Nakorn, Thai.*
Metformin hydrochloride (p.332·3).
Diabetes mellitus.

Mefac *Rowex, Irl.*
Mefenamic acid (p.51·2).
Musculoskeletal and joint disorders; pain.

Mefacap
Malayan, Hong Kong; MPF, Singapore.
Mefenamic acid (p.51·2).
Menstrual disorders; musculoskeletal and joint disorders; pain.

Mefalgic *Rolab, S.Afr.*
Mefenamic acid (p.51·2).
Now known as Rolab-Mefenamic acid.
Dysmenorrhoea; fever; pain.

Mefazil *Mayo, Mex.*
Indometacin (p.44·3).

Mefenacide *Streuli, Switz.*
Mefenamic acid (p.51·2).
Influenza symptoms; pain.

Mefenan *Greater Pharma, Thai.*
Mefenamic acid (p.51·2).
Pain.

Mefenix
Ranbaxy, Singapore; Ranbaxy, Thai.
Mefenamic acid (p.51·2).
Pain.

Mefic
Parke, Davis, Austral.; Alphapharm, Hong Kong.
Mefenamic acid (p.51·2).
Menorrhagia; pain; primary dysmenorrhoea.

Mefiron *Chew, Thai.*
Metronidazole (p.594·1).
Trichomoniasis.

Meflam *Trinity, UK.*
Mefenamic acid (p.51·2).
Fever; inflammation; pain.

Mefliam *Cipla-Medpro, S.Afr.*
Mefloquine hydrochloride (p.438·2).
Malaria.

Meformed *Medifive, Thai.*
Metformin hydrochloride (p.332·3).
Diabetes mellitus.

Mefoxin
Merck Sharp & Dohme, Austral.; Merck Sharp & Dohme, Belg.; Merck Sharp & Dohme, Braz.; Merck Frosst, Canad.; Merck Sharp & Dohme, Fin.; Merck Sharp & Dohme-Chibret, Fr.; Merck Sharp & Dohme, Hong Kong; Merck Sharp & Dohme, Irl.; Merck Sharp & Dohme, Ital.; Merck Sharp & Dohme, Neth.; Merck Sharp & Dohme, NZ; Merck Sharp & Dohme, Port.; Merck Sharp & Dohme, S.Afr.; Merck Sharp & Dohme, UK; Merck, USA.
Cefoxitin sodium (p.171·2).
Lignocaine [lidocaine] hydrochloride (p.1313·2) may be included in the intramuscular injection to alleviate the pain of injection.
Bacterial infections.

Mefoxitin
Merck Sharp & Dohme, Aust.; Merck Sharp & Dohme, Ger.; Merck

Mefoxitin (continued)
Sharp & Dohme, Norw.; Merck Sharp & Dohme, Spain; Merck Sharp & Dohme, Swed.; Merck Sharp & Dohme, Switz.
Cefoxitin sodium (p.171·2).
Lignocaine [lidocaine] hydrochloride (p.1313·2) may be included in the intramuscular injection to alleviate the pain of injection.
Bacterial infections.

Mefpa *Pharmasant, Thai.*
Methyldopa (p.927·3).
Hypertension.

Mefren Incolore *Novartis Consumer, Belg.*
Chlorhexidine gluconate (p.1635·3).
Disinfection of minor wounds; disinfection of the skin.

Mefren Pastilles *Novartis Consumer, Belg.*
Chlorhexidine hydrochloride (p.1138·2).
Mouth and throat infections.

Mega 65 *Arkopharma, Fr.*
Fish oil (p.949·3).
Nutritional supplement.

Mega Acidophilus *Bullivants, Austral.*
Lactic-acid-producing organisms (p.1626·3).
Maintenance of normal gastrointestinal flora.

Mega B
Sisu, Canad.; Quest, Canad.; Quest, UK; Arco, USA.
Vitamin B substances (p.1350·1).
Vitamin B deficiency.

Mega B Extra Strength *Cenovis, Austral.*
Vitamin B substances; ascorbic acid (p.1350·1).
Vitamin B deficiency.

Mega B Slow Release *Vitaglow, Austral.*
Vitamin B substances; ascorbic acid (p.1350·1).
Dietary supplement; premenstrual syndrome.

Mega Balance *Pharmavite, Canad.*
Multivitamin and mineral preparation (p.1350·1).

Mega C *Vitaglow, Austral.†*
Calcium ascorbate (p.1389·3); ascorbic acid (p.1389·3).
Vitamin C deficiency.

Mega Capsule *Quest, Canad.*
Multivitamin and mineral preparation (p.1350·1).

Mega E *Cenovis, Austral.*
dl-Alpha tocoferil acetate (p.1394·1).
Vitamin E supplement.

Mega Men *General Nutrition, Canad.*
Multivitamin and mineral preparation (p.1350·1).

Mega Multi *Cenovis, Austral.*
Vitamin and mineral preparation (p.1350·1).

Mega Stress Vitamins *Vita Pharm, Canad.*
Multivitamin and mineral preparation (p.1350·1).

Mega Vim *Jamieson, Canad.*
Multivitamin and mineral preparation (p.1350·1).

Mega VM *Nature's Bounty, USA.*
Multivitamin and mineral preparation (p.1350·1).

Megabyl *Martin, Fr.†*
Diisopromine hydrochloride (p.1222·2); sorbitol (p.1377·2).
Constipation; dyspepsia.

Mega-Cal *Jamieson, Hong Kong.*
Calcium (p.1187·3).
Calcium deficiency; calcium supplement.

Mega-Cal with Vit D *Jamieson, Hong Kong.*
Calcium (p.1187·3); vitamin D (p.1391·1).
Calcium deficiency; callcium supplement.

Mega-Calcium
Novartis, Aust.; Novartis, Fin.
Calcium lactate gluconate (p.1188·3); calcium carbonate (p.1215·1).
Calcium deficiency.

Megace
Bristol-Myers Squibb, Aust.; Bristol-Myers Squibb, Austral.; Bristol-Myers Squibb, Belg.; Bristol, Canad.; Bristol-Myers Squibb, Denm.; Bristol-Myers Squibb, Fin.; Bristol-Myers Squibb, Fr.; Bristol-Myers Squibb, Hong Kong; Bristol-Myers Squibb, Irl.; Bristol-Myers Squibb, Israel; Bristol-Myers Squibb, Ital.; Bristol-Myers Squibb, Mex.; Bristol-Myers Squibb, Neth.; Bristol-Myers Squibb, Norw.; Bristol-Myers Squibb, NZ; Bristol-Myers Squibb, Singapore; Bristol-Myers Squibb, Swed.; Bristol-Myers Squibb, Thai.; Bristol-Myers Squibb, UK; Bristol-Myers Squibb Oncology, USA.
Megestrol acetate (p.1481·2).
AIDS-associated and cancer-associated cachexia; breast cancer; endometrial cancer.

Megacillin
Note. This name is used for preparations of different composition.
Grunenthal, Aust.
Phenoxymethylpenicillin potassium (p.235·1).
Bacterial infections.

Frosst, Canad.†
Benzathine benzylpenicillin (p.156·2) or benzylpenicillin potassium (p.157·1).
Bacterial infections.

Megacillin oral *Grunenthal, Ger.*
Phenoxymethylpenicillin potassium (p.235·1).

Megacilline *Grunenthal, Switz.*
Injection: Clemizole penicillin (p.188·1).
Syrup; tablets: Phenoxymethylpenicillin potassium (p.235·1).
Bacterial infections.

Megacina *Reprefar, Port.†*
Ofloxacin (p.232·3).
Bacterial infections.

Megacort *Uno, Mex.*
Dexamethasone sodium phosphate (p.1067·1).
Musculoskeletal and joint disorders.

Megadin *Medipharma, Hong Kong.*
Cimetidine (p.1216·3).
Dyspepsia; gastritis; gastro-oesophageal reflux; peptic ulcer.

Megadose *Arco, USA.*
Multivitamin and mineral preparation (p.1350·1).

Megadoxa *Restan, S.Afr.*
Vitamin B substances (p.1350·1).

Megaflox *Baldacci, Port.*
Ciprofloxacin hydrochloride (p.182·3).
Bacterial infections.

Megafol *Alphapharm, Austral.*
Folic acid (p.1361·1).
Folic acid deficiency; megaloblastic anaemia.

Megagrisevit *Pharmacia Upjohn, Ger.*
Clostebol acetate (p.1466·3).
Anabolic.; fractures; osteoporosis.

Megal Simple *Andromaco, Mex.*
Dextromethorphan hydrobromide (p.1087·3).
Coughs.

Megalac *Krewel, Ger.*
Almasilate (p.1210·1) or hydrotalcite (p.1228·1).
Gastrointestinal hyperacidity.

Megalat *Agis, Israel.*
Nifedipine (p.940·1).
Angina pectoris; hypertension; Raynaud's syndrome.

Megalax *Propan, S.Afr.*
Bisacodyl (p.1212·2).
Bowel evacuation; constipation.

Megalocin *Kyorin, Jpn.*
Fleroxacin (p.206·3).
Bacterial infections.

Megalotect
Biotest, Fin.; Intra Pharma, Irl.; Biotest, Israel; Boehringer Ingelheim, Port.; Mednostica, S.Afr.; Leo, Swed.; Biotest, Thai.
A cytomegalovirus immunoglobulin (p.1536·1).
Passive immunisation.

Megamag *Mayoly-Spindler, Fr.*
Magnesium aspartate (p.1190·3).
Magnesium deficiency.

Megamilbedoce *Andromaco, Spain.*
Hydroxocobalamin (p.1388·1).
Vitamin B12 deficiency.

Megamox *Aspen, S.Afr.*
Ampicillin (p.150·3); cloxacillin (p.192·1).
Bacterial infections.

Megamylase *Leurquin, Fr.*
Amylase (p.1579·3).
Mouth and throat disorders.

Meganest *Clarben, Spain.*
Articaine.
Adrenaline [epinephrine] (p.829·1) is included in this preparation as a vasoconstrictor to diminish absorption and localise the effect of the local anaesthetic.
Local anaesthesia in dentistry.

Megapen
Note. This name is used for preparations of different composition.
Euroforma, Braz.
Benzylpenicillin potassium (p.157·1).
Bacterial infections.

Aspen, S.Afr.
Amoxicillin (p.149·2); flucloxacillin (p.207·1).
Bacterial infections.

Megapenil *Lakeside, Mex.*
Tablets: Phenoxymethylpenicillin potassium (p.235·1).
Injection: Clemizole penicillin (p.188·1).
Bacterial infections.

Megapenil Forte *Lakeside, Mex.*
Clemizole penicillin (p.188·1); benzylpenicillin sodium (p.157·2).
Lignocaine [lidocaine] hydrochloride (p.1313·2) is included in this preparation to alleviate the pain of injection.
Bacterial infections.

Mega-Prim *Hua, Thai.*
Co-trimoxazole (p.193·3).
Bacterial infections.

Megapyn *Compu, S.Afr.*
Syrup: Paracetamol (p.71·2); codeine phosphate (p.25·2); promethazine hydrochloride (p.423·2).
Fever; pain.
Tablets: Paracetamol (p.71·2); codeine phosphate (p.25·2); caffeine (p.761·3); meprobamate (p.691·1).
Pain and associated tension.

Megareal *Novartis Nutrition, Fr.*
Preparation for enteral nutrition (p.1350·1).

Megasin *Pierre Fabre, Braz.*
Ofloxacin (p.232·3).
Bacterial infections.

Megasthenyl *Byk, Fr.†*
Ribonucleic acid (p.1657·3); manganese gluconate (p.1371·3).
Tonic.

Megaton *Hyrex, USA.*
Vitamin B substances with minerals (p.1350·1).

Megavis *Volchem, Ital.*
Levocarnitine (p.1356·1).
Asthenia.

Megavites *ICN, Canad.*
Vitamin B substances and vitamin C (p.1350·1).

Megavix *Irex, Fr.*
Tetrazepam (p.708·1).
Skeletal muscle spasm.

Megefren *Pras, Spain.*
Megestrol acetate (p.1481·2).
Breast cancer; endometrial cancer.

Megestat
Bristol-Myers Squibb, Braz.; Bristol-Myers Squibb, Ger.; Bristol-Myers Squibb, Switz.
Megestrol acetate (p.1481·2).
Breast cancer; endometrial cancer.

Megestil *Roche, Ital.*
Megestrol acetate (p.1481·2).
AIDS-associated and cancer-associated cachexia; breast cancer; endometrial cancer.

Megestin
Nettopharma, Denm.; Leiras, Fin.
Megestrol acetate (p.1481·2).
Breast cancer; menopausal disorders; menstrual disorders.

Megestran *Novaquimica, Braz.*
Norethisterone (p.1485·1); mestranol (p.1482·2); pyridoxine.
Combined oral contraceptive.

Meggezones
Schering-Plough, Canad.; Schering-Plough, UK.
Menthol (p.1632·3).
Catarrh; cold symptoms; coughs; nasal congestion; sore throats.

Meglucon
Hexal, Aust.; Hexal, Ger.
Metformin hydrochloride (p.332·3).
Diabetes mellitus.

Megostat
Bristol-Myers Squibb, Austral.; Bristol-Myers Squibb, NZ; Squibb, Spain.
Megestrol acetate (p.1481·2).
AIDS-associated cachexia; breast cancer; endometrial cancer.

Megral *Glaxo Wellcome, Canad.*
Ergotamine tartrate (p.452·1); cyclizine hydrochloride (p.414·1); caffeine hydrate (p.761·3).
Migraine and other vascular headaches.

Meiact *Meiji, Jpn.*
Cefditoren pivoxil (p.165·3).
Bacterial infections.

Meicelin *Meiji, Jpn.*
Cefminox sodium (p.167·3).
Bacterial infections.

Meiclox *Meiji, Thai.*
Cloxacillin sodium (p.192·1).
Bacterial infections.

Meilax *Meiji, Jpn.*
Ethyl loflazepate (p.683·1).
Anxiety; sleep disorders.

Meinfusona *Mein, Spain†.*
Electrolyte infusion with vitamin B substances (p.1180·1)(p.1350·1).
Electrolyte depletion; vitamin B deficiency.

Meinvenil Fisiologico *Fresenius Kabi, Spain.*
Sodium chloride (p.1196·1).
Fluid and electrolyte disorders.

Meinvenil Glucosalina *Fresenius Kabi, Spain.*
Glucose (p.1364·1); sodium chloride (p.1196·1).
Carbohydrate source; fluid and electrolyte disorders.

Meixil *Meiji, Thai.*
Amoxicillin trihydrate (p.149·2).
Bacterial infections.

Mejoral
SmithKline Beecham, Mex.; SmithKline Beecham, Spain.
Aspirin (p.14·2).
Fever; musculoskeletal and joint disorders; pain; peri-articular disorders; thromboembolism prophylaxis.

Mejoral Cafeina *SmithKline Beecham, Spain.*
Aspirin (p.14·2); caffeine (p.761·3).
Fever; pain.

Mejorultra *SmithKline Beecham, Mex.*
Ibuprofen (p.43·2).

Mel Jatahy *Legrand, Braz.*
Sulfogaiacol (p.1101·1); sodium benzoate (p.1134·3); senega (p.1100·2); tolu balsam (p.1101·3); honey (p.1366·2); hymenaea courbarie.
Respiratory-tract congestion.

Melabon
Provita, Aust.; Lacer, Spain.
Paracetamol (p.71·2); propyphenazone (p.80·2); caffeine (p.761·3) or caffeine citrate (p.761·3).
Fever; pain.

Melabon Infantil *Lacer, Spain.*
Paracetamol (p.71·2).
Fever; pain.

Melabon K *Oramon, Ger.*
Aspirin (p.14·2); paracetamol (p.71·2); caffeine (p.761·3).
Fever; pain.

Melabon N *Agpharm, Switz.†.*
Aspirin (p.14·2); paracetamol (p.71·2); caffeine (p.761·3).
Cold symptoms; pain.

Melabon plus C *Oramon, Ger.*
Aspirin (p.14·2); ascorbic acid.
Cold symptoms; fever; pain.

Melactone *Clonmel, Irl.†.*
Spironolactone (p.973·2).
Heart failure; hepatic cirrhosis; hypertension; idiopathic oedema; nephrotic syndrome.

Meladinina *Chinoin, Mex.*
Methoxsalen (p.1118·3).
Psoriasis; vitiligo.

Meladinine
Chiesi, Fr.; Galderma, Ger.; Galderma, Neth.; Galderma, Switz.; Promedica, Thai.
Methoxsalen (p.1118·3).
Alopecia; mycosis fungoides; psoriasis; vitiligo.

Melagesic PM *Ascher, USA.*
Paracetamol (p.71·2); melatonin (p.1632·1).
Pain; sleep disorders.

Melagriao *Catarinense, Braz.*
Nasturtium officinale; aconite (p.1572·3); mikania glomerata; ipecacuanha (p.1093·1); senega (p.1100·2); tolu balsam (p.1101·3); honey (p.1366·2).
Respiratory-tract congestion.

Melanex
Note. This name is used for preparations of different composition.
Boehringer Mannheim, S.Afr.†.
Raubasine (p.967·2).
Vascular disorders.

Paraphar, Singapore; Neutrogena, USA.
Hydroquinone (p.1115·1).
Hyperpigmentation.

Melanex Duo
Paraphar, Fr.; Sofex, Port.†.
Hydroquinone (p.1115·1); alpha hydroxy acids.
Skin hyperpigmentation.

Melanox *Surya, Singapore.*
Hydroquinone (p.1115·1).
Skin hyperpigmentation.

Melaprugna *Lampugnani, Ital.*
Dietary fibre supplement (p.1214·2).

Melapure *Genzyme, Hong Kong.*
Melatonin (p.1632·1).
Insomnia associated with melatonin deficiency; jet lag.

Melaxose *Boehringer Ingelheim, Fr.*
Lactulose (p.1230·1); liquid paraffin (p.1407·1).
Constipation.

Melbetese *Clonmel, Irl.†.*
Glibenclamide (p.321·3).
Diabetes mellitus.

Melbin *Sumitomo, Hong Kong.*
Metformin hydrochloride (p.332·3).
Diabetes mellitus.

Mel-C *Fresenius Kabi, Aust.*
Sodium ascorbate (p.1390·1).
Vitamin C deficiency.

Meldopa *Clonmel, Irl.*
Methyldopa (p.927·3).
Hypertension.

Meleril *Novartis, Spain.*
Thioridazine (p.708·1) or thioridazine hydrochloride (p.708·1).
Anxiety; behaviour disorders; mixed anxiety depressive states; psychoses; sleep disorders.

Melex *Sankyo, Jpn†.*
Mexazolam (p.692·3).
Anxiety disorders; psychosomatic disorders; sleep disorders.

Melfen *Clonmel, Irl.*
Ibuprofen (p.43·2).
Musculoskeletal, joint, and peri-articular disorders; pain.

Melfiat *Numark, USA.*
Phendimetrazine tartrate (p.1513·3).
Obesity.

Melgisorb *Molnlycke, Fr.*
Calcium alginate (p.728·1); carmellose (p.1499·3).
Exudative wounds.

Mel-H
Fresenius Kabi, Aust.; Hafslund Nycomed, Thai.
Multivitamin and amino-acid preparation (p.1350·1).

Melhoral
SmithKline Beecham, Braz.; Sterling, Port.
Aspirin (p.14·2); caffeine (p.761·3).
Fever; pain.

Melhoral Infantil
SmithKline Beecham, Braz.; Sterling, Port.
Aspirin (p.14·2).
Fever; pain.

Meli Rephastasan *Repha, Ger.*
Melilotus officinalis.
Haemorrhoids; thrombophlebitis; venous insufficiency.

Meliane
Schering, Aust.; Schering, Belg.; Schering, Fin.; Schering, Fr.; Schering, Israel; Schering, Neth.; Schering, Singapore; Schering, Spain; Schering, Thai.
Gestodene (p.1479·1); ethinylestradiol (p.1476·2).
Combined oral contraceptive.

Melic *Pharmasant, Thai.*
Methandienone (p.1482·2).
Osteoporosis.

Melipramine *Boucher & Muir, Austral.*
Imipramine hydrochloride (p.291·1).
Depression.

Meliseptol *Braun, Ger.*
Propyl alcohol (p.1155·3); glyoxal (p.1145·3).
Surface disinfection.

Melisol *Max Ritter, Switz.†.*
Soya oil (p.1378·1); liquid paraffin (p.1407·1).
Dry skin.

Melissa comp. *Weleda, UK.*
Angelica root (p.1580·2); cinnamon (p.1595·3); melissa leaf (p.1632·2); nutmeg (p.1643·1); lemon oil (p.1628·2); coriander (p.1599·2); clove (p.1596·3).
Diarrhoea; dyspepsia; nausea; stomach pain.

Melissa Specie Composta *Dynacren, Ital.*
Valerian (p.1678·3); melissa (p.1632·2); lupulus (p.1629·3); peppermint (p.1243·2).

Melissa Tonic *Geistlich, Switz.†.*
Melissa (p.1632·2); monarda; rosemary; red-poppy petal (p.1029·1); hibiscus; valerian (p.1678·3); passion flower (p.1649·1).
Agitation; nervousness; sleep disorders.

Melissengeist
Note. This name is used for preparations of different composition.
Pharmonta, Aust.
Nutmeg oil (p.1643·1); clove oil (p.1597·1); cinnamon oil (p.1596·1); citronella oil (p.1596·3).
Digestive disorders; nausea; sleep disorders.

Hofmann & Sommer, Ger.
Melissa (p.1632·2); sage (p.1660·2); rosemary; thyme (p.1672·2); angelica (p.1580·2); nutmeg (p.1643·1); cinnamon (p.1595·3); clove (p.1596·3); lemon oil (p.1628·2); menthol (p.1632·3); citronella oil (p.1596·3); clove oil (p.1597·1); cinnamon oil (p.1596·1).
Gastrointestinal disorders; headache; neuralgia.

Melissin *Surf Ski International, UK.*
Guaifenesin (p.1092·2); menthol (p.1632·3); glycerol (p.1616·3); melissa (p.1632·2); benzoic acid (p.1134·2); citric acid (p.1596·2).
Colds; coughs.

Melival *Hofmann & Sommer, Ger.*
Valerian (p.1678·3).
Agitation; sleep disorders.

Melix
Lagap, Hong Kong; Pharmador, S.Afr.†; Lagap, Switz.
Glibenclamide (p.321·3).
Diabetes mellitus.

Melizid *Leiras, Fin.*
Glipizide (p.322·3).
Diabetes mellitus.

Melizide
Alphapharm, Austral.; Alphapharm, Singapore; Merck, Singapore; Merck, Thai.
Glipizide (p.322·3).
Diabetes mellitus.

Mellaril
Novartis, Canad.; Novartis, USA.
Thioridazine (p.708·1) or thioridazine hydrochloride (p.708·1).
Depression with anxiety; hyperactivity in children; insomnia; psychoses; severe behavioural problems in children.

Mellerette *Novartis, Ital.*
Thioridazine (p.708·1) or thioridazine hydrochloride (p.708·1).
Anxiety; behaviour disorders.

Melleretten
Novartis, Aust.; Asta Medica, Ger.; Sandoz, Ger.†; Novartis, Neth.
Thioridazine (p.708·1) or thioridazine hydrochloride (p.708·1).
Anxiety disorders; behaviour disorders; depression; sleep disorders.

Mellerettes *Novartis, Switz.*
Thioridazine hydrochloride (p.708·1).
Agitation; anxiety disorders; depression; psychoses; sleep disorders.

Melleril
Novartis, Aust.; Novartis, Austral.; Novartis, Belg.; Novartis, Braz.; Novartis, Denm.; Novartis, Fin.; Novartis, Fr.; Asta Medica, Ger.; Novartis, Hong Kong; Novartis, Irl.; Novartis, Israel; Novartis, Ital.; Novartis, Mex.; Novartis, Neth.; Novartis, Norw.; Novartis, NZ; Novartis, Port.; Novartis, S.Afr.; Novartis, Switz.; Novartis, UK.
Thioridazine (p.708·1) or thioridazine hydrochloride (p.708·1).
Alcohol withdrawal syndrome; agitation; anxiety disorders; behaviour disorders in children; insomnia; mixed anxiety depressive states; pain; psychoses; senile confusion.

Mellin AR *Mellin, Ital.*
Infant feed (p.1350·1).
Gastro-oesophageal reflux.

Mellin HA *Mellin, Ital.*
Infant feed (p.1350·1).
Food intolerance.

Mellitron *Cilag, Mex.*
Metformin; chlorpropamide (p.321·1).
Diabetes mellitus.

Melneurin *Hexal, Ger.*
Melperone hydrochloride (p.690·3).
Alcoholism; psychiatric disorders; sleep disorders.

Melocin *Curasan, Ger.†.*
Mezlocillin sodium (p.224·1).
Bacterial infections.

Meloden
Schering, Denm.; Schering, Switz.
Gestodene (p.1479·1); ethinylestradiol (p.1476·2).
Combined oral contraceptive.

Melodene
Schering, NZ; Schering, S.Afr.
21 Tablets, gestodene (p.1479·1); ethinylestradiol (p.1476·2); 7 tablets, inert.
Combined oral contraceptive.

Melodia *Schering, Fr.*
24 Tablets, gestodene (p.1479·1); ethinylestradiol (p.1476·2); 4 tablets, inert.
Combined oral contraceptive.

Melodil *Unipharm, Israel.*
Maprotiline hydrochloride (p.297·2).
Depression; mixed anxiety depressive states.

Meloids *Boots, Thai.*
Liquorice (p.1231·2); menthol (p.1632·3); cinnamon (p.1595·3); capsicum (p.1591·1).
Throat disorders.

Meloka *Lacer, Spain.*
Benfotiamine (p.1384·3); caffeine (p.761·3); codeine phosphate (p.25·2); paracetamol (p.71·2); propyphenazone (p.80·2).
Fever; pain.

Melol *Pharmasant, Thai.*
Metoprolol tartrate (p.931·2).
Angina pectoris; hypertension; myocardial infarction.

Melopat *Medopharm, Ger.*
Betahistine mesilate (p.1584·3).
Ménière's syndrome; vestibular disorders.

Melox Plus *Rhone-Poulenc Rorer, Mex.*
Aluminium hydroxide (p.1210·3); magnesium hydroxide (p.1233·1); dimethicone (p.1249·2).
Gastrointestinal disorders.

Melpaque HP *Stratus, USA†.*
Hydroquinone (p.1115·1).

Melpax *Orion, Fin.*
Melperone hydrochloride (p.690·3).
Alcohol withdrawal syndrome; anxiety disorders; pain; psychoses.

Melpaz *Profarb, Braz.*
Dipyrone (p.34·1); papaverine hydrochloride (p.1648·1).
Smooth muscle spasm.

Melperomerck *Merck dura, Ger.*
Melperone hydrochloride (p.690·3).
Alcoholism; psychiatric disorders; sleep disorders.

Mel-Puren *Isis Puren, Ger.*
Melperone hydrochloride (p.690·3).
Alcoholism; psychiatric disorders; sleep disorders.

Melquin HP *Stratus, USA†.*
Hydroquinone (p.1115·1).

Melrose *Roberts & Sheppey, UK.*
Hydrous wool fat (p.1411·2); yellow soft paraffin (p.1407·3); hard paraffin (p.1407·1).
Emollient.

Melrosum *Rhone-Poulenc Rorer, Neth.*
Honey (p.1366·2).
Coughs.

Melrosum Codein Hustensirup *Rhone-Poulenc Rorer, Ger.*
Codeine phosphate (p.25·2).
Coughs and catarrh.

Melrosum Extra Sterk *Rhone-Poulenc Rorer, Neth.*
Codeine phosphate (p.25·2); vegetable extracts.
Coughs.

Melrosum Hustensirup Forte *Rhone-Poulenc Rorer, Ger.*
Thyme (p.1672·2).
Bronchitis; catarrh; cough.

Melrosum Hustensirup N *Rhone-Poulenc Rorer, Ger.*
Grindelia (p.1618·2); pimpinella; cowslip root (p.1600·1); rose petals (p.1029·1); thyme (p.1672·2).
Catarrh.

Melrosum Medizinalbad *Rhone-Poulenc Rorer, Ger.*
Thyme oil (p.1672·3); oleum pini sylvestris.
Bath additive; respiratory-tract disorders.

Melsept
Braun, Ger.; Braun, Ital.
Formaldehyde (p.1144·2); glutaral (p.1145·2); glyoxal (p.1145·3).
Surface disinfection.

Melsept SF
Braun, Ger.; Braun, Ital.
Glutaral (p.1145·2); glyoxal (p.1145·3); didecyldimethylammonium chloride (p.1143·2).
Surface disinfection.

Melsept Spray *Braun, Ital.†.*
Alcohol (p.1130·3); glyoxal (p.1145·3).
Disinfection of minor wounds and surfaces.

Melsitt *Braun, Ger.*
Formaldehyde (p.1144·2); glutaral (p.1145·2); didecyldimethylammonium chloride (p.1143·2).
Surface disinfection.

Meltus Baby *SSL, UK.*
Dilute acetic acid (p.1571·2).
Coughs.

Meltus Cough Control *Seton, UK†.*
Dextromethorphan (p.1087·3).
Dry coughs.

Meltus Dry Cough *SSL, UK.*
Dextromethorphan hydrobromide (p.1087·3); pseudoephedrine hydrochloride (p.1099·2).
Coughs.

Meltus Expectorant *SSL, UK.*
Guaifenesin (p.1092·2); cetylpyridinium chloride (p.1138·1).
Coughs.

Meltus Expectorant with Decongestant *SSL, UK.*
Guaifenesin (p.1092·2); pseudoephedrine hydrochloride (p.1099·2).
Coughs; nasal and sinus congestion.

Meltus Honey & Lemon *SSL, UK.*
Guaifenesin (p.1092·2); honey (p.1366·2); glycerol (p.1616·3); terpeneless lemon oil (p.1628·2).
Coughs.

Meltus Junior Night Time *SSL, UK.*
Diphenhydramine hydrochloride (p.416·1); sodium citrate (p.1186·2).
Cold symptoms; coughs.

Meltus Night Time *SSL, UK.*
Diphenhydramine hydrochloride (p.416·1); ammonium chloride (p.1085·2); sodium citrate (p.1186·2).
Cold symptoms; coughs.

Melvit *Beta, Ital.*
Multivitamin and mineral preparation (p.1350·1).

Melxi *Hebron, Braz.*
Pineapple; honey (p.1366·2).
Respiratory-tract congestion.

Melzine *Clonmel, Irl.*
Thioridazine hydrochloride (p.708·1).
Agitation; anxiety disorders; childhood behaviour disorders; psychoses; senile confusion; tension.

Memac *Bracco, Ital.*
Donepezil hydrochloride (p.1417·2).
Alzheimer's disease.

Memonol *Utopian, Thai.*
Pyritinol hydrochloride (p.1657·1).
Mental function disorders.

Memo-Puren *Isis Puren, Ger.*
Piracetam (p.1652·1).
Mental function disorders.

Memoq *Parke, Davis, Ger.*
Nicergoline (p.1640·2).
Mental function disorders.

Memorandum *Lampugnani, Ital.*
Ginkgo biloba (p.1615·2); guarana (p.1681·1); levocarnitine (p.1356·1).
Mental function disorders.

Memorex *Provita, Ital.*
Amino-acid preparation with vitamins and minerals (p.1350·1).
Mental function disorders.

Memorfix *Heralds, Braz.*
Vitamin B substances, amino acids, and minerals (p.1350·1).

Memoril *Recordati, Ital.*
Levoglutamide (p.1365·2).
Mental function impairment.

Memorino *Vita, Spain.*
Piracetam (p.1652·1); pyritinol hydrochloride (p.1657·1).
Cerebrovascular disorders; mental function impairment.

Memorioglutan *Bunker, Braz.*
Multivitamin, mineral, and amino-acid preparation (p.1350·1).

Memoriol B6 *Baldacci, Braz.*
Levoglutamide; calcium glutamate; ditetraethylammonium phosphate; pyridoxine hydrochloride (p.1350·1).
Nutritional supplement.

Memorisan *Lopes, Braz.*
Phosphoric acid; saw palmetto; turnera aphrodisiaca; calcium phosphate; selenium (p.1350·1).
Tonic.

Memory Plus *Life Essence, UK.*
Becopa.
Memory impairment.

Memoserina S *Rhone-Poulenc Rorer, Ital.*
DL-Phosphoserine; levoglutamide (p.1365·2); cyanocobalamin (p.1388·1); protein hydrolysate (p.1350·1).
Tonic.

Memosprint *Searle, Ital.*
Pyridoxine phosphoserinate (p.1387·1).
Mental function impairment; tonic.

Memovigor *Euro-Pharma, Ital.*
Multivitamin and mineral preparation with phospholipids, acetylcarnitine, myrtillus, and ginkgo biloba (p.1350·1).
Mental function disorders.

Memovisus *Carlo Erba OTC, Ital.*
Myrtillus (p.1639·2); cobamamide (p.1388·3); DL-phosphoserine; aceglutamide (p.1571·2).
Tonic.

Memovit B12 *Magis, Ital.*
Levoglutamide (p.1365·2); DL-phosphoserine; cyanocobalamin (p.1388·1).
Tonic.

Memphil *General Drugs, Thai.*
Piracetam (p.1652·1).
Cerebrovascular disorders; mental function disorders.

Men Hormone *TP, Thai.*
Methyltestosterone (p.1482·3); vitamin E (p.1393·3).
Hypogonadism.

Menabil Complex *Menarini, Spain.*
Cynara (p.1601·3); boldine (p.1585·3); cyclobutyrol (p.1601·2); methionine phenylbutyrate; rhubarb (p.1248·1); bile salts (p.1585·1); fenipentol sodium hemisuccinate (p.1610·1); belladonna (p.463·1); cascara (p.1216·1).
Constipation; hepatobiliary disorders.

Menaderm *Menarini, Ital.*
Beclometasone dipropionate (p.1061·2); neomycin sulfate (p.228·1).
Infected skin disorders.

Menaderm Clio *Menarini, Spain.*
Beclometasone dipropionate (p.1061·2); clioquinol (p.190·2).
Infected skin disorders.

Menaderm Neomicina *Menarini, Spain.*
Beclometasone dipropionate (p.1061·2); neomycin sulfate (p.228·1).
Infected skin disorders.

Menaderm Otologico *Menarini, Spain.*
Beclometasone dipropionate (p.1061·2); clioquinol (p.190·2).
External ear disorders.

Menaderm Simple *Menarini, Spain.*
Beclometasone dipropionate (p.1061·2).
Skin disorders.

Menaderm Simplex *Menarini, Ital.*
Beclometasone dipropionate (p.1061·2).
Skin disorders.

Menadol *Rugby, USA.*
Ibuprofen (p.43·2).

Menalation *McGloin, Austral.*
Menthol (p.1632·3); pumilio pine oil (p.1656·3).
Cold symptoms.

Menalcol *Men, Spain.*
Alcohol (p.1130·3); chlorhexidine gluconate (p.1138·2).
Skin and wound disinfection.

Menalgil B6 *Menarini, Spain.*
Cyanocobalamin (p.1388·1); di-isopropylammonium dichloroacetate (p.874·3); monophosphothiamine (p.1385·2); pyridoxine hydrochloride (p.1386·3). Lignocaine [lidocaine] (p.1313·2) is included in the injection to alleviate the pain of injection.
Vitamin B deficiency.

Menalgon *Fidia, Ital.*
Monophosphothiamine (p.1385·2); cyanocobalamin (p.1388·1).
Neuritis.

Menalgon B6 *Fidia, Ital.*
Monophosphothiamine (p.1385·2); pyridoxine hydrochloride (p.1386·3); cyanocobalamin (p.1388·1).
Nerve and muscle pain and inflammation.

Menalmina *Montplet, Spain.*
Chlorhexidine gluconate (p.1138·2).
Skin and wound disinfection.

Menamin *PP Lab, Thai.*
Prosultiamine (p.1385·1).
Beri-beri; thiamine deficiency.

Menaven *Menarini, Spain.*
Heparin sodium (p.902·1).
Peripheral vascular disorders.

Mencalisvit *Menarini, Spain.*
Calcium lactate (p.1188·2); colecalciferol (p.1391·1).
Vitamin D and calcium deficiency.

Mencevax AC *SmithKline Beecham, Israel; SmithKline Beecham, Norw.; SmithKline Beecham, Singapore; SmithKline Beecham, Spain.*
A meningococcal vaccine (groups A and C) (p.1550·1).
Active immunisation.

Mencevax ACWY *SmithKline Beecham, Aust.; SmithKline Beecham, Austral.; SmithKline Beecham, Belg.; SmithKline Beecham, Ger.; SmithKline Beecham, Ital.; SmithKline Beecham, NZ.*
A meningococcal vaccine (groups A, C, W₁₃₅, and Y) (p.1550·1).
Active immunisation.

Mendrome *Bristol-Myers Squibb, S.Afr.†.*
Fluphenazine hydrochloride (p.684·3); bendrofluazide [bendroflumethiazide] (p.844·1).
Premenstrual syndrome.

Meneparol *Menarini, Spain.*
Amino acids (p.1350·1); cyanocobalamin (p.1388·1); liver extract.
Liver disorders.

Menest *Monarch, USA.*
Esterified oestrogens (p.1473·1).
Breast cancer; female castration; female hypogonadism; menopausal vasomotor symptoms; primary ovarian failure; prostatic cancer; vulval and vaginal atrophy.

Menfazona *Menarini, Spain.*
Nefazodone hydrochloride (p.300·3).
Depression.

Mengivac (A+C) *Aventis, Irl.; Pasteur Merieux, UK.*
A meningococcal vaccine (groups A and C) (p.1550·1).
Active immunisation.

Meni-D *Seatrace, USA.*
Meclozine hydrochloride (p.420·3).
Motion sickness; vertigo.

Meningitec *Wyeth, Irl.; Wyeth, UK.*
A meningococcal C conjugate vaccine (diphtheria CRM₁₉₇ protein conjugate) (p.1550·1).
Active immunisation.

Meningo A+C *Pasteur Merieux, Braz.*
A meningococcal vaccine (groups A and C) (p.1550·1).
Active immunisation.

Meningococcal A+C *Pasteur Merieux, Hong Kong; Pasteur Merieux, Thai.*
A meningococcal vaccine (groups A and C) (p.1550·1).
Active immunisation.

Meningokokken-Impfstoff A + C *Merieux, Ger.*
A meningococcal vaccine (groups A and C) (p.1550·1).
Active immunisation.

Meningovax A+C *Pasteur Merieux, Belg.; Pasteur Merieux, Denm.; Meda, Fin.; Pasteur Merieux, Neth.; Pasteur Merieux, Norw.; Pasteur Merieux, Swed.*
A meningococcal vaccine (groups A and C) (p.1550·1).
Active immunisation.

Menisole *Atlantic, Thai.*
Metronidazole (p.594·1).
Anaerobic bacterial infections.

Menjugate *Aventis, Irl.; Chiron, Irl.; Chiron, UK.*
A meningococcal conjugate vaccine (group C) (p.1550·1).
Active immunisation.

Menobiol *Yves Ponroy, Fr.*
Multivitamin and mineral preparation with fatty acids (p.1350·1).
Menopausal disorders.

Menocal *Korea Green Pharm, Singapore.*
Salcatonin (p.749·3).
Bone pain due to osteolysis; hypercalcaemia; osteoporosis; Paget's disease of bone; pancreatitis.

Meno-cyl Ho-Len-Complex *Liebermann, Ger.*
Homoeopathic preparation.

Menodoron *Weleda, Aust.; Weleda, UK.*
Shepherd's purse (p.1662·3); majorana; achillea (p.1572·2); oak (p.1643·2); urtica (p.1678·2).
Menstrual disorders.

Menofem *Pharmaton, Switz.*
Cimicifuga (p.1595·2).
Menopausal disorders.

Menoflush *Pharmaceutical Enterprises, S.Afr.*
Ethinylestradiol (p.1476·2); multivitamins (p.1350·1).
Menopausal disorders.

Menoflush + ¼ *Pharmaceutical Enterprises, S.Afr.†.*
Ethinylestradiol (p.1476·2); multivitamins (p.1350·1); phenobarbital (p.355·1).
Formerly known as Menoflush-Menogloed + ¼.
Menopausal disorders.

Menogen *Breckenridge, USA†.*
Esterified oestrogens (p.1473·1); methyltestosterone (p.1482·3).
Menopausal disorders.

Menogon *Ferring, Belg.; Ferring, Denm.; Ferring, Fin.; Ferring, Fr.; Ferring, Ger.; Ferring, Hong Kong; Ferring, Irl.; Ferring, Israel; Ferring, Ital.; Ferring, Neth.; Ferring, Singapore; Ferring, Swed.; Ferring, UK.*
Menotrophin (p.1288·2).
Male and female infertility.

Meno-Implant *Organon, Belg.; Organon, Neth.*
Estradiol (p.1473·1).
Oestrogen deficiency.

Meno-MPA *Antigen, Israel.*
16 Tablets, estradiol (p.1473·1); 12 tablets, estradiol; medroxyprogesterone acetate (p.1480·1).
Menopausal disorders; osteoporosis.

Menomune *CSL, Austral.; Pasteur Merieux, Ital.; Connaught, NZ; CSL, NZ; Pasteur Merieux, Singapore; Pasteur Merieux, USA.*
A meningococcal vaccine (groups A, C, Y and W-135) (p.1550·1).
Active immunisation.

Meno-Net *Antigen, Israel.*
16 Tablets, estradiol (p.1473·1); 12 tablets, estradiol; norethisterone (p.1485·1).
Menopausal disorders; osteoporosis.

Menopace *Vitabiotics, Hong Kong; Vitabiotics, UK.*
Multivitamin and mineral preparation (p.1350·1).
Menopausal disorders.

Meno-Patch *Hexal, Israel.*
Estradiol (p.1473·1).
Menopausal disorders; osteoporosis.

Menopause *Homeocan, Canad.*
Homoeopathic preparation.

Menopause L122 *Homeocan, Canad.*
Homoeopathic preparation.

Menopause Test *Electramed, Irl.*
Test for raised FSH in urine.

Menopax *Ache, Braz.*
Cyclofenil (p.1467·2).
Anovulatory infertility.

Menophase *Searle, Irl.†; Searle, UK†.*
15 Tablets, mestranol (p.1482·1); 13 tablets, mestranol; norethisterone (p.1485·1).
Menopausal disorders; osteoporosis.

Menoplex *Fiske, USA†.*
Paracetamol (p.71·2); phenyltoloxamine citrate (p.423·1).
Pain.

Menoprem *Wyeth-Ayerst, Austral.*
Maroon tablets, conjugated oestrogens (Premarin) (p.1467·1); blue tablets, medroxyprogesterone acetate (Provera) (p.1480·1).
Menopausal disorders; osteoporosis.
Wyeth, NZ.
28 Tablets, conjugated oestrogens (p.1467·1); 14 tablets, medroxyprogesterone acetate (p.1480·1).
Menopausal disorders; osteoporosis.

Menopur *Ferring, UK.*
Menotrophin (p.1288·2).
Male and female infertility.

Menorest *Rhone-Poulenc Rorer, Aust.; Novartis, Austral.; Rhone-Poulenc Rorer, Denm.†; Novartis, Fin.; Rhone-Poulenc Rorer, Fr.; Novartis, Ger.; Rhone-Poulenc Rorer, Irl.; Rhone-Poulenc Rorer, Ital.; Novartis, Neth.; Novartis, Norw.; Novartis, Port.; Rhone-Poulenc Rorer, S.Afr.†; Rhone-Poulenc Rorer, Spain; Novartis, Swed.; Rhone-Poulenc Rorer, Switz.; Novartis, UK.*
Estradiol (p.1473·1).
Menopausal disorders; osteoporosis.

Menoring *Galen, UK.*
Estradiol acetate.
Menopausal disorders.

Menosan *Bioforce, Switz.*
Homoeopathic preparation.

Menosedan *Haller, Braz.*
Conjugated oestrogens (p.1467·1).
Menopausal disorders.

Menoselect *Dreluso, Ger.†.*
Homoeopathic preparation.

Menosor *TP, Thai.*
Mebeverine hydrochloride (p.1233·3).
Smooth muscle spasm.

Menostress *Dansk-Flama, Braz.*
Chlordiazepoxide (p.659·2); conjugated oestrogens (p.1467·1).
Menopausal disorders.

Menotensil *Sintofarma, Braz.*
Chlordiazepoxide (p.659·2); conjugated oestrogens (p.1467·1).
Menopausal disorders.

Menovis *Teofarma, Ital.*
Estradiol benzoate (p.1473·1); progesterone (p.1488·3).
Menstrual disorders.

Menoxicor *Guidotti, Spain.*
Cloridarol (p.863·3).
Ischaemic heart disease.

Menpovax 4 *Chiron, Ital.; Chiron, Thai.*
A meningococcal vaccine (groups A, C, W, and Y) (p.1550·1).
Active immunisation.

Menpovax A+C *Chiron, Ital.; Chiron, Thai.*
A meningococcal vaccine (groups A and C) (p.1550·1).
Active immunisation.

Menpros *Continental, Spain†.*
Misoprostol (p.1446·1).
Peptic ulcer.

Menrium *Roche Products, USA†.*
Chlordiazepoxide (p.659·2); esterified oestrogens (p.1473·1).
Menopausal symptoms.

Mensiso *Menarini, Ital.*
Sisomicin sulfate (p.247·3).
Bacterial infections.

Mensoma *Baldacci, Port.*
Famotidine (p.1225·3).
Gastric hypersecretion; peptic ulcer.

Mensoton *Berlin-Chemie, Ger.*
Ibuprofen (p.43·2).
Pain.

Menstruasan *Bioforce, Switz.*
Homoeopathic preparation.

Mentacur *Asche, Ger.*
Peppermint oil (p.1243·3).
Irritable bowel syndrome.

Mental Alertness *Homeocan, Canad.*
Homoeopathic preparation.

Mentalgina *Novartis, Mex.*
Cetylpyridinium chloride (p.1138·1); oxybuprocaine hydrochloride (p.1318·1).
Mouth and throat disorders.

Mentamida *Kin, Spain.*
Benzydamine hydrochloride (p.20·1); hexetidine (p.1146·3).
Mouth and throat inflammation.

Mentax *Agis, Israel; Kaken, Jpn; Bertek, USA.*
Butenafine hydrochloride (p.381·1).
Fungal skin infections.

Menthacin *Mentholatum, USA.*
Capsaicin (p.23·1); menthol (p.1632·3).
Arthritis.

Menthodex *Bell, UK.*
Ammonium chloride (p.1085·2); sodium citrate (p.1186·2); menthol (p.1632·3).
Coughs.

Mentholatum Balm *Mentholatum, Israel.*
Menthol (p.1632·3); camphor (p.1589·3); eucalyptus oil (p.1609·2); pumilio pine oil (p.1656·3); methyl salicylate (p.55·1).
Cold and hayfever symptoms.

Mentholatum Cherry Chest Rub *Mentholatum, USA.*
Camphor (p.1589·3); menthol (p.1632·3); eucalyptus oil (p.1609·2).
Coughs and cold symptoms.

Mentholatum Cherry Ice *Mentholatum, USA.*
SPF 11: Padimate O (p.1518·2); dimethicone (p.1410·1).
Dry lips; sunscreen.

Mentholatum Cough Drops *Mentholatum, Canad.*
Eucalyptus oil (p.1609·2); menthol (p.1632·3).

Mentholatum Extra Strength Ointment *Mentholatum, Canad.*
Camphor (p.1589·3); eucalyptus oil (p.1609·2); menthol (p.1632·3).

Mentholatum Ibuprofen *Mentholatum, UK.*
Ibuprofen (p.43·2).
Musculoskeletal, joint, and soft-tissue disorders.

Mentholatum Nasal Inhaler
Mentholatum, Israel; Mentholatum, UK.
Menthol (p.1632·3); camphor (p.1589·3); methyl salicylate (p.55·1).
Nasal congestion.

Mentholatum Natural Ice *Mentholatum, USA.*
SPF 14: Padimate O (p.1518·2); dimethicone (p.1410·1).
Dry lips; sunscreen.

Mentholatum Natural Ice Lip Protectant
Mentholatum, USA.
Menthol (p.1632·3); camphor (p.1589·3).
Dry lips.

Mentholatum Ointment
Note.This name is used for preparations of different composition.
Mentholatum, Canad.; Mentholatum, Singapore.
Camphor (p.1589·3); menthol (p.1632·3).
Cold symptoms; skin disorders.

Mentholatum, USA.
Camphor (p.1589·3); menthol (p.1632·3); eucalyptus oil (p.1609·2).
Coughs and cold symptoms.

Mentholatum Rub *Mentholatum, UK.*
Menthol (p.1632·3); camphor (p.1589·3); eucalyptus oil (p.1609·2); pumilio pine oil (p.1656·3); methyl salicylate (p.55·1).
Catarrh; cold symptoms; hay fever; minor skin disorders; musculoskeletal and joint disorders.

Mentholatum Softlips *Mentholatum, USA.*
Dimethicone (p.1410·1).
Dry lips.

Mentholatum Softlips Lipbalm *Mentholatum, USA.*
Dimethicone (p.1410·1); padimate O (p.1518·2).
Dry lips.

Mentholatum Softlips Lipbalm (UV) *Mentholatum, USA.*
Octinoxate (p.1517·3); padimate O (p.1518·2); oxybenzone (p.1518·1); dimethicone (p.1410·1).
Dry lips; sunscreen.

Mentholease *Warner-Lambert, UK.*
Menthol (p.1632·3); eucalyptus oil (p.1609·2).
Hay fever.

Mentholon Original N *Schoning-Berlin, Ger.†*
Menthol (p.1632·3); camphor (p.1589·3); eucalyptus oil (p.1609·2).
Catarrh.

Mentho-lyptus *Warner-Lambert Confectionery, UK.*
Menthol (p.1632·3); eucalyptus oil (p.1609·2).
Cold symptoms; sore throat.

Menthoneurin
Note.This name is used for preparations of different composition.
Byk, Aust.; Byk, Neth.
Liniment: Glycol salicylate (p.42·2); benzyl nicotinate (p.20·2).
Formerly contained glycol salicylate, benzyl nicotinate, and methyl nicotinate in *Neth.*
Musculoskeletal, joint, peri-articular, and soft-tissue disorders; neuralgia.

Byk, Aust.; Byk, Neth.
Cream; ointment: Glycol salicylate (p.42·2); menthol (p.1632·3).
Headache; musculoskeletal, joint, peri-articular, and soft-tissue disorders; neuralgia.

Menthoneurin-Salbe *Roland, Ger.; Byk Gulden, Ger.*
Glycol salicylate (p.42·2); menthol (p.1632·3).
Muscular and neuromuscular disorders; rheumatic disorders; soft-tissue disorders.

Menthoneurin-Vollbad N *Tosse, Ger.†*
Glycol salicylate (p.42·2); benzyl nicotinate (p.20·2); methyl nicotinate (p.55·1).
Bath additive; musculoskeletal and joint disorders.

MenthoRub *Schein, USA†.*
Menthol (p.1632·3); camphor (p.1589·3).
Muscle, joint, and soft-tissue pain; neuralgia.

Menthymin mono *Chauvin ankerpharm, Ger.*
Thyme (p.1672·3).
Bronchitis; catarrh.

Mentis *Menarini, Spain.*
Pirisudanol maleate (p.1652·3).
Cerebrovascular impairment; senility.

Mentium *Guidotti, Ital.*
Pirisudanol maleate (p.1652·3).
Mental function disorders.

Mentobox *Edigen, Spain.*
Ointment: Camphor (p.1589·3); Cedrus deodora oil; eucalyptol (p.1609·2); methyl salicylate (p.55·1); thymol (p.1158·3); turpentine; menthol (p.1632·3).

Tablets†: Camphor (p.1589·3); tolu balsam (p.1101·3); eucalyptol (p.1609·2); drosera (p.1606·1); thyme (p.1672·2); menthol (p.1632·3); sodium benzoate (p.1134·3).

Upper respiratory-tract disorders.

Mentobox Antitusivo *Alcala, Spain†.*
Dextromethorphan hydrobromide (p.1087·3); benzocaine (p.1306·2); guaifenesin (p.1092·2); menthol (p.1632·3).
Respiratory-tract disorders.

Mentocaina R *Azevedos, Port.*
Tyrothricin (p.267·1); benzocaine (p.1306·2).
Mouth and throat disorders.

Mentofenol *Distriforma, Port.*
Zinc chloride (p.1398·1); menthol (p.1632·3).
Mouth disorders.

Mentolatun *EMS, Braz.*
Menthol (p.1632·3); eucalyptol (p.1609·2); thymol (p.1158·3); terpineol (p.1669·3); chlorophyll (p.1028·1).
Mouth and throat disorders.

Mento-O-Cap *Rekah, Israel.*
Turpentine oil (p.1676·3); eucalyptus oil (p.1609·2); pine oil; capsicum (p.1591·1); methyl salicylate (p.55·1); menthol (p.1632·3); camphor (p.1589·3).
Cold symptoms; musculoskeletal and joint disorders.

Mentopin
Note.This name is used for preparations of different composition.
Brady, Aust.
Lavender flower (p.1627·2); sage (p.1660·2); peppermint leaf (p.1243·2); paprika (p.1591·1); urtica (p.1678·2); pine; camphor (p.1589·3); menthol (p.1632·3); pumilio pine oil (p.1656·3); peppermint oil (p.1243·3).
Musculoskeletal and joint disorders; neuralgia.

Hermes, Ger.
Acetylcysteine (p.1082·3).
Coughs; respiratory disorders associated with viscid or excessive mucus.

Mentopin Echinacea *Hermes, Ger.†*
Echinacea purpura (p.1606·2).
Respiratory- and urinary-tract infections.

Mentopin Erkaltungsbalsam *Hermes, Ger.†*
Eucalyptus oil (p.1609·2); pine needle oil.
Cold symptoms.

Mentopin Gurgellosung *Hermes, Ger.†*
Chlorhexidine gluconate (p.1138·2).
Inflammation and infection of the mouth and throat.

Mentopin Hustenstiller *Hermes, Ger.*
Clobutinol hydrochloride (p.1087·1).
Catarrh; coughs.

Mentopin Nasenspray *Hermes, Ger.*
Xylometazoline hydrochloride (p.1102·2).
Nasal congestion; sinusitis.

Mentopin Vitamin C + ASS *Hermes, Ger.†*
Aspirin (p.14·2); ascorbic acid (p.1389·3).
Fever; pain.

Mentor *Lifeplan, UK.*
Ginkgo biloba (p.1615·2).

Menutil *Hoechst Marion Roussel, Belg.†*
Diethylpropion hydrochloride (p.1508·3).
Obesity.

Menzol *Schwarz, UK†.*
Norethisterone (p.1485·1).
Menstrual disorders.

Menzotil *Pharmasant, Thai.*
Tenoxicam (p.87·2).
Musculoskeletal, joint, and peri-articular disorders.

Meocil *Oftalder, Port.*
Prednisolone acetate (p.1078·1); neomycin sulfate (p.228·1); sulfacetamide sodium (p.250·3).
Infected eye disorders.

282 Mep *Lioh, Canad.*
Aspirin (p.14·2); caffeine citrate (p.761·3); codeine phosphate (p.25·2); meprobamate (p.691·1).
Anxiety; pain; skeletal muscle spasm.

Mepagyl *Nakorn, Thai.*
Metronidazole (p.594·1).
Amoebiasis; anaerobic bacterial infections; trichomoniasis.

Mepalax *ABC, Ital.*
Boldo (p.1585·3); rhubarb (p.1248·1); cascara (p.1216·1).
Constipation.

Mepastat *Orion, Fin.*
Medroxyprogesterone acetate (p.1480·1).
Malignant neoplasms.

Mepergan *Wyeth-Ayerst, USA.*
Pethidine hydrochloride (p.75·1); promethazine hydrochloride (p.423·2).
Premedication.

Mephamesone *Mepha, Switz.*
Dexamethasone sodium phosphate (p.1067·1).
Corticosteroid.

Mephanol
Mepha, Hong Kong; Mepha, Switz.; Mepha, Thai.
Allopurinol (p.397·2).
Gout; hyperuricaemia; renal calculi.

Mephaquin
Lessel, Braz.; Mepha, Hong Kong; Mepha, Israel; Mepha, Port.; Mepha, Singapore; Mepha, Thai.
Mefloquine hydrochloride (p.438·2).
Malaria.

Mephaquine *Mepha, Switz.*
Mefloquine hydrochloride (p.438·2).
Malaria.

Mephathiol *Mepha, Switz.*
Carbocisteine (p.1086·3).
Respiratory-tract disorders associated with increased mucus.

Mephatussine *Mepha, Switz.*
Prenoxdiazine hydrochloride (p.1099·2).
Coughs.

Mephatussine Compositum *Mepha, Switz.*
Prenoxdiazine hydrochloride (p.1099·2); guaifenesin (p.1092·2); terpin hydrate (p.1101·2).
Coughs.

Mephaxine *Mepha, Switz.†*
Prenoxdiazine hydrochloride (p.1099·2) or prenoxdiazine hibenzate (p.1099·2).
Coughs.

Mephaxine Compositum *Mepha, Switz.†*
Prenoxdiazine hydrochloride (p.1099·2); guaifenesin (p.1092·2); terpin hydrate (p.1101·2).
Coughs.

Mephyton *Merck, USA.*
Phytomenadione (p.1396·1).
Coagulation disorders due to faulty formation of factors II, VII, IX, and X.

Mepicain *Monico, Ital.*
Mepivacaine hydrochloride (p.1317·1).
Adrenaline [epinephrine] acid tartrate (p.829·2) is included in some injections as a vasoconstrictor to diminish absorption and localise the effect of the local anaesthetic.
Local anaesthesia.

Mepicaton
Weimer, Ger.†; Weimer, Switz.†; Weimer, Thai.
Mepivacaine hydrochloride (p.1317·1).
Local anaesthesia.

Mepident *Warner-Lambert, Ital.*
Mepivacaine hydrochloride (p.1317·1).
Adrenaline [epinephrine] acid tartrate (p.829·2) is included in some injections as a vasoconstrictor to diminish absorption and localise the effect of the local anaesthetic.
Local anaesthesia in dentistry.

Mepiforan *Clarmed, Ital.*
Mepivacaine hydrochloride (p.1317·1).
Adrenaline [epinephrine] acid tartrate (p.829·2) is included in some injections as a vasoconstrictor to diminish absorption and localise the effect of the local anaesthetic.
Local anaesthesia.

Mepihexal *Hexal, Ger.*
Mepivacaine hydrochloride (p.1317·1).
Local anaesthesia.

Mepi-Mynol *Molteni, Ital.*
Mepivacaine hydrochloride (p.1317·1).
Adrenaline [epinephrine] acid tartrate (p.829·2) is included in some injections as a vasoconstrictor to diminish absorption and localise the effect of the local anaesthetic.
Local anaesthesia.

Mepivastesin *Espe, Ger.*
Mepivacaine hydrochloride (p.1317·1).
Local anaesthesia.

Mepral *Bracco, Ital.*
Omeprazole (p.1239·1) or omeprazole sodium (p.1239·1).
Gastro-oesophageal reflux; peptic ulcer; Zollinger-Ellison syndrome.

Mepranix *Ashbourne, UK†.*
Metoprolol tartrate (p.931·2).
Angina pectoris; arrhythmias; hypertension; myocardial infarction.

Meprate *DDSA Pharmaceuticals, UK.*
Meprobamate (p.691·1).

Mepraz *Baldacci, Port.*
Omeprazole (p.1239·1).
Gastro-oesophageal reflux; peptic ulcer; Zollinger-Ellison syndrome.

Mepril *Kwizda, Aust.*
Enalapril maleate (p.883·3).
Heart failure; hypertension.

Meprizina *Pisa, Mex.*
Ampicillin (p.150·3).
Bacterial infections.

Mepro *Rekah, Israel.*
Meprobamate (p.691·1).
Anxiety; insomnia.

Meprodil *Streuli, Switz.*
Meprobamate (p.691·1).
Anxiety; muscle relaxant; sedative.

Meprofen *AGIPS, Ital.*
Ketoprofen (p.47·3).
Musculoskeletal, joint, peri-articular, and soft-tissue disorders.

Meprogesic *Propan, S.Afr.*
Paracetamol (p.71·2); codeine phosphate (p.25·2); meprobamate (p.691·1).
Pain; tension-type headache.

Meprolol *TAD, Ger.*
Metoprolol tartrate (p.931·2).
Arrhythmias; hypertension; ischaemic heart disease; migraine; myocardial infarction.

Mepromol *Propan, S.Afr.*
Paracetamol (p.71·2); codeine phosphate (p.25·2); caffeine (p.761·3); meprobamate (p.691·1).
Pain and associated tension.

Mepron
Glaxo Wellcome, Canad.; Glaxo Wellcome, USA.
Atovaquone (p.588·3).
Pneumocystis carinii pneumonia.

Mepronet *Nettopharma, Denm.*
Metoprolol tartrate (p.931·2).
Angina pectoris; arrhythmias; hypertension; hyperthyroidism; migraine; myocardial infarction.

Mepronizine *Sanofi Winthrop, Fr.*
Meprobamate (p.691·1); aceprometazine maleate (p.654·1).
Insomnia.

Meprosona-F *Sons, Mex.*
Prednisone (p.1079·2).
Corticosteroid.

Meprospan *Wallace, USA†.*
Meprobamate (p.691·1).
Anxiety.

Meptid
Wyeth, Ger.; Shire, Irl.; Monmouth, UK.
Meptazinol (p.53·1) or meptazinol hydrochloride (p.52·2).
Pain.

Meptidol *Wyeth Lederle, Aust.*
Meptazinol hydrochloride (p.52·2).
Pain.

Meptin
Otsuka, Hong Kong; Otsuka, Jpn; Otsuka, Singapore; Otsuka, Thai.
Procaterol hydrochloride (p.770·1).
Obstructive airways disease.

Mepyl *Molteni, Ital.*
Mepivacaine hydrochloride (p.1317·1).
Adrenaline [epinephrine] acid tartrate (p.829·2) is included in this preparation as a vasoconstrictor to diminish absorption and localise the effect of the local anaesthetic.
Local anaesthesia.

Mepyrimal *Propan, S.Afr.*
Mepyramine maleate (p.421·1).
Hypersensitivity reactions.

Meracilina *Asta Medica, Braz.*
Phenoxymethylpenicillin (p.235·1).
Bacterial infections.

Meracote *Sigma, Austral.*
Alginic acid (p.1498·3); aluminium hydroxide (p.1210·3); magnesium trisilicate (p.1233·3); sodium bicarbonate (p.1186·2).
Gastric reflux; heartburn.

Meralop
Merck Sharp & Dohme, Ital.; Thea, Spain.
Keracyanin (p.1626·1).
Eye disorders.

Meralops *Thea, Fr.†*
Keracyanin (p.1626·1).
Visual impairment.

Meramide *Hua, Thai.*
Metoclopramide hydrochloride (p.1235·2).
Gastrointestinal motility disorders; nausea and vomiting.

Merankol Pastiglie *Bruno, Ital.*
Dicyclomine [dicycloverine] hydrochloride (p.466·1); methylcellulose; sodium laurilsulfate; magnesium hydroxide (p.1233·1); dried aluminium hydroxide (p.1210·3); magnesium trisilicate (p.1233·3).
Gastrointestinal disorders.

Merasyn *Adcock Ingram, S.Afr.*
Aluminium hydroxide gel (p.1210·3); magnesium hydroxide (p.1233·1); simeticone (p.1249·2); methylcellulose (p.1502·2).
Formerly contained aluminium hydroxide gel, magnesium hydroxide, and simeticone.
Flatulence; hyperchlorhydria.

Merbentyl
Hoechst Marion Roussel, Austral.; Hoechst Marion Roussel, Irl.; Pharmaco, NZ; Adcock Ingram, S.Afr.; Florizel, UK.
Dicyclomine [dicycloverine] hydrochloride (p.466·1).
Gastrointestinal spasm.

Mercalm *Warner-Lambert, Fr.*
Caffeine (p.761·3); dimenhydrinate (p.415·2).
Motion sickness.

Mercap *Medac, Ger.†*
Mercaptopurine (p.552·2).
Acute lymphatic leukaemia; non-Hodgkin's lymphoma.

Mercaptina *Zambon, Braz.*
Mercaptopurine (p.552·2).
Inflammatory bowel disease; leukaemias; non-Hodgkin's lymphomas; polycythaemia vera; psoriatic arthritis.

Mercaptizol *Taro, Israel.*
Methimazole [thiamazole] (p.1525·1).
Hyperthyroidism; toxic adenoma.

Mercaptyl *Knoll, Switz.*
Penicillamine (p.1017·1).
Biliary cirrhosis; cystinuria; heavy-metal poisoning; hepatitis; pulmonary fibrosis; rheumatoid arthritis; scleroderma.

Merced *Menarini, Belg.*
Midecamycin acetate (p.224·3).
Bacterial infections.

Mercilon
Organon, Aust.; Organon, Belg.; Akzo, Braz.; Organon, Denm.; Organon, Fin.; Organon, Fr.; Organon, Hong Kong; Organon, Irl.; Organon, Israel; Organon, Ital.; Organon, Mex.; Organon, Neth.; Pharmaco, NZ; Organon, Port.; Danmed, S.Afr.; Organon, Singapore; Organon, Swed.; Organon, Switz.; Organon, Thai.; Organon, UK.
Desogestrel (p.1470·3); ethinylestradiol (p.1476·2).
28-Day packs also contain 7 inert tablets.
Combined oral contraceptive.

Merck-Cough Linctus *Xixia, S.Afr.*
Triprolidine hydrochloride (p.427·2); pseudoephedrine hydrochloride (p.1099·2); codeine phosphate (p.25·2).
Coughs.

Merck-Expectorant *Xixia, S.Afr.*
Triprolidine hydrochloride (p.427·2); pseudoephedrine hydrochloride (p.1099·2); codeine phosphate (p.25·2); guaifenesin (p.1092·2).
Coughs.

Merck-Fed *Xixia, S.Afr.*
Triprolidine hydrochloride (p.427·2); pseudoephedrine hydrochloride (p.1099·2).
Cold and influenza symptoms.

Merck-Flu *Xixia, S.Afr.*
Paracetamol (p.71·2); vitamin C (p.1389·3); phenylephrine hydrochloride (p.1097·1); chlorpheniramine

---

[chlorphenamine] maleate (p.412·1); caffeine (p.761·3).
Cold and influenza symptoms.

Merck-Gesic *Xixia, S.Afr.*
Paracetamol (p.71·2).
Fever; pain.

Mercodol with Decapryn *Hoechst Marion Roussel, Canad.*
Hydrocodone tartrate (p.42·2); etafedrine hydrochloride (p.1091·2); sodium citrate (p.1186·2); doxylamine succinate (p.417·1).
Coughs.

Mercromina *Lainco, Spain.*
Merbromin (p.1150·1).
Wound disinfection.

Mercrotona *Orravan, Spain.*
Merbromin sodium (p.1150·1); alcohol (p.1130·3).
Wound disinfection.

Mercryl *Menarini, Fr.*
Chlorhexidine gluconate (p.1138·2); benzalkonium chloride (p.1133·2).
Formerly known as Mercryl Lauryle and contained mercurobutol.
Skin and mucous membrane disinfection.

Mercryl Lauryle *Sanofi Synthelabo, Spain.*
Mercurobutol (p.1150·2).
Skin and mucous membrane disinfection.

Mercuchrom *Krewel, Ger.*
Merbromin (p.1150·1).
Burns; skin disinfection; skin ulceration; wounds.

Mercural *Berman, Mex.*
Thiomersal (p.1158·2).

Mercurin *Monik, Spain.*
Merbromin sodium (p.1150·1).
Wound disinfection.

Mercurio Cromo *Laborsil, Braz.*
Merbromin (p.1150·1).
Skin disinfection.

Mercuro Cromo *Greenpharma, Braz.*
Merbromin (p.1150·1).
Skin disinfection.

Mercurobromo *Spyfarma, Spain.*
Merbromin (p.1150·1).
Wound disinfection.

Mercutina Brota *Escaned, Spain.*
Merbromin (p.1150·1).
Wound disinfection.

Mercuval *Biosyn, Ger.*
Unithiol (p.1025·3).
Lead poisoning; mercury poisoning.

Meredazol *Wayne, Mex.*
Metronidazole (p.594·1).

Mereprine
Note.This name is used for preparations of different composition.
Hoechst Marion Roussel, Belg.†; Marion Merrell, Fr.; Cassella-med, Ger.; Hoechst Marion Roussel, Switz.†.
Doxylamine succinate (p.417·1).
Allergic disorders; restlessness and excitement in children; sleep disorders.

Inibsa, Port.
Captopril (p.853·3).
Heart failure; hypertension.

Meresa
Sanova, Aust.; Dolorgiet, Ger.
Sulpiride (p.706·1).
Depression; gastrointestinal disorders; psychoses; vertigo.

Meretek UBT *Meretek, USA.*
Carbon-13 (p.1591·3) labelled urea (Pranactin).
Diagnosis of Helicobacter pylori infection.

Merex *Tentan, Switz.*
Phenylpropanolamine hydrochloride (p.1098·1).
Obesity.

Merfen *Novartis Consumer, Switz.*
Chlorhexidine gluconate (p.1138·2) or chlorhexidine hydrochloride (p.1138·2); benzoxonium chloride (p.1135·2).
Skin and wound disinfection.

Merfene *Novartis Sante, Fr.*
Chlorhexidine gluconate (p.1138·2).
Formerly contained phenylmercuric borate.
Wound disinfection.

Merfluan Sali Dentali *Colgate-Palmolive, Ital.*
Sodium fluoride (p.1375·3); minerals.
Dental caries prophylaxis.

Mericomb
Novartis, Aust.; Novartis, Fin.; Novartis, Ger.; Novartis, Switz.
16 Tablets, estradiol valerate (p.1473·2); 12 tablets, estradiol valerate; norethisterone (p.1485·1).
Menopausal disorders; osteoporosis.

Meridia *Abbott, USA.*
Sibutramine hydrochloride (p.1514·3).
Obesity.

Meridol
Note.This name is used for preparations of different composition.
GABA, Fr.; Teva, Israel; Inibsa, Port.
Olaflur (p.1374·1); stannous fluoride (p.1379·3).
Dental caries prophylaxis; plaque prophylaxis.

Marion Merrell, Spain†.
Aluminium aspirin (p.13·3); caffeine (p.761·3); chlorpheniramine [chlorphenamine] maleate (p.412·1); paracetamol (p.71·2).
Influenza and cold symptoms; nasal congestion.

Meridol-D *Pharmaceutical Enterprises, S.Afr.†.*
Paracetamol (p.71·2); codeine phosphate (p.25·2); diphenhydramine (p.416·1).
Fever; pain.

Meriestra *Novartis, Spain.*
Estradiol valerate (p.1473·2).
Menopausal disorders.

Merieux Inactivated Rabies Vaccine *Pasteur Merieux, UK.*
An inactivated rabies vaccine (Wistar PM/WI 38 1503-3M strain) (p.1560·2).
Active immunisation.

Merigest
Novartis, Aust.; Novartis, Fin.; Novartis, Ger.; Novartis, Spain; Novartis, Switz.
Estradiol valerate (p.1473·2); norethisterone (p.1485·1).
Menopausal disorders; osteoporosis.

Merigest Combi *Novartis, Spain.*
16 Tablets, estradiol valerate (p.1473·2); 12 tablets, estradiol valerate; norethisterone (p.1485·1).
Menopausal disorders.

Merimono
Novartis, Fin.; Novartis, Ger.
Estradiol valerate (p.1473·2).
Menopausal disorders.

Merional *IBSA, Switz.*
Menotrophin (p.1288·2).
Female infertility.

Merislon
Eisai, Hong Kong; Eisai, Jpn; Eisai, Singapore; Eisai, Thai.
Betahistine mesilate (p.1584·3).
Ménière's disease; vertigo.

Meristel *Aqualab, Fr.*
Sea-water.
Nasal and skin irrigation.

Meritene
Sandoz Nutrition, Canad.†; Novartis Consumer, Ital.; Novartis, Norw.; Novartis Consumer, Port.; Novartis, Swed.; Wander Health Care, Switz.†; Novartis Nutrition, USA.
A range of preparations for enteral nutrition (p.1350·1).

Merlit *Ebewe, Aust.*
Lorazepam (p.688·3).
Anxiety disorders; sleep disorders.

Mermid *Merck, Mex.*
Dipyrone (p.34·1).
Fever; pain.

Merocaine *Seton, Irl.; SSL, UK.*
Benzocaine (p.1306·2); cetylpyridinium chloride (p.1138·1).
Adjunct in dental procedures; mouth and throat disorders.

Merocet *Hoechst Marion Roussel, UK†.*
Cetylpyridinium chloride (p.1138·1); alcohol (p.1130·3).
Oral cleansing.

Merocets *Seton, Irl.; SSL, UK.*
Cetylpyridinium chloride (p.1138·1).
Sore throat.

Merocets Plus *SSL, UK.*
Cetylpyridinium chloride (p.1138·1); menthol (p.1632·3); eucalyptus oil (p.1609·2).
Formerly known as Merothol.
Nasal congestion; sore mouth and throat.

Meroken New *Taro, Israel.*
Macrogol 3350 (p.1630·3); electrolytes (p.1180·1).
Bowel evacuation.

Merol *Medecine Vegetale, Fr.*
Pentoxyverine citrate (p.1096·3).
Formerly contained eucalyptus, bitter-orange, sulfogaiacol, and codeine.
Coughs.

Meromycin *Ratiopharm, Aust.*
Erythromycin (p.201·2), erythromycin ethyl succinate (p.201·2), or erythromycin stearate (p.201·3).
Bacterial infections.

Meronem
Zeneca, Belg.; AstraZeneca, Denm.; AstraZeneca, Fin.; Zeneca, Ger.; Grunenthal, Ger.; Zeneca, Hong Kong; Zeneca, Irl.; Zeneca, Israel; Zeneca, Neth.; AstraZeneca, Norw.; Zeneca, Port.; Zeneca, S.Afr.; AstraZeneca, Singapore; Zeneca, Spain; Zeneca, Swed.; Zeneca, Switz.; AstraZeneca, Thai.; AstraZeneca, UK.
Meropenem (p.222·1).
Bacterial infections.

Meropen *Sumitomo, Jpn.*
Meropenem (p.222·1).
Bacterial infections.

Merrem
Zeneca, Austral.; AstraZeneca, Canad.; Zeneca, Ital.; Zeneca, Mex.; AstraZeneca, NZ; Zeneca, USA.
Meropenem (p.222·1).
Bacterial infections.

MerSol *Ratiopharm, Ger.*
Note. A similar name is used for preparations of different composition (see below).
Nicotinamide (p.1372·3); folic acid (p.1361·1).
Photosensitivity.

Mersol *Century, USA.*
Note. A similar name is used for preparations of different composition (see above).
Thiomersal (p.1158·2).
Skin disinfection.

Mersyndol
Hoechst Marion Roussel, Austral.; Aventis, NZ.
Paracetamol (p.71·2); codeine phosphate (p.25·2); doxylamine succinate (p.417·1).
Fever; pain.

Mersyndol with Codeine *Hoechst Marion Roussel, Canad.*
Paracetamol (p.71·2); codeine phosphate (p.25·2); doxylamine succinate (p.417·1).
Cold symptoms; pain.

Mersyndol Daystrength *Hoechst Marion Roussel, Austral.*
Paracetamol (p.71·2); codeine phosphate (p.25·2).
Fever; pain.

Merthiolate
Note.This name is used for preparations of different composition.
Lilly, Braz.; Lilly, Mex.
Benzalkonium chloride (p.1133·2).
Skin disinfection.

Aspen, S.Afr.; Lilly, Thai.
Thiomersal (p.1158·2).
Skin disinfection; wounds.

Meruvax
Pasteur Merieux, Denm.; Pasteur Merieux, Swed.
A rubella vaccine (Wistar RA 27/3 strain) (p.1562·3).
Active immunisation.

Meruvax II
CSL, Austral.; Prodome, Braz.; Merck Sharp & Dohme, Hong Kong; Pro Vaccine, Switz.; Merck, USA.
A rubella vaccine (Wistar RA 27/3 strain) (p.1562·3).
Active immunisation.

Merxil *Merck, Mex.*
Diclofenac sodium (p.30·3).
Inflammation; musculoskeletal, joint and peri-articular disorders; pain.

Merz Spezial *Medra, Aust.*
Multivitamin and mineral preparation (p.1350·1).

Merz Spezial Dragees N *Merz, Ger.*
Multivitamin preparation with iron and acetylmethionine (p.1350·1).

Mesacol
Sun, Singapore; Sun, Thai.
Mesalazine (p.1234·1).
Inflammatory bowel disease.

Mesaflor *Fonten, Ital.*
Mesalazine (p.1234·1).
Crohn's disease; ulcerative colitis.

Mesantoin *Novartis, USA.*
Mephenytoin (p.353·2).
Epilepsy.

Mesasal
SmithKline Beecham, Austral.; SmithKline Beecham, Canad.; Sanofi Winthrop, Denm.; Sanofi Winthrop, Norw.; Tika, Swed.
Mesalazine (p.1234·1).
Inflammatory bowel disease.

Mescolor *Horizon, USA.*
Chlorpheniramine [chlorphenamine] maleate (p.412·1); pseudoephedrine hydrochloride (p.1099·2); hyoscine methonitrate (p.468·2).
Upper respiratory-tract symptoms.

Mescorit *Roche, Ger.*
Metformin hydrochloride (p.332·3).
Diabetes mellitus.

Mesid *Janssen-Cilag, Ital.†.*
Nimesulide (p.62·3).
Fever; inflammation; pain.

Mesigyna
Schering, Braz.; Schering, Mex.
Norethisterone enantate (p.1485·1); estradiol valerate (p.1473·2).
Injectable contraceptive.

Mesiken *Kener, Mex.*
Bromocriptine (p.1166·2).

Mesin *Unison, Thai.*
Albendazole (p.95·2).
Worm infections.

Mesitol *Laborsil, Braz.*
Methionine (p.1012·2); choline (p.1356·3); betaine (p.1584·3).
Liver disorders.

M-Eslon *Rhone-Poulenc Rorer, Canad.*
Morphine sulfate (p.56·1).
Pain.

Mesmerin *Novaquimica, Braz.*
Lorazepam (p.688·3).
Alcohol withdrawal syndrome; anxiety; epilepsy; insomnia; nausea and vomiting; premedication.

Mesnex *Bristol-Myers Squibb Oncology, USA.*
Mesna (p.1011·3).
Prevention of ifosfamide-induced haemorrhagic cystitis.

Mesnil *Asofarma, Mex.*
Mesna (p.1011·3).
Prevention of urotoxicity due to antineoplastic therapy.

Mesocaine *Pharmy, Fr.*
Lignocaine [lidocaine] hydrochloride (p.1313·2).
Local anaesthesia.

Mesolex *Shiwa, Thai.*
Metronidazole (p.594·1).
Amoebiasis; giardiasis; trichomoniasis.

Mespafin *Merckle, Ger.*
Doxycycline hyclate (p.200·1).
Bacterial infections.

Mesporin *Mepha, Port.*
Ceftriaxone sodium (p.177·1).
Bacterial infections.

Mestacine *Wyeth Lederle, Fr.*
Minocycline hydrochloride (p.224·3).
Bacterial infections.

Mestinon
ICN, Aust.; Dermatech, Austral.; Sanico, Belg.; Roche, Braz.; ICN, Canad.; Medilink, Denm.; Medilink, Fin.; CSP, Fr.; ICN, Ger.; ICN, Hong Kong; ICN, Irl.; Roche, Israel; ICN, Ital.; Roche, Mex.; ICN, Neth.†; Medilink, Norw.; Pacific, NZ; ICN, Port.; Pharmaco, S.Afr.; ICN, Singapore; ICN, Spain; Medilink, Swed.; ICN, Switz.; ICN, Thai.; ICN, UK; ICN, USA.
Pyridostigmine bromide (p.1423·3).
Flatulence; ileus; myasthenia gravis; paroxysmal tachycardia; removal of intestinal gas; reversal of competitive neuromuscular blockade; urinary retention.

Mestoranum
Schering, Denm.; Schering, Norw.†; Schering, Swed.
Mesterolone (p.1482·1).
Breast cancer; hypogonadism; metrorrhagia.

Mestrel *Lemery, Mex.*
Megestrol acetate (p.1481·2).
Breast cancer; endometrial cancer.

Mesulid
Therabel, Belg.; Ergha, Irl.; Rafa, Israel; Novartis, Ital.; Lakeside, Mex.
Nimesulide (p.62·3) or nimesulide betadex (p.62·3).
Fever; inflammation; musculoskeletal, joint, peri-articular, and soft-tissue disorders; pain.

Met *Betapharm, Ger.*
Metformin hydrochloride (p.332·3).
Diabetes mellitus.

Meta Franan *Oftalmiso, Spain.*
Metampicillin sodium (p.222·3).
Bacterial infections.

metabiarex *Meta Fackler, Ger.*
Homoeopathic preparation.

Metabolic Mineral Mixture
Scientific Hospital Supplies, Austral.; Scientific Hospital Supplies, UK.
Mineral and trace element preparation (p.1350·1).
Mineral supplementation for enteral diets.

Metabolicum *Novag, Spain.*
Sodium cytidine monophosphate; cobamamide (p.1388·3); hydroxocobalamin (p.1388·1).
Megaloblastic anaemias; neuritis; tonic.

Metabyn *Byk Gulden, Mex.*
Ispaghula (p.1229·1).

Metacaf *Chong Kun Dang, Ital.*
Cefmetazole sodium (p.167·2).
Lignocaine [lidocaine] hydrochloride (p.1313·2) is included in the intramuscular injection to alleviate the pain of injection.
Bacterial infections.

Metacen *Chiesi, Ital.*
Indometacin (p.44·3).
Musculoskeletal and joint disorders.

Metacuprol *Lemoine, Fr.*
Copper sulfate (p.1358·1).
Skin and mucous membrane infections.

Metadate *Medeva, USA.*
Methylphenidate hydrochloride (p.1511·3).
Attention deficit disorder; narcoleptic syndrome.

Metadoxil
Baldacci, Ital.; Baldacci, Port.; Eurodrug, Thai.
Metadoxine (p.1387·1).
Liver disorders.

Metadyne *Pharmavite, Canad.*
Povidone-iodine (p.1155·1).

Metafar *Lafare, Ital.*
Cefmetazole sodium (p.167·2).
Lignocaine [lidocaine] hydrochloride (p.1313·2) is included in the intramuscular injection to alleviate the pain of injection.
Bacterial infections.

metaginkgo *Meta Fackler, Ger.*
Homoeopathic preparation.

Metagliz *Almiral, Spain.*
Metoclopramide glycyrrhizinate (p.1236·3).
Aid in gastrointestinal examination; gastro-oesophageal reflux; gastroparesis; nausea and vomiting.

Metagliz Bismutico *Prodes, Spain†.*
Bismuth subnitrate (p.1213·2); metoclopramide glycyrrhizinate (p.1236·3).
Gastritis; peptic ulcer; vomiting.

Metagyl *Ranbaxy, S.Afr.*
Metronidazole (p.594·1).
Anaerobic bacterial infections; protozoal infections.

Metahydrin *Hoechst Marion Roussel, USA.*
Trichlormethiazide (p.987·1).
Hypertension; oedema.

Meta-K *Reuffer, Mex.*
Cefalexin (p.161·3).
Bacterial infections.

metakaveron *Meta Fackler, Ger.*
Homoeopathic preparation.

Metakelfin *Pharmacia Upjohn, Ital.*
Sulfametopyrazine (p.256·1); pyrimethamine (p.442·3).
Malaria.

Metakes *Inexfa, Spain.*
Metampicillin sodium (p.222·3).
Bacterial infections.

Metalax Leiras, Fin.
Bisacodyl (p.1212·2).
Constipation.

Metalcaptase
Heyl, Ger.; Knoll, S.Afr.
Penicillamine (p.1017·1).
Cystine calculi; cystinuria; heavy-metal poisoning; hepatitis; rheumatoid arthritis; scleroderma; Wilson's disease.

Metalon Caps, S.Afr.
Metoclopramide hydrochloride (p.1235·2).
Gastrointestinal motility disorders; vomiting.

Metalpha Ashbourne, UK†.
Methyldopa (p.927·3).

Metalyse
Boehringer Ingelheim, Austral.; Boehringer Ingelheim, UK.
Tenecteplase (p.979·3).
Myocardial infarction.

metamagnesol Meta Fackler, Ger.
Magnesium aspartate (p.1190·3).
Magnesium deficiency.

Metamide Pacific, NZ.
Metoclopramide hydrochloride (p.1235·2).
Gastrointestinal disorders.

Metamidol Sanofi Synthelabo, Port.
Diazepam (p.674·3).
Anxiety; febrile convulsions; insomnia; skeletal muscle spasm.

Metamucil
Procter & Gamble, Aust.; Procter & Gamble, Austral.; Procter & Gamble, Belg.†; Procter & Gamble, Braz.; Procter & Gamble, Canad.; Wick, Ger.; Searle, Hong Kong; Searle, Israel; Procter & Gamble, Mex.; Searle, Neth.; Procter & Gamble, NZ; Monsanto, Port.†; Searle, S.Afr.; Searle, Singapore; Procter & Gamble, Spain; Procter & Gamble, Swed.†; Procter & Gamble, Switz.; Searle, Thai.; Procter & Gamble, USA.
Ispaghula (p.1229·1).
Constipation; diverticular disease; irritable bowel syndrome; stool softener.

Metandren Novartis, Canad.†.
Methyltestosterone (p.1482·3).
Androgen replacement therapy; breast cancer.

Metanium
Bengue, Irl.; Roche Consumer, UK.
Titanium dioxide (p.1126·1); titanium peroxide (p.1126·1); titanium salicylate (p.1126·1).
Napkin rash and related disorders.

Metanor Asta Medica, Port.
Flupirtine maleate (p.41·1).
Pain.

metaossylen Meta Fackler, Ger.
Homoeopathic preparation.

Metapirona Allen, Mex.
Dipyrone (p.34·1).
Fever; pain.

Metaplex
Takeda, Hong Kong; Takeda, Thai.
Vitamin B substances (p.1350·1).
Vitamin deficiency.

Metaplexan
Rhone-Poulenc Rorer, Aust.; Pierre Fabre, Ger.
Mequitazine (p.421·2).
Hypersensitivity disorders.

Metaprel Novartis, USA†.
Orciprenaline sulfate (p.769·1).
Asthma; reversible bronchospasm.

Metasal Salus, Ital.
Cefmetazole sodium (p.167·2).
Lignocaine [lidocaine] hydrochloride (p.1313·2) is included in the intramuscular injection to alleviate the pain of injection.
Bacterial infections.

Metasedin Esteve, Spain.
Methadone hydrochloride (p.53·1).
Opioid withdrawal; pain.

metasolidago S Meta Fackler, Ger.
Homoeopathic preparation.

Metasolvens Hogapharm, Switz.†.
Bromhexine hydrochloride (p.1085·3).
Respiratory-tract disorders associated with increased mucus.

Metaspirine SmithKline Beecham Sante, Fr.
Aspirin (p.14·2); caffeine (p.761·3).
Fever; pain.

Metastron
Nycomed, Austral.; Amersham, Canad.†; Nycomed, Fr.; Amersham, Ital.; Amersham, Spain; Nycomed Amersham, UK; Medi-Physics, USA; Amersham, USA.
Strontium-89 chloride (p.1451·1).
Metastatic bone pain.

Metatensin Hoechst Marion Roussel, USA.
Trichlormethiazide (p.987·1); reserpine (p.967·3).
Hypertension.

Metatone
Warner-Lambert, Irl.; Warner-Lambert, UK.
Calcium glycerophosphate; manganese glycerophosphate; potassium glycerophosphate; sodium glycerophosphate; thiamine hydrochloride (p.1350·1).
Tonic.

metavirulent Meta Fackler, Ger.
Homoeopathic preparation.

Metax Sons, Mex.; Solfran, Mex.
Dexamethasone (p.1067·1).
Corticosteroid.

Metaxol Propan, S.Afr.; Covan, S.Afr.
Theophylline (p.777·2); codeine phosphate (p.25·2); mepyramine maleate (p.421·1).
Coughs.

Metazem
Bioglan, Hong Kong; Bioglan, Irl.; Clonmel, Irl.; Bioglan, Singapore; Bioglan, Thai.; Bioglan, UK.
Diltiazem hydrochloride (p.874·3).
Angina pectoris.

Metazin Clintex, Port.
Etodolac (p.35·2).
Gout; musculoskeletal and joint disorders; pain.

Metazinc 20th Century, Mex.
Zinc sulfate (p.1398·2).

Metazol
Note. This name is used for preparations of different composition.
CT, Ital.
Cefmetazole sodium (p.167·2).
Lignocaine [lidocaine] hydrochloride (p.1313·2) is included in the intramuscular injection to alleviate the pain of injection.
Bacterial infections.
Alliance, S.Afr.
Metronidazole (p.594·1).
Anaerobic bacterial infections; protozoal infections.

Metbay Bayer, Ital.
Metformin hydrochloride (p.332·3).
Diabetes mellitus.

Metblock Pharmacia Upjohn, Fin.
Metoprolol tartrate (p.931·2).
Angina pectoris; arrhythmias; hypertension; hyperthyroidism; migraine; myocardial infarction.

Metcon Docmed, S.Afr.†.
Metoclopramide hydrochloride (p.1235·2).
Gastrointestinal disorders; nausea and vomiting.

Meted
Medicis, Canad.; Dermapharm, Irl.; Dermapharm, UK; GenDerm, USA.
Salicylic acid (p.1122·3); sulfur (p.1123·3).
Scalp disorders.

Metenix 5 Borg, UK.
Metolazone (p.930·3).
Ascites; hypertension; oedema.

Meteophyt forte OTW, Ger.
Pancreatin (p.1646·1).
Pancreatic disorders.

Meteophyt N OTW, Ger.
Turmeric (p.1029·3).
Dyspepsia.

Meteophyt S OTW, Ger.
Chamomile (p.1593·2); peppermint leaf (p.1243·2); dried bitter-orange peel (p.1644·2); caraway (p.1591·2).
Dyspepsia; loss of appetite.

Meteoril Salvat, Spain.
Simeticone (p.1249·2); magnesium trisilicate (p.1233·3); aluminium glycinate (p.1210·3).
Formerly contained simeticone, magnesium trisilicate, aluminium glycinate, and metoclopramide hydrochloride.
Flatulence; gastrointestinal hyperacidity.

Meteosan Novartis Consumer, Ger.
Dimethicone (p.1249·2).
Gastrointestinal disorders associated with excess gas.

Meteospasmyl
Mayoly-Spindler, Fr.; Mayoly-Spindler, Hong Kong; Mayoly-Spindler, Singapore.
Alverine citrate (p.1211·3); simeticone (p.1249·2).
Formerly contained alverine citrate and methionine in Fr.
Dyspepsia; flatulence; irritable bowel syndrome.

Meteoxane Solvay, Fr.
Simeticone (p.1249·2); phloroglucinol (p.1650·3).
Formerly contained atropine, hyoscyamine, amobarbital, and dimethicone.
Gastrointestinal disorders.

Meteozym Novartis Consumer, Ger.
Pancreatin (p.1646·1); simeticone (p.1249·2).
Digestive-system disorders.

Meterfolic Durbin, UK.
Ferrous fumarate (p.1360·1); folic acid (p.1361·1).
Iron and folic acid deficiency in pregnancy; neural tube defect prophylaxis.

Metex Medac, Ger.
Methotrexate sodium (p.553·2).
Arthritis; psoriasis.

Metfirex Irex, Fr.
Metformin hydrochloride (p.332·3).
Diabetes mellitus.

Metfogamma Worwag, Ger.
Metformin hydrochloride (p.332·3).
Diabetes mellitus.

Metfor-500 Masa, Thai.
Metformin hydrochloride (p.332·3).
Diabetes mellitus.

Metforal Guidotti, Ital.
Metformin hydrochloride (p.332·3).
Diabetes mellitus.

Metforem Orion, Fin.
Metformin hydrochloride (p.332·3).
Diabetes mellitus.

Metfron Asian Pharm, Thai.
Metformin hydrochloride (p.332·3).
Diabetes mellitus.

Methabid Pharmador, S.Afr.†.
Indometacin (p.44·3).
Fever; musculoskeletal and joint disorders.

Methacin
Note. This name is used for preparations of different composition.
Mentholatum, Canad.
Menthol (p.1632·3); capsaicin (p.23·1).
Hovid, Singapore.
Indometacin (p.44·3).
Gout; musculoskeletal and soft-tissue pain.

Methaddict Addicare, Ger.
Methadone hydrochloride (p.53·1).
Opioid withdrawal.

Methadose
Rosemont, UK; Mallinckrodt, USA.
Methadone hydrochloride (p.53·1).
Opioid withdrawal; pain.

Methagual Gordon, USA.
Methyl salicylate (p.55·1); guaiacol (p.1092·1).
Muscle, joint, and soft-tissue pain; neuralgia.

Methalgen Alra, USA.
Methyl salicylate (p.55·1); menthol (p.1632·3); camphor (p.1589·3); mustard oil (p.1639·1).
Musculoskeletal and joint pain.

Methamax Garec, S.Afr.†.
Indometacin (p.44·3).
Gout; musculoskeletal and joint disorders.

Metharmon-F Zoki, Thai.
Pregnenolone; androstenedione (p.1465·2); androstenediol; testosterone (p.1492·1); estrone (p.1476·1); thyroid (p.1526·2).
Menopausal disorders; ovarian disorders.

Methatropic Goldline, USA.
Vitamin B substances with methionine (p.1350·1).

Methergin
Novartis, Aust.; Novartis, Belg.; Novartis, Braz.; Novartis, Denm.; Novartis, Fin.; Novartis, Fr.; Novartis, Hong Kong; Novartis, Israel; Novartis, Ital.; Novartis, Mex.; Novartis, Neth.; Novartis, Norw.†; Novartis, Port.; Novartis, Spain; Novartis, Swed.; Novartis, Switz.
Methylergometrine maleate (p.1635·1).
Menorrhagia; postpartum haemorrhage; postpartum uterine atony or subinvolution.

Methergine Novartis, USA.
Methylergometrine maleate (p.1635·1).
Postpartum atony; postpartum haemorrhage.

Methex Generics, UK.
Methadone hydrochloride (p.53·1).
Formerly known as Methodex.
Opioid withdrawal.

Methitoral Fuji, Jpn†.
Neticonazole hydrochloride (p.392·2).
Fungal infections.

Methnine Medical Research, Austral.
Methionine (p.1012·2).
Liver disorders; paracetamol overdosage.

Methoblastin
Pharmacia Upjohn, Austral.; Pharmacia Upjohn, Mex.; Pharmacia Upjohn, NZ; Pharmacia Upjohn, S.Afr.
Methotrexate (p.553·2) or methotrexate sodium (p.553·2).
Malignant neoplasms; psoriasis; rheumatoid arthritis.

Methoblastine Pharmacia Upjohn, Belg.
Methotrexate (p.553·2).
Malignant neoplasms.

Methocaps Caps, S.Afr.
Indometacin (p.44·3).
Gout; musculoskeletal and joint disorders.

Methocel
Ciba Vision, Canad.; Ciba Vision, Hong Kong; Ciba Vision, Ital.; Restan, S.Afr.; Ciba Vision, Singapore.
Hypromellose (p.1501·3) (p.1129·2).
Aid in eye examination; lubricating drops for use with contact lenses.

Methocel Dispersa Ciba Vision, Ger.†.
Hypromellose (p.1501·3) (p.1129·2).
Comfort solution for hard contact lenses.

Methopt
Sigma, Austral.; Sigma, NZ.
Hypromellose (p.1501·3).
Dry eyes.

Methorcon YF Chem, Thai.
Chlorpheniramine [chlorphenamine] maleate (p.412·1); dextromethorphan hydrobromide (p.1087·3); dl-methylephedrine hydrochloride (p.1094·3).
Coughs.

Methoxacet Technilab, Canad.
Methocarbamol (p.1329·3); paracetamol (p.71·2).

Methoxacet-C Technilab, Canad.
Methocarbamol (p.1329·3); paracetamol (p.71·2); codeine phosphate (p.25·2).

Methoxisal Technilab, Canad.
Methocarbamol (p.1329·3); aspirin (p.14·2).

Methoxisal-C Technilab, Canad.
Methocarbamol (p.1329·3); aspirin (p.14·2); codeine phosphate (p.25·2).

Methozane Taro, Israel.
Methotrimeprazine [levomepromazine] maleate (p.692·1).
Anxiety; pain; premedication; psychoses.

Methycobal
Eisai, Hong Kong; Eisai, Jpn; Eisai, Singapore; Eisai, Thai.
Mecobalamin (p.1388·3).
Megaloblastic anaemia; peripheral neuropathies.

Methyl Salicylate Compound Liniment McGloin, Austral.
Methyl salicylate (p.55·1); menthol (p.1632·3); eucalyptus oil (p.1609·2).
Muscle pain.

Methyl Salicylate Ointment Compound McGloin, Austral.
Methyl salicylate (p.55·1); menthol (p.1632·3); eucalyptol (p.1609·2); cajuput oil (p.1588·1).
Muscle pain.

Methylergobrevin Wernigerode, Ger.
Methylergometrine maleate (p.1635·1).
Postpartum haemorrhage; third-stage labour; uterine atony.

Methylin Mallinckrodt, USA.
Methylphenidate hydrochloride (p.1511·3).
Attention deficit hyperactivity disorder; minimal brain dysfunction; narcoleptic syndrome.

Methyment Pharmonta, Aust.
Aluminium acetotartrate (p.1578·2); aluminium formate; methylene blue [methylthioninium chloride] (p.1012·3).
Inflammation and infection of the mouth and throat.

Metibasol Sanobia, Port.
Methimazole [thiamazole] (p.1525·1).
Hyperthyroidism.

Meticel
Note. This name is used for preparations of different composition.
Sophia, Mex.
Hypromellose (p.1501·3).
Eye irritation.
Alter, Spain.
Ranitidine hydrochloride (p.1245·2).
Acid aspiration; gastro-oesophageal reflux; gastrointestinal haemorrhage; peptic ulcer; short-bowel syndrome; Zollinger-Ellison syndrome.

Meticortelone
Schering-Plough, Ital.; Schering-Plough, S.Afr.
Prednisolone (p.1077·3).
Corticosteroid.

Meticorten
Schering-Plough, Braz.; Schering-Plough, Mex.; Schering-Plough, Port.; Schering-Plough, S.Afr.; Schering, USA.
Prednisone (p.1079·2).
Corticosteroid.

Metifarma Merck, Spain.
Amoxicillin trihydrate (p.149·2).
Bacterial infections.

Metifarma Mucolit Merck, Spain.
Amoxicillin trihydrate (p.149·2); bromhexine hydrochloride (p.1085·3); guaifenesin (p.1092·2).
Respiratory-tract infections.

Metifex Cassella-med, Ger.
Ethacridine lactate (p.1130·3).
Diarrhoea; gastro-enteritis; spastic constipation.

Metifex-L Cassella-med, Ger.
Loperamide hydrochloride (p.1231·3).
Diarrhoea.

Metiguanide Pharmacia Upjohn, Ital.
Metformin hydrochloride (p.332·3).
Diabetes mellitus.

Metilbetasone Solubile SoSe, Ital.
Methylprednisolone acetate (p.1076·1).
Injectable corticosteroid.

Metilon Daiichi, Hong Kong.
Dipyrone (p.34·1).
Fever.

Metilpren Faulding, Port.
Methylprednisolone (p.1076·1).

Metilsedor Elofar, Braz.
Dipyrone (p.34·1); papaverine (p.1648·1).
Smooth muscle spasm.

Metimyd
Schering, Canad.†; Schering-Plough, Mex.; Schering-Plough, Swed.; Schering, USA.
Prednisolone acetate (p.1078·1); sulfacetamide sodium (p.250·3).
Ear infections; eye inflammation with bacterial infection.

Metina Fournier, Ital.
Carnitine hydrochloride (p.1356·2).
Carnitine deficiency; myocardial ischaemia.

Metinal-Idantoina Bayer, Ital.
Phenytoin (p.357·2); methylphenobarbital (p.353·3).
Epilepsy.

Metinal-Idantoina L Bayer, Ital.
Phenytoin (p.357·2); methylphenobarbital (p.353·3); phenobarbital (p.355·1).
Epilepsy.

Metindo Kenyaku, Thai.
Indometacin (p.44·3).
Gout; musculoskeletal, joint, and peri-articular disorders; polyneuritis; sciatic pain.

Metinet Nettopharma, Denm.†.
Cimetidine (p.1216·3).
Acid aspiration; gastro-oesophageal reflux; peptic ulcer; Zollinger-Ellison syndrome.

Metiocolin B12 Abbott, Braz.
Methionine (p.1012·2); choline chloride (p.1356·3); inositol (p.1623·3); vitamin B_{12} (p.1388·1).
Liver disorders.

Metiocolin Composto Abbott, Braz.
Acetylmethionine; choline citrate (p.1356·3); inositol (p.1623·3); vitamin B_{12} (p.1388·1).
Liver disorders.

Metionina Esfar, Port.
Choline (p.1356·3); inositol (p.1623·3); methionine (p.1012·2).

Metionina Composta Kanda, Braz.
Methionine (p.1012·2); choline (p.1356·3); inositol (p.1623·3); cynara (p.1601·3); boldo (p.1585·3); cascara (p.1216·1); carqueja amarga.
Liver disorders.

Metison Unison, Thai.
Cisapride (p.1220·1).
Constipation; dyspepsia; gastroparesis; gastro-oesophageal reflux.

Metisona Precimex, Mex.
Methylprednisolone (p.1076·1).

Metivirol Ripari-Gero, Ital.†
Inosine pranobex (p.627·2).
Viral infections.

Metixen Berlin-Chemie, Ger.
Metixene hydrochloride (p.470·2).
Drug-induced extrapyramidal disorders.

Metizol Glenwood, USA†.
Metronidazole (p.594·1).

Meto ABZ, Ger.; BASF, Ger.; Isis Puren, Ger.
Metoprolol tartrate (p.931·2).
Arrhythmias; hypertension; ischaemic heart disease; migraine; myocardial infarction.

Meto comp ABZ, Ger.
Metoprolol tartrate (p.931·2); hydrochlorothiazide (p.907·3).
Hypertension.

Metobeta Betapharm, Ger.
Metoprolol tartrate (p.931·2).
Arrhythmias; hypertension; ischaemic heart disease; migraine; myocardial infarction.

Metobeta comp Betapharm, Ger.
Metoprolol tartrate (p.931·2); hydrochlorothiazide (p.907·3).
Hypertension.

Metoblock Silom, Thai.
Metoprolol tartrate (p.931·2).
Angina pectoris; arrhythmias; hypertension; myocardial infarction.

Metocal Rottapharm, Ital.
Calcium carbonate (p.1215·1).
Calcium deficiency; calcium supplement.

Metoclan Medinfar, Port.
Metoclopramide hydrochloride (p.1235·2).
Gastrointestinal disorders.

Metoclor Pharmaland, Thai.
Metoclopramide hydrochloride (p.1235·2).
Gastrointestinal motility disorders; nausea and vomiting.

Meto-comp Ratiopharm, Ger.†
Metoprolol tartrate (p.931·2); hydrochlorothiazide (p.907·3).
Hypertension.

Metocor Rowa, Irl.
Metoprolol tartrate (p.931·2).
Angina pectoris; arrhythmias; hypertension; hyperthyroidism; migraine; myocardial infarction.

Metocyl
Rowa, Hong Kong; Rowa, Irl.; Rowa, Singapore.
Metoclopramide hydrochloride (p.1235·2).
Gastrointestinal disorders.

Metodine Searle, Mex.
Diiodohydroxyquinoline (p.590·2); metronidazole (p.594·1) or metronidazole benzoate (p.594·1).

Metodura Merck dura, Ger.
Metoprolol tartrate (p.931·2).
Arrhythmias; hypertension; ischaemic heart disease; migraine; myocardial infarction.

Metodura comp Merck dura, Ger.
Metoprolol tartrate (p.931·2); hydrochlorothiazide (p.907·3).
Hypertension.

Metogastron Hexal, Aust.
Metoclopramide hydrochloride (p.1235·2).
Nausea and vomiting; upper gastrointestinal motility disorders.

Metohexal
Hexal, Aust.; Hexal, Austral.; Hexal, Ger.
Metoprolol tartrate (p.931·2).
Angina pectoris; arrhythmias; hypertension; hyperthyroidism; migraine; myocardial infarction.

Metohexal comp Hexal, Ger.
Metoprolol tartrate (p.931·2); hydrochlorothiazide (p.907·3).
Hypertension.

Metolol
Ratiopharm, Aust.; Douglas, Austral.; Pharmaland, Thai.
Metoprolol tartrate (p.931·2).
Angina pectoris; arrhythmias; hypertension; hyperthyroidism; migraine; myocardial infarction.

Metolol compositum Ratiopharm, Aust.
Metoprolol tartrate (p.931·2); hydrochlorothiazide (p.907·3).
Hypertension.

Metolon Malaysia Chemist, Singapore.
Metoclopramide hydrochloride (p.1235·2).
Nausea and vomiting.

Metomerck Merck dura, Ger.
Metoprolol tartrate (p.931·2).
Arrhythmias; hypertension; ischaemic heart disease; migraine; myocardial infarction.

Metomide Grunenthal, Port.
Co-trimoxazole (p.193·3).
Bacterial infections.

Metomin Pacific, NZ.
Metformin hydrochloride (p.332·3).
Diabetes mellitus.

Metono Milano, Thai.
Metoclopramide hydrochloride (p.1235·2).
Nausea and vomiting.

Metop Gerard, Irl.
Metoprolol tartrate (p.931·2).
Angina pectoris; arrhythmias; hypertension; hyperthyroidism; migraine; myocardial infarction.

Metopiron
Novartis, Neth.; Novartis, Norw.†; Novartis, Swed.
Metyrapone (p.1635·3).
Cushing's syndrome; diagnosis of ACTH deficiencies or adrenocortical hyperfunction; hyperaldosteronism; oedema.

Metopirone
Novartis, Austral.; Novartis, Fr.; Novartis, Irl.; Novartis, NZ; Novartis, Switz.; Alliance, UK; Ciba-Geigy, USA.
Metyrapone (p.1635·3).
Cushing's syndrome; hyperaldosteronism; oedema; testing of hypothalamic-pituitary ACTH function.

Metoplex Jean-Marie, Hong Kong.
Dextromethorphan hydrobromide (p.1087·3); carbinoxamine maleate (p.411·1); bromhexine hydrochloride (p.1085·3); ephedrine hydrochloride (p.1090·1); caffeine (p.761·3); papaverine hydrochloride (p.1648·1).
Coughs; viscous bronchial secretions.

Metopram Leiras, Fin.
Metoclopramide hydrochloride (p.1235·2).
Adjunct in gastrointestinal investigations; gastro-oesophageal reflux; gastrointestinal motility disorders; nausea and vomiting.

Metopress
Agis, Israel; Ecosol, Switz.
Metoprolol tartrate (p.931·2).
Angina pectoris; arrhythmias; hypertension; hyperthyroidism; migraine; myocardial infarction.

Metoprin Bunker, Braz.
Co-trimoxazole (p.193·3).
Bacterial infections; Pneumocystis carinii pneumonia; protozoal infections.

Metoprin Balsamico Bunker, Braz.
Co-trimoxazole (p.193·3); guaifenesin (p.1092·2); ammonium chloride (p.1085·2).
Bacterial infections.

Metoproferm Fermenta, Swed.†
Metoprolol tartrate (p.931·2).
Cardiovascular disorders; migraine.

Metoprogamma Worwag, Ger.
Metoprolol tartrate (p.931·2).
Arrhythmias; hypertension; ischaemic heart disease; migraine; myocardial infarction.

Metoprolin Medinovum, Fin.
Metoprolol tartrate (p.931·2).
Angina pectoris; arrhythmias; hypertension; hyperthyroidism; migraine; myocardial infarction.

Metorene Sanofi Synthelabo, Spain.
Naftazone (p.739·2).
Peripheral vascular disorders.

Metorfan Fonten, Ital.
Dextromethorphan hydrobromide (p.1087·3).
Coughs.

Metoros Novartis, Aust.
Metoprolol fumarate (p.932·1).
Angina pectoris; hypertension.

Metostad Comp Stada, Ger.
Metoprolol tartrate (p.931·2); hydrochlorothiazide (p.907·3).
Hypertension.

Metosyn
Bioglan, Denm.; Zeneca, Irl.; Bioglan, Norw.; Bioglan, Singapore; Bioglan, UK.
Fluocinonide (p.1071·2).
Skin disorders.

Meto-Tablinen Sanorania, Ger.
Metoprolol tartrate (p.931·2).
Arrhythmias; hypertension; ischaemic heart disease; migraine; myocardial infarction.

meto-thiazid CT, Ger.
Metoprolol tartrate (p.931·2); hydrochlorothiazide (p.907·3).
Hypertension.

Metotyrol Tyrol, Aust.
Metoprolol tartrate (p.931·2).
Angina pectoris; arrhythmias; hypertension; hyperthyroidism; migraine; myocardial infarction.

Metoxiprim Rhein, Mex.
Co-trimoxazole (p.193·3).
Bacterial infections.

Metozoc Gea, Denm.; Gea, Fin.; Gea, Norw.
Metoprolol tartrate (p.931·2).
Angina pectoris; arrhythmias; hypertension; hyperthyroidism; migraine; myocardial infarction.

Metozzard Pizzard, Mex.
Metoprolol (p.932·1).

Metran Hoechst Marion Roussel, Spain.
Cefpirome sulfate (p.172·2).
Bacterial infections.

Metrazole
Docmed, S.Afr.†; General Drugs, Thai.
Metronidazole (p.594·1).
Anaerobic bacterial infections; protozoal infections.

Metrazone Boehringer de Angeli, Braz.
Feprazone (p.40·3).
Fever; musculoskeletal and joint disorders.

Metrecina Liferpal, Mex.
Oxytetracycline (p.234·1).
Bacterial infections.

Metreton Schering, Canad.
Prednisone acetate (p.1079·2); chlorpheniramine [chlorphenamine] maleate (p.412·1); ascorbic acid (p.1389·3).
Hypersensitivity disorders.

Metricom Protein, Mex.
Metronidazole (p.594·1).

Metrigen Fuerte Organon, Mex.
Estradiol benzoate (p.1473·1); progesterone (p.1488·3).
Menstrual disorders.

Metrim Siam Bheasach, Thai.
Co-trimoxazole (p.193·3).
Bacterial infections.

Metrine TP, Thai.
Methylergometrine maleate (p.1635·1).
Postpartum haemorrhage; postpartum uterine atony.

Metrizol Liferpal, Mex.
Metronidazole (p.594·1).
Protozoal infections.

Metro McGaw, USA.
Metronidazole (p.594·1).
Amoebiasis; anaerobic bacterial infections; trichomoniasis.

Metrocide Pharmaland, Thai.
Metronidazole (p.594·1).
Amoebiasis; trichomoniasis.

Metrocream
Galderma, Canad.; Galderma, USA.
Metronidazole (p.594·1).
Rosacea.

Metroderme Galderma, Port.
Metronidazole (p.594·1).
Rosacea.

Metrodin
Serono, Austral.; Serono, Braz.; Serono, Canad.†; Serono, Hong Kong; Serono, Irl.; Teva, Israel; Serono, Ital.; Serono, Neth.†; Serono, NZ; Serono, Port.; Serono, S.Afr.; Serono, Singapore; Serono, Switz.; Serono, Thai.; Serono, UK; Serono, USA.
Urofollitropin (p.1299·3).
Male and female infertility.

Metrodine Serono, Fr.†
Urofollitropin (p.1299·3).
Female infertility; ovarian stimulation for fertilisation in vitro.

Metrodiyod Serral, Mex.
Diiodohydroxyquinoline (p.590·2); metronidazole (p.594·1).
Amoebiasis; giardiasis; trichomoniasis.

Metrogel
Galderma, Canad.; Galderma, Denm.; Bioglan, Irl.; Galderma, Mex.; Boots Healthcare, Neth.; Novartis, UK; Galderma, UK; Galderma, USA.
Metronidazole (p.594·1).
Fungating malodorous tumours; rosacea.

Metrogel Vaginal 3M, USA.
Metronidazole (p.594·1).
Bacterial vaginosis.

Metrogyl
Alphapharm, Austral.; Alphapharm, Hong Kong; Teva, Israel; Unique, Thai.
Metronidazole (p.594·1) or metronidazole benzoate (p.594·1).
Anaerobic bacterial infections; protozoal infections.

Metrolex Siam Bheasach, Thai.
Metronidazole (p.594·1).
Amoebiasis; anaerobic bacterial infections; giardiasis; trichomoniasis.

Metrolyl Lagap, UK.
Metronidazole (p.594·1).
Anaerobic bacterial infections.

Metronide
Rhone-Poulenc Rorer, Austral.; Clonmel, Irl.
Metronidazole (p.594·1).
Anaerobic bacterial infections; protozoal infections.

Metronid-Puren Isis Puren, Ger.
Metronidazole (p.594·1).
Bacterial infections; trichomoniasis.

Metronil Sydenham, Mex.
Metronidazole benzoate (p.594·1).

Metronimerck Merck dura, Ger.
Metronidazole (p.594·1).
Bacterial infections; protozoal infections.

Metronix Opofarm, Braz.
Metronidazole (p.594·1).
Anaerobic bacterial infections; protozoal infections.

Metronom Ratiopharm, Aust.†
Propafenone hydrochloride (p.961·3).
Arrhythmias.

Metronour Nourypharma, Ger.
Metronidazole (p.594·1).
Bacterial infections; protozoal infections.

Metront Hexal, Ger.
Metronidazole (p.594·1).
Bacterial infections; protozoal infections.

Metroson Sons, Mex.
Metronidazole (p.594·1).
Amoebiasis; trichomoniasis.

Metrostat Propan, S.Afr.
Metronidazole (p.594·1).
Anaerobic bacterial infections; protozoal infections.

Metrotex Rhodia, Braz.
Methotrexate (p.553·2).
Malignant neoplasms.

Metrotop
Seton, Irl.; SSL, UK.
Metronidazole (p.594·1).
Malodorous fungating tumours; malodorous skin ulcers; rosacea.

Metrozine
Searle, Austral.†; Searle, Hong Kong.
Metronidazole (p.594·1).
Anaerobic bacterial infections; protozoal infections.

Metrozol Parkfields, UK.
Metronidazole (p.594·1).

Metrozole MPF, Singapore.
Metronidazole (p.594·1).
Anaerobic bacterial infections; protozoal infections.

Met-Rx Met-Rx, USA.
Preparations for enteral nutrition (p.1350·1).

Metsal
3M, Austral.; 3M, Hong Kong; 3M, NZ; 3M, Singapore.
Menthol (p.1632·3); eucalyptus oil (p.1609·2); methyl salicylate (p.55·1).
Musculoskeletal, joint, peri-articular, and soft-tissue disorders.

Metsal Analgesic 3M, Austral.
Trolamine salicylate (p.90·1); menthol (p.1632·3).
Muscle pain.

Metsal AR Analgesic 3M, Austral.
Trolamine salicylate (p.90·1).
Musculoskeletal and joint pain.

Metsal AR Heat Rub 3M, Austral.
Methyl salicylate (p.55·1); eucalyptus oil (p.1609·2); menthol (p.1632·3).
Musculoskeletal and joint pain.

Metsal Heat Rub 3M, Austral.
Methyl salicylate (p.55·1); eucalyptus oil (p.1609·2); menthol (p.1632·3).
Musculoskeletal and joint pain.

Metsal Liniment 3M, Austral.
Methyl salicylate (p.55·1).
Musculoskeletal and joint disorders.

Metsec TP, Thai.
Omeprazole (p.1239·1).
Gastro-oesophageal reflux; peptic ulcer; Zollinger-Ellison syndrome.

Met-Sil TP, Thai.
Metoclopramide hydrochloride (p.1235·2).
Gastrointestinal motility disorders; nausea and vomiting.

Metubine
Lilly, Canad.†; Dista, USA†.
Metocurine iodide (p.1337·2).
Competitive neuromuscular blocker.

Metussa Jean-Marie, Singapore.
Carbinoxamine maleate (p.411·1); dextromethorphan hydrobromide (p.1087·3).
Coughs.

Metussan Biomedis, Thai.; Great Eastern, Thai.
Dextromethorphan hydrobromide (p.1087·3); chlorpheniramine [chlorphenamine] maleate (p.412·1); guaifenesin (p.1092·2); sodium citrate (p.1186·2).
Coughs.

Metxaprim General Drugs, Thai.
Co-trimoxazole (p.193·3).
Bacterial infections.

Metypred Orion, Ger.
Methylprednisolone (p.1076·1), methylprednisolone acetate (p.1076·1), or methylprednisolone sodium succinate (p.1076·1).
Corticosteroid.

Metypresol Intramed, S.Afr.
Methylprednisolone sodium succinate (p.1076·1).
Corticosteroid.

Metysolon Dermapharm, Ger.
Methylprednisolone (p.1076·1).
Corticosteroid.

Mevacor
Merck Sharp & Dohme, Aust.; Merck Sharp & Dohme, Braz.; Merck Frosst, Canad.; Merck Sharp & Dohme, Denm.; Merck Sharp & Dohme, Fin.; Merck Sharp & Dohme, Hong Kong; Merck Sharp & Dohme, Mex.; Merck Sharp & Dohme, Norw.; Merck Sharp & Dohme, Spain; Merck, USA.
Lovastatin (p.922·3).
Atherosclerosis; hypercholesterolaemia.

Mevalon Guidotti, Ital.
Meglutol (p.926·1).
Hyperlipidaemia.

Mevalotin
Sankyo, Ger.; Sankyo, Jpn; Sankyo, Switz.; Sankyo, Thai.
Pravastatin sodium (p.957·3).
Hypercholesterolaemia.

Mevilin-L
Evans Medical, Israel; Medeva, UK†.
A measles vaccine (Schwarz strain) (p.1547·1).
Active immunisation.

Mevinacor
Merck Sharp & Dohme, Ger.; Merck Sharp & Dohme, Port.
Lovastatin (p.922·3).
Hypercholesterolaemia.

Mevlor *Monsanto, Port.*
Lovastatin (p.922·3).
Hypercholesterolaemia.

Mexalen *Ratiopharm, Aust.*
Paracetamol (p.71·2).
Fever; pain.

Mexan *Teva, Israel.*
Mesna (p.1011·3).
Prevention of ifosfamide or cyclophosphamide urothelial toxicity.

Mexasone *MPF, Singapore.*
Dexamethasone (p.1067·1).
Corticosteroid.

Mexa-Vit C *Ratiopharm, Aust.*
Paracetamol (p.71·2); ascorbic acid (p.1389·3).
Cold symptoms.

Mexcyn *Ofimex, Mex.*
Erythromycin (p.201·2).

Mexe N *Merckle, Ger.*
Codeine phosphate (p.25·2); paracetamol (p.71·2).
Pain.

Mexilen *Rafa, Israel.*
Mexiletine hydrochloride (p.932·2).
Ventricular arrhythmias.

Mexitil
Boehringer Ingelheim, Aust.; Boehringer Ingelheim, Austral.; Boehringer Ingelheim, Belg.; Boehringer de Angeli, Braz.; Boehringer Ingelheim, Canad.; Boehringer Ingelheim, Denm.; Boehringer Ingelheim, Fin.; Boehringer Ingelheim, Fr.; Boehringer Ingelheim, Ger.; Boehringer Ingelheim, Hong Kong; Boehringer Ingelheim, Irl.; Boehringer Ingelheim, Ital.; Boehringer Ingelheim, Mex.; Boehringer Ingelheim, Neth.†; Boehringer Ingelheim, Norw.; Boehringer Ingelheim, NZ; Boehringer Ingelheim, S.Afr.; Boehringer Ingelheim, Spain; Boehringer Ingelheim, Swed.; Boehringer Ingelheim, Switz.†; Boehringer Ingelheim, Thai.; Boehringer Ingelheim, UK; Boehringer Ingelheim, USA.
Mexiletine hydrochloride (p.932·2).
Ventricular arrhythmias.

Mexona *Orthos, Mex.*
Dexamethasone (p.1067·1).
Corticosteroid.

Mexsana *Schering-Plough, USA.*
Kaolin (p.1229·3); eucalyptus oil (p.1609·2); camphor (p.1589·3); corn starch (p.1379·3); lemon oil (p.1628·2); zinc oxide (p.1128·2).
Nappy rash.

Mezen *Errekappa, Ital.*
Promelase (p.1655·1).
Inflammation; oedema.

Mezenol *Pharmador, S.Afr.†*
Co-trimoxazole (p.193·3).
Bacterial infections.

Mezinc *Abigo, Swed.*
Zinc oxide (p.1128·2); zinc resin (p.1398·1).
Wound dressing.

Meziv *Euroderm, Ital.*
Methionine (p.1012·2); vitamin B substances (p.1350·1); zinc sulfate (p.1398·2).
Hair loss.

Mezlin *Bayer, USA.*
Mezlocillin sodium (p.224·1).
Bacterial infections.

Mezym F *Berlin-Chemie, Ger.*
Pancreatin (p.1646·1).
Pancreatic disorders.

MF 110 *Max Farma, Ital.†*
Nimesulide (p.62·3).
Fever; inflammation; pain.

MFV-Ject *Pasteur Merieux, UK.*
An inactivated influenza vaccine (split virion) (p.1544·3).
Active immunisation.

MG400 *Triton, USA.*
Salicylic acid (p.1122·3); sulfur (p.1123·3).
Seborrhoea.

MG 50 *Terapeutico, Ital.*
Magnesium proteinate.
Magnesium deficiency; magnesium supplement.

MG Cold Sore Formula *Outdoor Recreations, USA.*
Menthol (p.1632·3); lignocaine [lidocaine] (p.1313·2).

Mg 5-Granoral *Vifor, Switz.*
Magnesium aspartate (p.1190·3).
Magnesium deficiency; magnesium supplement.

Mg 5-Granulat *Artesan, Ger.; Cassella-med, Ger.*
Magnesium aspartate (p.1190·3).
Magnesium deficiency.

Mg 5-Longoral
Kolassa, Aust.; Artesan, Ger.; Cassella-med, Ger.; Vifor, Switz.
Magnesium aspartate (p.1190·3).
Magnesium deficiency; magnesium supplement.

MG217 Medicated *Triton, USA.*
Coal tar (p.1125·1).
MG217 Medicated shampoo and ointment formerly contained coal tar, salicylic acid, and colloidal sulfur.
Skin disorders.

MG217 Medicated Tar-Free *Triton, USA.*
Sulfur (p.1123·3); salicylic acid (p.1122·3).
Dandruff.

Mg 5-Oraleff *Vifor, Switz.*
Magnesium aspartate (p.1190·3).
Magnesium deficiency; magnesium supplement.

MG217 Sal-Acid *Triton, USA.*
Salicylic acid (p.1122·3).
Psoriasis.

Mg 5-Sulfat
Artesan, Ger.; Cassella-med, Ger.; Vifor International, Switz.
Magnesium sulfate (p.1191·1).
Arrhythmias; eclampsia; fetal hypotrophy; magnesium deficiency; myocardial infarction; pre-eclampsia; premature labour.

Mg-nor *Knoll, Ger.†*
Magnesium aspartate (p.1190·3).
Magnesium deficiency.

Miabene *Ratiopharm, Aust.*
Mianserin hydrochloride (p.298·1).
Depression.

Miacalcic
Novartis, Austral.; Novartis, Belg.; Novartis, Braz.; Novartis, Denm.; Novartis, Fin.; Novartis, Fr.; Novartis, Hong Kong; Novartis, Israel; LPB, Ital.; Novartis, Mex.; Novartis, Norw.; Novartis, NZ; Novartis, Port.; Novartis, S.Afr.; Novartis, Singapore; Novartis, Spain; Novartis, Swed.; Novartis, Switz.; Novartis, Thai.; Novartis, UK.
Salcatonin (p.749·3).
Acute pancreatitis; hypercalcaemia; hyperparathyroidism; osteolytic or osteopenic bone pain; osteoporosis; Paget's disease of bone; reflex sympathetic dystrophy; vitamin D intoxication.

Miacalcin
Novartis, Canad.; Novartis, USA.
Salcatonin (p.749·3).
Hypercalcaemia; osteoporosis; Paget's disease of bone.

Mi-Acid *Major, USA.*
Aluminium hydroxide (p.1210·3); magnesium hydroxide (p.1233·1); simeticone (p.1249·2).
Hyperacidity.

Mi-Acid Gelcaps *Major, USA.*
Calcium carbonate (p.1215·1); magnesium carbonate (p.1232·3).
Hyperacidity.

Miadenil *Francia, Ital.*
Salcatonin (p.749·3).
Hypercalcaemia; osteoporosis; Paget's disease of bone; reflex sympathetic dystrophy.

Mialgex *Cazi, Braz.*
Methyl salicylate (p.55·1); turpentine oil (p.1676·3); camphor (p.1589·3); menthol (p.1632·3).
Musculoskeletal and joint disorders.

Mialin *Biomedica, Ital.*
Alprazolam (p.654·2).
Anxiety disorders.

Miambutol *Wyeth Lederle, Ital.*
Ethambutol hydrochloride (p.205·1).
Tuberculosis.

Mianeurin *Hexal, Ger.*
Mianserin hydrochloride (p.298·1).
Depression.

Miantor *Pharmacia Upjohn, Mex.*
Etomidoline.

Miaxan *Orion, Fin.*
Mianserin hydrochloride (p.298·1).
Depression; insomnia.

Miazide *Cyanamid, Ital.†*
Ethambutol hydrochloride (p.205·1); isoniazid (p.215·3).
Tuberculosis.

Miazide B6 *Wyeth Lederle, Ital.*
Ethambutol hydrochloride (p.205·1); isoniazid (p.215·3); pyridoxine hydrochloride (p.1386·3).
Tuberculosis.

Mibazol *Precimex, Mex.*
Metronidazole (p.594·1).

Mibrox *Orion, Ger.*
Ambroxol hydrochloride (p.1084·3).
Respiratory disorders associated with viscid or excessive mucus.

Miburell *Sanorell, Ger.*
Homoeopathic preparation.

Mica *Epifarma, Ital.*
Heparin calcium (p.902·1).
Thromboembolic disorders.

Mical *Sam-On, Israel.*
Carbocisteine (p.1086·3).
Respiratory-tract disorders associated with viscous mucus.

Micane *Edol, Port.*
Miconazole nitrate (p.391·1).

Micanol
Schering, Aust.; Canderm, Canad.; Bioglan, Fin.; Bioglan, Ger.; Bioglan, Irl.; Bioglan, Israel; Bioglan, Norw.; CS, Port.; Bioglan, Singapore; Stiefel, Spain; Bioglan, Swed.; Bioglan, Thai.; Bioglan, UK; Bioglan, USA.
Dithranol (p.1113·3).
Psoriasis.

Micardis
Boehringer Ingelheim, Austral.; Boehringer Ingelheim, Belg.; Boehringer Ingelheim, Denm.; Boehringer Ingelheim, Fr.; Boehringer Ingelheim, Ger.; Glaxo Wellcome, Ger.; Boehringer Ingelheim, Irl.; Boehringer Ingelheim, Neth.; Boehringer Ingelheim, S.Afr.; Boehringer Ingelheim, Spain; Boehringer Ingelheim, Switz.; Boehringer Ingelheim, UK; Boehringer Ingelheim, USA.
Telmisartan (p.979·2).
Hypertension.

Micardis HCT *Boehringer Ingelheim, USA.*
Telmisartan (p.979·2); hydrochlorothiazide (p.907·3).
Hypertension.

Micarzin *AF, Mex.*
Ibuprofen (p.43·2).
Inflammation; musculoskeletal and joint disorders; pain.

Micatin
McNeil Consumer, Canad.; Advanced Care, USA.
Miconazole nitrate (p.391·1).
Fungal skin infections.

Micaveen
Note.This name is used for preparations of different composition.
Rydelle, Fr.
Avena (p.1583·1); undecenoic acid (p.395·3).
Fungal skin infections.

Johnson & Johnson, Ital.
Avena (p.1583·1).
Soap substitute.

Dermoteca, Port.†
Avena (p.1583·1); undecenoic acid (p.395·3); benzoic acid (p.1134·2).
Fungal skin infections.

Micazin *Chew, Thai.*
Miconazole (p.391·1).
Fungal skin and nail infections.

Miccil *Senosiain, Mex.*
Bumetanide (p.852·1).
Hypertension; oedema.

Micebrina *Synthelabo, Spain.*
A range of multivitamin preparations with or without minerals and ginseng (p.1350·1).

Micelle E *HSL, NZ.*
d-Alpha tocoferil acetate (p.1394·1).
Vitamin E supplement.

Micetal *Uriach, Spain.*
Flutrimazole (p.386·1).
Fungal skin infections.

Micetinoftalmina *Davi, Port.*
Chloramphenicol (p.179·1).
Bacterial eye infections.

Miciclin *Reuffer, Mex.*
Tetracycline (p.258·3).
Bacterial infections.

Micifrona *Iquinosa, Spain.*
Lespedeza capitata.
Uraemia.

Miclast *Pierre Fabre, Ital.*
Ciclopirox olamine (p.382·1).
Fungal skin and vaginal infections.

Micocid *Windson, Braz.*
Salicylic acid (p.1122·3); benzoic acid (p.1134·2); iodine (p.1522·3).
Fungal skin infections.

Micoderm *Kemyos, Ital.†*
Miconazole nitrate (p.391·1).
Fungal and bacterial infections.

Micoespec *Centrum, Spain.*
Econazole nitrate (p.382·3).
Fungal skin and nail infections.

Micofim *Elofar, Braz.*
Benzoic acid (p.1134·2); salicylic acid (p.1122·3); iodine (p.1522·3).
Fungal skin infections.

Micofoot *Zeta, Ital.*
Undecenoic acid (p.395·3); usnic acid (p.1678·3); salicylic acid (p.1122·3); aluminium acetate (p.1578·1).
Disinfection of skin, burns, and wounds; fungal skin infections.

Micogal *Galen, Mex.*
Ketoconazole (p.389·1).
Fungal infections.

Micogin *Crosara, Ital.†*
Econazole nitrate (p.382·3).
Fungal and bacterial infections.

Micogyn *Elofar, Braz.*
Miconazole (p.391·1).
Vulvovaginal candidiasis.

Micoisdin *Isdin, Spain.*
Tolnaftate (p.395·2).
Fungal skin and nail infections.

Micoless *Novaquimica, Braz.*
Miconazole nitrate (p.391·1).
Fungal skin infections.

Micolette
Dominion, Irl.; Dexcel, UK.
Sodium citrate (p.1186·2); sodium lauril sulfoacetate (p.1496·3); glycerol (p.1616·3).
Bowel evacuation; constipation.

Micoliv *Farmalab, Braz.*
Ciclopirox (p.382·1).
Fungal vulvovaginal infections.

Micomax *Max Farma, Ital.*
Miconazole pivoxil chloride (p.391·3).
Fungal infections; Gram-positive bacterial superinfections.

Micomicen *Sanofi Synthelabo, Ital.*
Ciclopirox olamine (p.382·1).
Vulvovaginal candidiasis.

Micomisan *Restan, S.Afr.*
Clotrimazole (p.382·1).
Fungal skin infections; vaginal candidiasis.

Miconal *Ecobi, Ital.*
Miconazole (p.391·1) or miconazole nitrate (p.391·1).
Fungal infections; secondary Gram-positive bacterial infections.

Miconan *Ativus, Braz.*
Ketoconazole (p.389·1).
Fungal infections.

Micoplex *Cazi, Braz.*
Tiabendazole (p.109·1); neomycin sulfate (p.228·1).
Skin infections.

Micoren *Novartis Consumer, Ital.*
Prethcamide (p.1514·2).
Respiratory insufficiency.

Micos *AGIPS, Ital.*
Econazole (p.383·1) or econazole nitrate (p.382·3).
Fungal infections; Gram-positive bacterial infections.

Micosan *Brasmedica, Braz.*
Undecenoic acid (p.395·3); triacetin (p.395·3); hexachlorophene (p.1146·1).
Skin disinfection.

Micoseptil *Reig Jofre, Spain†.*
Econazole nitrate (p.382·3).
Fungal skin and nail infections.

Micoser *Serral, Mex.*
Ketoconazole (p.389·1).
Fungal infections.

Micosid *Wayne, Mex.*
Miconazole (p.391·1).

Micosona *Schering, Spain.*
Naftifine hydrochloride (p.392·1).
Fungal skin and nail infections.

Micostatin
Bristol-Myers Squibb, Braz.; Bristol-Myers Squibb, Mex.
Nystatin (p.392·2).
Fungal infections.

Micostyl
Stiefel, Braz.; Stiefel, Mex.
Econazole (p.383·1) or econazole nitrate (p.382·3).
Fungal skin infections.

Micotar *Dermapharm, Ger.*
Miconazole (p.391·1) or miconazole nitrate (p.391·1).
Fungal infections.

Micotef *LPB, Ital.*
Miconazole (p.391·1) or miconazole nitrate (p.391·1).
Fungal infections; Gram-positive bacterial infections.

Micotiazol *Cazi, Braz.*
Benzoic acid (p.1134·2); salicylic acid (p.1122·3); iodine (p.1522·3).
Fungal skin infections.

Micoticum *Vita, Spain.*
Ketoconazole (p.389·1).
Fungal infections.

Micotissim *Stevia, Braz.*
Salicylic acid (p.1122·3); benzoic acid (p.1134·2); iodine (p.1522·3); sumatra benzoin (p.1668·3).
Fungal skin infections.

Micotrizol *Eurofarma, Braz.*
Clotrimazole (p.382·1).
Fungal skin infections.

Micoxolamina *Mastelli, Ital.*
Ciclopirox olamine (p.382·1).
Fungal infections.

Micoz *QIF, Braz.*
Undecenoic acid (p.395·3); sodium undecenoate (p.396·1); benzoic acid (p.1134·2); sumatra benzoin (p.1668·3).
Skin infections.

Micozole
Taro, Canad.; AFT, NZ.
Miconazole (p.391·1) or miconazole nitrate (p.391·1).
Vulvovaginal candidiasis.

Micrainin *Wallace, USA.*
Aspirin (p.14·2); meprobamate (p.691·1).
Pain.

Micral II *Roche Diagnostics, Irl.*
Test for microalbuminuria.

Micral Test II
Roche Diagnostics, Austral.; Lakeside, Mex.; Roche Diagnostics, UK.
Test for microalbuminuria in diagnosis of diabetic nephropathy.

Micral Test S *Lakeside, Mex.*
Test for microalbuminuria.

Micralax
Pharmacia Upjohn, Spain; Celltech, UK.
Sodium citrate (p.1186·2); sodium lauril sulfoacetate (p.1496·3).
Bowel evacuation; constipation; painful defaecation.

Micranet *Ogna, Ital.*
Propyphenazone (p.80·2); paracetamol (p.71·2); caffeine (p.761·3).
Migraine; toothache.

Micreme *Pacific, NZ.*
Miconazole nitrate (p.391·1).
Fungal balanitis; vulvovaginal candidiasis with Gram-positive superinfection.

Micreme H *Pacific, NZ.*
Miconazole nitrate (p.391·1); hydrocortisone (p.1073·3).
Infected skin disorders.

MICRhoGAM *Ortho Diagnostic, USA.*
An anti-D immunoglobulin (p.1532·1).
Prevention of rhesus sensitisation.

Micristin *OPW, Ger.†*
Aspirin (p.14·2).
Myocardial infarction; thrombosis prophylaxis; vascular disorders.

Micro + *Sabex, Canad.†*
A range of trace element preparations (p.1350·1).

Micro I *Sabex, Canad.†*
Sodium iodide (p.1522·3).
Trace element additive.

Micro Cr *Sabex, Canad.†*
Chromium trichloride (p.1357·1).
Trace element additive.

The symbol † denotes a preparation no longer actively marketed

Micro Cu *Sabex, Canad.†.*
Copper sulfate (p.1358·1).
Trace element additive.

Micro Mn *Sabex, Canad.†.*
Manganese sulfate (p.1371·3).
Trace element additive.

Micro Se *Sabex, Canad.†.*
Selenious acid (p.1375·2).
Trace element additive.

Micro Zn *Sabex, Canad.†.*
Zinc sulfate (p.1398·2).
Trace element additive.

Microalbustix *Bayer Diagnostics, Irl.*
Test for albumin and creatinine in urine.

Microbac *Propan, S.Afr.†.*
Co-trimoxazole (p.193·3).
Bacterial infections.

Microbactim *Pharmacos, Mex.*
Co-trimoxazole (p.193·3).
Bacterial infections.

Microbamat *Sanochemia, Aust.*
Meprobamate (p.691·1).
Anxiety disorders; sleep disorders.

Microbar-Colon *Bracco, Switz.*
Barium sulfate (p.1032·1).
Contrast medium for gastrointestinal radiography.

Microbar-HD (E-Z-HD) *Bracco, Switz.*
Barium sulfate (p.1032·1).
Contrast medium for gastrointestinal double-contrast radiography.

Microbumintest *Bayer Diagnostici, Ital.*
Test for albumin in urine.

Microcasen *Casen Fleet, Spain.*
Sodium lauril sulfoacetate (p.1496·3); sodium citrate (p.1186·2).
Bowel evacuation; constipation; painful defaecation.

Microcid
Bioglan, Denm.; Bioglan, Swed.
Hydrogen peroxide (p.1147·1).
Bacterial skin infections.

Microcidal *Aspen, S.Afr.*
Griseofulvin (p.386·2).
Fungal infections of the skin and nails.

Microclisma Evacuante AD-BB *Sofar, Ital.*
Glycerol (p.1616·3); chamomile (p.1593·2); mallow.

Microclismi Marco Viti *Boots, Ital.*
Glycerol (p.1616·3).
Bowel evacuation; constipation.

Microclismi Sella *Sella, Ital.*
Glycerol (p.1616·3).
Bowel evacuation; constipation.

Microdiol
Akzo, Braz.; Organon, Israel; Organon, Spain.
Desogestrel (p.1470·3); ethinylestradiol (p.1476·2).
Combined oral contraceptive; menstrual disorders.

Microdit *Kener, Mex.*
Ranitidine (p.1246·3).

Microdoine *Gomenol, Fr.*
Nitrofurantoin (p.230·3).
Cystitis.

Microgel *Restan, S.Afr.*
Oral suspension: Dicyclomine [dicycloverine] hydrochloride (p.466·1); aluminium hydroxide (p.1210·3); magnesium oxide (p.1233·2); simeticone (p.1249·2).
Tablets: Calcium carbonate (p.1215·1); magnesium carbonate (p.1232·3); magnesium trisilicate (p.1233·3); simeticone (p.1249·2); sodium hexametaphosphate.
Gastrointestinal disorders.

Microgest *Schering, Thai.*
21 Tablets, levonorgestrel (p.1486·2); ethinylestradiol (p.1476·2); 7 tablets, inert.
Combined oral contraceptive.

Microginon *Schering, Port.*
Levonorgestrel (p.1486·2); ethinylestradiol (p.1476·2).
Combined oral contraceptive.

Microgyn *Schering, Denm.*
Levonorgestrel (p.1486·2); ethinylestradiol (p.1476·2).
Combined oral contraceptive.

Microgynon
Schering, Aust.; Schering, Austral.; Schering, Belg.; Schering, Fin.; Schering, Ger.; Schering, Hong Kong; Schering, Israel; Schering, Ital.; Schering, Mex.; Schering, Neth.; Schering, Norw.; Schering, NZ; Schering, Singapore; Schering, Spain; Schering, Switz.; Schering, Thai.
Levonorgestrel (p.1486·2); ethinylestradiol (p.1476·2).
28-Day packs also contain 7 inert tablets.
Combined oral contraceptive.

Microgynon 30
Schering, Irl.; Schering, UK.
Levonorgestrel (p.1486·2); ethinylestradiol (p.1476·2).
28-Day packs also contain 7 inert tablets.
Combined oral contraceptive.

Micro-K *Wyeth-Ayerst, Canad.; Continental Ethicals, S.Afr.†; Robins, USA.*
Potassium chloride (p.1194·3).
Hypokalaemia; potassium depletion.

Micro-Kalium *Lannacher, Aust.*
Potassium chloride (p.1194·3).
Potassium deficiency.

Microklist
Pharmacia Upjohn, Aust.; Pharmacia Upjohn, Ger.; Pharmacia Upjohn, Switz.
Sodium citrate (p.1186·2); sodium lauril sulfoacetate (p.1496·3); sorbitol (p.1377·3).
Bowel evacuation; constipation.

Microlax
Note. This name is used for preparations of different composition.
Pharmacia Upjohn, Austral.; SmithKline Beecham Consumer, Belg.; Pharmacia Upjohn, Canad.; Pharmacia Upjohn, Fin.; Pharmacia Upjohn, Fr.; Pharmacia Upjohn, Hong Kong; Pharmacia Upjohn, Norw.; Pharmacia Upjohn, NZ; Pharmacia Upjohn, S.Afr.; Pharmacia Upjohn, Swed.; Pharmacia Upjohn, Switz.
Sodium citrate (p.1186·2); sodium lauril sulfoacetate (p.1496·3); sorbitol (p.1377·3).
Bowel evacuation; constipation.

Pharmacia Upjohn, Denm.; Pharmacia Upjohn, Irl.; Sanofi Winthrop, Mex.; Bonafarma, Port.; Pharmacia Upjohn, Singapore.
Sodium citrate (p.1186·2); sodium lauril sulfoacetate (p.1496·3).
Bowel evacuation; constipation.

Pharmacia Upjohn, Neth.
Sodium lauril sulfoacetate (p.1496·3); sorbitol (p.1377·3).
Bowel evacuation; constipation.

Microlet *Dexxon, Israel.*
Sodium citrate (p.1186·2); sodium lauril sulfoacetate (p.1496·3); glycerol (p.1616·3).
Constipation.

Microlev *Ida, Fr.*
Dried yeast (p.1398·1).
Vitamin B deficiency.

Microlipid *Sherwood, USA.*
High calorie preparation containing safflower oil (p.1375·1) for enteral nutrition (p.1350·1).

Microlite *Schering, Irl.*
Ethinylestradiol (p.1476·2); levonorgestrel (p.1486·2).
Combined oral contraceptive.

Microlut
Schering, Austral.; Schering, Belg.; Schering, Ger.; Schering, Ital.; Schering, Mex.; Schering, NZ; Schering, Switz.
Levonorgestrel (p.1486·2).
Progestogen-only oral contraceptive.

Microluton
Schering, Denm.; Schering, Fin.; Schering, Norw.
Levonorgestrel (p.1486·2).
Progestogen-only oral contraceptive.

Micronase *Pharmacia Upjohn, USA.*
Glibenclamide (p.321·3).
Diabetes mellitus.

microNefrin *Bird, USA.*
Racepinefrine hydrochloride (p.831·1).
Bronchospasm.

Micronoan *Ravizza, Ital.*
Diazepam (p.674·3).
Epilepsy; sedative.

Micronor
Janssen-Cilag, Austral.; Cilag, Braz.; Janssen-Ortho, Canad.; Janssen-Cilag, Irl.; Janssen-Cilag, UK; Ortho McNeil, USA.
Norethisterone (p.1485·1).
Progestogen-only oral contraceptive.

Micronor HRT *Janssen-Cilag, UK.*
Norethisterone (p.1485·1).
Menopausal disorders.

Micronovum
Janssen-Cilag, Aust.; Janssen-Cilag, Ger.†; Janssen-Cilag, S.Afr.†; Janssen-Cilag, Switz.
Norethisterone (p.1485·1).
Progestogen-only oral contraceptive.

Micropaque
Sanova, Aust.†; Codali, Belg.; Guerbet, Denm.; Guerbet, Fr.; Guerbet, Ger.; Guerbet, Neth.†; Nicholas, Port.; Pan Quimica, Spain; Guerbet, Switz.; Bioglan, UK†.
Barium sulfate (p.1032·1).
Contrast medium for gastrointestinal radiography.

Microphta *Europhta, Mon.*
Micronomicin sulfate (p.224·3).
Bacterial eye infections.

Microphyllin *Aventis, S.Afr.*
Theophylline (p.777·2).
Asthma; bronchospasm.

Micropirin
Dexcel, Israel; Generics, UK.
Aspirin (p.14·2).
Thromboembolism prophylaxis.

Micropur
Sirmeta, Austral.†; Katadyn, Fr.†.
Silver chloride complex (p.1664·1).
Water disinfection.

Microrgan *Liomont, Mex.*
Ciprofloxacin hydrochloride (p.182·3).
Bacterial infections.

Microsan N *Biosyn, Ger.*
Multivitamin and magnesium preparation (p.1350·1).

Microser *Formenti, Ital.*
Betahistine hydrochloride (p.1584·2).
Ménière's disease; vertigo; vestibular disorders.

Microshield 2, 4, 5, and 20 *Johnson & Johnson, Austral.*
Chlorhexidine gluconate (p.1138·2).
Skin, wound, and instrument disinfection.

Microshield Antiseptic *Johnson & Johnson, Austral.*
Cetrimide (p.1137·1); chlorhexidine gluconate (p.1138·2).
Skin, wound, burn, and instrument disinfection.

Microshield Handrub *Johnson & Johnson, Austral.*
Chlorhexidine gluconate (p.1138·2); alcohol (p.1130·3).
Skin disinfection.

Microshield PVP *Johnson & Johnson, Austral.*
Povidone-iodine (p.1155·1).
Skin disinfection.

Microshield PVP Plus *Johnson & Johnson, Austral.*
Povidone-iodine (p.1155·1); triclosan (p.1159·2).
Skin disinfection.

Microshield PVP-S *Johnson & Johnson, Austral.*
Povidone-iodine (p.1155·1).
Bacterial or fungal skin and mucous membrane infections; skin, wound, and burn disinfection.

Microshield T *Johnson & Johnson, Austral.*
Triclosan (p.1159·2).
Skin disinfection.

Microshield Tincture *Johnson & Johnson, Austral.*
Chlorhexidine gluconate (p.1138·2); alcohol (p.1130·3).
Skin, surface, and instrument disinfection.

Microsol *Herbaxt, Fr.*
A range of trace element and mineral preparations (p.1350·1).

Microstix-3 *Ames, Israel; Bayer, USA.*
Test for nitrite in urine and for bacterial growth.

Microstix Candida *Ames, Israel.*
Test for *Candida albicans* in vaginal flora.

Microtid *Kener, Mex.*
Ranitidine (p.1246·3).

Microtrast
Sanova, Aust.†; Guerbet, Fr.; Guerbet, Ger.; Nicholas, Port.
Barium sulfate (p.1032·1).
Contrast medium for throat and oesophageal radiography.

Microtrim *Rosen, Ger.*
Co-trimoxazole (p.193·3).
Bacterial infections.

Microval
Wyeth-Ayerst, Austral.; Wyeth Lederle, Belg.; Wyeth Lederle, Denm.; Wyeth Lederle, Fr.; Wyeth, NZ; Aspen, S.Afr.; Wyeth, UK.
Levonorgestrel (p.1486·2).
Progestogen-only oral contraceptive.

Microvlar *Schering, Braz.*
Ethinylestradiol (p.1476·2); levonorgestrel (p.1486·2).
Combined oral contraceptive.

Microxen *Rayere, Mex.*
Norfloxacin (p.232·1).
Urinary-tract infections.

Microzide *Watson, USA.*
Hydrochlorothiazide (p.907·3).
Hypertension; oedema.

Mictasol
Note. This name is used for preparations of different composition.
Medgenix, Belg.
Camphor monobromide; methenamine (p.223·1); mallow fruit.
Formerly contained camphor monobromide, methenamine, mallow fruit, esculoside, and rutoside.
Anorectal disorders; urogenital disorders.

Millet Roux, Braz.
Mallow; camphor monobromide.
Urinary-tract infections.

Martin, Fr.
Mallow; methenamine (p.223·1).
Formerly contained mallow, camphor monobromide, and methenamine.
Urinary-tract disorders.

Mictasol Bleu
Note. This name is used for preparations of different composition.
Martin, Fr.
Mallow; camphor monobromide; methylene blue [methylthioninium chloride] (p.1012·3).
Urinary-tract infections.

Formenti, Ital.
Malva purpurea; methylene blue [methylthioninium chloride] (p.1012·3).
Genito-urinary tract disorders; haemorrhoids.

Mictasol com Sulfa *Millet Roux, Braz.*
Mallow; sulfachlorpyridazine (p.251·1); camphor (p.1589·3).
Urinary-tract infections.

Mictasone *Formenti, Ital.*
Hydrocortisone acetate (p.1073·3); tetracycline hydrochloride (p.258·3); mallow flowers; mallow leaves.
Genito-urinary tract infections; haemorrhoids.

Mictonetten *Apogepha, Ger.*
Propiverine hydrochloride (p.473·3).
Bladder disorders; urinary incontinence.

Mictonorm *Apogepha, Ger.*
Propiverine hydrochloride (p.473·3).
Bladder disorders; urinary incontinence.

Mictral
Sanofi Winthrop, Irl.; Sanofi Winthrop, UK.
Nalidixic acid (p.227·1); sodium citrate (p.1186·2); citric acid (p.1599·2); sodium bicarbonate (p.1186·2).
Urinary-tract infections.

Mictrex *Heralds, Braz.*
Co-trimoxazole (p.193·3); phenazopyridine (p.78·1).
Urinary-tract infections.

Mictrin *Econo Med, USA.*
Hydrochlorothiazide (p.907·3).
Hypertension; oedema.

Micturol Sedante *Bioresearch, Spain.*
Phenazopyridine hydrochloride (p.77·3); sulfamethizole (p.253·3).
Urinary-tract infections.

Micutrin *Searle, Ital.*
Pyrrolnitrin (p.393·3).
Fungal skin infections.

Micutrin Beta *Searle, Ital.*
Pyrrolnitrin (p.393·3); betamethasone valerate (p.1063·2).
Inflammatory fungal skin infections; onychomycosis.

Midacina *Lensa, Spain.*
Fluocinolone acetonide (p.1071·1); gramicidin (p.213·3); neomycin (p.228·1).
Infected skin disorders.

Midalgan
Note. This name is used for preparations of different composition.
Welcker-Lyster, Canad.
Histamine hydrochloride (p.1619·2); methyl nicotinate (p.55·1); glycol salicylate (p.42·2); capsaicin (p.23·1).
Musculoskeletal and joint disorders.

Sanofi Synthelabo, Port.
Histamine hydrochloride (p.1619·2); methyl nicotinate (p.55·1); glycol salicylate (p.42·2).
Musculoskeletal and joint disorders.

SmithKline Beecham Consumer, Switz.
Histamine hydrochloride (p.1619·2); methyl nicotinate (p.55·1); glycol salicylate (p.42·2); capsicum (p.1591·1).
Musculoskeletal and joint disorders.

Midamor
Merck Sharp & Dohme, Aust.; Merck Sharp & Dohme, Austral.; Merck Frosst, Canad.; Merck Sharp & Dohme, Hong Kong; Merck Sharp & Dohme, Neth.†; Merck Sharp & Dohme, Norw.†; Merck Sharp & Dohme, NZ; Merck Sharp & Dohme, Swed.; Merck Sharp & Dohme, Switz.; Merck, USA.
Amiloride hydrochloride (p.835·1).
Heart failure; hypertension; liver cirrhosis with ascites; oedema.

Midarine
Glaxo Wellcome, Ital.; Wellcome, Switz.
Suxamethonium chloride (p.1340·1).
Depolarising neuromuscular blocker.

Midaten *Farmacusi, Spain†.*
Piretanide (p.956·2).
Hypertension; oedema.

Midchlor *Schein, USA†.*
Isometheptene mucate (p.1624·2); dichloralphenazone (p.682·1); paracetamol (p.71·2).
Tension and vascular headaches.

Midecamin
Merck, Braz.; Merck, Mex.
Midecamycin (p.224·3) or midecamycin acetate (p.224·3).
Upper respiratory-tract infections.

Midecin *Farmaka, Ital.*
Midecamycin (p.224·3).
Bacterial infections.

Midelin *Quimica y Farmacia, Mex.*
Dipyrone (p.34·1).
Fever; pain.

Miderm *Mendelejeff, Ital.*
Miconazole (p.391·1) or miconazole nitrate (p.391·1).
Fungal and Gram-positive bacterial infections.

Midium *Teofarma, Ital.*
Vitamin A palmitate (p.1383·2); tocoferil acetate (p.1394·1); pyridoxine hydrochloride (p.1386·3).
Metabolic disorders.

Midol *ICN, Hong Kong.*
Aspirin (p.14·2); caffeine (p.761·3); cinnamedrine hydrochloride.
Pain.

Midol Douche *Bayer, Canad.†.*
Acetic acid (p.1571·2).
Vaginal cleansing.

Midol Extra Strength *Bayer, Canad.*
Paracetamol (p.71·2); caffeine (p.761·3); mepyramine maleate (p.421·1).
Formerly contained paracetamol, pamabrom, mepyramine maleate.
Dysmenorrhoea.

Midol IB *Glenbrook, USA†.*
Ibuprofen (p.43·2).
Formerly known as Midol 200.
Fever; osteoarthritis; pain; rheumatoid arthritis.

Midol Maximum Strength Multi-Symptom Menstrual *Sterling Health, USA.*
Paracetamol (p.71·2); mepyramine maleate (p.421·1).
Pain.

Midol Multi-Symptom *Bayer, Canad.†.*
Paracetamol (p.71·2); caffeine (p.761·3); mepyramine maleate (p.421·1).
Backache; bloating; dysmenorrhoea; headache.

Midol Original *Bayer, Canad.†.*
Aspirin (p.14·2); cinnamedrine; caffeine (p.761·3).
Pain.

Midol PM *Sterling Health, USA.*
Paracetamol (p.71·2); diphenhydramine (p.416·1).

Midol PMS *Glenbrook, USA.*
Paracetamol (p.71·2); pamabrom (p.952·1); mepyramine maleate (p.421·1).
Pain.

Midol PMS Extra Strength *Bayer, Canad.*
Paracetamol (p.71·2); pamabrom (p.952·1); mepyramine maleate (p.421·1).
Premenstrual syndrome.

Midol Regular *Bayer, Canad.*
Aspirin (p.14·2); caffeine (p.761·3).
Pain.

Midol Traditional *Bayer, Canad.*
Aspirin (p.14·2); caffeine (p.761·3).
Dysmenorrhoea.

Midolam *Rafa, Israel.*
Midazolam (p.692·3).
General anaesthesia; premedication.

Midolen *Degorts, Mex.*
Aspirin (p.14·2).
Fever; inflammation; pain.

Midon *Shire, Irl.*
Midodrine hydrochloride (p.933·3).
Orthostatic hypotension.

Midoride *Amrad, Austral.*
Amiloride hydrochloride (p.835·1).
Ascites; hypertension; oedema.

Midotens
Boehringer Ingelheim, Denm.; Boehringer Ingelheim, Mex.; Boehringer Ingelheim, Swed.
Lacidipine (p.919·1).
Hypertension.

Midran *Novo Nordisk, S.Afr.†*
Aprotinin (p.725·3).
Antidote to fibrinolytics; haemorrhage; pancreatitis.

Midriati *Llorens, Spain.*
Atropine sulfate (p.461·1); hyoscine hydrobromide (p.468·2); phenylephrine hydrochloride (p.1097·1).
Eye disorders; production of mydriasis.

Midrid *Shire, Hong Kong; Manx, UK.*
Isometheptene mucate (p.1624·2); paracetamol (p.71·2).
Formerly contained dichloralphenazone, isometheptene mucate, and paracetamol in the UK.
Migraine.

Midrin *Women First, USA.*
Isometheptene mucate (p.1624·2); dichloralphenazone (p.682·1); paracetamol (p.71·2).
Tension and vascular headaches.

Midriodavi *Davi, Port.*
Cyclopentolate hydrochloride (p.465·2).
Production of mydriasis.

Midro
Note.This name is used for preparations of different composition.
Wolfs, Belg.
Senna (p.1248·2).
Constipation.

Vaillant, Ital.
Senna (p.1248·2); liquorice (p.1231·2); peppermint leaves (p.1243·2); caraway (p.1591·2).
Constipation.

Crefar, Port.
Senna (p.1248·2); liquorice (p.1231·2); peppermint leaf (p.1243·2); clove (p.1596·3); calcatrippae; mallow.
Constipation.

Midro Abfuhr *Midro, Ger.*
Senna (p.1248·2).
Constipation.

Midro Pico *Midro, Ger.*
Sodium picosulfate (p.1249·3).
Constipation.

Midro Tee
Note.This name is used for preparations of different composition.
Sanova, Aust.
Senna (p.1248·2); peppermint leaf (p.1243·2); caraway (p.1591·2); liquorice (p.1231·2); delphinium consolida; mallow flowers.
Bowel evacuation; constipation.

Midro, Ger.
Senna (p.1248·2).
Constipation.

Midro-Tea *Midro, Israel.*
Senna (p.1248·2); peppermint leaf (p.1243·2); caraway (p.1591·2); liquorice (p.1231·2); delphinium consolida flower; mallow flower.
Constipation.

Miduret *PP Lab, Thai.*
Amiloride hydrochloride (p.835·1); hydrochlorothiazide (p.907·3).
Hepatic cirrhosis with ascites; hypertension; oedema.

Midy Vitamine C *SmithKline Beecham Sante, Fr.*
Ascorbic acid (p.1389·3).
Tonic; vitamin C deficiency.

Midysalb *Sanofi Winthrop, Ger.†*
Glycol salicylate (p.42·2); methyl nicotinate (p.55·1); histamine hydrochloride (p.1619·2).
Musculoskeletal and joint disorders; neuralgia.

Miegel *SAN, Ital.†*
Honey (p.1366·2); royal jelly (p.1659·3).

Mielocol *Herbes Universelles, Canad.*
Guaifenesin (p.1092·2); aralia racemosa; eucalyptol (p.1609·2); honey (p.1366·2); poplar buds (p.1653·2); sanguinaria (p.1660·3); white pine; wild cherry (p.1680·3).

Mielogen *Schering-Plough, Ital.*
Molgramostim (p.738·3).
Neutropenia induced by antineoplastics, bone marrow transplant, or ganciclovir.

Mielomade *Esfar, Port.*
Gamma-aminobutyric acid (p.1613·1).
Hypertension; mental function disorders.

Mielucin *Zambon, Braz.*
Busulfan (p.513·3).
Malignant neoplasms.

Mifegyne
Exelgyn, Denm.; Exelgyn, Fr.; Exelgyn, Swed.; Cosan, Switz.; Farillon, UK.
Mifepristone (p.1483·1).
Termination of pregnancy.

Mifeprex *Danco, USA.*
Mifepristone (p.1483·1).
Termination of pregnancy.

Miflonide
Novartis, Denm.; Novartis, Ital.; Novartis, Port.
Budesonide (p.1064·2).
Asthma.

Miformin *Greater Pharma, Thai.*
Metformin hydrochloride (p.332·3).
Diabetes mellitus.

Migea *Gea, Denm.; Gea, Fin.*
Tolfenamic acid (p.88·3).
Migraine.

Migent *Wayne, Mex.*
Gentamicin (p.212·1).
Bacterial infections.

Migergot *G & W, USA†.*
Ergotamine tartrate (p.452·1); caffeine (p.761·3).

Miglucan *Roche, Fr.*
Glibenclamide (p.321·3).
Diabetes mellitus.

Migpriv
Sanofi Synthelabo, Belg.; Sanofi Winthrop, Denm.; Leiras Synthelabo, Fin.; Synthelabo, Fr.; Sanofi Synthelabo, Ital.; Astra, Swed.; Synthelabo, Switz.
Lysine aspirin (p.50·3); metoclopramide hydrochloride (p.1235·2).
Migraine.

Migracin *SmithKline Beecham, Ital.*
Amikacin sulfate (p.148·1).
Bacterial infections.

Migradon *Schmidgall, Aust.*
Propyphenazone (p.80·2); paracetamol (p.71·2); caffeine (p.761·3).
Fever; pain.

Migraeflux MCP *Hennig, Ger.*
Paracetamol (p.71·2); metoclopramide hydrochloride (p.1235·2).
Migraine.

Migraeflux N *Hennig, Ger.*
Orange tablets, dimenhydrinate (p.415·2); paracetamol (p.71·2); green tablets, paracetamol; codeine phosphate (p.25·2).
Migraine and other vascular headaches.

Migraeflux orange N *Hennig, Ger.*
Dimenhydrinate (p.415·2); paracetamol (p.71·2).
Migraine and other vascular headaches.

Migrafen *Chatfield Laboratories, UK.*
Ibuprofen (p.43·2).

Migrafin *Sanofi Synthelabo, Neth.*
Lysine aspirin (p.50·3); metoclopramide hydrochloride (p.1236·3).
Migraine.

Migraine Ice *Mentholatum, UK.*
Water-based gel compress.
Migraine and other severe headache.

Migraine-Kranit *Krewel, Switz.*
Paracetamol (p.71·2); caffeine (p.761·3); chlorpheniramine [chlorphenamine] maleate (p.412·1).
Migraine and other vascular headaches.

Migraine-Kranit Nova *Codali, Belg.*
Caffeine (p.761·3); paracetamol (p.71·2); propyphenazone (p.80·2).
Migraine.

Migral
Note.This name is used for preparations of different composition.
Glaxo Wellcome, Austral.
Ergotamine tartrate (p.452·1); cyclizine hydrochloride (p.414·1); caffeine (p.761·3).

QIF, Braz.
Phenylephrine hydrochloride (p.1097·1); caffeine (p.761·3); dexbrompheniramine (p.410·2).
Migraine.

Migralam *Lambda, USA†.*
Isometheptene mucate (p.1624·2); caffeine (p.761·3); paracetamol (p.71·2).
Tension and vascular headaches.

Migralave N *Temmler, Ger.*
Buclizine hydrochloride (p.411·1); paracetamol (p.71·2).
Migraine and other vascular headaches.

Migraleve
Note.This name is used for preparations of different composition.
Pfizer Consumer, Irl.; Charwell, Singapore; Pfizer Consumer, UK.
Pink tablets, buclizine hydrochloride (p.411·1); paracetamol (p.71·2); codeine phosphate (p.25·2); yellow tablets, paracetamol; codeine phosphate.
Migraine.

Charwell, Israel; Llorens, Spain.
Buclizine hydrochloride (p.411·1); paracetamol (p.71·2); codeine phosphate (p.25·2); docusate sodium (p.1223·1).
Migraine.

Pfizer, Port.; Unipharma, Switz.
Buclizine hydrochloride (p.411·1); paracetamol (p.71·2); codeine phosphate (p.25·2).
Migraine.

Migralgine *Martin, Fr.*
Paracetamol (p.71·2); codeine phosphate (p.25·2); caffeine (p.761·3).
Formerly contained phenazone, amylocaine hydrochloride, codeine, and caffeine.
Pain.

Migralift *Charwell Pharmaceuticals, UK†.*
Pink tablets, buclizine hydrochloride (p.411·1); paracetamol (p.71·2); codeine phosphate (p.25·2); yellow tablets, paracetamol; codeine phosphate.
Migraine.

Migramax *Elan, UK.*
Lysine aspirin (p.50·3); metoclopramide hydrochloride (p.1235·2).
Migraine.

Migranal
Novartis, Aust.; Novartis, Canad.; Novartis, Ital.; Novartis, Swed.; Novartis, UK†; Novartis, USA.
Dihydroergotamine mesilate (p.450·3).
Migraine.

Migranat *Rowa, Irl.*
Caffeine (p.761·3); ergotamine tartrate (p.452·1); pipoxolan hydrochloride (p.1651·3).
Migraine and other vascular headaches.

Migrane *Novaquimica, Braz.*
Aspirin (p.14·2); ergotamine tartrate (p.452·1); homatropine (p.468·1); caffeine (p.761·3).
Migraine.

Migrane-Gastreu R16 *Reckeweg, Ger.*
Homoeopathic preparation.

Migrane-Kranit Kombi *Krewel, Ger.*
Etaverine hydrochloride (p.1608·2); paracetamol (p.71·2); propyphenazone (p.80·2).
Headache including migraine.

Migrane-Kranit mono *Krewel, Ger.*
Phenazone (p.77·2).
Pain.

Migrane-Kranit N *Krewel, Ger.*
Paracetamol (p.71·2); propyphenazone (p.80·2); codeine phosphate (p.25·2).
Headache including migraine.

Migrane-Neuridal *Krewel, Ger.*
Paracetamol (p.71·2); metoclopramide hydrochloride (p.1235·2).
Migraine and other vascular headaches.

Migranerton *Dolorgiet, Ger.*
Paracetamol (p.71·2); metoclopramide hydrochloride (p.1235·2).
Migraine and other vascular headaches.

Migranin *Boots Healthcare, Ger.*
Phenazone (p.77·2); caffeine (p.761·3).
Migraine; pain.

Migraprim *Inverni della Beffa, Ital.*
Lysine aspirin (p.50·3); metoclopramide hydrochloride (p.1235·2).
Migraine.

Migrastick *Arkopharma, UK.*
Lavender oil (p.1627·2); peppermint oil (p.1243·3).
Migraine.

Migratan S *Berlin-Chemie, Ger.*
Ergotamine tartrate (p.452·1); propyphenazone (p.80·2).
Migraine and other vascular headaches.

Migratine *Major, USA.*
Isometheptene mucate (p.1624·2); dichloralphenazone (p.682·1); paracetamol (p.71·2).
Tension and vascular headaches.

Migravess *Bayer, UK†.*
Aspirin (p.14·2); metoclopramide hydrochloride (p.1235·2).
Migraine.

Migretil *Bial, Port.*
Belladonna (p.463·1); caffeine (p.761·3); ergotamine (p.453·1); paracetamol (p.71·2).
Migraine.

Migrexa
Note.This name is used for preparations of different composition.
Lichtenstein, Ger.
Ergotamine tartrate (p.452·1).
Cluster headache; migraine.

Sanorania, Switz.
Ergotamine tartrate (p.452·1); caffeine (p.761·3).
Dysmenorrhoea; migraine and other vascular headaches.

Migril
Note.This name is used for preparations of different composition.
Glaxo Wellcome, Aust.; Glaxo Wellcome, Hong Kong; Glaxo Wellcome, Irl.; Glaxo Wellcome, Neth.†; Glaxo Wellcome, NZ; Glaxo Wellcome, S.Afr.; Glaxo Wellcome, Singapore; Wellcome, Switz.; CP Pharmaceuticals, UK.
Ergotamine tartrate (p.452·1); cyclizine hydrochloride (p.414·1); caffeine hydrate (p.761·3).
Migraine.

Sintofarma, Braz.
Sumatriptan succinate (p.456·1).
Migraine.

Migristene
Rhone-Poulenc Rorer, Mex.; Rhone-Poulenc Rorer, Spain†.
Dimetotiazine mesilate (p.415·2).
Migraine.

Migwell *Glaxo Wellcome, Fr.*
Ergotamine tartrate (p.452·1); caffeine (p.761·3); cyclizine hydrochloride (p.414·1).
Migraine.

Mijal *Juste, Spain.*
Butibufen (p.22·2).
Musculoskeletal, joint, and peri-articular disorders; pain.

Mijex *Pickles, UK.*
Diethyltoluamide (p.1431·2).
Insect repellent.

Mijex Extra *Pickles, UK.*
Butylacetylamino propionate.
Insect repellent.

Mikacin *Julphar, UAE.*
Amikacin sulfate (p.148·1).
Bacterial infections.

Mikan *Bonincontro & Gazzone, Ital.*
Amikacin sulfate (p.148·1).
Gram-negative bacterial infections.

mikanil N *Mickan, Ger.*
Glycol salicylate (p.42·2); benzyl nicotinate (p.20·2); Norway spruce oil.
Muscle and joint pain; soft-tissue disorders.

Mikavir *Salus, Ital.*
Amikacin sulfate (p.148·1).
Gram-negative bacterial infections.

Mikazul *Ederka, Mex.*
Amikacin (p.147·3).
Bacterial infections.

Mikelan
Lipha Sante, Fr.; Otsuka, Hong Kong; Otsuka, Jpn; Aventis, S.Afr.; Otsuka, Spain.
Carteolol hydrochloride (p.855·1).
Angina pectoris; arrhythmias; glaucoma; hypertension; ocular hypertension.

Mi-Ke-Sons *Sons, Mex.*
Ketoconazole (p.389·1).
Fungal infections.

Miketos *Chinoin, Mex.*
Ketoconazole (p.389·1).

Mikostat *Julphar, UAE.*
Nystatin (p.392·2).
Candidiasis.

Mikozal *Julphar, UAE.*
Miconazole nitrate (p.391·1).
Fungal skin infections.

Mikro-30 *Wyeth, Ger.*
Levonorgestrel (p.1486·2).
Progestogen-only oral contraceptive.

Mikrobac *Bode, Ger.*
Benzalkonium chloride (p.1133·2); dodecylbispropylenetriamine.
Surface disinfection.

Mikrozid *Schulke & Mayr, Ger.*
Alcohol (p.1130·3); propyl alcohol (p.1155·3).
Surface disinfection.

Mikutan N *Streuli, Switz.*
Aluminium acetate (p.1578·1); zinc oxide (p.1128·2).
Skin disorders.

Mila-Asma *Milano, Thai.*
Theophylline (p.777·2); guaifenesin (p.1092·2).
Obstructive airways disease.

Mila-Cono *Milano, Thai.*
Codeine phosphate (p.25·2); guaifenesin (p.1092·2).
Coughs.

Milafed *Milano, Thai.*
Triprolidine hydrochloride (p.427·2); pseudoephedrine hydrochloride (p.1099·2).
Allergic rhinitis; cold symptoms; hay fever; nasal congestion.

Milagin *Milano, Thai.*
Paracetamol (p.71·2); phenylpropanolamine hydrochloride (p.1098·1); dextromethorphan hydrobromide (p.1087·3); chlorpheniramine [chlorphenamine] maleate (p.412·1).
Cold symptoms.

Milamet *Milano, Thai.*
Cimetidine (p.1216·3).
Peptic ulcer.

Milamox *Milano, Thai.*
Amoxicillin trihydrate (p.149·2).
Bacterial infections.

Milanidazole *Milano, Thai.*
Metronidazole (p.594·1).
Anaerobic bacterial infections.

Mila-Tercon *Milano, Thai.*
Codeine phosphate (p.25·2); guaifenesin (p.1092·2); terpin hydrate (p.1101·2).
Coughs.

Milavir *Novartis Consumer, Spain.*
Aciclovir (p.612·3).
Herpes simplex infections.

Milax *Berlin-Chemie, Ger.*
Glycerol (p.1616·3).
Bowel evacuation; constipation.

Milbedoce Anabolico *Andromaco, Spain.*
Cobamamide (p.1388·3); hydroxocobalamin acetate (p.1388·3).
Tonic.

Milcopen *Leiras, Fin.*
Phenoxymethylpenicillin calcium (p.235·1) or phenoxymethylpenicillin potassium (p.235·1).
Bacterial infections.

Mildison
Yamanouchi, Denm.; Yamanouchi, Fin.; Yamanouchi, Irl.; Yamanouchi, Neth.; Yamanouchi, Norw.; Yamanouchi, Swed.; Yamanouchi, Switz.
Hydrocortisone (p.1073·3).
Skin disorders.

Miles Nervine *Miles, USA.*
Diphenhydramine hydrochloride (p.416·1).
Insomnia.

The symbol † denotes a preparation no longer actively marketed

milgamma Worwag, Ger.
Benfotiamine (p.1384·3); pyridoxine hydrochloride (p.1386·3).
Neurological symptoms associated with vitamin B deficiency.

milgamma N Worwag, Ger.
Thiamine hydrochloride (p.1385·1); pyridoxine hydrochloride (p.1386·3); cyanocobalamin (p.1388·1).
Myalgia; neuralgia; neuritis; polyneuropathy.

milgamma-NA Worwag, Ger.
Benfotiamine (p.1384·3); pyridoxine hydrochloride (p.1386·3).
Neurological symptoms associated with vitamin B deficiency.

Milid Sanochemia, Aust.; Opfermann, Ger.; Rotta, Hong Kong; Rottapharm, Ital.; Delta, Port.; Rotta, Thai.
Proglumide (p.1244·3).
Gastrointestinal disorders.

Milidon MPF, Singapore.
Paracetamol (p.71·2).
Cold and influenza symptoms; fever; pain.

Milidon Compound MPF, Singapore.
Chlorpheniramine [chlorphenamine] maleate (p.412·1); paracetamol (p.71·2); phenylpropanolamine hydrochloride (p.1098·1).
Nasal and sinus congestion; rhinitis.

Miliken Mucol Med Retard Teofarma, Spain.
Ampicillin sodium (p.150·3); ampicillin benzathine (p.151·3); bromhexine hydrochloride (p.1085·3).
Lignocaine [lidocaine] hydrochloride (p.1313·2) is included in this preparation to alleviate the pain of injection.
Respiratory-tract infections.

Miliken Mucol Retard Teofarma, Spain.
Ampicillin sodium (p.150·3); ampicillin benzathine (p.151·3); bromhexine hydrochloride (p.1085·3); guaifenesin hydrochloride (p.1092·2).
Lignocaine [lidocaine] hydrochloride (p.1313·2) is included in this preparation to alleviate the pain of injection.
Respiratory-tract infections.

Miliken Mucolitico Teofarma, Spain.
Ampicillin sodium (p.150·3); bromhexine hydrochloride (p.1085·3); guaifenesin (p.1092·2).
Lignocaine [lidocaine] hydrochloride (p.1313·2) is included in this preparation to alleviate the pain of injection.
Respiratory-tract infections.

Milk of Magnesia SmithKline Beecham Consumer, Irl.; SmithKline Beecham Consumer, UK.
Magnesium hydroxide (p.1233·1).
Constipation; dyspepsia.

Milkinol Schwarz, USA†.
Liquid paraffin (p.1407·1).
Constipation.

Milla Ilex, Ital.
Chamomile (p.1593·2).

Millerspas Aspen, S.Afr.
Hyoscyamine sulfate (p.469·3); atropine sulfate (p.461·1); hyoscine hydrobromide (p.468·2); phenobarbital (p.355·1).
Peptic ulcer; reduction of respiratory and gastrointestinal secretions; renal and biliary colic.

Milli Anovlar Schering, Fr.†.
Norethisterone acetate (p.1485·1); ethinylestradiol (p.1476·2).
Combined oral contraceptive.

Millibar Lisapharma, Hong Kong; Lisapharma, Ital.; Lisapharma, Singapore.
Indapamide (p.913·1).
Hypertension.

Millicortene Novartis, Switz.
Dexamethasone (p.1067·1).
Corticosteroid.

Millicorten-Vioform Novartis, Ger.
Dexamethasone pivalate (p.1067·3); clioquinol (p.190·2).
Infected skin disorders.

Milligynon Schering, Fr.
Norethisterone acetate (p.1485·1).
Progestogen-only oral contraceptive.

Millisrol Kayaku, Jpn.
Glyceryl trinitrate (p.897·3).
Angina pectoris; heart failure; hypertension during surgery; maintenance of hypotension during surgery.

Millypar Adcock Ingram Self Medication, S.Afr.†.
Magnesium hydroxide (p.1233·1); liquid paraffin (p.1407·1).
Constipation.

Milneuron N Worwag, Ger.
Benfotiamine; cyanocobalamin; pyridoxine hydrochloride (p.1350·1).
Neuralgia; neuritis; neurological symptoms associated with vitamin B deficiency.

Milneuron Plus Worwag, Ger.
Benfotiamine; cyanocobalamin; pyridoxine hydrochloride (p.1350·1); propyphenazone (p.80·2).
Neuralgia; neuritis; neurological symptoms associated with vitamin B deficiency.

Miloderme Schering-Plough, Port.
Alclometasone dipropionate (p.1061·1).
Skin disorders.

Milophene Milex, USA†.
Clomifene citrate (p.1465·3).
Anovulatory infertility.

Milorex Remedica, Thai.
Amiloride hydrochloride (p.835·1); hydrochlorothiazide (p.907·3).
Hepatic cirrhosis with ascites; hypertension; oedema.

Miloride Pharmacia Upjohn, Fin.
Amiloride hydrochloride (p.835·1); hydrochlorothiazide (p.907·3).
Hypertension; liver cirrhosis with ascites; oedema.

Milpar SmithKline Beecham, Irl.
Magnesium hydroxide (p.1233·1); liquid paraffin (p.1407·1).

Mil-Par Merck Consumer, UK.
Magnesium hydroxide (p.1233·1); liquid paraffin (p.1407·1).
Constipation.

Milrila Yamanouchi, Jpn.
Milrinone (p.934·1).

Milrosina Biogalenica, Spain.
Resorcinol (p.1122·2); borax (p.1586·1).
Mouth ulcers.

Milrosina Nistatina Biogalenica, Spain.
Hydrocortisone hydrogen succinate (p.1074·1); nystatin (p.392·2).
Oral candidiasis.

Milsan Merck, Mex.
Preparation for enteral nutrition (p.1350·1).
Gastro-enteritis.

Milsana Milte, Ital.
Zinc oxide (p.1128·2).
Barrier cream; nappy rash.

Miltaun Byk, Aust.
Meprobamate (p.691·1).
Anxiety disorders; premedication; skeletal muscle spasticity; sleep disorders.

Miltex Asta Medica, Fin.; Asta Medica, Fr.; Asta Medica, Ger.; Pras, Spain; Asta Medica, Swed.
Miltefosine (p.557·3).
Skin metastases of breast cancer.

Miltina HA Milte, Port.
Infant feed (p.1350·1).
Food hypersensitivity.

Miltina IPO Milte, Ital.
Infant feed (p.1350·1).
Food intolerance.

Milton
Note. This name is used for preparations of different composition.
Procter & Gamble, Braz.; Lachartre, Fr.; Procter & Gamble, Irl.†; Procter & Gamble, Ital.; Procter & Gamble (H&B Care), UK.
Liquid: Sodium hypochlorite (p.1156·2).
Disinfection.

Lachartre, Fr.; Procter & Gamble, Irl.†; Procter & Gamble (H&B Care), UK.
Sterilising tablets: Sodium dichloroisocyanurate (p.1156·1).
Disinfection.

Milton Anti-Bacterial Procter & Gamble, Austral.
Sodium dichloroisocyanurate (p.1156·1) or sodium hypochlorite (p.1156·2).
Disinfection of infant feeding equipment; disinfection of surfaces and equipment.

Milton Infa-Care Procter & Gamble, Austral.†.
Soap substitute.

Milton Milgard Procter & Gamble, Austral.†.
Emollient cleanser.
Nappy rash.

Miltown Wallace, USA.
Meprobamate (p.691·1).
Anxiety.

Milumel AR Milupa, Fr.
Infant feed (p.1350·1).
Regurgitation.

Milumil Milupa, Ital.; Milupa, Port.
Infant feed (p.1350·1).
Gastro-oesophageal reflux.

Milupa Wyeth-Ayerst, Canad.†.
A range of foods for special diets (p.1350·1).

Milupa Biber-C Milupa, Ital.
Carbohydrate, amino-acid, lipid, and mineral preparation with vitamin C (p.1350·1).
Nutritional supplement.

Milupa Biberfrutta Milupa, Ital.
Carbohydrate, amino-acid, and lipid preparation with vitamin C and iron (p.1350·1).
Nutritional supplement.

Milupa GES Milupa, Aust.; Milupa, Ital.
Potassium chloride; sodium chloride; sodium bicarbonate; anhydrous glucose (p.1185·2).
Diarrhoea; oral rehydration therapy.

Milupa HIST Milupa, Ital.†.
Food for special diets (p.1350·1).
Histidinaemia.

Milupa Hn 25 Milupa, Ital.; Byk Gulden, Mex.
Food for special diets (p.1350·1).
Diarrhoea; gluten intolerance.

Milupa HOM Milupa, Ital.
Food for special diets (p.1350·1).
Homocystinuria.

Milupa lpd Milupa, Irl.; Milupa, UK.
Low protein drink for special diets (p.1350·1).
Inherited disorders of amino-acid metabolism in childhood.

Milupa Lpf Milupa, Ital.
Food for special diets (p.1350·1).
Protein metabolism disorders; renal impairment.

Milupa LYS Milupa, Ital.
Food for special diets (p.1350·1).
Hyperlysinaemia.

Milupa MSUD Milupa, Ital.
Food for special diets (p.1350·1).
Maple syrup urine disease.

Milupa OS Milupa, Ital.
Food for special diets (p.1350·1).
Methylmalonic aciduria; propionic acidaemia.

Milupa PKU Milupa, Irl.; Milupa, Ital.
Food for special diets (p.1350·1).
Hyperphenylaninaemia; phenylketonuria.

Milupa Pregomin Milupa, Ital.
Preparation for enteral nutrition (p.1350·1).
Diarrhoea; disorders of fructose and galactose metabolism; food hypersensitivity; gastrointestinal resection; milk and soya intolerance.

Milupa Som Milupa, Ital.
Food for special diets (p.1350·1).
Disaccharide deficiency; fructosaemia; galactosaemia; milk intolerance.

Milupa TYR Milupa, Ital.
Food for special diets (p.1350·1).
Hypertyrosinaemia.

Milupa UCD Milupa, Ital.
Food for special diets (p.1350·1).
Argininosuccinic aciduria; citrullinaemia; hyperammonaemia; hyperargininaemia; ornithinaemia.

Milurit Thiemann, Ger.; Egis, Hong Kong.
Allopurinol (p.397·2).
Gout; hyperuricaemia; renal calculi.

Milvane Schering, Denm.; Schering, Ital.; Schering, Switz.
Gestodene (p.1479·1); ethinylestradiol (p.1476·2).
Triphasic oral contraceptive.

Milyzer Mitsui, Jpn.
Nateplase.

Mimedran Esteve, Spain.
Piperazine sultamate (p.106·2).
Hyperlipidaemias.

Minac 50 Spirig, Switz.
Minocycline hydrochloride (p.224·3).
Acne.

Minachlor Esoform, Ital.
Tosylchloramide sodium (p.1159·1).
Disinfection of wounds, burns, and external genitalia.

Minadex Seven Seas, UK.
Multivitamin preparation with or without minerals (p.1350·1).

Minadex Mix Grifols, Spain.
Multivitamin and mineral preparation (p.1350·1).

Minadex Mix Ginseng Grifols, Spain.
Multivitamins and minerals (p.1350·1); ginseng (p.1615·3).

Minakne Hexal, Ger.
Minocycline hydrochloride (p.224·3).
Skin disorders.

Minalfene Bouchara, Fr.
Alminoprofen (p.13·2).
Inflammation; pain.

Minalgin Streuli, Switz.
Dipyrone (p.34·1).
Colic; fever; pain.

Minalka Cedar Health, UK.
Mineral preparation with vitamin D (p.1350·1).
Musculoskeletal and joint disorders.

Minamino
MPS, Austral.
Vitamins, minerals, and amino acids with liver, spleen, and gastric mucosa (p.1350·1).
Dietary supplement.

Aspen Consumer, S.Afr.
Amino acids; vitamin B substances; minerals; organ extracts (p.1350·1).
Tonic.

Cortecs, UK.
Vitamin B substances; amino acids; minerals (p.1350·1).

Minaphlex SHS, UK.
Food for special diets (p.1350·1).
Phenylketonuria.

Minard's Liniment SmithKline Beecham Consumer, Canad.
Camphor (p.1589·3); ammonium hydroxide; turpentine.

Minax
Alphapharm, Austral.; Alphapharm, Hong Kong.
Metoprolol tartrate (p.931·2).
Angina pectoris; hypertension; migraine; myocardial infarction.

Minaza British Dispensary, Thai.
Miconazole nitrate (p.391·1).
Fungal skin, hair, and nail infections; Gram-positive bacterial skin infections.

Mincifit Arkopharma, Fr.
Black currant leaves (p.1389·3); green tea (p.1681·1).
Obesity.

Mindac Eagle, Austral.
Bacopa monnieri; ginkgo biloba; centella asiatica; withania somnifera; schizandra chinensis; capsicum; glutamine; calcium glycerophosphate; nux vomica.
Tonic.

Mindiab Pharmacia Upjohn, Denm.; Pharmacia Upjohn, Fin.; Pharmacia Upjohn, Norw.; Pharmacia Upjohn, Swed.
Glipizide (p.322·3).
Diabetes mellitus.

Mindol Pacific, NZ.
Mebendazole (p.102·2).
Worm infections.

Mindol-Merck Bracco, Ital.
Propyphenazone (p.80·2); caffeine (p.761·3); ethylmorphine hydrochloride (dionina) (p.35·2).
Pain.

Mineral Volchem, Ital.
Mineral preparation (p.1350·1).

Minerasol Pharno-Wedropharm, Ger.
Emser salts.
Nasal congestion; rhinitis.

Minerell Sanorell, Ger.
Vitamin and mineral preparation (p.1350·1).

Minervicomplex Provita, Ital.
Multivitamin and mineral preparation (p.1350·1).

Minesse
Wyeth Lederle, Fr.; Wyeth, Irl.
24 Tablets, gestodene (p.1479·1); ethinylestradiol (p.1476·2); 4 tablets, inert.
Combined oral contraceptive.

Minestril Parke, Davis, Belg.
Norethisterone acetate (p.1485·1); ethinylestradiol (p.1476·2).
Combined oral contraceptive; gynaecological disorders.

Minestrin Parke, Davis, Canad.
Norethisterone acetate (p.1485·1); ethinylestradiol (p.1476·2).
28-Day packs also contain 7 inert tablets.
Combined oral contraceptive.

Minha Vifor, Switz.
Naphazoline nitrate (p.1095·1).
Eye disorders.

28 mini Jenapharm, Ger.
Levonorgestrel (p.1486·2).
Progestogen-only oral contraceptive.

Mini New Gen Roche, Ital.†.
Vitamin, mineral, and carbohydrate preparation (p.1350·1).
Nutritional supplement.

Mini Ovulo Lanzas Ipsen, Spain.
Benzalkonium chloride (p.1133·2).
Contraceptive.

Mini Pregnon Nourypharma, Neth.
22 Tablets, lynestrenol (p.1480·1); ethinylestradiol (p.1476·2); 6 tablets, inert.
Combined oral contraceptive.

Mini Pseudo BDI, USA.
Pseudoephedrine hydrochloride (p.1099·2).
Formerly known as Mini Thin Pseudo.
Nasal congestion.

Mini Two-Way Action BDI, USA.
Ephedrine hydrochloride (p.1090·1); guaifenesin (p.1092·2).
Formerly known as Mini Thin Asthma Relief.

Minias Farmades, Ital.
Lormetazepam (p.689·3).
Insomnia.

Miniasal OPW, Ger.
Aspirin (p.14·2).
Thromboembolism prophylaxis.

Minidalton Hoechst Marion Roussel, Ital.†.
Parnaparin sodium (p.952·2).
Thrombosis prophylaxis.

Minidex Alcon, Braz.
Dexamethasone (p.1067·1).
Eye disorders.

Minidiab Pharmacia Upjohn, Aust.; Pharmacia Upjohn, Austral.; Pharmacia Upjohn, Belg.; Carlo Erba, Braz.; Pharmacia Upjohn, Fr.; Pharmacia Upjohn, Hong Kong; Pharmacia Upjohn, Ital.; Pharmacia Upjohn, NZ; Pharmacia Upjohn, Port.; Pharmacia Upjohn, S.Afr.; Pharmacia Upjohn, Singapore; Pharmacia Upjohn, Thai.
Glipizide (p.322·3).
Diabetes mellitus.

Minidine Sigma, Austral.
Povidone-iodine (p.1155·1).
Herpes labialis; pre-operative antisepsis; sore throat; wounds.

Minidril Wyeth Lederle, Fr.
Levonorgestrel (p.1486·2); ethinylestradiol (p.1476·2).
Combined oral contraceptive.

Minidyne Pedinol, USA.
Povidone-iodine (p.1155·1).
Skin disinfection.

Minifom Astra, Denm.†; AstraZeneca, Fin.; AstraZeneca, Norw.; Draco, Swed.
Dimethicone (p.1249·2) (Antifoam M).
Adjunct to gastrointestinal radiography and endoscopy; colic; flatulence.

Mini-Gamulin Rh Armour, USA†.
An anti-D immunoglobulin (p.1532·1).
Prevention of rhesus sensitisation.

Minigeste *Schering, Port.*
Gestodene (p.1479·1); ethinylestradiol (p.1476·2).
Combined oral contraceptive.

Mini-Gravigard *SPA, Ital.†*
Copper (p.1357·3).
Intra-uterine contraceptive device.

Minihep
Leo, Irl.; Leo, Neth.; CSL, NZ; Leo, NZ; Leo, UK.
Heparin sodium (p.902·1).
Thromboembolic disorders.

Minilax
Note.This name is used for preparations of different composition.
Eurofarma, Braz.
Sorbitol (p.1377·3).
Constipation.

Sam-On, Israel.
Glycerol (p.1616·3).
Constipation.

Minima *Yung Shin, Thai.*
Prazosin hydrochloride (p.958·1).
Hypertension.

Minims Artificial Tears
Smith & Nephew, Austral.; Chauvin, Irl.; Chauvin, UK.
Hyetellose (p.1501·1); sodium chloride (p.1196·1).
Dry eyes.

Mini-Pe
Searle, Denm.; Searle, Swed.
Norethisterone (p.1485·1).
Progestogen-only oral contraceptive.

Miniphase *Schering, Fr.*
Norethisterone acetate (p.1485·1); ethinylestradiol (p.1476·2).
Biphasic oral contraceptive.

Mini-Pill *Searle, Fin.*
Norethisterone (p.1485·1).
Progestogen-only oral contraceptive.

Minipres
Pfizer, Mex.; Nostrum, Spain.
Prazosin hydrochloride (p.958·1).
Benign prostatic hyperplasia; heart failure; hypertension; Raynaud's syndrome.

Minipress
Pfizer, Aust.; Pfizer, Austral.; Roerig, Belg.; Pfizer, Braz.; Pfizer, Canad.; Pfizer, Fr.; Pfizer, Ger.; Pfizer, Hong Kong; Pfizer, Neth.; Pfizer, S.Afr.; Pfizer, Singapore; Pfizer, Swed.; Pfizer, Thai.; Pfizer, USA.
Prazosin hydrochloride (p.958·1).
Benign prostatic hyperplasia; heart failure; hypertension; Raynaud's syndrome.

Minirin
Sigmapharm, Aust.; Rhone-Poulenc Rorer, Austral.; Ferring, Belg.; Ferring, Denm.; Ferring, Fin.; Ferring, Fr.; Ferring, Ger.; Solvay, Ger.; Ferring, Hong Kong; Ferring, Israel; IQFA, Mex.; Ferring, Norw.; Aventis, NZ; Ferring, Singapore; Ferring, Swed.; Ferring, Switz.; Ferring, Thai.
Desmopressin acetate (p.1281·2).
Diabetes insipidus; haemophilia A; nocturnal enuresis; polydipsia; polyuria; stimulation of factor VIII activity; test of renal concentrating capacity; von Willebrand's disease.

Minirin/DDAVP *Ferring, Ital.*
Desmopressin acetate (p.1281·2).
Diabetes insipidus; haemophilia A; nocturnal enuresis; polydipsia; polyuria; renal function tests.

Miniscap *Vifor, Switz.*
Cathine hydrochloride (p.1507·1).
Obesity.

Mini-sintrom *Novartis, Fr.*
Nicoumalone [acenocoumarol] (p.940·1).
Thromboembolic disorders.

Minisiston *Jenapharm, Ger.*
Ethinylestradiol (p.1476·2); levonorgestrel (p.1486·2).
Combined oral contraceptive; menstrual disorders.

Minisol *Ederka, Mex.*
Ambroxol (p.1084·3).

Ministat
Organon, Belg.†; Organon, Neth.
Lynestrenol (p.1480·1); ethinylestradiol (p.1476·2).
Combined oral contraceptive.

Miniten *Utopian, Thai.*
Nitrendipine (p.947·1).
Hypertension.

Minitran
Byk, Aust.; 3M, Austral.; 3M, Belg.; 3M, Canad.; 3M, Fin.; 3M, Hong Kong; 3M, Ital.; Riker, Mex.; 3M, Neth.; 3M, Norw.; 3M, NZ; 3M, Spain; 3M, Swed.; 3M, Switz.; 3M, Thai.; Schering-Plough, UK; 3M, USA.
Glyceryl trinitrate (p.897·3).
Angina pectoris; maintenance of venous patency at peripheral infusion sites.

MinitranS *3M, Ger.*
Glyceryl trinitrate (p.897·3).
Angina pectoris.

Minit-Rub *Bristol-Myers Products, USA.*
Methyl salicylate (p.55·1); menthol (p.1632·3); camphor (p.1589·3).
Muscle, joint, and soft-tissue pain; neuralgia.

Minizide *Pfizer, USA.*
Prazosin hydrochloride (p.958·1); polythiazide (p.957·1).
Hypertension.

Mino-50 *Wyeth Lederle, Belg.*
Minocycline hydrochloride (p.224·3).
Acne.

Mino T *Wyeth, S.Afr.†*
Minocycline hydrochloride (p.224·3).
Acne; bacterial infections.

Minobese *Restan, S.Afr.*
Phentermine hydrochloride (p.1514·1).
Obesity.

Minocalve *Pharmacia Upjohn, Port.*
Minoxidil (p.934·2).

Minocin
Wyeth Lederle, Aust.; Wyeth Lederle, Belg.; Wyeth-Ayerst, Canad.; Lederle, Hong Kong; Lederle, Irl.; Lederle, Israel; Wyeth Lederle, Ital.; Wyeth, Mex.; Lederle, Neth.; Wyeth Lederle, Port.; Wyeth, Singapore; Cyanamid, Spain; Lederle, Switz.; Wyeth-Ayerst, Thai.; Wyeth, UK; Lederle, USA.
Minocycline hydrochloride (p.224·3).
Bacterial infections; intestinal amoebiasis.

Minoclin *Vitamed, Israel.*
Minocycline hydrochloride (p.224·3).
Bacterial infections.

Minoclir *Jenapharm, Ger.*
Minocycline hydrochloride (p.224·3).
Bacterial infections.

Minodiab
Pharmacia Upjohn, Mex.; Kenfarma, Spain; Pharmacia, UK.
Glipizide (p.322·3).
Diabetes mellitus.

Minofen *Liomont, Mex.*
Paracetamol (p.71·2).
Fever; pain.

Minogal *Galen, UK.*
Minocycline (p.225·3).

Minogalen *Galen, Ger.*
Minocycline hydrochloride (p.224·3).
Acne.

Minolis *Pharmascience, Fr.*
Minocycline hydrochloride (p.224·3).
Bacterial infections.

Minomax *Wyeth, Braz.*
Minocycline hydrochloride (p.224·3).
Bacterial infections.

Minomex *Liferpal, Mex.*
Paracetamol (p.71·2).
Fever; pain.

Minomycin
Lederle, Austral.; Lederle, NZ; Wyeth, S.Afr.
Minocycline hydrochloride (p.224·3).
Amoebiasis; bacterial infections; trachoma.

Minona *Orion, Fin.*
Minoxidil (p.934·2).
Hypertension.

Minoplus *Rosen, Ger.*
Minocycline hydrochloride (p.224·3).
Bacterial infections.

Minopres *Precimex, Mex.*
Pancuronium bromide (p.1338·2).
Competitive neuromuscular blocker.

Minoral *Liferpal, Mex.*
Dipyrone (p.34·1).
Fever; pain.

Minorplex *Abigo, Swed.*
Multivitamin preparation (p.1350·1).

Minostad *Stada, Aust.*
Minocycline hydrochloride (p.224·3).
Bacterial infections.

Minotab
Wyeth Lederle, Belg.; Wyeth, Neth.†
Minocycline hydrochloride (p.224·3).
Bacterial infections.

Minotabs
Wyeth, NZ; Hexal, S.Afr.
Minocycline hydrochloride (p.224·3).
Acne; bacterial infections.

Minoton *Madaus, Spain.*
Magaldrate (p.1232·2).
Dyspepsia; gastro-oesophageal reflux; peptic ulcer.

Minotrex *Hikma, Port.†*
Minocycline hydrochloride (p.224·3).
Bacterial infections.

Minovag *Novag, Mex.*
Secnidazole (p.602·1).
Amoebiasis; giardiasis; trichomoniasis.

Minovital *Terapeutico, Ital.*
Minoxidil (p.934·2).
Alopecia.

Min-Ovral *Wyeth-Ayerst, Canad.*
Levonorgestrel (p.1486·2); ethinylestradiol (p.1476·2).
28-Day packs also contain 7 inert tablets.
Combined oral contraceptive.

Mino-Wolff *Wolff, Ger.*
Minocycline hydrochloride (p.224·3).
Acne.

Minox
Note.This name is used for preparations of different composition.
Riva, Canad.; Oftalder, Port.
Minoxidil (p.934·2).
Alopecia androgenetica.

Rowex, Irl.
Minocycline (p.225·3).
Bacterial infections.

Minoxi *Trima, Israel.*
Minoxidil (p.934·2).
Alopecia androgenetica.

Minoxidine *Sanval, Braz.*
Minoxidil (p.934·2).
Alopecia androgenetica.

Minoxigaine *Kenral, Canad.†*
Minoxidil (p.934·2).
Alopecia androgenetica.

Minoximen *Menarini, Ital.*
Minoxidil (p.934·2).
Alopecia.

Minoxitrim
Trima, Singapore; Unipharm, Singapore; Trima, Thai.
Minoxidil (p.934·2).
Alopecia androgenetica.

Minozinan *Rhone-Poulenc Rorer, Switz.†*
Methotrimeprazine [levomepromazine] maleate (p.692·1).
Anxiety; asthma; excitement; hypersensitivity reactions; insomnia; psychoses.

Minprog
Pharmacia Upjohn, Aust.; Pharmacia Upjohn, Ger.
Alprostadil (p.1439·3).
Maintenance of ductus arteriosus patency.

Minprostin
Pharmacia Upjohn, Denm.; Pharmacia Upjohn, Fin.; Pharmacia Upjohn, Norw.; Pharmacia Upjohn, Swed.
Dinoprostone (p.1441·3).
Labour induction.

Minprostin E₂ *Pharmacia Upjohn, Ger.*
Dinoprostone (p.1441·3).
Labour induction; production of cervical dilatation.

Minprostin F₂α *Pharmacia Upjohn, Ger.*
Dinoprost trometamol (p.1441·2).
Uterine bleeding.

Minra *Nakorn, Thai.*
Brompheniramine maleate (p.410·2); phenylephrine hydrochloride (p.1097·1); phenylpropanolamine hydrochloride (p.1098·1).
Hay fever; rhinitis.

Minrin *Ferring, Neth.*
Desmopressin acetate (p.1281·2).
Diabetes insipidus; haemorrhagic disorders; nocturnal enuresis; polyuria; test of renal concentrating capacity; uraemia.

Mint Sensodyne *Block, USA†.*
Potassium nitrate (p.1154·3).
Hypersensitive teeth.

Mintec
Key, Austral.; Monmouth, UK.
Peppermint oil (p.1243·3).
Irritable bowel syndrome; spastic colon syndrome.

Mintetten Truw *Truw, Ger.†*
Cowslip rhizome (p.1600·1); drosera (p.1606·1); thyme (p.1672·2).
Catarrh; cough.

Mintezol
Merck Sharp & Dohme, Austral.; Merck Frosst, Canad.; Merck Sharp & Dohme, Irl.†; Merck Sharp & Dohme, UK†; Merck, USA.
Tiabendazole (p.109·1).
Worm infections.

Mint-Lysoform *Lysoform, Ger.*
Myrrh tincture (p.1639·2); peppermint oil (p.1243·3).
Formerly known as Fluomint and contained potassium fluoride, myrrh tincture, and peppermint oil.
Mouth and throat disorders.

Mintox *Major, USA.*
Aluminium hydroxide (p.1210·3); magnesium hydroxide (p.1233·1).
Hyperacidity.

Mintox Plus *Major, USA.*
Aluminium hydroxide (p.1210·3); magnesium hydroxide (p.1233·1); simeticone (p.1249·2).
Hyperacidity.

Minulet
Wyeth Lederle, Aust.; Wyeth, Austral.; Wyeth Lederle, Belg.; Wyeth, Braz.; Wyeth Lederle, Denm.; Wyeth Lederle, Fin.; Wyeth Lederle, Fr.; Wyeth, Ger.; Wyeth-Ayerst, Hong Kong; Wyeth, Irl.; Wyeth-Ayerst, Israel; Wyeth Lederle, Ital.; Wyeth, Mex.; Wyeth, Neth.; Wyeth, NZ; Wyeth Lederle, Port.; Wyeth, Singapore; Wyeth, Spain; Wyeth, Switz.; Wyeth-Ayerst, Thai.; Wyeth, UK.
Gestodene (p.1479·1); ethinylestradiol (p.1476·2).
28-Day packs also contain 7 inert tablets.
Combined oral contraceptive.

Minulette *Akromed, S.Afr.*
21 Tablets, gestodene (p.1479·1); ethinylestradiol (p.1476·2); 7 tablets, inert.
Combined oral contraceptive.

Minuric *Sanofi Synthelabo, S.Afr.*
Benzbromarone (p.399·3).
Gout; hyperuricaemia.

Minurin *Ferring, Spain.*
Desmopressin (p.1281·2) or desmopressin acetate (p.1281·2).
Diabetes insipidus; haemorrhage; nocturnal enuresis; test of renal concentrating capacity.

Minus Fat *Ocean Health, Singapore.*
L112 Absorbitol.
Reduction of fat and bile acid absorption.

Minus Fat Extra *Ocean Health, Singapore.*
Gymnema silvestre; chromium polynicotinate.
Dietary aid.

Minute-Gel *Oral-B, USA.*
Acidulated phosphate fluoride (p.1375·3).
Dental caries prophylaxis.

Minutil *Henkel, Ger.*
Formaldehyde (p.1144·2); glyoxal (p.1145·3); glutaral (p.1145·2).
Surface disinfection.

MinVitin *Wander Health Care, Switz.*
Food for special diets (p.1350·1).
Obesity.

Mio Relax *Belmac, Spain.*
Carisoprodol (p.1327·1).
Skeletal muscle spasm.

Miocacin *Roussel, Port.*
Midecamycin acetate (p.224·3).
Bacterial infections.

Miocamen *Menarini, Ital.*
Midecamycin acetate (p.224·3).
Bacterial infections.

Miocamycin *Meiji, Jpn.*
Midecamycin acetate (p.224·3).
Bacterial infections.

Miocardin *Magis, Ital.*
Carnitine (p.1356·1).
Carnitine deficiency; myocardial ischaemia.

Miocarpine *Ciba Vision, Canad.*
Pilocarpine hydrochloride (p.1422·3).
Open-angle glaucoma.

Miochol
Ciba Vision, Austral.; Bournonville, Belg.†; Ciba Vision, Canad.; Ciba Vision, Fin.; Iolab, Israel; Ciba Vision, NZ; MCM, S.Afr.; Ciba Vision, Swed.†; Ciba Vision, Switz.; General Drugs, Thai.; Novartis Ophthalmics, UK; Ciba Vision, USA.
Acetylcholine chloride (p.1415·1).
Production of miosis in eye surgery.

Miochole *Ciba Vision, Fr.*
Acetylcholine chloride (p.1415·1).
Production of miosis in eye surgery.

Miochol-E
Ciba Vision, Ger.; OMJ, Hong Kong; Ciba Vision, Ital.; Ciba Vision, Singapore.
Acetylcholine chloride (p.1415·1).
Production of miosis in eye surgery.

Miociclin *QIF, Braz.*
Tetracycline hydrochloride (p.258·3).
Bacterial infections.

Mio-Citalgan *Merck, Braz.*
Carisoprodol (p.1327·1); caffeine (p.761·3); vitamin B substances (p.1350·1); metamizole calcium (p.34·2).
Skeletal muscle spasm.

Miocor *Ecobi, Ital.*
Carnitine (p.1356·1).
Carnitine deficiency; myocardial ischaemia.

Miocrin
Rubio, Singapore; Rubio, Spain.
Sodium aurothiomalate (p.82·3).
Lupus erythematosus; rheumatoid arthritis; Still's disease.

Miocuril *Terapeutico, Ital.*
Sodium uridine triphosphate.
Heart failure; muscular disorders.

Miodaron *Biosintetica, Braz.*
Amiodarone hydrochloride (p.836·1).
Arrhythmias.

Miodene *Bioprogress, Ital.*
Ubidecarenone (p.1677·1).
Cardiac disorders.

Miodrina *Apsen, Braz.*
Ritodrine hydrochloride (p.1659·1).
Premature labour.

Miodrone *Alter, Port.*
Amiodarone hydrochloride (p.836·1).
Arrhythmias; heart failure.

Mioflex
Note.This name is used for preparations of different composition.
Sanofi Winthrop, Braz.
Carisoprodol (p.1327·1); paracetamol (p.71·2); phenylbutazone (p.78·1).
Skeletal muscle spasm.

Braun, Port.; Braun, Spain.
Suxamethonium chloride (p.1340·1).
Depolarising neuromuscular blocker.

Miokacin *FIRMA, Ital.*
Midecamycin acetate (p.224·3).
Bacterial infections.

Miokalium *Bama, Spain†.*
Magnesium chloride (p.1190·3); potassium aspartate (p.1195·2); potassium chloride (p.1194·3).
Potassium depletion.

Miol *Robert, Spain.*
Omeprazole (p.1239·1) or omeprazole sodium (p.1239·1).
Gastro-oesophageal reflux; peptic ulcer; Zollinger-Ellison syndrome.

Miolastan *Sanofi Winthrop, Mex.*
Tetrazepam (p.708·1).

Miolene *Lusofarmaco, Ital.*
Ritodrine hydrochloride (p.1659·1).
Premature labour; threatened abortion.

Mionevrasi *Roche, Ital.*
Cyanocobalamin (p.1388·1); pyridoxine hydrochloride (p.1386·3); cocarboxylase (p.1385·2).
Lignocaine [lidocaine] hydrochloride (p.1313·2) is included in this preparation to alleviate the pain of injection.
Neuralgia; neuritis; vitamin B deficiencies.

Mionevrix *Ache, Braz.*
Carisoprodol (p.1327·1); dipyrone (p.34·1); vitamin B substances (p.1350·1).
Skeletal muscle spasm.

Miopat *Polifarma, Ital.*
Metildigoxin (p.930·2).
Heart failure.

Miorel *Fornet, Fr.*
Thiocolchicoside (p.1330·2).
Skeletal muscle spasm.

The symbol † denotes a preparation no longer actively marketed

Mios INTES, Ital.
Pilocarpine hydrochloride (p.1422·3); carbachol (p.1416·1); paraoxon (p.1421·3); procaine hydrochloride (p.1319·1).
Raised intra-ocular pressure.

Miosal Technilab, Canad.
Trolamine salicylate (p.90·1).
Pain.

Miosen Belmac, Spain.
Dipyridamole (p.877·2).
Thromboembolism prophylaxis.

Miostat Alcon, Austral.; Alcon, Belg.; Alcon, Canad.; Alcon, Hong Kong; Alcon, Israel; Pacific, NZ; Alcon, Singapore; Alcon, Switz.; Alcon, Thai.; Alcon, USA.
Carbachol (p.1416·1).
Production of miosis.

Miostenil Bial, Port.
Magnesium aspartate (p.1190·3); potassium aspartate (p.1195·2).

Miotic Double Asta Medica, Belg.†.
Physostigmine salicylate (p.1421·3); pilocarpine hydrochloride (p.1422·3).
Glaucoma; herniated iris.

Mioticol Farmigea, Ital.
Carbachol (p.1416·1).
Production of miosis.

Miotin Meiji, Thai.
Midecamycin acetate (p.224·3).
Bacterial infections.

Miotonal Caber, Ital.
Carnitine (p.1356·1).
Carnitine deficiency; myocardial ischaemia.

Miotyn Ibirn, Ital.
Ubidecarenone (p.1677·1).
Cardiac disorders.

Miovisin Farmigea, Ital.
Acetylcholine chloride (p.1415·1).
Production of miosis in eye surgery.

Miowas G Wasserman, Spain.
Gallamine triethiodide (p.1337·1).
Competitive neuromuscular blocker.

Miozets Dermofarm, Spain.
Benzocaine (p.1306·2); tyrothricin (p.267·1).
Mouth and throat disorders.

Miphar Pharbita, Israel.
Frusemide [furosemide] (p.893·1).
Hypertension; oedema.

Mi-Pilo Fischer, Israel.
Pilocarpine hydrochloride (p.1422·3).
Glaucoma; production of miosis.

Mipralin Lennon, S.Afr.‡.
Imipramine hydrochloride (p.291·1).
Depression.

Mipraz Amrad, Austral.
Prazosin hydrochloride (p.958·1).
Benign prostatic hyperplasia; heart failure; hypertension; Raynaud's syndrome.

MIR Rafa, Israel.
Morphine sulfate (p.56·1).
Pain.

Mirabel Allergan-Frumtost, Braz.
Tetryzoline hydrochloride (p.1101·2); zinc sulfate (p.1398·2) methylene blue [methylthioninium chloride] (p.1012·3).
Ocular congestion.

Mirabol Volchem, Ital.
Preparation for enteral nutrition (p.1350·1).

Miracef Tosi, Ital.
Propylene glycol cefatrizine (p.164·3).
Bacterial infections.

Miracid Berlin Pharm, Thai.
Omeprazole (p.1239·1).
Gastro-oesophageal reflux; peptic ulcer; Zollinger-Ellison syndrome.

Miraclar Iquinosa, Spain.
Naphazoline hydrochloride (p.1095·1).
Eye disorders.

Miraclid Mochida, Jpn.
Ulinastatin (p.1677·1).
Circulatory failure; pancreatitis.

Miraclin Farmacologico Milanese, Ital.
Doxycycline hyclate (p.200·1).
Bacterial infections.

Miracorten Novartis Consumer, Austral.; Max Ritter, Switz.†.
Ulobetasol propionate (p.1081·3).
Skin disorders.

Miradol Durbin, UK.
Paracetamol (p.71·2).

Miradon Schering, USA.
Anisindione (p.840·2).
Thromboembolic disorders.

Miraflow Ciba Vision, Austral.; Ciba Vision, Canad.; Ciba Vision, NZ; Ciba Vision, USA.
Range of solutions for contact lenses (p.1129·2).

Mirafur Orion, Fin.
Carmofur (p.516·1).
Breast cancer; ovarian cancer.

Miral Leiras, Fin.
Potassium chloride (p.1194·3); magnesium hydroxide (p.1233·1).
Potassium and magnesium deficiency.

MiraLax Braintree, USA.
Macrogol 3350 (p.1630·3).
Bowel evacuation.

Miraluma Du Pont, USA.
Technetium-99m sestamibi (p.1451·1).
Breast imaging.

Miramycin Atlantic, Hong Kong; Atlantic, Singapore; Atlantic, Thai.
Gentamicin sulfate (p.210·1).
Bacterial infections.

Miranax Grunenthal, Aust.; Roche, Denm.; Roche, Fin.; Syntex, Swed.†.
Naproxen sodium (p.61·1).
Gout; inflammation; musculoskeletal, joint, and periarticular disorders; pain.

Miranova Schering, Ger.
Ethinylestradiol (p.1476·2); levonorgestrel (p.1486·2).
Combined oral contraceptive.

Mirantal Ciba Vision, Spain†.
Phenylephrine hydrochloride (p.1097·1); medrysone (p.1075·3); neomycin sulfate (p.228·1); zinc sulfate (p.1398·2).
Infected eye disorders.

Mirapex Boehringer Ingelheim, Canad.; Pharmacia Upjohn, USA.
Pramipexole hydrochloride (p.1176·1).
Parkinsonism.

Mirapexin Pharmacia Upjohn, Irl.; Pharmacia Upjohn, Ital.; Pharmacia Upjohn, Spain; Pharmacia, UK.
Pramipexole (p.1176·1) or pramipexole hydrochloride (p.1176·1).
Parkinsonism.

Mirapront Pfizer, Aust.†.
Phentermine resinate (p.1514·1).
Obesity.

Mirapront N Mack, Illert., Ger.; Mack, Hong Kong; Mack, Singapore; Mack, Thai.
Cathine (p.1507·1) or cathine polystyroldivinylbenzolsulfonic acid (p.1507·1).
Obesity.

MiraSept Alcon, USA.
Hydrogen peroxide (p.1147·1) (p.1129·2).
Disinfecting solution for soft contact lenses.

Mirax Berlin Pharm, Singapore; Berlin Pharm, Thai.
Domperidone (p.1224·1).
Delayed gastric emptying; dyspepsia; nausea and vomiting.

Miraxid Leo, Aust.; Lovens, Swed.†.
Pivampicillin (p.237·2); pivmecillinam (p.237·3) or pivmecillinam hydrochloride (p.237·3).
Bacterial infections.

Mirazul Fardi, Spain.
Phenylephrine hydrochloride (p.1097·1).
Eye irritation.

Mircette Organon, USA.
21 Tablets, desogestrel (p.1470·3); ethinylestradiol (p.1476·2); 5 tablets, ethinylestradiol; 2 tablets, placebo.
Sequential oral contraceptive.

Mircol Rhone-Poulenc Rorer, Belg.†; Rhone-Poulenc Rorer, Neth.†; Italfarmaco, Spain.
Mequitazine (p.421·2).
Hypersensitivity reactions.

Mirena Schering, Aust.; Schering, Belg.; Schering, Fr.; Schering, Ger.; Schering, Hong Kong; Schering, Irl.; Leiras, Israel; Schering, Israel; Schering, Ital.; Schering, Neth.; Schering, NZ; Schering, Port.; Schering, S.Afr.; Schering, Singapore; Schering, Swed.; Schering, UK; Berlex, USA.
Levonorgestrel (p.1486·2).
Menorrhagia; progestogen-releasing intra-uterine contraceptive device.

Miretic Utopian, Thai.
Amiloride hydrochloride (p.835·1); hydrochlorothiazide (p.907·3).
Hypertension; oedema.

Mireze Allergan, Canad.
Nedocromil sodium (p.768·3).
Allergic conjunctivitis.

Mirfat Merckle, Ger.
Clonidine hydrochloride (p.860·1).
Hypertension.

Mirfudorm Merckle, Ger.
Oxazepam (p.697·1).
Anxiety; sleep disorders.

Mirfulan Ratiopharm, Aust.; Merckle, Ger.
Cod-liver oil (p.1357·2); zinc oxide (p.1128·2); hamamelis (p.1618·3); urea (p.1127·3).
Burns; skin disorders; wounds.

Mirfulan Spray N Merckle, Ger.
Cod-liver oil (p.1357·2); zinc oxide (p.1128·2); levomenol (p.1629·1).
Burns; skin disorders; wounds.

Mirfusot Merckle, Ger.
Thyme (p.1672·2).
Coughs and associated respiratory-tract disorders.

Mirrorroidin Sedabel, Braz.
Rutoside (p.1611·2); hamamelis (p.1618·3); aesculus (p.1574·1); zinc (p.1398·1); menthol (p.1632·3); benzocaine (p.1306·2).
Haemorrhoids.

Miroton Knoll, Ger.
Squill (p.1100·3); convallaria (p.1599·1); oleander (p.1643·3); adonis vernalis (p.1573·3).
Cardiovascular disorders.

Miroton N Knoll, Ger.
Adonis vernalis (p.1573·3); convallaria (p.1599·1); squill (p.1100·3).
Cardiac disorders.

Mirpan Dolorgiet, Ger.
Maprotiline hydrochloride (p.297·2).
Depression.

Mirsol Permamed, Switz.†.
Zipeprol hydrochloride (p.1102·3).
Adjunct in bronchial examination; coughs.

Mirtex P DMG, Ital.
Vitamin, mineral, and lipid preparation with myrtillus (p.1350·1).
Nutritional supplement.

Mirtilene SIFI, Ital.
Myrtillus (p.1639·2); betacarotene (p.1355·1); dl-alpha tocoferil acetate (p.1394·1).
Capillary disorders; eye disorders.

Mirtilene Forte SIFI, Ital.
Myrtillus (p.1639·2).
Eye disorders.

Mirtilus Llorens, Spain.
Betacarotene (p.1355·1); myrtillus (p.1639·2).
Eye disorders.

Mirtilvedo C Fitobucaneve, Ital.
Vitamin preparation with betacarotene, myrtillus, carrot, and rose fruit (p.1350·1).
Nutritional supplement.

Mirtiros Pharmafar, Ital.
Hamamelis (p.1618·3); myrtillus (p.1639·2); crataegus (p.1600·2).
Skin disorders.

Mirtivit SIFI, Singapore.
Food supplement (p.1350·1).

Miscidon Torlan, Spain.
Spironolactone (p.973·2); hydrochlorothiazide (p.907·3).
Hypertension; oedema.

Misodex Sepharma, Ital.
Misoprostol (p.1446·1).
NSAID-induced peptic ulcer.

Misofenac Sefarma, Ital.
Diclofenac sodium (p.30·3).
Misoprostol (p.1446·1) is included in this preparation in an attempt to limit adverse effects on the gastrointestinal mucosa.
Musculoskeletal and joint disorders.

Misone PD, Thai.
Miconazole nitrate (p.391·1).
Fungal skin, hair, and nail infections.

Misovan TO-Chemicals, Thai.
Ambroxol hydrochloride (p.1084·3).
Respiratory-tract disorders associated with increased or viscous mucus.

Mission Prenatal Mission Pharmacal, USA.
A range of multivitamin and mineral preparations with iron and folic acid (p.1350·1).
Iron-deficiency anaemias; prenatal and postpartum supplement.

Mission Surgical Supplement Mission Pharmacal, USA.
Ferrous gluconate (p.1360·1); multivitamins and minerals (p.1350·1).
Dietary supplement for pre- and postsurgical patients; iron-deficiency anaemias.

Mistabron UCB, Aust.; Bios, Belg.; UCB, Hong Kong; UCB, Neth.; UCB, S.Afr.; UCB, Singapore; UCB, Switz.; UCB, Thai.
Mesna (p.1011·3).
Respiratory-tract disorders associated with increased or viscous mucus.

Mistabronco UCB, Ger.
Mesna (p.1011·3).
Respiratory-tract disorders.

Mistalin Galderma, Neth.
Mizolastine (p.421·3).
Allergic rhinoconjunctivitis; urticaria.

Mistaline Galderma, Fr.†.
Mizolastine (p.421·3).
Allergic rhinoconjunctivitis; urticaria.

Mistamine Galderma, Belg.; Galderma, Denm.; Galderma, Irl.; Galderma, Port.; Galderma, Spain; Galderma, Swed.; Galderma, UK.
Mizolastine (p.421·3).
Allergic conjunctivitis; allergic rhinitis; urticaria.

Mistel Curarina Harras-Curarina, Ger.
Mistletoe (p.1636·2).
Circulatory disorders.

Mistel-Krautertabletten Salushaus, Ger.
Mistletoe (p.1636·2).
Cardiovascular disorders.

Mistelol-Kapseln Twardy, Ger.
Mistletoe (p.1636·2).
Cardiovascular disorders.

Misteltropfen II Bio-Diat, Ger.
Mistletoe (p.1636·2).
Circulatory disorders.

Misteltropfen Hofmanns Hofmann & Sommer, Ger.
Mistletoe (p.1636·2).
Cardiovascular disorders.

Mistick Boots Healthcare, Ital.
Geranium oil (p.1615·1); citronella oil (p.1596·3); lavender oil (p.1627·2).
Insect repellent.

Mistosil McGloin, Austral.†.
Magnesium trisilicate (p.1233·3); calcium carbonate (p.1215·1); magnesium carbonate (p.1232·3).
Hyperacidity.

Mistral Mediolanum, Ital.
Dermatan sodium sulfate (p.867·1).
Thrombosis prophylaxis.

Misubar Farmachimici, Ital.
Barrier preparation.
Nappy nash.

Misulban Nuovo ISM, Ital.
Busulfan (p.513·3).
Chronic myeloid leukaemia.

Misura Searle, Ital.
Soya lecithin (p.1628·1).

Misurid Plus Farmachimici, Ital.
Barrier cream.

Mitan Toyo, Hong Kong.
Vitamin B substances (p.1350·1).
Neuralgias; vitamin B deficiencies.

Mitchell Expel Anti Lice Spray Mitchell, UK.
Carbaryl (p.1429·2).
Pediculosis.

Mite-X Fischer, Israel.
Permethrin (p.1436·1).
Scabies.

Mitexan Asta Medica, Braz.
Mesna (p.1011·3).
Prevention of urotoxicity due to oxazaphosphorine antineoplastics.

Mithen Fidia, Ital.
Magnesium; vitamin E (p.1350·1); hypericum (p.290·2).
Nutritional supplement.

Mithracin Pfizer, Neth.†; Pfizer, Norw.; Bayer, USA.
Plicamycin (p.565·2).
Hypercalcaemia of malignancy; hypercalciuria of malignancy; testicular cancer.

Mithracine Pfizer, Fr.
Plicamycin (p.565·2).
Hypercalcaemia of malignancy; malignant neoplasms.

Miticocan Asta Medica, Braz.
Benzyl benzoate (p.1428·2).
Pediculosis; scabies.

Mitiderma Milo, Spain.
Camphor (p.1589·3); eucalyptus oil (p.1609·2); methyl salicylate (p.55·1); oleum pini sylvestris; menthol (p.1632·3).
Coughs; muscular pain; nasal congestion.

Mitil Aspen, S.Afr.
Prochlorperazine maleate (p.701·2).
Migraine; nausea and vomiting; nonpsychotic mental disorders; vestibular disorders.

Mitocin Bristol-Myers Squibb, Braz.
Mitomycin (p.558·1).
Malignant neoplasms.

Mitocin-C Bristol-Myers Squibb, Mex.
Mitomycin (p.558·1).
Malignant neoplasms.

Mitocor Zambon, Ital.
Ubidecarenone (p.1677·1).
Cardiac disorders.

Mitocortyl Sanofi Synthelabo, Fr.
Hydrocortisone (p.1073·3).
Skin disorders.

Mitolem Lemery, Mex.
Mitomycin (p.558·1).
Malignant neoplasms.

Mito-medac Medac, Ger.
Mitomycin (p.558·1).
Malignant neoplasms.

Mitostat Orion, Fin.
Mitomycin (p.558·1).
Malignant neoplasms.

Mitosyl
Note.This name is used for preparations of different composition.
Sanofi Synthelabo, Belg.
Cod-liver oil (p.1357·2); zinc oxide (p.1128·2); methyl salicylate (p.55·1).
Burns; skin disorders; wounds.
Synthelabo, Fr.; Sanofi Synthelabo, Ger.; Sanofi Synthelabo, Port.
Cod-liver oil (p.1357·2); zinc oxide (p.1128·2).
Burns; skin disorders; wounds.
Synthelabo, Spain.
Colecalciferol (p.1391·1); vitamin A (p.1382·1); zinc oxide (p.1128·2).
Burns; skin disorders; wounds.

Mitoxana Asta Medica, UK.
Ifosfamide (p.546·1).
Malignant neoplasms.

Mitran Hauck, USA.
Chlordiazepoxide hydrochloride (p.659·2).
Alcohol withdrawal syndrome; anxiety.

Mitroken Kendrick, Mex.
Ciprofloxacin hydrochloride (p.182·3).
Bacterial infections.

Mitrolan Robins, USA.
Polycarbophil calcium (p.1244·2).
Constipation; diarrhoea.

Mitroxone Columbia, Mex.
Mitozantrone [mitoxantrone] hydrochloride (p.559·3).
Malignant neoplasms.

Mittoval Schering, Ital.
Alfuzosin hydrochloride (p.833·2).
Benign prostatic hyperplasia.

Mivacron
Glaxo Wellcome, Aust.; Glaxo Wellcome, Austral.; Glaxo Wellcome,
Belg.; Glaxo Wellcome, Canad.; Glaxo Wellcome, Denm.; Glaxo
Wellcome, Fin.; Glaxo Wellcome, Fr.; Glaxo Wellcome, Ger.; Zeneca,
Ger.; Glaxo Wellcome, Hong Kong; Wellcome, Irl.; Glaxo Wellcome,
Israel; Glaxo Wellcome, Ital.; Glaxo Wellcome, Mex.; Glaxo Well-
come, Neth.; Glaxo Wellcome, Norw.; Glaxo Wellcome, NZ; Well-
come, Port.; Glaxo Wellcome, S.Afr.; Glaxo Wellcome, Singapore;
Wellcome, Spain; Glaxo Wellcome, Swed.; Wellcome, Switz.; Glaxo
Wellcome, Thai.; Glaxo Wellcome, UK; Abbott, USA.
Mivacurium chloride (p.1337·3).
Competitive neuromuscular blocker.

mivitase 2000 Biosyn, Ger.
Multivitamin and mineral preparation (p.1350·1).

Mixavit Julphar, UAE.
Multivitamin preparation (p.1350·1).

Mixavit-M Julphar, UAE.
Multivitamin and mineral preparation (p.1350·1).

Mixed Vegetable Tablets Dorwest, UK.
Rorippa nasturtium aquaticum; celery seed and plant
(p.1592·3); horseradish (p.1620·1); parsley (p.1648·3).
*Cystitis; minor bladder disorders; musculoskeletal and
joint disorders.*

Mixer Biomedica, Ital.
Atenolol (p.841·3); nifedipine (p.940·1).
Angina pectoris; hypertension.

Mixobar
Astra Tech, Denm.; Astra Tech, Fin.; Byk Gulden, Ital.; Astra Tech,
Norw.; Astra Tech, Swed.
Barium sulfate (p.1032·1).
Contrast medium for gastrointestinal radiography.

Mixogen Donmed, S.Afr.
Injection: Estradiol benzoate (p.1473·1); estradiol phenylpropionate (p.1473·2); testosterone propionate
(p.1492·2); testosterone phenylpropionate (p.1492·2);
testosterone isocaproate (p.1492·2).
Oestrogen deficiency.
Tablets†: Ethinylestradiol (p.1476·2); methyltestosterone (p.1482·3).
Androgenic; oestrogenic.

Mixotone Teofarma, Ital.
Polymyxin B sulfate (p.238·1); neomycin sulfate
(p.228·1); hydrocortisone sodium succinate
(p.1074·1); lignocaine [lidocaine] hydrochloride
(p.1313·2).
Formerly contained tetracycline hydrochloride, polymyxin B sulfate, neomycin sulfate, hydrocortisone sodium succinate, tetryzoline hydrochloride, and
lignocaine [lidocaine] hydrochloride.
Bacterial infections of the ear.

Mixtard Novo Nordisk, Ger.
Mixture of insulin injection (porcine, highly-purified)
30% and isophane insulin (porcine, highly-purified)
70% (p.324·1).
A 50:50 mixture may be known as Initard.
Diabetes mellitus.

Mixtard 10/90, 20/80, 30/70, 40/60, 50/50
Novo Nordisk, Austral.; Novo Nordisk, Denm.; Novo Nordisk, Fin.;
Novo Nordisk, Neth.; Novo Nordisk, Norw.; Novo Nordisk, S.Afr.;
Novo Nordisk, Spain; Novo Nordisk, Swed.
Mixtures of insulin injection (human, recombinant
monocomponent) and isophane insulin injection (hu-
man, recombinant monocomponent) respectively in the
proportions indicated (p.324·1).
Diabetes mellitus.

Mixtard 10, 20, 30, 40, and 50 HM
Novo Nordisk, Fr.; Novo Nordisk, Hong Kong; Novo Nordisk, Port.;
Novo Nordisk, Singapore; Novo Nordisk, Thai.
Mixtures of insulin injection (human, monocompo-
nent) 10%, 20%, 30%, 40%, and 50% and isophane in-
sulin injection (human, monocomponent) 90%, 80%,
70%, 60%, and 50%, respectively (p.324·1).
Diabets mellitus.

Mixtard 10, 20, 30, 40, and 50
Novo Nordisk, Irl.; Novo Nordisk, NZ; Novo Nordisk, Spain.
Mixtures of insulin injection (human) 10%, 20%, 30%,
40%, and 50% and isophane insulin injection (human)
90%, 80%, 70%, 60%, and 50% respectively (p.324·1).
Formerly known as Human Mixtard in Irl.
Diabetes mellitus.

**Mixtard HM 10/90, 15/85, 20/80, 30/70, 40/
60, and 50/50**
Novo Nordisk, Aust.; Novo Nordisk, Belg.
Mixtures of insulin injection (human, monocomponent) and isophane insulin suspension (human, monocomponent) respectively in the proportions indicated
(p.324·1).
Diabetes mellitus.

Mixtard HM 10, 20, 30, 40, 50 Novo Nordisk, Switz.
Mixtures of insulin injection (human, monocomponent) 10%, 20%, 30%, 40%, and 50% and isophane insulin injection (human, monocomponent) 90%, 80%,
70%, 60%, and 50%, respectively (p.324·1).
Diabetes mellitus.

Mixtard Human Novo Nordisk, Ger.†
Mixture of soluble insulin (human) 30% and isophane
insulin (human) 70% (p.324·1).
A 50:50 mixture may be known as Initard.
Diabetes mellitus.

Mixtard 30 MC Novo Nordisk, Switz.
Mixture of insulin injection (porcine, monocomponent) 30% and isophane insulin injection (porcine,
monocomponent) 70% (p.324·1).
Diabetes mellitus.

Miya-BM Miyarisan, Jpn.
Clostridium butyricum.
Restoration of gastrointestinal flora.

Mizar Searle, Ital.
Flurithromycin ethyl succinate (p.207·3).
Bacterial infections.

Mizolen Synthelabo, Spain.
Mizolastine (p.421·3).
Allergic conjunctivitis; allergic rhinitis; urticaria.

Mizollen
Sanofi Synthelabo, Belg.; Sanofi Winthrop, Denm.; Leiras Synthelabo,
Fin.; Synthelabo, Fr.; Sanofi Synthelabo, Ger.; Sanofi Synthelabo, Ital.;
Sanofi Synthelabo, Neth.; Sanofi Synthelabo, Port.; Synthelabo,
Switz.; Schwarz, UK.
Mizolastine (p.421·3).
Allergic conjunctivitis; allergic rhinitis; urticaria.

Mizolmex Ofimex, Mex.
Mebendazole (p.102·2).

ML 20 Blackmores, Austral.
Magnesium phosphate (p.1191·1); dibasic potassium
phosphate (p.1193·1); dried yeast (p.1398·1); lecithin
(p.1628·1); d-alpha tocoferil acid succinate (p.1394·1).
Magnesium deficiency.

ML Cu 250 CCD, Fr.†
Copper-wound plastic (p.1357·3).
Intra-uterine contraceptive device.

ML Cu 375 CCD, Fr.†
Copper-wound plastic (p.1357·3).
Intra-uterine contraceptive device.

M-long Grunenthal, Ger.
Morphine sulfate (p.56·1).
Pain.

MM Diplovax Pasteur Merieux, Ger.
A measles and mumps vaccine (more attenuated End-
ers' and Jeryl Lynn strains, respectively) (p.1548·3).
Acitve immunisation.

MM Expectorante Farmasa, Braz.
Potassium iodide (p.1522·3); lobelia (p.1510·2); hyo-
scyamus (p.470·1).
Respiratory-tract congestion.

M-M Vax
Merck Sharp & Dohme, Aust.†; Chiron Behring, Ger.; Pro Vaccine,
Switz.
A measles and mumps vaccine (Enders' attenuated Ed-
monston and Jeryl Lynn (level B) strains respectively)
(p.1548·3).
Active immunisation.

MMR Pasteur Merieux, Denm.
A measles, mumps, and rubella vaccine (Enders Edmonston, Jeryl Lynn, and Wistar RA 27/3 strains, respectively) (p.1549·1).
Active immunisation.

MMR II
CSL, Austral.; Prodome, Braz.; Merck Frosst, Canad.; Merck Sharp &
Dohme, Hong Kong; Aventis, Irl.; Merck Sharp & Dohme, Israel; Pas-
teur Merieux, Ital.; Merck Sharp & Dohme, Mex.; Merck Sharp &
Dohme, NZ; Merck Sharp & Dohme, S.Afr.†; Merck Sharp & Dohme,
Singapore; Pasteur Merieux, Swed.; Pro Vaccine, Switz.; Merck Sharp
& Dohme, Thai.; Pasteur Merieux, UK; Merck, USA.
A measles, mumps, and rubella vaccine (Enders' atten-
uated Edmonston, Jeryl Lynn (B level), and Wistar RA
27/3 strains respectively) (p.1549·1).
Active immunisation.

MMR Triplovax Pasteur Merieux, Ger.
A measles, mumps, and rubella vaccine (More attenuated Enders', Jeryl Lynn, and Wistar RA 27/3 strains,
respectively) (p.1549·1).
Active immunisation.

MMR Vax
Merck Sharp & Dohme, Aust.; Pasteur Merieux, Belg.; Chiron Behring, Ger.
A measles, mumps, and rubella vaccine (Enders' attenuated Edmonston, Jeryl Lynn B, and Wistar RA 27/3
strains, respectively) (p.1549·1).
Active immunisation.

MND Malaysia Chemist, Singapore.
Metronidazole (p.594·1).
Amoebiasis; trichomoniasis.

Mnemo Organico Blue Cross, Ital.†
Royal jelly (p.1659·3); liver.
Nutritional supplement.

Mnesis Takeda, Ital.
Idebenone (p.1623·1).
Cerebrovascular disorders.

MN-Fusin Pisa, Mex.
Manganese (p.1371·3).

Moban
Du Pont, Hong Kong; Endo, USA.
Molindone hydrochloride (p.694·3).
Psychoses.

Mobec Boehringer Ingelheim, Ger.
Meloxicam (p.51·3).
Ankylosing spondylitis; rheumatoid arthritis.

Mobemide Unipharm, Israel.
Moclobemide (p.299·3).
Depression.

Moben Elofar, Braz.
Mebendazole (p.102·2).
Worm infections.

Mobic
Boehringer Ingelheim, Aust.; Boehringer Ingelheim, Belg.; Boehringer
Ingelheim, Denm.; Boehringer Ingelheim, Fin.; Boehringer Ingelheim,
Fr.; Boehringer Ingelheim, Hong Kong; Boehringer Ingelheim, Irl.; Boe-
hringer Ingelheim, Ital.; Boehringer Ingelheim, Norw.; Boehringer In-
gelheim, S.Afr.; Boehringer Ingelheim, Singapore; Boehringer

Ingelheim, Swed.; Boehringer Ingelheim, Thai.; Boehringer Ingelheim,
UK; Abbott, USA; Boehringer Ingelheim, USA.
Meloxicam (p.51·3).
Musculoskeletal and joint disorders.

Mobicox
Promeco, Mex.; Boehringer Ingelheim, Switz.
Meloxicam (p.51·3).
*Gout; inflammation; musculoskeletal, joint and peri-
articular disorders; pain.*

Mobidin Ascher, USA.
Magnesium salicylate (p.50·3).
Fever; inflammation; pain.

Mobiflex
Roche, Canad.; Roche, Irl.; Roche, UK.
Tenoxicam (p.87·2).
*Musculoskeletal, joint, peri-articular, and soft-tissue
disorders.*

Mobiforton Sanofi Synthelabo, Ger.
Tetrazepam (p.708·1).
Skeletal muscle spasm; spasticity.

Mobigesic Ascher, USA.
Magnesium salicylate (p.50·3); phenyltoloxamine cit-
rate (p.423·1).
Pain.

Mobilat
Note.This name is used for preparations of different composition.
Sankyo, Aust.; Sankyo, Belg.; Sankyo, Fin.; Sankyo, Hong Kong; Byk
Madaus, S.Afr.†; Sankyo, Singapore; Sankyo, Switz.†; Sankyo, Thai.
Supraadrenal extract (p.1080·1); a heparinoid (p.905·2);
salicylic acid (p.1122·3).
Musculoskeletal, joint, and soft-tissue disorders.

Luitpold, Braz.; Sankyo, Ger.; Byk Gulden, Mex.; Sankyo, Neth.
A heparinoid (p.905·2); salicylic acid (p.1122·3).
Peri-articular and soft-tissue disorders.

Luitpold, Ger.†
Tablets: Ibuprofen (p.43·2).
Fever; pain.

Sankyo, Ger.
Topical spray: Indometacin (p.44·3).
Musculoskeletal, joint, and soft-tissue disorders.

Sankyo, Ital.
Hydrocortisone (p.1073·3); a heparinoid (p.905·2); salicylic acid (p.1122·3).
*Musculoskeletal and joint trauma; peri-articular and
soft-tissue disorders.*

Sankyo, Port.†
Prednisolone (p.1077·3); a heparinoid (p.905·2); sali-
cylic acid (p.1122·3).
Peri-articular and soft-tissue disorders.

Mobilat N Sankyo, Switz.
A heparinoid (p.905·2); salicylic acid (p.1122·3).
Joint and soft-tissue disorders.

Mobilis
Alphapharm, Austral.; Alphapharm, Singapore; Merck, Singapore.
Piroxicam (p.79·1).
Musculoskeletal and joint disorders.

Mobilisin
Note.This name is used for preparations of different composition.
Sankyo, Aust.; Sankyo, Belg.; Sankyo, Ger.; Sankyo, Ital.; Sankyo,
Switz.
Flufenamic acid (p.41·1); glycol salicylate (p.42·2) or
salicylic acid (p.1122·3); a heparinoid (p.905·2).
*Musculoskeletal, joint, peri-articular, and soft-tissue
disorders; neuralgias.*

Sankyo, Port.
Cream: Flufenamic acid (p.41·1); a heparinoid
(p.905·2).
Topical gel: Flufenamic acid (p.41·1); salicylic acid
(p.1122·3); a heparinoid (p.905·2).
Musculoskeletal, joint, and peri-articular disorders.

Mobilisin Composto Luitpold, Braz.
Flufenamic acid (p.41·1); a heparinoid (p.905·2); gly-
col salicylate (p.42·2).
Musculoskeletal and joint disorders.

Mobilisin plus Sankyo, Aust.
Flufenamic acid (p.41·1); a heparinoid (p.905·2); ben-
zyl nicotinate (p.20·2).
Formerly contained flufenamic acid, a heparinoid, ben-
zyl nicotinate, and glycol salicylate.
Musculoskeletal and joint disorders.

Mobilyzer Omni, UK.
Green-lipped mussel (p.1618·2).
Nutritional supplement for joint care.

Mobisyl Ascher, USA.
Trolamine salicylate (p.90·1).
Muscle, joint, and soft-tissue pain; neuralgia.

Mobloc Astra, Ger.; Promed, Ger.
Felodipine (p.888·3); metoprolol succinate (p.932·1).
Hypertension.

Moclamine Roche, Fr.
Moclobemide (p.299·3).
Depression.

Moctanin Ethitek, USA.
Monoctanoin (p.1636·3).
Gallstones.

Mocydone Pharmasant, Thai.
Domperidone (p.1224·1).
Digestive disorders; dyspepsia; nausea and vomiting.

Mod IRBI, Ital.†
Domperidone (p.1224·1).
Gastrointestinal disorders.

Modal Rafa, Israel.
Sulpiride (p.706·1).
*Gastrointestinal disorders; peptic ulcer; psychiatric
disorders; vertigo.*

Modalim
Sanofi Synthelabo, Neth.; Sanofi Synthelabo, Singapore; Sanofi Win-
throp, UK.
Ciprofibrate (p.858·3).
Hyperlipidaemias.

Modalina Sanofi Synthelabo, Ital.
Trifluoperazine hydrochloride (p.710·3).
Psychiatric disorders.

Modamide Merck Sharp & Dohme-Chibret, Fr.
Amiloride hydrochloride (p.835·1).
Ascites; hypertension; oedema.

Modane
Note.This name is used for preparations of different composition.
Cooperation Pharmaceutique, Fr.
Calcium pantothenate (p.1374·1); senna (p.1248·2).
Formerly contained calcium pantothenate and dantron.
Constipation.

Reig Jofre, Spain.
Calcium sennoside A (p.1248·3); calcium sennoside B
(p.1248·3).
Constipation.

Savage, USA†.
Phenolphthalein (p.1244·1).
Constipation.

Modane Bulk Adria, USA.
Psyllium hydrophilic mucilloid (p.1229·1).
Constipation.

Modane Plus Adria, USA†.
Phenolphthalein (p.1244·1); docusate sodium
(p.1223·1).
Constipation.

Modane Soft Adria, USA.
Docusate sodium (p.1223·1).
Constipation.

Modantis Surf Ski International, UK.
Antazoline hydrochloride (p.408·3); titanium dioxide
(p.1126·1); allantoin (p.1110·1); cetrimide (p.1137·1).
Minor burns and scalds; sunburn.

Modaplate Berk, UK†.
Dipyridamole (p.877·2).
Thromboembolism prophylaxis.

Modasomil Ratiopharm, Aust.
Modafinil (p.1512·3).
Narcoleptic syndrome with or without cataplexy.

Modaton Armstrong, Mex.
Calcium pantothenate (p.1374·1); dantron (p.1221·3).
Constipation.

Modecate
Bristol-Myers Squibb, Austral.; Squibb, Canad.; Sanofi Winthrop, Fr.;
Bristol-Myers Squibb, Hong Kong; Bristol-Myers Squibb, Irl.; Bristol-
Myers Squibb, Israel; Bristol-Myers Squibb, Ital.; Bristol-Myers Squibb,
S.Afr.; Bristol-Myers Squibb, Singapore; Squibb, Spain; Bristol-Myers
Squibb, Thai.; Sanofi Winthrop, UK.
Fluphenazine decanoate (p.684·3).
Psychoses.

Modecate Acutum Bristol-Myers Squibb, S.Afr.†
Fluphenazine hydrochloride (p.684·3).
Psychoses.

Modenol
Note.This name is used for preparations of different composition.
Boehringer Mannheim, Aust.†
Butizide (p.853·1); reserpine (p.967·3); rescinnamine
(p.967·3); raubasine (p.967·2); potassium chloride
(p.1194·3).
Hypertension.

Roche, Ger.
Butizide (p.853·1); reserpine (p.967·3).
Hypertension.

Moderatan Theranol-Deglaude, Fr.†
Diethylpropion hydrochloride (p.1508·3).
Obesity.

Moderator Faes, Spain†.
Celiprolol hydrochloride (p.856·1).
Angina pectoris; hypertension.

Moderin Acne Pharmacia Upjohn, Spain.
Aluminium chlorohydrate (p.1110·2); sulfur
(p.1123·3); methylprednisolone acetate (p.1076·1).
Acne.

Moderine Uniao Quimica, Braz.
Mazindol (p.1510·3); diazepam (p.674·3).
Obesity.

Modern Herbals Cold & Catarrh Lane, UK.
Althaea (p.1577·1); echinacea (p.1606·2); sambucus
(p.1660·3).
Catarrh; sinus congestion.

Modern Herbals Cold & Congestion Lane, UK.
Lobelia (p.1510·2); tolu solution (p.1101·3).
*Catarrh; cold symptoms; congestion; hay fever; rhini-
tis.*

Modern Herbals Cough Mixture Lane, UK.
Ipecacuanha (p.1093·1); marrubium (p.1094·2); squill
vinegar (p.1100·3).
Catarrh; cold symptoms; coughs; sore throat.

Modern Herbals Laxative Lane, UK.
Senna (p.1248·2); aloin (p.1210·2); cascara (p.1216·2).
Constipation.

Modern Herbals Menopause Lane, UK.
Parsley (p.1648·3); vervain (p.1679·3); clivers
(p.1596·3); senna (p.1248·2).
Menopausal disorders.

Modern Herbals Muscular Pain Lane, UK.
Camphor (p.1589·3); menthol (p.1632·3); eucalyptus
oil (p.1609·2); methyl salicylate (p.55·1); turpentine oil
(p.1676·3).
Muscle pain.

Modern Herbals Pile *Lane, UK.*
Ointment: Hamamelis (p.1618·3); compound benzoin tincture; zinc oxide (p.1128·2).
Tablets: Cascara (p.1216·1); slippery elm (p.1665·1).
Haemorrhoids.

Modern Herbals Rheumatic Pain *Lane, UK.*
Celery leaf (p.1592·3); menyanthes (p.1633·1); cimicifuga (p.1595·2).
Musculoskeletal and joint pain.

Modern Herbals Sleep Aid *Lane, UK.*
Passion flower (p.1649·1).
Insomnia.

Modern Herbals Stress *Lane, UK.*
Motherwort (p.1637·3); valerian (p.1678·3); vervain (p.1679·3); passion flower (p.1649·1).
Irritability; stresses and strains.

Modern Herbals Trapped Wind & Indigestion *Lane, UK.*
Activated charcoal (p.1000·2).
Diarrhoea; dyspepsia; flatulence; heartburn.

Modern Herbals Water Retention *Lane, UK.*
Bearberry (p.1583·3); clivers (p.1596·3); lappa (p.1627·1).
Water retention.

Modicef *Ipso, Ital.*
Cefonicid sodium (p.168·1).
Lignocaine [lidocaine] hydrochloride (p.1313·2) is included in this preparation to alleviate the pain of injection.
Gram-negative bacterial infections.

Modicon
Janssen-Cilag, Neth.; Ortho McNeil, USA.
Norethisterone (p.1485·1); ethinylestradiol (p.1476·2).
28-Day packs also contain 7 inert tablets.
Combined oral contraceptive.

Modiem *Piam, Ital.*
Cefonicid sodium (p.168·1).
Lignocaine [lidocaine] hydrochloride (p.1313·2) is included in this preparation to alleviate the pain of injection.
Bacterial infections.

Modifast
Novartis Consumer, Austral.; Wander Health Care, Switz.
Food for special diets (p.1350·1).
Obesity.

Modifenac
Alpharma, Denm.; Alpharma, Norw.
Diclofenac sodium (p.30·3).
Inflammation; musculoskeletal and joint disorders.

Modifical *Gunther, Braz.*
Ondansetron hydrochloride (p.1241·3).
Nausea and vomiting induced by cytotoxics or radiotherapy.

Modified Seravit *Scientific Hospital Supplies, Austral.†*
Multivitamin and mineral preparation (p.1350·1).

Modil *General Drugs, Thai.*
Minoxidil (p.934·2).
Hypertension.

Modilac AR *Sodilac, Fr.†*
Infant feed (p.1350·1).
Regurgitation in infants.

Modilac HA *Sodilac, Fr.*
Infant feed (p.1350·1).
Milk-protein allergy.

Modilac sans Lactose *Sodilac, Fr.*
Infant feed (p.1350·1).
Diarrhoea; lactose intolerance.

ModimMunal *OM, Ger.*
Escherichia coli antigens.
Arthritis.

Modina *Pentafarma, Port.*
Nimodipine (p.946·1).
Neurological deficit following subarachnoid haemorrhage.

Modiodal
Lafon, Denm.; Lafon, Fr.; Nourypharma, Neth.; Aneid, Port.; CEPA, Spain.
Modafinil (p.1512·3).
Narcoleptic syndrome.

Modip *Promed, Ger.; Astra, Ger.*
Felodipine (p.888·3).
Hypertension.

Modisal *Lagap, UK.*
Isosorbide mononitrate (p.916·2).
Angina pectoris.

Modiscop *Brady, Aust.*
Morphine hydrochloride (p.56·1); ethylmorphine hydrochloride (p.35·2); hyoscine hydrobromide (p.468·2).
Pain.

Moditen
Squibb, Canad.; Sanofi Winthrop, Fr.; Bristol-Myers Squibb, Irl.†; Sanofi Winthrop, UK.
Fluphenazine enantate (p.684·3) or fluphenazine hydrochloride (p.684·3).
Anxiety; disturbed behaviour; psychoses.

Moditen Depot *Bristol-Myers Squibb, Ital.*
Fluphenazine decanoate (p.684·3).
Psychoses.

Modivid
Hoechst Marion Roussel, Irl.; Hoechst Marion Roussel, Ital.; Hoechst Marion Roussel, Mex.; Hoeport, Port.; Hoechst Marion Roussel, Thai.
Cefodizime sodium (p.167·3).
Lignocaine [lidocaine] hydrochloride (p.1313·2) or lignocaine [lidocaine] hydrochloride (p.1313·2) may be included in the

intramuscular injection to alleviate the pain of injection.
Bacterial infections.

Modizide *Amrad, Austral.*
Amiloride hydrochloride (p.835·1); hydrochlorothiazide (p.907·3).
Ascites; hypertension; oedema.

Modomed *Medifive, Thai.*
Domperidone (p.1224·1).
Digestive disorders; dyspepsia; heartburn; nausea and vomiting.

Modopar *Roche, Fr.*
Levodopa (p.1169·2); benserazide hydrochloride (p.1164·2).
Parkinsonism.

Modrasone
Dominion, Irl.; Dominion, UK.
Alclometasone dipropionate (p.1061·1).
Skin disorders.

Modrenal *Wanskerne, UK.*
Trilostane (p.1674·3).
Breast cancer; Cushing's syndrome; hyperaldosteronism.

Modual
Note.This name is used for preparations of different composition.
Mead Johnson, Austral.; Mead Johnson, NZ.
Maltodextrin (p.1371·2).
Carbohydrate supplement.

Mead Johnson, Port.; Mead Johnson Nutritionals, USA.
Glucose polymers (p.1350·1).
Carbohydrate supplement.

Moducren
Merck Sharp & Dohme-Chibret, Fr.; Merck Sharp & Dohme, Hong Kong; Merck Sharp & Dohme, Irl.; Merck Sharp & Dohme, Mex.; Merck Sharp & Dohme, Neth.†; Merck Sharp & Dohme, Port.; Merck Sharp & Dohme, S.Afr.; Merck Sharp & Dohme, Switz.; Merck Sharp & Dohme, UK.
Amiloride hydrochloride (p.835·1); hydrochlorothiazide (p.907·3); timolol maleate (p.982·1).
Hypertension.

Moducrin
Merck Sharp & Dohme, Aust.; Merck Sharp & Dohme, Ger.
Amiloride hydrochloride (p.835·1); hydrochlorothiazide (p.907·3); timolol maleate (p.982·1).
Hypertension.

Modula *Antonetto, Ital.*
Polycarbophil calcium (p.1244·2).
Constipation; diarrhoea.

Modulamin *Braun, Switz.*
Amino-acid infusion with or without electrolytes (p.1350·1).
Parenteral nutrition.

Modulanzime *Andromaco, Port.*
Bromopride (p.1215·1); dimethicone (p.1249·2); pepsin (p.1649·1); amylase (p.1579·3); fungal lipase.
Gastrointestinal disorders.

Modulator *Servier, Spain.*
Benfluorex hydrochloride (p.844·2).
Diabetes mellitus; hyerlipidaemias.

Modulen IBD *Nestle, Fr.*
Preparation for enteral nutrition (p.1350·1).
Crohn's disease.

Modulite *Eurorga, Fr.†*
Trimebutine (p.1675·1); sorbitol (p.1377·3).
Constipation.

Modulon
Axcan, Canad.; Parke, Davis, Fr.
Trimebutine maleate (p.1675·1).
Gastrointestinal disorders.

Modu-Puren *Isis Puren, Ger.*
Amiloride hydrochloride (p.835·1); hydrochlorothiazide (p.907·3).
Hypertension; oedema.

Moduret
Merck Frosst, Canad.; Du Pont, Irl.; Du Pont, UK.
Amiloride hydrochloride (p.835·1); hydrochlorothiazide (p.907·3).
These ingredients can be described by the British Approved Name Co-amilozide.
Ascites; heart failure; hypertension; oedema.

Moduretic
Merck Sharp & Dohme, Aust.; Merck Sharp & Dohme, Austral.; Merck Sharp & Dohme, Belg.; Prodome, Braz.; Merck Sharp & Dohme, Denm.; Merck Sharp & Dohme, Fin.; Du Pont, Fr.; Merck Sharp & Dohme, Hong Kong; Du Pont, Irl.; Merck Sharp & Dohme, Ital.; Merck Sharp & Dohme, Mex.; Merck Sharp & Dohme, Neth.; Merck Sharp & Dohme, NZ; Merck Sharp & Dohme, Port.; Merck Sharp & Dohme, S.Afr.; Merck Sharp & Dohme, Swed.; Merck Sharp & Dohme, Switz.; Merck Sharp & Dohme, Thai.; Du Pont, UK; Merck, USA.
Amiloride hydrochloride (p.835·1); hydrochlorothiazide (p.907·3).
These ingredients can be described by the British Approved Name Co-amilozide.
Ascites; heart failure; hypertension; oedema.

Moduretic Mite *Merck Sharp & Dohme, Norw.*
Amiloride hydrochloride (p.835·1); hydrochlorothiazide (p.907·3).
Hypertension; oedema.

Moduretik *Du Pont, Ger.*
Amiloride hydrochloride (p.835·1); hydrochlorothiazide (p.907·3).
Ascites; hypertension; oedema.

Modus *Almirall, Spain.*
Nimodipine (p.946·1).
Mental function impairment; neurological deficit following subarachnoid haemorrhage.

Modustatina *Sanofi Winthrop, Ital.*
Somatostatin acetate (p.1297·3).
Adjunct in gastrointestinal radiography; diabetic ketoacidosis; gastrointestinal haemorrhage; pancreatic disorders.

Modustatine
Sanofi Synthelabo, Belg.; Sanofi Winthrop, Fr.
Somatostatin acetate (p.1297·3).
Aid to gastrointestinal examinations; gastrointestinal haemorrhage; postoperative gastrointestinal fistulae.

Moex
Ercopharm, Denm.†; Schwarz, Fr.
Moexipril hydrochloride (p.935·3).
Hypertension.

Mofesal *Medice, Ger.*
Mofebutazone (p.55·3).
Rheumatism; superficial thrombophlebitis.

Mofesal N *Medice, Ger.*
Mofebutazone sodium (p.55·3).
Lignocaine [lidocaine] hydrochloride (p.1313·2) is included in this preparation to alleviate the pain of injection.
Rheumatism; superficial thrombophlebitis.

Mogadan *ICN, Ger.*
Nitrazepam (p.695·2).
Sleep disorders.

Mogadon
ICN, Aust.; Dermatech, Austral.; Sanico, Belg.; ICN, Canad.; Medilink, Denm.; CSP, Fr.; Roche, Hong Kong; ICN, Irl.; ICN, Ital.; ICN, Neth.†; Medilink, Norw.; Pharmaco, S.Afr.; Medilink, Swed.; ICN, Switz.; ICN, UK.
Nitrazepam (p.695·2).
Epilepsy; sleep disorders.

Mogasinte *CPH, Port.*
Domperidone (p.1224·1).
Adjunct in gastrointestinal examinations; dyspepsia; nausea and vomiting.

Mogetic *Azupharma, Ger.*
Morphine sulfate (p.56·1).
Pain.

Mohexal *Hexal, Austral.*
Moclobemide (p.299·3).
Depression.

Moist Again *Lake, USA.*
Vaginal lubricant.

Moi-Stir
Paladin, Canad.; Kingswood, USA.
Carmellose sodium (p.1499·3); electrolytes (p.1180·1); sorbitol (p.1377·3).
Dry mouth.

Moisture Drops
Note.This name is used for preparations of different composition.
Bausch & Lomb, Canad.
Hypromellose (p.1501·3); glycerol (p.1616·3); povidone (p.1503·2).
Dry eye; eye irritation.

Bausch & Lomb, USA.
Hypromellose (p.1501·3); dextran 70 (p.729·2); glycerol (p.1616·3).
Dry eyes.

Moisture Eyes *Co-Pharma, UK.*
Hypromellose (p.1501·3).
Keratoconjunctivitis sicca; lubrication of artificial eyes and hard contact lenses.

Moisture Shield *Avon, Canad.*
SPF 15: Octinoxate (p.1517·3); oxybenzone (p.1518·1).
Sunscreen.

Moisturel
Westwood-Squibb, Canad.
White soft paraffin (p.1407·3); dimethicone (p.1410·1).
Dry skin disorders.

Westwood-Squibb, USA.
Emollient.
Dry skin disorders.

Molax *Siam Bheasach, Thai.*
Domperidone (p.1224·1) or domperidone maleate (p.1224·1).
Gastrointestinal disorders.

Molcer *Wallace Mfg Chem., UK.*
Docusate sodium (p.1223·1).
Removal of ear wax.

Moldina *Juventus, Spain.*
Bifonazole (p.381·1).
Fungal skin and nail infections.

Molevac
Parke, Davis, Aust.; Parke, Davis, Ger.; Parke, Davis, Switz.†
Pyrvinium embonate (p.108·2).
Enterobiasis.

Molfenac *Amsa, Ital.*
Diclofenac epolamine (p.31·3).
Inflammation; musculoskeletal and joint disorders; pain.

Molipaxin
Hoechst Marion Roussel, Irl.; Aventis, S.Afr.; Hoechst Marion Roussel, UK.
Trazodone hydrochloride (p.310·1).
Depression; mixed anxiety depressive states.

Mol-Iron *Schering-Plough, USA†.*
Ferrous sulfate (p.1360·3).
Iron-deficiency anaemias.

Mollifene *Pfeiffer, USA.*
Urea hydrogen peroxide (p.1159·3).
Ear wax removal.

Mollipect *Tika, Swed.*
Bromhexine hydrochloride (p.1085·3); ephedrine hydrochloride (p.1090·1).
Coughs.

Molsi-Azu *Azupharma, Ger.*
Molsidomine (p.936·1).
Ischaemic heart disease.

Molsicor *Betapharm, Ger.*
Molsidomine (p.936·1).
Angina pectoris.

Molsidain *Hoechst Marion Roussel, Spain.*
Molsidomine (p.936·1).
Angina pectoris.

Molsidirex *Irex, Fr.*
Molsidomine (p.936·1).

Molsidolat *Hoechst Marion Roussel, Aust.*
Molsidomine (p.936·1).
Angina pectoris.

Molsihexal
Hexal, Aust.; Hexal, Ger.
Molsidomine (p.936·1).
Angina pectoris.

molsiket *Schwarz, Ger.*
Molsidomine (p.936·1).
Ischaemic heart disease.

Molsi-Puren *Isis Puren, Ger.*
Molsidomine (p.936·1).
Ischaemic heart disease.

Molybdene Injectable *Aguettant, Fr.*
Ammonium molybdate (p.1372·2).
Parenteral nutrition.

Molypen *American Pharmaceutical, USA.*
Ammonium molybdate (p.1372·2).
Parenteral nutrition.

Mom *Nestle, Mex.*
Nutritional supplement during pregnancy and lactation (p.1350·1).

Mom Gel *Candioli, Ital.*
Phenothrin (p.1436·2).
Pediculosis.

Mom Lozione Preventiva *Candioli, Ital.*
Benzyl benzoate (p.1428·2).
Insect repellent.

Mom Piretro Emulsione *Candioli, Ital.*
Tetramethrin (p.1437·3); piperonyl butoxide (p.1436·2).
Pediculosis.

Mom Shampoo Antiparassitario *Candioli, Ital.*
Tetramethrin (p.1437·3); phenothrin (p.1436·2).
Pediculosis.

Mom Shampoo Schiuma *Candioli, Ital.*
Phenothrin (p.1436·2).
Pediculosis.

Mom Zanzara *Candioli, Ital.*
Benzyl benzoate (p.1428·2); ethyl hexanediol.
Insect repellent.

Momendol *Angelini, Ital.*
Naproxen sodium (p.61·1).
Fever; inflammation; musculoskeletal and joint disorders; pain.

Moment *Angelini, Ital.*
Ibuprofen (p.43·2).
Fever; pain.

Momentol *Squibb, Spain.*
Co-trimoxazole (p.193·3).
Bacterial infections; Pneumocystis carinii pneumonia.

Momentum
Note.This name is used for preparations of different composition.
Wyeth Lederle, Aust.; Whitehall, Neth.
Paracetamol (p.71·2).
Fever; pain.

Whitehall, USA.
Aspirin (p.14·2); phenyltoloxamine citrate (p.423·1).
Backache.

Momentum Analgetikum *Much, Ger.†*
Paracetamol (p.71·2).
Fever; pain.

Momentum Muscular Backache Formula
Whitehall, USA.
Magnesium salicylate (p.50·3).
Pain.

Momicine *Farmacusi, Spain.*
Midecamycin acetate (p.224·3).
Bacterial infections.

Monafed *Monarch, USA.*
Guaifenesin (p.1092·2).
Coughs.

Monafed DM *Monarch, USA.*
Guaifenesin (p.1092·2); dextromethorphan hydrobromide (p.1087·3).
Coughs.

Mona-Lisa *Mona Lisa, Israel.*
Copper-wound plastic (p.1357·3).
Intra-uterine contraceptive device.

Monapax *Rhone-Poulenc Rorer, Ger.*
Homoeopathic preparation.

Monarc-M *American Red Cross, USA.*
A factor VIII preparation (p.734·1).
Haemorrhagic disorders.

Monaspor *Grunenthal, Aust.*
Cefsulodin sodium (p.174·2).
Pseudomonas aeruginosa infections.

The symbol † denotes a preparation no longer actively marketed

Monaxin Therabel, Belg.
Clarithromycin (p.186-2).
Bacterial infections.

Monazole Theramex, Mon.
Sertaconazole nitrate (p.393-3).
Vaginal candidiasis.

Monazole Technilab, Canad.
Miconazole nitrate (p.391-1).
Fungal vaginal infections.

Moneva Schering, Fr.
Gestodene (p.1479-1); ethinylestradiol (p.1476-2).
Combined oral contraceptive.

Moni BASF, Ger.; Sanponiog, Ger.
Isosorbide mononitrate (p.916-2).
Angina pectoris; heart failure; pulmonary hypertension.

Monicor Pierre Fabre, Fr.
Isosorbide mononitrate (p.916-2).
Angina pectoris; heart failure.

Monistat Chugai, Jpn.
Miconazole nitrate (p.391-1).
Fungal infections.

Monilac Chugai, Jpn.
Lactulose (p.1230-1).
Constipation; hyperammonaemia.

Monilen Recip, Swed.
Urea (p.1127-3).
Dry skin.

Monistat Janssen-Cilag, Austral.; McNeil Consumer, Canad.; Janssen-Cilag, Switz.; Advanced Care, USA.
Miconazole nitrate (p.391-1).
Fungal skin infections; vulvovaginal candidiasis.

Monit Sanofi Synthelabo, UK.
Isosorbide mononitrate (p.916-2).
Angina pectoris.

Monitan Wyeth-Ayerst, Canad.
Acebutolol hydrochloride (p.825-1).
Angina pectoris; hypertension.

Monit-Puren Isis Puren, Ger.
Isosorbide mononitrate (p.916-2).
Angina pectoris; hypertension.

mono corax corax, Ger.
Isosorbide mononitrate (p.916-2).
Heart failure; ischaemic heart disease; myocardial infarction; pulmonary hypertension.

Mono Demetrin Parke, Davis, Ger.
Prazepam (p.701-1).
Anxiety disorders; sleep disorders.

Mono Maycor Parke, Davis, Ger.; Godecke, Ger.
Isosorbide mononitrate (p.916-2).
Heart failure; ischaemic heart disease; myocardial infarction.

Mono Mack Pfizer, Austral.; Ger.; Mack, Hong Kong; Armstrong, Mex.; Mack, Neth.†; Mack, Singapore; Mack, Thai.
Isosorbide mononitrate (p.916-2).
Angina pectoris; heart failure; pulmonary hypertension.

Mono Praecimed Molimin, Ger.
Paracetamol (p.71-2).
Fever; pain.

Mono Wolff Wolff, Ger.
Isosorbide mononitrate (p.916-2).
Angina pectoris; heart failure; pulmonary hypertension.

Monobios CT, Ital.
Cefonicid sodium (p.168-1).
Bacterial infections.

Monobeta Betapharm, Ger.
Isosorbide mononitrate (p.916-2).
Angina pectoris; heart failure.

Monobac Bristol-Myers Squibb, Mex.
Aztreonam (p.154-2).
Gram-negative bacterial infections.

Monocal Mercian, USA.
Calcium carbonate (p.1215-1); monofluorophosphate.
Nutritional supplement.

Monocaps Freeda, USA.
Multivitamin and mineral preparation with iron and folic acid (p.1350-1).

Monocetin Novoquimica, Braz.
Tetracycline hydrochloride (p.258-3); bromelains (p.1586-3).
Bacterial infections.

Monocid SmithKline Beecham, Belg.; SmithKline Beecham, Hong Kong; Procter & Gamble, Ital.; Decomed, Port.; SmithKline, Spain; SmithKline Beecham, USA.
Cefonicid sodium (p.168-1).
Bacterial infections.

Mono & Disaccharide Free Diet Powder (Product 3232A) Mead Johnson, Austral.
Preparation for enteral nutrition (p.1350-1).
Impaired glucose transport; intractable diarrhoea; lactase, sucrase, or maltase deficiency; test for fructose utilisation.

Mono-Cedocard Byk, Neth.; Pharmacia Upjohn, UK†.
Isosorbide mononitrate (p.916-2).
Angina pectoris.

Monocilline Andeabol, Switz.†.
Phenoxymethylpenicillin potassium (p.235-1).
Bacterial infections.

Monocinque Isis, Ger.; CTI, Israel.
Isosorbide mononitrate (p.916-2).
Angina pectoris; heart failure; myocardial infarction.

Monoclair Hennig, Ger.
Isosorbide mononitrate (p.916-2).
Ischaemic heart disease; myocardial infarction; pulmonary hypertension.

Monoclate-P Centeon, Braz.; Centeon, Fr.; Centeon, Ger.; Centeon, Irl.; Centeon, Israel; Centeon, Mex.; Centeon, Spain; Centeon, Swed.; Aventis Behring, UK; Centeon, USA.
A factor VIII preparation (p.734-1).
Haemorrhagic disorders.

Monocline Dorms-Adrian, Fr.
Doxycycline hyclate (p.200-1).
Bacterial infections.

Monoclox Oclassen, USA.
Cloxacillin sodium (p.192-1).
Bacterial infections.

Monocor Medochemie, Hong Kong; Medochemie, Singapore; Medochemie, Thai.
Bisoprolol fumarate (p.850-1).
Angina pectoris; hypertension.

Monocord Dexxon, Israel.
Isosorbide mononitrate (p.916-2).
Angina pectoris; hypertension.

Monocordil Baldacci, Braz.
Isosorbide mononitrate (p.916-2).
Angina pectoris.

Monodox PMC, Austral.
Doxycycline (p.200-1).
Bacterial infections.

Monodoxin Crosara, Ital.†.
Doxycycline hyclate (p.200-1).
Bacterial infections.

Monodur Dexxon, Israel.
Isosorbide mononitrate (p.916-2).
Angina pectoris.

Monofed Aspen Consumer, S.Afr.
Pseudoephedrine hydrochloride (p.1099-2).
Upper respiratory-tract congestion.

Monofeme Wyeth-Ayerst, Austral.; Wyeth, NZ.
21 Tablets, levonorgestrel (p.1486-2); ethinylestradiol (p.1476-2); 7 tablets, inert.
Combined oral contraceptive.

Monoflam Lichtenstein, Ger.
Diclofenac sodium (p.30-3).
Gout; inflammation; musculoskeletal, joint, and soft-tissue disorders; pain.

Monofix-VF CSL, Austral.
A factor IX preparation (p.735-1).
Haemophilia B.

Monofocet Roussel Diamant, Fr.
Ofloxacin (p.232-3).
Bacterial infections.

Monofix CSL, NZ.
A factor IX preparation (p.735-1).
Haemophilia B.

Monoembolex Novartis, Ger.; rs Squibb, USA.
Certoparin sodium (p.856-2).
Postoperative thrombosis prophylaxis.

Monofoscin CEPA, Spain.
Fosfomycin trometamol (p.208-2).
Urinary-tract infections.

Mono-Jod Philopharm, Ger.
Potassium iodide (p.1522-3).
Iodine deficiency.

Mono-Gesic Schwarz, USA.
Salsalate (p.82-2).
Fever; osteoarthritis; pain; rheumatoid arthritis.

Monogen Scientific Hospital Supplies, Austral.; Nutricia, NZ; Scientific Hospital Supplies, NZ; Scientific Hospital Supplies, UK.
Preparation for enteral nutrition (p.1350-1).
Lipid and lymphatic disorders.

Monogestin Wyeth Lederle, Aust.
Gestodene (p.1479-1); ethinylestradiol (p.1476-2).
Combined oral contraceptive.

Monoket Gebro, Aust.; Chiesi, Ital.; Pharmacia Upjohn, Norw.; Neo-Farmaceutica, Port.; Pharmacia Upjohn, Swed.; Schwarz, USA.
Isosorbide mononitrate (p.916-2).
Angina pectoris; heart failure; myocardial infarction; pulmonary hypertension.

Monos Selvi, Ital.
Rufloxacin hydrochloride (p.247-3).
Bacterial infections.

Monopina Biondustria, Ital.
Amlodipine besilate (p.838-3).
Angina pectoris; hypertension.

Monores Valeas, Ital.
Clenbuterol hydrochloride (p.763-3).
Obstructive airways disease.

Monopront Fenna, Lynce, Port.
Isosorbide mononitrate (p.916-2).
Angina pectoris; heart failure; myocardial infarction; pulmonary hypertension.

Monopur Pohl, Ger.
Isosorbide mononitrate (p.916-2).
Angina pectoris; pulmonary hypertension.

Monoquin Zambon, Port.
Lomefloxacin hydrochloride (p.220-1).
Bacterial infections.

Monoprim Nycomed, Aust.
Trimethoprim (p.264-2).
Urinary and respiratory-tract bacterial infections.

Monopril comp Bristol-Myers Squibb, Swed.
Fosinopril sodium (p.892-3); hydrochlorothiazide (p.907-3).
Hypertension.

Monopril-HCT Bristol-Myers Squibb, USA.
Fosinopril sodium (p.892-3); hydrochlorothiazide (p.907-3).
Hypertension.

Monoplus Bristol-Myers Squibb, Austral.
Fosinopril sodium (p.892-3); hydrochlorothiazide (p.907-3).
Heart failure; hypertension.

Monopril Bristol-Myers Squibb, Austral.; Bristol-Myers Squibb, Canad.; Bristol-Myers Squibb, Denm.; Bristol-Myers Squibb, Ger.; Bristol-Myers Squibb, Hong Kong; Mead Johnson, Mex.; Bristol-Myers Squibb, Now, Bristol-Myers Squibb, S.Afr.; Bristol-Myers Squibb, Singapore; Bristol-Myers Squibb, Swed.; Bristol-Myers Squibb, Thai.; Bristol-Myers Squibb, USA.
Fosinopril sodium (p.892-3).
Heart failure; hypertension.

Monopress Bayer, Spain†.
Nitrendipine (p.947-1).
Angina pectoris; hypertension; Raynaud's syndrome.

Monosorb Dexcel, UK.
Isosorbide mononitrate (p.916-2).
Angina pectoris.

Monostenase Pharmonta, Aust.
Isosorbide mononitrate (p.916-2).
Angina pectoris.

MonoStep Asche, Ger.
Ethinylestradiol (p.1476-2); levonorgestrel (p.1486-2).
Combined oral contraceptive.

Monolin Biobras, Braz.
Isophane insulin injection (porcine, monocomponent) (p.324-1).
Diabetes mellitus.

Monolin NPH Biobras, Braz.
Isophane insulin injection (porcine, monocomponent) (p.324-1).
Diabetes mellitus.

Monolin Regular Biobras, Braz.
Neutral insulin injection (porcine, monocomponent) (p.324-1).
Diabetes mellitus.

Monolitum Salvat, Spain.
Lansoprazole (p.1230-3).
Gastro-oesophageal reflux; peptic ulcer.

Monolong Lusofarmaco, Ital.
Isosorbide mononitrate (p.916-2).
Angina pectoris; heart failure; pulmonary hypertension.

Monomax Trinity, UK.
Isosorbide mononitrate (p.916-2).
Angina pectoris.

Monomycin Grunenthal, Ger.
Erythromycin (p.201-2) or erythromycin ethyl succinate (p.201-2).
Bacterial infections.

Monomycine Grunenthal, Switz.
Erythromycin ethyl succinate (p.201-2).
Bacterial infections.

Mononine Centeon, Braz.; Centeon, Denm.; Centeon, Fr.; Centeon, Ger.; Centeon, Irl.; Centeon, Ital.; Aventis, Neth.; Centeon, Spain; Centeon, Swed.; Aventis Behring, UK; Centeon, USA.
A factor IX preparation (p.735-1).
Factor IX deficiency; haemophilia B.

Monoparin CP Pharmaceuticals, UK.
Heparin calcium (p.902-1), NZ; CP Pharmaceuticals, UK; or heparin sodium (p.902-1), CP Pharmaceuticals, UK.
Thromboembolic disorders.

Mononit Medis, Israel.
Isosorbide mononitrate (p.916-2).
Angina pectoris.

Mononitrat Verla, Ger.
Isosorbide mononitrate (p.916-2).
Heart failure; ischaemic heart disease; myocardial infarction; pulmonary hypertension.

Mononitril Baldacci, Port.
Isosorbide mononitrate (p.916-2).
Angina pectoris; heart failure; pulmonary hypertension.

Monotard Novo Nordisk, Austral.; Novo Nordisk, Denm.; Novo Nordisk, Fr.; Novo Nordisk, Ger.; Novo Nordisk, Irl.; Novo Nordisk, NZ; Novo Nordisk, Port.; Novo Nordisk, Spain; Novo Nordisk, Swed.
Insulin zinc suspension (amorphous 30%, crystalline 70%) (human, monocomponent) (p.324-1).
Formerly known as Human Monotard in Irl.

Monotard MC Novo Nordisk, Belg.; Novo Nordisk, Fr.; Novo Nordisk, Ger.; Novo Nordisk, Hong Kong; Novo Nordisk, NZ; Novo Nordisk, S.Afr.; Novo Nordisk, Switz.; Novo Nordisk, Thai.
Insulin zinc suspension (amorphous 30%, crystalline 70%) (porcine) (p.324-1).
Diabetes mellitus.

Monotard HM Novo Nordisk, Austral.; Novo Nordisk, Belg.; Novo Nordisk, Fr.; Novo Nordisk, ...
Insulin zinc suspension (amorphous 30%, crystalline 70%) (human, monocomponent) (p.324-1).
Diabetes mellitus.

Monotest Pasteur Merieux, Aust.; Aventis, S.Afr.; Pasteur Merieux, Fr.; Pasteur Merieux, Swed.
Tuberculin PPD (p.1675-3).
Tuberculosis test.

Mono-Tildiem Synthelabo, Fr.; Sanofi Synthelabo, Singapore; Sanofi Synthelabo, Switz.
Diltiazem hydrochloride (p.874-3).
Angina pectoris; hypertension.

Mono-Tridin Opfermann, Ger.
Sodium monofluorophosphate (p.1377-2).
Osteoporosis.

Monotrate Sun, Singapore; Sun, Thai.
Isosorbide mononitrate (p.916-2).
Angina pectoris; heart failure.

Monotren Gee, Denm.; Solvay, Irl.; Mono, S.Afr.†; Gea, Switz.; Solvay, UK.
Trimethoprim (p.264-2) or trimethoprim lactate (p.265-3).
Bacterial infections.

Monotrean Luiphil, Braz.; Sankyo, Ital.
Note. This name is used for preparations of different composition.
Papaverine (p.1648-1); quinine hydrochloride (p.445-1).
Diabetes mellitus.

Monovent Logap, UK.
Terbutaline sulfate (p.776-2).
Obstructive airways disease; premature labour.

Monovax Pasteur Merieux, Fr.
A BCG vaccine (p.1533-2).
Active immunisation.

Monovacc-Test Pasteur Merieux, USA.
Old tuberculin (p.1675-3).
Diagnosis of tuberculosis.

Mono-Vacc Test (O.T.) Pasteur Merieux, Belg.
Old tuberculin (p.1675-3).
Test for tuberculin sensitivity.

Monotussin Beige, S.Afr.
Codeine phosphate (p.25-2); mepyramine maleate (p.421-1); ephedrine hydrochloride (p.1090-1).
Coughs.

Monostop Synthelabo, Spain.
Bifonazole (p.381-1).
Fungal skin and nail infections.

Monphytol Laboratories for Applied Biology, UK.
Methyl undecenoate (p.396-1); propyl undecenoate (p.396-1); salicylic acid (p.1122-3); methyl salicylate (p.55-1); propyl salicylate; chlorobutanol (p.1141-2).
Fungal nail infections.

Montalen Pharmonta, Aust.
Magnesium trisilicate (p.1233-3); aluminium hydroxide (p.1210-3); peppermint oil (p.1243-3).
Gastrointestinal disorders associated with hyperacidity.

Montana Pharmonta, Aust.
Note. This name is used for preparations of different composition.
Lupulus (p.1629-3); gentian (p.1615-1); cinnamon (p.1595-3); bitter-orange peel (p.1623-2); caraway (p.1591-2); taraxacum (p.1669-1); peppermint oil (p.1243-3); pterocarpus santalinus.
Gastrointestinal disorders.

Montaned Montané, Aust.
Salverine hydrochloride (p.1660-3); propyphenazone (p.80-2); caffeine (p.761-3).
Pain.

Lignocaine [lidocaine] hydrochloride (p.1313-2) may be included in the intramuscular injection to alleviate the pain of injection.

Lignocaine [lidocaine] hydrochloride (p.1313-2) is included in this preparation to alleviate the pain of injection.

EGS, Ger.
Juniper (p.1625·2); caraway (p.1591·2); cardamom (p.1591·3); bitter-orange peel (p.1644·2); cinnamon (p.1595·3); peppermint oil (p.1243·3); senna (p.1248·2); menyanthes (p.1633·1); pterocarpus santalinus; sassafras; centaury (p.1593·1); absinthium (p.1571·1); calamus (p.1588·1); gentian (p.1615·3); valerian (p.1678·3); rhubarb (p.1248·1); aloes (p.1210·1); sarsaparilla (p.1661·1); aloes (p.1210·1).
Gastrointestinal disorders.

Montavon *Aerocid, Fr.†;*
Pilocarpine nitrate (p.1422·3); antimony potassium tartrate (p.97·1).
Alcohol withdrawal syndrome.

Montegen *Gentili, Ital.*
Montelukast sodium (p.768·1).
Asthma.

Montricin
Prospa, Belg.†; Asta Medica, Braz.; SPA, Ital.
Mepartricin sodium laurilsulfate (p.390·3).
Vulvovaginal candidiasis and trichomoniasis.

Monuril
Zambon, Aust.; Modasus, Belg.; Zambon, Braz.; Zambon, Fr.; Apogepha, Ger.; Pharmax, Irl.; Zambon, Ital.; Zambon, Neth.; Zambon, Port.; Inpharzam, Switz.; Pharmox, UK†;
Fosfomycin trometamol (p.208·2).
Urinary-tract infections.

Monydrin *Tika, Norw.†; Tika, Swed.†*
Phenylpropanolamine hydrochloride (p.1098·1).
Rhinitis.

Moorbad-Saar N *CPK, Ger.*
Salicylic acid (p.1122·3); sodium humate.
Bath additive; gynaecological disorders; musculoskeletal and joint disorders; neuralgia.

Moorland *Torbet Laboratories, UK.*
Bismuth aluminate (p.1213·1); magnesium trisilicate (p.1233·3); dried aluminium hydroxide gel (p.1210·3); heavy magnesium carbonate (p.1232·3); light kaolin (p.1229·3); calcium carbonate (p.1215·1).
Dyspepsia; flatulence; heartburn.

Moorlauge Bastian *Bastian, Ger.†;*
Medicinal mud.
Bath additive; rheumatic disorders.

Mopen *FIRMA, Ital.*
Amoxicillin trihydrate (p.149·2).
Bacterial infections.

Mopral
AstraZeneca, Fr.; Astra, Spain.
Omeprazole (p.1239·1) or omeprazole sodium (p.1239·1).
Gastro-oesophageal reflux; peptic ulcer; Zollinger-Ellison syndrome.

Mopsoralen *Wolfs, Belg.*
Methoxsalen (p.1118·3).
Mycosis fungoides; psoriasis; vitiligo.

Moradorm *Bouhon, Ger.*
Valerian (p.1678·3); passion flower (p.1649·1); diphenhydramine hydrochloride (p.416·1).
Nervous disorders; sleep disorders.

Moradorm S *Bouhon, Ger.*
Valerian (p.1678·3); passion flower (p.1649·1); lupulus (p.1629·3).
Nervous disorders; sleep disorders.

Morapid *Mundipharma, Aust.*
Morphine sulfate (p.56·1).
Pain.

Morcap *Faulding, UK.*
Morphine sulfate (p.56·1).
Pain.

Morde X *Vitaformo, Spain.*
Alcohol (p.1130·3); sucrose octa-acetate (p.1668·1).
Nail biting deterrent.

MoreDophilus *Freeda, USA.*
Acidophilus-carrot derivative (p.1626·3).
Dietary supplement.

Morfex *Tecnifar, Port.*
Flurazepam hydrochloride (p.685·3).
Insomnia.

Morgenxil *Llorente, Spain.*
Amoxicillin trihydrate (p.149·2).
Bacterial infections.

Morhulin
Seton, Irl.; SSL, UK.
Cod-liver oil (p.1357·2); zinc oxide (p.1128·2).
Skin disorders.

Moriamin *Hoechst Marion Roussel, Thai.*
Multivitamin and amino-acid preparation (p.1350·1).

Morniflu *Master Pharma, Ital.*
Morniflumate (p.56·1).
Fever; inflammation; pain.

Moronal *Bristol-Myers Squibb, Ger.*
Nystatin (p.392·2).
Fungal infections.

Moronal V *Bristol-Myers Squibb, Ger.*
Nystatin (p.392·2); triamcinolone acetonide (p.1080·1).
Skin disorders with fungal infection.

Morphalgin *Fawns & McAllan, Austral.*
Morphine hydrochloride (p.56·1); aspirin (p.14·2).
Pain.

Morphitec *Technilab, Canad.*
Morphine hydrochloride (p.56·1).
Pain.

Morrhulan *Streuli, Switz.*
Cod-liver oil (p.1357·2).
Minor skin lesions.

Morruetil *Quimioterápica, Braz.*
Vitamin A; vitamin D; eucalyptol; camphor (p.1350·1).
Nutritional supplement.

Morrugripe *Quimioterápica, Braz.*
Benzyl cinnamate; vitamin A; vitamin D (p.1350·1); eucalyptol (p.1609·2).
Cold and influenza symptoms.

Morstel *Clonmel, Irl.*
Morphine sulfate (p.56·1).
Pain.

Morton Salt Substitute *Morton Salt, USA.*
Low sodium dietary salt substitute (p.1350·1).

Morubel *Chiron, Ital.*
A measles and rubella vaccine (Schwarz and Wistar RA 27/3 strains respectively) (p.1549·1).
Active immunisation.

Moruman
Berna, Ital.†; Berna, Switz.†
A measles immunoglobulin (p.1547·1).
Passive immunisation.

Morupar *Chiron, Ital.*
A measles, mumps, and rubella vaccine (Schwarz, Urabe AM9, and Wistar RA 27/3 strains, respectively) (p.1549·1).
Active immunisation.

MoRu-Viraten
Berna, Canad.†; Berna, Switz.†
A measles (Edmonston-Zagreb strain) and rubella (Wistar RA 27/3 strain) vaccine (p.1549·1).
Active immunisation.

MOS *ICN, Canad.*
Morphine hydrochloride (p.56·1) or morphine sulfate (p.56·1).
Pain.

Mosco
Medtech, Canad.; Medtech, USA.
Salicylic acid (p.1122·3).
Hyperkeratosis.

Moscontin *Asta Medica, Fr.*
Morphine sulfate (p.56·1).
Pain.

Mosegor
Novartis, Ger.; Novartis, Spain; Novartis, Switz.; Novartis, Thai.
Pizotifen (p.455·1) or pizotifen malate (p.455·1).
Anorexia; migraine.

Mosil *Menarini, Fr.*
Midecamycin acetate (p.224·3).
Bacterial infections.

Moskizol *Moskizol, Fr.*
Solution: Permethrin (p.1436·1).
Topical gel: Diethyltoluamide (p.1431·2).
Insect repellent.

Motens
Boehringer Ingelheim, Belg.; Boehringer Ingelheim, Ger.; Glaxo Wellcome, Ger.; Boehringer Ingelheim, Neth.; Boehringer Ingelheim, Spain; Boehringer Ingelheim, Switz.; Boehringer Ingelheim, Thai.; Boehringer Ingelheim, UK.
Lacidipine (p.919·1).
Hypertension.

Mother's and Children's Vitamin Drops
Haghs Healthcare, UK.
Vitamins A, C, and D (p.1350·1).

Motiax *Neopharmed, Ital.*
Famotidine (p.1225·3).
Gastro-oesophageal reflux; peptic ulcer; Zollinger-Ellison syndrome.

Moticon *Condrugs, Thai.*
Domperidone (p.1224·1).
Dyspepsia; nausea and vomiting.

Motidine
Unison, Singapore; Unison, Thai.
Famotidine (p.1225·3).
Gastro-oesophageal reflux; peptic ulcer; Zollinger-Ellison syndrome.

Motidom *TO-Chemicals, Thai.*
Domperidone (p.1224·1).
Gastrointestinal motility disorders; nausea and vomiting.

Motifene
Sankyo, Belg.; Sankyo, Fin.; Sankyo, UK.
Diclofenac sodium (p.30·3).
Inflammation; musculoskeletal, joint, peri-articular and soft-tissue disorders; pain.

Motilex *Guidotti, Ital.*
Clebopride malate (p.1221·2).
Gastrointestinal disorders.

Motilidone *Technilab, Canad.*
Domperidone maleate (p.1224·1).

Motilium
Janssen-Cilag, Aust.; Janssen-Cilag, Austral.; Janssen-Cilag, Belg.; Janssen, Braz.; Janssen-Ortho, Canad.; Janssen-Cilag, Denm.; Janssen-Cilag, Fr.; Byk Gulden, Ger.; Janssen, Hong Kong; Janssen-Cilag, Irl.; Janssen-Cilag, Israel; Janssen-Cilag, Ital.; Janssen, Mex.; Janssen-Cilag, Neth.; Janssen-Cilag, NZ; Janssen-Cilag, S.Afr.; Janssen-Cilag, Singapore; Esteve, Spain; Janssen-Cilag, Switz.; Janssen, Thai.; Sanofi Winthrop, UK.
Domperidone (p.1224·1) or domperidone maleate (p.1224·1).
Adjunct in gastrointestinal radiology; delayed gastric emptying; dyspepsia; gastro-oesophageal reflux; hiccup; nausea and vomiting.

Motipress
Bristol-Myers Squibb, Irl.†; Sanofi Winthrop, UK.
Fluphenazine hydrochloride (p.684·3); nortriptyline hydrochloride (p.301·3).
Mixed anxiety depressive states.

Motival
Sanofi Winthrop, Fr.†; Bristol-Myers Squibb, Hong Kong; Bristol-Myers Squibb, Irl.; Bristol-Myers Squibb, S.Afr.; Bristol-Myers Squibb, Thai.; Sanofi Winthrop, UK.
Fluphenazine hydrochloride (p.684·3); nortriptyline hydrochloride (p.301·3).
Mixed anxiety depressive states.

Motivan
Faes, Spain.
Paroxetine hydrochloride (p.302·3).
Anxiety disorders; depression.

Motixal *Samokaephuegsij, Thai.*
Dimenhydrinate (p.415·2).
Motion sickness; nausea and vomiting; vestibular disorders.

Motivone *BASF, Ger.*
Fluoxetine (p.288·2).
Depression.

Motofen *Carnrick, USA.*
Difenoxin hydrochloride (p.1222·1).
Atropine sulfate (p.461·1) is included in this preparation to discourage abuse.
Diarrhoea.

Motosol *Europharma, Spain.*
Ambroxol hydrochloride (p.1084·3).
Respiratory-tract disorders.

Motozina *Biomedica, Ital.*
Dimenhydrinate (p.415·2).
Formerly contained cyclizine hydrochloride.
Motion sickness.

Motrim *Lannacher, Aust.*
Trimethoprim (p.264·2).
Bacterial infections.

Motrin
Pharmacia Upjohn, Belg.†; Pharmacia Upjohn, Braz.; McNeil Consumer, Canad.; Pharmacia Upjohn, Mex.; Pharmacia Upjohn, Port.†; Pharmacia Upjohn, Switz.†; Pharmacia, UK; McNeil Consumer, USA.
Ibuprofen (p.43·2).
Formerly known as Pediaprofen in the USA.
Fever; gout; inflammation; musculoskeletal, joint, peri-articular and soft-tissue disorders; pain.

Motrin IB Sinus *McNeil Consumer, USA.*
Pseudoephedrine hydrochloride (p.1099·2); ibuprofen (p.43·2).
Cold symptoms; sinusitis.

Mouthkote
Parnell, Irl.; Parnell, USA.
Artificial saliva.
Dry mouth.

MouthKote F/R *Parnell, USA†.*
Sodium fluoride (p.1375·3).

MouthKote O/R *Unimed, USA.*
Oral rinse: Benzyl alcohol (p.1135·2); menthol (p.1632·3).
Minor mouth or throat irritation.

MouthKote P/R *Unimed, USA.*
Ointment: Diphenhydramine hydrochloride (p.416·1).
Oral lesions.
Topical solution: Diphenhydramine (p.416·1); cetylpyridinium chloride (p.1138·1).
Minor mouth or throat irritation.

Mouthrinse *Arjo, Canad.†;*
Cetylpyridinium chloride (p.1138·1); sodium benzoate (p.1134·3).
Mouth and throat disorders; oral hygiene.

Mouthwash *National Care, Canad.*
Cetylpyridinium chloride (p.1138·1).

Mouthwash Antiseptic & Gargle *Lander, Canad.*
Alcohol (p.1130·3); eucalyptus oil (p.1609·2); menthol (p.1632·3); thymol (p.1158·3).
Oral hygiene.

Mouthwash & Gargle *Scott, Canad.†;*
Cetylpyridinium chloride (p.1138·1); domiphen bromide (p.1143·3).

Mouthwash Mint/Peppermint *Lander, Canad.†;*
Cetylpyridinium chloride (p.1138·1); domiphen bromide (p.1143·3).

Mova Nitrat *Lindopharm, Ger.*
Silver nitrate (p.1664·2).
Eye disorders.

Movalis
Boehringer Ingelheim, Aust.; Boehringer Ingelheim, Port.; Europharma, Spain.
Meloxicam (p.51·3).
Ankylosing spondylitis; osteoarthritis; rheumatoid arthritis.

Movatec *Boehringer de Angeli, Braz.*
Meloxicam (p.51·3).
Osteoarthritis; rheumatoid arthritis.

Movelat
Note. This name is used for preparations of different composition.
Sankyo, Austral.; Sankyo, Thai.; Sankyo, UK.
A heparinoid (p.905·2); salicylic acid (p.1122·3).
Formerly contained a heparinoid, adrenocortical extract, and salicylic acid in the UK.
Musculoskeletal, joint, and soft-tissue disorders.

Movens *Pharmofar, Ital.*
Meclofenamate sodium (p.51·1) or meclofenamic acid (p.51·1).
Musculoskeletal and joint disorders; pain.

Mover *Mitsubishi, Jpn.*
Actarit (p.11·2).
Rheumatoid arthritis.

Movergan *Orion, Ger.*
Selegiline hydrochloride (p.1177·2).
Parkinsonism.

Movex *Vitamed, Israel.*
Bromhexine hydrochloride (p.1085·3).
Bronchitis.

Movicard *Rovensberg, Ger.*
Magnesium aspartate (p.1190·3); potassium aspartate (p.1611·2).
Cardiac disorders.

Movicol
Norgine, Aust.; Norgine, Austral.; Norgine, Belg.; Norgine, Denm.; Sabora, Fin.; Norgine, Fr.; Norgine, Ger.; Norgine, Hong Kong; Norgine, Irl.; Norgine, Ital.; Norgine, S.Afr.; Norgine, Singapore; Stafford-Miller, Spain; Bioloc, Swed.; Norgine, Switz.; Norgine, UK.
Macrogol 3350 (p.1630·3); electrolytes (p.1180·1).
Constipation; faecal impaction.

Movicolon *Norgine, Neth.*
Macrogol 3350 (p.1630·3); electrolytes (p.1180·1).
Constipation.

Movicox *Boehringer Ingelheim, Neth.*
Meloxicam (p.51·3).
Ankylosing spondylitis; osteoarthritis; rheumatoid arthritis.

Moviflex
Sankyo, Aust.; Sankyo, Fin.; Sankyo, Switz.†;
Phenylephrine hydrochloride (p.1097·1); a heparinoid (p.905·2); glycol salicylate (p.42·2).
Musculoskeletal, joint, peri-articular, and soft-tissue disorders.

Movilat *Sankyo, Spain.*
A heparinoid (p.905·2); salicylic acid (p.1122·3); suprarenal extract (p.1080·1).
Rheumatic and muscular pain.

Movilisin
Sankyo, Hong Kong; Sankyo, Spain.
Flufenamic acid (p.41·1); a heparinoid (p.905·2); glycol salicylate (p.42·2) or salicylic acid (p.1122·3).
Musculoskeletal, joint, peri-articular, and soft-tissue disorders.

Movin *Neo-Farmaceutica, Port.*
Ticlopidine hydrochloride (p.981·1).
Thrombo-embolic disorders.

Movina *Pharmaton, Switz.*
Hypericum (p.290·2).
Depression.

Mowineuron *Rodisma, Ger.*
Vitamin B substances; vitamin E (p.1350·1).
Tonic.

Mowivit *Rodisma, Ger.*
d-Alpha tocopherol (p.1393·3).
Vitamin E deficiency.

Moxacef *Bristol-Myers Squibb, Belg.*
Cefadroxil (p.161·2).
Bacterial infections.

Moxacin *CSL, Austral.*
Amoxicillin sodium (p.149·2) or amoxicillin trihydrate (p.149·2).
Bacterial infections.

Moxadent *Vitoria, Port.*
Amoxicillin (p.149·2).
Bacterial infections.

Moxal *Julphar, UAE.*
Dried aluminium hydroxide (p.1210·3); magnesium hydroxide (p.1233·1).
Gastrointestinal hyperacidity.

Moxal II *Julphar, UAE.*
Aluminium hydroxide (p.1210·3); magnesium hydroxide (p.1233·1).
Gastro-oesophageal reflux; gastrointestinal hyperacidity.

Moxal Plus *Julphar, UAE.*
Aluminium hydroxide (p.1210·3); magnesium hydroxide (p.1233·1); simeticone (p.1249·2).
Flatulence; gastro-oesophageal reflux; gastrointestinal hyperacidity.

Moxaline *Bristol-Myers Squibb, Belg.*
Amoxicillin trihydrate (p.149·2).
Bacterial infections.

Moxan *Aspen, S.Afr.*
Amoxicillin (p.149·2).
Bacterial infections.

Moxapen *Olan-Kemed, Thai.*
Amoxicillin trihydrate (p.149·2).
Bacterial infections.

Moxcil *TP, Thai.*
Amoxicillin sodium (p.149·2) or amoxicillin trihydrate (p.149·2).
Bacterial infections.

Moxcin *General Drugs, Thai.*
Amoxicillin trihydrate (p.149·2).
Bacterial infections.

Moxicel *Welfer, Mex.*
Amoxicillin (p.149·2).
Bacterial infections.

Moxiclav *Medochemie, Hong Kong; Medochemie, Singapore.*
Amoxicillin trihydrate (p.149·2); potassium clavulanate (p.187·2).
Bacterial infections.

Moxilcap *Masa, Thai.*
Amoxicillin trihydrate (p.149·2).
Bacterial infections.

Moxilen *Medochemie, Singapore; Medochemie, Thai.*
Amoxicillin trihydrate (p.149·2).
Bacterial infections.

Moxilin *The Forty-Two, Thai.*
Amoxicillin trihydrate (p.149·2).
Bacterial infections.

Moximed *Unison, Thai.*
Amoxicillin trihydrate (p.149·2).
Bacterial infections.

Moxipan *Nakorn, Thai.*
Amoxicillin trihydrate (p.149·2).
Bacterial infections.

Moxipen *Sanofi Synthelabo, Port.; Xepa-Soul Pattinson, Singapore.*
Amoxicillin (p.149·2).
Bacterial infections.

Moxiral *Pharmacia Upjohn, Aust.*
Minoxidil (p.934·2).
Alopecia androgenetica.

Moxiren *Ist. Chim. Inter., Ital.*
Amoxicillin trihydrate (p.149·2).
Bacterial infections.

Moxlin *Pacific, Hong Kong; Merck, Mex.; Pacific, NZ.*
Amoxicillin trihydrate (p.149·2).
Bacterial infections.

Moxon *Solvay, Belg.; Solvay, Spain.*
Moxonidine (p.936·3).
Hypertension.

Moxydar *Grimberg, Fr.*
Aluminium hydroxide (p.1210·3); magnesium hydroxide (p.1233·1); aluminium phosphate (p.1211·3); guar gum (p.323·3).
Gastrointestinal disorders.

Moxymax *Parke-Med, S.Afr.†.*
Amoxicillin (p.149·2).
Bacterial infections.

Moxypen *Biogal, Israel; Aspen, S.Afr.*
Amoxicillin trihydrate (p.149·2).
Bacterial infections.

Moxyvit *Vitamed, Israel.*
Amoxicillin trihydrate (p.149·2).
Bacterial infections.

Moz-Bite *Hoe, Singapore.*
Crotamiton (p.1112·3).
Insect bites.

Mozzie Patch *Bioconcepts, UK.*
Citronella oil (p.1596·3).
Insect repellent.

MPA *Hexal, Ger.*
Medroxyprogesterone acetate (p.1480·1).
Breast cancer; endometrial cancer.

MPA Gyn *Hexal, Ger.*
Medroxyprogesterone acetate (p.1480·1).
Menopausal disorders; menstrual disorders.

MPA-beta *Betapharm, Ger.*
Medroxyprogesterone acetate (p.1480·1).
Breast cancer; endometrial cancer.

MPA-Noury *Nourypharma, Ger.*
Medroxyprogesterone acetate (p.1480·1).
Breast cancer; endometrial cancer.

M-P-Cil *Brovar, S.Afr.†.*
Ampicillin trihydrate (p.151·1).

M-Prednisol *Pasadena, USA.*
Methylprednisolone acetate (p.1076·1).
Corticosteroid.

Mr. Multy *Vitalia, UK.*
Multivitamin and mineral preparation (p.1350·1).

The symbol † denotes a preparation no longer actively marketed

Mrs Cullen's Powders *Cullen & Davison, UK.*
Aspirin (p.14·2); caffeine (p.761·3).
Fever; pain.

M-R-Vax II *Merck, USA.*
A measles and rubella vaccine (more attenuated Enders' attenuated Edmonston, and Wistar RA 27/3 strains respectively) (p.1549·1).
Active immunisation.

MRX *Mahdeen, Canad.*
Benzethonium chloride (p.1134·2); camphor (p.1589·3); alcohol (p.1130·3); benzoic acid (p.1134·2).

MS Contin *Mundipharma, Austral.; Asta Medica, Belg.; Purdue Frederick, Canad.; Asta Medica, Ital.; Asta Medica, Neth.; Purdue Frederick, USA.*
Morphine sulfate (p.56·1).
Pain.

MS Direct *Asta Medica, Belg.*
Morphine sulfate (p.56·1).
Pain.

MS Mono *Mundipharma, Austral.*
Morphine sulfate (p.56·1).
Pain.

MSI *Mundipharma, Ger.*
Morphine sulfate (p.56·1).
Pain.

MSIR *Purdue Frederick, Canad.; Purdue Frederick, USA.*
Morphine sulfate (p.56·1).
Pain.

MS/L *Richwood, USA†.*
Morphine sulfate (p.56·1).
Pain.

MS-Long *Janssen, Braz.*
Morphine sulfate (p.56·1).
Pain.

MSP *Rafa, Israel.*
Morphine sulfate (p.56·1).
Pain; sedative.

MSPD *Seroyal, Canad.*
Mineral preparation with vitamin C (p.1350·1).

MSR *Mundipharma, Ger.*
Morphine sulfate (p.56·1).
Pain.

MS/S *Richwood, USA†.*
Morphine sulfate (p.56·1).
Pain.

MST *Mundipharma, Ger.; Asta Medica, Port.*
Morphine sulfate (p.56·1) or morphine polistirex.
Pain.

MST Continus *Asta Medica, Braz.; Mundipharma, Hong Kong; Napp, Irl.; Columbia, Mex.; Douglas, NZ; Adcock Ingram, S.Afr.; Asta Medica, Singapore; Asta Medica, Spain; Mundipharma, Switz.; Napp, UK.*
Morphine sulfate (p.56·1).
Pain.

MSTA *Pasteur Merieux, USA.*
Mumps skin test (p.1638·1).
Assessment of cell-mediated immunity; detection of delayed hypersensitivity to mumps.

M-Stada *Stada, Ger.*
Morphine hydrochloride (p.56·1).
Pain.

MSUD III *Scientific Hospital Supplies, Irl.*
Food for special diets (p.1350·1).
Maple syrup urine disease.

MSUD Aid *Scientific Hospital Supplies, Austral.; Nutricia, NZ; Scientific Hospital Supplies, NZ; Scientific Hospital Supplies, UK.*
Food for special diets (p.1350·1).
Errors of branched-chain amino acid metabolism; maple syrup urine disease.

MSUD Analog *Scientific Hospital Supplies, Austral.*
Food for special diets (p.1350·1).
Maple syrup urine disease.

MSUD Diet *Mead Johnson, Hong Kong.*
Food for special diets (p.1350·1).
Disorders of branched-chain amino-acid metabolism; maple syrup urine disease.

MSUD Maxamaid *Scientific Hospital Supplies, Austral.; Scientific Hospital Supplies, Irl.*
Food for special diets (p.1350·1).
Maple syrup urine disease.

MSUD Maxamum *Scientific Hospital Supplies, Austral.*
Food for special diets (p.1350·1).
Maple syrup urine disease.

MTE *Fujisawa, Hong Kong; Baxter, NZ; American Pharmaceutical, USA.*
A range of trace element preparations (p.1350·1).
Additive for intravenous total parenteral nutrition solutions.

MTX *Hexal, Ger.; Choongwae, Singapore.*
Methotrexate (p.553·2) or methotrexate sodium (p.553·2).
Arthritis; malignant neoplasms; psoriasis.

Mucabrox *Streuli, Switz.*
Ambroxol hydrochloride (p.1084·3).
Respiratory-tract disorders associated with increased or viscous mucus.

Mucaderma S *Merz, Ger.*
Zinc oxide (p.1128·2); titanium dioxide (p.1126·1).
Ulcers; wounds.

Mucaine
Note.This name is used for preparations of different composition.
Whitehall, Austral.; Axcan, Canad.; Wyeth-Ayerst, Hong Kong; Wyeth, Irl.; Whitehall, NZ; Aspen Consumer, S.Afr.; Whitehall, Singapore; Whitehall, Thai.; Wyeth, UK.
Oral suspension: Aluminium hydroxide (p.1210·3); magnesium hydroxide (p.1233·1); oxetacaine (p.1317·3).
Gastritis; gastro-oesophageal reflux; heartburn; peptic ulcer.

Wyeth-Ayerst, Hong Kong; Whitehall, Singapore; Whitehall, Thai.
Tablets: Aluminium hydroxide (p.1210·3); magnesium carbonate (p.1232·3); oxetacaine (p.1317·3).
Gastritis; gastro-oesophageal reflux; heartburn; peptic ulcer.

Mucaine 2 in 1 *Whitehall, Austral.*
Aluminium hydroxide (p.1210·3); magnesium hydroxide (p.1233·1); simeticone (p.1249·2).
Dyspepsia; flatulence.

Mucal
Note.This name is used for preparations of different composition.
Bournonville, Belg†; OM, Port.
Aluminium silicate (p.1211·3); magnesium silicate (p.1502·1); calcium silicate (p.1189·1).
Gastrointestinal disorders.

Irex, Fr†.
Aluminium sodium silicate (p.1211·3); aluminium magnesium silicate (p.1499·1); aluminium calcium silicate (p.1211·3).
Gastrointestinal disorders.

OM, Ger.†
Aluminium magnesium silicate (p.1499·1); aluminium calcium silicate (p.1211·3).
Gastrointestinal disorders.

Mucantil *Serpero, Ital.†.*
Aerosol; elixir; oral drops: Iodinated glycerol (p.1092·3); phenylpropanolamine hydrochloride (p.1098·1).
Capsules: Iodinated glycerol (p.1092·3); phenylpropanolamine hydrochloride (p.1098·1); peppermint oil (p.1243·3).
Respiratory-tract disorders.

Mucasept-A *Merz, Ger.*
Isopropyl alcohol (p.1149·2); alcohol (p.1130·3).
Hand disinfection.

Mucedokehl *Sanum-Kehlbeck, Ger.*
Homoeopathic preparation.

Mucibron
Medley, Braz.; Novag, Mex.; Normon, Spain.
Ambroxol (p.1084·3) or ambroxol hydrochloride (p.1084·3).
Respiratory-tract congestion.

Muciclar
Note.This name is used for preparations of different composition.
Parke, Davis, Fr.
Carbocisteine (p.1086·3).
Respiratory-tract congestion.

Piam, Ital.
Ambroxol hydrochloride (p.1084·3).
Respiratory-tract disorders.

Mucidan *Solvay, Aust.†.*
Thiocyanate salt; ammonium chloride (p.1085·2); liquorice (p.1231·2).

Mucil *TO-Chemicals, Thai.*
Acetylcysteine (p.1082·3).
Respiratory-tract disorders associated with increased or viscous mucus.

Mucilar *Spirig, Switz.*
Ispaghula (p.1229·1).
Gastrointestinal disorders; obesity.

Mucilar Avena *Spirig, Switz.*
Ispaghula (p.1229·1); avena (p.1583·1).
Constipation; obesity.

Mucilax
Douglas, Austral.; Lincoln, NZ.
Ispaghula (p.1229·1).
Constipation.

Mucilin
Berlin Pharm, Singapore; Berlin Pharm, Thai.
Ispaghula (p.1229·1).
Constipation; dietary fibre supplement; stool softener.

Mucilloid *Lalco, Canad.†.*
Ispaghula (p.1229·1).

Mucine *Silom, Thai.*
Bromhexine hydrochloride (p.1085·3).
Respiratory-tract disorders associated with increased or viscous mucus.

Mucinol *Sanofi Synthelabo, Ger.*
Anethole trithione (p.1580·1).
Dry mouth.

Mucinum
Note.This name is used for preparations of different composition.
Pharmethic, Belg.
Bisacodyl (p.1212·2).
Formerly contained phenolphthalein, senna, cascara, boldo, aniseed, pancreas extract, erepsin, enterokinase, ox bile extract, belladonna, ipomoea resin, and dried magnesium sulfate.
Constipation.

Sabex, Canad.
Cascara (p.1216·1); senna (p.1248·2).
Formerly contained phenolphthalein and senna.
Constipation.

Innothera, Fr.†.
Phenolphthalein (p.1244·1); whole bile (p.1585·1); belladonna leaf (p.463·1); senna leaf (p.1248·2); fran-

gula bark (p.1227·1); boldo (p.1585·3); ipomoea (p.1228·3); aniseed (p.1580·2).
Constipation.

Innotech, Port.
Cascara (p.1216·1).
Constipation.

Mucinum a l'Extrait de Cascara *Innothera, Fr.*
Cascara (p.1216·1); senna leaf (p.1248·2); boldo (p.1585·3); aniseed (p.1580·2).
Constipation.

Mucinum Cascara *Innotech, Hong Kong.*
Senna (p.1248·2); boldo (p.1585·3); cascara (p.1216·1); aniseed (p.1580·2).
Constipation.

Muciplasma *Edigen, Spain.*
Methylcellulose (p.1502·2).
Constipation.

Mucipulgite *Ipsen, Belg.; Beaufour, Fr.; Beaufour, Switz.*
Activated attapulgite (p.1212·1); guar gum (p.323·3).
Gastrointestinal disorders.

Mucisol *Deca, Ital.*
Acetylcysteine (p.1082·3).
Respiratory-tract disorders.

Muciteran *Farmasan, Ger.*
Acetylcysteine (p.1082·3).
Ear and respiratory-tract disorders associated with increased or viscous mucus.

Mucitux *E Pharma, Fr.*
Eprazinone hydrochloride (p.1091·1).
Respiratory-tract congestion.

Mucivital *Frere, Belg.; Arkopharma, Fr.; Arkofarm, Ital.*
Ispaghula (p.1229·1).
Constipation; diarrhoea; stool softener.

Muclox *Sigma-Tau, Spain†.*
Famotidine (p.1225·3).
Gastro-oesophageal reflux; peptic ulcer; Zollinger-Ellison syndrome.

Muco4 *Sanofi Synthelabo, Ital.*
Neltenexine (p.1095·3).
Respiratory-tract disorders.

Muco Panoral *Lilly, Ger.*
Bromhexine hydrochloride (p.1085·3); cefaclor (p.161·1).
Bacterial infections of the respiratory tract.

Muco Sanigen *Thiemann, Ger.*
Acetylcysteine (p.1082·3).
Respiratory-tract disorders associated with increased or viscous mucus.

Muco-Aspecton *Krewel, Ger.*
Ambroxol hydrochloride (p.1084·3).
Respiratory-tract disorders associated with increased or viscous mucus.

Mucobene *Ratiopharm, Aust.*
Acetylcysteine (p.1082·3).
Respiratory-tract disorders associated with viscous mucus.

Mucobron *OFF, Ital.*
Ambroxol hydrochloride (p.1084·3).
Respiratory-tract disorders.

Mucobronchyl *Pharmacal, Switz.†.*
Isoprenaline sulfate (p.914·3); phenylephrine hydrochloride (p.1097·1).
Bronchitis.

Mucobroxol *Mundipharma, Ger.*
Ambroxol hydrochloride (p.1084·3).
Respiratory-tract disorders associated with increased or viscous mucus.

Mucocaps *Roche, S.Afr.*
Carbocisteine (p.1086·3).
Respiratory-tract disorders.

Mucocedyl *3M, Ger.*
Acetylcysteine (p.1082·3).
Respiratory-tract disorders associated with increased or viscous mucus.

Mucocef *Lilly, Mex.*
Cefalexin (p.161·3); bromhexine hydrochloride (p.1085·3).
Respiratory-tract infections with excessive mucus.

Mucocil
Novartis, Neth.; Utopian, Thai.
Acetylcysteine (p.1082·3).
Respiratory-tract disorders associated with increased or viscous mucus.

Mucocis *Fonten, Ital.*
Carbocisteine (p.1086·3).
Respiratory-tract congestion.

Muco-cyl Ho-Len-Complex *Liebermann, Ger.*
Homoeopathic preparation.

Muco-Dest *Klus, Switz.*
Peppermint oil (p.1243·3); camphor oil.
Nasal disorders.

Mucodestrol *Eurofarma, Braz.*
Carbocisteine (p.1086·3).
Respiratory-tract congestion.

Mucodex *Dexcel, Israel.*
Acetylcysteine (p.1082·3).
Respiratory-tract disorders associated with viscous mucus.

Mucodic *Progress, Thai.*
Ambroxol hydrochloride (p.1084·3).
Respiratory-tract disorders associated with increased or viscous mucus.

Mucodil Valeas, Ital.†.
Stepronin lysine (p.1101·1).
Respiratory-tract disorders.

Mucodox Delta, Port.
Cyclidrol (p.1100·3).
Respiratory-tract congestion.

Mucodrenol Medinfar, Port.
Ambroxol (p.1084·3).
Respiratory-tract congestion.

Mucodyne
Rhone-Poulenc Rorer, Hong Kong; Rhone-Poulenc Rorer, Irl.; Rhone-
Poulenc Rorer, Neth.; Rhone-Poulenc Rorer, UK.
Carbocisteine (p.1086·3).
*Respiratory-tract disorders associated with excessive
or viscous mucus.*

Mucofalk
Falk, Ger.; Falk, Hong Kong; Rhone-Poulenc Rorer, Port.; Falk, Singa-
pore; Falk, Thai.
Ispaghula (p.1229·1).
*Constipation; diarrhoea; inflammatory bowel disease;
irritable bowel syndrome; stool softener.*

Mucofan Whitehall, Braz.
Carbocisteine (p.1086·3).
Respiratory-tract congestion.

Muco-Fen Wakefield, USA.
Guaifenesin (p.1092·2).
Coughs.

Muco-Fen-DM Wakefield, USA.
Guaifenesin (p.1092·2); dextromethorphan hydrobro-
mide (p.1087·3).
Coughs.

Muco-Fen-LA Wakefield, USA.
Guaifenesin (p.1092·2).
Coughs.

Muco-Fips Lichtenstein, Ger.†.
Ambroxol hydrochloride (p.1084·3).
*Respiratory-tract disorders associated with increased
or viscous mucus.*

Mucoflem Xixia, S.Afr.
Carbocisteine (p.1086·3).
Respiratory-tract disorders.

Mucofluid
Note.This name is used for preparations of different composition.
UCB, Fr.; UCB, Ital.; UCB, Spain.
Mesna (p.1011·3).
Respiratory-tract disorders.

Spirig, Switz.
Acetylcysteine (p.1082·3).
Respiratory-tract disorders.

Mucoflux
Note.This name is used for preparations of different composition.
Merck, Braz.
Carbocisteine (p.1086·3).
Respiratory-tract congestion.

Rotta, Hong Kong; Rotta, Singapore; Rotta, Thai.
Sobrerol (p.1100·3).
*Respiratory-tract disorders associated with increased
or viscous mucus.*

Mucofor Vifor, Switz.
Erdosteine (p.1091·2).
*Respiratory-tract disorders associated with excess mu-
cus.*

Mucogel Pharmax, UK.
Aluminium hydroxide (p.1210·3); magnesium hydrox-
ide (p.1233·1).
These ingredients can be described by the British Ap-
proved Name Co-magaldrox.
Gastrointestinal hyperacidity.

Mucogen Antigen, Irl.
Carbocisteine (p.1086·3).
*Lower respiratory-tract disorders with excessive or
viscous mucus.*

Mucogeran Ogera, Switz.
Carbocisteine (p.1086·3).
Respiratory-tract congestion.

Mucojet Segix, Ital.
Carbocisteine (p.1086·3).
Respiratory-tract disorders.

Mucokehl Sanum-Kehlbeck, Ger.
Homoeopathic preparation.

Mucola Samakeephaesaj, Thai.
Bromhexine hydrochloride (p.1085·3).
*Respiratory-tract disorders associated with increased
or viscous mucus.*

Mucolair 3M, Belg.
Acetylcysteine (p.1082·3).
Adjuvant in respiratory-tract infections.

Mucolan Milano, Thai.
Ambroxol hydrochloride (p.1084·3).
Asthma; bronchitis.

Mucolase Lampugnani, Ital.
Carbocisteine (p.1086·3).
Respiratory-tract disorders.

Mucolator
Labina, Belg.†; Abbott, Fr.; Abbott, Hong Kong.
Acetylcysteine (p.1082·3).
*Paracetamol overdose; respiratory-tract disorders as-
sociated with excess or viscous mucus.*

Mucolavi Vitoria, Port.†.
Sobrerol (p.1100·3).

Mucolene Formenti, Ital.
Mesna (p.1011·3).
*Respiratory-tract disorders associated with excess or
viscous mucus.*

Mucoless Parke-Med, S.Afr.
Carbocisteine (p.1086·3).
Respiratory-tract disorders.

Mucolex
Warner-Lambert, Irl.; Warner-Lambert Consumer, Port.
Carbocisteine (p.1086·3).
*Respiratory-tract disorders with excessive or viscous
mucus.*

Mucolexin Pediatrica, Singapore.
Dextromethorphan hydrobromide (p.1087·3); guaifen-
esin (p.1092·2); sodium citrate (p.1186·2).
Coughs.

Mucolid Greater Pharma, Thai.
Ambroxol hydrochloride (p.1084·3).
Asthma; bronchitis.

Mucolin
Note.This name is used for preparations of different composition.
Knoll, Braz.
Ambroxol hydrochloride (p.1084·3).
Respiratory-tract congestion.

Sanofi Winthrop, Mex.
Carbocisteine (p.1086·3).

Mucolinct Propan, S.Afr.
Carbocisteine (p.1086·3).
Respiratory-tract disorders.

Mucolisil Sanofi Winthrop, Braz.
Carbocisteine (p.1086·3).
Respiratory-tract disorders.

Mucolit CTI, Israel.
Carbocisteine (p.1086·3).
*Respiratory-tract disorders associated with abnormal
or viscous mucus.*

Mucolitic Whitehall, Braz.
Carbocisteine (p.1086·3).
Respiratory-tract congestion.

Mucolitico Maggioni Sanofi Winthrop, Ital.†.
Domiodol (p.1089·1).
Respiratory-tract disorders.

Mucolix Xepa-Soul Pattinson, Hong Kong.
Bromhexine hydrochloride (p.1085·3).
Obstructive airways disease.

Mucolysin
Note.This name is used for preparations of different composition.
Durascan, Denm.
Acetylcysteine (p.1082·3).
Respiratory-tract congestion.

Farmila, Ital.; Interdelta, Switz.
Tiopronin (p.1025·1).
Respiratory-tract disorders.

Mucolyte Julphar, UAE.
Bromhexine hydrochloride (p.1085·3).
*Respiratory-tract disorders associated with viscous
mucus.*

Mucomed
Note.This name is used for preparations of different composition.
Medibrands, Israel.
Carbocisteine (p.1086·3).
*Respiratory-tract disorders associated with viscous
mucus.*

Medifive, Thai.
Ambroxol hydrochloride (p.1084·3).
*Respiratory-tract disorders associated with increased
or viscous mucus.*

Muco-Mepha Mepha, Switz.
Acetylcysteine (p.1082·3).
*Respiratory-tract disorders associated with increased
or viscous mucus.*

Mucomyst
Bristol-Myers Squibb, Aust.; Bristol-Myers Squibb, Austral.; Bristol-Myers Squibb, Belg.; Roberts, Canad.; AstraZeneca, Denm.; AstraZeneca, Fin.; UPSA, Fr.; Bristol-Myers Squibb, Israel; Bristol-Myers Squibb,
Neth.; AstraZeneca, Norw.; Draco, Swed.; Apothecon, USA.
Acetylcysteine (p.1082·3) or acetylcysteine sodium
(p.1083·1).
*Dry eyes; paracetamol poisoning; respiratory-tract
disorders associated with viscous mucus.*

Muconorm Prospa, Ital.
Telmesteine (p.1101·1).
Respiratory-tract disorders.

Mucopan Propan, S.Afr.†.
Carbocisteine (p.1086·3).
Respiratory-tract disorders.

Muco-Perasthman N Polypharm, Ger.†.
Acetylcysteine (p.1082·3).
*Respiratory-tract disorders associated with increased
or viscous mucus.*

Mucophlogat Azupharma, Ger.
Ambroxol hydrochloride (p.1084·3).
*Respiratory-tract disorders associated with increased
or viscous mucus.*

Mucoplexil Theraplix, Fr.†.
Carbocisteine (p.1086·3).
Respiratory-tract congestion.

Mucoporetta Pharmacia Upjohn, Fin.
Acetylcysteine (p.1082·3).
Respiratory-tract congestion.

Mucopront
Mack, Illert., Ger.; Madaus, S.Afr.†; Mack, Singapore; Mack, Thai.
Carbocisteine (p.1086·3) or carbocisteine sodium
(p.1086·3).
*Respiratory-tract disorders associated with increased
or viscous mucus.*

Mucoral Sanofi Synthelabo, Port.
Carbocisteine (p.1086·3).
Respiratory-tract disorders.

Mucorama Roche, Spain.
Phenylpropanolamine hydrochloride (p.1098·1); iodi-
nated glycerol (p.1092·3).
Obstructive airways disease.

Mucorama TS Roche, Spain.
Iodinated glycerol (p.1092·3); co-trimoxazole
(p.193·3).
Respiratory-tract infections.

Mucorex Almirall, Spain.
Citiolone (p.1596·2).
Respiratory-tract infections.

Mucorex Ampicilina
Almirall, Spain.
Capsules; tablets: Ampicillin (p.150·3); citiolone
(p.1596·2).
Respiratory-tract infections.

Berenguer Infale, Spain†.
Injection: Ampicillin sodium (p.150·3); ampicillin
benzathine (p.151·3); citiolone (p.1596·2).
Lignocaine [lidocaine] hydrochloride (p.1313·2) is included in this preparation to alleviate the pain of injection.
Respiratory-tract infections.

Mucorex Ciclin Almirall, Spain.
Citiolone (p.1596·2); tartaric acid (p.1669·2); tetracy-
cline hydrochloride (p.258·3).
Respiratory-tract infections.

Mucorhinyl Synthelabo, Belg.†.
Phenylephrine hydrochloride (p.1097·1); chlorpheniramine [chlorphenamine] maleate (p.412·1); sulfanilamide (p.256·2).
Rhinitis; rhinopharyngitis; sinusitis.

Mucosa compositum Heel, Ger.
Homoeopathic preparation.

Mucosan Boehringer Ingelheim, Spain.
Ambroxol hydrochloride (p.1084·3).
Respiratory-tract disorders.

Muco-Sana Klus, Switz.
Peppermint oil (p.1243·3); camphor oil; lavender oil
(p.1627·2).
Nasal disorders.

Mucoseptal Actipharm, Switz.†.
Carbocisteine (p.1086·3).
Respiratory-tract disorders.

Mucosil Dey, USA.
Acetylcysteine sodium (p.1083·1).
Mucolytic in bronchopulmonary disorders.

Mucosirop Roche, S.Afr.
Carbocisteine (p.1086·3).
Respiratory-tract disorders.

Mucosol Malaysia Chemist, Singapore.
Bromhexine hydrochloride (p.1085·3).
*Respiratory-tract disorders associated with increased
or viscous mucus.*

Mucosolvan
Boehringer Ingelheim, Aust.; Boehringer de Angeli, Braz.; Boehringer
Ingelheim, Ger.; Boehringer Ingelheim, Hong Kong; Boehringer Ingel-
heim, Ital.; Promeco, Mex.; Boehringer Ingelheim, Port.; Boehringer
Ingelheim, Singapore; Boehringer Ingelheim, Thai.
Ambroxol hydrochloride (p.1084·3).
*Neonatal respiratory distress syndrome; respiratory-
tract disorders associated with increased or viscous
mucus.*

Mucosolvan Compositum Promeco, Mex.
Ambroxol hydrochloride (p.1084·3); clenbuterol hy-
drochloride (p.763·3).
Respiratory-tract congestion.

Mucosolvon Boehringer Ingelheim, Switz.
Ambroxol hydrochloride (p.1084·3).
Respiratory-tract disorders.

Mucospas
Boehringer Ingelheim, Aust.; Boehringer Ingelheim, Port.
Ambroxol hydrochloride (p.1084·3); clenbuterol hy-
drochloride (p.763·3).
Respiratory-tract disorders.

Mucospect
Universal, Hong Kong; Triomed, S.Afr.
Carbocisteine (p.1086·3).
*Respiratory-tract disorders associated with increased
or viscous mucus.*

Mucospire Rosa-Phytopharma, Fr.
Acetylcysteine (p.1082·3).
Respiratory-tract disorders.

Mucosta Otsuka, Jpn.
Rebamipide (p.1247·3).
Gastric ulcer; gastritis.

Mucosteine Medgenix, Belg.
Carbocisteine (p.1086·3).
*Respiratory-tract disorders associated with viscous
mucus.*

Mucostop Mepha, Switz.
Acetylcysteine (p.1082·3).
*Respiratory-tract disorders associated with viscous
mucus.*

Mucosyt Bioprogress, Ital.
Tiopronin (p.1025·1).
*Respiratory-tract disorders associated with increased
or viscous mucus.*

Mucotablin Lichtenstein, Ger.
Ambroxol hydrochloride (p.1084·3).
*Respiratory-tract disorders associated with increased
or viscous mucus.*

Muco-Tablinen Sanorania, Ger.†.
Ambroxol hydrochloride (p.1084·3).
*Respiratory-tract disorders associated with increased
or viscous mucus.*

Mucotectan
Boehringer Ingelheim, Aust.; Boehringer Ingelheim, Ger.
Ambroxol hydrochloride (p.1084·3); doxycycline hy-
clate (p.200·1).
Bacterial infections of the respiratory tract.

Mucothera Therabel, Belg.
Erdosteine (p.1091·2).
Respiratory-tract disorders.

Mucotherm Lannacher, Aust.
Ethyl nicotinate (p.35·1).
Anorectal disorders; prostatitis.

Mucothiol
Theratech, Fr.; Geymonat, Ital.
Methyl diacetylcysteinate (p.1094·3).
Respiratory-tract congestion.

Mucotic Hua, Thai.
Acetylcysteine (p.1082·3).
Bronchitis associated with increased or viscous mucus.

Mucotoss Novaquimica, Braz.
Carbocisteine (p.1086·3).
Respiratory-tract congestion.

Mucotreis Ecobi, Ital.
Carbocisteine (p.1086·3).
Respiratory-tract disorders.

Muco-Trin Klus, Switz.
Xylometazoline hydrochloride (p.1102·2); peppermint
oil (p.1243·3); camphor oil.
Nasal congestion.

Mucotrophir Sanofi Winthrop, Fr.
Carbocisteine (p.1086·3).
Respiratory-tract disorders.

Mucovibrol Liomont, Mex.
Ambroxol hydrochloride (p.1084·3).
Respiratory-tract congestion.

Mucovibrol C Liomont, Mex.
Ambroxol hydrochloride (p.1084·3); clenbuterol hy-
drochloride (p.763·3).
Respiratory-tract congestion.

Mucovibrol T Liomont, Mex.
Ambroxol hydrochloride (p.1084·3).
Respiratory-tract congestion.

Mucovin Leiras, Fin.
Bromhexine hydrochloride (p.1085·3).
Respiratory-tract disorders.

Mucovital Almirall, Spain.
Carbocisteine lysine (p.1086·3).
Respiratory-tract congestion.

Mucoxin
Note.This name is used for preparations of different composition.
Wyeth Lederle, Ital.†.
Oral suspension: Oxetacaine (p.1317·3); aluminium
hydroxide (p.1210·3); magnesium oxide (p.1233·2).

Tablets: Oxetacaine (p.1317·3); algeldrate (p.1210·3);
magnesium carbonate (p.1232·3).

*Gastrointestinal disorders associated with hyperacidi-
ty.*

Pharmasant, Thai.
Bromhexine hydrochloride (p.1085·3).
*Respiratory-tract disorders associated with increased
or viscous mucus.*

Mucoxine-F Pharmasant, Thai.
Ambroxol hydrochloride (p.1084·3).
Respiratory-tract disorders.

Mucoxol Serral, Mex.
Ambroxol (p.1084·3).

Mucoza Pond's Chemical, Singapore.
Acetylcysteine (p.1082·3).
*Respiratory-tract disorders associated with increased
or viscous mucus.*

Mucozym Mucos, Ger.
Bromelains (p.1586·3).
Nasal inflammation.

Mucret
Astra, Aust.†; Stern, Ger.
Acetylcysteine (p.1082·3).
*Respiratory-tract disorders associated with increased
or viscous mucus.*

Mu-Cron
Novartis Consumer, Irl.; Novartis Consumer, UK†.
Paracetamol (p.71·2); phenylpropanolamine hydro-
chloride (p.1098·1).
Catarrh; fever; nasal congestion; sinus pain.

Mu-Cron Junior Zyma, UK†.
Phenylpropanolamine hydrochloride (p.1098·1); ipe-
cacuanha (p.1093·1).
Nasal congestion.

Mudd Acne Chattem, Canad.†.
Salicylic acid (p.1122·3).
Acne.

Mudrane ECR, USA.
Potassium iodide (p.1522·3); aminophylline (p.760·1);
phenobarbital (p.355·1); ephedrine hydrochloride
(p.1090·1).
Bronchospasm.

Mudrane GG ECR, USA.
Guaifenesin (p.1092·2); aminophylline (p.760·1); phenobarbital (p.355·1); ephedrine hydrochloride
(p.1090·1).
Bronchospasm.

Mudrane GG-2 ECR, USA.
Guaifenesin (p.1092·2); aminophylline (p.760·1).
Bronchospasm.

Muflex TO-Chemicals, Thai.
Carbocisteine (p.1086·3).
*Respiratory-tract disorders associated with increased
or viscous mucus.*

Mulgatol *Woelm, Ger.†.*
Multivitamin preparation (p.1350·1).

Mulgatol Gelee N *Woelm, Ger.†.*
Multivitamin and mineral preparation (p.1350·1).

Mulimen *Fides, Ger.*
Homoeopathic preparation.

Mulkine *Beaufour, Fr.*
Montmorillonite; guar gum (p.323·3).
Constipation.

Mulmicor *Lappe, Ger.*
Camphor (p.1589·3).
Hypotension.

Mulsal A Megadosis *Vitafarma, Spain.*
Vitamin A (p.1382·1).
Vitamin A deficiency.

Mulsal N *Mucos, Ger.*
Trypsin (p.1675·3); papain (p.1647·3); bromelains (p.1586·3).
Inflammation; musculoskeletal and joint disorders; oedema.

Mul-Tab *British Dispensary, Thai.*
Multivitamin preparation (p.1350·1).

Multene *Baxter, Fr.*
Amino-acid preparation (p.1350·1).
Parenteral nutrition.

Multe-Pak *SoloPak, USA.*
A range of trace element preparations (p.1350·1).
Parenteral nutrition.

Multi-12 *Sabex, Canad.*
A multivitamin preparation (p.1350·1).
Parenteral nutrition.

Multi II *Solgar, UK.*
Amino-acid, multivitamin, and mineral preparation (p.1350·1).

Multi II IV VI *Sisu, Canad.*
Multivitamin and mineral preparation (p.1350·1).

Multi 75 *Fibertone, USA.*
Multivitamin and mineral preparation (p.1350·1).

Multi 1000 *Sabex, Canad.†.*
Multivitamin preparation (p.1350·1).
Parenteral nutrition.

Multi B *Seroyal, Canad.*
Vitamin B substances (p.1350·1).

Multi B Complex *Quest, UK.*
Vitamin B and C preparation (p.1350·1).

Multi Cal-Mag *Seroyal, Canad.*
Vitamin and mineral preparation (p.1350·1).

Multi Formula for Men 50+ *Jamieson, Canad.*
Multivitamin and mineral preparation (p.1350·1).

Multi Forte 29 *Stanley, Canad.*
Multivitamin and mineral preparation (p.1350·1).

Multi Vit Drops with Iron *Barre-National, USA.*
Multivitamin preparation with iron (p.1350·1).

Multi for Women *Jamieson, Canad.*
Multivitamin and mineral preparation (p.1350·1).

Multi-B Forte *G.P. Laboratories, Austral.*
Vitamin B substances and vitamin C (p.1350·1).

Multi-B Strong *Vitabalans, Fin.*
Vitamin B substances (p.1350·1).

Multibionta
Merck, Aust.; Merck, Ger.; Merck, Irl.; Merck, Spain; Merck, Switz.; E. Merck, UK.
Multivitamin preparation (p.1350·1).
Parenteral nutrition.

Multibionta Complex Gins *Merck, Spain.*
Multivitamin and mineral preparation with ginseng (p.1350·1).

Multibionta Junior *Merck, Aust.*
Multivitamin preparation with calcium (p.1350·1).

Multibionta Mineral *Merck, Spain.*
Multivitamin and mineral preparation (p.1350·1).

Multibionta plus Mineral *Merck, Ger.*
Multivitamin and mineral preparation (p.1350·1).

Multibionta plus Mineralien *Merck, Aust.*
Multivitamin and mineral preparation (p.1350·1).

Multicebrina Efevit *Irisfarma, Spain.*
Multivitamin and mineral preparation (p.1350·1).

Multicentrum *Whitehall, Ital.*
Vitamin, mineral, and trace-element preparations (p.1350·1).
Nutritional supplement.

Multichew *Chew, Thai.*
Multivitamin preparation (p.1350·1).

Multi-Day *Nature's Bounty, USA.*
A range of vitamin preparations (p.1350·1).

Multiderm *Agis, Israel.*
Diflucortolone valerate (p.1069·3); chlorquinaldol (p.182·1).
Skin disorders.

Multifluorid *DMG, Ger.*
Sodium fluoride (p.1375·3); olaflur (p.1374·1); dectaflur (p.1359·1).
Dental caries prophylaxis; hypersensitive teeth.

Multifungin *Ebewe, Aust.†.*
Topical powder: Bromochlorosalicylanilide (p.381·1).
Topical solution; ointment: Bromochlorosalicylanilide (p.381·1); bamipine lactate (p.410·1) or bamipine salicylate (p.410·1).
Fungal skin and nail infections.

Multigen AL *Asta Medica, Braz.*
Allergen extracts of dust, pneumococcus, neisseria, streptococcus, *Haemophilus influenzae*, *Staphylococcus aureus*, and *Klebsiella pneumoniae* (p.1575·3).
Hyposensitisation.

Multiglyco *Seroyal, Canad.*
Vitamin B substances, vitamin C, and minerals (p.1350·1).

Multi-Gyn *Farmalight, Port.*
Preparations for vaginal hygiene and lubrication.

MultiHance
Bracco, Aust.; Byk, Belg.; Byk Gulden, Ger.; Bracco, Ital.; Byk, Neth.; Astra Tech, Swed.; Bracco, UK.
Meglumine gadobenate (p.1032·3).
Contrast medium for magnetic resonance imaging of the liver.

Multilase *Sigma-Tau, Ital.†.*
Anistreplase (p.840·2).
Myocardial infarction.

Multilens Solution *Agepha, Aust.*
Disinfection and storage solution for hard contact lenses (p.1129·2).

Multilex *Rugby, USA.*
A range of vitamin preparations (p.1350·1).

Multilim
Atlantic, Hong Kong; Atlantic, Thai.
Multivitamin preparation (p.1350·1).
Tonic; vitamin supplement.

Multilim RG *Atlantic, Thai.*
Ginseng (p.1615·3); royal jelly (p.1659·3); vitamins; minerals (p.1350·1).

Multilind
Bristol-Myers Squibb, Ger.; Niddapharm, Ger.; Bristol-Myers Squibb, Switz.
Nystatin (p.392·2); zinc oxide (p.1128·2).
Fungal infections.

Multiload
Organon, Austral.; Akzo, Braz.; Organon, Denm.†; Organon, Fr.; Nourypharma, Ger.; Organon, Hong Kong; Organon, Irl.; Multilan, Israel; Organon, Ital.; Organon, Mex.; Organon, Neth.; Pharmaco, NZ; Organon, Port.; Donmed, S.Afr.; Organon, Singapore; Organon, Switz.†; Organon, Thai.; Organon, UK.
Copper-wound plastic (p.1357·3).
Intra-uterine contraceptive device.

Multilyte *American Pharmaceutical, USA.*
A range of electrolyte preparations (p.1180·1).
Fluid and electrolyte disorders.

Multi-Min *GNLD, Austral.*
Mineral and trace element preparation with vitamin D (p.1350·1).

Multi-Min Electro *Quest, Canad.*
Mineral preparation with vitamins B_2 and C (p.1350·1).

Multi-Mins *Seroyal, Canad.*
Mineral preparation (p.1350·1).

Multi-Mulsin N *Mucos, Ger.*
Multivitamin preparation (p.1350·1).

Multiparin
CP Pharmaceuticals, Irl.; Artex, NZ; CP Pharmaceuticals, UK.
Heparin sodium (p.902·1).
Thromboembolic disorders.

Multipax *Rhone-Poulenc Rorer, Canad.†.*
Hydroxyzine hydrochloride (p.419·1).
Anxiety.

Multi-Phyto *Pharmavite, Canad.*
Multivitamin and mineral preparation (p.1350·1).

Multipore *Orion, Fin.*
Multivitamin and mineral preparation (p.1350·1).

Multiron *Vitabiotics, UK.*
Multivitamin and mineral preparation with ginseng (p.1350·1).

Multi-Sanasol *Vifor, Switz.*
Multivitamin and mineral preparation (p.1350·1).

Multi-Sanostol
Roland, Ger.
Multivitamin and mineral preparation (p.1350·1).
Byk Gulden, Hong Kong.
Multivitamin preparation (p.1350·1).

Multi-Sanosvit mit Eisen *Roland, Ger.*
Multivitamin preparation with minerals including iron (p.1350·1).

Multiselect 29 *Stanley, Canad.*
Multivitamin and mineral preparation (p.1350·1).

Multisoy *Dieterba, Ital.*
Infant feed (p.1350·1).
Milk intolerance.

Multistix
Bayer, Austral.; Bayer, Canad.†; Bayer Diagnostici, Ital.; Bayer, USA.
Test for glucose, protein, blood, ketones, bilirubin, urobilinogen, and pH in urine.

Multistix 2
Bayer, Canad.†; Bayer, USA.
Test for nitrites and leucocytes in urine.

Multistix 5
Bayer, Austral.; Bayer, Canad.†.
Test for glucose, blood, protein, nitrites, and leucocytes in urine.

Multistix 7
Bayer, Austral.†; Bayer, USA.
Test for glucose, protein, blood, ketones, nitrites, leucocytes, and pH in urine.

Multistix 9
Bayer, Austral.; Bayer, USA.
Test for pH, protein, glucose, ketones, bilirubin, blood, urobilinogen, nitrites, and leucocytes in urine.

Multistix GP *Bayer Diagnostics, UK.*
Test for specific gravity, pH, protein, glucose, ketones, blood, nitrites, and leucocytes in urine.

Multistix SG
Bayer, Austral.†; Bayer, Canad.†; Bayer Diagnostics, Irl.; Bayer Diagnostics, UK; Bayer, USA.
Test for pH, protein, glucose, ketones, bilirubin, blood, urobilinogen, and specific gravity in urine.

Multistix 8 SG
Bayer, Austral.†; Bayer, Canad.†; Bayer Diagnostics, Fr.; Bayer Diagnostics, UK; Bayer, USA.
Test for glucose, protein, blood, ketones, nitrites, leucocytes, pH, and specific gravity in urine.

Multistix 9 SG *Bayer, USA.*
Test for glucose, protein, blood, ketones, bilirubin, nitrites, leucocytes, pH, and specific gravity in urine.

Multistix 10 SG
Bayer, Austral.; Bayer, Canad.†; Bayer Diagnostics, Fr.; Bayer Diagnostics, Irl.; Bayer Diagnostici, Ital.; Bayer Diagnostics, Mex.; Bayer, Port.; Bayer Diagnostics, UK; Bayer, USA.
Test for pH, protein, glucose, ketones, bilirubin, blood, urobilinogen, nitrites, leucocytes, and specific gravity in urine.

Multi-Symptom Tylenol Cold *McNeil Consumer, USA.*
Chlorpheniramine [chlorphenamine] maleate (p.412·1); dextromethorphan hydrobromide (p.1087·3); paracetamol (p.71·2); pseudoephedrine hydrochloride (p.1099·2).
Coughs and cold symptoms.

Multi-Symptom Tylenol Cough *McNeil Consumer, USA.*
Dextromethorphan hydrobromide (p.1087·3); paracetamol (p.71·2).
Formerly known as Maximum Strength Tylenol Cough.
Coughs.

Multi-Symptom Tylenol Cough with Decongestant *McNeil Consumer, USA.*
Pseudoephedrine hydrochloride (p.1099·2); dextromethorphan hydrobromide (p.1087·3); paracetamol (p.71·2).
Formerly known as Maximum Strength Tylenol Cough with Decongestant.
Coughs and cold symptoms.

Multi-Tabs Neo *Ferrosan, Fin.*
Multivitamin and mineral preparation (p.1350·1).

Multi-Tar *ICN, Hong Kong.*
Pyrithione zinc (p.1122·1); tar (p.1125·1); cade oil (p.1124·3); coal tar (p.1125·1).
Scalp disorders.

Multi-Tar Plus *ICN, Canad.*
Cade oil (p.1124·3); tar (p.1125·1); coal tar (p.1125·1); pyrithione zinc (p.1122·1).
Seborrhoeic dermatitis.

Multitest
Serotherapeutiches, Aust.; Richter, Aust.; Pasteur Merieux, Belg.†; Pasteur Merieux, Braz.; Biosyn, Ger.
Tetanus antigen; diphtheria antigen; streptococcus antigen; tuberculin antigen (p.1675·3); candida albicans antigen; trichophyton antigen; proteus mirabilis antigen.
Assessment of cell-mediated immunity.

Multitest CMI
CSL, Austral.; Connaught, Canad.; Pasteur Merieux, Israel; Imtix, Neth.; CSL, NZ; Aventis, S.Afr.; Pasteur Merieux, USA†.
Tetanus antigen; diphtheria antigen; streptococcus antigen; tuberculin antigen (p.1675·3); candida albicans antigen; trichophyton antigen; proteus mirabilis antigen.
Assessment of cell-mediated immunity.

Multitest IMC
Imtix, Fr.; Imtix, Ital.; Rhone-Poulenc Rorer, Spain.
Tetanus antigen; diphtheria antigen; streptococcus antigen; tuberculin antigen (p.1675·3); candida albicans antigen; trichophyton antigen; proteus mirabilis antigen.
Assessment of cell-mediated immunity.

Multiton *Biochimici, Ital.*
Multivitamin and mineral preparation (p.1350·1).

Multitrace-5 Concentrate *American Regent, USA†.*
Trace element preparation (p.1350·1).

Multivac VR *Nikkho, Braz.*
Staphylococcus aureus; Streptococcus pyogenes; Streptococcus viridans; group D Streptococcus; *Moraxella catarrhalis; Corynebacterium diphtheroides; Streptococcus pneumoniae; Listeria monocytogenes; Klebsiella pneumoniae; Pseudomonas aeruginosa; Serratia marcesens* (p.1575·3).
Hyposensitisation.

Multi-Vi-Min *Sisu, Canad.*
Multivitamin and mineral preparation (p.1350·1).

Multivit Biovital *Roche, Switz.*
Multivitamin and mineral preparation with plant extracts (p.1350·1).

Multi-Vitamin Day & Night *Cenovis, Austral.*
Day tablets, vitamins and minerals (p.1350·1); night tablets, valerian (p.1678·3); passion flower (p.1649·1); chamomile (p.1593·2); crataegus (p.1600·2); vitamins and minerals.
Dietary supplement; insomnia; tonic.

Multivitamin Phytopharma V *OTW, Ger.*
Multivitamin preparation (p.1350·1).

Multivitamin-Aufbau-Kapseln *Wiedemann, Ger.*
Multivitamin and mineral preparation (p.1350·1).

Multivitamin-Dragees-Pascoe *Pascoe, Ger.†.*
Multivitamin preparation (p.1350·1).

Multivitamines *Gisand, Switz.*
Multivitamin and mineral preparation (p.1350·1).

Multivitaplex *Dumex-Alpharma, Singapore.*
Multivitamin preparation (p.1350·1).

Multivit-B *Lannacher, Aust.*
Vitamin B substances (p.1350·1).

Multi-Vite *Seroyal, Canad.*
Multivitamin and mineral preparation (p.1350·1).

Multivite Six *Boots, NZ.*
Multivitamin preparation (p.1350·1).

Multivitol *Hermes, Ger.*
Multivitamin and mineral preparation (p.1350·1).

Multodrin *Montavit, Aust.*
Dexamethasone (p.1067·1); diphenhydramine hydrochloride (p.416·1).
Skin disorders.

Multojod-Gastreu N R12 *Reckeweg, Ger.*
Homoeopathic preparation.

Multosin *Takeda, Ger.*
Estramustine meglumine phosphate or estramustine sodium phosphate (p.537·3).
Prostatic cancer.

Multovitan *Worwag, Ger.*
Vitamin B substances; ascorbic acid (p.1350·1).

Multum
Note. This name is used for preparations of different composition.
Rosen, Ger.
Chlordiazepoxide (p.659·2).
Anxiety disorders; sleep disorders.

Lampugnani, Ital.
Benzydamine hydrochloride (p.20·1).
Gynaecological disorders; mouth and throat disorders; musculoskeletal, joint, peri-articular, and soft-tissue disorders.

Mulvidren-F Softab *Stuart, USA.*
Sodium fluoride (p.1375·3) with multivitamins (p.1350·1).
Dental caries prophylaxis in children.

Mulvitin *Silom, Thai.*
Multivitamin preparation (p.1350·1).

Mumaten
Berna, Hong Kong†; Berna, Ital.†; Byk Madaus, S.Afr.; Berna, Switz.†; Berna, Thai.†.
A mumps vaccine (attenuated Rubini strain) (p.1551·1).
Active immunisation.

Mumpsvax
Merck Sharp & Dohme, Aust.†; Prodome, Braz.; Merck Frosst, Canad.; Pasteur Merieux, Denm.; Chiron Behring, Ger.; Pasteur Merieux, Irl.; Pasteur Merieux, Ital.†; Pro Vaccine, Switz.; Pasteur Merieux, UK; Merck, USA.
A mumps vaccine (Jeryl Lynn (B level) strain) (p.1551·1).
Active immunisation.

Mundicycline *Mundipharma, Aust.†.*
Doxycycline fosfatex (p.200·1).
Bacterial infections.

Mundidol *Mundipharma, Aust.*
Morphine sulfate (p.56·1).
Pain.

Mundil *Mundipharma, Ger.*
Captopril (p.853·3).
Heart failure; hypertension.

Mundiphyllin *Mundipharma, Aust.*
Aminophylline (p.760·1).
Respiratory-tract disorders.

Mundisal
Mundipharma, Aust.; Mundipharma, Ger.; Mundipharma, Switz.
Choline salicylate (p.24·3); cetalkonium chloride (p.1137·1).
Nasal and oropharyngeal pain and inflammation.

Mundisept *Mundipharma, Switz.*
Isopropyl alcohol (p.1149·2).
Hand disinfection.

Mundra *Zilly, Ger.*
Tormentil (p.1674·1); peppermint leaf (p.1243·2).
Mouth and throat disorders.

Municaps *Schwarzhaupt, Ger.*
Multivitamin preparation (p.1350·1).
Tonic.

Munitren H *Rabugen, Ger.*
Hydrocortisone (p.1073·3).
Anogenital pruritus; skin disorders.

Munleit *Hommel, Ger.*
Doxylamine succinate (p.417·1).
Insomnia.

Munobal
Hoechst Marion Roussel, Aust.; Hoechst Marion Roussel, Ger.; Hoechst Marion Roussel, Mex.; Hoechst Marion Roussel, Switz.
Felodipine (p.888·3).
Angina pectoris; hypertension.

Munolan *Allergan-Frumtost, Braz.*
Bacterial and fungal antigens (p.1575·3); muramidase hydrochloride (p.1638·1).
Immunostimulant.

Munostin *Atlantis, Mex.*
Lysates of *Streptococcus pneumoniae; Moraxella catarrhalis; Streptococcus pyogenes; Haemophilus influenzae* (p.0·0); *Staphylococcus aureus; Klebsiella pneumoniae.*
Respiratory-tract infections.

Munti-Vim Hua, Thai.
Multivitamin preparation (p.1350·1).

Munvatten Kabi, Swed.†.
Salol (p.82·2); terpineol (p.1669·3); menthol (p.1632·3).
Mouthwash.

Muphoran Servier, Aust.; Servier, Austral.; Servier, Fr.; Servier, Hong Kong; Servier, Israel.
Fotemustine (p.543·2).
Cerebral cancer; disseminated malignant melanoma.

Mupiderm Pharmafarm, Fr.
Mupirocin (p.226·1).
Bacterial skin infections.

Muraligne Murat, Fr.
Glucomannan (p.1616·2).
Obesity.

Murazyme Prospa, Belg.; Asta Medica, Braz.
Muramidase hydrochloride (p.1638·1).
Herpesvirus infections.

Murelax Wyeth, Austral.
Oxazepam (p.697·1).
Alcohol withdrawal syndrome; anxiety.

Muricalm Novartis, Braz.
Pimethixene (p.423·1).
Respiratory-tract disorders in children.

Murine
Note. This name is used for preparations of different composition.
Abbott, Austral.; Abbott, NZ.
Berberine chloride (p.1584·2).
Eye cleansing; eye irritation.

Abbott, Canad.; Ross, Ital.
Ear drops: Urea hydrogen peroxide (p.1159·3).
Removal of ear wax.

Abbott, Canad.; Abbott, Ross, USA.
Eye drops: Polyvinyl alcohol (p.1503·1); povidone (p.1503·2).
Dry eyes.

Abbott, Port.†; Abbott, UK.
Naphazoline hydrochloride (p.1095·1).
Eye irritation.

Murine Allergy Abbott, Austral.
Antazoline sulfate (p.408·3); xylometazoline hydrochloride (p.1102·2).
Allergic eye disorders.

Murine Clear Eyes Abbott, S.Afr.
Naphazoline hydrochloride (p.1095·1).
Eye irritation.

Murine Contact Abbott, Austral.
Hypromellose (p.1501·3); glycerol (p.1616·3).
Comfort drops for contact lenses.

Murine Plus Ross, USA.
Polyvinyl alcohol (p.1503·1); povidone (p.1503·2); tetryzoline hydrochloride (p.1101·2).
Minor eye irritation.

Murine Revital Eyes Abbott, Austral.
Polyvinyl alcohol (p.1503·1); povidone (p.1503·2).
Dry eyes; eye cleansing; eye irritation.

Murine Sore Eyes Abbott, Austral.
Tetryzoline hydrochloride (p.1101·2); polyvinyl alcohol (p.1503·1); povidone (p.1503·2).
Formerly contained tetryzoline hydrochloride and hypromellose.
Eye irritation.

Murine Supplemental Tears Abbott, Canad.
Artificial tears.

Murine Tears for Eyes Abbott, Austral.
Polyvinyl alcohol (p.1503·1); povidone (p.1503·2).
Dry eyes; eye cleansing; eye irritation.

Muro 128 Bausch & Lomb, Canad.; Bausch & Lomb, USA.
Sodium chloride (p.1196·1).
Corneal oedema.

Murocel Bausch & Lomb, Canad.; Bausch & Lomb, USA.
Methylcellulose (p.1502·2).
Dry eyes.

Murocoll-2 Bausch & Lomb, USA.
Hyoscine hydrobromide (p.468·2); phenylephrine hydrochloride (p.1097·1).
Induction of mydriasis and cycloplegia; uveitis.

Murode Teofarma, Spain.
Diflorasone diacetate (p.1069·2).
Skin disorders.

Muroptic Optopics, USA.
Sodium chloride (p.1196·1).
Corneal oedema.

Muro's Opcon Bausch & Lomb, USA†.
Naphazoline hydrochloride (p.1095·1); hypromellose (p.1501·3).
Minor eye irritation.

Murri Antidolorifico Bracco, Ital.
Aspirin (p.14·2); paracetamol (p.71·2); caffeine (p.761·3).
Fever; pain.

Musapam Krewel, Ger.
Tetrazepam (p.708·1).
Skeletal muscle tension and spasm.

Musaril Sanofi Synthelabo, Ger.
Tetrazepam (p.708·1).
Skeletal muscle spasm.

Muscadol Julphar, UAE.
Orphenadrine citrate (p.470·3); paracetamol (p.71·2).
Musculoskeletal pain.

Muscalax Polipharm, Thai.
Methyl salicylate (p.55·1); menthol (p.1632·3); eugenol (p.1609·3).
Musculoskeletal and joint pain; sprains; strains.

Muscaran Christiaens, Belg.
Bethanechol chloride (p.1415·3).
Urinary bladder atony; urinary retention.

Muscarsan Sanum-Kehlbeck, Ger.
Homoeopathic preparation.

Muscelax Hua, Thai.
Carisoprodol (p.1327·1); paracetamol (p.71·2).
Musculoskeletal and joint disorders; skeletal muscle spasm.

Muscinil Opus, UK.
Procyclidine hydrochloride (p.473·1).
Drug-induced extrapyramidal disorders; parkinsonism.

Muscle & Back Pain Relief Stanley, Canad.
Paracetamol (p.71·2); methocarbamol (p.1329·3).

Muscle Rub Schein, USA†.
Methyl salicylate (p.55·1); menthol (p.1632·3).
Muscle, joint, and soft-tissue pain; neuralgia.

Muscol
Teva, Israel; Teva, Thai.
Orphenadrine citrate (p.470·3); paracetamol (p.71·2).
Headache; musculoskeletal pain; neuralgia.

Muscoril Inverni della Beffa, Ital.
Thiocolchicoside (p.1330·2).
Muscle spasticity; neuromuscular pain; oedema; parkinsonism; soft-tissue disorders.

Muse
Vivus, Aust.; Astra, Austral.; Janssen-Ortho, Canad.; Vivus, Denm.; AstraZeneca, Fin.; Astra, Ger.; Janssen, Hong Kong; Astra, Irl.; Janssen-Cilag, Israel; Janssen, Mex.; AstraZeneca, NZ; Janssen-Cilag, S.Afr.; Janssen-Cilag, Singapore; Astra, Spain; Astra, Switz.; Janssen, Thai.; Abbott, UK; Vivus, USA.
Alprostadil (p.1439·3).
Erectile dysfunction.

Muskelat Azupharma, Ger.
Tetrazepam (p.708·1).
Skeletal muscle tension and spasm.

Muskol Schering-Plough, Canad.
SPF 6: Diethyltoluamide (p.1431·2); homosalate (p.1517·2); octinoxate (p.1517·3); octisalate (p.1518·1); oxybenzone (p.1518·1).
Insect repellent; sunscreen.

Musocan Sriprasit, Thai.
Ambroxol hydrochloride (p.1084·3).
Respiratory-tract disorders associated with increased or viscous mucus.

Musside Cosmofarma, Port.†.
Lindane (p.1434·1).
Pediculosis.

Mustargen Merck Sharp & Dohme, Aust.†; Merck Frosst, Canad.; Merck Sharp & Dohme, Israel; Merck Sharp & Dohme, Switz.; Merck, USA.
Mustine [chlormethine] hydrochloride (p.561·1).
Malignant neoplasms; mycosis fungoides; polycythaemia vera.

Musterole Schering-Plough, USA.
Methyl salicylate (p.55·1); menthol (p.1632·3); methyl nicotinate (p.55·1).
Muscle, joint, and soft-tissue pain; neuralgia.

Musterole Extra Schering-Plough, USA.
Methyl salicylate (p.55·1); camphor (p.1589·3); menthol (p.1632·3); mustard oil (p.1639·1).
Muscle, joint, and soft-tissue pain; neuralgia.

Musxan Pharmasant, Thai.
Methocarbamol (p.1329·3).
Skelatal muscle spasm.

Mutabase Schering-Plough, Spain.
Perphenazine (p.699·1); amitriptyline hydrochloride (p.273·3).
Depression.

Mutabon Schering-Plough, Ital.; Schering-Plough, Port.
Perphenazine (p.699·1); amitriptyline hydrochloride (p.273·3).
Psychiatric disorders.

Mutabon D Schering-Plough, Austral.†.
Perphenazine (p.699·1); amitriptyline hydrochloride (p.273·3).
Mixed anxiety depressive states.

Mutacol Berna, Canad.
A live oral attenuated cholera vaccine (CVD 103-HgR) (p.1535·2).
Active immunisation.

Mutaflor Emonta, Aust.; Ardeypharm, Ger.
Escherichia coli.
Gastrointestinal disorders.

Mutagrip Sanofi Synthelabo, Belg.; Pasteur Vaccins, Fr.; Pasteur Merieux, Ger.; Pasteur Merieux, Ital.; Sanofi Winthrop, Neth.†; Rhone-Poulenc Rorer, Spain; Pro Vaccine, Switz.
An influenza vaccine (p.1544·3).
Active immunisation.

Mutamycin Bristol, Canad.; Bristol-Myers Squibb, Fin.; Bristol-Myers Squibb, Norw.; Bristol-Myers Squibb, Swed.; Bristol-Myers Squibb Oncology, USA.
Mitomycin (p.558·1).
Malignant neoplasms.

Mutamycine Bristol-Myers Squibb, Switz.
Mitomycin (p.558·1).
Malignant neoplasms.

Mutan Lannacher, Aust.
Fluoxetine hydrochloride (p.284·2).
Anxiety disorders; bulimia nervosa; depression.

Mutellon Klein, Ger.
Lycopus europaeus; motherwort (p.1637·3); valerian (p.1678·3).
Hyperthyroidism.

Mutesa Wyeth Lederle, Fr.
Aluminium hydroxide (p.1210·3); magnesium oxide (p.1233·2); oxetacaine (p.1317·3).
Gastro-oesophageal pain.

Muthesa Whitehall, Belg.†; Wyeth, Switz.
Aluminium hydroxide (p.1210·3); magnesium hydroxide (p.1233·1), magnesium carbonate (p.1232·3), or magnesium oxide (p.1233·2); oxetacaine (p.1317·3).
Gastrointestinal disorders.

Muthesa N Whitehall, Neth.
Aluminium hydroxide (p.1210·3); magnesium hydroxide (p.1233·1).
Eructation; heartburn.

Muvial AGIPS, Ital.
Timonacic methyl hydrochloride (p.1673·2).
Otorhinolaryngeal disorders; respiratory-tract disorders.

Muxol
Note. This name is used for preparations of different composition.
Leurquin, Fr.; Andromaco, Mex.
Ambroxol hydrochloride (p.1084·3).
Respiratory-tract congestion.

Vifor, Switz.
Bisacodyl (p.1212·2).
Constipation.

MVI Rhone-Poulenc Rorer, Canad.; Grossman, Mex.; Aventis, NZ; Astra, USA.
Multivitamin infusion (p.1350·1).
Parenteral nutrition.

MVI-12 Rhone-Poulenc Rorer, Austral.; Rhone-Poulenc Rorer, Hong Kong; Armour, Israel.
Multivitamin preparation (p.1350·1).
Parenteral nutrition.

MVI Paediatric Rhone-Poulenc Rorer, Austral.
Multivitamin preparation (p.1350·1).
Parenteral nutrition.

MVI-Ped Armour, Israel.
Multivitamin preparation (p.1350·1).
Parenteral nutrition.

MVM Tyson, USA.
Multivitamin and mineral preparation (p.1350·1).

MXL Napp, Irl.; Napp, UK.
Morphine sulfate (p.56·1).
Pain.

Myacyne Schur, Ger.
Topical powder; ointment: Neomycin sulfate (p.228·1).
Infected skin disorders; infected wounds.

Topical powder spray†: Neomycin sulfate (p.228·1); tyrothricin (p.267·1).
Infected skin disorders.

Myadec Warner-Lambert, Austral.; Warner-Lambert, NZ; Parke, Davis, USA.
Multivitamin and mineral preparation (p.1350·1).

Myalgesic Wolfs, Belg.
Salicylamide (p.82·1); benzocaine (p.1306·2).
Musculoskeletal, joint, peri-articular, and joint disorders.

Myalgol N Robugen, Ger.
Glycol salicylate (p.42·2); benzyl nicotinate (p.20·2).
Formerly contained salicylic acid, camphor, glycol salicylate, benzyl nicotinate, and capsicum.
Circulatory disorders of the skin; muscle and joint pain; soft-tissue disorders.

Myambutol Wyeth Lederle, Aust.; Lederle, Austral.; Wyeth Lederle, Belg.; Wyeth-Ayerst, Canad.; Wyeth Lederle, Fr.; Lederle, Ger.; Lederle, Hong Kong; Wyeth, Irl.; Lederle, Israel; Wyeth, Mex.; Lederle, Neth.; Lederle, NZ; Wyeth, S.Afr.; Cyanamid, Spain; Wyeth Lederle, Swed.; Lederle, Switz.; Wyeth-Ayerst, Thai.; Wyeth, UK†; Lederle, USA.
Ethambutol hydrochloride (p.205·1).
Opportunistic mycobacterial infections; tuberculosis.

Myambutol-INH Wyeth Lederle, Aust.; Lederle, Ger.; Lederle, Switz.
Ethambutol hydrochloride (p.205·1); isoniazid (p.215·3).
Tuberculosis.

Myapap Gen-King, USA†.
Paracetamol (p.71·2).
Fever; pain.

Mybacin Greater Pharma, Thai.
Neomycin sulfate (p.228·1); bacitracin (p.155·2); amylocaine hydrochloride (p.1306·1).
Mouth and throat disorders.

Mybacin Dermic Greater Pharma, Thai.
Bacitracin (p.155·2); neomycin (p.228·1).
Infected skin disorders.

Mycardol Sanofi Winthrop, Irl.†; Sanofi Winthrop, UK†.
Pentaerithrityl tetranitrate (p.952·3).
Angina pectoris.

Mycatox Riemser, Ger.
Dequalinium chloride (p.1143·1); hexylresorcinol (p.1146·3); sage (p.1660·2).
Bath additive; fungal infections.

Mycel Sanus, Braz.
Isoconazole nitrate (p.387·2).
Fungal skin infections.

Mycelex Bayer, USA.
Clotrimazole (p.382·1).
Oral candidiasis.

Mycelex-3 Bayer, USA.
Butoconazole nitrate (p.381·2).
Vaginal candidiasis.

Mycelex-7 Bayer, USA.
Clotrimazole (p.382·1).
Vulvovaginal candidiasis.

Mycelex-G Bayer, USA†.
Clotrimazole (p.382·1).
Vulvovaginal candidiasis.

Mycella Silom, Thai.
Ketoconazole (p.389·1).
Fungal infections.

Mycetin Farmigea, Ital.
Chloramphenicol (p.179·1).
Bacterial eye infections.

Myciclid Wayne, Mex.
Carbenicillin (p.160·3).
Bacterial infections.

Mycidal Greater Pharma, Thai.
Glutaral (p.1145·2).
Instrument disinfection.

Mycifradin Pharmacia Upjohn, Canad.; Pharmacia Upjohn, Hong Kong; Pharmacia Upjohn, Irl.; Pharmacia Upjohn, S.Afr.†; Pharmacia Upjohn, UK†; Upjohn, USA.
Neomycin sulfate (p.228·1).
Hepatic coma; pre-operative bowel preparation.

Myciguent Pharmacia Upjohn, Canad.†; Upjohn, USA.
Neomycin sulfate (p.228·1).
Bacterial skin infections.

Mycil
Note. This name is used for preparations of different composition.
Boots, Austral.; Boots Healthcare, Irl.; Crookes Healthcare, UK.
Cream; ointment: Tolnaftate (p.395·2); benzalkonium chloride (p.1133·2).
Fungal skin infections.

Boots, Austral.; Boots Healthcare, Irl.; Crookes Healthcare, UK.
Topical powder: Tolnaftate (p.395·2); chlorhexidine hydrochloride (p.1138·2).
Fungal skin infections.

Roberts, Canad.
Chlorphenesin (p.381·3).
Fungal and bacterial skin infections.

Boots Healthcare, Irl.; Crookes Healthcare, UK.
Topical spray: Tolnaftate (p.395·2).
Fungal skin infections.

Mycil Gold Crookes Healthcare, UK.
Clotrimazole (p.382·1).
Fungal skin infections.

Mycinette Pfeiffer, USA.
Phenol (p.1152·3); alum (p.1577·2).
Sore throat.

Mycinettes Pfeiffer, USA.
Benzocaine (p.1306·2).
Sore throat.

Mycinopred Allergan, Switz.
Prednisolone acetate (p.1078·1); polymyxin B sulfate (p.238·1); neomycin sulfate (p.228·1).
Infected eye disorders.

Myci-Spray Misemer, USA.
Phenylephrine hydrochloride (p.1097·1); mepyramine maleate (p.421·1).
Nasal congestion.

Mycitracin Upjohn, USA.
Bacitracin (p.155·2); neomycin sulfate (p.228·1); polymyxin B sulfate (p.238·1).
Bacterial skin infections.

Mycitracin Plus Upjohn, USA†.
Bacitracin (p.155·2); neomycin sulfate (p.228·1); polymyxin B sulfate (p.238·1); lignocaine [lidocaine] (p.1313·2).
Bacterial skin infections.

Myclo-Derm Boehringer Ingelheim, Canad.
Clotrimazole (p.382·1).
Fungal skin infections.

Myclo-Gyne Boehringer Ingelheim, Canad.
Clotrimazole (p.382·1).
Vaginal candidiasis.

Mycoapaisyl Monot, Fr.
Econazole nitrate (p.382·3).
Formerly known as Furazanol.
Fungal skin infections.

Mycoban Adcock Ingram, S.Afr.
Clotrimazole (p.382·1).
Fungal skin infections; vulvovaginal candidiasis.

Myco-Biotic II Moore, USA.
Triamcinolone acetonide (p.1080·1); nystatin (p.392·3).
Skin disorders.

Mycobutin Pharmacia Upjohn, Aust.; Pharmacia Upjohn, Austral.; Pharmacia Upjohn, Belg.; Pharmacia Upjohn, Canad.; Pharmacia Upjohn, Ger.; Pharmacia Upjohn, Hong Kong; Pharmacia Upjohn, Israel; Pharmacia Upjohn, Ital.; Pharmacia Upjohn, Neth.; Pharmacia Upjohn, NZ; Pharmacia Upjohn, Port.; Pharmacia Upjohn, S.Afr.; Pharmacia Upjohn, Swed.; Pharmacia, UK; Pharmacia Upjohn, USA.
Rifabutin (p.242·1).
Opportunistic mycobacterial infections; tuberculosis.

Mycochlorin *Sermmitr, Thai.*
Chloramphenicol palmitate (p.179·2).
Bacterial infections.

Mycocide NS *Woodward, USA.*
Benzalkonium chloride (p.1133·2).
Skin disinfection.

Mycodecyl *Diepha, Fr.*
Cream: Undecenoic acid (p.395·3); zinc undecenoate (p.395·3).
Topical powder: Undecenoic acid (p.395·3); zinc undecenoate (p.395·3); calcium undecenoate (p.395·3).
Topical solution: Undecenoic acid (p.395·3).
Fungal skin infections.

Mycoderm *Ego, Austral.*
Cream: Salicylic acid (p.1122·3); undecenoic acid monoethanolamide (p.396·1); sodium propionate (p.393·2); butyl hydroxybenzoate (p.1148·1).
Fungal and bacterial skin infections.
Dusting powder: Salicylic acid (p.1122·3); sodium propionate (p.393·2); butyl hydroxybenzoate (p.1148·1).
Fungal skin infections.

Mycodermil *Vifor, Switz.*
Fenticonazole nitrate (p.383·2).
Fungal skin infections.

Mycodib *Diba, Mex.*
Ketoconazole (p.389·1).
Fungal infections.

Mycofen *Nycomed, Denm.*
Ciclopirox (p.382·1) or ciclopirox olamine (p.382·1).
Fungal skin and nail infections.

Mycofug *Hermal, Ger.*
Clotrimazole (p.382·1).
Fungal infections.

Mycogel *Saninter, Port.*
Copper pidolate; zinc pidolate; melaleuca oil (p.1631·3).
Fungal skin infections.

Mycogen II *Goldline, USA.*
Triamcinolone acetonide (p.1080·1); nystatin (p.392·2).
Skin disorders.

Mycohaug C *Betapharm, Ger.†*
Clotrimazole (p.382·1).
Fungal skin infections.

Myco-Hermal *Hermal, Israel; Hermal, Singapore.*
Clotrimazole (p.382·1).
Fungal skin infections.

Mycohexal *Hexal, S.Afr.*
Clotrimazole (p.382·1).
Vaginal candidiasis.

Mycol *Greater Pharma, Thai.*
Paracetamol (p.71·2); chlorpheniramine [chlorphenamine] maleate (p.412·1); phenylpropanolamine hydrochloride (p.1098·1).
Cold symptoms.

Mycolog *Note. This name is used for preparations of different composition.*
Sanofi Synthelabo, Belg.; Sanofi Synthelabo, Neth.; Sanofi Synthelabo, Switz.
Triamcinolone acetonide (p.1080·1); gramicidin (p.213·3); neomycin sulfate (p.228·1); nystatin (p.392·2).
Infected skin disorders.
Bristol-Myers Squibb, Fr.
Triamcinolone acetonide (p.1080·1); neomycin sulfate (p.228·1); nystatin (p.392·2).
Infected skin disorders.

Mycolog-II *Westwood-Squibb, USA.*
Triamcinolone acetonide (p.1080·1); nystatin (p.392·2).
Cutaneous candidiasis.

Mycomnes *Fumouze, Fr.†*
Nifuratel (p.598·1); nystatin (p.392·2).
Vaginal infections.

Myconel *Marnel, USA.*
Triamcinolone acetonide (p.1080·1); nystatin (p.392·2).
Skin disorders.

Mycopol *Nycomed, Aust.*
Undecenoic acid (p.395·3); benzoic acid (p.1134·2); isopropyl alcohol (p.1149·2).
Fungal infections.

Mycoral *Kalbe, Singapore.*
Ketoconazole (p.389·1).
Dandruff; fungal infections; seborrhoeic dermatitis.

Mycosamthong *Sermmitr, Thai.*
Co-trimoxazole (p.193·3).
Bacterial infections.

Mycospor
Note. This name is used for preparations of different composition.
Bayer, Austral.; Bayer, Belg.; Bayer, Denm.†; Bayer, Ger.; Bayer, Hong Kong; Bayer, Mex.; Bayer, Neth.; Bayer, Norw.; Bayer, Port.; Bayer, S.Afr.; Bayer, Spain; Bayer, Thai.
Bifonazole (p.381·1).
Fungal skin infections.
Bayer, Port.†
Ointment: Bifonazole (p.381·1); urea (p.1127·3).
Fungal nail infections.

Mycospor Carbamid
Bayer, Denm.†; Bayer, Norw.†
Bifonazole (p.381·1); urea (p.1127·3).
Fungal nail infections.

Mycospor Nagelset *Bayer, Ger.*
Bifonazole (p.381·1); urea (p.1127·3).
Fungal nail infections.

Mycospor Onicoset
Bayer, Mex.; Bayer, Spain.
Bifonazole (p.381·1); urea (p.1127·3).
Fungal nail infections.

Mycosporan *Bayer, Swed.*
Bifonazole (p.381·1).
Fungal skin infections.

Mycosporan Karbamid *Bayer, Swed.†*
Bifonazole (p.381·1); urea (p.1127·3).
Fungal nail infections.

Mycosporin *Bayer, Aust.†*
Bifonazole (p.381·1).
Fungal skin and nail infections.

Mycostatin
Bristol-Myers Squibb, Aust.; Bristol-Myers Squibb, Austral.; Squibb, Canad.; Bristol-Myers Squibb, Denm.; Bristol-Myers Squibb, Fin.; Bristol-Myers Squibb, Hong Kong; Bristol-Myers Squibb, Irl.; Bristol-Myers Squibb, Ital.; Bristol-Myers Squibb, Norw.; Bristol-Myers Squibb, NZ; Bristol-Myers Squibb, Port.; Bristol-Myers Squibb, S.Afr.; Bristol-Myers Squibb, Singapore; Squibb, Spain; Bristol-Myers Squibb, Swed.; Bristol-Myers Squibb, Thai.; Apothecon, USA; Mead Johnson Laboratories, USA; Westwood-Squibb, USA.
Nystatin (p.392·2).
Candidiasis.

Mycostatin V *Bristol-Myers Squibb, Aust.*
Triamcinolone acetonide (p.1080·1); neomycin sulfate (p.228·1); gramicidin (p.213·3); nystatin (p.392·2).
Infected skin disorders.

Mycostatine
Bristol-Myers Squibb, Fr.; Sanofi Synthelabo, Switz.
Nystatin (p.392·2).
Candidiasis.

Mycostatin-Zinkoxid *Bristol-Myers Squibb, Aust.*
Nystatin (p.392·2); zinc oxide (p.1128·2).
Candidiasis.

Mycoster *Pierre Fabre, Fr.*
Ciclopirox (p.382·1) or ciclopirox olamine (p.382·1).
Fungal infections of the skin and nails.

Myco-Synalar
Note. This name is used for preparations of different composition.
Grunenthal, Aust.; Grunenthal, Switz.
Cream: Fluocinolone acetonide (p.1071·1); chlormidazole hydrochloride (p.381·3).
Fungal skin infections.
Grunenthal, Aust.; Yamanouchi, Spain†; Grunenthal, Switz.
Topical solution: Fluocinolone acetonide (p.1071·1); chlormidazole hydrochloride (p.381·3); salicylic acid (p.1122·3).
Fungal skin infections.

Mycota
Note. This name is used for preparations of different composition.
Boots, Hong Kong; Reckitt Benckiser, S.Afr.; SSL, UK.
Cream; topical powder: Undecenoic acid (p.395·3); zinc undecenoate (p.395·3).
Fungal skin infections.
Reckitt Benckiser, S.Afr.; SSL, UK.
Topical spray: Undecenoic acid (p.395·3); dichlorophen (p.98·1).
Fungal skin infections.

Myco-Triacet II *Lemmon, USA.*
Triamcinolone acetonide (p.1080·1); nystatin (p.392·2).
Skin disorders.

Myco-Ultralan *Schering, Fr.*
Fluocortolone (p.1071·3); fluocortolone caproate (p.1071·3); nystatin (p.392·2); neomycin sulfate (p.228·1).
Infected skin disorders.

Mycozol *Warner-Lambert, Austral.†*
Salicylic acid (p.1122·3); benzoic acid (p.1134·2).
Fungal skin infections.

Mycrol *Rolab, S.Afr.†*
Ethambutol hydrochloride (p.205·1).
Tuberculosis.

Mycurium *Taro, Israel.*
Atracurium besilate (p.1333·1).
Competitive neuromuscular blocker.

Mydfrin
Alcon, Canad.; Alcon, Hong Kong; Alcon, Singapore; Alcon, USA.
Phenylephrine hydrochloride (p.1097·1).
Funduscopy; open-angle glaucoma; ophthalmic examination; pupil dilatation during surgery; refraction without cycloplegia; uveitis.

Mydocalm
Gebro, Aust.†; Strathmann, Ger.; Gedeon Richter, Hong Kong; Labatec, Switz.; Gedeon Richter, Thai.
Tolperisone hydrochloride (p.1330·3).
Lignocaine [lidocaine] hydrochloride (p.1313·2) may be included in the intravenous infusion.
Skeletal muscle spasm.

Mydocalm-A *Chinoin, Mex.*
Tolperisone hydrochloride (p.1330·3); paracetamol (p.71·2).
Skeletal muscle spasm and pain.

Mydosone *Condrugs, Thai.*
Tolperisone hydrochloride (p.1330·3).
Skeletal muscle spasm.

Mydral *Ocusoft, USA.*
Tropicamide (p.475·1).

Mydramide *Fischer, Israel.*
Tropicamide (p.475·1).
Production of mydriasis.

Mydriacil *Alcon, Irl.*
Tropicamide (p.475·1).
Production of mydriasis and cycloplegia.

Mydriacyl
Alcon, Austral.; Alcon, Braz.; Alcon, Canad.; Alcon, Denm.; Alcon, Hong Kong; Alcon, NZ; Alcon, S.Afr.; Alcon, Singapore; Alcon, Swed.; Alcon, Thai.; Alcon, UK; Alcon, USA.
Tropicamide (p.475·1).
Production of mydriasis and cycloplegia.

Mydrial-Atropin *Winzer, Ger.*
Tyramine hydrochloride (p.1676·3); atropine borate (p.462·1); adrenaline [epinephrine] acid tartrate (p.829·2).
Production of mydriasis.

Mydrian *Ciba Vision, Norw.*
Tropicamide (p.475·1).
Production of mydriasis.

Mydriaticum
Agepha, Aust.; Bournonville, Belg.†; Merck Sharp & Dohme-Chibret, Fr.; Stulln, Ger.; Ciba Vision, Hong Kong; Restan, S.Afr.; Ciba Vision, Switz.
Tropicamide (p.475·1).
Production of mydriasis and cycloplegia.

Mydrilate
Boehringer Ingelheim, Irl.; Intrapharm, UK.
Cyclopentolate hydrochloride (p.465·2).
Production of mydriasis and cycloplegia.

Mydrin-P *Santen, Hong Kong.*
Tropicamide (p.475·1); phenylephrine hydrochloride (p.1097·1).
Production of mydriasis and cycloplegia.

Mydrum *Chauvin ankerpharm, Ger.*
Tropicamide (p.475·1).
Aid in eye examination; production of mydriasis.

Myelobromol
Enzypharm, Aust.; Durbin, UK.
Mitobronitol (p.557·3).
Chronic myeloid leukaemia.

Myelostim *Italfarmaco, Ital.*
Lenograstim (p.738·1).
Mobilisation of autologous peripheral blood progenitor cells; neutropenia induced by bone-marrow transplantation or cytotoxic chemotherapy.

Myfedrine *Morton Grove, USA†.*
Paediatric liquid: Pseudoephedrine hydrochloride (p.1099·2).
Syrup: Pseudoephedrine hydrochloride (p.1099·2); guaifenesin (p.1092·2); dextromethorphan hydrobromide (p.1087·3).

Myfedrine Plus *Morton Grove, USA†.*
Pseudoephedrine hydrochloride (p.1099·2); chlorpheniramine [chlorphenamine] maleate (p.412·1).

Myfungar *Riemser, Ger.; Rhein, Mex.; Klinge, Switz.*
Oxiconazole nitrate (p.393·1).
Fungal and Gram-positive bacterial infections.

Mygale compositum *Weleda, Aust.*
Homoeopathic preparation.

Mygdalon *DDSA Pharmaceuticals, UK.*
Metoclopramide hydrochloride (p.1235·2).

Mygel *Geneva, USA.*
Aluminium hydroxide (p.1210·3); magnesium hydroxide (p.1233·1); simeticone (p.1249·2).
Hyperacidity.

Mygesal *Greater Pharma, Thai.*
Methyl salicylate (p.55·1).
Musculoskeletal and joint pain; sprains; strains.

Myidyl *Pharmaceutical Basics, USA†.*
Triprolidine hydrochloride (p.427·2).
Hypersensitivity reactions.

Myk *Cassenne, Fr.†.*
Sulconazole nitrate (p.393·3).
Fungal skin infections.

Myk-1
Will-Pharma, Belg.; Will-Pharma, Neth.
Sulconazole nitrate (p.393·3).
Fungal skin infections.

Myko Cordes
Note. This name is used for preparations of different composition.
Ichthyol, Ger.
Cream: Clotrimazole (p.382·1).
Paste: Clotrimazole (p.382·1); zinc oxide (p.1128·2).
Fungal skin infections.
Ichthyol, Ger.
Clotrimazole (p.382·1).
Fungal and corynebacterial skin infections.

Myko Cordes Plus *Ichthyol, Ger.*
Clotrimazole (p.382·1); zinc oxide (p.1128·2).
Fungal skin infections.

Mykoderm Heilsalbe *Engelhard, Ger.*
Nystatin (p.392·2).
Fungal skin infections.

Mykoderm Mund-Gel *Engelhard, Ger.*
Miconazole (p.391·1).
Fungal mouth infections.

Mykofungin *Riemser, Ger.*
Clotrimazole (p.382·1).
Fungal and bacterial infections of skin and genito-urinary tract.

Mykohaug *Betapharm, Ger.*
Clotrimazole (p.382·1).
Fungal and bacterial vaginal infections; vaginal trichomoniasis.

Mykontral *LAW, Ger.*
Tioconazole (p.395·1).
Fungal skin infections.

MykoPosterine N *Kade, Ger.*
Nystatin (p.392·2).
Anorectal fungal infections.

mykoproct sine *Bristol-Myers Squibb, Ger.†*
Nystatin (p.392·2); triamcinolone acetonide (p.1080·1).
Infected eczema.

Mykosert *Pfleger, Ger.*
Sertaconazole nitrate (p.393·3).
Fungal skin infections.

Mykotin mono *Ardeypharm, Ger.*
Miconazole nitrate (p.391·1).
Fungal skin infections.

Mykozem *Sanova, Aust.†*
Undecenoic acid (p.395·3); urea (p.1127·3); zinc stearate (p.1497·3).
Fungal skin infections.

Mykrox *Medeva, USA.*
Metolazone (p.930·3).
Formerly known as Microx.
Hypertension.

Mykundex *Biocur, Ger.*
Nystatin (p.392·2).
Fungal infections.

Mykundex Heilsalbe *Biocur, Ger.*
Nystatin (p.392·2); zinc oxide (p.1128·2).
Fungal infections.

Mykundex mono *Biocur, Ger.*
Nystatin (p.392·2).
Fungal infections.

Mylagen *Goldline, USA.*
Capsules: Calcium carbonate (p.1215·1); magnesium carbonate (p.1232·3).
Oral liquid: Aluminium hydroxide (p.1210·3); magnesium hydroxide (p.1233·1); simeticone (p.1249·2).
Hyperacidity.

Mylanta
Note. This name is used for preparations of different composition.
Warner-Lambert, Austral.; Janssen-Cilag, Belg.; Warner-Lambert, Canad.; Warner-Lambert, NZ.
Aluminium hydroxide (p.1210·3); magnesium hydroxide (p.1233·1); simeticone (p.1249·2).
Antacid; flatulence.
Johnson & Johnson, Hong Kong.
Oral liquid: Aluminium hydroxide (p.1210·3); magnesium hydroxide (p.1233·1); simeticone (p.1249·2).
Tablets: Magnesium hydroxide (p.1233·1); calcium carbonate (p.1215·1).
Dyspepsia; gastrointestinal hyperacidity.
J&J-Merck, USA.
Lozenges: Calcium carbonate (p.1215·1).
Hyperacidity.
Oral liquid; tablets: Aluminium hydroxide (p.1210·3); magnesium hydroxide (p.1233·1); simeticone (p.1249·2).
Flatulence; hyperacidity.

Mylanta AR Acid Reducer *J&J-Merck, USA.*
Famotidine (p.1225·3).
Dyspepsia; heartburn.

Mylanta Gas *J&J-Merck, USA.*
Simeticone (p.1249·2).
Flatulence.

Mylanta Gelcaps *J&J-Merck, USA.*
Calcium carbonate (p.1215·1); magnesium carbonate (p.1232·3).
Hyperacidity.

Mylanta Heartburn Relief
Note. This name is used for preparations of different composition.
Warner-Lambert, Austral.
Oral liquid: Aluminium hydroxide (p.1210·3); magnesium hydroxide (p.1233·1); calcium carbonate (p.1215·1); sodium bicarbonate (p.1186·2); alginic acid (p.1498·3).
Tablets: Magaldrate (p.1232·2); alginic acid (p.1498·3); sodium bicarbonate (p.1186·2).
Formerly known as Mylanta Plus.
Dyspepsia; gastro-oesophageal reflux.
Warner-Lambert, NZ.
Alginic acid (p.1498·3); calcium carbonate (p.1215·1); aluminium hydroxide (p.1210·3); magnesium hydroxide (p.1233·1); sodium bicarbonate (p.1186·2).
Antacid; gastro-oesophageal reflux.

Mylanta Natural Fiber *J&J-Merck, USA.*
Psyllium hydrophilic mucilloid (p.1229·1).

Mylanta Plain *Warner-Lambert, Canad.*
Aluminium hydroxide (p.1210·3); magnesium hydroxide (p.1233·1).
Gastrointestinal disorders associated with hyperacidity.

Mylanta Plus *Ache, Braz.*
Aluminium hydroxide (p.1210·3); magnesium hydroxide (p.1233·1); dimethicone (p.1249·2).
Flatulence; gastrointestinal hyperacidity.

Mylanta Rolltabs *Warner-Lambert, NZ.*
Calcium carbonate (p.1215·1); magnesium hydroxide (p.1233·1).
Antacid.

Mylepsinum *Zeneca, Ger.*
Primidone (p.363·3).
Epilepsy.

Myleran
Glaxo Wellcome, Aust.; Glaxo Wellcome, Austral.; Glaxo Wellcome,

Belg.; Glaxo Wellcome, Braz.; Glaxo Wellcome, Canad.; Glaxo Wellcome, Fr.; Glaxo Wellcome, Ger.; Glaxo Wellcome, Hong Kong; Glaxo Wellcome, Irl.; Glaxo Wellcome, Israel; Glaxo Wellcome, Ital.; Glaxo Wellcome, Mex.; Glaxo Wellcome, Neth.; Glaxo Wellcome, Norw.†; Glaxo Wellcome, NZ; Wellcome, Port.; Glaxo Wellcome, S.Afr.; Glaxo Wellcome, Singapore; Glaxo Wellcome, Swed.; Wellcome, Switz.; Glaxo Wellcome, Thai.; Glaxo Wellcome, UK; Glaxo Wellcome, USA.
Busulfan (p.513·3).
Bone-marrow transplantation; chronic myeloid leukaemia; essential thrombocythaemia; myelofibrosis; polycythaemia vera.

Myleuca Effimed, Fr.
Melaleuca oil (p.1631·3).
Adjunct in fungal skin infections; skin cleansing.

Mylicon Parke, Davis, Denm.; Warner-Lambert, Ital.; J&J-Merck, USA.
Simeticone (p.1249·2).
Adjunct in gastrointestinal investigations; flatulence; infant colic; meteorism.

Mylocel MGI, USA.
Hydroxyurea (p.544·2).
Malignant neoplasms.

Mylocort Triomed, S.Afr.
Hydrocortisone acetate (p.1073·3).
Skin disorders.

Mylol Boots, S.Afr.†
Topical liquid: Diethyltoluamide (p.1431·2); dimethyl phthalate (p.1431·3); dibutyl phthalate (p.1431·1).
Topical spray: Diethyltoluamide (p.1431·2).
Insect repellent.

Mylom Ranbaxy, Thai.
Simeticone (p.1249·2).
Flatulence.

Mylotarg Wyeth-Ayerst, USA.
Gemtuzumab ozogamicin (p.544·1).
Acute myeloid leukaemia.

Mylproin Desitin, Ger.
Valproic acid (p.366·2).
Epilepsy.

Mymin C Greater Pharma, Thai.
Vitamin C (p.1389·3).
Vitamin C deficiency.

Myminic Expectorant Morton Grove, USA†.
Phenylpropanolamine hydrochloride (p.1098·1); guaifenesin (p.1092·2).
Coughs.

Myminic Syrup Morton Grove, USA†.
Phenylpropanolamine hydrochloride (p.1098·1); chlorpheniramine [chlorphenamine] maleate (p.412·1).
Coughs.

Myminicol Morton Grove, USA†.
Phenylpropanolamine hydrochloride (p.1098·1); chlorpheniramine [chlorphenamine] maleate (p.412·1); dextromethorphan hydrobromide (p.1087·3).
Coughs and cold symptoms.

Mynah Wyeth, S.Afr.†.
Ethambutol hydrochloride (p.205·1); isoniazid (p.215·3).
Tuberculosis.

Mynatal ME Pharmaceuticals, USA.
Multivitamin and mineral preparation with iron and folic acid (p.1350·1).

Mynate 90 Plus ME Pharmaceuticals, USA.
Multivitamin and mineral preparation (p.1350·1).

Mynocine Wyeth Lederle, Fr.
Minocycline hydrochloride (p.224·3).
Bacterial infections.

Myo Hermes Organon, Spain.
Bethanechol chloride (p.1415·3).
Gastrointestinal motility disorders; urinary retention.

Myobloc Elan, USA.
Botulinum B toxin (p.1324·2).
Spasmodic torticollis.

Myocardon Byk, Aust.
Aminophylline hydrochloride (p.760·2); papaverine hydrochloride (p.1648·1); atropine methonitrate (p.461·1); glyceryl trinitrate (p.897·3).
Angina pectoris; heart failure; myocardial infarction.

Myocardon mono Byk, Aust.
Isosorbide mononitrate (p.916·2).
Angina pectoris; heart failure; myocardial infarction.

Myocardon N Byk Gulden, Ger.†.
Theophylline (p.777·2).
Formerly contained aminophylline hydrate, phenobarbital, papaverine hydrochloride, atropine methonitrate, and glyceryl trinitrate.
Cardiac disorders.

Myocet Elan, UK.
Liposomal doxorubicin citrate.
Breast cancer.

Myocholine Croma, Aust.; Glenwood, Ger.; Glenwood, Switz.
Bethanechol chloride (p.1415·3).
Antimuscarinic effects of tricyclic antidepressants; dysphagia; gastro-oesophageal reflux; urinary retention.

Myochrysine Prodome, Braz.; Rhone-Poulenc Rorer, Canad.; Merck, USA.
Sodium aurothiomalate (p.82·3).
Rheumatoid arthritis.

Myocin Shiwa, Thai.
Methocarbamol (p.1329·3).
Cramps; skelatal muscle spasm.

Myocrisin Rhone-Poulenc Rorer, Austral.; Aventis, Denm.; Rhone-Poulenc Rorer, Fin.; Rhone-Poulenc Rorer, Hong Kong; Rhone-Poulenc Rorer, Irl.;

Rhone-Poulenc Rorer, Norw.; Aventis, NZ; Aventis, S.Afr.; Rhone-Poulenc Rorer, Swed.; Rhone-Poulenc Rorer, Thai.; JHC Healthcare, UK.
Sodium aurothiomalate (p.82·3).
Juvenile idiopathic arthritis; rheumatoid arthritis.

Myodrine Charoen, Thai.
Orphenadrine citrate (p.470·3); paracetamol (p.71·2).
Muscle spasm; tension headache.

Myo-Echinacin Madaus, Aust.†.
Echinaceae purpureae (p.1606·2).
Urinary and respiratory-tract infections.

Myofedrin Apogepha, Ger.
Oxyfedrine hydrochloride (p.952·1).
Heart failure; ischaemic heart disease; myocardial infarction.

Myoflex
Note. This name is used for preparations of different composition.
Bayer, Canad.; Armstrong, Mex.; Fisons, USA.
Trolamine salicylate (p.90·1).
Muscle, joint, and soft-tissue pain; neuralgia.

Pharmacare Consumer, S.Afr.†.
Paracetamol (p.71·2); chlormezanone (p.660·1).
Pain and associated tension.

Siam Bheasach, Thai.
Orphenadrine citrate (p.470·3); paracetamol (p.71·2).
Musculoskeletal and joint pain; neuralgia.

Myoflex Ice Bayer, Canad.†.
Menthol (p.1632·3).
Pain.

Myoflex Ice Plus Bayer, Canad.
Trolamine salicylate (p.90·1); menthol (p.1632·3).
Muscle pain.

Myogeloticum N Hanosan, Ger.
Homoeopathic preparation.

Myogesic Lambda, USA†.
Magnesium salicylate (p.50·3); phenyltoloxamine citrate (p.423·1).

Myogit Pfleger, Ger.
Diclofenac sodium (p.30·3).
Inflammation; rheumatism.

Myolastan Sanofi Winthrop, Aust.; Sanofi Synthelabo, Belg.; Sanofi Winthrop, Fr.; Sanofi Synthelabo, Spain.
Tetrazepam (p.708·1).
Skeletal muscle spasm.

Myolax
Note. This name is used for preparations of different composition.
Shiwa, Thai.
Tolperisone hydrochloride (p.1330·3).
Parkinsonism; skeletal muscle spasm.

Siam Bheasach, Thai.
Carisoprodol (p.1327·1).
Skeletal muscle spasm.

Myolin Roberts, USA†; Hauck, USA†.
Orphenadrine citrate (p.470·3).
Musculoskeletal pain.

Myolosyx Syxyl, Ger.
Homoeopathic preparation.

Myomethol Abic, Thai.
Methocarbamol (p.1329·3).
Cramps; skelatal muscle spasm.

Myonac M & H, Thai.
Diclofenac diethylamine (p.30·2) or diclofenac sodium (p.30·3).
Gout; inflammation; musculoskeletal, joint, and peri-articular disorders.

Myonal Eisai, Jpn; Eisai, Singapore; Eisai, Thai.
Eperisone hydrochloride (p.1329·2).
Myotonias; skeletal muscle spasm.

Myonil Nycomed, Denm.
Diltiazem hydrochloride (p.874·3).
Angina pectoris; hypertension.

Myopar Ranbaxy, Thai.
Orphenadrine citrate (p.470·3); paracetamol (p.71·2).
Musculoskeletal and joint pain; tension headache.

Myopax Orion, Denm.
Atenolol (p.841·3).
Angina pectoris; arrhythmias; hypertension; myocardial infarction.

Myophen
Note. This name is used for preparations of different composition.
Charoen, Thai.
Carisoprodol (p.1327·1); phenylbutazone (p.78·1).
Musculoskeletal, joint, and peri-articular disorders.

Teral, USA†.
Orphenadrine citrate (p.470·3).

Myoplege Genevrier, Fr.
Thiocolchicoside (p.1330·2).
Skeletal muscle spasm.

Myoplegine Christiaens, Belg.
Suxamethonium chloride (p.1340·1).
Depolarising neuromuscular blocker.

Myoprin Desatnik, S.Afr.
Aspirin (p.14·2).
Fever; pain; thromboembolism prophylaxis.

Myoquin Fawns & McAllan, Austral.
Quinine bisulfate (p.445·1).
Malaria; nocturnal cramps.

Myoscain Sanochemia, Aust.
Guaifenesin (p.1092·2).
Coughs.

Myoscint Byk Gulden, Ital.†.
Indium-111 imciromab pentetate (p.1449·3).
Diagnosis of myocardial infarction.

Myosic M & H, Thai.
Orphenadrine citrate (p.470·3); paracetamol (p.71·2).
Musculoskeletal pain.

Myoson Strathmann, Ger.
Pridinol mesilate (p.1330·1).
Skeletal muscle spasm.

Myospasmal TAD, Ger.
Tetrazepam (p.708·1).
Skeletal muscle tension and spasm.

Myotenlis Pharmacia Upjohn, Ital.
Suxamethonium chloride (p.1340·1).
Depolarising neuromuscular blocker.

Myotonachol Glenwood, Canad.; Glenwood, USA.
Bethanechol chloride (p.1415·3).
Gastro-oesophageal reflux; neurogenic bladder; urinary retention.

Myotonine Glenwood, UK.
Bethanechol chloride (p.1415·3).
Gastro-oesophageal reflux; urinary retention.

Myoview Nycomed, Austral.; Nycomed, Fr.; Sorin, Ital.; Nycomed, Spain; Nycomed Amersham, UK.
Technetium-99m tetrofosmin (p.1451·1).
Myocardial perfusion imaging.

Myoviton Therabel, Fr.
Adenosine triphosphate, disodium salt (p.1573·3).
Formerly contained pyridoxine hydrochloride and adenosine triphosphate, disodium salt.
Pain.

Myoxam Menarini, Spain.
Midecamycin acetate (p.224·3).
Bacterial infections.

Myoxan TO-Chemicals, Thai.
Tolperisone hydrochloride (p.1330·3).
Parkinsonism; skeletal muscle spasm.

Mypaid Restan, S.Afr.
Ibuprofen (p.43·2); paracetamol (p.71·2).
Fever; pain.

Myphetane DC Morton Grove, USA†.
Phenylpropanolamine hydrochloride (p.1098·1); codeine phosphate (p.25·2); brompheniramine maleate (p.410·2).
Coughs and cold symptoms.

Myphetane DX Morton Grove, USA.
Pseudoephedrine hydrochloride (p.1099·2); brompheniramine maleate (p.410·2); dextromethorphan hydrobromide (p.1087·3).
Coughs and cold symptoms.

Myphetapp Morton Grove, USA†.
Phenylpropanolamine hydrochloride (p.1098·1); brompheniramine maleate (p.410·2).

Myprodol Adcock Ingram, S.Afr.
Ibuprofen (p.43·2); paracetamol (p.71·2); codeine phosphate (p.25·2).
Inflammation; pain.

Myproflam Adcock Ingram, S.Afr.
Ketoprofen (p.47·3).
Musculoskeletal, joint, and peri-articular disorders.

Myra 300-E Myra, Singapore.
Vitamin E (p.1393·3).
Vitamin E deficiency.

Myriacyl Alcon, Mex.
Tropicamide (p.475·1).
Production of mydriasis and cycloplegia.

Myrin
Wyeth, S.Afr.; Lederle, Thai.
Ethambutol hydrochloride (p.205·1); isoniazid (p.215·3); rifampicin (p.243·2).
Tuberculosis.

Myrin Plus Wyeth, S.Afr.
Ethambutol hydrochloride (p.205·1); isoniazid (p.215·3); rifampicin (p.243·2); pyrazinamide (p.240·1).
Tuberculosis.

Myrin-P Lederle, Thai.
Ethambutol hydrochloride (p.205·1); isoniazid (p.215·3); rifampicin (p.243·2); pyrazinamide (p.240·1).
Tuberculosis.

Myristoll Eagle, Austral.
Cetyl myristoleate.
Dietary supplement.

Myrol Dorom, Ital.†.
Dihydroergocryptine mesilate (p.1603·3).
Dementia; hyperprolactinaemia; lactation inhibition; parkinsonism; vascular headache.

Myrrhinil-Intest Repha, Ger.
Myrrh (p.1639·2); carbo coffeae (p.1681·2); chamomile (p.1593·2).
Gastrointestinal disorders.

Myrtaven IBSA, Switz.
Myrtillus (p.1639·2).
Peripheral vascular disorders.

Myrtilen Synpharma, Aust.
Myrtillus (p.1639·2); caraway (p.1591·2); rice starch (p.1379·3).
Diarrhoea.

Myser Mitsubishi, Jpn.
Diflupredonate (p.1069·3).
Skin disorders.

Mysial Douglas, Thai.; TTN, Thai.
Prazosin hydrochloride (p.958·1).
Hypertension.

Mysocort Greater Pharma, Thai.
Miconazole nitrate (p.391·1).
Fungal and Gram-positive bacterial skin infections.

Mysoline Zeneca, Aust.; Zeneca, Austral.; Zeneca, Belg.; Wyeth-Ayerst, Canad.; AstraZeneca, Denm.; AstraZeneca, Fin.; AstraZeneca, Fr.; Zeneca, Hong Kong; Zeneca, Irl.; SIT, Ital.; Zeneca, Mex.; Zeneca, Neth.; AstraZeneca, Norw.; AstraZeneca, NZ; Zeneca, Port.; Zeneca, S.Afr.; AstraZeneca, Singapore; Zeneca, Spain; Zeneca, Swed.; Zeneca, Switz.; AstraZeneca, UK; Athena Neurosciences, USA.
Primidone (p.363·3).
Epilepsy; essential tremor.

Mysolone-N Greater Pharma, Thai.
Prednisolone (p.1077·3); neomycin sulfate (p.228·1).
Burns; skin disorders; wounds.

Mysoven Greater Pharma, Thai.
Acetylcysteine (p.1082·3).
Respiratory-tract disorders associated with increased or viscous mucus.

Mysteclin
Note. This name is used for preparations of different composition.
Bristol-Myers Squibb, Aust.; Bristol-Myers Squibb, Ger.
Tetracycline (p.258·3); amphotericin B (p.377·2).
Vaginal infections.

Bristol-Myers Squibb, Austral.
Tetracycline hydrochloride (p.258·3).
Bacterial infections.

Mysteclin-V
Note. This name is used for preparations of different composition.
Bristol-Myers Squibb, Austral.
Tetracycline (p.258·3); nystatin (p.392·1).
Bacterial infections.

Bristol-Myers Squibb, S.Afr.†.
Tetracycline (p.258·3); amphotericin B (p.377·2).
Bacterial infections.

Mytancid Synco, Hong Kong.
Aluminium hydroxide (p.1210·3); magnesium hydroxide (p.1233·1); dimethicone (p.1249·2).
Flatulence; gastrointestinal hyperacidity.

Mytelase Sanofi Winthrop, Fr.; Sanofi Winthrop, Swed.; Sanofi Winthrop, USA.
Ambenonium chloride (p.1415·2).
Myasthenia gravis.

Mytex Morton Grove, USA†.
Phenylephrine hydrochloride (p.1097·1); phenylpropanolamine hydrochloride (p.1098·1); guaifenesin (p.1092·2).

Mytobrin Intramed, S.Afr.
Tobramycin sulfate (p.263·3).
Bacterial infections.

Mytrex Savage, USA.
Triamcinolone acetonide (p.1080·1); nystatin (p.392·1).
Skin disorders.

Mytussin Morton Grove, USA.
Guaifenesin (p.1092·2).
Coughs.

Mytussin AC Morton Grove, USA.
Codeine phosphate (p.25·2); guaifenesin (p.1092·2).
Coughs.

Mytussin CF Morton Grove, USA†.
Guaifenesin (p.1092·2); phenylpropanolamine hydrochloride (p.1098·1); dextromethorphan hydrobromide (p.1087·3).

Mytussin DAC Morton Grove, USA.
Pseudoephedrine hydrochloride (p.1099·2); guaifenesin (p.1092·2); codeine phosphate (p.25·2).
Coughs.

Mytussin DM Morton Grove, USA.
Dextromethorphan hydrobromide (p.1087·3); guaifenesin (p.1092·2).
Coughs.

Mytussin PE Morton Grove, USA.
Guaifenesin (p.1092·2); pseudoephedrine hydrochloride (p.1099·2).

My-Vitalife ME Pharmaceuticals, USA.
Multivitamin and mineral preparation (p.1350·1).

Myvlar Schering, Aust.
Gestodene (p.1479·1); ethinylestradiol (p.1476·2).
Combined oral contraceptive.

Myxofat Fatol, Ger.
Acetylcysteine (p.1082·3).
Respiratory-tract disorders associated with increased or viscous mucus.

MZM Ciba Vision, USA.
Methazolamide (p.927·1).

M-Zole Alpharma, USA.
Miconazole nitrate (p.391·1).
Vulvovaginal candidiasis.

N32 Collutorio Esoform, Ital.
Chlorhexidine gluconate (p.1138·2).
Oral disinfection.

N D Clear Seatrace, USA.
Pseudoephedrine hydrochloride (p.1099·2); chlorpheniramine [chlorphenamine] maleate (p.412·1).
Upper respiratory-tract symptoms.

Naabak Thea, Fr.
Sodium isospaglumate (p.1624·3).
Allergic conjunctivitis.

Naaprep
SmithKline Beecham, Belg.; SmithKline Beecham Consumer, Switz.
Sodium chloride (p.1196·1).
Cleansing of eyelids; nasal irrigation; rinsing solution for contact lenses.

Naaxia
Note. This name is used for preparations of different composition.
Allergan-Frumtost, Braz.; Thea, Fr.; Ciba Vision, Ital.; Ciba Vision, Port.; Ciba Vision, Spain.
Sodium isospaglumate (p.1624·3) or sodium spaglumate.
Allergic conjunctivitis.

Ciba Vision, Ger.†
Magnesium isospaglumate (p.1624·3).
Allergic conjunctivitis.

Restan, S.Afr.
Spaglumic acid; isospaglumic acid (p.1624·3).
Allergic conjunctivitis.

Ciba Vision, Switz.
Sodium isospaglumate (p.1624·3); spaglumate decahydrate.
Allergic keratoconjunctivitis.

Nabact Pharmador, S.Afr.†
Metronidazole (p.594·1).
Anaerobic bacterial infections.

Nabi-HB Nabi, USA.
A hepatitis B immunoglobulin (p.1542·1).
Passive immunisation.

Nabone TO-Chemicals, Thai.
Nabumetone (p.59·3).
Osteoarthritis; rheumatoid arthritis.

Nabucox Mayoly-Spindler, Fr.
Nabumetone (p.59·3).
Musculoskeletal and joint disorders.

Nabuser Geymonat, Ital.
Nabumetone (p.59·3).
Musculoskeletal, joint, and peri-articular disorders.

Nabutil Oberlin, Fr.
Loperamide hydrochloride (p.1231·3).
Diarrhoea.

NAC
CT, Ger.; ABZ, Ger.; Aliud, Ger.; Ratiopharm, Ger.; Stada, Ger.; Asta Medica, Thai.; Temmler, Thai.
Acetylcysteine (p.1082·3).
Paracetamol poisoning; respiratory-tract disorders associated with increased or viscous mucus.

Nacha Lineafarm, Spain.
A nonoxinol (p.1346·1).
Contraceptive.

Naclof
Ciba Vision, Neth.; Restan, S.Afr.; Ciba Vision, Swed.†; Ciba Vision, Thai.
Diclofenac sodium (p.30·3).
Eye inflammation; inhibition of intra-operative miosis; prevention of cystoid macular oedema following eye surgery.

Naclon Teofarma, Ital.
Sodium hypochlorite (p.1156·2).
Disinfection of skin, wounds, external genitalia, and drinking water.

Nacom Du Pont, Ger.
Carbidopa (p.1168·2); levodopa (p.1169·2).
Parkinsonism.

Nacor Merck, Spain.
Enalapril maleate (p.883·3).
Heart failure; hypertension.

Nacozil TO-Chemicals, Thai.
Isoconazole nitrate (p.387·2).
Fungal skin infections.

Nacro Investigaciones Filosoficas y Cientificas, Mex.
Nicotinamide (p.1372·3).

Nacton Pharmark, UK†.
Poldine metilsulfate (p.472·3).
Gastric hyperacidity; peptic ulcer.

Nad Medical, Spain.
Nadide (p.1639·3).
Vertigo.

Nadamen
Medochemie, Hong Kong; Medochemie, Singapore; Medochemie, Thai.
Tenoxicam (p.87·2).
Gout; inflammation; musculoskeletal, joint, peri-articular, and soft-tissue disorders.

Nadex
Zyma, Belg.†; Novartis, Switz.
Pirisudanol maleate (p.1652·3).
Asthenia; depression; mental function impairment.

Nadib Diba, Mex.
Glibenclamide (p.321·3).
Diabetes mellitus.

Nadinola Nadinola, Canad.
Hydroquinone (p.1115·1).

Nadione DMG, Ital.
Bioflavonoids; vitamin C; phytomenadione (p.1350·1).
Nutritional supplement.

Nadipinia Scherer, Hong Kong.
Nifedipine (p.940·1).
Heart failure; hypertension.

Nadiwil Willmar, Mex.
Nalidixic acid (p.227·1).

Nadopen-V Lioh, Canad.
Phenoxymethylpenicillin potassium (p.235·1).
Bacterial infections.

Nadostine
Nadeau, Canad.; Rougier, Hong Kong.
Nystatin (p.392·2).
Candidiasis.

Naetene Novartis, Braz.
Multivitamin and mineral preparation (p.1350·1).

Nafasol Aspen, S.Afr.
Naproxen (p.60·3).
Dysmenorrhoea; gout; musculoskeletal and joint disorders.

Nafazair Bausch & Lomb, USA.
Naphazoline hydrochloride (p.1095·1).
Minor eye irritation.

Nafazair A Bausch & Lomb, USA.
Naphazoline hydrochloride (p.1095·1); pheniramine maleate (p.422·3).
Eye irritation.

Nafcil Apothecon, USA†.
Nafcillin sodium (p.226·3).
Bacterial infections.

Nafcon A Alcon, Ital.
Naphazoline hydrochloride (p.1095·1); pheniramine maleate (p.422·3).
Conjunctivitis.

Naferon Sclavo, Ital.
Interferon beta (p.632·2).
Malignant neoplasms; viral infections.

Nafluryl Atlantis, Mex.
Flunarizine (p.418·2).
Migraine; peripheral vascular disorders.

NaFril Merckle, Ger.
Sodium fluoride (p.1375·3).
Osteoporosis.

Nafrine Schering, Canad.
Oxymetazoline hydrochloride (p.1096·2).

Naftazolina Bruschettini, Ital.
Naphazoline hydrochloride (p.1095·1).
Eye congestion; eye irritation.

Nafti CT, Ger.; Isis Puren, Ger.; Ratiopharm, Ger.
Naftidrofuryl oxalate (p.937·3).
Peripheral vascular disorders.

Naftifin Zinkpaste Biochemie, Aust.†.
Naftifine hydrochloride (p.392·1); zinc oxide (p.1128·2).
Fungal skin infections.

Naftilong Hexal, Ger.
Naftidrofuryl oxalate (p.937·3).
Peripheral vascular disorders.

Naftilux Therabel, Fr.
Naftidrofuryl oxalate (p.937·3).
Mental function impairment in the elderly; peripheral vascular and cerebrovascular disorders.

Naftin
Allergan, Canad.; Allergan, USA.
Naftifine hydrochloride (p.392·1).
Fungal skin infections.

Naftodril Arcana, Aust.
Naftidrofuryl oxalate (p.937·3).
Peripheral and cerebral vascular disorders.

Nagel Batrafen Hoechst Marion Roussel, Ger.
Ciclopirox (p.382·1).
Fungal nail infections.

Nail Batrafen Aventis, NZ.
Ciclopirox (p.382·1).
Fungal nail infections.

Nail Nutrition Cantassium Co., UK.
Multivitamins; minerals; amino acids (p.1350·1).

4 Nails Marlyn, USA.
Multivitamin, mineral, and amino-acid preparation (p.1350·1).

Nail-vit Pharmadass, UK.
Multivitamin, mineral, and trace element preparation (p.1350·1).

Nalador
Schering, Aust.; Schering, Fin.; Schering, Fr.; Schering, Ger.; Schering, Hong Kong; Schering, Ital.; Schering, Neth.; Schering, Singapore; Schering, Switz.; Schering, Thai.
Sulprostone (p.1447·2).
Labour induction in case of fetal death; postpartum haemorrhage; termination of pregnancy.

Nalapres Mediolanum, Ital.
Lisinopril (p.921·1); hydrochlorothiazide (p.907·3).
Hypertension.

Nalbu 20th Century, Mex.
Nalbuphine (p.60·2).

Nalcrom
Rhone-Poulenc Rorer, Canad.; Fisons, Irl.; Fisons, Israel; Rhone-Poulenc Rorer, Ital.; Rhone-Poulenc Rorer, Neth.; Aventis, NZ; Rhone-Poulenc Rorer, S.Afr.; Rhone-Poulenc Rorer, Spain†; Rhone-Poulenc Rorer, Switz.; Pantheon, UK.
Sodium cromoglicate (p.774·3).
Food allergies; inflammatory bowel disease.

Nalcron Rhone-Poulenc Rorer, Fr.
Sodium cromoglicate (p.774·3).
Food hypersensitivity.

Nalcryn Cryopharma, Mex.
Nalbuphine (p.60·2).
Pain.

Naldecon
Note. This name is used for preparations of different composition.
Bristol-Myers Squibb, Braz.
Phenylpropanolamine hydrochloride (p.1098·1); phenylephrine hydrochloride (p.1097·1); phenyltoloxamine citrate (p.423·1); carbinoxamine (p.411·1).
Nasal congestion.

Apothecon, USA†.
Phenylpropanolamine hydrochloride (p.1098·1); phenylephrine hydrochloride (p.1097·1); phenyltoloxamine citrate (p.423·1); chlorpheniramine [chlorphenamine] maleate (p.412·1).
Nasal congestion.

Naldecon CX Apothecon, USA†.
Phenylpropanolamine hydrochloride (p.1098·1); guaifenesin (p.1092·2); codeine phosphate (p.25·2).
Coughs and cold symptoms.

Naldecon DX Apothecon, USA†.
Phenylpropanolamine hydrochloride (p.1098·1); guaifenesin (p.1092·2); dextromethorphan hydrobromide (p.1087·3).
Coughs.

Naldecon EX Apothecon, USA†.
Phenylpropanolamine hydrochloride (p.1098·1); guaifenesin (p.1092·2).
Coughs and cold symptoms.

Naldecon Senior DX Apothecon, USA.
Guaifenesin (p.1092·2); dextromethorphan hydrobromide (p.1087·3).
Coughs.

Naldecon Senior EX Apothecon, USA.
Guaifenesin (p.1092·2).
Coughs and cold symptoms.

Naldelate DX Adult Barre-National, USA†.
Phenylpropanolamine hydrochloride (p.1098·1); dextromethorphan hydrobromide (p.1087·3); guaifenesin (p.1092·2).
Coughs.

Nalex Blansett, USA.
Pseudoephedrine hydrochloride (p.1099·2); guaifenesin (p.1092·2).

Nalex DH Blansett, USA.
Hydrocodone tartrate (p.42·2); phenylephrine hydrochloride (p.1097·1).

Nalex-A Blansett, USA.
Chlorpheniramine [chlorphenamine] maleate (p.412·1); phenyltoloxamine citrate (p.423·1); phenylephrine hydrochloride (p.1097·1).

Nalfan Novaquimica, Braz.
Vitamin A (p.1382·1).
Vitamin A deficiency.

Nalfon
Lilly, Aust.; Lilly, Canad.; Lilly, Denm.; Lilly, Mex.; Dista, USA.
Fenoprofen calcium (p.36·3).
Fever; gout; musculoskeletal and joint disorders; pain.

Nalgesic Lilly, Fr.
Fenoprofen calcium (p.36·3).
Pain.

Nalgest Major, USA†.
Phenylpropanolamine hydrochloride (p.1098·1); phenylephrine hydrochloride (p.1097·1); chlorpheniramine [chlorphenamine] maleate (p.412·1); phenyltoloxamine citrate (p.423·1).
Upper respiratory-tract symptoms.

Nalidin TAD, Ger.
Tilidate hydrochloride (p.88·2); naloxone hydrochloride (p.1014·3).
Pain.

Nalidixan Bioquimica, Mex.
Nalidixic acid (p.227·1).

Nalidixin NCSN, Ital.
Nalidixic acid (p.227·1).
Gram-negative genito-urinary tract infections.

Nalidoid Valdecasas, Mex.
Nalidixic acid (p.227·1).

Naligram Geymonat, Ital.
Nalidixic acid (p.227·1).
Gram-negative genito-urinary tract infections.

Naline Pharmaland, Thai.
Co-dergocrine mesilate (p.1597·3).
Cerebral and peripheral vascular disorders.

Nalion Vita Elan, Spain.
Norfloxacin (p.232·1).
Bacterial infections.

Nalissina Rhone-Poulenc Rorer, Ital.
Nalidixic acid (p.227·1).
Gram-negative urinary-tract infections.

Nalix Reuffer, Mex.
Nalidixic acid (p.227·1).

Nalixone Sons, Mex.
Nalidixic acid (p.227·1); phenazopyridine hydrochloride (p.77·3).
Urinary-tract infections and pain.

Nallpen SmithKline Beecham, USA†.
Nafcillin sodium (p.226·3).
Bacterial infections.

Nalone SERB, Fr.
Naloxone hydrochloride (p.1014·3).
Diagnosis of opioid dependence; diagnosis of toxic coma; opioid overdosage; opioid-induced respiratory depression.

Nalopril Siam Bheasach, Thai.
Enalapril maleate (p.883·3).
Heart failure; hypertension.

Nalorex
Schering-Plough, Fr.; Du Pont, Irl.; Du Pont, Ital.; Vitoria, Port.; Du Pont, UK.
Naltrexone hydrochloride (p.1016·1).
Alcohol withdrawal syndrome; opioid withdrawal.

Nalspan DX Morton Grove, USA†.
Phenylpropanolamine hydrochloride (p.1098·1); guaifenesin (p.1092·2); dextromethorphan hydrobromide (p.1087·3).

Nalspan Pediatric Morton Grove, USA†.
Phenylpropanolamine hydrochloride (p.1098·1); phenylephrine hydrochloride (p.1097·1); phenyltoloxamine citrate (p.423·1); chlorpheniramine [chlorphenamine] maleate (p.412·1).

Nalspan Senior DX Morton Grove, USA†.
Dextromethorphan hydrobromide (p.1087·3); guaifenesin (p.1092·2).

Nametone Pharmasant, Thai.
Nabumetone (p.59·3).
Osteoarthritis; rheumatoid arthritis.

Namic Atlantic, Thai.
Mefenamic acid (p.51·2).
Pain.

Namifen Novag, Mex.
Mefenamic acid (p.51·2).
Pain.

Nan HA
Nestle, Mex.; Nestle, Thai.
Infant feed (p.1350·1).
Cow's milk allergy.

NAN HA/AR Nestle, Port.
Infant feed (p.1350·1).
Gastro-oesophageal reflux.

Nan Sin Lactosa Nestle, Mex.
Food for special diets (p.1350·1).
Gastro-enteritis; lactose intolerance.

Nanafed PD, Thai.
Triprolidine hydrochloride (p.427·2); pseudoephedrine hydrochloride (p.1099·2).
Coughs; nasal congestion.

Nanbacine Rhone-Poulenc Rorer, Fr.†.
Xibornol (p.270·1).
Respiratory-tract disorders.

Nandain Ciba Vision, Port.†.
Nandrolone sodium sulfate (p.1484·2).
Corneal disorders.

Nandrol
Allergan-Frumtost, Braz.; Ciba Vision, Spain.
Nandrolone sodium sulfate (p.1484·2) or nandrolone sulfate (p.1484·3).
Corneal transplants; eye disorders.

Nani Pre Dental Alter, Spain.
Saffron (p.1029·1); guaiazulene (p.1618·3); lignocaine [lidocaine] hydrochloride (p.1313·2); myrrh (p.1639·2); menthol (p.1632·3).
Toothache.

Nanocoll Nycomed Amersham, UK.
Technetium-99m (p.1451·1) labelled albumin colloid.
Imaging of bone marrow and lymphatic system; scanning for inflammation.

Nanotiv
Pharmacia Upjohn, Norw.; Pharmacia Upjohn, Swed.
A factor IX preparation (p.735·1).
Haemorrhagic disorders.

Nansius Almirall, Spain.
Dipotassium clorazepate (p.670·3).
Anxiety; insomnia.

Napacod Propan, S.Afr.
Paracetamol (p.71·2); codeine phosphate (p.25·2).
Fever; pain.

Napageln Lederle, Jpn†.
Felbinac (p.36·1).
Inflammation; musculoskeletal, joint, and peri-articular disorders; pain.

Napamide
Douglas, Austral.; Douglas, Hong Kong; Douglas, NZ; Douglas, Singapore; Douglas, Thai.; TTN, Thai.
Indapamide (p.913·1).
Hypertension.

Napamol Propan, S.Afr.
Paracetamol (p.71·2).
Fever; pain.

Napan DHA, Hong Kong.
Mefenamic acid (p.51·2).
Musculoskeletal and joint disorders; pain.

Napflam Quatromed, S.Afr.
Naproxen (p.60·3).
Dysmenorrhoea; gout; musculoskeletal and joint disorders.

Napha Forte Medical Ophthalmics, USA.
Naphazoline hydrochloride (p.1095·1).

Naphacel Sophia, Mex.
Naphazoline hydrochloride (p.1095·1).
Eye irritation.

Naphasal Sam-On, Israel.
Naphazoline hydrochloride (p.1095·1).
Nasal congestion; rhinitis; sinusitis.

Naphazole-A Major, USA†.
Naphazoline hydrochloride (p.1095·1); pheniramine maleate (p.422·3).
Eye irritation.

Naphazoline Plus Parmed, USA.
Naphazoline hydrochloride (p.1095·1); pheniramine maleate (p.422·3).
Minor eye irritation.

Naphcon
Alcon, Austral.; Alcon, NZ; Alcon, Thai.; Alcon, USA.
Naphazoline hydrochloride (p.1095·1).
Eye irritation.

Naphcon Forte
Alcon, Canad.; Alcon, Israel.
Naphazoline hydrochloride (p.1095·1).
Conjunctivitis; eye congestion; nasal congestion.

Naphcon-A
Alcon, Austral.; Alcon, Canad.; Alcon, Hong Kong; Alcon, NZ; Alcon, Singapore; Alcon, Thai.; Alcon, USA.
Naphazoline hydrochloride (p.1095·1); pheniramine maleate (p.422·3).
Allergic or inflammatory eye disorders; eye congestion and irritation.

The symbol † denotes a preparation no longer actively marketed

Naphensyl *Propan, S.Afr.*
Phenylephrine hydrochloride (p.1097·1).
Respiratory-tract disorders.

Naphoptic-A *Optopics, USA.*
Naphazoline hydrochloride (p.1095·1); pheniramine maleate (p.422·3).
Eye irritation.

Napilene *Chinta, Thai.*
Benzalkonium chloride (p.1133·2); cetrimide (p.1137·1).
Minor burns and wounds; napkin rash.

Napiro *Brasmedica, Braz.*
Chlorpheniramine [chlorphenamine] (p.412·2); vitamin C (p.1389·3); guaifenesin (p.1092·2); dipyrone (p.34·1); eucalyptol (p.1609·2); terpineol (p.1669·3); chlorophyll (p.1028·1).
Cold and influenza symptoms.

Naplin *Pacific, NZ.*
Indapamide (p.913·1).
Hypertension.

Napmel *Clonmel, Irl.*
Naproxen (p.60·3).
Dysmenorrhoea; gout; musculoskeletal and joint disorders.

Nappy Rash Powder *Sigma, Austral.*
Chlorphenesin (p.381·3).
Chafing; nappy rash; prickly heat.

Nappy Rash Relief Cream *Brauer, Austral.*
Calendula (p.1589·2); clematis recta; hypericum (p.290·2); chamomile (p.1593·2); mezereum.
Nappy rash.

Nappy-Mate *Ethicare, Austral.*
Aluminium chlorohydrate (p.1110·2); zinc oxide (p.1128·2); benzoin tincture (p.1668·3); silicone (p.1410·1).
Nappy rash.

Napratec *Pharmacia, UK.*
Naproxen (p.60·3).
Misoprostol (p.1446·1) is included in this preparation in an attempt to limit adverse effects on the gastrointestinal mucosa.
Ankylosing spondylitis; osteoarthritis; rheumatoid arthritis.

Naprel *Brunel, S.Afr.*
Naproxen (p.60·3).
Dysmenorrhoea; gout; musculoskeletal and joint disorders.

Naprelan *Meda, Swed.†; Wyeth-Ayerst, USA.*
Naproxen sodium (p.61·1).
Gout; musculoskeletal, joint, and peri-articular disorders; pain.

Napren *Nycomed, Norw.; AFI, Norw.*
Naproxen (p.60·3).
Gout; musculoskeletal and joint disorders; pain.

Naprex
Note. This name is used for preparations of different composition.
Pinewood, Irl.; Curex, Israel.
Naproxen (p.60·3) or naproxen sodium (p.61·1).
Gout; musculoskeletal and joint disorders; pain.
Pediatrica, Singapore.
Paracetamol (p.71·2).
Fever; pain.

Naprilene *Sigma-Tau, Ital.; Sigma-Tau, Spain.*
Enalapril (p.883·3) or enalapril maleate (p.883·3).
Angina pectoris; heart failure; hypertension.

Naprina *Pisa, Mex.*
Noradrenaline [norepinephrine] (p.948·2).

Naprius *Aesculapius, Ital.*
Naproxen (p.60·3).
Fever; inflammation; musculoskeletal, joint, peri-articular, and soft-tissue disorders; pain.

Naprobene *Ratiopharm, Aust.*
Naproxen (p.60·3).
Gout; inflammation; musculoskeletal and joint disorders; pain.

Naprocet *Boniscontro & Gazzone, Ital.*
Naproxen cetrimonium (p.61·3).
Mouth and throat disorders.

Naprocoat *Roche, Neth.*
Naproxen (p.60·3).
Musculoskeletal and joint disorders.

Naprodil *Diba, Mex.*
Naproxen (p.60·3) or naproxen sodium (p.61·1).
Inflammation; musculoskeletal, joint and peri-articular disorders; pain.

Naprodol *Upsamedica, Ital.*
Naproxen sodium (p.61·1).
Pain.

Napro-Dorsch *Orion, Ger.*
Naproxen (p.60·3).
Inflammation; pain.

Naprogesic *Roche Consumer, Austral.; Roche, NZ.*
Naproxen sodium (p.61·1).
Dysmenorrhoea.

Naprokes *Inexfa, Spain.*
Naproxen (p.60·3).
Fever; gout; musculoskeletal and joint disorders; pain.

Naprometin *Roche, Fin.*
Naproxen (p.60·3).
Gout; inflammation; musculoskeletal and joint disorders; pain.

Napromex *Medinovum, Fin.*
Naproxen (p.60·3).
Gout; inflammation; musculoskeletal and joint disorders; pain.

Napronet *Nettopharma, Denm.†.*
Naproxen (p.60·3).
Musculoskeletal and joint disorders; pain.

Naprorex *Lampugnani, Ital.*
Naproxen sodium (p.61·1).
Inflammation; musculoskeletal and joint disorders; pain.

Naproscript *Ranbaxy, S.Afr.*
Naproxen (p.60·3).
Dysmenorrhoea; musculoskeletal and joint disorders.

Naprosian *Asian Pharm, Thai.*
Naproxen (p.60·3).
Musculoskeletal and joint disorders.

Naproso *M & H, Thai.*
Naproxen sodium (p.61·1).
Gout; musculoskeletal, joint, and peri-articular disorders; pain.

Naprosyn
Syntex, Austral.; Hoechst Marion Roussel, Braz.; Roche, Denm.; Roche, Fin.; Roche, Hong Kong; Roche, Irl.; Recordati, Ital.; Roche, Norw.; Roche, NZ; Janssen-Cilag, Port.; Roche, S.Afr.; Roche, Singapore; Syntex, Spain; Roche, Swed.; Roche, Switz.; Roche, Thai.; Roche, UK; Roche, USA.
Naproxen (p.60·3) or naproxen sodium (p.61·1).
Fever; gout; musculoskeletal, joint, peri-articular, and soft-tissue disorders; pain.

Naprosyne *Roche, Belg.; Grunenthal, Fr.; Roche, Neth.*
Naproxen (p.60·3).
Fever; gout; inflammation; musculoskeletal, joint, and peri-articular disorders; pain.

Naproval *Septa, Spain.*
Naproxen (p.60·3).
Fever; gout; musculoskeletal and joint disorders; pain.

Naprovite *Roche, Neth.*
Naproxen sodium (p.61·1).
Fever; gout; inflammation; musculoskeletal and joint disorders; pain.

Naproxi *Gerard, Israel.*
Naproxen (p.60·3).
Musculoskeletal and joint disorders; pain.

Napxen *Berlin Pharm, Thai.*
Naproxen (p.60·3).
Gout; musculoskeletal and joint disorders.

Naqua *Schering, USA.*
Trichlormethiazide (p.987·1).
Hypertension; oedema.

Naquinto *Makros, Braz.*
Sodium dibunate (p.1100·3); homatropine (p.468·1); bromoform (p.1587·1).
Coughs.

Naragran *Glaxo Wellcome, Denm.*
Naratriptan hydrochloride (p.454·3).
Migraine.

Naramig
Glaxo Wellcome, Aust.; Glaxo Wellcome, Austral.; Glaxo Wellcome, Belg.; Glaxo Wellcome, Fin.; Glaxo Wellcome, Fr.; Glaxo Wellcome, Ger.; Schwarz, Ger.; Glaxo Wellcome, Israel; Glaxo Wellcome, Mex.; Glaxo Wellcome, Neth.; Glaxo Wellcome, Norw.; Glaxo Wellcome, Port.; Glaxo Wellcome, S.Afr.; Glaxo Wellcome, Singapore; Glaxo Wellcome, Spain; Glaxo Wellcome, Swed.; Glaxo Wellcome, Switz.; Glaxo Wellcome, Thai.; Glaxo Wellcome, UK.
Naratriptan hydrochloride (p.454·3).
Migraine.

Naranocor *Pfluger, Ger.†.*
Crataegus (p.1600·2).
Arrhythmias; heart failure.

Naranocut H *Pfluger, Ger.*
Homoeopathic preparation.

Naranofem *Pfluger, Ger.*
Homoeopathic preparation.

Naranopect P *Pfluger, Ger.*
Hedera helix.
Respiratory-tract disorders.

Naranotox *Pfluger, Ger.*
Homoeopathic preparation.

Naranotox Plus *Pfluger, Ger.*
Homoeopathic preparation.

Narapril *Julphar, UAE.*
Enalapril maleate (p.883·3).
Heart failure; hypertension.

Narcan
Boots, Austral.; Du Pont, Belg.; Rhodia, Braz.; Du Pont, Canad.; Du Pont, Fr.; Du Pont, Hong Kong; Boots, Hong Kong; Boots, Irl.; Crinos, Ital.; Boots, NZ; Vitoria, Port.; Sanofi Synthelabo, S.Afr.; Du Pont, Singapore; Du Pont, Switz.; Boots, Thai.; Du Pont, Thai.; Du Pont, Endo, USA.
Naloxone hydrochloride (p.1014·3).
Opioid overdosage; reversal of opioid depression.

Narcanti
Torrex, Aust.; Du Pont, Denm.; Meda, Fin.; Du Pont, Ger.; Rhone-Poulenc Rorer, Mex.; Du Pont, Norw.; Meda, Swed.
Naloxone hydrochloride (p.1014·3).
Opioid overdosage; reversal of opioid depression.

Narcaricin
Heumann, Ger.; Heumann, Hong Kong; Ludwig, Singapore; Heumann, Thai.
Benzbromarone (p.399·3).
Gout; hyperuricaemia.

Narcaricina *Asta Medica, Braz.*
Benzbromarone (p.399·3).
Gout; hyperuricaemia.

Narcoral *Crinos, Ital.*
Naltrexone hydrochloride (p.1016·1).
Opioid overdosage; opioid withdrawal.

Narcotuss *Legrand, Braz.*
Guaifenesin (p.1092·2); ammonium chloride (p.1085·2).
Respiratory-tract disorders.

Narcozep *Roche, Fr.*
Flunitrazepam (p.683·2).
General anaesthesia; premedication.

Nardelzine *Parke, Davis, Belg.*
Phenelzine sulfate (p.303·2).
Depression.

Nardil
Parke, Davis, Austral.; Parke, Davis, Canad.; Hansam, Irl.; Warner-Lambert, Israel; Parke, Davis, NZ; Parke, Davis, UK; Parke, Davis, USA.
Phenelzine sulfate (p.303·2).
Depression; mixed anxiety depressive states.

Nardyl *Vifor, Switz.*
Promethazine hydrochloride (p.423·2); hyoscyamine sulfate (p.469·3); atropine sulfate (p.461·1); hyoscine hydrobromide (p.468·2).
Anxiety; neuroses; sleep disorders; tension.

Narfen *Alter, Spain†.*
Ibuprofen (p.43·2).
Fever; musculoskeletal, joint, and peri-articular disorders; pain.

Naribel *Sanofi Synthelabo, Ital.*
Sodium chloride (p.1196·1).
Nasal disorders.

Naricin *Sintofarma, Braz.*
Naphazoline hydrochloride (p.1095·1); mepyramine maleate (p.421·1).
Nasal congestion.

Naride *Amrad, Austral.*
Indapamide (p.913·1).
Hypertension.

Naridrin *EMS, Braz.*
Naphazoline hydrochloride (p.1095·1); mepyramine maleate (p.421·1); dexpanthenol (p.1602·3).
Nasal congestion.

Narifresh *Rappai, Switz.*
Sea salt (p.1196·1); chamomile (p.1593·2).
Nasal disorders.

Narilet *Fher, Spain†.*
Ipratropium bromide (p.766·1).
Rhinorrhoea.

Narine *Schering-Plough, Spain.*
Pseudoephedrine sulfate (p.1099·3); loratadine (p.420·1).
Allergic rhinitis.

Narisoro *Legrand, Braz.*
Sodium chloride (p.1196·1).
Nasal congestion.

Naristar *Vedim, Ital.; UCB, Ital.*
Cetirizine hydrochloride (p.411·2); pseudoephedrine hydrochloride (p.1099·2).
Conjunctivitis; rhinitis.

Naritec *TO-Chemicals, Thai.*
Enalapril maleate (p.883·3).
Heart failure; hypertension.

Narium
Hamilton, Austral.; Hamilton, NZ.
Sodium chloride (p.1196·1).
Nasal irritation and inflammation.

Narix *Honorterapica, Braz.*
Naphazoline (p.1095·1).
Nasal congestion.

Narixan *Wassermann, Ital.*
Pseudoephedrine hydrochloride (p.1099·2).
Rhinitis; upper respiratory-tract congestion.

Narizima *Baldacci, Port.*
Muramidase hydrochloride (p.1638·1); thonzylamine hydrochloride (p.426·2); isobenzidrine iodide.
Rhinitis; sinusitis.

Narizima Adulto *Baldacci, Braz.*
Muramidase hydrochloride (p.1638·1); ethylenediamine hydrochloride (p.1609·1); methylethylamine hydrochloride; oxymetazoline (p.1096·2); glycerol (p.1616·3).
Nasal congestion.

Narizima Pediatrico *Baldacci, Braz.*
Muramidase hydrochloride (p.1638·1); dimethylethylenediamine hydrochloride; oxyphenylmethylamine hydrochloride; glycerol (p.1616·3).
Nasal congestion.

Narlisim *Baldacci, Ital.*
Muramidase hydrochloride (p.1638·1); phenolpropamine iodide; thonzylamine hydrochloride (p.426·2).
Nasal congestion.

Narobic *Alliance, S.Afr.*
Metronidazole (p.594·1).
Anaerobic bacterial infections; protozoal infections.

Narocin *Teva, Israel.*
Naproxen sodium (p.61·1).
Fever; musculoskeletal and joint disorders; pain.

Narol *Almirall, Spain.*
Buspirone hydrochloride (p.657·2).
Anxiety.

Narop
Astra, Israel; Astra, Swed.
Ropivacaine hydrochloride (p.1320·2).
Local anaesthesia.

Naropeine *AstraZeneca, Fr.; Astra, Port.*
Ropivacaine hydrochloride (p.1320·2).
Local anaesthesia.

Naropin
Astra, Aust.; Astra, Austral.; Astra, Belg.; AstraZeneca, Canad.; Astra-Zeneca, Denm.; AstraZeneca, Fin.; Astra, Fr.; Astra, Hong Kong; Astra, Irl.; Astra, Mex.; Astra, Neth.; AstraZeneca, Norw.; AstraZeneca, NZ; Astra, S.Afr.; AstraZeneca, Singapore; Astra, Spain; Astra, Switz.; AstraZeneca, UK; Astra, USA.
Ropivacaine hydrochloride (p.1320·2).
Local anaesthesia.

Naropin with Fentanyl *AstraZeneca, Austral.*
Ropivacaine hydrochloride (p.1320·2); fentanyl citrate (p.37·1).
Epidural analgesia.

Naropina *Astra, Ital.*
Ropivacaine hydrochloride (p.1320·2).
Epidural anaesthesia; local anaesthesia; pain.

Narphen *Napp, UK†.*
Phenazocine hydrobromide (p.77·1).
Pain.

Nartap *Condrugs, Thai.*
Brompheniramine maleate (p.410·2); phenylephrine hydrochloride (p.1097·1); phenylpropanolamine hydrochloride (p.1098·1).
Nasal congestion; respiratory-tract disorders.

Narzen *Shiwa, Thai.*
Naproxen (p.60·3).
Musculoskeletal and joint disorders.

Nasa-12 *Glaxo Wellcome, Belg.*
Pseudoephedrine hydrochloride (p.1099·2).
Rhinitis.

Nasa Rhinathiol *Sanofi Synthelabo, Belg.*
Xylometazoline hydrochloride (p.1102·2).
Nasal congestion.

Nasabid *Jones, USA.*
Pseudoephedrine hydrochloride (p.1099·2); guaifenesin (p.1092·2).
Cough; nasal congestion.

Nasacor *Aventis, S.Afr.*
Triamcinolone acetonide (p.1080·1).
Allergic rhinitis.

Nasacort
Rhone-Poulenc Rorer, Aust.; Rhone-Poulenc Rorer, Canad.; Aventis, Denm.; Rhone-Poulenc Rorer, Fin.; Rhone-Poulenc Rorer, Fr.; Rhone-Poulenc Rorer, Ger.; Rhone-Poulenc Rorer, Irl.; Rhone-Poulenc Rorer, Ital.; Rhone-Poulenc Rorer, Mex.; Rhone-Poulenc Rorer, Neth.; Rhone-Poulenc Rorer, Norw.; Aventis, NZ; Rhone-Poulenc Rorer, Singapore; Rhone-Poulenc Rorer, Spain; Rhone-Poulenc Rorer, Swed.; Rhone-Poulenc Rorer, Switz.; Rhone-Poulenc Rorer, Thai.; Rhone-Poulenc Rorer, UK; Rhone-Poulenc Rorer, USA.
Triamcinolone acetonide (p.1080·1).
Allergic rhinitis.

Nasacort AQ *Rhone-Poulenc Rorer, Austral.*
Triamcinolone acetonide (p.1080·1).
Allergic rhinitis.

Nasahist B *Keene, USA†.*
Brompheniramine maleate (p.410·2).
Hypersensitivity reactions.

NaSal *Sterling Health, USA.*
Sodium chloride (p.1196·1).
Nasal congestion.

Nasal Inhaler *Pickles, UK.*
Eucalyptus (p.1609·2); menthol (p.1632·3); methyl salicylate (p.55·1); pumilio pine oil (p.1656·3).
Nasal congestion.

Nasal Jelly
Note. This name is used for preparations of different composition.
Thuna, Canad.
Ephedrine hydrochloride (p.1090·1); methyl salicylate (p.55·1); thymol (p.1158·3).
Kondon, USA.
Phenol (p.1152·3); camphor (p.1589·3); menthol (p.1632·3); eucalyptus oil (p.1609·2); lavender oil (p.1627·2).

Nasal Moist *Blairex, USA.*
Sodium chloride (p.1196·1).
Inflammation and dryness of nasal membranes.

Nasal Relief *Rugby, USA.*
Oxymetazoline hydrochloride (p.1096·2).
Nasal congestion.

Nasal & Sinus Relief *Stanley, Canad.*
Pseudoephedrine hydrochloride (p.1099·2).

Nasal Spray *Reese, USA.*
Oxymetazoline hydrochloride (p.1096·2).

Nasal Spray for Hayfever *Unichem, UK.*
Beclometasone dipropionate (p.1061·2).
Hayfever.

Nasalate *Paedpharm, Austral.*
Chlorhexidine (p.1138·2); phenylephrine hydrochloride (p.1097·1).
Epistaxis; nasal surgery; vestibulitis.

Nasal-Bec *Norton, UK.*
Beclometasone dipropionate (p.1061·2).
Rhinitis.

Nasalcrom *Pharmacia Upjohn, USA.*
Sodium cromoglicate (p.774·3).
Allergic rhinitis.

Nasal-Ease *Health Care Products, USA.*
Nasal gel: Zinc acetate (p.1398·1); aloe vera (p.1110·1); calendula (p.1589·2).
Nasal spray: Zinc gluconate (p.1398·2); sodium chloride (p.1196·1).
Inflammation and dryness of nasal membranes.

Nasalemed *SmithKline Beecham, Ital.†.*
Xylometazoline hydrochloride (p.1102·2); domiphen bromide (p.1143·3).
Nasal congestion.

Nasaleze *Healtheze, UK.*
Cellulose (p.1500·3).
Allergic rhinitis.

Nasalflu *Berna, Switz.*
An influenza vaccine (p.1544·3).
Active immunisation.

Nasalgen *Kenyaku, Thai.*
Syrup: Phenylpropanolamine hydrochloride (p.1098·1); carbinoxamine maleate (p.411·1).
Tablets: Phenylpropanolamine hydrochloride (p.1098·1); phenylephrine hydrochloride (p.1097·1); carbinoxamine maleate (p.411·1).
Hay fever; nasal congestion; rhinitis.

Nasalide *Cassenne, Fr.; Dura, USA.*
Flunisolide (p.1070·3).
Rhinitis.

Nasamine *Maxi, Thai.*
Dexchlorpheniramine maleate (p.412·1).
Hypersensitivity reactions.

Nasan *Hexal, Ger.*
Xylometazoline hydrochloride (p.1102·2).
Rhinitis.

Nasanal *Brady, Aust.*
Aluminium acetotartrate (p.1578·2); pumilio pine oil (p.1656·3).
Nasal disorders.

Nasapert *Searle, Belg.*
Brompheniramine maleate (p.410·2); phenylpropanolamine hydrochloride (p.1098·1).
Rhinitis.

Nasarel *Dura, USA.*
Flunisolide (p.1070·3).
Rhinitis.

Nasarox *Plough, Port.*
Oxymetazoline hydrochloride (p.1096·2).
Nasal congestion.

Nasatab LA *ECR, USA.*
Guaifenesin (p.1092·2); pseudoephedrine hydrochloride (p.1099·2).
Coughs.

Nasatuss *Abana, USA†.*
Hydrocodone tartrate (p.42·2); phenylephrine hydrochloride (p.1097·1); chlorpheniramine [chlorphenamine] maleate (p.412·1).
Coughs and congestion.

Nasben *Democal, Switz.*
Xylometazoline hydrochloride (p.1102·2).
Nasal congestion.

Nasben soft *Democal, Switz.*
Sodium chloride (p.1196·1).
Nasal disorders.

Nasciodine *Pharmadass, UK.*
Iodine (p.1522·3); menthol (p.1632·3); methyl salicylate (p.55·1); turpentine oil (p.1676·3); rectified camphor oil.
Musculoskeletal, joint, and soft-tissue disorders.

Nascobal *Schwarz, USA.*
Cyanocobalamin (p.1388·1).
Vitamin B₁₂ deficiency.

Nasdro *Adcock Ingram, S.Afr.*
Phenylephrine hydrochloride (p.1097·1); naphazoline nitrate (p.1095·1).
Nasal congestion.

Nasea *Yamanouchi, Jpn.*
Ramosetron hydrochloride (p.1245·2).
Nausea and vomiting induced by cytotoxic chemotherapy.

Nasello *Synpharma, Switz.†.*
Calcium levulinate (p.1188·3); camphor (p.1589·3); ephedrine hydrochloride (p.1090·1); menthol (p.1632·3); pheniramine maleate (p.422·3); procaine hydrochloride (p.1319·1); hydroxyquinoline (p.1622·2).
Rhinitis.

Nasengel *Ratiopharm, Ger.*
Xylometazoline hydrochloride (p.1102·2).
Catarrh; colds; sinusitis.

Nasengel AL *Aliud, Ger.*
Xylometazoline hydrochloride (p.1102·2).
Rhinitis.

Nasenspray AL *Aliud, Ger.*
Xylometazoline hydrochloride (p.1102·2).
Rhinitis.

Nasenspray E *Ratiopharm, Ger.*
Xylometazoline hydrochloride (p.1102·2).
Catarrh; rhinitis; sinusitis.

Nasenspray K *Ratiopharm, Ger.*
Xylometazoline hydrochloride (p.1102·2).
Catarrh; rhinitis; sinusitis.

Nasentropfen AL *Aliud, Ger.*
Xylometazoline hydrochloride (p.1102·2).
Rhinitis.

Nasentropfen E *Ratiopharm, Ger.*
Xylometazoline hydrochloride (p.1102·2).
Catarrh; rhinitis; sinusitis.

Nasentropfen K *Ratiopharm, Ger.*
Xylometazoline hydrochloride (p.1102·2).
Catarrh; rhinitis; sinusitis.

Nasentropfen-ratiopharm *Ratiopharm, Ger.*
Pine needle oil; peppermint oil (p.1243·3); pumilio pine oil (p.1656·3); eucalyptus oil (p.1609·2); thymol (p.1158·3).
Cold symptoms; nasal congestion.

Naseptin *Bioglan, Irl.; Genop, S.Afr.; Alliance, UK.*
Chlorhexidine hydrochloride (p.1138·2); neomycin sulfate (p.228·1).
Nasal carriage of staphylococci; staphylococcal infections.

Nasex
Note. This name is used for preparations of different composition.
Felton, Austral.
Oxymetazoline hydrochloride (p.1096·2); eucalyptol (p.1609·2); menthol (p.1632·3).
Nasal congestion.

Janssen-Cilag, Port.
Oxymetazoline hydrochloride (p.1096·2).

DP-Medica, Switz.
Phenylephrine hydrochloride (p.1097·1); cetylpyridinium chloride (p.1138·1).
Nasal disorders.

Nasic *Cassella-med, Ger.; Artesan, Ger.*
Xylometazoline hydrochloride (p.1102·2); dexpanthenol (p.1602·3).
Nasal congestion.

Nasicort *Bracco, Ital.*
Dexamethasone tebutate (p.1067·3); oxymetazoline hydrochloride (p.1096·2).
Nasal polyps; rhinitis; rhinopharyngitis; sinusitis.

Nasicur *Cassella-med, Ger.; Artesan, Ger.*
Dexpanthenol (p.1602·3).
Rhinitis sicca.

Nasil *Silom, Thai.*
Oxymetazoline hydrochloride (p.1096·2).
Nasal congestion.

Nasimild *Merck, Aust.*
Benzalkonium chloride (p.1133·2); polysorbate 80 (p.1347·3).
Nasal disorders.

Nasin *Tika, Swed.*
Oxymetazoline hydrochloride (p.1096·2).
Rhinitis; sinusitis.

Nasivin
Merck, Aust.; Merck, Braz.; Merck, Israel; Bracco, Ital.†; Merck, Neth.; Julphar, UAE.
Oxymetazoline hydrochloride (p.1096·2).
Nasal congestion; sinusitis.

Nasivin gegen Erkaltung Kinderbad *Merck, Ger.*
Eucalyptus oil (p.1609·2).
Respiratory-tract congestion.

Nasivin gegen Erkaltung N *Merck, Ger.*
Eucalyptus oil (p.1609·2); thyme oil (p.1672·3); camphor (p.1589·3).
Bath additive; catarrh.

Nasivin gegen Schnupfen *Merck, Ger.*
Oxymetazoline hydrochloride (p.1096·2).
Catarrh; otitis media; rhinitis.

Nasivin Intensiv-Bad N *Merck, Ger.*
Eucalyptus oil (p.1609·2); thyme oil (p.1672·3); camphor (p.1589·3).
Respiratory-tract congestion.

Nasivin Sanft *Merck, Ger.*
Oxymetazoline hydrochloride (p.1096·2).
Catarrh; nasal congestion; rhinitis.

Nasivine *Asta Medica, Switz.*
Oxymetazoline hydrochloride (p.1096·2).
Catarrh; rhinitis; sinusitis.

Nasivinetten gegen Schnupfen *Merck, Ger.*
Oxymetazoline hydrochloride (p.1096·2).
Catarrh; otitis media; rhinitis.

Nasivinettes *Asta Medica, Switz.*
Oxymetazoline hydrochloride (p.1096·2).
Formerly known as Nasivinetten.
Catarrh; rhinitis; sinusitis.

Naso Instil *Dinafarma, Braz.*
Tyrothricin (p.267·1); naphazoline hydrochloride (p.1095·1).
Nasal congestion.

Naso Pekamin *Medical, Spain.*
Phenylephrine hydrochloride (p.1097·1); kanamycin sulfate (p.218·1); trypsin (p.1675·3).
Nose and throat disorders.

Naso Prieulina *Medical, Port.*
Naphazoline hydrochloride (p.1095·1); ephedrine hydrochloride (p.1090·1); mepyramine maleate (p.421·1).
Rhinitis; sinusitis.

Nasobec
Baker Norton, Hong Kong; Norton Waterford, Irl.; Norton Healthcare, UK.
Beclometasone dipropionate (p.1061·2).
Rhinitis.

Nasobol *Sodip, Switz.*
Benzoic acid (p.1134·2); peru balsam (p.1650·2); verbena oil; eucalyptus oil (p.1609·2); lavender oil (p.1627·2); wild thyme oil.
Respiratory-tract disorders.

Naso-Calma *Salusif, Port.*
Ephedrine hydrochloride (p.1090·1); silver protein (p.1664·2).
Cold and influenza symptoms.

Nasocan *Protein, Mex.*
Naproxen sodium (p.61·1).

Nasocort *Teva, Israel.*
Budesonide (p.1064·2).
Rhinitis.

Nasoferm *Nordic, Swed.*
Xylometazoline hydrochloride (p.1102·2).
Rhinitis; sinusitis.

Nasoflux *IQB, Braz.*
Sodium chloride (p.1196·1).
Nasal congestion.

Nasogrip *Cazi, Braz.*
Phenylephrine hydrochloride (p.1097·1); paracetamol (p.71·2); mepyramine (p.421·1); caffeine (p.761·3).
Cold and influenza symptoms.

Nasolin
Note. This name is used for preparations of different composition.
Orion, Fin.
Xylometazoline hydrochloride (p.1102·2).
Allergic rhinitis.

Nakorn, Thai.
Triprolidine hydrochloride (p.427·2); pseudoephedrine hydrochloride (p.1099·2).
Allergic rhinitis; cold symptoms; hay fever; nasal congestion.

Nasolina *Salvat, Spain.*
Oxymetazoline hydrochloride (p.1096·2).
Nasal congestion.

Nasomet *Schering-Plough, Port.*
Mometasone furoate (p.1077·2).
Rhinitis.

Nasomixin
Note. This name is used for preparations of different composition.
Teofarma, Ital.
Phenylpropanolamine hydrochloride (p.1098·1); hydrocortisone (p.1073·3).
Formerly contained phenylephrine hydrochloride, phenylpropanolamine hydrochloride, hydrocortisone, and neomycin sulfate.
Cold symptoms; rhinitis; sinusitis.

Aventis, S.Afr.
Phenylephrine hydrochloride (p.1097·1); phenylpropanolamine hydrochloride (p.1098·1); hydrocortisone (p.1073·3); neomycin sulfate (p.228·1).
Rhinitis; sinusitis.

Nasonex
Schering-Plough, Austral.; Schering, Canad.; Schering-Plough, Denm.; Schering-Plough, Fin.; Schering-Plough, Fr.; Essex, Ger.; Schering-Plough, Hong Kong; Schering-Plough, Irl.; Schering-Plough, Israel; Schering-Plough, Ital.; Schering-Plough, Neth.; Schering-Plough, Norw.; Schering-Plough, S.Afr.; Schering-Plough, Singapore; Schering-Plough, Spain; Schering-Plough, Swed.; Essex, Switz.; Schering-Plough, Thai.; Schering-Plough, UK; Schering, USA.
Mometasone furoate (p.1077·2).
Allergic rhinitis.

Nasopan *Heralds, Braz.*
Naphazoline hydrochloride (p.1095·1); mepyramine maleate (p.421·1); dexpanthenol (p.1602·3).
Nasal congestion.

Nasopomada *Medical, Spain.*
Bismuth subgallate (p.1213·2); prednisolone (p.1077·3); rutoside (p.1611·2); sulfanilamide (p.256·2); tetracycline hydrochloride (p.258·3); urea; benzocaine (p.1306·2).
Nasal furunculosis; sinusitis.

Nasosil *Silom, Thai.*
Brompheniramine maleate (p.410·2); phenylephrine hydrochloride (p.1097·1); phenylpropanolamine hydrochloride (p.1098·1).
Nasal congestion.

Nasotic Oto *Juventus, Spain.*
Betamethasone valerate (p.1063·2); neomycin sulfate (p.228·1); papain (p.1647·3); polymyxin B sulfate (p.238·1).
Ear disorders; rhinitis.

Nasovalda *Sterling Health, Spain.*
Oxymetazoline hydrochloride (p.1096·2).
Nasal congestion.

Nastop *Democal, Switz.*
Dexpanthenol (p.1602·3); peppermint oil (p.1243·3); camphor (p.1589·3).
Nasal disorders.

Nastoren *Lepetit, Ital.*
Somatostatin acetate (p.1297·3).
Gastrointestinal haemorrhage; prevention of postoperative complications following pancreatic surgery.

Nasulind *Steierl, Ger.*
Peppermint oil (p.1243·3); thyme oil (p.1672·3).
Nasal congestion.

Natabec
Parke, Davis, Aust.; Warner-Lambert, Ger.; Warner-Lambert, Hong Kong; Warner-Lambert Consumer, Switz.
Multivitamin and mineral preparation (p.1350·1).

Natabec F *Warner-Lambert, Ger.*
Multivitamin and mineral preparation (p.1350·1) with sodium fluoride (p.1375·3).

Natabec-F.A. with Fluoride *Parke, Davis, S.Afr.†.*
Multivitamin and mineral preparation (p.1350·1).

NataChew *Warner Chilcott, USA.*
A multivitamin preparation with iron (p.1350·1).

Natacyn *Alcon, S.Afr.; Alcon, Singapore; Alcon, Thai.; Alcon, USA.*
Natamycin (p.392·1).
Fungal eye infections.

Natafort *Warner Chilcott, USA.*
Multivitamin and mineral preparation (p.1350·1).

Natafucin *Yamanouchi, Ital.*
Natamycin (p.392·1).
Fungal skin infections.

Natal Extra *Cypress, USA.*
Multivitamin and mineral preparation (p.1350·1).
Docusate sodium (p.1223·1) is included in this preparation to reduce the constipating effects of iron.

NatalCare *Ethex, USA.*
A range of multivitamin and multivitamin and mineral preparations (p.1350·1).

Natalin *Mead Johnson Nutritionals, USA.*
Multivitamin and mineral preparation with iron and folic acid (p.1350·1).
Dietary supplement during pregnancy and lactation.

Natalins *Mead Johnson, Hong Kong.*
Multivitamin and mineral preparation (p.1350·1).
Dietary supplement in pregnancy and lactation.

Natalins com Fluor *Bristol-Myers Squibb, Braz.*
Multivitamin and mineral preparation with iron, folic acid, and fluoride (p.1350·1).

Natalins Folico *Bristol-Myers Squibb, Braz.*
Multivitamin and mineral preparation with iron and folic acid (p.1350·1).

Nataral *Kenyaku, Thai.*
Multivitamin and mineral preparation (p.1350·1).

Natarex Prenatal *Major, USA.*
Multivitamin and mineral preparation with iron and folic acid (p.1350·1).

NataTab *Ethex, USA.*
Multivitamin and mineral preparation (p.1350·1).

Natavite *Schein, Canad.*
Multivitamin preparation with iron and folic acid (p.1350·1).

Natead *Lab Francais du Fractionnement, Fr.*
An anti-D immunoglobulin (p.1532·1).
Prevention of rhesus incompatibility.

Natecal *Italfarmaco, Spain.*
Calcium carbonate (p.1215·1).
Hypocalcaemia; osteoporosis.

Natecal D *Italfarmaco, Spain.*
Calcium carbonate (p.1215·1); colecalciferol (p.1391·1).
Calcium deficiency; osteoporosis.

Nathergen *PD, Thai.*
Methylergometrine maleate (p.1635·1).
Functional uterine bleeding; management of third stage of labour; postpartum haemorrhage; puerperal haemorrhage.

Naticardina *Asta Medica, Ital.*
Quinidine polygalacturonate (p.964·3).
Arrhythmias.

Nati-K *Centrapharm, Fr.*
Potassium tartrate (p.1195·1).
Hypokalaemia.

Natiken *Kener, Mex.*
Ibuprofen (p.43·2).

Natil *3M, Ger.*
Cyclandelate (p.865·2).
Cerebral metabolic and vascular disorders; migraine; retinopathy; vestibular disorders.

Natinate *Atlantic, Thai.*
Nicotinic acid (p.1372·3).
Pellagra.

Natisedina *Teofarma, Ital.*
Quinidine phenylethylbarbiturate (p.966·1).
Arrhythmias.

Natisedine
Note. This name is used for preparations of different composition.
Barrenne, Braz.
Quinidine (p.964·2).
Arrhythmias.

Sabex, Canad.†.
Quinidine phenylethylbarbiturate (p.966·1).
Nervous disorders with arrhythmia.

Procter & Gamble, Fr.†.
Phenobarbital (p.355·1); passion flower (p.1649·1).
Formerly contained quinidine phenylethylbarbiturate.
Anxiety; insomnia; palpitations.

Natispray
Procter & Gamble, Fr.; Teofarma, Ital.; Nativelle, Switz.†.
Glyceryl trinitrate (p.897·3).
Angina pectoris; pulmonary oedema.

Nativa HA *Guigoz, Ital.*
Infant feed (p.1350·1).
Milk intolerance.

Nativit *Novaquimica, Braz.*
Multivitamin and mineral preparation with iron (p.1350·1).

Na-To-Caps *SIT, Ital.*
Mixed tocopherols (p.1393·3).
Vitamin E deficiency.

Natopherol
Abbott, Hong Kong; Abbott, Singapore.
Vitamin E (p.1393·3).
Vitamin E supplement.

Natoss *Biologia, Braz.*
Sodium dibunate (p.1100·3); sodium benzoate (p.1134·3).
Coughs.

Natracalm *Peter Black, UK.*
Passion flower (p.1649·1).
Tension.

NatraFlex *Nutralife, UK.*
Capsaicin (p.23·1); dimethyl sulfone; boswellia serrata.
Joint pain.

The symbol † denotes a preparation no longer actively marketed

Natraleze *English Grains, UK.*
Slippery elm bark (p.1665·1); meadowsweet (p.1631·2); liquorice (p.1231·2).
Dyspepsia; flatulence; heartburn.

Natramid *Trinity, UK.*
Indapamide (p.913·1).
Hypertension.

Natrapel *Ardern, UK.*
Citronella oil (p.1596·3).
Insect repellent.

Natrasleep *Peter Black, UK.*
Lupulus (p.1629·3); valerian (p.1678·3).
Insomnia.

Natrecor *Scios, USA.*
Nesiritide (p.938·3).
Heart failure.

Natrilix
Servier, Austral.; Servier, Braz.; Servier, Denm.; Pharmacal, Fin.; Servier, Ger.; Servier, Hong Kong; Servier, Irl.; Servier, Ital.; Servier, NZ; Servier, S.Afr.; Servier, Singapore; Servier, Thai.; Servier, UK.
Indapamide (p.913·1).
Hypertension.

Natrioxen *Benedetti, Ital.†.*
Naproxen sodium (p.61·1).
Lignocaine [lidocaine] hydrochloride (p.1313·2) is included in the intramuscular injection to alleviate the pain of injection.
Inflammation; musculoskeletal and joint disorders; pain.

Natrocitral *Chemdorf, Spain.*
Oxetacaine (p.1317·3); sodium citrate (p.1186·2); aluminium glycinate (p.1210·3).
Gastrointestinal disorders.

Natrosteril *Orion, Fin.*
A range of sodium chloride infusions with or without glucose (p.1196·1).
Fluid and electrolyte disorders.

Natudolor *Duopharm, Ger.*
Potentilla anserina.
Dysmenorrhoea.

Natudophilus *Cantassium Co., UK.*
Lactobacillus acidophilus (p.1626·3); Bifidobacterium bifidum (p.1626·3).

Natudor *Plantes et Medecines, Fr.*
Crataegus (p.1600·2); passion flower (p.1649·1).
Anxiety; insomnia; palpitations.

Natu-fem *Rodisma, Ger.*
Cimicifuga (p.1595·2).
Menopausal disorders.

Natulan
Roche, Aust.†; Link, Austral.; Roche, Belg.†; Roche, Canad.†; Sigma-Tau, Fr.; Gry, Ger.; Roche, Israel; Roche, Ital.; Roche, Mex.; Sigma-Tau, Neth.; Roche, Norw.†; AFT, NZ; Roche, S.Afr.; Sigma-Tau, Spain; Roche, Switz.†; Cambridge, UK.
Procarbazine hydrochloride (p.566·2).
Now known as Procarbazine Capsules in the UK.
Malignant neoplasms.

Natulanar
Roche, Braz.; Roche, Swed.†.
Procarbazine hydrochloride (p.566·2).
Malignant neoplasms.

Natulax *Lichtenstein, Ger.†.*
Lactulose (p.1230·1).
Constipation; hepatic encephalopathy; salmonella enteritis.

Natura Medica *Dolisos, Fr.†.*
A range of herbal extracts.

Natura Viva *Novartis Consumer, Ital.*
Royal jelly (p.1659·3).
Nutritional supplement.

Natural Defense *Maybelline, Canad.*
Titanium dioxide (p.1126·1).
Sunscreen.

Natural Fibre *Cenovis, Austral.; Vitelle, Austral.*
Psyllium seed (p.1229·1).
Constipation; dietary fibre supplement.

Natural Herb Tablets *Dorwest, UK.*
Senna (p.1248·2); aloes (p.1210·1); cascara (p.1216·1); valerian (p.1678·3); taraxacum (p.1669·1).
Constipation.

Natural Horizons Solar Block Extreme *Mentholatum, Austral.*
SPF 30+: Octinoxate (p.1517·3); zinc oxide (p.1128·2).
Sunscreen.

Natural Horizons Solar Block Lotion *Mentholatum, Austral.*
SPF 15: Octinoxate (p.1517·3); avobenzone (p.1517·1); octil triazone; titanium dioxide (p.1126·1).
SPF 30+: Octinoxate (p.1517·3); zinc oxide (p.1128·2).
Sunscreen.

Natural Horizons Solar Block Toddler *Mentholatum, Austral.*
SPF 30+: Octinoxate (p.1517·3); zinc oxide (p.1128·2).
Sunscreen.

Natural Ice Extreme *Mentholatum, Canad.*
SPF 30: Avobenzone (p.1517·1); octinoxate (p.1517·3); octisalate (p.1518·1).
Sunscreen.

Natural Ice Lipbalm *Mentholatum, Canad.*
Octinoxate (p.1517·3); octisalate (p.1518·1).
Sunscreen.

Natural Source Laxative *Adams, Canad.*
Ispaghula (p.1229·1).
Constipation; fibre supplementation.

Natural Zanzy *Montefarmaco, Ital.*
Geranium oil (p.1615·1); lavender oil (p.1627·2); citronella oil (p.1596·3).
Insect repellent.

Naturalass *Naturmed, Ital.*
Lactulose (p.1230·1); mannitol (p.924·3); glycerol (p.1616·3); inulin (p.1624·1); plant fibre; minerals (p.1350·1).
Gastrointestinal disorders.

Naturalyte *Unico, USA.*
Glucose; electrolytes (p.1185·2).
Diarrhoea; oral rehydration therapy.

Naturcil *London Drugs, Canad.†.*
Ispaghula (p.1229·1).

Natures Own Acidophilus Plus *Bullivants, Austral.*
Lactobacillus acidophilus (p.1626·3); Lactobacillus bulgaricus (p.1626·3); apple pectin (p.1502·3).
Maintenance of normal gastrointestinal flora.

Natures Own Colds & Flu *Bullivants, Austral.*
Ferrous phosphate; potassium chloride (p.1194·3).
Cold and influenza symptoms.

Natures Own Digestive Enzymes *Bullivants, Austral.*
Pepsin (p.1649·3); bromelains (p.1586·3); peppermint oil (p.1243·3); pancreatin (p.1646·1); papain (p.1647·3).
Digestive disorders; dyspepsia; flatulence.

Natures Own Maxepa *Bullivants, Austral.*
Fish oil (p.949·3).
Dietary fatty acid supplement.

Natures Own Maxi B *Bullivants, Austral.*
Vitamin B substances (p.1350·1).
Vitamin B supplement.

Natures Own Mega-B + L-Tryptophan *Bullivants, Austral.*
Vitamin B substances; tryptophan; ginseng; fo-ti-tieng; rosehips; alfalfa (p.1350·1).
Tonic; vitamin B supplement.

Natures Own Super B Complex *Bullivants, Austral.*
Vitamin B substances; vitamin C; methionine; wheatgerm; lecithin (p.1350·1).
Tonic; vitamin B supplement.

Natures Remedy
Block, Canad.; SmithKline Beecham Consumer, USA.
Aloes (p.1210·1); cascara (p.1216·1).
Constipation.

Nature's Tears *Rugby, USA.*
Hypromellose (p.1501·3); dextran 70 (p.729·2).
Dry eyes.

Natures Way Acidophilus Plus *Roche Consumer, Austral.*
Lactobacillus acidophilus (p.1626·3); Bifidobacterium bifidum (p.1626·3).
Maintenance of normal gastrointestinal flora.

Natures Way All-in-One *Roche Consumer, Austral.*
Multivitamin and mineral preparation with ginseng (p.1350·1).

Natures Way Executive Formula *Roche Consumer, Austral.*
Vitamins; minerals; valerian; passion flower; chamomile (p.1350·1).
Stress; vitamin B supplement.

Natures Way Hi B Plus C *Roche Consumer, Austral.*
Vitamin B substances; ascorbic acid; minerals (p.1350·1).
Vitamin B and C deficiency.

Natures Way Lifespan Antioxidant *Roche Consumer, Austral.*
Multivitamin and mineral preparation (p.1350·1).

Natures Way Mega B *Roche Consumer, Austral.*
Vitamin B substances; ascorbic acid; minerals (p.1350·1).
Vitamin B supplement.

Natures Way Mega Multi *Roche Consumer, Austral.*
Multivitamin, mineral, and herbal preparation (p.1350·1).
Dietary supplement; tonic.

Natures Way Omega 3 *Roche Consumer, Austral.*
Omega-3 marine triglycerides (p.949·3).
Dietary fatty acid supplement.

Natures Way Omega 3 Complex *Roche Consumer, Austral.*
Omega-3 marine triglycerides; lecithin; garlic oil (p.1350·1).
Dietary supplement.

Natures Way Total C *Roche Consumer, Austral.*
Ascorbic acid (p.1389·3); hesperidin (p.1611·2); rutoside (p.1611·2); bioflavonoids (p.1611·1).
Cold and influenza symptoms.

Natures Way Total Calcium Plus *Roche Consumer, Austral.*
Calcium carbonate (p.1215·1); colecalciferol (p.1391·0).
Calcium and vitamin D supplement; osteoporosis.

Natures Way Total Zinc *Roche Consumer, Austral.*
Zinc amino acid chelate (p.1398·3); vitamin A palmitate (p.1383·2); pyridoxine hydrochloride (p.1386·3); magnesium phosphate (p.1191·1); manganese amino acid chelate.
Skin disorders; wounds.

Natures Way Womens All-in-One *Roche Consumer, Austral.*
Multivitamin and mineral preparation (p.1350·1).

Naturest
Note.This name is used for preparations of different composition.

Vitaglow, Austral.
Valerian (p.1678·3); passion flower (p.1649·1); skullcap (p.1664·3); vervain (p.1679·3); magnesium oxide (p.1233·2); calcium phosphate (p.1188·3).
Insomnia.

Lane, UK.
Passion flower (p.1649·1).
Insomnia.

Naturetin *Squibb, Canad.†; Apothecon, USA.*
Bendrofluazide [bendroflumethiazide] (p.844·1).
Hypertension; oedema.

Naturetti *Hoechst Marion Roussel, Mex.*
Senna (p.1248·2); cassia (p.1216·2); tamarind (p.1253·2); coriander (p.1599·2); liquorice (p.1231·2).
Constipation.

Naturgen terre silice *Marbot, Switz.†.*
Medicinal mud.
Bronchitis; coughs; musculoskeletal and joint disorders; phlebitis.

Naturgen terre volcanique *Marbot, Switz.†.*
Medicinal volcanic mud.
Digestive-system disorders.

Naturine *Leo, Fr.†.*
Bendrofluazide [bendroflumethiazide] (p.844·1).
Hypertension; oedema.

Naturland Entschlackung *Naturland, Aust.*
Parsley (p.1648·3); solidago virgaurea; ononis (p.1644·1).
Urinary-tract disorders.

Naturland Herz-Kreislauf *Naturland, Aust.*
Crataegus (p.1600·2); rosemary.
Cardiovascular disorders.

Naturland Rheuma-Tee *Naturland, Aust.*
Rosemary; urtica (p.1678·2); equisetum (p.1606·3); taraxacum (p.1669·1); salix (p.82·1).
Inflammation; pain.

Naturland Verdauungs *Naturland, Aust.*
Peppermint leaf (p.1243·2); gentian (p.1615·1); caraway (p.1591·2).
Gastrointestinal disorders.

Naturvite *Solgar, UK.*
Multivitamin and mineral preparation (p.1350·1).

Natus Gerin *Legrand, Braz.*
Multivitamin, mineral, and amino-acid preparation with ginseng (p.1350·1).

Natusan *Johnson & Johnson, Spain.*
Glyceroborate complex; boric acid (p.1586·1); borax (p.1586·1).
Skin irritation.

Natuscap retard *Vifor, Switz.*
Chlorpheniramine [chlorphenamine] maleate (p.412·1); codeine phosphate (p.25·2); phenylephrine hydrochloride (p.1097·1).
Coughs and associated respiratory-tract disorders.

Natuscilin *Natus, Braz.*
Ampicillin (p.150·3).
Bacterial infections.

Natusgel *Natus, Braz.*
Oral suspension: Aluminium hydroxide (p.1210·3).
Tablets: Aluminium hydroxide (p.1210·3); magnesium hydroxide (p.1233·1); calcium carbonate (p.1215·1).
Gastrointestinal hyperacidity.

Natuvit *Roche Nicholas, Fr.†.*
Dietary fibre supplement (p.1350·1).

Asta Medica, Neth.†.
Nutritional supplement (p.1350·1).

Natyl *Interdelta, Switz.†.*
Dipyridamole (p.877·2).
Thromboembolism prophylaxis.

Naudicelle
Key, Austral.; Swiss Herbal, Canad.; Bio-Oil Research, Irl.; Bio-Oil Research, UK.
Evening primrose oil (p.1613·2).
Dietary supplement.

Naudicelle Forte *Bio-Oil Research, UK.*
Borage oil (p.1613·1); marine fish oil (p.949·3).

Naudicelle Marine *Key, Austral.*
Evening primrose oil (p.1613·2); marine fish oil (p.949·3).
Dietary supplement.

Naudicelle Plus
Key, Austral.†; Bio-Oil Research, UK.
Evening primrose oil (p.1613·2); marine fish oil (p.949·3).
Dietary supplement.

Naudicelle SL *Bio-Oil Research, UK.*
Salmon oil (p.949·2); lecithin (p.1628·1).

Naudivite *Bio-Oil Research, UK.*
A range of vitamin, mineral, and nutritional supplements (p.1350·1).

Naupathon *Staufen, Ger.*
Homoeopathic preparation.

Naus-A-Way *Roberts, USA†.*
Glucose (p.1364·2); fructose (p.1363·3); phosphoric acid (p.1651·1).
Nausea and vomiting.

Nausea Relief *Brauer, Austral.*
Homoeopathic preparation.

Nauseatol *Sabex, Canad.*
Dimenhydrinate (p.415·2).
Nausea and vomiting.

Nausefe *Inibsa, Port.*
Dicyclomine [dicycloverine] hydrochloride (p.466·1); doxylamine succinate (p.417·1); pyridoxine hydrochloride (p.1386·3).
Nausea; vomiting.

Nausex *Asta Medica, Aust.; Nobel, Canad.†.*
Dimenhydrinate (p.415·2).
Ménière's disease; motion sickness; nausea and vomiting; vestibular disorders.

Nausicalm *Brothier, Fr.*
Dimenhydrinate (p.415·2).
Motion sickness; vertigo.

Nausigon *Mundipharma, Aust.*
Metoclopramide hydrochloride (p.1235·2).
Gastrointestinal ulcers; intractable hiccups; nausea and vomiting; upper gastrointestinal motility disorders.

Nausil *Siam Bheasach, Thai.*
Metoclopramide hydrochloride (p.1235·2).
Dyspepsia; flatulence; gastro-oesophageal reflux; nausea and vomiting; peptic ulcer.

Nausilen *Baldacci, Ital.*
Alizapride hydrochloride (p.1209·3).
Nausea and vomiting.

Nausyn *Weleda, Aust.; Weleda, UK.*
Homoeopathic preparation.

Nautamine *Synthelabo, Fr.*
Diphenhydramine di(acefyllinate) (p.416·1).
Motion sickness.

Nautisan *Sanova, Aust.†.*
Chlorobutanol (p.1141·2); caffeine (p.761·3).
Nausea and vomiting.

Nautrol *Precimex, Mex.*
Difenidol (p.1222·1).
Nausea and vomiting.

Nauzelin *Janssen-Cilag, Spain.*
Domperidone (p.1224·1).
Gastroparesis; nausea and vomiting.

Nauzine *Be-Tabs, S.Afr.*
Cyclizine hydrochloride (p.414·1).
Motion sickness; nausea and vomiting; vestibular disorders.

Navamed *Greater Pharma, Thai.*
Dimenhydrinate (p.415·2).
Motion sickness; nausea and vomiting.

Navamine *Greater Pharma, Thai.*
Dimenhydrinate (p.415·2).
Motion sickness; nausea and vomiting.

Navane
Pfizer, Austral.; Pfizer, Braz.; Pfizer, Canad.; Pfizer, Hong Kong; Pfizer, Neth.; Pfizer, Thai.; Pfizer, USA.
Tiotixene (p.709·2) or tiotixene hydrochloride (p.709·2).
Psychoses.

Navelbine
Boehringer Ingelheim, Aust.; Asta Medica, Austral.; Asta Medica, Braz.; Glaxo Wellcome, Canad.; Pierre Fabre, Denm.; Pierre Fabre, Fin.; Pierre Fabre, Fr.; Pierre Fabre, Ger.; Pierre Fabre, Israel; Pierre Fabre, Ital.; Schering-Plough, Mex.; Pierre Fabre, Norw.; Asta Medica, NZ; Pierre Fabre, Port.; Tema, S.Afr.; Orient, Singapore; Pierre Fabre, Singapore; Pierre Fabre, Spain; Pierre Fabre, Swed.; Robapharm, Switz.; Asta Medica, Thai.; Pierre Fabre, UK; Glaxo Wellcome, USA.
Vinorelbine tartrate (p.580·2).
Breast cancer; non-small cell lung cancer.

Navicalm
Note.This name is used for preparations of different composition.
UCB, Neth.
Hydroxyzine hydrochloride (p.419·1).
Anxiety; pruritus; urticaria.

Confar, Port.; UCB, Spain.
Meclozine (p.420·3) or meclozine hydrochloride (p.420·3).
Motion sickness.

Navidoxine
UCB, Hong Kong; UCB, Singapore.
Meclozine hydrochloride (p.420·3); pyridoxine hydrochloride (p.1386·3).
Nausea and vomiting.

Navidrex *Novartis, NZ; Goldshield, UK.*
Cyclopenthiazide (p.865·2).
Heart failure; hypertension; oedema.

Navispare
Novartis, Hong Kong; Novartis, Irl.; Novartis, UK.
Cyclopenthiazide (p.865·2); amiloride hydrochloride (p.835·1).
Hypertension.

Navixen *Mavi, Mex.*
Naproxen (p.60·3).

Navoban
Novartis, Aust.; Novartis, Austral.; Novartis, Braz.; Novartis, Denm.; Novartis, Fin.; Novartis, Fr.; Novartis, Ger.; Asta Medica, Ger.; Novartis, Hong Kong; Novartis, Irl.; Novartis, Israel; Novartis, Ital.; Novartis, Jpn; Novartis, Mex.; Novartis, Norw.; Novartis, Port.; Novartis, S.Afr.; Novartis, Spain; Novartis, Swed.; Novartis, Switz.; Novartis, Thai.; Novartis, UK.
Tropisetron (p.1253·3) or tropisetron hydrochloride (p.1253·3).
Nausea and vomiting induced by cytotoxic therapy; postoperative nausea and vomiting.

Naxen
Altimed, Canad.; Syntex, Mex.; Douglas, NZ; Rolab, S.Afr.
Naproxen (p.60·3).
Now known as Rolab-Naproxen in S.Afr.
Gout; musculoskeletal, joint, peri-articular, and soft-tissue disorders; pain.

Naxidine *Lilly, Neth.*
Nizatidine (p.1238·1).
Gastro-oesophageal reflux; peptic ulcer.

Naxil *Galen, Mex.*
Naproxen (p.60·3).

Naxilan-Plus *Rayere, Mex.*
Nalidixic acid (p.227·1); phenazopyridine (p.78·1).
Urinary-tract infections.

Naxo *Sons, Mex.*
Chloramphenicol (p.179·1).
Bacterial infections.

Naxodol *Syntex, Mex.*
Naproxen (p.60·3); carisoprodol (p.1327·1).
Musculoskeletal, joint, and peri-articular disorders.

Naxogil *Pharmacia Upjohn, Mex.*
Nimorazole (p.598·3).

Naxogin
Pharmacia Upjohn, Aust.; Pharmacia Upjohn, Belg.; Carlo Erba, Braz.; Pharmacia Upjohn, Hong Kong; Pharmacia, S.Afr.†; Pharmacia Upjohn, Thai.
Nimorazole (p.598·3).
Acute ulcerative gingivitis; amoebiasis; giardiasis; vaginal trichomoniasis.

Naxogin Composto *Carlo Erba, Braz.*
Nimorazole (p.598·3); chloramphenicol (p.179·1); nystatin (p.392·2).
Vulvovaginal infections.

Naxogyn *Pharmacia Upjohn, Fr.*
Nimorazole (p.598·3).
Trichomoniasis.

Naxolan *Faulding, Port.*
Naloxone hydrochloride (p.1014·3).

Naxopren *Pharmacia Upjohn, Fin.*
Naproxen (p.60·3).
Fever; gout; inflammation; musculoskeletal and joint disorders; pain.

Naxpa *Novag, Braz.*
Ambroxol hydrochloride (p.1084·3).
Respiratory-tract disorders.

Naxy *Sanofi Winthrop, Fr.*
Clarithromycin (p.186·2).
Bacterial infections.

Naxyn *Teva, Israel.*
Naproxen (p.60·3).
Dysmenorrhoea; gout; musculoskeletal, joint, and peri-articular disorders.

Nazalet *Stanley, Israel.*
Xylometazoline hydrochloride (p.1102·2).
Nasal congestion.

Nazene *Restan, S.Afr.*
Oxymetazoline hydrochloride (p.1096·2); zinc sulfate (p.1398·2).
Allergic rhinitis; nasal congestion; sinusitis.

Nazobel *Sedabel, Braz.*
Naphazoline (p.1095·1); neomycin (p.228·1).
Nasal disorders.

Nazobio *Luper, Braz.*
Naphazoline (p.1095·1); panthenol (p.1602·3); chlorobutanol (p.1141·2).
Nasal congestion.

Nazodin *Vitamed, Israel.*
Naphazoline hydrochloride (p.1095·1); diphenhydramine hydrochloride (p.416·1); neomycin sulfate (p.228·1).
Nasal congestion.

Nazolfarm *Continentales, Mex.*
Ketoconazole (p.389·1).

Nazophyl *Medecine Vegetale, Fr.†.*
Eucalyptus oil (p.1609·2); pine oil.
Nose and throat infections.

Nazotiran *Gilton, Braz.*
Naphazoline (p.1095·1); thiomersal (p.1158·2).
Nasal congestion.

NB-Tee N *Eu Rho, Ger.†.*
Birch leaf (p.1585·2); java tea (p.1625·1).
Urinary-tract disorders.

N-Combur Test *Roche Diagnostics, Austral.*
Test for nitrite, protein, glucose, and pH in urine.

ND Stat *Hyrex, USA†.*
Brompheniramine maleate (p.410·2).
Hypersensitivity reactions.

ND-Gesic *Hyrex, USA.*
Phenylephrine hydrochloride (p.1097·1); paracetamol (p.71·2); chlorpheniramine [chlorphenamine] maleate (p.412·1); mepyramine maleate (p.421·1).
Upper respiratory-tract symptoms.

Nealorin
Probios, Port.; Pras, Spain.
Carboplatin (p.515·1).
Malignant neoplasms.

Neat Effect *Neat Feat, NZ.*
Aluminium chlorohydrate (p.1110·2).
Hyperhidrosis.

Neat Feat *Neat Feat, NZ.*
Aluminium chlorohydrate (p.1110·2).
Hyperhidrosis.

Neat One *Neat Feat, NZ.*
Aluminium-zirconium tetrachlorohydrex glycine (p.1110·2).
Hyperhidrosis.

Neat Touch *Neat Feat, NZ.*
Aluminium chlorohydrate (p.1110·2).
Hyperhidrosis.

Neatenol *Fides Rottapharm, Spain.*
Atenolol (p.841·3).
Angina pectoris; arrhythmias; hypertension; myocardial infarction.

Neatenol Diu *Fides Rottapharm, Spain.*
Bendrofluazide [bendroflumethiazide] (p.844·1); atenolol (p.841·3).
Hypertension.

Neatenol Diuvas *Fides Rottapharm, Spain.*
Bendrofluazide [bendroflumethiazide] (p.844·1); hydralazine hydrochloride (p.905·3); atenolol (p.841·3).
Hypertension.

Nebacetin
Tyrol, Aust.; Byk, Braz.; Yamanouchi, Ger.; Byk Gulden, Hong Kong; Byk Gulden, S.Afr.†; Lundbeck, Swed.†; Eumedica, Switz.
Neomycin (p.228·1) or neomycin sulfate (p.228·1); bacitracin (p.155·2) or bacitracin zinc (p.155·2).
Bacterial infections.

Nebacetin N *Yamanouchi, Ger.*
Neomycin sulfate (p.228·1).
Burns; skin infections; wounds.

Nebacetina *Byk Gulden, Mex.*
Neomycin sulfate (p.228·1); bacitracin (p.155·2).
Bacterial skin infections.

Nebal *Reuffer, Mex.*
Hydroxocobalamin (p.1388·1).

Nebcin
Lilly, Austral.; Lilly, Canad.; Lilly, Hong Kong; Lilly, Irl.; Lilly, Israel; Lilly, NZ; Aspen, S.Afr.; Lilly, UK; Lilly, USA.
Tobramycin sulfate (p.263·3).
Bacterial infections.

Nebcina
Lilly, Denm.; Lilly, Fin.; Lilly, Norw.; Lilly, Swed.
Tobramycin sulfate (p.263·3).
Bacterial infections.

Nebcine *Lilly, Fr.*
Tobramycin sulfate (p.263·3).
Bacterial infections.

Nebicina *Lilly, Ital.*
Tobramycin sulfate (p.263·3).
Bacterial infections.

Nebilet
Janssen-Cilag, Aust.†; Berlin-Chemie, Ger.; Menarini, Irl.; Menarini, Neth.; Sanitas, Port.; Menarini, Switz.; Menarini, UK.
Nebivolol hydrochloride (p.938·2).
Hypertension.

Nebilox *Lusofarmaco, Ital.*
Nebivolol hydrochloride (p.938·2).
Hypertension.

Neblik *Knoll, Spain.*
Eformoterol [formoterol] fumarate (p.764·2).
Obstructive airways disease.

Nebris *Celafar, Ital.*
Olax dissitiflora; chamomile (p.1593·2).
Dry skin.

Nebulasma *Urbion, Spain.*
Sodium cromoglicate (p.774·3).
Asthma; bronchospasm.

Nebulcrom *Casen Fisons, Spain.*
Sodium cromoglicate (p.774·3).
Asthma; bronchospasm.

Nebulicina *Fher, Spain.*
Oxymetazoline hydrochloride (p.1096·2).
Formerly contained fenoxazoline hydrochloride.
Nasal congestion.

NebuPent *American Pharmaceutical, USA.*
Pentamidine isetionate (p.600·1).
Pneumocystis carinii pneumonia.

NEC *Essedi, Ital.*
Protein-free preparation for enteral nutrition (p.1350·1).
Renal disease.

Necamin *Ache, Braz.*
Mebendazole (p.102·2).
Worm infections.

Necid *New Research, Ital.*
Cefonicid sodium (p.168·1).
Lignocaine [lidocaine] hydrochloride (p.1313·2) is included in the intramuscular injection to alleviate the pain of injection.
Gram-negative bacterial infections.

Necon 0.5/35, 1/35 *Watson, USA.*
Norethisterone (p.1485·1); ethinylestradiol (p.1476·2).
28-Day packs also contain 7 inert tablets.
Combined oral contraceptive.

Necon 1/50 *Watson, USA.*
Norethisterone (p.1485·1); mestranol (p.1482·1).
28-Day packs also contain 7 inert tablets.
Combined oral contraceptive.

Necon 10/11 *Watson, USA.*
Norethisterone (p.1485·1); ethinylestradiol (p.1476·2).
28-Day packs also contain 7 inert tablets.
Biphasic oral contraceptive.

Necopen *Esteve, Spain.*
Cefixime (p.166·2).
Bacterial infections.

Necrohepat *Heralds, Braz.*
Methionine (p.1012·2); betaine tartrate (p.1584·3); choline (p.1356·3); inositol (p.1623·3); nicotinamide (p.1372·3); cynara (p.1601·3); liver extract.
Liver disorders.

Necroplex *Heralds, Braz.*
Citrulline (p.1357·2); ornithine (p.1374·1); arginine (p.1353·3); oxypurines.
Liver disorders.

Neatenol *Fides Rottapharm, Spain.*

Necyrane *Medeva, Fr.*
Ritiometan magnesium (p.1156·1).
Nose and throat infections.

Neda Fruchtewurfel
Note. This name is used for preparations of different composition.
Novartis Consumer, Aust.
Senna (p.1248·2); fig (p.1227·1); tamarind (p.1253·2).
Constipation.
Novartis Consumer, Ger.
Senna (p.1248·2).
Constipation.

Neda Lactiv Importal *Novartis Consumer, Ger.*
Lactitol (p.1230·1).
Constipation.

Nedeltran *Rhone-Poulenc Rorer, Neth.*
Trimeprazine [alimemazine] tartrate (p.426·2).
Hypersensitivity reactions; psychoses.

Nedios *Byk, Neth.*
Acipimox (p.827·3).
Hyperlipidaemias.

Nedolon P *Merck, Ger.*
Paracetamol (p.71·2); codeine phosphate (p.25·2).
Pain.

NEE 1/35 *Lexis, USA.*
Ethinylestradiol (p.1476·2); norethisterone (p.1485·1).
28-Day packs also contain 7 inert tablets.
Combined oral contraceptive.

Nefadar
Bristol-Myers Squibb, Denm.; Bristol-Myers Squibb, Fin.; Bristol-Myers Squibb, Ger.; Bristol-Myers Squibb, Norw.; Bristol-Myers Squibb, Swed.; Bristol-Myers Squibb, Switz.
Nefazodone hydrochloride (p.300·3).
Depression.

Nefadol *Zilliken, Ital.†.*
Nefopam hydrochloride (p.62·1).
Pain.

Nefam *Biagini, Ital.*
Nefopam hydrochloride (p.62·1).
Pain.

Nefluan *Molteni, Ital.*
Lignocaine [lidocaine] hydrochloride (p.1313·2); neomycin sulfate (p.228·1); fluocinolone acetonide (p.1071·1).
Endoscopy.

Nefrocarnit *Medice, Ger.*
Levocarnitine (p.1356·1).
Carnitine deficiency.

Nefrolactona *Vedim, Port.*
Spironolactone (p.973·2).
Hepatic cirrhosis; hyperaldosteronism; hypertension of pregnancy; hypokalaemia; hypomagnesaemia; oedema.

Nefroplasmal *Braun, Port.*
Amino-acid infusion (p.1350·1).
Parenteral nutrition in renal failure.

Nefro-Zinc *Medice, Ger.*
Zinc chloride (p.1398·1).
Zinc deficiency in dialysis patients.

Negaban *Beecham, Belg.†.*
Temocillin sodium (p.258·3).
Gram-negative bacterial infections.

Negacef *Julphar, UAE.*
Ceftazidime (p.174·3).
Bacterial infections.

Negatol
Byk, Fr.; Byk Gulden, Ital.; Juventus, Spain; Byk, Switz.
Metacresolsulfonic acid-formaldehyde (p.738·3).
Burns; gynaecological disorders; minor haemorrhage; ulcers; wounds.

Negatol Dental *Wild, Switz.*
Metacresolsulfonic acid-formaldehyde (p.738·3).
Aphthous stomatitis; gingival haemorrhage.

Negazole *Julphar, UAE.*
Metronidazole (p.594·1) or metronidazole benzoate (p.594·1).
Anaerobic bacterial infections; bacterial vaginosis; dracunculiasis; inflammatory bowel disease; protozoal infections.

NegGram
Sanofi Synthelabo, Canad.; Sanofi Winthrop, Israel; Sanofi Synthelabo, Ital.; Sanofi Winthrop, USA.
Nalidixic acid (p.227·1).
Gram-negative urinary-tract infections.

Negram
Sanofi Synthelabo, Austral.†; Sanofi Winthrop, Denm.†; Sanofi Winthrop, Fr.; Sanofi Winthrop, Irl.; Sanofi Winthrop, Norw.; Sanofi Winthrop, NZ; Sanofi Winthrop, Swed.†; Sanofi Winthrop, UK.
Nalidixic acid (p.227·1).
Gram-negative urinary- and gastrointestinal-tract infections.

Nehydrin *Sanochemia, Aust.*
Dihydroergocristine mesilate (p.1603·2).
Cerebrovascular disorders.

Nehydrin N *TAD, Ger.*
Co-dergocrine mesilate (p.1597·3).
Mental function disorders.

Neisvac-C *Baxter, UK.*
A meningococcal group C conjugate vaccine (tetanus toxoid protein conjugate) (p.1550·1).
Active immunisation.

Nekacin *New Research, Ital.*
Amikacin sulfate (p.148·1).
Gram-negative bacterial infections.

Nelapine *Berlin Pharm, Thai.*
Nifedipine (p.940·1).
Cardiac disorders; hypertension.

Nelex
Byk Gulden, Denm.†; Meda, Fin.; Byk, Port.; Byk Modaus, S.Afr.; Pharmacia Upjohn, Swed.†.
Metacresolsulfonic acid-formaldehyde (p.738·3).
Anogenital warts; burns; gynaecological disorders; haemorrhage; wounds.

Nelova 10/11 *Warner Chilcott, USA†.*
Norethisterone (p.1485·1); ethinylestradiol (p.1476·2).
28-Day packs also contain 7 inert tablets.
Biphasic oral contraceptive.

Nelova 0.5/35E and 1/35E *Warner Chilcott, USA†.*
Norethisterone (p.1485·1); ethinylestradiol (p.1476·2).
28-Day packs also contain 7 inert tablets.
Combined oral contraceptive.

Nelova 1/50M *Warner Chilcott, USA†.*
Norethisterone (p.1485·1); mestranol (p.1482·1).
28-Day packs also contain 7 inert tablets.
Combined oral contraceptive.

Nelsons Clikpak Series *Nelson, UK.*
A range of homoeopathic remedies.

Nemactil *Rhone-Poulenc Rorer, Spain.*
Pericyazine (p.698·3).
Anxiety; behaviour disorders; psychoses.

Nemapres *Precimex, Mex.*
Mebendazole (p.102·2).

Nemasol *ICN, Canad.*
Sodium aminosalicylate (p.148·3).
Tuberculosis.

Nembutal
Abbott, Canad.; Abbott, USA.
Pentobarbital sodium (p.698·2).
Epilepsy; insomnia; premedication; sedative.

Nemdyn *Hamilton, Austral.*
Neomycin undecylenate (p.228·1); bacitracin zinc (p.155·2).
Fungal or bacterial ear infections.

Nemesil *Synthelabo, Braz.*
Ketotifen fumarate (p.767·2).
Allergic conjunctivitis; allergic rhinitis; asthma; urticaria.

Nemestran
Hoechst Marion Roussel, Mex.; Hoechst Marion Roussel, Neth.; Hoechst Marion Roussel, Spain; Hoechst Marion Roussel, Switz.
Gestrinone (p.1479·2).
Endometriosis.

Nemexin
Torrex, Aust.; Du Pont, Ger.; Du Pont, Switz.
Naltrexone hydrochloride (p.1016·1).
Opioid withdrawal.

Nemodine *Kener, Mex.*
Ketotifen (p.767·2).

Nene Dent *Byk, Braz.*
Butoxycaine (p.1308·2); benzocaine (p.1306·2); ethacridine (p.1130·3); acriflavinium chloride (p.1130·2); myrrh (p.1639·2); chamomile (p.1593·2); menthol (p.1632·3).
Mouth disorders.

Nene-Lax *Dentinox, Ger.*
Glycerol (p.1616·3).
Bowel evacuation; constipation.

Neo *Neo Laboratories, UK.*
Cream: Cetrimide (p.1137·1); benzalkonium chloride (p.1133·2).
Napkin rash; skin irritation.
Oral mixture: Dill oil (p.1603·3); ginger (p.1227·2); sodium bicarbonate (p.1186·2).
Colic; teething.

Neo Analsona *Casen Fleet, Spain.*
Benzocaine (p.1306·2); fluocinolone acetonide (p.1071·1); neomycin (p.228·1); ruscogenin (p.1660·2).
Anorectal disorders.

Neo Aritmina *Solvay, Ital.†.*
Prajmalium bitartrate (p.957·2).
Arrhythmias.

Neo Artrol *Recordati, Spain.*
Flurbiprofen (p.41·2).
Musculoskeletal, joint, and peri-articular disorders; pain.

Neo Atromid *Zeneca, Spain.*
Clofibrate (p.859·1).
Hyperlipidaemias.

Neo Bace *Pharmavite, Canad.*
Bacitracin (p.155·2); polymyxin B sulfate (p.238·1).

Neo Bacitrin *Fides Rottapharm, Spain.*
Ointment: Bacitracin (p.155·2); neomycin sulfate (p.228·1); zinc oxide (p.1128·2).
Topical powder: Bacitracin (p.155·2); neomycin sulfate (p.228·1).
Burns; skin infections; ulcers; wounds.

Neo Bacitrin Hidrocortis *Fides Rottapharm, Spain.*
Bacitracin (p.155·2); hydrocortisone acetate (p.1073·3); neomycin sulfate (p.228·1); zinc oxide (p.1128·2).
Infected skin disorders.

Neo Borocillina *Wassermann, Ital.*
Dichlorobenzyl alcohol (p.1143·2); sodium benzoate (p.1134·3).
Mouth and throat disinfection.

Neo Borocillina Balsamica *Wassermann, Ital.*
Dichlorobenzyl alcohol (p.1143·2); terpin hydrate (p.1101·2); menglytate (p.1094·2).
Mouth and throat disinfection; respiratory-tract infections.

The symbol † denotes a preparation no longer actively marketed

Neo Borocillina C *Wassermann, Ital.*
Dichlorobenzyl alcohol (p.1143·3); ascorbic acid (p.1389·3).
Mouth and throat disinfection.

Neo Borocillina Collutorio *Wassermann, Ital.*
Dichlorobenzyl alcohol (p.1143·2).
Mouth and throat disinfection.

Neo Borocillina Spray *Wassermann, Ital.*
Dichlorobenzyl alcohol (p.1143·2).
Mouth and throat disinfection.

Neo Borocillina Tosse Compresse *Wassermann, Ital.*
Dextromethorphan hydrobromide (p.1087·3); guaifenesin (p.1092·2); menglytate (p.1094·3); dichlorobenzyl alcohol (p.1143·2).
Coughs; mouth and throat disinfection.

Neo Borocillina Tosse Sciroppo *Wassermann, Ital.*
Dextromethorphan hydrobromide (p.1087·3); guaifenesin (p.1092·2); menglytate (p.1094·3).
Coughs.

Neo Cal *Neolab, Canad.*
Calcium carbonate (p.1215·1).

Neo Cal D *Neolab, Canad.*
Calcium carbonate (p.1215·1); vitamin D (p.1391·1).

Neo Carbone Belloc *Vaillant, Ital.†*
Activated charcoal (p.1000·2).
Diarrhoea; flatulence.

Neo Cardiol *Francia, Ital.*
Carnitine (p.1356·1).
Carnitine deficiency; myocardial ischaemia.

Neo Cebetil *Searle, Braz.*
Vitamin B substances with vitamin C and fructose (p.1350·1).

Neo Cepacol Collutorio *Lepetit, Ital.†*
Cetylpyridinium chloride (p.1138·1); sodium phosphate; sodium diphosphate; disodium edetate; methyl salicylate; eucalyptol; cinnamon oil; mint oil; menthol.
Dental plaque prevention; mouth and throat disinfection.

Neo Cepacol Pastiglie *Hoechst Marion Roussel, Ital.*
Cetylpyridinium chloride (p.1138·1).
Mouth and throat disinfection.

Neo Citran
Novartis, Aust.; Novartis Consumer, Canad.; Novartis Consumer, Switz.
Paracetamol (p.71·2); pheniramine maleate (p.422·3); phenylephrine hydrochloride (p.1097·1); ascorbic acid (p.1389·3).
Cold symptoms.

Neo Citran A *Novartis Consumer, Canad.*
Phenylephrine hydrochloride (p.1097·1); pheniramine maleate (p.422·3); ascorbic acid (p.1389·3).

Neo Citran Calorie Reduced *Sandoz, Canad.*
Phenylephrine hydrochloride (p.1097·1); pheniramine maleate (p.422·3); paracetamol (p.71·2).
Formerly known as Neo Citran Nutrasweet.

Neo Citran Cough Cold & Flu *Novartis Consumer, Canad.*
Pseudoephedrine hydrochloride (p.1099·2); chlorpheniramine [chlorphenamine] maleate (p.412·1); dextromethorphan hydrobromide (p.1087·3); paracetamol (p.71·2).

Neo Citran Daycaps *Sandoz, Canad.†*
Pseudoephedrine hydrochloride (p.1099·2); dextromethorphan hydrobromide (p.1087·3); paracetamol (p.71·2).

Neo Citran DM *Novartis Consumer, Canad.*
Phenylephrine hydrochloride (p.1097·1); pheniramine maleate (p.422·3); dextromethorphan hydrobromide (p.1087·3).

Neo Citran Sinus *Novartis Consumer, Canad.*
Phenylephrine hydrochloride (p.1097·1); paracetamol (p.71·2).

Neo Citran Sore Throat & Cough *Novartis Consumer, Canad.*
Pseudoephedrine hydrochloride (p.1099·2); chlorpheniramine [chlorphenamine] maleate (p.412·1); dextromethorphan hydrobromide (p.1087·3); paracetamol (p.71·2).

Neo Coricidin *Schering-Plough, Ital.*
Chlorpheniramine [chlorphenamine] maleate (p.412·1); aspirin (p.14·2); caffeine (p.761·3).
Cold symptoms.

Neo Coricidin Gola *Schering-Plough, Ital.*
Cetylpyridinium chloride (p.1138·1).
Mouth and throat disinfection.

Neo Cystine *Sofex, Port.†*
Cystine; vitamin A (p.1350·1).
Hair and nail disorders.

Neo Decabutin *Inkeysa, Spain.*
Indometacin (p.44·3).
Gout; inflammation; musculoskeletal, joint, and peri-articular disorders; oedema; pain.

Neo Decapeptyl *Ache, Braz.*
Triptorelin (p.1299·1).
Prostatic cancer.

Neo Dohyfral *Solvay, Neth.*
Colecalciferol (p.1391·1).
Vitamin D deficiency.

Neo Dulceril *Codilab, Port.†*
Aspartame (p.1354·3).
Sugar substitute.

Neo Eblimon *Guidotti, Ital.*
Naproxen (p.60·3).
Inflammation; musculoskeletal and joint disorders; pain.

Neo Elixifilin *Morrith, Spain†.*
Theophylline (p.1140·1).
Heart failure; obstructive airways disease.

Neo Esoformolo *Esoform, Ital.*
Sodium *o*-phenylphenol (p.1152·1).
Disinfection of waste materials.

Neo Expectan *Wander OTC, Switz.†.*
Acetylcysteine (p.1082·3).
Respiratory-tract disorders associated with increased or viscous mucus.

Neo Fertinorm *Serono, Spain.*
Urofollitropin (p.1299·3).
Female infertility; male infertility.

Neo Fluostomygen *Stomygen, Ital.*
Sodium monofluorophosphate (p.1377·2).
Dental caries prophylaxis.

Neo Formitrol *Novartis Consumer, Ital.*
Cetylpyridinium chloride (p.1138·1).
Oral disinfection.

Neo Gastrausil *Searle, Ital.†*
Cimetidine (p.1216·3).
Gastrointestinal disorders associated with hyperacidity.

Neo Genyl *Meuse, Belg.*
Liver extract.
Vitamin B₁₂ deficiency.

Neo H2 *Boniscontro & Gazzone, Ital.*
Roxatidine acetate hydrochloride (p.1248·1).
Gastrointestinal disorders associated with hyperacidity.

Neo Hubber *Teofarma, Spain.*
Hydrocortisone acetate (p.1073·3); neomycin sulfate (p.228·1).
External ear disorders; rhinitis.

Neo Iloticina *Dista, Spain.*
Erythromycin estolate (p.201·2).
Bacterial infections.

Neo Kodan *Schulke & Mayr, Ger.*
Octenidine hydrochloride (p.1151·3); propyl alcohol (p.1155·3); isopropyl alcohol (p.1149·2).
Skin disinfection.

Neo Lacrim *Alcon Cusi, Spain.*
Phenylephrine hydrochloride (p.1097·1).
Eye irritation.

Neo Lactoflorene *Montefarmaco, Ital.*
Lactic-acid-producing organisms (p.1626·3); vitamins (p.1350·1).
Nutritional supplement.

Neo Lyndiol *Organon, Spain.*
Ethinylestradiol (p.1476·2); lynestrenol (p.1480·1).
Combined oral contraceptive; menstrual disorders.

Neo Makatussin N *Gebro, Switz.*
Dihydrocodeine hydrochloride (p.33·3); diphenhydramine hydrochloride (p.416·1).
Bronchitis; coughs.

Neo Melubrina *Hoechst Marion Roussel, Ital.*
Dipyrone (p.34·1).
Fever; pain.

Neo Moderin *Pharmacia Upjohn, Spain.*
Methylprednisolone acetate (p.1076·1); neomycin sulfate (p.228·1).
Infected skin disorders.

Neo Mom *Candioli, Ital.*
Tetramethrin (p.1437·3); phenothrin (p.1436·2).
Pediculosis.

Neo Nisidina C-Fher *Boehringer Ingelheim, Ital.†.*
Aspirin (p.14·2); paracetamol (p.71·2); ascorbic acid (p.1389·3).
Cold symptoms; pain.

Neo Nisidina-Fher *Boehringer Ingelheim, Ital.*
Aspirin (p.14·2); paracetamol (p.71·2); caffeine (p.761·3).
Cold symptoms; fever; pain.

neo OPT *Optimed, Ger.*
Bromazepam (p.656·3).
Anxiety; sleep disorders.

Neo Rinactive *Farmacusi, Spain.*
Budesonide (p.1064·2).
Rhinitis.

Neo Sampoon
Eisai, Hong Kong; Eisai, Singapore.
Menfegol (p.1346·1).
Spermicidal contraceptive.

Neo Sativan *Cibran, Braz.*
Salicylamide (p.82·1); ephedrine hydrochloride (p.1090·1); ascorbic acid (p.1389·3); garlic (p.1614·1).
Cold and influenza symptoms.

Neo Silvikrin *Doetsch, Grether, Switz.†.*
Wheat-germ oil; millet extract; keratin; L-cysteine; vitamins (p.1350·1).
Hair disorders.

Neo Soluzione Sulfo Balsamica *Deca, Ital.†.*
Sodium sulfide; sodium bromide (p.1587·1); eucalyptol (p.1609·2).
Catarrhal sore throat; rhinitis.

Neo Tomizol *Chemdorf, Spain.*
Carbimazole (p.1521·1).
Hyperthyroidism.

Neo Topico Giusto *Milupa, Ital.†.*
Benzethonium chloride (p.1134·2); hamamelis (p.1618·3).
Nipple care during breast feeding; wound disinfection.

Neo Uniplus *Angelini, Spain.*
Aspirin (p.14·2); paracetamol (p.71·2).
Cold symptoms; pain.

Neo Uniplus C *Angelini, Ital.*
Aspirin (p.14·2); paracetamol (p.71·2); ascorbic acid (p.1389·3).
Cold symptoms; pain.

Neo Urgenin
Neo-Farmaceutica, Port.†; Madaus, Spain.
Echinacea angustifolia (p.1606·2); pygeum africanum (p.1490·3); saw palmetto (p.1491·2).
Prostatic disorders.

Neo Vastrictol *Allergan-Frumtost, Braz.*
Antazoline mesilate (p.408·3); ephedrine hydrochloride (p.1090·1); ascorbic acid (p.1389·3); zinc sulfate (p.1398·2).
Nasal congestion.

Neo Visage *Otsuka, Spain.*
Sulfur (p.1123·3); dexpanthenol (p.1602·3); hexachlorophene (p.1146·1); hydrocortisone acetate (p.1073·3); placenta extract; basic zinc carbonate (p.1128·2).
Acne.

Neo Vitalisan *Zeller, Port.†.*
Ginseng (p.1615·3).
Tonic.

Neo Zeta-Foot *Zeta, Ital.†.*
Cream: Usnic acid (p.1678·2); salicylic acid (p.1122·3); undecenoic acid (p.395·3); aluminium acetate (p.1578·1).
Topical powder: Usnic acid (p.1678·2); undecenoic acid (p.395·3); aluminium oxide (p.1108·3); zinc stearate (p.1497·3); zinc oxide (p.1128·2); kaolin (p.1229·3); magnesium carbonate (p.1232·3); thyme oil (p.1672·3).
Foot infections.

Neo-Acarina *Upsifarma, Port.*
Benzyl benzoate (p.1428·2).
Pediculosis.

Neo-Alcos-Anal *Will-Pharma, Belg.*
Sodium oleate (p.1497·1); lauromacrogol 400 (p.1345·2).
Haemorrhoids.

Neo-Ampiplus *Menarini, Ital.*
Amoxicillin trihydrate (p.149·2).
Bacterial infections.

Neo-Angin
Note.This name is used for preparations of different composition.
Klosterfrau, Aust.
Gargle: Hexetidine (p.1146·3); anise oil (p.1580·3); clove oil (p.1597·1); peppermint oil (p.1243·3).
Pastilles: Dichlorobenzyl alcohol (p.1143·2); amylmetacresol (p.1133·2); anise oil (p.1580·3); peppermint oil (p.1243·3); menthol (p.1632·3).
Mouth and throat disorders.

Divapharma, Ger.†.
Hexetidine (p.1146·3); benzalkonium chloride (p.1133·2).
Mouth and throat infection and inflammation.

Neo-Angin au miel et citron *Doetsch, Grether, Switz.*
Dichlorobenzyl alcohol (p.1143·2); amylmetacresol (p.1133·2); honey (p.1366·2); lemon oil (p.1628·2); mint oil (p.1636·2).
Sore throat.

Neo-Angin avec vitamin C exempt de sucre
Doetsch, Grether, Switz.
Dichlorobenzyl alcohol (p.1143·2); amylmetacresol (p.1133·2); menthol (p.1632·3); ascorbic acid (p.1389·3).
Sore throat.

Neo-Angin exempt de sucre *Doetsch, Grether, Switz.*
Dichlorobenzyl alcohol (p.1143·2); amylmetacresol (p.1133·2); menthol (p.1632·3); anethole (p.1580·1); mint oil (p.1636·2); rectified camphor oil.
Sore throat.

Neo-Angin Lido *Doetsch, Grether, Switz.*
Cetylpyridinium chloride (p.1138·1); lignocaine [lidocaine] hydrochloride (p.1313·2); menthol (p.1632·3).
Mouth and throat disorders.

Neo-Angin N *Divapharma, Ger.*
Dichlorobenzyl alcohol (p.1143·2); menthol (p.1632·3); amylmetacresol (p.1133·2).
Mouth and throat disorders.

Neo-Audiocort *Teofarma, Ital.*
Triamcinolone acetonide hemisuccinate (p.1080·2); neomycin sulfate (p.228·1).
Ear disorders.

Neobac *Dermapharm, Ger.*
Neomycin sulfate (p.228·1); bacitracin (p.155·2).
Burns; fungal skin and nose infections; wounds.

Neobacigrin *Grin, Mex.*
Polymyxin B sulfate (p.238·1); neomycin sulfate (p.228·1); dexamethasone sodium phosphate (p.1067·1).
Infected eye disorders.

Neobacitracine *Erfa, Belg.*
Bacitracin (p.155·2); neomycin sulfate (p.228·1).
Bacterial infections.

Neo-Ballistol *Klever, Ger.*
Capsules: Potassium oleate; peppermint oil (p.1243·3); anise oil (p.1580·3); caraway oil (p.1591·2).
Oral liquid: Potassium oleate; ammonium oleate; peppermint oil (p.1243·3); anise oil (p.1580·3).
Gastrointestinal disorders.

Neobar *Merck, Braz.*
Barium sulfate (p.1032·1).
Contrast medium for gastrointestinal radiography.

Neobes *Medix, Mex.*
Diethylpropion hydrochloride (p.1508·2).
Obesity.

Neo-Bex *Neolab, Canad.*
Vitamin B substances (p.1350·1).

Neo-Bex Forte *Neolab, Canad.*
Vitamin B substances with ascorbic acid and zinc (p.1350·1).

Neobiphyllin *Trommsdorff, Ger.†.*
Diprophylline (p.764·1); proxyphylline (p.770·1); theophylline (p.777·2).
Cor pulmonale; obstructive airways disease.

Neo-Biphyllin *Zyma, Switz.†.*
Diprophylline (p.764·1); proxyphylline (p.770·1); theophylline (p.777·2).
Obstructive airways disease.

Neobiphyllin-Clys *Trommsdorff, Ger.†.*
Diprophylline (p.764·1); proxyphylline (p.770·1); theophylline (p.777·2).
Obstructive airways disease.

Neobloc *Unipharm, Israel.*
Metoprolol tartrate (p.931·2).
Angina pectoris; hypertension; migraine; myocardial infarction; reduction of paroxysmal tachycardia before cardiac catheterisation.

Neo-Boldolaxine *GNR, Fr.†.*
Senna (p.1248·2); docusate sodium (p.1223·1); boldo (p.1585·3).
Formerly contained bisacodyl, docusate sodium, boldo, aloin, and belladonna.
Constipation.

Neobonsen *Duopharm, Ger.*
Evening primrose oil (p.1613·2).
Eczema.

Neobradoral *Novartis Consumer, Port.*
Domiphen bromide (p.1143·3).
Mouth and throat infections.

Neobron *Pfizer, Switz.*
Multivitamin and mineral preparation (p.1350·1).

neo-bronchol *Divapharma, Ger.*
Ambroxol hydrochloride (p.1084·3).
Respiratory-tract disorders associated with increased or viscous mucus.

Neobros *Fidia, Ital.*
Phosphatidyl serine (p.1651·1); vitamin E (p.1350·1).
Mental function disorders.

Neobros 10 *Fidia, Ital.*
Phosphatidyl serine (p.1651·1); vitamins; minerals (p.1350·1).
Mental function disorders.

Neobrufen *Knoll, Austral.*
Ibuprofen (p.43·2).
Fever; musculoskeletal, joint, and peri-articular disorders; pain.

Neo-Bucosin *Synpharma, Switz.*
Dequalinium chloride (p.1143·1); lignocaine [lidocaine] hydrochloride (p.1313·2).
Mouth and throat disorders.

Neo-C *GNLD, Austral.*
Ascorbic acid (p.1389·3); Neo-Plex Concentrate (dried whole citrus juice; flavedo; mesocarp; endocarp; citrus protopectin; flavonoid complex); rutoside; hesperidin; lemon bioflavonoid complex.
Vitamin C deficiency.

Neocaina *Cristalia, Braz.*
Bupivacaine hydrochloride (p.1306·3).
Local anaesthesia.

Neo-Calglucon *Novartis, USA†.*
Calcium glubionate (p.1188·1).
Calcium deficiency; inadequate dietary calcium intake.

Neocapil *Spirig, Switz.*
Minoxidil (p.934·2).
Androgenic alopecia.

Neocate
Scientific Hospital Supplies, Austral.; Nutricia, Fin.; SHS, Fr.; Scientific Hospital Supplies, Irl.; Nutricia, Ital.; Nutricia, NZ; Scientific Hospital Supplies, NZ; Nutricia, Port.; SHS, Singapore; Scientific Hospital Supplies, UK.
Infant feed (p.1350·1).
Cow's milk allergy; gastrointestinal disorders; malabsorption; protein intolerance.

Neocate One + *SHS, USA.*
Preparation for enteral nutrition (p.1350·1).

Neocef *Atral, Port.*
Cefixime (p.166·2).
Bacterial infections.

Neocefal *Metapharma, Ital.*
Cefamandole nafate sodium (p.163·3).
Lignocaine [lidocaine] (p.1313·2) is included in this preparation to alleviate the pain of injection.
Bacterial infections.

Neocepacilina *CEPA, Spain†.*
Benzylpenicillin sodium (p.157·2); procaine penicillin [procaine benzylpenicillin] (p.239·2); benzathine benzylpenicillin (p.156·2).
Bacterial infections; rheumatic fever.

NeoCeuticals Clear Skin *Nuova ICT, Ital.*
Salicylic acid (p.1122·3); acetyl mandelic acid (p.221·2).
Acne.

Neoceuticals Clear Skin Solution *Hamilton, Austral.*
Salicylic acid (p.1122·3); alpha hydroxy acids.
Oily skin.

Neoceuticals PDS *Hamilton, Austral.*
Emollient.
Barrier cream; dry skin.

NeoCeuticals Spot Treatment *Nuova ICT, Ital.*
Glycolic acid (p.1115·1); acetyl mandelic acid (p.221·2); vitamin A (p.1382·1).
Acne.

Neoceuticals Therapeutic Shampoo *Hamilton, Austral.*
Piroctone olamine (p.1121·1).
Dandruff.

Neochinosol *Chinosolfabrik, Ger.*
Ethacridine lactate (p.1130·3).
Mouth and throat disorders.

Neocibalena *Novartis Consumer, Spain.*
Aspirin (p.14·2); caffeine (p.761·3); paracetamol (p.71·2).
Fever; pain.

Neo-Cibalgin *Novartis Consumer, Switz.*
Aspirin (p.14·2); paracetamol (p.71·2); caffeine (p.761·3).
Fever; pain.

Neo-Cibalgina *Zyma, Ital.; Novartis Consumer, Ital.*
Aspirin (p.14·2); paracetamol (p.71·2); caffeine (p.761·3).
Fever; pain.

Neociclina *Upsifarma, Port.*
Tetracycline hydrochloride (p.258·3).
Bacterial infections.

Neociclina Vitaminada *Upsifarma, Port.*
Tetracycline hydrochloride (p.258·3); vitamin B substances (p.1350·1).
Bacterial infections.

Neo-Cimexon *Cimex, Switz.*
Multivitamin and mineral preparation (p.1350·1).

Neo-Cimexon G *Cimex, Switz.*
Multivitamin and mineral preparation with ginseng (p.1350·1).

Neocin
Note. This name is used for preparations of different composition.
Fischer, Israel.
Neomycin sulfate (p.228·1).
Bacterial eye infections.

Ocusoft, USA.
Polymyxin B (p.238·3); neomycin (p.228·1); bacitracin (p.155·2).
Bacterial eye infections.

Neocinolon *Teuto, Braz.*
Neomycin sulfate (p.228·1); fluocinolone acetonide (p.1071·1).
Infected skin disorders.

Neocitran *Novartis Sante, Fr.†.*
Note. A similar name is used for preparations of different composition (see below).
Paracetamol (p.71·2); pseudoephedrine hydrochloride (p.1099·2).
Rhinitis.

NeoCitran *Sandoz, Ger.†.*
Note. A similar name is used for preparations of different composition (see above).
Paracetamol (p.71·2).
Fever; pain.

Neoclarityn *Schering-Plough, UK.*
Desloratadine (p.415·2).
Allergic rhinitis; urticaria.

Neo-Cleanse *GNLD, Austral.*
Senna leaf (p.1248·2); buckthorn bark (p.1215·1); liquorice root (p.1231·2); prune (p.1245·1); alfalfa leaf (p.1574·3); rhubarb root (p.1248·1); leptandra virginica root; blue malva flowers; asparagus; aniseed (p.1580·2).
Constipation.

Neoclym *Searle, Ital.*
Cyclofenil (p.1467·2).
Anovulatory infertility; menopausal disorders; menstrual disorders.

Neo-Codion
Note. This name is used for preparations of different composition.
Therabel, Belg.
Codeine camsilate (p.26·1); sulfogaiacol (p.1101·1).
Formerly contained codeine camsilate, ethylmorphine camsilate, and sulfogaiacol.
Coughs.

Bouchara, Fr.
Infant syrup: Sodium benzoate (p.1134·3); grindelia (p.1618·2); senega (p.1100·2).
Respiratory-tract congestion.
Paediatric syrup: Codeine camsilate (p.26·1); sodium benzoate (p.1134·3).
Coughs.
Suppositories; paediatric suppositories: Codeine camsilate (p.26·1); eucalyptol (p.1609·2).
Coughs.
Syrup: Codeine camsilate (p.26·1).
Coughs.
Tablets: Codeine camsilate (p.26·1); sulfogaiacol (p.1101·1); grindelia (p.1618·2).
Coughs.

Neo-Codion N *Bouchara, Switz.*
Syrup: Codeine camsilate (p.26·1); ascorbic acid (p.1389·3); ipecacuanha (p.1093·1); tolu balsam (p.1101·3).
Tablets: Codeine camsilate (p.26·1); sulfogaiacol (p.1101·1); grindelia (p.1618·2).
Coughs.

Neo-Codion NN *Fatol, Ger.*
Codeine camsilate (p.26·1).
Coughs.

Neocof *Masa, Thai.*
Codeine phosphate (p.25·2); guaifenesin (p.1092·2).
Coughs.

Neocolan *Seid, Spain.*
Dicyclomine [dicycloverine] hydrochloride (p.466·1); metochalcone (p.1635·3); procaine hydrochloride (p.1319·1).
Hepatobiliary disorders.

Neocon *Janssen-Cilag, Neth.*
Norethisterone (p.1485·1); ethinylestradiol (p.1476·2).
Combined oral contraceptive.

Neocones
Note. This name is used for preparations of different composition.
Austrodent, Aust.; Prats, Spain.
Amethocaine [tetracaine] hydrochloride (p.1305·2); neomycin (p.228·1) or neomycin sulfate (p.228·1); polymyxin B sulfate (p.238·1); tyrothricin (p.267·1).
Temporary dental filling.

Septodont, Switz.
Neomycin sulfate (p.228·1); benzocaine (p.1306·2).
Formerly contained amethocaine [tetracaine] hydrochloride, neomycin sulfate, polymyxin B sulfate, and tyrothricin.
Dental disorders.

Neocontrast *Bama, Spain†.*
Iopanoic acid (p.1035·2).
Contrast medium for biliary-tract radiography.

Neo-Cortef
Pharmacia Upjohn, Canad.; Pharmacia Upjohn, Irl.; Dominion, UK; Upjohn, USA†.
Hydrocortisone (p.1073·3) or hydrocortisone acetate (p.1073·3); neomycin sulfate (p.228·1).
Infected skin, eye, or ear disorders.

Neocortin *Llorens, Spain.*
Dexamethasone phosphate (p.1067·1); neomycin sulfate (p.228·1).
Infected eye and ear disorders.

Neo-Cortofen *Ripari-Gero, Ital.*
Dexamethasone (p.1067·1); neomycin sulfate (p.228·1).
Eczema; nasal mucosal inflammation; rhinitis.

Neo-Cranimal *Dagra, Neth.†.*
Ergotamine tartrate (p.452·1); caffeine monohydrate (p.761·3); meclozine hydrochloride (p.420·3).
Migraine and other vascular headaches.

Neo-Cratylen *Madaus, Aust.†; Madaus, Ger.†.*
Crataegus (p.1600·2).
Cardiac disorders.

Neo-Cromaton Bicomplesso *Menarini, Ital.*
Vitamin B substances (p.1350·1).
Deficiency states; macrocytic anaemias.

Neo-Cultol *Fisons, USA†.*
Liquid paraffin (p.1407·1).
Constipation.

Neo-Cutigenol *Centrapharm, Belg.*
Chlorhexidine acetate (p.1138·2); vitamin A palmitate (p.1383·2).
Formerly contained hydroxyquinoline sulfate, vitamin A palmitate, titanium dioxide, zinc oxide, and cod-liver oil.
Burns; skin disorders; wounds.

Neo-Cytamen *Pentaderm, Ital.*
Azelaic acid (p.1110·3); jaluramina.
Acne; seborrhoea.

Neo-Cytamen
DBL, Austral.; Medeva, Irl.; Teofarma, Ital.; Glaxo Wellcome, NZ; Celltech, UK.
Hydroxocobalamin (p.1388·1).
Leber's optic atrophy; macrocytic anaemias; tobacco amblyopia.

Neo-Dagracycline *Asta Medica, Neth.*
Doxycycline fosfatex (p.200·1).
Bacterial infections.

Neo-Davisolona *Davi, Port.*
Neomycin sulfate (p.228·1); prednisolone metasulfobenzoate sodium (p.1078·1).
Infected eye disorders.

Neo-Debiol AD3 *Meuse, Belg.*
Vitamin A acetate (p.1383·2); colecalciferol (p.1391·1).
Vitamin A and D deficiency.

Neo-Deca *Beacons, Singapore.*
Dexamethasone sodium phosphate (p.1067·1); neomycin sulfate (p.228·1).
Allergic and inflammatory eye disorders.

NeoDecadron *Merck Sharp & Dohme, Canad.†; Merck, USA.*
Dexamethasone sodium phosphate (p.1067·1); neomycin sulfate (p.228·1).
Inflammatory eye, ear, or skin disorders with bacterial infection.

Neo-Decongestine *Sanopharm, Switz.*
Kaolin (p.1229·3); glycerol (p.1616·3); guaiacol salicylate; methyl salicylate (p.55·1).
Soft-tissue disorders.

Neo-Delphicort *Wyeth Lederle, Aust.*
Triamcinolone acetonide (p.1080·1); neomycin sulfate (p.228·1).
Ear or eye infection and inflammation.

Neo-Dentocain *Taro, Israel.*
Phenylephrine hydrochloride (p.1097·1); benzocaine (p.1306·2); menthol (p.1632·3).
Gingivitis; local anaesthesia; stomatitis.

Neoderm
Note. This name is used for preparations of different composition.
Desbergers, Canad.
Zinc oxide (p.1128·2); zinc peroxide (p.1159·3).
Minor abrasions, wounds, and burns.

Propan, S.Afr.
Hydrocortisone acetate (p.1073·3); neomycin sulfate (p.228·1).
Skin disorders.

Tai Guk, Singapore.
Betamethasone dipropionate (p.1063·2); clotrimazole (p.382·1); gentamicin sulfate (p.210·1).
Infected skin disorders.

Neoderm Ginecologico *Crosara, Ital.†.*
Fluocinolone acetonide (p.1071·1).
Vulvovaginitis.

Neodesfila *Kin, Spain.*
Cresol (p.1142·3); eugenol (p.1609·3); hydroxyquinoline sulfate (p.1622·2); lignocaine [lidocaine] hydrochloride (p.1313·2).
Toothache.

Neo-Desogen *Rusch, Ital.*
Benzalkonium chloride (p.1133·2).
Instrument disinfection; skin, burn, and wound disinfection.

Neo-Destomygen *Stomygen, Ital.*
Chlorhexidine gluconate (p.1138·2).
Oral hygiene.

Neo-Dex (Improved)
Jean-Marie, Hong Kong; Jean-Marie, Singapore.
Dexamethasone (p.1067·1); chloramphenicol (p.179·1).
Inflammatory eye infections.

Neodexa *Llorens, Spain.*
Dexamethasone phosphate (p.1067·1); neomycin sulfate (p.228·1).
Infected eye disorders.

Neo-Dexair *Bausch & Lomb, USA†.*
Dexamethasone sodium phosphate (p.1067·1); neomycin sulfate (p.228·1).
Eye inflammation with bacterial infection.

Neo-Dexameth *Major, USA.*
Dexamethasone sodium phosphate (p.1067·1); neomycin sulfate (p.228·1).
Eye inflammation with bacterial infection.

Neodexasone *Medical Ophthalmics, USA.*
Dexamethasone phosphate (p.1067·1); neomycin (p.228·1).
Infected eye disorders.

Neodexon *Bournonville, Belg.†.*
Dexamethasone sodium phosphate (p.1067·1); neomycin sulfate (p.228·1).
Infected inflammatory eye disorders.

Neodextril 40 *Fresenius Kabi, Port.*
Dextran 40 (p.728·3) in glucose or sodium chloride.
Plasma volume expansion; thromboembolism prophylaxis.

Neodextril 70 *Fresenius Kabi, Port.*
Dextran 70 (p.729·2) in glucose or sodium chloride.
Plasma volume expansion; thromboembolism prophylaxis.

Neo-Diaral *Roberts, USA.*
Loperamide (p.1232·1).
Diarrhoea.

Neo-Diophen *Hamilton, Austral.*
Mepyramine maleate (p.421·1); phenylpropanolamine hydrochloride (p.1098·1); dextromethorphan hydrobromide (p.1087·3); atropine sulfate (p.461·1).
Asthma; bronchitis; coughs and cold symptoms; hay fever.

Neodol *Diba, Mex.*
Paracetamol (p.71·2).
Fever; pain.

Neodolito *Diba, Mex.*
Paracetamol (p.71·2).
Fever; pain.

Neodolpasse *Fresenius Kabi, Aust.*
Diclofenac sodium (p.30·3); orphenadrine citrate (p.470·2).
Inflammation; musculoskeletal and joint disorders; pain.

Neodone *Biochem, Ital.*
Paracetamol (p.71·2); aspirin (p.14·2); caffeine (p.761·3).
Fever; pain.

Neodorm SP *Knoll, Ger.†.*
Temazepam (p.707·2).
Sleep disorders.

Neodox *Rosen, Ger.*
Doxycycline hyclate (p.200·1).
Bacterial infections.

Neoduplamox *Procter & Gamble, Ital.*
Amoxicillin trihydrate (p.149·2); potassium clavulanate (p.187·2).
Bacterial infections.

Neo-Durabolic *Hauck, USA.*
Nandrolone decanoate (p.1484·2).
Anaemia in renal disease.

Neodyn *Sepharma, Ital.*
Sachets: Vitamin, mineral, and carbohydrate preparation with creatine (p.1350·1).
Tablets†: Carbohydrate, amino-acid, and fatty-acid preparation with creatine (p.1350·1).
Nutritional supplement.

Neo-Emedyl *Montavit, Aust.*
Dimenhydrinate (p.415·2); caffeine (p.761·3).
Motion sickness; nausea and vomiting; vestibular disorders.

Neo-Emocicatrol *Bouty, Ital.*
Tannic acid (p.1669·1); benzalkonium chloride (p.1133·2).

Neo-Emoform *Byk Gulden, Ital.*
Sodium monofluorophosphate (p.1377·2).
Gingivitis; oral hygiene.

Neo-Eparbiol *Ecobi, Ital.*
Inosine (p.1623·3); cyanocobalamin (p.1388·1).
Anaemias; tonic.

Neo-Eunomin *Grunenthal, Ger.*
Ethinylestradiol (p.1476·2); chlormadinone acetate (p.1465·3).
Acne; alopecia; biphasic oral contraceptive; hirsutism; seborrhoea.

Neo-Eunomine *Janssen-Cilag, Switz.*
Ethinylestradiol (p.1476·2); chlormadinone acetate (p.1465·3).
Biphasic oral contraceptive.

Neofarmotox *Brasmedica, Braz.*
Xanthine; methionine (p.1012·2); choline (p.1356·3).
Liver disorders.

Neofazol *Rubio, Spain.*
Cefazolin sodium (p.164·3).
Lignocaine [lidocaine] hydrochloride (p.1313·2) is included in this preparation to alleviate the pain of injection.
Bacterial infections.

Neofed *Propan, S.Afr.*
Triprolidine hydrochloride (p.427·2); pseudoephedrine hydrochloride (p.1099·2); guaifenesin (p.1092·2); codeine phosphate (p.25·2).
Coughs.

Neofenox *Boots Healthcare, Belg.*
Phenylephrine hydrochloride (p.1097·1); dichlorobenzyl alcohol (p.1143·2); naphazoline nitrate (p.1095·1).
Adjuvant in sinusitis; nasal congestion.

Neo-Fepramol *Istoria, Ital.*
Paracetamol (p.71·2).
Fever; pain.

Neo-Fer
Neolab, Canad.; Nycomed, Norw.
Ferrous fumarate (p.1360·1).
Iron deficiency; iron-deficiency anaemia.

Neoflogin *Neo Quimica, Braz.*
Benzydamine hydrochloride (p.20·1).
Fever; inflammation; pain.

Neofomiral *Silanes, Mex.*
Fluconazole (p.383·2).
Fungal infections.

Neo-fradin *Pharma Tek, USA.*
Neomycin sulfate (p.228·1).

Neofrin *Ocusoft, USA.*
Phenylephrine hydrochloride (p.1097·1).

Neofulvin *Chew, Thai.*
Griseofulvin (p.386·2).
Fungal infections.

Neo-Furadantin *Formenti, Ital.*
Nitrofurantoin (p.230·3).
Bacterial infections of the genito-urinary tract.

Neofyllin *Abigo, Denm.†.*
Proxyphylline (p.770·1).
Obstructive airways disease.

neogama *Hormosan, Ger.*
Sulpiride (p.706·1).
Psychiatric disorders; vestibular disorders.

neogama D novo *Hormosan, Ger.*
Sulpiride (p.706·1).
Depression.

Neogel *Masa, Thai.*
Piroxicam (p.79·1).
Musculoskeletal and joint disorders.

Neogentrol *Wyeth Lederle, Denm.*
Ethinylestradiol (p.1476·2); levonorgestrel (p.1486·2).
Combined oral contraceptive.

Neogest *Schering, UK.*
Norgestrel (p.1486·1).
Progestogen-only oral contraceptive.

Neo-Geynevral *Geymonat, Ital.*
Thiamine diphosphate hydrochloride; pyridoxine hydrochloride (p.1386·3); cyanocobalamin (p.1388·1).
Neuritis.

Neo-Gilurythmal *Giulini, Israel.*
Prajmalium bitartrate (p.957·2).
Arrythmias.

Neo-Gilurytmal
Solvay, Aust.; Solvay, Ger.; Lacer, Spain.
Prajmalium bitartrate (p.957·2).
Arrhythmias.

Neogluconin *Sanochemia, Aust.*
Glibenclamide (p.321·3).
Diabetes mellitus.

Neogobion *Pharos, Singapore.*
Ferrous gluconate (p.1360·1); manganese sulfate (p.1371·3); folic acid (p.1361·1); copper sulfate (p.1358·1); vitamin B₁₂ (p.1388·1).
Vitamin C (p.1389·3) is included in this preparation to increase the absorption and availability of iron.
Anaemias.

Neo-Golaseptine *SMB, Belg.*
Chlorhexidine (p.1138·2); benzethonium chloride (p.1134·2).
Mouth and throat disorders.

Neogram *SIFI, Ital.*
Neomycin sulfate (p.228·1); gramicidin (p.213·3).
Eye infections.

Neogynon
Schering, Aust.; Schering, Belg.; Schering, Denm.; Schering, Ger.; Schering, Hong Kong; Schering, Israel; Schering, Mex.; Schering, Neth.; Schering, Switz.
Levonorgestrel (p.1486·2); ethinylestradiol (p.1476·2).
28-Day packs contain 7 inert tablets.
Combined oral contraceptive; endometriosis; menstrual disorders.

Neogynona *Schering, Spain.*
Levonorgestrel (p.1486·2); ethinylestradiol (p.1476·2).
Combined oral contraceptive; menstrual disorders.

Neo-Heparbil *Montefarmaco, Ital.†.*
Fencibutirol (p.1610·1); frangula (p.1227·1); rhubarb (p.1248·1); cascara sagrada (p.1216·1); belladonna (p.463·1).
Constipation.

Neo-Hesna *Takeda, Thai.*
Carbazochrome sodium sulfonate (p.728·1).
Haemorrhagic disorders.

Neohexal *Riedel-Zabinka, Braz.*
Methenamine (p.223·1).
Bacterial urinary-tract infections.

Neo-Hydro *Streuli, Switz.*
Hydrocortisone acetate (p.1073·3); neomycin sulfate (p.228·1).
Inflammation and infection of the eye, nose, or ear.

Neo-Hytisone *Atlantic, Thai.*
Neomycin sulfate (p.228·1); hydrocortisone acetate (p.1073·3).
Bacterial skin infections.

Neo-Intol *Carlo Erba OTC, Ital.†.*
Cetrimonium tosilate (p.1137·3).
External genital disinfection.

Neoiodarsolo *Baldacci, Ital.*
Amino-acid preparation with vitamin B substances (p.1350·1).
Tonic.

Neokratin *Laevosan, Aust.; Fresenius Kabi, Aust.*
Paracetamol (p.71·2); propyphenazone (p.80·2); caffeine (p.761·3).
Fever; pain.

Neo-Lapitrypsin *Truw, Ger.†.*
Oleum pini sylvestris; pumilio pine oil (p.1656·3); melissa oil; spike lavender oil (p.1667·1); juniper oil (p.1625·2); fennel oil (p.1610·2); peppermint oil (p.1243·3).
Biliary disorders; gallstones; renal calculi.

Neo-Laryngobis *Technilab, Canad.*
Bismuth dipropylacetate (p.1214·1).
Sore throat.

Neo-Lidocaton
Weimer, Ger.†
Lignocaine [lidocaine] hydrochloride (p.1313·2).
Lypressin (p.1300·1) and noradrenaline [norepinephrine] (p.948·2) are included in this preparation as vasoconstrictors to diminish absorption and localise the effect of the local anaesthetic.
Local anaesthesia.

Weimer, Thai.
Lignocaine [lidocaine] hydrochloride (p.1313·2).
Vasopressin (p.1300·1) and noradrenaline [norepinephrine] (p.948·2) are included in this preparation as vasoconstrictors to diminish absorption and localise the effect of the local anaesthetic.
Local anaesthesia.

Neoloid
Bradley, Canad.; Kenwood, USA.
Castor oil (p.1592·1).
Bowel evacuation; constipation; diarrhoea.

Neo-Lotan *Neopharmed, Ital.*
Losartan potassium (p.921·3).
Hypertension.

Neo-Lotan Plus *Neopharmed, Ital.*
Losartan potassium (p.921·3); hydrochlorothiazide (p.907·3).
Hypertension.

Neomedil *Farmec, Ital.*
Benzalkonium chloride (p.1133·2); alcohol (p.1130·3).
Skin and wound disinfection.

Neo-Medrol
Note.This name is used for preparations of different composition.
Pharmacia Upjohn, Austral.; Pharmacia Upjohn, Israel; Pharmacia Upjohn, S.Afr.
Methylprednisolone acetate (p.1076·1); neomycin sulfate (p.228·1); aluminium chlorohydrate (p.1110·2); sulfur (p.1123·3).
Acne.

Pharmacia Upjohn, Singapore; Pharmacia Upjohn, Thai.
Methylprednisolone acetate (p.1076·1); neomycin sulfate (p.228·1); alcloxa (p.1109·3); sulfur (p.1123·3).
Acne; rosacea; seborrhoeic dermatitis.

Neo-Medrol Acne
Pharmacia Upjohn, Canad.; Pharmacia Upjohn, Hong Kong.
Methylprednisolone acetate (p.1076·1); neomycin sulfate (p.228·1); aluminium chlorohydrate (p.1110·2); colloidal sulfur (p.1123·3).
Acne; seborrhoeic dermatitis.

Neo-Medrol comp *Pharmacia Upjohn, Fin.*
Methylprednisolone acetate (p.1076·1); neomycin sulfate (p.228·1); aluminium chlorohydrate (p.1110·2); sulfur (p.1123·3).
Acne.

Neo-Medrol Veriderm
Pharmacia Upjohn, Canad.; Pharmacia Upjohn, Ital.
Methylprednisolone acetate (p.1076·1); neomycin sulfate (p.228·1).
Infected skin disorders.

Neo-Medrone *Pharmacia Upjohn, Irl.†.*
Cream: Methylprednisolone acetate (p.1076·1); neomycin sulfate (p.228·1).
Inflamed skin infections.

Topical lotion: Methylprednisolone acetate (p.1076·1); neomycin sulfate (p.228·1); aluminium chlorohydrate (p.1110·2); sulfur (p.1123·3).
Acne; rosacea; infected dermatitis.

Neo-Melubrina *Hoechst Marion Roussel, Mex.*
Dipyrone (p.34·1).
Fever; pain.

Neo-Mercazole
Roche, Austral.; Roche, Denm.; Nicholas, Fr.; Roche, Hong Kong; Roche, Irl.; Roche, Norw.; Roche, NZ; Aspen, S.Afr.; Roche, Singapore; Roche, Switz.; Roche, UK.
Carbimazole (p.1521·1).
Hyperthyroidism.

Neomercurochromo *SIT, Ital.*
Ointment; topical powder: Chlorhexidine gluconate (p.1138·2).
Wound disinfection.

Topical solution: Chloroxylenol (p.1142·1).
Skin disinfection.

Neomeritine *Janssen-Cilag, Belg.†.*
Ambucetamide hydrochloride (p.1578·3); aspirin (p.14·2); paracetamol (p.71·2); codeine phosphate (p.25·2); caffeine (p.761·3).
Gynaecological pain.

Neo-Meton *Jean-Marie, Singapore.*
Brompheniramine maleate (p.410·2).
Hypersensitivity reactions.

Neomicina Composta *Uniao Quimica, Braz.*
Neomycin (p.228·1); tyrothricin (p.267·1).
Mouth and throat infections.

Neomicol *Medix, Mex.*
Miconazole nitrate (p.391·1).
Fungal infections.

Neo-Mindol *Bracco, Ital.†.*
Ibuprofen (p.43·2).
Pain.

Neo-Minophagen C *Minophagen, Jpn†.*
Ammonium glycyrrhizinate (p.1085·2).
Liver disorders; skin disorders; stomatitis.

Neomite *M & H, Thai.*
Miconazole nitrate (p.391·1).
Fungal skin infections.

Neomixen *Pisa, Mex.*
Neomycin (p.228·1).

Neomixin *Hauck, USA†.*
Polymyxin B sulfate (p.238·1); neomycin sulfate (p.228·1); bacitracin (p.155·2).
Bacterial skin infections.

Neomonovar *Wyeth Lederle, Port.*
Levonorgestrel (p.1486·2); ethinylestradiol (p.1476·2).
Combined oral contraceptive.

Neo-Mune
Otsuka, Hong Kong; Thai Otsuka, Thai.
Preparation for enteral nutrition (p.1350·1).

Neo-Mydrial *Winzer, Ger.*
Phenylephrine hydrochloride (p.1097·1).
Formerly known as Mydrial.
Production of mydriasis.

Neomyrt Plus *Baif, Ital.*
Myrtillus (p.1639·2); fish-liver oil; centella (p.1112·2); selenium (p.1375·2).
Nutritional supplement.

Neo-NaClex
Glaxo Wellcome, NZ; Goldshield, UK.
Bendrofluazide [bendroflumethiazide] (p.844·1).
Hypertension; oedema.

Neo-NaClex-K *Goldshield, UK.*
Bendrofluazide [bendroflumethiazide] (p.844·1); potassium chloride (p.1194·3).
Hypertension; oedema.

Neonaxil *Galen, Mex.*
Naproxen (p.60·3).
Gout; musculoskeletal, joint, and peri-articular disorders; pain.

Neo-Nevral *Hoechst Marion Roussel, Ital.*
Paracetamol (p.71·2); aspirin (p.14·2); caffeine (p.761·3).
Fever; pain.

Neoniagar *Sintesa, Belg.†.*
Mebutizide (p.925·3).
Hypertension; oedema.

Neo-Optal *Olan-Kemed, Thai.*
Dexamethasone sodium phosphate (p.1067·1); neomycin sulfate (p.228·1).
Infected eye and ear disorders.

Neo-Optalidon *Novartis Consumer, Ital.*
Paracetamol (p.71·2); propyphenazone (p.80·2); caffeine (p.761·3).
Fever; pain.

NeoOstrogynal *Asche, Ger.*
Estradiol valerate (p.1473·2); estriol (p.1475·3).
Menopausal disorders; oestrogenic.

Neopan *Propan, S.Afr.*
Neomycin sulfate (p.228·1); sodium propionate (p.393·2).
Ear infections.

Neo-Panlacticos *Italmex, Mex.*
Lactic-acid-producing organisms (p.1626·3); vitamin B substances (p.1350·1).
Restoration of normal gastrointestinal flora.

Neo-Panlacticos Plus *Italmex, Mex.*
Lactic-acid-producing organisms (p.1626·3); vitamin B substances (p.1350·1); dimethicone (p.1249·2).
Flatulence; restoration of normal gastrointestinal flora.

Neopap *PolyMedica, USA.*
Paracetamol (p.71·2).
Fever; pain.

Neoparyl Framycetine *Ciba Vision, Fr.†.*
Phenylephrine and meglumine heparinate; framycetin sulfate (p.208·2).
Eye infections and burns.

Neopec *Propan, S.Afr.†.*
Kaolin (p.1229·3); pectin (p.1502·3); neomycin sulfate (p.228·1).
Diarrhoea.

Neopect *Masa, Thai.*
Codeine phosphate (p.25·2); guaifenesin (p.1092·2); phenylpropanolamine hydrochloride (p.1098·1).
Cold symptoms; coughs; nasal congestion.

Neopelle *Also, Ital.*
Collagen (p.1598·2).
Wound dressing.

Neopenyl *Grunenthal, Spain.*
Benzylpenicillin sodium (p.157·2); clemizole penicillin (p.188·1).
Lignocaine [lidocaine] hydrochloride (p.1313·2) is included in this preparation to alleviate the pain of injection.
Bacterial infections.

Neo-Pergonal *Serono, Fr.†.*
Menotrophin (p.1288·2).
Male and female infertility.

Neopermease *Novartis, Aust.*
Hyaluronidase (p.1620·3).
Adjunct with chemotherapy for malignant neoplasms.

Neophedan *Intramed, S.Afr.*
Tamoxifen citrate (p.571·1).
Breast cancer.

Neo-Phlogicid *Sanochemia, Aust.*
Aluminium acetotartrate (p.1578·2); camphor (p.1589·3); methyl salicylate (p.55·1); salicylic acid (p.1122·3); menthol (p.1632·3); eucalyptus oil (p.1609·2).
Frostbite; inflammation; musculoskeletal and joint disorders; sciatica.

Neo-Planotest *Organon, UK.*
Pregnancy test (p.1654·3).

Neo-Planotest Duoclon *Organon Teknika, Austral.†.*
Pregnancy test (p.1654·3).

Neoplatin *Bristol-Myers, Spain.*
Cisplatin (p.525·1).
Malignant neoplasms.

Neoplex *Austroplant, Aust.*
Albumin tannate (p.1209·3); liquorice (p.1231·2); magnesium trisilicate (p.1233·3).
Gastrointestinal disorders.

Neoplus *Terapeutico, Ital.*
Royal jelly (p.1659·3); pollen; ginseng (p.1615·3).
Nutritional supplement.

Neopolydex *Medical Ophthalmics, USA.*
Dexamethasone (p.1067·1); neomycin (p.228·1); polymyxin B (p.238·3).
Infected eye disorders.

Neopons *Baxenden, UK.*
A range of alkyl sulfates.

Neopred *PD, Thai.*
Neomycin sulfate (p.228·1); prednisolone (p.1077·3).
Allergic and inflammatory skin disorders.

Neo-Pregnosticon *Organon Teknika, Austral.†.*
Pregnancy test (p.1654·3).

Neo-Preocil *Oftalder, Port.*
Fluorometholone (p.1072·1); neomycin (p.228·1).
Infected eye disorders.

Neoprex *Sigma-Tau, Ital.*
Enalapril maleate (p.883·3); hydrochlorothiazide (p.907·3).
Hypertension.

Neo-Primovlar *Schering, Fin.*
Levonorgestrel (p.1486·2); ethinylestradiol (p.1476·2).
Combined oral contraceptive.

Neoproct *Schering, Fin.*
Fluocortolone pivalate (p.1071·3); lignocaine [lidocaine] hydrochloride (p.1313·2).
Anorectal disorders.

Neo-Prunex *Neolab, Canad.†.*
Phenolphthalein (p.1244·1).
Constipation.

Neopulmonier *Quimica y Farmacia, Mex.*
Dextromethorphan hydrobromide (p.1087·3).
Coughs.

Neo-Pyodron *Cassella-med, Ger.*
Zinc oxide (p.1128·2); almasilate (p.1210·1); dequalinium chloride (p.1143·1).
Infected skin disorders; pyoderma.

Neo-Pyrazon *United American, Singapore.*
Diclofenac sodium (p.30·3).
Musculoskeletal and joint disorders; pain.

Neopyrin *Riemser, Ger.*
Paracetamol (p.71·2); caffeine (p.761·3).
Pain.

Neoral
Novartis, Austral.; Novartis, Canad.; Novartis, Fr.; Novartis, Irl.; Novartis, Neth.; Novartis, NZ; Novartis, Switz.; Novartis, UK; Novartis, USA.
Ciclosporin (p.518·1).
Atopic dermatitis; nephrotic syndrome; prevention of graft-versus-host disease; psoriasis; rheumatoid arthritis; transplant rejection; uveitis.

Neoral-Sandimmun *Novartis, Belg.*
Ciclosporin (p.518·1).
Auto-immune disorders; transplant rejection.

NeoRecormon
Boehringer Mannheim, Aust.; Roche, Belg.; Roche, Denm.; Roche, Fin.; Roche, Fr.; Roche, Ger.; Roche, Irl.; Roche, Ital.; Roche, Norw.; Roche, Port.; Roche, Spain; Roche, Swed.; Roche, UK.
Epoetin beta (p.731·1).
Formerly known as Recormon in Swed.
Anaemias; autologous blood transfusion.

NeoRespin *Murdock, USA†.*
Ephedrine hydrochloride (p.1090·1); guaifenesin (p.1092·2).

Neorgine *Cantabria, Spain†.*
Cinnarizine (p.413·1); co-dergocrine mesilate (p.1597·3).
Cerebrovascular disorders.

Neo-Rinoleina *Sanofi Synthelabo, Ital.*
Xylometazoline hydrochloride (p.1102·2).
Nasal congestion.

Neorlest
Parke, Davis, Aust.†; Parke, Davis, Ger.
Ethinylestradiol (p.1476·2); norethisterone acetate (p.1485·1).
Combined oral contraceptive.

Neo-Rowachol *Rowa Wagner, Hong Kong.*
Menthol (p.1632·3); menthone; α-pinene; β-pinene; borneol; camphene; eucalyptol (p.1609·2).
Biliary disorders; gallstones; liver disorders.

Neo-Rowatinex *Rowa Wagner, Hong Kong.*
Camphene; borneol; fenchone; eucalyptol (p.1609·2); α-pinene; β-pinene; anethole (p.1580·1).
Urinary-tract disorders.

Neorutin *Helvepharm, Switz.*
Rutoside (p.1611·2).
Venous insufficiency.

Neorythmin *Unipharm, Israel.*
Prajmalium bitartrate (p.957·2).
Arrythmias.

neos nitro OPT *Optimed, Ger.*
Glyceryl trinitrate (p.897·3).
Angina pectoris.

Neo-Sabenyl *Qualiphar, Belg.*
Clorophene (p.1142·3); trolamine laurilsulfate (p.1496·3).
Disinfection of skin, hands, mucous membranes, instruments, and materials; irrigation in ear, nose, and throat procedures; skin disorders; wound irrigation.

Neosaldina *Knoll, Braz.*
Dipyrone (p.34·1); isometheptene (p.1624·2); caffeine (p.761·3).
Smooth muscle spasm.

Neosar *Adria, USA.*
Cyclophosphamide (p.527·3).
Malignant neoplasms.

Neosayomol *Cinfa, Spain.*
Diphenhydramine hydrochloride (p.416·1).
Allergic skin reactions.

Neosec *Masa, Thai.*
Paracetamol (p.71·2); orphenadrine citrate (p.470·3).
Pain.

Neosed *Advance, Hong Kong.*
Salicylamide (p.82·1); phenylephrine hydrochloride (p.1097·1); paracetamol (p.71·2); caffeine (p.761·3); brompheniramine maleate (p.410·2).
Cold and influenza symptoms.

Neoseptil *Dinafarma, Braz.*
Bismuth subgallate (p.1213·2); zinc oxide (p.1128·2).
Barrier preparation; skin disorders.

Neosidantoina *Squibb, Spain.*
Phenytoin sodium (p.357·2).
Epilepsy.

Neo-Sinedol *Wild, Switz.*
Lignocaine [lidocaine] hydrochloride (p.1313·2); dehydrated alcohol (p.1130·3).
Local anaesthesia.

Neo-Sinefrina
Sanofi Winthrop, Braz.; Sterling, Port.
Phenylephrine (p.1097·1) or phenylephrine hydrochloride (p.1097·1).
Nasal congestion.

Neo-Soyal *Nutricia, Ital.*
Infant feed (p.1350·1).
Galactosaemia; milk intolerance.

Neosporin
Note.This name is used for preparations of different composition.
Glaxo Wellcome, Austral.; Glaxo Wellcome, Hong Kong; Glaxo Wellcome, Irl.; Glaxo Wellcome, Mex.; Glaxo Wellcome, Singapore; Wellcome, Thai.; Glaxo Wellcome, Thai.; Dominion, UK; Monarch, USA.
Eye drops: Neomycin sulfate (p.228·1); polymyxin B sulfate (p.238·1); gramicidin (p.213·3).
Bacterial eye infections.

Glaxo Wellcome, Austral.; Glaxo Wellcome, Canad.; Glaxo Wellcome, Hong Kong; Glaxo Wellcome, Mex.; Glaxo Wellcome, S.Afr.; Warner-Lambert, USA; Monarch, USA.
Ointment; eye ointment: Neomycin sulfate (p.228·1); polymyxin B sulfate (p.238·1); bacitracin (p.155·2) or bacitracin zinc (p.155·2).
Bacterial eye or skin infections.

Glaxo Wellcome, Canad.
Bladder irrigation: Neomycin sulfate (p.228·1); polymyxin B sulfate (p.238·1).
Bacterial urinary-tract infections.

Cream; eye and ear drops: Neomycin sulfate (p.228·1); polymyxin B sulfate (p.238·1); gramicidin (p.213·3).
Bacterial eye and ear infections; bacterial skin infections.

Glaxo Wellcome, USA†.
Cream: Neomycin sulfate (p.228·1); polymyxin B sulfate (p.238·1).
Skin infections.

Neosporin GU Glaxo Wellcome, USA.
Neomycin sulfate (p.228·1); polymyxin B sulfate (p.238·1).
Prevention of catheter-associated urinary-tract infections.

Neosporin + Pain Relief Warner-Lambert, USA.
Cream: Neomycin (p.228·1); polymyxin B sulfate (p.238·1); pramocaine hydrochloride (p.1318·2).
Ointment: Neomycin (p.228·1); polymyxin B sulfate (p.238·1); bacitracin zinc (p.155·2); pramocaine hydrochloride (p.1318·2).

Neosporin Plus Glaxo Wellcome, USA.
Cream: Neomycin (p.228·1); polymyxin B sulfate (p.238·1); lignocaine [lidocaine] (p.1313·2).
Ointment†: Neomycin (p.228·1); polymyxin B sulfate (p.238·1); lignocaine [lidocaine] (p.1313·2); bacitracin zinc (p.155·2).

Neo-Stediril
Wyeth Lederle, Aust.; Wyeth Lederle, Belg.; Wyeth, Ger.; Wyeth, Neth.; Wyeth, S.Afr.; Wyeth, Ger.
Levonorgestrel (p.1486·2); ethinylestradiol (p.1476·2).
Combined oral contraceptive.

Neostigmine Min-I-Mix IMS, USA.
Neostigmine metilsulfate (p.1420·1).
Atropine sulfate (p.461·1) is included in this preparation to protect against muscarinic actions.
Reversal of competitive neuromuscular blockade.

Neostig-Reu Reusch, Ger.
Neostigmine metilsulfate (p.1420·1).
Myasthenia gravis; reversal of competitive neuromuscular blockade.

Neostil Novartis Consumer, Port.
Dimetindene maleate (p.415·3).
Hypersensitivity reactions.

Neostix-N Bayer, Austral.
Test for protein, glucose, blood, and nitrite in urine.

Neo-Stomygen Stomygen, Aust.
Mouthwash: Sodium monofluorophosphate (p.1377·2); cetylpyridinium chloride (p.1138·1); enoxolone (p.34·3); xylitol (p.1397·3).
Formerly contained chlorhexidine gluconate, cetylpyridinium chloride, and sodium monofluorophosphate.
Toothpaste: Sodium monofluorophosphate (p.1377·2); propolis (p.1655·1); enoxolone (p.34·3); cetylpyridinium chloride (p.1138·1).
Formerly contained chlorhexidine gluconate and cetylpyridinium chloride.
Oral disinfection; oral hygiene.

Neostrata
Hamilton, Austral.; Canderm, Canad.; Nuova ICT, Ital.
A range of preparations containing glycolic acid (p.1115·1) or gluconolactone.
Skin disorders.

Neostrata AHA NeoStrata, USA†.
Hydroquinone (p.1115·1).
Skin hyperpigmentation.

Neostrata AHA Astringent Acne Canderm, Canad.
Salicylic acid (p.1122·3).

Neostrata AHA Blemish Canderm, Canad.
Salicylic acid (p.1122·3); glycolic acid (p.1115·1).

Neostrata AHA Daytime Canderm, Canad.
SPF 15: Octinoxate (p.1517·3); oxybenzone (p.1518·1); glycolic acid (p.1115·1).

Neostrata AHA Light Canderm, Canad.
SPF 15: Octinoxate (p.1517·3); oxybenzone (p.1518·1); gluconolactone.

Neostrata AHA Smoothing and Moisturizing Canderm, Canad.
SPF 15: Octinoxate (p.1517·3); oxybenzone (p.1518·1); glycolic acid (p.1115·1).

Neostrata Daytime Protection Cream Hamilton, Austral.
Octinoxate (p.1517·3); oxybenzone (p.1518·1); titanium dioxide (p.1126·1).
Emollient; sunscreen.

Neostrata HQ Canderm, Canad.
Hydroquinone (p.1115·1).
Skin hyperpigmentation.

Neostrata Lip Conditioner Hamilton, Austral.
SPF 15: Octinoxate (p.1517·3); octisalate (p.1518·1).
Dry lips; sunscreen.

Neosulf
Alphapharm, Austral.; Pacific, NZ.
Neomycin sulfate (p.228·1).
Bowel sterilisation; hepatic encephalopathy.

Neosulin Lenta Biobras, Braz.
Insulin zinc suspension (porcine, monocomponent) (p.324·1).
Diabetes mellitus.

Neosulin NPH Biobras, Braz.
Isophane insulin injection (porcine, monocomponent) (p.324·1).
Diabetes mellitus.

Neosulin Regular Biobras, Braz.
Insulin injection (porcine, monocomponent) (p.324·1).
Diabetes mellitus.

Neo-Synalar Yamanouchi, Spain†.
Fluocinolone acetonide (p.1071·1); neomycin sulfate (p.228·1).
Infected skin disorders.

Neo-Synephrine
Sanofi Synthelabo, Austral.; Abbott, Austral.; Sanofi Synthelabo, Belg.; Sanofi Synthelabo, Canad.; Ciba Vision, Fr.; Merck Sharp & Dohme-Chibret, Fr.; Sanofi Winthrop, Israel; Teofarma, Ital.; Sanofi Winthrop, Swed.†; Sanofi Winthrop, USA.
Phenylephrine hydrochloride (p.1097·1).
Eye congestion; maintenance of blood pressure during surgery; paroxysmal supraventricular tachycardia; production of mydriasis; spinal and regional analgesia; vascular failure in shock or drug-induced hypotension or hypersensitivity.

Neo-Synephrine 12 Hour Sterling Health, USA.
Oxymetazoline hydrochloride (p.1096·2).
Nasal congestion.

Neosynephrin-POS Ursapharm, Ger.
Phenylephrine hydrochloride (p.1097·1).
Eye disorders.

Neo-Synodorm Synpharma, Switz.
Diphenhydramine (p.416·1).
Agitation; nervousness; sleep disorders.

Neo-Tabs Pharma Tek, USA†.
Neomycin sulfate (p.228·1).

Neotal Hauck, USA†.
Polymyxin B sulfate (p.238·1); neomycin sulfate (p.228·1); bacitracin zinc (p.155·2).
Eye infections.

Neotalem Lemery, Mex.
Mitozantrone [mitoxantrone] (p.754·1).
Malignant neoplasms.

NeoTect Diatide, USA.
Technetium-99m depreotide (p.1451·1).
Scintigraphic imaging for pulmonary malignancy.

Neotenol Biobras, Braz.
Atenolol (p.841·3).
Angina pectoris; arrhythmias; hypertension; myocardial infarction.

Neotensin CEPA, Spain.
Enalapril maleate (p.883·3).
Heart failure; hypertension.

Neotensin Diu CEPA, Spain.
Hydrochlorothiazide (p.907·3); enalapril maleate (p.883·3).
Hypertension.

Neotest Merieux, Fr.†.
Tuberculin PPD (p.1675·3).
Sensitivity testing.

Neotetranase Rottapharm, Ital.
Amoxicillin trihydrate (p.149·2).
Bacterial infections.

Neothyllin Metochem, Aust.†.
Diprophylline (p.764·1).
Heart failure; hypertension; obstructive airways disease.

Neothylline Lemmon, USA†.
Diprophylline (p.764·1).
Asthma; bronchospasm.

Neo-Thyreostat Herbrand, Ger.; Berlin-Chemie, Ger.
Carbimazole (p.1521·1).
Hyperthyroidism.

Neotica Nakorn, Thai.
Balm: Methyl salicylate (p.85·1); camphor (p.1589·3); menthol (p.1632·3); eucalyptus oil (p.1609·2); eugenol (p.1609·3).
Insect bites; muscle pain and inflammation; sports injuries; sprains.
Capsules: Piroxicam (p.79·1).
Gout; musculoskeletal and joint disorders.

Neotigason
Roche, Aust.; Roche, Austral.; Roche, Belg.; Roche, Denm.; Roche, Fin.; Roche, Ger.; Roche, Hong Kong; Roche, Irl.; Roche, Israel; Roche, Ital.; Roche, Neth.; Roche, Norw.; Roche, NZ; Roche, Port.; Roche, S.Afr.; Roche, Singapore; Roche, Spain; Roche, Swed.; Roche, Switz.; Roche, Thai.; Roche, UK.
Acitretin (p.1109·1).
Keratinisation disorders; psoriasis.

Neo-Tinic Neolab, Canad.
Multivitamins and iron (p.1350·1).

Neo-Tiroimade Esfar, Port.
Liothyronine sodium (p.1524·2).

Neo-Tizide Pharmacia Upjohn, Aust.†.
Methaniazide calcium (p.223·1).
Tuberculosis.

Neoton Searle, Ital.
Fosfocreatinine sodium (p.1612·3).
Cardiac disorders.

Neotopic
Technilab, Canad.; Technilab, Hong Kong.
Polymyxin B sulfate (p.238·1); bacitracin (p.155·2) or bacitracin zinc (p.155·2); neomycin sulfate (p.228·1).
Bacterial skin infections.

Neotrace American Pharmaceutical, USA.
Trace element preparation (p.1350·1).
Additive for intravenous total parenteral nutrition solutions.

Neotracin
Ciba Vision, Ger.; Ciba Vision, Switz.
Neomycin sulfate (p.228·1); bacitracin (p.155·2).
Bacterial eye infections.

Neotri Lilly, Ger.
Xipamide (p.999·2); triamterene (p.986·1).
Hypertension; oedema.

Neotricin Legrand, Braz.
Neomycin (p.228·1); bacitracin zinc (p.155·2).
Eye infections.

Neotricin HC Bausch & Lomb, USA.
Neomycin sulfate (p.228·1); bacitracin zinc (p.155·2); polymyxin B sulfate (p.238·1); hydrocortisone acetate (p.1073·3).
Eye inflammation with bacterial infection.

Neo-Trim Fibre GNLD, Austral.
Fibre blend (from oat bran, barley bran, soy bran, orange gibre, acacia, ispaghula husk) (p.1214·2); methylcellulose (p.1502·2).
Obesity.

Neo-Trim Meal Replacement GNLD, Austral.
Food for special diets (p.1350·1).
Obesity.

Neotrin Neo Quimica, Braz.
Co-trimoxazole (p.193·3).
Bacterial infections; Pneumocystis carinii pneumonia; protozoal infections.

Neotrin Balsamico Neo Quimica, Braz.
Co-trimoxazole (p.193·3); guaifenesin (p.1092·2); ammonium chloride (p.1085·2).
Bacterial infections.

Neotroparin Chinoin, Hung.
Drotaverine hydrochloride (p.1606·1); homatropine methylbromide (p.468·1).
Smooth muscle spasm.

Neo-Tuss Neolab, Canad.
Dextromethorphan hydrobromide (p.1087·3); chlorpheniramine [chlorphenamine] maleate (p.412·1); phenylephrine hydrochloride (p.1097·1); sodium citrate (p.1186·2); guaifenesin (p.1092·2).
Coughs; respiratory tract congestion.

NeoTussan Novartis Consumer, Ger.
Dextromethorphan polistirex (p.1088·2).
Coughs.

Neotyf Biocine, Ital.
A typhoid vaccine (p.1566·3).
Active immunisation.

Neo-Ulcoid Valdecasas, Mex.
Dextromethorphan (p.1087·3).

Neo-Uridixico Rimsa, Mex.
Nalidixic acid (p.227·1).

Neo-Urtisan Synpharma, Switz.†.
Pheniramine maleate (p.422·3); lignocaine [lidocaine] hydrochloride (p.1313·2); calcium gluconate (p.1188·2); chlortalidone gluconate (p.1138·2).
Hypersensitivity reactions of the skin.

Neo-Ustiol INTES, Ital.
Sodium citrate (p.1186·2); aminobenzoic acid (p.1516·3); procaine (p.1319·2); cod-liver oil (p.1357·2).
Ophthalmic burns.

Neovermim Neo Quimica, Braz.
Mebendazole (p.102·2); tiabendazole (p.109·1).
Worm infections.

Neovis Searle, Ital.
Vitamin, carbohydrate, and mineral preparation with creatine (p.1350·1).
Nutritional supplement.

Neovita
Savoy, Singapore; Wallace Mfg Chem., UK.
Multivitamin and ginseng preparation with or without minerals and lecithin (p.1350·1).

Neo-Vites Neolab, Canad.†.
Multivitamins or multivitamins and minerals (p.1350·1).

Neo-Vivactil Sanofi Winthrop, Switz.†.
Amino-acid, mineral, and vitamin C preparation (p.1350·1).

Neovlar Schering, Braz.
Ethinylestradiol (p.1476·2); levonorgestrel (p.1486·2).
Combined oral contraceptive.

Neovletta Schering, Swed.
Levonorgestrel (p.1486·2); ethinylestradiol (p.1476·2).
Combined oral contraceptive.

Neoxene Ecobi, Ital.
Chlorhexidine gluconate (p.1138·2).
Disinfection of skin, hands, wounds, burns, and vagina.

Neoxidil
Galderma, Belg.; Galderma, Braz.; Galderma, Fr.; Galderma, Hong Kong; Galderma, Singapore; Galderma, Thai.
Minoxidil (p.934·2).
Alopecia androgenetica.

Neoxil Galderma, Mex.
Minoxidil (p.934·2).

Neoxinal Farmec, Ital.
Chlorhexidine gluconate (p.1138·2).
Disinfection of skin, wounds, and burns.

Neo-Xylestesin Espe, Aust.
Lignocaine [lidocaine] hydrochloride (p.1313·2).
Adrenaline [epinephrine] hydrochloride (p.829·2) is included in this preparation as a vasoconstrictor to di-

minish absorption and localise the effect of the local anaesthetic.
Local anaesthesia in dentistry.

Neo-Xylestesin forte and Neo-Xylestesin special Espe, Aust.
Lignocaine [lidocaine] hydrochloride (p.1313·2).
Adrenaline [epinephrine] hydrochloride (p.829·2) and noradrenaline [norepinephrine] hydrochloride (p.948·2) are included in this preparation as vasoconstrictors to diminish absorption and localise the effect of the local anaesthetic.
Local anaesthesia in dentistry.

Neozep
Note. This name is used for preparations of different composition.
United American, Hong Kong.
Phenylpropanolamine hydrochloride (p.1098·1); paracetamol (p.71·2); salicylamide (p.82·1); chlorpheniramine [chlorphenamine] maleate (p.412·1); vitamin C (p.1389·3).
Cold and influenza symptoms; nasopharyngeal disorders.

Great Eastern, Thai.; Myra, Thai.
Paracetamol (p.71·2); phenylpropanolamine hydrochloride (p.1098·1); chlorpheniramine [chlorphenamine] maleate (p.412·1).
Allergic rhinitis; cold symptoms; hay fever; sinusitis.

Neozine
Note. This name is used for preparations of different composition.
Rhodia, Braz.
Methotrimeprazine [levomepromazine] (p.691·3).
Adjunct in general anaesthesia; pain; premedication; psychoses.

Sanofi Synthelabo, Port.
Oxymetazoline hydrochloride (p.1096·2).
Nasal congestion.

Neo-Zol Neolab, Canad.
Clotrimazole (p.382·1).

Neozolone British Dispensary, Thai.
Prednisolone (p.1077·3); neomycin (p.228·1).
Eczema; infected skin disorders; seborrhoeic dermatitis.

Nephlex Rx Nephro-Tech, USA.
Vitamin B substances and vitamin C (p.1350·1).

Nephosteril Fresenius, Thai.
Amino-acid infusion (p.1350·1).
Parenteral nutrition in renal disease.

NephPlex Nephro-Tech, USA.
Multivitamin preparation for dialysis patients (p.1350·1).

Nephral Pfleger, Ger.
Triamterene (p.986·1); hydrochlorothiazide (p.907·3).
Hypertension; oedema.

Nephramine
Fresenius Kabi, Fr.; Braun McGaw, Hong Kong; McGaw, NZ; Pharmacia Upjohn, Spain; Fresenius, UK†; R&D, USA.
Amino-acid infusion (p.1350·1).
Parenteral nutrition in renal impairment.

Nephrex
Rhone-Poulenc Rorer, Austral.; Fisons, Hong Kong.
Calcium acetate (p.1187·3).
Hyperphosphataemia.

Nephril
Pfizer, Irl.; Pfizer, UK.
Polythiazide (p.957·1).
Hypertension; oedema.

Nephrisan P Ziethen, Ger.
Squill (p.1100·3); crataegus (p.1600·2).
Heart failure.

Nephrisol mono Cesra, Ger.
Solidago virgaurea.
Urinary-tract disorders.

Nephro-Calci R&D, USA.
Calcium carbonate (p.1215·1).
Calcium deficiency; dietary supplement.

Nephrocaps Fleming, USA.
Vitamin B substances with vitamin C (p.1350·1).
Vitamin deficiency in renal dialysis.

Nephro-Derm R&D, USA†.
Emollient and moisturiser.

Nephro-Fer R&D, USA.
Ferrous fumarate (p.1360·1).
Iron-deficiency anaemias.

Nephro-Fer Rx R&D, USA.
Ferrous fumarate (p.1360·1); folic acid (p.1361·1).
Iron deficiency.

Nephrolith mono Biomo, Ger.
Solidago virgaurea.
Renal calculi.

Nephrolithol N Pfluger, Ger.†.
Homoeopathic preparation.

nephro-loges Loges, Ger.
Equisetum (p.1606·3); solidago virgaurea; ononis (p.1644·1); parsley root (p.1648·3).
Urinary-tract disorders.

Nephron Nephron, USA.
Racepinephrine hydrochloride (p.831·1).
Bronchospasm.

Nephron FA Nephro-Tech, USA.
Multivitamin preparation with iron and folic acid (p.1350·1).
Docusate sodium (p.1223·1) is included in this preparation to reduce the constipating effects of iron.

Nephronorm med APS, Ger.
Tablets: Java tea (p.1625·1).

Tea†: Silver birch (p.1585·2); solidago virgaurea; java tea (p.1625·1); ononis (p.1644·1); rose fruit (p.1389·3); centaurea cyanus; calendula (p.1589·2).
Urinary-tract disorders.

Nephro-Pasc *Pascoe, Ger.*
Solidago virgaurea; birch leaf (p.1585·2); java tea (p.1625·1).
Urinary-tract disorders.

Nephroplasmal N *Braun, Ger.†*
Amino-acid and glycerol infusion (p.1350·1).
Parenteral nutrition in renal disease.

Nephropur tri *Repha, Ger.*
Solidago virgaurea; birch leaf (p.1585·2); java tea (p.1625·1).
Urinary-tract disorders.

Nephroselect M *Dreluso, Ger.*
Solidago virgaurea; equisetum (p.1606·3); birch leaf (p.1585·2); ononis (p.1644·1); lovage (p.1629·3); tropaeolum majus (p.1584·2); saw palmetto (p.1491·2).
Urinary-tract disorders.

Nephrosolid N *Bioforce, Switz.*
Solidago virgaurea; silver birch (p.1585·2); ononis (p.1644·1); equisetum (p.1606·3).
Urinary-tract disorders.

Nephrosteril
Fresenius, Belg.†; Fresenius Kabi, Ital.; Fresenius Kabi, Switz.
Amino-acid infusion (p.1350·1).
Parenteral nutrition in renal disease.

Nephrotect *Fresenius Kabi, Ger.*
Amino-acid infusion (p.1350·1).
Parenteral nutrition in renal failure.

Nephrotrans
Medice, Ger.; Salmon, Switz.
Sodium bicarbonate (p.1186·2).
Metabolic acidosis.

Nephro-Vite *R&D, USA.*
Multivitamin preparations (p.1350·1).

Nephro-Vite +Fe *R&D, USA.*
Multivitamin preparation with iron (p.1350·1).

Nephrox *Fleming, USA.*
Aluminium hydroxide (p.1210·3).
Hyperacidity.

Nephrubin *Weber & Weber, Ger.†*
Herbal tea: Salix (p.82·1); aesculus (p.1574·1); sambucus (p.1660·3); tilia (p.1673·2); birch leaf (p.1585·2); parsley (p.1648·3); centaury (p.1593·1); herniaria (p.1619·2); guaiacum wood; celery (p.1592·3); java tea (p.1625·1).
Tablets: Birch leaf (p.1585·2); java tea (p.1625·1).
Urinary-tract disorders.

Nephulon G *Redel, Ger.†*
Guaifenesin (p.1092·2).
Cough and cold symptoms.

Nephur 4 *Roche Diagnostics, Irl.*
Test for pH, protein, glucose, and nitrite in urine.

Nephur 6 *Roche Diagnostics, Irl.*
Test for pH, protein, glucose, nitrite, blood, and leucocytes in urine.

Nephur 7 *Roche Diagnostics, Irl.*
Test for pH, protein, glucose, nitrite, blood, leucocytes, and ketones in urine.

Nephur-Test + Leucocytes
Roche Diagnostics, Austral.; Roche Diagnostics, UK.
Test for leucocytes, nitrites, pH, protein, glucose, and blood in urine.

Nepituss *Bioindustria, Ital.*
Nepinalone hydrochloride (p.1095·3).
Coughs.

Nepresol
Novartis, Aust.; Novartis, Belg.; Cristalia, Braz.; Novartis, Denm.; Novartis, Ger.; Novartis, Hong Kong; Novartis, Israel; Novartis, Neth.†; Novartis, Norw.; Novartis, S.Afr.; Novartis, Swed.; Novartis, Switz.; Novartis, Thai.
Dihydralazine (p.874·2), dihydralazine mesilate (p.874·2), or dihydralazine sulfate (p.874·2).
Heart failure; hypertension.

Nepressol *Ciba-Geigy, Fr.†*
Dihydralazine sulfate (p.874·2).
Heart failure; hypertension.

Nepro
Abbott, Austral.; Abbott, Canad.†; Abbott, Fin.; Abbott, Hong Kong; Abbott, Irl.; Abbott, NZ; Abbott, Thai.; Abbott Nutrition, UK; Ross, USA.
Preparation for enteral nutrition in renal dialysis patients (p.1350·1).

Neptal *Procter & Gamble, Ger.†*
Acebutolol hydrochloride (p.825·1).
Cardiac disorders; hypertension.

Neptazane
Lederle, Austral.; Wyeth-Ayerst, Canad.; Lederle, Israel; Wyeth-Ayerst, Thai.; Lederle, USA.
Methazolamide (p.927·1).
Glaucoma.

Nerdipina
OM, Port.; Ferrer, Spain.
Nicardipine hydrochloride (p.938·3).
Angina pectoris; cerebrovascular disorders; hypertension.

Nerdipine *Medochemie, Thai.*
Nicardipine (p.938·3).
Angina pectoris; hypertension.

Nerelid *New Research, Ital.*
Nimesulide (p.62·3).
Fever; inflammation; pain.

Nerex *Farmanova, Ital.*
Royal jelly (p.1659·3); honey (p.1366·2); myrtillus (p.1639·2); fructose.
Nutritional supplement.

Nergadan *Uriach, Spain.*
Lovastatin (p.922·3).
Atherosclerosis; hypercholesterolaemia.

Neribas
Schering, Ger.; Asche, Ger.; Schering, Switz.
Emollient.
Skin disorders.

Neribase
Schering, Denm.; Schering, Fin.; Schering, Fr.; Schering, Ital.; Schering, Port.
Basis for topical preparations; emollient.
Skin disorders.

Nericur *Schering, UK†.*
Benzoyl peroxide (p.1111·1).
Acne.

Neriderm *Pharma Clal, Israel.*
Diflucortolone valerate (p.1069·3).
Skin disorders.

Neriforte *Schering, Aust.*
Diflucortolone valerate (p.1069·3).
Skin disorders.

Neriquinol *Schering, Aust.*
Diflucortolone valerate (p.1069·3); chlorquinaldol (p.182·1).
Infected skin disorders.

Nerisalic
Stiefel, Canad.; Schering, Fr.
Diflucortolone valerate (p.1069·3); salicylic acid (p.1122·3).
Skin disorders.

Nerisona
Schering, Aust.; Schering, Belg.; Schering, Braz.; Schering, Denm.; Schering, Ger.; Asche, Ger.; Schering, Ital.; Schering, Mex.; Schering, Neth.; Schering, Port.; Schering, Switz.
Diflucortolone valerate (p.1069·3).
Skin disorders.

Nerisona C
Schering, Ger.; Asche, Ger.; Schering, Ital.; Schering, Port.
Diflucortolone valerate (p.1069·3); chlorquinaldol (p.182·1).
Infected skin disorders.

Nerisone
Stiefel, Canad.; Schering, Fr.; Schering, Hong Kong; Schering, NZ; Schering, S.Afr.; Schering, Singapore; Meadow, UK.
Diflucortolone valerate (p.1069·3).
Skin disorders.

Nerisone C
Schering, Fr.; Schering, Hong Kong; Schering, NZ; Schering, Singapore.
Diflucortolone valerate (p.1069·3); chlorquinaldol (p.182·1).
Infected skin disorders.

Nerofen *Boots Healthcare, Neth.†.*
Ibuprofen (p.43·2).
Fever; pain.

Nerolid *Sydenham, Mex.*
Diazepam (p.674·3).

Nerpemide *Morrith, Spain†.*
Proteolytic enzymes.
Herpesvirus infections; neuritis.

Nervade *Covan, S.Afr.*
Caffeine (p.761·3); sodium glycerophosphate (p.1617·3); magnesium glycerophosphate (p.1191·2); potassium glycerophosphate (p.1617·3); glycerophosphoric acid (p.1617·3); potassium citrate (p.1186·1); yeast extract.
Tonic.

Nervan *Rosch & Handel, Aust.*
Paracetamol (p.71·2); propyphenazone (p.80·2); caffeine citrate (p.761·3).
Fever; pain.

Nervatona *Brauer, Austral.*
Oral liquid: Anamirta cocculus; helonias (p.1619·1); passion flower (p.1649·1); ignatia; nux vomica; phosphoricum acidum; sepia; zincum metallicum.
Anxiety.

Oral spray: Homoeopathic preparation.

Nervatona Plus
Brauer, Austral.
Oral liquid: Anamirta cocculus; helonias (p.1619·1); ginseng (p.1615·3); passion flower (p.1649·1); ignatia; kali phosphoricum; magnesia phosphorica; nux vomica; phosphoricum acidum; sepia; valeriana; zincum metallicum.
Anxiety; stress.

Hamilton, Austral.
Oral spray; Tablets: Homoeopathic preparation.

Nerve Tonic *Hylands, Canad.*
Homoeopathic preparation.

Nervei *Rodisma, Ger.*
Hypericum (p.290·2).
Depression.

Nervencreme S *Fides, Ger.*
Peppermint oil (p.1243·3); eucalyptus oil (p.1609·2).
Pain.

Nervendragees
Note. This name is used for preparations of different composition.
Rosch & Handel, Aust.
Valerian (p.1678·3); lupulus (p.1629·3); melissa (p.1632·2).
Nervous disorders; sleep disorders.

Ratiopharm, Ger.
Valerian root (p.1678·3); passion flower (p.1649·1); lupulus (p.1629·3).
Anxiety disorders; insomnia.

Nerven-Dragees *Zeller, Israel.*
Crataegus (p.1600·2); passion flower (p.1649·1); lupulus (p.1629·3); valerian (p.1678·3).
Insomnia; nervous disorders.

Nervenja *OTW, Ger.*
Homoeopathic preparation.

Nervenruh *Klosterfrau, Aust.*
Valerian (p.1678·3); passion flower (p.1649·1); lupulus (p.1629·3).
Anxiety disorders; sleep disorders.

Nerventee *Smetana, Aust.*
Valerian (p.1678·3); lupulus (p.1629·3); hypericum (p.290·2); peppermint leaf (p.1243·2); calluna vulgaris; delphinium consolida.
Anxiety disorders; sleep disorders.

Nerven-Tee Stada N *Stada, Ger.†*
Passion flower (p.1649·1); peppermint leaf (p.1243·2); melissa (p.1632·2); valerian (p.1678·3).
Sedative; sleep disorders.

Nervfluid S *Fides, Ger.*
Camphor (p.1589·3); eucalyptus oil (p.1609·2); pumilio pine oil (p.1656·3).
Nerve, muscle, and joint pain.

Nervidox *Teral, USA†.*
Vitamin B_{12} (p.1388·1); vitamin B_1 (p.1385·2).

Nervidox 6 *Teral, USA†.*
Vitamin B_{12} (p.1388·1); vitamin B_1 (p.1385·2); vitamin B_6 (p.1386·3).

Nervifene *Interdelta, Switz.*
Cloral hydrate (p.669·3).
Agitation; insomnia.

Nervifloran *Bioflora, Aust.*
Valerian (p.1678·3); lupulus (p.1629·3); melissa (p.1632·2); orange flowers; rosemary.
Nervous disorders; sleep disorders.

Nervine *Mathieu, Canad.*
Aspirin (p.14·2); caffeine (p.761·3).

Nervinetten *Eurim, Ger.†.*
Valerian (p.1678·3); lupulus (p.1629·3).
Agitation; sleep disorders.

Nervinfant N *Rubiepharm, Ger.*
Lupulus (p.1629·3); passion flower (p.1649·1).
Agitation; sleep disorders.

Nervipan *Medopharm, Ger.†.*
Valerian (p.1678·3).
Anxiety.

Nervipane *Apotheke Roten Krebs, Aust.†.*
Valepotriates (p.1678·3).
Nervous disorders.

Nervita *Boiron, Canad.*
Homoeopathic preparation.

Nervium *De Mayo, Braz.*
Bromazepam (p.656·3).
Anxiety; insomnia.

nervo OPT N *Optimed, Ger.*
Diphenhydramine hydrochloride (p.416·1).
Sleep disorders.

Nervobion *Merck, Spain.*
Cyanocobalamin (p.1388·1); pyridoxine hydrochloride (p.1386·3); thiamine hydrochloride (p.1385·1) or thiamine nitrate (p.1385·1).

Nervocaine *Keene, USA.*
Lignocaine [lidocaine] hydrochloride (p.1313·2).
Local anaesthesia.

Nervoforcan *INQ, Braz.*
Iron (p.1366·3); sodium glycerophosphate; magnesium glycerophosphate; vitamin B substances (p.1350·1).
Iron deficiency; iron-deficiency anaemias.

Nervogastrol *Sanofi Synthelabo, Ger.*
Bismuth subnitrate (p.1213·2); bismuth subgallate (p.1213·2); heavy magnesium carbonate (p.1232·3); calcium carbonate (p.1215·1); sodium bicarbonate (p.1186·2); greater celandine (p.1618·1); condurango (p.1599·1); scopolia carniolica.
Gastrointestinal disorders.

Nervoject N *Syxyl, Ger.*
Homoeopathic preparation.

Nervonocton N *Pfluger, Ger.*
Kava (p.1625·3).
Nervous disorders.

Nervopax *Lehning, Fr.*
Homoeopathic preparation.

Nervoregin *Pfluger, Ger.*
Homoeopathic preparation.

Nervoregin forte *Pfluger, Ger.*
Valerian (p.1678·3); lupulus (p.1629·3); passion flower (p.1649·1).
Nervous disorders.

Nervoregin H *Pfluger, Ger.*
Homoeopathic preparation.

Nervosana *Hotz, Ger.*
Achillea (p.1572·2); liquorice (p.1231·2); melissa (p.1632·2); peppermint leaf (p.1243·2); rubus fruticosus; chamomille (p.1593·2); tilia (p.1673·2); valerian (p.1678·3); absinthium (p.1571·1).
Nervous disorders; sleep disorders.

Nervpin N *Schoning-Berlin, Ger.†.*
Menthol (p.1632·3); noble fir oil.
Nerve and joint pain; skin trauma; sprains.

Nervuton N *Cesra, Ger.*
Homoeopathic preparation.

Nesacain *Astra, Switz.*
Chloroprocaine hydrochloride (p.1308·3).
Local anaesthesia.

Nesacaine
AstraZeneca, Canad.; Astra, USA.
Chloroprocaine hydrochloride (p.1308·3).
Local anaesthesia.

Nesdonal
Rhone-Poulenc Rorer, Belg.†; Rhone-Poulenc Rorer, Neth.
Thiopental sodium (p.1269·1).
General anaesthesia.

Nesfare Antibiotico *Madaus, Spain.*
Framycetin sulfate (p.208·2); triamcinolone acetonide (p.1080·1); centella (p.1112·2).
Formerly contained human placenta, framycetin sulfate, triamcinolone acetonide, chamomile oil, and calendula oil.
Infected skin disorders.

Nesivine *Merck-Belgolabo, Belg.*
Oxymetazoline hydrochloride (p.1096·2).
Eustachian-tube inflammation; nasal congestion; otitis media; sinusitis.

Nesol *Orthos, Mex.*
Dipyrone (p.34·1).

Nesoro *Novaquimica, Braz.*
Sodium chloride (p.1196·2).
Nasal congestion.

Nestabs *Fielding, USA.*
Multivitamin and mineral preparation with iron and folic acid (p.1350·1).
Multivitamin and mineral supplement for pregnancy and lactation.

Nestargel
Nestle, Switz.; Nestle, UK.
Ceratonia (p.1500·3).
Infant feed thickener.

Nesthakchen *Schulke & Mayr, Aust.*
Fennel (p.1610·1); aniseed (p.1580·2); caraway (p.1591·2); chamomile (p.1593·2); liquorice (p.1231·2); fennel oil (p.1610·2); anise oil (p.1580·3); caraway oil (p.1591·2); chamomile oil.
Gastrointestinal disorders.

Nestic *Asian Pharm, Thai.*
Clotrimazole (p.382·1).
Trichomoniasis; vaginal fungal infections.

Nestosyl
Note. This name is used for preparations of different composition.
Pharmethic, Belg.
Pramocaine (p.1318·2); chlorhexidine hydrochloride (p.1138·2); zinc oxide (p.1128·2).
Formerly contained benzocaine, butyl aminobenzoate, resorcinol, and zinc oxide.
Minor wounds; skin disorders.

Synthelabo, Braz.
Benzocaine (p.1306·2); butyl aminobenzoate (p.1308·2); benzalkonium chloride (p.1133·2); zinc oxide (p.1128·2); hydroxyquinoline (p.1622·2).
Skin disorders.

Alpharma, Fr.
Benzocaine (p.1306·2); butyl aminobenzoate (p.1308·2); resorcinol (p.1122·2); hydroxyquinoline (p.1622·2); zinc oxide (p.1128·2).
Local anaesthesia; sunburn; superficial burns.

Nestum *Nestle, Port.*
Gluten-free food (p.1350·1).

Nethaprin Dospan *Mer-National, S.Afr.*
Bufylline (p.761·3); doxylamine succinate (p.417·1); etafedrine hydrochloride (p.1091·2); phenylephrine hydrochloride (p.1097·1).
Coughs; obstructive airways disease.

Nethaprin Expectorant *Mer-National, S.Afr.*
Bufylline (p.761·3); doxylamine succinate (p.417·1); etafedrine hydrochloride (p.1091·2); guaifenesin (p.1092·2).
Obstructive airways disease.

Netillin
Schering-Plough, Irl.; Schering-Plough, UK.
Netilmicin sulfate (p.229·3).
Bacterial infections.

Netilyn
Schering-Plough, Denm.; Schering-Plough, Fin.; Schering-Plough, Norw.; Schering-Plough, Swed.
Netilmicin sulfate (p.229·3).
Bacterial infections.

Netra *Sam-On, Israel.*
Calcium carbonate (p.1215·1); magnesium carbonate (p.1232·3).
Calcium supplement; gastrointestinal hyperacidity; heartburn.

Netrocin *Schering-Plough, Spain.*
Netilmicin sulfate (p.229·3).
Bacterial infections.

Netromicina
Schering-Plough, Braz.; Schering-Plough, Mex.; Schering-Plough, Port.
Netilmicin sulfate (p.229·3).
Bacterial infections.

Netromicine *Schering-Plough, Fr.*
Netilmicin sulfate (p.229·3).
Bacterial infections.

Netromycin
Schering-Plough, Austral.; Schering, Canad.; Schering-Plough, Hong Kong; Schering-Plough, NZ; Schering-Plough, S.Afr.; Schering-Plough, Thai.; Schering, USA.
Netilmicin sulfate (p.229·3).
Bacterial infections.

Netromycine *Schering-Plough, Belg.; Schering-Plough, Neth.; Essex, Switz.*
Netilmicin sulfate (p.229·3).
Bacterial infections.

Nettacin *Schering-Plough, Ital.*
Netilmicin sulfate (p.229·3).
Bacterial infections.

Nettinerv *Iso, Ger.*
Cinchona; conium; hamamelis; scrophularia; viscum album; pumilio pine oil (p.1656·3).
Neuralgia; pain; pruritus.

Nettle Rash L88 *Homeocan, Canad.*
Homoeopathic preparation.

Netux *Nicholas, Fr.*
Codeine (p.25·2); phenyltoloxamine (p.423·1).
Coughs.

Neu Viplex *Siam Bheasach, Thai.*
Vitamin B substances (p.1350·1).
Vitamin deficiency.

Neucare *Hoe, Singapore.*
Topical barrier preparation.

Neucor *CT, Ital.*
Nicardipine hydrochloride (p.938·3).
Angina pectoris; heart failure; hypertension.

Neuer
Daiichi, Hong Kong; Daiichi, Jpn.
Cetraxate hydrochloride (p.1216·2).
Gastritis; peptic ulcer.

Neufil *Bial, Port.*
Diprophylline (p.764·1).
Obstructive airways disease.

Neugal *Diba, Mex.*
Ranitidine hydrochloride (p.1245·2).
Gastro-oesophageal reflux; peptic ulcer; Zollinger-Ellison syndrome.

Neugen *Bioprogress, Ital.†*
Nicergoline (p.1640·2).
Cerebrovascular disorders.

Neugeron *Armstrong, Mex.*
Carbamazepine (p.342·2).
Epilepsy; neuralgias.

Neugra N *Hermes, Ger.†*
Multivitamin and mineral preparation (p.1350·1).

Neulactil
Rhone-Poulenc Rorer, Austral.; Aventis, Denm.; Rhone-Poulenc Rorer, Fin.; Rhone-Poulenc Rorer, Hong Kong; Rhone-Poulenc Rorer, Irl.; Rhone-Poulenc Rorer, Norw.†; Aventis, NZ; Aventis, S.Afr.; Rhone-Poulenc Rorer, Swed.†; JHC Healthcare, UK.
Pericyazine (p.698·3).
Anxiety disorders; behaviour disorders in children; psychoses.

Neuleptil
Rhone-Poulenc Rorer, Aust.; Rhone-Poulenc Rorer, Belg.†; Rhodia, Braz.; Rhone-Poulenc Rorer, Canad.; Rhone-Poulenc Rorer, Fr.; Rhone-Poulenc Rorer, Israel; Rhone-Poulenc Rorer, Ital.; Rhone-Poulenc Rorer, Neth.; Rhone-Poulenc Rorer, Switz.†
Pericyazine (p.698·3), pericyazine mesilate (p.698·3), or pericyazine tartrate (p.698·3).
Psychoses.

Neumega *Genetics Institute, USA.*
Oprelvekin (p.739·2).
Thrombocytopenia.

Neumobiot *Reig Jofre, Spain†.*
Benzylpenicillin sodium (p.157·2); niaouli oil (p.1640·2); guaifenesin (p.1092·2).
Lignocaine [lidocaine] hydrochloride (p.1313·2) is included in this preparation to alleviate the pain of injection.
Respiratory-tract infections.

Neumopectolina *Inkeysa, Spain.*
Guaifenesin (p.1092·2); sodium benzoate (p.1134·3); co-trimoxazole (p.193·3).
Respiratory-tract infections.

Neumoral *Medestea, Ital.*
Hypericum (p.290·2); magnesium oxide (p.1233·2).
Tonic.

Neupogen
Roche, Aust.; Amgen, Austral.; Amgen, Belg.; Amgen, Canad.; Amgen, Denm.; Amgen, Fin.; Roche, Fr.; Amgen, Ger.; Roche, Hong Kong; Amgen, Irl.; Roche, Israel; Dompe Biotec, Ital.; Roche, Mex.; Amgen, Neth.; Roche, Norw.; Roche, NZ; Amgen, Port.; Roche, S.Afr.; Roche, Singapore; Amgen, Spain; Amgen, Swed.; Roche, Switz.; Roche, Thai.; Amgen, UK; Amgen, USA.
Filgrastim (p.736·1).
Mobilisation of autologous peripheral blood progenitor cells; neutropenia.

Neupramir *Lusofarmaco, Ital.*
Pramiracetam sulfate (p.1654·2).
Mental function impairment.

Neuquinon *Eisai, Jpn.*
Ubidecarenone (p.1677·1).
Heart failure.

Neuraben *Pfizer, Ital.*
Thiamine Bezomil; pyridoxine hydrochloride (p.1386·3); cyanocobalamin (p.1388·1).
Joint disorders; neuritis.

Neuractiv *Novartis, Ital.†*
Oxiracetam (p.1645·3).
Mental function impairment.

Neuragon *Sriprasit, Thai.*
Perphenazine (p.699·1); amitriptyline hydrochloride (p.273·3).
Depression.

Neuralgietabletten N *Cosmochema, Ger.*
Homoeopathic preparation.

Neuralgietropfen CM *Cosmochema, Ger.*
Homoeopathic preparation.

Neuralgin *Pfleger, Ger.*
Aspirin (p.14·2); paracetamol (p.71·2); caffeine (p.761·3).
Pain.

Neuralgin ASS *Pfleger, Ger.*
Aspirin (p.14·2).
Fever; pain.

Neuralysan S *Steigerwald, Ger.*
Thiamine hydrochloride (p.1385·1); pyridoxine hydrochloride (p.1386·3).
Neuralgia; neuritis.

Neuramag P *CT, Ger.†*
Paracetamol (p.71·2); caffeine (p.761·3).
Pain.

Neuramate *Halsey, USA.*
Meprobamate (p.691·1).
Anxiety.

Neuramide Sherman *Difa, Ital.*
Neuramide.
Herpesvirus infections.

Neuramin *Orion, Fin.*
Thiamine hydrochloride (p.1385·1).
Thiamine deficiency; wernicke-korsakoff syndrome.

Neuramizone *Sriprasit, Thai.*
Belladonna alkaloids (p.463·1); ergotamine tartrate (p.452·1); phenobarbital (p.355·1).
Sedative.

Neur-Amyl *Sigma, Austral.*
Amobarbital (p.655·2).
Hypnotic; sedative.

Neuranidal *Stada, Ger.*
Aspirin (p.14·2); paracetamol (p.71·2); caffeine (p.761·3).
Pain.

Neuranidal Duo *LAW, Ger.†*
Aspirin (p.14·2); caffeine (p.761·3).
Fever; pain.

Neurapas *Pascoe, Ger.*
Hypericum (p.290·2); valerian (p.1678·3); passion flower (p.1649·1); larkspur; eschscholtzia.
Psychiatric disorders.

NeuRecover *NeuroGenesis, USA.*
A range of multivitamin, mineral, and amino-acid preparations (p.1350·1).

Neurex *Salus, Ital.*
Citicoline sodium (p.1596·1).
Cerebrovascular disorders; parkinsonism.

Neuriberi *Haller, Braz.*
Vitamin B₁; vitamin B₆; vitamin B₁₂ (p.1350·1).
Vitamin B deficiency.

Neuri-cyl N Ho-Len-Complex *Liebermann, Ger.*
Homoeopathic preparation.

Neuridon *Synthelabo, Belg.†*
Paracetamol (p.71·2).
Fever; pain.

Neuridon Forte *Sanofi Synthelabo, Belg.*
Paracetamol (p.71·2); propyphenazone (p.80·2); codeine phosphate (p.25·2).
Fever; pain.

Neuril *Sanova, Aust.*
Melperone hydrochloride (p.690·3).
Anxiety disorders; drug and alcohol withdrawal syndrome; psychoses; senile dementia; sleep disorders.

Neurinase *Rudefsa, Mex.*
Barbital sodium (p.656·2).
Sedative; sleep disorders.

Neuriplege *Genevrier, Fr.*
Cream: Chlorproethazine hydrochloride (p.660·1).
Ointment†: Chlorproethazine hydrochloride (p.660·1); cymene (p.26·2).
Painful skeletal muscle spasm.

Neurium *Hexal, Ger.*
Thioctic acid (p.1671·3) or ethylenediamine thioctate (p.1671·3).
Diabetic polyneuropathy.

Neuro *Stada, Ger.*
Thiamine hydrochloride (p.1385·1); pyridoxine hydrochloride (p.1386·3).
Nervous-system disorders.

Neuro B1-6-12 *Jean-Marie, Hong Kong.*
Vitamin B₁ (p.1385·2); vitamin B₆ (p.1387·1); vitamin B₁2 (p.1388·1).
Neuralgias; neuritis; vitamin B deficiencies.

Neuro B-12 *Lambda, USA†.*
Vitamin B₁₂ (p.1388·1); vitamin B₁ (p.1385·2).

Neuro B-12 Forte *Lambda, USA†.*
Vitamin B substances and ascorbic acid (p.1350·1).

Neuro Calme *Geistlich, Switz.*
Vitamin B substances and mineral preparation (p.1350·1).
Tonic.

Neuro Nutrients *Solgar, UK.*
Amino-acid preparation with vitamin B substances, vitamin C, and ginkgo biloba (p.1350·1).

Neuro uno *Stada, Ger.*
Benfotiamine (p.1384·3); pyridoxine hydrochloride (p.1386·3).
Nervous-system disorders.

Neuro-AS N *Teva, Ger.*
Thiamine hydrochloride (p.1385·1); pyridoxine hydrochloride (p.1386·3).
Vitamin B deficiency.

neuro-B forte *Biomo, Ger.*
Thiamine hydrochloride (p.1385·1); pyridoxine hydrochloride (p.1386·3).
Neurological system disorders.

Neurobex *British Dispensary, Thai.*
Vitamin B₁ (p.1385·2); vitamin B₆ (p.1387·1); vitamin B₁₂ (p.1388·1).
Lignocaine [lidocaine] hydrochloride (p.1313·2) is included in the injection to alleviate the pain of injection.
Anaemias; neurological disorders.

Neurobiol *Teofarma, Ital.*
Phenobarbital (p.355·1).
Formerly contained sodium bromide, phenobarbotone, passion flower, and crataegus.
Epilepsy; insomnia; sedative.

Neurobion
Merck, Aust.; Merck-Belgolabo, Belg.; Merck, Fin.; Merck, Ger.; Merck, Hong Kong; E. Merck, Irl.; Merck, Mex.; Merck, Neth.; Merck, Port.; Merck, S.Afr.; Merck, Singapore; Merck, Swed.; Merck, Thai.; Alba, USA†.
Vitamin B₁ (p.1385·2); vitamin B₆ (p.1387·1); vitamin B₁₂ (p.1388·1).
Neuralgia; neuritis; neuropathy; vitamin B deficiency.
Alba, USA†.
Injection: Cyanocobalamin (p.1388·1); thiamine hydrochloride (p.1385·1).

Neurobion N *Merck, Ger.*
Thiamine nitrate (p.1385·1) or thiamine disulfide (p.1385·2); pyridoxine hydrochloride (p.1386·3).
Neuralgia; neuritis.

Neurobionta *Bracco, Ital.*
Thiamine hydrochloride (p.1385·1); pyridoxine hydrochloride (p.1386·3); cyanocobalamin (p.1388·1).
Herpes zoster; neuralgias; neuritis.

NeuroBloc *Elan, UK.*
Botulinum B toxin (p.1324·2).
Spasmodic torticollis.

Neurocalcium *Biologiques de l'Ile-de-France, Fr.*
Syrup: Calcium bromide (p.1587·1); calcium chloride (p.1188·1); calcium gluconogluceptate.
Anxiety; insomnia.
Tablets: Calcium gluconate (p.1188·2); calcium bromide (p.1587·1); phenobarbital (p.355·1).
Anxiety; insomnia; palpitations.

Neurocardol *Produfarma, Port.*
Passion flower (p.1649·1); crataegus (p.1600·2); salix (p.82·1); valerian (p.1678·3).

Neurocatavin Dexa *Llorente, Spain.*
Vitamin B substances (p.1350·1); dexamethasone sodium phosphate (p.1067·1); suprarenal cortex (p.1080·1).
Lignocaine [lidocaine] (p.1313·2) is included in this preparation to alleviate the pain of injection.
Myalgia; neuralgia; neuritis; rheumatism.

Neurochol C *Merck, Ger.*
Greater celandine (p.1618·1); taraxacum (p.1669·1); absinthium (p.1571·1).
Biliary disorders; dyspepsia.

Neurocil *Bayer, Ger.*
Methotrimeprazine [levomepromazine] hydrochloride (p.691·3) or methotrimeprazine [levomepromazine] maleate (p.692·1).
Psychiatric disorders.

Neurodavur *Belmac, Spain.*
Vitamin B substances (p.1350·1).
Vitamin B deficiency.

Neurodavur Plus *Belmac, Spain.*
Vitamin B substances (p.1350·1); dexamethasone sodium phosphate (p.1067·1).
Lignocaine [lidocaine] hydrochloride (p.1313·2) is included in this preparation to alleviate the pain of injection.
Myalgia; neuralgia; neuritis.

Neurodep *Med. Prod. Panam., USA.*
Capsules: Vitamin B substances (p.1350·1).
Injection: Vitamin B substances and vitamin C (p.1350·1).

Neurodif *Vinas, Spain†.*
Lysine aspirin (p.50·3); vitamin B substances (p.1350·1).
Lignocaine [lidocaine] hydrochloride (p.1313·2) is included in the intramuscular injection to alleviate the pain of injection.
Musculoskeletal and joint disorders; neuritis.

Neuro-Do *Grasler, Ger.*
Homoeopathic preparation.

Neurodol Tissugel *IBSA, Switz.*
Lignocaine [lidocaine] (p.1313·2).
Post-herpetic neuralgia.

Neurodynamicum *Faes, Spain†.*
Citicoline sodium (p.1596·1).
Cerebrovascular disorders.

Neuro-Effekton B *Wyeth, Ger.*
Thiamine hydrochloride (p.1385·1); pyridoxine hydrochloride (p.1386·3).
Nervous-system disorders.

Neuro-Europan *Kwizda, Aust.†*
Ethenzamide (p.35·1); propyphenazone (p.80·2); vitamin B substances (p.1350·1).
Musculoskeletal and joint disorders; neuralgia; neuritis.

Neurofenac
Merck, Aust.; Merck, Hong Kong.
Diclofenac sodium (p.30·3); vitamin B substances (p.1350·1).
Gout; musculoskeletal, joint, and soft tissue disorders; neuralgia; neuritis; pain.

Neuro-Fibraflex N *Nycomed, Ger.†.*
Vitamin B substances (p.1350·1).
Vitamin B deficiency.

Neurofitol *Herals, Braz.*
Methyltestosterone (p.1482·3); vitamin E (p.1393·3); calcium magnesium phytate.
Erectile dysfunction.

Neuroflax *Hoechst Marion Roussel, Mex.*
Cobamamide (p.1388·3); thiocolchicoside (p.1330·2).
Musculoskeletal and joint disorders.

Neuroflorine *Fuca, Fr.*
Passion flower (p.1649·1); crataegus (p.1600·2); valerian (p.1678·3).
Anxiety; insomnia; palpitations.

Neurofor *Hoechst Marion Roussel, Mex.*
Cobamamide (p.1388·3).

Neuroforte *Beacons, Singapore.*
Vitamin B₁ (p.1385·2); vitamin B₆ (p.1387·1); vitamin B₁2 (p.1388·1).
Diabetic neuropathy; neuralgia; poluneuritis.

Neuroftal *INTES, Ital.*
Injection: Thiamine hydrochloride (p.1385·1); nicotinamide (p.1372·3); strychnine glycerophosphate.
Procaine hydrochloride (p.1319·1) is included in this preparation to alleviate the pain of injection.
Tablets: Thiamine hydrochloride (p.1385·1); riboflavin (p.1386·1); nicotinamide (p.1372·3); strychnine nitrate (p.1667·3); sodium glycerophosphate (p.1617·3).
Optic nerve atrophy.

Neurogamma *Worwag, Ger.*
Cyanocobalamin; pyridoxine hydrochloride; thiamine nitrate (p.1350·1).
Neuralgia; neuritis.

Neurogen-E *Imperial, Singapore.*
Vitamin B₁; vitamin B₆; vitamin B₁₂; vitamin E (p.1350·1).
Vitamin supplement.

Neuroglutamin *Pharmonta, Aust.*
Glutamic acid (p.1365·2).
Memory and concentration disorders.

Neurogobens *Normon, Spain†.*
Lysine aspirin (p.50·3); vitamin B substances (p.1350·1).
Lignocaine [lidocaine] hydrochloride (p.1313·2) is included in this preparation to alleviate the pain of injection.
Pain.

Neurogrisevit N *Pharmacia Upjohn, Ger.*
Thiamine nitrate (p.1385·1); pyridoxine hydrochloride (p.1386·3).
Nervous-system disorders.

Neurol
Note.This name is used for preparations of different composition.
SIT, Ital.
Sodium valerate; sodium glycerophosphate (p.1617·3).
Tonic.

Abigo, Swed.
Valerian (p.1678·3).
Insomnia; nervous disorders.

Neurolep *Promeco, Mex.*
Carbamazepine (p.342·2).

Neurolepsin *Kwizda, Aust.*
Lithium carbonate (p.292·1).
Depression; mania.

Neuro-Lichtenstein *Lichtenstein, Ger.*
Thiamine hydrochloride (p.1385·1); pyridoxine hydrochloride (p.1386·3); cyanocobalamin (p.1388·1).
Vitamin B deficiency.

Neuro-Lichtenstein N *Lichtenstein, Ger.*
Thiamine hydrochloride (p.1385·1); pyridoxine hydrochloride (p.1386·3).
Nervous-system disorders.

Neurolid *Recipe, Aust.†*
Lignocaine [lidocaine] hydrochloride (p.1313·2).
Local anaesthesia.

Neurolite
Du Pont, Belg.; Du Pont, Fr.; Du Pont, Spain.
Technetium-99m bicisate (p.1451·1).
Cerebral perfusion imaging.

Neurolithium
Labcatal, Fr.; Labcatal, Switz.
Lithium gluconate (p.296·2).
Bipolar disorder; hypomania; mania.

Neuromade *Teofarma, Spain.*
Cyanocobalamin (p.1388·1); thiamine hydrochloride (p.1385·1); pyridoxine hydrochloride (p.1386·3).
Lignocaine [lidocaine] hydrochloride (p.1313·2) is included in the intramuscular injection to alleviate the pain of injection.
Vitamin B deficiency.

Neuromax *Vitabalans, Fin.*
Vitamin B substances (p.1350·1).
Vitamin B deficiency.

Neuromet
Note.This name is used for preparations of different composition.
SmithKline Beecham, Ital.
Oxiracetam (p.1645·3).
Mental function impairment.

Merck, Thai.
Mecobalamin (p.1388·3).
Peripheral neuropathies; vitamin B₁₂ deficiency.

Neuromethyn *Sam Chun Dang, Singapore.*
Mecobalamin (p.1388·3).
Megaloblastic anaemia; peripheral neuropathies.

The symbol † denotes a preparation no longer actively marketed

Neuromultivit *Lannacher, Aust.*
Vitamin B substances (p.1350·1).
Neuropathy.

Neuronika *Klinge, Ger.*
Kawain (p.1625·3).
Alcohol withdrawal syndrome; psychiatric disorders.

Neurontin
Parke, Davis, Aust.; Parke, Davis, Austral.; Parke, Davis, Belg.; Parke, Davis, Canad.; Parke, Davis, Fin.; Parke, Davis, Fr.; Parke, Davis, Ger.; Parke, Davis, Hong Kong; Pfizer, Irl.; Parke, Davis, Israel; Parke, Davis, Ital.; Parke, Davis, Mex.; Parke, Davis, Neth.; Warner-Lambert, Norw.; Parke, Davis, NZ; Parke, Davis, Port.; Parke, Davis, S.Afr.; Parke, Davis, Singapore; Parke, Davis, Spain; Parke, Davis, Swed.; Parke, Davis, Switz.; Warner-Lambert, Thai.; Parke, Davis, UK; Parke, Davis, USA.
Gabapentin (p.350·2).
Epilepsy; neuropathic pain.

Neuropax *Labomed, Fr.*
Passion flower (p.1649·1); crataegus (p.1600·2).
Formerly contained passion flower, crataegus, and phe-
nobarbital.
Anxiety; insomnia.

Neuroplant *Spitzner, Ger.; Schwabe, Ger.*
Hypericum (p.290·2).
Anxiety; depression.

Neuro-ratiopharm *Ratiopharm, Ger.*
Thiamine hydrochloride (p.1385·1); pyridoxine hydro-
chloride (p.1386·3); cyanocobalamin (p.1388·1).
Nervous-system disorders.

Neuro-ratiopharm N *Ratiopharm, Ger.*
Thiamine hydrochloride (p.1385·1); pyridoxine hydro-
chloride (p.1386·3).
Nervous-system disorders.

Neurorubin *Mepha, Switz.*
Vitamin B substances (p.1350·1).
Neuralgias; neuritis; neuropathy.

Neurorubine
Mepha, Hong Kong; Mepha, Singapore.
Vitamin B₁ (p.1385·2); vitamin B₆ (p.1387·1); vitamin
B₁₂ (p.1388·1).
Lignocaine [lidocaine] hydrochloride (p.1313·2) may
be included in the injection to alleviate the pain of in-
jection.
*Neuralgia; neuritis; rheumatic pain; toxic lesions of
the nervous system.*

Neuroselect *Dreluso, Ger.*
Homoeopathic preparation.

Neurosine *Armstrong, Mex.*
Buspirone hydrochloride (p.657·2).
Anxiety disorders.

NeuroSlim *NeuroGenesis, USA; Matrix, USA.*
Multivitamin, mineral, and amino-acid preparation
(p.1350·1).

Neurosthenol *Richard, Fr.*
Glutamic acid; phosphoric acid; electrolytes
(p.1350·1).
Formerly contained cerebral cortex extract (pork),
glutamic acid, phosphoric acid, and electrolytes.
Tonic.

Neurostop *Lacer, Spain.*
Benfotiamine (p.1384·3).
Vitamin B1 deficiency.

Neurostop Complex *Lacer, Spain.*
Benfotiamine (p.1384·3); hydroxocobalamin acetate
(p.1388·3); pyridoxine hydrochloride (p.1386·3).
Vitamin B deficiency.

Neurotensyl *Sciencex, Fr.†.*
Crataegus (p.1600·2); passion flower (p.1649·1); vale-
rian (p.1678·3).
Anxiety; insomnia; palpitations.

Neurothioct *Knoll, Ger.*
Thioctic acid (p.1671·3).
Diabetic polyneuropathy.

Neurotisan *Hanosan, Ger.†.*
Hypericum (p.290·2).
Psychiatric disorders.

Neurotol *Orion, Fin.*
Carbamazepine (p.342·2).
*Alcohol withdrawal syndrome; bipolar disorder; epi-
lepsy; trigeminal neuralgia.*

Neuroton *NCSN, Ital.*
Citicoline sodium (p.1596·1).
Cerebrovascular disorders; parkinsonism.

Neurotonico *EMS, Braz.*
Minerals with vitamin B substances (p.1350·1).

Neurotop
Gerot, Ger.; Gerot, Singapore.
Carbamazepine (p.342·2).
*Alcohol withdrawal syndrome; bipolar disorder; dia-
betes insipidus; diabetic neuropathy; epilepsy; trigem-
inal neuralgia.*

Neurotrat
Knoll, Ger.; Knoll, Switz.
Thiamine hydrochloride (p.1385·1) or thiamine nitrate
(p.1385·1); pyridoxine hydrochloride (p.1386·3); cy-
anocobalamin (p.1388·1).
Neuralgias; neuritis; neuropathy.

Neurotrat B₁₂ *Knoll, Ger.*
Cyanocobalamin (p.1388·1).
Vitamin B₁₂ deficiency.

Neurotrat S *Knoll, Ger.*
Thiamine nitrate (p.1385·1); pyridoxine hydrochloride
(p.1386·3).
Nervous-system disorders.

neurotropan *Phonix, Ger.*
Choline citrate (p.1356·3).
Liver disorders.

Neurovegetalin *Verla, Ger.*
Hypericum (p.290·2).
Depression.

Neuro-Vibolex *Chephasaar, Ger.*
Injection: Thiamine hydrochloride (p.1385·1); pyridoxine hydrochloride (p.1386·3); cyanocobalamin
(p.1388·1).
Tablets: Thiamine hydrochloride (p.1385·1); pyridoxine hydrochloride (p.1386·3).
Neuralgia; neuritis; neuropathy.

Neurovitan
Note.This name is used for preparations of different composition.
Orion, Fin.
Thiamine nitrate (p.1385·1); pyridoxine hydrochloride
(p.1386·3); nicotinamide (p.1372·3); cyanocobalamin
(p.1388·1).
Vitamin B deficiency.
Fujisawa, Jpn.
Octotiamine (p.1385·1); riboflavin (p.1386·1); pyri-
doxine hydrochloride (p.1386·3); cyanocobalamin
(p.1388·1).
Vitamin B deficiency; vitamin B supplement.

Neuro-Wied *Wiedemann, Ger.*
Vitamin B substances (p.1350·1); di-isopropylammonium dichloroacetate (p.874·3); magnesium orotate
(p.1645·1).
*Mental function disorders; migraine; nerve pain; sleep
disorders.*

Neusinol *Labima, Belg.*
Naphazoline (p.1095·1).
Nasal congestion.

Neut *Abbott, USA.*
Sodium bicarbonate (p.1186·2).
*Neutralising additive solution for acidic intravenous
infusions.*

Neutracido *Medquimica, Braz.*
Sodium bicarbonate (p.1186·2); bismuth subcarbonate
(p.1213·1); kaolin (p.1229·3); magnesium hydroxide
(p.1233·1); calcium carbonate (p.1215·1); belladonna
(p.463·1).
Gastrointestinal hyperacidity.

Neutrafluor *Colgate Oral Care, Austral.*
Sodium fluoride (p.1375·3).
Fluoride supplement; sensitive teeth.

Neutrafort *Ariston, Braz.*
Magnesium hydroxide (p.1233·1); aluminium hydrox-
ide (p.1210·3); simeticone (p.1249·2).
Flatulence; gastrointestinal hyperacidity.

Neutragel *Propan, S.Afr.*
Dicyclomine [dicycloverine] hydrochloride (p.466·1);
dried aluminium hydroxide (p.1210·3); light magnesium oxide (p.1233·2).
Gastrointestinal hyperacidity.

Neutralca-S *Desbergers, Canad.*
Aluminium hydroxide (p.1210·3); magnesium hydrox-
ide (p.1233·1).
Gastric hyperacidity; peptic ulcer.

Neutralice *Key, Austral.*
Melaleuca oil (p.1631·3); lavender oil (p.1627·2).
Pediculosis.

Neutran *Prodotti, Braz.*
Aluminium hydroxide (p.1210·3); magnesium hydrox-
ide (p.1233·1).
Gastrointestinal hyperacidity.

Neutra-Phos *Alza, USA.*
Monobasic and dibasic sodium and potassium phos-
phates (p.1193·2) (p.1193·2) (p.1193·1) (p.1193·1).
Phosphorus supplement.

Neutra-Phos-K *Alza, USA.*
Monobasic and dibasic potassium phosphates
(p.1193·1) (p.1193·1).
Phosphorus supplement.

Neutrexin
*Lilly, Canad.; US Bioscience, Denm.; Ipsen Biotech, Fr.; Schering-
Plough, Hong Kong; Ipsen, Irl.; Ipsen, Ital.; Ipsen, Spain; Swedish Or-
phan, Swed.; Schering-Plough, Thai.; Ipsen, UK; US Bioscience, USA.*
Trimetrexate glucuronate (p.576·3).
Pneumocystis carinii pneumonia.

Neutro Bar *Darier, Mex.*
Glycerol (p.1616·3).

Neutrogena
Note.This name is used for preparations of different composition.
Faulding, Austral.
Trolamine (p.1675·1).
Soap substitute.
Neutrogena, Fr.
SPF 18.5: Octinoxate (p.1517·3); avobenzone
(p.1517·1); enzacamene (p.1517·2).
Sunscreen.
Johnson & Johnson, NZ.
Skin cleanser and emollient.
Neutrogena, USA.
SPF 8: Octinoxate (p.1517·3); methyl anthranilate; ti-
tanium dioxide (p.1126·1).
SPF 15: Octinoxate (p.1517·3); octisalate (p.1518·1);
methyl anthranilate; titanium dioxide (p.1126·1).
SPF 25: Octinoxate (p.1517·3); oxybenzone
(p.1518·1); octisalate (p.1518·1).
SPF 30: Octinoxate (p.1517·3); octocrilene (p.1518·1);
methyl anthranilate; zinc oxide (p.1128·2).
Sunscreen.
Neutrogena Dermatologics, USA.
Skin cleanser; emollient and moisturiser.

Neutrogena Acne Mask
*Faulding, Austral.; Professional Health, Canad.†; Neutrogena Derma-
tologics, USA.*
Benzoyl peroxide (p.1111·1).
Acne.

Neutrogena Acne Skin Cleanser *Faulding, Austral.*
Triclosan (p.1159·2).
Acne; oily skin.

Neutrogena Anti-Acne *Johnson & Johnson, Ital.*
Topical gel: Salicylic acid (p.1122·3).
Topical solution: Chamomile (p.1593·2); aloe
(p.1210·1).
Acne.

Neutrogena Antiseptic *Neutrogena, USA.*
Skin cleanser.

Neutrogena Chemical-Free *Neutrogena, USA.*
SPF 17: Titanium dioxide (p.1126·1).
Sunscreen.

Neutrogena Drying *Neutrogena Dermatologics, USA.*
Hamamelis (p.1618·3).

Neutrogena Glow *Neutrogena, USA.*
SPF 8: Octinoxate (p.1517·3).
Sunscreen.

Neutrogena Healthy Scalp Anti-Dandruff *Professional Health, Canad.*
Salicylic acid (p.1122·3).

Neutrogena Healthy Skin *Prof. Pharm. Corp., Canad.*
SPF 15: Octinoxate (p.1517·3); oxybenzone
(p.1518·1).
Sunscreen.

Neutrogena Intensified
Prof. Pharm. Corp., Canad.; Neutrogena, USA.
SPF 15: Octinoxate (p.1517·3); ensulizole (p.1517·2);
titanium dioxide (p.1126·1).
Sunscreen.

Neutrogena Lip *Neutrogena, USA.*
SPF 15: Octinoxate (p.1517·3); oxybenzone
(p.1518·1).
Sunscreen.

Neutrogena Long Lasting Dandruff Control
Johnson & Johnson, UK†.
Ketoconazole (p.389·1).
Dandruff.

Neutrogena Moisture
Note.This name is used for preparations of different composition.
Prof. Pharm. Corp., Canad.
SPF 15: Octinoxate (p.1517·3); octisalate (p.1518·1);
oxybenzone (p.1518·1).
Sunscreen.
Neutrogena, USA.
SPF 5: Octinoxate (p.1517·3).
SPF 15: Octinoxate (p.1517·3); oxybenzone
(p.1518·1).
Sunscreen.

**Neutrogena Norwegian Formula Dermato-
logical Cream** *Neutrogena, UK.*
Glycerol (p.1616·3).
Dry skin.

Neutrogena No-Stick *Neutrogena, USA.*
Octinoxate (p.1517·3); homosalate (p.1517·2); oxy-
benzone (p.1518·1); octisalate (p.1518·1).
Sunscreen.

Neutrogena No-Stick Sunblock *Professional
Health, Canad.*
SPF 30: Octinoxate (p.1517·3); homosalate
(p.1517·2); octisalate (p.1518·1); oxybenzone
(p.1518·1).
Sunscreen.

Neutrogena Oil-Free Sunblock *Prof. Pharm. Corp.,
Canad.*
SPF 30: Homosalate (p.1517·2); octinoxate
(p.1517·3); octisalate (p.1518·1); oxybenzone
(p.1518·1).
Sunscreen.

Neutrogena On-The-Spot Acne Lotion *Profes-
sional Health, Canad.†.*
Benzoyl peroxide (p.1111·1).
Acne.

Neutrogena Sunblock *Prof. Pharm. Corp., Canad.*
SPF 30: Meradimate (p.1517·3); octocrilene
(p.1518·1); octinoxate (p.1517·3); octisalate
(p.1518·1).
Sunscreen.

Neutrogena Sunblocker *Professional Health, Canad.*
SPF 17: Titanium dioxide (p.1126·1).
Sunscreen.

Neutrogena T/Derm *Neutrogena, USA.*
Coal tar (p.1125·1).
Skin disorders.

Neutrogena T/Gel
Faulding, Austral.; Professional Health, Canad.†; Neutrogena, USA.
Coal tar (p.1125·1).
Scalp disorders.

Neutrogena T/Sal
Faulding, Austral.; Neutrogena Dermatologics, USA.
Salicylic acid (p.1122·3); coal tar (p.1125·1).
Scalp disorders; seborrhoeic dermatitis.

Neutrogena T/Scalp *Neutrogena Dermatologics, USA.*
Hydrocortisone (p.1073·3).
Pruritus of the scalp.

Neutrogin *Chugai, Jpn.*
Lenograstim (p.738·1).
Neutropenia.

Neutrolac *Bayer, Ital.*
Aluminium hydroxide (p.1210·3); calcium carbonate
(p.1215·1); magnesium trisilicate (p.1233·3).
*Gastrointestinal disorders associated with hyperacidi-
ty.*

Neutromed *Kwizda, Aust.*
Cimetidine (p.1216·3).
*Acid aspiration; gastro-oesophageal reflux; gastroin-
testinal erosions; gastrointestinal haemorrhage; peptic
ulcer; Zollinger-Ellison syndrome.*

Neutronorm
Ebewe, Aust.; Ebewe, Hong Kong.
Cimetidine (p.1216·3).
*Gastro-oesophageal reflux; gastrointestinal erosions;
gastrointestinal haemorrhage; peptic ulcer; Zollinger-
Ellison syndrome.*

Neutrose S Pellegrino *Sanofi Synthelabo, Ital.*
Calcium carbonate (p.1215·1); magnesium carbonate
(p.1232·3); kaolin (p.1229·3); magnesium trisilicate
(p.1233·3).
*Gastrointestinal disorders associated with hyperacidi-
ty.*

Neutroses
Pharmethic, Belg.; DB, Fr.; DB, Switz.
Calcium carbonate (p.1215·1); magnesium carbonate
(p.1232·3); kaolin (p.1229·3); magnesium trisilicate
(p.1233·3).
Gastrointestinal disorders.

Neu-Up *Kyowa, Jpn†.*
Nartograstim (p.739·2).
Neutropenia.

Neuvita *Fujisawa, Jpn.*
Octotiamine (p.1385·1).
Vitamin B₁ deficiency.

Neuzym *Eisai, Hong Kong; Eisai, Jpn.*
Muramidase hydrochloride (p.1638·1).
*Chronic sinusitis; haemorrhage; respiratory-tract con-
gestion.*

Neuzyme *Eisai, Singapore.*
Muramidase hydrochloride (p.1638·1).
*Haemorrhage; respiratory-tract congestion and in-
flammation; sinusitis.*

Nevacort *Finderm, Ital.*
Hydrocortisone (p.1073·3); neomycin sulfate
(p.228·1).
Bacterial vaginal infections.

Neviran *Fonten, Ital.*
Aciclovir (p.612·3).
Herpesvirus infections.

Nevralgina *Climax, Braz.*
Dipyrone (p.34·1).
Fever; pain.

Nevramin
Takeda, Hong Kong; Takeda, Singapore; Takeda, Thai.
Fursultiamine (p.1384·3) or fursultiamine hydrochloride (p.1384·3); vitamin B₆ (p.1387·1); vitamin B₁₂
(p.1388·1).
Mepivacaine hydrochloride (p.1317·1) is included in
the intramuscular injection to alleviate the pain of injection.
*Anaemias; diabetic neuropathy; myelitis; neuralgia;
neuritis; paresis; rheumatic disorders.*

Nevril
Note.This name is used for preparations of different composition.
Amnol, Ital.
Cream: Hamamelis (p.1618·3); devil's claw root;
chamomile; mallow; calendula; salix; copper; zinc;
menthol (p.1632·3).
Skin disorders.
Tosi, Ital.†.
Injection: Thiamine phosphate monochloride
(p.1385·2); hydroxocobalamin (p.1388·1).
Megaloblastic anaemia; neuralgias; neuritis.

Nevril Crono *Amnol, Ital.*
Mutivitamin and mineral preparation with plant ex-
tracts (p.1350·1).
Nutritional supplement.

Nevrine Codeine *Pharmacobel, Belg.*
Paracetamol (p.71·2); caffeine hydrate (p.761·3); co-
deine phosphate (p.25·2).
Fever; pain.

Nevrosthenine Glycocolle Freyssinge
3M, Belg.; 3M, Fr.†.
Glycine; sodium glycerophosphate; potassium glycerophosphate; magnesium glycerophosphate (p.1350·1).
Tonic.

New Acute Cold Formula *Invamed, USA†.*
Chlorpheniramine [chlorphenamine] maleate
(p.412·1); phenylpropanolamine hydrochloride
(p.1098·1); dextromethorphan hydrobromide
(p.1087·3); paracetamol (p.71·2).

New Daigaku *Santen, Singapore.*
Boric acid (p.1586·1); d-borneol; menthol (p.1632·3);
zinc sulfate (p.1398·2).
Eye irritation.

New De Witt's Pills *Fleet, Austral.†.*
Bearberry (p.1583·3); buchu (p.1587·2).
Fluid retention.

New Decongestant Pediatric *Goldline, USA†.*
Phenylpropanolamine hydrochloride (p.1098·1); phenylephrine hydrochloride (p.1097·1); chlorpheniramine [chlorphenamine] maleate (p.412·1);
phenyltoloxamine citrate (p.423·1).
Upper respiratory-tract symptoms.

New Diatabs *Biomedis, Hong Kong.*
Attapulgite (p.1212·1).
Diarrhoea.

New Era Biochemic Tissue Salts *Seven Seas, UK.*
Homoeopathic preparation.

New Era Calm & Clear *Seven Seas, UK†.*
Dibasic potassium phosphate (p.1193·1).

New Era Combination Tissue Salts *Seven Seas, UK.*
Homoeopathic preparation.

New Era Elasto *Seven Seas, UK.*
Homoeopathic preparation.

New Era Hymosa *Seven Seas, UK†.*
Ferrous phosphate; potassium chloride (p.1194·3); potassium sulfate (p.1195·1); calcium sulfate (p.1589·1); silica (p.1503·3).
Wounds.

New Era Nervone *Seven Seas, UK.*
Homoeopathic preparation.

New Era Zief *Seven Seas, UK†.*
Iron phosphate; silica (p.1503·3); sodium phosphate; sodium sulfate (p.1250·1).
Rheumatic pain.

New Gen *Roche, Ital.*
Multivitamin and mineral preparation (p.1350·1).
Nutritional supplement.

New Hands *Johnson & Johnson, Canad.*
SPF 15: Octinoxate (p.1517·3); oxybenzone (p.1518·1).
Sunscreen.

New Patecs A *Daiichi, Hong Kong.*
Arnica (p.1581·3); glycol salicylate (p.42·2).
Musculoskeletal and joint disorders.

NewAce *Bristol-Myers Squibb, Neth.*
Fosinopril sodium (p.892·3).
Heart failure; hypertension.

Newderm *Wolfs, Belg.*
Zinc oxide (p.1128·2); vitamin A (p.1382·1); vitamin D (p.1391·1); cod-liver oil (p.1357·2).
Skin irritation.

Newral *Dojin Iyaku, Jpn†.*
Neticonazole hydrochloride (p.392·2).
Fungal skin infections.

Newrelax *Potter's, UK.*
Lupulus (p.1629·3); skullcap (p.1664·3); valerian (p.1678·3); vervain (p.1679·3).
Tension.

New-Skin *Medtech, USA.*
Topical barrier preparation.

Nexen *Therabel, Fr.*
Nimesulide (p.62·3).
Musculoskeletal and joint disorders.

Nexium
AstraZeneca, Austral.; AstraZeneca, Irl.; AstraZeneca, Swed.; Astra-Zeneca, UK; AstraZeneca, USA.
Esomeprazole magnesium (p.1225·2).
Gastro-oesophageal reflux; peptic ulcer.

NeyArthros (Revitorgan-Dilutionen Nr 43) *Vitorgan, Ger.*
Articuli fet.; cartilago; synovia.
Inflammatory and degenerative joint disorders.

NeyArthros-Liposome (Revitorgan Lp Nr 83) *Vitorgan, Ger.*
Cartilago articuli; synovia; articuli fet.; thymus fet.; funicul. umbilical.; metenolone acetate; prednisolone acetate; lipid extract of cartilago articuli/synovia/articuli fet.; zinc sulfate manganese sulfate; magnesium chloride; potassium chloride; calcium chloride; columna vertebralis fet.; capsula articuli fet.; musculi fet.; gland. suprarenal.
Inflammatory and degenerative joint disorders.

NeyCalm (Revitorgan-Dilutionen Nr 98, Revitorgan-Lingual Nr 98) *Vitorgan, Ger.*
Animal tissue extract: cortex cerebri; diencephalon; epiphysis; placenta mat.
Nervous disorders.

NeyChondrin N (Revitorgan-Dilutionen N Nr 68) *Vitorgan, Ger.*
Animal tissue extracts (NeyChondrin) (p.1631·2); metenolone acetate (p.1482·2); prednisolone acetate (p.1078·1); alpha tocoferil acetate (p.1394·1); procaine hydrochloride (p.1319·1).
Muscular, neuromuscular, and joint disorders.

NeyChondrin (Revitorgan-Dilutionen Nr 68) *Vitorgan, Ger.*
Thymus fet.; hypophysis; diencephalon; medulla spinal; gland. suprarenal.; testes juv.*; hepar; pancreas; musculi; columna vertebral. fet.; articuli fet.; ren; placenta; nucleus pulp.
Muscular, neuromuscular, and joint disorders.

NeyChondrin-Tropfen (Revitorgan-Lingual Nr 68) *Vitorgan, Ger.*
Animal tissue extracts (NeyChondrin); metenolone acetate; prednisolone acetate; alpha tocoferil acetate; procaine hydrochloride.
Muscular, neuromuscular, and joint disorders.

NeyCorenar (Revitorgan-Dilutionen Nr 6) *Vitorgan, Ger.*
Cor fet.
Cardiovascular disorders.

NeyDesib (Revitorgan-Dilutionen Nr 78) *Vitorgan, Ger.*
Thymus fet.; lien fet.; lymphonodi; gland. suprarenal.
Allergies; auto-immune disorders.

Neydin-F *Vitorgan, Ger.*
Placenta mat.; ovar; cutis fet.; amnion; hepar; gland. suprarenal.; liquor amnii.
Circulatory disorders of skin and soft tissue; skin ulcers; wounds.

Neydin-M *Vitorgan, Ger.*
Placenta mat.; testes; cutis fet.; amnion; hepar; gland. suprarenal.; liquor amnii; faex.
Hypersensitivity; inflammation.

NeyDop N (Revitorgan-Dilutionen N Nr 97) *Vitorgan, Ger.*
Cortex cerebri; diencephalon; cerebellum; placenta fet.; ascorbic acid (p.1389·3); lithium chloride (p.296·2); levodopa (p.1169·2).
Central nervous system disorders.

NeyDop (Revitorgan-Dilutionen Nr 97) *Vitorgan, Ger.*
Cortex cerebri; diencephalon; cerebellum; placenat fet.
Central nervous system disorders.

NeyDop-Tropfen (Revitorgan-Lingual Nr. 97) *Vitorgan, Ger.*
Animal tissue extracts (NeyDop N); ascorbic acid; lithium chloride; levodopa.
Central nervous system disorders.

NeyFaexan (Revitorgan-Dilutionen Nr 55) *Vitorgan, Ger.*
Mucosa intestinal.; muc. vesicae urinar.; mucosa vesicae felleae; muc. nasopharyngea.
Gastrointestinal disorders.

NeyFegan (Revitorgan-Dilutionen Nr 26) *Vitorgan, Ger.*
Liver extract.
Liver disorders.

NeyGeront N (Revitorgan-Dilutionen N Nr 64) *Vitorgan, Ger.*
Animal tissue extracts (NeyGeront); heparin (p.902·1); metenolone acetate (p.1482·2); liothyronine hydrochloride; vitamins (p.1350·1); procaine hydrochloride.
Tonic.

NeyGeront (Revitorgan-Dilutionen Nr 64) *Vitorgan, Ger.*
Embryo tot.; placenta; amnion; funiculus umbilical.; cor; ren; pancreas; mucosa intestinal.; lien; thymus juv.; gland. suprarenal.; gland. parathyreoid.; testes juv.; hypophysis; diencephalon; cort. cerebri.
Tonic.

NeyGeront-Tropfen (Revitorgan-Lingual Nr 64) *Vitorgan, Ger.*
Animal tissue extracts (NeyGeront); heparin; metenolone acetate; liothyronine hydrochloride; vitamins; procaine hydrochloride.
Tonic.

NeyGeront-Vitalkapseln *Vitorgan, Ger.*
Animal tissue extracts; heparin; metenolone acetate; liothyronine hydrochloride; procaine hydrochloride; lecithin; trace elements and vitamins.
Tonic.

NeyImmun (Revitorgan-Dilutionen Nr 73) *Vitorgan, Ger.*
Placenta mat.; funiculus umbilical.; thymus juv.
Tonic.

NeyNormin N (Revitorgan-Dilutionen N Nr 65) *Vitorgan, Ger.*
Animal tissue extracts (NeyNormin); prednisolone acetate (p.1078·1); liothyronine hydrochloride (p.1524·3); estradiol benzoate (p.1473·1); chorionic gonadotrophin (p.1279·2); alpha tocoferil acetate (p.1394·1); cyanocobalamin (p.1388·1).
Allergic diathesis; insufficiency of the diencephalon-pituitary-adrenal system; intestinal disorders; rheumatism; vegetative dystonias; virus infection.

NeyNormin (Revitorgan-Dilutionen Nr 65) *Vitorgan, Ger.*
Thymus fet.; gland. suprarenal.; lymphonodi; gland. parathyreoidea; hepar; ren; pancreas; lien; vasa fet.; funiculus umbilical.; hypophysis; diencephalon; mucosae miscae; cutis; medulla ossium.
Allergic diathesis; insufficiency of the diencephalon-pituitary-adrenal system; intestinal disorders; rheumatism; vegetative dystonias; virus infection.

NeyNormin-Tropfen (Revitorgan-Lingual Nr 65) *Vitorgan, Ger.*
Animal tissue extracts (NeyNormin); prednisolone acetate; liothyronine hydrochloride; estradiol benzoate; chorionic gonadotrophin; alpha tocoferil acetate; cyanocobalamin.
Allergic diathesis; insufficiency of the diencephalon-pituitary-adrenal system; intestinal disorders; rheumatism; vegetative dystonias; viral infections.

NeyParadent-Liposome *Vitorgan, Ger.*
Protein extracts from crista dentalis, placenta, and diencephalon; metenolone acetate; alpha tocoferil acetate; procaine hydrochloride; lipid extract from crista dentalis; sodium salicylate; ascorbic acid; chamomile; arnica; myrrh; sea salt.
Mouth disorders.

NeyPsorin (Revitorgan-Dilutionen Nr 5) *Vitorgan, Ger.*
Animal skin extract.
Skin disorders.

NeyPulpin N (Revitorgan-Dilutionen N Nr 10) *Vitorgan, Ger.*
Crista dentalis; placenta; diencephalon; metenolone acetate (p.1482·2); alpha tocoferil acetate (p.1394·1); ascorbic acid (p.1389·3); procaine hydrochloride (p.1319·1).
Dental disorders.

NeyPulpin (Revitorgan-Dilutionen Nr 10) *Vitorgan, Ger.*
Crista dental. fet.; placenta; diencephalon.
Dental disorders.

Neythymun *Vitorgan, Ger.*
Thymus extract.
Allergic disorders; immunosuppressant in rheumatic disorders; immunotherapy.

NeyTroph (Revitorgan-Dilutionen Nr 96) *Vitorgan, Ger.*
Musculi juv.; musculi fet.; cor fet.; thymus; medulla spinal.; cort. cerebri; epiphysis; diencephalon.
Muscular and nervous disorders.

NeyTroph-Tropfen (Revitorgan-Lingual Nr 96) *Vitorgan, Ger.*
Musculi juv.; musculi fet.; cor fet.; thymus; medulla spinal.; cort. cerebri; epiphysis; diencephalon.
Muscular and nervous disorders.

NeyTumorin N (Revitorgan-Dilutionen N Nr 66) *Vitorgan, Ger.*
Animal tissue extracts (NeyTumorin) (p.1631·2); metenolone acetate (p.1482·2); prednisolone acetate (p.1078·1); liothyronine hydrochloride (p.1524·3); alpha tocoferil acetate (p.1394·1); cyanocobalamin (p.1388·1).
Neoplasms.

NeyTumorin (Revitorgan-Dilutionen Nr 66) *Vitorgan, Ger.*
Diencephalon; placenta mat.; funiculus umbilical.; thymus juv.; epiphysis; testes juv.; gland. suprarenal.; gland. thyreoidea; medulla ossium; pulmo; hepar; pancreas; ren; lien; mucosa intestinal.
Neoplasms.

NeyTumorin-Tropfen (Revitorgan-Lingual Nr 66) *Vitorgan, Ger.*
Animal tissue extracts (NeyTumorin) (p.1631·2); metenolone acetate; prednisolone acetate; liothyronine hydrochloride; alpha tocoferil acetate; cyanocobalamin.
Neoplasms.

Nezeril
Astra, Denm.†; AstraZeneca, Fin.; Astra, Hong Kong; Draco, Swed.
Oxymetazoline hydrochloride (p.1096·2).
Nasal congestion; rhinitis; sinusitis.

NF Cough Syrup with Codeine *Technilab, Canad.*
Pseudoephedrine hydrochloride (p.1099·2); codeine phosphate (p.25·2); guaifenesin (p.1092·2).

NGT *Geneva, USA.*
Triamcinolone acetonide (p.1080·1); nystatin (p.392·2).
Skin disorders.

Nia *Novo Nordisk, Aust.*
Megestrol acetate (p.1481·2).
Breast cancer; endometrial cancer.

Nia-Bid *Roberts, USA†; Hauck, USA†.*
Nicotinic acid (p.1372·3).
Hyperlipidaemia (adjunct); nicotinic acid deficiency; pellagra.

Niacel *Medifarma, Mex.*
Metronidazole (p.594·1).

Niacels *Roberts, USA†.*
Nicotinic acid (p.1372·3).
Hyperlipidaemia (adjunct); nicotinic acid deficiency; pellagra.

Niacor *Upsher-Smith, USA.*
Nicotinic acid (p.1372·3).
Hyperlipidaemia (adjunct); nicotinic acid deficiency; pellagra.

Nialen *Novag, Spain.*
Ibuproxam (p.44·3).
Musculoskeletal, joint, peri-articular, and soft-tissue disorders; pain.

Niamid *Roerig, Belg.†*
Nialamide (p.301·3).
Depression.

Niar *Knoll, Braz.; Knoll, Mex.*
Selegiline hydrochloride (p.1177·2).
Parkinsonism.

Niaspan *KOS, USA.*
Nicotinic acid (p.1372·3).
Hyperlipidaemias.

Nibiol *Debat, Fr.*
Nitroxoline (p.231·3).
Bacterial infections of the urinary tract.

Nicabate
SmithKline Beecham Consumer, Austral.; SmithKline Beecham, NZ.
Nicotine (p.1640·3).
Aid to smoking withdrawal.

Nican *Uhlmann-Eyraud, Switz.*
Codeine (p.25·2); belladonna (p.463·1); drosera (p.1606·1); grindelia (p.1618·2); plantaginis; thyme (p.1672·2); sodium benzoate (p.1134·3).
Coughs.

Nicangin *Astra, Swed.*
Nicotinic acid (p.1372·3).
Hyperlipidaemias.

Nicant *Piam, Ital.*
Nicardipine hydrochloride (p.938·3).
Angina pectoris; heart failure; hypertension.

Nicaphlogyl *Vifor, Switz.*
Propyphenazone (p.80·2); ethenzamide (p.35·1).
Inflammation; pain.

Nicapress *Benedetti, Ital.*
Nicardipine hydrochloride (p.938·3).
Angina pectoris; heart failure; hypertension.

Nicardal *Italfarmaco, Ital.*
Nicardipine hydrochloride (p.938·3).
Angina pectoris; heart failure; hypertension.

Nicardium *Drug Research, Ital.*
Nicardipine hydrochloride (p.938·3).
Angina pectoris; heart failure; hypertension.

Nicarpin *San Carlo, Ital.*
Nicardipine hydrochloride (p.938·3).
Hypertension; ischaemic heart disease.

N'ice *SmithKline Beecham Consumer, USA.*
Lozenges: Menthol (p.1632·3).
Throat spray: Menthol (p.1632·3); glycerol (p.1616·3).
Sore throat.

N'ice 'n Clear *SmithKline Beecham Consumer, USA.*
Menthol (p.1632·3).

N'ice Vitamin C *SmithKline Beecham Consumer, USA.*
Ascorbic acid (p.1389·3).
Scurvy; vitamin C deficiency.

Nicef *Galen, UK.*
Cefradine (p.173·3).
Bacterial infections.

Nicene *Adcock Ingram, S.Afr.†.*
Nitroxoline (p.231·3); sulfamethizole (p.253·3); pyridoxine hydrochloride (p.1386·3).
Urinary-tract infections.

Nicene N *Adcock Ingram, S.Afr.*
Nitroxoline (p.231·3).
Urinary-tract infections.

Nicer *Ist. Chim. Inter., Ital.*
Nicergoline (p.1640·2).
Cerebrovascular disorders.

Nicergobeta *Betapharm, Ger.*
Nicergoline (p.1640·2).
Mental function disorders.

Nicerium *Hexal, Ger.*
Nicergoline (p.1640·2).
Cerebrovascular disorders.

Nicetile *Sigma-Tau, Ital.*
Acetylcarnitine hydrochloride (p.1572·1).
Cerebrovascular disorders; nerve disorders.

Nicholin *Wyeth Lederle, Ital.; Takeda, Jpn.*
Citicoline (p.1596·1).
Cerebrovascular disorders; pancreatitis; parkinsonism.

Nicizina *Pharmacia Upjohn, Ital.*
Isoniazid (p.215·3).
Tuberculosis.

Niclosan *Pharmasant, Thai.*
Niclosamide (p.104·2).
Diphyllobothriasis; hymenolepiasis; taeniasis.

Nico-400 *Jones, USA†.*
Nicotinic acid (p.1372·3).
Hyperlipidaemia (adjunct); nicotinic acid deficiency; pellagra.

Nico Hepatocyn *Uriach, Spain.*
Cynara (p.1601·3); aloes (p.1210·1); boldo (p.1585·3); cascara (p.1216·1).
Constipation.

Nicobid *Rhone-Poulenc Rorer, Hong Kong.*
Nicotinic acid (p.1372·3).
Hyperlipidaemias; nicotinic acid supplement.

Nicobid Tempules *Rorer, USA†.*
Nicotinic acid (p.1372·3).
Hyperlipidaemia (adjunct); nicotinic acid deficiency; pellagra.

Nicobion *AstraZeneca, Fr.; Merck, Ger.*
Nicotinamide (p.1372·3).
Nicotinamide deficiency; pellagra.

Nicobrevin *Pro-Health, NZ; Cedar Health, UK.*
Menthyl valerate; quinine (p.445·1); camphor (p.1589·3); eucalyptus oil (p.1609·2).
Aid to smoking withdrawal.

Nicodan *Wernigerode, Ger.*
Propyl nicotinate (p.80·2).
Musculoskeletal and joint pain; neuralgia; peripheral circulatory disorders.

Nicodan N *Wernigerode, Ger.*
Propyl nicotinate (p.80·2).
Musculoskeletal and joint pain; neuralgia; peripheral circulatory disorders.

Nicodent *Nicodent, Austral.†.*
Sodium monofluorophosphate (p.1377·2).
Dentifrice.

Nicoderm
Hoechst Marion Roussel, Canad.; SmithKline Beecham Consumer, USA.
Nicotine (p.1640·3).
Aid to smoking withdrawal.

Nicodisc *Lacer, Spain†.*
Nicotine (p.1640·3).
Aid to smoking withdrawal.

Nicogum *Pierre Fabre, Fr.*
Nicotine (p.1640·3).
Aid to smoking withdrawal.

Nicojuvel *Basi, Port.*
Tocoferil nicotinate (p.984·3).

Nicolan
Pharmacia Upjohn, Aust.; Biosintetica, Braz.; Meda, Swed.†.
Nicotine (p.1640·3).
Aid to smoking withdrawal.

Nicolar *Rhone-Poulenc Rorer, USA†.*
Nicotinic acid (p.1372·3).
Hyperlipidaemia (adjunct); nicotinic acid deficiency; pellagra.

Nicolip *Hennig, Ger.*
Inositol nicotinate (p.914·1).
Hyperlipidaemias.

Nicolmycetin *Unison, Thai.*
Chloramphenicol (p.179·1).
Bacterial infections.

The symbol † denotes a preparation no longer actively marketed

Nicolsint *Epifarma, Ital.*
Citicoline (p.1596·1).
Cerebrovascular disorders; parkinsonism.

Nicomax *Pensa, Spain.*
Nicotine (p.1640·3) or nicotine polacrilex (p.1641·3).
Aid to smoking withdrawal.

Niconil
Elan, Irl.; Elan, UK†.
Nicotine (p.1640·3).
Aid to smoking withdrawal.

Nicopatch *Pierre Fabre Sante, Fr.*
Nicotine (p.1640·3).
Aid to smoking withdrawal.

Nicopaverina *Enila, Braz.*
Nicotinic acid (p.1372·3); papaverine (p.1648·1).
Vasodilator.

Nicopaverina B6 *Enila, Braz.*
Nicotinic acid (p.1372·3); papaverine (p.1648·1); vitamin B_6 (p.1387·1).
Vasodilator.

Nicoprive
Note. This name is used for preparations of different composition.
Theranol-Deglaude, Fr.
Ascorbic acid (p.1389·3); crataegus (p.1600·2); vitamin B substances (p.1350·1).
Formerly contained quinine ascorbate, crataegus, and vitamins.
Aid to smoking withdrawal.

IFI, Ital.
Quinine ascorbate (p.1657·1); vitamins (p.1350·1); crataegus (p.1600·2).
Aid to smoking withdrawal.

Nicorette
Pharmacia Upjohn, Aust.; Pharmacia Upjohn, Austral.; Pharmacia Upjohn, Belg.; Hoechst Marion Roussel, Canad.; Pharmacia Upjohn, Denm.; Pharmacia Upjohn, Fin.; Pharmacia Upjohn, Fr.; Pharmacia Upjohn, Ger.; Pharmacia Upjohn, Hong Kong; Pharmacia Upjohn, Irl.; Pharmacia Upjohn, Israel; Carlo Erba OTC, Ital.; Hoechst Marion Roussel, Mex.; Pharmacia Upjohn, Neth.; Pharmacia Upjohn, Norw.; Pharmacia Upjohn, NZ; Pharmacia Upjohn, Port.; Pharmacia Upjohn, S.Afr.; Pharmacia Upjohn, Singapore; Pharmacia Upjohn, Spain; Pharmacia Upjohn, Swed.; Pharmacia Upjohn, Switz.; Pharmacia Upjohn, Thai.; Pharmacia, UK; SmithKline Beecham Consumer, USA.
Nicotine (p.1640·3), nicotine betadex (p.1640·3), or nicotine resin complex (p.1641·3).
Aid to smoking withdrawal.

Nicostop TTS *Drossapharm, Switz.†.*
Nicotine (p.1640·3).
Aid to smoking withdrawal.

Nicotibine *Aventis, Belg.*
Isoniazid (p.215·3).
Tuberculosis.

Nicotinell
Novartis Consumer, Aust.; Novartis Consumer, Austral.; Novartis Consumer, Belg.; Novartis, Denm.; Novartis, Fin.; Novartis Sante, Fr.; Novartis Consumer, Ger.; Novartis, Hong Kong; Novartis Consumer, Irl.; Novartis, Israel; Novartis Consumer, Neth.; Novartis, Norw.; Novartis, NZ; Novartis Nutrition, Singapore; Novartis Consumer, Spain; Novartis, Swed.; Novartis, Switz.; Novartis, Thai.; Novartis Consumer, UK.
Nicotine (p.1640·3), nicotine resin complex (p.1641·3), or nicotine tartrate (p.1641·3).
Aid to smoking withdrawal.

Nicotinell TTS
Novartis, Braz.; Novartis Consumer, Ital.; Novartis, Mex.; Novartis Consumer, Port.; Novartis Consumer, S.Afr.
Nicotine (p.1640·3).
Aid to smoking withdrawal.

Nicotinex *Fleming, USA.*
Nicotinic acid (p.1372·3).
Hyperlipidaemia (adjunct); nicotinic acid deficiency; pellagra.

Nicotinoid *Valdecasas, Mex.*
Nicotinamide (p.1372·3).

Nicotrans
Recordati, Ital.†; Pharmacia Upjohn, Spain†.
Nicotine (p.1640·3).
Aid to smoking withdrawal.

Nicotrol
Pharmacia Upjohn, Aust.; Johnson & Johnson, Canad.; Pharmacia Upjohn, Spain; McNeil Consumer, USA.
Nicotine (p.1640·3).
Aid to smoking withdrawal.

Nico-Vert *Edwards, USA†.*
Meclozine (p.420·3).
Formerly contained dimenhydrinate.
Motion sickness.

Nicovitol *Lannacher, Aust.*
Nicotinamide (p.1372·3).
Nicotinamide deficiency.

Nicozid *Piam, Ital.*
Isoniazid (p.215·3).
Tuberculosis.

NidaGel *3M, Canad.*
Metronidazole (p.594·1).
Bacterial vaginosis.

Nidal *Zerboni, Mex.*
Chlormadinone (p.1465·3).

Nidal AR *Nestle, Fr.*
Infant feed (p.1350·1).
Regurgitation in infants.

Nidal HA *Nestle, Fr.*
Infant feed (p.1350·1).
Potential hypersensitivity to cows milk.

Nidatron *Propan, S.Afr.†.*
Metronidazole (p.594·1).
Amoebiasis; anaerobic bacterial infections; giardiasis; trichomoniasis.

Nidazolem *Lemery, Mex.*
Metronidazole (p.594·1).

Nidazolin *Bunker, Braz.*
Nystatin (p.392·2).
Fungal infections.

Nide *Ibirn, Ital.*
Nimesulide (p.62·3).
Fever; inflammation; pain.

Nidex *Nestle, Ital.*
Maltodextrin (p.1371·2).
Nutritional supplement.

Nidina Confort *Nestle, Ital.*
Infant feed (p.1350·1).
Regurgitation.

Nidina HA
Nestle, Ital.; Nestle, Port.
Infant feed (p.1350·1).
Food hypersensitivity.

Nidina probiotico *Nestle, Ital.*
Infant feed (p.1350·1).
Gastrointestinal disorders.

Nidol
Eurodrug, Hong Kong; Damor, Ital.†; Eurodrug, Thai.
Nimesulide (p.62·3).
Fever; inflammation; pain.

Nidralon *Liferpal, Mex.*
Metronidazole (p.594·1).
Protozoal infections.

Nidran *Sankyo, Jpn.*
Nimustine hydrochloride (p.562·3).
Malignant neoplasms.

Nidrel *Schwarz, Fr.*
Nitrendipine (p.947·1).
Hypertension.

Nidrozol *Fustery, Mex.*
Metronidazole (p.594·1) or metronidazole benzoate (p.594·1).
Amoebiasis; giardiasis; trichomoniasis.

Nieral *Schuck, Ger.*
Solidago virgaurea.
Urinary-tract infections.

Nierano HM *Pfluger, Ger.*
Homoeopathic preparation.

Nieren-Elixier ST *Cosmochema, Ger.*
Homoeopathic preparation.

Nierentee *Smetana, Aust.*
Ononis (p.1644·1); equisetum (p.1606·3); herb. polygonii.
Urinary-tract disorders.

Nierentee 2000 *Sanofi Synthelabo, Ger.*
Birch leaf (p.1585·2); java tea (p.1625·1); juniper berry oil (p.1625·2); fennel oil (p.1610·2).
Urinary-tract disorders.

Nieron Blasen- und Nieren-Tee VI *Hoyer, Ger.*
Birch leaf (p.1585·2); java tea (p.1625·1); solidago virgaurea; peppermint leaf (p.1243·2); liquorice root (p.1231·2); ononis (p.1644·1).
Urinary-tract disorders.

Nieron S *Hoyer, Ger.*
Solidago virgaurea; taraxacum (p.1669·1).
Urinary-tract disorders.

Nieron-Tee N *Hoyer, Ger.*
Birch leaf (p.1585·2); equisetum (p.1606·3); taraxacum (p.1669·1); ononis (p.1644·1).
Urinary-tract disorders.

Nieroxin N *Hoyer, Ger.*
Maté leaf (p.1681·1); solidago virgaurea; juniper oil (p.1625·2).
Urinary-tract disorders.

Nifangin *Orion, Fin.*
Nifedipine (p.940·1).
Angina pectoris; hypertension; Raynaud's syndrome.

Nif-Atenil *Ecosol, Switz.*
Atenolol (p.841·3); nifedipine (p.940·1).
Hypertension.

Nifatenol *Hexal, Ger.*
Atenolol (p.841·3); nifedipine (p.940·1).
Hypertension.

Nifdemin *Medinovum, Fin.*
Nifedipine (p.940·1).
Angina pectoris; hypertension; Raynaud's syndrome.

Nife *CT, Ger.; ABZ, Ger.; BASF, Ger.; Isis Puren, Ger.; Wolff, Ger.*
Nifedipine (p.940·1).
Angina pectoris; hypertension; Raynaud's syndrome.

nife uno *CT, Ger.*
Nifedipine (p.940·1).
Hypertension.

nife-basan *Schonenberger, Switz.*
Nifedipine (p.940·1).
Hypertension; ischaemic heart disease.

Nifebene *Ratiopharm, Aust.*
Nifedipine (p.940·1).
Angina pectoris; hypertension; Raynaud's syndrome.

Nifecard
Asta Medica, Aust.; Sigma, Austral.; Lek, Hong Kong; Lek, Thai.
Nifedipine (p.940·1).
Angina pectoris; cardiomyopathy; heart failure; hypertension; pulmonary hypertension; Raynaud's syndrome.

Nifeclair *Hennig, Ger.*
Nifedipine (p.940·1).
Angina pectoris; hypertension; Raynaud's syndrome.

Nifecodan *Pharmacodane, Denm.*
Nifedipine (p.940·1).
Angina pectoris; hypertension; Raynaud syndrome.

Nifecor
Pharmacia Upjohn, Fin.; Betapharm, Ger.
Nifedipine (p.940·1).
Angina pectoris; hypertension; Raynaud's syndrome.

Nifed *Rowex, Irl.*
Nifedipine (p.940·1).
Angina pectoris; hypertension.

Nifedalat *Hexal, S.Afr.*
Nifedipine (p.940·1).
Angina pectoris; hypertension; Raynaud's syndrome.

Nifedate *Euro-Labor, Port.*
Nifedipine (p.940·1).
Hypertension; ischaemic heart disease; Raynaud's syndrome.

Nifedical *Teva, USA.*
Nifedipine (p.940·1).
Hypertension.

Nifedicor
Searle, Ital.; Streuli, Switz.
Nifedipine (p.940·1).
Hypertension; ischaemic heart disease; Raynaud's syndrome.

Nifedicron *Searle, Ital.*
Nifedipine (p.940·1).
Hypertension; ischaemic heart disease.

Nifedi-Denk *Denk, Singapore.*
Nifedipine (p.940·1).
Hypertension; ischaemic heart disease; Raynaud's syndrome.

Nifedigel *Pharmacaps, Mex.*
Nifedipine (p.940·1).

Nifedin *Benedetti, Ital.*
Nifedipine (p.940·1).
Hypertension; ischaemic heart disease; Raynaud's syndrome.

Nifedipat *Azupharma, Ger.*
Nifedipine (p.940·1).
Angina pectoris; hypertension.

Nifedipat uno *Azupharma, Ger.*
Nifedipine (p.940·1).
Angina pectoris; hypertension.

Nifedipres *Cryopharma, Mex.*
Nifedipine (p.940·1).
Angina pectoris; heart failure; hypertension.

Nifedipress *Berk, UK.*
Nifedipine (p.940·1).
Angina pectoris; hypertension.

Nifedotard *Bartholomew Rhodes, UK†.*
Nifedipine (p.940·1).
Angina pectoris; hypertension.

Nifehexal
Hexal, Aust.; Hexal, Austral.; Hexal, Ger.
Nifedipine (p.940·1).
Angina pectoris; hypertension; Raynaud's syndrome.

Nifehexal Sali *Hexal, Ger.†.*
Nifedipine (p.940·1); mefruside (p.926·1).
Hypertension.

Nifelat
Note. This name is used for preparations of different composition.
Biosintetica, Braz.
Nifedipine (p.940·1); atenolol (p.841·3).
Angina pectoris; hypertension.

TAD, Ger.; Remedica, Singapore; Remedica, Thai.
Nifedipine (p.940·1).
Angina pectoris; hypertension; Raynaud's syndrome.

Nifelease
Pinewood, Irl.; Lennon, UK†.
Nifedipine (p.940·1).
Angina pectoris; hypertension.

Nifensar *Rhone-Poulenc Rorer, Irl.†.*
Nifedipine (p.940·1).
Angina pectoris; hypertension.

Niferex
Landmark, Canad.; Tillomed, UK; Schwarz, USA.
Polysaccharide-iron complex (p.1374·3).
Iron-deficiency anaemia.

Niferex Daily *Schwarz, USA.*
Multivitamin and mineral preparation (p.1350·1).

Niferex Forte *Schwarz, USA.*
Polysaccharide-iron complex (p.1374·3); folic acid (p.1361·1); cyanocobalamin (p.1388·1).
Iron-deficiency anaemia; megaloblastic anaemia.

Niferex with Vitamin C *Schwarz, USA†.*
Polysaccharide-iron complex (p.1374·3).
Vitamin C (p.1389·3) is included in this preparation to increase the absorption and availability of iron.
Iron-deficiency anaemias.

Niferex-PN *Schwarz, USA.*
Multivitamin and mineral preparation with iron and folic acid (p.1350·1).

Nifesal *Salus, Ital.*
Nifedipine (p.940·1).
Angina pectoris; hypertension.

Nifetex *BPRL, Singapore.*
Atenolol (p.841·3); nifedipine (p.940·1).
Angina pectoris; hypertension.

Nifezzard *Pizzard, Mex.*
Nifedipine (p.940·1).
Angina pectoris; hypertension.

Nifical *Lichtenstein, Ger.*
Nifedipine (p.940·1).
Angina pectoris; hypertension; Raynaud's syndrome.

Nificard *Ranbaxy, Thai.*
Nifedipine (p.940·1).
Angina pectoris; hypertension; myocardial infarction.

Nifidine *Rolab, S.Afr.*
Nifedipine (p.940·1).
Angina pectoris.

Nifint
Ratiopharm, Aust.; Merckle, Ger.
Menthol (p.1632·3).
Upper respiratory-tract catarrh.

Niflactol *Upsamedica, Spain.*
Morniflumate (p.56·1) or niflumic acid (p.62·3).
Musculoskeletal, joint, peri-articular, and soft-tissue disorders; pain.

Niflam *Upsamedica, Ital.*
Capsules; cream; topical gel: Niflumic acid (p.62·3).
Suppositories: Morniflumate (p.56·1).
Inflammation; pain.

Niflan *Yoshitomi, Jpn†; Senju, Jpn†.*
Pranoprofen (p.80·1).
Fever; inflammation; pain.

Niflugel
Upsamedica, Belg.; UPSA, Fr.; Upsamedica, Switz.
Niflumic acid (p.62·3).
Musculoskeletal, joint, peri-articular and soft-tissue disorders.

Nifluril
Note. This name is used for preparations of different composition.
Upsamedica, Belg.; UPSA, Fr.; UPSA, Hong Kong; Bristol-Myers Squibb, Port.; Upsamedica, Switz.
Capsules; ointment: Niflumic acid (p.62·3).
Inflammation; musculoskeletal, joint, peri-articular, and soft-tissue disorders; pain.

UPSA, Fr.†; Bristol-Myers Squibb, Port.†.
Dental gel: Niflumic acid glycinamide (p.62·3); hexetidine (p.1146·3).
Gingivitis; inflammatory mouth disorders.

UPSA, Fr.; Upsamedica, Switz.
Suppositories: Morniflumate (p.56·1).
Inflammation; musculoskeletal, joint, and peri-articular disorders; pain.

Niflux *Alter, Port.*
Carbocisteine (p.1086·3); sobrerol (p.1100·3).
Respiratory-tract congestion.

Nifopress *Goldshield, UK.*
Nifedipine (p.940·1).
Angina pectoris; hypertension; Raynaud's syndrome.

Nifreal *Realpharma, Ger.†.*
Nifedipine (p.940·1).
Hypertension; ischaemic heart disease; Raynaud's syndrome.

Nif-Ten
Zeneca, Aust.; AstraZeneca, Fin.; Zeneca, Ger.; Zeneca, Hong Kong; Zeneca, Irl.; Zeneca, Ital.; Zeneca, Neth.; AstraZeneca, Singapore; Zeneca, Switz.
Atenolol (p.841·3); nifedipine (p.940·1).
Angina pectoris; hypertension.

Nifucin *Apogepha, Ger.†.*
Topical gel: Nitrofurazone (p.231·3).
Burns; wounds.
Topical liquid: Nitrofurazone (p.231·3); propipocaine hydrochloride (p.1319·3).
Bacterial skin infections; burns.

Nifur *Lafon, Fr.*
Nifuroxazide (p.230·2).
Now known as Nifuroxazide-Ratiopharm.
Diarrhoea.

Nifuran
Note. This name is used for preparations of different composition.
Jenapharm, Ger.
Furazolidone (p.592·1).
Vaginal infections.

Bamford, NZ.
Nitrofurantoin (p.230·3).
Urinary-tract infections.

Nifurantin *Apogepha, Ger.*
Nitrofurantoin (p.230·3).
Urinary-tract infections.

Nifurantin B 6 *Apogepha, Ger.*
Nitrofurantoin (p.230·3); pyridoxine hydrochloride (p.1386·3).
Urinary-tract infections.

Nifuretten *Apogepha, Ger.*
Nitrofurantoin (p.230·3).
Urinary-tract infections.

Nifurol *Reuffer, Mex.*
Nitrofurazone (p.231·3).

Nigersan *Sanum-Kehlbeck, Ger.*
Homoeopathic preparation.

Night Cold Comfort *Boots, UK.*
Paracetamol (p.71·2); pseudoephedrine hydrochloride (p.1099·2); diphenhydramine hydrochloride (p.416·1); pholcodine (p.1099·1).
Cold symptoms.

Night Leg Cramp Relief *Invamed, USA†.*
Quinine sulfate (p.445·1).

Night Nurse
SmithKline Beecham Consumer, Irl.; SmithKline Beecham Consumer, UK.
Paracetamol (p.71·2); promethazine hydrochloride (p.423·2); dextromethorphan hydrobromide (p.1087·3).
Cold and influenza symptoms.

Night Time *Healthcrafts, UK.*
Valerian (p.1678·3); lupulus (p.1629·3); passion flower (p.1649·1).
Sleep disturbances.

Night Time Cold/Flu Relief *Prometic, USA.*
Doxylamine succinate (p.417·1); dextromethorphan hydrobromide (p.1087·3); paracetamol (p.71·2); pseudoephedrine hydrochloride (p.1099·2).
Coughs and cold symptoms.

Nightcalm *Galpharm, UK.*
Diphenhydramine hydrochloride (p.416·1).
Insomnia.

Night-Care *CT, Ger.†.*
Pumilio pine oil (p.1656·3); thyme oil (p.1672·3); eucalyptus oil (p.1609·2); menthol (p.1632·3).
Catarrh.

Night-Time *WestCan, Canad.*
Pseudoephedrine hydrochloride (p.1099·2); menthol (p.1632·3).

Nighttime Cold & Flu *Stanley, Canad.*
Pseudoephedrine hydrochloride (p.1099·2); doxylamine succinate (p.417·1); dextromethorphan hydrobromide (p.1087·3); paracetamol (p.71·2).

Night-Time Effervescent Cold *Goldline, USA†.*
Phenylpropanolamine hydrochloride (p.1098·1); diphenhydramine citrate (p.416·1); aspirin (p.14·2).
Upper respiratory-tract symptoms.

Nighttime Pamprin *Chattem, USA.*
Diphenhydramine hydrochloride (p.416·1); paracetamol (p.71·2).
Insomnia.

NightTime Theraflu *Novartis, USA.*
Paracetamol (p.71·2); dextromethorphan hydrobromide (p.1087·3); pseudoephedrine hydrochloride (p.1099·2); chlorpheniramine [chlorphenamine] maleate (p.412·1).
Coughs and cold symptoms.

Nigrantyl *Lacteol du Dr Boucard, Fr.*
Black currant (p.1389·3); sodium citrate (p.1186·2).
Capillary fragility.

Nigroids *Ernest Jackson, UK.*
Liquorice (p.1231·2); menthol (p.1632·3).

Nikarin *TO-Chemicals, Thai.*
Miconazole nitrate (p.391·1).
Candidiasis.

Nikkho Vac *Nikkho, Braz.*
Allergen extracts (airborne proteins, food proteins, and respiratory-tract bacterial antigens) (p.1575·3).
Hyposensitisation.

Niklod *Savio, Ital.*
Disodium clodronate (p.751·2).
Hyperparathyroidism; multiple myeloma; osteolysis of malignancy; osteoporosis.

nikofrenon *Hefa, Ger.*
Nicotine (p.1640·3).
Aid to smoking withdrawal.

Nikorazol *Mavi, Mex.*
Ketoconazole (p.389·1).

Nikoril *Medinfar, Port.*
Nicorandil (p.939·2).
Angina pectoris.

Nikotugg *ACO, Swed.*
Nicotine resin (p.1641·3).
Aid to smoking withdrawal.

Nilandron *Hoechst Marion Roussel, USA.*
Nilutamide (p.562·3).
Prostatic cancer.

Nilcid *Abbott, Mex.*
Magaldrate (p.1232·2); simeticone (p.1249·2).
Gastrointestinal disorders.

Nilcid-MPS *Abbott, Hong Kong.*
Magaldrate (p.1232·2); simeticone (p.1249·2).
Flatulence; gastrointestinal hyperacidity; heartburn.

Nilevar *Laphal, Fr.*
Norethandrolone (p.1485·1).
Medullary aplasia.

Nilken *Kener, Mex.*
Buphenine hydrochloride (p.1587·3).

NilnOcen *Zeppenfeldt, Ger.*
Paracetamol (p.71·2).
Fever; pain.

Nilodor *Cussons, UK.*
A deodorant liquid for use with colostomies and ileostomies.

Nilstat *Wyeth-Ayerst, Austral.; Wyeth Lederle, Belg.; Technilab, Canad.; Wyeth, NZ; Lederle, USA.*
Nystatin (p.392·2).
Candidiasis.

Nimaz *EG, Fr.*
Loperamide hydrochloride (p.1231·3).
Diarrhoea.

Nimbex
Glaxo Wellcome, Aust.; Glaxo Wellcome, Austral.; Glaxo Wellcome, Belg.; Glaxo Wellcome, Canad.; Glaxo Wellcome, Denm.; Glaxo Wellcome, Fin.; Glaxo Wellcome, Fr.; Glaxo Wellcome, Ger.; Zeneca, Glaxo Wellcome, Hong Kong; Wellcome, Irl.; Glaxo Wellcome, Ital.; Glaxo Wellcome, Mex.; Glaxo Wellcome, Neth.; Glaxo Wellcome, Norw.; Wellcome, Port.; Glaxo Wellcome, S.Afr.; Glaxo Wellcome, Spain; Glaxo Wellcome, Swed.; Glaxo Wellcome, Switz.; Glaxo Wellcome, Thai.; Glaxo Wellcome, UK; Glaxo Wellcome, USA.
Cisatracurium besilate (p.1333·1).
Competitive neuromuscular blocker.

Nimbisan *Solvay, Ital.†.*
Brotizolam (p.657·2).
Insomnia.

Nimbus
Marco, Austral.; Biomerica, USA.
Pregnancy test (p.1654·3).

Nimed
Rhone-Poulenc Rorer, Fin.; Rhone-Poulenc Rorer, Port.
Nimesulide (p.62·3).
Fever; inflammation; pain.

Nimedex *Italfarmaco, Ital.*
Nimesulide betadex (p.62·3).
Fever; inflammation; pain.

Nimegen *Dong, Singapore.*
Isotretinoin (p.1115·3).
Acne.

Nimesil *Lusofarmaco, Ital.*
Nimesulide (p.62·3).
Fever; inflammation; pain.

Nimesulene *Guidotti, Ital.*
Nimesulide (p.62·3).
Fever; inflammation; pain.

Nimexan *Angelini, Ital.*
Nimesulide (p.62·3).
Fever; inflammation; pain.

Nimicon *Precimex, Mex.*
Miconazole (p.391·1).

Nimicor *Formenti, Ital.*
Nicardipine hydrochloride (p.938·3).
Angina pectoris; heart failure; hypertension.

Nimodrel *Opus, UK.*
Nifedipine (p.940·1).
Angina pectoris; hypertension.

Nimopect *Hevert, Ger.*
Thyme (p.1672·2).
Bronchitis; catarrh; coughs.

Nimotop
Bayer, Aust.; Bayer, Austral.; Bayer, Belg.; Bayer, Braz.; Bayer, Canad.; Bayer, Denm.; Bayer, Fin.; Bayer, Fr.; Bayer, Ger.; Bayer, Hong Kong; Bayer, Irl.; Bayer, Israel; Bayer, Ital.; Bayer, Mex.; Bayer, Neth.; Bayer, Norw.; Bayer, NZ; Bayer, Port.; Bayer, S.Afr.; Bayer, Singapore; Bayer, Spain; Bayer, Swed.; Bayer, Switz.; Bayer, Thai.; Bayer, UK; Bayer, USA.
Nimodipine (p.946·1).
Cerebral disorders in the elderly; neurological deficit following cerebral vasospasm or subarachnoid haemorrhage.

Nims *Caber, Ital.*
Nimesulide (p.62·3).
Fever; inflammation; pain.

Nina *Medichemie, Switz.*
Paracetamol (p.71·2).
Fever; pain.

Nina cum Diphenhydramino *Medichemie, Switz.†.*
Paracetamol (p.71·2); diphenhydramine hydrochloride (p.416·1).
Fever; pain.

Ninazol *TO-Chemicals, Thai.*
Ketoconazole (p.389·1).
Fungal infections.

Nindaxa *Ashbourne, UK.*
Indapamide (p.913·1).

Nine Rubbing Oils *Potter's, UK.*
Amber oil; clove oil (p.1597·1); eucalyptus oil (p.1609·2); linseed oil (p.1629·1); methyl salicylate (p.55·1); volatile mustard oil (p.1639·1); turpentine oil (p.1676·3); thyme oil (p.1672·3); peppermint oil (p.1243·3).
Musculoskeletal, joint, and soft-tissue disorders.

Ninlium *Chinta, Thai.*
Domperidone (p.1224·1).
Delayed gastric emptying; dyspepsia; nausea and vomiting.

Ni-No-Fluid N *Hotz, Ger.†.*
Peppermint oil (p.1243·3).
Cold symptoms; gastrointestinal disorders.

Niocitran *Novartis Consumer, Belg.*
Paracetamol (p.71·2); pseudoephedrine hydrochloride (p.1099·2).
Cold symptoms.

Niong retard *Rhone-Poulenc Rorer, Switz.*
Glyceryl trinitrate (p.897·3).
Angina pectoris; heart failure.

Niopam
E. Merck, Irl.; E. Merck, UK.
Iopamidol (p.1035·2).
Radiographic contrast medium.

Niotal *Sanofi Synthelabo, Ital.*
Zolpidem tartrate (p.712·2).
Insomnia.

Nipactrin *Heralds, Braz.*
Sulfamethoxypyridazine (p.256·1); nitrofurantoin (p.230·3); pyridine.
Urinary-tract infections.

Nipaxon *Pharmacia Upjohn, Swed.*
Noscapine (p.1096·1).
Coughs.

Nipent
Wyeth Lederle, Fr.; Lederle, Ger.; Parke, Davis, Ital.; Wyeth Lederle, Port.; Parke, Davis, Spain; Wyeth, UK; Supergen, USA.
Pentostatin (p.564·3).
Hairy-cell leukaemia.

Nipin *Lisapharma, Ital.*
Nifedipine (p.940·1).
Angina pectoris; hypertension.

Nipolept
Ebewe, Aust.; Rhone-Poulenc Rorer, Ger.
Zotepine (p.713·3).
Schizophrenia.

Nipride
Roche, Braz.; Roche, Canad.; Roche, Irl.; Roche, Israel; Roche, Neth.†; Roche, Swed.†.
Sodium nitroprusside (p.971·1).
Controlled hypotension; ergotamine intoxication; heart failure; hypertensive crisis.

Niprina *Pensa, Spain.*
Nitrendipine (p.947·1).
Angina pectoris; hypertension; Raynaud's syndrome.

Niprus *Schwarz, Israel.*
Sodium nitroprusside (p.971·1).
Hypertensive crisis.

Nipruss *Schwarz, Ger.*
Sodium nitroprusside (p.971·1).
Controlled hypotension; hypertension.

NiQuitin
SmithKline Beecham, Belg.; SmithKline Beecham, Denm.; SmithKline Beecham Sante, Fr.; SmithKline Beecham Consumer, Swed.; SmithKline Beecham Consumer, UK.
Nicotine (p.1640·3).
Aid to smoking withdrawal.

Niraben *Samchully, Singapore.*
Nifuroxazide (p.230·2).
Bacterial diarrhoea.

Nirason N *Ravensberg, Ger.*
Pentaerithrityl tetranitrate (p.952·3).
Ischaemic heart disease; myocardial infarction.

Nirolex for Chesty Coughs *Boots, UK.*
Guaifenesin (p.1092·2); ephedrine hydrochloride (p.1090·1); menthol (p.1632·3).
Coughs.

Nirolex for Dry Coughs *Boots, UK.*
Dextromethorphan hydrobromide (p.1087·3).
Coughs.

Nirox *Medici, Ital.†.*
Piroxicam (p.79·1).
Musculoskeletal and joint disorders.

Nirulid *Merck Sharp & Dohme, Denm.*
Amiloride hydrochloride (p.835·1).
Hypertension; oedema.

Nirvanil *Recordati, Ital.†.*
Valnoctamide (p.711·2).
Nervous disorders.

Nirvaxal *Teva, Israel.*
Chlordiazepoxide (p.659·2); clidinium bromide (p.465·1).
Nervous gastrointestinal disorders.

Nisaid *Alliance, S.Afr.*
Indometacin (p.44·3).
Gout; inflammation; musculoskeletal and joint disorders; pain.

Nisal *Epifarma, Ital.†.*
Nimesulide (p.62·3).
Fever; inflammation; pain.

Nisapulvol *Mayoly-Spindler, Fr.*
Benzyl hydroxybenzoate (p.1148·1).
Formerly contained methyl hydroxybenzoate, ethyl hydroxybenzoate, propyl hydroxybenzoate, benzyl hydroxybenzoate, and zinc oxide.
Pruritus.

Nisaseptol *Mayoly-Spindler, Fr.*
Benzyl hydroxybenzoate (p.1148·1).
Formerly contained propyl hydroxybenzoate and benzyl hydroxybenzoate.
Intertrigo; pruritus.

Nisasol *Mayoly-Spindler, Fr.*
Benzyl hydroxybenzoate (p.1148·1).
Formerly contained methyl hydroxybenzoate, ethyl hydroxybenzoate, and propyl hydroxybenzoate.
Infected skin disorders.

Nisicur *Apomedica, Aust.*
Ethenzamide (p.35·1); diphenhydramine hydrochloride (p.416·1); caffeine (p.761·3); ascorbic acid (p.1389·3).
Cold and influenza symptoms.

Nisis *Rhone-Poulenc Rorer, Fr.*
Valsartan (p.988·3).
Hypertension.

Nisisco *Rhone-Poulenc Rorer, Fr.*
Valsartan (p.988·3); hydrochlorothiazide (p.907·3).
Hypertension.

Nisita
Note. This name is used for preparations of different composition.
Engelhard, Ger.
Sodium chloride (p.1196·1); sodium bicarbonate (p.1186·2).
Nasal disorders.

Engelhard, Hong Kong.
Sodium iodide; sodium bromide; sodium chloride; lithium chloride; sodium bicarbonate; sodium sulfate; sodium phosphate; potassium sulfate (p.1180·1).
Nasal dryness.

Engelhard, Switz.†.
Sal ems.
Nasal disorders.

Nisolid *Chiesi, Ital.*
Flunisolide (p.1070·3).
Obstructive airways disease; rhinitis.

Nistaken *Kendrick, Mex.*
Propafenone hydrochloride (p.961·2).
Arrhythmias.

Nistan *Protein, Mex.*
Nystatin (p.392·2).

Nistaquim *Quimica y Farmacia, Mex.*
Nystatin (p.392·2).

Nisulid
Asta Medica, Braz.; Lederle, Switz.
Nimesulide (p.62·3).
Fever; inflammation; pain.

Nisylen *DHU, Ger.*
Homoeopathic preparation.

Nitan *Rekah, Israel.*
Pemoline (p.1513·1).
Attention deficit hyperactivity disorder; depression; fatigue.

Nite Time Cold Formula *Barre-National, USA.*
Pseudoephedrine hydrochloride (p.1099·2); dextromethorphan hydrobromide (p.1087·3); doxylamine succinate (p.417·1); paracetamol (p.71·2).
Coughs and cold symptoms.

Nitecall *Restan, S.Afr.*
Paracetamol (p.71·2); dextromethorphan hydrobromide (p.1087·3); chlorpheniramine [chlorphenamine] maleate (p.412·1); phenylpropanolamine hydrochloride (p.1098·1).
Cold and influenza symptoms.

Nitens *Pulitzer, Ital.*
Naproxen cetrimonium (p.61·3).
Gynaecological disorders; mouth and throat disorders.

Nitepax *Aspen Consumer, S.Afr.*
Noscapine (as resin complex) (p.1096·1).
Coughs.

Nitesco Smagliature *Pharmafar, Ital.*
Ruscus aculeatus; hedera helix; aesculus (p.1574·1); aescin (p.1574·1).
Formerly known as Nitesco S.
Stretch marks.

Nitlotion *Shantys, UK.*
Coconut oil (p.1409·1).
Pediculosis.

Nitoman
Virgo Healthcare, Austral.†; Roche, Canad.; Medilink, Denm.
Tetrabenazine (p.1669·3).
Drug-induced extrapyramidal disorders; hyperkinesis.

Nitopro *Maruishi, Jpn.*
Sodium nitroprusside (p.971·1).
Hypertension.

Nitorol
Eisai, Hong Kong; Eisai, Jpn.
Isosorbide dinitrate (p.915·2).
Angina pectoris; ischaemic heart disease; myocardial infarction.

Nitossil *Novartis Consumer, Ital.*
Cloperastine fendizoate (p.1087·2) or cloperastine hydrochloride (p.1087·2).
Coughs.

Nitradisc
Searle, Austral.; Searle, Braz.; Heumann, Ger.; Searle, Mex.; Searle, Norw.†; Monsanto, Port.; Searle, S.Afr.†; Monsanto, Spain; Searle, Thai.
Glyceryl trinitrate (p.897·3).
Angina pectoris; heart failure; myocardial infarction.

Nitrados
Douglas, NZ; Douglas, Singapore.
Nitrazepam (p.695·2).
Epilepsy; infantile spasm; insomnia.

Nitrangin *Isis, Ger.*
Glyceryl trinitrate (p.897·3).
Angina pectoris; coronary spasm; heart failure; myocardial infarction.

Nitrangin compositum *Isis, Ger.*
Glyceryl trinitrate (p.897·3); valerian (p.1678·3).
Angina pectoris; myocardial infarction.

Nitrangin forte *Wernigerode, Ger.†.*
Glyceryl trinitrate (p.897·3).
Angina pectoris; coronary spasm; myocardial infarction.

Nitrapamil *Orion, Fin.*
Diazepam (p.674·3); methylpropylpropanediol dinitrate.
Angina pectoris.

Nitrazadon *ICN, Canad.*
Nitrazepam (p.695·2).

Nitrazep *CT, Ger.†.*
Nitrazepam (p.695·2).
Insomnia.

Nitrazepan
Cristalia, Braz.; Prodes, Spain†.
Nitrazepam (p.695·2).
Epilepsy; insomnia.

Nitrazepol *Farmasa, Braz.*
Nitrazepam (p.695·2).
Epilepsy; insomnia.

Nitrazine Paper *Apothecon, USA.*
Test for pH in urine.

Nitregamma *Worwag, Ger.*
Nitrendipine (p.947·1).
Hypertension.

Nitrek *Bertek, USA.*
Glyceryl trinitrate (p.897·3).
Angina pectoris.

Nitren Lich *Lichtenstein, Ger.*
Nitrendipine (p.947·1).
Hypertension.

The symbol † denotes a preparation no longer actively marketed

Nitrencord *Biosintetica, Braz.*
Nitrendipine (p.947·1).
Hypertension.

Nitrendepat *Azupharma, Ger.*
Nitrendipine (p.947·1).
Hypertension.

Nitrendimerck *Merck dura, Ger.*
Nitrendipine (p.947·1).
Hypertension.

Nitrenpress *Sintofarma, Braz.*
Nitrendipine (p.947·1).
Hypertension.

Nitrensal *TAD, Ger.*
Nitrendipine (p.947·1).
Hypertension.

Nitrepress *Hexal, Ger.*
Nitrendipine (p.947·1).
Hypertension.

Nitre-Puren *Isis Puren, Ger.*
Nitrendipine (p.947·1).
Hypertension.

Nitrex *Essex, Ital.*
Isosorbide mononitrate (p.916·2).
Angina pectoris.

Nitriate *SERB, Fr.*
Sodium nitroprusside (p.971·1).
Controlled hypotension; heart failure; hypertensive crisis.

Nitriderm TTS *Novartis, Fr.*
Glyceryl trinitrate (p.897·3).
Angina pectoris.

Nitrileno *Libbs, Braz.*
Nitrofurazone (p.231·3); naphazoline hydrochloride (p.1095·1).
Nasal disorders.

Nitro *Orion, Fin.*
Glyceryl trinitrate (p.897·3).
Angina pectoris; controlled hypotension; heart failure; hypertension during cardiac surgery; myocardial infarction.

Nitro Mack
Pfizer, Aust.; Mack, Illert., Ger.; Mack, Hong Kong; Mack, Singapore; Mack, Switz.; Mack, Thai.
Glyceryl trinitrate (p.897·3).
Angina pectoris; controlled hypotension; coronary spasm; heart failure; hypertension; pulmonary hypertension.

Nitro Pohl
Sanova, Aust.; Pohl, Hong Kong; Pohl, Neth.
Glyceryl trinitrate (p.897·3).
Angina pectoris; heart failure; hypertension during coronary bypass; myocardial infarction pain.

Nitro Solvay *Solvay, Ger.*
Glyceryl trinitrate (p.897·3).
Angina pectoris; heart failure; myocardial infarction.

Nitrobaat *Nourypharma, Neth.†*
Glyceryl trinitrate (p.897·3).
Angina pectoris.

Nitro-Bid
Hoechst Marion Roussel, Austral.; Hoechst Marion Roussel, USA.
Glyceryl trinitrate (p.897·3).
Angina pectoris; controlled hypotension; heart failure; perioperative hypertension.

Nitrocine
Schwarz, Hong Kong; Schwarz, Irl.; Schwarz, Israel; Omnimed, S.Afr.; Schwarz, Thai.; Schwarz, UK.
Glyceryl trinitrate (p.897·3).
Angina pectoris; controlled hypotension; heart failure; hypertension during cardiac surgery; myocardial ischaemia during and after cardiovascular surgery.

Nitrocit *Genpharm, S.Afr.*
Potassium citrate (p.1186·1).
Urinary alkalinisation.

Nitrocod *Be-Tabs, S.Afr.*
Paracetamol (p.71·2); codeine phosphate (p.25·2).
Fever; pain.

Nitro-Crataegutt *Schwabe, Ger.*
Pentaerithrityl tetranitrate (p.952·3); crataegus (p.1600·2).
Heart failure.

Nitro-cum *Eu Rho, Ger.*
Glyceryl trinitrate (p.897·3); crataegus (p.1600·2); valerian (p.1678·3).
Angina pectoris; heart failure.

Nitroder *Keton, Mex.*
Glyceryl trinitrate (p.897·3).

Nitroderm
Novartis, Aust.; Novartis, Belg.; Novartis, NZ; Novartis, Thai.
Glyceryl trinitrate (p.897·3).
Angina pectoris; heart failure; prophylaxis of phlebitis and peripheral vein extravasation.

Nitro-Derm *Reuabuen, USA.*
Glyceryl trinitrate (p.897·3).
Angina pectoris.

Nitroderm TTS
Novartis, Braz.; Novartis, Ger.; Novartis, Hong Kong; Novartis, Israel; Novartis, Ital.; Novartis, Mex.; Novartis, Port.; Novartis, S.Afr.†; Novartis, Spain; Novartis, Switz.
Glyceryl trinitrate (p.897·3).
Angina pectoris; heart failure; prophylaxis of phlebitis and extravasation.

Nitrodex
Dexo, Fr.; Dexo, Switz.
Pentaerithrityl tetranitrate (p.952·3).
Angina pectoris; heart failure.

Nitrodisc *Roberts, USA.*
Glyceryl trinitrate (p.897·3).
Angina pectoris.

Nitro-Dur
Ebewe, Aust.; Schering-Plough, Austral.; Key, Canad.; Schering-Plough, Hong Kong; Schering-Plough, Irl.; Sigma-Tau, Ital.; Schering-Plough, Mex.; Schering-Plough, Neth.; Schering-Plough, Norw.; Schering-Plough, Port.; Schering-Plough, Spain; Essex, Switz.; Schering-Plough, UK; Key, USA.
Glyceryl trinitrate (p.897·3).
Angina pectoris; heart failure.

Nitro-Dyl *Bio-Therabel, Belg.*
Glyceryl trinitrate (p.897·3).
Angina pectoris.

Nitroflu *Beige, S.Afr.*
Aspirin (p.14·2); caffeine (p.761·3); ascorbic acid (p.1389·3); chlorpheniramine [chlorphenamine] maleate (p.412·1).
Cold and influenza symptoms.

Nitrofur-C *Leiras, Fin.*
Nitrofurantoin (p.230·3).
Urinary-tract infections.

Nitrogard *Forest Pharmaceuticals, USA.*
Glyceryl trinitrate (p.897·3).
Angina pectoris.

Nitroglyn
Kenwood, Hong Kong; Pharmacia, Swed.†; Kenwood, USA.
Glyceryl trinitrate (p.897·3).
Angina pectoris.

Nitroina *Teofarma, Spain.*
Acetic acid (p.1571·2); greater celandine (p.1618·1); salicylic acid (p.1122·3); iodine tincture (p.1522·3); thuja occidentalis (p.1672·1).
Warts.

Nitrokapseln-ratiopharm *Ratiopharm, Ger.*
Glyceryl trinitrate (p.897·3).
Angina pectoris.

Nitrokor *Robugen, Ger.*
Glyceryl trinitrate (p.897·3).
Angina pectoris; heart failure; myocardial infarction.

Nitrol
Note. This name is used for preparations of different composition.
Rhone-Poulenc Rorer, Canad.; Savage, USA.
Glyceryl trinitrate (p.897·3).
Angina pectoris.

SmithKline Beecham Sante, Fr.
Celandine (p.1618·1); thuja (p.1672·1); iodine (p.1522·3); salicylic acid (p.1122·3); glacial acetic acid (p.1571·2).
Warts.

Nitrolingual
Sanova, Aust.; Rhone-Poulenc Rorer, Austral.; Tramedico, Belg.; Rhone-Poulenc Rorer, Canad.; Pohl, Denm.; Pohl, Ger.; Pohl, Hong Kong; Lipha, Irl.; Pohl, Israel; Pohl, Neth.; Pohl, Norw.; Douglas, NZ; Mer-National, S.Afr.; Meda, Swed.; Pohl, Switz.; Merck, UK; Rhone-Poulenc Rorer, USA; Horizon, USA.
Glyceryl trinitrate (p.897·3).
Acute pulmonary oedema; angina pectoris; hypertensive crisis; smooth muscle spasm.

Nitromex
Dumex-Alpharma, Denm.; Dumex-Alpharma, Fin.; Alpharma, Norw.; Dumex-Alpharma, Swed.
Glyceryl trinitrate (p.897·3).
Angina pectoris; heart failure; hypertension during cardiac surgery; myocardial infarction.

Nitromidager *Streger, Mex.*
Metronidazole (p.594·1).
Amoebiasis; giardiasis; trichomoniasis.

Nitromin
Servier, Irl.; Servier, UK.
Glyceryl trinitrate (p.897·3).
Angina pectoris.

Nitromint
Rhone-Poulenc Rorer, Port.; Rhone-Poulenc Rorer, Switz.†.
Glyceryl trinitrate (p.897·3).
Angina pectoris; coronary artery spasm.

Nitronal
Sanova, Aust.; Pohl, Ger.†; Pohl, Hong Kong; Lipha, Irl.; Pohl, Israel; Douglas, NZ; Mer-National, S.Afr.†; Pohl, Switz.; Merck, UK.
Glyceryl trinitrate (p.897·3).
Angina pectoris; control of blood pressure during surgery; heart failure; myocardial infarction; pulmonary oedema.

Nitronasal *Eversil, Braz.*
Naphazoline hydrochloride (p.1095·1); nitrofurazone (p.231·3); panthenol (p.1602·3).
Nasal disorders.

Nitrong
Chemomedica, Aust.; Rhone-Poulenc Rorer, Belg.†; Rhone-Poulenc Rorer, Canad.; Ethicals, Denm.†; Orion, Swed.; Rhone-Poulenc Rorer, USA.
Glyceryl trinitrate (p.897·3).
Angina pectoris; heart failure.

Nitro-Obsidan *Isis, Ger.*
Pentaerithrityl tetranitrate (p.952·3); propranolol hydrochloride (p.962·3).
Angina pectoris; hypertension.

Nitropacin *Juste, Spain.*
Glyceryl trinitrate (p.897·3).
Angina pectoris; heart failure; myocardial infarction.

Nitro-Pflaster-ratiopharm TL *Ratiopharm, Ger.*
Glyceryl trinitrate (p.897·3).
Angina pectoris.

Nitroplast *Lacer, Spain.*
Glyceryl trinitrate (p.897·3).
Angina pectoris.

Nitro-Praecordin N *Roland, Ger.†.*
Glyceryl trinitrate (p.897·3); benzyl nicotinate (p.20·2).
Angina pectoris; coronary vascular disorders.

Nitropress *Abbott, USA.*
Sodium nitroprusside (p.971·1).
Controlled hypotension; hypertensive crisis.

Nitro-pro *Elan, USA.*
Lactose-free, gluten-free preparation for enteral nutrition (p.1350·1).
Formerly known as Nitrolan.

Nitroprussiat *Fides Rottapharm, Spain.*
Sodium nitroprusside (p.971·1).
Controlled hypotension; heart failure; hypertension.

Nitropulse *KV, Hong Kong.*
Glyceryl trinitrate (p.897·3).
Angina pectoris.

NitroQuick *Ethex, USA.*
Glyceryl trinitrate (p.897·3).
Angina pectoris.

Nitroretard *Dumex-Alpharma, Swed.†.*
Glyceryl trinitrate (p.897·3).
Angina pectoris.

Nitrosid *Pharmacal, Fin.*
Isosorbide dinitrate (p.915·2).
Angina pectoris; heart failure; myocardial infarction.

Nitrosorbide
Lusofarmaco, Ital.; Menarini, Singapore.
Isosorbide dinitrate (p.915·2).
Angina pectoris; cardiac disorders; ischaemic heart disease.

Nitrosorbon *Pohl, Ger.*
Isosorbide dinitrate (p.915·2).
Heart failure; ischaemic heart disease; myocardial infarction; pulmonary hypertension.

Nitrostat
Parke, Davis, Canad.; Parke, Davis, Hong Kong; Parke, Davis, Neth.; Parke, Davis, USA.
Glyceryl trinitrate (p.897·3).
Angina pectoris.

Nitrosylon *Knoll, Ital.*
Glyceryl trinitrate (p.897·3).
Angina pectoris.

NitroTab *Novopharm, USA.*
Glyceryl trinitrate (p.897·3).
Angina pectoris.

Nitro-Tablinen *Sanorania, Ger.†.*
Isosorbide dinitrate (p.915·2).
Cardiac disorders.

Nitrotard *Berenguer Infale, Spain†.*
Glyceryl trinitrate (p.897·3).
Angina pectoris; heart failure; myocardial infarction.

Nitro-Time *Time-Cap, USA.*
Glyceryl trinitrate (p.897·3).
Angina pectoris.

Nitrourean *Pras, Spain.*
Carmustine (p.516·1).
Malignant neoplasms.

Nitroven *Pohl, Norw.*
Glyceryl trinitrate (p.897·3).
Angina pectoris; blood pressure control during cardiac surgery; heart failure.

Nitrovis *CTI, Israel.*
Glyceryl trinitrate (p.897·3).
Angina pectoris; cardiac stenosis; myocardial infarction.

Nitrozell
Byk, Aust.†; Byk, Neth.†.
Glyceryl trinitrate (p.897·3).
Angina pectoris; myocardial infarction.

Nitrumon *Sintesa, Belg.*
Carmustine (p.516·1).
Malignant neoplasms.

Nitux *Inpharzam, Switz.*
Morclofone (p.1095·1).
Coughs.

Nivabetol *Alpharma, Fr.*
Betaine (p.1584·3); acetylmethionine; sorbitol (p.1377·3).
Constipation; dyspepsia.

Nivadil
Klinge, Ger.; Klinge, Irl.; Fujisawa, Jpn; Sanitas, Port.; Klinge, Switz.
Nilvadipine (p.946·1).
Hypertension.

Nivador *Menarini, Spain.*
Cefuroxime axetil (p.178·1).
Bacterial infections.

Nivagin *TP, Thai.*
Dipyrone (p.34·1).
Lignocaine [lidocaine] hydrochloride (p.1313·2) is included in the injection to alleviate the pain of injection.
Fever; pain.

Nivalin *Sanochemia, Aust.*
Galantamine hydrobromide (p.1419·1).
Alzheimer's disease; cerebrovascular disorders; glaucoma; myasthenia gravis; myelitis; neuritis; poliomyelitis; reversal of competitive neuromuscular blockade; smooth muscle atony.

Nivaquine
Rhone-Poulenc Rorer, Austral.†; Aventis, Belg.; Rhone-Poulenc Rorer, Fr.; Rhone-Poulenc Rorer, Irl.†; Rhone-Poulenc Rorer, Neth.; Aventis,

NZ; Aventis, S.Afr.; Rhone-Poulenc Rorer, Switz.; Rhone-Poulenc Rorer, UK.
Chloroquine sulfate (p.432·3).
Giardiasis; hepatic amoebiasis; light-sensitive skin conditions; lupus erythematosus; malaria; rheumatoid arthritis.

Nivaten *Cox, UK.*
Nifedipine (p.940·1).

Nivea *Beiersdorf, USA.*
A range of emollient, cleansing, and moisturising preparations.

Nivea Sun *Beiersdorf, USA.*
SPF 15: Octinoxate (p.1517·3); octisalate (p.1518·1); oxybenzone (p.1518·1); ensulizole (p.1517·2).
Sunscreen.

Nivea Visage *Beiersdorf, Canad.*
SPF 4: Octinoxate (p.1517·3); oxybenzone (p.1518·1).
SPF 15: Octinoxate (p.1517·3); oxybenzone (p.1518·1); ensulizole (p.1517·2).
Sunscreen.

Nivemycin *Waymade, UK.*
Neomycin sulfate (p.228·1).
Bowel preparation; hepatic coma.

Niven *Pulitzer, Ital.*
Nicardipine hydrochloride (p.938·3).
Angina pectoris; heart failure; hypertension.

Niver *Medeva, Fr.*
Codeine phosphate (p.25·2); grindelia (p.1618·2); thyme (p.1672·3); mallow.
Coughs.

Nivoflox
Andromaco, Mex.; Euro-Labor, Port.
Ciprofloxacin (p.182·3) or ciprofloxacin hydrochloride (p.182·3).
Bacterial infections.

Nix
Warner-Lambert, Austral.†; Warner-Lambert Consumer, Belg.; Warner-Lambert, Canad.; Glaxo Wellcome, Canad.; Warner-Lambert, Denm.; Warner-Lambert, Fin.; Warner-Lambert, Fr.; Warner-Lambert, Ital.; Warner-Lambert, Norw.; Warner-Lambert Consumer, Port.; Glaxo Wellcome, Swed.; Warner-Lambert, Swed.; Warner-Lambert, USA.
Permethrin (p.1436·1).
Pediculosis; scabies.

Nixal *Columbia, Mex.*
Naproxen sodium (p.61·1).
Fever; inflammation; pain.

Nixin *Mepha, Port.*
Ciprofloxacin hydrochloride (p.182·3).
Bacterial infections.

Nixyn *Organon, Spain.*
Capsules; suppositories: Isonixin (p.47·2).
Gout; musculoskeletal, joint, and peri-articular disorders; pain.
Cream: Isonixin (p.47·2); methyl salicylate (p.55·1).
Peri-articular and soft-tissue disorders.

Niyaplat *Precimex, Mex.*
Cisplatin (p.525·1).

Nizacol *Benedetti, Ital.*
Miconazole (p.391·1) or miconazole nitrate (p.391·1).
Fungal infections; Gram-positive bacterial infections.

Nizax
Lilly, Denm.; Lilly, Fin.; Lilly, Ger.; Lilly, Ital.; Lilly, Swed.
Nizatidine (p.1238·1).
Gastro-oesophageal reflux; peptic ulcer.

Nizaxid
Norgine, Fr.; Lilly, Port.
Nizatidine (p.1238·1).
Gastro-oesophageal reflux; peptic ulcer.

Nizcreme *Janssen-Cilag, S.Afr.*
Ketoconazole (p.389·1).
Fungal skin infections.

Nizole *Hovid, Singapore.*
Metronidazole (p.594·1).
Anaerobic bacterial infections; protozoal infections.

Nizoral
Janssen-Cilag, Aust.; Janssen-Cilag, Austral.; Janssen-Cilag, Belg.; Janssen, Braz.; McNeil Consumer, Canad.; Janssen-Ortho, Canad.; Janssen-Cilag, Denm.; Janssen-Cilag, Fin.; Janssen-Cilag, Fr.; Janssen-Cilag, Ger.; Janssen, Hong Kong; Janssen-Cilag, Irl.; Janssen-Cilag, Israel; Janssen-Cilag, Ital.; Janssen, Mex.; Janssen-Cilag, Neth.; Janssen-Cilag, NZ; Janssen-Cilag, Port.; Janssen-Cilag, S.Afr.; Janssen-Cilag, Singapore; Janssen-Cilag, Switz.; Janssen, Thai.; Janssen-Cilag, UK; Johnson & Johnson MSD Consumer, UK; Janssen, USA; McNeil Consumer, USA.
Ketoconazole (p.389·1).
Dandruff; fungal infections; seborrhoeic dermatitis.

Nizovules *Janssen-Cilag, S.Afr.*
Ketoconazole (p.389·1).
Vaginal candidiasis.

Nizshampoo *Janssen-Cilag, S.Afr.*
Ketoconazole (p.389·1).
Fungal scalp infections.

N-Labstix *Bayer Diagnostics, Irl.; Bayer Diagnostics, UK.*
Test for glucose, protein, pH, ketones, blood, and nitrites in urine.

N-Multistix *Bayer, Austral.†; Ames, Israel; Bayer, USA.*
Test for glucose, protein, blood, ketones, bilirubin, urobilinogen, nitrites, and pH in urine.

N-Multistix SG
Bayer, Austral.†; Bayer, Canad.†; Bayer Diagnostics, Irl.; Bayer Diagnostici, Ital.; Bayer Diagnostics, UK; Bayer, USA.
Test for specific gravity, glucose, protein, blood, ketones, bilirubin, urobilinogen, nitrite, and pH in urine.

No 440 *Herbes Universelles, Canad.*
Vitamins A, C, and D (p.1350·1).

No Doz *Key, Austral.*
Caffeine (p.761·3).
Fatigue.

No Doz Plus *Key, Austral.*
Caffeine (p.761·3); vitamin B substances (p.1350·1); glucose (p.1364·1).
Fatigue.

No Drowsiness Sinarest *Ciba, USA.*
Pseudoephedrine hydrochloride (p.1099·2); paracetamol (p.71·2).
Upper respiratory-tract symptoms.

No Gas *Key, Austral.*
Activated charcoal (p.1000·2); simeticone (p.1249·2).
Diarrhoea; drug poisoning; excess gastrointestinal gas.

No Grip *Vifor, Switz.†*
Salicylamide (p.82·1); noscapine hydrochloride (p.1096·1); mepyramine maleate (p.421·1); ascorbic acid (p.1389·3); hesperidin methyl chalcone (p.1611·2).
Cold symptoms.

No Grip C *Vifor, Switz.*
Paracetamol (p.71·2); ascorbic acid (p.1389·3).
Cold symptoms.

No Name Cough Lozenge *Sutton, Canad.†*
Menthol (p.1632·3).

No Pain-HP *Young Again Products, USA.*
Capsaicin (p.23·1).
Pain.

No-Acid *Infabra, Braz.*
Note. A similar name is used for preparations of different composition (see below).
Aluminium hydroxide (p.1210·3).
Gastrointestinal hyperacidity.

Noacid *OBA, Denm.*
Note. A similar name is used for preparations of different composition (see above).
Dihydroxyaluminum sodium carbonate (p.1222·1).
Gastritis; gastro-oesophageal reflux; peptic ulcer.

NO-AD Babies *Solar, Canad.*
SPF 30; SPF 45: Octinoxate (p.1517·3); octisalate (p.1518·1); oxybenzone (p.1518·1).
Sunscreen.

NO-AD Kids *Solar, Canad.*
SPF 30: Octinoxate (p.1517·3); octisalate (p.1518·1); oxybenzone (p.1518·1).
Sunscreen.

NO-AD Sport *Solar, Canad.*
SPF 15; SPF 30: Octinoxate (p.1517·3); octisalate (p.1518·1); oxybenzone (p.1518·1).
Sunscreen.

NO-AD Sunblock *Solar, Canad.*
SPF 15; SPF 30; SPF 45: Octinoxate (p.1517·3); octisalate (p.1518·1); oxybenzone (p.1518·1).
Sunscreen.

NO-AD Sunscreen *Solar, Canad.*
SPF 8: Octinoxate (p.1517·3); oxybenzone (p.1518·1).
Sunscreen.

Noalgil *Pharmacia Upjohn, Spain†.*
Ibuprofen (p.43·2).
Fever; inflammation; musculoskeletal, joint, and peri-articular disorders; pain.

Noalgos *Levofarma, Ital.*
Nimesulide (p.62·3).
Fever; inflammation; pain.

Noan
Farmasa, Braz.; Ravizza, Ital.
Diazepam (p.674·3).
Alcohol withdrawal syndrome; anxiety; epilepsy; insomnia; premedication; sedative; skeletal muscle spasm.

Nobacter *Boots Healthcare, Fr.†.*
Triclocarban (p.1159·2).
Skin cleansing and disinfection.

Nobec *Aspen Consumer, S.Afr.*
Beclometasone dipropionate (p.1061·2).
Allergic rhinitis.

Nobecutan *Astra, Ger.*
Thiram (p.1672·1).
Burns; wounds.

Nobecutane *Astra, Belg.†.*
Thiram (p.1672·1).
Antiseptic aerosol dressing.

Nobese *Farmedica, Braz.*
Fenproporex hydrochloride (p.1510·2).
Obesity.

Nobese No. 1 *Restan, S.Afr.*
Cathine hydrochloride (p.1507·1).
Obesity.

No-Bite *Brunel, S.Afr.*
Diethyltoluamide (p.1431·2); citronella oil (p.1596·3).
Mosquito bites.

Nobligan
Boehringer Mannheim, Aust.†; Grunenthal, Denm.; Janssen, Mex.; Grunenthal, Norw.; Searle, Swed.
Tramadol hydrochloride (p.89·1).
Pain.

Nobliten *Lacer, Spain†.*
A nonoxinol (p.1346·1).
Contraceptive.

Nobritol *Roche, Spain.*
Amitriptyline hydrochloride (p.273·3); medazepam (p.690·2).
Depression.

Nobrium *Roche, Neth.†.*
Medazepam (p.690·2).
Anxiety disorders.

Noceptin *Christiaens, Neth.*
Morphine sulfate (p.56·1).
Pain.

Nocertone
Sanofi Synthelabo, Belg.; Sanofi Winthrop, Fr.
Oxetorone fumarate (p.455·1).
Cluster headache; migraine.

Noctal *Abbott, Braz.*
Estazolam (p.682·3).
Insomnia.

Noctamid
Schering, Aust.; Schering, Belg.; Schering, Ger.; Asche, Ger.; Schering, Irl.; Schering, Neth.; Schering, NZ; Schering, Port.; Schering, S.Afr.; Schering, Spain; Schering, Swed.
Lormetazepam (p.689·3).
Premedication; sleep disorders.

Noctamide *Schering, Fr.*
Lormetazepam (p.689·3).
Insomnia.

Noctazepam *Hexal, Ger.*
Oxazepam (p.697·1).
Anxiety; sleep disorders.

Noctec *Bristol-Myers Squibb, UK†.*
Cloral hydrate (p.669·3).
Insomnia.

Noctirex *Irex, Fr.*
Zopiclone (p.713·1).
Insomnia.

Noctis *Bouty, Ital.*
Valerian (p.1678·3); passion flower (p.1649·1); crataegus (p.1600·2).
Sleep disorders.

Noctisan *Dolisos, Fr.†.*
Crataegus (p.1600·2); tilia (p.1673·2); valerian (p.1678·3).
Insomnia.

Noctran *Menarini, Fr.*
Dipotassium clorazepate (p.670·3); acepromazine (p.654·1); aceprometazine (p.654·1).
Insomnia.

Noctura *Nelson, UK.*
Homoeopathic preparation.

Nocturne *Wyeth, Austral.*
Temazepam (p.707·2).
Insomnia.

Nocturno *Unipharm, Israel.*
Zopiclone (p.713·1).
Insomnia.

Noctyl *Monot, Fr.*
Doxylamine succinate (p.417·1).
Insomnia.

Nocutil
Gebro, Switz.; Norgine, UK.
Desmopressin acetate (p.1281·2).
Diabetes insipidus; diagnosis of diabetes insipidus; nocturnal enuresis.

Nocvalene *Arkopharma, Fr.*
Crataegus (p.1600·2); red-poppy petal (p.1029·1); passion flower (p.1649·1).
Insomnia.

Node Tar *Piam, Ital.†.*
Coal tar (p.1125·1); cade oil (p.1124·3); selenium sulfide (p.1123·1); salicylic acid (p.1122·3).
Scalp disorders.

Nodepe
Euro-Labor, Port.; Andromaco, Spain.
Fluoxetine hydrochloride (p.284·2).
Bulimia; depression; obsessive-compulsive disorder.

Nodex *Brothier, Fr.*
Dextromethorphan hydrobromide (p.1087·3).
Coughs.

Nodoff *Potter's, UK.*
Oral liquid: Passion flower (p.1649·1); skullcap (p.1664·3); lupulus (p.1629·3); valerian (p.1678·3); Jamaica dogwood (p.1625·1).
Tablets: Passion flower (p.1649·1).
Insomnia.

Nodolfen *Lacer, Spain.*
Ibuprofen (p.43·2).
Fever; pain.

NoDoz *Bristol-Myers Products, USA.*
Caffeine (p.761·3).
Fatigue.

No-Drowsiness Allerest *Ciba, USA.*
Pseudoephedrine hydrochloride (p.1099·2); paracetamol (p.71·2).
Upper respiratory-tract symptoms.

Nodryl *Teva, Israel.*
Diphenhydramine hydrochloride (p.416·1); naphazoline hydrochloride (p.1095·1); neomycin sulfate (p.228·1).
Allergic rhinitis; nasal congestion.

Noemin N *Trommsdorff, Ger.*
Bismuth aluminate (p.1213·1).
Gastrointestinal disorders.

Nofagus *Sanus, Braz.*
Mazindol (p.1510·3); diazepam (p.674·3).
Obesity.

Nofedol *Rhone-Poulenc Rorer, Spain.*
Paracetamol (p.71·2).
Fever; pain.

Noflam *Pacific, NZ.*
Naproxen (p.60·3) or naproxen sodium (p.61·1).
Gout; musculoskeletal, joint, and peri-articular disorders; pain.

Noflam-N
Pacific, Hong Kong; Alphapharm, Singapore; Merck, Singapore.
Naproxen sodium (p.61·1).
Gout; musculoskeletal and joint disorders; pain.

No-Flu *Klinge, Switz.*
Paracetamol (p.71·2); dextromethorphan hydrobromide (p.1087·3); phenylephrine hydrochloride (p.1097·1).
Cold symptoms.

Nofum *Faes, Spain†.*
Lobeline sulfate (p.1510·3).
Aid to smoking withdrawal.

No-Gas *Giuliani, Ital.*
Dimethicone (p.1249·2); activated charcoal (p.1000·2).
Gastrointestinal disorders associated with excess gas.

No-Gravid *Irmed, Ital.*
Copper (p.1357·3).
Intra-uterine contraceptive device.

No-Hist *Dunhall, USA†.*
Phenylephrine hydrochloride (p.1097·1); phenylpropanolamine hydrochloride (p.1098·1); pseudoephedrine hydrochloride (p.1099·2).
Nasal congestion.

Noiafren *Hoechst Marion Roussel, Spain.*
Clobazam (p.668·1).
Alcohol withdrawal syndrome; anxiety; epilepsy.

Noivy *Hilarys, Canad.†.*
Calamine (p.1111·3); camphor (p.1589·3); menthol (p.1632·3); benzocaine (p.1306·2).

Nok *CTS, Israel.*
Permethrin (p.1436·1).
Pediculosis.

Nokid *Benedetti, Ital.*
Cefonicid sodium (p.168·1).
Lignocaine [lidocaine] hydrochloride (p.1313·2) is included in this preparation to alleviate the pain of injection.
Gram-negative bacterial infections.

Noktone *Gea, Norw.*
Ranitidine hydrochloride (p.1245·2).
Aspiration syndrome; gastro-oesophageal reflux; peptic ulcer; Zollinger-Ellison syndrome.

Nolac *Nestle, Ital.*
Infant feed (p.1350·1).
Intolerance to cow's milk, soya, egg, and gluten.

Nolahist *Carnrick, USA.*
Phenindamine tartrate (p.422·2).
Allergic rhinitis.

Nolamine *Carnrick, USA†.*
Phenindamine tartrate (p.422·2); chlorpheniramine [chlorphenamine] maleate (p.412·1); phenylpropanolamine hydrochloride (p.1098·1).
Nasal congestion.

Nolder *Searle, Ital.*
Amino-acid, carbohydrate, and phospholipid preparation with vitamins and selenium (p.1350·1).
Nutritional supplement.

Noleptan *Promeco, Mex.*
Fominoben (p.1091·3) or fominoben hydrochloride (p.1091·3).
Coughs.

Nolgen *Antigen, Irl.*
Tamoxifen citrate (p.571·1).
Breast cancer.

Nolipax *Salus, Ital.*
Fenofibrate (p.889·1).
Diabetic retinopathy; hyperlipidaemias; xanthomatosis.

Nolipid *Samil, Ital.†.*
Colextran hydrochloride (p.865·1).
Hyperlipidaemia.

Nolol *Docmed, S.Afr.*
Propranolol hydrochloride (p.962·3).
Angina pectoris; anxiety; arrhythmias; hypertension; hyperthyroidism; phaeochromocytoma.

Nolotil
Boehringer Ingelheim, Port.; Boehringer Ingelheim, Spain.
Metamizole magnesium (p.34·2).
Fever; pain.

Nolotil Compositum *Europharma, Spain.*
Metamizole magnesium (p.34·2); hyoscine butylbromide (p.468·2).
Gastrointestinal spasm; pain.

Nolvadex
Zeneca, Aust.; Zeneca, Austral.; Zeneca, Belg.; Glaxo Wellcome, Braz.; AstraZeneca, Canad.; AstraZeneca, Fin.; AstraZeneca, Fr.; Zeneca, Ger.; Zeneca, Hong Kong; Zeneca, Irl.; Zeneca, Israel; Zeneca, Ital.; Zeneca, Mex.; Zeneca, Neth.; AstraZeneca, Norw.; Astra-Zeneca, NZ; Zeneca, Port.; Zeneca, S.Afr.; AstraZeneca, Singapore; Zeneca, Spain; Zeneca, Swed.; Zeneca, Switz.; AstraZeneca, Thai.; AstraZeneca, UK; AstraZeneca, USA.
Tamoxifen citrate (p.571·1).
Anovulatory infertility; breast cancer; endometrial cancer.

Nomapam *Amrad, Austral.†.*
Temazepam (p.707·2).
Insomnia.

Nominfone *Atlantic, Thai.*
Dipyrone (p.34·1).
Fever; pain.

Nomon mono *Hoyer, Ger.*
Cucurbita (p.1601·1).
Urinary-tract disorders.

Nomopain *Aventis, S.Afr.*
Paracetamol (p.71·2); caffeine (p.761·3); doxylamine succinate (p.417·1); codeine phosphate (p.25·2).
Pain and associated tension.

Nomotec *Tecnofarma, Mex.*
Ketotifen (p.767·2).
Asthma; hypersensitivity.

Non Acid *FIRMA, Ital.†.*
Oral granules: Sodium citrate (p.1186·2); potassium citrate (p.1186·1); tribasic sodium phosphate (p.1193·3); tartaric acid (p.1669·2); sodium bicarbonate (p.1186·2).
Tablets: Sodium citrate (p.1186·2); potassium citrate (p.1186·1); tribasic sodium phosphate (p.1193·3).
Gastrointestinal disorders.

No-Name Dandruff Treatment *Sutton, Canad.†.*
Pyrithione zinc (p.1122·1).

Nonan
Baxter, Belg.; Aguettant, Fr.
Mineral preparation (p.1350·1).
Parenteral nutrition.

Nonavit *De Mayo, Braz.*
Multivitamin, amino-acid, and mineral preparation (p.1350·1).

Non-Drowsy Sudafed Dual Relief Max *Warner-Lambert, UK.*
Ibuprofen (p.43·2); pseudoephedrine hydrochloride (p.1099·2).
Nasal and sinus congestion.

Nonflamin *Yoshitomi, Jpn†.*
Tinoridine hydrochloride (p.88·3).
Inflammation; pain.

Non-Ovlon *Jenapharm, Ger.*
Ethinylestradiol (p.1476·2); norethisterone acetate (p.1485·1).
Combined oral contraceptive; menstrual disorders.

Noocetam *Pharmasant, Thai.*
Piracetam (p.1652·1).
Cerebral trauma; cerebrovascular disorders; chronic alcoholism; mental function impairment.

Noodipina *Apsen, Braz.*
Nimodipine (p.946·1).
Neurological deficit following subarachnoid haemorrhage.

Noodis *UCB, Belg.*
Piracetam (p.1652·1).
Childhood learning difficulties.

Noostan *UCB, Port.*
Piracetam (p.1652·1).
Alcohol withdrawal syndrome; dyslexia in children; mental function disorders; vertigo.

Nootron *Biosintetica, Braz.*
Piracetam (p.1652·1).
Alcoholism; behaviour disorders in children; cerebrovascular disorders; senile dementia; vertigo.

Nootrop *UCB, Ger.; Vedim, Ger.*
Piracetam (p.1652·1).
Mental function disorders.

Nootropil
UCB, Aust.; UCB, Belg.; Rhodia, Braz.; UCB, Fin.; UCB, Hong Kong; UCB, Ital.; UCB, Mex.; UCB, Neth.; Vedim, Port.; UCB, S.Afr.; UCB, Singapore; UCB, Spain; UCB, Swed.; UCB, Switz.; UCB, Thai.; UCB, UK.
Piracetam (p.1652·1).
Alcoholism; behaviour disorders in children; cerebrovascular disorders; myoclonus; senile dementia; vertigo.

Nootropyl *UCB, Fr.*
Piracetam (p.1652·1).
Dyslexia in children; mental function impairment in the elderly; stroke; vertigo.

Nopan *CTI, Israel.*
Buprenorphine (p.21·1) or buprenorphine hydrochloride (p.21·1).
Pain.

Nopar *Lilly, Ital.*
Pergolide mesilate (p.1175·1).
Parkinsonism.

Nopil *Mepha, Switz.*
Co-trimoxazole (p.193·3).
Bacterial infections; Pneumocystis carinii pneumonia.

Nopriken *Kendrick, Mex.*
Pefloxacin mesilate (p.234·3).
Bacterial infections.

Nopron
Genopharm, Fr.; Sanofi Synthelabo, Ital.
Niaprazine (p.422·1).
Insomnia.

Nopucid Composto *Hoechst Marion Roussel, Braz.*
Deltamethrin (p.1430·3); piperonyl butoxide (p.1436·2).
Pediculosis; scabies.

Nopyn *Rolab, S.Afr.*
Paracetamol (p.71·2); codeine phosphate (p.25·2); caffeine (p.761·3); meprobamate (p.691·1).
Pain associated with tension.

Noquema *Faes, Spain†.*
Cetylpyridinium chloride (p.1138·1); colecalciferol (p.1391·1); benzocaine (p.1306·2); vitamin A (p.1382·1).
Burns.

Nora *Nakorn, Thai.*
Ketoconazole (p.389·1).
Fungal infections; seborrhoeic dermatitis.

The symbol † denotes a preparation no longer actively marketed

Norabromol N *Michallik, Ger.*
Sodium 3,5-dibromo-4-hydroxybenzenesulfonate.
Wounds.

Noracin *Cibran, Braz.; Chew, Thai.*
Norfloxacin (p.232·1).
Bacterial infections.

Noradran *Norma, UK.*
Diphenhydramine hydrochloride (p.416·1); diprophylline (p.764·1); ephedrine hydrochloride (p.1090·1); guaifenesin (p.1092·2).
Coughs.

Norakin N *Hexal, Ger.*
Biperiden hydrochloride (p.464·2).
Blepharospasm; drug-induced extrapyramidal disorders; dystonias; parkinsonism; torticollis.

Noralget *Quatromed, S.Afr.*
Paracetamol (p.71·2); codeine phosphate (p.25·2); caffeine (p.761·3); meprobamate (p.691·1).
Pain and associated tension.

Noralone *Taro, Israel.*
Nandrolone phenylpropionate (p.1484·2).
Anabolic breast cancer; osteoporosis.

Nor-Anaesthol *Merz, Ger.†*
Lignocaine [lidocaine] hydrochloride (p.1313·2).
Noradrenaline [norepinephrine] (p.948·2) is included in this preparation as a vasoconstrictor to diminish absorption and localise the effect of the local anaesthetic.
Local anaesthesia.

Nora-ratiopharm *Ratiopharm, Ger.*
Ethinylestradiol (p.1476·2); norethisterone (p.1485·1).
Combined oral contraceptive.

Noravid *Hoechst Marion Roussel, Ital.*
Defibrotide (p.866·3).
Thromboembolic disorders.

Noraxin *TP, Thai.*
Norfloxacin (p.232·1).
Bacterial infections.

Norbactin *Ranbaxy, Singapore; Ranbaxy, Thai.*
Norfloxacin (p.232·1).
Bacterial infections.

Norbiline *Rhone-Poulenc Rorer, Fr.; Rhone-Poulenc Rorer, Ital.*
Prozapine hydrochloride (p.1655·2); sorbitol (p.1377·3).
Biliary-tract disorders; gastrointestinal disorders.

Norboral *Silanes, Mex.*
Glibenclamide (p.321·3).
Diabetes mellitus.

Norciden *Kendrick, Mex.*
Danazol (p.1468·3).
Breast cancer; endometriosis; hereditary angioedema; hypogonadism; hypopituitarism; mastalgia; osteoporosis; precocious puberty; suppression of lactation.

Norcin *The Forty-Two, Thai.; Utopian, Thai.*
Norfloxacin (p.232·1).
Bacterial infections.

Norco *Watson, USA.*
Hydrocodone tartrate (p.42·2); paracetamol (p.71·2).
Pain.

Norcolut *Gedeon Richter, Hong Kong; Gedeon Richter, Singapore.*
Norethisterone (p.1485·1).
Dysfunctional uterine bleeding; endometriosis; female infertility; lactation inhibition; menopausal disorders; menstrual disorders.

Norcuron
Organon Teknika, Aust.; Organon Teknika, Austral.; Organon Teknika, Belg.; Akzo, Braz.; Organon, Canad.; Organon Teknika, Denm.†; Organon Teknika, Fin.; Organon Teknika, Fr.; Organon Teknika, Ger.; Organon Teknika, Hong Kong; Organon Teknika, Irl.; Organon Teknika, Israel; Organon Teknika, Ital.; Organon Teknika, Mex.; Organon Teknika, Neth.; Organon Teknika, Norw.; Pharmaco, NZ; Organon, Port.; Sanofi Synthelabo, S.Afr.; Organon, Singapore; Organon Teknika, Spain; Organon Teknika, Swed.; Organon Teknika, Switz.; Organon, Thai.; Organon, UK; Organon, USA.
Vecuronium bromide (p.1343·2).
Competitive neuromuscular blocker.

Nordapanin N *Michallik, Ger.*
Benzocaine (p.1306·2); acriflavinium chloride (p.1130·2).
Mouth and throat disorders.

Nordathricin N *Michallik, Ger.*
Tyrothricin (p.267·1); cetylpyridinium chloride (p.1138·1); benzocaine (p.1306·2).
Mouth and throat disorders.

Nordaz *Bouchara, Fr.; Bouchara, Singapore.*
Nordazepam (p.696·1).
Alcohol withdrawal syndrome; anxiety.

Norden *Akzo, Braz.*
Multivitamins (p.1350·1); iron (p.1366·3).
Iron deficiency; iron-deficiency anaemias.

Nordet *Wyeth, Mex.*
Levonorgestrel (p.1486·2); ethinylestradiol (p.1476·2).
Combined oral contraceptive.

Nordette
Wyeth-Ayerst, Austral.; Wyeth, Braz.; Wyeth-Ayerst, Hong Kong; Wyeth-Ayerst, Israel; Wyeth, NZ; Aspen, S.Afr.; Wyeth, Singapore; Wyeth-Ayerst, Thai.; Wyeth-Ayerst, UK.
Levonorgestrel (p.1486·2); ethinylestradiol (p.1476·2).
28-Day packs also contain 7 inert tablets.
Combined oral contraceptive; menstrual disorders.

Nordiate *Hemasure, Denm.*
A factor VIII preparation (p.734·1).
Haemorrhagic disorders.

Nordicort *Ascot, Austral.†*
Hydrocortisone sodium succinate (p.1074·1).
Corticosteroid.

Nordimmun
Hemasure, Denm.; Hemasure, Swed.
A normal immunoglobulin (p.1551·3).
Hypogammaglobulinaemia; idiopathic thrombocytopenic purpura.

Nordiol
Wyeth-Ayerst, Austral.; Wyeth-Ayerst, Hong Kong; Wyeth, Mex.; Wyeth, NZ; Aspen, S.Afr.; Wyeth-Ayerst, Thai.
Levonorgestrel (p.1486·2); ethinylestradiol (p.1476·2).
28-Day packs also contain 7 inert tablets.
Combined oral contraceptive; menstrual disorders.

Norditropin
Novo Nordisk, Aust.; Novo Nordisk, Austral.; Novo Nordisk, Belg.; Novo Nordisk, Braz.; Novo Nordisk, Denm.; Novo Nordisk, Fin.; Novo Nordisk, Ger.; Novo Nordisk, Hong Kong; Novo Nordisk, Irl.; Novo Nordisk, Israel; Novo Nordisk, Ital.; Pisa, Mex.; Novo Nordisk, Neth.; Novo Nordisk, Norw.; Novo Nordisk, NZ; Novo Nordisk, Port.; Novo Nordisk, S.Afr.; Novo Nordisk, Spain; Novo Nordisk, Swed.; Novo Nordisk, UK; Novo Nordisk, USA.
Somatropin (p.1286·1).
Growth disorders in renal failure; growth hormone deficiency; Turner's syndrome.

Norditropine
Novo Nordisk, Fr.; Novo Nordisk, Switz.
Somatropin (p.1286·1).
Growth disorders in renal failure; growth hormone deficiency; Turner's syndrome.

Nordolce *Vegetal, Ital.*
Acero canadese.
Nutritional supplement.

Nordonil *Medinfar, Port.†*
Domperidone (p.1224·1).
Dyspepsia; nausea; vomiting.

Nordotol *Orion, Denm.*
Carbamazepine (p.342·2).
Alcohol withdrawal syndrome; diabetes insipidus; epilepsy; neuralgias.

Nordryl *Vortech, USA†.*
Diphenhydramine hydrochloride (p.416·1).
Insomnia; motion sickness; parkinsonism.

Nordyl *Rosemont, Thai.*
Promethazine hydrochloride (p.423·2); codeine phosphate (p.25·2).
Coughs.

Norebox *Pharmacia Upjohn, Spain.*
Reboxetine mesilate (p.308·1).
Depression.

Norecil *Maver, Mex.*
Metronidazole (p.594·1); diiodohydroxyquinoline (p.590·2).
Amoebiasis.

Norel *US Pharmaceutical, USA†.*
Phenylephrine hydrochloride (p.1097·1); phenylpropanolamine hydrochloride (p.1098·1); guaifenesin (p.1092·2).
Upper respiratory-tract symptoms.

Norel Plus *US Pharmaceutical, USA†.*
Phenylpropanolamine hydrochloride (p.1098·1); paracetamol (p.71·2); chlorpheniramine [chlorphenamine] maleate (p.412·1); phenyltoloxamine citrate (p.423·1).
Upper respiratory-tract symptoms.

Norethin 1/35E *Schiapparelli Searle, USA†.*
Norethisterone (p.1485·1); ethinylestradiol (p.1476·2).
28-Day packs also contain 7 inert tablets.
Combined oral contraceptive.

Norethin 1/50M *Schiapparelli Searle, USA†.*
Norethisterone (p.1485·1); mestranol (p.1482·1).
28-Day packs also contain 7 inert tablets.
Combined oral contraceptive.

Norfcin *SM, Thai.*
Norfloxacin (p.232·1).
Bacterial infections.

Norfemac *Hoechst Marion Roussel, Canad.*
Bufexamac (p.28·3).
Anorectal disorders; inflammatory skin disorders; phlebitis; vulval disorders.

Norfenazin *Reig Jofre, Spain.*
Nortriptyline hydrochloride (p.301·3).
Formerly contained nortriptyline hydrochloride and perphenazine.
Depression.

Norfenon *Knoll, Mex.*
Propafenone hydrochloride (p.961·3).
Arrhythmias.

Norflam T *3M, S.Afr.*
Ibuprofen (p.43·2).
Fever; pain.

Norflex
Sanova, Aust.†; 3M, Austral.; 3M, Belg.; 3M, Canad.; 3M, Denm.; 3M, Fin.; 3M, Ger.; Riker, Mex.; 3M, NZ; 3M, Port.†; 3M, S.Afr.; 3M, Singapore; 3M, Swed.; 3M, Switz.†; 3M, UK†; 3M, USA.
Orphenadrine citrate (p.470·3).
Drug-induced extrapyramidal disorders; hiccups; parkinsonism; skeletal muscle spasm; tension headache.

Norflex Co *3M, S.Afr.*
Orphenadrine citrate (p.470·3); paracetamol (p.71·2).
Fever; pain; skeletal muscle spasm.

Norflex Plus *Riker, Mex.*
Orphenadrine citrate (p.470·3); paracetamol (p.71·2).
Skeletal muscle spasm.

Norflo *Medifive, Thai.*
Norfloxacin (p.232·1).
Bacterial infections.

Norflocin
Mepha, Switz.; Polipharm, Thai.
Norfloxacin (p.232·1).
Bacterial infections.

Norflohexal *Hexal, Austral.*
Norfloxacin (p.232·1).
Bacterial infections.

Norflosal *TAD, Ger.*
Norfloxacin (p.232·1).
Urinary-tract infections.

Norflox *Virginia, Ital.*
Norfloxacin (p.232·1).
Urinary-tract infections.

Norflox-Azu *Azupharma, Ger.*
Norfloxacin (p.232·1).
Bacterial infections of the urinary tract.

Norfloxin *TO-Chemicals, Thai.*
Norfloxacin (p.232·1).
Bacterial infections.

Norforms *Fleet, USA.*
Pessaries: Vaginal deodorant.
Topical powder: Corn starch (p.1379·3); zinc oxide (p.1128·2).
Vaginal irritation.

Norgagil *Norgine, Fr.†*
Sterculia (p.1250·2); attapulgite (p.1212·1); meprobamate (p.691·1).
Gastrointestinal disorders.

Norgalax
Norgine, Belg.; Norgine, Fr.; Norgine, Ger.†; Norgine, Hong Kong; Norgine, Irl.; Norgine, Neth.; Norgine, Singapore; Norgine, Switz.; Norgine, UK.
Docusate sodium (p.1223·1).
Bowel evacuation; constipation.

Norgalax Miniklistier *Norgine, Ger.*
Docusate sodium (p.1223·1); glycerol (p.1616·3).
Bowel evacuation; constipation.

Norgesic
Note.This name is used for preparations of different composition.
Sanova, Aust.; 3M, Austral.; 3M, Fin.; 3M, Hong Kong; 3M, Irl.; 3M, Israel; 3M, NZ; 3M, Port.†; 3M, Singapore; 3M, Swed.; 3M, Switz.†; 3M, Thai.
Orphenadrine citrate (p.470·3); paracetamol (p.71·2).
Dysmenorrhoea; headache; skeletal muscle pain and spasm.

3M, Canad.; 3M, USA.
Orphenadrine citrate (p.470·3); aspirin (p.14·2); caffeine (p.761·3).
Musculoskeletal pain.

Norgesic N *3M, Ger.*
Orphenadrine citrate (p.470·3); propyphenazone (p.80·2).
Dysmenorrhoea; headache; musculoskeletal pain.

Norgeston *Schering, UK.*
Levonorgestrel (p.1486·2).
Progestogen-only oral contraceptive.

Norgic *Pond's, Thai.*
Orphenadrine citrate (p.470·3); paracetamol (p.71·2).
Skeletal muscle spasm.

Norglicem *Rottapharm, Spain.*
Glibenclamide (p.321·3).
Diabetes mellitus.

Norgotin *Helsinn Birex, Hong Kong.*
Chlorhexidine acetate (p.1138·2); ephedrine hydrochloride (p.1090·1); amethocaine [tetracaine] hydrochloride (p.1305·2).
Otitis.

Norica *Ottolenghi, Ital.*
Benzalkonium chloride (p.1133·2).
Room disinfection and deodorization.

Noricaven *Bionorica, Singapore.*
Asperula odorata; silybum marianum (p.1021·3); crataegus (p.1600·2); rue (p.1660·1); echinacea (p.1606·2).
Vascular disorders.

Noricaven novo *Bionorica, Ger.*
Aesculus (p.1574·1).
Venous insufficiency.

Noriclan *Lilly, Spain.*
Dirithromycin (p.199·2).
Bacterial infections.

Noriday
Searle, Austral.; Searle, Irl.; Searle, NZ; Pharmacia, UK.
Norethisterone (p.1485·1).
Progestogen-only oral contraceptive.

Norifortan *Hoechst Marion Roussel, S.Afr.†*
Avapyrazone; dipyrone (p.34·1).
Painful smooth muscle spasm.

Norilax *Ethimed, S.Afr.†*
Docusate sodium (p.1223·1); dantron (p.1221·3).
Constipation.

Noriline *Noristan, S.Afr.†*
Amitriptyline hydrochloride (p.273·3).
Depression; nocturnal enuresis.

Norimin
Monsanto, Austral.; Searle, Hong Kong; Searle, NZ; Pharmacia, UK.
Norethisterone (p.1485·1); ethinylestradiol (p.1476·2).
28-Day packs also contain 7 inert tablets.
Combined oral contraceptive.

Norimode
Quatromed, S.Afr.; Tillomed, UK.
Loperamide hydrochloride (p.1231·3).
Diarrhoea; ostomy management.

Norimox *Noristan, S.Afr.†*
Amoxicillin (p.149·2).
Bacterial infections.

Norincol *Volchem, Ital.*
Carbohydrate, lipid, amino-acid, and dietary fibre preparation (p.1350·1).
Nutritional supplement.

Norinyl *Searle, Mex.*
Norethisterone (p.1485·1); mestranol (p.1482·1).
28-Day packs also contain 7 inert tablets.
Combined oral contraceptive; menstrual disorders.

Norinyl-1
Searle, Austral.; Searle, Hong Kong; Searle, Irl.†; Searle, NZ; Pharmacia, UK.
Norethisterone (p.1485·1); mestranol (p.1482·1).
28-Day packs also contain 7 inert tablets.
Combined oral contraceptive; menstrual disorders.

Norinyl-1/28 *Syntex, S.Afr.*
21 Tablets, norethisterone (p.1485·1); mestranol (p.1482·1); 7 tablets, inert.
Combined oral contraceptive.

Norinyl 1 + 35 *Searle, USA.*
Norethisterone (p.1485·1); ethinylestradiol (p.1476·2).
28-Day packs also contain 7 inert tablets.
Combined oral contraceptive.

Norinyl 1 + 50 *Searle, USA.*
Norethisterone (p.1485·1); mestranol (p.1482·1).
28-Day packs also contain 7 inert tablets.
Combined oral contraceptive.

Norinyl 1/50 *Searle, Canad.*
Norethisterone (p.1485·1); mestranol (p.1482·1).
28-Day packs also contain 7 inert tablets.
Combined oral contraceptive.

Noripam *Compu, S.Afr.*
Oxazepam (p.697·1).
Alcohol withdrawal syndrome; anxiety disorders.

Noripurum *Byk, Braz.*
Iron polymaltose (p.1369·2).
Iron deficiency; iron-deficiency anaemias.

Noripurum Folico *Byk, Braz.*
Folic acid (p.1361·1); iron polymaltose (p.1369·2).
Iron deficiency; iron-deficiency anaemias.

Norisep *Noristan, S.Afr.†*
Co-trimoxazole (p.193·3).
Bacterial infections.

Norisodrine with Calcium Iodide *Abbott, USA.*
Isoprenaline sulfate (p.914·3); calcium iodide (p.1086·2).
Coughs.

Noristerat
Schering, Fr.; Schering, Ger.; Schering, Mex.; Schering, Singapore; Schering, Thai.; Schering, UK.
Norethisterone enantate (p.1485·1).
Progestogen-only injectable contraceptive.

Norit
Norit, Aust.; Wolfs, Belg.; Norit, Israel; Vemedia, Neth.
Activated charcoal (p.1000·2).
Diarrhoea; flatulence; treatment of poisoning.

Noritate
Dermik, Canad.; Kestrel, UK; Dermik, USA.
Metronidazole (p.594·1).
Acne; rosacea.

Norit-Carbomix
Norit, Aust.; Wolfs, Belg.
Activated charcoal (p.1000·2).
Diarrhoea; treatment of poisoning.

Noritet *Quatromed, S.Afr.*
Doxycycline hyclate (p.200·1).
Bacterial infections.

Noritrate *Dermik, Hong Kong.*
Metronidazole (p.594·1).
Anaerobic bacterial infections.

Noritren
Lundbeck, Denm.; Lundbeck, Fin.; Lundbeck, Ital.; Lundbeck, Norw.
Nortriptyline hydrochloride (p.301·3).
Depression.

Norivite *Aventis, S.Afr.*
Vitamin B substances (p.1350·1).

Norivite-12 *Aventis, S.Afr.*
Cyanocobalamin (p.1388·1).
Anaemias; tonic.

Norizal *EMS, Braz.*
Ketoconazole (p.389·1).
Fungal infections.

Norizine *Quatromed, S.Afr.*
Cyclizine hydrochloride (p.414·1).
Nausea and vomiting; vestibular disorders.

Norkotral Tema *Desitin, Ger.*
Temazepam (p.707·2).
Sleep disorders.

Norlevo *Besins-Iscovesco, Fr.*
Levonorgestrel (p.1486·2).
Postcoital contraceptive.

Norline *Pharmaland, Thai.*
Nortriptyline hydrochloride (p.301·3).
Depression.

Norlip *Unipharm, Israel.*
Bezafibrate (p.849·1).
Hyperlipidaemias.

Norlutate *Parke, Davis, Canad.*
Norethisterone acetate (p.1485·1).
Abnormal uterine bleeding; amenorrhoea; endometriosis.

Norluten *SmithKline Beecham, Fr.†*
Norethisterone (p.1485·1).
Endometriosis; fibromas; menstrual disorders.

Normabenzil *Farmoquimica, Braz.*
Benzathine benzylpenicillin (p.156·2).
Bacterial infections.

Normabrain *Hoechst Marion Roussel, Ger.*
Piracetam (p.1652·1).
Mental function disorders.

Normacidine *Synthelabo, Belg.†.*
Calcium carbonate (p.1215·1); aluminium glycinate
(p.1210·3).
Gastrointestinal disorders associated with hyperacidity.

Normacol
Note.This name is used for preparations of different composition.
Norgine, Belg.; Rivex, Canad.; Norgine, Fr.; Norgine, Hong Kong;
Norgine, Irl.; Norgine, Ital.; Norgine, Neth.; CSL, NZ; Norgine, NZ;
Norgine, S.Afr.; Norgine, Singapore; Norgine, Switz.; Norgine, UK.
Sterculia (p.1250·2).
Formerly known as Normacol Special in the *UK.*
Constipation.

Schering, Mex.
Bassorin; frangula bark (p.1227·1).
Constipation.

Normacol a la Bourdaine *Norgine, Fr.*
Sterculia (p.1250·2); frangula bark (p.1227·1).
Constipation.

Normacol Antispasmodique *Norgine, Belg.*
Sterculia (p.1250·2); alverine citrate (p.1211·3).
Constipation.

Normacol (avec bourdaine) *Norgine, Switz.*
Sterculia (p.1250·2); frangula (p.1227·1).
Constipation.

Normacol Forte *Rubio, Spain.*
Sterculia (p.1250·2); frangula bark (p.1227·1).
Constipation.

Normacol Lavement *Norgine, Fr.*
Monobasic sodium phosphate (p.1193·2); dibasic sodium phosphate (p.1193·2).
Bowel evacuation.

Normacol Plus
Norgine, Austral.; Norgine, Belg.; Norgine, Hong Kong; Norgine, Irl.;
CSL, NZ; Norgine, NZ; Helsinn, Port.; Norgine, S.Afr.; Norgine, Singapore; Norgine, UK.
Sterculia (p.1250·2); frangula (p.1227·1).
Formerly known as Normacol Standard in *Irl.* and the
UK.
Constipation; diverticular disease; ostomy management.

Normafibe *Norgine, Austral.*
Sterculia (p.1250·2).
Constipation; fibre supplement.

Normaform *Sodip, Switz.*
Phentermine resin (as an ion-exchange resin complex)
(p.1514·1).
Obesity.

Normagit *Synthelabo, Port.†.*
Tiapride hydrochloride (p.709·1).

Normagrin *QIF, Braz.*
Phenolphthalein (p.1244·1); bladderwrack (p.1585·2);
thyroid (p.1526·2); colecalciferol (p.1391·1); bile salts
(p.1585·1).
Constipation; obesity.

Normalax *Herbalia, Ital.†.*
Rhamnus alpinus; globularia vulgaris; chamomile
(p.1593·2); red-poppy petal (p.1029·1); liquorice
(p.1231·2); fennel (p.1610·1).
Constipation.

Normalene *Montefarmaco, Ital.*
Bisacodyl (p.1212·2).
Constipation.

Normalin *Noristan, S.Afr.†.*
Procaterol hydrochloride (p.770·1).
Bronchospasm.

NormaLine *Antonetto, Ital.*
Note. A similar name is used for preparations of different composition
(see below).
Glucomannan (p.1616·2).
Dietary supplement in diabetes mellitus and hyperlipidaemias; obesity.

Normaline *Apothecary, USA.*
Note. A similar name is used for preparations of different composition
(see below).
Sodium chloride (p.1196·1).
Sodium depletion.

Normalip pro *Knoll, Ger.*
Fenofibrate (p.889·1).
Hyperlipidaemias.

Normaloe *Tillomed, UK.*
Loperamide hydrochloride (p.1231·3).
Diarrhoea.

Normalol *Dexxon, Israel.*
Atenolol (p.841·3).
*Angina pectoris; hypertension; migraine; myocardial
infarction.*

Normamor *Uniao Quimica, Braz.*
Ethinylestradiol (p.1476·2); 13-beta-ethyl-17-alpha-
ethinyl-17-beta-hydroxygon-4-en-3-one.
Combined oral contraceptive.

Normase *Molteni, Ital.*
Lactulose (p.1230·1).
Constipation; gastrointestinal disorders; hepatic encephalopathy.

Normasol *Seton, Israel; SSL, UK.*
Sodium chloride (p.1196·1).
Irrigation solution.

Normastigmin *Sigmapharm, Aust.*
Neostigmine bromide (p.1419·3) or neostigmine metilsulfate (p.1420·1).
*Gastrointestinal atony; glaucoma; myasthenia gravis;
pre- and post-operative lowering of intra-ocular pressure; reversal of competitive neuromuscular blockade;
reversal of mydriasis and cycloplegia; urinary retention.*

Normastigmin mit Pilocarpin *Sigmapharm, Aust.*
Neostigmine bromide (p.1419·3); pilocarpine hydrochloride (p.1422·3).
*Glaucoma; pre- and post-operative lowering of intra-
ocular pressure; reversal of mydriasis and cycloplegia.*

Normaten *Xepa-Soul Pattinson, Singapore.*
Atenolol (p.841·3).
Angina pectoris; arrhythmias; hypertension; myocardial infarction.

Normatens *Solvay, Neth.*
Moxonidine (p.936·3).
Hypertension.

Normavom *Cryopharma, Mex.*
Difenidol hydrochloride (p.1222·1).
Nausea and vomiting; vertigo.

Normax *Celltech, UK.*
Dantron (p.1221·3); docusate sodium (p.1223·1).
These ingredients can be described by the British Approved Name Co-danthrusate.
Constipation.

Normegon *Organon, UK†.*
Human menopausal gonadotrophins (p.1288·2).
Infertility.

Normensan *Disperga, Aust.*
Papaverine hydrochloride (p.1648·1); hyoscyamine
(p.469·3); propyphenazone (p.80·2).
Dysmenorrhoea; migraine; smooth muscle spasm.

Normex *Heralds, Braz.*
Etynodiol (p.1477·2); ethinylestradiol (p.1476·2).
Combined oral contraceptive.

Normhydral *Gebro, Aust.*
Anhydrous glucose; sodium chloride; sodium citrate;
potassium chloride (p.1185·2).
Diarrhoea; oral rehydration therapy.

Normicina *Tedec Meiji, Spain.*
Midecamycin acetate (p.224·3).
Bacterial infections.

Normiflo *Wyeth-Ayerst, USA†.*
Ardeparin sodium (p.841·2).
Thrombosis prophylaxis.

Normin *Searle, Irl.†.*
Norethisterone (p.1485·1); ethinylestradiol (p.1476·2).
Combined oral contraceptive.

Normison
Wyeth, Austral.; Wyeth Lederle, Belg.; Wyeth Lederle, Denm.; Wyeth
Lederle, Fin.; Wyeth Lederle, Fr.; Wyeth, Irl.; Wyeth Lederle, Ital.;
Wyeth, Neth.; Wyeth, NZ; Wyeth Lederle, Port.; Aspen, S.Afr.;
Wyeth, Switz.; Wyeth, UK.
Temazepam (p.707·2).
Insomnia; premedication.

Normiten *Abic, Israel.*
Atenolol (p.841·3).
Angina pectoris; hypertension; myocardial infarction.

Normitrol *Searle, Mex.*
Difenidol (p.1222·1).

Normix *Wassermann, Ital.*
Rifaximin (p.246·3).
Gastrointestinal bacterial infections; hyperammonaemia.

Normo Gastryl *Sabex, Canad.*
Sodium bicarbonate (p.1186·2); sodium sulfate
(p.1250·1); sodium phosphate (p.1193·2).
Gastric hyperacidity.

Normo Nar *Zambon, Spain.*
Muramidase hydrochloride (p.1638·1); thonzylamine
hydrochloride (p.426·2); methylethylaminophenol hydriodide.
Nasal congestion; sinus congestion.

Normobren *Medosan, Ital.*
Acetylcarnitine hydrochloride (p.1572·1).
Cerebrovascular disorders.

Normoc *Merckle, Ger.*
Bromazepam (p.656·3).
Anxiety.

Normocir *Inkeysa, Spain.*
Ginkgo biloba (p.1615·2).
Cerebral and peripheral vascular disorders.

Normodiar *Hoechst Marion Roussel, Mex.*
Nifurzide (p.230·2).

Normodyne *Schering, USA.*
Labetalol hydrochloride (p.918·1).
Hypertension.

Normofenicol *Normon, Spain.*
Chloramphenicol (p.179·1) or chloramphenicol sodium succinate (p.179·2).
Lignocaine [lidocaine] hydrochloride (p.1313·2) is included in the injection to alleviate the pain of injection.
Bacterial infections.

Normofer *Magis, Ital.*
Iron acetylaspartilate-protein complex.
Anaemias; iron deficiency.

Normofundin *Braun, Ger.*
Electrolyte infusion with glucose (p.1180·1).
Carbohydrate source; fluid and electrolyte disorders.

Normofundin X *Braun, Ger.*
Electrolyte infusion with xylitol (p.1180·1).
Carbohydrate source; fluid and electrolyte disorders.

Normofundin G-5 *Braun, Ger.*
Electrolyte infusion with glucose (p.1180·1).
Carbohydrate source; fluid and electrolyte disorders.

Normofundin OP *Braun, Ger.*
Electrolyte infusion (p.1180·1).
Fluid and electrolyte disorders.

Normofundin sKG *Braun, Ger.*
Potassium-free electrolyte infusion with glucose
(p.1180·1).
Carbohydrate source; fluid and electrolyte disorders.

Normofusin *Fresenius Kabi, Ger.*
Electrolyte infusion with glucose.
Carbohydrate source; fluid and electrolyte disorders.

Normogam *ICT, Ital.*
Gamolenic acid (p.1613·1).
Gamolenic acid deficiency; nutritional supplement.

Normogamma *Nuovo ISM, Ital.*
A normal immunoglobulin (p.1551·3).
Passive immunisation.

Normogastryl
Note.This name is used for preparations of different composition.
Upsamedica, Belg.†.
Sodium bicarbonate (p.1186·2); sodium sulfate
(p.1250·1); sodium phosphate (p.1193·2); sodium bromide (p.1587·1); sodium benzoate (p.1134·3); sodium
citrate (p.1186·2).
Gastrointestinal disorders.

UPSA, Fr.; Upsamedica, Spain; Upsamedica, Switz.
Sodium bicarbonate (p.1186·2); sodium sulfate
(p.1250·1); sodium phosphate (p.1193·2).
Gastrointestinal disorders.

Normogin *Baldacci, Ital.*
Bacilli vaginalis culture.
Vaginal bacterial infections.

Normoglaucon
Tramedico, Belg.; Mann, Ger.; Mann, Neth.; Lepori, Port.; Mann, Singapore; Bausch & Lomb, Thai.; Mann, Thai.
Metipranolol hydrochloride (p.930·2); pilocarpine hydrochloride (p.1422·3).
Glaucoma; ocular hypertension.

Normoglucon *Klinge, Aust.*
Glibenclamide (p.321·3).
Diabetes mellitus.

Normolyt *Gebro, Aust.*
Anhydrous glucose; sodium chloride; sodium citrate;
potassium chloride (p.1185·2).
Diarrhoea; oral rehydration therapy.

Normolytoral *Gebro, Switz.*
Anhydrous glucose; sodium chloride; sodium citrate;
potassium chloride (p.1185·2).
Diarrhoea; oral rehydration therapy.

Normomensil *Sedabel, Braz.*
Progesterone (p.1488·3); estradiol (p.1473·1).
Menopausal disorders; menstrual disorders.

Normonal
Eisai, Ger.†; Eisai, Thai.
Tripamide (p.987·3).
Hypertension.

Normonsona *Normon, Spain†.*
Prednisolone (p.1077·3).
Corticosteroid.

Normoparin *Caber, Ital.*
Heparin sodium (p.902·1).
Thromboembolic disorders.

Normophasic *Nourypharma, Switz.*
7 Tablets, ethinylestradiol (p.1476·2); 15 tablets, ethinylestradiol; lynestrenol (p.1480·1).
Sequential-type oral contraceptive.

Normopresan *Rafa, Israel.*
Clonidine hydrochloride (p.860·1).
Hypertension.

Normopresil *Sanofi Synthelabo, Spain.*
Chlortalidone (p.857·1); atenolol (p.841·3).
Hypertension.

Normopress
Note.This name is used for preparations of different composition.
Caber, Ital.
Atenolol (p.841·3); indapamide (p.913·1).
Hypertension.

Alliance, S.Afr.
Methyldopa (p.927·3).
Hypertension.

Normopride Enzimatico *Sanofi Winthrop, Braz.*
Bromopride (p.1215·1); dimethicone (p.1249·2); lipase; cellulase (p.1593·1); amylase (p.1579·3).
Digestive-system disorders; nausea and vomiting.

Normo-real *Novartis Nutrition, Fr.*
A range of preparations for enteral nutrition (p.1350·1).

Normorix
Nycomed, Norw.; Nycomed, Swed.
Hydrochlorothiazide (p.907·3); amiloride hydrochloride (p.835·1).
Hypertension; liver cirrhosis with ascites; oedema.

Normosang
Leiras, Fin.; Orphan, Fr.; Falk, Ger.; Stauffacher, Switz.; Orphan, UK.
Haem arginate (p.1011·1).
Porphyria.

Normosol
Abbott, Hong Kong; Abbott, USA.
A range of electrolyte infusions with or without glucose (p.1180·1).
Fluid and electrolyte disorders.

Normosol M 900 Cal *Abbott, Ital.*
Electrolyte infusion with glucose and fructose
(p.1180·1).
Carbohydrate source; fluid and electrolyte disorders.

Normosol M Con Glucosio 5% *Abbott, Ital.*
Electrolyte infusion with glucose (p.1180·1).
Fluid and electrolyte disorders.

Normosol R *Abbott, Ital.*
Electrolyte infusion (p.1180·1).
Fluid and electrolyte disorders.

Normosol R Con Glucosio 5% *Abbott, Ital.*
Electrolyte infusion with glucose (p.1180·1).
Carbohydrate source; fluid and electrolyte disorders.

Normosol R/K Con Glucosio 5% *Abbott, Ital.*
Electrolyte infusion with glucose (p.1180·1).
Carbohydrate source; fluid and electrolyte disorders.

Normospor *Propan, S.Afr.*
Clotrimazole (p.382·1).
Fungal infections of the skin; vulvovaginal fungal infections.

Normosteril *Orion, Fin.*
Electrolyte infusion with glucose (p.1180·1).
Carbohydrate source; fluid and electrolyte disorders.

Normotensin *Hoechst Marion Roussel, Aust.*
Penbutolol sulfate (p.952·2); frusemide [furosemide]
(p.893·1).
Hypertension.

Normothen *Bioindustria, Ital.*
Doxazosin mesilate (p.883·2).
Hypertension.

Normotil *APS, Port.*
Captopril (p.853·3); hydrochlorothiazide (p.907·3).
Hypertension.

Normotin VI *OTW, Ger.†.*
Crataegus (p.1600·2).
Cardiac disorders.

Normotin-R *OTW, Ger.*
Etamivan (p.1509·3); norfenefrine hydrochloride
(p.949·1); heptaminol hydrochloride (p.1619·2).
Hypotension.

Normovite Antianemico *Normon, Spain.*
Folic acid (p.1361·1); ferrous gluceptate (p.1360·1).
Iron and folic acid deficiency.

Normovite Antianemico Inyectable *Normon,
Spain†.*
Folic acid (p.1361·1); ferrous gluceptate (p.1360·1).
Lignocaine [lidocaine] hydrochloride (p.1313·2) is included in this preparation to alleviate the pain of injection.
Anaemias; tonic.

Normovlar ED *Schering, S.Afr.†.*
21 Tablets, levonorgestrel (p.1486·2); ethinylestradiol
(p.1476·2); 7 tablets, inert.
Biphasic oral contraceptive; menstrual disorders.

Normoxidil *Medosan, Ital.*
Minoxidil (p.934·2).
Alopecia.

Normoxin *Asta Medica, Aust.*
Moxonidine (p.936·3).
Hypertension.

Normpress *Greater Pharma, Thai.*
Propranolol hydrochloride (p.962·3).
Angina pectoris; hypertension; myocardial infarction.

Normum *Serpero, Ital.†.*
Sulpiride (p.706·1).
Dysthymia; psychoses.

Norogil *Hoechst Marion Roussel, Braz.*
Dihydroergocristine mesilate (p.1603·2); lomifylline.
*Impaired mental function; migraine and other vascular
headaches; orthostatic hypotension; thrombosis
prophylaxis.*

No-Roma *Salts Healthcare, UK.*
A deodorant liquid for use with colostomies and ileostomies.
Formerly known as Saltair No-Roma.

Noroxin
Merck Sharp & Dohme, Austral.; Merck Frosst, Canad.; Merck Sharp
& Dohme, Fin.; Merck Sharp & Dohme, Ital.; Merck Sharp & Dohme,
Mex.; Merck Sharp & Dohme, Neth.; Merck Sharp & Dohme, NZ;
Merck Sharp & Dohme, Port.; Merck Sharp & Dohme, S.Afr.; Merck
Sharp & Dohme, Spain; Merck Sharp & Dohme, Switz.; Merck, USA;
Roberts, USA.
Norfloxacin (p.232·1).
Bacterial infections.

Noroxine *Merck Sharp & Dohme-Chibret, Fr.*
Norfloxacin (p.232·1).
*Bacterial infections of the urinary tract; gonococcal
cervicitis; gonococcal urethritis.*

Nor-Pa *Salus, Ital.*
Atenolol (p.841·3); indapamide (p.913·1).
Hypertension.

Norpace
Searle, Austral.; Roberts, Canad.†; Searle, Denm.†; Heumann, Ger.;
Searle, Hong Kong; Searle, S.Afr.; Searle, Switz.; Searle, Thai.; Searle,
USA.
Disopyramide phosphate (p.878·2).
Arrhythmias.

Norphen
Atlantic, Singapore; Atlantic, Thai.
Orphenadrine citrate (p.470·3); paracetamol (p.71·2).
Dysmenorrhoea; musculoskeletal pain; tension headache.

Norphyllin SR *Norton, UK.*
Aminophylline (p.760·1).
Bronchospasm.

Norpid *Greater Pharma, Thai.*
Gemfibrozil (p.896·2).
Hyperlipidaemias.

Norplant
Wyeth-Ayerst, Canad.; Discotrade, Israel; Sanofi Winthrop, Mex.;

Schering, Singapore; Leiras, Swed.; Schering, Thai.; Hoechst Marion Roussel, UK†; Wyeth-Ayerst, USA.
Levonorgestrel (p.1486·2).
Progestogen-only implantable contraceptive.

Norpramin
Note. This name is used for preparations of different composition.
Hoechst Marion Roussel, Canad.; Hoechst Marion Roussel, USA.
Desipramine hydrochloride (p.282·3).
Depression.

CEPA, Spain.
Omeprazole (p.1239·1).
Gastro-oesophageal reflux; peptic ulcer; Zollinger-Ellison syndrome.

Norpress Pacific, NZ.
Nortriptyline hydrochloride (p.301·3).
Depression.

Norpril Fustery, Mex.
Enalapril maleate (p.883·3).
Heart failure; hypertension.

Norpro Noristan, S.Afr.†.
Propranolol hydrochloride (p.962·3).
Anxiety disorders; cardiovascular disorders.

Norprolac
Novartis, Aust.; Novartis, Fin.; Novartis, Fr.; Novartis, Ger.; Novartis, Hong Kong; Novartis, Israel; Novartis, Mex.; Novartis, Neth.; Novartis, Norw.; Novartis, S.Afr.; Novartis, Spain; Novartis, Swed.; Novartis, Switz.; Novartis, UK.
Quinagolide hydrochloride (p.1176·2).
Hyperprolactinaemia.

Nor-QD Watson, USA.
Norethisterone (p.1485·1).
Progestogen-only oral contraceptive.

Norsa Shiwa, Thai.
Norfloxacin (p.232·1).
Bacterial infections.

Norset Riom, Fr.
Mirtazapine (p.299·1).
Depression.

Norsol Ecosol, Switz.
Norfloxacin (p.232·1).
Bacterial infections.

Nortase Asche, Ger.
Rizolipase; protease and amylase from *Aspergillus oryzae.*
Pancreatic insufficiency.

Nortem Norton Waterford, Irl.
Temazepam (p.707·2).
Insomnia.

Norterol Tecnifar, Port.
Nortriptyline hydrochloride (p.301·3).
Anxiety; depression; excitable states; insomnia.

Nor-Tet Vortech, USA†.
Tetracycline hydrochloride (p.258·3).
Bacterial infections.

Nortimil Chiesi, Ital.
Desipramine hydrochloride (p.282·3).
Depression; psychoses.

Norton Farmasa, Braz.
Nimodipine (p.946·1).
Neurological deficit following subarachnoid haemorrhage.

Nortrel Wyeth, Braz.
Levonorgestrel (p.1486·2).
Progestogen-only oral contraceptive.

Nortrilen
Lundbeck, Aust.; Lundbeck, Belg.; Lundbeck, Ger.; Lundbeck, Hong Kong; Lundbeck, Neth.; Lundbeck, Switz.; Lundbeck, Thai.
Nortriptyline hydrochloride (p.301·3).
Depression.

Nortrix Tecnifar, Port.†.
Nortriptyline hydrochloride (p.301·3).
Anxiety disorders; depression.

Nortron Dista, Spain.
Dirithromycin (p.199·2).
Bacterial infections.

Nortuss Rosemont, Thai.
Promethazine hydrochloride (p.423·2); codeine phosphate (p.25·2).
Coughs.

Nortussine
Note. This name is used for preparations of different composition.
Norgine, Belg.
Dextromethorphan hydrobromide (p.1087·3); mepyramine maleate (p.421·1); phenylephrine hydrochloride (p.1097·1); guaifenesin (p.1092·2).
Coughs.

Norgine, Fr.
Paediatric syrup: Dextromethorphan hydrobromide (p.1087·3); mepyramine maleate (p.421·1); guaifenesin (p.1092·2).
Syrup: Dextromethorphan hydrobromide (p.1087·3); mepyramine maleate (p.421·1).
Formerly contained dextromethorphan hydrobromide, mepyramine maleate, phenylephrine hydrochloride, and guaifenesin.
Coughs.

Nortyline Condrugs, Thai.
Nortriptyline hydrochloride (p.301·3).
Depression.

Norum Chew, Thai.
Aciclovir (p.612·3).
Herpes simplex infections of the skin and mucous membranes.

Noruxol Knoll, Ital.
Collagenase (p.1598·2).
Necrotic wounds and ulcers.

Norvas
Pfizer, Mex.; Pfizer Consumer, Spain.
Amlodipine besilate (p.838·3).
Angina pectoris; hypertension.

Norvasc
Pfizer, Aust.; Pfizer, Austral.; Pfizer, Braz.; Pfizer, Canad.; Pfizer, Denm.; Pfizer, Fin.; Pfizer, Ger.; Mack, Illert., Ger.; Pfizer, Hong Kong; Pfizer, Israel; Pfizer, Ital.; Pfizer, Neth.; Pfizer, Norw.; Douglas, NZ; Pfizer, Port.; Pfizer, S.Afr.; Pfizer, Singapore; Pfizer, Swed.; Pfizer, Switz.; Pfizer, Thai.; Pfizer, USA.
Amlodipine besilate (p.838·3).
Angina pectoris; hypertension.

Norvedan
Roche, Aust.; Helsinn, Port.
Fentiazac (p.40·2) or fentiazac calcium (p.40·2).
Fever; inflammation; musculoskeletal and joint disorders; pain.

Norvir
Abbott, Austral.; Abbott, Belg.; Abbott, Canad.; Abbott, Denm.; Abbott, Fin.; Abbott, Fr.; Abbott, Ger.; Abbott, Hong Kong; Abbott, Israel; Abbott, Ital.; Dainabot, Jpn; Abbott, Mex.; Abbott, Neth.; Norw.; Abbott, NZ; Abbott, Port.; Abbott, S.Afr.; Abbott, Spain; Abbott, Swed.; Abbott, Switz.; Abbott, Thai.; Abbott, UK; Abbott, USA.
Ritonavir (p.640·2).
HIV infection.

Norwich Extra Strength Procter & Gamble, USA.
Aspirin (p.14·2).
Fever; inflammation; myocardial infarction; pain; transient ischaemic attacks.

Norxacin Siam Bheasach, Thai.
Norfloxacin (p.232·1).
Bacterial infections.

Norxia Asian Pharm, Thai.
Norfloxacin (p.232·1).
Bacterial infections.

Norzac Norton Waterford, Irl.
Fluoxetine hydrochloride (p.284·2).
Bulimia; depression.

Norzetam IPFI, Ital.
Piracetam (p.1652·1).
Mental function impairment.

Norzine Purdue Frederick, USA†.
Thiethylperazine maleate (p.426·1).
Nausea and vomiting.

Norzol Rosemont, UK.
Metronidazole benzoate (p.594·1).
Bacterial infections.

Nos Dermoform, Spain.
Famotidine (p.1225·3).
Gastrointestinal hyperacidity.

NoSalt Norcliff Thayer, USA†.
Low sodium dietary salt substitute (p.1350·1).

Noscaflex Wolfs, Belg.
Paediatric syrup: Noscapine camsilate (p.1096·1).
Syrup: Noscapine hydrochloride (p.1096·1); guaifenesin (p.1092·2).
Tablets: Noscapine hydrochloride (p.1096·1).
Coughs.

Noscal Sankyo, Jpn†.
Troglitazone (p.337·1).
Diabetes mellitus.

Noscorex Interdelta, Switz.
Noscapine hydrochloride (p.1096·1); guaifenesin (p.1092·2).
Coughs; upper-respiratory-tract inflammation.

Nose Fresh Rappai, Switz.
Sea salt (p.1196·1).
Nasal disorders.

Nosebo Ottolenghi, Ital.
Sulfur (p.1123·3).
Acne; skin cleansing.

NoseEase Impharm, UK.
Jojoba oil; hyssop oil; artemisia oil (p.1609·2); peppermint oil (p.1243·3).
Nasal congestion.

Nosenil Farba, Ital.†.
Ginkgo biloba (p.1615·2); eleutherococcus (p.1615·3); kola (p.1681·1); equisetum (p.1606·3); urtica (p.1678·2).

Nositrol Cryopharma, Mex.
Hydrocortisone sodium succinate (p.1074·1).
Corticosteroid.

No-Sor Nose Balm Pickles, UK.
Dibrompropamidine isetionate (p.1143·1); wheat-germ oil; menthol (p.1632·3); eucalyptus (p.1609·2).

No-Sor Vapour Rub Pickles, UK.
Camphor (p.1589·3); turpentine; menthol (p.1632·3); eucalyptus oil (p.1609·2); nutmeg oil (p.1643·1); cedar wood oil; thymol (p.1158·3).
Upper respiratory-tract congestion.

No-Spa
Chinoin, Hung.; Sanofi Synthelabo, Thai.
Drotaverine hydrochloride (p.1606·1).
Peptic ulcer; smooth muscle spasm.

Nossacin Benedetti, Ital.
Cinoxacin (p.182·2).
Bacterial infections of the urinary tract.

Nostril
Note. This name is used for preparations of different composition.
Boehringer Ingelheim, Fr.
Chlorhexidine gluconate (p.1138·2); cetrimonium bromide (p.1137·3).
Nose and throat infections.

Ciba, USA.
Phenylephrine hydrochloride (p.1097·1).
Nasal congestion.

Nostrilla Ciba Consumer, USA.
Oxymetazoline hydrochloride (p.1096·2).
Nasal congestion.

Nostroline Co-Pharma, UK.
Menthol (p.1632·3); eucalyptol (p.1609·2); geranium oil (p.1615·1).
Nasal congestion.

Notakehl Sanum-Kehlbeck, Ger.
Homoeopathic preparation.

Noten
Alphapharm, Austral.; Merck, Thai.
Atenolol (p.841·3).
Angina pectoris; arrhythmias; hypertension; myocardial infarction.

Notensyl CTI, Israel.
Dicyclomine [dicycloverine] hydrochloride (p.466·1).
Irritable bowel syndrome.

Notezine Rhone-Poulenc Rorer, Fr.
Diethylcarbamazine citrate (p.98·1).
Filariasis.

Nothav Chiron, Ital.
A hepatitis A vaccine (p.1541·2).
Active immunisation.

Nottem Angelini, Ital.
Zolpidem tartrate (p.712·2).
Insomnia.

Notul Mendelejeff, Ital.
Cimetidine hydrochloride (p.1218·3).
Gastrointestinal disorders associated with hyperacidity.

Notuss Ache, Braz.
Paracetamol (p.71·2); diphenhydramine (p.416·1); pseudoephedrine (p.1099·2); dropropizine (p.1089·3).
Coughs.

Nourilax Chefaro, Neth.†.
Bisacodyl (p.1212·2).
Constipation.

Nourishake GNLD, Austral.
Nutritional supplement (p.1350·1).

Noury Hoofdlotion Alfaco, Neth.†.
Malathion (p.1434·2).
Pediculosis.

Nourymag Nourypharma, Ger.
Magnesium aspartate (p.1190·3).
Magnesium deficiency.

Nourytam Nourypharma, Ger.
Tamoxifen citrate (p.571·1).
Breast cancer.

Nova Derm Darier, Mex.
Cream; lotion; solution: Glycolic acid (p.1115·1).
Dry skin disorders.
Topical gel: Glycolic acid (p.1115·1); hydroquinone (p.1115·1).
Hyperpigmentation disorders.

Nova Perfecting Lotion Avon, Canad.†.
Salicylic acid (p.1122·3).
Acne.

Nova Rectal Sabex, Canad.†.
Pentobarbital sodium (p.698·2).
Insomnia; sedative.

Novaban
Novartis, Belg.; Novartis, Neth.
Tropisetron hydrochloride (p.1253·3).
Nausea and vomiting.

Novaboin Dermopen, Braz.
Aesculus (p.1574·1); menthol (p.1632·3); boric acid (p.1586·1); rutoside (p.1611·2); lignocaine [lidocaine] (p.1313·2); adrenaline [epinephrine] (p.829·1).
Haemorrhoids.

Novabritine SmithKline Beecham, Belg.
Amoxicillin sodium (p.149·2) or amoxicillin trihydrate (p.149·2).
Bacterial infections.

Novacef
Note. This name is used for preparations of different composition.
IFI, Ital.
Propylene glycol cefatrizine (p.164·3).
Bacterial infections.

Promeco, Mex.
Cefixime (p.166·2).
Bacterial infections.

Novacefrex Sanofi Synthelabo, Port.
Cefradine (p.173·3).
Bacterial infections.

Novacet Medicis, USA.
Sulfacetamide sodium (p.250·3); sulfur (p.1123·3).
Acne; seborrhoeic dermatitis.

Novacetol Pharmastra, Fr.
Aspirin (p.14·2); paracetamol (p.71·2); codeine hydrochloride (p.25·2).
Fever; pain.

Novaclens Johnson & Johnson, Austral.†.
Chlorhexidine gluconate (p.1138·2).
Skin disinfection; wounds.

Novacnyl Esseti, Ital.
Meclocycline sulfosalicylate (p.222·1).
Skin infections.

Novacol Johnson & Johnson, Austral.†.
Chlorhexidine gluconate (p.1138·2).
Skin, surface and instrument disinfection.

Novacort
Note. This name is used for preparations of different composition.
Ache, Braz.
Ketoconazole (p.389·1); neomycin sulfate (p.228·1); betamethasone (p.1063·1).
Infected skin disorders.

Syntex, Mex.
Cloprednol (p.1065·3).
Corticosteroid.

Nova-Dec Rugby, USA.
Multivitamin and mineral preparation with iron and folic acid (p.1350·1).

Novaderm Johnson & Johnson, Austral.†.
Triclosan (Irgasan DP300) (p.1159·2).
Skin disinfection.

Novadex Novag, Mex.
Naproxen (p.60·3).

Novadine Johnson & Johnson, Austral.†.
Povidone-iodine (p.1155·1).
Abrasions; burns; skin disinfection; skin infections.

Novadral
Parke, Davis, Aust.; Godecke, Ger.; Warner-Lambert, Switz.
Norfenefrine hydrochloride (p.949·1).
Hypotension.

Novafed A Hoechst Marion Roussel, USA.
Pseudoephedrine hydrochloride (p.1099·2); chlorpheniramine [chlorphenamine] maleate (p.412·1).
Upper respiratory-tract symptoms.

Novafur Novag, Mex.
Furazolidone (p.592·1).

Novagard Pharmacia Upjohn, UK†.
Copper-wound plastic (p.1357·3).
Intra-uterine contraceptive device.

Novagcilina Novag, Spain†.
Amoxicillin sodium (p.149·2) or amoxicillin trihydrate (p.149·2).
Bacterial infections.

Novagest Expectorant with Codeine Major, USA.
Guaifenesin (p.1092·2); pseudoephedrine hydrochloride (p.1099·2); codeine phosphate (p.25·2).
Coughs.

Novagon Novag, Mex.
Ispaghula (p.1229·1).
Constipation.

Novahaler 3M, Spain.
Beclometasone dipropionate (p.1061·2).
Asthma.

Novahistex C Hoechst Marion Roussel, Canad.
Codeine phosphate (p.25·2); phenylephrine hydrochloride (p.1097·1).
Coughs.

Novahistex DH Hoechst Marion Roussel, Canad.
Hydrocodone tartrate (p.42·2); phenylephrine hydrochloride (p.1097·1).
Coughs.

Novahistex DH Expectorant Hoechst Marion Roussel, Canad.
Phenylephrine hydrochloride (p.1097·1); hydrocodone tartrate (p.42·2); guaifenesin (p.1092·2).
Coughs.

Novahistex DM Buckley, Canad.
Dextromethorphan hydrobromide (p.1087·3).
Formerly contained dextromethorphan hydrobromide and pseudoephedrine hydrochloride.
Coughs.

Novahistex DM Decongestant Buckley, Canad.
Dextromethorphan hydrobromide (p.1087·3); pseudoephedrine hydrochloride (p.1099·2).
Coughs; respiratory-tract congestion.

Novahistex DM Decongestant Expectorant
Buckley, Canad.
Dextromethorphan hydrobromide (p.1087·3); pseudoephedrine hydrochloride (p.1099·2); guaifenesin (p.1092·2).
Coughs; respiratory-tract congestion.

Novahistex DM Expectorant Hoechst Marion Roussel, Canad.†.
Dextromethorphan hydrobromide (p.1087·3); guaifenesin (p.1092·2); pseudoephedrine hydrochloride (p.1099·2).
Formerly contained dextromethorphan hydrobromide, phenylephrine hydrochloride, and guaifenesin.
Coughs; nasal/sinus congestion.

Novahistex Expectorant Hoechst Marion Roussel, Canad.†.
Guaifenesin (p.1092·2); pseudoephedrine hydrochloride (p.1099·2).
Formerly contained phenylephrine hydrochloride and guaifenesin.
Respiratory-tract congestion.

Novahistine
Note. This name is used for preparations of different composition.
Buckley, Canad.
Phenylephrine hydrochloride (p.1097·1).
Nasal/sinus congestion.

SmithKline Beecham, USA†.
Phenylephrine hydrochloride (p.1097·1); chlorpheniramine [chlorphenamine] maleate (p.412·1).
Upper respiratory-tract symptoms.

Novahistine DH
Note. This name is used for preparations of different composition.
Hoechst Marion Roussel, Canad.
Hydrocodone tartrate (p.42·2); phenylephrine hydrochloride (p.1097·1).
Coughs.

SmithKline Beecham Consumer, USA.
Codeine phosphate (p.25·2); pseudoephedrine hydrochloride (p.1099·2); chlorpheniramine [chlorphenamine] maleate (p.412·1).
Coughs and cold symptoms; respiratory allergies.

Novahistine DM *Buckley, Canad.*
Dextromethorphan hydrobromide (p.1087·3).
Formerly contained dextromethorphan hydrobromide and pseudoephedrine hydrochloride.
Coughs.

Novahistine DM Decongestant *Buckley, Canad.*
Dextromethorphan hydrobromide (p.1087·3); pseudoephedrine hydrochloride (p.1099·2).
Coughs; respiratory-tract congestion.

Novahistine DM Decongestant Expectorant
Buckley, Canad.
Dextromethorphan hydrobromide (p.1087·3); pseudoephedrine hydrochloride (p.1099·2); guaifenesin (p.1092·2).
Coughs; respiratory-tract congestion.

Novahistine DM Expectorant *Hoechst Marion Roussel, Canad.†.*
Dextromethorphan hydrobromide (p.1087·3); guaifenesin (p.1092·2); pseudoephedrine hydrochloride (p.1099·2).
Formerly contained dextromethorphan hydrobromide, phenylephrine hydrochloride, and guaifenesin.
Coughs; nasal/sinus congestion.

Novahistine DMX *SmithKline Beecham Consumer, USA.*
Pseudoephedrine hydrochloride (p.1099·2); dextromethorphan hydrobromide (p.1087·3); guaifenesin (p.1092·2).
Coughs; nasal congestion.

Novahistine Expectorant *SmithKline Beecham, USA†.*
Codeine phosphate (p.25·2); pseudoephedrine hydrochloride (p.1099·2); guaifenesin (p.1092·2).
Coughs; respiratory congestion.

Novain *Agepha, Aust.*
Oxybuprocaine hydrochloride (p.1318·1).
Local anaesthesia.

Novalac AD *Novalac, Fr.*
Infant feed (p.1350·1).
Formerly known as Novalac Diarelac.
Diarrhoea.

Novalan *Orion, Fin.*
Emollient.
Skin disorders; vehicle for topical drugs.

Novalgin
Hoechst Marion Roussel, Aust.; Hoechst Marion Roussel, Ger.; Hoechst Marion Roussel, Israel; Hoechst Marion Roussel, Neth.; Hoechst Marion Roussel, Swed.; Hoechst Marion Roussel, Thai.
Dipyrone (p.34·1).
Fever; pain.

Novalgina
Hoechst Marion Roussel, Braz.; Hoechst Marion Roussel, Ital.; Hoeport, Port.
Dipyrone (p.34·1).
Fever; pain.

Novalgine
Aventis, Belg.; Hoechst, Fr.; Hoechst Marion Roussel, Switz.
Dipyrone (p.34·1).
Fever; pain.

Novalgrip *QIF, Braz.*
Dipyrone (p.34·1); ascorbic acid (p.1389·3); sodium camsilate; guaifenesin (p.1092·2); eucalyptol (p.1609·2).
Cold and influenza symptoms.

Novalm *LDM, Fr.†.*
Meprobamate (p.691·1).
Anxiety.

Novalucol Novum *Hassle, Swed.*
Calcium carbonate (p.1215·1); magnesium hydroxide (p.1233·1).
Heartburn.

Novaluzid
AstraZeneca, Denm.; AstraZeneca, Fin.; AstraZeneca, Norw.; Hassle, Swed.
Aluminium hydroxide (p.1210·3); magnesium hydroxide (p.1233·1); magnesium carbonate (p.1232·3).
Dyspepsia; gastritis; heartburn; hyperacidity; peptic ulcer.

Novamet
SmithKline Beecham, Denm.; SmithKline Beecham, Mex.
Cimetidine (p.1216·3).
Acid aspiration; gastro-oesophageal reflux; peptic ulcer; Zollinger-Ellison syndrome.

Novamilor *Novopharm, Canad.*
Amiloride hydrochloride (p.835·1); hydrochlorothiazide (p.907·3).
Hypertension; oedema.

Novamin *Bristol-Myers Squibb, Braz.*
Amikacin sulfate (p.148·1).
Bacterial infections.

Novamina *PQS, Spain.*
Benzalkonium chloride (p.1133·2).
Skin, mucous membrane, and wound disinfection.

Novamine *Clintec, USA.*
Amino-acid infusion (p.1350·1).
Parenteral nutrition.

Novaminsulfon
Lichtenstein, Ger.; Braun, Ger.; Ratiopharm, Ger.; Weimer, Ger.; Hong Kong.
Dipyrone (p.34·1).
Fever; pain.

Novamix
Orion, Fin.; Pharmalink, Swed.
Amino-acid, electrolyte, carbohydrate, and lipid (from safflower oil (p.1375·1) and soya oil (p.1378·1)) infusion (p.1350·1).
Parenteral nutrition.

Novamox *Ache, Braz.*
Amoxicillin trihydrate (p.149·2); potassium clavulanate (p.187·2).
Bacterial infections.

Novamoxin *Novopharm, Canad.*
Amoxicillin trihydrate (p.149·2).
Bacterial infections.

Novanaest *Gebro, Aust.*
Procaine hydrochloride (p.1319·1).
Local anaesthesia.

Novaneurina B12 *ISI, Ital.*
Monophosphothiamine monochloride (p.1385·2); cyanocobalamin (p.1388·1).
Neuritis; vitamin supplement.

Novanox *Pfleger, Ger.*
Nitrazepam (p.695·2).
Sleep disorders.

Novantron
Wyeth Lederle, Aust.; Lederle, Ger.; Lederle, Switz.
Mitozantrone [mitoxantrone] hydrochloride (p.559·3).
Malignant neoplasms.

Novantrone
Lederle, Austral.; Wyeth Lederle, Belg.; Wyeth, Braz.; Wyeth-Ayerst, Canad.; Wyeth Lederle, Denm.; Wyeth Lederle, Fin.; Wyeth Lederle, Fr.; Lederle, Hong Kong; Wyeth, Irl.; Lederle; Wyeth Lederle, Ital.; Wyeth, Mex.; Lederle, Neth.; Wyeth Lederle, Norw.; Lederle, NZ; Wyeth Lederle, Port.; Wyeth, S.Afr.; Wyeth, Singapore; Cyanamid, Spain; Wyeth Lederle, Swed.; Wyeth-Ayerst, Thai.; Wyeth, UK; Immunex, USA.
Mitozantrone [mitoxantrone] hydrochloride (p.559·3).
Malignant neoplasms.

Novapam
Note.This name is used for preparations of different composition.
Douglas, NZ.
Chlordiazepoxide hydrochloride (p.659·2).
Anxiety; premedication; skeletal muscle spasm.

Asian Pharm, Thai.
Dipyrone (p.34·1); paracetamol (p.71·2).
Fever; pain.

Novapamyl *Novalis, Fr.†.*
Verapamil hydrochloride (p.989·1).
Hypertension.

Novapen *Pinewood, Irl.*
Ampicillin (p.150·3).
Bacterial infections.

Novapirina *Novartis Consumer, Ital.*
Diclofenac sodium (p.30·3).
Fever; pain.

Novapres *Novag, Mex.*
Captopril (p.853·3).
Hypertension.

Novaprin *Pharmexco, UK.*
Ibuprofen (p.43·2).
Fever; pain.

Novapsyl *Novag, Mex.*
Benzonatate (p.1085·3).
Coughs.

Novarel *Ferring, USA.*
Chorionic gonadotrophin (p.1279·2).
Male and female infertility.

Novarok *Schering, Jpn†.*
Imidapril hydrochloride (p.912·3).
Hypertension.

Novarrutina *Zurita, Braz.*
Rutoside (p.1611·2); aesculus (p.1574·1).
Venous insufficiency.

Novasen *Novopharm, Canad.*
Aspirin (p.14·2).
Inflammation; pain.

Novasone *Schering-Plough, Austral.*
Mometasone furoate (p.1077·2).
Skin disorders.

Novasource Renal
Novartis Nutrition, Canad.; Novartis Nutrition, Hong Kong; Novartis Nutrition, USA.
Preparation for enteral nutrition in renal failure (p.1350·1).

Novasrub *Johnson & Johnson, Austral.†.*
Povidone-iodine (p.1155·1); triclosan (p.1159·2).
Skin disinfection.

Novastan *Mitsubishi, Jpn.*
Argatroban (p.841·3).
Thromboembolic disorders.

Novasten *Novag, Mex.*
Astemizole (p.409·1).
Hypersensitivity.

NovaStep *Asche, Ger.*
Levonorgestrel (p.1486·2); ethinylestradiol (p.1476·2).
Triphasic oral contraceptive.

Novasulfon *Terrier, Mex.*
Dapsone (p.196·1).

Nova-T
Berlex, Canad.†; Schering, Fr.; Schering, Ger.; Schering, Hong Kong; Schering, Israel; Schering, Ital.; Schering, Mex.; Schering, Neth.; Schering, NZ; Schering, S.Afr.; Schering, Singapore; Schering, Switz.; Schering, Thai.; Schering, UK.
Copper-wound plastic (p.1357·3) with a silver core (p.1664·1).
Intra-uterine contraceptive device.

Novatane *Johnson & Johnson, Austral.†.*
Chlorhexidine gluconate (p.1138·2).
Instrument disinfection; skin disinfection; wounds.

Novatec
Merck Sharp & Dohme, Belg.; Merck Sharp & Dohme, Neth.
Lisinopril (p.921·1).
Heart failure; hypertension; myocardial infarction.

Novatox *Pulitzer, Ital.†.*
Glutathione (p.1010·3).
Alcohol and drug poisoning; radiation trauma.

Novatrex *Wyeth Lederle, Fr.*
Methotrexate (p.553·2).
Psoriasis; rheumatoid arthritis.

Novatrim *Promeco, Mex.*
Brodimoprim (p.159·3).
Bacterial infections.

Novatropina *Searle, Braz.*
Homatropine methylbromide (p.468·1).
Smooth muscle spasm.

Novavir *Novag, Mex.*
Zidovudine (p.645·2).
HIV infection.

Novaxen *Novag, Mex.*
Naproxen (p.60·3).
Inflammation; musculoskeletal and joint disorders; pain.

Novazam *Pharmy, Fr.*
Diazepam (p.674·3).
Alcohol withdrawal syndrome; anxiety.

Novazyd
Merck Sharp & Dohme, Belg.; Merck Sharp & Dohme, Neth.
Lisinopril (p.921·1); hydrochlorothiazide (p.907·3).
Hypertension.

Novegam *Chinoin, Mex.*
Clenbuterol hydrochloride (p.763·3).
Obstructive airways disease.

Novel 1000 *Novel, Ital.*
Ginseng (p.1615·3).

Novel Ginkgo *Novel, Ital.*
Ginkgo biloba (p.1615·2).

Novel Jelly *Novel, Ital.*
Royal jelly (p.1659·3).
Nutritional supplement.

Novelciclina *Sabater, Spain.*
Doxycycline hyclate (p.200·1).
Bacterial infections.

Novelian *Almirall, Spain.*
Sumatriptan succinate (p.456·1).
Cluster headache; migraine.

Novelmin *Bunker, Braz.*
Mebendazole (p.102·2).
Worm infections.

Noveril
Novartis, Aust.; Novartis, Ger.; Du Pont, Ger.; Sandoz, S.Afr.†; Novartis, Switz.
Dibenzepin hydrochloride (p.283·2).
Depression; nocturnal enuresis.

Novesin
Ciba Vision, Hong Kong; Rentsch, S.Afr.; Ciba Vision, Singapore; Ciba Vision, Switz.; Ciba Vision, Thai.
Oxybuprocaine hydrochloride (p.1318·1).
Local anaesthesia.

Novesina *Novartis, Ital.*
Oxybuprocaine hydrochloride (p.1318·1).
Local anaesthesia.

Novesine
Bournonville, Belg.†; Merck Sharp & Dohme-Chibret, Fr.; Ciba Vision, Ger.; Novartis, Ger.
Oxybuprocaine hydrochloride (p.1318·1).
Local anaesthesia.

Novicarbon *CTI, Israel.*
Activated charcoal (p.1000·2); senna (p.1248·2); rhubarb (p.1248·1); fennel oil (p.1610·2).
Constipation; dyspepsia; flatulence.

Novid *Nycomed, Norw.*
Aspirin (p.14·2).
Fever; pain.

Novidol *Synpharma, Switz.*
Salicylamide (p.82·1); propyphenazone (p.80·2); caffeine (p.761·3).
Fever; pain.

Novidroxin *Fatol, Ger.*
Hydroxocobalamin acetate (p.1388·3).
Arteritis; arthritic and rheumatic pain; neuralgia; neuritis.

Noviform
Ciba Vision, Ger.; Meda, Swed.; Ciba Vision, Switz.
Bibrocathol (p.1585·1).
Eye disorders.

Noviforme-Blache *Chauvin Novopharma, Switz.*
Bibrocathol (p.1585·1).
Eye disorders.

Novifort *Ciba Vision, Ger.*
Bibrocathol (p.1585·1); hydrocortisone acetate (p.1073·3).
Allergic and inflammatory disorders of the eye.

Novilax *Europital, Ital.*
Sodium laurilsulfate (p.1496·3); sodium citrate (p.1186·2); glycerol (p.1616·3); sorbitol (p.1377·3).
Formerly known as Microlax.
Constipation.

Novim *Lalco, Canad.†.*
Multivitamin and mineral preparation (p.1350·1).

Novipec *Montavit, Aust.*
Salverine (p.1660·3); ephedrine (p.1090·1); spike lavender oil (p.1667·1).
Respiratory-tract disorders.

Novirasin *CTI, Israel.*
Phentermine resinate (p.1514·1).
Obesity.

Novirell B *Sanorell, Ger.*
Thiamine hydrochloride (p.1385·1); pyridoxine hydrochloride (p.1386·3); cyanocobalamin (p.1388·1).
Lignocaine [lidocaine] hydrochloride (p.1313·2) is included in this preparation to alleviate the pain of injection.
Dermatoses; neuralgia; neuritis; rheumatic disorders; spinal disorders.

Novitan *Theranol-Deglaude, Fr.†.*
Procaine hydrochloride (p.1319·1); haematoporphyrin (p.1618·3).
Tonic.

Novitropan *CTI, Israel.*
Oxybutynin hydrochloride (p.471·2).
Neurogenic bladder; nocturnal enuresis.

Novo AC and C *Novopharm, Canad.*
Aspirin (p.14·2); caffeine (p.761·3); codeine phosphate (p.25·2).
Pain.

Novo Aerofil Sedante *Reig Jofre, Spain.*
Dimethicone (p.1249·2); metoclopramide hydrochloride (p.1235·2); oxazepam (p.697·1).
Aerophagia; gastrointestinal dystonias; metorism.

Novo B *Novopharm, Canad.*
Vitamin B substances and vitamin C (p.1350·1).

Novo Dermoquinona *Llorente, Spain.*
Mequinol (p.1118·2).
Hyperpigmentation.

Novo E *Novopharm, Canad.*
d-Alpha tocoferil acetate (p.1394·1) or dl-alpha tocoferil acetate (p.1394·1).

Novo Mandrogallan N *Dolorgiet, Ger.†.*
Greater celandine (p.1618·1); taraxacum (p.1669·1); absinthium (p.1571·1).
Biliary-tract disorders; dyspepsia.

Novo Melanidina *Llorente, Spain.*
Psoralen.
Suntanning; vitiligo.

Novo Petrin *OTW, Ger.*
Paracetamol (p.71·2); propyphenazone (p.80·2); caffeine (p.761·3).
Fever; pain.

Novo Rino *Bunker, Braz.*
Naphazoline (p.1095·1); sodium chloride (p.1196·1).
Nasal congestion.

Novo V-K *Novo Nordisk, S.Afr.*
Phenoxymethylpenicillin potassium (p.235·1).
Bacterial infections.

Novo-Alprazol *Novopharm, Canad.*
Alprazolam (p.654·2).
Anxiety; sedative.

Novo-Atenol *Novopharm, Canad.*
Atenolol (p.841·3).
Angina pectoris; hypertension.

Novo-AZT *Novopharm, Canad.*
Zidovudine (p.645·2).
HIV infection.

Novobedouze *Therabel, Belg.*
Hydroxocobalamin acetate (p.1388·3).
Neuralgia; vitamin B₁₂ deficiency.

Novobiocyl *Francia, Ital.*
Cefoperazone sodium (p.168·2).
Lignocaine [lidocaine] hydrochloride (p.1313·2) is included in this preparation to alleviate the pain of injection.
Bacterial infections.

Novo-Butamide *Novopharm, Canad.†.*
Tolbutamide (p.336·3).
Diabetes mellitus.

Novo-Butazone *Novopharm, Canad.†.*
Phenylbutazone (p.78·1).
Arthritis; inflammation.

Novocain
Sanofi Synthelabo, Canad.; Hoechst Marion Roussel, Ger.; Abbott, USA.
Procaine hydrochloride (p.1319·1).
Local anaesthesia.

Novocalm *Vitamed, Israel.*
Paracetamol (p.71·2); salicylamide (p.82·1); caffeine (p.761·3); codeine phosphate (p.25·2).
Fever; pain.

Novo-Carbamaz *Novopharm, Canad.*
Carbamazepine (p.342·2).
Epilepsy.

Novocephal *Fresenius Kabi, Aust.*
Piracetam (p.1652·1).
Alcohol or opioid withdrawal syndrome; mental function disorders.

Novo-Cerusol *Chauvin Novopharma, Switz.*
Xylene (p.1406·3).
Ear wax removal.

Novocetam *Lilly, Ger.*
Piracetam (p.1652·1).
Mental function disorders.

Novo-Chlorocap *Novopharm, Canad.†.*
Chloramphenicol (p.179·1).
Bacterial infections.

Novo-Cholamine *Novopharm, Canad.*
Colestyramine (p.864·1).
Bile-acid induced diarrhoea; hypercholesterolaemia; pruritus associated with partial biliary obstruction.

Novocholin *Adler, Aust.*
Herba teucrii; agrimony herb (p.1574·3); rhubarb (p.1248·1); peppermint oil (p.1243·3).
Biliary disorders.

Novocilin *Ache, Braz.*
Note. A similar name is used for preparations of different composition (see below).
Amoxicillin (p.149·2).
Bacterial infections.

Novocilin Balsamico *Ache, Braz.*
Amoxicillin (p.149·2); bromhexine hydrochloride (p.1085·3).
Respiratory-tract infections.

Novocillin *Novo Nordisk, S.Afr.*
Note. A similar name is used for preparations of different composition (see above).
Procaine penicillin [procaine benzylpenicillin] (p.239·2).
Bacterial infections.

Novo-Cimetine *Novopharm, Canad.*
Cimetidine (p.1216·3).
Histamine H_2 receptor antagonist.

Novo-Clopamine *Novopharm, Canad.*
Clomipramine hydrochloride (p.282·1).
Depression; obsessive-compulsive disorder.

Novo-Clopate *Novopharm, Canad.*
Dipotassium clorazepate (p.670·3).
Anxiety; sedative.

Novo-Cloxin *Novopharm, Canad.*
Cloxacillin sodium (p.192·1).
Bacterial infections.

Novocortal *Novel, Ital.*
Hydrocortisone acetate (p.1073·3).
Skin disorders.

Novo-Cromolyn *Novopharm, Canad.*
Sodium cromoglicate (p.774·3).
Asthma.

Novo-Cycloprine *Novopharm, Canad.*
Cyclobenzaprine hydrochloride (p.1328·1).
Skeletal muscle spasm.

Novodentin *Faria, Braz.*
Sodium fluoride (p.1375·3).
Dental caries prophylaxis.

Novo-Difenac *Novopharm, Canad.*
Diclofenac potassium (p.30·2) or diclofenac sodium (p.30·3).
Inflammation; osteoarthritis; pain; rheumatoid arthritis.

Novodigal
Asta Medica, Aust.; Asta Medica, Belg.†; Lilly, Ger.
β-Acetyldigoxin (p.827·3) or digoxin (p.870·1).
Arrhythmias; heart failure.

Novodil
Note. This name is used for preparations of different composition.
Augot, Fr.†.
Cyclandelate (p.865·2).
Mental function impairment in the elderly.
OFF, Ital.†.
Dipyridamole (p.877·2).
Thromboembolic disorders.

Novo-Diltazem *Novopharm, Canad.*
Diltiazem hydrochloride (p.874·3).
Angina pectoris; hypertension.

Novo-Dimenate *Novopharm, Canad.*
Dimenhydrinate (p.415·2).
Nausea and vomiting; vertigo.

Novo-Dipam *Novopharm, Canad.†.*
Diazepam (p.674·3).

Novo-Dipiradol *Novopharm, Canad.*
Dipyridamole (p.877·2).
Cardiac disorders.

Novo-Doparil *Novopharm, Canad.†.*
Methyldopa (p.927·3); hydrochlorothiazide (p.907·3).
Hypertension.

Novo-Doxylin *Novopharm, Canad.*
Doxycycline hyclate (p.200·1).
Bacterial infections.

Novofen *Remedica, Thai.*
Tamoxifen citrate (p.571·1).
Anovulatory infertility; breast cancer.

Novofer *Ache, Braz.*
Ferrous sulfate (p.1360·3); vitamin B substances (p.1350·1).
Ascorbic acid (p.1389·3) is included in this preparation to increase the absorption and availability of iron.
Iron deficiency; iron-deficiency anaemias.

Novo-Ferrogluc *Novopharm, Canad.*
Ferrous gluconate (p.1360·1).
Iron-deficiency anaemia.

Novo-Ferrosulfate *Novopharm, Canad.*
Ferrous sulfate (p.1360·3).
Iron-deficiency anaemia.

Novo-Fibrate *Novopharm, Canad.†.*
Clofibrate (p.859·1).
Hyperlipidaemias.

Novo-Fibre *Novopharm, Canad.*
Grain and citrus fibre (p.1350·1).
Bowel disorders; constipation; fibre supplement.

Novofilin *Ferrer, Spain.*
Diprophylline (p.764·1); proxyphylline (p.770·1); theophylline (p.777·2).
Obstructive airways disease.

Novo-Flupam *Novopharm, Canad.†.*
Flurazepam hydrochloride (p.685·3).
Insomnia.

Novo-Flurazine *Novopharm, Canad.†.*
Trifluoperazine hydrochloride (p.710·3).

Novo-Flurprofen *Novopharm, Canad.*
Flurbiprofen (p.41·2).
Inflammation; pain.

Novo-Folacid *Novopharm, Canad.†.*
Folic acid (p.1361·1).
Anaemias.

Novo-Fumar *Novopharm, Canad.*
Ferrous fumarate (p.1360·1).
Iron deficiency anaemias.

Novo-Furantoin *Novopharm, Canad.*
Nitrofurantoin (p.230·3).
Bacterial infections of the urinary tract.

Novogel
Note. This name is used for preparations of different composition.
Morado, Ital.
Royal jelly (p.1659·3); liver extract.
Nutritional supplement.
Ford Medical, UK.
Hydrogel dressing.
Wounds.

Novogent *Temmler, Ger.*
Ibuprofen (p.43·2).
Fever; musculoskeletal and joint disorders.

Novo-Gesic *Novopharm, Canad.*
Paracetamol (p.71·2).
Fever; pain.

Novo-Gesic C *Novopharm, Canad.*
Paracetamol (p.71·2); caffeine (p.761·3); codeine phosphate (p.25·2).
Fever; pain.

Novogyn *Schering, Ital.*
Levonorgestrel (p.1486·2); ethinylestradiol (p.1476·2).
Combined oral contraceptive.

Novo-Helisen
Allergopharma, Ger.; Allergopharma, Switz.
Allergen extracts (p.1575·3).
Hyposensitisation.

Novo-Herklin 2000 *Armstrong, Mex.*
Permethrin (p.1436·1).
Pediculosis; scabies.

Novo-Hexidyl *Novopharm, Canad.†.*
Benzhexol [trihexyphenidyl] hydrochloride (p.463·3).

Novo-Hydrazide *Novopharm, Canad.†.*
Hydrochlorothiazide (p.907·3).
Hypertension; oedema.

Novo-Hydrocort *Novopharm, Canad.*
Hydrocortisone (p.1073·3).
Skin disorders.

Novo-Hylazin *Novopharm, Canad.*
Hydralazine hydrochloride (p.905·3).
Hypertension.

Novo-Ipramide *Novopharm, Canad.*
Ipratropium bromide (p.766·1).
Bronchodilator.

Novo-Keto *Novopharm, Canad.*
Ketoprofen (p.47·3).
Fever; pain.

Novolax *Medley, Braz.*
Liquorice (p.1231·2); cassia pulp (p.1216·2); coriander (p.1599·2); senna (p.1248·2); tamarind (p.1253·2).
Constipation.

Novo-Lexin *Novopharm, Canad.*
Cefalexin (p.161·3).
Bacterial infections.

Novolin 10/90, 20/80, 30/70, 40/60, 50/50 *Novo Nordisk, Canad.*
Mixtures of insulin injection (human, pyr) and isophane insulin injection (human) in the proportions indicated (p.324·1).
Diabetes mellitus.

Novolin 30/70 *Pisa, Mex.*
Mixture of insulin injection (human) and isophane insulin injection (human) respecively in the proportions indicated (p.324·1).
Diabetes mellitus.

Novolin 70/30
Novo Nordisk, Braz.; Novo Nordisk, USA.
Mixture of isophane insulin injection (human) 70% and insulin injection (human) 30% (p.324·1).
Diabetes mellitus.

Novolin L
Novo Nordisk, Braz.; Pisa, Mex.; Novo Nordisk, USA.
Insulin zinc suspension (human, monocomponent) (p.324·1).
Diabetes mellitus.

Novolin Lente *Novo Nordisk, Canad.*
Insulin zinc suspension (crystalline 70%) (human, pyr) (p.324·1).
Diabetes mellitus.

Novolin N
Novo Nordisk, Braz.; Pisa, Mex.; Novo Nordisk, USA.
Isophane insulin injection (human, monocomponent) (p.324·1).
Diabetes mellitus.

Novolin NPH *Novo Nordisk, Canad.*
Isophane insulin injection (human, pyr) (p.324·1).
Diabetes mellitus.

Novolin R
Novo Nordisk, Braz.; Pisa, Mex.; Novo Nordisk, USA.
Insulin injection (human, monocomponent) (p.324·1).
Diabetes mellitus.

Novolin Toronto *Novo Nordisk, Canad.*
Neutral insulin injection (human, pyr) (p.324·1).
Diabetes mellitus.

Novolin Ultralente *Novo Nordisk, Canad.*
Insulin zinc suspension (crystalline) (human, pyr) (p.324·1).
Diabetes mellitus.

NovoLog *Novo Nordisk, USA.*
Insulin aspart (p.329·2).
Diabetes mellitus.

Novo-Lorazem *Novopharm, Canad.*
Lorazepam (p.688·3).
Anxiety; sedative.

Novo-Medopa *Novopharm, Canad.*
Methyldopa (p.927·3).
Hypertension.

Novo-Medrone *Novopharm, Canad.*
Medroxyprogesterone acetate (p.1480·1).

Novo-Meprazine *Novopharm, Canad.*
Methotrimeprazine [levomepromazine] maleate (p.692·1).
Insomnia; nausea; pain; psychoses; vomiting.

Novo-Mepro *Novopharm, Canad.†.*
Meprobamate (p.691·1).
Anxiety.

Novomet *Novo Nordisk, Austral.*
Metformin hydrochloride (p.332·3).
Diabetes mellitus.

Novo-Methacin *Novopharm, Canad.*
Indometacin (p.44·3).
Inflammation; pain.

Novo-Metoprol *Novopharm, Canad.*
Metoprolol tartrate (p.931·2).
Angina pectoris; hypertension.

Novomin *Xepa-Soul Pattinson, Singapore.*
Dimenhydrinate (p.415·2).
Gastrointestinal disorders; Ménière's disease; motion sickness.

Novomint N *Demophorm, Switz.†.*
Cetylpyridinium chloride (p.1138·1); lignocaine [lidocaine] hydrochloride (p.1313·2); menthol (p.1632·3).
Mouth and throat disorders.

No-Vomit *IMA, Braz.*
Metoclopramide (p.1236·3).
Gastrointestinal motility disorders; nausea and vomiting.

Novo-Mucilax *Novopharm, Canad.*
Ispaghula (p.1229·1).
Constipation.

Novo-Naprox *Novopharm, Canad.*
Naproxen (p.60·3) or naproxen sodium (p.61·1).
Inflammation; pain.

Novonausin *Camps, Spain.*
Sodium citrate (p.1186·2); cerium oxalate (p.1216·2).
Nausea and vomiting.

Novo-Nidazol *Novopharm, Canad.*
Metronidazole (p.594·1).
Trichomoniasis.

Novo-Nifedin *Novopharm, Canad.*
Nifedipine (p.940·1).
Angina pectoris.

NovoNorm
Novo Nordisk, Aust.; Novo Nordisk, Austral.; Novo Nordisk, Denm.; Novo Nordisk, Fin.; Novo Nordisk, Fr.; Novo Nordisk, Ger.; Novo Nordisk, Irl.; Novo Nordisk, Ital.; Novo Nordisk, Neth.; Novo Nordisk, Norw.; Novo Nordisk, NZ; Novo Nordisk, S.Afr.; Novo Nordisk, Singapore; Novo Nordisk, Spain; Novo Nordisk, Swed.; Novo Nordisk, Thai.; Novo Nordisk, UK.
Repaglinide (p.334·1).
Diabetes mellitus.

Novopen *Novo Nordisk, S.Afr.*
Benzylpenicillin sodium (p.157·2).
Bacterial infections.

Novo-Pen-G *Novopharm, Canad.†.*
Benzylpenicillin potassium (p.157·1).
Bacterial infections.

Novo-Pen-VK *Novopharm, Canad.*
Phenoxymethylpenicillin potassium (p.235·1).
Bacterial infections.

Novo-Peridol *Novopharm, Canad.*
Haloperidol (p.686·3).
Nausea and vomiting; psychoses.

Novo-Pheniram *Novopharm, Canad.*
Chlorpheniramine [chlorphenamine] maleate (p.412·1).

Novopin MIG *Schoning-Berlin, Ger.†.*
Menthol (p.1632·3).
Headache including migraine.

Novo-Pindol *Novopharm, Canad.*
Pindolol (p.955·3).
Angina pectoris; hypertension.

Novo-Pirocam *Novopharm, Canad.*
Piroxicam (p.79·1).
Inflammation; pain.

Novoplat *Pharmacia Upjohn, Mex.*
Carboplatin (p.515·1).

Novoplatinum *Faulding, Port.*
Carboplatin (p.515·1).

Novo-Plus *Novopharm, Canad.†.*
Lactose (p.1370·2).
Placebo.

Novo-Poxide *Novopharm, Canad.*
Chlordiazepoxide hydrochloride (p.659·2).

Novo-Pramine *Novopharm, Canad.†.*
Imipramine hydrochloride (p.291·1).
Depression.

Novo-Pranol *Novopharm, Canad.†.*
Propranolol hydrochloride (p.962·3).
Cardiac disorders; hypertension; migraine headache; phaeochromocytoma.

Novo-Prazin *Novopharm, Canad.*
Prazosin hydrochloride (p.958·1).
Hypertension.

Novo-Profen *Novopharm, Canad.*
Ibuprofen (p.43·2).
Inflammation; pain.

Novo-Propamide *Novopharm, Canad.†.*
Chlorpropamide (p.321·1).
Diabetes mellitus.

Novo-Propoxyn *Novopharm, Canad.†.*
Dextropropoxyphene hydrochloride (p.27·1).
Pain.

Novoprotect *Merck dura, Ger.*
Amitriptyline hydrochloride (p.273·3).
Depression.

Novoptine *Thea, Fr.*
Cetylpyridinium chloride (p.1138·1).
Eye infections.

Novo-Purol *Novopharm, Canad.†.*
Allopurinol (p.397·2).

Novo-Pyrazone *Novopharm, Canad.†.*
Sulfinpyrazone (p.402·2).

Novoquin *Rayere, Mex.*
Ciprofloxacin (p.182·3).
Bacterial infections.

Novo-Ranidine *Novopharm, Canad.*
Ranitidine hydrochloride (p.1245·2).
Gastrointestinal disorders.

NovoRapid
Novo Nordisk, Austral.; Novo Nordisk, Denm.; Novo Nordisk, Fin.; Novo Nordisk, Fr.; Novo Nordisk, Irl.; Novo Nordisk, Neth.; Novo Nordisk, Swed.; Novo Nordisk, Switz.; Novo Nordisk, UK.
Insulin aspart (p.329·2).
Diabetes mellitus.

Novo-Renal *Novopharm, Canad.*
Multivitamin and mineral preparation for dialysis patients (p.1350·1).

Novo-Ridazine *Novopharm, Canad.†.*
Thioridazine hydrochloride (p.708·1).
Psychiatric disorders.

Novorutin *Negma, Israel.*
Troxerutin (p.1611·2).
Peripheral vascular disorders.

Novo-Rythro *Novopharm, Canad.*
Erythromycin (p.201·2).
Bacterial infections.

Novosal *Novartis Consumer, Ital.*
Low sodium dietary salt substitute (p.1350·1).

Novo-Salmol *Novopharm, Canad.*
Salbutamol (p.770·3) or salbutamol sulfate (p.770·3).
Obstructive airways disease.

Novo-Semide *Novopharm, Canad.†.*
Frusemide [furosemide] (p.893·1).
Oedema.

NovoSeven
Novo Nordisk, Aust.; Novo Nordisk, Austral.; Novo Nordisk, Denm.; Novo Nordisk, Fin.; Novo Nordisk, Fr.; Novo Nordisk, Ger.; Novo Nordisk, Irl.†; Novo Nordisk, Israel; Novo Nordisk, Ital.; Novo Nordisk, Neth.; Novo Nordisk, Norw.; Novo Nordisk, NZ; Novo Nordisk, S.Afr.; Novo Nordisk, Spain; Novo Nordisk, Swed.; Novo Nordisk, Switz.; Novo Nordisk, UK; Novo Nordisk, USA.
Activated eptacog alfa (p.733·3).
Haemorrhagic disorders.

Novo-Sorbide *Novopharm, Canad.†.*
Isosorbide dinitrate (p.915·2).
Angina pectoris.

Novo-Soxazole *Novopharm, Canad.†.*
Sulfafurazole (p.253·1).

Novo-Spiroton *Novopharm, Canad.*
Spironolactone (p.973·2).
Hyperaldosteronism.

Novo-Spirozine *Novopharm, Canad.*
Hydrochlorothiazide (p.907·3); spironolactone (p.973·2).
Hypertension; oedema.

Novospray *Peters, Fr.*
Mixed amphoteric and quaternary ammonium salts; polihexanide (p.1154·2); alcohol (p.1130·3); isopropyl alcohol (p.1149·2).
Disinfection.

Novostrep *Novo Nordisk, S.Afr.*
Streptomycin sulfate (p.249·1).
Bacterial infections.

Novo-Sucralate *Novopharm, Canad.*
Sucralfate (p.1250·2).
Peptic ulcer.

Novo-Sundac *Novopharm, Canad.*
Sulindac (p.85·3).
Inflammation; pain.

Novoter
Cusi, Hong Kong; Teofarma, Spain.
Fluocinonide (p.1071·2).
Skin disorders.

Novoter Gentamicin Cusi, Hong Kong.
Fluocinonide (p.1071·2); gentamicin sulfate (p.210·1).
Infected skin disorders.

Novoter Gentamicina Teofarma, Spain.
Fluocinonide (p.1071·2); gentamicin sulfate (p.210·1).
Infected skin disorders.

Novo-Tetra Novopharm, Canad.
Tetracycline hydrochloride (p.258·3).
Bacterial infections.

Novo-Thalidone Novopharm, Canad.†
Chlortalidone (p.857·1).
Hypertension; oedema.

Novo-Theophyl Novopharm, Canad.
Theophylline (p.777·2).

Novothyral
Merck, Aust.; Merck-Belgolabo, Belg.; Merck, Ger.; Merck, Switz.
Liothyronine sodium (p.1524·2); thyroxine [levothyroxine] sodium (p.1526·2).
Adjunct to antithyroid therapy; euthyroid goitre; hypothyroidism; thyroiditis.

Novo-Timol Novopharm, Canad.
Timolol maleate (p.982·1).
Angina pectoris; glaucoma; hypertension.

Novotiral Merck, Mex.
Liothyronine sodium (p.1524·2); thyroxine [levothyroxine] sodium (p.1526·2).
Adjunct to antithyroid therapy; euthyroid goitre; hypothyroidism.

Novotossil Zambon, Belg.
Cloperastine fendizoate (p.1087·2) or cloperastine hydrochloride (p.1087·2).
Coughs.

Novo-Triamzide Novopharm, Canad.
Triamterene (p.986·1); hydrochlorothiazide (p.907·3).
Hypertension; oedema.

Novo-Trimel Novopharm, Canad.
Co-trimoxazole (p.193·3).
Bacterial infections.

Novo-Triolam Novopharm, Canad.†
Triazolam (p.709·3).
Insomnia; sedative.

Novo-Triphyl Novopharm, Canad.†
Choline theophyllinate (p.763·3).

Novo-Tripramine Novopharm, Canad.
Trimipramine maleate (p.311·2).
Depression.

Novo-Triptyn Novopharm, Canad.†
Amitriptyline hydrochloride (p.273·3).
Depression.

Novotussan Gemballa, Braz.
Oxeladin (p.1096·2); diphenhydramine (p.416·1); ephedrine (p.1090·1); butamirate citrate (p.1086·2).
Coughs.

Novo-Veramil Novopharm, Canad.
Verapamil hydrochloride (p.989·1).
Angina pectoris; arrhythmias; hypertension.

Novo-Vites Novopharm, Canad.
Multivitamin preparation with or without iron (p.1350·1).

Novoxapam Novopharm, Canad.†
Oxazepam (p.697·1).

Novoxil Luper, Braz.
Amoxicillin (p.149·2).
Bacterial infections.

Novo-Zolamide Novopharm, Canad.†
Acetazolamide (p.826·1).

Novral Sintofarma, Braz.
Lisinopril (p.921·1).
Heart failure; hypertension.

Novuxol
Note. This name is used for preparations of different composition.
Knoll, Ger.
Enzymes from *Clostridium histolyticum.*
Cleansing of skin ulcers.

Nordmark, Neth.
Collagenase (p.1598·2).
Wound debridement.

Novynette Durascan, Denm.
Desogestrel (p.1470·3); ethinylestradiol (p.1476·2).
Combined oral contraceptive.

Noxacorn
Note. This name is used for preparations of different composition.
Dexxon, Israel.
Salicylic acid (p.1122·3); benzocaine (p.1306·2).
Corns; warts.

Roche Nicholas, Neth.†
Lignocaine [lidocaine] (p.1313·2); salicylic acid (p.1122·3).
Calluses; corns; warts.

Noxalide Lampugnani, Ital.
Nimesulide (p.62·3).
Fever; inflammation; pain.

Noxema 2-in-1 Procter & Gamble, Canad.
Salicylic acid (p.1122·3).
Acne.

Noxenur Disperga, Aust.
Atropine sulfate (p.461·1); ephedrine hydrochloride (p.1090·1); thiamine hydrochloride (p.1385·1).
Nocturnal enuresis.

Noxenur S Galenika, Ger.
Atropine sulfate (p.461·1).
Nocturnal enuresis.

Noxidil TO-Chemicals, Thai.
Minoxidil (p.934·2).
Hypertension.

Noxigram FIRMA, Ital.
Cinoxacin (p.182·2).
Bacterial infections of the urinary tract.

Noxigur Tegur, Mex.
Nitroxoline (p.231·3).

Noxine Sriprasit, Thai.
Norfloxacin (p.232·1).
Bacterial infections.

Noxinor Masa, Thai.
Norfloxacin (p.232·1).
Bacterial infections.

Noxitem Amrad, Austral.†
Tamoxifen citrate (p.571·1).
Breast cancer.

Noxom S Fides, Ger.
Homoeopathic preparation.

Noxotab Fides, Ger.†
Homoeopathic preparation.

Noxyflex Innothera, Fr.
Noxytiolin (p.1151·3).
Intraperitoneal infections.

Noxyflex S
Geistlich, Irl.; Geistlich, UK.
Noxytiolin (p.1151·3).
Fungal and bacterial infections.

Nozid Vitalpharma, Belg.
Aluminium hydroxide-magnesium carbonate co-dried gel (p.1211·2); magnesium hydroxide (p.1233·1) or magnesium oxide (p.1233·2).
Digestive disorders associated with hyperacidity.

Nozinan
Gerot, Aust.; Aventis, Belg.; Rhone-Poulenc Rorer, Canad.; Aventis, Denm.; Rhone-Poulenc Rorer, Fin.; Rhone-Poulenc Rorer, Fr.; Rhone-Poulenc Rorer, Irl.; Rhone-Poulenc Rorer, Israel; Rhone-Poulenc Rorer, Ital.; Rhone-Poulenc Rorer, Neth.; Pharmacia Upjohn, Norw.; Aventis, NZ; Vitoria, Port.; Rhone-Poulenc Rorer, Swed.; Rhone-Poulenc Rorer, Switz.; Link, UK.
Methotrimeprazine [levomepromazine] (p.691·3), methotrimeprazine [levomepromazine] embonate (p.692·1), methotrimeprazine [levomepromazine] hydrochloride (p.691·3), or methotrimeprazine [levomepromazine] maleate (p.692·1).
Tablets were formerly known as Veractil in the UK.
Alcohol withdrawal syndrome; anxiety; depression; hiccups; insomnia; pain; pruritus; psychoses; vomiting.

Nozolon ICN, Mex.
Gentamicin (p.212·1).
Bacterial infections.

NP-27 Thompson, USA†.
Tolnaftate (p.395·2).
Fungal skin infections.

NPH Iletin I Lilly, USA†.
Isophane insulin suspension (bovine and porcine) (p.324·1).
Diabetes mellitus.

NPH Iletin II Lilly, USA.
Isophane insulin suspension (porcine) (p.324·1).
Diabetes mellitus.

NSA CSL, Austral.†.
Human albumin (p.724·1).
Burns; cardiopulmonary bypass; haemodialysis; hypoproteinaemia; hypovolaemia; plasma exchange; respiratory distress syndrome; shock.

NTR Teofarma, Ital.
Phenylephrine hydrochloride (p.1097·1); thenyldiamine hydrochloride (p.425·3).
Cold symptoms.

NTS Hercon, USA†.
Glyceryl trinitrate (p.897·3).

NTZ Long Acting Nasal Sterling Health, USA.
Oxymetazoline hydrochloride (p.1096·2).
Nasal congestion.

Nu-Alpraz Nu-Pharm, Canad.
Alprazolam (p.654·2).
Anxiety; sedative.

Nu-Amilzide Nu-Pharm, Canad.
Hydrochlorothiazide (p.907·3); amiloride hydrochloride (p.835·3).
Hypertension; oedema.

Nu-Amoxi Nu-Pharm, Canad.
Amoxicillin trihydrate (p.149·2).
Bacterial infections.

Nu-Ampi Nu-Pharm, Canad.
Ampicillin trihydrate (p.151·1).
Bacterial infections.

Nuardin SmithKline Beecham, Belg.
Cimetidine (p.1216·3).
Gastrointestinal disorders associated with hyperacidity.

Nu-Atenol Nu-Pharm, Canad.
Atenolol (p.841·3).
Angina pectoris; hypertension.

Nu-Baclo Nu-Pharm, Canad.
Baclofen (p.1322·3).
Muscle relaxation; skeletal muscle spasticity.

Nubain
Torrex, Aust.; Du Pont, Canad.; Du Pont, Fr.; Du Pont, Ger.; Du Pont, Hong Kong; Boots, Hong Kong; Du Pont, Israel; Rhone-Poulenc Rorer, Mex.; Boots, NZ; Boots, S.Afr.†; Du Pont, Singapore; Du Pont, Switz.; Du Pont, Thai.; Du Pont, UK; Endo, USA.
Nalbuphine hydrochloride (p.60·1).
Adjunct to anaesthesia; pain; premedication.

Nubee Co Propan, S.Afr.†.
Vitamin B substances (p.1350·1).

Nubral
AB-Consult, Aust.; Galderma, Ger.
Urea (p.1127·3).
Dry skin.

Nubral 4 Galderma, Ger.
Urea (p.1127·3); sodium chloride (p.1196·1).
Dry skin.

Nubral Forte Galderma, Ger.
Urea (p.1127·3); sodium chloride (p.1196·1).
Skin disorders.

Nubral 4 HC Galderma, Ger.
Hydrocortisone (p.1073·3); urea (p.1127·3); sodium chloride (p.1196·1).
Skin disorders.

Nu-Cal Odan, Canad.
Calcium carbonate (p.1215·1).
Calcium deficiency.

Nu-Capto Nu-Pharm, Canad.
Captopril (p.853·3).
ACE inhibitor.

Nu-Cephalex Nu-Pharm, Canad.
Cefalexin (p.161·3).
Bacterial infections.

Nu-Cimet Nu-Pharm, Canad.
Cimetidine (p.1216·3).
Histamine H$_2$-receptor inhibitor.

Nucleo CMP
Note. This name is used for preparations of different composition.
Gross, Braz.
Disodium cytidine phosphate; trisodium uridine triphosphate; hydroxocobalamin (p.1388·1).
Neuritis.

Ferrer, Spain.
Sodium cytidine monophosphate; disodium uridine diphosphate; disodium uridilic acid; sodium uridine triphosphate.
Neuralgias; neuritis.

Nucleodoxina Baldacci, Port.
Taurine; adenosine monophosphate potassium; uridine monophosphate potassium; vitamin B$_6$; vitamin B$_{12}$ (p.1350·1).
Neuromuscular disorders.

Nucleserina Medea, Spain.
Pyridoxine hydrochloride (p.1386·3); ribonucleic acid (p.1657·3); phosphoserine; levoglutamide (p.1365·2).
Mental function disorders; tonic.

Nuclevit B$_{12}$ Synthelabo, Fr.†
Nucleotide preparation with cyanocobalamin (p.1388·1) (p.1350·1).
Tonic.

Nuclosina ICN, Spain.
Omeprazole (p.1239·1).
Gastro-oesophageal reflux; peptic ulcer; Zollinger-Ellison syndrome.

Nu-Cloxi Nu-Pharm, Canad.
Cloxacillin sodium (p.192·1).
Bacterial infections.

Nucoa Llorente, Spain.
Isopropyl myristate (p.1409·2).
Skin irritation; ulcers; wounds.

Nucofed Roberts, USA.
Codeine phosphate (p.25·2); pseudoephedrine hydrochloride (p.1099·2).
Coughs and cold symptoms.

Nucofed Expectorant Roberts, USA.
Codeine phosphate (p.25·2); pseudoephedrine hydrochloride (p.1099·2); guaifenesin (p.1092·2).
Coughs and cold symptoms.

Nucolox Sigma, Spain.
Ispaghula (p.1229·1); starch (p.1379·3).
Constipation.

Nucosef Sugar Free Pfizer, Austral.
Codeine phosphate (p.25·2); pseudoephedrine hydrochloride (p.1099·2).
Coughs; upper respiratory-tract congestion.

Nu-Cotrimox Nu-Pharm, Canad.
Co-trimoxazole (p.193·3).
Bacterial infections.

Nucotuss Expectorant Barre-National, USA.
Pseudoephedrine hydrochloride (p.1099·2); guaifenesin (p.1092·2); codeine phosphate (p.25·2).
Coughs.

Nuctalon Takeda, Fr.
Estazolam (p.682·3).
Insomnia.

Nuctane Armstrong, Mex.
Phenytoin sodium (p.357·2).
Epilepsy.

Nu-Diclo Nu-Pharm, Canad.
Diclofenac sodium (p.30·3).
Inflammation; pain.

Nu-Diltiaz Nu-Pharm, Canad.
Diltiazem hydrochloride (p.874·3).
Angina pectoris; hypertension.

Nudopa Douglas, Austral.†.
Methyldopa (p.927·3).
Hypertension.

Nuelin
3M, Austral.; 3M, Denm.; 3M, Fin.; 3M, Hong Kong; 3M, Irl.; 3M, Norw.; 3M, NZ; 3M, S.Afr.; 3M, Singapore; 3M, Thai.; 3M, UK.
Theophylline (p.777·2) or theophylline sodium glycinate (p.783·2).
Obstructive airways disease.

Nu-Gel
Note. This name is used for preparations of different composition.
Johnson & Johnson Medical, Fr.
Bandage: Povidone (p.1503·2).
Burns; wounds.

Johnson & Johnson Medical, Fr.; Johnson & Johnson, Israel.
Topical gel: Sodium alginate (p.1498·3).
Wounds.

Johnson & Johnson, Ger.
Sodium alginate (p.1498·3); carmellose (p.1499·3); hyetellose (p.1501·1).
Burns; skin ulcers; wounds.

Quatromed, S.Afr.
Dicyclomine [dicycloverine] hydrochloride (p.466·1); aluminium hydroxide (p.1210·3); light magnesium oxide (p.1233·2).
Gastrointestinal disorders.

Nuhair Polipharm, Thai.
Minoxidil (p.934·2).
Alopecia androgenetica.

Nu-Hydral Nu-Pharm, Canad.
Hydralazine hydrochloride (p.905·3).
Hypertension.

Nuicalm Stafford-Miller Continental, Belg.†
Diphenhydramine hydrochloride (p.416·1).
Insomnia.

Nuidor Monot, Fr.†
Phenobarbital (p.355·1); passion flower (p.1649·1); crataegus (p.1600·2).
Anxiety; insomnia.

Nu-Indo Nu-Pharm, Canad.
Indometacin (p.44·3).
Inflammation; pain.

Nu-Iron Merz, USA.
Polysaccharide-iron complex (p.1374·3).
Iron-deficiency anaemia.

Nu-Iron V Merz, USA.
Polysaccharide-iron complex (p.1374·3); folic acid (p.1361·1); vitamins and calcium (p.1350·1).
Iron-deficiency anaemias.

Nu-Iron Plus Merz, USA.
Polysaccharide-iron complex (p.1374·3); cyanocobalamin (p.1388·1); folic acid (p.1361·1).
Iron-deficiency anaemia.

Nujol
Schering-Plough, Canad.; Fumouze, Fr.
Liquid paraffin (p.1407·1).
Constipation.

Nulacin Goldshield, UK.
Magnesium trisilicate (p.1233·3); heavy magnesium oxide (p.1233·2); calcium carbonate (p.1215·1); heavy magnesium carbonate (p.1232·3); peppermint oil (p.1243·3).
Gastrointestinal hyperacidity.

Nulacin Fermentos Seid, Spain.
Amylolytic enzymes; proteolytic enzymes; lipolytic enzymes (p.1646·1); dehydrocholic acid (p.1602·2); procaine (p.1319·2).
Digestive enzyme deficiency.

Nulceran Euro-Labor, Port.
Famotidine (p.1225·3).
Gastro-oesophageal reflux; gastrointestinal bleeding; peptic ulcer; Zollinger-Ellison syndrome.

Nulcerin Andromaco, Spain.
Famotidine (p.1225·3).
Gastro-oesophageal reflux; peptic ulcer; Zollinger-Ellison syndrome.

Nuleron Teofarma, Ital.
Magnesium polygalacturonate; calcium pantothenate (p.1374·3); promethazine hydrochloride (p.423·2); dimethicone (p.1249·2).
Gastrointestinal disorders associated with excess gas.

NuLev Schwarz, USA.
Hyoscyamine sulfate (p.469·3).

Nu-Levocarb Nu-Pharm, Canad.
Levodopa (p.1169·2); carbidopa (p.1168·2).
Parkinsonism.

Nulicaine Kay, USA†.
Lignocaine [lidocaine] hydrochloride (p.1313·2).
Local anaesthesia.

Nullatuss Hofmann & Sommer, Ger.
Clobutinol hydrochloride (p.1087·1).
Coughs.

Nu-Loraz Nu-Pharm, Canad.
Lorazepam (p.688·3).
Anxiety; sedative.

Nu-Lotan Banyu, Jpn.
Losartan potassium (p.921·3).
Hypertension.

NuLytely
Asofarma, Mex.; Braintree, USA.
Macrogol 3350 (p.1630·3); electrolytes (p.1180·1).
Bowel evacuation.

Numatol Spyfarma, Spain.
Citicoline sodium (p.1596·1).
Cerebrovascular disorders; tonic.

Numbon Teva, Israel.
Nitrazepam (p.695·2).
Insomnia.

The symbol † denotes a preparation no longer actively marketed

Nu-Medopa Nu-Pharm, Canad.
Methyldopa (p.927·3).
Hypertension.

Numencial Armstrong, Mex.
Sulpiride (p.706·1); diazepam (p.674·3).
Mixed anxiety depressive states.

Nu-Metop Nu-Pharm, Canad.
Metoprolol tartrate (p.931·2).
Angina pectoris; hypertension.

Numidan Therabel, Ital.
Naproxen piperazine (p.61·3).
Musculoskeletal, joint, peri-articular, and soft-tissue disorders.

Numobid Teral, USA†.
Guaifenesin (p.1092·2).

Numobid DM Teral, USA†.
Guaifenesin (p.1092·2); dextromethorphan hydrobromide (p.1087·3).

Numonyl Teral, USA†.
Guaifenesin (p.1092·2); phenylephrine hydrochloride (p.1097·1).

Numorphan Du Pont, Canad.; Endo, USA.
Oxymorphone hydrochloride (p.71·1).
Adjunct to general anaesthesia; pain; premedication.

Numzident Goodys, USA.
Benzocaine (p.1306·2).
Oral lesions.

Numzit
Note. This name is used for preparations of different composition.
Beige, S.Afr.
Benzocaine (p.1306·2); menthol (p.1632·3).
Teething pain.

Goodys, USA.
Lotion: Benzocaine (p.1306·2); glycerol (p.1616·3).
Topical gel: Benzocaine (p.1306·2); clove oil (p.1597·1).
Oral lesions.

Nu-Naprox Nu-Pharm, Canad.
Naproxen (p.60·3).
Inflammation; pain.

Nu-Nifed Nu-Pharm, Canad.
Nifedipine (p.940·1).
Angina pectoris.

Nuomin Masa, Thai.
Multivitamin and mineral preparation (p.1350·1).

Nu-Oxybutyn Nu-Pharm, Canad.
Oxybutynin hydrochloride (p.471·2).

Nu-Pen-VK Nu-Pharm, Canad.
Phenoxymethylpenicillin potassium (p.235·1).
Bacterial infections.

Nupercainal
Note. This name is used for preparations of different composition.
Novartis, Braz.; Zyma, Switz.†; Eastern Pharmaceuticals, UK.
Cinchocaine hydrochloride (p.1309·1).
Anorectal disorders; skin irritation.

Novartis Consumer, Canad.
Cream: Cinchocaine (p.1309·1); domiphen bromide (p.1143·3).
Ointment: Cinchocaine (p.1309·1).
Pain; pruritus.

Ciba, USA.
Cream; ointment: Cinchocaine (p.1309·1).
Suppositories: Zinc oxide (p.1128·2).
Anorectal disorders.

Nupercaine Heavy Astra, Austral.
Cinchocaine hydrochloride (p.1309·1).
Spinal anaesthesia.

Nu-Pindol Nu-Pharm, Canad.
Pindolol (p.955·3).
Angina pectoris; hypertension.

Nu-Pirox Nu-Pharm, Canad.
Piroxicam (p.79·1).
Inflammation; pain.

Nu-Prazo Nu-Pharm, Canad.
Prazosin hydrochloride (p.958·1).
Hypertension.

Nuprilan Medinfar, Port.†.
Ibuprofen (p.43·2).
Fever; musculoskeletal, joint, peri-articular, and soft-tissue disorders; pain.

Nuprin Bristol-Myers Products, USA.
Ibuprofen (p.43·2).
Fever; osteoarthritis; pain; rheumatoid arthritis.

Nuprin Backache Bristol-Myers Products, USA.
Magnesium salicylate (p.50·3).
Pain.

Nu-Prochlor Nu-Pharm, Canad.
Prochlorperazine maleate (p.701·2).
Psychoses; vomiting.

Nuquin HP Stratus, USA†.
Cream: Hydroquinone (p.1115·1); dioxybenzone (p.1517·2); oxybenzone (p.1518·1).
Gel: Hydroquinone (p.1115·1); dioxybenzone (p.1517·2).

Nur I Tropfen Chlorhexidin One Drop Only, Ger.
Chlorhexidine gluconate (p.1138·2).
Mouth and throat disorders.

Nur I Tropfen medizinisches Mundwasser One Drop Only, Ger.
Peppermint oil (p.1243·3); clove oil (p.1597·1); menthol (p.1632·3); sumatra benzoin (p.1668·3).
Mouth and throat disorders.

Nu-Ranit Nu-Pharm, Canad.
Ranitidine hydrochloride (p.1245·2).
Histamine H₂-receptor antagonist.

Nurasic TO-Chemicals, Thai.
Orphenadrine citrate (p.470·3); paracetamol (p.71·2).
Musculoskeletal pain.

Nureflex Boots Healthcare, Fr.; Boots Healthcare, Spain.
Ibuprofen (p.43·2).
Fever; musculoskeletal, joint, and peri-articular disorders; pain.

Nuril Almirall, Spain.
Pipemidic acid (p.236·1).
Urinary-tract infections.

Nuriphasic Nourypharma, Ger.
7 Tablets, ethinylestradiol (p.1476·2); 15 tablets, lynestrenol (p.1480·1); ethinylestradiol.
Menorrhagia; menstrual disorders.

Nur-Isterate Schering, S.Afr.
Norethisterone enantate (p.1485·1).
Injectable contraceptive.

Nurocain Astra, Austral.; AstraZeneca, NZ.
Lignocaine [lidocaine] (p.1313·2) or lignocaine [lidocaine] hydrochloride (p.1313·2).
Adrenaline [epinephrine] (p.829·1) is included in this preparation as a vasoconstrictor to diminish absorption and localise the effect of the local anaesthetic.
Local anaesthesia.

Nurocain with Sympathin Astra, Austral.
Lignocaine [lidocaine] hydrochloride (p.1313·2).
Adrenaline [epinephrine] (p.829·1) and noradrenaline [norepinephrine] (p.948·2) are included in this preparation as vasoconstrictors to diminish absorption and localise the effect of the local anaesthetic.
Local anaesthesia.

Nurofen
Sanova, Aust.†; Boots, Austral.; Boots Healthcare, Belg.; Boots, Denm.†; Boots Healthcare, Fr.; Boots, Ger.; Boots, Hong Kong; Boots Healthcare, Irl.; Boots, Israel; Boots Healthcare, Ital.; Boots Healthcare, Neth.; Boots, NZ; Boots, S.Afr.; Boots, Singapore; Boots Healthcare, Spain; Astra, Swed.†; Boots, Switz.; Boots, Thai.; Crookes Healthcare, UK.
Ibuprofen (p.43·2) or ibuprofen sodium (p.44·1).
Formerly called Nerofen in Belg.
Fever; inflammation; pain.

Nurofen Advance Crookes Healthcare, UK.
Ibuprofen lysine (p.44·1).
Fever; pain.

Nurofen + Codeine Boots Healthcare, Belg.
Ibuprofen (p.43·2); codeine phosphate (p.25·2).
Fever; pain.

Nurofen Cold & Flu
Boots, Austral.; Boots Healthcare, Irl.; Boots, NZ; Boots, S.Afr.; Crookes Healthcare, UK.
Ibuprofen (p.43·2); pseudoephedrine hydrochloride (p.1099·2).
Cold and influenza symptoms.

Nurofen Plus
Boots, NZ; Crookes Healthcare, UK.
Ibuprofen (p.43·2); codeine phosphate (p.25·2).
Pain.

Nurofen Rhume Boots Healthcare, Fr.
Ibuprofen (p.43·2); pseudoephedrine hydrochloride (p.1099·2).
Cold symptoms.

Nurogrip Boots Healthcare, Spain.
Ibuprofen (p.43·2); pseudoephedrine hydrochloride (p.1099·2).
Cold and influenza symptoms.

Nuromax Glaxo Wellcome, Canad.; Glaxo Wellcome, USA.
Doxacurium chloride (p.1336·3).
Competitive neuromuscular blocker.

Nurse Harvey's Gripe Mixture
Note. This name is used for preparations of different composition.
Harvey Scruton, Israel.
Dill oil (p.1603·3); sodium bicarbonate (p.1186·2).
Infant colic.

Harvey-Scruton, UK.
Dill oil (p.1603·3); caraway oil (p.1591·2); sodium bicarbonate (p.1186·2).
Colic.

Nurse Sykes Balsam Anglian, UK.
Guaifenesin (p.1092·2).
Coughs.

Nurse Sykes Powders Anglian, UK.
Aspirin (p.14·2); paracetamol (p.71·2); caffeine (p.761·3).
Cold and influenza symptoms; fever; pain.

Nursoy
Wyeth-Ayerst, Canad.; Wyeth, Mex.; Wyeth, Singapore.
Soy protein infant feed (p.1350·1).
Galactokinase deficiency; galactosaemia; lactose intolerance.

Nurture Nourishing Heinz-Wattie, NZ.
Preparation for enteral nutrition in pregnancy and lactation (p.1350·1).

Nu-Salt Cumberland, USA.
Low sodium dietary salt substitute (p.1350·1).

Nu-Seals
Lilly, Irl.; Lilly, UK.
Aspirin (p.14·2).
Fever; inflammation; pain; thromboembolic disorders.

Nussidex Teva, Israel.
Dexchlorpheniramine maleate (p.412·1); pseudoephedrine hydrochloride (p.1099·2).
Allergic rhinitis; cold symptoms.

Nuta Osotspa, Thai.
Paracetamol (p.71·2); chlorpheniramine [chlorphenamine] maleate (p.412·1); phenylpropanolamine hydrochloride (p.1098·1).
Cold symptoms.

Nutacough Osotspa, Thai.
Dextromethorphan hydrobromide (p.1087·3); ammonium chloride (p.1085·2); chlorpheniramine [chlorphenamine] maleate (p.412·1).
Coughs.

Nutamol Osotspa, Thai.
Paracetamol (p.71·2).
Fever; pain.

Nu-Tears Optopics, USA.
Polyvinyl alcohol (p.1503·1).
Dry eyes.

Nu-Tears II Optopics, USA.
Polyvinyl alcohol (p.1503·1); macrogol 400 (p.1630·3).
Dry eyes.

Nu-Tetra Nu-Pharm, Canad.
Tetracycline hydrochloride (p.258·3).
Bacterial infections.

Nutilis Nutricia, Fr.; Nutricia, Irl.; Nutricia, Port.
Food thickener (p.1350·1).
Dysphagia.

Nutra Fibra Investigacion, Mex.
Multivitamin and mineral preparation with fibre (p.1350·1).

Nutra Nutrabain Galderma, Fr.†.
Soap substitute.
Dry skin.

Nutra Nutraderme Galderma, Fr.†.
Liquid paraffin (p.1407·1).
Dry skin.

Nutrabase Filorga, Fr.
Fructo-oligosaccharides; lactic-acid producing organisms; vitamins; magnesium (p.1350·1).
Restoration of normal gastrointestinal flora.

Nutrabeaute Filorga, Fr.
Fructo-oligosaccharides; lactic-acid producing organisms; vitamins; minerals; yeast; lappa; borage (p.1350·1).
Skin disorders.

Nutrabiotique Filorga, Fr.
Nutritional supplement (p.1350·1).

Nutracel
Note. This name is used for preparations of different composition.
Isdin, Spain.
Guanosine; inosine (p.1623·3); miconazole nitrate (p.391·1); vitamin F.
Skin disorders.

Baxter, UK.
Glucose and electrolyte infusion (p.1350·1).
Parenteral nutrition.

Nutracort
Galderma, Braz.; Orion, Fin.; Galderma, Mex.; Healthpoint, USA.
Hydrocortisone (p.1073·3) or hydrocortisone acetate (p.1073·3).
Skin disorders.

Nutra-D Galderma, Austral.
Emollient.

Nutraderm
Note. This name is used for preparations of different composition.
Galderma, Braz.; Galderma, Canad.; Orion, Fin.; Galderma, Mex.; Healthpoint, USA.
Emollient.
Skin disorders; vehicle for topical drugs.

Galderma, Singapore; Galderma, Thai.
Liquid paraffin (p.1407·1).
Dry skin; emollient.

Nutradex Fresenius Kabi, Swed.
Carbohydrate and electrolyte infusion (p.1350·1).
Parenteral nutrition.

Nutraflow Alcon, Fr.†.
Rinsing, neutralising, and storage solution for soft contact lenses (p.1129·2).

Nutraforme Filorga, Fr.
Fructo-oligosaccharides; lactic-acid producing organisms; vitamins; minerals; yeast; guarana (p.1350·1).
Tonic.

Nutraisdin Isdin, Port.
Dexpanthenol (p.1602·3); zinc oxide (p.1128·2); borage oil (p.1613·1); vitamin E (p.1394·1).
Napkin rash.

Nutraloric Nutraloric, USA.
Preparation for enteral nutrition (p.1350·1).

Nutrament Mead Johnson Nutritionals, USA.
Preparation for enteral nutrition (p.1350·1).

Nutramigen
Mead Johnson, Austral.; Mead Johnson Nutritionals, Fin.; Mead Johnson, Fr.; Mead Johnson, Hong Kong; Mead Johnson, Irl.; Mead Johnson, Israel; Mead Johnson, Ital.; Mead Johnson, NZ; Mead Johnson, Port.; Mead Johnson, Thai.; Mead Johnson Nutritionals, UK; Mead Johnson Nutritionals, USA.
Protein hydrolysate preparation (p.1350·1).
Abdominal colic; diarrhoea; galactokinase deficiency; galactosaemia; lactose or sucrose intolerance; protein sensitivity.

Nutra'Mix Beaufour, Fr.
Preparation for enteral nutrition (p.1350·1).

NutraMX Vita Health, Singapore.
Multivitamin and mineral preparation with ginkgo biloba, ginseng, glutamine, inositol, and lysine (p.1350·1).

Nutraplus
Galderma, Austral.; Galderma, Braz.; Galderma, Fr.; Galderma, Hong Kong; Galderma, Irl.; Galderma, Mex.; Galderma, NZ; Galderma, Singapore; Galderma, Switz.; Galderma, UK; Healthpoint, USA.
Urea (p.1127·3).
Formerly known as Nutra Nutraplus in Fr.
Dry skin; hyperkeratosis.

Nutrarepos Filorga, Fr.
Fructo-oligosaccharides; lactic-acid producing organisms; vitamins; calcium; hypericum; passion flower; valerian; melissa (p.1350·1).
Sleep disorders; stress.

Nutrasoothe Brimms, Israel.
Avena (p.1583·1).
Skin disorders.

Nutra-Soothe Pertussin, USA.
Emollient.

Nutrasorb
Note. This name is used for preparations of different composition.
Galderma, Austral.†.
Acrylate copolymer; glycerol (p.1616·3); menthol (p.1632·3).
Acne; oily skin.

Galderma, Mex.
Acrylate copolymer; glycerol (p.1616·3).
Acne; seborrhoea.

Nutravit Light Investigacion, Mex.
Protein, multivitamin and mineral supplement (p.1350·1).
Obesity.

Nutren Clintec, USA.
Lactose-free, gluten-free preparation for enteral nutrition (p.1350·1).

Nutr-E-Sol Advanced Nutritional Technology, USA.
Tocofersolan (p.1394·3).
Vitamin E supplement.

Nutrex Beta, Ital.†.
Royal jelly (p.1659·3); pollen; ginkgo biloba (p.1615·2); eleutherococcus (p.1615·3).
Nutritional supplement.

Nutri Concentrated Nutricia, Austral.
Preparation for enteral nutrition (p.1350·1).

Nutri 2000 (Nutrinaut) Nutricia, Ital.
Preparation for enteral nutrition (p.1350·1).

Nutri Twin Pharmacia Upjohn, Ger.
Amino-acid, electrolyte, and carbohydrate solution (p.1350·1).
Parenteral nutrition.

Nutri Yin-Nutri Yang Neom, Fr.
Nutritional supplement (p.1350·1).
Tonic.

Nu-Triazide Nu-Pharm, Canad.
Triamterene (p.986·1); hydrochlorothiazide (p.907·3).
Hypertension; oedema.

Nutribraun Braun, Port.
Amino-acid, electrolyte, and lipid (from soya oil (p.1378·1) and medium-chain triglycerides (p.1372·1)) (p.1350·1).
Parenteral nutrition.

Nutrical Nutricia, Ital.
Preparation for enteral nutrition (p.1350·1).

Baxter, NZ; Nutricia, NZ.
Nutritional supplement in renal and liver impairment (p.1350·1).

Nutricap Yves Ponroy, Fr.
Amino-acid, fatty-acid, vitamin, and mineral preparation (p.1350·1).
Hair and nail disorders.

Nutricomp Braun, Irl.†; Braun, Ital.†; Braun, UK.
A range of preparations for enteral nutrition (p.1350·1).

Nutricon Pasadena, USA.
Multivitamin and mineral preparation with iron and folic acid (p.1350·1).

Nutricremal Novartis Nutrition, Fr.
High-protein nutritional supplement (p.1350·1).

Nutrideen Bioceuticals, UK.
Marine protein extract with vitamin C and zinc (p.1350·1).

Nutridoral Novartis Nutrition, Fr.
High-protein nutritional supplement (p.1350·1).

Nutridrink
Nutricia, Austral.; Nutricia, Fin.; Nutricia, Fr.; Nutricia, Ital.; Baxter, NZ; Nutricia, NZ; Nutricia, Port.
Preparation for enteral nutrition (p.1350·1).

Nutriflex
Braun, Aust.; Braun, Belg.; Braun, Fr.; Braun, Ger.; Braun, Hong Kong; Braun, Norw.; Braun, Swed.; Braun, Switz.; Braun, UK.
A range of amino-acid, carbohydrate, and electrolyte infusions (p.1350·1).
Parenteral nutrition.

Nutriflex 1680 Braun, Switz.
Amino-acid, carbohydrate, lipid (from soya oil (p.1378·1)), and electrolyte infusion (p.1350·1).
Contains egg lecithin.
Parenteral nutrition.

Nutriflex Lipid
Note.This name is used for preparations of different composition.
Braun, Fin.
Amino-acid, carbohydrate, electrolyte, and lipid (from soyal oil (p.1378·1) and medium-chain triglycerides (p.1372·1)) infusion (p.1350·1).
Parenteral nutrition.

Braun, Ger.
An amino-acid, carbohydrate and lipid (from soya oil (p.1378·1)) infusion with or without electrolytes (p.1350·1).
Parenteral nutrition.

Braun, Port.
Amino-acid, carbohydrate, lipid, and electrolyte infusion (p.1350·1).
Parenteral nutrition.

Nutriflex Lipid N Braun, Swed.
Amino-acid, carbohydrate, electrolyte, and lipid (from soya oil (p.1378·1)) infusion (p.1350·1).
Parenteral nutrition.

Nutrigel Farbo, Ital.
Fructose; soya lecithin (p.1628·1); honey (p.1366·2); royal jelly (p.1659·3).

Nutrigene GNR, Fr.†.
Yellow tablets, deoxyribonucleic acid (p.1602·3); vitamin B substances (p.1350·1); alpha tocopherol acetate; blue tablets, ribonucleic acid (p.1657·3).
The yellow tablets were formerly brown, and the blue tablets formerly contained adenosine triphosphate, ribonucleic acid, magnesium iodide, and horse muscle extract.
Painful arthritic disorders.

Nutrigil Novartis Nutrition, Fr.
A range of preparations for enteral nutrition (p.1350·1).

Nutri-Junior
Nutricia, Fin.; Nutricia, Ital.
Infant feed (p.1350·1).
Cow's milk, soya protein and other food allergies.

Nutrilac Mellin, Ital.
Infant feed (p.1350·1).
Lactose intolerance.

Nutrilamine Braun, Fr.
Amino-acid infusion (p.1350·1).
Parenteral nutrition.

Nutrilan Galagen, USA.
Lactose-free preparation for enteral nutrition (p.1350·1).

Nutrilife Pro Nutrimed, Fr.
Nutritional supplement (p.1350·1).

Nutrilin Great Eastern, Thai.; Pediatrica, Thai.
Multivitamin preparation with iron (p.1350·1).

Nutrilon AR
Nutricia, Ital.; Nutricia, Port.
Infant feed (p.1350·1).
Gastro-oesophageal reflux.

Nutrilon Lactomin Nutricia, Port.
Infant feed (p.1350·1).
Lactose intolerance.

Nutrilon Pepti
Cow & Gate, Irl.; Nutricia, Ital.; Nutricia, Port.
Infant feed (p.1350·1).
Cow's milk intolerance.

Nutrilon Soja Nutricia, Port.
Infant feed (p.1350·1).
Diarrhoea.

Nutrilon Soya
Cow & Gate, Israel; Nutricia, Ital.
Infant feed (p.1350·1).
Cow's milk intolerance.

Nutrilyte American Regent, USA.
A range of electrolyte preparations (p.1180·1).
Fluid and electrolyte disorders.

Nutrimaiz SM Searle, Braz.
Vitamin B substances; glutamic acid; iron; magnesium; calcium phosphate (p.1350·1); buclizine (p.411·1); carnitine (p.1356·1).
Reduced appetite; tonic.

Nutrimed Nutrimed, Fr.
Preparation for enteral nutrition (p.1350·1).

Nutri-Mega American Health, Hong Kong.
Multivitamin and mineral preparation (p.1350·1).

Nutri-Min Chlorella, UK.
Mineral and trace element preparation (p.1350·1).

Nutrineal Baxter, Port.†.
Amino acids; sodium chloride; calcium chloride; magnesium chloride; sodium lactate (p.1184·1).
Peritoneal dialysis.

Nutrineal PD4
Baxter, Canad.; Baxter, Denm.; Baxter, Israel; Baxter, Spain; Baxter, Swed.; Baxter, Switz.; Baxter, UK.
Sodium chloride; calcium chloride; magnesium chloride; sodium lactate; amino acids (p.1184·1).
Peritoneal dialysis.

Nutrineal PD2 and PD4 Baxter, Ital.
Calcium chloride; magnesium chloride; sodium lactate; sodium chloride; amino acids (p.1184·1).
Peritoneal dialysis solution.

Nutrini
Nutricia, Fr.; Nutricia, Irl.; Baxter, NZ; Nutricia, NZ; Nutricia Clinical, UK.
A range of preparations for enteral nutrition (p.1350·1).

Nutriplasmal Braun, Spain.
Amino-acid, glucose, and lipid (from soya oil (p.1378·1)) infusion (p.1350·1).
Parenteral nutrition.

Nutri-Soija Nutricia, Fin.
Infant feed (p.1350·1).
Cow's milk allergy; lactose intolerance.

Nutrisol Green Cross Guangzhou, Singapore.
Amino-acid infusion (p.1350·1).
Parenteral nutrition.

Nutrison
Nutricia, Austral.; Nutricia, Fin.; Nutricia, Fr.; Nutricia, Irl.; Nutricia, Ital.; Baxter, NZ; Nutricia, NZ; Nutricia, Port.; Nutricia Clinical, UK.
A range of preparations for enteral nutrition (p.1350·1).
Formerly known as Fortison in the UK.

Nutrison MCT Nutricia Clinical, UK.
Gluten- and fructose-free, low-lactose preparation for enteral nutrition (p.1350·1).
Formerly known as Liquisorbon MCT.
Fat malabsorption.

Nutrison Pepti Nutricia Clinical, UK.
Gluten-free preparation for enteral nutrition (p.1350·1).
Formerly known as Pepti-2000 LF.

Nutrisource
Novartis Nutrition, Canad.; Novartis Nutrition, Port.†.
Preparation for enteral nutrition (p.1350·1).

Nutrisun Lait Solaire Insectifuge Charton, Canad.
SPF 8: Avobenzone (p.1517·1); octinoxate (p.1517·3); oxybenzone (p.1518·1).

SPF 16: Avobenzone (p.1517·1); octinoxate (p.1517·3); oxybenzone (p.1518·1).

SPF 30: Avobenzone (p.1517·1); octinoxate (p.1517·3); oxybenzone (p.1518·1); octisalate (p.1518·1).

Sunscreen.

NutriTwin G Fresenius Kabi, Aust.
Amino-acid, carbohydrate, and electrolyte infusion (p.1350·1).
Parenteral nutrition.

Nutrivit
Note.This name is used for preparations of different composition.
Makros, Braz.
Multivitamin and mineral preparation with lysine (p.1350·1).

Dynacren, Ital.
Brewer's yeast (p.1398·1).

Nutrizim Merck, Braz.
Pancreatin (p.1646·1); bromelains (p.1586·3); dimethicone (p.1249·2); ox bile (p.1585·1).
Digestive disorders.

Nutrizym
Note.This name is used for preparations of different composition.
Merck, Aust.
Pancreatin (p.1646·1); bromelains (p.1586·3); ox bile (p.1585·1).
Digestive disorders.

Merck, Irl.; E. Merck, UK.
Pancreatin (p.1646·1).
Pancreatic insufficiency.

Merck, Port.†.
Pancreatin (p.1646·1); bromelains (p.1586·3); ox bile (p.1585·1); dimethicone (p.1249·2).
Digestive disorders.

Nutrizym N Cascan, Ger.; Glaxo Wellcome, Ger.
Pancreatin (p.1646·1).
Pancreatic insufficiency.

Nutrodrip
Novartis, Fin.; Novartis Nutrition, Fr.; Novartis, Irl.; Novartis Consumer, Ital.; Novartis Consumer, UK.
A range of preparations for enteral nutrition (p.1350·1).

Nutrol A D Rolmex, Canad.
Vitamin A (p.1382·1); vitamin D (p.1391·1).

Nutrol C Rolmex, Canad.
Ascorbic acid (p.1389·3).

Nutrol E Rolmex, Canad.
d-Alpha tocoferil acetate (p.1394·1).

Nutrol E plus Zinc & Selenium Rolmex, Canad.
Vitamin E, zinc, and selenium (p.1350·1).

Nutrol No 1 Rolmex, Canad.
Multivitamin and mineral preparation (p.1350·1).

Nutrol V Rolmex, Canad.
Betacarotene, selenium, vitamin C, and vitamin E (p.1350·1).

Nutropin
Roche, Canad.; Genentech, USA.
Somatropin (p.1286·1).
Growth failure associated with renal insufficiency; growth hormone deficiency.

Nutroplex
United American, Hong Kong; United American, Singapore; Great Eastern, Thai.; United American, Thai.
Multivitamin and mineral preparation with iron (p.1350·1).
Iron-deficiency anaemia; nutritional supplement.

Nutroplex with Iron & Lysine
United American, Hong Kong; United American, Singapore.
Multivitamin and mineral preparation with iron and lysine (p.1350·1).
Tonic.

Nutroplex Lysine Great Eastern, Thai.; United American, Thai.
Multivitamin and mineral preparation with iron and lysine (p.1350·1).
Iron-deficiency anaemia; nutritional supplement.

Nutrox Tyson, USA.
Multivitamin, mineral, and amino-acid preparation (p.1350·1).

Nuvacthen Depot Padro, Spain.
Tetracosactide hexa-acetate (p.1298·2).
Adrenocorticotrophic hormone.

Nuvapen CEPA, Spain.
Ampicillin sodium (p.150·3) or ampicillin trihydrate (p.151·1).
Bacterial infections.

Nuvelle
Schering, Denm.; Schering, Irl.; Schering, Ital.; Schering, NZ; Schering, Port.; Schering, Spain; Schering, UK.
16 Tablets, estradiol valerate (p.1473·2); 12 tablets, estradiol valerate; levonorgestrel (p.1486·2).
Menopausal disorders; osteoporosis.

Nuvelle Continuous Schering, UK.
Estradiol (p.1473·1); norethisterone acetate (p.1485·1).
Menopausal disorders; osteoporosis.

Nuvelle TS
Farmades, Ital.; Schering, UK.
Phase I patches, estradiol (p.1473·1); phase II patches, estradiol; levonorgestrel (p.1486·2).
Menopausal disorders.

Nu-Verap Nu-Pharm, Canad.
Verapamil hydrochloride (p.989·1).
Angina pectoris; arrhythmias; hypertension.

Nuvit Pharmaland, Thai.
Vitamin B₁ (p.1385·2); vitamin B₆ (p.1387·1); vitamin B₁₂ (p.1388·1).
Anorexia; neurasthenia; neurological disorders; neuropathy; toxaemia of pregnancy.

Nuvorell Sanorell, Ger.
Homoeopathic preparation.

Nux ISO Iso, Ger.†.
Homoeopathic preparation.

Nux Med Complex Dynamit, Aust.
Homoeopathic preparation.

Nux vomica Oligoplex Madaus, Ger.
Homoeopathic preparation.

Nuxil Dolisos, Canad.†.
Homoeopathic preparation.

Nuzak Cipla-Medpro, S.Afr.
Fluoxetine hydrochloride (p.284·2).
Bulimia nervosa; depression; obsessive-compulsive disorder.

Nyaderm Taro, Canad.
Nystatin (p.392·2).
Fungal and bacterial infections.

Nyal Bronchitis SmithKline Beecham Consumer, Austral.
Ammonium chloride (p.1085·2); squill (p.1100·3); liquorice (p.1231·2); senega (p.1100·2).
Cough; upper respiratory-tract congestion.

Nyal Chesty Cough SmithKline Beecham Consumer, Austral.
Guaifenesin (p.1092·2); glucose (p.1364·1); treacle.
Coughs; upper respiratory-tract congestion.

Nyal Cold Sore SmithKline Beecham Consumer, Austral.
Cream: Menthol (p.1632·3); camphor (p.1589·3).
Cracked lips; herpes labialis.
Topical lotion†: Benzoin (p.1668·3); menthol (p.1632·3); camphor (p.1589·3).
Herpes labialis.

Nyal Decongestant SmithKline Beecham Consumer, Austral.
Phenylephrine hydrochloride (p.1097·1).
Nasal congestion.

Nyal Dry Cough SmithKline Beecham Consumer, Austral.
Pentoxyverine citrate (p.1096·3).
Coughs.

Nyal Medithroat Anaesthetic Lozenges SmithKline Beecham Consumer, Austral.
Hexylresorcinol (p.1146·3).
Sore mouth and throat.

Nyal Medithroat Gargle SmithKline Beecham Consumer, Austral.
Povidone-iodine (p.1155·1).
Sore throat.

Nyal Toothache Drops SmithKline Beecham Consumer, Austral.
Benzocaine (p.1306·2); phenol (p.1152·3).
Toothache.

Nycodol Nycomed, Aust.
Tramadol hydrochloride (p.89·1).
Pain.

Nycoflox
Nycomed, Denm.; Nycomed, Norw.
Fluoxetine hydrochloride (p.284·2).
Bulimia nervosa; depression.

Nycoheparin Leo, Norw.
Heparin sodium (p.902·1).
Thromboembolic disorders.

Nycopin
Nycomed, Denm.; Nycomed, Norw.
Nifedipine (p.940·1).
Angina pectoris; hypertension.

Nycopren
Nycomed, Aust.; Nycomed, Denm.†; Nycomed, Fin.; Sanofi Synthelabo, Neth.; Nycomed, Switz.; Ardern, UK.
Naproxen (p.60·3).
Fever; gout; inflammation; musculoskeletal and joint disorders; pain.

Nycovir Nycomed, Aust.
Aciclovir (p.612·3) or aciclovir sodium (p.612·3).
Herpes simplex infections; varicella-zoster infections.

Nydrazid Apothecon, USA.
Isoniazid (p.215·3).
Tuberculosis.

Nyefax
Douglas, Austral.; Douglas, NZ; Douglas, Thai.; TTN, Thai.
Nifedipine (p.940·1).
Angina pectoris; hypertension.

Nylax Crookes Healthcare, UK†.
Phenolphthalein (p.1244·1); senna leaf (p.1248·3); bisacodyl (p.1212·2).
Constipation.

Nylax with Senna Crookes Healthcare, UK.
Senna (p.1248·3).
Constipation.

Nymix Mucolytikum Dolorgiet, Ger.†.
Ambroxol hydrochloride (p.1084·3).
Respiratory-tract disorders associated with increased or viscous mucus.

Nyolol
Ciba Vision, Fr.; Ciba Vision, Hong Kong; Ciba Vision, Israel; Ciba Vision, Port.; Ciba Vision, Singapore; Ciba Vision, Spain†; Ciba Vision, Thai.
Timolol maleate (p.982·1).
Glaucoma; ocular hypertension.

Nyquil Procter & Gamble, Canad.
Dextromethorphan hydrobromide (p.1087·3); doxylamine succinate (p.417·1); pseudoephedrine hydrochloride (p.1099·2); paracetamol (p.71·2).
Coughs and cold symptoms.

NyQuil Hot Therapy Richardson-Vicks, USA.
Paracetamol (p.71·2); pseudoephedrine hydrochloride (p.1099·2); dextromethorphan hydrobromide (p.1087·3); doxylamine succinate (p.417·1).
Coughs and cold symptoms.

NyQuil Nighttime Cold/Flu Richardson-Vicks, USA.
Pseudoephedrine hydrochloride (p.1099·2); doxylamine succinate (p.417·1); dextromethorphan hydrobromide (p.1087·3); paracetamol (p.71·2).
Coughs and cold symptoms.

Nyrene Planta, Canad.†.
Melissa (p.1632·2); valerian (p.1678·3).
Insomnia.

Nysconitrine Bio-Therabel, Belg.
Glyceryl trinitrate (p.897·3).
Angina pectoris; heart failure.

Nyspes DDSA Pharmaceuticals, UK.
Nystatin (p.392·2).
Vaginal candidiasis.

Nystacid Aspen, S.Afr.
Nystatin (p.392·2).
Candidiasis.

Nystacortone Spirig, Switz.
Prednisolone acetate (p.1078·1); nystatin (p.392·2); chlorhexidine hydrochloride (p.1138·2).
Infected skin disorders.

Nystaderm Dermapharm, Ger.
Nystatin (p.392·2).
Fungal infections.

Nystaderm comp Dermapharm, Ger.
Nystatin (p.392·2); hydrocortisone acetate (p.1073·3).
Infected skin disorders.

Nystadermal Squibb, UK†.
Nystatin (p.392·2); triamcinolone acetonide (p.1080·1).
Inflammatory candidiasis.

Nystaform
Bayer, Irl.; Typharm, UK.
Nystatin (p.392·2); chlorhexidine hydrochloride (p.1138·2).
Fungal and bacterial skin infections.

Nystaform-HC
Bayer, Irl.; Typharm, UK.
Nystatin (p.392·2); chlorhexidine acetate (p.1138·2) or chlorhexidine hydrochloride (p.1138·2); hydrocortisone (p.1073·3).
Infected skin disorders.

Nystalocal
Nourypharma, Ger.; Medinova, Switz.
Dexamethasone (p.1067·1); chlorhexidine hydrochloride (p.1138·2); nystatin (p.392·2).
Infected skin disorders.

Nystamont Rosemont, UK.
Nystatin (p.392·2).
Formerly known as Arpistatin.
Candidiasis.

Nystan Squibb, UK.
Nystatin (p.392·2).
Fungal infections.

Nystasan Bioquimico, Mex.
Nystatin (p.392·2).

Nystatin-Dome Lagap, UK.
Nystatin (p.392·2).
Candidiasis.

Nystex Savage, USA.
Nystatin (p.392·2).
Candidiasis.

Nystin Polipharm, Thai.
Nystatin (p.392·2); diiodohydroxyquinoline (p.590·2); benzalkonium chloride (p.1133·2).
Vaginal infections.

Nystop Paddock, USA.
Nystatin (p.392·2).

Nytcold Medicine Rugby, USA.
Pseudoephedrine hydrochloride (p.1099·2); dextromethorphan hydrobromide (p.1087·3); doxylamine succinate (p.417·1); paracetamol (p.71·2).
Coughs and cold symptoms.

The symbol † denotes a preparation no longer actively marketed

Nytol *Stafford-Miller, Austral.; Block, Canad.; Block, Ger.; Stafford-Miller, Ital.; Searle, S.Afr.; Stafford-Miller, Spain; Stafford-Miller, UK; Block, USA.*
Diphenhydramine hydrochloride (p.416·1).
Insomnia.

Nytol Herbal *Stafford-Miller, UK.*
Lupulus (p.1629·3); Jamaica dogwood (p.1625·1); passion flower (p.1649·1); pulsatilla (p.1656·3); wild lettuce (p.1680·3).
Insomnia.

Nytol Natural Source *Block, Canad.*
Valerian (p.1678·3).
Insomnia.

O A R *Colgate Oral Care, Austral.*
Sodium nitrite (p.1023·1).
Rust prevention in disinfecting solutions. Not for use on human skin.

O-4 Cycline *Aspen, S.Afr.*
Oxytetracycline hydrochloride (p.234·1).
Bacterial infections.

Oasil Simes *Daker Farmasimes, Spain†.*
Meprobamate (p.691·1).
Anxiety; insomnia; skeletal muscle spasm.

Oat Milk Treatment Cream *Pierre Fabre, Hong Kong.*
Avena (p.1583·1); levomenol (p.1629·1).
Chapped skin; herpes labialis; skin irritation.

Obalan *Lannett, USA†.*
Phendimetrazine tartrate (p.1513·3).
Obesity.

Obaron *Mepha, Switz.*
Benzbromarone (p.399·3).
Gout; hyperuricaemia.

Obbekjaers *Bennett, UK.*
Peppermint oil (p.1243·3).
Irritable bowel syndrome.

Obeflorine *Lehning, Fr.*
Bladderwrack (p.1585·2); senna leaflets (p.1248·2); liquorice root (p.1231·2); ash leaves.
Constipation.

Obegyn Prenatal *Fleming, USA.*
Multivitamin preparation (p.1350·1).

Obelin *Bergamo, Braz.*
Tiratricol (p.1528·3).
Lipolytic.

Obe-Nix *Holloway, USA†.*
Phentermine hydrochloride (p.1514·1).
Obesity.

Obephen *Hauck, USA†.*
Phentermine hydrochloride (p.1514·1).
Obesity.

Obesan-X *Technikon, S.Afr.*
Phendimetrazine tartrate (p.1513·3).
Obesity.

Obesidex *Bunker, Braz.*
Phenolphthalein (p.1244·1); bladderwrack (p.1585·2); thyroid (p.1526·2).
Obesity.

Obesifran *Faria, Braz.*
Phenolphthalein (p.1244·1); bladderwrack (p.1585·2); thyroid (p.1526·2).
Obesity.

Obetine *Tecnobio, Spain.*
Almagate (p.1209·3).
Dyspepsia; gastritis; gastro-oesophageal reflux; peptic ulcer.

Obex-LA *Adcock Ingram, S.Afr.*
Phendimetrazine tartrate (p.1513·3).
Obesity.

Obifen *Ayrton, UK.*
Ibuprofen (p.43·2).

Obimin *Westmont, Hong Kong; Westmont, Singapore.*
Multivitamin and mineral preparation (p.1350·1).
Dietary supplement during pregnancy and lactation.

Obimin-AF *Great Eastern, Thai.; Westmont, Thai.*
Multivitamin and mineral preparation (p.1350·1).
Nutritional supplement.

Obimol *Ayrton, UK.*
Paracetamol (p.71·2).

Obinese *Pfizer, Mex.*
Chlorpropamide (p.321·1); metformin hydrochloride (p.332·3).
Diabetes mellitus.

Obiron Extra *Pfizer, Austral.*
Multivitamin and iron preparation (p.1350·1).

Obisin *Casmar, Mex.*
Fenproporex (p.1510·2).

Oblioser *Serono, Spain†.*
Morphine sulfate (p.56·1).
Pain.

Obliterol *Faes, Spain.*
Pantethine (p.952·1).
Hyperlipidaemias.

Oblivon *Doetsch, Grether, Switz.†.*
Methylpentynol (p.692·3).
Nervous disorders.

Obracin *Lilly, Braz.; Lilly, Neth.; Lilly, Switz.*
Tobramycin sulfate (p.263·3).
Bacterial infections.

Obsidan
Note.This name is used for preparations of different composition.
Verman, Fin.
Ferrous glycine sulfate (p.1360·2).
Iron deficiency; iron-deficiency anaemia.

Isis, Ger.
Propranolol hydrochloride (p.962·3).
Angina pectoris; anxiety; arrhythmias; hypertension; hyperthyroidism; migraine; myocardial infarction; tremor.

Obsidan comp *Verman, Fin.*
Ferrous glycine sulfate (p.1360·2); folic acid (p.1361·1).
Iron and folic acid deficiency.

Obsilazin N *Isis, Ger.*
Propranolol hydrochloride (p.962·3); dihydralazine sulfate (p.874·2).
Hypertension.

Obstar *Johnson & Johnson, Braz.*
Loperamide hydrochloride (p.1231·3).
Diarrhoea.

Obstilax *Sanico, Belg.†.*
Sodium picosulfate (p.1249·3).
Constipation.

Obstinol *Thiemann, Ger.†.*
Liquid paraffin (p.1407·1); phenolphthalein (p.1244·1).
Bowel evacuation; constipation.

Obstinol M *Thiemann, Ger.*
Liquid paraffin (p.1407·1).
Formerly known as Obstinol mild.
Bowel regulation.

Obus Form Therapeutic Heat *Mentholatum, Canad.*
Methyl salicylate (p.55·1); menthol (p.1632·3).

Obus Form Therapeutic Ice *Mentholatum, Canad.*
Menthol (p.1632·3).

Oby-Cap *Richwood, USA†.*
Phentermine hydrochloride (p.1514·1).
Obesity.

Oby-Trim 30 *Rexar, USA†.*
Phentermine hydrochloride (p.1514·1).
Obesity.

Ocadrik *Roussel Diamant, Fr.*
Verapamil (p.991·1); trandolapril (p.985·2).
Hypertension.

O-Cal FA *Pharmics, USA.*
Multivitamin and mineral preparation with iron and folic acid (p.1350·1).

Occhivit *Giuliani, Ital.*
Multivitamin and mineral preparation with myrtillus (p.1350·1).
Nutritional supplement.

Occidal *Ranbaxy, Thai.*
Ofloxacin (p.232·3).
Bacterial infections.

Occlucort *GenDerm, Canad.†.*
Betamethasone dipropionate (p.1063·2).
Skin disorders.

Occlusal
Medicis, Canad.; Dermapharm, Irl.; Dermapharm, UK; GenDerm, USA.
Salicylic acid (p.1122·3).
Warts.

Ocean *Fleming, USA.*
Sodium chloride (p.1196·1).
Nasal irritation.

Oceantone *Cantassium Co., UK.*
Green-lipped mussel (p.1618·2).

Oceral
Asta Medica, Aust.; Roche, Braz.; Medika, Switz.
Oxiconazole nitrate (p.393·1).
Fungal infections; mixed fungal and Gram-positive bacterial infections.

Oceral GB *Yamanouchi, Ger.*
Oxiconazole nitrate (p.393·1).
Fungal infections.

Ochozim *Italmex, Mex.*
Pepsin (p.1649·3); trypsin (p.1675·3); chymotrypsin (p.1595·1); amylase (p.1579·3); lipase; cellulase (p.1593·1); rennet; ox bile extract (p.1585·2); dimethicone (p.1249·2).
Gastrointestinal disorders.

OCL *Abbott, USA.*
Macrogol 3350 (p.1630·3); electrolytes (p.1180·1).
Bowel evacuation.

Ocsaar *Merck Sharp & Dohme, Israel.*
Losartan potassium (p.921·3).
Heart failure; hypertension.

Ocsaar Plus *Merck Sharp & Dohme, Israel.*
Losartan potassium (p.921·3); hydrochlorothiazide (p.907·3).
Hypertension.

Octacosanol *Cantassium Co., UK.*
Vitamin E (p.1393·3); octacosanol.

Octadon P *Thiemann, Ger.*
Paracetamol (p.71·2); caffeine (p.761·3).
Pain.

Octagam
Octapharma, Aust.; Octapharma, Ger.; Octapharma, Hong Kong; Octapharma, Norw.; Octapharma, Swed.; Octapharma, Switz.; Octapharma, UK.
A normal immunoglobulin (p.1551·3).
Bone marrow transplantation; hypogammaglobulinaemia; idiopathic thrombocytopenic purpura; immunodeficiency; Kawasaki disease; passive immunisation.

Octamide *Adria, USA.*
Metoclopramide hydrochloride (p.1235·2).
Nausea and vomiting.

Octanate *Octapharma, Ger.*
A factor VIII preparation (p.734·1).
Haemorrhagic disorders.

Octanine *Octapharma, Ger.*
A factor IX preparation (p.735·1).
Formerly known as Octanyne.
Haemorrhagic disorders.

Octanyne *Octapharma, Norw.*
A factor IX preparation (p.735·1).
Haemorrhagic disorders.

Octaplas
Octapharma, Aust.; Octapharma, Ger.; Octapharma, Switz.; Octapharma, UK.
Plasma (p.739·2).
Haemorrhagic disorders; reversal of oral anticoagulant effects; thrombocytopenic purpura.

Octatron *VAAS, Ital.*
Amino-acid, vitamin, and mineral preparation (p.1350·1).

Octavi
Octapharma, Ger.†; Octapharma, Norw.
A factor VIII preparation (p.734·1).
Haemorrhagic disorders.

Octenisept
Schulke & Mayr, Aust.; Schulke & Mayr, Ger.; Schulke & Mayr, Switz.
Octenidine hydrochloride (p.1151·3); phenoxyethanol (p.1153·3).
Skin and mucous membrane disinfection.

Octiban *Degorts, Mex.*
Co-trimoxazole (p.193·3).
Bacterial infections.

Octicair *Bausch & Lomb, USA.*
Hydrocortisone (p.1073·3); neomycin sulfate (p.228·1); polymyxin B (p.238·3).
Bacterial ear infections.

Octil *Genpharm, Israel.*
Timolol maleate (p.982·1).
Glaucoma; ocular hypertension.

Octilia
Bouty, Ital.; SIFI, Singapore.
Tetryzoline hydrochloride (p.1101·2).
Eye irritation and congestion.

Octim *Ferring, Fr.*
Desmopressin acetate (p.1281·2).
Haemorrhage.

Octinum *Knoll, Switz.*
Isometheptene hydrochloride (p.1624·2).
Migraine; smooth muscle spasm; vegetative dystonia.

Octocaine
Clarben, Spain; Novocol, USA.
Lignocaine [lidocaine] (p.1313·2) or lignocaine [lidocaine] hydrochloride (p.1313·2).
Adrenaline [epinephrine] (p.829·1) may be included in this preparation as a vasoconstrictor to diminish absorption and localise the effect of the local anaesthetic.
Local anaesthesia.

Octofene
Debat, Fr.; Hoechst Marion Roussel, Ital.; Fournier, Port.
Clofoctol (p.192·1).
Otorhinolaryngeal infections; respiratory-tract infections.

Octonativ-M
Pharmacia Upjohn, Norw.; Pharmacia Upjohn, Swed.
A factor VIII preparation (p.734·1).
Haemorrhagic disorders.

Octonox *Pharmethic, Belg.*
Lormetazepam (p.689·3).
Formerly contained phenobarbital sodium, secobarbital sodium, and amobarbital sodium.
Insomnia.

Octostim
Ferring, Aust.; Rhone-Poulenc Rorer, Austral.; Ferring, Canad.; Ferring, Denm.; Ferring, Fin.; Ferring, Hong Kong; Ferring, Israel; Ferring, Neth.; Ferring, Norw.; Aventis, NZ; Ferring, Singapore; Ferring, Swed.; Ferring, Switz.
Desmopressin acetate (p.1281·2).
Diabetes insipidus; haemorrhagic disorders; test of renal concentrating capacity.

Octotensina *Bioquimico, Mex.*
Civanetidine.

Octovit *Goldshield, UK.*
Multivitamin and mineral preparation (p.1350·1).

Octreoscan *Byk Gulden, Ital.*
Indium-111 pentetreotide (p.1449·3).
Detection and location of neuroendocrine tumours.

Octron *Lambda, USA†.*
Vitamin B substances and iron (p.1350·1).

Octron Plus *Lambda, USA†.*
Ferric cacodylate.

Octron₂ *Lambda, USA†.*
Vitamin B substances and iron (p.1350·1).

Ocubrax *Alcon Cusi, Spain.*
Tobramycin (p.263·3); diclofenac sodium (p.30·3).
Ocular inflammation following cataract surgery.

Ocu-Caine *Ocumed, USA.*
Proxymetacaine hydrochloride (p.1320·1).
Local anaesthesia.

OcuCaps *Akorn, USA.*
Antioxidant, vitamin, and mineral supplement (p.1350·1).

Ocu-Carpine *Ocumed, USA.*
Pilocarpine hydrochloride (p.1422·3).
Glaucoma; raised intra-ocular pressure; reversal of mydriasis.

Ocuclear
Schering, Canad.; Schering-Plough, Mex.; Schering-Plough, USA.
Oxymetazoline hydrochloride (p.1096·2).
Minor eye irritation.

Ocucoat
Note.This name is used for preparations of different composition.
Bausch & Lomb, Belg.; Storz, Israel; Storz, Swed.†; Storz, UK.
Hypromellose (p.1501·3).
Adjunct in ocular surgery.

Bausch & Lomb, USA.
Eye drops: Dextran 70 (p.729·2); hypromellose (p.1501·3).
Dry eyes.

Ocular syringe: Hypromellose (p.1501·3).
Adjunct in ocular surgery.

Ocufen
Allergan, Austral.; Allergan-Frumtost, Braz.; Allergan, Canad.; Allergan, Denm.; Allergan, Fr.; Allergan, Hong Kong; Allergan, Irl.; Allergan, Ital.; Allergan, Mex.; Allergan, NZ; Allergan, S.Afr.; Allergan, Singapore; Allergan, Thai.; Allergan, UK; Allergan, USA.
Flurbiprofen sodium (p.41·2).
Intra-operative miosis inhibition; postoperative anterior eye inflammation; prevention of cystoid macular oedema.

Ocuflox
Allergan, Austral.; Allergan, Canad.; Allergan, Mex.; Allergan, USA.
Ofloxacin (p.232·3).
Bacterial eye infections.

Ocuflur
Allergan, Aust.; Allergan, Belg.; Allergan, Ger.; Allergan, Port.; Allergan, Spain; Allergan, Switz.
Flurbiprofen sodium (p.41·2).
Intra-operative miosis inhibition; postoperative eye inflammation and pain; prevention of cystoid macular oedema following cataract surgery.

Ocufort *Farmila, Ital.*
Multivitamin and mineral preparation (p.1350·1).
Nutritional supplement.

Ocufri *Allergan, Norw.*
Polyvinyl alcohol (p.1503·1).
Dry eyes.

Ocugel *Asta Medica, Belg.*
Carbomer 974P (p.1499·2).

Ocugram *Charton, Canad.†.*
Gentamicin sulfate (p.210·1).
Bacterial infections.

Ocuhist *Pfizer Consumer, USA.*
Naphazoline hydrochloride (p.1095·1); pheniramine maleate (p.422·3).
Eye irritation and pruritus.

Oculac
Ciba Vision, Denm.; Ciba Vision, Fin.; Ciba Vision, Norw.; Ciba Vision, Swed.; Ciba Vision, Switz.
Povidone (p.1503·2) (p.1129·2).
Contact lens wetting solution; dry eyes.

Oculoforte *Restan, S.Afr.*
Zinc sulfate (p.1398·2); phenylephrine hydrochloride (p.1097·1); tetryzoline hydrochloride (p.1101·2).
Eye irritation.

Oculosan
Note.This name is used for preparations of different composition.
Ciba Vision, Hong Kong; Bausch & Lomb, S.Afr.; Ciba Vision, Thai.
Zinc sulfate (p.1398·2); naphazoline nitrate (p.1095·1).
Eye irritation.

Ciba Vision, Switz.
Zinc sulfate (p.1398·2); naphazoline nitrate (p.1095·1); hamamelis (p.1618·3); euphrasia (p.1609·3); neroli oil (p.1640·1); lavender oil (p.1627·2).
Eye irritation.

Oculosan forte *Ciba Vision, Switz.*
Zinc sulfate (p.1398·2); phenylephrine hydrochloride (p.1097·1); tetryzoline hydrochloride (p.1101·2); hamamelis (p.1618·3).
Eye irritation.

Oculosan N *Ciba Vision, Ger.*
Zinc sulfate (p.1398·2); naphazoline nitrate (p.1095·1).
Inflammatory and allergic disorders of the eye.

Oculotect
Note.This name is used for preparations of different composition.
Ciba Vision, Aust.; Ciba Vision, Neth.; Ciba Vision, Port.; Ciba Vision, Singapore; Ciba Vision, Spain; Novartis Ophthalmics, UK.
Povidone (p.1503·2) (p.1129·2).
Dry eyes; wetting solution for contact lenses.

Ciba Vision, Ger.
Eye drops: Vitamin A palmitate (p.1383·2); hypromellose (p.1501·3).
Dry eyes.

Ocular gel: Vitamin A palmitate (p.1383·2).
Eye disorders.

Ciba Vision, Switz.
Vitamin A palmitate (p.1383·2).
Corneal damage; dry eyes.

Oculotect Fluid *Ciba Vision, Ger.*
Povidone (p.1503·2).
Dry eyes.

Oculotect sine *Ciba Vision, Ger.*
Vitamin A palmitate (p.1383·2).
Eye disorders.

Oculube *Charton, Canad.†.*
White soft paraffin (p.1407·3); liquid paraffin (p.1407·1).
Dry eyes.

Oftrim Allergan-Frumtost, Braz.
Polymyxin B sulfate (p.238·1); framycetin sulfate (p.208·2); gramicidin (p.213·3).
Bacterial eye infections.

Oftyll Desoxydrop Omisan, Ital.†.
Disinfecting solution for contact lens (p.1129·2).

Ogamma Otsuka, Jpn.
Interferon gamma-n1 (p.634·1).

Ogast Takeda, Fr.
Lansoprazole (p.1230·3).
Gastro-oesophageal reflux; peptic ulcer; Zollinger-El-lison syndrome.

Ogasto Seber, Port.
Lansoprazole (p.1230·3).
Gastro-oesophageal reflux; peptic ulcer; Zollinger-El-lison syndrome.

Ogastro Abbott, Braz.; Abbott, Mex.
Lansoprazole (p.1230·3).
Gastro-oesophageal reflux; peptic ulcer; Zollinger-El-lison syndrome.

Ogen Pharmacia Upjohn, Austral.; Pharmacia Upjohn, Canad.; Pharmacia Upjohn, Mex.; Pharmacia Upjohn, USA.
Estropipate (p.1476·1).
Menopausal disorders; oestrogen deficiency; oste-oporosis.

Ogestane Besins-Iscovesco, Fr.†.
A vitamin, mineral, and fish oil preparation (p.1350·1).

Oglos Grunenthal, Spain.
Morphine hydrochloride (p.56·1).
Pain; premedication.

Ogyline Effik, Fr.
Norgestrienone (p.1487·2).
Progestogen-only oral contraceptive.

OH B12 Searle, Ital.; Jaba, Port.
Hydroxocobalamin (p.1388·1).
Anaemias; liver disorders; neuralgia; neuritis.

OH B12 B1 Poli, Ital.†.
Hydroxocobalamin (p.1388·1); monophosphothiamine chloride (p.1385·2).
Anaemias; neuralgia; neuritis.

Ohexine Greater Pharma, Thai.
Bromhexine hydrochloride (p.1085·3).
Respiratory-tract disorders associated with increased or viscous mucus.

OIF Otsuka, Jpn.
Interferon alfa (p.628·1).
Hepatitis; renal cancer.

Oil of Olay
Note.This name is used for preparations of different composition.
Procter & Gamble, Canad.
Octinoxate (p.1517·3); ensulizole (p.1517·2).
Sunscreen.

Procter & Gamble, USA.
SPF 15: Octinoxate (p.1517·3); titanium dioxide (p.1126·1); ensulizole (p.1517·2).
Sunscreen.

Oilatum
Note.This name is used for preparations of different composition.
Stiefel, Canad.; Stiefel, Ital.; Stiefel, Spain†.
Emollient.

Stiefel, Israel.
Soap substitute.

Stiefel, NZ.
Light liquid paraffin (p.1407·2).
Dry skin.

Oilatum Bar Stiefel, Austral.; Stiefel, Hong Kong; Stiefel, Singapore; Stiefel, Thai.
Liquid paraffin (p.1407·1).
Soap substitute.

Oilatum Bath Formula Stiefel, UK.
Light liquid paraffin (p.1407·2).
Dry skin disorders.

Oilatum Cream
Note.This name is used for preparations of different composition.
Stiefel, Fr.; Stiefel.
Light liquid paraffin (p.1407·2) or liquid paraffin (p.1407·1); white soft paraffin (p.1407·3).
Formerly contained arachis oil in the UK.
Dry skin disorders.

Stiefel, Hong Kong; Stiefel, Irl.; Stiefel, Singapore.
Arachis oil (p.1581·1).
Dry skin; skin irritation.

Oilatum Emollient
Note.This name is used for preparations of different composition.
Stiefel, Austral.; Stiefel, Irl.; Stiefel, UK.
Light liquid paraffin (p.1407·2) or liquid paraffin (p.1407·1); acetylated wool alcohols (p.1410·3).
Dry skin conditions.

Stiefel, Hong Kong; Stiefel, Singapore; Stiefel, Thai.
Light liquid paraffin (p.1407·2) or liquid paraffin (p.1407·1).
Dry skin disorders.

Oilatum Fragrance Free Stiefel, UK.
Light liquid paraffin (p.1407·2).
Dry skin disorders.

Oilatum Gel Stiefel, Hong Kong; Stiefel, Irl.; Stiefel, Singapore; Stiefel, UK.
Light liquid paraffin (p.1407·2) or liquid paraffin (p.1407·1).
Dry skin disorders.

Oilatum Jabon Stiefel, Mex.
Arachis oil (p.1581·1).
Dry skin disorders.

Oilatum Junior Stiefel, UK.
Bath additive: Light liquid paraffin (p.1407·2).
Cream: Light liquid paraffin (p.1407·2); white soft paraffin (p.1407·3).
Dry skin; pruritus.

Oilatum Junior Flare-Up
Stiefel, Irl.; Stiefel, UK.
Light liquid paraffin (p.1407·2); triclosan (p.1159·2); benzalkonium chloride (p.1133·2).
Infected eczema.

Oilatum Plus
Stiefel, Austral.; Stiefel, Hong Kong; Stiefel, NZ; Stiefel, S.Afr.; Stiefel, Singapore; Stiefel, Thai.; Stiefel, UK.
Light liquid paraffin (p.1407·2); triclosan (p.1159·2); benzalkonium chloride (p.1133·2).
Eczema.

Oilatum Shampoo Stiefel, UK.
Ciclopirox olamine (p.382·1).
Scalp disorders.

Oilatum Shower Gel Stiefel, Austral.
Light liquid paraffin (p.1407·2).
Dry skin.

Oilatum Skin Therapy Stiefel, UK†.
Light liquid paraffin (p.1407·2).
Dry skin.

Oilatum Soap
Note.This name is used for preparations of different composition.
Stiefel, UK.
Liquid paraffin (p.1407·1).
Dry skin disorders.

Stiefel, USA.
Skin cleanser.

Oil-Free Acne Wash Professional Health, Canad.†.
Salicylic acid (p.1122·3).
Acne.

Oil-Free Sunblock Clinique, Canad.
SPF 15: Octinoxate (p.1517·3); octocrilene (p.1518·1); octisalate (p.1518·1); oxybenzone (p.1518·1).
Sunscreen.

Oil-Free Sunscreen Avon, Canad.
SPF 15: Octinoxate (p.1517·3); octocrilene (p.1518·1); octisalate (p.1518·1).
Sunscreen.

Oil-Free Sunspray Estee Lauder, Canad.†.
SPF 10; SPF 15: Octinoxate (p.1517·3); homosalate (p.1517·2); octisalate (p.1518·1); oxybenzone (p.1518·1).
Sunscreen.

Ojensalve Neutral Ophtha, Denm.
Liquid paraffin (p.1407·1); white soft paraffin (p.1407·3).
Blepharitis; protection of eyelid and cornea.

Ojosbel Dermofarm, Spain.
Hamamelis water (p.1618·3); naphazoline hydrochloride (p.1095·1).
Eye irritation.

Ojosbel Azul Dermofarm, Spain.
Hamamelis water (p.1618·3); methylene blue [methyl-thioninium chloride] (p.1012·3); naphazoline hydrochloride (p.1095·1).
Eye irritation.

Okacin
Ciba Vision, Denm.; Ciba Vision, Fin.; Ciba Vision, Hong Kong; Ciba Vision, Irl.; Ciba Vision, Port.; Ciba Vision, Switz.; Ciba Vision, Thai.
Lomefloxacin hydrochloride (p.220·1).
Bacterial eye infections.

Okacyn
Restan, S.Afr.; Novartis Ophthalmics, UK.
Lomefloxacin hydrochloride (p.220·1).
Bacterial eye infections.

Okal Puerto Galiano, Spain.
Aspirin (p.14·2); caffeine (p.761·3).
Fever; pain.

Okal Infantil Puerto Galiano, Spain.
Aspirin (p.14·2).
Fever; musculoskeletal and joint disorders; pain; thrombosis prophylaxis.

Oki Dompe, Ital.
Ketoprofen lysine (p.48·1).
Inflammation; pain.

Okokit II Hughes & Hughes, UK.
Test for faecal occult blood.

Okoubarell Sanorell, Ger.
Homoeopathic preparation.

Okoubasan Sanum-Kehlbeck, Ger.
Homoeopathic preparation.

Okuzell Nycomed, Aust.
Hypromellose (p.1501·3).
Eye irritation.

O-Lac
Mead Johnson, Austral.; Mead Johnson, Fr.; Mead Johnson, Hong Kong; Mead Johnson, Ital.; Mead Johnson, NZ; Mead Johnson, Port.; Mead Johnson, Singapore; Mead Johnson Nutritionals, Thai.
Infant feed (p.1350·1).
Galactosaemia; lactose intolerance; sucrose intolerance.

Olamin P Delta BKB, Ital.
Piroctone olamine (p.1121·1).
Seborrhoeic dermatitis.

Ol-Amine Meuse, Belg.
Multivitamin and mineral preparation (p.1350·1).

Olan-Gin Olan-Kemed, Thai.
Dipyrone (p.34·1).
Lignocaine [lidocaine] (p.1313·2) is included in some injections to alleviate the pain of injection.
Fever; pain.

Olbad Cordes
Ichthyol, Aust.; Ichthyol, Ger.
Soya oil (p.1378·1).
Bath additive; skin disorders.

Olbad Cordes comp Ichthyol, Aust.
Soya oil (p.1378·1); shale oil.
Bath additive; skin disorders.

Olbad Cordes F Ichthyol, Ger.
Arachis oil (p.1581·1).
Bath additive; skin disorders.

Olbas
Note.This name is used for preparations of different composition.
Olbas, Ger.
Oil: Peppermint oil (p.1243·3); cajuput oil (p.1588·1); eucalyptus oil (p.1609·2); juniper oil (p.1625·2); sweet birch oil (p.55·2).
Cold symptoms; gastrointestinal disorders; headache; neuralgia; pain; rheumatism.
Pastilles: Peppermint oil (p.1243·3); cajuput oil (p.1588·1); eucalyptus oil (p.1609·2); juniper oil (p.1625·2); sweet birch oil (p.55·2).
Cold symptoms; mouth and throat disinfection.
Topical spray: Ethyl chloride (p.1312·1); menthol (p.1632·3).
Soft-tissue disorders; sports injuries.

Synpharma, Switz.
Inhaler: Peppermint oil (p.1243·3); eucalyptus oil (p.1609·2); menthol (p.1632·3); eucalyptol (p.1609·2).
Nasal congestion.
Oil: Peppermint oil (p.1243·3); eucalyptus oil (p.1609·2); cajuput oil (p.1588·1); sweet birch oil (p.55·2); juniper oil (p.1625·2); clove oil (p.1597·1).
Cold symptoms; nasal congestion.
Ointment: Peppermint oil (p.1243·3); eucalyptus oil (p.1609·2); cajuput oil (p.1588·1); sweet birch oil (p.55·2); turpentine oil (p.1676·3); clove oil (p.1597·1).
Cold symptoms; nasal congestion.

Lane, UK.
Inhaler: Cajuput oil (p.1588·1); menthol (p.1632·3); peppermint oil (p.1243·3); eucalyptus oil (p.1609·2).
Nasal congestion.
Oil: Cajuput oil (p.1588·1); eucalyptus oil (p.1609·2); sweet birch oil (p.55·2); clove oil (p.1597·1); juniper oil (p.1625·2); menthol (p.1632·3); dementholised mint oil (p.1636·2).
Nasal congestion.
Pastilles: Eucalyptus oil (p.1609·2); peppermint oil (p.1243·3); menthol (p.1632·3); juniper oil (p.1625·2); sweet birch oil (p.55·2); clove oil (p.1597·1).
Cold symptoms; coughs.

Olbemox Pharmacia Upjohn, Ger.
Acipimox (p.827·3).
Lipid disorders.

Olbetam
Pharmacia Upjohn, Aust.; Pharmacia Upjohn, Belg.; Carlo Erba, Braz.; Pharmacia Upjohn, Denm.; Pharmacia Upjohn, Hong Kong; Pharmacia Upjohn, Irl.; Farmitalia, Israel; Pharmacia Upjohn, Ital.; Pharmacia Upjohn, Mex.; Pharmacia Upjohn, NZ; Pharmacia Upjohn, S.Afr.; Pharmacia Upjohn, Singapore; Pharmacia Upjohn, Switz.; Pharmacia Upjohn, Thai.; Pharmacia, UK.
Acipimox (p.827·3).
Hyperlipidaemias.

Olbiacor Salus, Ital.
Fendiline hydrochloride (p.889·1).
Ischaemic heart disease; myocardial infarction.

Olcadil
Sanabo, Aust.†; Novartis, Braz.; Novartis, Port.
Cloxazolam (p.671·2).
Alcohol withdrawal syndrome; anxiety disorders; pre-medication; sleep disorders.

Olcam Irex, Fr.
Piroxicam (p.79·1).
Musculoskeletal and joint disorders.

Olcenon Lederle, Jpn†.
Tretinoin tocoferil.
Skin ulcers.

Oldamin Fuji, Jpn.
Monoethanolamine oleate (p.1636·3).
Oesophageal varices.

Oldan Europharma, Spain.
Acemetacin (p.11·2).
Musculoskeletal, joint, and peri-articular disorders.

Oleatum
Note.This name is used for preparations of different composition.
Stiefel, Ger.
Light liquid paraffin (p.1407·2).
Skin disorders.

Stiefel, Ital.
Emollient.

Oleatum Bar Stiefel, Fr.
Liquid paraffin (p.1407·1).
Dry skin.

Oleatum Emollient Stiefel, Fr.
Liquid paraffin (p.1407·1).
Dry skin.

Oleatum Gel Stiefel, Fr.
Liquid paraffin (p.1407·1).
Dry skin.

Oleo Dermosina Simples Davi, Port.
Zinc oxide (p.1128·2).
Skin disorders.

Oleo Eletrico QIF, Braz.
Camphor (p.1589·2); turpentine oil (p.1676·3); methyl salicylate (p.55·1).
Musculoskeletal and joint disorders.

Oleobal Pierre Fabre Dermo Kosmetik, Ger.
Soya oil (p.1378·1); light liquid paraffin (p.1407·2).
Bath additive; skin disorders.

Oleoban Medinfar, Port.
Sunflower oil (p.1381·2).
Skin cleansing; skin disorders.

Oleoban Composto Medinfar, Port.
Sunflower oil (p.1381·2); ichthammol (p.1115·2).
Skin disorders.

Oleoban Gel Medinfar, Port.
Sunflower oil (p.1381·2); liquid paraffin (p.1407·1).
Dry skin disorders.

Oleocal Mex-America, Mex.
Calcium hydroxide (p.1588·3).

Oleoderm Mex-America, Mex.
Calcium hydroxide (p.1588·3).
Skin disorders.

Oleoderm Plus Mex-America, Mex.
Calcium hydroxide (p.1588·3); avobenzone (p.1517·1); octinoxate (p.1517·3).
Sunscreen.

Oleomycetin
Agepha, Aust.; Winzer, Ger.
Chloramphenicol (p.179·1).
Bacterial eye infections.

Oleomycetin-Prednison
Agepha, Aust.; Winzer, Ger.
Chloramphenicol (p.179·1); prednisone (p.1079·2).
Infected eye disorders.

Oleosint Apomedica, Aust.
Diolamine oleate (p.1604·1); soya oil (p.1378·1).
Skin disorders.

Oleosorbate Bournonville, Belg.†.
Polysorbate 80 (p.1347·3).
Ear wax removal; rhinitis.

Oleovit Fresenius Kabi, Aust.
Vitamin A palmitate (p.1383·2); dexpanthenol (p.1602·3).
Eye disorders.

Oleovit A Fresenius Kabi, Aust.
Capsules: Vitamin A palmitate (p.1383·2).
Ear disorders; gastrointestinal disorders; hyperthy-roidism; respiratory-tract disorders; skin disorders; urogenital disorders.
Oral drops: Vitamin A (p.1382·1); betacarotene (p.1355·1).
Vitamin A deficiency.

Oleovit A + D Fresenius Kabi, Aust.
Capsules: Vitamin A palmitate (p.1383·2); colecalcif-erol (p.1391·1).
Oral drops: Vitamin A (p.1382·1); betacarotene (p.1355·1); colecalciferol (p.1391·1).
Rickets; vitamin A and D supplementation.

Oleovit A + D₃ Vitamed, Israel.
Vitamin A (p.1382·1); colecalciferol (p.1391·1).
Vitamin supplement.

Oleovit D₃ Fresenius Kabi, Aust.
Colecalciferol (p.1391·1).
Hypoparathyroidism; rickets.

Oleum Rhinale Weleda, UK.
Calendula (p.1589·2); merc. sulph.; peppermint oil (p.1243·3); eucalyptus oil (p.1609·2).
Catarrh; sinus congestion.

Olexin Rayere, Mex.
Omeprazole (p 1239·1).
Gastro-oesophageal reflux; peptic ulcer; Zollinger-El-lison syndrome.

Olf GNLD, Austral.
Reishi mushrooms; celery; avena; red sage; damiana; hypericum; astragalus; angelica; cinnamon; liquorice (p.1350·1).
Tonic.

Olfen
Mepha, Hong Kong; Mepha, Port.; Mepha, Singapore; Mepha, Switz.; Mepha, Thai.
Diclofenac sodium (p.30·3).
Lignocaine [lidocaine] (p.1313·2) or lignocaine [lido-caine] hydrochloride (p.1313·2) may be included in the intramuscular injection to alleviate the pain of injec-tion.
Gout; inflammation; musculoskeletal, joint, peri-artic-ular, and soft-tissue disorders; pain; renal and biliary colic.

Olfex Bial-Aristegui, Spain.
Budesonide (p.1064·2).
Asthma; insect bites; rhinitis; skin disorders.

Olibanum RA Zilly, Ger.
Indian frankincense.
Inflammation.

Olicard
Solvay, Ger.; Solvay, Spain.
Isosorbide mononitrate (p.916·2).
Angina pectoris; heart failure.

Olicardin Solvay, Aust.
Isosorbide mononitrate (p.916·2).
Angina pectoris; heart failure; myocardial infarction; pulmonary hypertension.

Olicide Cosmofarma, Port.†.
Malathion (p.1434·2).
Pediculosis.

Olidermil *Oftalder, Port.*
Zinc oxide (p.1128·2); almond oil (p.1576·3).
Dry skin.

Oligobs *CCD, Fr.*
A range of multivitamin and mineral preparations (p.1350·1).

Oligocean *Ido, Fr.*
Trace element and mineral preparation derived from shellfish (p.1350·1).
Tonic.

Oligocure *Labcatal, Fr.*
Manganese gluconate; copper gluconate; colloidal gold (p.1350·1).
Tonic.

Oligoderm *Labcatal, Fr.*
Manganese gluconate (p.1371·3); copper gluconate (p.1357·3).
Cracked nipples.

Oligoelementos *Braun, Port.*
Trace element preparation (p.1350·1).
Parenteral nutrition.

Oligo-elements Aguettant *Aguettant, Fr.*
Trace element preparation (p.1350·1).
Parenteral nutrition.

Oligo-Essentials *Richelet, Fr.*
A range of mineral and trace element preparations (p.1350·1).

Oligofer *Sabex, Canad.*
Mineral preparation with vitamin B_{12} (p.1350·1).

Oligoforme *Ido, Fr.*
A range of nutritional supplements (p.1350·1).

Oligogranul *Boiron, Fr.*
A range of trace element and mineral preparations (p.1350·1).

Oligophytum *Holistica, Fr.*
A range of mineral-rich plant extracts.

Oligoplex *Natural Touch, UK.*
A range of homoeopathic remedies.

Oligorhine *Monin, Fr.*
Copper; silver (p.1350·1).
Nasal irrigation.

Oligosol *Labcatal, Canad.; Labcatal, Fr.; Labcatal, Switz.*
A range of trace element and mineral preparations (p.1350·1).

Oligostim *Dolisos, Fr.*
A range of trace element and mineral preparations (p.1350·1).

Oliviase *UPSA, Fr.*
Olive leaves.
Diuresis.

Olivysat *Ysatfabrik, Ger.*
Olive leaves.
Prevention of atherosclerosis.

Olmifon *Lafon, Fr.*
Adrafinil (p.1506·2).
Mental function impairment in the elderly.

Olmoran *Novartis, Spain.*
Zafirlukast (p.785·3).
Asthma.

Olocynan *Makros, Braz.*
Cynara (p.1601·3); choline (p.1356·3).
Liver disorders.

Ologyn *Labatec, Switz.*
Levonorgestrel (p.1486·2); ethinylestradiol (p.1476·2).
Formerly contained norgestrel and ethinylestradiol.
Combined oral contraceptive.

Olohepat *Makros, Braz.*
Liver extract; iron (p.1366·3); choline (p.1356·3).
Liver disorders.

Oloprim *Rudefsa, Mex.*
Allopurinol (p.397·2).

Olren N *Heumann, Ger.*
Scopolia carniolica.
Urinary-tract disorders.

Oltens *Biotherapie, Fr.*
Captopril (p.853·3).
Diabetic nephropathy; heart failure; hypertension.

Olux *Connetics, USA.*
Clobetasol propionate (p.1065·2).
Scalp disorders.

Olympic Balm *ANB, Thai.*
Methyl salicylate (p.55·1); menthol (p.1632·3); eugenol (p.1609·3); eucalyptol (p.1609·2); cajuput oil (p.1588·1); peppermint oil (p.1243·3).
Musculoskeletal, joint, and peri-articular disorders.

Olynth *Parke, Davis, Aust.; Warner-Lambert, Ger.; Warner-Lambert Consumer, Switz.*
Xylometazoline hydrochloride (p.1102·2).
Nasal congestion.

Olynth Kombi *Warner-Lambert, Ger.*
Tripiolidine hydrochloride (p.427·2); pseudoephedrine hydrochloride (p.1099·2).
Rhinitis.

Olynth salin *Warner-Lambert, Ger.*
Sodium chloride (p.1196·1).
Nasal congestion.

Omacor *Pharmacia Upjohn, Norw.*
Omega-3 marine triglycerides (p.949·3).
Hyperlipidaemia.

Omadine *Erredici, Ital.*
Pyrithione disulfide (p.1122·1); urtica (p.1678·2).
Seborrhoeic dermatitis.

Omapren *Vita, Spain.*
Omeprazole (p.1239·1) or omeprazole sodium (p.1239·1).
Gastro-oesophageal reflux; peptic ulcers; Zollinger-Ellison syndrome.

Ombeta *Betapharm, Ger.*
Omeprazole (p.1239·1).
Gastro-oesophageal reflux; peptic ulcer; Zollinger-Ellison syndrome.

Ombolan *Allergan-Frumtost, Braz.*
Droxicam (p.34·2).
Fever; inflammation; pain.

Ombrelle *Dermtek, Canad.†*
SPF 30: Avobenzone (p.1517·1); octinoxate (p.1517·3); oxybenzone (p.1518·1).
Sunscreen.

Ombrelle Baume *Cosmair, Canad.*
SPF 30: Avobenzone (p.1517·1); octocrilene (p.1518·1); terephthalylidene dicamphor sulfonic acid; titanium dioxide (p.1126·1).
Sunscreen.

Ombrelle Creme Ecran *Cosmair, Canad.*
SPF 60: Avobenzone (p.1517·1); enzacamene (p.1517·2); terephthalylidene dicamphor sulfonic acid; titanium dioxide (p.1126·1).
Sunscreen.

Ombrelle Creme Kids *Cosmair, Canad.*
SPF 45: Avobenzone (p.1517·1); octocrilene (p.1518·1); enzacamene (p.1517·2); terephthalylidene dicamphor sulfonic acid; titanium dioxide.
Sunscreen.

Ombrelle Extreme *Cosmair, Canad.*
SPF 30: Avobenzone (p.1517·1); octinoxate (p.1517·3); oxybenzone (p.1518·1); titanium dioxide (p.1126·1).
Sunscreen.

Ombrelle for Kids *Cosmair, Canad.*
SPF 30: Avobenzone (p.1517·1); octinoxate (p.1517·3); ensulizole (p.1517·2); enzacamene (p.1517·2).
Sunscreen.

Ombrelle Lotion *Cosmair, Canad.*
SPF 15: Avobenzone (p.1517·1); octocrilene (p.1518·1); octisalate (p.1518·1).
SPF 30: Avobenzone (p.1517·1); enzacamene (p.1517·2); octinoxate (p.1517·3); ensulizole (p.1517·2).
Sunscreen.

Ombrelle, Ombrelle Sport Spray *Dermtek, Canad.†*
SPF 15: Avobenzone (p.1517·1); octinoxate (p.1517·3); oxybenzone (p.1518·1).
Sunscreen.

Ombrelle Vapo Sport *Cosmair, Canad.*
SPF 15: Avobenzone (p.1517·1); octocrilene (p.1518·1); octisalate (p.1518·1).
Sunscreen.

Omca *Bristol-Myers Squibb, Ger.*
Fluphenazine hydrochloride (p.684·3).
Psychoses.

Omcilon A *Bristol-Myers Squibb, Braz.*
Triamcinolone acetonide (p.1080·1); salicylic acid (p.1122·3).
Skin disorders.

Omcilon A Orabase *Bristol-Myers Squibb, Braz.*
Triamcinolone acetonide (p.1080·1).
Mouth ulceration.

Omcilon AM *Bristol-Myers Squibb, Braz.*
Triamcinolone acetonide (p.1080·1); neomycin (p.228·1); gramicidin (p.213·3); nystatin (p.392·2).
Infected skin disorders.

Omega *Schmidgall, Aust.*
Proxyphylline (p.770·1); crataegus (p.1600·2); convallaria (p.1599·1).
Cardiac disorders.

Omega-3 *Gisand, Switz.*
Omega-3 marine triglycerides (p.949·3).
Dietary supplement; hyperlipidaemia.

Omega 3+ *Proceane, Fr.*
Omega-3 marine triglycerides (p.949·3).
Dietary supplement.

Omegacoeur *Holistica, Fr.*
Omega-3 triglycerides (p.949·2); herbs (p.1350·1).
Circulatory disorders.

Omega-H3
Vitabiotics, Irl.
Multivitamin and mineral preparation (p.1350·1).

Vitabiotics, UK.
Multivitamin, mineral, and nutritional preparation (p.1350·1).

Omegaline *Holistica, Fr.*
Borage oil (p.1613·1).
Nutritional supplement.

Omegaven
Fresenius Kabi, Aust.; Fresenius Kabi, Fr.; Fresenius Kabi, Ger.; Fresenius Kabi, Irl.; Fresenius Kabi, Port.; Fresenius Kabi, Swed.; Fresenius Kabi, Switz.
Omega-3 marine triglycerides (p.949·3).
Lipid infusion for parenteral nutrition.

Ome-nerton *Dolorgiet, Ger.*
Omeprazole (p.1239·1).
Gastro-oesophageal reflux; peptic ulcer; Zollinger-Ellison syndrome.

Omep
UCI, Braz.; Hexal, Ger.
Omeprazole (p.1239·1).
Gastro-oesophageal reflux; peptic ulcer; Zollinger-Ellison syndrome.

Omepradex *Dexcel, Israel.*
Omeprazole (p.1239·1).
Gastro-oesophageal reflux; peptic ulcer; Zollinger-Ellison syndrome.

Omepral *Astra, Jpn.*
Omeprazole (p.1239·1).
Gastro-oesophageal reflux; peptic ulcer; Zollinger-Ellison syndrome.

Omeprasec *Hoechst Marion Roussel, Braz.*
Omeprazole (p.1239·1).
Gastro-oesophageal reflux; gastrointestinal hyperacidity; peptic ulcer.

Omeprazen *Malesci, Ital.*
Omeprazole (p.1239·1) or omeprazole sodium (p.1239·1).
Gastro-oesophageal reflux; peptic ulcer; Zollinger-Ellison syndrome.

Ome-Puren *Isis Puren, Ger.*
Omeprazole (p.1239·1).
Gastro-oesophageal reflux; peptic ulcer; Zollinger-Ellison syndrome.

Omeril *Bayer, Ger.†*
Mebhydrolin napadisilate (p.420·2).
Hypersensitivity reactions.

Omesan *Duomed, Switz.*
Omega-3 marine triglycerides (p.949·3).
Hyperlipidaemias.

Ometon *Clintex, Port.*
Omeprazole (p.1239·1).
Gastro-oesophageal reflux; peptic ulcer; Zollinger-Ellison syndrome.

Omezolan *Euro-Labor, Port.; Grunenthal, Port.*
Omeprazole (p.1239·1).
Gastro-oesophageal reflux; peptic ulcer; Zollinger-Ellison syndrome.

Omicite *Torrent, Thai.*
Clomifene citrate (p.1465·3).
Anovulatory infertility; male infertility.

Omida Gel Antirhumatismal *Omida, Switz.*
Homoeopathic preparation.

Omida Granules Relaxants *Omida, Switz.†*
Homoeopathic preparation.

Omida Spray Nasal *Omida, Switz.†*
Homoeopathic preparation.

Omifin
Hoechst Marion Roussel, Mex.; Marion Merrell, Spain†.
Clomifene citrate (p.1465·3).
Anovulatory infertility; male infertility.

Omix *Yamanouchi, Fr.*
Tamsulosin hydrochloride (p.978·3).
Benign prostatic hyperplasia.

Omnalio *Estedi, Spain.*
Chlordiazepoxide hydrochloride (p.659·2).
Alcohol withdrawal syndrome; anxiety; insomnia; skeletal muscle spasm.

Omneo *Nutricia, Port.*
A range of infant feeds (p.1350·1).
Gastrointestinal disorders.

Omniadiol *Montefarmaco, Ital.*
Propyphenazone (p.80·2); paracetamol (p.71·2); caffeine (p.1116·3).
Cold symptoms; pain.

Omniapharm *Merckle, Ger.*
Bromhexine hydrochloride (p.1085·3).
Respiratory-tract disorders associated with increased or viscous mucus.

Omnibionta
Merck, Aust.
Multivitamin infusion (p.1350·1).

Merck-Belgolabo, Belg.†; Merck, Swed.
Brown/red capsules, vitamins; yellow/ochre capsules minerals (p.1350·1).

Omnic
Yamanouchi, Denm.; Yamanouchi, Fin.; Yamanouchi, Ger.; Yamanouchi, Irl.; Yamanouchi, Ital.; Yamanouchi, Neth.; Yamanouchi, Norw.; Pharmaco, NZ; Yamanouchi, Port.; Yamanouchi, Spain.
Tamsulosin hydrochloride (p.978·3).
Benign prostatic hyperplasia.

Omnicare
Allergan, Aust.†; Allergan, Israel.
Solution, hydrogen peroxide (p.1147·1); tablets, catalase (p.1592·2) (p.1129·2).
Disinfecting and neutralising system for soft contact lenses.

Omnicare Daily Cleaner
Allergan, Austral.; Allergan, NZ.
Cleansing solution for soft contact lenses (p.1129·2).

Omnicare I Step
Allergan, Austral.; Allergan, NZ.
Solution, hydrogen peroxide (p.1147·1); tablets, catalase (p.1592·2) (p.1129·2).
Disinfecting and neutralising system for soft contact lenses.

Omnicef
Warner-Lambert, Thai.; Parke, Davis, USA.
Cefdinir (p.165·2).
Bacterial infections.

Omniderm *Face, Ital.*
Fluocinolone acetonide (p.1071·1).
Inflammatory skin disorders.

Omniflora *Novartis Consumer, Aust.*
Lactobacillus acidophilus (p.1626·3); Bifidobacterium bifidum (p.1626·3); Escherichia coli.
Gastrointestinal disorders.

Omniflora Akut *Novartis Consumer, Ger.*
Saccharomyces boulardii (p.1626·3).
Diarrhoea.

Omniflora N *Novartis Consumer, Ger.*
Lactobacillus gasseri; Bifidobacterium longum.
Gastrointestinal disorders.

Omnigel *CTS Dental, UK†.*
Stannous fluoride (p.1379·3).
Dental caries prophylaxis.

Omnigraf *Juste, Spain.*
Iohexol (p.1035·1).
Radiographic contrast medium.

OmniHIB *SmithKline Beecham, USA.*
A haemophilus influenzae conjugate vaccine (tetanus toxoid conjugate) (p.1540·2).
Active immunisation.

Omnihist LA *WE, USA.*
Phenylephrine hydrochloride (p.1097·1); chlorpheniramine [chlorphenamine] maleate (p.412·1); hyoscine methonitrate (p.468·2).
Upper respiratory-tract symptoms.

Omnilan *Schering, Aust.†.*
Fluocortolone pivalate (p.1071·3).
Skin disorders.

Omnipaque
Schering, Aust.; Nycomed, Austral.; Nycomed, Belg.; Sanofi Winthrop, Braz.; Nycomed Amersham, Canad.; Nycomed Imaging, Denm.; Nycomed, Fin.; Nycomed, Fr.; Schering, Ger.; Nycomed, Ital.; Nycomed, Neth.†; Nycomed Imaging, Norw.; Nycomed, NZ; Nycomed, Spain; Nycomed Amersham, Swed.; Schering, Switz.; Nycomed Amersham, UK; Nycomed, USA.
Iohexol (p.1035·1).
Radiographic contrast medium.

Omnipen
Wyeth, Mex.; Wyeth-Ayerst, USA.
Ampicillin (p.150·3) or ampicillin sodium (p.150·3).
Bacterial infections.

Omniplex *Vitaplex, Austral.*
Multivitamin and mineral supplement with herbs (p.1350·1).
Dietary supplement.

Omniscan
Nycomed, Austral.; Nycomed, Belg.; Nycomed Amersham, Canad.; Nycomed Imaging, Denm.; Nycomed, Fin.; Nycomed, Fr.; Nycomed, Ger.; Daiichi, Jpn; Nycomed, Neth.†; Nycomed Imaging, Norw.; Nycomed, NZ; Nycomed, Spain; Nycomed Amersham, Swed.; Nycomed, Switz.; Nycomed Amersham, UK; Sanofi Winthrop, USA.
Gadodiamide (p.1033·1).
Contrast medium for magnetic resonance imaging.

Omnisept *Monchpharma, Ger.*
Lactobacillus acidophilus (p.1626·3).
Diarrhoea.

Omnitrace *Lifeplan, UK.*
Trace element preparation (p.1350·1).

Omnitrast *Schering, Spain.*
Iohexol (p.1035·1).
Radiographic contrast medium.

Omni-Tuss *Rhone-Poulenc Rorer, Canad.*
Codeine resin (p.25·2); phenyltoloxamine resin (p.423·1); chlorpheniramine [chlorphenamine] resin (p.412·2); ephedrine resin (p.1090·1); guaiacol carbonate (p.1092·1).
Coughs.

Omnival *Knoll, Ger.*
Multivitamin and mineral preparation (p.1350·1).

Omnopon *Intramed, S.Afr.*
Papaveretum (p.70·1) (containing morphine hydrochloride, codeine hydrochloride, and papaverine hydrochloride).
Pain.

OMP *Chong Kun Dang, Thai.*
Omeprazole (p.1239·1).
Gastro-oesophageal reflux; peptic ulcer; Zollinger-Ellison syndrome.

Ompranyt *Roche, Spain.*
Omeprazole (p.1239·1).
Gastro-oesophageal reflux; peptic ulcer; Zollinger-Ellison syndrome.

Omr-IgG *Omrix, Israel.*
A normal immunoglobulin (p.1551·3).
Idiopathic thrombocytopenic purpura; immunodeficiency; passive immunisation.

Omrixate *Omrix, Israel.*
A factor VIII preparation (p.734·1).
Haemophilia A.

OMS Concentrate *Upsher-Smith, USA†.*
Morphine sulfate (p.56·1).
Pain.

Onagre *Sante Naturelle, Canad.*
Evening primrose oil (p.1613·2).

Onaka *Max Farma, Ital.*
Pidotimod (p.1651·3).
Immunostimulant.

Onapan *Alpharma, Mex.*
Diazepam (p.674·3).

Oncaspar
Rhone-Poulenc Rorer, Canad.; Medac, Ger.; Rhone-Poulenc Rorer, USA.
Pegaspargase (p.508·3).
Acute lymphoblastic leukaemia.

The symbol † denotes a preparation no longer actively marketed

Once-a-Day *Quest, Canad.; Quest, UK.*
Multivitamin and mineral preparation (p.1350·1).

Oncet *Wakefield, USA.*
Hydrocodone tartrate (p.42·2); paracetamol (p.71·2).
Cough and cold symptoms.

Onclast *Banyu, Jpn.*
Alendronate sodium (p.747·2).

Onco Tiotepa *Zambon, Braz.; Pras, Spain.*
Thiotepa (p.574·3).
Malignant neoplasms.

Onco-Carbide *Teofarma, Ital.*
Hydroxyurea [hydroxycarbamide] (p.544·2).
Chronic myeloid leukaemia; myelofibrosis; polycythaemia vera; thrombocythaemia.

Oncosal *Inibsa, Spain.*
Flutamide (p.542·3).
Prostatic cancer.

OncoScint CR 103 *CIS, Ital.; CIS, Spain.*
Indium-111 satumomab pendetide (p.1449·3).
Diagnosis of colorectal cancer.

OncoScint CR/OV *Cytogen, USA.*
Indium-111 satumomab pendetide (p.1449·3).
Detection of colorectal and ovarian metastases.

Oncotam *Mayoly-Spindler, Fr.*
Tamoxifen citrate (p.571·1).
Breast cancer.

OncoTICE *Organon Teknika, Aust.; Organon Teknika, Austral.; Organon Teknika, Canad.; Organon Teknika, Denm.; Organon Teknika, Fin.; Apogepha, Ger.; Organon Teknika, Hong Kong; Organon Teknika, Israel; Organon Teknika, Ital.; Organon Teknika, Neth.; Organon Teknika, Norw.; Pharmaco, NZ; Organon Teknika, Spain; Organon Teknika, Swed.; Organon Teknika, Switz.; Organon, UK.*
A BCG vaccine (p.1533·2).
Bladder cancer.

Oncovin *Lilly, Aust.; Lilly, Austral.; Lilly, Belg.; Lilly, Braz.; Lilly, Canad.†; Lilly, Denm.; Lilly, Fin.; Lilly, Fr.; Lilly, Irl.; Lilly, Israel; Lilly, Mex.; Lilly, Neth.†; Lilly, Norw.; Lilly, NZ; Lilly, Port.; Lilly, S.Afr.; Lilly, Swed.; Lilly, Switz.; Lilly, UK; Lilly, USA.*
Vincristine sulfate (p.578·3).
Idiopathic thrombocytopenic purpura; malignant neoplasms.

Oncovite *Mission Pharmacal, USA.*
Multivitamin preparation with zinc (p.1350·1).

Onctose *Monot, Fr.†.*
Diphenhydramine metilsulfate (p.416·2); lignocaine [lidocaine] hydrochloride (p.1313·2).
Pruritus.

Onctose a l'Hydrocortisone *Denolin, Belg.*
Hydrocortisone acetate (p.1073·3); diphenhydramine metilsulfate (p.416·2); lignocaine [lidocaine] hydrochloride (p.1313·2).
Cutaneous hypersensitivity reactions; insect stings; pruritus.

Onctose Hydrocortisone *Monot, Fr.†.*
Diphenhydramine metilsulfate (p.416·2); lignocaine [lidocaine] hydrochloride (p.1313·2); hydrocortisone acetate (p.1073·3).
Pruritus.

Ondolen *Sanitas, Port.*
Hydrochlorothiazide (p.907·3); spironolactone (p.973·2).
Ascites; hypertension; oedema.

Ondroly-A *Boffi, Ital.*
Peppermint oil (p.1243·3); clove oil (p.1597·1); menthol (p.1632·3); benzoin tincture (p.1662·3); phenol (p.1152·3).
Dentistry.

Ondrox *Unimed, USA.*
Multivitamin, mineral, and amino acid preparation (p.1350·1).

One A Day *Bayer, Canad.; Bayer, Ital.†; Bayer, Singapore; Miles Consumer Healthcare, USA.*
Vitamin, multivitamin, or multivitamin and mineral preparations (p.1350·1).

One Touch *Lifescan, Fr.; Lifescan, Irl.; Lifescan, Port.; Lifescan, USA.*
Test for glucose in blood (p.1616·3).

One-Alpha *Leo, Canad.; Leo, Hong Kong; Leo, Irl.; Leo, Israel; CSL, NZ; Adcock Ingram, S.Afr.; Leo, Singapore; Leo, Thai.; Leo, UK.*
Alfacalcidol (p.1391·1).
Hyperparathyroidism; hypocalcaemia; hypoparathyroidism; osteomalacia; osteoporosis; renal osteodystrophy; rickets.

One-Tablet-Daily *Goldline, USA.*
A range of vitamin preparations with or without minerals (p.1350·1).

Onglinex *Medinfar, Port.*
Cystine; pyridoxine hydrochloride (p.1350·1).
Hair and nail disorders.

Onguent Hemorrhoidal *Prodemdis, Canad.*
Pramocaine hydrochloride (p.1318·2); zinc sulfate (p.1398·2).
Haemorrhoids.

Onguent nasal Ruedi *Spirig, Switz.*
Mint oil (p.1636·3); camphor oil.
Nasal dryness.

Onico Fitex *Belmac, Spain.*
Borogallic acid; salicylic acid (p.1122·3).
Fungal nail infections.

Onkomorphin *Onkoworks, Ger.*
Morphine sulfate (p.56·1).
Pain.

Onkotrone *Asta Medica, Austral.; Asta Medica, Ger.; Asta Medica, UK.*
Mitozantrone [mitoxantrone] hydrochloride (p.559·3).
Malignant neoplasms.

Onkovertin *Braun, Aust.; Braun, Ger.†.*
Dextran 60 (p.729·2) in sodium chloride.
Plasma volume expansion; pre-operative haemodilution; thromboembolism prophylaxis.

Onkovertin N *Braun, Aust.; Braun, Ger.*
Dextran 40 (p.728·3) in sodium chloride.
Circulatory disorders; thromboembolism prophylaxis.

Only One *Sisu, Canad.*
Multivitamin and mineral preparation (p.1350·1).

Onofin-K *Rayere, Mex.*
Ketoconazole (p.389·1).
Fungal infections.

Onon *Ono, Jpn.*
Pranlukast (p.770·1).
Asthma.

Onopordon Comp B *Weleda, UK.*
Onopordon; cowslip (p.1600·1); hyoscyamus (p.470·1).
Cardiac disorders.

Onoprose *Ono, Jpn†; Alter, Port.*
Promelase (p.1655·1).
Inflammation; respiratory-tract congestion.

Onrectal *Herbes Universelles, Canad.*
Benzocaine (p.1306·2); bismuth subcarbonate (p.1213·1); bismuth subgallate (p.1213·2); hamamelis (p.1618·3); naphazoline hydrochloride (p.1095·1); zinc oxide (p.1128·2).
Haemorrhoids.

Onsia *Siam Bheasach, Thai.*
Ondansetron hydrochloride (p.1241·3).
Nausea and vomiting induced by cytotoxics or radiotherapy; postoperative nausea and vomiting.

Onsudil *Bonafarma, Port.*
Procaterol hydrochloride (p.770·1).
Obstructive airways disease.

Onsukil *Otsuka, Spain.*
Procaterol (p.770·1) or procaterol hydrochloride (p.770·1).
Obstructive airways disease.

Ontak *Ligand, USA.*
Denileukin diftitox (p.533·3).
T-cell lymphoma.

Ontosein *Tedec Meiji, Spain.*
Orgotein (p.86·3).
Arthropathies; cystitis; peri-articular disorders; secondary effects of radiotherapy.

Onxol *Zenith Goldline, USA.*
Paclitaxel (p.563·2).
Malignant neoplasms.

Onycho Phytex
Note.This name is used for preparations of different composition.
Rupertus, Aust.
Sorbic acid (p.1157·1); tannic acid (p.1669·1); methyl salicylate (p.55·1); salicylic acid (p.1122·3); acetic acid (p.1571·2).
Fungal nail infections.

UCB, Port.†.
Boric acid (p.1586·1).

Onychomal *Hermal, Ger.*
Urea (p.1127·3).
Nail disorders.

Ony-Clear *Pedinol, USA.*
Topical powder spray†: Miconazole nitrate (p.391·1).
Fungal skin infections.

Topical solution: Benzalkonium chloride (p.1133·2).
Formerly contained triacetin, cetylpyridinium chloride, and chloroxylenol.
Fungal nail infections.

Onysin *Lambda, USA†.*
Vitamin B substances and lysine (p.1350·1).

Opacist ER *Bracco, Ital.; Bracco, Switz.*
Meglumine iodamide (p.1034·1).
Contrast medium for urinary-tract radiography.

Opalgyne *Innothera, Fr.*
Benzydamine hydrochloride (p.20·1).
Vaginitis.

Opalia *Ecobi, Ital.†.*
Royal jelly (p.1959·3).
Nutritional supplement.

Opalmon *Ono, Jpn.*
Limaprost alfadex (p.1446·1).
Thromboangiitis obliterans.

Opamox *Orion, Fin.*
Oxazepam (p.697·1).
Anxiety disorders; depression; insomnia; psychoses.

Opas *Co-Pharma, UK.*
Sodium bicarbonate (p.1186·2); calcium carbonate (p.1215·1); magnesium carbonate (p.1232·3); magnesium trisilicate (p.1233·3).
Dyspepsia; flatulence; gastric hyperacidity; heartburn.

Opazimes *Co-Pharma, UK.*
Aluminium hydroxide (p.1210·3); light kaolin (p.1229·3); belladonna (p.463·1); morphine hydrochloride (p.56·1).
Diarrhoea; dyspepsia; gastro-enteritis.

Opcon-A *Bausch & Lomb, Canad.; Bausch & Lomb, USA.*
Naphazoline hydrochloride (p.1095·1); pheniramine maleate (p.422·3).
Allergic or inflammatory disorders of the eye.

Operand *Redi-Products, USA.*
Povidone-iodine (p.1155·1).
Skin disinfection; vaginal disorders.

Operidine *Janssen-Cilag, Austral.†.*
Phenoperidine hydrochloride (p.78·1).
Pain.

Operium *PP Lab, Thai.*
Loperamide hydrochloride (p.1231·3).
Diarrhoea.

Ophan *Chew, Thai.*
Chlorpheniramine [chlorphenamine] maleate (p.412·1); ammonium chloride (p.1085·2).
Coughs; nasal congestion.

Ophcillin N *Medicopharm, Aust.*
Benzylpenicillin sodium (p.157·2); sulfadiazine (p.251·1).

Ophdilvas N *Mann, Ger.*
Vincamine (p.1680·1).
Cerebral and peripheral vascular disorders; circulatory disorders of the eye.

Ophtacalm *Chauvin, Fr.*
Sodium cromoglicate (p.774·3).
Allergic eye disorders.

Ophtadil *Chauvin, Fr.*
Buphenine hydrochloride (p.1587·3); ethoxazorutoside (p.1611·2); sodium ascorbate (p.1390·1); d-alpha tocoferil acetate (p.1394·1).
Ocular vascular disorders.

Ophtagram *Chauvin, Fr.†; Chauvin ankerpharm, Ger.; Chauvin, Port.; Chauvin, Singapore; Chauvin Novopharma, Switz.*
Gentamicin sulfate (p.210·1).
Bacterial eye infections.

Ophtaguttal *Agepha, Aust.*
Naphazoline hydrochloride (p.1095·1); zinc sulfate (p.1398·2); boric acid (p.1586·1).
Conjunctival irritation.

Ophtal *Winzer, Ger.*
Idoxuridine (p.625·1).
Herpes infections of the eye.

Ophtalin *Ciba Vision, Ital.*
Sodium hyaluronate (p.1620·1).
Eye surgery.

Ophtalmin *Winzer, Ger.*
Oxedrine tartrate (p.950·3); naphazoline hydrochloride (p.1095·1); antazoline hydrochloride (p.408·3).
Eye disorders.

Ophtalmin N *Winzer, Ger.*
Tetryzoline hydrochloride (p.1101·2).
Eye disorders.

Ophtalmine *Cooperation Pharmaceutique, Fr.*
Boric acid (p.1586·1); borax (p.1586·1); red vine; rose water (p.1029·1); peppermint water (p.1243·2); hamamelis (p.1618·3).
Eye irritation.

Ophtalmotrim *Asta Medica, Belg.*
Trimethoprim (p.264·2); polymyxin B sulfate (p.238·1).
Bacterial eye infections.

Ophtamedine *Bournonville, Belg.†.*
Hexamidine isetionate (p.1146·2).
Eye disorders; otitis; rhinitis.

Ophtasiloxane *Alcon, Fr.*
Dimethicone (p.1410·1).
Corneal burns; prevention of corneal adhesions.

Ophtasone *Chauvin Novopharma, Switz.*
Betamethasone sodium phosphate (p.1063·2); gentamicin sulfate (p.210·1).
Infected eye disorders.

Ophtaxia *Chauvin, Fr.*
Sodium chloride; potassium chloride; calcium chloride; magnesium chloride (p.1180·1).
Eye irrigation.

Ophthaine *Bristol-Myers Squibb, Irl.†; Squibb, UK†; Apothecon, USA†; Squibb, USA†.*
Proxymetacaine hydrochloride (p.1320·1).
Local anaesthesia.

Ophthalgan *Wyeth-Ayerst, USA.*
Glycerol (p.1616·3).
Corneal oedema.

Ophthalin *Ciba Vision, Austral.; Ciba Vision, Hong Kong; Ciba Vision, NZ; Ciba Vision, Singapore; Ciba Vision, Thai.; Ciba Vision, UK.*
Sodium hyaluronate (p.1620·1).
Adjunct in ocular surgery.

Ophthetic *Allergan, Austral.; Allergan, Canad.; Allergan, NZ; Allergan, S.Afr.†; Allergan, USA.*
Proxymetacaine hydrochloride (p.1320·1).
Local anaesthesia.

Ophthiflour *Dellerht, USA.*
Fluorescein sodium (p.1612·1).
Ophthalmic diagnostic agent.

Ophtho-Bunolol *Altimed, Canad.*
Levobunolol hydrochloride (p.920·3).
Glaucoma.

Ophtho-Chloram *Altimed, Canad.*
Chloramphenicol (p.179·1).
Eye infections.

Ophthocort *Parke, Davis, Canad.†.*
Chloramphenicol (p.179·1); hydrocortisone acetate (p.1073·3); polymyxin B sulfate (p.238·1).
Infected eye disorders.

Ophtho-Sulf *Kenral, Canad.†.*
Sulfacetamide sodium (p.250·3).
Eye infections.

Ophtho-Tate *Altimed, Canad.*
Prednisolone acetate (p.1078·1).
Eye disorders.

Ophtim *Thea, Fr.*
Timolol maleate (p.982·1).
Glaucoma; ocular hypertension.

Ophtocain *Winzer, Ger.*
Amethocaine [tetracaine] hydrochloride (p.1305·2); naphazoline hydrochloride (p.1095·1).
Ophthalmic procedures.

Ophtocortin *Winzer, Ger.†.*
Medrysone (p.1075·3).
Inflammatory disorders of the eye.

Ophtol-A *Winzer, Ger.*
Vitamin A palmitate (p.1383·2).
Eye disorders.

Ophtopur-N *Winzer, Ger.*
Zinc borate (p.1586·2); naphazoline hydrochloride (p.1095·1).
Eye disorders.

Ophtosan *Winzer, Ger.*
Vitamin A palmitate (p.1383·2).
Eye disorders.

Ophtrivin-A *Ciba Vision, Canad.*
Xylometazoline hydrochloride (p.1102·2); antazoline sulfate (p.408·3).
Eye disorders.

Opidol *Norpharma, Denm.; Mundipharma, Fin.; Mundipharma, Swed.; Mundipharma, Switz.*
Hydromorphone hydrochloride (p.42·3).
Pain.

Opilon *Hansam, Irl.; Parke, Davis, UK.*
Thymoxamine [moxisylyte] hydrochloride (p.980·2).
Menière's disease; peripheral vascular disorders; Raynaud's syndrome.

Opino *Kolassa, Aust.*
Tablets: Buphenine hydrochloride (p.1587·3); aescin (p.1574·1).

Topical gel: Buphenine hydrochloride (p.1587·3); aescin (p.1574·1); rosemary oil (p.1659·3); pumilio pine oil (p.1656·3); melissa oil.
Vascular disorders.

opino N *Biomo, Ger.*
Aescin (p.1574·1).
Peripheral vascular disorders; soft-tissue disorders.

opino N spezial *Gepepharm, Ger.*
Buphenine hydrochloride (p.1587·3); aescin (p.1574·1).
Peripheral vascular disorders; soft-tissue disorders.

Opiren *Almirall, Spain.*
Lansoprazole (p.1230·3).
Gastro-oesophageal reflux; peptic ulcer.

Opnol *Tika, Swed.*
Dexamethasone sodium phosphate (p.1067·1).
Inflammatory eye disorders.

Opobyl
Note.This name is used for preparations of different composition.
Bailly, Fr.; Uriach, Spain.
Aloes (p.1210·1); boldo (p.1585·3).
Formerly contained bile and liver extracts, boldo, combretum, euonymine, aloes, belladonna, and hyoscyamus in Fr.
Constipation.

Interdelta, Switz.†.
Aloes (p.1210·1); boldo (p.1585·3); ox bile (p.1585·1).
Constipation.

Opobyl-phyto *Medipharma, Ger.*
Greater celandine (p.1618·1); turmeric (p.1029·3).
Biliary-tract disorders.

Oponaf *Juste, Spain.*
Lactitol (p.1230·1).
Constipation; hepatic encephalopathy.

Opoplex *Opofarm, Braz.*
Multivitamin, amino-acid, and mineral preparation (p.1350·1).

Opplin *Nakorn, Thai.*
Boric acid (p.1586·1); borax (p.1586·1); allantoin (p.1110·1); chlorobutanol (p.1141·2); salicylic acid (p.1122·3); zinc sulfate (p.1398·2); hamamelis (p.1618·3).
Eye irritation.

Oprad *Cryopharma, Mex.*
Amikacin sulfate (p.148·1).
Gram-negative bacterial infections.

Opragen *Lohmann, Ger.*
Collagen (p.1598·2).
Haemorrhage; skin ulcers; wounds.

Oprazole *Atlantic, Thai.*
Omeprazole (p.1239·1).
Gastro-oesophageal reflux; peptic ulcer; Zollinger-Ellison syndrome.

Opredsone *Greater Pharma, Thai.*
Prednisolone (p.1077·3).
Corticosteroid.

Opridan *Locatelli, Ital.†.*
Bromopride hydrochloride (p.1215·1).
Gastrointestinal disorders.

Oprimol *Taro, Israel.*
Opipramol hydrochloride (p.302·2).
Depression.

O'Prin *Dolisos, Canad.*
Homoeopathic preparation.

Oprisine *Opus, UK†.*
Azathioprine (p.509·3).
Chronic active hepatitis; dermatomyositis; haemolytic anaemia; idiopathic thrombocytopenic purpura; immunosuppressant in organ and tissue transplantation; pemphigus; polyarteritis nodosa; pyoderma gangrenosa; rheumatoid arthritis; systemic lupus erythematosus.

Opsacin *PD, Thai.*
Polymyxin B sulfate (p.238·1); neomycin sulfate (p.228·1); gramicidin (p.213·3).
Bacterial eye infections.

Opsa-His *PD, Thai.*
Antazoline hydrochloride (p.408·3); tetryzoline hydrochloride (p.1101·2).
Allergic eye disorders; conjunctivitis.

Opsar *PD, Thai.*
Sulfacetamide sodium (p.250·3).
Bacterial eye infections.

Opsaram *PD, Thai.*
Chloramphenicol (p.179·1).
Bacterial eye infections.

Opsardex *PD, Thai.*
Dexamethasone phosphate (p.1067·1); neomycin sulfate (p.228·1).
Bacterial eye and ear infections.

Opsil *Silom, Thai.*
Boric acid (p.1586·1); borax (p.1586·1); sodium chloride (p.1196·1).
Eye irritation.

Opsil Tears *Silom, Thai.*
Hypromellose (p.1501·3) (p.1129·2).
Dry eye; wetting solution for hard contact lenses.

Opsil-A *Silom, Thai.*
Tetryzoline hydrochloride (p.1101·2).
Allergic eye disorders.

Opsite
Smith & Nephew, Austral.; Smith & Nephew, Fr.; Smith & Nephew, S.Afr.; Smith & Nephew, UK.
Polyurethane dressing.
Wounds.

Opsonat *Pekana, Ger.*
Homoeopathic preparation.

Optacilin *Byk, Braz.*
Ampicillin benzathine (p.151·3); ampicillin sodium (p.150·3).
Bacterial infections.

Optacilin Balsamico *Byk, Braz.*
Ampicillin benzathine (p.151·3); ampicillin sodium (p.150·3); guaifenesin (p.1092·3); niaouli oil (p.1640·2); eucalyptol (p.1609·2).
Bacterial infections.

Optafen *Proge, Ital.*
Chloramphenicol (p.179·1).
Bacterial eye infections.

Optal *Olan-Kemed, Thai.*
Eye drops: Sulfacetamide sodium (p.250·3).
Bacterial eye infections.

Eye lotion: Boric acid (p.1586·1); borax (p.1586·1); chlorobutanol (p.1141·2); salicylic acid (p.1122·3).
Eye irritation.

Optalgin *Teva, Israel; Inibsa, Spain.*
Dipyrone (p.34·1).
Fever; pain.

Optalia *Boiron, Canad.*
Homoeopathic preparation.

Optalidon
Note. This name is used for preparations of different composition.
Novartis Consumer, Belg.; Novartis, Braz.; Novartis Consumer, Port.; Novartis Consumer, Spain†.
Propyphenazone (p.80·2); caffeine (p.761·3).
Fever; pain.

Novartis Consumer, Ger.
Ibuprofen (p.43·2).
Fever; pain.

Novartis Consumer, Ital.
Propyphenazone (p.80·2); caffeine (p.761·3); butalbital (p.658·3).
Pain.

Optalidon a la Noramidopyrine *Novartis, Fr.*
Caffeine (p.761·3); dipyrone (p.34·1).
Formerly contained caffeine, butalbital, and dipyrone.
Pain.

Optalidon N *Novartis Consumer, Ger.*
Propyphenazone (p.80·2); caffeine (p.761·3).
Pain.

Optalidon special NOC *Novartis, Ger.*
Dihydroergotamine mesilate (p.450·3); propyphenazone (p.80·2).
Vascular headache.

Optamid *Proge, Ital.*
Sulfacetamide sodium (p.250·3).
Bacterial eye infections.

Optamide *McGloin, Austral.*
Sulfacetamide sodium (p.250·3).
Bacterial eye infections.

Optamine *Theraplix, Fr.†.*
Co-dergocrine mesilate (p.1597·3).
Cerebral vascular disorders; mental function impairment in the elderly.

Optavite *Dioptic, Canad.; Akorn, Canad.*
Vitamin and mineral preparation (p.1350·1).

Optazine
Note. This name is used for preparations of different composition.
Whitehall, Austral.
Naphazoline hydrochloride (p.1095·1).
Eye irritation.

Uhlmann-Eyraud, Switz.†.
Naphazoline nitrate (p.1095·1); digitoxin (p.869·2); rutoside (p.1611·2); aesculus (p.1574·1); hamamelis (p.1618·3).
Eye irritation.

Optazine A *Whitehall, Austral.†.*
Naphazoline hydrochloride (p.1095·1); antazoline sulfate (p.408·3); zinc sulfate (p.1398·2).
Eye irritation.

Optazine Fresh *Whitehall, Austral.*
Tetryzoline hydrochloride (p.1101·2).
Eye irritation.

Opteron *Therabel, Ital.*
Ticlopidine hydrochloride (p.981·1).
Thrombosis prophylaxis.

Opthaflox *Grin, Mex.*
Ciprofloxacin hydrochloride (p.182·3).
Bacterial eye infections.

Opthavir *Grin, Mex.*
Aciclovir (p.612·3).
Herpes simplex eye infections.

Optibiol *Yves Ponroy, Fr.*
Nutritional supplement with fatty acids (p.1350·1).
Visual disorders.

Optical *Strallhofer, Aust.*
Multivitamin preparation with calcium carbonate (p.1350·1).

Optical mit Eisen *Strallhofer, Aust.*
Multivitamin preparation with calcium carbonate and ferrous gluconate (p.1350·1).

Opticare PMS *Standard Drug, USA.*
Multivitamin and mineral preparation with iron and folic acid (p.1350·1).

Opticef *Brahms, Ger.*
Cefodizime sodium (p.167·3).
Bacterial infections.

Opticide *Pharmaland, Thai.*
Praziquantel (p.106·3).
Trematode infections.

Opti-Clean
Alcon, Braz.; Alcon, USA.
Range of solutions for contact lenses (p.1129·2).

Opti-Clean II *Alcon, Canad.*
Cleaning solution for hard and soft contact lenses (p.1129·2).

Opticrom
Rhone-Poulenc Rorer, Aust.; Rhone-Poulenc Rorer, Austral.; Aventis, Belg.; Fisons, Braz.; Allergan, Canad.; Rhone-Poulenc Rorer, Ger.; Rhone-Poulenc Rorer, Hong Kong; Fisons, Irl.; Fisons, Israel; Rhone-Poulenc Rorer, Mex.; Rhone-Poulenc Rorer, Neth.; Aventis, NZ; Rhone-Poulenc Rorer, Port.; Aventis, S.Afr.; Fisons, Singapore; Rhone-Poulenc Rorer, Singapore; Rhone-Poulenc Rorer, Switz.; Rhone-Poulenc Rorer, Thai.; Rhone-Poulenc Rorer, UK; Allergan, USA.
Sodium cromoglicate (p.774·3).
Allergic conjunctivitis; vernal keratoconjunctivitis.

Opticron *Rhone-Poulenc Rorer, Fr.*
Sodium cromoglicate (p.774·3).
Allergic eye disorders.

Opticyl *Optopics, USA.*
Tropicamide (p.475·1).
Production of mydriasis and cycloplegia.

Optiderm
Hermal, Aust.; Hermal, Ger.; Boots Healthcare, Ital.; Boots Healthcare, Switz.
Urea (p.1127·3); lauromacrogol 400 (p.1345·2).
Dry and pruritic skin disorders.

Optiderme *Hermal, Port.†.*
Urea (p.1127·3); lauromacrogol 400 (p.1345·2).
Dry skin disorders; pruritus.

Optidorm *Dolorgiet, Ger.*
Zopiclone (p.713·1).
Sleep disorders.

Optifen *Spirig, Switz.*
Ibuprofen (p.43·2).
Fever; inflammation; musculoskeletal, joint, and periarticular disorders; pain.

Optifluor *Diba, Mex.*
Fluorescein sodium (p.1612·1).
Aid to eye examination.

Opti-Free
Alcon, Aust.; Alcon, Austral.; Alcon, Braz.; Alcon, Canad.; Alcon, Fr.; Alcon, Israel; Alcon, Mex.; Alcon, NZ; Alcon, UK; Alcon, USA.
A range of preparations for contact lens care (p.1129·2).

Optigen *Xepa-Soul Pattinson, Hong Kong.*
Gentamicin sulfate (p.210·1).
Bacterial eye infections.

Optigene *Pfeiffer, USA.*
Electrolytes (p.1180·1).
Eye irrigation.

Optigene 3 *Pfeiffer, USA.*
Tetryzoline hydrochloride (p.1101·2).
Minor eye irritation.

Opti-Genta *Vitamed, Israel.*
Gentamicin sulfate (p.210·1).
Bacterial eye infections.

Optiject
Codali, Belg.; Guerbet, Fr.
Ioversol (p.1037·1).
Radiographic contrast medium.

Optil *Opus, UK.*
Diltiazem hydrochloride (p.874·3).
Angina pectoris; hypertension.

Optilast *Asta Medica, UK.*
Azelastine hydrochloride (p.409·3).
Allergic conjunctivitis.

Optilax *Phytomed, Switz.*
Linseed (p.1629·1); senna (p.1248·2); frangula bark (p.1227·1); rhubarb (p.1248·1); malt extract (p.1371·1); chamomile (p.1593·2).
Constipation.

Optilets
Abbott, Hong Kong.
Multivitamin and mineral preparation (p.1350·1).

Abbott, USA.
Multivitamin preparation (p.1350·1).

Optilets-M *Abbott, USA.*
Multivitamin and mineral preparation with iron (p.1350·1).

Optilube *Dioptic, Canad.*
Wool fat (p.1410·3); liquid paraffin (p.1407·1); soft paraffin (p.1407·3).

Optilube PVA *Dioptic, Canad.*
Polyvinyl alcohol (p.1503·1).

Optima
Stanley, Canad.; Stanley, Israel.
Multivitamin and mineral preparation (p.1350·1).

Optima 50 Plus *Unichem, UK.*
Multivitamin preparation with ginkgo and ginseng (p.1350·1).

Opti-Mag *Dolisos, Ital.*
Vitamin B substances; magnesium; zinc (p.1350·1).

Optimal *Inibsa, Port.*
Dicyclomine [dicycloverine] hydrochloride (p.466·1).
Smooth muscle spasm.

Optimark *Mallinckrodt, Austral.*
Gadoversetamide.
Contrast medium for magnetic resonance imaging.

Optimax
Note. This name is used for preparations of different composition.
E. Merck, Irl.
Tryptophan (p.311·3); pyridoxine hydrochloride (p.1386·3); ascorbic acid (p.1389·3).
Depression.

E. Merck, UK.
Tryptophan (p.311·3).
Formerly contained tryptophan, pyridoxine hydrochloride, and ascorbic acid.
Depression.

Optimin
Note. This name is used for preparations of different composition.
Abbott, Mex.
Multivitamin and mineral preparation (p.1350·1).

Juste, Spain.
Loratadine (p.420·1).
Hypersensitivity reactions.

Optimine
Schering-Plough, Belg.; Schering, Canad.; Schering-Plough, Irl.; Schering-Plough, S.Afr.†; Schering-Plough, UK; Schering, USA.
Azatadine maleate (p.409·2).
Hypersensitivity reactions.

Optimoist *Colgate-Palmolive, USA.*
Hyetellose (p.1501·1); electrolytes (p.1180·1); sodium monofluorophosphate (p.1377·2); xylitol (p.1397·3).
Dry mouth.

Optimol
Alphapharm, Austral.; Santen, Denm.; Santen, Swed.
Timolol maleate (p.982·1).
Glaucoma; raised intra-ocular pressure.

Optimycin *Biochemie, Aust.†.*
Methacycline hydrochloride (p.222·3).
Bacterial infections.

Optimycin S *Biochemie, Aust.†.*
Methacycline hydrochloride (p.222·3); guaifenesin (p.1092·2).
Lower respiratory-tract bacterial infections.

Optimyd *Schering, USA†.*
Prednisolone sodium phosphate (p.1078·1); sulfacetamide sodium (p.250·3).
Eye inflammation with bacterial infection.

Optimyxin *Sabex, Canad.*
Eye ointment: Polymyxin B sulfate (p.238·1); bacitracin zinc (p.155·2).
Eye infections.

Eye/ear drops: Polymyxin B sulfate (p.238·1); gramicidin (p.213·3).
Eye or ear infections.

Optimyxin Plus *Sabex, Canad.*
Polymyxin B sulfate (p.238·1); gramicidin (p.213·3); neomycin sulfate (p.228·1).
Eye or ear infections.

Optinate
Hoechst Marion Roussel, Fin.; Hoechst Marion Roussel, Swed.
Risedronate sodium (p.755·2).
Osteoporosis; Paget's disease of bone.

Optinem *Zeneca, Aust.*
Meropenem (p.222·1).
Bacterial infections.

Optipect *Thiemann, Ger.†.*
Acetylcysteine (p.1082·3).
Respiratory-tract disorders with excess mucus.

Optipect Kodein *Thiemann, Ger.*
Codeine (p.25·2).
Coughs.

Optipect N *Thiemann, Ger.*
Camphor (p.1589·3); menthol (p.1632·3); peppermint oil (p.1243·3).
Respiratory-tract disorders.

Optipect Neo *Thiemann, Ger.*
Camphor (p.1589·3); menthol (p.1632·3); peppermint oil (p.1243·3).
Respiratory-tract disorders.

Opti-Plus
Alcon, Austral.; Alcon, Fr.†; Alcon, NZ.
Pancreatin (p.1646·1) (p.1129·2).
Cleaning solution for soft contact lenses.

OptiPranolol *Bausch & Lomb, USA.*
Metipranolol hydrochloride (p.930·2).
Glaucoma; ocular hypertension.

Optipyrin *Pfleger, Ger.*
Paracetamol (p.71·2); codeine phosphate (p.25·2).
Pain.

Optiray
Mallinckrodt, Aust.; Mallinckrodt, Austral.; Codali, Belg.; Mallinckrodt, Canad.; Mallinckrodt, Denm.; MAP, Fin.; Guerbet, Fr.; Mallinckrodt, Ger.; Guerbet, Israel; Byk Gulden, Ital.; Mallinckrodt, Port.; Mallinckrodt, Spain; Mallinckrodt, Swed.; Guerbet, Switz.; Mallinckrodt, USA.
Ioversol (p.1037·1).
Radiographic contrast medium.

Optisen *Allergan, Ital.†.*
Carbohydrate, vitamin, and mineral preparation (p.1350·1).
Antioxidant nutritional supplement.

Opti-Soak
Alcon, Aust.; Alcon, Austral.; Alcon, Canad.; Alcon, Fr.; Alcon, Israel; Alcon, Mex.; Alcon, NZ.
Wetting, soaking, and disinfecting solution for hard and gas-permeable contact lenses (p.1129·2).

Opti-Soft *Alcon, Canad.*
Rinsing and storage solution for soft contact lenses (p.1129·2).

Optisol *Fischer, Israel.*
Sulfacetamide sodium (p.250·3).
Bacterial eye infections.

Optison
Mallinckrodt, Aust.; Mallinckrodt, Denm.; Mallinckrodt, Ger.; Mallinckrodt, Port.; Mallinckrodt, Spain; Mallinckrodt, Swed.
Perflutren labelled albumin.
Contrast medium for echocardiography.

Opti-Tears
Alcon, Aust.; Alcon, Braz.; Alcon, Canad.; Alcon, Israel; Alcon, UK; Alcon, USA.
Comfort drops for contact lenses (p.1129·2).

Optivar *Muro, USA.*
Azelastine hydrochloride (p.409·3).
Allergic conjunctivitis.

Optivit *Leiras, Fin.*
Multivitamin and mineral preparation (p.1350·1).

Optivite PMT *Optimox, USA.*
Multivitamin and mineral preparation (p.1350·1).
Premenstrual syndrome.

Optizoline *Xepa-Soul Pattinson, Hong Kong.*
Tetryzoline hydrochloride (p.1101·2).
Eye irritation.

Optizor *Zicor, Fr.*
Glyceryl trinitrate (p.897·3).
Angina pectoris.

Opti-Zyme *Alcon, Canad.; Alcon, USA.*
Pancreatin (p.1646·1) (p.1129·2).
Contact lens cleaner.

Opto Vit-E *Democal, Switz.*
Alpha tocoferil acetate (p.1394·1).
Vitamin E deficiency.

Optocain *Molteni, Ital.*
Mepivacaine hydrochloride (p.1317·1).
Adrenaline [epinephrine] acid tartrate (p.829·2) is included in some preparations as a vasoconstrictor to diminish absorption and localise the effect of the local anaesthetic.
Local anaesthesia.

Optochinidin retard *Boehringer Mannheim, Ger.†.*
Quinidine sulfate (p.964·3).
Arrhythmias.

Optocillin *Bayer, Aust.; Bayer, Ger.*
Mezlocillin sodium (p.224·1); oxacillin sodium (p.233·2).
Bacterial infections.

Optocor *Kanoldt, Ger.†.*
Crataegus (p.1600·2).
Heart failure.

Optomicin *Grin, Mex.*
Erythromycin stearate (p.201·3).
Bacterial eye infections.

Optovit *Hermes, Ger.*
d-Alpha tocopherol (p.1393·3).
Vitamin E deficiency.

The symbol † denotes a preparation no longer actively marketed

Optovite B12 *Normon, Spain.*
Cyanocobalamin (p.1388·1).
Vitamin B₁₂ deficiency.

Optrelam *Boots Healthcare, Spain.*
Carmellose sodium (p.1499·3).
Dry eyes.

Optrex
Boots, Austral.; Schering-Plough, Canad.; Etris, Fr.; Boots Healthcare, Irl.; Boots Healthcare, Ital.; Boots, NZ; Inibsa, Port.; Optrex, Singapore; Boots Healthcare, Spain; Boots Healthcare, Switz.; Boots, Thai.; Crookes Healthcare, UK.
Hamamelis (p.1618·3).
Eye irritation.

Optrex Clear Eyes *Crookes Healthcare, UK.*
Hamamelis (p.1618·3); naphazoline hydrochloride (p.1095·1).
Formerly known as Optrex Clearine.
Eye irritation.

Optrex compresses *Boots Healthcare, Switz.*
Hamamelis (p.1618·3); allantoin (p.1110·1).
Eye irritation.

Optrex Hayfever Allergy
Boots, NZ; Crookes Healthcare, UK.
Sodium cromoglicate (p.774·3).
Allergic conjunctivitis.

Optrex Medicated *Boots, Austral.*
Hamamelis (p.1618·3); naphazoline hydrochloride (p.1095·1).
Eye irritation.

Optrex Red-Eye Relief *Boots, NZ.*
Hamamelis (p.1618·3); naphazoline hydrochloride (p.1095·1).
Eye irritation.

Optrol *Amrad, Austral.*
Salmeterol xinafoate (p.773·3).
Obstructive airways disease.

Optruma
Menarini, Ital.; Vitoria, Port.; Pensa, Spain.
Raloxifene hydrochloride (p.1491·1).
Osteoporosis.

Optryl *Teva, Israel.*
Naphazoline (p.1095·1); diphenhydramine hydrochloride (p.416·1).
Eye disorders.

Opturem *Kade, Ger.*
Ibuprofen (p.43·2).
Inflammation; musculoskeletal, joint, and soft-tissue disorders.

Opumide *Opus, UK†.*
Indapamide (p.913·1).
Hypertension.

Opustan *Opus, UK.*
Mefenamic acid (p.51·2).
Menorrhagia; pain.

OPV-Merieux *Aventis, S.Afr.*
An oral poliomyelitis vaccine (p.1558·2).
Active immunisation.

Ora *Masa, Thai.*
Lorazepam (p.688·3).
Anxiety.

ORA5 *McHenry, USA.*
Copper sulfate (p.1358·1); potassium iodide (p.1522·3); iodine (p.1522·3).
Minor mouth or throat irritation.

Orabase
Convatec, Austral.; Squibb, Canad.; Bristol-Myers Squibb, Irl.; Bristol-Myers Squibb, Israel; Convatec, UK.
Carmellose sodium (p.1499·3); pectin (p.1502·3); gelatin (p.737·2).
Oral and perioral lesions; stoma care.

Orabase Baby *Colgate-Hoyt, USA.*
Benzocaine (p.1306·2).
Mouth disorders.

Orabase Gel *Colgate Oral, USA.*
Benzocaine (p.1306·2).

Orabase HCA *Colgate-Hoyt, USA.*
Hydrocortisone acetate (p.1073·3).
Oral inflammatory and ulcerative lesions.

Orabase Lip *Colgate-Hoyt, USA.*
Benzocaine (p.1306·2); allantoin (p.1110·1); menthol (p.1632·3); camphor (p.1589·3); phenol (p.1152·3).
Minor irritation.

Orabase-B *Colgate-Palmolive, USA.*
Benzocaine (p.1306·2).
Oral lesions.

Orabet
Note.This name is used for preparations of different composition.
Fresenius Kabi, Aust.; Gea, Denm.; Gea, Norw.; Lagap, UK.
Metformin hydrochloride (p.332·3).
Diabetes mellitus.

Berlin-Chemie, Ger.
Tolbutamide (p.336·3).
Diabetes mellitus.

Orabolin *Donmed, S.Afr.†*
Ethylestrenol (p.1477·1).
Anabolic.

Oracef *Lilly, Ger.*
Cefalexin (p.161·3).
Bacterial infections.

Oracefal *UPSA, Fr.*
Cefadroxil (p.161·2).
Bacterial infections.

Oracilin *Legrand, Braz.*
Phenoxymethylpenicillin potassium (p.235·1).
Bacterial infections.

Oracilline
Aventis, Belg.; Schwarz, Fr.
Phenoxymethylpenicillin (p.235·1) or benzathine phenoxymethylpenicillin (p.157·1).
Bacterial infections.

Oracit *Carolina, USA.*
Sodium citrate (p.1186·2); citric acid (p.1596·2).
Chronic metabolic acidosis; urine alkalinising agent.

Oracort
Taro, Canad.; Taro, Israel; AFT, NZ; Taro, Thai.
Triamcinolone acetonide (p.1080·1).
Oral lesions.

Oracort E *Taro, Israel.*
Triamcinolone acetonide (p.1080·1); lignocaine [lidocaine] hydrochloride (p.1313·2).
Oral lesions.

Oracyclin *Wyeth Lederle, Aust.*
Minocycline hydrochloride (p.224·3).
Acne.

Oraday *Biolab, Thai.*
Atenolol (p.841·3).
Hypertension.

Oradexon
Organon, Belg.; Organon, Fin.; Nourypharma, Neth.; Organon, Port.; Donmed, S.Afr.; Organon, Switz.; Organon, Thai.
Dexamethasone (p.1067·1) or dexamethasone sodium phosphate (p.1067·1).
Corticosteroid.

Oradroxil *Lampugnani, Ital.*
Cefadroxil (p.161·2).
Bacterial infections.

Oradyne-Z *Stafford-Miller, Ital.†*
Benzalkonium saccharinate (p.1133·3); dodequinium bromide.
Oral disinfection.

Orafen *Technilab, Canad.*
Ketoprofen (p.47·3).
Musculoskeletal and joint disorders; pain.

Orafer Comp *Columbia, Mex.*
Ferrous sulfate (p.1360·3); cyanocobalamin (p.1388·1); folic acid (p.1361·1).
Iron deficiency; iron-deficiency anaemia.

Oragalin Espasmolitico *Lacer, Spain.*
Azintamide (p.1583·1); hyoscine methobromide (p.468·2).
Hepatobiliary disorders.

Ora-Gallin *Nycomed, Aust.*
Azintamide (p.1583·1); pancreatin (p.1646·1); cellulase (p.1593·1).
Liver and biliary disorders.

Ora-Gallin compositum *Nycomed, Aust.*
Azintamide (p.1583·1); papaverine hydrochloride (p.1648·1).
Gastrointestinal disorders; liver and biliary disorders.

Ora-Gallin purum *Nycomed, Aust.*
Azintamide (p.1583·1).
Liver and biliary disorders.

Oragallin S *Truw, Ger.†.*
Azintamide (p.1583·1); hyoscine methobromide (p.468·2).
Biliary disorders; diarrhoea; spastic constipation.

Oragard *Colgate-Palmolive, UK.*
Lignocaine [lidocaine] hydrochloride (p.1313·2); cetylpyridinium chloride (p.1138·1).
Mouth disorders.

Orageston *Akzo, Braz.*
Allylestrenol (p.1465·2).
Threatened abortion.

Oragrafin *Squibb Diagnostics, USA†.*
Sodium iopodate (p.1036·1).
Radiographic contrast medium for cholecystography.

Orahesive
Convatec, Austral.; Squibb, Canad.; Convatec, UK.
Carmellose sodium (p.1499·3); pectin (p.1502·3); gelatin (p.737·2).
Oral and perioral lesions; stoma care.

Oraica *Esfar, Port.*
Orotic acid (p.1645·1); orazamide (p.1644·2).
Gout; hyperuricaemia.

Orajel
Del, Canad.; Del, Switz.†; Del, USA.
Benzocaine (p.1306·2).
Minor mouth or throat irritation; toothache.

Orajel Mouth Aid
Note.This name is used for preparations of different composition.
Del, Canad.; Del, USA.
Topical gel: Benzocaine (p.1306·2); benzalkonium chloride (p.1133·2); zinc chloride (p.1398·1).
Mouth and lip sores.

Del, USA.
Topical liquid: Benzocaine (p.1306·2); cetylpyridinium chloride (p.1138·1).
Mouth and throat disorders.

Orajel Perioseptic *Del, USA.*
Urea hydrogen peroxide (p.1159·3).
Oral hygiene; oral inflammation.

Orakef *Leiras, Fin.*
Cefalexin (p.161·3).
Bacterial infections.

Oral Plan *Knoll, Canad.*
Triclosan (p.1159·2); cetylpyridinium chloride (p.1138·1); sodium fluoride (p.1375·3).
Oral hygiene.

Oral Rehidr Sal Farmasur *Farmasur, Spain.*
Glucose; potassium iodide; sodium bicarbonate; sodium chloride (p.1185·2).
Oral rehydration therapy.

Oral-Aid *Beacons, Singapore.*
Chlorhexidine hydrochloride (p.1138·2); triamcinolone acetonide (p.1080·1); lignocaine [lidocaine] (p.1313·2).
Mouth ulcers; sore gums; toothache.

Oralamid *CaDiGroup, Ital.†.*
Food for special diets (p.1350·1).
Diarrhoea.

Oralav *Braun, Ger.*
Macrogol 4000 (p.1630·3); electrolytes (p.1180·1).
Bowel evacuation.

Oral-B Anti-Bacterial with Fluoride *Oral-B, Canad.*
Cetylpyridinium chloride (p.1138·1); sodium fluoride (p.1375·3).

Oral-B Anti-Cavity Dental Rinse *Oral-B, Canad.*
Sodium fluoride (p.1375·3).

Oral-B Collutorio per la Protezione di Denti e Gengive *Oral-B, Ital.*
Cetylpyridinium chloride (p.1138·1); sodium fluoride (p.1375·3).
Prevention of dental disorders.

Oral-B Collutorio Protezione Anti-Carie Fluorine *Oral-B, Ital.*
Sodium fluoride (p.1375·3).
Dental caries prophylaxis.

Oral-B Sensitive *Oral-B, Austral.*
Potassium nitrate (p.1154·3); sodium fluoride (p.1375·3).
Dental caries prophylaxis; sensitive teeth.

Oralbalance *Ethical Research, Irl.†.*
Xylitol (p.1397·3).
Saliva substitute.

Oralbiotico *Sanofi Synthelabo, Port.*
Oral liquid: Tyrothricin (p.267·1); zinc chloride (p.1398·1).
Tablets: Tyrothricin (p.267·1); bacitracin zinc (p.155·2).
Mouth and throat infections.

Oralcer
Vitabiotics, Irl.; Vitabiotics, UK.
Clioquinol (p.190·2); ascorbic acid.
Mouth ulcers.

Oralcon
Alcon, Denm.; Alcon, Swed.
Diclofenamide (p.869·1).
Glaucoma; preoperative control of intra-ocular pressure.

Oralcrom *Monsanto, Spain.*
Sodium cromoglicate (p.774·3).
Gastrointestinal allergies; inflammatory bowel disease.

Oraldene
Warner-Lambert, Irl.; Warner-Lambert, UK.
Hexetidine (p.1146·3).
Mouth and throat infections; oral hygiene.

Oraldettes *Parke, Davis, S.Afr.†.*
Benzalkonium chloride (p.1133·2).
Mouth and throat infections.

Oraldine
Parke, Davis, S.Afr.; Warner-Lambert, Spain.
Hexetidine (p.1146·3).
Mouth and throat infections.

Oralesper *Pharmacia Upjohn, Spain.*
Magnesium chloride hexahydrate; potassium chloride; monobasic potassium phosphate; sodium chloride; sodium phosphate dodecahydrate; sodium lactate; glucose (p.1185·2).
Oral rehydration therapy.

Oralfene *Pierre Fabre Sante, Fr.*
Ibuprofen (p.43·2).
Fever; pain.

Oralgan *Pierre Fabre, Fr.†.*
Paracetamol (p.71·2).
Fever; pain.

Oralgan Codeine *Pierre Fabre, Fr.*
Paracetamol (p.71·2); codeine phosphate (p.25·2).
Fever; pain.

Oralgar *Marc-O, Canad.*
Benzocaine (p.1306·2); camphor (p.1589·3); chlorobutanol (p.1141·2).

Oralgen *Artu, Neth.*
Allergen extracts (p.1575·3).
Hyposensitisation.

Oralife Peppermint
Pharmacia Upjohn, Austral.
Peppermint oil (p.1243·3); chlorhexidine gluconate (p.1138·2).
Dry lips and mouth.

Pharmacia Upjohn, NZ.
Peppermint oil (p.1243·3); chlorhexidine gluconate (p.1138·2); wool fat (p.1410·3).
Dry, cracked lips.

Oral-K *Sclavo, Ital.†.*
dl-Potassium aspartate (p.1195·2); dl-magnesium aspartate (p.1190·3).

Oralmox *Pulitzer, Ital.*
Amoxicillin trihydrate (p.149·2).
Bacterial infections.

Oralone Dental *Thames, USA.*
Triamcinolone acetonide (p.1080·1).
Oral lesions.

Oralovite *Meda, Swed.*
Vitamin B substances with vitamin C (p.1350·1).
Alcoholism; polyneuropathy; vitamin deficiency.

Oralpadon
Leopold, Aust.†.
Glucose monohydrate; sodium chloride; potassium bicarbonate (p.1185·2).
Gastrointestinal disorders; oral rehydration therapy.

Niddapharm, Ger.; Helvepharm, Switz.
Glucose monohydrate; sodium chloride; potassium chloride; sodium acid citrate (p.1185·2).
Diarrhoea; oral rehydration therapy.

Oralsan *Bioprogress, Ital.*
Chlorhexidine hydrochloride (p.1138·2); sodium fluoride (p.1375·3); sodium monofluorophosphate (p.1377·2).
Oral disinfection.

Oralsone *Vinas, Spain.*
Hydrocortisone hydrogen succinate (p.1074·1).
Mouth ulcers.

Oralspray *Warner-Lambert, Spain.*
Hexetidine (p.1146·3).
Mouth and throat infections.

Oral-T *Silom, Thai.*
Triamcinolone acetonide (p.1080·1).
Oral lesions.

Oralten Troche *Agis, Israel.*
Clotrimazole (p.382·1).
Oropharyngeal candidiasis.

Oralvac *Bencard, Ger.*
Allergen extracts (p.1575·3).
Hyposensitisation.

Oral-Virelon *Chiron Behring, Ger.*
An oral poliomyelitis vaccine (p.1558·2).
Active immunisation.

Oramedy *Dong Kook, Singapore.*
Triamcinolone acetonide (p.1080·1).
Oral lesions.

Oramet *Gea, Fin.*
Metformin hydrochloride (p.332·3).
Diabetes mellitus.

Oramil *Ganassini, Ital.*
Rose honey (p.1366·2).
Oral disinfection.

Oraminax *Wyeth Lederle, Port.*
Amoxicillin (p.149·2).
Bacterial infections.

Oraminic II *Vortech, USA.*
Brompheniramine maleate (p.410·2).
Hypersensitivity reactions.

Oramorph
Boehringer Ingelheim, Aust.; Boehringer Ingelheim, Canad.; Boehringer Ingelheim, Irl.; Boehringer Ingelheim, Swed.; Boehringer Ingelheim, UK; Roxane, USA.
Morphine sulfate (p.56·1).
Pain.

Oramox *Antigen, Irl.*
Amoxicillin trihydrate (p.149·2).
Bacterial infections.

Orangel *Paraphar, Fr.*
Gelatin (p.737·2).
Hair and nail tonic.

Oranol *Piraud, Switz.†.*
Multivitamin and mineral preparation (p.1350·1).

Oranor *AF, Mex.*
Norfloxacin (p.232·1).
Bacterial infections.

Orap
Janssen-Cilag, Aust.; Janssen-Cilag, Austral.; Janssen-Cilag, Belg.; Janssen, Braz.; Janssen-Ortho, Canad.; Janssen-Cilag, Denm.; Janssen-Cilag, Fr.; Janssen-Cilag, Ger.; Janssen, Hong Kong; Janssen-Cilag, Irl.; Janssen-Cilag, Israel; Janssen-Cilag, Ital.; Janssen-Cilag, Neth.; Janssen-Cilag, Norw.; Janssen-Cilag, NZ; Janssen-Cilag, S.Afr.; Janssen-Cilag, Singapore; Janssen-Cilag, Spain; Janssen-Cilag, Swed.†; Janssen-Cilag, Switz.; Janssen, Thai.; Janssen-Cilag, UK; Gate, USA; Lemmon, USA.
Pimozide (p.699·3).
Behaviour disorders in children; psychoses; Tourette syndrome.

Oraphen-PD *Great Southern, USA.*
Paracetamol (p.71·2).
Fever; pain.

Orapred *Ascent, USA.*
Prednisolone (p.1077·3).
Corticosteroid.

Orascan *Germiphene, Canad.*
Tolonium chloride (p.1674·1).
Diagnosis of oral cancer.

Ora-Sed
Warner-Lambert, Austral.; Rosken, Hong Kong; Warner-Lambert, NZ; Rosken, Singapore.
Choline salicylate (p.24·3).
Mouth ulcers; sore gums; teething pain.

Orasept
Note.This name is used for preparations of different composition.
Silom, Thai.
Cetylpyridinium chloride (p.1138·1).
Mouth and throat disorders.

Pharmakon, USA.
Oral liquid: Tannic acid (p.1669·1); methylbenzethonium chloride (p.1150·3).

Throat spray: Benzocaine (p.1306·2); methylbenzethonium chloride (p.1150·3); menthol (p.1632·3).
Sore throat.

Oraseptic
Note. This name is used for preparations of different composition.
Prodemdis, Canad.
Domiphen bromide (p.1143·3).

Warner-Lambert, Ital.
Hexetidine (p.1146·3).
Mouth and throat disorders.

Oraseptic Gola *Warner-Lambert, Ital.*
Cetylpyridinium chloride (p.1138·1); dichlorobenzyl alcohol (p.1143·2).
Mouth and throat disorders.

Orasol *Goldline, USA.*
Benzocaine (p.1306·2); phenol (p.1152·3); alcohol (p.1130·3); povidone-iodine (p.1155·1).

Orasone *Solvay, USA†.*
Prednisone (p.1079·2).
Corticosteroid.

Orasorbil
Rottapharm, Ger.; Rottapharm, Ital.; Delta, Port.
Isosorbide mononitrate (p.916·2).
Angina pectoris.

Orastel *Clintec, Fr.†.*
Preparations for enteral nutrition (p.1350·1).

Orasthin *Hoechst Marion Roussel, Ger.*
Oxytocin (p.1294·1).
Induction and maintenance of labour; postpartum haemorrhage.

Orastina *Hoechst Marion Roussel, Braz.*
Oxytocin (p.1294·1).
Diagnosis of placental insufficiency or fetal distress; labour induction; lactation deficiency; postpartum haemorrhage.

Oratane
Douglas, Austral.; Douglas, NZ.
Isotretinoin (p.1115·3).
Acne.

Oratol *Codilab, Port.*
Salicylic acid (p.1122·3); zinc chloride (p.1398·1).
Mouth and throat disorders.

Oratol F *Codilab, Port.*
Sodium fluoride (p.1375·3).
Dental caries prophylaxis.

Oratrol
Alcon, Belg.; Alcon, Hong Kong; Alcon Cusi, Spain; Alcon, Switz.†.
Diclofenamide (p.869·2).
Glaucoma.

Oravil *Streuli, Switz.*
Vitamin A acetate (p.1383·2); *d*-alpha tocoferil acetate (p.1394·1).
Dietary supplement.

Oravir *SmithKline Beecham, Fr.*
Famciclovir (p.620·3).
Varicella-zoster infections.

Oraxim *Malesci, Ital.*
Cefuroxime axetil (p.178·1).
Bacterial infections.

Orazinc *Mericon, USA.*
Zinc sulfate (p.1398·2).
Dietary supplement.

Orbenil *Biogal, Israel.*
Cloxacillin sodium (p.192·1).
Gram-positive bacterial infections.

Orbenin
Beecham, Belg.†; SmithKline Beecham, Hong Kong; SmithKline Beecham, Irl.; SmithKline Beecham, Neth.; SmithKline Beecham, S.Afr.; SmithKline Beecham, Singapore; SmithKline Beecham, Spain; SmithKline Beecham, Thai.; Forley, UK†.
Cloxacillin sodium (p.192·1).
Bacterial infections.

Orbenine *Yamanouchi, Fr.*
Cloxacillin sodium (p.192·1).
Bacterial infections.

Orbifen *Orbis Consumer, UK.*
Ibuprofen (p.43·2).
Fever; musculoskeletal, joint, peri-articular, and soft-tissue disorders; pain.

Orchibion *Bittermedizin, Ger.*
Bovine testicular extract (p.1492·1).
Erectile dysfunction; male menopausal disorders.

Orcilone *Chew, Thai.*
Triamcinolone acetonide (p.1080·1).
Oral lesions.

Orcinol *Julphar, UAE.*
Clobutinol hydrochloride (p.1087·1); orciprenaline sulfate (p.769·1); ammonium chloride (p.1085·2).
Bronchitis; coughs.

Orcl *Shinyaku, Jpn.*
Actarit (p.11·2).
Musculoskeletal and joint disorders.

Orclor *Willmar, Mex.*
Orasulon.

Ordinal Forte *Asche, Ger.*
Octodrine camsilate (p.949·2); norfenefrine hydrochloride (p.949·1).
Circulatory disorders; hypotension.

Ordinator *Synthelabo, Fr.†.*
Fenozolone (p.1510·2).
Intellectual and physical impairment.

Ordine *Pharmacia Upjohn, Austral.*
Morphine hydrochloride (p.56·1).
Insomnia associated with pain; pain.

Ordov Chesty Cough *Or-Dov, Austral.*
Guaifenesin (p.1092·2); bromhexine hydrochloride (p.1085·3).
Coughs.

Ordov Congested Cough *Or-Dov, Austral.*
Guaifenesin (p.1092·2); pseudoephedrine hydrochloride (p.1099·2).
Respiratory-tract congestion.

Ordov Dry Tickly Cough *Or-Dov, Austral.*
Pholcodine (p.1099·1).
Coughs.

Ordov Extra Day & Night Cold and Flu *Or-Dov, Austral.*
16 Daytime tablets, codeine phosphate (p.25·2); paracetamol (p.71·2); pseudoephedrine hydrochloride (p.1099·2); 8 night-time tablets, paracetamol; pseudoephedrine hydrochloride; chlorpheniramine [chlorphenamine] maleate (p.412·1).
Cold and influenza symptoms.

Ordov Febrideine *Or-Dov, Austral.*
Paracetamol (p.71·2); codeine phosphate (p.25·2).
Fever; pain.

Ordov Febrigesic *Or-Dov, Austral.*
Paracetamol (p.71·2).
Pain.

Ordov Migradol *Or-Dov, Austral.*
Paracetamol (p.71·2); codeine phosphate (p.25·2); doxylamine succinate (p.417·1).
Pain.

Ordov Sinudec *Or-Dov, Austral.*
Oxymetazoline hydrochloride (p.1096·2).
Nasal congestion.

Ordov Sinus & Hayfever *Or-Dov, Austral.*
Paracetamol (p.71·2); pseudoephedrine hydrochloride (p.1099·2); chlorpheniramine [chlorphenamine] maleate (p.412·1).
Upper respiratory-tract disorders.

Ordrine AT Extended-Release *Eon, USA†.*
Phenylpropanolamine hydrochloride (p.1098·1); caramiphen edisilate (p.1086·2).
Coughs.

Oreda *Hua, Thai.*
Glucose; sodium chloride; potassium chloride; sodium citrate (p.1185·2).
Diarrhoea; oral rehydration therapy.

Orelox
Hoechst Marion Roussel, Austral.; Hoechst Marion Roussel, Denm.†; Roussel Diamant, Fr.; Hoechst Marion Roussel, Ger.; Hoechst Marion Roussel, Ital.; Hoechst Marion Roussel, Mex.; Hoechst Marion Roussel, Neth.; Aventis, S.Afr.; Roussel, Spain; Hoechst Marion Roussel, Swed.; Hoechst Marion Roussel, Switz.; Hoechst Marion Roussel, UK.
Cefpodoxime proxetil (p.172·3).
Bacterial infections.

Oretic *Abbott, USA.*
Hydrochlorothiazide (p.907·3).
Hypertension; oedema.

Oreton Methyl *Schering, USA†.*
Methyltestosterone (p.1482·3).
Androgen replacement therapy; breast cancer; male hypogonadism; postpartum breast engorgement; postpubertal cryptorchidism.

Orexin *Roberts, USA.*
Vitamin B preparation (p.1350·1).

Orfarin *Orion, Thai.*
Warfarin sodium (p.992·2).
Thromboembolic disorders.

Orfen *Wyeth, Austral.*
Aluminium hydroxide (p.1210·3); magnesium oxide (p.1233·2).
Hyperacidity.

Orfenace *Kinsmor, Canad.*
Orphenadrine citrate (p.470·3).
Skeletal muscle spasm.

Orfenal *Remedica, Thai.*
Orphenadrine hydrochloride (p.470·3).
Drug-induced extrapyramidal disorders; parkinsonism.

Orfidal *Wyeth, Spain.*
Lorazepam (p.688·3).
Alcohol withdrawal syndrome; anxiety; epilepsy; insomnia; nausea; vomiting.

Orfidora *Wyeth, Spain†.*
Indoramin (p.914·1).
Benign prostatic hyperplasia; hypertension.

Orfiril
Desitin, Denm.; Desitin, Fin.; Desitin, Ger.; Desitin, Hong Kong; Desitin, Norw.; Desitin, Singapore; Desitin, Swed.; Desitin, Switz.
Sodium valproate (p.366·3).
Formerly known as Orfilept in Swed.
Bipolar disorder; epilepsy.

Orflex *Chew, Thai.*
Orphenadrine citrate (p.470·3); paracetamol (p.71·2).
Pain; skeletal muscle spasm.

Orgafol *Organon, UK†.*
Urofollitropin (p.1299·3).
Fertility disorders.

Orgalutran *Organon, UK.*
Ganirelix (p.1283·3).
Adjunct in ovarian stimulation for assisted reproduction.

Orgametril
Organon, Aust.; Organon, Belg.; Organon, Denm.; Organon, Fin.; Organon, Fr.; Organon, Ger.; Organon, Neth.; Organon, Port.; Organon, Spain; Organon, Swed.; Organon, Switz.
Lynestrenol (p.1480·1).
Benign breast disorders; dysfunctional uterine bleeding; endometrial cancer; endometriosis; menstrual disorders; progestogen-only oral contraceptive.

Organex *Sante Naturelle, Canad.*
d-Alpha tocoferil acetate (p.1394·1).

Organidin NR *Wallace, USA.*
Guaifenesin (p.1092·2).
Formerly contained iodinated glycerol.
Coughs.

Organoneuro Cerebral *Gross, Braz.*
Gamma-aminobutyric acid; glutamic acid; calcium phosphate; vitamin B substances (p.1350·1).
Nutritional supplement.

Organoneuro Optico *Gross, Braz.*
Tryptophan; vitamin A; thiamine; riboflavin; ascorbic acid; tocopherol (p.1350·1).
Nutritional supplement.

Orgaplasma *Ardeypharm, Ger.*
Ginseng (p.1615·3).
Tonic.

Orgaran
Organon, Austral.; Organon, Canad.; Riom, Fr.; Thiemann, Ger.; Nourypharma, Neth.; Pharmaco, NZ; Organon, Swed.; Organon, UK; Organon, USA.
Danaparoid sodium (p.866·1).
Thromboembolic disorders.

Orgasuline 30/70 *Organon, Fr.*
Mixture of insulin injection (human, emp, highly purified) 30% and isophane insulin injection (human, emp, highly purified) 70% (p.324·1).
Diabetes mellitus.

Orgasuline NPH *Organon, Fr.*
Isophane insulin injection (human, emp, highly purified) (p.324·1).
Diabetes mellitus.

Orgasuline Rapide *Organon, Fr.*
Insulin injection (human, emp, highly purified) (p.324·1).
Diabetes mellitus.

Oribiox *Bohm, Spain.*
Oxolinic acid (p.233·3).
Urinary-tract infections.

Oributol *Orion, Fin.*
Ethambutol hydrochloride (p.205·1).
Tuberculosis.

Oricant *Luhr-Lehrs, Ger.*
Homoeopathic preparation.

Oricyclin *Orion, Fin.*
Tetracycline hydrochloride (p.258·3).
Bacterial infections.

Orifer F *Hoechst Marion Roussel, Canad.*
Multivitamin and mineral preparation (p.1350·1).
Prenatal supplement.

Original *Wassen, Ital.*
Multivitamin and mineral preparation (p.1350·1).
Nutritional supplement.

Original Alka-Seltzer Effervescent Tablets *Bayer, USA.*
Sodium bicarbonate (p.1186·2); citric acid (p.1596·2); aspirin (p.14·2).
Hyperacidity.

Original Cabdrivers Expectorant *Merck Consumer, UK.*
Dextromethorphan hydrobromide (p.1087·3); menthol (p.1632·3); terpin hydrate (p.1101·2); pumilio pine oil (p.1656·3); eucalyptus oil (p.1609·2).
Formerly known as Cabdrivers Adult Linctus.
Coughs.

Original Sensodyne *Block, USA.*
Strontium chloride (p.1667·2).
Hypersensitive teeth.

Original-Tinktur N Truw *Bilgast, Ger.*
Homoeopathic preparation.

Origlucon *Orion, Fin.*
Glibenclamide (p.321·3).
Diabetes mellitus.

Orimeten
Novartis, Aust.; Novartis, Belg.; Novartis, Braz.; Novartis, Ger.; Novartis, Irl.; Novartis, Ital.; Novartis, Neth.; Novartis, Norw.†; Novartis, S.Afr.; Novartis, Spain; Novartis, Swed.; Novartis, UK.
Aminoglutethimide (p.506·3).
Breast cancer; Cushing's syndrome; ectopic ACTH production; prostatic cancer.

Orimetene
Novartis, Fr.; Novartis, Hong Kong; Novartis, Israel; Novartis, Switz.
Aminoglutethimide (p.506·3).
Breast cancer; Cushing's syndrome; hyperaldosteronism; prostatic cancer.

Orimune *Lederle, USA.*
An oral poliomyelitis vaccine (p.1558·2).
Active immunisation.

Orinase *Hoechst Marion Roussel, Canad.†; Upjohn, USA.*
Tolbutamide (p.336·3).
Diabetes mellitus.

Orinase Diagnostic *Upjohn, USA.*
Tolbutamide sodium (p.336·3).
Diagnosis of pancreatic adenoma.

Oritaxim *Be-Tabs, S.Afr.*
Cefotaxime sodium (p.169·1).
Bacterial infections.

Orivan *Orion, Fin.*
Vancomycin hydrochloride (p.267·2).
Antibiotic-associated colitis; staphylococcal infections.

Orivir *Orion, Denm.*
Aciclovir (p.612·3).
Herpesvirus infections.

OrLAAM
Sipaco, Denm.†; Sipaco, Spain†; Britannia Pharmaceuticals, UK†; Roxane, USA.
Levacetylmethadol hydrochloride (p.49·3).
Opioid withdrawal syndrome.

Orlept *CP Pharmaceuticals, UK.*
Sodium valproate (p.366·3).
Epilepsy.

Orlest *Parke, Davis, Aust.†.*
Ethinylestradiol (p.1476·2); norethisterone acetate (p.1485·1).
Combined oral contraceptive.

Ormazine *Hauck, USA†.*
Chlorpromazine hydrochloride (p.660·2).
Acute intermittent porphyria; adjunct in tetanus; hiccups; nausea and vomiting; premedication; psychoses; severe behavioural disorders in children.

Ormigrein *Akzo, Braz.*
Paracetamol (p.71·2); ergotamine tartrate (p.452·1); caffeine (p.761·3); belladonna (p.463·1).
Migraine.

Ormobyl *Novartis Consumer, Ital.†.*
Phenolphthalein (p.1244·1); rhubarb (p.1248·1); boldo (p.1585·3).
Constipation.

Ormobyl CM *Novartis Consumer, Ital.*
Calcium sennoside A (p.1248·3); calcium sennoside B (p.1248·3); polycarbophil calcium (p.1244·2).
Constipation.

Ormodon *Pharmaceutical Enterprises, S.Afr.*
Nitrazepam (p.695·2).
Insomnia.

Ormox *Orion, Fin.*
Isosorbide mononitrate (p.916·2).
Angina pectoris; heart failure.

Ornade
Note. This name is used for preparations of different composition.
SmithKline Beecham, Belg.; SmithKline Beecham Consumer, Canad.†; Biosaude, Port.; SmithKline Beecham, USA.
Chlorpheniramine [chlorphenamine] maleate (p.412·1); phenylpropanolamine hydrochloride (p.1098·1).
Cold symptoms; nasal congestion; rhinitis; sinusitis.

Roche Nicholas, Spain.
Cinnarizine (p.413·1); phenylpropanolamine hydrochloride (p.1098·1); isopropamide iodide (p.470·1).
Nasal congestion.

Ornade Expectorant *SmithKline Beecham Consumer, Canad.†.*
Chlorpheniramine [chlorphenamine] maleate (p.412·1); phenylpropanolamine hydrochloride (p.1098·1); guaifenesin (p.1092·2).
Coughs and cold symptoms.

Ornade-DM *SmithKline Beecham Consumer, Canad.†.*
Chlorpheniramine [chlorphenamine] maleate (p.412·1); phenylpropanolamine hydrochloride (p.1098·1); dextromethorphan hydrobromide (p.1087·3).
Coughs and cold symptoms.

Ornatos *Procter & Gamble, Aust.†.*
Chlorpheniramine [chlorphenamine] maleate (p.412·1); phenylpropanolamine hydrochloride (p.1098·1).
Cold symptoms; hay fever.

Ornatrol *Enila, Braz.*
Diphenylpyraline hydrochloride (p.417·1); phenylpropanolamine hydrochloride (p.1098·1); isopropamide.
Nasal congestion.

Ornex
Note. This name is used for preparations of different composition.
ICN, Hong Kong.
Paracetamol (p.71·2); phenylpropanolamine hydrochloride (p.1098·1).
Cold and influenza symptoms; sinusitis.

Ascher, USA.
Paracetamol (p.71·2); pseudoephedrine hydrochloride (p.1099·2).
Upper respiratory-tract symptoms.

Ornicetil
Ebewe, Aust.; Chiesi, Fr.; Geymonat, Ital.; Sanofi Synthelabo, Spain; Inter.delta, Switz.
Ornithine oxoglurate (p.1374·1).
Hepatic encephalopathy; hyperammonaemia; nausea induced by cancer chemotherapy; pituitary function testing.

Ornicetil S *Geymonat, Ital.*
Ornithine oxoglurate (p.1374·1).
Mental function impairment.

Ornidyl *Marion Merrell Dow, USA.*
Eflornithine hydrochloride (p.591·1).
African trypanosomiasis.

Ornihepat *Faria, Braz.*
Arginine (p.1353·3); citrulline (p.1357·2); ornithine (p.1374·1).
Liver disorders.

Ornil *Volchem, Ital.*
L-Ornithine (p.1374·1).
Adjunct in dietary management of hypercholesterolaemia.

Ornil KG *Volchem, Ital.*
L-Ornithine oxoglurate (p.1374·1).
Stress.

Ornitaine *Schwarz, Fr.*
Ornithine hydrochloride (p.1374·1); betaine (p.1584·3); sorbitol (p.1377·3); citric acid monohydrate (p.1596·2); magnesium oxide (p.1233·2).
Dyspepsia.

Ornitargin *Baldacci, Braz.*
Arginine (p.1353·3); ornithine (p.1374·1); citrulline (p.1357·2).
Parenteral nutrition.

Oro B12 *Ripari-Gero, Ital.*
Orotic acid (p.1645·1); cyanocobalamin (p.1388·1); folic acid (p.1361·1).
Nutritional supplement.

Oroacid *Rosch & Handel, Aust.*
Betaine hydrochloride (p.1584·3); pepsin (p.1649·3).
Hypochlorhydria; loss of appetite.

Orobicin *Fulton, Ital.*
Bacitracin (p.155·2); neomycin sulfate (p.228·1).
Gastrointestinal infections; pre-operative bowel preparation.

Orocaine *Beige, S.Afr.*
Cetrimide (p.1137·1); benzocaine (p.1306·2).
Mouth and throat infections.

Orocal *Theramex, Mon.*
Calcium carbonate (p.1215·1).
Calcium deficiency; osteoporosis.

Orocal D₃ *Theramex, Mon.*
Calcium carbonate (p.1215·1); colecalciferol (p.1391·1).
Calcium and vitamin D deficiency.

Orochlor *Triomed, S.Afr.*
Benzocaine (p.1306·2); chlorhexidine gluconate (p.1138·2).
Mouth and throat disorders.

Orochol
CSL, Austral.; Pharmabroker, NZ; Berna, Switz.
An oral cholera vaccine (p.1535·2).
Active immunisation.

Orocholin *Rosch & Handel, Aust.*
Choline dihydrogen citrate (p.1356·3); calcium citrate (p.1188·1).
Adjuvant in surgery and radiotherapy; liver protection.

Oro-Clense *Germiphene, Canad.*
Chlorhexidine gluconate (p.1138·2).
Gingivitis.

Or-O-Derm *Giuliani, Ital.†.*
Vitamin and mineral preparation (p.1350·1).
Antioxidant nutritional supplement.

Orofar
Note. This name is used for preparations of different composition.
Novartis Consumer, Belg.
Benzoxonium chloride (p.1135·2).
Mouth and throat disorders.

Novartis Consumer, Port.; Novartis Consumer, Switz.; Novartis, Thai.
Benzoxonium chloride (p.1135·2); lignocaine [lidocaine] hydrochloride (p.1313·2).
Mouth and throat disorders.

Orofar Lidocaine *Novartis Consumer, Belg.*
Benzoxonium chloride (p.1135·2); lignocaine [lidocaine] hydrochloride (p.1313·2).
Mouth and throat disorders.

Orofen *Durascan, Denm.*
Ketoprofen (p.47·3).
Dysmenorrhoea; gout; inflammation; musculoskeletal and joint disorders.

Orofluor *Colgate Oral Care, Austral.†.*
Acidulated phosphate fluoride or sodium fluoride (p.1375·3).
Dental caries prophylaxis; sensitive teeth.

Orofungin *Asta Medica, Braz.*
Mepartricin (p.390·3).
Vulvovaginal candidiasis and trichomoniasis.

Oroken *Rhone-Poulenc Rorer, Fr.*
Cefixime (p.166·2).
Otitis media; pyelonephritis; respiratory-tract infections; urinary-tract infections.

Oromag *Theramex, Mon.*
Magnesium citrate (p.1232·3); magnesium lactate (p.1191·1).
Magnesium deficiency.

Oromedine *Sanofi Winthrop, Fr.*
Hexamidine isetionate (p.1146·2); amethocaine [tetracaine] hydrochloride (p.1305·2).
Mouth and throat disorders.

Oromone *Solvay, Fr.*
Estradiol (p.1473·1).
Menopausal disorders; osteoporosis.

Oro-NaF *Germiphene, Canad.*
Sodium fluoride (p.1375·3).
Dental caries prophylaxis.

Oro-Pivalone *Uhlmann-Eyraud, Switz.*
Tixocortol pivalate (p.1080·1); bacitracin zinc (p.155·2).
Mouth and throat disorders.

Oropivalone Bacitracine *Parke, Davis, Fr.*
Tixocortol pivalate (p.1080·1); bacitracin zinc (p.155·2).
Mouth and throat disorders.

Orosanyl *Berna, Ital.*
Sodium monofluorophosphate (p.1377·2); cetylpyridinium chloride (p.1138·1).
Gum disorders.

Orosept
Note. This name is used for preparations of different composition.
Triomed, S.Afr.
Chlorhexidine gluconate (p.1138·2).
Mouth disorders.

OroClean, Switz.†.
Isopropyl alcohol (p.1149·2); propyl alcohol (p.1155·3); didecyldiammonium chloride.
Hand disinfection.

Oroseptol *SmithKline Beecham Sante, Fr.†.*
Tablets: Dequalinium chloride (p.1143·1); amethocaine [tetracaine] hydrochloride (p.1305·2).
Throat spray: Hexamidine isetionate (p.1146·2); amethocaine [tetracaine] hydrochloride (p.1305·2).
Mouth and throat disorders.

Oroseptol Lysozyme *SmithKline Beecham Sante, Fr.*
Dequalinium chloride (p.1143·1); amethocaine [tetracaine] hydrochloride (p.1305·2); muramidase hydrochloride (p.1638·1).
Mouth and throat disorders.

Orostat *Gingi-Pak, Switz.†.*
Adrenaline [epinephrine] hydrochloride (p.829·2).
Dental haemorrhage and leakage of fluid from tissues.

Orostick *Ogna, Ital.*
Propolis (p.1655·1); allantoin (p.1110·1).
Emollient.

Orotric *Vita, Spain†.*
Succinimide (p.1668·1).
Hyperoxaluria; renal calculi.

Orotrix *San Carlo, Ital.*
Propylene glycol cefatrizine sulfate.
Bacterial infections.

Orovite
Seton, Irl.; SSL, UK.
Vitamin B substances with ascorbic acid (p.1350·1).

Orovite '7' *SSL, UK.*
Multivitamin preparation (p.1350·1).

Orovite Complement B₆ *SSL, UK.*
Pyridoxine hydrochloride (p.1386·3).
Isoniazid-induced peripheral neuritis; sideroblastic anaemia; vitamin B₆ deficiency.

Oroxadin
Sanofi Winthrop, Braz.; Sanofi Winthrop, Mex.
Ciprofibrate (p.858·3).
Hyperlipidaemias.

Oroxine
Glaxo Wellcome, Austral.; Glaxo Wellcome, Singapore.
Thyroxine [levothyroxine] sodium (p.1526·2).
Hypothyroidism; suppression of thyrotrophin.

Orpar *Pharmasant, Thai.*
Orphenadrine citrate (p.470·3); paracetamol (p.71·2).
Muscle pain.

Orpec *Orion, Switz.†.*
Ipecacuanha (p.1093·1).
Poisoning.

Orphengesic *Par, USA.*
Orphenadrine citrate (p.470·3); aspirin (p.14·2); caffeine (p.761·3).
Musculoskeletal pain.

Orphol *Opfermann, Ger.*
Co-dergocrine mesilate (p.1597·3).
Mental function disorders.

Orravina *Almirall, Spain.*
Aspirin (p.14·2).
Fever; musculoskeletal, joint, and peri-articular disorders; pain; thromboembolism prophylaxis.

Orsanil *Orion, Fin.*
Thioridazine hydrochloride (p.708·1).
Anxiety disorders; pain; psychoses.

Orset *Novartis, Israel.*
Oral rehydration solution (p.1185·2).
Diarrhoea; fluid and electrolyte depletion.

Orsinon *Rekah, Israel.*
Tolbutamide (p.336·3).
Diabetes mellitus.

Orstanorm
Novartis, Fin.; Novartis, Swed.
Dihydroergotamine mesilate (p.450·3).
Cluster headache; hypotension; migraine.

Ortenal *Specia, Fr.†.*
Phenobarbital (p.355·1); amfetamine sulfate (p.1506·3).
Epilepsy.

Ortensan *Cimex, Switz.†.*
Paracetamol (p.71·2).
Fever; pain.

Orthangin N *Roland, Ger.*
Crataegus (p.1600·2).
Cardiac disorders.

Orthangin novo *Roland, Ger.*
Crataegus (p.1600·2).
Cardiac disorders.

Ortho *Janssen-Cilag, Irl.*
Dienestrol (p.1471·1).
Atrophic vaginitis; kraurosis vulvae.

Ortho 0.5/35 *Janssen-Ortho, Canad.*
Norethisterone (p.1485·1); ethinylestradiol (p.1476·2).
28-Day packs also contain 7 inert tablets.
Combined oral contraceptive.

Ortho 1/35 *Janssen-Ortho, Canad.*
Norethisterone (p.1485·1); ethinylestradiol (p.1476·2).
28-Day packs also contain 7 inert tablets.
Combined oral contraceptive.

Ortho 7/7/7 *Janssen-Ortho, Canad.*
Norethisterone (p.1485·1); ethinylestradiol (p.1476·2).
28-Day packs also contain 7 inert tablets.
Triphasic oral contraceptive.

Ortho 10/11 *Janssen-Ortho, Canad.*
Norethisterone (p.1485·1); ethinylestradiol (p.1476·2).
28-Day packs also contain 7 inert tablets.
Biphasic oral contraceptive.

Ortho Cyclen *Janssen-Cilag, Israel; Ortho McNeil, USA.*
Norgestimate (p.1486·1); ethinylestradiol (p.1476·2).
28-Day packs also contain 7 inert tablets.
Combined oral contraceptive.

Ortho Gynest Depot *Janssen-Cilag, Ital.*
Estriol (p.1475·3).
Menopausal disorders.

Ortho Gyne-T *Janssen-Cilag, Irl.†.*
Copper-wound plastic (p.1357·3).
Intra-uterine contraceptive device.

Ortho Shields *Johnson & Johnson, Canad.*
Nonoxinol 9 (p.1346·1).
Contraceptive.

Ortho Tri-Cyclen *Ortho McNeil, USA.*
Norgestimate (p.1486·1); ethinylestradiol (p.1476·2).
28-Day packs also contain 7 inert tablets.
Triphasic oral contraceptive.

Orthocardon-N *Tosse, Ger.†.*
Crataegus (p.1600·2).
Cardiovascular disorders.

Ortho-Cept
Janssen-Ortho, Canad.; Ortho McNeil, USA.
Desogestrel (p.1470·3); ethinylestradiol (p.1476·2).
28-Day packs also contain 7 inert tablets.
Combined oral contraceptive.

Orthoclone OKT3
Janssen-Cilag, Austral.; Janssen-Cilag, Belg.; Janssen-Ortho, Canad.; Janssen-Cilag, Fin.; Janssen-Cilag, Fr.; Janssen-Cilag, Ger.; Cilag, Hong Kong; Janssen-Cilag, Israel; Janssen-Cilag, Ital.; Cilag, Mex.; Janssen-Cilag, Neth.; Janssen-Cilag, Norw.; Janssen-Cilag, NZ; Janssen-Cilag, Swed.; Janssen-Cilag, Switz.; Janssen, Thai.; Ortho Biotech, USA.
Muromonab-CD3 (p.560·3).
Acute renal, cardiac, or hepatic allograft rejection.

Ortho-Creme
Janssen-Cilag, Austral.; Janssen-Cilag, Irl.; Janssen-Cilag, UK.
Nonoxinol 9 (p.1346·1).
Contraceptive.

Ortho-Dienestrol *Ortho McNeil, USA.*
Dienestrol (p.1471·1).
Atrophic vaginitis; kraurosis vulvae.

Ortho-Dienoestrol
Janssen-Cilag, Belg.; Janssen-Cilag, Israel; Janssen-Cilag, UK†.
Dienestrol (p.1471·1).
Vulvovaginal disorders.

Ortho-Est
Janssen-Cilag, S.Afr.; Women First, USA.
Estropipate (p.1476·1).
Menopausal disorders; osteoporosis.

Orthoforms
Janssen-Cilag, Irl.; Janssen-Cilag, UK.
Nonoxinol 9 (p.1346·1).
Contraceptive.

Ortho-Gel *Janssen-Cilag, Ger.†.*
Nonoxinol 9 (p.1346·1).
Contraceptive.

Ortho-Gynest
Janssen-Cilag, Aust.; Janssen-Cilag, Belg.; Janssen-Cilag, Ger.; Janssen-Cilag, Irl.; Janssen-Cilag, Israel; Cilag, Mex.; Janssen-Cilag, Neth.†; Janssen-Cilag, Switz.; Janssen-Cilag, UK.
Estriol (p.1475·3).
Atrophic vaginitis; kraurosis vulvae; menopausal disorders; oestrogen deficiency.

Ortho-Gynol
Note. This name is used for preparations of different composition.
Janssen-Cilag, Austral.
An octoxinol (p.1346·3).
Contraceptive.

McNeil Consumer, Canad.†; Janssen-Cilag, Neth.†; Janssen-Cilag, NZ.
p-Di-isobutyl-phenoxypolyethoxyethanol (p.1344·2).
Contraceptive.

Advanced Care, USA.
Octoxinol 9 (p.1346·3).
Contraceptive.

Ortho-Gynol II *Johnson & Johnson, Canad.*
Nonoxinol 9 (p.1346·1).
Contraceptive.

Ortholan mit Salicylester *Medopharm, Ger.†.*
Glycol salicylate (p.42·2); benzyl nicotinate (p.20·2).
Musculoskeletal, joint, and soft-tissue disorders; peripheral vascular disorders.

Ortho-Maren retard *Lubapharm, Switz.*
Pholedrine sulfate (p.955·2); norfenefrine hydrochloride (p.949·1).
Hypotension.

Orthonett Novum *Janssen-Cilag, Swed.*
Norethisterone (p.1485·1); ethinylestradiol (p.1476·2).
Combined oral contraceptive.

Ortho-Novin *Janssen-Cilag, Irl.*
Norethisterone (p.1485·1); mestranol (p.1482·1).
Combined oral contraceptive.

Ortho-Novin 1/50 *Janssen-Cilag, UK†.*
Norethisterone (p.1485·1); mestranol (p.1482·1).
Combined oral contraceptive; menstrual disorders.

Ortho-Novum *Janssen-Cilag, Aust.*
Norethisterone (p.1485·1); mestranol (p.1482·1).
Combined oral contraceptive.

Ortho-Novum 1/35
Janssen-Cilag, Fr.; Cilag, Mex.; Ortho McNeil, USA.
Norethisterone (p.1485·1); ethinylestradiol (p.1476·2).
28-Day packs also contain 7 inert tablets.
Combined oral contraceptive.

Ortho-Novum 1/50
Janssen-Cilag, Belg.†; Janssen-Ortho, Canad.; Janssen-Cilag, Ger.†; Janssen-Cilag, Belg.†; Janssen-Cilag, Ger.†; Janssen-Cilag, Neth.†; Ortho McNeil, USA.
Norethisterone (p.1485·1); mestranol (p.1482·1).
28-Day packs also contain 7 inert tablets.
Combined oral contraceptive; endometriosis; menstrual disorders.

Ortho-Novum 7/7/7 *Ortho McNeil, USA.*
Norethisterone (p.1485·1); ethinylestradiol (p.1476·2).
28-Day packs also contain 7 inert tablets.
Triphasic oral contraceptive.

Ortho-Novum 10/11 *Ortho McNeil, USA.*
Norethisterone (p.1485·1); ethinylestradiol (p.1476·2).
28-Day packs also contain 7 inert tablets.
Biphasic oral contraceptive.

Ortho-Prefest *Ortho McNeil, USA.*
15 Tablets, estradiol (p.1473·1); 15 tablets, estradiol; norgestimate (p.1486·1).
Menopausal disorders; osteoporosis.

Orthosiphonblatter Indischer Nierentee
Fides, Ger.
Java tea (p.1625·1).
Urinary-tract disorders.

Orthovisc
Zimmer, Ger.; Anika, Israel; Zimmer, UK.
Sodium hyaluronate (p.1620·1).
Osteoarthritis.

Orthoxicol
Note. This name is used for preparations of different composition.
Pharmacia Upjohn, Belg.
Dextromethorphan hydrobromide (p.1087·3); methoxyphenamine hydrochloride (p.1094·3).
Coughs.

Pharmacia Upjohn, S.Afr.
Codeine phosphate (p.25·2); methoxyphenamine hydrochloride (p.1094·3); sodium citrate (p.1186·2).
Coughs.

Orthoxicol 5 and 7 *Johnson & Johnson, Austral.†.*
Guaifenesin (p.1092·2); pseudoephedrine hydrochloride (p.1099·2).
Chest congestion; nasal congestion.

Orthoxicol for Children Nightrest *Johnson & Johnson, Austral.†.*
Chlorpheniramine [chlorphenamine] maleate (p.412·1); dextromethorphan hydrobromide (p.1087·3).
Cold symptoms; coughs.

Orthoxicol Cold & Flu
Johnson & Johnson, Austral.; Johnson & Johnson, NZ.
Paracetamol (p.71·2); pseudoephedrine hydrochloride (p.1099·2); dextromethorphan hydrobromide (p.1087·3).
Cold and influenza symptoms.

Orthoxicol Congested Cough *Johnson & Johnson, Austral.†.*
Guaifenesin (p.1092·2); pseudoephedrine hydrochloride (p.1099·2).
Cold symptoms.

Orthoxicol Cough *Roberts, USA†.*
Phenylpropanolamine hydrochloride (p.1098·1); chlorpheniramine [chlorphenamine] maleate (p.412·1); dextromethorphan hydrobromide (p.1087·3).
Coughs and cold symptoms.

Orthoxicol Day & Night *Johnson & Johnson, NZ.*
Day caplets, paracetamol (p.71·2); pseudoephedrine hydrochloride (p.1099·2); dextromethorphan hydrobromide (p.1087·3); night caplets, paracetamol; chlorpheniramine [chlorphenamine] maleate (p.412·1); dextromethorphan hydrobromide.
Cold symptoms.

Orthoxicol Day & Night Cold & Flu *Johnson & Johnson, Austral.*
Daytime caplets, paracetamol (p.71·2); pseudoephedrine hydrochloride (p.1099·2); dextromethorphan hydrobromide (p.1087·3); night-time caplets, paracetamol; dextromethorphan hydrobromide; chlorpheniramine [chlorphenamine] maleate (p.412·1).
Cold and influenza symptoms.

Orthoxicol Dry Cough *Johnson & Johnson, Austral.†.*
Paracetamol (p.71·2); dextromethorphan hydrobromide (p.1087·3).
Cold symptoms.

Orthoxicol Headcold *Johnson & Johnson, Austral.†.*
Paracetamol (p.71·2); pseudoephedrine hydrochloride (p.1099·2).
Cold and influenza symptoms.

Orthoxicol Infant *Johnson & Johnson, Austral.†.*
Pseudoephedrine hydrochloride (p.1099·2).
Cold symptoms; nasal congestion.

Orthoxicol Night Cold & Flu *Johnson & Johnson, Austral.*
Paracetamol (p.71·2); chlorpheniramine [chlorphenamine] maleate (p.412·1); dextromethorphan hydrobromide (p.1087·3).
Cold and influenza symptoms.

Orti B *Seroyal, Canad.*
Vitamin B substances (p.1350·1).

Ortic C *Seroyal, Canad.*
Ascorbic acid (p.1389·3).

Ortisan
Note. This name is used for preparations of different composition.
Ortis, Ital.
Senna (p.1248·2); tamarind (p.1253·2).
Constipation.

Cedar Health, UK.
Fruit and fibre preparation.
Constipation.

Ortitruw *Truw, Ger.*
Homoeopathic preparation.

Orto Dermo P *Normon, Spain.*
Povidone-iodine (p.1155·1).
Burns; skin disinfection; wounds.

Orto Nasal *Normon, Spain.*
Eucalyptol (p.1609·2); oxymetazoline hydrochloride
(p.1096·2); menthol (p.1632·3).
Nasal congestion.

Ortociclina *Makros, Braz.*
Erythromycin (p.201·2).
Bacterial infections.

Ortocilin *Makros, Braz.*
Procaine penicillin [procaine benzylpenicillin]
(p.239·2); benzylpenicillin potassium (p.157·1); streptomycin (p.249·1); diphenhydramine (p.416·1).
Bacterial infections.

Ortodermina *Sofar, Ital.*
Lignocaine [lidocaine] hydrochloride (p.1313·2).
Surface anaesthesia of skin and mucous membranes.

Ortoflan *Medley, Braz.*
Diclofenac sodium (p.30·3).
*Gout; inflammation; musculoskeletal, joint, and peri-
articular disorders.*

Ortopsique *Psicofarma, Mex.*
Diazepam (p.674·3).
*Alcohol withdrawal syndrome; anxiety disorders; epi-
lepsy; skeletal muscle spasm.*

Ortoserpina *Makros, Braz.*
Reserpine (p.967·3).
Hypertension; Raynaud's syndrome.

Ortoton *Bastian, Ger.*
Methocarbamol (p.1329·3).
Skeletal muscle spasm and tension.

Ortoton Plus *Bastian, Ger.*
Methocarbamol (p.1329·3); aspirin (p.14·2).
Musculoskeletal, joint, and soft-tissue disorders.

Ortovermim *Makros, Braz.*
Piperazine (p.105·3).
Ascariasis; enterobiasis.

Ortrip *Pharmasant, Thai.*
Nortriptyline hydrochloride (p.301·3).
Depression.

Ortrizol *Farcoral, Mex.*
Metronidazole (p.594·1).
Ascariasis; giardiasis; trichomoniasis.

Or-Tyl *Ortega, USA.*
Dicyclomine [dicycloverine] hydrochloride (p.466·1).
Functional bowel/irritable bowel syndrome.

Orucote *Aventis, S.Afr.*
Ketoprofen (p.47·3).
Orucote Gel was formerly known as Orugel.
*Dysmenorrhoea; gout; musculoskeletal, joint, and
peri-articular disorders.*

Orudis
*Rhone-Poulenc Rorer, Austral.; Rhone-Poulenc Rorer, Canad.; Aventis,
Denm.; Rhone-Poulenc Rorer, Fin.; Rhone-Poulenc Rorer, Ger.; Rhone-
Poulenc Rorer, Hong Kong; Rhone-Poulenc Rorer, Irl.; Rhone-Poulenc
Rorer, Ital.; Rhone-Poulenc Rorer, Mex.; Rhone-Poulenc Rorer, Neth.;
Rhone-Poulenc Rorer, Norw.; Aventis, NZ; Rhone-Poulenc Rorer,
Spain; Rhone-Poulenc Rorer, Swed.; Rhone-Poulenc Rorer, Switz.†;
Hawgreen, UK; Wyeth-Ayerst, USA.*
Ketoprofen (p.47·3) or ketoprofen sodium (p.48·1).
*Gout; inflammation; musculoskeletal, joint, peri-artic-
ular, and soft-tissue disorders; pain.*

Orugesic *Rhone-Poulenc Rorer, Irl.*
Ketoprofen (p.47·3).
*Musculoskeletal, joint, peri-articular, and soft-tissue
disorders.*

Oruject *Aventis, S.Afr.*
Ketoprofen (p.47·3).
*Gout; musculoskeletal, joint, and peri-articular disor-
ders.*

Orulop *Llorente, Spain†.*
Loperamide hydrochloride (p.1231·3).
Diarrhoea.

Oruvail
*Rhone-Poulenc Rorer, Austral.; May & Baker, Canad.; Rhone-Poulenc
Rorer, Hong Kong; Rhone-Poulenc Rorer, Irl.; Rhone-Poulenc Rorer, Is-
rael; Aventis, NZ; Aventis, S.Afr.; Rhone-Poulenc Rorer, Singapore;
Rhone-Poulenc Rorer, Thai.; Rhone-Poulenc Rorer, UK; Wyeth-Ayerst,
USA.*
Ketoprofen (p.47·3).
*Gout; musculoskeletal, joint, peri-articular, and soft-
tissue disorders ; pain.*

Osa *Piraud, Switz.†.*
Salicylamide (p.82·1); lignocaine [lidocaine] hydrochloride (p.1313·2); calcium pantothenate (p.1374·1);
calcium phosphate (p.1188·3).
Gum pain.

Osa Gel de dentition aux plantes *Piraud, Switz.†.*
Mint oil (p.1636·2); chamomile oil; sage oil
(p.1660·2); clove oil (p.1597·1); propolis (p.1655·1).
Inflammatory dental disorders.

Osaline *Hua, Thai.*
Glucose; sodium chloride; potassium chloride; sodium
citrate (p.1185·2).
Diarrhoea; oral rehydration therapy.

Osangin *Antonetto, Ital.*
Dequalinium chloride (p.1143·1).
Mouth and throat disinfection.

Osanit *Zeppelfeldt, Ger.*
Homoeopathic preparation.

Os-Cal
*Wyeth-Ayerst, Canad.; Hoechst Marion Roussel, Hong Kong; Marion
Merrell Dow, Singapore; SmithKline Beecham Consumer, USA.*
Calcium carbonate (p.1215·1).
Calcium deficiency; calcium supplement.

Oscal *Aventis, NZ.*
Calcium carbonate (p.1215·1).
Calcium supplement.

Os-Cal D *Wyeth-Ayerst, Canad.*
Calcium carbonate (p.1215·1); colecalciferol
(p.1391·1).
Calcium and vitamin D supplement.

Oscal D *Aventis, NZ.*
Calcium carbonate (p.1215·1); vitamin D (p.1391·1).
Calcium supplement.

Os-Cal + D
*Hoechst Marion Roussel, Hong Kong; Marion Merrell Dow, Singa-
pore; SmithKline Beecham Consumer, USA.*
Calcium carbonate (p.1215·1); vitamin D (p.1391·1).
Calcium deficiency; calcium supplement.

Os-Cal Forte *SmithKline Beecham Consumer, USA.*
Multivitamin and mineral preparation with iron
(p.1350·1).

Os-Cal Fortified *SmithKline Beecham Consumer, USA.*
Multivitamin and mineral preparation with calcium
and iron (p.1350·1).

Os-Cal Plus *SmithKline Beecham, USA.*
Multivitamin and mineral preparation with iron
(p.1350·1).

Oscalcio *INQ, Braz.*
Vitamin B12; vitamin D; calcium phosphate (p.1350·1).
Nutritional supplement.

Oscevitin-A *Grasler, Ger.*
Calcium phosphate (p.1188·3); vitamin A acetate;
colecalciferol; ascorbic acid (p.1350·1).
Calcium deficiency; vitamin deficiency.

Oscillococcinum
Boiron, Canad.; Boiron, Fr.; Boiron, Port.; Boiron, Switz.
Homoeopathic preparation.

Oscorel *Rhone-Poulenc Rorer, Neth.*
Ketoprofen (p.47·3).
Musculoskeletal and joint disorders.

Osemin *Degorts, Mex.*
Frusemide [furosemide] (p.893·1).

Oseototal *Foes, Spain.*
Salcatonin (p.749·3).
*Hypercalcaemia; metastatic bone pain; Paget's dis-
ease of bone; postmenopausal osteoporosis.*

Oseum *Grossman, Mex.*
Salcatonin (p.749·3).
*Osteolysis of malignancy; osteoporosis; Paget's dis-
ease of bone; reflex sympathetic dystrophy.*

Osfolate *Asta Medica, Fr.; Mayoly-Spindler, Switz.†.*
Calcium folinate (p.1363·1).
*Drug-induced megaloblastic anaemias; folate defi-
ciency; prevention of folic-acid antagonist toxicity.*

Osfolato *Lusofarmaco, Ital.*
Calcium folinate (p.1363·1).
Folate deficiency; reversal of methotrexate toxicity.

O-Sid *Siam Bheasach, Thai.*
Omeprazole (p.1239·1).
*Gastro-oesophageal reflux; peptic ulcer; Zollinger-El-
lison syndrome.*

Osiren
Note. This name is used for preparations of different composition.
Hoechst Marion Roussel, Aust.
Injection: Potassium canrenoate (p.957·1).
Hyperaldosteronism.

Tablets: Spironolactone (p.973·2).
*Cardiac oedema; hyperaldosteronism; hypertension;
liver cirrhosis with ascites; nephrotic syndrome.*

Galen, Mex.
Omeprazole (p.1239·1).
*Gastro-oesophageal reflux; peptic ulcer; Zollinger-El-
lison syndrome.*

Osmil *Opfermann, Ger.*
16 Tablets, estradiol (p.1473·1); 12 tablets, estradiol;
medroxyprogesterone acetate (p.1480·1).
Menopausal disorders; osteoporosis.

Osmitrol *Baxter, Austral.; Baxter, Canad.; Baxter, USA.*
Mannitol (p.924·3).
*Cerebral oedema; early renal failure; forced diuresis;
raised intra-ocular pressure.*

Osmo *Nakorn, Thai.*
Multivitamin preparation with lysine (p.1350·1).

Osmo-Adalat *Pharma Clal, Israel.*
Nifedipine (p.940·1).
Angina pectoris; hypertension.

Osmofundin 10%
Braun, Aust.; Braun, Ger.
Mannitol (p.924·3); sodium acetate (p.1186·1); sodium
chloride (p.1196·1).
*Cataract surgery; cerebral oedema; forced diuresis;
oliguria; renal failure.*

Osmofundin 20% *Braun, Aust.*
Mannitol (p.924·3).
*Cataract surgery; cerebral oedema; forced diuresis;
oliguria; renal failure.*

Osmofundin 15% N *Braun, Ger.*
Mannitol (p.924·3).
Fluid retention; renal failure.

Osmofundina
Note. This name is used for preparations of different composition.
Braun, Port.
Mannitol (p.924·3).
*Forced diuresis; ocular hypertension; oedema; raised
intracranial pressure; renal failure.*

Braun, Spain.
Sodium bicarbonate (p.1186·2); sodium chloride
(p.1196·1); mannitol (p.924·3).

Osmofundina Concentrada *Braun, Spain.*
Mannitol (p.924·3).
*Ascites; cranial hypertension; glaucoma; oedema; ol-
iguria.*

Osmogel *Monot, Fr.*
Magnesium sulfate (p.1191·1); lignocaine [lidocaine]
hydrochloride (p.1313·2).
Soft-tissue disorders.

Osmogenol *INQ, Braz.*
Phenol (p.1152·3); amethocaine [tetracaine]
(p.1305·2); sodium bicarbonate (p.1186·2); sodium thiosulfate (p.1024·2).
Ear infections.

Osmoglyn *Alcon, USA.*
Glycerol (p.1616·3).
*Glaucoma; raised intra-ocular pressure before oph-
thalmic surgery.*

Osmohes *Laevosan, Aust.*
Pentastarch (p.732·3) in sodium chloride.
Hypovolaemic shock.

Osmolac *Sanofi Synthelabo, Ital.*
Lactulose (p.1230·1).
*Adjunct in gastrointestinal bacterial infections; consti-
pation; hepatic cirrhosis; hepatic encephalopathy.*

Osmoleine *Pharmethic, Belg.†.*
Precipitated sulfur (p.1123·3); boric acid (p.1586·1).
Rhinitis; sinusitis.

Osmolite
*Abbott, Austral.; Abbott, Braz.; Abbott, Fin.; Abbott, Fr.; Abbott,
Hong Kong; Abbott, Irl.; Abbott, Israel; Abbott, Ital.; Abbott, Switz.†;
Abbott Nutrition, UK; Ross, USA.*
A range of preparations for enteral nutrition (p.1350·1).

Osmolite HN *Abbott, Canad.*
Preparation for enteral nutrition (p.1350·1).

Osmopak-Plus *Technilab, Canad.*
Hydrated magnesium sulfate (p.1191·1); benzocaine
(p.1306·2).
Superficial inflammatory conditions.

Osmorich *Abbott, Ital.*
Preparation for enteral nutrition (p.1350·1).

Osmorol *Pisa, Mex.*
Mannitol (p.924·3).

Osmosal *Leiras, Fin.*
Sodium chloride; potassium chloride; sodium citrate;
glucose (p.1185·2).
Diarrhoea; oral rehydration solution.

Osmosteril 10% *Fresenius Kabi, Ger.*
Mannitol (p.924·3); sodium lactate (p.1186·2).
Fluid retention; renal failure.

Osmosteril 20% *Fresenius Kabi, Ger.*
Mannitol (p.924·3).
Forced diuresis; renal failure.

Osmotan G *Aguettant, Fr.*
Electrolyte infusion with glucose (p.1180·1).
Carbohydrate source; fluid and electrolyte disorders.

Osmotol *Chauvin, Fr.*
Resorcinol (p.1122·2); ephedrine hydrochloride
(p.1090·1).
Otitis externa.

Osmovist *Berlex, Canad.*
Iotrolan (p.1036·3).
Radiographic contrast medium.

Osnervan *Glaxo Wellcome, Ger.*
Procyclidine hydrochloride (p.473·1).
*Drug-induced extrapyramidal disorders; parkinson-
ism.*

Ospamox
*Tyrol, Aust.; Biochemie, Hong Kong; Normal, Port.; Biochemie, Singa-
pore.*
Amoxicillin (p.149·2) or amoxicillin trihydrate
(p.149·2).
Bacterial infections.

Ospen
*Biochemie, Aust.; Novartis, Fr.; Biochemie, Hong Kong; Biochemie,
Singapore; Novartis, Switz.*
Benzathine phenoxymethylpenicillin (p.157·1), phe-
noxymethylpenicillin (p.235·1), or phenoxymethyl-
penicillin potassium (p.235·1).
Bacterial infections.

Ospexin
Biochemie, Aust.; Biochemie, Hong Kong; Biochemie, Singapore.
Cefalexin (p.161·3).
Bacterial infections.

Ospocard *Unipack, Aust.*
Nifedipine (p.940·1).
Angina pectoris; hypertension; Raynaud's syndrome.

Ospolot
Ophthalmic Laboratories, Austral.; Desitin, Ger.; Desitin, Israel.
Sultiame (p.364·3).
Behavioural disorders; epilepsy.

Ospronim *Intramed, S.Afr.*
Pentazocine lactate (p.74·2).
Pain.

Ospur Ca *Henning, Ger.*
Calcium carbonate (p.1215·1).
Calcium deficiency; osteoporosis.

Ospur D₃ *Henning, Ger.*
Colecalciferol (p.1391·1).
Osteoporosis; vitamin D deficiency.

Ospur F *Henning, Ger.*
Sodium fluoride (p.1375·3).
Bone metastases; osteoporosis.

Osseans D3 *Sciencex, Fr.*
Calcium (p.1187·3); colecalciferol (p.1391·1).
Calcium and vitamin D deficiency; osteoporosis.

Osseocalcina *Normal, Port.†.*
Salcatonin (p.749·3).

Ossidal *Bilgast, Ger.*
Homoeopathic preparation.

Ossin
Note. This name is used for preparations of different composition.
Grunenthal, Ger.; Grunenthal, Switz.
Sodium fluoride (p.1375·3).
Osteoporosis.

Basi, Port.
Chondroitin sulfate A (p.1594·2).

Ossiplex *Gebro, Aust.; Henning, Ger.; Segix, Ital.; Aspen, S.Afr.*
Sodium fluoride (p.1375·3); ascorbic acid (p.1389·3).
Osteoporosis.

Ossiten *Roche, Ital.*
Disodium clodronate (p.751·2).
*Multiple myeloma; osteolytic tumours; postmenopau-
sal osteoporosis; primary hyperparathyroidism.*

Ossofluor *Streuli, Switz.*
Sodium fluoride (p.1375·3).
Osteoporosis.

Ossofortin *Strathmann, Ger.*
Calcium phosphate (p.1188·3); calcium gluconate
(p.1188·2); colecalciferol (p.1391·1).
Calcium and vitamin D deficiency; osteoporosis.

Ossofortin forte *Strathmann, Ger.*
Calcium carbonate (p.1215·1); colecalciferol
(p.1391·1).
Calcium and vitamin D₃ deficiency; osteoporosis.

Ossopan
*Germania, Aust.; Asta Medica, Braz.; Robapharm, Fr.; Pierre Fabre,
Ger.; Sanofi Winthrop, Irl.; Byk Gulden, Mex.; Pierre Fabre, Fr.; Ori-
ent, Singapore; Pierre Fabre, Singapore; Berna, Spain; Robapharm,
Switz.; Robapharm, Thai.; Sanofi Winthrop, UK.*
Microcrystalline hydroxyapatite (p.1622·1).
*Calcium and phosphorus deficiency; dental caries
prophylaxis; fractures; growth disorders; osteomala-
cia; osteoporosis; rickets.*

Osspulvit S *Madaus, Ger.*
Calcium phosphate (p.1188·3); colecalciferol
(p.1391·1).
Calcium deficiency.

Osspulvit S forte *Madaus, Ger.*
Calcium phosphate (p.1188·3); vitamins (p.1350·1).

Oss-regen *Pekana, Ger.*
Homoeopathic preparation.

OST Vit *Greater Pharma, Thai.*
Vitamin B₁; vitamin B₆; vitamin B₁₂ (p.1350·1).

Ostac
*Roche, Belg.; Asta Medica, Braz.; Roche, Canad.; Roche, Ger.; Roche,
Hong Kong; Boehringer Mannheim, Israel; Roche, Neth.; Roche,
Norw.; Roche, NZ; Boehringer Mannheim, Port.; Roche, S.Afr.; Roche,
Singapore; Roche, Swed.; Roche, Switz.*
Disodium clodronate (p.751·2).
*Hypercalcaemia of malignancy; osteolysis of malig-
nancy.*

Ostaren *Utopian, Thai.*
Diclofenac sodium (p.30·3).
Musculoskeletal and joint disorders.

Ostelin
Boots, Austral.; Teofarma, Ital.
Ergocalciferol (p.1391·2).
*Hypoparathyroidism; osteomalacia; rickets; vitamin D
deficiency.*

Osten *Takeda, Jpn.*
Ipriflavone (p.753·3).
Osteoporosis.

Ostenil *Chemedica, Ger.; Chemedica, Switz.*
Sodium hyaluronate (p.1620·1).
Osteoarthritis.

Osteo
Note. This name is used for preparations of different composition.
Quest, Canad.
Calcium, magnesium, vitamin C, vitamin D, and sili-
con (p.1350·1).

Healtheries, NZ.
Calcium carbonate (p.1215·1).
Calcium supplement.

Osteo Complex *Peter, Ital.*
Calcium; vitamin D; boron; fluoride; zinc; copper; eq-
uisetum; lupulus (p.1350·1).
Nutritional supplement for healthy bones.

Osteo D *Teva, Israel.*
Calcitriol (p.1391·1).
Renal osteodystrophy in chronic haemodialysis.

Osteo Support *Pharmagenics, UK.*
Hydroxyapatite (p.1622·1).
Bone disorders.

Osteoapatite with Boron *Nutrition Care, Austral.*
Calcium; manganese; zinc; copper; colecalciferol; bo-
ron (p.1350·1).
Osteoporosis.

Osteobion Merck, Spain.
Salcatonin (p.749·3).
Hypercalcaemia; metastatic bone pain; osteoporosis; Paget's disease of bone.

Osteocalcil Dolisos, Canad.
Homoeopathic preparation.

Osteocalcin
Eurodrug, Hong Kong; Tosi, Ital.; Eurodrug, Singapore; Eurodrug, Thai; Arcola, USA.
Salcatonin (p.749·3).
Hypercalcaemia; osteolytic bone pain; osteoporosis; Paget's disease of bone; reflex sympathetic dystrophy.

Osteocare Note.This name is used for preparations of different composition.
Vitabiotics, Hong Kong.
Calcium (p.1187·3); magnesium (p.1190·3); zinc (p.1398·1); vitamin D (p.1391·1).
Calcium deficiency; calcium supplement.

Vitabiotics, UK.
Calcium carbonate (p.1215·1); calcium lactate (p.1188·2); calcium citrate (p.1188·1); magnesium hydroxide (p.1233·1); zinc sulfate (p.1398·2); colecalciferol (p.1391·1).

Osteochondrin S Dyckerhoff, Ger.
Ribonucleic acids from cattle and yeast (p.1657·3).
Bone disorders.

Osteocynesine
Boiron, Canad.; Boiron, Fr.; Boiron, Port.
Homoeopathic preparation.

Osteodidronel Procter & Gamble, Belg.
Disodium etidronate (p.752·1).
Postmenopausal osteoporosis.

Osteofix Chiesi, Ital.
Ipriflavone (p.753·3).
Postmenopausal osteoporosis.

Osteofluor
Merck, Aust.; Lipha Sante, Fr.
Sodium fluoride (p.1375·3).
Osteoporosis.

Osteogen Richard, Fr.†.
Pyridoxine phosphate (p.1387·1); calcium ascorbate (p.1389·3); magnesium deoxyribonucleinate (p.1602·3); deoxyribonucleic acid (p.1602·3).
Osteopathies; senile debility.

Osteogenon Germania, Aust.
Hydroxyapatite (p.1622·1).
Calcium deficiency; fractures; osteoporosis.

Osteomerck Merck, Spain.
Calcium phosphate (p.1188·3); colecalciferol (p.1391·1).
Hypocalcaemia; osteoporosis.

Osteomin Byk Gulden, Mex.
Calcium carbonate (p.1215·1).
Calcium supplement; osteoporosis.

Osteoplex Vitaplex, Austral.
Mineral, vitamin, enzyme, and herb preparation (p.1350·1).
Calcium deficiency; osteoporosis.

Osteopor Pierre Fabre, Spain.
Hydroxyapatite (p.1622·1).
Calcium deficiency; osteoporosis.

Osteoporosis Mineral Plus Formula 9 Vitelle, Austral.†.
Calcium carbonate (p.1215·1); colecalciferol (p.1391·1).
Calcium deficiency; osteoporosis.

Osteopro Health Perception, UK.
Ipriflavone (p.753·3); calcium (p.1187·3); vitamins; minerals (p.1350·1).
Osteoporosis.

Osteos TAD, Ger.
Salcatonin acetate (p.750·2).
Hypercalcaemia; malignant osteolysis; osteoporosis; Paget's disease of bone; reflex sympathetic dystrophy.

Osteosil Ghimas, Ital.
Equisetum (p.1606·3).
Nutritional supplement.

Osteostabil Jenapharm, Hong Kong.
Salcatonin (p.749·3).
Hypercalcaemia; osteoporosis; Paget's disease of bone; reflex sympathetic dystrophy; tumour-related bone pain.

Osteoton Herbaline, Ital.†.
Food for special diets (p.1350·1).
Bone disorders.

Osteotonina Menarini, Ital.
Salcatonin (p.749·3).
Osteoporosis.

Osteovis NCSN, Ital.
Salcatonin (p.749·3).
Hypercalcaemia; osteoporosis; Paget's disease of bone; reflex sympathetic dystrophy.

Osteovit Pharmadass, UK.
Multivitamin, mineral, and trace element preparation (p.1350·1).

Osteral Silanes, Mex.
Piroxicam (p.79·1).
Gout; inflammation; musculoskeletal, joint, and periarticular disorders; pain.

Osteum Vinas, Spain.
Disodium etidronate (p.752·1).
Ectopic ossification; osteoporosis; Paget's disease of bone.

Ostiderm Pedinol, USA.
Lotion: Aluminium sulfate (p.1578·2); zinc oxide (p.1128·2).

Formerly contained aluminium sulfate and phenol.
Roll-on: Aluminium chlorohydrate (p.1110·2); camphor (p.1589·3).
Foot odour; hyperhidrosis.

Ostidil Garant, Ital.
Alfacalcidol (p.1391·1).
Hypoparathyroidism; osteomalacia; osteoporosis; renal osteodystrophy; rickets.

Ostine Lesvi, Spain.
Calcium carbonate (p.1215·1); colecalciferol (p.1391·1).
Calcium deficiency; osteoporosis.

Ostobon Coloplast, UK.
A deodorant powder for use with ostomies.

Ostochont Godecke, Ger.
Liniment: Glycol salicylate (p.42·2); benzyl nicotinate (p.20·2); nonivamide (p.63·1).
Musculoskeletal, joint, and soft-tissue disorders; neuralgia.

Ointment: Heparin sodium (p.902·1); glycol salicylate (p.42·2); benzyl nicotinate (p.20·2).
Inflammation; musculoskeletal and joint disorders.

Ostofen Shiwa, Thai.
Ibuprofen (p.43·2).
Inflammation; pain.

Ostoforte Merck Frosst, Canad.
Ergocalciferol (p.1391·2).
Hypoparathyroidism; phosphataemia; rickets.

Ostone-B12 TP, Thai.
Calcium (p.1187·3); ergocalciferol (p.1391·2); vitamin B₁₂ (p.1388·1).
Megaloblastic anaemia; osteomalacia; rickets.

Ostosalm Pharmacia Upjohn, Port.†.
Salcatonin (p.749·3).

Ostostabil
Jenapharm, Ger.; Jenapharm, Thai.
Salcatonin (p.749·3).
Hypercalcaemia; osteolytic bone pain; osteoporosis; Paget's disease of bone; reflex sympathetic dystrophy.

Ostram
Lipha Sante, Fr.; Merck, Mex.; Faes, Spain; Merck, Swed.; E. Merck, UK.
Calcium phosphate (p.1188·3).
Calcium deficiency; calcium supplement; osteoporosis.

Ostram Vitamine D₃ Lipha Sante, Fr.
Calcium phosphate (p.1188·3); colecalciferol (p.1391·1).
Calcium and vitamin D deficiencies; osteoporosis.

Ostram-D₃ Bracco, Ital.
Calcium phosphate (p.1188·3); colecalciferol (p.1391·1).
Calcium and vitamin D deficiency; osteoporosis.

Ostram-Vit D₃
Merck, Fin.; Merck, Swed.
Calcium phosphate (p.1188·3); colecalciferol (p.1391·1).
Calcium and vitamin D deficiency; osteoporosis.

Ostranorm Nycomed, Denm.
11 Tablets, estradiol (p.1473·1); 10 tablets, estradiol; norethisterone (p.1485·1).
Menopausal disorders; osteoporosis.

Ostrolut Schering, Ger.
Hydroxyprogesterone caproate (p.1479·3); estradiol benzoate (p.1473·1).
Secondary amenorrhoea.

Ostronara Asche, Ger.†.
16 Tablets, estradiol valerate (p.1473·2); 12 tablets, estradiol valerate; levonorgestrel (p.1486·2).
Menopausal disorders.

Ostro-Primolut Schering, Ger.†.
Norethisterone acetate (p.1485·1); ethinylestradiol (p.1476·2).
Menstrual disorders.

Osvical Alter, Spain†.
Ascorbic acid (p.1389·3); calcium hypophosphite; calcium levulinate (p.1188·3); colecalciferol (p.1391·1).
Bone and dental disorders; calcium deficiency; osteomalacia; rickets.

Osyrol Hoechst Marion Roussel, Ger.
Potassium canrenoate (p.957·1) or spironolactone (p.973·2).
Hyperaldosteronism; hypertension; liver cirrhosis and ascites; oedema.

Osyrol Lasix Hoechst Marion Roussel, Ger.
Spironolactone (p.973·2); frusemide [furosemide] (p.893·1).
Ascites; hyperaldosteronism; liver cirrhosis; oedema.

Otalgan Note.This name is used for preparations of different composition.
Willvonseder, Aust.; Wolfs, Belg.
Lignocaine [lidocaine] hydrochloride (p.1313·2); phenazone (p.77·2).
Formerly contained procaine hydrochloride and phenazone in *Belg.*

Sudmedica, Ger.; Berna, Ital.; Jaba, Port.; Berna, Spain; Medichemie, Switz.
Procaine hydrochloride (p.1319·1); phenazone (p.77·2).
Earache.

Vemedia, Neth.
Lignocaine [lidocaine] hydrochloride (p.1313·2).
Earache.

Otalgicin Sudmedica, Ger.
Xylometazoline hydrochloride (p.1102·2).
Ear disorders; nasal congestion.

Otarex Teva, Israel.
Hydroxyzine hydrochloride (p.419·1).
Anxiety; childhood behaviour disorders; premedication; pruritus.

Otazul Ottolenghi, Ital.†.
Benzalkonium chloride (p.1133·2); azulene (p.1583·2); hamamelis (p.1618·3).
Eye disinfection; eye irritation.

O-Tet Docmed, S.Afr.†.
Oxytetracycline hydrochloride (p.234·1).
Bacterial infections.

Otex Dendron, UK.
Urea hydrogen peroxide (p.1159·3).
Ear wax removal.

Otiborin Santen, Fin.
Boric acid (p.1586·1); alcohol (p.1130·3).
Ear infections.

Otic Domeboro Bayer, USA.
Acetic acid (p.1571·2); aluminium acetate (p.1578·1).
Superficial infections of the external auditory canal.

Otic-Care Parmed, USA.
Hydrocortisone (p.1073·3); neomycin sulfate (p.228·1); polymyxin B sulfate (p.238·1).
Bacterial ear infections.

Oticin HC Teral, USA†.
Polymyxin B sulfate (p.238·1); neomycin sulfate (p.228·1); hydrocortisone (p.1073·3).

Otidin Teva, Israel.
Phenazone (p.77·2); amethocaine [tetracaine] hydrochloride (p.1305·2).
Otitis externa; otitis media.

Otigent Allergan-Frumtost, Braz.
Gentamicin sulfate (p.210·1); lignocaine [lidocaine] hydrochloride (p.1313·2).
Ear disorders.

Oti-Med Hyrex, USA.
Pramocaine hydrochloride (p.1318·2); hydrocortisone (p.1073·3).
Ear disorders.

Otipax
Biodiphar, Belg.; Biocodex, Fr.; Merck, Port.; Inpharzam, Switz.
Lignocaine [lidocaine] hydrochloride (p.1313·2); phenazone (p.77·2).
Earache.

Otised Propan, S.Afr.
Phenazone (p.77·2); benzocaine (p.1306·2).
Ear infections.

Otitex Sudmedica, Ger.
Docusate sodium (p.1223·1).
Removal of ear wax.

OtiTricin Bausch & Lomb, USA.
Hydrocortisone (p.1073·3); neomycin sulfate (p.228·1); polymyxin B (p.238·3).
Bacterial ear infections.

Otix Farmacusi, Spain.
Dexamethasone phosphate (p.1067·1); polymyxin B sulfate (p.238·1); trimethoprim (p.264·2).
Otitis externa.

Oto Betnovate Glaxo Wellcome, Braz.
Betamethasone (p.1063·1); chlorphenesin (p.381·3); amethocaine [tetracaine] (p.1305·2).
Ear disorders.

Oto Difusor Medical, Spain.
Benzocaine (p.1306·2); hyaluronidase (p.1620·3); hydrocortisone acetate (p.1073·3); neomycin sulfate (p.228·1); sulfanilamide sodium mesilate (p.256·2).
Ear disorders.

Oto Neomicin Calm Ale, Spain†.
Benzocaine (p.1306·2); hydrocortisone acetate (p.1073·3); neomycin sulfate (p.228·1); sulfacetamide sodium (p.250·3).
Ear disorders.

Oto Xilodase Apsen, Braz.
Lignocaine [lidocaine] (p.1313·2); neomycin sulfate (p.228·1); hyaluronidase (p.1620·3).
Ear disorders.

Otobacid N Asche, Ger.
Dexamethasone (p.1067·1); cinchocaine hydrochloride (p.1309·1).
Ear disorders.

Otobel Sedabel, Braz.
Sulfathiazole (p.257·1); procaine hydrochloride (p.1319·1).
Ear infections.

Oto-Biotic Allergan-Frumtost, Braz.
Note. A similar name is used for preparations of different composition (see below).
Sulfacetamide sodium (p.250·3); chloramphenicol (p.179·1); amethocaine [tetracaine] hydrochloride (p.1305·2); boric acid (p.1586·1); urea (p.1127·3).
Ear infections.

Otobiotic Schering, USA.
Note. A similar name is used for preparations of different composition (see above).
Polymyxin B sulfate (p.238·1); hydrocortisone (p.1073·3).
Bacterial ear infections.

Otocain Abana, USA.
Benzocaine (p.1306·2).
Earache.

Otocalm Parmed, USA.
Benzocaine (p.1306·2); phenazone (p.77·2).
Earache.

Otocalma Salusif, Port.
Procaine hydrochloride (p.1319·1); phenazone (p.77·2); sulfanilamide (p.256·2).
Otitis.

Otocalmine Pharmacobel, Belg.
Phenazone (p.77·2); procaine hydrochloride (p.1319·1).
Ear disorders.

Oto-Cer Allergan-Frumtost, Braz.
Hydroxyquinoline borate (p.1622·2).
Ear infections.

Otoceril Sanitas, Port.
Paradichlorobenzene (p.1648·3); benzocaine (p.1306·2); chlorobutanol (p.1141·2).
Removal of ear wax.

Otocerum Reig Jofre, Spain.
Phenol (p.1152·3); chlorobutanol (p.1141·2); benzocaine (p.1306·2); turpentine oil (p.1676·3); castor oil (p.1592·1).
Removal of ear wax.

Otocomb Otic Bristol-Myers Squibb, Austral.
Triamcinolone acetonide (p.1080·1); neomycin sulfate (p.228·1); nystatin (p.392·2); gramicidin (p.213·3).
Otitis externa.

Otocort Note.This name is used for preparations of different composition.
Gemballa, Braz.
Fluocinolone acetonide (p.1071·1); polymyxin B (p.238·3); neomycin (p.228·1); lignocaine [lidocaine] (p.1313·2).

Lemmon, USA.
Hydrocortisone (p.1073·3); neomycin sulfate (p.228·1); polymyxin B (p.238·3).
Bacterial ear infections.

Oto-cyl Ho-Len-Complex Liebermann, Ger.
Homoeopathic preparation.

Otodex Qualimed, Austral.
Framycetin sulfate (p.208·2); gramicidin (p.213·3); dexamethasone (p.1067·1).
Ear disorders.

Otodol Farmion, Braz.
Nitrofurazone (p.231·3); neomycin sulfate (p.228·1); fludrocortisone (p.1070·1); lignocaine [lidocaine] (p.1313·2); dimethyl sulfoxide; menthol (p.1632·3).
Ear disorders.

Otodolor Ursapharm, Ger.
Phenazone (p.77·2); procaine hydrochloride (p.1319·1).
Inflammatory ear disorders.

Otofa
Bouchara, Fr.; Bouchara, Port.; Bouchara, Switz.
Rifamycin sodium (p.246·2).
Otitis.

Otofenicol-D Allergan-Frumtost, Braz.
Lignocaine [lidocaine] hydrochloride (p.1313·2); dexamethasone (p.1067·1); chloramphenicol (p.179·1).
Ear disorders.

Oto-Flexiole N Mann, Ger.†.
Amethocaine [tetracaine] hydrochloride (p.1305·2).
Earache; otitis.

Otoflogin Heralds, Braz.
Chloramphenicol (p.179·1); lignocaine [lidocaine] (p.1313·2).
Ear disorders.

Otofluor SIT, Ital.
Sodium fluoride (p.1375·3); calcium gluconate (p.1188·2).
Otosclerosis.

Otogen Calmante Belmac, Spain.
Benzalkonium chloride (p.1133·2); clove oil (p.1597·1); phenol (p.1152·3); amethocaine [tetracaine] hydrochloride (p.1305·2); menthol (p.1632·3).
Ear disorders.

Otoial Fidia, Ital.
Sodium hyaluronate (p.1620·1).
Tympanic membrane lesions.

Otolin Bergamo, Braz.
Neomycin (p.228·1); nitrofurazone (p.231·3); lignocaine [lidocaine] (p.1313·2).
Ear infections.

Otolitan N farblos 3M, Ger.
Dequalinium chloride (p.1143·1); lignocaine [lidocaine] hydrochloride (p.1313·2).
Earache; otitis.

Otolitan N mit Rivanol 3M, Ger.
Ethacridine lactate (p.1130·3); lignocaine [lidocaine] hydrochloride (p.1313·2).
Earache; otitis.

Otoloide Honorteropica, Braz.
Phenol (p.1152·3); procaine (p.1319·2).
Ear disorders.

Otolone Heralds, Braz.
Polymyxin B sulfate (p.238·1); neomycin sulfate (p.228·1); fluocinolone (p.1071·1).
Ear disorders.

Otolys Produfarma, Port.†.
Hydrocortisone (p.1073·3); lignocaine [lidocaine] (p.1313·2); neomycin (p.228·1); polymyxin B (p.238·3).

Otolysine Chauvin, Fr.
Trolamine caprylate.
Removal of ear wax.

Otomar-HC Marnel, USA.
Chloroxylenol (p.1142·1); hydrocortisone (p.1073·3); pramocaine hydrochloride (p.1318·2).
Ear disorders.

Otomicetina Deca, Ital.†.
Chloramphenicol (p.179·1); neomycin sulfate (p.228·1); tuaminoheptane sulfate (p.1102·2).
Ear infections.

Otomicina *Medley, Braz.*
Chloramphenicol (p.179·1); lignocaine [lidocaine] (p.1313·2).
Ear disorders.

Otomide *SERB, Fr.*
Hexamidine isetionate (p.1146·2); lignocaine [lidocaine] hydrochloride (p.1313·2).
Formerly contained sulfasuccinamide sodium and amylocaine hydrochloride.
Otitis.

Otomidone *SIT, Ital.*
Phenazone (p.77·2); procaine hydrochloride (p.1319·1).
Formerly contained aminophenazone, procaine hydrochloride, and chlorobutanol.
Earache.

Otomidrin *Fardi, Spain.*
Fluocinolone acetonide (p.1071·1); framycetin sulfate (p.208·2); lignocaine [lidocaine] hydrochloride (p.1313·2).
Ear disorders.

Otomixyn *EMS, Braz.*
Fluocinolone acetonide (p.1071·1); polymyxin B (p.238·3); neomycin sulfate (p.228·1); lignocaine [lidocaine] (p.1313·2).
Ear disorders.

Otomize *Stafford-Miller, Fin.; Stafford-Miller, Irl.; Stafford-Miller, Israel; Stafford-Miller, UK.*
Dexamethasone (p.1067·1); neomycin sulfate (p.228·1).
Otitis externa.

Otomycin *Taro, Israel.*
Neomycin sulfate (p.228·1); phenylephrine hydrochloride (p.1097·1); sodium propionate (p.393·2); benzocaine (p.1306·2); benzyl alcohol (p.1135·2).
Ear infections.

Otomycin-HPN *Misemer, USA.*
Hydrocortisone (p.1073·3); neomycin sulfate (p.228·1); polymyxin B (p.238·3).
Bacterial ear infections.

Otonal *Biochimico, Braz.*
Paracetamol (p.71·2); zinc bromide; valeric acid.
Vertigo.

Otonasal *Diftersa, Spain.*
Ephedrine hydrochloride (p.1090·1); procaine (p.1319·2); sulfanilamide (p.256·2).
Congestion and infection of the nose and ear.

Otonax *Sanval, Braz.*
Procaine hydrochloride (p.1319·1); phenol (p.1152·3).
Ear infections.

Otonina *Berna, Spain.*
Benzocaine (p.1306·2); neomycin sulfate (p.228·1); prednisolone (p.1077·3).
Ear disorders.

Otopax *Vaillant, Ital.*
Procaine hydrochloride (p.1319·1); phenazone (p.77·2).
Earache.

Otopen *Dinafarma, Braz.*
Chloramphenicol (p.179·1); lignocaine [lidocaine] hydrochloride (p.1313·2).
Ear disorders.

Oto-Phen *Adcock Ingram, S.Afr.*
Phenazone (p.77·2).
Earache; otitis.

Oto-Phen Forte *Adcock Ingram, S.Afr.*
Benzocaine (p.1306·2); ephedrine hydrochloride (p.1090·1); phenazone (p.77·2); potassium hydroxyquinoline sulfate (p.1654·2).
Earache; otitis.

Otoralgyl
Note.This name is used for preparations of different composition.
Aventis, Belg.; Martin, Fr.†.
Lignocaine [lidocaine] hydrochloride (p.1313·2).
Earache.

Martin, Switz.†.
Sulfasuccinamide sodium (p.256·3); lignocaine [lidocaine] hydrochloride (p.1313·2).
Earache; otitis.

Otoralgyl a la phenylephrine *Martin, Fr.*
Lignocaine [lidocaine] hydrochloride (p.1313·2); phenylephrine hydrochloride (p.1097·1); sodium propionate (p.393·2).
Otitis.

Otoralgyl sulfamide *Martin, Fr.†.*
Sulfasuccinamide sodium (p.256·3); lignocaine [lidocaine] hydrochloride (p.1313·2).
Earache; otitis externa.

Oto-Rinil *Faria, Braz.*
Prednazoline (p.1099·2).
Nasal disorders.

Otosan *Streuli, Switz.*
Procaine hydrochloride (p.1319·1); phenazone (p.77·2).
Ear disorders; earache.

Otosan Gocce Auricolari *Otosan, Ital.*
Almond oil (p.1576·3); alcohol (p.1130·3); cajuput oil (p.1588·1); geranium oil (p.1615·1); juniper oil (p.1625·2); chamomile (p.1593·2).
Ear wax removal.

Otosedol *Pensa, Spain.*
Phenazone (p.77·2); procaine hydrochloride (p.1319·1).
Earache.

Otosedol Biotico *Pensa, Spain.*
Chloramphenicol (p.179·1); benzocaine (p.1306·2); tyrothricin (p.267·1).
Ear disorders.

Otoseptil *Ethimed, S.Afr.†.*
Neomycin undecylenate (p.228·1); tyrothricin (p.267·1); hydrocortisone (p.1073·3).
Ear disorders.

Otosil *Silom, Thai.*
Chloramphenicol (p.179·1); prednisolone (p.1077·3).
Bacterial ear infections.

Otosporin
Note.This name is used for preparations of different composition.
Glaxo Wellcome, Aust.; Warner-Lambert Consumer, Belg.; Glaxo Wellcome, Braz.; Glaxo Wellcome, Ger.; Glaxo Wellcome, Hong Kong; Glaxo Wellcome, Irl.; Glaxo Wellcome, Israel; Glaxo Wellcome, Neth.; Glaxo Wellcome, S.Afr.; Glaxo Wellcome, Singapore; Wellcome, Spain; Wellcome, Switz.; Glaxo Wellcome, Thai.; Wellcome, UK; Calmic, USA.
Hydrocortisone (p.1073·3); neomycin sulfate (p.228·1); polymyxin B sulfate (p.238·1).
Bacterial ear infections.

Warner-Lambert, Ital.
Neomycin sulfate (p.228·1); polymyxin B sulfate (p.238·1).
Formerly contained hydrocortisone, neomycin sulfate, and polymyxin B sulfate.
Bacterial infections of the external ear.

Wellcome, Port.
Hydrocortisone (p.1073·3); neomycin sulfate (p.228·1); polymyxin B sulfate (p.238·1).

Otospray *Stafford-Miller, Switz.*
Neomycin sulfate (p.228·1); dexamethasone (p.1067·1).
Ear disorders.

Otosulf *Millet Roux, Braz.*
Sodium propionate (p.393·2); mafenide hydrochloride (p.221·2); benzethonium chloride (p.1134·2); benzocaine (p.1306·2).
Ear disorders.

Otosynalar *Hoechst Marion Roussel, Braz.*
Fluocinolone acetonide (p.1071·1); polymyxin B (p.238·3); neomycin (p.228·1); lignocaine [lidocaine] (p.1313·2); citric acid (p.1596·2).
Ear disorders.

Oto-Synalar N *Janssen-Cilag, Port.*
Fluocinolone acetonide (p.1071·1).

Otothricinol *Plan, Switz.*
Tyrothricin (p.267·1); phenazone (p.77·2); cetylpyridinium chloride (p.1138·1).
Ear disorders.

Otovowen *Weber & Weber, Ger.*
Homoeopathic preparation.

Otowaxol *Norgine, Ger.*
Docusate sodium (p.1223·1).
Removal of ear wax.

Otradrops *Manx, UK.*
Xylometazoline hydrochloride (p.1102·2).
Nasal congestion.

Otraspray *Manx, UK.*
Xylometazoline hydrochloride (p.1102·2).
Nasal congestion.

Otreon
Sankyo, Aust.; Sankyo, Ital.; Sankyo, Spain.
Cefpodoxime proxetil (p.172·3).
Bacterial infections.

O-trexat *Onkoworks, Ger.*
Methotrexate (p.553·2).
Malignant neoplasms.

Otrinol *Novartis, Israel; Novartis Consumer, Switz.*
Pseudoephedrine hydrochloride (p.1099·2).
Nasal congestion.

Otrisal *Novartis Consumer, Aust.; Novartis Consumer, Ger.*
Sodium chloride (p.1196·1).
Nasal and pharyngeal dryness; nasal congestion.

Otriven *Ciba Vision, Ger.*
Xylometazoline hydrochloride (p.1102·2).
Conjunctival disorders.

Otriven gegen Schnupfen *Novartis Consumer, Ger.*
Xylometazoline hydrochloride (p.1102·2).
Catarrh; nasal congestion; rhinitis.

Otriven H *Novartis Consumer, Ger.*
Sodium cromoglicate (p.774·3).
Allergic conjunctivitis; allergic rhinitis.

Otrivin
Novartis Consumer, Aust.; Novartis Consumer, Austral.; Novartis Consumer, Canad.; Novartis, Denm.; Novartis, Fin.; Novartis, Hong Kong; Novartis, Israel; Novartis Consumer, Ital.; Novartis Consumer, Neth.; Novartis, Norw.; Novartis Consumer, S.Afr.; Novartis Nutrition, Singapore; Novartis Consumer, Spain; Novartis, Swed.; Novartis Consumer, Switz.; Ciba Consumer, USA.
Xylometazoline hydrochloride (p.1102·2).
Aid in rhinoscopy; nasal congestion; otitis media; rhinitis; sinusitis.

Otrivin Menthol
Novartis, Denm.; Novartis, Fin.; Novartis, Swed.
Xylometazoline hydrochloride (p.1102·2); menthol (p.1632·3); eucalyptol (p.1609·2).
Rhinitis; sinusitis; upper repiratory-tract congestion.

Otrivina
Novartis, Braz.; Novartis Consumer, Port.
Xylometazoline hydrochloride (p.1102·2).
Nasal congestion.

Otrivine
Novartis Consumer, Belg.; Novartis Consumer, Irl.; Novartis, NZ; Novartis, Thai.; Novartis Consumer, UK.
Xylometazoline hydrochloride (p.1102·2).
Nasal congestion; otitis media; rhinitis; sinusitis.

Otrivine Menthol *Novartis, NZ.*
Xylometazoline hydrochloride (p.1102·2); menthol (p.1632·3); eucalyptus (p.1609·2).
Nasal congestion.

Otrivine Mu-Cron *Novartis Consumer, UK.*
Pseudoephedrine hydrochloride (p.1099·2); paracetamol (p.71·2).
Fever; nasal congestion; pain.

Otrivine-Antistin
Ciba Vision, Irl.; Ciba Vision, NZ; Novartis Consumer, UK.
Xylometazoline hydrochloride (p.1102·2); antazoline sulfate (p.408·3).
Allergic conjunctivitis.

Otrozol *Pisa, Mex.*
Metronidazole (p.594·1).
Amoebiasis; anaerobic bacterial infections.

Otsuka MV *Otsuka, Jpn.*
Multivitamin preparation (p.1350·1).
Parenteral nutrition.

Ottocid *Ottolenghi, Ital.*
Phenothrin (p.1436·2).
Acaricide.

Ottoclor *Ottolenghi, Ital.†.*
Tosylchloramide sodium (p.1159·1).
Wound disinfection.

Ottovis *Fitolife, Ital.*
Royal jelly (p.1659·3); ginseng (p.1615·3); wheatgerm oil; soya lecithin (p.1628·1); pollen.
Tonic.

Oturga *Legrand, Braz.*
Tyrothricin (p.267·1); salicylic acid (p.1122·3); boric acid (p.1586·1); procaine (p.1319·2).
Ear disorders.

Otylol *Bridoux, Fr.*
Procaine hydrochloride (p.1319·1); amethocaine [tetracaine] hydrochloride (p.1305·2); phenol (p.1152·3); ephedrine hydrochloride (p.1090·1); thyme oil (p.1672·3).
Ear disorders.

Ouate Hemostatique *Qualiphar, Belg.*
Ferric chloride (p.1610·3); phenazone (p.77·2).
Haemorrhage.

Out of Africa *Sutton, Canad.*
Pyrithione zinc (p.1122·1).

Outgro
Note.This name is used for preparations of different composition.
Medtech, Canad.

Whitehall-Robins, Canad.†; Whitehall, USA.
Tannic acid (p.1669·1); chlorobutanol (p.1141·2).
Ingrown toenails.

Out-of-Sorts *Potter's, UK.*
Senna (p.1248·2); aloes (p.1210·1); cascara (p.1216·1); taraxacum (p.1669·1); fennel (p.1610·1).
Constipation.

Ouvidonal *Neo Quimica, Braz.*
Chloramphenicol (p.179·1); lignocaine [lidocaine] (p.1313·2).
Ear disorders.

Ova-Mit
Remedica, Hong Kong; Remedica, Singapore; Remedica, Thai.
Clomifene citrate (p.1465·3).
Anovulatory infertility.

Ovanon
Organon, Aust.; Aaciphar, Belg.†; Organon, Fr.; Nourypharma, Ger.; Nourypharma, Neth.; Ercopharm, Switz.
7 Tablets, ethinylestradiol (p.1476·2); 15 tablets, ethinylestradiol; lynestrenol (p.1480·1).
28-Day packs also contain 6 inert tablets.
Sequential-type oral contraceptive.

Ovarell *Sanorell, Ger.*
Homoeopathic preparation.

Ovariuteran *Virtus, Braz.*
Cotton root bark; plumeria lancifolia; berberis laurina.
Dysmenorrhoea.

Ovastat *Medac, Ger.*
Treosulfan (p.576·2).
Ovarian cancer.

Ovcon 35 *Bristol-Myers Squibb, USA.*
Norethisterone (p.1485·1); ethinylestradiol (p.1476·2).
28-Day packs also contain 7 inert tablets.
Combined oral contraceptive.

Ovcon 50 *Bristol-Myers Squibb, USA.*
Norethisterone (p.1485·1); ethinylestradiol (p.1476·2).
28-Day packs also contain 7 inert tablets.
Combined oral contraceptive.

Overal *Lusofarmaco, Ital.*
Roxithromycin (p.247·2).
Bacterial infections.

Overoid *Valdecasas, Mex.*
Chlorosalicylamide.
Worm infections.

Overpon *Valdecasas, Mex.*
Piperazine (p.105·3).
Worm infections.

Ovesterin
Organon, Norw.; Organon, Swed.
Estriol (p.1475·3).
Vulvovaginal disorders due to oestrogen deficiency.

Ovestin
Organon, Aust.; Organon, Austral.; Organon, Denm.; Organon, Fin.; Organon, Ger.; Organon, Hong Kong; Organon, Irl.; Organon, Israel; Organon, Ital.; Organon, Neth.†; Organon, NZ; Organon, Port.; Organon, Singapore; Organon, Switz.; Organon, Thai.; Organon, UK.
Estriol (p.1475·3).
Female infertility; vulvovaginal disorders due to oestrogen deficiency.

Ovestinon *Organon, Spain.*
Estriol (p.1475·3).
Oestrogen deficiency.

Ovestrion *Akzo, Braz.*
Estriol (p.1475·3).
Menopausal disorders; osteoporosis.

Ovex *Johnson & Johnson MSD Consumer, UK.*
Mebendazole (p.102·2).
Enterobiasis.

Ovibion *Klinge, Aust.†.*
Porcine ovarian extract (p.1487·2).
Menopausal disorders; menstrual disorders.

Ovide *Medicis, USA.*
Malathion (p.1434·2).
Pediculosis.

Ovidol
Aaciphar, Belg.; Nourypharma, Neth.; Nourypharma, Switz.
7 Tablets, ethinylestradiol (p.1476·2); 15 tablets, ethinylestradiol; desogestrel (p.1470·3).
Sequential-type oral contraceptive.

Ovidrel *Serono, USA.*
Choriogonadotropin alfa (p.1279·2).
Female infertility.

Ovinum *Biolab, Thai.*
Clomifene citrate (p.1465·3).
Anovulatory infertility; male infertility.

Oviol *Nourypharma, Ger.*
7 Tablets, ethinylestradiol (p.1476·2); 15 tablets, ethinylestradiol; desogestrel (p.1470·3).
28-Day packs also contain 6 inert tablets.
Sequential-type oral contraceptive.

Ovis Neu *Warner-Lambert, Ger.*
Clotrimazole (p.382·1).
Fungal skin infections.

Ovitrelle *Serono, UK.*
Choriogonadotropin alfa (p.1279·2).
Formerly known as Ovidrelle
Female infertility.

Ovol
Carter Horner, Canad.; Carter Horner, Hong Kong; Carter Horner, Thai.
Simeticone (p.1249·2).
Bloating; flatulence; infant colic.

Ovoplex *Wyeth, Spain.*
Ethinylestradiol (p.1476·2); levonorgestrel (p.1486·2).
Combined oral contraceptive; menstrual disorders.

Ovoresta *Organon, Ger.†.*
Lynestrenol (p.1480·1); ethinylestradiol (p.1476·2).
Combined oral contraceptive; menstrual disorders.

Ovoresta M *Organon, Ger.*
Lynestrenol (p.1480·1); ethinylestradiol (p.1476·2).
Combined oral contraceptive; menstrual disorders.

Ovosiston *Jenapharm, Ger.*
Mestranol (p.1482·1); chlormadinone acetate (p.1465·3).
Combined oral contraceptive; menstrual disorders.

Ovostat
Organon, Belg.†; Organon, Neth.; Donmed, S.Afr.†; Organon, Switz.†.
Lynestrenol (p.1480·1); ethinylestradiol (p.1476·2).
28-Day packs also contain 7 inert tablets.
Combined oral contraceptive.

Ovo-Vinces *Wolff, Ger.*
Estriol (p.1475·3).
Menopausal disorders.

Ovral
Wyeth-Ayerst, Canad.; Wyeth-Ayerst, Hong Kong; Wyeth, Mex.; Wyeth, NZ; Aspen, S.Afr.; Wyeth-Ayerst, Thai.; Wyeth-Ayerst, USA.
Norgestrel (p.1486·1); ethinylestradiol (p.1476·2).
28-Day packs also contain 7 inert tablets.
Combined oral contraceptive; endometriosis; menstrual disorders.

Ovran
Wyeth, Irl.; Wyeth, UK.
Ethinylestradiol (p.1476·2); levonorgestrel (p.1486·2).
Combined oral contraceptive; endometriosis; menstrual disorders.

Ovran 30
Wyeth, Irl.; Wyeth, UK.
Ethinylestradiol (p.1476·2); levonorgestrel (p.1486·2).
Combined oral contraceptive.

Ovranet *Wyeth Lederle, Ital.*
Ethinylestradiol (p.1476·2); levonorgestrel (p.1486·2).
Combined oral contraceptive.

Ovranette
Wyeth Lederle, Aust.; Wyeth, Irl.; Wyeth, UK.
Ethinylestradiol (p.1476·2); levonorgestrel (p.1486·2).
Combined oral contraceptive; endometriosis; menstrual disorders.

Ovrette *Wyeth-Ayerst, USA.*
Norgestrel (p.1486·1).
Progestogen-only oral contraceptive.

OvuGen *BioGenex, USA.*
Fertility test (p.1654·3).

Ovukit
MediMar, UK; Monoclonal Antibodies, USA.
Fertility test (p.1654·3).

Ovulen Searle, Austral.†; Searle, Belg.†; Searle, Neth.†; Searle, Switz.†.
Etynodiol diacetate (p.1477·1); ethinylestradiol (p.1476·2).
28-Day packs also contain 7 inert tablets.
Combined oral contraceptive.

Ovules Sedo-Hemostatiques du Docteur Jouve Gerda, Fr.
Phenazone (p.77·2); calcium chloride (p.1188·1).
Minor gynaecological surgery.

Ovuplan Key, Austral.
Fertility test (p.1654·3).

Ovuquick
MediMar, UK; Monoclonal Antibodies, USA.
Fertility test (p.1654·3).

Ovysmen
Janssen-Cilag, Aust.; Janssen-Cilag, Belg.; Janssen-Cilag, Ger.; Janssen-Cilag, Irl.; Janssen-Cilag, Switz.; Janssen-Cilag, UK.
Norethisterone (p.1485·1); ethinylestradiol (p.1476·2).
Combined oral contraceptive.

Owbridges for Chesty Coughs Chefaro, UK.
Guaifenesin (p.1092·2).
Coughs.

oxa CT, Ger.
Oxazepam (p.697·1).
Anxiety disorders; sleep disorders.

Oxabenal Zerboni, Mex.
Oxyphenbutazone (p.71·1).

Oxabenz United Nordic, Denm.
Oxazepam (p.697·1).
Anxiety.

Oxacant N Klein, Ger.
Crataegus (p.1600·2); hypericum (p.290·2); convallaria (p.1599·1); adonis vernalis (p.1573·3); cereus (p.1593·1); scoparium (p.1661·2); melissa (p.1632·2); valerian (p.1678·3); motherwort (p.1637·3).
Cardiac disorders.

Oxacant-forte N Klein, Ger.
Crataegus (p.1600·2); convallaria (p.1599·1); adonis vernalis (p.1573·3); cereus (p.1593·1).
Cardiac disorders.

Oxacant-Khella N Klein, Ger.
Crataegus (p.1600·2); convallaria (p.1599·1); adonis vernalis (p.1573·3); cereus (p.1593·1); ammi visnaga (p.1579·1).
Cardiac disorders.

Oxacant-mono Klein, Ger.
Crataegus (p.1600·2).
Heart failure.

Oxacant-sedativ Klein, Ger.
Crataegus (p.1600·2); motherwort (p.1637·3); melissa (p.1632·2); valerian (p.1678·3).
Nervous cardiac disorders.

Oxacatin Taro, Israel.
Oxomemazine (p.422·2); sulfogaiacol (p.1101·1); sodium benzoate (p.1134·3).
Coughs.

Oxadilene Medeva, Fr.
Papaverine hydrochloride (p.1648·1).
Formerly contained butalamine hydrochloride and papaverine hydrochloride.
Cerebrovascular disorders.

Oxadol ISI, Ital.
Nefopam hydrochloride (p.62·1).
Pain.

Oxahexal Hexal, Aust.
Oxazepam (p.697·1).
Anxiety disorders; sleep disorders.

Oxaline Rolab, S.Afr.
Oxazepam (p.697·1).
Alcohol withdrawal syndrome; anxiety disorders.

Oxalyt Madaus, Aust.†.
Potassium sodium hydrogen citrate.
Renal calculi.

Oxamin Medinovum, Fin.
Oxazepam (p.697·1).
Anxiety disorders; depression; insomnia.

Oxandrin BTG, USA.
Oxandrolone (p.1487·2).
Bone pain associated with osteoporosis; protein catabolism; weight loss.

Oxanest Leiras, Fin.
Oxycodone hydrochloride (p.70·2).
Pain.

Oxapam Lilly, Ital.
Oxazepam (p.697·1).
Anxiety disorders.

Oxapax Durascan, Denm.
Oxazepam (p.697·1).
Anxiety.

Oxascand Enapharm, Swed.
Oxazepam (p.697·1).
Alcohol withdrawal syndrome; anxiety; sleep disorders.

Oxathos Medix, Mex.
Oxolamine (p.1096·2).
Respiratory-tract congestion.

Oxatokey Inkeysa, Austral.
Oxatomide (p.422·1).
Hypersensitivity reactions.

Oxbarukain Chauvin ankerpharm, Ger.
Oxybuprocaine hydrochloride (p.1318·1).
Local anaesthesia.

OxBipp Oxford Pharmaceuticals, UK.
Bismuth subnitrate (p.1213·2); iodoform (p.1149·1).

Oxcord Biosintetica, Braz.
Nifedipine (p.940·1).
Angina pectoris; hypertension; Raynaud's syndrome.

Oxelio Jaldes, Fr.
Vitamin and mineral preparation (p.1350·1).

Oxema Jean-Marie, Hong Kong.
Aluminium hydroxide (p.1210·2); magnesium carbonate (p.1232·3) or magnesium trisilicate (p.1233·3); oxetacaine (p.1317·3).
Gastrointestinal disorders.

Oxeol AstraZeneca, Fr.
Bambuterol hydrochloride (p.761·1).
Asthma.

Oxepa Abbott Nutrition, UK.
Preparation for enteral nutrition (p.1350·1).

Oxepam Wyeth Lederle, Fin.
Oxazepam (p.697·1).
Alcohol withdrawal syndrome; anxiety disorders.

Oxeprax Wyeth, Spain.
Tamoxifen citrate (p.571·1).
Breast cancer.

Oxeron Serono, Mex.
Hydroxyurea [hydroxycarbamide] (p.544·2).

Oxetine Pharmaland, Thai.
Fluoxetine hydrochloride (p.284·2).
Depression; obsessive-compulsive disorder.

Oxeze AstraZeneca, Canad.
Eformoterol [formoterol] fumarate (p.764·2).
Asthma.

Oxibran Prospa, Port.
Piracetam (p.1652·1).

Oxicam Bioprogress, Ital.
Piroxicam (p.79·1).
Musculoskeletal, joint, and peri-articular disorders.

Oxicanol Fustery, Mex.
Piroxicam (p.79·1).
Musculoskeletal, joint, peri-articular, and soft-tissue disorders; pain.

Oxiderma Galderma, Spain.
Benzoyl peroxide (p.1111·1).
Acne.

Oxidermiol Antihist Farmasur, Spain.
Benzocaine (p.1306·2); tyrothricin (p.267·1); triprelennamine hydrochloride (p.427·1).
Cutaneous hypersensitivity reactions.

Oxidermiol Enzima Farmasur, Spain.
Bacitracin (p.155·2); neomycin sulfate (p.228·1); trypsin (p.1675·3).
Skin infections; wounds.

Oxidermiol Fuerte Farmasur, Spain.
Fluocinolone acetonide (p.1071·1).
Skin disorders.

Oxidermiol Lassar Farmasur, Spain.
Starch; salicylic acid (p.1122·3); soft paraffin; zinc oxide (p.1128·2).
Skin disorders.

Oxido Amari Alcon Cusi, Spain.
Mercuric chloride (p.1633·3); mercuric oxide (p.1633·3).
Eye disorders.

Oxi-Freeda Freeda, USA.
Multivitamin, mineral, and amino-acid preparation (p.1350·1).

Oxifungol Armstrong, Mex.
Fluconazole (p.383·2).
Fungal infections.

Oxigen Biosintetica, Braz.
Nimodipine (p.946·1).
Neurological deficit following subarachnoid haemorrhage.

Oxiken Kendrick, Mex.
Dobutamine hydrochloride (p.880·2).
Heart failure; shock.

Oxiklorin Orion, Fin.
Hydroxychloroquine sulfate (p.437·2).
Light-sensitive skin disorders; lupus erythematosus; rheumatoid arthritis.

Oxilin
Allergan-Frumtost, Braz.; Allergan, Ital.
Oxymetazoline hydrochloride (p.1096·2).
Conjunctivitis; eye congestion.

Oxilium Labor, Aust.; Oxo, Switz.
Tetrachlorodecaoxide (p.1670·1).
Burns; skin disinfection; wounds.

Oximen Montplet, Spain.
Hydrogen peroxide (p.1147·1).
Haemostasis; skin and mucous membrane disinfection.

5-Oxin Torii, Hong Kong.
5-Oxyanthranilic acid; anthranilic acid; vitamin B substances; vitamin C (p.1350·1).
Constipation; diabetes; glaucoma.

Oxipor Medtech, Canad.
Coal tar (p.1125·1); salicylic acid (p.1122·3); benzocaine (p.1306·2).
Skin disorders.

Oxipor VHC Whitehall, USA.
Coal tar (p.1125·1).
Formerly contained coal tar, salicylic acid, and benzocaine.
Psoriasis.

Oxis
Astra, Aust.; Astra, Austral.; Astra, Belg.; AstraZeneca, Denm.; Astra-Zeneca, Fin.; Astra, Ger.; Stern, Ger.; Astra, Irl.; Teva, Israel; Astra-Zeneca, Ital.; Astra, Mex.; Astra, Neth.; AstraZeneca, Norw.;

AstraZeneca, NZ; Astra, Port.; Astra, S.Afr.; AstraZeneca, Singapore; Astra, Spain; Draco, Swed.; Astra, Switz.; AstraZeneca, Thai.; Astra-Zeneca, UK.
Eformoterol [formoterol] fumarate (p.764·2).
Asthma.

Oxistat
Glaxo Wellcome, Mex.; Glaxo Wellcome, USA.
Oxiconazole nitrate (p.393·1).
Fungal skin infections; mixed bacterial and fungal vaginal infections.

Oxi-Tabs C+E Ferrosan, Fin.
d-Alpha tocoferil acetate; ascorbic acid; selenium (p.1350·1).
Vitamins C and E and selenium deficiency.

Oxitopisa Pisa, Mex.
Oxytocin (p.1294·1).

Oxitover Llorente, Spain.
Mebendazole (p.102·2).
Worm infections.

Oxitraklin Atlantis, Mex.
Oxytetracycline (p.234·1).
Bacterial infections.

Oxiurazina UCI, Braz.
Piperazine (p.105·3).
Ascariasis; enterobiasis.

Oxivel
Zeller, Singapore; Zeller, Switz.
Ginkgo biloba (p.1615·2).
Tonic.

Oxivent
Boehringer Ingelheim, Aust.†; Boehringer Ingelheim, Belg.; Boehringer Ingelheim, Denm.†; Boehringer Ingelheim, Irl.; Boehringer Ingelheim, Ital.; Boehringer Ingelheim, UK.
Oxitropium bromide (p.769·2).
Obstructive airways disease.

Oxivite Neves, Port.
dl-Alpha tocoferil acetate (p.1394·1).
Vitamin E deficiency.

Oxizole
Note. This name is used for preparations of different composition.
Stiefel, Canad.
Oxiconazole nitrate (p.393·1).
Tinea pedis.

Orthos, Mex.
Mebendazole (p.102·2).

Oxleti Leti, Spain†.
Oxatomide (p.422·1).
Hypersensitivity reactions.

Oxobron Diba, Mex.
Oxolamine citrate (p.1096·2).
Coughs.

Oxodal Synthelabo, Spain.
Betaxolol hydrochloride (p.848·3).
Hypertension.

Oxoferin
Note. This name is used for preparations of different composition.
Yamanouchi, Ger.
Reaction product of sodium chlorite, sodium hypochlorite, sulfuric acid, potassium chlorate, sodium carbonate-hydrogen peroxide, and sodium peroxide.
Wounds.

Oxo, Thai.
Tetrachlorodecaoxide (p.1670·1).
Burns; ulcers; wounds.

Oxoinex Inexfa, Spain.
Oxolinic acid (p.233·3).
Urinary-tract infections.

Oxolam Diba, Mex.
Oxolamine (p.1096·2).

Oxomifer Reuffer, Mex.
Oxolamine (p.1096·2).

Oxopurin Dexxon, Israel.
Oxpentifylline [pentoxifylline] (p.950·3).
Vascular disorders.

Oxoquin Protermex, Mex.
Oxolamine citrate (p.1096·2).

Oxosint Medivis, Ital.
Co-tetroxazine (p.193·2).
Bacterial infections; Pneumocystis carinii pneumonia.

Oxoway Wayne, Mex.
Ambroxol (p.1084·3).

Ox-Pam Douglas, NZ.
Oxazepam (p.697·1).
Alcohol withdrawal syndrome; anxiety.

Oxsac Masa, Thai.
Fluoxetine hydrochloride (p.284·2).
Depression; obsessive-compulsive disorder.

Oxsoralen
Gerot, Aust.; Dermatech, Austral.; ICN, Canad.; ICN, Hong Kong; ICN, Israel; Italfarmaco, Ital.; ICN, Mex.; Elder, Neth.†; ICN, NZ; Restan, S.Afr.; ICN, Singapore; Galderma, Spain; ICN, USA.
Methoxsalen (p.1118·3).
Photosensitivity; psoriasis; vitiligo.

Oxsoralon Wolfs, Belg.†.
Methoxsalen (p.1118·3).
Psoriasis.

Oxy
Note. This name is used for preparations of different composition.
Reckitt & Colman, Austral.; SmithKline Beecham Consumer, Canad.; SmithKline Beecham OTC, Ger.; SmithKline Beecham, Hong Kong; SmithKline Beecham Consumer, UK; SmithKline Beecham Consumer, USA.
Benzoyl peroxide (p.1111·1).
Acne.

Triomed, S.Afr.†.
Oxytetracycline hydrochloride (p.234·1).
Bacterial infections.

Oxy Balance SmithKline Beecham, Hong Kong.
Salicylic acid (p.1122·3).
Acne.

Oxy Biciron S & K, Ger.
Oxytetracycline hydrochloride (p.234·1); tramazoline hydrochloride (p.1102·1).
Bacterial eye infections.

Oxy Clean Facial Scrub SmithKline Beecham Consumer, UK.
Borax (p.1586·1); triclosan (p.1159·2).
Acne.

Oxy Clean Medicated SmithKline Beecham, Israel.
Salicylic acid (p.1122·3); alcohol (p.1130·3).
Acne.

Oxy Clean Pore SmithKline Beecham Consumer, Canad.
Salicylic acid (p.1122·3).
Acne.

Oxy Cleanser SmithKline Beecham Consumer, UK.
Regular: Triclosan (p.1159·2); salicylic acid (p.1122·3); alcohol (p.1130·3).
Formerly called Oxy Clean Medicated Cleanser.
Sensitive: Salicylic acid (p.1122·3); alcohol (p.1130·3).
Acne.

Oxy Control SmithKline Beecham Consumer, Canad.†.
Salicylic acid (p.1122·3).
Acne.

Oxy Daily Facial Cleanser Regular SmithKline Beecham Consumer, Canad.
Triclosan (p.1159·2).
Acne.

Oxy Daily Skin Wash Reckitt Benckiser, NZ.
Triclosan (p.1159·2).
Acne.

Oxy Daily Wash SmithKline Beecham, Hong Kong.
Triclosan (p.1159·2).
Skin disorders.

Oxy Deep Pore SmithKline Beecham Consumer, Canad.
Salicylic acid (p.1122·3).
Acne.

Oxy Dots SmithKline Beecham Consumer, UK.
Salicylic acid (p.1122·3); triclosan (p.1159·2).
Spots.

Oxy Duo Pads SmithKline Beecham Consumer, UK.
Regular: Triclosan (p.1159·2); salicylic acid (p.1122·3); alcohol (p.1130·3).
Sensitive: Salicylic acid (p.1122·3); alcohol (p.1130·3).
Acne.

Oxy Facial Wash SmithKline Beecham Consumer, UK.
Triclosan (p.1159·2).
Formerly called Oxy Clean Facial Wash.
Skin disorders.

Oxy Fissan Fink, Ger.†; Zyma, Ger.†.
Benzoyl peroxide (p.1111·1).
Acne.

Oxy Gentle SmithKline Beecham Consumer, Canad.
Triclosan (p.1159·2).
Acne.

Oxy Medicated Pads SmithKline Beecham Consumer, Canad.
Salicylic acid (p.1122·3).
Formerly known as Oxy Power Pads.
Acne.

Oxy Medicated Soap
SmithKline Beecham Consumer, Canad.; SmithKline Beecham, USA.
Triclosan (p.1159·2).
Acne.

Oxy Night Watch
SmithKline Beecham Consumer, Canad.†; SmithKline Beecham Consumer, USA.
Salicylic acid (p.1122·3).
Acne.

Oxy ResiDon't SmithKline Beecham, USA†.
Triclosan (p.1159·2); diazolidinyl urea.
Acne.

Oxy Sensitive SmithKline Beecham, Israel.
Benzoyl peroxide (p.1111·1).
Acne.

Oxy Skin Wash Reckitt & Colman, Austral.
Triclosan (p.1159·2).
Acne; skin cleanser.

Oxyboldine Cooperation Pharmaceutique, Fr.
Boldine (p.1585·3); anhydrous sodium sulfate (p.1250·1); monobasic sodium phosphate (p.1193·2).
Dyspepsia.

Oxybugamma Worwag, Ger.
Oxybutynin hydrochloride (p.471·2).
Bladder instability; urinary incontinence.

Oxybuton Kanoldt, Ger.
Oxybutynin hydrochloride (p.471·2).
Bladder instability; urinary incontinence.

Oxybutyn ICN, Canad.
Oxybutynin hydrochloride (p.471·2).

Oxy-Care Agepha, Aust.
Hydrogen peroxide (p.1147·1); sodium chloride (p.1196·1).
Disinfecting, cleaning, and storage solution for hard and soft contact lenses.

Oxycel
Associated Hospital Supply, UK; Becton Dickinson, USA.
Oxidised cellulose (p.728·1).
Bleeding in surgical procedures.

Oxycline *General Drugs, Thai.*
Oxytetracycline hydrochloride (p.234·1).
Bacterial infections.

Oxycocet *Technilab, Canad.*
Oxycodone hydrochloride (p.70·2); paracetamol (p.71·2).
Fever; pain.

Oxycod *Rafa, Israel.*
Oxycodone hydrochloride (p.70·2).
Pain.

Oxycodan *Technilab, Canad.*
Oxycodone hydrochloride (p.70·2); aspirin (p.14·2).
Fever; inflammation; pain.

Oxycontin
Mundipharma, Austral.; Purdue Frederick, Canad.; Norpharma, Denm.; Mundipharma, Fin.; Napp, Irl.; Rafa, Israel; Asofarma, Mex.; Mundipharma, Swed.; Napp, UK; Purdue Frederick, USA.
Oxycodone hydrochloride (p.70·2).
Pain.

Oxyderm *ICN, Canad.*
Benzoyl peroxide (p.1111·1).
Hyperkeratosis.

Oxydermine *Wild, Switz.*
Zinc oxide (p.1128·2); lauromacrogol 400 (p.1345·2).
Burns; skin disorders; wounds.

Oxydess II *Vortech, USA†.*
Dexamfetamine sulfate (p.1507·3).
Attention deficit disorder with hyperactivity; narcoleptic syndrome; obesity.

Oxyfan *Coli, Ital.†.*
Oxitriptan (p.302·2).
Depression; nervous system disorders.

Oxyfast *Purdue Frederick, USA.*
Oxycodone hydrochloride (p.70·2).
Pain.

Oxyflux *Rayere, Mex.*
Clenbuterol (p.763·3).

Oxygeron
Boehringer Mannheim, Aust.†; Drossapharm, Switz.; Willpharma, Thai.
Vincamine (p.1680·1).
Cerebrovascular disorders; circulatory eye disorders; dizziness; headache; migraine.

Oxygesic *Mundipharma, Ger.*
Oxycodone hydrochloride (p.70·2).
Pain.

Oxygirex *Irex, Fr.*
Trimetazidine hydrochloride (p.987·3).
Angina pectoris; vascular eye disorders; vestibular disorders.

OxyIR *Purdue Frederick, USA.*
Oxycodone hydrochloride (p.70·2).
Pain.

Oxylim
Atlantic, Hong Kong; Atlantic, Singapore; Atlantic, Thai.
Oxytetracycline (p.234·1) or oxytetracycline hydrochloride (p.234·1).
Bacterial infections.

Oxylin
Allergan, Hong Kong; Allergan, Israel; Allergan, Mex.; Allergan, Port.; Allergan, S.Afr.; Allergan, Singapore; Allergan, Thai.
Oxymetazoline hydrochloride (p.1096·2).
Conjunctivitis; eye irritation.

Oxylin Liquifilm *Allergan, Neth.†.*
Oxymetazoline hydrochloride (p.1096·2).
Conjunctival irritation.

Oxymedin *Kade, Ger.*
Oxybutynin hydrochloride (p.471·2).
Neurogenic bladder; urinary incontinence.

Oxymet *Greater Pharma, Thai.*
Oxymetazoline hydrochloride (p.1096·2).
Nasal congestion; nasopharyngitis; rhinitis; sinusitis.

Oxymycin
Lennon, S.Afr.†; DDSA Pharmaceuticals, UK.
Oxytetracycline (p.234·1) or oxytetracycline hydrochloride (p.234·1).
Bacterial infections.

Oxyno *Milano, Thai.*
Oxyphencyclimine hydrochloride (p.472·1).
Gastrointestinal disorders; genito-urinary disorders.

Oxynorm
Mundipharma, Austral.; Norpharma, Denm.; Mundipharma, Fin.; Napp, Irl.; Mundipharma, Swed.; Napp, UK.
Oxycodone hydrochloride (p.70·2).
Pain.

Oxypan *Propan, S.Afr.*
Oxytetracycline hydrochloride (p.234·1).
Bacterial infections.

Oxypangam *Lichtenstein, Ger.*
Di-isopropylammonium dichloroacetate (p.874·3).
Hypoxia due to circulatory disorders.

Oxyperol *Lemoine, Fr.*
Peru balsam (p.1650·2); zinc oxide (p.1128·2).
Skin irritation.

Oxyplastine
Note.This name is used for preparations of different composition.
Bournonville, Belg.†.
Zinc oxide (p.1128·2); peru balsam (p.1650·2); calcium hydroxide (p.1588·3).
Barrier cream; skin disorders.

Parke, Davis, Fr.; Wild, Switz.
Zinc oxide (p.1128·2).
Skin disorders.

Oxyprenix *Ashbourne, UK†.*
Oxprenolol hydrochloride (p.951·3).
Angina pectoris; anxiety; hypertension.

Oxysept
Note.This name is used for preparations of different composition.
Allergan, Aust.†; Allergan, Israel.
Oxysept 1 solution, hydrogen peroxide (p.1147·1); Oxysept 2 solution, catalase (p.1592·2)(p.1129·2).
Disinfecting, neutralising, rinsing, and storage system for soft contact lenses.

Allergan, Austral.; Allergan, NZ.
Oxysept 1, hydrogen peroxide (p.1147·1); Oxysept 2, irrigating, neutralising, and storage solution (p.1129·2).
Disinfecting, rinsing, and storage system for soft contact lenses.

Allergan-Frumtost, Braz.; Allergan, USA.
Hydrogen peroxide (p.1147·1) (p.1129·2).
Disinfecting solution for soft contact lenses.

Allergan, Canad.
Cleaning and disinfecting solution for soft contact lenses (p.1129·2).

Allergan, Ger.†.
Oxysept 1, hydrogen peroxide (p.1147·1); Oxysept 2, disodium edetate (p.1008·1)(p.1129·2).
Disinfecting and neutralising system for soft contact lenses.

Allergan, Port.
Contact lens care solution (p.1129·2).

Oxysept Comfort
Allergan, Aust.†.; Allergan, Ger.†.
Solution, hydrogen peroxide (p.1147·1); tablets, catalase (p.1592·2) (p.1129·2).
Disinfecting and neutralising system for soft contact lenses.

Oxysept Quick *Allergan, Aust.†.*
Catalase (p.1592·2) (p.1129·2).
Neutralising tablet for soft contact lenses.

Oxytetral
Alpharma, Denm.; Alpharma, Norw.; Dumex-Alpharma, Swed.
Oxytetracycline hydrochloride (p.234·1).
Bacterial infections.

Oxytetramix *Ashbourne, UK.*
Oxytetracycline (p.234·1).
Bacterial infections.

Oxythyol *Richard, Fr.*
Zinc oxide (p.1128·2); ichthammol (p.1115·2).
Skin irritation.

Oxyzal *Gordon, USA.*
Hydroxyquinoline sulfate (p.1622·2); benzalkonium chloride (p.1133·2).
Minor skin infections.

Oyo *Polypharm, Ger.*
Sodium pangamate (p.1647·3).
Cerebral and peripheral vascular disorders; ischaemic heart disease; migraine.

Oysco *Rugby, USA.*
Calcium carbonate (p.1215·1).
Calcium deficiency; dietary supplement.

Oysco D *Rugby, USA.*
Calcium with vitamin D (p.1350·1).
Calcium deficiency; dietary supplement.

Oyst-Cal *Goldline, USA.*
Calcium carbonate (p.1215·1).
Calcium deficiency; dietary supplement.

Oyst-Cal-D *Goldline, USA.*
Calcium with vitamin D (p.1350·1).
Calcium deficiency; dietary supplement.

Oyster Calcium *Nature's Bounty, USA.*
Calcium with vitamins A and D (p.1350·1).
Calcium deficiency; dietary supplement.

Oyster Calcium with Vitamin D *Nion, USA.*
Calcium with vitamin D (p.1350·1).
Calcium deficiency; dietary supplement.

Oyster Shell Calcium *Vangard, USA.*
Calcium carbonate (p.1215·1).
Calcium deficiency; dietary supplement.

Oyster Shell Calcium with Vitamin D *Major, USA.*
Calcium with vitamin D (p.1350·1).
Calcium deficiency; dietary supplement.

Oystercal *Nature's Bounty, USA.*
Calcium carbonate (p.1215·1).
Calcium deficiency; dietary supplement.

Oystercal-D *Nature's Bounty, USA.*
Calcium with vitamin D (p.1350·1).
Calcium deficiency; dietary supplement.

Oz *Aleph, Ital.*
Zinc oxide (p.1128·2).
Skin disorders.

Ozex *Toyama, Jpn.*
Tosufloxacin tosilate (p.264·2).
Bacterial infections.

Ozidia *Pfizer, Fr.*
Glipizide (p.322·3).
Diabetes mellitus.

Ozoken *Kener, Mex.*
Omeprazole (p.1239·1).

Ozonol
Note.This name is used for preparations of different composition.
Bayer, Canad.
Phenol (p.1152·3); zinc oxide (p.1128·2).
Bites and stings; burns; cuts; skin irritation.

Sterling, Port.
Ibuprofen (p.43·2).

Ozonol Antibiotic Plus *Bayer, Canad.*
Polymyxin B (p.238·3); bacitracin (p.155·2); lignocaine [lidocaine] hydrochloride (p.1313·2).
Minor cuts and burns; skin irritation.

Ozonyl *Gross, Braz.*
Diphenhydramine (p.416·1); ammonium chloride (p.1085·2); sodium camsilate; guaifenesin (p.1092·2); eucalyptol (p.1609·2); niaouli oil (p.1640·2); menthol (p.1632·3).
Respiratory-tract congestion.

Ozopulmin *Geymonat, Ital.*
Injection: Verbenone.

Suppositories: Verbenone; pine oil.
Respiratory-system disorders.

Ozopulmin G *Geymonat, Ital.*
Suppositories: Verbenone; pine oil.
Respiratory system disorders.

Syrup: Verbenone; dextromethorphan hydrobromide (p.1087·3).
Coughs.

Topical gel: Verbenone.
Respiratory system disorders.

Ozothin *SmithKline Beecham, Ger.*
Injection; inhalation: Oxidation product of turpentine oil "Landes" (p.1676·3); terpin hydrate (p.1101·2).
Respiratory-tract disorders.

Suppositories: Paracetamol (p.71·2); oxidation product of turpentine oil "Landes" (p.1676·3); oleum pini sylvestris.
Fever and pain associated with respiratory-tract disorders.

Tablets: Diprophylline (p.764·3); oxidation products of turpentine oil "Landes" (p.1676·3).
Respiratory-tract disorders.

Ozothine *Laphal, Fr.*
Suppositories: Oxidation products of turpentine oil (p.1676·3).

Syrup: Oxidation products of turpentine oil (p.1676·3); sodium benzoate (p.1134·3).
Formerly contained oxidation products of turpentine oil, ethylmorphine hydrochloride, and sodium benzoate.
Respiratory-tract disorders.

Ozothine a la Diprophylline *Laphal, Fr.*
Oxidation products of turpentine oil (p.1676·3); diprophylline (p.764·1).
Respiratory-tract disorders.

Ozovit
Koch, Aust.; Pascoe, Ger.
Magnesium peroxide (p.1149·3).
Gastrointestinal disorders.

Ozym
Note.This name is used for preparations of different composition.
Procter & Gamble, Aust.†.
Amylase from *Aspergillus oryzae* (p.1579·3); papain (p.1647·3); fel suis (p.1585·1); pancreatin (p.1646·1).
Gastrointestinal disorders.

Trommsdorff, Ger.
Pancreatin (p.1646·1).
Pancreatic insufficiency.

P & S
Note.This name is used for preparations of different composition.
Baker Cummins, Canad.; Baker Cummins, USA.
Scalp application: Liquid phenol (p.1152·3).
Psoriasis; seborrhoeic dermatitis.

Baker Cummins, Canad.; Baker Cummins, USA.
Shampoo: Salicylic acid (p.1122·3).
Psoriasis; seborrhoea.

P & S Plus
Baker Cummins, Canad.; Baker Cummins, USA.
Coal tar (p.1125·1); salicylic acid (p.1122·3).
Psoriasis; seborrhoeic dermatitis.

P. Veinos *Augot, Fr.†.*
Aesculus (p.1574·1); cupressus sempervirens; hamamelis (p.1618·3).
Peripheral vascular disorders.

Pabafilm
Note.This name is used for preparations of different composition.
Alcon, Braz.
SPF 10; SPF 15: Padimate O (p.1518·2); benzophenone-6 (p.1517·1).
Sunscreen.

Galderma, Mex.
SPF10; SPF15: Padimate O (p.1518·2); oxybenzone (p.1518·1).
Sunscreen.

Pabalate *Robins, USA†.*
Sodium salicylate (p.84·2); sodium aminobenzoate.
Pain.

Pabanox *Surya, Singapore.*
Oxybenzone (p.1518·1); dioxybenzone (p.1517·2); padimate O (p.1518·2); titanium dioxide (p.1126·1).
Sunscreen.

Pabasol *Galderma, Mex.*
Padimate O (p.1518·2); oxybenzone (p.1518·1).
Sunscreen.

Pabasun *Alpharma, Fr.*
Aminobenzoic acid (p.1516·3).
Sunscreen.

Pabrinex
Link, Irl.; Link, UK.
Vitamin B and C substances (p.1350·1).
Vitamin deficiency.

P-A-C *Upjohn, USA.*
Aspirin (p.14·2); caffeine (p.761·3).
Pain.

Pac Merieux *Pasteur Merieux, Ger.*
An acellular pertussis vaccine (p.1555·3).
Active immunisation.

Pacaps *Lunsco, USA.*
Butalbital (p.658·3); caffeine (p.761·3); paracetamol (p.71·2).

Paceco *Malaysia Chemist, Singapore.*
Codeine phosphate (p.25·2); paracetamol (p.71·2).
Cold symptoms; fever; pain.

Paceflex *Gemballa, Braz.*
Carisoprodol (p.1327·1); paracetamol (p.71·2); caffeine (p.761·3).
Skeletal muscle spasm.

Pacemol
Gemballa, Braz.; Malaysia Chemist, Singapore.
Paracetamol (p.71·2).
Fever; pain.

Pacerone *Upsher-Smith, USA.*
Amiodarone hydrochloride (p.836·1).
Ventricular arrhythmias.

Pacetal *Rekah, Israel.*
Phenobarbital (p.355·1); paracetamol (p.71·2).
Fever; pain.

Paceum *Orion, Switz.*
Diazepam (p.674·3).
Convulsions; non-psychotic mental disorders; premedication; skeletal muscle spasm; sleep disorders.

Pacifen *Pacific, NZ.*
Baclofen (p.1322·3).
Skeletal muscle spasm and spasticity.

Pacifene *Sussex, UK.*
Ibuprofen (p.43·2).
Fever; pain.

Pacifenity *Vitaplex, Austral.*
Passion flower (p.1649·1); mistletoe (p.1636·2); avena (p.1583·1); valerian (p.1678·3); gentian (p.1615·1); lupulus (p.1629·3); skullcap (p.1664·3); motherwort (p.1637·3).
Herbal relaxant.

Pacimol *Nat Druggists, S.Afr.*
Paracetamol (p.71·2).
Fever; pain.

Pacinol
Schering-Plough, Denm.; Schering-Plough, Fin.; Schering-Plough, Swed.
Fluphenazine hydrochloride (p.684·3).
Psychoses.

Pacinone *Schering-Plough, Port.*
Halazepam (p.686·2).

Pacis
Biochem, Canad.; Urocor, USA.
A BCG vaccine (p.1533·2).
Bladder cancer.

Pacisyn *Syntetic, Denm.*
Nitrazepam (p.695·2).
Epilepsy; insomnia.

Pacium *Urioch, Spain.*
Diazepam (p.674·3).
Contains pyridoxine hydrochloride.
Alcohol withdrawal syndrome; anxiety; febrile convulsions; insomnia; skeletal muscle spasm.

Pacofen *DHA, Singapore.*
Codeine phosphate (p.25·2); paracetamol (p.71·2); caffeine (p.761·3).
Pain.

Pacopan *Pharmasant, Thai.*
Hyoscine butylbromide (p.468·2); paracetamol (p.71·2).
Smooth muscle spasm.

Pactens *Merck, Mex.*
Naproxen sodium (p.61·1).
Inflammation; pain.

Padamin *Fresenius Kabi, Aust.*
Amino-acid infusion (p.1350·1).
Parenteral nutrition.

Paderyl *Gerda, Fr.*
Syrup: Codeine phosphate (p.25·2).
Formerly contained papaverine hydrobromide, codeine hydrobromide, cinnamaverine hydrochloride, belladonna, hyoscyamus, and mistletoe.

Tablets: Codeine phosphate (p.25·2).
Formerly contained papaverine hydrobromide, codeine hydrobromide, cinnamaverine hydrochloride, belladonna, hyoscyamus, hyssop, and valerian.
Coughs.

Padiacrom *Padia, Ger.*
Sodium cromoglicate (p.774·3).
Asthma.

Padiafusin
Fresenius Kabi, Aust.; Pharmacia Upjohn, Ger.
Electrolyte infusion with glucose (p.1180·1).
Carbohydrate source; fluid and electrolyte disorders.

Padiafusin OP *Pharmacia Upjohn, Ger.*
Potassium-free electrolyte infusion with glucose (p.1180·1).
Carbohydrate source; fluid and electrolyte disorders.

Padiamol *Padia, Ger.*
Salbutamol sulfate (p.770·3).
Obstructive airways disease.

Padiamuc *Padia, Ger.*
Ambroxol hydrochloride (p.1084·3).
Respiratory-tract disorders.

Padiatifen *Padia, Ger.*
Ketotifen fumarate (p.767·2).
Asthma; bronchitis; hypersensitivity disorders.

The symbol † denotes a preparation no longer actively marketed

Padiken *Kener, Mex.*
Amantadine hydrochloride (p.1161·2).

Padma 28
Padma, Switz.; Padma, UK.
Aegle sepiar fructus; amomi fructus; aquilegiae herba; calendula flos; cardamomi fructus; caryophylli flos; costi amari radix; hedychii rhizoma; lactucae sativae herba; lichen islandicus; liquiritiae radix; meliae tousand fructus; myrobalani fructus; plantaginis herba; polygoni herba; potentillae aureae herba; santali rubri lignum; sidae cordifoliae herba; aconiti tuber; valerianae radix; calcium sulfate; camphor.
Circulatory disorders.

Padma-Lax *Padma, Switz.*
Aloes (p.1210·1); kaolin (p.1229·3); calumba radix (p.1589·2); condurango (p.1599·1); enulae radix; gentian (p.1615·1); myrobalan; sodium bicarbonate (p.1186·2); anhydrous sodium sulfate (p.1250·1); piper longum; frangula bark (p.1227·1); cascara (p.1216·1); rhubarb (p.1248·1); nux vomica (p.1643·1); ginger (p.1227·2).
Constipation.

Padrin *Fujisawa, Jpn.*
Prifinium bromide (p.473·1).
Gastrointestinal spasm; urinary-tract spasm.

Padutin
Bayer, Aust.; Bayer, Ger.
Kallidinogenase (Kallikrein) (p.1625·3).
Male infertility.

Paedamin *Paedpharm, Austral.*
Diphenhydramine hydrochloride (p.416·1); phenylephrine hydrochloride (p.1097·1).
Upper respiratory-tract disorders.

Paedialgon *Chephasaar, Ger.*
Paracetamol (p.71·2).
Fever; pain.

Paediasure *Abbott, Irl.; Abbott Nutrition, UK.*
Preparation for enteral nutrition (p.1350·1).

Paediathrocin *Abbott, Ger.*
Erythromycin (p.201·2) or erythromycin ethyl succinate (p.201·2).
Bacterial infections.

Paediatric Seravit
Scientific Hospital Supplies, Austral.; Scientific Hospital Supplies, UK.
Multivitamin and mineral preparation (p.1350·1).
Dietary supplement; metabolic disorders.

Paedisup *Chephasaar, Ger.*
Paracetamol (p.71·2); doxylamine succinate (p.417·1).
Fever; pain.

Paf *Lofarma, Ital.*
Bucarbetene.
Scabies.

Paftec *Boehringer Ingelheim, Port.*
Flunisolide (p.1070·3).
Asthma.

Pahtlisan *Bioquimico, Mex.*
Chlorothiazide (p.856·3).

Paididont *Metochem, Aust.*
Chamomile (p.1593·2); cetylpyridinium chloride (p.1138·1); lauromacrogol 400 (p.1345·2).
Teething pain.

Paidocin *Chiesi, Ital.*
Rokitamycin (p.247·1).
Bacterial infections.

Paidoflor *Ardeypharm, Ger.*
Lactobacillus acidophilus (p.1626·3).
Gastrointestinal disorders.

Paidomal *Malesci, Ital.*
Lysine theophyllinate (p.783·2).
Obstructive airways disease.

Paidorinovit *SIT, Ital.*
Ephedrine (p.1090·1); eucalyptol (p.1609·2); niaouli oil (p.1640·2).
Nasal congestion.

Paidoterin Descongestivo NF *Aldo, Spain.*
Chlorpheniramine [chlorphenamine] maleate (p.412·1); diphenhydramine hydrochloride (p.416·1); phenylephrine hydrochloride (p.1097·1).
Formerly known as Paidoterin Descongestivo and contained chlorpheniramine [chlorphenamine] maleate, diphenhydramine, phenylephrine hydrochloride, guaifenesin, choline salicylate, and sodium citrate.
Upper-respiratory-tract congestion.

Paidozim *Juventus, Spain.*
Amylase (p.1579·3); cellulase (p.1593·1); lipase; metoclopramide (p.1236·3); protease.
Digestive enzyme insufficiency; dyspepsia.

Paigastrol *Orravan, Spain†.*
Pancreatin (p.1646·1); pepsin (p.1649·3).
Digestive enzyme insufficiency.

Pain X *Ascher, USA†.*
Capsaicin (p.23·1); menthol (p.1632·3); camphor (p.1589·3).
Pain.

Pain Aid *Zee, Canad.*
Aspirin (p.14·2); caffeine (p.761·3).

Pain Aid Free *Zee, Canad.*
Paracetamol (p.71·2).

Pain Buster *Prodemdis, Canad.*
Methyl salicylate (p.55·1); camphor (p.1589·3); menthol (p.1632·3); eucalyptus oil (p.1609·2).

Pain Bust-R II *Continental, USA.*
Methyl salicylate (p.55·1); menthol (p.1632·3).
Musculoskeletal and joint disorders.

Pain Doctor *Fougera, USA.*
Capsaicin (p.23·1); methyl salicylate (p.55·1); menthol (p.1632·3).
Pain.

Pain And Fever Relief *Brauer, Austral.*
Homoeopathic preparation.

Pain Gel Plus *Mentholatum, USA†.*
Menthol (p.1632·3).
Pain.

Pain Patch *Mentholatum, USA†.*
Menthol (p.1632·3).
Musculoskeletal and joint pain.

Pain Relief Syrup for Children *Unichem, UK.*
Paracetamol (p.71·2).
Fever; pain.

Pain Reliever *Rugby, USA†.*
Paracetamol (p.71·2); aspirin (p.14·2); caffeine (p.761·3).
Pain.

Pain Relieving Ointment *Jamieson, Canad.*
Camphor (p.1589·3); menthol (p.1632·3); mentha arvensis; cajeput oil; cinnamon oil; clove oil.

Painagon *Be-Tabs, S.Afr.*
Syrup: Paracetamol (p.71·2); codeine phosphate (p.25·2); promethazine hydrochloride (p.423·2).
Fever; pain.
Tablets: Paracetamol (p.71·2); codeine phosphate (p.25·2); meprobamate (p.691·1); caffeine (p.761·3).
Pain; pain associated with tension.

Painamol *Be-Tabs, S.Afr.*
Paracetamol (p.71·2).
Fever; pain.

Painamol Plus *Be-Tabs, S.Afr.*
Paracetamol (p.71·2); codeine phosphate (p.25·2).
Fever; pain.

Paincod *Crown, S.Afr.*
Aspirin (p.14·2); paracetamol (p.71·2); codeine phosphate (p.25·2).

Painex *Confar, Port.*
Diclofenac sodium (p.30·3).
Inflammation; musculoskeletal, joint, and peri-articular disorders; pain.

Painnox *Charoen, Thai.*
Mefenamic acid (p.51·2).
Inflammation; pain.

Painrite *Columbia, S.Afr.†.*
Paracetamol (p.71·2); codeine phosphate (p.25·2); caffeine (p.761·3); meprobamate (p.691·1).
Pain and associated tension.

Painrite SA *Columbia, S.Afr.†.*
Paracetamol (p.71·2); codeine phosphate (p.25·2).
Fever; pain.

Pains-of *Eagle, Austral.*
Multivitamin and amino acid preparation (p.1350·1).
Pain.

Painstop *Paedpharm, Austral.*
Paracetamol (p.71·2); promethazine hydrochloride (p.423·2); codeine phosphate (p.25·2).
Pain.

Painza *Siam Bheasach, Thai.*
Methyl salicylate (p.55·1); menthol (p.1632·3); eugenol (p.1609·3).
Musculoskeletal pain.

Palacos
Schering-Plough, Neth.; Essex, Switz.†.
Methylmethacrylate/methylacrylate copolymer (p.1635·2).
Bone cement for orthopaedic surgery.

Palacos avec Garamycin *Essex, Switz.†.*
Methylmethacrylate co-polymer (p.1635·2); gentamicin sulfate (p.210·1).
Bone cement for orthopaedic surgery.

Palacos cum Gentamicin
Schering-Plough, Denm.; Schering-Plough, Norw.†; Schering-Plough, Swed.†.
Methylmethacrylate/methacrylate copolymer (p.1635·2); gentamicin sulfate (p.210·1).
Bone cement for orthopaedic surgery.

Palacos E with Garamycin *Schering-Plough, Austral.*
Methylmethacrylate methyl acrylate copolymer (p.1635·2); gentamicin sulfate (p.210·1).
Bone cement for orthopaedic surgery.

Palacos with Garamycin *Schering-Plough, NZ.*
Methylmethacrylate/methylacrylate copolymer (p.1635·2); gentamicin sulfate (p.210·1).
Bone cement for orthopaedic surgery.

Palacos LV avec Gentamicine *Schering-Plough, Fr.*
Methylmethacrylate/methacrylate copolymer (p.1635·2); gentamicin sulfate (p.210·1).
Bone cement for orthopaedic surgery.

Palacos LV with Gentamicin *Schering-Plough, UK.*
Methylmethacrylate/methylacrylate copolymer (p.1635·2); gentamicin sulfate (p.210·1).
Bone cement for orthopaedic surgery.

Palacos met gentamicine *Schering-Plough, Neth.*
Methylmethacrylate/methylacrylate copolymer (p.1635·2); gentamicin sulfate (p.210·1).
Bone cement for orthopaedic surgery.

Palacos R
Merck, Ger.; Schering-Plough, Port.†; Merck, Singapore; Merck, Thai.; Schering-Plough, UK.
Methylmethacrylate/methylacrylate copolymer (p.1635·2).
Bone cement for orthopaedic surgery.

Palacos R avec Gentamicine
Schering-Plough, Belg.; Schering-Plough, Fr.
Methylmethacrylate/methylacrylate copolymer (p.1635·2); gentamicin sulfate (p.210·1).
Bone cement for orthopaedic surgery.

Palacos R com Gentamicina *Schering-Plough, Port.†.*
Methylmethacrylate/methylacrylate copolymer (p.1635·2); gentamicin sulfate (p.210·1).
Bone cement.

Palacos R cum Gentamicin *Schering-Plough, Fin.*
Methylmethacrylate/methylacrylate copolymer (p.1635·2); gentamicin sulfate (p.210·1).
Bone cement for orthopaedic surgery.

Palacos R with Garamycin
Schering-Plough, Austral.; Schering-Plough, S.Afr.
Methylmethacrylate/methylacrylate copolymer (p.1635·2); gentamicin sulfate (p.210·1).
Bone cement for orthopaedic surgery.

Palacos R with Gentamicin
Schering-Plough, Irl.; Schering-Plough, UK.
Methylmethacrylate/methylacrylate copolymer (p.1635·2); gentamicin sulfate (p.210·1).
Bone cement for orthopaedic surgery.

Palacril *Warner-Lambert, Ger.*
Diphenhydramine hydrochloride (p.416·1); zinc oxide (p.1128·2).
Skin disorders.

Palafer *SmithKline Beecham, Canad.*
Ferrous fumarate (p.1360·1).
Iron deficiency; iron supplement; iron-deficiency anaemias.

Palafer CF *SmithKline Beecham, Canad.*
Ferrous fumarate (p.1360·1); folic acid (p.1361·1).
Ascorbic acid (p.1389·3) is included in this preparation to increase the absorption and availability of iron.
Prenatal supplement.

Palane *Cryopharma, Mex.*
Enalapril maleate (p.883·3).
Heart failure; hypertension.

Palaprin *Roche, Aust.*
Aloxiprin (p.13·2).
Pain.

Palatol *Pascoe, Ger.*
Peppermint oil (p.1243·3); niaouli oil (p.1640·2); cajuput oil (p.1588·1); eucalyptus oil (p.1609·2).
Catarrh.

Palatol N *Pascoe, Ger.*
Eucalyptus oil (p.1609·2); peppermint oil (p.1243·3); niaouli oil (p.1640·2); cajuput oil (p.1588·1); hamamelis (p.1618·3).
Catarrh.

Palcid *Pharmadica, Thai.*
Cisapride (p.1220·1).
Dyspepsia; gastro-oesophageal reflux; gastroparesis.

Palcol *Jofrain, Mex.*
Chloramphenicol (p.179·1).
Bacterial infections.

Paldesic *Rosemont, UK.*
Paracetamol (p.71·2).
Fever; pain.

Paleodina *Liferpal, Mex.*
Dipyrone (p.34·1).
Pain.

Palfium
Faulding, Austral.; Janssen-Cilag, Belg.†; Synthelabo, Fr.†; Antigen, Irl.; Asta Medica, Neth.; Roche, UK.
Dextromoramide tartrate (p.26·3).
Pain.

Palgic DS *Pan American, USA.*
Carbinoxamine maleate (p.411·1); pseudoephedrine hydrochloride (p.1099·2).
Rhinitis.

Palgic-D *Pan American, USA.*
Pseudoephedrine hydrochloride (p.1099·2); carbinoxamine maleate (p.411·1).
Upper respiratory-tract disorders.

Paliuryl *Richelet, Fr.*
Rhamnus paliurus.
Stimulation of renal water excretion.

Palladon *Mundipharma, Ger.*
Hydromorphone hydrochloride (p.42·3).
Pain.

Palladone
Napp, Irl.; Rafa, Israel; Napp, UK; Purdue Frederick, USA.
Hydromorphone hydrochloride (p.42·3).
Pain.

Pallia *SmithKline Beecham, Hong Kong.*
Cimetidine (p.1216·3).
Gastro-oesophageal reflux; peptic ulcer.

Pallidan *Berna, Spain†.*
Methaqualone (p.691·3).
Insomnia.

Pallidone *Douglas, NZ.*
Methadone hydrochloride (p.53·1).
Opioid dependence; pain.

Palmi *Medecine Vegetale, Fr.†.*
Boldo (p.1585·3); kinkeliba (p.1626·1); gentian (p.1615·1).
Digestive disorders.

Palmiclor *Universales, Mex.*
Chloramphenicol (p.179·1).
Bacterial infections.

Palmicol *Riemser, Ger.*
Heavy magnesium carbonate (p.1232·3).
Gastrointestinal disorders; magnesium deficiency.

Palmiffer *Reuffer, Mex.*
Chloramphenicol (p.179·1).
Bacterial infections.

Palmil *Cantabria, Spain.*
Castor oil (p.1592·1).
Bowel evacuation.

Palmisan *Hotz, Ger.*
Homoeopathic preparation.

Palmisol *Parggon, Mex.*
Chloramphenicol (p.179·1).
Bacterial infections.

Palmitate-A *Akorn, USA.*
Vitamin A (p.1382·1).

Palmolive UV *Palmolive Skincare, Austral.†.*
Octinoxate (p.1517·3); octisalate (p.1518·1); octocrilene (p.1518·1); avobenzone (p.1517·3).
Sunscreen.

Palon *Unison, Thai.*
Propranolol hydrochloride (p.962·3).
Angina pectoris; arrhythmias; hypertension; tremor.

Palpipax *Parke, Davis, Fr.*
Meprobamate (p.691·1); valerian (p.1678·3).
Formerly contained sparteine sulfate and meprobamate.
Nervous disorders.

Pals *Glenwood, USA.*
Chlorophyllin copper complex (p.1028·1).
Odour control in ostomy and incontinent patients.

Paludil *Farmoquimica, Braz.*
Quinine (p.445·1); methylene blue [methylthioninium chloride] (p.1012·3).
Babesiosis; leg cramps; malaria.

Paludrin *Zeneca, Israel.*
Proguanil hydrochloride (p.441·3).
Malaria.

Paludrine
Zeneca, Aust.; Zeneca, Austral.; Zeneca, Belg.; Wyeth-Ayerst, Canad.; Zeneca, Denm.; AstraZeneca, Fin.; AstraZeneca, Fr.; Zeneca, Ger.; Zeneca, Irl.; Zeneca, Ital.; Zeneca, Neth.; AstraZeneca, Norw.; AstraZeneca, NZ; Zeneca, Port.; Zeneca, S.Afr.; AstraZeneca, Singapore; Zeneca, Swed.; Zeneca, Switz.; AstraZeneca, UK.
Proguanil hydrochloride (p.441·3).
Malaria.

Paluken *Kener, Mex.*
Chloroquine (p.432·2).

Paluquina *Quimioterapica, Braz.*
Quinine (p.445·1).
Babesiosis; leg cramps; malaria.

Paluther *Rhone-Poulenc Rorer, Fr.*
Artemether (p.431·2).
Malaria.

Palux *Sanus, Braz.*
Chloroquine phosphate (p.432·3).
Hepatic amoebiasis; juvenile arthritis; lupus erythematosus; malaria; rheumatoid arthritis; solar urticaria.

Pamba *OPW, Ger.*
Aminomethylbenzoic acid (p.725·2).
Haemorrhage.

Pamecil
Medochemie, Hong Kong; Medochemie, Singapore.
Ampicillin (p.150·3) or ampicillin sodium (p.150·3).
Bacterial infections.

Pamedox *Medochemie, Hong Kong.*
Ampicillin trihydrate (p.151·1); cloxacillin sodium (p.192·1).
Bacterial infections.

Pamelor
Novartis, Braz.; Novartis, USA.
Nortriptyline hydrochloride (p.301·3).
Depression; narcoleptic syndrome; pain; panic disorder.

Pamergan *Cristalia, Braz.*
Promethazine hydrochloride (p.423·2).
Hypersensitivity reactions; insomnia; nausea and vomiting; pain; premedication; sedative.

Pamergan P100 *Martindale Pharmaceuticals, UK.*
Pethidine hydrochloride (p.75·1); promethazine hydrochloride (p.423·2).
NOTE. There is no connection between Martindale, The Complete Drug Reference and Martindale Pharmaceuticals.
Pain; premedication.

Pameton *SmithKline Beecham, UK†.*
Paracetamol (p.71·2); DL-methionine (p.1012·2).
These ingredients can be described by the British Approved Name Co-methiamol.
Fever; pain.

Pamid *CTI, Israel.*
Indapamide (p.913·1).
Hypertension; oedema.

Pamine *Kenwood, USA.*
Hyoscine methobromide (p.468·2).
Peptic ulcer (adjunct).

Pamocil *Uno, Ital.*
Amoxicillin trihydrate (p.149·2).
Bacterial infections.

Pamol
Nycomed, Denm.; Nycomed, Norw.; Warner-Lambert, NZ; Docmed, S.Afr.†.
Paracetamol (p.71·2).
Fever; pain.

Pamoxan *Uriach, Spain.*
Pyrvinium embonate (p.108·2).
Worm infections.

Pamprin
Chattem, Canad.; Chattem, USA.
Paracetamol (p.71·2); pamabrom (p.952·1); mepyramine maleate (p.421·1).
Pain; premenstrual syndrome.

Pan C *Freeda, USA.*
Hesperidin (p.1611·2); citrus bioflavonoids complex (p.1611·1); vitamin C (p.1389·3).
Capillary bleeding.

Panacef *Lilly, Ital.*
Cefaclor (p.161·1).
Bacterial infections.

Panacet *ECR, USA.*
Hydrocodone tartrate (p.42·2); paracetamol (p.71·2).

Panacod *Sanofi Winthrop, Fin.*
Paracetamol (p.71·2); codeine phosphate (p.25·2).
Pain.

Panacrearell *Sanorell, Ger.*
Homoeopathic preparation.

Panadeine
Note. This name is used for preparations of different composition.
Sanofi Synthelabo, Austral.; SmithKline Beecham Consumer, Austral.; Sanofi Winthrop, Hong Kong; SmithKline Beecham Consumer, Irl.; SmithKline Beecham, NZ; Sanofi Synthelabo, Singapore; Sterling Health, UK†.
Paracetamol (p.71·2); codeine phosphate (p.25·2).
Formerly known as Panadeine Co in the *UK.*
These ingredients can be described by the British Approved Name Co-codamol.
Fever; pain.

SmithKline Beecham, Belg.
Paracetamol (p.71·2); caffeine (p.761·3); codeine phosphate (p.25·2).
Fever; pain.

Panadeine Plus *SmithKline Beecham Consumer, Austral.*
Paracetamol (p.71·2); codeine phosphate (p.25·2); doxylamine succinate (p.417·1).
Fever; pain.

Panado *Restan, S.Afr.*
Paracetamol (p.71·2).
Fever; pain.

Panado-Co *Restan, S.Afr.*
Paracetamol (p.71·2); codeine phosphate (p.25·2).
Fever; pain.

Panadol
SmithKline Beecham Consumer, Austral.; SmithKline Beecham, Belg.; SmithKline Beecham Consumer, Canad.; SmithKline Beecham, Fin.; SmithKline Beecham Sante, Fr.; SmithKline Beecham, Hong Kong; SmithKline Beecham Consumer, Irl.; Maggioni, Ital.; SmithKline Beecham, Mex.; SmithKline Beecham Consumer, Neth.; SmithKline Beecham, NZ; Sterling, Port.; SmithKline Beecham, Singapore; SmithKline Beecham, Spain; SmithKline Beecham Consumer, Switz.; Sterling, Thai.; SmithKline Beecham Consumer, UK; Glenbrook, USA; Sterling Health, USA.
Paracetamol (p.71·2).
Fever; pain.

Panadol Allergy Sinus *SmithKline Beecham Consumer, Austral.*
Paracetamol (p.71·2); pseudoephedrine hydrochloride (p.1099·2); chlorpheniramine [chlorphenamine] maleate (p.412·1).
Allergic symptoms; pain; sinus congestion.

Panadol Children's Cold *SmithKline Beecham Consumer, Austral.*
Paracetamol (p.71·2); pseudoephedrine hydrochloride (p.1099·2); chlorpheniramine [chlorphenamine] maleate (p.412·1).
Cold symptoms; fever; pain.

Panadol Codeine
SmithKline Beecham, Belg.; SmithKline Beecham Sante, Fr.†.
Paracetamol (p.71·2); codeine phosphate (p.25·2).
Fever; pain.

Panadol Cold and Flu
Note. This name is used for preparations of different composition.
SmithKline Beecham Consumer, Austral.
Paracetamol (p.71·2); pseudoephedrine hydrochloride (p.1099·2); dextromethorphan hydrobromide (p.1087·3).
Cold and influenza symptoms.

SmithKline Beecham, Hong Kong.
Paracetamol (p.71·2); vitamin C (p.1389·3); phenylephrine hydrochloride (p.1097·1); noscapine (p.1096·1); caffeine (p.761·3); terpin hydrate (p.1101·2).
Cold and influenza symptoms.

Panadol for Cold & Flu *SmithKline Beecham, Singapore.*
Dextromethorphan hydrobromide (p.1087·3); pseudoephedrine hydrochloride (p.1099·2); paracetamol (p.71·2).
Cold and influenza symptoms.

Panadol for Cold Relief *SmithKline Beecham, Singapore.*
Pseudoephedrine hydrochloride (p.1099·2); paracetamol (p.71·2).
Cold and influenza symptoms.

Panadol Comp *SmithKline Beecham, Fin.*
Paracetamol (p.71·2); caffeine (p.761·3).
Fever; pain.

Panadol Elixir with Promethazine *SmithKline Beecham Consumer, Austral.†.*
Paracetamol (p.71·2); promethazine hydrochloride (p.423·2).
Fever; pain.

Panadol Extra
SmithKline Beecham, Hong Kong; SmithKline Beecham Consumer, Irl.; SmithKline Beecham, Singapore; SmithKline Beecham Consumer, UK.
Paracetamol (p.71·2); caffeine (p.761·3).
Fever; pain.

Panadol Hot *SmithKline Beecham, Fin.*
Paracetamol (p.71·2); menthol (p.1632·3).
Cold and influenza symptoms; fever; pain.

Panadol Night
SmithKline Beecham Consumer, Austral.; SmithKline Beecham Consumer, Irl.; SmithKline Beecham, NZ; SmithKline Beecham Consumer, UK.
Paracetamol (p.71·2); diphenhydramine hydrochloride (p.416·1).
Insomnia; pain.

Panadol Plus *SmithKline Beecham Consumer, Neth.*
Paracetamol (p.71·2); caffeine (p.761·3).
Fever; pain.

Panadol Sinus *SmithKline Beecham Consumer, Austral.*
Paracetamol (p.71·2); pseudoephedrine hydrochloride (p.1099·2).
Pain; sinus congestion.

Panadol Sinus Day/Night *SmithKline Beecham Consumer, Austral.*
Day caplets, paracetamol (p.71·2); pseudoephedrine hydrochloride (p.1099·2); night caplets, paracetamol; pseudoephedrine hydrochloride; chlorpheniramine [chlorphenamine] maleate (p.412·1).
Cold symptoms; fever.

Panadol Ultra *SmithKline Beecham Consumer, UK.*
Paracetamol (p.71·2); codeine phosphate (p.25·2). These ingredients can be described by the British Approved Name Co-codamol.
Pain.

Panadol-C *SmithKline Beecham Consumer, Switz.*
Paracetamol (p.71·2); ascorbic acid (p.1389·3).
Cold symptoms.

Panafcort
Rhone-Poulenc Rorer, Austral.; Propan, S.Afr.
Prednisone (p.1079·2).
Corticosteroid.

Panafcortelone
Rhone-Poulenc Rorer, Austral.; Fisons, Hong Kong.
Prednisolone (p.1077·3).
Corticosteroid.

Panafen *SmithKline Beecham, NZ.*
Ibuprofen (p.43·2).
Musculoskeletal and joint disorders; pain.

Panafil *Healthpoint, USA.*
Papain (p.1647·3); urea (p.1127·3); chlorophyllin copper complex sodium (p.1028·1).
Burns; ulcers; wounds.

Panafil-White *Rystan, USA.*
Papain (p.1647·3); urea (p.1127·3).
Burns; ulcers; wounds.

Panaflu *Malaysia Chemist, Singapore.*
Chlorpheniramine [chlorphenamine] maleate (p.412·1); paracetamol (p.71·2); phenylpropanolamine hydrochloride (p.1098·1).
Cold and influenza symptoms.

Panaflu Plus *Malaysia Chemist, Singapore.*
Chlorpheniramine [chlorphenamine] maleate (p.412·1); paracetamol (p.71·2); phenylpropanolamine hydrochloride (p.1098·1); caffeine (p.761·3).
Cold and influenza symptoms.

Panaleve *Pinewood, UK.*
Paracetamol (p.71·2).
Fever; pain.

Panalgesic *Sanofi Synthelabo, Austral.*
Paracetamol (p.71·2); codeine phosphate (p.25·2); doxylamine succinate (p.417·1).
Pain with agitation.

Panalgesic Gold *ECR, USA.*
Cream: Methyl salicylate (p.55·1); menthol (p.1632·3).
Liniment: Methyl salicylate (p.55·1); menthol (p.1632·3); camphor (p.1589·3).
Muscle, joint, and soft-tissue pain; neuralgia.

Panaline *Darier, Mex.*
Maize starch (p.1379·3).
Napkin rash.

Panamax *Sanofi Synthelabo, Austral.*
Paracetamol (p.71·2).
Fever; pain.

Panamax Co *Sanofi Synthelabo, Austral.*
Paracetamol (p.71·2); codeine phosphate (p.25·2).
Fever; pain.

Pan-Amin *Thai Otsuka, Thai.*
Amino-acid infusion (p.1350·1).
Parenteral nutrition.

Panamor *Aspen, S.Afr.*
Diclofenac sodium (p.30·3).
Gout; inflammation; musculoskeletal and joint disorders; pain.

Panasal *ECR, USA.*
Hydrocodone tartrate (p.42·2); aspirin (p.14·2).

Panasma *Propan, S.Afr.†.*
Aminophylline (p.760·1); ephedrine hydrochloride (p.1090·1); amobarbital (p.655·2).
Asthma.

Panasol-S *Seatrace, USA.*
Prednisone (p.1079·2).
Corticosteroid.

Panasorbe *Sanofi Synthelabo, Port.*
Paracetamol (p.71·2).
Fever; pain.

Panax *Willvonseder, Aust.*
Paracetamol (p.71·2); butetamate citrate (p.1086·2); caffeine (p.761·3).
Fever; pain.

Panax Complex *Blackmores, Austral.*
Avena (p.1583·1); fenugreek (p.1610·3); alfalfa (p.1574·3); ginseng (p.1615·3); multivitamins (p.1350·1).
Tonic.

Panax N *Medichemie, Switz.*
Ibuprofen (p.43·2).
Fever; pain.

Panaxid *Lilly, Belg.*
Nizatidine (p.1238·1).
Gastrointestinal disorders associated with hyperacidity.

Panbesy
Bio-Therabel, Belg.†; Eurodrug, Hong Kong; Eurodrug, Singapore; Eurodrug, Thai.
Phentermine hydrochloride (p.1514·1).
Obesity.

Pancardiol *Almirall, Spain†.*
Isosorbide mononitrate (p.916·2).
Angina pectoris; heart failure.

Pancebrin
Lilly, Aust.†; Lilly, Hong Kong; Aspen, S.Afr.; Lilly, Thai.
Multivitamin preparation (p.1350·1).

Pancenz *Nutrition Care, Austral.*
Pancreatin (p.1646·1).
Pancreatic insufficiency.

Panchelidon N *Kanoldt, Ger.*
Greater celandine (p.1618·1).
Smooth muscle spasms.

Pancholtruw N *Truw, Ger.†.*
Pancreatin (p.1646·1).
Pancholtruw formerly contained pancreatin, bromelains, dehydrocholic acid, chelidonium, and silybum marianum.
Digestive system disorders.

Pancillin *Durascan, Denm.*
Phenoxymethylpenicillin potassium (p.235·1).
Bacterial infections.

Panclasa *Atlantis, Mex.*
Phloroglucinol (p.1650·3); trimethylphloroglucinol (p.1650·3).
Smooth muscle spasm.

Pancof XP *Pan American, USA.*
Hydrocodone tartrate (p.42·2); guaifenesin (p.1092·2); pseudoephedrine hydrochloride (p.1099·2).
Coughs.

Pancof-HC *Pan American, USA.*
Hydrocodone tartrate (p.42·2); chlorpheniramine [chlorphenamine] maleate (p.412·1); pseudoephedrine hydrochloride (p.1099·2).
Coughs.

Pancof-XL *Pan American, USA.*
Hydrocodone bitartrate (p.42·2); guaifenesin (p.1092·2); pseudoephedrine hydrochloride (p.1099·2).
Coughs.

Pancreal Kirchner *Gerda, Fr.*
Pancreatin (porcine) (p.1646·1).
Dyspepsia.

Pancrease
Note. This name is used for preparations of different composition.
Janssen-Cilag, Austral.; Janssen-Cilag, Belg.; Janssen-Ortho, Canad.; Janssen-Cilag, Denm.; Janssen-Cilag, Fin.; McNeil, Israel; Janssen-Cilag, Ital.; Cilag, Mex.; Janssen-Cilag, Neth.; Janssen-Cilag, Norw.; Janssen-Cilag, NZ; Janssen-Cilag, Spain; Janssen-Cilag, Swed.; Janssen-Cilag, UK; Ortho McNeil, USA.
Pancrelipase (p.1647·2).
Cystic fibrosis; malabsorption; pancreatic insufficiency.

Janssen-Cilag, Irl.
Pancreatin (p.1646·1).
Pancreatic insufficiency.

Pancrease HL
Janssen-Cilag, Neth.; Janssen-Cilag, UK.
Pancreatin (p.1646·1).
Pancreatic insufficiency.

Pancrelase *DB, Fr.*
Pancreatin (porcine) (p.1646·1); fungal cellulase (p.1593·1).
Formerly contained pancreas (porcine), pancreatin (porcine), fungal cullulase, and tannic acid.
Dyspepsia; pancreatic insufficiency.

Pancreoflat *Solvay, Ital.*
Pancreatin (p.1646·1); dimethicone (p.1249·2).
Digestive system disorders.

Pancreolauryl-Test
Note. This name is used for preparations of different composition.
Sanova, Aust.; Pfizer Consumer, UK.
Combination pack: Blue capsules, fluorescein dilaurate (p.1612·1); red capsules, fluorescein sodium (p.1612·1).
Evaluation of pancreatic function.

Geymonat, Ital.†.
Fluorescein dilaurate (p.1612·1).
Evaluation of pancreatic function.

Pancreolauryl-Test N *Temmler, Ger.*
Combination pack: Blue capsules, fluorescein dilaurate (p.1612·1); red capsules, fluorescein sodium (p.1612·1).
Evaluation of pancreatic function.

Pancreon *Solvay, Ital.*
Pancreatin (p.1646·1).
Cystic fibrosis; malabsorption syndromes.

Pancreon Compositum *Solvay, Ital.†.*
Pancreatin (p.1646·1); ox bile extract (p.1585·1).
Digestive system disorders.

Pancresil *Edmond Pharma, Ital.*
Dimethicone (p.1249·2); pancreatin (p.1646·1).
Digestive system disorders.

Pancrex
Paines & Byrne, Irl.; LPB, Ital.; Paines & Byrne, NZ; Paines & Byrne, UK.
Pancreatin (p.1646·1).
Cystic fibrosis; malabsorption syndromes; pancreatic insufficiency.

Pancrezyme 4X *Vitaline, USA.*
Pancreatin (p.1646·1); pancrelipase (p.1647·2).
Pancreatic insufficiency.

Pancrin
Solvay, Aust.; Solvay, Ital.
Pancreatin (p.1646·1).
Cystic fibrosis; pancreatic insufficiency.

Pancrotanon *Geymonat, Ital.†.*
Pancreatin (p.1646·1).
Digestive system disorders.

Pancuron *Cristalia, Braz.*
Pancuronium bromide (p.1338·2).
Competitive neuromuscular blocker.

Pancurox *Faulding, Port.*
Pancuronium bromide (p.1338·2).
Competitive neuromuscular blocker.

Panda Baby Cream *Thornton & Ross, UK.*
Zinc oxide (p.1128·2); castor oil (p.1592·1).
Dry skin; nappy rash.

Pandel
Galderma, Ger.; Medinfar, Port.; Savage, USA.
Hydrocortisone buteprate (p.1074·2).
Skin disorders.

Panderm *Julphar, UAE.*
Nystatin (p.392·2); neomycin sulfate (p.228·1); gramicidin (p.213·3); triamcinolone acetonide (p.1080·1).
Infected skin disorders.

Pandermil *Oftalder, Port.*
Hydrocortisone (p.1073·3).
Skin disorders.

Panectyl *Rhone-Poulenc Rorer, Canad.*
Trimeprazine [alimemazine] tartrate (p.426·2).
Coughs; dyspnoea; pruritus.

Pan-Emecort *Merck, Braz.*
Fluprednidene acetate (p.1072·1); gentamicin sulfate (p.210·1); hydroxyquinoline (p.1622·2).
Skin disorders.

Pan-Enteral *Thai Otsuka, Thai.*
Preparation for enteral nutrition (p.1350·1).

Panerel *Cox, UK.*
Paracetamol (p.71·2); codeine phosphate (p.25·2). These ingredients can be described by the British Approved Name Co-codamol.
Fever; pain.

Panex *Roberts, USA†.*
Paracetamol (p.71·2).
Fever; pain.

Panfil G *Pan American, USA.*
Diprophylline (p.764·1); guaifenesin (p.1092·2).
Obstructive airways disease.

Panflavin *Chinosolfabrik, Ger.†.*
Acriflavinium chloride (p.1130·2).
Infections of the oropharynx.

Panflogin *Farmion, Braz.*
Benzydamine hydrochloride (p.20·1).
Fever; inflammation; pain.

Panfugan *Byk, Braz.*
Mebendazole (p.102·2).
Worm infections.

Pan-Fungex *Sanofi Synthelabo, Port.*
Clotrimazole (p.382·1).

Panfungol *Esteve, Spain.*
Ketoconazole (p.389·1).
Fungal infections.

Panfurex *Bouchara, Fr.*
Nifuroxazide (p.230·2).
Diarrhoea.

Pangamox *Synthelabo, Spain.*
Amoxicillin trihydrate (p.149·2); potassium clavulanate (p.187·2).
Bacterial infections.

Pangavit *Carter-Wallace, Mex.*
Cyanocobalamin (p.1388·1); thiamine hydrochloride (p.1385·1); pyridoxine hydrochloride (p.1386·3).
Neuralgias; neuritis; neuropathy; vitamin B deficiency.

Pangel *Pannoc, Belg.*
Benzoyl peroxide (p.1111·1).
Acne.

Pangen
Urgo, Fr.; Fournier, Ger.
Collagen (p.1598·2).
Haemorrhagic disorders.

Pangest *Farmasa, Braz.*
Cisapride (p.1220·1).
Gastro-oesophageal reflux; gastroparesis.

Panglobulin *American Red Cross, USA.*
A normal immunoglobulin (p.1551·3).

Pangon *LBS, Thai.*
Pentazocine hydrochloride (p.74·2) or pentazocine lactate (p.74·2).
Pain.

Pangrol *Berlin-Chemie, Ger.*
Pancreatin (p.1646·1).
Pancreatic insufficiency.

The symbol † denotes a preparation no longer actively marketed

Panhematin *Abbott, Austral.; Abbott, USA.*
Haematin (p.1011·1).
Porphyria.

Panimycin *Meiji, Jpn.*
Dibekacin sulfate (p.198·3).
Bacterial infections.

Paniodal *Adivar, Ital.*
Povidone-iodine (p.1155·1).
Skin and wound disinfection.

Paniodine *Angelini, Ital.*
Povidone-iodine (p.1155·1).
Skin and wound disinfection.

Panitol
Note.This name is used for preparations of different composition.
Cryopharma, Mex.
Propanidid (p.1265·3).
General anaesthesia.

Pharmaland, Thai.
Carbamazepine (p.342·2).
Epilepsy; trigeminal neuralgia.

Panitone *Wesley, USA.*
Paracetamol (p.71·2).
Fever; pain.

Panix *Research Labs, S.Afr.*
Alprazolam (p.654·2).
Anxiety disorders; mixed anxiety depressive states; panic attacks.

Pankreaden *Knoll, Ital.*
Pancrelipase (p.1647·2).
Pancreatic insufficiency.

Pankreaplex Neu *Schaper & Brummer, Ger.*
Silybum marianum (p.1021·3); syzygium jambolana; condurango (p.1599·1); sarsaparilla (p.1661·1).
Gastrointestinal disorders.

Pankrease *Janssen-Cilag, S.Afr.*
Pancrelipase (p.1647·2).
Pancreatic disorders.

Pankreatan *Novartis Consumer, Ger.*
Pancreatin (p.1646·1).
Digestive system disorders.

Pankreaticum *Hevert, Ger.*
Injection: Homoeopathic preparation.

Oral drops: Boldo (p.1585·3); curcuma (p.1029·3); eichhornia; myrtillus; okoubaka; quassia; syzygium; sanguinaria; tanacetum; taraxacum.
Biliary disorders; digestive disorders; pancreatitis.

Pankreoflat *Solvay, Aust.; Byk, Braz.; Solvay, Ger.; Solvay, Hong Kong; Solvay, Israel; Byk Gulden, Mex.; Solvay, Port.; Solvay, S.Afr.; Solvay, Spain.*
Pancreatin (p.1646·1); simeticone (p.1249·2).
Excess gastrointestinal gas; pancreatic insufficiency; preparation for gastrointestinal examinations.

Pankreon *Byk, Braz.; Solvay, Denm.; Solvay, Fin.; Solvay, Ger.; Solvay, Norw.; Solvay, Spain†; Solvay, Swed.*
Pancreatin (p.1646·1).
Cystic fibrosis; malabsorption; pancreatic insufficiency.

Pankreon compositum *Solvay, Aust.*
Pancreatin (p.1646·1); ox bile (p.1585·1).
Digestive system disorders; pancreatic insufficiency.

Pankreon forte *Solvay, Aust.*
Pancreatin (p.1646·1).
Digestive system disorders; pancreatic insufficiency.

Pankrevowen *Weber & Weber, Ger.†*
Homoeopathic preparation.

Panlem *Lemery, Mex.*
Pancuronium bromide (p.1338·2).
Competitive neuromuscular blocker.

Panlor DC *Pan American, USA.*
Paracetamol (p.71·2); caffeine (p.761·3); dihydrocodeine tartrate (p.33·1).
Pain.

Panmist JR *Pan American, USA.*
Pseudoephedrine (p.1099·2); guaifenesin (p.1092·2).
Coughs.

PanMist-DM *Pan American, USA.*
Pseudoephedrine hydrochloride (p.1099·2); dextromethorphan hydrobromide (p.1087·3); guaifenesin (p.1092·2).
Coughs.

Panmycin *Pharmacia Upjohn, NZ; Upjohn, USA.*
Tetracycline hydrochloride (p.258·3).
Bacterial infections.

Pannaz *Pan American, USA.*
Pseudoephedrine hydrochloride (p.1099·2); chlorpheniramine [chlorphenamine] maleate (p.412·1); hyoscine methonitrate (p.468·2).
Formerly contained phenylpropanolamine, chlorpheniramine [chlorphenamine], and hyoscine.
Upper respiratory-tract disorders.

Pannocort *Pannoc, Belg.*
Hydrocortisone acetate (p.1073·3).
Skin disorders.

Pannogel *CS, Fr.*
Benzoyl peroxide (p.1111·1).
Acne.

Panocaine *Hoechst Marion Roussel, Canad.†*
Benzocaine (p.1306·2); amethocaine [tetracaine] hydrochloride (p.1305·2).
Local anaesthesia in dentistry.

Panocod *Sanofi Winthrop, Swed.*
Paracetamol (p.71·2); codeine phosphate (p.25·2).
Pain.

Panodil
SmithKline Beecham, Denm.; SmithKline Beecham, Norw.; SmithKline Beecham Consumer, Swed.
Paracetamol (p.71·2).
Fever; pain.

Pan-Ophtal *Winzer, Ger.*
Dexpanthenol (p.1602·3).
Eye disorders.

Panoral *Lilly, Ger.*
Cefaclor (p.161·1).
Bacterial infections.

Panorex *Glaxo Wellcome, Ger.*
Edrecolomab (p.536·3).
Colorectal cancer.

Panos *Fornet, Fr.*
Tetrazepam (p.708·1).
Skeletal muscle spasm.

Panotil *Zambon, Braz.*
Polymyxin B sulfate (p.238·1); neomycin sulfate (p.228·1); fludrocortisone acetate (p.1070·1); lignocaine [lidocaine] hydrochloride (p.1313·2); nitrofurazone (p.231·3).
Ear disorders.

Panotile
Note.This name is used for preparations of different composition.
Zambon, Belg.; Zambon, Fr.; Zambon, Neth.; Inpharzam, Switz.
Polymyxin B sulfate (p.238·1); neomycin sulfate (p.228·1); fludrocortisone acetate (p.1070·1); lignocaine [lidocaine] hydrochloride (p.1313·2).
Ear disorders.

Zambon, Spain.
Polymyxin B sulfate (p.238·1); neomycin sulfate (p.228·1); fludrocortisone acetate (p.1070·1); furaltadone hydrochloride (p.208·3); lignocaine [lidocaine] hydrochloride (p.1313·2).
Ear disorders.

Panotile N *Zambon, Ger.*
Polymyxin B sulfate (p.238·1); fludrocortisone acetate (p.1070·1); lignocaine [lidocaine] hydrochloride (p.1313·2).
Ear disorders.

PanOxyl *Sanova, Aust.; Stiefel, Austral.; Stiefel, Canad.; Stiefel, Fin.; Stiefel, Fr.; Stiefel, Ger.; Stiefel, Hong Kong; Stiefel, Irl.; Stiefel, Israel; Stiefel, Ital.; Stiefel, Mex.; Stiefel, Norw.; Sparks, NZ; Stiefel, Port.; Stiefel, S.Afr.; Stiefel, Singapore; Stiefel, Spain; Stiefel, Switz.; Stiefel, Thai.; Stiefel, UK; Stiefel, USA.*
Benzoyl peroxide (p.1111·1).
Acne.

Panpeptal N *Philopharm, Ger.*
Pancreatin (p.1646·1).
Pancreatic insufficiency.

Panpur *Knoll, Ger.*
Porcine pancreatin (p.1646·1).
Digestive system disorders.

Panpurol *Shinyaku, Jpn; Shinyaku, Thai.*
Pipethanate ethobromide (p.472·2).
Benzyl alcohol (p.1135·2) may be included in the injection to alleviate the pain of injection.
Smooth muscle spasm.

Panquil *Warner-Lambert, Austral.*
Promethazine hydrochloride (p.423·2); paracetamol (p.71·2).
Fever; pain.

Panretin *Ligand, Canad.; Ligand, USA.*
Alitretinoin (p.506·2).
Kaposi's sarcoma.

Pansan *Solvay, Aust.*
Stomach enzymes (p.1649·3); glutamic acid hydrochloride (p.1365·2).
Gastrointestinal disorders.

Panscol *Baker Cummins, USA.*
Salicylic acid (p.1122·3).
Hyperkeratosis.

Pansebase *Sofex, Port.†*
Lecithin (p.1628·1); lactic acid (p.1626·2).
Seborrhoeic dermatitis.

Pansebase Composto *Sofex, Port.†*
Lecithin (p.1628·1); lactic acid (p.1626·2); ichthammol (p.1115·2).
Pruritus; psoriasis; seborrhoeic dermatitis.

Pansebase Solido *Sofex, Port.†*
Soap substitute.
Oily skin.

Pansecoff *Asta Medica, Aust.†*
Ergotamine tartrate (p.452·1); caffeine (p.761·3).
Migraine and other vascular headaches.

Pansements Coricides *Seton Scholl, Fr.*
Salicylic acid (p.1122·3).
Corns.

Panseptil *Gedis, Ital.*
Chlorhexidine gluconate (p.1138·2); cetrimide (p.1137·1); alcohol (p.1130·3); isopropyl alcohol (p.1149·2).
Surface disinfection.

Pansoral
Pierre Fabre Sante, Fr.; Pierre Fabre, Switz.†
Choline salicylate (p.24·3); cetalkonium chloride (p.1137·1).
Mouth disorders.

Pansporin *Takeda, Jpn.*
Cefotiam hydrochloride (p.171·1) or cefotiam hexetil hydrochloride (p.171·1).

Mepivacaine hydrochloride (p.1317·1) is included in the intramuscular injection to alleviate the pain of injection.
Bacterial infections.

Pansteryl *Sanofi Winthrop, Belg.†*
Benzalkonium chloride (p.1133·2).
Disinfection of instruments, materials, and hands; storage of sterile materials.

Pantacid *Finmedical, Ital.*
Cefonicid sodium (p.168·1).
Lignocaine [lidocaine] hydrochloride (p.1313·2) is included in this preparation to alleviate the pain of injection.
Gram-negative bacterial infections.

Pantecta *Ravizza, Ital.; Pharmacia Upjohn, Spain.*
Pantoprazole sodium (p.1243·2).
Gastro-oesophageal reflux; peptic ulcer.

Pantederm *Hexal, Ger.*
Zinc oxide (p.1128·2); dexpanthenol (p.1602·3).
Burns; wounds.

Pantelmin *Janssen-Cilag, Aust.; Cilag, Braz.; Janssen-Cilag, Port.*
Mebendazole (p.102·2).
Worm infections.

Pantenil *Quimica Medica, Spain.*
Calcium pantothenate (p.1374·1); mercuric chloride (p.1633·1); aminobenzoic acid (p.1516·3).
Hair, scalp, and skin disorders.

Panteston *Organon, Fin.; Pharmaco, NZ.*
Testosterone undecylate (p.1492·2).
Male hypogonadism; male infertility; osteoporosis in men.

Pantestone *Organon, Fr.*
Testosterone undecylate (p.1492·2).
Male hypogonadism.

Pantetina *Sanofi Synthelabo, Ital.*
Pantethine (p.952·1).
Hypertriglyceridaemia.

Pantevit *EMS, Braz.*
Pantothenic acid (p.1374·1); vitamin B₆ (p.1387·1); resorcinol (p.1122·2).
Psoriasis.

Panthenol *Jenapharm, Ger.; Alcon, Ger.; Braun, Ger.; Ratiopharm, Ger.; Riemser, Ger.; Lichtenstein, Ger.; Chauvin ankerpharm, Ger.; LAF, Ger.*
Dexpanthenol (p.1602·3).
Eye disorders; inflammatory disorders of the gastrointestinal tract; pantothenic acid deficiency; paraesthesias; paralytic ileus; postoperative gastrointestinal atony; respiratory-tract disorders; wounds.

Panthisone *Rekah, Israel.*
Panthenol (p.1602·3); hydrocortisone acetate (p.1073·3).
Anorectal disorders; skin disorders; wounds.

Panthoderm *Jones, USA.*
Dexpanthenol (p.1602·3).
Skin disorders.

Panthogenat *Azupharma, Ger.*
Dexpanthenol (p.1602·3).
Wounds.

Pantinol *Gerot, Aust.*
Aprotinin (p.725·3).
Hyperfibrinolysis; prevention of postoperative complications; shock.

Panto *Byk, Canad.*
Pantoprazole sodium (p.1243·2).
Gastrointestinal hyperacidity.

Pantobamin *Medix, Spain.*
Cyproheptadine (p.414·3); amino acids and vitamins (p.1350·1).
Anorexia; tonic.

Pantobionta *Merck, Spain.*
Multivitamin and mineral preparation (p.1350·1).

Pantobron *Abbott, Mex.*
Erythromycin (p.201·2) or erythromycin ethyl succinate (p.201·2); bromhexine hydrochloride (p.1085·3).
Respiratory-tract infections.

Pantoc *Byk, Port.*
Pantoprazole sodium (p.1243·2).
Gastro-oesophageal reflux; peptic ulcer.

Pantocarm *Byk Elmu, Spain.*
Pantoprazole sodium (p.1243·2).
Gastro-oesophageal reflux; peptic ulcer.

Pantocrinale *Simons, Ger.*
Hydrocortisone sodium phosphate (p.1074·1); salicylic acid (p.1122·3).
Scalp disorders.

Pantocycline *Chew, Thai.*
Tetracycline hydrochloride (p.258·3).
Bacterial infections.

Pantodrin *Abbott, Spain.*
Erythromycin (p.201·2).
Acne.

Pantogar
Medra, Aust.
Calcium pantothenate; cystine (p.1350·1).
Hair and nail disorders.

Cimex, Hong Kong.
Vitamins; medicinal yeast; keratin; aminobenzoic acid; cystine (p.1350·1).
Hair disorders.

Cimex, Singapore.
Thiamine; calcium pantothenate; medicinal yeast; cystine; keratin (p.1350·1).
Hair and nail disorders.

Agpharm, Switz.†
Thiamine nitrate; calcium pantothenate; medicinal yeast; cystine; keratin aminobenzoic acid (p.1350·1).
Hair and nail disorders.

Pantok *Lacer, Spain.*
Simvastatin (p.969·2).
Hypercholesterolaemia; ischaemic heart disease.

Pantolax *Schwabe-Curamed, Ger.*
Suxamethonium chloride (p.1340·1).
Depolarising neuromuscular blocker.

Pantoloc
Byk, Aust.; Solvay, Canad.; Byk, Canad.; Byk Gulden, Denm.; Byk Gulden, Hong Kong; Byk Madaus, S.Afr.; Nycomed, Swed.
Pantoprazole sodium (p.1243·2).
Gastro-oesophageal reflux; peptic ulcer.

Pantomicina
Abbott, Braz.; Abbott, Mex.; Abbott, Spain.
Erythromycin ethyl succinate (p.201·2), erythromycin lactobionate (p.201·3), or erythromycin stearate (p.201·3).
Bacterial infections.

Pantomin
Daiichi, Hong Kong; Daiichi, Jpn.
Pantethine (p.952·1).
Blood disorders; constipation; eczema; hyperlipidaemias; pantothenic acid deficiency; pantothenic acid supplement; streptomycin and kanamycin toxicity.

Pantonate *Eagle, Austral.*
Calcium pantothenate (p.1374·1).
Vitamin B₅ supplement.

PantoPAC *Byk, Ger.*
Tablets, pantoprazole sodium (p.1243·2); tablets, clarithromycin (p.186·2); tablets, amoxicillin trihydrate (p.149·2).
Peptic ulcer.

Pantopan *Pharmacia Upjohn, Ital.*
Pantoprazole sodium (p.1243·2).
Gastro-oesophageal reflux; peptic ulcer.

Pantopept *Biosintetica, Braz.*
Pepsin (p.1649·3); fermento amilolitico (p.1379·3).
Digestive disorders.

Pantopon *Roche, Austral.*
Hydrochlorides of mixed opium alkaloids (p.70·1).
Hypnotic; pain; sedative.

Pantorc *Byk Gulden, Ital.*
Pantoprazole sodium (p.1243·2).
Gastro-oesophageal reflux; peptic ulcer.

Pantostin *Simons, Ger.*
Estradiol (p.1473·1).
Alopecia androgenetica.

Pantothen
Note.This name is used for preparations of different composition.
Nycomed, Aust.
Panthenol (p.1602·3).
Alcoholism; gastrointestinal tract disorders; liver disorders; muscle cramps; neuropathies; respiratory-tract disorders; skin disorders; sweating.

Streuli, Switz.
Calcium pantothenate (p.1374·1).
Intestinal atony; pantothenic acid deficiency; sensation of burning in feet.

Pantovigar *Simons, Ger.*
Thiamine nitrate (p.1385·1); calcium pantothenate (p.1374·1); medicinal yeast (p.1398·1); cystine (p.1359·1); keratin; aminobenzoic acid (p.1516·3).
Disorders of the hair and nails.

Pantovit *Sanova, Aust.*
Multivitamin preparation (p.1350·1).

Pantovit Vital *Sanova, Aust.*
Multivitamin, iron, and mineral preparation (p.1350·1).

Pantozol
Byk, Belg.; Byk, Braz.; Byk Gulden, Ger.; Byk Gulden, Mex.; Byk, Neth.; Byk, Switz.
Pantoprazole (p.1243·1) or pantoprazole sodium (p.1243·2).
Gastro-oesophageal reflux; peptic ulcer; Zollinger-Ellison syndrome.

Pantozol-Rifun *Byk Gulden, Ger.; Schwarz, Ger.*
Pantoprazole sodium (p.1243·2).
Gastro-oesophageal reflux; peptic ulcer.

Pantrop *Lundbeck, Aust.*
Amitriptyline hydrochloride (p.273·3); chlordiazepoxide (p.659·2).
Depression; sleep disorders.

Pantyson *Orion, Fin.*
Hydrocortisone (p.1073·3); dexpanthenol (p.1602·3).
Skin disorders.

Panvit *Teuto, Braz.*
A range of multivitamin preparations with or without minerals (p.1350·1).

Panvitan-M
Takeda, Hong Kong; Takeda, Singapore; Takeda, Thai.
Multivitamin and mineral preparation (p.1350·1).

Panvitina BC *Neo Quimica, Braz.*
Multivitamin preparation (p.1350·1).

Panvitrop *Byk, Braz.*
Methionine (p.1012·2); choline tartrate (p.1356·3); sodium phenylethylacetate; liver extract; vitamin B substances; tocopherol (p.1350·1); rutoside (p.1611·2).
Liver disorders.

Panxeol *IPRAD, Fr.*
Eschscholtzia californica; passion flower (p.1649·1).
Insomnia; nervous disorders.

Panzid *Duncan, Ital.*
Ceftazidime (p.174·3).
Bacterial infections.

Panzynorm *Ebewe, Aust.*
Pancreatin (p.1646·1).

Panzynorm forte-N *Knoll, Ger.*
Porcine pancreatin (p.1646·1).
Pancreatic insufficiency.

Panzytrat
Knoll, Braz.; Knoll, Ger.; Knoll, Irl.; Nordmark, Neth.; Knoll, NZ; Knoll, Switz.
Pancreatin (p.1646·1).
Pancreatic insufficiency.

Papaine *DB, Fr.*
Carica papaya.
Dyspepsia.

Papase *Parke, Davis, Hong Kong.*
Prolase.
Inflammation; oedema.

Papaverine Hydrochloride *Boots, UK; Penn, UK; Martindale Pharmaceuticals, UK.*
Papaverine hydrochloride (p.1648·1).
NOTE. There is no connection between Martindale, The Complete Drug Reference and Martindale Pahrmaceuticals.
Erectile dysfunction.

Papaya Enzyme *Nature's Bounty, USA.*
Papain (p.1647·3); amylase (p.1579·3).
Gastrointestinal disorders.

Papaya Plus *Gerard House, UK.*
Charcoal (p.1000·3); papain (p.1647·3); slippery elm (p.1665·1); hydrastis (p.1621·1).
Digestive disorders.

Papayasanit-N *Weber & Weber, Ger.†*
Homoeopathic preparation.

Papilo Lisin *Mex-America, Mex.*
Podophyllum (p.1121·1).

Paps *Richard, Fr.*
Sulfur (p.1123·3); zinc undecenoate (p.395·3); bismuth subgallate (p.1213·2); menthol (p.1632·3); camphor (p.1589·3); salicylic acid (p.1122·3); zinc oxide (p.1128·2); boric acid (p.1586·1); lavender oil (p.1627·2).
Bacterial and fungal skin infections.

Papulex
Knoll, Austral.†; GenDerm, Canad.†; Helsinn Birex, Irl.; Pharmagenix, UK.
Nicotinamide (p.1372·3).
Acne.

Papytazyme *Anglo-French Drugs, Thai.*
Papain (p.1647·3); pepsin (p.1649·3); amylase (p.1579·3); pancreatin (p.1646·1); ox bile extract (p.1585·1); ginger oleoresin (p.1227·2); activated charcoal (p.1000·2).
Digestive disorders.

Par *Sanofi Winthrop, Braz.*
Paracetamol (p.71·2); dipyrone (p.34·1).
Fever; pain.

Par Glycerol *Par, USA.*
Iodinated glycerol (p.1092·3).
Coughs.

Para
Medgenix, Belg.; Medican, Canad.; SCAT, Denm.
Bioallethrin (p.1428·3); piperonyl butoxide (p.1436·2).
Pediculosis.

Para Lentes *Pharmygiene, Fr.*
Acetic acid (p.1571·2).
Pediculosis.

Para Plus
Medgenix, Belg.; Pharmygiene, Fr.; Rafa, Israel; Pacific, NZ.
Malathion (p.1434·2); permethrin (p.1436·1); piperonyl butoxide (p.1436·2).
Pediculosis.

Para Repulsif *Pharmygiene, Fr.*
Piperonal (p.1436·2).
Head lice repellent.

Para Special Poux *Pharmygiene, Fr.*
Bioallethrin (p.1428·3); piperonyl butoxide (p.1436·2).
Pediculosis.

Parabolan *Negma, Fr.†*
Trenbolone hexahydrobenzylcarbonate (p.1495·3).
Anabolic; osteoporosis.

Parabowl *Masa, Thai.*
Prazosin hydrochloride (p.958·1).
Hypertension.

Paracap *Masa, Thai.*
Paracetamol (p.71·2).
Fever; pain.

Paracare *PSM, NZ.*
Paracetamol (p.71·2).
Fever; pain.

Paracefan *Boehringer Ingelheim, Ger.*
Clonidine (p.861·1) or clonidine hydrochloride (p.860·1).
Alcohol withdrawal syndrome; opioid withdrawal syndrome; tics.

Paracet
Weifa, Norw.; Osotspa, Thai.
Paracetamol (p.71·2).
Fever; pain.

paracet comp *CT, Ger.*
Paracetamol (p.71·2); codeine phosphate (p.25·2).
Pain.

Paracetacod
Note. This name is used for preparations of different composition.
Ratiopharm, Ger.
Paracetamol (p.71·2); codeine phosphate (p.25·2).
Pain.

Adcock Ingram, S.Afr.
Paracetamol (p.71·2); codeine phosphate (p.25·2); ascorbic acid (p.1389·3).
Pain.

Paracetamol comp *Stada, Ger.*
Paracetamol (p.71·2); codeine phosphate (p.25·2).
Pain.

paracetamol plus *CT, Ger.*
Paracetamol (p.71·2); caffeine (p.761·3).
Cold symptoms; pain.

Paracetamolplus *Ratiopharm, Ger.*
Paracetamol (p.71·2); caffeine (p.761·3).
Pain.

Paracets *Sussex, UK.*
Paracetamol (p.71·2).
Fever; pain.

Paracets Cold Relief *Sussex, UK.*
Paracetamol (p.71·2); ascorbic acid (p.1389·3).
Cold and influenza symptoms.

Paracets Plus *Sussex, UK.*
Paracetamol (p.71·2); caffeine (p.761·3); phenylephrine hydrochloride (p.1097·1).
Cold and influenza symptoms.

Parachoc *Paedpharm, Austral.*
Methylcellulose (p.1502·2); liquid paraffin (p.1407·1).
Constipation.

Paracin *Chinta, Thai.*
Paracetamol (p.71·2); potassium citrate (p.1186·1); chlorpheniramine [chlorphenamine] maleate (p.412·1); phenylephrine hydrochloride (p.1097·1).
Cold and influenza symptoms; coughs.

Paraclear *Roche Consumer, UK.*
Paracetamol (p.71·2).

Paracod *Sam-On, Israel.*
Paracetamol (p.71·2); codeine phosphate (p.25·2).
Coughs; fever; pain.

Paracodin
Note. This name is used for preparations of different composition.
Ebewe, Aust.
Oral drops: Dihydrocodeine thiocyanate (p.33·3); thyme (p.1672·2).
Syrup: Dihydrocodeine tartrate (p.33·1); althaea (p.1577·1); grindelia (p.1618·2).
Tablets: Dihydrocodeine tartrate (p.33·1).
Coughs.

Knoll, Austral.; Knoll, Ger.; Knoll, Irl.; Knoll, S.Afr.; Knoll, Switz.
Dihydrocodeine tartrate (p.33·1) or dihydrocodeine thiocyanate (p.33·3).
Formerly contained dihydrocodeine tartrate, althaea, and grindelia in S.Afr.
Coughs; diarrhoea.

Paracodin N *Knoll, Ger.*
Dihydrocodeine tartrate (p.33·1) or dihydrocodeine thiocyanate (p.33·3).
Coughs.

Paracodin retard
Knoll, Ger.; Knoll, Switz.
Dihydrocodeine tartrate (p.33·1); dihydrocodeine resin (p.33·3).
Coughs; diarrhoea.

Paracodina
Knoll, Ital.; Knoll, Port.; Knoll, Spain.
Dihydrocodeine tartrate (p.33·1) or dihydrocodeine thiocyanate (p.33·3).
Coughs; pain.

Paracodine *Knoll, Belg.*
Syrup: Dihydrocodeine tartrate (p.33·1); grindelia (p.1618·2); althaea (p.1577·1).
Tablets: Dihydrocodeine tartrate (p.33·1).
Coughs.

Paracodol
Roche Consumer, Irl.; Roche Consumer, UK.
Paracetamol (p.71·2); codeine phosphate (p.25·2).
These ingredients can be described by the British Approved Name Co-codamol.
Fever; pain.

Paractol *Temmler, Ger.*
Chewable tablets: Simeticone (p.1249·2); aluminium hydroxide gel (p.1210·3).
Oral suspension: Simeticone (p.1249·2); aluminium hydroxide gel (p.1210·3); magnesium hydroxide (p.1233·1).
Gastrointestinal disorders.

Paradenton *Medicopharm, Aust.*
Myrrh (p.1639·2); sage leaf (p.1660·3); chamomile flowers (p.1593·2); tannic acid (p.1669·1).
Aphthous ulcers; bleeding gums; bruised gums; gingivitis; periodontitis.

Paraderm *Whitehall, Austral.*
Bufexamac (p.20·3).
Skin disorders.

Paraderm Plus *Whitehall, Austral.*
Chlorhexidine gluconate (p.1138·2); lignocaine [lidocaine] hydrochloride (p.1313·2); bufexamac (p.20·3).
Burns; insect bites; minor skin lesions; stings.

Paradex
Rhone-Poulenc Rorer, Austral.; PSM, NZ.
Dextropropoxyphene hydrochloride (p.27·1) or dextropropoxyphene napsilate (p.27·1); paracetamol (p.71·2).
Fever; pain.

Parador *Boehringer de Angeli, Braz.*
Paracetamol (p.71·2).
Fever; pain.

Paradote *Penn, UK.*
Paracetamol (p.71·2); DL-methionine (p.1012·2).

These ingredients can be described by the British Approved Name Co-methiamol.
Fever; pain.

Paradryl med efedrin *Ferrosan, Denm.*
Mefenidramium bromide; ephedrine hydrochloride (p.1090·1); ammonium chloride (p.1085·2).
Coughs.

Paraflex
AstraZeneca, Denm.; Janssen-Cilag, S.Afr.†; Astra, Swed.; McNeil Pharmaceutical, USA.
Chlorzoxazone (p.1327·3).
Musculoskeletal pain; skeletal muscle spasm.

Paraflex comp
AstraZeneca, Fin.; Astra, Swed.
Chlorzoxazone (p.1327·3); aspirin (p.14·2); dextropropoxyphene napsilate (p.27·1).
Musculoskeletal, joint, and peri-articular disorders.

Parafon
Janssen-Cilag, Aust.; Janssen-Cilag, Switz.†; Janssen, Thai.
Chlorzoxazone (p.1327·3); paracetamol (p.71·2).
Skeletal muscle pain and spasm.

Parafon Forte
Johnson & Johnson, Canad.; Cilag, Mex.
Chlorzoxazone (p.1327·3); paracetamol (p.71·2).
Skeletal muscle pain and spasm.

Parafon Forte C8 *Johnson & Johnson, Canad.*
Chlorzoxazone (p.1327·3); paracetamol (p.71·2); codeine phosphate (p.25·2).
Pain; skeletal muscle spasm.

Parafon Forte DSC *Ortho McNeil, USA.*
Chlorzoxazone (p.1327·3).
Musculoskeletal pain.

Paragar *Spirig, Switz.*
Liquid paraffin (p.1407·1); agar (p.1498·3); phenolphthalein (p.1244·1).
Constipation.

Paragard T380A *Ortho McNeil, USA.*
Copper-wound plastic (p.1357·3).
Intra-uterine contraceptive device.

Paraghurt *Leo, Denm.*
Enterococcus faecium (p.1626·3).
Diarrhoea.

Paragip *Boiron, Canad.*
Homoeopathic preparation.

Paragol *Streuli, Switz.*
Liquid paraffin (p.1407·1); phenolphthalein (p.1244·1).
Bowel evacuation; constipation.

Paragrippe
Boiron, Fr.; Boiron, Port.
Homoeopathic preparation.

Parahexal *Hexal, Austral.*
Paracetamol (p.71·2).
Fever; pain.

Para-Hist HD *Pharmics, USA.*
Phenylephrine hydrochloride (p.1097·1); chlorpheniramine [chlorphenamine] maleate (p.412·1); hydrocodone tartrate (p.42·3).
Coughs and cold symptoms.

Parahypon *Calmic, Irl.*
Paracetamol (p.71·2); caffeine (p.761·3); codeine phosphate (p.25·2).
Pain.

Parakapton *Strallhofer, Aust.*
Paracetamol (p.71·2).
Pain, fever.

Parake *Galen, UK.*
Paracetamol (p.71·2); codeine phosphate (p.25·2).
These ingredients can be described by the British Approved Name Co-codamol.
Pain.

Paral *Forest Pharmaceuticals, USA.*
Paraldehyde (p.697·3).
Sedative.

Paralergin *Vita, Spain.*
Astemizole (p.409·1).
Hypersensitivity reactions.

Paralgesic *Poythress, USA†.*
Methyl salicylate (p.55·1); menthol (p.1632·3); camphor (p.1589·3).

Paralgin
Note. This name is used for preparations of different composition.
Sigma, Austral.
Paracetamol (p.71·2).
Fever; pain.

Weifa, Norw.
Codeine phosphate (p.25·2); paracetamol (p.71·2).
Pain.

Paralice *Fleet, Austral.*
Bioallethrin (p.1428·3); piperonyl butoxide (p.1436·2).
Pediculosis.

Paralief *Clonmel, Irl.*
Paracetamol (p.71·2).
Fever; pain.

Paralink *Rice Steele, Irl.*
Paracetamol (p.71·2).
Fever; pain.

Paralyoc *Lafon, Fr.*
Paracetamol (p.71·2).
Fever; pain.

Paramax
Lorex Synthelabo, Irl.; SmithKline Beecham, NZ; Sanofi Synthelabo, UK.
Paracetamol (p.71·2); metoclopramide hydrochloride (p.1235·2).
Migraine.

Paramettes *Whitehall-Robins, Canad.*
Multivitamin and mineral preparation (p.1350·1).

Paramin *Wallis, UK.*
Paracetamol (p.71·2).
Fever; pain.

Paraminan *Alpharma, Fr.*
Aminobenzoic acid (p.1516·3).
Skin disorders.

Paramine *DHA, Singapore.*
Chlorpheniramine [chlorphenamine] maleate (p.412·1); paracetamol (p.71·2); phenylpropanolamine hydrochloride (p.1098·1).
Cold symptoms.

Paramol
Note. This name is used for preparations of different composition.
Galen, Irl.; SSL, UK.
Paracetamol (p.71·2); dihydrocodeine tartrate (p.33·1).
Coughs; fever; pain.

General Drugs, Thai.
Paracetamol (p.71·2).
Fever; pain.

Paramol TP *TP, Thai.*
Paracetamol (p.71·2).
Lignocaine [lidocaine] hydrochloride (p.1313·2) is included in the intramuscular injection to alleviate the pain of injection.
Fever; pain.

Paramol TP without Lignocaine *TP, Thai.*
Paracetamol (p.71·2).
Fever; pain.

Paramolan
Trima, Israel; Medinfar, Port.
Paracetamol (p.71·2).
Fever; pain.

Paramolan C *Medinfar, Port.*
Paracetamol (p.71·2); ascorbic acid (p.1389·3).
Fever; pain.

Paran *Noristan, S.Afr.†*
Paracetamol (p.71·2); codeine phosphate (p.25·2).
Pain.

Paranal *Siam Bheasach, Thai.*
Paracetamol (p.71·2).
Fever; pain.

Paranal-L *Siam Bheasach, Thai.*
Paracetamol (p.71·2).
Lignocaine [lidocaine] hydrochloride (p.1313·2) is included in this preparation to alleviate the pain of injection.
Fever; pain.

Paranico *Elerte, Fr.†.*
Nicotinamide (p.1372·3); quinine ascorbate (p.1657·1); thiamine hydrochloride (p.1385·1).
Aid to smoking withdrawal.

Paranorm *Wallace Mfg Chem., UK.*
Dextromethorphan hydrobromide (p.1087·3); ephedrine hydrochloride (p.1090·1); guaifenesin (p.1092·2).
Coughs.

Paranthil *Xixia, S.Afr.†.*
Albendazole (p.95·2).
Worm infections.

Parapaed
Pinewood, Irl.; Pinewood, UK.
Paracetamol (p.71·2).
Fever; pain.

Para-Pio *Franco, Port.*
Pyrethrin; piperonyl butoxide (p.1436·2).
Pediculosis.

Paraplatin
Bristol-Myers Squibb, Aust.; Bristol-Myers Squibb, Belg.; Bristol-Myers Squibb, Braz.; Bristol, Canad.; Bristol-Myers Squibb, Denm.; Bristol-Myers Squibb, Fin.; Bristol-Myers Squibb, Hong Kong; Bristol-Myers Squibb, Irl.; Bristol-Myers Squibb, Israel; Bristol-Myers Squibb, Ital.; Bristol-Myers Squibb, Mex.; Bristol-Myers Squibb, Neth.; Bristol-Myers Squibb, Norw.; Bristol-Myers Squibb, NZ; Bristol-Myers Squibb, S.Afr.; Bristol-Myers Squibb, Spain; Bristol-Myers Squibb, Swed.; Bristol-Myers Squibb, Thai.; Bristol-Myers Squibb, UK; Bristol-Myers Squibb Oncology, USA.
Carboplatin (p.515·1).
Malignant neoplasms.

Paraplatine
Bristol-Myers Squibb, Fr.; Bristol-Myers Squibb, Switz.
Carboplatin (p.515·1).
Malignant neoplasms.

Parapres *Almirall, Spain.*
Candesartan cilexetil (p.853·2).
Hypertension.

Parapsyllium *Iprad, Fr.*
Ispaghula (p.1229·1); light liquid paraffin (p.1407·2); sorbitol (p.1377·3).
Constipation.

Paraqueimol *Asta Medica, Braz.*
Sulfacetamide (p.250·3); trolamine (p.1675·1).
Skin infections.

Parartrin *Cazi, Braz.*
Ibuprofen (p.43·2).
Fever; inflammation; pain.

Parasidose *Gilbert, Fr.; Multichem, NZ.*
Phenothrin (p.1436·2).
Pediculosis.

Parasin *Ache, Braz.*
Albendazole (p.95·2).
Worm infections.

The symbol † denotes a preparation no longer actively marketed

Para-Speciaal *Byk, Neth.*
Bioallethrin (p.1428·3); piperonyl butoxide (p.1436·2).
Pediculosis.

Para-Suppo *Orion, Fin.*
Paracetamol (p.71·2).
Fever; pain.

Parat *Asian Pharm, Thai.*
Paracetamol (p.71·2).
Fever; pain.

Para-Tabs *Orion, Fin.*
Paracetamol (p.71·2).
Fever; pain.

Paratabs *PSM, NZ.*
Paracetamol (p.71·2).
Fever; pain.

Paratol *Chew, Thai.*
Paracetamol (p.71·2).
Fever; pain.

Paratosse *Heralds, Braz.*
Diphenhydramine (p.416·1); ammonium chloride (p.1085·2); sodium citrate (p.1186·2); menthol (p.1632·3).
Coughs.

Paratulle *SSL, UK.*
Yellow soft paraffin (p.1407·3).
Wounds.

Paravertebral LWS *Infirmarius-Rovit, Ger.*
Homoeopathic preparation.

Paraxin *Roche, Ger.*
Chloramphenicol sodium succinate (p.179·2).
Bacterial infections.

Parcaine *Ocusoft, USA.*
Proxymetacaine hydrochloride (p.1320·1).

Parcel *Novartis, Braz.*
Paracetamol (p.71·2); dihydroergotamine mesilate (p.450·3); caffeine (p.761·3).
Migraine.

Pardelprin *Cox, UK.*
Indometacin (p.44·3).
Dysmenorrhoea; musculoskeletal, joint, and peri-articular disorders.

Pa-Real *Lampugnani, Ital.*
Royal jelly (p.1659·3).
Nutritional supplement.

Parecid *Proge, Ital.*
Cefonicid sodium (p.168·1).
Lignocaine [lidocaine] hydrochloride (p.1313·2) is included in this preparation to alleviate the pain of injection.
Bacterial infections.

Paredrine *Pharmics, USA.*
Hydroxyamfetamine hydrobromide (p.1622·1).
Production of mydriasis.

Paregorique *Monot, Fr.*
Prepared opium (p.69·3); benzoic acid (p.1134·2); anise oil (p.1580·3); camphor (p.1589·3).
Diarrhoea.

Parelmin *QIF, Braz.*
Mebendazole (p.102·2).
Cestode infections; nematode infections.

Paremyd *Allergan, USA.*
Hydroxyamfetamine hydrobromide (p.1622·1); tropicamide (p.475·1).
Induction of mydriasis with partial cycloplegia.

Parenciclina *Hoechst Marion Roussel, Mex.*
Tetracycline (p.258·3).
Bacterial infections.

Parengesico *Hoechst Marion Roussel, Mex.*
Paracetamol (p.71·2).
Fever; pain.

Parentamin
Serag-Wiessner, Ger.; Fresenius Kabi, Ital.
Amino-acid infusion (p.1350·1).
Parenteral nutrition.

Parentamin E *Serag-Wiessner, Ger.*
Amino-acid and electrolyte infusion (p.1350·1).
Parenteral nutrition.

Parentamin X-E *Serag-Wiessner, Ger.*
Amino-acid, electrolyte, and xylitol infusion (p.1350·1).
Parenteral nutrition.

Parentamin EAS *Serag-Wiessner, Ger.*
Amino-acid infusion (p.1350·1).
Parenteral nutrition in renal impairment.

Parentamin G E *Serag-Wiessner, Ger.*
Amino-acid, electrolyte, and glucose infusion (p.1350·1).
Parenteral nutrition.

Parentamin GX E *Serag-Wiessner, Ger.*
Amino-acid, electrolyte, glucose, and xylitol infusion (p.1350·1).
Parenteral nutrition.

Parentamin-C-hepa *Serag-Wiessner, Ger.*
Amino-acid, electrolyte, and xylitol infusion (p.1350·1).
Parenteral nutrition in liver disease.

Parenteral *Serag-Wiessner, Ger.*
A range of electrolyte infusions (p.1180·1) with or without carbohydrate.
Fluid and electrolyte disorders.

Parenterin *Legrand, Braz.*
Neomycin sulfate (p.228·1); phthalylsulfathiazole (p.235·3); pectin (p.1502·3); aluminium hydroxide (p.1210·3).
Diarrhoea.

Parenzyme *Medley, Braz.*
Trypsin (p.1675·3); chymotrypsin (p.1595·1).
Inflammation.

Parenzyme Ampicilina *Medley, Braz.*
Trypsin (p.1675·3); chymotrypsin (p.1595·1); ampicillin (p.150·3).
Bacterial infections; inflammation.

Parenzyme Tetraciclina *Medley, Braz.*
Trypsin (p.1675·3); chymotrypsin (p.1595·1); tetracycline hydrochloride (p.258·3).
Bacterial infections; inflammation.

Pareox *Pharmadent, Fr.*
Chlorhexidine gluconate (p.1138·2).
Bacterial mouth infections.

Par-F *Pharmics, USA.*
Multivitamin and mineral preparation with iron and folic acid (p.1350·1).

Parfenac
Wyeth Lederle, Aust.; Whitehall, Fr.; Lederle, Ger.; Lederle, Neth.; Whitehall, Port.; Whitehall, S.Afr.†; Whitehall-Robins, Switz.
Bufexamac (p.20·3).
Burns; insect stings; skin disorders.

Parfenac Basisbad *Lederle, Ger.*
Arachis oil (p.1581·1); light liquid paraffin (p.1407·2).
Bath additive; dry, pruritic skin disorders.

Parfenal *Wyeth Lederle, Ital.*
Bufexamac (p.20·3).
Skin disorders.

Par-Gamma *Biagini, Ital.*
A mumps immunoglobulin (p.1551·1).
Passive immunisation.

Pargin *Metapharma, Ital.†*
Econazole nitrate (p.382·3).
Fungal infections.

Pargitan *Abigo, Swed.*
Benzhexol [trihexyphenidyl] hydrochloride (p.463·3).
Drug-induced extrapyramidal disorders; parkinsonism; spasms in children.

Pargo *Bio-Diat, Ger.*
Devil's claw root (p.26·3).
Biliary disorders; degenerative joint disorders; gastrointestinal disorders.

Parhist SR *Parmed, USA†.*
Phenylpropanolamine hydrochloride (p.1098·1); chlorpheniramine [chlorphenamine] maleate (p.412·1).
Upper respiratory-tract symptoms.

Pariet
Janssen-Cilag, Aust.; Janssen-Cilag, Denm.; Janssen-Cilag, Fin.; Janssen-Cilag, Fr.; Eisai, Ger.; Janssen-Cilag, Ger.; Janssen-Cilag, Irl.; Janssen-Cilag, Ital.; Eisai, Jpn; Janssen, Mex.; Janssen-Cilag, Neth.; Janssen-Cilag, Port.; Janssen-Cilag, Spain; Janssen-Cilag, Swed.; Eisai, Thai.; Eisai, UK; Eisai, UK.
Rabeprazole sodium (p.1245·1).
Gastro-oesophageal reflux; peptic ulcer; Zollinger-Ellison syndrome.

Parilac *Teva, Israel.*
Bromocriptine mesilate (p.1164·3).
Acromegaly; amenorrhoea; galactorrhoea; male and female infertility; parkinsonism; prolactinoma.

Paritrel *Trima, Israel.*
Amantadine hydrochloride (p.1161·2).
Drug-induced extrapyramidal disorders; influenza A; parkinsonism.

Parizac *Lacer, Spain.*
Omeprazole (p.1239·1) or omeprazole sodium (p.1239·1).
Gastro-oesophageal reflux; peptic ulcers; Zollinger-Ellison syndrome.

Parkadina *Basi, Port.*
Amantadine (p.1162·2).
Parkinsonism.

Parkelase *Parke, Davis, Spain†.*
Deoxyribonuclease (p.1089·1); fibrinolysin (p.890·1).
Wound healing.

Parkelase Chloromycetin *Parke, Davis, Spain†.*
Chloramphenicol (p.179·1); deoxyribonuclease (p.1089·1); fibrinolysin (p.890·1).
Abscesses; burns; cervicitis; ulcers; vaginitis.

Parkemed
Parke, Davis, Aust.; Parke, Davis, Ger.
Mefenamic acid (p.51·2).
Fever; inflammation; musculoskeletal and joint disorders; pain.

Parkinane *Wyeth Lederle, Fr.*
Benzhexol [trihexyphenidyl] hydrochloride (p.463·3).
Drug-induced extrapyramidal disorders; parkinsonism.

Parkinsan *Lundbeck, Ger.*
Budipine hydrochloride (p.1167·2).
Parkinsonism.

Parkipan
L'Arguenon, Fr.†
Topical solution: Trypan blue.
Viral infections of the skin and mucous membranes.

SERB, Fr.
Ointment: Trypan blue; amylocaine hydrochloride (p.1306·1); titanium dioxide (p.1126·1).
Viral skin infections.

Parkopan *Hexal, Ger.*
Benzhexol [trihexyphenidyl] hydrochloride (p.463·3).
Parkinsonism.

Parkotil *Lilly, Ger.*
Pergolide mesilate (p.1175·1).
Parkinsonism.

Parks *Hommel, Ger.*
Pridinol hydrochloride (p.1330·1).
Extrapyramidal disorders; parkinsonism.

Parlax *Labomed, Fr.*
Liquid paraffin (p.1407·1).
Constipation.

Parlodel
Novartis, Aust.; Novartis, Austral.; Novartis, Belg.; Novartis, Braz.; Novartis, Canad.; Novartis, Denm.; Novartis, Fin.; Novartis, Fr.; Novartis, Hong Kong; Novartis, Irl.; Novartis, Ital.; Sandoz, Jpn†; Novartis, Mex.; Novartis, Neth.; Novartis, Norw.; Novartis, NZ; Novartis, Port.; Novartis, S.Afr.; Novartis, Singapore; Novartis, Spain; Novartis, Switz.; Novartis, Thai.; Novartis, UK; Novartis, USA.
Bromocriptine mesilate (p.1164·3).
Acromegaly; benign breast disorders; fertility disorders; hyperprolactinaemia; lactation inhibition; menstrual disorders; parkinsonism; prolactinoma.

Parmecal
Geymonat, Ital.; Geymonat, Switz.
Food for special diets (p.1350·1).
Colic; diarrhoea.

Parmentier *Therabel, Belg.†*
Caffeine (p.761·3); phenazone (p.77·2).
Headache; migraine; pain.

Parmid *Lagap, UK.*
Metoclopramide hydrochloride (p.1235·2).
Gastrointestinal disorders; migraine.

Parmodalin *Sanofi Synthelabo, Ital.*
Tranylcypromine sulfate (p.309·3); trifluoperazine hydrochloride (p.710·3).
Depression.

Par-Natal Plus 1 Improved *Parmed, USA.*
Multivitamin and mineral preparation with iron and folic acid (p.1350·1).

Parnate
SmithKline Beecham, Austral.; Enila, Braz.; SmithKline Beecham, Canad.; Procter & Gamble, Ger.†; Goldshield, Irl.; SmithKline Beecham, NZ; SmithKline Beecham, S.Afr.; Sterling Health, Spain; Goldshield, UK; SmithKline Beecham, USA.
Tranylcypromine sulfate (p.309·3).
Depression.

Paro *Hoechst Marion Roussel, Ital.†*
Hydrocortisone acetate (p.1073·3).
Skin disorders.

Parocin *Almirall, Spain.*
Meloxicam (p.51·3).
Ankylosing spondylitis; osteoarthritis; rheumatoid arthritis.

Parodium *Pierre Fabre Sante, Fr.*
Chlorhexidine gluconate (p.1138·2); rhubarb (p.1248·1); formaldehyde (p.1144·2).
Gum disorders.

Parodontal *Serum-Werk Bernburg, Ger.*
Chamomile (p.1593·2); sage (p.1660·3); lignocaine [lidocaine] (p.1313·2).
Mouth inflammation.

Parodontal F5 med *Wernigerode, Ger.*
Salol (p.82·2); thymol (p.1158·3); mint oil (p.1636·2); eucalyptol (p.1609·2); clove oil (p.1597·1); sage oil (p.1660·2).
Mouth inflammation.

Parodontax
Note. This name is used for preparations of different composition.
Madaus, Aust.†
Mouthwash: Echinacea purpurea (p.1606·2); chamomile (p.1593·2); myrrh (p.1639·2); menthol (p.1632·3); clove oil (p.1597·1); caraway oil (p.1591·2); sage oil (p.1660·2); peppermint oil (p.1243·3); mint oil (p.1636·2).
Bleeding gums; inflammation of the mouth and gums; oral hygiene.
Toothpaste: Echinacea purpurea (p.1606·2); sodium bicarbonate (p.1186·2); chamomile (p.1593·2); myrrh (p.1639·2); rhatany root (p.1657·3); sage oil (p.1660·2); peppermint oil (p.1243·3).
Dental caries prophylaxis; oral hygiene.

Byk, Braz.
Echinacea purpurea (p.1606·2); sodium bicarbonate (p.1186·2); chamomile (p.1593·2); myrrh (p.1639·2); rhatany root (p.1657·3).
Oral hygiene.

Madaus, Israel.
Echinacea (p.1606·2); sodium bicarbonate (p.1186·2); chamomile (p.1593·2); myrrh (p.1639·2); rhatany (p.1657·3); sage oil (p.1660·2); peppermint oil (p.1243·3).
Dental disorders.

Parogencyl *Sanofi Synthelabo, Ital.*
Phermentol; provitamin B5.
Gum disorders.

Parol *Berman, Mex.*
Cyanocobalamin (p.1388·1).

Paronal *Christiaens, Belg.*
Asparaginase (p.508·3).
Acute leukaemia.

Paroven
Novartis Consumer, Austral.; Novartis Consumer, Irl.; Novartis, NZ; Novartis Consumer, S.Afr.; Novartis Consumer, UK.
Oxerutins (p.1611·2).
Chronic venous insufficiency; haemorrhoids; prevention of skin and mucosal reactions to radiotherapy.

Parsal *Wyeth, Ger.*
Ibuprofen (p.43·2).
Fever; gout; inflammation; musculoskeletal, joint, and soft-tissue disorders; pain.

Parsel
Note. This name is used for preparations of different composition.
Novartis, Mex.
Dihydroergotamine mesilate (p.450·3); paracetamol (p.71·2); caffeine (p.761·3).
Migraine.

Novartis Consumer, Port.
Paracetamol (p.71·2).
Fever; pain.

Parsilid *Crinos, Ital.*
Ticlopidine hydrochloride (p.981·1).
Thrombosis prophylaxis.

Parsitan *Rhone-Poulenc Rorer, Canad.*
Profenamine hydrochloride (p.473·2).
Drug-induced extrapyramidal disorders; parkinsonism.

Parstelin
SmithKline Beecham, Irl.; SmithKline Beecham, UK†.
Tranylcypromine sulfate (p.309·3); trifluoperazine hydrochloride (p.710·3).
Mixed anxiety depressive states.

Partamol *Atlantic, Thai.*
Paracetamol (p.71·2).
Fever; pain.

Partane *Taro, Israel.*
Benzhexol [trihexyphenidyl] hydrochloride (p.463·3).
Drug-induced extrapyramidal disorders; parkinsonism.

Partapp TD *Parmed, USA†.*
Phenylpropanolamine hydrochloride (p.1098·1); phenylephrine hydrochloride (p.1097·1); brompheniramine maleate (p.410·2).
Upper respiratory-tract symptoms.

Partobulin
Immuno, Aust.; Immuno, Ger.; Immuno, Hong Kong; Immuno, Ital.; Baxter, UK.
An anti-D immunoglobulin (p.1532·1).
Now known as Anti-D Immunoglobulin in the UK.
Prevention of rhesus sensitisation.

Partocon
Ferring, Israel; Ferring, Swed.†.
Oxytocin (p.1294·1).
Abortion induction; eclampsia; labour induction; pre-eclampsia; promotion of lactation.

Partogamma *Immuno, Braz.*
An anti-D immunoglobulin (p.1532·1).
Prevention of rhesus sensitisation.

Parto-Gamma *Biagini, Ital.*
An anti-D immunoglobulin (p.1532·1).
Prevention of rhesus sensitisation.

Partrim *Parke-Med, S.Afr.‡*
Co-trimoxazole (p.193·3).
Bacterial infections.

Partusisten
Boehringer Ingelheim, Ger.; Promeco, Mex.; Boehringer Ingelheim, Neth.; Vifor, Switz.†
Fenoterol hydrobromide (p.765·1).
Fetal distress; premature labour.

Partuss LA *Parmed, USA†.*
Phenylpropanolamine hydrochloride (p.1098·1); guaifenesin (p.1092·2).
Coughs.

Parulon *Proveedora Teknimex, Mex.*
Pancuronium bromide (p.1338·2).
Competitive neuromuscular blocker.

Paruman
Berna, Ital.†; Berna, Switz.†.
A mumps immunoglobulin (p.1551·1).
Passive immunisation.

Parvisedil *SIT, Ital.*
Aminohydroxybutyric acid (p.342·2); valerian (p.1678·3); passion flower (p.1649·1); chamomile (p.1593·2); crataegus (p.1600·2).
Restlessness and insomnia in infants.

Parvlex *Freeda, USA.*
Ferrous fumarate (p.1360·1); folic acid (p.1361·1); vitamin B substances with vitamin C (p.1350·1).
Iron-deficiency anaemias.

Parvolex
DBL, Austral.; Bioniche, Canad.; Faulding, Hong Kong; Evans Medical, Irl.; Baxter, NZ; Glaxo Wellcome, S.Afr.; Celltech, UK.
Acetylcysteine (p.1082·3).
Paracetamol overdosage; respiratory-tract congestion.

Pas Hain *Rudefsa, Mex.*
Isoniazid (p.215·3).

Pasaden *Farmades, Ital.*
Etizolam (p.683·1).
Anxiety; insomnia.

Pasalen *Pharmaland, Thai.*
Ketoconazole (p.389·1).
Fungal infections.

Pasalix *Marjan, Braz.*
Passion flower (p.1649·1); salix (p.82·1); crataegus (p.1600·2).
Sedative.

Pascallerg *Pascoe, Ger.*
Homoeopathic preparation.

Pascobilin novo *Pascoe, Ger.*
Peppermint leaf (p.1243·2); taraxacum (p.1669·1); cynara (p.1601·3).
Biliary-tract disorders.

Pascodolor Tropfen *Pascoe, Ger.*
Homoeopathic preparation.

Pascofemin *Pascoe, Ger.*
Homoeopathic preparation.

Pascohepan novo *Pascoe, Ger.*
Greater celandine (p.1618·1); silybum marianum (p.1021·3); taraxacum (p.1669·1).
Liver disorders.

Pascoletten N *Pascoe, Ger.*
Aloes (p.1210·1); chamomile (p.1593·2).
Constipation.

Pascoleucyn *Pascoe, Ger.*
Homoeopathic preparation.

Pascolibrin *Pascoe, Ger.*
Homoeopathic preparation.

Pascomag *Pascoe, Ger.*
Bismuth subnitrate (p.1213·2); chamomile (p.1593·2); linseed (p.1629·1).
Gastrointestinal disorders.

Pascomucil *Koch, Aust.; Pascoe, Ger.*
Ispaghula (p.1229·1).
Constipation; diarrhoea.

Pascoal forte Nerventropfen *Pascoe, Ger.*
Homoeopathic preparation.

Pasconal Nerventropfen *Pascoe, Ger.*
Homoeopathic preparation.

Pasconeural-Injektopas *Pascoe, Ger.*
Procaine hydrochloride (p.1319·1); caffeine (p.761·3).
Local anaesthesia.

Pasconeural-Injektopas 1% *Pascoe, Ger.†*
Procaine hydrochloride (p.1319·1).
Local anaesthesia.

Pascopankreat *Koch, Aust.*
Condurango (p.1599·1); silybum marianum (p.1021·3); fennel fruit (p.1610·1); caraway oil (p.1591·2); chamomile oil.
Gastrointestinal disorders.

Pascopankreat novo *Pascoe, Ger.*
Combination pack: Yellow tablets, absinthium (p.1571·1); condurango (p.1599·1); red tablets, pancreatin (porcine) (p.1646·1).
Digestive system disorders.
Oral drops: Caraway oil (p.1591·2); chamomile oil; condurango (p.1599·1); silybum marianum (p.1021·3); fennel (p.1610·1).
Gastrointestinal disorders.

Pascopankreat S *Pascoe, Ger.†*
Pancreatin; caraway oil (p.1591·2); chamomile oil; condurango; salicylaric; cholesterin.; menthol; ol. anisi; card. mar.; foenic.; syzyg. jamb.
Digestive system disorders.

Pascorenal *Pascoe, Ger.*
Homoeopathic preparation.

Pascosabal *Pascoe, Ger.*
Homoeopathic preparation.

Pascosedon *Pascoe, Ger.*
Valerian (p.1678·3); lupulus (p.1629·1); melissa (p.1632·2).
Anxiety; sleep disorders.

Pascotox *Pascoe, Ger.*
Oral drops: Echinacea (p.1606·2); baptisia; bryonia; eupator. perfol.; arnica; ferr. phosphoric.; thuja; china; lachesis; cupr. sulfuric.
Tablets: Echinacea (p.1606·2); baptisia; bryonia; eupatorium perfoliatum; thuja; lachesis.
Tonic.

Pascotox forte-Injektopas *Pascoe, Ger.*
Echinacea (p.1606·2).
Tonic.

Pascotox mono *Pascoe, Ger.*
Echinacea (p.1606·2).
Tonic.

Pascovegeton *Pascoe, Ger.*
Angelica (p.1580·2).
Gastrointestinal disorders.

Pascovenol novo *Pascoe, Ger.*
Aesculus (p.1574·1); melilotus; hamamelis (p.1618·3).
Thromboembolic disorders; vascular disorders.

Paser *Jacobus, USA.*
Aminosalicylic acid (p.148·3).
Tuberculosis.

Pas-Fatol N *Fatol, Ger.*
Sodium aminosalicylate (p.148·3).
Tuberculosis.

Pasgensin *Pascoe, Ger.*
Vitamins (p.1350·1); oxedrine tartrate (p.950·3).
Hypotension; tonic.

Pasisana *Hotz, Ger.*
Herbal and homoeopathic preparation.

Pasivital h *Hotz, Ger.*
Homoeopathic preparation.

Pasmolit *Jofrain, Mex.*
Homatropine (p.468·1).

Paspat
Note. This name is used for preparations of different composition.
Luitpold, Braz.
Staphylococcus aureus; Staphylococcus epidermidis; Staphylococcus viridans; Streptococcus haemolyticus; Streptococcus pneumoniae; Moraxella catarrhalis; Haemophilus influenzae; Candida albicans.
Immunotherapy.

Sankyo, Ger.; Byk Gulden, Mex.; Sankyo, Thai.
Lysate of *Staphylococcus aureus; Staphylococcus albus; Streptococcus viridans; Streptococcus haemolyticus; Streptococcus pneumoniae; Moraxella*

catarrhalis; Haemophilus influenzae; Candida albicans.
Eye and ear disorders; hypersensitivity reactions; respiratory-tract disorders.

Sankyo, Ital.
Lysate of *Staphylococcus aureus; Streptococcus mitis; Streptococcus pyogenes; Streptococcus pneumoniae; Klebsiella pneumoniae; Moraxella catarrhalis; Haemophilus influenzae.*
Respiratory-tract infections.

Paspat Oral *Sankyo, Port.*
Staphylococcus aureus; Streptococcus mitis; Streptococcus pyogenes; Streptococcus pneumoniae; Klebsiella pneumoniae; Moraxella catarrhalis; Haemophilus influenzae.
Respiratory-tract infections.

Paspertase *Solvay, Aust.; Solvay, Ger.*
Metoclopramide hydrochloride (p.1235·2); pancreatin (p.1646·1).
Gastrointestinal disorders.

Paspertin *Solvay, Aust.; Solvay, Ger.; Solvay, Switz.*
Metoclopramide (p.1236·3) or metoclopramide hydrochloride (p.1235·2).
Adjunct in gastrointestinal radiography; gastrointestinal disorders.

Pasrin *Aspen, S.Afr.*
Buspirone hydrochloride (p.657·2).
Anxiety; mixed anxiety depressive states.

Passagen *Durascan, Denm.*
Xylometazoline hydrochloride (p.1102·2).
Nasal congestion.

Passaja *Farmabraz, Braz.*
Thymol (p.1158·3); menthol (p.1632·3); camphor (p.1589·3); eugenol (p.1609·3); procaine hydrochloride (p.1319·1).
Oral hygiene.

Passaneuro *Bunker, Braz.*
Passion flower (p.1649·1); erythrina mulungu; chamomile (p.1593·2).
Sedative.

Passedan *Austroplant, Aust.*
Passion flower (p.1649·1); melissa leaf (p.1632·2).
Dystonias; menopausal disorders; sleep disorders.

Passedyl *Urgo, Fr.*
Sodium benzoate (p.1134·3); sulfogaiacol (p.1101·1).
Formerly contained drosera, grindelia, sodium benzoate, potassium bromide, sulfogaiacol, orange-flower water, terpin, tolu balsam, and senega.
Respiratory-tract congestion.

Passelyt *Smetana, Aust.*
Passion flower (p.1649·1); melissa leaf (p.1632·2).
Anxiety disorders; sleep disorders.

Passicarbone *Millet Roux, Braz.*
Vegetable charcoal (p.1000·3); passion flower (p.1649·1); crataegus (p.1600·2); salix alba (p.82·1).
Diarrhoea.

Passiflora *Tamar, Israel.*
Passion flower (p.1649·1); crataegus (p.1600·2); valerian (p.1678·3); orange flower.
Insomnia; nervousness; tension.

Passiflora Complex
Note. This name is used for preparations of different composition.
Blackmores, Austral.
Passion flower (p.1649·1); lupulus (p.1629·3); skullcap (p.1664·3); valerian (p.1678·3); multivitamins (p.1350·1).
Anxiety; insomnia; stress symptoms.

Dolisos, Canad.
Homoeopathic preparation.

Passiflora Compose *Boiron, Fr.*
Homoeopathic preparation.

Passiflora Composta *Luper, Braz.*
Passion flower (p.1649·1); erythrina mulungu; melissa (p.1632·2).
Sedative.

Passiflora Compound *Vitamed, Israel.*
Passion flower (p.1649·1); valerian (p.1678·3).
Anxiety; insomnia; tension.

Passiflora Curarina *Harras-Curarina, Ger.*
Passion flower (p.1649·1).
Agitation.

Passiflora GHL *Lehning, Fr.*
Homoeopathic preparation.

Passiflorin *Austroplant, Aust.*
Passion flower (p.1649·1).
Nervous disorders; sleep disorders.

Passiflorine
Note. This name is used for preparations of different composition.
Millet Roux, Braz.; Teofarma, Ital.; Wasserman, Spain.
Passion flower (p.1649·1); crataegus (p.1600·2); salix alba (p.82·1).
Anxiety; insomnia; menopausal disorders.

Theratech, Fr.
Passion flower (p.1649·1); crataegus (p.1600·2).
Insomnia; nervous disorders.

Passifuril *Millet Roux, Braz.*
Nifuroxazide (p.230·2).
Diarrhoea.

Passin *Simons, Ger.*
Crataegus (p.1600·2); passion flower (p.1649·1).
Anxiety; nervous gastrointestinal disorders; sleep disorders.

Passinevryl *Clement, Fr.*
Passion flower (p.1649·1); crataegus (p.1600·2); valerian (p.1678·3).

Formerly contained passion flower, willow, crataegus, and valerian.
Insomnia.

Passionflower Plus *Eagle, Austral.*
Passion flower (p.1649·1); valerian (p.1678·3); skullcap (p.1664·3); lupulus (p.1629·3).
Anxiety; insomnia.

Passiorin N *Simons, Ger.†*
Crataegus (p.1600·2); passion flower (p.1649·1).
Nervous disorders; sleep disorders.

Past Ail *Medecine Vegetale, Fr.†*
Garlic (p.1614·1).
Capillary fragility; circulatory disorders.

Pasta boli *Spirig, Switz.*
Salicylic acid (p.1122·3); eucalyptus oil (p.1609·2); peppermint oil (p.1243·3); methyl salicylate (p.55·1).
Musculoskeletal, joint, peri-articular, and soft-tissue disorders.

Pasta Cool *Apomedica, Aust.*
Heparin sodium (p.902·1); salicylic acid (p.1122·3).
Musculoskeletal and joint disorders; peri-articular disorders; soft-tissue injury.

Pasta d'Agua *Dermopen, Braz.; Medic, Braz.; Neckerman, Braz.; Stevia, Braz.*
Zinc oxide (p.1128·2); purified talc (p.1124·2); glycerol (p.1616·3); agua de cal.
Skin disorders.

Pasta De Lassar *Andromaco, Mex.*
Zinc oxide (p.1128·2).
Skin disorders.

Pasta Dicofarm *Dicofarm, Ital.*
Zinc oxide (p.1128·2); titanium dioxide (p.1126·1); vitamin E (p.1393·3); vitamin F.
Skin irritation.

Pasta Lactisol *Galactopharm, Ger.†*
Sour milk whey concentrate.
Skin disorders.

Pasta Lassar Imba *Calmante Vitaminado, Spain.*
Almond oil (p.1576·3); lanolin; zinc oxide (p.1128·2).
Burns; skin disorders; wounds.

Pasta Lassar Orravan *Orravan, Spain.*
Salicylic acid (p.1122·3); soft paraffin; zinc oxide (p.1128·2).
Burns; skin disorders; wounds.

Pasta Plumbi *Sanova, Aust.†*
Lead (p.1627·3).
Insect bites and stings.

Pasta Prura *Propan, S.Afr.†*
Coal tar (p.1125·1); zinc oxide (p.1128·2); calamine (p.1111·3).
Skin disorders.

Pasta rubra salicylata *Apomedica, Aust.*
Diethylamine salicylate (p.32·2); salicylic acid (p.1122·3); methyl salicylate (p.55·1).
Gout; rheumatism; sciatica; soft-tissue injury; tendinitis.

Pastiglie Valda *Valda, Ital.*
Cicliomenol; enoxolone (p.34·3); menthol (p.1632·3); eucalyptol (p.1609·2).
Catarrh; mouth and throat irritation.

Pastilhas Valda *Canonne, Braz.*
Menthol (p.1632·3); eucalyptol (p.1609·2).
Mouth disorders.

Pastillas Antisep Garg L *Procter & Gamble, Spain.*
Ascorbic acid (p.1389·3); cetylpyridinium chloride (p.1138·1); citric acid (p.1596·2); menthol (p.1632·3).
Throat irritation.

Pastillas Antisep Garg M *Procter & Gamble, Spain.*
Camphor (p.1589·3); benzyl alcohol (p.1135·2); tolu balsam (p.1101·3); thymol (p.1158·3); menthol (p.1632·3); eucalyptus (p.1609·2); cetylpyridinium chloride (p.1138·1).
Throat irritation.

Pastillas Dr Andreu *Roche Nicholas, Spain.*
Dextromethorphan hydrobromide (p.1087·3); sodium benzoate.
Coughs.

Pastillas Juanola *Farma Lepori, Spain.*
Eucalyptol (p.1609·2); liquorice (p.1231·2); terpineol (p.1669·2); menthol (p.1632·3).
Coughs; throat irritation.

Pastillas Koki Ment Tiro *Calmante Vitaminado, Spain.*
Benzocaine (p.1306·2); tyrothricin (p.267·1); menthol (p.1632·3).
Mouth and throat disorders.

Pastillas Pectoral Kely *Boots Healthcare, Spain.*
Eucalyptol (p.1609·2); niaouli (p.1640·2); senega (p.1100·2); liquorice (p.1231·2); sodium benzoate (p.1134·3); sulfogaiacol (p.1101·1); terpin monohydrate (p.1101·2).
Respiratory-tract disorders.

Pastillas d'Ems *Siemens, Switz.*
Sal ems.
Cold symptoms; upper-respiratory-tract inflammation.

Pastillas Medicinales Vicks *Lachartre, Fr.*
Camphor (p.1589·3); menthol (p.1632·3); eucalyptus oil (p.1609·2); thymol (p.1158·3); tolu balsam (p.1101·3); benzyl alcohol (p.1135·2).
Sore throats.

Pastilles Monleon *Toulade, Fr.*
Methylene blue [methylthioninium chloride] (p.1012·3); tolu balsam (p.1101·3); drosera (p.1606·1); hamamelis (p.1618·3).
Formerly contained methylene blue [methylthioninium chloride], tolu balsam, drosera, aconite, hamamelis, and ipecacuanha.
Mouth and throat disorders.

Pastilles pectorales Demo N *Democal, Switz.*
Drosera (p.1606·1); hedera helix; ipecacuanha (p.1093·1); plantain (p.1652·3); tolu balsam (p.1101·3); anise oil (p.1580·3); orange peel (p.1644·2); eucalyptus oil (p.1609·2); mint oil (p.1636·2); menthol (p.1632·3).
Coughs.

Pastilles pectorales formule 541 *Renapharm, Switz.*
Senega (p.1100·2); thyme (p.1672·3); drosera (p.1606·1); sage oil (p.1660·2); fennel oil (p.1610·2); star anise oil; menthol (p.1632·3); ephedrine hydrochloride (p.1090·1); eucalyptus oil (p.1609·2); liquorice (p.1231·2).
Coughs.

Pastilles pour la gorge no 535 *Renapharm, Switz.*
Dequalinium salicylate (p.1143·1).
Mouth and throat disorders.

Pastilles Valda *Valda, Fr.*
Guaiacol (p.1092·1); eucalyptol (p.1609·2); menthol (p.1632·3); terpin hydrate (p.1101·2); thymol (p.1158·3).

Pastimmun *Pasteur Merieux, Belg.†*
A BCG vaccine (p.1533·2).
Bladder cancer.

Pasuma-Dragees *Herchemie, Aust.†*
Methyltestosterone (p.1482·3); alpha tocoferil acetate (p.1394·1); yohimbine hydrochloride (p.1681·3); strychnine glycerophosphate; caffeine (p.761·3); oxedrine tartrate (p.950·3).

Patanol *Alcon, Canad.; Alcon, Singapore; Alcon, Thai.; Alcon, USA.*
Olopatadine hydrochloride (p.422·1).
Allergic conjunctivitis.

Pate a l'Eau Roche-Posay *Roche-Posay, Fr.*
Zinc oxide (p.1128·2); titanium dioxide (p.1126·1); borax (p.1586·1).
Eczema.

Pate d'Unna *Rougier, Canad.*
Zinc oxide (p.1128·2).

Pate Iodoforme du Prof Dr Walkhoff *Haupt, Switz.†*
Iodoform (p.1149·1); parachlorophenol (p.1152·1); camphor (p.1589·3); menthol (p.1632·3).
Dental inflammation.

Patector *AF, Mex.*
Algestone acetophenide (p.1465·1); estradiol enantate (p.1473·2).
Endometriosis; female infertility; injectable contraceptive; menstrual disorders.

Patentex *Medra, Aust.; Frere, Belg.; CCD, Fr.; PCR, Ger.; Brovar, S.Afr.†*
Nonoxinol 9 (p.1346·1).
Contraceptive.

Patentex Oval N
Patentex, Ger.; Patentex, Switz.
Nonoxinol 9 (p.1346·1).
Contraceptive.

Pates Pectorales *Oberlin, Fr.†*
Codeine (p.25·2); tolu balsam (p.1101·3); cherry-laurel.
Coughs.

Pathilon *Lederle, USA†.*
Tridihexethyl chloride (p.474·3).
Peptic ulcer (adjunct).

Pathocil *Wyeth-Ayerst, USA.*
Dicloxacillin sodium (p.199·1).
Bacterial infections.

Patriot *Agropharm, UK.*
Pyrethrins; piperonyl butoxide (p.1436·2).
Insecticide and repellent.

Patropin *Rekah, Israel.*
Papaverine hydrochloride (p.1648·1); atropine sulfate (p.461·1).
Smooth muscle spasm.

Patsolin *Leiras, Fin.*
Prazosin hydrochloride (p.958·1).
Heart failure; hypertension.

Patussol *Andreabal, Switz.†*
Oral drops: Dextromethorphan hydrobromide (p.1087·3); chlorpheniramine [chlorphenamine] maleate (p.412·1); ipecacuanha (p.1093·1); senega (p.1100·2).
Syrup: Dextromethorphan hydrobromide (p.1087·3); chlorpheniramine [chlorphenamine] maleate (p.412·1); ammonium chloride (p.1085·2); ipecacuanha (p.1093·1).
Coughs.

Patxen *Ehlinger, Mex.*
Naproxen (p.60·3).

Pausal *Theramex, Ital.*
11 Tablets, estradiol valerate (p.1473·2); 10 tablets, estradiol valerate; cyproterone acetate (p.1467·3).
Menopausal disorders.

Pausanol *Leiras, Fin.*
Estriol (p.1475·3).
Menopausal vaginal disorders; oestrogen deficiency.

Pausigin *Lepori, Port.*
Estriol (p.1475·3).
Vulvovaginal disorders.

Pavabid *Hoechst Marion Roussel, USA.*
Papaverine hydrochloride (p.1648·1).
Cerebral and peripheral ischaemia; smooth muscle spasm.

Pa-Vaccinol *Procter & Gamble, Ger.†*
A pertussis vaccine (p.1555·3).
Active immunisation.

Pavacol-D *Boehringer Ingelheim, UK.*
Pholcodine (p.1099·1).
Coughs.

Pavarine *Vortech, USA†.*
Papaverine hydrochloride (p.1648·1).
Cerebral and peripheral ischaemia; smooth muscle spasm.

Pavatine *Major, USA†.*
Papaverine hydrochloride (p.1648·1).
Cerebral and peripheral ischaemia; smooth muscle spasm.

Paveriwern *Wernigerode, Ger.*
Papaver somniferum.
Gastrointestinal spasm.

Paverolan *Lannett, USA†.*
Papaverine hydrochloride (p.1648·1).
Cerebral and peripheral ischaemia; smooth muscle spasm.

Paverysat forte *Ysatfabrik, Ger.*
Greater celandine (p.1618·1); turmeric (p.1029·3).
Biliary-tract spasm.

Pavitron *Alpha, Mex.*
Tetracycline (p.258·3).
Bacterial infections.

Pavulon
Organon Teknika, Aust.; Organon Teknika, Austral.; Akzo, Braz.; Organon, Canad.†; Organon Teknika, Denm.; Organon Teknika, Fin.; Organon Teknika, Fr.; Organon Teknika, Hong Kong; Organon Teknika, Irl.; Organon Teknika, Israel; Organon Teknika, Ital.; Organon Teknika, Mex.; Organon Teknika, Neth.; Organon Teknika, Norw.; Organon, Port.; Sanofi Synthelabo, S.Afr.; Organon, Singapore; Organon Teknika, Spain; Organon Teknika, Swed.; Organon Teknika, Switz.; Organon, Thai.; Organon, UK; Organon, USA.
Pancuronium bromide (p.1338·2).
Competitive neuromuscular blocker.

Pawa-Rutan *Hanosan, Ger.*
Homoeopathic preparation.

Pax *Aspen, S.Afr.*
Diazepam (p.674·3).
Alcohol withdrawal syndrome; anxiety; premedication.

Paxadorm *Alliance, S.Afr.*
Nitrazepam (p.695·2).
Insomnia.

Paxam *Alphapharm, Austral.*
Clonazepam (p.347·1).
Epilepsy.

Paxarel *Circle, USA.*
Acecarbromal.
Anxiety; insomnia; sedative; spastic colitis.

Paxate *Mead Johnson, Mex.*
Diazepam (p.674·3).

Paxeladine *Beaufour, Fr.*
Oxeladin citrate (p.1096·1).
Coughs.

Paxeladine Noctee *Beaufour, Fr.†.*
Oxeladin citrate (p.1096·1); promethazine hydrochloride (p.423·2).
Coughs.

Paxetil *Medibial, Port.*
Paroxetine hydrochloride (p.302·3).
Anxiety; depression; obsessive-compulsive disorder; panic disorders.

Paxical *Intramed, S.Afr.*
Droperidol (p.682·2).
Nausea and vomiting; neuroleptanalgesia; premedication.

Paxidal
Note. This name is used for preparations of different composition.
Propan, Israel.
Paracetamol (p.71·2); doxylamine succinate (p.417·1); caffeine (p.761·3); codeine phosphate (p.25·2).
Pain and associated tension.

Wallace Mfg Chem., UK.
Caffeine (p.761·3); meprobamate (p.691·1); paracetamol (p.71·2).

Paxidorm
Pharmaserve, Singapore; Norma, UK.
Diphenhydramine hydrochloride (p.416·1).
Insomnia.

Paxil
SmithKline Beecham, Canad.; SmithKline Beecham, Mex.; Glaxo-SmithKline, USA.
Paroxetine hydrochloride (p.302·3).
Anxiety; depression; obsessive-compulsive disorder; panic attacks; social phobia.

Paxilfar *Tecnifar, Port.*
Tramadol hydrochloride (p.89·1).
Pain.

Paxipam *Schering-Plough, Ital.*
Halazepam (p.686·2).
Anxiety.

Paxium *Jaba, Port.*
Chlordiazepoxide (p.659·2).
Alcohol withdrawal syndrome; anxiety; muscle spasm.

Paxtibi *Dista, Spain.*
Nortriptyline hydrochloride (p.301·3).
Depression.

Paxyl *Faulding, Austral.*
Lignocaine [lidocaine] (p.1313·2) or lignocaine [lidocaine] hydrochloride (p.1313·2); benzalkonium chloride (p.1133·2); allantoin (p.1110·1).
Burns; chapped skin; insect bites; skin abrasions; sunburn; windburn.

Pazbronquial *Cinfa, Spain.*
Codeine phosphate (p.25·2); ephedrine hydrochloride (p.1090·1); sodium benzoate (p.1134·3); sodium citrate

(p.1186·2); sulfogaiacol (p.1101·1); thiamine hydrochloride (p.1385·1); pyridoxine hydrochloride (p.1386·3); menthol (p.1632·3); drosera (p.1606·1); lobelia inflata (p.1510·2); thyme (p.1672·2); origanum vulgare; grindelia (p.1618·2).
Coughs.

Pazo *Bristol-Myers Products, USA.*
Benzocaine (p.1306·2); ephedrine sulfate (p.1090·2); zinc oxide (p.1128·2); camphor (p.1589·3).
Haemorrhoids.

Pazolam *Atral, Port.*
Alprazolam (p.654·2).
Anxiety.

Pazolini *Faria, Braz.*
Diazepam (p.674·3).
Alcohol withdrawal syndrome; anxiety; epilepsy; insomnia; premedication; sedative; skeletal muscle spasm.

PBZ *Geigy, USA.*
Tripelennamine citrate (p.427·1) or tripelennamine hydrochloride (p.427·1).
Hypersensitivity reactions.

PC Arthri-Spray *Procare, Austral.†.*
Copper salicylate; methyl salicylate (p.55·1).
Musculoskeletal, joint, and peri-articular disorders.

PC 30 N *Terra-Bio, Ger.*
Chamomile (p.1593·2).
Burns; skin disorders.

PC 30 V *Terra-Bio, Ger.*
Aesculus (p.1574·1); dexpanthenol (p.1602·3); chamomile (p.1593·2).
Skin disorders; ulcers; wounds.

PC Regulax *Procare, Austral.*
Peppermint leaf (p.1243·2); ispaghula (p.1229·1); slippery elm (p.1665·1); ginger (p.1227·2); pectin (p.1502·3).
Gastrointestinal disorders; haemorrhoids; hyperlipidaemias; varicose veins.

PC Rei-shi *Procare, Austral.*
Rei-shi; shi-taki.
Nutritional supplement.

PC-Cap *Alra, USA.*
Dextropropoxyphene hydrochloride (p.27·1); aspirin (p.14·2); caffeine (p.761·3).

PCE
Abbott, Canad.; Abbott, Hong Kong; Abbott, USA.
Erythromycin (p.201·2).
Bacterial infections.

PCF *Ritsert, Ger.*
Homoeopathic preparation.

PCL *Hoe, Singapore.*
Codeine phosphate (p.25·2); promethazine (p.423·2).
Coughs.

PD Cough *PD, Thai.*
Dextromethorphan hydrobromide (p.1087·3); pentoxyverine citrate (p.1096·3); phenylpropanolamine hydrochloride (p.1098·1); guaifenesin (p.1092·2).
Coughs.

PDP Liquid Protein *Wesley, USA.*
Tryptophan (p.311·3); hydrolysed animal collagen (p.1598·2).
Dietary supplement.

PE *Alcon, USA†.*
Pilocarpine hydrochloride (p.1422·3); adrenaline [epinephrine] acid tartrate (p.829·2).
Glaucoma; raised intra-ocular pressure.

Peacetime *Lifeplan, UK.*
Nutritional supplement (p.1350·1).

Peauline *Bipharma, Neth.†.*
Benzoyl peroxide (p.1111·1).
Acne.

Pebegal *Galen, Mex.*
Benzonatate (p.1085·3).
Coughs.

PEC *Universal, Hong Kong.*
Promethazine hydrochloride (p.423·2); ephedrine hydrochloride (p.1090·1); codeine phosphate (p.25·2).
Coughs.

Pe-Ce *Gebro, Aust.*
Turpentine oil (p.1676·3); eucalyptus oil (p.1609·2); nutmeg oil (p.1643·1); cedar leaf oil; camphor (p.1589·3); thymol (p.1158·3).
Coughs and cold symptoms.

Pe-Ce Ven N *Terra-Bio, Ger.*
Aescin (p.1574·1); heparin sodium (p.902·1).
Vascular disorders.

Pecram *Novartis Consumer, UK†.*
Aminophylline hydrate (p.760·1).
Bronchospasm; cardiac asthma and failure.

Pect Hustenloser *Rentschler, Ger.*
Ambroxol hydrochloride (p.1084·3).
Respiratory-tract disorders associated with increased or viscous mucus.

Pectal *Sedabel, Braz.*
Sodium dibunate (p.1100·3); aconite (p.1572·3); eucalyptol (p.1609·2); grindelia (p.1618·2); mikania glomerata; senega (p.1100·2).
Coughs.

Pectalin *EMS, Braz.*
Kaolin (p.1229·3); aluminium hydroxide (p.1210·3); pectin (p.1502·3).
Diarrhoea.

Pectamol *Alpharma, Norw.†.*
Oxeladin citrate (p.1096·1).
Coughs.

Pectapas *Pascoe, Ger.*
Homoeopathic preparation.

Pectikon *Be-Tabs, S.Afr.*
Light kaolin (p.1229·3); apple pectin (p.1502·3).
Diarrhoea.

Pectimax *Climax, Braz.*
Kaolin (p.1229·3); pectin (p.1502·3).
Diarrhoea.

Pectin-K *PD Pharm, S.Afr.*
Kaolin (p.1229·3); apple pectin (p.1502·3).
Diarrhoea.

Pecto-Baby *Pharmacal, Switz.*
Guaifenesin (p.1092·2); pholcodine (p.1099·1); chlorpheniramine [chlorphenamine] maleate (p.412·1).
Coughs.

Pectobal Dextro *Clariana, Spain.*
Dextromethorphan hydrobromide (p.1087·3); mepyramine maleate (p.421·1).
Respiratory-tract disorders.

Pectocalmine *Pharmacal, Switz.*
Codeine phosphate (p.25·2); guaifenesin (p.1092·2); ephedrine hydrochloride (p.1090·1); opium (p.69·3); senega (p.1100·2).
Coughs and associated respiratory-tract disorders.

Pectocalmine Junior N *Pharmacal, Switz.*
Codeine phosphate (p.25·2); tolu balsam (p.1101·3); red-poppy; anethole (p.1580·1).
Coughs and associated respiratory-tract disorders.

Pectocor N *LAW, Ger.*
Camphor (p.1589·3).
Cardiac disorders.

Pectoderme *Dolisos, Fr.*
α-Pinene; β-pinene; myrtol; lavender oil (p.1627·2); terpineol (p.1669·3); eugenol (p.1609·2); camphor (p.1589·3); eucalyptol (p.1609·2).
Respiratory-tract congestion.

Pectoids *Medeva, Fr.*
Liquorice (p.1231·2); menthol (p.1632·3).
Sore throat.

Pectojuvene *Cooperation Pharmaceutique, Fr.*
Carbocisteine (p.1086·3).
Respiratory-tract disorders.

Pectolin *Noristan, S.Afr.†.*
Kaolin (p.1229·3); apple pectin (p.1502·3); electrolytes (p.1185·2).
Diarrhoea.

Pectomucil *Qualiphar, Belg.*
Acetylcysteine (p.1082·3).
Paracetamol poisoning; respiratory-tract disorders associated with viscous secretions.

Pectoral
Note. This name is used for preparations of different composition.
Wenig, Aust.†.
Ephedrine hydrochloride (p.1090·1); α-phenylethylaceticacid-β-diethylaminoethanolester dihydrogen citrate.
Coughs.

Mepha, Hong Kong.
Ipecacuanha (p.1093·1); plantago lanceolata; cowslip (p.1600·1); quillaia (p.1348·2); thyme (p.1672·2); senega (p.1100·2).
Coughs.

Pectoral N *Mepha, Switz.*
Plantain (p.1652·3); cowslip (p.1600·1); senega (p.1100·2); thyme (p.1672·2).
Formerly contained ipecacuanha, plantain, primula, senega root, and thyme.
Cold symptoms; coughs.

Pectoral Brum *Brum, Spain†.*
Aconite (p.1572·3); tolu balsam (p.1101·3); ipecacuanha (p.1093·1); orange; sodium benzoate (p.1134·3); sulfogaiacol (p.1101·1).
Respiratory-tract disorders.

Pectoral Funk Antitus *Funk, Spain†.*
Carbocisteine (p.1086·3); chlorpheniramine [chlorphenamine] maleate (p.412·1); phenylephrine hydrochloride (p.1097·1); oxolamine citrate (p.1096·2).
Respiratory-tract disorders.

Pectosan *Cooperation Pharmaceutique, Fr.†.*
Sulfogaiacol (p.1101·1); codeine (p.25·2); bromoform (p.1587·1); sodium camsilate.
Formerly contained sulfogaiacol, pholcodine, ethylmorphine hydrochloride, belladonna, senega, and sodium benzoate.
Coughs.

Pectosan Ampicilina *Roche, Spain.*
Ampicillin trihydrate (p.151·1); ephedrine hydrochloride (p.1090·1).
Respiratory-tract infections.

Pectosan Expectorant *Cooperation Pharmaceutique, Fr.*
Carbocisteine (p.1086·3).
Coughs.

Pectosan Toux Seche *Cooperation Pharmaceutique, Fr.*
Pentoxyverine citrate (p.1096·3).
Coughs.

Pectosorin *Richter, Aust.*
Sulfogaiacol (p.1101·1).
Bronchitis; catarrh; coughs.

Pectoss *Heralds, Braz.*
Ipecacuanha (p.1093·1); sodium benzoate (p.1134·3); thyme (p.1672·2); poppy (p.1099·2); grindelia (p.1618·2).
Coughs.

Pectothymin *Planta, Canad.†.*
Aniseed (p.1580·2); thyme (p.1672·2); cowslip (p.1600·1).
Coughs.

Pectotussyl *Medeva, Fr.*
Terpin hydrate (p.1101·2).
Respirarory-tract disorders.

Pectox *Woelm, Ger.†; Italfarmaco, Spain; Piraud, Switz.†; Rhone-Poulenc Rorer, Thai.*
Carbocisteine (p.1086·3) or carbocisteine lysine (p.1086·3).
Respiratory-tract disorders associated with increased or viscous mucus.

Pectox Ampicilina *Italfarmaco, Spain†.*
Carbocisteine (p.1086·3); ampicillin (p.150·3).
Respiratory-tract infections.

Pectramin *Streuli, Switz.*
Diphenhydramine hydrochloride (p.416·1); ammonium chloride (p.1085·2); menthol (p.1632·3).
Coughs.

Pectrolyte *Restan, S.Afr.*
Kaolin (p.1229·3); pectin (p.1502·3); chloroform and morphine tincture (p.56·1); sodium lactate; potassium chloride; sodium chloride (p.1185·2).
Colic; diarrhoea.

Pectyl *Nycomed, Denm.*
Opium (p.69·3); benzoic acid (p.1134·2); camphor (p.1589·3); glycerol (p.1616·3).
Coughs.

Pedameth *Forest Pharmaceuticals, USA.*
Methionine (p.1012·2).
Control of odour, dermatitis, and ulceration in incontinent adults; nappy rash.

Ped-El
Pharmacia, Neth.†; Baxter, NZ; Kabi Pharmacia, NZ; Pharmacia, S.Afr.†; Pharmacia, Swed.†; KabiVitrum, UK.
Electrolyte (p.1180·1) and trace element (p.1350·1) preparation.
Parenteral nutrition.

Ped-Element *Darrow, Braz.*
Electrolyte (p.1180·1) and trace element (p.1350·1) preparation.
Parenteral nutrition.

PediaCare Allergy Formula *McNeil Consumer, USA.*
Chlorpheniramine [chlorphenamine] maleate (p.412·1).

PediaCare Cough-Cold *McNeil Consumer, USA.*
Pseudoephedrine hydrochloride (p.1099·2); chlorpheniramine [chlorphenamine] maleate (p.412·1); dextromethorphan hydrobromide (p.1087·3).
Coughs and cold symptoms.

PediaCare Infant's Decongestant *McNeil Consumer, USA.*
Pseudoephedrine hydrochloride (p.1099·2).
Nasal congestion.

PediaCare NightRest Cough-Cold Formula *McNeil Consumer, USA.*
Pseudoephedrine hydrochloride (p.1099·2); chlorpheniramine [chlorphenamine] maleate (p.412·1); dextromethorphan hydrobromide (p.1087·3).
Coughs and cold symptoms.

Pediacof *Sanofi Winthrop, USA.*
Codeine phosphate (p.25·2); phenylephrine hydrochloride (p.1097·1); chlorpheniramine [chlorphenamine] maleate (p.412·1); potassium iodide (p.1522·3).
Coughs.

Pedia-Col *Greater Pharma, Thai.*
Syrup: Paracetamol (p.71·2); phenylpropanolamine hydrochloride (p.1098·1); dextromethorphan hydrobromide (p.1087·3); chlorpheniramine [chlorphenamine] maleate (p.412·1).
Tablets: Paracetamol (p.71·2); phenylpropanolamine hydrochloride (p.1098·1); chlorpheniramine [chlorphenamine] maleate (p.412·1).
Allergic rhinitis; cold symptoms; hay fever; sinusitis.

Pediacon DX *Goldline, USA†.*
Phenylpropanolamine hydrochloride (p.1098·1); guaifenesin (p.1092·2); dextromethorphan hydrobromide (p.1087·3).
Coughs.

Pediacon EX *Goldline, USA†.*
Phenylpropanolamine (p.1098·1); guaifenesin (p.1092·2).
Coughs.

Pediaflor *Ross, USA.*
Sodium fluoride (p.1375·3).
Dental caries prophylaxis in children.

Pedialyte
Abbott, Austral.; Abbott, Braz.; Abbott, Canad.; Abbott, Hong Kong; Abbott, Ital.; Abbott, NZ; Abbott, Singapore; Abbott, Thai.; Ross, USA.
Electrolytes; glucose (p.1185·2).
Diarrhoea; oral rehydration therapy.

Pedialyte 90 *Abbott, Braz.*
Sodium chloride; potassium citrate; sodium citrate; glucose (p.1185·2).
Diarrhoea; oral rehydration therapy.

Pediaphyllin PL *Galephar, Neth.†.*
Theophylline (p.777·2).
Bronchospasm.

Pediapirin *Novartis, Spain†.*
Paracetamol (p.71·2).
Fever; pain.

Pediapred
Rhone-Poulenc Rorer, Canad.; Medeva, USA.
Prednisolone sodium phosphate (p.1078·1).
Corticosteroid.

PediaSure
Abbott, Austral.; Abbott, Canad.; Abbott, Fin.; Abbott, Hong Kong;

Abbott, Ital.; Abbott, Mex.; Abbott, NZ; Abbott, Singapore; Abbott, Thai.; Abbott, UK; Ross, USA.
Preparation for enteral nutrition in children (p.1350·1).

Pediatric Cough Syrup Technilab, Canad.
Pseudoephedrine hydrochloride (p.1099·2); dextromethorphan hydrobromide (p.1087·3).

Pediatric Electrolyte Pharmascience, Canad.
Glucose; fructose; potassium citrate; sodium chloride; sodium citrate (p.1185·2).
Diarrhoea; oral rehydration solution.

Pediatric Formula Reese, USA†.
Phenylpropanolamine hydrochloride (p.1098·1); guaifenesin (p.1092·2); dextromethorphan hydrobromide (p.1087·3).

Pediatrivite Seroyal, Canad.
Multivitamin and mineral preparation (p.1350·1).

Pediatrix Technilab, Canad.
Paracetamol (p.71·2).
Fever; pain.

Pediazole Abbott, Canad.; Abbott, Fr.; Abbott, Hong Kong; Abbott, Israel; Abbott, Mex.; Abbott, S.Afr.†; Abbott, Switz.†; Ross, USA.
Erythromycin ethyl succinate (p.201·2); acetyl sulfafurazole (p.253·1).
Otitis media.

Pedi-Bath Pedinol, USA†.
Emollient.

Pedi-Boro Soak Paks Pedinol, USA.
Aluminium sulfate (p.1578·2); calcium acetate (p.1187·3).
Skin irritation.

Pedi-Cort V Pedinol, USA†.
Hydrocortisone (p.1073·3); clioquinol (p.190·2).
Skin disorders.

Pedi-Dent Stanley, Canad.
Sodium fluoride (p.1375·3).
Dental caries prophylaxis.

Pedi-Dri Pedinol, USA.
Nystatin (p.392·2).
Candidiasis.

Pedigesic Parke-Med, S.Afr.†.
Paracetamol (p.71·2); codeine phosphate (p.25·2); promethazine hydrochloride (p.423·2).
Fever; pain.

Pedikurol Ratiopharm, Aust.
Clotrimazole (p.382·1).
Fungal skin and nail infections.

Pedil Salters, S.Afr.
Zinc undecenoate (p.395·3); undecenoic acid (p.395·3).
Fungal skin infections.

Pediletan Cimed, Braz.
Lindane (p.1434·1).
Pediculosis; scabies.

Pedimed Restan, S.Afr.
Aluminium oxide (p.1108·3); magnesium oxide (p.1233·2); methylpolysiloxane (p.1249·2).
Flatulence associated with hyperacidity.

Pediotic Monarch, USA.
Hydrocortisone (p.1073·3); neomycin sulfate (p.228·1); polymyxin B sulfate (p.238·1).
Bacterial ear infections.

Pedi-Pro Pedinol, USA.
Aluminium chlorohydrate (p.1110·2); chloroxylenol (p.1142·1); menthol (p.1632·3); zinc undecenoate (p.395·3).
Fungal skin infections; minor skin disorders.

Pediron ST, Thai.
Iron (p.1366·3).
Iron-deficiency anaemia.

Pedisafe BASF, Ger.
Clotrimazole (p.382·1).
Fungal infections.

Pedisol Fischer, Israel.
Cream: Triclosan (p.1159·2); panthenol (p.1602·3); chamomile (p.1593·2); wool fat (p.1410·3).
Dry skin; hard skin.

Topical spray: Undecenoic acid (p.395·3); aluminium chlorohydrate (p.1110·2); menthol (p.1632·3); purified talc (p.1124·2).
Foot odour.

Peditrace
Fresenius Kabi, Aust.; Fresenius Kabi, Denm.; Fresenius Kabi, Fin.; Pharmacia Upjohn, Ger.; Pharmacia Upjohn, Hong Kong; Pharmacia Upjohn, Irl.; Pharmacia Upjohn, Israel; Fresenius Kabi, Neth.; Fresenius Kabi, Norw.; Fresenius Kabi, Port.; Fresenius Kabi, S.Afr.; Fresenius Kabi, Swed.; Fresenius Kabi, Switz.; Fresenius, UK.
Trace element preparation (p.1350·1).
Parenteral nutrition.

Pedituss Cough Major, USA.
Phenylephrine hydrochloride (p.1097·1); chlorpheniramine [chlorphenamine] maleate (p.412·1); codeine phosphate (p.25·2); potassium iodide (p.1522·3).
Coughs.

Pedi-Vit-A Pedinol, USA.
Vitamin A (p.1382·1).
Irritated or dry skin.

Pedoc Ranbaxy, Thai.
Docusate sodium (p.1223·1).
Constipation.

Pedopur Jacoby, Aust.
Vitis vinifera.
Peripheral vascular disorders.

Pedoz Hamilton, Austral.
Tetrabromocresol (p.1158·1); undecenoic acid (p.395·3); zinc undecenoate (p.395·3); zinc oxide (p.1128·2).
Hyperhidrosis; skin irritation; tinea pedis.

Pedpain Aspen, S.Afr.
Paracetamol (p.71·2); codeine phosphate (p.25·2); promethazine hydrochloride (p.423·2).
Fever; pain.

Pedriachol Propan, S.Afr.
Phenobarbital (p.355·1); pipenzolate bromide (p.472·2).
Gastrointestinal disorders.

PedTE-PAK SoloPak, USA.
Trace element preparation (p.1350·1).
Parenteral nutrition.

Pedtrace American Pharmaceutical, USA.
Trace element preparation (p.1350·1).
Parenteral nutrition.

PedvaxHIB
CSL, Austral.; Merck Frosst, Canad.; Chiron Behring, Ger.; Merck Sharp & Dohme, Hong Kong; Merck Sharp & Dohme, Israel; Merck Sharp & Dohme, Mex.; Merck Sharp & Dohme, Neth.†; Merck Sharp & Dohme, Singapore; Pasteur Merieux, Swed.†; Merck Sharp & Dohme, Thai.; Merck, USA.
A haemophilus influenzae conjugate vaccine (meningococcal protein conjugate) (p.1540·2).
Active immunisation.

Pedvitin Greater Pharma, Thai.
Multivitamin preparation (p.1350·1).

PeeHoo Orion, Fin.
Aluminium hydroxide-magnesium carbonate co-dried gel (p.1211·2).
Gastric hyperacidity.

Peerless Composition Essence Potter's, UK.
Oak bark (p.1643·2); pinus canadensis; poplar bark (p.1653·2); prickly ash bark (p.1682·1); bayberry bark (p.1583·3).
Colds.

Peflacin
Rhodia, Braz.; Rhone-Poulenc Rorer, Ger.; Rhone-Poulenc Rorer, Ital.; Rhone-Poulenc Rorer, Neth.†.
Pefloxacin mesilate (p.234·3).
Bacterial infections.

Peflacina Rhone-Poulenc Rorer, Mex.
Pefloxacin mesilate (p.234·3).
Bacterial infections.

Peflacine
Rhone-Poulenc Rorer, Aust.; Aventis, Belg.; Rhone-Poulenc Rorer, Fr.; Rhone-Poulenc Rorer, Hong Kong; Rhone-Poulenc Rorer, Israel; Rhone-Poulenc Rorer, Port.; Rhone-Poulenc Rorer, Spain; Rhone-Poulenc Rorer, Thai.
Pefloxacin mesilate (p.234·3).
Bacterial infections.

Peflox Formenti, Ital.
Pefloxacin mesilate (p.234·3).
Bacterial infections.

Pefrakehl Sanum-Kehlbeck, Ger.
Homoeopathic preparation.

Pega Bailleul, Fr.
Potassium and arginine phosphocitroglutamate.
Asthenia.

Peganone Abbott, USA.
Ethotoin (p.348·3).
Epilepsy.

Pegina Potter's, UK.
Calumba (p.1589·2); calamus (p.1588·1); compound cardamom tincture (p.1591·3); magnesium sulfate (p.1191·1); magnesium trisilicate (p.1233·3); rhubarb (p.1248·1).
Dyspepsia; flatulence.

PegIntron
Schering-Plough, UK; Schering, USA.
Peginterferon alfa-2b (rbe) (p.630·1).
Chronic hepatitis C.

Peglyte
Note. This name is used for preparations of different composition.
Pharmascience, Canad.
Macrogol 3350 (p.1630·3); electrolytes (p.1180·1).
Bowel evacuation; constipation.

Pharmascience, Hong Kong.
Electrolytes (p.1180·1).
Gastrointestinal lavage.

Peinfort Ebewe, Aust.
Paracetamol (p.71·2).
Fever; pain.

Peitel Novag, Spain.
Prednicarbate (p.1077·3).
Skin disorders.

Peitoral Angico Pelotense CIF, Braz.
Iceland moss; althaea (p.1577·1); cuscuta umbellata; mallow; liquorice (p.1231·2); piptadenia colubrina; ammonium chloride (p.1085·2); tolu balsam (p.1101·3); sodium benzoate (p.1134·3).
Respiratory-tract congestion.

Pekamin Medical, Spain.
Benzylpenicillin sodium (p.157·2).
Bacterial infections.

Peking Ginseng Royal Jelly N Peking-Boell, Ger.
Ginseng (p.1615·3); honey; royal jelly.
Tonic.

Peking Royal Jelly N Peking-Boell, Ger.
Royal jelly (p.1659·3); codonopsis pilosulae; honey.
Tonic.

Pelamine Major, USA†.
Tripelennamine hydrochloride (p.427·1).
Hypersensitivity reactions.

Pelargon
Nestle, Fr.; Nestle, Ital.
Infant feed (p.1350·1).
Gastrointestinal disorders.

Peledox Novartis Consumer, Spain.
Doxycycline hyclate (p.200·1).
Bacterial infections; malaria.

Pelina MIP, Ger.
Dexpanthenol (p.1602·3).
Skin and mucous membrane lesions.

Peliphane Saninter, Port.†.
Piroctone olamine (p.1121·1); melaleuca oil (p.1631·3).
Seborrhoeic dermatitis.

Pellisal-Gel Woelm, Ger.†.
Diphenhydramine hydrochloride (p.416·1).
Allergic skin reactions; insect stings; minor burns; skin rashes; sunburn.

Pellit
Engelhard, Hong Kong; Asta Medica, Thai.
Diphenhydramine hydrochloride (p.416·1); diethyltoluamide (p.1431·2); dimethyl phthalate (p.1431·3).
Allergic skin reactions; insect bites; insect repellent.

Pellit dermal Wund- und Heilsalbe Engelhard, Ger.
Tyrothricin (p.267·1); fomocaine hydrochloride; diphenhydramine hydrochloride (p.416·1).
Infected skin disorders.

Pellit Insektenstich, Pellit Sonnenallergie Engelhard, Ger.†.
Diphenhydramine hydrochloride (p.416·1).
Allergic skin reactions; insect stings; minor burns.

Pellit Sonnenbrand Engelhard, Ger.†.
Hamamelis (p.1618·3).
Skin lesions and inflammation; sunburn.

Pelmic Breves, Braz.
Diphenylpyraline (p.417·1); methyl hydroxybenzoate (p.1148·1); propyl hydroxybenzoate (p.1148·2); alcohol (p.1130·3).
Skin disinfection.

Pelsana Med Schmidgall, Aust.
Bath oil: Sunflower oil (p.1381·2); undecenoic acid (p.395·3).
Ointment: Sunflower oil (p.1381·2); dexpanthenol (p.1602·3).
Topical powder: Zinc undecenoate (p.395·3).
Formerly known as Pelsano.
Skin disorders.

Pelsano
Note. This name is used for preparations of different composition.
Wolfs, Belg.†.
Undecenoic acid (p.395·3); zinc stearate (p.1497·3).
Skin disorders.

Iromedica, Switz.
Bath additive: Sunflower oil (p.1381·2); undecenoic acid (p.395·3).
Ointment: Sunflower oil (p.1381·2); dexpanthenol (p.1602·3).
Skin disorders.

Pelson Berenguer Infale, Spain†.
Nitrazepam (p.695·2).
Insomnia.

Peltazon Grelan, Jpn.
Pentazocine hydrochloride (p.74·2).
Fever; inflammation; pain.

Pelvichthol Ichthyol, Aust.†.
Ictasol (p.1115·3); benzyl nicotinate (p.20·2); homofenazine hydrochloride (p.688·2).
Urogenital disorders.

Pelvichthol N Ichthyol, Ger.
Ictasol (p.1115·3); benzyl nicotinate (p.20·2).
General pelvic symptoms.

Pelvo Magnesium 3M, Belg.
Onion (p.1644·1); magnesium carbonate (p.1232·3) or magnesium chloride (p.1190·3).
Painful pelvic congestion in females; prostate and micturition disorders in men.

PemADD Mallinckrodt, USA.
Pemoline (p.1513·1).
Attention-deficit hyperactivity disorder.

Pemine Lilly, Ital.
Penicillamine hydrochloride (p.1019·1).
Cystinuria; lead poisoning; rheumatoid arthritis; Wilson's disease.

PE-Mix Fresenius Kabi, Aust.
Amino-acid, carbohydrate, electrolyte, and lipid (as soya oil (p.1378·1)).
Contains egg lecithin.
Parenteral nutrition.

Pemix Prodes, Spain†.
Pirozadil (p.956·3).
Hyperlipidaemias.

Pen ABZ, Ger.
Phenoxymethylpenicillin potassium (p.235·1).
Bacterial infections.

Penaderm Johnson & Johnson, Ger.
Urea (p.1127·3).
Dry skin.

Penadur
Wyeth Lederle, Belg.; Wyeth Lederle, Port.; Wyeth, Singapore; Wyeth-Ayerst, Thai.
Benzathine benzylpenicillin (p.156·2).
Bacterial infections; prevention of acute flares of rheumatoid arthritis.

Penadur 6.3.3 Wyeth Lederle, Port.
Benzathine benzylpenicillin (p.156·2); benzylpenicillin potassium (p.157·1); procaine penicillin [procaine benzylpenicillin] (p.239·2).
Bacterial infections.

Penalta Bristol-Myers Squibb, Fin.
Amoxicillin trihydrate (p.149·2).
Bacterial infections.

Penamox
SmithKline Beecham, Mex.; Douglas, NZ; Tecnimede, Port.
Amoxicillin sodium (p.149·2) or amoxicillin trihydrate (p.149·2).
Bacterial infections.

Penamox M SmithKline Beecham, Mex.
Amoxicillin trihydrate (p.149·2); bromhexine (p.1085·3).
Respiratory-tract infections.

Penanyst Johnson & Johnson, Ger.
Zinc oxide (p.1128·2); nystatin (p.392·2).
Skin disorders with fungal infections.

Penaten
Note. This name is used for preparations of different composition.
Johnson & Johnson, Canad.
Hamamelis (p.1618·3); zinc oxide (p.1128·2).

Johnson & Johnson, Ger.
Thyme oil (p.1672·3).
Respiratory-tract disorders.

Penatoel Johnson & Johnson, Ger.
Soya oil (p.1378·1).
Dry skin; skin irritation.

Pen-BASF BASF, Ger.
Phenoxymethylpenicillin potassium (p.235·1).
Bacterial infections.

Penbene Ratiopharm, Aust.
Phenoxymethylpenicillin potassium (p.235·1).
Bacterial infections.

Penbeta Betapharm, Ger.
Phenoxymethylpenicillin potassium (p.235·1).
Bacterial infections.

Penbritin
Bencard, Belg.†; Wyeth-Ayerst, Canad.†; SmithKline Beecham, Hong Kong; SmithKline Beecham, Irl.; Hormona, Mex.; SmithKline Beecham, S.Afr.; SmithKline Beecham, Singapore; SmithKline Beecham, Thai.; SmithKline Beecham, UK.
Ampicillin (p.150·3), ampicillin sodium (p.150·3), or ampicillin trihydrate (p.151·1).
Bacterial infections.

Penclox Pisa, Mex.
Dicloxacillin (p.199·1).
Bacterial infections.

Pencotrex Hua, Thai.
Ampicillin trihydrate (p.151·1).
Bacterial infections.

Pendiben Compuesto Pisa, Mex.
Benzylpenicillin sodium (p.157·2); procaine penicillin [procaine benzylpenicillin] (p.239·2); benzathine benzylpenicillin (p.156·2).
Bacterial infections.

Pendramine Asta Medica, UK†.
Penicillamine (p.1017·1).
Cystinuria; heavy-metal poisoning; hepatitis; rheumatoid arthritis; Wilson's disease.

Pendysin Jenapharm, Ger.
Benzathine benzylpenicillin (p.156·2).
Lignocaine [lidocaine] hydrochloride (p.1313·2) is included in this preparation to alleviate the pain of injection.
Chronic streptococcal infections; syphilis.

Penecare Penederm, Canad.†; Reed & Carnrick, USA.
Emollient.

Penecort Allergan, USA.
Hydrocortisone (p.1073·3).
Skin disorders.

Penederm Penederm, Canad.
Cream: Lactic acid (p.1626·2); light liquid paraffin (p.1407·2).
Lotion: Lactic acid (p.1626·2).
Dry skin.

Penedil Teva, Israel.
Felodipine (p.888·3).
Angina pectoris; hypertension.

Pener Unison, Thai.
Phenoxymethylpenicillin (p.235·1).
Bacterial infections.

Penetran IMA, Braz.
Naphazoline (p.1095·1); diphenhydramine (p.416·1); neomycin (p.228·1).
Nasal congestion.

Penetrating Rub Golden Pride, Canad.†; Rawleigh, Canad.†.
Methyl salicylate (p.55·1); menthol (p.1632·3); eucalyptus oil (p.1609·2); cajuput oil (p.1588·1); expressed mustard oil (p.1639·1).

Penetrex Rhone-Poulenc Rorer, USA.
Enoxacin (p.201·1).
Gonorrhoea; urinary-tract infections.

Penetro Daudt, Braz.
Terpineol (p.1669·3); eucalyptol (p.1609·2); menthol (p.1632·3); benzoic acid (p.1134·2).
Respiratory-tract congestion.

Penetrol Seton, UK†.
Inhalation: Menthol (p.1632·3); cajuput oil (p.1588·1); lavender oil (p.1627·2); otto lavend; eucalyptus oil (p.1609·2); peppermint oil (p.1243·3).

The symbol † denotes a preparation no longer actively marketed

Lozenges: Ammonium chloride (p.1085·2); phenylephrine hydrochloride (p.1097·1); creosote (p.1087·3); menthol (p.1632·3).
Nasal congestion.

Penferm *Fermenta, Swed.†.*
Phenoxymethylpenicillin potassium (p.235·1).
Bacterial infections.

Pengesic *Hovid, Singapore.*
Tramadol hydrochloride (p.89·1).
Pain.

Pengesod *Lakeside, Mex.*
Benzylpenicillin sodium (p.157·2).
Bacterial infections.

Penglobe
Astra, Aust.; Astra, Belg.†; AstraZeneca, Canad.; Lundbeck, Denm.†; AstraZeneca, Fr.; Astra, Ger.; Astra, Hong Kong; Astra, Ital.; Astra, Mex.; AstraZeneca, Singapore; Astra, Spain; Astra, Swed.; AstraZeneca, Thai.
Bacampicillin hydrochloride (p.155·1).
Bacterial infections.

Penhexal *Hexal, Ger.*
Phenoxymethylpenicillin potassium (p.235·1).
Bacterial infections.

Penhexal VK *Hexal, Austral.*
Phenoxymethylpenicillin potassium (p.235·1).
Bacterial infections.

Penibiot *Normon, Spain.*
Benzylpenicillin sodium (p.157·2).
Bacterial infections.

Penibiot Lidocaina *Normon, Spain†.*
Benzylpenicillin sodium (p.157·2).
Lignocaine [lidocaine] hydrochloride (p.1313·2) is included in this preparation to alleviate the pain of injection.
Bacterial infections.

Penibrin *Biogal, Israel.*
Ampicillin (p.150·3).
Bacterial infections.

Penicil *Rimsa, Mex.*
Procaine penicillin [procaine benzylpenicillin] (p.239·2); benzylpenicillin sodium (p.157·2).
Bacterial infections.

Penicillat *Azupharma, Ger.*
Phenoxymethylpenicillin potassium (p.235·1).
Bacterial infections.

Penicilin Fortified *Vitamed, Israel.*
Procaine penicillin [procaine benzylpenicillin] (p.239·2); benzylpenicillin sodium (p.157·2).
Bacterial infections.

Penidural *Yamanouchi, Neth.*
Benzathine benzylpenicillin (p.156·2).
Bacterial infections.

Penidural D/F *Yamanouchi, Neth.*
Benzathine benzylpenicillin (p.156·2); procaine penicillin [procaine benzylpenicillin] (p.239·2); benzylpenicillin potassium (p.157·1).
Bacterial infections.

Penilan *Vitoria, Port.*
Amoxicillin trihydrate (p.149·2); potassium clavulanate (p.187·2).
Bacterial infections.

Penilente Forte *Novo Nordisk, S.Afr.*
Benzathine benzylpenicillin (p.156·2); procaine penicillin [procaine benzylpenicillin] (p.239·2); benzylpenicillin sodium (p.157·2).
Bacterial infections.

Penilente LA *Novo Nordisk, S.Afr.*
Benzathine benzylpenicillin (p.156·2).
Bacterial infections.

Penilevel *Ern, Spain.*
Capsules; oral sachets: Phenoxymethylpenicillin potassium (p.235·1).
Injection: Benzylpenicillin sodium (p.157·2).
Bacterial infections.

Penilevel Retard *Ern, Spain.*
Benzylpenicillin sodium (p.157·2); benzathine benzylpenicillin (p.156·2); phenoxymethylpenicillin calcium (p.235·1).
Bacterial infections; rheumatic fever.

Penimox *IBSA, Switz.*
Amoxicillin (p.149·2) or amoxicillin trihydrate (p.149·2).
Bacterial infections.

Peni-Oral *Wyeth Lederle, Belg.*
Phenoxymethylpenicillin potassium (p.235·1).
Bacterial infections.

Penipot *Antibioticos, Mex.*
Procaine penicillin [procaine benzylpenicillin] (p.239·2); benzylpenicillin sodium (p.157·1).
Bacterial infections.

Peniroger *UCB, Spain†.*
Benzylpenicillin sodium (p.157·2).
Bacterial infections.

Penisintex Bronquial *Jorba, Spain.*
Ampicillin sodium (p.150·3); ampicillin benzathine (p.151·3); bromhexine (p.1085·1).
Lignocaine [lidocaine] hydrochloride (p.1313·2) is included in this preparation to alleviate the pain of injection.
Respiratory-tract infections.

Penisodina *Pisa, Mex.*
Procaine penicillin [procaine benzylpenicillin] (p.239·2); benzylpenicillin sodium (p.157·1).
Bacterial infections.

Penisol *Ecosal, Switz.*
Phenoxymethylpenicillin potassium (p.235·1).
Bacterial infections.

Pen-Kera *Ascher, USA.*
Emollient and moisturiser.

Penlac *Dermik, USA.*
Ciclopirox (p.382·1).
Fungal nail infections.

Penles *Wyeth Lederle, Jpn.*
Lignocaine [lidocaine] (p.1313·2).
Pain of inserting intravenous needles.

Penlol *Pose, Thai.*
Oxpentifylline [pentoxifylline] (p.950·3).
Peripheral vascular disorders.

PenMix 10/90, 20/80, 30/70, 40/60, 50/50 *Novo Nordisk, UK†.*
Mixtures of insulin injection (human, pyr) and isophane insulin suspension (human, pyr) respectively in the proportions indicated (p.324·1).
Diabetes mellitus.

PenMix 10, 20, 30, 40, or 50 *Novo Nordisk, NZ.*
Mixtures of insulin injection (human) 10%, 20%, 30%, 40%, or 50% and isophane insulin (human) 90%, 80%, 70%, 60% or 50% respectively (p.324·1).
Diabetes mellitus.

Penmox *Compu, S.Afr.*
Amoxicillin (p.149·2).
Bacterial infections.

Pennsaid *Provalis, UK.*
Diclofenac sodium (p.30·3).
Osteoarthritis.

Penntuss *Rhone-Poulenc Rorer, Canad.†.*
Codeine polistirex (p.26·1); chlorpheniramine [chlorphenamine] polistirex (p.412·2).
Allergic rhinitis; coughs and cold symptoms.

Pen-Os *Biochemie, Aust.†.*
Benzathine phenoxymethylpenicillin (p.157·1).
Bacterial infections.

Penotran *Poli, Hong Kong.*
Hydrargaphen; potassium dinaphthylmethanedisulfonate.
Vaginal infections.

Penprocilina *Lakeside, Mex.*
Benzylpenicillin sodium (p.157·2); procaine penicillin [procaine benzylpenicillin] (p.239·2).
Bacterial infections.

Penrite *Columbia, S.Afr.†.*
Ampicillin trihydrate (p.151·1).
Bacterial infections.

Pensodital *Wayne, Mex.*
Thiopental (p.1269·3).

Penstad *Stada, Aust.*
Phenoxymethylpenicillin potassium (p.235·1).
Bacterial infections.

Penstapho
Bristol-Myers Squibb, Belg.; Bristol-Myers Squibb, Ital.
Oxacillin sodium (p.233·2).
Gram-positive bacterial infections.

Penstaphon *Bristol-Myers Squibb, Belg.*
Cloxacillin sodium (p.192·1).
Staphylococcal infections.
Formerly known as Penstapho N.

Pensulvit *SIFI, Ital.*
Tetracycline (p.258·3); sulfamethylthiazole (p.256·1).
Bacterial eye infections.

Penta 500 *Pediatrica, Singapore.*
Vitamin B substances; lysine hydrochloride (p.1350·1).
Tonic.

Penta-3B *Sabex, Canad.*
Thiamine hydrochloride (p.1385·1); pyridoxine hydrochloride (p.1386·3); cyanocobalamin (p.1388·1).
Alcoholism; neuritis; vitamin B supplement.

Penta-3B + C *Sabex, Canad.*
Thiamine hydrochloride (p.1385·1); pyridoxine hydrochloride (p.1386·3); cyanocobalamin (p.1388·1); ascorbic acid (p.1389·3).
Alcoholism; neuritis; vitamin supplement.

Penta-3B Plus *Sabex, Canad.*
Multivitamin preparation (p.1350·1).

Pentabil *OFF, Ital.*
Fenipentol (p.1610·1).
Hepatic and biliary-tract disorders.

Pentacard *Byk, Belg.†; Pacific, Thai.*
Isosorbide mononitrate (p.916·2).
Angina pectoris.

Pentacarinat
Gerot, Aust.; Rhone-Poulenc Rorer, Austral.†; Aventis, Belg.; Rhodia, Braz.; Rhone-Poulenc Rorer, Canad.; Aventis, Denm.; Rhone-Poulenc Rorer, Fin.; Rhone-Poulenc Rorer, Fr.; Rhone-Poulenc Rorer, Ger.; Glaxo Wellcome, Ger.; Rhone-Poulenc Rorer, Irl.; Rhone-Poulenc Rorer, Israel; Rhone-Poulenc Rorer, Ital.; Rhone-Poulenc Rorer, Neth.; Rhone-Poulenc Rorer, Norw.; Aventis, NZ; Rhone-Poulenc Rorer, Port.; Aventis, S.Afr.; Rhone-Poulenc Rorer, Spain; Rhone-Poulenc Rorer, Swed.; Rhone-Poulenc Rorer, Switz.; Rhone-Poulenc Rorer, Thai.; JHC Healthcare, UK; Aventis, USA.
Pentamidine isetionate (p.600·1).
African trypanosomiasis; leishmaniasis; Pneumocystis carinii pneumonia.

Pentacel *Connaught, Canad.*
Vial, a haemophilus influenzae conjugate vaccine (tetanus toxoid conjugate)(Act-HIB); ampoule, a diphtheria, tetanus, pertussis, and poliomyelitis vaccine (Quadracel) (p.1539·1).
Active immunisation.

Pentacine *Via, Switz.*
Pentamycin (p.393·2).
Vaginitis.

Pentacol *Sofar, Ital.*
Mesalazine (p.1234·1).
Crohn's disease; ulcerative colitis.

Pentacoq *Pasteur Merieux, Fr.*
Vial, a haemophilus influenzae conjugate vaccine (tetanus toxoid conjugate) (Act-HIB); syringe, a diphtheria, tetanus, pertussis, and poliomyelitis vaccine (Tetracoq) (p.1539·1).
Active immunisation.

Pentacort *Life, Ger.*
Betamethasone valerate (p.1063·2).
Skin disorders.

Pentacrom *Penta, Ger.*
Sodium cromoglicate (p.774·3).
Allergic eye disorders.

Pentact-HIB
Pasteur Merieux, Hong Kong; Pasteur Merieux, Israel; Pasteur Merieux, Thai.
A diphtheria, tetanus, pertussis, poliomyelitis, and haemophilus influenzae conjugate vaccine (p.1539·1).
Active immunisation.

Pentafen *Formenti, Ital.†.*
Pentazocine lactate (p.74·2).
Pain.

Pentagin *Sankyo, Jpn.*
Pentazocine hydrochloride (p.74·2).
Fever; inflammation; pain.

Pentaglobin
Biotest, Aust.; Biotest, Ger.; Biotest, Ital.; Precimex, Mex.; Mednostica, S.Afr.; Biotest, Spain; Biotest, Thai.
Immunoglobulins (M, A, and G) (p.1551·3).
Immunodeficiency; Kawasaki disease; passive immunisation; thrombocytopenia.

Pentaglucano *Biosan, Ital.*
Lactic-acid-producing organisms (p.1626·3); vitamin B substances (p.1350·1).
Maintenance of normal gastrointestinal flora.

Pental Forte *Cederroth, Spain.*
Benzalkonium chloride (p.1133·2); mafenide (p.221·2); sulfanilamide (p.256·2); zinc oxide (p.1128·2).
Skin infections.

Pentalgina *Pierrel, Ital.†.*
Pentazocine lactate (p.74·2).
Pain.

Pentalmicina *Cederroth, Spain†.*
Enoxolone (p.34·3); mafenide (p.221·2); neomycin sulfate (p.228·1); sulfanilamide (p.256·2).
Skin infections.

Pentalong *Isis, Ger.*
Pentaerithrityl tetranitrate (p.952·3).
Angina pectoris.

Pentam *Pisa, Mex.; American Pharmaceutical, USA.*
Pentamidine isetionate (p.600·1).
Leishmaniasis; Pneumocystis carinii pneumonia; trypanosomiasis.

Pentamina *Faulding, Port.*
Pentamidine isetionate (p.600·1).

Pentamol *Penta, Ger.*
Salbutamol sulfate (p.770·3).
Obstructive airways disease.

Pentamycetin *Sabex, Canad.*
Chloramphenicol (p.179·1).
Eye infections.

Pentamycetin-HC *Sabex, Canad.*
Chloramphenicol (p.179·1); hydrocortisone acetate (p.1073·3).
Eye and ear infections.

Pentasa
Ferring, Aust.; Ferring, Belg.; Ferring, Canad.; Ferring, Denm.; Ferring, Fin.; Ferring, Fr.; Ferring, Ger.; Ferring, Hong Kong; Ferring, Irl.; Ferring, Israel; Yamanouchi, Ital.; Kyorin, Jpn; Ferring, Neth.; Ferring, Norw.; Pharmaco, NZ; Ferring, Port.; Ferring, Singapore; Ferring, Swed.; Ferring, Switz.; Ferring, UK; Roberts, USA.
Mesalazine (p.1234·1).
Inflammatory bowel disease.

Pentaspan *Du Pont, Canad.; Rhone-Poulenc Rorer, Mex.; Boots, NZ; Geistlich, UK; Du Pont, USA.*
Pentastarch (p.732·3).
Leucopheresis; plasma volume expansion.

Penta-Thion *Sabex, Canad.*
Ascorbic acid (p.1389·3); thiamine hydrochloride (p.1385·1).
Vitamin supplement.

Pentatop *Life, Ger.*
Sodium cromoglicate (p.774·3).
Hypersensitivity reactions.

Pentavac
Pasteur Merieux, Fr.; Pasteur Merieux, Ger.; Procter & Gamble, Ger.; Pasteur Merieux, Ital.; Pasteur Merieux, Spain; Pasteur Merieux, Swed.
A diphtheria, tetanus, pertussis, poliomyelitis, and haemophilus influenzae vaccine (p.1539·1).
Active immunisation.

Penta-Vite Chewable Multi Vitamins with Minerals *Roche Consumer, Austral.*
Multivitamin and mineral preparation (p.1350·1).

Penta-Vite Childrens Vitamins with Iron *Roche Consumer, Austral.*
Multivitamin preparation with iron (p.1350·1).

Penta-Vite Infant Vitamins *Roche Consumer, Austral.*
Multivitamin preparation (p.1350·1).

Pentavitol *Nycomed, Aust.*
Multivitamin preparation (p.1350·1).

Pentazine *Century, USA†.*
Promethazine hydrochloride (p.423·2).
Hypersensitivity reactions; motion sickness; nausea; postoperative pain (adjunct); sedative; vomiting.

Pentazine VC with Codeine *Century, USA.*
Promethazine hydrochloride (p.423·2); codeine phosphate (p.25·2).
Coughs and cold symptoms.

Pentazole *Profarb, Braz.*
Mebendazole (p.102·2).
Worm infections.

Pentcillin *Toyama, Jpn.*
Piperacillin sodium (p.236·1).
Lignocaine [lidocaine] (p.1313·2) is included in the intramuscular injection to alleviate the pain of injection.
Bacterial infections.

Pent-HIBest *Pasteur Vaccins, Fr.*
Vial, a haemophilus influenzae conjugate vaccine (tetanus toxoid conjugate) (HIBest) (p.1540·2); syringe, a diphtheria, tetanus, pertussis, and poliomyelitis vaccine (DTCP) (p.1539·1).
Active immunisation.

Penthrane *Abbott, Austral.†.*
Methoxyflurane (p.1264·1).
General anaesthesia.

Pentibrom *Maver, Mex.*
Ampicillin trihydrate (p.151·1); bromhexine hydrochloride (p.1085·3).
Bacterial infections.

Pentibroxil *Maver, Mex.*
Amoxicillin (p.149·2); ambroxol (p.1084·3).
Bacterial infections.

Penticlox *Maver, Mex.*
Amoxicillin (p.149·2).
Bacterial infections.

Penticort *Wyeth Lederle, Fr.*
Amcinonide (p.1061·2).
Skin disorders.

Penticort Neomycine *Lederle, Fr.†.*
Amcinonide (p.1061·2); neomycin sulfate (p.228·1).
Infected skin disorders.

Pentilzeno *BA Farma, Port.†.*
Diltiazem hydrochloride (p.874·3).
Angina pectoris; arrhythmias; heart failure; hypertension.

Pentiver *Maver, Mex.*
Ampicillin (p.150·3).
Bacterial infections.

Pento *ABZ, Ger.*
Oxpentifylline [pentoxifylline] (p.950·3).
Peripheral vascular disorders.

Pentoflux *Bouchara, Fr.*
Oxpentifylline [pentoxifylline] (p.950·3).
Intermittent claudication; mental function impairment in the elderly.

Pentohexal *Hexal, Aust.; Hexal, Ger.*
Oxpentifylline [pentoxifylline] (p.950·3).
Peripheral vascular disorders.

Pentolair *Bausch & Lomb, USA.*
Cyclopentolate hydrochloride (p.465·2).

Pentomer *Ratiopharm, Aust.*
Oxpentifylline [pentoxifylline] (p.950·3).
Cerebral, ocular and peripheral vascular disorders; ear disorders.

Pento-Puren *Isis Puren, Ger.*
Oxpentifylline [pentoxifylline] (p.950·3).
Peripheral vascular disorders.

Pentostam
Glaxo Wellcome, Israel; Wellcome, UK.
Sodium stibogluconate (p.587·2).
Leishmaniasis.

Pentothal
Abbott, Austral.; Abbott, Belg.; Abbott, Canad.; Abbott, Denm.; Abbott, Fin.; Abbott, Hong Kong; Abbott, Israel; Abbott, Ital.; Abbott, Mex.; Abbott, Norw.; Abbott, NZ; Abbott, Singapore; Abbott, Spain; Abbott, Swed.; Abbott, Switz.; Abbott, Thai.; Abbott, USA.
Thiopental sodium (p.1269·1).
Convulsions; general anaesthesia; sedative.

Pentovena *Roche, Spain.*
Hidrosmin (p.1611·2).
Peripheral vascular disorders.

Pentox *Farmasa, Braz.; CT, Ital.*
Oxpentifylline [pentoxifylline] (p.950·3).
Peripheral vascular disorders.

Pentoxi *Genericon, Aust.; Mepha, Switz.*
Oxpentifylline [pentoxifylline] (p.950·3).
Vascular disorders.

Pentoxin *Medinovum, Fin.*
Oxpentifylline [pentoxifylline] (p.950·3).
Peripheral vascular disorders.

Pentoxy *Heumann, Ger.*
Oxpentifylline [pentoxifylline] (p.950·3).
Peripheral vascular disorders.

Pentran *Berk, UK†.*
Phenytoin sodium (p.357·2).
Epilepsy; trigeminal neuralgia.

Pentrax
Note. This name is used for preparations of different composition.

GenDerm, Canad.; Dermapharm, Irl.; Dermapharm, UK; GenDerm, USA.
Coal tar (Fractar) (p.1125·1).
Scalp disorders.

Johnson & Johnson, Ital.
Coal tar (Fractar) (p.1125·1); salicylic acid (p.1122·3).
Seborrhoeic dermatitis.

Pentrax Gold GenDerm, USA.
Coal tar (p.1125·1).
Scalp disorders.

Pentrexyl
Bristol-Myers Squibb, Belg.; Bristol-Myers Squibb, Denm.; Bristol-Myers Squibb, Hong Kong; Bristol-Myers Squibb, Israel; Bristol-Myers Squibb, Ital.; Bristol-Myers Squibb, Mex.; Bristol-Myers Squibb, Neth.; Bristol-Myers Squibb, Norw.; Bristol-Myers Squibb, Swed.; Bristol-Myers Squibb, Thai.
Ampicillin (p.150·3), ampicillin sodium (p.150·3), or ampicillin trihydrate (p.151·1).
Bacterial infections.

Pentrexyl Expec Bristol-Myers Squibb, Mex.
Ampicillin trihydrate (p.151·1); acebrophylline.
Bacterial infections of the repiratory tract.

Pentrones Rhone Poulenc Chemicals, UK.
A range of non-ionic and anionic surfactants.

Pentylan Lannett, USA†.
Pentaerithrityl tetranitrate (p.952·3).
Angina pectoris.

Pen-V
Genericon, Aust.; Atlantic, Hong Kong; Atlantic, Thai.; General Drugs, Thai.; Goldline, USA†.
Phenoxymethylpenicillin (p.235·1) or phenoxymethylpenicillin potassium (p.235·1).
Bacterial infections.

Pen-Vee Lioh, Canad.
Benzathine phenoxymethylpenicillin (p.157·1) or phenoxymethylpenicillin (p.235·1).
Bacterial infections.

Pen-Vee K Wyeth-Ayerst, USA.
Phenoxymethylpenicillin potassium (p.235·1).
Bacterial infections.

Pen-Ve-Oral Wyeth, Braz.
Phenoxymethylpenicillin potassium (p.235·1).
Bacterial infections.

Penvicilin Gemballa, Braz.
Amoxicillin (p.149·2).
Bacterial infections.

Pen-Vi-K Wyeth, Mex.
Phenoxymethylpenicillin potassium (p.235·1).
Bacterial infections.

Pen-V-Merck Merck dura, Ger.
Phenoxymethylpenicillin potassium (p.235·1).
Bacterial infections.

PEP Galpharm, UK.
Glucose (p.1364·1); caffeine (p.761·3).
Fatigue.

Pepcid
Amrad, Austral.; Merck Frosst, Canad.; Johnson & Johnson, Canad.; Pharmacia Upjohn, Fin.; Woelm, Ger.; Merck Sharp & Dohme, Hong Kong; Merck Sharp & Dohme, Irl.; Pharmacia Upjohn, Neth.; Pharmacia Upjohn, Norw.; Merck Sharp & Dohme, NZ; Merck Sharp & Dohme, S.Afr.; Abello, Spain; Pharmacia Upjohn, Swed.; Merck Sharp & Dohme, Switz.; Johnson & Johnson MSD Consumer, UK; J&J-Merck, USA; Merck, USA.
Famotidine (p.1225·3).
Dyspepsia; gastro-oesophageal reflux; heartburn; peptic ulcer; Zollinger-Ellison syndrome.

Pepcid Complete Johnson & Johnson, USA.
Famotidine (p.1225·3); calcium carbonate (p.1215·1); magnesium hydroxide (p.1233·1).
Gastrointestinal hyperacidity.

Pepcidac Martin, Fr.
Famotidine (p.1225·3).
Gastro-oesophageal reflux.

Pepcidduo Martin-Johnson & Johnson, Fr.
Famotidine (p.1225·3); magnesium hydroxide (p.1233·1); calcium carbonate (p.1215·1).
Gastro-oesophageal reflux.

Pepcidin
Merck Sharp & Dohme, Denm.; Merck Sharp & Dohme, Fin.; Merck Sharp & Dohme, Neth.; Merck Sharp & Dohme, Norw.; Merck Sharp & Dohme, Swed.
Famotidine (p.1225·3).
Gastro-oesophageal reflux; peptic ulcer; Zollinger-Ellison syndrome.

Pepcidina Merck Sharp & Dohme, Port.
Famotidine (p.1225·3).
Gastric hyperacidity; gastro-oesophageal reflux; peptic ulcer; Zollinger-Ellison syndrome.

Pepcidine
Merck Sharp & Dohme, Aust.; Merck Sharp & Dohme, Austral.; Merck Sharp & Dohme, Belg.; Merck Sharp & Dohme, Hong Kong; Merck Sharp & Dohme, Mex.; Merck Sharp & Dohme, NZ; Merck Sharp & Dohme, Singapore; Merck Sharp & Dohme, Switz.; Merck Sharp & Dohme, Thai.
Famotidine (p.1225·3).
Gastro-oesophageal reflux; peptic ulcer; Zollinger-Ellison syndrome.

Pepcidtwo Johnson & Johnson, UK.
Calcium carbonate (p.1215·1); magnesium hydroxide (p.1233·1); famotidine (p.1225·3).
Dyspepsia; heartburn.

Pepcine Masa, Thai.
Famotidine (p.1225·3).
Gastro-oesophageal reflux; peptic ulcer; Zollinger-Ellison syndrome.

Pepdine Merck Sharp & Dohme-Chibret, Fr.
Famotidine (p.1225·3).
Gastro-oesophageal reflux; peptic ulcer; Zollinger-Ellison syndrome.

Pepdite
Scientific Hospital Supplies, Irl.†; Scientific Hospital Supplies, UK.
Infant feed (p.1350·1).
Bowel disorders; malabsorption syndromes; protein or lactose intolerance.

Pepdul MSD Chibropharm, Ger.
Famotidine (p.1225·3).
Peptic ulcer; upper gastrointestinal haemorrhage; Zollinger-Ellison syndrome.

Pepevit Diba, Mex.
Nicotinic acid (p.1372·3).
Hypercholesterolaemia; pellagra.

Pepfamin Siam Bheasach, Thai.
Famotidine (p.1225·3).
Peptic ulcer; Zollinger-Ellison syndrome.

Pepleo Kayaku, Jpn†.
Peplomycin sulfate (p.565·1).
Malignant neoplasms.

Pepp Theranol-Deglaude, Fr.†.
Dimethicone (p.1249·2); aluminium hydroxide (p.1210·3); magnesium hydroxide (p.1233·1).
Gastrointestinal disorders.

Pep-Rani Medinfar, Port.
Ranitidine hydrochloride (p.1245·2).
Gastric hyperacidity; gastro-oesophageal reflux; peptic ulcer; Zollinger-Ellison syndrome.

Peprazol Libbs, Braz.
Omeprazole (p.1239·1).
Gastro-oesophageal reflux; gastrointestinal hyperacidity; peptic ulcer.

Pepsaletten N Riemser, Ger.
Glutamic acid hydrochloride (p.1365·2).
Gastrointestinal disorders.

Pepsamar
Sanofi Winthrop, Braz.; Lepori, Port.; Sanofi Synthelabo, Spain.
Aluminium hydroxide (p.1210·3).
Dyspepsia; gastro-oesophageal reflux; gastrointestinal hyperacidity; hyperphosphataemia.

Pepsane Rosa-Phytopharma, Fr.
Guaiazulene (p.1618·3); dimethicone (p.1249·2).
Gastrointestinal disorders.

Pepsitase Hua, Thai.
Pepsin (p.1649·3); amylase (p.1579·3); papain (p.1647·3); gentian (p.1615·1); pancreatin (p.1646·1); activated charcoal (p.1000·2); vitamin B₁.
Digestive disorders.

Pepsiton Unipack, Aust.
Pepsin (p.1649·3); absinthium (p.1571·1).
Gastrointestinal disorders.

Pepsivit Gemballa, Braz.
Carnitine (p.1356·1); buclizine (p.411·1); vitamin B substances (p.1350·1).
Reduced appetite; tonic.

Pepsogel Legrand, Braz.
Aluminium hydroxide (p.1210·3); magnesium hydroxide (p.1233·1); simeticone (p.1249·2).
Flatulence; gastrointestinal hyperacidity.

Pepsytoin Pond's, Thai.
Phenytoin sodium (p.357·2).
Epilepsy.

Peptab Rhone-Poulenc Rorer, Port.
Ranitidine hydrochloride (p.1245·2).
Gastro-oesophageal reflux; gastrointestinal haemorrhage; peptic ulcer; Zollinger-Ellison syndrome.

Peptac Baker Norton, UK.
Sodium alginate (p.1498·3); sodium bicarbonate (p.1186·2); calcium carbonate (p.1215·1).
Gastro-oesophageal reflux; heartburn; hiatus hernia.

Peptamen
Clintec, Irl.; Nestle, Ital.; Nestle, UK; Carnation, USA.
Preparation for enteral nutrition (p.1350·1).
Gastrointestinal disorders.

Peptavlon
Zeneca, Aust.†; Wyeth-Ayerst, Canad.†; Cambridge, Fr.; Zeneca, Swed.†; Zeneca, Switz.†; Cambridge, UK; Ayerst, USA†.
Pentagastrin (p.1649·3).
Now known as Pentagastrin Injection in the UK.
Test of gastric secretory function.

Peptazol Roche, Ital.
Pantoprazole sodium (p.1243·2).
Gastro-oesophageal reflux; peptic ulcer.

Pepti-2000
Nutricia, Austral.; Nutricia, Port.
Preparation for enteral nutrition (p.1350·1).
Malabsorption syndromes.

Pepti-2000 LF Nutricia, Irl.†.
Preparation for enteral nutrition (p.1350·1).

Peptic Guard Genpharm, Canad.
Famotidine (p.1225·3).

Peptic Relief Genpharm, Canad.
Ranitidine hydrochloride (p.1245·2).

Peptica Unison, Thai.
Cimetidine (p.1216·3).
Peptic ulcer; Zollinger-Ellison syndrome.

Peptichemio Nuovo ISM, Ital.†.
Multialchilpeptide (p.560·2).
Myeloproliferative disorders.

Pepticum Andromaco, Spain.
Omeprazole (p.1239·1).
Gastro-oesophageal reflux; peptic ulcer; Zollinger-Ellison syndrome.

Peptiditutteli Valio, Fin.
Infant feed (p.1350·1).
Cow's milk and soya protein intolerance.

Peptifar Tecnimede, Port.
Ranitidine hydrochloride (p.1245·2).

Pepti-Junior
Nutricia, Austral.; Nutricia, Fin.; Nutricia, Fr.; Cow & Gate, Irl.; Cow & Gate, Israel; Nutricia, Ital.; Nutricia, Port.; Cow & Gate, UK.
Food for special diets (p.1350·1).
Diarrhoea; food intolerance; malabsorption.

Peptimax Ashbourne, UK.
Cimetidine (p.1216·3).
Gastrointestinal disorders.

Peptinaut Nutricia, Ital.
Preparation for enteral nutrition (p.1350·1).

Peptireal Novartis Nutrition, Fr.
A range of preparations for enteral nutrition (p.1350·1).

Peptison
Nutricia, Ital.; Nutricia, Port.
Preparation for enteral nutrition (p.1350·1).

Peptisorb Pfrimmer Nutricia, Switz.
Range of preparations for enteral nutrition (p.1350·1).

Peptizole LSP, Thai.
Omeprazole (p.1239·1).
Gastro-oesophageal reflux; peptic ulcer; Zollinger-Ellison syndrome.

Pepto Diarrhea Control Procter & Gamble, USA.
Loperamide hydrochloride (p.1231·3).
Diarrhoea.

Pepto-Bismol
Note.This name is used for preparations of different composition.
Procter & Gamble, Canad.
Caplets; oral liquid: Bismuth salicylate (p.1213·1).
Tablets: Calcium carbonate (p.1215·1); bismuth salicylate (p.1213·1).
Diarrhoea; dyspepsia; nausea; upset stomach.

Procter & Gamble, Mex.; Procter & Gamble (H&B Care), UK; Procter & Gamble, USA.
Bismuth salicylate (p.1213·1).
Diarrhoea; dyspepsia; heartburn; nausea; upset stomach.

Peptoci Pharmasant, Thai.
Famotidine (p.1225·3).
Peptic ulcer; Zollinger-Ellison syndrome.

Peptol Carter Horner, Canad.
Cimetidine (p.1216·3).
Gastric acid hypersecretion.

Peptomet Remedica, Thai.
Domperidone (p.1224·1).
Delayed gastric emptying; gastro-oesophageal reflux.

Peptopancreasi Dansk-Flama, Braz.
Pepsin (p.1649·3); pancreatin (p.1646·1).
Digestive system disorders.

Pepto-Pancreasi SIT, Ital.
Pepsin (p.1649·3); pancreatin (p.1646·1).
Digestive system disorders.

Peptulan Farmasa, Braz.
Bismuth (p.1213·1).
Diarrhoea; gastrointestinal hyperacidity.

Pepzan
Douglas, Hong Kong; Douglas, NZ; Douglas, Singapore; Douglas, Thai.; TTN, Thai.
Famotidine (p.1225·3).
Peptic ulcer; Zollinger-Ellison syndrome.

Pepzitrat Berlin-Chemie, Ger.
Pepsin (p.1649·3); citric acid (p.1596·2).
Gastrointestinal disorders.

Peracel Monot, Fr.†.
Loperamide hydrochloride (p.1231·3).
Diarrhoea.

Peracil Boniscontro & Gazzone, Ital.
Piperacillin sodium (p.236·1).
Lignocaine [lidocaine] hydrochloride (p.1313·2) is included in this preparation to alleviate the pain of injection.
Bacterial infections.

Peracon Salvay, Aust.†; Solvay, Ger.†; Aventis, S.Afr.
Isoaminile citrate (p.1094·1) or isoaminile cyclamate (p.1094·1).
Coughs.

Peracon Expectorant Aventis, S.Afr.
Isoaminile cyclamate (p.1094·1); ammonium chloride (p.1085·2).
Coughs.

Peragit Gea, Denm.
Benzhexol [trihexyphenidyl] hydrochloride (p.463·3).
Drug-induced extrapyramidal disorders; parkinsonism.

Peralgin Infabra, Braz.
Phenylbutazone calcium (p.78·3).
Gout; musculoskeletal, joint, and peri-articular disorders.

Peran BASF, Ger.
Acemetacin (p.11·2).
Gout; inflammation; musculoskeletal, joint, and peri-articular disorders.

Perasian Asian Pharm, Thai.
Loperamide hydrochloride (p.1231·3).
Diarrhoea.

Perasthman N CHR, Ger.
Theophylline (p.777·2).
Obstructive airways disease.

Perative
Abbott, Austral.; Abbott, Hong Kong; Abbott, Irl.; Ross, Israel; Abbott Nutrition, UK.
Preparation for enteral nutrition (p.1350·1).

Peratsin Orion, Fin.
Perphenazine (p.699·1), perphenazine decanoate (p.699·1), or perphenazine enantate (p.699·1).
Psychoses.

Perazolin Zenyaku, Jpn†.
Sobuzoxane (p.569·1).
Leukaemia; lymphoma.

Perbilen Hoechst Marion Roussel, Spain.
Piretanide (p.956·2).
Hypertension; oedema.

Perchloracap Mallinckrodt, USA.
Potassium perchlorate (p.1525·2).
To reduce accumulation of pertechnetate by the choroid plexus, salivary glands, and thyroid.

Perclar Parke, Davis, Ital.
Mesoglycan sodium (p.1634·3).
Thrombosis prophylaxis.

Perclusone SERB, Fr.†.
Clofezone (p.25·1); clofexamide hydrochloride (p.25·1).
Musculoskeletal, joint, peri-articular, and soft-tissue disorders; superficial phlebitis.

Percocet
Du Pont, Canad.; Taro, Israel; Endo, USA.
Oxycodone hydrochloride (p.70·2); paracetamol (p.71·2).
Fever; pain.

Percodan
Note.This name is used for preparations of different composition.
Du Pont, Canad.
Oxycodone hydrochloride (p.70·2); aspirin (p.14·2).
Fever; inflammation; pain.

Taro, Israel; Endo, USA.
Oxycodone hydrochloride (p.70·2); oxycodone terephthalate (p.70·3); aspirin (p.14·2).
Pain.

Percoffedrinol N Passauer, Ger.
Caffeine (p.761·3).
Fatigue.

Percogesic Richardson-Vicks, USA.
Paracetamol (p.71·2); phenyltoloxamine citrate (p.423·1).
Fever; pain.

Percolone Endo, USA.
Oxycodone hydrochloride (p.70·2).
Pain.

Percorina Boehringer Ingelheim, Spain.
Isosorbide mononitrate (p.916·2).
Angina pectoris.

Percutafeine Pierre Fabre Sante, Fr.
Caffeine (p.761·3).
Obesity.

Percutalgine
Piette, Belg.; Besins-Iscovesco, Fr.; Piette, Thai.
Dexamethasone (p.1067·1) or dexamethasone acetate (p.1067·1); salicylamide (p.82·1); glycol salicylate (p.42·2); methyl nicotinate (p.55·1).
Musculoskeletal, joint, peri-articular, and soft-tissue disorders.

Percutalin Almirall, Spain†.
Dexamethasone (p.1067·1) or dexamethasone acetate (p.1067·1); salicylamide (p.82·1); glycol salicylate (p.42·2); methyl nicotinate (p.55·1).
Musculoskeletal, joint, peri-articular, and soft-tissue disorders.

Percutase N Godecke, Ger.†.
Glycol salicylate (p.42·2); benzyl nicotinate (p.20·2).
Formerly contained glycol salicylate, heparin, benzyl nicotinate, and nonivamide.
Musculoskeletal and joint disorders.

Percutol Dominion, UK.
Glyceryl trinitrate (p.897·3).
Angina pectoris.

Perderm
Schering-Plough, Hong Kong; Schering-Plough, Singapore.
Alclometasone dipropionate (p.1061·1).
Skin disorders.

Perdiem Novartis Consumer, USA.
Ispaghula (p.1229·1); senna (p.1248·2).
Constipation.

Perdiem Fiber Novartis Consumer, USA†.
Ispaghula (p.1229·1).
Constipation.

Perdiphen Spitzner, Ger.; Schwabe, Ger.
Ephedrine hydrochloride (p.1090·1); paracetamol (p.71·2); diphenylpyraline hydrochloride (p.417·1).
Influenza symptoms.

Perdiphen phyto Spitzner, Ger.†; Schwabe, Ger.†.
Cowslip rhizome (p.1600·1); thyme (p.1672·2).
Cold symptoms.

Perdipina Novartis, Ital.
Nicardipine hydrochloride (p.938·3).
Angina pectoris; heart failure; hypertension.

Perdipine Yamanouchi, Jpn.
Nicardipine hydrochloride (p.938·3).
Cerebrovascular disorders; heart failure; hypertension.

Perdix
Alpharma, Denm.; Alpharma, Fin.; Dumex-Alpharma, Swed.; Schwarz, UK.
Moexipril hydrochloride (p.935·3).
Hypertension.

Perdogrip *Janssen-Cilag, Belg.*
Paracetamol (p.71·2); vitamin C (p.1389·3).
Cold symptoms.

Perdolan *Janssen-Cilag, Belg.*
Suppositories (baby and child): Aspirin (p.14·2); paracetamol (p.71·2); codeine phosphate (p.25·2).
Tablets; suppositories (adult): Aspirin (p.14·2); paracetamol (p.71·2); caffeine (p.761·3); codeine phosphate (p.25·2).
Fever; pain.

Perdolan Duo *Janssen-Cilag, Belg.*
Paracetamol (p.71·2); codeine phosphate (p.25·2).
Pain.

Perdolan Mono *Janssen-Cilag, Belg.*
Paracetamol (p.71·2).
Fever; pain.

Perdolan Mono C *Janssen-Cilag, Belg.*
Paracetamol (p.71·2); ascorbic acid (p.1389·3).
Fever; pain.

Perduretas Codeina *Medea, Spain.*
Codeine phosphate (p.25·2).
Cough; diarrhoea; pain.

Perebron
Angelini, Ital.; Farma Lepori, Spain.
Oxolamine citrate (p.1096·2) or oxolamine phosphate (p.1096·2).
Adjunct in obstructive airways disease; coughs.

Pereflat *Solvay, Fr.*
Dimethicone (p.1249·2); pancreas extract (porcine).
Dyspepsia.

Peremesin
Bristol-Myers Squibb, Ger.; Meda, Norw.
Meclozine hydrochloride (p.420·3).
Formerly contained meclozine hydrochloride and caffeine in Norw.
Nausea; vertigo; vomiting.

Peremesin N *Bristol-Myers Squibb, Ger.*
Meclozine hydrochloride (p.420·3).
Formerly contained meclozine hydrochloride and caffeine.
Nausea; vertigo; vomiting.

Peremin *Novartis, Aust.*
Paracetamol (p.71·2); pheniramine maleate (p.422·3); phenylephrine hydrochloride (p.1097·1); ascorbic acid (p.1389·3).
Cold and influenza symptom.

Perenan
Sanofi Winthrop, Fr.; Sanofi Winthrop, Hong Kong; Sanofi Synthelabo, Singapore; Sanofi Synthelabo, Thai.
Co-dergocrine mesilate (p.1597·3).
Behavioural and psychological disorders in the elderly.

Perennia *Wyeth Lederle, Aust.*
Conjugated oestrogens (p.1467·1); medroxyprogesterone acetate (p.1480·1).
Menopausal disorders; osteoporosis.

Perenterol
Biodiphar, Belg.; Thiemann, Ger.; Biocodex, Switz.
Saccharomyces boulardii (p.1626·3).
Acne; diarrhoea; restoration of gastrointestinal flora; vitamin B deficiency-associated disorders.

Peresal
Henkel, Ger.; Henkel, Ital.
Hydrogen peroxide (p.1147·1); peracetic acid (p.1152·2).
Instrument disinfection.

Perfadex *Xvivo, Swed.*
Dextran 40 (p.728·3) in electrolytes.
Organ perfusion before transplantation.

Perfan
Aventis, Belg.; Hoechst Marion Roussel, Ger.; Hoechst Marion Roussel, Irl.; Lepetit, Ital.; Hoechst Marion Roussel, Neth.; Hoechst Marion Roussel, UK.
Enoximone (p.885·2).
Heart failure.

Perfane *Roussel Diamant, Fr.*
Enoximone (p.885·2).
Heart failure.

Perfarin *Wayne, Mex.*
Piroxicam (p.79·1).

Perfect Climate *Estee Lauder, Canad.*
Octinoxate (p.1517·3).
Sunscreen.

Perfectil
Vitabiotics, Hong Kong.
Multivitamin and mineral preparation with echinacea and lappa (p.1350·1).
Vitabiotics, UK.
Multivitamin, amino-acid, mineral, and herbal preparation (p.1350·1).

Perflux *Fresenius Kabi, Aust.*
Electrolyte infusion (p.1180·1).
Forced diuresis.

Perfolate *Asta Medica, Fr.*
Calcium folinate (p.1363·1).
Drug-induced megaloblastic anaemia; folate deficiency; prevention of methotrexate toxicity.

Perfolin *Gambar, Ital.*
Calcium folinate (p.1363·1).
Anaemias; antidote to folic acid antagonists; folate deficiency.

Perform *Schulke & Mayr, Ger.*
Potassium peroxymonosulfate.
Surface disinfection.

Perfudal *Astra, Spain.*
Felodipine (p.888·3).
Angina pectoris; hypertension.

Perfudan *Piam, Ital.*
Buflomedil hydrochloride (p.851·3).
Cerebral and peripheral vascular disorders.

Perfus Multivitaminico *Rius, Spain.*
Carbazochrome (p.728·1); vitamins (p.1350·1); electrolytes.
Haemorrhage; skeletal muscle disorders.

Perfusion de PAS *Bichsel, Switz.*
Sodium aminosalicylate (p.148·3).
Tuberculosis.

Perfusion mixte *Streuli, Switz.*
Sodium chloride (p.1196·1) infusion with glucose.
Dehydration.

Pergalen *Hoechst Marion Roussel, Braz.*
Sodium apolate (p.971·1); benzyl nicotinate (p.20·2).
Soft-tissue injuries.

Perganit *Astra, Ital.*
Glyceryl trinitrate (p.897·3).
Angina pectoris; hypertension; pulmonary oedema.

Pergastric *Prodes, Spain†.*
Dimethicone (p.1249·2).
Flatulence.

Perginol *Gambar, Ital.*
Sodium tetrachloroiodite.
Gynaecological infections.

Pergogreen
Serono, Ital.†; Serono, Swed.†; Serono, Switz.
Menotrophin (p.1288·2).
Male and female infertility.

Pergonal
Serono, Aust.†; Serono, Braz.; Serono, Canad.; Serono, Ger.; Serono, Hong Kong; Serono, Irl.; Teva, Israel; Serono, Neth.†; Serono, S.Afr.; Serono, Singapore; Serono, Spain; Serono, Swed.†; Serono, S.-serono, Thai.; Serono, UK†; Serono, USA.
Menotrophin (p.1288·2).
Male and female infertility.

Pergotime
Serono, Denm.; Serono, Fr.; Serono, Ger.†; Serono, Norw.; Serono, Swed.
Clomifene citrate (p.1465·3).
Anovulatory infertility.

Periactin
Merck Sharp & Dohme, Aust.; Merck Sharp & Dohme, Austral.; Merck Sharp & Dohme, Belg.; Johnson & Johnson, Canad.; Merck Sharp & Dohme, Denm.; Merck Sharp & Dohme, Hong Kong; Merck Sharp & Dohme, Irl.; Sigma-Tau, Ital.; Merck Sharp & Dohme, Neth.; Merck Sharp & Dohme, NZ; Merck Sharp & Dohme, Port.; Merck Sharp & Dohme, S.Afr.; Sigma-Tau, Spain; Merck Sharp & Dohme, Swed.; Merck Sharp & Dohme, Switz; Merck Sharp & Dohme, Thai.; Merck Sharp & Dohme, UK; Merck, USA.
Cyproheptadine hydrochloride (p.414·2).
Hypersensitivity reactions; migraine; pruritus; reduced appetite.

Periactine *Merck Sharp & Dohme-Chibret, Fr.*
Cyproheptadine hydrochloride (p.414·2).
Hypersensitivity reactions; pruritus.

Periamin *Fresenius Kabi, Spain.*
Amino-acid, carbohydrate, and electrolyte infusion (p.1350·1).
Parenteral nutrition.

Periamin X *Pharmacia Upjohn, Ger.*
Amino-acid, xylitol, and electrolyte infusion (p.1350·1).
Parenteral nutrition.

Periamin G
Fresenius Kabi, Spain.
Amino-acid, carbohydrate, and electrolyte infusion (p.1350·1).
Parenteral nutrition.
Pharmacia Upjohn, Ger.
Amino-acid, glucose, and electrolyte infusion (p.1350·1).
Parenteral nutrition.

Periatin *Prodome, Braz.*
Cyproheptadine hydrochloride (p.414·2).
Hypersensitivity reactions; migraine and other vascular headaches; reduced appetite.

Periatin BC *Prodome, Braz.*
Cyproheptadine hydrochloride (p.414·2); vitamins (p.1350·1).
Hypersensitivity reactions; migraine and other vascular headaches; reduced appetite.

Periavita *Prodome, Braz.*
Cyproheptadine hydrochloride (p.414·2); multivitamins (p.1350·1).
Hypersensitivity reactions; migraine and other vascular headaches; reduced appetite.

Peribilan *Lannacher, Aust.*
Ox bile (p.1585·1); pig bile (p.1585·1).
Constipation; gastrointestinal disorders.

Periblastine *Intramed, S.Afr.†.*
Vinblastine sulfate (p.577·3).
Malignant neoplasms.

Pericaina *Senese, Ital.*
Mepivacaine hydrochloride (p.1317·1).
Local anaesthesia.

Perical *Besins-Iscovesco, Fr.*
Calcium carbonate (p.1215·1).
Calcium deficiency; osteoporosis.

Pericam *Clonmel, Irl.*
Piroxicam (p.79·1).
Dysmenorrhoea; gout; musculoskeletal, joint, and peri-articular disorders.

Pericate *Unipharm, Israel.*
Haloperidol decanoate (p.686·3).
Schizophrenia.

Pericel *Pharmafar, Ital.*
Flavodate sodium (p.1611·1).
Vascular disorders.

Pericephal *Merck, Aust.*
Cinnarizine (p.413·1).
Cerebral and peripheral vascular disorders; vestibular disorders.

Peri-Colace
Roberts, Canad.; Roberts, USA.
Casanthranol (p.1216·1); docusate sodium (p.1223·1).
Constipation.

Pericristine *Teva, S.Afr.*
Vincristine sulfate (p.578·3).
Malignant neoplasms.

Perida *Codal Synto, Thai.*
Haloperidol (p.686·3).
Behaviour disorders in children; psychoses; stuttering; tics.

Peridal *Medley, Braz.*
Domperidone (p.1224·1).
Gastrointestinal motility disorders; nausea and vomiting.

Peridane *Columbia, Mex.*
Oxpentifylline [pentoxifylline] (p.950·3).
Cerebral and peripheral vascular disorders; thrombosis prophylaxis.

Peridex *Zila, Canad.; Procter & Gamble, USA.*
Chlorhexidine gluconate (p.1138·2).
Gingivitis.

Peridil *Cryopharma, Mex.*
Azapetine phosphate.
Peripheral vascular disorders.

Peridin-C *Beutlich, USA.*
Hesperidin methyl chalcone (p.1611·1); hesperidin complex (p.1611·2); ascorbic acid (p.1389·3).
Capillary bleeding.

Peridol *Technilab, Canad.*
Haloperidol (p.686·3).
Behaviour disorders; psychoses; Tourette syndrome.

Peridon *Italchimici, Ital.*
Domperidone (p.1224·1).
Gastrointestinal disorders.

Peridor *Unipharm, Israel.*
Haloperidol (p.686·3).
Hiccup; psychiatric disorders; Tourette syndrome; vomiting.

Peri-Dos Softgels *Goldline, USA.*
Docusate sodium (p.1223·1); casanthranol (p.1216·1).
Constipation.

Peridys *Robapharm, Fr.*
Domperidone (p.1224·1).
Dyspepsia; gastro-oesophageal reflux; nausea and vomiting.

Perifazo *Pharmacia Upjohn, Fr.†.*
Amino-acid infusion (p.1350·1).
Parenteral nutrition.

Perifem *Organon, Spain.*
11 Tablets, estradiol valerate (p.1473·2); 10 tablets, estradiol valerate (p.1473·2); medroxyprogesterone acetate (p.1480·1).
Menopausal disorders.

Perifer HI *BA Farma, Port.†.*
Astemizole (p.409·1).
Allergic conjunctivitis; allergic rhinitis; urticaria.

Periflex *Scientific Hospital Supplies, UK.*
Preparation for enteral nutrition (p.1350·1).

Perikliman *Kwizda, Aust.*
16 Tablets, estradiol (p.1473·1); 12 tablets, estradiol; norethisterone acetate (p.1485·1).
Menopausal disorders; osteoporosis.

Perikursal
Wyeth Lederle, Aust.; Wyeth, Ger.
Levonorgestrel (p.1486·2); ethinylestradiol (p.1476·2).
Biphasic oral contraceptive.

Perilax *Merck, Denm.*
Bisacodyl (p.1212·2).
Bowel evacuation; constipation.

Perilox *Drossapharm, Switz.*
Metronidazole (p.594·1).
Rosacea.

Perinal
Dermal Laboratories, Irl.; Dermal, Israel; Dermal Laboratories, UK.
Hydrocortisone (p.1073·3); lignocaine [lidocaine] hydrochloride (p.1313·2).
Anal and perianal pain and pruritus.

Perinorm *Nat Druggests, S.Afr.*
Metoclopramide hydrochloride (p.1235·2).
Gastrointestinal disorders.

Perio Chip *Perio, Israel.*
Chlorhexidine gluconate (p.1138·2).
Periodontitis.

Periochip
Procter & Gamble, UK; Astra, USA.
Chlorhexidine gluconate (p.1138·2).
Periodontal disease.

Periocline *Sunstar, Jpn.*
Minocycline hydrochloride (p.224·3).
Periodontitis.

Period Pain Relief *Herbal Concepts, UK.*
Alchemilla (p.1648·3); motherwort (p.1637·3); valerian (p.1678·3); pulsatilla (p.1656·3); vervain (p.1679·3); helonias (p.1619·1).
Dysmenorrhoea; premenstrual syndrome.

Periodentix *Germiphene, Israel.*
Chlorhexidine gluconate (p.1138·2).
Gingivitis; oral hygiene.

Periodine Anti-Malarico *Simoes, Braz.*
Sulfametopyrazine (p.256·1); pyrimethamine (p.442·3).
Malaria.

Periodontil *Rhodia, Braz.*
Spiramycin (p.248·3); metronidazole (p.594·1).
Bacterial infections; protozoal infections.

Periogard
Note. This name is used for preparations of different composition.
Colgate-Palmolive, Ital.; Asta Medica, Port.†
Mouthwash; oral drops: Sanguinaria (p.1660·3).
Gum disorders; halitosis; oral hygiene.
Colgate-Palmolive, Ital.; Asta Medica, Port.†
Toothpaste: Sanguinaria (p.1660·3); sodium monofluorophosphate (p.1377·2).
Gum disorders; halitosis; oral hygiene.
Colgate Oral, USA.
Chlorhexidine gluconate (p.1138·2).
Mouth disorders.

Periogard Chlorohex
Colgate Oral Care, Austral.; Colgate-Palmolive, Ger.; Colgate-Palmolive, Ital.; Asta Medica, Port.†.
Chlorhexidine (p.1138·2) or chlorhexidine gluconate (p.1138·2).
Mouth disorders; oral hygiene.

Periostat
Collagenex, UK; Collagenex, USA.
Doxycycline hyclate (p.200·1).
Bacterial infections.

Peripherin *Asta Medica, Aust.†*
Etofylline (p.765·1); theophylline hydrate (p.777·2); ephedrine (p.1090·1).
Cerebrovascular disorders.

Periphramine *Pharmacia Upjohn, Spain.*
Amino-acid infusion (p.1350·1).
Parenteral nutrition.

Periplasmal
Braun, Ger.; Braun, Switz.
Amino-acid, carbohydrate, and electrolyte infusion (p.1350·1).
Parenteral nutrition.

Periplasmal G *Braun, Spain.*
Amino-acid, carbohydrate, and electrolyte infusion (p.1350·1).
Parenteral nutrition.

Periplasmal XE *Braun, Spain.*
Amino-acid, xylitol, and electrolyte infusion (p.1350·1).
Parenteral nutrition.

Periplum *Italfarmaco, Ital.*
Nimodipine (p.946·1).
Cerebrovascular disorders.

Peripress
Pfizer, Denm.; Pfizer, Fin.; Pfizer, Swed.†.
Prazosin hydrochloride (p.958·1).
Benign prostatic hyperplasia; heart failure; hypertension; Raynaud's syndrome.

Peristaltine *Novartis Sante, Fr.*
Cascara (p.1216·1).
Constipation.

Peritoflex *Fresenius, Spain.*
Calcium chloride; anhydrous glucose; magnesium chloride; sodium chloride; sodium lactate (p.1184·1).
Peritoneal dialysis.

Peritofundin
Braun, Aust.; Braun, Braz.
Electrolytes; glucose or sorbitol (p.1184·1).
Peritoneal dialysis solution.

Peritofundinas *Braun, Port.*
Glucose; sodium chloride; calcium chloride; magnesium chloride; potassium chloride; sodium lactate (p.1184·1).
Peritoneal dialysis.

Peritol *Medphano, Ger.*
Cyproheptadine hydrochloride (p.414·2).
Hypersensitivity reactions; pruritus; reduced appetite.

Peritone *Blackmores, Austral.*
Aloes (p.1210·1); senna (p.1248·2); cascara (p.1216·1); ginger (p.1227·2); cardamom fruit (p.1591·3); peppermint oil (p.1243·3).
Constipation.

Peritrast
Kohler, Aust.; Kohler, Ger.
Lysine amidotrizoate (p.1032·1).
Radiographic contrast medium.

Peritrast comp *Kohler, Ger.*
Sodium amidotrizoate (p.1031·2); lysine amidotrizoate (p.1032·1).
Radiographic contrast medium.

Peritrast-Infusio 160/32% *Kohler, Ger.*
Lysine amidotrizoate (p.1032·1).
Radiographic contrast medium.

Peritrast-Infusio 180/31% *Kohler, Ger.*
Sodium amidotrizoate (p.1031·2); lysine amidotrizoate (p.1032·1).
Radiographic contrast medium.

Peritrast-Oral CT *Kohler, Ger.*
Lysine amidotrizoate (p.1032·1); sodium amidotrizoate (p.1031·2).
Contrast medium for computer tomography of the abdominal cavity.

Peritrast-Oral-GI *Kohler, Ger.*
Lysine amidotrizoate (p.1032·1).
Contrast medium for gastrointestinal radiography.

Peritrast-RE *Kohler, Ger.*
Lysine amidotrizoate (p.1032·1).
Contrast medium for rectal radiography.

Peritrate
Parke, Davis, Canad.†; Teofarma, Ital.; Parke, Davis, S.Afr.†; Warner-Lambert, Thai.
Pentaerithrityl tetranitrate (p.952·3).
Angina pectoris.

Perivar *Intersan, Ger.*
Troxerutin (p.1611·2); heptaminol hydrochloride (p.1619·2); ginkgo biloba (p.1615·2).
Vascular disorders.

Perivar Rosskaven *Intersan, Ger.*
Aesculus (p.1574·1).
Venous insufficiency.

Perivar Venensalbe *Intersan, Ger.*
Heparin sodium (p.902·1).
Soft-tissue injury; vascular disorders.

Perkamillon
Note.This name is used for preparations of different composition.
Robugen, Ger.; Medipharm, Switz.
Liquid: Chamomile (p.1593·2).
Inflammatory disorders of the skin or mucous membranes.

Medipharm, Switz.
Ointment: Chamomile (p.1593·2); hamamelis (p.1618·3).
Minor wounds.

Perketan *Inverni della Beffa, Ital.*
Ketanserin tartrate (p.917·2).
Hypertension.

Perkod *Biogalenique, Fr.*
Dipyridamole (p.877·2).
Thromboembolic disorders.

Perlax *UCI, Braz.*
Dantron (p.1221·3); dexpanthenol (p.1602·3).
Constipation.

Perles d'huile de foie de morue du Dr Geistlich *Geistlich, Switz.*
Cod-liver oil (p.1357·2); halibut-liver oil (p.1366·1).
Vitamin A and D deficiency.

Perlinganit
Nycomed, Aust.; Orion, Fin.; Schwarz, Ger.; Orion, Swed.; Schwarz, Switz.
Glyceryl trinitrate (p.897·3).
Cardiovascular disorders; controlled hypotension.

Perlinsol Cutaneo *Medea, Spain†.*
Acedoben sodium (p.1571·2); vitamin F.
Skin disorders.

Perlol *Asian Pharm, Thai.*
Propranolol hydrochloride (p.962·3).
Angina pectoris; arrhythmias; hypertension.

Perlutal *Promeco, Mex.*
Algestone acetophenide (p.1465·1); estradiol enantate (p.1473·2).
Endometriosis; female infertility; injectable contraceptive; menstrual disorders.

Perlutan *Boehringer de Angeli, Braz.*
Algestone acetophenide (p.1465·1); estradiol enantate (p.1473·2).
Injectable contraceptive.

Perlutex
Leo, Denm.; Leo, Norw.
Medroxyprogesterone acetate (p.1480·1).
Endometrial cancer; endometriosis; menopausal disorders; test of ovarian function.

Permadoze *Dumex, Port.*
Cyanocobalamin (p.1388·1).
Neuralgia; vitamin B_{12} deficiency.

Permapen *Roerig, USA.*
Benzathine benzylpenicillin (p.156·2).
Bacterial infections.

Permax
Lilly, Aust.; Lilly, Austral.; Lilly, Belg.; Draxis, Canad.; Lilly, Denm.; Lilly, Fin.; Lilly, Mex.; Lilly, Neth.; Lilly, NZ; Lilly, Port.; Lilly, S.Afr.; Lilly, Switz.; Athena Neurosciences, USA.
Pergolide mesilate (p.1175·1).
Parkinsonism.

Permease *Novartis, Aust.*
Hyaluronidase (p.1620·3).
Haematomas; increase absorption and reduce discomfort of injections; reduce viscosity of secretions and discharge.

Permitabs *Bioglan, UK.*
Potassium permanganate (p.1154·3).
Wound cleansing.

Permitil *Schering, USA.*
Fluphenazine hydrochloride (p.684·3).
Psychoses.

Permixon
Germania, Aust.; Pierre Fabre, Fr.; Pierre Fabre, Ital.; Schering-Plough, Mex.; Pierre Fabre, Port.; Orient, Singapore; Pierre Fabre, Singapore; Pierre Fabre, Spain; Pierre Fabre, Thai.
Saw palmetto (p.1491·2).
Benign prostatic hyperplasia; prostatic adenoma.

Permixon Novum *Robapharm, Switz.*
Saw palmetto (p.1491·2).
Prostatic hyperplasia.

Pernaemyl *Biosyn, Ger.†.*
Bovine liver extract (p.1388·1).
Liver disorders; megaloblastic anaemia; vitamin B_{12} deficiency.

Pernamed *Medifive, Thai.*
Perphenazine (p.699·1).
Nausea and vomiting; psychoses.

Pernazene *Synthelabo, Fr.†.*
Tymazoline hydrochloride (p.1102·2).
Nasal congestion.

Pernazine *Atlantic, Thai.*
Perphenazine (p.699·1).
Nausea and vomiting; psychoses.

Pernexin *Schering, Ital.*
Iron succinyl-protein complex (p.1369·3).
Anaemias; iron deficiency.

Pernionin *Krewel, Ger.*
Methyl salicylate (p.55·1); benzyl nicotinate (p.20·2); methyl nicotinate (p.55·1).
Musculoskeletal and joint disorders; peripheral vascular disorders.

Pernionin N *Krewel, Ger.*
Methyl salicylate (p.55·1); sage oil (p.1660·2).
Circulatory disorders.

Pernionin Teil-Bad *Krewel, Ger.*
Benzyl nicotinate (p.20·2).
Pernionin Teil-Bad N formerly contained methyl salicylate, benzyl nicotinate, and methyl nicotinate.
Bath additive; musculoskeletal and joint disorders; peripheral circulatory disorders.

Pernionin Voll-Bad N *Krewel, Ger.*
Norway spruce oil; benzyl nicotinate (p.20·2); methyl nicotinate (p.55·1).
Bath additive; musculoskeletal and joint disorders; peripheral circulatory disorders.

Pernox
Westwood-Squibb, Canad.; Westwood, USA.
Polyethylene granules (abrasive) (p.1108·3); sulfur (p.1123·3); salicylic acid (p.1122·3).
Acne; oily skin.

Pernutin *Grifols, Spain.*
Amino-acid, carbohydrate, electrolyte, and vitamin infusion (p.1350·1).
Parenteral nutrition.

Pernyzol *Recordati, Ital.†.*
Metronidazole benzoate (p.594·1).
Bacterial mouth infections.

Pero *Opfermann, Ger.*
Glycerol (p.1616·3); bleached wax.
Skin disorders.

Perocef *Pulitzer, Ital.†.*
Cefoperazone sodium (p.168·2).
Lignocaine [lidocaine] hydrochloride (p.1313·2) is included in this preparation to alleviate the pain of injection.
Bacterial infections.

Perocur *Biocur, Ger.*
Saccharomyces boulardii (p.1626·3).
Diarrhoea.

Perofen *Remedica, Thai.*
Ibuprofen (p.43·2).
Musculoskeletal, joint, peri-articular, and soft-tissue disorders; toothache.

Peroxacne *Isdin, Spain.*
Benzoyl peroxide (p.1111·1).
Acne.

Peroxiben *Isdin, Spain.*
Benzoyl peroxide (p.1111·1).
Acne.

Peroxin *Dermol, USA.*
Benzoyl peroxide (p.1111·1).
Acne.

Peroxyl
Colgate-Palmolive, UK; Colgate-Palmolive, USA.
Hydrogen peroxide (p.1147·1).
Oral lesions.

Perozon Erkaltungsbad *Sanova, Aust.*
Eucalyptus oil (p.1609·2); camphor (p.1589·3); menthol (p.1632·3).
Bath additive; cold symptoms; rheumatic disorders.

Perozon Heublumen *Sanova, Aust.*
Thyme oil (p.1672·3); hay flowers.
Bath additive.

Perozon Rosmarin-Olbad mono *Spitzner, Ger.*
Rosemary oil (p.1659·3).
Bath additive; peripheral vascular disorders.

Perpector *Grossmann, Switz.*
Codeine phosphate (p.25·2); ephedrine hydrochloride (p.1090·1); potassium iodide (p.1522·3); cowslip root (p.1600·1); valerian (p.1678·3).
Coughs.

Perphenan *Taro, Israel.*
Perphenazine (p.699·1).
Anxiety; nervous states; vomiting.

Perphyllon *Asta Medica, Aust.*
Etofylline (p.765·1); theophylline hydrate (p.777·2); papaverine hydrochloride (p.1648·1); atropine methonitrate (p.461·1).
Asthma; bronchitis; emphysema.

Persa-Gel *Ortho Dermatological, USA.*
Benzoyl peroxide (p.1111·1).
Acne.

Persantin
Boehringer Ingelheim, Aust.; Boehringer Ingelheim, Austral.; Boehringer de Angeli, Braz.; Boehringer Ingelheim, Denm.; Boehringer Ingelheim, Fin.; Boehringer Ingelheim, Ger.; Boehringer Ingelheim, Hong Kong; Boehringer Ingelheim, Irl.; Boehringer Ingelheim, Ital.; Boehringer Ingelheim, Mex.; Boehringer Ingelheim, Neth.; Boehringer Ingelheim, Norw.; Boehringer Ingelheim, NZ; Boehringer Ingelheim, Port.; Boehringer Ingelheim, S.Afr.; Boehringer Ingelheim, Singapore; Boe-
[continued]
hringer Ingelheim, Spain; Boehringer Ingelheim, Swed.; Boehringer Ingelheim, Switz.; Boehringer Ingelheim, UK; Boehringer Ingelheim, USA.
Dipyridamole (p.877·2) or dipyridamole hydrochloride (p.878·1).
Adjunct in myocardial thallium scanning; ischaemic heart disease; thromboembolic disorders.

Persantin Plus *Boehringer Ingelheim, Hong Kong.*
Dipyridamole (p.877·2); aspirin (p.14·2).
Thromboembolic disorders.

Persantin S *Boehringer de Angeli, Braz.*
Dipyridamole (p.877·2); aspirin (p.14·2).
Thrombosis prophylaxis.

Persantine
Boehringer Ingelheim, Belg.; Boehringer Ingelheim, Canad.; Boehringer Ingelheim, Fr.; Boehringer Ingelheim, Switz.; Boehringer Ingelheim, USA.
Dipyridamole (p.877·2).
Angina pectoris; thromboembolic disorders; vasodilator in myocardial perfusion imaging.

Persivate *Aspen, S.Afr.*
Betamethasone valerate (p.1063·2).
Skin disorders.

Perskindol
Singer, Hong Kong.
Menthol (p.1632·3); essential oils.
Muscle and joint pain.

Singer, Switz.†.
Menthol (p.1632·3).
Muscle and joint pain.

Persol
Note.This name is used for preparations of different composition.
Dreveny, Aust.†.
Hydrogen peroxide (p.1147·1) (p.1129·2).
Cleaning and disinfecting solution for hard and soft contact lenses.

Horner, Canad.†.
Benzoyl peroxide (p.1111·1); colloidal sulfur (p.1123·3).
Acne; rosacea.

Persolv Richter *Lepetit, Ital.*
Urokinase (p.988·1).
Thromboembolic disorders.

Personnel *Therapex, Canad.*
Bismuth salicylate (p.1213·1).

Personnelle Contre le Rhume *Therapex, Canad.*
Pseudoephedrine hydrochloride (p.1099·2); dextromethorphan hydrobromide (p.1087·3); paracetamol (p.71·2).
Coughs and associated respiratory-tract disorders.

Personnelle DM *Therapex, Canad.*
Pseudoephedrine hydrochloride (p.1099·2); dextromethorphan hydrobromide (p.1087·3).
Coughs and associated respiratory-tract disorders.

Persumbrax *Boehringer Ingelheim, Ital.†.*
Dipyridamole (p.877·2); oxazepam (p.697·1).
Cardiovascular disorders.

Pert Plus *Procter & Gamble, Canad.*
Pyrithione zinc (p.1122·1).
Seborrhoeic dermatitis.

Pertamin *Yauquimia, Mex.*
Vitamin A (p.1382·1).

Pertensal *Vinas, Spain.*
Nifedipine (p.940·1).
Angina pectoris; hypertension; Raynaud's syndrome.

Pertenso N *Fournier, Spain.*
Propranolol hydrochloride (p.962·3); hydralazine hydrochloride (p.905·3); bendrofluazide [bendroflumethiazide] (p.844·1).
Hypertension.

Pertil *Astra, Spain.*
Isosorbide mononitrate (p.916·2).
Angina pectoris.

Pertin *Solvay, Aust.†.*
Metoclopramide hydrochloride (p.1235·2).
Gastrointestinal motility disorders; nausea and vomiting.

Pertiroid *Piam, Ital.*
Potassium perchlorate (p.1525·2).
Hyperthyroidism.

Pertix *Hommel, Ger.*
Pentoxyverine (p.1096·3) or pentoxyverine citrate (p.1096·3).
Coughs and associated respiratory-tract disorders.

Pertix-Solo *Hommel, Ger.*
Menadiol calcium diphosphate.
Coughs.

Pertofran
Novartis, Aust.; Novartis, Austral.; Novartis, Belg.; Novartis, Fr.; Novartis, Ger.; Novartis, Neth.; Novartis, NZ; Ciba-Geigy, S.Afr.†; Novartis, UK†.
Desipramine hydrochloride (p.282·3).
Depression.

Pertofrane
Geigy, Canad.†; Rorer, USA†.
Desipramine hydrochloride (p.282·3).
Depression.

Pertoglobulin *Nuovo ISM, Ital.*
A pertussis immunoglobulin (p.1555·3).
Passive immunisation.

Pertranquil
Note.This name is used for preparations of different composition.
Hoechst Marion Roussel, Aust.†; Aventis, Belg.
Meprobamate (p.691·1).
Anxiety disorders; neurodermatitis; sedative; skeletal muscle spasm; sleep disorders.

Llorente, Spain.
Diazepam (p.674·3); aminohydroxybutyric acid (p.342·2).
Anxiety; insomnia.

Pertrim *Allergan-Frumtost, Braz.*
Polymyxin B sulfate (p.238·1); trimethoprim (p.264·2).
Bacterial eye infections.

Pertriptyl *Orion, Fin.*
Perphenazine (p.699·1); amitriptyline hydrochloride (p.273·3).
Anxiety disorders; depression; schizophrenia.

Pertrombon *Gerot, Aust.*
Sodium nicotinate; heparin (p.902·1).
Decubitus ulcer; promote resorption of excess fluid; soft-tissue injury; thrombophlebitis; ulcus cruris; varices.

Pertropin *Lannett, USA†.*
Linolenic acid, vitamin E substances, and essential fatty acids (p.1350·1).
Dietary supplement.

Pertudoron
Weleda, Aust.; Weleda, Fr.; Weleda, Ger.
Homoeopathic preparation.

Pertus-Gamma *Biagini, Ital.*
A human pertussis immunoglobulin (p.1555·3).
Passive immunisation.

Pertussex Compositum *Uhlmann-Eyraud, Switz.*
Codeine phosphate (p.25·2); ephedrine hydrochloride (p.1090·1); drosera; galeopsis; thyme; Iceland moss; cowslip.
Coughs and associated respiratory-tract disorders.

Pertussin *Pertussin, USA.*
Dextromethorphan hydrobromide (p.1087·3).
Coughs.

Pertuvac *Chiron Behring, Ger.†.*
A pertussis vaccine (p.1555·3).
Active immunisation.

Perubare *Mayoly-Spindler, Switz.*
Peru balsam (p.1650·2); thymol (p.1158·3); thyme oil (p.1672·3); rosemary oil (p.1659·3); lavender oil (p.1627·2).
Upper-respiratory-tract disorders.

Perubore
Note.This name is used for preparations of different composition.
ACP, Belg.
Peru balsam (p.1650·2); thyme oil (p.1672·3); rosemary oil (p.1659·3); thymol (p.1158·3).
Rhinitis; sinusitis.

Mayoly-Spindler, Fr.
Thyme oil (p.1672·3); rosemary oil (p.1659·3); lavender oil (p.1627·2); thymol (p.1158·3); peru balsam (p.1650·2).
Upper respiratory-tract congestion.

Perudent *Dreveny, Aust.*
Peru balsam (p.1650·2).
Dental preparation.

Peru-Lenicet *Athenstaedt, Ger.*
Aluminium diacetate hydroxide; aluminium hydroxide gel (p.1210·3); peru balsam (p.1650·2).
Skin disorders; wounds.

Perusliuos-K *Fresenius Kabi, Fin.*
Electrolyte infusion with glucose (p.1180·1).
Carbohydrate source; fluid and electrolyte disorders.

Pervasum *Lesvi, Spain.*
Cinnarizine (p.413·1).
Migraine and other vascular headaches; motion sickness; vestibular disorders.

Perviam *Janssen-Cilag, Belg.*
Ibuprofen lysine (p.44·1).
Fever; pain.

Pervincamine *Synthelabo, Fr.†.*
Vincamine (p.1680·1).
Formerly known as Pervincamine Forte.
Mental function impairment in the elderly.

Pervita *Lifeplan, UK.*
Betacarotene (p.1355·1).
Nutritional supplement.

Pervivo *Bittner, Aust.*
Manna, camphor; zedoary; angelica; myrrh; gentian; rowan; nutmeg; liquorice; helenin; centaury; clove; galanga; ginger; cnicus benedictus; ivae moschatae; theriac; iridus; verbascum; bitter orange peel; calamus; absinthium; aloes; cubeb; star anise; sweet orange peel; menyanthes.
Gastrointestinal disorders; tonic.

Perycit *Astra, Swed.*
Niceritrol (p.939·2).
Hyperlipidaemias.

Perzine *PP Lab, Thai.*
Perphenazine (p.699·1).
Nausea and vomiting; psychoses.

Pesendorfer *Iso, Ger.*
Homoeopathic preparation.

Pesex-R *Zimaia, Port.†.*
Fenproporex hydrochloride (p.1510·2).
Obesity.

Pesos *Valeas, Ital.†.*
Fenfluramine hydrochloride (p.1510·1).
Obesity.

Pessarios Profilaticos Rendel *CIF, Braz.*
Nonoxinol 10 (p.1346·2).
Vulvovaginal infections.

Pestarin *Provit, Mex.*
Rifampicin (p.243·2).
Bacterial infections.

Petadolex *Weber & Weber, Ger.*
Petasites officinalis.
Smooth muscle spasms.

Petadolor N *Bioforce, Switz.*
Petasites radix.
Migraine; smooth muscle spasm.

Petaforce V *Bioforce, Ger.*
Petasites officinalis.
Migraine; urinary-tract pain.

Pe-Tam *Qualiphar, Belg.*
Paracetamol (p.71·2).
Fever; pain.

Peteha *Fatol, Ger.*
Injection: Protionamide (p.239·3); nicotinamide (p.1372·3).
Tablets: Protionamide (p.239·3).
Tuberculosis.

Peter Pote's *Restan, S.Afr.*
Bismuth citrate (p.1213·1); potassium hydroxide (p.1654·1); pepsin (p.1649·3); belladonna (p.463·1); nux vomica (p.1643·1); ammonia solution (p.1579·1).
Gastrointestinal disorders.

Petercillin *Intramed, S.Afr.; Aspen, S.Afr.*
Ampicillin sodium (p.150·3) or ampicillin trihydrate (p.151·1).
Bacterial infections.

Peterkaien *Intramed, S.Afr.*
Lignocaine [lidocaine] hydrochloride (p.1313·2).
Arrhythmias; local anaesthesia.

Peterphyllin *Intramed, S.Afr.*
Aminophylline (p.760·1).
Heart failure; obstructive airways disease; oedema.

Peter's Sirop *Monot, Fr.†*
Ammoniated anise (p.1580·2); ethylmorphine hydrochloride (p.35·2); aconite (p.1572·3); belladonna (p.463·1); cherry laurel.
Respiratory-tract disorders.

Petidion *Gerot, Aust.; Gerot, Switz.*
Ethadione (p.348·1).
Absence seizures; myoclonic seizures.

Petiflog *Sanus, Braz.*
Benzydamine hydrochloride (p.20·1).
Fever; inflammation; pain.

Petina Compound *Jean-Marie, Hong Kong.*
Cyproheptadine hydrochloride (p.414·2); vitamins (p.1350·1).
Appetite loss; tonic.

Petinimid *Gerot, Aust.; Gerot, Switz.*
Ethosuximide (p.348·1).
Absence seizures.

Petinutin *Parke, Davis, Aust.; Parke, Davis, Ger.; Parke, Davis, Switz.*
Mesuximide (p.353·3).
Epilepsy.

Petites Pilules Carters *Fumouze, Fr.*
Boldine (p.1585·3); aloes (p.1210·1).
Constipation.

Petnidan *Desitin, Ger.*
Ethosuximide (p.348·1).
Absence seizures.

Petogen *Intramed, S.Afr.*
Medroxyprogesterone acetate (p.1480·1).
Injectable contraceptive.

Petrasch-Anthozym N *Reith & Petrasch, Ger.*
Rote beete; lactic acid (p.1626·2).
Adjuvant in radiotherapy and cytotoxic chemotherapy.

Petrolagar No. 2 *Whitehall, Irl.†*
Liquid paraffin (p.1407·1); light liquid paraffin (p.1407·2); phenolphthalein (p.1244·1).
Constipation.

Petrolagar with Phenolphthalein *Whitehall, Irl.*
Light liquid paraffin (p.1407·2); liquid paraffin (p.1407·1); phenolphthalein (p.1244·1).
Constipation.

Petroleum Med Complex *Dynamit, Aust.*
Homoeopathic preparation.

Petylyl *Dresden, Ger.; Temmler, Ger.*
Desipramine hydrochloride (p.282·3).
Depression.

Pevalip *Janssen-Cilag, Aust.*
Econazole (p.383·1).
Fungal skin and nail infections.

Pevaryl
Note.This name is used for preparations of different composition.
Janssen-Cilag, Aust.
Cream; lotion; shampoo; lipogel; topical solution; topical spray: Econazole (p.383·1) or econazole nitrate (p.382·3).
Paste; topical powder; topical powder spray: Econazole nitrate (p.382·3); zinc oxide (p.1128·2).
Fungal skin and nail infections; Gram-positive infections.
Dermatech, Austral.; Janssen-Cilag, Belg.; Janssen-Cilag, Denm.; Janssen-Cilag, Fin.; Janssen-Cilag, Fr.; Cilag, Hong Kong; Janssen-Cilag, Irl.; Janssen-Cilag, Israel; Janssen-Cilag, Ital.; Cilag, Mex.; Janssen-Cilag, Neth.; Janssen-Cilag, Norw.; ICN, NZ; Janssen-Cilag, Port.; Roche, S.Afr.; Janssen-Cilag, Singapore; Pensa, Spain; Janssen-Cilag, Swed.; Janssen-Cilag, UK.
Econazole (p.383·1) or econazole nitrate (p.382·3).
Fungal and Gram-positive bacterial infections.

Janssen-Cilag, Switz.
Cream; lipogel; lotion; shampoo; topical powder; topical solution; topical spray: Econazole (p.383·1) or econazole nitrate (p.382·3).
Fungal skin and scalp infections.
Paste: Econazole nitrate (p.382·3); zinc oxide (p.1128·2).
Fungal skin disorders.

Pevaryl TC *Janssen-Cilag, UK.*
Econazole nitrate (p.382·3); triamcinolone acetonide (p.1080·1).
Skin disorders with bacterial or fungal infection.

Pevidine *Rhone-Poulenc Rorer, Hong Kong.*
Povidone-iodine (p.1155·1).
Burns; disinfection of skin and mucous membranes; wounds.

Pevisone
Janssen-Cilag, Aust.; Janssen-Cilag, Belg.; Janssen-Cilag, Denm.; Janssen-Cilag, Fin.; Janssen-Cilag, Fr.; Cilag, Hong Kong; Janssen-Cilag, Israel; Janssen-Cilag, Ital.; Janssen-Cilag, Norw.; Janssen-Cilag, Port.; Roche, S.Afr.; Janssen-Cilag, Singapore; Janssen-Cilag, Swed.; Janssen-Cilag, Switz.; Janssen, Thai.
Econazole nitrate (p.382·3); triamcinolone acetonide (p.1080·1).
Infected skin disorders.

Pexan E *Worwag, Ger.*
d-Alpha tocopherol (p.1393·3) or alpha tocoferil acetate (p.1394·1).
Vitamin E deficiency.

Pexid *Sigma, Austral.; Hoechst Marion Roussel, Belg.†; Pharmaco, NZ.*
Perhexiline maleate (p.953·2).
Angina pectoris.

Pexsig *Sigma, Austral.*
Perhexiline maleate (p.953·2).
Angina pectoris.

Pfefferminz-Lysoform *Lysoform, Ger.†*
Formaldehyde (p.1144·2); peppermint oil (p.1243·3); menthol (p.1632·3).
Infections of the oropharynx.

Pfeiffer's Allergy *Pfeiffer, USA†.*
Chlorpheniramine [chlorphenamine] maleate (p.412·1).
Hypersensitivity reactions.

Pfeiffer's Cold Sore *Pfeiffer, USA.*
Sumatra benzoin (p.1668·3); camphor (p.1589·3); menthol (p.1632·3); eucalyptol (p.1609·2).
Oral lesions.

Pfeil *Stada, Ger.*
Ibuprofen (p.43·2).
Pain.

P-Fen *Masa, Thai.*
Ibuprofen (p.43·2).
Gout; musculoskeletal and joint disorders.

Pfizerpen *Pfizer, USA.*
Benzylpenicillin potassium (p.157·1).
Bacterial infections.

Pfizerpen-AS *Roerig, USA†.*
Procaine penicillin [procaine benzylpenicillin] (p.239·2).
Bacterial infections.

PG 53 *Bouty, Ital.†.*
Fertility test (p.1654·3).

pH 550 *Restan, S.Afr.*
Suspension: Dicyclomine [dicycloverine] hydrochloride (p.466·1); aluminium hydroxide gel (p.1210·3); magnesium oxide (p.1233·2); calcium carbonate (p.1215·1); dimethicone (p.1249·2).
Flatulence; gastric hyperacidity; hiatus hernia; peptic ulcer.
Tablets: Calcium carbonate (p.1215·1); magnesium carbonate (p.1232·3); magnesium trisilicate (p.1233·3).
Gastrointestinal disorders associated with hyperacidity.

PH maxi *Orion, Fin.*
Aluminium hydroxide (p.1210·3); magnesium hydroxide (p.1233·1); aluminium hydroxide-magnesium carbonate co-dried gel (p.1211·2).
Gastro-oesophageal reflux; hiatus hernia; peptic ulcer.

Phaeva *Schering, Fr.*
Gestodene (p.1479·1); ethinylestradiol (p.1476·2).
Triphasic oral contraceptive.

Phakan
Chauvin, Fr.
Combination pack: Oral solution, glycine (p.1365·3); glutamic acid (p.1365·2); pyridoxine hydrochloride (p.1386·3); capsules, cysteine hydrochloride (p.1358·3); ascorbic acid (p.1389·3).
Cataracts.
Chauvin, Port.
White capsules, glycine (p.1365·3); glutamic acid (p.1365·2); pyridoxine (p.1387·1); blue capsules, cysteine (p.1358·3); vitamin C (p.1389·3).
Cataracts.

Phakolen *Chauvin Novopharma, Switz.*
Combination pack: White capsules, glycine (p.1365·3); L-glutamic acid (p.1365·2); pyridoxine hydrochloride (p.1386·3); blue capsules, L-cysteine (p.1358·3); ascorbic acid (p.1389·3).
Prevention of cataract formation.

Phanacol *Pharmakon, USA†.*
Phenylpropanolamine hydrochloride (p.1098·1); dextromethorphan hydrobromide (p.1087·3); guaifenesin (p.1092·2); paracetamol (p.71·2).

Phanadex Cough *Pharmakon, USA†.*
Phenylpropanolamine hydrochloride (p.1098·1); dextromethorphan hydrobromide (p.1087·3); mepyramine maleate (p.421·1); guaifenesin (p.1092·2).
Coughs.

Phanalgin *Trima, Israel.*
Dipyrone (p.34·1).
Fever; pain.

Phanate *Pharmaland, Thai.*
Lithium carbonate (p.292·1).
Bipolar disorder.

Phanatuss Cough *Pharmakon, USA.*
Dextromethorphan hydrobromide (p.1087·3); guaifenesin (p.1092·2).
Coughs.

Phapax *Lehning, Fr.*
Homoeopathic preparation.

Phardol mono *Kreussler, Ger.*
Glycol salicylate (p.42·2).
Musculoskeletal, joint, soft-tissue, and nerve disorders.

Phardol Rheuma *Kreussler, Ger.*
Glycol salicylate (p.42·2); oleum pini sylvestris; benzyl nicotinate (p.20·2).
Musculoskeletal, joint, soft-tissue, and nerve disorders.

Pharken *Lilly, Spain.*
Pergolide mesilate (p.1175·1).
Parkinsonism.

Pharma Plus *Tanning Research, Canad.*
SPF 15: Octinoxate (p.1517·3); oxybenzone (p.1518·1).
SPF 30: Homosalate (p.1517·2); octinoxate (p.1517·3); octisalate (p.1518·1); oxybenzone (p.1518·1).
Sunscreen.

Pharma Plus Oil Free *Tanning Research, Canad.*
SPF 30: Octinoxate (p.1517·3); octisalate (p.1518·1); oxybenzone (p.1518·1).
Sunscreen.

Pharma Plus Sport *Tanning Research, Canad.*
SPF 30: Octinoxate (p.1517·3); octisalate (p.1518·1); oxybenzone (p.1518·1).
Sunscreen.

Pharmacare Aspec *PSM, NZ.*
Aspirin (p.14·2).
Thromboembolism prophylaxis.

Pharmacen *Alpharma, Mex.*
Paracetamol (p.71·2).
Fever; pain.

Pharmacetin *Olan-Kemed, Thai.*
Chloramphenicol (p.179·1).
Bacterial ear infections.

Pharmacilline *Monot, Fr.†*
Gramicidin (p.213·3).
Infections of the mouth, nose, and throat.

Pharmacists Creme *Reese, USA.*
Methyl salicylate (p.55·1); menthol (p.1632·3); capsicum oleoresin.

Pharmacists Lotion *Reese, USA.*
Methyl salicylate (p.55·1); menthol (p.1632·3); capsicum oleoresin.

Pharmacol DM *Therapex, Canad.†.*
Phenylpropanolamine hydrochloride (p.1098·1); pheniramine maleate (p.422·3); mepyramine maleate (p.421·1); dextromethorphan hydrobromide (p.1087·3).

Pharma-Col Junior *Warner-Lambert, Austral.*
Dextromethorphan hydrobromide (p.1087·3); pseudoephedrine hydrochloride (p.1099·2); paracetamol (p.71·2).
Coughs and cold symptoms.

Pharmacycare Barrier *Douglas, NZ.*
Dimethicone (p.1410·1).
Barrier cream.

Pharmacycare Bath Oil *Douglas, NZ.*
Hydrous wool fat (p.1410·3); liquid paraffin (p.1407·1).
Dry skin; pruritus.

Pharmacycare Cough *Douglas, NZ.*
Pholcodine (p.1099·1).
Coughs.

Pharmacycare Expectorant *Douglas, NZ.*
Choline theophyllinate (p.763·3); guaifenesin (p.1092·2).
Coughs.

Pharmacycare Hand & Body *Douglas, NZ.*
Hydrous wool fat (p.1410·3); liquid paraffin (p.1407·1).
Dry skin; pruritus.

Pharmadose alcool *Gilbert, Fr.*
Alcohol (p.1130·3).
Skin and wound disinfection.

Pharmadose mercuresceine *Gilbert, Fr.*
Merbromin (p.1150·1).
Wound and burn disinfection.

Pharmadose teinture d'arnica *Gilbert, Fr.*
Arnica (p.1581·3).
Ecchymoses.

Pharmaethyl *Austrodent, Aust.*
Cryofluorane (p.1199·1).
Local anaesthesia in dentistry.

Pharmaflam *Pharmador, S.Afr.†*
Diclofenac sodium (p.30·3).
Inflammation; musculoskeletal and joint disorders; pain.

Pharmaflex *Braun, Belg.*
Metronidazole (p.594·1).
Anaerobic bacterial infections; protozoal infections.

Pharmaflur *Pharmics, USA.*
Sodium fluoride (p.1375·3).
Dental caries prophylaxis.

Pharmalgen
ALK, Belg.; ALK, Denm.; ALK, Swed.†; Trimedal, Switz.; ALK, UK; ALK, USA.
Venoms of bee, wasp, hornet, yellow jacket, and mixed vespids (p.1575·3).
Hyposensitisation.

Pharmapress *Aspen, S.Afr.*
Enalapril maleate (p.883·3).
Heart failure; hypertension.

Pharmatex
Note.This name is used for preparations of different composition.
Innothera, Fr.
Pessaries; soap; tampons; vaginal cream: Benzalkonium chloride (p.1133·2).
Contraceptive; skin hygiene.
Topical gel: Hymetellose (p.1501·2); benzalkonium chloride (p.1133·2); glycerol (p.1616·3).
Vaginal lubricant.
Agis, Israel; Asta Medica, Port.
Benzalkonium chloride (p.1133·2).
Contraceptive.

Pharmaton
Boehringer Ingelheim, Austral.; Pharmaton, Ger.; Boehringer Ingelheim, NZ; Pharmaton, NZ; Boehringer Ingelheim, Port.; Boehringer Ingelheim Self Medication, UK.
Vitamins; minerals; ginseng; lecithin (p.1350·1).
Tonic.
Boehringer Ingelheim, Fr.; Boehringer Ingelheim, Irl.
Vitamins; minerals; deanol bitartrate; ginseng (p.1350·1).
Age-related disorders; tonic.
Boehringer Ingelheim, Hong Kong.
Ginseng; deanol bitartrate; rutoside; vitamins; minerals (p.1350·1).
Age-related disorders; tonic.
Promeco, Mex.; Pharmaton, Singapore.
Multivitamins; minerals; ginseng; lecithin; rutoside (p.1350·1).
Pharmaton, Thai.
Ginseng; deanol bitartrate; rutoside; lecithin; vitamins; minerals (p.1350·1).

Pharmaton Complex *Fher, Spain.*
Multivitamins and minerals (p.1350·1); ginseng; rutoside; lecithin; deanol bitartrate.
Tonic.

Pharmaton SA *Boehringer Ingelheim, S.Afr.*
Multivitamins and minerals (p.1350·1); ginseng; lecithin; rutoside.
Tonic.

Pharmatovit
Boehringer Ingelheim, Aust.; Pharmaton, Switz.
Multivitamin and mineral preparation (p.1350·1).
Pharmaton, Israel.
Multivitamins and mineral preparation with lecithin and rutoside (p.1350·1).

Pharmet *Pharmador, S.Afr.†.*
Methyldopa (p.927·3).
Hypertension.

Pharmetapp *Therapex, Canad.†.*
Phenylephrine hydrochloride (p.1097·1); phenylpropanolamine hydrochloride (p.1098·1); brompheniramine maleate (p.421·1).

Pharmilin-DM *Therapex, Canad.*
Dextromethorphan hydrobromide (p.1087·3).

Pharminicol DM *Therapex, Canad.*
Phenylpropanolamine hydrochloride (p.1098·1); pheniramine maleate (p.422·3); mepyramine maleate (p.421·1); dextromethorphan hydrobromide (p.1087·3).

Pharminil DM *Therapex, Canad.*
Dextromethorphan hydrobromide (p.1087·3).

Pharmitussin DM *Therapex, Canad.†.*
Dextromethorphan hydrobromide (p.1087·3); guaifenesin (p.1092·2).

Pharmorubicin
Pharmacia Upjohn, Austral.; Pharmacia Upjohn, Canad.; Pharmacia Upjohn, Hong Kong; Pharmacia Upjohn, Irl.; Pharmacia Upjohn, NZ; Pharmacia, UK.
Epirubicin hydrochloride (p.537·1).
Malignant neoplasms.

Pharmoxin *Pharmador, S.Afr.†.*
Amoxicillin trihydrate (p.149·2).
Bacterial infections.

Pharnax *Pharmaland, Thai.*
Alprazolam (p.654·2).
Mixed anxiety depressive states.

Pharo-Tus *Nakornpatana, Thai.*
Dextromethorphan hydrobromide (p.1087·3); phenylpropanolamine hydrochloride (p.1098·1); chlorpheniramine [chlorphenamine] maleate (p.412·1); guaifenesin (p.1092·2).
Coughs.

Pharyngine a la Vitamine C *Medeva, Fr.*
Tyrothricin (p.267·1); lignocaine [lidocaine] hydrochloride (p.1313·2); ascorbic acid (p.1389·3).
Formerly contained tyrothricin, amethocaine [tetracaine] hydrochloride, and ascorbic acid.
Infections of the mouth and throat.

Pharyngor *Rappai, Switz.*
Potassium chloride; sodium chloride; magnesium chloride; calcium chloride; potassium acid phosphate (p.1180·1); chamomile.
Dry mouth and throat.

Pharynx
DHA, Hong Kong; DHA, Singapore.
Cetylpyridinium chloride (p.1138·1); benzocaine (p.1306·2).
Mouth and throat infections.

Pharysyx N *Syxyl, Ger.*
Homoeopathic preparation.

Phatropine *Pharmaland, Thai.*
Benzatropine mesilate (p.463·2).
Drug-induced extrapyramidal disorders; parkinsonism.

Phazyme
Stafford-Miller, Austral.†; Reed & Carnrick, Canad.; Stafford-Miller, Spain; Reed & Carnrick, USA.
Simeticone (p.1249·2).
Aerophagia; dyspepsia; flatulence.

Phenacon *Teral, USA†.*
Phenylephrine hydrochloride (p.1097·1); chlorpheniramine [chlorphenamine] maleate (p.412·1); hyoscine methonitrate (p.468·2).
Coughs.

Phenadex Cough/Cold *Barre-National, USA†.*
Phenylpropanolamine hydrochloride (p.1098·1); dextromethorphan hydrobromide (p.1087·3); guaifenesin (p.1092·2).
Cough and cold symptoms.

Phenadex Senior *Barre-National, USA†.*
Dextromethorphan hydrobromide (p.1087·3); guaifenesin (p.1092·2).
Coughs.

Phenaemal *Desitin, Ger.*
Phenobarbital (p.355·1).
Epilepsy.

Phenaemaletten *Desitin, Ger.*
Phenobarbital (p.355·1).
Epilepsy.

Phenahist-TR *Williams, USA†.*
Phenylpropanolamine hydrochloride (p.1098·1); phenylephrine hydrochloride (p.1097·1); chlorpheniramine [chlorphenamine] maleate (p.412·1); hyoscyamine sulfate (p.469·3); hyoscine hydrobromide (p.468·2); atropine sulfate (p.461·1).
Upper respiratory-tract symptoms.

Phenameth *Major, USA†.*
Promethazine hydrochloride (p.423·2).
Hypersensitivity reactions; motion sickness; nausea; postoperative pain (adjunct); sedative; vomiting.

Phenameth DM *Major, USA.*
Promethazine hydrochloride (p.423·2); dextromethorphan hydrobromide (p.1087·3).
Coughs and cold symptoms.

Phenamin *Nycomed, Norw.*
Dexchlorpheniramine maleate (p.412·1).
Hypersensitivity reactions; pruritus.

Phenapap *Rugby, USA.*
Pseudoephedrine hydrochloride (p.1099·2); paracetamol (p.71·2).
Upper respiratory-tract disorders.

Phenapap Sinus Headache & Congestion *Rugby, USA.*
Pseudoephedrine hydrochloride (p.1099·2); paracetamol (p.71·2); chlorpheniramine [chlorphenamine] maleate (p.412·1).
Upper respiratory-tract symptoms.

Phenaphen with Codeine
Note. This name is used for preparations of different composition.
Wyeth-Ayerst, Canad.
Aspirin (p.14·2); phenobarbital (p.355·1); codeine phosphate (p.25·2).
Pain.

Robins, USA.
Paracetamol (p.71·2); codeine phosphate (p.25·2).
Pain.

Phenaseptic *Rugby, USA.*
Phenol (p.1152·3).
Minor mouth or throat irritation.

Phenate
Note. This name is used for preparations of different composition.
Pacific, NZ; Alphapharm, Singapore; Merck, Singapore.
Clomifene citrate (p.1465·3).
Anovulatory infertility.

Roberts, USA†; Hauck, USA†.
Phenylpropanolamine hydrochloride (p.1098·1); chlorpheniramine [chlorphenamine] maleate (p.412·1); paracetamol (p.71·2).
Upper respiratory-tract symptoms.

Phenazin *Faulding, Port.*
Fluphenazine hydrochloride (p.684·3).

Phenazine
Note. This name is used for preparations of different composition.
Pharmaland, Thai.
Fluphenazine decanoate (p.684·3).
Psychoses.

Keene, USA†.
Promethazine hydrochloride (p.423·2).
The name Phenazine has also been used for preparations containing phendimetrazine tartrate.
Hypersensitivity reactions; motion sickness; nausea; postoperative pain (adjunct); sedative; vomiting.

Phenazo *ICN, Canad.; CPC, Hong Kong.*
Phenazopyridine hydrochloride (p.77·3).
Urinary-tract pain.

Phenchlor SHA *Rugby, USA†.*
Phenylpropanolamine hydrochloride (p.1098·1); phenylephrine hydrochloride (p.1097·1); chlorpheniramine [chlorphenamine] maleate (p.412·1); hyoscyamine sulfate (p.469·3); atropine hydrobromide (p.468·2); atropine sulfate (p.461·1).
Upper respiratory-tract symptoms.

Phencodin *Medicap, Thai.*
Codeine phosphate (p.25·2); promethazine hydrochloride (p.423·2).
Coughs.

Phendex *Aspen Consumer, S.Afr.*
Triprolidine hydrochloride (p.427·2); pseudoephedrine hydrochloride (p.1099·2); guaifenesin (p.1092·2); codeine phosphate (p.25·2).
Coughs.

Phendiridine *TP, Thai.*
Phenazopyridine hydrochloride (p.77·3).
Urinary-tract pain.

Phendry *Lu Chem, USA†.*
Diphenhydramine hydrochloride (p.416·1).
Insomnia; motion sickness; parkinsonism.

Phenedrine *United American, Hong Kong.*
Theophylline (p.777·2).
Obstructive airways disease.

Phenerbel-S *Rugby, USA.*
Phenobarbital (p.355·1); ergotamine tartrate (p.452·1); belladonna (p.463·1).

Phenergan
Note. This name is used for preparations of different composition.
Rhone-Poulenc Rorer, Aust.; Rhone-Poulenc Rorer, Austral.; Aventis, Belg.; Rhone-Poulenc Rorer, Canad.; Rhone-Poulenc Rorer, Denm.; Medeva, Fr.; Rhone-Poulenc Rorer, Hong Kong; Rhone-Poulenc Rorer, Irl.; Rhone-Poulenc Rorer, Neth.; Rhone-Poulenc Rorer, Norw.; Aventis, NZ; Rhone-Poulenc Rorer, S.Afr.; Rhone-Poulenc Rorer, Singapore; Rhone-Poulenc Rorer, Switz.; Rhone-Poulenc Rorer, Thai.; Rhone-Poulenc Rorer, UK; Wyeth-Ayerst, USA.
Promethazine (p.423·2) or promethazine hydrochloride (p.423·2).
Hypersensitivity reactions; insomnia; motion sickness; nausea and vomiting; pain (adjunct); parkinsonism; premedication; sedative.

Rhone-Poulenc Rorer, S.Afr.†.
Cream: Promethazine (p.423·2); dibrompropamidine isetionate (p.1143·1).
Burns; insect bites; scalds; stings.

Phenergan with Codeine *Wyeth-Ayerst, USA.*
Promethazine hydrochloride (p.423·2); codeine phosphate (p.25·2).
Coughs and cold symptoms.

Phenergan with Dextromethorphan *Wyeth-Ayerst, USA.*
Promethazine hydrochloride (p.423·2); dextromethorphan hydrobromide (p.1087·3).
Coughs and cold symptoms.

Phenergan Expectorant
Note. This name is used for preparations of different composition.
Rhone-Poulenc Rorer, Belg.†.
Promethazine (p.423·2); sulfogaiacol (p.1101·1); ipecacuanha (p.1093·1).
Coughs.

Novartis Consumer, Canad.†.
Promethazine hydrochloride (p.423·2); sulfogaiacol (p.1101·1).
Coughs.

Rhone-Poulenc Rorer, Switz.
Promethazine hydrochloride (p.423·2); guaifenesin (p.1092·2); ipecacuanha (p.1093·1).
Coughs.

Phenergan Expectorant with Codeine *Novartis Consumer, Canad.†.*
Promethazine hydrochloride (p.423·2); sulfogaiacol (p.1101·1); codeine phosphate (p.25·2).
Coughs.

Phenergan VC *Wyeth-Ayerst, USA.*
Promethazine hydrochloride (p.423·2); phenylephrine hydrochloride (p.1097·1).
Cold symptoms; nasal congestion.

Phenergan VC with Codeine *Wyeth-Ayerst, USA.*
Promethazine hydrochloride (p.423·2); phenylephrine hydrochloride (p.1097·1); codeine phosphate (p.25·2).
Cold symptoms; coughs; nasal congestion.

Phenergan VC Expectorant *Novartis Consumer, Canad.†.*
Promethazine hydrochloride (p.423·2); phenylephrine hydrochloride (p.1097·1); sulfogaiacol (p.1101·1).
Coughs.

Phenergan VC Expectorant with Codeine *Novartis Consumer, Canad.†.*
Promethazine hydrochloride (p.423·2); phenylephrine hydrochloride (p.1097·1); sulfogaiacol (p.1101·1); codeine phosphate (p.25·2).
Coughs.

Phenetron *Lannett, USA†.*
Chlorpheniramine [chlorphenamine] maleate (p.412·1).
Hypersensitivity reactions.

Phenex
Abbott, Austral.; Ross, USA.
A range of phenylalanine-free preparations for enteral nutrition including an infant feed (p.1350·1).
Hyperphenylalaninaemia; phenylketonuria.

Phenexpect
Note. This name is used for preparations of different composition.
DHA, Hong Kong.
Diphenhydramine hydrochloride (p.416·1); ammonium chloride (p.1085·2); sodium citrate (p.1186·2).
Coughs.

DHA, Singapore.
Diphenhydramine hydrochloride (p.416·1); ammonium chloride (p.1085·2).
Coughs.

Phenexpect CD *DHA, Singapore.*
Diphenhydramine hydrochloride (p.416·1); codeine phosphate (p.25·2); ammonium chloride (p.1085·2).
Coughs.

Phenhalal *Halal, UK.*
Promethazine hydrochloride (p.423·2).

Phenhist DH with Codeine *Rugby, USA.*
Pseudoephedrine hydrochloride (p.1099·2); chlorpheniramine [chlorphenamine] maleate (p.412·1); codeine phosphate (p.25·2).
Coughs and cold symptoms.

Phenhist Expectorant *Rugby, USA.*
Pseudoephedrine hydrochloride (p.1099·2); guaifenesin (p.1092·2); codeine phosphate (p.25·2).
Coughs.

Phenhydan
Gerot, Aust.; Desitin, Ger.; Desitin, Switz.
Phenytoin (p.357·2) or phenytoin sodium (p.357·2).
Arrhythmias; epilepsy; trigeminal neuralgia.

Phenicol *Vitamed, Israel.*
Chloramphenicol (p.179·1).
Bacterial eye infections.

Phenimixin *Vitamed, Israel.*
Chloramphenicol (p.179·1); polymyxin B sulfate (p.238·1).
Bacterial eye infections.

Phenocillin *Streuli, Switz.*
Benzathine phenoxymethylpenicillin (p.157·1) or phenoxymethylpenicillin (p.235·1).
Bacterial infections.

Phenoject *Mayrand, USA†.*
Promethazine hydrochloride (p.423·2).
Hypersensitivity reactions; motion sickness; nausea; postoperative pain (adjunct); sedative; vomiting.

Phenolax *Upjohn, USA†.*
Phenolphthalein (p.1244·1).
Constipation.

Phenoptic *Optopics, USA.*
Phenylephrine hydrochloride (p.1097·1).
Funduscopy; open-angle glaucoma; ophthalmic examination; pupil dilatation during surgery; refraction without cycloplegia; uveitis.

Phenoris *Stickley, Canad.*
Clioquinol (p.190·2); allantoin (p.1110·1); phenol (p.1152·3).
Topical antiseptic.

Phenoro *Roche, Fr.*
Betacarotene (p.1355·1); canthaxanthin (p.1027·2).
Lupus erythematosus; photosensitivity.

Phenotal *Asian Pharm, Thai.*
Phenobarbital sodium (p.355·1).
Epilepsy; insomnia; sedative.

Phenoxine *Lannett, USA†.*
Phenylpropanolamine hydrochloride (p.1098·1).
Obesity.

Phenpro *Ratiopharm, Ger.*
Phenprocoumon (p.954·3).
Thromboembolic disorders.

Phensedyl
Note. This name is used for preparations of different composition.
Rhone-Poulenc Rorer, Austral.
Promethazine hydrochloride (p.423·2); pholcodine (p.1099·1); pseudoephedrine hydrochloride (p.1099·2).
Coughs.

Aventis, S.Afr.
Promethazine hydrochloride (p.423·2); codeine phosphate (p.25·2); ephedrine hydrochloride (p.1090·1).
Coughs.

Rhone-Poulenc Rorer, Singapore; Rhone-Poulenc Rorer, Thai.
Promethazine hydrochloride (p.423·2); codeine phosphate (p.25·2).
Cold symptoms; coughs.

Phensedyl Dry Family Cough *Aventis, NZ.*
Promethazine hydrochloride (p.423·2); pholcodine (p.1099·1); pseudoephedrine hydrochloride (p.1099·2).
Coughs.

Phensedyl Plus *Rhone-Poulenc Rorer, UK.*
Promethazine hydrochloride (p.423·2); pholcodine (p.1099·1); pseudoephedrine hydrochloride (p.1099·2).
Congestion; coughs; sore throats.

Phensic *Merck Consumer, UK.*
Aspirin (p.14·2); caffeine (p.761·3).
Fever; pain.

Phensic Dual Action *Merck Consumer, UK.*
Paracetamol (p.71·2); codeine phosphate (p.25·2); caffeine (p.761·3).
Cold and influenza symptoms; fever; pain.

Phensic Ibuprofen *Merck Consumer, UK.*
Ibuprofen (p.43·2).
Fever; pain.

Phenurone *Abbott, USA†.*
Phenacemide (p.354·3).
Epilepsy.

Phenylade *Taranis, Fr.*
Food for special diets (p.1350·1).
Phenylketonuria.

Phenyldrine *Rugby, USA†.*
Phenylpropanolamine hydrochloride (p.1098·1).
Obesity.

Phenylfenesin LA *Goldline, USA†.*
Phenylpropanolamine hydrochloride (p.1098·1); guaifenesin (p.1092·2).
Coughs.

Phenyl-Free
Mead Johnson, Hong Kong; Mead Johnson, Israel; Mead Johnson, Ital.; Mead Johnson, NZ.
Food for special diets (p.1350·1).
Disorders of phenylalanine metabolism; phenylketonuria.

Phenylgesic *Goldline, USA.*
Phenyltoloxamine citrate (p.423·1); paracetamol (p.71·2).
Upper respiratory-tract symptoms.

Phenyphrine-Azol *Vitamed, Israel.*
Mepyramine maleate (p.421·1); naphazoline hydrochloride (p.1095·1); phenylephrine hydrochloride (p.1097·1).
Nasal congestion.

Pheramin N *Kanoldt, Ger.*
Diphenhydramine hydrochloride (p.416·1).
Allergic disorders of the conjunctiva.

Pherarutin *Kanoldt, Ger.†.*
Troxerutin (p.1611·2).
Retinal disorders.

Pherazine with Codeine *Halsey, USA.*
Promethazine hydrochloride (p.423·2); codeine phosphate (p.25·2).
Coughs and cold symptoms.

Pherazine DM *Halsey, USA.*
Promethazine hydrochloride (p.423·2); dextromethorphan hydrobromide (p.1087·3).
Coughs and cold symptoms.

Pherazine VC *Halsey, USA.*
Promethazine hydrochloride (p.423·2); phenylephrine hydrochloride (p.1097·1).
Upper respiratory-tract symptoms.

Pherazine VC with Codeine *Halsey, USA.*
Promethazine hydrochloride (p.423·2); phenylephrine hydrochloride (p.1097·1); codeine phosphate (p.25·2).
Coughs and cold symptoms.

pH5-Eucerin
Beiersdorf, Ger.†; BDF, Mex.; Beiersdorf, Port.; Beiersdorf, Thai.
A range of skin cleansing and emollient preparations.

Phicon *Williams, USA.*
Pramocaine hydrochloride (p.1318·2); vitamin A (p.1382·1); vitamin E (p.1393·3).
Local anaesthesia.

Phicon-F *Williams, USA.*
Pramocaine hydrochloride (p.1318·2); undecenoic acid (p.395·3).
Fungal skin infections.

Philinal *Rekah, Israel.*
Suppositories: Diprophylline (p.764·1); phenobarbital (p.355·1).

Tablets: Diprophylline (p.764·1); diphenhydramine hydrochloride (p.416·1).
Obstructive airways disease.

Phillips' Chewable *Sterling, USA.*
Magnesium hydroxide (p.1233·1).
Hyperacidity.

Phillips Gelcaps *Bayer, Canad.†.*
Docusate sodium (p.1223·1); phenolphthalein (p.1244·1).
Constipation.

Phillips' Laxative Gelcaps *Sterling, USA†.*
Docusate sodium (p.1223·1); phenolphthalein (p.1244·1).

Phillips' Laxcaps *Glenbrook, USA†.*
Docusate sodium (p.1223·1); phenolphthalein (p.1244·1).
Constipation.

Phillips' Milk of Magnesia
Bayer, Canad.; Sterling Health, USA.
Magnesium hydroxide (p.1233·1).
Constipation; gastric hyperacidity.

Phillips P.T.Y. Yeast Tablets *Phillips Yeast, UK.*
Yeast (p.1398·1); vitamin B substances (p.1350·1).
Formerly known as Tonic Yeast.

Phimetin *BHR, UK†.*
Cimetidine (p.1216·3).
Gastrointestinal disorders associated with hyperacidity.

pHisoDerm
Note. This name is used for preparations of different composition.
SmithKline Beecham, Hong Kong.
Entsufon (p.1606·3).
Skin, scalp, and hair cleanser.

Cilag, UK†; Chattem, USA.
Skin cleanser.

pHisoHex
Sanofi Synthelabo, Canad.; Sanofi Winthrop, USA.
Entsufon sodium (p.1606·3); hexachlorophene (p.1146·1).
Skin cleansing; skin disinfection.

pHisoHex Face Wash *SmithKline Beecham Consumer, Austral.*
Triclosan (p.1159·2).
Acne; skin infections.

pHisoHex Reformulated
Note. This name is used for preparations of different composition.
Sanofi Winthrop, Hong Kong.
Triclosan (p.1159·2).
Acne; skin infections.

Sanofi Synthelabo, Singapore.
Triclosan (p.1159·2); pyrithione zinc (p.1122·1).
Skin cleanser.

pHiso-MED *Sanofi Synthelabo, UK.*
Chlorhexidine gluconate (p.1138·2).
Formerly contained hexachlorophene.
Skin disinfection.

Phlebocreme *Monot, Fr.*
Benzocaine (p.1306·2); dodeclonium bromide; esculoside (p.1574·1); enoxolone (p.34·3).

Phlebodril
Note.This name is used for preparations of different composition.
Pierre Fabre, Ger.
Ruscus aculeatus; trimethylhesperidin chalcone (p.1611·2).
Vascular disorders.

Robapharm, Switz.
Capsules†: Ruscus aculeatus; hesperidin methyl chalcone (p.1611·2); ascorbic acid (p.1389·3).
Vascular disorders.

Cream: Petit houx root; melilotus officinalis.
Venous insufficiency.

Phlebodril mono *Pierre Fabre, Ger.*
Ruscus aculeatus.
Vascular disorders.

Phlebodril N
Note.This name is used for preparations of different composition.
Pierre Fabre, Ger.
Ruscus aculeatus rhizome; melilotus officinalis; dextran sulfate (p.1603·1).
Vascular disorders.

Robapharm, Switz.
Ruscus aculeatus; hesperidin methyl chalcone (p.1611·2).
Haemorrhoids; venous insufficiency.

Phlebogel *Lipha Sante, Fr.*
Aescin (p.1574·1); buphenine hydrochloride (p.1587·3).
Peripheral vascular disorders.

Phlebosedol *Lehning, Fr.*
Aesculus (p.1574·1); hamamelis (p.1618·3); viburnum; alchemilla (p.1648·3); red wine.
Formerly contained aesculus, clematis vitalba, hamamelis, lesser celandine, viburnum, piscidia, frangula bark, senecio, and alchemilla.
Haemorrhoids; venous insufficiency.

Phlebostasin *Klinge, Switz.*
Aesculus (p.1574·1).
Peripheral vascular disorders.

Phlebostasin compositum *Klinge, Switz.*
Aesc in (p.1574·1); heparin sodium (p.902·1); glycol salicylate (p.42·2).
Oedema; phlebitis; soft-tissue disorders; venous insufficiency.

Phlebosup *Monot, Fr.*
Benzocaine (p.1306·2); dodeclonium bromide; esculoside (p.1574·1); enoxolone (p.34·3).
Anorectal disorders.

Phlexy
Scientific Hospital Supplies, Austral.; SHS, Fr.; Scientific Hospital Supplies, Irl.; Nutricia, NZ; Scientific Hospital Supplies, NZ.
Food for special diets (p.1350·1).
Phenylketonuria.

Phlexyvits
Scientific Hospital Supplies, Irl.; SHS, UK.
Multivitamin and mineral preparation (p.1350·1).

Phlogase *Godecke, Ger.†*
Oxyphenbutazone (p.71·1); heparin sodium (p.902·1).
Musculoskeletal and joint disorders; superficial phlebitis.

Phlogenzym
Mucos, Aust.; Mucos, Ger.; Romsa, Mex.
Bromelains (p.1586·3); trypsin (p.1675·3); rutoside (p.1611·2).
Inflammation; oedema; pain; soft-tissue disorders.

Phlogidermil *Vifor, Switz.†*
Ichthammol (p.1115·2); hamamelis (p.1618·3); guaiazulene (p.1618·3); cod-liver oil (p.1357·2); lavender oil (p.1627·2); zinc oxide (p.1128·2).
Inflammation; muscular pain.

Phlogont *Azupharma, Ger.*
Tablets†: Oxyphenbutazone (p.71·1).
Acute ankylosing spondylitis; gout.

Topical liquid: Glycol salicylate (p.42·2).
Musculoskeletal, joint, and soft-tissue disorders.

Phlogont Rheuma *Azupharma, Ger.*
Glycol salicylate (p.42·2).
Musculoskeletal, joint, and soft-tissue disorders.

Phlogont-Thermal *Azupharma, Ger.*
Glycol salicylate (p.42·2); benzyl nicotinate (p.20·2).
Muscle and joint disorders; sports injuries.

Phloctan *Aguettant, Fr.*
Glucose-1-phosphate disodium, tetrahydrate.
Hypophosphataemia; parenteral nutrition.

Pholcodyl *Medeva, Fr.*
Pholcodine (p.1099·1); erysimum.
Coughs.

Pholcolin *Antigen, Irl.*
Pholcodine (p.1099·1).
Coughs.

Pholcolinct *Propan, S.Afr.*
Pholcodine (p.1099·1).
Cough.

Pholcomed *Medo, UK†.*
Pholcodine (p.1099·1).

Formerly contained pholcodine and papaverine hydrochloride.
Coughs.

Pholco-Mereprine *OJG, Belg.*
Doxylamine succinate (p.417·1); pholcodine (p.1099·1); sulfogaiacol (p.1101·1); sodium benzoate (p.1134·3).
Respiratory-tract disorders.

Pholcones *Cooperation Pharmaceutique, Fr.†.*
Quinine sulfate (p.445·1); camphor (p.1589·3); eucalyptol (p.1609·2); pholcodine (p.1099·1); amylocaine hydrochloride (p.1306·1).
Coughs; respiratory disorders.

Pholcones Bismuth *Cooperation Pharmaceutique, Fr.*
Guaifenesin (p.1092·2); bismuth succinate (p.1214·1); eucalyptol (p.1609·2).
Respiratory-tract congestion.

Pholtex *3M, S.Afr.*
Pholcodine resin complex (p.1099·1); phenyltoloxamine resin complex (p.423·1).
Coughs.

Pholtrate *McGloin, Austral.*
Pholcodine (p.1099·1).
Coughs.

Phol-Tussil *Interdelta, Switz.*
Pholcodine (p.1099·1); sodium benzoate (p.1134·3); tolu balsam (p.1101·3).
Coughs.

Phol-Tux *Interdelta, Switz.*
Pholcodine (p.1099·1); ethylmorphine hydrochloride (p.35·2); sulfogaiacol (p.1101·1); belladonna (p.463·1); senega root (p.1100·2); sodium benzoate (p.1134·3).
Coughs.

Phonal *Reig Jofre, Spain.*
Lozenges: Bacitracin (p.155·2); benzocaine (p.1306·2); neomycin sulfate (p.228·1); polymyxin B sulfate (p.238·1).
Throat spray: Benzalkonium chloride (p.1133·2); dexamethasone sodium phosphate (p.1067·1).
Mouth and throat disorders.

Phonix Antitox *Phonix, Ger.*
Homoeopathic preparation.

Phonix Arthrophon *Phonix, Ger.*
Homoeopathic preparation.

Phonix Aurum III/012B *Phonix, Ger.*
Homoeopathic preparation.

Phonix Bronchophon *Phonix, Ger.*
Homoeopathic preparation.

Phonix Ferrum O32 A *Phonix, Ger.*
Homoeopathic preparation.

Phonix Gastriphon *Phonix, Ger.*
Artemisia abrotanum; absinthium (p.1571·1); centaury (p.1593·1); gentian (p.1615·1).
Gastrointestinal disorders.

Phonix Hydrargyrum II/027A *Phonix, Ger.*
Homoeopathic preparation.

Phonix Lymphophon *Phonix, Ger.*
Homoeopathic preparation.

Phonix Phonohepan *Phonix, Ger.*
Homoeopathic preparation.

Phonix Plumbum 024 A *Phonix, Ger.*
Homoeopathic preparation.

Phonix Solidago II/035 B *Phonix, Ger.*
Homoeopathic preparation.

Phonix Tartarus III/020 *Phonix, Ger.*
Homoeopathic preparation.

phono Arnica comp *Phonix, Ger.*
Homoeopathic preparation.

phono Chol *Phonix, Ger.*
Homoeopathic preparation.

phono Gripp *Phonix, Ger.*
Homoeopathic preparation.

phono Uren *Phonix, Ger.*
Homoeopathic preparation.

phono Ven *Phonix, Ger.*
Homoeopathic preparation.

Phor Pain *Goldshield, UK.*
Ibuprofen (p.43·2).
Muscle pain.

Phorpain *Goldshield, Irl.*
Ibuprofen (p.43·2).
Musculoskeletal, joint, and soft-tissue disorders; neuralgia.

Phos Kola *Phos-Kola, Braz.*
Calcium; medicinal plants (p.1350·1).
Nutritional supplement.

PhosChol *American Lecithin, USA.*
Phosphatidyl choline (p.1651·1).
Nutritional supplement.

Phoscortil *Kolassa, Aust.*
Prednisolone sodium metasulfobenzoate (p.1078·1); aluminium phosphate (p.1211·3).

Phosetamin *Kohler-Pharma, Ger.*
Calcium, magnesium, and potassium salts of phosphorylcolamine.
Electrolyte disorders.

Phos-Ex
Vitaline, Fin.; Vitaline, Norw.; Vitaline, Swed.; Vitaline, UK.
Calcium acetate (p.1187·3).
Hyperphosphataemia.

Phos-Flur
Colgate Oral Care, Austral.†.
Acidulated phosphate fluoride (p.1375·3).
Dental caries prophylaxis.

Colgate-Hoyt, USA.
Sodium fluoride (p.1375·3).
Dental caries prophylaxis.

Phosfo Enema *Cristalia, Braz.*
Monobasic sodium phosphate (p.1193·2); dibasic sodium phosphate (p.1193·2).
Bowel evacuation; constipation.

PhosLo *Braintree, USA.*
Calcium acetate (p.1187·3).
Hyperphosphataemia.

Phosoforme *Monin, Fr.*
Phosphoric acid (p.1651·1).
Urinary-tract disorders.

Phosphalugel
Kolassa, Aust.; Yamanouchi, Belg.; Yamanouchi, Fr.; Yamanouchi, Ger.; Yamanouchi, Port.; Boehringer Ingelheim, Switz.
Aluminium phosphate (p.1211·3).
Gastrointestinal disorders associated with hyperacidity.

Phospharome *Plantes et Medecines, Fr.†.*
Kola (p.1681·1); gentian (p.1615·1); cinchona (p.1595·3); minerals (p.1350·1).
Tonic.

Phosphate-Novartis *Novartis, Canad.*
Monobasic sodium phosphate (p.1193·2); potassium bicarbonate (p.1186·1).
Formerly known as Phosphate-Sandoz.
Electrolyte supplement; hypercalciuria.

Phosphates *Pharmascience, Canad.*
Monobasic sodium phosphate (p.1193·2); dibasic sodium phosphate (p.1193·2).
Bowel evacuation; constipation.

Phosphate-Sandoz
Novartis, Austral.; Novartis, Irl.†; Novartis, NZ; Novartis, S.Afr.; HK Pharma, UK.
Monobasic sodium phosphate (p.1193·2); sodium bicarbonate (p.1186·2); potassium bicarbonate (p.1186·1).
Hypercalcaemia; hypophosphataemia; rickets.

Phosphocalcina Iodada *CIF, Braz.*
Sodium carbonate; calcium hypophosphite; sodium hypophosphite; iodine; tannin (p.1185·2).
Oral rehydration therapy.

Phosphocholine *Yves Ponroy, Fr.*
Dibasic sodium phosphate (p.1193·2); choline citrate (p.1356·3); trisodium citrate (p.1186·2).
Dyspepsia.

Phosphocol *Mallinckrodt, USA.*
Phosphorus-32 (p.1450·3) in the form of chromic phosphate.
Malignant neoplasms.

Phospho-Lax *Sofar, Ital.*
Monobasic sodium phosphate (p.1193·2); dibasic sodium phosphate (p.1193·2).
Bowel evacuation; constipation.

Phospholine Iodide
Wyeth-Ayerst, Austral.; Wyeth Lederle, Belg.†; Wyeth-Ayerst, Canad.; Chiesi, Fr.; Wyeth-Ayerst, Israel; Wyeth, Neth.†; Dominion, UK; Wyeth-Ayerst, USA.
Ecothiopate iodide (p.1418·1).
Available on a named-patient basis only in the UK.
Convergent strabismus; glaucoma.

Phosphoneuros *Doms-Adrian, Fr.*
Phosphoric acid (p.1651·1); calcium dihydrogen phosphate (p.1588·2); dibasic sodium phosphate (p.1193·2); magnesium glycerophosphate (p.1191·1).
Hypercalciuria; hypophosphataemic rickets.

Phosphonorm
Medice, Ger.; Salmon, Switz.
Aluminium chlorohydrate (p.1110·2).
Hyperphosphataemia.

Phosphoprep *Pharmatel, Austral.*
Monobasic sodium phosphate (p.1193·2); dibasic sodium phosphate (p.1193·2).
Bowel evacuation.

Phosphoral
De Witt, Denm.; Ferring, Fin.; De Witt, Norw.; Ferring, Swed.
Monobasic sodium phosphate (p.1193·2); dibasic sodium phosphate (p.1193·2).
Bowel evacuation; constipation.

Phosphore-Sandoz *Novartis, Fr.†.*
Monoammonium phosphate (p.1579·2); monobasic potassium phosphate (p.1193·1); manganese glycerophosphate (p.1617·3).
Bone loss during immobilisation; hypercalciuria; osteoporosis; rickets.

Phosphorus Med Complex *Dynamit, Aust.*
Homoeopathic preparation.

Phospho-Soda *Baxter, NZ; Fleet, NZ.*
Monobasic sodium phosphate (p.1193·2); dibasic sodium phosphate (p.1193·2).
Bowel evacuation; constipation.

Phosphotec *Squibb Diagnostics, USA†.*
Technetium-99m pyrophosphate (p.1451·1).

Phostal
Stallergenes, Ital.; Stallergenes, Switz.
Allergen extracts (p.1575·3).
Hyposensitisation.

Photoderm *Bioderma, Fr.*
Capsules: Betacarotene; tomato oleoresin; fish oil; rape-seed oil; soya lecithin; vitamin E (p.1350·1).
Tablets: Lemon; tea; vitamin C; vitamin E (p.1350·1).

Photoderm Latte *Piam, Ital.†.*
Octinoxate (p.1517·3); avobenzone (p.1517·1).
Sunscreen.

Photoderm Max *Polaris, Ital.*
Cream: Octinoxate (p.1517·3); titanium dioxide (p.1126·1); avobenzone (p.1517·1); enzacamene (p.1517·2).
Topical milk: Octil octanoate; octinoxate (p.1517·3); titanium dioxide (p.1126·1); avobenzone (p.1517·1); octocrilene (p.1518·1); zinc oxide (p.1128·2).
Sunscreen.

Photoderm Mineral *Polaris, Ital.*
Octil octanoate; titanium dioxide (p.1126·1).
Sunscreen.

Photoderm Special *Polaris, Ital.*
Titanium dioxide (p.1126·1); octinoxate (p.1517·3); enzacamene (p.1517·2); avobenzone (p.1517·1); ensulizole (p.1517·2).
Sunscreen.

Photofrin
Ligand, Canad.; Ipsen, UK; Sanofi Winthrop, USA.
Porfimer sodium (p.566·1).
Non-small-cell lung cancer; oesophageal cancer; papillary bladder cancer.

Photoplex
Note.This name is used for preparations of different composition.
Allergan, Canad.
SPF 15: Avobenzone (p.1517·1); octisalate (p.1518·1); octocrilene (p.1518·1); oxybenzone (p.1518·1).
Sunscreen.

Allergan Herbert, USA†.
Avobenzone (p.1517·1); padimate O (p.1518·1).
Sunscreen.

Photoscreen *Ducray, Fr.*
SPF 60: Octinoxate (p.1517·3); octocrilene (p.1518·1); titanium dioxide (p.1126·1); zinc oxide (p.1128·2).
Sunscreen.

Phrenilin *Carnrick, USA.*
Butalbital (p.658·3); paracetamol (p.71·2).
Tension headache.

Phylarm *LCA, Fr.*
Sodium chloride (p.1196·1); borax (p.1586·1); boric acid (p.1586·1).
Eye wash.

Phyllocontin
Purdue Frederick, Canad.; Mundipharma, Hong Kong; Napp, Irl.; Pharmafrica, S.Afr.; Napp, UK; Purdue Frederick, USA†.
Aminophylline (p.760·1) or aminophylline hydrate (p.760·1).
Heart failure; obstructive airways disease.

Phyllosan *Seton, UK†.*
Multivitamin and mineral preparation (p.1350·1).

Phyllotemp
Mundipharma, Ger.; Mundipharma, Switz.
Aminophylline (p.760·1) or aminophylline hydrate (p.760·1).
Obstructive airways disease.

Phylorinol *Schaffer, USA.*
Mouthwash: Phenol (p.1152·3); methyl salicylate (p.55·1).
Minor mouth or throat irritation.

Topical solution: Phenol (p.1152·3); boric acid (p.1586·1); strong iodine solution (p.1522·3).
Oral wounds and infections.

Phymet DTF *Glaxo Wellcome, Irl.*
Methadone hydrochloride (p.53·1).
Opioid addiction.

Phymorax *Dong, Singapore.*
Hydroxyzine hydrochloride (p.419·1).
Alcohol withdrawal syndrome; anxiety; nausea and vomiting; premedication; skin disorders.

Physeptone
Glaxo Wellcome, Austral.; Glaxo Wellcome, Hong Kong; Wellcome, Irl.; Glaxo Wellcome, S.Afr.; Glaxo Wellcome, Singapore; Martindale, UK.
Methadone hydrochloride (p.53·1).
NOTE. There is no connection between Martindale, The Complete Drug Reference and Martindale Pharmaceuticals.
Cough; opioid withdrawal syndrome; pain.

Physex *Byk Elmu, Spain†.*
Chorionic gonadotrophin (p.1279·2).
Erectile dysfunction; male and female infertility; metrorrhagia; threatened or recurrent miscarriage.

Physiogel
Note.This name is used for preparations of different composition.
Stiefel, Hong Kong; Stiefel, Singapore.
Sodium cocoyl isetionate.
Soap substitute.

Braun, Switz.
Modified gelatin (p.737·2) with electrolytes.
Hypovolaemia.

Physiogesic *Hebert, Canad.*
Diethylamine salicylate (p.32·2).

Physiogine *Organon, Fr.*
Estriol (p.1475·3).
Oestrogen deficiency.

Physiolax *Medipharm, Switz.†.*
Aloes (p.1210·1); belladonna (p.463·1).
Constipation; stool softener.

Physiologica
Qualiphar, Belg.; Gifrer Barbezat, Fr.; Democal, Switz.
Sodium chloride (p.1196·1).
Eye wash; nasal irrigation.

Physiolyte *McGaw, USA.*
Electrolytes (p.1180·1).
Irrigation solution.

Physiomenthol *Hebert, Canad.*
Menthol (p.1632·3).

Physiomer
Sanofi Winthrop, Fr.; Ganassini, Ital.
Sea water (p.1196·1).
Nasal irrigation.

Physiomint *Koch, Aust.*
Mint oil (p.1636·2).
Gastrointestinal disorders; headache; migraine; respiratory-tract disorders; rheumatic disorders; soft-tissue and muscle injury.

Physiomycine *Laphal, Fr.*
Methacycline hydrochloride (p.222·3).
Bacterial infections.

Physioneal *Baxter, Denm.*
Anhydrous glucose; calcium chloride; magnesium chloride; sodium chloride; sodium bicarbonate; sodium lactate (p.1184·1).
Peritoneal dialysis.

Physiorhine *Aventis, Belg.*
Sodium chloride (p.1196·1).
Cleansing of nasal passages and eyelids.

Physio-Rub *Hebert, Canad.*
Methyl salicylate (p.55·1); menthol (p.1632·3); eucalyptol (p.1609·2).

Physiosoin
Chauvin, Fr.; Chauvin Novopharma, Switz.
Sodium chloride (p.1196·1).
Eye wash; nasal irrigation; wound irrigation.

PhysioSol *Abbott, USA.*
Electrolytes (p.1180·1).
Irrigation solution.

Physiostat *Organon, Fr.*
7 Tablets, ethinylestradiol (p.1476·2); 15 tablets, ethinylestradiol; lynestrenol (p.1480·1).
Sequential-type oral contraceptive.

Physiotens
Solvay, Denm.; Solvay, Fin.; Solvay, Fr.; Solvay, Ger.; Solvay, Norw.; Solvay, S.Afr.; Solvay, Swed.; Solvay, Switz.; Solvay, UK.
Moxonidine (p.936·3).
Hypertension.

Physiotherm *Arkopharma, Fr.*
Natural spring water of Berthemont-les-Bains (p.1180·1).
Nasal irrigation.

Physium *Boiron, Canad.*
Sodium chloride (p.1196·1).
Nasal congestion; nasal hygiene.

Phytat *Cochon, Fr.†.*
Sodium fytate (p.1023·1).
Hypercalciuria.

Phytemag *Lesourd, Fr.*
Magnesium glycerophosphate; apium root; buchu leaf; equisetum; ginger (p.1350·1).
Formerly contained magnesium silicate, magnesium glycerophosphate, chlorophyll, parsley, thyme and buchu powder, equisetum, wild celery and ginger powder, oxides of zinc, copper, and nickel.
Tonic.

Phytentielles *Bionatec, Fr.*
A range of herbal preparations.

Phytex
Note.This name is used for preparations of different composition.
Rupertus, Aust.
Sorbic acid (p.1157·1); tannic acid (p.1669·1); methyl salicylate (p.55·1); salicylic acid (p.1122·3); acetic acid (p.1571·2).
Fungal infections of the feet.

Pharmax, Irl.
Tannic acid (p.1669·1); boric acid (p.1586·1); salicylic acid (p.1122·3); methyl salicylate (p.55·1); acetic acid (p.1571·2).
Fungal skin and nail infections.

Wynlit, UK.
Borotannic complex (p.1669·1) (p.1586·1); salicylic acid (p.1122·3); methyl salicylate (p.55·1); acetic acid (p.1571·2).
Fungal skin and nail infections.

Phytic Acid *Crinos, Ital.*
Phytic acid (p.1023·1); glycolic acid (p.1115·1).
Hyperpigmentation disorders.

Phytoberidin *Synpharma, Switz.*
Valerian (p.1678·3); hypericum (p.290·2); passion flower (p.1649·1); guaiazulene (p.1618·3); lupulus (p.1629·3); melissa (p.1632·2).
Insomnia; nervous disorders.

Phytobronchin *Steigerwald, Ger.*
Cowslip rhizome (p.1600·1); thyme (p.1672·2).
Cold symptoms.

Phytocalm
Note.This name is used for preparations of different composition.
UPSA, Fr.
Valerian (p.1678·3); ballota; crataegus (p.1600·2); passion flower (p.1649·1).
Insomnia; nervous disorders.

Arkopharma, UK.
Passion flower (p.1649·1).
Insomnia; stress and strain.

Phytocean *Ido, Fr.*
Nutritional supplement (p.1350·1).

Phytocold *Arkopharma, UK.*
Echinacea (p.1606·2).
Colds.

Phytocortal *Steierl, Ger.*
Homoeopathic preparation.

Phytoderm Compositum *Teva, Israel.*
Tolnaftate (p.395·2); salicylic acid (p.1122·3); benzoic acid (p.1134·2).
Fungal skin infections.

Phytodolor
Madaus, Aust.; Steigerwald, Ger.
Populus tremula leaf and bark (p.1653·2); fraxinus excelsior bark; solidago virgaurea.
Musculoskeletal and joint disorders; neuralgia.

Phyto-Embryonnaire *Recherche Botanique, Fr.*
Crataegus; birch; black currant; rosa; ginkgo biloba; juglans regia (p.1350·1).
Gastrointestinal disorders.

Phytoestrol N *Muller Goppingen, Ger.*
Rhapontic rhubarb (p.1248·1).
Endometritis; juvenile oligomenorrhoea and dysmenorrhoea; menopausal disorders; primary and secondary amenorrhoea.

Phytofibre *Plantes et Medecines, Fr.†.*
Ispaghula (p.1229·1).
Constipation.

Phytogran
Note.This name is used for preparations of different composition.
Synpharma, Aust.
Valerian root (p.1678·3); lupulus (p.1629·3); melissa leaf (p.1632·2).
Anxiety; sleep disorders.

Grandel-Synpharma, Aust.
Lupulus (p.1629·3); hypericum (p.290·2).
Nervous disorders.

Phytohepar *Steigerwald, Ger.*
Silybum marianum (p.1021·3).
Liver disorders.

Phytohustil *Steigerwald, Ger.*
Althaea (p.1577·1).
Formerly known as Phytobronchin.
Coughs.

Phyto-Hypophyson C *Steierl, Ger.*
Homoeopathic preparation.

Phyto-Hypophyson L *Steierl, Ger.*
Homoeopathic preparation.

Phytolax
Note.This name is used for preparations of different composition.
Sante Naturelle, Canad.†.
Cascara (p.1216·1); phenolphthalein (p.1244·1); bile salts (p.1585·1); capsicum oleoresin (p.1591·1); papain (p.1647·3).

Synpharma, Switz.
Aloes (p.1210·1); frangula (p.1227·1); belladonna (p.463·1).
Constipation.

PhytoLaxin *Hanseler, Switz.*
Aloes (p.1210·1); frangula bark (p.1227·1); senna (p.1248·2).
Formerly known as Obducti laxativi vegetabiles S and contained aloes, belladonna, frangula bark, and senna.
Constipation.

Phytolife *Blackmores, Austral.*
Soya bean (p.1378·1); calcium (p.1187·3).
Calcium deficiency; menopausal disorders.

Phytolife Plus *Blackmores, UK.*
Calcium (p.1187·3); soya (p.1378·1).
Menopausal disorders.

Phytolithe *Phytosolba, Fr.*
Ichthammol (p.1115·2); cajuput oil (p.1588·1); cade oil (p.1124·3).
Seborrhoeic dermatitis.

Phytomed Cardio *Phytomed, Switz.†.*
Crataegus (p.1600·2); cereus (p.1593·1); passion flower (p.1649·1); rosemary.
Cardiac disorders.

Phytomed Gastro *Phytomed, Switz.†.*
Angelica (p.1580·2); centaury (p.1593·1); chamomile (p.1593·2); peppermint leaf (p.1243·2); caraway (p.1591·2); potato.
Digestive disorders.

Phytomed Hepato *Phytomed, Switz.*
Absinthium (p.1571·1); cynara (p.1601·3); peppermint leaf (p.1243·2); raphanus sativus var. nigra; silybum marianum (p.1021·3); taraxacum (p.1669·1).
Digestive disorders.

Phytomed Nephro *Phytomed, Switz.†.*
Silver birch (p.1585·2); solidago virgaurea; java tea (p.1625·1); juniper (p.1625·2); ononis (p.1644·1); taraxacum (p.1669·1).
Urinary-tract disorders.

Phytomed Prosta *Phytomed, Switz.*
Echinacea purpurea (p.1606·2); poplar buds (p.1653·2); saw palmetto (p.1491·2); solidago virgaurea.
Prostatic pain; urinary disorders.

Phytomed Rhino *Phytomed, Switz.†.*
Cinchona bark (p.1595·3); echinacea purpurea (p.1606·2); salix (p.82·1); solidago virgaurea.
Cold symptoms; sinusitis.

Phytomed Somni *Phytomed, Switz.*
Valerian (p.1678·3); passion flower (p.1649·1); lupulus (p.1629·3); lavandula angustifolia.
Sleep disorders.

Phytomelis *Lehning, Fr.*
Hamamelis (p.1618·3); aesculus (p.1574·1).
Haemorrhoids; peripheral vascular disorders.

Phytonoctu *Steigerwald, Ger.*
Melissa (p.1632·2); passion flower (p.1649·1); valerian (p.1678·3).
Nervous disorders; sleep disorders.

Phytonoxon N *Steigerwald, Ger.*
Corydalis cava; eschscholtzia california.
Sleep disorders.

Phytophanere *Phytosolba, Fr.*
Wheat-germ oil; carrot oil; borage oil (p.1613·1); rice-bran oil; salmon oil; yeast (p.1398·1); antilles cherries; fish roe.
Fragile hair and nails.

Phytopure *Lalco, Canad.*
Multivitamin and mineral preparation (p.1350·1).

Phytoslim *Arkopharma, UK.*
Kelp (p.1625·3).
Obesity.

Phytosyl Plus *Vita Health, Singapore.*
Fibre; *Lactobacillus* species; aloe vera (p.1350·1).
Dietary fibre supplement.

Phytotherapie Boribel no 8 *Dietetique et Sante, Fr.*
Tilia (p.1673·2); passion flower (p.1649·1); valerian (p.1678·3).
Insomnia; nervous disorders.

Phytotherapie Boribel no 9 *Dietetique et Sante, Fr.*
Fraxinus excelsior; bladderwrack (p.1585·2).
Obesity.

Phytotherapie Titree *Boiron, Fr.*
A range of herbal preparations.

Phytotux *Lehning, Fr.*
Tolu balsam (p.1101·3); Desessartz syrup.
Coughs.

Phytotux H *Homeocan, Canad.*
Homoeopathic preparation.

Phytovim *Sante Naturelle, Canad.*
Multivitamin and mineral preparation (p.1350·1).

Piascledine
Pharmascience, Fr.; ABC, Ital.
Avocado oil; soya oil (p.1378·1).
Gum disorders; musculoskeletal and joint disorders; phlebitis; skin disorders; skin ulceration.

Piat *Salus, Mex.*
Miconazole (p.391·1).
Fungal infections.

Piazofolina *Bracco, Ital.*
Morinamide hydrochloride (p.225·3).
Tuberculosis.

Picalm *Grunenthal, Port.*
Piketoprofen (p.78·3) or piketoprofen hydrochloride (p.78·3).
Musculoskeletal and joint disorders.

Picapan *DHA, Singapore.*
Paracetamol (p.71·2); caffeine (p.761·3).
Fever; pain.

Picariz *Picot, Fr.†.*
Food for special diets (p.1350·1).
Diarrhoea.

Picibanil *Chugai, Jpn.*
Lyophilised powder of *Streptococcus pyogenes*.
Malignant neoplasms.

Picillin
Laboratorio Farm., Israel; CT, Ital.
Piperacillin sodium (p.236·1).
Lignocaine [lidocaine] hydrochloride (p.1313·2) may be included in this preparation to alleviate the pain of injection.
Bacterial infections.

Pickles Antiseptic Cream *Pickles, UK.*
Dibromopropamide isetionate (p.1143·1).
Skin disinfection.

Pickles Chilblain Cream *Pickles, UK.*
Methyl nicotinate (p.55·1).

Pickles Corn Caps *Pickles, UK.*
Salicylic acid (p.1122·3); colophony (p.1598·3).

Pickles Foot Ointment *Pickles, UK.*
Salicylic acid (p.1122·3).
Calluses; corns.

Pickles Smelling Salts *Pickles, UK.*
Strong ammonia solution (p.1579·1); eucalyptus oil (p.1609·2); pine oil.
Headache; nasal congestion.

Pickles Toothache Tincture *Pickles, UK.*
Clove oil (p.1597·1); lignocaine [lidocaine] (p.1313·2).

Picolax
Note.This name is used for preparations of different composition.
Dendy, Austral.
Sodium picosulfate (p.1249·3); magnesium carbonate (p.1232·3); citric acid (p.1596·2).
Bowel evacuation; constipation.

Ferring, Irl.; Pharmia, Fin.
Sodium picosulfate (p.1249·3); magnesium citrate (p.1232·3).
Bowel evacuation.

Picolaxine *Pharmethic, Belg.*
Sodium picosulfate (p.1249·3).
Constipation.

Picolite *Picot, Fr.*
Maltodextrin; sucrose; sodium chloride; potassium citrate; citric acid (p.1185·2).
Diarrhoea; oral rehydration therapy.

Picolon *Medic, Denm.*
Sodium picosulfate (p.1249·3).
Constipation.

Picoprep *Pharmatel, Austral.*
Sodium picosulfate (p.1249·3); magnesium oxide (p.1233·2); citric acid (p.1596·2).
Bowel evacuation; constipation.

Pico-Salax
Ferring, Israel; Ferring, Norw.†; Ferring, Swed.†; Ferring, Switz.†.
Sodium picosulfate (p.1249·3); magnesium oxide (p.1233·2); citric acid (p.1596·2).
Bowel evacuation.

Picosyl *Synthelabo, Spain.*
Hydrocortisone acetate (p.1073·3).
Skin disorders.

Picot *Picot, Fr.*
Dextrin (p.1359·1); maltose (p.1371·2).
Sugar substitute.

Picot Sans Lactose *Picot, Fr.*
Infant feed (p.1350·1).
Lactose intolerance.

Pidilat *Solvay, Ger.*
Nifedipine (p.940·1).
Angina pectoris; hypertension; Raynaud's syndrome.

Pidocal *Sanofi Synthelabo, Switz.*
Calcium pidolate (p.1188·3); calcium carbonate (p.1215·1).
Calcium deficiency; osteoporosis.

Pidomag *Baldacci, Braz.*
Magnesium pidolate (p.1191·1).
Magnesium deficiency.

Pielograf
Darrow, Braz.; Juste, Spain.
Meglumine amidotrizoate (p.1031·2); sodium amidotrizoate (p.1031·2).
Radiographic contrast medium.

Pierami *Fournier, Ital.*
Amikacin sulfate (p.148·1).
Bacterial infections.

Pifrol *Arlex, Mex.*
Dipyrone (p.34·1).

Pigenil *Inverni della Beffa, Ital.*
Pygeum africanum (p.1490·3).
Prostatic hyperplasia.

Pigitil *Dorom, Ital.*
Pidotimod (p.1651·3).
Immunostimulant.

Pigmanorm
Note.This name is used for preparations of different composition.
Widmer, Ger.
Hydroquinone (p.1115·1); tretinoin (p.1126·2); hydrocortisone (p.1073·3).
Skin hyperpigmentation.

Widmer, Switz.
Hydroquinone (p.1115·1); tretinoin (p.1126·2); dexamethasone (p.1067·1); dexpanthenol (p.1602·3); octinoxate (p.1517·1); avobenzone (p.1517·1).
Skin hyperpigmentation.

Piketofen *Reuffer, Mex.*
Ketoprofen (p.47·3).

Pik-Gel *Tetido, Ital.*
Centella asiatica (p.1112·2); ginkgo biloba (p.1615·2); peppermint (p.1243·2); devil's claw root (p.26·3).
Skin disorders.

Pilagan *Allergan, USA†.*
Pilocarpine nitrate (p.1422·3).
Glaucoma; reversal of mydriasis.

Pilax *Agepha, Aust.*
Pilocarpine hydrochloride (p.1422·3).
Glaucoma; production of miosis.

Pilder *Quimifar, Spain.*
Gemfibrozil (p.896·2).
Hyperlipidaemias.

Pildoras Ferrug Sanatori *Santiveri, Spain.*
Sulfur (p.1123·3); ferrous sulfate (p.1360·3); cinchona (p.1595·3); rhubarb (p.1248·1).
Anaemias.

Pildoras Zeninas *Puerto Galiano, Spain.*
Aloes (p.1210·1); cascara (p.1216·1).
Formerly contained aloes, belladonna, cascara, jalap, podophyllum, phenolphthalein, and liquorice.
Constipation.

Pileabs *Lane, UK.*
Slippery elm bark (p.1665·1); cascara sagrada (p.1216·1).
Haemorrhoids.

Pilensar *IMA, Braz.*
Lindane (p.1434·1).
Pediculosis; scabies.

Piletabs *Potter's, UK.*
Pilewort (p.1651·3); agrimony (p.1574·3); cascara (p.1216·1); stone root (p.1667·1).
Haemorrhoids.

Pilewort Compound *Gerard House, UK.*
Pilewort (p.1651·3); senna leaf (p.1248·2); geum maculatum; cascara (p.1216·1).
Constipation.

Pil-Food
Vifor, Port.
Methionine; cystine; vitamins; millett (p.1350·1).
Hair and nail disorders.

Serra Pamies, Spain.
Multivitamins and amino acids; lactoalbumin; panicum miliaceum (p.1350·1).

Golaz, Switz.
Multivitamins and amino acids (p.1350·1); protein hydrolysate; millett.
Hair and nail disorders.

Pilfor P BASF, Ger.
Paracetamol (p.71·2); codeine phosphate (p.25·2).
Pain.

Pilison Schering, Aust.
Fluocortolone pivalate (p.1071·3); salicylic acid (p.1122·3).
Skin disorders.

Pilka Novartis Consumer, Aust.; Novartis, Israel; Ferrer, Spain.
Drosera (p.1606·1); thyme (p.1672·2).
Pilka suppositories formerly contained camphor, eucalyptol, drosera, niaouli oil, paracetamol, thyme, and cholesterol in Spain.
Bronchitis; coughs; throat disorders.

Novartis Consumer, Switz.
Drosera (p.1606·1); pinguiculae; thyme (p.1672·2).
Coughs.

Pilka F Novartis Consumer, Port.
Drosera (p.1606·1); wild thyme; pinguicula.
Coughs.

Pilka Forte Novartis Consumer, Aust.
Drosera (p.1606·1); thyme (p.1672·2); ephedrine hydrochloride (p.1090·1).
Coughs.

Pillole Fattori Ogna, Ital.
Cape aloes (p.1210·1); rhubarb (p.1248·1); cascara (p.1216·1).
Constipation.

Pilo Asta Medica, Belg.; Chauvin, Fr.; Grin, Mex.; Ciba Vision, Norw.; Chauvin Novopharma, Switz.
Pilocarpine hydrochloride (p.1422·3) or pilocarpine nitrate (p.1422·3).
Glaucoma; hernia of the iris; ocular hypertension; reversal of mydriasis and cycloplegia.

Pilobloc Farmila, Ital.
Pilocarpine hydrochloride (p.1422·3); timolol maleate (p.982·1).
Glaucoma; ocular hypertension.

Pilocar Ciba Vision, USA.
Pilocarpine hydrochloride (p.1422·3).
Glaucoma; raised intra-ocular pressure; reversal of mydriasis.

Pilocarcil Oftalder, Port.
Pilocarpine hydrochloride (p.1422·3).
Ocular hypertension; production of myosis.

Pilocarpol Winzer, Ger.
Pilocarpine (p.1422·2).
Glaucoma; production of miosis.

Pilodren Farmila, Ital.
Pilocarpine hydrochloride (p.1422·3); adrenaline [epinephrine] acid tartrate (p.829·2).
Open-angle glaucoma.

Pilo-Eserin Ciba Vision, Ger.
Pilocarpine hydrochloride (p.1422·3); physostigmine salicylate (p.1421·3).
Glaucoma; reversal of drug-induced mydriasis.

Pilof Nicolich Novag, Mex.
Pilocarpine (p.1422·2).

Piloftal Agepha, Aust.
Pilocarpine (p.1422·2).
Glaucoma; ophthalmic surgery.

Pilogel Alcon, Aust.; Alcon, Ger.; Alcon, Irl.; Alcon, Israel; Alcon, Ital.; Alcon, Neth.†; Alcon, S.Afr.; Alcon, Singapore; Alcon, Thai.; Alcon, UK.
Pilocarpine hydrochloride (p.1422·3).
Glaucoma; ocular hypertension.

Pilogel HS Alcon, Switz.†
Pilocarpine hydrochloride (p.1422·3).
Glaucoma.

Pilomann Mann, Ger.; Bausch & Lomb, Thai.; Mann, Thai.
Pilocarpine hydrochloride (p.1422·3).
Glaucoma; reversal of drug-induced mydriasis.

Pilomann-Ol Mann, Ger.
Pilocarpine (p.1422·2).
Glaucoma; reversal of drug-induced mydriasis.

Pilomed QIF, Braz.
Jaborandi.
Alopecia.

Pilopine HS Alcon, Canad.; Alcon, USA.
Pilocarpine hydrochloride (p.1422·3).
Glaucoma; raised intra-ocular pressure; reversal of mydriasis.

Piloplex Davi, Port.
Pilocarpine (p.1422·2).
Glaucoma; production of miosis.

Pilopos Ursapharm, Ger.
Pilocarpine nitrate (p.1422·3).
Glaucoma; reversal of drug-induced mydriasis.

Pilopt Sigma, Austral.; Pharmaco, NZ.
Pilocarpine hydrochloride (p.1422·3).
Glaucoma.

Piloptic Optopics, USA.
Pilocarpine hydrochloride (p.1422·3).
Glaucoma; reversal of mydriasis.

Pilopto-Carpine Lebeh, USA.
Pilocarpine hydrochloride (p.1422·3).
Glaucoma; raised intra-ocular pressure; reversal of mydriasis.

Pilostat Bausch & Lomb, USA.
Pilocarpine hydrochloride (p.1422·3).
Glaucoma; raised intra-ocular pressure; reversal of mydriasis.

Pilostigmin Puroptal Metochem, Aust.
Neostigmine bromide (p.1419·3); pilocarpine hydrochloride (p.1422·3).
Glaucoma; production of miosis.

Pilo-Stulln Stulln, Ger.
Pilocarpine hydrochloride (p.1422·3).
Glaucoma; reversal of drug-induced mydriasis.

Pilosuryl Pierre Fabre, Fr.
Pilosella; phyllanthus.
Water retention.

Pilotonina Farmila, Ital.
Pilocarpine hydrochloride (p.1422·3).
Ocular hypertension; production of miosis.

Pilovital Lesvi, Spain†.
Minoxidil (p.934·2).
Alopecia androgenetica.

Piloxil Golaz, Switz.
Minoxidil (p.934·2).
Alopecia androgenetica.

Pilulas De Witt's CIF, Braz.
Bearberry (p.1583·3); methylene blue [methylthioninium chloride] (p.1012·3); fabiana imbricata; juniper (p.1625·2); potassium nitrate (p.1154·3); parapetalifera betulina; cascara (p.1216·1); sodium salicylate (p.84·2).
Urinary-tract infections.

Pilulas Ross SmithKline Beecham, Braz.
Aloin (p.1210·2); oleoresin; ipecacuanha (p.1093·1); belladonna (p.463·1).
Constipation.

Pilules de Vichy Spiphar, Belg.†
Sodium picosulfate (p.1249·3); electrolytes (p.1180·1).
Formerly contained dantron and electrolytes.
Constipation.

Pilules Dupuis Synthelabo, Fr.†
Bisacodyl (p.1212·2); aloes (p.1210·1); frangula bark (p.1227·1).
Constipation.

Pilzcin Kolassa, Aust.; Merz, Ger.; Shionogi, Jpn.
Croconazole hydrochloride (p.382·3).
Fungal skin infections.

Pima Fleming, USA.
Potassium iodide (p.1522·3).
Respiratory-tract disorders.

Pima Biciron N S & K, Ger.
Natamycin (p.392·1).
Fungal eye infections.

Pimafucin Yamanouchi, Belg.†; Yamanouchi, Fin.; Galderma, Ger.
Natamycin (p.392·1).
Fungal infections; trichomoniasis.

Pimafucort Yamanouchi, Belg.; Yamanouchi, Fin.; Yamanouchi, Ger.; Yamanouchi, Neth.†; Pharmaco, NZ; Yamanouchi, Port.
Hydrocortisone (p.1073·3); natamycin (p.392·1); neomycin sulfate (p.228·1).
Infected skin disorders.

Pimexone Formenti, Ital.†
Mepixanox (p.1511·1).
Respiratory disorders.

Pinadone DTF Pinewood, Irl.
Methadone hydrochloride (p.53·1).
Opioid addiction.

Pinadrina Pisa, Mex.
Adrenaline [epinephrine] (p.829·1).

Pinal N Atzinger, Ger.
Zinc oxide (p.1128·2); N-(2-hydroxyethyl)-10-undecenamide; salicylic acid (p.1122·3).
Skin disorders.

Pin-Alcol Schoning-Berlin, Ger.†.
Menthol (p.1632·3); pine oil.
Neuromuscular and joint disorders; pruritus; soft-tissue injury.

Pinalgesic Pinewood, Irl.
Mefenamic acid (p.51·2).
Menorrhagia; pain.

Pinamet Pinewood, Irl.
Cimetidine (p.1216·3).
Gastric hyperacidity; peptic ulcer; Zollinger-Ellison syndrome.

Pinamox Pinewood, Irl.
Amoxicillin (p.149·2).
Bacterial infections.

Pindac Leo, Denm.†; Leo, Irl.†.
Pinacidil (p.955·3).
Hypertension.

Pinden Unipharm, Israel.
Pindolol (p.955·3).
Heart failure; hypertension.

Pindione Lipha Sante, Fr.
Phenindione (p.954·1).
Thromboembolic disorders.

Pindocor Pharmacia Upjohn, Fin.
Pindolol (p.955·3).
Angina pectoris; arrhythmias; hypertension.

Pindol Pacific, NZ.
Pindolol (p.955·3).
Angina pectoris; arrhythmias; hypertension.

Pindoptan Kanoldt, Ger.
Pindolol (p.955·3).
Glaucoma.

Pindoreal Realpharma, Ger.†.
Pindolol (p.955·3).
Arrhythmias; hypertension; ischaemic heart disease.

Pine OPC Eagle, Austral.
Pinus pinaster; myrtillus (p.1639·2).
Peripheral circulatory disorders; tonic.

Pineal Laborest, Ital.
Magnesium; nicotinic acid; tritofano (p.1350·1).
Depression.

Pinedrin Lisapharma, Ital.
Pumilio pine oil (p.1656·3); thyme (p.1672·2).
Respiratory system disorders.

Pinetarsol Ego, Austral.; Ego, Hong Kong; Ego, NZ; Ego, Singapore.
Pine tar (p.1125·1).
Skin disorders.

Pinex Alpharma, Denm.; Alpharma, Norw.
Paracetamol (p.71·2).
Fever; pain.

Pinex Comp Alpharma, Denm.
Paracetamol (p.71·2); codeine phosphate (p.25·2).
Pain.

Pinex Forte Alpharma, Norw.
Paracetamol (p.71·2); codeine phosphate (p.25·2).
Pain.

Pinex Major Alpharma, Norw.
Paracetamol (p.71·2); codeine phosphate (p.25·2).
Pain.

Pinifed Pinewood, Irl.
Nifedipine (p.940·1).
Hypertension; ischaemic heart disease.

Pinikehl Sanum-Kehlbeck, Ger.
Homoeopathic preparation.

Piniment Austroplant, Aust.
Balsam: Camphor (p.1589·3); eucalyptus oil (p.1609·2); oleum pini sylvestris; pumilio pine oil (p.1656·3); turpentine oil (p.1676·3); guaiazulene (p.1618·3).
Coughs; gastrointestinal spasm; musculoskeletal and joint disorders; respiratory-tract disorders.

Nasal ointment: Ephedrine hydrochloride (p.1090·1); camphor (p.1589·3); eucalyptus oil (p.1609·2); oleum pini sylvestris; pumilio pine oil (p.1656·3); turpentine oil (p.1676·3); sage oil (p.1660·2); sunflower oil (p.1381·2).
Nasal congestion.

Ointment: Camphor (p.1589·3); menthol (p.1632·3); eucalyptus oil (p.1609·2); oleum pini sylvestris; pumilio pine oil (p.1656·3); turpentine oil (p.1676·3).
Catarrh; cold and influenza symptoms; cough.

Piniment Piniol, Switz.
Camphor (p.1589·3); menthol (p.1632·3); orange oil (p.1644·1); pine cone oil; eucalyptus oil (p.1609·2); pumilio pine oil (p.1656·3); turpentine oil (p.1676·3); pine-needle oil.
Influenza; muscle and joint pain; neuralgia.

Piniment Erkaltungsbad Spitzner, Ger.
Camphor (p.1589·3); eucalyptus oil (p.1609·2); menthol (p.1632·3).
Bath additive; cold symptoms.

Piniment Erkaltungskapseln Spitzner, Ger.
Eucalyptus oil (p.1609·2).
Cold symptoms.

Piniment Erkaltungssalbe Spitzner, Ger.
Eucalyptus oil (p.1609·2); pine needle oil; menthol (p.1632·3).
Respiratory-tract disorders.

Piniment Liquidum Spitzner, Ger.
Eucalyptus oil (p.1609·2); pine needle oil; menthol (p.1632·3).
Neuralgia; respiratory-tract disorders; rheumatic disorders; skin ulcer prophylaxis.

Piniment N Spitzner, Ger.†; Piniol, Switz.
Eucalyptus oil (p.1609·2); pine needle oil; menthol (p.1632·3).
Cold symptoms.

Piniment Oral N Spitzner, Ger.†.
Anethole (p.1580·1); eucalyptol (p.1609·2); pumilio pine oil (p.1656·3).
Asthma; bronchitis.

Piniment S Spitzner, Ger.
Eucalyptus oil (p.1609·2); oleum pini sylvestris.
Respiratory-tract disorders.

Piniol Spitzner, Ger.
Naphazoline hydrochloride (p.1095·1).
Rhinitis.

Piniol Erkaltungsbalsam Spitzner, Ger.
Camphor (p.1589·3); eucalyptus oil (p.1609·2); oleum pini sylvestris.
Neuritis; respiratory-tract disorders; rheumatic disorders.

Piniol Nasensalbe Spitzner, Ger.
Camphor (p.1589·3); eucalyptus oil (p.1609·2); pine needle oil.
Cold symptoms.

Piniol Nasenspray Spitzner, Ger.
Naphazoline hydrochloride (p.1095·1).
Cold symptoms; hayfever.

Pink Biscoat Invamed, USA†.
Bismuth salicylate (p.1213·1).

Pink Bismuth Rose Technilab, Canad.
Bismuth salicylate (p.1213·1).

Pinloc Orion, Fin.
Pindolol (p.955·3).
Angina pectoris; arrhythmias; hypertension.

Pinorhinol Knoll, Fr.†.
Menthol (p.1632·3); camphor (p.1589·3); eucalyptol (p.1609·2).
Nose and throat infections.

Pinosil Sedar, Braz.
Sodium dibunate (p.1100·3); malt (p.1371·1); aconite (p.1572·3); lobelia (p.1510·2); pine oil; vitamin B₁; vitamin C; sulfogaiacol (p.1101·1); sodium benzoate (p.1134·3).
Coughs.

Pin-Rid Apothecary, USA.
Pyrantel embonate (p.108·1).

Pinselina Dr. Knapp Montefarmaco, Ital.
Benzocaine (p.1306·2); phenol (p.1152·3); thymol (p.1158·3); menthol (p.1632·3).
Mouth disorders.

Pinsken TO-Chemicals, Thai.
Pindolol (p.955·3).
Angina pectoris; arrhythmias; hypertension.

Pintacrom Diafarm, Spain†.
Merbromin (p.1150·1).
Wound disinfection.

Pin-X Effcon, USA.
Pyrantel embonate (p.108·1).

Piodermina Farmachimici, Ital.
Sodium fusidate (p.208·3); thyme (p.1672·2); mallow.
Bacterial skin infections.

Piodrex Bunker, Braz.
Lindane (p.1434·1).
Pediculosis; scabies.

Pioletal Delta, Braz.
Lindane (p.1434·1).
Pediculosis; scabies.

Pionax Sanval, Braz.
Lindane (p.1434·1).
Pediculosis; scabies.

Pioral Pasta Teofarma, Ital.
Chlorothymol (p.1142·1).
Oral disinfection.

Piorlis Diviser Aquilea, Spain.
Eucalyptol (p.1609·2); eugenol (p.1609·3); peppermint oil (p.1243·3); methyl salicylate (p.55·1); thymol (p.1158·3); tyrothricin (p.267·1).
Gingivitis; gum disinfection; mouth ulcers; pyorrhoea.

Pipcil Wyeth Lederle, Belg.; Lederle, Neth.
Piperacillin sodium (p.236·1).
Bacterial infections.

Pipeacid Tosi, Ital.
Pipemidic acid (p.236·1).
Urinary-tract infections.

Pipedac Teofarma, Ital.
Pipemidic acid (p.236·1).
Urinary-tract infections.

Pipedic Pharmasant, Thai.
Pipemidic acid (p.236·1).
Bacterial infections of the urinary tract.

Pipefort Lampugnani, Ital.
Pipemidic acid (p.236·1).
Urinary-tract infections.

Pipemed Tecnofarma, Mex.
Piperazine (p.105·3).

Pipemid Gentili, Ital.
Pipemidic acid (p.236·1).
Urinary-tract infections.

Pipemidol Quimica y Farmacia, Mex.
Pipemidic acid (p.236·1).
Urinary-tract infections.

Piperazil Allen, Mex.
Piperazine (p.105·3).
Ascariasis; enterobiasis.

Pipercream Usmed, Braz.
Piperazine (p.105·3).
Ascariasis; enterobiasis.

Piperilline Wyeth Lederle, Fr.†.
Piperacillin sodium (p.236·1).
Bacterial infections.

Piperital Ibi, Ital.
Piperacillin sodium (p.236·1).
Lignocaine [lidocaine] hydrochloride (p.1313·3) is included in this preparation to alleviate the pain of injection.
Bacterial infections.

Pipermed Medimport, Mex.
Piperazine citrate (p.105·3).
Ascariasis; enterobiasis.

Pipermel Basi, Port.
Piperazine (p.105·3).

Piperonil Lusofarmaco, Ital.
Pipamperone hydrochloride (p.700·3).
Psychiatric disorders.

Pipersal Uno, Ital.
Piperacillin sodium (p.236·1).
Lignocaine [lidocaine] hydrochloride (p.1313·2) is included in this preparation to alleviate the pain of injection.
Bacterial infections.

Pipertox Codilab, Ital.
Piperazine (p.105·3).
Worm infections.

Pipervermin Heralds, Braz.
Piperazine (p.105·3).
Ascariasis; enterobiasis.

Piperzam *Zambon, Spain†.*
Piperacillin sodium (p.236·1).
Bacterial infections.

Pipiol *Medeva, Fr.*
Menthol (p.1632·3); cloral hydrate (p.669·3); formaldehyde solution (p.1144·2).
Insect stings.

Piportil
Aventis, Belg.; Rhodia, Braz.; Rhone-Poulenc Rorer, Fr.; Rhone-Poulenc Rorer, Hong Kong; Rhone-Poulenc Rorer, Irl.; Rhone-Poulenc Rorer, Neth.; Aventis, NZ; Rhone-Poulenc Rorer, S.Afr.†; Rhone Poulenc Rorer, Singapore; Rhone-Poulenc Rorer, Switz.†; JHC Healthcare, UK.
Pipotiazine (p.700·3) or pipotiazine palmitate (p.700·3).
Psychoses.

Piportil L4
Rhone-Poulenc Rorer, Canad.; Rhone-Poulenc Rorer, Mex.
Pipotiazine palmitate (p.700·3).
Schizophrenia.

Pippen *Pharmaland, Thai.*
Ibuprofen (p.43·2).
Musculoskeletal and joint disorders.

Pipracil
Wyeth-Ayerst, Canad.; Lederle, Hong Kong; Wyeth-Ayerst, Thai.; Lederle, USA.
Piperacillin sodium (p.236·1).
Bacterial infections.

Pipracin *IRBI, Ital.†.*
Piperacillin sodium (p.236·1).
Lignocaine [lidocaine] hydrochloride (p.1313·2) is included in the intramuscular injection to alleviate the pain of injection.
Bacterial infections.

Pipralen *Lennon, S.Afr.†.*
Piperazine hydrate (p.106·1).
Ascariasis; enterobiasis.

Pipram
Rhone-Poulenc Rorer, Belg.†; Rhodia, Braz.; Rhone-Poulenc Rorer, Fr.; Rhone-Poulenc Rorer, Ital.; Rhone-Poulenc Rorer, Neth.
Pipemidic acid (p.236·1).
Urinary-tract infections.

Pipril
Wyeth Lederle, Aust.; Lederle, Austral.; Lederle, Ger.; Wyeth, Irl.; Lederle, Israel; Wyeth, NZ; Wyeth, S.Afr.; Cyanamid, Spain; Lederle, Switz.; Wyeth, UK†.
Piperacillin sodium (p.236·1).
Lignocaine [lidocaine] (p.1313·2) may be included in the intramuscular injection to alleviate the pain of injection.
Bacterial infections.

Piprine *Be-Tabs, S.Afr.*
Piperazine citrate (p.105·3).
Ascariasis; enterobiasis.

Piprol *Elfar, Spain.*
Ciprofloxacin hydrochloride (p.182·3).
Bacterial infections.

Piproxen *Nuovo ISM, Ital.*
Naproxen piperazine (p.61·3).
Gout; musculoskeletal, joint, and peri-articular disorders; neuralgia.

Piptalake P *Hoechst Marion Roussel, Braz.*
Piperidyl benzilate; phenobarbital (p.355·1).
Smooth muscle spasm.

Pipurin *NCSN, Ital.*
Pipemidic acid (p.236·1).
Urinary-tract infections.

Pipurol *Zambon, Braz.*
Pipemidic acid (p.236·1).
Urinary-tract infections.

Pirabene *Ratiopharm, Aust.*
Piracetam (p.1652·1).
Alcohol withdrawal syndrome; organic brain disorders.

Piracebral *Hexal, Ger.*
Piracetam (p.1652·1).
Mental function disorders.

Piracetam Complex *Almirall, Spain.*
Co-dergocrine mesilate (p.1597·3); piracetam (p.1652·1).
Cerebrovascular disorders.

Piracetrop *Holsten, Ger.*
Piracetam (p.1652·1).
Mental function disorders.

Pirafoid *Valdecasas, Mex.*
Pyrazinamide (p.240·1).

Pirafrin *Diba, Mex.*
Paracetamol (p.71·2); caffeine (p.761·3); phenylephrine hydrochloride (p.1097·1); chlorpheniramine [chlorphenamine] maleate (p.412·1).
Conjunctival congestion; fever; nasal congestion; pain; rhinitis.

Piraldin *Vitae, Mex.*
Paracetamol (p.71·2).
Fever; pain.

Piraldina *Bracco, Ital.*
Pyrazinamide (p.240·1).
Tuberculosis.

Piralgina *Diba, Mex.*
Paracetamol (p.71·2); caffeine (p.761·3); ephedrine hydrochloride (p.1090·1).
Congestion; fever; pain.

Piralone *Ferrer, Spain†.*
Lorazepam pivalate (p.689·2).
Alcohol withdrawal syndrome; anxiety; epilepsy; insomnia; nausea and vomiting.

Piram *General Drugs, Thai.*
Piroxicam (p.79·1).
Gout; musculoskeletal, joint, peri-articular, and soft-tissue disorders.

Piramagno *Pharmacos, Mex.*
Dipyrone (p.34·1).
Fever; pain.

Piram-D *Pacific, NZ.*
Piroxicam (p.79·1).
Gout; musculoskeletal and joint disorders; pain.

Piramin *Elofar, Braz.*
Paracetamol (p.71·2).
Fever; pain.

Pirandall *Randall, Mex.*
Dipyrone (p.34·1).
Fever; pain.

Pirantrim *Keton, Mex.*
Pyrantel embonate (p.108·1).

Piraside *Upsifarma, Port.*
Pyrazinamide (p.240·1).
Tuberculosis.

Piratam *Beacons, Singapore.*
Piracetam (p.1652·1).
Alcoholism; behaviour disorders in children; cerebral trauma; cerebrovascular disorders; senile dementia; sickle-cell disease; vertigo.

Pirawil *Willmar, Mex.*
Dipyrone (p.34·1).

Pirax
Note. This name is used for preparations of different composition.
Ecosol, Switz.
Piracetam (p.1652·1).
Mental function impairment.

Pharmaland, Thai.
Piroxicam (p.79·1).
Musculoskeletal and joint disorders.

Pirazer *Zerboni, Mex.*
Pyrazinamide (p.240·1).

Pirehexal *Hexal, Ger.†.*
Pirenzepine hydrochloride (p.472·2).
Gastrointestinal disorders.

piren-basan *Schonenberger, Switz.*
Pirenzepine hydrochloride (p.472·2).
Gastrointestinal disorders associated with hyperacidity.

Pirenex *Hoechst Marion Roussel, Switz.†.*
Piretanide (p.956·2) or piretanide sodium (p.956·2).
Hypertension; oedema; poisoning; renal disorders.

Pireuma *Noos, Ital.*
Propyphenazone (p.80·2).
Fever; pain.

Pirfalin *Farmigea, Ital.*
Pirenoxine sodium (p.1652·2).
Cataracts.

Piridasmin *Astra, Spain.*
Theophylline (p.777·2).
Obstructive airways disease.

Pirifedrina *Funk, Spain†.*
Codeine phosphate (p.25·2); ephedrine hydrochloride (p.1090·1); paracetamol (p.71·2).
Influenza and cold symptoms.

Pirifur *Sanofi Winthrop, Mex.*
Phenazopyridine hydrochloride (p.77·3); nalidixic acid (p.227·1).
Urinary-tract infections.

Piriject *Link, UK.*
Chlorpheniramine [chlorphenamine] maleate (p.412·1).
Formerly known as Piriton. Now known as Chlorphenamine Injection.
Hypersensitivity reactions.

Pirilene *Roussel Diamant, Fr.*
Pyrazinamide (p.240·1).
Tuberculosis.

Pirimat *Duopharma, Hong Kong.*
Chlorpheniramine [chlorphenamine] maleate (p.412·1).
Hypersensitivity reactions.

Pirinasol *Bayer, Spain.*
Paracetamol (p.71·2).
Fever; pain.

Pirinovag *Novag, Mex.*
Dipyrone (p.34·1).
Fever; pain.

Piriton
Boots, Austral.†; Glaxo Wellcome, Hong Kong; Stafford-Miller, Irl.; Glaxo Wellcome, Singapore; Glaxo Wellcome, Thai.; Stafford-Miller, UK.
Chlorpheniramine [chlorphenamine] maleate (p.412·1).
Hypersensitivity reactions.

Piriton Expectorant *Glaxo Wellcome, Thai.*
Chlorpheniramine [chlorphenamine] maleate (p.412·1); ammonium chloride (p.1085·2); sodium citrate (p.1186·2).
Coughs.

Piritosse *Bergamo, Braz.*
Diphenhydramine (p.416·1); ephedrine (p.1090·1); pentetrazol (p.1513·2); eucalyptol (p.1609·2); Desessartz syrup.
Cold and influenza symptoms.

Pirkam *Nycomed, Denm.*
Piroxicam (p.79·1).
Inflammation; musculoskeletal and joint disorders; pain.

Piro *ABZ, Ger.*
Piroxicam (p.79·1).
Musculoskeletal, joint, and soft-tissue disorders.

Piro KD *Kade, Ger.*
Piroxicam (p.79·1).
Musculoskeletal, joint, and soft-tissue disorders.

Pirobeta *Betapharm, Ger.*
Piroxicam (p.79·1).
Gout; musculoskeletal, joint, peri-articular, and soft-tissue disorders.

Pirocam
Ratiopharm, Aust.; Spirig, Switz.
Piroxicam (p.79·1).
Gout; inflammation; musculoskeletal and joint disorders; pain; peri-articular disorders.

Pirodax *Lemery, Mex.*
Piroxicam (p.79·1).
Inflammation; musculoskeletal and joint disorders; pain.

Piroflam
Lichtenstein, Ger.; Opus, UK.
Piroxicam (p.79·1).
Gout; musculoskeletal, joint, and soft-tissue disorders.

Piroftal *Bruschettini, Ital.*
Piroxicam (p.79·1).
Eye inflammation; ocular oedema.

Pirohexal-D *Hexal, Austral.*
Piroxicam (p.79·1).
Musculoskeletal and joint disorders.

Pirom
Note. This name is used for preparations of different composition.
Durascan, Denm.
Piroxicam (p.79·1).
Inflammation; musculoskeletal and joint disorders; pain.

Solmer, Switz.
Balm: Camphor (p.1589·3); menthol (p.1632·3); methyl salicylate (p.55·1); eucalyptus oil (p.1609·2); cinnamon oil (p.1596·1).
Headache; insect bites and stings; muscle and joint pain; sports injuries.
Embrocation: Camphor (p.1589·3); menthol (p.1632·3); methyl salicylate (p.55·1); eucalyptus oil (p.1609·2); sweet birch oil (p.55·2); citrus oil.
Cold symptoms; headache; insect bites and stings; muscle and joint pain; sports injuries.

Piromav *Mavi, Mex.*
Piroxicam (p.79·1).

Piromebrina *Degorts, Mex.*
Dipyrone (p.34·1).
Fever; pain.

Pironal *Wiener, Mex.*
Dipyrone (p.34·1).

Pironet *Nettopharma, Denm.†.*
Piroxicam (p.79·1).
Musculoskeletal and joint disorders; pain.

Pirongil *Arlex, Mex.*
Dipyrone (p.34·1).

Pirophen *Warner-Lambert, NZ.*
Aspirin (p.14·2); paracetamol (p.71·2); codeine phosphate (p.25·2).
Fever; pain.

Piro-Phlogont *Azupharma, Ger.*
Piroxicam (p.79·1).
Gout; musculoskeletal, joint, and soft-tissue disorders.

Piro-Puren *Isis Puren, Ger.*
Piroxicam (p.79·1).
Musculoskeletal, joint, and soft-tissue disorders.

Pirorheum
Hexal, Aust.; Hexal, Ger.
Piroxicam (p.79·1).
Gout; musculoskeletal, joint, peri-articular, and soft-tissue disorders; pain.

PirorheumA *Hexal, Ger.*
Piroxicam (p.79·1).
Musculoskeletal, joint, peri-articular, and soft-tissue disorders.

Pirosal *Teral, USA†.*
Sodium thiosalicylate (p.84·2).

Pirosol *Ecosol, Switz.*
Piroxicam (p.79·1).
Inflammation; musculoskeletal, joint, and peri-articular disorders; pain.

Pirox
G.P. Laboratories, Austral.; CT, Ger.; Alpharma, Norw.
Piroxicam (p.79·1).
Dysmenorrhoea; gout; musculoskeletal, joint, and soft-tissue disorders.

Piroxal *Alpharma, Fin.*
Piroxicam (p.79·1).
Dysmenorrhoea; musculoskeletal and joint disorders.

Piroxam *PP Lab, Thai.*
Piroxicam (p.79·1).
Gout; musculoskeletal and joint disorders.

Piroxan *Diba, Mex.*
Piroxicam (p.79·1).
Gout; inflammation; musculoskeletal, joint and peri-articular disorders; pain.

pirox-basan *Schonenberger, Switz.*
Piroxicam (p.79·1).
Gout; musculoskeletal and joint disorders; pain.

Piroxcin *Polipharm, Thai.*
Piroxicam (p.79·1).
Gout; musculoskeletal and joint disorders.

Piroxen *Ofimex, Mex.; Codal Synto, Thai.*
Piroxicam (p.79·1).
Gout; musculoskeletal and joint disorders.

Piroxene *Sintofarma, Braz.*
Piroxicam (p.79·1).
Dysmenorrhoea; gout; musculoskeletal, joint, and peri-articular disorders.

Piroxgel *Barcino, Spain.*
Coal tar (p.1125·1).
Dandruff; psoriasis; seborrhoeic dermatitis.

Piroxifen *Dansk-Flama, Braz.*
Piroxicam (p.79·1).
Dysmenorrhoea; gout; musculoskeletal, joint, and peri-articular disorders.

Piroxiflam *Luitpold, Braz.*
Piroxicam (p.79·1).
Dysmenorrhoea; gout; musculoskeletal, joint, and peri-articular disorders.

Piroxil *Sanval, Braz.*
Piroxicam (p.79·1).
Dysmenorrhoea; gout; musculoskeletal, joint, and peri-articular disorders.

Piroximerck *Merck, Ger.†.*
Piroxicam (p.79·1).
Gout; musculoskeletal and joint disorders.

Piroxin *Medinovum, Fin.*
Piroxicam (p.79·1).
Inflammation; pain; peri-articular and soft-tissue disorders.

Piroxiplus *Hebron, Braz.*
Piroxicam (p.79·1).
Dysmenorrhoea; gout; musculoskeletal, joint, and peri-articular disorders.

Piroxistad *Stada, Aust.*
Piroxicam (p.79·1).
Gout; musculoskeletal, joint, and peri-articular disorders; pain.

Piroxityrol *Tyrol, Aust.*
Piroxicam (p.79·1).
Gout; inflammation; musculoskeletal, joint, and peri-articular disorders; pain.

Piroxsil *Silom, Thai.*
Piroxicam (p.79·1).
Musculoskeletal and joint disorders.

Pirox-Spondyril *Orion, Ger.*
Piroxicam (p.79·1).
Gout; musculoskeletal, joint, and soft-tissue disorders.

Piroxy *Duopharma, Hong Kong.*
Piroxicam (p.79·1).
Ankylosing spondylitis; osteoarthritis; rheumatoid arthritis.

Pirozip *Ashbourne, UK.*
Piroxicam (p.79·1).
Gout; musculoskeletal and joint disorders.

Pirrolfungin *Esfar, Port.*
Pyrrolnitrin (p.393·3); salicylic acid (p.1122·3); diethyl sebacate.
Skin infections.

Pirxane *Lisapharma, Ital.*
Buflomedil pyridoxal phosphate compound (p.852·1).
Vascular disorders.

Pirzinol *Solfran, Mex.*
Piperazine (p.105·3).

Pisacaina *Pisa, Mex.*
Lignocaine [lidocaine] hydrochloride (p.1313·2).
Adrenaline [epinephrine] (p.829·1) is included in some injections as a vasoconstrictor to diminish absorption and localise the effect of the local anaesthetic.
Local anaesthesia; ventricular arrhythmias.

Pisatrina *Pisa, Mex.*
Co-trimoxazole (p.193·3).
Bacterial infections.

Pitocin
Parke, Davis, Aust.†; Warner-Lambert, Norw.; Parke, Davis, USA.
Oxytocin (p.1294·1) or oxytocin citrate (p.1294·3).
Incomplete or inevitable abortion; induction of labour; postpartum haemorrhage; uterine inertia.

Piton-S *Organon, Neth.†.*
Oxytocin (p.1294·1).
Labour induction; postpartum haemorrhage; promotion of lactation.

Pitressin
Parke, Davis, Austral.; Parke, Davis, Ger.; Goldshield, Irl.; Parke, Davis, NZ; Goldshield, UK; Parke, Davis, USA.
Argipressin (p.1300·1).
Aid in abdominal radiography; diabetes insipidus; postoperative abdominal distension; postoperative intestinal atony; variceal haemorrhage.

Pitrex
Taro, Canad.; Teva, Israel.
Tolnaftate (p.395·2).
Fungal skin infections.

Pitrion *Rafa, Israel.*
Miconazole nitrate (p.391·1).
Fungal skin and nail infections.

Pitrisan *Rekah, Israel.*
Ointment: Undecenoic acid (p.395·3); zinc undecenoate (p.395·3); allantoin (p.1110·1).

Topical solution: Undecenoic acid (p.395·3); salicylic acid (p.1122·3); benzoic acid (p.1134·2); chlorobutanol (p.1141·2); resorcinol (p.1122·2).
Fungal skin infections.

Pityval *Roche-Posay, Irl.*
Emollient.

Pivalone *Parke, Davis, Fr.; Dagra, Neth.†; Parke, Davis, Singapore; Uhlmann-Eyraud, Switz.*
Tixocortol pivalate (p.1080·1).
Nasal polyps; rhinitis.

Pivalone compositum *Uhlmann-Eyraud, Switz.*
Tixocortol pivalate (p.1080·1); neomycin sulfate (p.228·1).
Infected nasal disorders.

Pivalone Neomycin *Parke, Davis, Singapore*
Tixocortol pivalate (p.1080·1); neomycin sulfate (p.228·1).
Infected nasal polyps; rhinitis; sinusitis.

Pivalone Neomycine *Parke, Davis, Fr.*
Tixocortol pivalate (p.1080·1); neomycin sulfate (p.228·1).
Rhinitis; sinusitis.

Pivaloxicam *Chiesi, Ital.†*
Piroxicam pivalate (p.79·3).
Musculoskeletal and joint disorders.

Pivamiser *Serra Pamies, Spain.*
Pivampicillin hydrochloride (p.237·2).
Bacterial infections.

Pivanozolo *Benedetti, Ital.*
Miconazole pivoxil chloride (p.391·3).
Fungal infections; Gram-positive bacterial superinfections.

Pixfix *Hoernecke, Ger.*
Coal tar (p.1125·1).
Skin disorders.

Pixicam *Hexal, S.Afr.*
Piroxicam (p.79·1).
Gout; musculoskeletal and joint disorders.

Pixidin *Sanico, Belg.*
Chlorhexidine hydrochloride (p.1138·2).
Formerly contained tar, benzocaine, menthol, eucalyptol, senna, and red-poppy petal.
Mouth and throat disorders.

Pixol *Cortecs, UK†.*
Tar (p.1125·1); coal tar (p.1125·1); cade oil (p.1124·3).
Skin disorders.

Pixor Stick Anti-acne N *Doetsch, Grether, Switz.*
Salicylic acid (p.1122·3); triclosan (p.1159·2).
Acne.

Piz Buin *Novartis Consumer, UK.*
SPF 20: Octinoxate (p.1517·3); avobenzone (p.1517·1); titanium dioxide (p.1126·1).
Sunscreen.

Pizide *Pharmasant, Thai.*
Pimozide (p.699·3).
Psychoses.

Pizomed *Medifive, Thai.*
Pizotifen malate (p.455·1).
Anorexia; migraine.

PK Aid *Scientific Hospital Supplies, Austral.; Scientific Hospital Supplies, Irl.; Scientific Hospital Supplies, UK.*
Amino-acid preparation without phenylalanine (p.1350·1).
Phenylketonuria.

PK-Levo *Merz, Ger.*
Levodopa (p.1169·2); benserazide hydrochloride (p.1164·2).
Parkinsonism.

PK-Merz *Kolassa, Aust.; Merz, Ger.; Merz, Hong Kong; Megapharm, Israel; Merz, Switz.*
Amantadine sulfate (p.1161·2).
Coma; influenza; parkinsonism; postherpetic neuralgia.

PKU *Milupa, UK.*
Food for special diets (p.1350·1).
Phenylketonuria.

PKU 2 and 3 *Milupa, UK.*
Food for special diets (p.1350·1).
Phenylketonuria.

PKU 1 Mix *Milupa, Ital.*
Food for special diets (p.1350·1).
Hyperphenylalaninaemia; phenylketonuria.

Placatus *Pfizer Consumer, Ital.*
Nepinalone hydrochloride (p.1095·3).
Coughs.

Placentex *Mastelli, Ital.*
Polydeoxyribonucleotide (p.1602·3).
Inflammatory and degenerative disorders.

Placentina *INTES, Ital.†.*
Placenta extract.
Inflammation; rheumatic disorders.

Placidex *De Witt, UK.*
Paracetamol (p.71·2).
Fever; pain.

Placidyl *Abbott, USA.*
Ethchlorvynol (p.682·3).
Insomnia.

Placil *Alphapharm, Austral.*
Clomipramine hydrochloride (p.282·1).
Depression; narcoleptic syndrome; obsessive-compulsive disorder; phobias.

Placinoral *Robert, Spain.*
Lorazepam pivalate (p.689·2).
Alcohol withdrawal syndrome; anxiety; insomnia; nausea and vomiting; premedication.

Placis *Wasserman, Spain.*
Cisplatin (p.525·1).
Malignant neoplasms.

Plactidil *Novartis, Ital.*
Picotamide (p.955·2).
Thromboembolic disorders.

Plactosse *IMA, Braz.*
Sodium dibunate (p.1100·3); sodium benzoate (p.1134·3); guaifenesin (p.1092·2).
Coughs.

Plagon *De Mayo, Braz.*
Metoclopramide (p.1236·3); vitamin B_6 (p.1387·1).
Nausea and vomiting.

Plak *Byk Gulden, Ital.*
Chlorhexidine gluconate (p.1138·2).
Oral hygiene.

Plak Out *Byk, Aust.; Byk Gulden, Ital.; Inibsa, Port.*
Chlorhexidine gluconate (p.1138·2).
Mouth infections.

Plamet *Libbs, Braz.*
Bromopride (p.1215·1).
Nausea and vomiting.

Plamin *Apsen, Braz.*
Metoclopramide hydrochloride (p.1235·2).
Gastrointestinal motility disorders; nausea and vomiting.

Plan B *Womens Capital, USA.*
Levonorgestrel (p.1486·2).
Progestogen-only postcoital contraceptive.

Plander *Fresenius Kabi, Ital.*
Dextran 70 (p.729·2) in sodium chloride.
Plasma volume expansion.

Plander R *Fresenius Kabi, Ital.*
Dextran 40 (p.728·3) in sodium chloride.
Extracorporeal perfusion; plasma volume expansion; thrombosis prophylaxis.

Planizol *Solfran, Mex.*
Metronidazole (p.594·1).
Amoebiasis.

Planor *Effik, Fr.*
Norgestrienone (p.1487·2); ethinylestradiol (p.1476·2).
Combined oral contraceptive; endometriosis; mastalgia; menstrual disorders; polycystic ovary syndrome.

Planphylline *Asta Medica, Fr.†.*
Aminophylline (p.760·1).
Asthma; obstructive airways disease.

Plant Spray *Doliosis, Canad.*
Homoeopathic preparation.

Planta Lax *Hoeveler, Aust.*
Senna leaf and pod (p.1248·2); frangula bark (p.1227·1); blackberry leaf; chamomile flowers (p.1593·2); coriander (p.1599·2); fennel (p.1610·1).
Constipation.

Plantaben *Madaus, Spain.*
Ispaghula (p.1229·1).
Constipation.

Plantacard N *Madaus, Ger.*
Homoeopathic preparation.

Plantago Complex *Blackmores, Austral.†.*
Psyllium seed (p.1229·1); rhubarb (p.1248·1); whey; gentian (p.1615·1); cascara (p.1216·1).
Constipation.

Plantaguar *Madaus, Spain.*
Guar gum (p.323·3).
Diabetes mellitus.

Plantax *Farmion, Braz.*
Senna (p.1248·2); ispaghula (p.1229·1).
Constipation.

Planten *Whitehall, Israel; Whitehall, Ital.*
Ispaghula (p.1229·1).
Constipation; irritable bowel syndrome.

Plantiodine Plus *Blackmores, Austral.*
Bladderwrack (p.1585·2); alfalfa (p.1574·3); protibel yeast (p.1398·1); rose fruit (p.1389·3); lecithin (p.1628·1).
Tonic.

Plantival
Note. This name is used for preparations of different composition.
Farmasa, Mex.
Valerian (p.1678·3); melissa (p.1632·2).
Insomnia; nervous disorders.

Schwabe, Switz.†
Valerian (p.1678·3); passion flower (p.1649·1).
Anxiety disorders.

Plantival novo *Schwabe, Ger.*
Valerian (p.1678·3); melissa (p.1632·2).
Agitation; sleep disorders.

Plantmobil *Plantina, Ger.*
Camphor (p.1589·3); eucalyptus oil (p.1609·2); turpentine oil (p.1676·3).
Cold symptoms; musculoskeletal and joint disorders.

Plantocur *Biocur, Ger.*
Ispaghula (p.1229·1).
Constipation.

Plantoletten *Robugen, Ger.†.*
Rhubarb (p.1248·1); aloes (p.1210·1).
Constipation.

Planum
Note. This name is used for preparations of different composition.
Pharmacia Upjohn, Ger.; Pharmacia Upjohn, Switz.†.
Temazepam (p.707·2).
Sleep disorders.

Menarini, Ital.
Desogestrel (p.1470·3); ethinylestradiol (p.1476·2).
Combined oral contraceptive.

Plaqacide *Oral-B, Austral.*
Chlorhexidine gluconate (p.1138·2).
Oral disorders; prevention of dental plaque.

Plaquenil *Sanofi Winthrop, Aust.; Sanofi Synthelabo, Austral.; Sanofi Synthelabo, Belg.; Sanofi Synthelabo, Canad.; Sanofi Winthrop, Denm.; Sanofi Winthrop, Fin.; Sanofi Winthrop, Fr.; Sanofi Winthrop, Hong Kong; Sanofi Winthrop, Irl.; Sanofi Winthrop, Israel; Sanofi Synthelabo, Ital.; Sanofi Winthrop, Mex.; Sanofi Synthelabo, Neth.; Sanofi Winthrop, Norw.; Sanofi Winthrop, NZ; Sanofi Winthrop, Singapore; Sanofi Winthrop, Swed.; Sanofi Synthelabo, Switz.; Sanofi Synthelabo, Thai.; Sanofi Winthrop, UK; Sanofi Winthrop, USA.*
Hydroxychloroquine sulfate (p.437·2).
Lupus erythematosus; malaria; photodermatoses; rheumatoid arthritis; Sjögren's syndrome.

Plaquetal *Sanitas, Port.*
Ticlopidine hydrochloride (p.981·1).
Thrombosis prophylaxis.

Plaquinol *Sanofi Winthrop, Braz.; Sanofi Synthelabo, Port.*
Hydroxychloroquine sulfate (p.437·2).
Lupus erythematosus; malaria; photodermatoses; rheumatoid arthritis.

Plas-Amino *Otsuka, Jpn.*
Amino-acid and carbohydrate infusion (p.1350·1).
Parenteral nutrition.

Plasbumin *Bayer, Canad.; Bayer Biological, Hong Kong; Bayer, Israel; Bayer, Singapore; Bayer, Spain; Cutter, USA.*
Albumin (p.724·1).
Hypoalbuminaemia; hypoproteinaemia; hypovolaemia; neonatal hyperbilirubinaemia.

Plasil *Hoechst Marion Roussel, Braz.; Lepetit, Ital.; Hoechst Marion Roussel, Mex.; Hoechst Marion Roussel, Thai.*
Metoclopramide hydrochloride (p.1235·2).
Gastrointestinal motility disorders; nausea and vomiting.

Plasil Enzimatico *Hoechst Marion Roussel, Braz.; Hoechst Marion Roussel, Mex.*
Metoclopramide hydrochloride (p.1235·2); bromelains (p.1586·3); pancreatin (p.1646·1); sodium dehydrocholate (p.1602·3); simeticone (p.1249·2).
Gastrointestinal, biliary-tract and pancreatic disorders.

Plasimine *Isdin, Spain.*
Mupirocin (p.226·1).
Bacterial skin infections.

Plaskine Neomicina *Ipsen, Spain.*
Lysine acexamate (p.1572·2); neomycin undecenoate (p.228·1).
Burns; ulcers; wounds.

Plasma Marin Hypertonique *Aqualab, Fr.*
Mineral preparation (p.1350·1).

Plasmacair *Clintec, Fr.†.*
Dextran 40 (p.728·3) with electrolytes.
Haemodilution; hypotension; shock.

Plasmaclar *Lacer, Spain†.*
Xantinol nicotinate (p.999·1); pentosan polysulfate sodium (p.953·1).
Hyperlipidaemias.

Plasmafusin *Fresenius Kabi, Fin.*
Hetastarch (p.732·3) in sodium chloride.
Hypotension; hypovolaemia; shock.

Plasmafusin HES *Pharmacia Upjohn, Ger.*
Hetastarch (p.732·3) in sodium chloride.
Plasma volume expansion.

Plasmagel *Fresenius Kabi, Fr.*
Gelatin (p.737·2) with electrolytes or glucose.
Hypotension; shock.

Plasma-Lyte *Baxter, Austral.; Baxter, UK; Baxter, USA.*
A range of electrolyte infusions with or without glucose (p.1180·1).
Fluid and electrolyte disorders.

Plasma-Lyte IV *Baxter, NZ.*
A range of electrolyte infusions with or without glucose (p.1180·1).
Fluid and electrolyte disorders.

Plasma-Lyte 148 *Baxter, Spain.*
Electrolyte infusion (p.1180·1).
Fluid and electrolyte disorders.

Plasma-Lyte O *Baxter, NZ.*
Electrolyte solution (p.1180·1).
Diarrhoea; oral rehydration solution.

Plasmanate *Bayer, Canad.†; Bayer Biological, Hong Kong; Bayer, Israel; Bayer, Singapore; Cutter, USA.*
Plasma protein fraction (p.740·2).
Hypoproteinaemia; hypovolaemia.

Plasma-Plex *Armour, USA.*
Plasma protein fraction (p.740·2).
Hypoproteinaemia; hypovolaemia.

Plasmarine *Pharmadeveloppement, Fr.*
Mineral preparation (p.1350·1).
Tonic.

Plasmasteril *Fresenius Kabi, Aust.; Fresenius, Belg.†; Fresenius, Braz.; Fresenius Kabi, Ger.; Fresenius Kabi, Switz.*
Hetastarch (p.732·3) in sodium chloride.
Plasma volume expansion.

Plasmatein *Alpha Therapeutic, USA.*
Plasma protein fraction (p.740·2).
Hypoproteinaemia; hypovolaemia.

Plasmaviral *ISI, Ital.*
Plasma protein fraction (p.740·2).
Hypoproteinaemia; shock.

Plasmion *Fresenius Kabi, Fr.*
Gelatin (p.737·2) with electrolytes.
Hypotension; shock.

Plasmocolit *QIF, Braz.*
Furazolidone (p.592·1); homatropine methylbromide (p.468·1); pectin (p.1502·3).
Diarrhoea.

Plasmodex *Pharmalink, Norw.; Pharmalink, Swed.*
Dextran 60 (p.729·2) with electrolytes.
Plasma volume expansion.

Plasmonsoy *Plasmon, Ital.*
Infant feed (p.1350·1).
Cow's milk intolerance.

Plasmoquine *Medchem, S.Afr.*
Chloroquine sulfate (p.432·3).
Malaria.

Plasmotrim *Mepha, Thai.*
Sodium artesunate (p.431·2).
Malaria.

Plasonil *Heralds, Braz.*
Metoclopramide hydrochloride (p.1235·2); pyridoxine hydrochloride (p.1386·3).
Nausea and vomiting.

Plast Apyr Fisio Irrigac *Mein, Spain†.*
Sodium chloride (p.1196·1).
Urological irrigation.

Plast Apyr Fisiologico *Fresenius Kabi, Spain.*
Sodium chloride (p.1196·1).
Fluid and electrolyte disorders.

Plast Apyr Glucosado *Fresenius Kabi, Spain.*
Glucose (p.1364·1).
Carbohydrate source; fluid and electrolyte disorders.

Plast Apyr Glucosalino *Fresenius Kabi, Spain.*
Glucose (p.1364·1); sodium chloride (p.1196·1).
Carbohydrate source; fluid and electrolyte disorders.

Plastenan *Bournonville, Belg.†; Sanofi Winthrop, Braz.; Isopharm, Fr.†.*
Acexamic acid (p.1572·2) or sodium acexamate (p.1572·2).
Burns; leg ulcers; scars; wounds.

Plastenan Neomicina *CPH, Port.*
Sodium acexamate (p.1572·2); neomycin sulfate (p.228·1).
Burns; ulcers; wounds.

Plastenan Neomycine *Isopharm, Fr.†.*
Sodium acexamate (p.1572·2); neomycin sulfate (p.228·1).
Infected wounds and burns.

Plastesol *CPH, Port.*
Acexamic acid (p.1572·2).
Burns; wounds.

Plastistil *Pharmacia Upjohn, Mex.*
Cisplatin (p.525·1).

Plastranit *Bonafarma, Port.*
Glyceryl trinitrate (p.897·3).
Angina pectoris; heart failure.

Plastufer *Wyeth, Ger.*
Ferrous sulfate (p.1360·3).
Iron deficiency; iron-deficiency anaemia.

Plastulen N *Wyeth, Ger.*
Ferrous sulfate (p.1360·3); folic acid (p.1361·1).
Iron and folic acid deficiency.

Platamine *Pharmacia Upjohn, Ital.; Pharmacia Upjohn, NZ; Pharmacia Upjohn, S.Afr.*
Cisplatin (p.525·1).
Malignant neoplasms.

Platet *Nicholas, UK†.*
Aspirin (p.14·2).
Cardiovascular disorders.

Platiblastin *Pharmacia Upjohn, Aust.; Pharmacia Upjohn, Ger.*
Cisplatin (p.525·1).
Malignant neoplasms.

Platiblastin-S *Pharmacia Upjohn, Switz.*
Cisplatin (p.525·1).
Malignant neoplasms.

Platinex *Bristol-Myers Squibb, Ger.; Bristol-Myers Squibb, Israel; Bristol-Myers Squibb, Ital.; Bristol-Myers Squibb, UK.*
Cisplatin (p.525·1).
Malignant neoplasms.

Platinol *Bristol-Myers Squibb, Aust.; Bristol-Myers Squibb, Belg.; Bristol, Canad.; Bristol-Myers Squibb, Denm.; Bristol-Myers Squibb, Fin.; Bristol-Myers Squibb, Israel; Bristol-Myers Squibb, Mex.; Bristol-Myers Squibb, Neth.; Bristol-Myers Squibb, Norw.; Bristol-Myers Squibb, Swed.; Bristol-Myers Squibb, Switz.; Bristol-Myers Squibb, Thai.; Bristol-Myers Squibb Oncology, USA.*
Cisplatin (p.525·1).
Malignant neoplasms.

Platinum Years *General Nutrition, Canad.*
Multivitamin and mineral preparation (p.1350·1).

Platinwas *Wasserman, Spain.*
Carboplatin (p.515·1).
Malignant neoplasms.

Platiran *Bristol-Myers Squibb, Braz.*
Cisplatin (p.525·1).
Malignant neoplasms.

Platistil *Kenfarma, Spain.*
Cisplatin (p.525·1).
Malignant neoplasms.

Platistin
Pharmacia Upjohn, Norw.; Pharmacia Upjohn, Swed.†.
Cisplatin (p.525·1).
Malignant neoplasms.

Platistine
Pharmacia Upjohn, Belg.; Pharmacia Upjohn, Braz.
Cisplatin (p.525·1).
Malignant neoplasms.

Plato *Aspen, S.Afr.*
Dipyridamole (p.877·2).
Platelet function inhibition.

Platocillina *Crosara, Ital.†.*
Ampicillin (p.150·3).
Bacterial infections.

Platosin
Pharmachemie, Israel; Pharmachemie, S.Afr.; Pharmachemie, Thai.
Cisplatin (p.525·1).
Malignant neoplasms.

Plausital *Pharmacia Upjohn, Mex.*
Morclofone (p.1095·1).

Plausitin *Carlo Erba OTC, Ital.*
Morclofone (p.1095·1).
Coughs.

Plavix
Sanofi Winthrop, Aust.; Sanofi Synthelabo, Austral.; Sanofi Synthelabo, Belg.; Sanofi Synthelabo, Canad.; Bristol-Myers Squibb, Canad.; Sanofi, Denm.; Sanofi Winthrop, Fin.; Bristol-Myers Squibb, Fin.; Bristol-Myers Squibb, Fr.; Sanofi Winthrop, Fr.; Sanofi Synthelabo, Ger.; Bristol-Myers Squibb, Irl.; Sanofi Winthrop, Irl.; Sanofi Winthrop, Mex.; Bristol-Myers Squibb, Neth.; Sanofi Winthrop, Neth.; Sanofi Winthrop, Norw.; Bristol-Myers Squibb, Norw.; Sanofi Winthrop, NZ; Sanofi Synthelabo, Port.; Bristol-Myers Squibb, Singapore; Sanofi Synthelabo, Spain; Sanofi Winthrop, Swed.; Bristol-Myers Squibb, Swed.; Sanofi Synthelabo, Switz.; Sanofi Synthelabo, Switz.; Sanofi Winthrop, UK; Bristol-Myers Squibb, UK; Sanofi Winthrop, USA; Bristol-Myers Squibb, USA.
Clopidogrel bisulfate (p.863·1).
Atherosclerosis.

Plax
Note.This name is used for preparations of different composition.
Pfizer Consumer, Canad.
Sodium benzoate (p.1134·3); sodium laurilsulfate (p.1496·3); sodium salicylate (p.84·2).

Colgate-Palmolive, Ital.
Triclosan (p.1159·2); sodium fluoride (p.1375·3).
Dental plaque prevention.

Plazolit *Fustery, Mex.*
Omeprazole (p.1239·1).

Plebe *Pharmadeveloppement, Fr.†.*
Vitamin and mineral preparation (p.1350·1).
Tonic.

Plegicil *Pharmacia Upjohn, Denm.*
Acepromazine maleate (p.654·1).
Anxiety disorders; hiccup; nausea and vomiting.

Plegine
Wyeth Lederle, Ital.†; Wyeth-Ayerst, USA†.
Phendimetrazine tartrate (p.1513·3).
Obesity.

Plegisol
Abbott, Israel; Abbott, USA.
Electrolytes (p.1180·1).
Cardioplegic solution.

Plegivex *Ivex, UK.*
Electrolyte solution for coronary instillation (p.1180·1).
Induction of arrest during cardiothoracic surgery.

Pleiadon *Zambon, Braz.*
Domperidone (p.1224·1).
Gastrointestinal motility disorders; nausea and vomiting.

Pleiamide *Sanofi Synthelabo, Ital.*
Chlorpropamide (p.321·1); metformin hydrochloride (p.332·3).
Diabetes mellitus.

Plenacor *Armstrong, Mex.*
Atenolol (p.841·3); nifedipine (p.940·1).
Angina pectoris; hypertension.

Plenaer *Valeas, Ital.*
Salbutamol sulfate (p.770·3); flunisolide (p.1070·3).
Obstructive airways disease.

Plenax *Merck, Braz.*
Cefixime (p.166·2).
Bacterial infections.

Plendil
Astra, Aust.; Astra, Austral.; Astra, Belg.; AstraZeneca, Canad.; Astra-Zeneca, Denm.; AstraZeneca, Fin.; Astra, Hong Kong; Astra, Irl.; Astra, Ital., Mex.; Astra, Neth.; AstraZeneca, Norw.; AstraZeneca, NZ; Astra, S.Afr.; AstraZeneca, Singapore; Astra, Spain; Hassle, Swed.; Astra, Switz.; AstraZeneca, Thai.; AstraZeneca, UK; Astra, USA.
Felodipine (p.888·3).
Angina pectoris; hypertension.

Plenigraf
Darrow, Braz.; Juste, Spain.
Calcium amidotrizoate (p.1032·1); meglumine amidotrizoate (p.1031·2); sodium amidotrizoate (p.1031·2).
Radiographic contrast medium.

Plenish-K *Aspen, S.Afr.*
Potassium chloride (p.1194·3).
Potassium deficiencies.

Plenitude Excell A-3 *L'Oreal, Canad.*
SPF 8: Octinoxate (p.1517·3).
Sunscreen.

Plenocedan *Makros, Braz.*
Dipyrone (p.34·1); papaverine hydrochloride (p.1648·1); homatropine methylbromide (p.468·1).
Smooth muscle spasm.

Plenogripe *Farmoquimica, Braz.*
Dipyrone (p.34·1); sodium camsilate; guaifenesin (p.1092·2); eucalyptol (p.1609·2); niaouli oil (p.1640·2); lignocaine [lidocaine] (p.1313·2); vitamin C (p.1389·3); mepyramine (p.421·1).
Cold and influenza symptoms.

Plenolyt *Madaus, Spain.*
Ciprofloxacin hydrochloride (p.182·3).
Bacterial infections.

Plenomicina *Cibran, Braz.*
Erythromycin stearate (p.201·3).
Bacterial infections.

Plenosol N *Madaus, Ger.†.*
Mistletoe (p.1636·2).
Joint disorders.

Plenur *Ipsen, Spain.*
Lithium carbonate (p.292·1).
Bipolar disorder; depression; neutropenia.

Plenyl *Oberlin, Fr.*
Vitamin and mineral preparation (p.1350·1).

Pleo Vitamin *Inibsa, Spain.*
Multivitamins and minerals (p.1350·1); orotic acid, diethylaminoethanol salt; adenosine.
Tonic.

Pleocortex *Retrain, Spain.*
Suprarenal cortex (p.1080·1).
Adrenal insufficiency; tonic.

Pleocortex B6 *Retrain, Spain.*
Suprarenal cortex (p.1080·1); pyridoxine hydrochloride (p.1386·3).
Vomiting.

Pleomix-Alpha *Illa, Ger.*
Thioctic acid (p.1671·3) or trometamol thioctate (p.1675·2).
Diabetic polyneuropathy.

Pleomix-B *Trommsdorff, Ger.*
Thiamine hydrochloride (p.1385·1); pyridoxine hydrochloride (p.1386·3).
Nervous-system disorders.

Pleon *Lacer, Spain.*
Adenine; vitamin B substances; carnitine orotate; fructose diphosphate magnesium; potassium orotate; xanthine (p.1350·1).
Tonic.

Pleon RA *Henning, Ger.*
Sulfasalazine (p.1251·1).
Polyarthritis.

Plesmet
Link, Irl.; Link, UK.
Ferrous glycine sulfate (p.1360·2).
Iron-deficiency anaemia.

Pletaal
Otsuka, Jpn†; Otsuka, Thai.
Cilostazol (p.858·2).
Peripheral vascular disorders.

Pletal *Otsuka, USA.*
Cilostazol (p.858·2).
Intermittent claudication.

Pletil *Searle, Braz.*
Tinidazole (p.603·3).
Anaerobic bacterial infections; protozoal infections.

Plex Ton *Auad, Braz.*
Multivitamin and mineral preparation with lysine (p.1350·1).

Plexium *Lehning, Fr.*
Selenium (p.1375·2).
Muscular disorders; skin disorders.

Plexo Enterin *Sanval, Braz.*
Kaolin (p.1229·3); pectin (p.1502·3).
Diarrhoea.

Plexoton B12 *Fonten, Ital.*
Vitamin B substances (p.1350·1).
Anaemias; liver disorders; tonic.

Plexvita *Sedar, Braz.*
Multivitamin and mineral preparation (p.1350·1).

Pliagel
Alcon, Austral.; Alcon, Braz.; Alcon, NZ.
Poloxamer 407 (p.1347·1) (p.1129·2).
Cleaning solution for soft contact lenses.

Plidan *Rhein, Mex.*
Pargeverine hydrochloride.
Smooth muscle spasm.

Plidan Compuesto *Rhein, Mex.*
Pargeverine hydrochloride; clonixin lysine (p.25·1).
Smooth muscle pain and spasm.

Plinzene *Douglas, NZ.*
Fluoxetine hydrochloride (p.284·2).
Bulimia; depression; obsessive-compulsive disorder.

Plissamur *Ardeypharm, Ger.*
Aesculus (p.1574·1).
Venous insufficiency.

Plitican
Synthelabo, Fr.; Synthelabo, Hong Kong; Synthelabo, Port.†; Synthelabo, Switz.
Alizapride hydrochloride (p.1209·3).
Nausea; vomiting.

Plokon
Shinyaku, Hong Kong; Shinyaku, Thai.
Piprinhydrinate (p.1431·2).
Hypersensitivity reactions; Ménière's disease; motion sickness; urticaria.

Plumarol *Lacer, Spain.*
Miglitol (p.333·1).
Diabetes mellitus.

Pluravit
Bayer, Austral.; Bayer, NZ.
A range of multivitamin and mineral preparations (p.1350·1).

Pluravit Super B *Sterling Health, Austral.*
Vitamin B substances with ascorbic acid (p.1350·1).
Vitamin B supplement.

Plurexid *Medeva, Fr.*
Chlorhexidine gluconate (p.1138·2).
Disinfection of skin and mucous membranes.

Pluribios *Madariaga, Spain.*
Multivitamin preparation with cocarboxylase (p.1350·1).
Eye disorders.

Pluriderm *Guieu, Ital.†.*
Thyme (p.1672·2); carrot (p.1680·3); sage oil (p.1660·2); whey; lactic acid (p.1626·2).
Skin disinfection.

Pluridoxina *Asta Medica, Port.*
Doxycycline fosfatex (p.200·1).
Bacterial infections.

Plurifactor *Gomenol, Fr.†.*
Vitamin B substances; deoxyribonucleic acid; glycine (p.1350·1).
Tonic.

Plurilac *Chemitalia, Ital.*
Acacia; inulin; lactulose; mannitol; dimethicone; fennel; mallow; peppermint (p.1214·2).
Dietary fibre supplement; gastrointestinal disorders.

Plurimen *Asta Medica, Spain.*
Selegiline hydrochloride (p.1177·2).
Parkinsonism.

Plurisalina *Grifols, Spain.*
Electrolyte injection (p.1180·1) with sodium lactate (p.1186·2).
Fluid and electrolyte disorders.

Plurisan *Heralds, Braz.*
Lindane (p.1434·1).
Pediculosis; scabies.

Pluriverm *Medley, Braz.*
Mebendazole (p.102·2).
Worm infections.

Pluriviron mono *Stegropharm, Ger.*
Yohimbine hydrochloride (p.1681·3).
Erectile dysfunction.

50 Plus *Quest, Canad.*
Multivitamin preparation (p.1350·1).

Plus Kalium retard *Amino, Switz.*
Potassium chloride (p.1194·3).
Hypokalaemia.

Plus Sinus *Pfizer Consumer, Canad.*
Pseudoephedrine hydrochloride (p.1099·2).
Nasal congestion.

Plusapetit *IMA, Braz.*
Lysine; vitamin B12; calcium glycerophosphate (p.1350·1).
Nutritional supplement.

Pluviton *Sam-On, Israel.*
Multivitamin and mineral preparation (p.1350·1).

Pluviton B *Sam-On, Israel.*
Vitamin B substances with lysine (p.1350·1).

pM *Chiesi, Fr.*
Aluminium chlorohydrate (p.1110·2).
Hyperhidrosis.

PMB *Wyeth-Ayerst, USA†.*
Conjugated oestrogens (p.1467·1); meprobamate (p.691·1).
Menopausal disorders.

P-Mega-Tablinen *Sanorania, Ger.*
Phenoxymethylpenicillin potassium (p.235·1).
Bacterial infections.

PML Crono *SIFI, Ital.*
Nicotinamidel vitamin E; lutein (p.1350·1).

PMS *Homeocan, Canad.*
Homoeopathic preparation.

PMS L21 *Homeocan, Canad.*
Homoeopathic preparation.

PMS Support *Vitaplex, Austral.*
Vitamins; minerals (p.1350·1); viburnum; buchu (p.1587·2); ginger (p.1227·2); evening primrose oil (p.1613·2).
Muscular cramps; oedema.

PMS-Artificial Tears
Pharmascience, Canad.; Pharmascience, Hong Kong; Pharmascience, Singapore.
Polyvinyl alcohol (p.1503·1).
Dry eyes.

PMS-Artificial Tears Plus *Pharmascience, Canad.*
Polyvinyl alcohol (p.1503·1); povidone (p.1503·2).
Dry eyes.

PMS-Dicitrate *Pharmascience, Canad.*
Sodium citrate dihydrate (p.1186·2); citric acid monohydrate (p.1596·2).
Neutralising buffer; systemic alkaliniser.

PMS-Egozinc *Pharmascience, Canad.†.*
Zinc sulfate (p.1398·2).
Zinc supplement.

PMS-Egozinc-HC *Pharmascience, Canad.*
Zinc sulfate (p.1398·2); hydrocortisone acetate (p.1073·3).
Anorectal disorders.

PMS-Levazine *Pharmascience, Canad.†.*
Perphenazine (p.699·1); amitriptyline hydrochloride (p.273·3).
Depression; psychoses.

PMS-Phosphates *Pharmascience, Canad.†.*
Monobasic sodium phosphate (p.1193·2); dibasic sodium phosphate (p.1193·2).
Constipation.

PMT Complex
Note.This name is used for preparations of different composition.
Brauer, Austral.†.
Homoeopathic preparation.

Cenovis, Austral.; Vitelle, Austral.
Vitamins; minerals (p.1350·1); ginger (p.1227·2); viburnum; agnus castus (p.1574·2); cimicifuga (p.1595·2); bladderwrack (p.1585·2).
Premenstrual syndrome.

PMT Formula *Vitalia, UK.*
Evening primrose oil (p.1613·2); vitamins (p.1350·1); minerals; valerian (p.1678·3); passion flower (p.1649·1).
Premenstrual syndrome.

PMT Oral Spray *Brauer, Austral.*
Homoeopathic preparation.

PMT-EZE *Rhone-Poulenc Rorer, Austral.†.*
Vitamins, minerals (p.1350·1); bearberry (p.1583·3); parsley (p.1648·3); juniper (p.1625·2); viburnum opulus.
Premenstrual syndrome.

Pneucid *Divpharm, S.Afr.*
Sodium citrate (p.1186·2); citric acid monohydrate (p.1596·2).
Buffering agent for increasing gastric pH before anaesthesia.

Pneumaseptic *Cochon, Fr.†.*
Sulfogaiacol (p.1101·1); sodium benzoate (p.1134·3).
Respiratory-tract congestion.

Pneumo 23
Pasteur Merieux, Aust.; Pasteur Merieux, Braz.; Pasteur Merieux, Canad.; Pasteur Merieux, Fr.; Pasteur Merieux, Hong Kong; Pasteur Merieux, Ital.; Aventis, Port.; Pasteur Merieux, Singapore; Pasteur Merieux, Spain; Pasteur Merieux, Thai.
A pneumococcal vaccine (23-valent) (p.1557·2).
Active immunisation.

Pneumo 23 Imovax *Pasteur Merieux, Israel.*
A pneumococcal vaccine (23-valent) (p.1557·2).
Active immunisation.

Pneumoclar *Monot, Fr.*
Carbocisteine (p.1086·3).

Pneumodoron
Weleda, Aust.; Weleda, Ger.
A range of homoeopathic preparations.

Pneumogeine *Labomed, Fr.*
Theophylline sodium acetate (p.783·2).
Formerly contained theophylline, caffeine, potassium iodide, and sodium benzoate.
Asthma; obstructive airways disease.

Pneumogenol *Monot, Fr.*
Codeine (p.25·2).

Pneumolat *Farmion, Braz.*
Salbutamol sulfate (p.770·3).
Obstructive airways disease.

Pneumolat Expectorante *Farmion, Braz.*
Salbutamol sulfate (p.770·3); guaifenesin (p.1092·2).
Obstructive airways disease.

Pneumomist *ECR, USA.*
Guaifenesin (p.1092·2).

Pneumopan
Note.This name is used for preparations of different composition.
Gebro, Aust.
Thyme (p.1672·2); equisetum (p.1606·3); plantago lanceolata; sulfogaiacol (p.1101·1).
Coughs.

SmithKline Beecham Sante, Fr.
Codeine (p.25·2); chlorpheniramine [chlorphenamine] maleate (p.412·1).
Formerly contained codeine, chlorpheniramine [chlorphenamine] maleate, bromoform, and sodium benzoate.
Coughs.

Pneumopect *Gebro, Aust.*
Noscapine (p.1096·1); thyme (p.1672·2); viola.
Coughs.

Pneumopent *Rhone-Poulenc Rorer, Ital.*
Pentamidine isetionate (p.600·1).
Pneumocystis carinii pneumonia.

Pneumoplasme *Augot, Fr.†.*
Black-mustard-flour paper (p.1639·1).
Respiratory-tract congestion.

Pneumoplasme a l'Histamine *Augot, Fr.†.*
Black-mustard-flour paper (p.1639·1); histamine dihydrochloride (p.1619·2).
Respiratory-tract congestion.

Pneumopur *Chiron Behring, Ger.*
A pneumococcal vaccine (capsular polysaccharide, 23-valent) (p.1557·2).
Active immunisation.

Pneumorel
Eutherapie, Belg.†; Eutherapie, Fr.; Servier, Hong Kong; Stroder, Ital.; Servier, Port.
Fenspiride hydrochloride (p.765·3).
Respiratory-tract disorders.

Pneumotussin HC *ECR, USA.*
Hydrocodone tartrate (p.42·2); guaifenesin (p.1092·2).
Coughs.

The symbol † denotes a preparation no longer actively marketed

Pneumovax *Merck Sharp & Dohme, Aust.†; Pasteur Merieux, Denm.; Meda, Fin.; Pasteur Merieux, Norw.; Pasteur Merieux, Swed.*
A pneumococcal vaccine (23-valent) (p.1557·2).
Active immunisation.

Pneumovax II *Aventis, Irl.; Pasteur Merieux, UK.*
A pneumococcal vaccine (23-valent) (p.1557·2).
Active immunisation.

Pneumovax 23 *Merck Sharp & Dohme, Austral.; Pasteur Merieux, Belg.; Merck Frosst, Canad.; Pasteur Merieux, Ger.; Merck Sharp & Dohme, Hong Kong; Merck Sharp & Dohme, Israel; Pasteur Merieux, Neth.; Merck Sharp & Dohme, S.Afr.; Merck Sharp & Dohme, Singapore; Pro Vaccine, Switz.; Merck Sharp & Dohme, Thai.; Merck, USA.*
A pneumococcal vaccine (23-valent) (p.1557·2).
Active immunisation.

Pneumune *Wyeth Lederle, Belg.; Lederle, Neth.*
A pneumococcal vaccine (23-valent) (p.1557·2).
Active immunisation.

Pnu-Imune *Wyeth, Irl.; Wyeth Lederle, Norw.; Wyeth Lederle, Port.; Wyeth Lederle, Swed.; Wyeth, UK.*
A pneumococcal vaccine (23 valent) (p.1557·2).
Active immunisation.

Pnu-Imune 23 *Wyeth-Ayerst, Canad.; Wyeth Lederle, Fin.; Wyeth, Mex.; Lederle, Switz.; Lederle, USA.*
A pneumococcal vaccine (23-valent) (p.1557·2).
Active immunisation.

Pnu-Inmune *Cyanamid, Spain.*
A pneumococcal vaccine (23-valent) (p.1557·2).
Active immunisation.

P.O. 12 *Boehringer Ingelheim, Fr.*
Enoxolone (p.34·3).
Inflammatory skin disorders.

Po Antisseptico *Bunker, Braz.*
Boric acid (p.1586·1); salicylic acid (p.1122·3); benzoic acid (p.1134·2).
Skin disorders.

Pobrax *Pharmasant, Thai.*
Chlordiazepoxide (p.659·2); clidinium bromide (p.465·1).
Biliary dyskinesia; dysmenorrhoea; dyspepsia; irritable colon; peptic ulcer; ureteric spasm.

Pocin *Polipharm, Thai.*
Erythromycin stearate (p.201·3).
Bacterial infections.

PocketScan *Lifescan, Irl.*
Test for glucose in blood (p.1616·3).

Pockinal *Mauermann, Ger.†*
Hedera helix.
Bronchitis.

Poconeol *Dolisos, Fr.*
A range of homoeopathic preparations.

Pocophage *Pharmasant, Thai.*
Metformin hydrochloride (p.332·3).
Diabetes mellitus.

Pocyl *Lacer, Spain.*
Ibuprofen (p.43·2).
Fever; pain.

Podactin *Reese, USA.*
Cream: Miconazole nitrate (p.391·1).
Topical powder: Tolnaftate (p.395·2).

Podase *Pose, Thai.*
Serrapeptase (p.1662·1).
Inflammation; oedema.

Pod-Ben-25 *C & M, USA.*
Podophyllum resin (p.1121·1).
Warts.

Podertonic *Inkeysa, Spain.*
Ferrocholinate (p.1359·3).
Iron-deficiency anaemia.

Podine *Aspen Consumer, S.Afr.*
Povidone-iodine (p.1155·1).
Mouth and throat disorders; skin infections; wounds.

Podium *Torlan, Spain.*
Diazepam (p.674·3).
Contains pyridoxine hydrochloride.
Alcohol withdrawal syndrome; anxiety; febrile convulsions; insomnia; skeletal muscle spasm.

Podocon *Paddock, USA.*
Podophyllum resin (p.1121·1).
Genital warts.

Podofilia *Bustillos, Mex.*
Podophyllum resin (p.1121·1).
Keratosis; veruccas; warts.

Podofilm *Paladin, Canad.; Pharmascience, Hong Kong; Pharmascience, Singapore.*
Podophyllum resin (p.1121·1).
Warts.

Podofin *Syosset, USA.*
Podophyllum resin (p.1121·1).
Epitheliomatosis; genital warts; keratoses.

Podomexef *Sankyo, Ger.; Sankyo, Switz.*
Cefpodoxime proxetil (p.172·3).
Bacterial infections.

Pofol *Dong Kook, Singapore.*
Propofol (p.1265·3).
General anaesthesia; sedative.

Poikicholan *Lomapharm, Ger.*
Silybum marianum (p.1021·3).
Liver disorders.

Poikigastran N *Lomapharm, Ger.*
Algeldrate (p.1210·3); magnesium hydroxide (p.1233·1).
Gastrointestinal disorders.

Poikigeron *Lomapharm, Ger.*
Procaine hydrochloride; adenosine phosphate; haematoporphyrin; minerals; ginkgo biloba (p.1350·1).
Tonic.

Poikilocard Mono *Lomapharm, Ger.*
Crataegus (p.1600·2).
Cardiac disorders.

Poikiven T *Lomapharm, Ger.*
Homoeopathic preparation.

Point *Trima, Israel.*
Naproxen sodium (p.61·1).
Musculoskeletal, joint, and soft-tissue disorders; pain.

Point-Two *Colgate-Hoyt, USA.*
Sodium fluoride (p.1375·3).
Dental caries prophylaxis.

Poison Antidote Kit *Bowman, USA.*
Combination pack: Syrup, ipecacuanha (p.1093·1); suspension, charcoal (p.1000·2).
Emergency treatment of poisoning.

Poison Ivy/Oak *Hylands, Canad.*
Homoeopathic preparation.

Poladex *Major, USA†.*
Dexchlorpheniramine maleate (p.412·1).
Hypersensitivity reactions.

Polagen *Decomed, Port.*
Grass pollen extract (p.1575·3).
Hyposensitisation.

Polamin *Schering-Plough, Ital.*
Dexchlorpheniramine maleate (p.412·1).
Hypersensitivity reactions.

Polar Ice *Scott, Canad.*
Menthol (p.1632·3).
Musculoskeletal and joint pain.

Polaramin *Aesca, Aust.; Schering-Plough, Denm.; Schering-Plough, Ital.; Schering-Plough, Norw.; Schering-Plough, Swed.*
Dexchlorpheniramine maleate (p.412·1).
Hypersensitivity reactions; pruritus.

Polaramin Espettorante *Schering-Plough, Ital.*
Dexchlorpheniramine maleate (p.412·1); guaifenesin (p.1092·2); pseudoephedrine sulfate (p.1099·3).
Colds; coughs.

Polaramine *Schering-Plough, Austral.; Schering-Plough, Belg.; Schering-Plough, Braz.; Schering, Canad.; Schering-Plough, Fr.; Schering-Plough, Hong Kong; Schering-Plough, Mex.; Schering-Plough, Neth.; Schering-Plough, NZ; Schering-Plough, S.Afr.; Schering-Plough, Singapore; Schering-Plough, Spain; Essex, Switz.; Schering, USA.*
Dexchlorpheniramine maleate (p.412·1).
Hypersensitivity reactions; migraine; pruritus.

Polaramine Expec *Schering-Plough, Mex.*
Dexchlorpheniramine maleate (p.412·1); guaifenesin (p.1092·2); pseudoephedrine sulfate (p.1099·3).
Coughs; rhinitis.

Polaramine Expectorant *Schering-Plough, Belg.; Schering-Plough, Hong Kong; Schering-Plough, Singapore; Schering, USA.*
Dexchlorpheniramine maleate (p.412·1); guaifenesin (p.1092·2); pseudoephedrine sulfate (p.1099·3).
Asthma; cold symptoms; coughs; hay fever; rhinitis.

Polaramine Expectorante *Schering-Plough, Spain.*
Dexchlorpheniramine maleate (p.412·1); guaifenesin (p.1092·2); pseudoephedrine sulfate (p.1099·3).
Upper-respiratory-tract disorders.

Polaramine Pectoral *Schering-Plough, Fr.*
Dexchlorpheniramine maleate (p.412·1); guaifenesin (p.1092·2).
Formerly contained dexchlorpheniramine maleate, pseudoephedrine sulfate, guaifenesin, and sodium benzoate.
Coughs and cold symptoms; respiratory-tract disorders.

Polaramine Topico *Schering-Plough, Spain.*
Allantoin (p.1110·1); dexchlorpheniramine maleate (p.412·1).
Cutaneous hypersensitivity reactions.

Polaratyne *Schering-Plough, S.Afr.*
Loratadine (p.420·1).
Allergic rhinitis; urticaria.

Polaratyne D *Schering-Plough, S.Afr.*
Loratadine (p.420·1); pseudoephedrine sulfate (p.1099·3).
Upper respiratory-tract congestion.

Polaronil
Note.This name is used for preparations of different composition.
Aesca, Aust.; Essex, Ger.
Dexchlorpheniramine maleate (p.412·1).
Hypersensitivity reactions.
Schering-Plough, Belg.
Dexamethasone (p.1067·1); dexchlorpheniramine maleate (p.412·1); ascorbic acid (p.1389·3).
Hypersensitivity reactions.

Polase *Wyeth Lederle, Ital.*
Potassium aspartate hemihydrate (p.1195·2); magnesium aspartate tetrahydrate (p.1190·3).
Potassium and magnesium deficiency.

Polcortolon TC *Medphano, Ger.*
Triamcinolone acetonide (p.1080·1); tetracycline hydrochloride (p.258·3).
Infected skin disorders.

Poledin *Ciba Vision, Spain.*
Sodium cromoglicate (p.774·3).
Eye disorders.

Polery *Veyron-Froment, Fr.*
Paediatric syrup: Pholcodine (p.1099·1); erysimin
Formerly contained ethylmorphine hydrochloride, sodium bromide, sodium benzoate, codeine, belladonna, erysimin, and senega.
Syrup: Codeine (p.25·2); erysimin.
Formerly contained ethylmorphine hydrochloride, sodium bromide, sodium benzoate, codeine, aconite, belladonna, erysimin, senega, and cherry-laurel.
Coughs.

Poli ABE *Vita, Spain.*
Pyridoxine hydrochloride (p.1386·3); placenta extract; vitamin A palmitate (p.1383·2); tocoferil acetate (p.1394·1).
Deficiency of vitamins A and E.

Poli Miner Vit *QIF, Braz.*
Multivitamin and mineral preparation (p.1350·1).

Polial *Plasmon, Ital.; Ultrapharm, UK.*
Food for special diets (p.1350·1).
Egg intolerance; gluten intolerance; milk intolerance.

Poliantib *Alcon Cusi, Spain.*
Chlortetracycline hydrochloride (p.182·1); polymyxin B sulfate (p.238·1).
Bacterial eye infections.

Polibar *E-Z-EM, Belg.; E-Z-EM, Port.; E-Z-EM, UK.*
Barium sulfate (p.1032·1).
Formerly known as Polibar ACB in the UK.
Contrast medium for gastrointestinal radiography.

Polibar ACB *E-Z-EM, Israel; Bracco, Switz.*
Barium sulfate (p.1032·1).
Contrast medium for gastrointestinal radiography.

Polibar Rapid *E-Z-EM, UK.*
Barium sulfate (p.1032·1).
Contrast medium for gastrointestinal radiography.

Polibar Viscous *E-Z-EM, UK.*
Barium sulfate (p.1032·1).
Contrast medium for gastrointestinal radiography.

Polibatrim *Fustery, Mex.*
Co-trimoxazole (p.193·3).
Bacterial infections.

Poliben *Auad, Braz.*
Mebendazole (p.102·2); tiabendazole (p.109·1).
Worm infections.

Polibeta B12 *Ceccarelli, Ital.*
Vitamin B substances (p.1350·1).
Nutritional supplement.

Polibimbi *Searle, Ital.*
Electrolytes (p.1180·1).
Nasal irrigation.

Polibroxol *Polipharm, Thai.*
Ambroxol hydrochloride (p.1084·3).
Respiratory-tract disorders associated with increased or viscous mucus.

Polibutin *Juste, Spain.*
Trimebutine (p.1675·1) or trimebutine maleate (p.1675·1).
Gastrointestinal spasm; nausea and vomiting.

Poli-Cifloxin *Polipharm, Thai.*
Ciprofloxacin (p.182·3).
Bacterial infections.

Policol *Polipharm, Thai.*
Pseudoephedrine hydrochloride (p.1099·2); triprolidine hydrochloride (p.427·2).
Allergic rhinitis; cold symptoms; hay fever.

Policold *Polipharm, Thai.*
Pseudoephedrine hydrochloride (p.1099·2); triprolidine hydrochloride (p.427·2).
Cold symptoms; hay fever; hypersensitivity reactions; nasal congestion.

Policolinosil *Medea, Spain.*
Amino acids (p.1350·1); liver extract; pangamic acid (p.1647·3); ribonucleic acid (p.1657·3); thioctic acid (p.1671·3); inositol (p.1623·3); vitamin B substances (p.1350·1).
Liver disorders; tonic.

Poli-Cycline *Polipharm, Thai.*
Doxycycline hyclate (p.200·1).
Bacterial infections.

Polidasa *Almirall, Spain†.*
Amylase (p.1579·3); cellulase (p.1593·1); dimethicone (p.1249·2); tilactase (p.1673·2); lipase.
Digestive-system disorders.

Polideltaxin *Pharmacos, Mex.*
Dexamethasone (p.1067·1).

Polides *Farmigea, Ital.†.*
Polydeoxyribonucleotide (p.1602·3).
Gynaecological disorders.

Poli-Fibrozil *Polipharm, Thai.*
Gemfibrozil (p.896·2).
Hyperlipidaemias.

Poli-Flunarin *Polipharm, Thai.*
Flunarizine (p.418·2).
Cerebral and peripheral vascular disorders; irritability; memory impairment; migraine; sleep disorders.

Poli-Formin *Polipharm, Thai.*
Metformin hydrochloride (p.332·3).
Diabetes mellitus.

Poliginax *Sintofarma, Braz.*
Neomycin sulfate (p.228·1); polymyxin B (p.238·3); nystatin (p.392·2); tinidazole (p.603·3).
Vulvovaginal infections.

Poliglicol Anti Acne *Kin, Spain.*
Sulfur (p.1123·3); calamine (p.1111·3); resorcinol acetate (p.1122·2); triclosan (p.1159·2); zinc oxide (p.1128·2).
Acne.

Poligot *Polipharm, Thai.*
Dihydroergotamine mesilate (p.450·3).
Hypotension; migraine and other vascular headache.

Poligot-CF *Polipharm, Thai.*
Ergotamine tartrate (p.452·1); caffeine (p.761·3).
Migraine and other vascular headaches.

Polijodurato *Farmigea, Ital.*
Sodium iodide (p.1522·3); potassium iodide (p.1522·3); rubidium iodide (p.1660·1); calcium chloride (p.1188·1).
Cataracts.

Polilevo *Searle, Ital.*
Arginine hydrochloride (p.1353·3); ornithine hydrochloride (p.1374·1); citrulline (p.1357·2).
Formerly contained arginine hydrochloride, ornithine hydrochloride, citrulline, and vitamin B substances.
Liver disorders.

Polilevo N *Taurus, Ger.*
Arginine hydrochloride (p.1353·3); ornithine hydrochloride (p.1374·1); citrulline (p.1357·2).
Liver disorders.

Polimod *Searle, Ital.*
Pidotimod (p.1651·3).
Immunostimulant.

Polimoxil *Legrand, Braz.*
Amoxicillin (p.149·2).
Bacterial infections.

Polimucil *Searle, Ital.*
Carbocisteine (p.1086·3).
Formerly contained carbocisteine and sobrerol.
Respiratory-tract disorders.

Polinazolo *Guieu, Ital.*
Econazole nitrate (p.382·3).
Fungal and Gram-positive bacterial skin infections; vulvovaginal candidiasis.

Polineural *Biotekfarma, Ital.†.*
Citicoline sodium (p.1596·1).
Mental function impairment; parkinsonism.

Polinorm *Zeneca, Aust.*
Atenolol (p.841·3); chlortalidone (p.857·1); hydralazine hydrochloride (p.905·3).
Hypertension.

Polio Sabin *SmithKline Beecham, Ital.; SmithKline Beecham, Mex.; SmithKline Beecham, Thai.*
An oral poliomyelitis vaccine (p.1558·2).
Active immunisation.

Poliodine *Gifrer Barbezat, Fr.*
Povidone-iodine (p.1155·1).
Wound and skin disinfection.

PolioHib *SBL, Swed.*
A poliomyelitis and haemophilus influenzae vaccine.
Active immunisation.

poliomyelan *Feldhoff, Ger.*
Bovine testicular extract (p.1492·1); bovine placental extract.
Musculoskeletal disorders; peripheral circulatory disorders.

Polioral
Sclavo, Israel; Chiron, Ital.; Biovac, S.Afr.; Chiron, Thai.
An oral poliomyelitis vaccine (p.1558·2).
Active immunisation.

Polio-Vaccinol *Procter & Gamble, Ger.†*
An oral poliomyelitis vaccine (p.1558·2).
Active immunisation.

Poliovax-IN *Chiron, Ital.*
An inactivated poliomyelitis vaccine (p.1558·2).
Active immunisation.

Polipirox *Biologici Italia, Ital.*
Piroxicam (p.79·1).
Musculoskeletal and joint disorders.

Poliplex *Bristol-Myers Squibb, Braz.*
Multivitamin and mineral preparation (p.1350·1).

Polipred *Allergan-Frumtost, Braz.*
Prednisolone acetate (p.1078·1); neomycin sulfate (p.228·1); polymyxin B sulfate (p.238·1); polyvinyl alcohol (p.1503·1).
Infected eye disorders.

Poliptal *Sydenham, Ital.*
Pipenzolate (p.472·2).

Poli-Relaxane *Polipharm, Thai.*
Orphenadrine citrate (p.470·3); paracetamol (p.71·2).
Musculoskeletal pain; tension headache.

Polireumin *TRB, Braz.*
Sodium hyaluronate (p.1620·1).
Osteoarthritis.

Poliroxin *Polipharm, Thai.*
Roxithromycin (p.247·2).
Bacterial infections.

Polisan *Milana, Ital.*
Benzalkonium chloride (p.1133·2).
Surface disinfection.

Polised *Searle, Ital.*
Sulfogaiacol (p.1101·1); dextromethorphan hydrobromide (p.1087·3).
Coughs.

Polisilan Gel *Upsamedica, Spain†.*
Aluminium hydroxide (p.1210·3); dimethicone (p.1249·2); sorbitol (p.1377·3).
Gastrointestinal hyperacidity and flatulence.

Polisilon *Upsamedica, Ital.*
Aluminium hydroxide (p.1210·3); dimethicone (p.1249·2).
Aerophagia; gastrointestinal disorders associated with hyperacidity.

Polistin Pad *Trommsdorff, Ger.*
Carbinoxamine maleate (p.411·1).
Hypersensitivity reactions.

Polistin T-Caps *Trommsdorff, Ger.*
Carbinoxamine maleate (p.411·1).
Hypersensitivity reactions.

Polisulfade *Sanobia, Port.*
Polymyxin B sulfate (p.238·1); bacitracin zinc (p.155·2).
Skin infections.

Politelmin *Gilton, Braz.*
Mebendazole (p.102·2).
Worm infections.

Politifen *Polipharm, Thai.*
Ketotifen fumarate (p.767·2).
Asthma; bronchitis; hypersensitivity reactions.

Politosse *Searle, Ital.*
Cloperastine fendizoate (p.1087·2).
Coughs.

Poli-Uretic *Polipharm, Thai.*
Amiloride hydrochloride (p.835·1); hydrochlorothiazide (p.907·3).
Hepatic cirrhosis; hypertension; oedema.

Polivitaminico *CPH, Port.*
Multivitamin preparation (p.1350·1).

Poliwit *Radiumfarma, Ital.*
Multivitamin and mineral preparation (p.1350·1).

Polixan *Polipharm, Thai.*
Carisoprodol (p.1327·1); paracetamol (p.71·2).
Muscle pain and spasm.

Polixima *Sifarma, Ital.†.*
Cefuroxime sodium (p.178·2).
Bacterial infections.

Polixin *Sophia, Mex.*
Eye drops: Polymyxin B sulfate (p.238·1); neomycin sulfate (p.228·1); gramicidin (p.213·3).
Eye ointment: Polymyxin B sulfate (p.238·1); neomycin sulfate (p.228·1); bacitracin zinc (p.155·2).
Bacterial eye infections.

Polizep *Polipharm, Thai.*
Dipotassium clorazepate (p.670·3).
Anxiety; insomnia.

Pollalin *Hal, Neth.†.*
Grass pollen allergen extracts(p.1575·3).
Hyposensitisation.

Pollcapsan M *Alsitan, Ger.†.*
Pollen.
Tonic.

Pollen Royal *Ido, Fr.*
Pollen; propolis (p.1655·1); royal jelly (p.1659·3).
Nutritional supplement.

Pollenase Allergy *Peach, UK.*
Sodium cromoglicate (p.774·3).
Allergic eye disorders.

Pollenase Antihistamine *Peach, UK.*
Chlorpheniramine [chlorphenamine] (p.412·2).
Hypersensitivity reactions.

Pollenase Hayfever *Peach, UK.*
Beclometasone dipropionate (p.1061·2).
Hayfever.

Pollen-B *Wassen, UK.*
Pollen; dolomite.

Pollenna *Nelson, UK.*
Homoeopathic preparation.

Pollinex
Stallergenes, Belg.; Artu, Neth.; Allergy Therapeutics, UK.
Grass or tree pollen allergen extracts (p.1575·3).
Hyposensitisation.

Pollinex Quattro *Bencard, Ger.*
Pollen extracts(p.1575·3).
Hyposensitisation.

Pollinex-R *Bencard, Canad.*
Aqueous extract of short ragweed pollen(p.1575·3).
Hyposensitisation to ragweed pollen.

Pollingel *Bracco, Ital.*
Pollen; royal jelly (p.1659·3).
Nutritional supplement.

Pollingel con Ginkgo Biloba *Bracco, Ital.*
Pollen; ginkgo biloba (p.1615·2).
Nutritional supplement.

Pollinil *Dolisos, Canad.*
Homoeopathic preparation.

Pollinosan
Bioforce, Austral.; Bioforce, Switz.
Homoeopathic preparation.

Pollinose S *Alsitan, Ger.*
Pollen.
Pollen hypersensitivity.

Pollon-eze *Johnson & Johnson MSD Consumer, UK†.*
Astemizole (p.409·1).
Hay fever; urticaria.

Pollonis *Janssen-Cilag, Aust.†.*
Astemizole (p.409·1).
Hay fever.

Pollstimol *Strathmann, Ger.†.*
Grass pollen extracts.
Benign prostatic hyperplasia.

Pollyferm *Nordic, Swed.*
Sodium cromoglicate (p.774·3).
Allergic rhinitis and conjunctivitis.

Polocaine
AstraZeneca, Canad.; AstraZeneca, USA.
Mepivacaine hydrochloride (p.1317·1).
Corbadrine (p.1599·2) or corbadrine hydrochloride (p.1599·2) is included in some injections as a vasoconstrictor to diminish absorption and localise the effect of the local anaesthetic.
Local anaesthesia.

Poloral *Berna, Switz.†.*
An oral poliomyelitis vaccine (p.1558·2).
Active immunisation.

Poloren *Loren, Mex.*
Dipyrone (p.34·1).
Fever; inflammation; pain.

Poloris *Block, Ger.*
Coal tar (p.1125·1); allantoin (p.1110·1).
Psoriasis.

Poloris HC *Block, Ger.†.*
Coal tar (p.1125·1); allantoin (p.1110·1); hydrocortisone (p.1073·3).
Psoriasis.

Polvac *Teomed, Switz.*
Pollen allergen extracts (p.1575·3).
Hyposensitisation.

Polvos Wilfe *Calmante Vitaminado, Spain.*
Sulfanilamide (p.256·2); sulfathiazole (p.257·1).
Skin infections.

Poly Gel *Alcon, Austral.*
Carbomer (p.1499·2).
Dry eyes; eye irritation.

Poly Pred *Allergan, Spain.*
Neomycin sulfate (p.228·1); polymyxin B sulfate (p.238·1); prednisolone acetate (p.1078·1).
Infected eye disorders.

Poly Visc *Ioquin, Austral.*
Paraffin (p.1407·3); wool fat (p.1410·3).
Dry eyes.

Polyanion *Sigmapharm, Aust.*
Pentosan polysulfate sodium (p.953·1).
Hyperlipidaemias; thromboembolic disorders.

Polybactrin
Glaxo Wellcome, Aust.†; Wellcome, Irl.†.
Neomycin sulfate (p.228·1); polymyxin B sulfate (p.238·1); bacitracin (p.155·2) or bacitracin zinc (p.155·2).
Infected skin lesions.

Polybamycin *Shin Poong, Singapore.*
Bacitracin (p.155·2); neomycin sulfate (p.228·1); polymyxin B sulfate (p.238·1).
Bacterial skin infections.

Polybee *Chew, Thai.*
Vitamin B substances with yeast (p.1350·1).

Polybion
Merck, Fin.; Bracco, Ital.†; Meda, Swed.†.
Vitamin B substances (p.1350·1).
Alcoholism; polyneuropathy; vitamin B deficiency.

Polybion Forte *Merck, Ger.*
Vitamin B substances (p.1350·1).
Vitamin B deficiency.

Polybion N *Merck, Ger.*
Vitamin B substances (p.1350·1).
Vitamin B deficiency.

Polycal
Nutricia, Austral.; Nutricia, Irl.; Baxter, NZ; Nutricia, NZ; Nutricia Clinical, UK.
Food for special diets (p.1350·1).
Formerly known as Fortical in the *UK.*

Polycare *Alcon, Fr.*
Sodium dichloroisocyanurate (p.1156·1)(p.1129·2).
Soft contact-lens cleanser.

Polycidin *Ciba Vision, Canad.*
Eye ointment: Bacitracin zinc (p.155·2); polymyxin B sulfate (p.238·1).
Eye infections.
Eye/ear drops: Gramicidin (p.213·3); polymyxin B sulfate (p.238·1).
Eye and ear infections.

Polycillin *Apothecon, USA†.*
Ampicillin trihydrate (p.151·1).
Bacterial infections.

Polycillin-N *Apothecon, USA†.*
Ampicillin sodium (p.150·3).
Bacterial infections.

Polycillin-PRB *Apothecon, USA†.*
Ampicillin trihydrate (p.151·1).
Probenecid (p.401·3) is included in this preparation to reduce renal tubular excretion of ampicillin.
Bacterial infections.

Polycin *Nakornpatana, Thai.*
Nitrofurazone (p.231·3).
Burns; skin ulcers; wound infections.

Polycin-B *Ocusoft, USA.*
Bacitracin zinc (p.155·2); polymyxin B sulfate (p.238·1).
Bacterial eye infections.

Polycitra *Alza, USA.*
Potassium citrate (p.1186·1); sodium citrate (p.1186·2); citric acid monohydrate (p.1596·2).
Chronic metabolic acidosis; urine alkalinising agent.

Polycitra-K
Note.This name is used for preparations of different composition.
Alza, Canad.
Potassium citrate (p.1186·1).
Hypokalaemia.
Alza, USA.
Potassium citrate (p.1186·1); citric acid monohydrate (p.1596·2).
Chronic metabolic acidosis; urine alkalinising agent.

Polycitra-LC *Alza, USA.*
Potassium citrate (p.1186·1); sodium citrate (p.1186·2); citric acid monohydrate (p.1596·2).
Chronic metabolic acidosis; urine alkalinising agent.

Polyclean *Alcon, Fr.*
Cleansing solution for contact lenses (p.1129·2).

Polycleans *Alcon, Braz.*
Cleaning solution for contact lenses (p.1129·2).

Polyclens
Alcon, Austral.; Alcon, Mex.; Alcon, NZ.
Cleaning solution for contact lenses (p.1129·2).

Polyclox *Siam Bheasach, Thai.*
Ampicillin (p.150·3); cloxacillin (p.192·1).
Bacterial infections.

Polycolvit *Pharmasant, Thai.*
Ferrous fumarate (p.1360·1); vitamin B substances; vitamin C; calcium phosphate (p.1350·1).
Anaemias; vitamin B and C deficiency.

Polycose
Abbott, Austral.; Abbott, Canad.; Abbott, Fin.; Abbott, Hong Kong; Ross, Israel; Abbott, Ital.; Abbott, NZ; Abbott Nutrition, UK; Ross, USA.
Glucose polymers (p.1350·1).
Nutritional carbohydrate supplement.

Polycrol *Zurich, S.Afr.†.*
Aluminium hydroxide (p.1210·3); light magnesium oxide (p.1233·1); simeticone (p.1249·2).
Gastrointestinal hyperacidity.

Polycutan *Agis, Israel.*
Clotrimazole (p.382·1); dexamethasone acetate (p.1067·1); neomycin sulfate (p.228·1).
Infected skin disorders.

Polyderm *Taro, Canad.*
Bacitracin zinc (p.155·2); polymyxin B sulfate (p.238·1).
Burns; minor wounds.

Polydex *Pharmasant, Thai.*
Note. A similar name is used for preparations of different composition (see below).
Dextromethorphan hydrobromide (p.1087·3).
Coughs.

Poly-Dex *Ocusoft, USA.*
Note. A similar name is used for preparations of different composition (see above).
Dexamethasone (p.1067·1); neomycin sulfate (p.228·1); polymyxin B sulfate (p.238·1).
Infected eye disorders.

Polydexa
Therabel, Belg.; Bouchara, Fr.; Neo-Farmaceutica, Port.; Bouchara, Singapore; Bouchara, Switz.
Neomycin sulfate (p.228·1); polymyxin B sulfate (p.238·1); dexamethasone sodium metasulfobenzoate (p.1067·1).
Infected eye and ear disorders.

Polydexa a la Phenylephrine *Bouchara, Fr.*
Neomycin sulfate (p.228·1); polymyxin B sulfate (p.238·1); dexamethasone sodium metasulfobenzoate (p.1067·1); phenylephrine hydrochloride (p.1097·1).
Nose and throat disorders.

Polydiet *DHN, Fr.*
Preparation for enteral nutrition (p.1350·1).

Polydine
Note.This name is used for preparations of different composition.
Fischer, Israel; Century, USA.
Povidone-iodine (p.1155·1).
Skin and vaginal infections; skin disinfection.
Pharmasant, Thai.
Dextromethorphan hydrobromide (p.1087·3); brompheniramine maleate (p.410·2); phenylephrine hydrochloride (p.1097·1); ammonium chloride (p.1085·2).
Coughs.

Polydol *Pharmasant, Thai.*
Orphenadrine citrate (p.470·3); paracetamol (p.71·2).
Dysmenorrhoea; muscle pain; tension headache.

Polydona *Hexal, Ger.*
Povidone-iodine (p.1155·1).
Burns; skin ulcers; wounds.

Polyenzyme-I *Chew, Thai.*
Amylase (p.1579·3); papain (p.1647·3); pancreatin (p.1646·1); vitamin B substances (p.1350·1); diphenhydramine hydrochloride (p.416·1); homatropine methylbromide (p.468·1); simeticone (p.1249·2); activated charcoal (p.1000·2).
Digestive disorders.

Polyenzyme-N *Chew, Thai.*
Pancreatin (p.1646·1); simeticone (p.1249·2).
Digestive disorders.

Polyerga *Hor-Fer-Vit, Ger.*
Polypeptides derived from spleen.
Adjuvant tumour therapy.

Polyfax
Glaxo Wellcome, Hong Kong; Glaxo Wellcome, Irl.; Dominion, UK.
Polymyxin B sulfate (p.238·1); bacitracin zinc (p.155·2).
Bacterial infections of the skin and eye.

Polyfra *Alcon, Fr.*
Eye drops: Framycetin sulfate (p.208·2); polymyxin B sulfate (p.238·1); oxedrine hydrochloride (p.950·3).
Eye ointment: Framycetin sulfate (p.208·2); polymyxin B sulfate (p.238·1).
Formerly contained muramidase hydrochloride, framycetin sulfate, and polymyxin B sulfate.
Bacterial eye infections.

Polygam *NBI, S.Afr.; American Red Cross, USA.*
A normal immunoglobulin (p.1551·3).
Hypogammaglobulinaemia.

Polyglobin
Bayer, Spain; Bayer, Swed.
A normal immunoglobulin (p.1551·3).
Guillain-Barré syndrome; hypogammaglobulinaemia; idiopathic thrombocytopenic purpura; Kawasaki syndrome.

Polyglobin N *Bayer, Ger.†.*
A normal immunoglobulin (p.1551·3).
Hypogammaglobulinaemia; idiopathic thrombocytopenic purpura; passive immunisation.

Polygot *Pharmasant, Thai.*
Ergotamine tartrate (p.452·1); caffeine (p.761·3).
Migraine and other vascular headaches.

Polygynax
Darci, Belg.; Innothera, Fr.; UCB, Ger.; Innotech, Hong Kong; UCB, Port.; Innotech, Singapore.
Neomycin (p.228·1) or neomycin sulfate (p.228·1); nystatin (p.392·2); polymyxin B sulfate (p.238·1).
Vulvovaginal and cervical infections.

Polygynax Virgo *Innothera, Fr.*
Neomycin sulfate (p.228·1); nystatin (p.392·2); polymyxin B sulfate (p.238·1).
Vulvovaginitis.

Poly-Gynedron *Interpharm, S.Afr.†.*
Sulfisomidine (p.257·1); acetarsol sodium (p.587·2); borax (p.1586·1); diethylstilbestrol dipropionate (p.1471·2).
Vaginal infections.

Polyhadol *Pharmasant, Thai.*
Haloperidol (p.686·3).
Alcoholism; schizophrenia.

Poly-Histine *Sanofi Winthrop, USA.*
Phenyltoloxamine citrate (p.423·1); mepyramine maleate (p.421·1); pheniramine maleate (p.422·3).
Allergic rhinitis.

Poly-Histine CS *Sanofi Winthrop, USA†.*
Codeine phosphate (p.25·2); phenylpropanolamine hydrochloride (p.1098·1); brompheniramine maleate (p.410·2).
Coughs and cold symptoms.

Poly-Histine D *Sanofi Winthrop, USA†.*
Phenylpropanolamine hydrochloride (p.1098·1); phenyltoloxamine citrate (p.423·1); mepyramine maleate (p.421·1); pheniramine maleate (p.422·3).
Allergic rhinitis; nasal congestion.

Poly-Histine DM *Sanofi Winthrop, USA†.*
Dextromethorphan hydrobromide (p.1087·3); phenylpropanolamine hydrochloride (p.1098·1); brompheniramine maleate (p.410·2).
Coughs and cold symptoms.

Poly-Iron *Cypress, USA.*
Polysaccharide-iron complex (p.1374·3).
Iron deficiency.

Poly-Iron Forte *Cypress, USA.*
Polysaccharide-iron complex (p.1374·3); folic acid (p.1361·2); cyanocobalamin (p.1388·1).
Iron-deficiency anaemia; megaloblastic anaemia.

Poly-Joule *Sharpe, Austral.*
Dextrin (p.1359·1).
Nutritional supplement.

Poly-Karaya *Synthelabo, Fr.; Kramer, Switz.*
Sterculia (p.1250·2); povidone (p.1503·2).
Constipation; diarrhoea; meteorism.

Polymox *Mead Johnson, Mex.; Apothecon, USA†.*
Amoxicillin trihydrate (p.149·2).
Bacterial infections.

Polymycin *Medical Ophthalmics, USA.*
Eye drops: Neomycin (p.228·1); polymyxin B (p.238·3); gramicidin (p.213·3).
Eye ointment: Neomycin (p.228·1); polymyxin B (p.238·3); bacitracin (p.155·2).
Eye infections.

Polyoph *Seng, Thai.*
Neomycin sulfate (p.228·1); polymyxin B sulfate (p.238·1); gramicidin (p.213·3).
Bacterial eye infections.

Polypharm-Zahnungsgel N *Polypharm, Ger.†.*
Sage (p.1660·2); lignocaine [lidocaine] hydrochloride (p.1313·2).
Toothache.

Polyphed *Pharmasant, Thai.*
Theophylline (p.777·2); guaifenesin (p.1092·2).
Obstructive airways disease.

Polypirine *Lehning, Fr.*
Aspirin (p.14·2); caffeine citrate (p.761·3); meadowsweet (p.1631·2).
Formerly contained propyphenazone, phenicarbazide, phenacetin, caffeine citrate, cinnamon, ipecacuanha, and squill.
Fever; pain.

Polypred *Pharmasant, Thai.*
Note. *A similar name is used for preparations of different composition (see below).*
Prednisolone (p.1077·3).
Skin disorders.

Poly-Pred *Allergan, USA.*
Note. *A similar name is used for preparations of different composition (see above).*
Prednisolone acetate (p.1078·1); neomycin sulfate (p.228·1); polymyxin B sulfate (p.238·1).
Eye inflammation with bacterial infection.

Polypress
Note.This name is used for preparations of different composition.
Pfizer, Ger.
Prazosin hydrochloride (p.958·1); polythiazide (p.957·1).
Hypertension.

Pharmasant, Thai.
Prazosin hydrochloride (p.958·1).
Hypertension.

Polyrinse *Alcon, Fr.*
Sodium chloride (p.1196·1) (p.1129·2).
Rinsing and soaking solution for contact lenses.

Polyrinse Desinfektionssystem *Alcon, Aust.*
Sodium dichloroisocyanurate (p.1156·1)(p.1129·2).
Disinfection and rinsing of soft contact lenses.

Polyrinse-Aufnahmelosung *Alcon, Aust.*
Sodium chloride (p.1196·1)(p.1129·2).
Storage solution for soft contact lenses.

Polyrinse-Augenelement *Alcon, Aust.*
Sodium chloride (p.1196·1)(p.1129·2); boric acid (p.1586·1).
Comfort drops for contact lenses.

Poly-Rivitin *Clinced, Aust.*
Multivitamin preparation (p.1350·1).

Polysept *Dermapharm, Ger.*
Povidone-iodine (p.1155·1).
Bladder catheterisation; burns; skin and mucous membrane disinfection; skin ulcers; wounds.

Polyseptol *Qualiphar, Belg.*
Filtrate from culture of: *Staphylococcus aureus, Streptococcus pyogenes, Pseudomonas aeruginosa,* and *Escherichia coli;* sulfanilamide (p.256·2); cod-liver oil (p.1357·2).
Infected skin disorders.

Polysilane
Note.This name is used for preparations of different composition.
Synthelabo, Hong Kong; Sanofi Synthelabo, Singapore; Sanofi Synthelabo, Thai.
Aluminium hydroxide (p.1210·3); dimethicone (p.1249·2).
Dyspepsia; flatulence; gastritis; heartburn; pyrosis.

Upsamedica, Switz.
Dimethicone (p.1249·2).
Gastrointestinal disorders.

Polysilane Delalande *Synthelabo, Fr.*
Aluminium hydroxide (p.1210·3); simeticone (p.1249·2).
Gastrointestinal disorders.

Polysilane Joullie *Synthelabo, Fr.*
Chewable tablets/lozenges†: Simeticone (p.1249·2); aluminium hydroxide (p.1210·3).
Gastrointestinal disorders.
Paediatric oral granules: Simeticone (p.1249·2); ceratonia (p.1500·3).
Gastro-oesophageal reflux.

Polysilon *Upsamedica, Belg.*
Dimethicone (p.1249·2).
Gastrointestinal disorders associated with hyperacidity.

Polysorb *Fougera, USA.*
Emollient and moisturiser.

Polyspectran
Note.This name is used for preparations of different composition.
Alcon, Ger.; Thilo, Hong Kong.
Eye and ear drops: Polymyxin B sulfate (p.238·1); neomycin sulfate (p.228·1); gramicidin (p.213·3).
Bacterial infections of the eye and ear.

Alcon-Thilo, Ger.; Thilo, Hong Kong.
Ointment: Polymyxin B sulfate (p.238·1); bacitracin (p.155·2); neomycin sulfate (p.228·1).
Bacterial infections of the eye, ear, and nose.

Polyspectran B *Thilo, Neth.†*
Neomycin sulfate (p.228·1); polymyxin B sulfate (p.238·1); bacitracin (p.155·2).
Bacterial eye infections.

Polyspectran G *Thilo, Neth.†*
Neomycin sulfate (p.228·1); gramicidin (p.213·3); polymyxin B sulfate (p.238·1).
Bacterial eye infections.

Polyspectran HC *Alcon, Ger.*
Polymyxin B sulfate (p.238·1); bacitracin (p.155·2); hydrocortisone acetate (p.1073·3).
Bacterial and inflammatory eye disorders; otitis media; skin disorders.

Polysporin
Note.This name is used for preparations of different composition.
Warner-Lambert, Canad.
Cream; eye/ear drops: Polymyxin B sulfate (p.238·1); gramicidin (p.213·3).

Eye ointment; ointment: Polymyxin B sulfate (p.238·1); bacitracin (p.155·2).
Eye and ear infections; infected lesions.

Glaxo Wellcome, Fin.
Polymyxin B sulfate (p.238·1); neomycin sulfate (p.228·1); gramicidin (p.213·3).
Eye infections.

Glaxo Wellcome, S.Afr.
Polymyxin B sulfate (p.238·1); bacitracin zinc (p.155·2).
Burns; skin infections; wounds.

Warner-Lambert, USA; Monarch, USA.
Polymyxin B sulfate (p.238·1); bacitracin (p.155·2) or bacitracin zinc (p.155·2).
Eye infections; skin infections.

Polysporin Plus Pain Relief *Warner-Lambert, Canad.*
Polymyxin B sulfate (p.238·1); gramicidin (p.213·3); lignocaine [lidocaine] hydrochloride (p.1313·2).
Formerly known as Polysporin Burn Formula.
Infected burns; skin pain.

Polysporin Triple Antibiotic *Warner-Lambert, Canad.*
Polymyxin B sulfate (p.238·1); bacitracin (p.155·2); gramicidin (p.213·3).
Burns; minor wounds.

Polysporina *Wellcome, Port.†*
Polymyxin B sulfate (p.238·1); neomycin sulfate (p.228·1); gramicidin (p.213·3).
Eye infections.

Polytab *Pharmasant, Thai.*
Cyproheptadine hydrochloride (p.414·2).
Hypersensitivity reactions; pruritus; reduced appetite.

Polytabs-F *Major, USA.*
Multivitamin preparation with fluoride (p.1350·1)(p.1375·3).
Dental caries prophylaxis; dietary supplement.

Polytanol *Pharmasant, Thai.*
Amitriptyline hydrochloride (p.273·3).
Depression.

Polytar
Note.This name is used for preparations of different composition.
Stiefel, Austral.; Stiefel, Ger.; Stiefel, Hong Kong; Stiefel, Irl.; Stiefel, Israel; Stiefel, Mex.; Stiefel, NZ; Stiefel, S.Afr.; Stiefel, Singapore; Stiefel, Thai.
Tar (p.1125·1); cade oil (p.1124·3); coal tar (p.1125·1).
Skin and scalp disorders.

Stiefel, Canad.; Stiefel, Ital.†.
Wood tar (p.1125·1); mineral tar (p.1125·1).
Seborrhoeic dermatitis.

Stiefel, Spain.
Tar (p.1125·1); juniper oil (p.1625·2); coal tar (p.1125·1).
Skin and scalp disorders.

Stiefel, USA.
Coal tar solution; crude coal tar (p.1125·1).
Scalp and skin disorders.

Polytar AF
Note.This name is used for preparations of different composition.
Stiefel, Canad.
Coal tar (p.1125·1); pyrithione disulfide (p.1122·1); salicylic acid (p.1122·3); menthol (p.1632·3).
Scalp disorders.

Stiefel, UK.
Tar (p.1125·1); cade oil (p.1124·3); coal tar (p.1125·1); pyrithione zinc (p.1122·1).
Scalp disorders.

Polytar Emollient
Stiefel, Irl.; Stiefel, NZ; Stiefel, UK.
Tar (p.1125·1); cade oil (p.1124·3); coal tar (p.1125·1); liquid paraffin (p.1407·1).
Aid to ointment and paste removal in psoriasis; skin disorders.

Polytar Liquid *Stiefel, UK.*
Tar (p.1125·1); cade oil (p.1124·3); coal tar (p.1125·1).
Aid to ointment and paste removal in psoriasis; scalp disorders.

Polytar Plus
Stiefel, Hong Kong; Stiefel, Irl.†; Stiefel, NZ; Stiefel, UK.
Tar (p.1125·1); cade oil (p.1124·3); coal tar (p.1125·1).
Aid to ointment removal in psoriasis; scalp disorders.

Poly-Tears
Alcon, Austral.; Ioquin, Austral.; Alcon, NZ.
Hypromellose (p.1501·3); dextran 70 (p.729·2).
Dry eyes.

Polytinic *Pharmics, USA†.*
Ferrous fumarate (p.1360·1); folic acid (p.1361·1).
Ascorbic acid (p.1389·3) is included in this preparation to improve the absorption and availability of iron.

Polytonyl
Upsamedica, Belg.; UPSA, Fr.; Upsamedica, Switz.
Vitamin, mineral, and amino-acid preparation (p.1350·1).

Polytopic *Technilab, Canad.*
Cream: Polymyxin B sulfate (p.238·1); gramicidin (p.213·3).

Ointment: Polymyxin B sulfate (p.238·1); bacitracin (p.155·2).
Infected lesions.

Polytracin
Metapharma, Canad.†; Medical Ophthalmics, USA.
Bacitracin (p.155·2) or bacitracin zinc (p.155·2); polymyxin B (p.238·3).
Eye infections.

Polytrim
Glaxo Wellcome, Aust.; Glaxo Wellcome, Belg.; Allergan, Canad.; Glaxo Wellcome, Neth.; Glaxo Wellcome, S.Afr.; Dominion, UK; Allergan, USA.
Trimethoprim (p.264·2) or trimethoprim sulfate (p.265·3); polymyxin B sulfate (p.238·1).
Bacterial infections of the eyes and skin.

Polyvalent Snake Antivenom *CSL, Austral.*
A snake antiserum of king brown snake, tiger snake, brown snake, death adder, and taipan (p.1563·3).
Passive immunisation.

Poly-Vi-Flor
Mead Johnson Nutritionals, Canad.; Mead Johnson Nutritionals, Thai.; Mead Johnson Nutritionals, USA.
A range of vitamin preparations with fluoride (p.1350·1)(p.1375·3).
Dental caries prophylaxis; dietary supplement.

Poly-Vi-Fluor *Bristol-Myers Squibb, Braz.*
Multivitamin preparation (p.1350·1) with fluoride (p.1375·3).
Dietary supplement.

Poly-Vi-Sol
Mead Johnson Nutritionals, Canad.; Mead Johnson, Hong Kong; Mead Johnson Nutritionals, Thai.; Mead Johnson Nutritionals, USA.
A range of vitamin preparations (p.1350·1).

Polyvit
Note.This name is used for preparations of different composition.
Taro, Israel.
Oral drops: Multivitamin preparation (p.1350·1).
Tablets: Multivitamin and mineral preparation with ginseng (p.1350·1).

Propan, S.Afr.†.
Multivitamin preparation (p.1350·1).

Pharmasant, Thai.
Ferrous fumarate (p.1360·1); riboflavin; vitamin C; folic acid; citric acid (p.1350·1).
Anaemias; vitamin supplement.

Polyvit 30 Plus *Taro, Israel.*
Multivitamin and mineral preparation with ginseng and rutoside (p.1350·1).

Polyvita *Piette, Belg.†.*
Multivitamin, mineral, and amino-acid preparation (p.1350·1).

Poly-Vitamin Plus *Chephasaar, Ger.†.*
Multivitamin and mineral preparation (p.1350·1).

Polyxan *Ritsert, Ger.*
A range of homoeopathic preparations.

Polyxen *Pharmasant, Thai.*
Naproxen (p.60·3).
Gout; musculoskeletal and joint disorders.

Polyxicam *Pharmasant, Thai.*
Piroxicam (p.79·1).
Gout; musculoskeletal and joint disorders.

Polyxit *Pharmasant, Thai.*
Gemfibrozil (p.896·2).
Hyperlipidaemias.

Polyzalip *Pharmasant, Thai.*
Bezafibrate (p.849·1).
Hyperlipidaemias.

Polyzym
Alcon, Aust.; Alcon, Austral.; Alcon, Braz.; Alcon, Fr.; Alcon, Mex.; Alcon, NZ.
Pancreatin (p.1646·1)(p.1129·2).
Cleansing of hard and soft contact lenses.

Pomada Antibiotica *Knoll, Spain.*
Bacitracin (p.155·2); neomycin sulfate (p.228·1); polymyxin B sulfate (p.238·1).
Burns; skin infections; ulcers; wounds.

Pomada Balsamica *Alcala, Spain†.*
Camphor (p.1589·3); cedrus deodora oil; eucalyptol (p.1609·2); methyl salicylate (p.55·1); thymol (p.1158·3); turpentine.
Cold symptoms.

Pomada Blumen *Luper, Braz.*
Zinc (p.1398·1); boric acid (p.1586·1); zinc oxide (p.1128·2).
Skin disorders.

Pomada Heridas *Asens, Spain.*
Benzalkonium chloride (p.1133·2); phenazone (p.77·2); sulfanilamide (p.256·2); zinc oxide (p.1128·2).
Skin infections.

Pomada Infantil Vera *Labitec, Spain.*
Bismuth subnitrate (p.1213·2); boric acid (p.1586·1); talc (p.1124·2); zinc oxide (p.1128·2).
Skin irritation.

Pomada Minancora *Minancora, Braz.*
Benzalkonium chloride (p.1133·2); zinc oxide (p.1128·2); camphor (p.1589·3).
Skin disorders.

Pomada Revulsiva *Orravan, Spain†.*
Camphor (p.1589·3); capsicum oleoresin (p.1591·1); eugenol (p.1609·3); methyl salicylate (p.55·1); turpentine oil (p.1676·3).
Musculoskeletal, joint, peri-articular, and soft-tissue disorders.

Pomada Wilfe *Calmante Vitaminado, Spain.*
Sulfanilamide (p.256·2); sulfathiazole (p.257·1).
Skin infections.

Pomaglos *Merck, Port.*
Vitamin A; vitamin D (p.1350·1); cod-liver oil (p.1357·2); zinc oxide (p.1128·2).
Burns; skin irritation; wounds.

Pomaglos Pomada *EMS, Braz.*
Zinc oxide (p.1128·2); boric acid (p.1586·1).
Skin disorders.

Pomalgex *Uniao Quimica, Braz.*
Methacholine chloride (p.1419·3); methyl salicylate (p.55·1); menthol (p.1632·3); thymol (p.1158·3).
Musculoskeletal and joint disorders.

Pomata Midy HC *Maggioni, Ital.†.*
Benzocaine (p.1306·2); hamamelis (p.1618·3); aesculus (p.1574·1); hydrocortisone acetate (p.1073·3).
Anorectal disorders.

Pommade au The des Bois *Valma, Canad.*
Methyl salicylate (p.55·1); camphor (p.1589·3); menthol (p.1632·3); eucalyptol (p.1609·2).

Pommade Lelong *SmithKline Beecham Sante, Fr.†.*
Peru balsam (p.1650·2); sulfapyridine (p.256·3); vitamin A (p.1382·1).
Skin disorders.

Pommade Maurice *Cooperation Pharmaceutique, Fr.*
Yellow mercuric oxide (p.1633·3).
Eye infections.

Pommade Midy *Welcker-Lyster, Canad.*
Amylocaine hydrochloride (p.1306·1); benzocaine (p.1306·2); hamamelis (p.1618·3); aesculus (p.1574·1).
Haemorrhoids.

Pommade Mo Cochon *Tradiphar, Fr.*
Salicylic acid (p.1122·3).
Callus; corns; verrucae.

Pommade nasale Ruedi *Stotzer, Switz.†.*
Camphorated oil; mint oil (p.1636·2).
Nasal dryness.

Pommade Po-Ho N A Vogel *Bioforce, Switz.*
Hypericum (p.290·2); peppermint oil (p.1243·3); hamamelis (p.1618·3); peppermint leaf (p.1243·2); calendula (p.1589·2); lemon oil (p.1628·2).
Catarrh; cold and influenza symptoms; sinus disorders.

Ponac *Aspen Consumer, S.Afr.*
Mefenamic acid (p.51·2).
Musculoskeletal, joint, and soft-tissue disorders; pain.

Ponalar *Godecke, Ger.*
Mefenamic acid (p.51·2).
Inflammation; musculoskeletal, joint, and soft-tissue disorders; pain.

Ponalgic *Antigen, Irl.*
Mefenamic acid (p.51·2).
Menorrhagia; musculoskeletal and joint disorders; pain.

Pondarmett *Pond's, Thai.*
Cimetidine (p.1216·3).
Gastro-oesophageal reflux; peptic ulcer; Zollinger-Ellison syndrome.

Ponderal
Servier, Ital.†; Servier, Neth.†.
Fenfluramine hydrochloride (p.1510·1).
Obesity.

Ponderax *Servier, S.Afr.†.*
Fenfluramine hydrochloride (p.1510·1).
Obesity.

Pondicilina *Whitehall, Braz.*
Cetalkonium chloride (p.1137·1); cetylpyridinium chloride (p.1138·1).
Mouth and throat disorders.

Pondimin *Robins, USA†.*
Fenfluramine hydrochloride (p.1510·1).
Obesity.

Pondnoxcill *Pond's, Thai.*
Amoxicillin trihydrate (p.149·2).
Bacterial infections.

Pondocillin
Merck, Aust.†; Leo, Canad.; Leo, Denm.; Leo, Irl.†; Leo, Norw.; Adcock Ingram, S.Afr.†; Leo, Swed.; Leo, UK†.
Pivampicillin (p.237·2).
Bacterial infections.

Ponds Prevent *Lever Pond's, Canad.*
Cream: Octinoxate (p.1517·3); oxybenzone (p.1518·1).

SPF 15: Octinoxate (p.1517·3); ensulizole (p.1517·2).
Sunscreen.

Pondusvitam *IQB, Braz.*
Buclizine (p.411·1); vitamin B substances (p.1350·1).
Reduced appetite; tonic.

Ponmel *Clonmel, Irl.*
Mefenamic acid (p.51·2).
Pain.

Ponnac *Sriprasit, Thai.*
Mefenamic acid (p.51·2).
Pain.

Ponnesia *Asian Pharm, Thai.*
Mefenamic acid (p.51·2).
Pain.

Ponoxylan
Rhone-Poulenc Rorer, Austral.†; Aventis, NZ.
Polynoxylin (p.1154·2).
Bacterial and fungal skin infections.

Ponstan
Parke, Davis, Austral.; Ache, Braz.; Parke, Davis, Canad.; Parke, Davis, Fin.; Parke, Davis, Hong Kong; Elan, Irl.; Parke, Davis, Mex.; Parke, Davis, NZ; Parke, Davis, Port.; Parke, Davis, S.Afr.; Parke, Davis, Singapore; Parke, Davis, Switz.; Warner-Lambert, Thai.; Elan, UK; Chemidex, UK.
Mefenamic acid (p.51·2).
Dysmenorrhoea; fever; inflammation; menorrhagia; musculoskeletal, joint, peri-articular, and soft-tissue disorders; pain.

Ponstel
Parke-Med, S.Afr.; Parke, Davis, USA.
Mefenamic acid (p.51·2).
Fever; menorrhagia; pain.

Ponstyl *Parke, Davis, Fr.*
Mefenamic acid (p.51·2).
Pain.

Pontalon *Yung Shin, Thai.*
Mefenamic acid (p.51·2).
Pain.

Pontefix *Fimo, Ital.*
Zinc phosphate (p.1398·3).
Cement in dentistry.

Pontiride *Psicofarma, Mex.*
Sulpiride (p.706·1).
Anxiety disorders; schizophrenia; vertigo.

Pontocaine
Sanofi Synthelabo, Canad.; Sanofi Winthrop, Israel; Sanofi Winthrop, USA.
Amethocaine [tetracaine] (p.1305·2) or amethocaine [tetracaine] hydrochloride (p.1305·2).
Local anaesthesia.

Pontuc *Novartis, Aust.; Novartis, Ger.*
Co-dergocrine mesilate (p.1597·3); nifedipine (p.940·1).
Hypertension.

Pontyl *Malaysia Chemist, Singapore.*
Mefenamic acid (p.51·2).
Inflammation; pain.

Pool 8 *Fiori, Ital.*
Amino-acid preparation (p.1350·1).
Nutritional supplement.

Po-Pon-S *Shionogi, USA.*
Multivitamin and mineral preparation (p.1350·1).

POR 8
Ferring, Aust.; Rhone-Poulenc Rorer, Austral.; Sandoz, Ger.†; Aventis, NZ; Ferring, S.Afr.; Ferring, Switz.
Ornipressin (p.1293·3).
Reduction of bleeding during surgery; variceal haemorrhage.

Porazine *Pharmasant, Thai.*
Perphenazine (p.699·1).
Anxiety; nausea and vomiting.

Porcelana *Lavoris-Dep, Canad.; DEP, USA†.*
Hydroquinone (p.1115·1).
Hyperpigmentation.

Porcelana with Sunscreen
Note. This name is used for preparations of different composition.
Lavoris-Dep, Canad.
Hydroquinone (p.1115·1); octinoxate (p.1517·3).
DEP, USA†.
Hydroquinone (p.1115·1); padimate O (p.1518·2).
Hyperpigmentation.

Porcoll *MBP, Ger.*
Collagen (p.1598·2).
Haemorrhage.

Poremax-C *Orion, Fin.*
Ascorbic acid (p.1389·3).
Vitamin C deficiency; vitamin C supplement.

Porfirin 12 *Teofarma, Ital.*
Haematoporphyrin dihydrochloride (p.1618·3); cyanocobalamin (p.1388·1); inositol (p.1623·3).
Tonic.

Pork Actrapid *Novo Nordisk, UK.*
Insulin injection (porcine, highly purified) (p.324·1).
Diabetes mellitus.

Pork Insulatard *Novo Nordisk, UK.*
Isophane insulin injection (porcine, highly purified) (p.324·1).
Diabetes mellitus.

Pork Mixtard 30 *Novo Nordisk, UK.*
Mixture of neutral insulin injection (porcine, highly purified) 30% and isophane insulin injection (porcine, highly purified) 70% (p.324·1).
Formerly known as Mixtard 30/70.
Diabetes mellitus.

Porosis D *Cedar Health, UK.*
Calcium citrate (p.1188·1); magnesium citrate (p.1232·3); boron; vitamin D (p.1391·1).

Porostenina *Savio, Ital.†*
Salcatonin (p.749·3).
Hypercalcaemia; osteoporosis; Paget's disease of bone; reflex sympathetic dystrophy.

Porphyrocin *Medochemie, Hong Kong.*
Erythromycin stearate (p.201·3).
Bacterial infections.

Porriver *Ogna, Ital.*
Trichloroacetic acid (p.1674·3).
Verrucae; warts.

Portagen
Mead Johnson, Austral.; Mead Johnson Nutritionals, Canad.; Mead Johnson Nutritionals, Fin.; Mead Johnson, Hong Kong; Mead Johnson, Irl.; Mead Johnson, NZ; Mead Johnson, Port.; Bristol-Myers Squibb, S.Afr.; Mead Johnson, Singapore; Mead Johnson Nutritionals, USA.
Preparation for enteral nutrition (p.1350·1).
Disorders of fat digestion and absorption.

Portamin *Darrow, Braz.*
Amino-acid infusion (p.1350·1).
Parenteral nutrition.

Portolac
Novartis Consumer, Aust.; Novartis Consumer, Belg.; Novartis Consumer, Ital.; Shinyaku, Jpn.
Lactitol (p.1230·1).
Constipation; liver disorders.

Posalfilin
Norgine, Austral.; Norgine, Hong Kong; Norgine, Irl.; CSL, NZ; Norgine, NZ; Norgine, S.Afr.; Norgine, Singapore; Norgine, UK.
Podophyllum resin (p.1121·1); salicylic acid (p.1122·3).
Warts.

Posanin *Pose, Thai.*
Dipyridamole (p.877·2).
Ischaemic heart disease; thrombosis prophylaxis.

Posdrink *Catarinense, Braz.*
Aspirin (p.14·2); mepyramine (p.421·1); caffeine (p.761·3).

Aluminium hydroxide (p.1210·3) is included in this preparation in an attempt to limit adverse effects on the gastrointestinal mucosa.
Fever; pain.

Pose-Bac *Pose, Thai.*
Benzalkonium chloride (p.1133·2).
Disinfection.

Pose-CM *Pose, Thai.*
Cimetidine (p.1216·3).
Gastro-oesophageal reflux; hypersensitivity reactions; peptic ulcer; Zollinger-Ellison syndrome.

Posecus *Pose, Thai.*
Ambroxol hydrochloride (p.1084·3).
Respiratory-tract disorders associated with increased or viscous mucus.

Posedene *Pose, Thai.*
Piroxicam (p.79·1).
Musculoskeletal and joint disorders.

Pose-Dex *Pose, Thai.*
Glutaral (p.1145·2).
Instrument and surface disinfection.

Posedrine *Lasa, Spain†.*
Beclamide (p.342·2).
Epilepsy.

Poselium *Pose, Thai.*
Domperidone (p.1224·1).
Dyspepsia; nausea and vomiting.

Posicor
Roche, Austral.†; Roche, Irl.†; Roche, Neth.†; Roche, UK†; Roche, USA†.
Mibefradil hydrochloride (p.933·3).
Angina pectoris; hypertension.

Posicycline *Alcon, Fr.*
Oxytetracycline hydrochloride (p.234·1).
Bacterial eye infections.

Posidol *Pharmaland, Thai.*
Mebhydrolin napadisilate (p.420·2).
Hypersensitivity reactions.

Posifenicol *Ursapharm, Ger.*
Azidamfenicol (p.152·3).
Bacterial eye infections.

Posifenicol C *Ursapharm, Ger.*
Chloramphenicol (p.179·1).
Bacterial eye infections.

Posiformin *Ursapharm, Ger.*
Bibrocathol (p.1585·1).
Inflammatory eye disorders.

Posiject
Boehringer Ingelheim, Irl.; Alliance, S.Afr.; Boehringer Ingelheim, UK.
Dobutamine hydrochloride (p.880·2).
Agent for cardiac stress testing; heart failure.

Posilent *Ursapharm, Ger.*
Cytidine.
Muscular, accommodative, and nervous eye disorders.

Posine *Alcon, Fr.*
Oxedrine tartrate (p.950·3); chlorhexidine gluconate (p.1138·2).
Conjunctival irritation.

Posipen *Sanfer, Mex.*
Dicloxacillin sodium (p.199·1).
Bacterial infections.

Positivum *Sanova, Aust.*
Fluoxetine hydrochloride (p.284·2).
Depression; psychoses.

Positon *Iquinosa, Spain.*
Neomycin sulfate (p.228·1); nystatin (p.392·2); triamcinolone (p.1080·1) or triamcinolone acetonide (p.1080·1).
Infected skin disorders.

Posivil *Orion, Fin.*
Aspirin (p.14·2); caffeine (p.761·3); noscapine hydrochloride (p.1096·1); ascorbic acid (p.1389·3).
Cold and influenza symptoms; coughs.

Posmox *Pose, Thai.*
Amoxicillin trihydrate (p.149·2).
Bacterial infections.

Posnac *Pose, Thai.*
Diclofenac sodium (p.30·3).
Musculoskeletal and joint disorders.

Posorutin *Ursapharm, Ger.*
Troxerutin (p.1611·2).
Haemorrhoids; ophthalmic disorders; venous insufficiency.

Postacne *Dermik, Canad.*
Colloidal sulfur (p.1123·3).
Acne; oily skin.

Postacton *Ferring, Swed.†.*
Lypressin (p.1300·1).
Diabetes insipidus; haemorrhage; test of pituitary function.

Postadoxin N *Rodleben, Ger.*
Meclozine hydrochloride (p.420·3).
Motion sickness; nausea; vomiting.

Postadoxine *UCB, Belg.*
Meclozine (p.420·3); vitamin B₆ (p.1386·3).
Nausea and vomiting.

Postafen
Note. This name is used for preparations of different composition.
Rhodia, Braz.
Buclizine hydrochloride (p.411·1).
Reduced appetite.
UCB, Denm.; UCB, Fin.; UCB, Ger.; UCB, Norw.; UCB, Swed.
Meclozine (p.420·3) or meclozine hydrochloride (p.420·3).
Hypersensitivity reactions; motion sickness; nausea and vomiting; vertigo.

Postafene
Darci, Belg.; UCB, Hong Kong.
Meclozine hydrochloride (p.420·3).
Motion sickness; nausea and vomiting; vertigo.

Postafeno *UCB, Port.*
Buclizine (p.411·1).

Postap *Pose, Thai.*
Brompheniramine maleate (p.410·2); phenylephrine hydrochloride (p.1097·1); phenylpropanolamine hydrochloride (p.1098·1).
Coughs; hypersensitivity reactions; nasal congestion.

Postap Expectorant *Pose, Thai.*
Guaifenesin (p.1092·2); brompheniramine maleate (p.410·2); phenylephrine hydrochloride (p.1097·1); phenylpropanolamine hydrochloride (p.1098·1).
Coughs; hypersensitivity reactions; nasal congestion.

Postavit-B *Riker, Mex.*
Buclizine (p.411·1).

Posterine *Kade, Ger.*
Hamamelis (p.1618·3).
Anorectal disorders.

Posterine Corte *Kade, Ger.*
Hydrocortisone acetate (p.1073·3).
Anorectal disorders.

Posterisan
Mayrhofer, Aust.; Kade, Ger.; Knoll, S.Afr.
Cell contents and metabolic products of *Escherichia coli.*
Anorectal disorders.

Posterisan Forte
Kade, Ger.; Kade, Hong Kong.
Cell components and metabolic products of *Escherichia coli*; hydrocortisone (p.1073·3).
Anorectal disorders.

Posti N *Kade, Ger.*
Rutoside (p.1611·2); esculoside (p.1574·1).
Vascular disorders.

Postinor
Gedeon Richter, Singapore; Gedeon Richter, Thai.
Levonorgestrel (p.1486·2).
Postcoital oral contraceptive.

Postinor-2
Schering, NZ; Medimpex, UK.
Levonorgestrel (p.1486·2).
Available on a named-patient basis only in the UK.
Postcoital oral contraception.

PostMI *Ashbourne, UK.*
Aspirin (p.14·2).
Angina; ischaemic heart disease; myocardial infarction.

Postoval
Note. This name is used for preparations of different composition.
Wyeth, Braz.
White tablets, estradiol valerate (p.1473·2); orange tablets, estradiol valerate; levonorgestrel (p.1486·2).
Menopausal disorders; menstrual disorders.
Aspen, S.Afr.
11 Tablets, estradiol valerate (p.1473·2); 10 tablets, estradiol valerate; norgestrel (p.1486·1); 7 tablets, inert.
Menopausal disorders; menstrual disorders.

Posture *Whitehall, USA.*
Calcium phosphate (p.1188·3).
Calcium supplement.

Posture-D *Whitehall, USA.*
Calcium phosphate (p.1188·3); vitamin D (p.1391·1).
Calcium supplement.

Potaba
Croma, Aust.; Glenwood, Canad.; Glenwood, Ger.; Glenwood, Hong Kong; Glenwood, Switz.; Glenwood, UK; Glenwood, USA.
Potassium aminobenzoate (p.1653·3).
Dermatomyositis; linear scleroderma; morphoea; pemphigus; Peyronie's disease; scleroderma.

Potabex *Tegur, Mex.*
Potassium aminobenzoate (p.1653·3).

Potable Aqua *Wisconsin Pharmacal, USA†.*
Tetraglycine hydroperiodide (p.1158·2).
Disinfection of drinking water.

Potacol-R *Otsuka, Jpn.*
Carbohydrate and electrolyte infusion (p.1350·1).
Carbohydrate source; fluid and electrolyte disorders; metabolic acidosis.

Potasalan *Lannett, USA.*
Potassium chloride (p.1194·3).
Hypokalaemia; potassium depletion.

Potasi *Eagle, Austral.*
Dibasic potassium phosphate (p.1193·1); potassium citrate (p.1186·1); potassium amino acid chelate; potassium chloride (p.1194·3); potassium carbonate; potassium sulfate (p.1195·1).
Potassium supplement.

Potasion *Synthelabo, Spain.*
Potassium chloride (p.1194·3).
Potassium depletion.

Potasoral *Armstrong, Mex.*
Potassium gluconate (p.1194·3).
Hypokalaemia.

Potassion *Miba, Ital.*
Potassium succinate; potassium malate; potassium citrate (p.1186·1); potassium acid tartrate (p.1244·3); potassium bicarbonate (p.1186·1).
Acidosis; potassium deficiency.

Potassium Iodide and Stramonium Compound *McGloin, Austral.*
Potassium iodide (p.1522·3); stramonium (p.474·1); lobelia (p.1510·2); liquorice (p.1231·2).
Coughs; respiratory-tract congestion.

Potassium-Rougier *Rougier, Canad.*
Potassium gluconate (p.1194·3).
Potassium supplement.

Potassium-Sandoz *Sandoz, Canad.†*
Potassium chloride (p.1194·3); potassium bicarbonate (p.1186·1).
Potassium depletion; potassium load tests.

Potassride *General Drugs, Thai.*
Potassium chloride (p.1194·3).
Hypokalaemia.

Pota-Vi-Kin *Collins, Mex.*
Phenoxymethylpenicillin potassium (p.235·1).
Bacterial infections.

Potenciator *Iquinosa, Spain.*
Arginine aspartate (p.1354·1).
Tonic.

Potendal *Allen, Spain.*
Ceftazidime (p.174·3).
Bacterial infections.

Potensone *Pharmasant, Thai.*
Fluphenazine hydrochloride (p.684·3).
Anxiety.

Potent C *Vitaglow, Austral.†*
Ascorbic acid (p.1389·3).
Vitamin C deficiency.

Potentol *Orion, Fin.*
Methyltestosterone (p.1482·3); meprobamate (p.691·1); yohimbine hydrochloride (p.1681·3).
Erectile dysfunction.

Po-Trim *Polipharm, Thai.*
Co-trimoxazole (p.193·3).
Bacterial infections.

Potsilo *Stark, Ger.*
Bisacodyl (p.1212·2); docusate sodium (p.1223·1); calcium pantothenate (p.1374·1); benzyl mandelate.
Constipation.

Potter's Catarrh Pastilles *Ernest Jackson, UK.*
Oleum pini sylvestris; pumilio pine oil (p.1656·3); eucalyptus oil (p.1609·2); creosote (p.1087·3); menthol (p.1632·3); thymol (p.1158·3); althaea (p.1577·1).
Cough and cold symptoms.

Potters Children's Cough Pastilles *Ernest Jackson, UK.*
Ipecacuanha (p.1093·1); squill (p.1100·3); citric acid (p.1596·2); honey (p.1366·2).
Formerly known as Jacksons Childrens Cough Pastilles.
Coughs.

Potters Day & Night Cough Pastilles *Ernest Jackson, UK.*
Codeine phosphate (p.25·2); wild cherry bark (p.1680·3).
Formerly known as Night Cough Pastilles.
Coughs.

Potters Sugar Free Cough Pastilles *Ernest Jackson, UK.*
Liquorice (p.1231·2); menthol (p.1632·3); benzoin tincture (p.1668·3); anise oil (p.1580·3); clove oil (p.1597·1); peppermint oil (p.1243·3); capsicum oleoresin (p.1591·1).
Catarrh; cold symptoms; coughs.

Povadine *Hua, Thai.*
Povidone-iodine (p.1155·1).
Burns; wound disinfection.

Povanyl *Warner-Lambert, Fr.*
Pyrvinium embonate (p.108·2).
Enterobiasis.

Povid-Derme *Kinder, Braz.*
Povidone-iodine (p.1155·1).
Skin and wound disinfection.

Poviderm *Farmec, Ital.*
Povidone-iodine (p.1155·1).
Skin and wound disinfection.

Povidex *Morton Grove, USA†.*
Povidone-iodine (p.1155·1).

Powdered C *GNLD, Austral.*
Ascorbic acid and other vitamin C substances (p.1350·1).
Vitamin C deficiency.

Power Orot *Worwag, Ger.*
Magnesium orotate (p.1645·1).
Magnesium deficiency.

Power Rub *Pfizer, Mex.*
Methyl salicylate (p.55·1); menthol (p.1632·3); camphor (p.1589·3).
Musculoskeletal and joint disorders.

Powergel *Menarini, UK.*
Ketoprofen (p.47·3).
Inflammation; pain.

Powerin *Whitehall, UK†.*
Aspirin (p.14·2); caffeine (p.761·3); paracetamol (p.71·2).
Fever; pain.

PowerLean *Matley, UK.*
Conjugate linoleic acid (p.1613·2).
Nutritional supplement.

PowerMate *Green Turtle Bay Vitamin Co., USA.*
Vitamins; minerals; green tea extract; ginkgo biloba extract; glutathione; acetylcysteine; echinacea; golden seal root; pine bark extract (p.1350·1).
Tonic.

PowerSleep *Green Turtle Bay Vitamin Co., USA.*
Vitamins; minerals; passion flower; valerian; oxitriptan; melatonin (p.1350·1).
Tonic.

The symbol † denotes a preparation no longer actively marketed

PowerVites *Green Turtle Bay Vitamin Co., USA.*
Vitamins; minerals; aminobenzoic acid; inositol; bio-flavonoids; bee pollen; folic acid (p.1350·1).
Tonic.

Poxider *Martin, Spain†.*
Fluocinolone acetonide (p.1071·1); gramicidin (p.213·3); neomycin sulfate (p.228·1).
Infected skin disorders.

Pozapam *Pharmasant, Thai.*
Prazepam (p.701·1).
Anxiety.

Pozhexol *Pharmasant, Thai.*
Benzhexol [trihexyphenidyl] hydrochloride (p.463·3).
Parkinsonism.

PP-Cap *Alra, USA†.*
Dextropropoxyphene hydrochloride (p.27·1).

PPD Tine Test *Wyeth, S.Afr.†.*
Tuberculin (p.1675·3).
Diagnosis of tuberculosis.

PPG-5 *Fustery, Mex.*
Policosanol.
Hypercholesterolaemia.

PPS *Immuno, Ital.*
Plasma protein fraction (p.740·2).
Burns; hypovolaemia; shock.

PPSB Konzentrat S-TIM *Baxter, Ger.*
A factor IX preparation (p.735·1).
Haemorrhagic disorders.

PR 100 *Farmacologico Milanese, Ital.*
Desonide pivalate (p.1066·2).
Skin disorders.

PR 100-Cloressidina *Farmacologico Milanese, Ital.*
Desonide pivalate (p.1066·2); chlorhexidine (p.1138·2).
Skin disorders.

PR Freeze Spray *Crookes Healthcare, UK.*
Dimethyl ether (p.1199·1); dimethoxymethane (p.1604·1).
Formerly contained trichlorofluoromethane and dichlorodifluoromethane.
Muscular pain and stiffness.

PR Heat Spray *Crookes Healthcare, UK.*
Methyl salicylate (p.55·1); ethyl nicotinate (p.35·1); camphor (p.1589·3).
Bruises; muscular and rheumatic pain; sprains.

Prabioquim *Bioquimica, Mex.*
Prazosin (p.958·1).

Pra-Brexidol *Pharmacia Upjohn, Ger.*
Piroxicam (p.79·1).
Gout; musculoskeletal, joint, and soft-tissue disorders.

Pracem *Novag, Mex.*
Dipyridamole (p.877·2).

Practazin *Cardel, Fr.*
Spironolactone (p.973·2); altizide (p.835·1).
Hypertension; oedema.

Practil *Organon, Ital.*
Desogestrel (p.1470·3); ethinylestradiol (p.1476·2).
Combined oral contraceptive.

Practiser *Serral, Mex.*
Diclofenac (p.30·2).
Inflammation.

Practo-Clyss
Braun, Belg.; Fresenius Kabi, Ger.; Braun, Switz.
Monobasic sodium phosphate (p.1193·2); dibasic sodium phosphate (p.1193·2).
Bowel evacuation; constipation.

Practomil *Braun, Switz.*
Glycerol (p.1616·3).
Bowel evacuation; constipation.

Practon *Cardel, Fr.*
Spironolactone (p.973·2).
Hyperaldosteronism; hypertension; myasthenia; oedema.

Pradente *Dinafarma, Braz.*
Procaine hydrochloride (p.1319·1); phenol (p.1152·3).
Mouth and throat disorders.

Pradif
Boehringer Ingelheim, Ital.; Boehringer Ingelheim, Port.; Boehringer Ingelheim, Switz.
Tamsulosin hydrochloride (p.978·3).
Benign prostatic hyperplasia

Praecicor *Molimin, Ger.†.*
Verapamil hydrochloride (p.989·1).
Angina pectoris; arrhythmias; hypertension.

Praeciglucon *Pfleger, Ger.*
Glibenclamide (p.321·3).
Diabetes mellitus.

Praecineural *Pfleger, Ger.*
Aspirin (p.14·2); codeine phosphate (p.25·2).
Glycine (p.1365·3) is included in some preparations in an attempt to limit adverse effects on the gastrointestinal mucosa.
Pain; rheumatism.

Praecipect *Molimin, Ger.†.*
Thyme (p.1672·2); cowslip rhizome (p.1600·1).
Formerly contained thyme, cowslip rhizome, and ephedrine hydrochloride.
Respiratory-tract disorders.

Praecordin S *Roland, Ger.*
Strong camphor oil; menthol (p.1632·3); benzyl nicotinate (p.20·2).
Cardiac disorders.

Praedex *Fresenius Kabi, Aust.*
Dextran 1 (p.728·2).
Prevention of anaphylactic reactions to infusions of dextrans.

Praefeminon plus *Cesra, Ger.*
Ferric ammonium citrate (p.1359·2); pulsatilla pratensis; valeriana officinalis.
Gynaecological disorders.

Praesidin *Medopharm, Ger.*
Lignocaine [lidocaine] hydrochloride (p.1313·2); diphenhydramine metilsulfate (p.416·2); titanium dioxide (p.1126·1).
Skin disorders.

Pragman *Hoechst Marion Roussel, Aust.*
Tolpropamine hydrochloride (p.426·2).
Pruritus.

Pragmatar
Bioglan, Irl.; Alliance, UK.
Coal tar (p.1125·1); sulfur (p.1123·3); salicylic acid (p.1122·3).
Dandruff; skin disorders.

Prairie Gold *Larkhall Laboratories, UK.*
Vitamin E (p.1393·3).

Pralenal *Opus, UK.*
Enalapril maleate (p.883·3).
Angina pectoris; heart failure; hypertension.

Pralifan *Inibsa, Spain.*
Mitozantrone [mitoxantrone] hydrochloride (p.559·3).
Malignant neoplasms.

Pralol *Pharmasant, Thai.*
Propranolol hydrochloride (p.962·3).
Angina pectoris; anxiety; hypertension; migraine; myocardial infarction; tremor.

Pramace *Hassle, Swed.*
Ramipril (p.966·3).
Heart failure; hypertension.

PrameGel
Medicis, Canad.; GenDerm, USA.
Pramocaine hydrochloride (p.1318·2); menthol (p.1632·3).
Pruritus.

Pramet *Abbott, Port.†.*
Multivitmin and mineral preparation (p.1350·1).

Pramet FA *Abbott, Hong Kong.*
Multivitamin and mineral preparation with iron and folic acid (p.1350·1).

Pramidal *Chemia, Mex.*
Loperamide hydrochloride (p.1231·3).
Diarrhoea.

Pramide *Sanofi Synthelabo, Port.*
Pyrazinamide (p.240·1).
Tuberculosis.

Pramidin *Crinos, Ital.*
Metoclopramide hydrochloride (p.1235·2).
Gastrointestinal disorders.

Pramigel *Carnot, Mex.*
Metoclopramide hydrochloride (p.1235·2); aluminium hydroxide (p.1210·3); magnesium hydroxide (p.1233·1); dimethicone (p.1249·2).
Gastrointestinal disorders.

Pramilem *Lemery, Mex.*
Metoclopramide (p.1236·3).
Nausea and vomiting.

Pramilet FA
Abbott, Singapore; Abbott, Thai.; Ross, USA.
Multivitamin and mineral preparation with iron and folic acid (p.1350·1).

Pramin
Alphapharm, Austral.; Rafa, Israel.
Metoclopramide hydrochloride (p.1235·2).
Adjunct in gastrointestinal examination; dyspepsia; gastroparesis; hiccups; nausea and vomiting; peptic ulcer.

Pramino *Janssen-Cilag, Ger.*
Norgestimate (p.1486·1); ethinylestradiol (p.1476·2).
Acne; triphasic oral contraceptive.

Pramistar *FIRMA, Ital.*
Pramiracetam sulfate (p.1654·2).
Anxiety disorders; mental function impairment.

Pramosone *Ferndale, USA.*
Hydrocortisone acetate (p.1073·3); pramocaine hydrochloride (p.1318·2).
Skin disorders.

PramOtic *Cypress, USA.*
Chloroxylenol (p.1142·1); pramocaine hydrochloride (p.1318·2).
Bacterial infections of the external ear.

Pramotil *Pisa, Mex.*
Metoclopramide (p.1236·3).
Nausea and vomiting.

Pramox *Isdin, Spain.*
Pramocaine hydrochloride (p.1318·2).
Pruritus.

Pramox HC *Dermtek, Canad.*
Hydrocortisone acetate (p.1073·3); pramocaine hydrochloride (p.1318·2).
Skin disorders.

Prandase
Bayer, Canad.; Pharma Clal, Israel.
Acarbose (p.319·2).
Diabetes mellitus.

Prandin *Novo Nordisk, USA.*
Repaglinide (p.334·1).
Diabetes mellitus.

Prandin E₂ *Pharmacia Upjohn, S.Afr.*
Dinoprostone (p.1441·3).
Labour induction.

Pranolol *Alpharma, Norw.*
Propranolol hydrochloride (p.962·3).
Angina pectoris; arrhythmias; hypertension; hyperthyroidism; migraine; myocardial infarction; tremor.

Pranosine *Sanfer, Mex.*
Inosine pranobex (p.627·2).
Viral infections.

Pranox *Asta Medica, Belg.*
Pranoprofen (p.80·1).
Eye inflammation.

Pranoxen *Propan, S.Afr.†.*
Naproxen (p.60·3).
Dysmenorrhoea; gout; musculoskeletal and joint disorders.

Prantal
Schering-Plough, Austral.; Schering-Plough, Ital.; Schering-Plough, NZ.
Diphemanil metilsulfate (p.466·2).
Hyperhidrosis.

Pranzo *Vinas, Spain.*
Cyproheptadine hydrochloride (p.414·2); carnitine hydrochloride (p.1356·2); lysine hydrochloride (p.1370·3).
Anorexia; tonic.

Praquantel *Atlantic, Thai.*
Praziquantel (p.106·3).
Trematode infections.

Prareduct *Sankyo, Spain.*
Pravastatin sodium (p.957·3).
Atherosclerosis; hypercholesterolaemia.

Prasepine *Warner-Lambert, Thai.*
Prazepam (p.701·1).
Anxiety; skeletal muscle spasm.

Prasig *Sigma, Austral.*
Prazosin hydrochloride (p.958·1).
Benign prostatic hyperplasia; heart failure; hypertension; Raynaud's syndrome.

Prasikon *Polipharm, Thai.*
Praziquantel (p.106·3).
Trematode infections.

Prasterol *Malesci, Ital.*
Pravastatin sodium (p.957·3).
Arteriosclerosis; cardiovascular disorders; hypercholesterolaemia.

Praticef *Caber, Ital.*
Cefonicid sodium (p.168·1).
Lignocaine [lidocaine] hydrochloride (p.1313·2) is included in this preparation to alleviate the pain of injection.
Bacterial infections.

Pratsiol
Douglas, Austral.; Orion, Fin.; Douglas, Hong Kong; Douglas, NZ; Aspen, S.Afr.; Orion, Thai.
Prazosin hydrochloride (p.958·1).
Benign prostatic hyperplasia; heart failure; hypertension.

Prava
Note. This name is used for preparations of different composition.
Bristol-Myers Squibb, S.Afr.
Pravastatin sodium (p.957·3).
Hypercholesterolaemia.

Bristol-Myers Squibb, Switz.
Lomustine (p.550·2).
Malignant neoplasms.

Pravachol
Bristol-Myers Squibb, Aust.; Bristol-Myers Squibb, Austral.; Squibb, Canad.; Bristol-Myers Squibb, Denm.; Bristol-Myers Squibb, Fin.; Bristol-Myers Squibb, Hong Kong; Bristol-Myers Squibb, Norw.; Bristol-Myers Squibb, Singapore; Bristol-Myers Squibb, Swed.; Bristol-Myers Squibb, USA.
Pravastatin sodium (p.957·3).
Atherosclerosis; hypercholesterolaemia.

Pravacilin *Abbott, Braz.*
Metampicillin (p.222·3).
Bacterial infections.

Pravacol
Bristol-Myers Squibb, Braz.; Bristol-Myers Squibb, Mex.; Bristol-Myers Squibb, Port.
Pravastatin sodium (p.957·3).
Coronary atherosclerosis; hypercholesterolaemia.

Pravaselect *Menarini, Ital.*
Pravastatin sodium (p.957·3).
Arteriosclerosis; cardiovascular disorders; hypercholesterolaemia.

Pravasin *Bristol-Myers Squibb, Ger.*
Pravastatin sodium (p.957·3).
Hypercholesterolaemia.

Pravasine *Bristol-Myers Squibb, Belg.*
Pravastatin sodium (p.957·3).
Hypercholesterolaemia.

Pravidel
Novartis, Ger.; Novartis, Swed.
Bromocriptine mesilate (p.1164·3).
Acromegaly; amenorrhoea; breast disorders; galactorrhoea; hyperprolactinaemia; infertility; lactation inhibition; ovulation disorders; parkinsonism; premenstrual syndrome.

Prax *Ferndale, USA.*
Pramocaine hydrochloride (p.1318·2).
Local anaesthesia.

Praxel *Lemery, Mex.*
Paclitaxel (p.563·2).
Breast cancer; ovarian cancer.

Praxilene
Merck-Belgolabo, Belg.; Lipha Sante, Fr.; Lipha, Hong Kong; Lipha,

Irl.; Formenti, Ital.; Merck, Port.; Merck, Singapore; Merck-Lipha, Singapore; Faes, Spain; Lipha, Switz.; Merck, Thai.; Merck, UK.
Naftidrofuryl oxalate (p.937·3).
Cerebral and peripheral vascular disorders.

Praxinor *Lipha Sante, Fr.*
Theodrenaline hydrochloride (p.1671·3); cafedrine hydrochloride (p.853·1).
Hypotension.

Praxiten
Wyeth Lederle, Aust.; Wyeth, Ger.
Oxazepam (p.697·1).
Anxiety disorders; sleep disorders.

Prazac *Orion, Denm.*
Prazosin hydrochloride (p.958·1).
Heart failure; hypertension; Raynaud's syndrome.

Prazam *Euro-Labor, Port.*
Alprazolam (p.654·2).
Anxiety; depression; insomnia.

Prazene *Parke, Davis, Ital.*
Prazepam (p.701·1).
Anxiety disorders; psychoneurotic disorders.

Prazentol *Ferring, Port.*
Omeprazole (p.1239·1).
Gastro-oesophageal reflux; peptic ulcer; Zollinger-Ellison syndrome.

Prazidec *Tecnofarma, Mex.*
Omeprazole (p.1239·1).
Gastro-oesophageal reflux; peptic ulcer; Zollinger-Ellison syndrome.

Prazine
Wyeth Lederle, Belg.; Wyeth, Switz.
Promazine embonate (p.702·2) or promazine hydrochloride (p.702·2).
Behaviour disorders in children; hiccups; nausea; psychoses; sedative; tetany; vomiting.

Prazinil *Pierre Fabre, Fr.*
Carpipramine hydrochloride (p.659·2).
Anxiety; psychoses.

Prazite *Asian Pharm, Thai.*
Praziquantel (p.106·3).
Trematode infections.

Prazocor *Pharmacia Upjohn, Fin.*
Prazosin hydrochloride (p.958·1).
Heart failure; hypertension.

Prazohexal *Hexal, Austral.*
Prazosin hydrochloride (p.958·1).
Hypertension.

Prazoken *Kendrick, Mex.*
Megestrol (p.1481·3).

Prazolit *Fustery, Mex.*
Omeprazole (p.1239·1).
Gastro-oesophageal reflux; peptic ulcer; Zollinger-Ellison syndrome.

Pre Clor *Pfizer, Mex.*
Chloramphenicol (p.179·1); prednisone (p.1079·2).
Infected eye disorders.

Pre Natal *Cenovis, Austral.*
Omega-3 marine triglycerides (p.949·3); folic acid (p.1361·1).
Fatty-acid supplement; prevention of neural tube defects.

Pre Nutrison *Nutricia, Ital.*
Preparation for enteral nutrition (p.1350·1).

Preastig *Alfa Intes, Ital.*
Multivitamin and mineral preparation with glutathione (p.1350·1).
Nutritional supplement.

Pre-Attain *Sherwood, USA.*
Lactose-free preparation for enteral nutrition (p.1350·1).

Prebon *Alba, USA†.*
Multivitamin and mineral preparation (p.1350·1).

PreCare *Ther-Rx, USA.*
Multivitamin and mineral preparation (p.1350·1).

Precedex *Abbott, USA.*
Dexmedetomidine hydrochloride (p.674·3).
Sedation in mechanically ventilated patients.

Precef *Bristol-Myers Squibb, USA.*
Ceforanide (p.169·1); L-lysine.
Bacterial infections.

Precidona *Precimex, Mex.*
Dipyrone (p.34·1).

Precifen *Precimex, Mex.*
Paracetamol (p.71·2).
Fever; pain.

Precifenac *Precimex, Mex.*
Diclofenac (p.30·2).

Precileucin *Precimex, Mex.*
Folic acid (p.1361·1).

Precision
Wander, Ital.†; Sandoz Nutrition, USA.
A range of preparations for enteral nutrition (p.1350·1).

Precision Plus
Medisense, Austral.; Medica, NZ.
Test for glucose in blood (p.1616·3).

Precitene *Novartis Consumer, Port.*
A range of preparations for enteral nutrition (p.1350·1).

Precitene MCT 50 *Wander Health Care, Switz.†.*
Preparation for enteral nutrition (p.1350·1).

Preconceive *Lane, UK.*
Folic acid (p.1361·1).
Prevention of neural tube defects in pregnancy.

Precopen *Fides Rottapharm, Spain.*
Amoxicillin trihydrate (p.149·2).
Bacterial infections.

Precopen Mucolitico *Fides Rottapharm, Spain.*
Amoxicillin trihydrate (p.149·2); bromhexine hydrochloride (p.1085·3).
Respiratory-tract infections.

Precortalon aquosum *Organon, Swed.*
Prednisolone sodium succinate (p.1078·1).
Corticosteroid.

Precortisyl *Hoechst Marion Roussel, UK.*
Prednisolone (p.1077·3).
Corticosteroid.

Precosa
Biocodex, Denm.; AstraZeneca, Fin.; AstraZeneca, Norw.; Astra, Swed.
Saccharomyces boulardii (p.1626·3).
AIDS-related diarrhoea; antibiotic-associated diarrhoea.

Precose *Bayer, USA.*
Acarbose (p.319·2).
Diabetes mellitus.

Precosol *Wolfs, Belg.*
Macrogol 4000 (p.1630·3); electrolytes (p.1180·1).
Bowel evacuation.

Prectal *Artesan, Ger.; Cassella-med, Ger.*
Prednisolone acetate (p.1078·1).
Bronchitis; hypersensitivity reactions; laryngotracheal stenosis.

Precurgen *Knoll, Spain†.*
Cytosine inosinate.
Liver disorders.

Precyclan *Lisapharm, Fr.*
Meprobamate (p.691·1); bendrofluazide [bendroflumethiazide] (p.844·1); medroxyprogesterone acetate (p.1480·1).
Formerly contained meprobamate, bendrofluazide [bendroflumethiazide], and flumedroxone acetate.
Premenstrual syndrome.

Pred
Grin, Mex.; Allergan, Singapore; Alcon, USA.
Prednisolone acetate (p.1078·1) or prednisolone sodium phosphate (p.1078·1).
Inflammatory eye disorders.

Pred Fort *Allergan-Frumtost, Braz.*
Prednisolone acetate (p.1078·1).
Inflammatory eye disorders.

Pred Forte
Allergan, Belg.; Allergan, Canad.; Allergan, Fin.; Allergan, Hong Kong; Allergan, Irl.; Allergan, Neth.†; Allergan, NZ; Allergan, Spain; Allergan, Switz.; Allergan, Thai.; Allergan, UK; Allergan, USA.
Prednisolone acetate (p.1078·1).
Inflammatory eye disorders.

Pred G
Allergan, S.Afr.; Allergan, Switz.†; Allergan, USA.
Prednisolone acetate (p.1078·1); gentamicin sulfate (p.210·1).
Infected eye disorders.

Pred Mild
Allergan, Canad.; Allergan, Hong Kong; Allergan, Irl.; Allergan, NZ; Allergan, S.Afr.; Allergan, Switz.; Allergan, Thai.; Allergan, USA.
Prednisolone acetate (p.1078·1).
Corneal burns; inflammatory eye disorders.

Pred Oph *Seng, Thai.*
Prednisolone sodium phosphate (p.1078·1); gentamicin sulfate (p.210·1).
Infected eye and ear disorders.

Predalgic *Pred, Fr.*
Tramadol hydrochloride (p.89·1).
Pain.

Predalon *Organon, Ger.*
Chorionic gonadotrophin (p.1279·2).
Cryptorchidism; delayed puberty; stimulation of gonadal function.

Predalone *Forest Laboratories, USA.*
Prednisolone acetate (p.1078·1).
Corticosteroid.

Pred-Clysma
Leiras, Denm.; Leiras, Norw.; Schering, Swed.
Prednisolone sodium phosphate (p.1078·1).
Crohn's disease; proctosigmoiditis; ulcerative colitis.

Predcor *Hauck, USA.*
Prednisolone acetate (p.1078·1).
Corticosteroid.

Predeltilone *Noristan, S.Afr.†.*
Prednisolone (p.1077·3).
Corticosteroid.

Predeltin *Quatromed, S.Afr.*
Prednisone (p.1079·2).
Corticosteroid.

Predenema
Pharmax, Hong Kong; Pharmax, Irl.; Pharmax, UK.
Prednisolone metasulfobenzoate sodium (p.1078·1).
Ulcerative colitis.

Predesic *Pred, Fr.*
Articaine hydrochloride (p.1306·1).
Adrenaline [epinephrine] acid tartrate (p.829·2) is included in this preparation as a vasoconstrictor to diminish absorption and localise the effect of the local anaesthetic.
Local anaesthesia.

Predex *Rottapharm, Thai.*
Neomycin sulfate (p.228·1); prednisolone (p.1077·3).
Skin disorders.

Predfoam
Pharmax, Hong Kong; Pharmax, Irl.; Pharmax, UK.
Prednisolone metasulfobenzoate sodium (p.1078·1).
Proctitis; ulcerative colitis.

Predicor *Pisa, Mex.*
Prednisone (p.1079·2).
Corticosteroid.

Predicorten *Stiefel, Braz.*
Prednisone (p.1079·2).
Corticosteroid.

Predictor
Organon, Austral.†; Akzo, Braz.; Chefaro Ardeval, Fr.; Chefaro, Israel; Angelini, Ital.; Chefaro, UK.
Pregnancy test (p.1654·3).

Predisole *PP Lab, Thai.*
Prednisolone (p.1077·3).
Corticosteroid.

Predmicin *EMS, Braz.*
Polymyxin B sulfate (p.238·1); prednisolone (p.1077·3); butyl aminobenzoate (p.1308·2); hydroxyquinoline iodochloride (p.1622·2).
Skin disorders.

Predmix *Royal Childrens Hospital, Austral.*
Prednisolone sodium phosphate (p.1078·1).
Corticosteroid.

Predmycin
Allergan, Belg.; Allergan, Thai.
Prednisolone acetate (p.1078·1); polymyxin B sulfate (p.238·1); neomycin sulfate (p.228·1).
Infected eye disorders.

Predmycin-P *Allergan, Singapore.*
Prednisolone acetate (p.1078·1); polymyxin B sulfate (p.238·1); neomycin sulfate (p.228·1).
Infected eye disorders.

Predmycin-P Liquifilm *Allergan, Neth.†.*
Prednisolone acetate (p.1078·1); polymyxin B sulfate (p.238·1); neomycin sulfate (p.228·1).
Eye infections.

Prednabene *Merckle, Ger.*
Prednisolone sodium phosphate (p.1078·1).
Parenteral corticosteroid.

Prednefrin *Allergan, Austral.*
Prednisolone acetate (p.1078·1); phenylephrine hydrochloride (p.1097·1).
Eye inflammation.

Prednefrin SF *Allergan, Mex.*
Prednisolone acetate (p.1078·1).
Eye disorders.

Prednersone *General Drugs, Thai.*
Prednisolone (p.1077·3).
Corticosteroid.

Prednesol
Glaxo Wellcome, Irl.; Sovereign, UK†.
Prednisolone sodium phosphate (p.1078·1).
Corticosteroid.

Predni *Lichtenstein, Ger.*
Prednisolone acetate (p.1078·1).
Parenteral corticosteroid.

Predni Azuleno *Lacer, Spain.*
Chloramphenicol (p.179·1); guaiazulene (p.1618·3); prednisolone (p.1077·3).
Infected skin disorders.

Predni H *Lichtenstein, Ger.*
Prednisolone (p.1077·3) or prednisolone acetate (p.1078·1).
Corticosteroid.

Predni M *Lichtenstein, Ger.*
Methylprednisolone (p.1076·1).
Oral corticosteroid.

Predni Tablinen *Lichtenstein, Ger.*
Prednisone (p.1079·2).
Oral corticosteroid.

Prednicort *Continental Pharma, Belg.*
Prednisone (p.1079·2).
Corticosteroid.

Prednicortelone *Continental Pharma, Belg.*
Prednisolone (p.1077·3).
Corticosteroid.

Predniderma *Caldeira & Marques, Port.*
Prednisolone (p.1077·3); neomycin sulfate (p.228·1).
Skin disorders.

Prednidib *Diba, Mex.*
Prednisone (p.1079·2).
Corticosteroid.

Predni-F-Tablinen *Sanorania, Ger.†.*
Dexamethasone (p.1067·1).
Oral corticosteroid.

Predniftalmina *Davi, Port.*
Chloramphenicol (p.179·1); prednisolone (p.1077·3).
Infected eye disorders.

Predni-Helvacort *Helvepharm, Switz.†.*
Prednisolone (p.1077·3).
Corticosteroid.

Prednihexal
Hexal, Austral.; Hexal, Ger.
Prednisolone (p.1077·3) or prednisolone acetate (p.1078·1).
Corticosteroid.

Prednilem *Lemery, Mex.*
Methylprednisolone sodium succinate (p.1076·1).
Corticosteroid.

Predniment *Ferring, Denm.†; Ferring, Fin.*
Prednisolone sodium phosphate (p.1078·1).
Proctitis; ulcerative colitis.

Predniocil *Oftalder, Port.*
Prednisolone acetate (p.1078·1).
Eye disorders.

Predni-Ophtal *Winzer, Ger.*
Prednisolone acetate (p.1078·1).
Inflammatory eye disorders.

Predni-POS *Ursapharm, Ger.*
Prednisolone acetate (p.1078·1).
Inflammatory eye disorders.

Prednis Neomic *Alcon Cusi, Spain.*
Neomycin sulfate (p.228·1); prednisone (p.1079·2).
Infected eye disorders.

Prednisil *Silom, Thai.*
Cream: Prednisolone (p.1077·3).
Skin disorders.
Eye drops: Prednisolone sodium phosphate (p.1078·1); neomycin sulfate (p.228·1).
Infected eye disorders.

Prednisil-N *Silom, Thai.*
Prednisolone (p.1077·3); neomycin sulfate (p.228·1).
Infected skin disorders.

Prednisol *Pasadena, USA.*
Prednisolone tebutate (p.1078·2).
Corticosteroid.

Prednisolut *Jenapharm, Ger.*
Prednisolone hydrogen succinate (p.1078·1).
Parenteral corticosteroid.

Prednistyle *Fischer, Israel.*
Prednisolone ester (p.1077·3); sulfacetamide sodium (p.250·3).
Infected eye disorders.

Prednitone *Vitamed, Israel.*
Prednisone (p.1079·2).
Corticosteroid.

Prednitop
Hoechst Marion Roussel, Aust.; Knoll, Switz.
Prednicarbate (p.1077·3).
Inflammatory skin disorders.

Prednitracin
Ciba Vision, Ger.; Ciba Vision, Hong Kong; Ciba Vision, Switz.
Prednisolone acetate (p.1078·1); neomycin sulfate (p.228·1); bacitracin (p.155·2).
Infected eye disorders.

Predopa *Kyowa, Jpn†.*
Dopamine hydrochloride (p.881·3).
Shock.

Pred-Phosphate *Medical Ophthalmics, USA.*
Prednisolone phosphate (p.1078·3).
Eye disorders.

Predsol
Sigma, Austral.; Medeva, Irl.; Glaxo Wellcome, NZ; Glaxo Wellcome, S.Afr.; Celltech, UK.
Prednisolone sodium phosphate (p.1078·1).
Crohn's disease; inflammatory disorders of the ear or eye; proctitis; ulcerative colitis.

Predsol-N *Celltech, UK.*
Prednisolone sodium phosphate (p.1078·1); neomycin sulfate (p.228·1).
Inflammatory disorders of the ear or eye with bacterial infection.

Prefagyl *Oberlin, Fr.*
Magnesium chloride (p.1190·3); sodium bicarbonate (p.1186·2); anhydrous sodium sulfate (p.1250·1); dibasic sodium phosphate (p.1193·2).
Formerly contained magnesium chloride, sodium bicarbonate, sodium sulfate, dibasic sodium phosphate, and sodium bromide.
Gastrointestinal disorders.

Prefamone
Asta Medica, Belg†; Dexo, Thai.
Diethylpropion hydrochloride (p.1508·3).
Obesity.

Prefamone Chronules
Dexo, Fr.†; Dexo, Switz.
Diethylpropion hydrochloride (p.1508·3).
Obesity.

Preferid
Yamanouchi, Belg.†; Yamanouchi, Irl.; Yamanouchi, Ital.; Yamanouchi, Neth.†; Yamanouchi, Norw.†; Yamanouchi, Swed.†; Yamanouchi, Switz.†.
Budesonide (p.1064·2).
Skin disorders.

Preferred Remedies *Reese, USA.*
A range of homoeopathic preparations.

Prefil *Norgine, UK†.*
Sterculia (p.1250·2).
Obesity.

Prefin *Otsuka, Spain.*
Buprenorphine hydrochloride (p.21·1).
Pain.

Prefine *Pierre Fabre Sante, Fr.*
Sterculia (p.1250·2).
Obesity.

Preflex Daily Cleaner *Alcon, USA.*
Cleansing solution for soft contact lenses (p.1129·2).

Prefolic *Knoll, Ital.*
Calcium mefolinate (p.1363·2).
Antidote to folic acid antagonists; folate deficiency; reduction of aminopterin and methotrexate toxicity.

Preforms *Terrier, Mex.*
Nonoxinol (p.1346·1).

Prefrin
Allergan, Austral.; Allergan, Canad.; Allergan, Hong Kong; Allergan, Israel; Allergan, NZ; Allergan, S.Afr.; Allergan, Singapore.
Phenylephrine hydrochloride (p.1097·1).
Eye irritation.

Prefrin A
Allergan, Aust.; Allergan, Canad.; Allergan, S.Afr.†.
Mepyramine maleate (p.421·1); phenylephrine hydrochloride (p.1097·1).
Eye inflammation; eye irritation.

Prefrin Liquifilm
Allergan, Aust.; Allergan, USA.
Phenylephrine hydrochloride (p.1097·1).
Eye irritation.

Prefrin Z
Allergan, Aust.; Allergan, NZ.
Phenylephrine hydrochloride (p.1097·1); zinc sulfate (p.1398·2).
Eye irritation.

Pregaday *Celltech, UK.*
Ferrous fumarate (p.1360·1); folic acid (p.1361·1).
Prophylaxis of iron and folic acid deficiency in pregnancy.

Pregamal *Glaxo Wellcome, S.Afr.*
Folic acid (p.1361·1); ferrous fumarate (p.1360·1).
Anaemias.

Pregestimil
Mead Johnson, Austral.; Mead Johnson Nutritionals, Fin.; Mead Johnson, Fr.; Mead Johnson, Hong Kong; Mead Johnson, Irl.; Mead Johnson, Israel; Mead Johnson, Ital.; Mead Johnson, NZ; Mead Johnson, Port.; Mead Johnson, Singapore; Mead Johnson Nutritionals, Thai.; Mead Johnson Nutritionals, UK; Mead Johnson Nutritionals, USA.
Infant feed (p.1350·1).
Cystic fibrosis; diarrhoea; food hypersensitivity; galactokinase deficiency; galactosaemia; impaired fat absorption; lactose or sucrose and protein intolerance.

Preglandin *Ono, Jpn.*
Gemeprost (p.1445·1).
Termination of pregnancy.

Pregnacare *Vitabiotics, Hong Kong; Vitabiotics, UK.*
Multivitamin and mineral preparation (p.1350·1).
Dietary supplement in pregnancy and lactation.

Pregna-Cert *Merlin, UK.*
Pregnancy test (p.1654·3).

Pregnafort *Thompson, Austral.*
Multivitamin and mineral preparation (p.1350·1).

Pregnancy Formula *Eagle, Austral.*
Multivitamin, mineral, and amino-acid preparation with bioflavonoids, ginger and lecithin (p.1350·1).
Nutritional supplement.

Pregna-Sure HCG *Merlin, UK.*
Pregnancy test (p.1654·3).

Pregnatal *Scanpharm, Hong Kong.*
Multivitamin and mineral preparation (p.1350·1).
Dietary supplement in pregnancy and lactation.

Pregnavit *Ratiopharm, Aust.*
Multivitamin and iron preparation (p.1350·1).

Pregnavit F *Merckle, Ger.*
Multivitamin preparation (p.1350·1).

Pregnavite Forte F *Goldshield, UK.*
Dried ferrous sulfate (p.1360·3); folic acid (p.1361·1); vitamins (p.1350·1); calcium phosphate.
Prophylaxis of neural tube defects in pregnancy.

Pregnazon *Pharmadass, UK.*
Multivitamin, mineral, and trace element preparation (p.1350·1).

Pregnesin *Serono, Ger.*
Chorionic gonadotrophin (p.1279·2).
Cryptorchidism; delayed puberty in males; infertility in females and males.

Pregnifer *Weifa, Norw.*
Ferrous sulfate (p.1360·3); folic acid (p.1361·1).
Iron and folic acid deficiency.

Pregnon L *Nourypharma, Ger.*
Lynestrenol (p.1480·1); ethinylestradiol (p.1476·2).
Combined oral contraceptive.

Pregnosis
Key, Austral.; Roche, USA.
Pregnancy test (p.1654·3).

Pregnospia Duoclon *Organon, UK.*
Pregnancy test (p.1654·3).

Pregnosticon *Organon, Israel.*
Pregnancy test (p.1654·3).

Pregnyl
Organon, Aust.; Organon, Austral.; Organon, Belg.; Akzo, Braz.; Organon, Canad.; Organon, Denm.; Organon, Fin.; Organon, Hong Kong; Organon, Irl.; Organon, Israel; Organon, Ital.; Organon, Mex.; Organon, Neth.; Organon, Norw.; Organon, NZ; Organon, Port.; Donmed, S.Afr.; Organon, Singapore; Organon, Spain†; Organon, Swed.; Organon, Switz.; Organon, Thai.; Organon, UK; Organon, USA.
Chorionic gonadotrophin (p.1279·2).
Cryptorchidism; delayed puberty; hypogonadotrophic hypogonadism; male and female infertility; uterine haemorrhage.

Pregomin
Milupa, Singapore; Milupa, Switz.
Infant feed (p.1350·1).
Carbohydrate malabsorption syndromes; cow's-milk-protein intolerance; digestive system disorders; soya-milk-protein intolerance.

Pregomine *Milupa, Fr.*
Nutritional supplement (p.1350·1).
Gastrointestinal disorders.

Prehist *Marnel, USA.*
Phenylephrine hydrochloride (p.1097·1); chlorpheniramine [chlorphenamine] maleate (p.412·1).
Upper respiratory-tract symptoms.

The symbol † denotes a preparation no longer actively marketed

Prehist D *Marnel, USA.*
Phenylephrine hydrochloride (p.1097·1); chlorpheniramine [chlorphenamine] maleate (p.412·1); hyoscine methonitrate (p.468·2).
Upper respiratory-tract symptoms.

Prejomin *Milupa, Irl.; Milupa, UK.*
Gluten-free preparation for special diets (p.1350·1).
Galactokinase deficiency; galactosaemia; protein intolerance; sucrose, fructose, or lactose intolerance.

Prelac *Mead Johnson, Port.*
Nutritional supplement for pregnant and lactating women (p.1350·1).

Prelafel *Akromed, S.Afr.†*
Multivitamin and mineral preparation (p.1350·1).

Prelief *AkPharma, USA†.*
Calcium glycerophosphate (p.1188·2).
Dyspepsia.

Prelis *Novartis, Ger.*
Metoprolol tartrate (p.931·2).
Arrhythmias; hypertension; ischaemic heart disease; migraine; myocardial infarction.

Prelis comp *Novartis, Ger.*
Metoprolol tartrate (p.931·2); chlortalidone (p.857·1).
Hypertension.

Prelloran *Novartis, Hong Kong; Novartis Consumer, Switz.*
A heparinoid (p.905·2); glycol salicylate (p.42·2).
Haematomas; musculoskeletal pain and inflammation; peripheral vascular disorders; phlebitis.

Prelone *Muro, Israel; Adcock Ingram, S.Afr.; Muro, USA.*
Prednisolone (p.1077·3).
Corticosteroid.

Prelu-2 *Roxane, USA; Boehringer Ingelheim, USA.*
Phendimetrazine tartrate (p.1513·3).
Obesity.

Prelude *Rendell, UK.*
Nonoxinol 9 (p.1346·1).
Spermicidal contraceptive.

Prelus *Sanofi Winthrop, Port.†*
Isoprenaline hydrochloride (p.914·3); phenobarbital (p.355·1); ephedrine sulfate (p.1090·2); theophylline (p.777·2); potassium iodide (p.1522·3).
Asthma; bronchitis; coughs.

Premandol *Spirig, Switz.*
Prednisolone acetate (p.1078·1); almond oil (p.1576·3); zinc oxide (p.1128·2).
Skin disorders.

Premaril *Dexxon, Israel.*
Conjugated oestrogens (p.1467·1).
Menopausal disorders; osteoporosis.

Premaril MP *Dexxon, Israel.*
Conjugated oestrogens (p.1467·1); medroxyprogesterone acetate (p.1480·1).
Menopausal disorders; oestrogen deficiency.

Premaril Plus MP *Dexxon, Israel.*
28 Tablets, conjugated oestrogens (p.1467·1); 14 tablets, medroxyprogesterone acetate (p.1480·1).
Menopausal disorders; osteoporosis.

Premarin
Wyeth Lederle, Aust.; Wyeth-Ayerst, Austral.; Wyeth Lederle, Belg.; Wyeth, Braz.; Wyeth-Ayerst, Canad.; Wyeth Lederle, Denm.; Wyeth Lederle, Fin.; Wyeth-Ayerst, Fr.; Wyeth-Ayerst, Hong Kong; Wyeth, Irl.; Wyeth Lederle, Ital.; Wyeth, Mex.; Wyeth, Neth.; Wyeth, NZ; Wyeth, S.Afr.; Wyeth, Singapore; Wyeth, Spain; Wyeth, Switz.; Wyeth-Ayerst, Thai.; Wyeth, UK; Wyeth-Ayerst, USA.
Conjugated oestrogens (p.1467·1).
Breast cancer; dysfunctional uterine bleeding; menopausal disorders; oestrogen deficiency; osteoporosis; prostatic cancer.

Premarin compositum *Wyeth Lederle, Aust.*
16 Tablets, conjugated oestrogens (p.1467·1); 12 tablets, conjugated oestrogens; medrogestone (p.1480·1).
Oestrogen deficiency.

Premarin with Methyltestosterone *Wyeth-Ayerst, USA†.*
Conjugated oestrogens (p.1467·1); methyltestosterone (p.1482·3).
Menopausal disorders; postpartum breast engorgement.

Premarin Pak *Wyeth, Mex.*
21 Tablets, conjugated oestrogens (p.1467·1); 10 tablets, medrogestone (p.1480·1).
Menopausal disorders; osteoporosis.

Premarin Plus
Wyeth Lederle, Aust.; Wyeth, Neth.; Wyeth Lederle, Port.; Wyeth, Switz.
28 Tablets, conjugated oestrogens (p.1467·1); 12 tablets, medrogestone (p.1480·1).
Adjunct in vaginitis and cystitis; menopausal disorders; osteoporosis; ovarian insufficiency.

Premarina *Wyeth Lederle, Swed.*
Conjugated oestrogens (p.1467·1).
Hypogenitalism; menopausal disorders; osteoporosis.

Premarin-MPA *Wyeth Lederle, Aust.*
Conjugated oestrogens (p.1467·1); medroxyprogesterone acetate (p.1480·1).
Oestrogen deficiency.

Preme *Nakorn, Thai.*
Cyproterone acetate (p.1467·3); ethinylestradiol (p.1476·2).
Androgen-dependent acne, seborrhoea, alopecia, and hirsutism in females; oral contraceptive in women with androgenic symptoms.

Premella
Wyeth Lederle, Aust.†; Wyeth, Switz.
Conjugated oestrogens (p.1467·1); medroxyprogesterone acetate (p.1480·1).
Menopausal disorders; osteoporosis.

Premelle
Wyeth Lederle, Belg.; Wyeth-Ayerst, Hong Kong; Wyeth, Mex.; Wyeth, Neth.; Wyeth Lederle, Port.; Wyeth, S.Afr.; Wyeth, Singapore; Wyeth Lederle, Swed.
Conjugated oestrogens (p.1467·1); medroxyprogesterone acetate (p.1480·1).
Menopausal disorders; oestrogen deficiency; osteoporosis.

Wyeth, Spain.
28 Tablets, conjugated oestrogens (p.1467·1); 28 tablets, medroxyprogesterone acetate (p.1480·1).
Menopausal disorders; osteoporosis.

Premelle C *Wyeth Lederle, Ital.*
Conjugated oestrogens (p.1467·1); medroxyprogesterone acetate (p.1480·1).
Menopausal disorders; osteoporosis.

Premelle Ciclico *Wyeth, Spain.*
28 Tablets, conjugated oestrogens (p.1467·1); 14 tablets, medroxyprogesterone acetate (p.1480·1).
Menopausal disorders; osteoporosis.

Premelle Cycle
Wyeth-Ayerst, Hong Kong; Wyeth Lederle, Port.; Wyeth, Singapore.
14 Tablets, conjugated oestrogens (p.1467·1); 14 tablets, conjugated oestrogens; medroxyprogesterone acetate (p.1480·1).
Menopausal disorders; osteoporosis.

Wyeth, Neth.
28 Tablets, conjugated oestrogens (p.1467·1); 14 tablets, medroxyprogesterone acetate (p.1480·1).
Menopausal disorders; osteoporosis.

Premelle S *Wyeth Lederle, Ital.*
14 Tablets, conjugated oestrogens (p.1467·1); 14 tablets, conjugated oestrogens; medroxyprogesterone acetate (p.1480·1).
Menopausal disorders; osteoporosis.

Premelle Sekvens *Wyeth Lederle, Swed.*
14 Tablets, conjugated oestrogens (p.1467·1); 14 tablets, conjugated oestrogens; medroxyprogesterone acetate (p.1480·1).
Formerly known as Prempac Sekvens.
Oestrogen deficiency; osteoporosis.

Premence *Vitabiotics, Hong Kong; Vitabiotics, UK.*
Multivitamin and mineral preparation (p.1350·1).
Premenstrual syndrome.

PreMens *Zeller, Switz.*
Agnus castus (p.1574·2).
Premenstrual syndrome.

Prementaid *Potter's, UK.*
Vervain (p.1679·3); motherwort (p.1637·3); pulsatilla (p.1656·3); bearberry (p.1583·3); valerian (p.1678·3).
Premenstrual syndrome.

PremesisRx *Ther-Rx, USA.*
Vitamin $_6$ (p.1387·1); vitamin B$_{12}$ (p.1388·1); folic acid (p.1361·1); calcium (p.1187·3).
Nausea.

Premia *Wyeth, NZ.*
14 Tablets, conjugated oestrogens (p.1467·1); 14 tablets, conjugated oestrogens; medroxyprogesterone acetate (p.1480·1).
Menopausal disorders; osteoporosis.

Premia 5 *Wyeth-Ayerst, Austral.*
14 Tablets, conjugated oestrogens (p.1467·1); 14 tablets, conjugated oestrogens; medroxyprogesterone acetate (p.1480·1).
Menopausal disorders; osteoporosis.

Premia Continuous
Wyeth-Ayerst, Austral.; Wyeth, NZ.
Conjugated oestrogens (p.1467·1); medroxyprogesterone acetate (p.1480·1).
Menopausal disorders; osteoporosis.

Premid
Note.This name is used for preparations of different composition.
AstraZeneca, Denm.
Balsalazide sodium (p.1212·1).
Ulcerative colitis.

Grin, Mex.
Prednisolone acetate (p.1078·1); sulfacetamide sodium (p.250·3).
Infected eye disorders.

Premique *Wyeth, Irl.; Wyeth, UK.*
Conjugated oestrogens (p.1467·1); medroxyprogesterone acetate (p.1480·1).
Menopausal disorders; osteoporosis.

Premique Cycle *Wyeth, Irl.; Wyeth, UK.*
14 Tablets, conjugated oestrogens (p.1467·1); 14 tablets, conjugated oestrogens; medroxyprogesterone acetate (p.1480·1).
Menopausal disorders; osteoporosis.

Premium *Quest, Canad.*
Multivitamin and mineral preparation (p.1350·1).

Premium Prenatal *Quest, Canad.*
Multivitamin and mineral preparation (p.1350·1).

Premofil M *ZLB, Switz.*
A factor VIII preparation (p.734·1).
Haemorrhagic disorders.

Premella *Julphar, UAE.*
Metoclopramide (p.1236·3) or metoclopramide hydrochloride (p.1235·2).
Adjunct in gastrointestinal procedures; gastro-oesophageal reflux; gastrointestinal motility disorders; hiccup; nausea and vomiting.

Premox *Precimex, Mex.*
Pyrazinamide (p.240·1).

Prempak
Wyeth-Ayerst, Hong Kong; Wyeth-Ayerst, Thai.
21 Tablets, conjugated oestrogens (p.1467·1); 10 tablets, medrogestone (p.1480·1).
Menopausal disorders; oestrogen deficiency; osteoporosis.

Wyeth Lederle, Ital.
28 Tablets, conjugated oestrogens (p.1467·1); 12 tablets, medrogestone (p.1480·1).
Formerly contained conjugated oestrogens.
Atrophic urethritis; menopausal disorders; oestrogen deficiency; osteoporosis; vaginitis.

Prempak N *Wyeth, S.Afr.*
21 Tablets, conjugated oestrogens (p.1467·1); 10 tablets, medrogestone (p.1480·1).
28-Day packs also contain 7 inert tablets.
Menopausal disorders; osteoporosis.

Prempak-C
Wyeth, Irl.; Wyeth, Neth.; Wyeth, NZ; Wyeth, Singapore; Wyeth, UK.
28 Tablets, conjugated oestrogens (p.1467·1); 12 tablets, norgestrel (p.1486·1).
Menopausal disorders; oestrogen deficiency; osteoporosis.

Premphase *Wyeth-Ayerst, USA.*
Maroon tablets, conjugated oestrogens (p.1467·1); blue tablets, conjugated oestrogens; medroxyprogesterone acetate (p.1480·1).
Menopausal disorders; osteoporosis.

Premplus *Wyeth Lederle, Belg.*
28 Tablets, conjugated oestrogens (p.1467·1); 12 tablets, medrogestone (p.1480·1).
Oestrogen deficiency.

Prempro *Wyeth-Ayerst, USA.*
Conjugated oestrogens (p.1467·1); medroxyprogesterone acetate (p.1480·1).
Menopausal disorders; osteoporosis.

Premsyn PMS *Chattem, USA.*
Paracetamol (p.71·2); pamabrom (p.952·1); mepyramine maleate (p.421·1).
Pain.

Premus *Ciba Vision, Aust.†*
Storage and disinfecting solution for contact lenses (p.1129·2).

Prenacid *SIFI, Ital.*
Desonide sodium phosphate (p.1066·2).
Inflammatory eye disorders.

Prenafort *Cypress, USA.*
Multivitamin preparation with iron (p.1350·1).

Prenalex *Servier, Ger.*
Tertatolol hydrochloride (p.980·2).
Hypertension.

Prenatabs *Cypress, USA.*
A range of multivitamin and mineral preparations (p.1350·1).

Prenatal
Bio-Sante, Canad.; Jamieson, Canad.; Quest, Canad.; Stanley, Canad.; Stanley, Israel; Wyeth, Mex.; Wyeth Lederle, Port.; Ethex, USA.
A range of multivitamin and multivitamin and mineral preparations (p.1350·1).

Prenatal with Folic Acid *Geneva, USA.*
Multivitamin and mineral preparation with iron and folic acid (p.1350·1).

Prenatal Nutrients *Solgar, UK.*
Multivitamin and mineral preparation (p.1350·1).

Prenatal Plus *Zenith Goldline, USA.*
Multivitamin and mineral preparation with calcium and iron (p.1350·1).

Prenatal Plus Iron *Major, USA.*
Multivitamin and mineral preparation with iron (p.1350·1).

Prenatal Plus-Improved *Rugby, USA.*
Multivitamin and mineral preparation with iron and folic acid (p.1350·1).

Prenatal-S *Goldline, USA.*
Multivitamin and mineral preparation with iron and folic acid (p.1350·1).

Prenate *Sanofi Synthelabo, USA.*
Multivitamin and mineral preparation with iron and folic acid (p.1350·1).

Prenatex *Medix, Mex.*
Multivitamin and mineral preparation (p.1350·1).

Prenatol *Wyeth-Ayerst, Hong Kong.*
Amino acids; proteins (p.1350·1).
Prevention of stretch marks during pregnancy.

Prenavite
Roberts, Canad.
Multivitamin and mineral preparation (p.1350·1).
Dietary supplement during pregnancy and lactation.

Rugby, USA.
Multivitamin and mineral preparation with iron and folic acid (p.1350·1).

Prenefrin *Breves, Braz.*
Prednisolone (p.1077·3); phenylephrine (p.1097·1); mepyramine (p.421·1); neomycin (p.228·1).
Nasal disorders.

Prenilone *British Dispensary, Thai.*
Prednisolone (p.1077·3).
Corticosteroid.

Prenolol
Berlin Pharm, Singapore; Berlin Pharm, Thai.
Atenolol (p.841·3).
Angina pectoris; arrhythmias; hypertension; myocardial infarction.

Prenoxan au phenobarbital *Schering-Plough, Fr.†*
Phenobarbital (p.355·1); aspirin (p.14·2).
Fever; pain.

Prent
Gepepharm, Ger.; Bayer, Ital.; Bayer, Neth.†; Bayer, Port.
Acebutolol hydrochloride (p.825·1).
Arrhythmias; hypertension; ischaemic heart disease.

Pre-Nutrison *Nutricia, Port.*
Preparation for enteral nutrition (p.1350·1).

Prepacol
Sanova, Aust.†; Codali, Belg.; Guerbet, Fr.; Guerbet, Ger.
Combination pack: Tablets, bisacodyl (p.1212·2); oral solution, dibasic sodium phosphate (p.1193·2); monobasic sodium phosphate (p.1193·2).
Bowel evacuation.

Prepadine *Berk, UK.*
Dothiepin [dosulepin] hydrochloride (p.283·2).
Depression.

Pre-Par
Solvay, Belg.; Solvay, Fr.; Solvay, Ger.†; Solvay, Ital.†; Solvay, Neth.; Solvay, Port.; Solvay, Spain.
Ritodrine hydrochloride (p.1659·1).
Premature labour; prevention of fetal distress; relaxation of the uterus.

Preparacion H *Wyeth, Spain.*
Yeast extract (p.1398·1); shark-liver oil.
Haemorrhoids.

Preparado H *Whitehall, Braz.*
Live yeast (p.1398·1); cod-liver oil (p.1357·2); vitamin A (p.1382·1).
Haemorrhoids.

Preparation H
Note.This name is used for preparations of different composition.
Whitehall, Austral.; Whitehall-Robins, Canad.; Whitehall, Israel; Whitehall, Singapore; Whitehall, UK; Whitehall, USA.
Live yeast cell extract (p.1398·1); shark-liver oil.
Haemorrhoids.

Whitehall, Fr.
Rectal cream: Yeast (p.1398·1); halibut-liver oil (p.1366·1).
Suppositories: Butyl aminobenzoate (p.1308·2); yeast (p.1398·1); esculoside (p.1574·1); halibut-liver oil (p.1366·1).
Haemorrhoids.

Whitehall, Hong Kong; Whitehall, Thai.
Shark-liver oil; phenylephrine hydrochloride (p.1097·1).
Haemorrhoids.

Preparation H Cleansing Pads *Whitehall-Robins, Canad.*
Hamamelis (p.1618·3).
Anal and vaginal hygiene; anal irritation; haemorrhoids.

Preparation H Clear Gel *Whitehall, UK.*
Hamamelis (p.1618·3).
Haemorrhoids.

Preparation H Cooling Gel
Whitehall-Robins, Canad.; Whitehall-Robins, USA.
Hamamelis (p.1618·3); phenylephrine hydrochloride (p.1097·1).
Anorectal disorders.

Preparation H Hydrocortisone *Whitehall, USA†.*
Hydrocortisone (p.1073·3).
Anal pruritus.

Preparation H Sperti *Whitehall, Belg.†*
Dried yeast (p.1398·1).
Haemorrhoids.

Preparation H Veinotonic *Whitehall, Fr.*
Diosmin (p.1611·2).
Haemorrhoids.

Preparazione Antiemorroidaria *Giuliani, Ital.*
Hydrocortisone acetate (p.1073·3); benzocaine (p.1306·2).
Haemorrhoids.

Preparazione H *Whitehall, Ital.*
Yeast cell extract (p.1398·1); shark-liver oil.
Haemorrhoids.

Prepcare *Darrow, Braz.*
Povidone-iodine (p.1155·1).
Skin and wound disinfection.

Prepcat *Lafayette, USA.*
Barium sulfate (p.1032·1).
Contrast medium for gastrointestinal radiography.

Pre-Pen *Rivex, Canad.; Biolac, Swed.; Bayer, USA.*
Penicilloyl-polylysine (p.1649·2).
Diagnosis of penicillin hypersensitivity.

Prephen *Pharmacia Upjohn, NZ.*
Substituted phenols.
Disinfection.

Prepidil
Pharmacia Upjohn, Aust.; Pharmacia Upjohn, Belg.; Pharmacia Upjohn, Canad.; Pharmacia Upjohn, Fr.; Pharmacia Upjohn, Ger.; Pharmacia Upjohn, Hong Kong; Pharmacia Upjohn, Irl.; Pharmacia Upjohn, Israel; Pharmacia Upjohn, Ital.; Pharmacia Upjohn, Mex.; Pharmacia Upjohn, Neth.; Pharmacia Upjohn, NZ; Pharmacia Up-

john, S.Afr.; Pharmacia Upjohn, Spain; Pharmacia Upjohn, Switz.; Pharmacia Upjohn, UK†; Pharmacia Upjohn, USA.
Dinoprostone (p.1441·3).
Labour induction.

Prepulsid
Janssen-Cilag, Aust.; Janssen-Cilag, Austral.; Janssen-Cilag, Belg.; Janssen, Braz.; Janssen-Ortho, Canad.; Janssen-Cilag, Denm.; Janssen-Cilag, Fin.; Janssen-Cilag, Fr.; Janssen, Hong Kong; Janssen-Cilag, Irl.; Janssen-Cilag, Israel; Janssen-Cilag, Ital.; Janssen, Mex.; Janssen-Cilag, Neth.; Janssen-Cilag, Norw.; Janssen-Cilag, NZ; Janssen-Cilag, Port.; Janssen-Cilag, S.Afr.; Janssen-Cilag, Singapore; Janssen-Cilag, Spain; Janssen-Cilag, Swed.; Janssen-Cilag, Switz.; Janssen, Thai.; Janssen-Cilag, UK†.
Cisapride (p.1220·1) or cisapride tartrate (p.1221·1).
Dyspepsia; gastro-oesophageal reflux; impaired gastric motility.

Prepurex Glaxo Wellcome, Israel; Wellcome Diagnostics, UK.
Pregnancy test (p.1654·3).

Preran Hoechst Marion Roussel, Jpn.
Trandolapril (p.985·2).
Hypertension.

Pres Boehringer Ingelheim, Ger.
Enalapril maleate (p.883·3).
Heart failure; hypertension.

Pres iv Boehringer Ingelheim, Ger.
Enalaprilat (p.884·1).
Heart failure; hypertension.

Pres plus Boehringer Ingelheim, Ger.
Enalapril maleate (p.883·3); hydrochlorothiazide (p.907·3).
Hypertension.

Presalin Hauck, USA†.
Aspirin (p.14·2); paracetamol (p.71·2); salicylamide (p.82·1); aluminium hydroxide (p.1210·3).
Pain.

Prescaina Llorens, Spain.
Oxybuprocaine hydrochloride (p.1318·1).
Local anaesthesia.

Prescal
Novartis, Irl.†; Novartis, UK.
Isradipine (p.916·3).
Angina pectoris; hypertension.

Presco Polipharm, Thai.
Dextromethorphan hydrobromide (p.1087·3); bromhexine hydrochloride (p.1085·3).
Respiratory-tract disorders.

Prescol Atlantis, Mex.
Trimebutine (p.1675·1).
Gastrointestinal motility disorders.

Prescription Strength Desenex Ciba, USA†.
Cream: Clotrimazole (p.382·1).
Topical spray: Miconazole nitrate (p.391·1).
Fungal infections.

Presept
Ethicon, Ital.†; Johnson & Johnson Medical, UK.
Sodium dichloroisocyanurate (p.1156·1).
Instrument and surface disinfection.

Preservex UCB, UK.
Aceclofenac (p.11·1).
Musculoskeletal and joint disorders.

Presinol
Bayer, Aust.; Logosys, Ger.
Methyldopa (p.927·3).
Hypertension.

Preslow
Astra, Port.; Astra, Spain†.
Felodipine (p.888·3).
Angina pectoris; hypertension.

Presoken Kener, Mex.
Diltiazem (p.874·3).

Presol Cesam, Port.
SPF 20: Titanium dioxide (p.1126·1); zinc oxide (p.1128·2).
Sunscreen.

Presolol Alphapharm, Austral.
Labetalol hydrochloride (p.918·1).
Hypertension.

Presomen Solvay, Ger.
Extract from pregnant mare's urine.
Menopausal disorders.

Presomen compositum Kali-Chemie, Ger.
Combination pack: 10 Tablets, extract from pregnant mare's urine; 11 tablets, medrogestone (p.1480·1); extract from pregnant mare's urine.
Menopausal disorders; menstrual disorders.

Presoquim Kener, Mex.
Diltiazem (p.874·3).

Prespir Mex-America, Mex.
Aluminium chloride (p.1110·2).
Hyperhirosis.

Pressalolo Locatelli, Ital.†.
Labetalol hydrochloride (p.918·1).
Hypertension.

Pressalolo Diuretico Locatelli, Ital.†.
Labetalol hydrochloride (p.918·1); chlortalidone (p.857·1).
Hypertension.

Pressamina Teofarma, Ital.
Dimetofrine hydrochloride (p.877·2).
Hypotension.

Pressanol Propan, S.Afr.†.
Propranolol hydrochloride (p.962·3).
Cardiovascular disorders.

Presselin All Presselin, Ger.
Homoeopathic preparation.

Presselin Arterien K 5 P Presselin, Ger.
Crataegus (p.1600·2); hypericum (p.290·2); garlic (p.1614·1); barlauchkraut; java tea (p.1625·1); mistletoe (p.1636·2).
Circulatory disorders.

Presselin Blahungs K 4 N Presselin, Ger.
Peppermint leaf (p.1243·2); caraway (p.1591·2); fennel (p.1610·1); chamomile (p.1593·2); calamus (p.1588·1); absinthium (p.1571·1); sage (p.1660·2); melissa (p.1632·2).
Digestive-system disorders.

Presselin BN Nieren-Blasen Presselin, Ger.†.
Homoeopathic preparation.

Presselin Cpl 87 N Presselin, Ger.†.
Homoeopathic preparation.

Presselin Dysmen Olin 3 N Presselin, Ger.
Viburnum prunifolium: agnus castus (p.1574·2); anserina; shepherd's purse (p.1662·3); cimicifuga (p.1595·2).
Menopausal disorders; menstrual disorders.

Presselin Dyspeptikum Presselin, Ger.
Chamomile (p.1593·2); lavender (p.1627·2); sage (p.1660·2); caraway (p.1591·2); cardamom (p.1591·3); coriander (p.1599·2); fennel (p.1610·1); absinthium (p.1571·1); ginger (p.1227·2).
Biliary disorders; dyspepsia; liver disorders.

Presselin Gold N Presselin, Ger.
Homoeopathic preparation.

Presselin Heilozon P Presselin, Ger.
Magnesium citrate (p.1232·3).
Magnesium deficiency.

Presselin Hepaticum P Presselin, Ger.
Taraxacum (p.1669·1); greater celandine (p.1618·1); silybum marianum (p.1021·3).
Liver and biliary-tract disorders.

Presselin HK Herz-Kreislauf Presselin, Ger.
Homoeopathic preparation.

Presselin MIG F Presselin, Ger.
Homoeopathic preparation.

Presselin MIG M Presselin, Ger.
Homoeopathic preparation.

Presselin 218 N Presselin, Ger.†.
Homoeopathic preparation.

Presselin Nerven K I N Presselin, Ger.
Hypericum (p.290·2); valerian (p.1678·1); lupulus (p.1629·3); passion flower (p.1640·3).
Depression; nervous disorders; sleep disorders.

Presselin Nervennahrung N Presselin, Ger.
Homoeopathic preparation.

Presselin Nieren-Blasen K 3 Presselin, Ger.
Birch leaf (p.1585·2); java tea (p.1625·1); equisetum (p.1606·3); urtica root (p.1678·2); solidago virgaurea; lovage root (p.1629·3); ononis (p.1644·1).
Urinary-tract disorders.

Presselin Olin 5 Presselin, Ger.†.
Homoeopathic preparation.

Presselin Osteo Presselin, Ger.
Homoeopathic preparation.

Presselin Stoffwechsel-Tee Hapeka 225 N Presselin, Ger.
Chamomile (p.1593·2); stoechados; senna (p.1248·2); fennel (p.1610·1); juniper (p.1625·2); phaseolus (seed-free); equisetum (p.1606·3); couch-grass (p.1599·3).
Constipation.

Presselin VE Presselin, Ger.
Melilotus officinalis.
Venous disorders.

Pressimed Wild, Switz.†.
Dihydroergocristine mesilate (p.1603·2); bendrofluazide [bendroflumethiazide] (p.844·1); reserpine (p.967·3).
Hypertension.

Pressimedin Kwizda, Aust.
Dihydroergocristine mesilate (p.1603·2); bendrofluazide [bendroflumethiazide] (p.844·1); reserpine (p.967·3).
Hypertension.

Pressin
Alphapharm, Austral.; Utopian, Thai.
Prazosin hydrochloride (p.958·1).
Benign prostatic hyperplasia; heart failure; hypertension; Raynaud's syndrome.

Pressitan Iquinosa, Spain.
Enalapril maleate (p.883·3).
Heart failure; hypertension.

Pressitan Plus Iquinosa, Spain.
Enalapril maleate (p.883·3); hydrochlorothiazide (p.907·3).
Hypertension.

Pressolat Agis, Israel.
Nifedipine (p.940·1).
Hypertension.

Pressunic Compositum Unipharm, Israel.
Reserpine (p.967·3); dihydralazine (p.874·2).
Hypertension.

Pressural Polifarma, Ital.
Indapamide (p.913·1).
Hypertension.

Pressyn Ferring, Canad.
Vasopressin (p.1300·1).
Adjunct in abdominal radiography; diabetes insipidus; postoperative abdominal distension.

Prestim
Leo, Irl.; Leo, Neth.†; ICN, UK.
Timolol maleate (p.982·1); bendrofluazide [bendroflumethiazide] (p.844·1).
Hypertension.

Prestole Pharmafarm, Fr.
Triamterene (p.986·1); hydrochlorothiazide (p.907·3).
Hypertension.

Presun
Note.This name is used for preparations of different composition.
Westwood-Squibb, Canad.
Cream SPF 15†: Padimate O (p.1518·2); oxybenzone (p.1518·1).
Lotion SPF 15†: Aminobenzoic acid (p.1516·3); padimate O (p.1518·2); oxybenzone (p.1518·1).
SPF 15; SPF 27; SPF 30: Octinoxate (p.1517·3); octisalate (p.1518·1); oxybenzone (p.1518·1); avobenzone (p.1517·1).
SPF 21; SPF 28: Titanium dioxide (p.1126·1).
SPF 29: Octinoxate (p.1517·3); octisalate (p.1518·1); oxybenzone (p.1518·1).
SPF 39: Padimate O (p.1518·2); oxybenzone (p.1518·1).
Sunscreen.
Westwood, USA.
SPF 8; SPF 39: Padimate O (p.1518·2); oxybenzone (p.1518·1).
Cream SPF 15: Padimate O (p.1518·2); oxybenzone (p.1518·1).
Lotion SPF 15: Aminobenzoic acid (p.1516·3); padimate O (p.1518·2); oxybenzone (p.1518·1).
Sunscreen.

Presun Active Bristol-Myers Products, USA.
SPF 15; SPF 30: Octinoxate (p.1517·3); oxybenzone (p.1518·1); octisalate (p.1518·1).
Sunscreen.

Presun Facial Westwood, USA.
SPF 15: Padimate O (p.1518·2); oxybenzone (p.1518·1).
Sunscreen.

Presun for Kids Westwood, USA; Bristol-Myers Products, USA.
Octinoxate (p.1517·3); oxybenzone (p.1518·1); octisalate (p.1518·1).
Sunscreen.

Presun Lip Stick Westwood, USA.
SPF 15: Padimate O (p.1518·2); oxybenzone (p.1518·1).
Sunscreen.

Presun Moisturizing Bristol-Myers Products, USA.
SPF 46: Padimate O (p.1518·2); oxybenzone (p.1518·1).
Sunscreen.

Presun Moisturizing with Keri Bristol-Myers Products, USA.
SPF 15: Padimate O (p.1518·2); oxybenzone (p.1518·1).
SPF 25: Octinoxate (p.1517·3); oxybenzone (p.1518·1); octisalate (p.1518·1).
Sunscreen.

Presun Sensitive Skin Westwood, USA; Bristol-Myers Products, USA.
SPF 15; SPF 29: Octinoxate (p.1517·3); oxybenzone (p.1518·1); octisalate (p.1518·1).
Sunscreen.

Presun Spray Mist Bristol-Myers Products, USA.
SPF 23: Octinoxate (p.1517·3); padimate O (p.1518·2); oxybenzone (p.1518·1); octisalate (p.1518·1).
Sunscreen.

PreSun Ultra Westwood-Squibb, USA.
SPF 30: Avobenzone (p.1517·1); octinoxate (p.1517·3); octisalate (p.1518·1); oxybenzone (p.1518·1).
Sunscreen.

Preterax Therval, Fr.
Perindopril erbumine (p.953·2); indapamide (p.913·1).
Hypertension.

Pretts Diet Aid Milance, USA.
Alginic acid (p.1498·3); carmellose sodium (p.1499·3); sodium bicarbonate (p.1186·2).

Pretuval Roche, Switz.
Dextromethorphan hydrobromide (p.1087·3); pseudoephedrine hydrochloride (p.1099·2); paracetamol (p.71·2).
Cold symptoms.

Pretuval C Roche, Switz.
Dextromethorphan hydrobromide (p.1087·3); pseudoephedrine hydrochloride (p.1099·2); paracetamol (p.71·2); ascorbic acid (p.1389·3).
Cold symptoms.

Pretz
Note.This name is used for preparations of different composition.
Parnell, Irl.
Moisturising nasal spray.
Nasal dryness.
Parnell, USA.
Sodium chloride (p.1196·1).
Inflammation and dryness of nasal membranes.

Pretz-D Parnell, USA.
Ephedrine sulfate (p.1090·2).
Nasal congestion.

Prevacid
Abbott, Canad.; Takeda, Singapore; Takeda, Thai.; TAP, USA.
Lansoprazole (p.1230·3).
Gastro-oesophageal reflux; peptic ulcer; Zollinger-Ellison syndrome.

Prevagin-Premaril Dexxon, Israel.
Conjugated oestrogens (p.1467·1).
Menopausal vulvovaginal disorders.

Prevalin Chefaro, Neth.
Sodium cromoglicate (p.774·3).
Allergic conjunctivitis; allergic rhinitis.

Prevalite Upsher-Smith, USA.
Colestyramine (p.864·1).

Prevalon Abello, Spain.
Multivitamin and amino-acid preparation (p.1350·1).
Tonic.

Prevecilina Grunenthal, Port.
Clemizole penicillin (p.188·1); benzylpenicillin sodium (p.157·2).
Lignocaine [lidocaine] hydrochloride (p.1313·2) is included in the intramuscular injection to alleviate the pain of injection.
Bacterial infections.

Preven Gynetics, USA.
Levonorgestrel (p.1486·2); ethinylestradiol (p.1476·2).
Postcoital oral contraceptive.

Prevenar
Wyeth, Austral.; Wyeth, UK.
A pneumococcal conjugate vaccine (7-valent) (p.1557·2).
Active immunisation in infants and children.

Prevencal Lalco, Canad.†.
Calcium carbonate (p.1215·1).

Prevencal & D Lalco, Canad.†.
Calcium carbonate (p.1215·1); vitamin D (p.1391·1).

Prevencal & D & Fer Lalco, Canad.†.
Calcium carbonate (p.1215·1); vitamin D (p.1391·1); ferrous fumarate (p.1360·1).

Prevencal & D & Magnesium Lalco, Canad.†.
Calcium carbonate (p.1215·1); vitamin D (p.1391·1); magnesium oxide (p.1233·2).

Prevencor Almirall, Spain.
Atorvastatin calcium (p.842·3).
Hyperlipidaemias.

Prevent Agropharm, UK.
Pyrethrins; piperonyl butoxide (p.1436·2); d'lemonin.
Insecticide.

Prevex
Note.This name is used for preparations of different composition.
Trans Canaderm, Canad.
Cream: Cyclomethicone; yellow soft paraffin (p.1407·3).
Barrier cream for hands.
Lotion: Moisturiser.

AstraZeneca, Ital.
Felodipine (p.888·3).
Angina pectoris; hypertension.

Prevex B Trans Canaderm, Canad.
Betamethasone valerate (p.1063·2).
Skin disorders.

Prevex Diaper Rash Cream Trans Canaderm, Canad.†.
Zinc oxide (p.1128·2).
Barrier cream.

Prevex HC Trans Canaderm, Canad.
Hydrocortisone (p.1073·3).
Skin disorders.

Prevident Colgate Oral, USA.
Sodium fluoride (p.1375·3).
Dental caries prophylaxis.

Previgrip Chiron, It.
Inactivated influenza vaccine (p.1544·3).
Active immunisation.

Previscan Procter & Gamble, Fr.
Fluindione (p.892·1).
Thromboembolic disorders.

Previum Chefaro, Neth.†.
Aciclovir (p.612·3).
Herpes simplex infections.

Prevnar Wyeth-Ayerst, USA.
A pneumococcal conjugate vaccine (7-valent) (p.1557·2).
Active immunisation.

Prevpac TAP, USA.
Capsules, lansoprazole (Prevacid) (p.1230·3); capsules, amoxicillin trihydrate (Trimox) (p.149·2); tablets, clarithromycin (Biaxin) (p.186·2).
Duodenal ulcer associated with Helicobacter pylori infection.

Prewash Pharmacia Upjohn, Hong Kong.
Triclosan (p.1159·2).
Acne.

Prexan Lafare, Ital.
Naproxen (p.60·3).
Musculoskeletal, joint, peri-articular, and soft-tissue disorders; neuralgias.

Prexene Herbaline, Ital.†.
Garlic (p.1614·1); crataegus (p.1600·2); olive oil (p.1643·3); silver birch (p.1585·2).
Hypertension; tachycardia.

Prexidine Pred, Fr.
Chlorhexidine gluconate (p.1138·2).
Mouth infections.

Prezal Hoechst Marion Roussel, Neth.
Lansoprazole (p.1230·3).
Gastro-oesophageal reflux; peptic ulcer; Zollinger-Ellison syndrome.

Priadel
Sanofi Synthelabo, Belg.: Delandale, Irl.; Sanofi Synthelabo, Neth.;

The symbol † denotes a preparation no longer actively marketed

Bamford, NZ; Synthelabo, Port.; Sanofi Synthelabo, Singapore; Synthelabo, Switz.; Sanofi Synthelabo, UK.
Lithium carbonate (p.292·1) or lithium citrate (p.292·1).
Aggressive or self-mutilating behaviour; bipolar disorder; depression; mania.

Priamide Janssen-Cilag, Belg.†
Isopropamide iodide (p.470·1).
Diarrhoea; gastrointestinal spasm.

Priaxim Ravizza, Ital.
Flunoxaprofen (p.41·1).
Gynaecological inflammation; musculoskeletal, joint, peri-articular, and soft-tissue disorders; venous disorders.

Priciasol Labima, Belg.
Naphazoline nitrate (p.1095·1).
Nasal congestion.

Pricillin MPF, Singapore.
Ampicillin trihydrate (p.151·1).
Bacterial infections.

Prickly Heat Powder Carter-Wallace, Austral.
Zinc oxide (p.1128·2).
Chafed skin; eczema; heat rash; prickly heat.

Pridam Pisa, Mex.
Noradrenaline [norepinephrine] (p.948·2).

Pridana Novartis, Port.
Pirisudanol maleate (p.1652·3).
Mental function disorders.

Pridecil Farmalab, Braz.
Bromopride (p.1215·1).
Nausea and vomiting.

Pri-De-Sid Polipharm, Thai.
Cisapride (p.1220·1).
Dyspepsia; gastro-oesophageal reflux; gastrointestinal motility disorders; gastroparesis.

Pridinol Millet Roux, Braz.
Terfenadine (p.424·3).
Hypersensitivity reactions.

Pridio Quimifar, Spain.
Caffeine (p.761·3); chlorpheniramine [chlorphenamine] maleate (p.412·1); paracetamol (p.71·2); salicylamide (p.82·1).
Fever; nasal congestion; pain.

Priftin Hoechst Marion Roussel, USA.
Rifapentine (p.246·3).
Tuberculosis.

Prilace Hoechst Marion Roussel, Ital.
Ramipril (p.966·3); piretanide (p.956·2).
Hypertension.

Prilagin Gambar, Ital.
Miconazole (p.391·1) or miconazole nitrate (p.391·1).
Candidiasis; Gram-positive bacterial infections.

Prilosec Astra, USA.
Omeprazole (p.1239·1).
Gastro-oesophageal reflux; peptic ulcer; Zollinger-Ellison syndrome.

Prilovase CPH, Port.
Captopril (p.853·3).
Heart failure; hypertension.

Priltam Atache, Spain.
Capsaicin (p.23·1).
Muscle and joint pain.

Prima-Cal Prima, Thai.
Calcium carbonate (p.1215·1).
Calcium supplement.

Primacard Matara, Fr.
Pregnancy test (p.1654·3).

Primacin Boucher & Muir, Austral.
Primaquine phosphate (p.440·3).
Malaria.

Primacine Pinewood, Irl.
Erythromycin ethyl succinate (p.201·2) or erythromycin stearate (p.201·3).
Bacterial infections.

Primacor
Sanofi Synthelabo, Austral.; Sanofi Winthrop, Braz.; Sanofi Synthelabo, Canad.; Sanofi Winthrop, Hong Kong; Sanofi Winthrop, Israel; Sanofi Winthrop, NZ; Sanofi Synthelabo, Thai.; Sanofi Winthrop, UK; Sanofi Winthrop, USA.
Milrinone lactate (p.934·1).
Heart failure.

Primaderm-B Arrow, USA†.
Benzocaine (p.1306·2); zinc oxide (p.1128·2); cod-liver oil (p.1357·2).
Anorectal disorders.

Primafen Hoechst Marion Roussel, Spain.
Cefotaxime sodium (p.169·1).
Lignocaine [lidocaine] (p.1313·3) is included in the intramuscular injection to alleviate the pain of injection.
Bacterial infections.

Primahex Convatec, UK.
Chlorhexidine (p.1138·2); alcohol (p.1130·3).
Skin disinfection.

Primalan
Inava, Fr.; Rhone-Poulenc Rorer, Irl.†; Pierre Fabre, Ital.; Pierre Fabre, Port.; Rhone-Poulenc Sante, Thai.; May & Baker, UK†.
Mequitazine (p.421·2).
Hypersensitivity reactions; pruritus.

Primamed Sanofi Synthelabo, Ger.
Aluminium chlorohydrate (p.1110·2).
Burns; skin disorders; wounds.

Primanol Jamieson, Canad.
Evening primrose oil (p.1613·2).

Primanol-Borage Jamieson, Canad.†
A range of borage oil (p.1613·1) preparations.

Primasept Med Schulke & Mayr, Ger.
Propyl alcohol (p.1155·3); isopropyl alcohol (p.1149·2); orthophenylphenol (p.1152·1).
Hand disinfection.

Primasone Rhodia, Braz.
Mequitazine (p.421·2).
Hypersensitivity reactions.

Primaspan Orion, Fin.
Aspirin (p.14·2).
Musculoskeletal, joint and peri-articular disorders; pain; thromboembolism prophylaxis.

Primastick Matara, Fr.
Pregnancy test (p.1654·3).

Primatene Whitehall-Robins, USA.
Ephedrine hydrochloride (p.1090·1); guaifenesin (p.1092·2).
Formerly contained ephedrine hydrochloride and theophylline.
Bronchial asthma.

Primatene Dual Action Whitehall, USA†.
Theophylline (p.777·2); ephedrine hydrochloride (p.1090·1); guaifenesin (p.1092·2).
Asthma.

Primatene Mist Whitehall, USA.
Adrenaline [epinephrine] (p.829·1).
Bronchial asthma.

Primatene Mist Suspension Whitehall, USA.
Adrenaline [epinephrine] acid tartrate (p.829·2).
Bronchial asthma.

Primatime Matara, Fr.
Fertility test (p.1654·3).

Primatour Asta Medica, Neth.
Chlorcyclizine hydrochloride (p.411·3); cinnarizine (p.413·1).
Motion sickness.

Primatuss Cough Mixture 4 Rugby, USA.
Chlorpheniramine [chlorphenamine] maleate (p.412·1); dextromethorphan hydrobromide (p.1087·3).
Coughs and cold symptoms.

Primatuss Cough Mixture 4D Rugby, USA.
Pseudoephedrine hydrochloride (p.1099·2); dextromethorphan hydrobromide (p.1087·3); guaifenesin (p.1092·2).
Coughs.

Primavax Pasteur Merieux, Ital.
A diphtheria, tetanus, and hepatitis B vaccine.
Active immunisation.

Primaxin
Merck Sharp & Dohme, Austral.; Merck Frosst, Canad.; Merck Sharp & Dohme, NZ; Merck Sharp & Dohme, UK; Merck, USA.
Imipenem (p.214·1); cilastatin sodium (p.182·2).
Bacterial infections.

Primbactam Menarini, Ital.
Aztreonam (p.154·2).
Bacterial infections.

Primcillin AstraZeneca, Denm.
Phenoxymethylpenicillin potassium (p.235·1).
Bacterial infections.

Prime Time Quest, Canad.
Multivitamin and mineral preparation (p.1350·1).

Primene
Baxter, Canad.; Baxter, Fr.; Baxter, Ger.; Baxter, Irl.; Baxter, Spain; Baxter, UK.
Amino-acid infusion (p.1350·1).
Parenteral nutrition in infants.

Primer Unna Boot Glenwood, USA†.
Zinc oxide (p.1128·2); acacia; glycerol; castor oil; white soft paraffin.
Venous insufficiency.

Primeral
Note. This name is used for preparations of different composition.
Synthelabo, Braz.
Bromopride (p.1215·1); dimethicone (p.1249·2); pepsin (p.1649·3); α-amylase (p.1579·3); lipase.
Digestive disorders; nausea and vomiting.

Master Pharma, Ital.†
Naproxen sodium (p.61·1).
Musculoskeletal and joint disorders; pain.

Primesin LPB, Ital.
Fluvastatin sodium (p.892·1).
Hypercholesterolaemia.

Primil Francia, Ital.
Magnesium; potassium; vitamins (p.1350·1).
Nutritional supplement.

Primobolan
Schering, Aust.; Schering, Austral.; Schering, Ger.; Schering, Mex.; Schering, Norw.†; Schering, S.Afr.
Metenolone acetate (p.1482·2) or metenolone enantate (p.1482·2).
Anabolic; anaemias; breast cancer; female genital cancer; osteoporosis.

Primobolan Depot
Schering, Ital.†; Schering, Spain.
Metenolone enantate (p.1482·2).
Anabolic; anaemia in chronic renal failure; aplastic anaemia; breast cancer; osteoporosis.

Primobolan S Schering, Neth.
Metenolone acetate (p.1482·2).
Aplastic anaemia.

Primocef Julphar, UAE.
Cefotaxime sodium (p.169·1).
Bacterial infections.

Primodian Depot
Schering, Aust.†; Schering, Austral.†; Schering, S.Afr.; Schering, Thai.
Estradiol valerate (p.1473·2); testosterone enantate (p.1492·2).
Menopausal disorders; osteoporosis.

Primodium Janssen-Cilag, Swed.
Loperamide oxide (p.1232·1).
Diarrhoea.

Primofenac Streuli, Switz.
Diclofenac sodium (p.30·3).
Gout; inflammation; musculoskeletal, joint, and peri-articular disorders; pain.

Primogonyl Schering, Ger.
Chorionic gonadotrophin (p.1279·2).
Cryptorchidism, hypogonadism, and delayed puberty in males; infertility in females.

Primogyn Schering, Mex.
Estradiol valerate (p.1473·2).
Amenorrhoea; menorrhagia; oestrogen deficiency; uterine hypoplasia.

Primogyn Depot
Schering, Austral.; Schering, S.Afr.
Estradiol valerate (p.1473·2).
Amenorrhoea; menorrhagia; oestrogen deficiency; uterine hypoplasia.

Primolut Depot
Schering, Mex.; Schering, S.Afr.†
Hydroxyprogesterone caproate (p.1479·3).
Amenorrhoea; female infertility; threatened or recurrent miscarriage; uterine hypoplasia.

Primolut N
Schering, Austral.; Schering, Fin.; Schering, Hong Kong; Schering, Irl.; Schering, Neth.; Schering, Norw.; Schering, NZ; Schering, S.Afr.; Schering, Singapore; Schering, Swed.; Schering, Thai.; Schering, UK.
Norethisterone (p.1485·1).
Dysfunctional bleeding; endometriosis; mastopathy; menopausal disorders; menstrual disorders.

Primolut-Nor
Schering, Aust.; Schering, Belg.; Schering, Braz.; Schering, Fin.; Schering, Ger.; Schering, Israel; Schering, Ital.; Schering, Mex.; Schering, Port.; Schering, Spain; Schering, Swed.; Schering, Switz.
Norethisterone acetate (p.1485·1).
Benign breast disorders; breast cancer; dysfunctional uterine bleeding; endometriosis; fibromas; mastopathy; menstrual disorders; progestogen-only oral contraceptive; uterine hypoplasia.

Primonil Teva, Israel.
Imipramine hydrochloride (p.291·1).
Depression; nocturnal enuresis.

Primosept Andreabal, Switz.†
Trimethoprim (p.264·2).
Urinary-tract infections.

Primosiston
Note. This name is used for preparations of different composition.
Schering, Aust.; Schering, Braz.; Schering, Ger.; Schering, Spain; Schering, Switz.
Tablets: Norethisterone acetate (p.1485·1); ethinylestradiol (p.1476·2).
Menstrual disorders.

Schering, Mex.; Schering, Switz.
Injection: Hydroxyprogesterone caproate (p.1479·3); estradiol benzoate (p.1473·1).
Metrorrhagia.

Primostat Schering, Mex.
Gestonorone caproate (p.1479·1).
Benign prostatic hyperplasia; endometrial cancer.

Primoteston Depot
Schering, Austral.; Schering, Mex.; Schering, Norw.; Schering, NZ; Schering, UK.
Testosterone enantate (p.1492·2); testosterone propionate (p.1492·2).
Some injections contain only testosterone enantate.
Androgenic; aplastic anaemia; breast cancer; genital cancer in females; hypogonadism in males.

Primotussan Galenika, Yug.
Cowslip rhizome (p.1600·1); thyme (p.1672·2).
Cold symptoms.

Primover Alcon Cusi, Spain.
Sodium cromoglicate (p.774·3).
Allergic conjunctivitis.

Primovlar Schering, Braz.
Norgestrel (p.1486·1); ethinylestradiol (p.1476·2).
Combined oral contraceptive.

Primoxil Bayer, Ital.
Moexipril hydrochloride (p.935·3).
Hypertension.

Primperan
Sanofi Synthelabo, Belg.; Sanofi Winthrop, Denm.; Leiras Synthelabo, Fin.; Synthelabo, Fr.; Synthelabo, Hong Kong; Berk, Irl.†; Lorex Synthelabo, Neth.†; Sanofi Winthrop, Norw.; Sanofi Synthelabo, Port.; Roche, S.Afr.†; Sanofi Synthelabo, Singapore; Synthelabo, Spain; Tika, Swed.; Synthelabo, Switz.; Berk, UK.
Metoclopramide (p.1236·3) or metoclopramide hydrochloride (p.1235·2).
Adjunct in gastrointestinal examination; gastrointestinal disorders.

Primperan Complex Synthelabo, Spain†.
Dimethicone (p.1249·2); metoclopramide (p.1236·3); sorbitol (p.1377·3).
Aerophagia; dyspepsia; hiatus hernia; meteorism; vomiting.

Primperoxane Synthelabo, Fr.†.
Metoclopramide (p.1236·3); dimethicone (p.1249·2).
Dyspepsia.

Primsol Ascent, USA.
Trimethoprim hydrochloride (p.265·3).
Otitis media; urinary-tract infections.

Primyxine Alpharma, Fr.
Oxytetracycline hydrochloride (p.234·1); polymyxin B sulfate (p.238·1).
Skin and wound infections.

Prinachol Zurita, Braz.
Cynara (p.1601·3); boldo (p.1585·3).
Liver disorders.

Prinactizide Irex, Fr.
Altizide (p.835·1); spironolactone (p.973·2).
Hypertension; oedema.

Princi B1 + B6 Sanofi Synthelabo, Neth.
Thiamine hydrochloride (p.1385·1); pyridoxine hydrochloride (p.1386·3).
Vitamin B deficiency associated with alcoholism.

Princi-B
Note. This name is used for preparations of different composition.
Bournonville, Belg.†
Vitamin B substances (p.1350·1).
Alcoholism; cardiovascular disorders; drug intoxication; neurogenic pain; rheumatic pain.

SERP, Mon.
Pyridoxine hydrochloride; thiamine nitrate (p.1350·1).
Tonic.

Sanofi Synthelabo, Thai.
Vitamin B₁ (p.1385·2); vitamin B₆ (p.1387·1); vitamin B₁₂ (p.1388·1).
Beri-beri; neuritis.

Princi-B Fort
Sanofi Winthrop, Hong Kong; Sanofi Synthelabo, Singapore.
Vitamin B₁ (p.1385·2); vitamin B₆ (p.1387·1); vitamin B₁₂ (p.1388·1).
Neuralgias; neuritis; tonic; vitamin B deficiency.

Principen Apothecon, USA.
Ampicillin trihydrate (p.151·1).
Bacterial infections.

Princol Provit, Mex.
Lincomycin hydrochloride (p.219·2).
Bacterial infections.

Prindex Abbott, Mex.
Pseudoephedrine hydrochloride (p.1099·2); carbinoxamine maleate (p.411·1).
Upper respiratory-tract congestion.

Prinil Merck Sharp & Dohme, Switz.
Lisinopril (p.921·1).
Heart failure; hypertension.

Prinivil
Merck Sharp & Dohme, Aust.†; Amrad, Austral.; Prodome, Braz.; Merck Frosst, Canad.; Du Pont, Fr.; Merck Sharp & Dohme, Hong Kong; Du Pont, Ital.; Merck Sharp & Dohme, Mex.; Douglas, NZ; Merck Sharp & Dohme, Port.; Merck Sharp & Dohme, S.Afr.; Merck Sharp & Dohme, Singapore; Du Pont, Spain; Merck, USA.
Lisinopril (p.921·1).
Diabetic nephropathy; heart failure; hypertension; myocardial infarction.

Prinivil Plus Du Pont, Spain.
Lisinopril (p.921·1); hydrochlorothiazide (p.907·3).
Hypertension.

Prinsyl Coventry, UK.
Chloroxylenol (p.1142·1).

Printania Clintec, Fr.†
High protein nutritional supplement (p.1350·1).

Printol Coventry, UK.
Tar acids (p.1158·1).

Prinzide
Merck Sharp & Dohme, Aust.†; Prodome, Braz.; Merck Frosst, Canad.; Du Pont, Fr.; Du Pont, Ital.; Merck Sharp & Dohme, Mex.; Merck Sharp & Dohme, NZ; Merck Sharp & Dohme, Port.; Merck Sharp & Dohme, Switz.; Merck, USA.
Lisinopril (p.921·1); hydrochlorothiazide (p.907·3).
Hypertension.

Prioderm
Asta Medica, Belg.; Norpharma, Denm., Mundipharma, Fin.; Sarget, Fr.; Seton, Irl.; Seton, Israel; Asta Medica, Neth.; Norpharma, Norw.; Pharmaco, NZ; Abigo, Swed.; Mundipharma, Switz.; SSL, UK.
Malathion (p.1434·2).
Pediculosis; scabies.

Priorin
Roche, Aust.; Roche Nicholas, Ger.
Millet; calcium pantothenate; cystine (p.1350·1).
Hair and nail disorders.

Roche, Ital.†
Millet; calcium pantothenate; cystine; wheat-germ oil (p.1350·1).
Skin disorders.

Priorin Biotin Roche Nicholas, Ger.†
Biotin (p.1355·3).
Biotin deficiency.

Priorin N Roche, Switz.
Millet; calcium pantothenate; cystine; wheat-germ oil (p.1350·1).
Hair and nail disorders.

Priorix
SmithKline Beecham, Austral.; SmithKline Beecham, Belg.; SmithKline Beecham, Canad.; SmithKline Beecham, Fin.; SmithKline Beecham, Fr.; SmithKline Beecham, Ger.; SmithKline Beecham, Hong Kong; SmithKline Beecham, Irl.; SmithKline Beecham, Israel; SmithKline Beecham, Ital.; SmithKline Beecham, Mex.; SmithKline Beecham & French, Port.; SmithKline Beecham, Singapore; SmithKline Beecham, Spain; SBL, Swed.; SmithKline Beecham, Switz.; SmithKline Beecham, UK.
A measles, mumps, and rubella vaccine (attenuated Schwarz, Jeryl Lynn, and Wistar RA 27/3 strains respectively) (p.1549·1).
Active immunisation.

Priovit 12 SIT, Ital.
Multivitamin preparation (p.1350·1).

Pripsen
Note.This name is used for preparations of different composition.
Seton, Irl.
Piperazine phosphate (p.106·1); sennosides (p.1248·3).
Ascariasis; enterobiasis.

SSL, UK.
Elixir: Piperazine citrate (p.105·3).
Ascariasis; enterobiasis.
Oral powder: Piperazine phosphate (p.106·1); senna (p.1248·2).
Ascariasis; enterobiasis.
Tablets: Mebendazole (p.102·2).
Enterobiasis.

Priscol *Ciba Vision, Ger.*
Tolazoline hydrochloride (p.984·3).
Vascular eye disorders.

Priscoline
Novartis, Austral.†; Novartis, NZ; Ciba, USA.
Tolazoline hydrochloride (p.984·3).
Persistent pulmonary hypertension of the newborn.

Prisdal *Almirall, Spain.*
Citalopram hydrobromide (p.281·2).
Anxiety; depression.

Prisma
Note.This name is used for preparations of different composition.
Thiemann, Ger.
Mianserin hydrochloride (p.298·1).
Depression.

Mediolanum, Ital.; Medinfar, Port.
Mesoglycan sodium (p.1634·3).
Cerebral and peripheral vascular disorders; hyperlip-idaemias; thrombo-embolic disorders.

Prisoventril *Simoes, Braz.*
Phenolphthalein (p.1244·1); cascara (p.1216·1).
Constipation.

Pritor
Glaxo Wellcome, Austral.; Glaxo Wellcome, Fr.; Glaxo Wellcome, Ital.; Glaxo Wellcome, Port.; Glaxo Wellcome, Spain.
Telmisartan (p.979·2).
Hypertension.

Privacom *Typharm, UK.*
Clotrimazole (p.382·1).
Vaginal candidiasis.

Privin
Novartis, Aust.; Novartis, Ger.
Naphazoline nitrate (p.1095·1).
Aid to cystoscopy and rhinoscopy; nasal congestion.

Privina
Novartis, Braz.; Novartis, Spain†.
Naphazoline hydrochloride (p.1095·1) or naphazoline nitrate (p.1095·1).
Nasal congestion.

Privine *Ciba, USA.*
Naphazoline hydrochloride (p.1095·1).
Nasal congestion.

Privituss *Mitim, Ital.*
Cloperastine fendizoate (p.1087·2).
Coughs.

Prizem *Solfran, Mex.*
Diazepam (p.674·3).

Prizma *Unipharm, Israel.*
Fluoxetine hydrochloride (p.284·2).
Depression; obsessive-compulsive disorder.

Pro *Dunhall, USA†.*
Promethazine hydrochloride (p.423·2).
Hypersensitivity reactions; motion sickness; nausea; postoperative pain (adjunct); sedative; vomiting.

Pro Dorm *Synthelabo, Ger.†.*
Lorazepam (p.688·3).
Anxiety; sleep disorders.

Pro Skin *Marlyn, USA†.*
Multivitamin and mineral preparation (p.1350·1).

Pro Ulco *Vinas, Spain.*
Lansoprazole (p.1230·3).
Gastro-oesophageal reflux; peptic ulcer.

Proacid *Procare, Austral.†.*
Glycine (p.1365·3); calcium carbonate (p.1215·1); aloes (p.1210·1).
Gastric hyperacidity.

Pro-Actidil
Glaxo Wellcome, Aust.; Glaxo Wellcome, Israel; Wellcome, Spain.
Triprolidine hydrochloride (p.427·2).
Hypersensitivity reactions; skin disorders.

Proaf *Abic, Israel.*
Isoflupredone acetate (p.1075·3); ephedrine hydrochloride (p.1090·1); naphazoline nitrate (p.1095·1).
Rhinitis; sinusitis.

Proaller *Pekana, Ger.*
Homoeopathic preparation.

ProAmatine *Roberts, USA.*
Midodrine hydrochloride (p.933·3).
Orthostatic hypotension.

Proampi *Stafford-Miller, Fr.*
Pivampicillin (p.237·2).
Bacterial infections.

Proartinal *Provit, Mex.*
Ibuprofen (p.43·2).
Inflammation; pain.

Proasma-T *Progress, Thai.*
Terbutaline sulfate (p.776·2).
Obstructive airways disease; premature labour.

Probalan *Lannett, USA†.*
Probenecid (p.401·3).
Adjunct to beta-lactam antibacterials; gout.

The symbol † denotes a preparation no longer actively marketed

Pro-Banthine
Sigma, Austral.; Searle, Belg.†; Roberts, Canad.; Searle, Denm.†; Monsanto, Fr.†; Baker Norton, Irl.†; Searle, Israel; Searle, Neth.†; Pharmaco, NZ; Searle, S.Afr.; Searle, Swed.†; Searle, Switz.†; Hansam, UK; Schiapparelli Searle, USA.
Propantheline bromide (p.473·2).
Adjunct in gastrointestinal diagnostic procedures; cholecystitis; gastritis; gastrointestinal spasm; hyperhidrosis; inflammatory bowel disease; irritable bowel syndrome; pancreatitis; peptic ulcer; renal colic; urinary-tract disorders.

Probase 3 *Schering-Plough, UK.*
Emollient.
Dry skin.

Probax *Fischer, USA.*
Propolis (p.1655·1).
Skin disorders.

Probecid
AstraZeneca, Fin.; AstraZeneca, Norw.; Astra, Swed.
Probenecid (p.401·3).
Adjunct to beta-lactam antibacterials; gout.

Probecilin *Eurofarma, Braz.*
Procaine penicillin [procaine benzylpenicillin] (p.239·2).
Probenecid (p.401·3) is included in this preparation to reduce renal tubular excretion of the antibiotic.
Bacterial infections.

Probec-T *J&J-Merck, USA.*
Vitamin B substances with vitamin C (p.1350·1).

Proben *Quatromed, S.Afr.*
Probenecid (p.401·3).
Gout.

Proben-C *Rugby, USA†.*
Probenecid (p.401·3); colchicine (p.400·1).
Gout.

Probenzima *Farmoquimica, Braz.*
Ampicillin sodium (p.150·3).
Bacterial infections.

Probenzima Ampicilina *Farmoquimica, Braz.*
Ampicillin (p.150·3); trypsin (p.1675·3); chymotrypsin (p.1595·1).
Bacterial infections; inflammation.

Probenzima Analgesico *Farmoquimica, Braz.*
Paracetamol (p.71·2); trypsin (p.1675·3); chymotrypsin (p.1595·1).
Inflammation; pain.

Probeta *Allergan, Canad.*
Levobunolol hydrochloride (p.920·3); dipivefrine hydrochloride (p.1604·3).
Glaucoma; ocular hypertension.

Probeta LA *Trinity, UK.*
Propranolol hydrochloride (p.962·3).
Angina pectoris; hypertension.

Probi-Albumin *Probifasa, Mex.*
Albumin (p.724·1).
Acute barbiturate overdosage; burns; hypoproteinaemia; nephrotic syndrome; pancreatitis; plasma volume expansion; shock.

Probigol *Biohorma, Ital.*
Propolis (p.1655·1); echinacea (p.1606·2).
Oral hygiene.

Pro-Bionate *Natren, USA.*
Lactobacillus acidophilus (p.1626·3).
Dietary supplement.

Probiophyt V *OTW, Ger.*
Silybum marianum (p.1021·3).
Liver disorders.

Probiox *Baif, Ital.*
Vitamin B substances (p.1350·1); lactic-acid-producing organisms (p.1626·3).
Gastrointestinal disorders.

Probi-Rho D *Probifasa, Mex.*
An anti-D immunoglobulin (p.1532·1).
Prevention of rhesus sensitisation.

Probi-Tet *Probifasa, Mex.*
Tetanus immunoglobulin (p.1565·1).
Passive immunisation.

Probufen *Nakornpatana, Thai.*
Ibuprofen (p.43·2).
Musculoskeletal and joint disorders.

Pro-C *Procare, Austral.*
Ascorbic acid (p.1389·3).
Vitamin C supplement.

Pro-30C *Capo Sole, Ital.*
Propolis (p.1655·1).

Procadil *Recordati, Ital.*
Procaterol hydrochloride (p.770·1).
Obstructive airways disease.

Procal *Christiaens, Belg.*
Note. A similar name is used for preparations of different composition (see below).
Sodium fluoride (p.1375·3).
Osteoporosis.

Pro-Cal
Note. A similar name is used for preparations of different composition (see above).
Vitaflo, Irl.; Vitaflo, UK.
High energy and protein food fortifier (p.1350·1).

ProcalAmine
Braun McGaw, Hong Kong.
Amino-acid infusion (p.1350·1).
Parenteral nutrition.

Pisa, Mex.
Amino-acid, glycerol, and electrolyte preparation (p.1350·1).
Parenteral nutrition.

McGaw, NZ.
Amino-acid, carbohydrate, and electrolyte infusion (p.1350·1).
Parenteral nutrition.

McGaw, USA.
Amino-acid and electrolyte infusion (p.1350·1).
Parenteral nutrition.

Procal-D *Kato, Singapore.*
Calcium (p.1187·3); vitamin D (p.1391·1).
Calcium and vitamin D deficiency.

Procalmadiol *Hoechst Marion Roussel, Belg.†.*
Meprobamate (p.691·1).
Anxiety; insomnia; premedication; tension.

Pro-Cal-Sof *Vangard, USA†.*
Docusate calcium (p.1222·3).
Constipation.

Procamide
Zambon, Braz.; Zambon, Ital.†.
Procainamide hydrochloride (p.960·1).
Arrhythmias.

Procan *Parke, Davis, Canad.*
Procainamide hydrochloride (p.960·1).
Arrhythmias.

Procanbid *Monarch, USA.*
Procainamide hydrochloride (p.960·1).
Formerly called Procan SR.
Ventricular arrhythmias.

Procaneural *RAN, Ger.*
Procaine hydrochloride (p.1319·1).
Nervous system disorders.

Procaptan *Stroder, Ital.*
Perindopril erbumine (p.953·2).
Heart failure; hypertension.

Procardia *Pfizer, USA.*
Nifedipine (p.940·1).
Angina pectoris; hypertension.

Procardin *Medochemie, Singapore.*
Dipyridamole (p.877·2).
Thromboembolic disorders.

Pro-Cas *Milk Industries, Israel.*
Protein supplement (p.1350·1).

Procavit *EMS, Braz.*
Multivitamin, mineral, and amino-acid preparation (p.1350·1).

Procef
Bristol-Myers Squibb, Fin.; Bristol-Myers Squibb, Hong Kong; Dompe, Ital.; Mead Johnson, Mex.; Bristol-Myers Squibb, Port.; Bristol-Myers Squibb, Singapore; Grunenthal, Switz.; Bristol-Myers Squibb, Thai.
Cefprozil (p.173·2).
Bacterial infections.

Procephal *Provit, Mex.*
Erythromycin estolate (p.201·2).
Bacterial infections.

Prochol *Procare, Austral.*
Nicotinic acid (p.1372·3); oat bran (p.1214·2).
Hyperlipidaemias.

Prochor *Protein, Mex.*
Propranolol (p.963·1).

Prociclide *Crinos, Ital.*
Defibrotide (p.866·3).
Thrombosis prophylaxis.

Pro-Cid *Ophthalmic Laboratories, Austral.*
Probenecid (p.401·3).
Adjunct to beta-lactam antibacterials; gout; reduction of cidofovir-associated nephrotoxicity.

Procillin *Caps, S.Afr.*
Procaine penicillin [procaine benzylpenicillin] (p.239·2).
Bacterial infections.

Procimeti *Provit, Mex.*
Cimetidine (p.1216·3).
Peptic ulcer.

Procin *Schering-Plough, Braz.*
Ciprofloxacin hydrochloride (p.182·3).
Bacterial infections.

Proclim *Fournier, Canad.*
Medroxyprogesterone acetate (p.1480·1).
Menstrual disorders.

Proclimine *Progress, Thai.*
Oxyphencyclimine hydrochloride (p.472·1).
Gastrointestinal disorders; genito-urinary disorders.

Proclor *Pentafarma, Port.*
Omeprazole (p.1239·1).

Procloril *Provit, Mex.*
Chloramphenicol (p.179·1).
Bacterial infections.

Proclozine *Pharmasant, Thai.*
Prochlorperazine maleate (p.701·2).
Alcoholism; anxiety; mania; schizophrenia.

Procodin *DHA, Singapore.*
Codeine phosphate (p.25·2); promethazine hydrochloride (p.423·2).
Coughs.

Procof *Aspen, S.Afr.*
Diphenhydramine hydrochloride (p.416·1); pholcodine (p.1099·1); guaifenesin (p.1092·2).
Coughs.

Procol
SmithKline Beecham Consumer, Irl.†; SmithKline Beecham, UK†.
Phenylpropanolamine hydrochloride (p.1098·1).
Cold symptoms.

Procold *Procare, Austral.*
Ascorbic acid (p.1389·3); horseradish (p.1620·1); verbascum thapsus; euphorbia hirta (p.1609·3); garlic (p.1614·1).
Respiratory-tract disorders.

Pro-Coll *DMG, Ital.*
Amino acids, vitamin C, yeast, and minerals (p.1350·1).
Nutritional supplement.

Procomfrin *Planta, Canad.†.*
Comfrey (p.1598·3).
Bruises; sprains; wounds.

Procomvax *Chiron Behring, Ger.*
A haemophilus influenzae and hepatitis B vaccine (p.1541·1).
Active immunisation.

Procor
Note.This name is used for preparations of different composition.
Boehringer de Angeli, Braz.
Dipyridamole (p.877·2).
Ischaemic heart disease; thromboembolism prophylaxis.

Unipharm, Israel.
Amiodarone hydrochloride (p.836·1).
Angina pectoris; arrhythmias; heart failure; myocardial infarction.

Procor S *Boehringer de Angeli, Braz.*
Dipyridamole (p.877·2); salicylic acid (p.1122·3).
Thromboembolism prophylaxis.

Procordal Gold *Staufen, Ger.*
Homoeopathic preparation.

Procordal Weiss *Staufen, Ger.*
Homoeopathic preparation.

Procort *Roberts, USA.*
Hydrocortisone (p.1073·3).
Corticosteroid.

Procorum
Ebewe, Aust.; Knoll, Ger.; Knoll, Ital.; Knoll, Mex.; Knoll, Thai.
Gallopamil hydrochloride (p.896·2).
Angina pectoris; arrhythmias; hypertension; ischaemic heart disease; myocardial infarction.

Procoutol *Spirig, Switz.*
Triclosan (p.1159·2).
Skin disorders.

Procren
Abbott, Denm.; Abbott, Fin.; Abbott, Norw.; Abbott, Swed.
Leuprorelin acetate (p.1289·2).
Formerly known as Lupron in Swed.
Endometriosis; prostatic cancer; uterine fibroma.

Procrin *Abbott, Spain.*
Leuprorelin acetate (p.1289·2).
Endometriosis; precocious puberty; prostatic cancer; uterine fibroma.

Procrit *Ortho Biotech, USA.*
Epoetin alfa (p.731·1).
Anaemia in cancer patients on chemotherapy; anaemia in zidovudine-treated HIV-infected patients; anaemia of chronic renal failure; pre-operative anaemias.

Proctalgen *BC Lutz, Switz.*
Hamamelis (p.1618·3); diethylamine salicylate (p.32·2).
Anorectal disorders.

Proctase-P *Meiji, Thai.*
Proctase; pancreatin (p.1646·1).
Haematoma; inflammation; oedema; respiratory-tract congestion.

Proctena *Virginia, Ital.*
Hamamelis; aesculus; paeonia officinalis; cardiospermum halicacabum.

Proctidol *Novartis Consumer, Ital.*
Hydrocortisone acetate (p.1073·3); benzocaine (p.1306·2).
Haemorrhoids.

Proctil *Byk, Braz.*
Policresulen; cinchocaine hydrochloride (p.1309·1).
Haemorrhoids.

Proctium
Allergan-Frumtost, Braz.; Esteve, Spain.
Calcium dobesilate (p.1588·2); lignocaine [lidocaine] hydrochloride (p.1313·2); prednisolone (p.1077·3).
Anorectal disorders.

Procto *Cophar, Switz.*
Fluocinolone acetonide (p.1071·1); lignocaine [lidocaine] hydrochloride (p.1313·2).
Anorectal disorders.

Proctoacid *Byk Gulden, Mex.*
Policresulen; cinchocaine hydrochloride (p.1309·1).
Anorectal disorders.

Proctocort
Boehringer Ingelheim, Fr.; Monarch, USA.
Hydrocortisone (p.1073·3) or hydrocortisone acetate (p.1073·3).
Anorectal disorders; Crohn's disease; haemorrhagic colitis.

Proctocream HC
Note.This name is used for preparations of different composition.
Stafford-Miller, UK†.
Hydrocortisone acetate (p.1073·3); pramocaine hydrochloride (p.1318·2).
Anorectal disorders.

Schwarz, USA.
Hydrocortisone (p.1073·3).
Formerly contained hydrocortisone acetate and pramocaine.
Skin disorders.

Proctodan-HC *Odan, Canad.*
Pramocaine hydrochloride (p.1318·2); hydrocortisone acetate (p.1073·3); zinc sulfate (p.1398·2).
Anorectal disorders.

Proctofoam
Note.This name is used for preparations of different composition.
Searle, S.Afr.†.
Hydrocortisone acetate (p.1073·3); pramocaine hydrochloride (p.1318·2).
Anorectal disorders.

Schwarz, USA.
Pramocaine hydrochloride (p.1318·2).
Anorectal disorders.

Proctofoam-HC
Reed & Carnrick, Canad.; Stafford-Miller, Irl.; Stafford-Miller, Israel; Stafford-Miller, Ital.; Stafford-Miller, UK; Schwarz, USA.
Hydrocortisone acetate (p.1073·3); pramocaine hydrochloride (p.1318·2).
Anorectal disorders.

Procto-Glyvenol
Novartis, Aust.; Novartis, Braz.; Novartis, Israel; Novartis, Mex.; Novartis Consumer, Port.; Novartis Consumer, Switz.
Tribenoside (p.1674·2); lignocaine [lidocaine] (p.1313·2) or lignocaine [lidocaine] hydrochloride (p.1313·2).
Haemorrhoids.

Procto-Jellin *Grunenthal, Ger.*
Fluocinolone acetonide (p.1071·1); lignocaine [lidocaine] hydrochloride (p.1313·2).
Anorectal disorders.

Procto-Kaban *Asche, Ger.*
Clocortolone pivalate (p.1065·3); clocortolone caproate (p.1065·3); cinchocaine hydrochloride (p.1309·1).
Anorectal disorders.

Proctolog *Parke, Davis, Fr.; Sanitas, Port.; Parke, Davis, Singapore; Juste, Spain.*
Ruscogenin (p.1660·2); trimebutine (p.1675·1).
Anorectal disorders.

Proctolyn *Recordati, Ital.*
Fluocinolone acetonide (p.1071·1); ketocaine hydrochloride (p.1312·3).
Anorectal disorders.

Proctoparf *Whitehall-Much, Ger.*
Bufexamac (p.20·3); bismuth subgallate (p.1213·2); lignocaine [lidocaine] hydrochloride (p.1313·2); titanium dioxide (p.1126·1).
Anorectal disorders.

Proctor's Pineliptus *Ernest Jackson, UK.*
Eucalyptus oil (p.1609·2); menthol (p.1632·3); oleum pini sylvestris; siberian fir oil.
Coughs; throat irritation.

Proctosedyl
Note.This name is used for preparations of different composition.
Hoechst Marion Roussel, Austral.; Hoechst Marion Roussel, Israel; Aventis, NZ; Hoechst Marion Roussel, UK.
Cinchocaine hydrochloride (p.1309·1); hydrocortisone (p.1073·3).
Anorectal disorders.

Hoechst Marion Roussel, Canad.; Aventis, Denm.; Hoechst Marion Roussel, Fin.; Hoechst Marion Roussel, Hong Kong; Hoechst Marion Roussel, Irl.; Hoechst Marion Roussel, Norw.; Aventis, S.Afr.; Hoechst Marion Roussel, Singapore; Hoechst Marion Roussel, Swed.; Hoechst Marion Roussel, Thai.
Cinchocaine hydrochloride (p.1309·1); hydrocortisone (p.1073·3); framycetin sulfate (p.208·2); esculoside (p.1574·1).
Anorectal disorders.

Roche, Ital.
Ointment: Amylocaine (p.1306·1); benzocaine (p.1306·2); hydrocortisone acetate (p.1073·3); esculoside (p.1574·1).
Suppositories: Benzocaine (p.1306·2); hydrocortisone acetate (p.1073·3); esculoside (p.1574·1).
Anal pruritus; haemorrhoids.

Hoechst Marion Roussel, Neth.
Cinchocaine hydrochloride (p.1309·1); hydrocortisone (p.1073·3); framycetin sulfate (p.208·2).
Haemorrhoids.

Proctosoll *Wassermann, Ital.*
Benzocaine (p.1306·2); hydrocortisone acetate (p.1073·3); heparin sodium (p.902·1).
Haemorrhoids.

Proctosone
Note.This name is used for preparations of different composition.
Technilab, Canad.
Cinchocaine hydrochloride (p.1309·1); hydrocortisone acetate (p.1073·3); framycetin sulfate (p.208·2); esculoside (p.1574·1).
Formerly contained cinchocaine hydrochloride, hydrocortisone acetate, neomycin sulfate, and esculoside.
Anorectal disorders.

Technilab, Hong Kong.
Cinchocaine hydrochloride (p.1309·1); hydrocortisone acetate (p.1073·3); neomycin sulfate (p.228·1); esculoside (p.1574·1).
Haemorrhoids.

Proctospre
Hennig, Ger.; Sodip, Switz.
Cinchocaine (p.1309·1); chlorquinaldol (p.182·1); diphenylpyraline (p.417·1).
Anogenital disorders; anorectal disorders.

Proctosteroid *Aldo, Spain.*
Triamcinolone diacetate (p.1080·2).
Proctitis; proctosigmoiditis; ulcerative colitis.

Procto-Synalar
Note.This name is used for preparations of different composition.
Grunenthal, Aust.
Fluocinolone acetonide (p.1071·1); lignocaine [lidocaine] hydrochloride (p.1313·2).
Anorectal disorders.

Yamanouchi, Belg.
Fluocinolone acetonide (p.1071·1); lignocaine [lidocaine] hydrochloride (p.1313·2); bismuth subgallate (p.1213·2); menthol (p.1632·3).
Anorectal disorders.

Procto-Synalar N *Grunenthal, Switz.*
Fluocinolone acetonide (p.1071·1); lignocaine [lidocaine] hydrochloride (p.1313·2).
Procto-Synalar formerly contained fluocinolone acetonide, lignocaine [lidocaine] hydrochloride, menthol, and bismuth subgallate.
Anorectal disorders.

Proctozorin-N *Teva, Israel.*
Hydrocortisone (p.1073·3); allantoin (p.1110·1); benzocaine (p.1306·2); aluminium acetotartrate (p.1578·2); menthol (p.1632·3); zinc oxide (p.1128·2).
Anorectal disorders.

Proculin *Chauvin ankerpharm, Ger.*
Naphazoline hydrochloride (p.1095·1).
Conjunctivitis.

Procur *Douglas, Austral.*
Cyproterone acetate (p.1467·3).
Androgenisation in females; prostatic cancer; sexual deviation in males.

Pro-Cure *Merck Sharp & Dohme, Israel.*
Finasteride (p.1477·2).
Benign prostatic hyperplasia.

Procutan *Schering-Plough, S.Afr.*
Hydrocortisone (p.1073·3).
Skin disorders.

Pro-Cute *Ferndale, USA.*
Emollient and moisturiser.

ProCycle Gold *Cyclin, USA†.*
Multivitamin, mineral and nutritional preparation (p.1350·1).

Procyclid *ICN, Canad.*
Procyclidine hydrochloride (p.473·1).
Parkinsonism.

Procyclo *Organon, Ger.*
11 Tablets, estradiol valerate (p.1473·2); 10 tablets, estradiol valerate; medroxyprogesterone acetate (p.1480·1).
Menopausal disorders.

Procytox *Carter Horner, Canad.*
Cyclophosphamide (p.527·3).
Malignant neoplasms.

Pro-Dafalgan
Upsamedica, Belg.; Bristol-Myers Squibb, Fin.; UPSA, Fr.; Bristol-Myers Squibb, Port.; Upsamedica, Switz.
Propacetamol hydrochloride (p.80·1).
Fever; pain.

Prodafem
Pharmacia Upjohn, Aust.; Pharmacia Upjohn, Switz.
Medroxyprogesterone acetate (p.1480·1).
Amenorrhoea; endometriosis; menopausal disorders; menorrhagia.

Prodamox *Rubia, Spain.*
Proglumetacin maleate (p.80·1).
Musculoskeletal, joint, and peri-articular disorders.

Prodasone *Pharmacia Upjohn, Fr.*
Medroxyprogesterone acetate (p.1480·1).
Breast and endometrial cancers.

Prodazol *Protein, Mex.*
Mebendazole (p.102·2).

Prodeine *Sanofi Synthelabo, Austral.*
Paracetamol (p.71·2); codeine phosphate (p.25·2).
Fever; pain.

Prodep
Sun, Singapore; Sun, Thai.
Fluoxetine hydrochloride (p.284·2).
Depression; obsessive-compulsive disorder.

Proderm
Note.This name is used for preparations of different composition.
Darrow, Braz.
Triclosan (p.1159·2).
Skin disinfection.

Intra Pharma, Irl.
Barrier preparation.

Dow, USA.
Castor oil (p.1592·1); peru balsam (p.1650·2).
Decubitus ulcers.

Prodessal *Almirall, Spain.*
Cyanocobalamin (p.1388·1); cyclobutyrol (p.1601·2); cytidine; electrolytes (p.1180·1); uridine (p.1677·2).
Liver disorders; oral hygiene.

Pro-Diaban
Bayer, Aust.; Bayer, Ger.
Glisoxepide (p.323·2).
Diabetes mellitus.

Prodiarrhoea *Procare, Austral.†.*
Activated charcoal (p.1000·2).
Diarrhoea; flatulence.

Prodicard *Astra, Neth.*
Isosorbide dinitrate (p.915·2).
Angina pectoris.

Prodiem Plain *Novartis Consumer, Canad.*
Psyllium hydrophilic mucilloid (p.1229·1).
Constipation; fibre supplement.

Prodiem Plus *Novartis Consumer, Canad.*
Psyllium hydrophilic mucilloid (p.1229·1); senna pod (p.1248·2).
Constipation.

Prodifer *Provit, Mex.*
Ampicillin (p.150·3).
Bacterial infections.

Prodilantin *Parke, Davis, Fr.*
Fosphenytoin sodium (p.349·3).
Epilepsy.

Prodis *Procare, Austral.*
Multivitamins, amino acids, ginseng, and minerals (p.1350·1).
Dietary supplement.

Prodium
Note.This name is used for preparations of different composition.
Propan, S.Afr.
Loperamide hydrochloride (p.1231·3).
Diarrhoea; ostomy management.

Breckenridge, USA.
Phenazopyridine hydrochloride (p.77·3).
Irritation of the lower urinary tract.

Prodiuret *Biocur, Ger.*
Equisetum (p.1606·3).
Oedema; urinary-tract disorders.

Prodolina *Promeco, Mex.*
Dipyrone (p.34·1) or metamizole magnesium (p.34·2).
Fever; pain.

Prodon *Tika, Swed.*
Ketoprofen (p.47·3).
Musculoskeletal and joint disorders.

Prodop *Protein, Mex.*
Methyldopa (p.927·3).

Prodopa *Pacific, NZ.*
Methyldopa (p.927·3).
Hypertension.

Prodorol *Be-Tabs, S.Afr.*
Propranolol hydrochloride (p.962·3).
Angina pectoris; anxiety; arrhythmias; hypertension; hyperthyroidism; phaeochromocytoma.

Prodren *Alcon, Israel.*
Dipivefrine hydrochloride (p.1604·3).
Glaucoma.

Product Code 889 *Scientific Hospital Supplies, Austral.*
Preparation for enteral nutrition (p.1350·1).
Methylmalonic acidaemia; propionic acidaemia.

Proechina *Procare, Austral.†.*
Echinacea angustifolia (p.1606·2).

Pro-Efferalgan
Upsamedica, Ital.; Upsamedica, Spain.
Propacetamol hydrochloride (p.80·1).
Pain.

Proendotel *Fidia, Ital.*
Cloricromen hydrochloride (p.863·2).
Formerly called Cromocap.
Thrombotic disorders.

Pro-Epanutin
Parke, Davis, Denm.; Parke, Davis, Fin.; Parke, Davis, Irl.; Parke, Davis, Neth.; Warner-Lambert, Norw.; Parke, Davis, Port.; Parke, Davis, Swed.; Parke, Davis, UK.
Fosphenytoin sodium (p.349·3).
Epilepsy; seizures associated with neurosurgery and head trauma.

Proesten *Procare, Austral.*
Vitamins; minerals (p.1350·1); garlic (p.1614·1); cimicifuga (p.1595·2); viburnum opulus; passion flower (p.1649·1); sarsaparilla (p.1661·1).
Dietary supplement; menopausal disorders.

Profact *Hoechst Marion Roussel, Ger.*
Buserelin acetate (p.1278·1).
Prostatic cancer.

Profamid
Orion, Denm.; Orion, Fin.
Flutamide (p.542·3).
Prostatic cancer.

Profargil *Profarb, Braz.*
Metronidazole (p.594·1); vitamin B_1; vitamin B_2; vitamin B_6 (p.1350·1).
Alcoholism; protozoal infections.

Profasi
Serono, Aust.; Serono, Austral.; Serono, Denm.; Serono, Fin.; Serono, Hong Kong; Serono, Irl.; Serono, Mex.; Serono, Neth.; Serono, Norw.; Serono, NZ; Serono, S.Afr.; Serono, Singapore; Serono, Swed.; Serono, Switz.; Serono, Thai.; Serono, UK; Serono, USA.
Chorionic gonadotrophin (p.1279·2).
Cryptorchidism; hypogonadotrophic hypogonadism; male and female infertility; threatened or recurrent miscarriage.

Profasi HP
Serono, Braz.; Serono, Canad.; Serono, Ital.; Serono, Port.; Serono, Spain.
Chorionic gonadotrophin (p.1279·2).
Cryptorchidism; erectile dysfunction; hypogonadotrophic hypogonadism; male and female infertility; metrorrhagia; threatened or recurrent miscarriage.

Profed *Progress, Thai.*
Triprolidine hydrochloride (p.427·2); pseudoephedrine hydrochloride (p.1099·2).
Allergic rhinitis; cold symptoms; hay fever; nasal congestion.

Profelina *Farcoral, Mex.*
Dipyrone (p.34·1).

Profen *Wakefield, USA†.*
Phenylpropanolamine hydrochloride (p.1098·1); guaifenesin (p.1092·2).
Upper respiratory-tract symptoms.

Profen II *Wakefield, USA.*
Phenylpropanolamine hydrochloride (p.1098·1); guaifenesin (p.1092·2).
Coughs.

Profen II DM *Wakefield, USA.*
Pseudoephedrine hydrochloride (p.1099·2); guaifenesin (p.1092·2); dextromethorphan hydrobromide (p.1087·3).
Formerly contained phenylpropanolamine hydrochloride, guaifenesin, and dextromethorphan hydrobromide.
Coughs.

Profen Forte DM *Wakefield, USA.*
Pseudoephedrine hydrochloride (p.1099·2); dextromethorphan hydrobromide (p.1087·3); guaifenesin (p.1092·2).
Formerly contained phenylpropanolamine hydrochloride, dextromethorphan hydrobromide, and guaifenesin.
Coughs.

Profena *Pond's, Thai.*
Ibuprofen (p.43·2).
Musculoskeletal and joint disorders.

Profenal *Alcon, USA.*
Suprofen (p.87·1).
Inhibition of intra-operative miosis.

Profenda *Jamieson, Canad.*
Betacarotene, vitamin C, and vitamin E (p.1350·1).

Profenid
Rhone-Poulenc Rorer, Aust.; Rhodia, Braz.; Rhone-Poulenc Rorer, Fr.; Rhone-Poulenc Rorer, Israel; Rhone-Poulenc Rorer, Mex.; Vitoria, Port.; Rhone-Poulenc Rorer, Thai.
Ketoprofen (p.47·3).
Gout; inflammation; musculoskeletal, joint, peri-articular, and soft-tissue disorders; pain.

Profenil *Pascual, Hong Kong.*
Alverine citrate (p.1211·3).
Gastrointestinal spasm.

Profenzol *Farcoral, Mex.*
Mebendazole (p.102·2).
Worm infections.

Profer
Aesculapius, Ital.; Tedec Meiji, Spain†.
Ferritin (p.1359·3).
Iron deficiency; iron-deficiency anaemias.

Profiber *Sherwood, USA.*
Lactose-free preparation for enteral nutrition (p.1350·1).

Profil *Atral, Port.*
Amantadine (p.1162·2).

Profilasmim-Ped *Stiefel, Braz.*
Ketotifen fumarate (p.767·2).
Allergic conjunctivitis; allergic rhinitis; asthma; urticaria.

Profilate
Grifols, Ger.; Alpha, Israel.
A factor VIII preparation (p.734·1).
Haemorrhagic disorders.

Profilate HP, OSD *Alpha Therapeutic, USA†.*
A factor VIII preparation (p.734·1).
Haemophilia.

Profilnine
Alpha, Israel; Alpha Therapeutic, Singapore; Alpha Therapeutic, Thai.; Alpha Therapeutic, USA.
A factor IX complex (p.735·1).
Haemorrhagic disorders.

Profinal *Julphar, UAE.*
Ibuprofen (p.43·2).
Fever; inflammation; musculoskeletal, joint, peri-articular and soft-tissue disorders; pain.

Profiten *Pharma Clal, Israel.*
Ketotifen fumarate (p.767·2).
Hypersensitivity reactions.

Profium *De Mayo, Braz.*
Mebendazole (p.102·2); tiabendazole (p.109·1).
Worm infections.

Proflag *Salus, Mex.*
Metronidazole (p.594·1).

Proflam *Bristol-Myers Squibb, Braz.*
Aceclofenac (p.11·1).
Inflammation; pain.

Proflavanol *USANA, USA.*
Vitamin C (p.1389·3); flavonoids from grape seed (p.1611·1).
Nutritional supplement.

Proflex
Novartis Consumer, Irl.; Novartis Consumer, UK.
Ibuprofen (p.43·2).
Inflammation; musculoskeletal, joint, and peri-articular disorders; pain.

Proflo *Procare, Austral.*
Vitamins; minerals (p.1350·1); bioflavonoids (p.1611·1); ruscus aculeatus; aesculus (p.1574·1); hamamelis (p.1618·3); pulsatilla (p.1656·3).
Dietary supplement; peripheral vascular disorders.

Proflox *Pharmasant, Thai.*
Ciprofloxacin (p.182·3).
Bacterial infections.

Profluid *Procare, Austral.*
Taraxacum (p.1669·1); parsley piert (p.1648·3); bearberry (p.1583·3); juniper (p.1625·2).
Bladder disorders; cystitis; fluid retention.

Profol *Medley, Braz.*
Buclizine hydrochloride (p.411·1); lysine; tryptophan; vitamin B_6; vitamin B_{12} (p.1350·1).
Tonic.

ProFree *Allergan, USA.*
Papain (p.1647·3) (p.1129·2).
Cleansing solution for contact lenses.

Profrin-A *Allergan, Port.†.*
Mepyramine maleate (p.421·1); phenylephrine hydrochloride (p.1097·1); phenazone (p.77·2).
Eye irritation.

Profylac *ALK, Fin.*
Infant feed (p.1350·1).
Lactose intolerance; milk allergy; soya protein intolerance.

Progandol *Almirall, Spain.*
Doxazosin mesilate (p.883·2).
Benign prostatic hyperplasia; hypertension.

Progastrit *Hexal, Ger.*
Aluminium hydroxide (p.1210·3); magnesium hydroxide (p.1233·1).
Gastrointestinal disorders.

Progediol *Diba, Mex.*
Progesterone (p.1488·3); estradiol benzoate (p.1473·1).
Menstrual disorders.

Progeffik *Effik, Spain.*
Progesterone (p.1488·3).
Menopausal disorders; menstrual disorders.

Progenar *Sanitas, Port.*
Progesterone (p.1488·3).
Benign breast disorders.

Proger-F *Streger, Mex.*
Progesterone (p.1488·3); estradiol benzoate (p.1473·1).
Menstrual disorders.

Progeril *Sanofi Winthrop, Mex.; Sanofi Synthelabo, Switz.*
Co-dergocrine mesilate (p.1597·3).
Headache; peripheral and cerebral vascular disorders.

Progesic *Xepa-Soul Pattinson, Hong Kong.*
Note. A similar name is used for preparations of different composition (see below).
Paracetamol (p.71·2).
Pain.

Pro-gesic *Nastech, USA†.*
Note. A similar name is used for preparations of different composition (see above).
Trolamine salicylate (p.90·1).
Musculoskeletal and joint disorders.

Progest *Heralds, Braz.*
Estradiol benzoate (p.1473·1); progesterone (p.1488·3); hydroxyprogesterone (p.1479·3); ethinylestradiol (p.1476·2).
Menopausal disorders; menstrual disorders.

Progestan *Nourypharma, Neth.*
Progesterone (p.1488·3).
Hormone replacement therapy; menstrual disorders.

Progestasert *Theraplix, Fr.†; Alza, USA.*
Progesterone (p.1488·3).
Progestogen-only intra-uterine contraceptive device.

Progesteron-Depot *Jenapharm, Ger.*
Hydroxyprogesterone caproate (p.1479·3).
Female infertility; menstrual disorders; threatened or recurrent miscarriage.

Progesterone-retard Pharlon *Schering, Fr.*
Hydroxyprogesterone caproate (p.1479·3).
Female infertility; premature labour; progestogen; threatened or recurrent miscarriage.

Progestogel *Piette, Belg.; Besins-Iscovesco, Fr.; Kade, Ger.; Besins, Ger.; Lusofarmaco, Ital.; Quimedical, Port.; Seid, Spain; Besins-Iscovesco, Switz.; Piette, Thai.*
Progesterone (p.1488·3).
Benign breast disorders.

Progestol *Sanofi Synthelabo, Ital.*
Progesterone (p.1488·3).
Acne; seborrhoea; seborrhoeic alopecia.

Progestosol *Besins-Iscovesco, Fr.*
Progesterone (p.1488·3).
Hyperseborrhoea.

Progestrol *IBSA, Hong Kong†.*
Algestone acetophenide (p.1465·1); estradiol enantate (p.1473·2).
Endometriosis; injectable contraceptive; menstrual disorders.

Progevera *Pharmacia Upjohn, Spain.*
Medroxyprogesterone acetate (p.1480·1).
Endometriosis; female infertility; menometrorrhagia; menopausal disorders; menstrual disorders.

Progevera 250 *Pharmacia Upjohn, Spain.*
Medroxyprogesterone acetate (p.1480·1).
Breast cancer; endometrial cancer.

Progezzard *Pizzard, Mex.*
Medroxyprogesterone (p.1480·1).

Proginkgo *Procare, Austral.*
Ginkgo biloba (p.1615·2).
Cerebral and peripheral vascular disorders; tonic.

Proglan *Procare, Austral.*
Black currant seed oil.
Dietary supplement; source of polyunsaturated fatty acids.

Proglicem *Schering-Plough, Fr.; Essex, Ger.; Schering-Plough, Ital.; Schering-Plough, Neth.; Essex, Switz.*
Diazoxide (p.868·1).
Hypertension; hypoglycaemia.

Proglycem *Schering, Canad.; Baker Norton, USA.*
Diazoxide (p.868·1).
Hypoglycaemia.

Pro-Gola *Ghimas, Ital.*
Propolis (p.1655·1).

Progona *MIP, Ger.*
Glucosamine sulfate (p.1616·2).
Gonarthroses.

Progor *SMB, Belg.*
Diltiazem hydrochloride (p.874·3).
Hypertension.

Progout *Alphapharm, Austral.; Pacific, Hong Kong; Pacific, NZ; Alphapharm, Singapore; Merck, Singapore; CP Pharmaceuticals, UK.*
Allopurinol (p.397·2).
Gout; hyperuricaemia; renal calculi.

Prograf *Fujisawa, Aust.; Janssen-Cilag, Austral.; Fujisawa, Canad.; Fujisawa, Denm.; Fujisawa, Fin.; Fujisawa, Fr.; Fujisawa, Ger.; Fujisawa, Hong Kong; Fujisawa, Irl.; Fujisawa, Israel; Fujisawa, Ital.; Fujisawa, Jpn.; Cilag, Mex.; Fujisawa, Norw.; Janssen-Cilag, NZ; Neo-Farmaceutica, Port.; Janssen-Cilag, Singapore; Fujisawa, Spain; Fujisawa, Swed.; Fujisawa, Switz.; Janssen, Thai.; Fujisawa, UK; Fujisawa, USA.*
Tacrolimus (p.569·3).
Organ transplant rejection.

Prograft *Fujisawa, Belg.*
Tacrolimus (p.569·3).
Transplant rejection.

Progress *Procare, Austral.*
Ginseng; garlic; multivitamins; minerals; bladderwrack; cramp bark (p.1350·1).
Dietary supplement.

Proguval *Eberth, Ger.*
Plantago lanceolata.
Catarrh; mouth and throat inflammation.

Progyluton *Schering, Israel; Schering, Mex.; Schering, Port.; Schering, Singapore; Schering, Switz.*
11 Tablets, estradiol valerate (p.1473·2); 10 tablets, estradiol valerate; norgestrel (p.1486·1).
Menopausal disorders; menstrual disorders.

Progynon *Schering, Aust.; Schering, Denm.; Schering, Swed.; Schering, Thai.*
Estradiol valerate (p.1473·2).
Dysfunctional uterine bleeding; menopausal disorders; menstrual disorders; oestrogen deficiency; osteoporosis.

Progynon C *Schering, Aust.; Schering, Ger.; Schering, Israel.*
Ethinylestradiol (p.1476·2).
Endometrial hyperplasia; menstrual disorders; oestrogen deficiency.

Progynon Depot *Schering, Ital.; Schering, Switz.*
Estradiol valerate (p.1473·2).
Menstrual disorders; oestrogen deficiency.

Progynon Depot 10 *Schering, Ger.; Schering, Neth.; Schering, Switz.*
Estradiol valerate (p.1473·2).
Endometrial hyperplasia; menstrual disorders; oestrogen deficiency.

Progynova *Schering, Aust.; Schering, Austral.; Schering, Belg.; Schering, Fin.; Schering, Fr.; Schering, Ger.; Schering, Hong Kong; Schering, Israel; Schering, Ital.; Schering, Neth.; Schering, Norw.; Schering, NZ; Schering, S.Afr.; Schering, Singapore; Schering, Spain; CIC, Spain; Schering, Switz.; Schering, Thai.; Schering, UK.*
Estradiol (p.1473·1) or estradiol valerate (p.1473·2).
Menopausal disorders; oestrogen deficiency; osteoporosis.

Prohance *Bracco, Aust.; Byk, Belg.; Squibb Diagnostics, Canad.†; Bracco, Denm.; Byk, Fr.; Byk Gulden, Ger.; Bracco, Ital.; Byk, Neth.; Bracco, Norw.; Rovi, Spain; Astra Tech, Swed.; Bracco, Switz.; Bracco, UK; Bracco, USA.*
Gadoteridol (p.1033·2).
Contrast medium for magnetic resonance imaging.

Prohep *Aventis, S.Afr.*
Liver hydrolysate; vitamin B_{12} (p.1388·1); choline bitartrate (p.1356·3); cysteine (p.1358·3); inositol (p.1623·3).
Liver disorders.

Proheparum *Knoll, Thai.*
Cysteine (p.1358·3); choline bitartrate (p.1356·3); inositol (p.1623·3); liver hydrolysate.
Liver disorders.

ProHIBiT *Pasteur Merieux, Aust.; Pasteur Merieux, Swed.†; Berna, Switz.†; Pasteur Merieux, USA.*
A haemophilus influenzae conjugate vaccine (diphtheria toxoid conjugate) (p.1540·2).
Active immunisation.

ProHIBiT-DPT *Berna, Switz.†.*
A diphtheria, tetanus, pertussis, and Haemophilus influenzae vaccine (p.1538·3).
Active immunisation.

Prohist *Be-Tabs, S.Afr.*
Promethazine hydrochloride (p.423·2).
Hypersensitivity reactions; premedication; sedative.

Projuvex *Merck, Port.*
Co-dergocrine mesilate (p.1597·3); deanol acetamidobenzoate (p.1507·2); rutoside (p.1611·2); pyridoxine; vitamin E; potassium gluconate (p.1350·1).
Cerebral and peripheral vascular disorders; mental function disorders.

Proken M *Kendrick, Mex.*
Metoprolol tartrate (p.931·2).
Angina pectoris; hypertension; myocardial infarction.

Prokids *Procare, Austral.*
Multivitamin and mineral preparation (p.1350·1).

Prokinate *Julphar, UAE.*
Cisapride (p.1220·1).
Gastrointestinal motility disorders.

Prokinyl *Techni-Pharma, Mon.*
Metoclopramide hydrochloride (p.1235·2).
Aid to gastrointestinal examination; dyspepsia; nausea and vomiting.

Prol *Procare, Austral.*
Silybum marianum (p.1021·3).
Liver disorders.

Prolacam *Schering, Aust.*
Lisuride maleate (p.1174·1).
Acromegaly; amenorrhoea; female infertility; galactorrhoea; lactation inhibition; mastitis.

Proladone *Knoll, Austral.; Knoll, NZ.*
Oxycodone pectinate (p.70·3).
Pain.

Prolair *3M, Fr.*
Beclometasone dipropionate (p.1061·2).
Asthma.

Prolaken *Fustery, Mex.*
Metoprolol tartrate (p.931·2).
Angina pectoris; arrhythmias; hypertension.

Prolan *Procare, Austral.*
Multivitamin and mineral preparation (p.1350·1).
Anxiety; dietary supplement.

Prolastin *Bayer, Canad.; Bayer Biological, Hong Kong; Bayer, USA.*
Alpha₁-proteinase inhibitor (p.1576·3).
Congenital alpha₁ antitrypsin deficiency.

Prolastin HS *Bayer, Ger.*
Alpha₁-proteinase inhibitor (p.1576·3).
Alpha₁ antitrypsin deficiency.

Prolastina *Bayer, Ital.; Bayer, Spain.*
Alpha₁-proteinase inhibitor (p.1576·3).
Congenital alpha₁ antitrypsin deficiency.

Prolax *Procare, Austral.*
Note. A similar name is used for preparations of different composition (see below).
Senna (p.1248·2); prune (p.1245·2).
Constipation.

Pro-Lax *Rivex, Canad.†.*
Note. A similar name is used for preparations of different composition (see above).
Polyethylene glycol (p.1630·1); electrolytes (p.1180·1).
Constipation.

Prolert *Pensa, Spain.*
Caffeine (p.761·3).
Fatigue.

Proleukin *Fresenius Kabi, Aust.; CSL, Austral.; Ligand, Canad.; Chiron, Denm.; Chiron, Fr.; Chiron, Ger.; Chiron, Hong Kong; Chiron, Irl.; Chiron, Ital.; Asofarma, Mex.; Chiron, Neth.; Roche, Port.; Chiron, Singapore; Chiron, Spain; Roche, Switz.; Chiron, UK; Chiron, USA.*
Aldesleukin (p.547·3).
Metastatic melanoma; metastatic renal-cell carcinoma.

Prolidon *Carnot, Mex.*
Progesterone (p.1488·3).
Amenorrhoea; functional uterine haemorrhage; recurrent miscarriage.

Prolief *Propan, S.Afr.*
Paracetamol (p.71·2).
Fever; pain.

Prolifen *Chiesi, Ital.*
Clomifene citrate (p.1465·3).
Anovulatory infertility.

Prolipase *Janssen-Cilag, Aust.; Janssen-Cilag, Switz.*
Pancrelipase (p.1647·2).
Dyspepsia; pancreatic insufficiency.

Prolitrol *Millet Roux, Braz.*
Pygeum africanum (p.1490·3).
Benign prostatic hyperplasia.

Prolixan *Jacoby, Aust.; Asta Medica, Neth.; Neves, Port.; Siegfried, Switz.†.*
Azapropazone (p.19·1).
Gout; inflammation; musculoskeletal, joint, and periarticular disorders; pain.

Prolixana *Siegfried, Swed.†.*
Azapropazone (p.19·1).
Musculoskeletal and joint disorders.

Prolixin *Apothecon, USA; Princeton, USA.*
Fluphenazine decanoate (p.684·3), fluphenazine enantate (p.684·3), or fluphenazine hydrochloride (p.684·3).
Psychoses.

Prolmon *Tokyo Tanabe, Hong Kong.*
Protoporphyrin IX disodium (p.1655·2).
Cholecystitis; cholelithiasis.

Proloid *Parke, Davis, S.Afr.†.*
Thyroglobulin (p.1526·1).
Hypothyroidism.

Proloid S *Parke, Davis, Mex.*
Thyroxine [levothyroxine] sodium (p.1526·2); liothyronine sodium (p.1524·2).
Adjunct in hyperthyroidism; hypothyroidism.

Prolol *Dexxon, Israel; Atlantic, Thai.*
Propranolol hydrochloride (p.962·3).
Angina pectoris; arrhythmias; hypertension; hypertrophic subaortic stenosis; migraine; myocardial infarction; phaeochromocytoma.

Prolopa *Roche, Belg.; Roche, Braz.; Roche, Canad.*
Levodopa (p.1169·2); benserazide hydrochloride (p.1164·2).
Parkinsonism.

Proloprim *Glaxo Wellcome, Canad.; Glaxo Wellcome, USA.*
Trimethoprim (p.264·2).
Bacterial infections of the urinary tract.

Proluton *Schering, Aust.; Schering, Austral.; Schering, Thai.*
Progesterone (p.1488·3) or hydroxyprogesterone caproate (p.1479·3).
Amenorrhoea; female infertility; threatened or recurrent miscarriage.

Proluton Depot *Schering, Ger.; Schering, Hong Kong; Schering, Israel; Schering, Ital.; Schering, Neth.; Schering, Singapore; Schering, Spain†; Schering, Switz.; Schering, Thai.; Schering, UK.*
Hydroxyprogesterone caproate (p.1479·3).
Formerly known as Primolut Depot in the UK.
Amenorrhoea; female infertility; metrorrhagia; progestogen deficiency; threatened or recurrent miscarriage; uterine hypoplasia.

Promac *Provit, Mex.*
Nitrofurantoin (p.230·3).

Promahist *Propan, S.Afr.†.*
Promethazine hydrochloride (p.423·2).
Coughs; nausea; vomiting.

Promal *Propan, S.Afr.†.*
Chloroquine phosphate (p.432·3).
Malaria.

Promani *SmithKline Beecham, Canad.†.*
Triclosan (p.1159·2).
Dry or irritated skin.

Promanum N *Braun, Ger.*
Alcohol (p.1130·3); isopropyl alcohol (p.1149·2).
Hand disinfection.

Promatussin DM *Lioh, Canad.*
Promethazine hydrochloride (p.423·2); dextromethorphan hydrobromide (p.1087·3); pseudoephedrine (p.1099·2).
Coughs.

Promaxol *Otsuka, Spain.*
Procaterol hydrochloride (p.770·1).
Obstructive airways disease.

Promeal *Volchem, Ital.*
Preparation for enteral nutrition (p.1350·1).

Promecilina *Promeco, Mex.*
Ampicillin (p.150·3).
Bacterial infections.

Promedrol *Pharmacia Upjohn, Aust.†; Pharmacia Upjohn, Switz.†.*
Methylprednisolone suleptanate (p.1076·2).
Corticosteroid.

Promedyl *Beacons, Singapore.*
Codeine phosphate (p.25·2); promethazine hydrochloride (p.423·2); ephedrine hydrochloride (p.1090·1).
Coughs.

Promega *Parke, Davis, USA.*
Omega-3 marine triglycerides with vitamin E (p.949·3).
Dietary supplement.

Promelatonin *Laborest, Ital.*
Tryptophan; niacin; calcium; magnesium (p.1350·1).
Nutritional supplement; sleep disorders.

Promensil *Novogen, Austral.*
Red clover (p.1657·3).
Menopausal disorders.

Prometa *Muro, USA†.*
Orciprenaline sulfate (p.769·1).

Prometax *Medibial, Port.; Esteve, Spain.*
Rivastigmine hydrogen tartrate (p.1424·3).
Alzheimer's disease.

Prometh with Dextromethorphan *Barre-National, USA.*
Promethazine hydrochloride (p.423·2); dextromethorphan hydrobromide (p.1087·3).
Coughs and cold symptoms.

Prometh VC Plain *Warner Chilcott, USA; Goldline, USA; Barre-National, USA.*
Promethazine hydrochloride (p.423·2); phenylephrine hydrochloride (p.1097·1).
Allergic rhinitis; nasal congestion.

Promethawern *Wernigerode, Ger.*
Promethazine teoclate (p.423·2).
Anxiety; hypersensitivity reactions; nausea and vomiting; premedication; sleep disorders.

Promethazine Expectorants *Vitamed, Israel.*
Promethazine hydrochloride (p.423·2); ipecacuanha (p.1093·1); sulfogaiacol (p.1101·1).
Coughs.

Promethazine VC with Codeine *Warner Chilcott, USA.*
Promethazine hydrochloride (p.423·2); phenylephrine hydrochloride (p.1097·1); codeine phosphate (p.25·2).

Promethegan *G & W, USA†.*
Promethazine (p.423·2).

Promethist with Codeine *Rahslog, USA†.*
Phenylephrine hydrochloride (p.1097·1); codeine phosphate (p.25·2); promethazine hydrochloride (p.423·2).
Coughs and cold symptoms.

Prometrium *Schering, Canad.; Solvay, USA.*
Progesterone (p.1488·3).
Adjunct to oestrogen replacement therapy; amenorrhoea.

Promibasol *Rayere, Mex.*
Metronidazole (p.594·1).
Amoebiasis; giardiasis; trichomoniasis.

Promibasol-Plus *Rayere, Mex.*
Fluocinolone acetonide (p.1071·1); metronidazole (p.594·1); nystatin (p.392·2).
Vulvovaginal infections.

Promicturine *Ashbourne, UK†.*
Oxybutynin hydrochloride (p.471·2).
Neurogenic bladder; unstable bladder.

Promifen *Wiener, Mex.*
Prednisone (p.1079·2).
Corticosteroid.

Prominal
Sanofi Synthelabo, Austral.; Merck, Spain†; Sanofi Synthelabo, UK†.
Methylphenobarbital (p.353·3).
Epilepsy.

Promincil *Chefaro Ardeval, Fr.*
Capsules: Bladderwrack (p.1585·2); paullinia (p.1681·1); java tea (p.1625·1).
Formerly contained fucus, meadowsweet, and equisetum.
Topical gel: Hedera helix leaf; guarana (p.1681·1).
Herbal slimming preparation.

Prominol *MCR, USA.*
Butalbital (p.658·3); paracetamol (p.71·2).
Pain.

Promise
Wyeth, Mex.; Wyeth, Singapore.
Nutritional supplement for children (p.1350·1).

Promit
Torrex, Aust.; Fresenius Medical, Austral.; Pharmacia Upjohn, Fr.; Pharmalink, Ger.; Alliance, S.Afr.; Braun, Switz.; Pharmacia, USA.
Dextran 1 (p.728·2).
Prevention of anaphylactic reactions to infusions of dextrans.

Promiten
Pharmalink, Denm.; Pharmalink, Norw.; Pharmalink, Swed.
Dextran 1 (p.728·2).
Prevention of anaphylactic reactions to infusions of dextrans.

Promix *Capo Sole, Ital.*
Propolis (p.1655·1); agrumi; echinacea (p.1606·2); clove (p.1596·3).

Promix 3 *Capo Sole, Ital.*
Propolis (p.1655·1); myrtillus (p.1639·2); echinacea (p.1606·2); agrumi oil.

Promocard
Astra, Belg.; Astra, Neth.
Isosorbide mononitrate (p.916·2).
Angina pectoris.

ProMod
Abbott, Austral.; Abbott, Canad.; Abbott, Ital.; Abbott, NZ; Abbott, Singapore; Abbott Nutrition, UK; Ross, USA.
Dietary protein supplement (p.1350·1).

Promoxil *Medpro, S.Afr.*
Amoxicillin (p.149·2).
Bacterial infections.

Prompt *Procter & Gamble, Braz.*
Ispaghula (p.1229·1); senna (p.1248·2).
Constipation.

Promune *Procare, Austral.*
Multivitamin, amino-acid, and mineral preparation with thymus extract (p.1350·1).
Dietary supplement.

Pronaestin *Rekah, Israel.*
Benzocaine (p.1306·2); methylene blue [methylthioninium chloride] (p.1012·3); thymol (p.1158·3).
Gingivitis; mouth hygiene; stomatitis.

Pro-Nat *Pro-Nat, Fr.†.*
Note. A similar name is used for preparations of different composition (see below).
A range of organ extracts (bovine) (p.1631·2).

Pronat *Solfran, Mex.*
Note. A similar name is used for preparations of different composition (see above).
Naproxen (p.60·3).
Inflammation.

Pronaxen
Orion, Fin.; Orion, Swed.
Naproxen (p.60·3).
Gout; inflammation; musculoskeletal and joint disorders; pain.

Pronaxil *Streger, Mex.*
Naproxen (p.60·3).
Gout; musculoskeletal, joint, and peri-articular disorders.

Pronax-P *Kener, Mex.*
Naproxen sodium (p.61·3).

Pronemia Hematinic *Lederle, USA.*
Ferrous fumarate (p.1360·1); intrinsic factor concentrate; vitamin B$_{12}$ substances (p.1388·1); folic acid (p.1361·3).

Vitamin C (p.1389·3) is included in this preparation to increase the absorption and availability of iron.
Anaemias.

Pronerv *Gerot, Aust.*
Thiamine hydrochloride (p.1385·1) or thiamine mononitrate (p.1385·1); pyridoxine hydrochloride (p.1386·3); cyanocobalamin (p.1388·1).
Neuralgia; neuritis; neuropathies.

Pronervon Phyto *Lappe, Ger.*
Valerian (p.1678·3); passion flower (p.1649·1); melissa (p.1632·2).
Agitation; sleep disorders.

Pronervon T *Lappe, Ger.*
Temazepam (p.707·2).
Sleep disorders.

Pronestyl
Bristol-Myers Squibb, Austral.; Squibb, Canad.; Bristol-Myers Squibb, Hong Kong; Bristol-Myers Squibb, Irl.; Bristol-Myers Squibb, Israel; Bristol-Myers Squibb, Neth.; Bristol-Myers Squibb, NZ; Bristol-Myers Squibb, S.Afr.†; Bristol-Myers Squibb, Switz.; Bristol-Myers Squibb, Thai.; Bristol-Myers Squibb, UK; Apothecon, USA.
Procainamide hydrochloride (p.960·1).
Arrhythmias.

Proneurin *Hexal, Ger.*
Promethazine hydrochloride (p.423·2).
Anxiety; hypersensitivity reactions; sleep disorders; vomiting.

Pronicol *Bioresearch, Mex.*
Chloramphenicol (p.179·1).
Bacterial infections.

Pronitol *Fournier SA, Spain.*
Pygeum africanum (p.1490·3).
Benign prostatic hyperplasia.

Pronoctan *Schering, Denm.*
Lormetazepam (p.689·3).
Insomnia; premedication.

Pronosil *Silom, Thai.*
Propranolol hydrochloride (p.962·3).
Angina pectoris; arrhythmias; hypertension.

Pronovan *AFI, Norw.†.*
Propranolol hydrochloride (p.962·3).
Angina pectoris; arrhythmias; hypertension; hyperthyroidism; migraine; myocardial infarction; tremor.

Pronoxen *Farcoral, Mex.*
Naproxen (p.60·3).
Inflammation.

Prontalgin *GiEnne, Ital.*
Tramadol hydrochloride (p.89·1).
Pain.

Prontalgine *Boehringer Ingelheim, Fr.*
Paracetamol (p.71·2); codeine phosphate (p.25·2); caffeine (p.761·3).
Formerly contained paracetamol, dimethyl-*N*-octil-(β-benzoyl-ethyl) ammonium bromide, codeine phosphate, and caffeine.
Pain.

Prontamid *SIT, Ital.†.*
Sulfacetamide sodium (p.250·3).
Eye infections.

Pronto
Note. This name is used for preparations of different composition.
Del, Canad.
Pyrethrin; piperonyl butoxide (p.1436·2).

Del, USA.
Shampoo: Pyrethrins; piperonyl butoxide (p.1436·2).
Pediculosis.
Surface spray: Phenothrin (p.1436·2).
Lice infestation.

Pronto Emoform *Byk Gulden, Ital.†.*
Sodium monofluorophosphate (p.1377·2); sodium fluoride (p.1375·3).
Oral hygiene.

Pronto Platamine *Pharmacia Upjohn, Ital.*
Cisplatin (p.525·1).
Malignant neoplasms.

Prontoalivio *Laborsil, Braz.*
Methyl salicylate (p.55·1); turpentine oil (p.1676·3); camphor (p.1589·3).
Musculoskeletal and joint disorders.

Prontobario
Gerot, Aust.; Bracco, Ital.; Bracco, Port.
Barium sulfate (p.1032·1).
Simeticone (p.1249·2) is included in some preparations to eliminate gas from the gastrointestinal tract before radiography.
Contrast medium for gastrointestinal radiography.

Prontocid N *Braun, Ger.*
Formaldehyde (p.1144·2); glutaral (p.1145·2).
Instrument disinfection.

Prontofort *Wyeth, Mex.*
Tramadol hydrochloride (p.89·1).
Pain.

Prontogest *Amsa, Ital.*
Progesterone (p.1488·3).
Formerly known as Gestone.
Adjunct in gynaecological surgery; habitual abortion; menstrual disorders; postnatal depression; threatened or recurrent miscarriage.

Prontokef *Master Pharma, Ital.†.*
Cefoperazone sodium (p.168·2).
Lignocaine [lidocaine] hydrochloride (p.1313·3) is included in this preparation to alleviate the pain of injection.
Bacterial infections.

Prontolax *Streuli, Switz.*
Bisacodyl (p.1212·2).
Bowel evacuation; constipation.

Prontomixin *Farmila, Ital.*
Lactic-acid-producing organisms (p.1626·3); vitamin B substances; passion flower; pineapple; carrot (p.1350·1).
Maintenance of normal gastrointestinal flora.

Prontomucil *Francia, Ital.*
Guacetisal (p.1092·1).
Respiratory-tract congestion.

Prontopyrin plus *Mack, Illert., Ger.*
Paracetamol (p.71·2); caffeine (p.761·3).
Cold symptoms; pain.

Prontovent *Salus, Ital.*
Clenbuterol hydrochloride (p.763·3).
Obstructive airways disease.

Propa *Jean-Marie, Hong Kong.*
Propranolol (p.963·1).
Angina pectoris; anxiety; arrhythmias; essential tremor; hypertension; migraine; myocardial infarction.

Propa PH *Del, Canad.*
Salicylic acid (p.1122·3).
Acne.

Propabloc *Azupharma, Ger.*
Propranolol hydrochloride (p.962·3).
Angina pectoris; anxiety; arrhythmias; essential tremor; hypertension; hyperthyroidism; migraine.

Propac *Sherwood, USA.*
Dietary protein supplement (p.1350·1).

Propace *Protein, Mex.*
Metoclopramide (p.1236·3).

Propacet *Lemmon, USA.*
Dextropropoxyphene napsilate (p.27·1); paracetamol (p.71·2).
Pain.

Propacil *Halewood, Thai.*
Propylthiouracil (p.1525·3).
Hyperthyroidism.

Propaderm
Roberts, Canad.; Allen & Hanburys, S.Afr.†; Glaxo Wellcome, UK.
Beclometasone dipropionate (p.1061·2).
Skin disorders.

Propaderm-C *Allen & Hanburys, S.Afr.†.*
Beclometasone dipropionate (p.1061·2); clioquinol (p.190·2).
Infected skin disorders.

Propafen *BASF, Ger.*
Propafenone hydrochloride (p.961·3).
Arrhythmias.

Propagest *Carnrick, USA†.*
Phenylpropanolamine hydrochloride (p.1098·1).
Nasal congestion.

Propain
Note. This name is used for preparations of different composition.
Mer-National, S.Afr.
Syrup: Promethazine hydrochloride (p.423·2); paracetamol (p.71·2).
Tablets: Paracetamol (p.71·2); codeine phosphate (p.25·2); diphenhydramine hydrochloride (p.416·1); caffeine (p.761·3).
Pain and associated tension.

Sankyo, UK.
Paracetamol (p.71·2); codeine phosphate (p.25·2); diphenhydramine hydrochloride (p.416·1); caffeine (p.761·3).
Cold and influenza symptoms; fever; pain.

Propain Forte *Mer-National, S.Afr.*
Paracetamol (p.71·2); codeine phosphate (p.25·2); diphenhydramine (p.416·1); caffeine (p.761·3); phenobarbital (p.355·1).
Pain and associated tension.

Propal *Durascan, Denm.*
Propranolol hydrochloride (p.962·3).
Angina pectoris; hypertension; hyperthyroidism; migraine; myocardial infarction; tremor; variceal haemorrhage.

Propalem *Lemery, Mex.*
Propranolol (p.963·1).
Arrhythmias; hypertension.

Propalen *Zerboni, Mex.*
Propranolol (p.963·1).

Propalgin *Kener, Mex.*
Propranolol (p.963·1).

Propalgina Plus *Roche Nicholas, Spain.*
Ascorbic acid (p.1389·3); chlorpheniramine [chlorphenamine] maleate (p.412·1); dextromethorphan hydrobromide (p.1087·3); phenylephrine hydrochloride (p.1097·1); paracetamol (p.71·2).
Upper respiratory-tract disorders.

Propalgina PS Hot Lemon *Roche Nicholas, Spain.*
Dextromethorphan hydrobromide (p.1087·3); paracetamol (p.71·2); pseudoephedrine hydrochloride (p.1099·2).
Upper-respiratory-tract disorders.

Propam *Pacific, NZ.*
Diazepam (p.674·3).
Alcohol withdrawal syndrome; anxiety; epilepsy; premedication; skeletal muscle spasm; spasticity.

Propamerck *Merck dura, Ger.*
Propafenone hydrochloride (p.961·3).
Arrhythmias.

Propamide
Atlantic, Singapore; Atlantic, Thai.
Chlorpropamide (p.321·1).
Diabetes mellitus.

Propan
Note. This name is used for preparations of different composition.
UCI, Braz.
Buclizine hydrochloride (p.411·1); vitamin B substances; lysine hydrochloride; calcium phosphate (p.1350·1).
Tonic.

Rhone-Poulenc Rorer, Hong Kong.
Buclizine (p.411·1); vitamin B substances (p.1350·1).
Tonic.

Propan Gel-S *Propan, S.Afr.*
Aluminium hydroxide (p.1210·3); magnesium oxide (p.1233·2); dicyclomine [dicycloverine] hydrochloride (p.466·1); dimethicone (p.1249·2).
Gastrointestinal disorders associated with hyperacidity.

Propanix *Ashbourne, UK†.*
Propranolol hydrochloride (p.962·3).
Anxiety; cardiovascular disorders; essential tremor; migraine.

Propantel *Gastroenterologicas, Mex.*
Propantheline bromide (p.473·2).

Propanthel *ICN, Canad.*
Propantheline bromide (p.473·2).
Anticholinergic.

PropapH *Del, USA.*
Salicylic acid (p.1122·3).
Acne.

Propaphenin *Rodleben, Ger.*
Chlorpromazine hydrochloride (p.660·2).
Anxiety; hiccups; nausea; pain; premedication; pruritus; psychoses; sleep disorders; vomiting.

Proparakain-POS *Ursapharm, Ger.*
Proxymetacaine hydrochloride (p.1320·1).
Local anaesthesia.

Propargile *Holistica, Fr.*
Propolis (p.1655·1); pollen; clay.
Digestive disorders.

Proparin *Helber, Mex.*
Heparin sodium (p.902·1).
Thromboembolic disorders.

Propast *CaDiGroup, Ital.*
Zinc oxide (p.1128·2); propolis (p.1655·1); undecenoic acid (p.395·3).
Skin disorders.

Propastad *Stada, Ger.†.*
Propafenone hydrochloride (p.961·3).
Arrhythmias.

Propavan *Sanofi Winthrop, Swed.*
Propiomazine maleate (p.424·3).
Sleep disorders.

Propavente *Glaxo Wellcome, Port.*
Guaifenesin (p.1092·2); salbutamol (p.770·3).
Coughs.

Propecia
Merck Sharp & Dohme, Austral.; Merck Frosst, Canad.; Merck Sharp & Dohme, Denm.; Merck Sharp & Dohme, Fin.; Merck Sharp & Dohme-Chibret, Fr.; Merck Sharp & Dohme, Ger.; Merck Sharp & Dohme, Israel; Merck Sharp & Dohme, Ital.; Merck Sharp & Dohme, NZ; Merck Sharp & Dohme, Port.; Merck Sharp & Dohme, S.Afr.; Merck Sharp & Dohme, Singapore; Merck Sharp & Dohme, Spain; Merck Sharp & Dohme, Swed.; Merck Sharp & Dohme, Switz.; Merck Sharp & Dohme, Thai.; Merck Sharp & Dohme, UK; Merck, USA.
Finasteride (p.1477·2).
Alopecia androgenetica.

Propedil *Yauquimia, Mex.*
Pipenzolate (p.472·2).

Propeshia *Merck Sharp & Dohme, Mex.*
Finasteride (p.1477·2).
Alopecia androgenetica.

Propess
Ferring, Aust.; Ferring, Denm.†; Ferring, Fin.; Ferring, Fr.; Zeneca, Hong Kong; Ferring, Israel; Zeneca, Neth.; Ferring, Neth.; Ferring, Port.; Ferring, Spain; Ferring, Swed.; Ferring, Switz.; Ferring, UK.
Dinoprostone (p.1441·3).
Formerly known as Propess-RS in the UK.
Labour induction.

Prophage *Progress, Thai.*
Metformin hydrochloride (p.332·3).
Diabetes mellitus.

Prophedin *Siam Bheasach, Thai.*
Triprolidine hydrochloride (p.427·2); pseudoephedrine hydrochloride (p.1099·2).
Cold symptoms; hay fever; rhinitis; upper respiratory-tract congestion.

Pro-Phree *Ross, USA.*
Protein-free infant feed supplement (p.1350·1).

Prophthal *Procare, Austral.*
Myrtillus (p.1639·2); ginkgo biloba (p.1615·2).
Herbal supplement.

Prophyllin *Rystan, USA.*
Sodium propionate (p.393·2); chlorophyllin copper complex (p.1028·1).
Contact dermatoses; dermatophytosis; eczemas; minor burns.

Prophylux *Hennig, Ger.*
Propranolol hydrochloride (p.962·3).
Angina pectoris; anxiety; arrhythmias; essential tremor; migraine; myocardial infarction.

Propibay *Bayer, Mex.*
Propicillin potassium (p.239·3).
Bacterial infections.

Propiden *Durascan, Denm.*
Loperamide hydrochloride (p.1231·3).
Diarrhoea.

Propimex *Ross, USA.*
A range of methionine- and valine-free preparations for enteral nutrition including an infant feed (p.1350·1).
Methylmalonic acidaemia; propionic acidaemia.

Propine
Allergan, Austral.; Allergan, Belg.; Allergan-Frumtost, Braz.; Allergan, Canad.; Allergan, Denm.; Allergan, Fin.; Allergan, Fr.; Allergan, Hong Kong; Allergan, Irl.; Allergan, Israel; Allergan, Ital.; Allergan, Norw.; Allergan, NZ; Allergan, Port.; Allergan, S.Afr.; Allergan, Singapore; Allergan, Swed.; Allergan, Thai.; Allergan, UK; Allergan, USA.
Dipivefrine hydrochloride (p.1604·3).
Glaucoma; ocular hypertension.

Propiocine *Aventis, Fr.†.*
Erythromycin propionate (p.201·3).
Bacterial infections.

Propionat *Farmigea, Ital.*
Sodium propionate (p.393·2).
Eye disorders.

Propiral *Yauquimia, Mex.*
Dipyrone (p.34·1).

Proplex
Teva, Israel; Baxter, UK.
A factor IX preparation (p.735·1).
Haemorrhagic disorders.

Proplex T
Baxter-Hyland, Hong Kong; Baxter, Singapore; Baxter, Spain†; Baxter, USA.
A factor IX preparation (p.735·1).
Haemorrhagic disorders.

Pro-Plus *Roche Consumer, UK.*
Caffeine (p.761·3).
Fatigue.

Propofan *Marion Merrell, Fr.*
Dextropropoxyphene (p.27·1); paracetamol (p.71·2); caffeine (p.761·3).
Formerly contained dextropropoxyphene, carbasalate calcium, paracetamol, chlorpheniramine [chlorphenamine] maleate, and caffeine.
Pain.

Propol *Sydenham, Mex.*
Propranolol (p.963·1).

Propolcream *Bucaneve, Ital.*
Propolis (p.1655·1).

Propolisept Urtinktur *Johanser, Ger.*
Homoeopathic preparation.

Propolisept-Salbe *Johanser, Ger.*
Propolis (p.1655·1).
Skin disorders.

Propomill *CaDiGroup, Ital.*
Propolis (p.1655·1); chamomile (p.1593·2).
Skin disorders.

propra *CT, Ger.*
Propranolol hydrochloride (p.962·3).
Angina pectoris; arrhythmias; hypertension; hyperthyroidism; tremor.

Propra comp *Ratiopharm, Ger.*
Propranolol hydrochloride (p.962·3); triamterene (p.986·1); hydrochlorothiazide (p.907·3).
Hypertension.

Proprahexal *Hexal, Aust.*
Propranolol hydrochloride (p.962·3).
Angina pectoris; anxiety disorders; arrhythmias; hypertension; hyperthyroidism; migraine; phaeochromocytoma; tremor.

Propral *Orion, Fin.*
Propranolol hydrochloride (p.962·3).
Angina pectoris; arrhythmias; digitalis toxicity; essential tremor; hypertension; hyperthyroidism; migraine and cluster headache; myocardial infarction; phaeochromocytoma.

Propranet *Nettopharma, Denm.†.*
Propranolol hydrochloride (p.962·3).
Angina pectoris; arrhythmias; hypertension; hyperthyroidism; migraine; myocardial infarction; tremor; variceal haemorrhage.

Propranur *Stegropharm, Ger.*
Propranolol hydrochloride (p.962·3).
Angina pectoris; arrhythmias; hypertension; hyperthyroidism.

Propra-ratiopharm *Ratiopharm, Ger.*
Propranolol (p.963·1) or propranolol hydrochloride (p.962·3).
Angina pectoris; arrhythmias; hypertension; hyperthyroidism; tremor.

Pro-PS *Procare, Austral.*
Cream: Disodium fumarate (p.1114·3); cetrimide (p.1137·1); chlorhexidine gluconate (p.1138·2).
Tablets: Disodium fumarate (p.1114·3); fumaric acid (p.1114·3); vitamins; minerals (p.1350·1).
Psoriasis.

Propulm *Istoria, Ital.*
Procaterol hydrochloride (p.770·1).
Obstructive airways disease.

Propulsid *Janssen, USA†.*
Cisapride (p.1220·1).
Gastro-oesophageal reflux.

Propulsin *Janssen-Cilag, Ger.*
Cisapride (p.1220·1).
Gastrointestinal disorders.

Propycil
Solvay, Ger.; Solvay, Port.
Propylthiouracil (p.1525·3).
Hyperthyroidism.

Propyl *Sriprasit, Thai.*
Propylthiouracil (p.1525·3).
Hyperthyroidism.

Propy-Lacticare *Stiefel, Fr.*
Lactic acid (p.1626·2); propylene glycol (p.1655·1).
Dry skin disorders.

Propylthiocil *Teva, Israel.*
Propylthiouracil (p.1525·3).
Hyperthyroidism.

Propyl-Thyracil *Merck Frosst, Canad.*
Propylthiouracil (p.1525·3).
Hyperthyroidism.

Propyre T *Salvat, Spain.*
Aspirin (p.14·2); caffeine (p.761·3); theobromine (p.777·2).
Fever; inflammation; pain.

P-Roquine *PP Lab, Thai.*
Chloroquine phosphate (p.432·3).
Malaria.

Prorex *Hyrex, USA†.*
Promethazine hydrochloride (p.423·2).
Hypersensitivity reactions; motion sickness; nausea; postoperative pain (adjunct); sedative; vomiting.

Prorhinel
Note.This name is used for preparations of different composition.
Novartis Sante, Fr.; Stiefel, Ger.†.
Benzododecinium bromide (p.1135·1); polysorbate 80 (p.1347·3).
Rhinopharyngeal infections.

Interdelta, Switz.
Benzododecinium bromide (p.1135·1); sodium chloride (p.1196·1); polysorbate 80 (p.1347·3).
Nasal disorders.

Prorynorm *Hexal, Ger.*
Propafenone hydrochloride (p.961·3).
Arrhythmias.

Prosaid *BHR, UK†.*
Naproxen (p.60·3).
Musculoskeletal and joint disorders.

Proscar
Merck Sharp & Dohme, Aust.; Merck Sharp & Dohme, Austral.; Merck Sharp & Dohme, Belg.; Merck Sharp & Dohme, Braz.; Merck Frosst, Canad.; Merck Sharp & Dohme, Denm.; Merck Sharp & Dohme, Fin.; MSD Chibropharm, Ger.; Merck Sharp & Dohme, Hong Kong; Merck Sharp & Dohme, Irl.; Merck Sharp & Dohme, Ital.; Merck Sharp & Dohme, Mex.; Merck Sharp & Dohme, Neth.; Merck Sharp & Dohme, Norw.; Merck Sharp & Dohme, NZ; Merck Sharp & Dohme, Port.; Merck Sharp & Dohme, S.Afr.; Merck Sharp & Dohme, Singapore; Merck Sharp & Dohme, Spain; Merck Sharp & Dohme, Swed.; Merck Sharp & Dohme, Switz.; Merck Sharp & Dohme, Thai.; Merck Sharp & Dohme, UK; Merck, USA.
Finasteride (p.1477·2).
Benign prostatic hyperplasia.

Proscope *Tanabe, Jpn.*
Iopromide (p.1036·1).
Radiographic contrast medium.

Prosedar *Schering-Plough, Port.*
Quazepam (p.703·1).

Prosed/DS *Star, USA.*
Methenamine (p.223·1); salol (p.82·2); methylene blue [methylthioninium chloride] (p.1012·3); benzoic acid (p.1134·2); atropine sulfate (p.461·1); hyoscyamine sulfate (p.469·3).
Pain and discomfort of the urinary tract.

Prosed-X *Procare, Austral.*
Valerian (p.1678·3); lupulus (p.1629·3); passion flower (p.1649·1).
Anxiety; insomnia.

Proser *Ibirn, Ital.*
Saw palmetto (p.1491·2).
Prostatic hyperplasia.

Pro-Shape *Procare, Austral.*
Garcinia quaesita; chromium trichloride (p.1357·1); pectin (p.1502·3); methylcellulose (p.1502·2); magnesium amino acid chelate.
Dietary fibre supplement; obesity.

Prosicca *Agepha, Aust.*
Hypromellose (p.1501·3).
Eye irritation.

Prosiston *Schering, Ger.*
Norethisterone acetate (p.1485·1); ethinylestradiol (p.1476·2).
Menstrual disorders.

Proskin
Note.This name is used for preparations of different composition.
Procare, Austral.
Multivitamin and mineral preparation (p.1350·1).
Dietary supplement; skin disorders.

Upsamedica, Spain.
Dimethicone (p.1410·1); thiomersal (p.1158·2); zinc oxide (p.1128·2).
Skin disorders.

Julphar, UAE.
Zinc oxide (p.1128·2).
Skin disorders.

Proslender *Procare, Austral.*
Gymnema silvestre; dietary fibre (p.1214·2).
Obesity.

Proslim-Lipid *Procare, Austral.†.*
Purified bile extract (p.1585·1).
Obesity.

Prosobee
Mead Johnson, Austral.; Mead Johnson Nutritionals, Canad.†; Mead Johnson Nutritionals, Fr.; Mead Johnson, Ger.; Mead Johnson, Hong Kong; Mead Johnson, Irl.; Mead Johnson, Israel; Mead Johnson, Ital.; Mead Johnson, NZ; Mead Johnson, Port.; Mead Johnson, Singapore; Mead Johnson Nutritionals, Thai.; Mead Johnson Nutritionals, UK; Mead Johnson Nutritionals, USA.
Infant feed (p.1350·1).
Cow's milk intolerance; galactokinase deficiency; galactosaemia; gluten, lactose, or sucrose intolerance.

Pro-Sof Plus *Vangard, USA†.*
Docusate sodium (p.1223·1); casanthranol (p.1216·1).
Constipation.

ProSol *Baxter, USA†.*
Amino-acid infusion (p.1350·1).
Parenteral nutrition.

Prosom *Abbott, USA.*
Estazolam (p.682·3).
Insomnia.

Pro-Sope *Rougier, Canad.*
Sodium lauril ether sulfate (p.1496·3).
Instrument disinfection.

Prospan
Sanova, Aust.; Madaus, Fr.; Engelhard, Ger.; Engelhard, Switz.†.
Hedera helix.
Coughs and associated respiratory-tract disorders.

Prospec *Protein, Mex.*
Ambroxol (p.1084·3).

Prospervital *Provita, Aust.†.*
Deanol bitartrate (p.1507·2); orotic acid (p.1645·3); pentetrazol (p.1513·2); inositol nicotinate (p.914·1).

Prost-I *Procare, Austral.*
Vitamins; amino acids; minerals (p.1350·1); devil's claw root (p.26·3); yucca (p.1682·1); salix (p.82·1); green-lipped mussel (p.1618·2); bromelains (p.1586·3); papain (p.1647·3).
Dietary supplement; musculoskeletal and joint disorders.

Prost-2 *Procare, Austral.†.*
Vitamins; minerals (p.1350·1); green-lipped mussel (p.1618·2); bromelains (p.1586·3); papain (p.1647·3).
Dietary supplement.

Prosta *Procare, Austral.*
Saw palmetto (p.1491·2).
Benign prostatic hyperplasia.

Prosta Fink forte *SmithKline Beecham OTC, Ger.*
Cucurbita (p.1601·1).
Prostatic disorders.

Prosta Fink N *SmithKline Beecham OTC, Ger.*
Saw palmetto (p.1491·2); cucurbita (p.1601·1).
Prostatic disorders.

Prosta Urgenin Uno *Hoyer, Ger.*
Saw palmetto (p.1491·2).
Benign prostatic hyperplasia.

Prostabiol *Yves Ponroy, Fr.*
Cucurbita; red cherry; zinc gluconate; pollen (p.1350·1).
Urinary-tract disorders in men.

Prosta-Caps Chassot N *Mavena, Switz.*
Cucurbita (p.1601·1); cucurbita oil; saw palmetto (p.1491·2); echinacea angustifolia (p.1606·2); java tea (p.1625·1); ononis (p.1644·1).
Formerly contained cucurbita, cucurbita oil, saw palmetto, echinacea angustifolia, rubia tinctorum, java tea, and ononis.
Benign prostatic hyperplasia.

Prosta-Caps Fink *SmithKline Beecham Consumer, Switz.*
Cucurbita (p.1601·1); cucurbita oil; saw palmetto (p.1491·2).
Benign prostatic hyperplasia.

Prostacur *Pras, Spain.*
Flutamide (p.542·3).
Prostatic cancer.

Prostadilat *Pfizer, Aust.*
Doxazosin mesilate (p.883·2).
Benign prostatic hyperplasia; hypertension.

Prostadirex *Irex, Fr.*
Flutamide (p.542·3).
Prostatic cancer.

Prostaflor
Sanova, Aust.; Roche, Switz.
Pollen extracts.
Benign prostatic hyperplasia.

Prostaforton *Biocur, Ger.*
Urtica root (p.1678·2).
Prostatic disorders.

Prostagalen *Galenika, Ger.*
Urtica root (p.1678·2).
Prostatic disorders.

Prostagutt *Austroplant, Aust.*
Saw palmetto (p.1491·2); populi trem. (p.1653·3); urtica dioica (p.1678·2).
Bladder disorders; prostatic disorders.

Prostagutt forte *Schwabe, Ger.*
Sago palm; urtica root (p.1678·2).
Prostatic disorders.

Prostagutt mono *Schwabe, Ger.*
Sago palm.
Prostatic disorders.

Prostagutt uno *Schwabe, Ger.*
Sago palm.
Prostatic disorders.

Prostagutt-F *Schwabe, Switz.*
Saw palmetto (p.1491·2); urtica (p.1678·2).
Benign prostatic hyperplasia.

Prostaherb N *Cesra, Ger.*
Urtica root (p.1678·2).
Prostatic disorders.

Prostal
Note.This name is used for preparations of different composition.
Teikoku, Jpn.
Chlormadinone acetate (p.1465·3).
Prostatic cancer; prostatic hyperplasia.

Rolab, S.Afr.
Metoclopramide hydrochloride (p.1235·2).
Gastrointestinal disorders.

Prostalog *Byk Tosse, Ger.; Byk Gulden, Ger.*
Cucurbita (p.1601·1).
Prostatic disorders.

Prostamal *Almirall, Spain.*
Pygeum africanum (p.1490·3).
Benign prostatic hyperplasia.

Prostamed
Klein, Ger.; Distrifarma, Port.
Cucurbita (p.1601·1); solidago virgaurea; poplar buds (p.1653·2).
Prostatic disorders; urinary-tract disorders.

Prostamustin *Azupharma, Ger.*
Estramustine meglumine phosphate or estramustine sodium phosphate (p.537·3).
Metastatic prostatic cancer.

Prostan *Progress, Thai.*
Mefenamic acid (p.51·2).
Pain.

Prostandin *Ono, Jpn.*
Alprostadil alfadex (p.1440·1).
Peripheral vascular disorders.

Prostaneurin *Sanofi Synthelabo, Ger.*
Urtica root (p.1678·2).
Prostatic hyperplasia.

Prostap *Lederle, Irl.; Wyeth, UK.*
Leuprorelin acetate (p.1289·2).
Endometriosis; prostatic cancer; uterine fibroids.

Prostaphlin *Apothecon, USA†.*
Oxacillin sodium (p.233·2).
Bacterial infections.

Prostaphlin-A *Bristol-Myers Squibb, Israel.*
Cloxacillin sodium (p.192·1).
Staphylococcal infections.

Prostarell *Sanorell, Ger.*
Homoeopathic preparation.

Prostasal *TAD, Ger.*
Sitosterol (p.970·3).
Prostatic disorders.

Prostasan *Bioforce, Switz.*
Saw palmetto (p.1491·2).
Benign prostatic hyperplasia.

Prostaselect *Dreluso, Ger.†.*
Homoeopathic preparation.

Prostaserene *Therabel, Belg.*
Saw palmetto (p.1491·2).
Micturition disorders due to benign prostatic hyperplasia.

Prostasyx *Syxyl, Ger.*
Homoeopathic preparation.

Prostata *Stada, Ger.*
Urtica root (p.1678·2).
Prostatic disorders.

Prostata-Gastreu N R25 *Reckeweg, Ger.*
Homoeopathic preparation.

Prostata-Komplex N Ho-Fu-Complex *Liebermann, Ger.*
Homoeopathic preparation.

Prostata-Kurbis S *Twardy, Ger.*
Cucurbita (p.1601·1); cucurbita oil; sago palm.
Prostatic disorders; urinary-tract disorders.

Prostate Support *Reese, USA.*
Sitosterol (p.970·3); zinc citrate.

Prostatin F *Kanoldt, Ger.*
Bearberry (p.1583·3); urtica root (p.1678·2).
Prostatitis.

Prostatonin
Madaus, Aust.; Pharmaton, Switz.
Pygeum africanum (p.1490·3); urtica (p.1678·2).
Benign prostatic hyperplasia.

Prosta-Urgenin
Madaus, Belg.; Madaus, Ger.
Saw palmetto (p.1491·2).
Benign prostatic hyperplasia.

Prosta-Urgenine *Madaus, Switz.*
Saw palmetto (p.1491·2).
Benign prostatic hyperplasia.

Prostavasin
Gebro, Aust.; Schwarz, Ger.; Schwarz, Hong Kong; Schwarz, Ital.
Alprostadil alfadex (p.1440·1).
Peripheral arterial occlusion; thromboangiitis obliterans.

Prostawern *Wernigerode, Ger.*
Urtica root (p.1678·2).
Prostatic disorders.

Prostem *Baldacci, Braz.*
Pygeum africanum (p.1490·3).
Benign prostatic hyperplasia.

Prostem Plus *Baldacci, Braz.*
Pygeum africanum (p.1490·3); urtica (p.1678·2).
Benign prostatic hyperplasia.

Prosteo *Procare, Austral.*
Calcium gluconate (p.1188·2); calcium carbonate (p.1215·1); colecalciferol (p.1391·1); dolomite.
Calcium supplement.

Prostep
Glaxo Wellcome, Austral.†; Boehringer Ingelheim, Canad.†; Lederle, USA.
Nicotine (p.1640·3).
Aid to smoking withdrawal.

Prosteren Crinos, Ital.
Saw palmetto (p.1491·2).
Benign prostatic hyperplasia.

Prostess TAD, Ger.
Saw palmetto (p.1491·2).
Benign prostatic hyperplasia.

Prostetin Takeda, Jpn.
Oxendolone.
Prostatic hyperplasia.

Prostex Medix, Mex.
Saw palmetto (p.1491·2).
Benign prostatic hyperplasia.

Prostica TAD, Ger.
Flutamide (p.542·3).
Prostatic cancer.

Prostide
Libbs, Braz.; Sigma-Tau, Ital.
Finasteride (p.1477·2).
Benign prostatic hyperplasia.

Prostigmin
ICN, Aust.; Dermatech, Austral.; ICN, Canad.; ICN, Hong Kong; Roche, Irl.†; ICN, Neth.†; Medilink, Norw.†; ICN, Thai.; ICN, USA.
Neostigmine (p.1419·3), neostigmine bromide (p.1419·3), or neostigmine metilsulfate (p.1420·1).
Atonic constipation; heartburn and flatulence; meteorism; myasthenia gravis; postoperative intestinal atony and urinary retention; reversal of competitive neuromuscular blockade.

Prostigmina ICN, Ital.
Neostigmine metilsulfate (p.1420·1).
Gastrointestinal atony; myasthenia gravis; reversal of competitive neuromuscular blockade.

Prostigmine
Sanico, Belg.; Roche, Braz.; CSP, Fr.; Roche, Israel; Roche, Mex.; ICN, Port.; ICN, Spain; ICN, Switz.
Neostigmine (p.1419·3) or neostigmine metilsulfate (p.1420·1).
Ileus; meteorism; myasthenia gravis; postoperative intestinal atony; postoperative urinary retention; reversal of competitive neuromuscular blockade.

Prostin Pharmacia Upjohn, Singapore.
Dinoprostone (p.1441·3).
Labour induction.

Prostin E2
Pharmacia Upjohn, Aust.; Pharmacia Upjohn, Austral.; Pharmacia Upjohn, Belg.; Pharmacia Upjohn, Canad.; Pharmacia Upjohn, Hong Kong; Pharmacia Upjohn, Irl.; Pharmacia Upjohn, Israel; Pharmacia Upjohn, Ital.; Pharmacia Upjohn, Neth.; Pharmacia Upjohn, NZ; Pharmacia Upjohn, Port.; Pharmacia Upjohn, S.Afr.; Pharmacia Upjohn, Switz.; Pharmacia Upjohn, Thai.; Pharmacia, UK; Pharmacia Upjohn, USA.
Dinoprostone (p.1441·3).
Hydatidiform mole; labour induction; termination of pregnancy.

Prostin F2 Pharmacia Upjohn, Irl.
Dinoprost trometamol (p.1441·2).
Labour induction.

Prostin F2 Alpha
Pharmacia Upjohn, Austral.; Pharmacia Upjohn, Hong Kong; Pharmacia Upjohn, Israel; Pharmacia Upjohn, S.Afr.; Pharmacia Upjohn, UK†.
Dinoprost trometamol (p.1441·2).
Hydatidiform mole; labour induction; termination of pregnancy.

Prostin VR
Pharmacia Upjohn, Aust.; Pharmacia Upjohn, Belg.; Pharmacia Upjohn, Canad.; Pharmacia Upjohn, Hong Kong; Pharmacia Upjohn, Israel; Pharmacia Upjohn, Ital.; Pharmacia Upjohn, Neth.; Pharmacia Upjohn, NZ; Pharmacia Upjohn, Port.; Pharmacia Upjohn, S.Afr.; Pharmacia Upjohn, Switz.; Pharmacia Upjohn, Thai.; Pharmacia, UK; Upjohn, USA.
Alprostadil (p.1439·3).
Maintenance of patent ductus arteriosus.

Prostine E₂ Pharmacia Upjohn, Fr.
Dinoprostone (p.1441·3).
Hydatidiform mole; labour induction; termination of pregnancy.

Prostine F₂ Alpha Pharmacia Upjohn, Fr.†.
Dinoprost trometamol (p.1441·2).
Labour induction.

Prostine VR Pharmacia Upjohn, Fr.
Alprostadil (p.1439·3).
Maintenance of patent ductus arteriosus.

Prostinfenem
Pharmacia Upjohn, Denm.; Pharmacia Upjohn, Swed.
Carboprost trometamol (p.1441·1).
Intra-uterine death; postpartum haemorrhage; termination of pregnancy.

Prostin/15M
Pharmacia Upjohn, Belg.; Pharmacia Upjohn, Neth.; Pharmacia Upjohn, NZ.
Carboprost trometamol (p.1441·1).
Intra-uterine death; postpartum haemorrhage; termination of pregnancy.

Prostivas
Pharmacia Upjohn, Denm.; Pharmacia Upjohn, Fin.; Pharmacia Upjohn, Norw.; Pharmacia Upjohn, Swed.
Alprostadil (p.1439·3).
Maintenance of patent ductus arteriosus.

Prostogenat Azupharma, Ger.
Flutamide (p.542·3).
Prostatic cancer.

Prosturol Nexis, Spain.
Benzydamine hydrochloride (p.20·1); pygeum africanum (p.1490·3).
Prostatic adenoma.

Prost-X Homeocan, Canad.
Homoeopathic preparation.

Prosulf
CP Pharmaceuticals, Hong Kong; CP, Israel; CP Pharmaceuticals, UK.
Protamine sulfate (p.1021·1).
Neutralisation of heparin activity.

Prosymbioflor Peithner, Aust.
Autolysate of Escherichia coli; Enterococcus faecalis (p.1626·3).
Immunotherapy.

Pro-Symbioflor Symbiopharm, Ger.
Autolysates of: Escherichia coli; Enterococcus faecalis (p.1626·3).
Gastrointestinal disorders.

Protact Coloplast, Fr.
Barrier cream.
Formerly known as Conveen Protact.

Protactyl Hexal, Ger.
Promazine hydrochloride (p.702·2).
Anxiety; neurogenic pain; premedication; pruritus; psychoses; sleep disorders; vomiting.

Protagens Thilo, Neth.†.
Povidone (p.1503·2).
Dry eyes.

Protagent
Alcon, Aust.; Bournonville, Belg.†; Alcon, Ger.; Thilo, Hong Kong; Alcon, Ital.; Alcon, Switz.
Povidone (p.1503·2).
Dry eyes; eye irritation.

Protalgia Reig Jofre, Spain.
Fosfosal (p.42·1).
Fever; musculoskeletal, joint, and soft-tissue disorders; pain.

Protamide
Note. This name is used for preparations of different composition.
Therabel, Belg.†.
Stomach extract.
Postherpetic neuralgia.
Ferraz, Lynce, Port.†.
Amino-acids, peptones, and polypeptides (p.1350·1).

Protamine Zinc Insulin MC Novo Nordisk, Austral.†.
Protamine zinc insulin suspension (bovine, monocomponent) (p.324·1).
Diabetes mellitus.

Protan Protein, Mex.
Dextromethorphan (p.1087·3).

Protangix Expanpharm, Fr.
Dipyridamole (p.877·2).
Coronary disorders; thromboembolic disorders.

Protaphan Novo Nordisk, Fin.
Isophane insulin injection (human) (p.324·1).
Diabetes mellitus.

Protaphan HM Novo Nordisk, Ger.
Neutral isophane insulin injection (human) (p.324·1).
Diabetes mellitus.

Protaphane
Novo Nordisk, Austral.; Novo Nordisk, NZ.
Isophane insulin injection (human, monocomponent) (p.324·1).
Formerly known as Protaphane HM in Austral.
Diabetes mellitus.

Protaphane HM
Novo Nordisk, Hong Kong; Novo Nordisk, Ital.; Novo Nordisk, S.Afr.
Isophane insulin injection (human, monocomponent) (p.324·1).
Diabetes mellitus.

Protaphane MC
Novo Nordisk, Braz.; Novo Nordisk, Hong Kong.
Neutral isophane insulin injection (porcine, monocomponent) (p.324·1).
Diabetes mellitus.

Protar Protein Dermol, USA†.
Coal tar (p.1125·1).

Protarin Wayne, Mex.
Medroxyprogesterone (p.1480·1).

Protasol Alcon, Aust.
Comfort drops for hard contact lenses (p.1129·2).

Protat Potter's, UK.
Corn silk (p.1599·3); kava (p.1625·3).
Bladder discomfort.

Protaxil
Delta, Port.; Rottapharm, Spain.
Proglumetacin maleate (p.80·1).
Inflammation; musculoskeletal, joint, peri-articular, and soft-tissue disorders.

Protaxol Provit, Mex.
Co-trimoxazole (p.193·3).
Bacterial infections.

Protaxon
Sanofi Winthrop, Aust.; Opfermann, Ger.
Proglumetacin maleate (p.80·1).
Musculoskeletal and joint disorders; peri-articular disorders; soft-tissue disorders.

Proteamin Tanabe, Jpn†.
Amino-acid and carbohydrate infusion (p.1350·1).
Parenteral nutrition.

Protec Protec, UK.
Note. A similar name is used for preparations of different composition (see below).
Dioctyl adipate (p.1432·1).

Formerly known as Gurkha.
Insect repellent.

Pro-Tec Sport Allergan, Canad.
Note. A similar name is used for preparations of different composition (see above and below).
SPF 20: Octinoxate (p.1517·3); octisalate (p.1518·1); oxybenzone (p.1518·1).
Sunscreen.

Protec T Implementos Plasticos, Mex.
Note. A similar name is used for preparations of different composition (see above).
Copper-wound plastic (p.1357·3).
Intra-uterine contraceptive device.

ProTech Triton, USA.
Povidone-iodine (p.1155·1); lignocaine [lidocaine] hydrochloride (p.1313·2).
Burns; cuts.

Protecor Duopharm, Ger.
Crataegus (p.1600·2); magnesium complex with acid hydrolysate of corn starch; alpha tocoferil acetate (p.1394·1).
Cardiovascular disorders.

Protectaid
Axcan, Canad.; Axcan, Hong Kong; Sinclair, UK.
Nonoxinol 9 (p.1346·1); sodium cholate; benzalkonium chloride (p.1133·2).
Contraceptive.

Protecteur Levres Lancome, Canad.†.
SPF 15: Octinoxate (p.1517·3); titanium dioxide (p.1126·1).
Sunscreen.

Protecto National Care, Canad.
Benzethonium chloride (p.1134·2); zinc oxide (p.1128·2).
Barrier cream.

Protecto-Derm Ingram & Bell, Canad.†.
Silicone (p.1410·1).
Barrier cream.

Protectol Daniels, USA.
Calcium undecenoate (p.395·3).
Bromhidrosis; fungal skin infections; hyperhidrosis; minor skin irritation; nappy rash.

Protector Quimifar, Spain.
Loperamide (p.1232·1).
Formerly contained diphenoxylate hydrochloride.
Diarrhoea.

Protegra Lederle, USA†.
Multivitamin and mineral preparation (p.1350·1).

Proteika Leman, Fr.
Nutritional supplement (p.1350·1).

Protein Free Diet (Product 80056) Mead Johnson, Austral.
Preparation for infant enteral nutrition (p.1350·1).
Disorders of amino acid metabolism.

Protein Plus Nutricia, Austral.†.
High protein enteral feed (p.1350·1).

Protein-Free
Mead Johnson, Hong Kong; Mead Johnson, Ital.
Food for low-protein diets (p.1350·1).

Proteinsteril Hepa Fresenius, Belg.†.
Amino-acid infusion (p.1350·1).
Parenteral nutrition in liver failure.

Proteinsteril KE Fresenius, Belg.†.
Amino-acid infusion with electrolytes (p.1350·1).
Parenteral nutrition.

Protemp Procare, Austral.
Vitamins; minerals (p.1350·1); bearberry (p.1583·3); parsley piert (p.1648·3); juniper (p.1625·2); viburnum opulus.
Dietary supplement; dysmenorrhoea; premenstrual syndrome.

Proten Plus Fresenius Kabi, Port.
Preparation for enteral nutrition (p.1350·1).

Protenac Enila, Braz.
Preparation for enteral nutrition (p.1350·1).

Protenate
Baxter-Hyland, Hong Kong; Hyland, USA.
Plasma protein fraction (p.740·2).
Burns; hypoalbuminaemia; hypovolaemia.

Protensin-M Bristol-Myers Squibb, S.Afr.
Hydroflumethiazide (p.911·3); reserpine (p.967·3).
Hypertension.

Proteoferrina Bayer, Ital.
Iron succinyl-protein complex (p.1369·3).
Iron deficiency; iron-deficiency anaemia.

Proteozym Wiedemann, Ger.
Bromelains (p.1586·3).
Inflammation; oedema.

Proteval Protein, Mex.
Valproic acid (p.366·2).

Prothanon LAW, Ger.
Dioxopromethazine hydrochloride (p.424·1).
Skin disorders.

Prothanon cromo Chauvin ankerpharm, Ger.
Sodium cromoglicate (p.774·3).
Allergic conjunctivitis; allergic rhinitis.

Prothazin Rodleben, Ger.; Wernigerode, Ger.
Promethazine hydrochloride (p.423·2).
Allergic disorders; anxiety; biliary spasm; insomnia; premedication; psychoses; vomiting.

Prothazine Vortech, USA†.
Promethazine hydrochloride (p.423·2).
Hypersensitivity reactions; motion sickness; nausea; postoperative pain (adjunct); sedative; vomiting.

Prothiaden
Knoll, Austral.; Knoll, Belg.; Knoll, Denm.; Knoll, Fr.; Boots, Hong Kong; Knoll, Irl.; Knoll, Neth.; Knoll, NZ; Knoll, S.Afr.; Knoll, Singapore; Alter, Spain; Boots, Thai.; Knoll, UK.
Dothiepin [dosulepin] hydrochloride (p.283·2).
Depression; mixed anxiety depressive states.

Prothiazide Pacific, NZ.
Cyclopenthiazide (p.1525·3).
Heart failure; hypertension; oedema.

Prothiazine CTI, Israel.
Promethazine hydrochloride (p.423·2).
Anxiety; coughs; hypersensitivity reactions; insomnia; nausea; pain; parkinsonism; premedication.

Prothiazine Expectorant CTI, Israel.
Promethazine hydrochloride (p.423·2); guaifenesin (p.1092·2); ipecacuanha (p.1093·1).
Coughs.

Prothil Solvay, Ger.
Medrogestone (p.1480·1).
Menopausal disorders; progestagenic.

Prothiuncil Sanova, Aust.
Propylthiouracil (p.1525·3).
Hyperthyroidism; ulcerative colitis.

Prothrombinex CSL, NZ.
A factor IX preparation (p.735·1).
Haemorrhagic disorders.

Prothrombinkomplex BaWu Intersero, Ger.
A factor IX preparation (p.735·1).
Haemorrhagic disorders.

Prothromplex Immuno, UK.
A factor IX preparation (p.735·1).
Factor IX deficiency.

Prothromplex S-TIM 4
Immuno, Aust.; Immuno, Ger.†.
A factor IX preparation (p.735·1).
Haemorrhagic disorders.

Prothromplex Total S-TIM 4 Baxter, Switz.
A factor IX preparation (p.735·1).
Haemorrhagic disorders.

Prothromplex-T Immuno, Braz.
A factor IX preparation (p.735·1).
Haemorrhagic disorders.

Prothromplex-T TIM 4 Omnimed, S.Afr.
A factor IX preparation (p.735·1).
Haemorrhagic disorders.

Prothyrid
Mayrhofer, Aust.; Henning, Ger.
Thyroxine [levothyroxine] sodium (p.1526·2); liothyronine hydrochloride (p.1524·3).
Hypothyroidism; thyroiditis.

Prothyrysat Ysatfabrik, Ger.
Lycopus europaeus.
Hyperthyroidism.

Proti 5 Pharmygiene, Fr.
Nutritional supplement (p.1350·1).

Protiaden
Nordmark, Ital.; Knoll, Switz.
Dothiepin [dosulepin] hydrochloride (p.283·2).
Depression; mixed anxiety depressive states.

Protiadene Knoll, Port.
Dothiepin [dosulepin] hydrochloride (p.283·2).
Depression.

Protid Lunsco, USA.
Paracetamol (p.71·2); chlorpheniramine [chlorphenamine] maleate (p.412·1); phenylephrine hydrochloride (p.1097·1).

Protidiet Protidiet, Fr.
Nutritional protein supplement (p.1350·1).

Protifar
Nutricia, Austral.; Nutricia, Fin.; Nutricia, Fr.; Nutricia, Irl.; Nutricia, Ital.; Baxter, NZ; Nutricia, NZ; Nutricia, Thai.; Nutricia Clinical, UK.
Dietary protein supplement (p.1350·1).
Hypoproteinaemia; protein supplement.

Protifar Plus Nutricia, Port.
High protein nutritional supplement (p.1350·1).

Protifortf Pharmygiene, Fr.†.
Preparation for enteral nutrition (p.1350·1).

Protifortifiant Pharmygiene, Fr.
Preparation for enteral nutrition (p.1350·1).

Protil Diepal, Fr.†.
High protein nutritional supplement (p.1350·1).

Protilase Rugby, USA.
Pancrelipase (p.1647·2).
Pancreatic enzyme deficiency.

Protina G Torre, Ital.
Preparation for enteral nutrition (p.1350·1).

Protina Torre MP Torre, Ital.
Preparation for enteral nutrition (p.1350·1).

Protinin Probifasa, Mex.
Aprotinin (p.725·3).

Protinutril Pharmacia Upjohn, Fr.†.
Amino-acid, vitamin, and mineral infusion (p.1350·1).
Parenteral nutrition.

Protipharm DHN, Fr.
A range of nutritional supplements (p.1350·1).

Protireal Novartis Nutrition, Fr.
Preparation for enteral nutrition (p.1350·1).

Protium
Knoll, Irl.; Knoll, UK.
Pantoprazole sodium (p.1243·2).
Gastro-oesophageal reflux; peptic ulcer.

Protocide *Unipharm, Israel.*
Tinidazole (p.603·3).
Anaerobic bacterial infections; protozoal infections.

Protogyl
Xepa-Soul Pattinson, Hong Kong; Xepa-Soul Pattinson, Singapore.
Metronidazole (p.594·1).
Amoebiasis; genito-urinary-tract infections; trichomoniasis.

Protol *Procare, Austral.*
Vitamins; minerals (p.1350·1); garlic (p.1614·1).
Dietary supplement; viral infections.

Proton
Note.This name is used for preparations of different composition.
Heralds, Braz.
Vitamin B₁ (p.1385·2).
Vitamin B₁ deficiency; vitamin B₁ supplement.

Medinfar, Port.
Omeprazole (p.1239·1).
Gastro-oesophageal reflux; peptic ulcer; Zollinger-Ellison syndrome.

Protonix *Wyeth-Ayerst, USA.*
Pantoprazole sodium (p.1243·2).
Gastro-oesophageal reflux; Zollinger-Ellison syndrome.

Protopam
Wyeth-Ayerst, Canad.; Wyeth-Ayerst, USA.
Pralidoxime chloride (p.1020·1).
Anticholinesterase antagonist; organophosphorus insecticide poisoning.

Protopic *Fujisawa, USA.*
Tacrolimus (p.569·3).
Eczema.

Protosol *Kamada, Israel.*
Aprotinin (p.725·3).
Hyperfibrinolytic haemorrhagic; reduction of blood loss in cardiopulmonary bypass.

Protostat *Ortho Pharmaceutical, USA.*
Metronidazole (p.594·1).
Amoebiasis; anaerobic bacterial infections; trichomoniasis.

Protovit
Roche, Belg.; Roche, Braz.; Roche, Ital.; Roche Nicholas, Spain.
Multivitamin preparation (p.1350·1).

Protovit N *Roche, Port.*
Multivitamin preparation (p.1350·1).

Protozone *Technilab, Hong Kong.*
Hydrocortisone acetate (p.1073·3); cinchocaine hydrochloride (p.1309·1); neomycin sulfate (p.228·1); esculoside (p.1574·1).
Haemorrhoids.

Protraz *Propan, S.Afr.†.*
Nitrazepam (p.695·2).
Insomnia.

Protromplex TIM 3 *Immuno, Ital.*
Factor IX (p.735·1).
Deficiency of factors II, IX, and X.

Protropin
Roche, Canad.; Genentech, USA.
Somatrem (p.1286·1).
Growth hormone deficiency.

Protuss *Horizon, USA.*
Hydrocodone tartrate (p.42·2); sulfogaiacol (p.1101·1).
Coughs.

Protuss-D *Horizon, USA.*
Hydrocodone tartrate (p.42·2); pseudoephedrine hydrochloride (p.1099·2); sulfogaiacol (p.1101·1).
Coughs.

Protuss-DM *Horizon, USA.*
Guaifenesin (p.1092·2); pseudoephedrine hydrochloride (p.1099·2); dextromethorphan hydrobromide (p.1087·3).
Coughs.

Pro-Uro *Ghimas, Ital.†.*
Pipemidic acid (p.236·1).
Urinary-tract infections.

Provail *CCM, Singapore.*
Ketoprofen (p.47·3).
Musculoskeletal, joint, and peri-articular disorders.

Provames *Cassenne, Fr.*
Estradiol (p.1473·1).
Menopausal disorders; osteoporosis.

Provamicina *Rhone-Poulenc Rorer, Mex.*
Spiramycin (p.248·3).
Respiratory-tract infections; toxoplasmosis.

Provas *Schwarz, Ger.; Sanol, Ger.*
Valsartan (p.988·3).
Hypertension.

Provas comp *Schwarz, Ger.; Sanol, Ger.*
Valsartan (p.988·3); hydrochlorothiazide (p.907·3).
Hypertension.

Provascul *Gerot, Aust.*
Bamethan sulfate (p.843·1).
Peripheral vascular disorders.

Provatine *Duopharma, Hong Kong.*
Fluoxetine hydrochloride (p.284·2).
Depression.

Provax *Probios, Port.*
Lysates of *Staphylococcus aureus; Streptococcus pyogenes; Streptococcus viridans; Klebsiella pneumoniae; Klebsiella ozaenae; Streptococcus pneumoniae; Haemophilus influenzae; Moraxella cattarhalis.*
Respiratory-tract infections.

Provegol *SVR, Fr.*
Pyrithione zinc (p.1122·1).
Scalp disorders.

Provelle *Pharmacia Upjohn, Austral.*
28 Tablets, conjugated oestrogens (p.1467·1); 14 or 28 tablets, medroxyprogesterone acetate (p.1480·1).
Menopausal disorders; osteoporosis.

Provenal *Pulitzer, Ital.*
A heparinoid (p.905·2).
Vascular disorders with a risk of thrombosis.

Proveno N *Madaus, Ger.*
Aescin (p.1574·1).
Vascular disorders.

Pro-Vent *Wellcome, Irl.†.*
Theophylline (p.777·2).
Bronchospasm.

Proventil *Schering, USA.*
Salbutamol (p.770·3) or salbutamol sulfate (p.770·3).
Bronchospasm.

Provera
Pharmacia Upjohn, Aust.; Pharmacia Upjohn, Austral.; Pharmacia Upjohn, Belg.; Pharmacia Upjohn, Braz.; Pharmacia Upjohn, Canad.; Pharmacia Upjohn, Denm.; Pharmacia Upjohn, Fin.; Pharmacia Upjohn, Hong Kong; Pharmacia Upjohn, Irl.; Pharmacia Upjohn, Israel; Pharmacia Upjohn, Ital.; Pharmacia Upjohn, Mex.; Pharmacia Upjohn, Neth.; Pharmacia Upjohn, Norw.; Pharmacia Upjohn, NZ; Pharmacia Upjohn, Port.; Pharmacia Upjohn, S.Afr.; Pharmacia Upjohn, Singapore; Pharmacia Upjohn, Swed.; Pharmacia Upjohn, Switz.†; Pharmacia Upjohn, Thai.; Pharmacia, UK; Pharmacia Upjohn, USA.
Medroxyprogesterone acetate (p.1480·1).
Adjunct in oestrogen replacement therapy; amenorrhoea; breast cancer; dysfunctional uterine bleeding; endometrial cancer; endometriosis; menopausal disorders; renal cancer.

Provertin-UM TIM 3 *Immuno, Ital.*
Factor VII (p.733·3).
Factor VII deficiency.

Provetal *Protein, Mex.*
Valproic acid (p.366·2).

Provette Continuous *Pharmacia Upjohn, NZ.*
28 Tablets, conjugated oestrogens (p.1467·1); 28 tablets, medroxyprogesterone acetate (p.1480·1).
Menopausal disorders; osteoporosis.

Provette Sequential *Pharmacia Upjohn, NZ.*
28 Tablets, conjugated oestrogens (p.1467·1); 14 tablets, medroxyprogesterone acetate (p.1480·1).
Menopausal disorders; osteoporosis.

Provical *Stevia, Braz.*
Vitamin D; vitamin B₁₂; calcium chloride; calcium phosphate; fluoride; sorbitol (p.1350·1).
Nutritional supplement.

Provide *Rowa, Irl.†.*
Gluten-, lactose-, and milk-free food for special diets (p.1350·1).
Bowel disorders; nutritional supplement.

Providex *Baldassari, Braz.*
Neomycin (p.228·1); benzocaine (p.1306·2); chlorobutanol (p.1141·2).
Ear infections.

Providextra *Fresenius Kabi, Fin.*
Preparation for enteral nutrition (p.1350·1).

Provigil
Cephalon, Irl.; Cephalon, UK; Cephalon, USA.
Modafinil (p.1512·3).
Narcoleptic syndrome.

Provimin *Ross, USA.*
Preparation for enteral nutrition (p.1350·1).

Proviodine
Rougier, Canad.; Rougier, Hong Kong.
Povidone-iodine (p.1155·1).
Burns; skin and mucous membrane disinfection; vaginal infections; wounds.

Proviron
Schering, Aust.; Schering, Austral.; Schering, Belg.; Schering, Braz.; Schering, Fin.; Schering, Fr.†; Schering, Ger.; Schering, Hong Kong; Schering, Israel; Schering, Ital.; Schering, Mex.; Schering, Neth.; Schering, Port.; Schering, S.Afr.; Schering, Spain; Schering, Switz.; Schering, UK.
Mesterolone (p.1482·1).
Androgen deficiency; aplastic anaemia; erectile dysfunction; male hypogonadism; male infertility.

Provironum
Schering, Singapore; Schering, Thai.
Mesterolone (p.1482·1).
Androgen deficiency; erectile dysfunction; hypogonadism; male infertility.

Provisc
Alcon, Aust.†; Alcon, Austral.; Alcon, Belg.†; Alcon, Fr.; Alcon, Ger.; Alcon, Hong Kong; Alcon, Ital.; Alcon, NZ; Alcon, S.Afr.; Alcon, Singapore; Alcon, Swed.; Alcon, Thai.; Alcon, UK.
Sodium hyaluronate (p.1620·1).
Adjunct in eye surgery.

Provitamin A + D + E *Klein, Ger.*
Multivitamin preparation (p.1350·1).

Provitamin A-E *Cielle, Ital.*
Vitamin A (p.1382·1); vitamin E (p.1393·3); royal jelly (p.1659·3).
Nutritional supplement.

Provocholine
Methapharm, Canad.; Methapharm, USA.
Methacholine chloride (p.1419·3).
Diagnosis of bronchial hyperreactivity.

Provotest *Hoechst, Ger.†.*
Dichlorodifluoromethane (p.1199·1).
Diagnostic agent.

Prowess *Harley Street Supplies, UK.*
Yohimbine hydrochloride (p.1681·3); pemoline (p.1513·1); methyltestosterone (p.1482·3).
Erectile dysfunction.

Prowess Plain *Harley Street Supplies, UK.*
Yohimbine hydrochloride (p.1681·3).
Erectile dysfunction.

Pro-Whey *Milk Industries, Israel.*
Protein supplement (p.1350·1).

ProWohl *Eurim, Ger.†.*
Magaldrate (p.1232·2).
Gastrointestinal disorders.

Proxalin *Degorts, Mex.*
Naproxen (p.60·3).
Gout; inflammation; musculoskeletal, joint, and peri-articular disorders; pain.

Proxalyoc *Lafon, Fr.*
Piroxicam (p.79·1).
Musculoskeletal and joint disorders.

Proxen
Grunenthal, Aust.; Macarthur, Austral.; Syntex, Ger.; Roche, Ger.; Medochemie, Hong Kong; Garec, S.Afr.†; Almirall, Spain; Grunenthal, Switz.; Pharmaland, Thai.
Naproxen (p.60·3) or naproxen lysine (p.61·3).
Lignocaine [lidocaine] (p.1313·2) may be included in the injection to alleviate the pain of injection.
Fever; gout; musculoskeletal, joint, peri-articular, and soft-tissue disorders; pain.

Proxidin *Procare, Austral.*
Vitamins; minerals; garlic; eleutherococcus senticosis (p.1350·1).
Dietary supplement.

Proxigel *Reed & Carnrick, USA.*
Urea hydrogen peroxide (p.1159·3).
Oral inflammation.

Proxil *Rottapharm, Ital.*
Proglumetacin maleate (p.80·1).
Inflammation; pain.

Proxine *Del Saz & Filippini, Ital.†.*
Naproxen (p.60·3).
Musculoskeletal and joint disorders; pain.

Proxitec *Tecnofarma, Mex.*
Ciprofloxacin (p.182·3).
Bacterial infections.

Proxol *Sam-On, Israel.*
Dextropropoxyphene hydrochloride (p.27·1); paracetamol (p.71·2).
Fever; pain.

Proyeast *Procare, Austral.*
Garlic (p.1614·1); echinacea (p.1606·2); ascorbic acid (p.1389·3); chaparral (p.1593·3); zinc gluconate (p.1398·2); vitamin A (p.1382·1); pau d'arco.
Candidiasis.

Prozac
Lilly, Austral.; Lilly, Belg.; Lilly, Braz.; Lilly, Canad.; Lilly, Fr.; Lilly, Hong Kong; Dista, Irl.; Lilly, Irl.; Lilly, Israel; Lilly, Ital.; Lilly, Mex.; Lilly, Neth.; Lilly, NZ; Lilly, Port.; Lilly, S.Afr.; Lilly, Singapore; Dista, Spain; Lilly, Thai.; Lilly, UK; Dista, USA.
Fluoxetine hydrochloride (p.284·2).
Bulimia nervosa; depression; obsessive-compulsive disorder; premenstrual dysphoric disorder.

Prozamel *Clonmel, Irl.*
Fluoxetine hydrochloride (p.284·2).
Bulimia; depression; obsessive-compulsive disorder.

Prozatan *UCB, Irl.*
Fluoxetine hydrochloride (p.284·2).
Bulimia; depression; obsessive-compulsive disorder.

Prozef *Bristol-Myers Squibb, S.Afr.*
Cefprozil (p.173·2).
Bacterial infections.

Proziere *Ashbourne, UK.*
Prochlorperazine maleate (p.701·2).

Prozin *Lusofarmaco, Ital.*
Chlorpromazine hydrochloride (p.660·2).
Hiccups; pain; premedication; psychiatric disorders; vomiting.

Prozine
Note.This name is used for preparations of different composition.
Propan, S.Afr.†.
Carbamazepine (p.342·2).
Epilepsy; trigeminal neuralgia.

Utopian, Thai.
Chlorpromazine hydrochloride (p.660·2).
Psychoses.

Hauck, USA.
Promazine hydrochloride (p.702·2).
Psychoses.

Prozitel *Farcoral, Mex.*
Praziquantel (p.106·3).
Neurocysticercosis.

Prozolin *Liferpal, Mex.*
Metronidazole benzoate (p.594·1).

ProZone *Darier, Mex.*
SPF 30: Melanin; octinoxate (p.1517·3); octisalate (p.1518·1); oxybenzone (p.1518·1); butyl methoxycinnamate; homosalate (p.1517·2).
Sunscreen.

ProZone Body *Darier, Mex.*
SPF 25: Melanin; octinoxate (p.1517·3); oxybenzone (p.1518·1); avobenzone (p.1517·1); titanium dioxide (p.1126·1).
Sunscreen.

ProZone Face *Darier, Mex.*
SPF 25: Melanin; octinoxate (p.1517·3); oxybenzone (p.1518·1); octisalate (p.1518·1).
Sunscreen.

ProZone Ultra *Darier, Mex.*
SPF 80: Melanin; octocrilene (p.1518·1); octinoxate (p.1517·3); octisalate (p.1518·1); oxybenzone (p.1518·1); avobenzone (p.1517·1); titanium dioxide (p.1126·1).
Sunscreen.

Prozyme *Procare, Austral.*
Outer layer, pepsin (p.1649·3); bromelains (p.1586·3); glutamic acid hydrochloride (p.1365·2); inner layer, pancreatin (p.1646·1); papain (p.1647·3); bromelains.
Dyspepsia.

Prozyn *Adcock Ingram, S.Afr.†.*
Fluoxetine hydrochloride (p.284·2).
Bulimia nervosa; mixed anxiety depressive states; obsessive-compulsive disorder.

Pruina *Faes, Spain.*
Senna (p.1248·2); cassia fistula (p.1216·3); coriander (p.1599·2); tamarind (p.1253·2).
Constipation.

Prulet *Mission Pharmacal, USA†.*
Phenolphthalein (p.1244·1).
Constipation.

Prulit *Vinas, Spain.*
Menthol (p.1632·3).
Formerly known as Nopika.
Insect stings; muscle sprains and strains; pruritus.

Prunasine *Christiaens, Belg.*
Senna fruit (p.1248·2).
Constipation.

Prunodiet *DHN, Fr.*
Dietary fibre supplement (p.1350·1).
Constipation.

Prunogil *Novartis Nutrition, Fr.*
Dietary fibre supplement (p.1350·1).
Constipation.

Prunus-Bad *Weleda, Aust.*
Prunus spinosa.
Tonic.

Prurex *Agepha, Aust.*
Diphenhydramine hydrochloride (p.416·1).
Burns; hypersensitivity reactions; insect bites; pruritus; sunburn.

Pruridermase *Sofex, Port.†.*
Calamine (p.1111·3); diphenhydramine (p.416·1); menthol (p.1632·3); hamamelis (p.1618·3).
Pruritus; skin irritation.

Pruri-med *Permamed, Switz.*
Sodium sulfosuccinated undecenoic acid monoethanolamide (p.396·1); lauromacrogol 400 (p.1345·2).
Skin disorders.

Prurimix *Metochem, Aust.*
Talc (p.1124·2); zinc oxide (p.1128·2); lauromacrogol 400 (p.1345·2); menthol (p.1632·3); diphenylpyraline hydrochloride (p.417·1).
Skin disorders.

Pruritrat *Newlab, Braz.*
Lindane (p.1434·1).
Pediculosis; scabies.

Prurix *Stiefel, Mex.*
Camphor (p.1589·3); menthol (p.1632·3).
Pruritus.

Pryleugan *Dresden, Ger.; Temmler, Ger.*
Imipramine hydrochloride (p.291·1).
Depression; nocturnal enuresis; pain.

Pryndette *Aventis, NZ.*
Paracetamol (p.71·2); doxylamine succinate (p.417·1).
Fever; pain; sedative.

Prysma *UCB, Spain.*
Omeprazole (p.1239·1).
Gastro-oesophageal reflux; peptic ulcer; Zollinger-Ellison syndrome.

Prysoline *Rekah, Israel.*
Primidone (p.363·3).
Epilepsy.

Pselac *Fresenius Kabi, Aust.*
Lactitol (p.1230·1).
Constipation; hepatic encephalopathy.

Pserhofer's *Agepha, Aust.*
Aloes (p.1210·1); frangula (p.1227·1).
Constipation.

Pseudo *Major, USA.*
Pseudoephedrine hydrochloride (p.1099·2).
Nasal congestion.

Pseudo-Car DM *Geneva, USA.*
Pseudoephedrine hydrochloride (p.1099·2); carbinoxamine maleate (p.411·1); dextromethorphan hydrobromide (p.1087·3).
Coughs and cold symptoms.

Pseudocef
Grunenthal, Aust.; Takeda, Ger.
Cefsulodin sodium (p.174·2).
Lignocaine [lidocaine] hydrochloride (p.1313·2) may be included in the intramuscular injection to alleviate the pain of injection.
Bacterial infections.

Pseudo-Chlor *Geneva, USA; Major, USA.*
Pseudoephedrine hydrochloride (p.1099·2); chlorpheniramine [chlorphenamine] maleate (p.412·1).
Upper respiratory-tract symptoms.

Pseudofrin *Trianon, Canad.*
Pseudoephedrine hydrochloride (p.1099·2).
Congestion.

Pseudo-Gest *Major, USA.*
Pseudoephedrine hydrochloride (p.1099·2).
Nasal congestion.

Pseudo-Gest Plus *Major, USA.*
Pseudoephedrine hydrochloride (p.1099·2); chlorpheniramine [chlorphenamine] maleate (p.412·1).
Upper respiratory-tract symptoms.

Pseudono Milano, Thai.
Pseudoephedrine hydrochloride (p.1099·2).
Rhinitis; upper respiratory-tract congestion.

Pseudophage Servier, Fr.
Sodium alginate (p.1498·3); agar (p.1498·3).
Obesity.

Psico Blocan Estedi, Spain.
Chlordiazepoxide hydrochloride (p.659·2); hyoscine
methobromide (p.468·2).
Gastrointestinal spasm.

Psicocen Centrum, Spain.
Sulpiride (p.706·1).
Anxiety disorders; psychoses; vertigo.

Psicofar Sifarma, Ital.
Chlordiazepoxide hydrochloride (p.659·2).
Anxiety disorders; behaviour disorders in children.

Psicoglut Sanofi Winthrop, Braz.
Piracetam (p.1652·1); cyanocobalamin; levoglutamide;
DL-serine; iosine (p.1350·1).
Impaired mental function.

Psicosedin Farmasa, Braz.
Chlordiazepoxide (p.659·2).
*Adjuvant in general anaesthesia; alcohol withdrawal
syndrome; anxiety; panic attacks; tension headache;
tremor.*

Psicosoma Solucion Ferrer, Spain.
Magnesium glutamate hydrobromide (p.1631·1); pro-
methazine hydrochloride (p.423·2).
Insomnia; night terrors; sedative.

Psilo-Balsam N Stada, Ger.†.
Diphenhydramine hydrochloride (p.416·1); cetylpyridinium chloride (p.1138·1).
Formerly contained diphenhydramine hydrochloride,
cetylpyridinium chloride, and butoxycaine hydrochloride.
*First-degree burns; insect stings; nettle rash; skin irri-
tation; sunburn; wind burns.*

Psilumax Columbia, Mex.
Psyllium seed (p.1229·1); wheat fibre (p.1214·2).
Constipation.

Psipax Merck, Port.
Fluoxetine hydrochloride (p.284·2).
Depression.

Psiu Teuto, Braz.
Cetylpyridinium chloride (p.1138·1); ammonium chloride (p.1085·2); sodium citrate (p.1186·2); sodium benzoate (p.1134·3).
Respiratory-tract congestion.

Psodermil Oftalder, Port.
Betamethasone dipropionate (p.1063·2); salicylic acid
(p.1122·3).
Skin disorders.

Pso-Rad Pentamedical, Ital.
Mallow oil; lappa; aloe; badderwrack; calendula; lav-
ender; tormentil.
Skin disorders.

Psoraderm 5 Sun Life, Fr.†; Democal, Switz.
5-Methoxypsoralen (p.1120·3).
Psoriasis.

Psoradexan Procter & Gamble, Aust.†; Hermal, Ger.; Procter & Gamble, Switz.†.
Dithranol (p.1113·3); urea (p.1127·3).
Psoriasis.

Psoradrate Procter & Gamble, Irl.
Dithranol (p.1113·3); urea (p.1127·3).
Psoriasis.

Psoralon MT Hermal, Ger.
Dithranol (p.1113·3); salicylic acid (p.1122·3).
Psoriasis.

Psorantral Isdin, Spain.
Dithranol (p.1113·3); salicylic acid (p.1122·3).
Psoriasis.

Psor-a-set Hogil, USA.
Salicylic acid (p.1122·3).

Psor-Asist Sunspot, Aust.
Cream: Sulfur (p.1123·3); salicylic acid (p.1122·3);
coal tar (p.1125·1).
Lotion: Sulfur (p.1123·3); salicylic acid (p.1122·3); al-
oes (p.1210·1); urea (p.1127·3).
Psoriasis.

Psorasolv Potter's, UK.
Starch (p.1379·3); sublimed sulfur (p.1123·3); zinc ox-
ide (p.1128·2); pokeroot (p.1653·1); clivers (p.1596·3).
Psoriasis.

Psorcon Dermik, USA.
Diflorasone diacetate (p.1069·2).
Skin disorders.

Psorcutan Schering, Aust.; Schering, Ger.; Asche, Ger.; Schering, Ital.
Calcipotriol (p.1112·1).
Psoriasis.

Psorex Glaxo Wellcome, Braz.
Clobetasol propionate (p.1065·2).
Skin disorders.

Psoriacen Sanitas, Port.†.
Calaguala.
Dermatitis; psoriasis.

Psoriacreme Bradleys, NZ.
Coal tar (p.1125·1).
Eczema; psoriasis.

Psoriasdin Isdin, Spain.
Coal tar (p.1125·1).
Skin disorders.

Psoriasis-Bad Balneopharm, Ger.†.
Fumaric acid (p.1114·3); disodium fumarate
(p.1114·3).
Bath additive; psoriasis.

Psoriasis-Salbe M Balneopharm, Ger.†.
Fumaric acid (p.1114·3); coal tar (p.1125·1); allantoin
(p.1110·1); methyl salicylate (p.55·1); salicylic acid
(p.1122·3).
Psoriasis.

Psoriasis-Solution Balneopharm, Ger.†.
Disodium fumarate (p.1114·3).
Psoriasis.

Psoriasis-Sulfur L12 Homeocan, Canad.
Homoeopathic preparation.

Psoriasis-Tabletten Balneopharm, Ger.†.
Sodium fumarate (p.1114·3).
Psoriasis.

Psoriasol Lalco, Canad.†.
Tar (p.1125·1).
Psoriasis.

Psoricreme Schering-Plough, Neth.
Dithranol (p.1113·3).
Psoriasis.

Psoriderm
Note.This name is used for preparations of different composition.
Dermal Laboratories, Irl.; Dermal Laboratories, UK.
Coal tar (p.1125·1).
Psoriasis.
Istoria, Ital.
Dithranol (p.1113·3).
Psoriasis.

Psorigel Galderma, Austral.; Galderma, Canad.†; Galderma, Hong Kong; Gal-
derma, Irl.; Galderma, NZ; Galderma, S.Afr.†; Galderma, UK†;
Healthpoint, USA.
Coal tar (p.1125·1).
Eczema; psoriasis.

Psorigerb N Cesra, Ger.
Salicylic acid (p.1122·3); coal tar (p.1125·1); urea
(p.1127·3).
Eczema; psoriasis.

Psorimed Wolff, Ger.; Leo, Ger.
Salicylic acid (p.1122·3).
Scalp disorders.

Psorin Ayrton, UK.
Ointment: Dithranol (p.1113·3); salicylic acid
(p.1122·3); coal tar (p.1125·1).
Scalp gel: Dithranol (p.1113·3); salicylic acid
(p.1122·3); methyl salicylate (p.55·1).
Psoriasis.

Psorinase IDI, Ital.
Salicylic acid (p.1122·3); tretinoin (p.1126·2); betame-
thasone valero-acetate (p.1063·3).
Psoriasis.

Psorion ICN, USA†.
Betamethasone dipropionate (p.1063·2).

PsoriNail Summers, USA†.
Coal tar (p.1125·1).
Psoriasis.

Psychobald Sigmapharm, Aust.
Valerian (p.1678·3); bitter orange.
Anxiety disorders; sleep disorders.

Psychoneuroticum (Rowo-578) Pharmakon, Ger.
Homoeopathic preparation.
Lignocaine [lidocaine] hydrochloride (p.1313·2) is included in this preparation to alleviate the pain of injection.

Psychopax Sigmapharm, Aust.; Sigmapharm, Switz.
Diazepam (p.674·3).
*Anxiety disorders; skeletal muscle spasm; sleep disor-
ders.*

Psychotonin Madaus, Aust.; Steigerwald, Ger.
Hypericum (p.290·2).
Anxiety; depression.

Psychotonin M Steigerwald, Ger.
Hypericum (p.290·2).
Anxiety; depression.

Psychotonin-sed Steigerwald, Ger.
Hypericum (p.290·2); valerian (p.1678·3).
Anxiety; depression; sleep disorders.

Psycoton Esseti, Ital.
Piracetam (p.1652·1).
Mental function impairment.

Psylia Techni-Pharma, Mon.
Ispaghula (p.1229·1).
Constipation.

Psymion Declimed, Ger.
Maprotiline hydrochloride (p.297·2).
Depression.

Psyquil Sanofi Winthrop, Aust.; Sanofi Synthelabo, Ger.
Triflupromazine (p.711·1) or triflupromazine hydrochloride (p.711·1).
*Agitation; nausea and vomiting; neuroleptanalgesia;
premedication; schizophrenia; sedative.*

Psyrazine Condrugs, Thai.
Trifluoperazine (p.710·3).
Anxiety; nausea and vomiting; psychoses.

PSY-stabil Pekana, Ger.
Homoeopathic preparation.

PTE American Pharmaceutical, USA.
A range of trace element preparations (p.1350·1).
Parenteral nutrition.

Puamin Schwarzhaupt, Ger.†.
Lign. muira puama; yohimbe; nicametate citrate mono-
hydrate; alpha tocoferil acetate.
Erectile dysfunction; tonic.

Pudan-Lebertran-Zinksalbe Bano, Aust.
Zinc oxide (p.1128·2); peru balsam (p.1650·2); cod-
liver oil (p.1357·2).
Burns; decubitus ulcer; nappy rash; wounds.

Puernol Formenti, Ital.
Paracetamol (p.71·2).
Fever; pain.

Puersan Heralds, Braz.
Cichorium intybus; rhubarb (p.1248·1); fennel
(p.1610·1).
Gastrointestinal spasm.

Puerzym FIRMA, Ital.
Pepsinogen.
Digestive system disorders.

Pufolic Mavi, Ital.
Folic acid; magnesium; omega 6 and omega 3 triglyc-
erides (p.1350·1).
Nutritional supplement.

Pulbil Klinge, Ger.
Sodium cromoglicate (p.774·3).
Asthma.

Pulmadil 3M, Belg.†; 3M, Denm.†; 3M, Neth.†; 3M, S.Afr.†; 3M, UK†.
Rimiterol hydrobromide (p.770·2).
Bronchospasm.

Pulmarin NCSN, Ital.
Sulfogaiacol (p.1101·1); eucalyptol (p.1609·2); pine
oil; menthol (p.1632·3).
Catarrh.

Pulmax Zyma, Fr.†.
Peru balsam (p.1650·2); camphor (p.1589·3); eucalyp-
tus oil (p.1609·2); rosemary oil (p.1659·3).
Respiratory-tract congestion.

Pulmaxan Astra, Ital.
Budesonide (p.1064·2).
Asthma.

Pulmeno Novartis, Spain.
Theophylline (p.777·2).
*Heart failure; obstructive airways disease; paroxysmal
dyspnoea.*

Pulmex
Note.This name is used for preparations of different composition.
Novartis Consumer, Aust.; Novartis Consumer, Switz.
Peru balsam (p.1650·2); camphor (p.1589·3); eucalyp-
tus oil (p.1609·2); rosemary oil (p.1659·3).
Cold symptoms; coughs.
Novartis Consumer, Belg.
Benzyl benzoate (p.1428·2); benzyl cinnamate; peru
balsam (p.1650·2); camphor (p.1589·3); rosemary oil
(p.1659·3); eucalyptus oil (p.1609·2).
Cold symptoms.
Novartis, Israel.
Peru balsam (p.1650·2); camphor (p.1589·3).
Bronchitis; catarrh; cold symptoms; coughs.

Pulmex Baby
Note.This name is used for preparations of different composition.
Novartis Consumer, Belg.
Benzyl benzoate (p.1428·2); benzyl cinnamate; peru
balsam (p.1650·2); rosemary oil (p.1659·3); eucalyptus
oil (p.1609·2).
Cold symptoms.
Novartis Consumer, Switz.
Peru balsam (p.1650·2); eucalyptus oil (p.1609·2);
rosemary oil (p.1659·3).
Cold symptoms; coughs.

Pulmicort Astra, Aust.; Astra, Austral.; Astra, Belg.; AstraZeneca, Canad.; Astra-
Zeneca, Fin.; AstraZeneca, Fr.; Astra, Ger.; Stern, Ger.; Astra, Hong
Kong; Astra, Irl.; Astra, Mex.; Astra, Neth.; AstraZeneca, Norw.; As-
traZeneca, NZ; Astra, Port.; Astra, S.Afr.; AstraZeneca, Singapore;
Astra, Spain; Draco, Swed.; Astra, Switz.; AstraZeneca, Thai.; Astra-
Zeneca, UK; Astra, USA.
Budesonide (p.1064·2).
*Allergic rhinitis; asthma; croup; nasal polyps; ob-
structive airways disease.*

Pulmicret Stern, Ger.
Acetylcysteine (p.1082·3).
*Respiratory-tract disorders associated with increased
or viscous mucus.*

Pulmictan Faes, Spain.
Budesonide (p.1064·2).
Asthma.

Pulmidur Astra, Aust.; Stern, Ger.
Theophylline (p.777·2).
Obstructive airways disease.

Pulmilide Boehringer Ingelheim, Aust.
Flunisolide hemihydrate (p.1070·3).
Asthma.

Pulminflamatoria Faes, Spain.
Ampicillin sodium (p.150·3); ampicillin benzathine
(p.151·3); bromhexine hydrochloride (p.1085·3).
Respiratory-tract infections.

Pulmison Boehringer Ingelheim, S.Afr.
Prednisone (p.1079·2).
Obstructive airways disease.

Pulmo Bailly Bailly, Fr.; Bengue, Irl.†; Roche Consumer, UK.
Codeine (p.25·2) or codeine phosphate (p.25·2); guai-
acol (p.1092·1).
Coughs.

Pulmo Borbalan Spyfarma, Spain.
Amoxicillin trihydrate (p.149·2); bromhexine hydro-
chloride (p.1085·3).
Respiratory infections.

Pulmo Grey Balsam Orravan, Spain†.
Camphor (p.1589·3); allyl sulfide; eucalyptol
(p.1609·2); niaouli oil (p.1640·2); guaiacol (p.1092·1).
Respiratory disorders.

Pulmo Menal Alacan, Spain.
Bromhexine hydrochloride (p.1085·3); guaifenesin
(p.1092·2); sodium benzoate (p.1134·3); co-trimoxazole (p.193·3).
Respiratory-tract infections.

Pulmocare Abbott, Austral.; Abbott, Canad.; Ross, Hong Kong; Abbott, Irl.; Ross,
Israel; Abbott, Ital.; Abbott, NZ; Abbott, Singapore; Abbott, Thai.; Ab-
bott Nutrition, UK; Ross, USA.
Preparation for enteral nutrition (p.1350·1).
Respiratory system disorders.

Pulmocilin Eurofarma, Braz.
Benzylpenicillin potassium (p.157·1); procaine peni-
cillin [procaine benzylpenicillin] (p.239·2).
Bacterial infections.

Pulmoclase Bios, Belg.†; UCB, Fin.; UCB, Irl.; UCB, Neth.; UCB, Port.
Carbocisteine (p.1086·3).
*Respiratory-tract disorders associated with viscous
mucus.*

Pulmocod Warner-Lambert, Fr.
Codeine (p.25·2); sodium benzoate (p.1134·3); euca-
lyptol (p.1609·2).
Coughs.

Pulmocordio forte Hevert, Ger.
Ammi visnaga; belladonna; ipecacuanha; kalium jo-
dat.; thyme (p.1672·2); castanae; ephedrine hydrochloride (p.1090·1); sulfogaiacol (p.1101·1).
Coughs and associated respiratory-tract disorders.

Pulmocordio mite SL Hevert, Ger.
Anise oil (p.1580·3); fennel oil (p.1610·2); liquorice
(p.1231·2); thyme (p.1672·2).
Respiratory-tract disorders.

Pulmo-cyl Ho-Len-Complex Liebermann, Ger.
Homoeopathic preparation.

Pulmodex-C Baldassari, Braz.
Dipyrone (p.34·1); vitamin C (p.1389·3); eucalyptol
(p.1609·2); guaifenesin (p.1092·2).
Cold and influenza symptoms.

Pulmofasa Sabater, Spain.
Ammonium camphocarbonate diaminopyridine carboxylate (p.1507·1); calcium pantothenate (p.1374·1);
eucalyptol (p.1609·2); senega (p.1100·2); sodium benzoate (p.1134·3); sulfogaiacol (p.1101·1); tolu balsam
(p.1101·3); pinus sylvestris; anethole (p.1580·1).
Respiratory-tract disorders.

Pulmofasa Antihist Sabater, Spain.
Ammonium camphocarbonate (p.1507·1); calcium
pantothenate (p.1374·1); eucalyptol (p.1609·2);
diphenhydramine hydrochloride (p.416·1); sodium
benzoate (p.1134·3); sulfogaiacol (p.1101·1); senega
(p.1100·2); tolu balsam (p.1101·3); pinus sylvestris;
anethole (p.1580·1).
Upper respiratory-tract disorders.

Pulmofluide Simple Warner-Lambert, Fr.
Terpin (p.1101·2); eucalyptol (p.1609·2); sodium ben-
zoate (p.1134·3); guaifenesin (p.1092·2).
Formerly contained terpin, eucalyptol, sodium ben-
zoate, guaifenesin, codeine, and ipecacuanha.
Respiratory-tract congestion.

Pulmofor Vifor, Switz.
Dextromethorphan hydrobromide (p.1087·3).
Coughs.

Pulmoformil Uniao Quimica, Braz.
Guaifenesin (p.1092·2); ephedrine hydrochloride
(p.1090·1); homatropine methylbromide (p.468·1); lobelia (p.1510·2); grindelia (p.1618·2); tolu balsam
(p.1101·3).
Respiratory-tract congestion.

Pulmogripe Breves, Braz.
Sulfureto de alila; niaouli oil (p.1640·2); eucalyptol
(p.1609·2); benzyl cinnamate; camphor (p.1589·3).
Cold and influenza symptoms.

Pulmoiodo Bunker, Braz.
Belladonna (p.463·1); jaborandi; eucalyptus
(p.1609·2); ginger (p.1227·2); siparuna guyanensis;
lantana camara; mikania.
Respiratory-tract disorders.

Pulmoll SmithKline Beecham Sante, Fr.
Terpin (p.1101·2); menthol (p.1632·3); amylocaine hy-
drochloride (p.1306·1).
Throat disorders.

Pulmoll au menthol et a l'eucalyptus SmithKline
Beecham Sante, Fr.
Menthol (p.1632·3); peppermint oil (p.1243·3); euca-
lyptus oil (p.1609·2).
Throat disorders.

Pulmonal S Schaper & Brummer, Ger.†.
Ambroxol hydrochloride (p.1084·3).
*Respiratory-tract disorders associated with increased
or viscous mucus.*

Pulmonar
Rudefsa, Mex.
Lysate of *Streptococcus pneumoniae; Klebsiella pneu-
moniae; Streptococcus haemolyticus; Staphylococcus
aureus; Moraxella catarrhalis; Haemophilus influen-
zae.*
Respiratory-tract infections.
OM, Port.
Lysates of *Haemophilus influenzae; Streptococcus
pneumoniae; Klebsiella pneumoniae; Staphylococcus*

aureus; *Streptococcus pyogenes; Moraxella catarrhalis.*
Respiratory-tract infections.

Pulmonase *Monin, Fr.†.*
Codeine (p.25·2); sodium benzoate (p.1134·3); cherry-laurel; aconite root (p.1572·3); drosera (p.1606·1); tolu balsam (p.1101·3).
Coughs.

Pulmonilo Synergium *Aristegui, Spain†.*
Oxytetracycline (p.234·1); calcium guaiacolate; niaouli oil (p.1640·2); eucalyptol (p.1609·2).
Respiratory-tract infections.

Pulmonium N *Wala, Ger.†.*
Plantago lanceolata; Norway spruce; petasites officinalis.
Respiratory-tract disorders.

Pulmonix *Luper, Braz.*
Potassium iodide (p.1522·3); sulfogaiacol (p.1101·1); tolu balsam (p.1101·3).
Respiratory-tract congestion.

Pulmophyllin *Propan, S.Afr.*
Theophylline (p.777·2).
Obstructive airways disease.

Pulmophylline *Riva, Canad.†.*
Theophylline (p.777·2).
Bronchoconstriction.

Pulmorell *Sanorell, Ger.*
Homoeopathic preparation.

Pulmorex DM *Prodemdis, Canad.*
Diphenhydramine hydrochloride (p.416·1); dextromethorphan hydrobromide (p.1087·3); ammonium chloride (p.1085·2).

Pulmorphan *Riva, Canad.*
Dextromethorphan hydrobromide (p.1087·3); guaifenesin (p.1092·2); pheniramine maleate (p.422·3); phenylephrine hydrochloride (p.1097·1).
Coughs.

Pulmorphan Pediatrique *Riva, Canad.*
Dextromethorphan hydrobromide (p.1087·3); pheniramine maleate (p.422·3); phenylephrine hydrochloride (p.1097·1).
Coughs.

Pulmo-San *Zimaia, Port.*
Brovanexine hydrochloride (p.1086·1).
Coughs.

Pulmoserum *Bailly, Fr.*
Codeine (p.25·2); guaiacol (p.1092·1).
Formerly contained codeine, guaiacol, and phosphoric acid.
Coughs.

Pulmosin *Fresenius Kabi, Aust.*
Sodium cromoglicate (p.774·3).
Asthma.

Pulmosodyl *Bridoux, Fr.*
Pholcodine (p.1099·1); sodium benzoate (p.1134·3); tolu balsam (p.1101·3).
Formerly contained ethylmorphine hydrochloride, bromoform, sulfogaiacol, sodium benzoate, cherry-laurel, and tolu balsam.
Coughs.

Pulmospin *Spyfarma, Spain.*
Guaifenesin (p.1092·2); ampicillin trihydrate (p.151·1).
Respiratory-tract infections.

Pulmosterin Duo *Normon, Spain.*
Bromhexine (p.1085·3); guaifenesin (p.1092·2); co-trimoxazole (p.193·3).
Respiratory-tract infections.

Pulmosterin Meta *Normon, Spain†.*
Bromhexine (p.1085·3); guaifenesin (p.1092·2); metampicillin sodium (p.222·3).
Lignocaine [lidocaine] hydrochloride (p.1313·2) is included in this preparation to alleviate the pain of injection.
Respiratory-tract infections.

Pulmosterin Retard *Normon, Spain.*
Ampicillin sodium (p.150·3); ampicillin benzathine (p.151·3); guaifenesin (p.1092·2).
Respiratory-tract infections.

Pulmotide *Taro, Israel.*
Budesonide (p.1064·2).
Asthma.

Pulmo-Timelets
Temmler, Denm.; Temmler, Ger.
Theophylline (p.777·2).
Obstructive airways disease.

Pulmotin *Serum-Werk Bernburg, Ger.*
Thyme (p.1672·2); guaifenesin (p.1092·2).
Bronchitis; catarrh; coughs.

Pulmotin-N *Serum-Werk Bernburg, Ger.*
Anise oil (p.1580·3); camphor (p.1589·3); eucalyptus oil (p.1609·2); thyme oil (p.1672·3); conifer oil; thymol (p.1158·3).
Respiratory-tract disorders.

Pulmotosse *Delta, Braz.*
Diphenhydramine hydrochloride (p.416·1); ammonium chloride (p.1085·2).
Coughs.

Pulmotropic *Robert, Spain.*
Doxycycline guaiacolsulfonate (p.200·3); muramidase hydrochloride (p.1638·1).
Respiratory-tract infections.

Pulmovax *Merck Sharp & Dohme, Mex.*
A pneumococcal vaccine (23-valent) (p.1557·2).
Active immunisation.

Pulmovent *Boehringer Ingelheim, Aust.*
Acetylcysteine (p.1082·3).
Respiratory-tract disorders.

Pulmoverina *Prima, Braz.*
Sodium dibunate (p.1100·3); sulfogaiacol (p.1101·1); sodium benzoate (p.1134·3).
Coughs.

Pulmovirolo *Restiva, Ital.†.*
Sulfogaiacol (p.1101·1).
Respiratory-tract disorders.

Pulmozyme
Roche, Aust.; Roche, Austral.; Roche, Belg.; Roche, Braz.; Roche, Canad.; Roche, Denm.; Roche, Fin.; Roche, Fr.; Roche, Ger.; Roche, Irl.; Roche, Israel; Roche, Ital.; Roche, Mex.; Roche, Neth.; Roche, Norw.; Roche, NZ; Roche, Port.; Roche, S.Afr.; Roche, Spain; Roche, Swed.; Roche, Switz.; Roche, UK; Genentech, USA.
Dornase alfa (p.1089·1).
Cystic fibrosis; respiratory-tract disorders associated with increased or viscous mucus.

Pulpomixine *Septodont, Switz.*
Dexamethasone acetate (p.1067·1); framycetin sulfate (p.208·2); polymyxin B sulfate (p.238·1).
Dental disorders.

Pulsan *Yamanouchi, Jpn†.*
Indenolol hydrochloride (p.913·2).
Angina pectoris; arrhythmias; hypertension.

Pulsar *Medosan, Ital.*
Colextran hydrochloride (p.865·1).
Glucose metabolic disorders; hyperlipidaemia; obesity.

Pulsatilla Med Complex *Dynamit, Aust.*
Homoeopathic preparation.

Pulsit *Precimex, Mex.*
Haloperidol (p.686·3).

Pulsitil *Janssen-Cilag, Aust.*
Cisapride (p.1220·1).
Constipation; dyspepsia; gastro-oesophageal reflux; intestinal pseudo-obstruction.

Pulsol *Galen, Mex.*
Enalapril maleate (p.883·3).
Heart failure; hypertension.

Pulsor *Tecnimede, Port.*
Calcium pangamate (p.1647·3).

Pulsoton *Chinoin, Mex.*
Methyldopa (p.927·3).

Pulverizador Nasal *Collado, Spain†.*
Phenylephrine hydrochloride (p.1097·1).
Nasal congestion.

Pulvhydrops Mono *Lomapharm, Ger.*
Equisetum (p.1606·3).
Oedema; urinary-tract disorders.

Pulvicin *Biolab, Thai.*
Co-trimoxazole (p.193·3).
Bacterial infections.

Pulvis-3 *Bayer, Ital.†.*
Propoxur (p.1436·3).
Pediculosis.

Pulvispray *Peters, Fr.*
Mixed aldehydes; alcohol (p.1130·3); isopropyl alcohol (p.1149·2).
Disinfection.

Pulvo *Fournier, Ger.*
Catalase (p.1592·2); hexamidine isetionate (p.1146·2).
Ulcers; wounds.

Pulvo 47
Fournier, Belg.; Fournier, Fr.; Fournier, Thai.
Catalase (p.1592·2); hexamidine isetionate (p.1146·2).
Formerly contained catalase and hexachlorophene in Belg.
Burns; skin irritation; ulcers; wounds.

Pulvo Neomycin *Fournier, Ger.*
Catalase (p.1592·2); neomycin sulfate (p.228·1).
Burns; infected skin disorders; ulcers; wounds.

Pulvo Neomycine *Fournier, Belg.†.*
Catalase (p.1592·2); neomycin sulfate (p.228·1).
Burns; skin irritation; wounds.

Pulvo 47 Neomycine *Fournier, Fr.*
Catalase (p.1592·2); neomycin sulfate (p.228·1).
Infected wounds and burns.

Pumilen-N *Tosse, Ger.†.*
Eucalyptus oil (p.1609·2); pumilio pine oil (p.1656·3); oleum pini sylvestris; peppermint oil (p.1243·3); thymol (p.1158·3).
Colds; nasal congestion.

Pumilsan *Montefarmaco, Ital.*
Dequalinium chloride (p.1143·1).
Mouth and throat disinfection.

Pump-Hep *Leo, UK.*
Heparin sodium (p.902·1).
Now known as Heparin Sodium ampoules.
Thromboembolic disorders.

Puncto E *Asta Medica, Ger.*
d-Alpha tocopherol (p.1393·3).
Vitamin E deficiency.

Pungino *Whitehall, Ital.†.*
Vitamin B_1 (p.1385·2); citronella oil (p.1596·3).
Insect repellent.

Punktyl *Krewel, Ger.*
Lorazepam (p.688·3).
Anxiety; sleep disorders.

Puntual *Lainco, Spain.*
Calcium sennoside A (p.1248·3); calcium sennoside B (p.1248·3).
Constipation.

Puntualex *Lainco, Spain.*
Calcium sennoside A (p.1248·3); calcium sennoside B (p.1248·3).
Bowel evacuation.

Pupilla *Wassermann, Ital.*
Naphazoline nitrate (p.1095·1).
Inflammatory and allergic eye disorders.

Pupilla Antistaminico *Wassermann, Ital.*
Naphazoline nitrate (p.1095·1); thonzylamine hydrochloride (p.426·2).
Inflammatory and allergic eye disorders.

Pupilla Light *Wassermann, Ital.*
Benzalkonium chloride (p.1133·2); hypromellose; chamomile water; hyssop water; rose water; plantaginis water; mallow water; myrtillus water.
Eye disinfection; eye irritation.

Puralube
Note.This name is used for preparations of different composition.
Metapharma, Canad.
Liquid paraffin (p.1407·1); soft paraffin (p.1407·3).

Fougera, USA.
Eye drops: Polyvinyl alcohol (p.1503·1).
Eye ointment: White soft paraffin (p.1407·3); light liquid paraffin (p.1407·2).
Dry eyes.

Puran T4 *Sanofi Winthrop, Braz.*
Thyroxine [levothyroxine] sodium (p.1526·2).
Hypothyroidism.

Purata *Aspen, S.Afr.*
Oxazepam (p.697·1).
Alcohol withdrawal syndrome; anxiety.

Purazine *SA Druggists Self Med, S.Afr.†.*
Cinnarizine (p.413·1).
Nausea; vertigo; vomiting.

Purbac *Aspen, S.Afr.*
Co-trimoxazole (p.193·3).
Bacterial infections.

Pur-Bloka *Aspen, S.Afr.*
Propranolol hydrochloride (p.962·3).
Angina pectoris; arrhythmias; hypertension; hyperthyroidism; migraine; phaeochromocytoma.

Pure Omega *BritHealth, UK.*
Fish oil concentrate (p.949·2).

Pureduct *Rosen, Ger.*
Allopurinol (p.397·2).
Hyperuricaemia.

Puregon
Organon, Aust.; Organon, Austral.; Organon, Belg.; Organon, Canad.; Organon, Denm.; Organon, Fin.; Organon, Fr.; Organon, Ger.; Organon, Hong Kong; Organon, Irl.; Organon, Israel; Organon, Ital.; Organon, Mex.; Organon, Neth.; Organon, Norw.; Pharmaco, NZ; Organon, Port.; Organon, Singapore; Organon, Spain; Organon, Swed.; Organon, Switz.; Organon, Thai.; Organon, UK.
Follitropin beta (p.1283·1).
Female infertility.

Pureness Blemish Control *Shiseido, Canad.*
Sulfur (p.1123·3).
Acne.

Puresis *Aspen, S.Afr.*
Frusemide [furosemide] (p.893·1).
Hypertension; oedema.

Purethal
Hal, Ger.; Hal, Neth.
Modified allergen extracts of grass, tree and weed pollen(p.1575·3).
Hyposensitisation.

Purganol *Saunier-Daguin, Fr.†.*
Phenolphthalein (p.1244·1).
Constipation.

Purgante *Orravan, Spain†.*
Phenolphthalein (p.1244·1).
Constipation.

Purgazen *Agepha, Aust.*
Bisacodyl (p.1212·2); dimethicone (p.1249·2).
Bowel evacuation; constipation.

Purge *Fleming, USA.*
Castor oil (p.1592·1).
Constipation.

Purgestol *Blue Cross, Ital.†.*
Phenolphthalein (p.1244·1).
Constipation.

Purgoleite *Virtus, Braz.*
Phenolphthalein (p.1244·1); cascara (p.1216·1); calcium phosphate (p.1188·3).
Constipation.

Purgo-Pil *Qualiphar, Belg.*
Bisacodyl (p.1212·2).
Bowel evacuation; constipation.

Purgoxin *Aspen, S.Afr.*
Digoxin (p.870·1).
Cardiac disorders.

Purianta *Apomedica, Aust.†.*
Thyme (p.1672·2); guaifenesin (p.1092·2).
Coughs and cold symptoms.

Puricin *Shiwa, Thai.*
Allopurinol (p.397·2).
Gout; hyperuricaemia.

Puri-Clens *Sween, USA†.*
Methylbenzethonium chloride (p.1150·3).
Wound cleanser.

Puricos *Aspen, S.Afr.*
Allopurinol (p.397·2).
Gout; hyperuricaemia.

Puride *Polipharm, Thai.*
Allopurinol (p.397·2).
Gout; hyperuricaemia.

Purigoa *Wyeth Lederle, Aust.*
Bisacodyl (p.1212·2); docusate sodium (p.1223·1).
Constipation.

Puri-Nethol
Glaxo Wellcome, Aust.; Glaxo Wellcome, Austral.; Glaxo Wellcome, Belg.; Glaxo Wellcome, Braz.; Glaxo Wellcome, Canad.; Glaxo Wellcome, Fr.; Glaxo Wellcome, Ger.; Glaxo Wellcome, Hong Kong; Wellcome, Irl.; Glaxo Wellcome, Israel; Glaxo Wellcome, Ital.; Glaxo Wellcome, Mex.; Glaxo Wellcome, Neth.; Glaxo Wellcome, Norw.; Glaxo Wellcome, NZ; Glaxo Wellcome, S.Afr.; Glaxo Wellcome, Singapore; Glaxo Wellcome, Swed.; Wellcome, Switz.; Glaxo Wellcome, Thai.; Glaxo Wellcome, UK; Glaxo Wellcome, USA.
Mercaptopurine (p.552·2).
Leukaemias.

Purinol *Ratiopharm, Aust.; Pinewood, Irl.*
Allopurinol (p.397·2).
Gout; hyperuricaemia; prophylaxis of uric acid and calcium oxalate stones.

Puriphyl *Adam, Mon.*
Caprylylcollagenic acid.
Acne.

Purisole *Fresenius Kabi, Port.; Fresenius Kabi, Switz.†.*
Sorbitol (p.1377·3); mannitol (p.924·3).
Bladder irrigation.

Puritabs *Dermatech, Austral.*
Sodium dichloroisocyanurate (p.1156·1).
Water disinfection.

Purmolax *Hua, Thai.*
Phenolphthalein (p.1244·1).
Constipation.

Purmycin *Aspen, S.Afr.*
Erythromycin estolate (p.201·2).
Bacterial infections.

Purochin *Sclavo, Ital.*
Urokinase (p.988·1).
Thromboembolic disorders.

Purofilina *Rhein, Mex.*
Proxyphylline (p.770·1).

Purol *Bravir, Braz.*
Liquid paraffin (p.1407·1).
Constipation.

Puromylon *Aspen, S.Afr.*
Nalidixic acid (p.227·1).
Urinary-tract infections.

Puroptal *Metochem, Aust.†.*
Hypromellose (p.1501·3).
Eye irritation.

Purpose *Johnson & Johnson, USA; Merck, USA.*
A range of emollient, cleansing, and moisturising preparations.

Purpose Alpha Hydroxy *Johnson & Johnson, Canad.*
SPF 15: Octinoxate (p.1517·3); octisalate (p.1518·1); oxybenzone (p.1518·1).
Sunscreen.

Purpose Dual *Johnson & Johnson, Canad.*
SPF 15: Meradimate (p.1517·3); octinoxate (p.1517·3); titanium dioxide (p.1126·1).
Sunscreen.

Purpuralin *Alcon, Braz.; Alcon, Hong Kong.*
Anthocyanosides; betacarotene (p.1355·1).
Eye disorders.

Pur-Rutin *Andreabal, Switz.*
Troxerutin (p.1611·2).
Peripheral vascular disorders.

Pursana *Zeller, Switz.*
Sorbitol (p.1377·3); fig (p.1227·1).
Constipation.

Pursenid *Novartis Consumer, Spain†.*
Calcium sennoside A (p.1248·3); calcium sennoside B (p.1248·3).
Constipation.

Pursennid
Note.This name is used for preparations of different composition.
Novartis Consumer, Aust.; Novartis, Denm.; Novartis, Israel; Novartis Consumer, Ital.; Novartis, Norw.
Calcium sennoside A (p.1248·3); calcium sennoside B (p.1248·3).
Bowel evacuation; constipation.

Novartis, Fin.; Novartis, Swed.
Senna (p.1248·2).
Constipation.

Pursennid Complex *Novartis, Ital.†.*
Senna (p.1248·2); polycarbophil calcium (p.1244·2).
Constipation.

Pursennid Fibra *Novartis, Ital.†.*
Polycarbophil calcium (p.1244·2).
Constipation; diarrhoea.

Pursennide
Novartis Sante, Fr.; Novartis Consumer, Port.; Novartis Consumer, Switz.
Calcium sennosides (p.1248·3) (p.1248·3).
Constipation.

Pursept A *Merz, Ger.†.*
Alcohol (p.1130·3); glyoxal (p.1145·3); quaternary ammonium compounds.
Surface and instrument disinfection.

Puru-C *Vitabalans, Fin.*
Ascorbic acid (p.1389·3); sodium ascorbate (p.1390·1).
Vitamin C deficiency.

Pusiran *Atlantic, Hong Kong; Atlantic, Singapore; Vana, Thai.*
Dextromethorphan hydrobromide (p.1087·3).
Coughs.

Putaren *PD, Thai.*
Diclofenac sodium (p.30·3).
Musculoskeletal and joint disorders.

Putatone *Silom, Thai.*
Indometacin (p.44·3).
Gout; musculoskeletal and joint disorders.

Puvadin *Medochemie, Hong Kong.*
Trioxysalen (p.1127·2).
Vitiligo.

Puvasoralen *Crawford, UK.*
Methoxsalen (p.1118·3).
Available on a named-patient basis only.
Mycosis fungoides; psoriasis; vitiligo.

PV Carpine *Allergan, Austral.; Allergan, NZ; Allergan, S.Afr.†.*
Pilocarpine hydrochloride (p.1422·3) or pilocarpine nitrate (p.1422·3).
Glaucoma; reversal of mydriasis.

PVF *Frosst, Canad.†.*
Benzathine phenoxymethylpenicillin (p.157·1).
Bacterial infections.

PVFK *Lioh, Canad.*
Phenoxymethylpenicillin potassium (p.235·1).
Bacterial infections.

P-Vidine *PP Lab, Thai.*
Povidone-iodine (p.1155·1).
Skin, mucous membrane, and wound disinfection.

PVK *Lilly, Austral.*
Phenoxymethylpenicillin potassium (p.235·1).
Bacterial infections.

P-V-Tussin *Numark, USA.*
Syrup: Hydrocodone tartrate (p.42·2); pseudoephedrine hydrochloride (p.1099·2); chlorpheniramine [chlorphenamine] maleate (p.412·1).
Coughs and cold symptoms.
Tablets: Hydrocodone tartrate (p.42·2); phenindamine tartrate (p.422·2); guaifenesin (p.1092·2).
Coughs.

Pyal *Sanico, Belg.†.*
Sulfanilamide (p.256·2); sulfathiazole (p.257·1); cod-liver oil (p.1357·2); colecalciferol (p.1391·1).
Burns; wounds.

Pycnogenol Plus *Reese, USA.*
Bioflavonoids (p.1611·1); grape seed; pycnogenol (p.1611·2).

Pyelodion *Neo Quimica, Braz.*
Sulfacetamide (p.250·3); methenamine (p.223·1); belladonna (p.463·1).
Urinary-tract infections.

Pygmal *URPAC, Fr.*
2,4,5-Trichlorophenol complex with tri-isobutyl phosphate; zinc oxide (p.1128·2); zinc carbonate (p.1128·2).
Acne.

Pygosal *Salus, Mex.*
Ispaghula (p.1229·1).

Pykaryl T *Rodleben, Ger.*
Benzyl nicotinate (p.20·2).
Peripheral vascular disorders; rheumatic disorders; soft-tissue injuries.

Pykno *Procare, Austral.*
Vitis vinifera; myrtillus (p.1639·2).
Peripheral vascular disorders; tonic.

Pyknolepsinum *Desitin, Ger.†.*
Ethosuximide (p.348·1).
Absence seizures.

Pylobactell *Italchimici, Ital.; BSIA, UK.*
Carbon-13 (p.1591·3) labelled urea.
Diagnosis of Helicobacter pylori infection.

Pylorid *Glaxo Wellcome, Belg.; Glaxo Wellcome, Canad.; Glaxo Wellcome, Denm.; Glaxo Wellcome, Fin.; Glaxo Wellcome, Hong Kong; Glaxo Wellcome, Irl.; Glaxo Wellcome, Ital.; Glaxo Wellcome, Neth.; Glaxo Wellcome, Norw.; Glaxo Wellcome, Port.; Glaxo Wellcome, Singapore; Glaxo Wellcome, Spain; Glaxo Wellcome, Switz.; Glaxo Wellcome, Thai.; Glaxo Wellcome, UK.*
Ranitidine bismuth citrate (p.1247·2).
Peptic ulcer.

Pylorid-KA *Glaxo Wellcome, Austral.*
Combination pack: Tablets, ranitidine bismuth citrate (Pylorid) (p.1247·2); tablets, clarithromycin (Klacid) (p.186·2); capsules, amoxicillin trihydrate (Alphamox) (p.149·2).
Helicobacter pylori-associated peptic ulcer.

Pyloriset *Orion, USA.*
Test for gastrointestinal disorders.

Pylorisin *Glaxo Wellcome, Aust.*
Ranitidine bismuth citrate (p.1247·2).
Peptic ulcer.

Pynamic *Condrugs, Thai.*
Mefenamic acid (p.51·2).
Pain.

Pynmed *Medpro, S.Afr.*
Syrup: Paracetamol (p.71·2); codeine phosphate (p.25·2); promethazine hydrochloride (p.423·2).
Tablets: Paracetamol (p.71·2); codeine phosphate (p.25·2); caffeine (p.761·3); meprobamate (p.691·1).
Pain and associated tension.

Pynstop *Covan, S.Afr.*
Paracetamol (p.71·2); codeine phosphate (p.25·2); caffeine (p.761·3); doxylamine succinate (p.417·1).
Fever; pain and associated tension.

Pyocefal *Takeda, Fr.*
Cefsulodin sodium (p.174·2).
Lignocaine [lidocaine] (p.1313·2) is included in the intramuscular injection to alleviate the pain of injection.
Bacterial infections.

Pyocoline *Millet Roux, Braz.*
Ammonium chloride (p.1085·2); hydroxyquinoline hydrochloride; terpin hydrate (p.1101·2).
Urinary-tract infections.

Pyolysin *Serum-Werk Bernburg, Ger.*
Extract of staphylococci, streptococci, escherichia coli, pseudomonas aeruginosa, micrococcus-ovis-Buillon; zinc oxide (p.1128·2); salicylic acid (p.1122·3).
Burns; infected skin disorders; skin ulcers; wounds.

Pyoralene *Expanpharm, Fr.*
Maize (p.1379·3).
Mouth disorders.

Pyoredol *Roussel, Fr.†.*
Phenytoin sodium (p.357·2).
Gum disorders.

Pyorex *Bailly, Fr.*
Ethacridine lactate (p.1130·3); sodium ricinoleate.
Formerly contained ethacridine lactate, acetarsol lithium, and sodium ricinoleate.
Oral hygiene.

Pyostacine *Aventis, Belg.; Rhone-Poulenc Rorer, Fr.; Rhone-Poulenc Rorer, Israel.*
Pristinamycin (p.239·1).
Bacterial infections.

Pyracod *Propan, S.Afr.†.*
Sulfogaiacol (p.1101·1); mepyramine maleate (p.421·1); codeine phosphate (p.25·2); sodium citrate (p.1186·2).
Coughs.

Pyracon *Hua, Thai.*
Paracetamol (p.71·2).
Fever; pain.

Pyradol *Xixia, S.Afr.*
Paracetamol (p.71·2).
Fever; pain.

Pyrafat *Kolassa, Aust.; Fatol, Ger.; Fatol, Hong Kong.*
Pyrazinamide (p.240·1).
Tuberculosis.

Pyragesic *Noristan, S.Afr.†.*
Paracetamol (p.71·2).
Fever; pain.

Pyralin *Kenral, Austral.*
Sulfasalazine (p.1251·1).
Crohn's disease; rheumatoid arthritis; ulcerative colitis.

Pyralvex *Norgine, Aust.; Norgine, Austral.; Norgine, Belg.; Norgine, Fr.; Norgine, Ger.; Norgine, Irl.; Norgine, Ital.; Norgine, Neth.; Helsinn, Port.; Norgine, S.Afr.; Norgine, Singapore; Stafford-Miller, Spain; Norgine, Switz.; Norgine, UK.*
Rhubarb (p.1248·1); salicylic acid (p.1122·3).
Formerly known as Peralvex in the UK.
Mouth and throat disorders.

Norgine, Hong Kong, Thai.
Anthraquinone glycosides; salicylic acid (p.1122·3).
Mouth disorders.

Pyramine *Propan, S.Afr.†.*
Mepyramine maleate (p.421·1).
Hypersensitivity reactions.

Pyranol *Solfran, Mex.*
Dipyrone (p.34·1).
Pain.

Pyrantrin *Biolab, Hong Kong.*
Pyrantel embonate (p.108·1).
Worm infections.

Pyrapam *General Drugs, Thai.*
Pyrantel embonate (p.108·1).
Worm infections.

Pyratab *Shiwa, Thai.*
Pyrazinamide (p.240·1).
Tuberculosis.

Pyrazide *Aventis, S.Afr.*
Pyrazinamide (p.240·1).
Tuberculosis.

Pyrazol *Compu, S.Afr.†.*
Allopurinol (p.397·2).
Gout; hyperuricaemia.

Pyrcon *Krewel, Ger.*
Pyrvinium embonate (p.108·2).
Enterobiasis.

Pyreazid *Salvat, Spain†.*
Isoniazid (p.215·3).
Tuberculosis.

Pyrecol *Polipharm, Thai.*
Paracetamol (p.71·2); chlorpheniramine [chlorphenamine] maleate (p.412·1); phenylephrine hydrochloride (p.1097·1).
Cold symptoms; hay fever.

Pyreflor *Clement, Fr.*
Lotion: Permethrin (p.1436·1); piperonyl butoxide (p.1436·2); enoxolone (p.34·3).
Shampoo: Permethrin (p.1436·1); piperonyl butoxide (p.1436·2).
Pediculosis.

Pyreses *Berenguer Infale, Spain†.*
Aloglutamol (p.1210·2).
Gastrointestinal hyperacidity; peptic ulcer.

Pyretal *Shiwa, Thai.*
Paracetamol (p.71·2).
Fever; pain.

Pyrethane *Gerda, Fr.†.*
Dipyrone (p.34·1).
Pain.

Pyrethrum Spray *Nelson, UK.*
Homoeopathic preparation.

Pyribenzamine *Novartis Consumer, Canad.†.*
Tripelennamine hydrochloride (p.427·1).
Hypersensitivity reactions.

Pyriderm *Schering-Plough, Belg.†.*
Pyrethrum (p.1436·3); piperonyl butoxide (p.1436·2).
Pediculosis.

Pyridiate *Rugby, USA.*
Phenazopyridine hydrochloride (p.77·3).
Irritation of the lower urinary tract.

Pyridium *Ache, Braz.; Parke, Davis, Canad.; Parke, Davis, Hong Kong; Parke, Davis, S.Afr.; Warner Chilcott, USA.*
Phenazopyridine hydrochloride (p.77·3).
Pain and irritation of the urinary tract.

Pyridium Plus *Warner Chilcott, USA.*
Phenazopyridine hydrochloride (p.77·3); hyoscyamine hydrobromide (p.469·3); butalbital (p.658·3).
Urinary-tract pain and spasm, with apprehension.

Pyrifin *Hoechst Marion Roussel, S.Afr.†.*
Rifampicin (p.243·2); isoniazid (p.215·3); pyrazinamide (p.240·1).
Tuberculosis.

Pyrifoam *Dermatech, Austral.*
Permethrin (p.1436·1).
Pediculosis.

Pyril *Vitae, Mex.*
Dipyrone (p.34·1).
Fever; pain.

Pyrilax *Berlin-Chemie, Ger.*
Bisacodyl (p.1212·2).
Bowel evacuation; constipation.

Pyrinex *Ambix, USA.*
Pyrethrins; piperonyl butoxide (p.1436·2).
Pediculosis.

Pyrinyl II *Barre-National, USA.*
Pyrethrins; piperonyl butoxide technical (p.1436·2).
Pediculosis.

Pyrinyl Plus *Rugby, USA.*
Pyrethrins; piperonyl butoxide (p.1436·2).
Pediculosis.

Pyriped *Propan, S.Afr.†.*
Mepyramine maleate (p.421·1).
Antihistaminic.

Pyrisept *Weifa, Norw.*
Cetylpyridinium chloride (p.1138·1).
Disinfection of hands and skin; minor skin infections.

Pyritil *Biolab, Thai.*
Pyritinol hydrochloride (p.1657·1).
Organic brain disorders.

Pyrocaps *Be-Tabs, S.Afr.*
Piroxicam (p.79·1).
Gout; musculoskeletal and joint disorders.

Pyrogallic *Gordon, USA.*
Pyrogallol (p.1122·1).
Calluses; verrucas.

Pyrogastrone
Note. This name is used for preparations of different composition.
Sanofi Winthrop, Irl.; Sanofi Winthrop, UK.
Tablets: Carbenoxolone sodium (p.1215·3); alginic acid (p.1498·3); aluminium hydroxide (p.1210·3); magnesium trisilicate (p.1233·3); sodium bicarbonate (p.1186·2).
Gastro-oesophageal reflux.
Sanofi Winthrop, UK.
Oral suspension: Carbenoxolone sodium (p.1215·3); aluminium hydroxide (p.1210·3); sodium alginate (p.1498·3); potassium bicarbonate (p.1186·1).
Gastro-oesophageal reflux.

Pyrogenium N *Hanosan, Ger.*
Homoeopathic preparation.

Pyromed S *Sanofi Synthelabo, Ger.*
Paracetamol (p.71·2).
Fever; pain.

Pyron *Reuffer, Mex.*
Dipyrone (p.34·1).
Fever; pain.

Pyroxin *Rhone-Poulenc Rorer, Austral.*
Pyridoxine hydrochloride (p.1386·3).
Alcoholism; anaemias; homocystinuria; nausea and vomiting in pregnancy; premenstrual syndrome; radiation sickness.

Pyroxy *Shiwa, Thai.*
Piroxicam (p.79·1).
Gout; musculoskeletal, joint, peri-articular, and soft-tissue disorders.

Pyr-Pam *UCI, Braz.*
Pyrvinium embonate (p.108·2).
Enterobiasis.

Pyrvin *Orion, Fin.*
Pyrvinium embonate (p.108·2).
Worm infections.

Pytazen *Douglas, NZ.*
Dipyridamole (p.877·2).
Thromboembolic disorders.

Pytest *Tri-Med Specialties, USA.*
Carbon-14 (p.1449·1) labelled urea.
Diagnosis of Helicobacter pylori infection.

PZA *Hefa, Ger.; Biochemie, Singapore; Novartis, Thai.; Servipharm, Thai.*
Pyrazinamide (p.240·1).
Tuberculosis.

Q 10 *Asta Medica, Port.*
Ubidecarenone (p.1677·1).
Angina pectoris; drug-induced cardiotoxicity; heart failure; oedema.

Q200 *Pacific, NZ.*
Quinine sulfate (p.445·1).
Malaria; myotonia; nocturnal cramps.

Q300 *Pacific, NZ.*
Quinine sulfate (p.445·1).
Malaria; myotonia; nocturnal cramps.

Q-Age *Bracco, Ital.*
Vitamins; ubidecarenone (p.1350·1).

Qari *Mediolanum, Ital.*
Rufloxacin hydrochloride (p.247·3).
Bacterial infections.

Qiftrim *QIF, Braz.*
Co-trimoxazole (p.193·3).
Bacterial infections; Pneumocystis carinii pneumonia; protozoal infections.

Qinolon *Great Eastern, Thai.; Therapharma, Thai.*
Ofloxacin (p.232·3).
Bacterial infections.

QM Integratore *Mavi, Ital.*
Trace-element preparation with vitamin B substances and vitamin C (p.1350·1).
Nutritional supplement.

Q-Mazine *Seton, UK†.*
Promethazine hydrochloride (p.423·2).
Motion sickness; urticaria.

QT *Schering-Plough, USA.*
SPF 2: Octinoxate (p.1517·3); dihydroxyacetone (p.1113·2).
Sunscreen.

Q-Tech *Lifetech, Hong Kong.*
Phentolamine mesilate (p.954·3).
Peripheral vascular disorders.

QTest *Quidel, USA.*
Pregnancy test (p.1654·3).

QTest Ovulation *Quidel, USA.*
Fertility test (p.1654·3).

Quadblock *Hamilton, Austral.*
Cream SPF 30+; topical milk SPF 30+: Octinoxate (p.1517·3); titanium dioxide (p.1126·1); enzacamene (p.1517·2).
Stick SPF 30+: Oxybenzone (p.1518·1); octinoxate (p.1517·3); avobenzone (p.1517·1); titanium dioxide (p.1126·1).
Sunscreen.

Quadezyme *Pascual, Hong Kong.*
Muramidase hydrochloride (p.1638·1); dequalinium chloride (p.1143·1).
Allergic rhinitis; mouth and throat disorders; sinusitis.

Quadra Hist *Schein, USA†.*
Phenylpropanolamine hydrochloride (p.1098·1); phenylephrine hydrochloride (p.1097·1); chlorpheniramine [chlorphenamine] maleate (p.412·1); phenyltoloxamine citrate (p.423·1).
Upper respiratory-tract symptoms.

Quadracel *Connaught, Canad.*
A diphtheria, tetanus, pertussis and inactivated poliomyelitis vaccine (p.1539·1).
Active immunisation.

Quadra-Hist D *Ethex, USA†.*
Phenylpropanolamine hydrochloride (p.1098·1); phenyltoloxamine citrate (p.423·1); mepyramine maleate (p.421·1); pheniramine maleate (p.422·3).
Coughs and cold symptoms.

Quadramet *ARI, Austral.; CIS, Fr.; CIS, Ital.; Du Pont, USA.*
Samarium-153 lexidronam (p.1451·1).
Metastatic bone pain.

Quadrasa *Norgine, Fr.; Norgine, Ital.*
Sodium aminosalicylate (p.148·3).
Colorectal haemorrhage; ulcerative colitis.

Quadrax *Promeco, Mex.*
Ibuprofen (p.43·2).
Inflammation; pain.

Quadriderm *Schering-Plough, Braz.; Schering-Plough, Hong Kong; Schering-Plough, S.Afr.; Schering-Plough, Singapore; Essex, Switz.; Schering-Plough, Thai.*
Betamethasone valerate (p.1063·2); gentamicin sulfate (p.210·1); tolnaftate (p.395·2); clioquinol (p.190·2).
Infected skin disorders.

Quadriderm NF *Schering-Plough, Mex.*
Betamethasone dipropionate (p.1063·2); clotrimazole (p.382·1); gentamicin sulfate (p.210·1).
Infected skin disorders.

Quadriderme *Schering-Plough, Port.*
Betamethasone dipropionate (p.1063·2); clotrimazole (p.382·1); gentamicin sulfate (p.210·1).
Infected skin disorders.

Quadrilon *Neo Quimica, Braz.*
Betamethasone (p.1063·1); gentamicin (p.212·1); tolnaftate (p.395·2); clioquinol (p.190·2).
Infected skin disorders.

Quadrinal *Knoll, USA.*
Ephedrine hydrochloride (p.1090·1); phenobarbital (p.355·1); theophylline calcium salicylate (p.783·2); potassium iodide (p.1522·3).
Chronic respiratory disease.

Quadronal ASS comp *Asta Medica, Ger.*
Aspirin (p.14·2); caffeine (p.761·3).
Pain.

Quadronal comp *Asta Medica, Ger.*
Paracetamol (p.71·2); caffeine (p.761·3).
Pain.

Quadropril
Asta Medica, Aust.; Asta Medica, Ger.
Spirapril hydrochloride (p.973·2).
Hypertension.

Quait *SIT, Ital.†*
Lorazepam (p.688·3).
Anxiety disorders; premedication.

Qualiton *TO-Chemicals, Thai.*
Guaifenesin (p.1092·2); theophylline (p.777·2).
Coughs; obstructive airways disease.

Quam *Stada, Ger.*
Garlic (p.1614·1).
Lipid disorders; vascular disorders.

Quamatel *Gedeon Richter, Hong Kong.*
Famotidine (p.1225·3).
Gastro-oesophageal reflux; peptic ulcer; Zollinger-El-lison syndrome.

Quanil *Wyeth Lederle, Ital.*
Meprobamate (p.691·1).
Anxiety disorders.

Quantaffirm *Organon Teknika, USA.*
Test for infectious mononucleosis.

Quantalan
Bristol-Myers Squibb, Aust.; Bristol-Myers Squibb, Ger.; Bristol-Myers Squibb, Port.; Bristol-Myers Squibb, Switz.
Colestyramine (p.864·1).
Biliary-tract disorders; diarrhoea; hypercholestero-laemia; poisoning with phenprocoumon; pruritus asso-ciated with biliary obstruction.

Quantor *Almirall, Spain.*
Ranitidine hydrochloride (p.1245·2).
Acid aspiration; gastro-oesophageal reflux; gastroin-testinal haemorrhage; peptic ulcer; Zollinger-Ellison syndrome.

Quardin *Mepha, Port.*
Ranitidine hydrochloride (p.1245·2).
Acid aspiration; gastro-oesophageal reflux; gastroin-testinal haemorrhage; peptic ulcer; Zollinger-Ellison syndrome.

Quarelin *Chinoin, Hung.*
Dipyrone (p.34·1); caffeine (p.761·3); drotaverine hy-drochloride (p.1606·1).
Migraine.

Quark *Polifarma, Ital.*
Ramipril (p.966·3).
Heart failure; hypertension; myocardial infarction; re-nal insufficiency.

Quartamon Med *Schulke & Mayr, Ger.*
Benzalkonium chloride (p.1133·2).
Surface disinfection.

Quarzan *Roche, USA†.*
Clidinium bromide (p.465·1).
Peptic ulcer (adjunct).

Quasar *Ravizza, Ital.*
Verapamil hydrochloride (p.989·1).
Hypertension.

Quatohex *Braun, Ger.*
Didecyldimethylammonium chloride (p.1143·2); ben-zalkonium chloride (p.1133·2); biguanidinium acetate; polymeric biguanides.
Surface disinfection.

Quatro-Soda *Quatromed, S.Afr.*
Sodium citrate (p.1186·2); sodium bicarbonate (p.1186·2); tartaric acid (p.1669·2); citric acid (p.1596·2).
Gastrointestinal hyperacidity; urinary alkalisation.

Quatro-Virelon *Chiron Behring, Ger.*
A diphtheria, tetanus, pertussis, and poliomyelitis vac-cine (p.1539·1).
Active immunisation.

Quazium *Schering-Plough, Ital.*
Quazepam (p.703·1).
Insomnia.

Quefeno *Helfarma, Port.*
Ketotifen fumarate (p.767·2).
Allergic rhinitis; asthma; urticaria.

Quelacid *Enila, Braz.*
Aluminium and calcium chelate.
Gastrointestinal hyperacidity.

Quelicin
Abbott, Braz.; Abbott, Canad.; Abbott, USA.
Suxamethonium chloride (p.1340·1).
Depolarising neuromuscular blocker.

Quelidrine *Abbott, USA.*
Dextromethorphan hydrobromide (p.1087·3); chlor-pheniramine [chlorphenamine] maleate (p.412·1); ephedrine hydrochloride (p.1090·1); phenylephrine hy-drochloride (p.1097·1); ammonium chloride (p.1085·2); ipecac fluidextract (p.1093·1).
Coughs.

Quell P *Searle, S.Afr.†.*
Pyrethrum; piperonyl butoxide (p.1436·2).
Pediculosis.

Quellada
Note.This name is used for preparations of different composition.
Stafford-Miller, Austral.
Permethrin (p.1436·1).
Pediculosis; scabies.

Stafford-Miller Continental, Belg.†; Stafford-Miller, Irl.; Searle, S.Afr.
Lindane (p.1434·1).
Pediculosis; scabies.

Quellada H *Block, Ger.*
Lindane (p.1434·1).
Pediculosis.

Quellada P
Note.This name is used for preparations of different composition.
Block, Ger.
Pyrethrum flower (p.1436·3); piperonyl butoxide (p.1436·2).
Pediculosis.

Stafford-Miller, NZ.
Permethrin (p.1436·1).
Pediculosis; scabies.

Quellada-M *Stafford-Miller, UK.*
Malathion (p.1434·2).
Pediculosis; scabies.

Quelodin *Ariston, Braz.*
Menthol (p.1632·3); menthone; α-pinene; eucalyptol (p.1609·2); camphene; greater celandine (p.1618·1); phenylpropanol (p.1650·3); olive oil (p.1643·3).
Gallstones.

Quemicetina
Carlo Erba, Braz.; Pharmacia Upjohn, Mex.
Chloramphenicol (p.179·1), chloramphenicol palmi-tate (p.179·2), or chloramphenicol sodium succinate (p.179·2).
Bacterial infections.

Quenobilan *Estedi, Spain.*
Chenodeoxycholic acid (p.1594·1).
Gallstones.

Quenocol *Zambon, Spain.*
Chenodeoxycholic acid (p.1594·1).
Gallstones.

Quensyl *Sanofi Synthelabo, Ger.*
Hydroxychloroquine sulfate (p.437·2).
Chronic polyarthritis; lupus erythematosus; malaria.

Quentakehl *Sanum-Kehlbeck, Ger.*
Homoeopathic preparation.

Queratil *Reig Jofre, Spain.*
Eucalyptol (p.1609·2); ichthammol (p.1115·2); trini-trophenol (p.1675·1); ergocalciferol (p.1391·2); tannic acid (p.1669·1); zinc oxide (p.1128·2); vitamin A (p.1382·1).
Burns.

Quercetol Hemostatico *Ferrer, Spain.*
Carbazochrome (p.728·1); quercetin (p.1611·2); creat-inine sulfate.
Haemorrhage.

Quercetol K *Ferrer, Spain†.*
Ascorbic acid (p.1389·3); calcium gluconate (p.1188·2); carbazochrome (p.728·1); menadione sodi-um bisulfite (p.1395·3); quercetin (p.1611·2).
Capillary fragility; haemorrhage.

Querto *Byk Gulden, Ger.*
Carvedilol (p.855·2).
Angina pectoris; heart failure; hypertension.

Questran
Bristol-Myers Squibb, Austral.; Bristol-Myers Squibb, Belg.; Bristol-My-ers Squibb, Braz.; Bristol, Canad.; Bristol-Myers Squibb, Denm.; Bris-tol-Myers Squibb, Fin.; Bristol-Myers Squibb, Fr.; Bristol-Myers Squibb, Hong Kong; Bristol-Myers Squibb, Irl.; Bristol-Myers Squibb, Israel; Bristol-Myers Squibb, Ital.; Mead Johnson, Mex.; Bristol-Myers Squibb, Neth.; Bristol-Myers Squibb, Norw.; Bristol-Myers Squibb, S.Afr.; Bristol-Myers Squibb, Singapore; Bristol-Myers, Spain; Bristol-Myers Squibb, Swed.; Bristol-Myers Squibb, Thai.; Bristol-Myers Squibb, UK; Bristol-Myers Squibb, USA.
Colestyramine (p.864·1).
Adjunct in organophosphorus pesticide poisoning; di-arrhoea; hypercholesterolaemia; pruritus associated with biliary obstruction.

Quetzal *Smaller, Spain.*
Hypericum (p.290·2).
Tonic.

Quibron
Note.This name is used for preparations of different composition.
Bristol-Myers Squibb, Thai.
Theophylline (p.777·2).
Obstructive airways disease.

Apothecon, USA.
Theophylline (p.777·2); guaifenesin (p.1092·2).
Bronchospasm.

Quibron-T
Bristol, Canad.; Roberts, USA.
Theophylline (p.777·2).
Obstructive airways disease.

Quick Pep *Thompson, USA†.*
Caffeine (p.761·3).
Fatigue.

QuickCal
Vitaflo, Irl.; Vitaflo, UK.
High energy food fortifier (p.1350·1).

QuickVue *Quidel, USA.*
Pregnancy test (p.1654·3).

Quiedorm *Menarini, Spain.*
Quazepam (p.703·1).
Insomnia.

Quies *Quies, Fr.*
Eschscholtzia californica.
Nervous disorders.

Quiess *Forest Laboratories, USA†.*
Hydroxyzine hydrochloride (p.419·1).
Anxiety; hypersensitivity reactions.

Quiet Days *Cantassium Co., UK.*
Skullcap (p.1664·3); lupulus (p.1629·3); valerian (p.1678·3).

Quiet Life *Lane, UK.*
Motherwort (p.1637·3); wild lettuce (p.1680·3); lupu-lus (p.1629·3); passion flower (p.1649·1); valerian (p.1678·3); thiamine hydrochloride (p.1385·1); ribofla-vin (p.1386·1); nicotinamide (p.1372·3).
Insomnia; stresses and strains.

Quiet Nite *Cantassium Co., UK.*
Valerian (p.1678·3); lupulus (p.1629·3); lettuce (p.1680·3); passion flower (p.1649·1).
Insomnia.

Quiet Tyme *Cantassium Co., UK.*
Skullcap (p.1664·3); lupulus (p.1629·3); passion flow-er (p.1649·1); valerian (p.1678·3); gentian (p.1615·1); vitamin B substances (p.1350·1).

Quietan *Roche, Ital.†.*
Valerian (p.1678·3); passion flower (p.1649·1); cratae-gus (p.1600·2).
Insomnia.

Quietiline *Sciencex, Fr.*
Bromazepam (p.656·3).
Anxiety.

Quifloxona *Farmaco, Mex.*
Ciprofloxacin (p.182·3).
Bacterial infections.

Quik *Valeas, Ital.*
Cloperastine fendizoate (p.1087·2).
Coughs.

Quilagen *Randall, Mex.*
Gentamicin (p.212·1).
Bacterial infections.

Quilla simplex *Pharmacia Upjohn, Swed.*
Ammonium chloride (p.1085·2); quillaia (p.1348·2).
Respiratory-tract disorders.

Quilonorm
SmithKline Beecham, Aust.; Doetsch, Grether, Switz.
Lithium acetate (p.296·2) or lithium carbonate (p.292·1).
Bipolar disorder; depression; mania.

Quilonum
SmithKline Beecham, Austral.; SmithKline Beecham, Ger.; SmithKline Beecham, S.Afr.
Lithium acetate (p.296·2) or lithium carbonate (p.292·1).
Bipolar disorder; cluster headache; depression; ma-nia.

Quimefuran *Iqfasa, Mex.*
Furazolidone (p.592·1).

Quimio-Ped *Stiefel, Braz.*
Co-trimoxazole (p.193·3).
Bacterial infections; Pneumocystis carinii pneumonia; protozoal infections.

Quimio-Ped Balsamico *Stiefel, Braz.*
Co-trimoxazole (p.193·3); guaifenesin (p.1092·2); am-monium chloride (p.1085·2).
Bacterial infections.

Quimobrom *Maver, Mex.*
Erythromycin (p.201·2); bromhexine (p.1085·3).
Bacterial infections.

Quimocyclar *Grossman, Mex.*
Tetracycline (p.258·3).
Bacterial infections.

Quimodril *Italfarmaco, Spain.*
Trypsin (p.1675·3); chymotrypsin (p.1595·1); teclothi-azide potassium (p.979·2).
Oedema.

Quimolactona *Quimica y Farmacia, Mex.*
Spironolactone (p.973·2).
Hypertension.

Quimolauril *Maver, Mex.*
Erythromycin (p.201·2).
Bacterial infections.

Quimosporina *Quimica y Farmacia, Mex.*
Cefalexin (p.161·3).
Bacterial infections.

Quimotrase *Alcon Cusi, Spain.*
Chymotrypsin (p.1595·1).
Aid in cataract surgery.

Quimpe Amida *Quimpe, Spain.*
Sulfanilamide (p.256·2); zinc oxide (p.1128·2).
Bacterial skin infections.

Quimpe Antibiotico *Quimpe, Spain.*
Tetracycline hydrochloride (p.258·3).
Bacterial infections.

Quimpe Vitamin *Quimpe, Spain†.*
Vitamin B substances and amino-acid preparation (p.1350·1).

Quimpedor *Quimpe, Spain.*
Caffeine (p.761·3); phenazone (p.77·2); pyridoxine hy-drochloride (p.1386·3); propyphenazone (p.80·2); thia-mine hydrochloride (p.1385·1).
Fever; pain.

Quinaband *Seton Scholl, Austral.; SSL, UK.*
Calamine (p.1111·3); clioquinol (p.190·2); zinc oxide (p.1128·2).
Medicated bandage.

Quinaglute *Schering, S.Afr.; Berlex, USA.*
Quinidine gluconate (p.964·2).
Arrhythmias.

Quinalan *Lannett, USA†.*
Quinidine gluconate (p.964·2).
Arrhythmias.

Quinate
Note.This name is used for preparations of different composition.
Rhone-Poulenc Rorer, Austral.
Quinine sulfate (p.445·1).
Diagnosis of myasthenia gravis; malaria; muscle cramps; myotonia congenita.

Rougier, Canad.†.
Quinidine gluconate (p.964·2).
Arrhythmias.

Quinax
Alcon, Hong Kong; Alcon, Singapore; Alcon, Thai.
Azapentacene polysulfonate sodium.
Cataract.

Quinazide *Malesci, Ital.*
Quinapril hydrochloride (p.963·3); hydrochlorothi-azide (p.907·3).
Hypertension.

Quinazil *Malesci, Ital.*
Quinapril hydrochloride (p.963·3) or quinaprilat (p.964·1).
Heart failure; hypertension.

Quinbisul *Alphapharm, Austral.*
Quinine bisulfate (p.445·1).
Malaria; nocturnal leg cramps.

Quindoleina *Gastroenterologicos, Mex.*
Clioquinol (p.190·2).

Quineuron *Euromex, Mex.*
Quinidine (p.964·2).

Quinfamex *Ofimex, Mex.*
Quinfamide.

Quini *Astra, Mex.*
Quinidine bisulfate (p.964·2).
Arrhythmias.

Quinicardina *Berenguer Infale, Spain†.*
Quinidine sulfate (p.964·3).
Arrhythmias.

Quinicardine *Barrenne, Braz.*
Quinidine sulfate (p.964·3).
Arrhythmias.

Quinidex
Wyeth-Ayerst, Canad.; Robins, USA.
Quinidine sulfate (p.964·3).
Arrhythmias.

Quiniduran *Teva, Israel.*
Quinidine bisulfate (p.964·2).
Arrhythmias.

Quinidurule *AstraZeneca, Fr.*
Quinidine bisulfate (p.964·2).
Arrhythmias.

Quinimax *Sanofi Winthrop, Fr.*
Quinine gluconate (p.447·1) or quinine hydrochloride (p.445·1); quinidine gluconate (p.964·2) or quinidine hydrochloride (p.963·3); cinchonine hydrochloride; cinchonidine hydrochloride.
Formerly contained quinine-resorcinol dihydrochlo-ride, quinidine-resorcinol dihydrochloride, cincho-nine-resorcinol dihydrochloride, and cinchonidine-resorcinol dihydrochloride.
Malaria.

Quinisedine *Sodia, Fr.*
Quinine benzoate (p.447·1); crataegus (p.1600·2).
Formerly contained quinine valerianate, marrubium, crataegus, and phenobarbital.
Cramps.

Quinobarb *Rougier, Canad.†.*
Quinidine phenylethylbarbiturate (p.966·1).
Arrhythmias; sedative.

Quinoc *Douglas, NZ.*
Quinine sulfate (p.445·1).
Malaria; myotonia; nocturnal cramps.

Quinocarbine *GNR, Fr.*
Aluminium orthoxyquinoleate; activated charcoal (p.1000·2).
Diarrhoea; meteorism.

Quinocort
Quinoderm, Irl.; Adams, UK.
Potassium hydroxyquinoline sulfate (p.1654·2); hydro-cortisone (p.1073·3).
Infected skin disorders.

Quinoctal *Fawns & McAllan, Austral.*
Quinine sulfate (p.445·1).
Malaria; nocturnal leg cramps.

Quinoderm
Quinoderm, Irl.; Aventis, S.Afr.; Quinoderm, Switz.†; Adams, UK.
Benzoyl peroxide (p.1111·1); potassium hydroxyquin-oline sulfate (p.1654·2).
Acne; folliculitis; rosacea.

Quinoderm Antibacterial Face Wash *Adams, UK.*
Chlorhexidine gluconate (p.1138·2); cetrimide (p.1137·1); detergents.
Skin cleanser; soap substitute.

Quinoderm-H *Hoechst Marion Roussel, S.Afr.†.*
Benzoyl peroxide (p.1111·1); potassium hydroxyquin-oline sulfate (p.1654·2); hydrocortisone (p.1073·3).
Skin disorders.

Quinodermil *Oftalder, Port.*
Clioquinol (p.190·2).

Quinodis
Grunenthal, Aust.; Roche, Belg.†; Roche, Denm.; Roche, Ger.; Gru-nenthal, Ger.; Grunenthal, Switz.
Fleroxacin (p.206·3).
Bacterial infections.

The symbol † denotes a preparation no longer actively marketed

Quinoflex Mepha, Port.
Norfloxacin (p.232·1).
Bacterial infections.

Quinoflox
Uniao Quimica, Braz.; Diba, Mex.
Ciprofloxacin hydrochloride (p.182·3).
Bacterial infections.

Quinoform EMS, Braz.
Norfloxacin (p.232·1).
Bacterial infections.

Quinoforme Synthelabo, Fr.
Basic quinine formate (p.447·1).
Malaria.

Quinoped Adams, UK.
Benzoyl peroxide (p.1111·1); potassium hydroxyquin-
oline sulfate (p.1654·2).
Fungal skin infections.

Quinora Key, USA.
Quinidine sulfate (p.964·3).
Arrhythmias.

Quinortar Iquinosa, Spain.
Coal tar (p.1125·1); chlorquinaldol (p.182·1); titanium
dioxide (p.1126·1).
Skin disorders.

Quinox Labesfal, Port.†
Ciprofloxacin (p.182·3).
Bacterial infections.

Quinradon Hua, Thai.
Diiodohydroxyquinoline (p.590·2); boric acid
(p.1586·1); phosphoric acid (p.1651·1).
Vaginal infections.

Quinradon-N Hua, Thai.
Diiodohydroxyquinoline (p.590·2); nystatin (p.392·2);
boric acid (p.1586·1); phosphoric acid (p.1651·1).
Vaginal infections.

Quinsana Plus Mennen, USA.
Tolnaftate (p.395·2).
Fungal skin infections.

Quinsul Alphapharm, Austral.
Quinine sulfate (p.445·1).
Malaria; nocturnal leg cramps.

Quintabs Freeda, USA.
A range of vitamin preparations (p.1350·1).

Quintasa
Ferring, Canad.; Ferring, Spain.
Mesalazine (p.1234·1).
Inflammatory bowel disease.

Quintelmin EMS, Braz.
Mebendazole (p.102·2).
Worm infections.

Quintex Bio-Therabel, Belg.
Butamirate citrate (p.1086·2).
Formerly contained dioxethedrin hydrochloride, pro-
methazine hydrochloride, and codeine phosphate.
Coughs; respiratory-tract disorders.

Quintex Pediatrique Bio-Therabel, Belg.
Butamirate citrate (p.1086·2).
Formerly contained dioxethedrin hydrochloride, pro-
methazine hydrochloride pholcodine, and sulfogaiacol.
Coughs.

Quintonine SmithKline Beecham Sante, Fr.
Cinnamon (p.1595·3); kola (p.1681·1); dried bitter-orange peel (p.1644·2); cinchona bark (p.1595·3); quassia (p.1657·1); gentian (p.1615·1).
Formerly contained cinnamon, kola, dried bitter-orange peel, cinchona bark, quassia, gentian, calcium
glycerophosphate, and nux vomica.
Asthenia.

Quintopan SmithKline Beecham Sante, Fr.
Chlorpheniramine [chlorphenamine] maleate
(p.412·1); dextromethorphan hydrobromide
(p.1087·3); sodium benzoate (p.1134·3).
Formerly known as Quintopan Adult and contained codeine, ethylmorphine, bromoform, sodium benzoate,
grindelia, polygala, bryonia, and aconite.
Coughs.

Quintopan Enfant SmithKline Beecham Sante, Fr.†
Promethazine hydrochloride (p.423·2); pholcodine
(p.1099·1); sulfogaiacol (p.1101·1); dioxethedrin hydrochloride (p.1089·1).
Coughs.

Quipro Ciclum, Spain.
Ciprofloxacin hydrochloride (p.182·3).
Bacterial infections.

Quiralam Guidotti, Spain.
Dexketoprofen trometamol (p.47·3).
Pain.

Quiridil Formenti, Ital.†
Sulpiride (p.706·1).
Dysthymia; psychoses.

Quit Aspen Consumer, S.Afr.
Nicotine (p.1640·3).
Aid to smoking withdrawal.

Quitadrill Pierre Fabre Sante, Fr.
Mequitazine (p.421·2).
Hypersensitivity.

Quitaxon
Roche, Belg.; Ercopharm, Denm.†; Roche, Fr.
Doxepin hydrochloride (p.283·3).
Depression.

Quitoso Lepori, Port.
Pyrethrins; piperonyl butoxide (p.1436·2).
Pediculosis.

Quitt Meda, Swed.†.
Nicotine resin (p.1641·3).
Aid to smoking withdrawal.

Quixin Santen, USA.
Levofloxacin (p.219·1).
Bacterial conjunctivitis.

Quocel Rayere, Mex.
Quinfamide.
Amoebiasis.

Quocin Isdin, Spain.
Acetic acid (p.1571·2); salicylic acid (p.1122·3).
Callosities.

Quoderm Isdin, Spain.
Meclocycline sulfosalicylate (p.222·1).
Acne.

Quool Manx, UK.
Menthol (p.1632·3).
Muscular pain; sports injuries.

Quosten Ibi, Ital.
Salcatonin (p.749·3).
*Hypercalcaemia; osteoporosis; Paget's disease of
bone; reflex sympathetic dystrophy.*

Quotane Medeva, Fr.
Quinisocaine hydrochloride (p.1320·2).
Pruritus.

Quotivit O.E. Mayoly-Spindler, Fr.
Multivitamin and mineral preparation (p.1350·1).

QV
Ego, Austral.; Ego, Hong Kong; Ego, NZ; Ego, Singapore.
A range of emollients and soap substitutes.
Skin disorders.

QV Lip Balm
Ego, Austral.; Ego, Hong Kong; Ego, Singapore.
Avobenzone (p.1517·1); octinoxate (p.1517·3).
Dry, cracked, or chapped lips; sunscreen.

Qvar
3M, Austral.; 3M, Fr.; 3M, Irl.; 3M, Neth.; Aventis, NZ; 3M, S.Afr.;
3M, UK; 3M, USA.
Beclometasone dipropionate (p.1061·2).
Asthma.

Q-Vax CSL, Austral.
An inactivated Q fever vaccine (p.1560·1).
Active immunisation.

R 1406 Janssen-Cilag, Fr.†
Phenoperidine hydrochloride (p.78·1).
Analgesia in anaesthesia.

R & C
Reed & Carnrick, Canad.
Shampoo: Pyrethrins; piperonyl butoxide (p.1436·2).
Pediculosis.
Spray: Pyrethrins; piperonyl butoxide (p.1436·2).
Surface and textile insecticide.

Reed & Carnrick, USA.
Pyrethrins; piperonyl butoxide (p.1436·2).
Pediculosis.

R Calm Labima, Belg.
Diphenhydramine hydrochloride (p.416·1).
Bites and stings; skin disorders.

R Calm + B6 Labima, Belg.†
Dimenhydrinate (p.415·2); pyridoxine (p.1387·1).
Motion sickness; urticaria.

RA Lotion Medco, USA.
Resorcinol (p.1122·2); calamine (p.1111·3); borax
(p.1586·1).
Acne.

RA Morph Pharmacia Upjohn, NZ.
Morphine hydrochloride (p.56·1).
Pain.

Rabarbaroni Max Farma, Ital.
Rhubarb (p.1248·1); cinchona (p.1595·3); bitter orange
(p.1644·2); liquorice (p.1231·2).
Constipation.

RabAvert Chiron, USA.
A rabies vaccine (p.1560·2).
Active immunisation.

Rabies Gamma Biagini, Ital.
A rabies immunoglobulin (p.1560·2).
Passive immunisation.

Rabies-Imovax
Pasteur Merieux, Denm.; Meda, Fin.; Pasteur Merieux, Norw.; Pas-
teur Merieux, Swed.
A rabies vaccine (Wistar PM/WI 38-1503-3M)
(p.1560·2).
Active immunisation.

Rabigam NBI, S.Afr.
A rabies immunoglobulin (p.1560·2).
Passive immunisation.

Rabipur
Chiron Behring, Aust.; Chiron Behring, Ger.; Chiron, Thai.; Hoechst
Marion Roussel, Thai.; Masta, UK.
A rabies vaccine (Flury LEP strain) (p.1560·2).
Active immunisation.

Rabivac Chiron Behring, Ger.
A rabies vaccine (Pitman-Moore strain grown on hu-
man diploid cell cultures) (p.1560·2).
Active immunisation.

Raboldo IMO, Ital.
Cascara (p.1216·1); boldo (p.1585·3); rhubarb
(p.1248·1).
Constipation.

Rabro Vitafarma, Spain†.
Calcium carbonate (p.1215·1); frangula bark
(p.1227·1); liquorice (p.1231·2); magnesium oxide
(p.1233·2); dimethicone (p.1249·2).
Flatulence; gastritis; hyperchlorhydria; peptic ulcer.

Rabro N Fink, Ger.†
Calcium carbonate (p.1215·1); liquorice (p.1231·2);
magnesium oxide (p.1233·2).
Gastritis; hyperchlorhydria.

Rabuman
Kwizda, Aust.†; Berna, Hong Kong; Berna, Ital.; Berna, Switz.; Berna,
Thai.
A rabies immunoglobulin (p.1560·2).
Passive immunisation.

Racestyptin Austrodent, Aust.
Aluminium chloride (p.1110·2); hydroxyquinoline sul-
fate (p.1622·2).
Adjunct in dental procedures.

Racestyptine Septodont, Switz.
Solution: Aluminium chloride (p.1110·2).
Thread: Aluminium chloride (p.1110·2); lignocaine
[lidocaine] (p.1313·2); hydroxyquinoline (p.1622·2).
Dental and gum disorders.

Racetam Samjin, Singapore.
Piracetam (p.1652·1).
Cerebral trauma; cerebrovascular disorders.

Ra-Cliss Fresenius Kabi, Ital.
Monobasic sodium phosphate (p.1193·2); dibasic sodi-
um phosphate (p.1193·2).
Bowel evacuation; constipation.

Racovel Cryopharma, Mex.
Levodopa (p.1169·2); carbidopa (p.1168·2).
Parkinsonism.

Radalgin Streuli, Switz.
Nonivamide (p.63·1); methyl nicotinate (p.55·1); glycol salicylate (p.42·2); histamine hydrochloride
(p.1619·2).
Musculoskeletal pain; sports injuries.

Radan Marjan, Braz.
Ranitidine hydrochloride (p.1245·2).
*Gastro-oesophageal reflux; gastrointestinal haemor-
rhage; peptic ulcer; Zollinger-Ellison syndrome.*

Radanil Roche, Arg.
Benznidazole (p.589·2).
Protozoal infections.

Radecol Asta Medica, Ger.
Nicotinyl alcohol tartrate (p.939·3).
Hyperlipidaemias; vascular disorders.

Radedorm Asta Medica, Ger.
Nitrazepam (p.695·2).
Sleep disorders.

Radenarcon Asta Medica, Ger.
Etomidate (p.1259·2).
General anaesthesia.

Radepur Asta Medica, Ger.
Chlordiazepoxide (p.659·2).
Anxiety disorders; insomnia.

Radialar 280 Juste, Spain.
Meglumine amidotrizoate (p.1031·2).
Radiographic contrast medium.

Radian Roche, S.Afr.
Cream†: Menthol (p.1632·3); camphor (p.1589·3); methyl salicylate (p.55·1); capsicum oleoresin (p.1591·1);
camphor oil.
Liniment: Menthol (p.1632·3); aspirin (p.14·2); camphor (p.1589·3); methyl salicylate (p.55·1).
Pain.

Radian-B
Note.This name is used for preparations of different composition.
Roche Consumer, Austral.
Liniment: Menthol (p.1632·3); camphor (p.1589·3);
ammonium salicylate (p.14·1); methyl salicylate
(p.55·1); ethyl salicylate (p.35·1).
*Musculoskeletal and joint disorders; soft-tissue disor-
ders.*

Roche Consumer, Irl.; Roche Consumer, UK.
Liniment; topical spray: Menthol (p.1632·3); camphor
(p.1589·3); ammonium salicylate (p.14·1); salicylic
acid (p.1122·3).
Musculoskeletal and joint disorders; pain.

Radiol, Israel.
Liniment; topical spray: Aspirin (p.14·2); menthol
(p.1632·3); camphor (p.1589·3); methyl salicylate
(p.55·1).
Musculoskeletal and joint disorders.

Roche Consumer, Austral.; Radiol, Israel; Roche Consumer, UK.
Topical rub: Menthol (p.1632·3); camphor (p.1589·3);
methyl salicylate (p.55·1); capsicum oleoresin
(p.1591·1).
Musculoskeletal and joint disorders; pain.

Roche Consumer, Irl.
Topical rub: Menthol (p.1632·3); camphor (p.1589·3);
methyl salicylate (p.55·1); camphor oil; capsaicin
(p.23·1).
Musculoskeletal and soft-tissue disorders.

Radian-B Ibuprofen Roche Consumer, UK.
Ibuprofen (p.43·2).
Musculoskeletal pain; sports injuries.

Radikal
Note.This name is used for preparations of different composition.
Sandipro, Belg.
Malathion (p.1434·2).
Pediculosis.

Maurer, Ger.
Clotrimazole (p.382·1).
Fungal skin infections.

Radilem Lemery, Mex.
Methylprednisolone (p.1076·1).
Corticosteroid.

Radine Pond's, Thai.
Ranitidine hydrochloride (p.1245·2).
*Gastro-oesophageal reflux; peptic ulcer; Zollinger-El-
lison syndrome.*

Radio Salil Vinas, Spain.
Cream: Camphor (p.1589·3); methyl nicotinate
(p.55·1); methyl salicylate (p.55·1); salicylic acid
(p.1122·3); menthol (p.1632·3).
Spray: Camphor (p.1589·3); diethylamine salicylate
(p.32·2); menthol (p.1632·3).
*Musculoskeletal, joint, peri-articular, and soft-tissue
disorders.*

Radioced Interfarma, Ital.†
Dimethicone (p.1410·1).
Barrier preparation.

Radiogardase-Cs Heyl, Ger.
Prussian blue (p.1021·2).
Reduction in body-half-life of radiocaesium.

Radioselectan Schering, UK.
Sodium amidotrizoate (p.1031·3); meglumine amidot-
rizoate (p.1031·2).
Radiographic contrast medium.

Rado-Salil Will-Pharma, Belg.
Ethyl salicylate (p.35·1); methyl salicylate (p.55·1);
glycol salicylate (p.42·2); salicylic acid (p.1122·3);
camphor (p.1589·3); menthol (p.1632·3); capsicum
oleoresin (p.1591·1).
Lumbago; muscle and joint pain.

Raductil Knoll, Mex.
Sibutramine hydrochloride (p.1514·3).
Obesity.

Radyn Arlex, Mex.
Ranitidine (p.1246·3).

Rafapen V-K Rafa, Israel.
Phenoxymethylpenicillin (p.235·1).
Bacterial infections.

Rafapen Mega Rafa, Israel.
Phenoxymethylpenicillin (p.235·1).
Bacterial endocarditis prophylaxis.

Rafassal Rafa, Israel.
Mesalazine (p.1234·1).
Inflammatory bowel disease.

Rafathricin Rafa, Israel.
Tyrothricin (p.267·1).
Mouth and throat infections.

Rafathricin with Benzocaine Rafa, Israel.
Tyrothricin (p.267·1); benzocaine (p.1306·2).
Mouth and throat disorders.

Rafazocine Rafa, Israel.
Pentazocine (p.74·2).
Pain.

Rafazocine X Rafa, Israel.
Pentazocine hydrochloride (p.74·2); naloxone hydro-
chloride (p.1014·3).
Pain.

Rafen Alphapharm, Austral.
Ibuprofen (p.43·2).
*Dysmenorrhoea; musculoskeletal and joint disorders;
pain with inflammation; soft-tissue injuries.*

Raffreddoremed Iodosan, Ital.
Paracetamol (p.71·2); isopropamide iodide (p.470·1);
dimetofrine (p.877·2); caffeine (p.761·3); chlorpheniramine [chlorphenamine] maleate (p.412·1); ascorbic acid (p.1389·3).
Cold and influenza symptoms.

Rafton Ferring, Canad.
Alginic acid (p.1498·3) or sodium alginate (p.1498·3);
aluminium hydroxide (p.1210·3).
Heartburn.

Rafuzone Rafa, Israel.
Nitrofurazone (p.231·3).
Infected burns.

Ragaden Ganassini, Ital.
Cetylpyridinium chloride (p.1138·1).
Nipple disinfection.

Ragonil Roche, Ecuad.
Benznidazole (p.589·2).
Protozoal infections.

Ralgex
Seton, UK†.
Topical spray: Glycol monosalicylate (p.42·2); ethyl
salicylate (p.35·1); methyl salicylate (p.55·1); methyl
nicotinate (p.55·1).
Musculoskeletal and joint disorders; pain.

SSL, UK.
Cream: Glycol salicylate (p.42·2); methyl nicotinate
(p.55·1); capsicum oleoresin (p.1591·1).
Topical stick: Glycol salicylate (p.42·2); ethyl salicylate (p.35·1); methyl salicylate (p.55·1); capsicum
oleoresin (p.1591·1); menthol (p.1632·3).
Musculoskeletal and joint disorders; pain.

Ralgex Freeze Spray SSL, UK.
Isopentane; dimethyl ether (p.1199·1); glycol monosal-
icylate (p.42·2).
Musculoskeletal and joint disorders.

Ralgex Heat Spray (low-odour) SSL, UK.
Glycol monosalicylate (p.42·2); methyl nicotinate
(p.55·1).
Musculoskeletal and joint disorders; pain.

Ralicid Sanochemia, Aust.
Indometacin (p.44·3).
*Gout; inflammation; musculoskeletal, joint, and peri-
articular disorders; oedema; pain.*

Ralodantin Pharmacia Upjohn, Austral.
Nitrofurantoin (p.230·3).
Urinary-tract infections.

Ralofekt *Dresden, Ger.; Temmler, Ger.*
Oxpentifylline [pentoxifylline] (p.950·3).
Peripheral vascular disorders; vascular disorders of the eye or ear.

Ralogaine *Kenral, Austral.†.*
Minoxidil (p.934·2).
Alopecia androgenetica.

Ralopar *Hoeport, Port.*
Cefotaxime sodium (p.169·1).
Bacterial infections.

Ralovera *Kenral, Austral.*
Medroxyprogesterone acetate (p.1480·1).
Abnormal uterine bleeding; adjunct to oestrogen therapy; amenorrhoea; breast cancer; endometrial cancer; endometriosis; renal cancer.

Ralozam *Pharmacia Upjohn, Austral.*
Alprazolam (p.654·2).
Anxiety; panic disorders.

Ralsifen-X *Serral, Mex.*
Tamoxifen (p.572·2).
Breast cancer; renal cancer.

Ralur *Drossapharm, Switz.*
Heparin sodium (p.902·1); indometacin (p.44·3); lauromacrogol 400 (p.1345·2).
Musculoskeletal, joint, peri-articular, and soft-tissue disorders.

Ramace *Hoechst Marion Roussel, Austral.; Astra, Belg.; AstraZeneca, Denm.; AstraZeneca, Fin.; Astra, Mex.; Astra, S.Afr.*
Ramipril (p.966·3).
Heart failure; hypertension; myocardial infarction.

Ramavit *Leiras, Fin.*
Vitamin B substances with iron (p.1350·1).
Vitamin B and iron deficiency.

Ramend *Schieffer, Ger.*
Senna (p.1248·2).
Constipation.

Ramend Krauter *Schieffer, Ger.*
Senna (p.1248·2); maté (p.1681·1); coriander (p.1599·2); fennel (p.1610·1); aniseed (p.1580·2).
Constipation.

Ramet Cade *CS, Fr.*
Cade oil (p.1124·3).
Skin disorders.

Ramet Dalibour *CS, Fr.*
Copper sulfate (p.1358·1); zinc sulfate (p.1398·2).
Skin cleaning and disinfection.

Ramet Pain *CS, Fr.*
Copper sulfate (p.1358·1); zinc sulfate (p.1398·2).
Skin cleansing and disinfection.

Ramfin *Biolab, Thai.*
Rifampicin (p.243·2).
Gonorrhoea; tuberculosis.

Rami Slijmoplossende *Warner-Lambert, Neth.*
Carbocisteine (p.1086·3).
Coughs.

Rami-Dextromethorphan *Warner-Lambert, Neth.*
Dextromethorphan hydrobromide (p.1087·3).
Formerly contained codeine and antimony potassium tartrate.
Coughs.

Ramidox *Errekappa, Ital.*
Loperamide oxide (p.1232·1).
Diarrhoea.

Ramno-Flor *Medifood, Ital.*
Lactic-acid-producing organisms (p.1626·3).
Nutritional supplement.

Ramol *Nakornpatana, Thai.*
Paracetamol (p.71·2).
Pain.

Ramp *MediMar, UK.*
Pregnancy test (p.1654·3).

Rampicin *Shiwa, Thai.*
Rifampicin (p.243·2).
Gonorrhoea; leprosy; tuberculosis.

Ramses *Durex, Canad.; Schmid, USA.*
Nonoxinol 9 (p.1346·1).
Contraceptive.

Ramysis *Isis, UK.*
Doxycycline hyclate (p.200·1).
Bacterial infections.

Ran *Helsinn, Port.*
Ranitidine hydrochloride (p.1245·2).
Gastro-oesophageal reflux; peptic ulcer; Zollinger-Ellison syndrome.

Ran H2 *Seid, Spain.*
Ranitidine hydrochloride (p.1245·2).
Acid aspiration; gastro-oesophageal reflux; gastrointestinal haemorrhage; peptic ulcer; short-bowel syndrome; Zollinger-Ellison syndrome.

Ran Lich *Lichtenstein, Ger.*
Ranitidine hydrochloride (p.1245·2).
Acid aspiration; gastro-oesophageal reflux; gastrointestinal haemorrhage; peptic ulcer; Zollinger-Ellison syndrome.

Ranacid *Nycomed, Norw.†.*
Ranitidine hydrochloride (p.1245·2).
Acid aspiration syndrome; gastro-oesophageal reflux; peptic ulcer; Zollinger-Ellison syndrome.

Ranamp *Ranbaxy, S.Afr.*
Ampicillin trihydrate (p.151·1).
Bacterial infections.

Ranaps *Approved Prescription Services, UK†.*
Ranitidine hydrochloride (p.1245·2).
Acid aspiration; dyspepsia; gastro-oesophageal reflux; gastrointestinal haemorrhage; peptic ulcer; Zollinger-Ellison syndrome.

Ranceph *Ranbaxy, S.Afr.*
Cefalexin (p.161·3).
Bacterial infections.

Rancil *Ranbaxy, Thai.*
Amoxicillin trihydrate (p.149·2).
Bacterial infections.

Ranclav *Ranbaxy, S.Afr.*
Amoxicillin (p.149·2); clavulanic acid (p.187·2).
Bacterial infections.

Randa *Kayaku, Jpn†.*
Cisplatin (p.525·1).
Malignant neoplasms.

Randum *Hoechst Marion Roussel, Ital.*
Metoclopramide hydrochloride (p.1235·2).
Gastrointestinal disorders.

Ranepal *Liferpal, Mex.*
Ranitidine (p.1246·3).
Peptic ulcer.

Ranestol *Parke, Davis, Neth.†.*
Bevantolol hydrochloride (p.849·1).
Angina pectoris; hypertension.

Ranezide *Parke, Davis, Neth.†.*
Bevantolol hydrochloride (p.849·1); hydrochlorothiazide (p.907·3).
Hypertension.

Ranfen *Ranbaxy, S.Afr.*
Ibuprofen (p.43·2).
Fever; inflammation; musculoskeletal, joint, and soft-tissue disorders; pain.

Rani *ABZ, Ger.; BASF, Ger.; Isis Puren, Ger.*
Ranitidine hydrochloride (p.1245·2).
Acid aspiration; gastro-oesophageal reflux; gastrointestinal haemorrhage; peptic ulcer; Zollinger-Ellison syndrome.

Rani 2 *Alphapharm, Austral.*
Ranitidine hydrochloride (p.1245·2).
Gastro-oesophageal reflux; peptic ulcer; Zollinger-Ellison syndrome.

Raniben *FIRMA, Ital.*
Ranitidine hydrochloride (p.1245·2).
Gastrointestinal disorders associated with hyperacidity.

Raniberl *Berlin-Chemie, Ger.*
Ranitidine hydrochloride (p.1245·2).
Acid aspiration; gastro-oesophageal reflux; gastrointestinal haemorrhage; peptic ulcer; Zollinger-Ellison syndrome.

Ranibeta *Betapharm, Ger.*
Ranitidine hydrochloride (p.1245·2).
Acid aspiration; gastro-oesophageal reflux; gastrointestinal haemorrhage; peptic ulcer; Zollinger-Ellison syndrome.

Ranibloc
Wolff, Ger.; Glaxo Allen, Ital.
Ranitidine hydrochloride (p.1245·2).
Acid aspiration; gastro-oesophageal reflux; gastrointestinal haemorrhage; peptic ulcer; Zollinger-Ellison syndrome.

Ranic *Glaxo Wellcome, Belg.*
Ranitidine hydrochloride (p.1245·2).
Gastro-oesophageal reflux.

Ranicid *M & H, Thai.*
Ranitidine hydrochloride (p.1245·2).
Gastro-oesophageal reflux; peptic ulcer; Zollinger-Ellison syndrome.

Ranicodan *Pharmacodane, Denm.*
Ranitidine (p.1246·3).
Acid aspiration; gastro-oesophageal reflux; peptic ulcer; Zollinger-Ellison syndrome.

Ranicur *Pharmacia Upjohn, Fin.*
Ranitidine hydrochloride (p.1245·2).
Acid aspiration; gastro-oesophageal reflux; peptic ulcer; Zollinger-Ellison syndrome.

Ranicux *TAD, Ger.*
Ranitidine hydrochloride (p.1245·2).
Acid aspiration; gastro-oesophageal reflux; gastrointestinal haemorrhage; peptic ulcer; Zollinger-Ellison syndrome.

Ranidil *Menarini, Ital.*
Ranitidine hydrochloride (p.1245·2).
Gastrointestinal disorders associated with hyperacidity.

Ranidin
Uniao Quimica, Braz.; Faes, Spain.
Ranitidine hydrochloride (p.1245·2).
Acid aspiration; gastro-oesophageal reflux; gastrointestinal haemorrhage; peptic ulcer; short-bowel syndrome; Zollinger-Ellison syndrome.

Ranidine *Biolab, Thai.*
Ranitidine (p.1246·3).
Gastro-oesophageal reflux; peptic ulcer; Zollinger-Ellison syndrome.

Ranidura T *Merck dura, Ger.*
Ranitidine hydrochloride (p.1245·2).
Acid aspiration; gastro-oesophageal reflux; gastrointestinal haemorrhage; peptic ulcer; Zollinger-Ellison syndrome.

Ranifarma *Continentales, Mex.*
Ranitidine (p.1246·3).

Ranifur *Fustery, Mex.*
Ranitidine (p.1246·3) or ranitidine hydrochloride (p.1245·2).
Acid aspiration; gastro-oesophageal reflux; gastrointestinal haemorrhage; peptic ulcer; Zollinger-Ellison syndrome.

Ranihexal
Hexal, Austral.; Hexal, S.Afr.
Ranitidine hydrochloride (p.1245·2).
Acid aspiration; gastro-oesophageal reflux; peptic ulcer; Zollinger-Ellison syndrome.

Ranikur *Opco, Denm.*
Ranitidine (p.1246·3).
Acid aspiration; gastro-oesophageal reflux; peptic ulcer; Zollinger-Ellison syndrome.

Ranil *Gea, Fin.*
Ranitidine hydrochloride (p.1245·2).
Acid aspiration; dyspepsia; gastro-oesophageal reflux; peptic ulcer; Zollinger-Ellison syndrome.

Ranilonga *Synthelabo, Spain.*
Ranitidine hydrochloride (p.1245·2).
Acid aspiration; gastro-oesophageal reflux; gastrointestinal haemorrhage; peptic ulcer; short-bowel syndrome; Zollinger-Ellison syndrome.

Ranimed *Ecosol, Switz.*
Ranitidine hydrochloride (p.1245·2).
Gastro-oesophageal reflux; peptic ulcer; Zollinger-Ellison syndrome.

Ranimerck *Merck dura, Ger.*
Ranitidine hydrochloride (p.1245·2).
Acid aspiration; gastro-oesophageal reflux; gastrointestinal haemorrhage; peptic ulcer; Zollinger-Ellison syndrome.

Ranimex *Orion, Fin.*
Ranitidine hydrochloride (p.1245·2).
Gastrointestinal disorders associated with hyperacidity.

Rani-nerton *Dolorgiet, Ger.*
Ranitidine hydrochloride (p.1245·2).
Acid aspiration; gastro-oesophageal reflux; gastrointestinal haemorrhage; peptic ulcer; Zollinger-Ellison syndrome.

Raniplex *Fournier, Fr.*
Ranitidine hydrochloride (p.1245·2).
Gastro-oesophageal reflux; peptic ulcer; Zollinger-Ellison syndrome.

Raniprotect *Wyeth, Ger.*
Ranitidine hydrochloride (p.1245·2).
Acid aspiration; gastro-oesophageal reflux; gastrointestinal haemorrhage; peptic ulcer; Zollinger-Ellison syndrome.

Rani-Q *Scand Pharm, Swed.*
Ranitidine hydrochloride (p.1245·2).
Gastro-oesophageal reflux; heartburn.

Ranisen *Senosiain, Mex.*
Ranitidine hydrochloride (p.1245·2).
Acid aspiration; gastro-oesophageal reflux; gastrointestinal haemorrhage; peptic ulcer; Zollinger-Ellison syndrome.

Ranitic
Hexal, Ger.; Rowex, Irl.; Hexal, UK.
Ranitidine hydrochloride (p.1245·2).
Acid aspiration; chronic dyspepsia; gastro-oesophageal reflux; gastrointestinal haemorrhage; peptic ulcer; Zollinger-Ellison syndrome.

Ranitil *EMS, Braz.*
Ranitidine hydrochloride (p.1245·2).
Acid aspiration; gastro-oesophageal reflux; gastrointestinal haemorrhage; peptic ulcer; Zollinger-Ellison syndrome.

Ranitine *Azevedos, Port.*
Ranitidine hydrochloride (p.1245·2).
Gastro-oesophageal reflux; peptic ulcer; Zollinger-Ellison syndrome.

Ranivel *Duncan, Spain.*
Ranitidine hydrochloride (p.1245·2).
Gastrointestinal hyperacidity.

Ranix *Knoll, Spain.*
Ranitidine hydrochloride (p.1245·2).
Acid aspiration; gastro-oesophageal reflux; gastrointestinal haemorrhage; peptic ulcer; short-bowel syndrome; Zollinger-Ellison syndrome.

Ranixal *Medinovum, Fin.*
Ranitidine hydrochloride (p.1245·2).
Acid aspiration; gastro-oesophageal reflux; peptic ulcer; Zollinger-Ellison syndrome.

Ranmoxy *Ranbaxy, S.Afr.*
Amoxicillin trihydrate (p.149·2).
Bacterial infections.

Ranopine *Pinewood, Irl.*
Ranitidine hydrochloride (p.1245·2).
Gastric hyperacidity; gastro-oesophageal reflux; peptic ulcer; Zollinger-Ellison syndrome.

Ranoprin *Medinovum, Fin.*
Propranolol hydrochloride (p.962·3).
Angina pectoris; arrhythmias; essential tremor; glaucoma; hypertension; hyperthyroidism; hypertrophic obstructive cardiomyopathy; migraine; myocardial infarction.

Ranoxyl
Note. This name is used for preparations of different composition.
Douglas, Austral.
Ranitidine hydrochloride (p.1245·2).
Gastro-oesophageal reflux; petic ulcer; Zollinger-Ellison syndrome.

Ranbaxy, Singapore.
Amoxicillin trihydrate (p.149·2).
Bacterial infections.

Ranozol *ST, Thai.*
Miconazole nitrate (p.391·1).
Fungal skin infections.

Ranpuric *Triomed, S.Afr.*
Allopurinol (p.397·2).
Gout; hyperuricaemia.

Rantag *Julphar, UAE.*
Ranitidine hydrochloride (p.1245·2).
Acid aspiration; dyspepsia; gastro-oesophageal reflux; gastrointestinal haemorrhage; peptic ulcer; Zollinger-Ellison syndrome.

Rantec *Berk, UK.*
Ranitidine hydrochloride (p.1245·2).
Acid aspiration; dyspepsia; gastro-oesophageal reflux; gastrointestinal haemorrhage; peptic ulcer; Zollinger-Ellison syndrome.

Ranteen *Aspen, S.Afr.*
Ranitidine hydrochloride (p.1245·2).
Acid aspiration; gastro-oesophageal reflux; peptic ulcer; Zollinger-Ellison syndrome.

Ranthrocin *Ranbaxy, Singapore.*
Erythromycin ethyl succinate (p.201·2).
Bacterial infections.

Rantudil
Bayer, Ger.; Bayer, Mex.; Bial, Port.; Bayer, Singapore.
Acemetacin (p.11·2).
Gout; inflammation; musculoskeletal, joint, peri-articular, and soft-tissue disorders; pain; thrombophlebitis; vasculitis.

Ranuber *ICN, Spain.*
Ranitidine hydrochloride (p.1245·2).
Acid aspiration; gastro-oesophageal reflux; gastrointestinal haemorrhage; peptic ulcer; short-bowel syndrome; Zollinger-Ellison syndrome.

Ranulin *Pisa, Mex.*
Ranitidine (p.1246·3).

Ranvil *Gentili, Ital.*
Nicardipine hydrochloride (p.938·3).
Angina pectoris; heart failure; hypertension.

Ranzil *Tocogino, Mex.*
Ranitidine (p.1246·3).

Ranzol *Ranbaxy, S.Afr.*
Cefazolin sodium (p.164·3).
Bacterial infections.

Rapaid First Aid *Rye, Austral.*
Melaleuca oil (p.1631·3).
Bites; minor wounds; skin infections; skin irritation; stings.

Rapaid Medicated *Rye, Austral.*
Melaleuca oil (p.1631·3); zinc oxide (p.1128·2).
Skin disorders.

Rapako S *Bilgast, Ger.*
Homoeopathic preparation.

Rapako xylo *Bilgast, Ger.*
Xylometazoline hydrochloride (p.1102·2).
Rhinitis.

Rapamic *Cipan, Port.*
Ketoconazole (p.389·1).
Fungal infections.

Rapamune
Wyeth, UK; Wyeth-Ayerst, USA.
Sirolimus (p.568·2).
Renal transplant rejection.

Rap-eze *Roche Consumer, UK.*
Calcium carbonate (p.1215·1).
Dyspepsia; heartburn.

Raphanus S Potier *Pharmethic, Belg.*
Raphanus sativus niger.
Dyspepsia associated with biliary dyskinesia.

Rapicort *Malesci, Ital.†.*
Hydrocortisone sodium succinate (p.1074·1).
Shock.

Rapidal *Bial-Aristegui, Spain.*
Terfenadine (p.424·3).
Hypersensitivity reactions.

Rapidocaine *Sintetica, Switz.*
Lignocaine [lidocaine] hydrochloride (p.1313·2).
Adrenaline [epinephrine] hydrochloride (p.829·2) is included in some injections as a vasoconstrictor to diminish absorption and localise the effect of the local anaesthetic.
Arrhythmias; local anaesthesia.

Rapidol
Note. This name is used for preparations of different composition.
Pharmonta, Aust.
Paracetamol (p.71·2); propyphenazone (p.80·2); caffeine (p.761·3).
Fever; pain.

Ranbaxy, Singapore.
Paracetamol (p.71·2).
Fever; pain.

RapidVue *Quidel, USA.*
Pregnancy test (p.1654·3).

Rapifen
Janssen-Cilag, Aust.; Zeneca, Austral.; Janssen-Cilag, Belg.; Janssen, Braz.; Janssen-Cilag, Denm.; Orion, Fin.; Janssen-Cilag, Fr.; Janssen-Cilag, Ger.; Janssen, Hong Kong; Janssen-Cilag, Irl.; Janssen, Israel; Janssen, Mex.; Janssen-Cilag, Neth.; Janssen-Cilag, Norw.; Janssen-Cilag, NZ; Janssen, S.Afr.; Janssen-Cilag, Swed.; Janssen-Cilag, Switz.; Janssen-Cilag, UK.
Alfentanil hydrochloride (p.11·3).
Induction of general anaesthesia; pain during surgical procedures.

The symbol † denotes a preparation no longer actively marketed

Rapignost Basic Screen Plus *Hoechst Marion Roussel, Irl.*
Test for ascorbic acid, glucose, protein, blood, pH, and nitrites in urine.

Rapignost Diabetes Profile *Hoechst Marion Roussel, Irl.*
Test for ketones, ascorbic acid, and glucose in urine.

Rapignost Total Screen L *Hoechst Marion Roussel, Irl.*
Test for bilirubin, urobilinogen, pH, glucose, protein, ketones, blood, nitrite, ascorbic acid, and leucocytes in urine.

Rapilysin
Boehringer Mannheim, Aust.; Roche, Austral.; Roche, Belg.; Roche, Denm.; Roche, Fin.; Roche, Fr.; Roche, Ger.; Roche, Irl.; Roche, Ital.; Roche, Neth.; Roche, Norw.; Roche, NZ; Roche, Port.; Roche Diagnostics, Spain; Roche, Swed.; Roche, Switz.; Roche, UK.
Reteplase (p.968·2).
Myocardial infarction.

Rapi-snooze *Medinaturals, UK.*
Melatonin (p.1632·1); pyridoxine (p.1387·1); valerian (p.1678·3).

Rapitard *Novo Nordisk, Ger.†.*
Biphasic insulin injection (bovine with porcine, mono-component) (p.324·1).
Diabetes mellitus.

Rapitard MC
Novo Nordisk, Fr.†; Novo Nordisk, Switz.†; Novo Nordisk, UK†.
Biphasic insulin injection (bovine with porcine, mono-component) (p.324·1).
Diabetes mellitus.

Rapitil *Rhône-Poulenc Rorer, UK.*
Nedocromil sodium (p.768·3).
Allergic conjunctivitis; keratoconjunctivitis.

Rapitux *Boehringer Ingelheim, Ital.*
Levodropropizine (p.1089·3).
Coughs.

Rapivir *Glaxo Wellcome, Mex.*
Valaciclovir hydrochloride (p.643·1).
Herpes simplex infections; varicella-zoster infections.

Raplon *Organon, USA.*
Rapacuronium bromide (p.1339·2).
Competitive neuromuscular blocker.

Rapolyte *Helsinn Birex, Irl.*
Sodium chloride; potassium chloride; sodium citrate; glucose (p.1185·2).
Diarrhoea; oral rehydration therapy.

Rappell *Pfizer Consumer, UK.*
Piperonal (p.1436·2).
Head lice repellent.

Rapura *Globopharm, Switz.*
Peru balsam (p.1650·2); camphor (p.1589·3); thymol (p.1158·3); zinc oxide (p.1128·2).
Minor skin lesions.

Rarical *Cilag, Braz.*
Multivitamin and mineral preparation (p.1350·1).

Rariplex *União Química, Braz.*
Multivitamin and mineral preparation (p.1350·1).

RAS *Wiedemann, Ger.†.*
Antireticular serum (rabbit).
Tonic.

Rasal *Ipsen, Spain.*
Olsalazine sodium (p.1238·3).
Ulcerative colitis.

Rasilvax *Chiron, Ital.*
A rabies vaccine (human diploid cell) (p.1560·2).
Active immunisation.

Rastinon
Hoechst Marion Roussel, Aust.; Hoechst Marion Roussel, Austral.; Hoechst Marion Roussel, Belg.†; Hoechst, Ger.†; Hoechst Marion Roussel, Hong Kong; Hoechst Marion Roussel, Irl.†; Hoechst Marion Roussel, Ital.†; Hoechst Marion Roussel, Neth.; Hoechst Marion Roussel, Neth.†; Hoechst Marion Roussel, S.Afr.†; Hoechst Marion Roussel, Spain; Hoechst Marion Roussel, Switz.†; Hoechst Marion Roussel, UK†.
Tolbutamide (p.336·3).
Diabetes mellitus.

Ratacand *Astra, Ital.*
Candesartan cilexetil (p.853·2).
Hypertension.

Ratic *Atlantic, Thai.*
Ranitidine (p.1246·3).
Peptic ulcer; Zollinger-Ellison syndrome.

Ratica *LBS, Thai.*
Ranitidine (p.1246·3).
Gastro-oesophageal reflux; peptic ulcer.

ratioAllerg *Ratiopharm, Ger.*
Cream: Hydrocortisone (p.1073·3).
Skin disorders.

Nasal spray: Beclometasone dipropionate (p.1061·2).
Hayfever.

Topical gel: Diphenhydramine hydrochloride (p.416·1).
Hypersensitivity reactions.

ratioDolor *Ratiopharm, Ger.*
Ibuprofen lysine (p.44·1).
Fever; pain.

ratioGast *Ratiopharm, Ger.*
Capsules: Tormentil (p.1674·1).
Diarrhoea.

Oral drops: Anise oil (p.1580·3); fennel oil (p.1610·2); caraway oil (p.1591·2).
Dyspepsia.

ratioGrippal + C *Ratiopharm, Ger.*
Aspirin (p.14·2); paracetamol (p.71·2); ascorbic acid (p.1389·3).
Cold symptoms.

ratioHepar *Ratiopharm, Ger.*
Cynara (p.1601·3).
Biliary disorders.

ratioMobil *Ratiopharm, Ger.*
Piroxicam (p.79·1).
Musculoskeletal, joint, peri-articular, and soft-tissue disorders.

Rationale *Manetti Roberts, Ital.*
Colextran hydrochloride (p.865·1).
Hyperlipidaemias.

Rationasal *Ratiopharm, Spain.*
Xylometazoline hydrochloride (p.1102·2).
Nasal congestion; sinusitis.

ratiopyrin *Ratiopharm, Ger.*
Aspirin (p.14·2); paracetamol (p.71·2); caffeine (p.761·3).
Pain.

ratioSept *Ratiopharm, Ger.*
Rhatany root (p.1657·3).
Mouth inflammation.

Raudil *Novag, Mex.*
Ranitidine (p.1246·3).
Acid aspiration; gastro-oesophageal reflux; gastrointestinal haemorrhage; peptic ulcer; Zollinger-Ellison syndrome.

Raudopen *Alter, Spain.*
Amoxicillin trihydrate (p.149·2).
Bacterial infections.

Raufuncton N *Knoll, Ger.*
Rauwolfiae vomitoria (p.967·2); squill (p.1100·3); convallaria (p.1599·1); adonis vernalis (p.1573·3).
Arrhythmias; hypertension.

Rauserpin *Breves, Braz.*
Reserpine (p.967·3).
Hypertension; Raynaud's syndrome.

RauwolfiaViscomp *Schuck, Ger.*
Homoeopathic preparation.

Rauwolsan H *Pflüger, Ger.*
Homoeopathic preparation.

Rauwoplant *Schwabe, Ger.*
Rauwolfia (p.967·2); crataegus (p.1600·2).
Hypertension.

Rauzide *Apothecon, USA.*
Rauwolfia serpentina (p.967·2); bendroflumethiazide [bendrofluazide] (p.844·1).
Hypertension.

Ravalgen *SmithKline Beecham OTC, Ger.*
Garlic oil.
Arteriosclerosis.

Ravamil *Merck, S.Afr.*
Verapamil hydrochloride (p.989·1).
Angina pectoris; arrhythmias; hypertension.

Ravenol *Caber, Ital.*
A heparinoid (p.905·2).
Vascular disorders with a risk of thrombosis.

Raveron *Germania, Aust.; Asta Medica, Braz.*
Prostate extract.
Benign prostatic hyperplasia.

Ravigona *Roche Nicholas, Spain†.*
Vitamin A palmitate (p.1383·2); tocoferil acetate (p.1394·1).
Eye disorders; male infertility.

Ravocaine and Novocain *Cook-Waite, USA†.*
Propoxycaine hydrochloride (p.1319·2); procaine (p.1319·2).
Noradrenaline [norepinephrine] (p.948·2) is included as a vasoconstrictor to diminish absorption and localise the effect of the local anaesthetic.
Local anaesthesia.

Raxamida *Arlex, Mex.*
Loperamide (p.1232·1).

Raxar
Glaxo Wellcome, Aust.†; Glaxo Wellcome, Austral.†; Glaxo Wellcome, Canad.†; Glaxo Wellcome, Denm.†; Glaxo Wellcome, Israel†; Glaxo Wellcome, Mex.†; Glaxo Wellcome, Neth.†; Glaxo Wellcome, Switz.†.; Glaxo Wellcome, UK†; Glaxo Wellcome, USA†.
Grepafloxacin hydrochloride (p.214·1).
Bacterial infections.

Raxedin *Química y Farmacia, Mex.*
Loperamide (p.1232·1).

Ray Block *Del-Ray, USA.*
SPF 15: Padimate O (p.1518·2); oxybenzone (p.1518·1).
Sunscreen.

Rayepen *Rayere, Mex.*
Ampicillin (p.150·3).
Bacterial infections.

Rayetetra *Rayere, Mex.*
Tetracycline (p.258·3).
Bacterial infections.

Rayne *Fustery, Mex.*
Diazepam (p.674·3).

Rayvist *Schering, Switz.†.*
Meglumine ioglicate (p.1034·3) or meglumine ioglicate and sodium ioglicate (p.1034·3).
Radiographic contrast medium.

Rayvist 180 *Schering, Aust.*
Meglumine ioglicate (p.1034·3).
Radiographic contrast medium.

Razoxin *Cambridge, UK.*
Razoxane (p.567·2).
Now known as Razoxane Tablets.
Malignant neoplasms.

RBC *Rybar, Irl.; Co-Pharma, UK.*
Antazoline hydrochloride (p.408·3); calamine (p.1111·3); cetrimide (p.1137·1).
Insect stings; pruritus; skin irritation.

R-Cetate *GHP, Thai.*
Electrolyte infusion with or without glucose (p.1180·1).
Carbohydrate source; fluid and electrolyte disorders.

RCF *Ross, USA.*
Carbohydrate-free soy protein feed (p.1350·1).
Ketogenic diet; milk carbohydrate intolerance.

R-Den *Nakorn, Thai.*
21 Tablets, levonorgestrel (p.1486·2); ethinylestradiol (p.1476·2); 7 tablets, inert.
Combined oral contraceptive.

Reabilan
Nestle, Fr.; Clintec, Irl.†; Nestle, UK†; Galagen, USA.
A range of preparations for enteral nutrition (p.1350·1).

Reach Junior Fluoride *Johnson & Johnson, Irl.*
Sodium fluoride (p.1375·3).
Dental care.

Reactine *Pfizer Consumer, Canad.*
Cetirizine hydrochloride (p.411·2).
Allergic rhinitis; urticaria.

Reactine Plus *Pfizer Consumer, Canad.*
Tablets, cetirizine hydrochloride (p.411·2); extended-release capsules, pseudoephedrine hydrochloride (p.1099·2).
Allergic rhinitis; urticaria.

Reactivan *Merck, S.Afr.*
Fencamfamin hydrochloride (p.1509·3); vitamins (p.1350·1).
Tonic.

Reafix *Gemballa, Braz.*
Oral rehydration solution (p.1185·2).
Oral rehydration therapy.

Real Lemon Cold Powders *Sterwin, UK.*
Paracetamol (p.71·2); phenylephrine (p.1097·1); ascorbic acid (p.1389·3).
Cold symptoms.

Realderm *Reall, Switz.*
Zinc oxide (p.1128·2); glycerol (p.1616·3); aluminium acetotartrate (p.1578·2).
Nappy rash; skin irritation.

Realdrax *Liferpal, Mex.*
Ibuprofen (p.43·2).
Inflammation; pain.

Real-Vit *Solfran, Mex.*
Multivitamin preparation (p.1350·1).

Reapam *Parke, Davis, Neth.*
Prazepam (p.701·1).
Anxiety.

Reasec
Janssen-Cilag, Belg.†; Janssen-Cilag, Ger.†; Janssen-Cilag, Ital.†; Janssen-Cilag, Switz.
Diphenoxylate hydrochloride (p.1222·2).
Atropine sulfate (p.461·1) is included in this preparation to discourage abuse.
Diarrhoea.

Re-Azo *Reese, USA.*
Phenazopyridine hydrochloride (p.77·3).

Rebacil *New Research, Ital.*
Bacampicillin hydrochloride (p.155·1).
Bacterial infections.

ReBalance *Zeller, Switz.*
Hypericum (p.290·2).
Anxiety disorders; insomnia.

Rebetol
Schering-Plough, Aust.; Schering-Plough, Denm.; Schering-Plough, Fin.; Schering-Plough, Fr.; Essex, Ger.; Schering-Plough, Irl.; Schering-Plough, Ital.; Schering-Plough, Neth.; Schering-Plough, Port.; Schering-Plough, Spain; Schering-Plough, Swed.; Schering-Plough, UK.
Ribavirin (p.639·1).
For use in combination with interferon alfa-2b.
Hepatitis C.

Rebetron
Schering-Plough, Austral.; Schering, Canad.; Schering, USA.
Injection, interferon alfa-2b (Intron A) (p.628·1); capsules, ribavirin (Rebetol) (p.639·1).
Chronic hepatitis C.

Rebif
Serono, Aust.; Serono, Austral.; Serono, Canad.; Serono, Denm.; Serono, Fin.; Serono, Fr.; Serono, Ger.; Serono, Hong Kong; Serono, Irl.; ASI, Israel; Serono, Ital.; Serono, Mex.; Serono, Neth.; Serono, Norw.; Serono, Port.; Serono, Singapore; Serono, Spain; Serono, Swed.; Serono, Switz.; Serono, Thai.; Serono, UK.
Interferon beta-1a (p.632·2).
Multiple sclerosis.

Rebladerm *Dermoteca, Port.*
Urea (p.1127·3).
Dry skin disorders.

Reca *Cantabria, Spain.*
Enalapril maleate (p.883·3).
Heart failure; hypertension.

Recal *New Research, Ital.*
Calcium carbonate (p.1215·1).
Calcium deficiency.

Recalplex *Cazi, Braz.*
Vitamin B substances (p.1350·1).
Nutritional supplement.

Recarcin *Sanum-Kehlbeck, Ger.*
Bacillus firmus.
Immunotherapy; joint disorders; rheumatism; sciatica.

Recatol Algin *Riemser, Ger.*
Alginic acid (p.1498·3); carmellose sodium (p.1499·3).
Obesity.

Recatol mono *Riemser, Ger.*
Phenylpropanolamine hydrochloride (p.1098·1).
Obesity.

Recatol N *Riemser, Ger.*
Phenylpropanolamine hydrochloride (p.1098·1); thiamine hydrochloride (p.1385·1); pyridoxine hydrochloride (p.1386·3); ascorbic acid (p.1389·3).
Obesity.

Recef *Uno, Ital.*
Cefazolin sodium (p.164·3).
Bacterial infections.

Receptozine *Be-Tabs, S.Afr.*
Promethazine hydrochloride (p.423·2).
Hypersensitivity.

Recessan
Note.This name is used for preparations of different composition.
Provita, Aust.†.
Tyrothricin (p.267·1); thymol (p.1158·3); pancreatin (p.1646·1); lauromacrogol 400 (p.1345·2).
Infections and pain of the mouth and lips.

Kreussler, Ger.
Lauromacrogol 400 (p.1345·2).
Mouth and throat inflammation.

Recilugo *Ariston, Braz.*
Ethenzamide (p.35·1); nicotinylpyrazolone; orphenadrine (p.471·1).
Skeletal muscle spasm.

Recipect *Orion, Fin.*
Codeine phosphate (p.25·2); guaifenesin (p.1092·2).
Coughs.

Reclomide *Major, USA.*
Metoclopramide hydrochloride (p.1235·2).
Nausea and vomiting.

Recocef *Julphar, UAE.*
Cefaclor (p.161·1).
Bacterial infections.

Recofen *Reese, USA.*
Guaifenesin (p.1092·2); dextromethorphan hydrobromide (p.1087·3).

Recofen-D *Reese, USA.*
Guaifenesin (p.1092·2); dextromethorphan hydrobromide (p.1087·3).

Recofol
Leiras, Denm.†; Leiras, Fin.; Leiras, Israel; Schering, Israel; Pisa, Mex.; Leiras, Norw.; Organon, Port.; Leiras, Singapore; Schering, Spain; Schering, Swed.; Schering, Switz.
Propofol (p.1265·3).
General anaesthesia; sedative.

Recombinant H-B Vax II *Merck Sharp & Dohme, Israel.*
A hepatitis B vaccine (p.1542·2).
Active immunisation.

Recombinate
CSL, Austral.; Baxter, Belg.; Baxter, Canad.; Baxter, Denm.; Baxter, Fin.; Baxter, Fr.; Baxter, Ger.; Baxter, Ital.; Baxter, Jpn; Baxter, NZ; Baxter, Port.†; Baxter, Spain; Baxter, Swed.; ZLB, Switz.; Baxter, UK; Baxter, USA.
A factor VIII preparation (recombinant) (p.734·1).
Haemorrhagic disorders.

Recombivax HB
Merck Frosst, Canad.; Pasteur Merieux, Ital.; Aventis, Port.; Pasteur Merieux, Spain; Merck, USA.
A hepatitis B vaccine (recombinant DNA) (p.1542·2).
Active immunisation.

Reconovan *Fresenius, UK.*
Preparation for enteral nutrition (p.1350·1).

Recormon
Roche, Aust.; Boehringer Mannheim, Belg.†; Ercopharm, Denm.†; Boehringer Mannheim, Fr.†; Boehringer Mannheim, Ger.†; Roche, Hong Kong; Boehringer Mannheim, Irl.; Boehringer Mannheim, Israel; Lakeside, Mex.; Boehringer Mannheim, Neth.†; Boehringer Mannheim, Norw.†; Boehringer Mannheim, Port.†; Roche, S.Afr.; Roche, Singapore; Roche, Switz.; Roche, Thai.; Boehringer Mannheim, UK†.
Epoetin beta (p.1061·1).
Anaemias; autologous blood transfusions.

Recort Plus *Reese, USA.*
Hydrocortisone (p.1073·3).
Skin disorders.

Recoveron *Armstrong, Mex.*
Sodium acexamate (p.1572·2).
Burns; ulcers; wounds.

Recoveron N *Armstrong, Mex.*
Sodium acexamate (p.1572·2); neomycin sulfate (p.228·1).
Infected wounds; skin infections.

Recovery Food *Milupa, Irl.†.*
Food for special diet (p.1350·1).

Recozil *Recon, Singapore.*
Gemfibrozil (p.896·2).
Hyperlipidaemias.

Rectacaine *Reese, USA.*
Ointment: Phenylephrine hydrochloride (p.1097·1); shark-liver oil.

Suppositories: Phenylephrine hydrochloride (p.1097·1).

Rectagene II *Pfeiffer, USA†.*
Bismuth subgallate (p.1213·2); bismuth resorcinol compound (p.1214·1); benzyl benzoate (p.1428·2); zinc oxide (p.1128·2); bismuth oxyiodide (p.1214·1); calcium phosphate (p.1188·3); peru balsam (p.1650·2).
Haemorrhoids.

Rectagene Medicated Balm *Pfeiffer, USA.*
Yeast (p.1398·1); shark-liver oil.
Haemorrhoids.

Rectagene Medicated Rectal Balm *Pfeiffer, USA.*
Benzocaine (p.1306·2); phenylephrine hydrochloride (p.1097·1); bismuth subgallate (p.1213·2); zinc oxide (p.1128·2); mepyramine maleate (p.421·1).
Anorectal disorders.

Rectalad *Carter-Wallace, Austral.*
Docusate sodium (p.1223·1).
Bowel evacuation; constipation.

Rectamigdol *Diviser Aquilea, Spain.*
Bismuth camphocarbonate (p.1214·1).
Sore throat.

Rectanus *Herals, Braz.*
Tribenoside (p.1674·2); lignocaine [lidocaine] (p.1313·2).
Haemorrhoids.

Rectinol *G.P. Laboratories, Austral.*
Adrenaline [epinephrine] (p.829·1); benzocaine (p.1306·2); zinc oxide (p.1128·2).
Anorectal disorders.

Rectinol HC *Pfizer, Austral.*
Cinchocaine hydrochloride (p.1309·1); hydrocortisone (p.1073·3).
Anorectol disorders.

Rectiole *Caldeira & Metelo, Port.*
Glycerol (p.1616·3).
Bowel evacuation; constipation.

Recto Bronco Tosse *Labocor, Port.†*
Quinine sulfate (p.445·1); camphor (p.1589·3); niaouli oil (p.1640·2); terpin hydrate (p.1101·2).
Coughs.

Recto Menaderm *Menarini, Spain†.*
Beclometasone dipropionate (p.1061·2); clioquinol (p.190·2); heparin (p.902·1); cod-liver oil (p.1357·2); lignocaine [lidocaine] hydrochloride (p.1313·2).
Anorectal disorders.

Recto Menaderm NF *Merck, Spain.*
Beclometasone dipropionate (p.1061·2).
Anorectal disorders.

Recto Mugolio *Warner-Lambert, Ital.†*
Pumilio pine oil (p.1656·3).
Respiratory-tract disorders.

Rectocort
Welcker-Lyster, Canad.†; Rougier, Hong Kong.
Hydrocortisone acetate (p.1073·3).
Haemorrhoids.

Rectodelt *Trommsdorff, Ger.*
Prednisone (p.1079·2).
Rectal corticosteroid.

Rectogel *Riva, Canad.*
Benzocaine (p.1306·2); zinc sulfate (p.1398·2).
Anorectal disorders.

Rectogel HC *Riva, Canad.*
Benzocaine (p.1306·2); zinc sulfate (p.1398·2); hydrocortisone acetate (p.1073·3).
Anorectal disorders.

Rectogesic *Cellegy, Austral.*
Glyceryl trinitrate (p.897·3).
Anal fissure.

Rectopanbiline *Sarget, Fr.*
Bile extract (p.1585·1); gelatin (p.737·2); glycerol (p.1616·3).
Formerly contained bile extract, hepatica, and boldo.
Bowel evacuation; constipation.

Rectophedrol *Martin, Fr.†*
Eucalyptol (p.1609·2); guaiacol carbonate (p.1092·1); wild thyme oil; camphor (p.1589·3); ephedrine (p.1090·1); procaine hydrochloride (p.1319·1).
Respiratory-tract disorders.

Rectoplexil
Note. This name is used for preparations of different composition.
Rhone-Poulenc Rorer, Belg.
Oxomemazine (p.422·2); guaifenesin (p.1092·2); sodium benzoate (p.1134·3); paracetamol (p.71·2).
Coughs.

Theraplix, Fr.†.
Oxomemazine (p.422·2).
Formerly contained oxomemazine, guaifenesin, sodium benzoate, and paracetamol.
Coughs.

Rectopred *Jacoby, Aust.*
Prednisolone sodium phosphate (p.1078·1).
Croup.

Rectopulmo Adultos *Salusif, Port.*
Camphor (p.1589·3); eucalyptol (p.1609·2); niaouli oil (p.1640·2); quimica sulfate.
Respiratory tract disorders.

Rectopulmo Infantil *Salusif, Port.*
Camphor (p.1589·3); eucalyptol (p.1609·2); niaouli oil (p.1640·2).
Respiratory tract disorders.

Rectoquintyl *Sodip, Switz.*
Ethyl orthoformate (p.1091·3); wild thyme oil; eucalyptol (p.1609·2).
Coughs.

Rectoquintyl-Promethazine *Sodip, Switz.*
Ethyl orthoformate (p.1091·3); promethazine (p.423·2); wild thyme oil; eucalyptol (p.1609·2).
Coughs.

Rectoquotane *Medeva, Fr.*
Quinisocaine hydrochloride (p.1320·2); cetrimide (p.1137·1).

Formerly contained quinisocaine hydrochloride, esculoside, ephedrine hydrochloride, and cetrimonium bromide.
Anorectal disorders.

Recto-Reparil *Madaus, Ital.*
Aescin (p.1574·1); amethocaine [tetracaine] hydrochloride (p.1305·2).
Formerly contained aescin, belladonna, and amethocaine [tetracaine] hydrochloride.
Anorectal disorders.

Rectosan *Terramin, Aust.*
Naphazoline hydrochloride (p.1095·1); menthol (p.1632·3); benzocaine (p.1306·2).
Anorectal disorders.

Rectosan 'A' *Lennon, S.Afr.†*
Zinc oxide (p.1128·2); resorcinol (p.1122·2); bismuth subgallate (p.1213·2); peru balsam (p.1650·2); belladonna (p.463·1); benzocaine (p.1306·2).
Haemorrhoids.

Rectosellan *Mann, Ger.†.*
Aesculus (p.1574·1); melilotus officinalis.
Haemorrhoids.

Rectosellan H *Mann, Ger.†.*
Ointment: Lauromacrogol 400 (p.1345·2); zinc oxide (p.1128·2).
Anorectal disorders.
Suppositories: Zinc oxide (p.1128·2); benzocaine (p.1306·2).
Haemorrhoids.

Rectoseptal-Neo bismuthe *Actipharm, Switz.*
Bismuth succinate (p.1214·1); eucalyptol (p.1609·2); terpin hydrate (p.1101·2); potassium hydroxyquinoline sulfate hydrate (p.1654·2).
Pharyngeal disorders.

Rectoseptal-Neo Pholcodine *Actipharm, Switz.*
Guaiacol (p.1092·1); eucalyptol (p.1609·2); terpin hydrate (p.1101·2); pholcodine (p.1099·1).
Respiratory-tract disorders.

Rectoseptal-Neo simple *Actipharm, Switz.*
Guaiacol (p.1092·1); eucalyptol (p.1609·2); terpin hydrate (p.1101·2); potassium hydroxyquinoline sulfate hydrate (p.1654·2).
Respiratory-tract disorders.

Rectovalone
Jouveinal, Canad.†; Parke, Davis, Fr.†; Byk, Neth.; Juste, Spain.
Tixocortol pivalate (p.1080·1).
Haemorrhagic rectocolitis; ulcerative colitis; ulcerative proctitis.

Rectovasol *Qualiphar, Belg.*
Bismuth subgallate (p.1213·2); bismuth oxyiodogallate (p.1214·1); zinc oxide (p.1128·2); aesculus (p.1574·1); hamamelis (p.1618·3); amylocaine (p.1306·1); peru balsam (p.1650·2).
Haemorrhoids.

Rectozorin *Teva, Israel.*
Ointment: Bismuth oxychloride (p.1214·1); thymol iodide (p.1158·3); zinc oxide (p.1128·2); benzocaine (p.1306·2); menthol (p.1632·3).
Suppositories: Bismuth subgallate (p.1213·2); thymol iodide (p.1158·3); zinc oxide (p.1128·2); benzocaine (p.1306·2); menthol (p.1632·3); tannic acid (p.1669·1).
Haemorrhoids.

Recvalysat *Ysatfabrik, Ger.*
Valerian (p.1678·3).
Agitation; sleep disorders.

Recycline *Rekah, Israel.*
Tetracycline hydrochloride (p.258·3).
Bacterial eye and skin infections.

Red Away *Rivex, Canad.*
Naphazoline hydrochloride (p.1095·1).

Red Cross Canker Sore Medication *Mentholatum, USA†.*
Benzocaine (p.1306·2).
Canker sores.

Red Cross Toothache *Mentholatum, USA.*
Eugenol (p.1609·3).
Toothache.

Red Kooga *Peter Black, UK.*
Ginseng (p.1615·3).
Tonic.

Red Kooga Betalife *Peter Black, UK.*
Multivitamin preparation with ginseng, selenium, and fish oil (p.1350·1).

Red Kooga Co-Q-10 and Ginseng *Peter Black, UK.*
Ginseng (p.1615·3); ubidecarenone (p.1677·1).
Tonic.

Red Kooga Sport *English Grains, UK†.*
Multivitamin preparation with ginseng, iron, and glucose (p.1350·1).
Tonic.

Red Oil *Nella, UK.*
Methyl nicotinate (p.55·1); volatile mustard oil (p.1639·1); clove oil (p.1597·1); arachis oil (p.1581·1).
Muscle pain.

Red Point *Synpharma, Aust.*
Camphor (p.1589·3); citral; anise oil (p.1580·3); eucalyptus oil (p.1609·2); methyl salicylate (p.55·1); citronella oil (p.1596·3); niaouli oil (p.1640·2); rosemary oil (p.1243·3); thyme oil (p.1672·3); peppermint oil (p.1659·3); cayenne pepper (p.1591·1); mustard oil (p.1639·1); arnica (p.1581·3).
Musculoskeletal and joint disorders.

Red Seal Liquid Calcium *Ancient, Austral.*
Calcium carbonate (p.1215·1); ergocalciferol (p.1391·2).
Osteoporosis.

Redacid *Maver, Mex.*
Ranitidine (p.1246·3).
Peptic ulcer.

Redactiv
Wassermann, Ital.; Glaxo Wellcome, Mex.
Rifaximin (p.246·3).
Bacterial skin infections; gastrointestinal infections.

Redaflam *Maver, Mex.*
Nimesulide (p.62·3).
Fever; inflammation; pain.

Redalip *Maver, Mex.*
Bezafibrate (p.849·1).
Hypercholesterolaemia.

Redap *Galderma, Denm.*
Adapalene (p.1109·3).
Acne.

Redaxa fit *Hotz, Ger.*
Equisetum (p.1606·3).
Water retention.

Redaxa Lax *Palmical, Ger.†.*
Rhubarb (p.1248·1); aloes (p.1210·1).
Constipation.

Redeptin *Janssen-Cilag, Irl.*
Fluspirilene (p.686·1).
Schizophrenia.

Redergin *Lek, Thai.*
Co-dergocrine mesilate (p.1597·3).
Cerebrovascular disorders; hypertension; migraine and other vascular headache; peripheral vascular disorders.

Redergot *OM, Port.†.*
Co-dergocrine mesilate (p.1597·3).
Cerebral and peripheral vascular disorders.

Redipred
Rhone-Poulenc Rorer, Austral.; Aventis, NZ.
Prednisolone sodium phosphate (p.1078·1).
Corticosteroid.

Redisol *Unison, Thai.*
Cyanocobalamin (p.1388·1).
Schilling test; vitamin B$_{12}$ deficiency.

Redken Solve Acid Balance *Redken, Canad.*
Pyrithione zinc (p.1122·1).
Dandruff.

Redol Comp *Orion, Fin.*
Dextromethorphan hydrobromide (p.1087·1); salbutamol sulfate (p.770·3).
Respiratory-tract disorders.

Redolet *Solfran, Mex.*
Oxyphenbutazone (p.71·1).
Inflammation.

Redomex *Lundbeck, Belg.*
Amitriptyline hydrochloride (p.273·3).
Depression; pain.

ReDormin
Flordis, Austral.
Valerian (p.1678·3); lupulus (p.1629·3).
Sleep disorders.
Zeller, Switz.
Syrup: Valerian (p.1678·3).
Tablets: Valerian (p.1678·3); lupulus (p.1629·3).
Sleep disorders.

Redotex NF *Medix, Mex.*
Pseudoephedrine hydrochloride (p.1099·2); atropine sulfate (p.461·1); aloin (p.1210·2).
Obesity.

Redox-Injektopas *Pascoe, Ger.†.*
Multivitamin preparation (p.1350·1).
Procaine hydrochloride (p.1319·1) is included in this preparation to alleviate the pain of injection.

Redoxon
Note. This name is used for preparations of different composition.
Roche, Aust.; Roche Consumer, Austral.; Roche, Braz.; Roche, Canad.; Roche, Hong Kong; Roche Consumer, Irl.; Roche, Israel; Roche, Ital.; Roche, Mex.; Roche Consumer, Neth.; Roche, NZ; Roche, Port.; Roche, S.Afr.; Roche Consumer, Singapore; Roche Nicholas, Spain; Roche, Switz.; Roche, Thai.; Roche Consumer, UK.
Ascorbic acid (p.1389·3) or sodium ascorbate (p.1390·1).
Adjunct in iron supplementation; malabsorption syndromes; methaemoglobinaemia; vitamin C deficiency; vitamin C supplement.

Roche, Belg.
Effervescent tablets: Ascorbic acid (p.1389·3).
Methaemoglobinaemia; vitamin C deficiency; vitamin C supplement.
Injection: Sodium ascorbate (p.1390·1).
Methaemoglobinaemia; vitamin C deficiency; vitamin C supplement.
Tablets: Ascorbic acid (p.1389·3); calcium ascorbate (p.1389·3).
Gastrointestinal reabsorption disorders; methaemoglobinaemia; vitamin C deficiency.

Redoxon Calciovit *Roche Nicholas, Spain.*
Ascorbic acid (p.1389·3); calcium carbonate (p.1215·1); ergocalciferol (p.1391·2); pyridoxine hydrochloride.
Bone and dental disorders; calcium deficiency; osteomalacia; rickets.

Redoxon Complex *Roche Nicholas, Spain.*
Multivitamin and mineral preparation (p.1350·1).

Redoxon Double Action
Roche Consumer, Singapore; Roche Consumer, UK.
Vitamin C (p.1389·3); zinc (p.1398·1).
Vitamin C deficiency.

Redoxon Protector *Roche Consumer, UK.*
Multivitamin and mineral preparation (p.1350·1).

Redoxon-B *Roche, Canad.*
Ascorbic acid; vitamin B substances; magnesium salts (p.1350·1).
Nutritional supplement.

Redoxon-Cal *Roche, Canad.*
Ascorbic acid; ergocalciferol; pyridoxine hydrochloride; calcium carbonate (p.1350·1).
Bone and dental disorders; delayed wound and fracture healing; nutritional supplement; osteomalacia; osteoporosis.

Redrate *Sanofi Synthelabo, Port.*
Glucose; sodium chloride; sodium bicarbonate; potassium chloride (p.1185·2).
Diarrhoea; oral rehydration therapy.

Redrocin *Unison, Thai.*
Erythromycin ethyl succinate (p.201·2).
Bacterial infections.

Reducap *Casmar, Mex.*
Phentermine (p.1514·1).

Reducealin *Propan, S.Afr.*
Propylhexedrine (p.1514·2); vitamin B substances (p.1350·1).
Obesity.

Reducelle *Alsitan, Ger.†.*
Aloes (p.1210·1); birch leaf (p.1585·2); cascara (p.1216·1); ononis (p.1644·1); phaseolus vulgaris.
Bowel evacuation; constipation.

Reducol
Note. This name is used for preparations of different composition.
Prodome, Braz.
Lovastatin (p.922·3).
Hyperlipidaemias.
Saninter, Port.
Oxidised glycerol triester.
Cicatrisation; wounds.

Reductel *Degorts, Mex.*
Captopril (p.853·3).
Hypertension.

Reducterol *Elfar, Spain.*
Bezafibrate (p.849·1).
Hyperlipidaemias.

Reductil
Knoll, Ger.; Astra, Ger.; Knoll, S.Afr.; Knoll, Switz.; Knoll, UK.
Sibutramine hydrochloride (p.1514·3).
Obesity.

Reducto *Sanova, Aust.*
Monobasic potassium phosphate (p.1193·1); dibasic sodium phosphate dihydrate (p.1193·2).
Calcium oxalate stones; hypercalcaemia.

Reducto-special *Asta Medica, Switz.†.*
Monobasic potassium phosphate (p.1193·1); dibasic sodium phosphate dihydrate (p.1193·2).
Calcium oxalate stones; hypercalcaemia; phosphate supplement.

Reducto-spezial *Temmler, Ger.*
Monobasic potassium phosphate (p.1193·1); dibasic sodium phosphate dihydrate (p.1193·2).
Calcium oxalate stones; hypercalcaemia; phosphate supplement.

Redufen *Zollweiden, Switz.*
Ibuprofen (p.43·2).
Fever; pain.

Redupon *Aventis, S.Afr.*
Ephedrine hydrochloride (p.1090·1); caffeine (p.761·3); phenolphthalein (p.1244·1).
Obesity.

Redupres *Leti, Spain.*
Verapamil hydrochloride (p.989·1).
Angina pectoris; arrhythmias; hypertension.

Redurate *Alliance, S.Afr.*
Allopurinol (p.397·2).
Gout; hyperuricaemia.

Redusa *Jean-Marie, Hong Kong.*
Phentermine hydrochloride (p.1514·1).
Obesity.

Redusan *Farmalight, Port.*
Poliglusam; vitamin C.
Slimming aid.

Redutemp *International Ethical, USA.*
Paracetamol (p.71·2).

Reduterm *SFD, Port.*
Oxidised gycerol triester.
Burns; cicatrisation.

Redutona *Faes, Spain.*
Phenytoin (p.357·2); phenobarbital (p.355·1); aminohydroxybutyric acid (p.342·2); pyridoxine hydrochloride (p.1386·3).
Epilepsy.

Reduvit *Technikon, S.Afr.*
Multivitamin and mineral preparation (p.1350·1).

Reduxpain *Kenyaku, Thai.*
Methyl salicylate (p.55·1); menthol (p.1632·3); eugenol (p.1609·3).
Musculoskeletal, joint, and soft-tissue disorders.

Redvit *Bunker, Braz.*
Multivitamin, mineral, and amino-acid preparation (p.1350·1).

Reef Deep Sun Tan Oil *Boots, Austral.*
SPF6: Octinoxate (p.1517·3); oxybenzone (p.1518·1).
Sunscreen.

Reef Sun Tan Oil *Boots, Austral.*
SPF15: Octinoxate (p.1517·3); octocrilene (p.1518·1).
Sunscreen.

The symbol † denotes a preparation no longer actively marketed

Reef Sun'n Surf *Boots, Austral.*
SPF 15: Octinoxate (p.1517·3); oxybenzone (p.1518·1); titanium dioxide (p.1126·1).
Sunscreen.

Reef Tanning Lotion *Boots, Austral.†*
SPF6: Octinoxate (p.1517·3).

SPF15+: Octinoxate (p.1517·3); oxybenzone (p.1518·1).
Sunscreen.

Reemplazante Gastri Mein *Fresenius Kabi, Spain.*
Ammonium chloride; potassium chloride; sodium chloride (p.1180·1).
Fluid and electrolyte depletion.

Reemplazante Intesi *Mein, Spain†.*
Glucose; potassium chloride; sodium chloride; sodium lactate (p.1185·2).
Fluid depletion.

Reese's Pinworm *Reese, USA.*
Pyrantel embonate (p.108·1).
Worm infections.

ReFacto
Genetics Institute, Aust.; Wyeth Lederle, Belg.; Genetics Institute, Denm.; Wyeth Lederle, Fin.; Wyeth Lederle, Fr.; Wyeth, Ger.; Wyeth Lederle, Ital.; Wyeth Lederle, Port.; Wyeth, Spain; Wyeth Lederle, Swed.; Pharmacia Upjohn, Swed.; Wyeth, UK; Genetics Institute, USA.
A factor VIII preparation (recombinant) (p.734·1).
Haemorrhagic disorders.

Refenesen *Reese, USA.*
Guaifenesin (p.1092·2).

Refenesen Plus *Reese, USA.*
Guaifenesin (p.1092·2); pseudoephedrine hydrochloride (p.1099·2).

Refesan T *Hanosan, Ger.*
Homoeopathic preparation.

Reflex
Note.This name is used for preparations of different composition.
Boots Healthcare, Fr.†.
Picolamine salicylate (p.78·3).
Musculoskeletal and joint pain.

Boots Healthcare, Irl.
Camphor (p.1589·3); methyl salicylate (p.55·1); turpentine oil (p.1676·3); menthol (p.1632·3).
Rheumatic and muscle pain.

Reflexgel *Boots Healthcare, Belg.*
Methyl salicylate (p.55·1); camphor (p.1589·3); menthol (p.1632·3).
Muscle, joint, and peri-articular pain.

Reflexspray *Boots Healthcare, Belg.*
Methyl salicylate (p.55·1); turpentine oil (p.1676·3); camphor (p.1589·3); menthol (p.1632·3).
Muscle, joint, and peri-articular disorders.

Reflocheck *Roche Diagnostics, Ital.*
Test for glucose in blood (p.1616·3).

Reflotron *Roche Diagnostics, Irl.*
Test for a range of cardiac risk factors in blood, serum, or plasma.

Refludan
Hoechst Marion Roussel, Aust.; Aventis, Austral.; Aventis, Belg.; Aventis, Denm.; Hoechst Marion Roussel, Fin.; Hoechst, Fr.; Hoechst Marion Roussel, Ger.; Hoechst Marion Roussel, Hong Kong; Hoechst Marion Roussel, Ital.; Hoechst Marion Roussel, Neth.; Hoechst Marion Roussel, Norw.; Aventis, Port.; Hoechst Marion Roussel, Swed.; Hoechst Marion Roussel, Switz.; Hoechst Marion Roussel, UK; Hoechst Marion Roussel, USA.
Lepirudin (p.919·3).
Thromboembolic disorders in patients with heparin-associated thrombocytopenia.

Refludin *Aventis, S.Afr.*
Lepirudin (p.919·3).
Thromboembolic disorders in patients with heparin-associated thrombocytopenia.

Reflux *IPS, Neth.†.*
Methenamine mandelate (p.223·1).
Urinary-tract infections.

Refluxin *Orion, Fin.*
Sodium alginate (p.1498·3); sodium bicarbonate (p.1186·2); calcium carbonate (p.1215·1).
Gastro-oesophageal reflux; hiatus hernia.

Refluxine *Spirig, Switz.*
Alginic acid (p.1498·3); sodium bicarbonate (p.1186·2); aluminium hydroxide-magnesium carbonate co-dried gel (p.1211·2).
Gastro-oesophageal reflux.

Refobacin *Merck, Aust.; Merck, Ger.*
Gentamicin sulfate (p.210·1).
Bacterial infections.

Refobacin-Palacos R *Merck, Aust.; Merck, Ger.; Merck, Singapore; Merck, Thai.*
Gentamicin sulfate (p.210·1); methylmethacrylate/methylacrylate copolymer (p.1635·2).
Bone cement for orthopaedic surgery.

Refolinon *Pharmacia Upjohn, S.Afr.†; Pharmacia, UK.*
Calcium folinate (p.1363·1) or folinic acid (p.1363·1).
Antidote to folic acid antagonists; megaloblastic anaemia.

Refresh
Allergan, Austral.; Allergan, Canad.; Allergan, Fr.; Allergan, Israel; Allergan, NZ; Allergan, S.Afr.; Allergan, Singapore; Allergan, Thai.; Allergan, UK; Allergan, USA.
Polyvinyl alcohol (p.1503·3); povidone (p.1503·2).
Dry eyes; eye irritation.

Refresh Night Time *Allergan, UK†.*
White soft paraffin (p.1407·3); liquid paraffin (p.1407·1); wool alcohols (p.1410·3).
Dry eyes.

Refresh Plus *Allergan, USA.*
Carmellose sodium (p.1499·3).
Dry eyes.

Refresh PM *Allergan, USA.*
White soft paraffin (p.1407·3); liquid paraffin (p.1407·1); wool alcohols (p.1410·3).
Dry eyes.

Refresh Tears *Allergan, USA.*
Carmellose sodium (p.1499·3).
Dry eyes.

Refulgin *Spyfarma, Spain.*
Adenosine triphosphate (p.1573·3); hydroxocobalamin acetate (p.1388·3); pyritinol hydrochloride (p.1657·1); prosultiamine (p.1385·1).
Mental function disorders.

Refusal *Artu, Neth.*
Disulfiram (p.1605·1).
Chronic alcoholism.

Regadrin B *Berlin-Chemie, Ger.*
Bezafibrate (p.849·1).
Hyperlipidaemias.

Regain *R&D, USA.*
Note. A similar name is used for preparations of different composition (see below).
Nutritional supplement in renal failure (p.1350·1).

Regaine
Note. A similar name is used for preparations of different composition (see above).
Pharmacia Upjohn, Aust.; Pharmacia Upjohn, Austral.; Pharmacia Upjohn, Belg.; Pharmacia Upjohn, Braz.; Pharmacia Upjohn, Denm.; Pharmacia Upjohn, Fin.; Pharmacia Upjohn, Fr.; Pharmacia Upjohn, Hong Kong; Pharmacia Upjohn, Irl.; Pharmacia Upjohn, Israel; Pharmacia Upjohn, Ital.; Pharmacia Upjohn, Mex.; Pharmacia Upjohn, Neth.; Pharmacia Upjohn, Norw.; Pharmacia Upjohn, NZ; Pharmacia Upjohn, Port.; Pharmacia Upjohn, S.Afr.; Pharmacia Upjohn, Singapore; Pharmacia Upjohn, Spain; Pharmacia Upjohn, Swed.; Pharmacia Upjohn, Switz.; Pharmacia Upjohn, Thai.; Pharmacia, UK.
Minoxidil (p.934·2).
Alopecia androgenetica.

Regal *Cantabria, Spain†.*
Styrax tonkinensis tincture; myrrh tincture (p.1639·2); rhatany tincture (p.1657·3); resorcinol (p.1122·2); zinc chloride (p.1398·1); zinc phenolsulfonate (p.1128·3); methyl salicylate (p.55·1); menthol (p.1632·3).
Halitosis; mouth inflammation.

Regalen *Eisai, Jpn†.*
Chenodeoxycholic acid (p.1594·1).
Cholesterol gallstones.

Regalil *Farmoquimica, Braz.*
Ranitidine (p.1246·3).
Gastro-oesophageal reflux; gastrointestinal haemorrhage; peptic ulcer; Zollinger-Ellison syndrome.

Regard *Smith & Nephew, S.Afr.*
Glycerol (p.1616·3).
Lubrication.

Regasinum *Rowa, Ger.*
A range of homoeopathic preparations.

Regavasal N *Rowa, Ger.*
Homoeopathic preparation.

Regelan
Zeneca, Aust.; Zeneca, Switz.
Clofibrate (p.859·1).
Hyperlipidaemias.

Regelan N *Zeneca, Ger.†.*
Clofibrate (p.859·1).
Hyperlipidaemias.

Regenaplex *Regenaplex, Ger.*
A range of homoeopathic preparations.

Regender *Alacan, Spain.*
Polypodium leucotomos.
Skin disorders.

Regenerin *Sanova, Aust.*
Procaine hydrochloride (p.1319·1); vitamin A (p.1382·1); vitamin E (p.1393·3).
Reduced mental and physical capacity in the elderly.

Regenon
Sanova, Aust.†; Trenker, Belg.†; Temmler, Denm.†; Temmler, Ger.†; Asta Medica, Switz.
Diethylpropion hydrochloride (p.1508·3).
Obesity.

Regepar
Sanofi Winthrop, Aust.; Sodip, Switz.
Selegiline hydrochloride (p.1177·2).
Parkinsonism.

Regepithel
Alcon, Ger.
Vitamin A palmitate (p.1383·2); thiamine hydrochloride (p.1385·1); calcium pantothenate (p.1374·1).
Corneal defects.

Thilo, Hong Kong.
Vitamin A (p.1382·1); thiamine (p.1385·2); calcium pantothenate (p.1374·1).
Eye disorders.

Regibloc *Intramed, S.Afr.†.*
Bupivacaine hydrochloride (p.1306·3).
Local anaesthesia.

Regina Royal Concorde *Regina, UK.*
Royal jelly (p.1659·3); ginseng (p.1615·3); damiana aphrodisiaca (p.1602·1); saw palmetto (p.1491·2).

Regina Royal Five *Regina, UK.*
Royal jelly (p.1659·3); bee pollen; pure honey (p.1366·2).

Regina Royal One Hundred *Regina, UK.*
Royal jelly (p.1659·3).

Regitin *Novartis, Denm.*
Phentolamine mesilate (p.954·3).
Phaeochromocytoma.

Regitine
Novartis, Austral.; Novartis, Belg.; Novartis, Israel; Novartis, Neth.; Novartis, NZ; Novartis, S.Afr.; Novartis, Switz.; Novartis, USA.
Phentolamine mesilate (p.954·3).
Dermal necrosis and sloughing following intravenous administration of noradrenaline [norepinephrine]; phaeochromocytoma.

Regla pH
Note.This name is used for preparations of different composition.
Darci, Belg.
Algeldrate (p.1210·3); light magnesium oxide (p.1233·2).
Gastrointestinal disorders associated with hyperacidity.

UCB, Neth.

Chewable tablets: Aluminium hydroxide-magnesium carbonate co-dried gel (p.1211·2) magnesium hydroxide (p.1233·1).

Oral suspension: Aluminium hydroxide (p.1210·3); magnesium hydroxide (p.1233·1).
Gastritis; gastro-oesophageal reflux; heartburn; peptic ulcer.

UCB, Switz.†.

Suspension: Aluminium hydroxide (p.1210·3); light magnesium oxide (p.1233·2); aluminium hydroxide-magnesium carbonate co-dried gel (p.1211·2).

Tablets: Aluminium hydroxide-magnesium carbonate co-dried gel (p.1211·2); glycine (p.1365·3).
Gastric hyperacidity; peptic ulcer.

Regla pH Forte *Darci, Belg.*
Algeldrate (p.1210·3); light magnesium oxide (p.1233·2); aluminium hydroxide-magnesium carbonate co-dried gel(p.1211·2).
Gastric hyperacidity; peptic ulcer.

Reglan
Wyeth-Ayerst, Canad.; Sanofi Synthelabo, Port.; Robins, USA.
Metoclopramide hydrochloride (p.1235·2).
Adjunct in gastrointestinal procedures; diabetic gastroparesis; gastro-oesophageal reflux; nausea and vomiting.

Reglovar *Quimioterapica, Braz.*
Estradiol benzoate (p.1473·1).
Breast cancer; menopausal disorders; oestrogen deficiency; osteoporosis; prostatic cancer.

Reglusan *Novag, Mex.*
Glibenclamide (p.321·3).
Diabetes mellitus.

Regolact Plus *Naturmed, Ital.*
Lactic-acid-producing organisms (p.1626·3).
Maintenance of normal gastrointestinal flora.

Regolpause *Provita, Ital.*
Multivitamin and mineral preparation (p.1350·1).

Regomed *Interpharm, Aust.*
Enalapril maleate (p.883·3).
Heart failure; hypertension.

Regonol
Organon, Canad.†; Organon, USA.
Pyridostigmine bromide (p.1423·3).
Myasthenia gravis; reversal of competitive neuromuscular blockade.

Regran *Delta, Braz.*
Papaverine (p.1648·1); belladonna (p.463·1); viburnum prunifolium; Jamaica dogwood (p.1625·1); valerian (p.1678·3).
Dysmenorrhoea.

Regranex
Janssen-Ortho, Canad.; Janssen-Cilag, Fr.; Janssen-Cilag, Ger.; Janssen-Cilag, Israel; Cilag, Mex.; Janssen-Cilag, Singapore; Janssen-Cilag, Swed.; Janssen-Cilag, UK; Ortho McNeil, USA.
Becaplermin (p.1110·3).
Diabetic neuropathic ulcers.

Regro *DHA, Singapore.*
Minoxidil (p.934·2).
Alopecia androgenetica; alopecia areata.

Regroton *Rhone-Poulenc Rorer, USA.*
Chlortalidone (p.857·1); reserpine (p.967·3).
Hypertension.

Regubil *Riva, Canad.†.*
Biliary salts (p.1585·1); dehydrocholic acid (p.1602·2); deoxycholic acid.
Biliary-tract disorders.

Regucel *Terapia, Mex.*
Ferrous sulfate (p.1360·3).

Regufer *Terapia, Mex.*
Ferrous fumarate (p.1360·1).

Regulacin *Republic, USA.*
Docusate sodium (p.1223·1); casanthranol (p.1216·1).
Constipation.

Regulacor-POS *Ursapharm, Ger.*
Crataegus (p.1600·2).
Cardiac disorders.

Regulact *ICN, Mex.*
Lactulose (p.1230·1).
Constipation; hepatic encephalopathy.

Regulador Blumen *Luper, Braz.*
Cotton root bark; plumeria lancifolia; berberis laurina.
Dysmenorrhoea.

Regulador Gesteira *CIF, Braz.*
Paracetamol (p.71·2); viburnum prunifolium.
Dysmenorrhoea.

Regulan
Procter & Gamble, Irl.; Procter & Gamble (H&B Care), UK.
Ispaghula (p.1229·1).
Constipation; diverticular disease; irritable bowel syndrome.

Regular Iletin I *Lilly, USA†.*
Insulin injection (bovine and porcine) (p.324·1).
Diabetes mellitus.

Regular Iletin II *Lilly, USA.*
Insulin injection (porcine) (p.324·1).
Diabetes mellitus.

Regular Strength Anbesol *Whitehall, USA†.*
Benzocaine (p.1306·2); phenol (p.1152·3); alcohol (p.1130·3).
Dental pain.

Regular Strength Bayer *Sterling Health, USA.*
Aspirin (p.14·2).
Formerly known as Therapy Bayer.
Fever; inflammation; myocardial infarction; pain; transient ischaemic attacks.

Regular Strength Cold Daytime Relief *West-Can, Canad.*
Pseudoephedrine hydrochloride (p.1099·2); dextromethorphan hydrobromide (p.1087·3); paracetamol (p.71·2).

Regular Strength Cold Nighttime Relief *West-Can, Canad.*
Pseudoephedrine hydrochloride (p.1099·2); dextromethorphan hydrobromide (p.1087·3); paracetamol (p.71·2); chlorpheniramine [chlorphenamine] maleate (p.412·1).

Regular Strength Sinus *Stanley, Canad.*
Pseudoephedrine hydrochloride (p.1099·2); paracetamol (p.71·2).

Regulax *QIF, Braz.*
Cotton root bark; plumeria lancifolia; berberis laurina.
Dysmenorrhoea.

Regulax N *Krewel, Ger.*
Senna (p.1248·2).
Constipation.

Regulax Picosulfat *Krewel, Ger.*
Sodium picosulfate (p.1249·3).
Constipation.

Regulax SS *Republic, USA.*
Docusate sodium (p.1223·1).
Constipation.

Reguletts
Husler, Switz.†; Seton, UK†.
Phenolphthalein (p.1244·1).
Constipation.

Regulex *Whitehall-Robins, Canad.*
Docusate sodium (p.1223·1).
Constipation.

Regulex-D *Whitehall-Robins, Canad.†.*
Dantron (p.1221·3); docusate sodium (p.1223·1).
Constipation.

Regulim
Atlantic, Hong Kong; Atlantic, Singapore; Atlantic, Thai.
Phenolphthalein (p.1244·1).
Bowel evacuation; constipation.

Reguloid *Rugby, USA.*
Psyllium hydrophilic mucilloid (p.1229·1).
Constipation.

Regulose *Novartis Consumer, UK.*
Lactulose (p.1230·1).
Constipation.

Regulton
Knoll, Belg.; Knoll, Ger.†.
Amezinium metilsulfate (p.835·1).
Hypotension.

Regunon *Schering, Swed.*
Levonorgestrel (p.1486·2); ethinylestradiol (p.1476·2).
Combined oral contraceptive.

Regurin *Galen, UK.*
Trospium chloride (p.475·2).
Bladder instability.

Regutol *Schering-Plough, USA†.*
Docusate sodium (p.1223·1).
Constipation.

Rehalyt *SAD, Denm.*
Electrolyte infusion with glucose (p.1180·1).
Carbohydrate source; fluid and electrolyte disorders.

Rehidrat *Searle, Braz.*
Potassium chloride; sodium citrate dihydrate; sodium chloride; glucose (p.1185·2).
Diarrhoea; oral rehydration therapy.

Searle, Irl.; Pharmacia, UK.
Sodium chloride; potassium chloride; sodium bicarbonate; citric acid; glucose; sucrose; fructose (p.1185·2).
Diarrhoea; oral rehydration therapy.

Searle, Israel.
Sodium chloride; potassium chloride; sodium bicarbonate; citric acid; glucose (p.1185·2).
Diarrhoea; oral rehydration therapy.

Searle, S.Afr.
Sodium chloride; potassium chloride; sodium bicarbonate; glucose; sucrose (p.1185·2).
Diarrhoea; oral rehydration therapy.

Rehydralyte
Abbott, Canad.; Abbott, Thai.; Ross, USA.
Glucose; sodium citrate; sodium chloride; sodium citrate (p.1185·2).
Diarrhoea; oral rehydration therapy.

Rehydrex med glucos
Fresenius Kabi, Norw.; Fresenius Kabi, Swed.
Electrolyte infusion with glucose (p.1180·1).
Fluid and electrolyte disorders.

Rehydrex med Glucose *Fresenius Kabi, Denm.*
Electrolyte infusion with glucose (p.1180·1).
Carbohydrate source; fluid and electrolyte disorders.

Reidrax *Bonomelli, Ital.*
Electrolytes; glucose (p.1185·2).
Oral rehydration therapy.

Reise Superpep-K *Pharmacal, Switz.†*
Dimenhydrinate (p.415·2).
Motion sickness; nausea; vertigo; vomiting.

Reisedragee Eu Rho *Eu Rho, Ger.*
Diphenhydramine hydrochloride (p.416·1); 8-chlorotheophylline.
Nausea; vomiting.

Reisegold *Whitehall-Much, Ger.*
Sugar-coated tablets: Diphenhydramine hydrochloride (p.416·1); caffeine (p.761·3); 8-chlorotheophylline; pyridoxine hydrochloride (p.1386·3).
Tablets: Dimenhydrinate (p.415·2).
Motion sickness.

Reisetabletten-ratiopharm *Ratiopharm, Ger.*
Dimenhydrinate (p.415·2).
Motion sickness; nausea; vertigo; vomiting.

Rejuva *Stiefel, Canad.*
SPF 15: Avobenzone (p.1517·1); octinoxate (p.1517·3).
Sunscreen.

Rejuva-A *Stiefel, Canad.*
Tretinoin (p.1126·2).
Photodamaged skin.

Rejuvesol *Cytosol, Israel.*
Sodium pyruvate; inosine; adenine; dibasic sodium phosphate; monobasic sodium phosphate.
Extracorporeal rejuvenation.

Rekasitin *Rekah, Israel.*
Zinc oxide (p.1128·2); cod-liver oil (p.1357·3); allantoin (p.1110·1).
Barrier preparation; burns; nappy rash; skin disorders.

Rekawan
Solvay, Aust.; Rekawan, Ger.
Potassium chloride (p.1194·3).
Potassium deficiency.

Rekiv *Rekah, Israel.*
Magnesium carbonate (p.1232·3); bismuth subnitrate (p.1213·2); sodium bicarbonate (p.1186·2); frangula bark (p.1227·1); calamus (p.1588·1).
Gastritis; gastrointestinal hyperacidity; peptic ulcer.

Rekod *Rekah, Israel.*
Codeine phosphate (p.25·2).
Coughs; pain.

Rekont *Madaus, Aust.†*
Trospium chloride (p.475·2).
Bladder function disorders.

Rekord B12 *Sigma-Tau, Ital.*
Amino-acid and vitamin B substances (p.1350·1).
Tonic.

Rekord Ferro *Sigma-Tau, Ital.*
Iron succinyl-protein complex (p.1369·3).
Anaemias; iron-deficiency.

Relact *Kora, Irl.*
Lactic acid (p.1626·2).
Vaginal discharge.

Relafen *SmithKline Beecham, Canad.; SmithKline Beecham, USA.*
Nabumetone (p.59·3).
Osteoarthritis; rheumatoid arthritis.

Relapamil *Orion, Fin.*
Quinine hydrochloride (p.445·1); diazepam (p.674·3).
Muscle spasm.

Relar *Pharmaland, Thai.*
Orphenadrine citrate (p.470·3); paracetamol (p.71·2).
Muscle pain; tension headache.

Relasan *Bioquimico, Mex.*
Diazepam (p.674·3).

Relaten *Herbaline, Ital.†*
Chamomile (p.1593·2); crataegus (p.1600·2); eschscholtzia californica; red-poppy (p.1029·1).
Agitation; anxiety; insomnia.

Relatrac *Pisa, Mex.*
Atracurium besilate (p.1333·1).
Competitive neuromuscular blocker.

Relavit Fosforo *Seber, Port.*
Levoglutamide (p.1365·2); thiamine; inositol calcium phosphate; inositol magnesium phosphate.
Adjunct in epilepsy; depression; mental function disorders.

Relax *Zeller, Switz.*
Petasites; valerian (p.1678·3); passion flower (p.1649·1); melissa (p.1632·2).
Anxiety; sleep disorders.

Relax B+ *Vitalia, UK.*
Valerian (p.1678·3); lupulus (p.1629·3); passion flower (p.1649·1); vitamin B substances (p.1350·1).

Relax and Sleep *Jamieson, Canad.*
Cataria; lupulus (p.1629·3); passion flower (p.1649·1); valerian (p.1678·3).
Sleep disorders.

Relaxan *Gea, Denm.†*
Gallamine triethiodide (p.1337·1).
Competitive neuromuscular blocker.

Relaxaplex *Vitaplex, Austral.*
Valerian (p.1678·3); skullcap (p.1664·3); passion flower (p.1649·1); lupulus (p.1629·3); gentian (p.1615·2).
Herbal sedative.

Relaxar *Bouty, Ital.*
Mephenesin (p.1329·2); methyl nicotinate (p.55·1).
Neuromuscular pain; soft-tissue disorders.

Relaxa-Tabs *Woods, Austral.*
Mepyramine maleate (p.421·1).
Insomnia; nervous tension.

Relaxedans *Salvat, Spain†.*
Chlordiazepoxide (p.659·2); pyridoxine (p.1387·1).
Anxiety.

Relaxibys *Belmac, Spain.*
Carisoprodol (p.1327·1); paracetamol (p.71·2).
Musculoskeletal spasticity.

Relaxine
Trenker, Belg.; Warner-Lambert, Fr.
Valerian (p.1678·3).
Insomnia; nervous disorders.

Relaxin-P *Jean-Marie, Hong Kong.*
Chlorzoxazone (p.1327·3); paracetamol (p.71·2).
Painful skeletal muscle spasm.

Relaxit
Note. This name is used for preparations of different composition.
Abigo, Swed.
Sodium bicarbonate (p.1186·2); potassium acid tartrate (p.1244·3); calcium silicate (p.1189·1).
Constipation; faecal incontinence.

Crawford, UK.
Sodium citrate (p.1186·2); sodium laurilsulfate (p.1496·3); sorbic acid (p.1157·1); glycerol (p.1616·3); sorbitol (p.1377·3).
Constipation.

Relaxoddi *Leurquin, Fr.†*
Butacaine (p.1308·2); oleic acid (p.1409·3).
Dyspepsia.

Relaxyl
Note. This name is used for preparations of different composition.
Nycomed, Aust.
Dibasic sodium phosphate (p.1193·2); monobasic sodium phosphate (p.1193·2).
Bowel evacuation; constipation.

SSL, UK.
Alverine citrate (p.1211·3).
Irritable bowel syndrome.

Relazepam *Pisa, Mex.*
Diazepam (p.674·3).

Relcofen *Cox, UK.*
Ibuprofen (p.43·2).
Pain.

Releaf for PMS *Lake, USA.*
Pyridoxine hydrochloride (p.1386·3) in a base of natural herbs.
Premenstrual syndrome.

Relefact LH-RH
Hoechst Marion Roussel, Aust.; Hoechst Marion Roussel, Ger.; Hoechst Marion Roussel, Irl.†; Hoechst Marion Roussel, Israel; Hoechst Marion Roussel, Neth.; Hoechst Marion Roussel, UK†.
Gonadorelin (p.1283·3).
Diagnosis of hypothalamic-pituitary-gonadal dysfunction.

Relefact TRH
Hoechst Marion Roussel, Aust.; Hoechst Marion Roussel, Canad.; Hoechst Marion Roussel, Ger.; Hoechst Marion Roussel, Israel; Hoechst Marion Roussel, Neth.; Hoechst Marion Roussel, Switz.
Protirelin (p.1295·3).
Diagnosis of hypothalamic-pituitary-thyroid dysfunction.

Relenza
Glaxo Wellcome, Austral.; Glaxo Wellcome, Belg.; Glaxo Wellcome, Denm.; Glaxo Wellcome, Fin.; Glaxo Wellcome, Fr.; Glaxo Wellcome, Ger.; Cascan, Ger.; Glaxo Wellcome, Irl.; Glaxo Wellcome, Ital.; Glaxo Wellcome, Neth.; Glaxo Wellcome, Norw.; Glaxo Wellcome, NZ; Glaxo Wellcome, Port.; Glaxo Wellcome, Singapore; Glaxo Wellcome, Spain; Glaxo Wellcome, Swed.; Glaxo Wellcome, Switz.; Glaxo Wellcome, UK; Glaxo Wellcome, USA.
Zanamivir (p.644·3).
Influenza.

Reless *Scherax, Ger.*
Bee venom extract or wasp venom extract.
Hyposensitisation.

Relexic *Sunward, Singapore.*
Chlormezanone (p.660·1); paracetamol (p.71·2).
Pain; skeletal muscle spasm.

Reliberan *Geymonat, Ital.*
Chlordiazepoxide hydrochloride (p.659·2).
Anxiety disorders.

Relief *Allergan, USA.*
Phenylephrine hydrochloride (p.1097·1).
Minor eye irritation.

Relief Rub *Greenridge, Austral.*
Echinacea purpurea (p.1606·2); melaleuca oil (p.1631·3); eucalyptus oil (p.1609·2); thyme oil (p.1672·3); turpentine oil (p.1676·3); cajuput oil (p.1588·1); peppermint oil (p.1243·3).
Cold and influenza symptoms; musculoskeletal and joint pain.

Relief-Coff *PD Pharm, S.Afr.*
Diphenhydramine hydrochloride (p.416·1); ammonium chloride (p.1085·2); sodium citrate (p.1186·2).
Coughs.

Reliev *Darrow, Braz.*
Meglumine amidotrizoate (p.1031·2).
Radiographic contrast medium.

Relif *SmithKline, Spain.*
Nabumetone (p.59·3).
Osteoarthritis; rheumatoid arthritis.

Relifen *SmithKline Beecham, S.Afr.*
Nabumetone (p.59·3).
Musculoskeletal, joint, and soft-tissue disorders.

Relifex
SmithKline Beecham, Braz.; SmithKline Beecham, Denm.; SmithKline Beecham, Fin.; SmithKline Beecham, Hong Kong; SmithKline Beecham, Irl.; SmithKline Beecham, Israel; SmithKline Beecham, Mex.; SmithKline Beecham, Norw.; SmithKline Beecham, Singapore; SmithKline Beecham, Swed.; SmithKline Beecham, Thai.; SmithKline Beecham, UK.
Nabumetone (p.59·3).
Gout; inflammation; musculoskeletal and joint disorders.

Relisan *Xixia, S.Afr.*
Nabumetone (p.59·3).
Musculoskeletal and joint disorders.

Relisorm *Serono, Canad.†*
Gonadorelin acetate (p.1284·2).
Diagnosis of hypothalamic-pituitary-gonadal dysfunction.

Relisorm L
Serono, Braz.; Serono, Hong Kong; Serono, Mex.; Serono, Switz.
Gonadorelin acetate (p.1284·2).
Test of hypothalamic-pituitary-gonadal function.

Relitone *Aspen, S.Afr.*
Nabumetone (p.59·3).
Musculoskeletal and joint disorders.

Reliv *Recip, Swed.*
Paracetamol (p.71·2).
Fever; pain.

Relivora Komplex *Sanum-Kehlbeck, Ger.*
Homoeopathic preparation.

Relmus *Sanofi Synthelabo, Port.*
Thiocolchicoside (p.1330·2).
Neuromuscular pain; parkinsonism; skeletal muscle spasticity.

Relmus Compositum *Sanofi Synthelabo, Port.*
Thiocolchicoside (p.1330·2); aescin (p.1574·2).
Musculoskeletal and joint injury; phlebitis; thrombophlebitis.

Reloxyl
Note. This name is used for preparations of different composition.
RDC, Ital.
Benzoyl peroxide (p.1111·1).
Acne; skin disinfection.

Cheminova, Spain.
Amoxicillin trihydrate (p.149·2).
Bacterial infections.

Reloxyl Mucolitico *Cheminova, Spain.*
Amoxicillin trihydrate (p.149·2); guaifenesin (p.1092·2).
Respiratory-tract infections.

Relpax *Pfizer, UK.*
Eletriptan (p.451·3).
Migraine.

Relvene *Pharmascience, Fr.*
Oxerutins (p.1611·2).
Chronic venous insufficiency.

Remafen *Xepa-Soul Pattinson, Hong Kong; Xepa-Soul Pattinson, Singapore.*
Diclofenac sodium (p.30·3).
Gout; musculoskeletal and joint disorders.

Remcol Cold *Shionogi, USA†.*
Phenylpropanolamine hydrochloride (p.1098·1); chlorpheniramine [chlorphenamine] maleate (p.412·1); paracetamol (p.71·2).
Upper respiratory-tract symptoms.

Remcol-C *Shionogi, USA†.*
Chlorpheniramine [chlorphenamine] maleate (p.412·1); dextromethorphan hydrobromide (p.1087·3); paracetamol (p.71·2).
Coughs and cold symptoms.

Remdue *Biomedica, Ital.*
Flurazepam dihydrochloride (p.685·3).
Insomnia.

Remedacen *Rhone-Poulenc Rorer, Ger.*
Dihydrocodeine polistirex (p.33·3).
Coughs.

Remedeine *Napp, UK.*
Paracetamol (p.71·2); dihydrocodeine tartrate (p.33·1).
Pain.

Remederm *Widmer, Ger.*
Urea (p.1127·3); vitamin A palmitate (p.1383·2); alpha tocoferil acetate (p.1394·1); dexpanthenol (p.1602·3).
Skin disorders.

Remederm HC *Widmer, Ger.*
Hydrocortisone (p.1073·3).
Skin disorders.

Remedium Nervinum N EKF *Biomedica, Ger.*
Homoeopathic preparation.

Remedium Sinutale N EKF *Biomedica, Ger.*
Homoeopathic preparation.

Remedol *Remedica, Singapore.*
Paracetamol (p.71·2).
Fever; pain.

Remeflin *Recordati, Ital.*
Dimefline hydrochloride (p.1509·1).
Respiratory and circulatory disorders.

Remegel
Warner-Lambert, Irl.†; Warner-Lambert, Ital.†; SSL, UK.
Calcium carbonate (p.1215·1).
Gastric hyperacidity.

Remegel Wind Relief *SSL, UK.*
Calcium carbonate (p.1215·1); simeticone (p.1249·2).
Dyspepsia; flatulence; heartburn.

Remen *Parke, Davis, Ital.†*
Pramiracetam sulfate (p.1654·2).
Mental function impairment.

Remens *Bittner, Aust.*
Homoeopathic preparation.

Remergil *Organon, Ger.; Thiemann, Ger.*
Mirtazapine (p.299·1).
Depression.

Remeron
Organon, Aust.; Organon, Denm.; Organon, Fin.; Organon, Hong Kong; Organon, Israel; Organon, Ital.; Organon, Mex.; Nourypharma, Neth.; Organon, Port.; Donmed, S.Afr.; Organon, Singapore; Organon, Swed.; Organon, Thai.; Organon, USA.
Mirtazapine (p.299·1).
Depression.

Remestan
Wyeth Lederle, Aust.; Wyeth, Ger.
Temazepam (p.707·2).
Sleep disorders.

Remethan
Remedica, Singapore; Remedica, Thai.
Diclofenac diethylamine (p.30·2) or diclofenac sodium (p.30·3).
Gout; inflammation; musculoskeletal, joint, peri-articular, and soft-tissue disorders; pain.

Remethan R *Remedica, Hong Kong.*
Diclofenac sodium (p.30·3).
Gout; inflammation; musculoskeletal and joint disorders; pain.

Remexal *Lubapharm, Switz.*
Lauromacrogol 600 (p.1345·2); dimethyl sulfoxide (p.1402·2); glycol salicylate (p.42·2); dexpanthenol (p.1602·3); menthol (p.1632·3); camphor (p.1589·3).
Musculoskeletal, joint, and peri-articular disorders.

Remicade
Centocor, Denm.; Schering-Plough, Fin.; Schering-Plough, Fr.; Essex, Ger.; Schering-Plough, Irl.; Schering-Plough, Ital.; Schering-Plough, Neth.; Schering-Plough, Port.; Schering-Plough, Spain; Schering-Plough, Swed.; Schering-Plough, Switz.; Schering-Plough, UK; Centocor, USA.
Infliximab (p.1228·2).
Crohn's disease; rheumatoid arthritis.

Remicaine *Adcock Ingram Generics, S.Afr.*
Lignocaine [lidocaine] hydrochloride (p.1313·2).
Arrhythmias; local anaesthesia.

Remicard *Adcock Ingram Generics, S.Afr.*
Lignocaine [lidocaine] hydrochloride (p.1313·2).
Arrhythmias.

Remid *TAD, Ger.*
Allopurinol (p.397·2).
Gout; hyperuricaemia.

Remifemin
Schaper & Brummer, Ger.; Schaper & Brummer, Singapore; Asta Medica, Switz.†.
Cimicifuga (p.1595·2).
Menopausal and menstrual disorders.

Remifemin plus *Schaper & Brummer, Ger.*
Hypericum (p.290·2); cimicifuga (p.1595·2).
Menstrual and menopausal disorders.

Reminyl
Janssen-Cilag, Fr.; Shire, Irl.; Janssen-Cilag, Swed.; Shire, UK; Janssen, USA.
Galantamine hydrobromide (p.1419·1).
Alzheimer's disease.

Remiprostan uno *Schaper & Brummer, Ger.*
Saw palmetto (p.1491·2).
Benign prostatic hyperplasia.

Remisan *Vir, Spain.*
Amoxicillin trihydrate (p.149·2).
Bacterial infections.

Remisan Mucolitico *Vir, Spain.*
Amoxicillin trihydrate (p.149·2); bromhexine hydrochloride (p.1085·3).
Respiratory-tract infections.

Remnos *DDSA Pharmaceuticals, UK.*
Nitrazepam (p.695·2).
Insomnia.

Remodil *Remedica, Singapore.*
Diphenoxylate hydrochloride (p.1222·2).
Atropine sulfate (p.461·1) is included in this preparation to discourage abuse.
Diarrhoea.

Remontal *Vita, Spain.*
Nimodipine (p.946·1).
Cognitive impairment in the elderly; neurological deficit following subarachnoid haemorrhage.

Remoplexe *Lehning, Fr.†*
Copper gluconate (p.1357·3).
Musculoskeletal and joint disorders; viral infections.

Remotil *Azevedos, Port.*
Domperidone (p.1224·1).
Aid in gastrointestinal examination; dyspepsia; nausea; vomiting.

Remotiv
Flordis, Austral.; Bayer, Ger.; Knoll, Mex.; Zeller, Switz.
Hypericum (p.290·2).
Anxiety; depression; sleep disorders.

Remotrox *Pharmaceutical Enterprises, S.Afr.*
Dicycloverine [dicyclomine] hydrochloride (p.466·1); dried aluminium hydroxide gel (p.1210·3); light magnesium oxide (p.1233·2).
Gastrointestinal disorders.

The symbol † denotes a preparation no longer actively marketed

Remov Piam, Ital.
Nimesulide (p.62·3).
Fever; inflammation; pain.

Remove Smith & Nephew, Austral.
Dipropylene glycol methyl ether.
Adhesive remover.

Remular-S International Ethical, USA.
Chlorzoxazone (p.1327·3).
Musculoskeletal pain.

Remy Sella, Ital.
Camphor (p.1589·3); ethyl salicylate (p.35·1); menthol (p.1632·3); capsicum oleoresin (p.1591·1).
Rheumatism.

Remycin Remedica, Singapore.
Doxycycline (p.200·1).
Bacterial infections.

Remydrial Winzer, Ger.
Dapiprazole hydrochloride (p.1602·2).
Reversal of mydriasis.

Remysal N DCG, Swed.†
Diethylamine salicylate (p.32·2); benzyl nicotinate (p.20·2).
Topical pain relief.

Rena Pharmaland, Thai.
Orphenadrine citrate (p.470·3); paracetamol (p.71·2).
Muscle spasm; skeletal muscle spasm.

Renacidin Guardian, USA.
Anhydrous citric acid (p.1596·2); gluconic acid; magnesium carbonate (p.1232·3).
Renal calculi.

Renacor Dieckmann, Ger.
Enalapril maleate (p.883·3); hydrochlorothiazide (p.907·3).
Hypertension.

Renagel Genzyme, Fr.; Pinewood, Irl.; Genzyme, UK; Genzyme, USA.
Sevelamer hydrochloride (p.1021·2).
Hyperphosphataemia.

Renal Care Abbott, Ital.
Preparation for enteral nutrition in renal failure (p.1350·1).

Renalin Dialyzer Reprocessing Concentrate Renal Systems, USA†.
Hydrogen peroxide (p.1147·1); acetic acid (p.1571·2); peracetic acid (p.1152·2).

Renamel Clonmel, Irl.
Oxybutynin hydrochloride (p.471·2).
Neurogenic bladder; nocturnal enuresis; unstable bladder.

RenAmin Clintec, USA.
Amino-acid infusion (p.1350·1).
Parenteral nutrition in renal impairment.

Renapur Schering-Plough, Swed.
Anhydrous potassium citrate (p.1186·1); anhydrous sodium citrate (p.1186·2); anhydrous citric acid (p.1596·2).
Renal calculi.

Renase Pharmaland, Thai.
Amiloride hydrochloride (p.835·1); hydrochlorothiazide (p.907·3).
Hepatic cirrhosis with ascites and oedema; hypertension; oedema.

Renaton Korea United, Singapore.
Enalapril maleate (p.883·3).
Heart failure; hypertension.

Renax Everett, USA.
Multivitamin and mineral preparation in renal failure (p.1350·1).

Rendells Prisfar, Port.
Nonoxinol 9 (p.1346·1).
Contraceptive.

Rendells Plus NZ Medical & Scientific, NZ.
Nonoxinol 9 (p.1346·1).
Contraceptive.

Renedil
Aventis, Belg.; Hoechst Marion Roussel, Canad.; Hoechst Marion Roussel, Neth.
Felodipine (p.888·3).
Angina pectoris; hypertension.

Re/Neph Pisa, Mex.
Nutritional supplement in renal failure (p.1350·1).

Renese
Pfizer, Belg.; Pfizer, USA.
Polythiazide (p.957·1).
Hypertension; oedema.

Renese R Pfizer, USA.
Polythiazide (p.957·1); reserpine (p.967·3).
Hypertension.

Reneuron Juste, Spain.
Fluoxetine hydrochloride (p.284·2).
Bulimia; depression; obsessive-compulsive disorder.

Renezide Aspen, S.Afr.
Triamterene (p.986·1); hydrochlorothiazide (p.907·3).
Hypertension; oedema.

Renidur Merck Sharp & Dohme, Port.
Enalapril maleate (p.883·3); hydrochlorothiazide (p.907·3).
Hypertension.

Renilon Nutricia, Port.
Preparation for enteral nutrition (p.1350·1).
Renal or hepatic failure.

Renipril APS, Port.
Enalapril maleate (p.883·3).
Heart failure; hypertension.

Renitec
Merck Sharp & Dohme, Aust.; Merck Sharp & Dohme, Austral.; Merck Sharp & Dohme, Belg.; Merck Sharp & Dohme, Braz.; Merck Sharp & Dohme, Denm.; Merck Sharp & Dohme, Fin.; Merck Sharp & Dohme-Chibret, Fr.; Merck Sharp & Dohme, Hong Kong; Merck Sharp & Dohme, Mex.; Merck Sharp & Dohme, Neth.; Merck Sharp & Dohme, Norw.; Merck Sharp & Dohme, NZ; Merck Sharp & Dohme, Port.; Merck Sharp & Dohme, S.Afr.; Merck Sharp & Dohme, Singapore; Merck Sharp & Dohme, Spain; Merck Sharp & Dohme, Swed.; Merck Sharp & Dohme, Thai.
Enalapril (p.883·3), enalapril maleate (p.883·3), or enalaprilat (p.884·1).
Angina pectoris; heart failure; hypertension; myocardial infarction.

Renitec Comp
Merck Sharp & Dohme, Fin.; Merck Sharp & Dohme, Norw.; Merck Sharp & Dohme, Swed.
Enalapril maleate (p.883·3); hydrochlorothiazide (p.907·3).
Hypertension.

Renitec Plus
Merck Sharp & Dohme, Aust.; Merck Sharp & Dohme, Austral.; Merck Sharp & Dohme, Fin.; Merck Sharp & Dohme, Neth.
Enalapril maleate (p.883·3); hydrochlorothiazide (p.907·3).
Hypertension.

Renitecmax Merck Sharp & Dohme, Spain.
Enalapril maleate (p.883·3); hydrochlorothiazide (p.907·3).
Hypertension.

Reniten Merck Sharp & Dohme, Switz.
Enalapril maleate (p.883·3) or enalaprilat (p.884·1).
Heart failure; hypertension.

Reniten Plus Merck Sharp & Dohme, Switz.
Enalapril maleate (p.883·3); hydrochlorothiazide (p.907·3).
Hypertension.

Rennie
Roche, Belg.; Roche, Fin.; Roche Nicholas, Fr.; Roche Nicholas, Ger.; Roche, Hong Kong; Roche Nicholas, Israel; Roche, Ital.; Roche Consumer, Neth.; Roche Consumer, Singapore; Roche, Swed.; Roche, Switz.; Roche Consumer, UK.
Calcium carbonate (p.1215·1); magnesium carbonate (p.1232·3).
Dyspepsia; flatulence; heartburn.

Rennie Defarin Roche Nicholas, Ger.
Calcium carbonate (p.1215·1); heavy magnesium carbonate (p.1232·3); simeticone (p.1249·2).
Gastrointestinal disorders with meteorism.

Rennie Deflatine
Roche Nicholas, Fr.; Roche Consumer, Neth.; Roche, Switz.; Roche Consumer, UK.
Calcium carbonate (p.1215·1); magnesium carbonate (p.1232·3); simeticone (p.1249·2).
Dyspepsia; flatulence; heartburn.

Rennie Digestif Roche, Port.
Calcium carbonate (p.1215·1); magnesium carbonate (p.1232·3).
Dyspepsia; gastric hyperacidity.

Rennie Duo Roche Consumer, UK.
Calcium carbonate (p.1215·1); magnesium carbonate (p.1232·3); sodium alginate (p.1498·3).
Dyspepsia; heartburn.

Rennie Gold Roche Consumer, UK†.
Calcium carbonate (p.1215·1).
Dyspepsia; flatulence.

Rennie Rap-Eze Roche Consumer, Irl.
Calcium carbonate (p.1215·1).
Gastric hyperacidity; heartburn.

Rennie Refluxine Roche Nicholas, Fr.
Calcium carbonate (p.1215·1); light magnesium carbonate (p.1232·3); sodium alginate (p.1498·3).
Gastric hyperacidity; gastro-oesophageal reflux.

Renob Blasen- und Nierentee Pfleger, Ger.
Birch leaf (p.1585·2); couch-grass rhizome (p.1599·3); solidago virgaurea; ononis (p.1644·1); liquorice root (p.1231·2).
Urinary-tract disorders.

Renoclear Transphyto, Fr.
Cleansing, disinfection and soaking of soft contact lenses (p.1129·2).

Renofundina Braun, Port.
Glucose; calcium chloride; magnesium chloride; potassium chloride; sodium acetate; sodium chloride (p.1184·1).
Haemodialysis.

Renografin
Squibb Diagnostics, Canad.†; Squibb Diagnostics, USA.
Meglumine amidotrizoate (p.1031·2); sodium amidotrizoate (p.1031·2).
Radiographic contrast medium.

Reno-M
Squibb Diagnostics, Canad.†; Squibb Diagnostics, USA.
Meglumine amidotrizoate (p.1031·2).
Radiographic contrast medium.

Renoquid Glenwood, USA†.
Sulfacytine.
Bacterial infections.

Renorell Sanorell, Ger.
Homoeopathic preparation.

Renormax
Schering-Plough, Ital.; Italfarmaco, Spain.
Spirapril hydrochloride (p.973·2).
Hypertension.

Renova
Ortho Dermatological, Canad.; Janssen-Cilag, S.Afr.; Janssen, Thai.; Ortho Dermatological, USA.
Tretinoin (p.1126·2).
Photoageing of the skin; pigmentation disorders.

Renovist Squibb Diagnostics, USA†.
Meglumine amidotrizoate (p.1031·2); sodium amidotrizoate (p.1031·2).
Radiographic contrast medium.

Renovue Squibb Diagnostics, USA†.
Meglumine iodamide (p.1034·1).
Radiographic contrast medium.

Renpress ICN, Spain.
Spirapril hydrochloride (p.973·2).
Hypertension.

Rentamine Pediatric Major, USA.
Phenylephrine tannate (p.1097·3); ephedrine tannate (p.1090·3); chlorpheniramine [chlorphenamine] tannate (p.412·2); pentoxyverine tannate (p.1096·3).
Coughs and cold symptoms.

Rentibloc Fuisz, Ger.
Sotalol hydrochloride (p.972·2).
Arrhythmias.

Rentylin Fuisz, Ger.
Oxpentifylline [pentoxifylline] (p.950·3).
Peripheral and ocular vascular disorders.

Renu
Bausch & Lomb, Canad.; Bausch & Lomb, Fr.†; Bausch & Lomb, USA.
Range of solutions for soft contact lenses (p.1129·2).

Renu Enzymatic Cleaner Bausch & Lomb, USA.
Subtilisin-A (p.1129·2).
Cleansing solution for soft contact lenses.

Renu Multiplus Bausch & Lomb, UK.
Solution for cleansing, disinfecting, and removal of protein from contact lenses (p.1129·2).

Renutrin Heralds, Braz.
Ferrous fumarate (p.1360·1); vitamins (p.1350·1).
Iron deficiency; iron-deficiency anaemias.

Renutryl Germania, Aust.
Preparation for enteral nutrition (p.1350·1).

Renutryl 500 Nestle, Fr.
Nutritional supplement (p.1350·1).

Reocol Also, Ital.
Tartaric acid; sodium bicarbonate (p.1186·2); anhydrous citric acid; magnesium sulfate (p.1191·1).
Constipation; dyspepsia.

Reodyn Orion, Fin.
Carbocisteine (p.1086·3).
Respiratory-tract disorders.

Reoferol Zimaia, Port.
Tocoferil nicotinate (p.984·3).

Reoflus Pulitzer, Ital.
Heparin calcium (p.902·1).
Thromboembolic disorders.

Reolase Pulitzer, Ital.
Telmesteine (p.1101·1).
Respiratory-tract disorders.

Reolina IFI, Ital.†
Bile extract (p.1585·1); phenolphthalein (p.1244·1); cascara (p.1216·1); rhubarb (p.1248·1).
Constipation.

Reomax Pfizer, Ital.
Etacrynic acid (p.887·2) or sodium etacrynate (p.887·2).
Oedema.

Reomucil Astra, Ital.
Carbocisteine (p.1086·3).
Respiratory-tract congestion.

ReoPro
Centocor, Aust.; Lilly, Austral.; Lilly, Belg.; Lilly, Canad.; Centocor, Denm.; Lilly, Fin.; Lilly, Fr.; Lilly, Ger.; Lilly, Hong Kong; Lilly, Irl.; Centocor, Israel; Lilly, Ital.; Lilly, Neth.; Centocor, Norw.; Lilly, NZ; Lilly, S.Afr.; Lilly, Singapore; Lilly, Spain; Lilly, Swed.; Lilly, Switz.; Lilly, Thai.; Lilly, UK; Centocor, USA; Lilly, USA.
Abciximab (p.819·2).
Prevention of ischaemic cardiac complications during angioplasty or atherectomy; unstable angina pectoris.

Repalyte Rhone-Poulenc Rorer, Austral.
Sodium chloride; potassium chloride; sodium acid citrate; glucose (p.1185·2).
Diarrhoea; oral rehydration therapy.

Repan Everett, USA.
Butalbital (p.658·3); caffeine (p.761·3); paracetamol (p.71·2).
Pain.

Repan CF Everett, USA.
Paracetamol (p.71·2); butalbital (p.658·3).
Pain.

Reparil
Note.This name is used for preparations of different composition.
Madaus, Aust.; Madaus, Belg.†; Byk, Braz.; Madaus, Ger.†; Madaus, Ital.; Madaus, S.Afr.†; Madaus, Thai.
Injection: Sodium aescinate (p.1574·1).
Back pain; inflammation; oedema; peripheral vascular disorders.

Madaus, Aust.; Madaus, Belg.; Byk, Braz.; Madaus, Ger.; Madaus, Hong Kong; Madaus, Ital.; Madaus, Switz.; Madaus, Thai.
Tablets: Aescin (p.1574·1).
Inflammation; oedema; thrombophlebitis; venous insufficiency.

Madaus, Aust.; Byk Madaus, S.Afr.
Topical gel: Aescin (p.1574·1); diethylamine salicylate (p.32·2).
Soft-tissue injury; vascular disorders.

Madaus, Belg.; Byk, Braz.; Madaus, Fr.; Madaus, Hong Kong; Madaus, Switz.; Madaus, Thai.
Topical gel: Aescin (p.1574·1); sodium aescin polysulfate (p.1574·1); diethylamine salicylate (p.32·2).
Haematomas; inflammation; soft-tissue disorders; tenosynovitis; thrombophlebitis; varicose veins; venous insufficiency.

Madaus, Ital.
Topical gel: Aescin (p.1574·1); heparin sodium (p.902·1); diethylamine salicylate (p.32·2).
Soft-tissue disorders.

Reparil N Madaus, Switz.†
Aescin (p.1574·1); diethylamine salicylate (p.32·2).
Soft-tissue injury.

Reparil-Gel N, Reparil-Sportgel Madaus, Ger.
Aescin (p.1574·1); diethylamine salicylate (p.32·2).
Inflammation; soft-tissue disorders.

Repasma Pharmador, S.Afr.
Amobarbital (p.655·2); aminophylline (p.760·1); ephedrine hydrochloride (p.1090·1).
Asthma.

Repeltin Pierre Fabre, Ger.
Trimeprazine [alimemazine] (p.426·3).
Bronchial asthma or asthma-like complaints; pruritus.

Repervit IDI, Ital.
Vitamin A palmitate (p.1383·2).
Vitamin A deficiency.

Repha Orphon Repha, Ger.†
Java tea (p.1625·1).
Gout; rheumatism; urinary-tract disorders.

Rephacimin Repha, Ger.†
Homoeopathic preparation.

Rephacratin Repha, Ger.†
Crataegus (p.1600·2).
Cardiac disorders.

Rephahyval Repha, Ger.†
Hypericum (p.290·2).
Anxiety disorders; depression.

Rephalgin Repha, Ger.
Homoeopathic preparation.

Rephalysin C Repha, Ger.
Escherichia coli.
Gastrointestinal disorders.

Repha-Os Repha, Ger.
Tormentil root (p.1674·1); rhatany root (p.1657·3); myrrh (p.1639·2); eucalyptus oil (p.1580·3); peppermint oil (p.1243·3); clove oil (p.1597·1); menthol (p.1632·3).
Mouth and throat disorders.

Rephaprossan Repha, Ger.†
Homoeopathic preparation.

Rephastasan Repha, Ger.
Homoeopathic preparation.

Rephenyl Reese, USA†.
Guaifenesin (p.1092·2); phenylpropanolamine hydrochloride (p.1098·1).

Replavite Sussex, UK.
Oral rehydration solution (p.1185·2).
Diarrhoea.

Replenate BPL, UK.
A factor VIII preparation (p.734·1).
Formerly known as 8SM.
Haemophilia A.

Replenine
BPL, Singapore; BPL, UK.
A factor IX preparation (p.735·1).
Haemophilia B.

Replens
Note.This name is used for preparations of different composition.
Sanofi Synthelabo, Austral.; Wolfs, Belg.; Roberts, Canad.; Janssen-Cilag, Ital.; Sanofi Winthrop, Port.†; Adcock Ingram, S.Afr.; Ipsen, Spain; Meda, Swed.; Warner-Lambert, USA.
Polycarbophil (p.1244·2).
Vaginal dryness.

Solymes, Fr.; Ethical Research, Irl.†; Teva, Israel; Anglian, UK.
Vaginal lubricant.
Vaginal dryness; vaginal irritation.

Vifor, Switz.
Purified water (p.1680·2).
Vaginal dryness.

Replete Clintec, USA.
Lactose-free, gluten-free preparation for enteral nutrition (p.1350·1).

Replicare Smith & Nephew, UK.
Hydrocolloid dressing.
Burns; ulcers; wounds.

Reposans Wesley, USA.
Chlordiazepoxide hydrochloride (p.659·2).
Alcohol withdrawal syndrome; anxiety.

Reposo-Mono Medgenix, Belg.
Meprobamate (p.691·1).
Insomnia.

Reposton Provit, Mex.
Liver extract.
Anaemias.

Repotin Bioclones, S.Afr.
Epoetin (p.730·2).
Anaemias; autologous blood transfusions.

Repowine Truw, Ger.†
Scoparium (p.1661·2).
Cardiac disorders.

Repowinon Truw, Ger.†
Homoeopathic preparation.

Repriadol Nycomed, Denm.†.
Morphine sulfate (p.56·1).
Pain.

Repronex Ferring, USA.
Menotrophin (p.1288·2).
Infertility.

Reproven N Hanosan, Ger.
Homoeopathic preparation.

Reptilase
Disperga, Aust.; Pharmadeveloppement, Fr.; Difa, Ital.†; Neves, Port.; Llorente, Spain.
Haemocoagulase (p.726·3).
Haemorrhage.

Repursan M Boots, Ger.†.
Cort. yohimbe.; nuces colae; lign. muir. puam.; testes; vitamins; minerals (p.1350·1).
Tonic.

Repursan ST Biokanol, Ger.
Pausinystalia yohimbe; kola (p.1681·1); ephedra (p.1090·1); vitamins; minerals (p.1350·1).
Sexual fatigue.

Requiesan Klein, Ger.
Eschscholtzia californica; avena (p.1583·1).
Sleep disorders.

Requip
SmithKline Beecham, Aust.; SmithKline Beecham, Belg.; SmithKline Beecham, Canad.; SmithKline Beecham, Denm.; SmithKline Beecham, Fr.; SmithKline Beecham, Ger.; SmithKline Beecham, Hong Kong; SmithKline Beecham, Irl.; SmithKline Beecham, Israel; SmithKline Beecham, Ital.; SmithKline Beecham, Neth.; SmithKline Beecham, Norw.; Beecham, Port.; SmithKline Beecham, Spain; SmithKline Beecham, Swed.; SmithKline Beecham, Switz.; SmithKline Beecham, UK; SmithKline Beecham, USA.
Ropinirole hydrochloride (p.1177·1).
Parkinsonism.

Resaid Geneva, USA†.
Phenylpropanolamine hydrochloride (p.1098·1); chlorpheniramine [chlorphenamine] maleate (p.412·1).
Upper respiratory-tract symptoms.

Resalt Compu, S.Afr.
Sodium chloride; potassium chloride; glucose; sodium bicarbonate (p.1185·2).
Diarrhoea; oral rehydration therapy.

Resaltex
Procter & Gamble, Aust.; Procter & Gamble, Ger.†.
Hydrochlorothiazide (p.907·3); reserpine (p.967·3); triamterene (p.986·1).
Hypertension.

Resan Mucolitico Alacan, Spain.
Ampicillin sodium (p.150·3); bromhexine (p.1085·3).
Lignocaine [lidocaine] (p.1313·2) is included in this preparation to alleviate the pain of injection.
Respiratory-tract infections.

Resan Retard Alacan, Spain.
Ampicillin sodium (p.150·3); ampicillin benzathine (p.151·3); bromhexine hydrochloride (p.1085·3).
Lignocaine [lidocaine] hydrochloride (p.1313·2) is included in this preparation to alleviate the pain of injection.
Respiratory-tract infections.

Rescaps-D SR Geneva, USA†.
Phenylpropanolamine hydrochloride (p.1098·1); caramiphen edisilate (p.1086·2).
Coughs.

Rescon Capellon, USA.
Capsules: Pseudoephedrine hydrochloride (p.1099·2); chlorpheniramine [chlorphenamine] maleate (p.412·1).
Liquid†: Phenylpropanolamine hydrochloride (p.1098·1); chlorpheniramine [chlorphenamine] maleate (p.412·1).
Upper respiratory-tract symptoms.

Rescon-DM Capellon, USA.
Dextromethorphan hydrobromide (p.1087·3); pseudoephedrine hydrochloride (p.1099·2); chlorpheniramine [chlorphenamine] maleate (p.412·1).
Coughs and cold symptoms.

Rescon-ED Capellon, USA†.
Pseudoephedrine hydrochloride (p.1099·2); chlorpheniramine [chlorphenamine] maleate (p.412·1).
Upper respiratory-tract symptoms.

Rescon-GG Ion, USA.
Phenylephrine hydrochloride (p.1097·1); guaifenesin (p.1092·2).
Coughs.

Rescon-MX Capellon, USA.
Pseudoephedrine hydrochloride (p.1099·2); chlorpheniramine [chlorphenamine] maleate (p.412·1); hyoscine methonitrtae (p.468·2).
Upper respiratory-tract disorders.

Rescriptor
Pharmacia Upjohn, Austral.; Pharmacia Upjohn, Canad.; Pharmacia Upjohn, Mex.; Pharmacia Upjohn, USA.
Delavirdine mesilate (p.617·3).
HIV infection.

RescueFlow Biophausia, Denm.; Pharmalink, Swed.; IDIS, UK.
Dextran 70 (p.729·2) in sodium chloride.
Plasma volume expansion.

Rescula
Ueno, Jpn; Novartis, Mex.; Ciba Vision, Singapore; Ciba Vision, Thai.; Novartis Ophthalmics, USA.
Unoprostone isopropyl (p.1447·3).
Glaucoma; ocular hypertension.

Rescuvolin
Nettopharma, Denm.; Nycomed, Fin.; Medac, Ger.; Pharmachemie,
Israel; Nycomed, Norw.; Asta Medica, NZ; Pharmachemie, S.Afr.; Pharmachemie, Singapore; Nycomed, Swed.; Pharmachemie, Thai.
Calcium folinate (p.1363·1).
Adjunct to fluorouracil in colorectal cancer; antidote to folic acid antagonists; folic acid deficiency; megaloblastic anaemia; reduction of methotrexate toxicity.

Resdan Whitehall-Robins, Canad.†.
Cetrimide (p.1137·1).
Dandruff.

Resdan Rx Whitehall, Neth.†.
Coal tar (p.1125·1); menthol (p.1632·3).
Scalp disorders.

Resectal Fresenius Kabi, Aust.
Sorbitol (p.1377·3); mannitol (p.924·3).
Bladder and prostate surgery.

Resectisol
McGaw, NZ; Kendall McGaw, USA.
Mannitol (p.924·3).
Irrigation solution.

Reser TO-Chemicals, Thai.
Reserpine (p.967·3); hydralazine hydrochloride (p.905·3); hydrochlorothiazide (p.907·3).
Hypertension.

Reseril Mead Johnson, Ital.
Nefazodone hydrochloride (p.300·3).
Depression.

Reserpina British Dispensary, Thai.
Reserpine (p.967·3).
Hypertension; sedative.

Reset Biomedica, Ital.†.
Aniracetam (p.1580·2).
Mental function impairment.

Resfin Jofrain, Mex.
Paracetamol (p.71·2).
Fever; pain.

Resfolin Piam, Ital.
Calcium folinate (p.1363·1).
Anaemias; antidote to folic acid antagonists; folate deficiency; reduction of aminopterin and methotrexate toxicity.

Resfrialgina Farmedica, Braz.
Dipyrone (p.34·1); vitamin C (p.1389·3).
Cold and influenza symptoms.

Resfry Neo Quimica, Braz.
Salicylamide (p.82·1); chlorpheniramine [chlorphenamine] maleate (p.412·1); caffeine (p.761·3); ascorbic acid (p.1389·3).
Cold and influenza symptoms.

Resical Fresenius, Port.
Calcium polystyrene sulfonate (p.1002·3).
Hyperkalaemia.

Residex P55 Agropharm, UK.
Permethrin (p.1436·1).
Mosquito repellent for nets and clothing.

Resilar Orion, Fin.
Dextromethorphan hydrobromide (p.1087·3).
Coughs.

Resimatil Sanofi Synthelabo, Ger.
Primidone (p.363·3).
Epilepsy.

Resina Carbolica Dentilin Ghimas, Ital.
Guaiacol (p.1092·1); lignocaine [lidocaine] hydrochloride (p.1313·2); alcohol (p.1130·3); camphor (p.1589·3); thymol (p.1158·3).
Dental disinfection; dental pain.

Resincalcio Rubio, Spain.
Calcium polystyrene sulfonate (p.1002·3).
Hyperkalaemia.

Resincolestiramina
Rubio, Singapore; Rubio, Spain; Rubio, Thai.; TTN, Thai.
Colestyramine (p.864·1).
Diarrhoea; hypercholesterolaemia; pruritus associated with biliary stasis.

Resinol Mentholatum, USA.
Calamine (p.1111·3); zinc oxide (p.1128·2); resorcinol (p.1122·2).
Minor skin irritation.

Resinsodio
Rubio, Singapore; Rubio, Spain; Rubio, Thai.; TTN, Thai.
Sodium polystyrene sulfonate (p.1023·2).
Hyperkalaemia.

Resistan Lichtwer, Ger.
Homoeopathic preparation.

Resisten Retard Smaller, Spain.
Ampicillin sodium (p.150·3); ampicillin benzathine (p.151·3); bromhexine hydrochloride (p.1085·3).
Lignocaine [lidocaine] hydrochloride (p.1313·2) is included in this preparation to alleviate the pain of injection.
Respiratory-tract infections.

Resiston One Rhone-Poulenc Rorer, UK†.
Sodium cromoglicate (p.774·3); xylometazoline hydrochloride (p.1102·2).
Allergic rhinitis.

Resistone QD Rhone Poulenc Chemicals, UK.
Alkylaryltrialkylammonium chloride.
Disinfection.

Resivit Rhone-Poulenc Rorer, Spain†.
Multivitamin preparation (p.1350·1).

Resma UCB, Belg.
Zafirlukast (p.785·3).
Asthma.

Resnedal Byk Leo, Spain.
Chlortalidone (p.857·1); spironolactone (p.973·2); reserpine (p.967·3).
Hypertension.

Resochin
Bayer, Aust.; Bayer, Ger.; Bayer, Spain.
Chloroquine phosphate (p.432·3).
Amoebiasis; arthritis; malaria; systemic lupus erythematosus.

Resochina Bayer, Port.
Chloroquine phosphate (p.432·3).
Amoebiasis; lichen planus; lupus erythematosus; malaria; rheumatoid arthritis; rosacea.

Resochine Bayer, Switz.†.
Chloroquine phosphate (p.432·3).
Amoebiasis; lupus erythematosus; malaria; rheumatoid arthritis.

Resodermil Oftalder, Port.
Sulfur (p.1123·3); resorcinol (p.1122·2); zinc oxide (p.1128·2).
Acne.

Resoferon Ciba-Geigy, Belg.†; Novartis, Switz.
Ferrous sulfate (p.1360·3).
Succinic acid is included to increase the absorption and availability of iron.
Iron deficiency; iron-deficiency anaemia.

Resol
Note. This name is used for preparations of different composition.
Terramin, Aust.
Camphor (p.1589·3); terpineol (p.1669·3); eucalyptus oil (p.1609·2); pumilio pine oil (p.1656·3); menthol (p.1632·3); thymol (p.1158·3).
Catarrh; rheumatism.

Wyeth-Ayerst, USA.
Glucose; sodium chloride; potassium citrate; citric acid; sodium phosphate; magnesium chloride; calcium chloride; sodium citrate (p.1185·2).
Diarrhoea; oral rehydration therapy.

Resolution Phoenix Health, UK.
Nicotine (p.1640·3); vitamins (p.1350·1).
Aid to smoking withdrawal.

Resolutivo Regium Miquel Garriga, Spain.
Boldo (p.1585·3); chumbera; equisetum (p.1606·3); xanthium; sideritide; rosemary; cynodon; hepatica; saxifraga; arenaria; lithospermum; melissa (p.1632·2).
Formerly contained anethole, borneol, camphene, rubia tinctorum, oxidised terpenes, pinenes, fenchone, eucalyptol, atropine sulfate and papaverine hydrochloride.
Hyperuricaemia; renal calculi.

Resolve SSL, UK.
Paracetamol (p.71·2); anhydrous citric acid (p.1596·2); sodium bicarbonate (p.1186·2); potassium bicarbonate (p.1186·1); anhydrous sodium carbonate (p.1665·1); ascorbic acid (p.1389·3).
Headache with gastric upset.

Resolve Extra SSL, UK.
Paracetamol (p.71·2); sodium bicarbonate (p.1186·2); caffeine (p.761·3).
Dyspepsia; headache.

Resolve/GP Allergan, USA.
Cleansing solution for hard and gas permeable contact lenses (p.1129·2).

Resonium
Sanofi Winthrop, Denm.; Sanofi Synthelabo, Fin.; Sanofi Synthelabo, Port.; Sanofi Winthrop, Swed.
Sodium polystyrene sulfonate (p.1023·2).
Hyperkalaemia.

Resonium A
Sanofi Winthrop, Aust.; Sanofi Synthelabo, Austral.; Sanofi Synthelabo, Ger.; Sanofi Winthrop, Hong Kong; Sanofi Winthrop, Irl.; Sanofi Synthelabo, Neth.; Sanofi Winthrop, NZ; Sanofi Synthelabo, Switz.; Sanofi Synthelabo, Thai.; Sanofi Winthrop, UK.
Sodium polystyrene sulfonate (p.1023·2).
Hyperkalaemia.

Resonium Calcium
Sanofi Synthelabo, Canad.; Sanofi Winthrop, Denm.; Sanofi Winthrop, Norw.; Sanofi Winthrop, Swed.
Calcium polystyrene sulfonate (p.1002·3).
Hyperkalaemia.

Resorbane Spirig, Switz.
Eucalyptol (p.1609·2); camphor (p.1589·3); niaouli oil (p.1640·2).
Respiratory-tract disorders.

Resorborina Belmac, Spain.
Mouthwash: Benzalkonium chloride (p.1133·2); dexamethasone (p.1067·1); resorcinol (p.1122·2); amethocaine [tetracaine] hydrochloride (p.1305·2).
Throat spray: Benzalkonium chloride (p.1133·2); betamethasone valerate (p.1063·2); amethocaine [tetracaine] hydrochloride (p.1305·2).
Mouth and throat inflammation.

Resource
Novartis Nutrition, Canad.; Novartis, Fin.; Novartis Nutrition, Fr.; Novartis Nutrition, Hong Kong; Novartis Consumer, Port.; Novartis Nutrition, Singapore; Novartis Consumer, UK; Novartis Nutrition, USA.
A range preparations for enteral nutrition (p.1350·1).

Resource Benefiber
Note. This name is used for preparations of different composition.
Novartis Consumer, Ital.
Dietary fibre supplement (p.1214·2).

Novartis Consumer, UK.
Guar gum (p.323·3).
Nutritional supplement.

Resource Energy Novartis Consumer, Ital.
Preparation for enteral nutrition (p.1350·1).

Resource Fruit Novartis Consumer, Ital.
Preparation for enteral nutrition (p.1350·1).

Resource Gelificata Novartis Consumer, Ital.
Carrageenan (p.1500·1); xanthan gum (p.1504·3); guar gum (p.323·3).
Dysphagia.

Resource Thicken Up
Novartis, Irl.; Novartis Consumer, Ital.
Nutrtional supplement for thickening foods (p.1350·1).
Dysphagia.

Resp Murdock, USA†.
Ephedrine hydrochloride (p.1090·1).

Respa-ARM Respa, USA†.
Phenylephrine hydrochloride (p.1097·1); phenylpropanolamine hydrochloride (p.1098·1); chlorpheniramine [chlorphenamine] maleate (p.412·1); belladonna alkaloids (p.463·1).

Respacal
Bios, Belg.; UCB, UK†.
Tulobuterol hydrochloride (p.785·2).
Bronchospasm.

Respa-DM Respa, USA.
Dextromethorphan hydrobromide (p.1087·3); guaifenesin (p.1092·2).
Coughs; respiratory-tract congestion.

Respa-GF Respa, USA.
Guaifenesin (p.1092·2).

Respahist Respa, USA.
Pseudoephedrine hydrochloride (p.1099·2); brompheniramine maleate (p.410·2).

Respaire Laser, USA.
Pseudoephedrine hydrochloride (p.1099·2); guaifenesin (p.1092·2).
Coughs and cold symptoms; nasal congestion.

Respalis Nestle, Fr.
Preparation for enteral nutrition (p.1350·1).
Respiratory insufficiency.

Respalor
Mead Johnson, Hong Kong; Mead Johnson Nutritionals, Thai.; Mead Johnson Nutritionals, USA.
Preparation for enteral nutrition (p.1350·1).
Respiratory system disorders.

Respa-1st Respa, USA.
Pseudoephedrine hydrochloride (p.1099·2); guaifenesin (p.1092·2).
Respiratory-tract disorders associated with increased or viscous mucus.

Respatona Decongestant Formula Brauer, Austral.
Anise oil (p.1580·3); althaea (p.1577·1); bryonia (p.1587·2); iceland moss; chamomile (p.1593·2); thyme (p.1672·2); urtica (p.1678·2); ammonium causticum; aconitum napellus; coccus cacti; corallium rubrum; drosera rotundifolia; ipecacuanha; kali bich.; kreosotum; spongia tosta; sticta pulmonaria.
Coughs and cold symptoms.

Respatona Plus Bronchial Cough Relief Brauer, Austral.
Anise oil (p.1580·3); althaea (p.1577·1); bryonia (p.1587·2); iceland moss; echinacea angustifolia (p.1606·2); chamomile (p.1593·2); thyme (p.1672·2); urtica (p.1678·2); aconitum napellus; coccus cacti; corallium rubrum; drosera rotundifolia; ipecacuanha; kali bich.; kreosotum; spongia tosta; sticta pulmonaria.
Coughs.

Respax
Pharmacia Upjohn, Austral.; Pharmacia Upjohn, Hong Kong; Pharmacia Upjohn, NZ.
Salbutamol (p.770·3) or salbutamol sulfate (p.770·3).
Obstructive airways disease.

Respbid Boehringer Ingelheim, USA.
Theophylline (p.777·2).
Obstructive airways disease.

Respexil Prodome, Braz.
Norfloxacin (p.232·1).
Bacterial infections.

Respibien Cinfa, Spain.
Oxymetazoline hydrochloride (p.1096·2).
Nasal congestion.

Respicilin Haller, Braz.
Amoxicillin (p.149·2); bromhexine (p.1085·3).
Bacterial infections of the respiratory tract.

Respicort Mundipharma, Ger.
Budesonide (p.1064·2).
Obstructive airways disease.

Respicur
Byk, Aust.; Byk Gulden, Ital.
Theophylline (p.777·2).
Obstructive airways disease.

RespiGam Medimmune, USA.
Respiratory syncytial virus immunoglobulins (p.1562·1).
Passive immunisation.

Respilene
Note. This name is used for preparations of different composition.
Sanofi Winthrop, Fr.
Syrup: Pholcodine (p.1099·1).
Formerly contained zipeprol hydrochloride.
Respiratory-tract disorders.

Columbia, Mex.
Zipeprol (p.1102·3).
Coughs.

Respinol Pharmaceutical Enterprises, S.Afr.
Phenylephrine hydrochloride (p.1097·1); chlorpheniramine [chlorphenamine] maleate (p.412·1); hyoscine methonitrate (p.468·2).
Cold symptoms; sinusitis; vasomotor rhinitis.

Respinol Compound *Pharmaceutical Enterprises, S.Afr.*
Pholcodine (p.1099·1); pseudoephedrine hydrochloride (p.1099·2); chlorpheniramine [chlorphenamine] maleate (p.412·1); hyoscine methonitrate (p.468·2).
Cold symptoms; coughs; rhinitis; sinusitis.

Respir *Schering-Plough, Spain.*
Oxymetazoline hydrochloride (p.1096·2).
Nasal congestion.

Respir Balsamico *Schering-Plough, Spain†.*
Camphor (p.1589·3); eucalyptol (p.1609·2); oxymetazoline hydrochloride (p.1096·2); menthol (p.1632·3).
Nasal congestion.

Respiral *Sanofi Synthelabo, Port.*
Zipeprol hydrochloride (p.1102·3).
Coughs.

Respiro *Byk Gulden, Ital.*
Xylometazoline hydrochloride (p.1102·2).
Nasal congestion.

Respiroma *Fournier SA, Spain.*
Salbutamol sulfate (p.770·3).
Formerly contained iodinated glycerol and salbutamol sulfate.
Obstructive airways disease.

Respisniffers *Aspen Consumer, S.Afr.*
Eucalyptol (p.1609·2); pine oil; chloroxylenol (p.1142·1); turpentine oil (p.1676·3); menthol (p.1632·3).
Bronchitis; cold symptoms; nasal congestion.

Respitol *Cinfa, Spain.*
Sodium chloride (p.1196·1).
Nasal congestion.

Resplant *Spitzner, Ger.*
Echinacea purpurea (p.1606·2).
Respiratory- and urinary-tract infections.

Respocort
3M, Austral.; 3M, NZ.
Beclometasone dipropionate (p.1061·2).
Obstructive airways disease.

Respolin
3M, Austral.; 3M, Hong Kong; 3M, NZ; 3M, Singapore; 3M, Thai.
Salbutamol (p.770·3) or salbutamol sulfate (p.770·3).
Obstructive airways disease.

Responsar *Bayer, Ital.*
Cyfluthrin (p.1430·2).
Insecticide.

Respontin
Glaxo Wellcome, Norw.; Glaxo Wellcome, UK.
Ipratropium bromide (p.766·1).
Obstructive airways disease.

Resprim
Alphapharm, Austral.; Teva, Israel.
Co-trimoxazole (p.193·3).
Bacterial infections; Pneumocystis carinii pneumonia.

Resprin
Note. This name is used for preparations of different composition.
Johnson & Johnson, Braz.
Paracetamol (p.71·2); carbinoxamine (p.411·1); pentoxyverine citrate (p.1096·3); phenylephrine hydrochloride (p.1097·1).
Cold and influenza symptoms.

Rice Steele, Irl.
Aspirin (p.14·2).
Fever; inflammation; pain.

Restal *SFD, Port.*
Oxidised glycerol triester.
Cicatrisation; cracked lips.

Restameth-SR *Restan, S.Afr.*
Indometacin (p.44·3).
Gout; musculoskeletal and joint disorders.

Restandol
Organon, Denm.; Organon, Irl.; Organon, UK.
Testosterone undecylate (p.1492·2).
Male hypogonadism; osteoporosis.

Restaslim *Restan, S.Afr.*
Phenylpropanolamine hydrochloride (p.1098·1).
Obesity.

Restavit *Woods, Austral.*
Doxylamine succinate (p.417·1).
Insomnia.

Restenil *Recip, Swed.†.*
Meprobamate (p.691·1).
Anxiety; headache; skeletal muscle spasm; sleep disorders.

Restin *Restan, S.Afr.*
Valerian (p.1678·3); vitamin B substances (p.1350·1); ascorbic acid.
Nonpsychotic mental disorders.

Restore *InAgra, USA†.*
Psyllium hydrophilic mucilloid (p.1229·1).

Restoril
Novartis, Canad.; Novartis, USA.
Temazepam (p.707·2).
Insomnia.

Restovar
Organon, Aust.†; Organon, Swed.
Lynestrenol (p.1480·1); ethinylestradiol (p.1476·2).
Combined oral contraceptive.

Restrical *Monot, Fr.*
Liquid paraffin (p.1407·1).
Constipation.

Restwel *Covan, S.Afr.*
Doxylamine succinate (p.417·1).
Insomnia.

Resulax *Tika, Swed.*
Sorbitol (p.1377·3).
Bowel evacuation; constipation.

Resulin *Ist. Chim. Inter., Ital.*
Nimesulide (p.62·3).
Fever; inflammation; pain.

Resurmide *Ibi, Ital.*
Somatostatin acetate (p.1297·3).
Gastrointestinal haemorrhage.

Resyl
Novartis Consumer, Aust.; Novartis, Israel; Novartis Consumer, Ital.; Novartis, Swed.; Novartis Consumer, Switz.
Guaifenesin (p.1092·2).
Coughs; respiratory-tract congestion.

Resyl DM *Novartis Consumer, Ital.*
Guaifenesin (p.1092·2); dextromethorphan hydrobromide (p.1087·3).
Coughs.

Resyl mit Codein *Novartis Consumer, Aust.*
Guaifenesin (p.1092·2); codeine phosphate (p.25·2).
Coughs.

Resyl Plus *Novartis Consumer, Switz.*
Guaifenesin (p.1092·2); codeine phosphate (p.25·2).
Coughs.

Retabolin forte *Cimex, Switz.*
Vitamin B substances (p.1350·1).
Neuralgia; neuritis.

Retacillin *Jenapharm, Ger.*
Benzylpenicillin sodium (p.157·2); procaine penicillin [procaine benzylpenicillin] (p.239·2); benzathine benzylpenicillin (p.156·2).
Bacterial infections.

Retacnyl
Galderma, Fr.; Galderma, Hong Kong; Galderma, Mex.; Galderma, Singapore; Galderma, Thai.
Tretinoin (p.1126·2).
Acne; keratinisation disorders; photoageing of the skin.

Retafer
Orion, Fin.; Orion, Singapore.
Ferrous sulfate (p.1360·3).
Iron deficiency; iron-deficiency anaemia.

Retafyllin
Orion, Fin.; Orion, Singapore; Orion, Thai.
Theophylline (p.777·2).
Obstructive airways disease.

Retalzem *Lusofarmaco, Hong Kong.*
Diltiazem hydrochloride (p.874·3).
Hypertension; ischaemic heart disease.

Ret-A-Pres *Precimex, Mex.*
Tretinoin (p.1126·2).

Retardent *Periproducts, UK.*
Stabilised chlorine dioxide (CloSYS II).
Halitosis.

Retardex *Periproducts, UK.*
Stabilised chlorine dioxide (CloSYS II).
Halitosis.

Retardin *Janssen-Cilag, Denm.*
Diphenoxylate hydrochloride (p.1222·2).
Atropine sulfate (p.461·1) is included in this preparation to discourage abuse.
Diarrhoea.

Retarpen
Note. This name is used for preparations of different composition.
Biochemie, Aust.; Biochemie, Singapore.
Benzathine benzylpenicillin (p.156·2).
Bacterial infections.

Septa, Spain.
Ampicillin sodium (p.150·3); ampicillin benzathine (p.151·3).
Lignocaine [lidocaine] (p.1313·2) is included in this preparation to alleviate the pain of injection.
Bacterial infections.

Retarpen Balsamico *Septa, Spain.*
Ampicillin sodium (p.150·3); ampicillin benzathine (p.151·3); eucalyptol (p.1609·2); guaifenesin (p.1092·2).
Lignocaine [lidocaine] hydrochloride (p.1313·2) is included in this preparation to alleviate the pain of injection.
Respiratory-tract infections.

Retarpen compositum *Biochemie, Aust.*
Benzylpenicillin sodium (p.157·2); procaine penicillin [procaine benzylpenicillin] (p.239·2); benzathine benzylpenicillin (p.156·2).
Bacterial infections.

Retarpen Mucolitico *Septa, Spain.*
Ampicillin sodium (p.150·3); ampicillin benzathine (p.151·3); bromhexine hydrochloride (p.1085·3).
Lignocaine [lidocaine] hydrochloride (p.1313·2) is included in this preparation to alleviate the pain of injection.
Respiratory-tract infections.

Retavase
Crystaal, Canad.; Boehringer Mannheim, USA.
Reteplase (p.968·2).
Myocardial infarction.

Retavit *CTI, Israel.*
Tretinoin (p.1126·2).
Acne.

Retcin *DDSA Pharmaceuticals, UK.*
Erythromycin (p.201·2).

Retef *Galderma, Spain.*
Hydrocortisone aceponate (p.1074·2).
Skin disorders.

Retemic *Apsen, Braz.*
Oxybutynin (p.479·2).
Neurogenic bladder; urinary incontinence.

Retencal *UCB, Spain†.*
Imidazole oxoglurate (p.753·3).
Bone formation disorders; calcium metabolism disorders; osteoporosis; Paget's disease of bone; thromboembolic disorders.

Retens *Wasserman, Spain.*
Doxycycline hyclate (p.200·1).
Bacterial infections; malaria.

Reticulogen *Lilly, Ital.†.*
Cyanocobalamin (p.1388·1).
Megaloblastic anaemia; vitamin B₁₂ deficiency.

Reticulogen Fortificado *Lilly, Spain.*
Cyanocobalamin (p.1388·1).
Vitamin B₁₂ deficiency.

Reticus *Farmila, Ital.*
Desonide (p.1066·2).
Skin disorders.

Retimax *Alcon Cusi, Spain.*
Oxpentifylline [pentoxifylline] (p.950·3).
Cerebral and peripheral vascular disorders.

Retin-A
Janssen-Cilag, Aust.; Janssen-Cilag, Austral.; Cilag, Braz.; Ortho Dermatological, Canad.; Janssen-Cilag, Fr.; Cilag, Hong Kong; Janssen-Cilag, Irl.; Janssen-Cilag, Israel; Janssen-Cilag, Ital.; Cilag, Mex.; Janssen-Cilag, NZ; Janssen-Cilag, Port; Janssen-Cilag, S.Afr.; Janssen-Cilag, Singapore; Janssen-Cilag, Switz.; Janssen, Thai.; Janssen-Cilag, UK; Ortho Dermatological, USA.
Tretinoin (p.1126·2).
Acne; keratinisation disorders; photoageing of the skin.

Retinol *INTES, Ital.*
Myrtillus (p.1639·2).
Eye disorders.

Retinol-A *Young Again Products, USA.*
Vitamin A palmitate (p.1383·2).
Minor skin disorders.

Retinova
RoC, Belg.; RoC, Fr.; Janssen-Cilag, NZ; Johnson & Johnson, Spain; Johnson & Johnson, Swed.; Johnson & Johnson, UK.
Tretinoin (p.1126·2).
Acne; sunlight-induced skin damage.

Retirides *OTC, Spain.*
Tretinoin (p.1126·2).
Acne.

Retisdin *Isdin, Port.*
Vitamin A betadex.
UV-induced skin damage.

Retisol-A *Stiefel, Canad.*
Tretinoin (p.1126·2).
Acne.

Retitop *Roche-Posay, Fr.*
Tretinoin (p.1126·2).
Acne; keratinisation disorders.

Retodol Compositum *Rimsa, Mex.*
Hyoscine butylbromide (p.468·2); dipyrone (p.34·1).
Pain; smooth muscle spasm.

Retofar *Searle, Mex.*
Metronidazole (p.594·1).
Amoebiasis; anaerobic bacterial infections.

Retolen *Byk Elmu, Spain.*
Astemizole (p.409·1).
Hypersensitivity reactions.

ReTrieve *Dermatech, Austral.*
Tretinoin (p.1126·2).
Dry skin.

Retrovir
Glaxo Wellcome, Aust.; Glaxo Wellcome, Austral.; Glaxo Wellcome, Belg.; Glaxo Wellcome, Braz.; Glaxo Wellcome, Canad.; Glaxo Wellcome, Denm.; Glaxo Wellcome, Fin.; Glaxo Wellcome, Fr.; Glaxo Wellcome, Ger.; Glaxo Wellcome, Hong Kong; Wellcome, Irl.; Glaxo Wellcome, Israel; Glaxo Wellcome, Ital.; Glaxo Wellcome, Mex.; Glaxo Wellcome, Neth.; Glaxo Wellcome, Norw.; Glaxo Wellcome, NZ; Wellcome, Port.; Glaxo Wellcome, S.Afr.; Glaxo Wellcome, Singapore; Wellcome, Spain; Glaxo Wellcome, Swed.; Glaxo Wellcome, Switz.; Glaxo Wellcome, Thai.; Glaxo Wellcome, UK; Glaxo Wellcome, USA.
Zidovudine (p.645·2).
HIV infection.

Retrovir/3TC Post-HIV Exposure *Glaxo Wellcome, S.Afr.*
Capsules, zidovudine (Retrovir) (p.645·2); tablets, lamivudine (3TC) (p.635·1).
Prophylaxis of HIV infection.

Retterspitz Aerosol *Retterspitz, Ger.†.*
Ephedrine hydrochloride (p.1090·1); pumilio pine oil (p.1656·3); siberian fir oil; thyme oil (p.1672·3); eucalyptus oil (p.1609·2); menthol (p.1632·3).
Respiratory-tract infections.

Retterspitz Ausserlich *Retterspitz, Ger.†.*
Rosemary oil (p.1659·3); citric acid (p.1596·2); tartaric acid (p.1669·2); alum (p.1577·2); thymol (p.1158·3).
Inflammatory disorders.

Retterspitz Gelee *Retterspitz, Ger.†.*
Thymol (p.1158·3); allantoin (p.1110·1); rosemary oil (p.1659·3); tartaric acid (p.1669·2); alum (p.1577·2); citric acid (p.1596·2).
Skin disorders.

Retterspitz Heilsalbe *Retterspitz, Ger.†.*
Pumilio pine oil (p.1656·3); siberian fir oil; thymol (p.1158·3); allantoin (p.1110·1).
Haemorrhoids; skin disorders.

Retterspitz Innerlich *Retterspitz, Ger.†.*
Citric acid (p.1596·2); tartaric acid (p.1669·2); alum (p.1577·2); thyme oil (p.1672·3).
Gastrointestinal disorders.

Retterspitz Quick *Retterspitz, Ger.†.*
Rosemary oil (p.1659·3); camphor (p.1589·3); menthol (p.1632·3); thymol (p.1158·3).
Chest disorders; joint disorders; myalgia.

Reucam
CT, Ital.; Maver, Mex.
Piroxicam (p.79·1).
Inflammation; musculoskeletal, joint, and peri-articular disorders; pain.

Reudene *ABC, Ital.*
Piroxicam (p.79·1).
Musculoskeletal, joint, and peri-articular disorders.

Reufel *Ehlinger, Mex.*
Piroxicam (p.79·1).

Reufirron *Reuffer, Mex.*
Ferrous fumarate (p.1360·1).

Reuflodol *Nattermann, Spain†.*
Pinazone (p.40·3).
Musculoskeletal, joint, and peri-articular disorders; pain.

Reugast *Basi, Port.*
Fenbufen (p.36·2).

Reukamicin *Reuffer, Mex.*
Kanamycin (p.218·2).

Reumacort *Teofarma, Ital.*
Hydrocortisone acetate (p.1073·3); methyl gentisate (p.55·1).
Musculoskeletal and joint pain.

Reumadil *Heralds, Braz.*
Diclofenac (p.30·2).
Gout; inflammation; musculoskeletal, joint, and peri-articular disorders; pain.

Reumagel *Sanofi Winthrop, Mex.*
Etofenamate (p.35·3).

Reumagil *KBR, Ital.*
Piroxicam (p.79·1).
Musculoskeletal, joint, and peri-articular disorders.

Reumaless *Pharmaton, Ger.†.*
Balsam: Methyl salicylate (p.55·1); benzyl nicotinate (p.20·2).
Musculoskeletal, joint, and soft-tissue disorders; neuralgia.

Capsules: Urtica (p.1678·2).
Rheumatism.

Reumaren *QIF, Braz.*
Diclofenac sodium (p.30·3).
Gout; inflammation; musculoskeletal, joint, and peri-articular disorders; pain.

Reumatosil *Saba, Ital.*
Nifenazone (p.62·3).
Neuralgias; neuritis; rheumatic disorders.

Reumazine *Luper, Braz.*
Prednisolone (p.1077·3); oxyphenbutazone (p.71·1).
Inflammation.

Reumilase *MDM, Ital.*
Glucosamine hydrochloride; chondroitin calcium sulfate; collagen; devil's claw root; vitamins (p.1350·1).
Joint disorders.

Reumin *Willmar, Mex.*
Indometacin (p.44·3).

Reumix *Makros, Braz.*
Betamethasone (p.1063·1); phenylbutazone (p.78·1).
Aluminium glycinate (p.1210·3) is included in this preparation in an attempt to limit adverse effects on the gastrointestinal mucosa.
Inflammation.

Reumo *UCB, Spain.*
Indometacin (p.44·3).
Gout; inflammation; musculoskeletal, joint, and peri-articular disorders; pain.

Reumon *Biol, Port.*
Etofenamate (p.35·3).
Gout; inflammation; musculoskeletal, joint, and peri-articular, and soft-tissue disorders; pain.

Reumophan *Grisi, Mex.*
Ketoprofen (p.47·3); chlorzoxazone (p.1327·3).
Gout; musculoskeletal, joint, and peri-articular disorders.

Reumoquin *Nattermann, Spain†.*
Ketoprofen (p.47·3).
Gout; musculoskeletal, joint, and peri-articular disorders; pain.

Reumoxican *Medinfar, Port.*
Piroxicam (p.79·1).
Inflammation; pain.

Reupax *CPH, Port.*
Flurbiprofen (p.41·2).
Musculoskeletal, joint, and peri-articular disorders.

Reuplex *Farmasa, Braz.*
Ibuprofen (p.43·2); paracetamol (p.71·2).
Fever; inflammation; pain.

Reuprofen *Terapeutico, Ital.*
Ketoprofen (p.47·3).
Musculoskeletal, joint, peri-articular, and soft-tissue disorders.

Reusan *Reuffer, Mex.*
Dexamethasone (p.1067·1).
Corticosteroid.

Reusin *Sankyo, Spain.*
Indometacin (p.44·3).
Gout; inflammation; musculoskeletal, joint, peri-articular, and soft-tissue disorders; pain.

Reutenox Solvay, Spain.
Tenoxicam (p.87·2).
Calcium stones; musculoskeletal, joint, and peri-articular disorders.

Reutricam Liferpal, Mex.
Piroxicam (p.79·1).
Fever; musculoskeletal and joint disorders; pain.

Reuxen Tecnifar, Port.
Naproxen (p.60·3).
Fever; gout; inflammation; musculoskeletal, joint, peri-articular, and soft-tissue disorders; pain.

Revalid Geymonat, Ital.
Amino acids; millet; wheat-germ; dried yeast; soya protein; minerals; vitamins (p.1350·1).
Skin, hair, and nail disorders.

Vifor, Switz.
Multivitamins and minerals (p.1350·1); amino-acids; aminobenzoic acid; milii flavi; tritici embryonis; faex medicinal.
Hair and nail disorders.

Revanil Cambridge, UK.
Lisuride maleate (p.1174·1).
Parkinsonism.

Revapol AF, Mex.
Mebendazole (p.102·2).
Worm infections.

Revasc Rhone-Poulenc Rorer, Austral.; Rhone-Poulenc Rorer, Fin.; Rhone-Poulenc Rorer, Fr.; Rhone-Poulenc Rorer, Ger.; Novartis, Jpn.; Aventis, NZ; Rhone-Poulenc Rorer, Spain; Rhone-Poulenc Rorer, Swed.; Rhone-Poulenc Rorer, Switz.; Aventis, UK†.
Desirudin (p.867·2).
Thromboembolism prophylaxis.

Revaton Pharmco, S.Afr.†.
Haematoporphyrin (p.1618·3); vitamin B₁₂ (p.1388·1); ascorbic acid (p.1389·3); yeast extract (p.1398·1).
Tonic.

Revaxis Aventis, Fr.; Pasteur Merieux, Ger.
A diphtheria, tetanus, and poliomyelitis vaccine (p.1539·1).
Active immunisation.

Reve IMO, Ital.
Valerian (p.1678·3); passion flower (p.1649·1).
Insomnia.

Reveal BR Pharmaceuticals, UK.
Pregnancy test (p.1654·3).

Revelatest Pierre Fabre Sante, Fr.
Pregnancy test (p.1654·3).

Revenil Hoechst Marion Roussel, Braz.
Bufylline (p.761·3); doxylamine succinate (p.417·1); etafedrine hydrochloride (p.1091·2).
Bronchospastic disorders.

Revenil Dospan Hoechst Marion Roussel, Braz.
Bufylline (p.761·3); doxylamine succinate (p.417·1); etafedrine hydrochloride (p.1091·2); phenylephrine hydrochloride (p.1097·1).
Brochospastic disorders.

Revenil Expectorante Hoechst Marion Roussel, Braz.
Bufylline (p.761·3); doxylamine succinate (p.417·1); etafedrine hydrochloride (p.1091·2); guaifenesin (p.1092·2).
Bronchospastic disorders.

Reverin Hoechst Marion Roussel, Aust.†; Hoechst Marion Roussel, Canad.†; Hoechst Marion Roussel, S.Afr.†.
Rolitetracycline (p.247·1).
Bacterial infections.

Reversa AHA Dermtek, Canad.
Glycolic acid (p.1115·1).
Skin disorders requiring exfoliation.

Reversa AHA HQ Dermtek, Canad.
Glycolic acid (p.1115·1); hydroquinone (p.1115·1).
Skin disorders requiring exfoliation.

Reversol Organon, USA.
Edrophonium chloride (p.1418·2).
Diagnosis of myasthenia gravis; evaluation of emergency treatment of myasthenic crises; reversal of competitive neuromuscular blockade.

Revex Baxter, USA.
Nalmefene hydrochloride (p.1014·1).
Opioid poisoning.

Rev-Eyes Bausch & Lomb, USA.
Dapiprazole hydrochloride (p.1602·2).
Reversal of mydriasis.

Revia Torrex, Aust.; Orphan, Austral.; Du Pont, Canad.; Du Pont, Denm.; Meda, Fin.; Du Pont, Fr.; Du Pont, Irl.; Du Pont, Israel; Du Pont, Spain; Boots, Thai.; Du Pont, Thai.; Du Pont, USA.
Naltrexone hydrochloride (p.1016·1).
Alcohol withdrawal syndrome; opioid withdrawal syndrome.

Revic Alcon Cusi, Spain.
Carbomer (p.1499·2).
Dry eyes; eye irritation.

Revicain Wiedemann, Ger.
Procaine hydrochloride (p.1319·1); vitamins (p.1350·1).
Tonic.

Revicain comp Wiedemann, Ger.
Procaine hydrochloride (p.1319·1); aescin (p.1574·1); minerals (p.1350·1).
Tonic.

Revicain comp plus Wiedemann, Ger.
Procaine hydrochloride (p.1319·1); aescin (p.1574·1); haematoporphyrin (p.1618·3); vitamins; minerals (p.1350·1).
Tonic.

Revicon United American, Hong Kong; United American, Singapore; Great Eastern, Thai.; United American, Thai.
Multivitamin and mineral preparation with yeast and methionine (p.1350·1).
Dietary supplement.

Revit ICN, Canad.†.
Multivitamin preparation (p.1350·1).

Revital Basi, Port.
Multivitamin preparation (p.1350·1).

Revitaleyes Allergan, Canad.†.
Polyvinyl alcohol (p.1503·1).
Dry eyes.

Revitalizing Crinos, Ital.
Glycolic acid (p.1115·1).
Skin disorders.

Revitalose Darci, Fr.
Ampoule A, magnesium aspartate (p.1190·3); L-leucine (p.1370·3); L-lysine hydrochloride (p.1370·3); L-phenylalanine (p.1374·2); L-valine (p.1381·3); ampoule B, sodium ascorbate (p.1390·3).
Asthenia.

Revitalose C
Note. This name is used for preparations of different composition.
Rivex, Canad.
Ascorbic acid (p.1389·3).
Vitamin C supplement.

Darci, Belg.; UCB, Switz.
Amino acids; vitamin C (p.1350·1).
Tonic.

Revitam Sanus, Braz.
Vitamin and trace-element preparation (p.1350·1).

Revitan Ranbaxy, Thai.
Ginseng (p.1615·3); multivitamins and minerals (p.1350·1).
Tonic.

Revitex Gerbex, Canad.
Multivitamin preparation preparation with calcium and iron (p.1350·1).

Revitonil Lichtwer, UK.
Echinacea (p.1606·2); peppermint (p.1243·2); clove (p.1596·3); aniseed (p.1580·2); liquorice (p.1231·2); fennel (p.1610·1); eucalyptus (p.1609·2).
Cold symptoms.

Revitonus C Sabex, Canad.
Ascorbic acid (p.1389·3); suprarenal cortex extract (p.1080·1); testicular extract (p.1492·1); brain extract (p.1631·2).
Vitamin C supplement.

Revivan Zambon, Braz.; Astra, Ital.
Dopamine hydrochloride (p.881·3).
Heart failure; hypotension; shock.

Revive
Note. This name is used for preparations of different composition.
Pfizer, NZ.
Tetryzoline hydrochloride (p.1101·2); macrogol 400 (p.1630·3).
Eye irritation.

Allergan, UK.
Carmellose (p.1499·3) (p.1129·2).
Comfort drops for use with soft contact lenses.

Revivona Nycomed, Aust.
Multivitamin preparation (p.1350·1).

Revolyt Gunnar Kjems, Denm.
Glucose; potassium chloride; magnesium sulfate; sodium citrate; sodium chloride (p.1185·2).
Diarrhoea; oral rehydration therapy.

Revulsan Faria, Braz.
Papaverine diethylbarbiturate (p.1648·1); belladonna (p.463·1); pentetrazol (p.1513·2).
Smooth muscle spasm.

Rewodina Asta Medica, Ger.
Diclofenac sodium (p.30·3).
Gout; inflammation; musculoskeletal, joint, and soft-tissue disorders; pain.

Rex LPB, Ital.
Calcium lactate gluconate (p.1188·3); calcium carbonate (p.1215·1).
Bone disorders; hypocalcaemia.

Rexachlor Be-Tabs, S.Afr.†.
Paracetamol (p.72·2); chlormezanone (p.660·1).
Pain and associated tension.

Rexacin Unison, Thai.
Norfloxacin (p.232·1).
Bacterial infections.

Rexalgan Dompe, Ital.
Tenoxicam (p.87·2).
Musculoskeletal and joint disorders.

Rexan Ist. Chim. Inter., Ital.
Aciclovir (p.612·3).
Herpesvirus infections.

Rexer Organon, Spain.
Mirtazapine (p.299·1).
Depression.

Rexgenta Areu, Spain.
Gentamicin sulfate (p.210·1).
Bacterial infections.

Rexichlor Esoform, Ital.
Chlorhexidine gluconate (p.1138·2); benzalkonium chloride (p.1133·2).
Skin disinfection.

Rexigen Pharmador, S.Afr.†.
Propranolol hydrochloride (p.962·3).
Anxiety; cardiovascular disorders.

Rexigen Forte Ion, USA†.
Phendimetrazine tartrate (p.1513·3).

Rexilen Serra Pamies, Spain.
Doxycycline hyclate (p.200·1).
Bacterial infections; malaria.

Rexiluven S Novartis Consumer, Ger.
Aesculus (p.1574·1).
Venous insufficiency.

Reximide Duopharma, Hong Kong.
Loperamide hydrochloride (p.1231·3).
Diarrhoea; ostomy management.

Rexitene Roche, Aust.
Guanabenz acetate (p.900·2).
Hypertension.

Rexitol Rekah, Israel.
Chloroxylenol (p.1142·1); terpineol (p.1669·3).
Disinfection.

Rexophtal Chauvin Novopharma, Switz.
Chlorhexidine gluconate (p.1138·2); phenylephrine hydrochloride (p.1097·1).
Eye disorders.

Rexort Takeda, Fr.
Citicoline (p.1596·1).
Cerebrovascular disorders.

Rexorubia Homeocan, Canad.; Lehning, Fr.
Homoeopathic preparation.

Rezamid Summers, USA.
Resorcinol (p.1122·2); sulfur (p.1123·3).
Acne.

Rezine Marnel, USA†.
Hydroxyzine hydrochloride (p.419·1).

Rezulin Parke, Davis, Austral.†; Parke, Davis, Mex.; Parke, Davis, USA†.
Troglitazone (p.337·1).
Diabetes mellitus.

R-Flex Rolab, S.Afr.†.
Sulindac (p.85·3).
Musculoskeletal and joint disorders.

R-Gel Healthline, USA.
Capsaicin (p.23·1).

R-Gen Goldline, USA.
Iodinated glycerol (p.1092·3).
Coughs.

R-Gene Kabivitrum, USA.
Arginine hydrochloride (p.1353·3).
Test to assess pituitary reserve for growth hormone.

Rhabarex B Palmical, Ger.†.
Bisacodyl (p.1212·2).
Constipation; stool softener.

Rheaban Maximum Strength Pfizer, USA.
Activated attapulgite (p.1212·1).
Diarrhoea.

Rhefluin Kytta, Ger.†; Medika, Switz.
Amiloride hydrochloride (p.835·1); hydrochlorothiazide (p.907·3).
Ascites; hypertension; oedema.

Rheila Medicated Cough Drops Hilarys, Canad.†.
Liquorice (p.1231·2); menthol (p.1632·3).

Rheila Stringiet N Diedenhofen, Ger.†.
Benzalkonium chloride (p.1133·2).
Mouth and throat infections.

Rhemofenax Duopharma, Hong Kong.
Diclofenac sodium (p.30·3).
Musculoskeletal and joint disorders.

Rhenus med APS, Ger.
Ruscus aculeatus.
Haemorrhoids; venous insufficiency.

Rheobral Niverpharm, Fr.
Troxerutin (p.1611·2); vincamine (p.1680·1).
Mental function impairment in the elderly.

Rheoflux Niverpharm, Fr.
Troxerutin (p.1611·2).
Haemorrhoids; venous insufficiency.

Rheofusin Fresenius Kabi, Aust.
Dextran 40 (p.728·3) with electrolytes.
Microcirculatory disorders; thrombosis prophylaxis.

Rheogen
Note. This name is used for preparations of different composition.
Robugen, Ger.
Aloes (p.1210·1).
Formerly known as Rheogen N and contained rhubarb and aloes.
Constipation.

Robugen, Hong Kong.
Rhubarb (p.1248·1); aloes (p.1210·1); belladonna (p.463·1).
Constipation.

Rheohes Braun, Ger.
Pentastarch (p.732·3).
Circulatory disorders; plasma volume expansion.

Rheomacrodex Torrex, Aust.; Medical Specialties, Austral.; Braun, Braz.; Medisan, Canad.†; Pharmalink, Denm.; Pharmacia Upjohn, Fr.; Pharmalink, Ger.; Pharmacia Upjohn, Israel; Pisa, Mex.; Pharmalink, Norw.; Pharmacia Upjohn, S.Afr.; Antibioticos, Spain; Pharmalink, Swed.; Braun, Switz.; Cambridge, UK†; Pharmacia, USA.
Dextran 40 (p.728·3) in glucose or sodium chloride.
Extracorporeal circulation; plasma volume expansion; prophylaxis of surgical adhesions; thrombosis prophylaxis; vascular disorders.

rheotromb Curasan, Ger.
Urokinase (p.988·1).
Thromboembolic disorders.

Rhesogam Centeon, Aust.
An anti-D immunoglobulin (p.1532·1).
Prevention of rhesus sensitisation.

Rhesogamma Chiron Behring, Ger.; Centeon, Ger.; Centeon, Mex.; Centeon, Norw.; Centeon, Spain; Centeon, Swed.
An anti-D immunoglobulin (p.1532·1).
Prevention of rhesus sensitisation.

Rhesonativ Darrow, Braz.; Pharmacia Upjohn, Norw.; Pharmacia Upjohn, Swed.
An anti-D immunoglobulin (p.1532·1).
Prevention of rhesus sensitisation.

Rhesugam NBI, S.Afr.
An anti-D immunoglobulin (p.1532·1).
Prevention of rhesus sensitisation.

Rhesuman Berna, Belg.†; Berna, Hong Kong†; Berna, Ital.†; Berna, Port.†; Berna, Spain†; Berna, Switz.†; Berna, Thai.†.
An anti-D immunoglobulin (p.1532·1).
Prevention of rhesus sensitisation.

Rheu Vitasan, Aust.
Homoeopathic preparation.

Rheubalmin Hoernecke, Ger.†.
Diethylamine salicylate (p.32·2); benzyl nicotinate (p.20·2).
Musculoskeletal and joint disorders; neuralgia.

Rheubalmin Bad Hoernecke, Ger.
Methyl salicylate (p.55·1); isobornyl acetate; camphor (p.1589·3).
Bath additive; circulatory disorders; musculoskeletal, joint, and soft-tissue disorders; neuralgia; respiratory-tract disorders.

Rheubalmin Bad Nico Hoernecke, Ger.†.
Benzyl nicotinate (p.20·2).
Bath additive; circulatory disorders; musculoskeletal and joint disorders; neuralgia.

Rheubalmin Indo Hoernecke, Ger.
Indometacin (p.44·3).
Musculoskeletal, joint, peri-articular, and soft-tissue disorders.

Rheubalmin N Hoernecke, Ger.
Glycol salicylate (p.42·2).
Musculoskeletal and joint disorders; neuralgia.

Rheubalmin Thermo Hoernecke, Ger.
Ointment: Glycol salicylate (p.42·2); benzyl nicotinate (p.20·2).
Musculoskeletal, joint, and soft-tissue disorders; peripheral vascular disorders.

Topical solution†: Glycol salicylate (p.42·2); benzyl nicotinate (p.20·2); camphor (p.1589·3).
Musculoskeletal and joint disorders; neuralgia; peripheral vascular disorders.

Rheucastin Pfluger, Ger.
Homoeopathic preparation.

Rheucostan M Hanosan, Ger.
Homoeopathic preparation.

Rheufenac Helvepharm, Switz.
Diclofenac sodium (p.30·3).
Gout; inflammation; musculoskeletal, joint, and peri-articular disorders; oedema; pain; renal and biliary colic.

Rheuferm Phyto Wiedemann, Ger.
Devil's claw root (p.26·3).
Degenerative joint disorders.

Rheugesal Solvay, Aust.
Diethylamine salicylate (p.32·2); flufenamic acid (p.41·1); myrtecaine (p.1317·3).
Musculoskeletal, joint, peri-articular, and soft-tissue disorders.

Rheugesic Medpro, S.Afr.
Piroxicam (p.79·1).
Gout; musculoskeletal and joint disorders; pain.

Rheuma Weleda, Aust.
Aconitum napellus (p.1572·3); arnica (p.1581·3); betula folium (p.1585·2); mandragora radix; formica; rosemary oil (p.1659·3).
Musculoskeletal and joint disorders.

Rheuma Lindofluid Lindopharm, Ger.
Flufenamic acid (p.41·1).
Musculoskeletal, joint, peri-articular, and soft-tissue disorders.

Rheuma V + T Bad N Spitzner, Ger.
Glycol salicylate (p.42·2); diethylamine salicylate (p.32·2); oleum pini sylvestris.
Bath additive; cold symptoms; musculoskeletal, joint, peri-articular, and soft-tissue disorders; neuralgia.

Rheuma-Bad Eu Rho, Ger.
Glycol salicylate (p.42·2); benzyl nicotinate (p.20·2); camphor (p.1589·3); diethylamine salicylate (p.32·2).
Cold symptoms; musculoskeletal and joint disorders; neuralgia; peripheral vascular disorders.

Rheumabene Merckle, Ger.
Dimethyl sulfoxide (p.1402·2).
Musculoskeletal, joint, and peri-articular disorders.

The symbol † denotes a preparation no longer actively marketed

Rheumacin
Pacific, NZ; CP Pharmaceuticals, UK.
Indometacin (p.44·3).
Fever; gout; inflammation; musculoskeletal, joint, and peri-articular disorders; pain.

Rheumadoron
Weleda, Ger.
Homoeopathic preparation.

Weleda, UK.
Ointment: Aconitum napellus; arnica montana; betula alba; mandragora root; rosemary oil.
Oral drops: Aconitum napellus; arnica montana; betula alba; mandragora root.
Rheumatic and muscular pain.

Rheumadyn PMD Plantamed, Ger.
Homoeopathic preparation.

Rheuma-Gastreu R46 Reckeweg, Ger.
Homoeopathic preparation.

Rheuma-Gel Ratiopharm, Ger.
Etofenamate (p.35·3).
Musculoskeletal, joint, and soft-tissue disorders.

Rheuma-Hartkapseln Strathmann, Ger.
Urtica (p.1678·2).
Rheumatism.

Rheuma-Hek Strathmann, Ger.†
Urtica (p.1678·2).
Musculoskeletal and joint disorders.

Rheuma-Hevert Hevert, Ger.
Homoeopathic preparation.

Rheumajecta Enzypharm, Neth.
Sulfate adenyltransferase; chondroitin sulfotransferase; catalase (p.1592·2).
Rheumatic disorders.

Rheumakaps Steigerwald, Ger.
Salix (p.82·1).
Fever; headache; musculoskeletal and joint disorders.

Rheumalan Hilarys, Canad.
Methyl salicylate (p.55·1); camphor (p.1589·3); menthol (p.1632·3); belladonna (p.463·1); capsicum oleoresin (p.1591·1); croton oil (p.1221·3); eucalyptus oil (p.1609·2); expressed mustard oil (p.1639·1); salicylic acid (p.1122·3).

Rheumaliment N Galenika, Ger.
Camphor (p.1589·3); eucalyptus oil (p.1609·2); turpentine oil (p.1676·3).
Musculoskeletal and joint pain.

Rheuma-Liquidum Eu Rho, Ger.
Glycol salicylate (p.42·2); benzyl nicotinate (p.20·2); nonivamide (p.63·1).
Musculoskeletal, joint, peri-articular, and soft-tissue disorders; neuralgia; peripheral vascular disorders.

rheuma-loges Loges, Ger.
Homoeopathic preparation.

Rheumanox Charoen, Thai.
Ibuprofen (p.43·2).
Gout; musculoskeletal, joint, and peri-articular disorders.

Rheuma-Pasc Pascoe, Ger.
Homoeopathic preparation.

Rheuma-Pasc N Pascoe, Ger.†
Rosemary oil (p.1659·3); methyl salicylate (p.55·1); hamamelis (p.1618·3).
Neuralgia; neuritis.

Rheuma-Plantina Plantina, Ger.
Homoeopathic preparation.

Rheumaplast N Beiersdorf, Ger.
Cayenne pepper (p.1591·1).
Musculoskeletal and joint disorders.

Rheumasalbe CT, Ger.
Nonivamide (p.63·1); benzyl nicotinate (p.20·2); eucalyptus oil (p.1609·2).
Musculoskeletal, joint, and soft-tissue disorders; neuralgia.

Rheuma-Salbe
Note. This name is used for preparations of different composition.
Lichtenstein, Ger.
Glycol salicylate (p.42·2); benzyl nicotinate (p.20·2); camphor (p.1589·3).
Neuralgia; rheumatic pain; soft-tissue disorders; tenosynovitis.

Stada, Ger.
Glycol salicylate (p.42·2); benzyl nicotinate (p.20·2).
Musculoskeletal, joint, and soft-tissue disorders; peripheral vascular disorders.

Twardy, Ger.
Camphor (p.1589·3); menthol (p.1632·3); clove oil (p.1597·1).
Rheumatic disorders; sports injuries.

Rheumasan Kwizda, Aust.
Salicylic acid (p.1122·3); sodium humate; norway spruce oil; camphor (p.1589·3); eucalyptus oil (p.1609·2); menthol (p.1632·3).
Bath additive; cold symptoms; musculoskeletal and joint disorders.

Rheumasan Moor-Bad Sanofi Synthelabo, Ger.
Diethylamine salicylate (p.32·2); sodium humate.
Bath additive; musculoskeletal and joint disorders.

Rheumasan N Sanofi Synthelabo, Ger.
Ointment: Salicylic acid (p.1122·3); methyl nicotinate (p.55·1).
Bruising; muscle, joint, and nerve disorders.
Topical rub: Salicylic acid (p.1122·3); benzyl nicotinate (p.20·2).
Bruising; musculoskeletal, joint, and nerve disorders.

Rheumaselect Dreluso, Ger.
Homoeopathic preparation.

Rheuma-Sern Serturner, Ger.
Devil's claw root (p.26·3).
Musculoskeletal and joint disorders.

Rheumasit Medice, Ger.
Dexamethasone (p.1067·1); benzyl nicotinate (p.20·2).
Musculoskeletal, joint, peri-articular, and soft-tissue disorders; neuralgia.

Rheumasol Peter Black, UK.
Guaiacum resin (p.1618·2); prickly ash bark (p.1682·1).
Rheumatic and muscular pain and stiffness.

Rheumatab Salicis Schuck, Ger.
Salix (p.82·1).
Headache; rheumatic disorders.

Rheumatabletten N Cosmochema, Ger.
Homoeopathic preparation.

Rheumatac Waymade, UK.
Diclofenac sodium (p.30·3).
Gout; inflammation; musculoskeletal, joint, and peri-articular disorders; pain.

Rheuma-Teufelskralle HarpagoMega Twardy, Ger.†
Devil's claw root (p.26·3).
Appetite loss; dyspepsia; musculoskeletal and joint disorders.

Rheumatex Wampole, USA.
Test for rheumatoid factor in serum.

Rheumatic Pain Cantassium Co., UK.
Guaiacum resin (p.1618·2); taraxacum (p.1669·1); celery (p.1592·3); menyanthes (p.1633·1).
Muscle and joint pain.

Rheumatic Pain Relief Herbal Concepts, UK.
Menyanthes (p.1633·1); guaiacum resin (p.1618·2); capsicum (p.1591·1); capsicum oleoresin (p.1591·1); celery oil.
Musculoskeletal and joint pain.

Rheumatic Pain Remedy Potter's, UK.
Menyanthes (p.1633·1); lappa root (p.1627·1); achillea (p.1572·2); guaiacum resin (p.1618·2).
Rheumatic pain.

Rheumatic Pain Tablets Healthcrafts, UK.
Guaiacum resin (p.1618·2); menyanthes (p.1633·1); celery seed (p.1592·3).
Rheumatic pain.

Rheumatica Nelson, UK.
Homoeopathic preparation.

Rheumatism Rhus Tox Homeocan, Canad.
Homoeopathic preparation.

Rheumaton
Carter-Wallace, Switz.†; Wampole, USA.
Test for rheumatoid factor in serum or synovial fluid.

Rheumatrex
Wyeth-Ayerst, Canad.; Lederle, USA.
Methotrexate (p.553·2) or methotrexate sodium (p.553·2).
Psoriasis; rheumatoid arthritis.

Rheumatropfen N Cosmochema, Ger.
Homoeopathic preparation.

Rheumavincin Schur, Ger.†
Choline salicylate (p.24·3).
Musculoskeletal and joint disorders; pleuritis.

Rheumax Hoernecke, Ger.†
Methyl salicylate (p.55·1).
Musculoskeletal and joint disorders.

Rheumed Phytomed, Switz.
Homoeopathic preparation.

Rheumeda Madaus, Ger.
Homoeopathic preparation.

Rheumesser Gerot, Aust.
Kebuzone (p.47·2); salamidacetic acid (p.81·3); dexamethasone (p.1067·1); cyanocobalamin (p.1388·1) or hydroxocobalamin acetate (p.1388·3).
Lignocaine [lidocaine] (p.1313·2) is included in this preparation to alleviate the pain of injection.
Musculoskeletal and joint disorders.

Rheumex Gebro, Aust.
Glycol salicylate (p.42·2); benzyl nicotinate (p.20·2); allantoin (p.1110·1).
Musculoskeletal and joint disorders; sports injuries.

Rheumichthol Bad Ichthyol, Ger.†
Light ammonium bituminosulfonate (p.1115·2); glycol salicylate (p.42·2); diethylamine salicylate (p.32·2).
Bath additive; musculoskeletal and joint disorders.

Rheumitin Krewel, Ger.
Piroxicam (p.79·1).
Gout; musculoskeletal, joint, and soft-tissue disorders.

Rheumodoron Weleda, Ger.
A range of homoeopathic preparations.

Rheumox
Kolassa, Aust.; Bayer, Ger.; Drossapharm, Switz.
Etofenamate (p.35·3).
Inflammation; musculoskeletal, joint, peri-articular, and soft-tissue disorders; pain.

Rheumox
Goldshield, Irl.; Continental Ethicals, S.Afr.†; Lagamed, S.Afr.†; Goldshield, UK.
Azapropazone (p.19·1).
Acute gout; musculoskeletal and joint disorders.

Rheunervol N LAW, Ger.
Camphor (p.1589·3).
Musculoskeletal and joint disorders.

Rheutrop Kolassa, Aust.
Acemetacin (p.11·2).
Gout; inflammation; musculoskeletal and joint disorders; thrombophlebitis; vasculitis.

Rhewlin Beacons, Singapore.
Diclofenac diethylamine (p.30·2) or diclofenac sodium (p.30·3).
Inflammation; musculoskeletal, joint, and soft-tissue disorders; pain.

Rhinaaxia
Agepha, Aust.; Allergan-Frumtost, Braz.; Chiesi, Fr.; Zambon, Ital.; Inpharzam, Switz.
Magnesium isospaglumate (p.1624·3) or sodium spaglumate.
Allergic rhinitis.

Rhinadvil Whitehall, Fr.
Ibuprofen (p.43·2); pseudoephedrine hydrochloride (p.1099·2).
Fever; headache; rhinitis with nasal congestion.

Rhinalair Inava, Fr.†
Pseudoephedrine hydrochloride (p.1099·2).
Nasal congestion.

Rhinalar
Roche, Canad.; Roche, Hong Kong.
Flunisolide (p.1070·3).
Allergic rhinitis.

Rhinalene a la framycetine SmithKline Beecham Sante, Fr.†
Framycetin sulfate (p.208·2).
Nasal infections.

Rhinall Scherer, USA.
Phenylephrine hydrochloride (p.1097·1).
Nasal congestion.

Rhinamide
Note. This name is used for preparations of different composition.
Vitalpharma, Belg.
Diphenylpyraline hydrochloride (p.417·1); sulfanilamide (p.256·2); ephedrine hydrochloride (p.1090·1).
Nasal congestion.

Bailly, Fr.
Ephedrine hydrochloride (p.1090·1); benzoic acid (p.1134·2).
Formerly contained sulfanilamide, ephedrine hydrochloride, butacaine sulfate, and benzoic acid.
Congestion of the nose and throat.

Rhinar TP, Thai.
Carbinoxamine maleate (p.411·1); pseudoephedrine hydrochloride (p.1099·2).
Cold symptoms; rhinitis; upper respiratory-tract congestion.

Rhinaris Pharmascience, Canad.
Macrogol (p.1630·1); propylene glycol (p.1655·1).
Rhinitis.

Rhinatate Major, USA.
Phenylephrine tannate (p.1097·3); chlorpheniramine [chlorphenamine] tannate (p.412·2); mepyramine tannate (p.421·1).
Upper respiratory-tract symptoms.

Rhinathiol
Synthelabo, Fr.; Synthelabo, Hong Kong; Lorex Synthelabo, Neth.†; Sanofi Synthelabo, Singapore; Synthelabo, Switz.; Sanofi Synthelabo, Thai.
Carbocisteine (p.1086·3).
Respiratory-tract disorders associated with increased or viscous mucus.

Rhinathiol Antirhinitis Sanofi Synthelabo, Belg.
Phenylephrine hydrochloride (p.1097·1); chlorpheniramine [chlorphenamine] maleate (p.412·1).
Rhinitis; sinusitis.

Rhinathiol Antitussivum Sanofi Synthelabo, Belg.
Dextromethorphan hydrobromide (p.1087·3).
Coughs.

Rhinathiol Mucolyticum Sanofi Synthelabo, Belg.
Carbocisteine (p.1086·3).
Respiratory-tract disorders associated with abnormal mucus production.

Rhinathiol Promethazine
Synthelabo, Fr.; Synthelabo, Hong Kong; Sanofi Synthelabo, Singapore; Synthelabo, Switz.
Carbocisteine (p.1086·3); promethazine hydrochloride (p.423·2).
Coughs.

Rhinathiol Tosse Seca Sanofi Synthelabo, Port.
Dextromethorphan hydrobromide (p.1087·3).
Coughs.

Rhinathiol Toux Seche Synthelabo, Fr.
Dextromethorphan hydrobromide (p.1087·3).
Coughs.

RhinATP Aerocid, Fr.
Adenosine triphosphate, disodium salt (p.1573·3); sulfasuccinamide (p.256·3).
Infections of the nose and throat.

Rhinedrine Cooperation Pharmaceutique, Fr.
Benzododecinium bromide (p.1135·1).
Nose and throat infections.

Rhinedrine Lubricant Jamieson, Canad.
Carbowax; propylene glycol (p.1655·1).

Rhinedrine Moisturizing Jamieson, Canad.
Glycerol (p.1616·3); propylene glycol (p.1655·1).

Rhinex Werwigerode, Ger.
Naphazoline hydrochloride (p.1095·1).
Nasal congestion; rhinitis; sinusitis.

Rhinidine Warner-Lambert Consumer, Belg.
Xylometazoline hydrochloride (p.1102·2).
Nasal congestion and irritation.

Rhinipan Pharmacal, Switz.†
Phenylephrine hydrochloride (p.1097·1); dequalinium diacetate (p.1143·1); chlorhexidine gluconate (p.1138·2).
Catarrh; rhinitis; sinusitis.

Rhiniramine DHA, Singapore.
Dexchlorpheniramine maleate (p.412·1).
Hypersensitivity reactions.

Rhinirex Irex, Fr.
Beclometasone dipropionate (p.1061·2).
Rhinitis.

Rhinitisan Bioforce, Switz.
Homoeopathic preparation.

Rhinivict Klinge, Ger.
Beclometasone dipropionate (p.1061·2).
Rhinitis.

Rhinobiotal Martin, Fr.
Framycetin sulfate (p.208·2).
Nose and throat infections.

Rhinocap
Grossmann, Hong Kong; Grossmann, Switz.
Phenylephrine hydrochloride (p.1097·1); dimenhydrinate (p.415·2); caffeine (p.761·3).
Allergic rhinitis; cold symptoms; nasal congestion; sinus congestion.

Rhinocaps
Note. This name is used for preparations of different composition.
Vemedia, Neth.†
Camphor (p.1589·3); chlorothymol (p.1142·1); cineole (p.1609·2); menthol (p.1632·3); terpineol (p.1669·3).
Cold symptoms.

Ferndale, USA†.
Phenylpropanolamine hydrochloride (p.1098·1); aspirin (p.14·2); paracetamol (p.71·2).
Upper respiratory-tract symptoms.

Rhinocillin B Medicopharm, Aust.
Bacitracin (p.155·2).

Rhinoclir Agis, Israel.
Oxymetazoline hydrochloride (p.1096·2).
Nasal congestion.

Rhinocort
Note. This name is used for preparations of different composition.
AstraZeneca, Austral.; Astra, Belg.; AstraZeneca, Canad.; AstraZeneca, Denm.; AstraZeneca, Fin.; Astra, Hong Kong; Astra, Irl.; Astra, Ital.; Astra, Mex.; Astra, Neth.; AstraZeneca, Norw.; AstraZeneca, NZ; Astra, S.Afr.; AstraZeneca, Singapore; Astra, Spain; Tika, Swed.; Astra, Switz.; AstraZeneca, Thai.; AstraZeneca, UK; Astra, USA.
Budesonide (p.1064·2).
Nasal polyps; rhinitis.

Agis, Israel.
Beclometasone dipropionate (p.1061·2).
Rhinitis.

Rhinocortol Astra, Aust.
Budesonide (p.1064·2).
Nasal polyps; rhinitis.

Rhinocure Medibel, Switz.†
Polysorbate 80 (p.1347·3); sodium chloride (p.1196·1); matricaria (p.1593·2); benzethonium chloride (p.1134·2).
Rhinopharyngeal disorders.

Rhinocure Simplex Medibel, Switz.†
Polysorbate 80 (p.1347·3); sodium chloride (p.1196·1); benzethonium chloride (p.1134·2).
Rhinopharyngeal disorders.

Rhinodex INQ, Braz.
Naphazoline (p.1095·1); benzalkonium chloride (p.1133·2).
Nasal congestion.

Rhinodrin Montavit, Aust.
Diphenhydramine hydrochloride (p.416·1); naphazoline hydrochloride (p.1095·1).
Rhinitis.

Rhinofeb Martin, Fr.†
Paracetamol (p.71·2); chlorpheniramine [chlorphenamine] maleate (p.412·1); phenylpropanolamine hydrochloride (p.1098·1).
Cold symptoms.

Rhinofebral
Martin, Fr.; Martin, Switz.
Paracetamol (p.71·2); chlorpheniramine [chlorphenamine] maleate (p.412·1); ascorbic acid (p.1389·3).
Cold symptoms; rhinopharyngeal disorders.

Rhinofebryl Aventis, Belg.
Chlorpheniramine [chlorphenamine] maleate (p.412·1); paracetamol (p.71·2).
Rhinitis with fever and/or headache.

Rhinofed Noristan, S.Afr.†
Triprolidine hydrochloride (p.427·2); pseudoephedrine hydrochloride (p.1099·2).
Nasal congestion.

Rhinofluimucil Zambon, Fr.
Acetylcysteine (p.1082·3); tuaminoheptane sulfate (p.1102·2); benzalkonium chloride (p.1133·2).
Rhinopharyngeal congestion.

Rhino-Gastreu N R49 Reckeweg, Ger.
Homoeopathic preparation.

Rhinogen IBSA, Switz.
Sodium hyaluronate (p.1620·1).
Nasal dryness.

Rhinogesic Pal-Pak, USA†.
Phenylephrine hydrochloride (p.1097·1); paracetamol (p.71·2); chlorpheniramine [chlorphenamine] maleate (p.412·1); salicylamide (p.82·1).
Upper respiratory-tract symptoms.

Rhinoguttae Argenti diacetylotannici proteinici Leyh, Ger.
Silver protein acetyl tannate (p.1664·2).
Cold symptoms.

Rhinoguttae Dexamethasoni cum Naphazolino *Leyh, Ger.*
Dexamethasone (p.1067·1); naphazoline hydrochloride (p.1095·1).
Cold symptoms; rhinitis.

Rhinoguttae pro Infantibus *Leyh, Ger.*
Ephedrine hydrochloride (p.1090·1); silver protein acetyl tannate (p.1664·2).
Bacterial nose infections.

Rhinohist *Seng, Thai.*
Carbinoxamine maleate (p.411·1); pseudoephedrine hydrochloride (p.1099·2).
Allergic rhinitis; hay fever; upper respiratory-tract congestion.

Rhino-Lacteol *Lacteol du Dr Boucard, Fr.†.*
Lactobacillus acidophilus (p.1626·3).
Infections of the nose and throat.

Rhinolar-EX *McGregor, USA†.*
Phenylpropanolamine hydrochloride (p.1098·1); chlorpheniramine [chlorphenamine] maleate (p.412·1).
Upper respiratory-tract symptoms.

Rhinolast
Astra, Ger.†; Stern, Ger.†; Orion, Irl.; 3M, NZ; Mer-National, S.Afr.; Asta Medica, UK.
Azelastine hydrochloride (p.409·3).
Allergic rhinitis.

Rhinomer
Novartis Consumer, Ger.; Novartis Consumer, Port.; Novartis Consumer, Switz.
Isotonic sea water (p.1196·1).
Nasal disorders.

Novartis Consumer, UK.
Sodium chloride (p.1196·1).
Nasal congestion.

Rhino-Mex *Charton, Canad.*
Naphazoline hydrochloride (p.1095·1); amylocaine hydrochloride (p.1306·1).
Nasal congestion.

Rhino-Mex-N *Charton, Canad.†.*
Naphazoline hydrochloride (p.1095·1).
Nasal congestion.

Rhinon *Petrasch, Aust.*
Nasal ointment: Naphazoline hydrochloride (p.1095·1); sulfadiazine (p.251·1).
Rhinitis; sinusitis.

Nose drops: Naphazoline hydrochloride (p.1095·1).
Rhinitis.

Rhinoperd *Agepha, Aust.*
Naphazoline hydrochloride (p.1095·1).
Aid in rhinoscopy; rhinitis; sinusitis.

Rhinoperd comp *Agepha, Aust.*
Naphazoline hydrochloride (p.1095·1); diphenhydramine hydrochloride (p.416·1).
Cold symptoms; rhinitis.

Rhinophen-C *Maxi, Thai.*
Brompheniramine maleate (p.410·2); vitamin C (p.1389·3).
Hypersensitivity reactions.

Rhinopront
Note. This name is used for preparations of different composition.
Pfizer, Aust.; Vitalpharma, Belg.; Mack, Illert., Ger.; Mack, Hong Kong; Mack, Singapore; Mack, Switz.; Mack, Thai.
Capsules: Carbinoxamine maleate (p.411·1); phenylephrine hydrochloride (p.1097·1).
Cold symptoms; hay fever; rhinitis; sinusitis.

Pfizer, Aust.; Mack, Illert., Ger.; Mack, Hong Kong; Mack, Singapore; Mack, Switz.; Mack, Thai.
Syrup: Phenylpropanolamine polistirex (p.1098·3); carbinoxamine polistirex (p.411·1).
Cold symptoms; hay fever; rhinitis; sinusitis.

Mack, Illert., Ger.
Nasal spray: Tetryzoline hydrochloride (p.1101·2).
Catarrh; colds; hay fever.

Rhinopront Top *Mack, Switz.*
Tetryzoline hydrochloride (p.1101·2).
Rhinopharyngeal disorders.

Rhinopten *Debat, Fr.†.*
Antigens of: *Staphylococcus aureus* 634, 636; *Streptococcus* 147, 155 *Streptococcus pneumoniae* 209; *Moraxella catarrhalis* 987.
Disorders of the ear, nose, and throat.

Rhinosept *Delta, Braz.*
Naphazoline (p.1095·1); diphenhydramine (p.416·1); neomycin (p.228·1).
Nasal congestion.

Rhinosol *AstraZeneca, Denm.*
Budesonide (p.1064·2).
Hay fever.

Rhinosovil *Eu Rho, Ger.*
Naphazoline nitrate (p.1095·1); pheniramine maleate (p.422·3).
Nasal congestion; rhinitis.

Rhinospray
Boehringer Ingelheim, Belg.; Boehringer Ingelheim, Ger.; Boehringer Ingelheim, Neth.†; Boehringer Ingelheim, Port.; Fher, Spain.
Tramazoline hydrochloride (p.1102·1).
Nasal congestion.

Rhinospray Antialergico *Fher, Spain.*
Tramazoline hydrochloride (p.1102·1); chlorpheniramine [chlorphenamine] maleate (p.412·1).
Nasal congestion.

Rhinospray Atlantik *Boehringer Ingelheim, Ger.*
Sea water (p.1196·1).
Nasal disorders.

Rhinospray Plus
Boehringer Ingelheim, Aust.; Boehringer Ingelheim, Ger.
Tramazoline hydrochloride (p.1102·1); eucalyptol (p.1609·2); menthol (p.1632·3); camphor (p.1589·3).
Nasal congestion.

Rhino-stas *Stada, Ger.†.*
Xylometazoline hydrochloride (p.1102·2).
Rhinitis; sinusitis.

Rhino-Sulfuryl *Aerocid, Fr.*
Sodium thiosulfate (p.1024·2); ephedrine hydrochloride (p.1090·1).
Rhinopharyngeal congestion.

Rhinosyn *Great Southern, USA.*
Pseudoephedrine hydrochloride (p.1099·2); chlorpheniramine [chlorphenamine] maleate (p.412·1).
Upper respiratory-tract symptoms.

Rhinosyn-DM *Great Southern, USA.*
Pseudoephedrine hydrochloride (p.1099·2); chlorpheniramine [chlorphenamine] maleate (p.412·1); dextromethorphan hydrobromide (p.1087·3).
Coughs and cold symptoms.

Rhinosyn-DMX *Great Southern, USA.*
Dextromethorphan hydrobromide (p.1087·3); guaifenesin (p.1092·2).
Coughs.

Rhinosyn-X *Great Southern, USA.*
Pseudoephedrine hydrochloride (p.1099·2); dextromethorphan hydrobromide (p.1087·3); guaifenesin (p.1092·2).
Coughs.

Rhinothricinol *Plan, Switz.*
Tyrothricin (p.267·1); eucalyptus oil (p.1609·2).
Rhinopharyngeal infections.

Rhinotrophyl *Jolly-Jatel, Fr.*
Thenoate monoethanolamine (p.261·3); framycetin sulfate (p.208·2).
Infections of the nose and throat.

Rhinotussal
Note. This name is used for preparations of different composition.
Mack, Illert., Ger.; Madaus, S.Afr.†; Mack, Switz.
Capsules: Dextromethorphan hydrobromide (p.1087·3); phenylephrine hydrochloride (p.1097·1); carbinoxamine maleate (p.411·1).
Coughs and associated respiratory-tract disorders.

Mack, Illert., Ger.; Mack, Thai.
Oral liquid: Dextromethorphan polistirex (p.1088·2); phenylpropanolamine polistirex (p.1098·3); carbinoxamine polistirex (p.411·1).
Coughs and associated respiratory-tract disorders.

Ethimed, S.Afr.†.
Syrup: Dextromethorphan hydrobromide (p.1087·3); phenylpropanolamine hydrochloride (p.1098·1); carbinoxamine maleate (p.411·1).
Coughs.

Rhinovac *Darrow, Braz.*
Antigen extracts (p.1575·3).
Hyposensitisation.

Rhinovalon *Sintesa, Belg.*
Tixocortol pivalate (p.1080·1).
Rhinitis.

Rhinovalon Neomycine *Sintesa, Belg.*
Tixocortol pivalate (p.1080·1); neomycin sulfate (p.228·1).
Infective rhinitis.

Rhinovent *Boehringer Ingelheim, Switz.*
Ipratropium bromide (p.766·1).
Rhinitis.

Rhinovis *CTI, Israel.*
Carbinoxamine maleate (p.411·1); phenylephrine hydrochloride (p.1097·1).
Rhinitis; sinusitis.

Rhinox *Nycomed, Norw.*
Oxymetazoline hydrochloride (p.1096·2).
Nasal congestion.

Rhinureflex *Boots Healthcare, Fr.*
Ibuprofen (p.43·2); pseudoephedrine hydrochloride (p.1099·2).
Fever; headache; nasal congestion; rhinitis.

Rhinyl *Pierre Fabre Sante, Fr.*
Framycetin sulfate (p.208·2); sodium propionate (p.393·2).
Colds.

Rhodacine *Rhodiapharm, Canad.*
Indometacin (p.44·3).
Gout; musculoskeletal and joint disorders.

Rhodamer *Rhone-Poulenc Rorer, Mex.*
Methotrexate (p.553·2).

Rhodiaprox *Rhodiapharm, Canad.*
Naproxen (p.60·3).
Fever; inflammation; pain.

Rhodine *Rhone-Poulenc Rorer, Belg.†.*
Aspirin (p.14·2).
Dental pain; fever; headache; rheumatic pain.

Rhodis *Rhodiapharm, Canad.*
Ketoprofen (p.47·3).
Musculoskeletal and joint disorders.

Rhoditest-Tuberkulin *Pasteur Merieux, Swed.†.*
Tuberculin (PPD) (p.1675·3).
Sensitivity testing.

Rhodogil *Rhone-Poulenc Rorer, Spain.*
Spiramycin (p.248·3); metronidazole (p.594·1).
Bacterial infections.

RhoGAM
Ortho, Hong Kong; Ortho Diagnostic, USA.
An anti-D immunoglobulin (p.1532·1).
Prevention of rhesus sensitisation.

Rhoival *Byk Tosse, Ger.; Byk Gulden, Ger.*
Agrimony (p.1574·3); solidago virgaurea; hypericum (p.290·2); shepherd's purse (p.1662·3); arnica (p.1581·3); valerian (p.1678·3).
Urinary-tract disorders.

Rhonal
Rhone-Poulenc Rorer, Belg.†; Theraplix, Fr.†; Rhone-Poulenc Rorer, Israel; Rhone-Poulenc Rorer, Mex.; Nattermann, Neth.†; Rhone-Poulenc Rorer, Spain.
Aspirin (p.14·2).
Fever; musculoskeletal, joint and peri-articular disorders; pain; thromboembolism prophylaxis.

Rhonuracil *Rhone-Poulenc Rorer, Mex.*
Fluorouracil (p.540·2).

Rhophylac *ZLB, Switz.*
An anti-D immunoglobulin (p.1532·1).
Prevention of rhesus sensitisation.

Rhotral *Rhodiapharm, Canad.*
Acebutolol hydrochloride (p.825·1).
Angina pectoris; hypertension.

Rhotrimine *Rhodiapharm, Canad.*
Trimipramine maleate (p.311·2).
Depression.

Rhovail *Rho-Pharm, Canad.*
Ketoprofen (p.47·3).
Musculoskeletal and joint disorders.

Rhovane *Rhodiapharm, Canad.*
Zopiclone (p.713·1).
Insomnia.

Rhuaka *Anglian, UK.*
Cascara (p.1216·1); rhubarb (p.1248·1); senna (p.1248·2).
Constipation.

Rhuli Gel *Rydelle, USA.*
Benzyl alcohol (p.1135·2); menthol (p.1632·3); camphor (p.1589·3).
Minor skin irritation.

Rhuli Spray *Rydelle, USA.*
Calamine (p.1111·3); camphor (p.1589·3); benzocaine (p.1306·2).
Minor skin irritation.

Rhum Creosotado *Dansk-Flama, Braz.*
Creosote (p.1087·3); sodium hypophosphite; calcium hypophosphate.
Respiratory-tract congestion.

Rhumagrip *Cooperation Pharmaceutique, Fr.*
Paracetamol (p.71·2); pseudoephedrine hydrochloride (p.1099·2).
Cold symptoms.

Rhumalgan *Lagap, UK.*
Diclofenac sodium (p.30·3).
Gout; inflammation; musculoskeletal, joint, and peri-articular disorders; pain.

Rhumanol *TO-Chemicals, Thai.*
Diclofenac diethylamine (p.30·2).
Musculoskeletal, joint, and peri-articular disorders.

Rhumantin *Gea, Denm.†.*
Penicillamine (p.1017·1).
Cystinuria; heavy metal poisoning; rheumatoid arthritis; Wilson's disease.

Rhumatisme *Gerbex, Canad.*
Methyl salicylate (p.55·1); camphor (p.1589·3); capsicum oleoresin (p.1591·1); trimethylcyclohexanol.
Formerly known as Rheumatisme.

Rhus Med Complex *Dynamit, Aust.*
Homoeopathic preparation.

Rhus toxicodendron Oligoplex *Madaus, Ger.*
Homoeopathic preparation.

Rhus-Rheuma-Gel N *DHU, Ger.*
Rhus toxicodendron (p.1657·3); ledum; comfrey (p.1598·3).
Muscle and joint disorders.

Rhythmocor *Lannacher, Aust.*
Propafenone hydrochloride (p.961·3).
Arrhythmias.

Riabal
Chiesi, Fr.; Ibi, Ital.; Fujisawa, Thai.
Prifinium bromide (p.473·1).
Gastrointestinal disorders; renal calculi; smooth muscle spasm.

Riacen *Chiesi, Ital.*
Piroxicam (p.79·1).
Musculoskeletal, joint, and peri-articular disorders.

Riamet
Novartis, Switz.; Novartis, UK.
Artemether (p.431·2); lumefantrine (p.438·1).
Malaria.

Ribatran *Leurquin, Fr.*
Trypsin (p.1675·3); ribonuclease (p.1657·3); chymotrypsinogen.
Oedema following trauma or surgery.

Ribelfan *Pharmacia Upjohn, Ital.*
Propyphenazone (p.80·2); noscapine (p.1096·1).
Cold and influenza symptoms.

Ribex Flu *Pfizer Consumer, Ital.*
Diclofenac sodium (p.30·3).
Fever; influenza symptoms; pain.

Ribex Gola *Restiva, Ital.†.*
Benzethonium chloride (p.1134·2).
Mouth disinfection.

Ribex Nasale *Pfizer Consumer, Ital.*
Phenylephrine hydrochloride (p.1097·1).
Nasal congestion.

Ribex Tosse *Pfizer Consumer, Ital.*
Dropropizine (p.1089·3).
Coughs.

Ribexen con Espettorante *Pfizer Consumer, Ital.*
Dropropizine (p.1089·3); guaifenesin (p.1092·2).
Coughs.

Ribocarbo *Ribosepharm, Ger.*
Carboplatin (p.515·1).
Malignant neoplasms.

Ribociclina *Formenti, Ital.*
Doxycycline hyclate (p.200·1).
Bacterial infections.

Ribodoxo-L *Ribosepharm, Ger.*
Doxorubicin hydrochloride (p.534·3).
Malignant neoplasms.

Ribofluor *Ribosepharm, Ger.*
Fluorouracil (p.540·2).
Malignant neoplasms.

Ribofolin
Sanova, Aust.†; Ribosepharm, Ger.
Calcium folinate (p.1363·1).
Adjunct to fluorouracil therapy; methotrexate toxicity.

Ribolac *Gebro, Switz.*
Lactobacillus acidophilus (p.1626·3); vitamins (p.1350·1).
Diarrhoea.

Ribomicin *Farmigea, Ital.*
Gentamicin sulfate (p.210·1).
Bacterial eye infections.

Ribomunyl
Germania, Austral.; Inava, Fr.; Pierre Fabre, Ger.; Pierre Fabre, Port.; Pierre Fabre, Spain†; Robapharm, Switz.
Ribosomes of *Klebsiella pneumoniae*; *Streptococcus pneumoniae*; *Streptococcus pyogenes*; *Haemophilus influenzae*; membrane fraction of *Klebsiella pneumoniae*.
Respiratory-tract infections.

Ribomustin *Ribosepharm, Ger.*
Bendamustine hydrochloride.
Malignant neoplasms.

Ribon *Therabel, Belg.*
Riboflavin (p.1386·1).
Muscle cramps; vitamin B_2 deficiency.

Riboposid *Ribosepharm, Ger.*
Etoposide (p.538·1).
Malignant neoplasms.

Ribostat *Valeas, Ital.†.*
Ribostamycin sulfate.
Gastrointestinal infections.

Ribotrex *Pierre Fabre, Ital.*
Azithromycin (p.153·1).
Bacterial infections.

Ribovac *Schering-Plough, Mex.*
Ribosomal fractions of *Klebsiella pneumoniae*; *Streptococcus pneumoniae*; *Streptococcus pyogenes*; *Haemophilus influenzae*; membrane fraction of *Klebsiella pneumoniae*.
Respiratory-tract infections.

Ribovir *Plants, Ital.*
Royal jelly (p.1659·3); echinacea (p.1606·2); black currant (p.1389·3).
Nutritional supplement.

Ribo-Wied *Wiedemann, Ger.*
Spleen; liver; heart; placenta (p.1631·2).
Tonic.

Ribozym *Sofex, Port.†.*
Ribonucleic acids; glycerophosphates; kola; nicotinamide; thiamine; calcium; sodium (p.1350·1).
Tonic.

Ribrain *Yamanouchi, Ger.*
Betahistine mesilate (p.1584·3).
Ménière's disease.

Ribufen *Jofrain, Mex.*
Ibuprofen (p.43·2).

Ribujet *Wasserman, Spain.*
Budesonide (p.1064·2).
Asthma.

Ribusol *Wasserman, Spain†.*
Budesonide (p.1064·2).
Asthma; nasal polyps; rhinitis; skin disorders.

Rical *Rigers, Mex.*
Calcium gluconate (p.1188·2).

Riccomycine *Kropf, Switz.†.*
Neomycin sulfate (p.228·1); ichthammol (p.1115·2); matricaria (p.1593·2); vitamin A palmitate (p.1383·2); ergocalciferol (p.1391·2); hamamelis (p.1618·3).
Burns; superficial infected wounds.

Riccovitan *Kropf, Switz.*
Vitamin A palmitate (p.1383·2); ergocalciferol (p.1391·2); ichthammol (p.1115·2); hamamelis (p.1618·3); chamomile (p.1593·2); zinc oxide (p.1128·2).
Burns; skin inflammation; superficial wounds.

Ricerca System *Johnson & Johnson, Ital.*
Multivitamin, mineral, and amino-acid preparation (p.1350·1).
Skin, hair, and nail disorders.

Ricerca System Anagen *Dermoteca, Port.†.*
Vitamin, mineral, amino-acid, and lipid preparation (p.1350·1).
Hair and nail disorders.

Ricerca System Elios *Dermoteca, Port.†.*
Vitamin, mineral, amino-acid, and lipid preparation (p.1350·1).
Sunlight-induced skin disorders.

Ricerca System Hidra *Dermoteca, Port.†.*
Vitamins, minerals, amino-acids, and borage oil
(p.1350·1).
Emollient.

Ricerca System Iposeb *Dermoteca, Port.†.*
Vitamins, minerals, amino-acids, and cucurbita oil
(p.1350·1).
Acne; seborrhoeic dermatitis.

Ricilin *Galen, Mex.*
Rifampicin (p.243·2).

Ricin
Atlantic, Hong Kong; Atlantic, Thai.
Rifampicin (p.243·2).
Bacterial infections.

Ricinis
Atlantic, Hong Kong; Atlantic, Thai.
Rifampicin (p.243·2); isoniazid (p.215·3).
Tuberculosis.

Ricino Koki *Calmante Vitaminado, Spain.*
Castor oil (p.1592·1).
Bowel evacuation.

Ricobid *Rico, USA†.*
Chlorpheniramine [chlorphenamine] tannate (p.412·2);
phenylephrine tannate (p.1097·3).

Ricobid D *Rico, USA†.*
Phenylephrine tannate (p.1097·3).

Ricobid H *Rico, USA†.*
Chlorpheniramine [chlorphenamine] tannate (p.412·2).

Ricola *Cedar Health, UK.*
Menthol (p.1632·3); peppermint oil (p.1243·3).
Coughs; nasal congestion; sore throat.

Ricridene *Lipha Sante, Fr.*
Nifurzide (p.230·2).
Diarrhoea.

Ricura *Pekana, Ger.*
Homoeopathic preparation.

RID *Leeming, USA; Pfizer, USA.*
Pyrethrins; piperonyl butoxide (p.1436·2).
Pediculosis.

Ridamin *Unison, Thai.*
Loratadine (p.420·1).
Allergic rhinitis; allergic skin reactions.

Rid-a-Pain *Pfeiffer, USA.*
Benzocaine (p.1306·2); menthol (p.1632·3); eucalyptol
(p.1609·2).
Oral lesions.

Rid-a-Pain with Codeine *Pfeiffer, USA†.*
Codeine phosphate (p.25·2); paracetamol (p.71·2); caf-
feine (p.761·3); aspirin (p.14·2); salicylamide (p.82·1).
Pain.

Ridasa *Manuell, Mex.*
Ribonuclease (p.1657·3); dornase alfa (p.1089·1).
Viral infections.

Ridaura
*SmithKline Beecham, Aust.; SmithKline Beecham, Austral.; Ya-
manouchi, Belg.; SmithKline Beecham, Braz.; Pharmascience, Ca-
nad.; Goldshield, Denm.; SmithKline Beecham, Fin.; Yamanouchi,
Ger.; SmithKline Beecham, Hong Kong; Goldshield, Irl.; SmithKline
Beecham, Israel; Yamanouchi, Ital.; SmithKline Beecham, Mex.; Ya-
manouchi, Neth.; SmithKline Beecham, Norw.; SmithKline Beecham,
NZ; Yamanouchi, Port.; SmithKline Beecham, S.Afr.; SmithKline Bee-
cham, Singapore; Recordati, Spain; SmithKline Beecham, Swed.;
Doetsch, Grether, Switz.; SmithKline Beecham, Thai.; Yamanouchi,
UK; SmithKline Beecham, USA.*
Auranofin (p.18·2).
*Juvenile idiopathic arthritis; psoriatic arthritis; rheu-
matoid arthritis.*

Ridauran *Robapharm, Fr.*
Auranofin (p.18·2).
Rheumatoid arthritis.

Ridazin *Taro, Israel.*
Thioridazine hydrochloride (p.708·1).
Aggression; agitation; anxiety.

Ridazine
Rolab, S.Afr.†; Atlantic, Thai.
Thioridazine hydrochloride (p.708·1).
*Alcohol withdrawal syndrome; anxiety; depression;
psychoses.*

Ridene *Syntex, Mex.*
Nicardipine hydrochloride (p.938·3).
*Angina pectoris; cerebrovascular ischaemia; hyper-
tension.*

Ridenol *RID, USA.*
Paracetamol (p.71·2).

Rideril *DDSA Pharmaceuticals, UK.*
Thioridazine (p.708·1).
Schizophrenia.

Ridiodent *Ogna, Ital.*
Sodium fluoride (p.1375·3); cetylpyridinium chloride
(p.1138·1).
Dental caries prophylaxis.

Riduton Ergo *Francia, Ital.*
Carnitine; betacarotene; glutathione; vitamin C; vita-
min E (p.1350·1).
Nutritional supplement.

Ridutox *SoSe, Ital.*
Glutathione (p.1010·3).
Alcohol and drug poisoning; radiation sickness.

Riduvir *Francia, Ital.*
Aciclovir (p.612·3).
Herpesvirus infections.

Rielex *Sanval, Braz.*
Dipyrone (p.34·1); orphenadrine citrate (p.470·3); caf-
feine (p.761·3).
Skeletal muscle spasm.

Rifa *Grunenthal, Ger.*
Rifampicin (p.243·2) or rifampicin sodium (p.245·3).
Tuberculosis.

Rifacol *Formenti, Ital.*
Rifaximin (p.246·3).
*Adjuvant in hyperammonaemia; gastrointestinal infec-
tions.*

Rifadin
*Hoechst Marion Roussel, Austral.; Hoechst Marion Roussel, Canad.;
Hoechst Marion Roussel, Hong Kong; Hoechst Marion Roussel, Irl.;
Lepetit, Ital.; Hoechst Marion Roussel, Mex.; Hoechst Marion Rous-
sel, Neth.; Pharmacia Upjohn, Norw.†; Aventis, NZ; Aventis, Port.;
Aventis, S.Afr.; Hoechst Marion Roussel, Swed.; Hoechst Marion
Roussel, Thai.; Hoechst Marion Roussel, UK; Hoechst Marion Rous-
sel, USA.*
Rifampicin (p.243·2) or rifampicin sodium (p.245·3).
*Bacterial infections including tuberculosis and lepro-
sy; bacterial meningitis prophylaxis.*

Rifadine
Aventis, Belg.; Roussel Diamant, Fr.
Rifampicin (p.243·2) or rifampicin sodium (p.245·3).
*Bacterial infections including tuberculosis and lepro-
sy; bacterial meningitis prophylaxis.*

Rifafour *Aventis, S.Afr.*
Rifampicin (p.243·2); isoniazid (p.215·3); pyrazina-
mide (p.240·1); ethambutol (p.205·3).
Tuberculosis.

Rifagen
Llorente, Spain; General Drugs, Thai.
Rifampicin (p.243·2).
Meningitis; mycobacterial infections; tuberculosis.

Rifaldin
Hoechst Marion Roussel, Braz.; Hoechst Marion Roussel, Spain.
Rifampicin (p.243·2) or rifampicin sodium (p.245·3).
*Meningitis; mycobacterial infections; staphylococcal
infections.*

Rifam *Siam Bheasach, Thai.*
Rifampicin (p.243·2).
Bacterial infections.

Rifamate *Hoechst Marion Roussel, USA.*
Rifampicin (p.243·2); isoniazid (p.215·3).
Tuberculosis.

Rifamcilin *Galen, Mex.*
Rifampicin (p.243·2).

Rifamiso *Siam Bheasach, Thai.*
Rifampicin (p.243·2); isoniazid (p.215·3).
Tuberculosis.

Rifam-P *PP Lab, Thai.*
Rifampicin (p.243·2).
Gonorrhoea; leprosy; tuberculosis.

Rifanicozid *Piam, Ital.†.*
Rifampicin (p.243·2); isoniazid (p.215·3).
Tuberculosis.

Rifano *Milano, Thai.*
Rifampicin (p.243·2).
Gonorrhoea; leprosy; tuberculosis.

Rifapiam *Piam, Ital.*
Rifampicin (p.243·2).
Bacterial infections including tuberculosis.

Rifaprim *Hoechst Marion Roussel, Mex.*
Rifampicin (p.243·2); trimethoprim (p.264·2).
Bacterial infections.

Rifasynt
Medochemie, Hong Kong; Medochemie, Thai.
Rifampicin (p.243·2).
Bacterial infections including tuberculosis and leprosy.

Rifater
*Hoechst Marion Roussel, Aust.; Hoechst Marion Roussel, Canad.;
Roussel Diamant, Fr.; Grunenthal, Ger.; Hoechst Marion Roussel,
Hong Kong; Hoechst Marion Roussel, Irl.; Lepetit, Ital.; Hoechst Mar-
ion Roussel, Mex.; Aventis, Port.; Aventis, S.Afr.; Hoechst Marion
Roussel, Singapore; Hoechst Marion Roussel, Spain; Hoechst Marion
Roussel, Switz.; Hoechst Marion Roussel, Thai.; Hoechst Marion
Roussel, UK; Hoechst Marion Roussel, USA.*
Rifampicin (p.243·2); isoniazid (p.215·3); pyrazina-
mide (p.240·1).
Tuberculosis.

Rifcin *Rolab, S.Afr.*
Rifampicin (p.243·2).
Tuberculosis.

Rifedot *Alacan, Spain.*
Astemizole (p.409·1).
Hypersensitivity reactions.

Rifex *Sanofi Synthelabo, Port.*
Rifampicin (p.243·2).
Gram-positive bacterial infections; tuberculosis.

Rifinah
*Roussel Diamant, Fr.; Grunenthal, Ger.; Hoechst Marion Roussel,
Hong Kong; Hoechst Marion Roussel, Irl.; Lepetit, Ital.; Hoechst Mar-
ion Roussel, Mex.; Hoechst Marion Roussel, Neth.; Aventis, NZ;
Aventis, Port.; Aventis, S.Afr.; Hoechst Marion Roussel, Singapore;
Hoechst Marion Roussel, Spain; Hoechst Marion Roussel, Switz.;
Hoechst Marion Roussel, Thai.; Hoechst Marion Roussel, UK.*
Rifampicin (p.243·2); isoniazid (p.215·3).
Tuberculosis.

Rifocin
Hoechst Marion Roussel, Aust.; Lepetit, Ital.
Rifamycin sodium (p.246·2).
Lignocaine [lidocaine] hydrochloride (p.1313·2) may
be included in the intramuscular injection to alleviate
the pain of injection.
Bacterial infections.

Rifocina
Note.This name is used for preparations of different composition.
Hoechst Marion Roussel, Braz.; Aventis, Port.
Rifamycin (p.246·3) or rifamycin sodium (p.246·2).
Bacterial infections.

Marion Merrell, Spain†.
Rifampicin sodium (p.245·3).
*Asymptomatic carriers of Neisseria meningitidis; bac-
terial infections; tuberculosis.*

Rifocine
Aventis, Belg.; Marion Merrell, Fr.†.
Rifamycin (p.246·3).
Bacterial infections.

Rifocort *Medley, Braz.*
Rifamycin sodium (p.246·2); prednisolone acetate
(p.1078·1).
Skin disorders.

Rifocyna *Hoechst Marion Roussel, Mex.*
Rifamycin sodium (p.246·2).
Impetigo; infected burns and wounds.

Rifoldin *Hoechst Marion Roussel, Aust.*
Rifampicin (p.243·2).
*Asymptomatic Haemophilus influenzae carriers;
asymptomatic meningococcal carriers; brucellosis;
leprosy; staphylococcal infections; tuberculosis.*

Rifoldin INH *Hoechst Marion Roussel, Aust.*
Rifampicin (p.243·2); isoniazid (p.215·3).
Tuberculosis.

Rifoldine *Hoechst Marion Roussel, Switz.†.*
Rifampicin (p.243·2).
Bacterial infections including tuberculosis and leprosy.

Rifun *Schwarz, Ger.; Sanol, Ger.*
Pantoprazole sodium (p.1243·2).
Gastro-oesophageal reflux; peptic ulcer.

Riganpil *Rigers, Mex.*
Ampicillin (p.150·3).
Bacterial infections.

Riget *Biolab, Thai.*
21 Tablets, levonorgestrel (p.1486·2); ethinylestradiol
(p.1476·2); 7 tablets, inert.
Combined oral contraceptive.

Rigevidon
Gedeon Richter, Hong Kong; Gedeon Richter, Thai.
Levonorgestrel (p.1486·2); ethinylestradiol (p.1476·2).
28-Day packs also contain 7 inert tablets.
Combined oral contraceptive; menstrual disorders.

Rigidur
Ferring, Denm.; Ferring, Fin.
Alprostadil alfadex (p.1440·1).
Erectile dysfunction.

Rigidur Duo *Ferring, Swed.*
Alprostadil alfadex (p.1440·1).
Erectile dysfunction.

Rigoletten *Tendem, Neth.*
Aluminium hydroxide-magnesium carbonate co-dried
gel (p.1211·2); magnesium hydroxide (p.1233·1).
*Gastrointestinal disorders associated with hyperacidi-
ty.*

Rigoran *Vita, Spain.*
Ciprofloxacin hydrochloride (p.182·3) or ciprofloxacin
lactate (p.182·3).
Bacterial infections.

Riker Antibiotic-Spray *Sanova, Aust.†.*
Bacitracin zinc (p.155·2); neomycin sulfate (p.228·1);
polymyxin B sulfate (p.238·1).
Bacterial infections.

Riker Silicone-Spray *Sanova, Aust.†.*
Aluminium hydroxide (p.1210·3); allantoin
(p.1110·1); silicone (p.1410·1); cetylpyridinium chloride (p.1138·1).
Colostomy hygiene; decubitus ulcers; nappy rash.

Rikodeine *3M, Austral.*
Dihydrocodeine tartrate (p.33·1).
Coughs.

Rikoderm *3M, Austral.*
Light liquid paraffin (p.1407·2); dewaxed wool fat
(p.1410·3).
Dry skin disorders.

Rikospray *3M, Ital.*
Aldioxa (p.1109·3); cetylpyridinium chloride
(p.1138·1); terpineol (p.1669·3); dimethicone
(p.1410·1).
Barrier preparation; skin disinfection.

Rilamir *Gea, Denm.*
Triazolam (p.709·3).
Insomnia.

Rilan *UCI, Braz.*
Sodium cromoglicate (p.774·3).
Allergic rhinitis.

Rilaprost *Guidotti, Ital.*
Saw palmetto (p.1491·2).
Prostatic hyperplasia.

Rilaten *Guidotti, Ital.*
Rociverine (p.1659·2).
Smooth muscle spasm.

Rilatine *Novartis, Belg.*
Methylphenidate hydrochloride (p.1511·3).
*Attention deficit hyperactivity disorder; narcoleptic
syndrome.*

Rilcapton *Medochemie, Singapore.*
Captopril (p.853·3).
Heart failure; hypertension.

Rilex *Lindopharm, Ger.*
Tetrazepam (p.708·1).
Skeletal muscle spasticity; skeletal muscle tension.

Rilutek
*Rhone-Poulenc Rorer, Aust.; Aventis, Belg.; Aventis, Denm.; Rhone-
Poulenc Rorer, Fin.; Rhone-Poulenc Rorer, Fr.; Rhone-Poulenc Rorer,
Ger.; Rhone-Poulenc Rorer, Hong Kong; Rhone-Poulenc Rorer, Irl.;
Rhone-Poulenc Rorer, Israel; Rhone-Poulenc Rorer, Ital.; Rhone-Pou-
lenc Rorer, Jpn; Rhone-Poulenc Rorer, Mex.; Rhone-Poulenc Rorer,*

---

*Neth.; Rhone-Poulenc Rorer, Norw.; Aventis, Port.; Aventis, S.Afr.;
Rhone-Poulenc Rorer, Singapore; Rhone-Poulenc Rorer, Spain; Rhone-
Poulenc Rorer, Swed.; Rhone-Poulenc Rorer, Switz.; Rhone-Poulenc
Rorer, Thai.; Aventis, UK; Rhone-Poulenc Rorer, USA.*
Riluzole (p.1658·1).
Amyotrophic lateral sclerosis.

Rim *Bracco, Ital.†.*
Phenolphthalein (p.1244·1); sodium citrate (p.1186·2).
Constipation.

Rimacid *Rima, UK.*
Indometacin (p.44·3).

Rimacillin *Rima, UK.*
Ampicillin (p.150·3).
Bacterial infections.

Rimactan
*Biochemie, Aust.; Ciba-Geigy, Belg.†; Biochemie, Denm.; Novartis,
Fr.; Ciba, Ger.†; Novartis, Israel; Novartis, Mex.; Novartis, Neth.; Bi-
ochemie, Norw.; Novartis, Spain; Swedish Orphan, Swed.; Novartis,
Switz.*
Rifampicin (p.243·2) or rifampicin sodium (p.245·3).
*Bacterial infections including tuberculosis and lepro-
sy; prophylaxis of meningococcal meningitis.*

Rimactan + INH *Biochemie, Aust.*
Rifampicin (p.243·2); isoniazid (p.215·3).
Tuberculosis.

Rimactane
*Ciba, Canad.†; Novartis, Hong Kong; Swedish Orphan, Irl.; Rolab,
S.Afr.; Biochemie, Singapore; Novartis, Thai.; Biochemie, UK; Geneva,
USA.*
Rifampicin (p.243·2) or rifampicin sodium (p.245·3).
*Bacterial infections including tuberculosis and lepro-
sy; prophylaxis of meningococcal meningitis.*

Rimactazid
*Swedish Orphan, Irl.; Rolab, S.Afr.; Biochemie, Singapore; Novartis,
Spain; Novartis, Thai.; Biochemie, UK.*
Rifampicin (p.243·2); isoniazid (p.215·3).
Tuberculosis.

Rimactazide *Novartis, Switz.*
Rifampicin (p.243·2); isoniazid (p.215·3).
Tuberculosis.

Rimactazide + Z *Ciba, Switz.†.*
Tablets, rifampicin (p.243·2); isoniazid (p.215·3); tab-
lets, pyrazinamide (p.240·1).
Tuberculosis.

Rimafen *Rima, UK.*
Ibuprofen (p.43·2).

Rimafungol *Belmac, Spain†.*
Ciclopirox olamine (p.382·1).
Fungal infections.

Rimagrip *Belmac, Spain.*
Aspirin (p.14·2); ascorbic acid (p.1389·3); chlorpheniramine [chlorphenamine] maleate (p.412·1); kola
(p.1681·1).
Coughs; fever; nasal congestion; pain.

Rimapam *Rima, UK.*
Diazepam (p.674·3).

Rimapen
Note.This name is used for preparations of different composition.
Orion, Fin.
Rifampicin (p.243·2).
Tuberculosis.

Rima, UK†.
Phenoxymethylpenicillin potassium (p.235·1).

Rimapurinol *Rima, UK.*
Allopurinol (p.397·2).

Rimarin *Rima, UK.*
Chlorpheniramine [chlorphenamine] (p.412·1).

Rimasal *Rima, UK.*
Salbutamol (p.770·3).

Rimbol *Esteve, Spain†.*
Astemizole (p.409·1).
Hypersensitivity reactions.

Rimcure *Rolab, S.Afr.*
Rifampicin (p.243·2); isoniazid (p.215·3); pyrazina-
mide (p.240·1).
Tuberculosis.

Rimevax
*SmithKline Beecham, Aust.†; SmithKline Beecham, Austral.; SmithK-
line Beecham, Belg.; SmithKline Beecham, Israel; SmithKline Bee-
cham, Ital.†; SmithKline Beecham, Mex.; SmithKline Beecham, NZ;
SmithKline Beecham, S.Afr.; SmithKline Beecham, Spain; SmithKline Beecham,
Switz.; SmithKline Beecham, Thai.*
A measles vaccine (Schwarz strain) (p.1547·1).
Active immunisation.

Rimidol *UCB, Swed.*
Naphazoline hydrochloride (p.1095·1).
Eye irritation.

Rimifon
Laphal, Fr.; Roche, Spain; Labatec, Switz.; Cambridge, UK.
Isoniazid (p.215·3).
Now known as Isoniazid Ampoules in the UK.
Tuberculosis and other mycobacterial infections.

Rimoxallin *Rima, UK.*
Amoxicillin trihydrate (p.149·2).
Bacterial infections.

Rimoxyn *Rima, UK.*
Naproxen (p.60·3).

Rimsalin *Rima, Mex.*
Lincomycin hydrochloride (p.219·2).
Bacterial infections.

Rimso
*Roberts, Canad.; Britannia Pharmaceuticals, UK; Research Industries
Corp., USA.*
Dimethyl sulfoxide (p.1402·2).
Interstitial cystitis.

Rimycin *Alphapharm, Austral.*
Rifampicin (p.243·2).
Leprosy; prophylaxis of Haemophilus influenzae type B infection; prophylaxis of meningococcal infection; tuberculosis.

Rin Up *Farma Lepori, Spain.*
Phenylephrine hydrochloride (p.1097·1).
Upper respiratory-tract congestion.

Rinactive *Farmacusi, Spain†.*
Budesonide (p.1064·2).
Nasal polyps; rhinitis.

Rinade BID *Econo Med, USA.*
Pseudoephedrine hydrochloride (p.1099·2); chlorpheniramine [chlorphenamine] maleate (p.412·1).
Upper respiratory-tract symptoms.

Rinadine *Pharmaland, Thai.*
Cimetidine (p.1216·3).
Peptic ulcer; Zollinger-Ellison syndrome.

Rinafort *Schering-Plough, Belg.*
Dexbrompheniramine maleate (p.410·2); pseudoephedrine sulfate (p.1099·3).
Nasal congestion; rhinitis.

Rinantipiol *Antipiol, Ital.*
Silver protein (p.1664·2); resorcinol (p.1122·2); niaouli oil (p.1640·2); adrenaline [epinephrine] hydrochloride (p.829·2); procaine hydrochloride (p.1319·1).
Nasal congestion.

Rinatec *Boehringer Ingelheim, Irl.; Boehringer Ingelheim, UK.*
Ipratropium bromide (p.766·1).
Rhinitis.

Rinatrol *Windsor, Braz.*
Naphazoline (p.1095·1); panthenol (p.1602·3).
Nasal congestion.

Rinaze *Boehringer Ingelheim, S.Afr.*
Beclometasone dipropionate (p.1061·2).
Allergic rhinitis.

Rinazina *Maggioni, Ital.*
Naphazoline nitrate (p.1095·1).
Nasal congestion.

Rince Bouche Antiseptique *Atlas, Canad.*
Cetylpyridinium chloride (p.1138·1).

Rinedrone *Deca, Ital.†.*
Dexamethasone (p.1067·1); tonzonium bromide (p.1674·1).
Rhinitis; rhinosinusitis.

Rinelon *Malesci, Ital.; Schering-Plough, Mex.; Schering-Plough, Spain.*
Mometasone furoate (p.1077·2).
Rhinitis.

Rinerge *Atral, Port.*
Oxymetazoline hydrochloride (p.1096·2).
Nasal congestion.

Rinex *Triomed, S.Afr.*
Chlorpheniramine [chlorphenamine] maleate (p.412·1); phenylpropanolamine hydrochloride (p.1098·1); phenylephrine hydrochloride (p.1097·1).
Allergic rhinitis; cold and influenza symptoms.

Rinexin *Recip, Fin.; Recip, Norw.; Recip, Swed.*
Phenylpropanolamine hydrochloride (p.1098·1).
Rhinitis; sinusitis; urinary incontinence.

Ring N *Mack, Illert., Ger.*
Aspirin (p.14·2); caffeine (p.761·3); ascorbic acid.
Cold symptoms; fever; pain.

Ringersteril *Orion, Fin.*
Electolyte infusion with or without glucose (p.1180·1).
Fluid and electrolyte disorders.

Ringworm Ointment *Douglas, Austral.*
Tolnaftate (p.395·2).
Fungal skin infections.

Rinil *Recip, Swed.*
Sodium cromoglicate (p.774·3).
Allergic conjunctivitis; allergic rhinitis.

Rinilyn *Chefaro, Spain.*
Sodium cromoglicate (p.774·3).
Hay fever; rhinitis.

Rinisone *Medley, Braz.*
Fluprednisolone (p.1072·2); ephedrine (p.1090·1); naphazoline (p.1095·1).
Nasal disorders.

Rinnova *Sefarma, Ital.*
Calcium glycerophosphate; colecalciferol; soya isoflavones (p.1350·1).
Menopausal disorders.

Rino Calyptol *Rhone-Poulenc Rorer, Ital.*
Oxymetazoline hydrochloride (p.1096·2).
Nasal congestion.

Rino Clenil *Chiesi, Hong Kong; Chiesi, Ital.; Chiesi, Singapore.*
Beclometasone dipropionate (p.1061·2).
Rhinitis; sinusitis.

Rino Dexa *Synthelabo, Spain.*
Chlorpheniramine [chlorphenamine] maleate (p.412·1); dexamethasone sodium phosphate (p.1067·1); muramidase hydrochloride (p.1638·1); neomycin sulfate (p.228·1).
Rhinitis; rhinopharyngeal infection; sinusitis.

Rino Ebastel *Almirall, Spain.*
Pseudoephedrine hydrochloride (p.1099·2); ebastine (p.417·2).
Allergic rhinitis.

Rino Naftazolina *Bruschettini, Ital.*
Naphazoline hydrochloride (p.1095·1).
Nasal congestion.

Rino Spray *Heralds, Braz.*
Oxymetazoline (p.1096·2).
Nasal congestion.

Rinobalsamiche *Farmatre, Ital.; Iema, Ital.; Morigi, Ital.; Nova Argentia, Ital.; Ramini, Ital.; Sella, Ital.; Eugal, Ital.*
Menthol (p.1632·3); niaouli oil (p.1640·2).
Nasal congestion.

Rinobanedif *Roche Nicholas, Spain.*
Bacitracin zinc (p.155·2); phenylephrine hydrochloride (p.1097·1); neomycin sulfate (p.228·1); prednisolone (p.1077·3); eucalyptol (p.1609·2); niaouli oil (p.1640·2).
Formerly contained antazoline, bacitracin zinc, phenylephrine hydrochloride, neomycin sulfate, prednisolone, eucalyptol, and niaouli oil.
Upper respiratory-tract disorders.

Rinoblanco Dexa Antibio *Alcon Cusi, Spain.*
Dexamethasone sodium phosphate (p.1067·1); neomycin sulfate (p.228·1); xylometazoline hydrochloride (p.1102·2).
Upper respiratory-tract disorders.

Rinocidina *Valeas, Ital.*
Tyrothricin (p.267·1); naphazoline nitrate (p.1095·1).
Rhinitis; sinusitis.

Rinocorin *Synthelabo, Spain.*
Oxymetazoline hydrochloride (p.1096·2).
Nasal congestion.

Rinocron *Neo Quimica, Braz.*
Naphazoline (p.1095·1); tyrothricin (p.267·1); thiomersal (p.1158·2); nitrofurazone (p.231·3).
Nasal congestion.

Rinocusi Vitaminico *Synthelabo, Spain.*
Vitamin A (p.1382·1).
Nasal congestion; nasal irritation.

Rinodif *Roche Nicholas, Spain.*
Oxymetazoline hydrochloride (p.1096·2).
Nasal congestion.

Rinofen *Delta, Braz.*
Diosfenol; eucalyptol (p.1609·2); menthol (p.1632·3); sumatra benzoin (p.1668·3); lavender (p.1627·2).
Nasal congestion.

Rinofluimucil
Note.This name is used for preparations of different composition.
Zambon, Braz.
Acetylcysteine (p.1082·3); tuaminoheptane sulfate (p.1102·2); fludrocortisone (p.1070·1).
Rhinitis.

Zambon, Hong Kong; Zambon, Ital.; Zambon, Spain; Inpharzam, Switz.
Acetylcysteine (p.1082·3); tuaminoheptane sulfate (p.1102·2).
Formerly contained acetylcysteine, tuaminoheptane sulfate, and betamethasone in *Ital.*
Rhinitis; sinusitis.

Rinofluimucil-S *Zambon, Ger.*
Acetylcysteine (p.1082·3); tuaminoheptane sulfate (p.1102·2).
Rhinitis; sinusitis.

Rinoflux *IMA, Braz.*
Sodium chloride (p.1196·1).
Nasal congestion.

Rinofomentil *SIT, Ital.*
Silver protein (p.1664·2); naphazoline nitrate (p.1095·1); niaouli oil (p.1640·2).
Nasal disorders.

Rinofren *Carnot, Mex.*
Chlorpheniramine [chlorphenamine] maleate (p.412·1); phenylpropanolamine hydrochloride (p.1098·1); paracetamol (p.71·2); caffeine (p.761·3).
Cold and influenza symptoms.

Rinofrenal
Note.This name is used for preparations of different composition.
Searle, Ital.
Sodium cromoglicate (p.774·3); chlorpheniramine [chlorphenamine] maleate (p.412·1).
Rhinitis.

Sigma-Tau, Spain.
Sodium cromoglicate (p.774·3).
Hay fever; rhinitis.

Rinofrenal Plus *Sigma-Tau, Spain.*
Chlorpheniramine [chlorphenamine] maleate (p.412·1); sodium cromoglicate (p.774·3).
Hay fever; rhinitis.

Rinogan *Produfarma, Port.*
Chlorpheniramine [chlorphenamine] maleate (p.412·2); phenylpropanolamine (p.1098·1); ascorbic acid (p.1389·3).
Nasal congestion.

Rinoglin *Seber, Port.*
Chlorpheniramine [chlorphenamine] maleate (p.412·1); sodium cromoglicate (p.774·3).
Conjunctivitis; eye irritation; rhinitis.

Rinogutt Antiallergico Spray *Boehringer Ingelheim, Ital.*
Tramazoline hydrochloride (p.1102·1); chlorpheniramine [chlorphenamine] maleate (p.412·1).
Allergic rhinitis.

Rinogutt Eucalipto-Fher *Boehringer Ingelheim, Ital.*
Tramazoline hydrochloride (p.1102·1); eucalyptol (p.1609·2); menthol (p.1632·3); camphor (p.1589·3).
Nasal congestion.

Rinogutt Spray-Fher *Boehringer Ingelheim, Ital.*
Tramazoline hydrochloride (p.1102·1).
Nasal congestion.

Rinojet *Valeas, Ital.*
Betamethasone (p.1063·1); phenylephrine hydrochloride (p.1097·1).
Formerly contained betamethasone, neomycin sulfate, polymyxin B sulfate, and phenylephrine hydrochloride.
Rhinitis; rhinopharyngitis; sinusitis.

Rinojet SF *Valeas, Ital.*
Neomycin sulfate (p.228·1); polymyxin B sulfate (p.238·1).
Rinojet SF senza Fenilefrina formerly contained betamethasone, neomycin sulfate, and polymyxin B sulfate.
Infections of the upper-respiratory tract.

Rino-Lastin *Asta Medica, Braz.*
Azelastine hydrochloride (p.409·3).
Nasal congestion.

Rinomar *Cazi, Braz.*
Note.This name is used for preparations of different composition.
Janssen-Cilag, Belg.
Cinnarizine (p.413·1); phenylpropanolamine hydrochloride (p.1098·1); isopropamide iodide (p.470·1).
Rhinitis.

Recip, Fin.; Pharmacia Upjohn, Norw.†; Recip, Swed.
Cinnarizine (p.413·1); phenylpropanolamine hydrochloride (p.1098·1).
Nasal congestion; rhinitis.

Rinomax *Ern, Spain.*
Carbinoxamine maleate (p.411·1); pseudoephedrine (p.1099·2).
Nasal congestion.

Rinomicine *Fardi, Spain.*
Oral sachets: Ascorbic acid (p.1389·3); caffeine (p.761·3); chlorpheniramine [chlorphenamine] maleate (p.412·1); phenylephrine hydrochloride (p.1097·1); paracetamol (p.71·2); salicylamide (p.82·1).

Tablets: Caffeine (p.761·3); chlorpheniramine [chlorphenamine] maleate (p.412·1); phenylephrine hydrochloride (p.1097·1); paracetamol (p.71·2); salicylamide (p.82·1).
Influenza and cold symptoms; nasal congestion.

Rinomicine Activada *Fardi, Spain.*
Caffeine (p.761·3); chlorpheniramine [chlorphenamine] maleate (p.412·1); phenylephrine hydrochloride (p.1097·1); paracetamol (p.71·2); salicylamide (p.82·1).
Influenza and cold symptoms; nasal congestion.

Rinopaidolo *Deca, Ital.*
Niaouli oil (p.1640·2); eucalyptus oil (p.1609·2).
Nasal congestion.

Rinopanteina *DMG, Ital.*
Dexpanthenol (p.1602·3); vitamin A (p.1382·1).
Nasal hygiene.

Rinoretard *Pfizer Consumer, Spain.*
Carbinoxamine (p.411·1); phenylpropanolamine (p.1098·1).
Nasal congestion.

Rinos *Molteni, Ital.*
Xylometazoline hydrochloride (p.1102·2); thymol (p.1158·3); eucalyptol (p.1609·2).
Nasal congestion.

Rinosbon *Medley, Braz.*
Dexamethasone (p.1067·1); phenylephrine (p.1097·1); chlorpheniramine [chlorphenamine] (p.412·2).
Nasal disorders.

Rinosedin *Streuli, Switz.*
Xylometazoline hydrochloride (p.1102·2).
Adjunct in rhinoscopy; cold symptoms; otitis; sinus disorders.

Rinosil *Zeta, Ital.†.*
Cetylpyridinium chloride (p.1138·1); chlorobutanol; menthol; eucalyptol; camphor.
Nasal disinfection.

Rinosite *Sanval, Braz.*
Naphazoline (p.1095·1); diphenhydramine (p.416·1); neomycin (p.228·1).
Nasal congestion.

Rinosone *Faes, Spain.*
Fluticasone propionate (p.1072·2).
Nasal polyps; rhinitis.

Rinosoro *Farmasa, Braz.*
Sodium chloride (p.1196·1); benzalkonium chloride (p.1133·2).
Nasal congestion.

Rinospray *Recordati, Ital.†.*
Dequalinium chloride (p.1143·1); naphazoline hydrochloride (p.1095·1).
Disinfection and decongestion of the upper-respiratory tract.

Rinostil *Deca, Ital.*
Eucalyptus oil (p.1609·2); camphor (p.1589·3); thymol (p.1158·3); menthol (p.1632·3).
Rhinopharyngeal congestion.

Rinotil *Brasmedica, Braz.*
Sodium chloride (p.1196·1); benzalkonium chloride (p.1133·2).
Nasal congestion.

Rinotricina *SIT, Ital.*
Tyrothricin (p.267·1).
Rhinitis; sinusitis.

Rinovagos *Valeas, Ital.*
Ipratropium bromide (p.766·1).
Rhinitis.

Rinovel *Ern, Spain.*
Naphazoline nitrate (p.1095·1); neomycin sulfate (p.228·1); prednisolone (p.1077·3).
Congestion and infection of the nose and ear.

Rinovit *SIT, Ital.*
Ephedrine (p.1090·1); eucalyptol (p.1609·2); niaouli oil (p.1640·2).
Nasal congestion.

Rinovit Nube *SIT, Ital.†.*
Silver protein (p.1664·2); naphazoline nitrate (p.1095·1); niaouli oil (p.1640·2).
Congestion of the upper-respiratory tract.

Rinozin *QIF, Braz.*
Naphazoline hydrochloride (p.1095·1); dexpanthenol (p.1602·3).
Nasal congestion.

Rinsoderm *Nycomed, Norw.†.*
Pyrethrum extract (p.1436·3); piperonyl butoxide (p.1436·2).
Pediculosis.

Rinstead *Schering-Plough, UK.*
Contact pastille: Lignocaine [lidocaine] hydrochloride (p.1313·2).
Mouth irritation; mouth ulcers.

Pastilles: Menthol (p.1632·3); cetylpyridinium chloride (p.1138·1).
Mouth ulcers.

Topical gel: Benzocaine (p.1306·2); chloroxylenol (p.1142·1).
Mouth ulcers; teething pain.

Rinstead Teething Gel *Schering-Plough, UK.*
Lignocaine [lidocaine] (p.1313·2); cetylpyridinium chloride (p.1138·1).

Rinurel *Warner-Lambert, Fr.*
Phenylpropanolamine hydrochloride (p.1098·1); phenyltoloxamine citrate (p.423·1); paracetamol (p.71·2).
Disorders of the ear, nose, and throat.

Rinutan *Warner-Lambert, Fr.*
Paracetamol (p.71·2); phenylpropanolamine hydrochloride (p.1098·1); phenyltoloxamine citrate (p.423·1).
Disorders of the ear, nose, and throat.

Rio-Josipyrin N *CPF, Ger.*
Aspirin (p.14·2); paracetamol (p.71·2); caffeine (p.761·3).
Headache; influenza; neuralgia.

Riopan
Note.This name is used for preparations of different composition.
Byk, Aust.; Byk, Belg.; Byk, Braz.; Whitehall-Robins, Canad.; Byk, Fr.; Byk Gulden, Ger.; Roland, Ger.; Byk Gulden, Ital.; Byk, Neth.; Byk, Port.; Byk, Switz.; Whitehall, USA.
Magaldrate (p.1232·2).
Gastrointestinal disorders associated with hyperacidity.

Byk Gulden, Mex.
Magaldrate (p.1232·2); dimethicone (p.1249·2).
Gastrointestinal disorders associated with hyperacidity.

Riopan Plus *Byk, Braz.; Whitehall-Robins, Canad.; Whitehall, USA.*
Magaldrate (p.1232·2); simeticone (p.1249·2).
Gastrointestinal disorders.

Riopone *Akromed, S.Afr.†.*
Magaldrate (p.1232·2).
Gastrointestinal hyperacidity.

Riostatin *Mer-National, S.Afr.*
Tetracycline hydrochloride (p.258·3); nystatin (p.392·2); vitamin B substances (p.1350·1); ascorbic acid.
Bacterial infections.

Riotapen *Fermentaciones y Sintesis, Spain†.*
Amoxicillin sodium (p.149·2) or amoxicillin trihydrate (p.149·2).
Bacterial infections.

Rioven *Willmar, Mex.*
Vitamin B substances (p.1350·1).

Ripason *Knoll, Mex.*
Liver extract.

Riphenidate *Technilab, Canad.*
Methylphenidate hydrochloride (p.1511·3).

Ripix *Ciba Vision, Ital.; Ciba Vision, Switz.*
Metipranolol (p.930·2); pilocarpine hydrochloride (p.1422·3).
Glaucoma; ocular hypertension.

Risatarun *Ravensberg, Ger.*
Deanol aceglumate (p.1507·2).
Nervous system disorders.

Riscalon *Boehringer Mannheim, Spain†.*
Fentiazac (p.40·2).
Musculoskeletal, joint, peri-articular, and soft-tissue disorders.

Rischiaril *Piam, Ital.*
Deanol hemisuccinate (p.1507·2).
Mental function impairment.

Risek *Julphar, UAE.*
Omeprazole (p.1239·1).
Gastro-oesophageal reflux; peptic ulcer; Zollinger-Ellison syndrome.

Risicordin *Heumann, Ger.*
Spironolactone (p.973·2); hydrochlorothiazide (p.907·3).
Ascites; hyperaldosteronism; hypertension; liver cirrhosis; oedema.

Risidon *Merck, Port.*
Metformin hydrochloride (p.332·3).
Diabetes mellitus.

Risocalm *Medifive, Thai.*
Tolperisone hydrochloride (p.1330·3).
Skeletal muscle spasm.

The symbol † denotes a preparation no longer actively marketed

Risolid *Dumex-Alpharma, Denm.; Dumex-Alpharma, Fin.*
Chlordiazepoxide (p.659·2).
Alcohol withdrawal syndrome; anxiety disorders.

Risoltuss *Magis, Ital.†*
Cloperastine fendizoate (p.1087·2).
Coughs.

Risordan *Rhone-Poulenc Rorer, Fr.*
Isosorbide dinitrate (p.915·2).
Angina pectoris; heart failure; pulmonary oedema.

Risperdal
Janssen-Cilag, Aust.; Janssen-Cilag, Austral.; Janssen-Cilag, Belg.; Janssen, Braz.; Janssen-Ortho, Canad.; Janssen-Cilag, Denm.; Janssen-Cilag, Fin.; Janssen-Cilag, Fr.; Organon, Fr.; Janssen-Cilag, Ger.; Organon, Ger.; Janssen-Cilag, Hong Kong; Janssen-Cilag, Irl.; Janssen-Cilag, Israel; Janssen-Cilag, Ital.; Janssen-Kyowa, Jpn; Janssen, Mex.; Janssen-Cilag, Neth.; Janssen-Cilag, Norw.; Janssen-Cilag, NZ; Janssen-Cilag, Port.; Janssen-Cilag, S.Afr.; Janssen-Cilag, Singapore; Janssen-Cilag, Spain; Janssen-Cilag, Swed.; Organon, Swed.; Janssen-Cilag, Switz.; Janssen, Thai.; Janssen-Cilag, UK; Janssen, USA.
Risperidone (p.704·1) or risperidone tartrate.
Psychoses.

Rispolin *Janssen-Cilag, Aust.†*
Risperidone (p.704·1).
Psychoses.

Ristalen *Tedec Meiji, Spain.*
Enalapril maleate (p.883·3).
Heart failure; hypertension.

Risto *Progress, Thai.*
Triamcinolone acetonide (p.1080·1).
Skin disorders.

Risumic *Dainippon, Jpn†.*
Amezinium metilsulfate (p.835·1).
Hypotension.

Ritalin
Novartis, Aust.; Novartis, Austral.; Novartis, Canad.; Novartis, Denm.; Novartis, Ger.; Novartis, Hong Kong; Novartis, Israel; Novartis, Mex.; Novartis, Neth.; Novartis, Norw.; Novartis, NZ; Novartis, S.Afr.; Novartis, Singapore; Novartis, UK; Novartis, USA.
Methylphenidate hydrochloride (p.1511·3).
Attention-deficit hyperactivity disorder; narcoleptic syndrome.

Ritalina *Novartis, Braz.*
Methylphenidate hydrochloride (p.1511·3).
Attention-deficit hyperactivity disorder; narcoleptic syndrome.

Ritaline *Novartis, Fr.; Novartis, Switz.*
Methylphenidate hydrochloride (p.1511·3).
Attention-deficit hyperactivity disorder; narcoleptic syndrome.

Ritalmex *Alkaloida, Thai.*
Mexiletine (p.932·2).
Arrhythmias.

Riteban *Centrum, Spain.*
Minoxidil (p.934·2).
Alopecia androgenetica.

Rite-Diet
SHS, Irl.†; Nutricia, Irl.†; Nutricia Dietary, UK.
A range of gluten-free and low-protein foods (p.1350·1).
Gluten sensitivity; liver disorders; phenylketonuria; renal failure.

Rition *Piam, Ital.*
Glutathione sodium (p.1010·3).
Alcohol and drug poisoning; radiation trauma.

Ritmocor *Malesci, Ital.*
Quinidine polygalacturonate (p.964·3).
Arrhythmias.

Ritmodan *Hoechst Marion Roussel, Ital.; Roussel, Port.*
Disopyramide (p.878·2) or disopyramide phosphate (p.878·2).
Arrhythmias.

Ritmoforine *Hoechst Marion Roussel, Neth.*
Disopyramide phosphate (p.878·2).
Arrhythmias.

Ritmogel *Terapeutico, Ital.*
Royal jelly (p.1659·3).
Nutritional supplement.

Ritmolol *Cryopharma, Mex.*
Metoprolol tartrate (p.931·2).
Angina pectoris; arrhythmias; heart failure; hypertension; hyperthyroidism; migraine; myocardial infarction.

Ritmonorm *Knoll, Braz.*
Propafenone hydrochloride (p.961·3).
Arrhythmias.

Ritopar *Agis, Israel.*
Ritodrine hydrochloride (p.1659·1).
Fetal distress during labour; premature labour.

Ritro *Fournier, Ital.*
Flurithromycin ethyl succinate (p.207·3).
Bacterial infections.

Rituxan *IDEC, USA; Genentech, USA.*
Rituximab (p.567·3).
Non-Hodgkin's lymphoma.

Rivanase *Riva, Canad.*
Beclometasone dipropionate (p.1061·2).
Corticosteroid.

Rivanol *Chinosolfabrik, Ger.*
Ethacridine lactate (p.1130·3).
Antiseptic.

Rivasol *Riva, Canad.*
Zinc sulfate (p.1398·2).
Anorectal disorders.

Rivasol HC *Riva, Canad.*
Zinc sulfate (p.1398·2); hydrocortisone acetate (p.1073·3).
Anorectal disorders.

Rivasone *Riva, Canad.†*
Betamethasone valerate (p.1063·2).
Skin disorders.

Rivatril *Roche, Fin.*
Clonazepam (p.347·1).
Epilepsy.

Rivela *Beiersdorf, Ital.*
Pregnancy test (p.1654·3).

Rivescal Tar *Pergam, Ital.*
Coal tar (p.1125·1); salicylic acid (p.1122·3).
Seborrhoeic dermatitis.

Rivescal ZPT *Pergam, Ital.*
Pyrithione zinc (p.1122·1).
Seborrhoeic dermatitis.

Rividose *Rigers, Mex.*
Vitamin B substances (p.1350·1).

Rivitin BC *Lannacher, Aust.*
Vitamin B substances and vitamin C (p.1350·1).

Rivoltan *Lichtwer, Ger.*
Devil's claw root (p.26·3).
Degenerative joint disorders.

Rivopen-V *Rivopharm, Switz.†*
Phenoxymethylpenicillin potassium (p.235·1).
Bacterial infections.

Rivostatin *Rivopharm, Switz.†*
Nystatin (p.392·2).
Fungal infections.

Rivotril
Roche, Aust.; Roche, Austral.; Roche, Belg.; Roche, Braz.; Roche, Canad.; Roche, Denm.; Roche, Fr.; Roche, Ger.; Roche, Hong Kong; Roche, Irl.; Roche, Israel; Roche, Ital.; Roche, Mex.; Roche, Neth.; Roche, Norw.; Roche, NZ; Roche, Port.; Roche, S.Afr.; Roche, Singapore; Roche, Spain; Roche, Switz.; Roche, Thai.; Roche, UK.
Clonazepam (p.347·1).
Epilepsy; status epilepticus.

Rivovit *Rivopharm, Switz.*
Multivitamin preparation (p.1350·1).

Rivoxicillin *Rivopharm, Switz.†*
Amoxicillin (p.149·2).
Bacterial infections.

Rivozol *Rivopharm, Switz.*
Metronidazole (p.594·1) or metronidazole benzoate (p.594·1).
Anaerobic bacterial infections; protozoal infections.

Riwa Franzbranntwein *Gerlach, Ger.*
Camphor (p.1589·3); alcohol (p.1130·3).
Musculoskeletal, joint, and soft-tissue disorders; poor circulation.

α-Rix *SmithKline Beecham, Belg.*
An influenza vaccine (p.1544·3).
Active immunisation.

Rixapen *Menarini, Belg.*
Clometocillin potassium (p.192·1).
Bacterial infections.

Rizaben *Kissei, Jpn.*
Tranilast (p.785·2).
Allergic conjunctivitis; allergic rhinitis; asthma; atopic dermatitis; keloids.

Rizaliv *Neopharmed, Ital.*
Rizatriptan benzoate (p.455·2).
Migraine.

Rizalt *Merck Sharp & Dohme, Israel.*
Rizatriptan (p.455·3).
Migraine.

Rize *Yoshitomi, Jpn.*
Clotiazepam (p.671·1).
Anxiety states; autonomic disorders; premedication; sleep disorders.

Rizen *Formenti, Ital.*
Clotiazepam (p.671·1).
Anxiety disorders; sleep disorders.

RMS
Note. This name is used for preparations of different composition.
Reith & Petrasch, Ger.
Lactic acid (p.1626·2) or calcium lactate (p.1188·2).
Skin disorders.

Baxter, NZ; Upsher-Smith, USA.
Morphine sulfate (p.56·1).
Pain.

RN13 Regeneresen *Dyckerhoff, Ger.*
Ribonucleic acid (p.1657·3).
Tonic.

Roaccutan
Roche, Aust.; Roche, Denm.; Roche, Fin.; Roche, Ital.; Roche, Mex.; Roche, Port.
Isotretinoin (p.1115·3).
Acne.

Roaccutane
Roche, Austral.; Roche, Belg.; Roche, Fr.; Roche, Hong Kong; Roche, Irl.; Roche, Israel; Roche, Neth.; Roche, NZ; Roche, S.Afr.; Roche, Singapore; Roche, Switz.; Roche, Thai.; Roche, UK.
Isotretinoin (p.1115·3).
Acne.

Roacutan
Roche, Braz.; Roche, Spain.
Isotretinoin (p.1115·3).
Acne.

Ro-A-Vit
Roche, NZ; Cambridge, UK.
Vitamin A palmitate (p.1383·2).

Now known as Vitamin A Palmitate Ampoules in the UK.
Vitamin A deficiency.

Robafen AC Cough *Major, USA.*
Guaifenesin (p.1092·2); codeine phosphate (p.25·2).
Coughs.

Robafen CF *Major, USA†.*
Phenylpropanolamine hydrochloride (p.1098·1); dextromethorphan hydrobromide (p.1087·3); guaifenesin (p.1092·2).
Coughs.

Robafen DAC *Major, USA.*
Pseudoephedrine hydrochloride (p.1099·2); codeine phosphate (p.25·2); guaifenesin (p.1092·2).
Coughs.

Robafen DM *Major, USA.*
Dextromethorphan hydrobromide (p.1087·3); guaifenesin (p.1092·2).
Coughs.

Robatar *Rougier, Canad.*
Tar (p.1125·1).
Skin disorders of the scalp.

RoBathol *Pharmaceutical Specialties, USA.*
Emollient.

Robaxacet *Whitehall-Robins, Canad.*
Methocarbamol (p.1329·3); paracetamol (p.71·2).
Musculoskeletal, peri-articular, and soft-tissue pain.

Robaxacet-8 *Whitehall-Robins, Canad.*
Methocarbamol (p.1329·3); paracetamol (p.71·2); codeine phosphate (p.25·2).
Musculoskeletal pain.

Robaxifen *Wyeth, Mex.*
Methocarbamol (p.1329·3); paracetamol (p.71·2).
Musculoskeletal pain.

Robaxin
Whitehall-Robins, Canad.; Wyeth Lederle, Fin.; Robins, Hong Kong; Wyeth, Mex.; Aspen, S.Afr.; Ipsen, Spain; Wyeth Lederle, Swed.; Whitehall, Thai.; Shire, UK; Robins, USA.
Methocarbamol (p.1329·3).
Musculoskeletal pain; skeletal muscle spasm.

Robaxisal
Whitehall-Robins, Canad.; Shire, Irl.†; Wyeth, Mex.; Aspen, S.Afr.; Ipsen, Spain; Robins, USA.
Methocarbamol (p.1329·3); aspirin (p.14·2).
Musculoskeletal pain; skeletal muscle spasm.

Robaxisal Compuesto *Ipsen, Spain.*
Methocarbamol (p.1329·3); paracetamol (p.71·2).
Musculoskeletal pain.

Robaxisal Forte
Wyeth Lederle, Swed.; Shire, UK†.
Methocarbamol (p.1329·3); aspirin (p.14·2).
Musculoskeletal pain and spasm.

Robaxisal-C *Whitehall-Robins, Canad.*
Methocarbamol (p.1329·3); aspirin (p.14·2); codeine phosphate (p.25·2).
Musculoskeletal pain.

Roberfarin *Robert, Spain.*
Dequalinium chloride (p.1143·1); enoxolone (p.34·3); hydrocortisone acetate (p.1073·3); oxetacaine (p.1317·3); tyrothricin (p.267·1).
Mouth and throat inflammation.

Robervital *Robert, Spain.*
Oxaceprol (p.1645·2); tocoferil sodium succinate.
Dermatomyositis; musculoskeletal and joint disorders.

Robicillin VK *Robins, USA†.*
Phenoxymethylpenicillin potassium (p.235·1).
Bacterial infections.

Robidone *Wyeth-Ayerst, Canad.*
Hydrocodone tartrate (p.42·2).
Coughs.

Robidrine *Whitehall-Robins, Canad.*
Pseudoephedrine hydrochloride (p.1099·2).
Nasal congestion.

Robigesic *Whitehall-Robins, Canad.*
Paracetamol (p.71·2).
Fever; pain.

Robimycin Robitabs *Robins, USA.*
Erythromycin (p.201·2).
Bacterial infections.

Robinaz *Whitehall, Port.*
Oxymetazoline hydrochloride (p.1096·2).
Nasal congestion.

Robinia Med Complex *Dynamit, Aust.*
Homoeopathic preparation.

Robinia Ro-Plex (Rowo-99) *Pharmakon, Ger.†.*
Homoeopathic preparation.

Robinul
Wyeth Lederle, Aust.; Wyeth-Ayerst, Austral.; Wyeth Lederle, Belg.; Wyeth-Ayerst, Canad.; Wyeth Lederle, Denm.; Wyeth Lederle, Fin.; Wyeth, Ger.; Robins, Hong Kong; Antigen, Irl.; Wyeth, Neth.; Wyeth Lederle, Norw.; Wyeth, NZ; Aspen, S.Afr.; Wyeth Lederle, Swed.; Wyeth, Switz.; Anpharm, UK; Horizon, USA.
Glycopyrronium bromide (p.467·2).
Adjunct in peptic ulcer; intra-operative management of cardiac vagal reflexes; premedication; protection against muscarinic effects of anticholinesterases used to reverse neuromuscular blockade.

Anpharm, UK.
Powder for topical solution: Glycopyrronium bromide (p.467·2).
Hyperhidrosis.

Robinul-Neostigmin
Wyeth Lederle, Denm.; Wyeth Lederle, Fin.; Wyeth Lederle, Norw.; Wyeth Lederle, Swed.
Neostigmine metilsulfate (p.1420·1).

Glycopyrronium bromide (p.467·2) is included in this preparation to protect against the muscarinic actions.
Reversal of competitive neuromuscular blockade.

Robinul-Neostigmine
Wyeth Lederle, Belg.; Antigen, Irl.; Wyeth, Switz.; Anpharm, UK.
Neostigmine metilsulfate (p.1420·1).
Glycopyrronium bromide (p.467·2) is included in this preparation to protect against the muscarinic actions.
Reversal of competitive neuromuscular blockade.

Robitet Robicaps *Robins, USA†.*
Tetracycline hydrochloride (p.258·3).
Bacterial infections.

Robitussin
Whitehall, Austral.†; Whitehall-Robins, Canad.; Robins, Israel; Whitehall, Singapore; Wyeth, Spain; Whitehall, Swed.†; Whitehall, Thai.; Robins, USA.
Guaifenesin (p.1092·2).
Coughs; respiratory-tract congestion.

Robitussin AC
Note. This name is used for preparations of different composition.
Whitehall-Robins, Canad.
Guaifenesin (p.1092·2); pheniramine maleate (p.422·3); codeine phosphate (p.25·2).
Coughs.

Robins, USA.
Guaifenesin (p.1092·2); codeine phosphate (p.25·2).
Coughs.

Robitussin CF
Robins, Hong Kong; Robins, USA†.
Guaifenesin (p.1092·2); phenylpropanolamine hydrochloride (p.1098·1); dextromethorphan hydrobromide (p.1087·3).
Coughs.

Robitussin for Chesty Coughs *Whitehall, UK.*
Guaifenesin (p.1092·2).
Coughs.

Robitussin for Chesty Coughs with Congestion *Whitehall, UK.*
Guaifenesin (p.1092·2); pseudoephedrine hydrochloride (p.1099·2).
Formerly known as Robitussin Plus.
Coughs; nasal congestion.

Robitussin Childrens *Whitehall-Robins, Canad.*
Dextromethorphan hydrobromide (p.1087·3).
Formerly known as Robitussin Pediatric.
Coughs.

Robitussin Childrens Cough & Cold *Whitehall-Robins, Canad.*
Dextromethorphan hydrobromide (p.1087·3); pseudoephedrine hydrochloride (p.1099·2).
Formerly known as Robitussin Pediatric Cough & Cold.
Coughs and cold symptoms.

Robitussin with Codeine *Whitehall-Robins, Canad.*
Guaifenesin (p.1092·2); pheniramine maleate (p.422·3); codeine phosphate (p.25·2).
Coughs.

Robitussin Cold *Whitehall, Singapore.*
Guaifenesin (p.1092·2); pseudoephedrine hydrochloride (p.1099·2).
Coughs; nasal congestion.

Robitussin Cold & Cough
Whitehall, Singapore; Robins, USA.
Guaifenesin (p.1092·2); dextromethorphan hydrobromide (p.1087·3); pseudoephedrine hydrochloride (p.1099·2).
Coughs; nasal congestion.

Robitussin Cold, Cough & Flu *Whitehall, Singapore.*
Paracetamol (p.71·2); guaifenesin (p.1092·2); dextromethorphan hydrobromide (p.1087·3); pseudoephedrine hydrochloride (p.1099·2).
Cold and flu symptoms; coughs; nasal congestion.

Robitussin Cough Calmers *Robins, USA.*
Dextromethorphan hydrobromide (p.1087·3).
Coughs.

Robitussin Cough & Cold *Whitehall-Robins, Canad.*
Guaifenesin (p.1092·2); dextromethorphan hydrobromide (p.1087·3); pseudoephedrine hydrochloride (p.1099·2).
Coughs and cold symptoms.

Robitussin Cough Cold & Flu *Whitehall-Robins, Canad.*
Guaifenesin (p.1092·2); dextromethorphan hydrobromide (p.1087·3); pseudoephedrine hydrochloride (p.1099·2); paracetamol (p.71·2).
Cold and flu symptoms; coughs.

Robitussin Cough Drops *Robins, USA.*
Menthol (p.1632·3); eucalyptus oil (p.1609·2).

Robitussin Cough Soother *Whitehall, Irl.*
Dextromethorphan hydrobromide (p.1087·3).
Coughs.

Robitussin DAC *Robins, USA.*
Guaifenesin (p.1092·2); pseudoephedrine hydrochloride (p.1099·2); codeine phosphate (p.25·2).
Coughs.

Robitussin DM
Whitehall, Austral.; Whitehall-Robins, Canad.; Robins, Hong Kong; Robins, Israel; Wyeth, Mex.; Whitehall, Singapore; Whitehall, Thai.; Robins, USA.
Guaifenesin (p.1092·2); dextromethorphan hydrobromide (p.1087·3).

Robitussin DM Antitusivo *Wyeth, Spain.*
Dextromethorphan hydrobromide (p.1087·3).
Coughs.

Robitussin DM-P *Whitehall, Austral.*
Dextromethorphan hydrobromide (p.1087·3); pseudoephedrine hydrochloride (p.1099·2).
Coughs; nasal and sinus congestion.

Robitussin for Dry Coughs *Whitehall, UK.*
Dextromethorphan hydrobromide (p.1087·3).
Formerly known as Robitussin Cough Soother.
Coughs.

Robitussin DX *Whitehall, Austral.*
Dextromethorphan hydrobromide (p.1087·3).
Coughs.

Robitussin EX *Whitehall, Austral.*
Guaifenesin (p.1092·2).
Coughs.

Robitussin Expectorant
Note. This name is used for preparations of different composition.
Robins, Hong Kong; Whitehall, Irl.
Guaifenesin (p.1092·2).
Coughs.

Whitehall-Robins, Switz.
Acetylcysteine (p.1082·3).
Coughs with viscous mucus.

Robitussin Expectorant Plus *Whitehall, Irl.*
Guaifenesin (p.1092·2); pseudoephedrine hydrochloride (p.1099·2).
Coughs; nasal congestion.

Robitussin Junior *Whitehall, UK.*
Dextromethorphan hydrobromide (p.1087·3).
Coughs.

Robitussin Maximum Strength Cough *Robins, Hong Kong.*
Dextromethorphan hydrobromide (p.1087·3).
Coughs.

Robitussin Maximum Strength Cough & Cold *Robins, USA.*
Dextromethorphan hydrobromide (p.1087·3); pseudoephedrine hydrochloride (p.1099·2).
Coughs and cold symptoms.

Robitussin ME *Whitehall, Austral.*
Guaifenesin (p.1092·2); bromhexine hydrochloride (p.1085·3).
Coughs; respiratory-tract congestion.

Robitussin Night Relief *Robins, USA.*
Pseudoephedrine hydrochloride (p.1099·2); dextromethorphan hydrobromide (p.1087·3); mepyramine maleate (p.421·1); paracetamol (p.71·2).
Coughs and cold symptoms.

Robitussin Night-Time *Whitehall, UK.*
Brompheniramine maleate (p.410·2); codeine phosphate (p.25·2); pseudoephedrine hydrochloride (p.1099·2).
Coughs.

Robitussin PE
Robins, Hong Kong; Whitehall, Singapore; Whitehall, Thai.; Robins, USA.
Guaifenesin (p.1092·2); pseudoephedrine hydrochloride (p.1099·2).
Coughs; nasal congestion.

Robitussin Pediatric *Robins, USA.*
Dextromethorphan hydrobromide (p.1087·3).
Coughs.

Robitussin Pediatric Cough *Robins, Hong Kong.*
Dextromethorphan hydrobromide (p.1087·3).
Coughs.

Robitussin Pediatric Cough & Cold Formula *Robins, USA.*
Dextromethorphan hydrobromide (p.1087·3); pseudoephedrine hydrochloride (p.1099·2).
Coughs and cold symptoms.

Robitussin PS *Whitehall, Austral.*
Guaifenesin (p.1092·2); pseudoephedrine hydrochloride (p.1099·2).
Coughs; nasal congestion.

Robitussin Severe Congestion *Robins, USA.*
Guaifenesin (p.1092·2); pseudoephedrine hydrochloride (p.1099·2).
Coughs; nasal congestion.

Robovites *Vita Health, Singapore.*
Multivitamin preparation with or without iron or zinc (p.1350·1).

Robovites Multivitamin *Vita Health, Singapore.*
Multivitamins; cod-liver oil; evening primrose oil; echinacea; ginkgo biloba (p.1350·1).

Roburis *Ripari-Gero, Ital.*
Ubidecarenone (p.1677·1).
Cardiac disorders; coenzyme Q10 deficiency.

Roburvit *Echo, Ital.*
Royal jelly (p.1659·3).

Robuvalen *Robugen, Ger.*
Zinc oxide (p.1128·2).
Eczema; skin lesions.

RoC Sunscreen Stick *RoC, UK.*
Dibenzoylmethane (p.1517·1); a cinnamic ester.
Sunscreen.

RoC Total Sunblock *RoC, UK.*
SPF 25: Octinoxate (p.1517·3); avobenzone (p.1517·1); titanium dioxide (p.1126·1).
Sunscreen.

Rocaltrol
Roche, Aust.; Roche, Austral.; Roche, Belg.; Roche, Braz.; Roche, Canad.; Roche, Denm.; Roche, Fr.; Roche, Ger.; Roche, Hong Kong; Roche, Irl.; Roche, Ital.; Roche, Mex.; Roche, Neth.; Roche, Norw.; Roche, NZ; Roche, Port.; Roche, S.Afr.; Roche, Singapore; Roche,

Spain; Roche, Swed.; Roche, Switz.; Roche, Thai.; Roche, UK; Roche, USA.
Calcitriol (p.1391·1).
Hypoparathyroidism; hypophosphataemia; osteomalacia; osteoporosis; renal osteodystrophy; rickets; secondary hyperparathyroidism; vitamin D deficiency.

Rocanal Imediat *Medirel, Switz.†.*
Povidone-iodine (p.1155·1).
Dental disinfection.

Rocanal Permanent Gangrene *Medirel, Switz.†.*
Powder, hydrocortisone acetate (p.1073·3); paraformaldehyde (p.1152·2); zinc oxide (p.1128·2); zinc stearate (p.1497·3); zinc acetate (p.1398·1); liquid, eugenol (p.1609·3).
Dental infections.

Rocanal Permanent Vital *Medirel, Switz.†.*
Powder, paraformaldehyde (p.1152·2); zinc oxide (p.1128·2); zinc stearate (p.1497·3); zinc acetate (p.1398·1); liquid, eugenol (p.1609·3).
Dental disorders.

Rocap *Rolab, S.Afr.†.*
Oxytetracycline hydrochloride (p.234·1).
Bacterial infections.

Roccal *Sanofi Winthrop, Irl.; Schein, UK.*
Benzalkonium chloride (p.1133·2).
Skin disinfection.

Roccaxin *Nakorn, Thai.*
Piroxicam (p.79·1).
Musculoskeletal, joint, peri-articular, and soft-tissue disorders.

Rocefalin *Roche, Spain.*
Ceftriaxone sodium (p.177·1).
Lignocaine [lidocaine] (p.1313·2) is included in the intramuscular injection to alleviate the pain of injection.
Bacterial infections.

Rocefin *Roche, Braz.; Roche, Ital.*
Ceftriaxone sodium (p.177·1).
Lignocaine [lidocaine] hydrochloride (p.1313·2) may be included in the intramuscular injection to alleviate the pain of injection.
Bacterial infections.

Rocephalin *Roche, Denm.; Roche, Fin.; Roche, Norw.; Roche, Swed.*
Ceftriaxone sodium (p.177·1).
Lignocaine [lidocaine] hydrochloride (p.1313·2) may be included in some injections to alleviate the pain of injection.
Bacterial infections.

Rocephin
Biochemie, Aust.; Roche, Aust.; Roche, Austral.; Roche, Canad.; Roche, Ger.; Roche, Hong Kong; Roche, Irl.; Roche, Israel; Roche, Mex.; Roche, Neth.; Roche, NZ; Roche, Port.; Roche, S.Afr.; Roche, Singapore; Roche, Thai.; Roche, UK; Roche, USA.
Ceftriaxone sodium (p.177·1).
Lignocaine [lidocaine] hydrochloride (p.1313·2) may be included in the intramuscular injection to alleviate the pain of injection.
Bacterial infections.

Rocephine *Roche, Belg.; Roche, Fr.; Roche, Switz.*
Ceftriaxone sodium (p.177·1).
Lignocaine [lidocaine] hydrochloride (p.1313·2) is included in the intramuscular injection to alleviate the pain of injection.
Bacterial infections.

Roceron *Roche, Norw.*
Interferon alfa-2a (p.628·1).
Chronic active hepatitis B; chronic hepatitis C; malignant neoplasms.

Roceron-A *Roche, Denm.*
Interferon alfa-2a (p.628·1).
Chronic hepatitis B or C; malignant neoplasms.

Rocgel *Chiesi, Fr.*
Boehmite.
Gastrointestinal disorders.

Rochagan *Roche, Braz.*
Benznidazole (p.589·2).
American trypanosomiasis.

Roche *Syntex, Canad.†.*
Naproxen sodium (p.61·1).
Inflammation; pain.

Rochevit *Roche Nicholas, Spain.*
Multivitamin and mineral preparation (p.1350·1).

Rociclyn *Zambon, Neth.*
Tolfenamic acid (p.88·3).
Osteoarthritis; rheumatoid arthritis.

Rocid *Max Farma, Ital.*
Cefonicid sodium (p.168·1).
Lignocaine [lidocaine] hydrochloride (p.1313·2) is included in this preparation to alleviate the pain of injection.
Bacterial infections.

Rocilin *Rosco, Denm.; Rosco, Norw.*
Phenoxymethylpenicillin potassium (p.235·1).
Bacterial infections.

Rocillin *Rolab, S.Afr.*
Amoxicillin trihydrate (p.149·2).
Bacterial infections.

Rocmaline *Fresenius Kabi, Aust.; Chiesi, Fr.*
Arginine (p.1353·3); malic acid (p.1631·1).
Liver disorders.

Rocodin *Brunel, S.Afr.*
Paracetamol (p.71·2); codeine phosphate (p.25·2).
Fever; pain.

Rocof *Roche, Thai.*
Dextromethorphan hydrobromide (p.1087·3); chlorpheniramine [chlorphenamine] maleate (p.412·1); pseudoephedrine hydrochloride (p.1099·2).
Coughs.

Rocornal *Rodleben, Ger.; UCB, Ger.; Vedim, Ger.*
Trapidil (p.986·1).
Ischaemic heart disease.

Rodakin *Kener, Mex.*
Loratadine (p.420·1).

Rodase *Pond's, Thai.*
Serrapeptase (p.1662·1).
Inflammation; respiratory-tract congestion; wounds.

Rodavan *Laevosan, Aust.†; Asta Medica, Ger.*
Chlorphenoxamine hydrochloride (p.412·3); caffeine (p.761·3); 8-chlorotheophylline.
Motion sickness; nausea; vertigo; vomiting.

Rodazol *Novartis, Ger.*
Aminoglutethimide (p.506·3).
Breast cancer; Cushing's syndrome.

Rodermil *Oftalder, Port.*
Metronidazole (p.594·1).

Rodogyl *Rhone-Poulenc Rorer, Fr.*
Spiramycin (p.248·3); metronidazole (p.594·1).
Bacterial mouth infections.

RO-Dry Eyes *Richmond Ophthalmics, Canad.†.*
Polyvinyl alcohol (p.1503·1).
Dry eyes.

RO-Eye Drops *Richmond Ophthalmics, Canad.†.*
Tetryzoline hydrochloride (p.1101·2).

RO-Eyewash *Richmond Ophthalmics, Canad.†.*
Boric acid (p.1586·1).

Rofact *ICN, Canad.*
Rifampicin (p.243·2).
Tuberculosis.

Rofatuss *MIP, Ger.*
Clobutinol hydrochloride (p.1087·1).
Coughs.

Rofenid *Aventis, Belg.*
Ketoprofen (p.47·3).
Inflammation; musculoskeletal, joint, and peri-articular disorders; oedema; pain.

Rofepain *LBS, Thai.*
Ketoprofen (p.47·3).
Gout; musculoskeletal, joint, peri-articular, and soft-tissue disorders; pain.

Roferon-A
Roche, Aust.; Roche, Austral.; Roche, Belg.; Roche, Braz.; Roche, Canad.; Roche, Fin.; Roche, Fr.; Roche, Ger.; Roche, Hong Kong; Roche, Irl.; Roche, Ital.; Roche, Mex.; Roche, Neth.; Roche, NZ; Roche, Port.; Roche, S.Afr.; Roche, Singapore; Roche, Spain; Roche, Swed.; Roche, Switz.; Roche, Thai.; Roche, UK; Roche, USA.
Interferon alfa-2a (rbe) (p.628·1).
Formerly known as Receron-A in *Swed.*
Chronic hepatitis B and C; malignant neoplasms.

Roflatol Phyto (Rowo-146) *Pharmakon, Ger.†.*
Chamomile (p.1593·2); caraway oil (p.1591·2); fennel oil (p.1610·2); peppermint oil (p.1243·3).
Gastrointestinal disorders.

Rogaan *Abic, Israel.*
Dextropropoxyphene hydrochloride (p.27·1); aspirin (p.14·2); paracetamol (p.71·2); caffeine (p.761·3).
Cold symptoms; pain.

Rogaine
Pharmacia Upjohn, Aust.; Pharmacia Upjohn, Canad.; Pharmacia Upjohn, USA.
Minoxidil (p.934·2).
Alopecia androgenetica.

Rogal *Galen, Mex.*
Piroxicam (p.79·1).
Gout; musculoskeletal, joint, peri-articular, and soft-tissue disorders; pain.

Rogasti *Pacific, Israel.*
Famotidine (p.1225·3).
Duodenal ulcer; gastro-oesophageal reflux; Zollinger-Ellison syndrome.

Roge *Pastor Farina, Ital.*
Anhydrous citric acid (p.1596·2); magnesium carbonate (p.1232·3).
Constipation.

Rogitine
Novartis, Canad.; Alliance, UK.
Phentolamine mesilate (p.954·3).
Dermal necrosis and sloughing following intravenous administration of noradrenaline [norepinephrine]; phaeochromocytoma.

roha-Fenchel-Tee *Roha, Ger.*
Fennel (p.1610·1).
Gastrointestinal disorders.

rohasal *Roha, Ger.*
Absinthium (p.1571·1); aniseed (p.1580·2); kaolin (p.1229·3); calcium phosphate (p.1188·3); dried magnesium sulfate (p.1191·3); calcium carbonate (p.1215·1); heavy magnesium carbonate (p.1232·3); sodium bicarbonate (p.1186·2).
Gastrointestinal disorders.

rohasal N *Roha, Ger.*
Sodium bicarbonate (p.1186·2); calcium carbonate (p.1215·1); heavy magnesium carbonate (p.1232·3).
Gastrointestinal disorders.

Rohipnol *Roche, Spain.*
Flunitrazepam (p.683·2).
Anxiety; general anaesthesia; insomnia.

Rohypnol
Roche, Aust.; Roche, Austral.; Roche, Belg.; Roche, Braz.; Roche,

Denm.; Roche, Fr.; Roche, Ger.; Roche, Hong Kong; Roche, Irl.; Roche, Israel; Roche, Mex.; Roche, Neth.; Roche, Norw.; Roche, Port.; Roche, S.Afr.; Roche, Singapore; Roche, Switz.; Roche, Thai.; Roche, UK.
Flunitrazepam (p.683·2).
Insomnia; premedication.

Roical *Shin Poong, Singapore.*
Calcitriol (p.1391·1).
Hypoparathyroidism; osteomalacia; osteoporosis; renal osteodystrophy; rickets.

Roidhemo
Cusi, Hong Kong; Pan Quimica, Spain.
Aesculus (p.1574·1); benzyl phenol; benzyl salicylate; ephedrine hydrochloride (p.1090·1); hamamelis (p.1618·3); lactic acid (p.1626·2).
Anorectal disorders.

Roipnol *Roche, Ital.*
Flunitrazepam (p.683·2).
Insomnia.

Rojema *Self-Care Products, UK.*
Royal jelly (p.1659·3).

Rokacet *Taro, Israel.*
Paracetamol (p.71·2); caffeine (p.761·3); codeine phosphate (p.25·2).
Coughs fever; pain.

Rokacet Plus *Taro, Israel.*
Paracetamol (p.71·2); caffeine (p.761·3); codeine phosphate (p.25·2).
Coughs; fever; pain.

Rokal *Taro, Israel.*
Aspirin (p.14·2); caffeine (p.761·3); codeine phosphate (p.25·2).
Coughs; fever; pain; rheumatism.

Rokal Plus *Taro, Israel.*
Aspirin (p.14·2); caffeine (p.761·3); codeine phosphate (p.25·2).
Coughs; fever; pain; rheumatism.

Rokamol *Taro, Israel.*
Paracetamol (p.71·2).
Fever; pain.

Rokamol Plus Codeine *Taro, Israel.*
Paracetamol (p.71·2); codeine phosphate (p.25·2).
Coughs; fever; pain.

Rokan *Intersan, Ger.*
Ginkgo biloba leaf (p.1615·2).
Mental function disorders; peripheral circulatory disorders.

Rokanite *Taro, Israel.*
Aspirin (p.14·2); codeine phosphate (p.25·2).
Coughs; fever; pain.

Rokital *Formenti, Ital.*
Rokitamycin (p.247·1).
Bacterial infections.

Rolab-Antiflam *Rolab, S.Afr.*
Ibuprofen (p.43·2).
Formerly known as Rofen.
Fever; pain.

Rolaids *Warner-Lambert, Canad.*
Calcium carbonate (p.1215·1); magnesium hydroxide (p.1233·1).
Dyspepsia.

Rolar *Pharmaland, Thai.*
Codeine phosphate (p.25·2); guaifenesin (p.1092·2); phenylpropanolamine hydrochloride (p.1098·1).
Cold symptoms; coughs; nasal congestion.

Rolatuss Expectorant *Huckaby, USA.*
Phenylephrine hydrochloride (p.1097·1); codeine phosphate (p.25·2); chlorpheniramine [chlorphenamine] maleate (p.412·1); ammonium chloride (p.1085·2).
Coughs.

Rolatuss with Hydrocodone *Major, USA†.*
Phenylpropanolamine hydrochloride (p.1098·1); phenylephrine hydrochloride (p.1097·1); mepyramine maleate (p.421·1); pheniramine maleate (p.422·3); hydrocodone tartrate (p.42·2).
Coughs and cold symptoms.

Rolatuss Plain *Major, USA.*
Phenylephrine hydrochloride (p.1097·1); chlorpheniramine [chlorphenamine] maleate (p.412·1).
Upper respiratory-tract symptoms.

Rolazine *Rolab, S.Afr.*
Hydralazine hydrochloride (p.905·3).
Now known as Rolab-Hydralazine HCl.
Hypertension.

Roleca Wacholder *Serturner, Ger.*
Juniper oil (p.1625·2).
Diuretic.

Roleca-S *Medichemie Bioline, Switz.*
Juniper oil (p.1625·2).
Gastrointestinal disorders.

Rolene *Riva, Canad.†.*
Betamethasone dipropionate (p.1063·2).
Skin disorders.

Roliwol *Stada, Switz.†.*
Methyl salicylate (p.55·1); camphor (p.1589·3); methyl nicotinate (p.55·1); menthol (p.1632·3); turpentine oil (p.1676·3); eucalyptus oil (p.1609·2); mint oil (p.1636·2); thymol (p.1661·3); nutmeg oil (p.1643·1).
Musculoskeletal and joint pain; sports injuries.

Roliwol B *Stada, Switz.†.*
Glycol salicylate (p.42·2); camphor (p.1589·3); diethylamine salicylate (p.32·2); pine oil.
Musculoskeletal, joint, and peri-articular pain.

Roliwol S *Stada, Switz.†.*
Glycol salicylate (p.42·2); benzyl nicotinate (p.20·2); nonivamide (p.63·1).
Musculoskeletal, joint, and peri-articular disorders.

Roll-bene *Mepha, Switz.*
Heparin sodium (p.902·1); dimethyl sulfoxide (p.1402·2); dexpanthenol (p.1602·3).
Inflammation; musculoskeletal, joint, peri-articular, and soft-tissue disorders; pain; peripheral vascular disorders.

Roll-On *Shaklee, Canad.*
Aluminium chlorohydrate (p.1110·4).
Hyperhidrosis.

Roloken *Kendrick, Mex.*
Biperiden (p.464·2).

Romadin *Grunenthal, Spain.*
Astemizole (p.409·1).
Hypersensitivity reactions.

Romarene *Beaufour, Fr.*
Rosemary; taraxacum (p.1669·1); kinkeliba (p.1626·1); sodium potassium tartrate (p.1250·1); sodium citrate (p.1186·2).
Gastrointestinal disorders.

Romarinex *Aerocid, Fr.*
Rosemary; kinkeliba (p.1626·1).
Biliary-tract disorders.

Romarinex-Choline *Aerocid, Fr.†*
Rosemary; cynara (p.1601·3); boldo (p.1585·3); taraxacum (p.1669·1); kinkeliba (p.1626·1); choline citrate (p.1356·3).
Gastrointestinal disorders.

Romazicon *Roche, USA.*
Flumazenil (p.1008·3).
Formerly known as Mazicon.
Benzodiazepine overdosage; reversal of benzodiazepine-induced sedation.

Rombay *Apotheke Heiligen Dreifaltigkeit, Aust.*
Talc (p.1124·2); zinc oxide (p.1128·2); peru balsam (p.1650·2).
Skin irritation.

Rombellin *Simons, Ger.; Adroka, Switz.*
Biotin (p.1355·3).
Biotin deficiency.

Rombox *Glaxo Wellcome, Mex.*
Cefalexin (p.161·3); ambroxol hydrochloride (p.1084·3).
Respiratory-tract infections.

Romesa *Rhone-Poulenc Rorer, Mex.*
Warfarin sodium (p.992·2).

Romet *Mitsubishi, Jpn.*
Repirinast (p.770·2).
Asthma.

Romigal *Romigal, Ger.*
Aspirin (p.14·2).
Fever; inflammation; musculoskeletal, joint, and soft-tissue disorders; pain; thromboembolic disorders.

Romilar
Note. This name is used for preparations of different composition.
Roche, Ital.†
Dextromethorphan hydrobromide (p.1087·3); ammonium chloride (p.1085·2).
Coughs.

Roche, Mex.; Roche, Spain.
Dextromethorphan hydrobromide (p.1087·3).
Coughs.

Roche, Thai.
Dextromethorphan hydrobromide (p.1087·3); ammonium chloride (p.1085·2); dexpanthenol (p.1602·3).
Coughs.

Romilar AC *Scot-Tussin, USA.*
Codeine phosphate (p.25·2); guaifenesin (p.1092·2).
Coughs.

Romilar Antitussivum *Roche, Belg.*
Dextromethorphan hydrobromide (p.1087·3).
Coughs.

Romilar Mucolyticum *Roche, Belg.*
Carbocisteine (p.1086·3).
Respiratory-tract disorders associated with accumulation of mucus.

Romin *Rolab, S.Afr.*
Minocycline hydrochloride (p.224·3).
Now known as Rolab-Minocycline.
Acne; bacterial infections.

Romir *Diba, Mex.*
Captopril (p.853·3).
Heart failure; hypertension; myocardial infarction.

Rommix *Ashbourne, UK.*
Erythromycin (p.201·2).

Romozin *Glaxo Wellcome, UK†.*
Troglitazone (p.337·1).
Diabetes mellitus.

Romulin *Chew, Thai.*
Bromhexine hydrochloride (p.1085·3).
Respiratory-tract disorders associated with increased or viscous mucus.

Ronabin *Unimed, Israel.*
Dronabinol (p.1224·3).
Nausea and vomiting induced by cytotoxic therapy.

Ronal
Note. This name is used for preparations of different composition.
Rhodia, Braz.
Aspirin (p.14·2).
Fever; inflammation; pain; thromboembolism prophylaxis.

Durascan, Denm.
Flunitrazepam (p.683·2).
Insomnia.

Roname *Lacer, Spain.*
Glimepiride (p.322·3).
Diabetes mellitus.

RO-Naphz *Richmond Ophthalmics, Canad.†*
Naphazoline hydrochloride (p.1095·1).
Eye congestion.

Rondamine-DM *Major, USA.*
Pseudoephedrine hydrochloride (p.1099·2); dextromethorphan hydrobromide (p.1087·3); carbinoxamine maleate (p.411·1).
Coughs and cold symptoms.

Rondec
Note. This name is used for preparations of different composition.
Abbott, Ital.; Abbott, Spain†.
Carbinoxamine maleate (p.411·1); pseudoephedrine hydrochloride (p.1099·2).
Allergic and vasomotor rhinitis; nasal congestion.

Biovail, USA.
Oral drops: Carbinoxamine maleate (p.411·1); pseudoephedrine hydrochloride (p.1099·2).
Allergic and vasomotor rhinitis; nasal congestion.
Syrup: Brompheniramine maleate (p.410·2); pseudoephedrine hydrochloride (p.1099·2).
Upper respiratory-tract disorders.

Rondec-DM *Abbott, Thai.; Dura, USA.*
Carbinoxamine maleate (p.411·1); pseudoephedrine hydrochloride (p.1099·2); dextromethorphan hydrobromide (p.1087·3).
Coughs and cold symptoms; respiratory symptoms of allergy.

Rondimen *Asta Medica, Ger.*
Mefenorex hydrochloride (p.1511·1).
Obesity.

Rondomycin
Parke, Davis, Austral.†; Roerig, Swed.†.
Methacycline hydrochloride (p.222·3).
Bacterial infections.

Ronicol *Tillomed, UK†.*
Nicotinyl alcohol tartrate (p.939·3).
Peripheral vascular disorders.

Ronmix *Ashbourne, UK†.*
Erythromycin (p.201·2).

Ronpirin APCQ *Mitchell, UK.*
Paracetamol (p.71·2); aspirin (p.14·2); caffeine (p.761·3); quinine hydrochloride (p.445·1).

Ronpirin Cold Remedy *Mitchell, UK.*
Promethazine hydrochloride (p.423·2); dextromethorphan hydrochloride; paracetamol (p.71·2).
Cold symptoms.

Rontilona *Alter, Spain.*
Fluticasone propionate (p.1072·2).
Nasal polyps; rhinitis.

Ronvan *Asta Medica, Braz.*
Fosfestrol sodium (p.1478·3).
Breast cancer; prostatic cancer.

Ropect *Scherer, Thai.*
Codeine phosphate (p.25·2); guaifenesin (p.1092·2); phenylpropanolamine hydrochloride (p.1098·1).
Cold symptoms; coughs; nasal congestion.

Rophelin *Rolmex, Canad.*
Ammonium chloride (p.1085·2); tolu balsam (p.1101·3); white pine compound; wild cherry bark (p.1680·3).

R.O.R. *Pasteur Merieux, Fr.*
A measles, mumps, and rubella vaccine (Edmonston 749D, Jeryl Lynn, and Wistar RA 27/3 strains respectively) (p.1549·1).
Active immunisation.

Rosalgin
Lepori, Port.; Farma Lepori, Spain.
Benzydamine hydrochloride (p.20·1).
Cervicitis; vulvovaginitis.

Rosalox *Drossapharm, Switz.*
Metronidazole (p.594·1).
Rosacea.

Rosarthron *Steierl, Ger.*
Rosemary oil (p.1659·3); pumilio pine oil (p.1656·3).
Circulatory disorders; gout; musculoskeletal and joint disorders; neuritis; respiratory-tract disorders.

Rosarthron forte *Steierl, Ger.*
Rosemary oil (p.1659·3); methyl salicylate (p.55·1); benzyl nicotinate (p.20·2).
Circulatory disorders; gout; musculoskeletal and joint disorders; neuritis; respiratory-tract disorders.

Rosased *Pierre Fabre, Ital.*
Metronidazole (p.594·1).
Rosacea.

Roseliane Creme *Saninter, Port.*
Moisturiser.

Roseliane Lait *Saninter, Port.*
Soap substitute.

Rosets *Akorn, USA.*
Rose bengal sodium (p.1659·2).
Ophthalmic diagnostic agent.

Rosiced *Pierre Fabre, Fr.*
Metronidazole (p.594·1).
Formerly known as Rosaced.
Rosacea.

Rosiden *Shin Poong, Singapore.*
Piroxicam (p.79·1).
Gout; inflammation; musculoskeletal, joint, and peri-articular disorders; pain.

Rosig *Sigma, Austral.*
Piroxicam (p.79·1).
Ankylosing spondylitis; osteoarthritis; rheumatoid arthritis.

Rosilan *Aventis, Port.*
Deflazacort (p.1066·1).
Corticosteroid.

Rosils *Boots Healthcare, Belg.*
Noscapine (p.1096·3); phenylephrine hydrochloride (p.1097·1).
Coughs; upper respiratory-tract congestion.

Rosken Silk *Warner-Lambert, Austral.†.*
Octinoxate (p.1517·3); oxybenzone (p.1518·1); avobenzone (p.1517·1).
Emollient; sunscreen.

Rosken Skin Repair
Note. This name is used for preparations of different composition.
Warner-Lambert, Austral.
Dimethicone (p.1410·1).
Dermatitis; dry skin.

Warner-Lambert, NZ.
Diemthicone (p.1410·1); glycerol (p.1616·3).
Barrier cream; bedsores; dry skin.

Rosken Solar Block *Mentholatum, Austral.†.*
Lotion: Octinoxate (p.1517·3); avobenzone (p.1517·1); octil triazone; titanium dioxide (p.1126·1).
Sportstick: Octinoxate (p.1517·3); enzacamene (p.1517·2); avobenzone (p.1517·1).
Sunstick: Padimate O (p.1518·2); oxybenzone (p.1518·1); avobenzone (p.1517·1).
Sunscreen.

Rosken Solar Block Concentrated *Mentholatum, Austral.†.*
Padimate O (p.1518·2); enzacamene (p.1517·2); avobenzone (p.1517·1).
Sunscreen.

Rosken Solar Block Toddler *Mentholatum, Austral.†.*
Octinoxate (p.1517·3); avobenzone (p.1517·1); octil triazone; titanium dioxide (p.1126·1).
Sunscreen.

Rosol-Gamma *Biagini, Ital.*
A rubella immunoglobulin (p.1562·2).
Passive immunisation.

Rosone *Riva, Canad.†.*
Betamethasone dipropionate (p.1063·2).
Skin disorders.

Rosovax *Nuovo ISM, Ital.*
A rubella vaccine (Wistar RA 27/3 strain) (p.1562·3).
Active immunisation.

Rossepar *KBR, Ital.*
Ferric sodium gluconate (p.1360·2).
Iron deficiency; iron-deficiency anaemias.

Rossitrol *Hoechst Marion Roussel, Ital.*
Roxithromycin (p.247·2).
Bacterial infections.

Rossofolin *Errekappa, Ital.*
Multivitamin and mineral preparation (p.1350·1).

Ro-Strumal NEU (Rowo-221) *Pharmakon, Ger.*
Spongia tosta; ovi putamen tosta; magnesium hydrogen phosphate; anhydrous sodium phosphate; terra silicea purificata.
Hyperthyroidism.

RotaShield *Wyeth-Ayerst, USA†.*
A rotavirus vaccine (p.1562·2).
Active immunisation.

Roter
Four Macs, Austral.†; Boots Healthcare, Neth.†; Roter, Thai.
Bismuth subnitrate (p.1232·3); magnesium carbonate (p.1232·3); sodium bicarbonate (p.1186·2); frangula bark (p.1227·1).
Dyspepsia; gastric hyperacidity; gastritis; gastrointestinal spasm; heartburn; peptic ulcer.

Boots, S.Afr.‡.
Bismuth subcarbonate (p.1213·1); magnesium carbonate (p.1232·3); sodium bicarbonate (p.1186·2); frangula bark (p.1227·1).
Dyspepsia; peptic ulcer.

Roter APC *Boots Healthcare, Neth.†.*
Aspirin (p.14·2); paracetamol (p.71·2); caffeine (p.761·3).
Fever; pain.

Roter Complex *Farma Lepori, Spain†.*
Bismuth subnitrate (p.1213·2); magnesium carbonate (p.1232·3); sodium bicarbonate (p.1186·2); frangula bark (p.1227·1); calamus root (p.1588·1); sulpiride (p.706·1).
Duodenitis; gastritis; hyperchlorhydria; peptic ulcer.

Roter Keel *Boots Healthcare, Neth.†.*
Chlorhexidine hydrochloride (p.1138·2).
Sore throats.

Roter Noscapect *Boots Healthcare, Neth.†.*
Noscapine hydrochloride (p.1096·1).
Coughs.

Roter Paracof *Boots Healthcare, Neth.†.*
Paracetamol (p.71·2); caffeine (p.761·3).
Fever; pain.

Rotersept *Roterpharma, Irl.†.*
Chlorhexidine gluconate (p.1138·2).
Cracked nipples; mastitis.

Rotesan *Knoll, Spain.*
Roxithromycin (p.247·2).
Bacterial infections.

Rotet *Rolab, S.Afr.†.*
Tetracycline hydrochloride (p.258·3).
Bacterial infections.

Rothacin *Julphar, UAE.*
Indometacin (p.44·3).
Dysmenorrhoea; musculoskeletal, joint, and peri-articular disorders.

Rothricin *Siam Bheasach, Thai.*
Roxithromycin (p.247·2).
Bacterial infections.

Roth's RKT Tropfen *Infirmarius-Rovit, Ger.*
Homoeopathic preparation.

Roth's Ropulmin N *Infirmarius-Rovit, Ger.*
Homoeopathic preparation.

Roth's Rotacard *Infirmarius-Rovit, Ger.*
Homoeopathic preparation.

Rotilen *Terapeutico, Ital.*
Methacycline hydrochloride (p.222·3).
Bacterial infections.

Rotol *Jukunda, Ger.†.*
Hypericum (p.290·2).
Joint pain; nervous disorders; wounds.

Rotram *Schering-Plough, Braz.*
Roxithromycin (p.247·2).
Bacterial infections.

Rotramin *Medeva, Spain.*
Roxithromycin (p.247·2).
Bacterial infections.

Rotuss *Scherer, Thai.*
Codeine phosphate (p.25·2); guaifenesin (p.1092·2); phenylpropanolamine (p.1098·1).
Coughs; nasal congestion.

Roubac *Rougier, Canad.†.*
Co-trimoxazole (p.193·3).
Bacterial infections.

Rouhex-G *Rougier, Canad.*
Chlorhexidine gluconate (p.1138·2).
Acne; skin disinfection; surface and instrument disinfection.

Rounox *Rougier, Canad.*
Paracetamol (p.71·2).
Fever; pain.

Rouphylline
Rougier, Canad.; Rougier, Hong Kong.
Choline theophyllinate (p.763·3).
Obstructive airways disease.

Rouvax
Pasteur Merieux, Braz.; Pasteur Merieux, Fr.; Pasteur Merieux, Hong Kong; Pasteur Merieux, Israel; Pasteur Merieux, Ital.; Aventis, S.Afr.; Pasteur Merieux, Thai.
A measles vaccine (Schwarz strain) (p.1547·1).
Active immunisation.

Rovacor *Ranbaxy, Singapore.*
Lovastatin (p.922·3).
Hypercholesterolaemia.

Rovamicina *Rhodia, Braz.; Rhone-Poulenc Rorer, Ital.*
Spiramycin (p.248·3).
Bacterial infections.

Rovamycin
Gerot, Aust.; Aventis, Denm.; Rhone-Poulenc Rorer, Norw.; Rhone-Poulenc Rorer, Swed.†; Rhone-Poulenc Rorer, Thai.
Spiramycin (p.248·3).
Bacterial infections; toxoplasmosis.

Rovamycine
Aventis, Belg.; Rhone-Poulenc Rorer, Canad.; Rhone-Poulenc Rorer, Fr.; Rhone-Poulenc Rorer, Ger.; Rhone-Poulenc Rorer, Hong Kong; Rhone-Poulenc Rorer, Israel; Rhone-Poulenc Rorer, Neth.; Aventis, Port.; Rhone-Poulenc Rorer, Singapore; Rhone-Poulenc Rorer, Spain; Rhone-Poulenc Rorer, Switz.
Spiramycin (p.248·3) or spiramycin adipate (p.249·1).
Bacterial infections; cryptosporidiosis; prevention of flares of rheumatoid arthritis; toxoplasmosis.

Rovigon
Roche, Aust.; Roche, Belg.; Roche Nicholas, Fr.; Roche, Ital.; Roche, Port.; Roche, Switz.; Roche, Thai.
Vitamin A (p.1382·1) or vitamin A palmitate (p.1383·2); dl-alpha tocoferil acetate (p.1394·1).
Brittle hair and nails; deafness; menopausal disorders; mental and cardiovascular disorders in the elderly; male infertility; retinopathy; tinnitus.

Rovigon G *Roche Nicholas, Ger.*
Vitamin A palmitate (p.1383·2); alpha tocoferil acetate (p.1394·1).
Vitamin A and E deficiency.

Rowachol
Note. This name is used for preparations of different composition.
Rosch & Handel, Aust.; Rowa, Ger.; Rowa, Irl.
Menthol (p.1632·3); menthone; α-pinene; β-pinene; borneol; camphene; eucalyptol (p.1609·2).
Biliary tract disorders; liver disorders.

Rowa, Hong Kong; Rowa, Israel; Rowa, Thai.; Rowa, UK.
Menthol (p.1632·3); menthone; pinene; borneol; camphene; eucalyptol (p.1609·2).
Biliary tract disorders; liver disorders.

Diviser Aquilea, Spain.
Menthol (p.1632·3); pinenes; borneol; camphene; eucalyptol (p.1609·2); emodin; oxidised terpenes.
Anorexia; hepatobiliary disorders.

Rowachol comp *Rowa, Ger.*
Menthol (p.1632·3); menthone; α-pinene; β-pinene; borneol; camphene; eucalyptol (p.1609·2); deanol benzilate hydrochloride (p.1507·2).
Biliary-tract disorders.

Rowachol-Digestiv *Rowa, Ger.*
Menthol (p.1632·3); menthone; α-pinene; β-pinene; borneol; camphene; eucalyptol (p.1609·2).
Digestive system disorders; hepatobiliary disorders.

Rowaclimax *Rowa, Ger.*
Agnus castus; alchemilla; aletris farinosa; capsella bursa pastoris; chamomile; valerian.
Gynaecological disorders.

Rowadermat *Rosch & Handel, Aust.*
Carbenoxolone disodium (p.1215·3).
Aphthous ulcers; herpes labialis.

Rowalind
Rosch & Handel, Aust.; Rowa, Ger.†; Rowa, Irl.
Nicotinaldehyde; ammonium chloride (p.1085·2); ammonia solution (p.1579·1); camphor (p.1589·3); menthol (p.1632·3); rosemary oil (p.1659·3); lavender oil (p.1627·2).
Musculoskeletal, joint, and soft-tissue disorders; neuralgia; neuritis.

Rowanefrin *Diviser Aquilea, Spain.*
Anethole (p.1580·1); borneol; camphene; rubia tinctorum; oxidised terpenes; pinenes; fenchone; eucalyptol (p.1609·2).
Renal calculi; urinary-tract disorders.

Rowapraxin
Rowa, Ger.; Rowa, Hong Kong; Rowa, Irl.
Pipoxolan (p.1651·3) or pipoxolan hydrochloride (p.1651·3).
Smooth muscle spasm.

Rowarolan
Note. This name is used for preparations of different composition.
Rowa, Ger.†
Calcium carbonate (p.1215·1); colloidal silicon dioxide (p.1503·3).
Ulcers.

Rowa, Irl.
Calcium carbonate (p.1215·1).
Adsorbent in ulcers and sores.

Rowasa
Solvay, Fr.; Solvay, USA.
Mesalazine (p.1234·1).
Inflammatory bowel disease.

Rowatanal
Note. This name is used for preparations of different composition.
Rowa, Hong Kong; Rowa, Singapore.
Bismuth subgallate (p.1213·2); menthol (p.1632·3); zinc oxide (p.1128·2); calcium carbonate (p.1215·1).
Anorectal disorders.

Rowa, Irl.
Bismuth subgallate (p.1213·2); menthol (p.1632·3); zinc oxide (p.1128·2).
Anal irritation; haemorrhoids.

Rowatinex
Rosch & Handel, Aust.; Rowa, Ger.; Rowa, Irl.
α-Pinene; β-pinene; camphene; borneol; anethole (p.1580·1); fenchone; eucalyptol (p.1609·2).
Urinary-tract disorders.

Rowa, Hong Kong; Rowa, Israel; Rowa, Thai.; Monmouth, UK.
Pinene; camphene; borneol; anethole (p.1580·1); fenchone; eucalyptol (p.1609·2).
Urinary-tract disorders.

Rowo-52 *Pharmakon, Ger.†*
Homoeopathic preparation.
Lignocaine [lidocaine] hydrochloride (p.1313·2) is included in this preparation to alleviate the pain of injection.

Rowo-216 *Pharmakon, Ger.†*
Homoeopathic preparation.
Lignocaine [lidocaine] hydrochloride (p.1313·2) is included in this preparation to alleviate the pain of injection.

Rowo-298 *Pharmakon, Ger.*
Homoeopathic preparation.
Lignocaine [lidocaine] hydrochloride (p.1313·2) is included in this preparation to alleviate the pain of injection.

Rowo-629 *Pharmakon, Ger.*
Lignocaine [lidocaine] hydrochloride (p.1313·2).
Local anaesthesia.

Rowo-849 Echinacea Ro-Plex (Rowo-849)
Pharmakon, Ger.
Homoeopathic preparation.

Rowo Rytesthin Ro-Plex (Rowo-318) *Pharmakon, Ger.*
Homoeopathic preparation.

Rowo-778 Symphytum Ro-Plex T (Rowo-778) *Pharmakon, Ger.*
Homoeopathic preparation.

Rowo-Rytesthin (Rowo-576) *Pharmakon, Ger.†*
Homoeopathic preparation.

Rowo-Sedaphin 138 (Rowo-138) *Pharmakon, Ger.*
Homoeopathic preparation.

Roxalia *Boiron, Canad.*
Homoeopathic preparation.

Roxane
Hoechst Marion Roussel, Aust.; Hoechst Marion Roussel, Singapore.
Roxatidine acetate hydrochloride (p.1248·1).
Gastro-oesophageal reflux; peptic ulcer.

Roxanol *Roxane, USA.*
Morphine sulfate (p.56·1).
Pain.

Roxazin *Basi, Port.*
Piroxicam (p.79·1).

Roxcin *Biolab, Thai.*
Roxithromycin (p.247·2).
Bacterial infections.

Roxen *Hua, Thai.*
Naproxen (p.60·3).
Gout; musculoskeletal and joint disorders.

Roxene *Benedetti, Ital.*
Piroxicam (p.79·1).
Musculoskeletal, joint, peri-articular, and soft-tissue disorders.

Roxenil *Caber, Ital.*
Piroxicam (p.79·1).
Musculoskeletal, joint, and peri-articulr disorders.

Roxiam *Astra, Aust.†.*
Remoxipride hydrochloride (p.703·3).
Psychoses.

Roxibion *Leiras, Fin.*
Roxithromycin (p.247·2).
Bacterial infections.

Roxicam *Rolab, S.Afr.*
Piroxicam (p.79·1).
Inflammation; musculoskeletal and joint disorders; pain.

Roxicet
Boehringer Ingelheim, Canad.†; Roxane, USA.
Oxycodone hydrochloride (p.70·2); paracetamol (p.71·2).
Pain.

Roxicin *Atlantic, Thai.*
Roxithromycin (p.247·2).
Bacterial infections.

Roxicodone *Roxane, USA.*
Oxycodone hydrochloride (p.70·2).
Pain.

Roxiden *Pulitzer, Ital.*
Piroxicam (p.79·1).
Musculoskeletal, joint, and peri-articular disorders.

Roxifen *TO-Chemicals, Thai.*
Piroxicam (p.79·1).
Musculoskeletal, joint, and peri-articular disorders.

Roxilan *Olan-Kemed, Thai.*
Roxithromycin (p.247·2).
Bacterial infections.

Roxillin *Rowex, Irl.†.*
Amoxicillin trihydrate (p.149·2).
Bacterial infections.

Roxilox *Roxane, USA.*
Oxycodone hydrochloride (p.70·2); paracetamol (p.71·2).
Pain.

Roximin *Pharmaland, Thai.*
Roxithromycin (p.247·2).
Bacterial infections.

Roxine *Duopharma, Hong Kong.*
Dequalinium chloride (p.1143·1).
Mouth and throat disorders.

Roxiprin *Roxane, USA.*
Oxycodone hydrochloride (p.70·2); oxycodone terephthalate (p.70·3); aspirin (p.14·2).
Pain.

Roxit
Hoechst Marion Roussel, Ger.; Hoechst Marion Roussel, Ital.; Knoll, Neth.; Hoechst Marion Roussel, S.Afr.†.
Roxatidine acetate hydrochloride (p.1248·1).
Gastro-oesophageal reflux; peptic ulcer.

Roxitin *TP, Thai.*
Roxithromycin (p.247·2).
Bacterial infections.

Roxitrol *Ofimex, Mex.*
Roxithromycin (p.247·2).

Roxiwas *Wasserman, Spain.*
Roxatidine acetate (p.1248·2).
Gastro-oesophageal reflux; peptic ulcer.

Roxlecon *Pond's, Thai.*
Roxithromycin (p.247·2).
Bacterial infections.

Roxomycin *Silom, Thai.*
Roxithromycin (p.247·2).
Bacterial infections.

Roxthomed *Progress, Thai.*
Roxithromycin (p.247·2).
Bacterial infections.

Roxthrin *TO-Chemicals, Thai.*
Roxithromycin (p.247·2).
Bacterial infections.

Roxto *M & H, Thai.*
Roxithromycin (p.247·2).
Bacterial infections.

Roxtrocin *Greater Pharma, Thai.*
Roxithromycin (p.247·2).
Bacterial infections.

Roxy *Mer-National, S.Afr.*
Oxytetracycline hydrochloride (p.234·1).
Bacterial infections.

Roxycam *Greater Pharma, Thai.*
Piroxicam (p.79·1).
Gout; musculoskeletal and joint disorders.

Royal E *Cielle, Ital.*
Royal jelly (p.1659·3); vitamin E (p.1393·3).
Nutritional supplement.

Royal Galanol *Lifeplan, UK.*
Evening primrose oil (p.1613·3); royal jelly (p.1659·3).
Nutritional supplement.

Royal Life *Bioceuticals, UK.*
Multivitamin, mineral, and amino-acid preparation (p.1350·1).

Royalin *TO-Chemicals, Thai.*
Salbutamol sulfate (p.770·3); guaifenesin (p.1092·2).
Coughs; obstructive airways disease.

Roychlor *Waymar, Canad.*
Potassium chloride (p.1194·3).
Potassium deficiency.

Royen *Rubio, Spain.*
Calcium acetate (p.1187·3).
Hyperphosphataemia.

Royflex *Waymar, Canad.*
Trolamine salicylate (p.90·1).
Musculoskeletal and joint disorders.

Royl 6 *Covan, S.Afr.*
Vitamin B substances with vitamin C (p.1350·1).

Roytrin *Royton, Braz.*
Co-trimoxazole (p.193·3).
Bacterial infections; Pneumocystis carinii pneumonia; protozoal infections.

Royvac Kit *Waymar, Canad.*
Oral solution, magnesium citrate (p.1232·3); 3 tablets, bisacodyl (p.1212·2); 1 suppository, bisacodyl.
Bowel evacuation.

Rozacreme *Biorga, Fr.*
Metronidazole (p.594·1).
Rosacea.

Rozagel *Biorga, Fr.*
Metronidazole (p.594·1).
Rosacea.

Rozex
Galderma, Austral.; Galderma, Belg.; Galderma, Braz.; Galderma, Fr.; Galderma, Hong Kong; Galderma, Irl.; Galderma, Israel; Galderma, Ital.; Galderma, Neth.; Galderma, NZ; Galderma, S.Afr.; Galderma, Singapore; Galderma, Spain; Galderma, Swed.; Galderma, Switz.; Galderma, UK.
Metronidazole (p.594·1).
Rosacea.

Rozicel *Upsamedica, Ital.*
Cefprozil (p.173·2).
Bacterial infections.

Rozide *Rolab, S.Afr.*
Pyrazinamide (p.240·1).
Now known as Rolab-Pyrazinamide.
Tuberculosis.

RP-Pose *Pose, Thai.*
Rifampicin (p.243·2).
Bacterial infections including tuberculosis, leprosy, and gonorrhoea.

R/S Lotion *Summers, USA†.*
Sulfur (p.1123·3); resorcinol (p.1122·2).
Acne.

R-Tanna *Duramed, USA.*
Phenylephrine tannate (p.1097·3); mepyramine tannate (p.421·1).
Upper respiratory-tract disorders.

R-Tannamine *Qualitest, USA.*
Phenylephrine tannate (p.1097·3); chlorpheniramine [chlorphenamine] tannate (p.412·2); mepyramine tannate (p.421·1).
Upper respiratory-tract symptoms.

R-Tannate *Warner Chilcott, USA; Copley, USA; Schein, USA.*
Phenylephrine tannate (p.1097·3); chlorpheniramine [chlorphenamine] tannate (p.412·2); mepyramine tannate (p.421·1).
Allergic rhinitis; nasal congestion.

R-Tannic-S *Cypress, USA.*
Phenylephrine tannate (p.1097·3); mepyramine tannate (p.421·1).
Allergic rhinitis; cold symptoms; sinusitis.

Rubacina *Rubio, Spain.*
Famotidine (p.1225·3).
Gastro-oesophageal reflux; peptic ulcer; Zollinger-Ellison syndrome.

Rubeaten
Kwizda, Aust.; Berna, Hong Kong†; Berna, Ital.†; Berna, Port.; Byk Madaus, S.Afr.; Berna, Singapore; Berna, Spain; Berna, Switz.; Berna, Thai.
A rubella vaccine (attenuated Wistar RA 27/3 strain) (p.1562·3).
Active immunisation.

Rubegam *NBI, S.Afr.†.*
A rubella immunoglobulin (p.1562·2).
Passive immunisation.

Rubellovac *Chiron Behring, Ger.*
A rubella vaccine (Wistar RA 27/3 strain) (p.1562·3).
Active immunisation.

Rubesal
Hamilton, Austral.; Hamilton, Hong Kong.
Diethylamine salicylate (p.32·2); camphor (p.1589·3); menthol (p.1632·3).
Muscular pain.

Rubeuman
Berna, Ital.†; Berna, Switz.†.
A rubella immunoglobulin (p.1562·2).
Passive immunisation.

Rubex
Note. This name is used for preparations of different composition.
Bristol-Myers Squibb, Braz.; Bristol-Myers Squibb Oncology, USA.
Doxorubicin hydrochloride (p.534·3).
Malignant neoplasms.

Rice Steele, Irl.
Ascorbic acid (p.1389·3).
Vitamin C deficiency.

Rubia Paver *Medical, Spain.*
Atropine sulfate (p.461·1); papaverine hydrochloride (p.1648·1); rubia tinctorum.
Renal calculi.

Rubicalm *Julphar, UAE.*
Diethylamine salicylate (p.32·2); menthol (p.1632·3).
Musculoskeletal pain.

Rubicolan F *Syxyl, Ger.*
Homoeopathic preparation.

Rubi-Dex *Cazi, Braz.*
Methacholine chloride (p.1419·3); menthol (p.1632·3); methyl salicylate (p.55·1).
Musculoskeletal and joint disorders.

Rubidiosin Composto *SIT, Ital.*
Rubidium iodide (p.1660·1); potassium iodide (p.1522·3); testosterone hemisuccinate (p.1493·3); lignocaine [lidocaine] (p.1313·2); heparin sodium (p.902·1).
Cataracts.

RubieDorm *Rubiepharm, Ger.*
Valerian oil.
Agitation; sleep disorders.

RubieFol *Rubiepharm, Ger.*
Folic acid (p.1361·1).
Folic acid deficiency.

RubieMag + E *Rubiepharm, Ger.*
d-Alpha-Tocoferil acetate (p.1394·1); magnesium oxide (p.1233·2).
Vitamin E and magnesium deficiency.

RubieMen *Rubiepharm, Ger.*
Dimenhydrinate (p.415·2).
Motion sickness; nausea and vomiting; vertigo.

RubieMol *Rubiepharm, Ger.*
Paracetamol (p.71·2).
Fever; pain.

RubieNex mono *Rubiepharm, Ger.*
Ergotamine tartrate (p.452·1).
Headache; migraine.

RubieNex spezial *Rubiepharm, Ger.*
Ergotamine tartrate (p.452·1); propyphenazone (p.80·2).
Headache; migraine.

RubieSed *Rubiepharm, Ger.*
Valerian (p.1678·3); melissa (p.1632·2); passion flower (p.1649·1).
Agitation; sleep disorders.

Rubifen
Rubio, Singapore; Rubio, Spain.
Methylphenidate hydrochloride (p.1511·3).
Attention deficit hyperactivity disorder; depression; narcoleptic syndrome.

Rubifort *Kinder, Braz.*
Vitamin A; vitamin B₁₂; ergocalciferol; intrinsic factor (p.1350·1).
Anaemias.

Rubilax *Pharmachoice, S.Afr.*
Charcoal (p.1000·2); rhubarb (p.1248·1); senna (p.1248·2).
Constipation.

Rubilem *Lemery, Mex.*
Daunorubicin hydrochloride (p.533·1).
Malignant neoplasms.

Rubilin *Medeva, UK.*
A rubella vaccine (live attenuated Wistar RA 27/3) (p.1562·3).
Active immunisation.

Rubimycin *Pharmador, S.Afr.†.*
Erythromycin stearate (p.201·3).
Bacterial infections.

Rubio N *Worwag, Ger.*
Urea (p.1127·3).
Dry skin disorders.

Rubion *Desbergers, Canad.*
Cyanocobalamin (p.1388·1).
Anaemias.

Rubisan
DHU, Ger.; Omida, Switz.
Homoeopathic preparation.

Rubistenol *Fermenti, Ital.†.*
Rubidium iodide (p.1660·1); sodium iodide (p.1522·3); potassium iodide (p.1522·3); sodium formate (p.1612·3); strychnine glycerophosphate.
Eye disorders.

Rubiulcer *Rubio, Spain.*
Ranitidine hydrochloride (p.1245·2).
Acid aspiration; gastro-oesophageal reflux; gastrointestinal haemorrhage; peptic ulcer; short-bowel syndrome; Zollinger-Ellison syndrome.

Rubizon-Rheumagel *Makara, Aust.*
Glycol salicylate (p.42·2); camphor (p.1589·3); benzyl nicotinate (p.20·2); capsaicin (p.23·1).
Chillblains; musculoskeletal and joint disorders; neuralgia.

Rubjovit *SIFI, Ital.*
Rubidium iodide (p.1660·1); sodium iodide (p.1522·3); calcium formate (p.1612·3); sodium ascorbate (p.1390·1); thiamine hydrochloride (p.1385·1).
Cataracts.

Rublex D *Don, Israel.*
Menthol (p.1632·3); camphor (p.1589·3); methyl salicylate (p.55·1); salicylic acid (p.1122·3).
Musculoskeletal and joint disorders.

Rublex Massage Cream *Don, Israel.*
Menthol (p.1632·3); camphor (p.1589·3); methyl salicylate (p.55·1); capsicum oleoresin (p.1591·1).
Musculoskeletal and joint disorders.

Ruboderm *Labcatal, Fr.*
Zinc gluconate (p.1398·2); copper gluconate (p.1357·3).
Skin and hair disorders.

Ruboril *Darier, Mex.*
Barrier cream.

The symbol † denotes a preparation no longer actively marketed

Rubozinc *Labcatal, Fr.*
Zinc gluconate (p.1398·2).
Acne; acrodermatitis enteropathica.

Rubracobal *Medquimica, Braz.*
Vitamin B substances with amino acids and gastric mucosa extract (p.1350·1).

Rubragel *Adcock Ingram, S.Afr.†.*
Dried aluminium hydroxide gel (p.1210·3); magnesium oxide (p.1233·2); simeticone (p.1249·2).
Gastrointestinal hyperacidity with flatulence.

Rubralong *Dovalle, Braz.*
Ferrous fumarate (p.1360·1); vitamin B substances (p.1350·1).
Vitamin C (p.1389·3) is included in this preparation to increase the absorption and availability of iron.
Iron deficiency; iron-deficiency anaemias.

Rubramin *Squibb, Canad.*
Vitamin B₁₂ (p.1388·1).
Schilling test; vitamin B₁₂ deficiency.

Rubramin PC *Apothecon, USA†.*
Cyanocobalamin (p.1388·1).
Vitamin B₁₂ deficiency.

Rubranova *Bristol-Myers Squibb, Braz.*
Hydroxocobalamin (p.1388·1).
Megaloblastic anaemia; vitamin B₁₂ deficiency.

Rubrargil *IQB, Braz.*
Ferrous sulfate (p.1360·3); vitamin B₁; vitamin B₁₂; copper sulfate (p.1350·1).
Vitamin C (p.1389·3) is included in this preparation to increase the absorption and availability of iron.
Iron deficiency; iron-deficiency anaemias.

Rubratope *Squibb Diagnostics, USA†.*
Cobalt-58 (p.1449·2) as cyanocobalamin.

Rubriment
Note.This name is used for preparations of different composition.
Ebewe, Aust.
Benzyl nicotinate (p.20·2); nonivamide (p.63·1); glycol salicylate (p.42·2); salicylamide (p.82·1); camphor (p.1589·3); turpentine oil (p.1676·3).
Frostbite; joint, muscle, and nerve disorders; peripheral vascular disorders; sport massage.

Riemser, Ger.
Bath additive: Benzyl nicotinate (p.20·2).
Bath additive; peripheral vascular disorders; rheumatism.

Ointment: Benzyl nicotinate (p.20·2); nonivamide (p.63·1).
Inflammation; peripheral vascular disorders; rheumatism.

Rubriment-N *Riemser, Ger.*
Benzyl nicotinate (p.20·2); glycol salicylate (p.42·2); camphor (p.1589·3).
Frostbite; peripheral vascular disorders; rheumatism.

Rubrina *Solfran, Mex.*
Hydroxocobalamin (p.1388·1).

Rubrobion *Sintofarma, Braz.*
Ferric ammonium citrate (p.1359·2); vitamin B substances; inositol; liver extract (p.1350·1).
Iron deficiency; iron-deficiency anaemias.

Rubrocalcium *Caber, Ital.†.*
Calcium levulinate (p.1188·3).
Calcium deficiency.

Rubrociclina *DMG, Ital.*
Demeclocycline hydrochloride (p.198·2); erythromycin (p.201·2) or erythromycin estolate (p.201·2).
Bacterial infections.

Rubrocortin *Farma Lepori, Spain.*
Cyanocobalamin (p.1388·1); suprarenal cortex extract (p.1080·1); liver extract; inosine (p.1623·3).
Anaemias; tonic.

Rubroferrina *NCSN, Ital.*
Ferric sodium gluconate (p.1360·2).
Anaemias.

Rubus Complex *Blackmores, Austral.*
Raspberry leaf (p.1657·2); spirulina (p.1667·1); ascorbic acid; mitchella repens; hesperidin (p.1611·2); rutoside (p.1611·2); d-alpha tocoferil acid succinate; vitamin B substances (p.1350·1); choline bitartrate; inositol.
Obstetric and gynaecological disorders.

Rucaina *Rudefsa, Mex.*
Lignocaine (p.1313·2).

Rucin *General Drugs, Thai.*
Roxithromycin (p.247·2).
Bacterial infections.

RUDD-U *Frankin, Hong Kong.*
Oxyphencyclimine hydrochloride (p.472·1); methiosulfonium chloride (p.1635·1); aluminium hydroxide (p.1210·3); magnesium trisilicate (p.1233·3); simeticone (p.1249·2).
Dyspepsia; flatulence; gastrointestinal hyperacidity; stomach ache.

Rudesol *Pharmacos, Mex.*
Phenylbutazone (p.78·1).
Musculoskeletal and joint disorders.

Rudi-Rouvax
Merieux, Fr.†; Pasteur Merieux, Thai.
A measles and rubella vaccine (Schwarz and Wistar RA 27/3 strains respectively) (p.1549·1).
Active immunisation.

Rudistrol *Boiron, Canad.*
Homoeopathic preparation.

Rudivax
Pasteur Merieux, Braz.; Pasteur Merieux, Fr.; Pasteur Merieux, Hong Kong; Pasteur Merieux, Israel; Pasteur Merieux, Ital.; Aventis, S.Afr.; Pasteur Merieux, Singapore; Pasteur Merieux, Thai.
A live attenuated rubella vaccine (Wistar RA 27/3M strain) (p.1562·3).
Active immunisation.

Rudocaine *Streuli, Switz.*
Articaine hydrochloride (p.1306·1).
Adrenaline [epinephrine] hydrochloride (p.829·2) is included in this preparation as a vasoconstrictor to diminish absorption and localise the effect of the local anaesthetic.
Local anaesthesia.

Rudocycline *Streuli, Switz.*
Doxycycline hyclate (p.200·1).
Bacterial infections.

Rudolac *Streuli, Switz.*
Lactulose (p.1230·1).
Constipation; hepatic encephalopathy.

Rudotel *OPW, Ger.*
Medazepam (p.690·2).
Anxiety disorders.

Ru-Ef-Tb *Rudefsa, Mex.*
Isomicotin hydrazide.

Rufol *Debat, Fr.*
Sulfamethizole (p.253·3).
Bacterial infections of the urinary tract.

Ru-lets *Rugby, USA.*
A range of vitamin preparations (p.1350·1).

Rulicalcin *Hoechst Marion Roussel, Ital.*
Salcatonin (p.749·3).
Hypercalcaemia; osteoporosis; Paget's disease of bone; reflex sympathetic dystrophy.

Rulid
Aventis, Belg.; Hoechst Marion Roussel, Braz.; Roussel Diamant, Fr.; Hoechst Marion Roussel, Ger.; Hoechst Marion Roussel, Hong Kong; Hoechst Marion Roussel, Israel; Hoechst Marion Roussel, Ital.; Hoechst Marion Roussel, Mex.; Hoechst Marion Roussel, Singapore; Hoechst Marion Roussel, Switz.; Hoechst Marion Roussel, Thai.
Roxithromycin (p.247·2).
Bacterial infections.

Rulide
Hoechst Marion Roussel, Aust.; Hoechst Marion Roussel, Austral.; Hoechst Marion Roussel, Neth.; Aventis, NZ; Roussel, Port.; Aventis, S.Afr.; Hoechst Marion Roussel, Spain.
Roxithromycin (p.247·2).
Bacterial infections.

Rulivan *Europharma, Spain.*
Nefazodone hydrochloride (p.300·3).
Depression.

Rulofer G *Lomapharm, Ger.*
Ferrous gluconate (p.1360·1).
Iron deficiency.

Rulofer N *Lomapharm, Ger.*
Ferrous fumarate (p.1360·1).
Iron deficiency.

RuLox *Rugby, USA.*
Aluminium hydroxide (p.1210·3); magnesium hydroxide (p.1233·1).
Hyperacidity.

RuLox Plus *Rugby, USA.*
Aluminium hydroxide (p.1210·3); magnesium hydroxide (p.1233·1); simeticone (p.1249·2).
Hyperacidity.

Rulun *Lacer, Spain.*
Hydrochlorothiazide (p.907·3); rauwolfia (p.967·2); trichlormethiazide (p.987·1); xantinol nicotinate (p.999·1); pentosan polysulfate (p.953·1).
Hypertension.

Rumadene *Chew, Thai.*
Piroxicam (p.79·1).
Gout; musculoskeletal, joint, and peri-articular disorders.

Rumalon
Germania, Aust.†; Asta Medica, Braz.
Cartilage; bone marrow.
Degenerative joint disorders; inflammation.

Rumasian *Asian Pharm, Thai.*
Ibuprofen (p.43·2).
Musculoskeletal and joint disorders.

Rumatab *Pharmaland, Thai.*
Diclofenac sodium (p.30·3).
Gout; inflammation; musculoskeletal and joint disorders.

Rumatifen *Chew, Thai.*
Ibuprofen (p.43·2).
Dysmenorrhoea; gout; musculoskeletal and joint disorders.

Rumatifen-Plus *Chew, Thai.*
Ibuprofen (p.43·2); paracetamol (p.71·2).
Fever; pain.

Rumicine *Schering-Plough, Fr.*
Aspirin (p.14·2); chlorpheniramine [chlorphenamine] maleate (p.412·1); caffeine (p.761·3).
Fever; pain.

Rumitard *Zurich, S.Afr.†.*
Indometacin (p.44·3).
Musculoskeletal and joint disorders.

Rumitex *Beckerath, Ger.*
Homoeopathic preparation.

Rum-K *Fleming, USA.*
Potassium chloride (p.1194·3).
Hypokalaemia.

Rupan
Medochemie, Hong Kong; Medochemie, Thai.
Ibuprofen (p.43·2).
Dysmenorrhoea; musculoskeletal, joint, and soft-tissue disorders.

Rupton *Dexo, Thai.*
Brompheniramine maleate (p.410·2); phenylpropanolamine hydrochloride (p.1098·1).
Cold and flu symptoms; hay fever; sinusitis.

Rupton Chronules
Dexo, Fr.†; Dexo, Switz.
Brompheniramine maleate (p.410·2); phenylpropanolamine hydrochloride (p.1098·1).
Upper-respiratory-tract disorders.

Ruscorectal
Heumann, Ger.; Juste, Spain.
Ruscogenin (p.1660·2).
Anorectal disorders.

Ruscoroid *Inverni della Beffa, Ital.*
Ruscogenin (p.1660·2); amethocaine [tetracaine] hydrochloride (p.1305·2).
Anorectal disorders.

Ruscovarin *Alpinamed, Switz.†.*
Heparin (p.902·1).
Peripheral vascular disorders.

Ruscus *Llorens, Spain.*
Cinchocaine hydrochloride (p.1309·1); prednisolone (p.1077·3); ruscogenin (p.1660·2); zinc oxide (p.1128·2); menthol (p.1632·3).
Anorectal disorders.

Rusyde *CP Pharmaceuticals, UK.*
Frusemide [furosemide] (p.893·1).
Oedema.

Ruticalzon *Brady, Aust.*
Colecalciferol (p.1391·1); rutoside (p.1611·2); vitamin C (p.1389·3); calcium citrate (p.1188·1).
Haemorrhage; infections.

Ruticalzon VC *Stegropharm, Ger.*
Rutoside (p.1611·2); ascorbic acid (p.1389·3).
Haemorrhagic disorders.

Rutice Fuerte *Faes, Spain.*
Ascorbic acid (p.1389·3); rutoside (p.1611·2).
Vascular disorders.

Rutinice Fortissimo *Sanitas, Port.*
Rutoside (p.1611·2); ascorbic acid (p.1389·3).
Haemorrhage.

Rutinion *Biomo, Ger.*
Rutoside (p.1611·2).
Capillary impairment; venous insufficiency.

Rutisan CE *Carlo Erba OTC, Ital.*
Rutoside (p.1611·2); vitamin C (p.1389·3); vitamin E (p.1393·3).
Vascular disorders.

Rutiscorbin *Fresenius Kabi, Aust.*
Rutoside (p.1611·2); ascorbic acid (p.1389·3).
Haemorrhage; infections.

Rutisept extra *Henkel, Ger.*
Isopropyl alcohol (p.1149·2); triclosan (p.1159·2).
Hand disinfection.

Rutiviscal *Sanidom, Aust.*
Garlic (p.1614·1); crataegus (p.1600·2); mistletoe (p.1636·2); rutoside (p.1611·2).
Atherosclerosis.

Ru-Tuss *Boots, USA†.*
Oral liquid: Phenylephrine hydrochloride (p.1097·1); chlorpheniramine [chlorphenamine] maleate (p.412·1).
Tablets: Phenylephrine hydrochloride (p.1097·1); phenylpropanolamine hydrochloride (p.1098·1); chlorpheniramine [chlorphenamine] maleate (p.412·1); hyoscyamine sulfate (p.469·3); atropine sulfate (p.461·1); hyoscine hydrobromide (p.468·2).

Upper respiratory-tract symptoms.

Ru-Tuss II *Boots, USA†.*
Chlorpheniramine [chlorphenamine] maleate (p.412·1); phenylpropanolamine hydrochloride (p.1098·1).
Cold symptoms.

Ru-Tuss DE *Boots, USA†.*
Pseudoephedrine hydrochloride (p.1099·2); guaifenesin (p.1092·2).
Coughs.

Ru-Tuss Expectorant *Boots, USA†.*
Pseudoephedrine hydrochloride (p.1099·2); dextromethorphan hydrobromide (p.1087·3); guaifenesin (p.1092·2).
Coughs.

Ru-Tuss with Hydrocodone *Boots, USA†.*
Hydrocodone tartrate (p.42·2); phenylephrine hydrochloride (p.1097·1); phenylpropanolamine hydrochloride (p.1098·1); pheniramine maleate (p.422·3); mepyramine maleate (p.421·1).
Cough, cold, and hay fever symptoms.

RV Paque
Note.This name is used for preparations of different composition.
ICN, Canad.; ICN, Hong Kong; ICN, Singapore; ICN, USA.
Zinc oxide (p.1128·2); cinoxate (p.1517·1).
Sunscreen.

ICN, NZ.
Zinc oxide (p.1128·2); octinoxate (p.1517·3).
Sunscreen.

RVHB Maxamaid *Scientific Hospital Supplies, Austral.†.*
Food for special diets (p.1350·1).
Homocystinuria; hypermethioninaemia.

Ryccard *Propan, S.Afr.*
Cyclizine hydrochloride (p.414·1).
Nausea; vestibular disorders; vomiting.

Rydene *Yamanouchi, Belg.*
Nicardipine hydrochloride (p.938·3).
Angina pectoris; hypertension.

Rylosol *ICN, Canad.*
Sotalol hydrochloride (p.972·2).
Arrhythmias.

Rymed *Edwards, USA.*
Pseudoephedrine hydrochloride (p.1099·2); guaifenesin (p.1092·2).
Coughs.

Rymed-TR *Edwards, USA†.*
Phenylpropanolamine hydrochloride (p.1098·1); guaifenesin (p.1092·2).
Coughs.

Ryna *Wallace, USA.*
Pseudoephedrine hydrochloride (p.1099·2); chlorpheniramine [chlorphenamine] maleate (p.412·1).
Upper respiratory-tract symptoms.

Ryna-12 S *Wallace, USA.*
Mepyramine tannate (p.421·1); phenylephrine tannate (p.1097·3).
Nasal congestion; rhinitis.

Ryna-C *Wallace, USA.*
Pseudoephedrine hydrochloride (p.1099·2); chlorpheniramine [chlorphenamine] maleate (p.412·1); codeine phosphate (p.25·2).
Coughs and cold symptoms.

Rynacrom
Rhone-Poulenc Rorer, Austral.; Rhone-Poulenc Rorer, Canad.†; Fisons, Irl.; Rhone-Poulenc Rorer, Mex.; Aventis, NZ; Aventis, Port.; Aventis, S.Afr.; Fisons, Singapore; Rhone-Poulenc Rorer, Singapore; Rhone-Poulenc Rorer, Thai.; Pantheon, UK.
Sodium cromoglicate (p.774·3).
Allergic rhinitis.

Rynacrom Allergy *Pantheon, UK.*
Sodium cromoglicate (p.774·3); xylometazoline hydrochloride (p.1102·2).
Allergic rhinitis with associated nasal congestion.

Rynacrom Composto *Aventis, Port.*
Sodium cromoglicate (p.774·3); xylometazoline hydrochloride (p.1102·2).
Allergic rhinitis; nasal congestion.

Rynacrom Compound
Rhone-Poulenc Rorer, Hong Kong; Rhone-Poulenc Rorer, Irl.; Fisons, Singapore; Rhone-Poulenc Rorer, Singapore; Rhone-Poulenc Rorer, Thai.; Pantheon, UK.
Sodium cromoglicate (p.774·3); xylometazoline hydrochloride (p.1102·2).
Allergic rhinitis; nasal congestion.

Rynacrom M *Rhone-Poulenc Rorer, Hong Kong.*
Sodium cromoglicate (p.774·3).
Allergic rhinitis.

Ryna-CX *Wallace, USA.*
Pseudoephedrine hydrochloride (p.1099·2); guaifenesin (p.1092·2); codeine phosphate (p.25·2).
Coughs.

Rynatan *Wallace, USA.*
Azatadine maleate (p.409·2); pseudoephedrine sulfate (p.1099·3).
Formerly contained phenylephrine tannate, chlorpheniramine [chlorphenamine] tannate, and mepyramine tannate.
Cold symptoms.

Rynatuss *Wallace, USA.*
Pentoxyverine tannate (p.1096·3); chlorpheniramine [chlorphenamine] tannate (p.412·2); ephedrine tannate (p.1090·3); phenylephrine tannate (p.1097·3).
Coughs.

Ryped *Propan, S.Afr.*
Erythromycin estolate (p.201·2).
Bacterial infections.

Rythmex *Teva, Israel.*
Propafenone hydrochloride (p.961·3).
Arrhythmias.

Rythmical *Unipharm, Israel.*
Disopyramide phosphate (p.878·2).
Arrhythmias.

Rythmodan
Hoechst Marion Roussel, Aust.; Hoechst Marion Roussel, Austral.; Aventis, Belg.; Hoechst Marion Roussel, Canad.; Roussel Diamant, Fr.; Hoechst Marion Roussel, Irl.; Hoechst Marion Roussel, Neth.; Aventis, NZ; Aventis, S.Afr.; Borg, UK.
Disopyramide (p.878·2) or disopyramide phosphate (p.878·2).
Arrhythmias.

Rythmodul *Hoechst Marion Roussel, Ger.*
Disopyramide phosphate (p.878·2).
Arrhythmias.

Rythmol
Knoll, Canad.; Knoll, Fr.; Knoll, S.Afr.; Abbott, USA.
Propafenone hydrochloride (p.961·3).
Arrhythmias.

Rythocin *Masa, Thai.*
Erythromycin stearate (p.201·3).
Bacterial infections.

Rytmobeta *Knoll, Ital.*
Sotalol hydrochloride (p.972·2).
Arrhythmias.

Rytmogenat *Azupharma, Ger.*
Propafenone hydrochloride (p.961·3).
Arrhythmias.

Rytmonorm
Knoll, Belg.; Knoll, Denm.; Knoll, Fin.; Knoll, Ger.; Knoll, Hong Kong; Knoll, Ital.; Knoll, Neth.; Knoll, NZ; Knoll, Port.; Knoll, Singapore; Knoll, Spain; Knoll, Swed.; Knoll, Switz.; Knoll, Thai.
Propafenone hydrochloride (p.961·3).
Arrhythmias.

Rytmonorma *Ebewe, Aust.*
Propafenone hydrochloride (p.961·3).
Arrhythmias.

Rytmopasc *Pascoe, Ger.*
Homoeopathic preparation.

Rytmo-Puren *Isis Puren, Ger.*
Propafenone hydrochloride (p.961·3).
Arrhythmias.

Ry-Tuss *Cypress, USA.*
Pentoxyverine tannate (p.1096·3); chlorpheniramine
[chlorphenamine] tannate (p.412·2); ephedrine tannate
(p.1090·3); phenylephrine tannate (p.1097·3).
Coughs.

S-2 *Nephron, USA.*
Racepinefrine hydrochloride (p.831·1).
Bronchospasm.

S.8 *Chefaro, Ger.*
Diphenhydramine hydrochloride (p.416·1).
Sleep disorders.

S Amet *Europharma, Spain.*
Ademetionine (p.1573·1).
Depression; liver disorders.

S-26 AR *Wyeth Health, Austral.; Wyeth Lederle, Port.*
Infant feed (p.1350·1).
Gastro-oesophageal regurgitation.

S-26 LF *Wyeth Health, Austral.*
Infant feed (p.1350·1).
Lactose intolerance.

S-26 sem Lactose *Wyeth Lederle, Port.*
Infant feed (p.1350·1).
Lactose intolerance.

SAB *Parke, Davis, Aust.*
Simeticone (p.1249·2); magnesium hydroxide
(p.1233·1); aluminium hydroxide (p.1210·3).
Flatulence, dyspepsia; peptic ulcer.

SAB Simplex
Parke, Davis, Aust.; Parke, Davis, Ger.; Warner-Lambert, Switz.†.
Simeticone (p.1249·2).
Detergent intoxication; meteorism; reduction of intes-
tinal gas before or after gastrointestinal procedures.

Saba *Lampugnani, Ital.*
Saw palmetto (p.1491·2).
Prostatic hyperplasia.

Sabacur uno *Biocur, Ger.*
Saw palmetto (p.1491·2).
Benign prostatic hyperplasia.

Sabadilla Med Complex *Dynamit, Aust.*
Homoeopathic preparation.

Sabal
Note.This name is used for preparations of different composition.
Ducray, Fr.
Shampoo: Saw palmetto (p.1491·2); zinc salicylate.
Topical gel; topical emulsion: Saw palmetto
(p.1491·2); zinc pidolate; keluamid (p.1118·1).
Seborrhoea.

Duopharm, Ger.; Stada, Ger.
Saw palmetto (p.1491·2).
Benign prostatic hyperplasia.

Sabal uno *Apogepha, Ger.*
Saw palmetto (p.1491·2).
Benign prostatic hyperplasia.

Sabalia *Boiron, Canad.*
Homoeopathic preparation.

Sabalin *Lichtwer, UK.*
Saw palmetto (p.1491·2).
Male urinary discomfort.

Sabalvit *Bional, Ger.*
Saw palmetto (p.1491·2).
Benign prostatic hyperplasia.

Sabanotropico *Calmante Vitaminado, Spain.*
Bismuth subgallate (p.1213·2); dexamethasone sodium
phosphate (p.1526·2); phenol (p.1152·3); sulfathiazole
(p.257·1); tannic acid (p.1669·1); menthol (p.1632·3).
Chilblains; cold-induced skin damage.

Sabax Fosenema *Adcock Ingram, S.Afr.*
Monobasic sodium phosphate (p.1193·2); dibasic sodi-
um phosphate (p.1193·2).
Bowel evacuation.

Sabax Gentamix *Adcock Ingram, S.Afr.*
Gentamicin sulfate (p.210·1).
Bacterial infections.

Sabima *Atlantis, Mex.*
Secnidazole (p.602·1).
Amoebiasis; giardiasis; trichomoniasis.

Sabin *SmithKline Beecham, Belg.*
An oral poliomyelitis vaccine (p.1558·2).
Active immunisation.

Sabril
Hoechst Marion Roussel, Aust.; Hoechst Marion Roussel, Austral.;
Aventis, Belg.; Hoechst Marion Roussel, Braz.; Hoechst Marion Rous-
sel, Canad.; Marion Merrell, Fr.; Hoechst Marion Roussel, Ger.;
Hoechst Marion Roussel, Hong Kong; Hoechst Marion Roussel, Irl.;
Hoechst Marion Roussel, Ital.; Hoechst Marion Roussel, Mex.; Ya-
manouchi, Neth.; Aventis, NZ; Marion Merrell Dow, Port.; Aventis,
S.Afr.; Hoechst Marion Roussel, Spain.; Hoechst Marion Roussel,
Switz.; Hoechst Marion Roussel, UK.
Vigabatrin (p.370·1).
Epilepsy.

Sabrilan *Agis, Israel.*
Vigabatrin (p.370·1).
Epilepsy.

Sabrilex
Aventis, Denm.; Hoechst Marion Roussel, Fin.; Hoechst Marion Rous-

---

sel, Norw.; Hoechst Marion Roussel, Spain; Hoechst Marion Roussel,
Swed.
Vigabatrin (p.370·1).
Epilepsy.

Sabro *Senosiain, Mex.*
Aloglutamid (p.1210·2).
Gastrointestinal hyperacidity.

Saburgen-N *Weber & Weber, Ger.*
Homoeopathic preparation.

Sabutol *Malaysia Chemist, Singapore.*
Salbutamol sulfate (p.770·3).
Obstructive airways disease.

S-A-C *Lannett, USA†.*
Paracetamol (p.71·2); salicylamide (p.82·1); caffeine
(p.761·3).
Pain.

Sacnel
Note.This name is used for preparations of different composition.
URPAC, Fr.†.
Cream: Sublimed sulfur (p.1123·3); dithiosalicylic
acid (p.1113·3); hamamelis (p.1618·3); ethyl linoleate;
menthol (p.1632·3); cholesterol.
Lotion: Sublimed sulfur (p.1123·3); dithiosalicylic
acid (p.1113·3); zinc oxide (p.1128·2); titanium diox-
ide (p.1126·1); hamamelis (p.1618·3).
Acne.

Teofarma, Ital.
Colloidal sulfur (p.1123·3); zinc oxide (p.1128·2); titanium dioxide (p.1126·1); dithiosalicylic acid
(p.1113·3); hamamelis leaves (p.1618·3).
Acne; seborrhoeic dermatitis.

Sacolene *EG, Fr.*
Methylenated milk proteins.
Diarrhoea.

Sacsol *Eagle, Austral.*
Hexane (p.1403·3); camphor (p.1589·3).
Surgical cement solvent for stoma patients.

Sacsol NF *Eagle, Austral.*
Trichloroethane (p.1406·2); camphor (p.1589·3).
Non-flammable surgical cement solvent for stoma pa-
tients.

Sactabs *PSM, NZ.*
Saccharin (p.1374·3).
Artificial sweetener.

Sadefen *Roche Nicholas, Spain.*
Ibuprofen (p.43·2).
Fever; pain.

Sadol *Catarinense, Braz.*
Iron (p.1366·3); pyridoxine; nicotinamide; caffeine;
citric acid (p.1350·1).
Iron deficiency; iron-deficiency anaemias.

Saetil *Robapharm, Spain.*
Ibuprofen arginine (p.44·1).
Fever; musculoskeletal, joint, and peri-articular disor-
ders; pain.

Saf-Clens *Calgon Vestal, USA.*
Wound cleanser.

Safe Tussin 30 *Kramer, USA.*
Guaifenesin (p.1092·2); dextromethorphan hydrobro-
mide (p.1087·3).
Coughs.

Safeway Cough Lozenges *Sutton, Canad.†.*
Menthol (p.1632·3).

Safeway Nasal *Prodemdis, Canad.*
Sodium chloride (p.1196·1).

Sagamicin *Kyowa, Jpn.*
Micronomicin sulfate (p.224·3).
Bacterial infections.

Sagamicina *Tubilux, Ital.*
Micronomicin sulfate (p.224·3).
Bacterial eye infections.

Sagitta Kamillbad *BASF, Ger.*
Chamomile oil.
Bath additive; skin and mucous-membrane disorders.

Sagittacin N *BASF, Ger.†.*
Tetracycline hydrochloride (p.258·3).
Respiratory-tract infections.

Sagittacortin *BASF, Ger.*
Hydrocortisone (p.1073·3) or hydrocortisone acetate
(p.1073·3).
Skin disorders.

Sagittamuc *BASF, Ger.*
Ambroxol hydrochloride (p.1084·3); doxycycline hy-
clate (p.200·1).
Respiratory-tract infections.

Sagittaproct *BASF, Ger.*
Injection: Quinine dihydrochloride (p.445·1).
Haemorrhoids.
Suppositories; ointment: Hamamelis (p.1618·3); bis-
muth subgallate (p.1213·2).
Haemorrhoids.
Topical gel: Lignocaine [lidocaine] hydrochloride
(p.1313·2).
Local anaesthesia.

Sagittaproct S *BASF, Ger.*
Lauromacrogol 400 (p.1345·2); zinc oxide (p.1128·2);
bismuth subnitrate (p.1213·2).
Haemorrhoids.

Sagrada-Lax *Falqui, Ital.*
Cascara sagrada (p.1216·1).
Constipation.

Sagrosept *Schulke & Mayr, Ger.*
Lotion: Isopropyl alcohol (p.1149·2); propyl alcohol
(p.1155·3); lactic acid (p.1626·2).
Hand disinfection.

Medicated wipes: Isopropyl alcohol (p.1149·2); propyl
alcohol (p.1155·3); benzoic acid (p.1134·2); lactic acid
(p.1626·2).
Skin disinfection; surface disinfection; wounds.

Sagrotan Med *Schulke & Mayr, Ger.†.*
Benzalkonium chloride (p.1133·2).
Skin and wound disinfection.

Saintbois nouvelle formule *Vifor, Switz.*
Ethylmorphine hydrochloride (p.35·2); sulfogaiacol
(p.1101·1); sodium benzoate (p.1134·3); belladonna
(p.463·1); hyssopus officinalis; tolu balsam (p.1101·3).
Coughs; respiratory-tract disorders.

Sais Andrews *Sterling, Port.*
Citric acid (p.1596·2); magnesium sulfate (p.1191·1);
sodium bicarbonate (p.1186·2).

Sais de Frutos *Confar, Port.*
Tartaric acid (p.1669·2); sodium carbonate (p.1665·1).

Sais Zitos *Zimaia, Port.†.*
Tartaric acid (p.1669·2); sodium bicarbonate (p.1665·1);
sodium tartrate (p.1250·2).

Saizen
Serono, Aust.; Serono, Austral.; Serono, Braz.; Serono, Canad.; Serono,
Fin.; Serono, Fr.; Serono, Ger.; Serono, Hong Kong; Serono, Irl.; Serono,
Israel; Serono, Ital.; Serono, Mex.; Serono, Norw.; Serono, NZ; Serono,
Port.; Serono, S.Afr.; Serono, Singapore; Serono, Spain; Serono, Swed.;
Serono, Switz.; Serono, UK; Serono, USA.
Somatropin (p.1286·1).
Growth failure due to renal failure; growth hormone
deficiency; Turner's syndrome.

Sal de Andrews *SmithKline Beecham, Braz.*
Magnesium sulfate (p.1191·1); sodium bicarbonate
(p.1186·2); citric acid (p.1596·2).
Gastrointestinal hyperacidity.

Sal de Fruta Eno
SmithKline Beecham, Braz.
Sodium bicarbonate (p.1186·2); sodium carbonate
(p.1665·1).
Gastrointestinal hyperacidity.
SmithKline Beecham, Spain.
Citric acid (p.1596·2); sodium bicarbonate (p.1186·2);
sodium carbonate (p.1665·1).
Gastrointestinal hyperacidity.

Salac *Medicis, Canad.; GenDerm, USA.*
Salicylic acid (p.1122·3).
Acne.

Sal-Acid *Pedinol, USA.*
Salicylic acid (p.1122·3).
Warts.

Salact *Knoll, Austral.†.*
Salicylic acid (p.1122·3).
Acne.

Salactic Film *Pedinol, USA.*
Salicylic acid (p.1122·3).
Warts.

Salactol
Dermal Laboratories, Irl.; Dermal Laboratories, UK.
Salicylic acid (p.1122·3); lactic acid (p.1626·2).
Calluses; corns; verrucas; warts.

Salagen
Chiron, Aust.; Pharmacia Upjohn, Canad.; Chiron, Irl.; MGI, Israel;
Chiron, Ital.; Chiron, Neth.; Novartis Ophthalmics, UK; MGI, USA.
Pilocarpine hydrochloride (p.1422·3).
Radiation-induced xerostomia; Sjögren's syndrome.

Salagesic *Blackmores, Austral.*
Salix (p.82·1); wood betony; cimicifuga (p.1595·2);
phenylalanine; magnesium phosphate; glycine; iron
phosphate.
Pain.

Salamol
Norton Waterford, Irl.; Norton Healthcare, Singapore; Baker Norton,
UK.
Salbutamol (p.770·3) or salbutamol sulfate (p.770·3).
Asthma; bronchospasm.

Salapin *Pinewood, UK.*
Salbutamol sulfate (p.770·3).
Asthma.

Salatac
Dermal Laboratories, Irl.; Dermal, Israel.
Salicylic acid (p.1122·3); lactic acid (p.1626·2).
Calluses; corns; verrucas; warts.

Salatac Gel *Dermal Laboratories, UK.*
Salicylic acid (p.1122·3); lactic acid (p.1626·2).
Calluses; corns; verrucas; warts.

Salazine *CTI, Israel.*
Sulfasalazine (p.1251·1).
Ulcerative colitis.

Salazopirina *Jaba, Port.*
Sulfasalazine (p.1251·1).
Inflammatory bowel disease; rheumatoid arthritis.

Salazopyrin
Pharmacia Upjohn, Aust.; Pharmacia Upjohn, Austral.; Pharmacia
Upjohn, Canad.; Pharmacia Upjohn, Denm.; Pharmacia Upjohn, Fin.;
Pharmacia Upjohn, Hong Kong; Pharmacia Upjohn, Irl.; Pharmacia
Upjohn, Israel; Pharmacia Upjohn, Ital.; Pharmacia Upjohn, Norw.;
Pharmacia Upjohn, NZ; Pharmacia Upjohn, S.Afr.; Pharmacia Up-
john, Singapore; Pharmacia Upjohn, Swed.; Pharmacia Upjohn,
Switz.; Pharmacia Upjohn, Thai.; Pharmacia, UK.
Sulfasalazine (p.1251·1).
Inflammatory bowel disease; rheumatoid arthritis.

Salazopyrina *Pharmacia Upjohn, Spain.*
Sulfasalazine (p.1251·1).
Proctitis; ulcerative colitis.

Salazopyrine
Pharmacia Upjohn, Belg.; Pharmacia Upjohn, Fr.; Pharmacia Upjohn,
Neth.
Sulfasalazine (p.1251·1).
Inflammatory bowel disease; rheumatoid arthritis.

Salbei Curarina *Harras-Curarina, Ger.*
Sage (p.1660·2).
Mouth and throat inflammation.

Salbei-Halspastillen *Bioflora, Aust.*
Sage oil (p.1660·2); calcium pantothenate (p.1374·1);
chlorhexidine hydrochloride (p.1138·2).
Mouth and throat disorders.

Salbu *BASF, Ger.; Orion, Ger.; Fatol, Ger.*
Salbutamol (p.770·3) or salbutamol sulfate (p.770·3).
Obstructive airways disease.

Salbufax *Master Pharma, Ital.*
Salbutamol sulfate (p.770·3).
Asthma; bronchospastic disorders.

Salbuhexal *Hexal, Ger.*
Salbutamol (p.770·3) or salbutamol sulfate (p.770·3).
Obstructive airways disease.

Salbulair *3M, Ger.*
Salbutamol sulfate (p.770·3).
Obstructive airways disease.

Salbulin
3M, Denm.†; Riker, Mex.; 3M, S.Afr.; 3M, UK.
Salbutamol (p.770·3) or salbutamol sulfate (p.770·3).
Obstructive airways disease.

Salbumol *Glaxo Wellcome, Fr.*
Salbutamol sulfate (p.770·3).
Asthma; premature labour.

Salbupp *Pulmopharm, Ger.*
Salbutamol (p.770·3).
Obstructive airways disease.

Salbusian *Asian Pharm, Thai.*
Salbutamol sulfate (p.770·3).
Obstructive airways disease.

Salbutac *Polipharm, Thai.*
Salbutamol sulfate (p.770·3).
Obstructive airways disease.

Salbutalan *Quimica y Farmacia, Mex.*
Salbutamol (p.770·3).

Salbutalin *Hebron, Braz.*
Salbutamol (p.770·3).
Obstructive airways disease.

Salbutard
United Nordic, Denm.; Lusofarmaco, Ital.
Salbutamol sulfate (p.770·3).
Obstructive airways disease.

Salbuvent
Nycomed, Denm.; Leiras, Fin.; Nycomed, Norw.; Douglas, NZ.
Salbutamol (p.770·3) or salbutamol sulfate (p.770·3).
Obstructive airways disease.

Salcacam *Salvat, Spain.*
Piroxicam (p.79·1).
Gout; musculoskeletal, joint, and peri-articular disor-
ders; pain.

Salcat *Monsanto, Port.*
Salcatonin (p.749·3).
Hypercalcaemia; osteolysis of malignancy; osteoporo-
sis; Paget's disease of bone.

Salcedogen *Fardi, Spain.*
Citric acid (p.1596·2); magnesium chloride (p.1190·3);
sodium bicarbonate (p.1186·2); sodium citrate
(p.1186·2); mannitol (p.924·3).
Constipation; hepatobiliary disorders; hypomagnesae-
mia; lithiasis; uric acidaemia.

Salcedol *Fardi, Spain.*
Potassium sulfate (p.1195·1); sodium bicarbonate
(p.1186·2); sodium sulfate (p.1250·1); tartaric acid
(p.1669·2).
Constipation; digestive disorders; hepatobiliary disor-
ders.

Salcemetic *Fardi, Spain.*
Cyclobutyrol (p.1601·2); metoclopramide hydrochlo-
ride (p.1235·2); mannitol (p.924·3).
Gastrointestinal disorders.

Salceryl *Ranbaxy, Thai.*
Salbutamol sulfate (p.770·3); guaifenesin (p.1092·2).
Coughs; obstructive airways disease.

Sal-Clens *C & M, USA†.*
Salicylic acid (p.1122·3).
Acne.

Salco *Lisapharm, Israel.*
Salcatonin (p.749·3).
Hypercalcaemia; osteoporosis; Paget's disease of
bone.

Salcotan *Scherer, Hong Kong.*
Ubidecarenone (p.1677·1).
Cardiac disorders; cerebral metabolic disorders; mus-
cular disorders.

Saldac
Douglas, Austral.†; Douglas, NZ.
Sulindac (p.85·3).
Musculoskeletal, joint, and peri-articular disorders;
pain with inflammation.

Salder S *Medley, Braz.*
Salicylic acid (p.1122·3); sulfur (p.1123·3).
Acne.

Saldeva *Roche Nicholas, Spain.*
Caffeine (p.761·3); dimenhydrinate (p.415·2); para-
cetamol (p.71·2).
Dysmenorrhoea.

The symbol † denotes a preparation no longer actively marketed

Sales de Frutas P G *Calmante Vitaminado, Spain.*
Citric acid (p.1596·2); sodium bicarbonate (p.1186·2); tartaric acid (p.1669·2).
Constipation; gastrointestinal hyperacidity.

Sales Fruta Mag Viviar *Viviar, Spain.*
Magnesium carbonate (p.1232·3); sodium bicarbonate (p.1186·2); tartaric acid (p.1669·2).
Constipation; gastrointestinal hyperacidity.

Sales Orto *Normon, Spain†.*
Citric acid (p.1596·2); sodium bicarbonate (p.1186·2); tartaric acid (p.1669·2).
Gastrointestinal disorders.

Saleto *Roberts, USA.*
Paracetamol (p.71·2); aspirin (p.14·2); salicylamide (p.82·1); caffeine (p.761·3).
The name Saleto is also used for a preparation containing ibuprofen.
Pain.

Saleto-200 *Roberts, USA.*
Ibuprofen (p.43·2).
The name Saleto is also used for a preparation containing paracetamol, aspirin, salicylamide, and caffeine.
Fever; osteoarthritis; pain; rheumatoid arthritis.

Saleto-D *Roberts, USA†.*
Phenylpropanolamine hydrochloride (p.1098·1); paracetamol (p.71·2); caffeine (p.761·3); salicylamide (p.82·1).
Upper respiratory-tract symptoms.

Salflex *Carnrick, USA.*
Salsalate (p.82·2).
Musculoskeletal and joint disorders.

Salf-Pas *Salf, Ital.*
Sodium aminosalicylate (p.148·3).
Tuberculosis.

Salgydal a la noramidopyrine *Doms-Adrian, Fr.*
Dipyrone (p.34·1); paracetamol (p.71·2); codeine phosphate (p.25·2).
Pain.

Salhumin *Sanova, Aust.*
Bath additive: Sodium humate; salicylic acid (p.1122·3).
Rheumatic disorders.
Liniment: Sodium humate; capsicum (p.1591·1); salicylic acid (p.1122·3); eucalyptus oil (p.1609·2); rosemary oil (p.1659·3); turpentine oil (p.1676·3); camphor (p.1589·3).
Circulatory disorders; muscle, joint, and nerve pain.

Salhumin Gel *Bastian, Ger.*
Glycol salicylate (p.42·2).
Soft-tissue injury.

Salhumin Gel N *Bastian, Ger.†*
Glycol salicylate (p.42·2); benzyl nicotinate (p.20·2); camphor (p.1589·3).
Neuralgia; peripheral vascular disorders; rheumatism; sports injuries.

Salhumin Rheuma-Bad *Bastian, Ger.*
Salicylic acid (p.1122·3); sodium humate.
Bath additive; musculoskeletal and joint disorders.

Salhumin Sitzbad N *Bastian, Ger.*
Salicylic acid (p.1122·3); sodium humate.
Bath additive; gynaecological disorders.

Salhumin Teilbad N *Bastian, Ger.*
Salicylic acid (p.1122·3); sodium humate; esculoside (p.1574·1).
Bath additive; circulatory disorders.

Sali D'Achille *Terme di Salsomaggiore, Ital.*
Mineral salt preparation.
Sore feet.

Sali di Salsomaggiore *Terme di Salsomaggiore, Ital.*
Mineral salt preparation.
Gynaecological disorders; nose and throat disorders.

Sali Iodati di Montecatini *Terme di Montecatini, Ital.*
Mineral salt preparation.
Constipation.

Sali Lassativi di Chianciano *Terme di Chianciano, Ital.*
Mineral salt preparation.
Constipation; digestive-system disorders.

Sali Tamerici di Montecatini *Terme di Montecatini, Ital.*
Mineral salt preparation.
Constipation.

Sali-Adalat *Bayer, Ger.*
Nifedipine (p.940·1); mefruside (p.926·1).
Hypertension.

Sali-Aldopur *Kwizda, Aust.; Hormosan, Ger.*
Spironolactone (p.973·2); bendrofluazide [bendroflumethiazide] (p.844·1).
Hyperaldosteronism; hypertension; hypokalaemia; liver cirrhosis and ascites; oedema.

Salibra *Brothier, Fr.*
Monobasic calcium phosphate; monobasic magnesium phosphate; monobasic sodium phosphate; monobasic manganese phosphate; monobasic potassium phosphate; monobasic lithium phosphate (p.1350·1).
Tonic.

Salicairine *Aerocid, Fr.*
Salicaria.
Formerly contained salicaria and iron hydrate.
Diarrhoea.

Salicilato de Bismuto Composto *Simoes, Braz.*
Bismuth salicylate (p.1213·1); sodium bicarbonate (p.1186·2); magnesium oxide (p.1233·2); calcium carbonate (p.1215·1); belladonna (p.463·1).
Diarrhoea; gastrointestinal hyperacidity.

Salicin-C *Amnol, Ital.*
Salix; echinacea; minerals; vitamin C (p.1350·1).
Nutritional supplement.

Salicort-R *Kattwiga, Ger.*
Homoeopathic preparation.

Salicyl *Galderma, Denm.*
Salicylic acid (p.1122·3).
Keratinisation disorders.

Salicylcafeina *Sanitas, Port.*
Aspirin (p.14·2); caffeine (p.761·3).
Fever; pain.

Sali-Decoderm *Merck, Aust.; Hermal, Ger.*
Fluprednidene acetate (p.1072·1); salicylic acid (p.1122·3).
Scalp disorders; skin disorders.

Salidex *Braun, Norw.*
Anhydrous glucose (p.1364·1); sodium chloride (p.1196·1).
Carbohydrate source; fluid and electrolyte disorders.

Salidur *Almirall, Spain.*
Frusemide [furosemide] (p.893·1); triamterene (p.986·1).
Hypertension; oedema.

Salikaren *Rekah, Israel.*
Salicylic acid (p.1122·3).
Keratinisation disorders.

Saliker *Roche-Posay, Irl.*
Salicylic acid (p.1122·3); piroctone olamine (p.1121·1).
Dandruff; seborrhoeic dermatitis.

Salilax *Orion, Denm.; Orion, Swed.*
Magnesium oxide (p.1233·2).
Bowel evacuation.

Salimar-Bad L *Li-il, Ger.*
Sodium salicylate (p.84·2); salicylic acid (p.1122·3).
Bath additive; musculoskeletal and joint disorders.

Saliment *Vida, Hong Kong.*
Methyl salicylate (p.55·1); eucalyptus oil (p.1609·2); menthol (p.1632·3).
Musculoskeletal and joint pain.

Salimetin *Luper, Braz.*
Methyl salicylate (p.55·1); turpentine oil (p.1676·3); camphor (p.1589·3).
Musculoskeletal and joint disorders.

Salinal *Julphar, UAE.*
Simethicone (p.1249·2).
Adjunct in gastroscopy and bowel radiography; flatulence.

Salinex
Technilab, Canad.; Muro, USA.
Sodium chloride (p.1196·1).
Nasal hygiene.

Salinol *Technilab, Canad.*
Macrogol (p.1630·1); propylene glycol (p.1655·1).
Nasal lubricant.

Salipax *Mepha, Port.*
Fluoxetine hydrochloride (p.284·2).
Depression.

Salipran *Medeva, Fr.*
Benorilate (p.19·3).
Pain.

Sali-Prent *Bayer, Ger.*
Acebutolol hydrochloride (p.825·1); mefruside (p.926·1).
Hypertension.

Sali-Presinol *Bayer, Ger.†*
Methyldopa (p.927·3); mefruside (p.926·1).
Hypertension.

Sali-Puren *Isis Puren, Ger.*
Triamterene (p.986·1); hydrochlorothiazide (p.907·3).
Heart failure; hypertension; oedema.

Salisoap *Darrow, Braz.*
Salicylic acid (p.1122·3); sulfur (p.1123·3).
Seborrhoeic dermatitis.

Salisol *Rekah, Israel.*
Salicylic acid (p.1122·3); alcohol (p.1130·3).
Keratinisation disorders; skin disinfection.

Sali-Spiroctan *Roche, Switz.*
Spironolactone (p.973·2); butizide (p.853·1).
Hyperaldosteronism.

Salisteril *Fresenius Kabi, Switz.*
Electrolyte infusion (p.1180·1).
Fluid and electrolyte disorders.

Salistoperm *Ursapharm, Ger.*
Salicylamide (p.82·1); benzocaine (p.1306·2).
Musculoskeletal, joint, peri-articular, and soft-tissue disorders; neuralgia.

Salitanol Estreptomicina *Quimpe, Spain.*
Albumin tannate (p.1209·3); dihydrostreptomycin sulfate (p.199·2); sulfathiazole (p.257·1).
Gastrointestinal infections.

Saliton *Planta, Canad.†*
Salix (p.82·1).
Fever; pain.

Saliva medac *Medac, Ger.*
Mucin (porcine) (p.1501·1).
Saliva substitute.

Saliva Orthana
Note. This name is used for preparations of different composition.
Delta, Austral.
Mucins (p.1501·1); xylitol (p.1397·3); electrolytes (p.1180·1).
Saliva substitute.

A.S., UK.
Lozenges: Mucin (p.1501·1); xylitol (p.1397·3).
Oral spray: Mucin (p.1501·1); xylitol (p.1397·3); sodium fluoride (p.1375·3).
Saliva substitute.

Salivace *Penn, UK.*
Carmellose sodium (p.1499·3); xylitol (p.1397·3); electrolytes (p.1180·1).
Dry mouth.

Salivart
Gebauer, Canad.; Gebauer, Hong Kong; Gebauer, USA.
Carmellose sodium (p.1499·3); sorbitol (p.1377·3); electrolytes (p.1180·1).
Dry mouth.

Saliveze *Wyvern, UK.*
Electrolytes (p.1180·1).
Dry mouth.

Salivin *Kabi, Swed.†*
Malic acid (p.1631·1); xylitol (p.1397·3).
Saliva stimulation.

Salivix *Provalis, UK.*
Malic acid (p.1631·1); calcium lactate (p.1188·2); sodium phosphate (p.1193·2).
Dry mouth.

Salix *Scandinavian Natural Health & Beauty, USA.*
Artificial saliva.

Salmagne *Fardi, Spain.*
Magnesium citrate (p.1232·3); magnesium sulfate (p.1191·1); sodium bicarbonate (p.1186·2); tartaric acid (p.1669·2); mannitol (p.924·3).
Constipation; digestive disorders.

Salmetedur *Menarini, Ital.*
Salmeterol xinafoate (p.773·3).
Bronchospastic disorders.

Salmiak *Soldan, Ger.*
Ammonium chloride (p.1085·2); liquorice (p.1231·2); anise oil (p.1580·3).
Respiratory-tract disorders.

Salmocalcin *Ripari-Gero, Ital.†*
Salcatonin (p.749·3).
Hypercalcaemia; osteoporosis; Paget's disease of bone; reflex sympathetic dystrophy.

Salmocide *Atlantis, Mex.*
Furazolidone (p.592·1).
Gastrointestinal infections.

Salmofar *Lafare, Ital.*
Salcatonin (p.749·3).
Hypercalcaemia; osteoporosis; Paget's disease of bone; reflex sympathetic dystrophy.

Salmol
Atlantic, Hong Kong; Atlantic, Singapore; Atlantic, Thai.; Biolab, Thai.
Salbutamol sulfate (p.770·3).
Obstructive airways disease; premature labour.

Salmol Expectorant *Biolab, Thai.*
Salbutamol sulfate (p.770·3); guaifenesin (p.1092·2).
Obstructive airways disease.

Salmundin *Mundipharma, Ger.*
Salbutamol (p.770·3) or salbutamol sulfate (p.770·3).
Obstructive airways disease.

Salocol *Hauck, USA†.*
Aspirin (p.14·2); paracetamol (p.71·2); salicylamide (p.82·1); caffeine (p.761·3).
Pain.

Salodiur *Gerot, Aust.*
Triamterene (p.986·1); hydrochlorothiazide (p.907·3).
Hypertension; oedema.

Salofalk
Merck, Aust.; Axcan, Canad.; Falk, Ger.; Falk, Hong Kong; Antigen, Irl.; Knoll, Ital.; Farmasa, Mex.; Falk, Neth.; Aventis, Port.; Falk, Singapore; Phardi, Switz.; Falk, Thai.; Provalis, UK.
Mesalazine (p.1234·1).
Inflammatory bowel disease.

Sal-Oil-T *Syosset, USA.*
Coal tar (p.1125·1); salicylic acid (p.1122·3).
Seborrhoea.

Salomol *Clonmel, Irl.*
Salbutamol (p.770·3) or salbutamol sulfate (p.770·3).
Obstructive airways disease.

Salonair *Salonpas, UK.*
Methyl salicylate (p.55·1); menthol (p.1632·3); camphor (p.1589·3); benzyl nicotinate (p.20·2); glycol salicylate (p.42·2).
Muscle and joint pain.

Salongo *Biosarto, Spain.*
Oxiconazole nitrate (p.393·1).
Fungal infections.

Salonpas
Note. This name is used for preparations of different composition.
Formila, Ital.
Medicated bandage: Menthol (p.1632·3); methyl salicylate (p.55·1); camphor (p.1589·3); glycol salicylate (p.42·2); thymol (p.1158·3).
Topical spray: Methyl salicylate (p.55·1); menthol (p.1632·3); camphor (p.1589·3); benzyl nicotinate (p.20·2); glycol salicylate (p.42·2).
Musculoskeletal, joint, and soft-tissue pain.

Salonpas, UK.
Methyl salicylate (p.55·1); glycol salicylate (p.42·2).
Musculoskeletal and joint pain.

Salphenyl *Roberts, USA†; Hauck, USA†.*
Phenylephrine hydrochloride (p.1097·1); paracetamol (p.71·2); chlorpheniramine [chlorphenamine] maleate (p.412·1); salicylamide (p.82·1).
Upper respiratory-tract symptoms.

Sal-Plant *Pedinol, USA.*
Salicylic acid (p.1122·3).
Warts.

Salseb *Draxis, Canad.*
Salicylic acid (p.1122·3).

Salsitab *Upsher-Smith, USA.*
Salsalate (p.82·2).
Fever; inflammation; pain.

Salsyvase *Ipex, Swed.*
Salicylic acid (p.1122·3).
Formerly known as Salicylsyrevaselin.
Skin disorders.

Saltadol *Lindopharm, Ger.*
Potassium chloride; sodium chloride; sodium bicarbonate; glucose (p.1185·2).
Diarrhoea; oral rehydration therapy.

Saltamol *Ranbaxy, Thai.*
Salbutamol sulfate (p.770·3).
Obstructive airways disease.

Saltermox *Propan, S.Afr.*
Amoxicillin (p.149·2).
Bacterial infections.

Salterpyn *Propan, S.Afr.*
Syrup: Paracetamol (p.71·2); codeine phosphate (p.25·2); promethazine hydrochloride (p.423·2).
Fever; pain.
Tablets: Paracetamol (p.71·2); codeine phosphate (p.25·2); caffeine (p.761·3); meprobamate (p.691·1).
Pain with tension.

Saltrates *Uhlmann-Eyraud, Switz.*
Cream: Triclosan (p.1159·2); methylchloroisothiazolinone (p.1149·3); menthol (p.1632·3); chamomile oil; hypericum oil (p.290·3); melissa oil; lavender oil (p.1627·2).
Dry or painful feet.
Topical gel: Sodium hydroxide (p.1665·3); trometamol (p.1675·2).
Calluses; corns.

Saltrates Rodell *Uhlmann-Eyraud, Switz.*
Chamomile (p.1593·2); hypericum (p.290·2); sodium bicarbonate (p.1186·2); anhydrous sodium carbonate (p.1665·1); sodium sesquicarbonate; sodium perborate (p.1156·3).
Foot disorders.

Sal-Tropine *Hope, USA.*
Atropine sulfate (p.461·1).

Saltucin
Roche, Aust.; Boehringer Mannheim, Ger.†
Butizide (p.853·1).
Diabetes insipidus; heart failure; hypertension; oedema; renal calculi.

Saltucin Co *Boehringer Mannheim, S.Afr.†*
Butizide (p.853·1); reserpine (p.967·3); rescinnamine (p.967·3); raubasine (p.967·2); potassium chloride (p.1194·3).
Hypertension.

Salube *Colgate Oral Care, Austral.†*
Artificial saliva.
Reduced salivary flow.

Salucur *Salus, Fr.*
Urtica (p.1678·2); saw palmetto (p.1491·2); cucurbita (p.1601·1); vitamin B substances; vitamin C (p.1350·1).
Prostatic disorders; urinary-tract disorders.

Saludopin *SIT, Ital.*
Methyldopa (p.927·3); butizide (p.853·1).
Hypertension.

Salugliben *Salus, Mex.*
Glibenclamide (p.321·3).
Diabetes mellitus.

Saluket-H I *Salus, Mex.*
Ketotifen (p.767·2).
Asthma.

Salures *Pharmacia Upjohn, Swed.*
Bendrofluazide [bendroflumethiazide] (p.844·1).
Hypertension; oedema; renal calculi.

Salures-K *Pharmacia Upjohn, Swed.*
Bendrofluazide [bendroflumethiazide] (p.844·1); potassium chloride (p.1194·3).
Hypertension; oedema; renal calculi.

Saluretin *Zeneca, Switz.*
Spironolactone (p.973·2); bendrofluazide [bendroflumethiazide] (p.844·1).
Hyperaldosteronism; hypertension; oedema.

Saluric *Merck Sharp & Dohme, Irl.†; Merck Sharp & Dohme, UK†.*
Chlorothiazide (p.856·3).
Hypertension; oedema.

Salurin *Julphar, UAE.*
Frusemide [furosemide] (p.893·1).
Hypertension; oedema.

Saluron *Apothecon, USA.*
Hydroflumethiazide (p.911·3).
Hypertension; oedema.

Salus *Salushaus, Ger.†*
Devil's claw root (p.26·3).
Tonic.

Salus Abfuhr-Tee Nr. 2 *Salushaus, Ger.†*
Rose fruit (p.1389·3); chamomile (p.1593·2); calendula (p.1589·2); buckthorn (p.1215·1); senna (p.1248·2); fennel (p.1610·1).
Constipation.

Salus Augenschutz-Kapseln N *Salushaus, Ger.*
Myrtillus (p.1639·2); vitamin A palmitate (p.1383·2); riboflavin sodium phosphate (p.1386·1).
Hypersensitivity to light; night blindness.

Salus Bronchial-Tee Nr.8 *Salushaus, Ger.†.*
Fennel (p.1610·1); calendula (p.1589·2); Iceland moss; verbascum; tilia (p.1673·2); cowslip flower (p.1600·1); lamium album; thyme (p.1672·2); knotgrass; raspberry leaf (p.1657·2).
Coughs and associated respiratory-tract disorders.

Salus Herz-Schutz-Kapseln *Salushaus, Ger.*
Crataegus (p.1600·2); alpha tocoferil acetate (p.1394·1); magnesium complex with acid hydrolysate of maize starch.
Tonic.

Salus Leber-Galle-Tee Nr.18 *Salushaus, Ger.†.*
Cynara (p.1601·3); fennel (p.1610·1); chamomile (p.1593·2); taraxacum (p.1669·1); stoechados; calendula (p.1589·2); achillea (p.1572·2); peppermint leaf (p.1243·2).
Liver and biliary disorders.

Salus Mistel-Tropfen *Salushaus, Ger.*
Mistletoe (p.1636·2).
Arteriosclerosis.

Salus Multi-Vitamin-Energetikum *Salushaus, Ger.*
Multivitamin preparation with plant extracts (p.1350·1).
Tonic; vitamin deficiency.

Salus Nerven-Schlaf-Tee Nr.22 *Salushaus, Ger.†.*
Chamomile (p.1593·2); bellis perennis; paeonia officinalis; stoechados; fennel (p.1610·1); lupulus (p.1629·3); hypericum (p.290·2); lavender (p.1627·2); melissa (p.1632·2); citrus sinensis.
Nervous disorders.

Salus Rheuma-Tee Krautertee Nr. 12 *Salushaus, Ger.†.*
Birch leaf (p.1585·2); urtica (p.1678·2); fennel (p.1610·1); taraxacum (p.1669·1); calendula (p.1589·2); equisetum (p.1606·3); achillea (p.1572·2); juniper (p.1625·2).
Rheumatic disorders.

Salus Venen Krauter Dragees N *Salushaus, Ger.*
Aesculus (p.1574·1); melilotus.
Vascular disorders.

Salus Zinnkraut *Salushaus, Ger.*
Equisetum (p.1606·3).
Oedema.

Salusan *Salushaus, Ger.†.*
Crataegus (p.1600·2); mistletoe (p.1636·2); ammi visnaga fruit (p.1579·1); equisetum (p.1606·3); dried bitter-orange peel (p.1644·2); lemon peel; passion flower (p.1649·1); melissa (p.1632·2); valerian (p.1678·3); hypericum (p.290·2); lupulus (p.1629·3); rosemary; cymbopogon citratus; bearberry (p.1583·3); wheat germ; tinct. germen. hordeoli.
Cardiovascular disorders.

Salutensin *Roberts, USA.*
Hydroflumethiazide (p.911·3); reserpine (p.967·3).
Hypertension.

Salutina *Bergamo, Braz.*
Kola (p.1681·1); carqueja; iodine (p.1522·3); potassium iodide (p.1522·3); calcium dihydrogen phosphate (p.1588·2); glycerol; alcohol.

Salva Infantes *Camps, Spain.*
Magnesium carbonate (p.1232·3); magnesium sulfate (p.1191·1); betanaphthyl benzoate (p.97·2).
Gastrointestinal disorders.

Salvacam *Salvat, Spain.*
Piroxicam (p.79·1).
Gout; musculoskeletal, joint, peri-articular, and soft-tissue disorders; pain.

Salvacolina NF *Salvat, Spain.*
Loperamide hydrochloride (p.1231·3).
Salvacolina formerly contained albumin tannate and opium.
Diarrhoea.

Salvacolon *Salvat, Spain.*
Bacillus subtilis; vitamins and amino acids (p.1350·1).
Cystitis; gastrointestinal disorders; restoration of the gastrointestinal flora.

Salvalion *Norman, Spain.*
Raubasine (p.967·2); almitrine (p.1506·2).
Cerebrovascular disorders; vestibular disorders.

Salvapen *Salvat, Spain.*
Amoxicillin trihydrate (p.149·2).
Bacterial infections.

Salvapen Mucolitico *Salvat, Spain.*
Amoxicillin trihydrate (p.149·2); bromhexine hydrochloride (p.1085·3).
Respiratory-tract infections.

Salvarina *Salvat, Spain.*
Caffeine (p.761·3); dimenhydrinate (p.415·2); ibuprofen (p.43·2).
Dysmenorrhoea.

Salvatrim *Salvat, Spain.*
Co-trimoxazole (p.193·3).
Bacterial infections; Pneumocystis carinii pneumonia.

Salvent *Wolff, Ger.*
Salbutamol (p.770·3).
Obstructive airways disease.

Salvesept *Cederroth, Spain.*
Alcohol (p.1130·3); chlorhexidine hydrochloride (p.1138·2).
Wound disinfection.

salvi CAL E-G *Baxter, Ger.*
Glucose and electrolyte infusion (p.1350·1).
Parenteral nutrition.

salvi CAL GX *Baxter, Ger.*
Glucose monohydrate (p.1364·2); xylitol (p.1397·3).
Parenteral nutrition.

salviamin X-E *Baxter, Ger.*
Amino-acid, xylitol, and electrolyte infusion (p.1350·1).
Parenteral nutrition.

salviamin G-E *Baxter, Ger.*
Amino-acid, glucose, and electrolyte infusion (p.1350·1).
Parenteral nutrition.

salviamin GX-E *Baxter, Ger.*
Amino-acid, glucose, xylitol, and electrolyte infusion (p.1350·1).
Parenteral nutrition.

salviamin hepar *Baxter, Ger.*
Amino-acid and electrolyte infusion (p.1350·1).
Parenteral nutrition in liver disease.

Salviathymol N *Galenika, Ger.*
Sage oil (p.1660·2); eucalyptus oil (p.1609·2); peppermint oil (p.1243·3); cinnamon oil (p.1596·1); clove oil (p.1597·1); fennel oil (p.1610·2); anise oil (p.1580·3); menthol (p.1632·3); thymol (p.1158·3).
Mouth and throat disorders.

Salvibest *CT, Ger.*
Rhatany root (p.1657·3).
Mouth and gum disorders.

Salviette H *Whitehall, Ital.*
Hamamelis water (p.1618·3); glycerol (p.1616·3).
Anal cleansing; haemorrhoids.

salvilipid *Baxter, Ger.*
Soya oil (p.1378·1).
Contains egg lecithin.
Lipid infusion for parenteral nutrition.

Salvital *Reckitt & Colman, Austral.*
Magnesium sulfate (p.1191·1); sodium bicarbonate (p.1186·2); tartaric acid (p.1669·2).
Dyspepsia; nausea.

Salvituss *FIRMA, Ital.*
Levodropropizine (p.1089·3).
Coughs.

Salvyl *Petrasch, Aust.*
Undecenoic acid (p.395·3) sulfur (p.1123·3) complex; betanaphthol (p.97·2); salicylic acid (p.1122·3).
Acne; erythrasma; fungal skin infections.

Salvysat *Mayrhofer, Aust.; Ysatfabrik, Ger.*
Sage leaf (p.1660·2).
Hyperhidrosis; mouth and throat inflammation.

Salycilina *Upsifarma, Port.*
Aspirin (p.14·2).
Fever; pain.

Salzone *Wallace Mfg Chem., UK.*
Paracetamol (p.71·2).
Fever; pain.

Sambil *Lacer, Spain†.*
Boldine (p.1585·3); hydroxymethylnicotinamide (p.1622·2).
Digestive-system disorders.

Sambuco (Specie Composta) *Dynacren, Ital.*
Tilia (p.1673·2); sambucus (p.1660·3); spiraea (p.1631·2); rose fruit (p.1389·3).
Respiratory-tract disorders.

Sambucol *Biopura, Port.*
Sambucus (p.1660·3).
Cold and influenza symptoms.

Sambucus Complex *Blackmores, Austral.*
Sambucus (p.1660·3); euphrasia (p.1609·3); echinacea angustifolia (p.1606·2); hydrastis (p.1621·1); euphorbia hirta (p.1609·3); d-alpha tocoferil acid succinate (p.1394·1); vitamin A acetate (p.1383·2).
Conjunctivitis; otorrhoea; upper respiratory-tract disorders.

Same Plast *Savoma, Ital.*
Emollient.

Same-Seb *Savoma, Ital.*
Colloidal sulfur (p.1123·3); salicylic acid (p.1122·3).
Acne; seborrhoea.

Samilstin *LPB, Ital.*
Octreotide (p.1292·1).
Acromegaly; diarrhoea associated with immunodeficiency; endocrinal tumours of the gastrointestinal tract; pancreatic fistula; postoperative complications of pancreatic surgery; variceal haemorrhage.

Samyr *Knoll, Ital.; Knoll, Mex.*
Ademetionine sulfate tosilate (p.1573·1).
Depression; liver disorders.

Sanabronchiol *Falqui, Ital.*
Dextromethorphan hydrobromide (p.1087·3).
Coughs.

Sanaco *PD, Thai.*
Chlorophyll (p.1028·1); benzalkonium chloride (p.1133·2).
Personal hygiene; vaginal douche.

Sanacol *SmithKline Beecham, Braz.*
Aspirin (p.14·2); cinnamedrine hydrochloride; caffeine (p.761·3).
Smooth muscle spasm.

Sanaden Reforzado *Calmante Vitaminado, Spain.*
Creosote (p.1087·3); benzocaine (p.1306·2); niaouli oil (p.1640·2).
Toothache.

Sanaderm *Herbaline, Ital.†.*
Echinacea (p.1606·2); calendula (p.1589·2); viola tricolor; helichrysum italicum; bergamot oil (p.1584·2); lavender oil (p.1627·2); thyme oil (p.1672·3); geranium oil (p.1615·1).
Burns; skin irritation; wounds.

Sanadermil *Vifor, Switz.*
Hydrocortisone acetate (p.1073·3).
Skin disorders.

Sanador *Virtus, Braz.*
Methyl salicylate (p.55·1); turpentine oil (p.1676·3); camphor (p.1589·3); menthol (p.1632·3); chlorophyll (p.1028·1).
Musculoskeletal and joint disorders.

Sanadorn *Jacoby, Aust.†.*
Crataegus (p.1600·2).
Heart disorders.

Sanaform *Esoform, Ital.*
Benzalkonium chloride (p.1133·2).
Surface disinfection.

Sanalepsi N *Roche, Switz.*
Doxylamine succinate (p.417·1).
Hypersensitivity reactions; nervous disorders.

Sanalgin *Boehringer Ingelheim, Neth.; Gebro, Switz.*
Paracetamol (p.71·2); propyphenazone (p.80·2); caffeine (p.761·3).
Fever; pain.

Sanamidol *Inkeysa, Spain.*
Omeprazole (p.1239·1).
Gastro-oesophageal reflux; peptic ulcer; Zollinger-Ellison syndrome.

Sanaprav *Sankyo, Aust.; Sankyo, Ital.; Sankyo, Port.*
Pravastatin sodium (p.957·3).
Atherosclerosis; hypercholesterolaemia.

Sanasepton *Pharbita, Ger.*
Erythromycin (p.201·2), erythromycin estolate (p.201·2), or erythromycin ethyl succinate (p.201·2).
Bacterial infections.

Sana-Sol *Nycomed, Fin.*
Multivitamin preparation (p.1350·1).

Sanasthmax *Glaxo Wellcome, Ger.*
Beclometasone dipropionate (p.1061·2).
Asthma; bronchitis.

Sanasthmyl *Glaxo Wellcome, Ger.*
Beclometasone dipropionate (p.1061·2).
Asthma; bronchitis; tracheitis.

Sanation Mono *Taurus, Ger.*
Hydrocortisone (p.1073·3).
Burns; skin disorders.

Sanatogen *Key, Austral.*
Food for special diets (p.1350·1).
Protein supplementation.

Roche, Hong Kong; Roche Consumer, Irl.; Roche, S.Afr.†; Roche Consumer, Singapore; Roche Consumer, UK.
A range of vitamin, mineral, and nutritional preparations (p.1350·1).

Sanato-Rhev *Hotz, Ger.†.*
Camphor (p.1589·3); isopropyl alcohol (p.1149·2).
Muscle and joint pain; soft-tissue disorders; superficial circulatory disorders.

Sanaven *Sankyo, Ger.*
A heparinoid (p.905·2); phenylephrine hydrochloride (p.1097·1).
Venous disorders.

Sanaven Venentabletten *Sankyo, Ger.*
Aesculus (p.1574·1).
Venous disorders.

Sanavitan S *Bottger, Ger.*
dl-Alpha tocoferil acetate (p.1394·1).
Vitamin E deficiency.

Sanaxin *Tyrol, Aust.*
Cefalexin (p.161·3).
Bacterial infections.

Sancago *Chinta, Thai.*
Indometacin (p.44·3); methocarbamol (p.1329·3).
Gout; musculoskeletal and joint disorders.

Sanderson's Throat Specific *Sandersons, UK.*
Mixture: Acetic acid (p.1571·2); quassia (p.1657·1); squill (p.1100·3); capsicum (p.1591·1).
Pastilles: Honey (p.1366·2); squill vinegar (p.1100·3); capsicum (p.1591·1); tolu (p.1101·3); menthol (p.1632·3); cinnamic acid (p.1142·2); benzoic acid (p.1134·2); eucalyptus oil (p.1609·2).
Catarrh; sore throat.

Sandimmun *Novartis, Aust.; Novartis, Austral.; Novartis, Belg.; Novartis, Braz.; Novartis, Denm.; Novartis, Fin.; Novartis, Fr.; Novartis, Ger.; Novartis, Hong Kong; Novartis, Irl.; Novartis, Israel; Novartis, Ital.; Novartis, Mex.; Novartis, Norw.; Novartis, NZ; Novartis, Port.; Novartis, S.Afr.; Novartis, Spain; Novartis, Swed.; Novartis, Switz.; Novartis, Thai.; Novartis, UK.*
Ciclosporin (p.518·1).
Atopic dermatitis; graft-versus-host disease; nephrotic syndrome; psoriasis; rheumatoid arthritis; transplant rejection; uveitis.

Sandimmun Neoral *Novartis, Singapore.*
Ciclosporin (p.518·1).
Atopic dermatitis; nephrotic syndrome; psoriasis; rheumatoid arthritis; transplant rejection; uveitis.

Sandimmune *Novartis, Canad.; Novartis, Neth.; Novartis, USA.*
Ciclosporin (p.518·1).
Graft-versus-host disease; nephrotic syndrome; psoriasis; rheumatoid arthritis; transplant or graft rejection.

Sandocal
Novartis Consumer, Austral.; Novartis, Fr.; Novartis, Irl.; Novartis Consumer, Port.; Novartis Consumer, UK.
Calcium lactate gluconate (p.1188·3); calcium carbonate (p.1215·1).
Formerly contained sodium and potassium in the UK.
Hypocalcaemia; osteoporosis.

Sandocal-D *Novartis, Ger.*
Calcium carbonate (p.1215·1); colecalciferol (p.1391·1).
Calcium and vitamin D deficiency; osteoporosis.

Sandoglobulin
Novartis, Aust.; Novartis, Austral.; Novartis, Fin.; Novartis, Ger.; Novartis, Irl.; Novartis, Israel; Novartis, Norw.†; Novartis, NZ; Sandoz, S.Afr.†; Novartis, Swed.; Novartis, UK; Novartis, USA.
A normal immunoglobulin (p.1551·3).
Bone marrow transplantation; Guillain-Barré syndrome; hypogammaglobulinaemia; idiopathic thrombocytopenic purpura; immunodeficiency; Kawasaki disease; passive immunisation.

Sandoglobulina
Novartis, Braz.; Novartis, Ital.; Novartis, Mex.; Novartis, Port.
A normal immunoglobulin (p.1551·3).
Auto-immune disorders; hypogammaglobulinaemia; idiopathic thrombocytopenic purpurea; Kawasaki disease; passive immunisation.

Sandoglobuline
Novartis, Belg.; Novartis, Fr.; Novartis, Switz.
A normal immunoglobulin (p.1551·3).
Guillain-Barré syndrome; hypogammaglobulinaemia; idiopathic thrombocytopenic purpura; immunodeficiency; Kawasaki disease; neuropathies; passive immunisation.

Sando-K
Novartis, Irl.†; HK Pharma, UK.
Potassium bicarbonate (p.1186·1); potassium chloride (p.1194·3).
Hypokalaemia.

Sandolanid *Novartis, Aust.*
Acetyldigoxin (p.827·3).
Arrhythmias.

Sandomigran
Novartis, Aust.; Novartis, Austral.; Novartis, Belg.; Novartis, Braz.; Novartis, Canad.; Novartis, Ger.; Novartis, Hong Kong; Novartis, Israel; Novartis, Ital.; Novartis, Neth.; Novartis, NZ; Novartis, S.Afr.; Novartis, Spain.
Pizotifen malate (p.455·1).
Cluster headache; migraine and other vascular headaches.

Sandomigrin
Novartis, Denm.; Novartis, Norw.†; Novartis, Swed.
Pizotifen malate (p.455·1).
Cluster headache; migraine.

Sandonorm
Novartis, Aust.; Novartis, Switz.
Bopindolol malonate (p.850·3).
Angina pectoris; hypertension.

Sandoparin *Novartis, Aust.*
Certoparin sodium (p.856·2).
Thrombosis prophylaxis.

Sandoparine *Novartis, Switz.*
Certoparin sodium (p.856·2).
Thrombosis prophylaxis.

Sandopart *Sandoz, Ital.†.*
Demoxytocin (p.1281·1).
Induction of labour; post-partum uterine involution; prevention of breast engorgement and mastitis; stimulation of lactation.

Sandopril *Sandoz, Aust.†.*
Spirapril hydrochloride (p.973·2).
Hypertension.

Sandoretic *Novartis, Switz.*
Bopindolol malonate (p.850·3); chlortalidone (p.857·1).
Hypertension.

Sandosource
Novartis, Irl.; Novartis Consumer, Ital.; Novartis Consumer, UK.
Preparation for enteral nutrition (p.1350·1).
Gastrointestinal disorders.

Sandosource GI Control *Novartis, Fin.*
Preparation for enteral nutrition (p.1350·1).

Sandosource Peptide *Novartis Nutrition, Canad.*
Preparation for enteral nutrition (p.1350·1).

Sandostatin
Novartis, Aust.; Novartis, Austral.; Novartis, Braz.; Novartis, Canad.; Novartis, Denm.; Novartis, Fin.; Novartis, Ger.; Novartis, Hong Kong; Novartis, Irl.; Novartis, Israel; Novartis, Norw.; Novartis, NZ; Novartis, S.Afr.; Novartis, Singapore; Novartis, Spain; Novartis, Swed.; Novartis, Thai.; Novartis, UK; Novartis, USA.
Octreotide (p.1292·1) or octreotide acetate (p.1291·2).
Acromegaly; AIDS-associated refractory diarrhoea; gastrointestinal endocrine tumours; prevention of complications following pancreatic surgery; variceal haemorrhage.

Sandostatina
Novartis, Ital.; Novartis, Mex.; Novartis, Port.
Octreotide (p.1292·1).
Acromegaly; gastrointestinal endocrine tumours; oesophageal haemorrhage; pancreatic fistulae; prevention of complications following pancreatic surgery; refractory diarrhoea associated with HIV infection.

Sandostatine
Novartis, Belg.; Novartis, Fr.; Novartis, Neth.; Novartis, Switz.
Octreotide (p.1292·1) or octreotide acetate (p.1291·2).
Acromegaly; complications following pancreatic surgery; external fistulae of the pancreas and small intestine; gastrointestinal neoplasms; refractory diarrhoea associated with HIV infection.

Sandothal *Sandoz, S.Afr.†.*
Thiopental sodium (p.1269·1).
General anaesthesia.

Sandovac *Novartis, Aust.*
An inactivated influenza vaccine (p.1544·3).
Active immunisation.

Sandoven *Novartis, Aust.*
Dihydroergocristine mesilate (p.1603·2); esculoside
(p.1574·1); rutoside (p.1611·2).
Thrombophlebitic disorders; venous insufficiency.

Sandoz Calcium-C *Novartis Consumer, S.Afr.*
Calcium lactate gluconate (p.1188·3); calcium carbon-
ate (p.1215·1); vitamin C (p.1389·3).
Vitamin C and calcium supplement.

Sandrena
*Organon, Austral.; Organon, Denm.; Organon, Ger.; Organon, Ital.;
Organon, Neth.; Pharmaco, NZ; Organon, Switz.; Organon, UK.*
Estradiol (p.1473·1).
Menopausal disorders; osteoporosis.

Sanein *Almirall, Spain.*
Aceclofenac (p.11·1).
*Musculoskeletal, joint, and peri-articular disorders;
pain.*

Sanelor *Chefaro, Belg.*
Loratadine (p.420·1).
Allergic rhinitis; urticaria.

Sangcya *Sangstat, UK†.*
Ciclosporin (p.518·1).
*Atopic dermatitis; graft-versus-host disease; nephrotic
syndrome; psoriasis; rheumatoid arthritis; transplant
rejection.*

Sangen Casa *Boots Healthcare, Ital.*
Liquid: Benzethonium chloride (p.1134·2); benzalko-
nium chloride (p.1133·2).
Spray: Orthophenylphenol (p.1152·1); benzalkonium
chloride (p.1133·2).
Surface disinfection.

Sangen Medical *Boots Healthcare, Ital.*
Benzalkonium chloride (p.1133·2).
Personal hygiene.

Sangen Sapone Disinfettante *Boots Healthcare, Ital.*
Triclocarban (p.1159·2).
Skin disinfection.

Sangenor *Mundipharma, Aust.*
Arginine aspartate (p.1354·1).
Tonic.

Sangerol *Novartis Consumer, Switz.*
Lignocaine [lidocaine] hydrochloride (p.1313·2); muramidase hydrochloride (p.1638·1); tyrothricin
(p.267·1).
Mouth and throat disorders.

Sangobion
Merck, Singapore; Merck, Thai.
Ferrous gluconate (p.1360·1); folic acid (p.1361·1); vi-
tamin B₁₂ (p.1388·1); minerals (p.1350·1).
Vitamin C (p.1389·3) is included in this preparation to
increase the absorption and availability of iron.
Anaemias.

Sangotone *Gemballa, Braz.*
Ferrous citrate; choline citrate; copper gluconate; vita-
min B substances (p.1350·1).
Iron deficiency; iron-deficiency anaemias.

Sanguisan N *Coradol, Ger.*
Homoeopathic preparation.

Sanguisorbis F *Madaus, Ger.*
Homoeopathic preparation.

Sangur-Test *Roche Diagnostics, Austral.*
Test for blood in urine.

Sanhelios 333 *Pharmacia Upjohn, Switz.*
Garlic (p.1614·1).
Atherosclerosis.

Sanhelios Capsules a la vitamine A *Pharmacia
Upjohn, Switz.*
Vitamin A palmitate (p.1383·2); wheat-germ oil.
Vitamin A deficiency.

Sanhelios Einschlaf *Bregenzer, Aust.*
Valerian root (p.1678·3); lupulus (p.1629·3).
Sleep disorders.

Sanhelios Leber-Galle *Bregenzer, Aust.*
Silybum marianum (p.1021·3); turmeric (p.1029·3).
Digestive disorders; hepatobiliary disorders.

Sanhelios Venen *Pharmacia Upjohn, Switz.*
Aesculus (p.1574·1).
Venous insufficiency.

Sanhelios-Entwasserungsdragees *Bregenzer, Aust.*
Silver birch (p.1585·2).
Urinary-tract disorders.

Sanicel *Squibb, Spain.*
Amphotericin B (p.377·2); tetracycline hydrochloride
(p.258·3).
Vulvovaginal infections.

Sanicolax *Sanico, Belg.†.*
Phenolphthalein (p.1244·1); podophyllum (p.1121·1);
aloin (p.1210·2); belladonna (p.463·1) hyoscyamus
(p.470·1); nux vomica (p.1643·1).
Constipation.

Sanicopyrine *Sanico, Belg.*
Paracetamol (p.71·2).
Fever; pain.

Sanieb *Puerto Galiano, Spain.*
Glycine (p.1365·3); arginine (p.1353·3); brassica oler-
acea.
Gastritis; gastrointestinal hyperacidity; peptic ulcer.

Sanifer *Esseti, Ital.*
Ferric sodium gluconate (p.1360·2).
Anaemias; oligohaemia in infants.

Saniflor Dentifricio *Esseti, Ital.*
Benzydamine hydrochloride (p.20·1).
Gingivitis.

Saniflor Vena *Esseti, Ital.*
Benzydamine hydrochloride (p.20·1).
Peripheral vascular disorders.

Sanifolin *Esseti, Ital.*
Calcium folinate (p.1363·1).
*Anaemias; antidote to folic acid antagonists; folate de-
ficiency; reduction of aminopterin and methotrexate
toxicity.*

Sanifug *Wolff, Ger.*
Loperamide hydrochloride (p.1231·3).
Diarrhoea.

Saniquiet *Sanitalia, Ital.*
Passion flower; tilia; birch; magnesium; lithium; manganese (p.1350·1).

Sani-Supp *G & W, USA.*
Glycerol (p.1616·3).
Constipation.

Sanivit *Scherer, Thai.*
Multivitamin and mineral preparation with procaine
hydrochloride, royal jelly, and lecithin (p.1350·1).

Sankombi *Sanum-Kehlbeck, Ger.*
Homoeopathic preparation.

Sanmigran *Novartis, Fr.*
Pizotifen malate (p.455·1).
Migraine.

Sano Tuss *Welti, Switz.*
Emetine hydrochloride (p.591·3); ethylmorphine hydrochloride (p.35·2); ephedrine hydrochloride
(p.1090·1); codeine phosphate (p.25·2); guaifenesin
(p.1092·2); cherry-laurel; tolu balsam (p.1101·3).
Catarrh; coughs.

Sanobamat *Sanico, Belg.†.*
Meprobamate (p.691·1).
Anxiety disorders; sleep disorders.

Sanoclorofila *Veafarm, Braz.*
Iodine (p.1522·3); salicylic acid (p.1122·3); menthol
(p.1632·3); chlorophyll (p.1028·1).
Fungal skin infections.

Sanodin *Byk Leo, Spain.*
Carbenoxolone sodium (p.1215·3).
Gingivitis; mouth ulcers.

Sanoformine *Mayoly-Spindler, Fr.†.*
Anhydrous copper sulfate (p.1358·1); sodium fluoride
(p.1375·3).
Disinfection of mucous membranes.

Sanogyl *Pharmascience, Fr.*
Pink toothpaste: Sodium monofluorophosphate
(p.1377·2); sodium fluoride (p.1375·3).
White toothpaste: Sodium fluoride (p.1375·3).
Formerly contained sodium fluoride and sodium
monofluorophosphate.
Oral hygiene.

Sanogyl Bianco *Berna, Ital.†.*
Sodium monofluorophosphate (p.1377·2); acetarsol
sodium (p.587·2).
Gingivitis; oral hygiene.

Sanogyl Fluo *Pharmascience, Fr.*
Sodium monofluorophosphate (p.1377·2); sodium flu-
oride (p.1375·3).
Dental caries prophylaxis.

Sanogyl Junior *Pharmascience, Fr.*
Sodium monofluorophosphate (p.1377·2); sodium flu-
oride (p.1375·3).
Dental caries prophylaxis.

Sanoma *Heilit, Ger.*
Carisoprodol (p.1327·1).
Skeletal muscle spasm.

Sanomigran
Novartis, Irl.; Novartis, UK.
Pizotifen malate (p.455·1).
Migraine and other vascular headaches.

Sanopinwern *Wernigerode, Ger.*
Eucalyptus oil (p.1609·2); oleum pini sylvestris.
Cold symptoms.

Sanor *Biolab, Thai.*
Dipotassium clorazepate (p.670·3).
Anxiety.

Sanoral
Note. This name is used for preparations of different composition.
Novartis, Aust.
Tyrothricin (p.267·1); muramidase hydrochloride
(p.1638·1); lignocaine [lidocaine] hydrochloride
(p.1313·2).
Mouth and throat inflammation.
Bioprogress, Ital.
Chlorhexidine gluconate (p.1138·2).
Mouth disinfection.

Sanorex
Novartis, Canad.; Sandoz, Jpn†; Novartis, Mex.; Novartis, USA†.
Mazindol (p.1510·3).
Obesity.

Sanostol *Schmidgall, Aust.*
Multivitamin preparation (p.1350·1).

Sanoxit *Galderma, Ger.*
Benzoyl peroxide (p.1111·1).
Acne.

Sanoyodo *Cinfa, Spain.*
Povidone-iodine (p.1155·1).
Skin and wound disinfection.

Sans-Acne *Galderma, Canad.*
Erythromycin (p.201·2); alcohol (p.1130·3).
Acne.

Sansacne *Galderma, Mex.*
Erythromycin (p.201·2).
Acne.

Sansanal *Rottapharm, Ger.*
Captopril (p.853·3).
Heart failure; hypertension.

Sansert
Novartis, Canad.; Novartis, USA.
Methysergide maleate (p.454·1).
Vascular headache.

Sansudor *Boehringer Ingelheim, Switz.*
Aluminium chlorohydrex (p.1110·2).
Hyperhidrosis; intertrigo.

Santa Flora S *Madaus, Ger.*
Homoeopathic preparation.

Santaherba
Homeocan, Canad.; Lehning, Fr.
Homoeopathic preparation.

Santalyt *Asche, Ger.*
Sodium chloride; glucose; potassium chloride; sodium
bicarbonate (p.1185·2).
Diarrhoea; oral rehydration therapy.

Santane A₄ *Iphym, Fr.*
Meadowsweet flowers (p.1631·2); black currant leaf;
salix leaf (p.82·1); heather flowers; orange leaf; juniper
berry (p.1625·2); chamomile flowers (p.1593·2); matricaria flowers; vervain leaf (p.1679·3).
Musculoskeletal disorders.

Santane C₆ *Iphym, Fr.*
Frangula bark (p.1227·1); senna leaf (p.1248·3); boldo
leaf (p.1585·3); vervain leaf (p.1679·3); peppermint
leaf (p.1243·2); mallow flowers; centaurea cyanus
flowers; pale rose flowers; caraway seed (p.1591·2).
Constipation.

Santane D₅ *Iphym, Fr.*
Melissa leaf (p.1632·2); origanum flowers; peppermint
leaf (p.1243·2); fennel seed (p.1610·1); aniseed
(p.1580·2); lupulus flowers (p.1629·3); matricaria
flowers (p.1593·2); thyme flowers (p.1672·2); rosemary leaf; caraway seed (p.1591·2); cinnamon bark
(p.1595·3).
Gastrointestinal disorders.

Santane F₁₀ *Iphym, Fr.*
Boldo leaf (p.1585·3); box leaf; peppermint leaf
(p.1243·2); tetragonum leaf; calendula flower
(p.1589·2); rosemary leaf; chamomile flower
(p.1593·2); caraway seed (p.1591·2); cinnamon bark
(p.1595·3).
Hepato-biliary insufficiency.

Santane H₇ *Iphym, Fr.*
Mistletoe leaf (p.1636·2); olive leaf; crataegus flower
and leaf (p.1600·2); melilot flower; calendula flower
(p.1589·2); myrtillus berry (p.1639·2); peppermint leaf
(p.1243·2); vervain leaf (p.1679·3); broom flower
(p.1661·2); fennel seed (p.1610·1); sweet orange peel.
Hypertension.

Santane N₉ *Iphym, Fr.*
Tilia flowers (p.1673·2); crataegus flowers and leaves
(p.1600·2); pale rose flowers; peppermint leaf
(p.1243·2); melissa leaf (p.1632·2); bitter-orange
leaves and buds; origanum flowers; lupulus flowers
(p.1629·3); lavender flowers (p.1627·2).
Nervous disorders.

Santane O₁ *Iphym, Fr.*
Heather flowers; bearberry leaf (p.1583·3); peppermint
leaf (p.1243·2); pulegium (p.1655·3); meadowsweet
flowers (p.1631·2); rosemary leaf; mallow flowers; tilia
flowers (p.1673·2); eucalyptus leaf (p.1609·2); laurel
leaf; caraway seed (p.1591·2); bitter orange leaves.
Nutritional disorders.

Santane R₈ *Iphym, Fr.*
Bearberry leaf (p.1583·3); heather flowers; black currant leaf; rosemary leaf; peppermint leaf (p.1243·2);
broom flowers (p.1661·2); lavender flowers (p.1627·2);
juniper berry (p.1625·2); thyme flowers (p.1672·2);
meadowsweet flowers (p.1631·2); cinnamon bark
(p.1595·3).
Kidney disorders.

Santane V₃ *Iphym, Fr.*
Artemisia leaf; peppermint leaf (p.1243·2); sage leaf
(p.1660·2); crataegus flowers and leaf (p.1600·2);
broom flowers (p.1661·2); green tea flowers
(p.1681·1); cupressus sempervirens leaf; melilotus officinalis flower and leaf; sweet orange peel (p.1644·2);
citrus aurantium leaf.
Vascular disorders.

Santasal N *Merckle, Ger.*
Aspirin (p.14·2).
Fever; pain.

Santasapina *Bioforce, Switz.*
Pine buds.
Upper-respiratory-tract disorders.

Santasapina V *Bioforce, Ger.*
Pine needle.
Catarrh.

Santax S *Asche, Ger.*
Saccharomyces boulardii (p.1626·3).
Diarrhoea.

Santenol *Coop. Farm., Ital.*
Lefetamine hydrochloride (p.49·3).
Lignocaine [lidocaine] hydrochloride (p.1313·2) is in-
cluded in this preparation to alleviate the pain of injec-
tion.
Pain.

Santussal *Novartis, Braz.*
Pimethixene (p.423·1); proxyphylline (p.770·1); am-
monium chloride (p.1085·2).
Coughs.

Santyl
Knoll, Canad.; Knoll, USA.
Collagenase (p.1598·2).
Debridement of dermal ulcers and severe burns.

Sanukehl D6 and D7 *Sanum-Kehlbeck, Ger.*
Homoeopathic preparation.

Sanutri Osseo *Novartis Nutrition, Port.†.*
Calcium-enriched nutritional supplement (p.1350·1).
Osteoporosis.

Sanuvis *Sanum-Kehlbeck, Ger.*
Homoeopathic preparation.

Sanvita Bronchial *Sanamed, Aust.*
Eucalyptus oil (p.1609·2); peppermint oil (p.1243·3);
thyme oil (p.1672·3).
Catarrh; coughs.

Sanvita Enerlecit *Sanamed, Aust.*
Lecithin; vitamins (p.1350·1).
Tonic.

Sanvita Enerlecit-Tonikum mit Rosmarin *San-
amed, Aust.†.*
Lecithin (p.1628·1); rosemary.
Tonic.

Sanvita Entschlackungstonikum *Strallhofer, Aust.†.*
Parsley (p.1648·3); silver birch (p.1585·2); ononis
(p.1644·1).
Diuresis.

Sanvita Herz *Sanamed, Aust.†.*
Crataegus (p.1600·2); rosemary.
Cardiovascular disorders.

Sanvita Leber-Galle *Sanamed, Aust.*
Cynara (p.1601·3); turmeric (p.1029·3); taraxacum
(p.1669·1).
Hepatobiliary disorders.

Sanvita Magen *Sanamed, Aust.*
Ginger (p.1227·2); caraway oil (p.1591·2); gentian root
(p.1615·1).
Dyspepsia; motion sickness; nausea; vomiting.

Sanvita Verdauungstropfen *Strallhofer, Aust.†.*
Peppermint leaf (p.1243·2); gentian root (p.1615·1);
caraway fruit (p.1591·2).
Gastrointestinal disorders.

Sanxon *Mayo, Mex.*
A multivitamin preparation (p.1350·1).

Sanyrene *Urgo, Fr.*
Barrier preparation.

Sanytol *Ideal, Fr.*
Permethrin (p.1436·1); phenothrin (p.1436·2); benzyl
benzoate (p.1428·2); didecyldimethylammonium chloride (p.1143·2); triclosan (p.1159·2).
Formerly contained bis(aminopropyl) lauryllamine and
permethrin.
House dust mite acaricide.

Sanzur *Aspen, S.Afr.*
Fluoxetine hydrochloride (p.284·2).
Anxiety disorders; bulimia nervosa; depression.

Sanzyme-S *Sankyo, Thai.*
Cellulase (p.1593·1); lipase; pancreatin (p.1646·1);
sanzyme-N.
Digestive disorders.

Sapec *Lichtwer, Ger.*
Garlic (p.1614·1).
Hyperlipidaemias.

Sapoderm
Note. This name is used for preparations of different composition.
Reckitt & Colman, Austral.
Triclosan (p.1159·2).
Skin cleansing.
Ingram & Bell, Canad.†.
Hexachlorophene (p.1146·1).
Antisepsis.

Sapresta *Taiho, Jpn.*
Aranidipine (p.841·2).
Hypertension.

Sapriken *Kener, Mex.*
Cisapride (p.1220·1).

Saquat *Ramini, Ital.*
Benzalkonium chloride (p.1133·2).
Disinfection of wounds and burns.

Sara *Nakorn, Thai.*
Paracetamol (p.71·2).
Fever; pain.

Sarafem *Lilly, USA.*
Fluoxetine hydrochloride (p.284·2).
Premenstrual dysphoric disorder.

Sarapin *High Chemical, USA.*
Sarracenia purpurea distillate (p.82·3).
Neuromuscular or neuralgic pain.

Saratoga *Blair, USA.*
Zinc oxide (p.1128·2); boric acid (p.1586·1); eucalyp-
tol (p.1609·2); peru balsam (p.1650·2).
Minor skin irritation.

Sarcoderma *Produfarma, Port.*
Lindane (p.1434·1).
Pediculosis; scabies.

Sarcoton *Medley, Braz.*
Disulfiram (p.1605·1); metronidazole (p.594·1).
Alcoholism.

Sarf *Julphar, UAE.*
Ciprofloxacin hydrochloride (p.182·3).
Bacterial infections.

Sargenor
Sarget, Fr.; Asta Medica, Ital.; Asta Medica, Port.; Asta Medica, Spain.
Arginine aspartate (p.1354·1).
Tonic.

Sargenor a la Vitamine C Sarget, Fr.
Arginine aspartate (p.1354·1); vitamin C (p.1389·3).
Tonic.

Sargepirine Asta Medica, Fr.†
Aspirin (p.14·2).
Glycine (p.1365·3) is included in this preparation in an attempt to limit adverse effects on the gastrointestinal mucosa.
Fever; pain.

Saridine Atlantic, Thai.
Sulfasalazine (p.1251·1).
Ulcerative colitis.

Saridon
Note.This name is used for preparations of different composition.
Roche, Aust.; Roche, Belg.; Roche, Braz.; Roche Nicholas, Ger.; Roche, Hong Kong; Roche, Ital.; Roche Consumer, Neth.; Roche Nicholas, Spain; Roche, Switz.
Paracetamol (p.71·2); propyphenazone (p.80·2); caffeine (p.761·3).
Fever; pain.

Roche, Mex.
Paracetamol (p.71·2); caffeine (p.761·3).
Fever; pain.

Roche, Thai.
Paracetamol (p.71·2).
Fever; pain.

Saridon N Roche, Port.
Paracetamol (p.71·2); propyphenazone (p.80·2); caffeine (p.761·3).
Pain.

Sarilen Normon, Spain.
Roxatidine acetate (p.1248·2).
Gastro-oesophageal reflux; peptic ulcer.

Sarna
Stiefel, Austral.; Stiefel, Singapore; Stiefel, Thai.
Camphor (p.1589·3); menthol (p.1632·3); phenol (p.1152·3).
Dry skin; pruritus.

Sarna Anti-Itch Stiefel, USA.
Camphor (p.1589·3); menthol (p.1632·3).
Poison ivy; poison oak; pruritus; sunburn.

Sarna HC Stiefel, Canad.
Hydrocortisone (p.1073·3).
Skin disorders.

Sarna-P Stiefel, Canad.
Pramocaine hydrochloride (p.1318·2); camphor (p.1589·3); menthol (p.1632·3).
Skin irritation.

Sarnapin Dovalle, Braz.
Lindane (p.1434·1).
Pediculosis; scabies.

Sarnigal QIF, Braz.
Benzyl benzoate (p.1428·2).
Pediculosis; scabies.

Sarnisan Eurofarma, Braz.
Benzyl benzoate (p.1428·2).
Pediculosis; scabies.

Sarnodex Bunker, Braz.
Benzyl benzoate (p.1428·2).
Pediculosis; scabies.

Sarnol Stiefel, Fr.
Camphor (p.1589·3); menthol (p.1632·3).
Skin disorders.

Saroten
Lundbeck, Aust.; Lundbeck, Denm.; Lundbeck, Fin.; Bayer, Ger.; Lundbeck, S.Afr.; Lundbeck, Swed.; Lundbeck, Switz.
Amitriptyline hydrochloride (p.273·3).
Depression; insomnia; nocturnal enuresis; pain.

Sarotex
Lundbeck, Neth.; Lundbeck, Norw.
Amitriptyline hydrochloride (p.273·3).
Depression; nocturnal enuresis; pain.

Sarpiol INQ, Braz.
Lindane (p.1434·1).
Pediculosis; scabies.

Sarpul Toyama, Jpn.
Aniracetam (p.1580·2).
Cerebral infarction.

Sarsaparol Uro Madaus, Ger.
Homoeopathic preparation.

Sarsapsor Ysatfabrik, Ger.†
Sarsaparilla (p.1661·1).
Psoriasis.

Sartol Stiefel, Spain.
Menthol (p.1632·3); camphor (p.1589·3).
Insect bites; pruritus; urticaria.

SAS ICN, Canad.
Sulfasalazine (p.1251·1).
Ulcerative colitis.

Saspryl Inibsa, Spain.
Aspirin (p.14·2).
Fever; musculoskeletal, joint and peri-articular disorders; pain; thromboembolism prophylaxis.

Sastid
Note.This name is used for preparations of different composition.
Stiefel, Canad.; Stiefel, Hong Kong; Stiefel, Mex.; Stiefel, S.Afr.; Stiefel, Singapore; Stiefel, Thai.
Sulfur (p.1123·3); salicylic acid (p.1122·3).
Acne; pityriasis versicolor; seborrhoea.

Stiefel, USA.
Precipitated sulfur (p.1123·3).
Formerly contained precipitated sulfur and salicylic acid.

Sasulen Faes, Spain.
Piroxicam (p.79·1).
Gout; musculoskeletal, joint, peri-articular, and soft-tissue disorders; pain.

Satedon Protein, Mex.
Azathioprine (p.509·3).

Satinique Anti-Dandruff Amway, Canad.
Pyrithione zinc (p.1122·1).

Sativol Boiron, Canad.
Homoeopathic preparation.

Saugella Salviettine Guieu, Ital.
Sage (p.1660·2); lactic acid (p.1626·2).
Personal hygiene.

Saugella Uomo Guieu, Ital.
Helichrysum italicum; clove (p.1596·3).
Male personal hygiene.

Sauran Abello, Spain.
Citicoline (p.1596·1) or citicoline sodium (p.1596·1).
Cerebrovascular disorders.

Savacol Mouth and Throat Rinse Colgate Oral Care, Austral.
Chlorhexidine gluconate (p.1138·2).
Minor oral infections; mouth ulcers.

Savarine AstraZeneca, Fr.
Proguanil hydrochloride (p.441·3); chloroquine phosphate (p.432·3).
Malaria.

Savecal Ibirn, Ital.
Calcium carbonate (p.1215·1).
Calcium deficiency; calcium supplement.

Saventrine
Pharmax, Hong Kong; Pharmax, Irl.; Restan, S.Afr.†; Pharmax, Singapore; Pharmax, UK.
Isoprenaline hydrochloride (p.914·3).
Bradycardia; cardiogenic or endotoxic shock; evaluation of congenital heart defects; heart block; Stokes-Adams syndrome.

Savex Sabex, Canad.
Camphor (p.1589·3); menthol (p.1632·3).

Savex 15 Sabex, Canad.
SPF 15: Octinoxate (p.1517·3); oxybenzone (p.1518·1); camphor (p.1589·3).
Sunscreen.

Savex with PABA Sabex, Canad.
Padimate O (p.1518·2); camphor (p.1589·3); menthol (p.1632·3); salicylic acid (p.1122·3).
Sunscreen.

Savex Sunblock Sabex, Canad.
SPF 15: Padimate O (p.1518·2); oxybenzone (p.1518·1).
Sunscreen.

Savex with Sunscreen Sabex, Canad.
Camphor (p.1589·3); menthol (p.1632·3); salicylic acid (p.1122·3).
Sunscreen.

Savior Abic, Israel.
Chlorhexidine gluconate (p.1138·2); cetrimide (p.1137·1).
Burns; skin disinfection; wounds.

Savlodil AstraZeneca, Canad.
Cetrimide (p.1137·1); chlorhexidine gluconate (p.1138·2).
Wound disinfection.

Savlon
Note.This name is used for preparations of different composition.
AstraZeneca, Canad.; Novartis Consumer, Irl.; Boots, NZ; Zeneca, Port.; Pharmedica, S.Afr.; Johnson & Johnson, Singapore.
Cetrimide (p.1137·1); chlorhexidine gluconate (p.1138·2).
Formerly known as Savlon Hospital Concentrate in Canad.
Burns; disinfection; wounds.

Whitehall-Robins, Canad.†
Cetrimide (p.1137·1).
Skin disorders.

Savlon Antiseptic Boots, Austral.
Cream; topical liquid: Cetrimide (p.1137·1); chlorhexidine (p.1138·2).
Skin abrasions; wounds.

Topical powder; liquid treatment: Povidone-iodine (p.1155·1).
Burns; fungal skin infections; skin abrasions; wounds.

Savlon Concentrated Antiseptic Novartis Consumer, UK.
Cetrimide (p.1137·1); chlorhexidine gluconate (p.1138·2).
Skin disinfection.

Savlon Cream Novartis Consumer, UK.
Cetrimide (p.1137·1); chlorhexidine gluconate (p.1138·2).
Skin disinfection.

Savlon Dry Novartis Consumer, UK.
Povidone-iodine (p.1155·1).
Skin disinfection.

Savlon Natural Antiseptic Novartis Consumer, UK.
Melaleuca oil (p.1631·3).
Skin irritation.

Savlon Natural First Aid for Bruises Novartis Consumer, UK.
Arnica (p.1581·3).
Bruises.

Savlon Natural First Aid for Burns Novartis Consumer, UK.
Calendula (p.1589·2); echinacea (p.1606·2); hypericum (p.290·2); urtica (p.1678·2).
Burns.

Savlon Natural First Aid for Cuts & Sores Novartis Consumer, UK.
Calendula (p.1589·2); hypericum (p.290·2).
Minor wounds.

Savlon Natural First Aid for Insect Bites & Stings Novartis Consumer, UK.
Hypericum (p.290·2); yellow dock (p.1681·3); echinacea angustifolia (p.1606·2); ledum palustre; calendula (p.1589·2); arnica (p.1581·3); pyrethrum (p.1436·3).
Insect bites and stings.

Savlon Wound Wash Novartis Consumer, UK.
Chlorhexidine gluconate (p.1138·2).
Formerly known as Savlon Junior.
Skin disinfection.

Savoral Novartis Nutrition, Fr.
Preparation for enteral nutrition (p.1350·1).

Savorix T Cesam, Port.
Piroctone olamine (p.1121·1); sulfur (p.1123·3).
Dandruff; seborrhoeic dermatitis.

Sayomol Cinfa, Spain†.
Promethazine hydrochloride (p.423·2).
Cutaneous hypersensitivity reactions.

SBOB Nadon, Thai.
Loperamide hydrochloride (p.1231·3).
Diarrhoea.

SC-300 Hamilton, Austral.
Coconut oil derivatives.
Barrier cream; skin cleansing.

Scabecid Stiefel, Fr.
Lindane (p.1434·1).
Pediculosis; scabies.

Scabene
Note.This name is used for preparations of different composition.
Medican, Canad.
Esdepallethrine (p.1432·2); piperonyl butoxide (p.1436·2).
Scabies.

Stiefel, Mex.
Lindane (p.1434·1).

Scabicin
Fischer, Israel; Cosmofarma, Port.†
Crotamiton (p.1112·3).
Pruritus; scabies.

Scabiex Rekah, Israel.
Benzyl benzoate (p.1428·2).
Scabies.

Scabisan Chinoin, Mex.
Lindane (p.1434·1).
Pediculosis; scabies.

Scabisan Plus Chinoin, Mex.
Lindane (p.1434·1); benzyl benzoate (p.1428·2).
Scabies.

Scadan Miles, USA.
Trimethyltetradecylammonium bromide (p.1137·2); stearyl dimethyl benzyl ammonium chloride.
Seborrhoea.

Scaflam Schering-Plough, Braz.
Nimesulide (p.62·3).
Fever; inflammation; pain.

Scalid Uniao Quimica, Braz.
Nimesulide (p.62·3).
Fever; inflammation; pain.

Scalpicin
Note.This name is used for preparations of different composition.
Combe, Ital.
Hydrocortisone (p.1073·3); menthol (p.1632·3).
Skin irritation.

Combe, USA.
Salicylic acid (p.1122·3); menthol (p.1632·3).
Formerly contained hydrocortisone, and menthol.

Scalpicin Anti-Dandruff Anti-Itch Coombe, Canad.
Menthol (p.1632·3); salicylic acid (p.1122·3).

Scalpicin Capilar Combe, Spain.
Hydrocortisone (p.1073·3).
Skin disorders.

Scalpvit Kemiprogress, Ital.
Vitamins, selenium, yeast, and amino acids (p.1350·1).
Nutritional supplement.

Scandicain
Astra, Aust.; Astra, Ger.; Astra, Switz.
Mepivacaine hydrochloride (p.1317·1).
Adrenaline [epinephrine] acid tartrate (p.829·2) is included in some injections as a vasoconstrictor to diminish absorption and localise the effect of the local anaesthetic.
Local anaesthesia.

Scandicaine
Astra, Belg.; Astra, Neth.
Mepivacaine hydrochloride (p.1317·1).
Adrenaline [epinephrine] acid tartrate (p.829·2) is included in some injections as a vasoconstrictor to diminish absorption and localise the effect of the local anaesthetic.
Local anaesthesia.

Scandine
Zambon, Belg.; Zambon, Ital.; Zambon, Port.
Ibopamine hydrochloride (p.912·1).
Heart failure.

Scandinibsa
Inibsa, Port.; Inibsa, Spain.
Mepivacaine hydrochloride (p.1317·1).
Adrenaline [epinephrine] (p.829·1) or adrenaline [epinephrine] acid tartrate (p.829·2) is included in some injections as a vasoconstrictor to diminish absorption and localise the effect of the local anaesthetic.
Local anaesthesia.

Scandishake
Nutricia, Fin.; Scientific Hospital Supplies, Irl.; Scandipharm, Israel; Scientific Hospital Supplies, UK.
Preparation for enteral nutrition (p.1350·1).

Scandonest
Austrodent, Aust.; Dentsply, Austral.; Septodont, Denm.; Ogna, Ital.; Dental Warehouse, S.Afr.; Septodont, Switz.
Mepivacaine hydrochloride (p.1317·1).
Adrenaline [epinephrine] (p.829·1) or noradrenaline [norepinephrine] acid tartrate (p.948·2) is included in some injections as a vasoconstrictor to diminish absorption and localise the effect of the local anaesthetic.
Local anaesthesia.

Scannotrast Gerot, Aust.
Barium sulfate (p.1477·2).
Radiographic contrast medium for CT scanning.

Scavenger Aesculapius, Ital.
Glutathione (p.1010·3).
Alcohol or drug poisoning; ionising radiation trauma.

SCF Searle, Austral.†
Sucralfate (p.1250·2).
Peptic ulcers.

Schamill Ritsert, Ger.
Achillea (p.1572·2).
Dyspepsia.

Scheinpharm Artificial Tears Schein, Canad.
Polyvinyl alcohol (p.1503·1).

Scheinpharm Artificial Tears Plus Schein, Canad.
Polyvinyl alcohol (p.1503·1); povidone (p.1503·2).

Scheinpharm Testone-Cyp Schein, Canad.†
Testosterone cipionate (p.1492·1).
Androgen.

Scheinpharm Triamcine-A Schein, Canad.†
Triamcinolone acetonide (p.1080·1).
Corticosteroid.

Scheribase Schering, Port.
Emollient.
Pharmaceutical diluent; skin disorders.

Schericur
Schering, Aust.; Schering, Spain.
Hydrocortisone (p.1073·3).
Skin disorders.

Scheriderm Schering, Mex.
Diflucortolone valerate (p.1069·3); isoconazole nitrate (p.387·2); neomycin sulfate (p.228·1).
Infected skin disorders.

Schering Base Schering, Canad.
Emollient.
Dry skin; topical diluent.

Schering PC4 Schering, UK†.
Norgestrel (p.1486·1); ethinylestradiol (p.1476·2).
Postcoital oral contraceptive.

Scheriproct
Note.This name is used for preparations of different composition.
Schering, Aust.; Schering, Ger.; Asche, Ger.; Schering, Irl.; Schering, Mex.; Schering, Norw.; Schering, Port.; Schering, S.Afr.; Schering, Switz.; Schering, UK.
Prednisolone caproate (p.1078·1); cinchocaine hydrochloride (p.1309·1).
Formerly contained prednisolone caproate, clemizole undecylate, and cinchocaine hydrochloride.
Anorectal disorders.

Schering, Austral.; Schering, Belg.; Schering, Fin.; Schering, Thai.
Prednisolone caproate (p.1078·1); cinchocaine hydrochloride (p.1309·1); clemizole undecylate (p.413·3).
Anorectal disorders.

Schering, Spain.
Prednisolone (p.1077·3); cinchocaine hydrochloride (p.1309·1); menthol (p.1632·3).
Anorectal disorders.

Scheriproct N Schering, Swed.
Prednisolone caproate (p.1078·1); cinchocaine hydrochloride (p.1309·1).
Anorectal disorders.

Scherogel
Schering, Aust.; Schering, Belg.; Asche, Ger.; Schering, Ital.
Benzoyl peroxide (p.1111·1).
Acne.

Schias-Amaro Medicinale AFOM, Ital.
Rhubarb (p.1248·1); boldo (p.1585·3); cascara (p.1216·1).
Constipation; digestive disorders.

Schiwalys Hemofiltration Althin, Swed.
Electrolyte solution for haemofiltration (p.1184·1).
Some solutions also contain glucose.

Schlaf- und Nerventee Bad Heilbrunner, Ger.
Valerian (p.1678·3); melissa (p.1632·2); lupulus (p.1629·3).
Nervous disorders.

SchlafTabs Ratiopharm, Ger.
Doxylamine succinate (p.417·1).
Sleep disorders.

Schlehepar N Hanosan, Ger.
Homoeopathic preparation.

Schleimhaut-Komplex Ho-Fu-Complex Liebermann, Ger.
Homoeopathic preparation.

The symbol † denotes a preparation no longer actively marketed

Schmerz-Dolgit *Dolorgiet, Ger.*
Ibuprofen (p.43·2).
Fever; pain; rheumatism.

Schneckensaft N *Hotz, Ger.†*
Thyme (p.1672·2); castanea vulgaris; limacin.
Bronchitis; coughs.

Schneckensirup *Alsitan, Ger.*
Alfalfa (p.1574·3); thyme (p.1672·2).
Cold symptoms.

schnupfen endrine *Asche, Ger.*
Xylometazoline hydrochloride (p.1102·2).
Nasal congestion.

Scholl Athlete's Foot *SSL, UK.*
Tolnaftate (p.395·2).
Tinea pedis.

Scholl Athlete's Foot Preparations *Schering-Plough, Canad.*
Tolnaftate (p.395·2).
Tinea pedis.

Scholl Callous Removal *SSL, UK.*
Salicylic acid (p.1122·3).
Calluses.

Scholl Callus Remover *Schering-Plough, Canad.*
Salicylic acid (p.1122·3).
Calluses; corns.

Scholl Clear Away *Schering-Plough, Canad.*
Salicylic acid (p.1122·3).
Warts.

Scholl Corn & Callous Removal Liquid *SSL, UK.*
Salicylic acid (p.1122·3); camphor (p.1589·3).
Calluses; corns.

Scholl Corn, Callus Plaster Preparation *Schering-Plough, Canad.†*
Salicylic acid (p.1122·3).
Calluses; corns.

Scholl Corn Removal *SSL, UK.*
Salicylic acid (p.1122·3).
Corns.

Scholl Corn Remover *Schering-Plough, Canad.*
Salicylic acid (p.1122·3).
Calluses; corns.

Scholl Corn Salve *Schering-Plough, Canad.†*
Salicylic acid (p.1122·3).
Calluses; corns.

Scholl Corn/Callous Removers *Scholl, Israel.*
Salicylic acid (p.1122·3).
Corns.

Scholl 2-Drop Corn Remedy *Schering-Plough, Canad.*
Salicylic acid (p.1122·3).
Calluses; corns.

Scholl Dry Antiperspirant Foot Spray *Schering-Plough, Canad.*
Aluminium chlorohydrate (p.1110·2).
Foot odour; foot perspiration.

Scholl One Step *Schering-Plough, Canad.*
Salicylic acid (p.1122·3).
Calluses; corns; warts.

Scholl Seal & Heal *SSL, UK.*
Salicylic acid (p.1122·3); camphor (p.1589·3).
Verrucas.

Scholl Verucca Removal *SSL, UK.*
Salicylic acid (p.1122·3).
Warts.

Scholl Wart Remover *Schering-Plough, Canad.*
Salicylic acid (p.1122·3).
Warts.

Scholl Zino *Scholl, Canad.*
Salicylic acid (p.1122·3).
Corns.

Schoolife *Lifeplan, UK.*
Multinutrient preparation (p.1350·1).

Schoum *Pharmygiene, Fr.*
Fumitory (p.1612·3); ononis (p.1644·1); Jamaica dogwood (p.1625·1); sorbitol (p.1377·3); alverine citrate (p.1211·3).
Gastrointestinal and kidney disorders.

Schrundensalbe Dermi-cyl *Liebermann, Ger.*
Salicylic acid (p.1122·3).
Skin disorders.

Schufen *Kenyaku, Thai.*
Ibuprofen (p.43·2).
Fever; inflammation; pain.

Schupps Baldrian Sedativbad *Schupp, Ger.†*
Valerian (p.1678·3); valerian oil; citronella oil (p.1596·3); lupulus (p.1629·3).
Bath additive; nervous disorders; sleep disorders.

Schupps Fichte-Menthol Olbad *Schupp, Ger.†*
Norway spruce oil; eucalyptus oil (p.1609·2); menthol (p.1632·3).
Bath additive; catarrh.

Schupps Heilkrauter Erkaltungsbad *Schupp, Ger.*
Eucalyptus oil (p.1609·2); thyme oil (p.1672·3); peppermint oil (p.1243·3).
Bath additive; cold symptoms.

Schupps Heilkrauter Rheumabad *Schupp, Ger.*
Methyl salicylate (p.55·1); camphor (p.1589·3); rosemary oil (p.1659·3); Norway spruce oil; sage oil (p.1660·2); juniper oil (p.1625·2).
Bath additive; musculoskeletal and joint disorders.

Schupps Kohlensaurebad *Schupp, Ger.*
Sodium bicarbonate (p.1186·2); aluminium sulfate (p.1578·2).
Bath additive; circulatory disorders; hypertension.

Schupps Latschenkiefer Olbad *Schupp, Ger.†*
Pumilio pine oil (p.1656·3); pine-needle oil; Norway spruce oil; turpentine oil (p.1676·3); juniper oil (p.1625·2).
Bath additive; musculoskeletal and joint disorders; nervous disorders.

Schupps Melissen Olbad *Schupp, Ger.*
Citronella oil (p.1596·3).
Bath additive; nervous disorders.

Schwarze-Salbe *Lichtenstein, Ger.†*
Ichthammol (p.1115·2).
Skin disorders.

Schwarzwalder Heublumen-Extrakt *Schupp, Ger.*
Hay flowers.
Rheumatism.

Schwedenjorg mild *Mayrhofer, Aust.†*
Aloes (p.1210·1); angelica root (p.1580·2); gentian root (p.1615·1); imperatoria root; galanga root; zedoary root; rosemary leaf; nutmeg (p.1643·1).
Gastrointestinal disorders.

Schwedentrunk *Infirmarius-Rovit, Ger.†*
Aloes (p.1210·1); senna (p.1248·2); manna (p.1233·3); myrrh (p.1639·2); angelica (p.1580·2); carlina; gentian (p.1615·1); zedoary; camphor (p.1589·3); saffron (p.1029·1); theriacale; vitamin C (p.1389·3).
Gastrointestinal disorders.

Schwedentrunk der Echte Elixier *Infirmarius-Rovit, Ger.*
Angelica (p.1580·2); gentian (p.1615·1); cardamom fruit (p.1591·3); cinnamon (p.1595·3); valerian (p.1678·3).
Digestive-system disorders.

Schwedentrunk mit Ginseng *Infirmarius-Rovit, Ger.†*
Aloes (p.1210·1); senna (p.1248·2); manna (p.1233·3); myrrh (p.1639·2); angelica (p.1580·2); carlina; gentian (p.1615·1); zedoary; camphor (p.1589·3); saffron (p.1029·1); theriacale; vitamin C (p.1389·3); ginseng (p.1615·3).
Gastrointestinal disorders.

Schwefelbad Dr Klopfer
Note. This name is used for preparations of different composition.
Austroplant, Aust.; Protina, Ger.
Sulfur (p.1123·3); sodium thiosulfate (p.1024·2).
Bath additive; musculoskeletal and joint disorders; skin disorders.

Protina, Switz.†
Zinc sulfide; sodium sulfite (p.1157·2); sodium bisulfite (p.1157·2); colloidal sulfur (p.1123·3); pine oil; turpentine oil (p.1676·3).
Formerly known as Bain Soufre du Dr Klopfer.
Circulatory disorders; hyperhidrosis; musculoskeletal and joint disorders; skin disorders.

Schwefelbad-Saar *CPF, Ger.*
Sulfurated potash (p.1124·1).
Bath additive; rheumatic disorders; skin disorders.

Schwefel-Diasporal *Protina, Ger.*
Cream: Sulfur (p.1123·3).

Topical solution: Sulfur (p.1123·3); camphor (p.1589·3).
Skin disorders.

Schwohepan S *Schworer, Ger.*
Silybum marianum (p.1021·3); greater celandine (p.1618·1).
Biliary and gastrointestinal spasm; liver disorders.

Schwoneural *Schworer, Ger.*
Homoeopathic preparation.

Schworocard *Schworer, Ger.*
Homoeopathic preparation.

Schworocor *Schworer, Ger.*
Homoeopathic preparation.

Schworosin *Schworer, Ger.*
Homoeopathic preparation.

Schworotox *Schworer, Ger.*
Homoeopathic preparation.

Sciargo *Potter's, UK.*
Shepherd's purse (p.1662·3); wild carrot (p.1680·3); clivers (p.1596·3); bearberry (p.1583·3); juniper berry oil (p.1625·2).
Lumbago; sciatica.

Scillacor *Steigerwald, Ger.*
Homoeopathic preparation.

Scillase N *Ziethen, Ger.*
Squill (p.1100·3).
Heart failure; kidney disorders.

Scintadren *Nycomed Amersham, UK.*
Selenium-75 (p.1451·1) in the form of 6β-(methyl(^{75}Se)seleno)methyl-19-norcholest-5(10)-en-3β-ol.
Adrenal gland imaging.

Sciroppo Berta *Berta, Ital.*
Liquorice (p.1231·2); sulfogaiacol (p.1101·1).
Catarrh; coughs.

Sciroppo Fenoglio *AFOM, Ital.*
Ferric ammonium citrate (p.1359·2).
Anaemias.

Sciroppo Merck all'Efetonina *Bracco, Ital.*
Racephedrine hydrochloride (Efetonina) (p.1090·3); thyme (p.1672·2).
Coughs; respiratory-tract disorders.

Scitropin *Biotechnology, Singapore.*
Somatropin (p.1286·1).
Growth hormone deficiency; Turner's syndrome.

Sclane *Llorente, Spain.*
Betamethasone acetate (p.1063·1); betamethasone sodium phosphate (p.1063·2).
Corticosteroid.

Scleramin *Ibirn, Ital.*
Vinburnine phosphate (p.1680·1).
Cerebrovascular disorders.

Scleremo *Therica, Fr.*
Chrome alum (p.1594·2); glycerol (p.1616·3).
Varicose veins.

Scleril *AGIPS, Ital.*
Fenofibrate (p.889·1).
Hyperlipidaemias.

Sclerocalcine *Lehning, Fr.*
Homoeopathic preparation.

Scleromate *Palisades, USA.*
Sodium morrhuate (p.1666·1).
Varicose veins.

Sclerovein *Resinag, Switz.*
Lauromacrogol 600 (p.1345·2); alcohol (p.1130·3).
Variceal sclerosis.

S-Coaltar *Ducray, Fr.†*
Coal tar (p.1125·1); salicylic acid (p.1122·3).
Dandruff.

Scoline
DBL, Austral.; Glaxo Wellcome, S.Afr.; Medeva, UK†.
Suxamethonium chloride (p.1340·1).
Depolarising neuromuscular blocker.

Scolybil *Windson, Braz.*
Acetylmethionine; choline citrate (p.1356·3); sorbitol (p.1377·3).
Liver disorders.

Scopace *Hope, USA.*
Hyoscine hydrobromide (p.468·2).
Parkinsonism.

Scopas *Asian Pharm, Thai.*
Hyoscine butylbromide (p.468·2).
Gastro-duodenitis; nausea and vomiting; peptic ulcer; smooth muscle spasm.

Scope
Note. This name is used for preparations of different composition.
Procter & Gamble, Canad.
Cetylpyridinium chloride (p.1138·1); domiphen bromide (p.1143·3).
Formerly known as Scope with Oraseptate.
Oral hygiene.

Procter & Gamble, USA.
Cetylpyridinium chloride (p.1138·1).
Minor mouth or throat irritation.

Scopex *Propan, S.Afr.; Restan, S.Afr.*
Hyoscine butylbromide (p.468·2).
Dysmenorrhoea; smooth muscle spasm.

Scopex Co *Propan, S.Afr.†*
Hyoscine butylbromide (p.468·2); dipyrone (p.34·1).
Gastrointestinal spasm; urinary-tract spasm.

Scopinal *Julphar, UAE.*
Hyoscine butylbromide (p.468·2).
Smooth muscle spasm.

Scopoderm
Novartis, Aust.; Novartis, Denm.; Novartis, Fin.; Novartis, Norw.; Novartis, Swed.
Hyoscine (p.468·2).
Motion sickness.

Scopoderm TTS
Novartis, Fr.; Novartis, Ger.; Novartis Consumer, Neth.; Novartis, NZ; Ciba-Geigy, S.Afr.†; Novartis Nutrition, Singapore; Novartis, Switz.; Novartis Consumer, UK.
Hyoscine (p.468·2).
Intractable cough in terminal illness; motion sickness.

Scorbex *Aspen Consumer, S.Afr.*
Vitamin C (p.1389·3).
Vitamin C deficiency.

Scordal *Kattwiga, Ger.*
Capsules: Herba teucrii.

Oral drops: Herba teucrii; magnesium chloride (p.1190·3).
Cardiovascular disorders; gastrointestinal disorders.

Scorotox *Kattwiga, Ger.*
Homoeopathic preparation.

Scottopect *Nycomed, Aust.*
Gel: Turpentine oil (p.1676·3); eucalyptus oil (p.1609·2); thyme oil (p.1672·3); menthol (p.1632·3); camphor (p.1589·3).

Oral drops: Thyme (p.1672·2).

Oral liquid: Thyme (p.1672·2); wild thyme; plantago lanceolata.
Bronchitis; catarrh.

Scott's Cod Liver *SmithKline Beecham, Thai.*
Vitamins A and D (p.1350·1).

Scott's Emulsion
Note. This name is used for preparations of different composition.
SmithKline Beecham Consumer, UK.
Cod-liver oil (p.1357·2); calcium hypophosphite; sodium hypophosphite.

SmithKline Beecham, USA.
Vitamins A and D (p.1350·1).

Scott's Emulsion Orange *SmithKline Beecham, Hong Kong.*
Cod-liver oil (p.1357·2); calcium hypophosphite.
Dietary supplement.

Scott's Emulsion Original *SmithKline Beecham, Hong Kong.*
Cod-liver oil; capelin oil; calcium hypophosphite; sodium hypophosphite (p.1350·1).
Dietary supplement.

Scot-Tussin Allergy *Scot-Tussin, USA.*
Diphenhydramine hydrochloride (p.416·1).

Scot-Tussin DM *Scot-Tussin, USA.*
Chlorpheniramine [chlorphenamine] maleate (p.412·1); dextromethorphan hydrobromide (p.1087·3).
Coughs and cold symptoms.

Scot-Tussin DM Cough Chasers *Scot-Tussin, USA.*
Dextromethorphan hydrobromide (p.1087·3).
Coughs.

Scot-Tussin Expectorant *Scot-Tussin, USA.*
Guaifenesin (p.1092·2).
Coughs.

Scot-Tussin Original 5-Action *Scot-Tussin, USA.*
Phenylephrine hydrochloride (p.1097·1); pheniramine maleate (p.422·3); sodium citrate (p.1186·2); sodium salicylate (p.84·2); caffeine citrate (p.761·3).
Upper respiratory-tract symptoms.

Scot-Tussin Senior Clear *Scot-Tussin, USA.*
Guaifenesin (p.1092·2); dextromethorphan hydrobromide (p.1087·3).
Coughs.

SCR *Pickles, UK.*
Salicylic acid (p.1122·3).
Cradle cap.

Scriptogesic *Propan, S.Afr.†*
Paracetamol (p.71·2); codeine phosphate (p.25·2); caffeine (p.761·3); meprobamate (p.691·1).
Pain.

Scriptolyte *Propan, S.Afr.*
Potassium chloride; sodium chloride; sodium citrate; glucose (p.1185·2).
Diarrhoea; oral rehydration therapy.

Scripto-Metic *Propan, S.Afr.*
Prochlorperazine maleate (p.701·2).
Anxiety disorders; migraine; nausea and vomiting; vestibular disorders.

Scriptopam *Propan, S.Afr.†*
Diazepam (p.674·3).
Alcohol withdrawal syndrome; anxiety; premedication.

Scriptozone *Pharmagen, S.Afr.†*
Phenylbutazone (p.78·1).
Ankylosing spondylitis.

Scullcap & Gentian Tablets *Dorwest, UK.*
Skullcap (p.1664·3); valerian (p.1678·3); vervain (p.1679·3); gentian (p.1615·1).
Anxiety; insomnia; irritability.

SD-Hermal *Hermal, Ger.*
Clotrimazole (p.382·1).
Pityriasis versicolor; seborrhoeic dermatitis.

SDL *Bencard, Ger.*
Allergen extracts (p.1575·3).
Hyposensitisation.

SDV *Teomed, Switz.*
Pollen allergen extracts (p.1575·3).
Hyposensitisation.

Sea Breeze *Bristol-Myers Squibb, Canad.†*
Alcohol (p.1130·3); camphor (p.1589·3); benzoic acid (p.1134·2).
Skin cleansing.

Sea-Cal *Bioceuticals, UK.*
Calcium carbonate (p.1215·1).

Seacor *SPA, Ital.*
Omega-3 triglycerides (p.949·2).
Hypertriglyceridaemia.

Sealdin *Lacer, Spain.*
Sertraline hydrochloride (p.308·3).
Depression; obsessive-compulsive disorder; panic disorder.

Sea-Legs
Boots, NZ; SSL, UK.
Meclozine hydrochloride (p.420·3).
Motion sickness.

Seale's Lotion *C & M, USA.*
Sulfur (p.1123·3); borax (p.1586·1); zinc oxide (p.1128·2).
Acne.

Seal-On *Beta Healthcare, UK.*
Calcium oxidised cellulose (p.728·2); sodium oxidised cellulose (p.728·2).
Capillary haemorrhage.

SeaMist *Schein, USA.*
Sodium chloride (p.1196·1).
Inflammation and dryness of nasal membranes.

Sea-Omega *Rugby, USA.*
Omega-3 marine triglycerides with vitamin E (p.949·3).
Dietary supplement.

Search *Stafford-Miller, UK†.*
Cetylpyridinium chloride (p.1138·1).
Oral hygiene.

Seatone *Peter Black, UK.*
Green-lipped mussel (p.1618·2).

Sebaklen *Fumouze, Fr.†*
Xenysalate hydrochloride (p.1128·2).
Seborrhoeic dermatitis.

Sebamed
Sebapharma, Hong Kong; Sebapharma, Thai.
A range of skin cleansers and emollients.

Sebamed Suncream *Sebapharma, Thai.*
Octinoxate (p.1517·3); avobenzone (p.1517·1); enzacamene (p.1517·2).
Sunscreen.

Sebamed Sunlotion *Sebapharma, Thai.*
SPF 20: Octinoxate (p.1517·3); avobenzone (p.1517·1); enzacamene (p.1517·2).
Sunscreen.

Seba-Nil *Healthpoint, USA.*
Skin cleanser.
Acne.

Sebaquin *Summers, USA.*
Diiodohydroxyquinoline (p.590·2).
Scalp disorders.

Sebase *Westbrook, UK.*
A self-emulsifying base.

Sebasorb *Summers, USA.*
Sulfur (p.1123·3); salicylic acid (p.1122·3).
Acne.

Sebaveen
Rydelle, Ital.†; Dermoteca, Port.†.
Avena (p.1583·1); salicylic acid (p.1122·3); carbocisteine (p.1086·3).
Seborrhoeic dermatitis.

Sebcur *Dermtek, Canad.*
Salicylic acid (p.1122·3).
Seborrhoea of the scalp.

Sebcur/T *Dermtek, Canad.*
Salicylic acid (p.1122·3); coal tar (p.1125·1).
Psoriasis of the scalp.

Sebercim *SmithKline Beecham, Ital.*
Norfloxacin (p.232·1).
Urinary-tract infections.

Sebex *Rugby, USA.*
Salicylic acid (p.1122·3); sulfur (p.1123·3).
Seborrhoea.

Sebexol *Devesa, Ger.*
Emollient.
Skin disorders.

Sebexol cum urea *Devesa, Ger.*
Urea (p.1127·3).
Skin disorders.

Sebex-T *Rugby, USA.*
Coal tar (p.1125·1); sulfur (p.1123·3); salicylic acid (p.1122·3).
Seborrhoea.

Sebirinse
Ego, Austral.; Ego, NZ.
Diacetyldimonium chloride; dexpanthenol (p.1602·3); phenethyl alcohol (p.1152·2).
Dry scalp and hair disorders.

Sebitar
Ego, Austral.; Ego, Hong Kong; Ego, NZ; Ego, Singapore.
Tar (p.1125·1); coal tar (p.1125·1); salicylic acid (p.1122·3); undecylenamide (p.396·1).
Skin and scalp disorders.

Sebium K2 *Polaris, Ital.*
Salicylic acid (p.1122·3).
Acne.

Sebizole
Douglas, Austral.; Douglas, NZ.
Ketoconazole (p.389·1).
Dandruff; seborrhoeic dermatitis.

Sebizon *Schering, USA.*
Sulfacetamide sodium (p.250·3).
Bacterial skin infections; seborrhoeic dermatitis of the scalp.

Sebo *Chew, Thai.*
Betamethasone valerate (p.1063·2).
Scalp disorders.

Sebo Concept D/A *Marcel, Canad.*
Resorcinol (p.1122·2); salicylic acid (p.1122·3); sulfur (p.1123·3).

Sebo Creme *Widmer, Switz.*
Vitamins (p.1350·1); urea (p.1127·3); triclosan (p.1159·2).
Acne; seborrhoea.

Sebo Shampooing *Widmer, Switz.*
Pyrithione zinc (p.1122·1); sodium sulfosuccinated undecenoic acid monoethanolamide (p.396·1); triclosan (p.1159·2).
Scalp disorders.

Sebolith *Widmer, Switz.*
Econazole (p.383·1).
Pityriasis versicolor.

Sebophane *Saninter, Port.*
Abietic acid; copper pidolate; zinc pidolate.
Seborrhoeic dermatitis.

Sebo-Psor *Widmer, Switz.*
Dexamethasone (p.1067·1); tretinoin (p.1126·2); urea (p.1127·3).
Scalp disorders.

Seborrol
Ego, Austral.; Ego, Hong Kong; Ego, NZ.
Salicylic acid (p.1122·3); resorcinol (p.1122·2); undecylenamide (p.396·1).
Scalp disorders.

Sebosel
Taro, Israel; Taro, Thai.
Selenium sulfide (p.1123·1).
Scalp disorders.

Sebosquam *Paraphar, Fr.*
Ictasol (p.1115·3); cade oil (p.1124·3); climbazole.
Seborrhoeic dermatitis.

Sebrane *Menarini, Fr.*
Dextromethorphan hydrobromide (p.1087·3).
Coughs.

Sebrane Rhume *Menarini, Fr.*
Phenylpropanolamine hydrochloride (p.1098·1); brompheniramine maleate (p.410·2).
Cold symptoms.

Sebryl *Bioclon, Mex.*
Allantoin (p.1110·1); clioquinol (p.190·2); coal tar (p.1125·1).
Dandruff; seborrhoeic dermatitis.

Sebryl Plus *Bioclon, Mex.*
Allantoin (p.1110·1); clioquinol (p.190·2); coal tar (p.1125·1); triclosan (p.1159·2).
Dandruff; seborrhoeic dermatitis.

Sebucare *Westwood-Squibb, USA.*
Salicylic acid (p.1122·3).
Seborrhoea.

Sebulex
Westwood-Squibb, Canad.; Westwood-Squibb, USA.
Sulfur (p.1123·3); salicylic acid (p.1122·3).
Scalp disorders.

Sebulon
Westwood-Squibb, Canad.; Westwood-Squibb, USA†.
Pyrithione zinc (p.1122·1).
Scalp disorders.

Sebumselen *Llorente, Spain.*
Benzalkonium chloride (p.1133·2); selenium sulfide (p.1123·1).
Skin and scalp disorders.

Sebutone
Westwood-Squibb, Canad.; Westwood, Singapore; Westwood-Squibb, USA†.
Coal tar (p.1125·1); salicylic acid (p.1122·3); sulfur (p.1123·3).
Scalp disorders.

Secabiol *Norman, Spain.*
Carnitine (p.1356·1).
Cardiac disorders; carnitine deficiency.

Secadine *Xixia, S.Afr.*
Cimetidine (p.1216·3).
Gastrointestinal disorders.

Secadrex
Rhone-Poulenc Rorer, Hong Kong; Rhone-Poulenc Rorer, Irl.†; Rhone-Poulenc Rorer, Neth.; Aventis, S.Afr.; Italfarmaco, Spain; Aventis, UK.
Acebutolol hydrochloride (p.825·1); hydrochlorothiazide (p.907·3).
Hypertension.

Secalan *Max Ritter, Switz.†.*
Chlorhexidine gluconate (p.1138·2); isopropyl alcohol (p.1149·2).
Minor skin lesions; skin disinfection.

Secale (Hevertoplex 147) *Hevert, Ger.†.*
Homoeopathic preparation.

Secale Med Complex *Dynamit, Aust.*
Homoeopathic preparation.

Secalip
Biotherapie, Fr.; Fournier SA, Spain.
Fenofibrate (p.889·1).
Hyperlipidaemias.

Secalosan N *Hanosan, Ger.*
Homoeopathic preparation.

Secalysat EM *Ysatfabrik, Ger.†.*
Ergometrine maleate (p.1607·1).
Gynaecological bleeding.

Secamin *Lab, Port.*
Co-dergocrine mesilate (p.1597·3).
Cerebral and peripheral vascular disorders; mental function disorders.

Secaris *Pharmascience, Canad.*
Macrogol (p.1630·1); propylene glycol (p.1655·1).
Rhinitis.

Seclodin *Much, Ger.†.*
Ibuprofen (p.43·2).
Fever; pain.

Secnidal
Rhodia, Braz.; Rhone-Poulenc Rorer, Mex.
Secnidazole (p.602·1).
Amoebiasis; giardiasis; trichomoniasis.

Secni-Plus *Farmoquimica, Braz.*
Secnidazole (p.602·1).
Amoebiasis; giardiasis.

Seconal
Lilly, Canad.†; Lilly, Irl.†; Lilly, S.Afr.†; Lilly, UK; Lilly, USA.
Secobarbital sodium (p.705·2).
Insomnia; sedative.

Secotex *Promeco, Mex.*
Tamsulosin hydrochloride (p.978·3).
Benign prostatic hyperplasia.

Secpel *Medinfar, Port.*
Lactic acid (p.1626·2); lecithin (p.1628·1).
Seborrhoeic dermatitis of the scalp.

Secpel Composto *Medinfar, Port.*
Ichthammol (p.1115·2); lactic acid (p.1626·2); lecithin (p.1628·1).
Dermatitis of the scalp; psoriasis.

Secran *Scherer, USA.*
Multivitamin preparation (p.1350·1).

Secrelux *Goldham, Ger.*
Secretin hydrochloride (p.1661·3).
Diagnosis of Zollinger-Ellison syndrome; test of pancreatic function.

Secrepat *Knoll, Spain.*
Aluminium hydroxide (p.1210·3); calcium carbonate (p.1215·1); magnesium trisilicate (p.1233·3); aluminium glycinate (p.1210·3).
Gastrointestinal hyperacidity.

Secrepina *Synthelabo, Spain.*
Omeprazole (p.1239·1) or omeprazole sodium (p.1239·1).
Gastro-oesophageal reflux; peptic ulcer; Zollinger-Ellison syndrome.

Secresol *Permamed, Switz.*
Acetylcysteine (p.1082·3).
Respiratory-tract disorders associated with increased or viscous mucus.

Secretil *Caber, Ital.*
Ambroxol hydrochloride (p.1084·3).
Respiratory-tract congestion.

Secron *De Witt, UK.*
Ephedrine hydrochloride (p.1090·1); Ipecacuanha (p.1093·1).
Nasal congestion.

Sectam *Locatelli, Ital.†.*
Latamoxef disodium (p.218·3).
Bacterial infections.

Sectral
Rhone-Poulenc Rorer, Aust.; Aventis, Belg.; Rhone-Poulenc Rorer, Canad.; Rhone-Poulenc Rorer, Fr.; Rhone-Poulenc Rorer, Hong Kong; Rhone-Poulenc Rorer, Irl.; Rhone-Poulenc Rorer, Israel; Rhone-Poulenc Rorer, Ital.; Rhone-Poulenc Rorer, Neth.; Aventis, S.Afr.; Rhone-Poulenc Rorer, Singapore; Italfarmaco, Spain; Rhone-Poulenc Rorer, Switz.; Aventis, UK; Wyeth-Ayerst, USA.
Acebutolol hydrochloride (p.825·1).
Angina pectoris; arrhythmias; hypertension; hyperthyroidism; myocardial infarction; obstructive cardiomyopathy.

Sectrazide *Aventis, Belg.*
Acebutolol hydrochloride (p.825·1); hydrochlorothiazide (p.907·3).
Hypertension.

Secubar *Vita Elan, Spain.*
Lisinopril (p.921·1).
Diabetic nephropathy; heart failure; hypertension; myocardial infarction.

Secubar Diu *Vita Elan, Spain.*
Lisinopril (p.921·1); hydrochlorothiazide (p.907·3).
Hypertension.

Secuentex-21 *Searle, Mex.*
15 Tablets, mestranol (p.1482·1); 6 tablets, chlormadinone acetate (p.1465·3); mestranol.
Sequential oral contraceptive.

Se-Cure *Everett, USA.*
Shark cartilage; vitamin E; vitamin C; zinc oxide; selenium (p.1350·1).
Nutritional supplement.

Securgin *Menarini, Ital.*
Desogestrel (p.1470·3); ethinylestradiol (p.1476·2).
Combined oral contraceptive.

Securon *Knoll, UK.*
Verapamil hydrochloride (p.989·1).
Angina pectoris; arrhythmias; hypertension; myocardial infarction.

Securopen
Bayer, Aust.; Bayer, Ger.; Bayer, Irl.; Bayer, Ital.†; Bayer, Norw.†; Bayer, UK†.
Azlocillin sodium (p.154·1).
Bacterial infections.

Securpres *Searle, Ital.*
Indenolol hydrochloride (p.913·2).
Angina pectoris; arrhythmias; hypertension.

Seda Kneipp N *Kneipp, Ger.†.*
Valerian (p.1678·3); lupulus (p.1629·3).
Nervous disorders; sleep disorders.

Sedabarb *Be-Tabs, S.Afr.*
Phenobarbital (p.355·1).

Sedacalman *Schwarzwalder, Ger.*
Homoeopathic preparation.

Sedacollyre *Cooperation Pharmaceutique, Fr.*
Oxedrine tartrate (p.950·3); berberine hydrochloride (p.1584·2); benzododecinium bromide (p.1135·1).
Eye disorders.

Sedacoron
Ebewe, Aust.; Ebewe, Hong Kong.
Amiodarone hydrochloride (p.836·1).
Arrhythmias.

Sedactrim *Sedar, Braz.*
Co-trimoxazole (p.193·3).
Bacterial infections; Pneumocystis carinii pneumonia; protozoal infections.

Sedactrim Balsamico *Sedar, Braz.*
Co-trimoxazole (p.193·3); guaifenesin (p.1092·2); ammonium chloride (p.1085·2).
Bacterial infections.

Sedacur *Schaper & Brummer, Ger.*
Valerian (p.1678·3); lupulus (p.1629·3); melissa (p.1632·2).
Nervous disorders; sleep disorders.

Seda-Do *Grasler, Ger.*
Homoeopathic preparation.

Seda-Gel *Key, Austral.*
Lotion: Lignocaine [lidocaine] (p.1313·2).
Mouth ulcers; teething and denture pain.
Oral gel: Choline salicylate (p.24·3); menthol (p.1632·3).
Painful mouth disorders.

Sedagin *Biocontrolfarm, Ital.†.*
Eschscholtzia californica.

Seda-Grandelat *Synpharma, Aust.*
Lupulus (p.1629·3); melissa leaf (p.1632·2).
Anxiety disorders.

Sedagripe *Novaquimica, Braz.*
Chlorpheniramine [chlorphenamine] maleate (p.412·1); aspirin (p.14·2); methoxyphenamine (p.1094·3); caffeine (p.761·3).
Cold and influenza symptoms.

Sedagul *Wild, Switz.*
Lignocaine [lidocaine] hydrochloride (p.1313·2).
Local anaesthesia.

Sedahopf *Hennig, Ger.†.*
Valerian (p.1678·3); lupulus (p.1629·3).
Nervous disorders; sleep disorders.

Sedakatt *Kottwig, Ger.*
Homoeopathic preparation.

Sedalen Cort *Montefarmaco, Ital.*
Hydrocortisone acetate (p.1073·3); benzocaine (p.1306·2); hamamelis (p.1618·3); aesculus (p.1574·1).
Anorectal disorders.

Sedalene *Gunther, Braz.*
Dipyrone (p.34·1); homatropine methylbromide (p.468·1); papaverine (p.1648·1); adiphenine.
Smooth muscle spasm.

Sedalin
Note.This name is used for preparations of different composition.
Dinafarma, Braz.
Passion flower (p.1649·1); erythrina mulungu; crataegus (p.1600·2).
Sedative.
Chi Sheng, Thai.
Ceftriaxone sodium (p.177·1).
Bacterial infections.

Sedalint Baldrian *Madaus, Ger.*
Valerian root (p.1678·3).
Nervous disorders; sleep disorders.

Sedalint Kava *Madaus, Ger.*
Kava (p.1625·3).
Anxiety disorders.

Sedalipid *Steigerwald, Ger.*
Magnesium-pyridoxal-5′-phosphate-glutaminate.
Hyperlipidaemias.

Sedalito *Merck, Mex.*
Paracetamol (p.71·2).
Fever; pain.

Sedalmerck
Note.This name is used for preparations of different composition.
Merck, Mex.
Paracetamol (p.71·2); caffeine (p.761·3); psuedoephedrine hydrochloride (p.1099·2).
Fever; nasal congestion; pain; rhinitis; sinusitis.
Merck, Spain.
Caffeine (p.761·3); ephedrine hydrochloride (p.1090·1); ethylmorphine hydrochloride (p.35·2); propyphenazone (p.80·2).
Pain.

Sedalmerck TH *Merck, Mex.*
Paracetamol (p.71·2); pseudoephedrine hydrochloride (p.1099·2); dextromethorphan hydrobromide (p.1087·3).
Coughs; fever; nasal congestion; pain; rhinitis; sinusitis.

Sedalozia *Iphym, Fr.*
Crataegus (p.1600·2); eschscholtzia californica; valerian (p.1678·3).
Insomnia; nervous disorders.

Sedalpan *Teofarma, Ital.*
Methyl nicotinate (p.55·1); diethylamine salicylate (p.32·2).
Musculoskeletal, joint, and soft-tissue disorders.

Sedans *Ganassini, Ital.*
Amitriptyline hydrochloride (p.273·3); chlordiazepoxide hydrochloride (p.659·2).
Nervous disorders.

Sedantol *Dovalle, Braz.*
Valerian (p.1678·3); melissa (p.1632·2); passion flower (p.1649·1).
Sedative.

Sedapain *Aspen Consumer, S.Afr.*
Paracetamol (p.71·2); doxylamine succinate (p.417·1); caffeine (p.761·3); codeine phosphate (p.25·2).
Pain with tension.

Sedapap *Merz, USA.*
Paracetamol (p.71·2); butalbital (p.658·3).
Tension headache.

Sedaplaie *Medeva, Fr.*
Dodeclonium bromide; amylocaine hydrochloride (p.1306·1).
Burns; wounds.

Seda-Plantina *Plantina, Ger.*
Valerian (p.1678·3); lupulus (p.1629·3); melissa (p.1632·2); passion flower (p.1649·1); rosemary.
Agitation; sleep disorders.

Sedaplus *Chephasaar, Ger.; Rosen, Ger.*
Doxylamine succinate (p.417·1).
Hypersensitivity reactions; nervous disorders; nocturnal enuresis; sleep disorders.

Seda-Rash *Key, Austral.*
Zinc oxide (p.1128·2); castor oil (p.1592·1).
Eczema; heat rash; intertrigo; nappy rash.

Sedarene *Theratech, Fr.*
Paracetamol (p.71·2); codeine phosphate (p.25·2).
Fever; pain.

Sedariston *Steiner, Ger.*
Valerian root (p.1678·3); hypericum (p.290·3); melissa leaf (p.1632·2).
Nervous disorders.

The symbol † denotes a preparation no longer actively marketed

Sedariston Konzentrat *Steiner, Ger.*
Hypericum (p.290·2); valerian root (p.1678·3).
Anxiety disorders; sleep disorders.

Sedartryl *Oberlin, Fr.*
Methyl nicotinate (p.55·1); amyl salicylate (p.14·1); menthol (p.1632·3).
Formerly contained methyl nicotinate, amyl salicylate, salicylic acid, menthol, camphor, turpentine oil, and volatile mustard oil.
Musculoskeletal and joint pain.

Sedaselect *Dreluso, Ger.*
Homoeopathic preparation.

Sedaselect N *Dreluso, Ger.*
Lupulus (p.1629·3); valerian (p.1678·3); passion flower (p.1649·1); melissa (p.1632·2).
Nervous disorders; sleep disorders.

Sedasept
Note. This name is used for preparations of different composition.
Michaux, Belg.
Chlorhexidine gluconate (p.1138·2); lignocaine [lidocaine] hydrochloride (p.1313·2).
Formerly contained acetarsol sodium, sulfanilamide, and thymol.
Mouth and throat disorders.

Sanico, Switz.
Eucalyptol (p.1609·2); peppermint oil (p.1243·3); thyme oil (p.1672·3); menthol (p.1632·3); thymol (p.1158·3); methyl salicylate (p.55·1).
Dental inflammation; oral hygiene.

Sedaspir *Bride, Fr.*
Codeine phosphate (p.25·2); caffeine (p.761·3); aspirin (p.14·2).
Pain.

Sedasyx *Syxyl, Ger.*
Valerian (p.1678·3); lupulus (p.1629·3); melissa (p.1632·2).
Nervous disorders; sleep disorders.

Sedatif PC *Boiron, Canad.; Boiron, Fr.; Boiron, Port.; Boiron, Switz.*
Homoeopathic preparation.

Sedatif Tiber *Medecine Vegetale, Fr.*
Crataegus (p.1600·2); passion flower (p.1649·1); potassium bromide; sodium bromide (p.1587·1).
Anxiety; insomnia.

Sedatol *Bonomelli, Ital.*
Capsules: Passion flower (p.1649·1); valerian (p.1678·3); crataegus (p.1600·2); chamomile (p.1593·2); piscidia (p.1625·1).
Syrup: Passion flower (p.1649·1); chamomile (p.1593·2); crataegus (p.1600·2); piscidia (p.1625·1); melissa (p.1632·2).
Insomnia.

Sedatonyl *Lipha Sante, Fr.†*
Phenobarbital (p.355·1); crataegus (p.1600·2).
Anxiety; insomnia.

Sedatoss *Cilag, Braz.*
Fedrilate (p.1091·3).
Coughs.

Sedatruw S *Truw, Ger.†*
Valerian (p.1678·3); lupulus (p.1629·3); melissa (p.1632·2).
Nervous disorders; sleep disorders.

Sedatuss *Trianon, Canad.†*
Dextromethorphan hydrobromide (p.1087·3); chlorpheniramine [chlorphenamine] maleate (p.412·1); guaiacol (p.1092·1); pseudoephedrine hydrochloride (p.1099·2).
Coughs.

Sedatuss DM *Trianon, Canad.*
Dextromethorphan hydrobromide (p.1087·3).

Sedatux *EMS, Braz.*
Potassium iodide (p.1522·3); lobelia (p.1510·2); hyoscyamus (p.470·1).
Respiratory-tract congestion.

Sedauric *Laborsil, Braz.*
Tyrothricin (p.267·1); urea (p.1127·3).
Ear infections.

Sedergine *Upsamedica, Belg.; Bristol-Myers Squibb, Port.†; Upsamedica, Spain.*
Aspirin (p.14·2).
Fever; musculoskeletal, joint and peri-articular disorders; pain; thromboembolism prophylaxis.

Sedergine C *Upsamedica, Belg.; Princeton, Spain.*
Aspirin (p.14·2); ascorbic acid (p.1389·3).
Fever; pain.

Sedermyl *Cooperation Pharmaceutique, Fr.*
Isothipendyl hydrochloride (p.419·2).
Insect stings; pruritus.

Sedex *Janssen-Cilag, Port.†*
Flunitrazepam (p.683·2).

Sediat *Pfleger, Ger.*
Diphenhydramine hydrochloride (p.416·1).
Sleep disorders.

Sedibaine *Marion Merrell, Fr.†*
Phenobarbital (p.355·1); crataegus (p.1600·2); ballota; valerian (p.1678·3).
Formerly contained strophanthus, phenobarbital, hyoscyamus, crataegus, ballota, valerian, and belladonna.
Nervous disorders.

Sedicepan *Almirall, Spain.*
Lorazepam (p.688·3).
Alcohol withdrawal syndrome; anxiety; insomnia; nausea; premedication; vomiting.

Sediel *Sumitomo, Jpn.*
Tandospirone citrate (p.707·1).
Anxiety; depression; phobias; sleep disorders.

Sedilene Procto *Montefarmaco, Ital.*
Benzocaine (p.1306·2); aesculus (p.1574·1); hamamelis (p.1618·3).
Anorectal disorders.

Sedilix *Xepa-Soul Pattinson, Singapore.*
Codeine phosphate (p.25·2); promethazine hydrochloride (p.423·2); ephedrine hydrochloride (p.1090·1).
Coughs.

Sedilix DM
Xepa-Soul Pattinson, Hong Kong; Xepa-Soul Pattinson, Singapore.
Dextromethorphan hydrobromide (p.1087·3); pseudoephedrine hydrochloride (p.1099·2); promethazine hydrochloride (p.423·2).
Coughs; nasal congestion.

Sedilor *Dolisos, Canad.*
Homoeopathic preparation.

Sedinal *Melisana, Belg.*
Crataegus (p.1600·2); ballota; passion flower (p.1649·1).
Nervous disorders.

Sedinfant N *Biocur, Ger.*
Valerian (p.1678·3); melissa (p.1632·2); passion flower (p.1649·1).
Agitation; excitability; sleep disorders.

Sedinol *Aspen Consumer, S.Afr.*
Doxylamine succinate (p.417·1); paracetamol (p.71·2); codeine phosphate (p.25·2); caffeine (p.761·3).
Pain and associated pain.

Sedioton *Wyeth Lederle, Port.†*
Ambutonium bromide; oxazepam (p.697·1).

Sedisan *Bioquimico, Mex.*
Trifluoperazine (p.710·3).

Sediten *Taro, Israel.*
Fluphenazine hydrochloride (p.684·3).
Anxiety.

Sediver *Maver, Mex.*
Diazepam (p.674·3).
Anxiety; muscle spasm; sedative.

Sedizepan *Septa, Spain†.*
Lorazepam (p.688·3).
Alcohol withdrawal syndrome; anxiety; epilepsy; insomnia; nausea; vomiting.

Sedo *Rapide, Spain†.*
Methadone (p.54·2).
Diamorphine detoxification; opioid withdrawal; pain.

Sedobex *Ecobi, Ital.†.*
Sodium dibunate (p.1100·3); grindelia (p.1618·2); cardamom (p.1591·3); lattuca sativa; sodium benzoate (p.1134·3).
Bronchial disorders; coughs.

Sedobion *Sintofarma, Braz.*
Dipyrone (p.34·1); hyoscine methobromide (p.468·2).
Smooth muscle spasm.

Sedobrina *Vinas, Spain†.*
Lormetazepam (p.689·3).
Insomnia.

Sedocalcio *Deca, Ital.*
Calcium lactate (p.1188·2); sodium benzoate (p.1134·3).
Mouth and throat disorders.

Sedocardin *Pfluger, Ger.*
Homoeopathic preparation.

Sedodermil *Vifor, Switz.†.*
Methyl anthranilate; pentyl valerate; bornyl salicylate (p.20·3); laurus nobilis oil; menthol (p.1632·3).
Musculoskeletal and joint pain.

Sedofan *Julphar, UAE.*
Triprolidine hydrochloride (p.427·2); pseudoephedrine hydrochloride (p.1099·2).
Upper respiratory-tract congestion.

Sedofan II *Julphar, UAE.*
Pseudoephedrine hydrochloride (p.1099·2).
Nasal congestion; otitis media; sinusitis.

Sedofan DM *Julphar, UAE.*
Triprolidine hydrochloride (p.427·2); pseudoephedrine hydrochloride (p.1099·2); dextromethorphan hydrobromide (p.1087·3).
Upper respiratory-tract disorders.

Sedofarin *Pensa, Spain.*
Dequalinium chloride (p.1143·1); dexamethasone (p.1067·1); benzocaine (p.1306·2); tyrothricin (p.267·1).
Mouth and throat disorders.

Sedogelat *Metochem, Aust.*
Valerian root (p.1678·3); lupulus (p.1629·3); passion flower (p.1649·1).
Formerly contained valerian root, melissa leaf, and passion flower.
Anxiety disorders; sleep disorders.

Sedogelat forte *Metochem, Aust.*
Valerian (p.1678·3); passion flower (p.1649·1).
Formerly contained valerian and melissa.
Anxiety disorders; sleep disorders.

Sedol *OFF, Ital.*
Propyphenazone (p.80·2); caffeine (p.761·3).
Fever; influenza symptoms; neuralgia.

Sedonium *Lichtwer, Ger.*
Valerian (p.1678·3).
Agitation; insomnia.

Sedopal *Lehning, Fr.*
Crataegus (p.1600·2); eschscholtzia californica; melilotus officinalis.
Insomnia; nervous disorders.

Sedophon *Mayoly-Spindler, Fr.*
Ethylmorphine hydrochloride (p.35·2); aconite (p.1572·3); guaifenesin (p.1092·2).
Coughs.

Sedopretten *Schoning-Berlin, Ger.†*
Diphenhydramine hydrochloride (p.416·1).
Insomnia.

Sedopuer F *SIT, Ital.*
Passion flower (p.1649·1); valerian (p.1678·3); crataegus (p.1600·2); calcium glycerophosphate (p.1188·2).
Insomnia; nervous disorders.

Sedorrhoide *Cooperation Pharmaceutique, Fr.*
Dodec!onium; benzocaine (p.1306·2); esculoside (p.1574·1); enoxolone (p.34·3).
Anorectal disorders.

Sedosan *Grossmann, Switz.*
Crataegus (p.1600·2); passion flower (p.1649·1).
Nervous disorders.

Sedosil *Vifor, Switz.†*
Pimethixene (p.423·1).
Nervous disorders.

Sedotime *Iquinosa, Spain.*
Ketazolam (p.688·2).
Anxiety; insomnia; skeletal muscle spasm.

Sedotusse *Helfarma, Port.*
Codeine phosphate (p.25·2); ephedrine hydrochloride (p.1090·1).
Coughs.

Sedotussin
Note. This name is used for preparations of different composition.
UCB, Aust.; UCB, Ger.; Rodleben, Ger.; Vedim, Ger.
Pentoxyverine (p.1096·3), pentoxyverine citrate (p.1096·3), or pentoxyverine hydrochloride (p.1096·3).
Coughs.

UCB, Switz.
Oral drops: Pentoxyverine citrate (p.1096·3); terpin hydrate (p.1101·2); eucalyptol (p.1609·2); menthol (p.1632·3); thymol (p.1158·3); guaifenesin (p.1092·2).
Suppositories: Pentoxyverine (p.1096·3); terpin hydrate (p.1101·2); terpineol (p.1669·3); eucalyptol (p.1609·2); guaifenesin (p.1092·2).
Syrup†: Pentoxyverine citrate (p.1096·3); terpin hydrate (p.1101·2); eucalyptol (p.1609·2); menthol (p.1632·3); thyme (p.1672·2).
Coughs and associated respiratory-tract disorders.

Sedotussin Efeu *Vedim, Ger.; Rodleben, Ger.; UCB, Ger.*
Hedera helix.
Bronchitis; catarrh.

Sedotussin Expectorans *UCB, Ger.†*
Oral drops: Pentoxyverine citrate (p.1096·3); terpin (p.1101·2); eucalyptol (p.1609·2); menthol (p.1632·3); thymol (p.1158·3); guaifenesin (p.1092·2).
Syrup: Pentoxyverine citrate (p.1096·3); terpin (p.1101·2); eucalyptol (p.1609·2); menthol (p.1632·3); thyme (p.1672·2).
Coughs and associated respiratory-tract disorders.

Sedotussin muco *UCB, Ger.; Rodleben, Ger.; Vedim, Ger.*
Carbocisteine (p.1086·3).
Respiratory-tract disorders with excess or viscous mucus.

Sedotussin plus *UCB, Ger.; Rodleben, Ger.; Vedim, Ger.*
Pentoxyverine citrate (p.1096·3); chlorpheniramine [chlorphenamine] maleate (p.412·1).
Coughs.

Sedovegan *Wolff, Ger.*
Hypericum (p.290·2).
Depression.

Sedovegan Novo *Wolff, Ger.*
Diphenhydramine hydrochloride (p.416·1).
Insomnia.

Sedovent *Schworer, Ger.*
Cinchona bark (p.1595·3); cinnamon (p.1595·3); dried bitter-orange peel (p.1644·2); achillea (p.1572·2); calamus (p.1588·1); gentian (p.1615·1).
Gastrointestinal disorders.

Sedoxil *Medibial, Port.*
Mexazolam (p.692·3).
Anxiety disorders; premedication.

Sedral *Banyu, Jpn†.*
Cefadroxil (p.161·2).
Bacterial infections.

Sedural *Rekah, Israel.*
Phenazopyridine hydrochloride (p.77·3).
Urinary-tract pain and irritation.

Seduspan *QIF, Braz.*
Buspirone hydrochloride (p.657·2).
Anxiety.

Sefaretic *Unison, Thai.*
Amiloride hydrochloride (p.835·1); hydrochlorothiazide (p.907·3).
Heart failure; hepatic cirrhosis with ascites; hypertension.

Seferin *General Drugs, Thai.*
Aspirin (p.14·2).
Inflammation; musculoskeletal and joint disorders; pain.

Sefmal
Unison, Singapore; Unison, Thai.
Tramadol hydrochloride (p.89·1).
Pain.

Sefmex *Unison, Thai.*
Selegiline hydrochloride (p.1177·2).
Alzheimer's disease; parkinsonism.

Sefmic *Unison, Thai.*
Mefenamic acid (p.51·2).
Pain.

Seforman *Valdecasas, Mex.*
Furazolidone (p.592·1).

Sefril *Bristol-Myers Squibb, Aust.†*
Cefradine (p.173·3).
Bacterial infections.

Seftem *Shionogi, Jpn.*
Ceftibuten (p.176·1).
Bacterial infections.

Seftil *Unison, Thai.*
Tenoxicam (p.87·2).
Gout; inflammation; musculoskeletal and joint disorders.

Sefulken *Kendrick, Mex.*
Diazoxide (p.868·1).
Hypertension.

Segel *Diba, Mex.*
Aluminium hydroxide (p.1210·3); glycine (p.1365·3); calcium carbonate (p.1215·1); dimethicone (p.1249·2).
Gastrointestinal hyperacidity.

Seglor
Schwarz, Fr.; Pharmafar, Ital.; Sanofi Synthelabo, Port.
Dihydroergotamine mesilate (p.450·3).
Headache; migraine; orthostatic hypotension; peripheral vascular disorders; vertigo.

Segmentocut Thermo *Redel, Ger.†*
Glycol salicylate (p.42·2); benzyl nicotinate (p.20·2).
Musculoskeletal, joint, and soft-tissue pain; superficial vascular disorders.

Seguril *Hoechst Marion Roussel, Spain.*
Frusemide [furosemide] (p.893·1).
Forced diuresis; heart failure; hypertension; nephrotic syndrome; oedema; oliguria; renal failure.

Sejungin B *Bock, Ger.†*
Homoeopathic preparation.

Seki
Zambon, Braz.; Zambon, Ital.
Cloperastine fendizoate (p.1087·2) or cloperastine hydrochloride (p.1087·2).
Coughs.

Sekin *Sintesa, Belg.*
Cloperastine fendizoate (p.1087·2) or cloperastine hydrochloride (p.1087·2).
Coughs.

Sekisan *Almirall, Spain.*
Cloperastine fendizoate (p.1087·2) or cloperastine hydrochloride (p.1087·2).
Coughs.

Sekretolin *Hoechst, Ger.*
Secretin hydrochloride (p.1661·3).
Diagnosis of pancreatic disorders and Zollinger-Ellison syndrome.

Sekretovit
Boehringer Ingelheim, Aust.; Promeco, Mex.
Ambroxol hydrochloride (p.1084·3).
Respiratory-tract congestion.

Sekretovit Amoxi *Promeco, Mex.*
Ambroxol hydrochloride (p.1084·3); amoxicillin trihydrate (p.149·2).
Respiratory-tract infections.

Sekucid
Note. This name is used for preparations of different composition.
Paragerm, Fr.
Glutaral (p.1145·2).
Instrument disinfection.

Henkel, Ital.
Glutaral (p.1145·2); isopropyl alcohol (p.1149·2).
Instrument disinfection.

Sekucid konz *Henkel, Ital.*
Glutaral (p.1145·2); isopropyl alcohol (p.1149·2); ethylhexanal.
Instrument disinfection.

Sekudrill
Henkel, Ger.; Henkel, Ital.
Potassium hydroxide (p.1654·1); propylene glycol (p.1655·1).
Instrument disinfection.

Sekugerm *Henkel, Ital.†*
Glutaral (p.1145·2); glyoxal (p.1145·3).
Disinfection of fibre-optic equipment; endoscope disinfection.

Sekumatic D *Henkel, Ital.*
Glutaral (p.1145·2); alcohol (p.1130·3); chloroform; acetone.
Instrument disinfection.

Sekumatic FD *Henkel, Ger.*
Glutaral (p.1145·2).
Instrument disinfection.

Sekumatic FDR *Henkel, Ger.*
Glucoprotamine; didecylmethylpoly(oxyethyl) ammonium propionate; tributyltetradecylphosphonium chloride.
Surface and instrument disinfection.

Sekusept *Henkel, Ger.*
Sodium perborate (p.1156·3); tetraacetyl ethylenediamine.
Instrument and surface disinfection.

Sekusept Extra N
Henkel, Ger.; Henkel, Ital.
Benzalkonium chloride (p.1133·2); glutaral (p.1145·2).
Instrument disinfection.

Sekusept forte *Henkel, Ger.*
Formaldehyde (p.1144·2); glyoxal (p.1145·3); glutaral (p.1145·2); benzalkonium chloride (p.1133·2).
Instrument disinfection.

Sekusept forte S Henkel, Ger.
Formaldehyde (p.1144·2); glutaral (p.1145·2).
Instrument disinfection.

Sekusept N Henkel, Ital.
Sodium perborate (p.1156·3).
Instrument disinfection.

Sekusept Plus Henkel, Ger.
Glucoprotamine.
Instrument disinfection.

Sel D Pharmadeveloppement, Fr.
Sodium chloride; sodium phosphate; sodium sulfate; sodium iodide; sodium bromide (p.1350·1).
Dietary salt substitute.

Sel d'Ems Siemens, Switz.
Natural sels d'Ems.
Upper-respiratory-tract disorders.

Selan Iquinosa, Spain.
Cefuroxime axetil (p.178·1).
Bacterial infections.

Selanac Whitehall, Braz.
Magaldrate (p.1232·2).
Gastrointestinal hyperacidity.

Selax Odan, Canad.
Docusate sodium (p.1223·1).
Constipation.

Selbex Eisai, Jpn; Eisai, Thai.
Teprenone (p.1253·2).
Gastric ulcer; gastritis.

Sel'bis Expanpharm, Fr.
Potassium chloride (p.1350·1); ammonium chloride; calcium formate; glutamic acid.
Dietary salt substitute.

Seldane Hoechst Marion Roussel, Canad.†; Hoechst Marion Roussel, UK†; Merrell Dow, USA†.
Terfenadine (p.424·3).
Hypersensitivity reactions.

Seldane-D Marion Merrell Dow, USA†.
Pseudoephedrine hydrochloride (p.1099·2); terfenadine (p.424·3).
Upper respiratory-tract symptoms.

Selecid Leo, Port.
Pivmecillinam hydrochloride (p.237·3).
Salmonella enteritis; urinary-tract infections.

Selecim Cimex, Switz.
Selegiline hydrochloride (p.1177·2).
Parkinsonism.

Select 1/35 Dispensapharm, Canad.
Norethisterone (p.1485·1); ethinylestradiol (p.1476·2).
Combined oral contraceptive.

Selectadoce Diba, Mex.
Thiamine (p.1385·2); pyridoxine (p.1387·1); hydroxocobalamin (p.1388·1).
Anaemias; neuritis.

Selectadril Diba, Mex.
Metoprolol tartrate (p.931·2).
Hypertension; myocardial infarction.

Selectafer N Dreluso, Ger.
Iron sucrose (p.1937·1); cyanocobalamin (p.1388·1); folic acid (p.1361·1).
Primary and secondary anaemias; tonic.

Selecten Unipharm, Israel.
Fluphenazine hydrochloride (p.684·3).
Anxiety; psychoses.

Selectin Bristol-Myers Squibb, Ital.
Pravastatin sodium (p.957·3).
Arteriosclerosis; cardiovascular disorders; hypercholesterolaemia.

Selecto Diba, Mex.
Pancreatin (p.1646·1).
Pancreatic insufficiency.

Selectocalcio Asta Medica, Braz.
Calcium chloride; ergocalciferol; calcium phosphate; cyanocobalamin; sodium fluoride (p.1350·1).
Nutritional supplement.

Selecto-D Diba, Mex.
Pancreatin (p.1646·1); dimethicone (p.1249·2).
Gastrointestinal disorders.

Selectofen Diba, Mex.
Diclofenac sodium (p.30·3).
And soft-tissue disorders; gout; inflammation; musculoskeletal, joint; pain.

Selectofur Diba, Mex.
Frusemide [furosemide] (p.893·1).
Hypertension; oedema.

Selectografin Schering, Ital.†
Sodium amidotrizoate (p.1031·2); meglumine amidotrizoate (p.1031·2).
Contrast medium for urography and angiography.

Selectol
Gerot, Aust.; Pharmacia Upjohn, Belg.; Leiras, Fin.; Pharmacia Upjohn, Ger.; Rhone-Poulenc Rorer, Hong Kong; Rhone-Poulenc Rorer, Irl.; Shinyaku, Jpn; Aventis, NZ; Rhone-Poulenc Rorer, Switz.
Celiprolol hydrochloride (p.856·1).
Angina pectoris; arrhythmias; hypertension.

Selectomycin Grunenthal, Ger.
Spiramycin (p.248·3).
Bacterial infections; toxoplasmosis.

Selectovit Diba, Mex.
Vitamin B substances (p.1350·1).

Selecturon Gerot, Aust.
Celiprolol hydrochloride (p.856·1); chlortalidone (p.857·1).
Hypertension.

Seledat Master Pharma, Ital.
Selegiline hydrochloride (p.1177·2).
Psychiatric disorders.

Selefusin Pisa, Mex.
Selenium (p.1375·2).

Selegam Hexal, Ger.
Selegiline hydrochloride (p.1177·2).
Parkinsonism.

Selegel Ducray, Fr.
Selenium sulfide (p.1123·1).
Seborrhoeic dermatitis.

Selegil Diba, Mex.
Metronidazole (p.594·1) or metronidazole benzoate (p.594·1).
Amoebiasis; giardiasis; trichomoniasis.

Selegos
Medochemie, Hong Kong; Medochemie, Singapore.
Selegiline (p.1178·1) or selegiline hydrochloride (p.1177·2).
Parkinsonism.

Selektine Bristol-Myers Squibb, Neth.
Pravastatin sodium (p.957·3).
Hypercholesterolaemia.

Selemax Novartis Consumer, Ital.
Selenium; betacarotene; vitamin E; vitamin C; zinc; copper (p.1350·1).
Antioxidant nutritional supplement.

Selemerck Merck dura, Ger.
Selegiline hydrochloride (p.1177·2).
Parkinsonism.

Selemite-B Blackmores, Austral.
Selenomethionine.
Selenium deficiency.

Selemix Provita, Ital.
Vitamins; minerals; ubidecarenone (p.1350·1).

Selemycin Medochemie, Singapore.
Amikacin sulfate (p.148·1).
Bacterial infections.

Selen Fresenius Kabi, Aust.; Kabi, Swed.†
Sodium selenite (p.1375·2).
Dietary supplement.

Selen + E Kabi, Swed.†
Sodium selenite (p.1375·2); dl-alpha tocoferil acetate (p.1394·1).
Dietary supplement.

Selenarell Sanorell, Ger.
Homoeopathic preparation.

selenase Biosyn, Ger.
Sodium selenite (p.1375·2).
Selenium deficiency.

Selenica Nikken, Jpn†.
Sodium valproate (p.366·3).
Epilepsy.

Selenion Labcatal, Fr.
Selenium (p.1375·2).
Muscular disorders; skin disorders.

Selenium E Biomedica, Austral.
Selenomethionine; d-alpha tocoferil acid succinate (p.1394·1).
Dietary supplement.

Selenium Med Complex Dynamit, Aust.
Homoeopathic preparation.

Selenium Plus Sisu, Canad.
Selenium (p.1375·2); methionine (p.1012·2).

Selenium-ACE
Richelet, Fr.; Helsinn, Port.; Wassen, UK.
Selenium yeast (p.1375·2); vitamins A, C, and E (p.1350·1).

Selenix Novartis Consumer, Port.
Selenium sulfide (p.1123·1).
Dandruff; pityriasis versicolor.

Seleno-6 Solgar, UK.
Selenomethionine.
Dietary supplement.

Selenokehl Sanum-Kehlbeck, Ger.
Homoeopathic preparation.

Selenol Merck, Denm.
Selenium sulfide (p.1123·1).
Pityriasis versicolor; seborrhoeic dermatitis.

Selen-Wied Wiedemann, Ger.
Homoeopathic preparation.

Sele-Pak Smith & Nephew SoloPak, USA.
Selenious acid (p.1375·2).
Parenteral nutrition.

Seleparina Italfarmaco, Ital.
Nadroparin calcium (p.937·2).
Thrombosis prophylaxis.

Selepark Betapharm, Ger.
Selegiline hydrochloride (p.1177·2).
Parkinsonism.

Selepen
Fujisawa, Hong Kong; American Pharmaceutical, USA.
Selenious acid (p.1375·2).
Parenteral nutrition.

Seleplus Chemedica, Switz.
Selenium yeast; vitamins A, C, and E (p.1350·1).
Selenium deficiency.

Seles Beta Schwarz, Ital.
Atenolol (p.841·3).
Angina pectoris; hypertension.

Selexid
Leo, Aust.; Leo, Belg.; Leo, Canad.; Leo, Denm.; Leo, Fin.; Leo, Fr.; Leo, Norw.; Leo, Swed.; Leo, UK.
Mecillinam (p.221·3), pivmecillinam (p.237·3), or pivmecillinam hydrochloride (p.237·3).
Bacterial infections of the urinary tract.

Selezen Teofarma, Ital.
Imidazole salicylate (p.44·3).
Fever; inflammation; pain.

Selg Promefarm, Ital.
Macrogol 4000 (p.1630·3); electrolytes (p.1180·1).
Bowel evacuation; constipation.

Selgene
Alphapharm, Austral.; Pacific, NZ; Merck, Thai.
Selegiline hydrochloride (p.1177·2).
Parkinsonism.

Selg-Esse Promefarm, Ital.
Macrogol 4000 (p.1630·3); simeticone (p.1249·2); electrolytes (p.1180·1).
Bowel evacuation.

Selgimed Hennig, Ger.
Selegiline hydrochloride (p.1177·2).
Parkinsonism.

Selgine Teofarma, Fr.
Sodium chloride (p.1196·3); sel marin.
Mouth disorders.

Seline Berlin Pharm, Thai.
Selegiline hydrochloride (p.1177·2).
Parkinsonism.

Selinol Orion, Swed.
Atenolol (p.841·3).
Angina pectoris; arrhythmias; hypertension.

Selipran Bristol-Myers Squibb, Aust.; Bristol-Myers Squibb, Switz.
Pravastatin sodium (p.957·3).
Hypercholesterolaemia.

Selit Biosyn, Ger.
Sodium selenite (p.1375·2).
Selenium deficiency.

Selm Precimex, Mex.
Methyldopa (p.927·3).

Selobloc Logap, Switz.
Atenolol (p.841·3).
Angina pectoris; arrhythmias; hypertension.

Selocomp ZOC Searle, Fin.
Metoprolol succinate (p.932·1); hydrochlorothiazide (p.907·3).
Hypertension.

Selokeen Astra, Neth.
Metoprolol succinate (p.932·1) or metoprolol tartrate (p.931·2).
Angina pectoris; arrhythmias; hypertension; hyperthyroidism; migraine; myocardial infarction.

Seloken
Astra, Aust.; Astra, Belg.; Astra, Braz.; AstraZeneca, Denm.; AstraZeneca, Fr.; Astra, Ital.; Astra, Jpn; Astra, Mex.; Astra, Norw.†; AstraZeneca, Norw.; Astra, Spain; Hassle, Swed.
Metoprolol (p.932·1), metoprolol succinate (p.932·1), or metoprolol tartrate (p.931·2).
Angina pectoris; arrhythmias; cardiomyopathy; hypertension; hyperthyroidism; migraine; myocardial infarction.

Seloken retard Plus Astra, Aust.
Metoprolol succinate (p.932·1); hydrochlorothiazide (p.907·3).
Hypertension.

Seloken ZOC
AstraZeneca, Fin.; Hassle, Swed.
Metoprolol succinate (p.932·1).
Angina pectoris; arrhythmias; hypertension; migraine; myocardial infarction.

Seloken ZOC/ASA
AstraZeneca, Fin.; Hassle, Swed.
Tablets, metoprolol succinate (p.932·1); tablets, aspirin (p.14·2).
Angina pectoris; myocardial infarction.

Selokomb Astra, Neth.
Metoprolol succinate (p.932·1) or metoprolol tartrate (p.931·2); hydrochlorothiazide (p.907·3).
Hypertension.

Selon Serturner, Ger.
Valerian (p.1678·3); lupulus (p.1629·3).
Agitation; sleep disorders.

Selopral Orion, Fin.
Metoprolol tartrate (p.931·2).
Angina pectoris; arrhythmias; hypertension; migraine; myocardial infarction.

Selopres Astra, Mex.
Metoprolol succinate (p.932·1); hydrochlorothiazide (p.907·3).
Hypertension.

Selopresin Astra, Spain.
Metoprolol tartrate (p.931·2); hydrochlorothiazide (p.907·3).
Hypertension.

Selopress Astra, Braz.
Metoprolol (p.932·1); hydrochlorothiazide (p.907·3).
Hypertension.

Selozide Astra, Belg.; Astra, Ital.
Metoprolol tartrate (p.931·2); hydrochlorothiazide (p.907·3).
Hypertension.

Selo-Zok
Astra, Belg.; AstraZeneca, Denm.; AstraZeneca, Norw.
Metoprolol succinate (p.932·1).
Angina pectoris; arrhythmias; hypertension; hyperthyroidism; migraine; myocardial infarction; tremor.

Selpar Therabel, Ital.†
Selegiline hydrochloride (p.1177·2).
Parkinsonism.

Selpiran Diba, Mex.
Hyoscine butylbromide (p.468·2); dipyrone (p.34·1).
Smooth muscle spasm and pain.

Selpiran-S Diba, Mex.
Hyoscine butylbromide (p.468·2).
Smooth muscle spasm.

Sels Calcaires Nutritifs Weleda, Fr.
Combination pack: Homoeopathic preparation.

Selso Luchon, Fr.
Sodium chloride (p.1196·3); sulfur (p.1123·3).
Nasal irrigation.

Selsun
Abbott, Aust.; Abbott, Austral.; Abbott, Belg.; Abbott, Braz.; Abbott, Canad.; Abbott, Denm.; Abbott, Fin.; Abbott, Fr.; Abbott, Ger.; Abbott, Hong Kong; Abbott, Irl.; Abbott, Israel; Abbott, Norw.; Abbott, NZ; Abbott, Port.; Abbott, S.Afr.; Abbott, Swed.; Abbott, Switz.; Abbott, Thai.; Abbott, UK; Ross, USA.
Selenium sulfide (p.1123·1).
Dandruff; pityriasis versicolor; seborrhoeic dermatitis of the scalp.

Selsun Blu Abbott, Ital.
Selenium sulfide (p.1123·1).
Seborrhoeic dermatitis.

Selsun Plus Abbott, Ital.
Selenium sulfide (p.1123·1); menthol (p.1632·3).
Dandruff.

Selsun with Provitamin B₅ Abbott, Canad.
Selenium sulfide (p.1123·1); panthenol (p.1602·3).

Selsun-R Abbott, Neth.
Selenium sulfide (p.1123·1).
Pityriasis versicolor.

Seltoc Apomedica, Aust.
Ethenzamide (p.35·1); diphenhydramine hydrochloride (p.416·1); quinine hydrochloride (p.445·1); ascorbic acid (p.1389·3).
Cold symptoms.

Seltomylon Diba, Mex.
Nalidixic acid (p.227·1).
Urinary-tract infections.

Seltouch Wyeth Lederle, Jpn.
Felbinac (p.36·1).
Inflammation; musculoskeletal, joint, and peri-articular disorders; pain.

Seltrans Niddapharm, Ger.
Sodium selenite (p.1375·2).
Selenium deficiency.

Selukos
Ipex, Aust.; Ipex, Fin.; Ipex, Ger.; Ipex, Norw.; Ipex, Swed.
Selenium sulfide (p.1123·1).
Dandruff; pityriasis versicolor; seborrhoeic dermatitis of the scalp.

Selvigon
Asta Medica, Aust.; Asta Medica, Braz.; Sanfer, Mex.
Pipazetate hydrochloride (p.1099·1).
Coughs.

Selvigon Hustensaft Asta Medica, Ger.
Pipazetate hydrochloride (p.1099·1).
Coughs.

Selvigon Rhone-Poulenc Rorer, Ital.
Pipazetate hydrochloride (p.1099·1).
Coughs.

Semap
Janssen-Cilag, Aust.; Janssen-Cilag, Belg.; Janssen, Braz.; Janssen-Cilag, Denm.; Janssen-Cilag, Fr.; Janssen-Cilag, Israel; Janssen, Mex.; Janssen-Cilag, Neth.; Janssen-Cilag, Switz.
Penfluridol (p.698·1).
Psychoses.

Sembrina
Boehringer Mannheim, Ger.†; Boehringer Mannheim, Neth.†
Methyldopa (p.927·3).
Hypertension.

Semeth Greater Pharma, Thai.
Simeticone (p.1249·2).
Flatulence; meteorism; preparation of gastrointestinal tract for radiological examination or gastroscopy.

Semibiocin Orion, Ger.
Erythromycin ethyl succinate (p.201·2).
Bacterial infections.

Semicid Theraplix, Fr.†; Whitehall, USA.
Nonoxinol 9 (p.1346·1).
Contraceptive.

Semi-Daonil
Hoechst Marion Roussel, Austral.; Hoechst Marion Roussel, Hong Kong; Hoechst Marion Roussel, Irl.; Aventis, NZ; Hoeport, Port.; Hoechst Marion Roussel, S.Afr.†; Hoechst Marion Roussel, Switz.; Hoechst Marion Roussel, UK.
Glibenclamide (p.321·3).
Diabetes mellitus.

Semi-Euglucon
Roche, Aust.; Hoechst Marion Roussel, Aust.; Roche, Fin.; Roche, Hong Kong; Boehringer Mannheim, Neth.†; Roche, Port.; Roche, Switz.; Roche, Thai.
Glibenclamide (p.321·3).
Diabetes mellitus.

The symbol † denotes a preparation no longer actively marketed

Semi-Euglucon N *Roche, Ger.; Hoechst Marion Roussel, Ger.*
Glibenclamide (p.321·3).
Diabetes mellitus.

Semi-Gliben-Puren N *Isis Puren, Ger.*
Glibenclamide (p.321·3).
Diabetes mellitus.

Semilente *Novo Nordisk, Ger.*
Insulin zinc suspension (porcine, monocomponent) (p.324·1).
Diabetes mellitus.

Semilente MC
Novo Nordisk, Fr.†; Novo Nordisk, Switz.
Insulin zinc suspension (amorphous) (porcine, monocomponent) (p.324·1).
Diabetes mellitus.

Semipenil *Magis, Ital.*
Piperacillin sodium (p.236·1).
Lignocaine [lidocaine] hydrochloride (p.1313·2) is included in this preparation to alleviate the pain of injection.
Bacterial infections.

Semitard MC *Novo Nordisk, UK†.*
Insulin zinc suspension (amorphous) (porcine, monocomponent) (p.324·1).
Diabetes mellitus.

Semper *Semper, Fin.*
Range of nutritional preparations (p.1350·1).

Sempera *Janssen-Cilag, Ger.; Glaxo Wellcome, Ger.*
Itraconazole (p.387·2).
Fungal infections.

Semprex
Glaxo Wellcome, Aust.; Warner-Lambert, Denm.†; Warner-Lambert, Fin.; Glaxo Wellcome, Hong Kong; Glaxo Wellcome, Ital.; Glaxo Wellcome, Neth.; Glaxo Wellcome, S.Afr.; Glaxo Wellcome, Singapore; Glaxo Wellcome, Swed.; Glaxo Wellcome, Switz.; Glaxo Wellcome, Thai.; Wellcome, UK.
Acrivastine (p.408·2).
Allergic conjunctivitis; allergic rhinitis; allergic skin disorders.

Semprex-D *Medeva, USA.*
Acrivastine (p.408·2); pseudoephedrine hydrochloride (p.1099·2).
Allergic rhinitis.

Senagar *Sigma, Austral.*
Senega (p.1100·2) and ammonia mixture, chloroform free.
Coughs.

Sendoxan
Asta, Denm.; Asta Medica, Fin.; Asta Medica, Norw.; Asta Medica, Swed.
Cyclophosphamide (p.527·3).
Immune system disorders; malignant neoplasms.

Senecard *Metochem, Aust.†.*
Crataegus (p.1600·2).
Heart disorders.

Senecion *Klein, Ger.†.*
Senecio (p.1661·3); ascorbic acid (p.1389·3).
Haemorrhagic disorders.

Senefor *Pierre Fabre, Ital.†.*
Phosphatidyl serine (p.1651·1).
Mental function impairment.

Senega *Kabi, Swed.†.*
Senega (p.1100·2); ammonium chloride (p.1085·2).
Coughs; sore throats.

Senega and Ammonia *McGloin, Austral.*
Ammonium bicarbonate (p.1085·1); camphor (p.1589·3); liquorice (p.1231·2); senega root (p.1100·2); ammonia solution (p.1579·1).
Cold symptoms.

Seneuval *Qualiphar, Belg.*
Valerian (p.1678·3); passion flower (p.1649·1); crataegus (p.1600·2).
Formerly contained valerian and melissa.
Insomnia; nervousness.

Senexon *Rugby, USA.*
Senna (p.1248·2).
Constipation.

Senicor *Duopharm, Ger.*
Crataegus (p.1600·2).
Cardiac disorders.

Senikolp *Leiras, Fin.*
Sodium estrone sulfate; estradiol (p.1473·1); broxyquinoline.
Menopausal disorders; oestrogen deficiency.

Senilezol *Edwards, USA.*
Vitamin B substances with iron (p.1350·1).

Senior *Strathmann, Ger.†.*
Pemoline (p.1513·1).
Mental function disorders.

Senior Formula *Pharmavite, Canad.*
Multivitamin and mineral preparation (p.1350·1).

Senioral *Belmac, Spain.*
Clocinizine hydrochloride (p.413·3); phenylpropanolamine hydrochloride (p.1098·1).
Formerly contained buzepide metiodide, clocinizine hydrochloride, and pholcodine.
Upper respiratory-tract congestion.

Seniovita aktiv *Cesra, Ger.*
Homoeopathic preparation.

Senlax *Intercare, UK.*
Senna (p.1248·2).
Constipation.

Senna-Gen *Goldline, USA.*
Senna (p.1248·2).
Constipation.

Sennapur *Pharmia, Fin.*
Senna (p.1248·2).
Constipation.

Senna-Specie Composta *Dynacren, Ital.*
Senna (p.1248·2); peppermint (p.1243·2); chamomile (p.1593·2); fennel (p.1610·1).
Constipation.

Sennatural *G & W, USA†.*
Senna (p.1248·2).
Constipation.

Sennesoft *Herron, Austral.*
Docusate sodium (p.1223·1); sennosides (p.1248·3).
Constipation.

Sennetabs *Herron, Austral.*
Sennosides (p.1248·3).
Constipation.

Sennocol *Asta Medica, Neth.*
Senna (p.1248·2).
Constipation.

Senociclin *Senosiain, Mex.*
Tetracycline (p.258·3).
Bacterial infections.

Senodin-AN *Bristol-Myers Squibb, Ital.*
Pheniramine maleate (p.422·3); codeine phosphate (p.25·2).
Coughs.

Senokot
Note.This name is used for preparations of different composition.
Reckitt & Colman, Austral.; Reckitt Benckiser, Irl.; Columbia, Mex.; Reckitt Benckiser, NZ; Reckitt Benckiser, S.Afr.; Reckitt & Colman, Thai.
Sennosides A and B (p.1248·3).
Bowel evacuation; constipation.

Reckitt & Colman, Belg.; Purdue Frederick, Canad.; Sarget, Fr.; Reckitt & Colman, Hong Kong; Nycomed, Norw.; Reckitt & Colman, Singapore; Reckitt & Colman, UK; Purdue Frederick, USA.
Senna (p.1248·2).
Bowel evacuation; constipation.

Senokot-S
Purdue Frederick, Canad.; Purdue Frederick, USA.
Senna (p.1248·2); docusate sodium (p.1223·1).
Constipation.

Senokotxtra *Purdue Frederick, USA.*
Senna (p.1248·2).
Constipation.

Senol
Note.This name is used for preparations of different composition.
Gembalia, Braz.
Allantoin (p.1110·1); aminoacridine (p.1130·3); cinchocaine hydrochloride (p.1309·1); benzocaine (p.1306·2); hydroxyquinoline sulfate (p.1622·2).
Skin disorders.

Bier, Ital.
Cetrimonium bromide (p.1137·3).
Nipple disinfection.

Senolax
Neolab, Canad.†.
Sennosides A and B (p.1248·3).

Schein, USA†.
Senna (p.1248·2).
Constipation.

Senophile
Note.This name is used for preparations of different composition.
Prima, Braz.
Bismuth subnitrate (p.1213·2); bismuth subgallate (p.1213·2); boric acid (p.1586·1); zinc oxide (p.1128·2); magnesium trisilicate (p.1233·3).
Skin disorders.

Braun, Fr.
Zinc oxide (p.1128·2); cholesteryl benzoate.
Skin disorders.

Senorm *Sun, Thai.*
Haloperidol decanoate (p.686·3).
Schizophrenia.

Senosan Crema *Cos Farma, Ital.*
Emollient.

Senro *Biosarto, Spain.*
Norfloxacin (p.232·1).
Genito-urinary tract infections.

Sensaval *Lundbeck, Swed.*
Nortriptyline hydrochloride (p.301·3).
Depression.

Sensibit *Liomont, Mex.*
Loratadine (p.420·1).
Hypersensitivity.

Sensicutan *Harras-Curarina, Ger.*
Levomenol (p.1629·1); heparin sodium (p.902·1).
Skin disorders.

Sensifluid
Ducray, Fr.; Pierre Fabre, Hong Kong.
Avena (p.1583·1).
Soap substitute.

Sensifluor *Warner-Lambert, Ital.†.*
Sodium fluoride (p.1375·3).
Dental caries prophylaxis; dental hypersensitivity.

Sensigel *Pergam, Ital.*
Allantoin (p.1110·1); vitamin A; vitamin E; lactic acid (p.1626·2).
Vaginal lubricant.

Sensinerv forte *Cesra, Ger.*
Valerian root (p.1678·3); lupulus (p.1629·1).
Nervous disorders; sleep disorders.

Sensiotin *Steigerwald, Ger.*
Homoeopathic preparation.

Sensit
Organon, Aust.; Thiemann, Ger.; Organon, Switz.†.
Fendiline hydrochloride (p.889·1).
Ischaemic heart disease.

Sensitex *Kinder, Braz.*
Betamethasone (p.1063·2).
Skin disorders.

Sensit-F *Organon, Ital.*
Fendiline hydrochloride (p.889·1).
Ischaemic heart disease; myocardial infarction.

Sensitiner *Statens Serum Institut, Denm.*
Antigens from *Mycobacterium* spp. (p.1575·3).
Diagnosis of mycobacterial infections.

Sensitive Care *Asta Medica, Port.†.*
Potassium citrate (p.1186·1); sodium monofluorophosphate (p.1377·2).
Dental caries prophylaxis; dental hypersensitivity.

Sensitive Eyes
Bausch & Lomb, Canad.; Bausch & Lomb, USA.
Range of solutions for contact lenses (p.1129·2).

Sensitivity Protection Crest *Procter & Gamble, USA.*
Potassium nitrate (p.1154·3); sodium fluoride (p.1375·3).
Sensitive teeth.

Sensivision au plantain *Chauvin, Fr.*
Plantain (p.1652·3).
Eye disorders.

Sensodent *Stafford-Miller, Switz.*
Strontium chloride (p.1667·2).
Hypersensitive teeth.

Sensodyne *Block, Canad.*
Strontium chloride (p.1667·2).
Hypersensitive teeth.

Sensodyne med *Block, Aust.*
Strontium chloride (p.1667·2).
Hypersensitive teeth.

Sensodyne-F
Note.This name is used for preparations of different composition.
Block, Canad.; Block, USA.
Potassium nitrate (p.1154·3); sodium fluoride (p.1375·3) or sodium monofluorophosphate (p.1377·2).
Hypersensitive teeth.

Stafford-Miller, UK.
Potassium chloride (p.1194·3); sodium fluoride (p.1375·3); triclosan (p.1159·2).
Dental caries prophylaxis; hypersensitive teeth.

Sensodyne-SC *Block, USA.*
Strontium chloride (p.1667·2).
Hypersensitive teeth.

SensoGARD *Block, USA.*
Benzocaine (p.1306·2).
Mouth and throat disorders.

Sensorcaine
AstraZeneca, Canad.; Astra, USA.
Bupivacaine hydrochloride (p.1306·3).
Adrenaline [epinephrine] (p.829·1) or adrenaline [epinephrine] acid tartrate (p.829·2) is included in some injections as a vasoconstrictor to diminish absorption and localise the effect of the local anaesthetic.
Local anaesthesia.

Sentril *Biomedis, Thai.; Great Eastern, Thai.*
Dequalinium chloride (p.1143·1); cetylpyridinium chloride (p.1138·1); ascorbic acid (p.1389·3).
Mouth and throat infections.

Sepan *Janssen-Cilag, Denm.*
Cinnarizine (p.413·1).
Allergic rhinitis; hay fever; motion sickness; urticaria.

Sepatren *Sumitomo, Jpn.*
Cefpiramide sodium (p.172·1).
Bacterial infections.

Sepazon
Sankyo, Hong Kong; Sankyo, Jpn†.
Cloxazolam (p.671·2).
Anxiety states; premedication; sleep disorders.

Sepcen *Centrum, Spain.*
Ciprofloxacin hydrochloride (p.182·3).
Bacterial infections.

Sepdine *PD, Thai.*
Chlorhexidine gluconate (p.1138·2); cetrimide (p.1137·1).
Skin, instrument, and wound disinfection.

Sepexin *Schering-Plough, S.Afr.*
Ceftibuten (p.176·1).
Bacterial infections.

Sepfadine *Nakorn, Thai.*
Povidone-iodine (p.1155·1).
Burns; skin and soft-tissue disinfection; wounds.

Se-Power *Cantassium Co, UK.*
Selenium yeast (p.1375·2); myrtillus (p.1639·2); euphrasia (p.1609·3); vitamin E (p.1393·3); zinc gluconate (p.1398·2); vitamin A (p.1382·1); riboflavin (p.1386·1).

Seprafilm *Genzyme, UK.*
Sodium hyaluronate (p.1620·1); carmellose (p.1499·3).
Prevention of surgical adhesions.

Sepram *Bayer, USA.*
Citalopram hydrobromide (p.281·2).
Depression.

Sepsilem *Lemery, Mex.*
Cefotaxime (p.169·1).
Bacterial infections.

Sepso J *Hofmann & Sommer, Ger.*
Povidone-iodine (p.1155·1).
Burns; infected skin disorders; skin, hand, and mucous membrane disinfection; wounds.

Septa *Circle, USA†.*
Polymyxin B sulfate (p.238·1); neomycin sulfate (p.228·1); bacitracin (p.155·2).
Bacterial skin infections.

Septacare *Teva, Israel.*
Chlorhexidine acetate (p.1138·2); cetrimide (p.1137·1).
Burns; genito-urinary disinfection; skin disinfection; wounds.

Septacef *Septa, Spain.*
Cefradine (p.173·3).
Bacterial infections.

Septacin *Chinoin, Mex.*
Ambroxol hydrochloride (p.1084·3).
Respiratory-tract congestion.

Septacin Amoxi *Chinoin, Mex.*
Ambroxol hydrochloride (p.1084·3); amoxicillin trihydrate (p.149·2).
Respiratory-tract infections.

Septacin Ex *Chinoin, Mex.*
Ambroxol hydrochloride (p.1084·3); clenbuterol hydrochloride (p.763·3).
Respiratory-tract disorders.

Septacord *Muller Goppingen, Ger.*
Potassium aspartate (p.1195·2); magnesium aspartate (p.1190·3); crataegus (p.1600·2).
Cardiac disorders.

Septadine
Note.This name is used for preparations of different composition.
Floris, Israel.
Alcohol (p.1130·3); chlorhexidine (p.1138·2).
Skin disinfection.

Be-Tabs, S.Afr.
Povidone-iodine (p.1155·1).
Minor throat infections; skin infections; wound and burn disinfection.

Septal *Teva, Israel.*
Chlorhexidine gluconate (p.1138·2).
Skin disinfection; wounds.

Septalibour *Ducray, Fr.*
Avena (p.1583·1); copper sulfate (p.1358·1); zinc sulfate (p.1398·2).
Cleansing of atopic skin.

Septalone *Teva, Israel.*
Chlorhexidine gluconate (p.1138·2).
Burns; disinfection in obstetrics; skin and instrument disinfection; wounds.

Septanest
Ogna, Ital.; Septodont, Switz.; Deproco, UK.
Articaine hydrochloride (p.1306·1).
Adrenaline [epinephrine] acid tartrate (p.829·2) is included in this preparation as a vasoconstrictor to diminish absorption and localise the effect of the local anaesthetic.
Local anaesthesia.

Septeal *Sinbio, Fr.*
Chlorhexidine gluconate (p.1138·2).
Skin and wound disinfection.

Septicol
Note.This name is used for preparations of different composition.
Willmar, Mex.
Thiomersal (p.1158·2).

Streuli, Switz.
Chloramphenicol (p.179·1).
Bacterial eye infections.

Septicon *Ciba Vision, Aust.*
Combination pack: Lensept, hydrogen peroxide (p.1147·1); Lensrins NT, storage and rinsing solution (p.1129·2).
Care of soft contact lenses.

Septicortin *Streuli, Switz.†.*
Cortisone acetate (p.1065·3); chloramphenicol (p.179·1).
Inflammatory eye infections.

Septidiaryl *Martin-Johnson & Johnson, Fr.*
Nifuroxazide (p.230·2).

Septidine *Osoth, Thai.*
Povidone-iodine (p.1155·1).
Burns; skin disinfection; wounds.

Septidron *Aventis, S.Afr.*
Pipemidic acid (p.236·1).
Urinary-tract infections.

Septil *Azevedos, Port.*
Povidone-iodine (p.1155·1).
Burns; skin disinfection; skin infections; ulcers; wounds.

Septilisin *Grin, Mex.*
Polymyxin B sulfate (p.238·1); neomycin sulfate (p.228·1); gramicidin (p.213·3).
Bacterial eye infections.

Septiolan *Climax, Braz.*
Co-trimoxazole (p.193·3).
Bacterial infections; Pneumocystis carinii pneumonia; protozoal infections.

Septiolan Balsamico *Climax, Braz.*
Co-trimoxazole (p.193·3); guaifenesin (p.1092·2); ammonium chloride (p.1085·2).
Bacterial infections.

Septirose *Sudo, Singapore.*
Serrapeptase (p.1662·1).
Inflammation; respiratory-tract congestion.

Septisan *Cederroth, Spain.*
Chlorhexidine gluconate (p.1138·2).
Disinfection of skin, burns, and wounds.

Septisept *Chefaro Ardeval, Fr.*
Cetrimide (p.1137·1).

Formerly known as Asepto 7.
Burns; wounds.

Septi-Soft *Calgon Vestal, USA.*
Triclosan (p.1159·2).
Skin cleanser.

Septisol
Note. This name is used for preparations of different composition.
Monot, Fr.†.
Salicylic acid (p.1122·3).
Chronic conjunctivitis.

Calgon Vestal, USA.
Foam: Hexachlorophene (p.1146·1).
Skin disinfection.
Solution: Triclosan (p.1159·2).
Skin cleanser; skin disinfection.

Septison *Orion, Fin.*
Prednisolone (p.1077·3); dequalinium chloride (p.1143·1).
Skin disorders.

Septisooth *Pharmachoice, S.Afr.*
Povidone-iodine (p.1155·1).
Burns; skin infections; ulcers; wounds.

Septivon *Chefaro Ardeval, Fr.*
Triclocarban (p.1159·2); detergents.
Skin and mucous membrane disinfection.

Septivon N *Scholl, Switz.*
Triclocarban (p.1159·2); cetrimonium chloride (p.1137·3).
Hand disinfection; minor skin lesions.

Septocaine *Septodont, USA.*
Articaine hydrochloride (p.1306·1).
Adrenaline [epinephrine] (p.829·1) is included in this preparation as a vasoconstrictor to reduce absorption and localise the effect of the local anaesthetic.
Local anaesthesia.

Septocipro *Lesvi, Spain.*
Ciprofloxacin hydrochloride (p.182·3) or ciprofloxacin lactate (p.182·3).
Bacterial infections.

Septol *Teva, Israel.*
Chlorhexidine gluconate (p.1138·2).
Skin disinfection.

Septolit *Henkel, Ger.*
Benzalkonium chloride (p.1133·2); oligo(di(iminoimidocarbonyl)iminohexamethylene).
Surface disinfection.

Septomandolo *IPA, Ital.*
Cefamandole nafate (p.163·3).
Lignocaine [lidocaine] hydrochloride (p.1313·2) is included in the intramuscular injection to alleviate the pain of injection.
Bacterial infections.

Septomixine *Septodont, Switz.*
Hydrocortisone acetate (p.1073·3); framycetin sulfate (p.208·2).
Formerly contained dexamethasone, polymyxin B sulfate, tyrothricin, and neomycin sulfate.
Dental infections.

Septone *Shiwa, Thai.*
Chlorhexidine gluconate (p.1138·2); cetrimide (p.1137·1).
Burns; skin and instrument disinfection; wounds.

Septonsil *Pekana, Ger.*
Homoeopathic preparation.

Septopal
Merck, Aust.; Biomet, Austral.; Mediplant, Belg.; Merck, Braz.; Merck, Denm.; Merck, Fin.; Merck, Ger.; Merck, Hong Kong; Merck, Irl.; Ortomed, Neth.; Merck, Norw.; Merck, S.Afr.; Merck, Singapore; Anatomica, Swed.; Merck, Switz.; Merck, Thai.; E. Merck, UK.
Gentamicin sulfate (p.210·1); polymethylmethacrylate-methylmethacrylate copolymer (p.1635·2).
Bacterial infections of bone and soft tissues.

Septoprin *Medley, Braz.*
Co-trimoxazole (p.193·3).
Bacterial infections; Pneumocystis carinii pneumonia; protozoal infections.

Septoral *Merck, Port.*
Cetylpyridinium chloride (p.1138·1).

Septosan *Stiefel, Fr.*
Triclocarban (p.1159·2); triclosan (p.1159·2).
Disinfection.

Septosol *Xeragen, S.Afr.*
Phenol (p.1152·3).
Sore throat.

Septra *Glaxo Wellcome, Canad.; Monarch, USA.*
Co-trimoxazole (p.193·3).
Bacterial infections; Pneumocystis carinii pneumonia.

Septran *Glaxo Wellcome, S.Afr.*
Co-trimoxazole (p.193·3).
Bacterial infections.

Septrin
Glaxo Wellcome, Austral.; Glaxo Wellcome, Hong Kong; Glaxo Wellcome, Irl.; Glaxo Wellcome, Israel; Glaxo Wellcome, Mex.; Wellcome, Port.; Glaxo Wellcome, Singapore; Medeva, Spain; Glaxo Wellcome, Thai.; Glaxo Wellcome, UK.
Co-trimoxazole (p.193·3).
Bacterial infections; nocardiosis; Pneumocystis carinii pneumonia; toxoplasmosis.

Sepurin *Gross, Braz.*
Methenamine (p.223·1); methylene blue [methylthioninium chloride] (p.1012·3).
Vulvovaginal infections.

Sequennia *Wyeth Lederle, Aust.*
14 Tablets, conjugated oestrogens (p.1467·1); 14 tablets, medroxyprogesterone acetate (p.1480·1).
Menopausal disorders.

Sequilar
Schering, Aust.; Schering, Ger.; Schering, Switz.†.
Levonorgestrel (p.1486·2); ethinylestradiol (p.1476·2).
28-Day packs also contain 7 inert tablets.
Biphasic oral contraceptive.

Sequilar ED *Schering, Austral.*
21 Tablets, levonorgestrel (p.1486·2); ethinylestradiol (p.1476·2); 7 tablets, inert.
Biphasic oral contraceptive.

Sequilarum *Schering, Swed.†.*
Levonorgestrel (p.1486·2); ethinylestradiol (p.1476·2).
Biphasic oral contraceptive.

Sequostat *Jenapharm, Ger.*
6 Tablets, ethinylestradiol (p.1476·2); 15 tablets, ethinylestradiol (p.1476·2); norethisterone acetate (p.1485·1).
Sequential oral contraceptive.

Seracalm *Demopharm, Switz.†.*
Valerian (p.1678·3); melissa (p.1632·2); neroli oil (p.1640·1); lavender oil (p.1627·2).
Sleep disorders.

Seracin *Pharmaland, Thai.*
Ofloxacin (p.232·3).
Bacterial infections.

Seractil *Gebro, Aust.*
Dexibuprofen (p.44·1).
Fever; inflammation; musculoskeletal and joint disorders; pain.

Serad *Pfizer Consumer, Ital.*
Sertraline hydrochloride (p.308·3).
Depression.

Serag BSS *Serag-Wiessner, Ger.*
Electrolyte solution (p.1180·1).
Eye irrigation.

Serag-HAES *Serag-Wiessner, Ger.*
Pentastarch (p.732·3) in sodium chloride.
Hypovolaemia; plasma volume expansion.

Seralbuman *ISI, Ital.†.*
Albumin (p.724·1).
Hypoalbuminaemia.

Seralbumin *Probifasa, Mex.*
Albumin (p.724·1).
Hypoalbuminaemia; plasma volume expansion; shock.

Seralgan *Lundbeck, Aust.†.*
Citalopram hydrobromide (p.281·2).
Pain.

Seramed *Medifive, Thai.*
Serrapeptase (p.1662·1).
Inflammation; respiratory-tract congestion.

Seranex sans codeine *Democal, Switz.*
Phenazone (p.77·2); propyphenazone (p.80·2); ethenzamide (p.35·1); benzyl mandelate; caffeine (p.761·3).
Pain.

Ser-Ap-Es
Novartis, Canad.†; Novartis, Thai.; Ciba, USA.
Reserpine (p.967·3); hydralazine hydrochloride (p.905·3); hydrochlorothiazide (p.907·3).
Hypertension.

Serasa *Serono, Mex.*
Asparaginase (p.508·3).

Seravit
SHS, Fr.; Scientific Hospital Supplies, Irl.; Scientific Hospital Supplies, UK.
A range of multivitamin and mineral preparations (p.1350·1).

Serax *Wyeth-Ayerst, Canad.; Wyeth-Ayerst, USA.*
Oxazepam (p.697·1).
Alcohol withdrawal syndrome; anxiety.

Serc
Solvay, Austral.; Solvay, Canad.; Solvay, Fr.; Solvay, Irl.; Byk Gulden, Mex.; Solvay, NZ; Solvay, S.Afr.; Solvay, Spain; Solvay, Thai.; Solvay, UK.
Betahistine hydrochloride (p.1584·2).
Ménière's disease; vestibular disorders.

Serdolect
Lundbeck, Aust.; Lundbeck, Denm.†; Lundbeck, Ger.; Lundbeck, Irl.†; Lundbeck, Neth.†; Lundbeck, Norw.; Lundbeck, Switz.; Lundbeck, UK†.
Sertindole (p.705·3).
Schizophrenia.

Serebon *Sankyo, Hong Kong.*
Oxazolam (p.697·2).
Anxiety; depression; premedication; sleep disorders.

Serecid *Lincoln, NZ.*
Hydroxyzine hydrochloride (p.419·1).
Anxiety; nausea and vomiting.

Serecor *Synthelabo, Fr.*
Hydroquinidine hydrochloride (p.912·1).
Arrhythmias.

Seredyn *Degorts, Mex.*
Diazepam (p.674·3).

Sereine *Optikem, USA.*
Range of solutions for hard contact lenses (p.1129·2).

Sere-Mit *Mitim, Ital.*
Saw palmetto (p.1491·2).
Prostatic hyperplasia.

Seren Vita *Synthelabo, Ital.†.*
Chlordiazepoxide hydrochloride (p.659·2).
Alcohol withdrawal syndrome; anxiety.

Serenace
Sigma, Austral.; Searle, Hong Kong; Baker Norton, Irl.; Pharmaco, NZ; Searle, S.Afr.; Searle, Singapore; Searle, Thai.; Baker Norton, UK.
Haloperidol (p.686·3).
Agitation; alcohol withdrawal syndrome; anxiety; childhood behaviour disorders; intractable hiccup;

---

nausea and vomiting; neuroleptanalgesia; psychoses; Tourette syndrome.

Serenade *Alter, Spain.*
Nitrazepam (p.695·2).
Insomnia.

Serenal
Note. This name is used for preparations of different composition.
Sankyo, Jpn†.
Oxazolam (p.697·2).
Anxiety states; premedication; sleep disorders.

Wyeth Lederle, Port.
Oxazepam (p.697·1).

Serenase
Note. This name is used for preparations of different composition.
Sintesa, Belg.
Lorazepam (p.688·3).
Anxiety; insomnia; premedication.

QIF, Braz.
Passion flower (p.1649·1); chamomile (p.1593·2); erythrina mulungu.
Sedative.

Janssen-Cilag, Denm.; Orion, Fin.; Lusofarmaco, Ital.
Haloperidol (p.686·3) or haloperidol decanoate (p.686·3).
Alcohol withdrawal syndrome; disturbed behaviour; hiccups; movement disorders; pain; psychoses; vomiting.

Serene *Pharmaland, Thai.*
Dipotassium clorazepate (p.670·3).
Anxiety.

Serenelfi *Lusofarmaco, Port.*
Haloperidol (p.686·3).

Serenex *Sintofarma, Braz.*
Zopiclone (p.713·1).
Insomnia.

Serenight *Montefarmaco, Ital.*
Vitamin B₆; magnesium; kava; lupulus; eschscholtzia (p.1350·1).

Serenival *Chefaro Ardeval, Fr.†.*
Crataegus (p.1600·2); passion flower (p.1649·1); valerian (p.1678·3).
Insomnia; nervous disorders.

Serenoa Complex *Blackmores, Austral.*
Equisetum (p.1606·3); saw palmetto (p.1491·2); buchu (p.1587·2); d-alpha tocoferil acid succinate (p.1394·1); zinc amino acid chelate (p.1398·3).
Prostate disorders; urinary-tract disorders.

Serenoa-C *Wassen, UK.*
Saw palmetto (p.1491·2); vitamins; minerals (p.1350·1).

Serenol *Dolisos, Canad.*
Homoeopathic preparation.

Serentil
Novartis, Canad.†; Boehringer Ingelheim, USA.
Mesoridazine besilate (p.691·2).
Alcohol withdrawal syndrome; behavioural and personality disorders; psychoses.

Serenus *Sanus, Braz.*
Passion flower (p.1649·1); crataegus (p.1600·2); adonis vernalis (p.1573·3).
Sedative.

Serepax
Wyeth, Austral.; Wyeth Lederle, Denm.; Wyeth Lederle, Norw.; Wyeth, NZ; Aspen, S.Afr.; Wyeth Lederle, Swed.†.
Oxazepam (p.697·1).
Alcohol withdrawal syndrome; anxiety disorders; insomnia.

Serepress *Formenti, Ital.*
Ketanserin tartrate (p.917·2).
Hypertension.

Sereprile *Sanofi Synthelabo, Ital.*
Tiapride hydrochloride (p.709·1).
Gastrointestinal dyskinesia; movement and behaviour disorders.

Sereprostat *Robapharm, Spain.*
Saw palmetto (p.1491·2).
Prostatic disorders.

Seresis *Pharmaton, Switz.*
Vitamins; lycopene; proanthocyanidines; selenium (p.1350·1).

Seresta
Wyeth Lederle, Belg.; Wyeth Lederle, Fr.; Wyeth, Neth.; Wyeth, Switz.
Oxazepam (p.697·1).
Alcohol withdrawal syndrome; anxiety; sleep disorders.

Seretaide *Glaxo Wellcome, Port.*
Salmeterol xinafoate (p.773·3); fluticasone propionate (p.1072·2).
Asthma.

Seretide
Glaxo Wellcome, Aust.; Glaxo Wellcome, Austral.; Glaxo Wellcome, Denm.; Glaxo Wellcome, Fin.; Allen & Hanburys, Irl.; Glaxo Wellcome, Neth.; Glaxo Wellcome, Norw.; Glaxo Wellcome, Singapore; Glaxo Wellcome, Spain; Glaxo Wellcome, Swed.; Glaxo Wellcome, Switz.; Allen & Hanburys, UK.
Salmeterol xinafoate (p.773·3); fluticasone propionate (p.1072·2).
Asthma.

Sereupin *Ravizza, Ital.*
Paroxetine hydrochloride (p.302·3).
Depression; obsessive-compulsive disorder; panic disorders.

Serevent
Glaxo Wellcome, Aust.; Allen & Hanburys, Austral.; Glaxo Wellcome, Belg.; Glaxo Wellcome, Braz.; Glaxo Wellcome, Canad.; Glaxo Well-

---

come, Denm.; Glaxo Wellcome, Fin.; Glaxo Wellcome, Fr.; Glaxo Wellcome, Ger.; Cascan, Ger.; Glaxo Wellcome, Hong Kong; Allen & Hanburys, Irl.; Glaxo Wellcome, Israel; Glaxo Wellcome, Ital.; Glaxo Wellcome, Mex.; Glaxo Wellcome, Neth.; Glaxo Wellcome, Norw.; Glaxo Wellcome, NZ; Glaxo Wellcome, Port.; Allen & Hanburys, S.Afr.; Glaxo Wellcome, Singapore; Glaxo Wellcome, Spain; Glaxo Wellcome, Swed.; Glaxo Wellcome, Switz.; Allen & Hanburys, UK; Glaxo Wellcome, USA.
Salmeterol xinafoate (p.773·3).
Obstructive airways disease.

Serfabiotic *Serra Pamies, Spain.*
Metampicillin sodium (p.222·3).
Bacterial infections.

Serfinato *Basi, Port.†.*
Reserpine (p.967·3).
Hypertension.

Serformin *Novartis, Thai.; Servipharm, Thai.*
Metformin hydrochloride (p.332·3).
Diabetes mellitus.

Serfoxide *Beecham, Spain.*
Pyridoxine phosphoserinate (p.1387·1).
Chronic alcoholism; vitamin B₆ deficiency.

Sergast *Serturner, Ger.*
Turmeric (p.1029·3).
Digestive system disorders.

Seriglutan B12 *Serpero, Ital.†.*
Amino-acid and vitamin B₁₂ preparation (p.1350·1).
Tonic.

Serlain *Roerig, Belg.*
Sertraline hydrochloride (p.308·3).
Depression; obsessive-compulsive disorder; panic disorders.

Serless *Serturner, Ger.*
Urtica root (p.1678·2).
Benign prostatic hyperplasia.

Sermaka *Lilly, Ger.*
Flurandrenolone [fludroxycortide] (p.1072·2).
Skin disorders.

Sermetrol *Serral, Mex.*
Metoprolol (p.932·1).

Sermion
Pharmacia Upjohn, Aust.; Carlo Erba, Braz.; Rhone-Poulenc Rorer, Fr.; Pharmacia Upjohn, Ger.; Pharmacia Upjohn, Hong Kong; Pharmacia Upjohn, Ital.; Pharmacia Upjohn, Mex.; Pharmacia Upjohn, Port.; Kenfarma, Spain; Pharmacia Upjohn, Switz.; Pharmacia Upjohn, Thai.
Nicergoline (p.1640·2) or nicergoline tartrate (p.1640·2).
Cerebral and peripheral vascular disorders; headache; hypertension.

Sermonil *Pharmaland, Thai.*
Imipramine hydrochloride (p.291·1).
Depression; nocturnal enuresis.

Serobif *Serono, Ital.*
Interferon beta (p.632·2).
Malignant neoplasms; viral infections.

Serocalcin *Serono, Mex.*
Calcitonin (p.749·2).

Serocion *Sanwa, Jpn†.*
Propagermanium (p.639·1).
Hepatitis B.

Serocryptin *Serono, Hong Kong; Serono, Mex.; Serono, Singapore; Serono, Switz.; Serono, Thai.*
Bromocriptine mesilate (p.1164·3).
Acromegaly; benign breast disorders; female infertility; galactorrhoea; lactation inhibition; male hypogonadism; menstrual disorders; parkinsonism; pituitary adenoma.

Serocytol *Serolab, Switz.*
A range of equine antisera raised against body tissues and organs.

Serodox *Serono, Mex.*
Doxorubicin.

Serofene *Serono, Braz.; Serono, Ital.; Serono, Mex.*
Clomifene citrate (p.1465·3).
Anovulatory infertility; functional uterine haemorrhage; male infertility; polycystic ovary syndrome.

Serofusine *Braun, Switz.*
Electrolyte infusion with or without glucose (p.1180·1).
Fluid and electrolyte disorders.

Seroglubin *Probifasa, Mex.*
A normal immunoglobulin (p.1551·3).
Passive immunisation.

Seromex *Medinovum, Ital.*
Fluoxetine hydrochloride (p.284·2).
Bulimia nervosa; depression; obsessive-compulsive disorder.

Seromida *Serono, Mex.*
Ifosfamide (p.546·1).

Seromycin
Lilly, Canad.†; Lilly, Hong Kong; Dura, USA.
Cycloserine (p.195·3).
Tuberculosis; urinary-tract infections.

Seronex *Medix, Mex.*
Domperidone (p.1224·1).
Gastrointestinal motility disorders; nausea and vomiting.

Seronil *Orion, Fin.*
Fluoxetine hydrochloride (p.284·2).
Bulimia nervosa; depression; obsessive-compulsive disorder.

Serophene
Serono, Aust.; Serono, Austral.; Serono, Canad.; Serono, Hong Kong;

The symbol † denotes a preparation no longer actively marketed

Serono, Irl.; Serono, Neth.; Serono, NZ; Serono, S.Afr.; Serono, Singapore; Serono, Switz.; Serono, Thai.; Serono, UK†; Serono, USA.
Clomifene citrate (p.1465·3).
Anovulatory infertility; male infertility.

Serophy Monal, Fr.†; Interdelta, Switz.
Sodium chloride (p.1196·1).
Nasal disorders.

Seroplatin Serono, Mex.
Cisplatin (p.525·1).

Seroposide Serono, Mex.
Etoposide (p.538·1).

Seropram Lundbeck, Aust.; Lundbeck, Fr.; Lundbeck, Ital.; Organon, Mex.; Lundbeck, Spain; Lundbeck, Switz.
Citalopram (p.281·2), citalopram hydrobromide (p.281·2), or citalopram hydrochloride (p.281·2).
Anxiety disorders; depression; panic disorder.

Seroquel Zeneca, Austral.; AstraZeneca, Canad.; AstraZeneca, Fin.; Zeneca, Hong Kong; AstraZeneca, Irl.; AstraZeneca, Ital.; Zeneca, Mex.; AstraZeneca, NZ; Zeneca, S.Afr.; AstraZeneca, Singapore; AstraZeneca, Thai.; AstraZeneca, UK; Zeneca, USA.
Quetiapine fumarate (p.703·2).
Psychoses.

Seroscand Scand Pharm, Swed.
Fluoxetine hydrochloride (p.284·2).
Depression.

Serostim Serono, Canad.; Serono, Singapore; Serono, USA.
Somatropin (p.1286·1).
AIDS-related cachexia.

Serotabir Serono, Mex.
Cytarabine (p.530·1).

Serotone Yoshitomi, Jpn.
Azasetron hydrochloride (p.1212·1).
Nausea and vomiting associated with antineoplastic therapy.

Serotron Serono, Mex.
Mitozantrone [mitoxantrone].

Serotulle SSL, UK.
Chlorhexidine acetate (p.1138·2).
Wounds.

Serovidina Serono, Mex.
Zidovudine (p.645·2).

Serovin Serono, Mex.
Vinblastine.

Seroxat SmithKline Beecham, Aust.; SmithKline Beecham, Belg.; SmithKline Beecham, Denm.; SmithKline Beecham, Fin.; SmithKline Beecham, Ger.; SmithKline Beecham, Hong Kong; SmithKline Beecham, Irl.; SmithKline Beecham, Israel; SmithKline Beecham, Ital.; SmithKline Beecham, Neth.; SmithKline Beecham, Norw.; Beecham, Port.; SmithKline Beecham, Singapore; SmithKline Beecham, Spain; SmithKline Beecham, Swed.; SmithKline Beecham, Thai.; SmithKline Beecham, UK.
Paroxetine hydrochloride (p.302·3).
Depression; obsessive-compulsive disorder; panic disorders; post-traumatic stress disorder; social anxiety disorder.

Serpalan Lannett, USA†.
Reserpine (p.967·3).
Hypertension; psychoses.

Serpasil Ciba, Canad.†.
Reserpine (p.967·3).
Hypertension; psychoses.

Serpax Wyeth Lederle, Ital.
Oxazepam (p.697·1).
Alcohol withdrawal syndrome; anxiety; depression; insomnia.

Serpens Lisapharma, Ital.
Saw palmetto (p.1491·2).
Prostatic hyperplasia.

Serradase Siam Bheasach, Thai.
Serrapeptase (p.1662·1).
Inflammation; respiratory-tract congestion; wounds.

Serranit Serral, Mex.
Ranitidine (p.1246·3).
Peptic ulcer.

Serrano M & H, Thai.
Serrapeptase (p.1662·1).
Breast engorgement; cystitis; epididymitis; inflammation; oedema; sinusitis.

Serrao Masa, Thai.
Serrapeptase (p.1662·1).
Inflammation; respiratory-tract congestion; wounds.

Serrapep Asian Pharm, Thai.
Serrapeptase (p.1662·1).
Inflammation; respiratory-tract congestion; wounds.

Serrason Unison, Thai.
Serrapeptase (p.1662·1).
Breast engorgement; cystitis; epididymitis; inflammation; sinusitis; wisdom tooth pericoronitis; wounds.

Serratol Serral, Mex.
Difenidol (p.1222·1).
Nausea and vomiting; vertigo.

Serrazyme Shin Poong, Singapore.
Serrapeptase (p.1662·1).
Inflammation; respiratory-tract congestion.

Sertalia Theramex, Mon.
Copper-wound polyethylene (p.1357·3).
Intra-uterine contraceptive device; postcoital contraceptive.

Serterol Serral, Mex.
Probucol (p.959·2).
Hypercholesterolaemia.

Sertidine Serral, Mex.
Famotidine (p.1225·3).
Peptic ulcer.

Sertrixen Serral, Mex.
Naproxen (p.60·3).
Inflammation; pain.

Serum-Cholinesterase Centeon, Ger.†
Acetylcholinesterase (p.1000·2).
Antidote to suxamethonium chloride; organophosphorus poisoning.

Serutan Menley & James, USA.
Psyllium seed (p.1229·1).
Constipation.

Servambutol Novartis, Thai.; Servipharm, Thai.
Ethambutol hydrochloride (p.205·1).
Tuberculosis.

Servamox Novartis, Mex.; Servipharm, Switz.†; Novartis, Thai.; Servipharm, Thai.
Amoxicillin (p.149·2) or amoxicillin trihydrate (p.149·2).
Bacterial infections.

Servamox CLV Novartis, Mex.
Amoxicillin trihydrate (p.149·2); potassium clavulanate (p.187·2).
Bacterial infections.

Servamox-F Novartis, Mex.
Amoxicillin trihydrate (p.149·2).
Bacterial infections.

Servanolol Novartis, Thai.; Servipharm, Thai.
Propranolol hydrochloride (p.962·3).
Angina pectoris; hypertension; myocardial infarction.

Servatrin Aspen, S.Afr.
Timolol maleate (p.982·1); amiloride hydrochloride (p.835·1); hydrochlorothiazide (p.907·3).
Hypertension.

Servetinal
Note.This name is used for preparations of different composition.
Salusif, Port.
Bismuth salicylate (p.1213·1); belladonna (p.463·1); calcium carbonate (p.1215·1); magnesium hydroxide (p.1233·1); peppermint oil (p.1243·3); sodium bicarbonate (p.1186·2).
Gastric hyperacidity.
Seid, Spain†.
Aluminium hydroxide (p.1210·3); belladonna (p.463·1); calcium carbonate (p.1215·1); magnesium hydroxide (p.1233·1); sodium bicarbonate (p.1186·2).
Gastritis; gastrointestinal hyperacidity.

Servicef
Note.This name is used for preparations of different composition.
Novartis, Mex.
Cefalexin (p.161·3).
Bacterial infections.
Servipharm, Switz.†.
Cefazolin sodium (p.164·3).
Bacterial infections.

Servicillin Novartis, Thai.; Servipharm, Thai.
Ampicillin trihydrate (p.151·1).
Bacterial infections.

Servicimet Novartis, Thai.; Servipharm, Thai.
Cimetidine (p.1216·3).
Gastro-oesophageal reflux; peptic ulcer; Zollinger-Ellison syndrome.

Serviclazide Novartis, Thai.; Servipharm, Thai.
Gliclazide (p.322·2).
Diabetes mellitus.

Serviclox Novartis, Thai.; Servipharm, Thai.
Cloxacillin sodium (p.192·1).
Bacterial infections.

Servicol Novartis, Thai.; Servipharm, Thai.
Chloramphenicol (p.179·1) or chloramphenicol palmitate (p.179·2).
Bacterial infections.

Servicyclin Novartis, Thai.; Servipharm, Thai.
Oxytetracycline hydrochloride (p.234·1).
Bacterial infections.

Servidapsone Novartis, Thai.; Servipharm, Thai.
Dapsone (p.196·1).
Dermatitis herpetiformis; leprosy.

Servidiclox Novartis, Thai.; Servipharm, Thai.
Dicloxacillin sodium (p.199·1).
Bacterial infections.

Servidipine Novartis, Thai.; Servipharm, Thai.
Nifedipine (p.940·1).
Hypertension; ischaemic heart disease.

Servidopa Novartis, Thai.; Servipharm, Thai.
Methyldopa (p.927·3).
Hypertension.

Servidoxyne Servipharm, Hong Kong; Servipharm, Singapore; Novartis, Thai.; Servipharm, Thai.
Doxycycline hyclate (p.200·1).
Bacterial infections.

Servidrat Servipharm, Singapore; Novartis, Thai.; Servipharm, Thai.
Glucose; electrolytes (p.1185·2).
Diarrhoea; oral rehydration therapy.

Serviflox Novartis, Thai.
Ciprofloxacin (p.182·3).
Bacterial infections.

Servigenta Novartis, Mex.; Servipharm, Switz.†; Novartis, Thai.; Servipharm, Thai.
Gentamicin sulfate (p.210·1).
Bacterial infections.

Servin Condrugs, Thai.
Mianserin hydrochloride (p.298·1).
Depression.

Servinadine Novartis, Thai.; Servipharm, Thai.
Terfenadine (p.424·3).
Allergic conjunctivitis; allergic rhinitis.

Servinaprox Servipharm, Switz.†.
Naproxen (p.60·3).
Inflammation; pain.

Servindomet Novartis, Thai.; Servipharm, Thai.
Indometacin (p.44·3).
Gout; musculoskeletal and joint disorders; pain.

Servipen-V Novartis, Thai.; Servipharm, Thai.
Phenoxymethylpenicillin potassium (p.235·1).
Bacterial infections.

Servipep Servipharm, Hong Kong; Servipharm, Singapore; Novartis, Thai.; Servipharm, Thai.
Famotidine (p.1225·3).
Gastro-oesophageal reflux; peptic ulcer; Zollinger-Ellison syndrome.

Serviprofen Servipharm, Switz.†; Novartis, Thai.; Servipharm, Thai.
Ibuprofen (p.43·2).
Fever; gout; inflammation; musculoskeletal and joint disorders; pain.

Serviproxan Novartis, Thai.; Servipharm, Thai.
Naproxen sodium (p.61·1).
Gout; musculoskeletal and joint disorders; pain.

Serviradine Novartis, Thai.; Servipharm, Thai.
Ranitidine hydrochloride (p.1245·2).
Acid aspiration; gastro-oesophageal reflux; gastrointestinal haemorrhage; peptic ulcer; Zollinger-Ellison syndrome.

Servispor Servipharm, Switz.†; Novartis, Thai.; Servipharm, Thai.
Cefalexin (p.161·3).
Bacterial infections.

Servitamol Servipharm, Switz.†; Novartis, Thai.; Servipharm, Thai.
Salbutamol (p.770·3).
Obstructive airways disease.

Servitenol Servipharm, Switz.†.
Atenolol (p.841·3).
Angina pectoris; hypertension; myocardial infarction.

Servitet Novartis, Thai.; Servipharm, Thai.
Tetracycline hydrochloride (p.258·3).
Bacterial infections.

Servithiazid Novartis, Thai.; Servipharm, Thai.
Hydrochlorothiazide (p.907·3).
Hypertension; oedema.

Servitifen Novartis, Thai.; Servipharm, Thai.
Ketotifen (p.767·2).
Allergic bronchitis; asthma; hay fever.

Servitrim Novartis, Mex.; Novartis, Thai.; Servipharm, Thai.
Co-trimoxazole (p.193·3).
Bacterial infections; Pneumocystis carinii pneumonia.

Servitrocin Servipharm, Hong Kong; Servipharm, Singapore; Servipharm, Switz.†; Novartis, Thai.; Servipharm, Thai.
Erythromycin ethyl succinate (p.201·2) or erythromycin stearate (p.201·3).
Bacterial infections.

Servium Teva, Israel.
Chlordiazepoxide (p.659·2).
Anxiety; insomnia; premedication; sedative.

Servizol Novartis, Mex.; Servipharm, Singapore; Servipharm, Switz.†; Novartis, Thai.; Servipharm, Thai.
Metronidazole (p.594·1) or metronidazole benzoate (p.594·1).
Anaerobic infections; protozoal infections.

Serzone Bristol-Myers Squibb, Austral.; Bristol-Myers Squibb, Braz.; Bristol-Myers Squibb, Canad.; Bristol-Myers Squibb, Hong Kong; Bristol-Myers Squibb, Mex.; Bristol-Myers Squibb, NZ; Bristol-Myers Squibb, S.Afr.; Bristol-Myers Squibb, Singapore; Bristol-Myers Squibb, Thai.; Bristol-Myers Squibb, USA.
Nefazodone hydrochloride (p.300·3).
Depression.

Serzonil Bristol-Myers Squibb, Israel.
Nefazodone hydrochloride (p.300·3).
Depression.

Sesal Ophtha, Denm.
Antazoline hydrochloride (p.408·3); naphazoline hydrochloride (p.1095·1).
Allergic conjunctivitis.

Sesalgin Willmar, Mex.
Dipyrone (p.34·1).

Sesame Street McNeil Consumer, USA.
A range of vitamin preparations (p.1350·1).

Sesden Tanabe, Jpn; Tanabe, Singapore.
Timepidium bromide (p.474·2).
Premedication for examination of the gastrointestinal or urinary tract; smooth muscle spasm.

Sessoforte Denk, Hong Kong.
Vitamins; methyltestosterone; kola; damiana; yohimbine; strychnos; ephedra; testis extract (p.1350·1).
Tonic.

Setamol Reckitt & Colman, Austral.; Hovid, Singapore.
Paracetamol (p.71·2).
Fever; pain.

Setin Alliance, S.Afr.
Metoclopramide hydrochloride (p.1235·2).
Gastrointestinal disorders.

Setlers Stafford-Miller, UK.
Calcium carbonate (p.1215·1).
Dyspepsia; flatulence; heartburn; nausea.

Setlers Extra Strength Stafford-Miller, UK†.
Aluminium hydroxide (p.1210·3); magnesium hydroxide (p.1233·1).
These ingredients can be described by the British Approved Name Co-magaldrox.

Setlers Heartburn & Indigestion Liquid Stafford-Miller, UK.
Calcium carbonate (p.1215·1); sodium bicarbonate (p.1186·2); sodium alginate (p.1498·3).
Dyspepsia; gastro-oesophageal reflux; heartburn.

Setlers Tums SmithKline Beecham Consumer, Irl.
Calcium carbonate (p.1215·1).
Dyspepsia; flatulence; heartburn; nausea.

Setlers Wind-eze Stafford-Miller, UK.
Simeticone (p.1249·2).
Flatulence.

Setrilan Essex, Ital.
Spirapril hydrochloride (p.973·2).
Hypertension.

Setron Agis, Israel.
Granisetron (p.1227·3).
Nausea and vomiting induced by cytotoxic therapy.

Setux Hoechst Marion Roussel, Braz.
Codeine resinate; phenyltoloxamine resinate.
Coughs.

Setux Expectorante Hoechst Marion Roussel, Braz.
Codeine resinate; guaifenesin (p.1092·2); phenyltoloxamine resinate.
Coughs.

Seudotabs Parmed, USA.
Pseudoephedrine hydrochloride (p.1099·2).
Nasal congestion.

Seven Seas British Cod Liver Oils, Hong Kong; Seven Seas, Singapore; Merck, Thai.; Seven Seas, UK.
A range of vitamin, mineral, and nutritional preparations (p.1350·1).

Sevenal Chinoin, Mex.
Phenobarbital sodium (p.355·1).

Sevenaleta Chinoin, Mex.
Phenobarbital sodium (p.355·1).

Severin Chinoin, Mex.
Nimesulide (p.62·3).
Fever; inflammation; pain.

Sevinol Schering-Plough, Belg.
Fluphenazine hydrochloride (p.684·3).
Anxiety; nausea; psychosis; vomiting.

Sevorane Abbott, Aust.; Abbott, Austral.; Abbott, Belg.; Abbott, Canad.; Abbott, Denm.; Abbott, Fin.; Abbott, Fr.; Abbott, Ger.; Abbott, Hong Kong; Abbott, Irl.; Abbott, Israel; Abbott, Ital.; Abbott, Mex.; Abbott, Neth.; Abbott, Norw.; Abbott, NZ; Abbott, Singapore; Abbott, Spain; Abbott, Swed.; Abbott, Thai.; Abbott, UK.
Sevoflurane (p.1267·3).
General anaesthesia.

Sevorex Tika, Swed.
Precipitated sulfur (p.1123·3); salicylic acid (p.1122·3).
Scalp disorders.

Sevredol Asta Medica, Fr.; Mundipharma, Ger.; Napp, Irl.; Asta Medica, Neth.; Douglas, NZ; Asta Medica, Spain; Mundipharma, Switz.; Napp, UK.
Morphine sulfate (p.56·1).
Pain.

Sevre-Long Mundipharma, Switz.
Morphine sulfate (p.56·1).
Pain.

Sevrium Vinas, Spain.
Tetrabamate.
Alcohol withdrawal syndrome.

Sexadien Leo, Denm.
Dienestrol (p.1471·1).
Vulvovaginal disorders.

Sexormom INQ, Braz.
Methyltestosterone (p.1482·3); yohimbine (p.1681·3); caffeine (p.761·3); tocopherol (p.1393·3); ephedrine (p.1090·1).
Erectile dysfunction.

SF Gel Cypress, USA.
Sodium fluoride (p.1375·3).
Dental caries prophylaxis.

SFC Lotion Stiefel, USA.
Stearyl alcohol (p.1410·2).
Skin cleanser.

S/Gel Neutrogena, Fr.
Salicylic acid (p.1122·3).
Scalp disorders.

Sguardi Farmigea, Ital.
Benzalkonium chloride (p.1133·2).
Eye disorders.

SH-206 Pharmascience, Canad.
Acetic acid (p.1571·2); camphor (p.1589·3).
Pediculosis.

Shade
Note.This name is used for preparations of different composition.
Schering-Plough, Canad.†.
SPF 15: Octinoxate (p.1517·3); oxybenzone (p.1518·1).
SPF 25: Oxybenzone (p.1518·1); octinoxate (p.1517·3); octisalate (p.1518·1).
SPF 30: Oxybenzone (p.1518·1); octinoxate (p.1517·3); homosalate (p.1517·2); octisalate (p.1518·1).
SPF 45: Octinoxate (p.1517·3); octocrilene (p.1518·1); octisalate (p.1518·1); oxybenzone (p.1518·1).
Sunscreen.
Schering-Plough, USA.
SPF 15: Octinoxate (p.1517·3); oxybenzone (p.1518·1).
Gel SPF 30: Octinoxate (p.1517·3); oxybenzone (p.1518·1); homosalate (p.1517·2).
Lotion SPF 30; stick SPF 30: Octinoxate (p.1517·3); oxybenzone (p.1518·1); homosalate (p.1517·2); octisalate (p.1518·1).
SPF 45: Octinoxate (p.1517·3); oxybenzone (p.1518·1); octocrilene (p.1518·1); octisalate (p.1518·1).
Sunscreen.

Shade UVAGuard Schering-Plough, USA.
Octinoxate (p.1517·3); avobenzone (p.1517·1); oxybenzone (p.1518·1).
Sunscreen.

Shak Iso Clintec, Fr.†.
Preparation for enteral nutrition (p.1350·1).

Shaklee Dandruff Control Shaklee, Canad.
Pyrithione zinc (p.1122·1).

Shaklee Lip Protection Stick Shaklee, Canad.
SPF 15: Padimate O (p.1518·2); oxybenzone (p.1518·1).
Sunscreen.

Shaklee Sunscreen Shaklee, Canad.†.
SPF 30: Octinoxate (p.1517·3); octisalate (p.1518·1); oxybenzone (p.1518·1).
Sunscreen.

Shamday Antiforfora Euroderm, Ital.
Piroctone olamine (p.1121·1); urtica (p.1678·2).
Seborrhoeic dermatitis.

Shampoo SDE Tar Essex, Ital.
Coal tar (p.1125·1).
Scalp disorders.

Shampoo SDE Zinc Essex, Ital.
Pyrithione zinc (p.1122·1).
Seborrhoeic dermatitis.

Shampoo Tersa-Tar Dermaclin, Mex.
Coal tar (p.1125·1).
Scalp disorders.

Shampooing Anti-Pelliculaire Atlas, Canad.
Pyrithione zinc (p.1122·1).

Shampooing extra-doux Widmer, Switz.
Triclosan (p.1159·2).
Scalp disorders.

Shampoux Qualiphar, Belg.†.
Permethrin (p.1436·1); piperonyl butoxide (p.1436·2).
Pediculosis.

Shampoux Repel Qualiphar, Belg.†.
(N-Butyl-N-acetyl)-3-ethylaminopropionate.
Pediculosis.

Sheik Durex, Canad.
Nonoxinol 9 (p.1346·1).
Contraceptive.

Sheik Elite Schmid, USA.
Nonoxinol 9 (p.1346·1).
Contraceptive.

Shemol Grin, Mex.
Timolol maleate (p.982·1).
Glaucoma; ocular hypertension.

Shepard's Dermik, USA.
Emollient and moisturiser.

Shii-ta-ker Holistica, Fr.
Lentinus edodes.
Immunostimulant.

Shin-Biofermin S Takeda, Hong Kong.
Bifidobacterium bifidum (p.1626·3); Lactobacillus acidophilus (p.1626·3); Enterococcus faecalis (p.1626·3).
Constipation; diarrhoea; meteorism.

Shinbit Schering, Jpn.
Nifekalant hydrochloride (p.946·1).
Arrhythmias.

Shincort Yung Shin, Thai.
Triamcinolone acetonide (p.1080·1).
Musculoskeletal, joint, and peri-articular disorders; skin disorders.

Shingles Pain Relief Procare, Austral.
Capsicum (p.1591·1).
Arthritic and rheumatic pain; postherpetic neuralgia.

Shiomarin Shionogi, Jpn.
Latamoxef sodium (p.218·3).
Lignocaine [lidocaine] (p.1313·2) is included in the intramuscular injection to alleviate the pain of injection.
Bacterial infections.

Shiseido Benefiance Daytime Shiseido, Canad.
Cream: Octinoxate (p.1517·3); oxybenzone (p.1518·1).
Emulsion: Octinoxate (p.1517·3).
Sunscreen.

Shiseido Sun Block Stick Shiseido, Canad.
Octinoxate (p.1517·3); titanium dioxide (p.1126·1).
Sunscreen.

Shiseido Sun Protection Shiseido, Canad.
SPF 8: Octinoxate (p.1517·3).
Sunscreen.

Shiseido Sunblock Shiseido, Canad.
SPF 19: Octinoxate (p.1517·3); oxybenzone (p.1518·1).
Sunscreen.

Shiseido Sunblock Face Cream Shiseido, Canad.
Octinoxate (p.1517·3); oxybenzone (p.1518·1); ensulizole (p.1517·2); titanium dioxide (p.1126·1).
Sunscreen.

Shiseido Sunblock Lip Treatment Shiseido, Canad.
Octinoxate (p.1517·3).
Sunscreen.

Shiseido Tanning Shiseido, Canad.†.
SPF 4: Octinoxate (p.1517·3).
Sunscreen.

Shiseido Translucent Sun Block Shiseido, Canad.
Octinoxate (p.1517·3); oxybenzone (p.1518·1); titanium dioxide (p.1126·1).
Sunscreen.

Shiseido Vital-Perfection Shiseido, Canad.
Cream: Octinoxate (p.1517·3); oxybenzone (p.1518·1); titanium dioxide (p.1126·1).
Stick: Octinoxate (p.1517·3).
Sunscreen.

Shur-Seal Milex, USA.
Nonoxinol 9 (p.1346·1).
Contraceptive.

Siadocin Siam Bheasach, Thai.
Doxycycline hyclate (p.200·1).
Bacterial infections.

Sialexin Siam Bheasach, Thai.
Cefalexin (p.161·3).
Bacterial infections.

Sialin Sigmapharm, Aust.
Carmellose sodium (p.1499·3); electrolytes (p.1180·1).
Saliva substitute.

Sialor Solvay, Canad.
Anethole trithione (p.1580·1).
Dry mouth.

Siamdopa Siam Bheasach, Thai.
Methyldopa (p.927·3).
Hypertension.

Siamformet Siam Bheasach, Thai.
Metformin hydrochloride (p.332·3).
Diabetes mellitus.

Siamidine Siam Bheasach, Thai.
Cimetidine (p.1216·3).
Gastric hyperacidity; gastro-oesophageal reflux; peptic ulcer.

Siamik Siam Bheasach, Thai.
Amikacin sulfate (p.148·1).
Bacterial infections.

Sia-Mox Siam Bheasach, Thai.
Amoxicillin trihydrate (p.149·2).
Bacterial infections.

Siampicil Siam Bheasach, Thai.
Ampicillin trihydrate (p.151·2).
Bacterial infections.

Siampraxol Siam Bheasach, Thai.
Alprazolam (p.654·2).
Anxiety; mixed anxiety depressive states.

Siarizine Siam Bheasach, Thai.
Cinnarizine (p.413·1).
Cerebrovascular disorders; migraine; motion sickness; peripheral vascular disorders; vestibular disorders.

Siaten Italfarmaco, Spain.
Zopiclone (p.713·1).
Insomnia.

Sibelium
Janssen-Cilag, Aust.; Janssen-Cilag, Belg.; Janssen, Braz.; Pharmascience, Canad.; Janssen-Cilag, Denm.; Janssen-Cilag, Fr.; Janssen-Cilag, Ger.; Janssen, Hong Kong; Janssen-Cilag, Irl.; Janssen-Cilag, Ital.; Janssen, Mex.; Janssen-Cilag, Neth.; Janssen-Cilag, Port.; Janssen-Cilag, S.Afr.; Janssen-Cilag, Singapore; Esteve, Spain; Janssen-Cilag, Switz.; Janssen, Thai.
Flunarizine hydrochloride (p.418·1).
Migraine; vestibular disorders.

Sibicort Orion, Fin.
Hydrocortisone (p.1073·3); chlorhexidine gluconate (p.1138·2).
Infected skin disorders.

Siblin Warner-Lambert, USA†.
Ispaghula (p.1229·1).
Constipation.

Sical
Rottapharm, Ital.; Rottapharm, Spain.
Salcatonin (p.749·3).
Hypercalcaemia; metastatic bone pain; osteoporosis; Paget's disease of bone.

Sicazine Smith & Nephew, Fr.; Inibsa, Port.
Sulfadiazine silver (p.251·3).
Burns; wounds.

Siccafluid
Thea, Fr.; Farmila, Ital.; Thea, Spain.
Carbomer (p.1499·2).
Dry eyes; eye irritation.

Siccagent Bournonville, Belg.†.
Povidone (p.1503·2).
Dry eyes.

Siccalix Drossapharm, Switz.
Sea salt (p.1196·3); dexpanthenol (p.1602·3).
Nasal dryness.

Siccapos Ursapharm, Ger.
Carbomer 980 (p.1499·2).
Dry eyes.

Siccaprotect
Croma, Aust.; Ursapharm, Ger.
Dexpanthenol (p.1602·3); polyvinyl alcohol (p.1503·1).
Dry eyes.

Sicca-Stulln Stulln, Ger.
Hypromellose (p.1501·3).
Dry eyes.

Siccatears Allergan, Neth.†.
White paraffin (p.1407·3); liquid paraffin (p.1407·1); Amerchol CAB.
Dry eyes.

Sicco Asta Medica, Ger.
Indapamide (p.913·1).
Hypertension.

Siccoral Sanova, Aust.
Acetylcysteine (p.1082·3).
Respiratory-tract disorders associated with viscous mucus.

Sicef Kemyos, Ital.
Cefazolin sodium (p.164·3).
Lignocaine [lidocaine] hydrochloride (p.1313·2) is included in this preparation to alleviate the pain of injection.
Bacterial infections.

Si-Cliss SIFRA, Ital.†.
Sorbitol (p.1377·3); sodium citrate (p.1186·2); sodium lauril sulfoacetate (p.1496·3).
Constipation.

Sico Relax Rottapharm, Spain.
Diazepam (p.674·3).
Alcohol withdrawal syndrome; anxiety; epilepsy; premedication; skeletal muscle spasticity; sleep disorders.

Sicobal Siam Bheasach, Thai.
Mecobalamin (p.1388·3).
Peripheral neuropathies.

Sicombyl Christiaens, Belg.
Salicylic acid (p.1122·3).
Hygiene of the umbilicus in neonates.

Sic-Ophtal Winzer, Ger.
Hypromellose (p.1501·3).
Dry eyes.

Sicorten
Novartis Consumer, Aust.; Novartis Consumer, Belg.; Novartis, Ger.; Novartis, Hong Kong; Novartis, Israel; Novartis, Neth.; Novartis Consumer, Port.; Geminis, Spain; Novartis, Switz.
Halometasone (p.1073·2).
Skin disorders.

Sicorten Plus
Novartis, Ger.; Novartis, Hong Kong; Novartis, Israel; Novartis Consumer, Port.; Novartis, Spain; Novartis, Switz.
Halometasone (p.1073·2); triclosan (p.1159·2).
Infected skin disorders.

Sideril Senosiain, Mex.
Trazodone (p.311·1).

Sideroglobina Pharmacia Upjohn, Ital.
Ferritransferrin.
Iron-deficiency anaemia.

Sidroga Brust-Husten-Tee Jacoby, Aust.
Althaea (p.1577·1); plantago lanceolata; thyme leaf (p.1672·2); aniseed (p.1580·2); orange flowers.
Catarrh; coughs.

Sidroga Erkaltungstee Jacoby, Aust.
Rose fruit (p.1389·3); wild thyme; chamomile flower (p.1593·2); sambucus (p.1660·3); tilia (p.1673·2).
Respiratory tract disorders.

Sidroga Herz-Kreislauf-Tee Jacoby, Aust.
Crataegus (p.1600·2); melissa leaf (p.1632·2); rosemary leaf; orange flowers; spearmint (p.1666·3).
Anxiety disorders; cardiac disorders.

Sidroga Kindertee Jacoby, Aust.
Fennel (p.1610·1); chamomile flower (p.1593·2); melissa leaf (p.1632·2); peppermint leaf (p.1243·2); tilia (p.1673·2).
Gastrointestinal disorders; sleep disorders.

Sidroga Leber-Galle-Tee Jacoby, Aust.
Taraxacum (p.1669·1); silybum marianum fruit (p.1021·3); achillea (p.1572·2); peppermint leaf (p.1243·2); caraway (p.1591·2).
Gastrointestinal and biliary disorders.

Sidroga Magen-Darm-Tee Jacoby, Aust.
Calamus root (p.1588·1); centaury (p.1593·1); chamomile flower (p.1593·2); achillea (p.1572·2); melissa leaf (p.1632·2); spearmint (p.1666·3).
Gastrointestinal disorders.

Sidroga Nerven- und Schlaftee Jacoby, Aust.
Lupulus (p.1629·3); melissa leaf (p.1632·2); valerian root (p.1678·3); spearmint (p.1666·3); orange flowers.
Anxiety disorders; sleep disorders.

Sidroga Nieren- und Blasentee Jacoby, Aust.
Bearberry leaf (p.1583·3); silver birch leaf (p.1585·2); solidago virgaurea; java tea (p.1625·1); couch-grass (p.1599·3); peppermint leaf (p.1243·2).
Urinary-tract disorders.

Sidroga Stoffwechseltee Jacoby, Aust.
Spearmint (p.1666·3); taraxacum (p.1669·1); urtica (p.1678·2); prunus spinosa.
Digestive disorders; renal disorders.

Siduol Eisai, Thai.
Alpha tocoferil calcium succinate; phytomenadione (p.1396·1); rutoside (p.1611·2); muramidase hydrochloride (p.1638·1); pluronic F-68.
Haemorrhoids.

Siduro Ipex, Swed.
Ketoprofen (p.47·3).
Musculoskeletal pain.

Siepex Nattermann, Spain.
Dextromethorphan hydrobromide (p.1087·3).
Cough.

Siero Antiofidico Sclavo, Ital.
European viper venom antiserum (p.1563·3).
European viper bite.

Sies Senosiain, Mex.
Hidrosmin (p.1611·2).
Capillary fragility; haemorrhoids; oedema; venous insufficiency.

Siesta-1 Welti, Switz.
Anhydrous citric acid (p.1596·2); tartaric acid (p.1669·2); magnesium sulfate (p.1191·1); sodium bicarbonate (p.1186·2).
Constipation.

Siete Mares Higado Bacal Grifols, Spain†.
Cod-liver oil (p.1357·2); tocopherol.
Vitamin A and D deficiencies.

Sifaclor Siam Bheasach, Thai.
Cefaclor (p.161·1).
Bacterial infections.

Sifamic SIFI, Ital.†.
Amikacin sulfate (p.148·1).
Eye infections.

Sificetina SIFI, Ital.
Chloramphenicol (p.179·1).
Eye infections.

Sificrom SIFI, Ital.; SIFI, Singapore.
Sodium cromoglicate (p.774·3).
Conjunctivitis; keratoconjunctivitis.

Sifiviral SIFI, Ital.
Aciclovir (p.612·3).
Herpes simplex keratitis.

Siframin Fresenius Kabi, Ital.
Amino-acid infusion (p.1350·1).
Parenteral nutrition.

Sifrol
Boehringer Ingelheim, Denm.; Boehringer Ingelheim, Fin.; Boehringer Ingelheim, Ger.; Boehringer Ingelheim, Neth.; Boehringer Ingelheim, Norw.; Boehringer Ingelheim, Swed.; Boehringer Ingelheim, Switz.
Pramipexole hydrochloride (p.1176·1).
Parkinsonism.

Sigabloc Dumex, Ger.
Atenolol (p.841·3); chlortalidone (p.857·1).
Hypertension.

Sigabroxol Dumex, Ger.
Ambroxol hydrochloride (p.1084·3).
Respiratory-tract disorders with increased or viscous mucus.

Sigacalm Dumex, Ger.
Oxazepam (p.697·1).
Anxiety; sleep disorders.

Sigacap Cor Dumex, Ger.
Captopril (p.853·3).
Heart failure; hypertension.

Sigacefal Dumex, Ger.
Cefaclor (p.161·1).
Bacterial infections.

Sigacimet Dumex, Ger.
Cimetidine (p.1216·3).
Acid aspiration; gastro-oesophageal reflux; peptic ulcer; Zollinger-Ellison syndrome.

Sigacora Dumex, Ger.
Isosorbide mononitrate (p.916·2).
Angina pectoris; heart failure; pulmonary hypertension.

Sigadoc Dumex, Ger.
Indometacin (p.44·3).
Musculoskeletal, joint, and soft-tissue disorders; sports injuries.

Sigadoxin
Jacoby, Aust.; Dumex, Ger.; Neves, Port.; Medika, Switz.
Doxycycline (p.200·1) or doxycycline hyclate (p.200·1).
Bacterial infections.

Sigafam Rhein, Mex.
Famotidine (p.1225·3).
Gastro-oesophageal reflux; peptic ulcer; Zollinger-Ellison syndrome.

Sigafenac Dumex, Ger.
Diclofenac sodium (p.30·3).
Gout; inflammation; musculoskeletal, joint, and soft-tissue disorders; pain.

Sigamopen Dumex, Ger.
Amoxicillin trihydrate (p.149·2).
Bacterial infections.

Sigamuc Dumex, Ger.
Doxycycline hyclate (p.200·1); ambroxol hydrochloride (p.1084·3).
Bacterial infections of the respiratory tract.

Sigamucil Dumex, Ger.
Acetylcysteine (p.1082·3).
Respiratory-tract disorders associated with increased or viscous mucus.

Sigaperidol *Dumex, Ger.; Medika, Switz.*
Haloperidol (p.686·3).
Hyperactivity; pain; psychiatric disorders; vomiting.

Sigaprim *Dumex, Ger.; Medika, Switz.*
Co-trimoxazole (p.193·3).
Bacterial infections; Pneumocystis carinii pneumonia.

Sigaprolol *Dumex, Ger.*
Metoprolol tartrate (p.931·2).
Arrhythmias; hypertension; ischaemic heart disease; migraine; myocardial infarction.

Sigapurol *Medika, Switz.; Siegfried, Thai.*
Allopurinol (p.397·2).
Gout; hyperuricaemia; renal calculi.

Sigasalur *Dumex, Ger.*
Frusemide [furosemide] (p.893·1).
Hypertension; oedema.

Sigma Liquid Antacid *Sigma, Austral.*
Aluminium hydroxide (p.1210·3); magnesium hydroxide (p.1233·1); simeticone (p.1249·2).
Dyspepsia; flatulence; heartburn.

Sigma Relief *Sigma, Austral.; Sigma, Hong Kong.*
Dextromethorphan hydrobromide (p.1087·3); pseudoephedrine hydrochloride (p.1099·2); guaifenesin (p.1092·2).
Coughs; respiratory-tract congestion.

Sigma Relief Junior *Sigma, Austral.; Sigma, Hong Kong.*
Dextromethorphan hydrobromide (p.1087·3); pseudoephedrine hydrochloride (p.1099·2).
Coughs; respiratory-tract congestion.

Sigmacort *Sigma, Austral.*
Hydrocortisone acetate (p.1073·3).
Inflammatory skin disorders.

Sigmafon *Lafare, Ital.*
Mebutamate (p.925·3).
Hypertension.

Sigmalin B₆ *Sigmapharm, Aust.*
Salicylamide (p.82·1); paracetamol (p.71·2); caffeine (p.761·3); pyridoxine hydrochloride (p.1386·3).
Fever; pain.

Sigmalin B₆ forte *Sigmapharm, Aust.*
Salicylamide (p.82·1); paracetamol (p.71·2); dextropropoxyphene hydrochloride (p.27·1); caffeine (p.761·3); pyridoxine hydrochloride (p.1386·3).
Fever; pain.

Sigmalin B₆ ohne Coffein *Sigmapharm, Aust.*
Salicylamide (p.82·1); paracetamol (p.71·2); pyridoxine hydrochloride (p.1386·3).
Fever; pain.

Sigman-Haustropfen *Sigmapharm, Aust.*
Peppermint oil (p.1243·3); caraway oil (p.1591·2); dexpanthenol (p.1602·3); chamomile flower (p.1593·2); condurango bark (p.1599·1); senna leaf (p.1248·2); frangula bark (p.1227·1); liquorice root (p.1231·2); absinthium (p.1571·1); gentian root (p.1615·1); bitter orange peel (p.1644·2).
Gastrointestinal and biliary-tract disorders.

Sigmart *Chugai, Jpn.*
Nicorandil (p.939·2).
Angina pectoris.

Sigmetadine *Sigma, Austral.*
Cimetidine (p.1216·3).
Gastro-oesophageal reflux; peptic ulcer; Zollinger-Ellison syndrome.

Signal *Green Turtle Bay Vitamin Co., USA.*
Omega triglycerides (p.1350·1).
Tonic.

Sigtab-M *Roberts, USA.*
Multivitamin and mineral preparation (p.1350·1).

Siguent Hycor *Sigma, Austral.*
Hydrocortisone acetate (p.1073·3).
Inflammatory eye disorders.

Siguent Neomycin *Sigma, Austral.*
Neomycin sulfate (p.228·1).
Topical skin infections.

Silace *Tanta, Canad.; Silarx, USA.*
Docusate sodium (p.1223·1).
Constipation.

Silace-C *Silarx, USA.*
Casanthranol (p.1216·1); docusate sodium (p.1223·1).
Constipation.

SilaClean 20/20 *Professional Supplies, USA†.*
Cleansing solution for hard contact lenses (p.1129·2).

Silact *Sofar, Ital.*
Tilactase (p.1673·2).
Lactose intolerance.

Siladryl *Silarx, USA.*
Diphenhydramine hydrochloride (p.416·1).
Hypersensitivity reactions.

Silafed *Silarx, USA.*
Pseudoephedrine hydrochloride (p.1099·2); triprolidine hydrochloride (p.427·2).
Upper respiratory-tract symptoms.

Silain *Teva, Israel.*
Simeticone (p.1249·2); aluminium oxide-magnesium carbonate co-dried gel (p.1211·2).
Flatulence; gastrointestinal hyperacidity.

Silaminic Cold *Silarx, USA†.*
Phenylpropanolamine hydrochloride (p.1098·1); chlorpheniramine [chlorphenamine] maleate (p.412·1).
Cold symptoms.

Silaminic Expectorant *Silarx, USA†.*
Phenylpropanolamine hydrochloride (p.1098·1); guaifenesin (p.1092·2).
Coughs.

Sil-A-Mox *Silom, Thai.*
Amoxicillin trihydrate (p.149·2).
Bacterial infections.

Silan *Smith & Nephew, Denm.*
Dimethicone (p.1410·1); zinc oxide (p.1128·2).
Dry skin.

Silapap *Silarx, USA.*
Paracetamol (p.71·2).
Fever; pain.

Silarine *Vir, Spain.*
Silymarin (p.1021·3).
Toxic hepatitis.

Silastic *Dow Corning, UK.*
Liquid silicone (p.1410·1); stannous octoate.
Open granulating wounds.

Silaxon *Restan, S.Afr.*
Sennosides A and B (p.1248·3).
Constipation.

Silbar *Sigma, Austral.†.*
Barrier cream.

Silberne *Brady, Aust.*
Cascara (p.1216·3); rhubarb (p.1248·1); ox bile (p.1585·1).
Constipation.

Silcon *Faulding, Austral.*
Dimethicone (p.1410·1); wool fat (p.1410·3).
Barrier preparation.

Sildec-DM *Silarx, USA.*
Oral drops: Carbinoxamine maleate (p.411·1); pseudoephedrine hydrochloride (p.1099·2); dextromethorphan hydrobromide (p.1087·3).
Syrup: Brompheniramine maleate (p.410·2); pseudoephedrine hydrochloride (p.1099·2); dextromethorphan hydrobromide (p.1087·3).
Coughs.

Sildicon-E *Silarx, USA†.*
Phenylpropanolamine hydrochloride (p.1098·1); guaifenesin (p.1092·2).
Coughs.

Silencium *Hoechst Marion Roussel, Braz.*
Dextromethorphan hydrobromide (p.1087·3); doxylamine succinate (p.417·1); sodium citrate (p.1186·2).
Coughs.

Silentan *Krewel, Ger.*
Nefopam hydrochloride (p.62·1).
Formerly contained diazepam and aspirin.
Pain.

Silepar *Ibirn, Ital.*
Silymarin (p.1021·3).
Liver disorders.

Silettum *Jaldes, Fr.*
Equisetum; hydolysed sesame protein; vitamin B substances (p.1350·1).
Hair disorders.

Silfedrine *Silarx, USA.*
Pseudoephedrine hydrochloride (p.1099·2).
Nasal congestion.

Silflam *Silom, Thai.*
Diclofenac diethylamine (p.30·2).
Musculoskeletal, joint, and peri-articular disorders.

Silgel *Nagor, UK.*
Silicone (p.1410·1).
Hypertrophic and keloid scars.

Silibene *Merckle, Ger.*
Silybum marianum (p.1021·3).
Liver disorders.

Silic *Ego, NZ.*
Dimethicone (p.1410·1); glycerol (p.1616·3).
Barrier agent.

Silic 15 *Ego, Austral.; Ego, Hong Kong; Ego, Singapore.*
Dimethicone (p.1410·1).
Barrier preparation; dry skin.

Silica L11 *Homeocan, Canad.*
Homoeopathic preparation.

Silicic Complex *Procare, Austral.*
Equisetum (p.1606·3); silica (p.1503·3); calcium (p.1187·3); potassium (p.1194·3).
Brittle nails and hair; tissue repair.

Silicin *Greater Pharma, Thai.*
Cinnarizine (p.413·1).
Cerebrovascular disorders; migraine; motion sickness; peripheral vascular disorders; vestibular disorders.

Silicur *Biocur, Ger.*
Silybum marianum (p.1021·3).
Liver disorders.

Silidermil *Fides Rottapharm, Spain.*
Ointment: Dimethicone (p.1410·1); zinc oxide (p.1128·2).
Topical powder: Cetylpyridinium chloride (p.1138·1); dimethicone (p.1410·1); zinc oxide (p.1128·2).
Skin disorders.

Silidron *Enila, Braz.*
Dimethicone (p.1249·2).
Flatulence.

Siligaz *Bio-Sante, Canad.; Arkomedika, Fr.*
Dimethicone (p.1249·2).
Abdominal distension; flatulence; gastro-oesophageal reflux.

Siligel *Enila, Braz.*
Aluminium hydroxide (p.1210·3); magnesium trisilicate (p.1233·3); dimethicone (p.1249·2).
Flatulence; gastrointestinal hyperacidity.

Silimag *Faes, Spain.*
Magnesium trisilicate (p.1233·3).
Dyspepsia; peptic ulcer.

Silimalon *Nikkho, Braz.*
Methionine (p.1012·3); silymarin (p.1021·3).
Liver disorders.

Silimarin *Benedetti, Ital.*
Silymarin (p.1021·3).
Liver disorders.

Silimarit *Bionorica, Ger.*
Silybum marianum (p.1021·3).
Liver disorders.

Silimazu *Farmasur, Spain.*
Silymarin (p.1021·3).
Toxic hepatitis.

Sili-Met-San
Note. This name is used for preparations of different composition.
Bio-Therabel, Belg.; UCB, Switz.
Tablets: Dimethicone (p.1249·2); calcium pantothenate (p.1374·1).
Aid to radiologic examination; flatulence.
UCB, Switz.
Oral suspension: Dimethicone (p.1249·2).
Aid to radiological examination; flatulence.

Siliprele *Herboxt, Fr.*
Equisetum (p.1606·3).
Gastrointestinal and renal disorders.

Silirex *Lampugnani, Ital.*
Silymarin (p.1021·3).
Liver disorders.

Silisan *Lipha, Ital.*
Simeticone (p.1249·2); calcium pantothenate (p.1374·1).
Gastrointestinal disorders associated with excess gas; preparation of the stomach for endoscopy and surgery.

Siliver *Abbott, Braz.*
Silymarin (p.1021·3).
Liver disorders.

Silkonol *Pharmacia Upjohn, Aust.†.*
Dimethicone (p.1249·2); zinc oxide (p.1128·2).
Barrier preparation.

Silliver *Abbott, Braz.*
Silymarin (p.1021·3).
Liver disorders.

Sillix *Giuliani, Ital.*
Dried yeast (p.1398·1); vitamin B substances (p.1350·1).

Sillix Donna *Giuliani, Ital.†.*
Minerals; dried yeast; vitamin E; vitamin B₆; folic acid (p.1350·1).
Nutritional supplement.

Silmar *Hennig, Ger.†.*
Silybum marianum (p.1021·3).
Liver disorders.

Silmycetin *Silom, Thai.*
Chloramphenicol (p.179·1).
Bacterial eye or ear infections.

Sil-Norboral *Silanes, Mex.*
Glibenclamide (p.321·3); metformin.
Diabetes mellitus.

Silomat
Note. This name is used for preparations of different composition.
Boehringer Ingelheim, Aust.; Boehringer Ingelheim, Belg.; Boehringer de Angeli, Braz.; Boehringer Ingelheim, Fin.; Boehringer Ingelheim, Ger.; Boehringer Ingelheim, Port.; Boehringer Ingelheim, Singapore; Boehringer Ingelheim, Thai.
Clobutinol hydrochloride (p.1087·1).
Coughs.
Boehringer Ingelheim, Fr.
Syrup: Clobutinol hydrochloride (p.1087·1); sodium benzoate (p.1134·3).
Formerly contained clobutinol hydrochloride, ammonium chloride, and sodium benzoate.
Tablets; oral solution; injection: Clobutinol hydrochloride (p.1087·1).
Coughs.

Silomat Compositum
Boehringer Ingelheim, Swed.†; Boehringer Ingelheim, Thai.
Clobutinol hydrochloride (p.1087·1); orciprenaline sulfate (p.769·1).
Coughs.

Silomat DA *Boehringer Ingelheim, S.Afr.*
Clobutinol hydrochloride (p.1087·1); orciprenaline sulfate (p.769·1).
Formerly known as Silomat Composit.
Coughs.

Silomat Plus *Boehringer de Angeli, Braz.*
Clobutinol hydrochloride (p.1087·1); doxylamine succinate (p.417·1).
Coughs.

Silomat-Fher *Boehringer Ingelheim, Ital.*
Clobutinol hydrochloride (p.1087·1).
Coughs.

Silon *Smith & Nephew, Swed.*
Dimethicone (p.1410·1); zinc oxide (p.1128·2).
Barrier cream.

Silox-50 *Jean-Marie, Hong Kong.*
Aluminium hydroxide (p.1210·3); magnesium trisilicate (p.1233·3); simeticone (p.1249·2).
Flatulence; gastritis; gastrointestinal hyperacidity; heartburn.

Siloxan *Nycomed, Norw.*
Dimethicone (p.1249·2).
Flatulence; postoperative intestinal gas retention.

Silphen *Silarx, USA.*
Diphenhydramine hydrochloride (p.416·1).

Silphen DM *Silarx, USA.*
Dextromethorphan hydrobromide (p.1087·3).
Coughs.

Silpin *Laborsil, Braz.*
Co-trimoxazole (p.193·3).
Bacterial infections; Pneumocystis carinii pneumonia; protozoal infections.

Siltapp *Silarx, USA†.*
Brompheniramine maleate (p.410·2); phenylpropanolamine hydrochloride (p.1098·1); dextromethorphan hydrobromide (p.1087·3).
Upper respiratory-tract symptoms.

Sil-Tex *Silarx, USA†.*
Phenylephrine hydrochloride (p.1097·1); phenylpropanolamine hydrochloride (p.1098·1); guaifenesin (p.1092·2).
Coughs.

Siltussin
Note. This name is used for preparations of different composition.
Silom, Thai.
Guaifenesin (p.1092·2); ammonium chloride (p.1085·2); menthol (p.1632·3).
Coughs.
Silarx, USA.
Guaifenesin (p.1092·2).
Coughs.

Siltussin DM *Silarx, USA.*
Guaifenesin (p.1092·2); dextromethorphan hydrobromide (p.1087·3).
Coughs.

Siltussin-CF *Silarx, USA†.*
Guaifenesin (p.1092·2); phenylpropanolamine hydrochloride (p.1098·1); dextromethorphan hydrobromide (p.1087·3).
Coughs.

Silubin
Andromaco, Spain; Grunenthal, Switz.
Buformin (p.321·1) or buformin hydrochloride (p.321·1).
Diabetes mellitus.

Siludrox *Whitehall, Braz.*
Dimethicone (p.1249·2); aluminium hydroxide (p.1210·3); magnesium hydroxide (p.1233·1).
Flatulence; gastrointestinal hyperacidity.

Silvadene *Rhone-Poulenc Rorer, Mex.; Hoechst Marion Roussel, Switz.†; Hoechst Marion Roussel, USA.*
Sulfadiazine silver (p.251·3).
Infected burns; skin ulcers.

Silvana *Molteni, Ital.*
Benzalkonium chloride (p.1133·2); glacial acetic acid (p.1571·2).
Skin disinfection.

Silvaysan *Sanum-Kehlbeck, Ger.*
Silybum marianum (p.1021·3).
Liver disorders.

Silvazine
Smith & Nephew, Austral.; Smith & Nephew, NZ; Smith & Nephew, Singapore.
Sulfadiazine silver (p.251·3); chlorhexidine gluconate (p.1138·2).
Infected burns, ulcers, and pressure sores.

Silvederma *Aldo, Spain.*
Sulfadiazine silver (p.251·3).
Burns; skin ulcers; wounds.

Silvedine *Silvestre, Braz.*
Povidone-iodine (p.1155·1).
Disinfection of skin, mucous membranes, wounds, and instruments.

Silver Clove Medicated Balm *Sportbalm, Austral.*
Clove bud oil (p.1597·1); menthol (p.1632·3); cajuput oil (p.1588·1); peppermint oil (p.1243·3); camphor (p.1589·3).
Musculoskeletal and joint pain.

Silvercef *Tosi, Ital.*
Cefonicid sodium (p.168·1).
Lignocaine [lidocaine] hydrochloride (p.1313·2) is included in this preparation to alleviate the pain of injection.
Gram-negative bacterial infections.

Silverol
Abic, Hong Kong; Abic, Israel; Abic, Thai.
Sulfadiazine silver (p.251·3).
Infected burns; infected skin ulcers; infected wounds.

Silvertone *Resinag, Switz.*
Sulfadiazine silver (p.251·3).
Infected burns; infected wounds.

Silybum Complex *Blackmores, Austral.*
Silybum marianum (p.1021·3); garlic (p.1614·1); taraxacum (p.1669·1); nicotinic acid (p.1372·3); sodium sulfate (p.1250·1).
Hypercholesterolaemia; liver and biliary-tract disorders.

Silyhexal *Hexal, Aust.*
Silybum marianum (p.1021·3).
Liver disorders.

Silymarin Phytosome *Eagle, Austral.*
Silybum marianum (p.1021·3).
Digestive disorders.

Silzolin *Tosi, Ital.*
Cefazolin sodium (p.164·3).

Lignocaine [lidocaine] hydrochloride (p.1313·2) is included in this preparation to alleviate the pain of injection.
Bacterial infections.

Simaal Gel 2 Schein, USA.
Aluminium hydroxide (p.1210·3); magnesium hydroxide (p.1233·1); simeticone (p.1249·2).
Hyperacidity.

Simacort Siam Bheasach, Thai.
Triamcinolone acetonide (p.1080·1).
Musculoskeletal, joint, and peri-articular disorders; skin disorders.

Simagel
Note. This name is used for preparations of different composition.
Philopharm, Ger.
Almasilate (p.1210·1).
Gastrointestinal disorders.
Atlantic, Thai.
Dried aluminium hydroxide gel (p.1210·3); magnesium hydroxide (p.1233·1); simeticone (p.1249·2).
Flatulence; gastric hyperacidity; gastritis; heartburn; peptic ulcer.

Simaglen Unison, Thai.
Cimetidine (p.1216·3).
Gastro-oesophageal reflux; peptic ulcer.

Simaphil Philopharm, Ger.
Magaldrate (p.1232·2).
Gastrointestinal disorders.

Simar Ofimex, Mex.
Rifampicin (p.243·2).

Simatin Chemomedica, Aust.
Ethosuximide (p.348·1).
Absence seizures.

Simcone TO-Chemicals, Thai.
Simeticone (p.1249·2).
Infant flatulence.

Simdax Orion, Swed.
Levosimendan (p.920·3).
Heart failure.

Simeco
Note. This name is used for preparations of different composition.
Whitehall, Austral.†; Whitehall, Singapore; Whitehall, Thai.; Wyeth, UK.
Oral suspension: Aluminium hydroxide (p.1210·3); magnesium hydroxide (p.1233·1); simeticone (p.1249·2).
Dyspepsia; flatulence.
Wyeth-Ayerst, Hong Kong; Whitehall, Singapore; Whitehall, Thai.; Wyeth, UK.
Tablets: Aluminium hydroxide-magnesium carbonate co-dried gel (p.1211·2); magnesium hydroxide (p.1233·1); simeticone (p.1249·2).
Dyspepsia; flatulence.

Simeco Plus Wyeth, Braz.
Aluminium hydroxide (p.1210·3); magnesium hydroxide (p.1233·1); dimethicone (p.1249·2).
Flatulence; gastrointestinal hyperacidity.

Simecon Chinta, Thai.
Simeticone (p.1249·2).
Infant flatulence.

Simegel-F Medipharma, Hong Kong.
Aluminium hydroxide (p.1210·3); magnesium hydroxide (p.1233·1); simeticone (p.1249·2).
Dyspepsia; flatulence; gastrointestinal hyperacidity; peptic ulcer.

Simepar
Mepha, Hong Kong; Mepha, Singapore; Mepha, Switz.
Silymarin (p.1021·3); vitamin B substances (p.1350·1).
Liver disorders.

Simetac Vida, Hong Kong.
Ranitidine hydrochloride (p.1245·2).
Gastro-oesophageal reflux; peptic ulcer.

Simex Hua, Thai.
Cimetidine (p.1216·3).
Peptic ulcer; Zollinger-Ellison syndrome.

Simic Zyma, Switz.†.
Urtica root (p.1678·2).
Benign prostatic hyperplasia.

Simicol CTI, Israel.
Simeticone (p.1249·2).
Colic; flatulence; griping pain.

Simil NF Labima, Belg.†.
Ethenzamide (p.35·1).
Fever; pain.

Similac Ross, USA.
Low-mineral infant feed (p.1350·1).
For infants predisposed to hypocalcaemia or requiring low mineral levels.

Similac Isomil Abbott, Israel.
Infant feed (p.1350·1).
Cows milk protein sensitivity.

Similac LF
Abbott, Israel; Abbott, Hong Kong; Abbott, Ital.; Abbott, Thai.
Lactose-free infant feed (p.1350·1).
Lactose intolerance.

Similac RA Abbott, Ital.
Infant feed (p.1350·1).
Hypersensitivity.

Similasan 1 Ocusoft, USA.
Artificial tears.

Simoph Tears Siam Bheasach, Thai.
Hypromellose (p.1501·3) (p.1129·2).
Dry eye; wetting solution for hard contact lenses.

Simovil Merck Sharp & Dohme, Israel.
Simvastatin (p.969·2).
Hyperlipidaemias.

Simoxil Virginia, Ital.
Amoxicillin trihydrate (p.149·2).
Bacterial infections.

Simoyiam Siam Bheasach, Thai.
Flunarizine hydrochloride (p.418·1).
Cerebrovascular disorders; migraine.

Simp Esoform, Ital.
Chlorhexidine gluconate (p.1138·2); benzalkonium chloride (p.1133·2).
Skin and wound disinfection.

Simple Agepha, Aust.
Disinfection and storage solution for contact lenses (p.1129·2).

Simple Cleaner Agepha, Aust.
Cleaning solution for contact lenses (p.1129·2).

Simplene
Chauvin, Irl.†; Smith & Nephew, S.Afr.†; Chauvin, UK†.
Adrenaline [epinephrine] (p.829·1).
Open-angle glaucoma.

Simplet Major, USA.
Pseudoephedrine hydrochloride (p.1099·2); chlorpheniramine [chlorphenamine] maleate (p.412·1); paracetamol (p.71·2).
Upper respiratory-tract symptoms.

Simplex Nycomed, Norw.
Liquid paraffin (p.1407·1); white soft paraffin (p.1407·3).
Sore and dry skin in the eyelid area.

Simplex-Fieberblasen Nycomed, Aust.
Aciclovir (p.612·3).
Herpes labialis.

Simplicity Stanley, Canad.
Pregnancy test and fertility test (p.1654·3).

Simplotan
G.P. Laboratories, Austral.; Pfizer, Ger.; Pierre Fabre, Ger.
Tinidazole (p.603·3).
Anaerobic bacterial infections; protozoal infections.

Simpottantacinque Esoform, Ital.
Benzalkonium chloride (p.1133·2); chlorhexidine gluconate (p.1138·2); alcohol (p.1130·3).
Disinfection of skin, hands, and wounds.

Simprox Areu, Spain.
Astemizole (p.409·1).
Hypersensitivity reactions.

Simpsons Medico-Biological Laboratories, UK.
Zinc stearate (p.1497·3); zinc oxide (p.1128·2); sublimed sulfur (p.1123·3); salicylic acid (p.1122·3).
Skin disorders.

Simron SmithKline Beecham, USA†.
Ferrous gluconate (p.1360·1).
Iron-deficiency anaemias.

Simron Plus SmithKline Beecham, USA.
Vitamin B substances with vitamin C, iron, and folic acid (p.1350·1).

Simulcium G3 Gandhour, Fr.
Monomethyltrisilanol mannuronate.
Skin disorders.

Simulect
Novartis, Austral.; Novartis, Belg.; Novartis, Denm.; Novartis, Fin.; Novartis, Fr.; Novartis, Ger.; Novartis, Hong Kong; Novartis, Irl.; Novartis, Ital.; Novartis, Mex.; Novartis, Neth.; Novartis, Norw.; Novartis, NZ; Novartis, Port.; Novartis, S.Afr.; Novartis, Singapore; Novartis, Spain; Novartis, Swed.; Novartis, Switz.; Novartis, Thai.; Novartis, UK; Novartis, USA.
Basiliximab (p.511·1).
Renal transplant rejection.

Simusol Siam Bheasach, Thai.
Ambroxol hydrochloride (p.1084·3).
Respiratory-tract disorders associated with increased or viscous mucus.

Simvast Julphar, UAE.
Simvastatin sodium (p.970·2).
Atherosclerosis; hypercholesterolaemia.

Sin Mareo x 4 Calmante Vitaminado, Spain.
Dimenhydrinate (p.415·2); belladonna (p.463·1).
Nausea; vertigo; vomiting.

Sinacarb Amrad, Austral.
Levodopa (p.1169·2); carbidopa (p.1168·2).
Parkinsonism.

Si-Nade SmithKline Beecham, S.Afr.
Paracetamol (p.71·2); phenylpropanolamine hydrochloride (p.1098·1).
Cold and influenza symptoms; sinusitis.

Sinadrin Plus Reese, USA.
Paracetamol (p.71·2); pseudoephedrine hydrochloride (p.1099·2); dexbrompheniramine maleate (p.410·2).

Sinaf Taro, Israel.
Oxymetazoline hydrochloride (p.1096·2); phenylephrine hydrochloride (p.1097·1).
Nasal congestion.

Sinalfa
Abbott, Denm.; Abbott, Norw.; Abbott, Swed.
Terazosin hydrochloride (p.980·1).
Benign prostatic hyperplasia; hypertension.

Sinapause Organon, Mex.
Estriol (p.1475·3) or estriol succinate (p.1475·3).
Genito-urinary tract disorders associated with oestrogen deficiency.

Sinapils Pfeiffer, USA†.
Phenylpropanolamine hydrochloride (p.1098·1); chlorpheniramine [chlorphenamine] maleate (p.412·1); paracetamol (p.71·2); caffeine (p.761·3).
Upper respiratory-tract symptoms.

Sinapisme Rigollot Chefaro Ardeval, Fr.
Defatted black mustard paper (p.1639·1).
Respiratory-tract congestion.

Sinaplin Rimsa, Mex.
Ampicillin (p.150·3), ampicillin sodium (p.150·3), or ampicillin trihydrate (p.151·1).
Bacterial infections.

Sinapsan Rodleben, Ger.; Vedim, Ger.
Piracetam (p.1652·1).
Organic brain disorders.

Sinaqua Sofex, Port.†.
Barrier preparation.

Sinarest Ciba, USA.
Pseudoephedrine hydrochloride (p.1099·2); chlorpheniramine [chlorphenamine] maleate (p.412·1); paracetamol (p.71·2).
Upper respiratory-tract symptoms.

Sinarona Kener, Mex.
Amiodarone hydrochloride (p.836·1).

Sinartrol SPA, Ital.
Piroxicam cinnamate (p.79·3).
Musculoskeletal and joint disorders.

Sinaryl Homberger, Ger.
Homoeopathic preparation.

Sinase Douglas, NZ.
Beclometasone dipropionate (p.1061·2).
Allergic rhinitis.

Sinaspril-Paracetamol Roche Consumer, Neth.
Paracetamol (p.71·2).
Fever; pain.

Sinaxial TRB, Braz.
Polysiagoside.
Cerebrovascular disorders.

Sincerck Salus, Mex.
Praziquantel (p.106·3).

Sincon Tika, Swed.
Polyvinyl alcohol (p.1503·1).
Dry eyes.

Sincosan Omisan, Ital.†.
Benzalkonium chloride (p.1133·2).
Surface disinfection.

Sincrivit AGIPS, Ital.
Multivitamin preparation (p.1350·1).

Sindopa Pacific, NZ.
Carbidopa (p.1168·2); levodopa (p.1169·2).
Parkinsonism.

Sindrat Windson, Braz.
Oral rehydration solution (p.1185·2).
Diarrhoea; oral rehydration therapy.

Sine-Aid IB McNeil Consumer, USA.
Pseudoephedrine (p.1099·2); ibuprofen (p.43·2).

Sine-Aid Maximum Strength McNeil Consumer, USA.
Paracetamol (p.71·2); pseudoephedrine hydrochloride (p.1099·2).
Sinus headache.

Sinecod
Novartis Consumer, Belg.; Novartis Consumer, Port.; Novartis Consumer, Switz.; Novartis, Thai.
Butamirate citrate (p.1086·2).
Coughs.

Sinecod Bocca Zyma, Ital.†.
Benzoxonium chloride (p.1135·2).
Oral antiseptic.

Sinecod Tosse Fluidificante Novartis Consumer, Ital.
Carbocisteine (p.1086·3).
Catarrh; coughs.

Sinecod Tosse Sedativo Novartis Consumer, Ital.
Butamirate citrate (p.1086·2).
Formerly known as Sinecod Tosse.
Coughs.

Sinedal Synpharma, Switz.
Propyphenazone (p.80·2); paracetamol (p.71·2); caffeine (p.761·3).
Fever; pain.

Sinedol Italmex, Mex.
Paracetamol (p.71·2).
Fever; pain.

Sinedyston Steiner, Ger.†.
Co-dergocrine mesilate (p.1597·3); hypericum (p.290·2).
Mental function disorders.

Sinefricol Sanofi Synthelabo, Spain.
Caffeine (p.761·3); phenylephrine hydrochloride (p.1097·1); paracetamol (p.71·2); thenyldiamine hydrochloride (p.425·3).
Catarrh; influenza symptoms.

Sinegastrin
Note. This name is used for preparations of different composition.
Novag, Mex.
Cimetidine (p.1216·3).
Peptic ulcer.
Ferrer, Spain.
Almasilate (p.1210·1).
Dyspepsia; gastritis; gastro-oesophageal reflux; peptic ulcer.

Sinemet
Merck Sharp & Dohme, Aust.; Merck Sharp & Dohme, Austral.; Merck Sharp & Dohme, Belg.; Prodome, Braz.; Du Pont, Canad.; Merck Sharp & Dohme, Denm.; Merck Sharp & Dohme, Fin.; Du Pont, Fr.; Merck Sharp & Dohme, Hong Kong; Du Pont, Irl.; Merck Sharp & Dohme, Israel; Du Pont, Ital.; Merck Sharp & Dohme, Mex.; Merck Sharp & Dohme, Neth.; Merck Sharp & Dohme, Norw.; Merck Sharp & Dohme, NZ; Merck Sharp & Dohme, Port.; Merck Sharp & Dohme, S.Afr.; Merck Sharp & Dohme, Singapore; Du Pont, Spain; Merck Sharp & Dohme, Swed.; Merck Sharp & Dohme, Switz.; Merck Sharp & Dohme, Thai.; Du Pont, UK; Du Pont, USA.
Carbidopa (p.1168·2); levodopa (p.1169·2).

These ingredients can be described by the British Approved Name Co-careldopa.
Drug-induced extrapyramidal disorders; parkinsonism.

Sine-Off Allergy SmithKline Beecham Consumer, Canad.†.
Paracetamol (p.71·2); chlorpheniramine [chlorphenamine] maleate (p.412·1); phenylpropanolamine hydrochloride (p.1098·1).

Sine-Off Maximum Strength Allergy/Sinus SmithKline Beecham, USA.
Paracetamol (p.71·2); chlorpheniramine [chlorphenamine] maleate (p.412·1); pseudoephedrine hydrochloride (p.1099·2).
Upper respiratory-tract symptoms.

Sine-Off Maximum Strength No Drowsiness Formula SmithKline Beecham Consumer, USA.
Paracetamol (p.71·2); pseudoephedrine hydrochloride (p.1099·2).
Upper respiratory-tract symptoms.

Sine-Off ND SmithKline Beecham Consumer, Canad.†.
Paracetamol (p.71·2); phenylpropanolamine hydrochloride (p.1098·1).

Sine-Off Sinus Medicine SmithKline Beecham Consumer, USA†.
Aspirin (p.14·2); chlorpheniramine [chlorphenamine] maleate (p.412·1); phenylpropanolamine hydrochloride (p.1098·1).
Upper respiratory-tract symptoms.

Sinepress Rolab, S.Afr.
Methyldopa (p.927·3).
Known as Rolab-Methyldopa.
Hypertension.

Sinequan
Pfizer, Aust.; Pfizer, Austral.; Pfizer, Belg.; Pfizer, Canad.; Pfizer, Denm.; Pfizer, Fr.†; Pfizer, Hong Kong; Pfizer, Irl.; Pfizer, Mex.; Pfizer, Neth.; Pfizer, Norw.; Farmasierra, Spain; Pfizer, Thai.; Pfizer, UK; Pfizer, USA.
Doxepin hydrochloride (p.283·3).
Anxiety disorders; depression.

Sinerbe Plough, Port.
Dexchlorpheniramine maleate (p.412·1); pseudoephedrine sulfate (p.1099·3); guaifenesin (p.1092·2).
Coughs and associated respiratory-tract disorders.

Sinergina Faes, Spain.
Phenytoin (p.357·2).
Epilepsy.

Sinertec Merck Sharp & Dohme, Ital.
Enalapril maleate (p.883·3); hydrochlorothiazide (p.907·3).
Hypertension.

Sinesalin Zeneca, Switz.†.
Bendrofluazide [bendroflumethiazide] (p.844·1).
Hypertension; oedema.

Sinestron Medix, Mex.
Lorazepam (p.688·3).
Axiety; mixed anxiety depressive states.

Sinevrile Serpero, Ital.†.
Hydroxocobalamin (p.1388·1); monophosphothiamine chloride (p.1385·2).
Lignocaine [lidocaine] hydrochloride (p.1313·2) is included in this preparation to alleviate the pain of injection.
Alcoholic neuritis; diabetic neuritis; neuritis; polyneuritis; sciatica; trigeminal neuralgia.

Sinex
Note. This name is used for preparations of different composition.
Lachartre, Fr.†.
Oxymetazoline hydrochloride (p.1096·2); menthol (p.1632·3); camphor (p.1589·3).
Congestion of the upper respiratory tract.
Richardson-Vicks, Mex.
Phenylephrine hydrochloride (p.1097·1).
Nasal congestion.

Sinfrontal Muller Goppingen, Ger.
Homoeopathic preparation.

Singlet SmithKline Beecham Consumer, USA.
Pseudoephedrine hydrochloride (p.1099·2); chlorpheniramine [chlorphenamine] maleate (p.412·1); paracetamol (p.71·2).
Upper respiratory-tract symptoms.

Singulair
Merck Sharp & Dohme, Aust.; Merck Sharp & Dohme, Austral.; Merck Sharp & Dohme, Belg.; Merck Frosst, Canad.; Merck Sharp & Dohme, Denm.; Dieckmann, Ger.; Merck Sharp & Dohme, Fin.; Merck Sharp & Dohme, Hong Kong; Merck Sharp & Dohme, Irl.; Merck Sharp & Dohme, Israel; Merck Sharp & Dohme, Ital.; Merck Sharp & Dohme, Mex.; Merck Sharp & Dohme, Neth.; Merck Sharp & Dohme, Norw.; Merck Sharp & Dohme, NZ; Merck Sharp & Dohme, Port.; Merck Sharp & Dohme, S.Afr.; Merck Sharp & Dohme, Singapore; Merck Sharp & Dohme, Spain; Merck Sharp & Dohme, Swed.; Merck Sharp & Dohme, Switz.; Merck Sharp & Dohme, Thai.; Merck Sharp & Dohme, UK; Merck, USA.
Montelukast sodium (p.768·1).
Asthma.

Sinhcloran Vitae, Mex.
Ranitidine (p.1246·3).
Peptic ulcer.

Siniphen Singer, Switz.†.
Suppositories: Salicylamide (p.82·1); propyphenazone (p.80·2); caffeine (p.761·3); lignocaine [lidocaine] hydrochloride (p.1313·2).
Tablets: Salicylamide (p.82·1); propyphenazone (p.80·2); caffeine (p.761·3).
Fever; pain.

Sinketol Locatelli, Ital.†.
Ketoprofen (p.47·3).
Gout; musculoskeletal, joint, and peri-articular disorders.

Sinkron Ripari-Gero, Ital.
Citicoline sodium (p.1596·1).
Cerebrovascular disorders; mental function disorders.

Sinmol Maxfarma, Spain.
Paracetamol (p.71·2).
Fever; pain.

Sinogan
Rhone-Poulenc Rorer, Mex.; Rhone-Poulenc Rorer, Spain.
Methotrimeprazine [levomepromazine] hydrochloride (p.691·3) or methotrimeprazine [levomepromazine] maleate (p.692·1).
Anxiety; depression; pain; psychoses; sleep disorders.

Sinografin
Squibb Diagnostics, Canad.†; Squibb Diagnostics, USA.
Meglumine amidotrizoate (p.1031·2); meglumine adiipiodone (p.1031·1).
Contrast medium for hysterosalpingography.

Sinolax-Milder Synpharma, Aust.
Fig (p.1227·1); fennel (p.1610·1); manna (p.1233·3).
Constipation; stool softener.

Sinophenin Rodleben, Ger.
Promazine hydrochloride (p.702·2).
Anxiety disorders; pain; pre- and postoperative sedative; pruritus; psychoses; sleep disorders; vomiting; withdrawal symptoms.

Sinoral Biolab, Thai.
Tenoxicam (p.87·2).
Gout; musculoskeletal, joint, and peri-articular disorders.

Sinotar Lane, UK.
Althaea (p.1577·1); echinacea (p.1606·2); sambucus (p.1660·3).
Blocked sinuses; catarrh.

Sinovula Asche, Ger.
Norethisterone (p.1485·1); ethinylestradiol (p.1476·2).
Combined oral contraceptive; menstrual disorders.

Sinoxis Hosbon, Spain†.
Buflomedil hydrochloride (p.851·3).
Vascular disorders.

Sinozzard Cryopharma, Mex.
Prazosin hydrochloride (p.958·1).
Hypertension.

Sinquan Pfizer, Ger.
Doxepin hydrochloride (p.283·3).
Anxiety; depression; sleep disorders; withdrawal syndromes.

Sinquane Pfizer, Switz.
Doxepin hydrochloride (p.283·3).
Anxiety disorders; depression.

Sinsurrene Parke, Davis, Ital.†.
Hydrocortisone sodium hemisuccinate (p.1074·1); desoxycortone sodium hemisuccinate (corticosterone) (p.1066·3); aldosterone sodium hemisuccinate (p.1061·2); prasterone sodium sulfate (p.1488·2).
Adrenal insufficiency.

Sintalgin Sintofarma, Braz.
Nimesulide (p.62·3).
Fever; inflammation; pain.

Sintamin Fresenius Kabi, Ital.
Amino-acid infusion (p.1350·1).
Parenteral nutrition.

Sintenyl Sintetica, Switz.
Fentanyl citrate (p.37·1).
Pain.

Sinteroid Breves, Braz.
A heparinoid (p.905·2); clofibrate (p.859·1).
Hyperlipidaemias.

Sinthrome Alliance, UK.
Nicoumalone [acenocoumarol] (p.940·1).
Thromboembolic disorders.

Sintisone
Pharmacia Upjohn, Hong Kong; Pharmacia Upjohn, Port.; Pharmacia, Swed.†.
Prednisolone steaglate (p.1078·2).
Corticosteroid.

Sintobil Molteni, Ital.†.
Fencibutirol (p.1610·1); boldo (p.1585·3); cascara (p.1216·1); frangula (p.1227·1).
Constipation.

Sintocalcin Biagini, Ital.†.
Elcatonin (p.749·2).
Hypercalcaemia; osteoporosis; Paget's disease of bone; reflex sympathetic dystrophy.

Sintocef Pulitzer, Ital.
Cefonicid sodium (p.168·1).
Lignocaine [lidocaine] hydrochloride (p.1313·2) is included in the intramuscular injection to alleviate the pain of injection.
Bacterial infections.

Sintoclar Pulitzer, Ital.
Citicoline (p.1596·1).
Cerebrovascular disorders; mental function disorders.

Sintodian Pharmacia Upjohn, Ital.
Droperidol (p.682·2).
Anaesthesia; psychoses.

Sintolatt Lampugnani, Ital.
Lactulose (p.1230·1).
Constipation; disturbances in intestinal flora.

Sintomicetina Medley, Braz.
Chloramphenicol (p.179·1).
Bacterial infections.

Sintomodulina Italfarmaco, Ital.
Thymopentin (p.1672·3).
Immunodeficiency.

Sintonal Europharma, Spain.
Brotizolam (p.657·2).
Insomnia.

Sintopen Magis, Ital.
Amoxicillin trihydrate (p.149·2).
Bacterial infections.

Sintoplus PH&T, Ital.
Piperacillin sodium (p.236·1).
Lignocaine [lidocaine] hydrochloride (p.1313·2) is included in this preparation to alleviate the pain of injection.
Bacterial infections.

Sintotrat Bracco, Ital.
Hydrocortisone acetate (p.1073·3).
Skin disorders.

Sintozima Sintofarma, Braz.
Pancreatin (p.1646·1); metoclopramide hydrochloride (p.1235·2); bromelains (p.1586·3); dehydrocholic acid (p.1602·2); cellulase (p.1593·1); dimethicone (p.1249·2).
Digestive disorders.

Sintrogel Roche Nicholas, Spain.
Aluminium hydroxide (p.1210·3); magnesium carbonate (p.1232·3); magnesium oxide (p.1233·2).
Gastrointestinal hyperacidity.

Sintrom
Novartis, Aust.; Novartis, Belg.; Novartis, Canad.; Novartis, Fr.; Novartis, Israel; Novartis, Ital.; Novartis, Mex.; Novartis, Port.; Novartis, Spain; Novartis, Switz.
Nicoumalone [acenocoumarol] (p.940·1).
Thromboembolic disorders.

Sintrom Mitis Novartis, Neth.
Nicoumalone [acenocoumarol] (p.940·1).
Thromboembolic disorders.

Sinuberase Rudefsa, Mex.
Lactic-acid-producing organisms (p.1626·3).

Sinuc Biocur, Ger.
Hedera helix.
Bronchitis; catarrh.

Sinuclear Aspen, S.Afr.
Paracetamol (p.71·2); phenylpropanolamine hydrochloride (p.1098·1).
Upper respiratory-tract congestion.

Sinuclear P Garec, S.Afr.
Paracetamol (p.71·2); triprolidine hydrochloride (p.427·2); pseudoephedrine hydrochloride (p.1099·2).
Cold and influenza symptoms; nasal congestion.

Sinucon Salters, S.Afr.
Paracetamol (p.71·2); ephedrine hydrochloride (p.1090·1); caffeine (p.761·3); chlorpheniramine [chlorphenamine] maleate (p.412·1).
Cold and influenza symptoms; hay fever; sinus congestion.

Sinufed Trima, Israel.
Pseudoephedrine hydrochloride (p.1099·2).
Nasal congestion; sinus congestion.

Sinufed Timecelles Roberts, USA.
Pseudoephedrine hydrochloride (p.1099·2); guaifenesin (p.1092·2).
Coughs and cold symptoms; nasal congestion.

Sinuforce Bioforce, Switz.
Homoeopathic preparation.

Sinuforton Sanofi Synthelabo, Ger.
Capsules: Anise oil (p.1580·3); cowslip rhizome (p.1600·1); thyme (p.1672·2).
Sinusitis.
Oral drops: Anise oil (p.1580·3); eucalyptus oil (p.1600·2); thyme (p.1672·2).
Sinusitis.
Oral liquid: Cowslip rhizome (p.1600·1); thyme (p.1672·2).
Cold symptoms.

Sinugex Frega, Canad.†.
Diphenylpyraline hydrochloride (p.417·1); paracetamol (p.71·2); caffeine (p.761·3).

Sinulin
Note. This name is used for preparations of different composition.
Flordis, Austral.
Gentian (p.1615·1); primrose.
Respiratory-tract infections; sinusitis.
Carnrick, USA†.
Paracetamol (p.71·2); chlorpheniramine [chlorphenamine] maleate (p.412·1); phenylpropanolamine hydrochloride (p.1098·1).
Cold symptoms; nasal congestion.

Sinumax Janssen-Cilag, S.Afr.
Paracetamol (p.71·2); pseudoephedrine hydrochloride (p.1099·2).
Cold symptoms.

Sinumax Allergy Sinus Janssen-Cilag, S.Afr.
Paracetamol (p.71·2); pseudoephedrine hydrochloride (p.1099·2); chlorpheniramine [chlorphenamine] maleate (p.412·1).
Cold symptoms; nasal congestion.

Sinumed Triomed, S.Afr.
Pseudoephedrine hydrochloride (p.1099·2).
Upper respiratory-tract congestion.

Sinumine Maxi, Thai.
Carbinoxamine maleate (p.411·1).
Hypersensitivity reactions.

Sinumist-SR Hauck, USA.
Guaifenesin (p.1092·2).
Coughs.

Sinupan Ion, USA.
Guaifenesin (p.1092·2); phenylephrine hydrochloride (p.1097·1).
Coughs and cold symptoms; nasal congestion.

Sinupas N Pascoe, Ger.
Homoeopathic preparation.

Sinupret
Austroplant, Aust.; Bionorica, Ger.; Bionorica, Hong Kong; Bionorica, Singapore; Bionorica, Switz.; Bionorica, Thai.
Gentian root (p.1615·1); cowslip flower (p.1600·1); rumex acetosa (p.1681·3); sambucus flower (p.1660·3); vervain (p.1679·3).
Respiratory-tract inflammation; sinusitis.

Sinus Homeocan, Canad.
Homoeopathic preparation.

Sinus & Congestion Relief WestCan, Canad.†.
Pseudoephedrine hydrochloride (p.1099·2); paracetamol (p.71·2).

Sinus Excedrin Bristol-Myers Squibb, USA.
Paracetamol (p.71·2); pseudoephedrine hydrochloride (p.1099·2).
Nasal congestion.

Sinus and Hayfever Vitaglow, Austral.
Horseradish (p.1620·1); fenugreek (p.1610·3); ascorbic acid (p.1389·3); betacarotene (p.1355·1); zinc amino acid chelate (p.1398·3).
Hay fever; sinusitis; upper respiratory-tract congestion.

Sinus Inhalaciones Boots Healthcare, Spain.
Camphor (p.1589·3); eucalyptol (p.1609·2); peppermint oil (p.1243·3); oleum pini sylvestris; menthol (p.1632·3); eucalyptus oil (p.1609·2).
Nasal congestion.

Sinus Medication Stanley, Canad.†.
Pseudoephedrine hydrochloride (p.1099·2); paracetamol (p.71·2).

Sinus Pain & Nasal Congestion Relief WestCan, Canad.
Pseudoephedrine hydrochloride (p.1099·2); paracetamol (p.71·2).

Sinus Relief Brauer, Austral.
Homoeopathic preparation.

Sinusaid Sriprasit, Thai.
Triprolidine hydrochloride (p.427·2); pseudoephedrine hydrochloride (p.1099·2).
Nasal congestion.

Sinusal Sam-On, Israel.
Paracetamol (p.71·2); phenylpropanolamine hydrochloride (p.1098·1).
Cold symptoms; nasal congestion; rhinitis; sinus congestion; sinusitis.

Sinusalia Boiron, Canad.
Homoeopathic preparation.

Sinuselect Dreluso, Ger.
Homoeopathic preparation.

Sinusitis Hevert N Hevert, Ger.
Homoeopathic preparation.

Sinusitis PMD Plantamed, Ger.
Homoeopathic preparation.

Sinusitis-Komplex N Staufen, Ger.
Homoeopathic preparation.

Sinusitis-Sellplex Weber & Weber, Ger.
Homoeopathic preparation.

Sinusol Richter, Aust.
Gentian root (p.1615·1); cowslip flower (p.1600·1); vervain (p.1679·3).
Catarrh.

Sinusol-B Kay, USA†.
Brompheniramine malcate (p.410·2).
Hypersensitivity reactions.

Sinusol-Schleimlosender Tee Richter, Aust.
Cowslip flower (p.1600·1); sambucus flower (p.1660·3); vervain (p.1679·3).
Catarrh.

Sinuspax
Homeocan, Canad.; Lehning, Fr.
Homoeopathic preparation.

Sinus-Relief Major, USA.
Pseudoephedrine hydrochloride (p.1099·2); paracetamol (p.71·2).
Upper respiratory-tract symptoms.

Sinustat Xixia, S.Afr.
Paracetamol (p.71·2); phenylpropanolamine hydrochloride (p.1098·1).
Cold and influenza symptoms.

Sinustop Adcock Ingram Self Medication, S.Afr.†.
Nasal spray: Oxymetazoline hydrochloride (p.1096·2).
Nasal congestion.
Tablets: Paracetamol (p.71·2); phenylpropanolamine hydrochloride (p.1098·1); phenyltoloxamine citrate (p.423·1).
Cold and flu symptoms.

Sinustop with Codeine Adcock Ingram Self Medication, S.Afr.†.
Paracetamol (p.71·2); phenylpropanolamine hydrochloride (p.1098·1); phenyltoloxamine citrate (p.423·1); codeine phosphate (p.25·2).
Cold and flu symptoms.

Sinustop Pro Murdock, USA.
Pseudoephedrine hydrochloride (p.1099·2).
Nasal congestion.

Sinustrat Zurita, Braz.
Lufta operculata; sodium chloride (p.1196·1).
Nasal congestion.

Sinusyx Syxyl, Ger.
Homoeopathic preparation.

Sinutab
Note. This name is used for preparations of different composition.
Warner-Lambert Consumer, Belg.; Ache, Braz.; Warner-Lambert, Hong Kong.
Paracetamol (p.71·2); phenylpropanolamine hydrochloride (p.1098·1); phenyltoloxamine citrate (p.423·1).
Cold symptoms; sinusitis.
Warner-Lambert, Irl.; Warner-Lambert, UK.
Paracetamol (p.71·2); phenylpropanolamine hydrochloride (p.1098·1).
Headache; nasal and sinus congestion.
Parke, Davis, S.Afr.
Nasal spray†: Xylometazoline hydrochloride (p.1102·2).
Nasal congestion.
Tablets; sustained-release tablets: Paracetamol (p.71·2); phenylpropanolamine hydrochloride (p.1098·1); phenyltoloxamine citrate (p.423·1).
Cold and influenza symptoms; sinus headache.
Warner-Lambert, Spain†.
Chlorpheniramine [chlorphenamine] maleate (p.412·1); paracetamol (p.71·2); pseudoephedrine hydrochloride (p.1099·2).
Fever; influenza and cold symptoms; pain.

Sinutab II Warner-Lambert Consumer, Port.
Paracetamol (p.71·2); pseudoephedrine hydrochloride (p.1099·2).
Nasal congestion; sinusitis.

Sinutab with Codeine
Note. This name is used for preparations of different composition.
Warner-Lambert, Canad.
Paracetamol (p.71·2); pseudoephedrine hydrochloride (p.1099·2); chlorpheniramine [chlorphenamine] maleate (p.412·1); codeine (p.25·2).
Cold symptoms; nasal congestion.
Parke, Davis, S.Afr.
Paracetamol (p.71·2); phenylpropanolamine hydrochloride (p.1098·1); phenyltoloxamine citrate (p.423·1); codeine phosphate (p.25·2).
Cold and influenza symptoms; sinus headache.

Sinutab Extra Strength Warner-Lambert, Canad.†.
Paracetamol (p.71·2); pseudoephedrine hydrochloride (p.1099·2); chlorpheniramine [chlorphenamine] maleate (p.412·1).
Cold symptoms; nasal congestion.

Sinutab Extra Strength Daytime/Nightime Warner-Lambert, Canad.
Tablets (Daytime), pseudoephedrine hydrochloride (p.1099·2); paracetamol (p.71·2); tablets (Nightime), pseudoephedrine hydrochloride; paracetamol; diphenhydramine hydrochloride (p.416·1).
Cold symptoms; rhinitis; sinusitis.

Sinutab Maximum Strength Sinus Allergy Warner-Lambert, Canad.
Pseudoephedrine hydrochloride (p.1099·2); chlorpheniramine [chlorphenamine] maleate (p.412·1); paracetamol (p.71·2).
Upper respiratory-tract symptoms.

Sinutab ND Parke, Davis, S.Afr.
Paracetamol (p.71·2); phenylpropanolamine hydrochloride (p.1098·1).
Cold and influenza symptoms.

Sinutab Nightime
Note. This name is used for preparations of different composition.
Warner-Lambert, Canad.
Paracetamol (p.71·2); diphenhydramine hydrochloride (p.416·1); pseudoephedrine hydrochloride (p.1099·2).
Formerly contained paracetamol, chlorpheniramine [chlorphenamine], and pseudoephedrine.
Cold symptoms; nasal congestion.
Warner-Lambert, UK.
Paracetamol (p.71·2); phenylpropanolamine hydrochloride (p.1098·1); phenyltoloxamine citrate (p.423·1).
Congestion.

Sinutab Non-Drying Warner-Lambert, USA.
Pseudoephedrine hydrochloride (p.1099·2); guaifenesin (p.1092·2).
Coughs.

Sinutab Sinus & Allergy Warner-Lambert, Canad.
Paracetamol (p.71·2); pseudoephedrine hydrochloride (p.1099·2); chlorpheniramine [chlorphenamine] maleate (p.412·1).
Formerly known as Sinutab Regular.
Cold symptoms; nasal congestion.

Sinutab Sinus & Allergy 12 Hour Warner-Lambert, Canad.†.
Paracetamol (p.71·2); phenylpropanolamine hydrochloride (p.1098·1); phenyltoloxamine citrate (p.423·1).
Formerly known as Sinutab SA.
Cold symptoms; nasal congestion.

Sinutab Sinus Allergy & Pain Relief Warner-Lambert, Austral.; Warner-Lambert, NZ.
Paracetamol (p.71·2); pseudoephedrine hydrochloride (p.1099·2); chlorpheniramine [chlorphenamine] maleate (p.412·1).
Allergic rhinitis; cold symptoms; sinus headache.

Sinutab Sinus (Daytime) Non Drowsy Warner-Lambert, Canad.
Paracetamol (p.71·2); pseudoephedrine hydrochloride (p.1099·2).
Formerly known as Sinutab ND Daytime Formula.
Cold symptoms; nasal congestion.

Sinutab Sinus Non Drowsy Warner-Lambert, Canad.
Paracetamol (p.71·2); pseudoephedrine hydrochloride (p.1099·2).

Formerly known as Sinutab No Drowsiness.
Cold symptoms; nasal congestion.

Sinutab Sinus & Pain Relief
Warner-Lambert, Austral.; Warner-Lambert, NZ.
Paracetamol (p.71·2); pseudoephedrine hydrochloride (p.1099·2).
Cold symptoms; sinus headache.

Sinutab Sinus Relief *Warner-Lambert, Austral.†.*
Pseudoephedrine hydrochloride (p.1099·2).
Formerly known as Sinutab Decongestant.
Sinus disorders.

Sinutab Without Drowsiness *Warner-Lambert, USA.*
Pseudoephedrine hydrochloride (p.1099·2); paracetamol (p.71·2).
Upper respiratory-tract symptoms.

Sinutrex Extra Strength *Schein, USA†.*
Pseudoephedrine hydrochloride (p.1099·2); chlorpheniramine [chlorphenamine] maleate (p.412·1); paracetamol (p.71·2).
Upper respiratory-tract symptoms.

SINUvent *WE, USA†.*
Phenylpropanolamine hydrochloride (p.1098·1); guaifenesin (p.1092·2).
Coughs and cold symptoms; nasal congestion.

Sinuzin-D
Biolab, Singapore; Biolab, Thai.
Chlorpheniramine [chlorphenamine] maleate (p.412·1); paracetamol (p.71·2); phenylpropanolamine hydrochloride (p.1098·1).
Cold symptoms; rhinitis; upper respiratory-tract disorders.

Sinvacor *Merck Sharp & Dohme, Ital.*
Simvastatin (p.969·2).
Coronary atherosclerosis; hypercholesterolaemia.

Siofor *Berlin-Chemie, Ger.*
Metformin hydrochloride (p.332·3).
Diabetes mellitus.

Siopel
Bioglan, Irl.; Genop, S.Afr.; Bioglan, UK.
Cetrimide (p.1137·1); dimethicone 1000 (p.1410·1).
Barrier cream; napkin rash.

Siosol *Febena, Ger.*
Greater celandine (p.1618·1).
Biliary and gastrointestinal spasm.

Siozwo N *Febena, Ger.*
Nasal ointment: Naphazoline hydrochloride (p.1095·1); peppermint oil (p.1243·3).
Catarrh; nasal congestion; rhinitis.
Ointment: Bismuth subgallate (p.1213·2); hamamelis (p.1618·3); zinc oxide (p.1128·2).
Burns; skin disorders; wounds.

Sipam *Siam Bheasach, Thai.*
Diazepam (p.674·3).
Anxiety; insomnia.

Sipental *Siam Bheasach, Thai.*
Oxpentifylline [pentoxifylline] (p.950·3).
Cerebral, ocular, and peripheral vascular disorders.

Siprofen *Labima, Belg.*
Ibuprofen (p.43·2).
Fever; pain.

Siqualine *Bristol-Myers Squibb, Mex.*
Fluphenazine (p.684·3).

Siqualone
Bristol-Myers Squibb, Denm.; Bristol-Myers Squibb, Fin.; Bristol-Myers Squibb, Norw.; Bristol-Myers Squibb, Swed.
Fluphenazine decanoate (p.684·3) or fluphenazine hydrochloride (p.684·3).
Alcohol withdrawal syndrome; anxiety; nausea and vomiting; psychoses; senile agitation and confusion.

Siquial *Merck, Mex.*
Fluoxetine hydrochloride (p.284·2).
Bulimia nervosa; depression; obsessive compulsive disorder.

Siquil *Bristol-Myers Squibb, Neth.†.*
Triflupromazine hydrochloride (p.711·1).
Bipolar disorder; psychoses.

Siran
Temmler, Ger.; Temmler, Israel.
Acetylcysteine (p.1082·3).
Respiratory-tract disorders associated with increased or viscous mucus.

Sirani *Ofimex, Mex.*
Ranitidine (p.1246·3).

Sirben *Searle, Braz.*
Mebendazole (p.102·2).
Worm infections.

Sirdalud
Novartis, Austral.; Novartis, Belg.; Novartis, Braz.; Novartis, Denm.; Novartis, Fin.; Sanofi Synthelabo, Ger.; Novartis, Ital.; Novartis, Mex.; Novartis, Neth.; Novartis, Port.; Novartis, Spain; Novartis, Switz.; Novartis, Thai.
Tizanidine hydrochloride (p.1330·2).
Skeletal muscle spasm; spasticity.

Sirepar *Gedeon Richter, Thai.*
Liver extract.
Liver disorders.

Sirigen *Adivar, Ital.*
Benzalkonium chloride (p.1133·2).
Disinfection of wounds and burns.

Sirmia Abfuhrkapseln *Niedermaier, Ger.†.*
Senna (p.1248·2); peppermint oil (p.1243·3); caraway oil (p.1591·2).
Constipation.

Sirmia Artischockenelixier N *Niedermaier, Ger.*
Cynara (p.1601·3); taraxacum (p.1669·1).
Hepatobiliary disorders.

Sirmia Knoblauchsaft N *Niedermaier, Ger.†.*
Garlic (p.1614·1).
Hyperlipidaemia.

Sirmiosta Nervenelixier N *Niedermaier, Ger.†.*
Melissa (p.1632·2); passion flower (p.1649·1); valerian (p.1678·3).
Agitation; insomnia.

Sirodina *Clariana, Spain.*
Pyridoxine (p.1387·1); sulpiride (p.706·1).
Nervous disorders; vertigo.

Sirolax *Pharbita, Israel.*
Lactulose (p.1230·1).
Constipation; hepatic coma.

Sirop antitussif Wyss a base de codeine *Wyss, Switz.†.*
Codeine phosphate (p.25·2); cherry-laurel; ipecacuanha (p.1093·1); senega root (p.1100·2); althaea (p.1577·1).
Coughs.

Sirop Boin *Picot, Fr.†.*
Codeine (p.25·2); menthol (p.1632·3); adrenaline [epinephrine] (p.829·1); guaiacol (p.1092·1); aconite (p.1572·3); cherry laurel.
Respiratory disorders.

Sirop Cocillana Codeine *Atlas, Canad.*
Codeine phosphate (p.25·2); cocillana (p.1087·2); euphorbia (p.1609·3); senega (p.1100·2); squill (p.1100·3); wild lettuce (p.1680·3).

Sirop contre la toux nouvelle formule *Zeller, Switz.*
Hedera helix.
Bronchial disorders with viscous mucus.

Sirop Dentition *Sabex, Canad.*
Benzocaine (p.1306·2).

Sirop Des Vosges *SmithKline Beecham Sante, Fr.*
Pholcodine (p.1099·1).
Formerly known as Sirop Des Vosges Caze.
Coughs.

Sirop des Vosges Expectorant *SmithKline Beecham Sante, Fr.*
Carbocisteine (p.1086·3).
Respiratory-tract congestion.

Sirop DM *Marc-O, Canad.*
Dextromethorphan hydrobromide (p.1087·3).

Sirop Expectorant *Marc-O, Canad.*
Guaifenesin (p.1092·2).

Sirop Passi-Par *Parsenn, Switz.*
Passion flower (p.1649·1); crataegus (p.1600·2).
Anxiety; insomnia.

Sirop Pectoral adulte *Oberlin, Fr.†.*
Ethylmorphine hydrochloride (p.35·2); aconite (p.1572·3); bromoform (p.1587·1); sodium benzoate (p.1134·3); sulfogaiacol (p.1101·1); cherry laurel; belladonna (p.463·1); drosera (p.1606·1); eucalyptus oil (p.1609·2); senega (p.1100·2); ipecacuanha (p.1093·1) tolu balsam (p.1101·3).
Coughs.

Sirop pectoral DP1 *DP-Medica, Switz.†.*
Guaifenesin (p.1092·2); codeine phosphate (p.25·2); ephedrine hydrochloride (p.1090·1); sodium benzoate (p.1134·3); althaea (p.1577·1); tolu balsam (p.1101·3); plantain (p.1652·3); thyme (p.1672·2); pine buds; pectoral syrup.
Bronchitis; catarrh; coughs.

Sirop pectoral DP2, DP3 *DP-Medica, Switz.†.*
Guaifenesin (p.1092·2); codeine phosphate (p.25·2); ephedrine hydrochloride (p.1090·1); sodium benzoate (p.1134·3); belladonna (p.463·1); althaea (p.1577·1); tolu balsam (p.1101·3); plantain (p.1652·3); thyme (p.1672·2); pine buds; pectoral syrup.
Bronchitis; catarrh; coughs.

Sirop Pectoral enfant *Oberlin, Fr.†.*
Sodium benzoate (p.1134·3); sulfogaiacol (p.1101·1); sodium bromide (p.1587·1); drosera (p.1606·1); eucalyptus oil (p.1609·2); frangula (p.1227·1); ethylmorphine hydrochloride (p.35·2); tolu balsam (p.1101·3).
Coughs.

Sirop Pectoral Vicks *Lachartre, Fr.*
Pentoxyverine citrate (p.1096·3).
Formerly contained pentoxyverine citrate, guaifenesin, and sodium citrate.
Coughs.

Sirop pour le sommeil *Zeller, Switz.*
Valerian (p.1678·3).
Sleep disorders.

Sirop S contre la toux et la bronchite *Synpharma, Switz.*
Codeine phosphate (p.25·2); drosera (p.1606·1); hyoscyamus (p.470·1); liquorice (p.1231·2) cowslip root (p.1600·1).
Coughs.

Sirop Teyssedre *Therica, Fr.*
Calcium bromide (p.1587·1); cloral hydrate (p.669·3); calamint.
Sleep disorders in children.

Sirop Toux du Larynx *Qualiphar, Belg.†.*
Codeine phosphate (p.25·2); belladonna (p.463·1); aconite (p.1572·3); lobelia (p.1510·2); cherry-laurel water; drosera (p.1606·1); erysimin.
Coughs.

Sirop Wyss contre la toux *Wyss, Switz.†.*
Cherry-laurel; ipecacuanha (p.1093·1); senega root (p.1100·2); althaea (p.1577·1).
Coughs.

Siros *Janssen-Cilag, Ger.*
Itraconazole (p.387·2).
Vulvovaginal candidiasis.

Siroxyl
Aventis, Belg.; Sopar, Neth.†.
Carbocisteine (p.1086·3).
Respiratory-tract disorders associated with retention of bronchial secretions.

Sirtal
Sanofi Winthrop, Aust.†; Merck dura, Ger.
Carbamazepine (p.342·2).
Alcohol withdrawal syndrome; bipolar disorder; diabetes insipidus; diabetic neuropathy; epilepsy; multiple sclerosis; neuralgia.

Sisare *Nourypharma, Ger.*
11 Tablets, estradiol valerate (p.1473·2); 10 tablets, estradiol valerate; medroxyprogesterone acetate (p.1480·1).
Menopausal disorders.

Sisare mono *Nourypharma, Ger.*
Estradiol (p.1473·1).
Menopausal disorders.

Sisomina *Schering-Plough, Spain†.*
Sisomicin sulfate (p.247·3).
Bacterial infections.

Sita *Hoyer, Ger.*
Saw palmetto (p.1491·2).
Benign prostatic hyperplasia.

Sito-Lande *Sanofi Synthelabo, Ger.*
Sitosterol (p.970·3).
Hyperlipidaemias.

Sitriol *Alphapharm, Austral.*
Calcitriol (p.1391·1).
Hypocalcaemia; osteoporosis.

Situalin *Formenti, Ital.†.*
Dexamethasone linoleate (p.1067·3).
Inflammatory skin disorders.

Situalin Antibiotico *Formenti, Ital.†.*
Dexamethasone linoleate (p.1067·3); bekanamycin sulfate (p.156·1).
Infected skin disorders.

Sitzmarks *Konsyl, USA.*
Polyvinyl chloride.
Contrast medium for gastrointestinal radiography.

Sivastin *Sigma-Tau, Ital.*
Simvastatin (p.969·2).
Coronary arteriosclerosis; hypercholesterolaemia; ischaemic heart disease.

SJ Liniment *International Dermatologicals, Canad.*
Methyl salicylate (p.55·1); menthol (p.1632·3); ammonia (p.1579·1); coal tar (p.1125·1).

Skaelud *Merck, Denm.*
Pyrithione zinc (p.1122·1).
Pityriasis versicolor; seborrhoeic dermatitis.

Skeeter Stik *Triton, USA.*
Lignocaine [lidocaine] (p.1313·2); phenol (p.1152·3).
Skin disorders.

Skelan *Great Eastern, Thai.; Therapharma, Thai.*
Ibuprofen (p.43·2); paracetamol (p.71·2).
Pain.

Skelan IB *Biomedis, Thai.; Great Eastern, Thai.*
Ibuprofen (p.43·2).
Gout; musculoskeletal, joint, and peri-articular disorders; pain.

Skelaxin *Carnrick, USA.*
Metaxalone (p.1329·3).
Painful musculoskeletal conditions.

Skelid
Sanofi Winthrop, Aust.†; Sanofi Synthelabo, Austral.; Sanofi Synthelabo, Ger.; Sanofi Winthrop, Fin.; Sanofi Winthrop, Fr.; Sanofi Synthelabo, Ger.; Sanofi Synthelabo, Neth.; Sanofi Winthrop, Spain; Sanofi Winthrop, Swed.; Sanofi Synthelabo, Switz.; Sanofi Winthrop, UK; Sanofi Winthrop, USA.
Tiludronate sodium (p.756·2).
Paget's disease of bone.

Skema *Pentamedical, Ital.*
Cream: Zinc oxide (p.1128·2); titanium dioxide (p.1126·1).
Lotion: Octinoxate (p.1517·3); avobenzone (p.1517·1).
Sunscreen.

Skenan
Upsamedica, Belg.; UPSA, Fr.; Ethypharm, Ital.; Bristol-Myers Squibb, Neth.; Upsamedica, Spain.
Morphine sulfate (p.56·1).
Pain.

Skezide *Masa, Thai.*
Hydrochlorothiazide (p.907·3); triamterene (p.986·1).
Hypertension; oedema.

SK-F, BIC-F *Fresenius Medical, Switz.*
Acidic and basic haemodialysis concentrates (p.1184·1).

Skiacol *Alcon, Fr.*
Cyclopentolate hydrochloride (p.465·2).
Ophthalmic procedures.

Skiatropine *Chauvin Novopharma, Switz.*
Atropine sulfate (p.461·1).
Eye disorders; production of mydriasis and cycloplegia.

Skid *Lichtenstein, Ger.*
Minocycline hydrochloride (p.224·3).

Skid E *Lichtenstein, Ger.†.*
Erythromycin (p.201·1).
Acne.

Skilax *Almirall, Spain.*
Sodium picosulfate (p.1249·3).
Constipation.

Skin Bond Cement *Smith & Nephew, Austral.*
Appliance adhesive.

Skin Cap *Medix, Mex.*
Pyrithione zinc (p.1122·1).

Skin Cleanser & Deodorizer *Arjo, Canad.*
Benzethonium chloride (p.1134·2).
Skin hygiene in incontinent patients.

Skin Cleansing *Cantassium Co., UK.*
Lappa (p.1627·1); senna (p.1248·2); fumitory (p.1612·3); clivers (p.1596·3).

Skin Clear *Potter's, UK.*
Ointment: Starch (p.1379·3); sublimed sulfur (p.1123·3); zinc oxide (p.1128·2); melaleuca oil (p.1631·3).
Tablets: Echinacea root (p.1606·2).
Skin disorders.

Skin Conditioner & Bath Oil *Arjo, Canad.†.*
Light liquid paraffin (p.1407·2).
Dry skin; pruritus.

Skin Cure *Young Again Products, USA.*
Pyrithione zinc (p.1122·1).
Skin disorders.

Skin Dry *Darier, Mex.*
Aluminium tetrachlorohydrate (p.1110·2).

Skin Eruptions Mixture *Potter's, UK.*
Blue flag (p.1624·3); lappa root (p.1627·1); yellow dock (p.1681·3); sarsaparilla (p.1661·1); buchu (p.1587·2); cascara (p.1216·1).
Skin disorders.

Skin Healing Cream *Brauer, Austral.*
Calendula (p.1589·2); hypericum (p.290·2).
Bruised fingers and toes; cuts and abrasions; insect bites; skin irritation.

Skin Prep *Smith & Nephew, Austral.*
Film dressing.

Skin Repair
Rosken, Hong Kong; Rosken, Singapore.
Dimethicone (p.1410·1).
Cracked and dry skin; eczema.

Skin Repair Daily Care *Rosken, Singapore.*
Emollient and barrier preparation.

Skin Shield
Del, Canad.†; Del, USA.
Dyclonine hydrochloride (p.1311·3); benzethonium chloride (p.1134·2).
Liquid bandage.

Skin So Soft Antibacterial *Avon, Canad.*
Lotion: Triclosan (p.1159·2).
Topical gel: Alcohol (p.1130·3).

Skinat *Teofarma, Ital.*
Collagen (p.1598·2).
Prevention of scarring.

Skincalm
Boots, NZ; Noristan, S.Afr.†.
Hydrocortisone (p.1073·3) or hydrocortisone acetate (p.1073·3).
Skin disorders.

Skinicles *Skinicles, Canad.*
Hydroquinone (p.1115·1); padimate O (p.1518·2).

Skinman Intensiv *Henkel, Ger.†.*
Alcohol (p.1130·3); chlorhexidine gluconate (p.1138·2).
Skin disinfection.

Skinman Soft *Henkel, Ger.*
Isopropyl alcohol (p.1149·2); benzalkonium chloride (p.1133·2); undecenoic acid (p.395·3).
Skin disinfection.

Skinoderm *Pharma Clal, Israel.*
Azelaic acid (p.1110·3).
Acne.

Skinoren
Schering, Aust.; Schering, Austral.; Schering, Belg.; Schering, Denm.; Schering, Fin.; Schering, Fr.; Schering, Ger.; Asche, Ger.; Schering, Hong Kong; Schering, Ital.; Schering, Norw.; Schering, NZ; Schering, Port.; Schering, S.Afr.; Schering, Singapore; Schering, Spain; Schering, Swed.; Schering, Switz.; Schering, Thai.; Schering, UK.
Azelaic acid (p.1110·3).
Acne; pigmentation disorders.

Skinsept F *Henkel, Ger.*
Isopropyl alcohol (p.1149·2); chlorhexidine gluconate (p.1138·2); hydrogen peroxide (p.1147·1).
Skin disinfection.

Skinsept G *Henkel, Ger.*
Alcohol (p.1130·3); isopropyl alcohol (p.1149·2).
Skin disinfection.

Skinsept mucosa *Henkel, Ger.*
Alcohol (p.1130·3); hydrogen peroxide 30% (p.1147·2); chlorhexidine gluconate (p.1138·2).
Mucous membrane disinfection.

Skintex *Lloyd, Aimee, UK.*
Chloroxylenol (p.1142·1); camphor (p.1589·3).
Skin disorders.

Skin-vit *Pharmadass, UK.*
Multivitamin, mineral, and trace element preparation (p.1350·2).

Sklerofibrat *Merckle, Ger.*
Bezafibrate (p.849·1).
Hyperlipidaemias.

Sklerosol *Febena, Ger.*
Colloidal silicon dioxide (p.1503·3).
Atherosclerosis; silicon deficiency.

Sklerovenol N *Febena, Ger.*
Aesculus (p.1574·1); rutoside sodium sulfate (p.1611·2).
Vascular disorders.

The symbol † denotes a preparation no longer actively marketed

Sklerovitol *Lannacher, Aust.*
Vitamin B substances (p.1350·1); rutoside (p.1611·2).
Peripheral vascular disorders; reduced mental and physical capacity in the elderly; tonic.

Sleep Aid
Tanta, Canad.; Stanley, Canad.; Technilab, Canad.; Galpharm, UK.
Diphenhydramine hydrochloride (p.416·1).
Insomnia.

Sleep Complex *Brauer, Austral.†*
Homoeopathic preparation.

Sleepeaze *Galpharm, UK.*
Diphenhydramine hydrochloride (p.416·1).
Insomnia.

Sleep-Ettes D *Reese, USA.*
Diphenhydramine hydrochloride (p.416·1).
Insomnia.

Sleep-eze 3 *Whitehall, USA.*
Diphenhydramine hydrochloride (p.416·1).
Insomnia.

Sleep-Eze D *Medtech, Canad.*
Diphenhydramine hydrochloride (p.416·1).
Insomnia.

Sleep-Eze V Natural *Medtech, Canad.*
Valerian (p.1678·3).
Sleep disorders.

Sleepia *Pfizer Consumer, UK†.*
Diphenhydramine hydrochloride (p.416·1).
Insomnia.

Sleeplessness & Insomnia Relief *Brauer, Austral.*
Homoeopathic preparation.

Sleepwell 2-nite *Rugby, USA.*
Diphenhydramine hydrochloride (p.416·1).
Insomnia.

Slepan *Staufen, Ger.*
Homoeopathic preparation.

Slim Mint
Note. This name is used for preparations of different composition.
Stella, Canad.
Benzocaine (p.1306·2); methylcellulose (p.1502·2).
Obesity.

Thompson, USA†.
Benzocaine (p.1306·2).
Obesity.

Slim 'n Trim *Covan, S.Afr.*
Cathine (p.1507·1).
Obesity.

Slimase *Sessa, Ital.*
Ananas.
Inflammation.

SlimLinea *Bifarma, Ital.†.*
Bladderwrack (p.1585·2); betula (p.1585·2).

Slimmer *Baif, Ital.*
Piscidia erythrina; bladderwrack; ananas sativa; equi-setum arvense; betula alba; ononis spinosa; centella asiatica; orthosiphon stamineus; ruscus aculeatus; lespedeza capitata (p.1350·1).
Nutritional supplement.

Slimomin *Eurodrug, Hong Kong.*
Phenylpropanolamine hydrochloride (p.1098·1).
Obesity.

Slippery Elm Stomach Tablets *Potter's, UK.*
Slippery elm bark (p.1665·1); cinnamon oil (p.1596·1); anise oil (p.1580·3); peppermint oil (p.1243·3).
Dyspepsia; flatulence.

Sloan *Warner-Lambert, Ital.*
Capsicum oleoresin (p.1591·1); glycol monosalicylate (p.42·2); white camphor oil; pine oil; menthol (p.1632·3); eucalyptus oil (p.1609·2); benzyl nicotinate (p.20·2).
Musculoskeletal, joint, and soft-tissue pain.

Sloan Baume *Soma, Switz.†.*
Ethyl nicotinate (p.35·1); menthol (p.1632·3); camphor (p.1589·3); methyl salicylate (p.55·1); capsicum oleoresin (p.1591·1); eucalyptus oil (p.1609·2); pine oil; turpentine oil (p.1676·3).
Musculoskeletal and joint disorders.

Sloan Liniment *Soma, Switz.†.*
Camphor (p.1589·3); methyl salicylate (p.55·1); capsicum oleoresin (p.1591·1); pine oil; turpentine oil (p.1676·3).
Musculoskeletal and joint disorders.

Sloan's balsem *Warner-Lambert, Neth.*
Capsicum (p.1591·1); camphor (p.1589·3); benzyl nicotinate (p.20·2); glycol salicylate (p.42·2).
Muscle and joint pain.

Sloan's liniment *Parke, Davis, Swed.†.*
Capsicum oleoresin (p.1591·1); methyl salicylate (p.55·1); camphor oil; pine oil; ammonia solution (p.1579·1); turpentine oil (p.1676·3).
Muscle pain.

Slo-Bid
Rhone-Poulenc Rorer, Canad.; Rhone-Poulenc Rorer, Hong Kong; Rhone-Poulenc Rorer, Mex.; Rhone-Poulenc Rorer, USA.
Theophylline (p.777·2).
Obstructive airways disease.

Slofedipine *Sanofi Winthrop, UK.*
Nifedipine (p.940·1).
Angina pectoris; hypertension.

Slofenac *Sterwin, UK.*
Diclofenac sodium (p.30·3).

Slo-Indo *Generics, UK.*
Indometacin (p.44·3).
Inflammation; pain.

Slo-Morph *Helsinn Birex, Irl.*
Morphine sulfate (p.56·1).
Pain.

Slo-Niacin *Upsher-Smith, USA.*
Nicotinic acid (p.1372·3).
Hyperlipidaemia (adjunct); nicotinic acid deficiency; pellagra.

Slo-Phyllin
Rhone-Poulenc Rorer, Irl.; Merck, UK; Rhone-Poulenc Rorer, USA.
Theophylline (p.777·2).
Obstructive airways disease.

Slo-Phyllin GG *Rhone-Poulenc Rorer, USA.*
Theophylline (p.777·2); guaifenesin (p.1092·2).
Asthma; bronchospasm.

Slo-Salt-K *Mission Pharmacal, USA.*
Sodium chloride (p.1196·1); potassium chloride (p.1194·3).
Dehydration; heat prostration; sodium depletion; volume depletion.

Slow Deralin *Abic, Israel.*
Propranolol hydrochloride (p.962·3).
Angina pectoris; hypertension; migraine.

Slow Fe with Folic Acid *Novartis Consumer, USA.*
Dried ferrous sulfate (p.1360·3); folic acid (p.1361·1).
Iron and folic acid deficiency.

Slow Release Mega C *Vitaglow, Austral.*
Calcium ascorbate (p.1389·3); ascorbic acid (p.1389·3).
Bruising; cold and influenza symptoms; maintenance of oral health; vitamin supplement; wounds.

Slow Release Mega Multi *Vitaglow, Austral.*
Multivitamin and mineral preparation (p.1350·1).

Slow-Fe
Novartis Consumer, Canad.; Novartis, Israel; Novartis Consumer, UK; Novartis Consumer, USA.
Dried ferrous sulfate (p.1360·3).
Iron deficiency; iron-deficiency anaemia.

Slow-Fe Folic
Novartis Consumer, Canad.; Novartis, Israel; Novartis Consumer, UK.
Dried ferrous sulfate (p.1360·3); folic acid (p.1361·1).
Iron and folic acid deficiency in pregnancy and the puerperium.

Slow-K
Novartis, Austral.; Allergan-Frumtost, Braz.; Novartis, Canad.; Novartis, Hong Kong; Novartis, Irl.; Novartis, Israel; Novartis, Neth.; Novartis, NZ; Novartis, S.Afr.; Alliance, UK; Summit, USA.
Potassium chloride (p.1194·3).
Hypokalaemia; potassium supplement.

Slow-Lopresor
Novartis, Belg.; Novartis, NZ.
Metoprolol tartrate (p.931·2).
Angina pectoris; arrhythmias; hypertension; hyperthyroidism; migraine; myocardial infarction.

Slow-Mag
Roberts, Canad.; Merck, S.Afr.; Roberts, USA.
Magnesium chloride (p.1190·3).
Magnesium deficiency; magnesium supplement.

Slow-Sodium
Novartis, Austral.; Novartis, Irl.; HK Pharma, UK.
Sodium chloride (p.1196·1).
Hyponatraemia.

Slow-Trasicor
Novartis, Canad.; Novartis, Irl.; Novartis, NZ; Novartis, Switz.; Sovereign, UK.
Oxprenolol hydrochloride (p.951·3).
Angina pectoris; anxiety; arrhythmias; hypertension; myocardial infarction.

Slow-Trasitensine *Novartis, Switz.*
Oxprenolol hydrochloride (p.951·3); chlortalidone (p.857·1).
Hypertension.

Slozem *Merck, UK.*
Diltiazem hydrochloride (p.874·3).
Angina pectoris; hypertension.

SLT *C & M, USA.*
Coal tar (p.1125·1); salicylic acid (p.1122·3); lactic acid (p.1626·2).
Seborrhoea.

Slumber *Seven Seas, UK.*
Lupulus (p.1629·3); piscidia (p.1625·1); passion flower (p.1649·1); wild lettuce (p.1680·3).
Insomnia.

SM-33 *Roche Consumer, Austral.*
Salicylic acid (p.1122·3); lignocaine [lidocaine] (p.1313·2); tannic acid (p.1669·1); menthol (p.1632·3); thymol (p.1158·3); glycerol; alcohol.
Mouth ulcers; oral abrasions; teething and denture pain.

SM-33 Adult Formula *Roche Consumer, Austral.*
Lignocaine [lidocaine] (p.1313·2); salicylic acid (p.1122·3); tannins; alcohol; rhubarb (p.1248·1).
Mouth ulcers; oral abrasions.

SMA AR *Wyeth, Mex.*
Infant feed (p.1350·1).
Gastro-oesaphageal reflux.

SMA LF *SMA Nutrition, Irl.*
Infant feed (p.1350·1).
Lactose intolerance.

SMA Sin Lactosa *Wyeth, Mex.*
Infant feed (p.1350·1).
Lactose intolerance.

Smart Fizz *Thompson, Austral.*
A range of multivitamin and mineral preparations (p.1350·1).

Smecta
Beaufour, Fr.; Beaufour-Ipsen, Hong Kong; Beaufour-Ipsen, Singapore; Emerging Pharma, Singapore; Beaufour-Ipsen, Thai.
Dioctahedral smectite.
Diarrhoea; gastro-enteritis; gastro-oesophageal reflux; irritable bowel syndrome.

Smok Quits *Eagle, Austral.*
Homoeopathic preparation.

Smoke-Eze *Brauer, Austral.*
Homoeopathic preparation.

Smokeless *Inibsa, Spain.*
Lobeline sulfate (p.1510·3).
Aid to smoking withdrawal.

Smokerette *Medinex, Canad.†.*
Silver acetate (p.1664·1).
Aid to smoking withdrawal.

Smoking Withdrawal Support *Homeocan, Canad.*
Homoeopathic preparation.

SMZ-TMP *Apothecon, USA.*
Co-trimoxazole (p.193·3).

Snake Bite *CSL, Austral.*
A range of monovalent and polyvalent snake antisera (brown snake, tiger snake, death adder, taipan, black snake) (p.1563·3).
Passive immunisation.

Snap Skin Cleanser Normal *Stella, Canad.*
Isopropyl alcohol (p.1149·2); hamamelis (p.1618·3).

Snap Skin Cleanser Sensitive *Stella, Canad.*
Hamamelis (p.1618·3).

Snaplets-D *Baker Norton, USA†.*
Phenylpropanolamine hydrochloride (p.1098·1); chlorpheniramine [chlorphenamine] maleate (p.412·1).
Upper respiratory-tract symptoms.

Snaplets-DM *Baker Cummins, USA†.*
Phenylpropanolamine hydrochloride (p.1098·1); dextromethorphan hydrobromide (p.1087·3).
Coughs and cold symptoms.

Snaplets-EX *Baker Cummins, USA†.*
Phenylpropanolamine hydrochloride (p.1098·1); guaifenesin (p.1092·2).
Coughs.

Snaplets-FR *Baker Cummins, USA†.*
Paracetamol (p.71·2).
Pain.

Snaplets-Multi *Baker Cummins, USA†.*
Phenylpropanolamine hydrochloride (p.1098·1); dextromethorphan hydrobromide (p.1087·3); chlorpheniramine [chlorphenamine] maleate (p.412·1).
Coughs and cold symptoms.

Sno Phenicol *Chauvin, UK.*
Chloramphenicol (p.179·1).
Bacterial eye infections.

Sno Pilo *Chauvin, UK†.*
Pilocarpine hydrochloride (p.1422·3).
Glaucoma; reduction of intra-ocular pressure before surgery; reversal of mydriasis.

Sno Pro *Scientific Hospital Supplies, Irl.*
Low-protein, low-phenylalanine food for special diets (p.1350·1).
Disorders of amino-acid metabolism; milk substitute.

Sno Strips
Smith & Nephew, Irl.; Akorn, USA.
Test for tear production.

Sno Tears
Chauvin, Irl.; Chauvin, UK.
Polyvinyl alcohol (p.1503·1).
Dry eyes.

Snooze Fast *BDI, USA.*
Diphenhydramine hydrochloride (p.416·1).
Insomnia.

Sno-Pro *Piam, Ital.*
Food for special diets (p.1350·1).
Phenylketonuria; renal failure.

Snor-Away *Medicines International, UK.*
Almond oil (p.1576·3); olive oil (p.1643·3); peppermint oil (p.1243·3); sesame oil (p.1662·2); sunflower oil (p.1381·2); vitamins.
Snoring.

Snore Eze *Brauer, Austral.*
Homoeopathic preparation.

Snorenz *Passion for Life, UK.*
Peppermint oil (p.1243·3); olive oil (p.1643·3); sunflower oil (p.1381·2); sesame oil (p.1662·2); almond oil (p.1576·3); vitamins E, C, and B$_6$ (p.1350·1).
Snoring.

Snowfire *Pickles, UK.*
Benzoin (p.1668·3); citronella (p.1596·3); thyme oil (p.1672·3); lemon thyme (p.1672·2); clove oil (p.1597·1); cade oil (p.1124·3).
Chapped hands; chilblains.

SNP *Quatromed, S.Afr.*
Sodium nitroprusside hydrochloride.
Hypertension; production of controlled hypotension during surgery.

Snufflebabe *Pickles, UK.*
Menthol (p.1632·3); thyme oil (p.1672·3); eucalyptus oil (p.1609·2).
Congestion.

Soaclens
Alcon, Austral.; Alcon, Braz.; Alcon, Canad.; Alcon, Fr.†; Alcon, NZ; Alcon, USA.
Wetting, soaking, and storage solution for hard and gas-permeable contact lenses (p.1129·2).

Soapex *Darrow, Braz.*
Triclosan (p.1159·2); triclocarban (p.1159·2).
Skin disinfection.

Sobelin
Note. This name is used for preparations of different composition.
Pharmacia Upjohn, Ger.
Clindamycin hydrochloride (p.188·1), clindamycin palmitate hydrochloride (p.188·1) or clindamycin phosphate (p.188·2).
Bacterial infections.

TO-Chemicals, Thai.
Flunarizine (p.418·2).
Cerebrovascular disorders; migraine; motion sickness; peripheral vascular disorders; vestibular disorders.

Sobrepin *Abbott, Braz.; Roche, Ital.; Tedec Meiji, Spain.*
Sobrerol (p.1100·3).
Respiratory-tract disorders.

Sobrepina *Baldacci, Port.*
Nimodipine (p.946·1).
Cerebral ischaemia; cerebral vasospasm following subarachnoid haemorrhage.

Sobril *Pharmacia Upjohn, Norw.; Pharmacia Upjohn, Swed.*
Oxazepam (p.697·1).
Alcohol withdrawal syndrome; anxiety disorders; insomnia; premedication.

Socian *Synthelabo, Braz.; Sanofi Synthelabo, Port.*
Amisulpride (p.655·1).
Depression; psychoses.

Socloxin *Olan-Kemed, Thai.*
Cloxacillin sodium (p.192·1).
Bacterial infections.

Soden *DHA, Singapore.*
Naproxen sodium (p.61·1).
Gout; musculoskeletal and joint disorders; pain.

Soderm *Dermapharm, Ger.*
Betamethasone valerate (p.1063·2).
Skin disorders.

Sodex N *Woelm, Ger.†.*
Calcium carbonate (p.1215·1); magnesium hydroxide (p.1233·1).
Sodex formerly contained calcium carbonate, magnesium hydroxide, and bismuth subnitrate.
Gastrointestinal disorders.

Sodexx *Kwizda, Aust.*
Cimetidine (p.1216·3).
Gastro-oesophageal reflux; peptic ulcer; Zollinger-Ellison syndrome.

Sodibic *Rhone-Poulenc Rorer, Austral.*
Sodium bicarbonate (p.1186·2).
Bicarbonate replacement in renal failure.

Sodical Plus *Blackmores, Austral.†.*
Sodium phosphate (p.1193·2); iron phosphate; calcium phosphate (p.1188·3).

Sodiclo *Brissenco, S.Afr.†.*
Diclofenac sodium (p.30·3).
Inflammation; rheumatic disorders.

Sodinon *Boehringer Mannheim, Aust.†.*
Alginic acid (p.1498·3); aluminium hydroxide (p.1210·3); magnesium trisilicate (p.1233·3); sodium bicarbonate (p.1186·2).
Dyspepsia with reflux.

Sodiofolin *Medac, UK.*
Sodium folinate (p.1363·2).
Adjunct to fluorouracil in colorectal cancer; methotrexate toxicity.

Sodiopen *CEPA, Spain.*
Benzylpenicillin sodium (p.157·2).
Bacterial infections.

Sodioral *CaDiGroup, Ital.†.*
Glucose; sodium chloride (p.1185·2).
Diarrhoea.

Sodioral with Inulina *CaDiGroup, Ital.*
Oral rehydration solution with inulin (p.1185·2).
Diarrhoea.

Sodipen *Antibioticos, Mex.*
Benzylpenicillin sodium (p.157·2).
Bacterial infections.

Sodipental *Pisa, Mex.*
Thiopental sodium (p.1269·1).
Convulsions; general anaesthesia.

Sodip-phylline *Sodip, Switz.*
Theophylline (p.777·2).
Obstructive airways disease.

Sodipryl retard *Sodip, Switz.*
Naftidrofuryl oxalate (p.937·3).
Peripheral and cerebral vascular disorders.

Sodium Sulamyd *Schering, Canad.; Schering, USA.*
Sulfacetamide sodium (p.250·3).
Eye infections.

Sodixen *Rayere, Mex.*
Naproxen sodium (p.61·1).
Fever; musculoskeletal and joint disorders; pain.

Sodol Compound *Major, USA.*
Aspirin (p.14·2); carisoprodol (p.1327·1).
Musculoskeletal pain.

Sodolac *Sofex, Port.†.*
Etodolac (p.35·2).
Gout; musculoskeletal, joint, and peri-articular disorders; pain.

Sofargen *Sofar, Ital.*
Sulfadiazine silver (p.251·3).
Bacterial skin infections; burns; wounds.

Sofenol *C & M, USA.*
Emollient and moisturiser.

Soffodex *Dexxon, Israel.*
Dibasic sodium phosphate (p.1193·2); monobasic sodium phosphate (p.1193·2).
Bowel evacuation; constipation.

Sofilex *Xepa-Soul Pattinson, Singapore.*
Cefalexin (p.161·3).
Bacterial infections.

Soflax
Note.This name is used for preparations of different composition.
Pharmascience, Canad.
Docusate sodium (p.1223·1).
Constipation.

Julphar, UAE.
Lactulose (p.1230·1).
Constipation; hepatic encephalopathy.

Soflax EX *Pharmascience, Canad.*
Bisacodyl (p.1212·2).
Constipation.

Soflax Fleet *Fleet, USA†.*
Docusate sodium (p.1223·1).
Stool softener.

Soflax Overnight *Fleet, USA†.*
Docusate sodium (p.1223·1); casanthranol (p.1216·1).
Constipation; stool softener.

Sofloran *Pisa, Mex.*
Isoflurane (p.1261·1).
General anaesthesia.

Sof/Pro Clean *Sherman, Israel; Sherman, USA†.*
Cleansing solution for soft contact lenses (p.1129·2).

Sofracort *Hoechst Marion Roussel, Belg.*
Framycetin sulfate (p.208·2); gramicidin (p.213·3); dexamethasone (p.1067·1).
Ear disorders; eye disorders.

Sofradex
Hoechst Marion Roussel, Austral.; Aventis, Denm.; Hoechst Marion Roussel, Fin.; Hoechst Marion Roussel, Hong Kong; Hoechst Marion Roussel, Irl.; Hoechst Marion Roussel, Neth.; Hoechst Marion Roussel, Norw.; Hoechst Marion Roussel, NZ; Aventis, S.Afr.; Hoechst Marion Roussel, Singapore; Hoechst Marion Roussel, Swed.; Hoechst Marion Roussel, Switz.; Hoechst Marion Roussel, Thai.; Florizel, UK.
Dexamethasone (p.1067·1) or dexamethasone sodium metasulfobenzoate (p.1067·1); framycetin sulfate (p.208·2); gramicidin (p.213·3).
Infected eye disorders; otitis externa.

Sofraline *Aventis, Belg.*
Framycetin sulfate (p.208·2); naphazoline nitrate (p.1095·1).
Respiratory-tract disorders.

Soframycin
Note.This name is used for preparations of different composition.
Hoechst Marion Roussel, Austral.; Hoechst Marion Roussel, Canad.; Roussel, Irl.; Hoechst Marion Roussel, Neth.; Aventis, NZ; Hoechst Marion Roussel, S.Afr.†; Hoechst Marion Roussel, Singapore; Hoechst Marion Roussel, Switz.; Florizel, UK.
Eye/ear drops; eye/ear ointment: Framycetin sulfate (p.208·2).
Bacterial eye and ear infections.

Hoechst Marion Roussel, Austral.; Hoechst Marion Roussel, Canad.; Hoechst Marion Roussel, Irl.; Aventis, NZ; Hoechst Marion Roussel, UK†.
Ointment: Framycetin sulfate (p.208·2); gramicidin (p.213·3).
Bacterial skin infections.

Hoechst Marion Roussel, Canad.†.
Nasal spray: Framycetin sulfate (p.208·2); gramicidin (p.213·3); phenylephrine hydrochloride (p.1097·1).
Bacterial nasal infections; nasal congestion.

Soframycine
Aventis, Belg.; Roussel, Fr.
Framycetin sulfate (p.208·2).
Bacterial nose and throat infections.

Soframycine Hydrocortisone *Roussel, Fr.*
Framycetin sulfate (p.208·2); hydrocortisone (p.1073·3).
Bacterial nose and throat infections with inflammation.

Soframycine Naphazoline *Roussel, Fr.*
Framycetin sulfate (p.208·2); naphazoline nitrate (p.1095·1).
Congestion and bacterial infection of the nose and throat.

Sofrasolone *Aventis, Belg.*
Prednisolone acetate (p.1078·1); framycetin sulfate (p.208·2); naphazoline nitrate (p.1095·1).
Allergy or infections of the respiratory-tract.

Sofra-Tull
Hoechst Marion Roussel, Aust.; Hoechst Marion Roussel, Ger.
Framycetin sulfate (p.208·2).
Burns; skin infections; ulcers; wounds.

Sofra-Tulle
Hoechst Marion Roussel, Austral.; Hoechst Marion Roussel, Canad.; Hoechst Marion Roussel, Denm.†; Hoechst Marion Roussel, Fr.; Hoechst Marion Roussel, Hong Kong; Hoechst Marion Roussel, Irl.; Hoechst Marion Roussel, Israel; Hoechst Marion Roussel, Neth.; Hoechst Marion Roussel, Norw.; Aventis, NZ; Aventis, S.Afr.; Hoechst Marion Roussel, Singapore; Hoechst Marion Roussel, Swed.; Hoechst Marion Roussel, Switz.; Hoechst Marion Roussel, Thai.; Hoechst Marion Roussel, UK.
Framycetin sulfate (p.208·2).
Burns; infected skin disorders; medicated dressing; skin ulcers; wounds.

The symbol † denotes a preparation no longer actively marketed

SOF-T *Doetsch, Grether, Switz.†*
Copper-wound plastic (p.1357·3).
Intra-uterine contraceptive device.

Soft Lips *Mentholatum, Canad.*
SPF 17: Octinoxate (p.1517·3); oxybenzone (p.1518·1); padimate O (p.1518·2); dimethicone (p.1410·1).
Sunscreen.

Soft Lips Sparkle *Mentholatum, Canad.*
SPF 10: Octinoxate (p.1517·3).
Sunscreen.

Soft Mate
Barnes Hind, NZ; Pilkington Barnes-Hind, USA.
A range of solutions for soft contact lenses (p.1129·2).

Soft Mate Comfort Drops *Allergan, Austral.†.*
Lubricating and cleansing solution (p.1129·2).
Irritation and dryness occurring during contact lens wear.

Soft Mate Consept *Pilkington Barnes-Hind, USA.*
Hydrogen peroxide (p.1147·1) (p.1129·2).
Disinfecting solution for soft contact lenses.

Soft Mate Consept I
Willvonseder, Aust.; Allergan, Austral.†.
Hydrogen peroxide (p.1147·1) (p.1129·2).
Cleansing and disinfecting solution for contact lenses.

Soft Mate Consept 2
Willvonseder, Aust.; Allergan, Austral.†.
Rinsing and neutralising solutions for contact lenses (p.1129·2).

Soft Mate Daily Cleaning Solution *Allergan, Austral.†.*
Cleansing solution for soft contact lenses (p.1129·2).

Soft Mate Enzyme Plus Cleaner *Pilkington Barnes-Hind, USA.*
Subtilisin-A (p.1129·2).
Cleansing solution for soft contact lenses.

Soft Rinse 250 *SoftRinse, USA†.*
Sodium chloride (p.1196·1)(p.1129·2).
Rinsing and storage solution for soft contact lenses.

Softa Man
Braun, Ger.; Braun, Ital.
Alcohol (p.1130·3); propyl alcohol (p.1155·3).
Hand disinfection.

Softab
Alcon, Austral.†; Alcon, NZ.
Sodium dichloroisocyanurate (p.1156·1) (p.1129·2).
Cleansing and sterilisation of soft contact lenses.

Softasept N *Braun, Ger.*
Alcohol (p.1130·3); isopropyl alcohol (p.1149·2).
Skin disinfection.

Softene *Melisana, Belg.*
Docusate sodium (p.1223·1); bisacodyl (p.1212·2).
Constipation.

Softin *Dexcel, Israel.*
Vaginal lubricant.

Softon *Banner, Hong Kong.*
Docusate sodium (p.1223·1).
Constipation.

Softon Plus *Banner, Hong Kong.*
Docusate sodium (p.1223·1); casanthranol (p.1216·1).
Constipation.

Softwash *Palmolive Skincare, Austral.†.*
Triclosan (p.1159·2).
Hand disinfection.

Softwear
Ciba Vision, Austral.; Ciba Vision, Canad.; Ciba Vision, NZ.
Sodium chloride (p.1196·1) (p.1129·2).
Rinsing and storage solution for soft contact lenses.

Sogoon *Steiner, Ger.*
Devil's claw root (p.26·3).
Joint disorders.

Soijatutteli *Valio, Fin.*
Infant feed (p.1350·1).
Cow's milk allergy; lactose intolerance.

Soker *Medecine Vegetale, Fr.†.*
Aniseed (p.1580·2); star anise; condurango (p.1599·1); sodium hydrogen phosphate (p.1193·2); calcium carbonate (p.1215·1); magnesium oxide (p.1233·2).
Gastrointestinal disorders.

Soklinal *Allergan, Ger.†.*
Phenylmercuric nitrate (p.1154·1) (p.1129·2).
Storage and rinsing solution for contact lenses.

Sol Schoum *Expancience, Spain.*
Boldo (p.1585·3); fumitory (p.1612·3); hamamelis (p.1618·3); melissa (p.1632·2); rhubarb (p.1248·1); piscidia (p.1625·1); peppermint oil (p.1243·3); hydrastis canadensis (p.1621·1); ethyl alcohol; glycerol.
Hepatobiliary disorders.

Sola Stick Broad Spectrum *Hamilton, Austral.†.*
SPF15+: Octinoxate (p.1517·3); avobenzone (p.1517·1).
Sunscreen.

Solacap *SAT, Spain.*
Fluconazole (p.383·2).
Fungal infections.

Solacy *Grimberg, Fr.*
Cystine (p.1359·1); sulfur (p.1123·3); vitamin A acetate (p.1383·2); yeast (p.1398·1).
Upper respiratory-tract disorders.

Solamin *Pharmacia Upjohn, Ital.*
Amino-acid infusion (p.1350·1).
Parenteral nutrition.

Solan-M *Winzer, Ger.*
Vitamin A palmitate (p.1383·2).
Eye disorders.

Solantal *Fujisawa, Jpn.*
Tiaramide hydrochloride (p.88·2).
Inflammation; pain.

Solaquin
Note.This name is used for preparations of different composition.
ICN, Hong Kong; ICN, Singapore; ICN, USA.
Hydroquinone (p.1115·1).
Skin hyperpigmentation.

ICN, Mex.
Hydroquinone (p.1115·1); padimate O (p.1518·2); octinoxate (p.1517·3); oxybenzone (p.1518·1).
Skin hyperpigmentation.

Solaquin Forte
Note.This name is used for preparations of different composition.
ICN, Canad.
Hydroquinone (p.1115·1); roxadimate (p.1518·3); dioxybenzone (p.1517·2); oxybenzone (p.1518·1).
Skin hyperpigmentation.

ICN, USA.
Cream: Hydroquinone (p.1115·1); padimate O (p.1518·2); dioxybenzone (p.1517·2); oxybenzone (p.1518·1).
Topical gel: Hydroquinone (p.1115·1); padimate O (p.1518·2); dioxybenzone (p.1517·2).
Skin hyperpigmentation.

Solaraze
Bioglan, UK; Skye, USA.
Diclofenac sodium (p.30·3).
Actinic keratoses.

Solarcaine
Note.This name is used for preparations of different composition.
Schering-Plough, Canad.; Schering-Plough, Hong Kong; Schering-Plough, USA.
Benzocaine (p.1306·2); triclosan (p.1159·2).
Minor skin lesions and burns; skin irritation.

Schering-Plough, Spain.
Benzocaine (p.1306·2); hexachlorophene (p.1146·1).
Burns; insect stings; skin disorders.

Democal, Switz.
Lignocaine [lidocaine] (p.1313·2).
Minor skin lesions and burns.

Schering-Plough, UK.
Cream; lotion; topical spray: Benzocaine (p.1306·2); triclosan (p.1159·2).
Minor skin injuries; sunburn.
Topical gel: Aloe vera (p.1110·1); lignocaine [lidocaine] (p.1313·2).
Cuts; insect bites; sunburn.

Solarcaine Aloe Extra Burn Relief *Schering-Plough, USA.*
Lignocaine [lidocaine] (p.1313·2); aloe vera (p.1110·1).
Local anaesthesia.

Solarcaine Lidocaine *Schering-Plough, Canad.*
Lignocaine [lidocaine] (p.1313·2) or lignocaine [lidocaine] hydrochloride (p.1313·2).
Sunburn; wounds.

Solarcaine Stop Itch *Schering-Plough, Canad.*
Papain (p.1647·3).
Skin pain and irritation.

Solart *Pfizer, Ital.*
Acemetacin (p.11·2).
Musculoskeletal and joint disorders.

Solaskil *Specia, Fr.†.*
Levamisole hydrochloride (p.101·2).
Worm infections.

Solatran
SmithKline Beecham, Belg.; SmithKline Beecham, S.Afr.; Doetsch, Grether, Switz.
Ketazolam (p.688·2).
Anxiety disorders; nervous disorders; sedative; skeletal muscle spasm.

Solaurit *Polcopharma, Austral.*
Homoeopathic preparation.

Solaxin *Eisai, Hong Kong.*
Chlorzoxazone (p.1327·3).
Painful skeletal muscle spasm.

SolBar
Note.This name is used for preparations of different composition.
Person & Covey, Canad.
SPF 50: Octocrilene (p.1518·1); octinoxate (p.1517·3); oxybenzone (p.1518·1).
Sunscreen.

Person & Covey, USA.
SPF 15: Octinoxate (p.1517·3); oxybenzone (p.1518·1).
SPF 30; SPF 50: Octocrilene (p.1518·1); octinoxate (p.1517·3); oxybenzone (p.1518·1).
Sunscreen.

SolBar Plus *Person & Covey, Canad.†.*
SPF 15: Oxybenzone (p.1518·1); roxadimate (p.1518·3).
Sunscreen.

Solblastin *Faulding, Port.*
Vinblastine sulfate (p.577·3).

Solciclina *Solfran, Mex.*
Amoxicillin trihydrate (p.149·2).
Bacterial infections.

Solclin *Solfran, Mex.*
Tetracycline (p.258·3).
Bacterial infections.

Solcode *Reckitt & Colman, Austral.*
Aspirin (p.14·2); codeine phosphate (p.25·2).
Fever; pain.

Solcoderm
Solco, Hong Kong; Solco, Switz.
Nitric acid (p.1642·3); glacial acetic acid (p.1571·2); oxalic acid dihydrate (p.1645·2); lactic acid (p.1626·2); copper nitrate trihydrate.
Benign skin growths.

Solco-Derman *Galderma, Ger.*
Glacial acetic acid (p.1571·2); oxalic acid (p.1645·2); nitric acid (p.1642·3); lactic acid (p.1626·2); copper nitrate.
Skin disorders.

Solcogyn *Solco, Switz.*
Nitric acid (p.1642·3); glacial acetic acid (p.1571·2); oxalic acid dihydrate (p.1645·2); zinc nitrate hexahydrate.
Benign cervical lesions.

Solcoseryl
Solco, Aust.; Solco, Hong Kong; Asta Medica, Ital.†; Asta Medica, Neth.; Swisspharm, S.Afr.†; Diafarm, Spain; Solco, Switz.; Merck, Thai.; Solco, Thai.
Protein-free calf blood extract.
Burns; cerebral and peripheral vascular disorders; eye disorders; mouth and throat disorders; peptic ulcer; skin ulceration; wounds.

Solcoseryl Dental
Solco, Aust.; Solco, Ger.; Solco, Hong Kong; Solco, Switz.; Merck, Thai.; Solco, Thai.
Protein-free calf blood extract; lauromacrogol 400 (p.1345·2).
Formerly known as Solcoseryl comp in Aust.
Dental adhesive; mouth disorders.

Solcosplen *Strathmann, Ger.*
Calf spleen extract.
Menopausal disorders.

Solco-Trichovac
Solco, Hong Kong; Solco, Switz.
Lactobacillus acidophilus (p.1626·3).
Vaginal infections.

Soldactone
Searle, Belg.; Searle, Denm.; Searle, Fin.; Searle, Neth.; Searle, Norw.; Searle, Swed.; Searle, Switz.
Potassium canrenoate (p.957·1).
Ascites; hyperaldosteronism; hypokalaemia; oedema.

Soldermil Ecran Total *Edol, Port.*
SPF 8; SPF 15: Zinc oxide (p.1128·2); titanium dioxide (p.1126·1).
Sunscreen.

Soldesam *Farmacologico Milanese, Ital.*
Dexamethasone sodium phosphate (p.1067·1).
Corticosteroid.

Soldrin *Columbia, Mex.*
Ear drops: Hydrocortisone (p.1073·3); chloramphenicol (p.179·1); benzocaine (p.1306·2).
Otitis externa.
Eye drops: Dexamethasone sodium phosphate (p.1067·1); neomycin sulfate (p.228·1).
Infected eye disorders.

Solecin *Echo, Ital.*
Soya lecithin (p.1628·1); wheat germ; gelatin (p.737·2); glycerol (p.1616·3); betacarotene (p.1355·1).
Nutritional supplement.

Soledum *Cassella-med, Ger.*
Eucalyptol (p.1609·2).
Bronchitis; sinusitis.

Soledum Balsam *Cassella-med, Ger.*
Eucalyptol (p.1609·2).
Respiratory-tract disorders.

Soledum Hustensaft *Cassella-med, Ger.*
Thyme (p.1672·2).
Bronchitis; catarrh; coughs.

Soledum Hustentropfen *Cassella-med, Ger.*
Thyme (p.1672·2).
Bronchitis; catarrh; coughs.

Soledum med *Cassella-med, Ger.*
Chamomile oil.
Nasal congestion; rhinitis.

Solex A15 *Dermol, USA.*
Padimate O (p.1518·2); oxybenzone (p.1518·1).
Sunscreen.

Soleze *Pickles, UK.*
Dibrompropamidine isetionate (p.1143·1); hydroviton.
Burns; sunburn.

Solfa *Takeda, Jpn.*
Amlexanox (p.760·3).
Allergic rhinitis; asthma.

Solfac EW *Bayer, Ital.*
Cyfluthrin (p.1430·2).
Insecticide.

Solfen *Antigen, Irl.*
Ibuprofen (p.43·2).
Fever; pain.

Solfomucil *Locatelli, Ital.†.*
Carbocisteine (p.1086·3).
Otorhinolaryngeal disorders; respiratory-tract congestion.

Solfoton *ECR, USA.*
Phenobarbital (p.355·1).
Epilepsy; insomnia; sedative.

Solfranicol *Solfran, Mex.*
Chloramphenicol (p.179·1); tetracycline (p.258·3).
Bacterial infections.

Solfurol *Solfran, Mex.*
Furazolidone (p.592·1); clioquinol (p.190·2).
Diarrhoea.

Solganal
Schering, Canad.; Schering-Plough, Israel; Schering, USA.
Aurothioglucose (p.18·3).
Rheumatoid arthritis.

Solgeretik Bristol-Myers Squibb, Aust.
Nadolol (p.937·1); bendrofluazide [bendroflumethiazide] (p.844·1).
Hypertension.

Solgol
Bristol-Myers Squibb, Aust.; Bristol-Myers Squibb, Ger.; Sanofi Synthelabo, Spain.
Nadolol (p.937·1).
Angina pectoris; arrhythmias; hypertension; migraine.

Solian
Synthelabo, Fr.; Sanofi Synthelabo, Ger.; Lorex, Irl.; Sanofi Synthelabo, Singapore; Synthelabo, Switz.; Sanofi Synthelabo, UK.
Amisulpride (p.655·1).
Psychoses.

Solibay Bayer, Mex.
Bezafibrate (p.849·1).
Hyperlipidaemias.

Solicam SMB, Belg.
Piroxicam (p.79·1).
Gout; musculoskeletal and joint disorders; pain.

Solidago M Pilsensee, Ger.
Solidago virgaurea.
Urinary-tract disorders.

Solidagoren N Klein, Ger.
Solidago virgaurea; potentilla anserina; equisetum (p.1606·3).
Renal disorders.

Solidagosan N Hanosan, Ger.
Homoeopathic preparation.

Solinase Yamanouchi, Jpn.
Pamiteplase.

Solinitrina Almirall, Spain.
Glyceryl trinitrate (p.897·3).
Angina pectoris; heart failure; induction of hypotension in surgery; myocardial infarction.

Solipid Laevosan, Aust.
Soya oil (p.1378·1).
Some preparations contain egg lecithin.
Lipid infusion for parenteral nutrition.

Solisan Synpharma, Aust.
Ononis root (p.1644·1); taraxacum (p.1669·1); centaury (p.1593·1).
Formerly contained ononis root, bearberry, and centaury.
Urinary-tract disorders.

Solitab Hermes, Ger.†
Magnesium trisilicate (p.1233·3).
Gastrointestinal disorders associated with hyperacidity.

Solivito N
Pharmacia Upjohn, Irl.; Fresenius, UK.
Multivitamin preparation (p.1350·1).
Parenteral nutrition.

Sol-Jod Ecobi, Ital.
Iodine (p.1522·3).
Oral antisepsis.

Solkan Solfran, Mex.
Kanamycin (p.218·2).
Bacterial infections.

Sollival Sirval, Ital.
Emollient.

Solmag Ecosol, Switz.
Magnesium aspartate (p.1190·3).
Arrhythmias; magnesium deficiency; magnesium supplement; myocardial infarction.

Solmucaine IBSA, Switz.
Acetylcysteine (p.1082·3); tyrothricin (p.267·1); lignocaine [lidocaine] hydrochloride (p.1313·2).
Upper respiratory-tract disorders with viscous mucus.

Solmucalm IBSA, Switz.
Acetylcysteine (p.1082·3); chlorpheniramine [chlorphenamine] maleate (p.412·1).
Coughs.

Solmucol
Genevrier, Fr.; IBSA, Hong Kong; Fidia, Ital.; Aspen Consumer, S.Afr.; IBSA, Switz.
Acetylcysteine (p.1082·3).
Eye disorders; paracetamol overdosage; respiratory-tract disorders.

Solmux Westmont, Hong Kong.
Carbocisteine (p.1086·3).
Respiratory-tract disorders associated with increased or viscous mucus.

Solo-care
Ciba Vision, Austral.; Ciba Vision, Canad.
Cleansing, rinsing, disinfecting, and storage solution for soft contact lenses (p.1129·2).

Solocare Ciba Vision, NZ.
Cleaning, disinfecting, rinsing, and storage solution for soft contact lenses (p.1129·2).

Solo-care Hard
Ciba Vision, Aust.
Rinsing, storage, and disinfecting solution for hard contact lenses (p.1129·2).

Ciba Vision, Canad.
Cleansing, rinsing, conditioning, storage, and wetting solution for hard and gas permeable contact lenses (p.1129·2).

Solo-care Soft Ciba Vision, Aust.
Rinsing, storage, and disinfecting solution for soft contact lenses (p.1129·2).

Solomet Orion, Fin.
Methylprednisolone (p.1076·1), methylprednisolone acetate (p.1076·1), or methylprednisolone sodium succinate (p.1076·1).
Corticosteroid.

Solomet c bupivacain hydrochlorid Orion, Fin.
Methylprednisolone acetate (p.1076·1); bupivacaine hydrochloride (p.1306·3).
Musculoskeletal, joint, and peri-articular disorders.

Solone Fawns & McAllan, Austral.
Prednisolone (p.1077·3).
Corticosteroid.

Solosa Hoechst Marion Roussel, Ital.
Glimepiride (p.322·3).
Diabetes mellitus.

Solosin Hoechst Marion Roussel, Ger.
Theophylline (p.777·2).
Obstructive airways disease.

SoloSite Smith & Nephew, Austral.
Carmellose sodium (p.1499·3); allantoin (p.1110·1).
Wounds.

Solotrim Fresenius Kabi, Aust.
Trimethoprim (p.264·2).
Bacterial infections.

Solovite Solgar, U.K.
Multivitamin and mineral preparation (p.1350·1).

Solpadeine
SmithKline Beecham Consumer, Irl.; SmithKline Beecham Consumer, UK.
Paracetamol (p.71·2); codeine phosphate (p.25·2); caffeine (p.761·3).
Fever; pain.

Solpadeine Max SmithKline Beecham Consumer, UK.
Paracetamol (p.71·2); codeine phosphate (p.25·2).
These ingredients can be described by the British Approved Name Co-codamol.
Pain.

Solpadol
Sanofi Winthrop, Irl.; Sanofi Winthrop, UK.
Paracetamol (p.71·2); codeine phosphate (p.25·2).
These ingredients can be described by the British Approved Name Co-codamol 30/500.
Pain.

Solpaflex
Note. This name is used for preparations of different composition.
SmithKline Beecham, Denm.
Ibuprofen (p.43·2).
Inflammation; musculoskeletal and joint disorders; pain.

SmithKline Beecham Consumer, UK.
Tablets: Ibuprofen (p.43·2); codeine phosphate (p.25·2).
Fever; pain.
Topical gel†: Ketoprofen (p.47·3).
Oedema; pain; peri-articular and soft-tissue disorders.

Solphyllex Adcock Ingram, S.Afr.
Theophylline (p.777·2); etofylline (p.765·1); diphenylpyraline hydrochloride (p.417·1); ammonium chloride (p.1085·2); sodium citrate (p.1186·2).
Coughs.

Solphyllin Adcock Ingram, S.Afr.
Theophylline (p.777·2); etofylline (p.765·1).
Obstructive airways disease.

Solpic Medical, Port.
Mepyramine maleate (p.421·1); calamine (p.1111·3); benzocaine (p.1306·2).
Skin irritation.

Solplex 40 Fresenius Kabi, Ital.
Dextran 40 (p.728·3) in sodium chloride.
Plasma volume expansion.

Solplex 70 Fresenius Kabi, Ital.
Dextran 70 (p.729·2) in sodium chloride.
Plasma volume expansion; thrombosis prophylaxis.

Solprene Farmigea, Ital.
Prednisolone sodium phosphate (p.1078·1); neomycin sulfate (p.228·1).
Infected eye disorders.

Solprin
Reckitt & Colman, Austral.
Aspirin (p.14·2).
Fever; inhibition of platelet aggregation; pain.

Reckitt Benckiser, NZ.
Calcium aspirin (p.14·2).
Inflammation; pain.

Solsavit Solfran, Mex.
Vitamin B$_{12}$; vitamin B$_6$ (p.1350·1).

Solsolona Cryopharma, Mex.
Methylprednisolone acetate (p.1076·1).
Corticosteroid.

Soltamox Rosemont, UK.
Tamoxifen citrate (p.571·1).
Anovulatory infertility; breast cancer.

Soltice Chattem, USA.
Methyl salicylate (p.55·1); camphor (p.1589·3); menthol (p.1632·3).
Muscle, joint, and soft-tissue pain; neuralgia.

Soltric ICN, Mex.
Mebendazole (p.102·2).

Soltrim Almirall, Spain.
Sulfamethoxazole lysine (p.255·2); trimethoprim (p.264·2).
Bacterial infections; Pneumocystis carinii pneumonia.

Solubacter
Boots Healthcare, Fr.; Innotech, Port.
Triclocarban (p.1159·2).
Disinfection of skin and mucous membranes.

Solubeol
Note. This name is used for preparations of different composition.
Piette, Belg.
Guaifenesin (p.1092·2); phenoxyethanol (p.1153·3).
Solvent for painful intramuscular injections.

Azevedos, Port.
Cypress oil; eucalyptus oil (p.1609·2); hyssop oil; lavender oil (p.1627·2); oleum pini sylvestris.
Respiratory-tract disorders.

Solu-Biloptin Schering, UK.
Calcium iopodate (p.1035·3).
Contrast medium for biliary-tract radiography.

Solubitrat Sanova, Aust.
Silver birch leaf (p.1585·2); solidago virgaurea; java tea (p.1625·3); fennel oil (p.1610·2).
Urinary-tract disorders.

Solucalcine Prima, Braz.
Calcium chloride (p.1188·1).
Hypocalcaemia.

Solucamphre
Note. This name is used for preparations of different composition.
Synthelabo, Belg.†
Codeine (p.25·2); ethylmorphine (p.35·2); ephedrine (p.1090·1); piperazine hydrate (p.106·1); camsylic acid; aconite (p.1572·3); belladonna (p.463·1); ipecacuanha (p.1093·1); senna (p.1248·2).
Coughs.

Synthelabo, Fr.†
Piperazine camsilate (p.106·2).
Hypotension.

Synthelabo, Switz.†
Codeine camsilate (p.26·1); ethylmorphine camsilate (p.35·2); ephedrine camsilate (p.1090·3); belladonna (p.463·1); ipecacuanha (p.1093·1).
Coughs.

Solucao Aminon JP, Braz.
Amino-acid infusion (p.1350·1).
Parenteral nutrition.

Solucao Aminorin JP, Braz.
Amino-acid infusion (p.1350·1).
Parenteral nutrition.

Solucao Anticoagulante Hypofarma, Braz.
Citric acid (p.1596·2); glucose (p.1364·1); sodium citrate (p.1186·2).
Anticoagulant for blood transfusions.

Solucao Nasal de Nafazolina Bergamo, Braz.
Naphazoline (p.1095·1); nitrofurazone (p.231·3); panthenol (p.1602·3).
Nasal congestion.

Solucao Stago Merck, Port.
Boldo (p.1585·3); comfrey (p.1598·3); chamomile (p.1593·2); cinchona bark (p.1595·3); sarsaparilla (p.1661·1); black pine; euonymus (p.1225·3); buchu (p.1587·2); junco.
Dyspepsia.

Solucaps Medix, Mex.
Mazindol (p.1510·3).
Obesity.

Soluciel Stiefel, Spain.
Benzoyl peroxide (p.1111·1).
Acne.

Solu-Celestan Aesca, Aust.
Betamethasone disodium phosphate (p.1063·2).
Corticosteroid.

Soluchrom Cooperation Pharmaceutique, Fr.
Merbromin sodium (p.1150·1).
Skin, burn and wound disinfection.

Solucion DP Pisa, Mex.
Glucose; sodium chloride; calcium chloride; magnesium chloride; sodium lactate (p.1184·1).
Peritoneal dialysis.

Solucion Fisio PQS, Spain; Cinfa, Spain.
Sodium chloride (p.1196·1).
Nasal congestion.

Solucionic Diviser Aquilea, Spain†.
Povidone-iodine (p.1155·1).
Bacterial vaginosis.

Solucis Aesculapius, Ital.
Carbocisteine (p.1086·3).
Respiratory-tract congestion.

Solucol PSM, NZ.
Sodium bicarbonate (p.1186·2); tartaric acid (p.1669·2); thymol (p.1158·3).
Oral hygiene.

Solucort Merck Sharp & Dohme-Chibret, Fr.
Prednisolone sodium phosphate (p.1078·1).
Corticosteroid.

Solu-Cortef
Pharmacia Upjohn, Austral.; Pharmacia Upjohn, Belg.; Rhodia, Braz.; Pharmacia Upjohn, Canad.; Pharmacia Upjohn, Denm.; Pharmacia Upjohn, Fin.; Pharmacia Upjohn, Hong Kong; Pharmacia Upjohn, Irl.; Pharmacia Upjohn, Israel; Pharmacia Upjohn, Ital.; Pharmacia Upjohn, Neth.; Pharmacia Upjohn, Norw.; Pharmacia Upjohn, NZ; Pharmacia Upjohn, S.Afr.; Pharmacia Upjohn, Singapore; Pharmacia Upjohn, Swed.; Pharmacia Upjohn, Switz.; Pharmacia, UK; Upjohn, USA.
Hydrocortisone sodium succinate (p.1074·1).
Corticosteroid.

Solu-Crom Sabex, Canad.
Sodium cromoglicate (p.774·3).
Allergic conjunctivitis.

Solu-Dacortin Merck, Aust.
Prednisolone sodium succinate (p.1078·2).
Corticosteroid.

Soludacortin Bracco, Ital.
Prednisolone sodium succinate (p.1078·2).
Corticosteroid.

Solu-Dacortin H Merck, Spain†.
Prednisolone sodium succinate (p.1078·2).
Corticosteroid.

Solu-Dacortina Merck, Port.
Prednisolone sodium succinate (p.1078·2).
Corticosteroid.

Solu-Dacortine
Merck-Belgolabo, Belg.; Merck, Switz.
Prednisolone sodium succinate (p.1078·2).
Corticosteroid.

Soludactone Monsanto, Fr.
Potassium canrenoate (p.957·1).
Ascites; hyperaldosteronism; hypokalaemia; oedema.

Soludecadron Merck Sharp & Dohme-Chibret, Fr.†.
Dexamethasone sodium phosphate (p.1067·1).
Corticosteroid.

Solu-Decortin-H Merck, Ger.
Prednisolone sodium succinate (p.1078·2).
Parenteral corticosteroid.

Soluderme Schering-Plough, Port.
Betamethasone dipropionate (p.1063·2).
Skin disorders.

Soludial Soludia, Fr.
Sodium bicarbonate (p.1186·2).
Haemodialysis.

Soludor Lehning, Fr.
Homoeopathic preparation.

Solufen
Note. This name is used for preparations of different composition.
Galephar, Fr.; Brovar, S.Afr.†; Whitehall-Robins, Switz.
Ibuprofen (p.43·2).
Fever; pain.

Rigers, Mex.
Chloramphenicol (p.179·1).
Bacterial infections.

Solufena UCB, Spain.
Ibuprofen (p.43·2).
Fever; pain.

Solufilina BOI, Spain.
Etamiphylline hydrochloride (p.765·1).
Angina pectoris; heart failure; myocardial infarction; obstructive airways disease.

Solufilina Sedante BOI, Spain†.
Etamiphylline hydrochloride (p.765·1); phenobarbital (p.355·1).
Obstructive airways disease; precordial pain.

Solufilina Simple BOI, Spain.
Etamiphylline hydrochloride (p.765·1).
Angina pectoris; heart failure; myocardial infarction; obstructive airways disease.

Solu-Flur Germiphene, Canad.†.
Sodium fluoride (p.1375·3).
Dental caries prophylaxis.

Solufos Busto, Spain.
Fosfomycin calcium (p.208·2) or fosfomycin sodium (p.208·2).
Lignocaine [lidocaine] (p.1313·3) is included in the intramuscular injection to alleviate the pain of injection.
Bacterial infections.

Solugastril
Sanova, Aust.; Heumann, Ger.
Aluminium hydroxide (p.1210·3); calcium carbonate (p.1215·1).
Gastrointestinal disorders.

Solugel
Note. This name is used for preparations of different composition.
Johnson & Johnson, Austral.
Hydrogel dressing.
Burns; wounds.

Stiefel, Canad.; Stiefel, Mex.
Benzoyl peroxide (p.1111·1).
Acne.

Solulexin Duopharma, Hong Kong.
Cefalexin (p.161·3).
Bacterial infections.

Solumag
Note. This name is used for preparations of different composition.
Kolassa, Aust.; Boehringer Ingelheim, Fr.; Geymonat, Ital.
Magnesium pidolate (p.1191·1).
Anxiety related hyperventilation; dysmenorrhoea; eclampsia; magnesium deficiency; premature labour.

Hexal, S.Afr.
Magnesium oxide (p.1233·2).
Magnesium deficiency.

Solu-Medrol
Pharmacia Upjohn, Aust.; Pharmacia Upjohn, Austral.; Pharmacia Upjohn, Belg.; Pharmacia Upjohn, Braz.; Pharmacia Upjohn, Canad.; Pharmacia Upjohn, Denm.; Pharmacia Upjohn, Fin.; Pharmacia Upjohn, Hong Kong; Pharmacia Upjohn, Israel; Pharmacia Upjohn, Ital.; Pharmacia Upjohn, Mex.; Pharmacia Upjohn, Neth.; Pharmacia Upjohn, Norw.; Pharmacia Upjohn, NZ; Pharmacia Upjohn, Port.; Pharmacia Upjohn, S.Afr.; Pharmacia Upjohn, Singapore; Pharmacia Upjohn, Swed.; Pharmacia Upjohn, Switz.; Pharmacia Upjohn, Thai.; Pharmacia Upjohn, USA.
Methylprednisolone sodium succinate (p.1076·1).
Corticosteroid.

Pharmacia Upjohn, Fr.
Methylprednisolone hydrogen succinate (p.1076·1).
Corticosteroid.

Solu-Medrone
Pharmacia Upjohn, Irl.; Pharmacia, UK.
Methylprednisolone sodium succinate (p.1076·1).
Corticosteroid.

Solumidazol Diba, Mex.
Metronidazole (p.594·1).
Amoebiasis; trichomoniasis.

Solu-Moderin *Pharmacia Upjohn, Spain.*
Methylprednisolone sodium succinate (p.1076·1).
Corticosteroid.

Solumol *C & M, USA.*
Vehicle for topical preparations.

Solupen *Bial-Aristegui, Spain.*
Doxycycline hyclate (p.200·1).
Bacterial infections; malaria.

Solupen Enzimatico *Bial-Aristegui, Spain.*
Doxycycline hyclate (p.200·1); chymotrypsin (p.1595·1); trypsin (p.1675·3).
Bacterial infections.

Solupen-D *Winzer, Ger.*
Oxedrine tartrate (p.950·3); naphazoline hydrochloride (p.1095·1); dexamethasone sodium phosphate (p.1067·1).
Rhinitis; sinusitis.

Solupred *Aventis, Fr.*
Prednisolone metasulfobenzoate sodium (p.1078·1).
Corticosteroid.

Soluprick SQ *ALK, Denm.; ALK, Fin.; ALK, Swed.*
Allergen extracts (p.1575·3).
Diagnosis of hypersensitivity.

Solupsa *Upsamedica, Belg.*
Carbasalate calcium (p.23·3).
Cardiovascular disorders.

Solupsan *UPSA, Fr.*
Carbasalate calcium (p.23·3).
Fever; pain; rheumatic disorders.

Solurex *Hyrex, USA.*
Dexamethasone acetate (p.1067·1) or dexamethasone sodium phosphate (p.1067·1).
Corticosteroid.

Solurin *JP, Braz.*
Electrolytes (p.1184·1).
Haemodialysis solution.

Solurrinol *Teofarma, Spain.*
Potassium chlorate (p.1654·1); sodium bicarbonate (p.1186·2); sodium chloride (p.1196·3).
Upper-respiratory-tract disorders.

Solurutine Papaverine F. Retard *Synthelabo, Fr.†.*
Ethoxazorutoside (p.1611·2); ascorbic acid (p.1389·3); papaverine hydrochloride (p.1648·1).
Cerebral and peripheral vascular disorders.

Solus *Lifeplan, UK.*
Multivitamin, mineral, and nutritional preparation (p.1350·1).

Solusprin *Knoll, Spain.*
Lysine aspirin (p.50·3).
Fever; musculoskeletal, joint and peri-articular disorders; pain; thromboembolism prophylaxis.

Solusteril *Urgo, Fr.†.*
Sodium dichloroisocyanurate (p.1156·1).
Infant feeding equipment disinfection.

Soluston *Rafa, Israel.*
Chenodeoxycholic acid (p.1594·1).
Cholesterol gallstones.

Solustrep *Caps, S.Afr.*
Streptomycin sulfate (p.249·1).
Tuberculosis.

Solutina *Alcon, Mex.*
Pheniramine maleate (p.422·3); naphazoline hydrochloride (p.1095·1).
Conjunctivitis.

Solutio Cordes *Ichthyol, Aust.; Ichthyol, Ger.*
Ictasol (p.1115·3).
Scalp disorders.

Solutio Cordes Dexa N *Ichthyol, Ger.*
Dexamethasone (p.1067·1).
Scalp disorders.

Solution ChKM du Prof Dr Walkhoff *Haupt, Switz.†.*
Parachlorophenol (p.1152·1); camphor (p.1589·3); menthol (p.1632·3).
Dental inflammation.

Solution Stago Diluee *Pharmadeveloppement, Fr.*
Boldo (p.1585·3); chamomile (p.1593·2); kinkeliba (p.1626·1); golden rod.
Digestive disorders.

Solutrast *Byk Gulden, Ger.*
Iopamidol (p.1035·2).
Radiographic contrast medium.

Solutricine *Schieffer, Switz.†.*
Tyrothricin (p.267·1); ascorbic acid (p.1389·3).
Mouth and throat disorders.

Solutricine Maux de Gorge *Theraplix, Fr.*
Amethocaine [tetracaine] hydrochloride (p.1305·2); hexamidine isetionate (p.1146·2).
Mouth and throat disorders.

Solutricine Tetracaine *Theraplix, Fr.*
Tyrothricin (p.267·1); amethocaine [tetracaine] hydrochloride (p.1305·2).
Mouth and throat disorders.

Solutricine Vitamine C *Theraplix, Fr.*
Tyrothricin (p.267·1); ascorbic acid (p.1389·3).
Mouth and throat infections.

Soluver *Dermtek, Canad.*
Salicylic acid (p.1122·3).
Verrucas.

Soluver Plus *Dermtek, Canad.*
Salicylic acid (p.1122·3).
Warts.

Soluvit *Pharmacia Upjohn, Belg.†; Fresenius Kabi, Denm.; Fresenius Kabi, Fin.; Fresenius Kabi, Fr.; Fresenius Kabi, Ital.; Fresenius Kabi, Norw.; Fresenius Kabi, S.Afr; Fresenius Kabi, Spain; Fresenius Kabi, Swed.; Fresenius Kabi, Switz.*
Multivitamin preparation (p.1350·1).
Parenteral nutrition.

Soluvit N *Hamilton, Austral.†; Pharmacia Upjohn, Ger.; Pharmacia Upjohn, Hong Kong; Pharmacia Upjohn, Israel; Pharmacia Upjohn, Neth.; Baxter, NZ; Nutricia, NZ; Fresenius Kabi, Port.; Fresenius Kabi, Singapore; Pharmacia Upjohn, Thai.*
Multivitamin preparation (p.1350·1).
Parenteral nutrition.

Soluvit Neu *Fresenius Kabi, Aust.*
Multivitamin preparation (p.1350·1).
Parenteral nutrition.

Soluvite *Pharmics, USA.*
Multivitamin preparation with fluoride (p.1375·3)(p.1350·1).
Dental caries prophylaxis; dietary supplement.

Solu-Volon A *Bristol-Myers Squibb, Aust.*
Triamcinolone acetonide dipotassium phosphate (p.1080·2).
Corticosteroid.

Soluzione Composta Alcoolica Saponosa di Coaltar *Bruni, Ital.†.*
Coal tar (p.1125·1); quillaia (p.1348·2); methyl salicylate (p.55·1); alcohol (p.1130·3).
Eczema.

Soluzione Darrow *Diaco, Ital.*
Electrolytes (p.1185·2).
Infantile diarrhoea.

Soluzione Schoum *Rhone-Poulenc Rorer, Ital.*
Fumitory (p.1612·3); ononis (p.1644·1); piscidia (p.1625·1).
Painful spasm of the urinary and biliary tracts.

Solvazinc *Cortecs, UK.*
Zinc sulfate (p.1398·2).
Zinc deficiency.

Solvex *Teva, Israel.*
Bromhexine hydrochloride (p.1085·3).
Respiratory-tract congestion.

Solvezink *Astra, Aust.; AstraZeneca, Denm.; AstraZeneca, Fin.; Stern, Ger.; AstraZeneca, Norw.; Tika, Swed.*
Zinc sulfate (p.1398·2).
Acne; acrodermatitis enteropathica; leg ulcer; zinc deficiency.

Solviflu *Boots Healthcare, Ital.*
Ibuprofen (p.43·2); pseudoephedrine hydrochloride (p.1099·2).
Cold and influenza symptoms.

Solving *Finmedical, Ital.*
Nimesulide (p.62·3).
Fever; inflammation; pain.

Solvipect *Nycomed, Norw.*
Guaifenesin (p.1092·2); liquorice (p.1231·2).
Coughs.

Solvipect comp *Nycomed, Norw.*
Guaifenesin (p.1092·2); liquorice (p.1231·2); ethylmorphine hydrochloride (p.35·2).
Coughs.

Solvisol *Solfran, Mex.*
Multivitamin preparation (p.1350·1).

Solvium *Chefaro, Spain.*
Ibuprofen (p.43·2).
Musculoskeletal, joint, and peri-articular disorders.

Solvobil
Note. This name is used for preparations of different composition.
Abbott, Braz.
Cynara (p.1601·3); boldo (p.1585·3); cascara (p.1216·1); belladonna (p.463·1); peppermint leaf (p.1243·2).
Liver disorders.

Recordati, Ital.
Sodium cholate; nicotinamide (p.1372·3); boldo (p.1585·3); cascara (p.1216·1).
Constipation.

Solvolin *Genera, Switz.†.*
Bromhexine hydrochloride (p.1085·3).
Respiratory-tract disorders with viscous mucus.

Solvomed *Kwizda, Aust.*
Acetylcysteine (p.1082·3).
Bronchitis.

Solvopret *Bionorica, Thai.*
Thyme (p.1672·2); hedera helix.
Bronchitis.

Solvopret TP *Bionorica, Thai.*
Thyme (p.1672·2); cowslip rhizome (p.1600·1).
Bronchitis.

Solyptol *Faulding, Austral.*
Cream: Benzalkonium chloride (p.1133·2); allantoin (p.1110·1).
Abrasions; burns; cuts; insect bites.
Soap: Triclosan (Irgasan) (p.1159·2).
Abrasions; cuts; insect bites.
Topical liquid: Pine oil; chloroxylenol (p.1142·1).
Abrasions; cuts; insect bites.

Som *Satori, Port.*
A range of nutritional supplements (p.1350·1).

Soma
Note. This name is used for preparations of different composition.
Novaquimica, Braz.
Ampicillin benzathine (p.151·3); ampicillin sodium (p.150·3).
Bacterial infections.

Carter Horner, Canad.; Wallace, USA.
Carisoprodol (p.1327·1).
Musculoskeletal disorders.

Soma Balsamico *Novaquimica, Braz.*
Ampicillin benzathine (p.151·3); ampicillin sodium (p.150·3); guaifenesin (p.1092·2); eucalyptol (p.1609·2); niaouli oil (p.1640·2).
Lignocaine [lidocaine] (p.1313·2) is included in this preparation to alleviate the pain of injection.
Bacterial infections.

Soma Complex *Teofarma, Ital.*
Carisoprodol (p.1327·1); dipyrone (p.34·1).
Musculoskeletal and joint pain and spasm.

Soma Compound *Wallace, USA.*
Carisoprodol (p.1327·1); aspirin (p.14·2).
Musculoskeletal disorders.

Soma Compound with Codeine *Wallace, USA.*
Carisoprodol (p.1327·1); aspirin (p.14·2); codeine phosphate (p.25·2).
Musculoskeletal disorders.

Somac *Pharmacia Upjohn, Austral.; Pharmacia Upjohn, Fin.; Byk Gulden, Norw.; Pharmacia Upjohn, NZ.*
Pantoprazole sodium (p.1243·2).
Gastro-oesophageal reflux; peptic ulcer; Zollinger-Ellison syndrome.

Somadril *Dumex-Alpharma, Denm.; Alpharma, Norw.; Dumex-Alpharma, Swed.*
Carisoprodol (p.1327·1).
Pain; skeletal muscle spasm.

Somadril Comp *Dumex-Alpharma, Fin.; Dumex-Alpharma, Swed.*
Carisoprodol (p.1327·1); paracetamol (p.71·2); caffeine (p.761·3).
Musculoskeletal and joint disorders; pain.

Somaflex *Novaquimica, Braz.*
Carisoprodol (p.1327·1); dipyrone (p.34·1).
Skeletal muscle spasm.

Somagerol *Wyeth, Ger.*
Lorazepam (p.688·3).
Anxiety disorders; premedication; sleep disorders.

Somalgesic *Carter-Wallace, Mex.*
Naproxen (p.60·3); carisoprodol (p.1327·1).
Musculoskeletal, joint, and peri-articular disorders.

Somalgin *Novaquimica, Braz.*
Aspirin (p.14·2).
Aluminium glycinate (p.1210·3) and magnesium carbonate (p.1232·3) are included in this preparation in an attempt to limit adverse effects on the gastrointestinal mucosa.
Fever; inflammation; pain.

Somalgit *Inibsa, Spain†.*
Carisoprodol (p.1327·1).
Skeletal muscle spasm.

Somalium *Ache, Braz.*
Bromazepam (p.656·3).
Anxiety; insomnia.

Somanol *Braun, Swed.†.*
Sorbitol (p.1377·3); mannitol (p.924·3).
Urological irrigation.

Somanol + Ethanol *Braun, Fin.*
Sorbitol (p.1377·3); mannitol (p.924·3); alcohol (p.1130·3).
Urological irrigation.

Somapam *Pacific, NZ.*
Temazepam (p.707·2).
Insomnia; premedication.

Somaplus *Cazi, Braz.*
Diazepam (p.674·3).
Alcohol withdrawal syndrome; anxiety; epilepsy; insomnia; premedication; sedative; skeletal muscle spasm.

Somarexin *Lalco, Canad.*
Vitamin B substances and iron (p.1350·1).

Somarexin & C *Lalco, Canad.*
Vitamin B substances, vitamin C, calcium, and iron (p.1350·1).

Somasedin *Heralds, Braz.*
Papaverine hydrochloride (p.1648·1); homatropine methylbromide (p.468·1); adiphenine hydrochloride.
Smooth muscle spasm.

Somatarax *Vedim, Spain.*
Brallobarbital calcium (p.656·3); hydroxyzine dihydrochloride (p.419·1); secobarbital sodium (p.705·2).
Insomnia.

Somatin *Torrex, Aust.*
Somatostatin acetate (p.1297·3).
Gastrointestinal haemorrhage; prevention of complications following pancreatic surgery.

Somatobiss *Bissendorf, Neth.†.*
Somatorelin acetate (p.1297·2).
Test for growth hormone deficiency.

Somatofalk *Falk, Neth.*
Somatostatin acetate (p.1297·3).
Gastrointestinal haemorrhage.

Somatolan *Lannacher, Aust.*
Somatostatin acetate (p.1297·3).
Gastrointestinal haemorrhage; prevention of complications following pancreatic surgery.

Somatoline *Manetti Roberts, Ital.*
Thyroxine [levothyroxine] (p.1528·1); aescin (p.1574·1).
Adipose states with cellulite.

Somatosan *Curamed, Thai.*
Somatostatin acetate (p.1297·3).
Gastrointestinal haemorrhage; pancreatic and duodenal fistulae; prevention of complications following pancreatic surgery.

Somatrel *Ferring, Denm.*
Somatorelin acetate (p.1297·2).
Test for growth hormone deficiency.

Somatron *Volchem, Ital.*
L-Arginine (p.1353·3); L-ornithine (p.1374·1).
Nutritional supplement.

Somatulina *Ipsen, Port.; Ipsen, Spain.*
Lanreotide acetate (p.1289·2).
Acromegaly; neuroendocrine tumours.

Somatuline *Ipsen, Aust.; Ipsen, Belg.; Ipsen, Fin.; Ipsen Biotech, Fr.; Beaufour-Ipsen, Hong Kong; Ipsen, Irl.; Ipsen, UK.*
Lanreotide acetate (p.1289·2).
Acromegaly; neuroendocrine tumours.

Somatyl *Teofarma, Ital.*
Betaine sodium aspartate (p.1584·3).
Digestive disorders.

Somazina *Novag, Mex.; CPH, Port.; Ferrer, Spain.*
Citicoline (p.1596·1).
Asthenia; cerebrovascular disorders.

Somelin *Sankyo, Jpn†.*
Haloxazolam (p.688·1).
Insomnia.

Somese *Pharmacia Upjohn, Singapore.*
Triazolam (p.709·3).
Insomnia.

Somiaton *Serono, Spain.*
Somatostatin acetate (p.1297·3).
Pancreatic fistulae; variceal haemorrhage.

Sominex
Note. This name is used for preparations of different composition.
EMS, Braz.
Passion flower (p.1649·1); crataegus (p.1600·2); valerian (p.1678·3).
Sedative.

SmithKline Beecham Consumer, Canad.; SmithKline Beecham Consumer, USA.
Diphenhydramine hydrochloride (p.416·1).
Insomnia.

SSL, UK.
Promethazine hydrochloride (p.423·2).
Insomnia.

Sominex Pain Relief *SmithKline Beecham Consumer, USA.*
Diphenhydramine hydrochloride (p.416·1); paracetamol (p.71·2).
Insomnia.

Somnil *Aspen Consumer, S.Afr.*
Doxylamine succinate (p.417·1).
Insomnia.

Somnipar *Rolab, S.Afr.*
Nitrazepam (p.695·2).
Now known as Rolab-Nitrazepam.
Insomnia.

Somnite *Norgine, Irl.; Norgine, UK.*
Nitrazepam (p.695·2).
Insomnia.

Somnium *Fresenius Kabi, Aust.; Medichemie, Switz.*
Lorazepam (p.688·3); diphenhydramine hydrochloride (p.416·1).
Sleep disorders.

Somnol *Carter Horner, Canad.*
Flurazepam monohydrochloride (p.685·3).
Insomnia.

Somnosan *Hormosan, Ger.*
Zopiclone (p.713·1).
Sleep disorders.

Somnovit *Hoechst Marion Roussel, Spain.*
Loprazolam (p.688·3).
Insomnia.

Somnubene *Ratiopharm, Aust.*
Flunitrazepam (p.683·2).
Sleep disorders.

Somnuvis S *Bilgast, Ger.*
Valerian (p.1678·3); lupulus (p.1629·3); passion flower (p.1649·1); kava (p.1625·3).
Nervous disorders; sleep disorders.

Somonal *Juste, Spain.*
Somatostatin acetate (p.1297·3).
Bleeding oesophageal varices; pancreatic fistulas.

Somsanit *Kohler, Ger.*
Sodium oxybate (p.1268·2).
General anaesthesia.

Sonacide *Wyeth-Ayerst, Canad.†.*
Glutaral (p.1145·2).
Instrument disinfection.

Sonata *Wyeth Lederle, Belg.; Wyeth Lederle, Denm.; Wyeth Lederle, Fin.; Wyeth, Ger.; Wyeth, Irl.; Wyeth Lederle, Ital.; Wyeth Lederle, Swed.; Wyeth, Switz.; Wyeth, UK; Wyeth-Ayerst, USA.*
Zaleplon (p.711·2).
Insomnia.

Sondalis *Nestle, Fr.; Clintec, Ital.; Nestle, UK.*
A range of preparations for enteral nutrition (p.1350·1).

Sone Fawns & McAllan, Austral.
Prednisone (p.1079·2).
Corticosteroid.

Sonebon Novaquimica, Braz.
Nitrazepam (p.695·2).
Epilepsy; insomnia.

Soneriper Pharmasant, Thai.
Tolperisone hydrochloride (p.1330·3).
Skeletal muscle spasm.

Soneryl Rhone-Poulenc Rorer, Austral.†; Hansam, UK.
Butobarbital (p.659·1).
Insomnia.

Songar Valeas, Ital.
Triazolam (p.709·3).
Insomnia.

Songha Boehringer Ingelheim, Port.
Valerian (p.1678·3); melissa (p.1632·2).
Insomnia.

Songha Day Pharmaton, Switz.
Kava (p.1625·3).
Anxiety.

Songha Night Pharmaton, Switz.
Valerian (p.1678·3); melissa (p.1632·2).
Sedative.

Sonicur Solvay, Spain.
Anethole trithione (p.1580·1).
Dry mouth.

Sonifilan Kaken, Jpn.
Sizofiran (p.568·3).
Radiotherapy enhancement for uterine cervical cancer.

Sonin
Note.This name is used for preparations of different composition.
Asta Medica, Braz.
Pimethixene (p.423·1).
Respiratory-tract disorders in children.

Merck, Ger.
Loprazolam (p.688·3).
Sleep disorders.

Soni-Slo Helsinn Birex, Irl.; Lipha, Irl.; Lipha, UK†.
Isosorbide dinitrate (p.915·2).
Angina pectoris.

Sonnenbraun Twardy, Ger.
Betacarotene (p.1355·1); biotin (p.1355·3); calcium pantothenate (p.1374·1).
Sunburn.

Sonodor Vitafarma, Spain.
Diphenhydramine hydrochloride (p.416·1).
Formerly contained diphenhydramine hydrochloride and pyrithyldione.
Insomnia.

Sonofit Arkochim, Spain.
Crataegus (p.1600·2); eschscholtzia californica; passion flower (p.1649·1).
Insomnia; nervous disorders.

SonoRx Bracco, USA.
Simeticone coated cellulose (p.1249·2).
Adjunct in ultrasound imaging.

Sonotrat Medley, Braz.
Nitrazepam (p.695·2).
Epilepsy; insomnia.

Sonotryl Singer, Switz.†.
Propyphenazone (p.80·2); paracetamol (p.71·2); caffeine (p.761·3); drofenine hydrochloride (p.466·3).
Painful smooth muscle spasm.

Sonrisal SmithKline Beecham, Braz.
Aspirin (p.14·2); sodium carbonate anhydrous (p.1665·1); sodium bicarbonate (p.1186·2); citric acid (p.1596·2).
Dyspepsia; pain.

Sons Piral Sons, Mex.
Paracetamol (p.71·2).
Fever; pain.

Sonsuur Rolab, S.Afr.
Cimetidine (p.1216·3).
Now known as Rolab-Cimetidine.
Gastrointestinal disorders.

Sontedril Willmar, Mex.
Diphenhydramine (p.416·1).

Soolan Julphar, UAE.
Chlorpheniramine [chlorphenamine] maleate (p.412·1); phenylephrine hydrochloride (p.1097·1); guaifenesin (p.1092·2).
Coughs.

Soor-Gel Engelhard, Ger.†.
Dequalinium salicylate (p.1143·1).
Fungal and bacterial mouth and throat infections.

Soorphenesin Kade, Ger.
Chlorphenesin (p.381·3).
Fungal and bacterial infections of the vagina.

Sootha Nelson, UK.
Homoeopathic preparation.

Soothaderm Pharmakon, USA.
Mepyramine maleate (p.421·1); benzocaine (p.1306·2); zinc oxide (p.1128·2).
Pruritus.

Soothake Toothache Gel Pickles, UK.
Clove oil (p.1597·1).
Formerly contained benzocaine and clove oil.
Toothache.

Soothe Alcon, USA†.
Tetryzoline hydrochloride (p.1101·2).
Minor eye irritation.

Soothe Aid Zee, Canad.
Hexylresorcinol (p.1146·3).

Soothelip Bayer, UK.
Aciclovir (p.612·3).
Herpes labialis.

Soothe'n Heal Mentholatum, Austral.
Hydrous wool fat (p.1411·2); chlorocresol (p.1141·3); benzyl alcohol (p.1135·2).
Formerly contained trolamine oleate, hydrous wool fat, and glycerol.
Dry skin.

Soothex Jamieson, Canad.
Allantoin (p.1110·1).

Soov Bite
Note.This name is used for preparations of different composition.
Ego, Austral.; Ego, Singapore.
Lignocaine [lidocaine] hydrochloride (p.1313·2); cetrimide (p.1137·1); menthol (p.1632·3).
Insect bites and stings.

Ego, Hong Kong.
Lignocaine [lidocaine] hydrochloride (p.1313·2); cetrimide (p.1137·1); phenoxyisopropanol (p.1153·3).
Insect bites; pruritus; stings.

Soov Burn Ego, Austral.
Lignocaine [lidocaine] hydrochloride (p.1313·2); cetrimide (p.1137·1).
Minor burns; minor cuts; sunburn.

Soov Cream Ego, Austral.; Ego, Singapore.
Lignocaine [lidocaine] hydrochloride (p.1313·2); cetrimide (p.1137·1); chlorhexidine gluconate (p.1138·2).
Haemorrhoids; minor cuts, abrasions, and burns; sunburn.

Soov Prickly Heat Ego, Austral.; Ego, Hong Kong; Ego, Singapore.
Salicylic acid (p.1122·3); zinc oxide (p.1128·2); liquid paraffin (p.1407·1) or light liquid paraffin (p.1407·2).
Heat rash.

Sopalamin 3B Melisana, Belg.
Vitamin B substances (p.1350·1).
Alcoholism; neurogenic pain; vitamin B deficiency.

Sopalamine 3B Technilab, Canad.
Vitamin B substances (p.1350·1).
Vitamin B deficiency.

Sopalamine 3B Plus Charton, Canad.†.
Multivitamin preparation (p.1350·1).

Sopalamine 3B Plus C Technilab, Canad.
Multivitamin preparation (p.1350·1).

Sopax Zimaia, Port.
Nordazepam (p.696·1).
Anxiety.

Sophidone UPSA, Fr.
Hydromorphone hydrochloride (p.42·3).
Pain.

Sophipren Sophia, Mex.
Prednisolone acetate (p.1078·1).
Eye disorders.

Sophixen Sophia, Mex.
Ciprofloxacin hydrochloride (p.182·3).
Bacterial eye infections.

Sophtal Alcon, Fr.
Eye drops: Salicylic acid (p.1122·3); chlorhexidine gluconate (p.1138·2).

Eye lotion: Salicylic acid (p.1122·3); borax (p.1586·1); rose water.
Eye disorders.

Sophtal-POS N Ursapharm, Ger.
Salicylic acid (p.1122·3).
Eye irritation; inflammatory eye disorders.

Soporin Herbamed, Switz.
Valerian (p.1678·3); passion flower (p.1649·1); lupulus (p.1629·3); melissa (p.1632·2).
Sleep disorders.

Soprol Wyeth Lederle, Fr.; Helsinn Birex, Irl.
Bisoprolol fumarate (p.850·1).
Angina pectoris; hypertension.

Soproxen Berlin Pharm, Singapore; Berlin Pharm, Thai.
Naproxen sodium (p.61·1).
Gout; musculoskeletal, joint, and soft-tissue inflammation; pain.

Sopulmin Scharper, Ital.
Sobrerol (p.1100·3).
Respiratory-tract disorders.

Soraderm Stafford-Miller, Norw.
Coal tar (p.1125·1).
Psoriasis; seborrhoeic dermatitis.

Soramin Darrow, Braz.
Amino-acid infusion (p.1350·1).
Parenteral nutrition.

Sorbalgon Hartmann, Fr.
Calcium alginate (p.728·1).
Ulcers; wounds.

Sorbangil
Pharmacia Upjohn, Norw.; Pharmacia Upjohn, Swed.
Isosorbide dinitrate (p.915·2).
Angina pectoris; heart failure.

Sorbecal QIF, Braz.
Calcium phosphate; calcium pantothenate; ergocalciferol; vitamin B_{12} (p.1350·1).
Nutritional supplement.

Sorbenor Casen Fleet, Spain.
Arginine aspartate (p.1354·1).
Tonic.

Sorbichew AstraZeneca, UK†.
Isosorbide dinitrate (p.915·2).
Angina pectoris.

Sorbiclis SIT, Ital.
Sorbitol (p.1377·3); docusate sodium (p.1223·1).
Constipation.

Sorbid AstraZeneca, UK†.
Isosorbide dinitrate (p.915·2).
Angina pectoris.

Sorbidilat
Astra, Austral.; Astra, Switz.
Isosorbide dinitrate (p.915·2).
Angina pectoris; heart failure; hypertension; myocardial infarction.

Sorbidin
Alphapharm, Austral.; Merck, Thai.
Isosorbide dinitrate (p.915·2).
Angina pectoris; heart failure; ischaemic heart disease.

Sorbidon Hydrate Gordon, USA.
Emollient.
Dry skin; hyperkeratosis.

Sorbifer Astra, Hong Kong.
Ferrous sulfate (p.1360·3).
Iron deficiency; iron-deficiency anaemia.

Sorbilax Pharmacia Upjohn, Austral.
Sorbitol (p.1377·3).
Constipation.

Sorbimon Ratiopharm, Aust.
Isosorbide mononitrate (p.916·2).
Angina pectoris; heart failure; myocardial infarction; pulmonary hypertension.

Sorbisal
Allergan, Austral.†; Allergan, NZ.
Irrigation and rinsing solution for contact lenses (p.1129·2).

Sorbisterit
Fresenius, Aust.; Fresenius Medical, Ger.; Fresenius Medical, Switz.
Calcium polystyrene sulfonate (p.1002·3).
Hyperkalaemia.

Sorbitrate
Zeneca, Belg.†; AstraZeneca, Thai.; AstraZeneca, UK†; Zeneca, USA.
Isosorbide dinitrate (p.915·2).
Angina pectoris; heart failure.

Sorbitur Baxter, Swed.†.
Sorbitol (p.1377·3).
Bladder irrigation.

Sorbon Unipharm, Israel.
Buspirone hydrochloride (p.657·2).
Anxiety disorders.

Sorbsan
Seton Scholl, Austral.; Braun, Fr.; Braun, Ital.; Steriseal, UK.
Calcium alginate (p.728·1).
Burns; skin ulceration; wounds.

Sorcal Wyeth, Braz.
Calcium polystyrene sulfonate (p.1002·3).
Hypercalcaemia.

Sorciclina Inexfa, Spain.
Doxycycline hyclate (p.200·1); prolase.
Bacterial infections.

Sordinol Lundbeck, Ital.†.
Clopenthixol hydrochloride (p.714·2).
Anxiety; mental function disorders; psychoses.

Sore Mouth Gel Boots, Thai.
Lignocaine [lidocaine] (p.1313·2); cetylpyridinium chloride (p.1138·1); menthol (p.1632·3); eucalyptol (p.1600·2).
Oral pain.

Sore Throat Chewing Gum Or-Dov, Austral.
Dichlorobenzyl alcohol (p.1143·2); amylmetacresol (p.1133·2); vitamin C (p.1389·3).
Sore throat.

Sore Throat L39 Homeocan, Canad.
Homoeopathic preparation.

Sore Throat Lozenges Sutton, Canad.
Benzocaine (p.1306·2); menthol (p.1632·3).

Sore Throat Relief Brauer, Austral.
Homoeopathic preparation.

Sorebral Condrugs, Thai.
Cinnarizine (p.413·1).
Cerebrovascular disorders; migraine; peripheral vascular disorders; vestibular disorders.

Soren Daewon, Hong Kong.
Naproxen sodium (p.61·1).
Gout; musculoskeletal, joint, and peri-articular disorders; pain.

Sorgoa Scheurich, Ger.†.
Tolnaftate (p.395·2).
Fungal skin infections.

Sorgoran Sanova, Aust.
Tolnaftate (p.395·2).
Fungal skin and nail infections.

Soriatane
Roche, Canad.; Roche, Fr.; Roche, USA.
Acitretin (p.1109·1).
Keratinisation disorders; psoriasis.

Soriflor Nycomed, Swed.†.
Diflorasone diacetate (p.1069·2).
Skin disorders.

Sorine Adulto Ache, Braz.
Benzalkonium chloride (p.1133·2); sodium chloride (p.1196·1); naphazoline (p.1095·1).
Nasal congestion.

Sorine Infantil Ache, Braz.
Benzalkonium chloride (p.1133·2); sodium chloride (p.1196·1).
Nasal congestion.

Sormodren
Ebewe, Aust.; Knoll, Ger.; Ravizza, Ital.; Knoll, Mex.
Bornaprine hydrochloride (p.464·3).
Drug-induced extrapyramidal disorders; hyperhidrosis; parkinsonism.

Sormon Gerard, Irl.
Isosorbide mononitrate (p.916·2).
Angina pectoris.

Sornil Utopian, Thai.
Isosorbide dinitrate (p.915·2).
Angina pectoris.

Soro de Manutencao H Labesfal, Port.
Electrolyte infusion with glucose (p.1180·1).
Carbohydrate source; fluid and electrolyte disorders.

Soronal Cimed, Braz.
Sodium chloride (p.1196·1); benzalkonium chloride (p.1133·2).
Nasal congestion.

Soropon Purdue Frederick, Canad.
Tyrothricin (p.267·1); trolamine polypeptide cocoate condensate (p.1675·2).
Scalp disorders.

Sorot
Petrasch, Aust.; Ravensberg, Ger.
Dequalinium chloride (p.1143·1).
Mouth and throat infections.

Sorquetan Basotherm, Ger.†.
Tinidazole (p.603·3).
Bacterial or protozoal infections.

Sortis
Parke, Davis, Aust.; Parke, Davis, Ger.; Godecke, Ger.; Pfizer, Ger.; Mack, Illert., Ger.; Warner-Lambert, Switz.
Atorvastatin calcium (p.842·3).
Hyperlipidaemias.

Sosegon
Yamanouchi, Jpn; Sanofi Synthelabo, Port.; Sanofi Synthelabo, Spain; Sanofi Synthelabo, Thai.
Pentazocine (p.74·2), pentazocine hydrochloride (p.74·2), or pentazocine lactate (p.74·2).
Pain.

Sosenol Adcock Ingram, S.Afr.
Pentazocine (p.74·2).
Pain.

Sostenon Organon, Mex.
Testosterone propionate (p.1492·2); testosterone phenylpropionate (p.1492·2); testosterone isocaproate (p.1492·2); testosterone decanoate (p.1492·2).
Androgen deficiency.

Sostilar Pharmacia Upjohn, Belg.
Cabergoline (p.1167·3).
Hyperprolactinaemia.

Sostril Cascan, Ger.; Glaxo Wellcome, Ger.
Ranitidine hydrochloride (p.1245·2).
Acid aspiration; gastro-oesophageal reflux; gastrointestinal haemorrhage; gastrointestinal hyperacidity; peptic ulcer; Zollinger-Ellison syndrome.

Sota ABZ, Ger.
Sotalol hydrochloride (p.972·2).
Arrhythmias.

Sota Lich Lichtenstein, Ger.
Sotalol hydrochloride (p.972·2).
Arrhythmias.

Sotab Douglas, Austral.
Sotalol hydrochloride (p.972·2).
Ventricular arrhythmias.

Sotabet Gea, Denm.
Sotalol hydrochloride (p.972·2).
Arrhythmias.

Sotabeta Betapharm, Ger.
Sotalol hydrochloride (p.972·2).
Arrhythmias.

Sotacor
Bristol-Myers Squibb, Aust.; Bristol-Myers Squibb, Austral.; Bristol-Myers Squibb, Braz.; Bristol, Canad.; Bristol-Myers Squibb, Denm.; Bristol-Myers Squibb, Fin.; Bristol-Myers Squibb, Hong Kong; Bristol-Myers Squibb, Irl.; Bristol-Myers Squibb, Israel; Bristol-Myers Squibb, Jpn; Bristol-Myers Squibb, Neth.; Bristol-Myers Squibb, Norw.; Bristol-Myers Squibb, NZ; Bristol-Myers Squibb, S.Afr.; Bristol-Myers Squibb, Singapore; Bristol-Myers Squibb, Swed.; Bristol-Myers Squibb, Thai.; Bristol-Myers Squibb, UK.
Sotalol hydrochloride (p.972·2).
Angina pectoris; arrhythmias; hypertension; hyperthyroidism; myocardial infarction.

Sotacor/ASA Bristol-Myers Squibb, Swed.†.
Tablet I, sotalol hydrochloride (p.972·2); tablet II , aspirin (p.14·2).
Angina pectoris.

Sotagamma Worwag, Ger.
Sotalol hydrochloride (p.972·2).
Arrhythmias.

Sota-Gry Teva, Ger.
Sotalol hydrochloride (p.972·2).
Arrhythmias.

Sotahexal
Hexal, Austral.; Hexal, Ger.; Hexal, S.Afr.
Sotalol hydrochloride (p.972·2).
Angina pectoris; arrhythmias; hypertension; hyperthyroidism; myocardial infarction.

Sotalex *Bristol-Myers Squibb, Belg.; Bristol-Myers Squibb, Fr.; Bristol-Myers Squibb, Ger.; Bristol-Myers Squibb, Ital.; Bristol-Myers Squibb, Switz.*
Sotalol hydrochloride (p.972·2).
Angina pectoris; arrhythmias; hypertension; myocardial infarction.

Sotalin *Medinovum, Fin.*
Sotalol hydrochloride (p.972·2).
Arrhythmias.

Sotamed *S Med, Aust.*
Sotalol hydrochloride (p.972·2).
Arrhythmias.

Sotamol *Technilab, Canad.*
Sotalol hydrochloride (p.972·2).
Arrhythmias.

Sotaper *Mead Johnson, Mex.*
Sotalol (p.972·3).

Sotapor *Bristol-Myers, Spain.*
Sotalol hydrochloride (p.972·2).
Arrhythmias.

Sota-Puren *Isis Puren, Ger.*
Sotalol hydrochloride (p.972·2).
Arrhythmias.

Sotaryt *Azupharma, Ger.*
Sotalol hydrochloride (p.972·2).
Arrhythmias.

Sota-saar *Rosen, Ger.*
Sotalol hydrochloride (p.972·2).
Arrhythmias.

Sotastad *Stada, Aust.; Stada, Ger.*
Sotalol hydrochloride (p.972·2).
Arrhythmias.

Sotazide *Bristol-Myers Squibb, S.Afr.†*
Sotalol hydrochloride (p.972·2); hydrochlorothiazide (p.907·3).
Hypertension.

Sotaziden N *Bristol-Myers Squibb, Ger.*
Nadolol (p.937·1); bendrofluazide [bendroflumethiazide] (p.844·1).
Hypertension.

Sotilen
Medochemie, Hong Kong; Medochemie, Singapore; Medochemie, Thai.
Piroxicam (p.79·1).
Gout; musculoskeletal and joint disorders.

Sotradecol *Elkins-Sinn, USA.*
Sodium tetradecyl sulfate (p.1497·2).
Varicose veins.

Soufrane *Sanofi Winthrop, Fr.*
Thenoate sodium (p.261·3).
Nasopharyngeal infections.

Soufrol *Gebro, Switz.*
Mesulphen (p.1118·3).
Bath additive; musculoskeletal and joint disorders; skin disorders.

Soufrol TP *Gebro, Switz.*
Medicinal mud; sulfur (p.1123·3).
Musculoskeletal and joint disorders.

Soufrol ZNP *Gebro, Switz.*
Sulfur (p.1123·3); pyrithione zinc (p.1122·1).
Scalp disorders.

Sovarel *Normon, Spain†.*
Almitrine (p.1506·2).
Respiratory depression.

Sovel *Novartis, Ger.*
Norethisterone acetate (p.1485·1).
Menstrual disorders.

Soventol
Ebewe, Aust.; Knoll, Ger.; Knoll, Mex.; Knoll, Neth.†.
Bamipine (p.410·1), bamipine hydrochloride (p.410·1), or bamipine lactate (p.410·1).
Burns; frostbite; hay fever; insect and jellyfish stings; pruritus; sunburn; urticaria.

Soventol Hydrocortison *Knoll, Ger.*
Hydrocortisone acetate (p.1073·3).
Insect stings; itchy eczema; sunburn; urticaria.

Soy Forte with Block Cohosh *Cenovis, Austral.*
Soya (p.1378·1); cimicifuga (p.1595·2); calcium hydrogen phosphate (p.1188·2); colecalciferol (p.1391·1); magnesium oxide (p.1233·2).
Menopausal disorders; osteoporosis.

Soyacal
Grifols, Spain; Alpha Therapeutic, UK†.
Soya oil (p.1378·1).
Contains egg phospholipids.
Lipid infusion for parenteral nutrition.

Soyalac *Nutricia-Luma Lindar, USA.*
Lactose-free soy protein infant feed (p.1350·1).

Soyaloid *Serral, Mex.*
Soya flour (p.1378·1); povidone (p.1503·2).
Bath aditive; skin disorders.

Soyaven *Delicias, Mex.*
Food for special diets (p.1350·1).
Food allergies; lactose and cow's milk intolerance.

Soydex *Darier, Mex.*
Soya flour (p.1378·1); povidone (p.1503·2).
Bath additive; skin disorders.

SP *Sussex, UK.*
Paracetamol (p.71·2); caffeine (p.761·3); phenylephrine hydrochloride (p.1097·1).

SP54 *Bene-Chemie, Hong Kong.*
Pentosan polysulfate sodium (p.953·1).
Thromboembolic disorders.

SP Betaisodona *Mundipharma, Ger.†*
Povidone-iodine (p.1155·1).
Hand disinfection; skin and mucous membrane disinfection.

SP Cream *Curacel, Austral.*
Melaleuca oil (p.1631·3); salicylic acid (p.1122·3); solanum lycopersicum; urea (p.1127·3).
Keratoses; sunspots; warts.

SP Troches *Meiji, Singapore.*
Dequalinium chloride (p.1143·1).
Mouth and throat disorders.

Spaciclina *SPA, Ital.†*
Tetracycline hydrochloride (p.258·3).
Bacterial and protozoal infections.

Spagall *Sanova, Aust.*
Tolynol nicotinate (p.1674·1); naphthylacetic acid (p.1639·3); caroverine (p.1591·3).
Hepatobiliary disorders.

Spagulax *Pharmafarm, Fr.*
Ispaghula (p.1229·1).
Constipation.

Spagulax au Citrate de Potassium *Pharmafarm, Fr.*
Ispaghula (p.1229·1); potassium citrate (p.1186·1).
Constipation.

Spagulax au Sorbitol *Pharmafarm, Fr.*
Ispaghula (p.1229·1); sorbitol (p.1377·3).
Constipation.

Spagymun *Spagyros, Switz.*
Echinacea angustifolia flowers and roots; echinacea purpura flowers and roots (p.1606·2); eupatorium perfoliatum.
Immune stimulant.

Spagyrom *Spagyros, Switz.*
Echinacea angustifolia flowers and roots; echinacea purpura flowers and roots (p.1606·2); clove oil (p.1597·1); cinnamon oil (p.1596·1); juniper oil (p.1625·2); lavender oil (p.1627·2); chamomile oil; peppermint oil (p.1243·3); rosemary oil (p.1659·3); savory oil; thyme oil (p.1672·3).
Common cold; mouth and throat disorders.

Spai *INTES, Ital.*
Sodium chloride; potassium chloride; calcium chloride; magnesium chloride; sodium acetate; sodium citrate (p.1180·1).
Adjunct in otorhinolaryngeal procedures; cleaning solution for contact lens; ocular irrigation.

Spalgin *SPA, Ital.†*
Pipethanate ethobromide (p.472·2).
Premedication; smooth muscle spasticity.

Spalt
Note.This name is used for preparations of different composition.
Sanova, Aust.
Phenazone salicylate (p.77·2); salicylamide (p.82·1); caffeine (p.761·3).
Pain.

Much, Ger.†.
Aspirin (p.14·2).
Cold symptoms; fever; pain.

Spalt N
Note.This name is used for preparations of different composition.
Whitehall, Swed.†.
Phenazone (p.77·2).
Fever; pain.

Whitehall-Robins, Switz.
Paracetamol (p.71·2).
Fever; pain.

Spalt Schmerz-Gel *Whitehall-Much, Ger.*
Diisopropanolamine felbinac (p.36·1).
Musculoskeletal, joint, and soft-tissue disorders.

Spalt Schmerztabletten *Whitehall-Much, Ger.*
Aspirin (p.14·2); paracetamol (p.71·2).
Pain.

Span C *Freeda, USA.*
Citrus bioflavonoids complex (p.1611·1); ascorbic acid (p.1389·3).
Capillary bleeding.

Spancap No. I *Vortech, USA†.*
Dexamfetamine sulfate (p.1507·3).
Attention deficit disorder with hyperactivity; narcoleptic syndrome; obesity.

Span-FF *Lexis, USA†.*
Ferrous fumarate (p.1360·1).
Iron-deficiency anaemias.

Spanidin *Kayaku, Jpn.*
Gusperimus hydrochloride (p.544·1).
Renal transplant rejection.

Spanish Tummy Mixture *Potter's, UK.*
Blackberry root bark; catechu (p.1592·2).
Diarrhoea.

Span-K
Rhone-Poulenc Rorer, Austral.; Fisons, Hong Kong; Aventis, NZ.
Potassium chloride (p.1194·3).
Potassium deficiency.

Spanor *Biotherapie, Fr.*
Doxycycline hyclate (p.200·1).
Bacterial infections.

Spara *Dainippon, Jpn.*
Sparfloxacin (p.248·1).
Bacterial infections.

Sparaplaie *Urgo, Fr.*
Benzalkonium chloride (p.1133·2).
Burns; wounds.

Sparine
Wyeth, Austral.†; Wyeth Lederle, Denm.; Wyeth Lederle, Fin.; Wyeth, Irl.; Akromed, S.Afr.†; Genus, UK; Wyeth-Ayerst, USA†.
Promazine embonate (p.702·2) or promazine hydrochloride (p.702·2).
Agitation; alcohol withdrawal syndrome; hiccups; nausea and vomiting; pain; premedication; psychoses; sedative.

Spark *Medecine Vegetale, Fr.†.*
Frangula bark (p.1227·1); boldo leaf (p.1585·3); aloes (p.1210·1).
Constipation.

Sparkal
Gea, Denm.; Gea, Fin.; Gea, Swed.
Amiloride hydrochloride (p.835·1); hydrochlorothiazide (p.907·3).
Hypertension; liver cirrhosis with ascites; oedema.

Sparkles *Lafayette, USA.*
Sodium bicarbonate (p.1186·2); citric acid (p.1596·2); simeticone (p.1249·2).
Adjunct in endoscopy; flatulence.

Sparksol *Asta Medica, Ital.*
Amino-acid preparation with vitamin B₆ (p.1350·1).

Spartiol *Klein, Ger.*
Sarothamnus scoparius (p.1661·2).
Arrhythmias.

Spartocine
Darci, Belg.; UCB, Fin.
Ferrous aspartate (p.1359·3).
Iron deficiency; iron-deficiency anaemias.

Spartocine N *UCB, Ger.*
Ferrous aspartate (p.1359·3).
Iron-deficiency anaemias.

Spasen *FIRMA, Ital.*
Suppositories: Otilonium bromide (p.1645·2); lignocaine [lidocaine] hydrochloride (p.1313·2).
Gastrointestinal spasm.
Tablets: Otilonium bromide (p.1645·2).
The name Spasen was formerly used for a preparation containing fenalamide and aminopropylone.
Gastrointestinal pain and spasm.

Spasen Somatico *FIRMA, Ital.*
Otilonium bromide (p.1645·2); diazepam (p.674·3).
Gastrointestinal pain and spasm.

Spasfon
Bio-Therabel, Belg.; Lafon, Fr.
Phloroglucinol (p.1650·3); trimethylphloroglucinol (p.1650·3).
Smooth muscle spasm.

Spasfon-Lyoc *Lafon, Fr.*
Phloroglucinol (p.1650·3).
Smooth muscle spasm.

Spasgone *Chew, Thai.*
Paracetamol (p.71·2); hyoscine butylbromide (p.468·2).
Smooth muscle spasm.

Spasgone-H *Chew, Thai.*
Hyoscine butylbromide (p.468·2).
Smooth muscle spasm.

Spasma *Stella, Belg.*
Morphine hydrochloride (p.56·1); hyoscine hydrobromide (p.468·2).
Biliary and renal colic; pain; premedication.

Spasmag *Grimberg, Fr.*
Capsules; oral solution: Magnesium sulfate (p.1191·1); dried yeast (p.1398·1).
Magnesium deficiency.
Injection: Magnesium sulfate (p.1191·1).
Eclampsia; magnesium deficiency.

Spasmalgan *Apogepha, Ger.*
Denaverine hydrochloride.
Smooth muscle spasm.

Spasmalgin *Sam-On, Israel.*
Atropine sulfate (p.461·1); papaverine hydrochloride (p.1648·1); paracetamol (p.71·2); codeine phosphate (p.25·2).
Smooth muscle spasm.

Spasman *Merckle, Ger.*
Demelverine hydrochloride; benzhexol [trihexyphenidyl] hydrochloride (p.463·3).
Smooth muscle spasm.

Spasman scop *Merckle, Ger.*
Hyoscine butylbromide (p.468·2).
Smooth muscle spasm.

Spasmaverine *Theraplix, Fr.*
Suppositories: Alverine (p.1212·1); benzocaine (p.1306·2).
Smooth muscle spasm.
Tablets: Alverine citrate (p.1211·3).
Smooth muscle spasm.

Spasmend *Restan, S.Afr.*
Paracetamol (p.71·2); mephenesin (p.1329·2).
Pain; skeletal muscle spasm.

Spasmeridan *UCB, Ital.*
Diazepam (p.674·3); hyoscine methobromide (p.468·2).
Gastrointestinal pain and spasm.

Spasmex
Note.This name is used for preparations of different composition.
Pfleger, Ger.
Trospium chloride (p.475·2).
Smooth muscle spasms; urinary incontinence.

Scharper, Ital.
Injection: Phloroglucinol (p.1650·3).
Tablets: Phloroglucinol (p.1650·3); trimethylphloroglucinol (p.1650·3).
Painful spasm of the biliary and urinary tracts.

Spasmidenal *Jolly-Jatel, Fr.*
Crataegus (p.1600·2); valerian (p.1678·3); phenobarbital (p.355·1).
Insomnia; nervous disorders.

Spasmine
Note.This name is used for preparations of different composition.
Norgine, Belg.
Alverine citrate (p.1211·3).
Irritable bowel syndrome.

Jolly-Jatel, Fr.
Valerian (p.1678·3); crataegus (p.1600·2).
Insomnia; nervous disorders.

Spasmium *Sanova, Aust.*
Caroverine (p.1591·3) or caroverine hydrochloride (p.1591·3).
Smooth muscle spasm; tinnitus.

Spasmium comp *Sanova, Aust.*
Caroverine (p.1591·3); metamizole calcium (p.34·2).
Painful smooth muscle spasm.

Spasmo Claim *Apomedica, Aust.*
Turmeric (p.1029·3); benzyl mandelate; tolynol (p.1674·1); peppermint oil (p.1243·3); caraway oil (p.1591·2); fennel oil (p.1610·2); lemon oil (p.1628·2); camphor (p.1589·3); thymol (p.1158·3); guaiazulene (p.1618·3).
Gastrointestinal disorders.

spasmo gall sanol mint *Sanol, Ger.; Schwarz, Ger.*
Peppermint oil (p.1243·3).
Biliary-tract spasm.

spasmo gallo sanol *Sanol, Ger.*
Greater celandine (p.1618·1); turmeric (p.1029·3).
Biliary and gastrointestinal disorders.

Spasmo Gallo Sanol N *Sanol, Ger.†.*
Xenytropium bromide (p.475·3); ox bile (p.1585·1); aloes (p.1210·1).
Biliary disorders.

Spasmo Gallosanol *Mayrhofer, Aust.†.*
Xenytropium bromide (p.475·3); ox bile (p.1585·1); aloes (p.1210·1).
Biliary-tract disorders.

Spasmo Inalgon Neu *Fresenius Kabi, Aust.*
Dipyrone (p.34·1).
Painful smooth muscle spasm.

Spasmo Nil *Duchesnay, Canad.†.*
Aluminium hydroxide (p.1210·3); magnesium trisilicate (p.1233·3); dicyclomine [dicycloverine] hydrochloride (p.466·1); simeticone (p.1249·2).

Spasmo-Barbamin *Streuli, Switz.†.*
Propyphenazone (p.80·2); adiphenine hydrochloride; diphenhydramine hydrochloride (p.416·1).
Painful smooth muscle spasm.

Spasmo-Barbamine compositum *Streuli, Switz.†.*
Propyphenazone (p.80·2); adiphenine hydrochloride; diphenhydramine hydrochloride (p.416·1); codeine phosphate (p.25·2).
Painful smooth muscle spasm.

Spasmo-Bomaleb *Hevert, Ger.†.*
Homoeopathic preparation.

Spasmo-Canulase
Novartis Consumer, S.Afr.; Novartis Consumer, Switz.
Metixene hydrochloride (p.470·2); dimethicone (p.1249·2); pancreatin (p.1646·1); cellulase (p.1593·1); pepsin (p.1649·3); glutamic acid hydrochloride (p.1365·2); sodium dehydrocholate (p.1602·2).
Gastrointestinal disorders.

Spasmo-Cibalgin *Novartis Consumer, Switz.*
Propyphenazone (p.80·2); drofenine hydrochloride (p.466·3).
Painful smooth muscle spasm.

Spasmo-Cibalgin comp *Novartis Consumer, Switz.*
Propyphenazone (p.80·2); drofenine hydrochloride (p.466·3); codeine phosphate (p.25·2).
Painful smooth muscle spasm.

Spasmo-Cibalgin compositum S *Novartis, Ger.*
Propyphenazone (p.80·2); drofenine hydrochloride (p.466·3); codeine phosphate (p.25·2).
Smooth muscle spasm.

Spasmo-Cibalgin S *Novartis, Ger.*
Propyphenazone (p.80·2); drofenine hydrochloride (p.466·3).
Smooth muscle spasm.

Spasmo-Cibalgina *Novartis, Ital.*
Propyphenazone (p.80·2); drofenine hydrochloride (p.466·3).
Painful smooth muscle spasm.

Spasmo-Cibalgine *Ciba-Geigy, Belg.†.*
Propyphenazone (p.80·2); drofenine hydrochloride (p.466·3).
Dysmenorrhoea; smooth muscle spasm.

Spasmocor *Asta Medica, Aust.*
Glyceryl trinitrate (p.897·3); pentaerythrityl tetranitrate (p.952·3); nicotinic acid (p.1372·3); benzyl mandelate.
Angina pectoris; heart failure; peripheral vascular spasm.

Spasmoctyl *Guidotti, Spain.*
Otilonium bromide (p.1645·2).
Gastrointestinal spasm; irritable bowel syndrome.

Spasmocyclon *3M, Ger.*
Cyclandelate (p.865·2).
Cerebrovascular disorders; migraine; vestibular disorders.

Spasmodene *Edochim, Ital.*
Pipethanate ethobromide (p.472·2).
Biliary and urinary-tract spasm and dyskinesia; gastrointestinal spasm; premedication for endoscopy and radiography.

The symbol † denotes a preparation no longer actively marketed

Spasmodex Crinex, Fr.
Dihexyverine hydrochloride (p.466·2).
Gastrointestinal disorders.

Spasmodil ABC, Ital.
Pipethanate ethobromide (p.472·2).
Gastrointestinal spasm and hypermotility; premedication for endoscopy and radiography; urinary and biliary spasm and dyskinesia.

Spasmofen Abigo, Swed.
Hyoscine methonitrate (p.468·2); papaverine hydrochloride (p.1648·1); morphine hydrochloride (p.56·1); noscapine hydrochloride (p.1096·1); codeine hydrochloride (p.25·2).
Pain; smooth muscle spasm.

Spasmofides S Fides, Ger.
Homoeopathic preparation.

Spasmoflex Rolab, S.Afr.†
Paracetamol (p.71·2); chlormezanone (p.660·1).
Pain and associated tension.

Spasmogel Alliance, S.Afr.
Dicyclomine [dicycloverine] hydrochloride (p.466·1); light magnesium oxide (p.1233·2); aluminium hydroxide (p.1210·3).
Dyspepsia; flatulence; gastritis; gastro-oesophageal reflux; heartburn; peptic ulcer.

Spasmo-Granobil-Krampf- und Reizhusten
Synpharma, Aust.
Aniseed (p.1580·2); helianthus annuus; thyme (p.1672·2).
Coughs.

Spasmoliv Xepa-Soul Pattinson, Singapore.
Hyoscine butylbromide (p.468·2).
Smooth muscle spasm.

Spasmolyt Madaus, Aust.
Trospium chloride (p.475·2).
Bladder function disorders; smooth muscle spasm.

Spasmo-Lyt
Madaus, Ger.; Madaus, Thai.
Trospium chloride (p.475·2).
Bladder function disorders.

Spasmomen Menarini, Belg.; Menarini, Hong Kong; Menarini, Ital.
Otilonium bromide (p.1645·2).
Gastrointestinal spasm; irritable bowel syndrome; premedication for gastrointestinal procedures.

Spasmomen Somatico Menarini, Ital.
Otilonium bromide (p.1645·2); diazepam (p.674·3).
Gastrointestinal spasm.

Spasmo-Mucosolvan Boehringer Ingelheim, Ger.
Clenbuterol hydrochloride (p.763·3); ambroxol hydrochloride (p.1084·3).
Respiratory-tract disorders.

Spasmonal
Note.This name is used for preparations of different composition.
Trenker, Belg.
Mebeverine hydrochloride (p.1233·3).
Irritable bowel syndrome.

Norgine, Hong Kong; Norgine, Irl.; Norgine, Singapore; Norgine, Thai.; Norgine, UK.
Alverine citrate (p.1211·3).
Smooth muscle spasm.

Spasmonal Fibre Norgine, UK.
Sterculia (p.1250·2); alverine citrate (p.1211·3).
Formerly known as Alvercol.
Hypertonic colon; irritable bowel syndrome.

Spasmo-Nervogastrol Abbott Synthelabo, Ger.
Butinoline phosphate (p.1587·3); calcium carbonate (p.1215·1); bismuth subnitrate (p.1213·2).
Gastrointestinal disorders.

Spasmo-Oxepam Wyeth Lederle, Fin.
Oxazepam (p.697·1); ambutonium bromide (p.468·1).
Anxiety disorders; gastrointestinal motility disorders.

Spasmoplus
Note.This name is used for preparations of different composition.
Novartis, Aust.; Novartis, Belg.
Propyphenazone (p.80·2); drofenine hydrochloride (p.466·3); codeine phosphate (p.25·2).
Painful smooth muscle spasm.

Novartis, Ital.
Propyphenazone (p.80·2); codeine phosphate (p.25·2).
Pain.

Spasmopriv
Note.This name is used for preparations of different composition.
Irex, Fr.
Mebeverine hydrochloride (p.1233·3).
Gastrointestinal and biliary-tract spasm.

Lusofarmaco, Ital.†; Senosiain, Mex.; Eurodrug, Singapore; Eurodrug, Thai.
Fenoverine (p.1610·3).
Smooth muscle spasm.

Spasmo-Rhoival TC Byk Tosse, Ger.; Byk Gulden, Ger.
Trospium chloride (p.475·2).
Bladder function disorders.

Spasmosarto Biosarto, Spain†.
Trospium chloride (p.475·2).
Urinary incontinence.

Spasmosedine
Note.This name is used for preparations of different composition.
Pharmethic, Belg.†
Crataegus (p.1600·2); phenobarbital (p.355·1); quinine hydrobromide (p.445·1); meprobamate (p.691·1).
Arrhythmias; vascular spasm.

Theranol-Deglaude, Fr.
Crataegus (p.1600·2).
Formerly contained crataegus and phenobarbital.
Cardiac disorders; nervous disorders.

Spasmosol Streuli, Switz.
Morphine hydrochloride (p.56·1); codeine hydrochloride (p.25·2); noscapine hydrochloride (p.1096·1); atropine sulfate (p.461·1); papaverine hydrochloride (p.1648·1).
Pain.

Spasmo-Solugastril Sanova, Aust.; Heumann, Ger.
Aluminium hydroxide (p.1210·3); butinoline phosphate (p.1587·3); calcium carbonate (p.1215·1).
Gastrointestinal disorders.

Spasmosyx F Syxyl, Ger.
Homoeopathic preparation.

Spasmotropin Legrand, Braz.
Dipyrone (p.34·1); papaverine (p.1648·1); homatropine (p.468·1).
Smooth muscle spasm.

Spasmo-Urgenin
Madaus, Aust.; Neo-Farmaceutica, Port.; Byk Madaus, S.Afr.; Madaus, Spain; Madaus, Thai.
Trospium chloride (p.475·2); echinacea (p.1606·2); saw palmetto (p.1491·2).
Prostatic and urinary-tract spasm and pain.

Spasmo-Urgenin TC Madaus, Ger.
Trospium chloride (p.475·2).
Bladder function disorders.

Spasmo-Urgenine Neo Madaus, Switz.
Trospium chloride (p.475·2).
Spasmo-Urgenine formerly contained trospium chloride, echinacea angustifolia, and saw palmetto.
Urinary-tract disorders.

Spasmo-Urolong Organon, Aust.†
Nitrofurantoin (p.230·3); camylofin hydrochloride (p.1590·1).
Urinary-tract infection with pain.

Spasmowern Wernigerode, Ger.
Hyoscine butylbromide (p.468·2).
Smooth muscle spasm.

Spassirex Irex, Fr.
Phloroglucinol (p.1650·3).
Smooth muscle pain and spasm.

Spastrex Propan, S.Afr.
Oxyphenonium bromide (p.472·1).
Gastrointestinal and urinary-tract spasm.

Spasuret Sanofi Synthelabo, Ger.
Flavoxate hydrochloride (p.467·1).
Urinary-tract disorders.

Spasuri Pharmasant, Thai.
Flavoxate hydrochloride (p.467·1).
Urinary-tract disorders.

Spasyt TAD, Ger.
Oxybutynin hydrochloride (p.471·2).
Bladder instability; urinary incontinence.

Speciafoldine Rhone-Poulenc Rorer, Fr.
Folic acid (p.1361·1).
Nutritional deficiency; prevention of neural tube disorders.

Special Defense Sun Block Clinique, Canad.
SPF 25: Titanium dioxide (p.1126·1).
Sunscreen.

Speci-Chol Pekana, Ger.
Homoeopathic preparation.

Species Carvi comp Weleda, Aust.
Aniseed (p.1580·2); urtica (p.1678·2); fennel (p.1610·1); caraway (p.1591·2).
Flatulence; gastrointestinal cramp.

Species nervinae Kwizda, Aust.
Hypericum (p.290·2); valerian (p.1678·3); melissa leaf (p.1632·2); peppermint leaf (p.1243·2).
Anxiety disorders; sleep disorders.

Spec-T
Note.This name is used for preparations of different composition.
Apothecon, USA.
Dextromethorphan hydrobromide (p.1087·3); benzocaine (p.1306·2).
Coughs.

Squibb, USA.
Benzocaine (p.1306·2).
Sore throat.

Spec-T Sore Throat/Decongestant Apothecon, USA†.
Phenylpropanolamine hydrochloride (p.1098·1); phenylephrine hydrochloride (p.1097·1); benzocaine (p.1306·2).
Upper respiratory-tract symptoms.

Spectazole Ortho Dermatological, USA.
Econazole nitrate (p.382·3).
Fungal skin infections.

Spectraban
Note.This name is used for preparations of different composition.
Stiefel, Mex.
SPF 20: Oxybenzone (p.1518·1); homosalate (p.1517·2); octinoxate (p.1517·3).
Sunscreen.

Stiefel, S.Afr.†
SPF 4: Padimate O (p.1518·2).
Sunscreen.

Stiefel, Thai.
SPF 19: Zinc oxide (p.1128·2).
Sunscreen.

Stiefel, UK.
SPF 25: Padimate O (p.1518·2); aminobenzoic acid (p.1516·3).
Sunscreen.

Spectraban Ultra
Stiefel, Mex.
SPF 17(UVB); SPF 6(UVA): Padimate O (p.1518·2); oxybenzone (p.1518·1); avobenzone (p.1517·1); titanium dioxide (p.1126·1).
Sunscreen.

Stiefel, Thai.
SPF 28+: Padimate O (p.1518·2); avobenzone (p.1517·1); oxybenzone (p.1518·1); titanium dioxide (p.1126·1).
Sunscreen.

Stiefel, UK.
Padimate O (p.1518·2); avobenzone (p.1517·1); oxybenzone (p.1518·1); titanium dioxide (p.1126·1).
Sunscreen.

Spectracef TAP, USA.
Cefditoren pivoxil (p.165·3).
Bacterial infections.

Spectracil Alliance, S.Afr.
Ampicillin trihydrate (p.151·1).
Bacterial infections.

Spectramedryn Allergan, Ger.
Medrysone (p.1075·3).
Allergic and inflammatory disorders of the eye.

Spectramox Alliance, S.Afr.
Amoxicillin trihydrate (p.149·2).
Bacterial infections.

Spectrapain Alliance, S.Afr.
Paracetamol (p.71·2); codeine phosphate (p.25·2).
Pain.

Spectrapain Forte Alliance, S.Afr.
Paracetamol (p.71·2); codeine phosphate (p.25·2); caffeine (p.761·3); meprobamate (p.691·1).
Pain and associated tension.

Spectrasone Alliance, S.Afr.
Erythromycin estolate (p.201·2).
Bacterial infections.

Spectratet Alliance, S.Afr.
Oxytetracycline (p.234·1).
Bacterial infections.

Spectrim Alliance, S.Afr.
Co-trimoxazole (p.193·3).
Bacterial infections.

Spectro Derm Spectropharm, Canad.
Skin cleanser.
Cleansing of abraded and irritated skin.

Spectro Gluvs Spectropharm, Canad.
Barrier cream.

Spectro Gram Spectropharm, Canad.
Chlorhexidine gluconate (p.1138·2).
Disinfection of skin and hands.

Spectro Jel Spectropharm, Canad.
Skin cleanser.

Spectro Tar Spectropharm, Canad.
Shampoo: Chlorhexidine gluconate (p.1138·2); coal tar (p.1125·1).
Scalp disorders.
Skin wash: Coal tar (p.1125·1).
Eczema; psoriasis.

Spectrobid Pfizer, USA†.
Bacampicillin hydrochloride (p.155·1).
Bacterial infections.

Spectrocin Iquinosa, Spain.
Gramicidin (p.213·3); neomycin sulfate (p.228·1).
Infected burns; infected wounds; skin infections; superficial eye infections.

Spectrocin Plus Numark, USA.
Neomycin sulfate (p.228·1); polymyxin B sulfate (p.238·1); bacitracin (p.155·2); lignocaine [lidocaine] (p.1313·2).
Bacterial skin infections.

Spectro-Jel Recsei, USA.
Soap-free skin cleanser.

Spectroxyl Ecosol, Switz.
Amoxicillin (p.149·2).
Bacterial infections.

Spectrum
Note.This name is used for preparations of different composition.
KSL, Canad.†
Multivitamin and mineral preparation (p.1350·1).

Sigma-Tau, Ital.
Ceftazidime (p.174·3).
Bacterial infections.

Johnson & Johnson Medical, UK.
Alcohol (p.1130·3); quaternary ammonium compounds.
Formerly contained alcohol, chlorhexidine gluconate, and quaternary ammonium compounds.
Surface disinfection.

Specyton cartilage-parathyroide Menarini, Fr.
Cartilage and parathyroid antisera.
Arthritis.

Spedifen Inpharzam, Switz.
Ibuprofen (p.43·2).
Fever; inflammation; pain.

Spedralgin sans codeine Democal, Switz.
Paracetamol (p.71·2); phenazone (p.77·2); propyphenazone (p.80·2); caffeine (p.761·3).
Fever; pain.

Spedro Demopharm, Switz.†
Codeine phosphate (p.25·2); ephedrine hydrochloride (p.1090·1); belladonna (p.463·1); ipecacuanha (p.1093·1); guaifenesin (p.1092·2); sodium benzoate (p.1134·3); terpin hydrate (p.1101·2).
Coughs and associated respiratory-tract disorders.

Spektramox
AstraZeneca, Denm.; AstraZeneca, Fin.; Astra, Swed.
Amoxicillin trihydrate (p.149·2); potassium clavulanate (p.187·2).
Bacterial infections.

Spencer's Bronchitis McGloin, Austral.
Ammonium chloride (p.1085·2); codeine phosphate (p.25·2); phenylpropanolamine hydrochloride (p.1098·1).
Cold symptoms; throat irritation.

Spenglersan Apotheke Roten Krebs, Aust.
An antisera.
Active and passive immunisation.

Spenglersan Kolloid Meckel, Ger.
Homoeopathic preparation.

Spersacarbachol Ciba Vision, Switz.
Carbachol (p.1416·1).
Glaucoma; ocular hypertension.

Spersacarpin Ciba Vision, Switz.
Pilocarpine hydrochloride (p.1422·3).
Glaucoma; reversal of mydriasis.

Spersacarpine
Ciba Vision, Hong Kong; Ciba Vision, Singapore; Ciba Vision, Swed.†; Ciba Vision, Switz.
Pilocarpine hydrochloride (p.1422·3) or pilocarpine nitrate (p.1422·3).
Glaucoma; ocular hypertension.

Spersacet
Ciba Vision, Hong Kong; Ciba Vision, Switz.
Sulfacetamide sodium (p.250·3).
Bacterial eye infections; dacryocystitis.

Spersacet C
Ciba Vision, Hong Kong; Restan, S.Afr.; Ciba Vision, Switz.; Ciba Vision, Thai.
Sulfacetamide sodium (p.250·3); chloramphenicol (p.179·1).
Eye infections; lachrymo-nasal irrigation.

Spersadex
Ciba Vision, Ger.; Ciba Vision, Hong Kong; Ciba Vision, Norw.; Restan, S.Afr.; Ciba Vision, Switz.
Dexamethasone sodium phosphate (p.1067·1).
Inflammatory eye disorders.

Spersadex Comp
Ciba Vision, Denm.; Ciba Vision, Ger.; Ciba Vision, Hong Kong; Restan, S.Afr.; Ciba Vision, Singapore; Ciba Vision, Switz.
Dexamethasone sodium phosphate (p.1067·1); chloramphenicol (p.179·1).
Inflammatory eye infections.

Spersadex med kloramfenikol Ciba Vision, Norw.
Dexamethasone sodium phosphate (p.1067·1); chloramphenicol (p.179·1).
Inflammatory eye infections.

Spersadexolin Ciba Vision, Ger.
Dexamethasone sodium phosphate (p.1067·1); chloramphenicol (p.179·1); tetryzoline hydrochloride (p.1101·2).
Eye disorders.

Spersadexoline
Ciba Vision, Hong Kong; Restan, S.Afr.; Ciba Vision, Singapore; Ciba Vision, Thai.
Dexamethasone sodium phosphate (p.1067·1); chloramphenicol (p.179·1); tetryzoline hydrochloride (p.1101·2).
Inflammatory eye infections.

Spersallerg
Ciba Vision, Ger.; Ciba Vision, Hong Kong; Ciba Vision, Norw.; Restan, S.Afr.; Ciba Vision, Singapore; Ciba Vision, Switz.; Ciba Vision, Thai.
Antazoline hydrochloride (p.408·3); tetryzoline hydrochloride (p.1101·2).
Allergic conjunctivitis.

Spersamide Restan, S.Afr.
Sulfacetamide sodium (p.250·3).
Eye infections.

Spersanicol
Ciba Vision, Hong Kong; Novartis, Mex.; Restan, S.Afr.; Ciba Vision, Singapore; Ciba Vision, Switz.
Chloramphenicol (p.179·1).
Eye infections; lachrymo-nasal irrigation.

Spersapolymyxin
Ciba Vision, Hong Kong; Ciba Vision, Switz.; Ciba Vision, Thai.
Polymyxin B sulfate (p.238·1); neomycin sulfate (p.228·1).
Bacterial eye infections.

Spersatear Restan, S.Afr.
Hypromellose (p.1501·3).
Dry eyes.

Spersatropine Restan, S.Afr.†
Atropine sulfate (p.461·1).
Ophthalmic diagnostic procedures.

Spersin Sigma, Austral.†
Ointment: Neomycin sulfate (p.228·1); bacitracin (p.155·2); polymyxin B sulfate (p.238·1).
Topical powder: Polymyxin B sulfate (p.238·1); neomycin sulfate (p.228·1).
Skin infections.

Sperti Preparation H
Wyeth Lederle, Aust.; Whitehall-Much, Ger.
Yeast (p.1398·1); shark-liver oil.
Haemorrhoids.

Sperti Preparacao H Whitehall, Port.
Yeast (p.1398·1); shark-liver oil.
Anorectal disorders.

Sperti Preparation H
Whitehall, Neth.; Whitehall-Robins, Switz.
Yeast (p.1398·1); shark-liver oil.
Haemorrhoids.

Spesicor *Leiras, Fin.*
Metoprolol succinate (p.932·1) or metoprolol tartrate (p.931·2).
Angina pectoris; arrhythmias; hypertension; hyperthyroidism; migraine; myocardial infarction.

Speton *Temmler, Port.†.*
Halazone (p.1145·3).

Spevin *Expanpharm, Fr.*
Cascara sagrada (p.1216·1); quassia amara (p.1657·1).
Constipation.

Spherex *Pharmacia Upjohn, Ger.*
Amilomer 25-45.
Adjuvant to antineoplastics in liver cancer.

Spherulin *ALK, USA.*
Coccidioidin (p.1597·2).
Skin test for coccidioidomycosis.

S.P.H.P. *Cantassium Co., UK.*
Prostate gland; spinal cord (p.1631·2); calcium hypophosphite; nicotinamide (p.1372·3); lecithin (p.1628·1); wheat germ; kola (p.1681·1); vitamin A (p.1382·1); vitamin D (p.1391·1).

Spicline *Socopharm, Fr.†.*
Minocycline hydrochloride (p.224·3).
Bacterial infections.

Spidifen *Zambon, Belg.*
Ibuprofen (p.43·2).
Fever; musculoskeletal and joint disorders; pain.

Spilacnet *Nettopharma, Denm.†.*
Spironolactone (p.973·2).
Hyperaldosteronism; hypertension; oedema.

Spilan *Kanoldt, Ger.*
Hypericum (p.290·2).
Anxiety disorders; depression.

Spir *Inava, Fr.*
Beclometasone dipropionate (p.1061·2).
Asthma.

Spiractin *Alphapharm, Austral.; Aspen, S.Afr.*
Spironolactone (p.973·2).
Heart failure; hepatic cirrhosis with ascites and oedema; hirsutism in females; hypertension; hyperaldosteronism; nephrotic syndrome.

Spiralgin *Spirig, Switz.*
Mefenamic acid (p.51·2).
Fever; inflammation; pain.

Spiraphan *Kattwiga, Ger.*
Homoeopathic preparation.

Spiravet *Merial, Denm.†.*
Spiramycin (p.248·3).
Bacterial infections.

Spirbon *Fresenius Kabi, Aust.*
Chlorphenoxamine hydrochloride (p.412·1); ephedrine hydrochloride (p.1090·1); emetine hydrochloride (p.591·3).
Respiratory-tract disorders.

Spiresis *Orion, Fin.*
Spironolactone (p.973·2).
Hyperaldosteronism; hypertension; liver cirrhosis with ascites; oedema.

Spiretic *DDSA Pharmaceuticals, UK.*
Spironolactone (p.973·2).

Spirial *SVR, Fr.; SVR, Ital.*
Aluminium chlorohydrate (p.1110·2).
Hyperhidrosis.

Spiricort *Spirig, Switz.*
Prednisolone (p.1077·3).
Corticosteroid.

Spiridazide *SIT, Ital.*
Spironolactone (p.973·2); hydrochlorothiazide (p.907·3).
Hyperaldosteronism.

Spiridon *Orion, Singapore.*
Spironolactone (p.973·2).
Heart failure; hyperaldosteronism; hypertension; liver cirrhosis; nephrotic syndrome; oedema.

Spirix *Nycomed, Denm.; Nycomed, Fin.; Nycomed, Norw.; Nycomed, Swed.*
Spironolactone (p.973·2).
Hyperaldosteronism; hypertension; liver cirrhosis with ascites; oedema.

spiro *CT, Ger.*
Spironolactone (p.973·2).
Ascites; hyperaldosteronism; oedema.

Spiro comp *Ratiopharm, Ger.*
Spironolactone (p.973·2); frusemide [furosemide] (p.893·1).
Ascites; hyperaldosteronism; liver cirrhosis; nephrotic syndrome; oedema.

Spirobene *Ratiopharm, Aust.*
Spironolactone (p.973·2).
Hyperaldosteronism; hypertension; oedema.

Spiro-Co *Norton, UK.*
Spironolactone (p.973·2); hydroflumethiazide (p.911·3).
These ingredients are present in such proportions that together they can be described by the British Approved Name Co-flumactone.
Heart failure.

Spirocort *AstraZeneca, Denm.*
Budesonide (p.1064·2).
Asthma.

Spiroctan *Roche, Fr.; Roche, Switz.; Roche, UK†.*
Potassium canrenoate (p.957·1) or spironolactone (p.973·2).
Adjuvant in myasthenia; ascites; heart failure; hyperaldosteronism; hypertension; oedema.

Spiroctan-M *Boehringer Mannheim, UK†.*
Potassium canrenoate (p.957·1).
Ascites; hyperaldosteronism; oedema.

Spiroctazine *Roche, Ital.*
Spironolactone (p.973·2); altizide (p.835·1).
Hypertension; oedema.

Spiro-D *Lichtenstein, Ger.*
Spironolactone (p.973·2); frusemide [furosemide] (p.893·1).
Ascites; heart failure; hyperaldosteronism; hypertension; oedema.

Spiroderm *Searle, Ital.*
Spironolactone (p.973·2).
Acne.

Spirofur *Bruno, Ital.*
Spironolactone (p.973·2); frusemide [furosemide] (p.893·1).
Hypertension; oedema.

Spirogel *Worndli, Switz.†.*
Camphor (p.1589·3); phenol (p.1152·3); cinnamic acid (p.1142·2); cinnamaldehyde; guaiacol (p.1092·1); phenazone (p.77·2); chlorobutanol (p.1141·2); thymol iodide (p.1158·3); thymol (p.1158·3); anethole (p.1580·1); safrole; eugenol (p.1609·3).
Dental disorders.

Spirohexal *Hexal, Aust.*
Spironolactone (p.973·2).
Hyperaldosteronism; hypertension; oedema.

Spirolair *3M, Belg.*
Pirbuterol acetate (p.769·3).
Asthma; bronchitis; emphysema.

Spirolang *SIT, Ital.*
Spironolactone (p.973·2).
Hyperaldosteronism.

Spirolone *Berk, UK†.*
Spironolactone (p.973·2).
Ascites; heart failure; nephrotic syndrome; oedema; primary hyperaldosteronism.

Spirolept *Transphyto, Fr.*
An inactivated leptospirosis vaccine (p.1546·2).
Active immunisation.

Spirometon *Belmac, Spain.*
Bendrofluazide [bendroflumethiazide] (p.844·1); spironolactone (p.973·2).
Hypertension; oedema.

Spiron *Orion, Denm.*
Spironolactone (p.973·2).
Ascites; hyperaldosteronism; oedema.

Spironex *PP Lab, Thai.*
Spironolactone (p.973·2).
Ascites; hypertension; oedema; primary aldosteronism.

Spirono *Isis Puren, Ger.*
Spironolactone (p.973·2).
Ascites; hyperaldosteronism; oedema.

Spirono comp *Genericon, Aust.*
Spironolactone (p.973·2); frusemide [furosemide] (p.893·1).
Hyperaldosteronism; oedema.

Spironol *Pharbita, Israel.*
Spironolactone (p.973·2).
Heart failure; hepatic cirrhosis; hypertension; hypokalaemia; oedema; primary hyperaldosteronism.

Spironolacton Plus *Heumann, Ger.*
Spironolactone (p.973·2) frusemide [furosemide] (p.893·1).
Ascites; oedema.

Spironone *EG, Fr.*
Spironolactone (p.973·2).
Adjuvant in myasthenia; hyperaldosteronism; hypertension; oedema.

Spironothiazid *Henning, Ger.; Synthelabo, Switz.*
Spironolactone (p.973·2); hydrochlorothiazide (p.907·3).
Ascites; hyperaldosteronism; hypertension; oedema.

Spiropal *Nycomed, Norw.*
Spironolactone (p.973·2).
Hyperaldosteronism; hypertension; oedema.

Spiropent *Boehringer Ingelheim, Aust.; Boehringer Ingelheim, Ger.; Boehringer Ingelheim, Ital.; Promeco, Mex.; Europharma, Spain.*
Clenbuterol hydrochloride (p.763·3).
Obstructive airways disease.

Spiroscand *Enapharm, Swed.*
Spironolactone (p.973·2).
Hyperaldosteronism; hypertension; liver cirrhosis with ascites; oedema.

Spirospare *Ashbourne, UK.*
Spironolactone (p.973·2).
Ascites; heart failure; nephrotic syndrome; oedema; primary hyperaldosteronism.

Spirostada comp *Stada, Ger.*
Spironolactone (p.973·2); bendrofluazide [bendroflumethiazide] (p.844·1).
Ascites; hyperaldosteronism; hypertension; oedema.

Spiro-Tablinen *Sanorania, Ger.†.*
Spironolactone (p.973·2).
Ascites; hyperaldosteronism; oedema.

Spirotone *Pacific, NZ.*
Spironolactone (p.973·2).
Aldosteronism; heart failure; hepatic cirrhosis with ascites; hirsutism; hypertension; hypokalaemia; nephrotic syndrome; oedema.

Spirox *Agepha, Aust.*
Spironolactone (p.973·2).
Hyperaldosteronism; hypertension; nephrotic syndrome; oedema.

Spirsa *Alter, Spain.*
Chlorpheniramine [chlorphenamine] maleate (p.412·1); phenylephrine hydrochloride (p.1097·1); paracetamol (p.71·2).
Cold and influenza symptoms.

Spitacid *Henkel, Ger.*
Alcohol (p.1130·3); isopropyl alcohol (p.1149·2); benzyl alcohol (p.1135·2).
Hand disinfection.

Spitaderm *Paragerm, Fr.; Henkel, Ital.*
Isopropyl alcohol (p.1149·2); chlorhexidine gluconate (p.1138·2); hydrogen peroxide (p.1147·1).
Skin disinfection.

Spitalen *Erfa, Belg.*
Virginiamycin (p.269·3); neomycin sulfate (p.228·1).
Bacterial infections.

Spizef *Grunenthal, Aust.; Takeda, Ger.*
Cefotiam hydrochloride (p.171·1).
Lignocaine [lidocaine] hydrochloride (p.1313·2) may be included in the intramuscular injection to alleviate the pain of injection.
Bacterial infections.

SPL *Delmont, USA.*
Two strains of lysed *Staphylococcus aureus* in solution (p.1565·1).
Staphylococcal infection.

Splendil *Astra, Braz.; Astra, Jpn.*
Felodipine (p.888·3).
Angina pectoris; hypertension; Raynaud's syndrome.

Splenocarbine *Lesourd, Fr.*
Activated charcoal (p.1000·2).
Gastrointestinal disorders.

Splen-Uvocal *Stroschein, Ger.†.*
Spleen extract.
Immunotherapy.

Spolera *OTW, Ger.*
Acmella ciliata.
Insect stings; soft-tissue injuries.

Spondylon *Wyeth, Ger.*
Capsules: Ketoprofen (p.47·3).
Gout; inflammation; musculoskeletal, joint, and soft-tissue disorders; pain.
Embrocation: Methyl nicotinate (p.55·1); camphor (p.1589·3).
Muscular and neuromuscular disorders.

Spondylonal *Wyeth, Ger.*
Multivitamin preparation (p.1350·1).

Spondyvit *Wyeth, Ger.*
d-Alpha tocoferil acetate (p.1394·1).
Vitamin E deficiency.

Spongostan *Johnson & Johnson, Aust.†; Ethicon, Ital.†; Novo Nordisk, S.Afr.†.*
Absorbable gelatin sponge (p.737·2).
Haemostatic.

Sponsin *Farmasan, Ger.*
Co-dergocrine mesilate (p.1597·3).
Adjuvant for mental function disorders; cervical disc syndrome; hypertension.

Sponwiga *Kattwiga, Ger.*
Homoeopathic preparation.

Sporacid *IMS, Ital.*
Glutaral (p.1145·2).
Instrument disinfection.

Sporal *Janssen, Thai.*
Itraconazole (p.387·2).
Fungal infections.

Sporanox *Janssen-Cilag, Aust.; Janssen-Cilag, Austral.; Janssen-Cilag, Belg.; Janssen, Braz.; Janssen-Ortho, Canad.; Janssen-Cilag, Denm.; Janssen-Cilag, Fin.; Janssen-Cilag, Fr.; Janssen, Hong Kong; Janssen-Cilag, Irl.; Janssen-Cilag, Israel; Janssen-Cilag, Ital.; Janssen, Mex.; Janssen-Cilag, Norw.; Janssen-Cilag, NZ; Janssen-Cilag, Port.; Janssen-Cilag, S.Afr.; Janssen-Cilag, Singapore; Janssen, Spain; Janssen-Cilag, Swed.; Janssen-Cilag, Switz.; Janssen-Cilag, UK; Janssen, USA.*
Itraconazole (p.387·2).
Fungal infections.

Sporasec *Janssen, Mex.*
Itraconazole (p.387·2); secnidazole (p.602·1).
Bacterial and fungal vaginosis.

Sporcid *Fresenius Kabi, Ger.*
Glutaral (p.1145·2); formaldehyde (p.1144·2).
Formerly contained 2-alkoxi-3,4-dihydro-2-H-pyran aldehyde adduct, formaldehyde, glyoxal, ricinoleic acid propylamidotrimethylammonium methosulfate, and oleylaminooxyethylate.
Instrument disinfection.

Sporex
Note. This name is used for preparations of different composition.
Rougier, Canad.
Formaldehyde (p.1144·2); benzalkonium chloride (p.1133·2); sodium nitrite (p.1023·1).
Instrument sterilisation.

IMS, Ital.
Glutaral (p.1145·2).
Instrument disinfection.

Sporicef *Ranbaxy, Thai.*
Cefalexin (p.161·3).
Bacterial infections.

Sporicidin *IMS, Ital.*
Glutaral-phenate complex (p.1145·3).
Instrument and surface disinfection.

Sporidex *Ranbaxy, Singapore.*
Cefalexin (p.161·3).
Bacterial infections.

Sporiline *Schering-Plough, Fr.*
Tolnaftate (p.549·2).
Fungal skin infections.

Sporinex *Medochemie, Thai.*
Tinidazole (p.603·3).
Amoebiasis; giardiasis; trichomoniasis.

Sporostatin *Schering-Plough, Braz.*
Griseofulvin (p.386·2).
Fungal infections.

Sport Sunblock *Avon, Canad.*
SPF 30: Octinoxate (p.1517·3); octisalate (p.1518·1); oxybenzone (p.1518·1).
Sunscreen.

Sportenine
Boiron, Canad.; Boiron, Port.
Homoeopathic preparation.

Sportino *Harras-Curarina, Ger.*
Heparin sodium (p.902·1).
Soft-tissue injury; superficial vascular disorders.

Sportino Akut
Harras-Curarina, Aust.; Harras-Curarina, Ger.
Glycol salicylate (p.42·2); arnica (p.1581·3).
Musculoskeletal, joint, and soft-tissue disorders.

Sportium Emgel *Lyron, Switz.*
Heparin sodium (p.902·1); allantoin (p.1110·1); dexpanthenol (p.1602·3).
Soft-tissue injuries; venous insufficiency.

Sports Eze Bruising Relief *Brauer, Austral.*
Oral spray: Homoeopathic preparation.
Topical gel: Arnica (p.1581·3).
Soft-tissue injuries.

Sports Eze Joint & Muscle *Brauer, Austral.*
Homoeopathic preparation.

Sports Multi *Cenovis, Austral.*
Multivitamin and mineral preparation (p.1350·1).

Sportscreme *Thompson, USA.*
Trolamine salicylate (p.90·1).
Muscle, joint, and soft-tissue pain; neuralgia.

Sportscreme Ice *Thompson, USA.*
Menthol (p.1632·3).
Muscle, joint, and soft-tissue pain; neuralgia.

Sportsman Rub *Salters, S.Afr.*
Capsicum oleoresin (p.1591·1); methyl nicotinate (p.55·1); methyl salicylate (p.55·1).
Musculoskeletal pain.

Sportsmega *Cantassium Co., UK.*
Multivitamin and mineral preparation (p.1350·1).

Sportupac N *Terra-Bio, Ger.*
Aesculus (p.1574·1); aescin (p.1574·1); heparin sodium (p.902·1).
Myopathy; soft-tissue injuries.

Sportsual *Permamed, Switz.*
Lauromacrogol 400 (p.1345·2); dimethyl sulfoxide (p.1402·2); heparin sodium (p.902·1); glycol salicylate (p.42·2); dexpanthenol (p.1602·3).
Soft-tissue trauma; superficial thrombophlebitis; varices.

Sportsual Spray sine heparino *Permamed, Switz.*
Lauromacrogol 400 (p.1345·2); dimethyl sulfoxide (p.1402·2); glycol salicylate (p.42·2); dexpanthenol (p.1602·3); menthol (p.1632·3); camphor (p.1589·3).
Soft-tissue disorders.

Sportz Sunscreen *Scott, Canad.*
SPF 15: Octinoxate (p.1517·3); octisalate (p.1518·1); oxybenzone (p.1518·1).
Sunscreen.

Spotof *CCD, Fr.*
Tranexamic acid (p.742·2).
Haemorrhage.

Spotoway *Food Supplement, UK.*
Chlorhexidine (p.1138·2).
Skin irritation and spots.

Spozal *Chong Kun Dang, Singapore.*
Ketoconazole (p.389·1).
Dandruff; fungal scalp infections.

Spray Auto-Bronzant *Clarins, Canad.*
SPF 15: Avobenzone (p.1517·1); octocrilene (p.1518·1); octinoxate (p.1517·3); octisalate (p.1518·1); oxybenzone (p.1518·1).
Sunscreen.

Spray Solaire Bronzage Rapide *Clarins, Canad.*
SPF 6: Avobenzone (p.1517·1); octinoxate (p.1517·3).
Sunscreen.

Spray Solaire Bronzage Securite *Clarins, Canad.*
SPF 15: Octocrilene (p.1518·1); octinoxate (p.1517·3); octisalate (p.1518·1); oxybenzone (p.1518·1).
Sunscreen.

Spraychrome *Beige, S.Afr.*
Merbromin (p.1150·1).
Minor wound disinfection.

Spray-n-Wake *Caprice Greystoke, USA†.*
Caffeine (p.761·3).

Spray-on Bande *Eagle, Austral.*
Povidone and vinyl acetate copolymer.
Plastic skin preparation for colostomies and ileostomies.

Spray-Pax *Pharmygiene, Fr.*
Pyrethrum (p.1436·3); piperonyl butoxide (p.1436·2).
Pediculosis.

Spray-Tish *Boehringer Ingelheim, Austral.*
Tramazoline hydrochloride (p.1102·1).
Nasal congestion.

Spray-ur-Cold *Caprice Greystoke, USA†.*
Phenylpropanolamine hydrochloride (p.1098·1); dextromethorphan (p.1087·3); chlorpheniramine [chlorphenamine] (p.412·2).

Spray-U-Thin *Caprice Greystoke, USA†.*
Phenylpropanolamine hydrochloride (p.1098·1).

Spregal
Note. This name is used for preparations of different composition.
Pharmygiene, Fr.; Medpro, S.Afr.
Esdepallethrine (p.1432·2); piperonyl butoxide (p.1436·2).
Scabies.

Wolff, Ger.
Bioallethrin (p.1428·3); piperonyl butoxide (p.1436·2).
Scabies.

Spren *Sigma, Austral.*
Aspirin (p.14·2).
Fever; inhibition of platelet aggregation; pain.

Spreor *Inava, Fr.*
Salbutamol (p.770·3).
Obstructive airways disease.

Sprilon *Smith & Nephew, Irl.; Smith & Nephew Healthcare, UK.*
Dimethicone (p.1410·1); zinc oxide (p.1128·2).
Barrier preparation; eczema; pressure sores; skin fissures; skin ulcers.

Sprinsol *Fortune, Hong Kong.*
Chlorpheniramine [chlorphenamine] maleate (p.412·1).
Hypersensitivity reactions.

SPS *Carolina, USA.*
Sodium polystyrene sulfonate (p.1023·2).
Hyperkalaemia.

S-P-T *Fleming, USA†.*
Thyroid (porcine) (p.1526·2).
Hypothyroidism; thyroid cancer.

SPZ *Douglas, NZ.*
Sulfinpyrazone (p.402·2).
Gout; thromboembolic disorders.

Squad *Irex, Fr.†.*
Flavodate sodium (p.1611·1).
Menorrhagia; peripheral vascular disorders.

Squamasol *Ichthyol, Aust.; Ichthyol, Ger.*
Salicylic acid (p.1122·3).
Scalp disorders.

Squa-med *Permamed, Switz.*
Pyrithione zinc (p.1122·1); sodium undecylamide MEA-sulfosuccinate; urea (p.1127·3).
Scalp disorders.

Squaphane *Saninter, Port.*
Lotion: Malic acid (p.1631·1); piroctone olamine (p.1121·1); cade oil (p.1124·3).

Shampoo: Malic acid (p.1631·1); resorcinol (p.1122·2); piroctone olamine (p.1121·1); cade oil (p.1124·3).
Scalp disorders.

Squibb-HC *Bristol-Myers Squibb, Austral.*
Hydrocortisone acetate (p.1073·3).
Skin disorders.

Sqworm *Norgine, Austral.†.*
Mebendazole (p.102·2).
Enterobiasis.

SRC Expectorant *Edwards, USA.*
Pseudoephedrine hydrochloride (p.1099·2); guaifenesin (p.1092·2); hydrocodone tartrate (p.42·2).
Coughs.

Srilane *Merck-Belgolabo, Belg.; Lipha Sante, Fr.; Lipha, Hong Kong.*
Idrocilamide (p.1329·2).
Skeletal muscle spasm; superficial phlebitis.

SRM-Rhotard *Alliance, S.Afr.; Ethical, Singapore.*
Morphine sulfate (p.56·1).
Pain.

SSD *Knoll, Canad.; Par, USA.*
Sulfadiazine silver (p.251·3).
Burns; wounds.

SSKI *Upsher-Smith, USA.*
Potassium iodide (p.1522·3).
Respiratory-tract disorders.

SST *Sinclair, UK.*
Sorbitol (p.1377·3); macrogol (p.1630·1); malic acid (p.1631·1); sodium citrate (p.1186·2).
Dry mouth.

SS-Tab *Alra, USA†.*
Sulfafurazole (p.253·1).

ST-52 *Asta Medica, Fr.*
Fosfestrol sodium (p.1478·3).
Prostatic cancer.

ST 37 *Menley & James, USA.*
Hexylresorcinol (p.1146·3).
Antiseptic.

St Bonifatius-Tee *Kolassa, Aust.*
Equisetum (p.1606·3); frangula bark (p.1227·1); senna leaf (p.1248·2); valerian root (p.1678·3); citrus auranti-

---

um; tilia flower (p.1673·2); boldo leaf (p.1585·3); juniper wood (p.1625·3); rhubarb (p.1248·1).
Diuretic; gastrointestinal motility disorders.

S-T Cort *Scot-Tussin, USA.*
Hydrocortisone (p.1073·3).
Skin disorders.

S-T Forte *Scot-Tussin, USA†.*
Hydrocodone tartrate (p.42·2); phenylephrine hydrochloride (p.1097·1); phenylpropanolamine hydrochloride (p.1098·1); pheniramine maleate (p.422·3); guaifenesin (p.1092·2).
Coughs and cold symptoms; nasal congestion.

S-T Forte 2 *Scot-Tussin, USA.*
Chlorpheniramine [chlorphenamine] maleate (p.412·1); hydrocodone tartrate (p.42·2).
Coughs and cold symptoms.

St. Jakobs-Balsam Mono *Riemser, Ger.*
Zinc oxide (p.1128·2).
Burns; skin disorders; wounds.

St James Balm *Medico-Biological Laboratories, UK.*
Zinc oxide (p.1128·2); ichthammol (p.1115·2); salicylic acid (p.1122·3); urea (p.1127·3).
Skin disorders.

St Johnswort Compound *Potter's, UK.*
Juniper oil (p.1625·2); hypericum (p.290·2); salix (p.82·1); cimicifuga (p.1595·2); skullcap (p.1664·3).
Sciatica.

St. Joseph Adult Chewable *Schering-Plough, USA.*
Aspirin (p.14·2).

St. Joseph Aspirin-Free for Children *Plough, USA†.*
Paracetamol (p.71·2).
Fever; pain.

St. Joseph Cold Tablets For Children *Schering-Plough, USA†.*
Phenylpropanolamine hydrochloride (p.1098·1); paracetamol (p.71·2).
Upper respiratory-tract symptoms.

St. Joseph Cough Suppressant *Schering-Plough, USA.*
Dextromethorphan hydrobromide (p.1087·3).
Coughs.

St Luke's Oil *British Dispensary, Thai.*
Methyl salicylate (p.55·1); menthol (p.1632·3); camphor (p.1589·3); thyme oil (p.1672·3).
Muscle pain; soft-tissue injury.

St Luke's Sports Oil *British Dispensary, Thai.*
Methyl salicylate (p.55·1); menthol (p.1632·3); camphor (p.1589·3); eucalyptus oil (p.1609·2).
Muscle pain; soft-tissue injury.

St Mary's Thistle Plus *Eagle, Austral.*
Silybum marianum (p.1021·3); myrtillus (p.1639·2); taraxacum (p.1669·1).
Liver tonic; peripheral vascular disorders; psoriasis.

St Radegunder Abfuhrtee mild *Synpharma, Aust.*
Prunus spinosa; cichorium intybus; fennel (p.1610·1); mallow flower.
Constipation.

St Radegunder Beruhigungs- und Einschlaftee *Synpharma, Aust.*
Valerian root (p.1678·3); lupulus (p.1629·3); citrus aurantium; melissa leaf (p.1632·2).
Anxiety disorders; sleep disorders.

St Radegunder Blahungstreibender Tee *Synpharma, Aust.*
Fennel (p.1610·1); caraway (p.1591·2); peppermint leaf (p.1243·2); chamomile flower (p.1593·2).
Dyspepsia; flatulence.

St Radegunder Bronchialtee *Synpharma, Aust.*
Fennel (p.1610·1); thyme (p.1672·2); eucalyptus leaf (p.1609·2); veronica officinalis; verbascum flower.
Catarrh.

St Radegunder Entschlackungs-Elixier *Synpharma, Aust.*
Taraxacum (p.1669·1); pansy; manna (p.1233·3); bitter orange peel (p.1644·2); rose fruit (p.1389·3).
Diuretic.

St Radegunder Entwasserungs-Elixier *Synpharma, Aust.*
Silver birch (p.1585·2); equisetum (p.1606·3); urtica (p.1678·2).
Urinary-tract disorders.

St Radegunder Entwasserungstee *Synpharma, Aust.*
Ononis root (p.1644·1); silver birch (p.1585·2); equisetum (p.1606·3); urtica (p.1678·2).
Urinary-tract disorders.

St Radegunder Fiebertee *Synpharma, Aust.*
Tilia flower (p.1673·2); sambucus flower (p.1660·3); chamomile flower (p.1593·2); melissa leaf (p.1632·2).
Cold symptoms.

St Radegunder Herz-Kreislauf-Tonikum *Synpharma, Aust.*
Crataegus (p.1600·2); melissa leaf (p.1632·2); rosemary leaf.
Cardiac disorders.

St Radegunder Herz-Kreislauf-unterstutzender Tee *Synpharma, Aust.*
Crataegus (p.1600·2); rosemary leaf; melissa leaf (p.1632·2); lavender flower (p.1627·2).
Cardiac disorders.

St Radegunder Hustentee *Synpharma, Aust.*
Wild thyme; plantago lanceolata; althaea (p.1577·1); galeopsis ochroleuca; mallow flower.
Coughs.

St Radegunder Leber-Galle-Tee *Synpharma, Aust.*
Cichorium intybus root; taraxacum (p.1669·1); marrubium vulgare root (p.1094·2); peppermint leaf (p.1243·2).
Gastrointestinal and biliary-tract disorders.

St Radegunder Magenberuhigungstee *Synpharma, Aust.*
Melissa leaf (p.1632·2); peppermint leaf (p.1243·2); fennel fruit (p.1610·1); mallow flower.
Gastrointestinal disorders.

St Radegunder Nerventee *Synpharma, Aust.*
Melissa leaf (p.1632·2); valerian root (p.1678·3); lupulus (p.1629·3); delphinium consolida flower.
Nervous disorders; sleep disorders.

St Radegunder Nerven-Tonikum *Synpharma, Aust.*
Valerian root (p.1678·3); lupulus (p.1629·3); melissa leaf (p.1632·2).
Nervous disorders; sleep disorders.

St Radegunder Nierentee *Synpharma, Aust.*
Bearberry (p.1583·3); equisetum (p.1606·3); herniaria (p.1619·2); ononis (p.1644·1).
Urinary-tract disorders.

St Radegunder Reizmildernder Magentee *Synpharma, Aust.*
Chamomile flower (p.1593·2); mallow; fennel (p.1610·1); melissa leaf (p.1632·2).
Gastrointestinal disorders.

St Radegunder Rosmarin-Wein *Synpharma, Aust.*
Rosemary leaf; melissa leaf (p.1632·2).
Circulatory disorders.

St Radegunder Tee gegen Durchfall *Synpharma, Aust.*
Hamamelis leaf (p.1618·3); strawberry; chamomile flower (p.1593·2); juglans regia; fennel (p.1610·1).
Diarrhoea.

St Radegunder Thorasan-Krauterhustensaft *Synpharma, Aust.*
Cowslip root (p.1600·1); thyme (p.1672·2); plantago lanceolata.
Catarrh; coughs.

St Radegunder Verdauungstee *Synpharma, Aust.*
Absinthium (p.1571·2); centaury (p.1593·1); bitter orange peel (p.1644·2); caraway (p.1591·2); gentian root (p.1615·1).
Gastrointestinal disorders.

Stabicilline *Vifor, Switz.*
Phenoxymethylpenicillin potassium (p.235·1).
Bacterial infections.

Stablon *Ardix, Fr.; Sanfer, Mex.; Servier, Port.; Servier, Thai.*
Tianeptine (p.309·2) or tianeptine sodium (p.309·2).
Depression; mixed anxiety depressive states.

Stacer *Atral, Port.*
Ranitidine hydrochloride (p.1245·2).
Gastro-oesophageal reflux; peptic ulcer.

Stacho-Zym N *Kattwiga, Ger.†.*
Pancreatin (p.1646·1); enzymes from Aspergillus.
Digestive system disorders.

Stacort-A *Standard, Hong Kong.*
Triamcinolone acetonide (p.1080·1).
Corticosteroid.

Stadaglicin *Stada, Hong Kong; Stada, Singapore; Stada, Thai.*
Sodium cromoglicate (p.774·3).
Allergic rhinitis; conjunctivitis.

Stadalax *Stada, Ger.*
Bisacodyl (p.1212·2).
Constipation.

Stadol *Bristol-Myers Squibb, Canad.; Bristol-Myers Squibb, Israel; Bristol-Myers Squibb, Mex.; Bristol-Myers Squibb, USA; Cephalon, USA.*
Butorphanol (p.22·3) or butorphanol tartrate (p.22·2).
Pain.

Staficilin N *Bristol-Myers Squibb, Braz.*
Oxacillin sodium (p.233·2).
Bacterial infections.

Staficyn *FIRMA, Ital.*
Meticillin sodium (p.223·3).
Staphylococcal infections.

Stafilon *AGIPS, Ital.*
Methacycline hydrochloride (p.222·3).
Bacterial infections.

Staflocil *Orion, Fin.*
Cloxacillin sodium (p.192·1).
Bacterial infections.

Stafoxil *Yamanouchi, Irl.†; Yamanouchi, Neth.; Yamanouchi, UK†.*
Flucloxacillin sodium (p.207·1).
Bacterial infections.

Stagesic *Huckaby, USA.*
Hydrocodone tartrate (p.42·2); paracetamol (p.71·2).
Pain.

Stagid *Lipha Sante, Fr.; Merck, Port.*
Metformin embonate (p.332·3).
Diabetes mellitus.

Stago *Synthelabo, Switz.*
Greater celandine (p.1618·1); turmeric (p.1029·3); cynara scolymus (p.1601·3); boldo (p.1585·3).
Biliary-tract disorders; constipation; nausea.

Stahist *Huckaby, USA.*
Pseudoephedrine hydrochloride (p.1099·2); phenylephrine hydrochloride (p.1097·1); chlorpheniramine [chlorphenamine] maleate (p.412·1); hyoscyamine sulfate (p.469·3); hyoscine hydrobromide (p.468·2); atropine sulfate (p.461·1).

Formerly contained phenylpropanolamine hydrochloride, phenylephrine hydrochloride, chlorpheniramine [chlorphenamine] maleate, hyoscyamine sulfate, hyoscine hydrobromide, and atropine sulfate.
Upper respiratory-tract symptoms.

Stalcin *Locatelli, Ital.†.*
Salcatonin (p.749·3).
Hypercalcaemia; osteoporosis; Paget's disease.

Stallergenes MRV *Stallergenes, Fr.†.*
Staphylococcus aureus; Staphylococcus albus; Streptococcus spp.; Streptococcus pneumoniae; Haemophilus influenzae; Klebsiella pneumoniae; Moraxella catarrhalis.
Respiratory-tract infections.

Staloral *Stallergenes, Ital.; Stallergenes, Switz.*
Allergen extracts (p.1575·3).
Hyposensitisation.

Staltor *Bayer, Fr.†.*
Cerivastatin (p.856·1).
Hypercholesterolaemia.

Stamaril *CSL, Austral.; Pasteur Merieux, Belg.; Pasteur Merieux, Denm.; Meda, Fin.; Pasteur Vaccins, Fr.; Pasteur Merieux, Ger.; Aventis, Irl.; Pasteur Merieux, Ital.; Pasteur Merieux, Neth.; Pasteur Merieux, Norw.; Aventis, S.Afr.; Pasteur Merieux, Singapore; Pasteur Merieux, Swed.; Pro Vaccine, Switz.; Aventis, UK.*
A yellow fever vaccine (17D strain) (p.1568·3).
Active immunisation.

Stamina *Chi Sheng, Thai.*
Vitamin B substances with glucose (p.1350·1).

Stamoist E *Huckaby, USA.*
Pseudoephedrine hydrochloride (p.1099·2); guaifenesin (p.1092·2).
Coughs.

Stamoist LA *Huckaby, USA†.*
Phenylpropanolamine hydrochloride (p.1098·1); guaifenesin (p.1092·2).
Coughs and cold symptoms; nasal congestion.

Stancare *Stanley, Canad.†.*
Wool fat (p.1410·3); liquid paraffin (p.1407·1).

Standacillin *Biochemie, Aust.; Biochemie, Singapore.*
Ampicillin sodium (p.150·3) or ampicillin trihydrate (p.151·1).
Bacterial infections.

Standard III *Aguettant, Fr.*
Electrolyte preparation (p.1180·1).
Parenteral nutrition.

Stangyl *Rhone-Poulenc Rorer, Aust.; Rhone-Poulenc Rorer, Ger.*
Trimipramine (p.311·2), trimipramine maleate (p.311·2), or trimipramine mesilate (p.311·3).
Depression; pain.

Stanhexidine *Stanley, Canad.*
Chlorhexidine (p.1138·2).

Stanilo *Pharmacia Upjohn, Ger.*
Spectinomycin hydrochloride (p.248·2).
Gonorrhoea.

Stanno-Bardane *Pharmacobel, Belg.†.*
Tin (p.1673·2); lappa (p.1627·1).
Staphylococcal infections.

Stapenor *Bayer, Aust.; Bayer, Ger.*
Oxacillin sodium (p.233·2).
Staphylococcal infections.

Staphcillin *Apothecon, USA†.*
Meticillin sodium (p.223·3).
Bacterial infections.

Staphlex *Pacific, NZ.; Alphapharm, Singapore; Merck, Singapore.*
Flucloxacillin (p.207·1) or flucloxacillin sodium (p.207·1).
Bacterial infections.

Staphycid *SmithKline Beecham, Belg.*
Flucloxacillin magnesium (p.207·1) or flucloxacillin sodium (p.207·1).
Bacterial infections.

Staphylase *Prima, Braz.*
Dried yeast (p.1398·1); white wine; glycerol.
Digestive disorders.

Staphylex *Alphapharm, Austral.; SmithKline Beecham, Ger.*
Flucloxacillin magnesium (p.207·1) or flucloxacillin sodium (p.207·1).
Bacterial infections.

Staphylomycine *SmithKline Beecham, Fr.†.*
Virginiamycin (p.269·3).
Bacterial infections.

Staphypan *Berna, Switz.*
Staphylococci.
Staphylococcal infections.

Staporos *Hoechst Marion Roussel, Braz.*
Calcitonin (pork) (p.749·2).
Hypercalcaemia; osteoporosis; Paget's disease of bone.

Starasid *Kayaku, Jpn†.*
Cytarabine ocfosfate (p.531·1).
Malignant neoplasms.

Starcef *FIRMA, Ital.*
Ceftazidime (p.174·3).
Bacterial infections.

Starem *Hoechst, Fr.*
Dextropropoxyphene hydrochloride (p.27·1); paracetamol (p.71·2).
Pain.

Staril Squibb, UK.
Fosinopril sodium (p.892·3).
Heart failure; hypertension.

Starkungs- und Kraftigungstee Sanova, Aust.
Achillea bitter orange peel; gentian; rosemary leaf; rose fruit.
Tonic.

Starlep Farma Lepori, Spain.
Metoclopramide glycyrrhizinate (p.1236·3); sodium bicarbonate (p.1186·2); tartaric acid (p.1669·2).
Gastritis, nausea; gastrointestinal hyperacidity; hepatobiliary disorders; vomiting.

Starlix Novartis, UK; Novartis, USA.
Nateglinide (p.333·2).
Diabetes mellitus.

Starogyn Leiras, Fin.
Broxyquinoline.
Vaginal infections.

Star-Otic Stellar, USA.
Glacial acetic acid (p.1571·2); aluminium acetate (p.1578·1); boric acid (p.1586·1).
Ear infection.

Star-Pen Tyrol, Aust.
Benzathine phenoxymethylpenicillin (p.157·1) or phenoxymethylpenicillin potassium (p.235·1).
Bacterial infections.

Startonyl Wyeth Lederle, Aust.; Seber, Port.
Citicoline (p.1596·1).
Cerebrovascular disorders; head injury.

Stas Akut Stada, Ger.†.
Acetylcysteine (p.1082·3).
Respiratory-tract disorders with excess mucus.

stas Erkaltungssalbe Stada, Ger.
Camphor (p.1589·3); eucalyptus oil (p.1609·2); pine needle oil.
Cold symptoms.

stas Erkaltungssalbe mild Stada, Ger.
Eucalyptus oil (p.1609·2); pine needle oil.
Cold symptoms.

Stas Gurgellosung Stada, Ger.†
Hexetidine (p.1146·3).
Inflammatory disorders and infections of the oropharynx.

stas Halsschmerz-Tabletten Stada, Ger.
Cetylpyridinium chloride(p.1138·1); dequalinium chloride (p.1143·1).
Bacterial infections of the mouth and throat.

stas Nasentropfen, Nasenspray Stada, Ger.
Xylometazoline hydrochloride (p.1102·2).
Nasal congestion; rhinitis.

stas-Hustenloser Stada, Ger.
Ambroxol hydrochloride (p.1084·3).
Respiratory-tract disorders associated with increased or viscous mucus.

stas-Hustenstiller N Stada, Ger.
Clobutinol hydrochloride (p.1087·1).
Coughs.

Statcillin Pharmador, S.Afr.†.
Ampicillin trihydrate (p.151·1).
Bacterial infections.

Stat-Crit Wampole, USA.
Test for haematocrit/haemoglobin measurement.

Statex Paladin, Canad.; Pharmascience, Singapore.
Morphine sulfate (p.56·1).
Pain.

Staticin Westwood-Squibb, Canad.; Westwood, USA.
Erythromycin (p.201·2).
Acne.

Staticine Bristol-Myers Squibb, Switz.
Erythromycin (p.201·2).
Acne.

Staticum Uriach, Spain.
Glisentide (p.323·2).
Diabetes mellitus.

Statiflex G Braun, Switz.
Electrolyte infusion with glucose (p.1180·1).
Carbohydrate source; fluid and electrolyte disorders.

Statinclyne Cazi, Braz.
Tetracycline hydrochloride (p.258·3).
Bacterial infections.

Stativa Chiesi, Ital.
Cerivastatin sodium (p.856·1).
Hypercholesterolaemia.

Statrol
Note.This name is used for preparations of different composition.
Alcon, Belg.; Alcon, Thai.
Neomycin sulfate (p.228·1); polymyxin B sulfate (p.238·1).
Bacterial eye infections.

Alcon Cusi, Spain.
Neomycin sulfate (p.228·1); polymyxin B sulfate (p.238·1); phenylphrine hydrochloride (p.1097·1).
Eye infections.

Statuss Expectorant Huckaby, USA†.
Phenylpropanolamine hydrochloride (p.1098·1); codeine phosphate (p.25·2); guaifenesin (p.1092·2).
Coughs.

Statuss Green Huckaby, USA†.
Pheniramine maleate (p.422·3); mepyramine maleate (p.421·1); phenylephrine hydrochloride (p.1097·1);

phenylpropanolamine hydrochloride (p.1098·1); hydrocodone tartrate (p.42·2).
Coughs and cold symptoms.

Staurodorm Modasa, Belg.
Flurazepam (p.685·3).
Insomnia.

Staurodorm Neu Dolorgiet, Ger.
Flurazepam (p.685·3).
Sleep disorders.

Stay Alert Apothecary, USA.
Caffeine (p.761·3).
Fatigue.

Stay Moist Lip Conditioner Stanback, USA†.
Padimate O (p.1518·2); oxybenzone (p.1518·1); aloe vera (p.1110·1); vitamin E (p.1393·3).
Skin disorders.

Stay Trim Schering-Plough, USA†.
Phenylpropanolamine (p.1098·1).

Stay-Wet 3 Sherman, USA.
Cleansing, wetting, and soaking solution for gas permeable contact lenses (p.1129·2).

Stay-Wet 4 Sherman, USA.
Wetting solutions for hard contact lenses (p.1129·2).

STD Faulding, Austral.†; Intramed, S.Afr.†.
Sodium tetradecyl sulfate (p.1497·2).
Varicose veins.

Steclin Bristol-Myers Squibb, Aust.†.
Tetracycline hydrochloride (p.258·3).

Stediril
Note.This name is used for preparations of different composition.
Wyeth Lederle, Belg.†; Wyeth Lederle, Fr.; Wyeth, Ger.
Norgestrel (p.1486·1); ethinylestradiol (p.1476·2).
Combined oral contraceptive; endometriosis; menstrual disorders.

Wyeth, Neth.
Levonorgestrel (p.1486·2); ethinylestradiol (p.1476·2).
Combined oral contraceptive.

Stediril 30
Wyeth Lederle, Belg.; Wyeth, Ger.; Wyeth, Switz.
Levonorgestrel (p.1486·2); ethinylestradiol (p.1476·2).
28-Day packs also contain 7 inert tablets.
Combined oral contraceptive.

Stediril D
Wyeth Lederle, Aust.; Wyeth Lederle, Belg., Ger.; Wyeth, Switz.
Levonorgestrel (p.1486·2); ethinylestradiol (p.1476·2).
Combined oral contraceptive; endometriosis; menstrual disorders.

Steicardin N Steigerwald, Ger.
Homoeopathic preparation.

Steicorton Steigerwald, Ger.
Crataegus (p.1600·2).
Heart failure.

Steigal Steigerwald, Ger.
Turmeric (p.1029·3); greater celandine (p.1618·1).
Biliary colic.

Steiprostat Steigerwald, Ger.
Saw palmetto (p.1491·2).
Benign prostatic hyperplasia.

Steirocall Steierl, Ger.
Homoeopathic preparation.

Steiroplex Steierl, Ger.
Homoeopathic preparation.

Steitonit Lopes, Braz.
Podophyllum (p.1121·1); rhubarb (p.1248·1); senna (p.1248·2); olive oil (p.1643·3); peppermint leaf (p.1243·2); castor oil (p.1592·1).
Calculi.

Stelabid Procter & Gamble, Aust.†; SmithKline Beecham, Canad.; SmithKline Beecham, Irl.; SmithKline Beecham, Mex.; SmithKline Beecham, S.Afr.†.
Isopropamide iodide (p.470·1); trifluoperazine hydrochloride (p.710·3).
Gastrointestinal disorders.

Stelapar Enila, Braz.
Trifluoperazine hydrochloride (p.710·3); tranylcypromine hydrochloride (p.309·3).
Psychoses.

Stelazine SmithKline Beecham, Austral.; Enila, Braz.; SmithKline Beecham, Braz.; SmithKline Beecham, Canad.; Goldshield, Irl.; SmithKline Beecham, Mex.; SmithKline Beecham, NZ; SmithKline Beecham, S.Afr.; SmithKline Beecham, UK; SmithKline Beecham, USA.
Trifluoperazine hydrochloride (p.710·3).
Agitation; alcohol withdrawal syndrome; anxiety; nausea and vomiting; psychoses.

Stella Jean-Marie, Hong Kong.
Prochlorperazine mesilate (p.701·2).
Anxiety; nausea.

Stellamicina Pierrel, Ital.†.
Erythromycin estolate (p.201·2).
Bacterial infections.

Stellatropine Stella, Belg.
Atropine sulfate (p.461·1).
Arrhythmias; cholinesterase inhibitor intoxication; premedication.

Stellisept Beiersdorf, Switz.
Orthophenylphenol (p.1152·1); sodium laurilsulfate (p.1496·3).
Skin and hand disinfection.

Stellorphinad Stella, Belg.
Morphine hydrochloride (p.56·1).
Pain.

Stellorphine Stella, Belg.
Morphine hydrochloride (p.56·1).
Acute pulmonary oedema; pain; premedication; severe trauma.

Stemetil Rhone-Poulenc Rorer, Austral.; Rhone-Poulenc Rorer, Canad.; Aventis, Denm.; Rhone-Poulenc Rorer, Fin.; Rhone-Poulenc Rorer, Hong Kong; Rhone-Poulenc Rorer, Irl.; Rhone-Poulenc Rorer, Ital.; Rhone-Poulenc Rorer, Neth.; Rhone-Poulenc Rorer, Norw.; Aventis, NZ; Aventis, S.Afr.; Rhone-Poulenc Rorer, Singapore; Rhone-Poulenc Rorer, Swed.; Rhone-Poulenc Rorer, Thai.; Castlemead, UK.
Prochlorperazine (p.701·1), prochlorperazine maleate (p.701·2), or prochlorperazine mesilate (p.701·2).
Alcohol and opioid withdrawal syndromes; anxiety; migraine; nausea and vomiting; psychoses; vestibular disorders.

Stemgen Amgen, Austral.
Ancestim.
Mobilisation of autologous peripheral blood progenitor cells.

Stemzine Rhone-Poulenc Rorer, Austral.
Prochlorperazine maleate (p.701·2).
Nausea and vomiting; vertigo.

Sten Atlantis, Mex.
Prasterone (p.1488·2); testosterone propionate (p.1492·2); testosterone cipionate (p.1492·1).
Androgenic; breast cancer; erectile dysfunction; hypogonadism.

Stenobronchial Giovanardi, Ital.
Sulfogaiacol (p.1101·1); wild thyme; tolu balsam (p.1101·3).
Coughs, catarrh.

Stenocrat Schwabe, Ger.
Ammi visnaga fruit (p.1579·1); crataegus leaves, flowers, and fruit (p.1600·2).
Angina pectoris.

steno-loges N Loges, Ger.
Ammi visnaga (p.1579·1).
Cardiac disorders; obstructive airways disease.

Stenoptin Knoll, Ger.†.
Verapamil hydrochloride (p.989·1); isosorbide dinitrate (p.915·2).
Cardiac disorders.

Stenox Atlantis, Mex.
Fluoxymesterone (p.1478·2).
Androgenic; erectile dysfunction; hypogonadism.

Steocar Christiaens, Belg.
Calcium carbonate (p.1215·1).
Calcium deficiency; calcium supplement; osteoporosis.

Steocin SoSe, Ital.
Salcatonin (p.749·3).
Hypercalcaemia; osteoporosis; Paget's disease of bone.

Step 2
Note.This name is used for preparations of different composition.
Candioli, Ital.
Extract of Triticum sativum.
Aid to removal of lice eggs.

GenDerm, USA†.
Benzyl alcohol (p.1135·2); formic acid (p.1612·3).
Aid to removal of lice eggs.

Sterac
Note.This name is used for preparations of different composition.
Ivex, UK.
Sterile water (p.1680·2).
Diluent for antiseptic solutions; wounds.

Ivex, UK.
Sodium chloride (p.1196·1).
Irrigation solution.

Steramin Formenti, Ital.
Benzalkonium chloride (p.1133·2).
Disinfection of wounds, burns, and mucous membranes.

Steramina G Formenti, Ital.
Benzalkonium chloride (p.1133·2).
Disinfection of wounds, burns, vagina, hands, instruments, surfaces, and skin.

Steranabol Ritardo Pharmacia Upjohn, Ital.†.
Oxabolone cipionate (p.1487·2).
Osteoporosis.

Steranios Anios, Fr.
Glutaral (p.1145·2).
Instrument disinfection.

Sterapred Merz, USA.
Prednisone (p.1079·2).
Corticosteroid.

Sterax Galderma, Belg.; Galderma, Ger.; Galderma, Switz.
Desonide (p.1066·2).
Skin disorders.

Ster-Dex Ciba Vision, Fr.
Oxytetracycline (p.234·1); dexamethasone (p.1067·1).
Eye disorders.

Sterecyt Pharmacia, Swed.†.
Prednimustine (p.566·2).
Malignant neoplasms.

Sterets SSL, UK.
Isopropyl alcohol (p.1149·2).
Skin disinfection.

Sterets H Seton, Israel; SSL, UK.
Isopropyl alcohol (p.1149·2); chlorhexidine acetate (p.1138·2) or chlorhexidine gluconate (p.1138·2).
Skin disinfection.

Sterets Unisept SSL, UK.
Chlorhexidine gluconate (p.1138·2).
Skin disinfection.

Sterex International Dermatologicals, Canad.
Coal tar (p.1125·1); salicylic acid (p.1122·3); sulfur (p.1123·3).

Sterexidine Ivex, UK.
Chlorhexidine gluconate (p.1138·2).
Antiseptic irrigation solution.

Steridol Biocure, Ital.
Chlorhexidine gluconate (p.1138·2); cetrimide (p.1137·1).
Disinfection.

Steridrolo Molteni, Ital.
Tosylchloramide sodium (p.1159·1).
Disinfection of wounds, burns, and external genitals.

Steridrolo a rapida idrolisi Molteni, Ital.
Halazone (p.1145·3).
Water purification.

Sterigel SSL, UK.
Hemicellulose (p.1500·2).
Ulcers; wounds.

Sterijet Seton, UK†.
Sodium chloride (p.1196·1).
Wound irrigation.

Steril Zeta Zeta, Ital.
Cream: Triclosan (p.1159·2); usnic acid (p.1678·2); hamamelis (p.1618·3); cod-liver oil (p.1357·2).
Insect stings; wound disinfection.
Topical powder: Triclosan (p.1159·2); usnic acid (p.1678·2); zinc oxide (p.1128·2); zinc stearate (p.1497·3).
Wound disinfection.

Sterilent SIFI, Ital.†.
Sterilising solution for hard contact lenses (p.1129·2).

Sterilite Coventry, UK.
Tar acids (p.1158·1).

Sterilix Restiva, Ital.†.
Benzalkonium chloride (p.1133·2).
Disinfection wounds and burns.

Sterillium Bode, Aust.; Rivadis, Fr.; Bode, Ger.
Mecetronium etilsulfate (p.1150·1); isopropyl alcohol (p.1149·2); propyl alcohol (p.1155·3).
Skin disinfection.

Sterillium Virugard Bode, Ger.
Alcohol (p.1130·3).
Hand disinfection.

Sterilon Boots Healthcare, Belg.; Boots Healthcare, Neth.; Boots, Spain†.
Chlorhexidine gluconate (p.1138·2) or chlorhexidine hydrochloride (p.1138·2).
Skin and wound disinfection.

Sterilys B 84 Pharmalink, Swed.†.
Electrolyte solution (p.1184·1).
Haemodialysis.

Sterimar Fumouze, Fr.; Intra Pharma, Irl.; Fumouze, Israel; Asta Medica, Port.; Carter-Wallace, UK.
Sea water (p.1196·1).
Nasal hygiene.

Sterimycine Ciba Vision, Fr.
Kanamycin sulfate (p.218·1); polymyxin B sulfate (p.238·1).
Eye infections.

SteriNail Dr. Nordyke, USA†.
Undecenoic acid (p.395·3); tolnaftate (p.395·2).
Fungal nail infections.

Steri-Neb Cromogen Norton Waterford, Irl.
Sodium cromoglicate (p.774·3).
Asthma.

Steri-Neb Salamol Norton Waterford, Irl.
Salbutamol sulfate (p.770·3).
Obstructive airways disease.

Sterinet Consol, Ital.
Cetylpyridinium chloride (p.1138·1).
Skin and hand disinfection.

Sterinor Heumann, Ger.; ABC, Ital.†.
Co-tetroxazine (p.193·2).
Bacterial infections.

Sterinova Medentech, Irl.†.
Sodium dichloroisocyanurate (p.1156·1).
Sterilisation of infant feeding equipment.

Steripaste SSL, UK.
Zinc oxide (p.1128·2).
Ulcers.

Steripod Blue SSL, UK.
Sodium chloride (p.1196·1).
Irrigation solution.

Steripod Chlorhexidine Gluconate SSL, UK.
Chlorhexidine gluconate (p.1138·2).
Formerly known as Steripod Pink.
Skin disinfection.

Steripod Chlorhexidine Gluconate with Cetrimide SSL, UK.
Chlorhexidine gluconate (p.1138·2); cetrimide (p.1137·1).
Formerly known as Steripod Yellow.
Skin disinfection.

Sterisol Warner-Lambert, NZ.
Hexetidine (p.1146·3).
Mouth and throat infections.

Steri/Sol Warner-Lambert, Canad.
Hexetidine (p.1146·3).
Mouth and throat disorders.

The symbol † denotes a preparation no longer actively marketed

Stomagel N *CPF, Ger.*
Aluminium hydroxide gel (p.1210·3); magnesium oxide (p.1233·2).
Gastritis; gastrointestinal hyperacidity; peptic ulcer.

Stomahesive
Note. This name is used for preparations of different composition.
Convatec, Austral.
Topical paste: Butyl monoester polymer with ethanol.
Colostomies and ileostomies.
Convatec, Austral.; Bristol-Myers Squibb, NZ; Convatec, UK.
Topical wafer: Carmellose sodium (p.1499·3); gelatin (p.737·2); pectin (p.1502·3); polyisobutylene.
Stoma care.
Convatec, Fr.
Barrier paste.
Fistulae; stoma care.

Stomakon *Searle, Braz.*
Cimetidine (p.1216·3).
Acid aspiration; gastro-oesophageal reflux; gastrointestinal haemorrhage; peptic ulcer; Zollinger-Ellison syndrome.

Stomasal Med *Mauermann, Ger.*
Aluminium hydroxide (p.1210·3); magnesium oxide (p.1233·2); lupulus (p.1629·3); peppermint leaf (p.1243·2); agrimony (p.1574·3); calamus (p.1588·1); chlorophyllin (p.1028·1).
Gastrointestinal disorders.

Stomax *Hope, USA†.*
Bismuth subgallate (p.1213·2).
Control of ostomy odour.

Stomedine *SmithKline Beecham Sante, Fr.*
Cimetidine (p.1216·3).
Gastro-oesophageal reflux.

Stomet *Farmoquimica, Braz.; Sark, Ital.*
Cimetidine (p.1216·3).
Gastro-oesophageal reflux; gastrointestinal haemorrhage; peptic ulcer; Zollinger-Ellison syndrome.

Stomidros *Stomygen, Ital.†*
Calcium hydroxide (p.1588·3).
Dental capping; infection of the dental canal.

Stomigen *Steiner, Ger.*
Magnesium hydroxide (p.1233·1); calcium carbonate (p.1215·1).
Gastrointestinal hyperacidity; peptic ulcer.

Stomosan *Vicente, Spain.*
Bismuth subnitrate (p.1213·2); marrubium vulgare (p.1094·2); sodium bromide (p.1587·1); sodium citrate (p.1186·2).
Gastritis; gastrointestinal hyperacidity; peptic ulcer.

Stomygen *Stomygen, Ital.*
Sodium monofluorophosphate (p.1377·2); cetylpyridinium chloride (p.1138·1).
Oral hygiene.

Stongel *Cazi, Braz.*
Aluminium hydroxide (p.1210·3); magnesium hydroxide (p.1233·1).
Gastrointestinal hyperacidity.

Stop
Oral-B, UK.; Oral-B, USA.
Stannous fluoride (p.1379·3).
Dental caries prophylaxis.

Stop Espinilla Normaderm *Capilares, Spain.*
Benzoyl peroxide (p.1111·1).
Acne.

Stop Hemo
Brothier, Fr.; Brothier, Switz.†; G-B-M, UK†.
Calcium alginate (p.728·1).
Superficial haemorrhage.

Stop Itch *Dermatech, Austral.*
Papain (p.1647·3).
Insect bites; jelly fish stings; minor burns; skin rashes.

Stopain
Note. This name is used for preparations of different composition.
Mundogen, Spain.
Paracetamol (p.71·2).
Fever; pain.
Chew, Thai.
Cream: Methyl salicylate (p.55·1); menthol (p.1632·3); eugenol (p.1609·3); thymol (p.1158·3); eucalyptus oil (p.1609·2); turpentine oil (p.1676·3).
Topical gel: Menthol (p.1632·3).
Musculoskeletal pain.

Stopayne *Adcock Ingram, S.Afr.*
Syrup: Paracetamol (p.71·2); codeine phosphate (p.25·2); promethazine hydrochloride (p.423·2).
Tablets; capsules: Paracetamol (p.71·2); codeine phosphate (p.25·2); caffeine (p.761·3); meprobamate (p.691·1).
Fever; pain.

Stopcold *Vedim, Spain.*
Cetirizine hydrochloride (p.411·2); pseudoephedrine hydrochloride (p.1099·2).
Allergic rhinitis.

Stopex *Medical, Port.*
Sulfathiazole (p.257·1).
Vaginal infections.

Stopit *Rafa, Israel.*
Loperamide hydrochloride (p.1231·3).
Diarrhoea.

Stopitch *Restan, S.Afr.*
Hydrocortisone acetate (p.1073·3).
Skin disorders.

Stoppers *Charwell Pharmaceuticals, UK.*
Nicotine (p.1640·3).
Aid to smoking withdrawal.

Storzfen *Lederle, USA†.*
Phenylephrine hydrochloride (p.1097·1).
Aid in eye examination; glaucoma; production of mydriasis.

Storzine *Lederle, USA†.*
Pilocarpine hydrochloride (p.1422·3).
Glaucoma; production of miosis; raised intra-ocular pressure.

Storz-N-D *Lederle, USA†.*
Neomycin (p.228·1); dexamethasone sodium phosphate (p.1067·1).
Infected eye disorders.

Storz-N-P-D *Lederle, USA†.*
Neomycin (p.228·1); polymyxin B (p.238·3); dexamethasone (p.1067·1).
Infected eye disorders.

Storz-Sulf *Lederle, USA†.*
Sulfacetamide sodium (p.250·3).
Eye infections.

Stovalid N *Cesra, Ger.*
Peppermint leaf (p.1243·2); absinthium (p.1571·1); fennel (p.1610·1); chamomile (p.1593·2); aniseed (p.1580·2); caraway (p.1591·2); angelica root (p.1580·2); calamus root (p.1588·1); gentian root (p.1615·1).
Appetite loss; dyspepsia.

Stoxil
Dermatech, Austral.; ICN, Hong Kong; ICN, Singapore.
Idoxuridine (p.625·1).
Herpes simplex infections of the skin and mucous membranes.

Strafortin *Strathmann, Ger.*
Calcium carbonate (p.1215·1); colecalciferol (p.1391·1).
Osteoporosis.

Strains Ointment *Nelson, UK.*
Homoeopathic preparation.

Stranoval *Teofarma, Ital.*
Betamethasone valerate (p.1063·2); dextran sulfate (p.1603·1).
Peripheral vascular disorders; soft-tissue disorders.

Stratene *Gerda, Fr.*
Cetiedil citrate (p.856·3).
Intermittent claudication.

Strefen *Crookes Healthcare, UK.*
Flurbiprofen (p.41·2).
Sore throat.

Strength *Potter's, UK.*
Damiana (p.1602·1); kola (p.1681·1); saw palmetto (p.1491·2).
Tonic.

Strepfen
Boots, Austral.; Boots, NZ.
Flurbiprofen (p.41·2).
Sore throat.

Strepsils
Boots, Austral.; Boots Healthcare, Belg.; Schering-Plough, Canad.; Boots, Denm.; Boots, Fin.; Boots Healthcare, Fr.; Boots, Hong Kong; Boots Healthcare, Irl.; Boots, Israel; Boots Healthcare, Neth.; Boots, NZ; Boots, S.Afr.; Boots, Singapore; Boots Healthcare, Spain; Astra, Swed.; Crookes Healthcare, UK.
Dichlorobenzyl alcohol (p.1143·2); amylmetacresol (p.1133·2).
Sore throat.

Strepsils I *Schering-Plough, Canad.*
Amylmetacresol (p.1133·2).
Sore throat.

Strepsils Anaesthetic *Boots, Austral.†.*
Lignocaine [lidocaine] hydrochloride (p.1313·2); dichlorobenzyl alcohol (p.1143·2); amylmetacresol (p.1133·2).
Mouth ulcers; sore throat.

Strepsils con Anestesico *Boots Healthcare, Spain.*
Dichlorobenzyl alcohol (p.1143·2); amylmetacresol (p.1133·2); lignocaine [lidocaine] (p.1313·2).
Mouth and throat disorders.

Strepsils con Vitamina C *Boots Healthcare, Spain.*
Sodium ascorbate (p.1390·1); ascorbic acid (p.1389·3); dichlorobenzyl alcohol (p.1143·2); amylmetacresol (p.1133·2).
Sore throat.

Strepsils Cough
Boots, NZ; Crookes Healthcare, UK.
Dextromethorphan hydrobromide (p.1087·3).
Coughs.

Strepsils Cough Relief *Boots, Austral.*
Dextromethorphan hydrobromide (p.1087·3).
Coughs.

Strepsils Dual Action
Boots Healthcare, Irl.; Boots, Singapore.
Amylmetacresol (p.1133·2); dichlorobenzyl alcohol (p.1143·2); lignocaine [lidocaine] (p.1313·2) or lignocaine [lidocaine] hydrochloride (p.1313·2).
Sore throat.

Strepsils Eucalyptus Menthol *Boots, S.Afr.*
Dichlorobenzyl alcohol (p.1143·2); amylmetacresol (p.1133·2); menthol (p.1632·3).
Sore throat.

Strepsils Extra
Boots, Austral.; Crookes Healthcare, UK.
Hexylresorcinol (p.1146·3).
Mouth and throat disorders.

Strepsils Lidocaine *Boots, Fr.*
Amylmetacresol (p.1133·2); dichlorobenzyl alcohol (p.1143·2); lignocaine [lidocaine] hydrochloride (p.1313·2).
Sore throat.

Strepsils + Lidocaine *Boots Healthcare, Belg.*
Dichlorobenzyl alcohol (p.1143·2); amylmetacresol (p.1133·2); lignocaine [lidocaine] (p.1313·2).
Sore throat.

Strepsils Menthol
Boots Healthcare, Belg.; Boots, Fin.
Dichlorobenzyl alcohol (p.1143·2); amylmetacresol (p.1133·2); menthol (p.1632·3).
Mouth and throat disorders; nasal congestion.

Strepsils Menthol en Eucalyptus *Boots Healthcare, Neth.*
Amylmetacresol (p.1133·2); dichlorobenzyl alcohol (p.1143·2); menthol (p.1632·3); eucalyptus oil (p.1609·2).
Sore throat.

Strepsils Miel-Citron *Boots Healthcare, Fr.*
Amylmetacresol (p.1133·2); dichlorobenzyl alcohol (p.1143·2).
Sore throat.

Strepsils Orange-C *Boots, S.Afr.*
Dichlorobenzyl alcohol (p.1143·2); amylmetacresol (p.1133·2); ascorbic acid (p.1389·3); menthol (p.1632·3).
Sore throat.

Strepsils Pain Relief Plus *Crookes Healthcare, UK.*
Lignocaine [lidocaine] (p.1313·2); dichlorobenzyl alcohol (p.1143·2); amylmetacresol (p.1133·2).
Formerly known as Strepsils Dual Action.
Sore throat.

Strepsils Pain Relief Spray *Crookes Healthcare, UK.*
Lignocaine [lidocaine] hydrochloride (p.1313·2).
Formerly known as Strepsils Direct Action Spray.
Sore throat.

Strepsils Plus
Boots, Austral.; Boots, Israel; Boots, S.Afr.
Dichlorobenzyl alcohol (p.1143·2); amylmetacresol (p.1133·2); lignocaine [lidocaine] hydrochloride (p.1313·2).
Sore throat.

Strepsils Plus Anaesthetic
Boots, NZ; Boots, Thai.
Dichlorobenzyl alcohol (p.1143·2); amylmetacresol (p.1133·2); lignocaine [lidocaine] hydrochloride (p.1313·2).
Sore throat.

Strepsils Plus Vit C *Boots, Thai.*
Dichlorobenzyl alcohol (p.1143·2); amylmetacresol (p.1133·2); vitamin C (p.1389·3).
Sore throat.

Strepsils Sinaasappel en Vitamine C *Boots Healthcare, Neth.*
Dichlorobenzyl alcohol (p.1143·2); amylmetacresol (p.1133·2); ascorbic acid (p.1389·3).
Sore throat.

Strepsils Soothing Honey & Lemon *Boots, S.Afr.*
Dichlorobenzyl alcohol (p.1143·2); amylmetacresol (p.1133·2).
Sore throat.

Strepsils Sugar Free *Boots, Thai.*
Amylmetacresol (p.1133·2); dichlorobenzyl alcohol (p.1143·2).
Sore throat.

Strepsils Vit C *Boots Healthcare, Belg.*
Dichlorobenzyl alcohol (p.1143·2); amylmetacresol (p.1133·2); ascorbic acid (p.1389·3); sodium ascorbate (p.1390·1).
Sore throat.

Strepsils Vitamin C *Boots Healthcare, Irl.*
Dichlorobenzyl alcohol (p.1143·2); amylmetacresol (p.1133·2); vitamin C (p.1389·3).
Sore throat.

Strepsils with Vitamin C
Boots, Israel; Boots, NZ; Crookes Healthcare, UK.
Dichlorobenzyl alcohol (p.1143·2); amylmetacresol (p.1133·2); ascorbic acid (p.1389·3) or sodium ascorbate (p.1390·1).
Sore throat.

Strepsils Vitamine C *Boots Healthcare, Fr.*
Amylmetacresol (p.1133·2); dichlorobenzyl alcohol (p.1143·2); ascorbic acid (p.1389·3); sodium ascorbate (p.1390·1).
Sore throat.

Strepsils Zinc Cold Relief *Boots, Austral.*
Zinc gluconate (p.1398·2); sodium ascorbate (p.1390·1); ascorbic acid (p.1389·3).
Cold symptoms.

Strepsils Zinc Defence *Crookes Healthcare, UK.*
Zinc gluconate (p.1398·2); ascorbic acid (p.1389·3).

Strepsilspray Lidocaine *Boots Healthcare, UK.*
Amylmetacresol (p.1133·2); dichlorobenzyl alcohol (p.1143·2); lignocaine [lidocaine] (p.1313·2).
Mouth and throat infections.

Streptase
Hoechst Marion Roussel, Aust.; Hoechst Marion Roussel, Austral.; Aventis, Belg.; Hoechst Marion Roussel, Braz.; Hoechst Marion Roussel, Canad.; Aventis, Denm.; Hoechst Marion Roussel, Fin.; Hoechst, Fr.; Hoechst Marion Roussel, Ger.; Hoechst Marion Roussel, Hong Kong; Hoechst Marion Roussel, Irl.; Hoechst Marion Roussel, Israel; Hoechst Marion Roussel, Ital.; Hoechst Marion Roussel, Mex.; Behring, Neth.; Hoechst Marion Roussel, Norw.; Aventis, NZ; Hoechst Marion Roussel, Port.; Aventis, S.Afr.; Hoechst Marion Roussel, Singapore; Hoechst Marion Roussel, Spain; Hoechst Marion Roussel, Swed.; Hoechst Marion Roussel, Switz.; Hoechst Marion Roussel, Thai.; Aventis Behring, UK; Astra, USA.
Streptokinase (p.975·3).
Thromboembolic disorders.

Strepto *General Drugs, Thai.*
Streptomycin sulfate (p.249·1).
Bacterial infections including tuberculosis.

Streptocol *Molteni, Ital.†.*
Streptomycin sulfate (p.249·1).
Bacterial infections of the gastrointestinal tract.

Strepto-Fatol *Fatol, Ger.*
Streptomycin sulfate (p.249·1).
Bacterial infections including tuberculosis.

Strepto-Hefa *Hefa, Ger.*
Streptomycin sulfate (p.249·1).
Bacterial infections including tuberculosis.

Streptomagma *Wyeth Lederle, Ital.*
Oral suspension: Dried aluminium hydroxide (p.1210·3); heavy kaolin (p.1229·3); pectin (p.1502·3).
Tablets: Activated attapulgite (p.1212·3); pectin (p.1502·3); dried aluminium hydroxide (p.1210·3).
Diarrhoea.

Strepto-Plus *Molteni, Ital.†.*
Co-trimoxazole (p.193·3).
Bacterial infections.

Streptosil con Neomicina-Fher *Boehringer Ingelheim, Ital.*
Neomycin sulfate (p.228·1); sulfathiazole (p.257·1).
Bacterial skin infections.

Streptosil L PMC *Fher, Ital.*
Benzalkonium chloride (p.1133·2).
Skin, hand, and wound disinfection.

Streptozyme
Carter-Wallace, Switz.†; Wampole, USA.
Test for streptococcal extracellular antigens in blood, plasma, and serum.

Stresam *Biocodex, Fr.*
Etifoxine hydrochloride (p.683·1).
Anxiety.

Stress *Homeocan, Canad.*
Homoeopathic preparation.

Stress 600 *Nion, USA.*
Multivitamin and mineral preparation (p.1350·1).

Stress B Complex
Pharmavite, Canad.; Moore, USA.
A range of vitamin preparations with or without minerals (p.1350·1).

Stress Formula
Wampole, Canad.; Nature's Bounty, USA.
A range of vitamin preparations with or without minerals (p.1350·1).
Nutritional supplement.

Stress Formula B Compound plus Vitamin C *Quest, Canad.*
Vitamin B substances and vitamin C (p.1350·1).

Stress Plex C *Jamieson, Canad.*
Vitamin B substances, vitamin C, and zinc (p.1350·1).

Stress Relief *Brauer, Austral.*
Homoeopathic preparation.

Stress Tab *Shoppers Drug Mart, Canad.*
Vitamin B substances and vitamin C (p.1350·1).

Stress Tab with Iron *Shoppers Drug Mart, Canad.*
Multivitamin preparation with iron (p.1350·1).

Stress Tab with Zinc *Shoppers Drug Mart, Canad.*
Multivitamin preparation with zinc (p.1350·1).

Stress Tablets *Drug Trading, Canad.†.*
Vitamin B substances and vitamin C (p.1350·1).

Stresscaps
Gilton, Braz.
Vitamin B substances (p.1350·1).
Nutritional supplement.
Lederle, USA†.
Vitamin B substances with vitamin C (p.1350·1).

Stressease *Jamieson, Canad.*
Multivitamin and mineral preparation (p.1350·1).

Stressen *Medosan, Ital.*
Amino-acid and vitamin preparation (p.1350·1).
Tonic.

StressForm "605" with Iron *Nature's Bounty, USA.*
Multivitamin preparation with iron (p.1350·1).

Stresson
Note. This name is used for preparations of different composition.
Boehringer Ingelheim, Aust.†.
Bunitrolol hydrochloride (p.852·3).
Angina pectoris; arrhythmias; heart failure.
Nutricia, Austral.; Nutricia, Irl.; Nutricia, Ital.
Preparations for enteral nutrition (p.1350·1).

Stresstabs
Prodome, Braz.; Whitehall-Robins, Canad.; Lederle, Hong Kong; Wyeth, Mex.; Whitehall, Port.; Whitehall, Thai.; Lederle, USA.
A range of vitamin preparations with or without minerals (p.1350·1).

Stresstabs with Zinc *Lederle, Israel.*
Multivitamin and mineral preparation (p.1350·1).

Stresstein *Sandoz Nutrition, USA.*
Preparation for enteral nutrition (p.1350·1).
Stress.

Striaton *Knoll, Ger.*
Levodopa (p.1169·2); carbidopa (p.1168·2).
Parkinsonism.

Striatridin *Opfermann, Ger.*
Cetostearyl octanoate; amino acids; ethyl nicotinate (p.35·1).
Skin disorders.

Stri-Dex Antibacterial Cleansing *Sterling, USA.*
Triclosan (p.1159·2).

Stri-Dex Clear *Sterling, USA.*
Salicylic acid (p.1122·3).

The symbol † denotes a preparation no longer actively marketed

Stri-Dex Face Wash *Sterling Health, USA.*
Triclosan (p.1159·2).
Skin cleanser.

Stri-Dex Pads *Glenbrook, USA.*
Salicylic acid (p.1122·3); alcohol (p.1130·3).
Acne.

Stringan *Strallhofer, Aust.*
Polyphloretin phosphate; phenylephrine (p.1097·1).
Nasal congestion.

Strocain *Eisai, Hong Kong; Eisai, Jpn; Eisai, Singapore; Eisai, Thai.*
Oxetacaine (p.1317·3).
Gastrointestinal disorders.

Strodival *Herbert, Ger.*
Ouabain (p.950·2).
Cardiac disorders.

Strogen *Strathmann, Ger.*
Saw palmetto (p.1491·2).
Benign prostatic hyperplasia.

Stromba *Sanofi Synthelabo, Belg.; Sanofi Winthrop, Irl.; Sanofi Synthelabo, Neth.; Sanofi Winthrop, UK.*
Stanozolol (p.1491·3).
Angioedema; Behçet's disease; cutaneous vasculitis; osteoporosis; Raynaud's syndrome; scleroderma; thromboembolic disorders.

Strombaject *Sanofi Synthelabo, Belg.*
Stanozolol (p.1491·3).
Anabolic.

Stromectol *Merck Sharp & Dohme, Austral.; Merck Sharp & Dohme-Chibret, Fr.; Merck, USA.*
Ivermectin (p.99·3).
Onchocerciasis; strongyloidiasis.

Stromic *Strathmann, Ger.†*
Solidago virgaurea.
Urinary-tract disorders.

217 Strong *Frosst, Canad.†*
Aspirin (p.14·2); caffeine citrate (p.761·3).
Fever; inflammation; pain.

StrongStart *Savage, USA.*
Multivitamin and mineral preparation (p.1350·1).

Strongus *Franconpharm, Ger.*
Garlic (p.1614·1).
Hyperlipidaemia.

Strophantab *Fides, Ger.*
Homoeopathic preparation.

Strophanthin-Herztabletten compositum *Cosmochema, Ger.*
Homoeopathic preparation.

Strophanthus *Phytomed, Switz.*
Homoeopathic preparation.

Stropheupas-forte *Pascoe, Ger.*
Homoeopathic preparation.

Strophocor N *Hennig, Ger.†*
Ouabain (p.950·2).
Cardiac disorders.

Strotan *Strathmann, Ger.*
Agnus castus (p.1574·2).
Mastalgia; menstrual disorders.

Strovite *Everett, USA.*
A range of vitamin and mineral preparations (p.1350·1).

Structolipid *Fresenius Kabi, Fin.; Fresenius Kabi, Port.; Fresenius Kabi, Swed.*
Soya oil (p.1378·1); coconut oil (p.1409·1) or palm oil triglycerides.
Contains egg phospholipid.
Lipid infusion for parenteral nutrition.

Structolipide *Fresenius Kabi, Fr.*
Triglycerides from coconut oil (p.1409·1) and soya oil (p.1378·1).
Contains egg lecithin.
Lipid infusion for parenteral nutrition.

Structum *Pierre Fabre, Fr.; Robapharm, Switz.*
Sodium chondroitin sulfate A (p.1594·2).
Arthritis.

Strumazol *Christiaens, Belg.; Nourypharma, Neth.*
Methimazole [thiamazole] (p.1525·1).
Hyperthyroidism.

Strumedical 400 *Henning, Ger.*
Diiodotyrosine (p.1522·3).
Iodine-deficiency disorders.

Strumex *Robugen, Ger.*
Sodium iodide (p.1522·3).
Iodine-deficiency disorders.

Stryphnasal *Serturner, Ger.*
Adrenalone hydrochloride (p.1574·1).
Formerly known as Stryphonasal.
Epistaxis.

Stryphnon *Salus, Denm.*
Adrenalone hydrochloride (p.1574·1).
Haemorrhage.

Stuart Formula *J&J-Merck, USA.*
Multivitamin and mineral preparation with iron and folic acid (p.1350·1).

Stuart Prenatal *Wyeth-Ayerst, USA.*
Multivitamin and mineral preparation with folic acid and iron (p.1350·1).
Dietary supplement in pregnancy.

Stuartinic *J&J-Merck, USA†.*
Ferrous fumarate (p.1360·1); vitamin B substances with vitamin C (p.1350·1).
Iron-deficiency anaemias.

Stuartnatal 1+1 *Wyeth-Ayerst, USA.*
Multivitamin and mineral preparation with iron and folic acid (p.1350·1).
Dietary supplement in pregnancy.

Stuartnatal Plus *Wyeth-Ayerst, USA.*
Multivitamin and mineral preparation (p.1350·1).

Stubit *Pickles, UK†.*
Nicotine (p.1640·3).
Aid to smoking withdrawal.

Stud 100 *Key, Austral.; Trupharm, Israel.*
Lignocaine [lidocaine] (p.1313·2).
Premature ejaculation.

Stugeron *Janssen-Cilag, Belg.; Janssen, Braz.; Janssen, Hong Kong; Janssen-Cilag, Irl.; Janssen-Cilag, Ital.; Janssen, Mex.; Janssen-Cilag, Port.; Janssen-Cilag, S.Afr.; Janssen, Singapore; Esteve, Spain; Janssen-Cilag, Switz.; Janssen, Thai.; Janssen-Cilag, UK; Johnson & Johnson MSD Consumer, UK.*
Cinnarizine (p.413·1).
Cerebral and peripheral vascular disorders; migraine; motion sickness; nausea and vomiting; vestibular disorders.

Stullmaton *Stulln, Ger.*
Centaury (p.1593·1); arnica (p.1581·3); melissa (p.1632·2); chamomile (p.1593·2); absinthium (p.1571·1); spruce tips; trace elements.
Gastrointestinal disorders.

Stunarone *Janssen-Cilag, Israel.*
Cinnarizine (p.413·1).
Vestibular disorders.

Stutgeron *Janssen-Cilag, Aust.; Janssen-Cilag, Ger.†.*
Cinnarizine (p.413·1).
Cerebral and peripheral vascular disorders; vestibular disorders.

Stye *Del, USA.*
Yellow mercuric oxide (p.1633·3).
Minor eye infections.

Stylo Sport *Lancome, Canad.†.*
SPF 15: Octinoxate (p.1517·3); titanium dioxide (p.1126·1).
Sunscreen.

stypro *Curasan, Ger.*
Gelatin (p.737·2).
Haemostatic.

Styptanon *Organon, Aust.*
Estriol sodium succinate (p.1475·3).
Capillary haemorrhage.

Akzo, Braz.
Estriol succinate (p.1475·3).
Haemorrhage; thrombocytopenia.

Stypto-Caine *Pedinol, USA.*
Aluminium chloride (p.1110·2); amethocaine [tetracaine] (p.1305·2); hydroxyquinoline sulfate (p.1622·2).
Bleeding in minor wounds.

Styptysat *Ysatfabrik, Ger.*
Shepherd's purse (p.1662·3).
Haemorrhagic disorders.

Suadian *Schering, Ger.*
Naftifine hydrochloride (p.392·1).
Fungal skin and nail infections.

Sualyn *Vita, Spain†.*
Bismuth subnitrate (p.1213·2); magnesium carbonate (p.1232·3); metoclopramide hydrochloride (p.1235·2); sorbitol (p.1377·3).
Gastric spasms; gastritis; nausea; peptic ulcer; vomiting.

Suamoxil *Cantabria, Spain.*
Amoxicillin trihydrate (p.149·2).
Bacterial infections.

Suavit Calcio *Dinafarma, Braz.*
Vitamin B₁₂; ergocalciferol; calcium chloride (p.1350·1).
Nutritional supplement.

Suaviter *Boehringer Mannheim, Ital.*
Aspartame (p.1354·3).
Sugar substitute.

Suavuret *Organon, Spain.*
Ethinylestradiol (p.1476·2); desogestrel (p.1470·3).
Combined oral contraceptive; menstrual disorders.

Sub Tensin *Byk Elmu, Spain.*
Nitrendipine (p.947·1).
Hypertension.

Subcutin N *Ritsert, Ger.*
Benzocaine (p.1306·2).
Gastrointestinal disorders; mouth and throat disorders.

Subdue *Mead Johnson Nutritionals, Canad.; Mead Johnson, NZ.*
Preparation for enteral nutrition (p.1350·1).

Subitan *Eurofarma, Braz.*
Potassium iodide (p.1522·3); ammonium chloride (p.1085·2); mepyramine maleate (p.421·1); ephedrine hydrochloride (p.1090·1); lobelia (p.1510·2); hyoscyamus (p.470·1).
Respiratory-tract congestion.

Sublimaze *Janssen-Cilag, Austral.; Janssen-Ortho, Canad.†; Janssen-Cilag, Irl.;*
Janssen-Cilag, NZ; Janssen-Cilag, S.Afr.; Janssen-Cilag, UK; Janssen, USA.
Fentanyl citrate (p.37·1).
Adjunct to general anaesthesia; analgesia in anaesthesia; neuroleptanalgesia.

Sublivac *Hal, Ger.*
Allergen extracts of pollen, fungi, house dust mites, and skin (p.1575·3).
Hyposensitisation.

Sublivac B.E.S.T. *Hal, Neth.*
Allergen extracts (glycerolinated) (p.1575·3).
Hyposensitisation.

Subreum *Byk, Aust.; Byk Tosse, Ger.; Byk Gulden, Ger.; OM, Port.*
Escherichia coli extract.
Chronic polyarthritis.

Substi *Abbott, Fr.*
Preparation for enteral nutrition (p.1350·1).

Substitol *Note. This name is used for preparations of different composition.*
Mundipharma, Aust.
Morphine sulfate (p.56·1).
Substitution therapy in opiate dependence.

Solvay, Aust.†
Estradiol (p.1473·1).
Oestrogen deficiency.

Subutex *Reckitt Benckiser, Austral.; Schering-Plough, Denm.; Schering-Plough, Fin.; Schering-Plough, Fr.; Essex, Ital.; Schering-Plough, Port.; Schering-Plough, Swed.; Essex, Switz.; Schering-Plough, UK.*
Buprenorphine hydrochloride (p.21·1).
Opioid withdrawal syndrome.

Sucadermil *Oftalder, Port.*
Salicylic acid (p.1122·3); sulfur (p.1123·3); cade oil (p.1124·3).

Sucari *Jean-Marie, Hong Kong.*
Sucralfate (p.1250·2).
Gastritis; peptic ulcer.

Sucaryl *Note. This name is used for preparations of different composition.*
Abbott, Austral.; Abbott, Fr.; Abbott, NZ.
Calcium cyclamate (p.1358·3) or sodium cyclamate (p.1358·3); saccharin sodium (p.1375·1).
Sugar substitute.

Abbott, Braz.
Sodium cyclamate (p.1358·3).
Sugar substitute.

Abbott, Canad.
Sodium cyclamate (p.1358·3) with or without glucose.
Sugar substitute.

Succi Pharmacetin *Olan-Kemed, Thai.*
Chloramphenicol sodium succinate (p.179·2).
Bacterial infections.

Succicaptal *SERB, Fr.*
Succimer (p.1024·3).
Mercury and lead poisoning.

Succicuran *Rodleben, Ger.*
Suxamethonium chloride (p.1340·1).
Depolarising neuromuscular blocker.

Succilate *Aspen, S.Afr.*
Erythromycin estolate (p.201·2).
Bacterial infections.

Succin *Abbott, S.Afr.*
Erythromycin ethyl succinate (p.201·2).
Bacterial infections.

Succinolin *Amino, Switz.*
Suxamethonium chloride (p.1340·1).
Depolarising neuromuscular blocker.

Succinyl *Taro, Israel.; Dagra, Neth.†; Asta Medica, Thai.*
Suxamethonium chloride (p.1340·1).
Depolarising neuromuscular blocker.

Succosa *Tika, Swed.†.*
Sucralfate (p.1250·2).
Peptic ulcer.

Succus Cineraria Maritima *Walker Pharmacal, USA.*
Senecio (p.1661·3); hamamelis (p.1618·3); boric acid (p.1586·1).
Cataract opacity.

Sucontral *Harras-Curarina, Ger.*
Coutarea latiflora.
Diabetes mellitus (adjuvant).

Sucrabest *Hexal, Ger.†.*
Sucralfate (p.1250·2).
Peptic ulcer.

Sucrafen *LSP, Thai.*
Sucralfate (p.1250·2).
Gastritis; gastro-oesophageal reflux; peptic ulcer.

Sucrager *Ripari-Gero, Ital.*
Sucralfate (p.1250·2).
Gastritis; gastro-oesophageal reflux; peptic ulcer.

Sucraid *Orphan Medical, USA.*
Sacrosidase (p.1660·2).
Sucrase deficiency.

Sucral *Bioprogress, Ital.; Ranbaxy, Thai.*
Sucralfate (p.1250·2).
Gastritis; gastro-oesophageal reflux; peptic ulcer.

Sucralan *Lannacher, Aust.*
Sucralfate (p.1250·2).
Gastro-oesophageal reflux; peptic ulcer.

Sucralbene *Ratiopharm, Aust.*
Sucralfate (p.1250·2).
Peptic ulcer.

Sucralfin *Inverni della Beffa, Ital.*
Sucralfate (p.1250·2).
Gastritis; gastro-oesophageal reflux; peptic ulcer.

Sucralose *Julphar, UAE.*
Sucralfate (p.1250·2).
Gastro-oesophageal reflux; peptic ulcer.

Sucralstad *Stada, Aust.*
Sucralfate (p.1250·2).
Peptic ulcer.

Sucralum *Inibsa, Port.*
Sucralfate (p.1250·2).
Gastritis; gastro-oesophageal reflux; peptic ulcer.

Sucramal *Sanofi Synthelabo, Ital.*
Sucralfate (p.1250·2).
Gastritis; gastro-oesophageal reflux; peptic ulcer.

Sucramed *S Med, Aust.*
Sucralfate (p.1250·2).
Peptic ulcer.

Sucraphil *Philopharm, Ger.*
Sucralfate (p.1250·2).
Gastro-oesophageal reflux; peptic ulcer.

Sucrate *Lisapharma, Ital.; Lisapharma, Thai.*
Sucralfate (p.1250·2).
Gastritis; gastro-oesophageal reflux; peptic ulcer.

Sucrato *Armstrong, Mex.*
Tripotassium dicitratobismuthate (p.1213·2).
Peptic ulcer.

Sucredulcor *Pierre Fabre Sante, Fr.*
Saccharin (p.1374·3).
Sugar substitute.

Sucret *Sintofarma, Braz.*
Aspartame (p.1354·3).
Sugar substitute.

Sucrets *Note. This name is used for preparations of different composition.*
SmithKline Beecham Consumer, Canad.; SmithKline Beecham Consumer, USA.
Dyclonine hydrochloride (p.1311·3).
Sore throat.

SmithKline Beecham, Israel.
Hexylresorcinol (p.1146·3).
Sore throat.

Sucrets Children's Formula *SmithKline Beecham, Israel.*
Dyclonine hydrochloride (p.1311·3).
Sore throat.

Sucrets Cough Control *SmithKline Beecham Consumer, Canad.; SmithKline Beecham, USA.*
Dextromethorphan (p.1087·3) or dextromethorphan hydrobromide (p.1087·3).
Coughs; sore throat.

Sucrets Extra Strength *SmithKline Beecham Consumer, Canad.*
Hexylresorcinol (p.1146·3).
Sore throat.

Sucrets 4-Hour Cough *SmithKline Beecham Consumer, USA.*
Dextromethorphan (p.1087·3).
Coughs.

Sucrets for Kids *SmithKline Beecham Consumer, Canad.*
Dyclonine hydrochloride (p.1311·3).

Sucrets Maximum Strength *SmithKline Beecham, Israel.*
Dyclonine hydrochloride (p.1311·3).
Sore throat.

Sucrets Sore Throat *SmithKline Beecham Consumer, USA.*
Hexylresorcinol (p.1146·3).
Sore throat.

Sucrin *Rafa, Israel.*
Sodium cyclamate (p.1358·3); saccharin sodium (p.1375·1).
Sugar substitute.

Sucroral *Sofar, Ital.*
Sucralfate (p.1250·2).
Gastrointestinal disorders.

Suczulen mono *Knoll, Ger.*
Liquorice (p.1231·2).
Peptic ulcer.

Sudafed *Glaxo Wellcome, Fr.; Glaxo Wellcome, Hong Kong; Calmic, Irl.; Warner-Lambert, Ital.; Glaxo Wellcome, Mex.; Warner-Lambert Consumer, Port.; Glaxo Wellcome, S.Afr.; Glaxo Wellcome, Singapore; Warner-Lambert, UK; Warner-Lambert, USA.*
Pseudoephedrine hydrochloride (p.1099·2).
Upper respiratory-tract congestion.

Sudafed for Children *Warner-Lambert, NZ.*
Pseudoephedrine hydrochloride (p.1099·2).
Nasal congestion.

Sudafed Co *Warner-Lambert, UK.*
Pseudoephedrine hydrochloride (p.1099·2); paracetamol (p.71·2).
Cold and influenza symptoms.

Sudafed Cold & Allergy *Warner-Lambert, USA.*
Pseudoephedrine hydrochloride (p.1099·2); chlorpheniramine [chlorphenamine] maleate (p.412·1).

Sudafed Cold & Cough *Note. This name is used for preparations of different composition.*
Warner-Lambert, Canad.
Pseudoephedrine hydrochloride (p.1099·2); dextromethorphan hydrobromide (p.1087·3); paracetamol (p.71·2).
Coughs and cold symptoms.

Warner-Lambert, USA.
Pseudoephedrine hydrochloride (p.1099·2); dextromethorphan hydrobromide (p.1087·3); paracetamol (p.71·2); guaifenesin (p.1092·2).
Coughs and cold symptoms.

Sudafed Cold & Flu *Warner-Lambert, Canad.*
Paracetamol (p.71·2); dextromethorphan (p.1087·3); guaifenesin (p.1092·2); pseudoephedrine hydrochloride (p.1099·2).
Coughs and cold symptoms.

Sudafed Cold & Sinus *Warner-Lambert, USA.*
Pseudoephedrine hydrochloride (p.1099·2); paracetamol (p.71·2).
Nasal congestion.

Sudafed Day/Nightime Relief *Warner-Lambert, NZ.*
Day tablets, pseudoephedrine hydrochloride (p.1099·2); paracetamol (p.71·2); night tablets, pseudoephedrine hydrochloride; paracetamol; triprolidine hydrochloride (p.427·2).
Cold and influenza symptoms.

Sudafed Decongestant *Warner-Lambert, Canad.*
Pseudoephedrine hydrochloride (p.1099·2).
Nasal congestion.

Sudafed DM *Warner-Lambert, Canad.†*
Pseudoephedrine hydrochloride (p.1099·2); dextromethorphan hydrobromide (p.1087·3).
Cold symptoms; nasal congestion.

Sudafed Dual Relief *Warner-Lambert, UK.*
Paracetamol (p.71·2); phenylephrine hydrochloride (p.1097·1); caffeine (p.761·3).
Cold and influenza symptoms.

Sudafed Expectorant
Glaxo Wellcome, Hong Kong; Calmic, Irl.; Glaxo Wellcome, S.Afr.; Glaxo Wellcome, Singapore; Warner-Lambert, UK.
Pseudoephedrine hydrochloride (p.1099·2); guaifenesin (p.1092·2).
Coughs; upper respiratory-tract congestion.

Sudafed Head Cold & Sinus *Warner-Lambert, Canad.*
Pseudoephedrine hydrochloride (p.1099·2); paracetamol (p.71·2).
Cold symptoms; sinus pain.

Sudafed 12 Hour Relief *Warner-Lambert, NZ.*
Pseudoephedrine hydrochloride (p.1099·2).
Nasal congestion.

Sudafed Linctus *Warner-Lambert, UK.*
Pseudoephedrine hydrochloride (p.1099·2); dextromethorphan hydrobromide (p.1087·3).
Coughs; upper respiratory-tract congestion.

Sudafed Nasal Spray *Warner-Lambert, UK.*
Oxymetazoline hydrochloride (p.1096·2).
Nasal congestion.

Sudafed Non-Drying Sinus *Warner-Lambert, USA.*
Pseudoephedrine hydrochloride (p.1099·2); guaifenesin (p.1092·2).
Coughs and cold symptoms.

Sudafed Plus
Note.This name is used for preparations of different composition.
Warner-Lambert, UK.
Pseudoephedrine hydrochloride (p.1099·2); triprolidine hydrochloride (p.427·2).
Allergic rhinitis.

Wellcome, USA.
Pseudoephedrine hydrochloride (p.1099·2); chlorpheniramine [chlorphenamine] maleate (p.412·1).
Upper respiratory-tract symptoms.

Sudafed Severe Cold *Warner-Lambert, USA.*
Pseudoephedrine hydrochloride (p.1099·2); dextromethorphan hydrobromide (p.1087·3); paracetamol (p.71·2).
Coughs and cold symptoms.

Sudafed Sinus *Warner-Lambert, USA.*
Pseudoephedrine hydrochloride (p.1099·2); paracetamol (p.71·2).
Nasal congestion.

Sudafed Sinus & Nasal Decongestant
Warner-Lambert, Austral.; Warner-Lambert, NZ.
Pseudoephedrine hydrochloride (p.1099·2).
Nasal and sinus congestion.

Sudafed Sinus Pain & Allergy Relief *Warner-Lambert, Austral.*
Pseudoephedrine hydrochloride (p.1099·2); paracetamol (p.71·2); triprolidine hydrochloride (p.427·2).
Formerly known as Sudafed Plus.
Sinus disorders.

Sudafed Sinus Pain Relief
Warner-Lambert, Austral.; Warner-Lambert, NZ.
Pseudoephedrine hydrochloride (p.1099·2); paracetamol (p.71·2).
Nasal congestion; sinus pain and congestion.

Sudagesic *Glaxo Wellcome, S.Afr.*
Pseudoephedrine hydrochloride (p.1099·2); paracetamol (p.71·2).
Cold and influenza symptoms.

Sudal *Atley, USA.*
Pseudoephedrine hydrochloride (p.1099·2); guaifenesin (p.1092·2).
Coughs.

Suda-Tussin *Reese, USA†.*
Phenylpropanolamine hydrochloride (p.1098·2); guaifenesin (p.1092·2); dextromethorphan hydrobromide (p.1087·3).

Sudex *Roberts, USA†.*
Pseudoephedrine hydrochloride (p.1099·2).
Formerly contained pseudoephedrine hydrochloride and guaifenesin.
Nasal congestion.

Sudocrem *Tosara, Irl.†; Tosara, UK.*
Zinc oxide (p.1128·2); benzyl benzoate (p.1428·2); benzyl cinnamate; benzyl alcohol (p.1135·2).
Acne; bed sores; burns; chilblains; eczema; napkin rash; sunburn; wounds.

Sudodrin *ICN, Canad.†.*
Pseudoephedrine hydrochloride (p.1099·2).

Sudol *Coventry, UK.*
Tar acids (p.1158·1).

Sudomyl *PSM, NZ.*
Pseudoephedrine hydrochloride (p.1099·2).
Nasal congestion.

Sudosian *Asian Pharm, Thai.*
Pseudoephedrine hydrochloride (p.1099·2).
Nasal congestion; obstructive airways disease; rhinitis.

Sudosin *Medea, Spain.*
Formaldehyde (p.1144·2); lindane (p.1434·1); aminobenzoic acid (p.1516·3); salicylic acid (p.1122·3); talc; thymol (p.1158·3); lavender essence.
Skin disorders.

Suero Fisiologico *Cinfa, Spain.*
Sodium chloride (p.1196·1).
Nasal congestion.

Suero Glucosado Vitulia *Ern, Spain.*
Glucose (p.1364·1).
Carbohydrate source; fluid depletion.

Suero Glucosalino Vitulia *Ern, Spain.*
Sodium chloride (p.1196·1); glucose (p.1364·1).
Carbohydrate source; fluid and electrolyte depletion.

Suero Levulosado Vitulia *Ern, Spain.*
Fructose (p.1363·3).
Carbohydrate source; fluid depletion.

Suero Potassico Bieffe ME *Bieffe, Spain.*
Potassium chloride (p.1194·3); sodium chloride (p.1196·1).
Diabetic ketoacidosis; hypokalaemia.

Suero Ringer Braun *Braun, Spain.*
Electrolyte infusion (p.1180·1).
Fluid and electrolyte depletion.

Suero Ringer Lactato Vitulia *Ern, Spain.*
Electrolyte infusion (p.1180·1).
Fluid and electrolyte depletion.

Sueroral *Casen Fleet, Spain.*
Glucose; potassium chloride; sodium citrate; sodium chloride (p.1185·2).
Diarrhoea; oral rehydration therapy; vomiting.

Sueroral Hiposodico *Casen Fleet, Spain.*
Glucose; potassium chloride; sucrose; sodium bicarbonate; sodium chloride (p.1185·2).
Diarrhoea; oral rehydration therapy; vomiting.

Suevitine *Augot, Fr.*
Vitamin, mineral, and trace element preparation (p.1350·1).

Sufenta
Janssen-Cilag, Aust.; Janssen-Cilag, Belg.; Janssen-Ortho, Canad.; Janssen-Cilag, Denm.; Janssen-Cilag, Fin.; Janssen-Cilag, Fr.; Janssen-Cilag, Ger.; Janssen-Cilag, Neth.; Janssen-Cilag, Norw.; Janssen-Cilag, S.Afr.; Janssen-Cilag, Swed.; Janssen-Cilag, Switz.; Taylor, USA.
Sufentanil citrate (p.84·3).
Analgesia in anaesthesia; general anaesthesia; pain.

Sufil *Elfar, Spain.*
Mebendazole (p.102·2).
Worm infections.

Sufisal *Silanes, Mex.*
Oxpentifylline [pentoxifylline] (p.950·3).
Vascular disorders.

Sufortan *Sanfer, Mex.*
Penicillamine (p.1017·1).
Cystinuria; heavy-metal poisoning; rheumatoid arthritis; Wilson's disease.

Sufortanon *Asta Medica, Spain.*
Penicillamine (p.1017·1).
Cystinuria; heavy-metal poisoning; rheumatoid arthritis; Wilson's disease.

Sufralem *Solvay, Port.*
Anethole trithione (p.1580·1).
Dry eyes; dry mouth.

Sufrexal
Janssen-Cilag, Belg.; Janssen-Cilag, Ital.; Janssen-Cilag, Port.; Janssen, Thai.
Ketanserin tartrate (p.917·2).
Hypertension.

Janssen, Mex.
Ketanserin (p.917·3).
Burns; skin ulcers; wounds.

Sugar *Uno, Ital.*
Sucralfate (p.1250·2).
Gastritis; gastro-oesophageal reflux; peptic ulcer.

Sugar Bloc *Cantassium Co., UK.*
Gymnema silvestre; chromium orotate (p.1645·1).
Diet aid.

Sugarbil *Novag, Spain.*
Cyclobutyrol sodium (p.1601·2); magnesium sulfate (p.1191·1); sorbitol (p.1377·3).
Constipation; hepatobiliary disorders.

Sugarceton *Novag, Spain†.*
Calcium fructose diphosphate; hydroxocobalamin hydrochloride (p.1388·3); promethazine hydrochloride (p.423·2); thiamine phosphate (p.1385·2); trometamol acephyllinate (p.1675·2); trometamol thioctate (p.1675·2); sorbitol (p.1377·3); glucose (p.1364·1).
Acetonaemia; acidosis.

Sugarless C *Cenovis, Austral.; Vitelle, Austral.*
Ascorbic acid (p.1389·3); sodium ascorbate (p.1390·1).
Vitamin C supplement.

Sugast *Selvi, Ital.*
Sucralfate (p.1250·2).
Gastritis; gastro-oesophageal reflux; peptic ulcer.

Sugiran *Pensa, Spain.*
Alprostadil alfadex (p.1440·1).
Peripheral vascular disease.

Sugril *Siam Bheasach, Thai.*
Glibenclamide (p.321·3).
Diabetes mellitus.

Suguan *Hoechst Marion Roussel, Ital.*
Glibenclamide (p.321·3); phenformin hydrochloride (p.333·2).
Diabetes mellitus.

Suguan M *Hoechst Marion Roussel, Ital.*
Glibenclamide (p.321·3); metformin hydrochloride (p.332·3).
Diabetes mellitus.

Suiflox *Novartis, Mex.*
Ciprofloxacin hydrochloride (p.182·3).
Bacterial infections.

Sukepar *Biochimico, Braz.*
Liver extract.
Liver disorders.

Sukir *Brasifa, Braz.*
Saccharin sodium (p.1375·1).
Sugar substitute.

Sukolin *Orion, Fin.*
Suxamethonium chloride (p.1340·1).
Depolarising neuromuscular blocker.

Sulamid *Baldacci, Ital.*
Amisulpride (p.655·1).
Depression.

Sular
Zeneca, Belg.; Zeneca, Mex.; Zeneca, Neth.; Zeneca, Spain; Zeneca, USA.
Nisoldipine (p.946·3).
Angina pectoris; hypertension.

Sulartrene *NCSN, Ital.*
Sulindac (p.85·3).
Gout; musculoskeletal, joint, peri-articular, and soft-tissue disorders.

Sulazine *Chatfield Laboratories, UK.*
Sulfasalazine (p.1251·1).
Inflammatory bowel disease; rheumatoid arthritis.

Sulbacta *Olan-Kemed, Thai.*
Co-trimoxazole (p.193·3).
Bacterial infections.

Sulcain
Shinyaku, Hong Kong; Shinyaku, Singapore; Shinyaku, Thai.
Ethyl *p*-piperidinoacetylaminobenzoate (p.1312·1); magcerin (magnesia alumina hydrate).
Gastric pain; gastritis; nausea; pyrosis.

Shinyaku, Jpn.
Ethyl *p*-piperidinoacetylaminobenzoate (p.1312·1).
Gastritis.

Sulcrate *Hoechst Marion Roussel, Canad.*
Sucralfate (p.1250·2).
Gastrointestinal haemorrhage; peptic ulcer.

Sulen *Farmacologica Milanese, Ital.*
Sulindac (p.85·3).
Gout; musculoskeletal, joint, and peri-articular disorders.

Suleo-C *Seton, UK†.*
Carbaryl (p.1429·2).
Pediculosis.

Suleo-M *SSL, UK.*
Malathion (p.1434·2).
Pediculosis.

Sulf-10 *Ciba Vision, USA.*
Sulfacetamide sodium (p.250·3).
Eye infections.

Sulfa 10 *Asta Medica, Belg.*
Sulfacetamide sodium (p.250·3).
Bacterial eye infections.

Sulfa Cloran *Grin, Mex.*
Chloramphenicol (p.179·1); sulfacetamide sodium (p.250·3).
Bacterial eye infections.

Sulfa Hidro *Grin, Mex.*
Hydrocortisone acetate (p.1073·3); sulfacetamide sodium (p.250·3).
Infected eye disorders.

Sulfac *Ocusoft, USA.*
Sulfacetamide sodium (p.250·3).
Bacterial eye infections.

Sulfacet *Llorens, Spain†.*
Sulfacetamide sodium (p.250·3).
Bacterial eye infections.

Sulfacetam *Medical, Spain.*
Sulfacetamide sodium (p.250·3).
Eye infections.

Sulfacet-R
Dermik, Canad.; Dermik, USA.
Sulfacetamide sodium (p.250·3); sulfur (p.1123·3).
Acne; rosacea; seborrhoeic dermatitis.

Sulfacid *Fischer, Israel.*
Sulfacetamide sodium (p.250·3).
Eye infections.

Sulfafer *Protein, Mex.*
Ferrous sulfate (p.1360·3).

Sulfagine *Tocogino, Mex.*
Sulfathiazole (p.257·1).

Sulfalax Calcium *Major, USA†.*
Docusate calcium (p.1222·3).
Constipation.

Sulfamethoprim *Quad, USA†.*
Co-trimoxazole (p.193·3).
Bacterial infections; Pneumocystis carinii pneumonia.

Sulfamide *Medical Ophthalmics, USA.*
Prednisolone acetate (p.1078·1); sulfacetamide sodium (p.250·3).
Infected eye disorders.

Sulfamylon *Bertek, USA.*
Mafenide acetate (p.221·2).
Burns.

Sulfanil *Allergan-Frumtost, Braz.*
Sulfacetamide (p.250·3).
Bacterial eye infections.

Sulfarlem
Solvay, Belg.†; Solvay, Canad.; Solvay, Fr.; Solvay, Hong Kong; Hoechst Marion Roussel, S.Afr.†; Solvay, Switz.
Anethole trithione (p.1580·1).
Biliary-tract disorders; dry eye; dry mouth; hypersensitivity reactions; liver disorders.

Sulfarlem Choline *Solvay, Belg.*
Anethole trithione (p.1580·1); choline bitartrate (p.1356·3).
Liver disorders; steatosis.

Sulfarlem S 25 *Solvay, Belg.*
Anethole trithione (p.1580·1).
Dry mouth.

Sulfaryl *Zeneca, Belg.†*
Acetarsol (p.587·2); sulfanilamide (p.256·2); sodium perborate (p.1156·3).
Mouth disorders.

Sulfatrex *QIF, Braz.*
Co-trimoxazole (p.193·3); guaifenesin (p.1092·2); ammonium chloride (p.1085·2).
Bacterial infections.

Sulfatril *Hua, Thai.*
Sulfadiazine (p.251·1); sulfadimidine (p.252·2); sulfamerazine (p.253·3).
Bacterial infections.

Sulfatrim
Vitamed, Israel; Schein, USA.
Co-trimoxazole (p.193·3).
Bacterial infections; Pneumocystis carinii pneumonia.

Sulfawal *Novag, Mex.*
Co-trimoxazole (p.193·3).
Bacterial infections.

Sulfestrep *Pisa, Mex.*
Streptomycin (p.249·1).
Bacterial infections.

Sulfex
Charton, Canad.†; Xepa-Soul Pattinson, Hong Kong.
Sulfacetamide sodium (p.250·3).
Bacterial eye infections.

Sulfile *Searle, Ital.*
Arginine timonacicate (p.1354·1).
Liver disorders.

Lepori, Port.
Arginine tidiacicate (p.1354·1).
Liver disorders.

Sulfinona *Basi, Port.*
Sulfinpyrazone (p.402·2).

Sulfintestin Neom *Hosbon, Spain†.*
Formosulfathiazole (p.207·3); neomycin sulfate (p.228·1).
Gastrointestinal infections.

Sulfintestin Neomicina *Normon, Spain.*
Dihydrostreptomycin sulfate (p.199·2); formosulfathiazole (p.207·3); neomycin sulfate (p.228·1).
Gastrointestinal infections.

Sulfiselen *Diviser Aquilea, Spain.*
Selenium sulfide (p.1123·1); thiram disulfide (p.1672·1).
Dandruff.

Sulfix *Allo Pro, Aust.*
Methylmethacrylate/polymethylmethacrylate (p.1635·2).
Bone cement.

Sulfizax *Remir, Mex.*
Sulfafurazole (p.253·1).
Bacterial infections.

Sulfoam *Bradley, USA.*
Sulfur (p.1123·3).
Formerly contained salicylic acid.
Dandruff; seborrhoea.

Sulfoid Trimetho *Valdecasas, Mex.*
Co-trimoxazole (p.193·3).
Bacterial infections.

Sulfoil *C & M, USA.*
Soap-free skin cleanser.

Sulfometh *Hua, Thai.*
Co-trimoxazole (p.193·3).
Bacterial infections.

Sulfona
Zimaia, Port.; Orsade, Spain.
Dapsone (p.196·1).
Leprosy.

Sulfo-Olbad Cordes *Ichthyol, Ger.*
Shale oil; soya oil (p.1378·1).
Bath additive; skin disorders.

Sulfopino *Schoning-Berlin, Ger.†*
Colloidal sulfur (p.1123·3).
Bath additive; joint disorders; neuralgia; skin disorders.

Sulforcin *Healthpoint, USA.*
Sulfur (p.1123·3); resorcinol (p.1122·2).
Acne.

Sulfort *Alpha, Mex.*
Co-trimoxazole (p.193·3).
Bacterial infections.

Sulfo-Salicyl *Life, Israel.*
Salicylic acid (p.1122·3); sulfur (p.1123·3); Dead Sea
minerals.
Psoriasis; seborrhoea.

Sulfo-Schwefelbad *Strallhofer, Aust.*
Sulfur (p.1123·3); sodium hydroxide (p.1665·3).
Musculoskeletal and joint disorders; skin disorders.

Sulfo-Selenium *Asta Medica, Belg.†*
Hydrocortisone (p.1073·3); selenium disulfide
(p.1123·1).
Squamous blepharitis.

Sulfosol *Sanochemia, Aust.†*
Sulfur (p.1123·3).
Inflammatory gynaecological disorders; musculoskeletal and joint disorders; skin disorders.

Sulfotrim *Gea, Denm.*
Co-trimoxazole (p.193·3).
Bacterial infections; Pneumocystis carinii pneumonia.

Sulfoxyl *Stiefel, Stiefel, USA.*
Benzoyl peroxide (p.1111·1); sulphur (p.1123·3).
Acne.

Sulfredox *Rubiepharm, Ger.*
Oral granules: Aluminium sodium silicate (p.1211·3);
sulfur (p.1123·3); calcium carbonate (p.1215·1); magnesium oxide (p.1233·2); sodium ascorbate; trace elements.
Tablets: Aluminium sodium silicate (p.1211·3); sulfur
(p.1123·3); calcium carbonate (p.1215·1); sodium
ascorbate; trace elements.
Digestive system disorders.

Sulfur Med Complex *Dynamit, Aust.*
Homoeopathic preparation.

Sulfurell *Sanorell, Ger.*
Homoeopathic preparation.

Sulfuretten *Stulln, Ger.*
Sulfur (p.1123·3); sodium thiosulfate (p.1691·2).
Dermatoses; lead, arsenic, or mercury poisoning; metabolic disorders.

Sulfuryl *Aerocid, Fr.*
Bath additive: Sulfurated aluminium sodium silicate
(p.1211·3); precipitated sulphur (p.1123·3).
Arthroses; skin disorders.
Chewable tablets; inhalation tablets: Sulfurated aluminium sodium silicate (p.1211·3).
Respiratory-tract congestion.
Soap: Sulfurated aluminium sodium silicate
(p.1211·3); precipitated sulphur (p.1123·3).
Skin disorders.

Sulgan *Doetsch, Grether, Switz.*
Ointment; suppositories: Ethyl linoleate; ethyl linolenate; lignocaine [lidocaine] hydrochloride
(p.1313·2); dichlorobenzyl alcohol (p.1143·2);
hamamelis (p.1618·3); camphor (p.1589·3); menthol
(p.1632·3); triclosan (p.1159·2).
Wipes: Dichlorobenzyl alcohol (p.1143·2); lignocaine
[lidocaine] hydrochloride (p.1313·2); chamomile
(p.1593·2); hamamelis (p.1618·3); camphor
(p.1589·3); menthol (p.1632·3).
Anorectal disorders.

Sulgan 99 *Klosterfrau, Aust.*
Ointment; suppositories: Ethyl linoleate; ethyl linolenate; benzocaine (p.1306·2); dichlorobenzyl alcohol
(p.1143·2); aluminium chlorohydrate (p.1110·2);
hamamelis (p.1618·3); camphor (p.1589·3); menthol
(p.1632·3); zinc oxide (p.1128·2).
Rectal wipes: Benzocaine (p.1306·2); dichlorobenzyl
alcohol (p.1143·2); hamamelis (p.1618·3); chamomile
water (p.1593·2); camphor (p.1589·3); menthol
(p.1632·3).
Anorectal disorders.

Sulic *Crosara, Ital.†*
Sulindac (p.85·3) or sulindac sodium (p.86·2).
Gout; musculoskeletal, joint, and peri-articular disorders; neuritis; sciatica.

Sulidamor *Damor, Ital.*
Nimesulide (p.62·3).
Fever; inflammation; pain.

Sulide *Virginia, Ital.*
Nimesulide (p.62·3).
Fever; inflammation; pain.

Sulimed *Inibsa, Port.*
Nimesulide (p.62·3).
Inflammation; musculoskeletal, joint, and peri-articular disorders; pain.

Sulindal *Chibret, Spain.*
Sulindac (p.85·3).
Gout; inflammation; musculoskeletal, joint, and peri-articular disorders; pain.

Sulindor *Millet Roux, Braz.*
Dipyrone (p.34·1); isometheptene (p.1624·2); caffeine
(p.761·3).
Smooth muscle spasm.

Sulinol *ICT, Ital.†*
Sulindac (p.85·3).
Gout; musculoskeletal, joint, and peri-articular disorders; neuritis; sciatica.

Sulmasque *C & M, USA.*
Sulfur (p.1123·3).
Acne.

Sulmetin *Sanofi Synthelabo, Spain.*
Magnesium sulfate (p.1191·1).
Procaine hydrochloride (p.1319·1) is included in the
intramuscular injection to alleviate the pain of injection.
Convulsions; tachycardia; vertigo.

Sulmetin Papaver *Sanofi Synthelabo, Spain.*
Atropine methobromide (p.460·3); magnesium sulfate
(p.1191·1); papaverine hydrochloride (p.1648·1); propyphenazone (p.80·2).
Pain due to smooth muscle spasm.

Sulmetin Papaverina *Sanofi Synthelabo, Spain.*
Injection: Magnesium sulfate (p.1191·1); papaverine
hydrochloride (p.1648·1).
Procaine hydrochloride (p.1319·1) is included in the
intramuscular injection to alleviate the pain of injection.
*Convulsions; hypertension; smooth muscle spasm;
tachycardia.*
Tablets: Atropine methobromide (p.460·3); magnesium gluconate (p.1190·3); papaverine hydrochloride
(p.1648·1); propyphenazone (p.80·2).
Pain due to smooth muscle spasm.

Sulmycin
Aesca, Aust.; Essex, Ger.
Gentamicin sulfate (p.210·1).
Bacterial infections.

Sulmycin mit Celestan-V *Essex, Ger.*
Gentamicin sulfate (p.210·1); betamethasone valerate
(p.1063·2).
Infected skin disorders.

Sulmyn *Sons, Mex.*
Kanamycin (p.218·2).
Bacterial infections.

Sulnil *Allergan-Frumtost, Braz.*
Chloramphenicol (p.179·1); sulfacetamide (p.250·3).
Bacterial eye infections.

Sulobil *Atlantis, Mex.*
Chenodeoxycholic acid (p.1594·1).
Cholesterol gallstones.

Sulorane *Zeneca, Israel.*
Desflurane (p.1257·2).
General anaesthesia.

Suloves *Lampugnani, Ital.†*
A heparinoid (p.905·2).
Thrombosis prophylaxis.

Sulp *Hexal, Ger.*
Sulpiride (p.706·1).
Depression; schizophrenia; vestibular disorders.

Sulpan *Synthelabo, Braz.*
Sulpiride (p.706·1); bromazepam (p.656·3).
Depression.

Sulparex *Bristol-Myers Squibb, UK†.*
Sulpiride (p.706·1).
Schizophrenia.

Sulperazon
Pfizer, Hong Kong; Pfizer, Thai.
Sulbactam (p.250·1) or sulbactam sodium (p.250·1);
cefoperazone (p.168·2) or cefoperazone sodium
(p.168·2).
Bacterial infections.

Sulphamide *Vitamed, Israel.*
Sulfacetamide sodium (p.250·3).
Bacterial eye infections.

Sulpho-Lac *Doak, USA.*
Sulfur (p.1123·3); zinc sulfate (p.1398·2).
Acne.

Sulphonated Lauryls *Ronsheim & Moore, UK.*
A range of alkyl sulfates.

Sulpiren *Medochemie, Hong Kong.*
Sulpiride (p.706·1).
Gastrointestinal disorders.

Sulpitil *Pharmacia, UK.*
Sulpiride (p.706·1).
Schizophrenia.

Sulpivert *Hennig, Ger.*
Sulpiride (p.706·1).
Depression; schizophrenia; vertigo.

Sulpor *Rosemont, UK.*
Sulpiride (p.706·1).

Sulpril *AstraZeneca, Denm.*
Sulpiride (p.706·1).
Schizophrenia.

Sulprim *Berman, Mex.*
Co-trimoxazole (p.193·3).
Bacterial infections.

Sulpyrin *CCPC, Hong Kong.*
Dipyrone (p.34·1).
Fever.

Sulquibron *Bohm, Spain.*
Ampicillin (p.150·3); citiolone (p.1596·2).
Respiratory-tract infections.

Sulquipen *Bohm, Spain.*
Cefalexin (p.161·3).
Bacterial infections.

Sulster *Akorn, USA†.*
Sulfacetamide sodium (p.250·3); prednisolone sodium
phosphate (p.1078·1).
Infected eye disorders.

Sultanol
Glaxo Wellcome, Aust.; Glaxo Wellcome, Ger.; Cascan, Ger.
Salbutamol sulfate (p.770·3).
Obstructive airways disease.

Sulterline *TP, Thai.*
Terbutaline sulfate (p.776·2).
Obstructive airways disease.

Sulton *Geymonat, Ital.*
Calcium folinate (p.1363·1).
*Anaemias; antidote to folic acid antagonists; reduction
of aminopterin and methotrexate toxicity.*

Sultrin
*Janssen-Cilag, Austral.; Janssen-Cilag, Belg.; Janssen-Ortho, Canad.;
Janssen-Cilag, Port.; Janssen-Cilag, S.Afr.; Janssen-Cilag, UK; Ortho McNeil, USA.*
Sulfabenzamide (p.250·2); sulfacetamide (p.250·3);
sulfathiazole (p.257·1).
Bacterial vaginitis and cervicitis.

Sultroquin *Farcoral, Mex.*
Clioquinol (p.190·2); homatropine (p.468·1); phthalylsulfathiazole (p.235·3).
Gastrointestinal disorders.

Sumacal *Sherwood, USA.*
Glucose polymers (p.1350·1).
Carbohydrate source.

Sumapen *Great Eastern, Thai.; Westmont, Thai.*
Ampicillin trihydrate (p.151·1).
Bacterial infections.

Sumax *Libbs, Braz.*
Sumatriptan (p.457·2).
Migraine.

Sumedium *Milano, Thai.*
Phenazopyridine hydrochloride (p.77·3).
Urinary-tract pain.

Sumial *Zeneca, Spain.*
Propranolol hydrochloride (p.962·3).
*Angina pectoris; arrhythmias; gastrointestinal haemorrhage; hypertension; hyperthyroidism; migraine;
myocardial infarction; obstructive cardiomyopathy;
phaeochromocytoma; tremor.*

Sumidin *Pharmaland, Thai.*
Serrapeptase (p.2381·1).
Inflammation; oedema; respiratory-tract congestion.

Sumigrene *Sigma-Tau, Ital.*
Sumatriptan succinate (p.456·1).
Cluster headache; migraine.

Summavit *Bioprogress, Ital.*
Multivitamin preparation (p.1350·1).

Summers Eve *Fleet, USA.*
A range of feminine hygiene preparations.

Summers Eve Disposable
Note. This name is used for preparations of different composition.
Fleet, Austral.
Fresh Scent: Phenol (p.1152·3).
Herbal Scented†; White Flowers†; Hint of Musk†: Octoxinol 9 (p.1346·3).
Vinegar and Water: Vinegar (p.1571·2).
Vaginal cleanser.
Fleet, USA.
Regular solution: Sodium citrate (p.1186·2); citric acid
(p.1596·2); sodium benzoate (p.1134·3).
Scented solution: Sodium citrate (p.1186·2); citric acid
(p.1596·2); sodium benzoate (p.1134·3); octoxinol 9
(p.1346·3).
Solution: Vinegar (p.1571·2).
Vaginal disorders.

Summers Eve Feminine
Fleet, Austral.
Bath additive; topical liquid; topical spray: Soap substitute.
Vaginal hygiene.
Topical powder: Octoxinol 9 (p.1346·3); benzethonium chloride (p.1134·2).
Intertrigo; vaginal irritation.
Towelettes: Octoxinol 9 (p.1346·3).
Vaginal hygiene.

Summers Eve Medicated
Fleet, Singapore; Fleet, USA.
Povidone-iodine (p.1155·1).
Vaginal disorders.

Summers Eve Post-Menstrual *Fleet, USA.*
Sodium laurilsulfate (p.1496·3); monobasic sodium
phosphate (p.1193·2); dibasic sodium phosphate
(p.1193·2); sodium chloride (p.1196·1); edetic acid
(p.1008·3).
Vaginal disorders.

Sumycin *Apothecon, USA.*
Tetracycline hydrochloride (p.258·3).
Bacterial infections.

Sun Buffer *Clinique, Canad.*
SPF 15: Octinoxate (p.1517·3).
Sunscreen.

Sun Defense Lip Block *Norman, Canad.*
SPF 15: Octinoxate (p.1517·3); oxybenzone
(p.1518·1).
Sunscreen.

Sun Defense Sunblock *Norman, Canad.*
SPF 25: Octinoxate (p.1517·3); homosalate
(p.1517·2); octisalate (p.1518·1); oxybenzone
(p.1518·1).
Sunscreen.

Sun Defense Sunscreen *Norman, Canad.*
SPF 8: Octinoxate (p.1517·3); oxybenzone (p.1518·1).
Sunscreen.

Sun Management Extensive Protection *Kay,
Canad.*
Octinoxate (p.1517·3); octisalate (p.1518·1); oxybenzone (p.1518·1).
Sunscreen.

Sun Management Intensive Protection *Kay,
Canad.*
SPF 20: Octinoxate (p.1517·3); octisalate (p.1518·1);
oxybenzone (p.1518·1).
Sunscreen.

Sun Management Lip Protection *Kay, Canad.*
SPF 15: Octinoxate (p.1517·3); oxybenzone
(p.1518·1).
Sunscreen.

Sun Management Sensible Protection *Kay, Canad.*
Octinoxate (p.1517·3); oxybenzone (p.1518·1).
Sunscreen.

Sun Pacer *Amway, Canad.*
SPF 8; SPF 15: Octinoxate (p.1517·3); oxybenzone
(p.1518·1).
SPF 30: Octocrilene (p.1518·1); octinoxate (p.1517·3);
octisalate (p.1518·1); oxybenzone (p.1518·1).
Sunscreen.

Sun Pacer Protective *Amway, Canad.†*
SPF 8: Oxybenzone (p.1518·1); padimate O
(p.1518·2).
SPF 15: Octinoxate (p.1517·3); oxybenzone
(p.1518·1); padimate O (p.1518·2).
SPF 30: Octinoxate (p.1517·3); oxybenzone
(p.1518·1); padimate O (p.1518·2); titanium dioxide
(p.1126·1).
Sunscreen.

Sun Pacer Sunless Tanning *Amway, Canad.*
SPF 15: Octinoxate (p.1517·3); octisalate (p.1518·1);
oxybenzone (p.1518·1).
Sunscreen.

Sun Tanning *Solar, Canad.*
SPF 4: Octinoxate (p.1517·3).
Sunscreen.

Sun-Benz *Sun, Canad.*
Benzydamine hydrochloride (p.20·1).
Oropharyngeal mucositis; sore throat.

Sunblock *Estee Lauder, Canad.*
SPF 15; SPF 25: Titanium dioxide (p.1126·1).
Sunscreen.

Suncodin
Aventis, S.Afr.
Tablets: Paracetamol (p.71·2); codeine phosphate
(p.25·2); phenyltoloxamine citrate (p.423·1); caffeine
(p.761·3).
Fever; pain; sinus congestion.
Noristan, S.Afr.†.
Syrup: Paracetamol (p.71·2); codeine phosphate
(p.25·2).
Fever; pain.

Sundays Maximum Protection *Nutri-Metics, Canad.†.*
SPF 15: Avobenzone (p.1517·1); octinoxate
(p.1517·3).
Sunscreen.

Sundown
Johnson & Johnson, Austral.; Johnson & Johnson, USA.
SPF 8; SPF 15; SPF 30: Octinoxate (p.1517·3); octisalate (p.1518·1); oxybenzone (p.1518·1); titanium dioxide (p.1126·1).
Sunscreen.

Sundown Active *Johnson & Johnson, Austral.*
SPF 15: Titanium dioxide (p.1126·1); zinc oxide
(p.1128·2).
Sunscreen.

Sundown with Insect Repellent *Johnson & Johnson,
Austral.*
SPF 15+: Octinoxate (p.1517·3); avobenzone
(p.1517·1); titanium dioxide (p.1126·1); di-N-propyl
isocinchomeronate; piperonyl butoxide (p.1436·2); N-
octylbicycloheptene dicarboximide; pyrethrins.
Sunscreen and insect repellent.

Sundown Sport *Johnson & Johnson, USA.*
SPF 15: Zinc oxide (p.1128·2); titanium dioxide
(p.1126·1).
Sunscreen.

Sundown Toddler *Johnson & Johnson, Austral.†.*
SPF 15+: Octinoxate (p.1517·3); oxybenzone
(p.1518·1); octisalate (p.1518·1); avobenzone
(p.1517·1).
Sunscreen.

SuNerven *Modern Health Products, UK.*
Motherwort (p.1637·3); vervain (p.1679·3); valerian
(p.1678·3); passion flower (p.1649·1).
Stresses and strains.

Sunfilter *Estee Lauder, Canad.†.*
SPF 15: Avobenzone (p.1517·1); octinoxate
(p.1517·3); titanium dioxide (p.1126·1).
Sunscreen.

Sun-Glizide *Sunward, Singapore.*
Gliclazide (p.322·2).
Diabetes mellitus.

Suniderma *Farmacusi, Spain.*
Hydrocortisone aceponate (p.1074·2).
Skin disorders.

Sunkist *Ciba, USA.*
Ascorbic acid (p.1389·3).

Sunnie *Green Turtle Bay Vitamin Co., USA.*
Vitamins; minerals; glutamine; hypericum; betaine;
ginkgo biloba (p.1350·1).
Tonic.

Sunprox *Sunward, Singapore.*
Naproxen sodium (p.61·1).
Gout; musculoskeletal, joint, and peri-articular disorders; pain.

SUNPRuF C & M, USA†.
SPF 15: Octinoxate (p.1517·3); oxybenzone (p.1518·1).
SPF 17: Octinoxate (p.1517·3); octisalate (p.1518·1).
Sunscreen.

Sunrythm Suntory, Jpn.
Pilsicainide hydrochloride (p.955·3).
Arrhythmias.

Sunsan-Heillotion Richter, Aust.
Diphenhydramine hydrochloride (p.416·1); dexpanthenol (p.1602·3); allantoin (p.1110·1).
Inflammatory skin disorders; skin irritation.

Sunscreen Hamilton, Austral.†.
Cream SPF 15+: Octinoxate (p.1517·3); avobenzone (p.1517·1); octisalate (p.1518·1).
Lotion-spray SPF 15+: Octinoxate (p.1517·3); avobenzone (p.1517·1); oxybenzone (p.1518·1).
Milky lotion SPF 15+: Enzacamene (p.1517·2); octinoxate (p.1517·3); avobenzone (p.1517·1).
Sunscreen.

Sunscreen Lotion
Norwood, Canad.
SPF 8; SPF 15: Octinoxate (p.1517·3); oxybenzone (p.1518·1); titanium dioxide (p.1126·1).
SPF 25; SPF 30: Octinoxate (p.1517·3); octisalate (p.1518·1); oxybenzone (p.1518·1); titanium dioxide (p.1126·1).
SPF 45: Octinoxate (p.1517·3); octocrilene (p.1518·1); octisalate (p.1518·1); oxybenzone (p.1518·1).
Sunscreen.

Therapex, Canad.
SPF 15: Avobenzone (p.1517·1); octinoxate (p.1517·3); oxybenzone (p.1518·1).
SPF 30: Avobenzone (p.1517·1); octinoxate (p.1517·3); oxybenzone (p.1518·1); titanium dioxide (p.1126·1).
Sunscreen.

Sunscreen Lotion Ecran Prodemdis, Canad.
SPF 15: Avobenzone (p.1517·1); octinoxate (p.1517·3); oxybenzone (p.1518·1).
SPF 30: Avobenzone (p.1517·1); enzacamene (p.1517·2); octinoxate (p.1517·3); ensulizole (p.1517·2).
Sunscreen.

Sunseekers Avon, Canad.
SPF 15: Octinoxate (p.1517·3); oxybenzone (p.1518·1).
SPF 6; SPF30: Octinoxate (p.1517·3); octisalate (p.1518·1); oxybenzone (p.1518·1).
Sunscreen.

Sunsense
Note.This name is used for preparations of different composition.
Ego, Austral.†.
SPF 15+: Titanium dioxide (p.1126·1); oxybenzone (p.1518·1); octinoxate (p.1517·3); avobenzone (p.1517·1).
Sunscreen.

Ego, Hong Kong; Ego, Singapore.
Cream SPF30+; Ultra SPF 30+; Face Milk SPF 30+: Octinoxate (p.1517·3); oxybenzone (p.1518·1); titanium dioxide (p.1126·1).
Sunscreen.

Ego, NZ.
SPF 15+: Titanium dioxide (p.1126·1); oxybenzone (p.1518·1); avobenzone (p.1517·1); ethylhexyl cinnamate.
Sunscreen.

Sunsense Aftersun Ego, Austral.
Emollient.
Dry skin.

Sunsense Daily Face
Note.This name is used for preparations of different composition.
Ego, Austral.; Ego, Hong Kong.
SPF 30+: Octinoxate (p.1517·3); titanium dioxide (p.1126·1); enzacamene (p.1517·2).
Sunscreen.

Ego, Singapore.
SPF 30+: Octinoxate (p.1517·3); titanium dioxide (p.1126·1); enzacamene (p.1517·2); oxybenzone (p.1518·1).
Sunscreen.

Sunsense LIF Ego, Austral.†.
Octinoxate (p.1517·3); titanium dioxide (p.1126·1); avobenzone (p.1517·1).
Sunscreen.

Sunsense Lip Balm
Ego, Austral.; Ego, Hong Kong.
SPF 30+: Octinoxate (p.1517·3); oxybenzone (p.1518·1); titanium dioxide (p.1126·1); avobenzone (p.1517·1).
Sunscreen.

Sunsense Low Irritant
Ego, Austral.; Ego, Hong Kong; Ego, Singapore.
SPF 20: Titanium dioxide (p.1126·1).
Sunscreen.

Sunsense Sport
Ego, Austral.; Ego, Hong Kong; Ego, Singapore.
SPF 30+: Octinoxate (p.1517·3); oxybenzone (p.1518·1); titanium dioxide (p.1126·1); enzacamene (p.1517·2).
Sunscreen.

Sunsense and Sunsense Ultra Ego, Austral.
SPF 30+: Octinoxate (p.1517·3); oxybenzone (p.1518·1); titanium dioxide (p.1126·1).
Sunscreen.

Sunsense Toddler Milk
Ego, Austral.; Ego, Hong Kong; Ego, Singapore.
SPF 30+: Octinoxate (p.1517·3); oxybenzone (p.1518·1); titanium dioxide (p.1126·1); amiloxate (p.1516·3).
Sunscreen.

Sunsense Ultra Lagap, UK.
Octinoxate (p.1517·3); oxybenzone (p.1518·1); titanium dioxide (p.1126·1).
Sunscreen.

Sunsmackers Bonne Bell, Canad.†.
SPF 6; SPF 30: Octinoxate (p.1517·3); oxybenzone (p.1518·1); padimate O (p.1518·2).
Sunscreen.

Sunspot
Note.This name is used for preparations of different composition.
Sunspot, Austral.
Salicylic acid (p.1122·3).
Hard skin; solar keratoses.

Surf Ski International, UK.
Camphor (p.1589·3); benzoin (p.1668·3); ethyl glycol.; benzalkonium chloride (p.1133·2); allantoin (p.1110·1); isopropyl alcohol (p.1149·2).
Herpes labialis.

Supa C Vitaplex, Austral.
Calcium ascorbate (p.1389·3).
Vitamin C deficiency.

Supa-Boost Vitaplex, Austral.
Multivitamin and mineral preparation with rutoside (p.1350·1).

Supac Mission Pharmacal, USA†.
Paracetamol (p.71·2); aspirin (p.14·2); caffeine (p.761·3).
Pain.

Supadol Whitehall, Fr.
Paracetamol (p.71·2); codeine phosphate (p.25·2).
Formerly contained paracetamol, papaverine hydrochloride, papaverine nicotinate, codeine hydrobromide, and homatropine methylbromide.
Pain.

Supartz Smith & Nephew, UK.
Sodium hyaluronate (p.1620·1).
Synovial fluid replacement.

Super Active Multi Quest, Canad.
Multivitamin and mineral preparation (p.1350·1).

Super AO Formula Seroyal, Canad.
Betacarotene, selenium, vitamin C, vitamin D, and zinc (p.1350·1).

Super B Vitaglow, Austral.
Vitamin B substances with ascorbic acid (p.1350·1).
Dietary supplement.

Super B Complex Sisu, Canad.
Vitamin B substances (p.1350·1).
Nutritional supplement.

Super B Extra Roche Consumer, Austral.†.
Vitamin B substances with ascorbic acid and minerals (p.1350·1).
Dietary supplement.

Super B Plus Vitaglow, Austral.
Vitamin B substances; vitamin C; lysine hydrochloride; magnesium oxide; potassium sulfate; zinc amino acid chelate (p.1350·1).
Dietary supplement; tonic.

Super B Plus Liver Tonic Vitaglow, Austral.
Silybum marianum (p.1021·3); vitamins; minerals (p.1350·1).
Dietary supplement; digestive system disorders.

Super B Stress Roche Consumer, Austral.
Vitamin B substances; vitamin C; minerals; passion flower (p.1350·1).
Dietary supplement.

Super Banish Smith & Nephew, Austral.
Silver nitrate (p.1664·2); ethylene thiourea.
Ostomy deodorant.

Super C Jamieson, Canad.; Quest, Canad.; Swiss Herbal, Canad.
Ascorbic acid (p.1389·3).

Super Cal-C Bio Eagle, Austral.
Calcium ascorbate (p.1389·3); bioflavonoids (p.1611·1).
Vitamin C deficiency.

Super Cal-Mag Seroyal, Canad.
Mineral preparation with vitamin D (p.1350·1).

Super Citro Cee Marlyn, USA†.
Lemon bioflavonoids (p.1611·1); rutoside (p.1611·2); ascorbic acid (p.1389·3); rose hips (p.1389·3).
Capillary bleeding.

Super Cold Tabs Reese, USA†.
Paracetamol (p.71·2); phenylpropanolamine hydrochloride (p.1098·1); chlorpheniramine [chlorphenamine] (p.412·2).
Cold symptoms.

Super Complex C Approved Drug, USA†.
Hesperidin (p.1611·2); citrus bioflavonoids complex (p.1611·1); rutoside (p.1611·2); ascorbic acid (p.1389·3); rose hips (p.1389·3); red cherry (p.1029·1).
Capillary bleeding.

Super Cromer Orto Normon, Spain.
Merbromin (p.1150·1).
Wound disinfection.

Super D Perles Roberts, USA.
Vitamins A and D (p.1350·1).

Super Daily Lee-Adams, Canad.
Multivitamin and mineral preparation (p.1350·1).

Super Energex Plus Sante Naturelle, Canad.
Vitamin B substances, minerals, kola, and liver extract (p.1350·1).

Super 28 Formula Reese, USA.
Multivitamin, mineral, and herbal preparation (p.1350·1).

Super Galanol Lifeplan, UK.
Borage oil (p.1613·1).
Nutritional supplement.

Super Gamma Oil with Vitamin E Quest, Canad.
Evening primrose oil (p.1613·2); vitamin E (p.1394·1).

Super GammaOil Marine Quest, UK.
Evening primrose oil (p.1613·2); borage oil (p.1613·1); concentrated fish oil (p.949·3).

Super GLA Cantassium Co., UK.
Gamma linolenic acid (from vegetable oils) (p.1613·1).

Super Hi Potency Nion, USA.
Multivitamin and mineral preparation (p.1350·1).

Super Ivy Dry Ivy Corp, USA.
Zinc acetate (p.1398·1); benzyl alcohol (p.1135·2).
Minor skin irritation.

Super Malic Optimox, USA†.
Malic acid (p.1··); magnesium (p.1190·3).

Super Mega B+C Quest, UK.
Vitamin B and C substances (p.1350·1); valerian (p.1678·3); passion flower (p.1649·1); peppermint oil (p.1243·3); wood betony; cimicifuga root (p.1595·2); skullcap (p.1664·3); lupulus (p.1629·3); ginger root (p.1227·2).

Super Once A Day
Quest, Canad.; Quest, UK.
Multivitamin and mineral preparation (p.1350·1).

Super Orti-Vite Seroyal, Canad.
Multivitamin and mineral preparation (p.1350·1).

Super Plenamins
3M, Irl.; 3M, UK.
Multivitamin and mineral preparation (p.1350·1).

Super Quints Freeda, USA.
Vitamin B substances (p.1350·1).

Super Soluble Maxipro HBV Scientific Hospital Supplies, Austral.
Preparation for enteral nutrition (p.1350·1).
Hypoproteinaemia.

Super Strength Sinadrin Reese, USA†.
Paracetamol (p.71·2); phenylpropanolamine hydrochloride (p.1098·1); chlorpheniramine [chlorphenamine] (p.412·2).

Super Stress Mega B plus Vitamin C Quest, Canad.
Vitamin B substances and vitamin C (p.1350·1).

Super Vikaps Reese, USA.
Multivitamin and mineral preparation (p.1350·1).

Super Vita Vim
Jamieson, Canad.; Jamieson, Hong Kong.
Multivitamin and mineral preparation (p.1350·1).

Super Vitalex Carmaran, Canad.†.
Vitamin B substances and iron (p.1350·1).

Super Wate-On DDD, UK.
Nutritional supplement with vitamins (p.1350·1).

Superan Synthelabo, Braz.
Alizapride hydrochloride (p.1209·3).
Nausea and vomiting.

Superdophilus Natren, USA.
Lactobacillus acidophilus (p.1626·3).
Dietary supplement.

SuperEPA Advanced Nutritional Technology, USA.
Omega-3 marine triglycerides (p.949·3).
Dietary supplement.

Superfade Sunspot, Austral.
Hydroquinone (p.1115·1); salicylic acid (p.1122·3); dexpanthenol (p.1602·3); padimate O (p.1518·2); vitamin E.
Skin hyperpigmentation.

Supergan Sanochemia, Aust.
Dihydroergocristine mesilate (p.1603·2); reserpine (p.967·3); hydrochlorothiazide (p.907·3).
Hypertension.

Superhist Whitehall, Braz.
Phenindamine (p.422·2); ascorbic acid (p.1389·3); aspirin (p.14·2); caffeine (p.761·3).
Aluminium hydroxide-magnesium carbonate co-dried gel (p.1211·2) is included in this preparation in an attempt to limit adverse effects on the gastrointestinal mucosa.
Cold and influenza symptoms.

Superlipid Almirall, Spain.
Probucol (p.959·2).
Hyperlipidaemias.

Supermin Vitaglow, Austral.
Mineral and trace element preparation with vitamin D and lecithin (p.1350·1).

Supero Italfarmaco, Ital.
Cefuroxime sodium (p.178·2).
Lignocaine [lidocaine] hydrochloride (p.1313·3) is included in the intramuscular injection to alleviate the pain of injection.
Bacterial infections.

Superol Tendem, Neth.
Hydroxyquinoline sulfate (p.1622·2).
Sore throat.

Superpeni Roussel, Spain†.
Amoxicillin trihydrate (p.149·2).
Bacterial infections.

Superpeni Mucolitico Roussel, Spain†.
Amoxicillin trihydrate (p.149·2); bromhexine hydrochloride (p.1085·2).
Respiratory-tract infections.

Superpep
Hermes, Ger.; Democal, Switz.
Dimenhydrinate (p.415·2).
Motion sickness; nausea; vertigo; vomiting.

Superplex-T Major, USA.
Vitamin B substances with vitamin C (p.1350·1).

Supersan Merck, Port.
Cyproheptadine hydrochloride (p.414·2).
Appetite stimulant.

SuperSkin Medlogic, UK.
Enbucrilate (p.1601·2).
Barrier preparation.

Supertendin 2000 N Thiemann, Ger.
Dexamethasone (p.1067·1); lignocaine [lidocaine] hydrochloride (p.1313·2).
Painful inflammatory musculoskeletal and joint disorders.

Supertendin-Depot Thiemann, Ger.
Dexamethasone acetate (p.1067·1); lignocaine [lidocaine] hydrochloride (p.1313·2).
Musculoskeletal, joint, and peri-articular disorders; neuritis.

Superthiol Francia, Ital.
Carbocisteine (p.1086·3) or carbocisteine sodium (p.1086·3).
Respiratory-tract congestion.

Supertonic Diafarm, Spain.
Amino-acid preparation with cyanocobalamin (p.1350·1).
Tonic.

Supervit QIF, Braz.
Vitamin B substances (p.1350·1).
Nutritional supplement.

Supeudol Sabex, Canad.
Oxycodone hydrochloride (p.70·2).
Pain.

Suplac
Biolab, Singapore; Biolab, Thai.
Bromocriptine mesilate (p.1164·3).
Amenorrhoea; female and male infertility; galactorrhoea; lactation inhibition.

Suplasyn
Paladin, Canad.; Dominion, UK.
Sodium hyaluronate (p.1620·1).
Osteoarthritis of the knee; synovial fluid replacement following arthrocentesis.

Supledin S Luper, Braz.
Multivitamin, amino-acid, and mineral preparation (p.1350·1).

Suplena
Abbott, Austral.; Abbott, Canad.†; Abbott, Hong Kong; Abbott, Irl.; Ross, Israel; Abbott, NZ; Ross, USA.
Preparation for enteral nutrition in renal failure (p.1350·1).
Formerly known as Replena in the *USA.*

Suplevit
EMS, Braz.; Riva, Canad.
Multivitamin and mineral preparation (p.1350·1).

Supo Gliz Calmante Vitaminado, Spain.
Glycerol (p.1616·3).
Constipation; laxative dependence.

Supo Kristal CEPA, Spain†.
Glycerol (p.1616·3).
Constipation; laxative dependence.

Supofen Basi, Port.
Paracetamol (p.71·2).
Fever; pain.

Supositorios Senosiain Senosiain, Mex.
Glycerol (p.1616·3).
Constipation.

Suppap Raway, USA†.
Paracetamol (p.71·2).
Pain.

Supla-Cal NCI, USA†.
Supplemental nutrition bar (p.1350·1).

Supplamins F 3M, Israel.
Multivitamin and mineral preparation (p.1350·1).

Supplemaman Yves Ponroy, Fr.†.
Vitamin B substances, fatty acids, magnesium, and iron (p.1350·1).
Nutritional supplement during pregnancy.

Suppletive Dermoteca, Port.
Moisturiser.
Dry skin.

Supplevit Magnum Woelm, Ger.†.
Magnesium oxide (p.1233·2); alpha tocoferil acetate (p.1394·1).
Vitamin E or magnesium deficiency.

Suppomaline Solvay, Fr.
Belladonna (p.463·1); codeine phosphate (p.25·2); caffeine (p.761·3); paracetamol (p.71·2).
Fever; pain.

Supportan
Fresenius Kabi, Fin.; Fresenius Kabi, Ital.; Fresenius Kabi, Port.
Preparation for enteral nutrition (p.1350·1).

Supprelin Roberts, USA.
Histrelin acetate (p.1288·2).
Precocious puberty.

Suppress
Note.This name is used for preparations of different composition.
Stanley, Canad.
Diphenhydramine hydrochloride (p.416·1); codeine phosphate (p.25·2); ammonium chloride (p.1085·2).

The symbol † denotes a preparation no longer actively marketed

Ferndale, USA.
Dextromethorphan hydrobromide (p.1087·3).
Coughs.

Supra *ICN, Mex.*
Lidamidine hydrochloride (p.1231·2).
Gastrointestinal disorders.

Supraalox *Rhone-Poulenc Rorer, Spain.*
Aluminium hydroxide (p.1210·3); magnesium hydroxide (p.1233·1).
Dyspepsia; peptic ulcer.

Supracaine *Hoechst Marion Roussel, Canad.†*
Amethocaine [tetracaine] (p.1305·2).
Oral soft-tissue pain; reduction of gag reflex.

Supracef *Orion, Fin.*
Cefixime (p.166·2).
Bacterial infections.

Supracid *Asta Medica, Aust.*
Spironolactone (p.973·2); hydrochlorothiazide (p.907·3).
Hyperaldosteronism; hypertension; oedema.

Supracombin *Grunenthal, Aust.; Grunenthal, Ger.; Grunenthal, Switz.*
Co-trimoxazole (p.193·3).
Bacterial infections; Pneumocystis carinii pneumonia.

Supracream *Boots, Thai.; Hermal, Thai.*
Emollient barrier cream.
Dry skin; nappy rash.

Supracyclin *Grunenthal, Aust.; Grunenthal, Ger.*
Doxycycline (p.200·1) or doxycycline hyclate (p.200·1).
Bacterial infections.

Supracycline *Grunenthal, Switz.*
Doxycycline (p.200·1).
Bacterial infections.

Supradol *Liomont, Mex.*
Ketorolac trometamol (p.48·2).
Pain.

Supradyn *Roche, Aust.; Roche Consumer, Austral.; Roche, Belg†; Roche, Braz.; Roche Nicholas, Ger.; Roche, Hong Kong; Roche, Ital.; Roche, Mex.; Roche Consumer, Neth.; Roche, NZ; Roche, Port.; Roche, S.Afr.†; Roche Consumer, Singapore; Roche, Switz.; Roche, Thai.; Roche Consumer, UK.*
Multivitamin and mineral preparation (p.1350·1).

Supradyn Junior *Roche, Aust.*
Multivitamin and mineral preparation (p.1350·1).
Formerly known as Supradyn + Mineralien + Spurenelementen.

Supradyn N *Roche, Israel.*
Multivitamin and mineral preparation (p.1350·1).

Supradyne *Roche Nicholas, Fr.*
Multivitamin and mineral preparation (p.1350·1).

Supradynvital *Roche Nicholas, Fr.*
Multivitamin and mineral preparation with ginseng (p.1350·1).

Supragesic *Pharmaceutical Enterprises, S.Afr.*
Capsules: Paracetamol (p.71·2); codeine phosphate (p.25·2); caffeine (p.761·3); meprobamate (p.691·1).
Pain.
Syrup: Paracetamol (p.71·2); codeine phosphate (p.25·2).
Fever; pain.

Supralan *Siam Bheasach, Thai.*
Fluocinolone acetonide (p.1071·1).
Skin disorders.

Supralan-N *Siam Bheasach, Thai.*
Fluocinolone acetonide (p.1071·1); neomycin sulfate (p.228·1).
Infected skin disorders.

Supralef *Martin, Spain†.*
Hydrocortisone acetate (p.1073·3).
Skin disorders.

Supralip *Fournier, UK.*
Fenofibrate (p.889·1).
Hyperlipidaemias.

Supralox *Aventis, Fr.†; Rhone-Poulenc Rorer, Ger.†*
Aluminium hydroxide (p.1210·3); magnesium hydroxide (p.1233·1).
Gastrointestinal disorders.

Supramol *Sam-On, Israel.*
Paracetamol (p.71·2).
Fever; pain.

Supramox *Grunenthal, Aust.; Grunenthal, Switz.*
Amoxicillin (p.149·2) or amoxicillin trihydrate (p.149·2).
Bacterial infections.

Supramycin *Grunenthal, Ger.*
Tetracycline hydrochloride (p.258·3).
Bacterial infections.

Supran *Teva, Israel.*
Cefixime (p.166·2).
Bacterial infections.

Suprane *Pharmacia Upjohn, Aust.; Zeneca, Austral.; Pharmacia Upjohn, Belg.; AstraZeneca, Canad.; Baxter, Denm.; Baxter, Fin.; Pharmacia Upjohn, Ger.; Pharmacia Upjohn, Irl.; Pharmacia Upjohn, Ital.; Zeneca, Mex.; Pharmacia Upjohn, Neth.; Pharmacia Upjohn, Norw.†; AstraZeneca, NZ; Zeneca, S.Afr.; AstraZeneca, Singapore; Pharmacia Upjohn, Spain; Baxter, Swed.; Pharmacia Upjohn, Switz.; Baxter, UK; Ohmeda, USA.*
Desflurane (p.1257·2).
General anaesthesia.

Suprapen *SmithKline Beecham, S.Afr.*
Amoxicillin (p.149·2); flucloxacillin (p.207·1).
Bacterial infections.

Supraproct-S *Julphar, UAE.*
Betamethasone valerate (p.1063·2); cinchocaine hydrochloride (p.1309·1).
Anorectal disorders.

Suprarenin *Hoechst Marion Roussel, Aust.; Hoechst Marion Roussel, Ger.*
Adrenaline [epinephrine] hydrochloride (p.829·2).
Adjunct to local anaesthesia; circulatory collapse; hypersensitivity reactions; shock.

Suprasten *Gross, Braz.*
Suprarenal cortex (p.1080·1); ascorbic acid (p.1389·3); pentetrazol (p.1513·2).
Impaired mental function.

Suprastin *EGIS, Hung.*
Chloropyramine hydrochloride (p.412·1).
Hypersensitivity reactions.

Supratonin *Grunenthal, Ger.*
Amezinium metilsulfate (p.835·1).
Hypotension.

Supra-Vir *Trima, Israel.*
Aciclovir (p.612·3).
Herpesvirus infections.

Supraviran *Grunenthal, Ger.*
Aciclovir (p.612·3) or aciclovir sodium (p.612·3).
Herpesvirus infections.

Supravite
Nobel, Canad.
Vitamin B substances and iron (p.1350·1).

Pharmavite, Canad.†.
A range of vitamin preparations with or without minerals (p.1350·1).

Supravite C *Nobel, Canad.*
Vitamin B substances, vitamin C, and iron (p.1350·1).

Suprax
Rhone-Poulenc Rorer, Canad.; Klinge, Ger.; Rhone-Poulenc Rorer, Irl.; Wyeth Lederle, Ital.; Rhone-Poulenc Rorer, UK; Lederle, USA.
Cefixime (p.166·2).
Bacterial infections.

Suprecur
Hoechst Marion Roussel, Aust.; Aventis, Denm.; Hoechst Marion Roussel, Fin.; Hoechst Marion Roussel, Ger.; Hoechst Marion Roussel, Hong Kong; Hoechst Marion Roussel, Irl.; Hoechst Marion Roussel, Neth.; Hoechst Marion Roussel, Norw.; Hoechst Marion Roussel, S.Afr.†; Hoechst Marion Roussel, Singapore; Hoechst Marion Roussel, Swed.; Shire, UK.
Buserelin acetate (p.1278·1).
Endometriosis; ovulation induction.

Suprefact
Hoechst Marion Roussel, Aust.; Aventis, Belg.; Hoechst Marion Roussel, Braz.; Hoechst Marion Roussel, Canad.; Aventis, Denm.; Hoechst Marion Roussel, Fin.; Hoechst, Fr.; Hoechst Marion Roussel, Hong Kong; Hoechst Marion Roussel, Irl.; Hoechst Marion Roussel, Israel; Hoechst Marion Roussel, Ital.; Hoechst Marion Roussel, Neth.; Hoechst Marion Roussel, Norw.; Aventis, NZ; Hoeport, Port.; Aventis, S.Afr.; Hoechst Marion Roussel, Singapore; Hoechst Marion Roussel, Spain; Hoechst Marion Roussel, Swed.; Hoechst Marion Roussel, Switz.; Hoechst Marion Roussel, Thai.; Shire, UK.
Buserelin acetate (p.1278·1).
Endometriosis; ovulation induction; precocious puberty; prostatic cancer; uterine fibroids.

Suprenoat *Roche, Aust.*
Spironolactone (p.973·2); butizide (p.853·1); reserpine (p.967·3).
Hypertension.

Supres *Merck Frosst, Canad.*
Methyldopa (p.927·3); chlorothiazide (p.856·3).
Hypertension.

Supressin *Pfizer, Aust.*
Doxazosin mesilate (p.883·2).
Benign prostatic hyperplasia; hypertension.

Suprexon
Ciba Vision, Denm.†; Ciba Vision, Ger.; Ciba Vision, Neth.; Ciba Vision, Switz.†.
Guanethidine monosulfate (p.901·1); adrenaline [epinephrine] (p.829·1).
Glaucoma.

Sup-Rhinite *SmithKline Beecham Sante, Fr.*
Chlorpheniramine [chlorphenamine] maleate (p.412·1); phenylephrine hydrochloride (p.1097·1).
Rhinopharyngeal congestion.

Suprim
Note.This name is used for preparations of different composition.
Degorts, Mex.
Dipyrone (p.34·1).
Fever; pain.
Hovid, Singapore.
Co-trimoxazole (p.193·3).
Bacterial infections; protozoal infections.

Suprimal *IPS, Neth.†.*
Meclozine hydrochloride (p.420·3).
Motion sickness.

Suprin *Invamed, USA†.*
Aspirin (p.14·2); aluminium hydroxide (p.1210·3); magnesium oxide (p.1233·2).

Supristol
Note.This name is used for preparations of different composition.
Knoll, Mex.
Co-trimoxazole (p.193·3).
Bacterial infections.
Noristan, S.Afr.†.
Co-trifamole (p.193·3).
Bacterial infections.

Suprium *Leiras Synthelabo, Fin.*
Sulpiride (p.706·1).
Depression; psychoses.

Suprotide *Torre, Ital.*
Nutritional supplement (p.1350·1).

Suralgan *Searle, Ital.*
Tiaprofenic acid (p.88·1).
Inflammation; pain.

Surazem *Pharmacia Upjohn, Neth.*
Diltiazem hydrochloride (p.874·3).
Hypertension.

Surbex
Abbott, Canad.; Abbott, USA.
A range of vitamin preparations (p.1350·1).

Surbex with C *Abbott, Hong Kong.*
Vitamin B substances with vitamin C (p.1350·1).
Vitamin B and C deficiencies.

Surbex plus Iron *Abbott, Canad.*
Vitamin B substances with ascorbic acid and ferrous sulfate (p.1350·1).
Nutritional supplement.

Surbex plus Zinc
Abbott, Canad.
Vitamin B substances with ascorbic acid and zinc sulfate (p.1350·1).
Nutritional supplement.

Abbott, Singapore.
Vitamin B substances; vitamin C; vitamin E; zinc (p.1350·1).

Surbex T
Abbott, Hong Kong; Abbott, S.Afr.†; Abbott, Singapore; Abbott, Thai.
Vitamin B substances with vitamin C (p.1350·1).
Vitamin B and C deficiencies.

Surbex with Zinc *Abbott, Hong Kong.*
Multivitamin preparation with zinc (p.1350·1).
Nutritional supplement.

Surbronc
Boehringer Ingelheim, Belg.; Boehringer Ingelheim, Fr.
Ambroxol hydrochloride (p.1084·3).
Respiratory-tract congestion.

Surbu-Gen-T *Goldline, USA.*
Vitamin B substances with vitamin C (p.1350·1).

Surdolin *Ofimex, Mex.*
Tiaprofenic acid (p.88·1).

Sure Lax *Islacan, Spain.*
Phenolphthalein (p.1244·1).
Constipation.

SureLac *Caraco, USA.*
Tilactase (p.1673·2).
Lactose intolerance.

Sure-Lax *English Grains, UK†.*
Yellow phenolphthalein (p.1244·1).
Constipation.

Sure-Lax (Herbal) *Peter Black, UK.*
Aloes (p.1210·1); fennel (p.1610·1); valerian (p.1678·3); cnicus benedictus (p.1597·2).
Constipation.

Surelen *Roche Nicholas, Fr.*
Nutritional supplement (p.1350·1).
Tonic.

Surem *Roche, Spain†.*
Butalamine hydrochloride (p.853·1).
Vascular disorders.

Sureptil
Synthelabo, Braz.; Synthelabo, Fr.
Cinnarizine (p.413·1); heptaminol acephyllinate (p.765·3).
Mental function impairment; vascular disorders.

Sureskin *Euromedex, Fr.*
Carmellose sodium (p.1499·3); pectin (p.1502·3).
Burns; ulcers; wounds.

Suretin *Recordati, Ital.*
Tazarotene (p.1125·3).
Psoriasis.

Surfa-Base *Rougier, Canad.*
Emollient and vehicle.

Surfactal *Boehringer Ingelheim, Ital.*
Ambroxol hydrochloride (p.1084·3).
Neonatal surfactant deficiency; prevention of bronchopulmonary complications following surgery.

Surfacten *Tokyo Tanabe, Jpn.*
Bovine pulmonary extract (p.1655·3).
Respiratory distress syndrome.

Surfactil *Farmion, Braz.*
Ambroxol hydrochloride (p.1084·3).
Respiratory-tract congestion.

Surfak
Hoechst Marion Roussel, Canad.; Upjohn, USA.
Docusate calcium (p.1222·3).
Constipation.

Surfexo Neonatal *Glaxo Wellcome, Fr.*
Colfosceril palmitate (p.1656·1).
Respiratory distress syndrome in premature infants.

Surfol *Stiefel, USA.*
Emollient.

Surfolase *Searle; Lepori, Port.*
Ambroxol acefyllinate (p.1084·3).
Obstructive airways disease.

Surfont *Ardeypharm, Ger.*
Mebendazole (p.102·2).
Worm infections.

Surfortan *Diepha, Fr.*
Amino acid, mineral, and vitamin preparation (p.1350·1).
Tonic.

Surgam
Hoechst Marion Roussel, Austral.; Tramedico, Belg.; Hoechst Marion Roussel, Canad.; Roussel Diamant, Fr.; Hoechst Marion Roussel, Ger.; Hoechst Marion Roussel, Irl.; Hoechst Marion Roussel, Mex.; Hoechst Marion Roussel, Neth.; Aventis, NZ; Aventis, Port.; Aventis, S.Afr.; Hoechst Marion Roussel, Switz.†; Hoechst Marion Roussel, Thai.; Florizel, UK.
Tiaprofenic acid (p.88·1) or tiaprofenic acid, trometamol salt (p.88·2).
Gout; inflammation; musculoskeletal, joint, peri-articular and soft-tissue disorders; pain.

Surgamic *Roussel, Spain.*
Tiaprofenic acid (p.88·1).
Inflammation; musculoskeletal, joint, and peri-articular disorders; pain.

Surgamyl
Aventis, Denm.; Hoechst Marion Roussel, Fin.; Scharper, Ital.
Tiaprofenic acid (p.88·1).
Lignocaine [lidocaine] (p.1313·2) may be included in the intramuscular injection to alleviate the pain of injection.
Inflammation; musculoskeletal and joint disorders; pain.

Surgel *Ulmer, USA.*
Carmellose sodium (p.1499·3); propylene glycol (p.1655·1); glycerol (p.1616·3).
Vaginal lubricant.

Surgestone
Cassenne, Fr.; Roussel, Port.
Promegestone (p.1490·3).
Fibroids; mastalgia; menopausal disorders; menstrual disorders.

Surgicel
Ethicon, Fr.; Johnson & Johnson Medical, UK; Johnson & Johnson Medical, USA.
Oxidised cellulose (p.728·1).
Haemorrhage.

Surgicoll *MBP, Ger.†; Biodynamics, Ger.†*
Collagen (p.1598·2).
Haemorrhage.

Surgident *Mini, Switz.†.*
Adrenaline [epinephrine] hydrochloride (p.829·2).
Gingival haemorrhage.

Surifarm *Reig Jofre, Spain.*
Aluminium hydroxide (p.1210·3); dimethicone (p.1249·2); magnesium trisilicate (p.1233·3); metoclopramide (p.1236·3).
Aerophagia; digestive disorders; meteorism.

Suril *Ibirn, Ital.*
Sucralfate (p.1250·2).
Gastritis; gastro-oesophageal reflux; peptic ulcer.

Sur-Lax
Jean-Marie, Hong Kong; Jean-Marie, Singapore.
Sodium picosulfate (p.1249·3).
Constipation; stool softener.

Surlid
Aventis, Denm.; Hoechst Marion Roussel, Fin.; Hoechst Marion Roussel, Mex.; Hoechst Marion Roussel, Swed.
Roxithromycin (p.247·2).
Bacterial infections.

Surmenalit *Foes, Spain.*
Sulbutiamine (p.1385·1).
Vitamin B1 deficiency.

Surmontil
Rhone-Poulenc Rorer, Austral.; Aventis, Belg.; Rhone-Poulenc Rorer, Canad.; Aventis, Denm.; Rhone-Poulenc Rorer, Fin.; Rhone-Poulenc Rorer, Fr.; Rhone-Poulenc Rorer, Hong Kong; Rhone-Poulenc Rorer, Irl.; Rhone-Poulenc Rorer, Israel; Rhone-Poulenc Rorer, Ital.; Rhone-Poulenc Rorer, Neth.; Rhone-Poulenc Rorer, NZ; Vitoria, Port.; Aventis, S.Afr.; Rhone-Poulenc Rorer, Spain; Rhone-Poulenc Rorer, Swed.; Rhone-Poulenc Rorer, Switz.; Aventis, UK; Wyeth-Ayerst, USA.
Trimipramine (p.311·2), trimipramine maleate (p.311·2), or trimipramine mesilate (p.311·3).
Anxiety; depression; irritable bowel syndrome; pain; peptic ulcer; sleep disorders.

Surmouroine *Bournonville, Belg.†*
Cod-liver oil (p.1357·2).
Osteomalacia; osteoporosis; rickets; vitamin A and D deficiency.

Surnox *Hoechst Marion Roussel, Spain.*
Ofloxacin (p.232·3) or ofloxacin hydrochloride (p.233·1).
Bacterial infections.

Suronit *Ehlinger, Mex.*
Ranitidine (p.1246·3).

Surpass *Wrigley, USA.*
Calcium carbonate (p.1215·1).
Dyspepsia; heartburn.

Surquina *Innotech, Fr.*
Quinine hydrochloride (p.445·1).
Malaria.

Sursum *Abiogen, Ital.*
Alpha tocopherol (p.1394·1).
Vitamin E deficiency.

Survanta
Abbott, Aust.; Abbott, Austral.; Abbott, Belg.; Abbott, Braz.; Abbott, Canad.; Abbott, Fr.; Abbott, Ger.; Ross, Hong Kong; Abbott, Mex.; Abbott, Neth.; Abbott, NZ; Abbott, S.Afr.; Abbott, Singapore; Abbott, Spain; Abbott, Switz.; Abbott, Thai.; Abbott, UK; Ross, USA.
Beractant (p.1655·3).
Neonatal respiratory distress syndrome.

Survanta-Vent *Abbott, Norw.; Abbott, Swed.*
Beractant (p.1655·3).
Neonatal respiratory distress syndrome.

Survector *Servier, Braz.; Eutherapie, Fr.†; Stroder, Ital.†; Teravix, Port.†; Danval, Spain†.*
Amineptine hydrochloride (p.273·2).
Depression.

Survimed *Fresenius Kabi, Ital.; Fresenius Kabi, Port.; Fresenius Kabi, Switz.*
Range of preparations for enteral nutrition (p.1350·1).

Survitine *Roche Nicholas, Fr.†*
Multivitamin and mineral preparation (p.1350·1).
Nutritional disorders.

Susano *Halsey, USA.*
Atropine sulfate (p.461·1); hyoscine hydrobromide (p.468·2); hyoscyamine hydrobromide (p.469·3) or hyoscyamine sulfate (p.469·3); phenobarbital (p.355·1).
Gastrointestinal disorders.

Suscard *Pharmax, Irl.; AstraZeneca, Norw.; Hassle, Swed.; Pharmax, UK.*
Glyceryl trinitrate (p.897·3).
Angina pectoris; heart failure.

Sus-Phrine *Forest Pharmaceuticals, USA.*
Adrenaline [epinephrine] (p.829·1).
Asthma; bronchospasm.

Suss *Hoechst Marion Roussel, Braz.*
Co-trimoxazole (p.193·3).
Bacterial infections; Pneumocystis carinii pneumonia; protozoal infections.

Suss Balsamico *Hoechst Marion Roussel, Braz.*
Co-trimoxazole (p.193·3); guaifenesin (p.1092·2); ammonium chloride (p.1085·2).
Bacterial infections.

Sustac *Pharmax, Irl.; Pharmax, UK.*
Glyceryl trinitrate (p.897·3).
Angina pectoris.

Sustacal *Mead Johnson, Austral.; Mead Johnson Nutritionals, Canad.†; Mead Johnson, Hong Kong; Mead Johnson, Israel; Mead Johnson Nutritionals, Thai.; Mead Johnson Nutritionals, USA.*
A range of preparations for enteral nutrition (p.1350·1).

Sustagen *Mead Johnson, Austral.; Mead Johnson, Hong Kong; Mead Johnson, NZ; Mead Johnson Nutritionals, Thai.; Mead Johnson Nutritionals, USA.*
A range of preparations for enteral nutrition (p.1350·1).

Sustained Release Buffered C *Blackmores, Austral.*
Vitamin C (p.1389·3); bioflavonoids (p.1611·1); hesperidin (p.1611·2); rose fruit (p.1389·3); rutoside (p.1611·2).
Vitamin C supplement.

Sustained Release Executive B Plus Herbs *Blackmores, Austral.*
Vitamins; minerals; passion flower; avena (p.1350·1).
Nutritional supplement; stress.

Sustaire *Pfizer, USA.*
Theophylline (p.777·2).
Asthma; bronchospastic disorders.

Sustamycin *Boehringer Mannheim, UK†.*
Tetracycline hydrochloride (p.258·3).
Bacterial infections.

Sustanon *Organon, Belg.; Organon, Hong Kong; Organon, Ital.; Pharmaco, NZ.*
Testosterone propionate (p.1492·2); testosterone phenylpropionate (p.1492·2); testosterone isocaproate (p.1492·2); testosterone decanoate (p.1492·2).
Androgen deficiency; male hypogonadism.

Sustanon 100 *Organon, Austral.; Organon, Irl.; Organon, Neth.; Organon, UK.*
Testosterone propionate (p.1492·2); testosterone phenylpropionate (p.1492·2); testosterone isocaproate (p.1492·2).
Androgen deficiency; female breast cancer; male hypogonadism; osteoporosis.

Sustanon 250 *Organon, Austral.; Organon, Fin.; Organon, Irl.; Organon, Israel; Organon, Neth.; Donmed, S.Afr.; Organon, Singapore; Organon, UK.*
Testosterone propionate (p.1492·2); testosterone phenylpropionate (p.1492·2); testosterone isocaproate (p.1492·2); testosterone decanoate (p.1492·2).
Androgen deficiency; female breast cancer; male hypogonadism; osteoporosis.

Sustemial *Malesci, Ital.*
Ferrous gluconate (p.1360·1).
Anaemias; iron deficiency.

Sustenium *Menarini, Ital.*
Fosfocreatinine disodium (p.1612·3).
Muscle disorders.

Susteron 250 *Organon, Port.*
Testosterone propionate (p.1492·2); testosterone phenylpropionate (p.1492·2); testosterone decanoate (p.1492·2).
Male hypogonadism; osteoporosis.

Sustiva *Du Pont, Canad.; Du Pont, Fr.; Du Pont, Ger.; Du Pont, Irl.; Du Pont, Ital.; Du Pont, Spain; Du Pont, UK; Du Pont, USA.*
Efavirenz (p.620·1).
HIV infection.

Sustrate *Bristol-Myers Squibb, Braz.*
Propatylnitrate (p.962·3).
Angina pectoris.

Sutril *Novag, Spain.*
Torasemide (p.985·1) or torasemide sodium (p.985·2).
Hypertension; oedema.

Su-Tuss DM *Cypress, USA.*
Dextromethorphan hydrobromide (p.1087·3); guaifenesin (p.1092·2).
Coughs.

Su-Tuss HD *Cypress, USA.*
Hydrocodone tartrate (p.42·2); pseudoephedrine hydrochloride (p.1099·2); guaifenesin (p.1092·2).
Coughs.

Suvipen *Thera, Fr.†.*
Metampicillin sodium (p.222·3).
Bacterial infections.

Suxar *Sanus, Braz.*
Salbutamol (p.770·3).
Obstructive airways disease.

Suxidina *Seid, Spain.*
Aspergillus oryzae; dimethicone (p.1249·2); metoclopramide hydrochloride (p.1235·2); oxazepam hemisuccinate (p.697·2).
Aerophagia; digestive disorders; meteorism.

Suxilep *Jenapharm, Ger.*
Ethosuximide (p.348·1).
Absence seizures.

Suxinutin *Parke, Davis, Aust.; Parke, Davis, Fin.; Parke, Davis, Ger.; Parke, Davis, Swed.; Parke, Davis, Switz.*
Ethosuximide (p.348·1).
Absence seizures.

Svedocain Sin Vasoconstr *Inibsa, Spain.*
Bupivacaine hydrochloride (p.1306·3).
Local anaesthesia.

SVR 50B *SVR, Fr.*
SPF 50: Titanium dioxide (p.1126·1); zinc oxide (p.1128·2).
Sunscreen.

Swarm *Pickles, UK.*
Hamamelis (p.1618·3); dibrompropamidine isetionate (p.1143·1); calamine (p.1111·3).
Insect bites and stings.

Sweatosan N *Novartis Consumer, Ger.*
Sage (p.1660·2).
Hyperhidrosis.

Sween *Coloplast, UK.*
A deodorant for stoma care.

Sween Cream *Coloplast, USA.*
Barrier cream.

Sweet Touch *Farmacologico Milanese, Ital.*
Aspartame (p.1354·3).
Sugar substitute.

Sweetabb *Pose, Thai.*
Aspartame (p.1354·3).
Sugar substitute.

Sweetex *Boots, NZ.*
Saccharin sodium (p.1375·1).
Sweetening agent.

Swiff *Berlin Pharm, Thai.*
Monobasic sodium phosphate (p.1193·2); dibasic sodium phosphate (p.1193·2).
Bowel evacuation; constipation.

Swim-Ear *Metapharma, Canad.; Co-Pharma, UK; Fougera, USA.*
Isopropyl alcohol (p.1149·2); glycerol (p.1616·3).
Removal of trapped ear water.

Swiss Herb Cough Drops *Ricola, Canad.*
Althaea (p.1577·1); burnet (p.1587·3); horehound (p.1094·2); mallow; menthol (p.1632·3); parsley piert (p.1648·3); peppermint oil (p.1243·3); plantago cordata; thyme (p.1672·2); veronica officinalis with or without ascorbic acid (p.1389·3).

Swiss One *Swiss Herbal, Canad.*
Multivitamin and mineral preparation (p.1350·1).

Swiss-Kal Eff *Byk Madaus, S.Afr.†.*
Potassium citrate (p.1186·1); potassium bicarbonate (p.1186·1).
Hypokalaemia in hyperchloraemic acidosis.

Swiss-Kal SR *Byk Madaus, S.Afr.*
Potassium chloride (p.1194·3).

SX Carduus *Schwabe Extracta, Ger.*
Silybum marianum (p.1021·3).
Liver disorders.

SX Mentha *Schwabe Extracta, Ger.*
Peppermint oil (p.1243·3).
Irritable bowel syndrome.

SX Sabal *Schwabe Extracta, Ger.*
Saw palmetto (p.1491·2).
Benign prostatic hyperplasia.

SX Valeriana comp *Schwabe Extracta, Ger.*
Valerian (p.1678·3); melissa (p.1632·2).
Agitation; sleep disorders.

Sycold *Siam Bheasach, Thai.*
Phenylpropanolamine hydrochloride (p.1098·1); paracetamol (p.71·2); chlorpheniramine [chlorphenamine] maleate (p.412·1).
Cold and influenza symptoms; hay fever; sinusitis; upper respiratory-tract disorders.

Sydolil *Columbia, Mex.*
Ergotamine tartrate (p.452·1); caffeine (p.761·3); aspirin (p.14·2).
Headache including migraine.

Sygen *TRB, Braz.*
Monosialoganglioside sodium (p.1614·1); electrolytes.
Cerebrovascular disorders.

Sykofen *Silom, Thai.*
Ketotifen fumarate (p.767·2).
Asthma; bronchitis; hypersensitivity reactions.

Sylador *Sanofi Winthrop, Braz.*
Tramadol hydrochloride (p.89·1).
Pain.

Syllact *Wallace, USA.*
Ispaghula (p.1229·1).
Constipation.

Syllamalt *Wallace, USA†.*
Malt extract (p.1371·1); ispaghula (p.1229·1).
Constipation.

Symadal M *Chauvin ankerpharm, Ger.*
Dimethicone 200 (p.1410·1).
Barrier preparation.

Symax *Capellon, USA.*
Hyoscyamine sulfate (p.469·3).
Control of gastrointestinal secretions; cystitis; gastrointestinal spasm; heart block; parkinsonism; renal colic; rhinitis.

Symbial *Galderma, Neth.*
Urea (p.1127·3); sodium chloride (p.1196·1).
Skin disorders.

Symbicort *AstraZeneca, UK.*
Budesonide (p.1064·2); eformoterol [formoterol] fumarate (p.764·2).
Asthma.

Symbioflor I *Peithner, Aust.*
Live cells and autolysate of *Enterococcus faecalis* (p.1626·3).
Gastrointestinal disorders; infections.

Symbioflor 1 *Symbiopharm, Ger.*
Cells and autolysate of *Enterococcus faecalis* (p.1626·3).
Immunotherapy.

Symbioflor II *Peithner, Aust.*
Live cells and autolysate of *Escherichia coli.*
Gastrointestinal disorders; infections.

Symbioflor 2 *Symbiopharm, Ger.*
Cells and autolysate of *Escherichia coli.*
Gastrointestinal disorders; infections.

Symbioflor-Antigen *Symbiopharm, Ger.*
Escherichia coli.
Immunotherapy.

Symfona N *Medichemie, Switz.*
Ginkgo biloba (p.1615·2).
Cerebrovascular disorders.

Symmetrel *Novartis, Austral.; Du Pont, Canad.; Novartis, Hong Kong; Novartis, Irl.; Novartis, Israel; Novartis, Neth.; Novartis, NZ; Novartis, S.Afr.; Novartis, Singapore; Novartis, Switz.; Alliance, UK; Endo, USA.*
Amantadine hydrochloride (p.1161·2).
Drug-induced extrapyramidal disorders; herpes zoster; influenza A; parkinsonism.

Symoron *Yamanouchi, Neth.*
Methadone hydrochloride (p.53·1).
Opioid addiction; pain.

Sympal *Berlin-Chemie, Ger.*
Dexketoprofen trometamol (p.47·3).
Pain.

Sympalept *Streuli, Switz.*
Oxedrine tartrate (p.950·3).
Circulatory disorders; hypotension.

Sympaneurol *Lemoine, Fr.†.*
Phenobarbital (p.355·1); crataegus (p.1600·2); passion flower (p.1649·1); valerian (p.1678·3).
Anxiety; sleep disorders.

Sympathyl *Innothera, Fr.*
Crataegus (p.1600·2); eschscholtzia californica; magnesium oxide (p.1233·2).
Formerly contained phenobarbital and crataegus.
Anxiety; sleep disorders.

Sympatol *Boehringer Ingelheim, Aust.; Boehringer Ingelheim, Ger.†; Boehringer Ingelheim, Ital.*
Oxedrine tartrate (p.950·3).
Hypotension.

Sympavagol *Novartis Sante, Fr.*
Passion flower (p.1649·1); crataegus (p.1600·2).
The tablets formerly contained phenobarbital.
Nervous disorders; sleep disorders.

Symphocal *Abic, Israel.*
Oxolamine citrate (p.1096·2).
Coughs.

Symphytum Ro-Plex (Rowo-776) *Pharmakon, Ger.*
Homoeopathic preparation.

Symphytum-Komplex N *Rodler, Ger.*
Homoeopathic preparation.

Symptofed *Propan, S.Afr.*
Pseudoephedrine hydrochloride (p.1099·2).
Upper respiratory-tract congestion.

Syn MD *Synthelabo, Belg.†; Kramer, Switz.*
Sorbitol (p.1377·3).
Bowel evacuation; constipation; dyspepsia.

Synacol CF *Roberts, USA.*
Dextromethorphan hydrobromide (p.1087·3); guaifenesin (p.1092·2).
Coughs.

Synacort *Syntex, USA.*
Hydrocortisone (p.1073·3).
Skin disorders.

Synacthen *Novartis, Aust.; Novartis, Austral.; Novartis, Belg.; Novartis, Denm.; Novartis, Ger.; Novartis, Irl.; Novartis, Israel; Novartis, Ital.; Novartis, Neth.; Novartis, Norw.†; Novartis, NZ; Novartis, Port.; Novartis, Swed.; Novartis, Switz.; Alliance, UK.*
Tetracosactide (p.1298·2), tetracosactide hexa-acetate (p.1298·2), or tetracosactide-zinc complex (p.1298·2).
Adrenocorticotrophic hormone; diagnosis of adrenocortical insufficiency; hypsarrhythmia; infantile spasms; multiple sclerosis.

Synacthen Depot *Novartis, Canad.; Novartis, Ger.; Novartis, S.Afr.; Alliance, UK.*
Tetracosactide acetate zinc phosphate complex (p.1298·2).
Adrenocorticotrophic hormone; diagnosis of adrenocortical insufficiency.

Synacthen Retard *Novartis, Switz.*
Tetracosactide hexaacetate zinc complex (p.1298·2).
Adrenocorticotrophic hormone.

Synacthene *Novartis, Fr.*
Tetracosactide (p.1298·2).
Adrenocorticotrophic hormone; diagnosis of adrenocortical insufficiency; infantile spasms.

Syn-A-Gen *Pharmacal, Switz.†.*
Nonoxinol 9 (p.1346·2).
Contraceptive.

Synagis *Abbott, Austral.; Abbott, Denm.; Abbott, Fin.; Abbott, Ital.; Abbott, Neth.; Abbott, Norw.; Abbott, NZ; Abbott, Singapore; Abbott, Swed.; Abbott, UK; Medimmune, USA.*
Palivizumab (p.1562·1).
Respiratory syncytial virus infections.

Synalar *Grunenthal, Aust.; Yamanouchi, Belg.; Hoechst Marion Roussel, Braz.; Medicis, Canad.; Bioglan, Denm.; Cassenne, Fr.†; Bioglan, Irl.; Syntex, Mex.; Yamanouchi, Neth.†; Bioglan, Norw.; AstraZeneca, NZ; Janssen-Cilag, Port.†; Genop, S.Afr.; Bioglan, Singapore; Yamanouchi, Spain; Bioglan, Swed.; Grunenthal, Switz.; Grunenthal, Thai.; Sanofi Synthelabo, Thai.; Bioglan, UK; Medicis, USA.*
Fluocinolone acetonide (p.1071·1).
Skin disorders.

Synalar Bi-Otic *Yamanouchi, Belg.; Yamanouchi, Neth.*
Fluocinolone acetonide (p.1071·1); neomycin sulfate (p.228·1); polymyxin B sulfate (p.238·1).
Inflammatory ear infections.

Synalar C *Bioglan, Irl.; Syntex, Mex.; Genop, S.Afr.; Bioglan, Singapore; Bioglan, UK.*
Fluocinolone acetonide (p.1071·1); clioquinol (p.190·2).
Infected skin disorders.

Synalar + DBO *Syntex, Neth.†.*
Fluocinolone acetonide (p.1071·1); broxyquinoline.
Skin disorders.

Synalar med Chinoform *Bioglan, Denm.; Bioglan, Norw.*
Fluocinolone acetonide (p.1071·1); clioquinol (p.190·2).
Infected skin disorders.

Synalar N *Note.This name is used for preparations of different composition.*
Grunenthal, Aust.; Bioglan, Irl.; Genop, S.Afr.; Bioglan, Singapore; Grunenthal, Switz.; Grunenthal, Thai.; Sanofi Synthelabo, Thai.; Bioglan, UK.
Fluocinolone acetonide (p.1071·1); neomycin sulfate (p.228·1).
Infected skin disorders.

Syntex, Mex.
Fluocinolone acetonide (p.1071·1); polymyxin B sulfate (p.238·1); neomycin sulfate (p.228·1); phenylephrine hydrochloride (p.1097·1).
Nasal and sinus disorders.

Synalar Nasal *Yamanouchi, Spain.*
Phenylephrine hydrochloride (p.1097·1); fluocinolone acetonide (p.1071·1); neomycin (p.228·1); polymyxin B sulfate (p.238·1).
Nasal congestion and infection.

Synalar Neo *Syntex, Mex.*
Fluocinolone acetonide (p.1071·1); neomycin sulfate (p.228·1).
Infected skin disorders.

Synalar Neomicina *Yamanouchi, Spain.*
Fluocinolone acetonide (p.1071·1); neomycin sulfate (p.228·1).
Infected skin disorders.

Synalar Neomycine *Cassenne, Fr.†.*
Fluocinolone acetonide (p.1071·1); neomycin sulfate (p.228·1).
Infected skin disorders.

Synalar O *Syntex, Mex.*
Fluocinolone acetonide (p.1071·1); polymyxin B sulfate (p.238·1); neomycin sulfate (p.228·1); lignocaine [lidocaine] hydrochloride (p.1313·2).
Otitis externa.

Synalar Oftalmico *Syntex, Mex.*
Fluocinolone acetonide (p.1071·1); polymyxin B sulfate (p.238·1); neomycin sulfate (p.228·1).
Infected eye disorders.

Synalar Otico *Yamanouchi, Spain.*
Fluocinolone acetonide (p.1071·1); neomycin sulfate (p.228·1); polymyxin B sulfate (p.238·1).
Ear disorders.

Synalar Rectal *Janssen-Cilag, Port.; Yamanouchi, Spain.*
Bismuth subgallate (p.1213·2); fluocinolone acetonide (p.1071·1); lignocaine [lidocaine] hydrochloride (p.1313·2); menthol (p.1632·3).
Anorectal disorders.

Synalar Rectal Simple *Yamanouchi, Spain.*
Fluocinolone acetonide (p.1071·1).
Anorectal disorders.

Synaleve *Mer-National, S.Afr.*
Capsules: Paracetamol (p.71·2); codeine phosphate (p.25·2); meprobamate (p.691·1).
Pain and associated tension.

Syrup†: Paracetamol (p.71·2); codeine phosphate (p.25·2); promethazine hydrochloride (p.423·2).
Fever; pain.

Tablets†: Paracetamol (p.71·2); codeine phosphate (p.25·2); caffeine (p.761·3); meprobamate (p.691·1).
Pain and associated tension.

Synalgo *Geymonat, Ital.*
Naproxen aminobutanol (p.61·3).
Gout; musculoskeletal and joint disorders; neuralgia; sciatica.

Synalgos-DC *Wyeth-Ayerst, USA.*
Dihydrocodeine tartrate (p.33·1); aspirin (p.14·2); caffeine (p.761·3).
Pain.

Synap *Restan, S.Afr.*
Paracetamol (p.71·2); dextropropoxyphene napsilate (p.27·1); diphenhydramine hydrochloride (p.416·1); caffeine (p.761·3).
Pain.

Synapausa *Organon, Port.*
Estriol succinate (p.1475·3).
Oestrogen deficiency.

Synapause *Donmed, S.Afr.; Organon, Spain.*
Estriol succinate (p.1475·3).
Oestrogen deficiency.

Synapause E *Nourypharma, Ger.*
Estriol (p.1475·3).
Menopausal disorders.

Synapause-E₃ *Organon, Neth.*
Estriol (p.1475·3).
Adjunct in cervical smear tests; menopausal disorders; oestrogen deficiency.

Synarel
Searle, Austral.; Searle, Belg.; Searle, Canad.; Monsanto, Fr.; Searle, Hong Kong; Searle, Irl.; Searle, Israel; Searle, Mex.; Searle, Neth.; Searle, NZ; Searle, S.Afr.; Searle, Spain; Pharmacia, UK; Searle, USA.
Nafarelin acetate (p.1291·1).
Endometriosis; ovarian stimulation; precocious puberty; uterine fibroids.

Synarela
Searle, Denm.; Searle, Fin.; Heumann, Ger.; Searle, Norw.; Searle, Swed.
Nafarelin acetate (p.1291·1).
Endometriosis; ovarian stimulation for in-vitro fertilisation; uterine fibroids.

Synastone *Auden McKenzie, UK.*
Methadone hydrochloride (p.53·1).

Synbetamine *Synco, Hong Kong.*
Betamethasone (p.1063·1); dexchlorpheniramine maleate (p.412·1).
Hypersensitivity reactions; inflammatory eye disorders.

Synbrozil *Synco, Hong Kong.*
Gemfibrozil (p.896·2).
Hyperlipidaemias.

Syncarpin *Winzer, Ger.*
Pilocarpine borate (p.1422·3); neostigmine bromide (p.1419·3); naphazoline hydrochloride (p.1095·1).
Glaucoma.

Synchlolim *Atlantic, Thai.*
Chloramphenicol sodium succinate (p.179·2).
Bacterial infections.

Synchrorose *Dermoteca, Port.*
Silymarin (p.1021·3); acetyl glucosamine; *dl*-alpha tocoferil acetate (p.1394·1); hyaluronic acid (p.1620·1).
High skin coloration.

Syncillin *Infectopharm, Ger.*
Azidocillin sodium (p.153·1).
Bacterial infections.

Synco-CFN *Synco, Hong Kong.*
Clotrimazole (p.382·1); fluocinolone acetonide (p.1071·1); neomycin sulfate (p.228·1).
Infected skin disorders.

Syncoforte *Synco, Hong Kong.*
Vitamin B substances (p.1350·1).
Vitamin B deficiencies.

Syncomet *Synco, Hong Kong.*
Cimetidine (p.1216·3).
Gastritis; gastro-oesophageal reflux; peptic ulcer.

Syncoquin *Synco, Hong Kong.*
Chloroquine phosphate (p.432·3).
Amoebic hepatitis; lupus erythematosus; malaria; rheumatoid arthritis.

Syncortyl *Roussel Diamant, Fr.*
Desoxycortone acetate (p.1066·3).
Mineralocorticoid deficiency.

Syndette *Adcock Ingram, S.Afr.*
Paracetamol (p.71·2); doxylamine succinate (p.417·1).
Fever; pain; sedative.

Syndol
Note. This name is used for preparations of different composition.
Seton, Irl.; Adcock Ingram, S.Afr.; SSL, UK.
Tablets: Paracetamol (p.71·2); codeine phosphate (p.25·2); doxylamine succinate (p.417·1); caffeine (p.761·3).
Pain and associated tension.

Mer-National, S.Afr.†
Syrup: Paracetamol (p.71·2); doxylamine succinate (p.417·1); codeine phosphate (p.25·2).
Fever; pain with tension.

Syndopa *Sun, Thai.*
Carbidopa (p.1168·2); levodopa (p.1169·2).
Parkinsonism.

Synedil *Yamanouchi, Fr.*
Sulpiride (p.706·1).
Nervous disorders; psychoses.

Synemol *Medicis, USA.*
Fluocinolone acetonide (p.1071·1).
Skin disorders.

Synerbiol *Nutergia, Fr.*
Marine fish oil (p.949·3).
Nutritional supplement.

Synercid
Rhone-Poulenc Rorer, Austral.; Rhone-Poulenc Rorer, Fin.; Aventis, Fr.; Aventis, UK; Rhone-Poulenc Rorer, USA.
Quinupristin (p.241·3) or quinupristin mesilate (p.241·2); dalfopristin (p.241·3) or dalfopristin mesilate (p.241·2).
Bacterial infections.

Synerga *Laves, Ger.*
Cell-free lysate of *Escherichia coli*.
Allergies; neurodermatitis.

Synergistic Manganese *Quest, Canad.*
Manganese, vitamin A, and vitamin C (p.1350·1).

Synergistic Selenium *Quest, Canad.*
Selenium, vitamin C, and vitamin E (p.1350·1).

Synergomycin *Abbott, Ger.*
Erythromycin (p.201·2) or erythromycin ethyl succinate (p.201·2); bromhexine hydrochloride (p.1085·3).
Bacterial infections of the respiratory tract.

Synergon *Lipha Sante, Fr.*
Progesterone (p.1488·3); estrone (p.1476·1).
Amenorrhoea.

Synergyl *Monsanto, Fr.†*
Multivitamin and mineral preparation (p.1350·1).

Synermox *Douglas, NZ.*
Amoxicillin trihydrate (p.149·2); potassium clavulanate (p.187·2).
Bacterial infections.

Synerpril
Merck Sharp & Dohme, Denm.; Merck Sharp & Dohme, Swed.
Enalapril maleate (p.883·3); hydrochlorothiazide (p.907·3).
Hypertension.

Syneudon *Krewel, Ger.*
Amitriptyline hydrochloride (p.273·3).
Depression; pain.

Synfase *Searle, Norw.; Searle, Swed.*
Norethisterone (p.1485·1); ethinylestradiol (p.1476·2).
28-Day packs also contain 7 inert tablets.
Triphasic oral contraceptive.

Synflex
Altimed, Canad.; Roche, Hong Kong; Roche, Irl.; Recordati, Ital.; Syntex, NZ; Roche, S.Afr.; Roche, Singapore; Roche, Thai.; Roche, UK.
Naproxen sodium (p.61·1).
Gout; musculoskeletal, joint, peri-articular, and soft-tissue disorders; pain.

Syngel *Will-Pharma, Belg.*
Aluminium hydroxide-magnesium carbonate co-dried gel (p.1211·2); magnesium hydroxide (p.1233·1); magnesium trisilicate (p.1233·3); lignocaine [lidocaine] hydrochloride (p.1313·2).
Gastritis; gastro-oesophageal reflux.

Syngynon *Jenapharm, Ger.*
Hydroxyprogesterone caproate (p.1479·3); estradiol benzoate (p.1473·1).
Menstrual disorders.

Synkapton *Strallhofer, Aust.*
Ergotamine tartrate (p.452·1); dimenhydrinate (p.415·2); caffeine (p.761·3).
Migraine and other vascular headaches.

Synkavit *Cambridge, UK.*
Menadiol sodium phosphate (p.1395·3).
Factor VII deficiency; hypoprothrombinaemia.

Synobel *Yamanouchi, Spain.*
Clioquinol (p.190·2); fluocinolone acetonide (p.1071·1).
Infected skin disorders.

Synogin *Chinta, Thai.*
Naproxen (p.60·3).
Gout; musculoskeletal and joint disorders.

Synoxicam *Synco, Hong Kong.*
Piroxicam (p.79·1).
Gout; inflammation; musculoskeletal and joint disorders; pain.

SynPharma Bronchial *Synpharma, Aust.*
Anise oil (p.1580·3); eucalyptus oil (p.1609·2); thyme oil (p.1672·3).
Catarrh; coughs.

Synpharma Instant-Blasen-und-Nierentee
Synpharma, Aust.
Silver birch (p.1585·2); equisetum (p.1606·3); urtica (p.1678·2).
Urinary-tract disorders.

Synpharma Instant-Brust- und Hustentee
Synpharma, Aust.
Althaea (p.1577·1); cowslip (p.1600·1); thyme (p.1672·2).
Respiratory-tract disorders.

Synpharma Instant-Nerventee *Synpharma, Aust.*
Valerian (p.1678·3); melissa leaf (p.1632·2); orange.
Nervous disorders; sleep disorders.

Synphase *Searle, Hong Kong; Pharmacia, UK.*
Ethinylestradiol (p.1476·2); norethisterone (p.1485·1).
Triphasic oral contraceptive.

Synphasec *Grunenthal, Ger.*
Ethinylestradiol (p.1476·2); norethisterone (p.1485·1).
Triphasic oral contraceptive.

Synphasic *Searle, Austral.; Searle, Canad.; Searle, NZ.*
Ethinylestradiol (p.1476·2); norethisterone (p.1485·1).
28-Day packs also contain 7 inert tablets.
Triphasic oral contraceptive.

Synrelina *Searle, Switz.*
Nafarelin acetate (p.1291·1).
Endometriosis.

Syn-Rx *Medeva, USA.*
Dark blue tablets, pseudoephedrine hydrochloride (p.1099·2); guaifenesin (p.1092·2); light green tablets, guaifenesin.
Respiratory-tract congestion.

Syn-Rx DM *Medeva, USA.*
Light blue tablets, pseudoephedrine hydrochloride (p.1099·2); guaifenesin (p.1092·2); yellow tablets, dextromethorphan hydrobromide (p.1087·3); guaifenesin.
Coughs; nasal congestion.

Syntaris
Roche, Aust.; Roche, Belg.; Dermapharm, Ger.; Roche, Irl.; Recordati, Ital.; Roche, Neth.; Roche, S.Afr.†; Roche, Switz.; Roche, UK.
Flunisolide (p.1070·3).
Allergic rhinitis; asthma; bronchitis.

Syntestan *Syntex, Ger.; Roche, Ger.*
Cloprednol (p.1065·3).
Asthma; polyarthritis.

Synthamin
Baxter, Austral.; Baxter, Irl.; Baxter, NZ; Fresenius Kabi, S.Afr.; Baxter, Switz.; Baxter, UK.
Amino-acid infusion with or without electrolytes (p.1350·1).
Parenteral nutrition.

Synthamin V *Baxter, Ger.*
Amino-acid infusion (p.1350·1).
Parenteral nutrition.

Synthamin V E *Baxter, Ger.*
Amino-acid and electrolyte infusion (p.1350·1).
Parenteral nutrition.

Synthamin Reform Sin Ele *Baxter, Spain.*
Amino-acid infusion (p.1350·1).
Parenteral nutrition.

Synthamin Reformulado *Baxter, Spain.*
Amino-acid and electrolyte infusion (p.1350·1).
Parenteral nutrition.

Synthol
Bournonville, Belg†; SmithKline Beecham Sante, Fr.
Cloral hydrate (p.669·3); menthol (p.1632·3); resorcinol (p.1122·2); salicylic acid (p.1612·3); veratrol.
Mouth and throat disorders; soft-tissue trauma.

Synthomycin *Rekah, Israel.*
Chloramphenicol (p.179·1).
Eye infections.

Synthomycine *Abic, Israel.*
Chloramphenicol (p.179·1) or chloramphenicol sodium succinate (p.179·2).
Bacterial infections.

Synthroid *Knoll, Canad.; Abbott, USA.*
Thyroxine [levothyroxine] sodium (p.1526·2).
Diagnosis of hyperthyroidism; hypothyroidism; thyroid-stimulating hormone suppression.

Syntidine *Synco, Hong Kong.*
Ranitidine hydrochloride (p.1245·2).
Dyspepsia; gastro-oesophageal reflux; oesophagitis; peptic ulcer; Zollinger-Ellison syndrome.

Syntocaine *Sintetica, Switz.†*
Procaine hydrochloride (p.1319·1).
Local anaesthesia.

Syntocinon
Novartis, Aust.; Novartis, Austral.; Novartis, Belg.; Novartis, Braz.; Novartis, Denm.; Novartis, Fin.; Novartis, Fr.; Novartis, Ger.; Novartis, Hong Kong; Janssen-Cilag, Irl.; Novartis, Israel; Novartis, Ital.; Novartis, Mex.; Novartis, Neth.; Novartis, Norw.; Novartis, NZ; Novartis, Port.; Novartis, S.Afr.; Novartis, Singapore; Novartis, Spain; Novartis, Swed.; Novartis, Switz.; Novartis, Thai.; Alliance, UK; Novartis, USA†.
Oxytocin (p.1294·1).
Caesarean section; incomplete abortion; induction and maintenance of labour; lactation disorders; postpartum haemorrhage; postpartum uterine atony.

Syntoclox *Codal Synto, Thai.*
Cloxacillin sodium (p.192·1).
Bacterial infections.

Syntofene *SmithKline Beecham Sante, Fr.*
Ibuprofen (p.43·2).
Soft-tissue disorders.

Syntometrin *Novartis, Ger.*
Methylergometrine maleate (p.1635·1); oxytocin (p.1294·1).
Delivery of the placenta; postpartum haemorrhage.

Syntometrine
Novartis, Austral.; Novartis, Hong Kong; Novartis, Irl.; Novartis, Israel; Novartis, NZ; Novartis, S.Afr.; Alliance, UK.
Ergometrine maleate (p.1607·1); oxytocin (p.1294·1).
Management of third-stage labour; postpartum haemorrhage.

Syntonol *Codal Synto, Thai.*
Propranolol hydrochloride (p.962·3).
Angina pectoris; anxiety; arrhythmias; hypertension; phaeochromocytoma; tremor.

Syntopressin *Novartis, Irl.; Sandoz, UK†.*
Lypressin (p.1300·1).
Diabetes insipidus.

Synuretic *DDSA Pharmaceuticals, UK.*
Hydrochlorothiazide (p.907·3); amiloride hydrochloride (p.835·1).
These ingredients can be described by the British Approved Name Co-amilozide.
Ascites; heart failure; hypertension.

Synureticum *Medisa, Switz.†.*
Spironolactone (p.973·2); hydrochlorothiazide (p.907·3).
Heart failure; hypertension; nephrotic syndrome; oedema.

Synvisc
Bayer, Austral.; Biomatrix, Canad.; Boehringer Ingelheim, Fr.; Wyeth, Ger.; Biomatrix, Hong Kong; Biomatrix, Israel; Bayer, NZ; Roche, S.Afr.; Bayer, Singapore; Roche, Swed.; Biomatrix, UK; Wyeth-Ayerst, USA.
Hylan G-F 20 (p.1620·1).
Osteoarthritis of the knee; synovial fluid replacement.

Synvomin *Synco, Hong Kong.*
Promethazine teoclate (p.423·2).
Nausea and vomiting.

Syprine *Merck, USA.*
Trientine dihydrochloride (p.1025·3).
Formerly known as Cuprid.
Wilson's disease.

Syprol *Rosemont, UK.*
Propranolol hydrochloride (p.962·3).

Syracol CF *Roberts, USA.*
Guaifenesin (p.1092·2); dextromethorphan hydrobromide (p.1087·3).
Coughs.

Syraprim *Galen, Mex.*
Co-trimoxazole (p.193·3).
Bacterial infections.

Syrea *Medac, Ger.*
Hydroxyurea [hydroxycarbamide] (p.544·2).
Malignant neoplasms.

Syrup DM *Therapex, Canad.*
Dextromethorphan hydrobromide (p.1087·3).

Syrup DM-D *Therapex, Canad.*
Dextromethorphan hydrobromide (p.1087·3); pseudoephedrine hydrochloride (p.1099·2).

Syrup DM-D-E *Therapex, Canad.*
Dextromethorphan hydrobromide (p.1087·3); pseudoephedrine hydrochloride (p.1099·2); guaifenesin (p.1092·2).

Syrup DM-E *Therapex, Canad.*
Dextromethorphan hydrobromide (p.1087·3); guaifenesin (p.1092·2).

Syrvite *Barre-National, USA; Major, USA; Moore, USA.*
Multivitamin preparation (p.1350·1).

Syscor
Bayer, Aust.; Bayer, Belg.; Bayer, Fin.; Bayer, Ital.; Zeneca, Mex.; Zeneca, Neth.; Zeneca, S.Afr.; Zeneca, Spain; Bayer, Swed.†; Zeneca, Switz.; Pharmax, UK.
Nisoldipine (p.946·3).
Angina pectoris; heart failure; hypertension.

Systen
Janssen-Cilag, Aust.; Janssen-Cilag, Belg.; Janssen-Cilag, Fr.; Janssen-Cilag, Ital.; Cilag, Mex.; Janssen-Cilag, Neth.; Janssen-Cilag, Switz.
Estradiol (p.1473·1).
Menopausal disorders; oestrogen deficiency; osteoporosis.

Systen Conti *Janssen-Cilag, Switz.*
Estradiol (p.1473·1); norethisterone acetate (p.1485·1).
Menopausal disorders.

Systen Sequi *Janssen-Cilag, Switz.*
4 Patches, estradiol (p.1473·1) (Systen); 4 patches, estradiol; norethisterone acetate (p.1485·1) (Systen Conti).
Menopausal disorders.

Systepin *Klinge, Irl.*
Nifedipine (p.940·1).
Hypertension; ischaemic heart disease.

Systodin *Nycomed, Norw.†.*
Quinidine sulfate (p.964·3).
Arrhythmias.

Systral
Fresenius Kabi, Aust.; Asta Medica, Ger.; Asta Medica, Hong Kong; Dagra, Port.†; Asta Medica, Thai.
Chlorphenoxamine hydrochloride (p.412·3).
Allergic skin disorders; asthma; dysmenorrhoea; migraine; motion sickness; nausea; rhinitis; skin irritation.

Systral C *Asta Medica, Aust.; Asta Medica, Ger.*
Chlorphenoxamine hydrochloride (p.412·3); caffeine (p.761·3).
Asthma; dysmenorrhoea; hypersensitivity reactions; migraine; motion sickness; nausea; rhinitis.

Systral Hydrocort *Asta Medica, Ger.*
Hydrocortisone (p.1073·3).
Skin disorders.

Systrason *Asta Medica, Aust.*
Chlorphenoxamine (p.412·3); hydrocortisone acetate (p.1073·3).
Skin disorders.

Sytron *Link, UK.*
Sodium feredetate (p.1375·3).
Iron-deficiency anaemia.

Syviman N *Muller Goppingen, Ger.*
Comfrey (p.1598·3); mistletoe (p.1636·2).
Joint disorders.

Syxal *Syxyl, Ger.*
Hypericum (p.290·2).
Depression.

Syxyl-Vitamin-Comb *Syxyl, Ger.†*
Vitamin B substances (p.1350·1).
Vitamin B deficiency.

Szillosan forte *Henk, Ger.†*
Squill (p.1100·3); crataegus (p.1600·2).
Heart failure.

T. Polio *Pasteur Merieux, Fr.*
A tetanus and poliomyelitis (inactivated) vaccine (p.1566·2).
Active immunisation.

T & T Antioxidant *Procare, Austral.*
Silybum marianum (p.1021·3); camellia sinensis (p.1681·1).
Adjunct in detoxification regimens; exposure to chemical and environmental toxins and tobacco smoke; inflammation.

TA Baumpollen *Bencard, Ger.*
Allergen extracts of tree pollen(p.1575·3).
Hyposensitisation.

TA Graserpollen *Bencard, Ger.*
Allergen extracts of grass pollen (p.1575·3).
Hyposensitisation.

TA MIX *Bencard, Ger.*
Allergen extracts of mixed pollens(p.1575·3).
Hyposensitisation.

Tab Vaccine *Berna, Singapore†.*
Salmonella typhi.
Active immunisation.

Tabalon
Hoechst Marion Roussel, Ger.; Hoechst Marion Roussel, Mex.
Ibuprofen (p.43·2).
Gout; fever; inflammation; musculoskeletal, joint, and soft-tissue disorders; pain.

Tabarell *Sanorell, Ger.*
Homoeopathic preparation.

Tab-A-Vite *Major, USA.*
A range of vitamin preparations (p.1350·1).

Tabcin *Bayer, Aust.*
Ibuprofen (p.43·2).
Pain.

Tabletas Quimpe *Quimpe, Spain.*
Atropine methonitrate (p.461·1); codeine phosphate (p.25·2); diphenhydramine hydrochloride (p.416·1); ephedrine hydrochloride (p.1090·1); phenazone (p.77·2); propyphenazone (p.80·2).
Upper respiratory-tract disorders.

Tabletes Valda *Canonne, Braz.*
Menthol (p.1632·3); eucalyptol (p.1609·2); terpineol (p.1669·3); thymol (p.1158·3).
Mouth and throat disorders.

Taborcil *Lacer, Spain†.*
Gemfibrozil (p.896·2).
Hyperlipidaemias.

Tabotamp
Johnson & Johnson, Ger.†; Ethicon, Ital.†.
Oxidised cellulose (p.728·1).
Surgical haemorrhage.

Tabritis *Potter's, UK.*
Sambucus (p.1660·3); achillea (p.1572·2); prickly ash bark (p.1682·1); lappa (p.1627·1); clivers (p.1596·3); poplar bark (p.1653·2); bearberry (p.1583·3); senna (p.1248·2).
Musculoskeletal and joint disorders.

Tac *Parnell, USA.*
Triamcinolone acetonide (p.1080·1).
Corticosteroid.

TAC Esofago *Bracco, Ital.*
Barium sulfate (p.1032·1).
Contrast medium for computerised tomography of the oesophagus.

Tacaryl *Westwood-Squibb, USA†.*
Methdilazine (p.421·2) or methdilazine hydrochloride (p.421·3).
Nasal allergies; pruritus.

Tace
Marion Merrell, Spain†; Marion Merrell Dow, USA†.
Chlorotrianisene (p.1465·3).
Menopausal disorders; oestrogen deficiency; prostatic cancer.

Tacef *Grunenthal, Aust.; Takeda, Ger.†.*
Cefmenoxime hydrochloride (p.167·1).
Bacterial infections.

Tacex *Galen, Mex.*
Ceftriaxone sodium (p.177·1).
Bacterial infections.

Tachidol *Angelini, Ital.*
Paracetamol (p.71·2); codeine phosphate (p.25·2).
Fever; pain.

Tachipirina *Angelini, Ital.*
Paracetamol (p.71·2).
Fever; pain.

Tachmalcor *Asta Medica, Ger.*
Detajmium bitartrate.
Arrhythmias.

Tachmalin *Dresden, Ger.†.*
Ajmaline (p.833·1).
Arrhythmias.

TachoComb
Nycomed, Aust.; Nycomed, Ger.; Nycomed, Hong Kong; Hafslund Nycomed, Thai.
Collagen (p.1598·2); fibrinogen (p.736·1); thrombin (p.741·3); aprotinin (p.725·3).
Haemorrhage.

Tacholiquin
Sigmapharm, Aust.; Bene, Ger.
Tyloxapol (p.1349·3).
Respiratory-tract disorders associated with increased or viscous mucus.

Tachotop N *Nycomed, Ger.*
Collagen (p.1598·2).
Haemorrhage.

Tachydaron *Asta Medica, Ger.*
Amiodarone hydrochloride (p.836·1).
Arrhythmias.

Tachyfenon *Dresden, Ger.†.*
Propafenone hydrochloride (p.961·3).
Arrhythmias.

Tachynerg N *Eberth, Ger.*
Testosterone propionate (p.1492·2); benzyl nicotinate (p.20·2); camphor (p.1589·3); menthol (p.1632·3); lemon oil (p.1628·2).
Cardiac disorders.

Tachystin *Chauvin ankerpharm, Ger.*
Dihydrotachysterol (p.1391·2).
Hypoparathyroidism; pseudohypoparathyroidism.

Tachytalol *Asta Medica, Ger.*
Sotalol hydrochloride (p.972·2).
Arrhythmias.

Tacid-4 *Roche, S.Afr.†.*
Aluminium hydroxide-magnesium carbonate co-dried gel (p.1211·2); calcium carbonate (p.1215·1); magnesium hydroxide (p.1233·1); sodium bicarbonate (p.1186·2).
Hyperchlorhydria.

Tacidina *Sedar, Braz.*
Aspirin (p.14·2); caffeine (p.761·3).
Fever; pain.

Tacinol *Polipharm, Thai.*
Triamcinolone acetonide (p.1080·1).
Skin disorders.

Tacrinal *Biosintetica, Braz.*
Tacrine (p.1425·3).
Alzheimer's disease.

Tacron
Note.This name is used for preparations of different composition.
Korea United, Singapore.
Ticlopidine hydrochloride (p.981·1).
Atherosclerosis; peripheral vascular disease.
Farmasierra, Spain.
Naproxen (p.60·3).
Fever; gout; musculoskeletal and joint disorders; pain.

Tacryl *Abigo, Denm.*
Methdilazine (p.421·2).
Hay fever; rhinitis; urticaria.

tactu-nerval *Feldhoff, Ger.*
Bovine testicular extract (p.1492·1); bovine placental extract.
Musculoskeletal disorders; peripheral circulatory disorders.

TAD
Biomedica, Hong Kong; Biomedica, Ital.
Glutathione (p.1010·3) or glutathione sodium (p.1010·3).
Alcohol or drug poisoning; liver disorders; radiation injury.

TAD+ *Seroyal, Canad.*
Multivitamins with zinc (p.1350·1).

Tadenan
Roche, Aust.; Debat, Fr.; Debat, Hong Kong; Fournier, Ital.; Fournier, Port.; Fournier, Switz.; Debat, Thai.
Pygeum africanum (p.1490·3).
Benign prostatic hyperplasia.

Tadex *Orion, Fin.*
Tamoxifen citrate (p.571·1).
Breast cancer.

Tafenil *Asofarma, Mex.*
Flutamide (p.542·3).

Tafil
Pharmacia Upjohn, Denm.; Pharmacia Upjohn, Ger.; Pharmacia Upjohn, Mex.
Alprazolam (p.654·2).
Alcohol withdrawal syndrome; anxiety disorders.

Taflox *Fariberica, Port.*
Norfloxacin (p.232·1).
Bacterial infections.

Tagadine *Duopharma, Hong Kong.*
Cimetidine (p.1216·3).
Gastro-oesophageal reflux; gastrointestinal haemorrhage; peptic ulcer; Zollinger-Ellison syndrome.

Tagagel *SmithKline Beecham, Ger.†.*
Cimetidine (p.1216·3).
Gastro-oesophageal reflux; peptic ulcer; Zollinger-Ellison syndrome.

Tagal *Galen, Mex.*
Ceftazidime (p.174·3).
Bacterial infections.

Tagamet
SmithKline Beecham, Austral.; SmithKline Beecham, Belg.; SmithKline Beecham, Braz.; SmithKline Beecham, Canad.; SmithKline Beecham, Denm.; SmithKline Beecham, Fr.; SmithKline Beecham, Ger.; SmithKline Beecham, Hong Kong; SmithKline Beecham, Irl.; SmithKline Beecham, Israel; SmithKline Beecham, Ital.; SmithKline Beecham, Mex.; SmithKline Beecham, Neth.; SmithKline Beecham, Norw.; SmithKline

Beecham, NZ; Smith Kline & French, Port.; SmithKline Beecham, S.Afr.; SmithKline Beecham, Singapore; SmithKline Beecham, Spain; SmithKline Beecham, Swed.; SmithKline Beecham, Switz.; SmithKline Beecham, Thai.; SmithKline Beecham, UK; SmithKline Beecham, USA.
Cimetidine (p.1216·3) or cimetidine hydrochloride (p.1218·3).
Acid aspiration; adjunct in pancreatic insufficiency; dyspepsia; gastro-oesophageal reflux; gastrointestinal haemorrhage; peptic ulcer; Zollinger-Ellison syndrome.

Tagamet Dual Action *SmithKline Beecham Consumer, UK†.*
Cimetidine (p.1216·3); sodium alginate (p.1498·3).
Heartburn.

TAGG *Eagle, Austral.*
Benzalkonium chloride (p.1133·1); lauromacrogol 400 (p.1345·2).
Formerly contained benzododecinium chloride.
Deodorant detergent for ostomies.

Tagonis *Janssen-Cilag, Ger.*
Paroxetine hydrochloride (p.302·3).
Depression.

Tagozzard *Pizzard, Mex.*
Psyllium seed (p.1229·1).

Taguinol *Spyfarma, Spain.*
Loperamide hydrochloride (p.1231·3).
Diarrhoea.

Taharmayim *Medentech, Israel.*
Sodium dichloroisocyanurate (p.1156·1).
Water purification.

Taharsept *Medentech, Israel.*
Sodium dichloroisocyanurate (p.1156·1).
Instrument, surface, and equipment disinfection.

Tahartaf *Medentech, Israel.*
Sodium dichloroisocyanurate (p.1156·1).
Equipment disinfection.

Tahor *Parke, Davis, Fr.*
Atorvastatin calcium (p.842·3).
Hypercholesterolaemia.

Tai Ginseng N *Poehlmann, Switz.*
Ginseng (p.1615·3); crataegus (p.1600·2); hypericum (p.290·2); vitamins (p.1350·1).
Tonic.

Taingel *Ghimas, Ital.*
Royal jelly; pollen; ginseng; eleutherococcus (p.1350·1).
Nutritional supplement.

Tairal *Rottapharm, Spain.*
Famotidine (p.1225·3).
Gastro-oesophageal reflux; peptic ulcer; Zollinger-Ellison syndrome.

Taka-Diastase *Warner-Lambert, Ital.†.*
Pepsin (p.1649·3); pancreatin (p.1646·1).
Formerly contained amylitic enzymes of *Aspergillus oryzae.*
Dyspepsia.

Takadispep Complex *Cantabria, Spain†.*
Amylase (p.1579·3); dimethicone (p.1249·2); pancreatin (p.1646·1); papain (p.1647·3).
Aerophagia; digestive enzyme deficiency; dyspepsia; meteorism.

Takata *Madariaga, Spain.*
Aloin (p.1210·2); belladonna (p.463·1); phenolphthalein (p.1244·1).
Constipation.

Takepron
Takeda, Hong Kong; Takeda, Jpn.
Lansoprazole (p.1230·3).
Gastro-oesophageal reflux; peptic ulcer; Zollinger-Ellison syndrome.

Takesulin *Takeda, Jpn.*
Cefsulodin sodium (p.174·2).
Mepivacaine hydrochloride (p.1317·1) is included in the intramuscular injection to alleviate the pain of injection.
Pseudomonal infections.

Taketiam *Takeda, Fr.*
Cefotiam hexetil hydrochloride (p.171·1).
Formerly known as Pansporine.
Bacterial infections.

Taks *Codal Synto, Thai.*
Diclofenac sodium (p.30·3).
Musculoskeletal and joint disorders.

Takus *Pharmacia Upjohn, Ger.*
Ceruletide tris(diethylamine) (p.1593·2).
Diagnostic agent; paralytic ileus; postoperative atony.

Talacen *Sanofi Winthrop, USA.*
Pentazocine hydrochloride (p.74·2); paracetamol (p.71·2).
Pain.

Talavir *Duncan, Ital.*
Valaciclovir hydrochloride (p.643·1).
Herpes zoster infections.

Talcid
Bayer, Aust.; Bayer, Ger.; Bayer, Mex.; Bayer, Spain; Bayer, Swed.†.
Hydrotalcite (p.1228·1).
Gastrointestinal disorders.

Talco Antihistam Calber *Pentafarm, Spain.*
Calamine (p.1111·3); zinc oxide (p.1128·2); bismuth subnitrate (p.1213·2); kaolin; diphenhydramine hydrochloride (p.416·1); menthol (p.1632·3); talc (p.1124·2).
Cutaneous hypersensitivity reactions.

Talgo Odontalgico *Ern, Spain†.*
Ethyl chloride (p.1312·1); trichloroethylene (p.1270·2).
Dental pain.

Talidat
Merck, Ger.; Merck, Spain.
Hydrotalcite (p.1228·1).
Gastrointestinal disorders associated with hyperacidity.

Talis *Organon, Ger.†.*
Metaclazepam hydrochloride (p.691·3).
Psychiatric disorders.

Talizer *Serral, Mex.*
Talomida.
Adjunct in HIV infection; leprosy.

Talkosona *Vita, Spain†.*
Benzalkonium chloride (p.1133·2); bismuth subnitrate (p.1213·2); dexamethasone (p.1067·1); talc; tannic acid (p.1669·1); zinc oxide (p.1128·2).
Skin infections with inflammation.

Talofen *Fournier, Ital.*
Promazine hydrochloride (p.702·2).
Anxiety; pain; psychoses; vomiting.

Talofilina *Novartis, Braz.*
Theophylline (p.777·2).
Obstructive airways disease.

Talohexal *Hexal, Austral.*
Citalopram hydrobromide (p.281·2).
Depression.

Taloxa
Aesca, Aust.; Schering-Plough, Belg.; Schering-Plough, Fr.; Essex, Ger.; Schering-Plough, Ital.; Schering-Plough, Neth.; Schering-Plough, Norw.; Schering-Plough, Port.; Schering-Plough, Spain; Schering-Plough, Swed.; Essex, Switz.
Felbamate (p.349·1).
Formerly known as Taloxoral in Norw.
Epilepsy; Lennox-Gastaut syndrome.

Talpramin *Psicofarma, Mex.*
Imipramine hydrochloride (p.291·1).
Depression; nocturnal enuresis; parasomnias.

Talquis Cusi *Synthelabo, Spain.*
Diphenhydramine hydrochloride (p.416·1); zinc oxide (p.1128·2); talc (p.1124·2).
Allergic skin disorders.

Talquissar *Vita, Spain†.*
Bismuth subnitrate (p.1213·2); boric acid (p.1586·1); calamine (p.1111·3); talc (p.1124·2); tannic acid (p.1669·1).
Skin disorders.

Talquistina *Vita, Spain.*
Calamine (p.1111·3); diphenhydramine hydrochloride (p.416·1).
Formerly contained bismuth subnitrate, boric acid, calamine, diphenhydramine hydrochloride, talc, and tannic acid.
Insect bites; pruritus.

Talso
Sanofi Winthrop, Aust.†; Sanofi Synthelabo, Ger.
Saw palmetto (p.1491·2).
Benign prostatic hyperplasia.

Talsutin
Bristol-Myers Squibb, Braz.; Bristol-Myers Squibb, Hong Kong.
Tetracycline hydrochloride (p.258·3); amphotericin B (p.377·2).
Bacterial and fungal vaginal infections.

Taludon *Novaquimica, Braz.*
Phenytoin (p.357·2); glutamic acid (p.1365·2).
Epilepsy.

Talusin
Knoll, Austral.; Knoll, Fin.; Knoll, Ger.; Knoll, S.Afr.†; Knoll, Switz.
Proscillaridin (p.963·3).
Heart failure.

Talval *Lipha, Switz.*
Idrocilamide (p.1329·2).
Musculoskeletal and joint disorders.

Talvosilen
Sigmapharm, Aust.; Bene, Ger.
Codeine phosphate (p.25·2); paracetamol (p.71·2).
Pain.

Talvosilene *Milupa, Switz.*
Codeine phosphate (p.25·2); paracetamol (p.71·2).
Pain.

Talwin
Sanofi Synthelabo, Canad.; Sanofi Winthrop, Israel; Abbott, Ital.; Abbott, Singapore; Sanofi Synthelabo, Singapore; Sanofi Winthrop, USA.
Pentazocine hydrochloride (p.74·2) or pentazocine lactate (p.74·2).
Adjunct to general anaesthesia; pain; premedication.

Talwin Compound *Sanofi Winthrop, USA.*
Pentazocine hydrochloride (p.74·2); aspirin (p.14·2).
Pain.

Talwin NX
Sanofi Winthrop, Israel; Sanofi Winthrop, USA.
Pentazocine hydrochloride (p.74·2).
Naloxone hydrochloride (p.1014·3) is included in this preparation to discourage abuse.
Pain.

Talwin-Tab *Abbott, Ital.*
Pentazocine hydrochloride (p.74·2).
Pain.

Tam *Alacan, Spain.*
Ciprofloxacin hydrochloride (p.182·3).
Bacterial infections.

Tamagon
Medochemie, Hong Kong; Medochemie, Thai.
Terfenadine (p.581·3).
Allergic skin disorders; hay fever; rhinitis; rhinoconjunctivitis.

Tamanybonsan *Salushaus, Ger.†.*
Salix (p.82·1).
Fever; headache; rheumatic disorders.

The symbol † denotes a preparation no longer actively marketed

Tamaril *Marjan, Braz.*
Senna (p.1248·2); tamarind (p.1253·2); cassia pulp (p.1216·2); liquorice (p.1231·2); coriander (p.1599·2).
Constipation.

Tamarine
Note.This name is used for preparations of different composition.
SmithKline Beecham, Belg.; Barrenne, Braz.; Whitehall, Ital.; Whitehall-Robins, Switz.†.
Tamarind (p.1253·2); cassia (p.1216·2); senna (p.1248·2); coriander (p.1599·2); liquorice (p.1231·2).
Constipation.

SmithKline Beecham Sante, Fr.
Tamarind (p.1253·2); senna (p.1248·2).
Constipation.

Tamarix *Hebron, Braz.*
Tamarind (p.1253·2); cassia pulp (p.1216·2); senna (p.1248·2); liquorice (p.1231·2).
Constipation.

Tamax *Fresenius Kabi, Aust.*
Tamoxifen citrate (p.571·1).
Breast cancer; endometrial cancer.

Tamaxin *Orion, Swed.†.*
Tamoxifen citrate (p.571·1).
Breast cancer.

Tambocor
3M, Austral.; 3M, Belg.; 3M, Canad.; 3M, Denm.; 3M, Fin.; 3M, Ger.; 3M, Hong Kong; 3M, Irl.; 3M, Israel; Riker, Mex.; 3M, Neth.; 3M, Norw.; 3M, NZ; 3M, S.Afr.; 3M, Singapore; 3M, Swed.; 3M, Switz.; 3M, Thai.; 3M, UK; 3M, USA.
Flecainide acetate (p.890·1).
Arrhythmias.

Tambutec *Tecnofarma, Mex.*
Ethambutol (p.205·3).

Tameran *Sanofi Synthelabo, Spain.*
Famotidine (p.1225·3).
Gastro-oesophageal reflux; peptic ulcer; Zollinger-Ellison syndrome.

Tametin *Caber, Ital.†.*
Cimetidine (p.1216·3).
Gastric hyperacidity; peptic ulcer; Zollinger-Ellison syndrome.

Tamexin *Medinovum, Fin.*
Tamoxifen citrate (p.571·1).
Breast cancer.

Tamifen *Medochemie, Hong Kong.*
Tamoxifen citrate (p.571·1).
Anovulatory infertility; breast cancer.

Tamiflu
Roche, Austral.; Roche, NZ; Roche, USA.
Oseltamivir or oseltamivir phosphate (p.638·1).
Influenza.

Tamigen *Solfran, Mex.*
Gentamicin (p.212·1).
Bacterial infections.

Tamik
EG, Fr.; Marcofina, Hong Kong.
Dihydroergotamine mesilate (p.450·3).
Migraine; orthostatic hypotension; venous insufficiency.

Tamin *Merck Sharp & Dohme, Spain.*
Famotidine (p.1225·3).
Gastro-oesophageal reflux; peptic ulcer; Zollinger-Ellison syndrome.

Tamine SR *Geneva, USA†.*
Phenylpropanolamine hydrochloride (p.1098·1); phenylephrine hydrochloride (p.1097·1); brompheniramine maleate (p.410·2).
Upper respiratory-tract symptoms.

Tamizam *Zambon, Belg.*
Tamoxifen citrate (p.571·1).
Breast cancer; endometrial cancer.

Tamobeta *Betapharm, Ger.*
Tamoxifen citrate (p.571·1).
Breast cancer.

Tamofen
Schering, Aust.; Rhodia, Braz.; Rhone-Poulenc Rorer, Canad.; Aventis, Denm.; Leiras, Fin.; Rhone-Poulenc Rorer, Ger.; Douglas, Hong Kong; Pharmacia Upjohn, Irl.; Leiras, Israel; Rhone-Poulenc Rorer, Mex.; Leiras, Norw.; Douglas, NZ; Leiras, Singapore; Douglas, Thai.; TTN, Thai.; Pharmacia, UK.
Tamoxifen citrate (p.571·1).
Anovulatory infertility; breast cancer; endometrial cancer.

Tamofene *Rhone-Poulenc Rorer, Fr.*
Tamoxifen citrate (p.571·1).
Breast cancer.

Tamokadin *Kade, Ger.*
Tamoxifen citrate (p.571·1).
Breast cancer.

Tamone *Pharmacia Upjohn, Canad.†.*
Tamoxifen citrate (p.571·1).
Breast cancer.

Tamophar *Julphar, UAE.*
Tamoxifen citrate (p.571·1).
Anovulatory infertility; breast cancer.

Tamoplex
Nycomed, Aust.; Pharmachemie, Israel; Pharmachemie, S.Afr.; Pharmachemie, Singapore; Pharmachemie, Thai.
Tamoxifen citrate (p.571·1).
Breast cancer; endometrial cancer.

Tamosin *Sigma, Austral.*
Tamoxifen citrate (p.571·1).
Breast cancer.

Tamox
ABZ, Ger.; Gry, Ger.; Isis Puren, Ger.; Rowex, Irl.
Tamoxifen citrate (p.571·1).
Breast cancer; endometrial cancer.

Tamoxan
Kener, Mex.; Tecnimede, Port.
Tamoxifen citrate (p.571·1).

Tamoxasta *Asta Medica, Ger.*
Tamoxifen citrate (p.571·1).
Breast cancer.

Tamoxen
Douglas, Austral.; CTI, Israel.
Tamoxifen citrate (p.571·1).
Breast cancer.

Tamoxi *Generics, Israel.*
Tamoxifen citrate (p.571·1).
Breast cancer.

Tamoxigenat *Azupharma, Ger.*
Tamoxifen citrate (p.571·1).
Breast cancer.

Tamoximerck *Merck dura, Ger.*
Tamoxifen citrate (p.571·1).
Breast cancer.

Tamoxistad *Stada, Ger.*
Tamoxifen citrate (p.571·1).
Breast cancer.

Tampo *Nakorn, Thai.*
Co-trimoxazole (p.193·3).
Bacterial infections.

Tamposit N *Lappe, Ger.*
Lauromacrogol 400 (p.1345·2) zinc oxide (p.1128·2); bismuth subnitrate (p.1213·2).
Anorectal disorders.

Tampositorien H *Lappe, Ger.*
Hamamelis (p.1618·3).
Anorectal disorders.

Tampositorien mit Belladonna *Provita, Aust.*
Belladonna (p.463·1); guaiazulene (p.1618·3); hamamelis (p.1618·3).
Anorectal disorders.

Tampovagan *Co-Pharma, UK.*
Diethylstilbestrol (p.1471·2); lactic acid (p.1626·2).
Postmenopausal vaginitis.

Tampovagan c Acid lact *Sanofi Synthelabo, Ger.*
Lactic acid (p.1626·2).
Vaginitis.

Tamuc *TAD, Ger.†.*
Acetylcysteine (p.1082·3).
Respiratory-tract disorders associated with increased or viscous mucus.

Tamyl *Farmatrading, Ital.*
Propylene glycol cefatrizine (p.164·3).
Bacterial infections.

Tan Express *Banana Boat, Canad.*
SPF 4: Octinoxate (p.1517·3); octisalate (p.1518·1); oxybenzone (p.1518·1).
Sunscreen.

Tanac
Note.This name is used for preparations of different composition.
Del, Canad.
Topical gel: Allantoin (p.1110·1); dyclonine hydrochloride (p.1311·3).
Topical liquid: Benzocaine (p.1306·2); benzalkonium chloride (p.1133·2); tannic acid (p.1669·1).

Del, USA.
Lipstick: Benzocaine (p.1306·2); benzalkonium chloride (p.1133·2); tannic acid (p.1669·1).
Sore lips.
Topical gel: Allantoin (p.1110·1); dyclonine hydrochloride (p.1311·3).
Herpes labialis.
Topical liquid: Benzocaine (p.1306·2); benzalkonium chloride (p.1133·2).
Mouth ulcers; sore gums.

Tanac Dual Core *Del, USA.*
Benzocaine (p.1306·2); tannic acid (p.1669·1); allantoin (p.1110·1); benzalkonium chloride (p.1133·2); padimate O (p.1518·2).
Oral lesions.

Tanacet
Ashbury, Canad.; Herbal Laboratories, UK.
Feverfew (p.453·3).
Migraine.

Tanadopa *Tanabe, Jpn.*
Docarpamine (p.881·2).
Heart failure.

Tanafed *Horizon, USA.*
Chlorpheniramine [chlorphenamine] tannate (p.412·2); pseudoephedrine tannate (p.1100·1).
Upper respiratory-tract symptoms.

Tanagel *Durban, Spain.*
Belladonna (p.463·1); gelatin tannate; opium (p.69·3).
Colitis; diarrhoea; gastroenteritis.

Tanagel Papeles *Durban, Spain.*
Gelatin tannate.
Diarrhoea.

Tanakan
Knoll, Braz.; Beaufour, Fr.; Beaufour-Ipsen, Hong Kong; Knoll, Mex.; Beaufour-Ipsen, Singapore; Emerging Pharma, Singapore; Beaufour-Ipsen, Thai.
Ginkgo biloba (p.1615·2).
Deafness; mental function impairment; vascular disorders.

Tanakene
Sanofi Synthelabo, Spain; Intersan, Switz.
Ginkgo biloba (p.1615·2).
Vascular disorders.

Tanalbina *Knoll, Port.*
Albumin tannate (p.1209·3).
Diarrhoea.

Tanalone *Labima, Belg.*
Albumin tannate (p.1209·3); pectin (p.1502·3).
Diarrhoea.

Tanasid *Pfizer Consumer, Spain.*
Aluminium hydroxide (p.1210·3); sodium carbonate (p.1665·2).
Gastrointestinal hyperacidity.

Tanatril
Gerot, Aust.; Algol, Fin.; Beaufour, Fr.; Hormosan, Ger.; Rottapharm, Ital.; Tanabe, Jpn; Tanabe, Singapore; Tanabe, Thai.; Trinity, UK.
Imidapril hydrochloride (p.912·3).
Hypertension.

Tandax *Novartis, Mex.*
Naproxen sodium (p.61·1).
Inflammation; pain.

Tandem Icon *Britpharm, UK.*
Pregnancy test (p.1654·3).

Tanderil *Ciba Vision, Aust.*
Oxyphenbutazone (p.71·1).
Eye disorders.

Tanderon *Pharmaland, Thai.*
Tolperisone hydrochloride (p.1330·3).
Skeletal muscle spasm.

Tandial *Solfran, Mex.*
Diazepam (p.674·3).

Tandix *Azevedos, Port.*
Indapamide (p.913·1).
Hypertension.

Tandorene *Vitae, Mex.*
Oxyphenbutazone (p.71·1).
Inflammation; musculoskeletal and joint disorders.

Tandrex *Sintofarma, Braz.*
Oxyphenbutazone (p.71·1).
Aluminium hydroxide (p.1210·3) and magnesium trisilicate (p.1233·3) are included in this preparation in an attempt to limit adverse effects on the gastrointestinal mucosa.
Musculoskeletal and joint disorders.

Tandrex A *Sintofarma, Braz.*
Oxyphenbutazone (p.71·1); paracetamol (p.71·2).
Aluminium hydroxide (p.1210·3) and magnesium trisilicate (p.1233·3) are included in this preparation in an attempt to limit adverse effects on the gastrointestinal mucosa.
Musculoskeletal and joint disorders.

Tandrexin *Sintofarma, Braz.*
Ampicillin (p.150·3).
Bacterial infections.

Tandrilax *Ache, Braz.*
Paracetamol (p.71·2); carisoprodol (p.1327·1); diclofenac sodium (p.30·3); caffeine (p.761·3).
Skeletal muscle spasm.

Tanganil *Pierre Fabre, Fr.*
Acetylleucine (p.1572·1).
Vertigo.

Tangenol *Bucca, Spain.*
Eugenol (p.1609·3); procaine hydrochloride (p.1319·1); tannic acid (p.1669·1).
Dental disorders.

Tanidina *Robert, Spain.*
Ranitidine hydrochloride (p.1245·2).
Acid aspiration; gastro-oesophageal reflux; gastrointestinal haemorrhage; peptic ulcer; short-bowel syndrome; Zollinger-Ellison syndrome.

Tannacomp *Knoll, Ger.*
Albumin tannate (p.1209·3); ethacridine lactate (p.1130·3).
Diarrhoea.

Tannalbin
Ebewe, Aust.; Knoll, Austral.†; Knoll, Ger.; Knoll, Neth.
Albumin tannate (p.1209·3).
Diarrhoea.

Tannic-12 *Cypress, USA.*
Pentoxyverine tannate (p.1096·3); chlorpheniramine [chlorphenamine] tannate (p.412·2).
Coughs.

Tannidin Plus *GD, Ital.*
Betacarotene (p.1355·1); selenium (p.1375·2); vitamin E (p.1393·3).
Antioxidant.

Tannisol *GD, Ital.*
Betacarotene (p.1355·1).
Sunscreen.

Tannolact *Galderma, Ger.*
Condensation product of urea-sodium cresolsulfonic acid.
Hyperhidrosis; skin disorders.

Tannolil *Li-il, Ger.*
Tannic acid (p.1669·1); aluminium sulfate (p.1578·2).
Haemorrhoids; hyperhidrosis; skin irritation.

Tannopon *Orion, Fin.*
Opium (p.69·3); belladonna (p.463·1); bismuth salicylate (p.1213·1); albumin tannate (p.1209·3).
Diarrhoea.

Tannosynt
Note.This name is used for preparations of different composition.
Hermal, Aust.
2,6-Bis-N′ (2-hydroxy-3-sulfo-(ev. 5-methyl-)benzyl)-ureidomethyl-phenol(ev. p-cresol) disodium.
Skin disorders.

Hermal, Ger.
Tannic acid (p.1669·1).
Burns; hyperhidrosis; skin disorders.

Hermal, Port.
Dimethyl urea; phenol (p.1152·3); sodium phenolsulfonate.
Skin disorders.

Boots Healthcare, Switz.
Phenol cresol sulfonic acid-formaldehyde condensation product.
Formerly contained tannic acid or sodium tannate.
Skin disorders.

Tanoral *Parmed, USA.*
Phenylephrine tannate (p.1097·3); chlorpheniramine [chlorphenamine] tannate (p.412·2); mepyramine tannate (p.421·1).
Upper respiratory-tract symptoms.

Tanrix
SmithKline Beecham, Aust.†; SmithKline Beecham, Ital.
An adsorbed tetanus vaccine (p.1565·2).
Active immunisation.

Tantacol DM *Tanta, Canad.†.*
Phenylpropanolamine hydrochloride (p.1098·1); pheniramine maleate (p.422·3); mepyramine maleate (p.421·1); dextromethorphan hydrobromide (p.1087·3).
Cold symptoms; coughs.

Tantafed *Tanta, Canad.*
Pseudoephedrine hydrochloride (p.1099·2).

Tantaphen *Tanta, Canad.*
Paracetamol (p.71·2).
Fever; pain.

Tantapp *Tanta, Canad.†.*
Phenylpropanolamine hydrochloride (p.1097·1); phenylpropanolamine hydrochloride (p.1098·1); brompheniramine maleate (p.410·2).

Tantol Skin Cleanser *Quatromed, S.Afr.†.*
Triclosan (p.1159·2); phenonip; phenoxyethanol (p.1153·3).
Skin disinfection.

Tantol Skin Lotion *Quatromed, S.Afr.†.*
Soap substitute.

Tantum
Note.This name is used for preparations of different composition.
CSC, Aust.; 3M, Ger.; Angelini, Ital.; Chefaro, Neth.†; Lepori, Port.; Donmed, S.Afr.†.
Benzydamine hydrochloride (p.20·1).
Gynaecological disorders; inflammation; mouth and throat disorders; pain; peri-articular and soft-tissue disorders; phlebitis; venous insufficiency.

Farma Lepori, Spain.
Ointment; cream: Benzydamine hydrochloride (p.20·1).
Peri-articular and soft-tissue disorders.
Throat spray: Benzydamine hydrochloride (p.20·1); hexamidine di-isetionate (p.1146·2).
Mouth and throat disorders.

Tantum Ciclina *Farma Lepori, Spain.*
Benzydamine hydrochloride (p.20·1); tetracycline hydrochloride (p.258·3).
Acne; bacterial infections.

Tantum Rosa *Lepori, Port.*
Benzydamine hydrochloride (p.20·1); trimethylcetylammonium toluenesulfonate.
Vulvovaginal infections.

Tantum Verde
Note.This name is used for preparations of different composition.
Solvay, Aust.; Farma Lepori, Spain.
Benzydamine hydrochloride (p.20·1).
Mouth and throat disorders.

Lepori, Port.
Nebuliser solution; oral liquid: Benzydamine hydrochloride (p.20·1).
Mouth and throat inflammation.
Pastilles: Benzydamine hydrochloride (p.20·1); benzocaine (p.1306·2).
Mouth and throat pain and inflammation.

Tanyl *Intramed, S.Afr.*
Fentanyl citrate (p.37·1).
Adjunct to general anaesthesia; pain.

Tanzal *Iquinosa, Spain.*
Oxatomide (p.422·1).
Hypersensitivity reactions.

TAO *Pfizer, USA.*
Troleandomycin (p.266·1).
Bacterial infections.

Tapanol *Republic, USA.*
Paracetamol (p.71·2).
Fever; pain.

Tapazol
Lilly, Braz.; Lilly, Mex.
Methimazole [thiamazole] (p.1525·1).
Hyperthyroidism.

Tapazole
Lilly, Canad.; Lilly, Hong Kong; Lilly, Israel; Lilly, Ital.; Lilly, S.Afr.†; Dista, Switz.; Lilly, Thai.; Lilly, USA.
Methimazole [thiamazole] (p.1525·1).
Hyperthyroidism.

Taponoto *Teoforma, Spain.*
Potassium carbonate.
Removal of ear wax.

Taporin *Galen, Mex.*
Cefotaxime sodium (p.169·1).
Bacterial infections.

Taprodex *Provit, Mex.*
Dexamethasone (p.1067·1).
Corticosteroid.

Tapzol *Rayere, Mex.*
Kaolin (p.1229·3); pectin (p.1502·3).
Diarrhoea.

Tapzol Con Neomicina *Rayere, Mex.*
Kaolin (p.1229·3); pectin (p.1502·3); neomycin (p.228·1).
Diarrhoea.

Tar Doak *Trans Canaderm, Canad.†*
Coal tar (p.1125·1).
Skin disorders.

Tar Isdin Champu *Isdin, Spain.*
Coal tar (p.1125·1).
Scalp disorders.

Tar Isdin Plus *Isdin, Spain.*
Coal tar (p.1125·1); salicylic acid (p.1122·3).
Scalp disorders.

Tara *Polipharm, Thai.*
Miconazole nitrate (p.391·1).
Fungal skin, hair, and nail infections.

Tara Abfuhrsirup *Disperga, Aust.*
Senna (p.1248·2).
Bowel evacuation; constipation; stool softener.

Taradyl *Roche, Belg.*
Ketorolac trometamol (p.48·2).
Pain.

Taraleon *Zilly, Ger.*
Taraxacum (p.1669·1).
Biliary-tract disorders; diuretic; dyspepsia; loss of appetite.

Taraphilic *Medco, USA.*
Coal tar (p.1125·1).
Skin disorders.

Tara-Plus *Polipharm, Thai.*
Miconazole nitrate (p.391·1); triamcinolone acetonide (p.1080·1).
Fungal skin and nail infections.

Taraten *Polipharm, Thai.*
Clotrimazole (p.382·1).
Fungal skin infections.

Taraxacum Med Complex *Dynamit, Aust.*
Homoeopathic preparation.

Taraxin *TO-Chemicals, Thai.*
Hydroxyzine hydrochloride (p.419·1).
Allergic skin disorders; pruritus; sedative.

Tarband *Seton Scholl, Austral.; SSL, UK.*
Coal tar (p.1125·1); zinc oxide (p.1128·2).
Leg ulcers; medicated bandage; skin disorders.

Tarcil *SmithKline Beecham, Austral.†*
Ticarcillin sodium (p.262·3).
Bacterial infections.

Tarcortin *Stafford-Miller, UK†.*
Hydrocortisone (p.1073·3); coal tar (p.1125·1).
Skin disorders.

Tardan *Odan, Canad.*
Salicylic acid (p.1122·3); coal tar (p.1125·1).
Seborrhoea.

Tardigal *Lilly, Ger.*
Digitoxin (p.869·2).
Heart failure.

Tardocillin *Bayer, Ger.*
Benzathine benzylpenicillin (p.156·2).
Tolycaine hydrochloride (p.1321·1) is included in this preparation to alleviate the pain of injection.
Long-term treatment of rheumatic fever.

Tardotol *Orion, Denm.†.*
Carbamazepine (p.342·2).
Alcohol withdrawal syndrome; diabetes insipidus; epilepsy; trigeminal neuralgia.

Tardurol *Procter & Gamble, Aust.†.*
Propranolol hydrochloride (p.962·3); triamterene (p.986·1); hydrochlorothiazide (p.907·3).
Hypertension.

Tardyferon
Germania, Aust.; Robapharm, Fr.; Robapharm, Switz.
Ferrous sulfate (p.1360·3); mucoproteose.
Ascorbic acid (p.1389·3) may be included in this preparation to increase the absorption and availability of iron.
Iron deficiency; iron-deficiency anaemias.

Pierre Fabre, Ger.; Knoll, Mex.; Pierre Fabre, Port.; Pierre Fabre, Spain.
Ferrous sulfate (p.1360·3).
Ascorbic acid (p.1389·3) may be included in this preparation to increase the absorption and availability of iron.
Iron-deficiency; iron-deficiency anaemias.

Tardyferon B₉ *Robapharm, Fr.*
Ferrous sulfate (p.1360·3); folic acid (p.1361·1); mucoproteose.
Ascorbic acid (p.1389·3) is included in this preparation to increase the absorption and availability of iron.
Iron and folic acid deficiency.

Tardyferon-Fol
Germania, Aust.
Ferrous sulfate (p.1360·3); folic acid (p.1361·1); mucoprotease.
Folic acid deficiency; iron-deficiency anaemias.

Pierre Fabre, Ger.; Pierre Fabre, Port.
Ferrous sulfate (p.1360·3); folic acid (p.1361·1).

The symbol † denotes a preparation no longer actively marketed

Ascorbic acid (p.1389·3) may be included in this preparation to increase the absorption and availability of iron.
Iron and folic acid deficiency; iron-deficiency anaemias.

Tareg
Novartis, Fr.; Novartis, Ital.
Valsartan (p.988·3).
Hypertension.

Targel *Odan, Canad.*
Coal tar (p.1125·1).
Psoriasis.

Targel SA *Odan, Canad.*
Coal tar solution (p.1125·1); salicylic acid (p.1122·3).
Psoriasis.

Target
Note. This name is used for preparations of different composition.
Wyeth Lederle, Aust.; Whitehall-Much, Ger.; Lederle, Switz.†.
Felbinac (p.36·1) or felbinac iminopropanol salt (p.36·1).
Musculoskeletal, joint, peri-articular, and soft-tissue disorders.

Lisapharma, Hong Kong; Lisapharma, Ital.
Atenolol (p.841·3); chlortalidone (p.857·1).
Hypertension.

Targifor *Hoechst Marion Roussel, Braz.*
Arginine aspartate (p.1354·1).
Nutritional supplement.

Targifor C *Hoechst Marion Roussel, Braz.*
Arginine aspartate (p.1354·1); ascorbic acid (p.1389·3).
Nutritional supplement.

Targocid
Wyeth Lederle, Aust.; Hoechst Marion Roussel, Austral.; Aventis, Belg.; Hoechst Marion Roussel, Braz.; Aventis, Denm.; Hoechst Marion Roussel, Fin.; Roussel Diamant, Fr.; Hoechst Marion Roussel, Ger.; Hoechst Marion Roussel, Hong Kong; Hoechst Marion Roussel, Irl.; Hoechst Marion Roussel, Israel; Hoechst Marion Roussel, Jpn; Hoechst Marion Roussel, Mex.; Hoechst Marion Roussel, Neth.; Hoechst Marion Roussel, Norw.; Aventis, NZ; Aventis, S.Afr.; Hoechst Marion Roussel, Singapore; Marion Merrell, Spain; Hoechst Marion Roussel, Swed.; Hoechst Marion Roussel, Switz.; Hoechst Marion Roussel, Thai.; Hoechst Marion Roussel, UK.
Teicoplanin (p.257·3).
Gram-positive bacterial infections.

Targosid
Lepetit, Ital.; Aventis, Port.
Teicoplanin (p.257·3).
Gram-positive bacterial infections.

Targretin *Ligand, USA.*
Bexarotene (p.511·2).
Cutaneous T-cell lymphoma.

Tarisdin *Isdin, Spain†.*
Coal tar (p.1125·1); salicylic acid (p.1122·3).
Skin disorders.

Taritux *Monot, Fr.*
Dextromethorphan hydrobromide (p.1087·3).
Coughs.

Tarivid
Hoechst Marion Roussel, Aust.; Aventis, Belg.; Aventis, Denm.; Hoechst Marion Roussel, Fin.; Hoechst Marion Roussel, Ger.; Daiichi, Hong Kong; Hoechst Marion Roussel, Irl.; Hoechst Marion Roussel, Israel; Daiichi, Jpn; Santen, Jpn; Hoechst Marion Roussel, Mex.; Hoechst Marion Roussel, Neth.; Hoechst Marion Roussel, Norw.; Hoeport, Port.; Aventis, S.Afr.; Daiichi, Singapore; Hoechst Marion Roussel, Spain; Hoechst Marion Roussel, Swed.; Hoechst Marion Roussel, Switz.; Daiichi, Thai.; Hoechst Marion Roussel, UK.
Ofloxacin (p.232·3) or ofloxacin hydrochloride (p.233·1).
Bacterial infections.

Tarjen *Samakeephaesaj, Thai.*
Diclofenac sodium (p.30·3).
Musculoskeletal, joint, peri-articular, and soft-tissue disorders.

Tarjena *Samakeephaesaj, Thai.*
Diclofenac sodium (p.30·3).
Gout; musculoskeletal and joint disorders.

Tarka
Knoll, Denm.; Knoll, Fin.; Knoll, Fr.; Knoll, Ger.; Procter & Gamble, Ger.; Knoll, Ital.; Knoll, Mex.; Knoll, Neth.; Knoll, S.Afr.; Knoll, Spain; Knoll, Swed.; Knoll, Switz.; Knoll, UK; Abbott, USA.
Trandolapril (p.985·2); verapamil hydrochloride (p.989·1).
Hypertension.

Tarlene *Medco, USA.*
Coal tar (p.1125·1); salicylic acid (p.1122·3).
Seborrhoea.

Tarmed
Stiefel, Ger.; Stiefel, Ital.†; Stiefel, Mex.; Stiefel, Spain.
Coal tar (p.1125·1).
Scalp disorders.

Taro Gel
Taro, Canad.
Sterile lubricating jelly.

Taro, Israel.
Propylene glycol (p.1655·1); glycerol (p.1616·3).
Lubricating gel.

Tarocidin *Taro, Israel.*
Chloramphenicol (p.179·1); polymyxin B sulfate (p.238·1).
Blepharitis; conjunctivitis.

Tarocidin D *Taro, Israel.*
Chloramphenicol (p.179·1); polymyxin B sulfate (p.238·1); dexamethasone sodium phosphate (p.1067·1).
Blepharitis; conjunctivitis.

Taroctyl *Taro, Israel.*
Chlorpromazine hydrochloride (p.660·2).
Psychiatric disorders; vomiting.

Tarocyn *Taro, Israel.*
Oxytetracycline hydrochloride (p.234·1); polymyxin B sulfate (p.238·1).
Bacterial infections.

Tarodent *Taro, Israel.*
Chlorhexidine gluconate (p.1138·2).
Mouth disorders.

Tarodex *Taro, Israel.*
Dextromethorphan hydrobromide (p.1087·3).
Coughs.

Tarophed *Taro, Israel.*
Pseudoephedrine hydrochloride (p.1099·2).
Aural and nasal congestion.

Tarophenicol *Taro, Israel.*
Chloramphenicol (p.179·1).
Blepharitis; conjunctivitis.

Taro-Sone *Taro, Canad.*
Betamethasone dipropionate (p.1063·2).
Skin disorders.

Tarseb *Draxis, Canad.*
Tar (p.1125·1).

Tarsum *Summers, USA.*
Coal tar (p.1125·1); salicylic acid (p.1122·3).
Seborrhoea.

Tartar Control Listerine *Warner-Lambert, UK.*
Zinc chloride (p.1398·1).
Tooth tartar.

Tartephedreel *Peithner, Aust.*
Homoeopathic preparation.

Tartrina *Mead Johnson, Mex.*
Dextromethorphan (p.1087·3).

Tasedan *Hormona, Mex.*
Estazolam (p.682·3).
Insomnia; premedication.

Tasep *IPS, Spain.*
Cefazolin sodium (p.164·3).
Bacterial infections.

Tasmaderm *Roche, Switz.*
Motretinide (p.1121·3).
Acne.

Tasmar
Roche, Aust.; Roche, Denm.†; Roche, Hong Kong; Roche, Irl.†; Roche, Mex.; Roche, Norw.; Roche, NZ; Roche, S.Afr.; Roche, Singapore; Roche, Swed.†; Roche, Switz.; Roche, Thai.; Roche, UK†; Roche, USA.
Tolcapone (p.1179·2).
Parkinsonism.

Tasnon *Kolassa, Aust.†.*
Piperazine citrate (p.105·3).

Tasty C *Nutrition Care, Austral.*
Vitamin C (p.1389·3); vitamin E; betacarotene; rutoside; zinc amino-acid chelate (p.1350·1).
Vitamin C deficiency.

Tathion *Yamanouchi, Jpn†.*
Reduced glutathione (p.1010·3).
Corneal disorders; hepatic disorders; leucopenia due to radiotherapy or chemotherapy; poisoning; radiation-induced inflammation of oral mucosa; skin disorders; vomiting.

Tatig *Bioindustria, Ital.*
Sertraline hydrochloride (p.308·3).
Depression.

Tationil *Roche, Ital.*
Glutathione sodium (p.1010·3).
Alcohol or drug poisoning; radiation trauma.

Tau Kit *Isomed, Spain.*
Carbon-13 labelled urea (p.1591·3).
Test for gastrointestinal Helicobacter pylori infection.

Taucor *Sigma-Tau, Spain.*
Lovastatin (p.922·3).
Hyperlipidaemias.

Tauglicolo
SIT, Ital.
Bromhexine hydrochloride (p.1085·3); sulfogaiacol (p.1101·1).
Respiratory-tract congestion.

IBI, Thai.
Bromhexine hydrochloride (p.1085·3); guaifenesin (p.1092·2).
Respiratory-tract disorders associated with increased or viscous mucus.

Tauliz *Hoechst Marion Roussel, Ital.*
Piretanide (p.956·2).
Hypertension; oedema.

Tauma *IMO, Ital.*
Salix (p.82·1); passion flower (p.1649·1); crataegus (p.1600·2).
Insomnia.

Taurargin *Baldacci, Braz.*
Arginine; taurine; ditetraethylammonium phosphate (p.1350·1).
Nutritional supplement.

Tauredon
Byk, Aust.; Byk Tosse, Ger.; Byk Gulden, Ger.; Byk, Port.; Byk, Switz.
Sodium aurothiomalate (p.82·3).
Juvenile idiopathic arthritis; psoriatic arthritis; rheumatoid arthritis.

Tauro *Ravizza, Ital.*
Tauroursodeoxycholic acid (p.1677·3).
Gallstones.

Taurobetina *Zambon, Spain.*
Adenosine phosphate dipotassium (p.1573·3); cyanocobalamin (p.1388·1); pyridoxine hydrochloride (p.1386·3); uridine phosphate (p.1677·2); taurine (p.1669·3).
Lignocaine [lidocaine] hydrochloride (p.1313·2) is included in the intramuscular injection to alleviate the pain of injection.
Neuromuscular metabolic disorders.

Taurolin
Chemomedica, Aust.; Hoechst Marion Roussel, Ger.; Geistlich, Switz.
Taurolidine (p.257·2).
Bacterial infections.

Taurovit *Bruschettini, Ital.*
Mineral and vitamin preparation with taurine (p.1350·1).
Nutritional supplement.

Tautoss *Sigma-Tau, Spain.*
Levodropropizine (p.1089·3).
Coughs.

Tauval *Sigma-Tau, Spain.*
Valerian (p.1678·3).
Anxiety; insomnia.

Tauxolo *SIT, Ital.*
Ambroxol hydrochloride (p.1084·3).
Respiratory-tract congestion.

Tavanic
Hoechst Marion Roussel, Aust.; Aventis, Belg.; Hoechst Marion Roussel, Fin.; Roussel Diamant, Fr.; Hoechst Marion Roussel, Ger.; Hoechst Marion Roussel, Irl.; Hoechst Marion Roussel, Ital.; Hoechst Marion Roussel, Mex.; Hoechst Marion Roussel, Neth.; Aventis, Port.; Aventis, S.Afr.; Hoechst Marion Roussel, Spain; Hoechst Marion Roussel, Swed.; Hoechst Marion Roussel, Switz.; Hoechst Marion Roussel, UK.
Levofloxacin (p.219·1).
Bacterial infections.

Tavan-SP 54 *Aventis, S.Afr.*
Pentosan polysulfate sodium (p.953·1).
Hyperlipidaemias; thromboembolic disorders.

Tavegil
Novartis Consumer, Ger.; Novartis, Irl.; Novartis Consumer, Ital.; Novartis Consumer, Neth.; Novartis, Spain; Novartis Consumer, UK.
Clemastine fumarate (p.413·2).
Hypersensitivity reactions; insect bites; pruritus; sunburn.

Tavegyl
Novartis, S.Afr.; Novartis, Denm.; Novartis, Norw.†; Novartis Consumer, Port.; Novartis Consumer, S.Afr.; Novartis, Swed.; Novartis Consumer, Switz.
Clemastine fumarate (p.413·2).
Hypersensitivity reactions; skin disorders.

Taver *Medochemie, Thai.*
Carbamazepine (p.342·2).
Epilepsy; glossopharyngeal neuralgia; trigeminal neuralgia.

Tavidan *Baldacci, Ital.*
Suleparoid (p.978·2).
Thrombosis prophylaxis.

Tavipec *Montavit, Aust.; Montavit, Thai.*
Spike lavender oil (p.1667·1).
Respiratory-tract disorders.

Tavist
Novartis Consumer, Canad.; Novartis, Mex.; Novartis Consumer, Port.; Novartis, USA.
Clemastine fumarate (p.413·2).
Hypersensitivity reactions.

Tavist Allergy *Novartis, USA.*
Clemastine fumarate (p.413·2).
Formerly known as Tavist-1.
Allergic rhinitis.

Tavist-D
Novartis Consumer, Canad.†; Novartis, Mex.; Novartis, USA†.
Clemastine fumarate (p.413·2); phenylpropanolamine hydrochloride (p.1098·1).
Allergic rhinitis; nasal congestion.

Tavolax *Singer, Switz.†.*
Aloes (p.1210·1); belladonna (p.463·1); matricaria (p.1593·2); cascara (p.1216·1); senna (p.1248·2); bisacodyl (p.1212·2); docusate sodium (p.1223·1).
Bowel evacuation; constipation.

Tavolax nouvelle formule *Singer, Switz.*
Bisacodyl (p.1212·2).
Bowel evacuation; constipation.

Tavonin *VSM, Neth.*
Ginkgo biloba (p.1615·2).
Peripheral vascular disorders.

Tavor
Note. This name is used for preparations of different composition.
Wyeth, Ger.; Wyeth Lederle, Ital.
Lorazepam (p.688·3).
Anxiety; epilepsy; insomnia; premedication.

Asoforma, Mex.
Oxybutynin chloride (p.471·2).
Neurogenic bladder.

Taxifur *Fustery, Mex.*
Ceftazidime (p.174·3).
Bacterial infections.

Taxilan
Lundbeck, Ger.; Byk, Neth.†.
Perazine dimalonate (p.698·3).
Agitation; depression; mania; psychoses.

Taxol
Bristol-Myers Squibb, Aust.; Bristol-Myers Squibb, Austral.; Bristol-Myers Squibb, Belg.; Bristol-Myers Squibb, Braz.; Bristol-Myers Squibb, Canad.; Bristol-Myers Squibb, Denm.; Bristol-Myers Squibb, Fin.; Bristol-Myers Squibb, Fr.; Bristol-Myers Squibb, Ger.; Bristol-Myers

Squibb, Hong Kong; Bristol-Myers Squibb, Irl.; Bristol-Myers Squibb, Israel; Bristol-Myers Squibb, Ital.; Bristol-Myers Squibb, Jpn; Bristol-Myers Squibb, Neth.; Bristol-Myers Squibb, Norw.; Bristol-Myers Squibb, NZ; Bristol-Myers Squibb, Port.; Bristol-Myers Squibb, S.Afr.; Bristol-Myers Squibb, Singapore; Bristol-Myers Squibb, Spain; Bristol-Myers Squibb, Swed.; Bristol-Myers Squibb, Switz.; Bristol-Myers Squibb, Thai.; Bristol-Myers Squibb, UK; Bristol-Myers Squibb Oncology, USA.
Paclitaxel (p.563·2).
AIDS-related Kaposi's sarcoma; breast cancer; non-small cell lung cancer; ovarian cancer.

Taxotere
Sanova, Aust.; Rhone-Poulenc Rorer, Austral.; Aventis, Belg.; Rhodia, Braz.; Rhone-Poulenc Rorer, Canad.; Aventis, Denm.; Rhone-Poulenc Rorer, Fin.; Aventis, Fr.; Rhone-Poulenc Rorer, Ger.; Rhone-Poulenc Rorer, Hong Kong; Rhone-Poulenc Rorer, Irl.; Rhone-Poulenc Rorer, Israel; Rhone-Poulenc Rorer, Ital.; Rhone-Poulenc Rorer, Jpn; Rhone-Poulenc Rorer, Neth.; Rhone-Poulenc Rorer, Norw.; Aventis, NZ; Aventis, Port.; Aventis, S.Afr.; Rhone-Poulenc Rorer, Singapore; Rhone-Poulenc Rorer, Spain; Rhone-Poulenc Rorer, Swed.; Rhone-Poulenc Rorer, Switz.; Rhone-Poulenc Rorer, Thai.; Aventis, UK; Rhone-Poulenc Rorer, USA.
Docetaxel (p.534·1).
Breast cancer; non-small-cell lung cancer; ovarian cancer.

Taxus Asofarma, Mex.
Tamoxifen citrate (p.571·1).
Breast cancer; endometrial cancer; prostatic cancer.

Taxyl Solfran, Mex.
Dexamethasone (p.1067·1).
Corticosteroid.

Tazac Lilly, Austral.
Nizatidine (p.1238·1).
Gastro-oesophageal reflux; peptic ulcer.

Tazicef SmithKline Beecham, USA; Bristol-Myers Squibb, USA.
Ceftazidime (p.174·3).
Bacterial infections.

Tazidem Eurofarma, Braz.
Ceftazidime (p.174·3).
Bacterial infections.

Tazidime Lilly, Canad.; Lilly, USA.
Ceftazidime (p.174·3).
Bacterial infections.

Taziken Kendrick, Mex.
Terbutaline sulfate (p.776·2).
Obstructive airways disease; premature labour.

Tazobac Lederle, Ger.; IRBI, Ital.†; Wyeth Lederle, Port.; Lederle, Switz.
Piperacillin sodium (p.236·1); tazobactam sodium (p.257·2).
Bacterial infections.

Tazocel Cyanamid, Spain.
Piperacillin sodium (p.236·1); tazobactam sodium (p.257·2).
Bacterial infections.

Tazocilline Wyeth Lederle, Fr.
Piperacillin sodium (p.236·1); tazobactam sodium (p.257·2).
Bacterial infections.

Tazocin
Lederle, Austral.; Wyeth Lederle, Belg.; Wyeth-Ayerst, Canad.; Wyeth Lederle, Denm.; Lederle, Hong Kong; Lederle, Irl.; Lederle, Israel; Wyeth Lederle, Ital.; Lederle, Neth.; Lederle, NZ; Wyeth, S.Afr.; Wyeth, Singapore; Wyeth Lederle, Swed.; Wyeth-Ayerst, Thai.; Wyeth, UK.
Piperacillin sodium (p.236·1); tazobactam sodium (p.257·2).
Lignocaine [lidocaine] hydrochloride (p.1313·2) may be included in the intramuscular injection to alleviate the pain of injection.
Bacterial infections.

Tazonam Wyeth Lederle, Aust.
Piperacillin sodium (p.236·1); tazobactam sodium (p.257·2).
Bacterial infections.

Tazorac Allergan, Canad.; Allergan, USA.
Tazarotene (p.1125·3).
Acne; psoriasis.

T-BMP Seroyal, Canad.
Vitamin B₁ and choline tartrate (p.1350·1).

TBV Seroyal, Canad.
Vitamin B₁, vitamin B₃, and magnesium (p.1350·1).

3TC
Glaxo Wellcome, Austral.; Glaxo Wellcome, Canad.; Glaxo Wellcome, Hong Kong; Glaxo Wellcome, Mex.; Glaxo Wellcome, S.Afr.; Glaxo Wellcome, Switz.
Lamivudine (p.635·1).
HIV infection.

TCO Seroyal, Canad.
Vitamin and mineral preparation (p.1350·1).

TCP Pfizer Consumer, UK.
Cream: Chloroxylenol (p.1142·1); triclosan (p.1159·2); halogenated phenols; phenol (p.1152·3); sodium salicylate (p.84·2).
Minor skin disorders; skin disinfection.
Liquid: Halogenated phenols; phenol (p.1152·3).
Formerly contained halogenated phenols, phenol, and sodium salicylate.
Minor skin disorders; mouth ulcers; sore throat.
Lozenges: Hexylresorcinol (p.1146·3).
Sore throat.
Ointment: Iodine (p.1522·3); phenol (p.1152·3); sodium salicylate (p.84·2); methyl salicylate (p.55·1); precipitated sulfur (p.1123·3); tannic acid (p.1669·1); camphor (p.1589·3); salicylic acid (p.1122·3).
Haemorrhoids; minor skin disorders; pruritus.

TD Spray Iso Mack Mack, Illert., Ger.
Isosorbide dinitrate (p.915·2).
Ischaemic heart disease.

Td-Impfstoff Pasteur Merieux, Ger.
An adsorbed diphtheria and tetanus vaccine (p.1537·1).
Active immunisation of older children and adults.

Td-Polio Connaught, Canad.
An adsorbed diphtheria, tetanus, and inactivated poliomyelitis vaccine (p.1539·1).
Active immunisation.

Td-pur Chiron Behring, Aust.; Chiron Behring, Ger.
An adsorbed diphtheria and tetanus vaccine (p.1537·1).
Active immunisation of older children and adults.

Td-Rix SmithKline Beecham, Ger.
An adsorbed diphtheria and tetanus vaccine (p.1537·1).
Active immunisation of older children and adults.

T-Dry Jones, USA†.
Pseudoephedrine hydrochloride (p.1099·2); chlorpheniramine [chlorphenamine] maleate (p.412·1).
Cold symptoms.

Td-Vaccinol Procter & Gamble, Ger.
An adsorbed diphtheria and tetanus vaccine (p.1537·1).
Active immunisation of older children and adults.

Te Anatoxal
Kwizda, Aust.; Berna, Hong Kong; Pharmabroker, NZ; Berna, Singapore; Berna, Thai.; Berna, USA.
An adsorbed tetanus vaccine (p.1565·2).
Active immunisation.

Tea Tree & Witch Hazel Cream Lane, UK.
Hamamelis (p.1618·3); eucalyptus oil (p.1609·2); methyl salicylate (p.55·1); camphor (p.1589·3); melaleuca oil (p.1631·3); zinc oxide (p.1128·2).
Skin disorders.

Tealine Arkopharma, Fr.
Java tea (p.1625·1); green tea (p.1681·1).
Slimming aid.

Tear Drop Parmed, USA†.
Polyvinyl alcohol (p.1503·1).
Dry eyes.

Teardrops
Ciba Vision, Austral.; Ciba Vision, Canad.; Ciba Vision, NZ.
Polyvinyl alcohol (p.1503·1); povidone (p.1503·2).
Dry eyes.

TearGard Lee, USA.
Hyetellose (p.1501·1).
Artificial tears.

Tear-Gel Novartis Ophthalmics, Canad.
Carbomer 940 (p.1499·2).
Dry eyes.

Teargel Restan, S.Afr.
Carbomer (p.1499·2).
Dry eyes.

Teargen Goldline, USA.
Artificial tear solution.
Dry eyes.

Tearisol Ciba Vision, USA.
Hypromellose (p.1501·3).
Dry eyes.

Tears Again Ocusoft, USA.
Eye drops: Polyvinyl alcohol (p.1503·1).
Eye ointment: White soft paraffin (p.1407·3); liquid paraffin (p.1407·1).
Dry eyes.

Tears Again MC Ocusoft, USA.
Hypromellose (p.1501·3).
Dry eyes.

Tears Encore Dioptic, Canad.
Polysorbate 80 (p.1347·3).
Dry eyes.

Tears Humectant Alcon Cusi, Spain.
Dextran 70 (p.729·2); hypromellose (p.1501·3).
Dry eyes.

Tears Lubricante Alcon Cusi, Spain.
Wool fat (p.1410·3); white soft paraffin (p.1407·3).
Formerly known as Tears Gel.
Dry eyes.

Tears Naturale
Alcon, Austral.; Alcon, Belg.; Alcon, Canad.; Alcon, Hong Kong; Alcon, Irl.; Alcon, Israel; Alcon, NZ; Alcon, Port.; Alcon, S.Afr.; Alcon, Singapore; Alcon, Swed.; Alcon, Switz.; Alcon, Thai.; Alcon, UK; Alcon, USA.
Dextran 70 (p.729·2); hypromellose (p.1501·3).
Dry eyes.

Tears Night & Day Ocusoft, USA.
Carmellose sodium (p.1499·3); povidone (p.1503·2).
Dry eyes.

Tears Plus
Allergan, Austral.; Allergan, Canad.; Allergan, Neth.†; Allergan, NZ; Allergan, S.Afr.; Allergan, Switz.; Allergan, USA.
Polyvinyl alcohol (p.1503·1); povidone (p.1503·2).
Dry eyes.

Tears Renewed Akorn, USA.
Eye drops: Dextran 70 (p.729·2); hypromellose (p.1501·3).
Eye ointment: White soft paraffin (p.1407·3); light liquid paraffin (p.1407·2).
Dry eyes.

Teatrois Theranol-Deglaude, Fr.
Tiratricol (p.1528·3).
Thyroid disorders.

Tebamide G & W, USA.
Trimethobenzamide hydrochloride (p.426·3).
Nausea and vomiting.

Tebasedan Windson, Braz.
Dipyrone (p.34·1); homatropine methylbromide (p.468·1); papaverine hydrochloride (p.1648·1).
Smooth muscle spasm.

Tebege-Tannin Fresenius Kabi, Aust.
Tannic acid (p.1669·1); acriflavinium chloride (p.1130·2).
Anal fissures; burns; frostbite; infected skin disorders; sunburn; ulcers.

Tebertin Berenguer Infale, Spain†.
Inosine (p.1623·3).
Digitalis intoxication; heart failure; hepatitis; radiation toxicity.

tebesium Hefa, Ger.
Isoniazid (p.215·3).
Pyridoxine hydrochloride (p.1386·3) is included in this preparation for the prophylaxis of peripheral neuropathy.
Tuberculosis.

tebesium-s Hefa, Ger.
Isoniazid (p.215·3).
Tuberculosis.

Tebetane Composto Ferraz, Lynce, Port.
Alanine (p.1353·3); glycine (p.1365·3); glutamic acid (p.1365·2); prunus arborea.

Tebetane Compuesto Elfar, Spain.
Alanine (p.1353·3); glycine (p.1365·3); glutamic acid (p.1365·2); pygeum africanum (p.1490·3).
Prostatic disorders.

Tebezide Be-Tabs, S.Afr.
Pyrazinamide (p.240·1).
Tuberculosis.

Tebloc Lafare, Ital.
Loperamide hydrochloride (p.1231·3).
Diarrhoea.

Tebofortan Austroplant, Aust.
Ginkgo biloba (p.1615·2).
Cerebral and peripheral vascular disorders.

Tebofortin Schwabe, Switz.
Ginkgo biloba (p.1615·2).
Tonic.

Tebokan Beaufour-Ipsen, Singapore; Emerging Pharma, Singapore.
Ginkgo biloba (p.1615·2).
Vascular disorders.

Tebonin
Austroplant, Aust.; Byk, Braz.; Schwabe, Ger.; Farmasa, Mex.
Ginkgo biloba (p.1615·2).
Cerebral and peripheral vascular disorders; tinnitus; vertigo.

Teboven Farmasa, Mex.
Troxerutin (p.1611·2).
Venous insufficiency.

Te-Br Provit, Mex.
Tetracycline hydrochloride (p.258·3).
Bacterial infections.

Tebraxin Bracco, Ital.
Rufloxacin hydrochloride (p.247·3).
Bacterial infections.

Tebrazid
Continental Pharma, Belg.; ICN, Canad.
Pyrazinamide (p.240·1).
Tuberculosis.

Tecelac Biotest, Ger.
Plasma protein fraction (p.740·2).
Heart transplantation.

Tecfazolina Bohm, Spain.
Cefazolin sodium (p.164·3).
Lignocaine [lidocaine] hydrochloride (p.1313·2) is included in this preparation to alleviate the pain of injection.
Bacterial infections.

Techneplex Squibb Diagnostics, USA†.
Technetium-99m pentetate (p.1451·2).

TechneScan HDP
Mallinckrodt, Spain; Mallinckrodt, USA.
Technetium-99m oxidronate (p.1451·3).
Bone scanning agent.

TechneScan MAG3
Byk Gulden, Ital.; Mallinckrodt, Spain.
Technetium-99m betiatide (p.1451·2).
Contrast medium for renal imaging.

Tecnal Technilab, Canad.
Butalbital (p.658·3); caffeine (p.761·3); aspirin (p.14·2).
Pain; tension.

Tecnal C Technilab, Canad.
Butalbital (p.658·3); caffeine (p.761·3); aspirin (p.14·2); codeine phosphate (p.25·2).
Pain; tension.

Tecnemab K1 Amersham, Spain.
Antimelanoma antibody.
Diagnosis of melanoma.

Tecnofen Columbia, Mex.
Tamoxifen citrate (p.571·1).
Breast cancer.

Tecnoflut Gunther, Braz.
Flutamide (p.542·3).
Prostatic cancer.

Tecnolip Tecnifar, Port.
Lovastatin (p.922·3).
Atherosclerosis; hypercholesterolaemia.

Tecnoplatin Columbia, Mex.
Cisplatin (p.525·1).
Malignant neoplasms.

Tecnosal Tecnifar, Port.
Triflusal (p.987·2).
Thromboembolic disorders.

Tecnotax Gunther, Braz.
Tamoxifen (p.572·2).
Breast cancer.

Tecnovorin Gunther, Braz.
Calcium folinate (p.1363·1).
Adjunct to fluorouracil in colorectal cancer; antidote to folic acid antagonists; megaloblastic anaemias.

Teconam Asian Pharm, Thai.
Tenoxicam (p.87·2).
Gout; musculoskeletal and joint disorders.

Tecyn Jofrain, Mex.
Tetracycline (p.258·3).
Bacterial infections.

Teczem Hoechst Marion Roussel, USA.
Enalapril maleate (p.883·3); diltiazem malate (p.876·2).
Hypertension.

Tedec Profer Tedec Meiji, Spain.
Ferritin (p.1359·3).
Iron-deficiency anaemia.

Tediprima Estedi, Spain.
Trimethoprim (p.264·2).
Genito-urinary infections.

Tedipulmo Estedi, Spain.
Terbutaline sulfate (p.776·2).
Obstructive airways disease.

Tedivax SmithKline Beecham, Belg.
An adsorbed diphtheria and tetanus vaccine (p.1537·1).
Active immunisation.

Tedol Oftalder, Port.
Ketoconazole (p.389·1).
Fungal infections.

Tedral
Parke, Davis, Canad.†; Parke, Davis, S.Afr.†.
Theophylline (p.777·2); ephedrine hydrochloride (p.1090·1); phenobarbital (p.355·1).
Asthma.

Tedralan SERP, Mon.
Theophylline (p.777·2).
Formerly contained theophylline, racephedrine hydrochloride, and phenobarbital.
Asthma; bronchospasm.

Tedrigen Goldline, USA.
Theophylline (p.777·2); ephedrine hydrochloride (p.1090·1); phenobarbital (p.355·1).
Bronchospasm.

Tee gegen Durchfall Sanova, Aust.
Tormentil root (p.1674·1); chamomile flower (p.1593·2); fragaria vesca; rubus fruticosus; raspberry leaf (p.1657·2).
Diarrhoea.

Teedex Rice Steele, Irl.
Paracetamol (p.71·2); diphenhydramine hydrochloride (p.416·1).
Fever; pain.

Teejel
Asta Medica, Belg.; Purdue Frederick, Canad.; Seton, Irl.; Rafa, Israel.
Choline salicylate (p.24·3).
Gum and mouth pain.

Teekanne Blasen- und Nierentee Teekanne, Aust.
Equisetum (p.1606·3); silver birch (p.1585·2); solidago virgaurea; ononis (p.1644·1); peppermint leaf (p.1243·2).
Urinary tract disorders.

Teekanne Erkaltungstee Teekanne, Aust.
Sambucus (p.1660·3); tilia (p.1673·2); thyme (p.1672·2).
Cold symptoms.

Teekanne Herz- und Kreislauftee Teekanne, Aust.
Crataegus (p.1600·2); rosemary; fennel (p.1610·1); spearmint (p.1666·3).
Cardiac disorders.

Teekanne Husten- und Brusttee Teekanne, Aust.
Fennel (p.1610·1); aniseed (p.1580·2); wild thyme; sage leaf (p.1660·2); thyme (p.1672·2).
Coughs.

Teekanne Leber- und Galletee Teekanne, Aust.
Fennel (p.1610·1); curcuma zanthorrhiza; chamomile (p.1593·2); taraxacum (p.1669·2).
Liver and biliary disorders.

Teekanne Magen- und Darmtee Teekanne, Aust.
Chamomile (p.1593·2); peppermint leaf (p.1243·2); cinnamon (p.1595·3); melissa leaf (p.1632·2).
Gastrointestinal disorders.

Teekanne Schlaf- und Nerventee Teekanne, Aust.
Lavender (p.1627·2); peppermint leaf (p.1243·2); melissa (p.1632·2); valerian (p.1678·3).
Sleep disorders.

Teen Formula Avon, Canad.
Multivitamin and mineral preparation (p.1350·1).

Teen Midol Sterling, USA.
Paracetamol (p.71·2); pamabrom (p.952·1).

Teen Vitamins Adams, Canad.
Multivitamin and mineral preparation (p.1350·1).

Teenstick Arkopharma, Fr.
Clove oil (p.1597·1); geranium oil (p.1615·1); palmarosa oil; melaleuca oil (p.1631·3); ylang ylang oil; Dixeol.
Acne.

Teer-Linola-Fett *Wolff, Ger.*
Coal tar (p.1125·1).
Skin disorders.

Teerol *Max Ritter, Switz.†.*
Coal tar (p.1125·1).
Skin disorders.

Teerol-H *Max Ritter, Switz.†.*
Coal tar (p.1125·1); allantoin (p.1110·1); triclosan (p.1159·2).
Scalp disorders.

Teeth Tough *Vitamed, Israel.*
Sodium fluoride (p.1375·3).
Dental caries.

Teetha *Nelson, UK.*
Homoeopathic preparation.
Formerly known as Teething Granules.

Teething *Hylands, Canad.*
Homoeopathic preparation.

Teething Relief *Brauer, Austral.*
Homoeopathic preparation.

Tefaclor *TO-Chemicals, Thai.*
Cefaclor (p.161·1).
Bacterial infections.

Tefamin *Recordati, Ital.*
Aminophylline (p.760·1) or theophylline (p.777·2).
Asthma; bronchospasm.

Tefavinca *Bohm, Spain.*
Vincamine (p.1680·1).
Cerebral trauma; cerebrovascular disorders; circulatory disorders of the eye, ear, nose, and throat; vestibular disorders.

Tefilin *Hermal, Ger.*
Tetracycline hydrochloride (p.258·3).
Bacterial skin infections.

Tefizox *Teva, Israel.*
Ceftizoxime sodium (p.176·3).
Bacterial infections.

Tegasorb *3M, Fr.*
Carmellose (p.1499·3).
Burns; ulcers.

Tega-Vert *Ortega, USA†.*
Dimenhydrinate (p.415·2).
Motion sickness.

Tegeline *Lab Francais du Fractionnement, Fr.*
A normal immunoglobulin (p.1551·3).
Hypogammaglobulinaemia; idiopathic thrombocytopenic purpura; Kawasaki disease; passive immunisation; retinochoroiditis.

Tegens *Inverni della Beffa, Ital.*
Myrtillus (p.1639·2).
Capillary disorders.

Tegisec *Roussel, Port.†; Roussel, Spain.*
Fenproporex (p.1510·2) or fenproporex hydrochloride (p.1510·2).
Obesity.

Tegison *Roche, USA†.*
Etretinate (p.1114·2).
Psoriasis.

Tego 2000 *Goldschmidt, UK.*
1-alkyl-1,5-diazapentane.
Surface disinfection.

Tegodor *Goldschmidt, UK.*
Benzalkonium chloride (p.1133·2); glutaral (p.1145·2); formaldehyde (p.1144·2).
Surface and instrument disinfection.

Tegopen *Bristol, Canad.; Apothecon, USA†.*
Cloxacillin sodium (p.192·1).
Bacterial infections.

Tegra *Hermes, Ger.; Sanapharm, Ger.*
Garlic oil.
Hyperlipidaemias.

Tegreen *Pharmanex, USA.*
Green tea (p.1681·1).
Dietary supplement.

Tegretal *Novartis, Ger.*
Carbamazepine (p.342·2).
Alcohol withdrawal syndrome; bipolar disorder; epilepsy; neuralgias; neuropathies.

Tegretard *Cristalia, Braz.*
Carbamazepine (p.342·2).
Alcohol withdrawal syndrome; bipolar disorder; diabetes insipidus; epilepsy; neuralgias; psychoses.

Tegretol *Novartis, Aust.; Novartis, Austral.; Novartis, Belg.; Novartis, Braz.; Novartis, Canad.; Novartis, Denm.; Novartis, Fin.; Novartis, Fr.; Novartis, Hong Kong; Novartis, Irl.; Novartis, Israel; Novartis, Ital.; Novartis, Mex.; Novartis, Neth.; Novartis, Norw.; Novartis, NZ; Novartis, Port.; Novartis, S.Afr.; Novartis, Singapore; Novartis, Spain; Novartis, Swed.; Novartis, Switz.; Novartis, Thai.; Novartis, UK; Novartis, USA.*
Carbamazepine (p.342·2).
Alcohol withdrawal syndrome; bipolar disorder; diabetes insipidus; diabetic neuropathy; epilepsy; glossopharyngeal neuralgia; mania; trigeminal neuralgia.

Tegrin Note. This name is used for preparations of different composition.
Block, Canad.; Reedco, USA.
Coal tar (p.1125·1).
Skin and scalp disorders.

Stafford-Miller, Port.†.
Allantoin (p.1110·1); coal tar (p.1125·1).
Psoriasis.

Tegrin Medicated *Block, USA.*
Coal tar (p.1125·1).
Skin disorders.

Tegrin-HC *Block, USA.*
Hydrocortisone (p.1073·3).
Skin disorders.

Tegrin-LT *Block, USA.*
Pyrethrins; piperonyl butoxide (p.1436·2).

Tegunal *CEPA, Spain.*
Dimethicone (p.1410·1); benzethonium chloride (p.1134·2); talc (p.1124·2); zinc oxide (p.1128·2).
Skin disorders.

Teguran *Tegur, Mex.*
Nitrofurantoin (p.230·3).

Teicomid *Hoechst Marion Roussel, Ital.†.*
Teicoplanin (p.257·3).
Gram-positive bacterial infections.

Tejuntivo *Iquinosa, Spain.*
Oxaceprol (p.1645·2).
Musculoskeletal, joint, and peri-articular disorders; osteoporosis; soft tissue injury.

Telachlor *Major, USA†.*
Chlorpheniramine [chlorphenamine] maleate (p.412·1).
Hypersensitivity reactions.

Teladar *Dermol, USA.*
Betamethasone dipropionate (p.1063·2).
Skin disorders.

Telament *Adcock Ingram Self Medication, S.Afr.†.*
Chewable tablets: Simeticone (p.1249·2); atropine methobromide (p.460·3); magnesium carbonate (p.1232·3); dried aluminium hydroxide gel (p.1210·3).
Dyspepsia; flatulence.

Mer-National, S.Afr.
Oral drops: Simeticone (p.1249·2).
Colic; gripe.

Telbibur N *Fatol, Ger.*
Cyanocobalamin (p.1388·1); nicotinamide (p.1372·3); pyridoxine hydrochloride (p.1386·3).
Lignocaine [lidocaine] hydrochloride (p.1313·2) is included in this preparation to alleviate the pain of injection.
Liver disorders.

Telbon *Novartis, Braz.*
Sulfogaiacol (p.1101·1); chlorpheniramine [chlorphenamine] maleate (p.412·1).
Respiratory-tract congestion.

Teldafed *Albert-Roussel, Aust.†.*
Terfenadine (p.424·3); pseudoephedrine hydrochloride (p.1099·2).
Allergic rhinitis.

Teldafen *Hoechst Marion Roussel, Belg.†; Hoechst Marion Roussel, Braz.*
Terfenadine (p.424·3); pseudoephedrine hydrochloride (p.1099·2).
Allergic rhinitis.

Teldane *Hoechst Marion Roussel, Austral.; Hoechst Marion Roussel, Braz.; Marion Merrell, Fr.†; Hoechst Marion Roussel, Ger.; Hoechst Marion Roussel, Hong Kong; Lepetit, Ital.†; Hoechst Marion Roussel, Mex.; Hoechst Marion Roussel, Switz.†.*
Terfenadine (p.424·3).
Hypersensitivity reactions.

Teldanex *Aventis, Denm.; Hoechst Marion Roussel, Fin.; Hoechst Marion Roussel, Norw.; Hoechst Marion Roussel, Swed.*
Terfenadine (p.424·3).
Hypersensitivity reactions.

Teldrin *SmithKline Beecham Consumer, USA.*
Chlorpheniramine [chlorphenamine] maleate (p.412·1).
Hypersensitivity reactions.

Telebar *Guerbet, Braz.*
Barium sulfate (p.1032·1).
Dimethicone (p.1249·2) is included in this preparation to eliminate gas from the gastrointestinal tract before radiography.
Contrast medium for gastrointestinal radiography.

Telebrix *Sanova, Aust.†; Codali, Belg.; Mallinckrodt, Canad.; Guerbet, Denm.†; Guerbet, Israel.*
Meglumine ioxitalamate (p.1037·2) and/or sodium ioxitalamate (p.1037·2).
Radiographic contrast medium.

Telebrix 12 *Guerbet, Fr.; Guerbet, Neth.†; Guerbet, Port.; Guerbet, Switz.*
Sodium ioxitalamate (p.1037·2).
Radiographic contrast medium.

Telebrix 30 *Guerbet, Braz.; Guerbet, Fr.; Guerbet, Ital.†; Guerbet, Neth.†; Guerbet, Switz.*
Meglumine ioxitalamate (p.1037·2).
Radiographic contrast medium.

Telebrix 35 *Guerbet, Fr.; Guerbet, Switz.*
Meglumine ioxitalamate (p.1037·2); sodium ioxitalamate (p.1037·2).
Radiographic contrast medium.

Telebrix 38 *Guerbet, Braz.; Guerbet, Ital.†.*
Meglumine ioxitalamate (p.1037·2); sodium ioxitalamate (p.1037·2).
Radiographic contrast medium.

Telebrix 350 *Guerbet, Neth.†; Guerbet, Port.*
Meglumine ioxitalamate (p.1037·2); sodium ioxitalamate (p.1037·2).
Radiographic contrast medium.

Telebrix Coronar *Guerbet, Braz.*
Meglumine ioxitalamate (p.1037·2); sodium ioxitalamate (p.1037·2).
Radiographic contrast medium.

Telebrix Gastro *Codali, Belg.; Guerbet, Fr.; Guerbet, Ger.; Guerbet, Israel; Guerbet, Neth.†; Guerbet, Port.; Guerbet, Switz.*
Meglumine ioxitalamate (p.1037·2).
Contrast medium for gastrointestinal radiography.

Telebrix Hystero *Codali, Belg.; Guerbet, Fr.; Guerbet, Port.*
Meglumine ioxitalamate (p.1037·2).
Contrast medium for hysterosalpingography and uretrography.

Telebrix N 180 and 300 *Guerbet, Ger.*
Meglumine ioxitalamate (p.1037·2).
Contrast medium for urinary-tract radiography.

Telebrix Polyvidone *Guerbet, Neth.†.*
Meglumine ioxitalamate (p.1037·2); povidone.
Formerly known as Vasurix-Polyvidone.
Contrast medium for hysterosalpingography and urinary-tract radiography.

Telebrix TC *Guerbet, Braz.*
Meglumine ioxitalamate (p.1037·2).
Radiographic contrast medium.

Telen *Yamanouchi, Ger.*
Tripotassium dicitratobismuthate (p.1213·2).
Duodenal ulcer.

Telepaque *Nycomed, Austral.; Sanofi Winthrop, Braz.; Sanofi Winthrop, Canad.†; Sanofi Winthrop, UK†; Nycomed, USA.*
Iopanoic acid (p.1035·2).
Contrast medium for biliary-tract radiography.

Telergon II *Codit, Ital.*
Royal jelly (p.1659·3).
Nutritional supplement.

Telesol *Ipsen, Spain.*
Oxitriptan (p.302·2).
Depression; epilepsy.

Tele-Stulln *Stulln, Ger.*
Actinoquinol sodium (p.1573·1); naphazoline nitrate (p.1095·1).
Blepharitis; conjunctivitis.

Telfast *Hoechst Marion Roussel, Aust.; Hoechst Marion Roussel, Austral.; Aventis, Belg.; Aventis, Denm.; Marion Merrell, Fr.; Hoechst Marion Roussel, Ger.; Procter & Gamble, Ger.; Hoechst Marion Roussel, Hong Kong; Hoechst Marion Roussel, Irl.; Lepetit, Ital.; Hoechst Marion Roussel, Neth.; Hoechst Marion Roussel, Norw.; Aventis, NZ; Aventis, Port.; Aventis, S.Afr.; Hoechst Marion Roussel, Spain; Hoechst Marion Roussel, Swed.; Orion, Swed.; Hoechst Marion Roussel, Switz.; Hoechst Marion Roussel, Thai.; Hoechst Marion Roussel, UK.*
Fexofenadine hydrochloride (p.417·3).
Allergic rhinitis; urticaria.

Telfast Decongestant *Hoechst Marion Roussel, Austral.; Aventis, NZ.*
Fexofenadine hydrochloride (p.417·3); pseudoephedrine hydrochloride (p.1099·2).
Allergic rhinitis.

Teline *Hauck, USA†.*
Tetracycline hydrochloride (p.258·3).
Bacterial infections.

Telmitin *Nakornpatana, Thai.*
Niclosamide (p.104·2).
Cestode infections.

Telo Cypro *Relax, Ital.*
Copper wire (p.1357·3).
Headache; insomnia; muscle spasm; musculoskeletal and joint disorders; pain.

Telos *Merckle, Ger.*
Lornoxicam (p.50·2).
Musculoskeletal and joint disorders.

Teltonal *Schuck, Ger.*
Devil's claw root (p.26·3).
Joint disorders.

Temaco *Nakornpatana, Thai.*
Theophylline (p.777·2).
Obstructive airways disease.

Temador *Sanico, Belg.†.*
Temazepam (p.707·2).
Anxiety disorders; premedication; sleep disorders.

Temaze *Alphapharm, Austral.*
Temazepam (p.707·2).
Insomnia.

temazep *CT, Ger.*
Temazepam (p.707·2).
Sleep disorders.

Temazin Cold *Trenier, USA†.*
Phenylpropanolamine hydrochloride (p.1098·1); chlorpheniramine [chlorphenamine] maleate (p.412·1).
Upper respiratory-tract symptoms.

Temazine *Pinewood, Irl.†.*
Temazepam (p.707·2).
Insomnia.

Temesta *Wyeth Lederle, Aust.; Wyeth Lederle, Belg.; Wyeth Lederle, Denm.;*
Wyeth Lederle, Fin.; Wyeth Lederle, Fr.; Wyeth, Neth.; Wyeth Lederle, Swed.; Wyeth, Switz.
Lorazepam (p.688·3).
Alcohol withdrawal syndrome; anxiety; insomnia; nausea and vomiting; premedication; status epilepticus.

Temetex *Roche, Ital.*
Diflucortolone valerate (p.1069·3).
Skin disorders.

Temgesic *Aesca, Aust.; Reckitt & Colman, Austral.; Schering-Plough, Belg.; Schering-Plough, Braz.; Schering-Plough, Denm.; Schering-Plough, Fin.; Schering-Plough, Fr.; Essex, Ger.; Reckitt & Colman, Hong Kong; Reckitt Benckiser, Irl.; Schering-Plough, Ital.; Schering-Plough, Mex.; Schering-Plough, Neth.; Reckitt & Colman, Norw.; Reckitt Benckiser, NZ; Schering-Plough, S.Afr.; Reckitt & Colman, Singapore; Schering-Plough, Singapore; Schering-Plough, Swed.; Essex, Switz.; Schering-Plough, Thai.; Schering-Plough, UK.*
Buprenorphine hydrochloride (p.21·1).
Pain.

Temgesic-nX *Reckitt Benckiser, NZ.*
Buprenorphine hydrochloride (p.21·1).
Naloxone hydrochloride (p.1014·3) is included in this preparation to discourage abuse.
Pain.

Temic *Uno, Ital.*
Cimetidine (p.1216·3).
Gastric hyperacidity; gastro-oesophageal reflux; gastrointestinal haemorrhage; peptic ulcer; Zollinger-Ellison syndrome.

Temigran *Teva, Israel.*
Ergotamine tartrate (p.452·1); chlorcyclizine (p.411·3); caffeine (p.761·3); codeine phosphate (p.25·2).
Vascular headache.

Temodal *Schering-Plough, Aust.; Schering-Plough, Austral.; Schering-Plough, Denm.; Schering-Plough, Fin.; Schering-Plough, Fr.; Essex, Ger.; Schering-Plough, Neth.; Schering-Plough, NZ; Schering-Plough, Port.; Schering-Plough, Spain; Schering-Plough, Swed.; Schering-Plough, UK.*
Temozolomide (p.573·3).
Astrocytoma; glioblastoma multiforme; malignant glioma.

Temodar *Schering, USA.*
Temozolomide (p.573·3).
Anaplastic astrocytoma.

Temol *Rolab, S.Afr.*
Paracetamol (p.71·2).
Fever; pain.

Temolan *Olan-Kemed, Thai.*
Paracetamol (p.71·2).
Lignocaine [lidocaine] hydrochloride (p.1313·2) is included in this preparation to alleviate the pain of injection.
Fever; pain.

Temopen *Bencard, UK†.*
Temocillin sodium (p.258·3).
Bacterial infections.

Temovate *Glaxo Wellcome, USA.*
Clobetasol propionate (p.1065·2).
Skin disorders.

Temoxol *Schering-Plough, S.Afr.*
Temozolomide (p.573·3).
Malignant glioma.

Temperal *Allen, Mex.; Diviser Aquilea, Spain.*
Paracetamol (p.71·2).
Fever; pain.

Tempil *Temmler, Ger.*
Ibuprofen (p.43·2).
Fever; pain.

Tempil N *Temmler, Ger.*
Diphenylpyraline hydrochloride (p.417·1); metamfepramone hydrochloride (p.1634·3); aspirin (p.14·2).
Cold symptoms.

Tempo *Thompson, USA.*
Aluminium hydroxide (p.1210·3); magnesium hydroxide (p.1233·1); simeticone (p.1249·2); calcium carbonate (p.1215·1).
Hyperacidity.

Tempodia *SmithKline Beecham Sante, Fr.†.*
Ascorbic acid (p.1389·3).
Vitamin C deficiency.

Tempolax *Hommel, Ger.*
Bisacodyl (p.1212·2).
Bowel evacuation; constipation.

Temporinolo *Hoechst Marion Roussel, Ital.*
Phenylpropanolamine hydrochloride (p.1098·1); chlorpheniramine [chlorphenamine] maleate (p.412·1).
Nasal congestion.

Temporol *Orion, Irl.; SMP, S.Afr.†.*
Carbamazepine (p.342·2).
Alcohol withdrawal syndrome; deafferentation pain; epilepsy; trigeminal neuralgia.

Temposil *Wyeth-Ayerst, Canad.†.*
Calcium carbimide (p.1588·2).
Alcoholism.

Tempra *Mead Johnson, Austral.; Bristol-Myers Squibb, Belg.; Mead Johnson Nutritionals, Canad.; Mead Johnson, Mex.; Mead Johnson, Singapore; Upsamedica, Spain; Mead Johnson Nutritionals, Thai.; Mead Johnson Nutritionals, USA.*
Paracetamol (p.71·2).
Fever; pain.

Mead Johnson, Mex.
Injection: Propacetamol hydrochloride (p.80·1).
Fever; pain.

Tempra CD *Mead Johnson, Mex.*
Paracetamol (p.71·2); codeine phosphate (p.25·2).
Pain.

Temprin *Continentales, Mex.*
Paracetamol (p.71·2).
Fever; pain.

Temtabs *Wyeth, Austral.*
Temazepam (p.707·2).
Insomnia.

Tenacid *Sigma-Tau, Ital.*
Imipenem (p.214·1); cilastatin sodium (p.182·2).
Lignocaine [lidocaine] hydrochloride (p.1313·2) is included in the intramuscular injection to alleviate the pain of injection.
Bacterial infections.

Tenadren *Wyeth, Braz.*
Propranolol hydrochloride (p.962·3); hydrochlorothiazide (p.907·3).
Hypertension.

Tenadrin *Hua, Thai.*
Diphenhydramine hydrochloride (p.416·1); ammonium chloride (p.1085·2); sodium citrate (p.1186·2); menthol (p.1632·3).
Coughs; nasal congestion.

Tenat *Helvepharm, Switz.*
Atenolol (p.841·3).
Angina pectoris; arrhythmias; hypertension; myocardial infarction.

Tenax *Siam Bheasach, Thai.*
Tenoxicam (p.87·2).
Gout; musculoskeletal, joint, and peri-articular disorders.

Tenben *Galen, UK.*
Atenolol (p.841·3); bendrofluazide [bendroflumethiazide] (p.844·1).
Hypertension.

Ten-Bloka *Aspen, S.Afr.*
Atenolol (p.841·3).
Angina pectoris; hypertension.

Tencef *Tedec Meiji, Spain.*
Cefminox sodium (p.167·3).
Bacterial infections.

Tencet *Hauck, USA.*
Paracetamol (p.71·2); butalbital (p.658·3); caffeine (p.761·3).
Formerly known as G-1.
Pain.

Tenchlor
Berk, Irl.†; Aspen, S.Afr.; Berk, UK.
Atenolol (p.841·3); chlortalidone (p.857·1).
These ingredients can be described by the British Approved Name Co-tenidone.
Hypertension.

Tencon *International Ethical, USA.*
Paracetamol (p.71·2); butalbital (p.658·3).

Tender Age *Jamieson, Canad.*
Multivitamin preparation (p.1350·1).

TenderWet *IVF, Switz.*
Xanthan gum (p.1504·3).
Wounds.

Tendosimol *Tendem, Neth.†.*
Albumin tannate (p.1209·3).
Diarrhoea.

Tendrin *Pisa, Mex.*
Ephedrine (p.1090·1).

Tenelid *Allergan-Frumtost, Braz.*
Guanabenz acetate (p.900·2).
Hypertension.

Teneretic *Zeneca, Ger.*
Atenolol (p.841·3); chlortalidone (p.857·1).
Hypertension.

Tenex *Robins, USA.*
Guanfacine hydrochloride (p.901·3).
Hypertension.

Tenibex *Lemery, Mex.*
Albendazole (p.95·2).

Tenidon *Gerard, Denm.*
Atenolol (p.841·3); chlortalidone (p.857·1).
Hypertension.

Tenif
Zeneca, Belg.; AstraZeneca, UK.
Atenolol (p.841·3); nifedipine (p.940·1).
Angina pectoris; hypertension.

Teniken *Kener, Mex.*
Praziquantel (p.106·3).

Tenitran *Pfizer, Ital.*
Tenitramine (p.980·1).
Cardiac stenosis; ischaemic heart disease.

Teniverme *Basi, Port.*
Flubendazole (p.99·2).

Ten-K *Summit, USA.*
Potassium chloride (p.1194·3).
Hypokalaemia; potassium depletion.

Tenkafruse *CP Pharmaceuticals, UK.*
Frusemide [furosemide] (p.893·1).
Hypercalcaemia; hypertension; oedema; oliguria.

Tenlol *Amrad, Austral.*
Atenolol (p.841·3).
Angina pectoris; arrhythmias; hypertension; myocardial infarction.

Teno *BASF, Ger.*
Atenolol (p.841·3).
Arrhythmias; hypertension; ischaemic heart disease.

Tenoblock *Leiras, Fin.*
Atenolol (p.841·3).
Angina pectoris; arrhythmias; hypertension; hyperthyroidism; myocardial infarction.

Tenocam *M & H, Thai.*
Tenoxicam (p.87·2).
Gout; musculoskeletal and joint disorders.

Tenolin *Technilab, Canad.*
Atenolol (p.841·3).
Angina pectoris; hypertension.

Tenolol *Siam Bheasach, Thai.*
Atenolol (p.841·3).
Angina pectoris; arrhythmias; hypertension.

Tenolone *Lusofarmaco, Ital.*
Atenolol (p.841·3); chlortalidone (p.857·1).
Hypertension.

Tenol-Plus *Vortech, USA†.*
Paracetamol (p.71·2); aspirin (p.14·2); caffeine (p.761·3).
Pain.

Tenomax *Boniscontro & Gazzone, Ital.*
Atenolol (p.841·3).
Angina pectoris; arrhythmias; hypertension; myocardial infarction.

Tenon *Biolab, Thai.*
Astemizole (p.409·1).
Allergic conjunctivitis; allergic rhinitis; hypersensitivity reactions; pruritus; urticaria.

Tenoprin *Medinovum, Fin.*
Atenolol (p.841·3).
Angina pectoris; arrhythmias; hypertension; hyperthyroidism; myocardial infarction.

Tenopt *Sigma, Austral.*
Timolol maleate (p.982·1).
Glaucoma; ocular hypertension.

Tenordate *AstraZeneca, Fr.*
Nifedipine (p.940·1); atenolol (p.841·3).
Hypertension.

Tenoret
Zeneca, Hong Kong; Zeneca, Irl.; AstraZeneca, NZ; Zeneca, S.Afr.†; AstraZeneca, Singapore; AstraZeneca, UK.
Atenolol (p.841·3); chlortalidone (p.857·1).
These ingredients can be described by the British Approved Name Co-tenidone.
Hypertension.

Tenoretic
Zeneca, Aust.; Zeneca, Belg.; Zeneca, Braz.; AstraZeneca, Canad.; Searle, Denm.; AstraZeneca, Fr.; Zeneca, Hong Kong; Zeneca, Irl.; Zeneca, Ital.; Zeneca, Mex.; Zeneca, Neth.; AstraZeneca, NZ; Zeneca, Port.; Zeneca, S.Afr.; AstraZeneca, Singapore; Zeneca, Spain; Zeneca, Switz.; AstraZeneca, Thai.; AstraZeneca, UK; Zeneca, USA.
Atenolol (p.841·3); chlortalidone (p.857·1).
These ingredients can be described by the British Approved Name Co-tenidone.
Hypertension.

Tenormin
Zeneca, Aust.; Zeneca, Austral.; Zeneca, Belg.; AstraZeneca, Canad.; Searle, Denm.; Zeneca, Ger.; Zeneca, Hong Kong; Zeneca, Irl.; Zeneca, Ital.; Zeneca, Mex.; Zeneca, Neth.; Searle, Norw.; Astra-Zeneca, NZ; Zeneca, Port.; AstraZeneca, S.Afr.; AstraZeneca, Singapore; Zeneca, Spain; Searle, Swed.; Zeneca, Switz.; AstraZeneca, Thai.; AstraZeneca, UK; Zeneca, USA.
Atenolol (p.841·3).
Angina pectoris; arrhythmias; hypertension; hyperthyroidism; migraine; myocardial infarction.

Tenormine *AstraZeneca, Fr.*
Atenolol (p.841·3).
Angina pectoris; hypertension; myocardial infarction.

Ten-O-Six *Bonne Bell, Canad.†.*
Salicylic acid (p.1122·3).
Acne.

Tenox
Note. This name is used for preparations of different composition.
Orion, Fin.; Orion, Irl.
Temazepam (p.707·2).
Anxiety; insomnia; premedication.

Charoen, Thai.
Tenoxicam (p.87·2).
Gout; musculoskeletal, joint, and peri-articular disorders.

Tenoxen *Biosintetica, Braz.*
Tenoxicam (p.87·2).
Musculoskeletal, joint, and peri-articular disorders.

Tenoxil *Olan-Kemed, Thai.*
Tenoxicam (p.87·2).
Musculoskeletal, joint, and peri-articular disorders.

Tenoxol *Pulitzer, Ital.*
Neltenexine (p.1095·3).
Respiratory-tract disorders.

Tens *Boehringer Ingelheim, Port.*
Lacidipine (p.919·1).
Hypertension.

Tensadiur *Crinos, Ital.*
Benazepril hydrochloride (p.843·2); hydrochlorothiazide (p.907·3).
Hypertension.

Tensan *Klinge, Aust.*
Nilvadipine (p.946·1).

Tensanil *Crinos, Ital.*
Benazepril hydrochloride (p.843·2).

Tensazol *Tecnifar, Port.*
Enalapril maleate (p.883·3).
Heart failure; hypertension; ischaemic heart disease; myocardial infarction.

Tensidol *Kenyaku, Thai.*
Haloperidol (p.686·3).
Anxiety; psychiatric disorders.

Tensig *Sigma, Austral.*
Atenolol (p.841·3).
Angina pectoris; arrhythmias; hypertension; myocardial infarction.

Tensigradyl *Lipha Sante, Fr.†.*
Guabenxan sulfate (p.900·2); bemetizide (p.843·2).
Hypertension.

Tensikey *Inkeysa, Spain.*
Lisinopril (p.921·1).
Diabetic nephropathy; heart failure; hypertension; myocardial infarction.

Tensil *Sintofarma, Braz.*
Chlordiazepoxide (p.659·2).
Alcohol withdrawal syndrome; anxiety; tension headache; tremor.

Tensilon
ICN, Canad.†; Roche, S.Afr.†; ICN, USA.
Edrophonium chloride (p.1418·2).
Diagnosis of myasthenia gravis; reversal of competitive neuromuscular blockade.

Tensin *Rolab, S.Afr.*
Spironolactone (p.973·2).
Ascites; oedema.

Tensiocomplet *Medea, Spain.*
Hydralazine hydrochloride (p.905·3); hydrochlorothiazide (p.907·3); reserpine (p.967·3).
Hypertension.

Tensiomin
Thiemann, Ger.; Egis, Hong Kong; Egis, Thai.
Captopril (p.853·3).
Heart failure; hypertension.

Tensiomin-Cor *Thiemann, Ger.*
Captopril (p.853·3).
Heart failure; hypertension.

Tensionorme *Leo, Fr.*
Bendrofluazide [bendroflumethiazide] (p.844·1); reserpine (p.967·3).
Hypertension.

Tensipine *Genus, UK.*
Nifedipine (p.940·1).
Angina pectoris; hypertension.

Tensiplex *Francia, Ital.*
Vinburnine phosphate (p.1680·1).
Cerebrovascular disorders; mental function impairment.

Tensitruw *Truw, Ger.†.*
Crataegus (p.1600·2).
Cardiac disorders.

Tensium *DDSA Pharmaceuticals, UK.*
Diazepam (p.674·3).
Alcohol withdrawal syndrome; anxiety; epilepsy; insomnia; premedication; skeletal muscle spasm.

Tenso Stop *Esteve, Spain.*
Fosinopril sodium (p.892·3).
Heart failure; hypertension.

Tenso Stop Plus *Esteve, Spain.*
Fosinopril sodium (p.892·3); hydrochlorothiazide (p.907·3).
Hypertension.

Tensobon
Schwarz, Ger.; Upsamedica, Switz.
Captopril (p.853·3).
Diabetic nephropathy; heart failure; hypertension.

Tensobon comp
Schwarz, Ger.; Upsamedica, Switz.
Captopril (p.853·3); hydrochlorothiazide (p.907·3).
Heart failure; hypertension.

Tensocardil *Esteve, Spain.*
Fosinopril sodium (p.892·3).
Heart failure; hypertension.

Tensoderm *Ferraz, Lynce, Port.*
Zinc oxide (p.1128·2); sulfur (p.1123·3); camphor (p.1589·3).
Acne; seborrhoea.

Tensoflux *Hennig, Ger.*
Bendrofluazide [bendroflumethiazide] (p.844·1); amiloride hydrochloride (p.835·1).
Ascites; hypertension; oedema; renal calculi.

Tensogard *Mead Johnson, Ital.*
Fosinopril sodium (p.892·3).
Heart failure; hypertension.

Tensogradal *Almirall, Spain.*
Nitrendipine (p.947·1).
Hypertension.

Tensolve *Aspen, S.Afr.*
Paracetamol (p.71·2); diphenhydramine hydrochloride (p.416·1); codeine phosphate (p.25·2); caffeine (p.761·3).
Pain.

Tensoprel
Rubio, Singapore; Rubio, Spain.
Captopril (p.853·3).
Diabetic nephropathy; heart failure; hypertension; myocardial infarction.

Tensopril
Note. This name is used for preparations of different composition.
Norton Waterford, Irl.; Sanofi Synthelabo, Port.; Medimpex, UK.
Captopril (p.853·3).
Heart failure; hypertension.

Merck Sharp & Dohme, Israel.
Lisinopril (p.921·1).
Heart failure; hypertension.

Tensopyn *Parke-Med, S.Afr.†.*
Paracetamol (p.71·2); codeine phosphate (p.25·2); doxylamine succinate (p.417·1); caffeine (p.761·3).
Pain and associated tension.

Tensostad *Stada, Ger.*
Captopril (p.853·3).
Heart failure; hypertension.

Tensotin *Julphar, UAE.*
Atenolol (p.841·3).
Angina pectoris; arrhythmias; hypertension.

Tensozide *Mead Johnson, Ital.*
Fosinopril sodium (p.892·3); hydrochlorothiazide (p.907·3).
Hypertension.

Tenstaten *Beaufour, Fr.*
Cicletanine hydrochloride (p.857·3).
Hypertension.

Tenston *Covan, S.Afr.*
Sustained-release capsules; sustained-release tablets:
Paracetamol (p.71·2); caffeine (p.761·3); codeine phosphate (p.25·2); meprobamate (p.691·1).
Fever; pain.
Syrup: Promethazine hydrochloride (p.423·3); paracetamol (p.71·2); codeine phosphate (p.25·2).
Fever; pain.
Tablets: Aspirin (p.14·2); paracetamol (p.71·2); caffeine (p.761·3); codeine phosphate (p.25·2); meprobamate (p.691·1).
Pain.

Tensuril *Cristalia, Braz.*
Diazoxide (p.868·1).
Hypertension; hypoglycaemia.

Tenuate
Hoechst Marion Roussel, Austral.; Hoechst Marion Roussel, Canad.; Hoechst Marion Roussel, USA.
Diethylpropion hydrochloride (p.1508·3).
Obesity.

Tenuate Dospan
Hoechst Marion Roussel, Belg.†; Marion Merrell, Fr.†; Bruno, Ital.†; Hoechst Marion Roussel, Mex.; Aventis, NZ; Mer-National, S.Afr.
Diethylpropion hydrochloride (p.1508·3).
Obesity.

Tenuate Retard
Artegodan, Ger.†; Hoechst Marion Roussel, Switz.
Diethylpropion hydrochloride (p.1508·3).
Obesity.

Tenuatina *Rottapharm, Spain†.*
Dihydroergotamine mesilate (p.450·3).
Circulatory disorders; migraine; orthostatic hypotension.

Tenutex *Recip, Swed.*
Disulfiram (p.1605·1); benzyl benzoate (p.1428·2).
Pediculosis; scabies.

Tenzone *Tocogino, Mex.*
Methyldopa (p.927·3).

Teobid *Vita, Ital.*
Theophylline (p.777·2).
Asthma; bronchospasm.

Teodelin *Leti, Spain†.*
Theophylline (p.777·2).
Heart failure; obstructive airways disease; paroxysmal dyspnoea.

Teodrin *Prodotti, Braz.*
Aminophylline (p.760·1); ephedrine (p.1090·1).
Obstructive airways disease.

Teofylamin *Medic, Denm.*
Aminophylline (p.760·1).
Obstructive airways disease.

Teolixir *Biogalenica, Spain.*
Theophylline (p.777·2).
Heart failure; obstructive airways disease; paroxysmal dyspnoea.

Teolixir Compositum *Biogalenica, Spain.*
Guaifenesin (p.1092·2); prednisolone (p.1077·3); theophylline (p.777·2).
Obstructive airways disease.

Teolong
Knoll, Braz.; Knoll, Mex.
Theophylline (p.777·2).
Obstructive airways disease.

Teonibsa *Inibsa, Port.†.*
Theophylline (p.777·2).
Heart failure; obstructive airways disease; pulmonary oedema.

Teonim *Mipharm, Ital.*
Nimesulide (p.62·3).
Fever; inflammation; pain.

Teonova *Corvi, Ital.†.*
Theophylline (p.777·2).
Obstructive airways disease.

Teoptic
Ciba Vision, Irl.; Ciba Vision, Neth.; Restan, S.Afr.; Novartis Ophthalmics, UK.
Carteolol hydrochloride (p.855·1).
Glaucoma; ocular hypertension.

Teoremac *Sanfer, Mex.*
Glucametacin (p.42·1).
Inflammation; pain.

Teoremin *Asta Medica, Braz.*
Glucametacin (p.42·1).
Musculoskeletal and joint disorders.

Teovent
Pharmacia Upjohn, Norw.; Pharmacia Upjohn, Swed.
Choline theophyllinate (p.763·3).
Obstructive airways disease.

Schering-Plough, Port.
Theophylline (p.777·2).

Teovit Inexfa, Spain.
Aceglutamide (p.1571·2); hydroxocobalamin acetate (p.1388·3); pyridoxine hydrochloride (p.1386·3); thiamine phosphate (p.1385·2).
Vitamin B deficiency.

Tepam BASF, Ger.
Tetrazepam (p.708·1).
Skeletal muscle tension and spasticity.

Tepavil Almirall, Spain.
Sulpiride (p.706·1).
Anxiety; psychoses; vertigo.

Tepazepan Almirall, Spain.
Diazepam (p.674·3); pyridoxine (p.1387·1); sulpiride (p.706·1).
Anxiety; neurosis; psychoses; psychosomatic disorders.

Tepilta Wyeth Lederle, Aust.; Wyeth, Ger.; Wyeth, Spain†.
Aluminium hydroxide (p.1210·3); light magnesium carbonate (p.1232·3) or magnesium hydroxide (p.1233·1); oxetacaine (p.1317·3).
Gastrointestinal disorders.

Tepox Cal Solvay, Spain.
Calcium pidolate (p.1188·3).
Calcium deficiency.

Tequin Bristol-Myers Squibb, Austral.; Bristol-Myers Squibb, USA.
Gatifloxacin (p.209·3).
Bacterial infections.

Teradyl Hua, Thai.
Codeine phosphate (p.25·2); promethazine hydrochloride (p.423·2).
Coughs.

Teragran Junior Bristol-Myers Squibb, Braz.
Multivitamin preparation (p.1350·1).

Teragran M Bristol-Myers Squibb, Braz.
Multivitamin and mineral preparation (p.1350·1).

Terak Akorn, USA.
Oxytetracycline hydrochloride (p.234·1); polymyxin B sulfate (p.238·1).
Bacterial eye infections.

Teralithe Rhone-Poulenc Rorer, Fr.
Lithium carbonate (p.292·1).
Bipolar disorder; psychoses.

Teranic Biolab, Thai.
Terfenadine (p.424·3).
Allergic conjunctivitis; allergic rhinitis; urticaria.

Teraprost Malesci, Ital.
Terazosin hydrochloride (p.980·1).
Benign prostatic hyperplasia.

Terazol Janssen-Cilag, Canad.; Janssen-Cilag, Denm.†; Janssen-Cilag, S.Afr.†; Janssen-Cilag, Swed.†; Ortho McNeil, USA.
Terconazole (p.395·1).
Vulvovaginal candidiasis.

Terbac Syntex, Mex.
Ceftriaxone sodium (p.177·1).
Bacterial infections.

Terbasmin Astra, Spain.
Terbutaline sulfate (p.776·2).
Obstructive airways disease.

Terbasmin Expectorante Astra, Spain.
Guaifenesin (p.1092·2); terbutaline sulfate (p.776·2).
Obstructive airways disease.

Terbolan
Hoechst Marion Roussel, Aust.†; Hoechst Marion Roussel, Braz.
Frusemide [furosemide] (p.893·1); reserpine (p.967·3).
Hypertension.

Terbosil Silom, Thai.
Terbutaline sulfate (p.776·2); guaifenesin (p.1092·2).
Coughs; obstructive airways disease.

Terbron Biolab, Thai.
Terbutaline sulfate (p.776·2).
Obstructive airways disease.

Terbron Expectorant Biolab, Thai.
Terbutaline sulfate (p.776·2); guaifenesin (p.1092·2).
Obstructive airways disease.

Terbuken Kener, Mex.
Terbutaline sulfate (p.776·2).

Terbul Hexal, Ger.
Terbutaline sulfate (p.776·2).
Obstructive airways disease.

Terbulin
Vitamed, Israel; Chinta, Thai.; Great Eastern, Thai.; Westmont, Thai.
Terbutaline sulfate (p.776·2).
Obstructive airways disease; premature labour.

Terbulin Expectorant Chinta, Thai.
Terbutaline sulfate (p.776·2); guaifenesin (p.1092·2).
Obstructive airways disease.

Terbuno Milano, Thai.
Terbutaline sulfate (p.776·2).
Obstructive airways disease.

Terbuturmant Pulmopharm, Ger.
Terbutaline sulfate (p.776·2).
Obstructive airways disease.

Tercian
Rhone-Poulenc Rorer, Fr.; Vitoria, Port.
Cyamemazine (p.674·1) or cyamemazine tartrate (p.674·1).
Anxiety; depression; psychoses; withdrawal syndromes.

Terco-C Hua, Thai.
Codeine phosphate (p.25·2); guaifenesin (p.1092·2); terpin hydrate (p.1101·2).
Coughs.

Terco-D Hua, Thai.
Dextromethorphan hydrobromide (p.1087·3); guaifenesin (p.1092·2); terpin hydrate (p.1101·2).
Coughs.

Terden Shiwa, Thai.
Terfenadine (p.424·3).
Allergic skin disorders; hay fever; rhinitis; rhinoconjunctivitis.

Terdine Silom, Thai.
Terfenadine (p.424·3).
Allergic conjunctivitis; allergic rhinitis; allergic skin disorders; hay fever; urticaria.

Terelit Farmasan, Ger.
Doxycycline hyclate (p.200·1); ambroxol hydrochloride (p.1084·3).
Respiratory-tract infections associated with increased or viscous mucus.

Terfadine Samakeephaesaj, Thai.
Terfenadine (p.424·3).
Allergic conjunctivitis; allergic rhinitis; allergic skin disorders.

Terfedura Merck dura, Ger.
Terfenadine (p.424·3).
Hypersensitivity disorders.

Terfegen General Drugs, Thai.
Terfenadine (p.424·3).
Allergic rhinitis; allergic skin disorders.

Terfemundin Mundipharma, Ger.
Terfenadine (p.424·3).
Hypersensitivity disorders.

Terfen Siam Bheasach, Thai.
Terfenadine (p.424·3).
Allergic conjunctivitis; allergic rhinitis; urticaria.

Terfenor Norton, S.Afr.
Terfenadine (p.424·3).
Allergic rhinitis; allergic skin disorders.

Terfenor Antihistamine Norton, UK.
Terfenadine (p.424·3).
Allergic rhinitis; allergic skin disorders.

Terfex Ciba Vision, Swed.†; Penn, UK†.
Terfenadine (p.424·3).
Hypersensitivity reactions.

Terfium Hexal, Ger.†.
Terfenadine (p.424·3).
Hypersensitivity reactions.

Terfluzine
ICN, Canad.†; Aventis, Fr.†; Rhone-Poulenc Rorer, Israel; Rhone-Poulenc Rorer, Neth.
Trifluoperazine hydrochloride (p.710·3).
Agitation; psychoses.

Tergynan Bouchara, Fr.†.
Ternidazole (p.603·2); neomycin sulfate (p.228·1); nystatin (p.392·2); prednisolone metasulfobenzoate sodium (p.1078·1).
Vaginitis.

Tericin AT Ativus, Braz.
Tetracycline (p.258·3); amphotericin B (p.377·2).
Bacterial and fungal vulvovaginal infections.

Teril
Alphapharm, Austral.; Alphapharm, Hong Kong; Taro, Israel; Pacific, NZ; Taro, UK.
Carbamazepine (p.342·2).
Alcohol withdrawal syndrome; bipolar disorder; diabetes insipidus; diabetic neuropathy; epilepsy; neuralgia.

Terivalidin
Gerot, Aust.; Noristan, S.Afr.†.
Terizidone (p.258·3).
Bacterial infections.

Terlane Mundipharma, Aust.
Terfenadine (p.424·3).
Hypersensitivity reactions.

Terlomexin Effik, Fr.
Fenticonazole nitrate (p.383·2).
Candidiasis.

Termalgin
Novartis, Spain; Novartis Consumer, Switz.
Paracetamol (p.71·2).
Fever; pain.

Termalgin Codeina Novartis, Spain.
Codeine phosphate (p.25·2); paracetamol (p.71·2).
Pain.

Termigripe C Luper, Braz.
Chlorpheniramine [chlorphenamine] (p.412·2); ascorbic acid (p.1389·3); caffeine (p.761·3); salicylamide (p.82·1).
Cold and influenza symptoms.

Termizol Fustery, Mex.
Ketoconazole (p.389·1).
Fungal infections.

Termonil Liferpal, Mex.
Dipyrone (p.34·1).
Fever; pain.

Termosan Dom, Spain.
Camphor (p.1589·3); capsicum oleoresin (p.1591·1); methyl salicylate (p.55·1); salicylic acid (p.1122·3); turpentine oil (p.1676·3); menthol (p.1632·3); lavender oil (p.1627·2); thyme oil (p.1672·3); eucalyptus oil (p.1609·2).
Muscle pain; soft-tissue disorders; upper respiratory-tract disorders.

Termotrin Loren, Mex.
Paracetamol (p.71·2).
Fever; pain.

Ternadin Cantabria, Spain.
Terfenadine (p.424·3).
Hypersensitivity reactions.

Ternalin Agis, Israel.
Terfenadine (p.424·3).
Allergic rhinitis; allergic skin disorders.

Ternalin-D Agis, Israel.
Terfenadine (p.424·3); pseudoephedrine (p.1099·2).
Allergic rhinitis.

Ternelin Sandoz, Jpn†.
Tizanidine hydrochloride (p.1330·2).
Myotonia; spastic paralysis.

Terneurine Bristol-Myers Squibb, Fr.†.
Vitamin B substances (p.1350·1).
Asthenia.

Terocaps Medix, Mex.
Garcinia cambogia.
Hypercholesterolaemia; obesity.

Terol Mavi, Mex.
Paracetamol (p.71·2).
Fever; pain.

Terolut Solvay, Fin.
Dydrogesterone (p.1472·3).
Endometriosis; menopausal disorders; menstrual disorders.

Teronac
Novartis, Israel; Novartis, Neth.†; Novartis, Singapore; Novartis, Switz.
Mazindol (p.1510·3).
Obesity.

Terpalate Ferrer, Spain†.
Aluminium hydroxide (p.1210·3); attapulgite (p.1212·1); enoxolone aluminium (p.1225·2); magnesium oxide (p.1233·2); sodium citrate (p.1186·2).
Gastritis; gastrointestinal hyperacidity; peptic ulcer.

Terpestrol H Medopharm, Ger.
Turpentine oil (p.1676·3).
Respiratory-tract disorders.

Terpine des Monts-Dore Centrapharm, Fr.
Terpin (p.1101·2).
Respiratory-tract congestion.

Terpine Gonnon
Monot, Fr.
Tablets: Terpin (p.1101·2); codeine (p.25·2).
Respiratory-tract disorders.

Pharminter, Fr.†.
Oral liquid: Terpin (p.1101·2); tolu balsam (p.1101·3).
Respiratory-tract disorders.

Terpoin Houghs Healthcare, UK.
Codeine phosphate (p.25·2); menthol; eucalyptol.
Coughs.

Terpone Rosa-Phytopharma, Fr.
Terpin (p.1101·2); Siberian fir oil; niaouli oil (p.1640·2); eucalyptus oil (p.1609·2).
Formerly contained semisynthetic oxide derivatives of terpene oils terpin, and quinine camsilate.
Respiratory-tract disorders.

Terponil Vitafarma, Spain.
Oxidised terpenes; terpin (p.1101·2).
Respiratory-tract disorders.

Terposen Vir, Spain.
Ranitidine hydrochloride (p.1245·2).
Acid aspiration; gastro-oesophageal reflux; gastrointestinal haemorrhage; peptic ulcer; short-bowel syndrome; Zollinger-Ellison syndrome.

Terra-Cortril
Note. This name is used for preparations of different composition.
Pfizer, Aust.†; Pfizer, Belg.; Pfizer, Braz.; Pfizer, Fin.; Pfizer, Irl.; Pfizer, Neth.†; Pfizer, Norw.; Pfizer, S.Afr.; Farmasierra, Spain; Pfizer, UK.
Ointment: Oxytetracycline hydrochloride (p.234·1); hydrocortisone (p.1073·3) or hydrocortisone acetate (p.1073·3).
Infected inflammatory skin disorders.

Pfizer, Belg.; Pfizer, S.Afr.; Farmasierra, Spain.
Ear/eye ointment; ear/eye drops: Oxytetracycline hydrochloride (p.234·1); hydrocortisone acetate (p.1073·3); polymyxin B sulfate (p.238·1).
Infected inflammatory ear or eye disorders.

Pfizer, USA.
Oxytetracycline hydrochloride (p.234·1); hydrocortisone acetate (p.1073·3).
Eye inflammation with bacterial infection.

Terracortril
Note. This name is used for preparations of different composition.
Pfizer, Ger.; Pfizer, Switz.
Cream; ointment; topical spray: Oxytetracycline hydrochloride (p.234·1); hydrocortisone (p.1073·3); polymyxin B sulfate (p.238·1).
Infected skin disorders.

Pfizer, Ger.; Pfizer, Switz.
Eye/ear drops; eye ointment: Oxytetracycline hydrochloride (p.234·1); hydrocortisone acetate (p.1073·3); polymyxin B sulfate (p.238·1).
Ear infections; inflammatory disorders of the eye.

Pfizer, Swed.
Oxytetracycline hydrochloride (p.234·1); hydrocortisone (p.1073·3).
Infected skin disorders; otitis externa.

Terra-Cortril com Polimixina B Pfizer, Braz.
Oxytetracycline hydrochloride (p.234·1); hydrocortisone (p.1073·3); polymyxin B sulfate (p.238·1).
Infected skin disorders.

Terra-Cortril Gel Steraject met polymyxine-B Pfizer, Neth.
Oxytetracycline calcium (p.234·1); hydrocortisone (p.1073·3); polymyxin B sulfate (p.238·1).
Sinusitis.

Terracortril med polymyxin B Pfizer, Swed.
Oxytetracycline hydrochloride (p.234·1); hydrocortisone acetate (p.1073·3); polymyxin B sulfate (p.238·1).
Infected ear and eye disorders; otitis externa.

Terra-Cortril met polymyxine-B Pfizer, Neth.
Oxytetracycline calcium (p.234·1); hydrocortisone acetate (p.1073·3); polymyxin B sulfate (p.238·1).
Blepharitis squamosa; inflammatory ear infections.

Terra-Cortril mit Gentamicin Pfizer, Aust.†.
Oxytetracycline calcium (p.234·1); gentamicin sulfate (p.210·1); hydrocortisone acetate (p.1073·3).
Bacterial infections and inflammation of the nose or genito-urinary tract.

Terra-Cortril mit Polymyxin B-Sulfat Pfizer, Aust.†.
Oxytetracycline calcium (p.234·1) or oxytetracycline hydrochloride (p.234·1); polymyxin B sulfate (p.238·1); hydrocortisone (p.1073·3).
Bacterial infections and inflammation of the nose and sinuses.

Terra-Cortril Nystatin
Pfizer, Irl.; Pfizer, UK.
Oxytetracycline calcium (p.234·1); hydrocortisone (p.1073·3); nystatin (p.392·2).
Infected skin disorders.

Terra-Cortril P Pfizer, Fin.
Oxytetracycline hydrochloride (p.234·1); hydrocortisone acetate (p.1073·3); polymyxin B sulfate (p.238·1).
Infected ear and eye disorders; infected eye disorders.

Terra-Cortril Polymyxin B Pfizer, Norw.
Oxytetracycline hydrochloride (p.234·1); hydrocortisone (p.1073·3); polymyxin B sulfate (p.238·1).
Ear disorders.

Terradermina Flopen, Braz.
Salicylic acid (p.1122·3); sulfur (p.1123·3).
Acne.

Terrados Pfizer, Mex.
Oxytetracycline (p.234·1).
Bacterial infections.

Terrafor Claytone, Fr.
Octalite.
Gastrointestinal disorders.

Terralin Schulke & Mayr, Ger.
Benzalkonium chloride (p.1133·2); phenoxypropanol (p.1153·3).
Surface disinfection.

Terramicina
Note. This name is used for preparations of different composition.
Pfizer, Braz.; Pfizer, Mex.; Farmasierra, Spain.
Capsules; eye ointment; injection; tablets: Oxytetracycline (p.234·1) or oxytetracycline hydrochloride (p.234·1).
Lignocaine [lidocaine] (p.1313·2) is included in the injection to alleviate the pain of injection.
Bacterial infections.

Pfizer, Mex.; Farmasierra, Spain.
Eye ointment; ointment: Oxytetracycline (p.234·1) or oxytetracycline hydrochloride (p.234·1); polymyxin B sulfate (p.238·1).
Bacterial infections.

Terramicina Polimixina B Pfizer, Braz.
Oxytetracycline hydrochloride (p.234·1); polymyxin B sulfate (p.238·1).
Bacterial skin infections.

Terramycin
Note. This name is used for preparations of different composition.
Pfizer, Ger.; Pfizer, Israel; Pfizer, S.Afr.; Pfizer, Singapore; Pfizer, Thai.
Eye ointment; ointment; pessaries: Oxytetracycline (p.234·1) or oxytetracycline hydrochloride (p.234·1); polymyxin B (p.238·3) or polymyxin B sulfate (p.238·1).
Bacterial infections.

Pfizer, Hong Kong; Pfizer, S.Afr.†; Pfizer, Singapore; Pfizer, Thai.; Pfizer, UK; Pfizer, USA.
Capsules; injection; tablets: Oxytetracycline (p.234·1) or oxytetracycline hydrochloride (p.234·1).
Lignocaine [lidocaine] (p.1313·2) may be included in the injection to alleviate the pain of injection.
Bacterial infections.

Terramycin met polymyxine-B Pfizer, Neth.†.
Oxytetracycline hydrochloride (p.234·1); polymyxin B sulfate (p.238·1).
Bacterial infections.

Terramycin mit Polymyxin-B-Sulfat Pfizer, Aust.†.
Oxytetracycline hydrochloride (p.234·1); polymyxin B sulfate (p.238·1).
Bacterial infections of the eye or skin.

Terramycin with Polymyxin B
Pfizer, Hong Kong; Pfizer, USA.
Oxytetracycline hydrochloride (p.234·1); polymyxin B sulfate (p.238·1).
Bacterial eye and skin infections.

Terramycin Polymyxin B
Pfizer, Denm.; Pfizer, Norw.; Pfizer, Swed.
Oxytetracycline hydrochloride (p.234·1); polymyxin B sulfate (p.238·1).
Bacterial skin and eye infections.

Terramycine
Pfizer, Belg.; Pfizer, Switz.†.
Oxytetracycline hydrochloride (p.234·1); polymyxin B sulfate (p.238·1).
Eye infections; skin infections.

Terramycine Solu-Retard *Pfizer, Fr.†.*
Oxytetracycline (p.234·1).
Lignocaine [lidocaine] (p.1313·2) is included in this preparation to alleviate the pain of injection.
Bacterial infections.

Terranilo *Bial-Aristegui, Spain.*
Chymotrypsin (p.1595·1); tetracycline hydrochloride (p.258·3).
Bacterial infections.

Terranumonyl *Sanofi Winthrop, Mex.*
Tetracycline (p.258·3).
Bacterial infections.

Terrasil *Silom, Thai.*
Oxytetracycline (p.234·1); polymyxin B sulfate (p.238·1).
Eye infections.

Terricil *Oftalder, Port.*
Oxytetracycline hydrochloride (p.234·1).
Bacterial eye infections.

Tersac *Trans Canaderm, Canad.*
Salicylic acid (p.1122·3); triclosan (p.1159·2).
Acne.

Tersaseptic
Note. This name is used for preparations of different composition.
Trans Canaderm, Canad.
Triclosan (p.1159·2).
Skin cleanser; skin disorders.

Dermaclin, Mex.
Soap substitute.
Acne.

Doak, USA.
Soap substitute.

Tersa-Tar *Trans Canaderm, Canad.*
Coal tar (p.1125·1).
Psoriasis; seborrhoea.

Tersatar *Doak, Hong Kong.*
Tar (p.1125·1).
Feminine hygiene; skin and scalp disorders.

Tersigat *3M, Fr.*
Oxitropium bromide (p.769·2).
Obstructive airways disease.

Tertensif *Servier, Spain.*
Indapamide (p.913·1).
Hypertension; oedema.

Tertroxin
Boots, Austral.; Glaxo Wellcome, NZ; Glaxo Wellcome, S.Afr.; Glaxo Wellcome, Thai.; Goldshield, UK.
Liothyronine sodium (p.1524·2).
Hyperthyroidism; hypothyroidism; myxoedema coma.

Terzolin
Janssen-Cilag, Ger.; Janssen-Cilag, Switz.
Ketoconazole (p.389·1).
Scalp disorders.

Tesacof *Novartis, Mex.*
Bromhexine hydrochloride (p.1085·3).
Respiratory-tract congestion.

Tesalon *Novartis, Mex.*
Benzonatate (p.1085·3).
Coughs.

Tesamone *Dunhall, USA†.*
Testosterone (p.1492·1).
Androgen replacement therapy; delayed puberty.

Teslac *Bristol-Myers Squibb Oncology, USA.*
Testolactone (p.574·2).
Breast cancer.

Teslascan
Nycomed, Aust.; Nycomed, Belg.; Nycomed Imaging, Denm.; Nycomed, Fin.; Nycomed, Fr.; Nycomed, Ger.; Nycomed Imaging, Norw.; Nycomed, NZ; Nycomed, Spain; Nycomed Amersham, Swed.; Nycomed Amersham, UK; Nycomed, USA.
Mangafodipir trisodium (p.1037·3).
Contrast medium for magnetic resonance imaging of the liver.

Tesopalmed Forte cum Yohimbine *Trima, Israel.*
Yohimbine hydrochloride (p.1681·3); strychnine nitrate (p.1667·3).
Erectile dysfunction.

Tesoprel *Thiemann, Ger.*
Bromperidol (p.657·1) or bromperidol lactate (p.657·1).
Schizophrenia.

Tesor-C *Segix, Ital.*
Estradiol (p.1473·1); norethisterone acetate (p.1485·1).
Menopausal disorders; osteoporosis.

Tesos *Byk Elmu, Spain.*
Tetridamine maleate (p.87·3).
Vaginitis.

Tespamin *Sumitomo, Jpn†.*
Thiotepa (p.574·3).
Malignant neoplasms.

Tessalon *Forest Pharmaceuticals, USA.*
Benzonatate (p.1085·3).
Coughs.

Tessifol *Esfar, Port.*
Atenolol (p.841·3).
Angina pectoris; arrhythmias; hypertension; myocardial infarction.

Tessofort *Bustillos, Mex.*
Multivitamin preparation (p.1350·1).

Test Pack Plus *Abbott, UK.*
Pregnancy test (p.1654·3).

Testac *Medac, Ger.†.*
Flutamide (p.542·3).
Prostatic cancer.

Testandro *Redur, USA†.*
Testosterone (p.1492·1).
Androgen replacement therapy; delayed puberty.

Tes-Tape
Lilly, Austral.; Lilly, Canad.; Lilly, Irl.; Lilly, Ital.; Lilly, NZ; Lilly, S.Afr.†; Lilly, Switz.
Test for glucose in urine (p.1616·3).

testasa e *Chefaro, Ger.*
Yohimbe extract.
Male sexual exhaustion.

Testerell *Sanorell, Ger.*
Homoeopathic preparation.

Test-Estro *Rugby, USA†.*
Estradiol cipionate (p.1473·2); testosterone cipionate (p.1492·1).
Menopausal vasomotor symptoms; prevention of postpartum breast engorgement.

Testex *Byk Elmu, Spain.*
Testosterone cipionate (p.1492·1) or testosterone propionate (p.1492·2).
Aplastic anaemia; female breast cancer; lactation inhibition; male hypogonadism and androgen deficiency; osteoporosis.

Testiculi *Disperga, Aust.*
Testis extract (p.1492·1).
Androgen deficiency; hypogonadism.

Testinfex *Flopen, Braz.*
Neomycin (p.228·1); sulfamethoxypyridazine (p.256·1); sulfadiazine (p.251·1); sulfaguanidine (p.253·2).
Diarrhoea.

Testiormina *Sanval, Braz.*
Testosterone cipionate (p.1492·1).
Androgen; breast cancer in females; delayed puberty; male hypogonadism.

Testo *Baldassari, Braz.*
Guarana; erythroxylon catuaba; ginseng; arginine; lysine; ptychopetalum uncinatum; gelatin; testis extract; wheat germ; kola (p.1350·1).

Testoderm
Ferring, Aust.; Ferring, Belg.; Ferring, Ger.; Ferring, Neth.; Ferring, UK†; Alza, USA.
Testosterone (p.1492·1).
Hypogonadism; testosterone deficiency.

Testo-Enant *Geymonat, Ital.*
Testosterone enantate (p.1492·2).
Androgenic; breast cancer; fibroids.

Testofran *Faria, Braz.*
Yohimbine (p.1681·3); vitamin B₁; vitamin E; calcium inositohexaphosphate; magnesium inositohexaphosphate; magnesium stearate.
Erectile dysfunction.

Testonus *Profarb, Braz.*
Methyltestosterone (p.1482·3); vitamin B₁; vitamin E.
Breast cancer in females; cryptorchidism; delayed puberty in males; erectile dysfunction; hypogonadism in males.

Testopel *Bartor Pharmacal, USA.*
Testosterone (p.1492·1).
Androgen deficiency; delayed puberty.

Testosterone Implants *Organon, UK.*
Testosterone (p.1492·1).
Male hypogonadism.

Testotard *Chephasaar, Ger.*
Flutamide (p.542·3).
Prostatic cancer.

Testotonic B *Sam-On, Israel.*
Methyltestosterone (p.1482·3).
Erectile dysfunction.

Testotop *Stada, Aust.†.*
Testosterone (p.1492·1).
Testosterone deficiency.

Testoviron 100 *Schering, Aust.; Schering, Thai.*
Testosterone propionate (p.1492·2); testosterone enantate (p.1492·2).
Aplastic anaemia in men; erectile dysfunction; female breast cancer; male hypogonadism.

Testoviron 250 *Schering, Aust.; Schering, Thai.*
Testosterone enantate (p.1492·2).
Aplastic anaemia in men; erectile dysfunction; female breast cancer; male hypogonadism.

Testoviron Depot
Schering, Belg.; Schering, Hong Kong; Schering, Irl.†; Schering, Neth.; Schering, Port.; Schering, Singapore; Schering, Swed.; Schering, Switz.
Testosterone enantate (p.1492·2).
Aplastic anaemia; erectile dysfunction; female breast cancer; male hypogonadism.

Schering, Israel; Schering, Ital.
Testosterone enantate (p.1492·2); testosterone propionate (p.1492·2).
Aplastic anaemia; breast cancer; endometrial cancer; erectile dysfunction; male hypogonadism.

Testoviron Depot 50 *Schering, Ger.*
Testosterone enantate (p.1492·2); testosterone propionate (p.1492·2).
Hypogonadism in men.

Testoviron Depot 100 *Schering, Ger.; Schering, Spain.*
Testosterone enantate (p.1492·2); testosterone propionate (p.1492·2).
Female breast cancer; haematopoietic disorders; hepatic cirrhosis; male hypogonadism and androgen deficiency; male infertility; osteoporosis.

Testoviron Depot 135 *Schering, Denm.*
Testosterone enantate (p.1492·2); testosterone propionate (p.1492·2).
Breast cancer; male hypogonadism.

Testoviron Depot 250
Schering, Denm.; Schering, Ger.; Schering, Spain.
Testosterone enantate (p.1492·2).
Female breast cancer; haematopoietic disorders; hepatic cirrhosis; male hypogonadism and androgen deficiency; male infertility; osteoporosis.

Testovis *SIT, Ital.*
Methyltestosterone (p.1482·3) or testosterone propionate (p.1492·2).
Androgenic; breast disorders; fibroids; menstrual disorders.

Testozzard *Pizzard, Mex.*
Testosterone (p.1492·1).

Testpack hCG-Urine *Abbott, Irl.*
Pregnancy test (p.1654·3).

TestPack Plus hCG-Urine *Abbott, USA.*
Pregnancy test (p.1654·3).

Testred *ICN, USA.*
Methyltestosterone (p.1482·3).
Androgen replacement therapy; breast cancer.

Tesuloid *Squibb Diagnostics, USA†.*
Technetium-99m sulfur colloid (p.1451·1).

Tesurene *A Natureza, Braz.*
Testosterone propionate (p.1492·2); vitamin E (p.1393·3).
Androgenic; breast cancer in females; lichen sclerosus.

Teta Extra *Fresenius Kabi, Ger.*
Didecyldimethylammonium chloride (p.1143·2); polihexanide (p.1154·2).
Disinfectant.

Tetabulin
Immuno, Aust.; Immuno, Hong Kong; Immuno, Irl.; Immuno, Ital.; Hyland Immuno, UK.
A tetanus immunoglobulin (p.1565·1).
Formerly known as Humotet in the UK.
Passive immunisation.

Tetabuline
Baxter, Belg.; Immuno, Switz.†.
A tetanus immunoglobulin (p.1565·1).
Passive immunisation.

Tetagam
Centeon, Aust.; NBI, S.Afr.
A tetanus immunoglobulin (p.1565·1).
Passive immunisation.

Tetagam N *Centeon, Ger.; Chiron Behring, Ger.*
A tetanus immunoglobulin (p.1565·1).
Passive immunisation.

Tetagamma *Nuovo ISM, Ital.*
A tetanus immunoglobulin (p.1565·1).
Passive immunisation.

Tetaglobulina *Pasteur Merieux, Braz.*
A tetanus immunoglobulin (p.1565·1).
Passive immunisation.

Tetaglobuline *Pasteur Merieux, Israel.*
A tetanus immunoglobulin (p.1565·1).
Passive immunisation.

Tetagrip *Pasteur Merieux, Fr.*
A tetanus and influenza vaccine (p.1566·2).
Active immunisation.

Tetamer *Pasteur Merieux, Belg.†.*
An adsorbed tetanus vaccine (p.1565·2).
Active immunisation.

Tetamun SSW *SmithKline Beecham, Ger.*
A tetanus vaccine (p.1565·2).
Active immunisation.

Tetanobulin
Immuno, Braz.; Immuno, Mex.
A tetanus immunoglobulin (p.1565·1).
Passive immunisation.

Tetanogamma
Centeon, Braz.; Centeon, Mex.
A tetanus immunoglobulin (p.1565·1).
Passive immunisation.

Tetanol
Chiron Behring, Aust.; Chiron Behring, Ger.
An adsorbed tetanus vaccine (p.1565·2).
Active immunisation.

Tetanosimultan *Immuno, Aust.*
A tetanus immunoglobulin (p.1565·1).
Passive immunisation.

Tetanus-Gamma *Biagini, Ital.*
A tetanus immunoglobulin (p.1565·1).
Passive immunisation.

Teta-S *Fresenius Kabi, Ger.*
Didecylmethylalkoxiammonium propionate; cocospropylenediamineguanidinium diacetate; polihexanide (p.1154·2).
Surface disinfection.

Tetasorbat SSW *SmithKline Beecham, Ger.*
An adsorbed tetanus vaccine (p.1565·2).
Active immunisation.

Tetatox *Berna, Ital.*
An adsorbed tetanus vaccine (p.1565·2).
Active immunisation.

Tetavax
Merieux, Fr.†; Pasteur Merieux, Ger.†; Pasteur Merieux, Hong Kong; Pasteur Merieux, Neth.; Aventis, S.Afr.; Pasteur Merieux, Thai.; Pasteur Merieux, UK.
An adsorbed tetanus vaccine (p.1565·2).
Active immunisation.

Tetaven *Immuno, Ital.*
A tetanus immunoglobulin (p.1565·1).
Passive immunisation.

Tetavenin *Immuno, Aust.*
A tetanus immunoglobulin (p.1565·1).
Passive immunisation.

Tetefit Vitamin E *Medra, Aust.*
Alpha tocopherol (p.1394·1).
Tonic.

Tetesept
Note. This name is used for preparations of different composition.
Kolassa, Aust.
Balsam: Camphor (p.1589·3); menthol (p.1632·3); eucalyptus oil (p.1609·2); pumilio pine oil (p.1656·3); turpentine oil (p.1676·3); rosemary oil (p.1659·3); sage oil (p.1660·2).
Coughs and cold symptoms.

Pastilles: Dequalinium chloride (p.1143·1); cetylpyridinium chloride (p.1138·1); hesperidin methyl chalcone (p.1611·2); ascorbic acid (p.1389·3).
Bacterial infections of the mouth and throat.

Medra, Aust.
Oral liquid: Plantago lanceolata.
Catarrh; coughs.

Tetesept Calcium *Medra, Aust.*
Calcium carbonate (p.1215·1).
Calcium supplement.

Tetesept Magnesium *Medra, Aust.*
Magnesium carbonate (p.1232·3).
Magnesium deficiency.

Tetesept Vitamin C *Medra, Aust.*
Ascorbic acid (p.1389·3).
Vitamin C deficiency.

Tethexal *Hexal, Ger.*
Tetrazepam (p.708·1).
Skeletal muscle tension and spasticity.

Tetinox *Silanes, Mex.*
A tetanus vaccine (p.1565·2).
Active immunisation.

Tetmosol
Zeneca, Braz.; Zeneca, Mex.; Zeneca, S.Afr.; AstraZeneca, Singapore.
Sulfiram (p.1437·2).
Scabies.

Tetra *Atlantis, Mex.*
Tetracycline (p.258·3).
Bacterial infections.

Tetra Caplets *Reese, USA†.*
Paracetamol (p.71·2); phenylpropanolamine hydrochloride (p.1098·1).

Tetra Hubber *ICN, Spain.*
Tetracycline hydrochloride (p.258·3).
Bacterial infections.

Tetra Tripsin *Torlan, Spain.*
Novobiocin (p.232·2); protease; tetracycline phosphate (p.259·1).
Bacterial infections.

Tetrabioptal *Farmila, Ital.*
Tetracycline (p.258·3) or tetracycline hydrochloride (p.258·3).
Bacterial infections of the eye.

Tetrabronco *Flopen, Braz.*
Potassium iodide (p.1522·3); guaifenesin (p.1092·2); oxeladin (p.1096·2).
Respiratory-tract congestion.

Tetracap *Circle, USA.*
Tetracycline hydrochloride (p.258·3).
Bacterial infections.

Tetracem *Crown, S.Afr.*
Oxytetracycline (p.234·1).
Bacterial infections.

Tetrachel *Berk, UK†.*
Tetracycline hydrochloride (p.258·3).
Amoebiasis; bacterial infections.

Tetracoq
Pasteur Merieux, Belg.; Pasteur Merieux, Braz.; Pasteur Merieux, Fr.; Pasteur Merieux, Hong Kong; Pasteur Merieux, Israel; Pasteur Merieux, Thai.
An adsorbed diphtheria, tetanus, pertussis, and poliomyelitis (inactivated) vaccine (p.1539·1).
Active immunisation.

Tetract-HIB
Pasteur Merieux, Belg.; Pasteur Merieux, Israel; Pasteur Merieux, Ital.†; Pasteur Merieux, Singapore; Pasteur Merieux, Spain; Pasteur Merieux, Thai.
A diphtheria, tetanus, pertussis, and haemophilus influenzae conjugate vaccine (p.1538·3).
Active immunisation.

Tetracyn *Pfizer, Canad.†.*
Tetracycline hydrochloride (p.258·3).
Bacterial infections.

Tetradin *Caldeira & Metelo, Port.*
Disulfiram (p.1565·1).
Chronic alcoholism.

Tetradox
Ranbaxy, Singapore; Ranbaxy, Thai.
Doxycycline hyclate (p.200·1).
Bacterial infections.

Tetrafluor *Stomygen, Ital.†.*
Ammonium fluoride (p.1376·2); potassium fluoride (p.1376·2); sodium fluoride (p.1375·3); sodium monofluorophosphate (p.1377·2).
Oral hygiene.

Tetrafosammina *FIRMA, Ital.*
Tetracycline phosphate complex (p.259·1).
Bacterial infections.

Tetra-Gelomyrtol *Sanova, Aust.; Pohl, Ger.*
Oxytetracycline hydrochloride (p.234·1); myrtol.
Bronchitis; sinusitis.

Tetragynon *Schering, Denm.; Schering, Fr.; Schering, Ger.; Schering, Norw.; Schering, Port.; Schering, Swed.†; Schering, Switz.*
Levonorgestrel (p.1486·2); ethinylestradiol (p.1476·2).
Postcoital oral contraceptive.

Tetrahelmin *Luper, Braz.*
Mebendazole (p.102·2).
Worm infections.

Tetralan *Lannett, USA†.*
Tetracycline hydrochloride (p.258·3).
Bacterial infections.

Tetralim *Vana, Thai.*
Tetracycline phosphate complex (p.259·1).
Bacterial infections.

Tetralution *Merckle, Ger.*
Tetracycline hydrochloride (p.258·3).
Bacterial infections.

Tetralysal *AB-Consult, Aust.; Galderma, Belg.; Galderma, Denm.; Galderma, Fin.; Galderma, Fr.; Galderma, Irl.; Galderma, Norw.; Galderma, S.Afr.; Galderma, Swed.; Galderma, UK.*
Lymecycline (p.221·1).
Bacterial infections.

Tetram *Nycomed, Norw.*
Piroxicam (p.79·1).
Dysmenorrhoea; musculoskeletal and joint disorders.

Tetra-Mag *Cypress, USA.*
Magnesium salicylate (p.50·3); phenyltoloxamine citrate (p.423·1).

Tetramdura *Merck dura, Ger.*
Tetrazepam (p.708·1).
Skeletal muscle spasm.

Tetramel *Aspen, S.Afr.*
Oxytetracycline hydrochloride (p.234·1).
Bacterial infections.

Tetramil *Farmigea, Ital.*
Tetryzoline hydrochloride (p.1101·2); pheniramine maleate (p.422·3).
Conjunctivitis; eye irritation and congestion.

Tetramizol Composto *Iodo Suma, Braz.*
Tetramisole (p.108·3); tiabendazole (p.109·1).
Nematode infections.

Tetramizotil *Osorio de Moraes, Braz.*
Tetramisole (p.108·3).
Nematode infections.

Tetramune *Wyeth-Ayerst, Canad.†; Wyeth-Ayerst, Hong Kong; Wyeth, Mex.; Lederle, NZ; Wyeth, Singapore; Lederle, Switz.; Lederle, USA†.*
A diphtheria, tetanus, pertussis, and haemophilus influenzae vaccine (p.1538·3).
Active immunisation.

Tetrana *Vana, Thai.*
Tetracycline (p.258·3).
Bacterial infections.

Tetranase *Rottapharm, Fr.*
Oxytetracycline hydrochloride (p.234·1).
Formerly contained oxytetracycline hydrochloride and bromelains.
Bacterial infections.

Tetranovax *Pisa, Mex.*
Tetracycline (p.258·3).
Bacterial infections.

Tetrapres *Precimex, Mex.*
Tetracycline (p.258·3).
Bacterial infections.

Tetraprocyn *Protein, Mex.*
Tetracycline (p.258·3).
Bacterial infections.

Tetrapulmo *Medley, Braz.*
Sodium camsilate; chlorpheniramine [chlorphenamine] maleate (p.412·1); dipyrone (p.34·1); guaifenesin (p.1092·2).
Cold and influenza symptoms.

Tetrarco *Richter, Aust.†.*
Tetracycline hydrochloride (p.258·3).

Tetra-saar *Chephasaar, Ger.*
Tetrazepam (p.708·1).
Skeletal muscle tension and spasticity.

Tetrasan *CEPA, Spain†.*
Doxycycline hyclate (p.200·1).
Bacterial infections.

Tetraseptine *Andreabal, Switz.†.*
Tetracycline hydrochloride (p.258·3).
Bacterial infections.

Tetrasine *Optopics, USA.*
Tetryzoline hydrochloride (p.1101·2).
Minor eye irritation.

Tetrasine Extra *Optopics, USA.*
Tetryzoline hydrochloride (p.1101·2); macrogol 400 (p.1630·1).
Minor eye irritation.

Tetra-Tablinen *Wenig, Aust.†; Sanorania, Ger.†.*
Oxytetracycline hydrochloride (p.234·1).
Bacterial infections.

TetraTITER *Wyeth, S.Afr.*
A diphtheria, tetanus, pertussis, and haemophilus influenzae vaccine (p.1538·3).
Active immunisation.

Tetratoss *Heralds, Braz.*
Sodium camsilate; eucalyptol (p.1609·2); menthol (p.1632·3); guaifenesin (p.1092·2); oxeladin citrate (p.1096·1).
Respiratory-tract congestion.

Tetravac *Pasteur Merieux, Belg.; Pasteur Merieux, Fr.; Pasteur Merieux, Ger.*
A diphtheria, tetanus, pertussis, and poliomyelitis vaccine (p.1539·1).
Active immunisation.

Tetrazep *ABZ, Ger.; CT, Ger.*
Tetrazepam (p.708·1).
Skeletal muscle tension and spasticity.

Tetrazil *Arlex, Mex.*
Tetracycline (p.258·3).
Bacterial infections.

Tetrerba *Pharmacia Upjohn, Mex.*
Tetracycline (p.258·3).
Bacterial infections.

Tetrex *Bristol-Myers Squibb, Austral.; Bristol-Myers Squibb, Braz.; Bristol-Myers Squibb, Mex.; Bristol-Myers Squibb, S.Afr.†.*
Tetracycline hydrochloride (p.258·3) or tetracycline phosphate complex (p.259·1).
Adjunct in amoebiasis; bacterial infections; malaria.

Tetrex-F *Bristol-Myers Squibb, S.Afr.†.*
Tetracycline hydrochloride (p.258·3); nystatin (p.392·2).
Bacterial infections; candidiasis.

Tetrilin *MIP, Ger.*
Tetryzoline hydrochloride (p.1101·2).
Nasal congestion.

Tetrisal *MIP, Ger.*
Sodium chloride (p.1196·1).
Dry nose; nasal congestion.

Tetroid *Ache, Braz.*
Thyroxine [levothyroxine] sodium (p.1526·2).
Hypothyroidism.

Tet-Tox *CSL, Austral.; CSL, NZ.*
An adsorbed tetanus vaccine (p.1565·2).
Active immunisation.

Tetuman *Kwizda, Aust.†; Berna, Belg.†; Berna, Hong Kong; Berna, Ital.; Berna, Port.; Byk Madaus, S.Afr.; Berna, Spain; Berna, Switz.; Berna, Thai.*
A tetanus immunoglobulin (p.1565·1).
Passive immunisation.

Teutonico *Teuto, Braz.*
Ferrous sulfate (p.1360·3); phosphoric acid (p.1651·1).
Iron deficiency; iron-deficiency anaemias.

Teutoss *Teuto, Braz.*
Potassium iodide (p.1522·3); ephedrine hydrochloride (p.1090·1); belladonna (p.463·1); stramonium (p.474·1).
Respiratory-tract congestion.

Teutrin *Teuto, Braz.*
Co-trimoxazole (p.193·3).
Bacterial infections; Pneumocystis carinii pneumonia; protozoal infections.

Teutrin Balsamico *Teuto, Braz.*
Co-trimoxazole (p.193·3); guaifenesin (p.1092·2); ammonium chloride (p.1085·2).
Bacterial infections.

Tevacaine *Teva, Israel.*
Mepivacaine hydrochloride (p.1317·1).
Local anaesthesia.

Tevacor *Teva, Israel.*
Oxprenolol hydrochloride (p.951·3).
Angina pectoris; arrhythmias; hypertension.

Tevacycline *Teva, Israel.*
Tetracycline hydrochloride (p.258·3).
Bacterial infections.

Tevax *SmithKline Beecham, Belg.*
An adsorbed tetanus vaccine (p.1565·2).
Active immunisation.

Teveten *Solvay, Austral.; Solvay, Denm.; Orion, Fin.; Solvay, Ger.; Hoechst Marion Roussel, Ger.; Solvay, Irl.; SmithKline Beecham, Neth.; Solvay, Port.; Solvay, Swed.; Solvay, UK; SmithKline Beecham, USA.*
Eprosartan mesilate (p.886·1).
Hypertension.

Tevetens *SmithKline Beecham, Spain.*
Eprosartan mesilate (p.886·1).
Hypertension.

Texacort *GenDerm, Canad.†; GenDerm, USA.*
Hydrocortisone (p.1073·3).
Skin disorders.

Texate *Columbia, Mex.*
Methotrexate (p.553·2).
Malignant neoplasms.

Texodil *Cassenne, Fr.*
Cefotiam hexetil hydrochloride (p.171·1).
Bacterial infections of the respiratory-tract.

Texoven *Tecnofarma, Mex.*
Benzonatate (p.1085·3).
Coughs.

Texx *Krewel, Ger.*
Hypericum (p.290·2).
Anxiety; depression.

TFE *Seroyal, Canad.*
Vitamin A, vitamin E, and zinc (p.1350·1).

TFT *Alcon, Ger.; Bausch & Lomb, S.Afr.*
Trifluridine (p.642·2).
Herpes simplex keratitis.

TFT Ophtiole *Tramedico, Belg.; Mann, Neth.*
Trifluridine (p.642·2).
Viral eye infections.

T/Gel
Note. This name is used for preparations of different composition.
Neutrogena, Fr.
Salicylic acid (p.1122·3); piroctone olamine (p.1121·1).
Scalp and hair disorders.

Neutrogena, Israel; Neutrogena, UK.
Coal tar (p.1125·1).
Scalp disorders.

T-Gen *Goldline, USA.*
Trimethobenzamide hydrochloride (p.426·3).
Nausea and vomiting.

T-Gesic *Williams, USA.*
Paracetamol (p.71·2); hydrocodone tartrate (p.42·2).
Pain.

THA *Woods, Austral.*
Tacrine hydrochloride (p.1425·1).
Postoperative respiratory stimulant; reversal of competitive neuromuscular blockade.

Thacapzol *Recip, Swed.*
Methimazole [thiamazole] (p.1525·1).
Hyperthyroidism.

Thaden *Aspen, S.Afr.; Trinity, UK.*
Dothiepin [dosulepin] hydrochloride (p.283·2).
Depression; mixed anxiety depressive states.

Thais *Besins-Iscovesco, Fr.*
Estradiol (p.1473·1).
Menopausal disorders.

Thalamonal *Janssen-Cilag, Aust.†; Janssen-Cilag, Belg.†; Janssen-Cilag, Ger.†; Janssen-Cilag, Neth.†.*
Droperidol (p.682·2); fentanyl citrate (p.37·1).
General anaesthesia; neuroleptanalgesia; pain; premedication.

Thalaris *Technilab, Canad.*
Sodium chloride (p.1196·1).
Oral hygiene.

Thalitone *Monarch, USA.*
Chlortalidone (p.857·1).
Hypertension; oedema.

Thalomid *Celgene, USA.*
Thalidomide (p.1670·2).
Erythema nodosum leprosum.

Tham *Abbott, Austral.; Kohler, Ger.*
Trometamol (p.1675·2).
Metabolic acidosis.

Thamacetat *Bellon, Fr.†.*
Trometamol (p.1675·2).
Metabolic acidosis.

Thamesol *Diaco, Ital.*
Trometamol (p.1675·2).
Metabolic acidosis.

t/h-basan *Schonenberger, Switz.*
Triamterene (p.986·1); hydrochlorothiazide (p.907·3).
Hypertension; oedema.

Thé Brioni *Husler, Switz.*
Sambucus (p.1660·3); melissa (p.1632·2); peppermint leaf (p.1243·2); senna (p.1248·2); fennel (p.1610·1); agrimony (p.1574·3).
Constipation.

The Chambard-Tee *Brady, Aust.*
Senna leaf (p.1248·2); althaea leaf (p.1577·1); peppermint leaf (p.1243·2); melissa leaf (p.1632·2); hyssopus officinalis; anthyllidis flower; calendula (p.1589·2); cyanae flower.
Bowel evacuation; constipation; stool softener.

Thé Franklin *Noveal, Aust.†.*
Senna (p.1248·2); couch-grass (p.1599·3); fennel (p.1610·1); melissa (p.1632·2); boldo (p.1585·3); hyssopus officinalis; cuminum cyminum; peppermint leaf (p.1243·2); aniseed (p.1580·2).
Constipation.

The Ginseng King *Codit, Ital.*
Fish milk; fish brain extract; cod-liver extract; myrtillus; acacia honey; fructose; ginseng (p.1350·1).
Nutritional supplement.

Thé laxatif Solubilax *Heumann, Switz.†.*
Senna (p.1248·2); frangula bark (p.1227·1).
Bowel evacuation; constipation.

Thedox *Mer-National, S.Afr.†.*
Doxycycline polyphosphate sodium complex (p.200·1).
Bacterial infections.

Theinol *Bailly, Fr.*
Paracetamol (p.71·2); caffeine (p.761·3).
Formerly contained sodium salicylate, phenazone, and caffeine.
Fever; pain.

theo *CT, Ger.*
Theophylline hydrate (p.777·2) or theophylline sodium glycinate (p.783·2).
Obstructive airways disease.

Theo₂ *Galphar, Neth.†.*
Theophylline (p.777·2).
Bronchospasm.

Theo-24 *Searle, UK; UCB, USA.*
Theophylline (p.777·2).
Obstructive airways disease.

Theo Max *Desarrollo, Spain.*
Theophylline (p.777·2).
Heart failure; obstructive airways disease; paroxysmal dyspnoea.

Theobid Duracaps *Russ, USA.*
Theophylline (p.777·2).
Asthma; chronic bronchitis; emphysema.

Theo-Bronc *Rougier, Canad.*
Guaifenesin (p.1092·2); potassium iodide (p.1522·3); theophylline (p.777·2); mepyramine maleate (p.421·1).
Obstructive airways disease.

Theocaradrin *Loevosan, Aust.†.*
Proscillaridin (p.963·3); theophylline hydrate (p.777·2).
Heart failure.

Theochron *Riva, Canad.; Inwood, USA; Lemmon, USA.*
Theophylline (p.777·2).
Obstructive airways disease.

Theoclear *Schwarz, USA.*
Theophylline (p.777·2).
Asthma; bronchospasm.

Theocol *Beige, S.Afr.*
Diphenhydramine hydrochloride (p.416·1); ammonium chloride (p.1085·2); sodium citrate (p.1186·2); menthol (p.1632·3).
Coughs.

Theodrine *Rugby, USA.*
Theophylline (p.777·2); ephedrine hydrochloride (p.1090·1); phenobarbital (p.355·1).
Bronchospasm.

Theo-Dur *Astra, Austral.; Astra, Belg.; AstraZeneca, Canad.; AstraZeneca, Denm.; AstraZeneca, Fin.; Astra, Hong Kong; Astra, Irl.; Recordati, Ital.; AstraZeneca, Norw.; AstraZeneca, NZ; Astra, S.Afr.; AstraZeneca, Singapore; Pharmacia Upjohn, Spain; Draco, Swed.; AstraZeneca, Thai.; AstraZeneca, UK; Key, USA.*
Theophylline (p.777·2).
Heart failure; obstructive airways disease; paroxysmal dyspnoea.

Theofol *Leiras, Fin.*
Theophylline (p.777·2).
Obstructive airways disease.

Theofol Comp *Leiras, Fin.*
Theophylline (p.777·2); guaifenesin (p.1092·2).
Obstructive airways disease.

Theogel *SAN, Ital.†.*
Royal jelly (p.1659·3).

Theohexal *Hexal, Ger.*
Theophylline (p.777·2).
Obstructive airways disease.

Theolair *3M, Belg.; 3M, Canad.; 3M, Fr.; 3M, Ger.; 3M, Ital.; 3M, Neth.; 3M, Spain; 3M, Switz.; 3M, USA.*
Theophylline (p.777·2).
Heart failure; obstructive airways disease; paroxysmal dyspnoea.

Theolan *Elan, Irl.*
Theophylline (p.777·2).
Bronchospasm.

Theo-Lanicor *Boehringer Mannheim, Aust.†.*
Digoxin (p.870·1); theophylline (p.777·2); theobromine (p.777·2).
Heart failure.

Theo-Lanitop *Boehringer Mannheim, Aust.†.*
Theophylline (p.777·2); metildigoxin (p.930·1).
Heart failure.

Theolin *Astra, Neth.; Beacons, Singapore.*
Theophylline (p.777·2).
Obstructive airways disease.

Theolong *Eisai, Jpn.*
Theophylline (p.777·2).
Obstructive airways disease.

Theomax DF *Barre-National, USA; Schein, USA.*
Theophylline (p.777·2); ephedrine sulfate (p.1090·2); hydroxyzine hydrochloride (p.419·1).
Bronchospasm.

Theophar *Julphar, UAE.*
Theophylline (p.777·2).
Obstructive airways disease.

Theophen *Aspen Consumer, S.Afr.*
Theophylline (p.777·2); etofylline (p.765·1).
Obstructive airways disease.

Theophen Comp *Aspen Consumer, S.Afr.*
Theophylline (p.777·2); etofylline (p.765·1); diphenylpyraline hydrochloride (p.417·1); ammonium chloride (p.1085·2).
Coughs.

Theophyllaminum *Leiras, Fin.*
Aminophylline hydrate (p.760·1).
Obstructive airways disease.

Theophyllard *Byk, Belg.; OPW, Ger.†.*
Theophylline (p.777·2).
Obstructive airways disease.

Theoplus *Germania, Aust.; Byk Madaus, S.Afr.; Pierre Fabre, Spain.*
Theophylline (p.777·2).
Heart failure; obstructive airways disease; paroxysmal dyspnoea.

Theosal *Ranbaxy, Thai.*
Theophylline (p.777·2); salbutamol (p.770·3).
Obstructive airways disease.

Theospan-SR *Laser, USA.*
Theophylline (p.777·2).

The symbol † denotes a preparation no longer actively marketed

Theospirex *Gebro, Aust.*
Theophylline (p.777·2) or theophylline sodium glycinate (p.783·2).
Obstructive airways disease.

Theo-SR *Rhone-Poulenc Rorer, Canad.†*
Theophylline (p.777·2).
Obstructive airways disease.

Theostat
Note.This name is used for preparations of different composition.
Inava, Fr.
Theophylline hydrate (p.777·2).
Asthma; obstructive airways disease.

Logamed, S.Afr.†
Etofylline (p.765·1).
Obstructive airways disease.

Laser, USA†.
Theophylline (p.777·2).
Asthma; bronchospasm.

Theo-Talusin *Knoll, Switz.*
Proscillaridin (p.963·3); etofylline (p.765·1).
Cardiac disorders.

Theotard *CTI, Israel.*
Theophylline (p.777·2).
Obstructive airways disease.

Theotex *Terapeutico, Ital.*
Metalkonium chloride.
Personal hygiene; skin disinfection.

Theotrim *Trima, Israel; Trima, Thai.*
Theophylline (p.777·2).
Obstructive airways disease.

Theovent
Schering-Plough, Hong Kong; Schering, USA.
Theophylline (p.777·2).
Asthma; reversible bronchospasm.

Theo-X *Carnrick, USA.*
Theophylline (p.777·2).
Obstructive airways disease.

Thephorin *Sinclair, Irl.; Sinclair, UK†.*
Phenindamine tartrate (p.422·2).
Hypersensitivity reactions.

Theprubicine *Rhone-Poulenc Rorer, Fr.*
Pirarubicin (p.565·1).
Breast cancer.

Thera Hematinic *Major, USA.*
Ferrous fumarate (p.1360·1); folic acid (p.1361·1); multivitamins and minerals (p.1350·1).
Iron-deficiency anaemias.

Therabid *Mission Pharmacal, USA.*
Multivitamin preparation (p.1350·1).

Therac *C & M, USA.*
Sulfur (p.1123·3); salicylic acid (p.1122·3).
Acne.

Theracap *Nycomed Amersham, UK.*
Iodine-131 (p.1450·1) as sodium iodide.
Hyperthyroidism; thyroid cancer.

Theracaps *Reese, USA†.*
Paracetamol (p.71·2); phenylpropanolamine hydrochloride (p.1098·1); mepyramine maleate (p.421·1); dextromethorphan hydrobromide (p.1087·3).

Theraclox *Great Eastern, Thai.; Therapharma, Thai.*
Cloxacillin (p.192·1).
Bacterial infections.

Theracof Plus *Reese, USA.*
Paracetamol (p.71·2); phenylephrine hydrochloride (p.1097·1); guaifenesin (p.1092·2); diphenhydramine hydrochloride (p.416·1).

TheraCys *Pasteur Merieux, USA.*
A BCG vaccine (p.1533·2).
Bladder cancer.

Theradol *Knoll, Neth.*
Tramadol hydrochloride (p.89·1).
Pain.

TheraFlu *Novartis, Mex.*
Paracetamol (p.71·2); pseudoephedrine hydrochloride (p.1099·2); chlorpheniramine [chlorphenamine] maleate (p.412·1).
Cold and influenza symptoms.

TheraFlu Flu and Cold *Novartis, USA.*
Chlorpheniramine [chlorphenamine] maleate (p.412·1); pseudoephedrine hydrochloride (p.1099·2); paracetamol (p.71·2).
Cold and flu symptoms.

TheraFlu Flu, Cold & Cough
Sandoz, Canad.†; Novartis, USA.
Chlorpheniramine [chlorphenamine] maleate (p.412·1); pseudoephedrine hydrochloride (p.1099·2); paracetamol (p.71·2); dextromethorphan hydrobromide (p.1087·3).
Coughs and cold symptoms.

Thera-Flur *Colgate-Hoyt, USA.*
Sodium fluoride (p.1375·3).
Dental caries prophylaxis.

Theragen *Reese, USA.*
Capsaicin (p.23·1).

Theragenerix *Goldline, USA.*
A range of vitamin preparations (p.1350·1).

Theragenerix-H *Goldline, USA.*
Ferrous fumarate (p.1360·1); folic acid (p.1361·1); multivitamins and minerals (p.1350·1).
Iron-deficiency anaemias.

Thera-gesic *Mission Pharmacal, USA.*
Methyl salicylate (p.55·1); menthol (p.1632·3).
Musculoskeletal and joint pain.

Theragran *Mead Johnson Nutritionals, USA.*
A range of vitamin preparations (p.1350·1).

Theragran AntiOxidant *Bristol-Myers Squibb, USA.*
Vitamins A, C, and E with minerals (p.1350·1).

Theragran Hematinic *Apothecon, USA.*
Multivitamin and mineral preparation with iron and folic acid (p.1350·1).
Iron-deficiency anaemias.

Theragran-M
Bristol-Myers Squibb, S.Afr.†; Bristol-Myers Squibb, Thai.
Multivitamin and mineral preparation (p.1350·1).

Thera-Hist *Major, USA†.*
Phenylpropanolamine hydrochloride (p.1098·1); chlorpheniramine [chlorphenamine] maleate (p.412·1).
Upper respiratory-tract symptoms.

Theralen *Rhone-Poulenc Rorer, Swed.*
Trimeprazine [alimemazine] tartrate (p.426·2).
Anxiety; behaviour disorders; hypersensitivity reactions; premedication; sleep disorders; vomiting.

Theralene
Aventis, Belg.; Medeva, Fr.
Trimeprazine [alimemazine] (p.426·3) or trimeprazine [alimemazine] tartrate (p.426·2).
Cough; cramps; dystonias; hypersensitivity reactions; insomnia; premedication; pruritus; psychiatric disorders; tics.

Theralene Pectoral *Rhone-Poulenc Rorer, Belg†.*
Trimeprazine [alimemazine] tartrate (p.426·2); ethylmorphine hydrochloride (p.35·2); ephedrine hydrochloride (p.1090·1); ammonium acetate (p.1085·1).
Coughs.

Theralene Pectoral Nourrisson *Medeva, Fr.*
Trimeprazine [alimemazine] tartrate (p.426·2); ammonium acetate (p.1085·1); tolu balsam (p.1101·3).
Formerly contained trimeprazine [alimemazine] tartrate, ammonium acetate, sodium benzoate, magnesium sulfate, and tolu balsam.
Coughs.

Thera-M *Major, USA.*
Multivitamin preparation with minerals and folic acid (p.1350·1).

Theramycin Z *Medicis, USA.*
Erythromycin (p.201·2).
Acne.

Theranal *Roche Consumer, Neth.*
Bismuth subnitrate (p.1213·2); zinc oxide (p.1128·2); lignocaine [lidocaine] (p.1313·2).
Haemorrhoids.

Theranyl *Abigo, Swed.*
Nicotinic acid (p.1372·3); salicylic acid (p.1122·3).
Musculoskeletal and joint disorders.

TheraPatch Cold Sore *Lectec, USA.*
Lignocaine [lidocaine] (p.1313·2); camphor (p.1589·3).
Herpes labialis.

Therapeutic Bath *Goldline, USA.*
Emollient and moisturiser.

Therapeutic Bath Oil
Avant Garde, Canad.
Liquid paraffin (p.1407·1).

Scott, Canad.
Liquid paraffin (p.1407·1); wool fat (p.1410·3).

Therapeutic Mineral Ice *Bristol-Myers Products, USA.*
Menthol (p.1632·3).
Muscle, joint, and soft-tissue pain; neuralgia.

Therapeutic Skin Lotion *Scott, Canad.*
Lanolin oil (p.1410·3); liquid paraffin (p.1407·1).

Therapeutic Soothing Ice *Jamieson, Canad.*
Methyl salicylate (p.55·1); camphor (p.1589·3); menthol (p.1632·3); eucalyptus oil (p.1609·2).

Theraplex T *Medicis, USA.*
Coal tar (p.1125·1).
Scalp disorders.

Theraplex Z *Medicis, USA.*
Pyrithione zinc (p.1122·1).
Dandruff; seborrhoeic dermatitis.

Therarubicin *Meiji, Jpn†.*
Pirarubicin hydrochloride (p.565·1).
Malignant neoplasms.

Therasa *Therabel, Belg.*
Aspirin (p.14·2).
Thromboembolic disorders.

Theravee *Vangard, USA.*
A range of vitamin preparations (p.1350·1).

Theravee Hematinic *Vangard, USA.*
Iron (p.1366·3); folic acid (p.1361·1); multivitamins and minerals (p.1350·1).
Iron-deficiency anaemias.

Theravim *Nature's Bounty, USA.*
A range of vitamin preparations (p.1350·1).

Theravite *Barre-National, USA.*
Multivitamin preparation (p.1350·1).

Therems *Rugby, USA.*
A range of vitamin preparations (p.1350·1).

Therevac Plus *Jones, USA.*
Docusate sodium (p.1223·1); glycerol (p.1616·3); benzocaine (p.1306·2); soft soap (p.1496·1).
Constipation.

Therevac SB *Jones, USA.*
Docusate sodium (p.1223·1); glycerol (p.1616·3); soft soap (p.1496·1).
Constipation.

Therma Ayoral *Rayere, Mex.*
Dipyrone (p.34·1).
Fever; pain.

Thermal
Provita, Aust.; Alpharma, Norw.
Ethyl nicotinate (p.35·1); diethylamine salicylate (p.32·2).
Stiff and painful muscles and joints.

Thermalife *Thermalife, Austral.†.*
Protein and trace metal complex (Peptophen).
Arthritic pain; bath additive; bed sores; emollient; muscular pain.

Thermalife C *Thermalife, Austral.†.*
Protein/trace metal complex (Peptophen); capsicum oleoresin (p.1591·1).
Arthritic pain; muscular pain.

Thermazene *Sherwood, USA.*
Sulfadiazine silver (p.251·3).
Infected burns.

Thermo Burger *Ysatfabrik, Ger.*
Capsicum (p.1591·1).
Musculoskeletal, joint, and soft-tissue disorders; neuralgia.

Thermo Mobilisin *Sankyo, Ger.*
Flufenamic acid (p.41·1); a heparinoid (p.905·2); benzyl nicotinate (p.20·2).
Musculoskeletal and joint disorders; neuralgia.

Thermo Rub *Rolmex, Canad.*
Methyl salicylate (p.55·1); menthol (p.1632·3); eucalyptol (p.1609·2).

Thermocutan *Streuli, Switz.*
Nonivamide (p.63·1); ethyl nicotinate (p.35·1); benzyl nicotinate (p.20·2); aminophenazone salicylate (p.13·3).
Chilblains; musculoskeletal, joint, peri-articular, and soft-tissue disorders.

Thermodent *Mentholatum, Austral.†.*
Potassium nitrate (p.1154·3); sodium monofluorophosphate (p.1377·2).
Desensitising toothpaste.

Thermo-Gel *Prodemdis, Canad.*
Camphor (p.1589·3); menthol (p.1632·3); benzocaine (p.1306·2); thymol (p.1158·3).

Thermogene *Montefarmaco, Ital.*
Capsicum oleoresin (p.1591·1).
Musculoskeletal and joint pain.

thermo-loges *Loges, Ger.*
Benzyl nicotinate (p.20·2); pine needle oil; rosemary oil (p.1659·3).
Circulatory disorders; musculoskeletal, joint, and soft-tissue disorders.

Thermo-Menthoneurin *Byk Gulden, Ger.; Roland, Ger.*
Glycol salicylate (p.42·2); benzyl nicotinate (p.20·2).
Musculoskeletal, joint, and peri-articular disorders; neuralgia.

Thermo-Menthoneurin Bad *Tosse, Ger.†.*
Glycol salicylate (p.42·2); benzyl nicotinate (p.20·2); methyl nicotinate (p.55·1).
Bath additive; musculoskeletal and joint disorders; peripheral circulatory disorders.

Thermo-Rheumon
Kolassa, Aust.; Bayer, Ger.
Etofenamate (p.35·3); benzyl nicotinate (p.20·2).
Musculoskeletal, joint, peri-articular disorders, and soft-tissue disorders.

Thermo-Rub *Propan, S.Afr.*
Methyl salicylate (p.55·1).
Muscular pain; rheumatism.

Thermosenex *Wyeth, Ger.*
Camphor (p.1589·3); glycol salicylate (p.42·2); benzyl nicotinate (p.20·2).
Musculoskeletal and joint disorders; neuralgia; sprains.

Thesit *Gepepharm, Ger.*
Lauromacrogol 400 (p.1345·2); mepivacaine hydrochloride (p.1317·1); benzalkonium chloride (p.1133·2).
Burns; insect stings; skin disorders.

Thesit P *Gepepharm, Ger.*
Lauromacrogol 400 (p.1345·2); promethazine hydrochloride (p.423·2); prednisolone acetate (p.1078·1).
Skin disorders.

Thevier *Glaxo Wellcome, Ger.*
Thyroxine [levothyroxine] sodium (p.1526·3).
Hypothyroidism.

Thex Forte *Lee, USA.*
Vitamin B and C preparation (p.1350·1).

Thiaben *UCI, Braz.*
Tiabendazole (p.109·1).
Nematode infections.

Thiabena *UCI, Braz.*
Tiabendazole (p.109·1); neomycin sulfate (p.228·1).
Skin infections.

Thiabet *Wolff, Ger.*
Metformin hydrochloride (p.332·3).
Diabetes mellitus.

Thiamcin *General Drugs, Thai.*
Thiamphenicol (p.261·3).
Bacterial infections.

Thiamilate *Tyson, USA†.*
Thiamine hydrochloride (p.1385·1).
Thiamine deficiency.

Thiaminose *Climax, Braz.*
Ascorbic acid (p.1389·3); thiamine hydrochloride (p.1385·1).
Nutritional supplement.

Thiaton *Hokuriku, Jpn†.*
Tiquizium bromide (p.1673·3).
Smooth muscle spasm and hypermotility.

Thiavit *Julphar, UAE.*
Thiamine hydrochloride (p.1385·1).
Vitamin B_1 deficiency.

Thiazid-comp *Wolff, Ger.*
Triamterene (p.986·1); hydrochlorothiazide (p.907·3).
Hypertension; oedema.

Thick & Easy
American Institutional, Hong Kong; American Institutional, Singapore.
Food thickener (p.1350·1).
Dysphagia.

Thierry *Makara, Aust.*
Fennel oil (p.1610·2); purified honey (p.1366·2).
Catarrh; colds; coughs.

Thilo Tears *Bournonville, Belg.†.*
Carbomer (p.1499·2).
Dry eyes.

Thilo Wet *Alcon, Aust.*
A wetting solution for contact lenses (p.1129·2).

Thiloadren *Alcon, Aust.*
Dipivefrine hydrochloride (p.1604·3); pilocarpine hydrochloride (p.1422·3).
Glaucoma.

Thiloadren N *Alcon, Ger.*
Dipivefrine hydrochloride (p.1604·3); pilocarpine hydrochloride (p.1422·3).
Glaucoma.

Thilocanfol *Alcon, Ger.*
Azidamfenicol (p.152·3).
Bacterial eye infections.

Thilocanfol C *Alcon, Ger.*
Chloramphenicol (p.179·1).
Bacterial eye infections.

Thilocombin *Alcon, Aust.*
Theophylline (p.777·2); heptaminol (p.1619·2) or heptaminol hydrochloride (p.1619·2); nicotinyl alcohol (p.939·3) or nicotinyl alcohol tartrate (p.939·3).
Angina pectoris; migraine; peripheral, coronary, and cerebral vascular disorders; thromboembolic disorders.

Thilodigon
Alcon, Aust.; Alcon, Ger.
Guanethidine monosulfate (p.901·1); dipivefrine hydrochloride (p.1604·3).
Glaucoma.

Thilorbin *Alcon, Ger.*
Oxybuprocaine hydrochloride (p.1318·1); fluorescein sodium (p.1612·1).
Ophthalmic procedures.

Thilo-Tears
Alcon, Ger.; Thilo, Neth.†; Alcon, Switz.†.
Carbomer (p.1499·2).
Dry eyes.

Thinz *Aspen Consumer, S.Afr.*
Cathine hydrochloride (p.1507·1).
Obesity.

Thiobitum *Riemser, Ger.*
Ichthammol (p.1115·2).
Skin disorders.

Thioctacid *Asta Medica, Ger.*
Thioctic acid (p.1671·3) or trometamol thioctate (p.1675·2).
Diabetic neuropathy.

Thiocyl *Alba, USA†.*
Sodium thiosalicylate (p.84·2).

Thiodantol *Rekah, Israel.*
Isothipendyl hydrochloride (p.419·2).
Skin irritation.

Thiodeol *Breves, Braz.*
Sulfogaiacol (p.1101·1); iodine (p.1522·3); sodium methylarsinate (p.1666·1); calcium glycerophosphate (p.1188·2); neroli oil (p.1640·1).
Respiratory-tract disorders.

Thioderon *Shionogi, Jpn.*
Mepitiostane (p.1482·1).
Breast cancer; renal anaemia.

Thiogamma *Worwag, Ger.*
Meglumine thioctate or thioctic acid (p.1671·3).
Diabetic neuropathy.

Thiola
Santen, Hong Kong; Coop. Farm., Ital.; Mission Pharmacal, USA.
Tiopronin (p.1025·1).
Cataract; liver disorders; mercury poisoning; prevention of cystine renal calculi.

Thiomed *Medifive, Thai.*
Thioridazine hydrochloride (p.708·1).
Anxiety; mania; schizophrenia.

Thionembutal *Abbott, Braz.*
Thiopental (p.1269·3).
General anaesthesia.

Thiophenicol *Sanofi Winthrop, Fr.*
Thiamphenicol (p.261·3) or thiamphenicol glycinate hydrochloride (p.262·1).
Bacterial infections.

Thioplex
Wyeth Lederle, Ital.; Immunex, USA.
Thiotepa (p.574·3).
Malignant neoplasms.

Thiopon *Amido, Fr.†*
Thiophene oil.
Respiratory-tract inflammation.

Thiopon Balsamique *Amido, Fr.†*
Thiophene oil; eucalyptus oil (p.1609·2); pine oil; niaouli oil (p.1640·2).
Upper respiratory-tract infections.

Thiopon Pantothenique *Amido, Fr.†*
Thiophene oil; calcium pantothenate (p.1374·1).
Respiratory-tract inflammation.

Thioprine *Alphapharm, Austral.; Pacific, NZ.*
Azathioprine (p.509·3).
Auto-immune disorders; transplant rejection.

Thiorubrol *Adroka, Switz.*
Bath additive: Sodium thioricinol sulfonate; sodium thiosulfate (p.1024·2); sodium sulfate (p.1250·1).
Bath oil: Trolamine thioricinol sulfate.
Musculoskeletal and joint disorders; skin disorders.

Thiosan *Azevedos, Port.*
Sulfiram (p.1437·2).
Pediculosis; scabies.

Thiosedal *Zyma, Fr.†*
Ethylmorphine hydrochloride (p.35·2); hyoscyamus (p.470·1); sulfogaiacol (p.1101·1).
Coughs.

Thiosept *Terrapharm, Aust.*
Shale oil.
Hyperhidrosis; inflammation; musculoskeletal and joint disorders; peripheral vascular disorders; skin disorders.

Thiosia *Asian Pharm, Thai.*
Thioridazine hydrochloride (p.708·1).
Anxiety; depression.

Thiosol *Coop. Farm., Ital.*
Tiopronin (p.1025·1).
Respiratory-tract congestion.

Thiosulfil Forte *Wyeth-Ayerst, USA†.*
Sulfamethizole (p.253·3).
Urinary-tract infections.

Thiovalone *Parke, Davis, Fr.*
Tixocortol pivalate (p.1080·1); chlorhexidine acetate (p.1138·2).
Inflammation of the mouth and throat.

Thioxene *Esseti, Ital.*
Glutathione sodium (p.1010·3).
Alcohol or drug poisoning; ionising radiation damage.

Thiozine *Pinewood, Irl.*
Thioridazine hydrochloride (p.708·1).
Anxiety; behaviour disorders; psychoses; senile confusion; tension.

Thirial *Dolisos, Fr.*
Garlic (p.1614·1).
Circulatory disorders.

Thiuretic *Warner Chilcott, USA†.*
Hydrochlorothiazide (p.907·3).
Hypertension; oedema.

Thixit *Lincoln, NZ.*
Tiotixene hydrochloride (p.709·2).
Psychoses.

Thixo-Flur *Colgate Oral Care, Austral.†.*
Fluoride.

Thohelur I *Truw, Ger.†.*
Mineral preparation (p.1350·1).

Thohelur II *Truw, Ger.†.*
Mineral preparation with colecalciferol (p.1350·1).

Thomaeamin X E *Delta, Ger.*
Amino-acid, electrolyte, and xylitol infusion (p.1350·1).
Parenteral nutrition.

Thomaeamin GX E *Delta, Ger.†.*
Amino-acid, electrolyte, glucose, and xylitol infusion (p.1350·1).
Parenteral nutrition.

Thomaeamin hepar *Delta, Ger.*
Amino-acid infusion (p.1350·1).
Parenteral nutrition in liver failure.

Thomaeamin n *Delta, Ger.*
Amino-acid and vitamin infusion with or without electrolytes (p.1350·1).
Parenteral nutrition.

Thomaeamin Pad *Delta, Ger.†.*
Amino-acid infusion (p.1350·1).
Parenteral nutrition.

Thomaedex 40 *Delta, Ger.*
Dextran 40 (p.728·3) in sodium chloride.
Plasma volume expansion; thrombosis prophylaxis; vascular disorders.

Thomaedex 60 *Delta, Ger.*
Dextran 60 (p.729·2) in sodium chloride.
Plasma volume expansion; thrombosis prophylaxis.

Thomaegelin *Delta, Ger.*
Gelatin polysuccinate (p.737·2) in Ringer acetate.
Hypovolaemia.

Thomaejonin *Delta, Ger.*
A range of electrolyte infusions with or without carbohydrate (p.1180·1).
Fluid and electrolyte disorders.

Thomaemannit *Delta, Ger.*
Mannitol (p.924·3).
Fluid retention; renal failure.

Thomapyrin *Boehringer Ingelheim, Aust.; Boehringer Ingelheim, Ger.*
Aspirin (p.14·2); paracetamol (p.71·2); caffeine (p.761·3).
Cold symptoms; fever; inflammation; pain.

Thomapyrin akut *Boehringer Ingelheim, Ger.*
Aspirin (p.14·2).
Fever; pain.

Thomapyrin C *Boehringer Ingelheim, Ger.*
Aspirin (p.14·2); paracetamol (p.71·2); ascorbic acid (p.1389·3).
Cold symptoms; fever; inflammation; pain.

Thomapyrin mit Vitamin C *Boehringer Ingelheim, Aust.*
Aspirin (p.14·2); paracetamol (p.71·2); ascorbic acid (p.1389·3).
Cold symptoms.

Thomapyrine *Boehringer Ingelheim, Switz.*
Aspirin (p.14·2); paracetamol (p.71·2); caffeine (p.761·3).
Fever; pain.

Thomasin *Apogepha, Ger.*
Etilefrine hydrochloride (p.888·1).
Cardiovascular disorders; dumping syndrome.

Thombran *Boehringer Ingelheim, Ger.*
Trazodone hydrochloride (p.310·1).
Depression.

Thorazine *SmithKline Beecham, USA.*
Chlorpromazine (p.660·2) or chlorpromazine hydrochloride (p.660·2).
Acute intermittent porphyria; adjunct in tetanus; bipolar disorder; hiccups; nausea and vomiting; premedication; psychoses; severe behavioural disorders in children.

Thoxaprim *Pharmagen, S.Afr.†.*
Co-trimoxazole (p.193·3).
Bacterial infections.

THR *Seroyal, Canad.*
Vitamin E, magnesium, and potassium (p.1350·1).

Threamine DM *Barre-National, USA†.*
Phenylpropanolamine hydrochloride (p.1098·1); chlorpheniramine [chlorphenamine] maleate (p.412·1); dextromethorphan hydrobromide (p.1087·3).
Coughs and cold symptoms.

Threolone *Abic, Israel.*
Prednisolone (p.1077·3); chloramphenicol (p.179·1).
Infected skin disorders.

Thriazol *Alpharma, Mex.*
Co-trimoxazole (p.193·3).
Bacterial infections.

Throat *Dumex-Alpharma, Denm.*
Benzoic acid (p.1134·2); lignocaine [lidocaine] (p.1313·2); menthol (p.1632·3).
Stomatitis.

Throat Discs *SmithKline Beecham, USA.*
Capsicum (p.1591·1); peppermint oil (p.1243·3); liquid paraffin (p.1407·1).
Sore throat.

Throat Lozenges
Note. This name is used for preparations of different composition.
Novopharm, Canad.
Benzocaine (p.1306·2); cetylpyridinium chloride (p.1138·1).
Novopharm, Canad.
Cetylpyridinium chloride (p.1138·1).
Stanley, Canad.
Hexylresorcinol (p.1146·3).

Throaties Catarrh Pastilles *Ernest Jackson, UK†.*
Menthol (p.1632·3); lemon oil (p.1628·2); eucalyptus (p.1609·2); honey (p.1366·2).

Throaties Family Cough Linctus *Ernest Jackson, UK†.*
Ipecacuanha (p.1093·1); glycerol (p.1616·3); honey (p.1366·2); terpeneless lemon oil (p.1628·2); citric acid (p.1596·2).
Coughs.

Thromabate *Bayer, USA.*
Antithrombin III (p.725·2).
Antithrombin III deficiency.

Thrombace *Drossapharm, Switz.†.*
Aloxiprin (p.13·2).
Thromboembolic disorders.

Thrombace Neo *Drossapharm, Switz.*
Aspirin (p.14·2).
Thromboembolism prophylaxis.

Thrombareduct *Azupharma, Ger.*
Heparin sodium (p.902·1).
Soft-tissue disorders; soft-tissue injury.

Thrombate *Bayer, Canad.; Bayer Biological, Hong Kong.*
Antithrombin III (p.725·2).
Antithrombin III deficiency.

Thrombate III *Bayer, USA.*
Antithrombin III (p.725·2).
Antithrombin III deficiency.

Thrombhibin *Immuno, Aust.*
Antithrombin III (p.725·2).
Antithrombin III deficiency.

Thrombinar *Rhone-Poulenc Rorer, Austral.†; Jones, USA.*
Thrombin (p.741·3).
Minor haemorrhage.

Thrombo ASS *Lannacher, Aust.*
Aspirin (p.14·2).
Thrombosis prophylaxis.

Thrombocid
Note. This name is used for preparations of different composition.
Sigmapharm, Aust.; Bene, Ger.; Neo-Farmaceutica, Port.; Milupa, Switz.
Ointment: Pentosan polysulfate sodium (p.953·1); guaiazulene (p.1618·3); thymol (p.1158·3).
Burns; insect bites; soft-tissue disorders; superficial vascular disorders.
Bene, Ger.
Suppositories: Pentosan polysulfate sodium (p.953·1); aluminium monostearate; guaiazulene (p.1618·3).
Anorectal disorders.
Bene, Ger.; Neo-Farmaceutica, Port.; Milupa, Switz.
Topical gel: Pentosan polysulfate sodium (p.953·1); rosemary oil (p.1659·3); pumilio pine oil (p.1656·3); melissa oil.
Soft-tissue disorders; superficial vascular disorders.
Bene-Chemie, Hong Kong.
Pentosan polysulfate sodium (p.953·1); guaiazulene (p.1618·3).
Haemorrhoids; insect stings; sunburn; superficial phlebitis; venous insufficiency.
Neo-Farmaceutica, Port.
Suppositories: Pentosan polysulfate sodium (p.953·1); guaiazulene (p.1618·3).
Anorectal disorders.
Lacer, Spain.
Pentosan polysulfate sodium (p.953·1); thymol (p.1158·3).
Burns; haemorrhoids; peripheral vascular disorders; soft-tissue disorders.

Thrombocoll *Johnson & Johnson, Ger.†.*
Thrombin (p.741·3).
Haemorrhage.

Thrombodine *Lannacher, Aust.*
Ticlopidine hydrochloride (p.981·1).
Thrombosis prophylaxis.

Thrombogen *Johnson & Johnson Medical, USA.*
Thrombin (p.741·3).
Bleeding from small blood vessels.

Thrombophob
Note. This name is used for preparations of different composition.
Ebewe, Aust.; Hoechst Marion Roussel, S.Afr.†.
Ointment: Heparin (p.902·1) or heparin sodium (p.902·1); benzyl nicotinate (p.20·2).
Muscular pain; soft-tissue injury; superficial vascular disorders.
Ebewe, Aust.; Aventis, S.Afr.
Topical gel: Heparin (p.902·1) or heparin sodium (p.902·1).
Soft-tissue injuries; superficial vascular disorders.
Knoll, Ger.
Heparin sodium (p.902·1).
Soft-tissue injury; thromboembolic disorders.

Thrombophob-S *Ebewe, Aust.*
Heparin sodium (p.902·1).
Soft-tissue injury; superficial vascular disorders.

Thrombosantin *Boehringer Ingelheim, Aust.*
Dipyridamole (p.877·2); aspirin (p.14·2).
Thromboembolic disorders.

Thrombostat *Parke, Davis, Austral.; Parke, Davis, Canad.; Parke, Davis, NZ; Parke, Davis, Singapore; Parke, Davis, USA.*
Thrombin (p.741·3).
Minor haemorrhage.

Thrombotrol *CSL, NZ.*
Antithrombin III (p.725·2).
Antithrombin III deficiency.

Thrombotrol-VF *CSL, Austral.*
Antithrombin III (p.725·2).
Antithrombin III deficiency.

Thuja Med Complex *Dynamit, Aust.*
Homoeopathic preparation.

Thuja Oligoplex *Madaus, Ger.*
Homoeopathic preparation.

Thunas Bilettes *Thuna, Canad.†.*
Aloin (p.1210·2); cascara (p.1216·1); phenolphthalein (p.1244·1).

Thunas Eye Drops *Thuna, Canad.*
Boric acid (p.1586·1); borax (p.1586·1).

Thunas Hyperacidity Tablets *Thuna, Canad.*
Magnesium hydroxide (p.1233·1); aluminium hydroxide-magnesium carbonate co-dried gel (p.1211·2); simeticone (p.1249·2).

Thunas Laxative *Thuna, Canad.*
Cascara (p.1216·1); senna (p.1248·2); bryony; fennel (p.1610·1); liquorice (p.1231·2); juglans; leptandra.

Thunas Pile *Thuna, Canad.*
Benzocaine (p.1306·2); bismuth subcarbonate (p.1213·1); ephedrine sulfate (p.1090·2); zinc oxide (p.1128·2).
Haemorrhoids.

Thunas Salve for Rheumatic Pains *Thuna, Canad.*
Methyl salicylate (p.55·1); camphor (p.1589·3); menthol (p.1632·3).

Thunas Tab for Menstrual Pain *Thuna, Canad.*
Motherwort (p.1637·3); senecio (p.1661·3); sodium salicylate (p.84·2); teucrium scorodonia; viburnum.

Thybon *Henning, Ger.*
Liothyronine hydrochloride (p.1524·3).
Hypothyroidism.

Thycapzol *Gea, Denm.*
Methimazole [thiamazole] (p.1525·1).
Hyperthyroidism.

Thymi Syrup *Vitamed, Israel.*
Thyme (p.1672·2).
Coughs.

Thymian Erkaltungs-Bad *Li-il, Ger.*
Thyme (p.1672·3).
Bath additive; respiratory-tract disorders; skin disorders.

Thymi-Fips *Lichtenstein, Ger.†.*
Thyme (p.1672·2).
Respiratory-tract disorders.

Thymipin N *Novartis Consumer, Ger.*
Cream: Thyme (p.1672·2); camphor (p.1589·3); eucalyptus oil (p.1609·2).
Syrup; oral drops; suppositories: Thyme (p.1672·2).
Bronchitis; catarrh; coughs.

Thymiverlan *Verla, Ger.*
Thyme (p.1672·2).
Respiratory-tract disorders.

Thymodrosin *Gubler, Switz.†.*
Guaifenesin (p.1092·2); codeine phosphate (p.25·2); thyme (p.1672·2); drosera (p.1606·1); plantaginis; castanea vulgaris; ipecacuanha (p.1093·1); belladonna (p.463·1); liquorice (p.1231·2).
Coughs.

Thymodrosin N *Gubler, Switz.*
Guaifenesin (p.1092·2); thyme (p.1672·2); drosera (p.1606·1); plantaginis; liquorice (p.1231·2).
Respiratory-tract disorders.

Thymo-Glanduretten *Biosyn, Ger.*
Bovine thymus extract.
Immunotherapy.

Thymoglobulin *Imtix, Ger.*
An antithymocyte immunoglobulin (p.508·2).
Immunosuppressive therapy.

Thymoglobuline *Imtix, Belg.; Pasteur Merieux, Braz.; Imtix, Denm.; Imtix, Fr.; Pasteur Merieux, Hong Kong; Pasteur Merieux, Israel; Aventis, S.Afr.; Imtix, Switz.; Pasteur Merieux, Thai.*
An antithymocyte immunoglobulin (rabbit) (p.508·2).
Aplastic anaemia; graft-versus-host disease; transplant rejection.

Thymoject *Biosyn, Ger.*
Bovine thymus extract.
Immunological disorders.

Thymol Mouthwash Red *Pharmacia Upjohn, Austral.*
Thymol (p.1158·3); menthol (p.1632·3).
Dry mouth; oral hygiene.

Thymophysin *CytoChemia, Ger.*
Thymus extract.
Immunotherapy.

Thymorell *Sanorell, Ger.*
Homoeopathic preparation.

Thymoval *Smetana, Aust.*
Cowslip (p.1600·1); valerian (p.1678·3); thyme (p.1672·2).
Coughs.

Thymowied *Wiedemann, Ger.*
Thymus.
Immunotherapy.

Thymunes *Eagle, Austral.*
Thymus.

Thym-Uvocal *Strathmann, Ger.*
Calf thymus extract.
Immunotherapy.

Thypinone *Abbott, USA.*
Protirelin (p.1295·3).
Diagnostic assessment of thyroid function.

Thyradin-S *Teikoku, Jpn.*
Thyroxine [levothyroxine] sodium (p.1526·2).
Goitre; hypothyroidism.

Thyrar *Rhone-Poulenc Rorer, USA†.*
Thyroid (bovine) (p.1526·2).
Hypothyroidism; thyroid cancer.

Thyrax *Organon, Belg.; Nourypharma, Neth.; Organon, Port.; Organon, Spain.*
Thyroxine [levothyroxine] sodium (p.1526·2).
Diagnostic suppression of thyroid activity; hypothyroidism; thyroid cancer.

Thyrefact *Aventis, Denm.; Hoechst Marion Roussel, Swed.*
Protirelin (p.1295·3).
Test of thyroid or pituitary-hypothalamic function; thyroid disorders.

Thyrel-TRH *Ferring, USA.*
Protirelin (p.1295·3).
Formerly called Relefact TRH.
Diagnosis of thyroid dysfunction.

Thyreocomb N *Berlin-Chemie, Ger.*
Thyroxine [levothyroxine] (p.1528·1); potassium iodide (p.1522·3).
Iodine-deficiency disorders.

Thyreogutt *Austroplant, Aust.*
Motherwort (p.1637·3); lycopus europaeus.
Hyperthyroidism; mastalgia; tachycardia.

Thyreogutt mono *Schwabe, Ger.*
Motherwort (p.1637·3).
Mastalgia; mild hyperthyroidism.

thyreo-loges comp *Loges, Ger.*
Homoeopathic preparation.

thyreo-loges N *Loges, Ger.*
Lycopus europaeus.
Hyperthyroidism; mastalgia.

Thyreo-Pasc N *Pascoe, Ger.*
Homoeopathic preparation.

Thyreostat II Herbrand, Ger.; Berlin-Chemie, Ger.
Propylthiouracil (p.1525·3).
Hyperthyroidism.

Thyreotom Berlin-Chemie, Ger.
Liothyronine (p.1524·3); thyroxine [levothyroxine] (p.1528·1).
Hypothyroidism.

Thyrex Biochemie, Aust.
Thyroxine [levothyroxine] sodium (p.1526·2).
Hypothyroidism.

Thyro-Block Carter Horner, Canad.; Wallace, USA.
Potassium iodide (p.1522·3).
Blockade of thyroid uptake of radioiodine.

Thyrogen Genzyme, USA.
Thyrotropin alfa (p.1298·3).
Measurement of serum thyroglobulin.

Thyrolar Forest Pharmaceuticals, USA.
Liothyronine sodium (p.1524·2); thyroxine [levothyroxine] sodium (p.1526·2).
Evaluation of thyroid function; hypothyroidism; TSH suppression.

Thyroliberin Merck, Ger.
Protirelin (p.1295·3).
Assessment of pituitary and thyroid function.

Thyronajod Henning, Ger.
Thyroxine [levothyroxine] sodium (p.1526·2); potassium iodide (p.1522·3).
Hypothyroidism.

Thyrosit Sriprasit, Thai.
Thyroxine [levothyroxine] sodium (p.1526·2).
Hypothyroidism.

Thyrotardin N Henning, Ger.
Liothyronine hydrochloride (p.1524·3).
Hypothyroidism.

Thyrozol
Merck, Ger.; Merck, Singapore.
Methimazole [thiamazole] (p.1525·1).
Hyperthyroidism.

Thytropar
USV, Israel; Armour, USA†.
Thyrotrophin (p.1298·3).
Diagnosis of thyroid disorders.

TI Baby Natural Fischer, USA.
SPF 16: Titanium dioxide (p.1126·1).
Sunscreen.

TI Lite Fischer, USA.
SPF 15: Octinoxate (p.1517·3); titanium dioxide (p.1126·1).
Sunscreen.

TI Screen Pedinol, USA.
SPF 8; SPF 15: Octinoxate (p.1517·3); oxybenzone (p.1518·1).
SPF 30: Octinoxate (p.1517·3); oxybenzone (p.1518·1); octisalate (p.1518·1); octocrilene (p.1518·1).
Sunscreen.

TI Screen Natural Pedinol, USA.
SPF 16: Titanium dioxide (p.1126·1).
Sunscreen.

TI Screen Sunless Pedinol, USA.
SPF 17; SPF 23: Octinoxate (p.1517·3); oxybenzone (p.1518·1).
Sunscreen.

Tia Doce Alba, USA†.
Cyanocobalamin (p.1388·1); thiamine hydrochloride (p.1385·1).

Tiabiose UCI, Braz.
Tiabendazole (p.109·1).
Nematode infections.

Tiabrenolo NCSN, Ital.
Tiadenol (p.980·3).
Hyperlipidaemias.

Tiacid Draxis, Canad.
Salicylic acid (p.1122·3); lactic acid (p.1626·2).

Tiaden Malesci, Ital.
Tiadenol (p.980·3).
Hyperlipidaemias.

Tiadil
Zambon, Neth.; Basi, Port.
Diltiazem hydrochloride (p.874·3).
Hypertension.

Tiadilon Crinex, Fr.
Arginine tidiacicate (p.1354·1).
Liver disorders.

Tiadipona Knoll, Spain.
Bentazepam (p.656·3).
Anxiety; insomnia.

Tiakem Vita, Ital.
Diltiazem hydrochloride (p.874·3).
Hypertension; ischaemic heart disease.

Tiamate Hoechst Marion Roussel, USA.
Diltiazem malate (p.876·2).
Angina pectoris; hypertension.

Tiaminal B₁₂ Silanes, Mex.
Cyanocobalamin (p.1388·1); thiamine hydrochloride (p.1385·1).
Lignocaine [lidocaine] hydrochloride (p.1313·2) is included in this preparation to alleviate the pain of injection.
Neuralgia; neuritis; vitamin B deficiencies.

Tiaminal B₁₂ Trivalente Silanes, Mex.
Cyanocobalamin (p.1388·1) or hydroxocobalamin (p.1388·1); thiamine hydrochloride (p.1385·1); pyridoxine hydrochloride (p.1386·3).
Neuralgia; neuritis; pernicious anaemia; vitamin B deficiencies.

Tiamol Spectropharm, Canad.
Fluocinonide (p.1071·2).
Skin disorders.

Tiamon Mono Temmler, Ger.
Dihydrocodeine tartrate (p.33·1).
Coughs.

Tiapridal
Sanofi Synthelabo, Belg.; Synthelabo, Braz.; Synthelabo, Fr.; Synthelabo, Hong Kong; Sanofi Synthelabo, Neth.; Sanofi Synthelabo, Port.; Sanofi Synthelabo, Singapore; Synthelabo, Switz.
Tiapride hydrochloride (p.709·1).
Aggression; alcohol withdrawal syndrome; anxiety; behaviour disorders; choreic movements; dyskinesia.

Tiapridex Sanofi Synthelabo, Ger.
Tiapride hydrochloride (p.709·1).
Parkinsonism and other hyperkinetic disorders.

Tiaprizal Synthelabo, Spain.
Tiapride hydrochloride (p.709·1).
Anxiety; behaviour disorders; movement disorders; nausea and vomiting.

Tiaprofen Bioprogress, Ital.
Tiaprofenic acid (p.88·1).
Inflammation; pain.

Tiaprorex Lampugnani, Ital.†
Tiaprofenic acid (p.88·1).
Inflammation; pain.

Tiase Vedim, Ital.†
Stepronin (p.1101·1).
Liver disorders.

Tiatral 100 SR Novartis, Switz.
Aspirin (p.14·2).
Thromboembolic disorders.

Tiazac
Crystaal, Canad.; Forest Pharmaceuticals, USA.
Diltiazem hydrochloride (p.874·3).
Angina pectoris; hypertension.

Tiazen Bioprogress, Ital.†
Diltiazem hydrochloride (p.874·3).
Hypertension; ischaemic heart disease.

Tiazolidin Solvay, Ital.†
Timonacic (p.1673·2).
Liver disorders.

Tiba Pharmaland, Thai.
Gemfibrozil (p.896·2).
Hyperlipidaemias.

Tiberal
Roche, Belg.; Roche, Fr.; Roche, Israel; Roche, Ital.; Roche, Mex.; Roche, NZ; Roche, Switz.
Ornidazole (p.599·1).
Anaerobic bacterial infections; protozoal infections.

Tibinide Recip, Swed.
Isoniazid (p.215·3).
Tuberculosis.

Tibirim Ranbaxy, Thai.
Rifampicin (p.243·2).
Tuberculosis.

Tiblex Fournier SA, Spain†.
Sucralfate (p.1250·2).
Gastrointestinal haemorrhage; peptic ulcer.

Tiburon Monot, Fr.†
Ibuprofen (p.43·2).
Fever; musculoskeletal and joint disorders; pain; soft-tissue disorders.

Ticalma Kelemata, Ital.
Valerian root (p.1678·3).
Sedative.

Ticar
SmithKline Beecham, Canad.†; Link, UK†; SmithKline Beecham, USA.
Ticarcillin sodium (p.262·3).
Bacterial infections.

Ticarpen
SmithKline Beecham, Fr.; SmithKline Beecham, Neth.; SmithKline Beecham, Spain.
Ticarcillin sodium (p.262·3).
Bacterial infections.

Tice Organon, USA.
A BCG vaccine (p.1533·2).
Active immunisation; bladder cancer.

Ticillin CSL, Austral.†.
Ticarcillin sodium (p.262·3).
Bacterial infections.

Ticlid
Roche, Austral.; Sanofi Synthelabo, Belg.; Sanofi Winthrop, Braz.; Roche, Canad.; Sanofi Winthrop, Fr.; Sanofi Winthrop, Hong Kong; Syntex, Mex.; Sanofi Winthrop, Norw.; Roche, NZ; Sanofi Synthelabo, S.Afr.; Sanofi Synthelabo, Singapore; Sanofi Winthrop, Swed.; Sanofi Winthrop, Switz.†; Sanofi Synthelabo, Thai.; Sanofi Winthrop, UK; Roche, USA.
Ticlopidine hydrochloride (p.981·1).
Intermittent claudication; maintenance of extracorporeal circulation; stroke prophylaxis; thromboembolism prophylaxis.

Ticlidil CTI, Israel.
Ticlopidine hydrochloride (p.981·1).
Stroke prophylaxis.

Ticlodix Vitoria, Port.
Ticlopidine hydrochloride (p.981·1).
Thromboembolism prophylaxis.

Ticlodone
Sanofi Winthrop, Aust.†; Sigma-Tau, Ital.; Almirall, Spain.
Ticlopidine hydrochloride (p.981·1).
Thromboembolism prophylaxis.

Ticlogi Ibirn, Ital.
Ticlopidine hydrochloride (p.981·1).
Thrombosis prophylaxis.

Ticloproge Proge, Ital.
Ticlopidine hydrochloride (p.981·1).
Thrombosis prophylaxis.

Ticoflex Uno, Ital.
Naproxen aminobutanol (p.61·3).
Gout; musculoskeletal, joint, peri-articular, and soft-tissue disorders; neuralgias.

Ticolcin Tecnofarma, Mex.
Colchicine (p.400·1).
Gout; liver cirrhosis.

Ticon Hauck, USA.
Trimethobenzamide hydrochloride (p.426·3).
Nausea and vomiting.

Ticovac Baxter, Fr.
A tick-borne encephalitis vaccine (p.1539·3).
Active immunisation.

Tiddy Sriprasit, Thai.
Multivitamin and mineral preparation with lysine (p.1350·1).

Tielle
Johnson & Johnson, Ger.; Johnson & Johnson Medical, UK.
Foamed hydrogel.
Skin ulcers; wounds.

Tiempe DDSA Pharmaceuticals, UK.
Trimethoprim (p.264·2).

Tienam
Merck Sharp & Dohme, Belg.; Merck Sharp & Dohme, Braz.; Merck Sharp & Dohme, Denm.; Merck Sharp & Dohme, Fin.; Merck Sharp & Dohme-Chibret, Fr.; Merck Sharp & Dohme, Hong Kong; Merck Sharp & Dohme, Israel; Merck Sharp & Dohme, Ital.; Merck Sharp & Dohme, Mex.; Merck Sharp & Dohme, Neth.; Merck Sharp & Dohme, Norw.; Merck Sharp & Dohme, Port.; Merck Sharp & Dohme, S.Afr.; Merck Sharp & Dohme, Singapore; Merck Sharp & Dohme, Spain; Merck Sharp & Dohme, Swed.; Merck Sharp & Dohme, Switz.; Merck Sharp & Dohme, Thai.
Imipenem (p.214·1); cilastatin sodium (p.182·2).
Lignocaine [lidocaine] hydrochloride (p.1313·2) may be included in the intramuscular injection to alleviate the pain of injection.
Bacterial infections.

Tienor Farmaka, Ital.
Clotiazepam (p.671·1).
Anxiety; insomnia; nervous disorders.

Tifell Bucca, Spain.
Eucalyptol (p.1609·2); cresol (p.1142·3); eugenol (p.1609·3); formaldehyde (p.1144·2).
Mouth infections.

Tifenso Clinced, Aust.
Benzyl nicotinate (p.20·2); choline salicylate (p.24·3).

Tiffy
Note.This name is used for preparations of different composition.
Medochemie, Hong Kong.
Paracetamol (p.71·2).
Fever; pain.

Nakorn, Thai.
Syrup: Paracetamol (p.71·2); phenylpropanolamine hydrochloride (p.1098·1); chlorpheniramine [chlorphenamine] maleate (p.412·1); phenylephrine hydrochloride (p.1097·1).
Tablets: Paracetamol (p.71·2); chlorpheniramine [chlorphenamine] maleate (p.412·1); phenylpropanolamine hydrochloride (p.1098·1).
Cold and flu symptoms; hay fever.

Tiffyrub Nakorn, Thai.
Menthol (p.1632·3); camphor (p.1589·3); turpentine oil (p.1676·3); eucalyptus oil (p.1609·2); nutmeg oil (p.1643·1).
Cold symptoms; coughs; nasal congestion.

Tifox Chong Kun Dang, Ital.
Cefoxitin sodium (p.171·2).
Lignocaine [lidocaine] hydrochloride (p.1313·2) is included in the intramuscular injection to alleviate the pain of injection.
Gram-negative bacterial infections.

Tigan
Note.This name is used for preparations of different composition.
SmithKline Beecham, Mex.
Trimethobenzamide (p.427·1).

Roberts, USA.
Capsules; injection: Trimethobenzamide hydrochloride (p.426·3).
Suppositories: Trimethobenzamide hydrochloride (p.426·3); benzocaine (p.1306·2).
Nausea and vomiting.

Tigason
Roche, Braz.; Roche, Ital.†.
Etretinate (p.1114·2).
Keratinisation disorders; psoriasis.

Tiger Balm Liquid LRC Products, UK†.
Cajuput oil (p.1588·1); camphor (p.1589·3); cinnamon oil (p.1596·1); clove oil (p.1597·1); menthol (p.1632·3); peppermint oil (p.1243·3).
Muscle ache.

Tiger Balm Red
Note.This name is used for preparations of different composition.
Felton, Austral.†.
Cajuput oil (p.1588·1); camphor (p.1589·3); cassia oil (p.1592·1); clove oil (p.1597·1); menthol (p.1632·3).
Muscular aches and pains.

Haw Par, Canad.
Camphor (p.1589·3); menthol (p.1632·3); cajuput oil (p.1588·1); cinnamon oil (p.1596·1); clove oil (p.1597·1); peppermint oil (p.1243·3).

SSL, UK.
Cajuput oil (p.1588·1); camphor (p.1589·3); clove oil (p.1597·1); menthol (p.1632·3).
Muscle pain.

Tiger Balm White
Felton, Austral.†.
Cajuput oil (p.1588·1); camphor (p.1589·3); clove oil (p.1597·1); menthol (p.1632·3); dementholised mint oil (p.1636·2).
Muscular aches and pains.

Haw Par, Canad.
Camphor (p.1589·3); menthol (p.1632·3); cajuput oil (p.1588·1); clove oil (p.1597·1); peppermint oil (p.1243·3).

Tiger Balsam Rot Klosterfrau, Aust.
Camphor (p.1589·3); menthol (p.1632·3); cajuput oil (p.1588·1); peppermint oil (p.1243·3); clove oil (p.1597·1); cinnamon oil (p.1596·1).
Muscle pain.

Tiger Liniment DHA, Canad.
Methyl salicylate (p.55·1); menthol (p.1632·3); eucalyptus oil (p.1609·2).

Tigridol Phytomedica, Fr.
Camphor (p.1589·3); menthol (p.1632·3); clove oil (p.1597·1); eucalyptus oil (p.1609·2); peppermint oil (p.1243·3); cinnamon oil (p.1596·1).
Pain.

Tikacillin Tika, Swed.
Phenoxymethylpenicillin potassium (p.235·1).
Bacterial infections.

Tiklid
Sanofi Winthrop, Aust.; Sanofi Synthelabo, Ital.; Sanofi Synthelabo, Spain.
Ticlopidine hydrochloride (p.981·1).
Thromboembolism prophylaxis.

Tiklyd
Sanofi Synthelabo, Ger.; Sanofi Synthelabo, Port.
Ticlopidine hydrochloride (p.981·1).
Thrombosis prophylaxis.

Tikosyn Pfizer, USA.
Dofetilide (p.881·2).
Arrhythmias.

Tilad Rhone-Poulenc Rorer, Spain.
Nedocromil sodium (p.768·3).
Asthma.

Tilade
Sanova, Aust.; Rhone-Poulenc Rorer, Austral.; Fisons, Braz.; Rhone-Poulenc Rorer, Canad.; Fisons, Denm.; Rhone-Poulenc Rorer, Fin.; Rhone-Poulenc Rorer, Fr.; Rhone-Poulenc Rorer, Ger.; Rhone-Poulenc Rorer, Hong Kong; Fisons, Irl.; Fisons, Israel; Rhone-Poulenc Rorer, Ital.; Rhone-Poulenc Rorer, Neth.; Aventis, NZ; Aventis, S.Afr.; Rhone-Poulenc Rorer, Switz.; Pantheon, UK; Rhone-Poulenc Rorer, USA.
Nedocromil sodium (p.768·3).
Asthma.

Tilaire Rhone-Poulenc Rorer, Mex.
Nedocromil sodium (p.768·3).
Obstructive airways disease.

Tilarin
Sanova, Aust.; Rhone-Poulenc Rorer, Fin.; Rhone-Poulenc Rorer, Ital.; Aventis, NZ; Rhone-Poulenc Rorer, Switz.; Rhone-Poulenc Rorer, UK†.
Nedocromil sodium (p.768·3).
Allergic rhinitis.

Tilatil Roche, Braz.
Tenoxicam (p.87·2).
Musculoskeletal, joint, and peri-articular disorders.

Tilavist
Sanova, Aust.; Fisons, Denm.; Rhone-Poulenc Rorer, Fin.; Rhone-Poulenc Rorer, Fr.; Fisons, Irl.; Fisons, Israel; Rhone-Poulenc Rorer, Ital.; Rhone-Poulenc Rorer, Neth.; Fisons, Norw.; Aventis, NZ; Aventis, Port.; Fisons, Singapore; Rhone-Poulenc Rorer, Singapore; Rhone-Poulenc Rorer, Spain; Rhone-Poulenc Rorer, Swed.; Rhone-Poulenc Rorer, Switz.
Nedocromil sodium (p.768·3).
Allergic conjunctivitis.

Tilazem
Parke, Davis, Mex.; Parke, Davis, S.Afr.
Diltiazem hydrochloride (p.874·3).
Angina pectoris; hypertension.

Tilcotil
Roche, Aust.; Roche, Austral.; Roche, Belg.; Roche, Denm.; Roche, Fin.; Roche, Fr.; Roche, Hong Kong; Roche, Irl.; Roche, Ital.; Roche, Mex.; Roche, Neth.; Roche, NZ; Roche, Port.; Roche, S.Afr.; Roche, Singapore; Roche, Spain; Roche, Switz.; Roche, Thai.
Tenoxicam (p.87·2).
Gout; inflammation; musculoskeletal, joint, peri-articular, and soft-tissue disorders; pain.

Tildiem
Sanofi Synthelabo, Belg.; Synthelabo, Fr.; Synthelabo, Hong Kong; Lorex, Irl.; Sanofi Synthelabo, Neth.; Sanofi Synthelabo, Singapore; Synthelabo, Switz.; Sanofi Synthelabo, Thai.; Sanofi Synthelabo, UK.
Diltiazem hydrochloride (p.874·3).
Angina pectoris; arrhythmias; hypertension; myocardial ischaemia.

Tilene Francia, Ital.
Fenofibrate (p.889·1).
Hyperlipidaemias.

Tilexim Select, Ital.†.
Cefuroxime axetil (p.178·1).
Bacterial infections.

Tilfilin *Funk, Spain†.*
Carbocisteine (p.1086·3); chlorpheniramine [chlorphenamine] maleate (p.412·1); phenylephrine hydrochloride (p.1097·1); choline theophyllinate (p.763·3).
Obstructive airways disease.

Tili *ABZ, Ger.*
Tilidate hydrochloride (p.88·2).
Naloxone hydrochloride (p.1014·3) is included in this preparation to discourage abuse.
Pain.

Tilicomp *Betapharm, Ger.*
Tilidate hydrochloride (p.88·2).
Naloxone hydrochloride (p.1014·3) is included in this preparation to discourage abuse.
Pain.

Tilidalor *Hexal, Ger.*
Tilidate hydrochloride (p.88·2).
Naloxone hydrochloride (p.1014·3) is included in this preparation to discourage abuse.
Pain.

Tilidin comp *Bayer, Ger.; Heumann, Ger.; Stada, Ger.*
Tilidate hydrochloride (p.88·2).
Naloxone hydrochloride (p.1014·3) is included in this preparation to discourage abuse.
Pain.

Tilidin N *BASF, Ger.; Lichtenstein, Ger.*
Tilidate hydrochloride (p.88·2).
Naloxone hydrochloride (p.1014·3) is included in this preparation to discourage abuse.
Pain.

Tilidin plus *Ratiopharm, Ger.*
Tilidate hydrochloride (p.88·2).
Naloxone hydrochloride (p.1014·3) is included in this preparation to discourage abuse.
Pain.

Tilidin-saar *Chephasaar, Ger.*
Tilidate hydrochloride (p.88·2).
Naloxone hydrochloride (p.1014·3) is included in this preparation to discourage abuse.
Pain.

Tiligetic *Azupharma, Ger.*
Tilidate hydrochloride (p.88·2).
Naloxone hydrochloride (p.1014·3) is included in this preparation to discourage abuse.
Pain.

Tilimerck *Merck dura, Ger.*
Tilidate hydrochloride (p.88·2).
Naloxone hydrochloride (p.1014·3) is included in this preparation to discourage abuse.
Pain.

Tili-Puren *Isis Puren, Ger.*
Tilidate hydrochloride (p.88·2).
Naloxone hydrochloride (p.1014·3) is included in this preparation to discourage abuse.
Pain.

Tilitrate *Parke, Davis, Spain†.*
Tilidate hydrochloride (p.88·2).
Pain.

Tilker *Sanofi Winthrop, Denm.; Sanofi Winthrop, Norw.; Synthelabo, Spain.*
Diltiazem hydrochloride (p.874·3).
Angina pectoris; hypertension.

Till *Amnol, Ital.*
Triclosan (p.1159·2); alkylamidobetaine.
Personal hygiene.

tilnalox *CT, Ger.*
Tilidate hydrochloride (p.88·2).
Naloxone hydrochloride (p.1014·3) is included in this preparation to discourage abuse.
Pain.

Tilodene *Alphapharm, Austral.*
Ticlopidine hydrochloride (p.981·1).
Thromboembolism prophylaxis.

Tiloptic *Merck Sharp & Dohme, Israel.*
Timolol maleate (p.982·1).
Glaucoma; ocular hypertension.

Tiloryth *Tillomed, UK.*
Erythromycin (p.201·2).
Bacterial infections.

Tilosin *Wayne, Mex.*
Hyoscine butylbromide (p.468·2).

Ti-Lub *Draxis, Canad.*
Liquid paraffin (p.1407·1) or light liquid paraffin (p.1407·2).

Tilur *Drossapharm, Switz.*
Acemetacin (p.11·2).
Musculoskeletal and joint disorders; superficial thrombophlebitis.

TIM *Seroyal, Canad.*
Vitamins A, C, and E, and zinc (p.1350·1).

Timabak *Agepha, Aust.; Thea, Fr.; Thea, Hong Kong; Pharmacia Upjohn, Singapore.*
Timolol maleate (p.982·1).
Glaucoma; ocular hypertension.

Timacar *Merck Sharp & Dohme, Denm.*
Timolol maleate (p.982·1).
Angina pectoris; glaucoma; hypertension; migraine; myocardial infarction.

Timacor *Merck Sharp & Dohme-Chibret, Fr.*
Timolol maleate (p.982·1).
Angina pectoris; hypertension; myocardial infarction.

Tim-Ak *Dioptic, Canad.*
Timolol maleate (p.982·1).
Raised intra-ocular pressure.

Time Action B Complex with C *Hall, Canad.*
Vitamins B and C (p.1350·1).

Time Release Ester C *Swiss Herbal, Canad.*
Vitamin C substances (p.1389·3).

Time Released Balanced B *Lee-Adams, Canad.*
Vitamin B substances (p.1350·1).

Timecef *Hoechst Marion Roussel, Aust.; Hoechst Marion Roussel, Braz.; Hoechst Marion Roussel, Ital.; Hoechst Marion Roussel, UK†.*
Cefodizime sodium (p.167·3).
Lignocaine [lidocaine] hydrochloride (p.1313·2) may be included in some intramuscular injections to alleviate the pain of injection.
Bacterial infections.

Timed Action Balanced B *Hall, Canad.*
Vitamin B substances (p.1350·1).

Timed Release C *Jamieson, Canad.*
Ascorbic acid (p.1389·3).

Timed Release Mega Men *General Nutrition, Canad.*
Multivitamin and mineral preparation (p.1350·1).

Timed Release Swiss One *Swiss Herbal, Canad.*
Multivitamin and mineral preparation (p.1350·1).

Timed Release Ultra Mega *General Nutrition, Canad.*
Range of multivitamin and mineral preparations (p.1350·1).

Timed Release Vita-Vim *Jamieson, Canad.*
Multivitamin and mineral preparation (p.1350·1).

Timed Release Womens Ultra Mega *General Nutrition, Canad.*
Multivitamin and mineral preparation (p.1350·1).

Timelit *Lundbeck, Ital.*
Lofepramine hydrochloride (p.297·1).
Depression.

Timenten *SmithKline Beecham, Aust.†; SmithKline Beecham, Switz.*
Ticarcillin sodium (p.262·3); potassium clavulanate (p.187·2).
Bacterial infections.

Timentin *SmithKline Beecham, Austral.; SmithKline Beecham, Belg.; SmithKline Beecham, Braz.; SmithKline Beecham, Canad.; SmithKline Beecham, Hong Kong; SmithKline Beecham, Irl.; SmithKline Beecham, Israel; SmithKline Beecham, Ital.; SmithKline Beecham, Mex.; SmithKline Beecham, Neth.; SmithKline Beecham, NZ; SmithKline Beecham, UK; SmithKline Beecham, USA.*
Ticarcillin sodium (p.262·3); potassium clavulanate (p.187·2).
Lignocaine [lidocaine] hydrochloride (p.1313·2) may be included in the intramuscular injection to alleviate the pain of injection.
Bacterial infections.

Timicolid *Pfizer Consumer, Ital.*
Dithranol (p.1113·3).
Psoriasis.

Timicon *Merck Sharp & Dohme, Ital.*
Timolol maleate (p.982·1); pilocarpine hydrochloride (p.1422·3).
Glaucoma; ocular hypertension.

Timisol *Ecosol, Switz.*
Timolol maleate (p.982·1).
Glaucoma; ocular hypertension.

T-Immun *Immuno, Aust.; Immuno, Ger.†.*
A tetanus vaccine (p.1565·2).
Active immunisation.

Timo-COMOD *Ursapharm, Ger.; Ursapharm, Neth.*
Timolol maleate (p.982·1).
Glaucoma; ocular hypertension.

Timodine *Reckitt Benckiser, Irl.; Reckitt & Colman, UK.*
Nystatin (p.392·2); hydrocortisone (p.1073·3).
Infected skin disorders.

Timodrop *Biolab, Thai.*
Timolol maleate (p.982·1).
Glaucoma; ocular hypertension.

TimoEDO *Mann, Ger.*
Timolol maleate (p.982·1).
Glaucoma; ocular hypertension.

Timoftal *Agepha, Aust.*
Timolol maleate (p.982·1).
Glaucoma; ocular hypertension.

Timoftol *Merck Sharp & Dohme, Spain.*
Timolol maleate (p.982·1).
Glaucoma; ocular hypertension.

Timoglau *Oftalder, Port.*
Timolol maleate (p.982·1).
Ocular hypertension.

Timoglau Plus *Oftalder, Port.*
Timolol maleate (p.982·1); pilocarpine hydrochloride (p.1422·3).
Glaucoma.

Timohexal *Hexal, Aust.; Hexal, Ger.*
Timolol maleate (p.982·1).
Cataracts; glaucoma; ocular hypertension.

Timolen *Davi, Port.*
Timolol maleate (p.982·1).
Glaucoma; ocular hypertension.

Timolide *Merck Frosst, Canad.; Merck, USA.*
Timolol maleate (p.982·1); hydrochlorothiazide (p.907·3).
Hypertension.

Timomann *Mann, Ger.*
Timolol maleate (p.982·1).
Glaucoma; ocular hypertension.

Timonil *Desitin, Ger.; Desitin, Hong Kong; Desitin, Israel; Desitin, Switz.; CP Pharmaceuticals, UK.*
Carbamazepine (p.342·2).
Alcohol withdrawal syndrome; bipolar disorder; diabetes insipidus; diabetic neuropathy; epilepsy; mania; trigeminal neuralgia.

Tim-Ophtal *Agepha, Aust.; Winzer, Ger.*
Timolol maleate (p.982·1).
Glaucoma; ocular hypertension.

Timoptic *Merck Sharp & Dohme, Aust.; Merck Frosst, Canad.; Merck Sharp & Dohme, Switz.; Merck, USA.*
Timolol maleate (p.982·1).
Glaucoma; ocular hypertension.

Timoptol *Frosst, Austral.; Merck Sharp & Dohme, Belg.; Merck Sharp & Dohme, Braz.; Merck Sharp & Dohme-Chibret, Fr.; Merck Sharp & Dohme, Hong Kong; Merck Sharp & Dohme, Irl.; Merck Sharp & Dohme, Ital.; Merck Sharp & Dohme, Mex.; Merck Sharp & Dohme, Neth.; Merck Sharp & Dohme, NZ; Chibret, Port.; Merck Sharp & Dohme, S.Afr.; Merck Sharp & Dohme, Singapore; Merck Sharp & Dohme, Thai.; Merck Sharp & Dohme, UK.*
Timolol maleate (p.982·1).
Glaucoma; ocular hypertension.

Timoptol-XE *Merck Sharp & Dohme, Austral.*
Timolol maleate (p.982·1).
Glaucoma; ocular hypertension.

Timosan *Note. This name is used for preparations of different composition.*
Funda Paiva, Braz.
Thymus polypeptides (bovine) (p.1672·3).
Immunotherapy.
Santen, Fin.
Timolol maleate (p.982·1).
Glaucoma; ocular hypertension.

Timosil *Silom, Thai.*
Timolol maleate (p.982·1).
Glaucoma; ocular hypertension.

Timosin *Sclavo, Ital.†.*
Thymalfasin (p.1672·1).
Influenza in immunodeficient patients.

Timosine *Chibret, Ger.*
Timolol maleate (p.982·1).
Glaucoma; ocular hypertension.

Timo-Stulln *Stulln, Ger.*
Timolol maleate (p.982·1).
Glaucoma; ocular hypertension.

Timozzard *Pizzard, Mex.*
Timolol (p.982·2).
Glaucoma.

Timpanol *QIF, Braz.*
Procaine hydrochloride (p.1319·1); phenol (p.1152·3).
Ear infections; earache.

Timpilo *Merck Sharp & Dohme, Aust.; Merck Sharp & Dohme, Austral.; Merck Frosst, Canad.; Merck Sharp & Dohme, Denm.; Merck Sharp & Dohme, Fin.; Merck Sharp & Dohme-Chibret, Fr.; Chibret, Ger.; Merck Sharp & Dohme, Hong Kong; Merck Sharp & Dohme, Israel; Merck Sharp & Dohme, Mex.; Merck Sharp & Dohme, Neth.; Merck Sharp & Dohme, Norw.; Merck Sharp & Dohme, NZ; Merck Sharp & Dohme, Singapore; Merck Sharp & Dohme, Swed.; Merck Sharp & Dohme, Switz.*
Timolol maleate (p.982·1); pilocarpine hydrochloride (p.1422·3).
Glaucoma; ocular hypertension.

Timpron *Berk, UK.*
Naproxen (p.60·3).
Gout; musculoskeletal and joint disorders.

Timunox *Janssen-Cilag, Ital.*
Thymopentin (p.1672·3).
Immunodeficiency.

Tina *Biolab, Thai.*
Cyproterone acetate (p.1467·3); ethinylestradiol (p.1476·2).
Androgen-dependent acne, alopecia, and hirsutism in females; oral contraceptive in women with androgenic symptoms.

Tinactin *Schering, Canad.; Schering-Plough, USA.*
Tolnaftate (p.395·2).
Fungal skin infections.

Tinaderm *Schering-Plough, Austral.; Schering-Plough, Irl.; Schering-Plough, Ital.; Schering-Plough, Mex.; Schering-Plough, NZ; Schering-Plough, S.Afr.; Schering-Plough, Singapore; Schering-Plough, Spain; Schering-Plough, UK.*
Tolnaftate (p.395·2).
Fungal skin, hair, and nail infections.

Tinaderm Extra *Schering-Plough, Austral.*
Clotrimazole (p.382·1).
Fungal skin infections.

Tinaderme *Plough, Port.*
Tolnaftate (p.395·2).
Fungal skin and nail infections.

Tinaderm-M *Schering-Plough, Irl.; Schering-Plough, UK.*
Tolnaftate (p.395·2); nystatin (p.392·2).
Fungal skin and nail infections.

Tinagel *Schering-Plough, Belg.; Schering-Plough, Neth.†.*
Benzoyl peroxide (p.1111·1).
Acne.

Tinaroc-Combi *Orion, Fin.*
Tablets (morning), phenylpropanolamine hydrochloride (Tinaroc) (p.1098·1); tablets (evening), phenylpro-

panolamine hydrochloride; carbinoxamine maleate (Tinaroc-A) (p.411·1).
Allergic rhinitis.

Tinasol *Fischer, Israel.*
Tolnaftate (p.395·2).
Fungal skin infections.

Tinatox *Riemser, Ger.*
Tolnaftate (p.395·2).
Fungal skin infections.

Tinazole *General Drugs, Thai.*
Tinidazole (p.603·3).
Amoebiasis; giardiasis; trichomoniasis.

TinBen *Ferndale, USA.*
Barrier preparation.

TinCoBen *Ferndale, USA.*
Barrier preparation.

Tinctura Justi *Pascoe, Ger.†.*
Homoeopathic preparation.

Tine Test PPD *Lederle, USA.*
Tuberculin purified protein derivative (p.1675·3).
Diagnosis of tuberculosis.

Tineafax *Note. This name is used for preparations of different composition.*
Glaxo Wellcome, Aust.†.
Ointment: Zinc undecenoate (p.395·3); zinc naphthenate; mesulphen (p.1118·3); methyl salicylate (p.55·1); terpineol (p.1669·3).
Topical powder: Zinc undecenoate (p.395·3); methyl salicylate (p.55·1); eucalyptus oil (p.1609·2).
Douglas, Austral.
Tolnaftate (p.395·2).
Tinea pedis.

Tinerol *Roche, Spain.*
Ornidazole (p.599·1).
Amoebiasis; anaerobic bacterial infections; giardiasis.

Ting *Ciba, USA.*
Miconazole nitrate (p.391·1).
Formerly contained tolnaftate.
Fungal skin infections.

Tini *Codal Synto, Thai.*
Tinidazole (p.603·3).
Amoebiasis; anaerobic bacterial infections; giardiasis; trichomoniasis.

Tiniazol *Liferpal, Mex.*
Ketoconazole (p.389·1).
Fungal skin, nail, and vaginal infections.

Tinnitin *Sanova, Aust.*
Caroverine hydrochloride (p.1591·3).
Smooth muscle spasm; tinnitus.

Tinset *Janssen-Cilag, Aust.; Janssen-Cilag, Belg.; Janssen-Cilag, Fr.; Janssen-Cilag, Ger.†; Cilag, Hong Kong; Formenti, Ital.; Janssen, Mex.; Taxandria, Neth.; Janssen-Cilag, Port.; Janssen-Cilag, S.Afr.; Janssen, Thai.*
Oxatomide (p.422·1).
Hypersensitivity reactions.

Tintorine *Bipharma, Neth.*
Salicylic acid (p.1122·3); lactic acid (p.1626·2).
Warts.

Tintu. Mertiolato Asens *Asens, Spain†.*
Thiomersal (p.1158·2); monoethanolamine.
Skin disinfection.

Tintura Benjui *Orion, Fin.*
Camphor (p.1589·3); menthol (p.1632·3).
Respiratory-tract congestion.

Tintura de Salsa Caroba e Manaca *Dansk-Flama, Braz.*
Parsley (p.1648·3); jacaranda caroba; brunfelsia hopeana; sassafras; sarsaparilla (p.1661·1).

Tintus *Orion, Fin.*
Guaifenesin (p.1092·2).
Coughs.

Tinver *Pilkington Barnes-Hind, USA.*
Sodium thiosulfate (p.1024·2); salicylic acid (p.1122·3); isopropyl alcohol (p.1149·2).
Pityriasis versicolor.

Tiobarbital *Braun, Spain.*
Thiopental sodium (p.1269·1).
Epilepsy; general anaesthesia.

Tiobec *Pharma-Natura, Ital.*
Thioctic acid (p.1671·3); vitamins (p.1350·1).
Neuropathies; nutritional supplement.

Tiocalmina *Ottolenghi, Ital.*
Sulfogaiacol (p.1101·1); dropropizine (p.1089·3).
Coughs.

Tiocosol *OFF, Ital.*
Sulfogaiacol (p.1101·1); sodium benzoate (p.1134·3).
Formerly contained sulfogaiacol, sodium benzoate, tolu balsam, and grindelia.
Bronchial congestion; coughs.

Tioctan *Note. This name is used for preparations of different composition.*
Rothpharma, Ital.; Fujisawa, Jpn.
Thioctic acid (p.1671·3).
Diabetic neuropathy; subacute necrotising encephalomyelopathy; thioctic acid supplement; vestibular deafness.
Leiras, Fin.
Vitamin B substances (p.1350·1).
Vitamin B deficiency.

Tioctidasi *ISI, Ital.†.*
Ethylenediamine thioctate (p.1671·3).
Liver disorders.

Tiof *Novag, Mex.*
Timolol (p.982·2).

Tiofeniclin *Sanofi Winthrop, Mex.*
Thiamphenicol (p.261·3).
Bacterial infections.

Tioguaialina *Montefarmaco, Ital.*
Sulfogaiacol (p.1101·1).
Catarrh; coughs.

Tionamil *Ogna, Ital.*
Sulfogaiacol (p.1101·1); sodium benzoate (p.1134·3);
terpin hydrate (p.1101·2).
Coughs.

Tioner *Grunenthal, Spain.*
Tramadol hydrochloride (p.89·1).
Pain.

Tiorfan *Bioprojet, Fr.*
Racecadotril (p.1245·2).
Diarrhoea.

Tiosalprin *Salus, Mex.*
Azathioprine (p.509·3).

Tioscina *Inverni della Beffa, Ital.†*
Aescin (p.1574·1); thiocolchicoside (p.1330·2).
Inflammation; musculoskeletal and soft-tissue disorders.

Tiosol *União Quimica, Braz.*
Sulfiram (p.1437·2).
Scabies.

Tioten *Therabel, Ital.†*
Stepronin sodium (p.1101·1).
Respiratory-tract congestion.

Tiotil *Abigo, Swed.*
Propylthiouracil (p.1525·3).
Hyperthyroidism.

Tiovalone *Juste, Spain.*
Tixocortol pivalate (p.1080·1).
Nasal polyps; rhinitis.

Tioxal *Solfran, Mex.*
Vitamin B₁₂; vitamin B₆ (p.1350·1).

TIP *Farmalider, Spain.*
Dextromethorphan hydrobromide (p.1087·3).
Coughs.

Tiparol *Astra, Swed.*
Tramadol hydrochloride (p.89·1).
Pain.

Tiperal *Clonmel, Irl.*
Propranolol hydrochloride (p.962·3).
Angina pectoris; anxiety; arrhythmias; essential tremor; hypertension; migraine; myocardial infarction; obstructive cardiomyopathy; phaeochromocytoma.

Tipidin *DHA, Singapore.*
Ticlopidine hydrochloride (p.981·1).
Intermittent claudication; stroke prophylaxis.

Tipkin *TP, Thai.*
Amikacin sulfate (p.148·1).
Gram-negative bacterial infections.

Tiplac *Euro-Labor, Port.*
Lysine aspirin (p.50·3).
Thrombosis prophylaxis.

Tipodex *Ern, Spain.*
Famotidine (p.1225·3).
Gastro-oesophageal reflux; peptic ulcer; Zollinger-Ellison syndrome.

Tiprocin *Clonmel, Irl.*
Erythromycin ethyl succinate (p.201·2).
Bacterial infections.

Tipuric *Clonmel, Irl.*
Allopurinol (p.397·2).
Gout; prophylaxis of uric acid and calcium oxalate stones.

Tiq'Aouta *Clement, Fr.*
Diethyltoluamide (p.1431·2); dimethyl phthalate (p.1431·3); enoxolone (p.34·3).
Insect repellent.

Tiracaspa *QIF, Braz.*
Cetrimonium bromide (p.1137·3).
Seborrhoeic dermatitis.

Tiracrin *Geymonat, Ital.*
Thyroxine [levothyroxine] sodium (p.1526·2).
Formerly contained iodothyreoglobulin.
Hypothyroidism.

Tirakallos *Dakota, Braz.*
Salicylic acid (p.1612·3); lactic acid (p.1626·2).
Keratinisation disorders.

Tirend *SmithKline Beecham, USA†.*
Caffeine (p.761·3).
Fatigue.

Tirgon N *Woelm, Ger.*
Bisacodyl (p.1212·2).
Constipation.

Tirocal *Cryopharma, Mex.*
Calcitriol (p.1391·1).
Hypocalcaemia; hypoparathyroidism; osteoporosis; renal osteodystrophy; rickets.

Tirocular *Angelini, Ital.*
Acetylcysteine (p.1082·3).
Corneal disorders; dry eyes.

Tirodril *Estedi, Spain.*
Methimazole [thiamazole] (p.1525·1).
Hyperthyroidism.

Tiroide Amsa *Amsa, Ital.*
Thyroxine [levothyroxine] sodium (p.1526·2); liothyronine sodium (p.1524·2).
Hypothyroidism.

Tiroidine *Rudefsa, Mex.*
Thyroxine [levothyroxine] sodium (p.1526·2).
Hypothyroidism.

Tirolaxo *Edigen, Spain†.*
Docusate sodium (p.1223·1).
Constipation.

Tiroler Steinol *Tiroler, Aust.*
Yellow soft paraffin (p.1407·3); yellow beeswax (p.1408·2); hydrous wool fat (p.1411·2); white soft paraffin (p.1407·3).
Skin disorders.

Tirosint *Amsa, Ital.*
Thyroxine [levothyroxine] sodium (p.1526·2).
Hypothyroidism.

Tirs *Difa, Ital.*
Benzalkonium chloride (p.1133·2); hypromellose (p.1501·3).
Dry eyes; eye disinfection.

Tisamid *Orion, Fin.*
Pyrazinamide (p.240·1).
Tuberculosis.

Tisana Arnaldi *Arnaldi-Uscio, Ital.†.*
Senna (p.1248·2); frangula bark (p.1227·1); liquorice (p.1231·2); boldo leaves (p.1585·3); chinese rhubarb (p.1248·1); greater celandine (p.1618·1); couch-grass root (p.1599·3); saponaria root; dulcamara (p.1606·2); melissa leaves (p.1632·2); angelica root (p.1580·2); viola tricolor flowers.
Constipation.

Tisana Cisbey *Geymonat, Ital.†.*
Rhubarb (p.1248·1); liquorice (p.1231·2); couch-grass (p.1599·3); peppermint leaf (p.1243·2); parietaria; melissa (p.1632·2); fennel (p.1610·1); coriander (p.1599·2); mallow.
Digestive disorders; sleep disorders.

Tisana Kelemata *Kelemata, Ital.*
Tablets; granules: Senna (p.1248·2).
Teabags; tea: Senna (p.1248·2); couch-grass (p.1599·3); guaiacum; hyssop; parietaria; peppermint (p.1243·2); sarsaparilla (p.1661·1); aniseed (p.1580·2); melissa (p.1632·2).
Constipation.

Tisane Antibiliaire et Stomachique *Denolin, Belg.*
Senna (p.1248·2); frangula bark (p.1227·1); althaea (p.1577·1); peppermint leaf (p.1243·2); cnicus benedictus (p.1597·2); rosemary; melilotus officinalis (p.1231·2); calendula flower (p.1589·2); mallow flower; fennel (p.1610·1); aniseed (p.1580·2); tilia (p.1673·2).
Biliary-tract congestion; digestive disorders.

Tisane antiflatulente pour les enfants *Sidroga, Switz.*
Fennel (p.1610·1); chamomile (p.1593·2); tilia (p.1673·2); melissa (p.1632·2); peppermint leaf (p.1243·2); vervain (p.1679·3).
Flatulence.

Tisane antirhumatismale *Sidroga, Switz.*
Spearmint (p.1666·3); passion flower (p.1649·1); salix (p.82·1); stevia rebaudiana.
Rheumatism.

Tisane calmante pour les enfants *Sidroga, Switz.*
Valerian (p.1678·3); lupulus (p.1629·3); melissa (p.1632·2); orange flowers; passion flower (p.1649·1).
Nervous excitement; sleep disorders.

Tisane Clairo *Weleda, Fr.†.*
Aniseed (p.1580·2); clove (p.1596·3); peppermint leaf (p.1243·2); senna leaflets (p.1248·2).
Constipation.

Tisane Contre la Tension *Denolin, Belg.*
Mistletoe (p.1636·2); frangula bark (p.1227·1); crataegus (p.1600·2); orthosiphonis stamineus (p.1625·1); bearberry (p.1583·3); curcuma zanthorrhiza; passion flower (p.1649·1); olive leaf; star anise; peppermint leaf (p.1243·2).
Hypertension.

Tisane contre les refroidissements *Sidroga, Switz.*
Rose fruit (p.1389·3); sambucus (p.1660·3); chamomile (p.1593·2); tilia (p.1673·2); wild thyme.
Cold symptoms.

Tisane Depurative "les 12 Plantes" *Denolin, Belg.*
Sarsaparilla (p.1661·1); lappa (p.1627·1); fumitory (p.1612·3); parietaria; saponaria; senna (p.1248·2); frangula bark (p.1227·1); liquorice (p.1231·2); peppermint leaf (p.1243·2); mallow flower; calendula flower (p.1589·2); fennel (p.1610·1); angelica (p.1580·2); star anise.
Digestive disorders; kidney disorders; skin eruptions.

Tisane des Familles *Monot, Fr.*
Equisetum (p.1606·3); tilia (p.1673·2); senna (p.1248·2); peppermint (p.1243·2); althaea (p.1577·1); liquorice (p.1231·2); parietaria; fennel (p.1610·1); melissa (p.1632·2); caraway (p.1591·2); sambucus (p.1660·3); ash; vervain (p.1679·3); cynara (p.1601·3); boldo (p.1585·3); aniseed (p.1580·2); frangula (p.1227·1); meadowsweet (p.1631·2).
Constipation.

Tisane Digestive Weleda *Weleda, Fr.†.*
Achillea (p.1572·2); aniseed (p.1580·2); caraway (p.1591·2); fennel (p.1610·1); chamomile (p.1593·2).
Gastrointestinal disorders.

Tisane Diuretique
Note. This name is used for preparations of different composition.
Denolin, Belg.
Bearberry (p.1583·3); juniper (p.1625·2); meadowsweet (p.1631·2); fraxinus excelsior; cynodontis root; liquorice (p.1231·2); calendula flower (p.1589·2); star anise; calluna; angelica (p.1580·2); fennel (p.1610·1); tritici root.
Kidney and urinary disorders.

Sidroga, Switz.
Birch (p.1585·2); bean pods; urtica (p.1678·2); equisetum (p.1606·3).
Urinary-tract disorders.

Tisane favorisant l'allaitement *Sidroga, Switz.*
Aniseed (p.1580·2); fennel (p.1610·1); caraway (p.1591·2); melissa (p.1632·2).
Lactation stimulant.

Tisane Grande Chartreuse *Aerocid, Fr.*
Marjoram; althaea (p.1577·1); liquorice (p.1231·2); senna (p.1248·2); frangula (p.1227·1); melissa (p.1632·2); peppermint (p.1243·2); ash; parietaria; coriander (p.1599·2).
Constipation; skin disorders of digestive origin.

Tisane Hepatique de Hoerdt *Wieger, Fr.*
Absinthium (p.1571·1); achillea (p.1572·2); agrimony (p.1574·3); boldo (p.1585·3); centaury (p.1593·1); couch-grass (p.1599·3); menyanthes (p.1633·1); sage (p.1660·2).
Liver and biliary-tract disorders.

Tisane hepatique et biliaire *Sidroga, Switz.*
Cynara (p.1601·3); boldo (p.1585·3); taraxacum (p.1669·1); silybum marianum (p.1021·3); peppermint leaf (p.1243·2); achillea (p.1572·2).
Digestive system disorders.

Tisane laxative *Sidroga, Switz.*
Frangula bark (p.1227·1); fennel (p.1610·1); senna (p.1248·2); star anise; liquorice (p.1231·2).
Constipation.

Tisane laxative H nouvelle formulation *Hanseler, Switz.*
Sambucus (p.1660·3); senna (p.1248·2); aniseed (p.1580·2); fennel (p.1610·1); mint (p.1666·3).
Constipation.

Tisane laxative Natterman no 13 *Piraud, Switz.†*
Senna (p.1248·2); aniseed (p.1580·2); caraway (p.1591·2); coriander (p.1599·2); fennel (p.1610·1); juniper (p.1625·2); liquorice (p.1231·2).
Constipation.

Tisane laxative Natterman no 13 instant *Piraud, Switz.†.*
Senna (p.1248·2); liquorice (p.1231·2).
Constipation.

Tisane Mexicaine *Medecine Vegetale, Fr.†*
Red vine leaf; boldo leaf (p.1585·3); frangula bark (p.1227·1); hyssop; rosemary; ash leaf; senna leaf (p.1248·2).
Venous-lymphatic insufficiency.

Tisane Orientale Soker *Medecine Vegetale, Fr.†.*
Arenaria; parietaria; couch-grass root (p.1599·3); bearberry leaves (p.1583·3); corn silk (p.1599·3).
Urinary infections; water retention.

Tisane Pectorale *Denolin, Belg.*
Poppy capsule (p.1099·2); star anise; liquorice (p.1231·2); carrageenan (p.1500·1); hedera terrestris (p.1618·2); hyssop; angelica (p.1580·2); althaea (p.1577·1); mallow flower; calendula flower (p.1589·2); tilia (p.1673·2).
Coughs.

Tisane pectorale et antitussive *Sidroga, Switz.*
Sage (p.1660·2); althaea (p.1577·1); fennel (p.1610·1); iceland moss; red-poppy petal (p.1029·1); plantaginis; star anise; liquorice (p.1231·2); thyme (p.1672·2).
Coughs and congestion.

Tisane pectorale pour les enfants *Sidroga, Switz.*
Althaea (p.1577·1); cowslip flower (p.1600·1); plantain (p.1652·3); liquorice (p.1231·2); thyme (p.1672·2).
Cold symptoms.

Tisane pour Dormir *Denolin, Belg.*
Poppy capsule (p.1099·2); citrus aurantium; chamomile (p.1593·2); crataegus (p.1600·2); star anise; sage (p.1660·2); peppermint leaf (p.1243·2).
Insomnia; nervous disorders.

Tisane pour le coeur et la circulation *Sidroga, Switz.*
Birch (p.1585·2); motherwort (p.1637·3); spearmint (p.1666·3); melissa (p.1632·2); crataegus (p.1600·2).
Cardiac and circulatory disorders.

Tisane pour le Foie *Denolin, Belg.*
Curcuma zanthorrhiza; fabianae imbricatae; boldo (p.1585·3); cynara scolymus (p.1601·3); kinkeliba (p.1626·1); senna (p.1248·2); peppermint leaf (p.1243·2); melissa (p.1632·2); aniseed (p.1580·2); vervain (p.1679·3); liquorice (p.1231·2); tilia (p.1673·2); calendula flower (p.1589·2).
Biliary-tract congestion; digestive disorders.

Tisane pour le sommeil et les nerfs *Sidroga, Switz.*
Valerian (p.1678·3); lupulus (p.1629·3); spearmint (p.1666·3); melissa (p.1632·2); orange flower.
Nervousness; sleep disorders.

Tisane pour les enfants *Sidroga, Switz.†.*
Fennel (p.1610·1); matricaria (p.1593·2); tilia (p.1673·2); melissa (p.1632·2); peppermint leaf (p.1243·2); vervain (p.1679·3).
Agitation; muscular contractures; sleep disorders.

Tisane pour les reins et la vessie *Sidroga, Switz.*
Bearberry (p.1583·3); birch (p.1585·2); Java tea (p.1625·1); lovage root (p.1629·3); peppermint leaf (p.1243·2); juniper (p.1625·2).
Formerly contained bearberry, birch, boldo, angelica, rose fruit, lovage, tilia, mallow flowers, orthosiphon, peppermint leaf, equisetum, juniper, and juglans regia.
Urinary-tract disorders.

Tisane pour l'estomac *Sidroga, Switz.*
Calamus (p.1588·1); matricaria (p.1593·2); spearmint (p.1666·3); melissa (p.1632·2); achillea (p.1572·2); centaury (p.1593·1).
Gastrointestinal disorders.

Tisane Purgative *Denolin, Belg.*
Senna (p.1248·2); frangula bark (p.1227·1); peppermint leaf (p.1243·2); althaea (p.1577·1); fennel (p.1610·1); aniseed (p.1580·2); calendula flower

(p.1589·2); mallow flower; angelica (p.1580·2); liquorice (p.1231·2); melissa (p.1632·2).
Constipation; digestive disorders.

Tisane relaxante *Sidroga, Switz.*
Valerian (p.1678·3); achillea (p.1572·2); lavender flower (p.1627·2); melissa (p.1632·2); passion flower (p.1649·1).
Nervous tension.

Tisane Sedative Weleda *Weleda, Fr.†.*
Lavender (p.1627·2); valerian (p.1678·3); mallow flowers.
Insomnia; nervous disorders.

Tisane Touraine *Pharmacie Principale, Fr.†.*
Ash; vervain (p.1679·3); asperule; parietaria; meadowsweet (p.1631·2); melissa (p.1632·2); peppermint (p.1243·2); melissa (p.1632·2); frangula (p.1227·1); centaurea cyanus; senna (p.1248·2).
Constipation.

Tisanes de l'Abbe Hamon no 3 *Aerocid, Fr.*
Frangula (p.1227·1); viola; convallaria (p.1599·1); equisetum (p.1606·3); ash; meadowsweet (p.1631·2); maize (p.1599·3); centaurea cyanus; hazel.
Arthritis; gout; pain; sciatica.

Tisanes de l'Abbe Hamon no 6 *Aerocid, Fr.*
Asperule; oranger; passion flower (p.1649·1); waterlily; sage (p.1660·2); calendula (p.1589·2); mistletoe (p.1636·2); tilia (p.1673·2); lyciet.
Nervous disorders.

Tisanes de l'Abbe Hamon no 11 *Aerocid, Fr.*
Bladderwrack (p.1585·2); yellow dock (p.1681·3); couch-grass (p.1599·3); liquorice (p.1231·2); hazel.
Obesity.

Tisanes de l'Abbe Hamon no 14 *Aerocid, Fr.†.*
Groundsel; achillea (p.1572·2); viburnum; shepherd's purse (p.1662·3); oak (p.1643·2); cupressus sempervirens; lemon verbena (p.1628·3); asperule; liquorice (p.1231·2); hazel; calendula (p.1589·2); centaurea cyanus; euphorbia (p.1609·3).
Circulatory disorders.

Tisanes de l'Abbe Hamon no 15 *Aerocid, Fr.†.*
Elecampane (p.1089·3); comfrey (p.1598·3); erysimum; marrube (p.1094·2); borage (p.1586·1); bugloss; eucalyptus (p.1609·2); hazel; sticta pulmonaria.
Respiratory-tract disorders.

Tisanes de l'Abbe Hamon no 16 *Aerocid, Fr.†.*
Lappa (p.1627·1); carrot; centaury (p.1593·1); thistle-roland; scoparium (p.1661·2); gratiola; convallaria (p.1599·1); hazel; liquorice (p.1231·2).
Liver disorders.

Tisanes de l'Abbe Hamon no 17 *Aerocid, Fr.†.*
Globulaire; frangula (p.1227·1); mint (p.1666·3); mercurial; hazel; rhapontic rhubarb (p.1248·1).
Constipation.

Tisatin *Arlex, Mex.*
Phenylbutazone (p.78·1).

Tisept *Seton, Israel; SSL, UK.*
Cetrimide (p.1137·1); chlorhexidine gluconate (p.1138·2).
Skin, burn, and wound disinfection.

Tisercin *Thiemann, Ger.†.*
Methotrimeprazine [levomepromazine] (p.691·3) or methotrimeprazine [levomepromazine] maleate (p.692·1).
Pain; psychoses.

Tisit *Pfeiffer, USA.*
Pyrethrins; piperonyl butoxide (p.1436·2).
Pediculosis.

TiSol *Parnell, USA.*
Benzyl alcohol (p.1135·2); menthol (p.1632·3).
Minor mouth or throat irritation.

Tisplal *Rhone-Poulenc Rorer, Mex.*
Cisplatin (p.525·1).

Tispol Ibu-DD *Woelm, Ger.*
Ibuprofen lysine (p.44·1).
Fever; pain.

Tispol S *Woelm, Ger.†*
Propyphenazone (p.80·2); paracetamol (p.71·2).
Toothache.

Tisseel
Baxter, Canad.; Immuno, Hong Kong; Immuno, Irl.; Immuno, Israel; Adcock-Ingram Critical Care, S.Afr.; Baxter, UK.
1 Vial, fibrinogen (p.736·1); fibronectin (p.1611·1); factor XIII (p.735·3); plasminogen (p.956·3); 1 vial, aprotinin (p.725·3); 1 vial, calcium chloride (p.1188·1); 2 vials, thrombin (p.741·3).
On mixing this forms a fibrin glue (p.735·3).
Wounds.

Tisseel Duo Quick
Baxter, Denm.; Baxter, Fin.; Baxter, Swed.
1 Vial, fibrinogen (p.736·1); fibronectin (p.1611·1); factor XIII (p.735·3); plasminogen (p.956·3); aprotinin (p.725·3); albumin (p.724·1); 1 vial, thrombin (p.741·3); plasma protein (p.740·2); calcium chloride (p.1188·1).
On mixing this forms a fibrin glue (p.735·3).
Haemorrhage.

Tissucol
Immuno, Aust.; Baxter, Belg.; Immuno, Braz.; Baxter, Fr.; Immuno, Ital.; Immuno, Spain; Baxter, Switz.
1 Vial, fibrinogen (p.736·1); fibronectin (p.1611·1); factor XIII (p.735·3); plasminogen (p.956·3); 1 vial, aprotinin (p.725·3); 2 vials, thrombin (p.741·3); 1 vial, calcium chloride (p.1188·1).
On mixing this forms a fibrin glue (p.735·3).
Haemorrhage; wounds.

Tissucol Duo Quick *Immuno, Aust.*
1 Vial, fibrinogen (p.736·1); fibronectin (p.1611·1); factor XIII (p.735·3); plasminogen (p.956·3); aprotinin (p.725·3); 1 vial, thrombin (p.741·3); calcium chloride

(p.1188·1)
On mixing this forms a fibrin glue (p.735·3).
Wounds.

Tissucol Duo S *Immuno, Ger.; Baxter, Switz.*
1 Vial, plasma protein (p.740·2); fibrinogen (p.736·1); fibronectin (p.1611·1); aprotinin (p.725·3); factor XIII (p.735·3); plasminogen (p.956·3); 1 vial, thrombin (p.741·3); calcium chloride (p.1188·1)
On mixing this forms a fibrin glue (p.735·3).
Haemorrhage.

Tissucol Fibrinkleber tiefgefroren *Immuno, Ger.†.*
1 Ampoule: plasma protein fraction (p.740·2); fibrinogen (p.736·1); fibronectin (p.1611·1); factor XIII (p.735·3); plasminogen (p.956·3); 1 application set: aprotinin (p.725·3); calcium chloride (p.1188·1); lotion: calcium chloride; thrombin (p.741·3)
On mixing this forms a fibrin glue (p.735·3).
Wounds.

Tissucol-Kit *Immuno, Ger.*
1 Ampoule: plasma protein fraction (p.740·2); fibrinogen (p.736·1); fibronectin (p.1611·1); factor XIII (p.735·3); plasminogen (p.956·3); 1 ampoule: aprotinin (p.725·3); 2 ampoules: thrombin (p.741·3); 1 ampoule: calcium chloride (p.1188·1)
On mixing this forms a fibrin glue (p.735·3).
Wounds.

TissuVlies *Immuno, Ger.†.*
Collagen (p.1598·2).
Haemorrhage.

Tisuderma *Cinfa, Spain.*
Hydrocortisone acetate (p.1073·3); neomycin sulfate (p.228·1).
Skin infections with inflammation.

Tis-U-Sol *Baxter, USA.*
Electrolytes (p.1180·1).
Irrigation solution.

Titan
Note.This name is used for preparations of different composition.
Durex, Canad.
Nonoxinol 9 (p.1346·1).
Contraceptive.

Pilkington Barnes-Hind, USA.
Cleansing solution for hard contact lenses (p.1129·2).

Titanorein *Abello, Spain.*
Carrageenan (p.1500·1); titanium dioxide (p.1126·1); lignocaine [lidocaine] (p.1313·2).
Haemorrhoids.

Titanoreine *Martin, Fr.; Martin, Switz.*
Cream; ointment: Carrageenan (p.1500·1); titanium dioxide (p.1126·1); zinc oxide (p.1128·2); lignocaine [lidocaine] (p.1313·2).
Anorectal disorders.

Martin, Fr.; Martin, Switz.
Suppositories: Carrageenan (p.1500·1); titanium dioxide (p.1126·1); zinc oxide (p.1128·2).
Anorectal disorders.

Tition *Pharmazam, Spain.*
Reduced glutathione (p.1010·3).
Hepatitis.

Titmus Losung 1 *Ciba Vision, Aust.*
Hydrogen peroxide (p.1147·1) (p.1129·2).
Disinfection and storage of contact lenses.

Titmus Losung 2 *Ciba Vision, Aust.*
Catalase (p.1592·2) (p.1129·2).
Neutralisation and rinsing of contact lenses.

Titralac
3M, Austral.; 3M, Hong Kong; 3M, NZ; 3M, S.Afr.; 3M, UK.
Calcium carbonate (p.1215·1); glycine.
Calcium supplement; dyspepsia; gastrointestinal hyperacidity; heartburn; hyperphosphataemia; peptic ulcer.

3M, Canad.†; Nycomed, Norw.
Calcium carbonate (p.1215·1).
Gastrointestinal disorders associated with hyperacidity.

Titralac Extra Strength *3M, USA.*
Calcium carbonate (p.1215·1).
Hyperacidity.

Titralac Plus *3M, USA.*
Calcium carbonate (p.1215·1); simeticone (p.1249·2).
Hyperacidity.

Titralac-Sil
3M, Austral.; 3M, NZ; 3M, Singapore.
Calcium carbonate (p.1215·1); simeticone (p.1249·2); glycine.
Dyspepsia; flatulence; gastric hyperacidity; gastritis; heartburn; peptic ulcer.

Titralgan *Berlin-Chemie, Ger.*
Phenazone (p.77·2); paracetamol (p.71·2); caffeine (p.761·3).
Fever; pain.

Titrane *CEPA, Spain†.*
Isosorbide mononitrate (p.916·2).
Angina pectoris; heart failure.

Ti-Tre *Teofarma, Ital.*
Liothyronine sodium (p.1524·2).
Hypothyroidism.

Titretta *Berlin-Chemie, Ger.*
Propyphenazone (p.80·2); codeine phosphate (p.25·2).
Pain.

Ti-U-Lac *Draxis, Canad.*
Urea (p.1127·3).

Ti-U-Lac HC *Spectropharm, Canad.*
Hydrocortisone (p.1073·3); urea (p.1127·3).
Skin disorders.

Ti-UVA-B *Draxis, Canad.*
SPF 22: Octinoxate (p.1517·3); oxybenzone (p.1518·1).
Sunscreen.

Tivitis *Llorens, Spain.*
Gramicidin (p.213·3); methylene blue [methylthioninium chloride] (p.1012·3); neomycin sulfate (p.228·1); polymyxin B sulfate (p.238·1); tetryzoline hydrochloride (p.1101·2).
Bacterial eye infections.

Tixair *Byk, Fr.*
Acetylcysteine (p.1082·3).
Mucolytic in respiratory-tract disorders.

Tixobar *Astra, Austral.*
Barium sulfate (p.1032·1).
Radiography of gastrointestinal tract.

Tixycolds *Novartis Consumer, UK.*
Diphenhydramine hydrochloride (p.416·1); pseudoephedrine hydrochloride (p.1099·2).
Cold and influenza symptoms.

Tixycolds Cold and Allergy *Novartis Consumer, UK.*
Xylometazoline hydrochloride (p.1102·2).
Nasal congestion; rhinitis.

Tixycolds Cold and Hayfever *Novartis Consumer, UK.*
Camphor (p.1589·3); menthol (p.1632·3); turpentine oil (p.1676·3); eucalyptus oil (p.1609·2).
Formerly known as Tixylix Inhalant.
Nasal congestion.

Tixylix
Note.This name is used for preparations of different composition.
Intercare, Irl.†.
Promethazine hydrochloride (p.423·2); pholcodine citrate (p.1099·1); phenylpropanolamine hydrochloride (p.1098·1).
Coughs.

Aventis, NZ.
Promethazine hydrochloride (p.423·2); pholcodine citrate (p.1099·1).
Coughs.

Aspen Consumer, S.Afr.
Promethazine hydrochloride (p.423·2); pholcodine (p.1099·1).
Formerly contained promethazine hydrochloride, pholcodine, and phenylpropanolamine hydrochloride.
Coughs and cold symptoms.

Tixylix Baby Syrup *Novartis Consumer, UK.*
Glycerol (p.1616·3).
Coughs.

Tixylix Catarrh *Novartis Consumer, UK†.*
Diphenhydramine hydrochloride (p.416·1); menthol (p.1632·3).
Nasal congestion.

Tixylix Chest Rub
Rhone-Poulenc Rorer, Austral.; Aventis, NZ.
Eucalyptol (p.1609·2); pine oil; rosemary oil (p.1659·3); thyme oil (p.1672·3); terpineol (p.1669·3).
Nasal congestion.

Tixylix Chesty Cough
Novartis Consumer, Irl.; Novartis Consumer, UK.
Guaifenesin (p.1092·2).
Coughs.

Tixylix Cough & Cold *Novartis Consumer, UK.*
Pseudoephedrine hydrochloride (p.1099·2); chlorpheniramine [chlorphenamine] maleate (p.412·1); pholcodine (p.1099·1).
Coughs and cold symptoms.

Tixylix Daytime
Note.This name is used for preparations of different composition.
Rhone-Poulenc Rorer, Austral.†.
Pseudoephedrine hydrochloride (p.1099·2).
Upper respiratory-tract congestion.

Novartis Consumer, UK.
Pholcodine (p.1099·1).
Coughs.

Tixylix Flu *Quatromed, S.Afr.*
Triprolidine hydrochloride (p.427·2); pseudoephedrine hydrochloride (p.1099·2).
Nasal congestion.

Tixylix Nightime
Rhone-Poulenc Rorer, Austral.; Rhone-Poulenc Rorer, Hong Kong.
Promethazine hydrochloride (p.423·2); pholcodine (p.1099·1).
Coughs.

Tixylix Night-Time *Novartis Consumer, UK.*
Promethazine hydrochloride (p.423·2); pholcodine (p.1099·1).
Formerly known as Tixylix Original.
Coughs.

Tixymol *Novartis Consumer, UK.*
Paracetamol (p.71·2).
Fever; pain.

T-KI *Seroyal, Canad.*
Vitamin A and vitamin C (p.1350·1).

T-Koff *Williams, USA†.*
Phenylpropanolamine hydrochloride (p.1098·1); phenylephrine hydrochloride (p.1097·1); chlorpheniramine [chlorphenamine] maleate (p.412·1); codeine phosphate (p.25·2).
Coughs and cold symptoms.

T-LI *Seroyal, Canad.*
Vitamin B substances, vitamin C, copper, and iron (p.1350·1).

TLM *Seroyal, Canad.*
Vitamin C and minerals (p.1350·1).

T-LU *Seroyal, Canad.*
Vitamins A, C, and E (p.1350·1).

T-MA *Seroyal, Canad.*
Vitamin A, vitamin E, and zinc (p.1350·1).

T-Medevax *Ribosepharm, Ger.†.*
An adsorbed tetanus vaccine (p.1565·2).
Active immunisation.

TMP *Pacific, NZ.*
Trimethoprim (p.264·2).
Bacterial infections of the urinary tract.

TMP-ratiopharm *Ratiopharm, Ger.*
Trimethoprim (p.264·2).
Bacterial infections of the urinary tract.

TMS *TAD, Ger.*
Co-trimoxazole (p.193·3).
Bacterial infections.

TNKase *Genentech, USA.*
Tenecteplase (p.979·3).
Myocardial infarction.

Toallet Benzal *Terrier, Mex.*
Benzalkonium.

Tobedoce *Jofrain, Mex.*
Vitamin B substances (p.1350·1).

Tobi
Amrad, Austral.; Pathogenesis, Canad.; Pathogenesis, UK; Pathogenesis, USA.
Tobramycin (p.263·3) or tobramycin sulfate (p.263·3).
Pseudomonal infections in cystic fibrosis.

Tobispray *Boehringer Ingelheim, Austral.†.*
Tramazoline hydrochloride (p.1102·1); dexamethasone isonicotinate (p.1067·1).
Allergic rhinitis.

Tobitil *Ranbaxy, S.Afr.*
Tenoxicam (p.87·2).
Dysmenorrhoea; gout; musculoskeletal, joint, and peri-articular disorders.

Tobra *Lilly, Mex.*
Tobramycin sulfate (p.263·3).
Bacterial infections.

Tobra Gobens *APS, Port.; Normon, Spain.*
Tobramycin sulfate (p.263·3).
Bacterial infections.

Tobra-cell *Cell Pharm, Ger.*
Tobramycin sulfate (p.263·3).
Bacterial infections.

Tobracil *Oftalder, Port.*
Tobramycin sulfate (p.263·3).
Bacterial eye infections.

Tobradex
Alcon, Belg.; Alcon, Braz.; Alcon, Canad.; Alcon, Fr.; Alcon, Hong Kong; Alcon, Ital.; Alcon, Neth.†; Alcon, NZ; Alcon, S.Afr.; Alcon, Singapore; Alcon Cusi, Spain; Alcon, Switz.; Alcon, Thai.; Alcon, UK; Alcon, USA.
Tobramycin (p.263·3); dexamethasone (p.1067·1).
Ear disorders; infected eye disorders.

Tobradistin *Dista, Spain.*
Tobramycin sulfate (p.263·3).
Bacterial infections.

Tobrafen *Alcon, Switz.*
Diclofenac sodium (p.30·3); tobramycin (p.263·3).
Postoperative eye inflammation.

Tobral *Alcon, Ital.*
Tobramycin (p.263·3).
Bacterial infections of the eye and external ear.

Tobralex
Alcon, Irl.; Alcon, UK†.
Tobramycin (p.263·3).
Bacterial eye infections.

Tobramaxin *Alcon, Ger.*
Tobramycin (p.263·3).
Bacterial infections.

Tobramina *Lilly, Braz.*
Tobramycin sulfate (p.263·3).
Bacterial infections.

Tobrasix *Lilly, Aust.*
Tobramycin sulfate (p.263·3).
Bacterial infections.

Tobrasol *Ocusoft, USA.*
Tobramycin (p.263·3).
Bacterial eye infections.

Tobrasone *Alcon, NZ.*
Tobramycin (p.263·3); fluorometholone acetate (p.1072·1).
Infected inflammatory eye disorders.

Tobrex
Alcon, Aust.; Alcon, Austral.; Alcon, Belg.; Alcon, Braz.; Alcon, Canad.; Alcon, Denm.; Alcon, Fin.; Alcon, Fr.; Alcon, Hong Kong; Alcon, Israel; FIRMA, Ital.; Alcon, Mex.; Alcon, Neth.†; Alcon, NZ; Alcon, Port.; Alcon, S.Afr.; Alcon, Singapore; Alcon Cusi, Spain; Alcon, Swed.; Alcon, Switz.; Alcon, Thai.; Alcon, UK; Alcon, USA.
Tobramycin (p.263·3) or tobramycin sulfate (p.263·3).
Bacterial eye infections.

Tobridavi *Davi, Port.*
Tobramycin (p.263·3).
Bacterial eye infections.

Tobutol *General Drugs, Thai.*
Ethambutol hydrochloride (p.205·1).
Tuberculosis.

Tocalfa
Note.This name is used for preparations of different composition.
Cipharm, Fr.†.
dl-Alpha tocoferil acetate (p.1394·1).
Vitamin E deficiency.

Asta Medica, Ital.
dl-Alpha tocoferil acetate (p.1394·1); vitamin A esters (p.1382·1).
Vitamin A and E deficiency.

Tocid *TO-Chemicals, Singapore.*
Aluminium hydroxide-magnesium carbonate co-dried gel (p.1211·2); dicyclomine [dicycloverine] hydrochloride (p.466·1); simeticone (p.1249·2).
Duodenitis; dyspepsia; flatulence; gastric hyperacidity; gastritis; gastro-oesophageal reflux; gastrointestinal motility disorders; heartburn; peptic ulcer; pylorospasm.

Toclase *UCB, Denm.; UCB, Fin.; UCB, Hong Kong; UCB, Norw.; Vedim, Port.†; UCB, Swed.; UCB, Thai.*
Pentoxyverine (p.1096·3), pentoxyverine citrate (p.1096·3), or pentoxyverine hydrochloride (p.1096·3).
Coughs.

Toclase Expectorant
Note.This name is used for preparations of different composition.
UCB, Fin.
Pentoxyverine citrate (p.1096·3); terpin hydrate (p.1101·2).
Coughs.

Darci, Fr.
Carbocisteine (p.1086·3).
Respiratory-tract disorders.

Toclase Toux Seche *Darci, Fr.*
Pentoxyverine citrate (p.1096·3).
Coughs.

Toco *Pharma 2000, Fr.*
Alpha tocoferil acetate (p.1394·1).
Hyperlipidaemia.

Tocodrine *Medichemie, Switz.*
Buphenine hydrochloride (p.1587·3).
Inhibition of uterine contraction.

Tocogen *Abiogen, Ital.*
d-Alpha tocoferil acetate (p.1394·1).
Cardiac stenosis; diabetes mellitus; disorders of the female reproductive system; muscular dystrophy; peripheral vascular disorders.

Tocogestan *Theramex, Mon.*
Hydroxyprogesterone enantate (p.1479·3); progesterone (p.1488·3); dl-alpha tocoferil palmitate (p.1394·3).
Premature labour; threatened abortion.

Tocolion *Sciencex, Fr.*
Alpha tocoferil acetate (p.1394·1).
Hyperlipidaemias.

Tocomine *Parke, Davis, Fr.*
dl-Alpha tocoferil acetate (p.1394·1).
Vitamin E deficiency.

Tocomizol *Tocogino, Mex.*
Ketoconazole (p.389·1).
Fungal infections.

Toconal *Cryopharma, Mex.*
Ketoconazole (p.389·1).
Fungal infections.

Tocopa *Arkopharma, Fr.*
Alpha tocoferil acetate (p.1394·1).
Formerly known as Tocophan.
Hyperlipidaemias.

Tocorell *Sanorell, Ger.*
d-Alpha tocopherol (p.1393·3) or d-α-tocoferil acetate (p.1394·1).
Formerly contained d-alpha tocopherol.
Vitamin E deficiency.

Tocovenos *Fresenius, Ger.†.*
dl-Alpha tocoferil acetate (p.1394·1).
Vitamin E deficiency.

Tocovid *Hovid, Singapore.*
Vitamin E; squalene; phytosterol complex; phyto-carotenoid complex; ubidecarenone (p.1350·1).
Vitamin E supplement.

Tocovital *Steigerwald, Ger.*
d-Alpha tocoferil acetate (p.1394·1).
Vitamin E deficiency.

Todalgil *Aldo, Spain†.*
Ibuprofen (p.43·2).
Fever; musculoskeletal, joint, and peri-articular disorders; pain.

Today *Wyeth, UK; Whitehall, USA†.*
Nonoxinol 9 (p.1346·1).
Contraceptive.

Todolac *Leo, Denm.*
Etodolac (p.35·2).
Gout; inflammation; musculoskeletal and joint disorders.

Toepedo *Dendron, UK.*
Benzoic acid (p.1134·2); salicylic acid (p.1122·3).
Fungal skin infections.

Tofen *Utopian, Thai.*
Ibuprofen (p.43·2).
Inflammation; musculoskeletal and joint disorders; pain.

Toflex *TO-Chemicals, Thai.*
Cefalexin (p.161·3).
Bacterial infections.

Tofranil
Novartis, Aust.; Novartis, Austral.; Novartis, Belg.; Novartis, Braz.; Novartis, Canad.; Novartis, Fr.; Novartis, Ger.; Novartis, Hong Kong; Novartis, Irl.; Novartis, Israel; Novartis, Ital.; Novartis, Mex.; Novartis, Neth.; Novartis, Norw.†; Novartis, Port.; Novartis, S.Afr.; Novartis,

---

The symbol † denotes a preparation no longer actively marketed

Spain; Novartis, Swed.; Novartis, Switz.; Novartis, Thai.; Novartis, UK; Geigy, USA.
Imipramine (p.291·1), imipramine embonate (p.291·1), or imipramine hydrochloride (p.291·1).
Depression; nocturnal enuresis; pain; panic attacks.

Tofranil-PM Novartis, USA.
Imipramine embonate (p.291·1).
Depression.

Togal
Note. This name is used for preparations of different composition.
Sanova, Aust.; Togal, Ger.
Tablets: Aspirin (p.14·2); lithium citrate (p.292·1); quinine dihydrochloride (p.445·1).
Fever; inflammation; pain.

Togal, Ger.
Suppositories: Paracetamol (p.71·2).
Fever; pain.

Togal ASS
Togal, Ger.; Togal, Switz.
Aspirin (p.14·2).
Fever; inflammation; pain.

Togal Kopfschmerzbrause + Vit C Togal, Ger.
Aspirin (p.14·2); ascorbic acid (p.1389·3); caffeine (p.761·3).
Pain.

Togal Mobil Rheuma-Bad Togal, Ger.
Camphor (p.1589·3); benzyl nicotinate (p.20·2); Norway spruce oil; rosemary oil (p.1659·3).
Bath additive; circulatory disorders; musculoskeletal, joint, peri-articular, and soft-tissue disorders.

Togal Mobil-Gel Togal, Ger.
Glycol salicylate (p.42·2); benzyl nicotinate (p.20·2).
Musculoskeletal and soft-tissue disorders.

Togal N Togal, Ger.
Ibuprofen (p.43·2).
Fever; pain.

Togamycin Pharmacia Upjohn, Israel.
Spectinomycin hydrochloride (p.248·2).
Gonorrhoea.

Togasan Togal, Ger.
dl-Alpha tocopherol (p.1394·1) or dl-alpha tocoferil acetate (p.1394·1).
Vitamin E deficiency.

Togrisol Solfran, Mex.
Aspirin (p.14·2); caffeine (p.761·3).
Cold symptoms.

Toilax Orion, Denm.; Ercopharm, Fin.; Orion, Irl.; Orion, Norw.; Orion, Swed.
Bisacodyl (p.1212·2).
Bowel evacuation; constipation.

Tokovitan Orion, Fin.
d-Alpha tocoferil acetate (p.1394·1).
Vitamin E deficiency.

Tolan Solfran, Mex.
Methyl salicylate (p.55·1).

Tolanase Pharmacia Upjohn, Irl.†; Pharmacia Upjohn, UK†.
Tolazamide (p.336·2).
Diabetes mellitus.

Tolbin Unison, Singapore.
Terbutaline sulfate (p.776·2).
Obstructive airways disease; premature labour.

Tolchicine TO-Chemicals, Thai.
Colchicine (p.400·1).
Gout.

Toldex Bial, Port.
Aspirin (p.14·2).

Tolecen Centrum, Spain.
Hypericum (p.290·2).
Asthenia; sleep disorders.

Tolectin Janssen-Cilag, Aust.; Janssen-Cilag, Belg.; Janssen-Ortho, Canad.; Janssen-Cilag, Denm.; Janssen-Cilag, Fr.; Janssen-Cilag, Ital.; Janssen-Cilag, Mex.; Janssen-Cilag, Neth.; Janssen-Cilag, S.Afr.†; Janssen-Cilag, Switz.; Janssen-Cilag, UK†; Ortho McNeil, USA.
Tolmetin (p.89·1) or tolmetin sodium (p.88·3).
Inflammation; musculoskeletal, joint, peri-articular, and soft-tissue disorders; pain.

Tolerex Novartis Nutrition, Canad.; Novartis, Israel; Procter & Gamble, USA.
Preparation for enteral nutrition (p.1350·1).

Toleriane Roche-Posay, Irl.
Emollient.
Dry skin.

Tolexine Biorga, Fr.; Biorga, Hong Kong.
Doxycycline (p.200·1).
Bacterial infections.

Tolfrinic Ascher, USA.
Ferrous fumarate (p.1360·1); cyanocobalamin (p.1388·1).
Ascorbic acid (p.1389·3) is included in this preparation to increase the absorption and availability of iron.
Iron-deficiency anaemias.

Tolid Dolorgiet, Ger.
Lorazepam (p.688·3).
Anxiety; sleep disorders.

Toliman Scharper, Ital.
Cinnarizine (p.413·1).
Cerebral and peripheral vascular disorders.

Tolimed Medifive, Thai.
Mianserin hydrochloride (p.298·1).
Depression.

Tolinase Upjohn, Neth.†; Pharmacia Upjohn, Swed.†; Upjohn, USA.
Tolazamide (p.336·2).
Diabetes mellitus.

Tolindol Meuse, Belg.
Proglumetacin (p.80·1).
Musculoskeletal, joint, and peri-articular disorders.

Tollwutglobulin Pasteur Merieux, Ger.†
A rabies immunoglobulin (p.1560·2).
Passive immunisation.

Tollwut-Impfstoff (HDC) Pasteur Merieux, Ger.
A rabies vaccine (human diploid cell) (p.1560·2).
Active immunisation.

Tolmicen Pharmacia Upjohn, Hong Kong; Pharmacia Upjohn, Ital.; Pharmacia Upjohn, NZ; Pharmacia Upjohn, Port.†
Tolciclate (p.395·2).
Fungal skin infections.

Tolmicol Carlo Erba, Braz.
Tolciclate (p.395·2).
Fungal skin infections.

Tolmin Durascan, Denm.
Mianserin hydrochloride (p.298·1).
Depression.

Tolnaderm Quimica y Farmacia, Mex.
Tolnaftate (p.395·2).

Tolodina Estedi, Spain.
Amoxicillin trihydrate (p.149·2).
Bacterial infections.

Toloxim Merck, Port.
Mebendazole (p.102·2).
Worm infections.

Toloxin Searle, Braz.
Note. This name is used for preparations of different composition.
Metamizole magnesium (p.34·2).
Fever; pain.

TO-Chemicals, Thai.
Digoxin (p.870·1).
Arrhythmias; heart failure.

Tol-Tab Alra, USA.
Tolbutamide (p.336·3).

Toluidinblau Kohler, Ger.
Tolonium chloride (p.1674·1).
Methaemoglobinaemia.

Tolu-Sed DM Scherer, USA.
Dextromethorphan hydrobromide (p.1087·3); guaifenesin (p.1092·2).
Coughs.

Tolusil INQ, Braz.
Potassium iodide (p.1522·3); sodium benzoate (p.1134·3); ephedrine hydrochloride (p.1090·1).
Respiratory-tract congestion.

Tolvin Organon, Aust.
Mianserin hydrochloride (p.298·1).
Depression.

Tolvon Organon, Aust.; Organon, Austral.; Akzo, Braz.; Organon, Denm.; Organon, Fin.; Organon, Hong Kong; Organon, Irl.; Organon, Mex.; Nourypharma, Neth.; Organon, Norw.; Pharmaco, NZ; Organon, Port.; Organon, Singapore; Organon, Swed.; Organon, Switz.; Organon, Thai.
Mianserin hydrochloride (p.298·1).
Depression.

Tolyprin Du Pont, Ger.
Azapropazone (p.19·1).
Acute gout; inflammation; pain; rheumatism; soft-tissue disorders.

Tomabef Salus, Ital.
Cefoperazone sodium (p.168·2).
Lignocaine [lidocaine] hydrochloride (p.1313·2) is included in this preparation to alleviate the pain of injection.
Bacterial infections.

Tomcin General Drugs, Thai.
Erythromycin estolate (p.201·2) or erythromycin stearate (p.201·3).
Bacterial infections.

Tomevis Brasifa, Braz.
Multivitamin and mineral preparation (p.1350·1).

Tomevit Spyfarma, Spain.
Adenosine triphosphate; arginine aspartate; glutathione; hydroxocobalamin acetate; lysine hydrochloride; pyritinol hydrochloride (p.1350·1).
Tonic.

Tomiron Toyama, Jpn.
Cefteram pivoxil (p.176·1).
Bacterial infections.

Tomocat Lafayette, USA.
Barium sulfate (p.1032·1).
Contrast medium for gastrointestinal radiography.

Tomudex Zeneca, Aust.; Zeneca, Austral.; Zeneca, Belg.; AstraZeneca, Canad.; AstraZeneca, Fr.; Zeneca, Irl.; Zeneca, Ital.; Zeneca, Neth.; AstraZeneca, Norw.; Zeneca, S.Afr.; Zeneca, Spain; Zeneca, Switz.; AstraZeneca, UK.
Raltitrexed (p.567·1).
Colorectal cancer.

Tomycin Orion, Fin.
Tobramycin sulfate (p.263·3).
Bacterial infections.

Tomycine Ciba Vision, Canad.
Tobramycin (p.263·3).
Bacterial eye infections.

Ton Was Wasserman, Spain.
Vitamin B substances (p.1350·1); ginseng (p.1615·3).
Tonic.

Tonactil Arkopharma, Fr.
Kola (p.1681·1); ginseng (p.1615·3).
Asthenia.

Tonactiv Herbaline, Ital.†
Angelica (p.1580·2); fennel (p.1610·1); laurus nobilis; aniseed (p.1580·2).
Depression; hypotension; tonic.

Tonamil Ecobi, Ital.
Thonzylamine (p.426·2).
Conjunctivitis; rhinitis; skin irritation.

Tonaton Luitpold, Braz.
Yohimbine (p.1681·3); fevillea trilobata; labiadas; ephedrine hydrochloride (p.1090·1); atropine methonitrate (p.461·1).
Erectile dysfunction.

Toncard-Do Grasler, Ger.
Homoeopathic preparation.

Toncils Vitabalans, Fin.
Chlorhexidine hydrochloride (p.1138·2); benzocaine (p.1306·2).
Mouth and throat disorders.

Tondex Hormona, Mex.
Gentamicin sulfate (p.210·1).
Bacterial infections.

Tondinel H Pfluger, Ger.
Homoeopathic preparation.

Tonerg Angelini, Ital.†
Pivagabine (p.307·3).
Depression.

Toness Angelini, Ital.
Proxazole citrate (p.1655·2).
Smooth muscle relaxant; vascular disorders.

Tonex Boehringer Ingelheim, Switz.
Amethocaine [tetracaine] hydrochloride (p.1305·2); chamomile (p.1593·2); sage (p.1660·2); aluminium formate; mint oil (p.1636·2); menthol (p.1632·3).
Minor skin lesions; mouth disorders.

Tonexis Clintec, Fr.†; Clintec, Irl.†; Clintec, Ital.†; Nestle, UK†.
A range of preparations for enteral nutrition (p.1350·1).

Tonexis HP Clintec, Fr.†
High-protein nutritional supplement (p.1350·1).

Tonexol Krug, Aust.†
Amethocaine [tetracaine] hydrochloride (p.1305·2); ethacridine lactate (p.1130·3).
Local anaesthesia.

Tongill Novartis, Aust.
Tyrothricin (p.267·1); muramidase hydrochloride (p.1638·1); lignocaine [lidocaine] hydrochloride (p.1313·2).
Mouth and throat disorders.

Tonible Novartis Consumer, Braz.†
Multivitamin and mineral preparation (p.1350·1).

Tonibral GNR, Port.
Deanol hemisuccinate (p.1507·2).
Tonic.

Tonibral Adulte GNR, Fr.
Deanol hemisuccinate (p.1507·2).
Tonic.

Tonicalcium Therabel, Belg.†; Bouchara, Fr.
DL-Lysine ascorbate; calcium ascorbate (p.1389·3).
Tonic; vitamin C deficiency.

Tonice Produfarma, Port.
Oral liquid: Deanol pyroglutamate (p.1507·2); magnesium aminobenzoate; ascorbic acid.

Syrup: Deanol pyroglutamate (p.1507·2); calcium gluceptate; lysine glutamate.
Tonic.

Tonico Juventus Juventus, Spain.
Cyproheptadine hydrochloride (p.414·2); cobamamide (p.1388·3).
Tonic.

Tonico No 1 QIF, Braz.
Ferrous sulfate (p.1360·3); phosphoric acid (p.1651·1).
Iron deficiency; iron-deficiency anaemias.

Tonico Prata Uniao Quimica, Braz.
Manganese sulfate; sodium glycerophosphate; ferric ammonium citrate (p.1359·2).
Iron deficiency; iron-deficiency anaemias.

Tonicol & ADC Multi-Pro, Canad.
Multivitamin and iron preparation (p.1350·1).

Tonicum Petrasch, Aust.
Vitamins (p.1350·1); caffeine; lactic acid.
Tonic.

SIT, Ital.
Amino-acid and vitamin preparation (p.1350·1).

Tonid Milano, Thai.
Tinidazole (p.603·3).
Amoebiasis; anaerobic bacterial infections; giardiasis; trichomoniasis.

Tonilax Monot, Fr.
Frangula bark (p.1227·1); aloes (p.1210·1).

Tonimol Herbes Universelles, Canad.
Multivitamin preparation (p.1350·1).

Tonipan Alpharma, Norw.
Vitamin B substances with manganese (p.1350·1).
Vitamin B deficiency.

Tonique D Democal, Switz.
Multivitamin and minerals with plant extracts (p.1350·1).
Tonic.

Tonique Vegetal Lehning, Fr.
Homoeopathic preparation.

Tonisan Dolisos, Fr.†
Ginseng (p.1615·3); black tea (p.1681·1).
Tonic.

Tonizin Betapharm, Ger.
Hypericum (p.290·2).
Anxiety; depression; nervous disorders.

Tono Milano, Thai.
Tolnaftate (p.395·2).
Fungal skin infections.

Tonocalcin Searle, Ital.; Merck, Mex.; Alfa Wassermann, Thai.
Salcatonin (p.749·3).
Hypercalcaemia; osteoporosis; Paget's disease of bone; reflex sympathetic dystrophy.

Tonocaltin Zambon, Port.; Zambon, Spain.
Salcatonin (p.749·3).
Hypercalcaemia; metastatic bone pain; osteolysis of malignancy; osteoporosis; Paget's disease of bone.

Tonocard AstraZeneca, Canad.; Astra, Hong Kong; Astra, Irl.; Astra, Neth.; Hassle, Swed.; AstraZeneca, Thai.; AstraZeneca, UK†; Astra, USA.
Tocainide hydrochloride (p.983·3).
Ventricular arrhythmias.

Tonofolin Teofarma, Ital.
Calcium folinate (p.1363·1).
Megaloblastic anaemias.

Tonoftal Essex, Ital.
Tolnaftate (p.395·2).
Fungal skin infections.

Tonogen ABC, Ital.
Haematoporphyrin hydrochloride (p.1618·3); cyanocobalamin (p.1388·1).
Tonic.

Tonoglutal Roche, Switz.
Glutamic acid; sodium hydroxybenzylphosphinate; ascorbic acid; magnesium glycerophosphate; thiamine nitrate (p.1350·1).
Tonic.

Tonoklen Farmabraz, Braz.
Ptychopetalum uncinatum; erythroxylon catuaba.
Tonic.

Tonopan Novartis, Aust.; Novartis, Braz.; Novartis, Mex.; Novartis, Spain; Novartis Consumer, Switz.
Caffeine (p.761·3); dihydroergotamine mesilate (p.450·3); propyphenazone (p.119·2).
Migraine and other vascular headaches.

Tonopaque Lafayette, USA.
Barium sulfate (p.1032·1).
Contrast medium for gastrointestinal radiography.

Tonoplantin Mono Palmicol, Ger.†
Crataegus (p.1600·2).
Heart failure.

Tonoplus ABC, Ital.
Arginine oxoglurate (p.1354·1); aceglutamide (p.1571·2).
Tonic.

Tonopres Boehringer Ingelheim, Ger.†
Dihydroergotamine mesilate (p.450·3).
Hypotension; migraine and other vascular headaches.

Tonoprotect Dumex, Ger.
Atenolol (p.841·3).
Angina pectoris; arrhythmias; hypertension.

Tonosai QIF, Braz.
Ferric ammonium citrate (p.1359·2); vitamins (p.1350·1); liver extract; calcium glycerophosphate.
Iron deficiency; iron-deficiency anaemias.

Tonosol Unifa, Port.
Multivitamin preparation (p.1350·1).

Tonovin Windson, Braz.
Multivitamin and mineral preparation (p.1350·1).

Tonovix Sedabel, Braz.
Vitamin B substances with lysine (p.1350·1).

Tonsan akut Bittner, Aust.
Homoeopathic preparation.

Tonsan chronisch Bittner, Aust.
Homoeopathic preparation.

Tonsicur Agepha, Aust.
Tyrothricin (p.267·1); benzalkonium chloride (p.1133·2).
Mouth and throat disorders.

Tonsilase dolo Medice, Ger.†
Benzocaine (p.1306·2); cetylpyridinium chloride (p.1138·1).
Mouth and throat disorders.

Tonsildrops Eversil, Braz.
Cetylpyridinium chloride (p.1138·1); benzocaine (p.1306·2).
Mouth and throat disorders.

Tonsilgon N Bionorica, Ger.
Althaea (p.1577·1); chamomile (p.1593·2); equisetum (p.1606·3); juglans regia; achillea (p.1572·2); oak bark (p.1643·2); taraxacum (p.1669·1).
Respiratory-tract infections.

Tonsillitis PMD Plantamed, Ger.
Homoeopathic preparation.

Tonsillol *Ratiopharm, Aust.*
Dequalinium chloride (p.1143·1).
Mouth and throat infections.

Tonsillopas *Pascoe, Ger.*
Homoeopathic preparation.

Tonsillosyx *Syxyl, Ger.*
Homoeopathic preparation.

Tonsiotren H *DHU, Ger.*
Homoeopathic preparation.

Tonterin *Fortune, Hong Kong.*
Caffeine (p.761·3); propyphenazone (p.80·2); thiamine (p.1385·2).
Fever; pain.

Tonum *Almirall, Spain.*
Ketorolac trometamol (p.48·2).
Pain.

Tonus *Lab, Port.*
Distigmine bromide (p.1417·1).

Tonus-forte-Tablinen *Sanorania, Ger.†*
Etilefrine hydrochloride (p.888·1).
Hypotension.

Toose *Juventus, Spain†.*
Co-trimoxazole (p.193·3).
Bacterial infections.

Toothache Drops *ICN, NZ.*
Phenol (p.1152·3); benzocaine (p.1306·2); camphor (p.1589·3); peppermint oil (p.1243·3); clove oil (p.1597·1).
Toothache.

Toothache Gel *Roberts, USA.*
Benzocaine (p.1306·2); clove oil (p.1597·1).
Toothache.

3 in 1 Toothache Relief *Dent, USA.*
Benzocaine (p.1306·2).

Top Calcium *Esseti, Ital.*
Calcium carbonate (p.1215·1).
Calcium depletion; calcium supplement.

Top dent fluor *Pharmalink, Swed.*
Sodium fluoride (p.1375·3).
Dental caries prophylaxis.

Top Marks *Lifeplan, UK.*
Multinutrient preparation (p.1350·1).

Topaal *Pierre Fabre, Fr.*
Alginic acid (p.1498·3); colloidal aluminium hydroxide (p.1210·3); magnesium carbonate (p.1232·3); silicon dioxide (p.1503·3).
Gastro-oesophageal reflux.

Topadol *Teva, Israel.*
Ketorolac trometamol (p.48·2).
Pain.

Topal *Ceuta, UK.*
Aluminium hydroxide (p.1210·3); light magnesium carbonate (p.1232·3); alginic acid (p.1498·3).
Gastic hyperacidity; gastritis; gastro-oesophageal reflux.

Topalgic *Hoechst, Fr.*
Tramadol hydrochloride (p.89·1).
Pain.

Topamax *Janssen-Cilag, Aust.; Janssen-Cilag, Austral.; Janssen-Cilag, Belg.; Janssen-Ortho, Canad.; Janssen-Cilag, Ger.; Janssen, Hong Kong; Janssen-Cilag, Irl.; Janssen-Cilag, Israel; Janssen-Cilag, Ital.; Cilag, Mex.; Janssen-Cilag, Neth.; Janssen-Cilag, NZ; Janssen-Cilag, Port.; Janssen-Cilag, S.Afr.; Janssen-Cilag, Singapore; Janssen-Cilag, Spain; Janssen-Cilag, Switz.; Janssen, Thai.; Janssen-Cilag, UK; Ortho McNeil, USA.*
Topiramate (p.365·2).
Epilepsy.

Toparal *Novag, Mex.*
Methyldopa (p.927·3).
Hypertension.

Topasel *Europharma, Spain.*
Algestone acetophenide (p.1465·1); estradiol enantate (p.1473·2).
Combined injectable contraceptive.

Top-Dal *Randall, Mex.*
Loperamide hydrochloride (p.1231·3).
Diarrhoea.

Topfena *Alpharma, Fr.*
Ketoprofen (p.47·3).
Formerly known as Topfen.
Musculoskeletal, joint, peri-articular, and soft-tissue disorders; pain.

Topher-E *Scherer, Hong Kong.*
α-Tocopherol (p.1393·3).
Vitamin E supplement.

Topialyse *SVR, Ital.*
Gamolenic acid (p.1613·1); borage oil (p.1613·1).
Nutritional supplement.

Topic *Syntex, USA.*
Benzyl alcohol (p.1135·2); camphor (p.1589·3); menthol (p.1632·3).
Pruritus.

Topicaina
Note. This name is used for preparations of different composition.
Braun, Spain.
Butyl aminobenzoate hydrochloride; benzocaine (p.1306·2); amethocaine [tetracaine] hydrochloride (p.1305·2).
Local anaesthesia.

Organon Teknika, Spain.
Benzalkonium chloride (p.1133·2); butacaine sulfate (p.1308·2); butyl aminobenzoate (p.1308·2); cetrimide (p.1137·3); benzocaine (p.1306·2); amethocaine [tetracaine] hydrochloride (p.1305·2).
Local anaesthesia.

Topicaine
Colgate Oral Care, Austral.†; Hoechst Marion Roussel, Canad.†.
Benzocaine (p.1306·2).
Local anaesthesia.

Topical *Tecnimede, Port.*
Bifonazole (p.381·1).
Fungal infections.

Topicil *Douglas, NZ.*
Clindamycin phosphate (p.188·2).
Acne.

Topico Denticion Vera *Labitec, Spain.*
Sodium bromide (p.1587·1); borax (p.1586·1); ethylene glycol; musk; anemone pulsatilla; menthol.
Toothache.

Topicort
Hoechst Marion Roussel, Canad.; Medicis, USA.
Desoximetasone (p.1066·2).
Skin disorders.

Topicorte
Hoechst Marion Roussel, Belg.†; Roussel, Fr.†; Hoechst Marion Roussel, Neth.; Hoechst Marion Roussel, Singapore; Hoechst Marion Roussel, Thai.
Desoximetasone (p.1066·2).
Skin disorders.

Topicorten V *Trima, Israel.*
Flumetasone pivalate (p.1070·3); clioquinol (p.190·2).
Infected skin disorders.

Topicorten-Tar *Trima, Israel.*
Flumetasone pivalate (p.1070·3); coal tar (p.1125·1); salicylic acid (p.1122·3).
Skin disorders.

Topicrem
Note. This name is used for preparations of different composition.
Nigy, Singapore.
Urea (p.1127·3); glycerol (p.1616·3).
Dry skin disorders.

Rhone-Poulenc Rorer, Spain.
Trolamine salicylate (p.90·1).
Peri-articular and soft-tissue disorders.

Topicycline *Shire, Irl.; Monmouth, UK; Procter & Gamble, USA.*
Tetracycline hydrochloride (p.258·3).
Acne.

Topidexa *Kinder, Braz.*
Dexamethasone (p.1067·1); nandrolone (p.1484·2); chlorhexidine (p.1138·2).
Skin disorders.

Topifram *Roussel, Fr.†; Hoechst Marion Roussel, Singapore; Hoechst Marion Roussel, Thai.*
Desoximetasone (p.1066·2); framycetin sulfate (p.208·2); gramicidin (p.213·3).
Infected skin disorders.

Topilene *Technilab, Canad.; Technilab, Hong Kong.*
Betamethasone dipropionate (p.1063·2).
Skin disorders.

Topilone *Chew, Thai.*
Triamcinolone acetonide (p.1080·1).
Skin disorders.

Topimax *Janssen-Cilag, Denm.; Janssen-Cilag, Fin.; Janssen-Cilag, Norw.; Janssen-Cilag, Swed.*
Topiramate (p.365·2).
Epilepsy.

Topionic *Diviser Aquilea, Spain.*
Povidone-iodine (p.1155·1).
Instrument disinfection; mouth and throat infections; skin, burn, and wound disinfection.

Topisalen *Trima, Israel.*
Flumetasone pivalate (p.1070·3); salicylic acid (p.1122·3).
Skin disorders.

Topisolon
Note. This name is used for preparations of different composition.
Hoechst Marion Roussel, Aust.; Hoechst Marion Roussel, Irl.†; Hoechst Marion Roussel, S.Afr.†; Knoll, Switz.
Desoximetasone (p.1066·2).
Burns; skin disorders.

Hoechst Marion Roussel, Ger.
Ointment; lotion; fatty ointment: Desoximetasone (p.1066·2).
Burns; skin disorders.
Topical solution: Desoximetasone (p.1066·2); salicylic acid (p.1122·3).
Scalp disorders; skin disorders.

Topisolon mit Salicylsaure *Hoechst Marion Roussel, Aust.*
Desoximetasone (p.1066·2); salicylic acid (p.1122·3).
Skin disorders.

Topisone *Technilab, Canad.*
Betamethasone dipropionate (p.1063·2).
Skin disorders.

Topivate *Xeragen, S.Afr.*
Betamethasone valerate (p.1063·2).
Skin disorders.

Toplexil
Note. This name is used for preparations of different composition.
Aventis, Belg.; Rhodia, Braz.
Oxomemazine (p.422·2); guaifenesin (p.1092·2); paracetamol (p.71·2); sodium benzoate (p.1134·3).
Coughs.

Theraplix, Fr.
Oxomemazine (p.422·2); guaifenesin (p.1092·2).
Formerly contained oxomemazine, guaifenesin, sodium benzoate, and paracetamol.
Coughs.

Rhone-Poulenc Rorer, Israel; Rhone-Poulenc Rorer, Neth.; Rhone-Poulenc Rorer, Switz.
Oxomemazine (p.422·2); guaifenesin (p.1092·2); sodium benzoate (p.1134·3).
Coughs.

Top-Mag *Genevrier, Fr.*
Magnesium pidolate (p.1191·1).
Magnesium deficiency.

Top-Nitro *Schering-Plough, Ital.*
Glyceryl trinitrate (p.897·3).
Angina pectoris.

Topo Worth *Dermopen, Braz.*
Cod-liver oil (p.1357·2); zinc oxide (p.1128·2); boric acid (p.1586·1).
Barrier preparation; skin disorders.

Topoderm N *Gepepharm, Ger.*
Diphenylpyraline hydrochloride (p.417·1); hydrocortisone (p.1535·3); neomycin sulfate (p.228·1).
Haemorrhoids; infected skin disorders; skin disorders.

Toposar *Pharmacia, USA.*
Etoposide (p.538·1).
Small-cell lung cancer; testicular cancer.

Topramine *Condrugs, Thai.*
Imipramine (p.291·1).
Depression; nocturnal enuresis.

Toprec *Theraplix, Fr.*
Ketoprofen (p.47·3).
Fever; pain.

Toprek *Rhone-Poulenc Rorer, Aust.; Aventis, Belg.; Rhone-Poulenc Rorer, Ital.*
Ketoprofen (p.47·3).
Musculoskeletal, joint and peri-articular disorders; pain.

Toprilem *Lemery, Mex.*
Captopril (p.853·3).
Hypertension.

Toprim *Nakorn, Thai.*
Co-trimoxazole (p.193·3).
Bacterial infections.

Toprol XL *Astra, USA.*
Metoprolol succinate (p.932·1).
Angina pectoris; heart failure; hypertension.

Topromel *Clonmel, Irl.*
Metoprolol tartrate (p.931·2).
Angina pectoris; arrhythmias; hyperthyroidism; migraine; myocardial infarction.

Topron *Chinoin, Mex.*
Nifuroxazide (p.230·2).
Gastro-enteritis.

Topsiton *Triomed, S.Afr.*
Vitamins; anhydrous caffeine; calcium gluconate; calcium citrate (p.1350·1).
Tonic.

Topster *Valeas, Ital.*
Beclometasone dipropionate (p.1061·2).
Inflammatory bowel disease.

Topsym *Grunenthal, Aust.; Grunenthal, Ger.; Grunenthal, Switz.*
Fluocinonide (p.1071·2).
Skin disorders.

Topsym polyvalent
Note. This name is used for preparations of different composition.
Grunenthal, Aust.; Grunenthal, Switz.
Fluocinonide (p.1071·2); gramicidin (p.213·3); neomycin sulfate (p.228·1); nystatin (p.392·2).
Infected skin disorders.

Grunenthal, Ger.
Fluocinonide (p.1071·2); neomycin sulfate (p.228·1); nystatin (p.392·2).
Infected skin disorders.

Topsymin *Grunenthal, Switz.*
Fluocinonide (p.1071·2).
Skin disorders.

Topsymin F *Grunenthal, Aust.*
Fluocinonide (p.1071·2).
Skin disorders.

Topsyn *Medicis, Canad.; Teofarma, Ital.; Syntex, Mex.*
Fluocinonide (p.1071·2).
Skin disorders.

Topsyne *Cassenne, Fr.†; Yamanouchi, Neth.*
Fluocinonide (p.1071·2).
Skin disorders.

Topsyne Neomycine *Cassenne, Fr.†.*
Fluocinonide (p.1071·2); neomycin sulfate (p.228·1).
Infected skin disorders.

Topsyn-Y *Syntex, Mex.*
Fluocinonide (p.1071·2); clioquinol (p.190·2).
Infected skin disorders.

Toptabs *Sussex, UK.*
Aspirin (p.14·2); caffeine (p.761·3).

Toquilone compositum *Medichemie, Switz.*
Methaqualone (p.691·3); diphenhydramine hydrochloride (p.416·1).
Sleep disorders.

Toradiur *Roche, Ital.*
Torasemide (p.985·2).
Ascites; heart failure; oedema; renal failure.

Toradol
Syntex, Austral.; Roche, Canad.; Roche, Denm.; Roche, Fin.; Roche, Hong Kong; Roche, Norw.; Roche, Port.; Roche, Singapore; Roche, Spain; Roche, Swed.; Roche, UK; Roche, USA.
Ketorolac (p.49·2) or ketorolac trometamol (p.48·2).
Pain.

Tora-Dol
Recordati, Ital.; Roche, S.Afr.; Roche, Switz.
Ketorolac trometamol (p.48·2).
Pain.

Toraseptol *Lesvi, Spain.*
Azithromycin (p.153·1).
Bacterial infections.

Torbetol
Note. This name is used for preparations of different composition.
Torbet, Irl.
Cetrimide (p.1137·1); benzalkonium chloride (p.1133·2); hexachlorophene (p.1146·1).
Acne.

Torbet Laboratories, UK.
Cetrimide (p.1137·1); chlorhexidine gluconate (p.1138·2).
Formerly contained hexachlorophene.
Acne.

Torecan
Novartis, Aust.; Novartis, Ger.; Novartis, Ital.; Novartis, Mex.; Sandoz, Neth.†; Novartis, Spain; Novartis, Swed.; Novartis, Switz.; Roxane, USA.
Thiethylperazine (p.426·1), thiethylperazine malate (p.426·1), or thiethylperazine maleate (p.426·1).
Nausea; vestibular disorders; vomiting.

Torem
Berlin-Chemie, Ger.; Boehringer Mannheim, Neth.†; Roche, Swed.; Roche, Switz.; Roche, UK.
Torasemide (p.985·1) or torasemide sodium (p.985·2).
Heart failure; hypertension; oedema; renal failure.

Torental
Aventis, Belg.; Hoechst, Fr.
Oxpentifylline [pentoxifylline] (p.950·3).
Intermittent claudication; mental function impairment in the elderly; vascular disorders.

Torfan *Abbott, Ital.*
Dextromethorphan hydrobromide (p.1087·3); guaifenesin (p.1092·2); carbinoxamine maleate (p.411·1).
Coughs.

Toriac *Rhone-Poulenc Rorer, Belg.†.*
Loperamide hydrochloride (p.1231·3).
Diarrhoea.

Toriol *Vita, Spain.*
Ranitidine hydrochloride (p.1245·2).
Acid aspiration; gastro-oesophageal reflux; gastrointestinal haemorrhage; peptic ulcer; short-bowel syndrome; Zollinger-Ellison syndrome.

Torlanbulina Antitetani *Torlan, Spain†.*
A tetanus immunoglobulin (p.1565·1).
Passive immunisation.

Torlasporin *Torlan, Spain.*
Cefalexin (p.161·3).
Bacterial infections.

Tornalate *Dura, USA.*
Bitolterol mesilate (p.761·2).
Asthma; bronchospasm.

Tornix *Steierl, Ger.*
Crataegus (p.1600·2); valerian (p.1678·3); passion flower (p.1649·1); rutoside (p.1611·2).
Cardiac disorders.

Torrat *Roche, Aust.; Roche, Ger.; Roche, Hong Kong.*
Metipranolol (p.930·2); butizide (p.853·1).
Hypertension.

Torrem *Boehringer Mannheim, Belg.*
Torasemide (p.985·1).
Hypertension; oedema.

Torvast *Pfizer, Ital.*
Atorvastatin calcium (p.842·3).
Hyperlipidaemias.

Torymycin *Chinta, Thai.*
Doxycycline hyclate (p.200·1).
Bacterial infections.

Toryxil *Baer, Ger.*
Diclofenac sodium (p.30·3).
Inflammation; rheumatism.

T-OS *Seroyal, Canad.*
Calcium, molybdenum, phosphorus, and vitamin D (p.1350·1).

Tos Mai *Edigen, Spain.*
Dextromethorphan hydrobromide (p.1087·3); benzocaine (p.1306·2); guaiacol (p.1092·1); sodium benzoate (p.1134·3).
Respiratory-tract disorders.

Toscal *Abbott, Spain†.*
Syrup: Ammonium chloride (p.1085·2); tolu balsam (p.1101·3); dextromethorphan hydrobromide (p.1087·3); ephedrine hydrochloride (p.1090·1); ipecacuanha (p.1093·1).
Tablets: Carbinoxamine maleate (p.411·1); dextromethorphan hydrobromide (p.1087·3).
Respiratory-tract disorders.

Toscal Compositum *Abbott, Spain†.*
Ammonium chloride (p.1085·2); tolu balsam (p.1101·3); carbinoxamine maleate (p.411·1); dextromethorphan hydrobromide (p.1087·3); ephedrine hydrochloride (p.1090·1); ipecacuanha (p.1093·1).
Upper respiratory-tract disorders.

Tosdetan *Martin, Spain†.*
Citiolone (p.1596·2); co-trimoxazole (p.193·3).
Respiratory-tract infections.

Tosdiazina *Clariana, Spain.*
Tolu balsam (p.1101·3); erythromycin stearate (p.201·3); guaifenesin (p.1092·2).
Respiratory-tract infections.

Tosdrope *Schering-Plough, Port.*
Dexchlorpheniramine maleate (p.412·1); pseudoephe-
drine sulfate (p.1099·3); guaifenesin (p.1092·2).
Coughs.

Toseina NF *Italfarmaco, Spain.*
Codeine phosphate (p.25·2).
Coughs; diarrhoea; pain.

Tosfriol *Synthelabo, Spain.*
Dextromethorphan hydrobromide (p.1087·3).
Coughs.

Tosidrin *Fardi, Spain.*
Dihydrocodeine tartrate (p.33·1).
Coughs.

Tosifar *Bial-Aristegui, Spain.*
Fominoben hydrochloride (p.1091·3).
Respiratory-tract disorders.

Tosion Retard *Boots Healthcare, Neth.†*
Dextromethorphan polistirex (p.1088·2).
Coughs.

Tossamine *Novartis Consumer, Switz.*
Codeine phosphate (p.25·2); noscapine (p.1096·1).
Coughs.

Tossamine plus *Novartis Consumer, Switz.*
White capsules, codeine phosphate (p.25·2); noscapine
(p.1096·1); methylephedrine hydrochloride (p.1094·3);
blue capsules, codeine phosphate; noscapine; diphenhydramine hydrochloride (p.416·1).
Coughs.

Tossarel *Aerocid, Fr.†*
Elecampane (p.1089·3); marrubium (p.1094·2); terpin
(p.1101·2); sodium benzoate (p.1134·3).
Coughs.

Tossbel *Riedel-Zabinka, Braz.*
Diphenhydramine hydrochloride (p.416·1); dextromethorphan hydrobromide (p.1087·3); ammonium
chloride (p.1085·2).
Coughs.

Tossefedrin *Leofarma, Braz.*
Ephedrine hydrochloride (p.1090·1); bromoform
(p.1587·1); sodium dibunate (p.1100·3).
Respiratory-tract congestion.

Tossefin *IQB, Braz.*
Sodium dibunate (p.1100·3); sulfogaiacol (p.1101·1).
Coughs.

Tosseina *Bergamo, Braz.*
Umbauba; sodium benzoate (p.1134·3); ipecacuanha
(p.1093·1); mikania glomerata; carqueja; eucalyptus
(p.1609·2); lobelia (p.1510·2).
Coughs.

Tossemed *Iodosan, Ital.*
Dextromethorphan hydrobromide (p.1087·3); guaifen-
esin (p.1092·2).
Coughs.

Tosseque *Lab, Port.*
Bromhexine hydrochloride (p.1085·3).
Respiratory-tract congestion.

Tossestop *IMA, Braz.*
Diphenhydramine (p.416·1); ammonium chloride
(p.1085·2).
Coughs.

Tossilerg *Bunker, Braz.*
Diphenhydramine hydrochloride (p.416·1); ammoni-
um chloride (p.1085·2).
Coughs.

Tossoral *Recordati, Ital.*
Dextromethorphan hydrobromide (p.1087·3).
Coughs.

Tosuman
Berna, Ital.†; Berna, Switz.†.
A pertussis immunoglobulin (p.1555·3).
Passive immunisation.

Totacef
Bristol-Myers Squibb, Israel; Bristol-Myers Squibb, Ital.
Cefazolin sodium (p.164·3).
Bacterial infections.

Totacide *Adams, Thai.*
Glutaral (p.1145·2).
Instrument disinfection.

Totacillin *SmithKline Beecham, USA.*
Ampicillin trihydrate (p.151·1).
Bacterial infections.

Totacillin-N *SmithKline Beecham, USA†.*
Ampicillin sodium (p.150·3).
Bacterial infections.

Totaforte
Asta Medica, Belg.†; Asta Medica, Neth.; Asta Medica, Port.
Multivitamin and mineral preparation (p.1350·1).

Total
Note. This name is used for preparations of different composition.
Allergan, Canad.
Polyvinyl alcohol (p.1503·1) (p.1129·2).
*Cleansing, wetting, and soaking solution for hard and
gas permeable contact lenses.*

Allergan, Israel; Allergan, Port.; Allergan, USA.
Cleansing, soaking and wetting solution for contact
lenses (p.1129·2).

Total Care *Allergan, Austral.*
A range of preparations for care of hard and gas permeable contact lenses (p.1129·2).

Total Cover Sunblock *Clinique, Canad.*
SPF 30: Octinoxate (p.1517·3); homosalate
(p.1517·2); octisalate (p.1518·1); oxybenzone
(p.1518·1).
Sunscreen.

Total Eclipse *Triangle, USA.*
SPF 15: Padimate O (p.1518·2); oxybenzone
(p.1518·1); lisadimate (p.1517·3).
Sunscreen.

Total Eclipse Moisturizing *Triangle, USA.*
SPF 15: Padimate O (p.1518·2); oxybenzone
(p.1518·1); octisalate (p.1518·1).
Sunscreen.

Total Formula *Vitaline, USA.*
A range of vitamin preparations (p.1350·1).

Total Woman *Vitaglow, Austral.*
A range of multivitamin and mineral preparations
(p.1350·1).
Dietary supplement.

Totalbloc *Australis, Austral.†.*
SPF15+: Padimate O (p.1518·2); oxybenzone
(p.1518·1); avobenzone (p.1517·1).
Sunscreen.

Totalbloc Maximum Protection *Creative Brands,
Austral.*
SPF 15+: Escalol 507; oxybenzone (p.1518·1);
avobenzone (p.1517·1).
Sunscreen.

TotalCare *Allergan, Ger.†.*
Disinfecting, storage, and moistening solution for contact lenses (p.1129·2).

Totalens *Allergan-Frumtost, Braz.*
Polyvinyl alcohol (p.1503·1) (p.1129·2).
Cleaning solution for contact lenses.

Totalip *Guidotti, Ital.*
Atorvastatin calcium (p.842·3).
Hyperlipidaemias.

Totamine *Baxter, Fr.*
Amino-acid, electrolyte, and vitamin infusion
(p.1350·1).
Parenteral nutrition.

Totamol *CP Pharmaceuticals, UK.*
Atenolol (p.841·3).
Now known as Atenolol tablets.
Angina pectoris; arrhythmias; hypertension.

Totapen
Riedel-Zabinka, Braz.; Bristol-Myers Squibb, Fr.
Ampicillin (p.150·3), ampicillin sodium (p.150·3), or
ampicillin trihydrate (p.151·1).
Bacterial infections.

Totaretic *CP Pharmaceuticals, UK.*
Atenolol (p.841·3); chlortalidone (p.857·1).
These ingredients can be described by the British Ap-
proved Name Co-tenidone.
Hypertension.

Totatrom *Tocogino, Mex.*
Erythromycin (p.201·2).
Bacterial infections.

Totavit *Seton, UK†.*
Multivitamin, mineral, and amino acid preparation
(p.1350·1).

Totephan *Paraphar, Fr.*
Cream: Glycerol; cholesterol; oleic acid; urea
(p.1350·1).
Oral powder: Plant proteins; vitamins; minerals
(p.1350·1).
Hair and nail tonic.

Tot'Hema
Innothera, Fr.
Ferrous gluconate (p.1360·1); manganese gluconate;
copper gluconate (p.1350·1).
Anaemia.

Innotech, Port.
Ferrous gluconate (p.1360·1); manganese gluconate;
copper gluconate; cobalt glutamate; vitamin B$_{12}$
(p.1350·1).
Anaemia.

Totipen *Liferpal, Mex.*
Ampicillin (p.150·3).
Bacterial infections.

Totocortin *Winzer, Ger.*
Dexamethasone sodium phosphate (p.1067·1).
Eye disorders.

Totonik *Pharmaceutical Enterprises, S.Afr.*
Vitamins; potassium glycerophosphate; caffeine; fer-
rous sulfate (p.1350·1).
Tonic.

Toularynx *Qualiphar, Belg.*
Codeine phosphate (p.25·2).
Coughs.

Toulumad *Ceninter, Spain.*
Magnesium polygalacturonate.
Gastric hyperacidity; peptic ulcer.

Touristil *Janssen-Cilag, Belg.*
Cinnarizine (p.413·1); domperidone maleate
(p.1224·1).
*Dyspepsia; motion sickness; nausea; sleep disorders;
vertigo; vomiting.*

Touro A & H *Dartmouth, USA.*
Pseudoephedrine hydrochloride (p.1099·2); bromphe-
niramine maleate (p.410·2).
Allergic rhinitis; nasal congestion.

Touro Allergy *Dartmouth, USA.*
Pseudoephedrine hydrochloride (p.1099·2); bromphe-
niramine maleate (p.410·2).
Rhinitis; upper respiratory-tract congestion.

Touro CC *Dartmouth, USA.*
Pseudoephedrine hydrochloride (p.1099·2); dextromethorphan hydrobromide (p.1087·3); guaifenesin
(p.1092·2).
Coughs; nasal congestion.

Touro DM *Dartmouth, USA.*
Dextromethorphan hydrobromide (p.1087·3); guaifen-
esin (p.1092·2).
Coughs.

Touro Ex *Dartmouth, USA.*
Guaifenesin (p.1092·2).
Coughs.

Touro LA *Dartmouth, USA.*
Pseudoephedrine hydrochloride (p.1099·2); guaifenes-
in (p.1092·2).
Coughs and cold symptoms.

Touxium *SMB, Belg.†*
Dextromethorphan hydrobromide (p.1087·3).
Coughs.

Tovene *Solvay, Ger.*
Diosmin (p.1611·1).
Venous insufficiency.

Toverine *TO-Chemicals, Thai.*
Drotaverine hydrochloride (p.1606·1).
Smooth muscle spasm.

T.O.Vir *TO-Chemicals, Thai.*
Zidovudine (p.645·2).
HIV infection.

Toxal *Rayere, Mex.*
Oxolamine (p.1096·2).
Coughs.

Toxanal *Columbia, Mex.*
A tetanus vaccine (p.1565·2).
Active immunisation.

Toxepasi *Roche, Ital.*
Cogalactoisomerase sodium (p.1598·1).
Hyperbilirubinaemia.

Toxex *Pekana, Ger.*
Homoeopathic preparation.

Toxicerna *Fides, Ger.*
Homoeopathic preparation.

Toxicol *Eagle, Austral.*
Vitamin B substances with mineral, herbal, and nutritional agents (p.1350·1).

toxi-L 90 N *Loges, Ger.*
Homoeopathic preparation.

toxi-loges *Loges, Ger.*
Homoeopathic preparation.

toxi-loges N *Loges, Ger.*
Homoeopathic preparation.

Toximer *Ratiopharm, Aust.*
Suppositories: Paracetamol (p.71·2); codeine phos-
phate (p.25·2).
Pain.
Tablets: Propyphenazone (p.80·2); paracetamol
(p.71·2); codeine phosphate (p.25·2).
Fever; pain.

Toximer C *Merckle, Ger.*
Paracetamol (p.71·2); caffeine (p.761·2).
Pain.

Toxiselect *Dreluso, Ger.*
Homoeopathic preparation.

Toxogonin
*Merck, Aust.; Merck, Denm.; Merck, Ger.; Merck, Neth.; Merck,
S.Afr.; Merck, Swed.*
Obidoxime chloride (p.1016·3).
Organophosphorus poisoning.

Toxogonine *Merck, Switz.†.*
Obidoxime chloride (p.1016·3).
Organophosphorus poisoning.

TP-1
Serono, Braz.; Serono, Ital.†; Serono, Spain.
Thymostimulin (p.1672·3).
Immunotherapy.

T-PA *Seroyal, Canad.†*
Vitamin D and minerals (p.1350·1).

TPE 1800 GX *Pharmacia Upjohn, Ger.*
Amino-acid, carbohydrate, and electrolyte infusion
(p.1350·1).
Parenteral nutrition.

TPH *Baxter, Ital.*
Amino-acid infusion (p.1350·1).
Parenteral nutrition for neonates and infants.

T-Phyl *Purdue Frederick, USA.*
Theophylline (p.777·2).
Asthma; bronchospasm.

TPN Additive *DBL, Austral.*
Electrolytes (p.1180·1).
Parenteral nutrition.

TP-Ophtal *Winzer, Ger.*
Pilocarpine hydrochloride (p.1422·3); timolol maleate
(p.982·1).
Glaucoma; ocular hypertension.

Trabar *Mepha, Israel.*
Tramadol hydrochloride (p.89·1).
Pain.

Trabit
Note. This name is used for preparations of different composition.
Mepha, Hong Kong.
Injection: 1 Ampoule, phenylbutazone sodium
(p.78·3) orthocarbamoylphenoxyacetate sodium; dexamethasone (p.1067·1); 1 ampoule, vitamin B$_{12}$
(p.1388·1).
Lignocaine [lidocaine] hydrochloride (p.1313·2) is included in this preparation to alleviate the pain of injection.
Rectal capsules: Phenylbutazone (p.78·1); dexamethasone (p.1067·1); vitamin B12 (p.1388·1).

Tablets: Phenylbutazone (p.78·1); dexamethasone
(p.1067·1); vitamin B$_1$; vitamin B12 (p.1388·1).
Aluminium glycinate (p.1210·3) is included in this
preparation in an attempt to limit adverse effects on the
gastrointestinal mucosa.
Rheumatism.

Mepha, Thai.
Injection: Ampoule A, phenylbutazone sodium
(p.78·3); salamidacetic acid (p.81·3); dexamethasone
(p.1067·1); ampoule B, vitamin B$_{12}$ (p.1388·1).
Lignocaine [lidocaine] hydrochloride (p.1313·2) is included in each ampoule to alleviate the pain of injection.
Rectal capsules: Phenylbutazone (p.78·1); dexamethasone (p.1067·1); vitamin B$_{12}$ (p.1388·1).
Musculoskeletal and joint disorders.

Trabona *Leiras, Fin.*
Diclofenac potassium (p.30·2) or diclofenac sodium
(p.30·3).
*Inflammation; musculoskeletal and joint disorders;
pain.*

Trac Tabs 2X *Hyrex, USA.*
Methenamine (p.223·1); salol (p.82·2); atropine sulfate
(p.461·1); hyoscyamine sulfate (p.469·3); benzoic acid
(p.1134·2); methylene blue [methylthioninium chlo-
ride] (p.1012·3).
Urinary-tract infections.

Tracel
*Fresenius Kabi, Denm.; Fresenius Kabi, Fin.; Fresenius Kabi, Norw.;
Fresenius Kabi, Swed.*
Trace element infusion (p.1350·1).
Parenteral nutrition.

Tracelyte *American Pharmaceutical, USA†.*
A range of trace element and electrolyte preparations
(p.1180·1).
Parenteral nutrition.

Tracemate *Pharmy, Fr.†.*
Disodium edetate (p.1008·1).
Hypocalcaemia provocation test.

Tracer bG *Boehringer Mannheim, USA†.*
Test for glucose in blood (p.1616·3).

Tracer Glucose *Boehringer Mannheim, Fr.†.*
Test for glucose in blood (p.1616·3).

Tracheo Fresh *Rappai, Switz.*
Sea salt (p.1196·1); macrogol 300 (p.1630·3).
Tracheal lubricant; tracheostomy care.

Trachiform *Philopharm, Ger.*
Cetylpyridinium chloride (p.1138·1); benzocaine
(p.1306·2); mint oil (p.1636·2); menthol (p.1632·3).
Mouth and throat disorders.

Trachisan
Note. This name is used for preparations of different composition.
Engelhard, Ger.; Engelhard, Singapore.
Gargle: Chlorhexidine gluconate (p.1138·2); ligno-
caine [lidocaine] hydrochloride (p.1313·2).
Mouth and throat disorders.

Engelhard, Ger.; Engelhard, Singapore; Engelhard, Switz.†.
Lozenges: Chlorhexidine gluconate (p.1138·2); lignocaine [lidocaine] (p.1313·2) or lignocaine [lidocaine]
hydrochloride (p.1313·2); tyrothricin (p.267·1).
Mouth and throat disorders.

Trachitol *Engelhard, Ger.*
Lignocaine [lidocaine] hydrochloride (p.1313·2); propyl hydroxybenzoate (p.1148·2); alum (p.1577·2).
*Infections of the upper-respiratory tract; inflammatory
disorders of the oropharynx.*

Trachyl *Monal, Fr.†.*
Ethylmorphine hydrochloride (p.35·2).
Coughs.

Tracin *Berman, Mex.*
Oxytetracycline (p.234·1).
Bacterial infections.

Tracitrans plus *Fresenius Kabi, Denm.*
Electrolyte and trace element preparation (p.1350·1).
Parenteral nutrition.

Tracleer *Actelion, USA.*
Bosentan (p.850·3).
Pulmonary hypertension.

Traconal *Ache, Braz.*
Itraconazole (p.387·2).
Fungal infections.

Tracrium
*Glaxo Wellcome, Aust.; Glaxo Wellcome, Austral.; Glaxo Wellcome,
Belg.; Glaxo Wellcome, Braz.; Glaxo Wellcome, Canad.; Glaxo Well-
come, Denm.; Glaxo Wellcome, Fin.; Glaxo Wellcome, Fr.; Glaxo
Wellcome, Ger.; Glaxo Wellcome, Hong Kong; Wellcome, Irl.; Glaxo
Wellcome, Israel; Glaxo Wellcome, Ital.; Glaxo Wellcome, Mex.;
Glaxo Wellcome, Neth.; Glaxo Wellcome, Norw.; Glaxo Wellcome,
NZ; Wellcome, Port.; Glaxo Wellcome, S.Afr.; Glaxo Wellcome, Sin-
gapore; Wellcome, Spain; Glaxo Wellcome, Swed.; Glaxo Wellcome,
Switz.; Glaxo Wellcome, Thai.; Glaxo Wellcome, UK; Glaxo Well-
come, USA.*
Atracurium besilate (p.1333·1).
Competitive neuromuscular blocker.

Tractocile
Ferring, Denm.; Ferring, Fin.; Ferring, Irl.; Ferring, UK.
Atosiban acetate (p.1278·1).
Premature labour.

Tractoven
Amnol, Ital.
Capsules: Centella; melilot; rutoside; vitamin E
(p.1350·1).
Nutritional supplement.
Cream: Hedera; birch; aesculus; equisetum; myrtillus;
centella; vitamin E (p.1350·1).

Tractur *Damor, Ital.*
Pipemidic acid (p.236·1).
Bacterial infections of the urinary tract.

Tracutil Braun, Ger.
Trace-element preparation (p.1350·1).
Parenteral nutrition.

Braun, Switz.
Mineral preparation (p.1350·1).
Parenteral nutrition.

Tradelia Wolff, Ger.
Estradiol (p.1473·1).
Menopausal disorders.

Tradol Isis Puren, Ger.; Rowa, Irl.; Lakeside, Mex.; Shin Poong, Singapore.
Tramadol hydrochloride (p.89·1).
Pain.

Tradolan Lannacher, Aust.; Lannacher, Denm.; Nordic, Swed.
Tramadol hydrochloride (p.89·1).
Pain.

Tradon Lilly, Ger.
Pemoline (p.1513·1).
Hyperactivity in older children.

Tradonal Asta Medica, Belg.; Asta Medica, Ital.; Asta Medica, Spain; Asta Medica, Thai.
Tramadol hydrochloride (p.89·1).
Pain.

Trafloxal Tramedico, Belg.; Mann, Neth.
Ofloxacin (p.232·3).
Bacterial eye infections.

Tralen Pfizer, Braz.
Tioconazole (p.395·1).
Fungal skin infections.

Tralgiol Ciclum, Spain.
Tramadol hydrochloride (p.89·1).
Pain.

Trama ABZ, Ger.; BASF, Ger.; Kade, Ger.
Tramadol hydrochloride (p.89·1).
Pain.

Tramabene Ratiopharm, Aust.
Tramadol hydrochloride (p.89·1).
Pain.

Tramabeta Betapharm, Ger.
Tramadol hydrochloride (p.89·1).
Pain.

Tramadex Dexcel, Israel.
Tramadol hydrochloride (p.89·1).
Pain.

Tramadin Medinovum, Fin.
Tramadol hydrochloride (p.89·1).
Pain.

Tramadol-Dolgit Dolorgiet, Ger.
Tramadol hydrochloride (p.89·1).
Pain.

Tramadolor Hexal, Ger.; Mepha, Switz.†.
Tramadol hydrochloride (p.89·1).
Pain.

Trama-Dorsch Orion, Ger.
Tramadol hydrochloride (p.89·1).
Pain.

Tramadura Merck dura, Ger.
Tramadol hydrochloride (p.89·1).
Pain.

Tramagetic Azupharma, Ger.; Christiaens, Neth.
Tramadol hydrochloride (p.89·1).
Pain.

Tramagit Krewel, Ger.
Tramadol hydrochloride (p.89·1).
Pain.

Tramake Galen, Irl.; Galen, UK.
Tramadol hydrochloride (p.89·1).
Pain.

Tramal Grunenthal, Aust.; CSL, Austral.; Carlo Erba, Braz.; Grunenthal, Ger.; Grunenthal, Hong Kong; Sanofi Winthrop, Hong Kong; Grunenthal, Neth.; CSL, NZ; Grunenthal, Port.; Janssen-Cilag, S.Afr.; Grunenthal, Singapore; Sanofi Synthelabo, Singapore; Grunenthal, Switz.; Grunenthal, Thai.; Sanofi Synthelabo, Thai.
Tramadol hydrochloride (p.89·1).
Pain.

Tramalan Olan-Kemed, Thai.
Tramadol hydrochloride (p.89·1).
Pain.

Tramamed Medifive, Thai.
Tramadol hydrochloride (p.89·1).
Pain.

Tramamerck Merck dura, Ger.
Tramadol hydrochloride (p.89·1).
Pain.

Tramedphano Medphano, Ger.†.
Tramadol hydrochloride (p.89·1).
Pain.

Tramex Antigen, Irl.
Tramadol hydrochloride (p.89·1).
Pain.

Tramil
Note. This name is used for preparations of different composition.
Whitehall, Irl.
Paracetamol (p.71·2); caffeine (p.761·3).
Fever; pain.

Whitehall, UK†.
Paracetamol (p.71·2).
Fever; pain.

Tramisal URPAC, Fr.
Ginkgo biloba (p.1615·2).
Mental function impairment in the elderly; peripheral vascular disorders.

Tramo Jean-Marie, Hong Kong.
Tramadol hydrochloride (p.89·1).
Pain.

Tramoda LBS, Thai.
Tramadol hydrochloride (p.89·1).
Pain.

Tramol Orion, Fin.
Tramadol hydrochloride (p.89·1).
Pain.

Tramsilione Greater Pharma, Thai.
Triamcinolone acetonide (p.1080·1).
Skin disorders.

Tramundal Mundipharma, Aust.
Tramadol hydrochloride (p.89·1).
Pain.

Tramundin Mundipharma, Ger.
Tramadol hydrochloride (p.89·1).
Pain.

Trancap TP, Thai.
Dipotassium clorazepate (p.670·3).
Anxiety; insomnia.

Tranclor Siam Bheasach, Thai.
Dipotassium clorazepate (p.670·3).
Anxiety.

Trancon Condrugs, Thai.
Dipotassium clorazepate (p.670·3).
Anxiety.

Trancopal Sanofi Winthrop, Aust.†; Sanofi Winthrop, Neth.†; Sanofi Winthrop, Swed.†; Sanofi Winthrop, Switz.†; Sanofi Winthrop, USA†.
Chlormezanone (p.660·1).
Anxiety; musculoskeletal pain and spasm.

Trancopal compositum Sanofi Winthrop, Aust.†; Sanofi Winthrop, Switz.†.
Chlormezanone (p.660·1); paracetamol (p.71·2).
Musculoskeletal pain and spasm.

Trancopal Dolo Sanofi Synthelabo, Ger.
Flupirtine maleate (p.41·1).
Pain.

Trandate Glaxo Wellcome, Aust.; Glaxo Wellcome, Austral.; Glaxo Wellcome, Belg.; Roberts, Canad.; Glaxo Wellcome, Denm.; Glaxo Wellcome, Fr.; Glaxo Wellcome, Hong Kong; Medeva, Irl.; Glaxo Wellcome, Israel; Teofarma, Ital.; Glaxo Wellcome, Neth.; Glaxo Wellcome, Norw.; Glaxo Wellcome, NZ; Glaxo Wellcome, Port.; Glaxo Wellcome, S.Afr.; Glaxo Wellcome, Singapore; Duncan, Spain; Glaxo Wellcome, Swed.; Glaxo Wellcome, Switz.; Celltech, UK; Faro, USA.
Labetalol hydrochloride (p.918·1).
Angina pectoris; controlled hypotension during anaesthesia; hypertension.

Trandiur Teofarma, Ital.
Labetalol hydrochloride (p.918·1); chlortalidone (p.857·1).
Hypertension.

Trandor Lilly, Braz.
Fenoprofen calcium (p.36·3).
Gout; inflammation; musculoskeletal, joint, and peri-articular disorders; pain.

Trandrozine Asian Pharm, Thai.
Hydroxyzine hydrochloride (p.419·1).
Anxiety; pruritus.

Tranex Malesci, Ital.
Tranexamic acid (p.742·2).
Hyperfibrinolytic haemorrhage.

Trangorex Sanofi Synthelabo, Spain.
Amiodarone hydrochloride (p.836·1).
Arrhythmias.

Trankimazin Pharmacia Upjohn, Spain.
Alprazolam (p.654·2).
Anxiety.

Tran-Qil Rolab, S.Afr.†.
Lorazepam (p.688·3).
Anxiety.

Tranqipam Aspen, S.Afr.
Lorazepam (p.688·3).
Alcohol withdrawal syndrome; anxiety; premedication; sedative.

Tranquase Azupharma, Ger.
Diazepam (p.674·3).
Anxiety; premedication; skeletal muscle spasm.

Tranquax Berk, UK†.
Clomipramine hydrochloride (p.282·1).
Depression; narcoleptic syndrome; obsessive-compulsive disorder.

Tranquil Pharmadass, UK.
Crataegus (p.1600·2); tilia flower (p.1673·2); viburnum; hawthorn oil (p.1600·2).

Tranquilyn Genus, UK.
Methylphenidate.

Tranquiplex Vitaplex, Austral.†.
Vitamins and minerals (p.1350·1); passion flower (p.1649·1); skullcap (p.1664·3); valerian (p.1678·3).

Tranquirit Rhone-Poulenc Rorer, Ital.
Diazepam (p.674·3).
Anxiety; epilepsy; insomnia; psychoses.

Tranquital Novartis Sante, Fr.
Valerian (p.1678·3); crataegus (p.1600·2).
Insomnia; nervous disorders.

Tranquo Boehringer Ingelheim, Belg.
Oxazepam (p.697·2).
Anxiety disorders.

Transacalm Norgine, Fr.
Trimebutine maleate (p.1675·1).
Formerly called Transicalm.
Gastrointestinal disorders.

Transact Boots, S.Afr.
Flurbiprofen (p.41·2).
Formerly known as Trans Act_LAT_.
Musculoskeletal and joint disorders.

Transact Lat Ravizza, Ital.; Knoll, Port.
Flurbiprofen (p.41·2).
Musculoskeletal, joint, peri-articular, and soft-tissue disorders.

Transamin Nikkho, Braz.; Daiichi, Hong Kong; Daiichi, Jpn; Daiichi, Thai.
Tranexamic acid (p.742·2).
Haemorrhagic disorders.

Transannon Pharmacia Upjohn, Ger.
21 Tablets, conjugated oestrogens (p.1467·1); 7 tablets, inert.
Menopausal disorders; osteoporosis.

Pharmacia Upjohn, Switz.
Conjugated oestrogens (p.1467·1).
Menopausal disorders.

Transbilix Codali, Belg.†; Guerbet, Fr.†.
Meglumine adipiodone (p.1031·1).
Contrast medium for biliary-tract radiography.

Transbronchin Asta Medica, Ger.
Carbocisteine (p.1086·3) or carbocisteine sodium (p.1086·3).
Respiratory-tract disorders associated with increased or viscous mucus.

Transbronquina Lab, Port.
Codeine (p.25·2); trolamine (p.1675·1).
Coughs.

Transbronquina Rectal Lab, Port.
Camphor (p.1589·3); quinine (p.445·1).

Transcop Recordati, Ital.
Hyoscine (p.468·2).
Motion sickness.

TransCyte Smith & Nephew, USA.
Bioengineered human skin equivalent (p.1123·2).
Burns.

Transderm Scop Novartis Consumer, USA.
Hyoscine (p.468·2).
Motion sickness.

Transdermal-NTG Warner Chilcott, USA.
Glyceryl trinitrate (p.897·3).
Angina pectoris.

Transderm-Nitro Novartis, Canad.; Novartis, USA.
Glyceryl trinitrate (p.897·3).
Angina pectoris.

Transderm-V Novartis, Canad.
Hyoscine (p.468·2).
Motion sickness.

Transene Sanofi Winthrop, Ital.
Dipotassium clorazepate (p.670·3).
Anxiety; insomnia; nervous disorders.

Transferal Ferrer, Spain†.
Tocofibrate (p.984·3).
Hyperlipidaemias.

Transfert Piam, Ital.
Carnitine (p.1356·1).
Carnitine deficiency.

Transidern-Nitro
Novartis, Austral.; Novartis, Denm.; Novartis, Fin.; Novartis, Irl.; Novartis, Neth.; Novartis, Norw.; Novartis, Swed.; Novartis, UK.
Glyceryl trinitrate (p.897·3).
Angina pectoris; prophylaxis of phlebitis and extravasation.

Transilane Innotech, Fr.
Ispaghula (p.1229·1).
Constipation.

Transipeg Roche, Belg.; Nicholas, Fr.; Syntex, Mex.; Roche, Switz.
Macrogol 3350 (p.1630·3); electrolytes (p.1180·1).
Constipation.

Transitol Schwarz, Fr.
White soft paraffin (p.1407·3); light liquid paraffin (p.1407·2).
Constipation.

Transix Christiaens, Belg.
Senna (p.1248·2).
Bowel evacuation; constipation.

Translet Franklin Medical, UK.
Barrier cream.

Translet Plus One Rusch, UK.
A deodorant liquid for use with colostomies and ileostomies.

Translet Plus Two Rusch, UK.
A deodorant liquid for use with colostomies and ileostomies.

Translight Merck Sharp & Dohme-Chibret, Fr.†.
Tyloxapol (p.1349·3)(p.1129·2).
Hard contact lens cleaner.

Transmer Tradiphar, Fr.
Promethazine hydrochloride (p.423·2); ephedrine hydrochloride (p.1090·1).
Motion sickness.

Transmetil Knoll, Ital.
Ademetionine butanedisulfonate (p.1573·1).
Liver disorders.

Transoak Pabisch, Aust.
A rinsing and storage solution for hard and gas permeable contact lenses (p.1129·2).

Transoddi Lipha Sante, Fr.
Cinametic acid (p.1595·3).
Gastrointestinal disorders.

Transol Pabisch, Aust.
A wetting solution for hard and gas permeable contact lenses (p.1129·2).

Transoxyl Ferraz, Lynce, Port.
Almitrine dimesilate (p.1506·2); raubasine (p.967·2).

Trans-Plantar Westwood-Squibb, Canad.
Salicylic acid (p.1122·3).
Plantar warts.

Transpulmin Asta Medica, Thai.
Pipazetate hydrochloride (p.1099·1).
Coughs.

Transpulmin Baby Asta Medica, Ger.
Eucalyptus oil (p.1609·2); pine needle oil.
Cold symptoms.

Transpulmin Balsam Asta Medica, Ger.
Eucalyptol (p.1609·2); menthol (p.1632·3); camphor (p.1589·3).
Bronchitis; catarrh.

Transpulmin Balsamo Asta Medica, Braz.
Camphor (p.1589·3); guaiacol (p.1092·1); eucalyptol (p.1609·2); menthol (p.1632·3).
Respiratory-tract congestion.

Transpulmin Kinderbalsam S Asta Medica, Ger.
Eucalyptus oil (p.1609·2); pine needle oil.
Cold symptoms.

Transpulmin Supositorio Asta Medica, Braz.
Camphor (p.1589·3); guaiacol (p.1092·1); eucalyptol (p.1609·2); menthol (p.1632·3).
Respiratory-tract congestion.

Transpulmin Xarope Asta Medica, Braz.
Guaifenesin (p.1092·2); oxeladin (p.1096·2); eucalyptol (p.1609·2); menthol (p.1632·3); sodium camsilate.
Respiratory-tract congestion.

Transpulmina Dogra, Port.
Camphor (p.1589·3); eucalyptol (p.1609·2); menthol (p.1632·3).
Respiratory-tract disorders.

Transpulmina Gola Bayer, Ital.
Dequalinium chloride (p.1143·1); menthol (p.1632·3); eucalyptol (p.1609·2).
Mouth and throat infections.

Transpulmina Tosse Bayer, Ital.
Pastilles: Guaifenesin (p.1092·2); menthol (p.1632·3); eucalyptol (p.1609·2); camphor (p.1589·3).
Syrup: Guaifenesin (p.1092·2); menthol (p.1632·3); eucalyptol (p.1609·2).
Catarrh; coughs.

Transulose Schwarz, Fr.
Lactulose (p.1230·1); liquid paraffin (p.1407·1); white soft paraffin (p.1407·3).
Constipation.

Transvane Promedis, Belg.†.
Thurfyl salicylate (p.88·1); hexyl nicotinate (p.42·2); ethyl nicotinate (p.35·1); benzocaine (p.1306·2).
Musculoskeletal, joint, and soft-tissue disorders.

Transvasin
Seton, Irl.; Seton, NZ; Sparks, NZ; Meda, Swed.†.
Ethyl nicotinate (p.35·1); hexyl nicotinate (p.42·2); thurfyl salicylate (p.88·1).
Formerly contained thurfyl salicylate, ethyl nicotinate, hexyl nicotinate, and benzocaine in Irl.
Rheumatic and muscular pain; sprains; strains.

Transvasin Heat Rub SSL, UK.
Ethyl nicotinate (p.35·1); hexyl nicotinate (p.42·2); thurfyl salicylate (p.88·1).
Rheumatic and muscular pain; sprains; strains.

Transvasin Heat Spray SSL, UK.
Glycol salicylate (p.42·2); diethylamine salicylate (p.32·2); methyl nicotinate (p.55·1).
Rheumatic and muscular pain.

Transvercid Pierre Fabre Sante, Fr.
Salicylic acid (p.1122·3).
Warts.

Trans-Ver-Sal
Westwood-Squibb, Canad.; Difa, Ital.; Darier, Mex.
Salicylic acid (p.1122·3).
Calluses; verrucas; warts.

Trans-Ver-Sal AdultPatch Doak, USA.
Salicylic acid (p.1122·3).
Verrucas.

Trans-Ver-Sal PediaPatch Doak, USA.
Salicylic acid (p.1122·3).
Formerly known as PediaPatch.
Warts.

Trans-Ver-Sal PlantarPatch Doak, USA.
Salicylic acid (p.1122·3).
Formerly known as Trans-Plantar.
Warts.

Transzone Par, USA.
Melatonin (p.1632·1).

Trantalol Pinewood, Irl.
Atenolol (p.841·3).
Angina pectoris; arrhythmias; hypertension; myocardial infarction.

Trantil Rudefsa, Mex.
Carbamazepine (p.342·2).

The symbol † denotes a preparation no longer actively marketed

Tranxal CTI, Israel.
Dipotassium clorazepate (p.670·3).
Alcohol withdrawal syndrome; anxiety.

Tranxen Searle, Denm.†.
Dipotassium clorazepate (p.670·3).
Alcohol withdrawal syndrome; anxiety.

Tranxene
Glaxo Wellcome, Austral.†; Sanofi Synthelabo, Belg.; Abbott, Canad.; Sanofi Winthrop, Fr.; Sanofi Winthrop, Hong Kong; Boehringer Ingelheim, Irl.; Sanofi Winthrop, Mex.; Sanofi Synthelabo, Neth.; Sanofi Synthelabo, Port.; Sanofi Synthelabo, S.Afr.; Sanofi Synthelabo, Singapore; Sanofi Synthelabo, Thai.; Boehringer Ingelheim, UK; Abbott, USA.
Dipotassium clorazepate (p.670·3).
Alcohol withdrawal syndrome; anxiety; disturbed behaviour; epilepsy; premedication; sleep disorders; tetany.

Tranxilene Sanofi Winthrop, Braz.
Dipotassium clorazepate (p.670·3).
Alcohol withdrawal syndrome; anxiety; epilepsy.

Tranxilium
Sanofi Winthrop, Aust.; Sanofi Synthelabo, Ger.; Sanofi Synthelabo, Spain; Sanofi Synthelabo, Switz.
Dipotassium clorazepate (p.670·3).
Agitation; anxiety; premedication; sleep disorders.

Tranxilium N Sanofi Winthrop, Ger.
Nordazepam (p.696·1).
Anxiety; sleep disorders.

Trapanal Byk Gulden, Ger.
Thiopental sodium (p.1269·1).
General anaesthesia.

Traqueobron Medquimica, Braz.
Cetylpyridinium; ammonium chloride (p.1085·2); sodium benzoate (p.1134·3).
Respiratory-tract congestion.

Traquivan Llorente, Spain.
Dihydrocodeine tartrate (p.33·1); co-trimoxazole (p.193·3).
Respiratory-tract infections.

Trasedal Elerte, Fr.
Tramadol hydrochloride (p.89·1).
Pain.

Trasicor
Novartis, Aust.; Novartis, Belg.; Novartis, Canad.; Novartis, Denm.; Novartis, Fr.; Novartis, Ger.; Novartis, Irl.; Novartis, Israel; Novartis, Neth.; Novartis, NZ; Novartis, S.Afr.; Novartis, Spain; Novartis, Switz.; Sovereign, UK.
Oxprenolol hydrochloride (p.951·3).
Angina pectoris; anxiety; arrhythmias; hypertension; hyperthyroidism; myocardial infarction; obstructive cardiomyopathy.

Trasidrex
Novartis, Irl.; Novartis, S.Afr.; Novartis, UK.
Oxprenolol hydrochloride (p.951·3); cyclopenthiazide (p.865·2).
These ingredients can be described by the British Approved Name Co-prenozide.
Hypertension.

Trasipressol Novartis, Fr.†.
Oxprenolol hydrochloride (p.951·3); dihydralazine sulfate (p.874·2).
Hypertension.

Trasitensin
Novartis, Aust.; Novartis, Ger.; Novartis, Ital.; Novartis, Spain.
Oxprenolol hydrochloride (p.951·3); chlortalidone (p.857·1).
Hypertension.

Trasitensine
Novartis, Fr.; Novartis, Switz.
Oxprenolol hydrochloride (p.951·3); chlortalidone (p.857·1).
Hypertension.

Trasylol
Bayer, Aust.; Bayer, Austral.; Bayer, Belg.; Bayer, Canad.; Bayer, Denm.; Bayer, Fin.; Bayer, Fr.; Bayer, Ger.; Bayer, Hong Kong; Bayer, Ital.†; Bayer, Mex.; Bayer, Neth.; Bayer, NZ; Bayer, S.Afr.; Bayer, Singapore; Bayer, Swed.; Bayer, Switz.; Bayer, Thai.; Bayer, UK; Bayer, USA.
Aprotinin (p.725·3).
Hyperfibrinolytic haemorrhage; reduction of blood loss in open heart surgery; shock; thrombolytic therapy complications.

Tratocoli IMA, Braz.
Furazolidone (p.592·1); phthalylsulfathiazole (p.235·3); pectin (p.1502·3).
Diarrhoea.

Tratoderm IMA, Braz.
Triclosan (p.1159·2); allantoin (p.1110·1).
Skin disorders.

Tratul Gerot, Aust.
Diclofenac (p.30·2) or diclofenac diethylamine (p.30·2) or diclofenac sodium (p.30·3).
Fever; gout; inflammation; musculoskeletal, joint, and peri-articular disorders; pain.

Trauma Relief Brauer, Austral.
Homoeopathic preparation.

Traumac Catarinense, Braz.
Benzocaine (p.1306·2); camphor (p.1589·3); lavender (p.1627·2); turpentine oil (p.1676·3); menthol (p.1632·3); methyl salicylate (p.55·1).
Musculoskeletal and joint disorders.

TraumaCal
Mead Johnson, Austral.; Mead Johnson, NZ; Mead Johnson, Singapore; Mead Johnson Nutritionals, Thai.; Mead Johnson Nutritionals, USA.
Preparation for enteral nutrition (p.1350·1).

Trauma-cyl Liebermann, Ger.
Chamomile oil; sage oil (p.1660·2); arnica (p.1581·3); aesculus (p.1574·1); hamamelis (p.1618·3).
Soft-tissue injury; vascular disorders.

Trauma-cyl N Complex Liebermann, Ger.
Homoeopathic preparation.

Trauma-Dolgit Dolorgiet, Ger.
Ibuprofen (p.43·2).
Musculoskeletal and joint disorders; sports injuries.

Traumadyn Plantamed, Ger.
Homoeopathic preparation.

Traumafusin Fresenius Kabi, Aust.
Amino-acid and electrolyte infusion (p.1350·1).
Parenteral nutrition.

Traumagel Sanval, Braz.
Methyl salicylate (p.55·1); camphor (p.1589·3); turpentine oil (p.1676·3); menthol (p.1632·3).
Musculoskeletal and joint disorders.

Trauma-kuhlend Mayrhofer, Aust.
Methyl salicylate (p.55·1); camphor (p.1589·3); menthol (p.1632·3).
Musculoskeletal, joint, and soft-tissue disorders.

Traumal Novartis Consumer, Ital.
Oxerutins (p.1611·2); a heparinoid (p.905·2).
Bruises; sprains.

Traumalgyl Pharmadeveloppement, Fr.
Mephenesin (p.1329·2); diethylamine salicylate (p.32·2); lignocaine [lidocaine] (p.1313·2).
Formerly contained phenylbutazone, mephenesin, diethylamine salicylate, and lignocaine [lidocaine].
Musculoskeletal, joint, peri-articular, and soft-tissue disorders.

Traumalitan 3M, Ger.
Heparin sodium (p.902·1).
Skin trauma; thromboembolic disorders.

Traumalix Drossapharm, Switz.
Etofenamate (p.35·3).
Musculoskeletal, joint, peri-articular, and soft-tissue disorders.

Traumanase
Rhone-Poulenc Rorer, Ger.; Rhone-Poulenc Rorer, Switz.
Bromelains (p.1586·3).
Inflammation with oedema.

Traumaparil Madaus, Aust.†.
Aescin (p.1574·1).
Soft-tissue disorders.

Traumaplant Harras-Curarina, Ger.
Comfrey (p.1598·3).
Musculoskeletal and joint disorders; sports injuries; wounds.

Trauma-Puren Isis Puren, Ger.
Heparin sodium (p.902·1); menthol (p.1632·3); glycol salicylate (p.42·2).
Haematoma; inflammation; phlebitis.

Traumasalbe Provita, Aust.
Capsicum (p.1591·1); methyl salicylate (p.55·1); turpentine oil (p.1676·3).
Musculoskeletal, joint, peri-articular, and soft-tissue disorders.

Trauma-Salbe Rodler 301 N Woelm, Ger.
Camphor (p.1589·3); menthol (p.1632·3); methyl salicylate (p.55·1).
Cold symptoms; joint, muscular, and neuromuscular pain.

Trauma-Salbe Rodler 302 N Woelm, Ger.
Camphor (p.1589·3); turpentine oil (p.1676·3); eucalyptus oil (p.1609·2).
Muscle and joint injuries.

Trauma-Salbe Rodler 303 N Woelm, Ger.†.
Camphor (p.1589·3).
Formerly contained cayenne pepper, camphor, menthol, and methyl salicylate.
Muscle and joint disorders.

Traumasenex Riemser, Ger.
Glycol salicylate (p.42·2).
Rheumatism; soft-tissue disorders.

Traumasept Wolff, Ger.
Povidone-iodine (p.1155·1).
Burns; skin disinfection; ulcers; vaginal infections; wounds.

Traumasive Hexal, Ger.
Hydrocolloid dressing.
Burns; wounds.

Traumasport IBSA, Switz.
Diclofenac epolamine (p.31·3).
Musculoskeletal, joint, peri-ariacular and soft-tissue injuries.

Traumasteril kohlenhydratfrei Fresenius, Ger.
Amino-acid and electrolyte infusion (p.1350·1).
Parenteral nutrition.

Traumatociclina Biomedica, Ital.
Meclocycline sulfosalicylate (p.222·1).
Bacterial skin infections.

Trauma-warmend Mayrhofer, Aust.
Methyl salicylate (p.55·1); capsicum (p.1591·1); turpentine oil (p.1676·3).
Musculoskeletal, joint, and soft-tissue disorders.

Traumazol Chinoin, Mex.
Ethyl chloride (p.1312·1).
Local anaesthesia.

Traumeel
Peithner, Aust.; Heel, USA.
Homoeopathic preparation.

Traumeel S
Heel, Ger.; Heel, S.Afr.
Homoeopathic preparation.

Traumicid Darec, Ital.
Methylbenzethonium chloride (p.1150·3); chlorothymol (p.1142·1).
Wound disinfection.

Traumon
Kolassa, Aust.; Bayer, Ger.
Etofenamate (p.35·3).
Musculoskeletal, joint, peri-articular, and soft-tissue disorders.

Traumox Medpro, S.Afr.
Naproxen (p.60·3).
Dysmenorrhoea; gout; musculoskeletal and joint disorders.

Trausan Vitoria, Port.
Citicoline (p.1596·1).
Cerebrovascular disorders; movement disorders; speech disorders; vertigo.

Trautil CEPA, Spain.
Cisapride (p.1220·1).
Gastro-oesophageal reflux; gastroparesis.

Travacalm Hamilton, Austral.
Dimenhydrinate (p.415·2); hyoscine hydrobromide (p.468·2); caffeine (p.761·3).
Motion sickness.

Travacalm HO Hamilton, Austral.
Hyoscine hydrobromide (p.468·2).
Motion sickness.

Travacalm Natural Hamilton, Austral.
Ginger (p.1227·2).
Motion sickness.

Travad Baxter, Austral.
Anhydrous monobasic sodium phosphate (p.1193·2); anhydrous dibasic sodium phosphate (p.1193·2).
Bowel evacuation; constipation.

Travahex Baxter, Fin.
Chlorhexidine acetate (p.1138·2).
Skin, wound, and mucous membrane disinfection.

Travamin Rekah, Israel.
Dimenhydrinate (p.415·2).
Motion sickness; radiation sickness.

Travamine ICN, Canad.
Dimenhydrinate (p.415·2).

Travasept
Baxter, Israel; Baxter, UK.
Cetrimide (p.1137·1); chlorhexidine acetate (p.1138·2).
Skin, burn, and wound disinfection.

Travasol
Baxter, Canad.; Clintec, USA.
A range of amino-acid infusions with or without carbohydrate and electrolytes (p.1350·1).
Parenteral nutrition.

Travasorb Clintec, USA.
A range of preparations for enteral nutrition (p.1350·1).

Travatan
Alcon, UK; Alcon, USA.
Travoprost (p.1447·3).
Glaucoma; ocular hypertension.

Travel Aid WestCan, Canad.
Dimenhydrinate (p.415·2).
Nausea; vomiting.

Travel Calm Boots, UK; Unichem, UK.
Hyoscine hydrobromide (p.468·2).
Motion sickness.

Travel Sickness Cantassium Co., UK.
Ginger (p.1227·2).

Travel Sickness Cocculus Homeocan, Canad.
Homoeopathic preparation.

Travel Tabs WestCan, Canad.
Dimenhydrinate (p.415·2).
Motion sickness.

Travel Well Farmalider, Spain.
Dimenhydrinate (p.415·2).
Motion sickness.

Travelaide Yauyip, Austral.
Ginger (p.1227·2); cardamom (p.1591·3); slippery elm (p.1665·1).
Motion sickness.

Travelbac Co-Pharma, UK.
Bacterial extracts; vitamin B substances; yeast (p.1350·1).
Dietary supplement for travellers.

Travel-Caps English Grains, UK.
Ginger (p.1227·2); calumba (p.1589·2); chamomile (p.1593·2).

Travelgum
Asta Medica, Hong Kong; Asta Medica, Ital.
Dimenhydrinate (p.415·2).
Motion sickness.

Travel-Gum
Asta Medica, Aust.; Asta Medica, Port.†.
Dimenhydrinate (p.415·2).
Motion sickness; vestibular disorders.

Travella Nelson, UK.
Homoeopathic preparation.
Formerly known as Travel Sickness Tablets.

Travellers Phillips Yeast, UK.
Ginger (p.1227·2).
Motion sickness.

Travello
Pharmacia Upjohn, Denm.; Pharmacia Upjohn, Norw.; Pharmacia Upjohn, Swed.
Loperamide hydrochloride (p.1231·3).
Diarrhoea.

Travelmate Shoppers Drug Mart, Canad.†.
Dimenhydrinate (p.415·2).

Traveltabs Stanley, Canad.
Dimenhydrinate (p.415·2).
Nausea; vomiting.

Travert
Pharmacia Upjohn, Norw.†; Baxter, USA.
Invert sugar (p.1366·2); electrolytes (p.1180·1).
Carbohydrate source; fluid and electrolyte disorders.

Travex Asta Medica, Port.
Tramadol hydrochloride (p.89·1).
Pain.

Travisco Master Pharma, Ital.
Trapidil (p.986·1).
Ischaemic heart disease; prevention of restenosis following angioplasty.

Travocort
Schering, Aust.; Schering, Belg.; Schering, Ger.; Asche, Ger.; Schering, Hong Kong; Schering, Irl.; Schering, Ital.; Schering, Port.; Schering, S.Afr.; Schering, Singapore; Schering, Switz.; Schering, Thai.
Isoconazole nitrate (p.387·2); diflucortolone valerate (p.1069·3).
Inflamed fungal skin infections.

Travogen
Schering, Aust.; Schering, Belg.; Schering, Ger.; Asche, Ger.; Schering, Hong Kong; Schering, Ital.; Schering, Singapore; Schering, Switz.; Schering, Thai.
Isoconazole (p.387·1) or isoconazole nitrate (p.387·2).
Erythrasma; fungal infections of the skin, nail, vulva, and vagina.

Travogyn Schering, UK†.
Isoconazole nitrate (p.387·2).
Fungal vaginal infections.

Trawell Asta Medica, Switz.
Dimenhydrinate (p.415·2).
Motion sickness.

Traxam
Whitehall, Irl.; Wyeth Lederle, Ital.; Goldshield, UK.
Felbinac (p.36·1).
Inflammation; musculoskeletal, joint, peri-articular, and soft-tissue disorders; pain.

Traxaton Steigerwald, Ger.
Oak bark (p.1643·2).
Diarrhoea.

Trazidex Sophia, Mex.
Tobramycin sulfate (p.263·3); dexamethasone (p.1067·1).
Infected eye disorders.

Trazil Sophia, Mex.
Tobramycin sulfate (p.263·3).
Bacterial eye infections.

Trazinac Sophia, Mex.
Diclofenac sodium (p.30·3); tobramycin sulfate (p.263·3).
Adjunct to eye surgery; bacterial eye infections.

Trazodil Unipharm, Israel.
Trazodone hydrochloride (p.310·1).
Depression.

Trazograf
Darrow, Braz.; Juste, Spain.
Meglumine amidotrizoate (p.1031·2); sodium amidotrizoate (p.1031·2).
Radiographic contrast medium.

Trazolan
Continental Pharma, Belg.; Searle, Neth.
Trazodone hydrochloride (p.310·1).
Depression.

Trazone Tecnifar, Port.
Trazodone hydrochloride (p.310·1).
Depression.

Trazorel ICN, Canad.
Trazodone hydrochloride (p.310·1).
Depression.

Trazyl Angelini, Ital.
Ibopamine hydrochloride (p.912·1).
Diagnosis of glaucoma; postoperative ocular hypotension; production of mydriasis.

TRCS-Verorab Pasteur Merieux, Thai.
A rabies vaccine (p.1560·2).
Active immunisation.

Trecalmo Bayer, Ger.†.
Clotiazepam (p.671·1).
Anxiety; sleep disorders.

Trecator Wyeth-Ayerst, USA.
Ethionamide (p.206·1).
Tuberculosis.

Treda Sanfer, Mex.
Neomycin sulfate (p.228·1); pectin (p.1502·3); kaolin (p.1229·3).
Gastro-enteritis.

Tredalat Bayer, Ger.
Nifedipine (p.940·1); acebutolol hydrochloride (p.825·1).
Angina pectoris; hypertension.

Tredemine Rhone-Poulenc Rorer, Fr.
Niclosamide (p.104·2).
Taeniasis.

Tredol Quimica y Farmacia, Mex.
Dipyrone (p.34·1).

Trefovital Vaillant, Ital.†.
Royal jelly (p.1659·3).
Nutritional supplement.

tregor Hormosan, Ger.
Amantadine sulfate (p.1161·2).
Parkinsonism.

Treloc Astra, Ger.; Promed, Ger.
Metoprolol tartrate (p.931·2); hydrochlorothiazide (p.907·3); hydralazine hydrochloride (p.905·3).
Hypertension.

Trelstar Pharmacia Upjohn, USA.
Triptorelin embonate (p.1299·1).
Prostatic cancer.

Tremaril LPB, Ital.
Metixene hydrochloride (p.470·2).
Parkinsonism.

Tremarit Asta Medica, Ger.
Metixene hydrochloride (p.470·2).
Parkinsonism and other hyperkinetic disorders.

Tremblex Janssen-Cilag, Belg.; Janssen-Cilag, Neth.
Dexetimide hydrochloride (p.465·3).
Drug-induced extrapyramidal disorders.

Tremoforat Klein, Ger.
Belladonna (p.463·1).
Parkinsonism.

Tremoquil Astra, Swed.
Metixene hydrochloride (p.470·2).
Parkinsonism.

Tremorex Durascan, Denm.
Selegiline hydrochloride (p.1177·2).
Parkinsonism.

Trenantone Takeda, Aust.; Takeda, Ger.
Leuprorelin acetate (p.1289·2).
Prostatic cancer.

Trendar PMS Whitehall-Robins, Canad.
Paracetamol (p.71·2); pamabrom (p.952·1); mepyramine maleate (p.421·1).
Premenstrual syndrome.

Trendinol Vita Elan, Spain.
Nitrendipine (p.947·1).
Hypertension.

Trenelone Schering-Plough, Port.
Dexchlorpheniramine maleate (p.412·1).

Trenlin CCM, Singapore.
Oxpentifylline [pentoxifylline] (p.950·3).
Cerebral and peripheral vascular disorders.

Trentadil Christiaens, Belg.; Medeva, Fr.
Bamifylline hydrochloride (p.761·2).
Asthma; obstructive airways disease.

Trental Hoechst Marion Roussel, Aust.; Hoechst Marion Roussel, Austral.; Hoechst Marion Roussel, Braz.; Hoechst Marion Roussel, Canad.; Aventis, Denm.; Hoechst Marion Roussel, Fin.; Hoechst Marion Roussel, Ger.; Hoechst Marion Roussel, Hong Kong; Hoechst Marion Roussel, Irl.; Hoechst Marion Roussel, Israel; Hoechst Marion Roussel, Ital.; Hoechst Marion Roussel, Mex.; Hoechst Marion Roussel, Neth.; Hoechst Marion Roussel, Norw.; Aventis, NZ; Hoeport, Port.; Aventis, S.Afr.; Hoechst Marion Roussel, Singapore; Hoechst Marion Roussel, Switz.; Hoechst Marion Roussel, Thai.; Borg, UK; Hoechst Marion Roussel, USA.
Oxpentifylline [pentoxifylline] (p.950·3).
Angioneurotic disorders; cerebral and ocular vascular disorders; disorders of the inner ear; peripheral vascular disorders.

Treo Pharmacia Upjohn, Aust.†; Lundbeck, Denm.; Pharmacia Upjohn, Fin.; Pharmacia Upjohn, Swed.
Note. This name is used for preparations of different composition.
Aspirin (p.14·2); caffeine (p.761·3).
Fever; pain.

Biopharm, USA.
SPF 8; SPF 15; SPF 30: Octocrilene (p.1518·1); octinoxate (p.1517·3); oxybenzone (p.1518·1); octisalate (p.1518·1); citronella oil (p.1596·3).
Sunscreen.

Treo comp Pharmacia Upjohn, Swed.
Aspirin (p.14·2); codeine phosphate (p.25·2); caffeine (p.761·3).
Pain.

Treomycin Chew, Thai.
Thiamphenicol (p.261·3).
Bacterial infections.

Treparin NCSN, Ital.
A heparinoid (p.905·2).
Thrombosis prophylaxis.

Trepidan Max Farma, Ital.
Prazepam (p.701·1).
Anxiety.

Trepiline Aspen, S.Afr.
Amitriptyline hydrochloride (p.273·3).
Mixed anxiety depressive states.

Trepol Lemery, Mex.
Dipyridamole (p.877·2).

Trepress Novartis, Aust.; Novartis, Ger.; Ciba, Switz.†.
Oxprenolol hydrochloride (p.951·3); hydralazine hydrochloride (p.905·3); chlortalidone (p.857·1).
Hypertension.

Tres Orix Forte Almirall, Hong Kong; Almirall, Spain.
Cyproheptadine orotate (p.414·3); amino acids and vitamins (p.1350·1).
Anorexia; tonic; weight loss.

Tresal Tremedic, Swed.†.
Sodium chloride (p.1196·1).
Irrigation solution.

Tresium Prodes, Spain†.
Bromhexine hydrochloride (p.1085·3); co-trimoxazole (p.193·3).
Respiratory-tract infections.

Tresleen Pfizer, Aust.
Sertraline hydrochloride (p.308·3).
Anxiety disorders; depression.

Tresos B Eagle, Austral.
Multivitamin, amino-acid, and mineral preparation (p.1350·1).
Dietary supplement.

Tretinoine Widmer, Switz.†.
Tretinoin (p.1126·2); urea (p.1127·3); triclosan (p.1159·2).
Acne.

Tretinoine Kefrane RoC, Fr.
Tretinoin (p.1126·2).
Acne.

Tretinon Wayne, Mex.
Tretinoin (p.1126·2).

Treupel comp Asta Medica, Ger.
Codeine phosphate (p.25·2); paracetamol (p.71·2).
Fever; pain.

Treupel mono Asta Medica, Ger.
Paracetamol (p.71·2).
Fever; pain.

Treupel N Asta Medica, Switz.†.
Paracetamol (p.71·2).
Fever; pain.

Treupel sans codeine Asta Medica, Switz.
Aspirin (p.14·2); paracetamol (p.71·2).
Fever; pain.

Treupel simplex Asta Medica, Switz.
Aspirin (p.14·2); paracetamol (p.71·2); ascorbic acid (p.1389·3).
Fever; pain.

Treuphadol Treupha, Switz.
Paracetamol (p.71·2).
Fever; pain.

Treuphadol Plus Treupha, Switz.
Paracetamol (p.71·2); codeine phosphate (p.25·2).
Fever; pain.

Trevilor Wyeth, Ger.
Venlafaxine hydrochloride (p.312·2).
Depression.

Trevina Orion, Denm.
70 Tablets, estradiol valerate (p.1473·2); *14 tablets,* estradiol valerate; medroxyprogesterone acetate (p.1480·1); *7 tablets,* inert.
Menopausal disorders; osteoporosis.

Trevis Kabi, Swed.†.
4 Strains of *Lactobacillus* (p.1626·3).
Diarrhoea.

Trewilor Wyeth Lederle, Aust.
Venlafaxine hydrochloride (p.312·2).
Depression.

Trexall Barr, USA.
Methotrexate (p.553·2).
Malignant neoplasms; psoriasis; rheumatoid arthritis.

Trexan Orion, Fin.
Note. This name is used for preparations of different composition.
Methotrexate (p.553·2).
Malignant neoplasms.

Du Pont, Hong Kong; Boots, Hong Kong; Du Pont, Singapore; Du Pont, USA.
Naltrexone hydrochloride (p.1016·1).
Opioid dependence.

Trexeron Serono, Mex.
Methotrexate (p.553·2).

Trexofin Cheil, Singapore.
Ceftriaxone sodium (p.177·1).
Bacterial infections.

Trexyl Ranbaxy, Thai.
Terfenadine (p.424·3).
Allergic eye disorders; allergic rhinitis; allergic skin disorders.

TRH UCB, Belg.; Berlin-Chemie, Ger.; Ferring, Ger.; Ferring, Israel; Roche, Israel; Cambridge, UK.
Protirelin (p.1295·3).
Now known as Protirelin in the UK.
Diagnosis of hypothalamic-pituitary-thyroid dysfunction.

TRH Prem Novartis Consumer, Spain.
Protirelin (p.1295·3).
Evaluation of thyroid function.

Tri Hachemina Medea, Spain.
Inositol (p.1623·3); calcium pantothenate (p.1374·1); aminobenzoic acid (p.1516·3) or sodium aminobenzoate.
Infertility; skin disorders.

Tri Vit with Fluoride Barre-National, USA.
Multivitamin preparation with fluoride (p.1375·3)(p.1350·1).
Dental caries prophylaxis; dietary supplement.

Triac Ache, Braz.
Tiratricol (p.1528·3).
Thyroid disorders.

Triacana Laphal, Fr.
Tiratricol (p.1528·3).
Thyroid disorders; treatment of cellulite.

Triacelluvax Chiron, Ital.
A diphtheria, tetanus, and acellular pertussis vaccine (p.1537·3).

Formerly known as Acelluvax DTP.
Active immunisation.

Triacet Lemmon, USA.
Triamcinolone acetonide (p.1080·1).
Skin disorders.

Triacilline Beecham, Belg.†.
Ticarcillin sodium (p.262·3).
Bacterial infections.

Triacomb Technilab, Canad.; Technilab, Hong Kong.
Triamcinolone acetonide (p.1080·1); nystatin (p.392·2); neomycin sulfate (p.228·1); gramicidin (p.213·3).
Anal and vulvar pruritus; infected skin disorders.

Triactin Prometic, USA†.
Phenylpropanolamine hydrochloride (p.1098·1); chlorpheniramine [chlorphenamine] maleate (p.412·1).
Upper respiratory-tract disorders.

Triad Forest Pharmaceuticals, USA.
Butalbital (p.658·3); paracetamol (p.71·2); caffeine (p.761·3).
Tension headache.

Triadapin Novopharm, Canad.†.
Doxepin hydrochloride (p.283·3).
Depression.

Tri-Adcortyl Squibb, UK.
Nystatin (p.392·2); triamcinolone acetonide (p.1080·1); neomycin sulfate (p.228·1); gramicidin (p.213·3).
Bacterial and fungal skin infections.

Triadene Schering, UK.
Ethinylestradiol (p.1476·2); gestodene (p.1479·1).
Triphasic oral contraceptive.

Triaderm Taro, Canad.
Triamcinolone acetonide (p.1080·1).
Skin disorders.

Triafed Schein, USA†.
Pseudoephedrine hydrochloride (p.1099·2); triprolidine hydrochloride (p.427·2).
Upper respiratory-tract symptoms.

Triafed with Codeine Schein, USA†.
Pseudoephedrine hydrochloride (p.1099·2); triprolidine hydrochloride (p.427·2); codeine phosphate (p.25·2).
Coughs.

Triaformo Cusi, Hong Kong.
Clioquinol (p.190·2); triamcinolone acetonide (p.1080·1).
Infected skin disorders.

Triagynon Schering, Spain.
Levonorgestrel (p.1486·2); ethinylestradiol (p.1476·2).
Triphasic oral contraceptive.

Triaken Kendrick, Mex.
Ceftriaxone sodium (p.177·1).
Lignocaine [lidocaine] hydrochloride (p.1313·2) is included in the intramuscular injection to alleviate the pain of injection.
Bacterial infections.

Trialix Hoechst Marion Roussel, Aust.; Hoechst Marion Roussel, Irl.; Hoechst Marion Roussel, Spain.
Ramipril (p.966·3); piretanide (p.956·2).
Hypertension.

Trialmin Menarini, Spain.
Gemfibrozil (p.896·2).
Hyperlipidaemias.

Trialona Alter, Spain.
Fluticasone propionate (p.1072·2).
Asthma.

Trialone Janssen-Cilag, S.Afr.
Miconazole nitrate (p.391·1); triamcinolone acetonide (p.1080·1); neomycin sulfate (p.228·1).
Infected skin disorders.

Trialyn DM Trianon, Canad.
Dextromethorphan hydrobromide (p.1087·3); diphenhydramine hydrochloride (p.416·1); ammonium chloride (p.1085·2).
Coughs.

Triam Lichtenstein, Ger.
Triamcinolone acetonide (p.1080·1).
Corticosteroid.

Hyrex, USA.
Triamcinolone diacetate (p.1080·2).
Corticosteroid.

Triama Samakeephaesaj, Thai.
Triamcinolone acetonide (p.1080·1).
Skin disorders.

Triam-A Hyrex, USA.
Triamcinolone acetonide (p.1080·1).
Corticosteroid.

Triamaxco Ashbourne, UK.
Triamterene (p.986·1); hydrochlorothiazide (p.907·3).
These ingredients can be described by the British Approved Name Co-triamterzide.
Hypertension; oedema.

Triam-Co Baker Norton, Hong Kong.
Hydrochlorothiazide (p.907·3); triamterene (p.986·1).
Hypertension; oedema.

Triamco Baker Norton, UK.
Hydrochlorothiazide (p.907·3); triamterene (p.986·1).
These ingredients can be described by the British Approved Name Co-triamterzide.
Hypertension; oedema.

Triamcort Helvepharm, Switz.
Triamcinolone acetonide (p.1080·1).
Corticosteroid.

TriamCreme Lichtenstein, Ger.
Triamcinolone acetonide (p.1080·1).
Skin disorders.

Triamer Pasteur Merieux, Belg.
An adsorbed diphtheria, tetanus, and pertussis vaccine (p.1537·3).
Active immunisation of infants and young children.

Triamgalen Galen, Ger.
Triamcinolone acetonide (p.1080·1).
Allergic and inflammatory skin disorders.

Triamhexal Hexal, Ger.
Triamcinolone acetonide (p.1080·1).
Corticosteroid.

Triami Sandoz, S.Afr.†.
Phenylpropanolamine hydrochloride (p.1098·1); pheniramine maleate (p.422·3); mepyramine maleate (p.421·1); caffeine (p.761·3).
Nasal congestion; rhinitis; sinusitis.

Triaminic
Note. This name is used for preparations of different composition.
Sandoz, Canad.†; Novartis Consumer, S.Afr.
Phenylpropanolamine hydrochloride (p.1098·1); pheniramine maleate (p.422·3); mepyramine maleate (p.421·1).
Hayfever; nasal congestion; rhinitis; sinusitis.

Novartis Sante, Fr.†.
Phenylpropanolamine hydrochloride (p.1098·1); pheniramine maleate (p.422·3).
Formerly contained phenylpropanolamine hydrochloride, mepyramine maleate, and pheniramine maleate.
Allergic and congestive disorders of the upper respiratory tract.

Novartis Consumer, Ital.
Nasal spray: Chlorpheniramine [chlorphenamine] maleate (p.412·1); oxymetazoline hydrochloride (p.1096·2).
Nasal congestion.
Tablets: Phenylpropanolamine hydrochloride (p.1098·1); pheniramine maleate (p.422·3); mepyramine maleate (p.421·1); caffeine (p.761·3).
Cold symptoms.

Novartis Consumer, USA†.
Phenylpropanolamine hydrochloride (p.1098·1); chlorpheniramine [chlorphenamine] maleate (p.412·1).
Formerly contained mepyramine maleate, pheniramine maleate, and phenylpropanolamine hydrochloride.
Upper respiratory-tract symptoms.

Triaminic-12 Novartis Consumer, USA†.
Phenylpropanolamine hydrochloride (p.1098·1); chlorpheniramine [chlorphenamine] maleate (p.412·1).
Cold symptoms.

Triaminic Allergy Novartis Consumer, USA†.
Phenylpropanolamine hydrochloride (p.1098·1); chlorpheniramine [chlorphenamine] maleate (p.412·1).
Upper respiratory-tract symptoms.

Triaminic AM Cough & Decongestant Formula Novartis Consumer, USA.
Pseudoephedrine hydrochloride (p.1099·2); dextromethorphan hydrobromide (p.1087·3).

Triaminic AM Decongestant Formula Novartis Consumer, USA.
Pseudoephedrine hydrochloride (p.1099·2).

Triaminic Chewable Novartis Consumer, USA†.
Phenylpropanolamine hydrochloride (p.1098·1); chlorpheniramine [chlorphenamine] maleate (p.412·1).
Upper respiratory-tract symptoms.

Triaminic Cold Novartis Consumer, USA†.
Phenylpropanolamine hydrochloride (p.1098·1); chlorpheniramine [chlorphenamine] maleate (p.412·1).
Cold symptoms.

Triaminic Cold & Allergy Novartis Consumer, Canad.†; Novartis, USA†.
Phenylpropanolamine hydrochloride (p.1098·1); chlorpheniramine [chlorphenamine] maleate (p.412·1).
Nasal and sinus congestion.

Triaminic Cold & Cough Novartis, USA.
Pseudoephedrine hydrochloride (p.1099·2); dextromethorphan hydrobromide (p.1087·3); chlorpheniramine [chlorphenamine] maleate (p.412·1).
Coughs and cold symptoms.

Triaminic Cold & Fever Novartis Consumer, Canad.
Pseudoephedrine hydrochloride (p.1099·2); dextromethorphan hydrobromide (p.1087·3); paracetamol (p.71·2).

Triaminic Decongestant & Expectorant Sandoz, Canad.†.
Pseudoephedrine hydrochloride (p.1099·2); guaifenesin (p.1092·2).

Triaminic DM Novartis Consumer, USA†.
Phenylpropanolamine hydrochloride (p.1098·1); dextromethorphan hydrobromide (p.1087·3).
Coughs and cold symptoms.

Triaminic DM Daytime Novartis Consumer, Canad.†.
Dextromethorphan hydrobromide (p.1087·3); phenylpropanolamine hydrochloride (p.1098·1); guaifenesin (p.1092·2).
Coughs and cold symptoms.

Triaminic DM Expectorant Novartis Consumer, Canad.
Dextromethorphan hydrobromide (p.1087·3); pseudoephedrine hydrochloride (p.1099·2); chlorpheniramine [chlorphenamine] maleate (p.412·1); guaifenesin (p.1092·2).
Formerly contained dextromethorphan hydrobromide, phenylpropanolamine hydrochloride, pheniramine maleate, mepyramine maleate, and guaifenesin.
Coughs; nasal congestion.

The symbol † denotes a preparation no longer actively marketed

Triaminic DM Nighttime Novartis Consumer, Canad.
Dextromethorphan hydrobromide (p.1087·3); chlorpheniramine [chlorphenamine] maleate (p.412·1); pseudoephedrine hydrochloride (p.1099·2).
Coughs; nasal congestion.

Triaminic DM-D Sandoz, Canad.†
Dextromethorphan hydrobromide (p.1087·3); pseudoephedrine hydrochloride (p.1099·2).
Coughs; nasal and sinus congestion.

Triaminic Expectorant
Note.This name is used for preparations of different composition.
Novartis Consumer, Canad.
Pseudoephedrine hydrochloride (p.1099·2); chlorpheniramine [chlorphenamine] maleate (p.412·1); guaifenesin (p.1092·2).
Formerly contained phenylpropanolamine hydrochloride, pheniramine maleate, mepyramine maleate, and guaifenesin.
Coughs; nasal congestion.

Novartis Consumer, USA†.
Phenylpropanolamine hydrochloride (p.1098·1); guaifenesin (p.1092·2).
Coughs.

Triaminic Expectorant with Codeine Novartis Consumer, USA†.
Codeine phosphate (p.25·2); phenylpropanolamine hydrochloride (p.1098·1); guaifenesin (p.1092·2).
Coughs.

Triaminic Expectorant DH
Sandoz, Canad.†; Novartis Consumer, USA†.
Hydrocodone tartrate (p.42·2); phenylpropanolamine hydrochloride (p.1098·1); pheniramine maleate (p.422·3); mepyramine maleate (p.421·1); guaifenesin (p.1092·2).
Coughs.

Triaminic Infant Oral Decongestant Novartis, USA.
Pseudoephedrine hydrochloride (p.1099·2).
Nasal congestion.

Triaminic Long Lasting DM Novartis Consumer, Canad.
Dextromethorphan hydrobromide (p.1087·3).
Formerly known as Triaminic DM.
Coughs.

Triaminic Night Time Rub Sandoz, Canad.†
Camphor (p.1589·3); eucalyptus oil (p.1609·2); menthol (p.1632·3).

Triaminic Nite Light Novartis Consumer, USA.
Pseudoephedrine hydrochloride (p.1099·2); chlorpheniramine [chlorphenamine] maleate (p.412·1); dextromethorphan hydrobromide (p.1087·3).
Coughs and cold symptoms.

Triaminic Oral Infant Novartis Consumer, USA†.
Phenylpropanolamine hydrochloride (p.1098·1); mepyramine maleate (p.421·1); pheniramine maleate (p.422·3).
Upper respiratory-tract symptoms.

Triaminic Pediatric Drops Novartis Consumer, Canad.
Pseudoephedrine hydrochloride (p.1099·2).

Triaminic Severe Cold & Fever Novartis, USA.
Paracetamol (p.71·2); pseudoephedrine hydrochloride (p.1099·2); dextromethorphan hydrobromide (p.1087·3); chlorpheniramine [chlorphenamine] maleate (p.412·1).
Coughs and cold symptoms.

Triaminic Softchews Novartis, USA.
Pseudoephedrine hydrochloride (p.1099·2); chlorpheniramine [chlorphenamine] maleate (p.412·1).
Upper respiratory-tract disorders.

Triaminic Sore Throat Formula Novartis Consumer, USA.
Pseudoephedrine hydrochloride (p.1099·2); dextromethorphan hydrobromide (p.1087·3); paracetamol (p.71·2).
Coughs and cold symptoms.

Triaminic Throat Pain & Cough Novartis, USA.
Paracetamol (p.71·2); pseudoephedrine (p.1099·2); dextromethorphan hydrobromide (p.1087·3).
Coughs; sore throat.

Triaminicflu Novartis Consumer, Ital.
Paracetamol (p.71·2); pheniramine maleate (p.422·3); phenylephrine hydrochloride (p.1097·1).
Cold and influenza symptoms.

Triaminicin Novartis Consumer, Canad.†
Phenylpropanolamine hydrochloride (p.1098·1); mepyramine maleate (p.421·1); pheniramine maleate (p.422·3); paracetamol (p.71·2); caffeine (p.761·3).
Cold symptoms.

Triaminicin Cold, Allergy, Sinus Novartis Consumer, USA†.
Phenylpropanolamine hydrochloride (p.1098·1); chlorpheniramine [chlorphenamine] maleate (p.412·1); paracetamol (p.71·2).
Upper respiratory-tract symptoms.

Triaminicol DM Novartis Consumer, Canad.
Pseudoephedrine hydrochloride (p.1099·2); chlorpheniramine [chlorphenamine] maleate (p.412·1); dextromethorphan hydrobromide (p.1087·3).
Formerly contained phenylpropanolamine hydrochloride, mepyramine maleate, pheniramine maleate, and dextromethorphan hydrobromide.
Coughs; nasal congestion.

Triaminicol Multi-Symptom Cough and Cold Novartis Consumer, USA†.
Phenylpropanolamine hydrochloride (p.1098·1); chlorpheniramine [chlorphenamine] maleate (p.412·1); dextromethorphan hydrobromide (p.1087·3).
Coughs and cold symptoms.

Triaminicol Multi-Symptom Relief Novartis Consumer, USA†.
Phenylpropanolamine hydrochloride (p.1098·1); chlorpheniramine [chlorphenamine] maleate (p.412·1); dextromethorphan hydrobromide (p.1087·3).
Coughs and cold symptoms.

Triam-Injekt Sanorania, Ger.
Triamcinolone acetonide (p.1080·1).
Corticosteroid.

Triamizide Pacific, NZ.
Hydrochlorothiazide (p.907·3); triamterene (p.986·1).
Hypertension.

Triamolone Forest Pharmaceuticals, USA†.
Triamcinolone diacetate (p.1080·2).
Corticosteroid.

Triamonide Forest Pharmaceuticals, USA.
Triamcinolone acetonide (p.1080·1).
Corticosteroid.

Triam-oral Lichtenstein, Ger.
Triamcinolone (p.1080·1).
Corticosteroid.

Triampur Asta Medica, Ger.
Triamterene (p.986·1); hydrochlorothiazide (p.907·3).
Heart failure; hypertension; oedema.

TriamSalbe Lichtenstein, Ger.
Triamcinolone acetonide (p.1080·1).
Skin disorders.

Triamsicort Diba, Mex.
Triamcinolone (p.1080·1).
Corticosteroid.

Triamteren comp
Generricon, Aust.; Ratiopharm, Ger.
Triamterene (p.986·1); hydrochlorothiazide (p.907·3).
Heart failure; hypertension; oedema.

Triamteren-H 3M, Ger.
Triamterene (p.986·1); hydrochlorothiazide (p.907·3).
Heart failure; hypertension; oedema.

Triamteren/HCT Aliud, Ger.
Triamterene (p.986·1); hydrochlorothiazide (p.907·3).
Heart failure; hypertension; oedema.

Triam-Tiazida R Normal, Port.
Triamterene (p.986·1); hydrochlorothiazide (p.907·3).
Hypertension.

Trianal
Note.This name is used for preparations of different composition.
Will-Pharma, Belg.; Will-Pharma, Neth.
Triamcinolone acetonide (p.1080·1); lignocaine [lidocaine] hydrochloride (p.1313·2).
Anal eczema and pruritus; haemorrhoids.

Trianon, Canad.
Aspirin (p.14·2); caffeine (p.761·3); butalbital (p.658·3).
Pain; sedative.

Trianal C Trianon, Canad.
Aspirin (p.14·2); caffeine (p.761·3); butalbital (p.658·3); codeine phosphate (p.25·2).
Pain; sedative.

Tri-Anemul Medopharm, Ger.†
Triamcinolone acetonide (p.1080·1).
Skin disorders.

Triapin
Hoechst Marion Roussel, Neth.; Hoechst Marion Roussel, UK.
Felodipine (p.888·3); ramipril (p.966·3).
Hypertension.

Triaprin Dunhall, USA†.
Paracetamol (p.71·2); butalbital (p.658·3).
Pain.

Triapten LAW, Ger.; Wyeth, Ger.
Foscarnet sodium (p.621·2).
Local herpes simplex virus infections.

Tri-Aqua Pfeiffer, USA.
Caffeine (p.761·3); buchu (p.1587·2); bearberry (p.1583·3); maize (p.1599·3); triticum.
Oedema associated with premenstrual syndrome.

Triarese Hexal, Ger.
Triamterene (p.986·1); hydrochlorothiazide (p.907·3).
Heart failure; hypertension; oedema.

Triasox Berna, Spain.
Tiabendazole (p.109·1).
Worm infections.

Triasporin Italfarmaco, Ital.
Itraconazole (p.387·2).
Fungal infections.

Triastad HCT Stada, Aust.
Triamterene (p.986·1); hydrochlorothiazide (p.907·3).
Hypertension; oedema.

Triastonal Hoyer, Ger.
Sitosterol (p.1373·3).
Benign prostatic hyperplasia.

Triatec
Hoechst Marion Roussel, Braz.; Aventis, Denm.; Hoechst, Fr.; Hoechst Marion Roussel, Ital.; Hoechst Marion Roussel, Norw.; Hoeport, Port.; Hoechst Marion Roussel, Swed.; Hoechst Marion Roussel, Switz.
Ramipril (p.966·3).
Heart failure; hypertension; myocardial infarction; renal insufficiency.

Triatec-8 Trianon, Canad.
Paracetamol (p.71·2); codeine phosphate (p.25·2); caffeine citrate (p.761·3).
Coughs; fever; pain.

Triatec-30 Trianon, Canad.
Paracetamol (p.71·2); codeine phosphate (p.25·2).
Coughs; fever; pain.

Triatec Comp
Aventis, Denm.; Hoechst Marion Roussel, Swed.; Hoechst Marion Roussel, Switz.
Ramipril (p.966·3); hydrochlorothiazide (p.907·3).
Hypertension.

Triatec Composto Hoeport, Port.
Ramipril (p.966·3); hydrochlorothiazide (p.907·3).
Hypertension.

Triatec HCT Hoechst Marion Roussel, Ital.
Ramipril (p.966·3); hydrochlorothiazide (p.907·3).
Hypertension.

Triatop
Janssen-Cilag, Ital.; Janssen, Thai.
Ketoconazole (p.389·1).
Scalp disorders.

Triaval Orion, Switz.
70 Tablets, estradiol valerate (p.1473·2); 14 tablets, estradiol valerate; medroxyprogesterone acetate (p.1480·1); 7 tablets, inert.
Menopausal disorders; osteoporosis.

Triavil Merck Frosst, Canad.; Lotus, USA.
Perphenazine (p.699·1); amitriptyline hydrochloride (p.273·1).
Mixed anxiety depressive states; schizophrenia.

Tri-A-Vite F Major, USA.
Multivitamin preparation with fluoride (p.1350·1).

Triaxin Eurofarma, Braz.
Ceftriaxone (p.177·1).
Bacterial infections.

Triaxone Julphar, UAE.
Ceftriaxone sodium (p.177·1).
Bacterial infections.

Triaz Medicis, USA.
Benzoyl peroxide (p.1111·1).
Acne.

triazid CT, Ger.
Triamterene (p.986·1); hydrochlorothiazide (p.907·3).
Heart failure; hypertension; oedema.

Triazine Aspen Consumer, S.Afr.
Cyclizine hydrochloride (p.414·1).
Motion sickness; vertigo.

Triazol Sanus, Braz.
Fluconazole (p.383·2).
Fungal infections.

Tri-B3 Rhone-Poulenc Rorer, Austral.†.
Nicotinic acid (p.1372·3).
Hyperlipidaemias.

Tribakin Farcoral, Mex.
Co-trimoxazole (p.193·3).
Bacterial infections.

Triban
Note.This name is used for preparations of different composition.
Solfran, Mex.
Vitamin B₁₂; vitamin B₁ (p.1350·1).

Great Southern, USA.
Trimethobenzamide hydrochloride (p.426·3); benzocaine (p.1306·2).

Tribedex Medifarma, Mex.
Vitamin B substances (p.1350·1).

Tribedoxyl Hoechst Marion Roussel, Mex.
Capsules: Cyanocobalamin (p.1388·1); benfotiamine (p.1384·3); pyridoxine hydrochloride (p.1386·3).
Injection: Hydroxocobalamin acetate (p.1388·3); thiamine hydrochloride (p.1385·1); pyridoxine hydrochloride (p.1386·3).
Lignocaine [lidocaine] hydrochloride (p.1313·2) is included in this preparation to alleviate the pain of injection.
Anaemias; neuralgias; neuritis; neuropathies.

Tribemin Sam-On, Israel.
Vitamin B₁ (p.1385·2); vitamin B₆ (p.1387·1); vitamin B₁₂ (p.1388·1).
Megaloblastic anaemia; neuralgias.

Tribesian Asian Pharm, Thai.
Vitamin B₁ (p.1385·2); vitamin B₆ (p.1387·1); vitamin B₁₂ (p.1388·1).
Anaemias; migraine; neuralgia; neuritis.

Tribeton Chemedica, Switz.
Cyanocobalamin (p.1388·1) or hydroxocobalamin (p.1388·1); thiamine hydrochloride (p.1385·1); pyridoxine hydrochloride (p.1386·3).
Lignocaine [lidocaine] hydrochloride (p.1313·2) is included in the injections to alleviate the pain of injection.
Alcoholism; nerve pain; neuritis; pain; vitamin B deficiency.

Tribiot Grin, Mex.
Neomycin sulfate (p.228·1); polymyxin B sulfate (p.238·1); bacitracin zinc (p.155·2).
Bacterial eye infections.

Tribiotic Plus Thompson, USA†.
Polymyxin B sulfate (p.238·1); neomycin sulfate (p.228·1); bacitracin (p.155·2); lignocaine [lidocaine] (p.1313·2).

Tri-Biozene Reese, USA.
Bacitracin (p.155·2); polymyxin B sulfate (p.238·1); neomycin sulfate (p.228·1); pramocaine hydrochloride (p.1318·2).

Tribonat
Fresenius Kabi, Norw.; Fresenius Kabi, Swed.
Trometamol (p.1675·2); electrolytes (p.1180·1).
Buffer; metabolic and respiratory acidosis.

Tri-Cal Medical Research, Hong Kong.
Calcium hydrogen phosphate (p.1188·2); calcium carbonate (p.1215·1); calcium gluconate (p.1188·2); vitamin D (p.1391·1); zinc oxide (p.1128·2); magnesium oxide (p.1233·2).
Calcium supplement; osteoporosis.

Tricalcio com Fluor Bergamo, Braz.
Vitamin and mineral preparation (p.1350·1).

Trican Teva, Israel.
Fluconazole (p.383·2).
Fungal infections.

Tricandil
Prospa, Belg.; SPA, Ital.; Prospa, Port.
Mepartricin (p.390·3).
Candidiasis; trichomoniasis.

Tricangine-A Asta Medica, Braz.
Mepartricin (p.390·3); tetracycline (p.258·3).
Bacterial and fungal vulvovaginal infections.

Tricef
Merck, Aust.; Bialfar, Port.; Astra, Swed.
Cefixime (p.166·2).
Bacterial infections.

Eurofarmaco, Ital.
Propylene glycol cefatrizine (p.164·3).
Bacterial infections.

Tricen Alter, Spain.
Verapamil hydrochloride (p.989·1); trandolapril (p.985·2).
Hypertension.

Tricephin Atlantic, Thai.
Ceftriaxone sodium (p.177·1).
Bacterial infections.

Tricept Cuprocept, S.Afr.
Copper-wound plastic (p.1357·3).
Intra-uterine contraceptive device.

Tricerol
Searle, Braz.; Armstrong, Mex.
Etofibrate (p.888·2).
Atherosclerosis; hyperlipidaemias.

Trichazole Intramed, S.Afr.; Aspen, S.Afr.
Metronidazole (p.594·1).
Anaerobic bacterial infections; protozoal infections.

Trichex Gerot, Aust.
Metronidazole (p.594·1).
Gardnerella vaginalis infections; trichomoniasis.

Tri-Chlor Gordon, USA.
Trichloroacetic acid (p.1674·3).
Warts.

Trichlorol Lysoform, Ger.
Tosylchloramide sodium (p.1159·1).
Surface and hand disinfection.

Trichobiol Therasophia, Fr.
Amino-acid, mineral, vitamin, and herbal preparation (p.1350·1).
Hair and nail disorders.

Trichonas Pharmasant, Thai.
Tinidazole (p.603·3).
Amoebiasis; anaerobic bacterial infections; giardiasis; trichomoniasis.

Trichotine Reed & Carnrick, USA.
Powder: Sodium laurilsulfate (p.1496·3); sodium perborate (p.1156·3); sodium chloride (p.1196·1).
Solution: Sodium laurilsulfate (p.1496·3); borax (p.1586·1); alcohol (p.1130·3).
Vaginal disorders.

Trichozole Pacific, NZ.
Metronidazole (p.594·1).
Anaerobic bacterial infections; protozoal infections.

Triciclor Wyeth, Spain.
Levonorgestrel (p.1486·2); ethinylestradiol (p.1476·2).
Triphasic oral contraceptive.

Tricidine Warner-Lambert Consumer, Belg.
Tyrothricin (p.267·1); lignocaine [lidocaine] hydrochloride (p.1313·2).
Mouth and throat disorders.

TriCilest
Janssen-Cilag, Aust.; Janssen-Cilag, S.Afr.
Norgestimate (p.1486·1); ethinylestradiol (p.1476·2).
Formerly known as Ortrel in Aust.
28-Day packs contain 7 inert tablets.
Triphasic oral contraceptive.

Triclin Solfran, Mex.
Tetracycline (p.258·3).
Bacterial infections.

Triclonam CTI, Israel.
Triclofos sodium (p.710·2).
Insomnia; sedative.

Tricloryl Galen, Irl.
Triclofos (p.710·2).
Hypnotic; sedative.

Triclose ICT, Israel.
Azanidazole (p.589·2).
Vaginal trichomoniasis.

Tri-Co Garec, S.Afr.
Co-trimoxazole (p.193·3).
Bacterial infections.

Tricocel UCI, Braz.
Oxypyrantel.
Worm infections.

Tricodein
Solco, Aust.; Solco, Ger.; Solco, Switz.
Codeine phosphate (p.25·2).
Coughs.

Tricodene Cough & Cold Pfeiffer, USA.
Mepyramine maleate (p.421·1); codeine phosphate (p.25·2).
Coughs and cold symptoms.

Tricodene Forte *Pfeiffer, USA†.*
Phenylpropanolamine hydrochloride (p.1098·1); chlorpheniramine [chlorphenamine] maleate (p.412·1); dextromethorphan hydrobromide (p.1087·3).
Coughs and cold symptoms.

Tricodene NN *Pfeiffer, USA†.*
Phenylpropanolamine hydrochloride (p.1098·1); chlorpheniramine [chlorphenamine] maleate (p.412·1); dextromethorphan hydrobromide (p.1087·3).
Coughs and cold symptoms.

Tricodene Pediatric Cough & Cold *Pfeiffer, USA†.*
Phenylpropanolamine hydrochloride (p.1098·1); dextromethorphan hydrobromide (p.1087·3).
Coughs and cold symptoms.

Tricodene Sugar Free *Pfeiffer, USA.*
Chlorpheniramine [chlorphenamine] maleate (p.412·1); dextromethorphan hydrobromide (p.1087·3).
Coughs and cold symptoms.

Tricogyn *Pharmaland, Thai.*
Tinidazole (p.603·3).
Amoebiasis; giardiasis.

Tricol Softgels *Ram, USA†.*
Omega-3 marine triglycerides (p.949·3).

Tricolam *Farmasierra, Spain.*
Tinidazole (p.603·3).
Anaerobic bacterial infections; protozoal infections.

Tri-Cold *Labima, Belg.†.*
Note. A similar name is used for preparations of different composition (see below).
Diphenylpyraline hydrochloride (p.417·1); phenylephrine hydrochloride (p.1097·1); terpin hydrate (p.1101·2).
Cold symptoms; hay fever; hypersensitivity reactions; nasal congestion; sinusitis.

Tricold *Agis, Israel.*
Note. A similar name is used for preparations of different composition (see above).
Paracetamol (p.71·2); phenylephrine hydrochloride (p.1097·1); dextromethorphan hydrobromide (p.1087·3).
Coughs and cold symptoms.

Tricolpex *Bunker, Braz.*
Metronidazole (p.594·1); nystatin (p.392·2); urea (p.1127·3).
Vulvovaginal infections.

Tricom *Nutripharm, USA†.*
Pseudoephedrine hydrochloride (p.1099·2); chlorpheniramine [chlorphenamine] maleate (p.412·1); paracetamol (p.71·2).
Upper respiratory-tract symptoms.

Tricomed *Hua, Thai.*
Metronidazole (p.594·1).
Trichomoniasis.

Tricomox *Pinewood, Irl.†.*
Co-trimoxazole (p.193·3).
Bacterial infections.

Tricor *Abbott, USA.*
Fenofibrate (p.889·1).
Hyperlipidaemias.

Tricorex *Provita, Ital.*
Amino-acid, vitamin, and mineral preparation (p.1350·1).
Nutritional supplement.

Tricortin *Fidia, Ital.*
Phosphatides (p.1628·1); cyanocobalamin (p.1388·1).
Lignocaine [lidocaine] hydrochloride (p.1313·2) is included in this preparation to alleviate the pain of injection.
Peripheral and central nervous system disorders.

Fidia, Ital.
Phospholipids; pyridoxine hydrochloride (p.1386·3); cyanocobalamin (p.1388·1).
Metabolic and circulatory disorders of the brain.

Tricosal *Invamed, USA†.*
Choline magnesium trisalicylate (p.24·3).

Tricosten *Farmion, Braz.*
Clotrimazole (p.382·1).
Fungal skin and vaginal infections.

Tricovivax *Medinfar, Port.*
Minoxidil (p.934·2).
Alopecia androgenetica.

Tricowas B *Wasserman, Spain.*
Metronidazole (p.594·1).
Anaerobic bacterial infections; protozoal infections.

Tricoxidil *Pfizer Consumer, Ital.*
Minoxidil (p.934·2).
Alopecia androgenetica.

Tricozone *Hua, Thai.*
Tinidazole (p.603·3).
Amoebiasis; giardiasis; trichomoniasis.

Tri-Cyclen *Janssen-Ortho, Canad.*
Norgestimate (p.1486·1); ethinylestradiol (p.1476·2).
Triphasic oral contraceptive.

Tridelta *Ceccarelli, Ital.*
Colecalciferol (p.1391·1).
Vitamin D deficiency.

Trident *Adams, Canad.*
Xylitol (p.1397·3).
Dental caries prophylaxis.

Triderm
Note.This name is used for preparations of different composition.

Schering-Plough, Hong Kong; Schering-Plough, Israel; Schering-Plough, Singapore; Essex, Switz.
Betamethasone dipropionate (p.1063·2); clotrimazole (p.382·1); gentamicin sulfate (p.210·1).
Infected skin disorders.

Del-Ray, USA.
Triamcinolone acetonide (p.1080·1).
Skin disorders.

Triderm 5 Bio Nike *ICIM, Ital.*
Barrier preparation.

Triderm Zeta *ICIM, Ital.*
Zinc oxide (p.1128·2).
Skin disorders.

Tridesilon
Note.This name is used for preparations of different composition.
Bayer, Canad.; Bayer, USA.
Cream; ointment: Desonide (p.1066·2).
Skin disorders.

Bayer, USA.
Ear drops: Desonide (p.1066·2); acetic acid (p.1571·2).
Superficial ear infections with inflammation.

Tridesonit *CS, Fr.*
Desonide (p.1066·2).
Skin disorders.

Tridestra
Orion, Irl.; Orion, UK.
70 Tablets, estradiol valerate (p.1473·2); 14 tablets, estradiol valerate; medroxyprogesterone acetate (p.1480·1); 7 tablets, inert.
Menopausal disorders; osteoporosis.

Tridil
Du Pont, Canad.†; Du Pont, Hong Kong; Boots, Hong Kong; Du Pont, Irl.†; Sanofi Synthelabo, S.Afr.; Faulding, USA.
Glyceryl trinitrate (p.897·3).
Control of blood pressure during surgery; heart failure; ischaemic heart disease.

Tridin *Opfermann, Ger.*
Sodium monofluorophosphate (p.1377·2); calcium gluconate (p.1188·2); calcium citrate (p.1188·1).
Osteoporosis.

Rotta, Hong Kong; Rottapharm, Ital.
Levoglutamide monofluorophosphate; calcium gluconate (p.1188·2); calcium citrate (p.1188·1).
Osteoporosis.

Triditol-G *Advance, Hong Kong.*
Triamcinolone acetonide (p.1080·1); gentamicin sulfate (p.210·1); diphenhydramine hydrochloride (p.416·1); tolnaftate (p.395·2).
Inflamed bacterial and fungal skin infections.

Tridocemine *Aventis, Port.*
Injection: Vitamin B₁₂ (p.1388·1).
Anaemia; neuralgia; neuritis; tonic.
Tablets: Benfotiamine (p.1384·3); pyridoxine hydrochloride (p.1386·3); hydroxocobalamin (p.1388·1).
Neuralgia; neuritis; tonic.

Tridomose *Aventis, S.Afr.*
Gestrinone (p.1479·2).
Endometriosis.

Tridrate Bowel Evacuant Kit *Lafayette, USA†.*
Combination pack: Magnesium citrate solution (p.1232·3); 3 bisacodyl tablets (p.1212·2); 1 bisacodyl suppository (p.1212·2).
Constipation.

Tridyl *Condrugs, Thai.*
Benzhexol [trihexyphenidyl] hydrochloride (p.463·3).
Drug-induced extrapyramidal disorders; parkinsonism.

Triella *Janssen-Cilag, Fr.*
Norethisterone (p.1485·1); ethinylestradiol (p.1476·2).
Triphasic oral contraceptive.

Triene *Wassermann, Ital.*
Polyenacid.
Barrier preparation; burns; skin irritation; wounds.

Triette *LAW, Ger.*
Levonorgestrel (p.1486·2); ethinylestradiol (p.1476·2).
Triphasic oral contraceptive.

Trifacta *Nikkho, Braz.*
Injection: Vitamin B substances (p.1350·1); anti-anaemic fraction G.
Anaemias.
Tablets: Vitamin B substances (p.1350·1); anti-anaemic fraction G; ferrous sulfate (p.1360·3); copper chloride; manganese chloride.
Anaemias; dietary supplement.

Trifed
Nakornpatana, Thai.; Geneva, USA†.
Pseudoephedrine hydrochloride (p.1099·2); triprolidine hydrochloride (p.427·2).
Allergic rhinitis; cold symptoms; hay fever; nasal congestion.

Trifed-C Cough *Geneva, USA.*
Pseudoephedrine hydrochloride (p.1099·2); codeine phosphate (p.25·2); triprolidine hydrochloride (p.427·2).
Coughs and cold symptoms.

Trifedrin *Glaxo Wellcome, Braz.*
Pseudoephedrine hydrochloride (p.1099·2); triprolidine hydrochloride (p.427·2); sulfogaiacol (p.1101·1).
Hypersensitivity disorders.

Trifeme
Wyeth-Ayerst, Austral.; Wyeth, NZ.
21 Tablets, ethinylestradiol (p.1476·2); levonorgestrel (p.1486·2); 7 tablets, inert.
Triphasic oral contraceptive.

Tri-Femoden *Schering, Fin.*
Gestodene (p.1479·1); ethinylestradiol (p.1476·2).
Triphasic oral contraceptive.

Trifen *Be-Tabs, S.Afr.*
Triprolidine hydrochloride (p.427·2); pseudoephedrine hydrochloride (p.1099·2); codeine phosphate (p.25·2); guaifenesin (p.1092·2).
Coughs.

Trifene *Medinfar, Port.*
Ibuprofen (p.43·2).
Fever; pain.

Triferon *Salus, Ital.*
Thiamine hydrochloride (p.1385·1); pyridoxine hydrochloride (p.1386·3); hydroxocobalamin (p.1388·1).
Neuralgia; neuritis; post-infection paresis; vitamin B deficiency.

Trifibra Mix *Sanofi Winthrop, Braz.*
Bran (p.1214·2).
Constipation; dietary supplement.

Tri-Filena *Organon, Aust.*
White tablets, estradiol valerate (p.1473·2); blue tablets, estradiol valerate; medroxyprogesterone acetate (p.1480·1); yellow tablets, inert.
Menopausal disorders; osteoporosis.

Tri-Flor-Vite with Fluoride *Everett, USA†.*
Multivitamin and fluoride preparation (p.1375·3) (p.1350·1).

Triflucan
Pfizer, Fr.; Pfizer, Israel.
Fluconazole (p.383·2).
Fungal infections.

Trifluid *Otsuka, Jpn.*
Carbohydrate and electrolyte infusion (p.1350·1).
Parenteral nutrition.

Triflumann *Mann, Ger.*
Trifluridine (p.642·2).
Herpesvirus keratitis.

Triflumed *Medifive, Thai.*
Trifluoperazine (p.710·3).
Anxiety; nausea and vomiting; psychoses.

Triflux *Scharper, Ital.*
Triflusal (p.987·2).
Thromboembolic disorders.

Trifolium Complex *Blackmores, Austral.*
Yellow dock (p.1681·3); taraxacum (p.1669·1); red clover (p.1657·3); lappa (p.1627·1); zinc amino acid chelate (p.1398·3); vitamin A acetate (p.1383·2).
Skin disorders.

Trifosfaneurina *Lepori, Port.*
Cocarboxylase chloride (p.1385·2).
Acidosis; cardiopathy; diabetes mellitus; eclampsia; headache; neuralgia; neuritis; neuromuscular disorders; tonic; vomiting of pregnancy.

Trifosfaneurina B6 *Farma Lepori, Spain.*
Cyanocobalamine; pyridoxal phosphate; riboflavin; thiamine phosphate (p.1350·1).
Lignocaine [lidocaine] hydrochloride (p.1313·2) is included in this preparation to alleviate the pain of injection.
Vitamin B deficiency.

Trifosfaneurina B2 B12 *Farma Lepori, Spain.*
Cyanocobalamin; riboflavin phosphate sodium; thiamine phosphate (p.1350·1).
Vitamin B deficiency.

Trifyba
Sanofi Winthrop, Irl.; Sanofi Winthrop, UK.
Wheat grain extract (p.1214·2).
Bowel disorders; constipation; haemorrhoids; stoma management.

Trigastril
Sanova, Aust.; Heumann, Ger.
Aluminium hydroxide gel (p.1210·3); magnesium hydroxide (p.1233·1); calcium carbonate (p.1215·1).
Gastrointestinal disorders.

Tri-Gel *Vida, Hong Kong.*
Triamcinolone acetonide (p.1080·1); lignocaine [lidocaine] (p.1313·2); cetrimide (p.1137·1).
Mouth lesions.

Trigesic *Squibb, USA†.*
Paracetamol (p.71·2); aspirin (p.14·2); caffeine (p.761·3).
Pain.

Trigger *Poliforma, Ital.†.*
Ranitidine hydrochloride (p.1245·2).
Gastric hyperacidity; gastro-oesophageal reflux; peptic ulcer; Zollinger-Ellison syndrome.

Triglicen *Prospa, Ital.*
Omega-3 triglycerides (p.949·2).
Dietary supplement; hypertriglyceridaemia.

Triglobe
Astra, Aust.; Astra, Braz.; Astra, Ger.; AstraZeneca, Singapore; Astra, Spain†.
Sulfadiazine (p.251·1); trimethoprim (p.264·2).
Bacterial infections.

Trigoa *Wyeth, Ger.; Lederle, Ger.*
Levonorgestrel (p.1486·2); ethinylestradiol (p.1476·2).
Triphasic oral contraceptive.

Trigogine
Atlantic, Hong Kong; Atlantic, Singapore; Atlantic, Thai.
Co-dergocrine mesilate (p.1597·3).
Cerebral and peripheral vascular disorders; mental function impairment.

Trigon Depot *Squibb, Spain.*
Triamcinolone acetonide (p.1080·1).
Corticosteroid.

Trigon Rectal *Squibb, Spain.*
Lignocaine [lidocaine] (p.1313·2); triamcinolone acetonide (p.1080·1).
Anorectal disorders.

Trigon Topico *Squibb, Spain.*
Amphotericin B (p.377·2); gramicidin (p.213·3); neomycin sulfate (p.228·1); triamcinolone acetonide (p.1080·1).
Infected skin disorders.

Tri-Gynera *Schering, Port.*
Gestodene (p.1479·1); ethinylestradiol (p.1476·2).
Triphasic oral contraceptive.

Trigynon
Schering, Aust.; Schering, Belg.; Schering, Ital.; Schering, Neth.
Levonorgestrel (p.1486·2); ethinylestradiol (p.1476·2).
Triphasic oral contraceptive.

Trigynovin *Schering, Spain.*
Gestodene (p.1479·1); ethinylestradiol (p.1476·2).
Triphasic oral contraceptive.

TriHEMIC *Lederle, USA.*
Ferrous fumarate (p.1360·1); vitamin B₁₂ substances (p.1388·1); intrinsic factor concentrate; folic acid (p.1361·1); vitamin E.
Vitamin C (p.1389·3) is included in this preparation to increase the absorption and availability of ferrous fumarate; docusate sodium (p.1223·1) is included to reduce the constipating effects of ferrous fumarate.
Anaemias.

Triherpine
Ciba Vision, Fr.; Ciba Vision, Hong Kong; Ciba Vision, Ital.; Ciba Vision, Switz.; Ciba Vision, Thai.
Trifluridine (p.642·2).
Herpes simplex infections of the eye.

Trihexy *Geneva, USA.*
Benzhexol [trihexyphenidyl] hydrochloride (p.463·3).
Parkinsonism.

TriHIBit *Pasteur Merieux, USA.*
A diphtheria, tetanus, acellular pertussis, and haemophilus influenzae vaccine (p.1538·3).
Active immunisation.

Trihistalex *Wolfs, Belg.*
Diphenhydramine hydrochloride (p.416·1); cinchocaine hydrochloride (p.1309·1); nicotinamide (p.1372·3).
Cutaneous hypersensitivity reactions; pain.

Trihistan
Gea, Denm.; Weifa, Norw.
Chlorcyclizine hydrochloride (p.411·3).
Hypersensitivity reactions; motion sickness; nausea; vertigo.

Trihist-CS *Cypress, USA†.*
Codeine phosphate (p.25·2); phenylpropanolamine hydrochloride (p.1098·1); brompheniramine maleate (p.410·2).

Trihist-D *Cypress, USA†.*
Phenylpropanolamine hydrochloride (p.1098·1); phenyltoloxamine citrate (p.423·1); mepyramine maleate (p.421·1); pheniramine maleate (p.422·3).
Allergic rhinitis; sinusitis.

Trihist-DM *Cypress, USA†.*
Phenylpropanolamine hydrochloride (p.1098·1); brompheniramine maleate (p.410·2); dextromethorphan hydrobromide (p.1087·3).

Tri-Hydroserpine *Rugby, USA.*
Hydrochlorothiazide (p.907·3); reserpine (p.967·3); hydralazine hydrochloride (p.905·3).
Hypertension.

Tri-Immunol
Wyeth-Ayerst, Canad.†; Lederle-Praxis, USA†.
An adsorbed diphtheria, tetanus and pertussis vaccine (p.1537·3).
Active immunisation of infants and young children.

Triiodothyronine Injection *Medeva, UK.*
Liothyronine sodium (p.1524·2).
Myxoedema coma.

Tri-K *Century, USA.*
Potassium acetate (p.1194·3); potassium bicarbonate (p.1186·1); potassium citrate (p.1186·1).
Hypokalaemia; potassium depletion.

Trikacide *Pharmascience, Canad.†.*
Metronidazole (p.594·1).
Bacterial infections; protozoal infections.

Trikof-D *Respa, USA†.*
Guaifenesin (p.1092·2); dextromethorphan hydrobromide (p.1087·3); phenylpropanolamine hydrochloride (p.1098·1).
Coughs; nasal congestion.

Tri-Kort *Keene, USA.*
Triamcinolone acetonide (p.1080·1).
Corticosteroid.

Trikozol *Orion, Fin.*
Metronidazole (p.594·1).
Anaerobic bacterial infections; antibiotic-associated colitis; Crohn's disease; eradication of Helicobacter pylori in peptic ulcer; protozoal infections.

Trikvilar *Schering, Fin.*
Levonorgestrel (p.1486·2); ethinylestradiol (p.1476·2).
Triphasic oral contraceptive.

Trilafon
Schering-Plough, Belg.; Schering, Canad.; Schering-Plough, Denm.; Schering-Plough, Ital.; Schering-Plough, Mex.; Schering-Plough, Neth.; Schering-Plough, Norw.; Schering-Plough, S.Afr.; Schering-Plough, Swed.; Essex, Switz.; Schering, USA.
Perphenazine (p.699·1), perphenazine decanoate (p.699·1), or perphenazine enantate (p.699·1).
Alcohol withdrawal syndrome; anxiety; hiccup; nausea; pain; premedication; pruritus; psychoses; vomiting.

The symbol † denotes a preparation no longer actively marketed

Trilam *Gerard, Irl.*
Triazolam (p.709·3).
Insomnia.

Trileptal *Novartis, Aust.; Novartis, Austral.; Novartis, Braz.; Novartis, Denm.; Novartis, Fin.; Novartis, Fr.; Novartis, Hong Kong; Novartis, Irl.; Novartis, Ital.; Novartis, Mex.; Novartis, Neth.; Novartis, S.Afr.; Novartis, Switz.; Novartis, UK; Novartis, USA.*
Oxcarbazepine (p.354·1).
Epilepsy.

Trileptin *Novartis, Israel.*
Oxcarbazepine (p.354·1).
Epilepsy.

Tri-Levlen *Berlex, USA.*
Levonorgestrel (p.1486·2); ethinylestradiol (p.1476·2). 28-Day packs also contain 7 inert tablets.
Triphasic oral contraceptive.

Trilifan *Schering-Plough, Fr.*
Perphenazine enantate (p.699·1).
Psychoses.

Trilisate *Purdue Frederick, Canad.; Purdue Frederick, USA.*
Choline magnesium trisalicylate (p.24·3).
Musculoskeletal and joint disorders.

Trillium Complex *Blackmores, Austral.*
Trillium erectum; geranium maculatum; hydrastis (p.1621·1); ginseng (p.1615·3); d-alpha tocoferil acid succinate (p.1394·1).
Menorrhagia.

Triloc *Astra, Aust.*
Metoprolol tartrate (p.931·2); hydrochlorothiazide (p.907·3); hydralazine hydrochloride (p.905·3).
Hypertension.

Trilog *Hauck, USA.*
Triamcinolone acetonide (p.1080·1).
Corticosteroid.

Trilombrin *Farmasierra, Spain.*
Pyrantel embonate (p.108·1).
Worm infections.

Trilone *Hauck, USA.*
Triamcinolone diacetate (p.1080·2).
Corticosteroid.

Trilosil *Silom, Thai.*
Triamcinolone acetonide (p.1080·1).
Skin disorders.

Trilosil N *Silom, Thai.*
Triamcinolone acetonide (p.1080·1) neomycin sulfate (p.228·1).
Infected skin disorders.

Triludan *Hoechst Marion Roussel, Aust.; Aventis, Belg.; Hoechst Marion Roussel, Irl.; Hoechst Marion Roussel, Ital.†; Hoechst Marion Roussel, Neth.; Aventis, Port.; Aventis, S.Afr.; Marion Merrell, Spain†; Hoechst Marion Roussel, Switz.†; Hoechst Marion Roussel, UK†.*
Terfenadine (p.424·3).
Hypersensitivity reactions.

Trilufen *Marion Merrell Dow, Port.†.*
Terfenadine (p.424·3); pseudoephedrine hydrochloride (p.1099·2).
Allergic rhinitis.

Trim *M & H, Thai.*
Triamcinolone acetonide (p.1080·1).
Oral lesions.

Trimadiaz Antrima *Doms-Adrian, Fr.†.*
Co-trimazine (p.193·2).
Formerly known as Antrima.
Bacterial infections; Pneumocystis carinii pneumonia.

Trimag *Uniao Quimica, Braz.*
Tiratricol (p.1528·3).
Thyroid disorders.

Trimasone *Pharmaland, Thai.*
Triamcinolone acetonide (p.1080·1).
Skin disorders.

Trimate-Ace *Sankyo, Thai.*
Vitamin B substances with vitamin E (p.1350·1).

Trimaze *Aspen, S.Afr.*
Clotrimazole (p.382·1).
Fungal skin infections.

Trimazide *Major, USA.*
Trimethobenzamide hydrochloride (p.426·3).
Nausea and vomiting.

Trimedal *Allergan-Frumtost, Braz.*
Dimetindene maleate (p.415·3); rutoside (p.1611·2); paracetamol (p.71·2); ascorbic acid (p.1389·3); phenylephrine (p.1097·1).
Cold and influenza symptoms.

Trimedat *Italfarmaco, Ital.*
Trimebutine maleate (p.1675·1).
Gastrointestinal spasm; irritable bowel disease; oesophageal motility disorders.

Trimedil *Novartis Consumer, Aust.*
Paracetamol (p.71·2); phenylephrine hydrochloride (p.1097·1); dimetindene maleate (p.415·3); ascorbic acid (p.1389·3); oxerutins (p.1611·2).
Cold symptoms.

Trimel *Douglas, NZ.*
Co-trimoxazole (p.193·3).
Bacterial infections; nocardiosis; Pneumocystis carinii pneumonia; toxoplasmosis.

Trim-Elim *Reese, USA.*
Caffeine (p.761·3); potassium salicylate; salicylamide (p.82·1).

Trimesul *Universales, Mex.*
Co-trimoxazole (p.193·3).
Bacterial infections.

Trimesuxol *Ofimex, Mex.*
Co-trimoxazole (p.193·3).
Bacterial infections.

Trimetabol
Note. This name is used for preparations of different composition.
Dansk-Flama, Braz.
Cyproheptadine acephyllinate (p.414·3); lysine; carnitine; vitamin B₁; vitamin B₁₂ (p.1350·1).
Reduced appetite; tonic.
Zimaia, Port.
Cyproheptadine acephyllinate (p.414·3).
Appetite stimulant.
Uriach, Spain.
Cyproheptadine acephyllinate (p.414·3); amino acids and vitamins (p.1350·1).
Anorexia; tonic; weight loss.

Trimetho comp *Strallhofer, Aust.*
Co-trimoxazole (p.193·3).
Bacterial infections.

Trimethox *Caps, S.Afr.*
Co-trimoxazole (p.193·3).
Bacterial infections.

Trimetin *Vitabalans, Fin.*
Trimethoprim (p.264·2).
Urinary-tract infections.

Trimetin Duplo *Vitabalans, Fin.*
Sulfadiazine (p.251·1); trimethoprim (p.264·2).
Respiratory-tract and urinary-tract infections.

Trimetoger *Streger, Mex.*
Co-trimoxazole (p.193·3).
Bacterial infections.

Trimeton *Schering-Plough, Ital.*
Chlorpheniramine [chlorphenamine] maleate (p.412·1).
Hypersensitivity reactions.

Trimetoprim Balsamico *Prodotti, Braz.*
Co-trimoxazole (p.193·3); guaifenesin (p.1092·2); ammonium chloride (p.1085·2).
Bacterial infections.

Trimetoprim-Sulfa *Selena, Swed.†.*
Co-trimoxazole (p.193·3).
Bacterial infections; Pneumocystis carinii pneumonia.

Trimetox *Rimsa, Mex.*
Co-trimoxazole (p.193·3).
Bacterial infections.

Trimex *Medinovum, Fin.*
Trimethoprim (p.264·2).
Urinary-tract infections.

Trimexazol *Sanofi Winthrop, Braz.; ICN, Mex.*
Co-trimoxazole (p.193·3).
Bacterial infections; Pneumocystis carinii pneumonia; protozoal infections.

Trimexazol Balsamico *Sanofi Winthrop, Braz.*
Co-trimoxazole (p.193·3); guaifenesin (p.1092·2); ammonium chloride (p.1085·2).
Bacterial infections.

Trimexazole *Pharmasant, Thai.*
Co-trimoxazole (p.193·3).
Bacterial infections.

Trimexine *ICN, Mex.*
Ambroxol hydrochloride (p.1084·3).
Respiratory-tract congestion.

Trimexole *Rayere, Mex.*
Co-trimoxazole (p.193·3).
Bacterial infections.

Trimexole Compositum *Rayere, Mex.*
Co-trimoxazole (p.193·3); guaifenesin (p.1092·2).
Respiratory-tract infections.

Trimezole *MPF, Singapore.*
Co-trimoxazole (p.193·3).
Bacterial infections.

Tri-Micon *Beacons, Singapore.*
Betamethasone valerate (p.1063·2); miconazole nitrate (p.391·1); gentamicin sulfate (p.210·1).
Infected skin disorders.

Trimin sulfa *Astra, Swed.*
Sulfadiazine (p.251·1); trimethoprim (p.264·2).
Urinary-tract infections.

Triminol Cough *Rugby, USA†.*
Phenylpropanolamine hydrochloride (p.1098·1); chlorpheniramine [chlorphenamine] maleate (p.412·1); dextromethorphan hydrobromide (p.1087·3).
Coughs and cold symptoms.

Tri-Minulet *Wyeth Lederle, Aust.; Wyeth-Ayerst, Austral.; Wyeth Lederle, Belg.; Wyeth Lederle, Denm.; Wyeth Lederle, Fin.; Wyeth Lederle, Fr.; Wyeth, Irl.; Wyeth Lederle, Neth.; Wyeth Lederle, Port.; Akromed, S.Afr.; Wyeth, Spain; Wyeth, Switz.; Wyeth, UK.*
Gestodene (p.1479·1); ethinylestradiol (p.1476·2). 28-Day packs also contain 7 inert tablets.
Triphasic oral contraceptive.

Trimiron *Organon, Swed.*
Desogestrel (p.1470·3); ethinylestradiol (p.1476·2). 28-Day packs also contain 7 inert tablets.
Triphasic oral contraceptive.

TriMix E *Fresenius Kabi, Aust.*
Amino-acid, carbohydrate, lipid (from soya oil (p.1378·1)), and electrolyte infusion (p.1350·1). Contains egg lecithin.
Parenteral nutrition.

Trimogal *Lagap, UK.*
Trimethoprim (p.264·2).
Bronchitis; urinary-tract infections.

Trimoks *Docmed, S.Afr.†.*
Co-trimoxazole (p.193·3).
Bacterial infections.

Trimol *Julphar, UAE.*
Co-trimoxazole (p.193·3).
Bacterial infections; nocardiosis; Pneumocystis carinii pneumonia; toxoplasmosis.

Trimolex *Zurich, S.Afr.†.*
Amiloride hydrochloride (p.835·1); hydrochlorothiazide (p.907·3).
Hypertension; oedema.

Trimonase *Tosi, Ital.*
Tinidazole (p.603·3).
Amoebiasis; giardiasis; trichomoniasis.

Trimonil *Desitin, Denm.; Desitin, Fin.; Desitin, Norw.; Desitin, Swed.*
Carbamazepine (p.342·2).
Alcohol withdrawal syndrome; bipolar disorder; diabetes insipidus; diabetic neuropathy; epilepsy; mania; trigeminal neuralgia.

Trimono *Procter & Gamble, Ger.†.*
Trimethoprim (p.264·2).
Bacterial infections of the urinary tract.

Trimopan *Orion, Denm.; Orion, Fin.; Berk, UK.*
Trimethoprim (p.264·2).
Urinary- and respiratory-tract infections.

Trimo-San *Milex, USA.*
Hydroxyquinoline sulfate (p.1622·2); boric acid (p.1586·1); borax (p.1586·1); sodium laurilsulfate (p.1496·3); glycerol (p.1616·3).
Vaginal deodoriser.

Trimovate *Glaxo Wellcome, UK.*
Clobetasone butyrate (p.1065·2); oxytetracycline calcium (p.234·1); nystatin (p.392·2).
Skin disorders with bacterial or fungal infection.

Trimovax *Pasteur Merieux, Braz.; Pasteur Merieux, Hong Kong; Pasteur Merieux, Ital.†; Aventis, S.Afr.; Pasteur Merieux, UK†.*
A measles, mumps, and rubella vaccine (Schwarz, Urabe AM9, and Wistar RA27/3M strains, respectively) (p.1549·1).
Active immunisation.

Trimox
Note. This name is used for preparations of different composition.
Pose, Thai.
Co-trimoxazole (p.193·3).
Bacterial infections.
Apothecon, USA.
Amoxicillin trihydrate (p.149·2).
Bacterial infections.

Trimoxazole *Biochemie, Austral.*
Co-trimoxazole (p.193·3).
Bacterial infections.

Trimoxol *Yamanouchi, Neth.*
Co-trimoxazole (p.193·3).
Bacterial infections; Pneumocystis carinii pneumonia.

Trimoxzol *Olan-Kemed, Thai.*
Co-trimoxazole (p.193·3).
Bacterial infections.

Trimpex *Roche, USA.*
Trimethoprim (p.264·2).
Urinary-tract infections.

Trimstat *Laser, USA†.*
Phendimetrazine tartrate (p.1513·3).
Obesity.

Trim-Vit *Vitae, Mex.*
Co-trimoxazole (p.193·3).
Bacterial infections.

Trimzol
Randall, Mex.; Schwulst, S.Afr.†.
Co-trimoxazole (p.193·3).
Bacterial infections.

Trinaderm *Schering, Braz.*
Tolnaftate (p.395·2).
Fungal skin infections.

Trinagesic *Propan, S.Afr.*
Meprobamate (p.691·1); paracetamol (p.71·2); codeine phosphate (p.25·2).
Pain and associated tension.

Trinalgen *Eurofarma, Braz.*
Hydroxocobalamin (p.1388·1); thiamine hydrochloride (p.1385·1); pyridoxine hydrochloride (p.1386·3). Lignocaine [lidocaine] hydrochloride (p.1313·2) is included in this preparation to alleviate the pain of injection.
Megaloblastic anaemia; vitamin B deficiency.

Trinalin *Schering, Canad.; Schering-Plough, Mex.; Key, USA.*
Azatadine maleate (p.409·2); pseudoephedrine sulfate (p.1099·3).
Allergic rhinitis; Eustachian tube congestion; nasal congestion.

Trinalion *Neo-Farmaceutica, Port.*
Nimodipine (p.946·1).
Cerebral ischaemia; cerebral vasospasm following subarachnoid haemorrhage.

Tri-Nasal *Muro, USA.*
Triamcinolone acetonide (p.1080·1).
Allergic rhinitis.

Trind *Mead Johnson Nutritionals, USA†.*
Phenylpropanolamine hydrochloride (p.1098·1); chlorpheniramine [chlorphenamine] maleate (p.412·1).
Upper respiratory-tract symptoms.

Tri-Nefrin Extra Strength *Pfeiffer, USA†.*
Phenylpropanolamine hydrochloride (p.1098·1); chlorpheniramine [chlorphenamine] maleate (p.412·1).
Upper respiratory-tract symptoms.

Trinelax *Protein, Mex.*
Co-trimoxazole (p.193·3).
Bacterial infections.

Trinergot *Atlantis, Mex.*
Caffeine (p.761·3); ergotamine tartrate (p.452·1).
Migraine and other vascular headaches.

Trinestril *Hoechst Marion Roussel, Braz.*
Estradiol hexahydrobenzoate (p.1473·2); testosterone hexahydrobenzoate (p.1493·3); hydroxyprogesterone (p.1479·3).

Trineurin *Orion, Fin.*
Vitamin B substances (p.1350·1).
Vitamin B deficiency.

Trinevral *Eurofarma, Braz.*
Hydroxocobalamin (p.1388·1); thiamine hydrochloride (p.1385·1); pyridoxine hydrochloride (p.1386·3).
Megaloblastic anaemia; vitamin B deficiency.

Trinevrina B6 *Guidotti, Ital.*
Thiamine hydrochloride (p.1385·1); pyridoxine hydrochloride (p.1386·3); cyanocobalamin (p.1388·1). Lignocaine [lidocaine] hydrochloride (p.1313·2) is included in the intramuscular injection to alleviate the pain of injection.
Neuralgias; neuritis; radiation sickness; toxicosis.

Triniagar *Almirall, Spain.*
Mebutizide (p.925·3); triamterene (p.986·1).
Hypertension; oedema.

Trinidex *Diaco, Ital.*
Glucose and vitamin infusion (p.1350·1).
Parenteral nutrition.

Triniol *Syntex, Spain†.*
Paramethasone acetate (p.1077·2); paramethasone disodium phosphate (p.1077·2).
Corticosteroid.

Trinipatch *Fournier, Belg.; Sanofi Synthelabo, Canad.; Synthelabo, Fr.; Laviphorm, Israel; Sanofi Synthelabo, Neth.; Synthelabo, Spain.*
Glyceryl trinitrate (p.897·3).
Angina pectoris.

Triniplas *Novartis, Ital.*
Glyceryl trinitrate (p.897·3).
Angina pectoris.

Triniscon *Lilly, Hong Kong.*
Liver and stomach concentrate; cobalamin (p.1388·1); ferrous fumarate (p.1360·1); folic acid (p.1361·1). Vitamin C (p.1389·3) is included in this preparation to increase the absorption and availability of iron.
Anaemias; iron deficiency.

Triniton *Apogepha, Ger.*
Dihydralazine sulfate (p.874·2); hydrochlorothiazide (p.907·3); reserpine (p.967·3).
Hypertension.

Trinitrina *Pharmacia Upjohn, Ital.*
Glyceryl trinitrate (p.897·3).
Angina pectoris.

Triniton *Apogepha, Ger.*

Triniton *Sodip, Switz.*
Glyceryl trinitrate (p.897·3).
Angina pectoris; heart failure; pulmonary oedema.

Trinitrosan *Merck, Ger.*
Glyceryl trinitrate (p.897·3).
Angina pectoris; controlled hypotension; heart failure; hypertensive crisis; myocardial infarction.

Trinizol *UCI, Braz.*
Tinidazole (p.603·3).
Anaerobic bacterial infections; protozoal infections.

Trinizol M *UCI, Braz.*
Tinidazole (p.603·3); miconazole nitrate (p.391·1).
Vulvovaginal infections.

Trinordiol *Wyeth Lederle, Aust.; Wyeth Lederle, Belg.; Wyeth, Braz.; Wyeth Lederle, Denm.; Wyeth Lederle, Fin.; Wyeth Lederle, Fr.; Wyeth, Ger.; Wyeth-Ayerst, Hong Kong; Wyeth, Irl.; Wyeth-Ayerst, Israel; Wyeth Lederle, Ital.; Wyeth, Mex.; Wyeth, Neth.; Wyeth Lederle, Norw.; Wyeth, Singapore; Wyeth Lederle, Swed.; Wyeth, Switz.; Wyeth-Ayerst, Thai.; Wyeth, UK.*
Levonorgestrel (p.1486·2); ethinylestradiol (p.1476·2). 28-Day packs also contain 7 inert tablets.
Triphasic oral contraceptive.

Tri-Norinyl *Searle, USA.*
Norethisterone (p.1485·1); ethinylestradiol (p.1476·2). 28-Day packs also contain 7 inert tablets.
Triphasic oral contraceptive.

Trinorm *Nycomed, Denm.*
18 Tablets, estradiol (p.1473·1); 10 tablets, estradiol; norethisterone (p.1485·1).
Menopausal disorders; osteoporosis.

TRI-Normin *Zeneca, Ger.*
Atenolol (p.841·3); chlortalidone (p.857·1); hydralazine hydrochloride (p.905·3).
Hypertension.

Trinotrex *Faria, Braz.*
Tetracycline (p.258·3); muramidase (p.1638·1).
Bacterial infections.

Trinovum *Janssen-Cilag, Aust.; Janssen-Cilag, Belg.; Cilag, Braz.; Janssen-Cilag, Denm.; Janssen-Cilag, Ger.; Cilag, Hong Kong; Janssen-Cilag, Irl.; Janssen-Cilag, Ital.; Janssen-Cilag, Neth.; Janssen-Cilag, S.Afr.; Janssen-Cilag, Swed.; Janssen-Cilag, Switz.; Janssen-Cilag, UK.*
Norethisterone (p.1485·1); ethinylestradiol (p.1476·2). 28-Day packs also contain 7 inert tablets.
Triphasic oral contraceptive.

Trinsicon *Lilly, Aust.†; Lilly, S.Afr.†; Lilly, Thai.; UCB, USA.*
Ferrous fumarate (p.1360·1); vitamin B₁₂ substances (p.1388·1); intrinsic factor (liver-stomach preparation); folic acid (p.1361·1).
Ascorbic acid (p.1389·3) is included in this preparation to increase the absorption and availability of iron.
Anaemias.

Trio D *LED, Fr.*
Liquorice (p.1231·2).
Hyperpigmentation disorders.

TrioBe *Recip, Swed.*
Folic acid; cyanocobalamin; pyridoxine (p.1350·1).
Vitamin B and folic acid deficiency.

Triocalcio *Heralds, Braz.*
Calcium carbonate (p.1215·1); vitamins A, C, and D (p.1350·1).

Triocaps *Vifor, Switz.*
Chlorpheniramine [chlorphenamine] maleate (p.412·1); phenylephrine hydrochloride (p.1097·1).
Upper-respiratory-tract disorders.

Triocetin *OFF, Ital.*
Troleandomycin (p.266·1).
Bacterial infections.

Triodeen *Schering, Neth.*
Gestodene (p.1479·1); ethinylestradiol (p.1476·2).
Triphasic oral contraceptive.

Trioden ED *Schering, Austral.*
21 Tablets, gestodene (p.1479·1); ethinylestradiol (p.1476·2); 7 tablets, inert.
Triphasic oral contraceptive.

Triodena *Schering, Aust.*
Gestodene (p.1479·1); ethinylestradiol (p.1476·2).
Triphasic oral contraceptive.

Triodene *Schering, Belg.; Schering, Irl.; Schering, S.Afr.*
Gestodene (p.1479·1); ethinylestradiol (p.1476·2).
28-Day packs also contain 7 inert tablets.
Triphasic oral contraceptive.

Triodurin *Pharmacia Upjohn, Aust.†.*
Polyestriol phosphate (p.1488·2).
Mepivacaine hydrochloride (p.1317·1) is included in this preparation to alleviate the pain of injection.
Menopausal disorders; oestrogen deficiency.

Triofan *Vifor, Switz.*
Xylometazoline hydrochloride (p.1102·2); carbocisteine (p.1086·3).
Upper-respiratory-tract disorders.

Triofed *Pharmasant, Thai.; Barre-National, USA.*
Triprolidine hydrochloride (p.427·2); pseudoephedrine hydrochloride (p.1099·2).
Allergic rhinitis; cold symptoms; hayfever; nasal congestion.

Triogene *Medecine Vegetale, Fr.*
Kola (p.1681·1); gentian (p.1615·1); magnesium chloride (p.1190·3); ferrous gluconate (p.1360·1).
Tonic.

Triogesic *Novartis Consumer, Irl.; Novartis Consumer, UK†.*
Phenylpropanolamine hydrochloride (p.1098·1); paracetamol (p.71·2).
Nasal and sinus congestion.

Triogestena *Schering, Aust.*
Gestodene (p.1479·1); ethinylestradiol (p.1476·2).
Triphasic oral contraceptive.

Triogestin *Wyeth Lederle, Aust.*
Gestodene (p.1479·1); ethinylestradiol (p.1476·2).
Triphasic oral contraceptive.

Triolax *Herbes Universelles, Canad.†.*
Aloin (p.1210·2); cascara (p.1216·1); phenolphthalein (p.1244·1); bile salts (p.1585·1).

Triolip *Sofar, Ital.*
Omega-3 triglycerides (p.949·2).
Dietary supplement.

TRI-OM *OM, Switz.*
Aluminium magnesium silicate (p.1499·1); aluminium calcium silicate (p.1211·3).
Gastrointestinal disorders.

Triomar *Pharmagic, Ital.; Prism, UK.*
Omega-3 marine triglycerides (p.949·3).
Hyperlipidaemias; joint disorders; skin disorders.

Triomer *Vifor, Switz.*
Sterile sea water (p.1196·1).
Nasal disorders.

Triomin *Triomed, S.Afr.*
Minocycline hydrochloride (p.224·3).
Bacterial infections.

Triominic
Note.This name is used for preparations of different composition.
Novartis Consumer, Irl.; Novartis Consumer, UK†.
Phenylpropanolamine hydrochloride (p.1098·1); pheniramine maleate (p.422·3).
Allergic rhinitis; nasal congestion.

Novartis, Spain†.
Phenylpropanolamine hydrochloride (p.1098·1); pheniramine maleate (p.422·3); mepyramine maleate (p.421·1).
Nasal congestion.

Trionetta *Schering, Norw.; Schering, Swed.*
Levonorgestrel (p.1486·2); ethinylestradiol (p.1476·2).
28-Day packs also contain 7 inert tablets.
Triphasic oral contraceptive.

Trioplex *Triomed, S.Afr.†.*
Multivitamin and mineral preparation (p.1350·1).

Triospan *Extractum, Hung.*
Isopropamide iodide (p.470·1); drotaverine hydrochloride (p.1606·1); phenobarbital (p.355·1).
Smooth muscle spasm.

Triostat *Jones, USA.*
Liothyronine sodium (p.1524·2).
Evaluation of thyroid function; hypothyroidism.

Triotann *Invamed, USA; Duramed, USA.*
Phenylephrine tannate (p.1097·3); mepyramine tannate (p.421·1); chlorpheniramine [chlorphenamine] tannate (p.412·2).
Allergic rhinitis; nasal congestion.

Tri-Otic *Pharmics, USA.*
Chloroxylenol (p.1142·1); pramocaine hydrochloride (p.1318·2); hydrocortisone (p.1073·3).
Inflammatory ear infections.

Triotonico *Heralds, Braz.*
Multivitamin and mineral preparation (p.1350·1).

Triovit *Lane, UK.*
A vitamin A, C, and D preparation (p.1350·1).

Tri-P *Cypress, USA†.*
Phenylpropanolamine hydrochloride (p.1098·1); pheniramine maleate (p.422·3); mepyramine maleate (p.421·1).

Tripac-Cyano *Covan, S.Afr.*
4 Vials, sodium thiosulfate (p.1024·2); 2 vials, sodium nitrite (p.1023·1); 6 vials, amyl nitrite (p.1002·1).
Cyanide poisoning.

Tripacel *CSL, Austral.; Connaught, Canad.†; Pasteur Merieux, Hong Kong; CSL, NZ; Pasteur Merieux, Singapore; Pasteur Merieux, Thai.*
An adsorbed diphtheria, tetanus, and acellular pertussis vaccine (p.1537·3).
Active immunisation.

Tri-Pain *Ferndale, USA†.*
Paracetamol (p.71·2); aspirin (p.14·2); salicylamide (p.82·1); caffeine (p.761·3).
Pain.

Tripalgen Cold *Barre-National, USA†.*
Phenylpropanolamine hydrochloride (p.1098·1); chlorpheniramine [chlorphenamine] maleate (p.412·1).
Upper respiratory-tract symptoms.

Triparen *Otsuka, Jpn.*
Carbohydrate and electrolyte infusion (p.1350·1).
Parenteral nutrition.

Triparsean *Tecnobio, Spain.*
Piketoprofen (p.78·3) or piketoprofen hydrochloride (p.78·3).
Peri-articular and soft-tissue disorders.

Tripe P *Universal, Hong Kong.*
Promethazine hydrochloride (p.423·2); pholcodine (p.1099·1); phenylpropanolamine hydrochloride (p.1098·1).
Coughs and cold symptoms.

Tripedia *Pasteur Merieux, USA.*
A diphtheria, tetanus, and acellular pertussis vaccine (p.1537·3).
Active immunisation of infants and young children.

Triperidol *Janssen-Cilag, Fr.†; Janssen-Cilag, Ger.†.*
Trifluperidol hydrochloride (p.711·1).
Psychoses.

Triphacycline *Tripharma, Switz.*
Tetracycline hydrochloride (p.258·3).
Bacterial infections.

Triphasil *Wyeth-Ayerst, Austral.; Wyeth-Ayerst, Canad.; Wyeth, NZ; Aspen, S.Afr.; Wyeth-Ayerst, USA.*
Levonorgestrel (p.1486·2); ethinylestradiol (p.1476·2).
28-Day packs also contain 7 inert tablets.
Triphasic oral contraceptive.

Tri-Phen-Chlor TR *Rugby, USA†.*
Phenylpropanolamine hydrochloride (p.1098·1); phenylephrine hydrochloride (p.1097·1); chlorpheniramine [chlorphenamine] maleate (p.412·1); phenyltoloxamine citrate (p.423·1).
Upper respiratory-tract symptoms.

Triphenyl *Rugby, USA†.*
Phenylpropanolamine hydrochloride (p.1098·1); chlorpheniramine [chlorphenamine] maleate (p.412·1).
Upper respiratory-tract symptoms.

Triphenyl Expectorant *Rugby, USA†.*
Phenylpropanolamine hydrochloride (p.1098·1); guaifenesin (p.1092·2).
Coughs.

Triphosmag *Boehringer Ingelheim, Fr.†.*
Phosphoric acid; dibasic sodium phosphate; magnesium chloride; magnesium glycerophosphate (p.1350·1).
Tonic.

Triple X *Carter-Wallace, USA.*
Pyrethrins; piperonyl butoxide (p.1436·2).
Pediculosis.

Triple Antibiotic *Dixon-Shane, USA†; Geneva, USA†; Marsam, USA†; Goldline, USA†; Lannett, USA†; Moore, USA†; NMC, USA†; Parmed, USA†; Rugby, USA†.*
Polymyxin B sulfate (p.238·1); neomycin sulfate (p.228·1); bacitracin (p.155·2).
Bacterial skin infections.

Triple Antigen *CSL, Austral.; Commonwealth Serum, Hong Kong.*
An adsorbed diphtheria, tetanus, and pertussis vaccine (p.1537·3).
Active immunisation.

Triple Care Cleanser
Note.This name is used for preparations of different composition.
Smith & Nephew, Austral.
Emollient and skin cleanser.
Skin disorders associated with incontinence.

Smith & Nephew, Canad.
Emollient and skin cleanser in ostomy care.

Smith & Nephew, USA†.
Benzethonium chloride (p.1134·2); glycerol (p.1616·3); aloe vera (p.1110·1).
Removal of urine and faeces.

Triple Care Cream *Smith & Nephew, Canad.*
Zinc oxide (p.1128·2).

Triple Care Extra Protective Cream *Smith & Nephew, USA†.*
Zinc oxide (p.1128·2); soft paraffin (p.1407·3); chloroxylenol (p.1142·1).
Protection of skin from incontinence.

Triple Care Protective Cream *Smith & Nephew, USA†.*
Zinc oxide (p.1128·2); aloe vera (p.1110·1); allantoin (p.1110·1).
Protection of skin from incontinence.

Triple Protection *Beiersdorf, Canad.*
SPF 15: Octinoxate (p.1517·3); octisalate (p.1518·1); oxybenzone (p.1518·1).
Sunscreen.

Triple Sulfa *Fougera, USA; Goldline, USA; Major, USA; NMC, USA; Rugby, USA.*
Sulfathiazole (p.257·1); sulfacetamide (p.250·3); sulfabenzamide (p.250·2).
Vaginitis due to Gardnerella vaginalis.

Tri-Plen *Aventis, S.Afr.*
Ramipril (p.966·3); felodipine (p.888·3).
Hypertension.

Triplex *Sriprasit, Thai.*
Trifluoperazine hydrochloride (p.710·3).
Anxiety; nausea and vomiting; psychoses.

Tripo *Hua, Thai.*
Triprolidine hydrochloride (p.427·2); pseudoephedrine hydrochloride (p.1099·2).
Cold symptoms; hayfever; rhinitis; upper respiratory-tract congestion.

Triposed *Halsey, USA.*
Pseudoephedrine hydrochloride (p.1099·2); triprolidine hydrochloride (p.427·2).
Upper respiratory-tract symptoms.

Tripress *Pacific, NZ.*
Trimipramine maleate (p.311·2).
Depression.

Triprim
Note.This name is used for preparations of different composition.
Ratiopharm, Aust.; Glaxo Wellcome, Austral.; Glaxo Wellcome, NZ; Roche, S.Afr.
Trimethoprim (p.264·2).
Bacterial infections of the urinary tract.

Pharmaland, Thai.
Co-trimoxazole (p.193·3).
Bacterial infections.

Triprimix *Ashbourne, UK†.*
Trimethoprim (p.264·2).
Bacterial infections.

Triprodrine *Asian Pharm, Thai.*
Triprolidine hydrochloride (p.427·2); pseudoephedrine hydrochloride (p.1099·2).
Cold symptoms; hayfever; respiratory-tract congestion; rhinitis.

Triprofed *ICN, Canad.†.*
Pseudoephedrine hydrochloride (p.1099·2); triprolidine hydrochloride (p.427·2).

Tri-Profen *3M, Austral.*
Ibuprofen (p.43·2).
Inflammation; musculoskeletal and joint disorders; pain.

Tri-Profen Cold & Flu *3M, Austral.*
Ibuprofen (p.43·2); pseudoephedrine hydrochloride (p.1099·2).
Cold and influenza symptoms.

Tripsor *Orion, Fin.*
Trioxysalen (p.1127·2).
Lichen obtusus; lichen planus; psoriasis.

Tripta *Atlantic, Singapore; Atlantic, Thai.*
Amitriptyline hydrochloride (p.273·3).
Depression.

Triptafen *Goldshield, Irl.†; Forley, UK.*
Amitriptyline hydrochloride (p.273·3); perphenazine (p.699·1).
Mixed anxiety depressive states.

Triptil *Merck Frosst, Canad.*
Protriptyline hydrochloride (p.307·3).
Depression.

Triptizol *Merck Sharp & Dohme, Ital.*
Amitriptyline hydrochloride (p.273·3).
Depression.

Tript-OH *Sigma-Tau, Ital.; Sigma-Tau, Switz.*
Oxitriptan (p.302·2).
Depression; Down's syndrome; epilepsy; headache; insomnia; migraine; movement disorders; pain; parkinsonism; phenylketonuria.

Triptone *Del, USA.*
Dimenhydrinate (p.415·2).
Motion sickness.

Triptyl *Orion, Fin.*
Amitriptyline hydrochloride (p.273·3).
Depression; insomnia.

Triptyline *Medifive, Thai.*
Amitriptyline hydrochloride (p.273·3).
Depression.

Tripulmin *QIF, Braz.*
Ointment: Camphor (p.1589·3); eucalyptol (p.1609·2); menthol (p.1632·3); guaiacol (p.1092·1).
Syrup: Sodium camsilate; oxeladin citrate (p.1096·1); guaifenesin (p.1092·2); menthol (p.1632·3); eucalyptol (p.1609·2).
Respiratory-tract congestion.

Triquilar *Schering, Austral.; Schering, Braz.; Berlex, Canad.; Schering, Denm.; Schering, Ger.; Schering, Hong Kong; Schering, Mex.; Schering, NZ; Schering, Port.; Schering, Singapore; Schering, Switz.; Schering, Thai.*
Levonorgestrel (p.1486·2); ethinylestradiol (p.1476·2).
28-Day packs also contain 7 inert tablets.
Triphasic oral contraceptive.

Tri-Regol *Gedeon Richter, Hong Kong.*
Levonorgestrel (p.1486·2); ethinylestradiol (p.1476·2).
Triphasic oral contraceptive.

Tririnol *Biomedica, Ital.†.*
Xylometazoline hydrochloride (p.1102·2); dequalinium chloride (p.1143·1).
Cold symptoms; sinusitis.

Trirubin *Uniao Quimica, Braz.*
Vitamin B₁₂ (p.1388·1); vitamin B₁ (p.1385·2); vitamin B₆ (p.1387·1).
Megaloblastic anaemia; vitamin B deficiency.

Trirutin *Strathmann, Ger.†.*
Heparin sodium (p.902·1).
Skin trauma; vascular disorders.

Trirutin N *Strathmann, Ger.†.*
Troxerutin (p.1611·2).
Formerly contained troxerutin and etofylline.
Vascular disorders.

Tris *Fresenius Kabi, Aust.; Braun, Ger.*
Trometamol (p.1675·2).
Citrate intoxication following blood transfusion; metabolic acidosis; respiratory acidosis.

Trisalgina *Molteni, Ital.*
Dipyrone (p.34·1).
Fever; pain.

Trisdazol *Riedel-Zabinka, Braz.*
Metronidazole (p.594·1); nystatin (p.392·2); muramidase (p.1638·1).
Vulvovaginal infections.

Trisdine *Delta, Austral.†.*
Chlorhexidine gluconate (p.1138·2).
Urinary catheter care.

Trisekvens *Novo Nordisk, Denm.; Novo Nordisk, Fin.; Novo Nordisk, Norw.; Novo Nordisk, Swed.*
18 Tablets, estradiol (p.1473·1); 10 tablets, estradiol; norethisterone acetate (p.1485·1).
Menopausal disorders; osteoporosis.

Trisenox *Cell Therapeutics, USA.*
Arsenic trioxide (p.1582·1).
Acute promyelocytic leukaemia.

Triseptil
Note.This name is used for preparations of different composition.
Gedis, Ital.
Chlorhexidine gluconate (p.1138·2).
Hand disinfection.

Degorts, Mex.
Tinidazole (p.603·3).
Amoebiasis; giardiasis; trichomoniasis.

Trisequens *Novo Nordisk, Aust.; Novo Nordisk, Austral.; Novo Nordisk, Belg.; Rhone-Poulenc Rorer, Fr.; Novo Nordisk, Hong Kong; Novo Nordisk, Irl.; Novo Nordisk, Israel; Novo Nordisk, Ital.; Novo Nordisk, Neth.; Novo Nordisk, NZ; Novo Nordisk, Port.; Novo Nordisk, S.Afr.; Novo Nordisk, Singapore; Isdin, Spain; Novo Nordisk, Switz.; Novo Nordisk, Thai.; Novo Nordisk, UK.*
18 Tablets, estradiol (p.1473·1); 10 tablets, estradiol; norethisterone acetate (p.1485·1).
Formerly contained estradiol and estriol, and estradiol, estriol, and norethisterone acetate.
Menopausal disorders; osteoporosis.

Novo Nordisk, Ger.
16 Tablets, estradiol (p.1473·1); 12 tablets, estradiol; norethisterone acetate (p.1485·1).
Menopausal disorders; osteoporosis.

Tri-Sinerge *Atral, Port.*
Neomycin sulfate (p.228·1); streptomycin sulfate (p.249·1); bacitracin (p.155·2).
Bowel sterilisation; gastrointestinal infections.

Trisiston *Jenapharm, Ger.*
Ethinylestradiol (p.1476·2); levonorgestrel (p.1486·2).
Triphasic oral contraceptive.

Trisofort *Westmont, Hong Kong.*
Isoniazid (p.215·3).
Vitamin B substances (p.1350·1) are included in this preparation for the prophylaxis of peripheral neuropathy.
Tuberculosis.

Trisolvit *Chauvin, Fr.†.*
Tocofersolan (p.1394·3); sodium ascorbate (p.1390·1); ethoxazorutoside (p.1611·2).
Vascular eye disorders.

The symbol † denotes a preparation no longer actively marketed

Trisoralen *Dermatech, Austral.†; ICN, Canad.; ICN, Hong Kong; Lifepharma, Ital.†; Restan, S.Afr.†; ICN, USA.*
Trioxysalen (p.1127·2).
Intolerance to sunlight; vitiligo.

Trisorcin *Merckle, Ger.*
Penicillamine (p.1017·1).
Cystinuria; heavy-metal poisoning; polyarthritis; scleroderma; Wilson's disease.

Trisporal *Janssen-Cilag, Neth.*
Itraconazole (p.387·2).
Fungal infections.

Trissil *Piam, Ital.†*
Silymarin (p.1021·3).
Liver disorders.

Tri-Statin II *Rugby, USA.*
Triamcinolone acetonide (p.1080·1); nystatin (p.392·2).
Skin disorders.

TriStep *Asche, Ger.*
Levonorgestrel (p.1486·2); ethinylestradiol (p.1476·2).
Triphasic oral contraceptive.

Tristoject *Mayrand, USA.*
Triamcinolone diacetate (p.1080·2).
Corticosteroid.

Trisufin *Loren, Mex.*
Co-trimoxazole (p.193·3).
Bacterial infections.

Trisul *Pacific, NZ.*
Co-trimoxazole (p.193·3).
Bacterial infections; nocardiosis; Pneumocystis carinii pneumonia; toxoplasmosis.

Trisulfamid *Weifa, Norw.†*
Sulfadiazine (p.251·1); sulfadimidine(p.252·2); sulfacarbamide (p.250·2).
Bacterial infections of the urinary tract.

Trisulfaminic *Shepherd, Canad.†*
Phenylpropanolamine hydrochloride (p.1098·1); pheniramine maleate (p.422·3); mepyramine maleate (p.421·1); sulfadiazine (p.251·1); sulfamerazine (p.253·3); sulfadimidine (p.252·2).
Congestion and infections of the upper respiratory-tract.

Trisyn *Baker Cummins, Canad.†*
Fluocinonide (p.1071·2); procinonide (p.1079·3); ciprocinonide (p.1065·2).
Skin disorders.

Tritace
Hoechst Marion Roussel, Aust.; Aventis, Austral.; Aventis, Belg.; Hoechst Marion Roussel, Hong Kong; Hoechst Marion Roussel, Irl.; Hoechst Marion Roussel, Israel; Hoechst Marion Roussel, Mex.; Hoechst Marion Roussel, Neth.; Aventis, S.Afr.; Hoechst Marion Roussel, Singapore; Hoechst Marion Roussel, Thai.; Aventis, UK.
Ramipril (p.966·3).
Diabetic nephropathy; heart failure; hypertension; myocardial infarction; primary prophylaxis of atherosclerotic complications.

Tritan *Eon, USA.*
Chlorpheniramine [chlorphenamine] tannate (p.412·2); mepyramine tannate (p.421·1); phenylephrine tannate (p.1097·3).
Allergic rhinitis; nasal congestion.

Tri-Tannate *Rugby, USA.*
Phenylephrine tannate (p.1097·3); chlorpheniramine [chlorphenamine] tannate (p.412·2); mepyramine tannate (p.421·1).
Upper respiratory-tract symptoms.

Tri-Tannate Plus Pediatric *Rugby, USA.*
Phenylephrine tannate (p.1097·3); ephedrine tannate (p.1090·3); chlorpheniramine [chlorphenamine] tannate (p.412·2); pentoxyverine tannate (p.1096·3).
Coughs and cold symptoms.

Tritanrix *SmithKline Beecham, Ital.†*
A diphtheria, tetanus, and pertussis vaccine (p.1537·3).
Active immunisation.

Tritanrix HB
SmithKline Beecham, Spain; SmithKline Beecham, Thai.
A diphtheria, tetanus, pertussis, and hepatitis B vaccine (p.1538·3).
Active immunisation of infants and young children.

Tritanrix-DTPw *SmithKline Beecham, Aust.†*
A diphtheria, tetanus and pertussis vaccine (p.1537·3).
Active immunisation.

Tritazide
Hoechst Marion Roussel, Aust.; Aventis, Belg.; Hoechst Marion Roussel, Mex.; Hoechst Marion Roussel, Neth.
Ramipril (p.966·3); hydrochlorothiazide (p.907·3).
Hypertension.

Tritec *Glaxo Wellcome, USA.*
Ranitidine bismuth citrate (p.1247·2).
Peptic ulcer.

Tritet *Akromed, S.Afr.†*
Tetracycline hydrochloride (p.258·3); chlortetracycline hydrochloride (p.182·1); demeclocycline hydrochloride (p.198·2).
Bacterial infections.

Tri-Thiazid *Stada, Ger.*
Triamterene (p.986·1); hydrochlorothiazide (p.907·3).
Heart failure; hypertension; oedema.

Tri-Thiazid Reserpin *Stada, Ger.*
Triamterene (p.986·1); hydrochlorothiazide (p.907·3); reserpine (p.967·3).
Hypertension.

Triticum *Lepori, Port.*
Trazodone hydrochloride (p.310·1).
Depression.

Tri-Torrat *Roche, Ger.*
Metipranolol (p.930·2); butizide (p.853·1); dihydralazine sulfate (p.874·2).
Hypertension.

Trittico
CSC, Aust.; Angelini, Hong Kong; Angelini, Ital.; ACRAF, Switz.
Trazodone hydrochloride (p.310·1).
Depression; neuroleptanalgesia; pain; premedication.

Triv *Boyle, USA.*
Hydroxyquinoline sulfate (p.1622·2); alkyl aryl sulfonate; edetic acid (p.1008·3); sodium sulfate (p.1250·1).
Vaginal disorders.

Trivacuna *Leti, Spain.*
A diphtheria, tetanus, and pertussis vaccine (p.1537·3).
Active immunisation of infants and young children.

Trivagel N *Marjan, Braz.*
Dexamethasone acetate (p.1067·1); neomycin sulfate (p.228·1); nystatin (p.392·2); tyrothricin (p.267·1).
Vulvovaginal disorders.

Trivanex *Pharmasant, Thai.*
Griseofulvin (p.386·2).
Fungal infections.

Trivastal
Servier, Braz.; Eutherapie, Fr.; Servier, Ger.; Servier, Port.; Servier, Singapore; Servier, Thai.
Piribedil (p.1175·3) or piribedil mesilate (p.1175·3).
Mental function impairment in the elderly; parkinsonism; peripheral vascular disorders; vascular eye disorders.

Trivastan *Stroder, Ital.*
Piribedil (p.1175·3).
Vascular disorders.

Trivax *Wellcome, Irl.†*
A diphtheria, tetanus, and pertussis vaccine (p.1537·3).
Active immunisation.

Trivax-AD
Wellcome, Irl.†; Evans, UK.
An adsorbed diphtheria, tetanus, and pertussis vaccine (p.1537·3).
Active immunisation of infants and young children.

Trivax-Hib *SmithKline Beecham, UK†.*
A diphtheria, tetanus, pertussis, and haemophilus influenzae vaccine (p.1538·3).
Active immunisation.

Trive *Baxter, Fr.; Baxter, Spain; Baxter, Thai.; Clintec, Thai.*
Amino-acid, carbohydrate, and lipid (from soya oil (p.1378·1)) infusion (p.1350·1).
Parenteral nutrition.

Trivemil *Clintec, Ital.*
An amino-acid, lipid, and carbohydrate preparation (p.1350·1).
Parenteral nutrition.

Trivermon *Bergamo, Braz.*
Piperazine (p.105·3).
Ascariasis; enterobiasis.

Tri-Vi-Flor
Mead Johnson Nutritionals, Canad.; Mead Johnson Nutritionals, USA.
A range of vitamin preparations with fluoride (p.1375·3)(p.1350·1).
Dental caries prophylaxis; dietary supplement.

Tri-Vi-Fluor *Bristol-Myers Squibb, Braz.*
Multivitamin preparation with fluoride (p.1350·1)(p.1375·3).
Dental caries prophylaxis; dietary supplement.

Triviken *Kener, Mex.*
Vitamin B substances (p.1350·1).

Trivina
Pharmacia Upjohn, Belg.; Aspen, S.Afr.; Orion, Swed.
White tablets, estradiol valerate (p.1473·2); blue tablets estradiol valerate; medroxyprogesterone acetate (p.1480·1); yellow tablets, inert.
Menopausal disorders; osteoporosis.

Triviraten
Berna, Hong Kong; Berna, Ital.; Pharmabroker, NZ; Berna, Port.; Byk Madaus, S.Afr.; Berna, Spain; Berna, Switz.; Berna, Thai.
A measles, mumps, and rubella vaccine (Edmonston-Zagreb, Rubini, and Wistar RA 27/3 strains, respectively) (p.1549·1).
Active immunisation.

Tri-Vi-Sol
Bristol-Myers Squibb, Braz.; Mead Johnson Nutritionals, Canad.; Mead Johnson, Hong Kong; Mead Johnson, Mex.; Mead Johnson Nutritionals, USA.
Multivitamin preparation (p.1350·1).

Tri-Vi-Sol with Fluoride *Mead Johnson Nutritionals, Canad.*
Multivitamin preparation (p.1350·1) with fluoride (p.1375·3).
Dental caries prophylaxis; vitamin supplement.

Tri-Vi-Sol with Iron *Mead Johnson Nutritionals, USA.*
Multivitamin preparation with iron (p.1350·1).

Tri-Vitamin *Schein, USA.*
Vitamins A, C, and D (p.1350·1).

Trivitamin Fluoride Drops *Schein, USA.*
Multivitamin preparation with fluoride (p.1375·3)(p.1350·1).

Trivitan *Merck, Spain†.*
Pyridoxine (p.1387·1); vitamin A (p.1382·1); tocopherol (p.1394·1).
Hyperkeratosis; keratoconjunctivitis; rhinitis; tonic; xerophthalmia.

Trivit-B *TP, Thai.*
Vitamin B$_1$ (p.1385·2); vitamin B$_6$ (p.1387·1); vitamin B$_{12}$ (p.1388·1).
Neuritis; vitamin B deficiency.

Trivitol *Agepha, Aust.*
Vitamins (p.1350·1); caffeine; kola.
Tonic.

Trivon *Great Eastern, Thai.; Therapharma, Thai.*
Vitamin B$_1$; vitamin B$_6$; vitamin B$_{12}$ (p.1350·1).
Tonic.

Trivora *Watson, USA.*
Levonorgestrel (p.1486·2); ethinylestradiol (p.1476·2). 28-Day packs also contain 7 inert tablets.
Triphasic oral contraceptive.

Tri-Wycillina *Pharmacia Upjohn, Ital.*
Benzathine benzylpenicillin (p.156·2); benzylpenicillin potassium (p.157·1); procaine penicillin [procaine benzylpenicillin] (p.239·2).
Bacterial infections.

Trixidine *Asta Medica, Ital.†*
Propylene glycol cefatrizine (p.164·3).
Bacterial infections.

Trixilan *Pulitzer, Ital.*
Propylene glycol cefatrizine (p.164·3).
Bacterial infections.

Trixilem *Lemery, Mex.; Lemery, Thai.*
Methotrexate (p.553·2).
Malignant neoplasms; mycosis fungoides; rheumatoid arthritis.

Trixone *LBS, Thai.*
Ceftriaxone sodium (p.177·1).
Bacterial infections.

Trixzol *Great Eastern, Thai.; Westmont, Thai.*
Co-trimoxazole (p.193·3).
Bacterial infections.

Triyodisan *Bioquimica, Mex.*
Liothyronine (p.1524·3).

Triyotex *Medix, Mex.*
Liothyronine sodium (p.1524·2).
Hypothyroidism.

Triz *Indoco, Thai.*
Cetirizine hydrochloride (p.411·2).
Allergic conjunctivitis; allergic rhinitis; allergic skin disorders.

Trizele *Choongwae, Hong Kong.*
Metronidazole (p.594·1).
Anaerobic bacterial infections.

Trizid
Douglas, Hong Kong; Douglas, NZ.
Triamterene (p.986·1); hydrochlorothiazide (p.907·3).
Hypertension; oedema.

Trizina *Francia, Ital.*
Propylene glycol cefatrizine (p.164·3).
Bacterial infections.

Trizivir
Glaxo Wellcome, UK; Glaxo Wellcome, USA.
Abacavir sulfate (p.612·2); lamivudine (p.635·1); zidovudine (p.645·2).
HIV infection.

Trizol Balsamico *Riedel-Zabinka, Braz.*
Co-trimoxazole (p.193·3); guaifenesin (p.1092·2).
Bacterial infections.

Trizolin
Remedica, Singapore; Remedica, Thai.
Norfloxacin (p.232·1).
Bacterial infections.

Trobicin
Pharmacia Upjohn, Aust.; Pharmacia Upjohn, Austral.; Pharmacia Upjohn, Belg.; Pharmacia Upjohn, Braz.; Pharmacia Upjohn, Canad.†; Pharmacia Upjohn, Hong Kong; Pharmacia Upjohn, Irl.†; Pharmacia Upjohn, Ital.; Pharmacia Upjohn, Mex.; Pharmacia Upjohn, Port.; Pharmacia Upjohn, S.Afr.; Pharmacia Upjohn, Singapore; Pharmacia Upjohn, Swed.†; Pharmacia Upjohn, Switz.; Pharmacia Upjohn, Thai.; Pharmacia Upjohn, UK†; Pharmacia, USA†.
Spectinomycin hydrochloride (p.248·2).
Gonorrhoea.

Trobicine *Pharmacia Upjohn, Fr.*
Spectinomycin hydrochloride (p.248·2).
Gonorrhoea.

Troca Cationi *Pharma-Natura, Braz.*
Magnesium; potassium; zinc (p.1180·1).
Mineral deficiencies; stress; viral infections.

Troca Flu *Laborest, Ital.*
Zinc; magnesium; vitamin C; vitamin A (p.1350·1).
Candidiasis; viral infections.

Trocacin *Nakornpatana, Thai.*
Tyrothricin (p.267·1); benzocaine (p.1306·2).
Mouth and throat disorders.

Trocaine *Roberts, USA.*
Benzocaine (p.1306·2).
Obesity; sore throat.

Trocal *Roberts, USA.*
Dextromethorphan hydrobromide (p.1087·3).
Coughs.

Trochain *Propan, S.Afr.*
Cetrimide (p.1137·1); benzocaine (p.1306·2).
Mouth and throat disorders.

Trofalgon *Madariaga, Spain.*
Cyanocobalamin (p.1388·1); muramidase hydrochloride (p.1638·1).
Anorexia; tonic; weight loss.

Trofen *TP, Thai.*
Ibuprofen (p.64·2).
Fever; musculoskeletal and joint disorders; pain.

Troferit *Chinoin, Mex.*
Dropropizine (p.1089·3).
Coughs.

Trofesil *Solfran, Mex.*
Multivitamin preparation (p.1350·1).

Trofi Milina *Europharma, Spain†.*
Capsules: Phospholipids; pyridoxine hydrochloride (p.1386·3).
Injection: Cyanocobalamin (p.1388·1); phospholipids. Lignocaine [lidocaine] hydrochloride (p.1313·2) is included in this preparation to alleviate the pain of injection.
Dystonia; tonic.

Troficardil *Sintofarma, Braz.*
Inosine (p.1623·3).
Cardiovascular disorders.

Trofinerv *Fidia, Ital.*
Omega-3 marine triglycerides (p.949·3); vitamins (p.1350·1).
Nutritional supplement.

Trofinerv Antiox *Fidia, Ital.*
Omega-3 triglycerides (p.949·2); gamolenic acid (p.1613·1); vitamins; minerals (p.1350·1).
Nutritional supplement.

Trofo 5 *Uniderm, Ital.*
Zinc oxide (p.1128·2); cod-liver oil (p.1357·2); hyaluronic acid (p.1620·1); chamomile oil.
Skin disorders.

Trofocalcium *Fournier, Ital.*
Vitamin D and calcium preparation (p.1350·1).
Calcium depletion; metabolic bone disorders.

Trofodermin
Carlo Erba, Braz.; Carlo Erba OTC, Ital.; Pharmacia Upjohn, Thai.
Clostebol acetate (p.1466·3); neomycin sulfate (p.228·1).
Skin infections; wounds.

Trofodermin-S *Pharmacia Upjohn, Mex.*
Clostebol (p.1466·3).
Skin disorders.

Trofomed *Trofomed, Ital.†*
Royal jelly (p.1659·3).

Troforex Pepsico *Reig Jofre, Spain.*
Cyproheptadine hydrochloride (p.414·2); amino acids and hydroxocobalamin (p.1350·1); pepsin (p.1649·3).
Anorexia; tonic; weight-loss.

Trofoseptine *Boehringer Ingelheim, Fr.*
Sodium acexamate (p.1572·2); neomycin sulfate (p.228·1).
Formerly contained clostebol acetate and neomycin sulfate.
Infected ulcers.

Trojan *Carter Horner, Canad.*
Nonoxinol 9 (p.1346·1).
Contraceptive.

Troliber *Randall, Mex.*
Dextropropoxyphene (p.27·1).

Trolic *Garec, S.Afr.†*
Prednisone (p.1079·2).
Corticosteroid.

Trolovol
Dexo, Fr.; Asta Medica, Ger.
Penicillamine (p.1017·1).
Chronic polyarthritis; cystinuria; heavy-metal poisoning; rheumatoid arthritis; scleroderma; Wilson's disease.

Tromadil *Biolab, Thai.*
Bromhexine hydrochloride (p.1085·3).
Respiratory-tract disorders associated with increased or viscous mucus.

Tromalyt *Madaus, Spain.*
Aspirin (p.14·2).
Thrombosis prophylaxis.

Tromasin SA *Parke, Davis, S.Afr.†*
Papain (p.1647·3).
Inflammation; oedema.

Trombenox *Menarini, Ital.*
Enoxaparin sodium (p.885·1).
Thromboembolic disorders.

Trombofob *Knoll, Braz.*
Ointment: Heparin sodium (p.902·1); benzyl nicotinate (p.20·2).
Soft-tissue injury; superficial vascular disorders.
Topical gel: Heparin sodium (p.902·1).
Superficial vascular disorders.

Trombolisin *Proge, Ital.*
Heparin calcium (p.902·1).
Thromboembolic disorders.

Trombolysin *Nordic Healthcare, Denm.*
Urokinase (p.988·1).
Myocardial infarction.

Trombopat *Pentafarma, Port.*
Ticlopidine hydrochloride (p.981·1).

Trombosol *Orion, Fin.*
Heparin sodium (p.902·1).
Thromboembolic disorders.

Trombovar *Therapex, Canad.; Chiesi, Fr.; Bouty, Ital.*
Sodium tetradecyl sulfate (p.1497·2).
Cysts; oesophageal varices; varicose veins.

Trombyl *Pharmacia Upjohn, Swed.*
Aspirin (p.14·2).
Angina pectoris; myocardial infarction; prevention of cerebrovascular ischaemia.

Tromcardin *Trommsdorff, Ger.*
Potassium aspartate (p.1195·2); magnesium aspartate (p.1190·2).
Arrhythmias; heart failure; myocardial infarction; potassium and magnesium deficiency.

Tromgallol *Jacoby, Aust.*†.
Cyclobutyrol sodium (p.1601·2); cynarine (p.1602·1); sorbitol (p.1377·3); magnesium sulfate dihydrate (p.1191·1).
Hepatobiliary disorders.

Tromicol *Willmar, Mex.*
Tetracycline (p.258·3).
Bacterial infections.

Tromigal *Galen, Mex.*
Erythromycin (p.201·2).
Bacterial infections.

Tromir *Ibirn, Ital.*
Suleparoid (p.978·2).
Thrombosis prophylaxis.

Tromlipon *Trommsdorff, Ger.*
Thioctic acid (p.1671·3) or trometamol thioctate (p.1675·2).
Diabetic neuropathy.

Trommcardin *Jacoby, Aust.*
Potassium aspartate (p.1195·2); magnesium aspartate (p.1190·3).
Arrhythmias; digitalis intoxication; heart failure; myocardial infarction; potassium and magnesium deficiency.

Trompersantin *Boehringer Ingelheim, Mex.*
Dipyridamole (p.877·2).
Thromboembolic disorders.

Tromphyllin *Trommsdorff, Ger.*
Theophylline (p.777·2).
Obstructive airways disease.

Tronan *Roche, Ital.*
Suleparoid (p.978·2).
Thrombosis prophylaxis.

Troneo *Nakorn, Thai.*
Tyrothricin (p.267·1); benzocaine (p.1306·2).
Mouth and throat infections.

Tronex *Tocogino, Mex.*
Ampicillin (p.150·3).
Bacterial infections.

Tronolane *Ross, USA.*
Cream: Pramocaine hydrochloride (p.1318·2); zinc oxide (p.1128·2).
Suppositories†: Pramocaine hydrochloride (p.1318·2); pramocaine (p.1318·2); zinc oxide (p.1128·2).
Haemorrhoids.

Tronotene *Abbott, Ital.*
Pramocaine hydrochloride (p.1318·2).
Burns; haemorrhoids; pruritus.

Tronothane
Abbott, Fr.; Abbott, USA.
Pramocaine hydrochloride (p.1318·2).
Anal pain and pruritus; local anaesthesia.

Tronoxal *Pras, Spain.*
Ifosfamide (p.546·1).
Malignant neoplasms.

Tropargal *Synthelabo, Spain.*
Diazepam (p.674·3); nortriptyline hydrochloride (p.301·3).
Depression with anxiety or agitation.

Troparin *Biochemie, Aust.*†.
Certoparin sodium (p.856·2).
Thromboembolism prophylaxis.

Troparin compositum *Biochemie, Aust.*†.
Certoparin sodium (p.856·2); dihydroergotamine mesilate (p.450·3).
Lignocaine [lidocaine] hydrochloride (p.1313·2) is included in this preparation to alleviate the pain of injection.
Thromboembolism prophylaxis.

Tropax *Noristan, S.Afr.*†.
Phenobarbital (p.355·1); hyoscyamine sulfate (p.469·3); atropine sulfate (p.461·1); hyoscine hydrobromide (p.468·2).
Gastrointestinal disorders; urinary-tract spasm.

Tropergen *Goldshield, UK.*
Diphenoxylate hydrochloride (p.1222·2).
Atropine sulfate (p.461·1) is included in this preparation to discourage abuse.
These ingredients can be described by the British Approved Name Co-phenotrope.
Diarrhoea.

Tropex
Rowa, Irl.
Phenazone (p.77·2).
Ear wax removal; otitis media.

Rowa, Singapore.
Phenazone (p.77·2); glycerol (p.1616·3).
Ear wax removal; otitis media.

Trophamine
Braun McGaw, Hong Kong; Pisa, Mex.; McGaw, NZ; Pharmacia Upjohn, Spain; McGaw, USA.
Amino-acid infusion (p.1350·1).
Parenteral nutrition.

Trophicard *Kohler-Pharma, Ger.; Kohler, Ger.*
Potassium aspartate (p.1195·2); magnesium aspartate (p.1190·3).
Cardiac disorders; magnesium or potassium deficiency.

Trophicreme *Sanofi Winthrop, Fr.*
Estriol (p.1475·3).
Postmenopausal vulvovaginal disorders.

Trophiderm *Brothier, Fr.*†.
Calcium alginate (p.728·1).
Ulcers.

Trophigil *Sanofi Winthrop, Fr.*
Lactobacillus caseivar rhamnosus (p.1626·3); estriol (p.1475·3); progesterone (p.1488·3).
Atrophic vaginitis; pre- and postoperative gynaecological care.

Trophires
Note.This name is used for preparations of different composition.
Sanofi Winthrop, Fr.
Suppositories: Eucalyptus oil (p.1609·2); thenoate sodium (p.261·3).
Formerly contained camphor, myrtle oil, eucalyptus oil, and thenoate sodium.
Respiratory-tract disorders.

Syrup: Pholcodine (p.1099·1); thenoate sodium (p.261·3); eucalyptus oil (p.1609·2).
Coughs.

Sanofi Synthelabo, Spain.
Nasal drops: Eucalyptol (p.1609·2); cypress oil; myrtle oil; thenoate sodium (p.261·3).
Nasal cleansing.

Sanofi Winthrop, Spain†.
Suppositories; syrup: Pholcodine (p.1099·1).
Cough.

Sanofi Winthrop, Spain†.
Capsules: Thenoate sodium (p.261·3).
Bronchitis.

Trophires Compose *Sanofi Winthrop, Fr.*
Paracetamol (p.71·2); eucalyptus oil (p.1609·2); thenoate sodium (p.261·3).
Formerly contained camphor, myrtle oil, eucalyptus oil, thenoate sodium, paracetamol, and pholcodine.
Fever; respiratory-tract disorders.

Trophobolene *Theramex, Mon.*†.
Estrapronicate (p.1475·3); nandrolone undecylate (p.1484·2); hydroxyprogesterone enantate (p.1479·3).
Anabolic; osteoporosis.

Trophoseptine *Sanofi Synthelabo, Port.*
Promestriene (p.1490·3); chlorquinaldol (p.182·1).
Vaginal infections.

Trophysan *Baxter, Fr.*
Amino-acid, carbohydrate, mineral, and vitamin infusion (p.1350·1).
Enteral and parenteral nutrition.

Tropicacyl *Akorn, USA.*
Tropicamide (p.475·1).
Induction of mydriasis and cycloplegia.

Tropical Blend *Schering-Plough, Canad.*†.
Oxybenzone (p.1518·1).
Sunscreen.

Tropical Blend Dark Tanning *Schering-Plough, USA.*
SPF 2: Homosalate (p.1517·2).
Lotion SPF 4: Octinoxate (p.1517·3); oxybenzone (p.1518·1).
Oil SPF 4: Padimate O (p.1518·2); oxybenzone (p.1518·1).
Sunscreen.

Tropical Blend Dry Oil *Schering-Plough, USA.*
SPF 2: Homosalate (p.1517·2).
SPF 4: Homosalate (p.1517·2); oxybenzone (p.1518·1).
Sunscreen.

Tropical Blend Tan Magnifier *Schering-Plough, USA.*
SPF 2; SPF 4: Trolamine salicylate (p.90·1).
Sunscreen.

Tropical Gold Dark Tanning *Goldline, USA.*
SPF 2: Octinoxate (p.1517·3); padimate O (p.1518·2).
SPF 4: Octinoxate (p.1517·3); oxybenzone (p.1518·1).
Sunscreen.

Tropical Gold Sunblock *Goldline, USA.*
SPF 15: Octinoxate (p.1517·3); oxybenzone (p.1518·1).
SPF 30: Octinoxate (p.1517·3); octisalate (p.1518·1); homosalate (p.1517·2); oxybenzone (p.1518·1).
Sunscreen.

Tropical Gold Sunscreen *Goldline, USA.*
SPF 8: Octinoxate (p.1517·3); oxybenzone (p.1518·1).
Sunscreen.

Tropicil Top *Oftalder, Port.*
Tropicamide (p.475·1).
Production of mydriasis and cycloplegia.

Tropico *Calmante Vitaminado, Spain.*
Menthol (p.1632·3); eucalyptus oil (p.1609·2).
Nasal congestion.

Tropicol *Bournonville, Belg.*†.
Tropicamide (p.475·1).
Production of mydriasis.

Tropimil *Farmigea, Ital.*
Tropicamide (p.475·1).
Production of mydriasis and cycloplegia.

Tropinal *Novaquimica, Braz.*
Dipyrone (p.34·1); homatropine methylbromide (p.468·1); hyoscyamine sulfate (p.469·3); hyoscine hydrobromide (p.468·2).
Smooth muscle spasm.

Tropiovent *Ashbourne, UK.*
Ipratropium bromide (p.766·1).
Obstructive airways disease.

Tropisol *Protein, Mex.*
Captopril (p.853·3).

Tropi-Storz *Lederle, USA*†.
Tropicamide (p.475·1).
Production of mydriasis and cycloplegia.

Tropium *DDSA Pharmaceuticals, UK.*
Chlordiazepoxide hydrochloride (p.659·2).
Alcohol withdrawal syndrome; anxiety.

Tropoderm *Kolassa, Aust.*
Neomycin sulfate (p.228·1); diphenylpyraline hydrochloride (p.417·1); buphenine hydrochloride (p.1587·3); hydrocortisone (p.1073·3).

Tropyn Z *Zafiro, Mex.*
Atropine sulfate (p.461·1).
Gastrointestinal disorders; organophosphorus pesticide poisoning; premedication.

Trosic *General Drugs, Thai.*
Tramadol hydrochloride (p.89·1).
Pain.

Trosid *Pfizer Consumer, Spain.*
Tioconazole (p.395·1).
Fungal skin and nail infections; vulvovaginal candidiasis.

Trospi *Medac, Ger.*
Trospium chloride (p.475·2).
Urinary-tract disorders.

Trosycort *Pfizer, Fin.*
Tioconazole (p.395·1); hydrocortisone acetate (p.1073·3).
Inflammatory fungal skin infections with secondary bacterial infection.

Trosyd
Pfizer, Aust.; Pfizer Consumer, Canad.; Pfizer, Fin.; Pfizer, Fr.†*; Pfizer, Hong Kong; Roerig, Ital.; Pfizer, NZ; Farminova, Port.; Pfizer, S.Afr.; Pfizer, Singapore; Pfizer, Switz.; Pfizer, Thai.*
Tioconazole (p.395·1).
Fungal and Gram-positive bacterial infections of the skin, nails, and vagina; vaginal trichomoniasis.

Trosyl
Pfizer, Irl.; Pfizer, UK.
Tioconazole (p.395·1).
Fungal and bacterial infections of the nails.

Trova *Pfizer, Israel.*
Alatrofloxacin mesilate (p.147·3).
Bacterial infections.

Trovan
Pfizer, Aust.†*; Pfizer, Austral.; Pfizer, Canad.; Pfizer, Swed.*†*; Pfizer, Mex.; Pfizer, Swed.*†*; Pfizer, USA.*
Injection: Alatrofloxacin mesilate (p.147·3).
Bacterial infections.

Pfizer, Aust.†*; Pfizer, Austral.; Pfizer, Canad.; Pfizer, Hong Kong; Pfizer, Mex.; Pfizer, Swed.*†*; Pfizer, USA.*
Tablets: Trovafloxacin mesilate (p.266·3).
Bacterial infections.

Troxazole *Propan, S.Afr.*†.
Co-trimoxazole (p.193·3).
Bacterial infections.

Troxeven *Kreussler, Ger.*
Troxerutin (p.1611·2).
Venous disorders.

Troymycetin *Noristan, S.Afr.*†.
Chloramphenicol (p.179·1).
Bacterial infections.

Trozocina *Sigma-Tau, Ital.*
Azithromycin (p.153·1).
Bacterial infections.

True Illusion *Maybelline, Canad.*
Cream SPF 10: Titanium dioxide (p.1126·1).
Liquid SPF 10: Octinoxate (p.1517·3).
Sunscreen.

True Test
ALK, Denm.; Abello, Ger.†*; CSL, NZ; Alk-Abello, NZ; Glaxo Wellcome, USA.*
A range of allergen-impregnated patches (p.1575·3).
Diagnosis of allergic contact dermatitis.

Trufree
Cantassium Co., UK.
Gluten-free, wheat-free flours for special diets (p.1350·1).
Gluten sensitivity.

Cantassium Co., UK.
Tablets: Multivitamin and mineral preparation (p.1350·1).

Trumsal *Centrum, Spain.*
Diltiazem hydrochloride (p.874·3).
Angina pectoris; hypertension.

Truphylline *G & W, USA.*
Aminophylline (p.760·1).
Asthma; bronchospasm.

Truquil *Lundbeck, Israel.*
Chlorprothixene hydrochloride (p.667·3).
Psychoses.

Trusopt
Merck Sharp & Dohme, Aust.; Merck Sharp & Dohme, Austral.; Merck Sharp & Dohme, Belg.; Merck Frosst, Canad.; Merck Sharp & Dohme, Denm.; Merck Sharp & Dohme, Fin.; Merck Sharp & Dohme-Chibret, Fr.; Chibret, Ger.; Merck Sharp & Dohme, Hong Kong; Merck Sharp & Dohme, Irl.; Merck Sharp & Dohme, Israel; Merck Sharp & Dohme, Ital.; Merck Sharp & Dohme, Mex.; Merck Sharp & Dohme, Neth.; Merck Sharp & Dohme, Norw.; Merck Sharp & Dohme, NZ; Chibret, Port.; Merck Sharp & Dohme, S.Afr.; Merck Sharp & Dohme, Singapore; Merck Sharp & Dohme, Swed.; Merck Sharp & Dohme, Switz.; Merck Sharp & Dohme, Thai.; Merck Sharp & Dohme, UK.
Dorzolamide hydrochloride (p.883·1).
Glaucoma; ocular hypertension.

Truxal
Lundbeck, Aust.; Lundbeck, Denm.; Lundbeck, Fin.; Lundbeck, Ger.; Lundbeck, Neth.; Lundbeck, Norw.; Lundbeck, Swed.; Lundbeck, Switz.
Chlorprothixene (p.667·3), chlorprothixene acetate (p.667·3), chlorprothixene citrate (p.667·3), or chlorprothixene hydrochloride (p.667·3).
Alcohol and drug withdrawal syndromes; anxiety disorders; behaviour disorders in children; depression; mania; neuroses; pain; psychoses; sedative; sleep disorders; vomiting.

Truxaletten
Lundbeck, Aust.; Lundbeck, Switz.
Chlorprothixene (p.667·3) or chlorprothixene hydrochloride (p.667·3).
Alcohol and drug withdrawal syndromes; anxiety disorders; behaviour disorders in children; neuroses; pain; sleep disorders; vomiting.

Try *Nicholas, Fr.*
Vaginal lubricant.

Tryasol *Wernigerode, Ger.*
Codeine phosphate (p.25·2).
Coughs.

Trycam *Douglas, NZ.*
Triazolam (p.709·3).
Insomnia.

Tryptal *Unipharm, Israel.*
Amitriptyline hydrochloride (p.273·3).
Depression; nocturnal enuresis.

Tryptan *ICN, Canad.*
Tryptophan (p.311·3).
Adjunct in treatment of depression.

Tryptanol
Merck Sharp & Dohme, Austral.; Prodome, Braz.; Merck Sharp & Dohme, Hong Kong; Merck Sharp & Dohme, Mex.; Merck Sharp & Dohme, NZ; Merck Sharp & Dohme, S.Afr.; Merck Sharp & Dohme, Thai.
Amitriptyline (p.273·3), amitriptyline embonate (p.273·3), or amitriptyline hydrochloride (p.273·3).
Depression; nocturnal enuresis.

Tryptil *Cristalia, Braz.*
Amitriptyline (p.273·3).
Depression; nocturnal enuresis.

Tryptine *Amrad, Austral.*
Amitriptyline hydrochloride (p.273·3).
Depression; nocturnal enuresis.

Tryptizol
Merck Sharp & Dohme, Aust.; Merck Sharp & Dohme, Belg.; Merck Sharp & Dohme, Denm.; Morson, Irl.; Merck Sharp & Dohme, Neth.; Merck Sharp & Dohme, Norw.; Merck Sharp & Dohme, Port.; Merck Sharp & Dohme, Spain; Merck Sharp & Dohme, Swed.; Merck Sharp & Dohme, Switz.; Merck Sharp & Dohme, UK†.
Amitriptyline embonate (p.273·3) or amitriptyline hydrochloride (p.273·3).
Bulimia; depression; nocturnal enuresis; postherpetic neuralgia.

Tryptoferm *Gaschler, Ger.*
Pancreatin (p.1646·1).
Inflammatory disorders.

Trysul *Savage, USA*†.
Sulfathiazole (p.257·1); sulfacetamide (p.250·3); sulfabenzamide (p.250·2).
Vaginitis due to Gardnerella vaginalis.

T-Stat
Westwood-Squibb, Canad.; Bristol-Myers Squibb, Mex.; Westwood, Singapore; Westwood-Squibb, USA.
Erythromycin (p.201·2).
Acne.

TTC *Investigaciones Filosoficas y Cientificas, Mex.*
Thiamine (p.1385·2).

TTD-B₃-B₄ *AJC, Fr.*
Disulfiram (p.1605·1); nicotinamide (p.1372·3); adenine (p.1573·2).
Alcoholism.

Tubarine *Glaxo Wellcome, Israel.*
Tubocurarine chloride (p.1343·1).
Competitive neuromuscular blocker.

Tuberen *Upsifarma, Port.*
Rifampicin (p.243·2); isoniazid (p.215·3); pyrazinamide (p.240·1).
Tuberculosis.

Tubergen-Test *Chiron Behring, Ger.*
Tuberculin (p.1675·3).
Sensitivity test.

Tuberol *Rolab, S.Afr.*†.
Ethambutol hydrochloride (p.205·1); isoniazid (p.215·3).
Tuberculosis.

Tubersol
Connaught, Canad.; CSL, NZ; Connaught, NZ; Pasteur Merieux, USA.
Tuberculin purified protein derivative (p.1675·3).
Diagnosis of tuberculosis.

Tubersol PPD *Parisis, Spain.*
Tuberculins (p.1675·3).
Diagnostic agent.

Tubetam *Bioquimica, Mex.*
Ethambutol (p.205·3).

Tubilysin *Orion, Fin.*
Isoniazid (p.215·3).
Tuberculosis.

Tucks
Warner-Lambert, Canad.; Warner-Lambert, USA.
Hamamelis (p.1618·3); glycerol (p.1616·3).
Perianal cleansing; skin cleansing.

Tuclase
Bios, Belg.; UCB, Ital.; UCB, Neth.
Pentoxyverine citrate (p.1096·3) or pentoxyverine hydrochloride (p.1096·3).
Coughs.

Tudcabil *Pharmacia Upjohn, Ital.*
Tauroursodeoxycholic acid (p.1677·3).
Biliary disorders.

Tueor *Sofar, Ital.*
Barrier cream.

Tufemin *Ravensberg, Ger.†*
Multivitamin preparation with iron (p.1350·1).
Anaemias; iron and vitamin deficiency.

Tuinal
Lilly, Canad.†; Lilly, Irl.†; Lilly, UK; Lilly, USA.
Secobarbital sodium (p.705·2); amobarbital sodium (p.655·2).
Insomnia; sedative.

Tukol *Atlantis, Mex.*
Guaifenesin (p.1092·2).
Coughs.

Tukson *Sons, Mex.*
Oxolamine (p.1096·2).
Coughs.

Tulgrasum Antibiotico *Knoll, Spain.*
Bacitracin zinc (p.155·2) neomycin sulfate (p.228·1); polymyxin B sulfate (p.238·1).
Burns; skin disorders; skin ulcers; wounds.

Tulgrasum Cicatrizante *Knoll, Spain.*
Glycine; benzyl benzoate (p.1428·2); benzalkonium chloride (p.1133·2); amino acids.
Burns; skin disorders; skin ulcers; wounds.

Tulip *Pharmacia Upjohn, Spain.*
Flurbiprofen (p.41·2).
Musculoskeletal, joint, and peri-articular disorders; pain.

Tulle Gras Lumiere
Solvay, Belg.; Solvay, Fr.; Hefa, Ger.†
Peru balsam (p.1650·2).
Burns; wounds.

Tulotract *Ardeypharm, Ger.*
Lactulose (p.1230·1).
Constipation; hepatic encephalopathy; salmonella enteritis.

Tumarol
Note.This name is used for preparations of different composition.
Robugen, Ger.
Eucalyptus oil (p.1609·2); camphor (p.1589·3); menthol (p.1632·3).
Cold symptoms.

Renapharm, Switz.
Camphor (p.1589·3); menthol (p.1632·3); cedar atlant. oil; eucalyptus oil (p.1609·2); turpentine oil (p.1676·3); thymol (p.1158·3).
Cold symptoms.

Tumarol Kinderbalsam *Robugen, Ger.*
Eucalyptus oil (p.1609·2); oleum pini sylvestris.
Cold symptoms.

Tumarol-N *Robugen, Ger.*
Camphor (p.1589·3); menthol (p.1632·3); eucalyptus oil (p.1609·2).
Cold symptoms.

Tumax *Sriprasit, Thai.*
Chlordiazepoxide hydrochloride (p.659·2); clidinium bromide (p.465·1).
Gastrointestinal disorders; peptic ulcer.

Tumdi *Sriprasit, Thai.*
Paracetamol (p.71·2).
Fever; pain.

Tums
SmithKline Beecham, Braz.; SmithKline Beecham Consumer, Canad.; SmithKline Beecham, Israel; SmithKline Beecham Consumer, UK; SmithKline Beecham Consumer, USA.
Calcium carbonate (p.1215·1).
Calcium supplement; gastric hyperacidity.

Tums Plus *SmithKline Beecham, USA.*
Calcium carbonate (p.1215·1); simeticone (p.1249·2).

Tundrax *Tecnobio, Spain.*
Pseudoephedrine hydrochloride (p.1099·2); ebastine (p.417·2).
Allergic rhinitis.

Tuneluz *Baldacci, Port.*
Fluoxetine hydrochloride (p.284·2).
Bulimia; depression.

Tunitol-BX *Streger, Mex.*
Ambroxol hydrochloride (p.1084·3).
Respiratory-tract congestion.

Tuosomin *Leiras, Thai.*
Tamoxifen citrate (p.571·1).
Anovulatory infertility; breast cancer; endometrial cancer.

Turbatherm *Torfwerk Einfeld, Ger.†*
Peat.
Gastrointestinal disorders; musculoskeletal and joint disorders.

Turbinal *Valeas, Ital.*
Beclometasone dipropionate (p.1061·3).
Rhinitis.

Turbocalcin
SmithKline Beecham, Braz.; SmithKline Beecham, Ital.
Elcatonin (p.749·2).
Hypercalcaemia; osteoporosis; Paget's disease of bone; reflex sympathetic dystrophy.

Turexan Capilla *Turimed, Switz.*
Cetrimonium bromide (p.1137·3); urea (p.1127·3); dexpanthenol (p.1602·3).
Scalp disorders.

Turexan Creme *Turimed, Switz.*
Undecenoic acid (p.395·3); zinc undecenoate (p.395·3).
Barrier cream; skin disorders.

Turexan Douche *Turimed, Switz.*
Undecenoic acid (p.395·3).
Skin disorders; soap substitute.

Turexan Emulsion *Turimed, Switz.*
Undecenoic acid (p.395·3); zinc undecenoate (p.395·3); triclosan (p.1159·2).
Skin disorders; soap substitute.

Turexan Lotion *Turimed, Switz.*
Urea (p.1127·3); dexpanthenol (p.1602·3).
Skin disorders.

Turfa *Worwag, Ger.*
Triamterene (p.986·1); hydrochlorothiazide (p.907·3).
Hypertension; oedema.

Turicard *Jenapharm, Ger.†*
Glyceryl trinitrate (p.897·3).
Cardiac disorders.

Turifarm *Reuffer, Mex.*
Rifampicin (p.243·2).

Turimonit *Jenapharm, Ger.*
Isosorbide mononitrate (p.916·2).
Cardiac disorders.

Turimycin *Jenapharm, Ger.*
Clindamycin hydrochloride (p.188·1).
Bacterial infections.

Turinal
Gedeon Richter, Hong Kong; Gedeon Richter, Singapore.
Allylestrenol (p.1465·2).
Premature labour; threatened or recurrent miscarriage.

Turineurin *Jenapharm, Ger.*
Hypericum (p.290·2).
Anxiety; depression.

Turiplex *Jenapharm, Ger.*
Cucurbita (p.1601·1).
Urinary-tract disorders.

Turisan *Turimed, Switz.*
Cetrimonium bromide (p.1137·3).
Skin disinfection; skin infections.

Turisteron *Jenapharm, Ger.*
Ethinylestradiol propanesulfonate (p.1476·2).
Prostatic cancer.

Turixin *SmithKline Beecham, Ger.*
Calcium mupirocin (p.226·2).
Nasal carriage of staphylococci.

Turkadon *Bioiberica, Spain†.*
Chondroitin sulfate (p.1594·2).
Arteriosclerosis; thromboembolic disorders.

Turoptin
Ciba Vision, Ital.; Ciba Vision, Switz.
Metipranolol (p.930·2).
Glaucoma; ocular hypertension.

Turpentine White Liniment *McGloin, Austral.*
Turpentine oil (p.1676·3); camphor (p.1589·3).
Muscle pain.

Turresis *Sanofi Synthelabo, Port.*
Ethambutol hydrochloride (p.205·1).
Tuberculosis.

Tusben *Benedetti, Ital.*
Dimemorfan phosphate (p.1089·1).
Coughs.

Tuscalman
Note.This name is used for preparations of different composition.
Kwizda, Aust.; Berna, Switz.
Oral drops; suppositories: Noscapine hydrochloride (p.1096·1); guaifenesin (p.1092·2).
Respiratory-tract disorders.

Kwizda, Aust.
Syrup: Noscapine hydrochloride (p.1096·1); guaifenesin (p.1092·2); althaea (p.1577·1); sambucus (p.1660·3).
Catarrh; coughs.

Berna, Ital.
Oral drops; suppositories: Noscapine hydrochloride (p.1096·1); guaifenesin (p.1092·2).
Coughs.

Berna, Spain.
Syrup; infant suppositories: Noscapine hydrochloride (p.1096·1).
Coughs.

Berna, Switz.
Syrup: Noscapine hydrochloride (p.1096·1); guaifenesin (p.1092·2); althaea (p.1577·1).
Respiratory-tract disorders.

Tusco *Hua, Thai.*
Dextromethorphan hydrobromide (p.1087·3).
Coughs.

Tuscolgen *Great Eastern, Thai.; Westmont, Thai.*
Dextromethorphan hydrobromide (p.1087·3); guaifenesin (p.1092·2); chlorpheniramine [chlorphenamine] maleate (p.412·1).
Coughs.

Tusehli *Ehlinger, Mex.*
Benzonatate (p.1085·3).

Tuselin Descongestivo *Reig Jofre, Spain.*
Dextromethorphan hydrobromide (p.1087·3); phenylephrine hydrochloride (p.1097·1).
Coughs; nasal congestion.

Tuselin Expectorante *Reig Jofre, Spain.*
Alloclamide hydrochloride (p.1084·3); ammonium chloride (p.1085·2); carbocisteine (p.1086·3); phenylephrine hydrochloride (p.1097·1); ipecacuanha (p.1093·1).
Respiratory-tract disorders.

Tuseran *Medichem, Hong Kong.*
Dextromethorphan hydrobromide (p.1087·3); guaifenesin (p.1092·2); phenylpropanolamine hydrochloride (p.1098·1); chlorpheniramine [chlorphenamine] maleate (p.412·1); paracetamol (p.71·2).
Coughs and cold symptoms.

Tusibron
Note.This name is used for preparations of different composition.
Kener, Mex.
Ambroxol (p.1084·3).

Kenwood, Mex.
Guaifenesin (p.1092·2).
Coughs.

Tusibron-DM *Kenwood, USA.*
Guaifenesin (p.1092·2); dextromethorphan hydrobromide (p.1087·3).
Coughs.

Tusical *Andromaco, Mex.*
Benzonatate (p.1085·3).
Coughs.

Tusigen *Liomont, Mex.*
Zipeprol hydrochloride (p.1102·3).
Coughs.

Tusilen *Allen, Mex.*
Dextromethorphan hydrobromide (p.1087·3); guaifenesin (p.1092·2); phenylephrine hydrochloride (p.1097·1).
Coughs; respiratory-tract congestion.

Tusilen Pediatrico *Allen, Mex.*
Dextromethorphan hydrobromide (p.1087·3); guaifenesin (p.1092·2); paracetamol (p.71·2).
Coughs; fever.

Tusitato *Fustery, Mex.*
Benzonatate (p.1085·3).
Coughs.

Tusitinas *Pensa, Spain.*
Dextromethorphan hydrobromide (p.1087·3).
Coughs.

Tusno *Milano, Thai.*
Dextromethorphan hydrobromide (p.1087·3); guaifenesin (p.1092·2); bromhexine hydrochloride (p.1085·3).
Coughs.

Tusofren *Almirall, Spain.*
Dropropizine (p.1089·3).
Coughs.

Tusol *Rhone-Poulenc Rorer, Mex.*
Oxolamine citrate (p.1096·2).
Coughs.

Tusorama *Quimifar, Spain.*
Dextromethorphan hydrobromide (p.1087·3).
Coughs.

Tusquelin *Circle, USA†.*
Phenylpropanolamine hydrochloride (p.1098·1); dextromethorphan hydrobromide (p.1087·3); phenylephrine hydrochloride (p.1097·1); chlorpheniramine [chlorphenamine] maleate (p.412·1); ipecacuanha (p.1093·1); sulfogaiacol (p.1101·1).
Coughs and cold symptoms.

Tusquit *Xixia, S.Afr.*
Diphenhydramine hydrochloride (p.416·1); ammonium chloride (p.1085·2).
Coughs.

Tuss *Disperga, Aust.*
Wild thyme; castanea vulgaris.
Coughs and viscous mucus.

Tuss Hustenstiller *Rentschler, Ger.*
Dextromethorphan hydrobromide (p.1087·3).
Coughs.

Tussa *Silom, Thai.*
Guaifenesin (p.1092·2).
Coughs.

Tussafed *Everett, USA.*
Carbinoxamine maleate (p.411·1); pseudoephedrine hydrochloride (p.1099·2); dextromethorphan hydrobromide (p.1087·3).
Coughs and cold symptoms.

Tussafed HC *Everett, USA.*
Hydrocodone tartrate (p.42·2); phenylephrine hydrochloride (p.1097·1); guaifenesin (p.1092·2).
Coughs.

Tussafed-LA *Everett, USA.*
Guaifenesin (p.1092·2); pseudoephedrine hydrochloride (p.1099·2); dextromethorphan hydrobromide (p.1087·3).
Coughs; respiratory-tract congestion.

Tussafin Expectorant *Rugby, USA.*
Pseudoephedrine hydrochloride (p.1099·2); guaifenesin (p.1092·2); hydrocodone tartrate (p.42·2).
Coughs.

Tussafug *Robugen, Ger.; Medipharm, Switz.*
Benproperine embonate (p.1085·2) or benproperine phosphate (p.1085·2).
Coughs.

Tuss-Allergine Modified TD *Rugby, USA†.*
Phenylpropanolamine hydrochloride (p.1098·1); caramiphen edisilate (p.1086·2).
Coughs.

Tussamag
Note.This name is used for preparations of different composition.
Montavit, Aust.
Ointment: Spike lavender oil (p.1667·1); eucalyptus oil (p.1609·2); turpentine oil (p.1676·3); camphor (p.1589·3).
Oral liquid: Thyme (p.1672·3); castanea vulgaris.
Bronchitis; catarrh; coughs.

Teofarma, Ital.
Wild thyme; castanea leaves.
Respiratory-tract congestion.

Tussamag Codeintropfen *CT, Ger.†*
Codeine phosphate (p.25·2).
Coughs.

Tussamag Complex *Teofarma, Ital.*
Wild thyme; dropropizine (p.1089·3).
Coughs.

Tussamag Erkaltungsbalsam N *CT, Ger.*
Eucalyptus oil (p.1609·2); pine needle oil.
Catarrh.

Tussamag Halstabletten *CT, Ger.†*
Benzocaine (p.1306·2); menthol (p.1632·3); peppermint oil (p.1243·3); eucalyptus oil (p.1609·2).
Pain, inflammation, and infection of the mouth and throat.

Tussamag Hustensaft N *CT, Ger.*
Thyme (p.1672·2).
Bronchitis; catarrh; coughs.

Tussamag Hustentropfen N *CT, Ger.*
Thyme (p.1672·2).
Bronchitis; catarrh; coughs.

Tussamed *Hexal, Ger.†*
Clobutinol hydrochloride (p.1087·1).
Coughs.

Tussaminic C *Sandoz, Canad.†*
Codeine phosphate (p.25·2); phenylpropanolamine hydrochloride (p.1098·1); mepyramine maleate (p.421·1); pheniramine maleate (p.422·3).
Coughs.

Tussaminic DH *Sandoz, Canad.†*
Hydrocodone tartrate (p.42·2); phenylpropanolamine hydrochloride (p.1098·1); mepyramine maleate (p.421·1); pheniramine maleate (p.422·3).
Coughs.

Tussanil Compositum *Vifor, Switz.*
Noscapine (p.1096·1); drosera (p.1606·1); liquorice (p.1231·2); eucalyptus oil (p.1609·2); peppermint oil (p.1243·3).
Coughs.

Tussanil DH *Misemer, USA.*
Syrup: Phenylephrine hydrochloride (p.1097·1); chlorpheniramine [chlorphenamine] maleate (p.412·1); hydrocodone tartrate (p.42·2).
Coughs and cold symptoms.
Tablets†: Phenylpropanolamine hydrochloride (p.1098·1); hydrocodone tartrate (p.42·2); guaifenesin (p.1092·2).
Coughs.

Tussanil N *Vifor, Switz.*
Noscapine hydrochloride (p.1096·1).
Coughs.

Tussanil Plain *Misemer, USA.*
Phenylephrine hydrochloride (p.1097·1); chlorpheniramine [chlorphenamine] maleate (p.412·1).
Upper respiratory-tract symptoms.

Tussantiol *Medisa, Switz.*
Carbocisteine (p.1086·3).
Respiratory-tract disorders with increased mucus.

Tussanyl *Giovanardi, Ital.*
Sulfogaiacol (p.1101·1); grindelia (p.1618·2).
Catarrh; coughs.

Tussar-2 *Rhone-Poulenc Rorer, USA.*
Codeine phosphate (p.25·2); guaifenesin (p.1092·2); pseudoephedrine hydrochloride (p.1099·2).
Coughs.

Tussar DM *Rhone-Poulenc Rorer, USA.*
Dextromethorphan hydrobromide (p.1087·3); chlorpheniramine [chlorphenamine] maleate (p.412·1); pseudoephedrine hydrochloride (p.1099·2).
Coughs and cold symptoms.

Tussar SF *Rhone-Poulenc Rorer, USA.*
Codeine phosphate (p.25·2); guaifenesin (p.1092·2); pseudoephedrine hydrochloride (p.1099·2).
Coughs.

Tussa-Tablinen *Sanorania, Ger.†*
Pentoxyverine citrate (p.1096·3).
Coughs.

Tusscodin *Lannacher, Aust.*
Nicocodine hydrochloride (p.1095·3).
Coughs.

Tuss-DM *Hyrex, USA.*
Dextromethorphan hydrobromide (p.1087·3); guaifenesin (p.1092·2).
Coughs.

Tussed *Hexal, Ger.†*
Clobutinol hydrochloride (p.1087·1).
Coughs.

Tusselix *Propan, S.Afr.†*
Terpin hydrate (p.1101·2); tolu syrup (p.1101·3); squill (p.1100·3).
Coughs.

Tussend *Monarch, USA.*
Hydrocodone tartrate (p.42·2); pseudoephedrine hydrochloride (p.1099·2); chlorpheniramine [chlorphenamine] maleate (p.412·1).
Coughs.

Tussgen *Goldline, USA†.*
Hydrocodone tartrate (p.42·2); pseudoephedrine hydrochloride (p.1099·2).
Coughs and cold symptoms.

Tuss-Genade Modified *Goldline, USA†.*
Phenylpropanolamine hydrochloride (p.1098·1); caramiphen edisilate (p.1086·2).
Coughs.

Tussi-12 *Wallace, USA.*
Pentoxyverine tannate (p.1096·3); chlorpheniramine [chlorphenamine] tannate (p.412·2); phenylephrine tannate (p.1097·3).
Coughs.

Tussibron *Sella, Ital.*
Oxolamine citrate (p.1096·2).
Coughs.

Tussicare *ST, Thai.*
Guaifenesin (p.1092·2); dextromethorphan hydrobromide (p.1087·3).
Coughs.

Tussicon *The Forty-Two, Thai.*
Syrup: Dextromethorphan hydrobromide (p.1087·3); guaifenesin (p.1092·2); sodium citrate (p.1186·2).
Tablets: Dextromethorphan hydrobromide (p.1087·3); phenylpropanolamine hydrochloride (p.1098·1); chlorpheniramine [chlorphenamine] maleate (p.412·1).
Bronchitis; coughs; respiratory-tract disorders.

Tussidermil N *Li-il, Ger.*
Eucalyptus oil (p.1609·2).
Catarrh; musculoskeletal and joint disorders.

Tussidex *Xepa-Soul Pattinson, Singapore.*
Dextromethorphan hydrobromide (p.1087·3).
Coughs.

Tussidoron *Weleda, Fr.*
Thyme (p.1672·2); drosera (p.1606·1).
Coughs.

Tussidrill *Pierre Fabre, Spain.*
Dextromethorphan hydrobromide (p.1087·3).
Coughs.

Tussidyl *Tika, Swed.*
Dextromethorphan hydrobromide (p.1087·3).
Coughs.

Tussifed *Warner-Lambert, Fr.†.*
Triprolidine hydrochloride (p.427·2); dextromethorphan hydrobromide (p.1087·3).
Formerly contained triprolidine hydrochloride, pseudoephedrine hydrochloride, and dextromethorphan hydrobromide.
Coughs.

Tussifen *QIF, Braz.*
Belladonna (p.463·1); jaborandi; eucalyptus (p.1609·2); ginger (p.1227·2); siparuna guyanensis; lantana camara.
Respiratory-tract congestion.

Tussiflex *Kemyos, Ital.†.*
Oxeladin citrate (p.1096·1); terpin hydrate (p.1101·2).
Coughs.

Tussiflex D *Abbott, Braz.*
Dropropizine (p.1089·3).
Coughs.

Tussiflorin forte *Pascoe, Ger.*
Hedera helix; cowslip root (p.1600·1); thyme (p.1672·2).
Asthma; bronchitis.

Tussiflorin Hustensaft *Pascoe, Ger.*
Vogelknöterichkraut; sanikelkraut; hohlzahnkraut; cowslip root (p.1600·1).
Asthma; bronchitis; coughs.

Tussiflorin Hustenstiller *Pascoe, Ger.*
Thyme (p.1672·2); drosera (p.1606·1).
Cold symptoms; coughs.

Tussiflorin Hustentropfen *Pascoe, Ger.*
Vogelknöterichkraut; sanikelkraut; hohlzahnkraut; cowslip root (p.1600·1).
Asthma; bronchitis; coughs.

Tussiflorin N *Pascoe, Ger.*
Knotgrass; sanicula europaea; galeopsis ochroleuca; equisetum (p.1606·3); cowslip rhizome (p.1600·1).
Coughs and associated respiratory-tract disorders.

Tussigon *Daniels, USA.*
Hydrocodone tartrate (p.42·2); homatropine methylbromide (p.468·1).
Coughs and cold symptoms.

Tussilene *Alpharma, Fr.*
Carbocisteine (p.1086·3).
Respiratory-tract disorders.

Tussilinct *Restan, S.Afr.*
Diphenhydramine hydrochloride (p.416·1); codeine phosphate (p.25·2); ammonium chloride (p.1085·2); sodium citrate (p.1186·2).
Coughs.

Tussils
Note. This name is used for preparations of different composition.
Boots, Hong Kong.
Dextromethorphan hydrobromide (p.1087·3); phenylephrine hydrochloride (p.1097·1).
Coughs.

Boots, Singapore; Boots, Thai.
Dextromethorphan hydrobromide (p.1087·3).
Coughs.

Tussimag Codein *Montavit, Aust.*
Codeine phosphate (p.25·2); aesculus (p.1574·1); ephedrine hydrochloride (p.1090·1).
Formerly known as Tussamag mit Codein und Ephedrin. Formerly known as Tussamag mit Codein.
Bronchitis; catarrh; coughs.

Tussimed *Propan, S.Afr.†.*
Diphenhydramine hydrochloride (p.416·1); codeine phosphate (p.25·2); ammonium chloride (p.1085·2); sodium citrate (p.1186·2); menthol (p.1632·3).
Coughs.

Tussimed Expectorant *Propan, S.Afr.†.*
Diphenhydramine hydrochloride (p.416·1); ammonium chloride (p.1085·2); sodium citrate (p.1186·2); menthol (p.1632·3).
Coughs.

Tussimont *Pharmonta, Aust.*
Ointment: Camphor (p.1589·3); menthol (p.1632·3); eucalyptus oil (p.1609·2).
Coughs and cold symptoms.

Oral drops: Ammonium chloride (p.1085·2); thyme (p.1672·2); plantago lanceolata.
Coughs.

Oral liquid: Senega (p.1100·2); thyme (p.1672·2).
Coughs.

Tussin Antitussive *Stanley, Canad.*
Dextromethorphan hydrobromide (p.1087·3).

Tussin Antitussive, Expectorant, Decongestant *Stanley, Canad.*
Pseudoephedrine hydrochloride (p.1099·2); dextromethorphan hydrobromide (p.1087·3); guaifenesin (p.1092·2).

Tussin Children's DM *Stanley, Canad.*
Pseudoephedrine hydrochloride (p.1099·2); dextromethorphan hydrobromide (p.1087·3).

Tussin Expectorant *Stanley, Canad.*
Guaifenesin (p.1092·2).

TUSSinfant N *Rubiepharm, Ger.*
Cowslip root (p.1600·1); thyme (p.1672·2).
Cold symptoms.

Tussinol *G.P. Laboratories, Austral.*
Pholcodine (p.1099·1).
Coughs.

Tussinol Cough & Cold *Pfizer Consumer, Austral.*
Chlorpheniramine [chlorphenamine] maleate (p.412·1); dextromethorphan hydrobromide (p.1087·3); pseudoephedrine hydrochloride (p.1099·2).
Coughs and cold symptoms.

Tussinol Day-Time Cough & Cold *Pfizer Consumer, Austral.*
Dextromethorphan hydrobromide (p.1087·3); pseudoephedrine hydrochloride (p.1099·2).
Coughs and cold symptoms.

Tussinol for Dry Coughs *Pfizer Consumer, Austral.*
Dextromethorphan hydrobromide (p.1087·3).
Coughs.

Tussinol Expectorant *Pfizer Consumer, Austral.*
Bromhexine hydrochloride (p.1085·3); guaifenesin (p.1092·2).
Coughs.

Tussin-Pinho *Gilton, Braz.*
Potassium iodide (p.1522·3); guaifenesin (p.1092·2).
Respiratory-tract congestion.

Tussionex *Rhone-Poulenc Rorer, Canad.*
Hydrocodone resin complex; phenyltoloxamine resin complex (p.423·1).
Coughs.

Tussionex Pennkinetic *Medeva, USA.*
Hydrocodone polistirex (p.42·3); chlorpheniramine [chlorphenamine] polistirex (p.412·2).
Coughs and cold symptoms.

Tussi-Organidin DM NR *Wallace, USA.*
Guaifenesin (p.1092·2); dextromethorphan hydrobromide (p.1087·3).
Tussi-Organidin DM formerly contained iodinated glycerol and dextromethorphan hydrobromide.
Coughs.

Tussi-Organidin NR *Wallace, USA.*
Codeine phosphate (p.25·2); guaifenesin (p.1092·2).
Tussi-Organidin formerly contained codeine phosphate and iodinated glycerol.
Coughs.

Tussipax *Therica, Fr.*
Oral solution: Ethylmorphine hydrochloride (p.35·2); codeine (p.25·2).
Formerly contained ethylmorphine hydrochloride, codeine, bromoform, and maidenhair fern.
Syrup: Ethylmorphine hydrochloride (p.35·2); codeine (p.25·2); tolu balsam (p.1101·3); pectoral concentrate.
Formerly contained ethylmorphine hydrochloride, codeine, bromoform, tolu balsam, and pectoral concentrate.
Tablets: Ethylmorphine hydrochloride (p.35·2); codeine (p.25·2).
Formerly contained ethylmorphine hydrochloride, codeine, bromoform, drosera, and maidenhair fern.
Coughs.

Tussipax a l'Euquinine *Therica, Fr.†.*
Ethylmorphine hydrochloride (p.35·2); codeine (p.25·2); pine oil; eucalyptus oil (p.1609·2); quinine ethyl carbonate (p.445·1).
Coughs.

Tussipect
Note. This name is used for preparations of different composition.
Qualiphar, Belg.
Dextromethorphan hydrobromide (p.1087·3).
Coughs.

Beiersdorf-Lilly, Ger.†.
Thyme (p.1672·2); liquorice (p.1231·2); saponin; cetylpyridinium chloride (p.1138·1); peppermint oil (p.1243·3); menthol (p.1632·3); anethole (p.1580·1); eucalyptus oil (p.1609·2); camphor (p.1589·3).
Coughs and associated respiratory-tract disorders.

Tussiphane *Medeva, Belg.*
Dextromethorphan hydrobromide (p.1087·3).
Coughs.

Tussiplex *Vifor, Switz.*
Chlorpheniramine [chlorphenamine] maleate (p.412·1); phenylephrine hydrochloride (p.1097·1); pholcodine (p.1099·1); guaifenesin (p.1092·2).
Coughs.

Tussirex *Scot-Tussin, USA.*
Codeine phosphate (p.25·2); pheniramine maleate (p.422·3); phenylephrine hydrochloride (p.1097·1); sodium citrate (p.1186·2); sodium salicylate (p.84·2); caffeine citrate (p.761·3); menthol (p.1632·3).
Coughs.

Tussis
Note. This name is used for preparations of different composition.
OM, Port.†.
Bibenzonium bromide (p.1085·3).
Coughs.

Berlin Pharm, Thai.
Diphenhydramine hydrochloride (p.416·1); ammonium chloride (p.1085·2); sodium citrate (p.1186·2); glycerol (p.1616·3); menthol (p.1632·3).
Coughs; nasal congestion.

Tussisana N *Muller Goppingen, Ger.*
Homoeopathic preparation.

Tussisedal *Elerte, Fr.*
Noscapine (p.1096·1); promethazine (p.423·2); polysorbate 85 (Tween 85).
Coughs.

Tussistin *DHU, Ger.*
Homoeopathic preparation.

Tussistin N *DHU, Ger.*
Homoeopathic preparation.

Tussitot *Restan, S.Afr.*
Diphenhydramine hydrochloride (p.416·1); codeine phosphate (p.25·2); ammonium chloride (p.1085·2); sodium citrate (p.1186·2).
Coughs.

Tussiverlan *Verla, Ger.*
Acetylcysteine (p.1082·3).
Respiratory-tract disorders with viscous mucus.

Tuss-LA *Hyrex, USA.*
Pseudoephedrine hydrochloride (p.1099·2); guaifenesin (p.1092·2).
Coughs.

Tusso *BASF, Ger.*
Ambroxol hydrochloride (p.1084·3).
Respiratory-tract disorders with increased or viscous mucus.

Tussocal *Agis, Israel.*
Dextromethorphan hydrobromide (p.1087·3); phenylephrine hydrochloride (p.1097·1).
Coughs; nasal congestion.

Tussodan DM *Odan, Canad.*
Dextromethorphan hydrobromide (p.1087·3); pseudoephedrine hydrochloride (p.1099·2).
Coughs.

Tussodina *Dovalle, Braz.*
Sodium dibunate (p.1100·3); sodium benzoate (p.1134·3); sulfogaiacol (p.1101·1).
Coughs.

Tusso-DM *Everett, USA†.*
Dextromethorphan hydrobromide (p.1087·3); iodinated glycerol (p.1092·3).
Coughs.

Tussogest Extended-Release *Major, USA†.*
Phenylpropanolamine hydrochloride (p.1098·1); caramiphen edisilate (p.1086·2).
Coughs.

Tussol
Note. This name is used for preparations of different composition.
Amnol, Ital.
Myrtillus (p.1639·2); thyme (p.1672·2); tilia (p.1673·2); liquorice (p.1231·2).
Respiratory-tract disorders.

Nycomed, Norw.†.
Guaifenesin (p.1092·2); ammonium chloride (p.1085·2); liquorice (p.1231·2); ammonium glycyrrhizinate (p.1085·2).
Coughs.

Tussolvina *Pfizer, Ital.*
Nepinalone hydrochloride (p.1095·3).
Coughs.

Tussophedrine *Trima, Israel.*
Ephedrine hydrochloride (p.1090·1); codeine phosphate (p.25·2); sulfogaiacol (p.1101·1); sodium benzoate (p.1134·3).
Coughs.

Tussoret *Klinge, Ger.*
Codeine phosphate (p.25·2).
Formerly known as Tussoretard SN.
Coughs.

Tussoretardin *Klinge, Aust.*
White day capsules, pentoxyverine citrate (p.1096·3); methylephedrine hydrochloride (p.1094·3); blue night capsules, pentoxyverine citrate; diphenhydramine hydrochloride (p.416·1).
Coughs.

Tuss-Ornade *SmithKline Beecham, USA†.*
Caramiphen edisilate (p.1086·2); phenylpropanolamine hydrochloride (p.1098·1).
Coughs and cold symptoms.

Tussosedan *Teva, Israel.*
Pheniramine maleate (p.422·3); ephedrine hydrochloride (p.1090·1); codeine phosphate (p.25·2); ammonium chloride (p.1085·2).
Coughs.

Tuss-Tan *Econolab, USA.*
Pentoxyverine tannate (p.1096·3); chlorpheniramine [chlorphenamine] tannate (p.412·2); ephedrine tannate (p.1090·3).
Upper respiratory-tract symptoms.

Tusstat *Century, USA.*
Diphenhydramine hydrochloride (p.416·1).
Coughs.

Tussycalm *Rhone-Poulenc Rorer, Ital.*
Dextromethorphan hydrobromide (p.1087·3).
Coughs.

Tutiverm *Elofar, Braz.*
Tiabendazole (p.109·1).
Nematode infections.

Tutofusin *Fresenius Kabi, Aust.*
Electrolyte infusion with glucose (p.1180·1).
Carbohydrate source; fluid and electrolyte disorders.

Pharmacia Upjohn, Ger.
Electrolyte infusion (p.1180·1).
Fluid and electrolyte disorders; peritoneal irrigation.

Tutofusin B *Pharmacia Upjohn, Ger.*
Electrolyte solution with glucose (p.1180·1).
Carbohydrate source; fluid and electrolyte disorders.

Tutofusin BX *Pharmacia Upjohn, Ger.*
Electrolyte infusion with xylitol (p.1180·1).
Carbohydrate source; fluid and electrolyte disorders.

Tutofusin G5 *Pharmacia Upjohn, Ger.*
Electrolyte infusion with glucose (p.1180·1).
Carbohydrate source; fluid and electrolyte disorders.

Tutofusin H G5 *Pharmacia Upjohn, Ger.*
Electrolyte infusion with glucose (p.1180·1).
Carbohydrate source; fluid and electrolyte disorders.

Tutofusin K 10 *Pharmacia Upjohn, Ger.*
Electrolyte infusion (p.1180·1).
Fluid and electrolyte disorders.

Tutofusin K 80 *Pharmacia Upjohn, Ger.*
Electrolyte infusion with xylitol and glucose (p.1180·1).
Potassium deficiency in cardiac disorders.

Tutofusin NS X *Pharmacia Upjohn, Ger.*
Electrolyte infusion with xylitol (p.1180·1).
Fluid and electrolyte disorders.

Tutofusin OP *Pharmacia Upjohn, Ger.*
Electrolyte infusion (p.1180·1).
Fluid and electrolyte disorders.

Tutofusin OP X *Pharmacia Upjohn, Ger.*
Electrolyte infusion with xylitol (p.1180·1).
Carbohydrate source; fluid and electrolyte disorders.

Tutofusin OP G *Pharmacia Upjohn, Ger.*
Electrolyte infusion with glucose (p.1180·1).
Carbohydrate source; fluid and electrolyte disorders.

Tutofusin S *Pharmacia Upjohn, Ger.*
Sodium chloride (p.1196·1); sodium acetate (p.1186·1); sorbitol (p.1377·3).
Fluid retention; renal failure.

Tutoplast Dura *Tutogen, Ger.*
Absorbable collagen from dehydrated human dura mater (p.1598·2).
Repair or closure of body tissue.

Tutoplast Fascia lata *Tutogen, Ger.*
Dehydrated human fascia lata (p.1598·2).
Repair of joints and tendons.

Tutoseral *Streuli, Switz.*
Electrolyte infusion (p.1180·1).
Fluid and electrolyte disorders.

Tuttozem N *Strathmann, Ger.†.*
Dexamethasone (p.1067·1).
Burns; skin disorders.

Tux *Warner-Lambert Consumer, Belg.*
Ethylmorphine hydrochloride (p.35·2); codeine phosphate (p.25·2); ephedrine hydrochloride (p.1090·1); guaifenesin (p.1092·2); sodium benzoate (p.1134·3); sodium camsilate; senega (p.1100·2); senna (p.1248·2); tolu balsam (p.1101·3).
Colds; coughs; respiratory disorders.

Tuxi *Leiras, Fin.; Weifa, Norw.*
Pholcodine (p.1099·1).
Coughs.

Tuxidrin *Weifa, Norw.*
Pholcodine (p.1099·1); ephedrine (p.1090·1).
Coughs.

Tuxium *Galephar, Fr.*
Dextromethorphan hydrobromide (p.1087·3).
Coughs.

Tuzanil *Bohm, Spain.*
Pygeum africanum (p.1490·3).
Benign prostatic hyperplasia.

Tuzo *Brasifa, Braz.*
Sodium benzoate (p.1134·3); ammonium chloride (p.1085·2); potassium iodide (p.1522·3); ephedrine hydrochloride (p.1090·1).
Respiratory-tract congestion.

TVC-2 Dandruff Shampoo *Dermol, USA†.*
Pyrithione zinc (p.1122·1).

T-Vites *Freeda, USA.*
Multivitamin preparation with minerals (p.1350·1).

Twice-A-Day *Major, USA.*
Oxymetazoline hydrochloride (p.1096·2).
Nasal congestion.

Twilite *Pfeiffer, USA.*
Diphenhydramine hydrochloride (p.416·1).
Insomnia.

Twin-K *Boots, USA.*
Potassium gluconate (p.1194·3); potassium citrate (p.1186·1).
Hypokalaemia; potassium depletion.

Twinrix
SmithKline Beecham, Aust.; SmithKline Beecham, Austral.; SmithKline Beecham, Belg.; SmithKline Beecham, Canad.; SmithKline Beecham, Denm.; SmithKline Beecham, Fin.; SmithKline Beecham, Fr.; SmithKline Beecham, Ger.; SmithKline Beecham, Irl.; SmithKline Beecham, Israel; SmithKline Beecham, Ital.; SmithKline Beecham, Mex.; SmithKline Beecham, Neth.; SmithKline Beecham, Norw.; SmithKline Beecham, NZ; Smith Kline & French, Port.; SmithKline Beecham, Singapore; SmithKline Beecham, Spain; SmithKline Beecham, Swed.;

The symbol † denotes a preparation no longer actively marketed

SmithKline Beecham, Switz.; SmithKline Beecham, UK; SmithKline Beecham, USA.
An inactivated hepatitis A and recombinant hepatitis B vaccine (p.1544·2).
Separate preparations are available for infants and children and for adults.
Active immunisation.

Two Cal HN Abbott, Austral.; Abbott, NZ.
Preparation for enteral nutrition (p.1350·1).

Twocal Abbott, Ital.
Preparation for enteral nutrition (p.1350·1).

Twocal HN Ross, USA.
High calorie, high nitrogen lactose-free preparation for enteral nutrition (p.1350·1).

Two-Dyne Hyrex, USA†.
Paracetamol (p.71·2); caffeine (p.761·3); butalbital (p.658·3).
Pain.

Tybikin M & H, Thai.
Amikacin sulfate (p.148·1).
Gram-negative bacterial infections.

Ty-Cold Major, USA†.
Chlorpheniramine [chlorphenamine] maleate (p.412·1); dextromethorphan hydrobromide (p.1087·3); paracetamol (p.71·2); pseudoephedrine hydrochloride (p.1099·2).
Coughs and cold symptoms.

Tydamine Aspen, S.Afr.
Trimipramine (p.311·2).
Anxiety disorders; depression; nocturnal enuresis.

Tylenol
Johnson & Johnson, Aust.; Johnson & Johnson, Austral.; Cilag, Braz.; McNeil Consumer, Canad.; Johnson & Johnson, Hong Kong; Johnson & Johnson, Irl.; Janssen, Mex.; Johnson & Johnson, Port.; Janssen-Cilag, S.Afr.; Abello, Spain; Janssen-Cilag, Switz.; Janssen, Thai.; McNeil Consumer, USA.
Paracetamol (p.71·2).
Fever; pain.

Tylenol Aches & Strains McNeil Consumer, Canad.
Chlorzoxazone (p.1327·3); paracetamol (p.71·2).
Muscular aches and strains.

Tylenol Allergy Sinus
Johnson & Johnson, Austral.; McNeil Consumer, Canad.
Paracetamol (p.71·2); chlorpheniramine [chlorphenamine] maleate (p.412·1); pseudoephedrine hydrochloride (p.1099·2).
Allergy symptoms; sinus pain and congestion.

Tylenol with Codeine
McNeil Consumer, Canad.; Janssen, Thai.; Ortho McNeil, USA.
Paracetamol (p.71·2); codeine phosphate (p.25·2).
Fever; pain.

Tylenol with Codeine No 1, No 2, or No 3
McNeil, Canad.
Paracetamol (p.71·2); caffeine (p.761·3); codeine phosphate (p.25·2).
Fever; pain.

Tylenol with Codeine No 4 McNeil, Canad.
Paracetamol (p.71·2); codeine phosphate (p.25·2).
Fever; pain.

Tylenol Cold & Flu
Note. This name is used for preparations of different composition.
Johnson & Johnson, Austral.
Paracetamol (p.71·2); chlorpheniramine [chlorphenamine] maleate (p.412·1); pseudoephedrine hydrochloride (p.1099·2); dextromethorphan hydrobromide (p.1087·3).
Cold and influenza symptoms.

Janssen-Cilag, S.Afr.
Paracetamol (p.71·2); chlorpheniramine [chlorphenamine] maleate (p.412·1); pseudoephedrine hydrochloride (p.1099·2).
Allergic rhinitis; cold symptoms.

Tylenol Cold & Flu Non-Drowsy Johnson & Johnson, Austral.
Paracetamol (p.71·2); pseudoephedrine hydrochloride (p.1099·2); dextromethorphan hydrobromide (p.1087·3).
Cold and influenza symptoms.

Tylenol Cold and Flu Powder McNeil Consumer, Canad.
Paracetamol (p.71·2); chlorpheniramine [chlorphenamine] maleate (p.412·1); pseudoephedrine hydrochloride (p.1099·2); dextromethorphan hydrobromide (p.1087·3).
Cold symptoms.

Tylenol Cold Medication McNeil Consumer, Canad.
Paracetamol (p.71·2); chlorpheniramine [chlorphenamine] maleate (p.412·1); pseudoephedrine hydrochloride (p.1099·2).
Cold symptoms.

Tylenol Cold Medication (Daytime) McNeil Consumer, Canad.
Paracetamol (p.71·2); pseudoephedrine hydrochloride (p.1099·2); dextromethorphan hydrobromide (p.1087·3).
Cold symptoms.

Tylenol Cold Medication DM McNeil Consumer, Canad.
Paracetamol (p.71·2); chlorpheniramine [chlorphenamine] maleate (p.412·1); pseudoephedrine hydrochloride (p.1099·2); dextromethorphan hydrobromide (p.1087·3).
Cold symptoms.

Tylenol Cold Medication (Nighttime) McNeil Consumer, Canad.
Paracetamol (p.71·2); chlorpheniramine [chlorphenamine] maleate (p.412·1); pseudoephedrine hydrochlo-

ride (p.1099·2); dextromethorphan hydrobromide (p.1087·3).
Cold symptoms.

Tylenol Cold No Drowsiness McNeil Consumer, USA.
Paracetamol (p.71·2); pseudoephedrine hydrochloride (p.1099·2); dextromethorphan hydrobromide (p.1087·3).
Coughs and cold symptoms.

Tylenol Cold Severe Congestion McNeil Consumer, USA.
Paracetamol (p.71·2); pseudoephedrine hydrochloride (p.1099·2); dextromethorphan hydrobromide (p.1087·3); guaifenesin (p.1092·2).
Coughs and cold symptoms.

Tylenol Cough McNeil Consumer, Canad.
Paracetamol (p.71·2); dextromethorphan hydrobromide (p.1087·3).
Coughs; fever; pain; sore throat.

Tylenol Cough with Decongestant McNeil Consumer, Canad.†
Paracetamol (p.71·2); dextromethorphan hydrobromide (p.1087·3); pseudoephedrine hydrochloride (p.1099·2).
Coughs; fever; nasal congestion; pain; sore throat.

Tylenol Decongestant McNeil Consumer, Canad.
Paracetamol (p.71·2); pseudoephedrine hydrochloride (p.1099·2).
Cold and influenza symptoms.

Tylenol Flu McNeil Consumer, Canad.
Paracetamol (p.71·2); pseudoephedrine hydrochloride (p.1099·2); diphenhydramine hydrochloride (p.416·1).
Influenza symptoms.

Tylenol Flu Night Time McNeil Consumer, USA.
Paracetamol (p.71·2); diphenhydramine hydrochloride (p.416·1); pseudoephedrine hydrochloride (p.1099·2).
Influenza symptoms.

Tylenol Flu No Drowsiness McNeil Consumer, USA.
Paracetamol (p.71·2); dextromethorphan hydrobromide (p.1087·3); pseudoephedrine hydrochloride (p.1099·2).
Influenza symptoms.

Tylenol Menstrual McNeil Consumer, Canad.
Paracetamol (p.71·2); pamabrom (p.952·1); mepyramine maleate (p.421·1).
Premenstrual syndrome.

Tylenol Night Pain Janssen-Cilag, S.Afr.
Paracetamol (p.71·2); diphenhydramine hydrochloride (p.416·1).
Insomnia with pain.

Tylenol Severe Allergy McNeil Consumer, USA.
Paracetamol (p.71·2); diphenhydramine hydrochloride (p.416·1).
Hypersensitivity symptoms.

Tylenol Sinus Johnson & Johnson, Austral.
Paracetamol (p.71·2); pseudoephedrine hydrochloride (p.1099·2).
Sinus and nasal congestion; sinus pain.

Tylenol Sinus Medication McNeil Consumer, Canad.
Paracetamol (p.71·2); pseudoephedrine hydrochloride (p.1099·2).
Cold symptoms; sinus.

Tylephen IQB, Braz.
Paracetamol (p.71·2).
Fever; pain.

Tylex
Note. This name is used for preparations of different composition.
Cilag, Braz.; Schwarz, Irl.; Schwarz, UK.
Paracetamol (p.71·2); codeine phosphate (p.25·2).
These ingredients can be described by the British Approved Name Co-codamol 30/500.
Pain.

Cilag, Mex.
Paracetamol (p.71·2).
Fever; pain.

Tylex CD Cilag, Mex.
Paracetamol (p.71·2); codeine phosphate (p.25·2).
Pain.

Tylex Flu Cilag, Mex.
Paracetamol (p.71·2); pseudoephedrine hydrochloride (p.1099·2); chlorpheniramine [chlorphenamine] maleate (p.412·1); dextromethorphan hydrobromide (p.1087·3).
Cold and influenza symptoms; coughs.

Tylox Ortho McNeil, USA.
Oxycodone hydrochloride (p.70·2); paracetamol (p.71·2).
Pain.

Tymelyt
Lundbeck, Aust.; Lundbeck, Belg.†; Lundbeck, Denm.; Lundbeck, Swed.
Lofepramine hydrochloride (p.297·1).
Depression.

Tymol Pharmaland, Thai.
Paracetamol (p.71·2).
Fever; pain.

Tympagesic Savage, USA.
Phenylephrine hydrochloride (p.1097·1); phenazone (p.77·2); benzocaine (p.1306·2).
Earache.

Tympalgine Therabel, Belg.
Phenazone (p.77·2); procaine hydrochloride (p.1319·1).
Otitis.

Typherix
SmithKline Beecham, Aust.; SmithKline Beecham, Austral.; SmithKline Beecham, Belg.; SmithKline Beecham, Fin.; SmithKline Beecham, Fr.; SmithKline Beecham, Ger.; SmithKline Beecham, Irl.; SmithKline

Beecham, Ital.; SmithKline Beecham, NZ; SmithKline Beecham, Swed.; SmithKline Beecham, UK.
A typhoid vaccine (Vi capsular polysaccharide) (p.1566·3).
Active immunisation.

Typhim Vi
Pasteur Merieux, Aust.; CSL, Austral.; Pasteur Merieux, Belg.; Connaught, Canad.; Pasteur Merieux, Denm.; Meda, Fin.; Pasteur Vaccins, Fr.; Pasteur Merieux, Ger.; Pasteur Merieux, Hong Kong; Aventis, Irl.; Pasteur Merieux, Israel; Pasteur Merieux, Ital.; Pasteur Merieux, Neth.; Pasteur Merieux, Norw.; CSL, NZ; Aventis, S.Afr.; Pasteur Merieux, Singapore; Pasteur Merieux, Spain; Pasteur Merieux, Swed.; Pasteur Merieux, Thai.; Pasteur Merieux, UK; Pasteur Merieux, USA.
A typhoid vaccine (Vi capsular polysaccharide) (p.1566·3).
Active immunisation.

Typhoral L Chiron Behring, Ger.
A live oral typhoid vaccine (p.1566·3).
Active immunisation.

Typh-Vax
CSL, Austral.; CSL, NZ.
An oral typhoid vaccine (attenuated Ty21a Berna strain) (p.1566·3).
Active immunisation.

Tyrazol Yamanouchi, Fin.
Carbimazole (p.1521·1).
Hyperthyroidism.

Tyrcine Oberlin, Fr.
Tyrothricin (p.267·1); amethocaine [tetracaine] hydrochloride (p.1305·2).
Mouth and throat disorders.

Tyrex Ross, USA.
Phenylalanine- and tyrosine-free preparation for enteral nutrition (p.1350·1).
Tyrosinaemia type II.

Tyrocaine Synco, Hong Kong.
Tyrothricin (p.267·1); benzocaine (p.1306·2).
Mouth and throat infections.

Tyrocombine Synpharma, Switz.
Ointment: Tyrothricin (p.267·1); neomycin sulfate (p.228·1); benzethonium chloride (p.1134·2).
Infected skin disorders; infected wounds.
Topical powder: Tyrothricin (p.267·1); neomycin sulfate (p.228·1); benzethonium chloride (p.1134·2).
Formerly contained tyrothricin, neomycin sulfate, benzethonium chloride, and sulfathiazole.
Infected skin disorders.

Tyrodone Ross, USA.
Hydrocodone tartrate (p.42·2); pseudoephedrine hydrochloride (p.1099·2).

Tyro-Drops Centrapharm, Belg.
Tyrothricin (p.267·1); lignocaine [lidocaine] hydrochloride (p.1313·2).
Mouth and throat disorders.

Tyrogel Mer-National, S.Afr.†
Tyrothricin (p.267·1); hydroxypolyethoxy dodecan (p.1345·2).
Burns; wounds.

Tyromex Ross, USA.
Methionine-, phenylalanine-, and tyrosine-free infant feed (p.1350·1).
Tyrosinaemia type I.

Tyroneomicin Alcala, Spain†.
Bacitracin zinc (p.155·2); benzocaine (p.1306·2); hydrocortisone acetate (p.1073·2); neomycin sulfate (p.228·1); potassium chlorate (p.1654·1).
Mouth and throat disorders.

Tyroplus Enila, Braz.
Liothyronine sodium (p.1524·2); thyroxine [levothyroxine] (p.1528·1).
Thyroid disorders.

Tyroqualine Spirig, Switz.
Tyrothricin (p.267·1); dequalinium chloride (p.1143·1); lignocaine [lidocaine] hydrochloride (p.1313·2).
Mouth and throat disorders.

Tyroseng Eagle, Austral.
Tyrosine (p.1381·3); eleutherococcus senticosis (p.1615·3); calcium glycerophosphate (p.1188·2); phosphatidyl choline (p.1651·1); vitamin B substances (p.1350·1).
Dietary supplement.

Tyrosin S Bencard, Ger.
Mixed allergen extracts (p.1575·3).
Hyposensitisation.

Tyrosolvetten Roland, Ger.; Byk Gulden, Ger.
Cetylpyridinium chloride (p.1138·1); benzocaine (p.1306·2).
Mouth and throat disorders.

Tyrosolvetten-C Roland, Ger.; Byk Gulden, Ger.
Cetylpyridinium chloride (p.1138·1); ascorbic acid (p.1389·3).
Mouth and throat infections.

Tyrosolvin Lundbeck, Aust.†
Tyrothricin (p.267·1); cetylpyridinium chloride (p.1138·1).
Bacterial infections.

Tyrosum Summers, USA.
Skin cleanser.

Tyrosur
Note. This name is used for preparations of different composition.
Engelhard, Ger.
Topical gel: Tyrothricin (p.267·1); cetylpyridinium chloride (p.1138·1).
Topical powder: Tyrothricin (p.267·1).
Infected skin disorders; infected wounds and burns.

Engelhard, Hong Kong.
Tyrothricin (p.267·1).
Infected skin disorders; infected wounds.

Tyrothricin Streuli, Switz.
Tyrothricin (p.267·1); ethacridine lactate (p.1130·3); lignocaine [lidocaine] hydrochloride (p.1313·2); menthol (p.1632·3); mint oil (p.1636·2).
Mouth and throat disorders.

Tyrothricin Co Jean-Marie, Hong Kong.
Tyrothricin (p.267·1); codeine phosphate (p.25·2); benzocaine (p.1306·2).
Throat disorders.

Tyrothricin comp Provita, Aust.
Tyrothricin (p.267·1); neomycin sulfate (p.228·1); benzalkonium chloride (p.1133·2); benzocaine (p.1306·2).
Mouth and throat disorders.

Tyrothricine + Gramicidine Demochal, Switz.
Tyrothricin (p.267·1); gramicidin (p.213·3); amethocaine [tetracaine] hydrochloride (p.1305·2); benzethonium chloride (p.1134·2).
Mouth and throat disorders.

Tyrothricine Lafran Lafran, Fr.†
Tyrothricin (p.267·1); butyl aminobenzoate (p.1308·2).
Mouth and throat disorders.

Tyrozets
Merck Sharp & Dohme, Irl.; Merck Sharp & Dohme, Port.†; Johnson & Johnson MSD Consumer, UK.
Tyrothricin (p.267·1); benzocaine (p.1306·2).
Mouth and throat disorders.

Tyzine
Pfizer, Denm.; Pfizer, Ger.; Pfizer, Switz.†; Kenwood, USA.
Tetrazoline hydrochloride (p.1101·2).
Conjunctivitis; eye irritation; nasal congestion; rhinitis; sinusitis.

T-ZA Siam Bheasach, Thai.
Zidovudine (p.645·2).
HIV infection.

Tzoali Kendrick, Mex.
Diphenhydramine hydrochloride (p.416·1).
Insomnia.

U Lactin Cosmofarma, Port.†
Urea (p.1127·3); alpha hydroxy acids.
Dry skin disorders.

UAA Econo Med, USA.
Methenamine (p.223·1); salol (p.82·2); atropine sulfate (p.461·1); hyoscyamine sulfate (p.469·3); benzoic acid (p.1134·2); methylene blue [methylthioninium chloride] (p.1012·3).
Urinary-tract infections.

UAD-Otic UAD, USA.
Hydrocortisone (p.1073·3); neomycin sulfate (p.228·1); polymyxin B sulfate (p.238·1).
Bacterial ear infections.

Ubenzima Pentafarma, Port.
Ubidecarenone (p.1677·1).

Ubicarden Locatelli, Ital.†
Ubidecarenone (p.1677·1).
Cardiac disorders; coenzyme Q10 deficiency.

Ubicardio Tosi, Ital.
Ubidecarenone (p.1677·1).
Cardiac disorders; coenzyme Q10 deficiency.

Ubicondrial Medicamed, Port.
Ubidecarenone (p.1677·1).
Cardiac disorders.

Ubicor Magis, Ital.
Ubidecarenone (p.1677·1).
Cardiac disorders; coenzyme Q10 deficiency.

Ubidenone Esseti, Ital.
Ubidecarenone (p.1677·1).
Cardiac disorders; coenzyme Q10 deficiency.

Ubidex OFF, Ital.
Ubidecarenone (p.1677·1).
Cardiac disorders; coenzyme Q10 deficiency.

Ubifactor San Carlo, Ital.
Ubidecarenone (p.1677·1).
Cardiac disorders; coenzyme Q10 deficiency.

Ubilab Del Saz & Filippini, Ital.†
Ubidecarenone (p.1677·1).
Cardiac disorders.

Ubimaior Chiesi, Ital.
Ubidecarenone (p.1677·1).
Cardiac disorders; coenzyme Q10 deficiency.

Ubisint Francia, Ital.†
Ubidecarenone (p.1677·1).
Coenzyme Q10 deficiency: cardiac disorders.

Ubistesin
Espe, Aust.; Espe, Ger.; Espe, Ital.; Espe, Switz.
Articaine hydrochloride (p.1306·1).
Adrenaline [epinephrine] hydrochloride (p.829·2) is included in this preparation as a vasoconstrictor to diminish absorption and localise the effect of the local anaesthetic.
Local anaesthesia.

Ubiten Lifepharma, Ital.
Ubidecarenone (p.1677·1).
Cardiac disorders; coenzyme Q10 deficiency.

Ubivis AGIPS, Ital.
Ubidecarenone (p.1677·1).
Cardiac disorders; coenzyme Q10 deficiency.

Ubizol Alter, Port.
Fluticasone propionate (p.1072·2).
Skin disorders.

Ubretid
Nycomed, Aust.; Rhone-Poulenc Rorer, Austral.†; Nycomed, Fin.; Nycomed, Ger.; Nycomed, Hong Kong; Rhone-Poulenc Rorer, Irl.†; Chris-

Ulkusal TAD, Ger.†
Cimetidine (p.1216·3).
Acid aspiration; gastro-oesophageal reflux; peptic ulcer; Zollinger-Ellison syndrome.

Ullus Blasen-Nieren-Tee N Polypharm, Ger.
Birch leaf (p.1585·2); solidago virgaurea; ononis (p.1644·1).
Urinary-tract disorders.

Ullus Galle-Tee N Polypharm, Ger.
Taraxacum (p.1669·1); peppermint leaf (p.1243·2); cynara (p.1601·3).
Gastrointestinal spasm.

Ullus Kapseln N Polypharm, Ger.
Liquorice (p.1231·2); chamomile (p.1593·2).
Gastrointestinal disorders.

Ullus Magen-Tee N Polypharm, Ger.
Fennel (p.1610·1); peppermint leaf (p.1243·2).
Dyspepsia.

Ulmet Ace, S.Afr.†
Cimetidine (p.1216·3).
Gastrointestinal disorders.

Ulogen Fustery, Mex.
Cimetidine (p.1216·3).

Ulone 3M, Canad.
Clofedanol hydrochloride (p.1087·1).
Coughs.

Ulpax Hormona, Mex.
Lansoprazole (p.1230·3).
Gastro-oesophageal reflux; peptic ulcer; Zollinger-Ellison syndrome.

Ulprazole Polipharm, Thai.
Omeprazole (p.1239·1).
Gastro-oesophageal reflux; peptic ulcer; Zollinger-Ellison syndrome.

ULR-LA Geneva, USA†.
Phenylpropanolamine hydrochloride (p.1098·1); guaifenesin (p.1092·2).
Coughs and cold symptoms; nasal congestion.

Ulsal Gebro, Aust.
Ranitidine hydrochloride (p.1245·2).
Acid aspiration; gastro-oesophageal reflux; gastrointestinal haemorrhage; peptic ulcer; stress-related ulcer; Zollinger-Ellison syndrome.

Ulsanic
Chugai, Hong Kong; Tava, Israel; Aspen Consumer, S.Afr.; Chugai, Thai.
Sucralfate (p.1250·2).
Gastritis; gastro-oesophageal reflux; peptic ulcer.

Ulsaven Collins, Mex.
Ranitidine hydrochloride (p.1245·2).
Gastro-oesophageal reflux; hyperchlorhydria; peptic ulcer; Zollinger-Ellison syndrome.

Ulsen Senosiain, Mex.
Omeprazole (p.1239·1).
Gastro-oesophageal reflux; peptic ulcer; Zollinger-Ellison syndrome.

Ulserral Serral, Mex.
Cimetidine (p.1216·3).
Peptic ulcer.

Ultacit Hoechst Marion Roussel, Neth.
Hydrotalcite (p.1228·1).
Gastrointestinal disorders associated with hyperacidity.

Ultacite Roche Nicholas, Fr.†.
Hydrotalcite (p.1228·1).
Gastrointestinal disorders.

Ultane
Abbott, S.Afr.; Abbott, USA.
Sevoflurane (p.1267·3).
General anaesthesia.

Ultec
Teva, Hong Kong; Berk, UK.
Cimetidine (p.1216·3).
Dyspepsia; heartburn; peptic ulcer.

Ultexiv Alcon, Ger.
Triamcinolone acetonide (p.1080·1); neomycin sulfate (p.228·1); gramicidin (p.213·3).
Eye disorders.

Ultidin Pharmacaps, Mex.
Famotidine (p.1225·3).

Ultilac N Bittermedizin, Ger.
Almasilate (p.1210·1); calcium carbonate (p.1215·1); skimmed milk powder.
Gastrointestinal disorders.

Ultimag Mirren, S.Afr.
Magnesium chloride (p.1190·3); zinc oxide (p.1128·2).
Magnesium and zinc supplement.

Ultiva
Glaxo Wellcome, Aust.; Glaxo Wellcome, Austral.; Glaxo Wellcome, Belg.; Glaxo Wellcome, Canad.; Glaxo Wellcome, Denm.; Glaxo Wellcome, Fin.; Glaxo Wellcome, Fr.; Glaxo Wellcome, Ger.; Zeneca, Ger.; Glaxo Wellcome, Israel; Glaxo Wellcome, Ital.; Glaxo Wellcome, Mex.; Glaxo Wellcome, Neth.; Glaxo Wellcome, Norw.; Glaxo Wellcome, NZ; Glaxo Wellcome, Port.; Glaxo Wellcome, S.Afr.; Glaxo Wellcome, Singapore; Glaxo Wellcome, Spain; Glaxo Wellcome, Swed.; Glaxo Wellcome, Switz.; Elan, UK; Glaxo Wellcome, USA.
Remifentanil hydrochloride (p.80·3).
Analgesia in anaesthesia.

Ultra Medgenix, Belg.
Sulfacetamide sodium (p.250·3).
Infected skin lesions.

Ultra Adsorb Lainco, Spain.
Activated charcoal (p.1000·2).
Diarrhoea.

Ultra Augenschutz Provita, Aust.
Actinoquinol sodium (p.1573·1).
Protection of the eyes from ultraviolet radiation.

Ultra Derm Reese, USA.
Emollient and moisturiser.

Ultra Heartburn Relief Galpharm, UK.
Famotidine (p.1225·3).
Dyspepsia; heartburn.

Ultra Mide
Baker Cummins, Canad.; Baker Cummins, USA.
Urea (p.1127·3).
Dry skin; hyperkeratosis.

Ultra Strength Megadophilus Bullivants, Austral.
Lactobacillus acidophilus (p.1626·3); Bifidobacterium bifidum (p.1626·3).
Maintenance of normal gastrointestinal flora.

Ultra Tears
Alcon, Switz.†; Alcon, USA.
Hypromellose (p.1501·3).
Dry eyes.

Ultra Vita Time Nature's Bounty, USA.
Multivitamin and mineral preparation with iron and folic acid (p.1350·1).

Ultrabas Schering, Ger.†.
Emollient.
Diluent for Ultralan ointment.

Ultrabase
Schering, S.Afr.; Schering, UK.
Emollient.
Dry skin; pharmaceutical diluent.

Ultrabeta Vitoria, Port.
Salmeterol xinafoate (p.773·3).
Asthma.

Ultrabion Sabater, Spain.
Ampicillin sodium (p.150·3); ampicillin benzathine (p.151·3).
Bacterial infections.

Ultrabion Balsamico Sabater, Spain.
Ampicillin sodium (p.150·3); ampicillin benzathine (p.151·3); niaouli oil (p.1640·2); guaifenesin (p.1092·2).
Respiratory-tract infections.

ULTRAbrom WE, USA.
Pseudoephedrine hydrochloride (p.1099·2); brompheniramine maleate (p.410·2).
Upper respiratory-tract symptoms.

Ultracain
Hoechst Marion Roussel, Ger.; Normon, Spain.
Articaine hydrochloride (p.1306·1).
Adrenaline [epinephrine] (p.829·1) may be included in this preparation as a vasoconstrictor to diminish absorption and localise the effect of the local anaesthetic.
Local anaesthesia.

Ultracain Dental Hoechst Marion Roussel, Aust.
Articaine hydrochloride (p.1306·1).
Adrenaline [epinephrine] hydrochloride (p.829·2) is included in this preparation as a vasoconstrictor to diminish absorption and localise the effect of the local anaesthetic.
Local anaesthesia.

Ultracain D-S
Hoechst Marion Roussel, Ger.; Novaxa, Ital.; Hoechst Marion Roussel, Neth.
Articaine hydrochloride (p.1306·1).
Adrenaline [epinephrine] hydrochloride (p.829·2) is included in this preparation as a vasoconstrictor to diminish absorption and localise the effect of the local anaesthetic.
Local anaesthesia.

Ultracain D-Suprarenin Hoechst Marion Roussel, Fin.
Articaine hydrochloride (p.1306·1).
Adrenaline [epinephrine] hydrochloride (p.829·2) is included in this preparation as a vasoconstrictor to diminish absorption and localise the effect of the local anaesthetic.
Local anaesthesia.

Ultracain Hyperbaar Hoechst Marion Roussel, Neth.
Articaine hydrochloride (p.1306·1).
Local anaesthesia.

Ultracain hyperbar Hoechst Marion Roussel, Ger.
Articaine hydrochloride (p.1306·1).
Local anaesthesia.

Ultracaine D-S
Hoechst Marion Roussel, Canad.; Hoechst Marion Roussel, Switz.
Articaine hydrochloride (p.1306·1).
Adrenaline [epinephrine] (p.829·1) or adrenaline [epinephrine] hydrochloride (p.829·2) is included in this preparation as a vasoconstrictor to diminish absorption and localise the effect of the local anaesthetic.
Local anaesthesia.

Ultracaine-Suprarenin Hoechst Marion Roussel, Ger.
Articaine hydrochloride (p.1306·1).
Adrenaline [epinephrine] hydrochloride (p.829·2) is included in this preparation as a vasoconstrictor to diminish absorption and localise the effect of the local anaesthetic.
Local anaesthesia.

Ultracal
Mead Johnson, Austral.; Mead Johnson, Hong Kong; Mead Johnson, NZ; Mead Johnson Nutritionals, Thai.; Mead Johnson Nutritionals, USA.
Preparation for enteral nutrition (p.1350·1).

Ultracarbon
Merck, Ger.; Merck, Singapore; Merck, Thai.
Activated charcoal (p.1000·2).
Diarrhoea; flatulence; poisoning.

UltraCare
Note. A similar name is used for preparations of different composition (see below).
Allergan, Canad.; Allergan, USA.
Disinfecting solution, hydrogen peroxide 3% (p.1147·1); neutralising tablets, catalase (p.1592·2) (p.1129·2).
Contact lens care.

Ultracare Optident, UK.
Note. A similar name is used for preparations of different composition (see above).
Benzocaine (p.1306·2).
Local anaesthesia.

UltraCare Daily Cleaner Allergan, Canad.
Cleaning solution for soft contact lenses (p.1129·2).

Ultracef
Note. This name is used for preparations of different composition.
Bristol-Myers Squibb, Ter.
Cefadroxil (p.161·2).
Bacterial infections.

Promeco, Mex.
Ceftizoxime (p.176·3).
Bacterial infections.

Ultracet Johnson, USA.
Tramadol hydrochloride (p.89·1); paracetamol (p.71·2).
Pain.

Ultracillin Caps, S.Afr.
Benzathine benzylpenicillin (p.156·2); benzylpenicillin sodium (p.157·2); procaine penicillin [procaine benzylpenicillin] (p.239·2).
Bacterial infections.

Ultra-Clear-A-Med Procter & Gamble, Aust.
Benzoyl peroxide (p.1111·1).
Acne.

Ultracorten H Novartis, Israel.
Prednisolone sodium tetrahydrophthalate (p.1078·3).
Hypersensitivity reactions; shock.

Ultracortene-H Novartis, Switz.
Prednisolone sodium tetrahydrophthalate (p.1078·3).
Corticosteroid.

Ultracortenol
Ciba Vision, Aust.; Ciba Vision, Denm.; Ciba Vision, Fin.; Ciba Vision, Ger.; Ciba Vision, Hong Kong; Ciba Vision, Israel; Ciba Vision, Neth.; Ciba Vision, Norw.; Ciba Vision, Swed.; Ciba Vision, Switz.
Prednisolone acetate (p.1078·1) or prednisolone pivalate (p.1078·1).
Inflammatory eye disorders.

Ultra-Demoplas Godecke, Ger.
Dexamethasone (p.1067·1); prednisolone (p.1077·3); lignocaine [lidocaine] hydrochloride (p.1313·2).
Musculoskeletal and joint disorders.

Ultraderm Ecobi, Ital.
Fluocinolone acetonide (p.1071·1).
Skin disorders.

Ultraderme Richelet, Fr.
Saccharomyces boulardii (p.1626·3).
Seborrhoea.

Ultradina Brasmedica, Braz.
Silver (p.1664·1).
Diarrhoea.

Ultradol Procter & Gamble, Canad.
Etodolac (p.35·2).
Osteoarthritis; pain; rheumatoid arthritis.

Ultrafort H-3 Brasmedica, Braz.
Multivitamin, amino-acid, and mineral preparation (p.1350·1).

Ultra-Freeda Freeda, USA.
Multivitamin and mineral preparation (p.1350·1).

Ultra-K Melisana, Belg.
Potassium gluconate (p.1194·3).
Potassium depletion.

Ultralan
Note. This name is used for preparations of different composition.
Schering, Aust.; Schering, Ger.; Asche, Ger.; Schering, Ital.; Schering, Mex.
Cream; lotion: Fluocortolone caproate (p.1071·3); fluocortolone pivalate (p.1071·3).
Skin disorders.

Schering, Aust.; Schering, Fr.; Schering, Ger.; Asche, Ger.; Schering, Hong Kong; Schering, Ital.; Schering, Mex.
Ointment; topical spray: Fluocortolone (p.1071·3); fluocortolone caproate (p.1071·3).
Skin disorders.

Schering, Aust.; Schering, Ger.; Asche, Ger.; Schering, Israel; Schering, Ital.
Tablets: Fluocortolone (p.1071·3).
Corticosteroid.

Schering, Israel.
Cream; ointment: Fluocortolone (p.1071·3); fluocortolone caproate (p.1071·3).
Skin disorders.

Schering, Neth.
Fluocortolone (p.1071·3) or fluocortolone pivalate (p.1071·3); fluocortolone caproate (p.1071·3).
Skin disorders.

Schering, Switz.†.
Fluocortolone (p.1071·3) or fluocortolone pivalate (p.1071·3); fluocortolone caproate (p.1071·3).
Skin disorders.

Galagen, USA.
Lactose-free, gluten-free preparation for enteral nutrition (p.1350·1).

Ultralan M Schering, Spain.
Fluocortolone (p.1071·3).
Skin disorders.

Ultralan-crinale Schering, Ger.†.
Fluocortolone pivalate (p.1071·3); salicylic acid (p.1122·3).
Scalp disorders; skin disorders.

Ultralanum Schering, Swed.†.
Fluocortolone (p.1071·3) or fluocortolone pivalate (p.1071·3); fluocortolone caproate (p.1071·3).
Skin disorders.

Ultralanum Plain Meadow, UK.
Fluocortolone (p.1071·3) or fluocortolone pivalate (p.1071·3); fluocortolone caproate (p.1071·3).
Skin disorders.

Ultralente
Novo Nordisk, Ger.†; Novo Nordisk, USA.
Insulin zinc suspension (crystalline) (bovine, monocomponent) (p.324·1).
Diabetes mellitus.

Ultralente MC
Novo Nordisk, Austral.†; Novo Nordisk, Belg.†; Novo Nordisk, Fr.†; Novo Nordisk, Switz.†.
Insulin zinc suspension (crystalline) (bovine, monocomponent) (p.324·1).
Diabetes mellitus.

Ultra-Levura Upsamedica, Spain.
Saccharomyces boulardii (p.1626·3).
Restoration of the gastrointestinal flora.

Ultra-Levure
Biocodex, Fr.; Biocodex, Switz.
Saccharomyces boulardii (p.1626·3).
Diarrhoea.

Ultram Ortho McNeil, USA.
Tramadol hydrochloride (p.89·1).
Pain.

Ultra-Mag Germania, Aust.
Magnesium gluconate (p.1190·3).
Magnesium deficiency.

Ultra-Mg Melisana, Belg.
Magnesium gluconate (p.1190·3).
Magnesium deficiency; neuromuscular hyperexcitability.

Ultramicina
Note. This name is used for preparations of different composition.
Lisapharma, Ital.
Fosfomycin calcium (p.208·2) or fosfomycin disodium (p.208·2).
Lignocaine [lidocaine] hydrochloride (p.1313·2) is included in the intramuscular injection to alleviate the pain of injection.
Bacterial infections.

Dom, Spain.
Ciprofloxacin hydrochloride (p.182·3).
Bacterial infections.

Ultramidol Sanofi Synthelabo, Port.
Bromazepam (p.656·3).
Anxiety.

Ultramol Sanofi Winthrop, UK.
Paracetamol (p.71·2); codeine phosphate (p.25·2); caffeine (p.761·3).
Fever; pain.

Ultramop Canderm, Canad.
Methoxsalen (p.1118·3).
Psoriasis; vitiligo.

Ultramox Restan, S.Afr.†.
Amoxicillin trihydrate (p.149·2).
Bacterial infections.

Ultran Randall, Mex.
Ranitidine (p.1246·3).
Acid aspiration; gastric hypersecretion; gastro-oesophageal reflux; gastrointestinal haemorrhage; peptic ulcer; Zollinger-Ellison syndrome.

Ultra-Natal Ethex, USA.
Multivitamin and mineral preparation with carbonyl iron (p.1366·3) (p.1350·1).
Nutritional supplement in pregnancy and postnatal period.

Ultrapenil Vir, Spain.
Ampicillin sodium (p.150·3); ampicillin benzathine (p.151·3).
Bacterial infections.

Ultraplex 31 Presselin, Ger.†.
Homoeopathic preparation.

Ultraproct
Note. This name is used for preparations of different composition.
Schering, Aust.; Schering, Austral.; Schering, Belg.; Schering, Braz.; Schering, Hong Kong.
Fluocortolone pivalate (p.1071·3); fluocortolone caproate (p.1071·3); cinchocaine hydrochloride (p.1309·1); clemizole undecylate (p.413·3).
Anorectal disorders.

Schering, Fr.; Schering, Ger.; Asche, Ger.; Schering, Irl.; Schering, Ital.; Schering, Mex.; Schering, Neth.†; Schering, NZ; Schering, Switz.†; Meadow, UK.
Fluocortolone pivalate (p.1071·3); fluocortolone caproate (p.1071·3); cinchocaine hydrochloride (p.1309·1).
Formerly contained fluocortolone pivalate, fluocortolone caproate, cinchocaine hydrochloride, and clemizole undecylate in Irl. and Ital.
Anorectal disorders.

Schering, Port.
Fluocortolone pivalate (p.1071·3); lignocaine [lidocaine] hydrochloride (p.1313·2).
Ultraproct cream formerly contained fluocortolone pivalate, lignocaine [lidocaine] hydrochloride, and chlorquinaldol.
Anorectal disorders.

Ultraquin *Canderm, Canad.*
Hydroquinone (p.1115·1); padimate O (p.1518·2); ox-
ybenzone (p.1518·1).
Skin hyperpigmentation; sunscreen.

Ultraquin Plain *Canderm, Canad.*
Hydroquinone (p.1115·1).
Skin hyperpigmentation.

Ultraquinol *Schering, Aust.†*
Fluocortolone pivalate (p.1071·3); fluocortolone
caproate (p.1071·3); chlorquinaldol (p.182·1).
Infected skin disorders.

Ultra-R *Therapex, Canad.†*
Barium sulfate (p.1032·1).
Contrast medium for radiography of the small bowel.

Ultra-Rich *Pierre Fabre, Hong Kong.*
Avena (p.1583·1).
Bath additive; skin irritation.

Ultrase
Axcan, Canad.; Axcan, USA.
Pancrelipase (p.1143·3).
Pancreatic enzyme deficiency.

Ultrasep *Rivadis, Fr.†*
Glutaral (p.1145·2); didecyldimethylammonium chlo-
ride (p.1143·2).
Surface disinfection.

Ultrasept *Genpharm, S.Afr.*
Co-trimoxazole (p.193·3).
Bacterial infections.

Ultrasine *Schering, Ger.*
Emollient base.
Diluent for Ultralan lotion.

Ultrasol-F *Fresenius Kabi, Ger.*
Formaldehyde (p.1144·2); glyoxal (p.1145·3); glutaral
(p.1145·2); benzalkonium chloride (p.1133·2).
Surface disinfection.

Ultrasol-S *Fresenius, Ger.†*
Formaldehyde (p.1144·2); glyoxal (p.1145·3); glutaral
(p.1145·2); benzalkonium chloride (p.1133·2).
Surface disinfection.

Ultratard
Novo Nordisk, Austral.; Novo Nordisk, Fin.; Novo Nordisk, Irl.; Novo Nordisk, Ital.; Novo Nordisk, Neth.; Novo Nordisk, Norw.; Novo Nordisk, NZ; Novo Nordisk, Port.; Novo Nordisk, Spain; Novo Nordisk, Swed.
Insulin zinc suspension (crystalline) (human, mono-
component) (p.324·1).
Formerly known as Human Ultratard in *Irl.*
Diabetes mellitus.

Ultratard HM
Novo Nordisk, Aust.; Novo Nordisk, Belg.; Novo Nordisk, Fr.; Novo Nordisk, Ger.; Novo Nordisk, Hong Kong; Novo Nordisk, S.Afr.; Novo Nordisk, Singapore; Novo Nordisk, Switz.; Novo Nordisk, Thai.
Insulin zinc suspension (recombinant, human, mono-
component) (p.324·1).
Diabetes mellitus.

Ultrathon *3M, UK.*
Diethyltoluamide (p.1431·2).
Insect repellent.

Ultravate
Westwood-Squibb, Canad.; Westwood-Squibb, USA.
Ulobetasol propionate (p.1081·3).
Skin disorders.

Ultra-Vinca *Tecnimede, Port.*
Vinpocetine (p.1680·1).

Ultraviro C *Covan, S.Afr.*
Aspirin (p.14·2); caffeine (p.761·3); ascorbic acid
(p.1389·3); chlorpheniramine [chlorphenamine]
maleate (p.412·1).
Cold symptoms; fever; pain.

Ultravisin *Farmigea, Ital.*
Myrtillus (p.1639·2); *dl*-alpha tocoferil acetate
(p.1394·1).
Vascular retinopathy; vision disorders.

Ultravist
Schering, Aust.; Schering, Austral.; Schering, Belg.; Berlex, Canad.; Schering, Denm.; Schering, Fin.; Schering, Fr.; Schering, Ger.; Schering, Israel; Schering, Ital.; Schering, Neth.; Schering, Norw.; Schering, NZ; Schering, Port.; Schering, S.Afr.; Schering, Spain; Schering, Swed.; Schering, Switz.; Schering, UK; Berlex, USA.
Iopromide (p.1036·1).
Radiographic contrast medium.

Ultravite with Minerals *Stanley, Canad.*
Multivitamin and mineral preparation (p.1350·1).

Ultrazole *Rolab, S.Afr.*
Co-trimoxazole (p.193·3).
Bacterial infections.

Ultrazon N *Douglas, NZ.*
Betamethasone acetate (p.1063·1); neomycin sulfate
(p.228·1).
Infected eye and ear disorders.

Ultrazyme
Allergan, Austral.; Allergan-Frumtost, Braz.; Allergan, Canad.; Allergan, Irl.; Allergan, NZ; Allergan, Port.; Allergan, USA.
Subtilisin-A (p.1129·2).
Cleanser for soft contact lenses.

Ultren *Sanova, Aust.*
Vitamin A acetate (p.1383·2); ascorbic acid (p.1389·3).
Cold and influenza symptoms; vitamin deficiency.

Ultreon *Pfizer, Ger.*
Azithromycin (p.153·1).
Mycobacterial infections.

Ulxit *Tyrol, Aust.*
Nizatidine (p.1238·1).
Gastro-oesophageal reflux; peptic ulcer.

UM Instante *Farmabraz, Braz.*
Amethocaine [tetracaine] (p.1305·2); eugenol
(p.1609·3); phenol (p.1152·3); menthol (p.1632·3).
Mouth disorders.

Umadren *Montavit, Aust.†*
Skin wash: Undecenoic acid polydiethanolamide
(p.396·1).
Topical gel: Undecenoic acid monoethanolamide
(p.396·1); diphenhydramine hydrochloride (p.416·1).
Topical powder: Undecenoic acid polydiethanolamide
(p.396·1); diphenhydramine hydrochloride (p.416·1);
paraformaldehyde (p.1152·2).
Fungal skin infections.

Uman-Big *Biagini, Ital.*
A hepatitis B immunoglobulin (p.1542·1).
Passive immunisation.

Uman-Cig *Biagini, Ital.*
A cytomegalovirus immunoglobulin (p.1536·1).
Passive immunisation.

Uman-Complex *Nuovo ISM, Ital.*
A factor IX preparation (p.735·1).
Deficiency of factors II, IX or X.

Uman-Cry DI *Nuovo ISM, Ital.*
Factor VIII (p.734·1).
Factor VIII deficiency.

Uman-Fibrin *Biagini, Ital.†*
Fibrinogen (p.736·1).
Hypofibrinogenaemia.

Uman-Gal E *Biagini, Ital.†*
Antilymphocyte immunoglobulin (horse) (p.508·2).
Immunosuppressant therapy.

Uman-Gamma *Biagini, Ital.*
A normal immunoglobulin (p.1551·3).
Hypogammaglobulinaemia; passive immunisation.

Uman-Serum *Biagini, Ital.*
Plasma protein fraction (p.740·2).
Hypoproteinaemia; shock.

Uman-Vzig *Biagini, Ital.*
A varicella-zoster immunoglobulin (p.1567·3).
Passive immunisation.

Umatrope *Lilly, Fr.*
Somatropin (p.1286·1).
Growth hormone deficiency; Turner's syndrome.

Umbradol *Salvat, Spain.*
Salsalate (p.82·2).
Musculoskeletal, joint, and peri-articular disorders.

Umbrium *Kwizda, Aust.*
Diazepam (p.674·3).
Anxiety disorders; skeletal muscle spasm; sleep disor-
ders.

Umckaloabo *Iso, Ger.*
Pelargonium reniforme/sidoides.
Upper respiratory-tract infections.

Umine
Douglas, NZ; Douglas, Singapore.
Phentermine hydrochloride (p.1514·1).
Obesity.

Umizan *Zerboni, Mex.*
Phenazopyridine (p.78·1).

Umoril *Synthelabo, Ital.†*
Toloxatone (p.309·2).
Depression.

Umprel *Novartis, Aust.*
Bromocriptine mesilate (p.1164·3).
Parkinsonism.

Umuline Profil 10, 20, 30, 40, and 50 *Lilly, Fr.*
Mixtures of neutral insulin injection (human, prb)
10%, 20%, 30%, 40%, and 50% and isophane insulin
injection (human, prb) 90%, 80%, 70%, 60%, and 50%
respectively (p.324·1).
Diabetes mellitus.

Umuline Protamine Isophane (NPH) *Lilly, Fr.*
Isophane insulin injection (human, prb) (p.324·1).
Diabetes mellitus.

Umuline Rapide *Lilly, Fr.*
Neutral insulin injection (human, prb) (p.324·1).
Diabetes mellitus.

Umuline Zinc *Lilly, Fr.*
Insulin zinc suspension (human, prb) (crystalline)
(p.324·1).
Diabetes mellitus.

Umuline Zinc Compose *Lilly, Fr.*
Insulin zinc suspension (human, prb) (amorphous 30%,
crystalline 70%) (p.324·1).
Diabetes mellitus.

Unacid *Pfizer, Ger.*
Sulbactam sodium (p.250·1); ampicillin sodium
(p.150·3).
Bacterial infections.

Unacid PD *Pfizer, Ger.*
Sultamicillin (p.257·2) or sultamicillin tosilate
(p.257·2).
Bacterial infections.

Unacil *FIRMA, Ital.*
Doxycycline hyclate (p.200·1).

Unacim
Jouveinal, Fr.†
Tablets: Sultamicillin tosilate (p.257·2).
Bacterial infections.

Parke, Davis, Fr.
Injection: Sulbactam sodium (p.250·1); ampicillin sodium (p.150·3).

Lignocaine [lidocaine] hydrochloride (p.1313·2) is included in the intramuscular injection to alleviate the
pain of injection.
Bacterial infections.

Unakalm
Pharmacia Upjohn, Belg.; Pharmacia Upjohn, Neth.; Tecnifar, Port.
Ketazolam (p.688·2).
Anxiety.

Un-Alfa *Leo, Fr.*
Alfacalcidol (p.1391·1).
Hypocalcaemia; hypoparathyroidism; renal osteodys-
trophy; rickets.

Unamol *Senosiain, Mex.*
Cisapride (p.1220·1).
Constipation; dyspepsia; gastro-oesophageal reflux;
gastroparesis.

Unasyn
Pfizer, Aust.; Pfizer, Hong Kong; Pfizer, Ital.; Pfizer, Singapore; Farmasierra, Spain; Pfizer, Thai.; Pfizer, USA.
Injection: Ampicillin sodium (p.150·3); sulbactam so-
dium (p.250·1).
Lignocaine [lidocaine] hydrochloride (p.1313·2) may
be included in the intramuscular injection to alleviate
the pain of injection.
Bacterial infections.

Pfizer, Aust.; Pfizer, Hong Kong; Pfizer, Ital.; Pfizer, Singapore; Farmasierra, Spain; Pfizer, Thai.
Tablets; oral suspension: Sultamicillin (p.257·2) or
sultamicillin tosilate (p.257·2).
Bacterial infections.

Unasyna *Pfizer, Mex.*
Injection: Sulbactam sodium (p.250·1); ampicillin so-
dium (p.150·3).
Tablets; oral suspension: Sultamicillin (p.257·2).
Bacterial infections.

Unat
Roche, Ger.; Roche, Hong Kong; Lakeside, Mex.; Roche, S.Afr.
Torasemide (p.985·1) or torasemide sodium (p.985·2).
Hypertension; oedema; renal insufficiency.

Unatol *Streuli, Switz.*
Vitamin A palmitate (p.1383·2); dexpanthenol
(p.1602·3); allantoin (p.1110·1).
Nasal disorders.

Undecyl *Rekah, Israel.*
Zinc undecenoate (p.395·3); undecenoic acid
(p.395·3).
Fungal skin infections.

Undelenic *Gordon, USA.*
Undecenoic acid (p.395·3).
Fungal skin infections.

Undestor
Organon, Belg.; Organon, Swed.
Testosterone undecylate (p.1492·2).
Male hypogonadism; osteoporosis associated with an-
drogen deficiency.

Unergol *Poli, Ital.†*
Dihydroergocristine mesilate (p.1603·2).
Hyperprolactinaemia; inhibition of lactation.

Unex Amarum *Repha, Ger.*
Gentian (p.1615·1); absinthium (p.1571·1); ginger
(p.1227·2).
Appetite loss; dyspepsia; meteorism.

Unexym MD *Repha, Ger.*
Pancreatin (p.1646·1); papain (p.1647·3); betaine hy-
drochloride (p.1584·3).
Digestive disorders.

Unexym mono *Repha, Ger.*
Pancreatin (p.1646·1).
Pancreatic disorders.

Ung Vernleigh *Propan, S.Afr.*
Sulfanilamide (p.256·2); merbromin (p.1150·1); peru
balsam (p.1650·2); cod-liver oil (p.1357·2).
Burns; wounds.

Unguentacid *Mucos, Ger.*
Linoleic acid triglyceride; vitamin A palmitate
(p.1383·2); *dl*-alpha tocoferil acetate (p.1394·1).
Skin disorders; ulcers; wounds.

Unguentine *Mentholatum, USA.*
Phenol (p.1152·3); zinc oxide (p.1128·2); eucalyptus
oil (p.1609·2); thyme oil (p.1672·3).
Pain in minor burns.

Unguentine Plus *Mentholatum, USA.*
Lignocaine [lidocaine] hydrochloride (p.1313·2); chlo-
roxylenol (p.1142·1); phenol (p.1152·3).
Skin disorders.

Unguento Callicida Naion *Puerto Galiana, Spain.*
Lactic acid (p.1626·2); salicylic acid (p.1122·3).
Callosities.

Unguento Morry *Teofarma, Spain.*
Salicylic acid (p.1122·3).
Calluses.

Unguentolan *Heyl, Ger.*
Cod-liver oil (p.1357·2).
Anorectal disorders; burns; ulcers; wounds.

Unguentum Bossi *Doak, USA.*
Ammoniated mercury (p.1118·3); methenamine sul-
fosalicylate (p.1125·1); coal tar (p.1125·1).
Skin disorders.

Unguentum Lactisol *Galactopharm, Ger.†*
Lactic acid (p.1626·2).
Skin disorders; wounds.

Unguentum lymphaticum *PGM, Ger.*
Hemlock (p.401·2); colchicum (p.401·2); digitalis (p.869·1); podophyllum (p.1121·1); hyoscyamus (p.470·1); calendula (p.1589·2).
Lymphatic disorders.

Unguentum M
Boots Healthcare, Irl.; Crookes Healthcare, UK.
Emollient.
Formerly known as Unguentum Merck.
Dry skin disorders; nappy rash; pharmaceutical dilu-
ent.

Unguentum Truw *Truw, Ger.†*
Homoeopathic preparation.

Ungvita
Note.This name is used for preparations of different composition.
Roche Consumer, Austral.
Cream: Zinc oxide (p.1128·2).
Formerly contained vitamin A palmitate, calamine, and
a dimethicone.
Minor cuts and abrasions; skin disorders.
Ointment: Fish-liver oil; vitamin A palmitate
(p.1383·2).
Traumatic skin disorders.

Roche, NZ.
Cream: Vitamin A palmitate (p.1383·2); calamine
(p.1111·3); dimethicone (p.1410·1).
Skin abrasions; skin irritation.
Ointment: Vitamin A palmitate (p.1383·2).
Dry skin; minor burns.

Uni Masdil *Esteve, Spain.*
Diltiazem hydrochloride (p.874·3).
Angina pectoris; hypertension.

Uni Mist *Asta Medica, Spain.*
Morphine sulfate (p.56·1).
Pain.

Uni Salve *Smith & Nephew, Austral.*
Soft paraffin (p.1407·3).
Barrier cream; minor skin irritations.

Uni-Ace *URL, USA.*
Paracetamol (p.71·2).

Unibac *Lilly, Belg.*
Dirithromycin (p.199·2).
Bacterial infections.

Unibar *Therapex, Canad.†*
Barium sulfate (p.1032·1).
Radiographic contrast medium.

Unibaryt
Note.This name is used for preparations of different composition.
Procter & Gamble, Aust.†
Barium sulfate (p.1032·1).
Contrast medium for gastrointestinal radiography.

Goldham, Ger.†
Sodium bicarbonate (p.1186·2); anhydrous citric acid
(p.1596·2); simeticone (p.1249·2).
Adjuvant to double contrast radiography; diagnostic
agent.

Unibase *Warner Chilcott, USA.*
Vehicle for topical preparations.

Uni-Bent Cough *URL, USA.*
Diphenhydramine hydrochloride (p.416·1).

Unibloc *Roche, Neth.†*
Atenolol (p.841·3).
Angina pectoris; arrhythmias; hypertension; myocar-
dial infarction.

Unicaine *Bournonville, Belg.†*
Oxybuprocaine hydrochloride (p.1318·1).
Local anaesthesia.

Unicap
Pharmacia Upjohn, Hong Kong; Upjohn, UK; Upjohn, USA.
A range of vitamin preparations (p.1350·1).

Unicap M *Pharmacia Upjohn, Hong Kong.*
Multivitamin and mineral preparation (p.1350·1).

Unicap Pre-Natal F *Pharmacia Upjohn, Braz.*
Multivitamin and mineral preparation (p.1350·1).

Unicap T *Pharmacia Upjohn, Braz.*
Multivitamin and mineral preparation (p.1350·1).

Unicef *Ripari-Gero, Ital.†*
Cefonicid sodium (p.168·1).
Lignocaine [lidocaine] hydrochloride (p.1313·2) is in-
cluded in this preparation to alleviate the pain of injec-
tion.
Bacterial infections.

Unichew *Ranbaxy, Thai.*
Dried aluminium hydroxide gel (p.1210·3); magnesi-
um hydroxide (p.1233·1).
Gastric hyperacidity; peptic ulcer.

Unichol *Merck, Aust.*
Hymecromone (p.1622·3).
Biliary-tract disorders.

Unicid *Prospa, Ital.*
Cefonicid sodium (p.168·1).
Lignocaine [lidocaine] hydrochloride (p.1313·2) is in-
cluded in the intramuscular injection to alleviate the
pain of injection.
Bacterial infections.

Unicide *Unison, Thai.*
Niclosamide (p.104·2).
Cestode infections.

Unicilin *Universales, Mex.*
Ampicillin (p.150·3).
Bacterial infections.

Unicilina *Antibioticos, Spain.*
Benzylpenicillin sodium (p.157·2).
Bacterial infections.

Uniclor *Solfran, Mex.*
Chloramphenicol (p.179·1).
Bacterial infections.

Uni-Colex *Universal, Hong Kong.*
Guaifenesin (p.1092·2).
Coughs.

The symbol † denotes a preparation no longer actively marketed

Unicomplex-T & M *Rugby, USA.*
Multivitamin and mineral preparation with iron and folic acid (p.1350·1).

Unicontin *Asta Medica, Port.*
Theophylline (p.777·2).
Obstructive airways disease.

Unicordium *Riom, Fr.*
Bepridil hydrochloride (p.844·3).
Angina pectoris.

Uni-Decon *URL, USA†.*
Phenylpropanolamine hydrochloride (p.1098·1); phenylephrine hydrochloride (p.1097·1); chlorpheniramine [chlorphenamine] maleate (p.412·1); phenyltoloxamine citrate (p.423·1).
Upper respiratory-tract symptoms.

Uniderm
Note.This name is used for preparations of different composition.
Smith & Nephew, Austral.
Moisturiser.

Schering-Plough, Denm.; Schering-Plough, Fin.; Schering-Plough, Swed.
Hydrocortisone (p.1073·3).
Skin disorders.

Unison, Singapore.
Clobetasol propionate (p.1065·2).
Skin disorders.

Unidermo *Uniderm, Ital.*
Lactic acid (p.1626·2); collagen (p.1598·2).
Skin cleansing.

Unidie *Fournier SA, Spain.*
Cefonicid sodium (p.168·1).
Bacterial infections.

Unidipin *Pharmacia Upjohn, Aust.†.*
Nifedipine (p.940·1).
Angina pectoris; hypertension.

Unidixina *Universales, Mex.*
Nalidixic acid (p.227·1).
No indications.

Unidor *Synthelabo, Spain.*
Aspirin (p.14·2); caffeine (p.761·3).
Fever; pain.

Unidose *Endoterapica, Braz.*
Etynodiol diacetate (p.1477·1); ethinylestradiol (p.1476·2).
Combined oral contraceptive.

Unidox *Yamanouchi, Belg.; Yamanouchi, Neth.*
Doxycycline (p.200·1).
Bacterial infections.

Uni-Dur *Recordati, Ital.; Schering-Plough, Mex.; Schering-Plough, S.Afr.; Key, USA.*
Theophylline (p.777·2).
Obstructive airways disease.

Unif *Medicap, Thai.*
Triamcinolone acetonide (p.1080·1).
Skin and scalp disorders.

Uni-Febrin *Universal, Hong Kong.*
Paracetamol (p.71·2).
Fever; pain.

Uni-Fedra Compound *Universal, Hong Kong.*
Triprolidine hydrochloride (p.427·2); pseudoephedrine hydrochloride (p.1099·2); codeine phosphate (p.25·2).
Coughs; nasal congestion.

Unifer *Tosi, Ital.*
Iron sucrose (p.1370·1).
Iron deficiency anaemias.

Grossman, Mex.
Iron carbonyl.
Iron deficiency anaemia.

Unifiber *Niche, USA.*
Powdered cellulose (p.1500·3).
Constipation.

Unifibre *Niche, Singapore.*
Dietary fibre supplement (p.1350·1).
Constipation.

Uniflex *Xepa-Soul Pattinson, Singapore.*
Betamethasone valerate (p.1063·2).
Skin disorders.

Uniflex-N *Xepa-Soul Pattinson, Singapore.*
Betamethasone valerate (p.1063·2); neomycin sulfate (p.228·1).
Infected skin disorders.

Uniflox *Besins-Iscovesco, Fr.*
Ciprofloxacin hydrochloride (p.182·3).
Cystitis; gonococcal urethritis.

Uniflu with Gregovite C *Unigreg, UK.*
Uniflu tablets, phenylephrine hydrochloride (p.1097·1); caffeine (p.761·3); codeine phosphate (p.25·2); diphenhydramine hydrochloride (p.416·1); paracetamol (p.71·2); Gregovite C tablets, ascorbic acid (p.1389·3).
Cold and influenza symptoms; nasal cogestion.

Uniflu & Gregovite C *Unigreg, Irl.†.*
Uniflu tablets, paracetamol (p.71·2); codeine phosphate (p.25·2); caffeine (p.761·3); diphenhydramine hydrochloride (p.416·1); phenylephrine hydrochloride (p.1097·1); Gregovite C tablets, ascorbic acid (p.1389·3).
Colds and influenza symptoms.

Unifyl *Mundipharma, Aust.; Mundipharma, Switz.*
Theophylline (p.777·2).
Obstructive airways disease.

Unigam *Norgine, UK†.*
Evening primrose oil (p.1613·2).
Atopic eczema; mastalgia.

Unigamol *Norgine, Ger.*
Evening primrose oil (p.1613·2).
Atopic eczema.

Unigan *Unison, Thai.*
Hyoscine butylbromide (p.468·2); paracetamol (p.71·2).
Smooth muscle spasm.

Unigest *Unigreg, UK†.*
Aluminium hydroxide (p.1210·3); dimethicone (p.1249·2).
Gastrointestinal disorders.

Uni-Gold hCG *Kora, Irl.*
Pregnancy test (p.1654·3).

Unigyn *Uniderm, Ital.*
Lactic acid (p.1626·2).
Personal hygiene; vaginal douche.

Unihep *Leo, Irl.; Leo, UK†.*
Heparin sodium (p.902·1).
Thromboembolic disorders.

Uni-Kaotin *Universal, Hong Kong.*
Kaolin (p.1229·3); pectin (p.1502·3).
Diarrhoea.

Uniket *Lacer, Spain.*
Isosorbide mononitrate (p.916·2).
Angina pectoris; heart failure.

Unik-Zoru *Therapex, Canad.†.*
Tartaric acid (p.1669·2); sodium bicarbonate (p.1186·2).
Diagnostic agent.

Unilair *3M, Ger.; 3M, Neth.†.*
Theophylline (p.777·2).
Obstructive airways disease.

Unilan *Merck, Port.*
Alprazolam (p.654·2).
Anxiety.

Unilarm *Ciba Vision, Fr.*
Sodium chloride (p.1196·1).
Dry eye.

Unilax *Ascher, USA†.*
Docusate sodium (p.1223·1); phenolphthalein (p.1244·1).
Constipation.

Uniloc *Nycomed, Denm.; Nycomed, Fin.; Nycomed, Norw.; Nycomed, Swed.*
Atenolol (p.841·3).
Angina pectoris; arrhythmias; hypertension; hyperthyroidism; migraine; myocardial infarction.

Unilong *Byk Elmu, Spain.*
Theophylline (p.777·2).
Heart failure; obstructive airways disease; paroxysmal dyspnoea.

Unilux *Goldham, Ger.*
Iopamidol (p.1035·2).
Radiographic contrast medium.

Uni-Ma *Unison, Thai.*
Monobasic sodium phosphate (p.1193·2); dibasic sodium phosphate (p.1193·2).
Bowel evacuation; constipation.

Unimaalox *Rhone-Poulenc Rorer, Spain.*
Aluminium hydroxide (p.1210·3); magnesium hydroxide (p.1233·1).
Dyspepsia; gastrointestinal hyperacidity.

Unimax *AstraZeneca, Fin.; Astra, Ger.; Promed, Ger.; Astra, Switz.*
Felodipine (p.888·3); ramipril (p.966·3).
Hypertension.

Unimest *Astra, Spain.*
Felodipine (p.888·3); ramipril (p.966·3).
Hypertension.

Unimezol *Ranbaxy, Thai.*
Metronidazole (p.594·1).
Amoebiasis; anaerobic bacterial infections; giardiasis; trichomoniasis.

Unimol *Unison, Thai.*
Paracetamol (p.71·2).
Fever; pain.

Unimox *Propan, S.Afr.†; Unison, Thai.*
Amoxicillin (p.149·2) or amoxicillin trihydrate (p.149·2).
Bacterial infections.

Uniparin *Rhone-Poulenc Rorer, Austral.; CP Pharmaceuticals, Irl.; CP Pharmaceuticals, UK†.*
Heparin calcium (p.902·1) or heparin sodium (p.902·1).
Thromboembolic disorders.

Unipen *Wyeth-Ayerst, USA†.*
Nafcillin sodium (p.226·3).
Bacterial infections.

Unipexil *Gifrer Barbezat, Fr.*
Minoxidil (p.934·2).
Alopecia androgenetica.

Uni-Phen *Universal, Hong Kong.*
Ammonium chloride (p.1085·2); sodium citrate (p.1186·2); diphenhydramine hydrochloride (p.416·1); menthol (p.1632·3).
Coughs; nasal congestion.

Uni-Pholco *Universal, Hong Kong.*
Pholcodine (p.1099·1).
Coughs.

Uniphyl *Purdue Frederick, Canad.; Mundipharma, Hong Kong; Adcock Ingram, S.Afr.; Purdue Frederick, USA.*
Theophylline (p.777·2).
Obstructive airways disease.

Uniphyllin *Mundipharma, Ger.*
Theophylline (p.777·2) or theophylline sodium glycinate (p.783·2).
Obstructive airways disease.

Uniphyllin Continus *Napp, Irl.; Napp, UK.*
Theophylline (p.777·2).
Asthma; bronchospasm; heart failure; obstructive airways disease.

Unipine XL *Genus, UK†.*
Nifedipine (p.940·1).
Hypertension.

Uniplus *Angelini, Ital.*
Oxolamine citrate (p.1096·2); propyphenazone (p.80·2).
Influenza symptoms; oral inflammation; otorhinolaryngeal inflammation; tracheobronchitis.

Unipril *Astra, Ital.*
Ramipril (p.966·3).
Heart failure; hypertension; renal insufficiency.

Uniquin *Biochemie, Aust.; Wassermann, Ital.; Medinfar, Port.; Searle, S.Afr.*
Lomefloxacin hydrochloride (p.220·1).
Bacterial infections.

Uni-Ramine *Universal, Hong Kong.*
Chlorpheniramine [chlorphenamine] maleate (p.412·1).
Antihistamine.

Uni-Ramine CE *Universal, Hong Kong.*
Codeine phosphate (p.25·2); ephedrine hydrochloride (p.1090·1); ammonium chloride (p.1085·2); chlorpheniramine [chlorphenamine] maleate (p.412·1).
Coughs.

Uni-Ramine Expectorant *Universal, Hong Kong.*
Chlorpheniramine [chlorphenamine] maleate (p.412·1); ammonium chloride (p.1085·2); sodium citrate (p.1186·2).
Coughs.

Uniren
Unison, Singapore; Unison, Thai.
Diclofenac diethylamine (p.30·2) or diclofenac sodium (p.30·3).
Musculoskeletal, joint, peri-articular, and soft-tissue disorders.

Uniretic *Schwarz, USA.*
Moexipril hydrochloride (p.935·3); hydrochlorothiazide (p.907·3).
Hypertension.

Unirhinol *Union, Singapore.*
Chlorpheniramine [chlorphenamine] maleate (p.412·1); paracetamol (p.71·2); phenylpropanolamine hydrochloride (p.1098·1).
Cold symptoms.

Uniroid *Unigreg, UK†.*
Hydrocortisone (p.1073·3); neomycin sulfate (p.228·1); polymyxin B sulfate (p.238·1); cinchocaine hydrochloride (p.1309·1).
Anorectal disorders.

Uniroid-HC *Chemidex, UK.*
Cinchocaine hydrochloride (p.1309·1); hydrocortisone (p.1073·3).
Anorectal disorders.

Unisal *Merck Sharp & Dohme, Switz.*
Diflunisal (p.32·2).
Inflammation; pain.

Uniscrub
Seton, Israel; SSL, UK.
Chlorhexidine gluconate (p.1138·2).
Skin disinfection.

Unisedil *Merck, Port.*
Diazepam (p.674·3).
Alcohol withdrawal syndrome; anxiety disorders; skeletal muscle spasm.

Unisedyl *Union, Singapore.*
Codeine phosphate (p.25·2); promethazine hydrochloride (p.423·2); ephedrine hydrochloride (p.1090·1).
Coughs.

Unisept *Seton, Israel.*
Chlorhexidine gluconate (p.1138·2).
Disinfection of burns, mucous membranes, skin, and wounds.

Unisoil *Therapex, Canad.†.*
Castor oil (p.1592·1).
Constipation.

Unisol
Agepha, Aust.
Disinfecting and storage solution for contact lenses (p.1129·2).

Alcon, USA.
Rinsing and storage solutions for soft contact lenses (p.1129·2).

Unisolve *Smith & Nephew, Austral.*
Dipropylene glycol methyl ether; isopropyl alcohol (p.1606·3); isoparaffin.
Medical adhesive remover.

Unisom
Note.This name is used for preparations of different composition.
Pfizer, Austral.; Pfizer, Canad.
Diphenhydramine hydrochloride (p.416·1).
Insomnia.

Pfizer, Israel; Rovifarma, Spain.
Doxylamine succinate (p.417·1).
Insomnia.

Unisom-2 *Pfizer, Canad.*
Doxylamine succinate (p.417·1).
Insomnia.

Unisom Natural Source *Pfizer Consumer, Canad.*
Valerian (p.1678·3).
Insomnia.

Unisom with Pain Relief *Pfizer Consumer, USA.*
Paracetamol (p.71·2); diphenhydramine hydrochloride (p.416·1).
Insomnia; pain.

Unisom SleepTabs *Pfizer Consumer, USA.*
Doxylamine succinate (p.417·1).
Insomnia.

Unisom-C *Pfizer, Canad.†.*
Diphenhydramine hydrochloride (p.416·1).
Insomnia.

Unisomnia *Unigreg, UK†.*
Nitrazepam (p.695·2).
Insomnia.

Unison Enema *Unison, Thai.*
Macrogol (p.1630·1); sodium chloride.
Constipation.

Unison Ointment *Unison, Thai.*
Chloramphenicol (p.179·1).
Bacterial skin infections.

Unistep hCG *Orion, USA.*
Pregnancy test (p.1654·3).

Unitable *INQ, Braz.*
Multivitamin and mineral preparation (p.1350·1).

United Soft Guard *Smith & Nephew, Austral.†.*
Carmellose (p.1499·3); polyisobutylene; pectin (p.1502·3).
Skin protection; wounds.

Unithroid *Stevens, USA.*
Thyroxine [levothyroxine] sodium (p.1526·2).
Hypothyroidism.

Unitifed *Union, Singapore.*
Triprolidine hydrochloride (p.427·2); pseudoephedrine hydrochloride (p.1099·2).
Allergic rhinitis; cold symptoms; coughs; nasal and upper respiratory-tract congestion; sinusitis.

Unitifed Compound *Union, Singapore.*
Codeine phosphate (p.25·2); triprolidine hydrochloride (p.427·2); pseudoephedrine hydrochloride (p.1099·2).
Allergic rhinitis; cold symptoms; coughs; nasal and upper respiratory-tract congestion; sinusitis.

Unitimoftol *Merck Sharp & Dohme, Spain.*
Timolol maleate (p.982·1).
Glaucoma; ocular hypertension.

Unitone *Darier, Mex.*
Betacarotene (p.1355·1); octinoxate (p.1517·3); avobenzone (p.1517·1).
Skin hyperpigmentation.

Uni-Tranxene *Sanofi Synthelabo, Belg.*
Dipotassium clorazepate (p.670·3).
Anxiety; mixed anxiety depressive states.

Unitril *Kener, Mex.*
Dimenhydrinate (p.415·2).

Unitrim *Master Pharma, Ital.†.*
Brodimoprim (p.159·3).
Otorhinolaryngeal infections; respiratory-tract infections.

Unitrol *Republic, USA†.*
Phenylpropanolamine hydrochloride (p.1098·1).
Obesity.

Unitul Complex *Bama, Spain.*
Sodium acexamate (p.1572·2); sulfadiazine silver (p.251·3).
Burns; ulcers; wounds.

Unitulle
Hoechst Marion Roussel, Austral.; Cassenne, Fr.†.
White soft paraffin (p.1407·3).
Burns; skin ulcers; wounds.

Unituss HC *URL, USA.*
Hydrocodone tartrate (p.42·2); phenylephrine hydrochloride (p.1097·1); chlorpheniramine [chlorphenamine] maleate (p.412·1).
Upper respiratory-tract symptoms.

Uni-tussin *URL, USA.*
Guaifenesin (p.1092·2).
Coughs.

Uni-tussin DM *URL, USA.*
Dextromethorphan hydrobromide (p.1087·3); guaifenesin (p.1092·2).
Coughs.

Univasc *Schwarz, USA.*
Moexipril hydrochloride (p.935·3).
Hypertension.

Uni-Vasin *Universal, Hong Kong.*
Chlorpheniramine [chlorphenamine] maleate (p.412·1); phenylephrine hydrochloride (p.1097·1); phenylpropanolamine hydrochloride (p.1098·1).
Upper respiratory-tract symptoms.

Univate *Xepa-Soul Pattinson, Singapore.*
Clobetasol propionate (p.1065·2).
Skin disorders.

Univer *Elan, UK.*
Verapamil hydrochloride (p.989·1).
Angina pectoris; hypertension.

Universal Concentration Tablets *Universal, S.Afr.†.*
Caffeine (p.761·3).
Fatigue.

Universal Earache Drops *Propan, S.Afr.*
Phenazone (p.77·2); procaine hydrochloride (p.1319·1); potassium hydroxyquinoline sulfate (p.1654·2).
Ear disorders.

Universal Eye Drops *Propan, S.Afr.*
Phenylephrine hydrochloride (p.1097·1); boric acid (p.1586·1).
Eye inflammation; eye irritation.

Universal Nasal Drops *Propan, S.Afr.*
Phenylephrine hydrochloride (p.1097·1); naphazoline nitrate (p.1095·1).
Allergic rhinitis; sinusitis.

Universal Throat Lollies *Propan, S.Afr.*
Cetylpyridinium chloride (p.1138·1).
Mouth and throat infections.

Univol *Carter Horner, Canad.*
Aluminium hydroxide (p.1210·3); magnesium hydroxide (p.1233·1).
Gastrointestinal disorders associated with hyperacidity.

Uniwash *Smith & Nephew, Austral.*
Skin cleanser.

UniXan *Norpharma, Denm.*
Theophylline (p.777·3).
Obstructive airways disease.

Unixime *FIRMA, Ital.*
Cefixime (p.166·2).
Bacterial infections.

Unizen *Unison, Singapore; Unison, Thai.*
Serrapeptase (p.1662·1).
Alveolar abscess; breast engorgement; cystitis; epididymitis; inflammation; respiratory-tract congestion; sinusitis; wisdom tooth pericoronitis; wounds.

Unizink *Kohler, Ger.; Kohler-Pharma, Ger.*
Zinc aspartate.
Zinc deficiency.

Unizuric *Quimica y Farmacia, Mex.*
Allopurinol (p.397·2).
Hyperuricaemia.

Unizyme *Ciba Vision, Canad.*
Subtilisin (p.1129·2).
Protein removal from contact lenses.

UnoCardil *Orion, Denm.*
Diltiazem hydrochloride (p.874·3).
Hypertension.

Uno-Ciclo *Biochimico, Braz.*
Algestone acetophenide (p.1465·1); estradiol enantate (p.1473·2).
Injectable contraceptive.

Uno-Enantone *Takeda, Ger.*
Leuprorelin acetate (p.1289·2).
Prostatic cancer.

Uno-Lin *3M, Denm.*
Theophylline hydrate (p.777·2).
Obstructive airways disease.

Unoprost *Guidotti, Ital.*
Terazosin hydrochloride (p.980·1).
Benign prostatic hyperplasia.

Unotex N feminin *Bilgast, Ger.†.*
Homoeopathic preparation.

Unotex N masculin *Bilgast, Ger.†.*
Homoeopathic preparation.

Uno-Vit *Wiedemann, Ger.*
dl-Alpha tocopherol (p.1394·1).
Vitamin E deficiency.

Untigex *Herals, Braz.*
Menthol (p.1632·3); methyl salicylate (p.55·1).
Musculoskeletal and joint disorders.

Uonin *Unison, Thai.*
Roxithromycin (p.247·2).
Bacterial infections.

Up Mep *Cimed, Braz.*
Cimetidine (p.1216·3).
Gastro-oesophageal reflux; gastrointestinal haemorrhage; peptic ulcer; Zollinger-Ellison syndrome.

Upelva *Pekana, Ger.*
Homoeopathic preparation.

Upfen *UPSA, Fr.*
Ibuprofen (p.43·2).
Fever; pain.

Uprima *Abbott, UK.*
Apomorphine hydrochloride (p.1163·1).
Erectile dysfunction.

U-Proxyn *Unison, Thai.*
Naproxen (p.60·3).
Gout; musculoskeletal and joint disorders.

Upsa C *Upsamedica, Belg.; Upsamedica, Spain.*
Ascorbic acid (p.1389·3).
Adjunct in treatment of iron supplementation; methaemoglobinaemia; vitamin C deficiency.

Upsa Plus *Upsamedica, Ital.*
Oxolamine citrate (p.1096·2); propyphenazone (p.80·2).
Influenza symptoms; respiratory-tract inflammation.

Upsadex *Upsamedica, Spain.*
Doxylamine succinate (p.417·1); sodium bromide; dibasic sodium phosphate; sodium sulfate (p.1180·1).
Anxiety disorders; insomnia.

Upsalgin C *Upsamedica, Switz.*
Aspirin (p.14·2); ascorbic acid (p.1389·3).
Fever; pain.

Upsalgina *Upsamedica, Ital.; Upsamedica, Spain†.*
Aspirin (p.14·2).
Fever; inflammation; pain; thrombosis prophylaxis.

Upsalgine *Upsamedica, Belg.*
Carbasalate calcium (p.23·3).
Fever; pain.

Upsavit C *Upsamedica, Belg.*
Ascorbic acid (p.1389·3).
Methaemoglobinaemia; vitamin C deficiency.

Upset Stomach *Homeocan, Canad.*
Homoeopathic preparation.

Uracid
Note. This name is used for preparations of different composition.
Hassle, Swed.†.
Aluminium hydroxide (p.1210·3); calcium carbonate (p.1215·1).
Heartburn; hyperphosphataemia; peptic ulcer.

Wesley, USA.
Methionine (p.1012·2).
Odour, dermatitis, and ulceration in incontinent adults.

Uracil *Pharmasant, Thai.*
Propylthiouracil (p.1525·3).
Hyperthyroidism.

Uractazide *Prospa, Belg.*
Hydrochlorothiazide (p.907·3); spironolactone (p.973·2).
Hypertension; oedema.

Uractone
Prospa, Belg.; SPA, Ital.
Spironolactone (p.973·2).
Hyperaldosteronism; hypertension; oedema.

Uractonum *Medochemie, Singapore.*
Spironolactone (p.973·2).
Heart failure; hyperaldosteronism; hypertension; liver cirrhosis with oedema; nephrotic syndrome.

Ural
Abbott, Austral.; Abbott, NZ.
Sodium bicarbonate (p.1186·2); anhydrous sodium citrate (p.1186·2); anhydrous citric acid (p.1596·2); tartaric acid (p.1669·2).
Gastric hyperacidity; urinary alkalinisation.

Uralgin *Ceccarelli, Ital.*
Nalidixic acid (p.227·1).
Gram-negative bacterial infections of the urinary tract.

Uralyt *Madaus, Spain†.*
Arnica (p.1581·3); convallaria (p.1599·1); equisetum arvense (p.1606·3); rubia tinctorum; solidago virgaurea; echinacea angustifolia (p.1606·2); magnesium phosphate (p.1191·1).
Renal calculi.

Uralyt Urato *Madaus, Spain.*
Citric acid (p.1596·2); potassium citrate (p.1186·1).
Formerly contained citric acid, aescin, potassium citrate, ruberitric acid, and sodium citrate.
Hypocitraturia; renal calculi; renal tubular acidosis.

Uralyt-U
Madaus, Aust.; Madaus, Belg.; Hoyer, Ger.; Madaus, Israel; Ibi, Ital.; Neo-Farmaceutica, Port.; Byk Madaus, S.Afr.; Madaus, Switz.; Madaus, Thai.
Potassium sodium hydrogen citrate.
Cystinuria; porphyria cutanea tarda; renal calculi; urinary alkalinisation.

Uramox *Taro, Israel.*
Acetazolamide (p.826·1).
Drug-induced oedema; epilepsy; glaucoma; heart failure.

Urantin *Xixia, S.Afr†.*
Nitrofurantoin (p.230·3).
Urinary-tract infections.

Urantoin *Rafa, Israel; DDSA Pharmaceuticals, UK.*
Nitrofurantoin (p.230·3).
Genito-urinary-tract infections.

Uraplex *Madaus, Spain.*
Trospium chloride (p.475·2).
Urinary incontinence.

Urapro *Eagle, Austral.*
Saw palmetto (p.1491·2); lycopersicon esculentum; hydrastis (p.1621·1); urtica (p.1678·2); zinc gluconate (p.1398·2); nickel; ferrous phosphate.
Nutritional supplement.

Urarthone *Homeocan, Canad.; Lehning, Fr.*
Homoeopathic preparation.

Urasal *Carter Horner, Canad.*
Methenamine (p.223·1).
Urinary-tract infections.

Urasin *Nakorn, Thai.*
Frusemide [furosemide] (p.893·1).
Forced diuresis; heart failure; oedema.

Urbadan *Hoechst Marion Roussel, Mex.; Roussel, Neth.†.*
Clobazam (p.668·1).
Anxiety.

Urbal *Merck, Spain.*
Sucralfate (p.1250·2).
Gastrointestinal haemorrhage; peptic ulcer.

Urbanil
Hoechst Marion Roussel, Braz.; Aventis, Port.
Clobazam (p.668·1).
Anxiety; epilepsy.

Urbanol *Sanofi Synthelabo, S.Afr.*
Clobazam (p.668·1).
Alcohol withdrawal syndrome; anxiety; premedication.

Urbanyl
Synthelabo, Fr.; Hoechst Marion Roussel, Switz.
Clobazam (p.668·1).
Alcohol withdrawal syndrome; anxiety; epilepsy.

Urbason
Hoechst Marion Roussel, Aust.; Hoechst Marion Roussel, Ger.; Hoechst Marion Roussel, Ital.; Hoechst Marion Roussel, Spain; Hoechst Marion Roussel, Switz.
Methylprednisolone (p.1076·1), methylprednisolone acetate (p.1076·1), or methylprednisolone sodium succinate (p.1076·1).
Corticosteroid.

Urdes *Errekappa, Ital.*
Ursodeoxycholic acid (p.1677·2).
Biliary disorders.

Urdox *CP Pharmaceuticals, UK.*
Ursodeoxycholic acid (p.1677·2).
Cholesterol gallstones.

Urdrim *Urbion, Spain.*
Astemizole (p.409·1).
Hypersensitivity reactions.

Ureacin *Pedinol, USA.*
Urea (p.1127·3).
Dry skin; hyperkeratosis.

Ureadin 10 and 20 *Isdin, Port.*
Urea (p.1127·3).
Dry skin; hyperkeratotic skin disorders.

Ureadin 30 *Isdin, Port.*
Urea (p.1127·3); glycolic acid (p.1115·1); salicylic acid (p.1122·3).
Hyperkeratotic skin disorders.

Ureadin Facial *Isdin, Port.*
SPF 10: Urea (p.1127·3); glycerol (p.1616·3); borage oil (p.1613·1); sunscreens.
Dry skin.

Ureadin Maos *Isdin, Port.*
Urea (p.1127·3); glycerol (p.1616·3); lactic acid (p.1626·2).
Dry skin.

Ureadin 10 Plus *Isdin, Port.*
Urea (p.1127·3); dexpanthenol (p.1602·3).
Dry skin disorders.

Ureaphil *Abbott, USA.*
Urea (p.1127·3).
Cerebral oedema; raised intra-ocular pressure.

Ureata S *Fides, Ger.*
Urea (p.1127·3); alpha tocoferil acetate (p.1394·1).
Skin disorders; ulcers.

Urecare *Pharmacia Upjohn, Austral.; Pharmacia Upjohn, Singapore.*
Urea (p.1127·3).
Dry skin disorders.

Urecholine *Merck Sharp & Dohme, Austral.; Merck Frosst, Canad.; Merck Sharp & Dohme, Israel; Merck Sharp & Dohme, Ital.†; Merck Sharp & Dohme, S.Afr.; Merck Sharp & Dohme, Thai.; Merck, USA†.*
Bethanechol chloride (p.1415·3).
Congenital megacolon; gastro-oesophageal reflux; neurogenic bladder; postoperative abdominal distension; urinary retention.

Urecrem *Stiefel, Fr.*
Urea (p.1127·3).
Dry skin disorders.

Urederm
Hamilton, Austral.; Hamilton, Hong Kong.
Urea (p.1127·3).
Dry skin; skin irritation.

Uredimin *Andreabal, Switz.†.*
Allopurinol (p.397·2).
Gout; hyperuricaemia; renal calculi.

Uree *Riva, Canad.*
Urea (p.1127·3).

Uregyt *Medphano, Ger.†.*
Etacrynic acid (p.887·2).
Refractory oedema.

Ureina *Produfarma, Port.*
Parietaria officinalis.

Urelium Neu *Europharm, Aust.*
Ammi visnaga fruit (p.1579·1); solidago virgaurea; taraxacum (p.1669·1); aescin (p.1574·1).
Renal calculi.

Urem *Kade, Ger.*
Ibuprofen (p.43·2) or ibuprofen sodium (p.44·1).
Fever; inflammation; musculoskeletal, joint, and soft-tissue disorders; pain.

Uremiase *Nogues, Fr.†.*
Kinkeliba (p.1626·1); calcium carbonate (p.1215·1).
Formerly contained silica, cholesterol, tricalcium phosphate, dibasic sodium phosphate, sodium chloride, kidney extract, combretum micranthum, heavy chalk.
Gastrointestinal disorders.

Uremide
Alphapharm, Austral.; Propan, S.Afr.
Frusemide [furosemide] (p.893·1).
Hypertension; oedema.

Uremol *Trans Canaderm, Canad.*
Urea (p.1127·3).
Skin disorders.

Uremol-HC *Trans Canaderm, Canad.*
Hydrocortisone acetate (p.1073·2); urea (p.1127·3).
Skin disorders.

Ureotop *Dermapharm, Ger.*
Urea (p.1127·3).
Skin disorders.

Ureotop + VAS *Dermapharm, Ger.*
Urea (p.1127·3); tretinoin (p.1126·2).
Keratinisation disorders.

Uretil *Uniao Quimica, Braz.*
Phenazopyridine hydrochloride (p.77·3); nitrohydroxyquinoline.
Urinary-tract infections.

Uretren Comp *Orion, Fin.*
Triamterene (p.986·1); trichlormethiazide (p.987·1).
Hypertension; oedema.

Uretrim *TAD, Ger.†.*
Trimethoprim (p.264·2).
Urinary-tract infections.

Urex
Note. This name is used for preparations of different composition.
Fawns & McAllan, Austral.; Fawns & McAllan, Hong Kong.
Frusemide [furosemide] (p.893·1).
Hypertension; oedema; renal failure.

3M, USA.
Methenamine hippurate (p.223·1).
Urinary-tract infections.

Urfadyn PL *Zambon, Belg.*
Nifurtoinol (p.230·2).
Urinary-tract infections.

Urfadyne *Inpharzam, Switz.†.*
Nifurtoinol (p.230·2).
Urinary-tract infections.

Urfamycin
Zambon, Spain; Sermmitr, Thai.; Zambon, Thai.
Thiamphenicol (p.261·3) or thiamphenicol glycinate hydrochloride (p.262·1).
Bacterial infections.

Urfamycine
Zambon, Belg.; Inpharzam, Switz.
Thiamphenicol (p.261·3) or thiamphenicol glycinate hydrochloride (p.262·1).
Bacterial infections.

Urgenin
Note. This name is used for preparations of different composition.
Madaus, Aust.; Polcopharma, Austral.; Madaus, Belg.; Madaus, Hong Kong; Madaus, Israel.
Echinacea (p.1606·2); saw palmetto (p.1491·2).
Prostatic and urinary-tract disorders.

Madaus, Spain.
Echinacea angustifolia (p.1606·2); saw palmetto (p.1491·2); esculoside (p.1574·1).
Prostatic and urinary-tract disorders.

Urgenin Cucurbitae oleum *Hoyer, Ger.*
Cucurbita seed oil.
Benign prostatic hyperplasia; urinary-tract disorders.

Urgenine *Madaus, Switz.†.*
Echinacea purpurea (p.1606·2); saw palmetto (p.1491·2).
Bladder irritability; prostatitis.

Urgo Pangen *Madaus, Aust.†.*
Collagen (p.1598·2).
Haemorrhage.

Urgocall *Fournier SA, Spain.*
Salicylic acid (p.1122·3).
Calluses; corns.

Urgomed *Urgo, Fr.*
Carmellose (p.1499·3).
Burns; wounds.

Urgo-N Huhneraugenpflaster *Fournier, Ger.*
Salicylic acid (p.1122·3).
Calluses; corns.

Uriage
Note. This name is used for preparations of different composition.
Biorga, Fr.
SPF 25: Octinoxate (p.1517·3); titanium dioxide (p.1126·1); dibenzoylmethane (p.1517·1).
Sunscreen.

Saniniter, Port.
A range of emollients, moisturisers, and soap substitutes.

Uriage Ecran Mineral
Note. This name is used for preparations of different composition.
Biorga, Fr.
SPF 100: Octinoxate (p.1517·3); titanium dioxide (p.1126·1); zinc oxide (p.1128·2).
Sunscreen.

Biorga, Fr.
SPF 100: Titanium dioxide (p.1126·1); zinc oxide (p.1128·2).
Sunscreen.

Saniniter, Port.
SPF 60: Titanium dioxide (p.1126·1); zinc oxide (p.1128·2).
Sunscreen.

Uriage Ecran Total
Note. This name is used for preparations of different composition.
Biorga, Fr.
SPF 35: Octinoxate (p.1517·3); titanium dioxide (p.1126·1).
Sunscreen.

Saniniter, Port.
SPF20; SPF25: Dibenzoylmethane (p.1517·1); cinnamate; titanium dioxide (p.1126·1).
Sunscreen.

Uriage Ecran Total Mineral *Biorga, Fr.*
SPF 28: Titanium dioxide (p.1126·1).
Sunscreen.

Uriage Extreme
*Note.*This name is used for preparations of different composition.
Biorga, Fr.
SPF 90: Octinoxate (p.1517·3); titanium dioxide (p.1126·1).
Sunscreen.

Saninter, Port.
SPF60: Cinnamate; titanium dioxide (p.1126·1).
Sunscreen.

Uriage IP 90 *Saninter, Port.*
Octinoxate (p.1517·3); titanium dioxide (p.1126·1); zinc oxide (p.1128·2).
Sunscreen.

Uri-Alk *Medchem, S.Afr.*
Sodium citrate (p.1186·2); sodium bicarbonate (p.1186·2); tartaric acid (p.1669·2); anhydrous citric acid (p.1596·2).
Gastrointestinal hyperacidity; urinary alkalinisation.

Uribac *Precimex, Mex.*
Pipemidic acid (p.236·1).

Uriben *Rosemont, UK.*
Nalidixic acid (p.227·1).
Urinary-tract infections.

Uribenz *RAN, Ger.*
Allopurinol (p.397·2).
Gout; hyperuricaemia.

Uricad *Great Eastern, Thai.; Westmont, Thai.*
Allopurinol (p.397·2).
Gout; hyperuricaemia; renal calculi.

Uricemil *Cristalia, Braz.; Molteni, Ital.*
Allopurinol (p.397·2).
Gout; hyperuricaemia; renal calculi.

Uricodue *IFI, Ital.*
Allopurinol (p.397·2); benziodarone (p.400·1).
Hyperuricaemia.

Uriconorme *Streuli, Switz.*
Allopurinol (p.397·2).
Gout; hyperuricaemia; renal calculi.

Uricovac *Sanofi Winthrop, Aust.*
Benzbromarone (p.399·3).
Gout; hyperuricaemia; psoriasis; psoriatic arthritis.

Uricozyme
Sanofi Winthrop, Fr.; Sanofi Synthelabo, Ital.
Urate oxidase (p.403·3).
Hyperuricaemia.

Urideal *Dolisos, Fr.*
Pilosella.
Gastrointestinal disorders; renal disorders.

Uridion *Gentili, Ital.†*
Isobromindione (p.401·2).
Gout; hyperuricaemia.

Uridon Modified *Rugby, USA.*
Methenamine (p.223·1); salol (p.82·2); atropine sulfate (p.461·1); hyoscyamine sulfate (p.469·3); benzoic acid (p.1134·2); methylene blue [methylthioninium chloride] (p.1012·3).
Urinary-tract infections.

Uridoz *Therabel, Fr.*
Fosfomycin trometamol (p.208·2).
Cystitis.

Uriflex C *SSL, UK.*
Chlorhexidine gluconate (p.1138·2).
Urinary catheter care.

Uriflex G *SSL, UK.*
Citric acid (p.1596·2); sodium bicarbonate (p.1186·2); light magnesium oxide (p.1233·2); disodium edetate (p.1008·3).
Urinary catheter care.

Uriflex R *SSL, UK.*
Citric acid (p.1596·2); light magnesium carbonate (p.1232·3); gluconolactone; disodium edetate (p.1008·3).
Urinary catheter care.

Uriflex S *SSL, UK.*
Sodium chloride (p.1196·3).
Urinary catheter care.

Uriflex W *SSL, UK.*
Sterile pyrogen free water (p.1680·2).
Urinary catheter care.

Uri-Flor *AGIPS, Ital.*
Nalidixic acid (p.227·1).
Gram-negative bacterial infections of the urinary tract.

Urifron *Probiomed, Mex.*
Interferon alfa-2b (p.628·1).
Hepatitis B; hepatitis C; malignant neoplasms.

Uriginex Urtica *Repha, Ger.†*
Urtica (p.1678·2).
Rheumatic disorders.

Urigram *Trima, Israel.*
Nalidixic acid (p.227·1).
Gram-negative bacterial urinary-tract infections.

Urihesive *Convatec, Austral.*
Medical adhesive.

Urikal *Rafa, Israel.*
Sodium citrate (p.1186·2); sodium bicarbonate (p.1186·2); citric acid (p.1596·2); sodium carbonate (p.1665·1).
Urinary-tract infections.

Uriken *Kener, Mex.*
Pipemidic acid (p.236·1).

Urilin *Faria, Braz.*
Oxolinic acid (p.233·3).
Urinary-tract infections.

Urimar-T *Marnel, USA.*
Methenamine (p.223·1); monobasic sodium phosphate (p.1193·2); salol (p.82·2); methylene blue [methylthioninium chloride] (p.1012·3); hyoscyamine sulfate (p.469·3).
Urinary-tract infections.

Urimax *Integrity, USA.*
Methenamine (p.223·1); monobasic sodium phosphate (p.1193·2); salol (p.82·2); methylene blue [methylthioninium chloride] (p.1012·3); hyoscyamine sulfate (p.469·3).
Lower urinary-tract disorders.

Urinase *Eagle, Austral.*
Saw palmetto (p.1491·2); echinacea (p.1606·2); maize (p.1599·3); buchu (p.1587·2); hydrastis (p.1621·1); sassafras; bearberry (p.1583·3); minerals.
Prostatitis; urinary bladder disorders.

Urinex (nouvelle formule) *Kern, Switz.*
Birch (p.1585·2); buchu (p.1587·2); barbiflore; bearberry (p.1583·3); haricot bean; equisetum (p.1606·3); solidago virgaurea; meadowsweet (p.1631·2); calamus (p.1588·1); calendula (p.1589·2).
Urinary-tract disorders.

Urinol *Lennon, S.Afr.†*
Allopurinol (p.397·2).
Gout; hyperuricaemia.

Urinorm *Sanofi Winthrop, Spain.*
Benzbromarone (p.399·3).
Hyperuricaemia.

Urinox *Charoen, Thai.*
Norfloxacin (p.232·1).
Bacterial infections.

Urion
Zambon, Fr.; Byk Gulden, Ger.
Alfuzosin hydrochloride (p.833·2).
Benign prostatic hyperplasia.

Uripiser *Serral, Mex.*
Pipemidic acid (p.236·1).
Urinary-tract infections.

Uri-Plus Rubia *Homeocan, Canad.*
Homoeopathic preparation.

Uriprim *Bial, Port.*
Allopurinol (p.397·2).
Gout; hyperuricaemia.

Uripurinol *Azupharma, Ger.*
Allopurinol (p.397·2).
Gout; hyperuricaemia.

Urirex-K *Aspen, S.Afr.*
Hydrochlorothiazide (p.907·3); potassium chloride (p.1194·3).
Hypertension; oedema.

Urisan *Tedec Meiji, Spain.*
Pipemidic acid (p.236·1).
Urinary-tract infections.

Uriscreen *Medical Industries, Austral.*
Test for bacteriuria, haematuria, and pyuria.

Urisec *Odan, Canad.*
Urea (p.1127·3).
Dry skin conditions.

Urised *PolyMedica, USA.*
Methenamine (p.223·1); salol (p.82·2); methylene blue [methylthioninium chloride] (p.1012·3); benzoic acid (p.1134·2); atropine sulfate (p.461·1); hyoscyamine sulfate (p.469·3).
Lower urinary-tract infection or spasm.

Urisedamine *PolyMedica, USA.*
Methenamine mandelate (p.223·1); hyoscyamine (p.469·3).
Urinary-tract infections.

Urispadol *Abigo, Denm.*
Flavoxate hydrochloride (p.467·1).
Neurogenic bladder.

Urispas
Byk, Aust.; Byk, Belg.; Paladin, Canad.; Negma, Fr.; Shire, Hong Kong; Shire, Irl.; Byk, Neth.; Synthelabo, Port.; Searle, S.Afr.; Galenica, Switz.; Shire, UK; SmithKline Beecham, USA.
Flavoxate hydrochloride (p.467·1).
Urinary-tract disorders.

Uristix
Bayer, Austral.; Bayer, Canad.†; Bayer Diagnostics, Irl.; Bayer Diagnostics, UK; Bayer, USA.
Test for glucose and protein in urine.

Uristix 2 *Bayer Diagnostici, Ital.*
Test for leucocytes and nitrites in urine.

Uristix 4
Bayer, Canad.†; Bayer, USA.
Test for glucose, protein, nitrite, and leucocytes in urine.

Uritest *Bayer Diagnostics, Fr.*
Test for glucose, protein, nitrite, and leucocytes in urine.

Uritest 2 *Bayer Diagnostics, Fr.*
Test for leucocytes and nitrites in urine.

Uri-Tet *American Urologicals, USA†.*
Oxytetracycline hydrochloride (p.234·1).
Bacterial infections.

Uritrat NF *Libbs, Braz.*
Norfloxacin (p.232·1).
Bacterial infections.

Uritrate *Parke, Davis, Belg.*
Oxolinic acid (p.233·3).
Gram-negative bacterial infections of the urinary tract.

Urival *Zerboni, Mex.*
Nitrohydroxyquinoletina.
Urinary-tract infections.

Urizal *Novaquimica, Braz.*
Co-trimoxazole (p.193·3); phenazopyridine (p.78·1).
Urinary-tract infections.

Urizide *Rolab, S.Afr.*
Triamterene (p.986·1); hydrochlorothiazide (p.907·3).
Now known as Rolab-Triamterene/Hydrochlorothiazide.
Hypertension; oedema.

Urizine
Unison, Singapore; Unison, Thai.
Cinnarizine (p.413·1).
Cerebal and peripheral vascular disorders; migraine; motion sickness; vestibular disorders.

Urizone *Mer-National, S.Afr.*
Fosfomycin trometamol (p.208·2).
Urinary-tract Escherichia coli infections.

Urlix *Precimex, Mex.*
Nalidixic acid (p.227·1).

Urmidin *Ofimex, Mex.*
Pipemidic acid (p.236·1).

Uro 3000 *Aguettant, Fr.†*
Sodium chloride (p.1196·1), water, or glycine (p.1365·3) for irrigation.

Uro Angiografin *Schering, Spain.*
Meglumine amidotrizoate (p.1031·2).
Radiographic contrast medium.

Uro Bac Septin *Gilton, Braz.*
Co-trimoxazole (p.193·3); phenazopyridine (p.78·1).
Urinary-tract infections.

Uro Bactrim *Roche, Braz.*
Co-trimoxazole (p.193·3); phenazopyridine (p.78·1).
Urinary-tract infections.

Uro Batrox *Bergamo, Braz.*
Co-trimoxazole (p.193·3); phenazopyridine (p.78·1).
Urinary-tract infections.

Uro Duoctrim *Haller, Braz.*
Co-trimoxazole (p.193·3); phenazopyridine (p.78·1).
Urinary-tract infections.

Uro Fink *Fink, Ger.†*
Silver birch leaf (p.1585·2); solidago virgaurea; java tea (p.1625·1); black currant leaf; bearberry (p.1583·3).
Urinary-tract disorders.

Uro Furan *Bunker, Braz.*
Nitrofurantoin (p.230·3).
Urinary-tract infections.

Uro Heractrim *Heralds, Braz.*
Co-trimoxazole (p.193·3); phenazopyridine (p.78·1).
Urinary-tract infections.

Uro Septoprin *Medley, Braz.*
Co-trimoxazole (p.193·3); phenazopyridine (p.78·1).
Urinary-tract infections.

Urobac *Ofimex, Mex.*
Nitrofurantoin (p.230·3).

Urobacid
Tyrol, Aust.; Biochemie, Singapore.
Norfloxacin (p.232·1).
Bacterial infections.

Urobactam *Bristol-Myers, Spain.*
Aztreonam (p.154·2).
Bacterial infections.

Uro-Bacteracin *Teuto, Braz.*
Co-trimoxazole (p.193·3); phenazopyridine (p.78·1).
Urinary-tract infections.

Urobactrex *Sintofarma, Braz.*
Co-trimoxazole (p.193·3); phenazopyridine (p.78·1).
Urinary-tract infections.

Urobak *Shionogi, USA†.*
Sulfamethoxazole (p.254·1).
Bacterial infections.

Uro-Baxapril *Brasmedica, Braz.*
Co-trimoxazole (p.193·3); phenazopyridine (p.78·1).
Urinary-tract infections.

Uro-Beniktol N *Byk, Switz.†*
Neomycin sulfate (p.228·1).
Uro-Beniktol formerly contained neomycin sulfate and sulfamethizole.

Urobine *Eshcol, Singapore.*
Yohimbine hydrochloride (p.1681·3).

Urobioctrin *Cazi, Braz.*
Co-trimoxazole (p.193·3); phenazopyridine (p.78·1).
Urinary-tract infections.

Urobiotic *QIF, Braz.*
Phenazopyridine hydrochloride (p.77·3); ampicillin (p.150·3).
Urinary-tract infections.

Urobiotic-250 *Pfizer, USA.*
Oxytetracycline hydrochloride (p.234·1); sulfamethizole (p.253·3); phenazopyridine hydrochloride (p.77·3).
Genito-urinary infections.

Uroc *Lampugnani, Ital.*
Cinoxacin (p.182·2).
Urinary-tract infections.

Urocalun *Shinyaku, Singapore.*
Quercus stenophylla (p.1643·2).
Renal calculi.

Urocarb *Hamilton, Austral.*
Bethanechol chloride (p.1415·3).
Neurogenic bladder; urinary retention.

Urocarf *SPA, Ital.†*
Carfecillin sodium (p.160·3).
Urinary-tract infections.

Urocaudal *Pan Quimica, Spain.*
Triamterene (p.986·1).
Obesity; oedema.

Urocaudal Tiazida *Pan Quimica, Spain.*
Hydrochlorothiazide (p.907·3); triamterene (p.986·1).
Hypertension; oedema.

Uro-Cephoral *Merck, Ger.*
Cefixime (p.166·2).
Bacterial infections.

Urocit-K
Orphan, Austral.; Mission Pharmacal, Singapore; Mission Pharmacal, USA.
Potassium citrate (p.1186·1).
Renal calculi; urinary alkalinising agent.

Urocrasina *Sanobia, Port.*
Methenamine (p.223·1); piperazine hydrate (p.106·1); lithium benzoate (p.1629·1).
Urinary-tract disorders.

Urocridin *Fresenius, Ger.†*
Ethacridine lactate (p.1130·3).
Bladder irrigation for urinary-tract infections.

Uroctal *Almirall, Braz.*
Norfloxacin (p.232·1).
Urinary-tract infections.

Uroctrim *Legrand, Braz.*
Co-trimoxazole (p.193·3); phenazopyridine (p.78·1).
Urinary-tract infections.

Urodene *OFF, Ital.*
Pipemidic acid (p.236·1).
Urinary-tract infections.

Urodie *Abbott, Ital.*
Terazosin hydrochloride (p.980·1).
Benign prostatic hyperplasia.

Urodil Blasen-Nieren Arzneitee *Selz, Ger.†*
Java tea (p.1625·1); ononis (p.1644·1); birch leaf (p.1585·2); solidago virgaurea; fennel (p.1610·1); rose fruit (p.1389·3); peppermint leaf (p.1243·2); calendula (p.1589·2); liquorice (p.1231·2).
Urinary-tract disorders.

Urodil phyto *Selz, Ger.*
Birch leaf (p.1585·2); solidago virgaurea; java tea (p.1625·1).
Urinary-tract disorders.

Urodin *Streuli, Switz.*
Nitrofurantoin (p.230·3).
Urinary-tract infections.

Urodine *Interstate Drug Exchange, USA†; Schein, USA†.*
Phenazopyridine hydrochloride (p.77·3).
Irritation of the lower urinary tract.

Urodonal *Farmabraz, Braz.*
Theobromine (p.777·2); methenamine (p.223·1).
Hyperuricaemia.

Urodyn *Bionorica, Ger.†*
Solidago virgaurea.
Urinary-tract disorders.

Urofar *Elofar, Braz.*
Co-trimoxazole (p.193·3); phenazopyridine (p.78·1).
Urinary-tract infections.

Urofen *Teuto, Braz.*
Sulfamethoxypyridazine (p.256·1); nitrofurantoin (p.230·3); phenazopyridine hydrochloride (p.77·3).
Urinary-tract infections.

Uroflan *Biocur, Ger.*
Birch leaf (p.1585·2).
Urinary-tract disorders.

Uroflo *Abbott, Aust.*
Terazosin hydrochloride (p.980·1).
Benign prostatic hyperplasia.

Uroflox
Farmion, Braz.; Bial, Port.
Norfloxacin (p.232·1).
Bacterial infections.

Urofossat *Dreluso, Ger.*
Homoeopathic preparation.

Urogal *Galen, Mex.*
Pipemidic acid (p.236·1).
Urinary-tract infections.

Urogen *Prodotti, Braz.*
Nitrofurantoin (p.230·3).
Urinary-tract infections.

Urogesic
Atlantic, Singapore; Edwards, USA.
Phenazopyridine hydrochloride (p.77·3).
Irritation of the lower urinary tract.

Urogesic Blue *Edwards, USA.*
Methenamine (p.223·1); monobasic sodium phosphate (p.1193·2); salol (p.82·2); methylene blue [methylthioninium chloride] (p.1012·3); hyoscyamine sulfate (p.469·3).
Urinary-tract infections.

Urogliss *Montavit, Neth.*
Chlorhexidine hydrochloride (p.1138·2); lignocaine [lidocaine] hydrochloride (p.1313·2).
Catheterisation.

Urogliss-S *Montavit, Neth.*
Chlorhexidine hydrochloride (p.1138·2).
Catheterisation.

Urogobens Antiespasmo *Normon, Spain†.*
Phenazopyridine hydrochloride (p.77·3); nitrofurantoin (p.230·3); hyoscine butylbromide (p.468·2).
Urinary-tract infections; urinary-tract spasm.

Urografin *Schering, Aust.; Schering, Denm.; Schering, Ger.; Schering, Israel; Schering, Neth.; Schering, NZ; Schering, S.Afr.; Schering, Spain; Schering, Swed.; Schering, Switz.; Schering, UK.*
Meglumine amidotrizoate (p.1031·2); sodium amidotrizoate (p.1031·2).
Radiographic contrast medium.

Urografin Meglumin *Schering, Denm.*
Meglumine amidotrizoate (p.1031·2).
Radiographic contrast medium.

Urografina *Schering, Braz.; Schering, Port.*
Meglumine amidotrizoate (p.1031·2); sodium amidotrizoate (p.1031·2).
Radiographic contrast medium.

Urografine *Schering, Belg.*
Meglumine amidotrizoate (p.1031·2); sodium amidotrizoate (p.1031·2).
Radiographic contrast medium.

Urogram *FIRMA, Ital.*
Nalidixic acid (p.227·1).
Gram-negative bacterial infections of the genito-urinary tract.

Urogutt *Farmasa, Mex.; TTN, Thai.; Willmar, Thai.*
Saw palmetto (p.1491·2).
Benign prostatic hyperplasia.

Uro-KP-Neutral *Star, USA.*
Mineral preparation (p.1350·1).
Phosphorus supplement.

Urol mono *Hoyer, Ger.*
Solidago virgaurea.
Urinary-tract disorders.

uro-L 90 N *Loges, Ger.*
Homoeopathic preparation.

Urolene Blue *Star, USA.*
Methylene blue [methylthioninium chloride] (p.1012·3).
Cyanide poisoning; cystitis: urethritis; drug-induced methaemoglobinaemia.

Uro-Leotrim *Leoforma, Braz.*
Co-trimoxazole (p.193·3); phenazopyridine (p.78·1).
Urinary-tract infections.

Urolithico *Dansk-Flama, Braz.*
Persea americana; juglans regia; samambaia; phyllanthus niruri.
Urinary-tract disorders.

Urologicum PMD *Plantamed, Ger.*
Homoeopathic preparation.

Urologicum-Echtroplex *Weber & Weber, Ger.*
Homoeopathic preparation.

Urologin *Delta, Braz.*
Phenazopyridine hydrochloride (p.77·3).
Urinary-tract disorders.

Urolong *Organon, Aust.†.*
Nitrofurantoin (p.230·3).
Bacterial infections of the urinary tract.

Urolosin *Fher, Spain.*
Tamsulosin hydrochloride (p.978·3).
Benign prostatic hyperplasia.

Urolucosil *Lundbeck, Aust.†.*
Sulfamethizole (p.253·3).
Bacterial infections of the urinary tract.

Urolux Retro *Goldham, Ger.*
Meglumine amidotrizoate (p.1031·2); sodium amidotrizoate (p.1031·2).
Contrast medium for urinary-tract radiography.

Uro-Mag *Blaine, USA.*
Magnesium oxide (p.1233·2).
Hyperacidity; magnesium deficiency.

Urombrine *Dagra, Neth.†.*
Meglumine iodamide (p.1034·1).
Radiographic contrast medium.

Urombrine 420 *Dagra, Neth.†.*
Meglumine iodamide (p.1034·1); sodium iodamide (p.1034·1).
Pyelography.

Urometron *Pharmagen, S.Afr.†.*
Metronidazole (p.594·1).
Anaerobic bacterial infections; protozoal infections.

Uromil *IPRAD, Fr.*
Bearberry (p.1583·3); green tea (p.1681·1).
Formerly contained piperazine, methenamine, anhydrous dibasic sodium phosphate, morpholine mandelate, and theophylline.
Urinary-tract disorders.

Uromiro *Gerot, Aust.; Bracco, Port.; Bracco, Switz.*
Meglumine iodamide (p.1034·1).
Radiographic contrast medium.

Uromiro 24%, 36%, and 300 *Bracco, Ital.*
Meglumine iodamide (p.1034·1).
Radiographic contrast medium.

Uromiro 340 and 420 *Bracco, Ital.*
Meglumine iodamide (p.1034·1); sodium iodamide (p.1034·1).
Radiographic contrast medium.

Uromiro 300 Sodico *Bracco, Ital.*
Sodium iodamide (p.1034·1).
Radiographic contrast medium.

Uromiron *Schering, Braz.*
Meglumine iodamide (p.1034·1).
Radiographic contrast medium.

Uromitexan *Asta Medica, Aust.; Asta Medica, Austral.; Asta Medica, Belg.; Bristol, Canad.; Asta, Denm.; Asta Medica, Fin.; Asta Medica, Fr.; Asta Medica, Ger.; Asta Medica, Hong Kong; Asta Medica, Irl.; Asta Medica, Ital.; Sanfer, Mex.; Asta Medica, Neth.; Asta Medica, Norw.; Asta Medica, NZ; Asta Medica, Port.; Aventis, S.Afr.; Asta Medica, Singapore; Pras, Spain; Asta Medica, Swed.; Asta Medica, Switz.; Asta Medica, Thai.; Asta Medica, UK.*
Mesna (p.1011·3).
Prevention of urotoxicity due to oxazaphosphorine antineoplastics.

Uromix *Breves, Braz.*
Sulfamethizole (p.253·3); phenazopyridine (p.78·1); sulfacetamide (p.250·3).
Urinary-tract infections.

Uromont *Montavit, Aust.*
Dexamethasone (p.1067·1); chlorhexidine hydrochloride (p.1138·2); lignocaine [lidocaine] hydrochloride (p.1313·2).
Stricture prevention following transurethral procedures.

Uro-Munal *OM, Ger.*
Escherichia coli.
Urinary-tract infections.

Uromykol *Hoyer, Ger.*
Clotrimazole (p.382·1).
Fungal infections of skin and genito-urinary tract.

Uronalin *Vitae, Mex.*
Nalidixic acid (p.227·1).
Urinary-tract infections.

Uro-Nebacetin N *Byk Gulden, Ger.*
Neomycin sulfate (p.228·1).
Urinary-tract infections.

Uronefrex *Therabel, Belg†; Cassenne, Fr.; Robert, Spain.*
Acetohydroxamic acid (p.1571·3).
Adjunct in urinary-tract infections with urea-splitting organisms; renal calculi due to bacterial urease.

Uroneotrim *Neo Quimica, Braz.*
Co-trimoxazole (p.193·3); phenazopyridine (p.78·1).
Urinary-tract infections.

Uronid *Recordati, Ital.*
Flavoxate hydrochloride (p.467·1).
Urinary-tract disorders.

Uronor *Kanoldt, Ger.*
Potassium citrate (p.1186·1); potassium bicarbonate (p.1186·1); anhydrous citric acid (p.1596·2).
Renal calculi.

Uronorm *Wassermann, Ital.*
Cinoxacin (p.182·2).
Urinary-tract infections.

Uronovag *Novag, Mex.*
Pipemidic acid (p.236·1).

Uropac *EMS, Braz.*
Sulfamethoxypyridazine (p.256·1); nitrofurantoin (p.230·3); phenazopyridine hydrochloride (p.77·3).
Urinary-tract infections.

Uro-Pasc *Pascoe, Ger.*
Solidago virgaurea; taraxacum (p.1669·1).
Urinary-tract disorders.

Uro-pH Control *Apothecary, USA†.*
Cranberry (p.1600·2); vitamin C (p.1389·3).

Uro-Phosphate *ECR, USA.*
Methenamine (p.223·1); monobasic sodium phosphate (p.1193·2).
Urinary-tract infections.

Urophytum *Arkomedika, Fr.*
Buchu (p.1587·2); bearberry (p.1583·3).
Urinary-tract disorders.

Uropielon *Legrand, Braz.*
Ampicillin (p.150·3); phenazopyridine (p.78·1).
Urinary-tract infections.

Uropimid *CT, Ital.*
Pipemidic acid (p.236·1).
Urinary-tract infections.

Uropipedil *Fournier SA, Spain†.*
Pipemidic acid (p.236·1).
Urinary-tract infections.

Uropipemid *AF, Mex.*
Pipemidic acid (p.236·1).
Urinary-tract infections.

Uropirite *INQ, Braz.*
Phenazopyridine (p.78·1); methenamine (p.223·1).
Urinary-tract infections.

Uroplant forte *Biomo, Ger.*
Solidago virgaurea.
Urinary-tract disorders.

Uroplex *Sintofarma, Braz.*
Norfloxacin (p.232·1).
Bacterial infections.

Uroplus
Note. This name is used for preparations of different composition.
Kwizda, Aust.†.
Allopurinol (p.397·2); benzbromarone (p.399·3).
Gout; hyperuricaemia.
Shionogi, USA†.
Co-trimoxazole (p.193·3).
Bacterial infections; Pneumocystis carinii pneumonia.

Uropol *IMA, Braz.*
Co-trimoxazole (p.193·3); phenazopyridine (p.78·1).
Urinary-tract infections.

Uro-POS *Ursapharm, Ger.*
Urtica (p.1678·2).
Prostatic hyperplasia.

Uro-Pract *Ebewe, Aust.*
Sodium chloride (p.1196·1).
Bladder irrigation; maintenance of bladder catheters.

Uro-Pract N *Fresenius, Ger.†.*
Sodium chloride (p.1196·1).
Maintenance of bladder catheters.

Uropurat *Kwizda, Aust.*
Bearberry (p.1583·3); herniaria (p.1619·2); equisetum (p.1606·3); ononis (p.1644·1).
Urinary-tract disorders.

Uropyrine *Pharmacobel, Belg.*
Phenazopyridine hydrochloride (p.77·3).
Urinary-tract infections.

Uroqid-Acid *Beach, USA.*
Methenamine mandelate (p.223·1); monobasic sodium phosphate monohydrate (p.1193·2).
Urinary-tract infections.

Uroquidan *Serono, Spain.*
Urokinase (p.988·1).
Intra-ocular haemorrhage; thromboembolic disorders.

Uroquina *Rhone-Poulenc Rorer, Mex.*
Pefloxacin (p.234·3).

Urorenal *Schwabe, Ger.*
Birch leaf (p.1585·2).
Urinary-tract disorders.

Uro-Ripirin *Pharmacia Upjohn, Ger.*
Emepronium carrageenate (p.466·3).
Urinary-tract disorders.

Urosalin *Heralds, Braz.*
Methenamine (p.223·1); methylene blue [methylthioninium chloride] (p.1012·3).
Urinary-tract infections.

Urosan *AGIPS, Ital.*
Pipemidic acid (p.236·1).
Urinary-tract infections.

Uroseptin *Gilton, Braz.*
Phenazopyridine (p.78·1); methylene blue [methylthioninium chloride] (p.1012·3); methenamine mandelate (p.223·1); papaverine (p.1648·1).
Urinary-tract infections.

Uro-Septiolan *Climax, Braz.*
Co-trimoxazole (p.193·3); phenazopyridine (p.78·1).
Urinary-tract infections.

Uroseptol *Fresenius Kabi, Ger.*
Ethacridine lactate (p.1130·3).
Urinary-tract infections.

Urosetic *Finmedical, Ital.*
Pipemidic acid (p.236·1).
Urinary-tract infections.

Urosin *Roche, Aust.; Boehringer Mannheim, Ger.†.*
Allopurinol (p.397·2).
Gout; hyperuricaemia; renal calculi.

Urosiphon *Pierre Fabre Sante, Fr.*
Java tea (p.1625·1).
Diuretic; slimming aid.

Urospasmon *Heumann, Ger.*
Nitrofurantoin (p.230·3); sulfadiazine (p.251·1); phenazopyridine hydrochloride (p.77·3).
Urinary-tract infections.

Urospasmon sine *Heumann, Ger.*
Nitrofurantoin (p.230·3); sulfadiazine (p.251·1).
Urinary-tract infections.

Urospasmon sine phenazopyridino *Sanova, Aust.†.*
Nitrofurantoin (p.230·3); sulfadiazine (p.251·1).

Urostei *Steigerwald, Ger.*
Birch leaf (p.1585·2); solidago virgaurea; java tea (p.1625·1).
Urinary-tract disorders.

Uro-Stilloson *Farco, Ger.*
Dexamethasone (p.1067·1); lignocaine [lidocaine] hydrochloride (p.1313·2); chlorhexidine gluconate (p.1138·2).
Urinary-tract disorders.

Uro-Tablinen *Lichtenstein, Ger.*
Nitrofurantoin (p.230·3).
Urinary-tract infections.

Uro-Tainer
Note. This name is used for preparations of different composition.
Braun, Belg.
Chlorhexidine acetate (p.1138·2).
Urinary catheter care; urinary-bladder lavage.
Isramedcom, Israel.
Sodium chloride (p.1196·1).
Maintenance of indwelling urinary catheters.

Uro-Tainer M *CliniMed, UK.*
Sodium chloride (p.1196·1).
Vehicle for intravesical administration of drugs.

Uro-Tainer Solutio R *Vifor Medical, Switz.†.*
Citric acid monohydrate (p.1596·2); gluconolactone; light magnesium carbonate (p.1232·3).
Urinary catheter care.

Uro-Tainer Solution R *CliniMed, UK.*
Citric acid (p.1596·2); gluconolactone; light magnesium carbonate (p.1232·3).
Urinary catheter care.

Uro-Tainer Suby G *Vifor Medical, Switz.†; CliniMed, UK.*
Citric acid (p.1596·2); light magnesium oxide (p.1233·2); sodium bicarbonate (p.1186·2).
Urinary catheter care.

Urotal *Lemery, Mex.*
Pipemidic acid (p.236·1).

Uro-Tarivid *Hoechst Marion Roussel, Ger.*
Ofloxacin (p.232·3).
Urinary-tract infections.

Uro-Teutrim *Teuto, Braz.*
Co-trimoxazole (p.193·3); phenazopyridine (p.78·1).
Urinary-tract infections.

Uro-Trac *Apothecary, USA†.*
Phenazopyridine hydrochloride (p.77·3).

Urotractan *Klinge, Ger.*
Methenamine hippurate (p.223·1).
Urinary-tract infections.

Urotractin *Eurodrug, Hong Kong; SmithKline Beecham, Ital.; Eurodrug, Singapore; Eurodrug, Thai.*
Pipemidic acid (p.236·1).
Urinary-tract infections.

Urotrate *Parke, Davis, Fr.†.*
Oxolinic acid (p.233·3).
Urinary-tract infections.

Urotril *QIF, Braz.*
Nitroxoline (p.231·3); phenazopyridine hydrochloride (p.77·3).
Urinary-tract infections.

Urotrol *Almirall, Spain.*
Tolterodine tartrate (p.474·2).
Bladder instability.

Urotruw S *Truw, Ger.†.*
Homoeopathic preparation.

Uroval *FIRMA, Ital.*
Pipemidic acid (p.236·1).
Genito-urinary-tract infections.

Uro-Vaxom *Sanofi Synthelabo, Ger.; Knoll, Mex.; OM, Port.; OM, Switz.*
Escherichia coli.
Urinary-tract infections.

Urovison *Schering, Aust.; Schering, Ger.; Schering, Neth.*
Meglumine amidotrizoate (p.1031·2); sodium amidotrizoate (p.1031·2).
Radiographic contrast medium.

Urovist *Berlex, USA†.*
Meglumine amidotrizoate (p.1031·2) or sodium amidotrizoate (p.1031·2).
Radiographic contrast medium.

Uroxacin *Malesci, Ital.*
Cinoxacin (p.182·2).
Urinary-tract infections.

Uroxate *General Drugs, Thai.*
Flavoxate hydrochloride (p.467·1).
Urinary-tract disorders.

UroXatral *Sanofi Synthelabo, Ger.*
Alfuzosin hydrochloride (p.833·2).
Benign prostatic hyperplasia.

Uroxazol *Bunker, Braz.*
Co-trimoxazole (p.193·3); phenazopyridine (p.78·1).
Urinary-tract infections.

Uroxin
Note. This name is used for preparations of different composition.
Unison, Singapore.
Ciprofloxacin hydrochloride (p.182·3).
Bacterial infections.

Unison, Thai.
Ciprofloxacin (p.182·3).
Bacterial infections.

Julphar, UAE.
Norfloxacin (p.232·1).
Bacterial infections.

Uroxina *Farmalab, Braz.*
Pipemidic acid (p.236·1).
Urinary-tract infections.

Urozyl-SR *Restan, S.Afr.†.*
Allopurinol (p.397·2).
Gout; hyperuricaemia.

Urprosan *Biohorm, Spain†.*
Finasteride (p.1477·2).
Benign prostatic hyperplasia.

Ursacol *Zambon, Braz.; Zambon, Ital.*
Ursodeoxycholic acid (p.1677·2).
Biliary-tract disorders.

Ursilon *Ibi, Ital.*
Ursodeoxycholic acid (p.1677·2).
Biliary-tract disorders.

Ursinus Inlay-Tabs *Novartis, USA.*
Pseudoephedrine hydrochloride (p.1099·2); aspirin (p.14·2).
Upper respiratory-tract symptoms.

Urso *Axcan, Canad.; Heumann, Ger.; Tokyo Tanabe, Jpn†; Axcan, USA.*
Ursodeoxycholic acid (p.1677·2).
Biliary-tract disorders; cholesterol gallstones; gastrointestinal disorders; hepatic disorders; hyperlipidaemia.

Urso Mix *Niddapharm, Ger.*
Chenodeoxycholic acid (p.1594·1); ursodeoxycholic acid (p.1677·2).
Cholesterol gallstones.

Ursobil *ABC, Ital.*
Ursodeoxycholic acid (p.1677·2).
Biliary-tract disorders.

Ursobilane *Estedi, Spain.*
Ursodeoxycholic acid (p.1677·2).
Gallstones.

The symbol † denotes a preparation no longer actively marketed

Ursochol *Zambon, Belg.; Zambon, Ger.; Zambon, Neth.; Zambon, Spain; In-pharzam, Switz.*
Ursodeoxycholic acid (p.1677·2).
Cholesterol gallstones; primary biliary cirrhosis.

Ursodamor *Damor, Ital.*
Sodium succinate ursodeoxycholate (p.1677·3).
Biliary-tract disorders.

Ursodiol *Bioprogress, Ital.*
Ursodeoxycholic acid (p.1677·2).
Biliary-tract disorders.

Ursofalk *Merck, Aust.; Orphan, Austral.; Codali, Belg.; Jouveinal, Canad.†; Falk, Ger.; Falk, Hong Kong; Antigen, Irl.; Knoll, Ital.; Farmasa, Mex.; Falk, Neth.; Rhone-Poulenc Rorer, Port.; Falk, Singapore; Meda, Swed.; Phardi, Switz.; Falk, Thai.; Cortecs, UK.*
Ursodeoxycholic acid (p.1677·2).
Cholesterol gallstones; liver disorders; primary biliary cirrhosis.

Ursofalk + Chenofalk *Falk, Ger.*
White capsules, ursodeoxycholic acid (Ursofalk) (p.1677·2); yellow-orange capsules, chenodeoxycholic acid (Chenofalk) (p.1594·1).
Cholesterol gallstones.

Ursoflor *SoSe, Ital.*
Ursodeoxycholic acid (p.1677·2).
Biliary-tract disorders.

Ursogal *Galen, UK.*
Ursodeoxycholic acid (p.1677·2).
Cholesterol gallstones.

Ursolac *Biomedica, Ital.*
Ursodeoxycholic acid (p.1677·2).
Biliary-tract disorders.

Ursolisin *Magis, Ital.*
Ursodeoxycholic acid (p.1677·2).
Biliary-tract disorders.

Ursolit *CTI, Israel.*
Ursodeoxycholic acid (p.1677·2).
Gallstones; liver disorders.

Ursolite *Vita, Spain.*
Ursodeoxycholic acid (p.1677·2).
Gallstones.

Ursolvan *Synthelabo, Fr.; Synthelabo, Hong Kong; Sanofi Synthelabo, Singapore.*
Ursodeoxycholic acid (p.1677·2).
Cholestasis; cholesterol gallstones.

Urson *Ripari-Gero, Ital.*
Sodium succinate ursodeoxycholate (p.1677·3).
Biliary-tract disorders.

Ursoproge *Proge, Ital.*
Ursodeoxycholic acid (p.1677·2).
Biliary-tract disorders.

Ursosan *Tokyo Tanabe, Hong Kong.*
Ursodeoxycholic acid (p.1677·2).
Biliary disorders; cholesterol gallstones; liver disorders.

Ursotan *Aventis, S.Afr.*
Ursodeoxycholic acid (p.1677·2).
Cholesterol gallstones.

Urtias *BASF, Ger.†*
Allopurinol (p.397·2).
Gout; hyperuricaemia.

Urtica Plus *Europharm, Aust.*
Urtica (p.1678·2).
Urinary-tract disorders.

Urtica Plus N *Hoyer, Ger.†*
Urtica (p.1678·2).
Benign prostatic hyperplasia.

Urticalcin *Bioforce, Canad.†; Bioforce, Ger.; Bioforce, Switz.*
Homoeopathic preparation.

Urticaprostat uno *Azupharma, Ger.*
Urtica (p.1678·2).
Benign prostatic hyperplasia.

Urticur *Biocur, Ger.†*
Urtica (p.1678·2).
Benign prostatic hyperplasia.

Urtigen *Sons, Mex.*
Astemizole (p.409·1).
Hypersensitivity.

Urtipret *Bionorica, Ger.; Bionorica, Thai.*
Urtica (p.1678·2).
Benign prostatic hyperplasia.

Urtivac *Darrow, Braz.*
Allergen extracts (p.1575·3).
Hyposensitisation.

Urtivit *Bional, Ger.*
Urtica (p.1678·2).
Benign prostatic hyperplasia.

Urupan *Merckle, Ger.*
Dexpanthenol (p.1602·3).
Wounds.

Useton *Farmedica, Braz.*
Buclizine (p.411·1); carnitine; lysine; gamma-aminobutyric acid; vitamin B substances (p.1350·1).
Reduced appetite; tonic.

Uskan *Desitin, Ger.; Cimex, Switz.†*
Oxazepam (p.697·1).
Anxiety; sleep disorders.

Usneabasan *Sanum-Kehlbeck, Ger.*
Homoeopathic preparation.

U-Spa *Sriprasit, Thai.*
Flavoxate hydrochloride (p.467·1).
Urinary-tract disorders.

Ustilakehl *Sanum-Kehlbeck, Ger.*
Homoeopathic preparation.

Ustimon *Sigmapharm, Aust.; Lacer, Spain†.*
Hexobendine hydrochloride (p.905·3).
Cardiac disorders.

Ustiosan *Kelemata, Ital.*
Procaine hydrochloride (p.1319·1); lignocaine [lidocaine] hydrochloride (p.1313·2); hydroxyquinoline sulfate (p.1622·2).
Minor wounds; skin irritation.

Utabon *Uriach, Spain.*
Oxymetazoline hydrochloride (p.1096·2).
Nasal congestion.

Utefos *Almirall, Spain.*
Tegafur (p.573·2).
Malignant neoplasms.

Uteplex *Wyeth Lederle, Fr.*
Trisodium uridine triphosphate.
Musculoskeletal disorders.

Uterovarol *Simoes, Braz.*
Viburnum prunifolium; hydrastis (p.1621·1); valerian (p.1678·3); potassium bromide.
Dysmenorrhoea.

Uticox *Squibb, Spain.*
Meloxicam (p.51·3).
Ankylosing spondylitis osteoarthritis; rheumatoid arthritis.

Utidol *Diba, Mex.*
Dipyrone (p.34·1).
Fever; pain.

Utilin *Sanum-Kehlbeck, Ger.*
Bacillus subtilis.
Immunotherapy.

Utilin N *Sanum-Kehlbeck, Ger.*
Bacillus subtilis.
Gout; musculoskeletal and joint disorders; skin disorders.

Utilin S *Sanum-Kehlbeck, Ger.*
Mycobacterium phlei.
Immunotherapy.

Utin *Cipla-Medpro, S.Afr.*
Norfloxacin (p.232·1).
Urinary-tract infections.

Utinor *Neopharmed, Ital.; Merck Sharp & Dohme, UK.*
Norfloxacin (p.232·1).
Bacterial infections of the urinary tract.

utk *TAD, Ger.*
Urtica (p.1678·2).
Benign prostatic hyperplasia.

Utovlan *Pharmacia, UK.*
Norethisterone (p.1485·1).
Breast cancer; endometriosis; menstrual disorders.

Utrim *Sanofi Winthrop, Braz.*
Co-trimoxazole (p.193·3); phenazopyridine (p.78·1).
Urinary-tract infections.

Utrogest *Kade, Ger.; Besins, Ger.*
Progesterone (p.1488·3).
Menopausal disorders.

Utrogestan *Asta Medica, Aust.; Piette, Belg.; Besins-Iscovesco, Fr.; Besins, Hong Kong; Hoechst Marion Roussel, Irl.; Besins-Iscovesco, Israel; Jaba, Port.; Scientific, S.Afr.; Besins-Iscovesco, Singapore; Seid, Spain; Besins-Iscovesco, Switz.; Piette, Thai.*
Progesterone (p.1488·3).
Benign breast disorders; dysfunctional uterine bleeding; endometriosis; female infertility; menopausal disorders; menstrual disorders; premature labour; threatened or recurrent miscarriage.

UV Face Broad Spectrum *Boots, Austral.†*
SPF 15+: Octinoxate (p.1517·3); ensulizole (p.1517·2); titanium dioxide (p.1126·1).
Sunscreen.

UV Protectant *Norwood, Canad.*
SPF 15: Avobenzone (p.1517·1); octinoxate (p.1517·3); oxybenzone (p.1518·1).
Sunscreen.

UV Sport Gel *Boots, Austral.*
SPF 15+: Octinoxate (p.1517·3); octisalate (p.1518·1); octocrilene (p.1518·1); avobenzone (p.1517·1).
Sunscreen.

UV Triplegard *Boots, Austral.*
SPF 15: Octinoxate (p.1517·3); oxybenzone (p.1518·1); titanium dioxide (p.1126·1).
SPF 30+: Octinoxate (p.1517·3); enzacamene (p.1517·2); zinc oxide (p.1128·2).
Sunscreen.

UV Triplegard Broad Spectrum - Water Resistant *Palmolive Skincare, Austral.†*
Stick SPF 15+: Octinoxate (p.1517·3); oxybenzone (p.1518·1); avobenzone (p.1517·1).
Sunscreen.

UV Triplegard Clear *Boots, Austral.†*
Octinoxate (p.1517·3); octisalate (p.1518·1); oxybenzone (p.1518·1).
Sunscreen.

UV Triplegard Hydrating Face Lotion *Boots, Austral.*
SPF 20: Octinoxate (p.1517·3); zinc oxide (p.1128·2); enzacamene (p.1517·2).
Sunscreen.

UV Triplegard Kids *Boots, Austral.*
SPF 30+: Octinoxate (p.1517·3); enzacamene (p.1517·2); zinc oxide (p.1128·2).
Sunscreen.

UV Triplegard Low Allergenic *Boots, Austral.†*
SPF 15+: Titanium dioxide (p.1126·1).
Sunscreen.

UV Triplegard Sensitive Skin *Boots, Austral.*
SPF 20: Titanium dioxide (p.1126·1).
Sunscreen.

UV Triplegard Sunscreen Cream - Water Resistant *Boots, Austral.†*
SPF 15+: Octinoxate (p.1517·3); oxybenzone (p.1518·1); titanium dioxide (p.1126·1).
Sunscreen.

UV Triplegard Sunstick & Lip Balm *Boots, Austral.*
SPF 30+: Octinoxate (p.1517·3); octocrilene (p.1518·1); zinc oxide (p.1128·2).
Sunscreen.

UV Triplegard Toddler Block Broad Spectrum Lotion - Water Resistant *Boots, Austral.†*
SPF 15+: Octinoxate (p.1517·3); oxybenzone (p.1518·1); titanium dioxide (p.1126·1).
Sunscreen.

UV Triplegard Watersports *Boots, Austral.*
SPF 30 +: Octinoxate (p.1517·3); titanium dioxide (p.1126·1).
Sunscreen.

UV Ultrablock *Colgate Palmolive, NZ.*
SPF 15+; SPF 50+: Padimate O (p.1518·2); oxybenzone (p.1518·1).
Sunscreen.

Uvacin *Lichtwer, UK.*
Taraxacum (p.1669·1); bearberry (p.1583·3).
Female bladder discomfort.

Uvadex *Therakos, USA.*
Methoxsalen (p.1118·3).
T-cell lymphoma.

Uvalysat *Ysatfabrik, Ger.*
Bearberry leaf (p.1583·3).
Urinary-tract infections.

Uvamin *Mepha, Israel.*
Nitrofurantoin (p.230·3).
Urinary-tract infections.

Uvamine retard *Mepha, Switz.*
Nitrofurantoin (p.230·3).
Urinary-tract infections.

Uva-Ursi Complex *Blackmores, Austral.*
Taraxacum (p.1669·1); galium aparine (p.1596·3); bearberry (p.1583·3); buchu (p.1587·2).
Bloating; dysuria; fluid retention; prostatitis; renal calculi; urethritis.

Uva-Ursi Plus *Eagle, Austral.*
Bearberry (p.1583·3); parsley (p.1648·3); taraxacum (p.1669·1); zanthoxylum (p.1682·1).
Cystitis; fluid retention.

Uvavit *Kolassa, Aust.*
Multivitamin and mineral preparation (p.1350·1).
Nutritional supplement in pregnancy.

Uvedose *Crinex, Fr.*
Colecalciferol (p.1391·1).
Vitamin D deficiency.

Uvega *Hormona, Mex.*
Lignocaine [lidocaine] hydrochloride (p.1313·2).
Otitis externa.

Uveline *Martin, Fr.*
Methylhydroxyquinoline metilsulfate (p.1635·2).
Eye disorders.

Uvestat *Bournonville, Belg.†*
Methylhydroxyquinoline metilsulfate (p.1635·2).
Light-induced eye irritation.

Uvesterol *Crinex, Fr.*
Multivitamin preparation (p.1350·1).

Uvesterol D *Crinex, Fr.*
Ergocalciferol (p.1391·2).
Vitamin D deficiency.

UVGuard *Schering-Plough, Canad.†*
Octinoxate (p.1517·3); avobenzone (p.1517·1); oxybenzone (p.1518·1).
Sunscreen.

Uvicin *Steigerwald, Ger.*
Homoeopathic preparation.

Uvicol *Monot, Fr.*
Actinoquinol (p.1573·1); oxedrine hydrochloride (p.950·3).
Eye disorders.

Uvimag B₆ *Lophal, Fr.*
Magnesium glycerophosphate (p.1191·1); pyridoxine hydrochloride (p.1386·3).
Vitamin and mineral supplementation.

Uvirgan mono *Kanoldt, Ger.*
Cucurbita (p.1601·1).
Urinary-tract disorders.

Uvirgan N *Kanoldt, Ger.*
Urtica (p.1678·2); cucurbita (p.1601·1); ononis (p.1644·1).
Urinary-tract disorders.

Uvistat *Windsor, UK.*
SPF 6; SPF 8: Mexenone (p.1517·3); octinoxate (p.1517·3).
SPF 10: Mexenone (p.1517·3); octinoxate (p.1517·3); avobenzone (p.1517·1); titanium dioxide (p.1126·1).

SPF 15: Octinoxate (p.1517·3); avobenzone (p.1517·1).
Sunscreen.

Uvistat Babysun Cream *Windsor, UK.*
SPF 12: Mexenone (p.1517·3); octinoxate (p.1517·3).
Sunscreen.

Uvistat Lipscreen *Boehringer Ingelheim, Irl.*
SPF 25; SPF 30: Avobenzone (p.1517·1); titanium dioxide (p.1126·1).
Sunscreen.

Uvistat Lotion *Boehringer Ingelheim, Irl.*
SPF 15; SPF 20; SPF 30; SPF 50: Octinoxate (p.1517·3); avobenzone (p.1517·1); titanium dioxide (p.1126·1).
Sunscreen.

Uvistat UV Protectant *Windsor, Irl.†*
SPF 6; SPF 8; SPF 15: Mexenone (p.1517·3); octinoxate (p.1517·3); avobenzone (p.1517·1); titanium dioxide (p.1126·1).
Sunscreen.

Uvistik *Air Link, Austral.†*
Octinoxate (p.1517·3); avobenzone (p.1517·1).
Sunscreen.

Uxicolin *Pisa, Mex.*
Suxamethonium chloride (p.1340·1).
Depolarising neuromuscular blocker.

3V *Julphar, UAE.*
Thiamine nitrate (p.1385·1); pyridoxine hydrochloride (p.1386·3); cyanocobalamin (p.1388·1).
Migraine; neuralgia; neuritis; neuropathy; rheumatic pain.

V Day 1612 *PP Lab, Thai.*
Prosultiamine; vitamin B₆; vitamin B₁₂ (p.1350·1).
Vitamin B deficiency.

V Day Lozenges *PP Lab, Thai.*
Dequalinium chloride (p.1143·1).
Mouth and throat infections.

V Day Milk *PP Lab, Thai.*
Aluminium hydroxide (p.1210·3); magnesium hydroxide (p.1233·1); simeticone (p.1249·2).
Gastric hyperacidity.

V Day Zepam *PP Lab, Thai.*
Diazepam (p.674·3).
Anxiety; insomnia.

V Infusionslosung *Baxter, Ger.*
Electrolyte infusion (p.1180·1).
Fluid and electrolyte disorders.

Vaben *Rafa, Israel.*
Oxazepam (p.697·1).
Agitation; anxiety.

Vabeta *Oftalder, Port.*
Betamethasone valerate (p.1063·2).
Skin disorders.

Vabicin *Vana, Thai.*
Spectinomycin hydrochloride (p.248·2).
Gonorrhoea.

Vabon *Biolab, Thai.*
Danazol (p.1468·3).
Benign breast disorders; endometriosis; gynaecomastia; hereditary angioedema; mennorhagia; precocious puberty.

Vac Antigrip Frac *Berna, Spain; Leti, Spain.*
An influenza vaccine (p.1544·3).
Active immunisation.

Vac Antimeningococic A+C *Pasteur Merieux, Spain.*
A meningococcal vaccine (groups A and C) (p.1550·1).
Active immunisation.

Vac Antiparotiditis *Pasteur Merieux, Spain†.*
A mumps vaccine (p.1551·1).
Active immunisation.

Vac Antipolio Or *Medeva, Spain; Alcala, Spain.*
An oral poliomyelitis vaccine (p.1558·2).
Active immunisation.

Vac Antipolio Oral *Glaxo Wellcome, Spain†.*
An oral poliomyelitis vaccine (p.1558·2).
Active immunisation.

Vac Antirrabica *Pasteur Merieux, Spain.*
A rabies vaccine (p.1560·2).
Active immunisation.

Vac Antirrubeola *Evans, Spain; Pasteur Merieux, Spain; SmithKline Beecham, Spain.*
A rubella vaccine (RA 27/3) (p.1562·3).
Active immunisation.

Vac Antitetanica *Medeva, Spain.*
A tetanus vaccine (p.1565·2).
Active immunisation.

Vac Antitifica Or *Medeva, Spain.*
An oral typhoid vaccine (inactivated strain Ty21a) (p.1566·3).
Active immunisation.

Vac Polio Sabin *SmithKline, Spain.*
An oral poliomyelitis vaccine (p.1558·2).
Active immunisation.

Vac Poliomielitica *Berna, Spain.*
A poliomyelitis vaccine (p.1558·2).
Active immunisation.

Vac Triple MSD *Pasteur Merieux, Spain.*
A measles, mumps, and rubella vaccine (attenuated Enders, Jeryl Lynn, and Wistar RA 27/3 strains respectively) (p.1549·1).
Active immunisation.

Vacanyl *Vana, Thai.*
Terbutaline sulfate (p.776·2).
Obstructive airways disease.

Vaccin Catarrhal Berna, Belg.†
An inactivated vaccine containing: pneumococci; *Staphylococcus aureus; Staphylococcus albus;* streptococci; *Klebsiella pneumoniae; Moraxella catarrhalis; Haemophilus influenzae.*
Upper respiratory-tract infections.

Vaccin DTCP Pasteur Vaccins, Fr.
An adsorbed diphtheria, tetanus, pertussis, and poliomyelitis (inactivated) vaccine (p.1539·1).
Active immunisation.

Vaccin DTP Pasteur Vaccins, Fr.
A diphtheria, tetanus, and poliomyelitis (inactivated) vaccine (p.1539·1).
Active immunisation.

Vaccin Tab Berna, Switz.†
A typhoid vaccine (p.1566·3).
Active immunisation.

Vaccin TP Pasteur Vaccins, Fr.
A tetanus and poliomyelitis (inactivated) vaccine (p.1566·2).
Active immunisation.

Vaccino Antipiogeno Bruschettini, Ital.
A vaccine prepared from *Staphylococcus aureus, Pseudomonas aeruginosa, Escherichia coli, Streptococcus pyogenes,* and *Streptococcus pneumoniae.*
Active immunisation against pyogenic bacterial infections.

Vaccino Antipneumocatarrale Bruschettini, Ital.
A vaccine prepared from *Streptococcus pneumoniae, Streptococcus pyogenes, Haemophilus influenzae,* and *Moraxella catarrhalis.*
Bacterial infections of the respiratory tract.

Vaccino Difto Tetano ISI, Ital.
An adsorbed diphtheria and tetanus vaccine (p.1537·1).
Active immunisation.

Vaccino DPT ISI, Ital.
An adsorbed diphtheria, tetanus, and pertussis vaccine (p.1537·3).
Active immunisation.

Vaccino Tab Te Nuovo ISM, Ital.†
A typhoid, paratyphoid A and B, and tetanus vaccine.
Active immunisation.

Vacillin Vana, Thai.
Ampicillin trihydrate (p.151·1).
Bacterial infections.

Vacina Antipiogenica Sanus, Braz.
A vaccine prepared from: *Streptococcus pyogenes; Streptococcus pneumoniae; Staphylococcus aureus; Pseudomonas aeruginosa; Escherichia coli.*
Active immunisation against pyogenic bacterial infections.

Vacina Antipneumocatarral Sanus, Braz.
A vaccine prepared from *Streptococcus pyogenes; Streptococcus pneumoniae; Haemophilus influenzae; Moraxella catarrhalis.*
Bacterial infections of the respiratory tract.

Vacina Catarral Berna, Port.†
Pneumococci; *Staphylococcus aureus; Staphylococcus albus;* streptococci; *Klebsiella pneumoniae; Moraxella catarrhalis; Haemophilus influenzae.*

Vacina Dupla DT Butantan, Braz.
A diphtheria and tetanus vaccine (p.1537·1).
Active immunisation.

Vacina Triplice DPT Butantan, Braz.
A diphtheria, tetanus, and pertussis vaccine (p.1537·3).
Active immunisation.

Vacinolone Vana, Thai.
Triamcinolone acetonide (p.1080·1).
Skin disorders.

Vaclox Vana, Thai.
Cloxacillin (p.192·1).
Bacterial infections.

Vacolax Vana, Thai.
Bisacodyl (p.1212·2).
Constipation.

Vacontil
Medochemie, Singapore; Medochemie, Thai.
Loperamide hydrochloride (p.1231·3).
Diarrhoea.

Vacopan
Atlantic, Singapore; Vana, Thai.
Hyoscine butylbromide (p.468·2).
Gastro-duodenitis; nausea and vomiting; peptic ulcer; smooth muscle spasm.

Vacrax Samchully, Singapore.
Aciclovir (p.612·3).
Herpesvirus infections.

Vacudol Xixia, S.Afr.
Paracetamol (p.71·2); codeine phosphate (p.25·2); promethazine hydrochloride (p.423·2).
Fever; pain.

Vacudol Forte Xixia, S.Afr.
Paracetamol (p.71·2); codeine phosphate (p.25·2); caffeine (p.761·3); meprobamate (p.691·1).
Pain and associated tension.

Vaculin Biolab, Thai.
Co-dergocrine mesilate (p.1597·3).
Mental function disorders.

Vacuna Antigripal Leti, Spain.
Inactivated polyvalent influenza vaccines (whole virion or split virion) (p.1544·3).
Active immunisation.

Pasteur Merieux, Spain.
An influenza vaccine (p.1544·3).
Active immunisation.

Vadarex Bell, UK.
Methyl salicylate (p.55·1); menthol (p.1632·3).
Musculoskeletal pain.

Vademin-Z Roberts, USA; Hauck, USA.
Multivitamin and mineral preparation (p.1350·1).

Vadicate Inkeysa, Spain.
Vincamine hydrochloride (p.1680·1).
Cerebral trauma; cerebrovascular disorders; circulatory disorders of the eye, ear, nose, and throat; vestibular disorders.

Vadilex
Synthelabo, Fr.; Synthelabo, Hong Kong; Sanofi Synthelabo, Singapore.
Ifenprodil tartrate (p.912·3).
Cerebral and peripheral vascular disorders; premature labour; threatened abortion.

Vadinar Serral, Mex.
Dipyridamole (p.877·2).

Vadol Phyteia, Switz.†
Aspirin (p.14·2); caffeine (p.761·3).
Fever; pain.

Vadolax Ogna, Ital.
Cascara (p.1216·1); cynara (p.1601·3).
Constipation.

Vadosilan Mead Johnson, Mex.
Isoxsuprine (p.1625·1).
Peripheral and cerebral vascular disorders; premature labour.

Vag Oral IQB, Braz.
Allergen extracts (p.1575·3).
Hyposensitisation.

Vagaka Vana, Thai.
Mebendazole (p.102·2).
Worm infections.

Vagantin Riemser, Ger.
Methanthelinium bromide (p.470·2).
Gastrointestinal disorders.

Vagarsol Aspen, S.Afr.
Diiodohydroxyquinoline (p.590·2); cetylpyridinium chloride (p.1138·1); aminoacridine hydrochloride (p.1130·2); boric acid (p.1586·1).
Vaginal infections.

Vagi Biotic Honorterapica, Braz.
Nystatin (p.392·2); metronidazole (p.594·1); benzalkonium chloride (p.1133·2); urea (p.1127·3); muramidase (p.1638·1).
Vulvovaginal infections.

Vagi-C Artesan, Ger.; Cassella-med, Ger.; Taurus, Ger.
Ascorbic acid (p.1389·3).
Vaginal disorders.

Vagicillin Schur, Ger.
Neomycin sulfate (p.228·1).
Vaginal infections.

Vagicin Charoen, Thai.
Diiodohydroxyquinoline (p.590·2); nystatin (p.392·2); chloramphenicol (p.179·1).
Vaginal infections.

Vagifem
Novo Nordisk, Aust.; Novo Nordisk, Austral.; Novo Nordisk, Belg.; Novo Nordisk, Denm.; Novo Nordisk, Fin.; Novo Nordisk, Ger.; Novo Nordisk, Irl.; Novo Nordisk, Israel; Novo Nordisk, Ital.; Novo Nordisk, Neth.; Novo Nordisk, NZ; Novo Nordisk, Port.; Novo Nordisk, S.Afr.; Novo Nordisk, Singapore; Novo Nordisk, Swed.; Novo Nordisk, Switz.; Novo Nordisk, Thai.; Novo Nordisk, UK; Novo Nordisk, USA.
Estradiol (p.1473·1).
Atrophic vaginitis.

Isdin, Spain.
Estradiol (p.1473·1).
Menopausal disorders; osteoporosis.

Vagiflor Asche, Ger.
Lactobacillus acidophilus (p.1626·3).
Disorders of the vaginal flora; vaginitis.

Vagi-Gard Medicated Cream Lake, USA.
Benzocaine (p.1306·2); benzalkonium chloride (p.1133·2).
Vaginal irritation.

Vagi-Gard Medicated Disposable Douche
Lake, USA.
Octoxinol 9 (p.1346·3).
Vaginal irritation and discharge.

Vagi-Gard Personal Lubricating Gel Lake, USA.
Vaginal lubricant.

Vagi-Hex
Pierre Fabre, Ger.; Drossapharm, Switz.
Hexetidine (p.1146·3).
Vaginitis.

Vagil PP Lab, Thai.
Metronidazole (p.594·1).
Anaerobic bacterial infections.

Vagilen Farmigea, Ital.
Metronidazole (p.594·1).
Trichomoniasis.

Vagimax Prodotti, Braz.
Metronidazole (p.594·1); nystatin (p.392·2).
Vulvovaginal infections.

Vagimid Apogepha, Ger.
Metronidazole (p.594·1).
Anaerobic bacterial infections; protozoal infections.

Vaginex
Schmid, Canad.†; QHP, USA.
Tripelennamine hydrochloride (p.427·1).
External vaginal irritation.

Vaginyl DDSA Pharmaceuticals, UK.
Metronidazole (p.594·1).

Vagisan Wolff, Ger.
Lactic acid (p.1626·2); sodium lactate (p.1186·2).
Vaginitis.

Vagisil
Note. This name is used for preparations of different composition.
Combe, Canad.; Combe, Israel.
Benzocaine (p.1306·2); resorcinol (p.1122·2).
Vaginal irritation.

Combe, Ital.
Lignocaine [lidocaine] (p.1313·2); chlorothymol (p.1142·1).
Anal and vulvar pruritus.

Combe, UK.
Lignocaine [lidocaine] (p.1313·2).
Vaginal and rectal pruritus.

Combe, USA.
Cream: Benzocaine (p.1306·2); resorcinol (p.1122·2).
Skin disorders.

Topical powder: Aloes (p.1210·1); liquid paraffin (p.1407·1); benzethonium chloride (p.1134·2).
Vaginal disorders.

Vagistat Bristol-Myers Squibb, USA.
Tioconazole (p.395·1).
Vulvovaginal candidiasis.

Vagitrene Ache, Braz.
Wheat germ.
Vulvovaginal disorders.

Vagitrin-N Bunker, Braz.
Dexamethasone (p.1067·1); nystatin (p.392·2); neomycin sulfate (p.228·1); tyrothricin (p.267·1); sodium propionate (p.393·2); boric acid (p.1586·1).
Vulvovaginal infections.

Vagitrol-V Syntex, Mex.
Fluocinolone acetonide (p.1071·1); metronidazole (p.594·1); nystatin (p.392·2).
Cervicitis; vaginitis; vulvitis.

Vagmicor Zerboni, Mex.
Ketoconazole (p.389·1).

Vagmycin Bristol-Myers Squibb, S.Afr.
Tetracycline (p.258·3); amphotericin B (p.377·2).
Vaginal infections.

Vagoclyss Grossmann, Switz.
Lactic acid (p.1626·2).
Vaginal infections and irritation.

Vagolisal Biotekfarma, Ital.†
Cimetidine (p.1216·3).
Gastritis and duodenitis associated with acid hypersecretion; peptic ulcer.

Vagomine Qualiphar, Belg.
Dimenhydrinate (p.415·2).
Motion sickness; nausea; vertigo; vomiting.

Vagopax Jaba, Port.
Propinox.
Smooth muscle spasm.

Vagoplex Makros, Braz.
Reserpine (p.967·3); homatropine methylbromide (p.468·1); hyoscine hydrobromide (p.468·2).
Smooth muscle spasm.

Vagostabyl Leurquin, Fr.
Crataegus (p.1600·2); calcium lactate (p.1188·2); melissa (p.1632·2); magnesium thiosulfate (p.1024·2).
Nervous disorders.

Vagostal Cantabria, Spain.
Famotidine (p.1225·3).
Gastro-oesophageal reflux; peptic ulcer; Zollinger-Ellison syndrome.

Vagostesyl Gross, Braz.
Atropine sulfate (p.461·1); papaverine hydrochloride (p.1648·1); phenobarbital (p.355·1); leptolobium elegans; passion flower (p.1649·1).
Smooth muscle spasm.

Vagotrope-S Sanofi Synthelabo, Port.
Hyoscine butylbromide (p.468·2).

Vagyl Vana, Thai.
Metronidazole (p.594·1).
Amoebiasis; giardiasis; trichomoniasis.

Valamin 12 Pisa, Mex.
Hydroxocobalamin (p.1388·1).

Valatux Farmacologico Milanese, Ital.†
Dextromethorphan hydrobromide (p.1087·3).
Coughs.

Valavir Orion, Fin.
Valaciclovir hydrochloride (p.643·1).
Herpesvirus infections.

Valaxona United Nordic, Denm.
Diazepam (p.674·3).
Alcohol withdrawal syndrome; anxiety; spasticity.

Valbet Biolab, Thai.
Betamethasone valerate (p.1063·2).
Skin disorders.

Valbet-N Biolab, Thai.
Betamethasone (p.1063·1); neomycin (p.228·1).
Infected skin disorders.

Valbil
CHR, Ger.; CPH, Port.
Febuprol (p.1610·1).
Biliary-tract dyskinesia; dyspepsia.

Valcaps Pharmacaps, Mex.
Valproic acid (p.366·2).

Valclair Durbin, UK.
Diazepam (p.674·3).
Alcohol withdrawal syndrome; anxiety; epilepsy; premedication; skeletal muscle spasm.

Valcyte Roche, USA.
Valganciclovir hydrochloride (p.643·2).
Cytomegalovirus retinitis.

Valda
Bayer, Canad.
Menthol (p.1632·3); eucalyptol (p.1609·2); thymol (p.1158·3); terpin hydrate (p.1101·2); guaiacol (p.1092·1).
Coughs.

SmithKline Beecham Sante, Fr.; SmithKline Beecham, Hong Kong; SmithKline Beecham Consumer, Irl.; Sterling, Port.; Sterling Health, UK†.
Menthol (p.1632·3); eucalyptol (p.1609·2); thymol (p.1158·3); terpineol (p.1669·3); guaiacol (p.1092·1).
Upper respiratory-tract disorders.

Valda F3 Sterling Midy, Ital.†
Potassium fluoride (p.1376·2); sodium fluoride (p.1375·3); cicliomenol; enoxolone (p.34·3).
Dental disorders.

Valda Septol SmithKline Beecham Sante, Fr.†
Menthol (p.1589·3); eucalyptol (p.1609·2); enoxolone (p.34·3); cicliomenol.
Mouth and throat infections.

Valdatos Sterling Health, Spain.
Dextromethorphan hydrobromide (p.1087·3).
Coughs.

Valdefer Valdecasas, Mex.
Ferrous sulfate (p.1360·3).
Iron deficiency anaemia.

Valderma
Roche Consumer, Irl.; Roche Consumer, UK.
Cream: Potassium hydroxyquinoline sulfate (p.1654·2); chlorocresol (p.1141·3).
Acne.

Roche Consumer, Irl.; Roche Consumer, UK.
Soap: Triclocarban (p.1159·2).
Acne.

Valderma Active Roche Consumer, UK†.
Benzoyl peroxide (p.1111·1).
Acne.

Valdig-N Burger Ysatfabrik, Ger.
Convallaria (p.1599·1).
Heart failure.

Valdispert
Solvay, Belg.; Solvay, Ger.; Solvay, Neth.; Solvay, Port.; Solvay, Spain; Solvay, Switz.
Valerian (p.1678·3).
Insomnia; nervous disorders.

Valdispert comp Solvay, Ger.
Valerian (p.1678·3); lupulus (p.1629·3).
Anxiety; sleep disorders.

Valdorm Valeas, Ital.
Flurazepam monohydrochloride (p.685·3).
Insomnia.

Valeans Valeas, Ital.
Alprazolam (p.654·2).
Anxiety.

Valecid Depofarma, Ital.
Cefonicid sodium (p.168·1).
Lignocaine [lidocaine] hydrochloride (p.1313·2) is included in this preparation to alleviate the pain of injection.
Gram-negative bacterial infections.

Valena N Spreewald, Ger.
Hypericum (p.290·2); passion flower (p.1649·1); valerian (p.1678·3).
Anxiety; depression.

Valenium Kenyaku, Thai.
Diazepam (p.674·3).
Anxiety.

Valerbe Bride, Fr.
Valerian (p.1678·3); vitamins (p.1350·1).
Aid to smoking withdrawal.

Valerecen Abigo, Swed.
Valerian (p.1678·3).
Sedative.

Valergen Hyrex, USA.
Estradiol valerate (p.1473·2).
Female castration; female hypogonadism; menopausal vasomotor symptoms; prevention of breast engorgement; primary ovarian failure; prostatic cancer; vulval and vaginal atrophy.

Valerial Zambon, Belg.†
Valerian (p.1678·3).
Sleep disorders.

Valerian Vitaplex, Austral.
Motherwort (p.1637·3); valerian (p.1678·3); skullcap (p.1664·3); populus (p.1653·2); capsicum (p.1591·1).
Herbal sedative.

Valerian Plus Herbal Plus Formula 12 Vitelle, Austral.
Valerian (p.1678·3); passion flower (p.1649·1); dibasic potassium phosphate (p.1193·1); magnesium oxide (p.1233·2).
Insomnia; smooth muscle spasm.

Valeriana comp Hevert, Ger.
Diphenhydramine hydrochloride (p.416·1); pericarpium aurantii (p.1644·2); chamomile (p.1593·2); lupulus (p.1629·3); kava (p.1625·3); valerian (p.1678·3); peppermint oil (p.1243·3).
Nervous disorders; sleep disorders.

Valeriana forte Hevert, Ger.
Diphenhydramine hydrochloride (p.416·1); valerian (p.1678·3); lupulus (p.1629·3).
Sedative.

Valeriana mild *Hevert, Ger.*
Valerian (p.1678·3); passion flower (p.1649·1); lupulus (p.1629·3).
Nervous disorders; sleep disorders.

Valeriana Orto *Normon, Spain.*
Valerian (p.1678·3).
Insomnia; nervous disorders.

Valeric
Atlantic, Singapore; Vana, Thai.
Allopurinol (p.397·2).
Gout; hyperuricaemia.

Valerina Day Time *Lichtwer, UK.*
Valerian (p.1678·3); melissa (p.1632·2).
Strain; stress.

Valerina Night-Time *Lichtwer, UK.*
Valerian (p.1678·3); lupulus (p.1629·3); melissa (p.1632·2).
Insomnia.

Valerocalma *Piam, Ital.*
Centranthus ruber.
Insomnia; sedative.

Valertest *Hyrex, USA.*
Estradiol valerate (p.1473·2); testosterone enantate (p.1492·2).
Menopausal vasomotor symptoms; prevention of post-partum breast engorgement.

Valesono *Neves, Port.*
Valerian (p.1678·3); passion flower (p.1649·1).
Alcohol withdrawal syndrome; anxiety disorders; insomnia; smoking cessation.

Valeton *Rekah, Israel.*
Valerian (p.1678·3).
Nervous disorders.

Valette *Jenapharm, Ger.*
Ethinylestradiol (p.1476·2); dienogest (p.1471·2).
Androgen-dependent acne, seborrhoea, hirsutism, and alopecia in females; combined oral contraceptive.

Valherpes *Pensa, Spain.*
Valaciclovir hydrochloride (p.643·1).
Herpesvirus infections.

Valin Baldrian *Sanova, Aust.*
Valerian (p.1678·3); citronella oil (p.1596·3).
Nervous disorders; sleep disorders.

Valinor *Baxter, Fr.*
Amino-acid infusion (p.1350·1).
Parenteral nutrition.

Valiquid *Roche, Ger.*
Diazepam (p.674·3).
Anxiety disorders; muscular disorders; premedication; sleep disorders.

Valisone
Schering, Canad.; Schering, USA.
Betamethasone valerate (p.1063·2).
Scalp and skin disorders.

Valisone-G *Schering, Canad.*
Betamethasone valerate (p.1063·2); gentamicin sulfate (p.210·1).
Infected skin disorders.

Valium
Roche, Aust.; Roche, Austral.; Roche, Belg.; Roche, Braz.; Roche, Canad.; Roche, Fin.; Roche, Fr.; Roche, Ger.; Roche, Gr.; Roche, Israel; Roche, Ital.; Roche, Mex.; Roche, Neth.; Roche, Norw.; Roche, Port.; Roche, S.Afr.; Roche, Singapore; Roche, Spain; Roche, Swed.†; Roche, Switz.; Roche, Thai.; Roche, UK; Roche, USA.
Diazepam (p.674·3).
Alcohol withdrawal syndrome; anxiety disorders; cerebral spasticity; eclampsia; epilepsy; febrile convulsions; panic attacks; parasomnias; premedication; sedative; skeletal muscle spasm; sleep disorders; status epilepticus; tetanus.

Valken *Kener, Mex.*
Valproic acid (p.366·2).

Vallergan
Rhone-Poulenc Rorer, Austral.; Rhone-Poulenc Rorer, Denm.†; Rhone-Poulenc Rorer, Hong Kong; Rhone-Poulenc Rorer, Irl.; Rhone-Poulenc Rorer, Norw.; Aventis, NZ; Aventis, S.Afr.; Castlemead, UK.
Trimeprazine [alimemazine] tartrate (p.426·2).
Premedication; pruritus; sleep disorders; urticaria.

Valmane
Note.This name is used for preparations of different composition.
Medicopharm, Aust.; Byk, Braz.
Valepotriates (p.1678·3).
Anxiety disorders.
Solvay, Ger.; Vemedia, Neth.†.
Valerian (p.1678·3).
Anxiety disorders; nervous disorders; sleep disorders.

Valmarin Bad N *Hoernecke, Ger.†.*
Citronella oil (p.1596·3).
Bath additive; insomnia; nervous disorders.

Valocordin-Diazepam *Krewel, Ger.*
Diazepam (p.674·3).
Anxiety disorders; sleep disorders.

Valoid
Glaxo Wellcome, Hong Kong; Wellcome, Irl.; Glaxo Wellcome, NZ; Glaxo Wellcome, S.Afr.; CeNeS, UK.
Cyclizine (p.414·1), cyclizine hydrochloride (p.414·1), or cyclizine lactate (p.414·1).
Acid aspiration; nausea; vestibular disorders; vomiting.

Valontan *Recordati, Ital.*
Dimenhydrinate (p.415·2).
Motion sickness.

Valopride *Pharmafar, Ital.*
Bromopride (p.1215·1).
Gastrointestinal disorders.

Valoran
Medochemie, Hong Kong; Medochemie, Thai.
Cefotaxime sodium (p.169·1).
Bacterial infections.

Valoron
Parke, Davis, Belg.; Parke, Davis, S.Afr.; Parke, Davis, Switz.
Tilidate hydrochloride (p.88·2).
Pain.

Valoron N *Godecke, Ger.*
Tilidate hydrochloride (p.88·2).
Naloxone hydrochloride (p.1014·3) is included in this preparation to discourage abuse.
Pain.

Valpakine *Sanofi Winthrop, Braz.*
Sodium valproate (p.366·3).
Bipolar disorder; epilepsy.

Valparin *Torrent, Thai.*
Sodium valproate (p.366·3).
Epilepsy.

Valpeda *Roche Consumer, UK.*
Halquinol (p.214·1).
Skin infections.

Valpiform *General Dietary, UK.*
A range of gluten-free foods (p.1350·1).

Valpinax *Crinos, Ital.*
Octatropine methylbromide (p.470·3); diazepam (p.674·3).
Gastrointestinal spasm.

Val-Plus *Edmond Pharma, Ital.*
Valerian (p.1678·3); passion flower (p.1649·1).
Insomnia; sedative.

Valporal *Teva, Israel.*
Valproic acid (p.366·2) or sodium valproate (p.366·3).
Epilepsy.

Valpression *Menarini, Ital.*
Valsartan (p.988·3).
Hypertension.

Valpridol *Alonga, Spain.*
Valaciclovir hydrochloride (p.643·1).
Herpesvirus infections.

Valpro
Alphapharm, Austral.; Alphapharm, Hong Kong.
Sodium valproate (p.366·3).
Epilepsy.

Valprosid *Armstrong, Mex.*
Valproic acid (p.366·2) or sodium valproate (p.366·3).
Epilepsy.

Valrian *Leiras, Fin.*
Valerian (p.1678·3).
Nervous disorders; sleep disorders.

Vals *Esteve, Spain.*
Valsartan (p.988·3).
Hypertension.

Valsera *Polifarma, Ital.*
Flunitrazepam (p.683·2).
Insomnia.

Valstar *Medeva, USA.*
Valrubicin (p.577·2).
Bladder cancer.

Valtran *Parke, Davis, Belg.*
Tilidate hydrochloride (p.88·2).
Naloxone hydrochloride (p.1014·3) is included in this preparation to discourage abuse.
Pain.

Valtrax *Valeas, Ital.*
Diazepam (p.674·3); isopropamide iodide (p.470·1).
Gastrointestinal spasm.

Valtrex
Glaxo Wellcome, Aust.; Glaxo Wellcome, Austral.; Glaxo Wellcome, Canad.; Glaxo Wellcome, Fin.; Glaxo Wellcome, Ger.; Cascan, Ger.; Glaxo Wellcome, Hong Kong; Wellcome, Irl.; Glaxo Wellcome, Israel; Glaxo Wellcome, Norw.; Glaxo Wellcome, Singapore; Wellcome, Spain; Glaxo Wellcome, Swed.; Wellcome, Switz.; Glaxo Wellcome, Thai.; Wellcome, UK; Glaxo Wellcome, USA.
Valaciclovir hydrochloride (p.643·1).
Herpesvirus infections.

Val-Uno *Edmond Pharma, Ital.*
Valerian (p.1678·3).
Insomnia; sedative.

Valverde boutons de fievre creme *Novartis Consumer, Switz.*
Melissa (p.1632·2).
Herpes simplex or labialis.

Valverde Dragees laxatives *Novartis Consumer, Switz.*
Fig (p.1227·1); senna (p.1248·2); petasites root.
Constipation.

Valverde Dragees pour la detente *Novartis Consumer, Switz.*
Petasites root; passion flower (p.1649·1); valerian (p.1678·3); melissa (p.1632·2).
Nervous disorders.

Valverde Dragees pour le coeur *Novartis Consumer, Switz.*
Crataegus leaves and fruit (p.1600·2); passion flower (p.1649·1); lupulus (p.1629·3); valerian root (p.1678·3).
Cardiac disorders.

Valverde Dragees pour le sommeil *Novartis Consumer, Switz.*
Lupulus (p.1629·3); valerian root (p.1678·3).
Sleep disorders.

Valverde Efeu *Novartis Consumer, Ger.*
Hedera helix.
Bronchitis; catarrh.

Valverde Gouttes pour le coeur *Novartis Consumer, Switz.*
Crataegus leaves and fruit (p.1600·2); passion flower (p.1649·1).
Cardiac disorders.

Valverde Hyperval *Zyma, Switz.†.*
Hypericum (p.290·2).
Anxiety; tension.

Valverde prostate capsules *Novartis Consumer, Switz.*
Urtica (p.1678·2).
Prostate disorders.

Valverde regulateur du transit intestinal granules *Novartis Consumer, Switz.*
Ispaghula (p.1229·1).
Constipation.

Valverde Sabal *Novartis Consumer, Ger.*
Saw palmetto (p.1491·2).
Benign prostatic hyperplasia.

Valverde Sirop contre la toux *Novartis Consumer, Switz.*
Hedera helix.
Respiratory-tract disorders associated with excess mucus.

Valverde Sirop laxatif *Novartis Consumer, Switz.*
Fig (p.1227·1); senna (p.1248·2).
Constipation.

Valverde Sirop pour le sommeil *Novartis Consumer, Switz.*
Valerian (p.1678·3).
Sleep disorders.

Valverde Tablettes contre la toux *Novartis Consumer, Switz.*
Hedera helix.
Respiratory-tract disorders associated with excess mucus.

Valverde Traubensilberkerze *Novartis Consumer, Ger.*
Cimicifuga (p.1595·2).
Menopausal disorders.

Valverde Vitalite *Novartis Consumer, Switz.*
Ginkgo biloba (p.1615·2).
Tonic.

Vamazole *Nakornpatana, Thai.*
Clotrimazole (p.382·1).
Fungal skin infections.

Vamin
Fresenius Kabi, Aust.; Fresenius Medical, Austral.; Pharmacia Upjohn, Belg.†; Baxter, Canad.; Fresenius Kabi, Denm.; Pharmacia Upjohn, Hong Kong; Pharmacia Upjohn, Irl.†; Pharmacia Upjohn, Neth.; Fresenius Kabi, Norw.; Baxter, NZ; Kabi Pharmacia, NZ; Fresenius Kabi, Port.; Fresenius Kabi, S.Afr.; Fresenius Kabi, Swed.; Fresenius, UK.
Amino-acid infusion with or without electrolytes (p.1350·1).
Parenteral nutrition.

Vamin con Glucosa *Pharmacia Upjohn, Spain.*
Amino-acid infusion with glucose and electrolytes (p.1350·1).
Parenteral nutrition.

Vamin EF *Fresenius Kabi, Ital.*
Amino-acid infusion (p.1350·1).
Parenteral nutrition.

Vamin 18EF *Fresenius Kabi, Singapore.*
Amino-acid infusion (p.1350·1).
Parenteral nutrition.

Vamin Glucose
Fresenius Medical, Austral.; Pharmacia Upjohn, Belg.†; Pharmacia Upjohn, Hong Kong; Pharmacia Upjohn, Irl.; Pharmacia Upjohn, Israel; Pharmacia Upjohn, Neth.; Fresenius Kabi, S.Afr.; Fresenius Kabi, Singapore; Pharmacia Upjohn, Thai.; Fresenius, UK.
Amino-acid, glucose, and electrolyte infusion (p.1350·1).
Parenteral nutrition.

Vamin Glukos
Fresenius Kabi, Denm.; Fresenius Kabi, Fin.; Fresenius Kabi, Norw.; Fresenius Kabi, Swed.
Amino-acid, glucose, and electrolyte infusion (p.1350·1).
Parenteral nutrition.

Vamin Glukos Combi *Fresenius Kabi, Fin.*
1 infusion, amino-acid, glucose, and electrolyte infusion (Vamin Glukos) (p.1350·1); 1 infusion, soya oil (Intralipid) (p.1378·1).
Parenteral nutrition.

Vamin mit Glukose *Fresenius Kabi, Aust.*
Amino-acid, glucose, and electrolyte infusion (p.1350·1).
Parenteral nutrition.

Vamin N *Fresenius Medical, Austral.*
Amino-acid and electrolyte infusion (p.1350·1).
Parenteral nutrition.

Vamin N/I *Fresenius Kabi, Fin.*
Amino-acid infusion (p.1350·1).
Parenteral nutrition.

Vamina *Fresenius Kabi, Switz.*
Amino-acid infusion (p.1350·1).
Parenteral nutrition.

Vamina Glucose *Fresenius Kabi, Switz.*
Amino-acid, carbohydrate, and electrolyte infusion (p.1350·1).
Parenteral nutrition.

Vamine *Fresenius Kabi, Fr.*
Amino-acid and electrolyte infusion with or without glucose (p.1350·1).
Parenteral nutrition.

Vaminolac
Fresenius Kabi, Denm.; Fresenius Kabi, Fin.; Fresenius Kabi, Norw.; Fresenius Kabi, Swed.
Amino-acid infusion (p.1350·1).
Parenteral nutrition.

Vaminolact
Fresenius Kabi, Aust.; Pharmacia Upjohn, Belg.†; Fresenius Kabi, Fr.; Pharmacia Upjohn, Hong Kong; Pharmacia Upjohn, Irl.; Pharmacia Upjohn, Neth.; Baxter, NZ; Kabi Pharmacia, NZ; Fresenius Kabi, Port.; Fresenius Kabi, Singapore; Fresenius Kabi, Switz.; Pharmacia Upjohn, Thai.; Fresenius, UK.
Amino-acid infusion (p.1350·1).
Parenteral nutrition.

Vanadiol *Farmavy, Braz.*
Vitamin B substances (p.1350·1).
Vitamin B deficiency; vitamin B supplement.

Vanafen *Vana, Thai.*
Chloramphenicol (p.179·1).
Bacterial eye or ear infections.

Vanafen-S
Atlantic, Hong Kong; Atlantic, Singapore.
Chloramphenicol (p.179·1).
Eye infections.

Vancenase
Schering, Canad.; Schering, USA.
Beclometasone dipropionate (p.1061·2).
Nasal polyps; rhinitis.

Vanceril
Schering, Canad.; Schering, USA.
Beclometasone dipropionate (p.1061·2).
Asthma.

VANCO *Cell Pharm, Ger.; Azupharma, Ger.*
Vancomycin hydrochloride (p.267·2).
Bacterial infections.

Vancocin
Lilly, Austral.; Lilly, Belg.; Lilly, Canad.; Lilly, Denm.; Lilly, Fin.; Lilly, Hong Kong; Lilly, Irl.; Lilly, Israel; Lilly, Mex.; Lilly, Neth.; Lilly, Norw.; Lilly, NZ; Lilly, S.Afr.; Lilly, Swed.; Lilly, Switz.; Lilly, Thai.; Lilly, UK; Lilly, USA.
Vancomycin hydrochloride (p.267·2).
Antibiotic-associated colitis; bacterial infections.

Vancocina
Lilly, Braz.; Lilly, Ital.; Lilly, Port.
Vancomycin hydrochloride (p.267·2).
Bacterial infections.

Vancocine *Lilly, Fr.*
Vancomycin hydrochloride (p.267·2).
Bacterial infections.

Vancoled
Lederle, Austral.; Lederle, Israel; Lederle, Switz.; Lederle, USA.
Vancomycin hydrochloride (p.267·2).
Bacterial infections.

Vancolin *Julphar, UAE.*
Vancomycin hydrochloride (p.267·2).
Bacterial infections.

Vanco-saar *Chephasaar, Ger.*
Vancomycin hydrochloride (p.267·2).
Bacterial infections.

Vancoscand *Scand Pharm, Swed.*
Vancomycin hydrochloride (p.267·2).
Gram-positive bacterial infections.

Vanco-Teva
Abic, Hong Kong; Teva, Israel.
Vancomycin hydrochloride (p.267·2).
Antibiotic-associated colitis; bacterial infections.

Vancox *Lemery, Mex.*
Vancomycin (p.269·1).
Bacterial infections.

Vanderbumin *Grossman, Mex.*
Albumin (p.724·1).
Barbiturate overdosage; burns; cerebral oedema; hypoproteinaemia; hypovolaemia; shock.

Vanderm *Agis, Israel.*
Methylprednisolone aceponate (p.1076·2).
Eczema; neurodermatitis.

Vandol *Schering-Plough, S.Afr.*
Vitamin A (p.1382·1); vitamin D (p.1391·1).
Skin disorders.

Vandral *Wyeth, Spain.*
Venlafaxine hydrochloride (p.312·2).
Depression.

Vanesten *Vana, Thai.*
Clotrimazole (p.382·1).
Fungal skin infections.

Vanex Expectorant *Abana, USA.*
Pseudoephedrine hydrochloride (p.1099·2); guaifenesin (p.1092·2); hydrocodone tartrate (p.42·2).
Coughs.

Vanex Forte *Abana, USA†.*
Phenylpropanolamine hydrochloride (p.1098·1); phenylephrine hydrochloride (p.1097·1); chlorpheniramine [chlorphenamine] maleate (p.412·1); mepyramine maleate (p.421·1).
Upper respiratory-tract symptoms.

Vanex Forte-R *Jones, USA†.*
Phenylpropanolamine hydrochloride (p.1098·1); chlorpheniramine [chlorphenamine] maleate (p.412·1).
Upper respiratory-tract disorders.

Vanex Grape *Abana, USA†.*
Dihydrocodeine tartrate (p.33·1); phenylephrine hydrochloride (p.1097·1); phenylpropanolamine hydrochloride (p.1098·1); chlorpheniramine [chlorphenamine] maleate (p.412·1).
Coughs and congestion.

Vanex-HD *Abana, USA.*
Phenylephrine hydrochloride (p.1097·1); chlorphe-niramine [chlorphenamine] maleate (p.412·1); hydrocodone tartrate (p.42·2).
Coughs and cold symptoms.

Vanicream *Pharmaceutical Specialties, USA.*
Vehicle for topical preparations.

Vanidene *Asta Medica, Belg.†*
Cyclovalone (p.1601·3).
Liver disorders; skin disorders; vomiting with ketonuria.

Vanilone *Tradiphar, Fr.*
Cyclovalone (p.1601·3).
Dyspepsia.

Vaniqa *Bristol-Myers Squibb, USA.*
Eflornithine hydrochloride (p.591·1).
Reduction of unwanted facial hair in women.

Vanmicina *Pisa, Mex.*
Vancomycin hydrochloride (p.267·2).
Antibiotic-associated colitis due to Clostridium difficile; bacterial infections.

Vanocin *Stratus, USA.*
Sulfacetamide sodium (p.250·3).
Acne; rosacea; seborrhoeic dermatitis.

Vanoxide *Dermik, USA.*
Benzoyl peroxide (p.1111·1).
Acne.

Vanoxide-HC *Dermik, USA.*
Benzoyl peroxide (p.1111·1); hydrocortisone (p.1073·3).
Acne; seborrhoea.

Vanquin *Warner-Lambert, Canad.; Parke, Davis, Denm.; Warner-Lambert, Ital†; Warner-Lambert, Norw.; Parke, Davis, Swed.*
Pyrvinium embonate (p.108·2).
Enterobiasis.

Vanquish *Glenbrook, USA.*
Aspirin (p.14·2); paracetamol (p.71·2); caffeine (p.761·3).
Aluminium hydroxide (p.1210·3) and magnesium hydroxide (p.1233·1) are included in this preparation in an attempt to limit adverse effects on the gastrointestinal mucosa.
Pain.

Vansil *Pfizer, USA†.*
Oxamniquine (p.105·1).
Schistosomiasis.

Vantaggio *Gazzoni, Ital.†*
Aspartame (p.1354·3).
Sugar substitute.

Vantal *Grossman, Mex.*
Benzydamine hydrochloride (p.20·1).
Inflammatory disorders.

Vantin *Pharmacia Upjohn, USA.*
Cefpodoxime proxetil (p.172·3).
Bacterial infections.

Vanzor *Tocogino, Mex.*
Diazepam (p.674·3).

Vap Air *Drug Trading, Canad.†.*
Camphor (p.1589·3); eucalyptus oil (p.1609·2); menthol (p.1632·3); pumilio pine oil (p.1656·3); thymol (p.1158·3).

Vapex
Roche, Hong Kong.
Menthol (p.1632·3); linalyl acetate; eucalyptus oil (p.1609·2); bornyl acetate (p.1586·3); camphor oil.
Nasal congestion.

Roche Consumer, Singapore.
Menthol (p.1632·3); linalyl acetate; eucalyptus oil (p.1609·2); bornyl acetate (p.1586·3); camphor oil; lavender oil (p.1627·2).
Nasal congestion.

Vapin *Lacer, Spain.*
Octatropine methylbromide (p.470·3).
Adjunct in peptic ulcer; gastrointestinal spasm; irritable bowel syndrome.

Vapin Complex *Lacer, Spain.*
Dipyrone (p.34·1); octatropine methylbromide (p.470·3).
Gastrointestinal spasm; pain.

Vapio *Millet Roux, Braz.*
Bioallethrin (p.1428·3); piperonyl butoxide (p.1436·2).
Pediculosis.

Vapo-Myrtol *Marion Merrell, Fr.†.*
Borneol; menthol (p.1632·3); myrtle oil; niaouli oil (p.1640·2); thyme oil (p.1672·3); eucalyptol (p.1609·2).
Respiratory-tract congestion.

Vaponefrin
Rhone-Poulenc Rorer, Canad.; Fisons, USA†.
Racemethorphine (p.831·1) or racepinefrine hydrochloride (p.831·1).
Bronchospasm.

Vapor Flay *Chimicor, Ital.*
Cymbopogon nardus oil; geranium oil (p.1615·1); pinus sylvestris oil; verbena citriodora oil; peppermint oil (p.1243·3).
Insect repellent.

Vapores Pyt *Fardi, Spain.*
Peru balsam (p.1650·2); cupressus sempervirens; eucalyptus (p.1609·2); niaouli oil (p.1640·2); diplotaxis tenuifolia; abies pectinata; pinus sylvestris; beech.
Upper respiratory-tract congestion.

Vaporil *Medical, Port.*
Belladonna (p.463·1); eucalyptus oil (p.1609·2); benzoin (p.1668·3); thyme oil (p.1672·3); lavender oil (p.1627·2); camphor (p.1589·3).
Catarrh.

Vaporisateur Medicamente
Note.This name is used for preparations of different composition.

Alsi, Canad.
Camphor (p.1589·3); eucalyptol (p.1609·2); menthol (p.1632·3); thymol (p.1158·3).

Multi-Pro, Canad.
Camphor (p.1589·3); eucalyptus oil (p.1609·2); menthol (p.1632·3); thymol (p.1158·3).

Vaporisateur Nasal Decongestionnant *Prodemdis, Canad.*
Xylometazoline hydrochloride (p.1102·2).

Vaporizing Colds Rub *Scott, Canad.*
Camphor (p.1589·3); eucalyptus oil (p.1609·2); menthol (p.1633·3).

Vaporizing Ointment *Prodemdis, Canad.*
Camphor (p.1589·3); cedar; eucalyptus oil (p.1609·2); menthol (p.1632·3); nutmeg oil (p.1643·1); thymol (p.1158·3); turpentine.

Vapour Rub
Note.This name is used for preparations of different composition.
Mentholatum, UK.
Menthol (p.1632·3); camphor (p.1589·3); methyl salicylate (p.55·1).
Nasal congestion; rheumatic and muscular pain; skin irritation.

Numark, UK.
Eucalyptus oil (p.1609·2); camphor (p.1589·3); menthol (p.1632·3).

VAQTA
CSL, Austral.; Pasteur Merieux, Belg.; Merck Frosst, Canad.; Pasteur Merieux, Fr.; Pasteur Merieux, Ger.; Chiron Behring, Ger.; Merck Sharp & Dohme, Hong Kong; Aventis, Irl.; Pasteur Merieux, Ital.; Merck Sharp & Dohme, Mex.; Merck Sharp & Dohme, NZ; Merck Sharp & Dohme, Singapore; Pasteur Merieux, Spain; Pasteur Merieux, Swed.; Pro Vaccine, Switz.; Merck Sharp & Dohme, Thai.; Pasteur Merieux, UK; Merck, USA.
A hepatitis A vaccine (p.1541·2).
Separate preparations are available for children and adolescents and for adults.
Active immunisation.

Varemoid
Novartis, Austral.†; Novartis Consumer, S.Afr.†; Zyma, Switz.†; Novartis, Thai.
Oxerutins (p.1611·2).
Anorectal disorders.

Varfine *Lusofarmaco, Port.*
Warfarin sodium (p.992·2).

Variargil *Italfarmaco, Spain.*
Trimeprazine [alimemazine] tartrate (p.426·2).
Hypersensitivity reactions.

Varibiotic *Cyanamid, Spain.*
Demeclocycline hydrochloride (p.198·2); streptodornase (p.1667·2); streptokinase (p.975·3).
Bacterial infections.

Varicella *SmithKline Beecham, Aust.*
A varicella-zoster vaccine (OKA strain) (p.1568·1).
Active immunisation.

Varicellon *Centeon, Ger.; Chiron Behring, Ger.*
A varicella-zoster immunoglobulin (p.1567·3).
Passive immunisation.

Varicex *Lohmann, Ital.*
Zinc oxide (p.1128·2).
Medicated dressing.

Varicogel *Wassermann, Ital.*
Aesculus (p.1574·1); hamamelis (p.1618·3).
Peripheral vascular disorders.

Varicose Ointment *Potter's, UK.*
Cade oil (p.1124·3); hamamelis (p.1618·3); zinc oxide (p.1128·2).
Skin irritation due to varicosity.

Varicylum *Chemosan, Aust.*
Hamamelis (p.1618·3); chamomile oil; arnica (p.1581·3).
Skin disorders; soft-tissue disorders.

Varicylum N *Liebermann, Ger.*
Homoeopathic preparation.

Varicylum-S *Liebermann, Ger.*
Chamomile oil; sage oil (p.1660·2); arnica (p.1581·3); aesculus (p.1574·1); hamamelis (p.1618·3).
Haemorrhoids; soft-tissue injury; vascular disorders.

Varidasa
Wyeth, Mex.; Wyeth Lederle, Port.; Cyanamid, Spain.
Streptokinase (p.975·3); streptodornase (p.1667·2).
Inflammation; local removal of blood clots; oedema; tissue damage.

Varidase
Wyeth Lederle, Aust.; Lederle, Austral.; Wyeth Lederle, Belg.; Wyeth Lederle, Denm.; Wyeth Lederle, Fin.; Lederle, Ger.; Lederle, Irl.; Lederle, Israel; Wyeth Lederle, Ital.; Lederle, Neth.; Wyeth Lederle, Norw.; Lederle, NZ; Wyeth, S.Afr.; Wyeth Lederle, Swed.; Wyeth, UK.
Streptokinase (p.975·3); streptodornase (p.1667·2).
Inflammation; local removal of blood clots, fibrin, and necrotic material; oedema.

Varidoid *General Drugs, Thai.*
A heparinoid (p.905·2).
Haematoma; oedema; phleitis; scars; sunburn; thrombosis; varicose veins.

Varigerm *Heralds, Braz.*
Tyrothricin (p.267·1); hydroxyquinoline sulfate (p.1622·2); menthol (p.1632·3); mallow; lactic acid (p.1626·2).
Skin disorders.

Varigloban *Kreussler, Ger.*
Sodium iodide (p.1522·3); iodine (p.1522·3).
Haemorrhoids; varicose veins.

Variglobin *Globopharm, Switz.*
Sodium iodide (p.1522·3); iodine (p.1522·3).
Varicose veins.

Varihes
Laevosan, Aust.; Fresenius Kabi, Switz.
Hetastarch (p.732·3).
Hypovolaemia.

Varihesive
Convatec, Port.
Carmellose sodium (p.1499·3); gelatin (p.737·2); pectin (p.1502·3).
Skin ulcers; wounds.

Convatec, UK†.
Carmellose sodium (p.1499·3); gelatin (p.737·2); pectin (p.1502·3); polyisobutylene.
Leg ulcers.

Varihesive Hydroactive *Convatec, Switz.†.*
Carmellose sodium (p.1499·3); gelatin (p.737·2); pectin (p.1502·3).
Burns; skin ulcers; wounds.

Varilisin *Knoll, Belg.*
Collagenase (p.1598·2).
Debridement of necrotic ulcers.

Varilrix
SmithKline Beecham, Aust.; SmithKline Beecham, Austral.; SmithKline Beecham, Belg.; SmithKline Beecham, Denm.; SmithKline Beecham, Fin.; SmithKline Beecham, Ger.; Dresden, Ger.; SmithKline Beecham, Hong Kong; SmithKline Beecham, Irl.; SmithKline Beecham, Mex.; SmithKline Beecham, Norw.; SmithKline Beecham, NZ; SmithKline Beecham, Singapore; SmithKline Beecham, Spain; SmithKline Beecham, Swed.; SmithKline Beecham, Switz.; SmithKline Beecham, Thai.
A live attenuated varicella-zoster vaccine (OKA strain) (p.1568·1).
Active immunisation.

Varimine *Atral, Port.*
Multivitamin and mineral preparation (p.1350·1).

Variplastic *Virtus, Braz.*
Digitoxin (p.869·2).
Arrhythmias; heart failure.

Varison *Euro-Labor, Port.*
Myrtillus (p.1639·2).
Haemorrhoids; metrorrhagia; venous insufficiency.

Varitan N *Godecke, Ger.*
Bismuth subgallate (p.1213·2); zinc oxide (p.1128·2); lauromacrogol 400 (p.1345·2).
Anorectal disorders.

Varitect
Biotest, Aust.; Biotest, Ger.; Biotest, Hong Kong; Intra Pharma, Irl.; Biotest, Israel; Biotest, Ital.; Boehringer Ingelheim, Port.; Biotest, Singapore; Biotest, Switz.; Biotest, Thai.
A varicella-zoster immunoglobulin (p.1567·3).
Passive immunisation.

Variton *Hormona, Mex.*
Diosmin (p.1611·1); hesperidin (p.1611·2).
Haemorrhoids; venous insufficiency.

Varivax
CSL, Austral.; Merck Frosst, Canad.; Merck Sharp & Dohme, Hong Kong; Merck Sharp & Dohme, Singapore; Merck, USA.
A live varicella-zoster vaccine (Oka/Merck) (p.1568·1).
Active immunisation.

Varizol *Simoes, Braz.*
Rutoside (p.1611·2); panthenol (p.1602·3); aesculus (p.1574·1); hamamelis (p.1618·3); lignocaine [lidocaine] (p.1313·2).
Haemorrhoids.

Varlane *Schering, Belg.*
Fluocortin butyl (p.1071·3).
Burns; skin disorders; stings.

Varnoline *Organon, Fr.*
Desogestrel (p.1470·3); ethinylestradiol (p.1476·2).
28-Day packs also contain 7 inert tablets.
Combined oral contraceptive.

Varson *Almirall, Spain.*
Nicergoline (p.1640·2).
Vascular disorders.

Vartmedel *Kabi, Swed.†.*
Salicylic acid (p.1122·3); lactic acid (p.1626·2).
Warts.

Var-Zeta *Alfa Biotech, Ital.†.*
A varicella-zoster immunoglobulin (p.1567·3).
Passive immunisation.

Vas
Note.This name is used for preparations of different composition.
Elexsam, Austral.†.
Methyl nicotinate (p.55·1).
Peripheral vascular disorders.

Geymonat, Ital.
Suleparoid (p.978·2).
Thrombosis prophylaxis.

Vasactife *Ferring, Port.*
Ginkgo biloba (p.1615·2).
Vascular disorders.

Vasa-Gastreu N R63 *Reckeweg, Ger.*
Homoeopathic preparation.

Vascace
Roche, Irl.; Roche, Israel; Roche, UK.
Cilazapril (p.858·1).
Heart failure; hypertension.

Vascace Plus *Roche, Israel.*
Cilazapril (p.858·1); hydrochlorothiazide (p.907·3).
Hypertension.

Vascal *Schwarz, Ger.*
Isradipine (p.916·3).
Hypertension.

Vascard *Parke-Med, S.Afr.*
Nifedipine (p.940·1).
Angina pectoris; hypertension.

Vascase
Roche, Braz.; Roche, Neth.; Pharmacia Upjohn, Port.
Cilazapril (p.858·1).
Heart failure; hypertension.

Vascase Plus
Roche, Neth.; Pharmacia Upjohn, Port.
Cilazapril (p.858·1); hydrochlorothiazide (p.907·3).
Hypertension.

Vascocitrol *Alpharma, Fr.*
Citroflavonoids (p.1611·1); ascorbic acid (p.1389·3); light magnesium carbonate (p.1232·3).
Venous insufficiency.

Vascoman *Takeda, Ital.*
Manidipine hydrochloride (p.924·3).
Hypertension.

Vascor *Ortho McNeil, USA.*
Bepridil hydrochloride (p.844·3).
Angina pectoris.

Vascoray *Mallinckrodt, USA†.*
Meglumine iothalamate (p.1036·2); sodium iothalamate (p.1036·2).
Radiographic contrast medium.

Vascoten
Medochemie, Hong Kong; Medochemie, Singapore; Medochemie, Thai.
Atenolol (p.841·3).
Angina pectoris; arrhythmias; hypertension; myocardial infarction.

Vasculat
Boehringer Ingelheim, Aust.†; Boehringer de Angeli, Braz.; Boehringer Ingelheim, Spain.
Bamethan sulfate (p.843·1).
Cerebral and peripheral vascular disorders.

Vasculene *Finmedical, Ital.*
Flunarizine hydrochloride (p.418·1).
Migraine; vascular disorders; vertigo.

Vasculine *Desbergers, Canad.*
Multivitamin and mineral preparation (p.1350·1).

Vascunormyl *Alcon, Fr.*
Cyclandelate (p.865·2).
Intermittent claudication; vascular eye disorders.

Vasdalat *Kalbe, Singapore.*
Nifedipine (p.940·1).
Angina pectoris; hypertension.

Vasdilat *MDM, Ital.*
Isosorbide mononitrate (p.916·2).
Ischaemic heart disease.

Vaselatum *Stiefel, Spain.*
Paraffin (p.1407·1); benzalkonium chloride (p.1133·2); triclosan (p.1159·2).
Eczema.

Vaselina Boricada *Brum, Spain; Calmante Vitaminado, Spain; Orravan, Spain; Puerto Galiano, Spain.*
Boric acid (p.1586·1); white soft paraffin (p.1407·3).
Skin disorders; urethral or rectal lubricant.

Vaselina Mentolada
Note.This name is used for preparations of different composition.
Brum, Spain.
White soft paraffin (p.1407·3); menthol (p.1632·3); peppermint oil (p.1243·3).
Skin disorders; urethral or rectal lubricant.

Puerto Galiano, Spain.
White soft paraffin (p.1407·3); menthol (p.1632·3).
Skin disorders; urethral or rectal lubricant.

Vaseline
Lever Pond's, Canad.; Chesebrough-Pond's, UK.
White soft paraffin (p.1407·3).
Barrier preparation; dry skin.

Vaseline Gomenolee *Gomenol, Fr.*
Niaouli oil (p.1640·2); white soft paraffin.
Nasal disoreders.

Vaseline Intensive Care *Chesebrough-Pond's, USA.*
SPF4; SPF 8; SPF 15: Octinoxate (p.1517·3); oxybenzone (p.1518·1).

SPF 25: Octinoxate (p.1517·3); oxybenzone (p.1518·1); octisalate (p.1518·1).

SPF 30: Octinoxate (p.1517·3); oxybenzone (p.1518·1); octisalate (p.1518·1); titanium dioxide (p.1126·1).

Sunscreen.

Vaseline Intensive Care Active Sport *Chesebrough-Pond's, USA.*
SPF 8; SPF 15: Octinoxate (p.1517·3); oxybenzone (p.1518·1).
Sunscreen.

Vaseline Intensive Care Baby *Chesebrough-Pond's, USA.*
SPF 15: Titanium dioxide (p.1126·1); zinc oxide (p.1128·2).

SPF 30+: Octinoxate (p.1517·3); oxybenzone (p.1518·1); octisalate (p.1518·1); titanium dioxide (p.1126·1).
Sunscreen.

Vaseline Intensive Care Blockout *Chesebrough-Pond's, USA.*
SPF 40: Padimate (p.1518·2); octinoxate (p.1517·3); oxybenzone (p.1518·1); octisalate (p.1518·1); titanium dioxide (p.1126·1).
Sunscreen.

Vaseline Intensive Care No Burn No Bite *Chesebrough-Pond's, USA.*
SPF 8; SPF 15: Octinoxate (p.1517·3); oxybenzone (p.1518·1).
Sunscreen.

Vaseline Intensive Care-Total Care *Lever Pond's, Canad.*
SPF 15: Octinoxate (p.1517·3); oxybenzone (p.1518·1).
Sunscreen.

Vaseline Lip Therapy *Lever Pond's, Canad.*
SPF 15: Octinoxate (p.1517·3); oxybenzone (p.1518·1); white soft paraffin.
Sunscreen.

Vaseretic *Merck Frosst, Canad.; Merck, USA.*
Enalapril maleate (p.883·3); hydrochlorothiazide (p.907·3).
Hypertension.

Vasesana-Vasoregulans *Hotz, Ger.*
Aesculus (p.1574·1); mistletoe (p.1636·2); crataegus (p.1600·2); hamamelis (p.1618·3); arnica (p.1581·3); silybum marianum (p.1021·3).
Haemorrhoids; vascular disorders.

Vasian *Asian Pharm, Thai.*
Co-dergocrine mesilate (p.1597·3).
Mental function disorders.

Vasican *DHA, Hong Kong; DHA, Singapore.*
Bromhexine hydrochloride (p.1085·3).
Respiratory-tract disorders associated with increased or viscous mucus.

Vasil *Pharmasant, Thai.*
Metoclopramide hydrochloride (p.1235·2).
Nausea and vomiting.

Vasilium *Medinfar, Port.*
Flunarizine hydrochloride (p.418·1).
Migraine; vertigo.

Vaslan *Faes, Spain†.*
Isradipine (p.916·3).
Hypertension.

Vaslip *Ferrer, Spain.*
Cerivastatin sodium (p.856·1).
Hyperlipolaemia.

Vasobrain *Errekappa, Ital.*
Phospholipids; vitamin E; ginkgo biloba (p.1615·2) (p.1350·1).
Mental function disorders.

Vasobral *Chiesi, Fr.; Logeais, Hong Kong; Geymonat, Ital.*
Dihydroergocryptine mesilate (p.1603·3); caffeine (p.761·3).
Cerebral and peripheral vascular disorders; headache.

Vasobrix *Guerbet, Braz.*
Monoethanolamine ioxitalamate (p.1037·2); meglumine ioxitalamate (p.1037·2).
Radiographic contrast medium.

Vasocardol *Hoechst Marion Roussel, Austral.*
Diltiazem hydrochloride (p.874·3).
Angina pectoris; hypertension.

Vasocedine *Qualiphar, Belg.*
Naphazoline nitrate (p.1095·1).
Nasal congestion.

Vasocedine Pseudoefedrine *Qualiphar, Belg.*
Pseudoephedrine hydrochloride (p.1099·2).
Rhinitis.

Vasocet *Cipharm, Fr.†.*
Cetiedil citrate (p.856·3).
Vascular disorders.

Vasocidin *Ciba Vision, Canad.; Ciba Vision, USA.*
Prednisolone acetate (p.1078·1) or prednisolone sodium phosphate (p.1078·1); sulfacetamide sodium (p.250·3).
Formerly contained prednisolone sodium phosphate, phenylephrine hydrochloride, and sulfacetamide sodium in *Canad.*
Eye inflammation with bacterial infection.

Vasocine *Ciba Vision, USA.*
Prednisolone acetate (p.1078·1); sulfacetamide sodium (p.250·3).
Infected eye disorders.

VasoClear *Ciba Vision, USA.*
Naphazoline hydrochloride (p.1095·1); polyvinyl alcohol (p.1503·1).
Minor eye irritation.

VasoClear A *Ciba Vision, USA.*
Naphazoline hydrochloride (p.1095·1); zinc sulfate (p.1398·2).
Eye irritation.

Vasocon *Ciba Vision, Canad.; Ciba Vision, USA.*
Naphazoline hydrochloride (p.1095·1).
Eye irritation.

Vasocon Ant *Ciba Vision, Spain.*
Naphazoline nitrate (p.1095·1); neomycin sulfate (p.228·1); zinc sulfate (p.1398·2).
Eye congestion; eye infections.

Vasocon-A *Ciba Vision, Canad.; Ciba Vision, USA.*
Naphazoline hydrochloride (p.1095·1); antazoline phosphate (p.408·3).
Eye irritation.

Vasoconstr *Ciba Vision, Spain.*
Naphazoline nitrate (p.1095·1); zinc sulfate (p.1398·2).
Eye irritation.

Vasoconstrictor Pensa *Pensa, Spain.*
Naphazoline hydrochloride (p.1095·1).
Nasal congestion.

Vasoderm *Taro, USA†.*
Fluocinonide (p.1071·2).
Skin disorders.

Vasodexa *Llorens, Spain.*
Dexamethasone sodium succinate (p.1067·3); tetryzoline hydrochloride (p.1101·2).
Inflammatory eye disorders.

Vasodil *Byk Gulden, Mex.*
Ginkgo biloba (p.1615·2).
Vascular disorders.

Vasodilan *Apothecon, USA.*
Isoxsuprine hydrochloride (p.1624·3).
Cerebrovascular disorders; peripheral vascular disorders.

Vaso-Dilatan *Agepha, Aust.*
Tolazoline hydrochloride (p.984·3).
Vascular disorders.

Vasodin *Teofarma, Ital.*
Nicardipine hydrochloride (p.938·3).
Angina pectoris; heart failure; hypertension.

Vasodip *Dexcel, Israel.*
Lercanidipine hydrochloride (p.920·2).
Hypertension.

Vaso-E-Bion *Rodisma, Ger.*
Troxerutin (p.1611·2); *dl*-alpha tocoferil acetate (p.1394·1).
Vascular disorders.

Vasofed *Antigen, Irl.; Garec, S.Afr.*
Nifedipine (p.940·1).
Angina pectoris; hypertension.

Vasofen *Tubilux, Ital.*
Chloramphenicol sodium hemisuccinate (p.179·2); phenylephrine (p.1097·1); mepyramine maleate (p.421·1).
Eye disorders.

Vasofluina *Zambon, Braz.*
Raubasine hydrochloride (p.967·2); dihydroergocristine mesilate (p.1603·2); dihydroergotamine mesilate (p.450·3).
Vascular disorders.

Vasoforte N *Krugmann, Ger.*
Aesculus (p.1574·1).
Vascular disorders.

Vasofrinic *Trianon, Canad.*
Chlorpheniramine [chlorphenamine] maleate (p.412·1); pseudoephedrine hydrochloride (p.1099·2).
Respiratory congestion.

Vasofrinic Plus *Trianon, Canad.*
Dextromethorphan hydrobromide (p.1087·3); guaifenesin (p.1092·2); chlorpheniramine [chlorphenamine] maleate (p.412·1); pseudoephedrine hydrochloride (p.1099·2).
Coughs; respiratory congestion.

Vasofyl *Fustery, Mex.*
Oxpentifylline [pentoxifylline] (p.950·3).
Cerebral, ocular, and peripheral vascular disorders.

Vasogen
Pharmax, Irl.; Pharmax, UK.
Dimethicone (p.1410·1); zinc oxide (p.1128·2); calamine (p.1111·3).
Barrier cream; bedsores; nappy rash; ostomy management.

Vasolan
Note.This name is used for preparations of different composition.
Dexxon, Israel.
Isoxsuprine hydrochloride (p.1624·3).
Cerebral and peripheral vascular disorders; dysmenorrhoea; premature labour.
Eisai, Jpn†.
Verapamil hydrochloride (p.989·1).
Angina pectoris; arrhythmias; ischaemic heart disease; myocardial infarction.

Vasolastine *Enzypharm, Neth.†.*
Triacylglycerol lipase; acyl-CoA-dehydrogenase; amine oxidase.
Vascular disorders.

Vasolator *Sanwa, Jpn†.*
Glyceryl trinitrate (p.897·3).
Angina pectoris.

Vasolipid
Note.This name is used for preparations of different composition.
Braun, Denm.†.
Soya oil (p.1378·1).
Contains egg phospholipid.
Lipid infusion for parenteral nutrition.
Braun, Fin.; Braun, Norw.; Braun, Swed.
Soya oil (p.1378·1); medium-chain triglycerides (p.1372·1).
Contains egg lecithin.
Lipid infusion for parenteral nutrition.

Vasomil *Aspen, S.Afr.*
Verapamil hydrochloride (p.989·1).
Angina pectoris; arrhythmias.

Vasomotal *Solvay, Ger.*
Betahistine hydrochloride (p.1584·2).
Ménière's disease; vertigo; vestibular disorders.

Vasonase *Yamanouchi, Spain.*
Nicardipine hydrochloride (p.938·3).
Angina pectoris; cerebrovascular disorders; hypertension.

Vasonett *INTES, Ital.*
Vincamine (p.1680·1).
Cerebrovascular insufficiency.

Vasonorm *NCSN, Ital.*
Nicardipine hydrochloride (p.938·3).
Angina pectoris; heart failure; hypertension.

Vasopos N *Ursapharm, Ger.*
Tetryzoline hydrochloride (p.1101·2).
Eye disorders.

Vasopresina *Novartis, Spain†.*
Lypressin (p.1300·1).
Diabetes insipidus.

Vasopressin
Sandoz, Ger.†; Sandoz, S.Afr.†.
Lypressin (p.1300·1).
Diabetes insipidus.

Vasopressine *Sandoz, Neth.†.*
Lypressin (p.1300·1).
Diabetes insipidus; variceal haemorrhage.

Vasopril *Bristol-Myers Squibb, Israel.*
Fosinopril sodium (p.892·3).
Heart failure; hypertension.

Vasopten *Torrent, Thai.*
Verapamil hydrochloride (p.989·1).
Angina pectoris; arrhythmias; myocardial infarction.

Vasorbate *Arcana, Aust.*
Isosorbide dinitrate (p.915·2).
Angina pectoris; heart failure; myocardial infarction.

Vasorema *Inverni della Beffa, Ital.*
Suleparoid (p.978·2).
Thrombosis prophylaxis.

Vasoretic *Merck Sharp & Dohme, Ital.*
Enalapril maleate (p.883·3); hydrochlorothiazide (p.907·3).
Hypertension.

Vasorinil *Farmila, Ital.*
Tetryzoline hydrochloride (p.1101·2).
Nasal congestion.

Vasosan *Felgentrager, Ger.*
Colestyramine (p.864·1).
Hyperlipidaemias.

Vasosterone *Angelini, Ital.*
Hydrocortisone (p.1073·3); tetryzoline hydrochloride (p.1101·2).
Nasal congestion.

Vasosterone Antibiotico *Angelini, Ital.*
Hydrocortisone acetate (p.1073·3); tetryzoline hydrochloride (p.1101·2); neomycin sulfate (p.228·1); gramicidin (p.213·3).
Rhinitis.

Vasosterone Collirio *Angelini, Ital.*
Hydrocortisone acetate (p.1073·3); tetryzoline hydrochloride (p.1101·2); neomycin sulfate (p.228·1).
Eye disorders.

Vasosterone Oto *Angelini, Ital.*
Flumetasone pivalate (p.1070·3); gentamicin sulfate (p.210·1).
Formerly contained hydrocortisone, tetryzoline hydrochloride, neomycin sulfate, and gramicidin.
Otitis externa.

Vasosulf *Ciba Vision, Canad.†; Ciba Vision, USA.*
Sulfacetamide sodium (p.250·3); phenylephrine hydrochloride (p.1097·1).
Bacterial eye infections.

Vasosuprina Ilfi *Lusofarmaco, Ital.*
Isoxsuprine hydrochloride (p.1624·3).
Premature labour; threatened abortion.

Vasotec *Merck Frosst, Canad.; Merck, USA.*
Enalapril maleate (p.883·3) or enalaprilat (p.884·1).
Heart failure; hypertension.

Vasoton *NCSN, Ital.*
Dihydroergocristine mesilate (p.1603·2).
Cerebral and peripheral vascular disorders; dopamine deficiency; headache; hypertension; migraine.

Vasotonin *Merz, Ger.*
Capsules: Aesculus (p.1574·1).
Haemorrhoids; vascular disorders.
Topical gel: Arnica (p.1581·3).
Musculoskeletal, joint, and soft-tissue disorders; superficial thrombophlebitis.

Vasotonin forte *Merz, Ger.†.*
Aesculus (p.1574·1); mofebutazone (p.55·3).
Superficial thrombophlebitis.

Vasovitol *Lannacher, Aust.*
Vitamin A palmitate (p.1383·2); alpha tocoferil acetate (p.1394·1).
Vitamin A and E deficiency.

Vasoxine *Glaxo Wellcome, Aust.†; Wellcome, Irl.; Glaxo Wellcome, UK.*
Methoxamine hydrochloride (p.927·2).
Hypotension.

Vasoxyl *Glaxo Wellcome, Canad.; Glaxo Wellcome, USA.*
Methoxamine hydrochloride (p.927·2).
Control of blood pressure during surgery; postoperative collapse; supraventricular tachycardia.

Vasperdil *Lacer, Spain†.*
Etamivan (p.1509·3); etofylline (p.765·1); hexobendine hydrochloride (p.905·3).
Cerebrovascular disorders; circulatory disorders.

Vaspit *Asche, Ger.; Schering, Ital.; Schering, Spain.*
Fluocortin butyl (p.1071·3).
Burns; insect stings; skin disorders.

Vastarel *Servier, Denm.; Biopharma, Fr.; Servier, Hong Kong; Servier, Irl.; Stroder, Ital.; Servier, Port.; Servier, Singapore; Servier, Thai.*
Trimetazidine hydrochloride (p.987·3).
Angina pectoris; vascular eye disorders; vestibular disorders.

Vasten *Rhone-Poulenc Rorer, Fr.*
Pravastatin sodium (p.957·3).
Hypercholesterolaemia.

Vastensium *Salvat, Spain.*
Nitrendipine (p.947·1).
Hypertension.

Vastin *Astra, Austral.; AstraZeneca, NZ.*
Fluvastatin sodium (p.892·1).
Atherosclerosis; hypercholesterolaemia.

Vastinol *TO-Chemicals, Thai.*
Trimetazidine hydrochloride (p.987·3).
Ischaemic heart disease.

Vastribil *Farmasan, Ger.*
Troxerutin (p.1611·2).
Vascular disorders.

Vastrictol *Allergan-Frumtost, Braz.*
Naphazoline nitrate (p.1095·1); zinc sulfate (p.1398·2).
Ocular congestion.

Vasurix Polividona *Guerbet, Braz.*
Meglumine ioxitalamate (p.1037·2); povidone.
Radiographic contrast medium.

Vasylox *Douglas, Austral.*
Oxymetazoline hydrochloride (p.1096·2); eucalyptol (p.1609·2); menthol (p.1632·3).
Nasal congestion.

Vasylox Junior *Douglas, Austral.†.*
Methoxamine hydrochloride (p.927·2).
Nasal congestion; rhinitis.

Vatran *Valeas, Ital.*
Diazepam (p.674·3).
Anxiety; eclampsia; epilepsy; premedication; psychosomatic disorders; skeletal muscle spasm.

Vatrasin *Sanofi Synthelabo, Spain.*
Nicardipine hydrochloride (p.938·3).
Angina pectoris; cerebrovascular disorders; hypertension.

Vatrem *Kener, Mex.*
Piroxicam (p.79·1).

Vatrix-S *Bioclon, Mex.*
Metronidazole (p.594·1).

Vaxar *Glaxo Wellcome, Ger.†; Cascan, Ger.†.*
Grepafloxacin hydrochloride (p.214·1).
Bacterial infections.

Vaxem Hib *Chiron, Ital.*
A Haemophilus influenzae conjugate vaccine (p.1540·2).
Active immunisation.

Vaxicoq *Pasteur Merieux, Fr.*
An adsorbed pertussis vaccine (p.1555·3).
Active immunisation.

Vaxicum N *Worwag, Ger.*
Camphor oil; rosemary oil (p.1659·3); lauromacrogol 400 (p.1345·2).
Musculoskeletal, joint, peri-articular, and soft-tissue disorders; neuralgia.

Vaxidina *VAAS, Ital.†.*
Chlorhexidine gluconate (p.1138·2).
Skin disinfection; wound disinfection.

Vaxigrip *Pasteur Merieux, Aust.; CSL, Austral.; Pasteur Merieux, Belg.; Pasteur Merieux, Braz.; Connaught, Canad.; Pasteur Merieux, Denm.; Meda, Fin.; Pasteur Merieux, Fr.; Pasteur Merieux, Hong Kong; Pasteur Merieux, Israel; Pasteur Merieux, Ital.; Pasteur Merieux, Neth.; Pasteur Merieux, Norw.; Aventis, NZ; Vedim, Port.; Aventis, S.Afr.; Pasteur Merieux, Singapore; Meda, Swed.; Pasteur Merieux, Thai.*
An inactivated influenza vaccine (split virion) (p.1544·3).
Active immunisation.

Vaxipar *Chiron, Ital.*
A mumps vaccine (Urabe strain) (p.1551·1).
Active immunisation.

Vaxitiol *Bouty, Ital.*
Lactobacillus sporogenes; Lactobacillus acidophilus (p.1626·3); *Streptococcus thermophilus* (p.1626·3); *Bifidobacterium bifidum* (p.1626·3); vitamins; minerals (p.1350·1).
Maintenance of normal gastrointestinal flora.

Vazigam *NBI, S.Afr.*
A varicella-zoster immunoglobulin (p.1567·3).
Passive immunisation.

Vcanalare *Vebas, Ital.*
Orthophenylphenol (p.1152·1).
Root canal disinfection.

VCF *Apothecus, Hong Kong; Apothecus, USA.*
Nonoxinol 9 (p.1346·1).
Contraceptive.

V-Cil-K *Lilly, S.Afr.†.*
Phenoxymethylpenicillin potassium (p.235·1).
Bacterial infections.

V-Cillin K *Lilly, Canad.†; Lilly, USA†.*
Phenoxymethylpenicillin potassium (p.235·1).
Bacterial infections.

V-Crima *Vitamed, Israel.*
Povidone (p.1503·2); hypromellose (p.1501·3).
Dry eyes.

V-Dec-M *Seatrace, USA.*
Pseudoephedrine hydrochloride (p.1099·2); guaifenesin (p.1092·2).
Coughs.

Ve *Tecnifar, Port.*
Vitamin E (p.1394·1).
Atherosclerosis; growth disorders; infertility; menstrual disorders; myasthenia gravis; recurrent miscarriage.

Veafer *Veafarm, Braz.*
Ferric ammonium citrate (p.1359·2); vitamin B substances (p.1350·1).
Iron deficiency; iron-deficiency anaemias.

Veclam *Malesci, Ital.*
Clarithromycin (p.186·2).
Bacterial infections.

Vectarion *Servier, Belg.; Servier, Braz.; Servier, Denm.; Eutherapie, Fr.; Servier, Ger.; Servier, Irl.; Servier, Port.; Servier, Spain.*
Almitrine dimesilate (p.1506·2).
Obstructive airways disease; respiratory insufficiency.

Vectavir *SmithKline Beecham Consumer, Austral.; SmithKline Beecham, Belg.; SmithKline Beecham, Denm.; SmithKline Beecham, Fin.; SmithKline Beecham, Ger.; SmithKline Beecham, Hong Kong; SmithKline Beecham, Israel; SmithKline Beecham, Ital.; SmithKline Beecham, NZ; SmithKline Beecham, Spain; SmithKline Beecham, Norw.; SmithKline Beecham Consumer, UK; Novartis, UK.*
Penciclovir (p.638·1).
Herpes labialis.

Vectrin *Warner Chilcott, USA.*
Minocycline hydrochloride (p.224·3).
Bacterial infections.

Vectrine *Pharma 2000, Fr.*
Erdosteine (p.1091·2).
Respiratory-tract congestion.

Vedrin *Poliforma, Ital.*
Xantinol nicotinate (p.999·1).
Peripheral vascular disorders.

Veekay *Pharmador, S.Afr.†.*
Phenoxymethylpenicillin potassium (p.235·1).
Bacterial infections.

Veenac *Progress, Thai.*
Diclofenac sodium (p.30·3).
Gout; inflammation; musculoskeletal and joint disorders; pain.

Veetids *Apothecon, USA.*
Phenoxymethylpenicillin potassium (p.235·1).
Bacterial infections.

Vega *Ono, Jpn†.*
Ozagrel hydrochloride (p.1645·3).
Asthma.

Vegadeine *Warner-Lambert, Fr.*
Aspirin (p.14·2); paracetamol (p.71·2); codeine phosphate (p.25·2).
Fever; pain.

Vegal *Jofrain, Mex.*
Dipyrone (p.34·1).

Veganin *Note. This name is used for preparations of different composition. Parke, Davis, Aust.†; Warner-Lambert, Hong Kong; Warner-Lambert, Irl.; Warner-Lambert, Spain†; Warner-Lambert, UK.*
Aspirin (p.14·2); paracetamol (p.71·2); codeine phosphate (p.25·2).
Fever; pain.

Warner-Lambert, Austral.
Aspirin (p.14·2); codeine phosphate (p.25·2).
Fever; pain.

Veganin 3 *Aspen, S.Afr.*
Aspirin (p.14·2); paracetamol (p.71·2); codeine phosphate (p.25·2).
Fever; pain.

Veganine *Note. This name is used for preparations of different composition. Warner-Lambert Consumer, Belg.†; Warner-Lambert Consumer, Port.†.*
Aspirin (p.14·2); paracetamol (p.71·2); codeine phosphate (p.25·2).
Fever; pain.

Warner-Lambert, Fr.
Paracetamol (p.71·2); caffeine (p.761·3).
Formerly contained aspirin, paracetamol and codeine phosphate.
Fever; pain.

Vege Swiss One *Swiss Herbal, Canad.*
Multivitamin and mineral preparation (p.1350·1).

Vegebaby *Clintec, Fr.†.*
Infant feed (p.1350·1).
Milk intolerance.

Vegebom *Jessel, Fr.*
Eucalyptol (p.1609·2); cajuput oil (p.1588·1); sassafras oil (p.1661·1); cedar oil; camphor (p.1589·3); menthol (p.1632·3); nutmeg oil (p.1643·1); bay-laurel oil.
Musculoskeletal, joint, and peri-articular disorders.

Vegebyl *Roche, Ital.†.*
Boldo (p.1585·3); cynara (p.1601·3); rhubarb (p.1248·1); cascara (p.1216·1); chamomile (p.1593·2).
Constipation; digestive disorders.

Vegelact *Diepal, Fr.†.*
Infant feed (p.1350·1).
Milk intolerance.

Vegelax *Biologiques de l'Ile-de-France, Fr.*
Senna (p.1248·2); boldo (p.1585·3); cynara (p.1601·3).
Formerly contained frangula, cascara, senna, boldo, cynara, belladonna, aloes, scammony, and rhubarb.
Constipation.

Vegelose *Clintec, Fr.†.*
Gluten-free, milk-free nutritional supplement (p.1350·1).

Vegesan *Mack, Switz.*
Nordazepam (p.696·1).
Anxiety disorders.

Vegetable Cough Remover *Potter's, UK.*
Capsicum (p.1591·1); cimicifuga (p.1595·2); ipecacuanha (p.1093·1); lobelia (p.1510·2); pleurisy root (p.1653·1); skullcap (p.1664·3); skunk cabbage (p.1664·3); valerian (p.1678·3); elecampane (p.1089·3); marrubium (p.1094·2); hyssop; anise oil (p.1580·3); liquorice (p.1231·2).
Coughs.

Vegetal Tonic *Homeocan, Canad.*
Homoeopathic preparation.

Vegetalin *Genove, Spain.*
Bearberry (p.1583·3); senna (p.1248·2); coriander (p.1599·2); hyssop; sage (p.1660·2).
Constipation.

Vegetallumina *Recordati, Ital.*
Camphor (p.1589·3); aluminium subacetate (p.1578·2); methyl salicylate (p.55·1); thyme oil (p.1672·3).
Soft-tissue and peri-articular disorders.

Vegetarian Protein Supplement *GNLD, Austral.*
Nutritional supplement (p.1350·1).

Vegetex *Lane, UK.*
Celery (p.1592·3); menyanthes (p.1633·1); cimicifuga (p.1595·2).
Muscular pain.

Vegetoserum *Alpharma, Fr.*
Ethylmorphine hydrochloride (p.35·2); grindelia (p.1618·2).
Formerly contained ethylmorphine hydrochloride, aconite, belladonna, grindelia, and cherry-laurel.
Coughs.

Vegicap Vegetarian *Solgar, UK.*
Multivitamin and mineral preparation (p.1350·1).

Vehem *Sandoz, Fr.†.*
Teniposide (p.574·1).
Malignant neoplasms.

Veil *Blake, UK.*
A covering cream.
Concealment of birth marks, scars, and disfiguring skin disease.

Veinamitol *Negma, Belg.; Negma, Fr.*
Troxerutin (p.1611·2).
Haemorrhoids; venous insufficiency.

Veineva *CCD, Fr.*
Diosmin (p.1611·1).
Capillary disorders; haemorrhoids; venous insufficiency.

Veinobiase *Fournier, Fr.; Quimifar, Spain.*
Black currant (p.1389·3); ruscus; ascorbic acid (p.1389·3).
Haemorrhoids; venous insufficiency.

Veinoconfort *Yves Ponroy, Fr.†.*
Vitamin C substances (p.1350·1).
Circulatory disorders.

Veino-Gouttes-N *Phytomed, Switz.*
Aesculus (p.1574·1); mellilot; ruscus aculeatus.
Venous insufficiency.

Veinophytum *Arkopharma, Fr.*
Aesculus (p.1574·1); red vine.
Capillary disorders; haemorrhoids; venous insufficiency.

Veinosane *Dolisos, Fr.†.*
Melilotus officinalis; red vine leaf.
Haemorrhoids; venous insufficiency.

Veinostase *Richelet, Fr.*
Aesculus (p.1574·1); hamamelis (p.1618·3); cupressus sempervirens; ascorbic acid (p.1389·3).
Haemorrhoids; vascular disorders.

Veinotonyl *Lipha Sante, Fr.*
Aesculus (p.1574·1); meteseculetol sodium (p.1635·1).
Peripheral vascular disorders.

Velamox *SmithKline Beecham, Ital.*
Amoxicillin sodium (p.149·2) or amoxicillin trihydrate (p.149·2).
Bacterial infections.

Velasulin *Novo Nordisk, Ger.*
Neutral insulin injection (crystalline) (porcine, highly-purified) (p.324·1).
Diabetes mellitus.

Velasulin Human *Novo Nordisk, Ger.*
Insulin injection (human) (p.324·1).
Diabetes mellitus.

Velasulin MC *Novo Nordisk, Ger.*
Insulin injection (porcine, monocomponent) (p.324·1).
Diabetes mellitus.

Velaten *Hoechst Marion Roussel, Ital.†.*
Sulfamethoxypyridazine (p.256·2); trimethoprim (p.264·2).
Bacterial infections; Pneumocystis carinii pneumonia.

Velbacil *Farmasierra, Spain.*
Bacampicillin hydrochloride (p.155·1).
Bacterial infections.

Velban *Lilly, Braz.; Lilly, USA.*
Vinblastine sulfate (p.577·3).
Malignant neoplasms.

Velbe *Lilly, Aust.; Lilly, Austral.; Lilly, Belg.; Lilly, Canad.; Lilly, Denm.; Lilly, Fin.; Lilly, Fr.; Lilly, Ger.; Lilly, Hong Kong; Lilly, Israel; Lilly, Ital.; Lilly, Mex.; Lilly, Neth.; Lilly, Norw.; Lilly, Port.; Lilly, Swed.; Lilly, Switz.; Lilly, UK.*
Vinblastine sulfate (p.577·3).
Malignant neoplasms.

Veliten *Laphal, Fr.*
Vitamins (p.1350·1); rutoside (p.1611·2).
Vascular disorders.

Vellutan *Abiogen, Ital.*
Tacalcitol (p.1124·2).
Psoriasis.

Velmonit *Esteve, Spain.*
Ciprofloxacin hydrochloride (p.182·3) or ciprofloxacin lactate (p.182·3).
Bacterial infections.

Velocef *Squibb, Braz.*
Cefradine (p.173·3).
Bacterial infections.

Velodan *Vita, Spain.*
Loratadine (p.420·1).
Hypersensitivity reactions.

Velonarcon *Asta Medica, Ger.*
Ketamine hydrochloride (p.1262·2).
General anaesthesia; pain; status asthmaticus.

velopural *Optimed, Ger.*
Hydrocortisone acetate (p.1073·3).
Skin disorders.

Velorin *Remedica, Hong Kong; Remedica, Singapore; Remedica, Thai.*
Atenolol (p.841·3).
Angina pectoris; arrhythmias; hypertension; myocardial infarction.

Velosef *Bristol-Myers Squibb, Belg.; Bristol-Myers Squibb, Hong Kong; Bristol-Myers Squibb, Irl.; Bristol-Myers Squibb, Israel; Bristol-Myers Squibb, Neth.; Bristol-Myers Squibb, NZ; Bristol-Myers Squibb, Port.; Squibb, UK; Apothecon, USA.*
Cefradine (p.173·3).
Bacterial infections.

Velosulin *Novo Nordisk, Denm.; Novo Nordisk, Fin.; Novo Nordisk, Neth.; Novo Nordisk, Norw.; Novo Nordisk, Swed.*
Insulin injection (human, monocomponent) (p.324·1).
Diabetes mellitus.

Novo Nordisk, UK†; Glaxo Wellcome, UK†.
Insulin injection (porcine, highly purified) (p.324·1).
Diabetes mellitus.

Velosulin HM *Novo Nordisk, Aust.; Novo Nordisk, Switz.*
Insulin injection (human, monocomponent) (p.324·1).
Diabetes mellitus.

Velosulin Human BR *Novo Nordisk, USA.*
Insulin injection (human, emp) (p.324·1).
Diabetes mellitus.

Velosulin MC *Novo Nordisk, Switz.†.*
Insulin injection (porcine, monocomponent) (p.324·1).
Diabetes mellitus.

Velosuline Humanum *Novo Nordisk, Belg.*
Insulin injection (human, emp) (p.324·1).
Diabetes mellitus.

Veloudiet *DHN, Fr.*
Preparation for enteral nutrition (p.1350·1).

Velpro *Alpharma, Mex.*
Benzonatate (p.1085·3).
Coughs.

Velsay *Sons, Mex.*
Naproxen (p.60·3).
Musculoskeletal and joint disorders.

Veltane *Lannett, USA†.*
Brompheniramine maleate (p.410·2).
Hypersensitivity reactions.

Veltex *Restan, S.Afr.*
Diclofenac sodium (p.30·3).
Gout; inflammation; musculoskeletal and joint disorders; pain.

Velutrix *Eversil, Braz.*
Tetracycline phosphate complex (p.259·1); muramidase hydrochloride (p.1638·1).
Bacterial infections.

Velvachol *Healthpoint, USA.*
Vehicle for topical preparations.

Velvelan *Merck Sharp & Dohme, Canad.†; Frosst, Canad.†.*
Urea (p.1127·3).
Dry skin disorders.

Vemol *PP Lab, Thai.*
Paracetamol (p.71·2).
Fever; pain.

Venachlor *Lennon, S.Afr.†.*
Atenolol (p.841·3); chlortalidone (p.857·1).
Hypertension.

Venacol *Llorens, Spain.*
Aescin (p.1574·1); esculoside (p.1574·1); heparin sodium (p.902·1); ruscogenin (p.1660·2).
Oedema; peripheral vascular disorders.

Venactive *Formila, Ital.*
Bioflavonoids (p.1611·1); omega-3 triglycerides (p.949·2); centella (p.1112·2).
Vascular disorders.

Venacton *Klein, Ger.*
Aesculus (p.1574·1); scoparium (p.1661·2); hypericum (p.290·2); silybum marianum (p.1021·3); hamamelis (p.1618·3).
Haemorrhoids; paraesthesias; vascular disorders.

Venactone *Benedetti, Ital.*
Potassium canrenoate (p.957·1).
Hyperaldosteronism; hypertension.

Venalisin *AGIPS, Ital.*
Tribenoside (p.1674·2).
Haemorrhoids; thrombophlebitis; varicose veins.

Venalitan *3M, Ger.*
Heparin sodium (p.902·1).
Skin trauma.

Venalot *Note. This name is used for preparations of different composition.*
Byk, Braz.; Byk Gulden, Mex.
Coumarin (p.1599·3); troxerutin (p.1611·2).
Haemorrhoids; oedema; venous insufficiency.

Schaper & Brummer, Ger.
Sustained-release tablets: Coumarin (p.1599·3); troxerutin (p.1611·2).
Haemorrhoids; vascular disorders.
Tablets†: Melilotus.
Formerly contained melilotus and rutoside.
Haemorrhoids; venous insufficiency.

Asta Medica, Switz.†.
Liniment: Melilotus; heparin (p.902·1).
Peripheral vascular disorders.
Sustained-release tablets: Coumarin (p.1599·3).
Formerly contained coumarin and troxerutin.
Lymphoedema.

Venalot H *Byk, Braz.*
Coumarin (p.1599·3); heparin (p.902·1).
Soft-tissue injury.

Venalot mono *Schaper & Brummer, Ger.*
Coumarin (p.1599·3).
Soft-tissue injury.

Venalot N *Schaper & Brummer, Ger.*
Coumarin (p.1599·3); rutoside sodium sulfate (p.1611·2).
Vascular disorders.

Venalot novo *Schaper & Brummer, Ger.*
Aesculus (p.1574·1).
Peripheral vascular disorders.

Venapulse *Lennon, S.Afr.†.*
Atenolol (p.841·3).
Angina pectoris; hypertension.

Venastat *Promeco, Mex.; Pharmaton, Switz.*
Aesculus (p.1574·1).
Chronic venous insufficiency.

Venbig *Biagini, Ital.*
A hepatitis B immunoglobulin (p.1542·1).
Passive immunisation.

Vencipon N *Artesan, Ger.*
Ephedrine hydrochloride (p.1090·1); phenolphthalein (p.1244·1).
Obesity.

Vendal *Lannacher, Aust.*
Morphine hydrochloride (p.56·1).
Pain.

Ven-Detrex *Therabel, Belg.*
Diosmin (p.1611·1).
Peripheral vascular disorders.

Venelbin *Hoechst, Ger.†.*
Dihydroergotamine mesilate (p.450·3); troxerutin (p.1611·2).
Vascular disorders.

Venelbin N *Hoechst, Ger.†.*
Heparin sodium (p.902·1).
Superficial vascular disorders.

Venelbin ruscus *Biocur, Ger.*
Ruscus aculeatus.
Chronic venous insufficiency; haemorrhoids.

Venen-Dragees *CT, Ger.*
Aesculus (p.1574·1).
Venous insufficiency.

Venen-Fluid *CT, Ger.*
Aesculus (p.1574·1).
Phlebitis; soft-tissue injury; varices.

Venengel *Ratiopharm, Ger.*
Heparin sodium (p.902·1); arnica (p.1581·3); aesculus (p.1574·1).
Soft-tissue injury; vascular disorders.

Venen-Salbe *Eu Rho, Ger.*
Aesculus (p.1574·1); arnica (p.1581·3).
Haemorrhoids; soft-tissue injury; venous insufficiency.

Venen-Salbe N *CT, Ger.*
Aesculus (p.1574·1); esculoside (p.1574·1).
Bruising; oedema; varices.

Venen-Tabletten *Stada, Ger.*
Aesculus (p.1574·1).
Venous insufficiency.

Venentabs *Ratiopharm, Ger.*
Aesculus (p.1574·1).
Venous insufficiency.

Venen-Tropfen *Eu Rho, Ger.*
Aesculus (p.1574·1).
Haemorrhoids; thrombosis prophylaxis; venous insufficiency.

Venen-Tropfen N *Bioforce, Ger.*
Aesculus (p.1574·1).
Venous insufficiency.

Venex *Decomed, Port.*
Diosmin (p.1611·1).
Capillary fragility; haemorrhoids; menstrual disorders; orthostatic hypotension; venous insufficiency.

Venimmun *Centeon, Aust.; Centeon, Ger.; Centeon, Ital.*
A normal immunoglobulin (p.1551·3).
Hypogammaglobulinaemia; idiopathic thrombocytopenic purpura; passive immunisation.

Venirene *Irex, Fr.*
Diosmin (p.1611·1).
Capillary disorders; haemorrhoids; venous insufficiency.

Veniten *Whitehall-Robins, Switz.†*
Troxerutin (p.1611·2).
Peripheral vascular disorders.

Venitrin *Astra, Ital.*
Glyceryl trinitrate (p.897·3).
Angina pectoris; hypertensive crises; left-ventricular failure; myocardial infarction.

Venium *Lubapharm Phlebologie, Switz.†*
Coumarin (p.1599·3).
Lymphoedema.

Veno *Sanochemia, Aust.*
Troxerutin (p.1611·2); dihydroergotamine tartrate (p.450·3).
Chronic venous insufficiency.

Veno SL *Ursapharm, Ger.*
Troxerutin (p.1611·2).
Vascular disorders.

Venobene *Ratiopharm, Aust.*
Heparin sodium (p.902·1); dexpanthenol (p.1602·3).
Anorectal disorders; soft-tissue injury; superficial vascular disorders.

Venobiase *Fournier, Ger.*
Ruscus aculeatus rhizome; black currant (p.1389·3).
Vascular disorders.

Venobiase mono *Fournier, Ger.*
Ruscus aculeatus rhizome.
Haemorrhoids; venous insufficiency.

veno-biomo *Biomo, Ger.*
Aesculus (p.1574·1).
Thromboembolic disorders; venous insufficiency.

Venocaina *Braun, Spain†.*
Procaine hydrochloride (p.1319·1).
Local anaesthesia.

Venocur Triplex *Knoll, Braz.*
Rutoside (p.1611·2); aesculus (p.1574·1); miroton.
Venous insufficiency.

Venodin *Tosi, Ital.†*
Tribenoside (p.1674·2).
Haemorrhoids; thrombophlebitis; varicose veins.

Venofer *Therabel, Fr.; Fresenius, Ger.; Vifor, Hong Kong; Vifor, Israel; Ferraz, Lynce, Port.; Vifor International, Israel.; SPB, Thai.; Vifor, Thai.; Syner-Med, UK; American Regent, USA.*
Iron sucrose (p.1370·1).
Iron deficiency; iron-deficiency anaemia.

Venoferrum *Byk Gulden, Mex.*
Iron sucrose (p.1370·1).
Iron-deficiency anaemia.

Venofit *Arkochim, Spain.*
Ruscus aculeatus; melilotus officinalis; hamamelis (p.1618·3).
Peripheral vascular disorders.

Venofortan *Ariston, Braz.*
Aescin (p.1574·1); vitamin B$_1$ (p.1385·2).
Venous insufficiency.

Venogal *Chinosolfabrik, Ger.*
Aesculus (p.1574·1).
Venous insufficiency.

Venogamma *Veripalvelu, Fin.*
A normal immunoglobulin (p.1551·3).
Hypogammaglobulinaemia; idiopathic thrombocytopenic purpura.

Venogamma Anti-Rho (D) *Alfa Biotech, Ital.†.*
An anti-D immunoglobulin (p.1532·1).
Prevention of rhesus sensitisation.

Venogamma Polivalente *Wassermann, Ital.*
A normal immunoglobulin (p.1551·3).
Hypogammaglobulinaemia; passive immunisation.

Venoglobulin *Alpha, Israel; Alpha Therapeutic, Singapore; Alpha Therapeutic, USA.*
A normal immunoglobulin (p.1551·3).
Idiopathic thrombocytopenic purpura; immunodeficiency; Kawasaki disease.

Venoglobulin-S *Alpha, Hong Kong; Alpha Therapeutic, Thai.*
A normal immunoglobulin (p.1551·3).
Idiopathic thrombocytopenic purpura; immunodeficiency; Kawasaki disease.

Venogyl *Teva, Israel.*
Metronidazole (p.594·1).
Anaerobic bacterial infections.

Veno-Hexanicit *Promed, Ger.†.*
Inositol nicotinate (p.914·1); heptaminol hydrochloride (p.1619·2); troxerutin (p.1611·2).
Inflammation; oedema; vascular disorders; vascular headache.

Veno-Kattwiga N *Kattwiga, Ger.*
Aescin (p.1574·1); procaine hydrochloride (p.1319·1).
Vascular disorders.

veno-L 90 N *Loges, Ger.*
Homoeopathic preparation.

Venolen *Pharma Line, Ital.*
Troxerutin (p.1611·2).
Haemorrhoids; varicose veins.

Venolep *Farma Lepori, Spain.*
Hidrosmin (p.1611·2).
Venous insufficiency.

Venomenhal *Hal, Ger.*
Allergen extracts of bee venom and wasp venom (p.1575·3).
Hyposensitisation.

Venomhal *Hal, Neth.†.*
Aqueous bee venom and wasp venom(p.1575·3).
Hyposensitisation.

Venomil *Bencard, Ger.; Miles, USA.*
Venoms of bee, wasp, hornet, yellow jacket, and mixed vespids (p.1575·3).
Hyposensitisation.

Venoparil *Neo-Farmaceutica, Port.*
Tablets: Aescin (p.1574·1).
Haemorrhoids; joint pain; oedema; venous insufficiency.
Topical gel: Aescin (p.1574·1); diethylamine salicylate (p.32·2).
Musculoskeletal, joint, and soft-tissue injury; thrombophlebitis; varices.

Venoplant *Note.This name is used for preparations of different composition.*
Australplant, Aust.†; Schwabe, Ger.
Aesculus (p.1574·1).
Inflammation; menstrual disorders; thromboembolic disorders; venous insufficiency.
Also, Ital.†.
Injection: Aesculus (p.1574·1).
Tablets: Aesculus (p.1574·1); silybum marianum (p.1021·3); hamamelis (p.1618·3).
Varicose veins.
Schwabe, Neth.†.
Aesculus (p.1574·1); hamamelis (p.1618·3); silybum marianum (p.1021·3).
Vascular disorders.
Sanofi Synthelabo, Spain; Schwabe, Spain.
Tablets; oral drops: Silybum marianum (p.1021·3); aesculus (p.1574·1); hamamelis (p.1618·3).
Vascular disorders.
Ointment: Aesculus (p.1574·1); hamamelis (p.1618·3); heparin (p.902·1).
Peripheral vascular disorders.

Venoplant AHS *Schwabe, Ger.*
Aescin (p.1574·1); heparin sodium (p.902·1); glycol salicylate (p.42·2).
Soft-tissue injury; venous insufficiency.

Venoplant comp *Schwabe, Switz.*
Aescin (p.1574·1); heparin sodium (p.902·1); glycol salicylate (p.42·2).
Musculoskeletal, joint, and soft-tissue injuries; scars; venous insufficiency.

Venoplant N *Schwabe, Switz.†.*
Aesculus (p.1574·1); heparin (p.902·1).
Vascular disorders.

Venoplant top *Schwabe, Ger.*
Hamamelis (p.1618·3).
Skin inflammation; varices.

Venoplus *Also, Ital.*
Aesculus (p.1574·1); hamamelis (p.1618·3); silybum marianum (p.1021·3).
Alterations in capillary permeability; varicose veins; venous dilatation.

Venopyronum *Knoll, Ger.*
Delayed-release tablets: Aesculus (p.1574·1).
Venous insufficiency.

Venopyronum N *Knoll, Ger.*
Aesculus (p.1574·1).
Venous insufficiency.

Venopyronum N triplex *Minden, Ger.†.*
Aesculus (p.1574·1); squill (p.1100·3); convallaria (p.1599·1); oleander (p.1643·3); adonis vernalis (p.1573·3).
Venopyronum triplex formerly contained aesculus, squill, convallaria, oleander, adonis vernalis, and rutoside.
Vascular disorders.

Venorell *Sanorell, Ger.*
Homoeopathic preparation.

Venoruton *Note.This name is used for preparations of different composition.*
Novartis Consumer, Aust.; Novartis Consumer, Belg.; Novartis, Denm.; Novartis Consumer, Ger.; Novartis, Hong Kong; Novartis, Is-
rael; *Novartis Consumer, Ital.; Novartis Consumer, Neth.; Novartis Consumer, Port.; Novartis Consumer, Spain; Novartis Consumer, Switz.*
Oxerutins (p.1611·2).
Chronic venous insufficiency; diabetic retinopathy; haemorrhoids; soft-tissue injury.
Allergan-Frumtost, Braz.; Novartis, Thai.
Troxerutin (p.1611·2).
Chronic venous insufficiency; haemorrhoids.

Venoruton Emulgel *Novartis Consumer, Ger.*
Heparin sodium (p.902·1).
Formerly known as Venoruton Heparin.
Superficial vascular disorders.

Venos Cough Mixture *SmithKline Beecham Consumer, UK.*
Glucose (p.1364·1); treacle.
Coughs.

Venos Expectorant *SmithKline Beecham Consumer, Irl.; SmithKline Beecham Consumer, UK.*
Guaifenesin (p.1092·2); glucose (p.1364·2); treacle.
Coughs.

Venos Honey & Lemon *SmithKline Beecham Consumer, UK.*
Glucose (p.1364·1); honey (p.1366·2); lemon juice.
Formerly contained ammonium chloride and ipecacuanha.
Coughs.

Venosan *Binesa, Spain; Mack, Switz.†.*
Inositol nicotinate (p.914·1); pholedrine sulfate (p.955·2); troxerutin (p.1611·2).
Vascular disorders.

Venoselect N *Dreluso, Ger.*
Homoeopathic preparation.

Venosin *Klinge, Aust.*
Capsules; ointment; oral drops: Aesculus (p.1574·1).
Chronic venous insufficiency; haemorrhoids; oedema; superficial vascular disorders; thrombosis prophylaxis.
Topical gel: Aescin (p.1574·1); heparin sodium (p.902·1); glycol salicylate (p.42·2).
Chronic venous insufficiency; oedema; soft-tissue disorders.

Venosmil *Vitoria, Port.; Faes, Spain.*
Hidrosmin (p.1611·2).
Cerebral and ocular vascular disorders; venous insufficiency; vestibular disorders.

Venosmine *Geymonat, Ital.*
Diosmin (p.1611·1).
Peripheral vascular disorders.

Venostasin *Note.This name is used for preparations of different composition.*
Klinge, Aust.; Ariston, Braz.; Klinge, Ger.
Controlled-release capsules; ointment: Aesculus (p.1574·1).
Inflammation; venous insufficiency.
Klinge, Ger.
Topical gel: Aescin (p.1574·1); heparin sodium (p.902·1); glycol salicylate (p.42·2).
Soft-tissue injury; vascular disorders.

Venostasin Composto *Ariston, Braz.*
Heparin sodium (p.902·1); aescin (p.1574·1); glycol salicylate (p.42·2).
Oedema; venous insufficiency.

Veno-Tebonin N *Schwabe, Ger.*
Ginkgo biloba (p.1615·2); heptaminol hydrochloride (p.1619·2); troxerutin (p.1611·2).
Haemorrhoids; vascular disorders.

Venotop *Novartis, Aust.*
Dihydroergotamine tartrate (p.450·3); troxerutin (p.1611·2).
Chronic venous insufficiency.

Venotrauma *Also, Ital.*
Aesculus (p.1574·1); hamamelis (p.1618·3); heparin sodium (p.902·1).
Soft-tissue disorders.

Venotrulan *Bilgast, Ger.*
Hamamelis (p.1618·3); collinsonia canad.; paeonia offic.
Haemorrhoids; vascular disorders.

Venotrulan N *Truw, Ger.†.*
Aesculus (p.1574·1).
Venous insufficiency.

Veno-V *Inibsa, Port.*
Diosmin (p.1611·1).
Oedema; vascular disorders.

Venovit *Vaillant, Ital.*
Ruscus; hamamelis (p.1618·3); aesculus (p.1574·1).
Venous insufficiency.

Vent Retard *BOI, Spain.*
Theophylline (p.777·2).
Heart failure; obstructive airways disease; paroxysmal dyspnoea.

Ventadur *Medeva, Spain.*
Salbutamol sulfate (p.770·3).
Obstructive airways disease.

Ventamol *Pinewood, Irl.*
Salbutamol (p.770·3).
Obstructive airways disease.

Venterol *Greater Pharma, Thai.*
Salbutamol sulfate (p.770·3).
Obstructive airways disease.

Venteze *Aspen, S.Afr.*
Salbutamol (p.770·3) or salbutamol sulfate (p.770·3).
Obstructive airways disease.

Ventide *Glaxo Wellcome, Aust.; Glaxo Wellcome, Hong Kong; Glaxo Wellcome, Mex.; Glaxo Wellcome, Singapore; Glaxo Wellcome, Thai.; Allen & Hanburys, UK.*
Salbutamol (p.770·3) or salbutamol sulfate (p.770·3); beclometasone dipropionate (p.1061·2).
Obstructive airways disease.

Ventilan *Note.This name is used for preparations of different composition.*
Sintofarma, Braz.
Clenbuterol hydrochloride (p.763·3).
Obstructive airways disease.
Glaxo Wellcome, Port.
Salbutamol (p.770·3) or salbutamol sulfate (p.770·3).
Obstructive airways disease; premature labour.

Ventilat *Boehringer Ingelheim, Ger.*
Oxitropium bromide (p.769·2).
Obstructive airways disease.

Ventimax *Norton, S.Afr.*
Salbutamol (p.770·3).
Obstructive airways disease.

Ventisol *Fustery, Mex.*
Ketotifen fumarate (p.767·2).
Asthma; hypersensitivity.

Ventmax *Trinity, UK.*
Salbutamol sulfate (p.770·3).
Obstructive airways disease.

Ventnaze *Aspen, S.Afr.*
Beclometasone dipropionate (p.1061·2).
Hayfever; rhinitis.

Ventodisk *Glaxo Wellcome, Canad.; Glaxo Wellcome, NZ; Glaxo Wellcome, S.Afr.; Glaxo Wellcome, Switz.; Glaxo Wellcome, Thai.*
Salbutamol sulfate (p.770·3).
Obstructive airways disease.

Ventodisks *Glaxo Wellcome, Fr.; Glaxo Wellcome, Hong Kong; Allen & Hanburys, Irl.; Allen & Hanburys, UK.*
Salbutamol sulfate (p.770·3).
Bronchospasm; obstructive airways disease.

Ventolair *3M, Ger.*
Beclometasone dipropionate (p.1061·2).
Asthma.

Ventolase *Juste, Spain.*
Clenbuterol hydrochloride (p.763·3).
Obstructive airways disease.

Ventoliber *Tecnimede, Port.*
Ambroxol hydrochloride (p.1084·3); clenbuterol hydrochloride (p.763·3).

Ventolin *Allen & Hanburys, Austral.; Glaxo Wellcome, Austral.; Glaxo Wellcome, Belg.; Glaxo Wellcome, Canad.; Glaxo Wellcome, Hong Kong; Allen & Hanburys, Irl.; Glaxo Wellcome, Israel; Glaxo Wellcome, Ital.; Glaxo Wellcome, Mex.; Glaxo Wellcome, Neth.; Glaxo Wellcome, NZ; Glaxo Wellcome, S.Afr.; Glaxo Wellcome, Singapore; Glaxo Wellcome, Spain; Glaxo Wellcome, Switz.; Glaxo Wellcome, Thai.; Allen & Hanburys, UK; Glaxo Wellcome, USA.*
Salbutamol (p.770·3) or salbutamol sulfate (p.770·3).
Obstructive airways disease; premature labour; status asthmaticus.

Ventolin Espettorante *Glaxo Wellcome, Ital.*
Salbutamol sulfate (p.770·3); guaifenesin (p.1092·2).
Bronchial congestion; bronchospasm.

Ventolin Expectorant *Glaxo Wellcome, Hong Kong; Glaxo Wellcome, Thai.*
Salbutamol sulfate (p.770·3); guaifenesin (p.1092·2).
Obstructive airways disease.

Ventolin Flogo *Glaxo Wellcome, Ital.*
Beclometasone dipropionate (p.1061·2); salbutamol (p.770·3).
Obstructive airways disease.

Ventoline *Glaxo Wellcome, Denm.; Glaxo Wellcome, Fin.; Glaxo Wellcome, Fr.; Glaxo Wellcome, Norw.; Glaxo Wellcome, Swed.*
Salbutamol (p.770·3) or salbutamol sulfate (p.770·3).
Obstructive airways disease; premature labour.

Ventox *Leiras, Fin.*
Oxitropium bromide (p.769·2).
Obstructive airways disease.

Ventracid N *Repha, Ger.*
Sodium bicarbonate (p.1186·2); pancreatin (p.1646·1); curcuma (p.1029·3).
Gastrointestinal disorders.

Ventre Livre *CIF, Braz.*
Cascara (p.1216·1); docusate sodium (p.1223·1).
Constipation.

Ventricon N *Syxyl, Ger.*
Bismuth subnitrate (p.1213·2); calcium carbonate (p.1215·1); magnesium oxide (p.1233·2).
Gastrointestinal disorders.

Ventrigutt N *Hanosan, Ger.*
Homoeopathic preparation.

ventri-loges *Loges, Ger.*
Homoeopathic preparation.

Ventrimarin novo *Steigerwald, Ger.*
Absinthium (p.1571·1); gentian (p.1615·1); angelica (p.1580·2).
Appetite loss; dyspepsia; meteorism.

Ventrux *Cernelle, Switz.*
Enterococcus faecium (p.1626·3).
Gastrointestinal disorders; restoration of intestinal flora.

Ventzone *Aspen, S.Afr.*
Beclometasone dipropionate (p.1061·2).
Asthma.

Venucreme *Lubapharm, Switz.*
Heparin sodium (p.902·1); glycol salicylate (p.42·2); dimethyl sulfoxide (p.1402·2); lauromacrogol 600 (p.1345·2); dexpanthenol (p.1602·3).
Phlebitis; soft-tissue disorders; venous insufficiency.

Venugel *Lubapharm, Switz.*
Heparin sodium (p.902·1); glycol salicylate (p.42·2); dimethyl sulfoxide (p.1402·2); lauromacrogol 600 (p.1345·2); dexpanthenol (p.1602·3).
Phlebitis; soft-tissue disorders; venous insufficiency.

Venustas Lozione Antiforfora *BPR, Ital.*
Cinchona succirubra (p.1595·3).
Seborrhoeic dermatitis.

Venustas Lozione Caduta *BPR, Ital.*
Arnica (p.1581·3).
Alopecia.

Venustas Shampoo per Capelli con Forfora e/o Grassi *BPR, Ital.*
Urtica (p.1678·2).
Seborrhoeic dermatitis.

Venyl *Dolisos, Fr.*
Ruscus aculeatus; hesperidin methyl chalcone (p.1611·2); ascorbic acid (p.1389·3).
Haemorrhoids; peripheral vascular disorders.

Vepar *Savio, Ital.†*
Suleparoid (p.978·2).
Peripheral vascular disorders.

Vepenicillin *Scand Pharm, Swed.†*
Phenoxymethylpenicillin potassium (p.235·1).
Bacterial infections.

Vepesid
Bristol-Myers Squibb, Aust.; Bristol-Myers Squibb, Austral.; Bristol-Myers Squibb, Belg.; Bristol-Myers Squibb, Braz.; Bristol, Canad.; Bristol-Myers Squibb, Denm.; Bristol-Myers Squibb, Fin.; Bristol-Myers Squibb, Ger.; Bristol-Myers Squibb, Hong Kong; Bristol-Myers Squibb, Irl.; Bristol-Myers Squibb, Israel; Bristol-Myers Squibb, Ital.; Bristol-Myers Squibb, Mex.; Bristol-Myers Squibb, Neth.; Bristol-Myers Squibb, Norw.; Bristol-Myers Squibb, NZ; Bristol-Myers Squibb, S.Afr.; Bristol-Myers Squibb, Singapore; Bristol-Myers Squibb, Spain; Bristol-Myers Squibb, Swed.; Bristol-Myers Squibb, Switz.; Bristol-Myers Squibb, Thai.; Bristol-Myers Squibb, UK; Bristol-Myers Squibb Oncology, USA.
Etoposide (p.538·1).
Malignant neoplasms.

Vepeside *Novartis, Fr.*
Etoposide (p.538·1).
Malignant neoplasms.

Vepicombin *Nycomed, Denm.*
Phenoxymethylpenicillin potassium (p.235·1).
Bacterial infections.

Vera *ABZ, Ger.; CT, Ger.; Heumann, Ger.; BASF, Ger.*
Verapamil hydrochloride (p.989·1).
Angina pectoris; arrhythmias; hypertension.

Verabeta *Betapharm, Ger.*
Verapamil hydrochloride (p.989·1).
Angina pectoris; arrhythmias; hypertension.

Veracaps *Sigma, Austral.*
Verapamil hydrochloride (p.989·1).
Angina pectoris; hypertension.

Veracapt *Ebewe, Aust.*
Verapamil hydrochloride (p.989·1); captopril (p.853·3).
Hypertension.

Veracef *Bristol-Myers Squibb, Mex.*
Cefradine (p.173·3).
Bacterial infections.

Veracim *Cimex, Switz.†*
Verapamil hydrochloride (p.989·1).
Arrhythmias; ischaemic heart disease.

Veracolate
Note. This name is used for preparations of different composition.
Aspen, S.Afr.
Cascara sagrada (p.1216·1); phenolphthalein (p.1244·1).
Formerly contained bile salts, cascara sagrada, phenolphthalein, and capsicum oleoresin.
Constipation.
Warner-Lambert, Thai.
Bile salt (p.1585·1); cascara (p.1216·1); phenolphthalein (p.1244·1); capsicum oleoresin (p.1591·1).
Biliary-tract disorders; intestinal motility disorders.
Numark, USA†.
Cascara (p.1216·1); phenolphthalein (p.1244·1); capsicum oleoresin (p.1591·1).

Veracor *Dexxon, Israel.*
Verapamil hydrochloride (p.989·1).
Angina pectoris; arrhythmias; hypertension.

Veracoron *Cibran, Braz.*
Verapamil hydrochloride (p.989·1).
Angina pectoris; arrhythmias; hypertension.

Veracur *Typharm, Irl.†; Typharm, UK.*
Formaldehyde (p.1144·2).
Warts.

Veragamma *Worwag, Ger.*
Verapamil hydrochloride (p.989·1).
Angina pectoris; arrhythmias; hypertension.

Veragel
United American, Hong Kong; Great Eastern, Thai.; United American, Thai.
Aluminium hydroxide-magnesium carbonate co-dried gel (p.1211·2); dimethicone (p.1249·2); dicyclomine [dicycloverine] hydrochloride (p.466·1).
Dyspepsia; gastric hyperacidity; gastritis; heartburn; peptic ulcer.

Veragel DMS *United American, Singapore.*
Aluminium hydroxide-magnesium carbonate co-dried gel (p.1211·2); dimethicone (p.1249·2); dicyclomine [dicycloverine] hydrochloride (p.466·1).
Duodenitis; dyspepsia; flatulence; gastric hyperacidity; gastritis; gastro-oesophageal reflux; gastrointestinal motility disorders; heartburn; peptic ulcer; pylorospasm.

Verahexal
Hexal, Austral.; Hexal, Ger.; Hexal, S.Afr.†
Verapamil hydrochloride (p.989·1).
Angina pectoris; arrhythmias; hypertension.

Verakard *Nycomed, Norw.*
Verapamil hydrochloride (p.989·1).
Angina pectoris; arrhythmias; hypertension.

Veraken *Kener, Mex.*
Verapamil (p.991·1).

Veralan *Quimica y Farmacia, Mex.*
Verapamil hydrochloride (p.989·1).
Angina pectoris; arrhythmias; hypertension.

Vera-Lich *Lichtenstein, Ger.*
Verapamil hydrochloride (p.989·1).
Angina pectoris; arrhythmias; hypertension.

Veraligral *Searle, Mex.*
Veralipride (p.711·2).
Menopausal disorders.

Veralipril *Sanofi Synthelabo, Ital.*
Veralipride (p.711·2).
Menopausal disorders.

Veraloc
Orion, Denm.; Orion, Swed.
Verapamil hydrochloride (p.989·1).
Angina pectoris; arrhythmias; hypertension; myocardial infarction.

Veramex *Sanofi Synthelabo, Ger.*
Verapamil hydrochloride (p.989·1).
Angina pectoris; arrhythmias; hypertension; myocardial infarction.

Veramil *Orion, Irl.*
Verapamil hydrochloride (p.989·1).
Angina pectoris; arrhythmias; hypertension.

Veramon
Note. This name is used for preparations of different composition.
Schering-Plough, Braz.
Aspirin (p.14·2); paracetamol (p.71·2); caffeine (p.761·3).
Fever; pain.
Sofar, Ital.
Propyphenazone (p.80·2); paracetamol (p.71·2).
Fever; pain.

Veranorm *Isis Puren, Ger.*
Verapamil hydrochloride (p.989·1).
Angina pectoris; arrhythmias; hypertension.

Verapabene *Ratiopharm, Aust.*
Verapamil hydrochloride (p.989·1).
Angina pectoris; arrhythmias; heart failure; hypertension; hypertrophic obstructive cardiomyopathy.

Verapin *Berlin Pharm, Thai.*
Verapamil hydrochloride (p.989·1).
Angina pectoris; arrhythmias; hypertension.

Verapress
Dexcel, Israel; Dexcel, UK.
Verapamil hydrochloride (p.989·1).
Angina pectoris; hypertension.

Verasal *TAD, Ger.*
Verapamil hydrochloride (p.989·1).
Angina pectoris; arrhythmias; hypertension.

Verasifar *Siphar, Switz.*
Verapamil hydrochloride (p.989·1).
Hypertension.

Veratensin *Farma Lepori, Spain.*
Verapamil hydrochloride (p.989·1).
Angina pectoris; arrhythmias; hypertension.

Veratide *Procter & Gamble, Ger.*
Verapamil hydrochloride (p.989·1); triamterene (p.986·1); hydrochlorothiazide (p.907·3).
Hypertension.

Veratran *Murat, Fr.*
Clotiazepam (p.671·1).
Alcohol withdrawal syndrome; anxiety.

Veratrum Med Complex *Dynamit, Aust.*
Homoeopathic preparation.

Verax
Tosi, Hong Kong; Tosi, Ital.
Benzydamine hydrochloride (p.20·1).
Mouth and throat disorders; phlebitis; venous insufficiency; vulvovaginal disorders.

Verazinc *Forest Pharmaceuticals, USA.*
Zinc sulfate (p.1398·2).
Dietary supplement.

Verbalem *Lemery, Mex.*
Paracetamol (p.71·2).
Fever; pain.

Verbascum Complex *Blackmores, Austral.*
Verbascum thapsus; marrubium vulgare (p.1094·2); pleurisy root (p.1653·1); liquorice (p.1231·2); ascorbic acid (p.1389·3); vitamin A acetate (p.1383·2).
Respiratory system disorders.

Verbesol *ICT, Ital.†*
L-Verbenone.
Respiratory-tract disorders.

Verbex *Istoria, Ital.†*
L-verbenone.
Respiratory-tract disorders.

Verboril *Select, Ital.†*
L-Verbenone.
Respiratory-tract disorders.

Vercef
Faulding, Austral.; Ranbaxy, S.Afr.; Ranbaxy, Singapore; Ranbaxy, Thai.
Cefaclor (p.161·1).
Bacterial infections.

Vercite *Abbott, Ital.*
Pipobroman (p.565·1).
Chronic myeloid leukaemia; polycythaemia vera.

Vercyte *Abbott, Ital.*
Pipobroman (p.565·1).
Polycythaemia vera.

Verdal *Falqui, Ital.*
Aspirin (p.14·2); paracetamol (p.71·2); caffeine (p.761·3).
Fever; influenza symptoms; pain.

Verecolene CM *Maggioni, Ital.*
Bisacodyl (p.1212·2).
Constipation.

Verecolene Complesso *Maggioni, Ital.†*
Fencibutirol (p.1610·1); frangula (p.1227·1); rhubarb (p.1248·1); cascara (p.1216·1); phenolphthalein (p.1244·1).
Constipation.

Verel *Yamanouchi, Ital.*
Salicylic acid (p.1122·3); lactic acid (p.1626·2).
Hard skin; verrucas; warts.

Verelait *Bouty, Ital.*
Lactulose (p.1230·1).
Constipation.

Verelan
Wyeth-Ayerst, Canad.; Elan, Irl.; Schwarz, USA.
Verapamil hydrochloride (p.989·1).
Hypertension.

Verexamil *Fresenius Kabi, Aust.*
Verapamil hydrochloride (p.989·1).
Angina pectoris; arrhythmias; hypertension.

Verfid *Continentales, Mex.*
Piperazine (p.105·3).

Vergentan *Sanofi Synthelabo, Ger.*
Alizapride hydrochloride (p.1209·3).
Nausea and vomiting; radiation sickness.

Vergeturine *Bailleul, Fr.*
Vitamins (p.1350·1).
Skin disorders.

Vergon *Marnel, USA.*
Meclozine hydrochloride (p.420·3).

Vericaps *Ovelle, Irl.*
Salicylic acid (p.1122·3).
Warts.

Vericardine *Biologiques de l'Ile-de-France, Fr.*
Phenobarbital (p.355·1); crataegus (p.1600·2).
Formerly contained papaverine hydrochloride, quinine hydrobromide, phenobarbital, and crataegus.
Anxiety; insomnia; nervous disorders.

Veriderm *Lachifarma, Ital.†*
Sulfur (p.1123·3).
Seborrhoea.

Veriga *Frega, Canad.†*
Piperazine citrate (p.105·3).

Verimex *Vachon, Canad.*
Piperazine citrate (p.105·3).

Verintex *Pekana, Ger.*
Homoeopathic preparation.

Verintex N *Pekana, Ger.*
Homoeopathic preparation.

Veripaque *Sanofi Winthrop, UK†.*
Oxyphenisatine (p.1243·1).
Barium enema adjunct; bowel evacuation.

Verisan *Knoll, Mex.*
Aesculus (p.1574·1).
Venous insufficiency.

Veriscal D *Faes, Spain.*
Calcium carbonate (p.1215·1); colecalciferol (p.1391·1).
Calcium deficiency; osteoporosis.

Verisop *Gerard, Irl.*
Verapamil hydrochloride (p.989·1).
Angina pectoris; hypertension; supraventricular tachycardia.

Verizym *Bittermedizin, Ger.*
Papain (p.1647·3).

Verladyn *Verla, Ger.*
Dihydroergotamine mesilate (p.450·3).
Hypotension; migraine and related vascular headaches.

Verla-Lipon *Verla, Ger.*
Thioctic acid (p.1671·3) or ethylenediamine thioctate (p.1671·3).
Diabetic polyneuropathy.

Verlim 3 *Saninter, Port.*
Collodion.
Verrucas.

Verlin *Sanval, Braz.*
Procaine hydrochloride (p.1319·1); zinc sulfate (p.1398·2); boric acid (p.1586·1).
Eye disorders.

Vermepen *Dinafarma, Braz.*
Mebendazole (p.102·2).
Worm infections.

Vermex *Hua, Thai.*
Piperazine citrate (p.105·3).
Ascariasis; enterobiasis.

Vermi *Quimpe, Spain.*
Piperazine adipate (p.105·3).
Worm infections.

Vermicol *Degorts, Mex.*
Mebendazole (p.102·2).
Worm infections.

Vermidil *Diba, Mex.*
Mebendazole (p.102·2).
Worm infections.

Vermifran *Faria, Braz.*
Piperazine hydrate (p.106·1).
Ascariasis; enterobiasis.

Vermifuge *Sorin-Maxim, Fr.*
Piperazine hydrate (p.106·1).
Formerly contained piperazine hydrate and sodium bromide.
Intestinal nematode infections.

Vermilan *Quimica y Farmacia, Mex.*
Albendazole (p.95·2).
Worm infections.

Vermilen *Quimioterapica, Braz.*
Piperazine (p.105·3).
Ascariasis; enterobiasis.

Vermin
Note. This name is used for preparations of different composition.
Medinovum, Fin.
Verapamil hydrochloride (p.989·1).
Angina pectoris; arrhythmias; hypertension; myocardial infarction.
Streger, Mex.
Piperazine (p.105·3).
Worm infections.

Vermin-Dazol *Streger, Mex.*
Mebendazole (p.102·2).
Worm infections.

Vermine *Pharmasant, Thai.*
Verapamil hydrochloride (p.989·1).
Angina pectoris; arrhythmias; hypertension.

Vermin-Plus *Streger, Mex.*
Albendazole (p.95·2).
Intestinal nematode infections.

Vermirax *Johnson & Johnson, Braz.*
Mebendazole (p.102·2).
Worm infections.

Vermisen *Novag, Mex.*
Albendazole (p.95·2).
Worm infections.

Vermital *Elofar, Braz.*
Albendazole (p.95·2).
Worm infections.

Vermixide *Polipharm, Thai.*
Albendazole (p.95·2).
Worm infections.

Vermizol *Kinder, Braz.*
Tetramisole (p.108·3); pyrvinium embonate (p.108·2).
Nematode infections.

Vermol *Faria, Braz.*
Mebendazole (p.102·2); tiabendazole (p.109·1).
Worm infections.

Vermonon *Brasifa, Braz.*
Mebendazole (p.102·2).
Worm infections.

Vermoplex *Honorterapica, Braz.*
Mebendazole (p.102·2).
Worm infections.

Vermoral *Legrand, Braz.*
Mebendazole (p.102·2).
Worm infections.

Vermox
Janssen-Cilag, Austral.; Janssen-Cilag, Belg.; Janssen-Ortho, Canad.; Janssen-Cilag, Denm.; Janssen-Cilag, Ger.; Janssen, Hong Kong; Janssen-Cilag, Irl.; Janssen-Cilag, Israel; Janssen-Cilag, Ital.; Janssen, Mex.; Janssen-Cilag, Neth.; Janssen-Cilag, Norw.; Janssen-Cilag, NZ; Janssen-Cilag, S.Afr.; Janssen-Cilag, Swed.; Janssen-Cilag, Switz.; Janssen-Cilag, UK; Janssen, USA.
Mebendazole (p.102·2).
Worm infections.

Vernacycline-V *Propan, S.Afr.†*
Oxytetracycline hydrochloride (p.234·1); vitamin B substances (p.1350·1).
Bacterial infections.

Vernarin *Nakornpatana, Thai.*
Cinnarizine (p.413·1).
Cerebral and peripheral vascular disorders; migraine; motion sickness; vestibular disorders.

Vernausin *Ofimex, Mex.*
Difenidol (p.1222·1).

Vernelan *Verla, Ger.*
Magnesium aspartate hydrobromide (p.690·2).
Nervous disorders; sleep disorders.

Vernies *Davis, Spain.*
Glyceryl trinitrate (p.897·3).
Angina pectoris; heart failure; myocardial infarction.

Vernleigh Baby Cream *Propan, S.Afr.; Covan, S.Afr.*
Zinc oxide (p.1128·2); starch.
Skin disorders.

Vernthol *Propan, S.Afr.†*
Theophylline (p.777·2).
Obstructive airways disease.

Verolax *Angelini, Ital.*
Glycerol (p.1616·3).
Constipation.

The symbol † denotes a preparation no longer actively marketed

Veroptinstada *Stada, Ger.*
Verapamil hydrochloride (p.989·1).
Angina pectoris; arrhythmias; hypertension.

Verorab *Aventis, S.Afr.*
Rabies vaccine (p.1560·2).
Formerly known as Imovax Rabies Vero.
Active immunisation.

verospiron *Hormosan, Ger.*
Spironolactone (p.973·2).
Oedema.

Verotina *Libbs, Braz.*
Fluoxetine (p.288·2).
Depression; obsessive-compulsive disorder.

Veroven *Lepori, Port.*
Hidrosmin (p.1611·2).
Cerebrovascular disorders; haemorrhoids; venous insufficiency.

Veroxil *Baldacci, Ital.*
Indapamide (p.913·1).
Hypertension.

Verpacor *Pharmacia Upjohn, Fin.*
Verapamil hydrochloride (p.989·1).
Angina pectoris; arrhythmias; hypertension; myocardial infarction.

Verpamil *Orion, Fin.; Pacific, NZ; Rolab, S.Afr.; Orion, Singapore.*
Verapamil (p.991·1) or verapamil hydrochloride (p.989·1).
Now known as Rolab-Verapamil HCl in S.Afr.
Angina pectoris; arrhythmias; hypertension; myocardial infarction.

Verra-med *Permamed, Switz.*
Tretinoin (p.1126·2); salicylic acid (p.1122·3); dimethyl sulfoxide (p.1402·2).
Warts.

Verr-Canth *C & M, USA†; Palisades, USA†.*
Cantharidin (p.1590·3).
Removal of benign epithelial growths.

Verrex *C & M, USA†; Palisades, USA†.*
Salicylic acid (p.1122·3); podophyllum resin (p.1121·1).
Removal of benign epithelial growths.

Verruca Treatment *Numark, UK.*
Salicylic acid (p.1122·3).

Verrucare *Medinfar, Port.*
Salicylic acid (p.1122·3); lactic acid (p.1626·2); fluorouracil (p.540·2).
Warts.

Verrucid *Galen, Ger.*
Salicylic acid (p.1122·3).
Calluses; corns; warts.

Verrucosal *Monal, Fr.†.*
Salicylic acid (p.1122·3).
Warts.

Verrufilm *Biorga, Fr.; Isopharm, Hong Kong; Medinfar, Port.*
Lactic acid (p.1626·2); salicylic acid (p.1122·3).
Warts.

Verrugon *Pickles, UK.*
Salicylic acid (p.1122·3).
Hard skin; warts.

Verrulyse-Methionine
Bournonville, Belg.†.
Magnesium oxide (p.1233·2); methionine (p.1012·2); calcium glycerophosphate (p.1188·2); ferric glycerophosphate (p.1617·3); manganese glycerophosphate (p.1617·3); magnesium glycerophosphate (p.1191·1).
Warts.

CS, Fr.
Magnesium oxide (p.1233·2); methionine (p.1012·2); calcium glycerophosphate (p.1188·2); ferric glycerophosphate (p.1617·3); manganese glycerophosphate (p.1617·3).
Warts.

Verrumal
Note.This name is used for preparations of different composition.
Hermal, Ger.; Hermal, Hong Kong; Hermal, Israel; Hermal, Singapore; Boots Healthcare, Switz.; Boots, Thai.; Hermal, Thai.
Fluorouracil (p.540·2); salicylic acid (p.1122·3); dimethyl sulfoxide (p.1402·2).
Warts.

Hermal, Port.
Fluorouracil (p.540·2); salicylic acid (p.1122·3).
Solar keratoses; warts.

Verrupan *Pharmadeveloppement, Fr.*
Thuja (p.1672·1); salicylic acid (p.1122·3); lactic acid (p.1626·2).
Warts.

Verrupatch *Vinas, Spain.*
Salicylic acid (p.1122·3).
Warts.

Verruplan *Vinas, Spain.*
Salicylic acid (p.1122·3).
Warts.

Verrupor *Sella, Ital.*
Trichloroacetic acid (p.1674·3).
Hard skin; verrucas; warts.

Verrux *Novaquimica, Braz.*
Lactic acid (p.1626·2); salicylic acid (p.1122·3).
Hard skin; keratinisation disorders; warts.

Versacaps *Seatrace, USA.*
Pseudoephedrine hydrochloride (p.1099·2); guaifenesin (p.1092·2).
Coughs.

Versal
Schering-Plough, Denm.; Nycomed, Norw.†; Pro Medica, Swed.
Loratadine (p.420·1).
Allergic conjunctivitis; allergic rhinitis; urticaria.

Versamiv *Novag, Mex.*
Diiodohydroxyquinoline (p.590·2).
Amoebiasis.

Versan *Sanfer, Mex.*
Dextromethorphan (p.1087·3).

Versed
Roche, Canad.; Roche, USA.
Midazolam hydrochloride (p.692·3).
Premedication; sedative.

Versel *Trans Canaderm, Canad.*
Selenium sulfide (p.1123·1).
Fungal skin infections.

Versiclear *Hope, USA.*
Sodium thiosulfate (p.1024·2); salicylic acid (p.1122·3).
Fungal infections.

Versigen *Chew, Thai.*
Gentamicin (p.212·1).
Bacterial skin infections.

Versol
Note.This name is used for preparations of different composition.
Gerbex, Canad.†.
Piperazine (p.105·3).

Aguettant, Fr.
Sodium chloride (p.1196·1) or water for irrigation.

Verstadol *Bristol-Myers, Spain†.*
Butorphanol tartrate (p.22·2).
Pain; premedication.

Versus *CSC, Aust.; Angelini, Ital.*
Bendazac (p.19·3).
Skin disorders.

Vertab
Note.This name is used for preparations of different composition.
Dexcel, UK.
Verapamil hydrochloride (p.989·1).
Angina pectoris; hypertension.

UAD, USA†.
Dimenhydrinate (p.415·2).

Vertebralon N *Rentschler, Ger.*
Glycol salicylate (p.42·2); nonivamide (p.63·1); salicylic acid (p.1122·3).
Musculoskeletal, joint, and soft-tissue disorders.

Vertel *Bial, Port.*
Pyrantel embonate (p.108·1).

Vertex *Carnot, Mex.*
Mebendazole (p.102·2).
Worm infections.

Vertigirex *Irex, Fr.*
Betahistine hydrochloride (p.1584·2).
Vestibular disorders.

Vertigoheel
Heel, Ger.; Heel, S.Afr.; Heel, USA.
Homoeopathic preparation.

Vertigo-Hevert *Hevert, Ger.*
Homoeopathic preparation.

Vertigo-Meresa *Dolorgiet, Ger.*
Sulpiride (p.706·1).
Ménière's disease.

Vertigon *Gerard, Irl.*
Betahistine hydrochloride (p.1584·2).
Formerly contained prochlorperazine maleate.
Ménière's disease.

vertigo-neogama *Hormosan, Ger.*
Sulpiride (p.706·1).
Vertigo.

Vertigopas *Pascoe, Ger.*
Homoeopathic preparation.

Vertigo-Vomex *Yamanouchi, Ger.*
Dimenhydrinate (p.415·2).
Vertigo; vestibular disorders.

Vertigum *Liade, Spain†.*
Dixyrazine (p.682·1); inositol nicotinate (p.914·1); pyridoxine hydrochloride (p.1386·3).
Vertigo.

Vertin *Alba, USA†.*
Meclozine hydrochloride (p.420·3).

Vertipam *Orion, Fin.*
Diazepam (p.674·3); cyclizine hydrochloride (p.414·1); nicotinic acid (p.1372·3).
Vestibular disorders.

Vertirosan *Sigmapharm, Aust.*
Dimenhydrinate (p.415·2).
Migraine; motion sickness; nausea and vomiting; vestibular disorders.

Vertirosan Vitamin B₆ *Sigmapharm, Aust.*
Dimenhydrinate (p.415·2); pyridoxine hydrochloride (p.1386·3).
Migraine; motion sickness; nausea and vomiting; vestibular disorders.

Vertisal *Silanes, Mex.*
Metronidazole (p.594·1) or metronidazole benzoate (p.594·1).
Amoebiasis; anaerobic bacterial infections; giardiasis; trichomoniasis.

Vertiserc *Solvay, Ital.*
Betahistine hydrochloride (p.1584·2).
Vestibular disorders.

Vertix *Ache, Braz.*
Flunarizine hydrochloride (p.418·1).
Vertigo.

Vertizine D *Ache, Braz.*
Dihydroergocristine mesilate (p.1603·2); flunarizine hydrochloride (p.418·1).
Vertigo.

Vertizole *Rayere, Mex.*
Mebendazole (p.102·2).
Worm infections.

Verucasep *Galen, Irl.†; Galen, UK†.*
Glutaral (p.1145·2).
Warts.

Verucca Removal System *SSL, UK.*
Salicylic acid (p.1122·3).
Verrucas.

Verucid
Note.This name is used for preparations of different composition.
Galderma, Denm.; Yamanouchi, Ital.; Galderma, Norw.
Salicylic acid (p.1122·3); lactic acid (p.1626·2).
Hard skin; verrucas; warts.

Agis, Israel.
Salicylic acid (p.1122·3); fluorouracil (p.540·2); dimethyl sulfoxide (p.1402·2).
Warts.

Verufil *Stiefel, Spain.*
Lactic acid (p.1626·2); salicylic acid (p.1122·3).
Warts.

Verunec 3 *Savoma, Ital.*
Salicylic acid (p.1122·3); lactic acid (p.1626·2); urea (p.1127·3).
Hard skin; verrucas; warts.

Verutal *Stiefel, Fr.*
Glutaral (p.1145·2).
Warts.

Verutex *Roche, Braz.*
Fusidic acid (p.208·3).
Bacterial skin infections.

Verytracin *Diba, Mex.*
Erythromycin (p.201·2).
Bacterial infections.

Vesadol *Janssen-Cilag, Fr.*
Haloperidol (p.686·3); buzepide metiodide (p.465·1).
Gastrointestinal spasms associated with anxiety.

Vesagex *Rybar, Irl.; Co-Pharma, UK.*
Cetrimide (p.1137·1).
Skin injuries, irritation, and inflammation.

Vesalium *Janssen-Cilag, Aust.; Janssen-Cilag, Belg.†.*
Haloperidol (p.686·3); isopropamide iodide (p.470·1).
Anxiety; psychosomatic disorders.

Vesanoid
Roche, Aust.; Roche, Austral.; Roche, Belg.; Roche, Canad.; Roche, Fin.; Roche, Fr.; Roche, Ger.; Roche, Hong Kong; Roche, Israel; Roche, Ital.; Roche, Mex.; Roche, Neth.; Roche, Norw.†; Roche, NZ; Roche, Port.; Roche, S.Afr.; Roche, Singapore; Roche, Swed.†; Roche, Switz.; Roche, UK; Roche, USA.
Tretinoin (p.1126·2).
Acute promyelocytic leukaemia.

Vesdil
Astra, Ger.; Promed, Ger.; Astra, Switz.
Ramipril (p.966·3).
Heart failure; hypertension; myocardial infarction.

Vesdil plus *Astra, Ger.; Promed, Ger.*
Ramipril (p.966·3); hydrochlorothiazide (p.907·3).
Hypertension.

Vesibil *Flopen, Braz.*
Choline (p.1356·3); vitamin B substances (p.1350·1).
Liver disorders.

Vesiherb *Cesra, Ger.*
Cucurbita (p.1601·1).
Formerly known as Prostaherb Cucurbitae.
Prostatic disorders.

Vesilax *Frega, Canad.†.*
Cascara (p.1216·1); phenolphthalein (p.1244·1); bile salts (p.1585·1); pancreatin (p.1646·1); papain (p.1647·3).

Vesirig *Aguettant, Fr.*
Sodium chloride (p.1196·1).
Lavage and irrigation.

Vesix *Nycomed, Fin.*
Frusemide [furosemide] (p.893·1).
Hypertension; oedema.

Vesparax
UCB, Belg.†; UCB, Neth.; UCB, Port.†; UCB, S.Afr.†.
Hydroxyzine (p.419·2); brallobarbital (p.656·3); secobarbital (p.705·2).
Insomnia.

Vesprin *Apothecon, USA.*
Triflupromazine hydrochloride (p.711·1).
Nausea; psychoses; vomiting.

Vessel *Farmion, Braz.*
Cinnarizine (p.413·1).
Peripheral vascular disorders; vertigo.

Vessel Due F *Wassermann, Ital.*
Sulodexide (p.978·3).
Thrombosis prophylaxis.

Vesselvite *Bajamar, USA.*
Folic acid; vitamin B₆; vitamin B₁₂; vitamin E (p.1350·1).

Vessiflex *Wassermann, Ital.*
Sulodexide (p.978·3); aminopropylone (p.13·3).
Inflammation; injuries associated with pain and swelling.

Vetedol *Robert, Spain†.*
Benorilate (p.19·3).
Fever; musculoskeletal, joint, and peri-articular disorders; pain.

Vethoine *Wolfs, Belg.*
Phenytoin (p.357·2); phenobarbital (p.355·1); cascara (p.1216·1).
Epilepsy.

Vetren *Byk, Aust.; Byk Gulden, Ger.; Roland, Ger.*
Heparin sodium (p.902·1).
Soft tissue injury; superficial vascular disorders.

Vetuss HC *Cypress, USA†.*
Hydrocodone tartrate (p.42·2); phenylephrine hydrochloride (p.1097·1); phenylpropanolamine hydrochloride (p.1098·1); mepyramine maleate (p.421·1); pheniramine maleate (p.422·3).
Coughs and related respiratory-tract disorders.

Vexol *Alcon, Aust.; Alcon, Canad.; Alcon, Denm.; Alcon, Fin.; Alcon, Fr.; Alcon, Ger.; Alcon, Irl.; Alcon, Ital.; Alcon, Port.; Alcon Cusi, Spain; Alcon, Swed.; Alcon, Switz.; Alcon, UK; Alcon, USA.*
Rimexolone (p.1079·3).
Inflammatory eye disorders.

Vexolon *Alcon, Norw.*
Rimexolone (p.1079·3).
Inflammatory eye disorders.

Veybirol-Tyrothyricine *Veyron-Froment, Fr.*
Solution A: formaldehyde (p.1144·2); solution B: tyrothricin (p.267·1).
Mouth infections.

Via Mal *Byk Gulden, Ital.*
Aspirin (p.14·2); caffeine (p.761·3).
Aluminium hydroxide (p.1210·3) is included in this preparation in an attempt to limit the adverse effects of aspirin on the gastrointestinal mucosa.
Fever; pain.

Via Mal Trauma Gel *Byk Gulden, Ital.*
Diethylamine salicylate (p.32·2); heparin sodium (p.902·1); menthol (p.1632·3).
Soft-tissue disorders.

Viabom *CPH, Port.*
Dimenhydrinate (p.415·2).
Motion sickness.

Viacin *Aspen, S.Afr.*
Doxycycline hyclate (p.200·1).
Bacterial infections.

Viadent
Note.This name is used for preparations of different composition.
Carter Horner, Canad.
Mouthwash: Sanguinaria (p.1660·3).

Colgate-Palmolive, Canad.
Toothpaste: Sanguinaria (p.1660·3); sodium monofluorophosphate (p.1377·2).
Dental plaque; gingivitis.

Viaderm-KC *Taro, Canad.*
Triamcinolone acetonide (p.1080·1); neomycin sulfate (p.228·1); nystatin (p.392·2); gramicidin (p.213·3).
Infected skin disorders.

Viadetres *Alacan, Spain.*
Hydroxocobalamin (p.1388·1); pyritinol hydrochloride (p.1657·1); prosultiamine (p.1385·1).
Vitamin B deficiency.

Viadur *Alza, USA.*
Leuprorelin acetate (p.1289·2).
Prostatic cancer.

Viafen *Novartis Consumer, Ital.*
Bufexamac (p.20·3).
Dermatitis; insect stings; pruritus.

Viaggio *Vifor, Switz.†.*
Dimenhydrinate (p.415·2); atropine sulfate (p.461·1); hyoscyamine sulfate (p.469·3); hyoscine hydrobromide (p.468·2); caffeine (p.761·3).
Motion sickness; nausea; vomiting.

Viagra
Pfizer, Aust.; Pfizer, Austral.; Pfizer, Belg.; Pfizer, Canad.; Pfizer, Denm.; Pfizer, Fin.; Pfizer, Fr.; Pfizer, Ger.; Pfizer, Hong Kong; Pfizer, Irl.; Pfizer, Israel; Pfizer, Ital.; Pfizer, Mex.; Pfizer, Norw.; Douglas, NZ; Pfizer, Port.; Pfizer, S.Afr.; Pfizer, Singapore; Pfizer Consumer, Spain; Pfizer, Swed.; Pfizer, Switz.; Pfizer, Thai.; Pfizer, UK; Pfizer, USA.
Sildenafil citrate (p.1662·3).
Erectile dysfunction.

Vial's tonischer Wein *Eberth, Ger.*
Calcium phospholactate; beef extract; cinchonine; wine.
Tonic.

Viamon *Nadeau, Canad.*
Multivitamin and mineral preparation (p.1350·1).

Viani *Glaxo Wellcome, Ger.; Cascan, Ger.*
Salmeterol; fluticasone propionate (p.1072·2).
Asthma.

Viapres *Zambon, Ital.*
Lacidipine (p.919·1).
Hypertension.

Viarex *Schering-Plough, Israel.*
Beclometasone dipropionate (p.1061·2).
Asthma.

Viarox
Byk Gulden, Ger.; Schering-Plough, S.Afr.
Beclometasone dipropionate (p.1061·2).
Asthma; rhinitis.

Viartril
Note.This name is used for preparations of different composition.
Rotta, Hong Kong; Rotta, Thai.
Capsules; oral powder: Glucosamine sulfate (p.1616·2).
Musculoskeletal and joint disorders.

Rotta, Hong Kong; Rotta, Thai.
Injection: Glucosamine sulfate (p.1616·2); glucosamine hydriodide (p.1616·2).
Lignocaine [lidocaine] hydrochloride (p.1313·2) is included in this preparation to alleviate the pain of injection.
Musculoskeletal and joint disorders.

Viartril S
Rottapharm, Ital.; Delta, Port.
Glucosamine sulfate (p.1616·2).
Lignocaine [lidocaine] hydrochloride (p.1313·2) is included in this preparation to alleviate the pain of injection.
Musculoskeletal and joint disorders.

Viaspan
Du Pont, Canad.; Du Pont, Singapore.
Solution for flushing and cold storage of donor organs.

ViATIM Aventis, UK.
An inactivated hepatitis A and typhoid (Vi polysaccharide) vaccine (p.1544·2).
Active immunisation.

Viatine Essex, Spain.
Loratadine (p.420·1).
Hypersensitivity reactions.

Viavent Byk Madaus, S.Afr.†.
Salbutamol sulfate (p.770·3).
Obstructive airways disease.

Viaxol Maver, Mex.
Ambroxol (p.1084·3).
Respiratory-tract disorders.

Viazem
Biovail, Denm.; Gea, Swed.; Du Pont, UK.
Diltiazem hydrochloride (p.874·3).
Angina pectoris; hypertension.

Vibalgan Doms-Adrian, Fr.†.
Hydroxocobalamin acetate (p.1388·3); cobamamide (p.1388·3).
Vitamin B₁₂ deficiency.

Vibeden Gea, Denm.
Hydroxocobalamin (p.1388·1).
Megaloblastic anaemia; vitamin B₁₂ deficiency.

Vibee Biolab, Singapore.
Vitamin B₁; vitamin B₆; vitamin B₁₂ (p.1350·1).
Vitamin B deficiency.

Viberol Tirotricina Organon, Spain.
Formaldehyde (p.1144·2); tyrothricin (p.267·1).
Mouth and throat inflammation; oral hygiene.

Vibetrat Honorterapica, Braz.
Vitamin B₁ (p.1385·2); vitamin B₆ (p.1387·1); vitamin B₁₂ (p.1388·1).
Vitamin B deficiency.

Vibetrat Dexa Honorterapica, Braz.
Dexamethasone acetate (p.1067·1); vitamin B₁ (p.1385·2); vitamin B₆ (p.1387·1); vitamin B₁₂ (p.1388·1).
Neuritis.

Vibion Jean-Marie, Hong Kong.
Vitamin B substances (p.1350·1).
Neuralgias; neuritis; neuropathies; vitamin B deficiencies.

Vibolex E MIP, Ger.
d-Alpha tocoferil acetate (p.1394·1) or dl-alpha tocoferil acetate (p.1394·1).
Vitamin E deficiency.

Vibrabron Pfizer, Aust.†.
Doxycycline hyclate (p.200·1); ambroxol hydrochloride (p.1084·3).
Bacterial infections of the respiratory tract.

Vibracare Pfizer, Belg.†.
Doxycycline carrageenate (p.200·3).
Bacterial infections.

Vibracina Invicta, Spain.
Doxycycline hyclate (p.200·1).
Bacterial infections; malaria.

Vibradox Durascan, Denm.
Doxycycline (p.200·1).
Bacterial infections.

Vibral Sintofarma, Braz.
Dropropizine (p.1089·3).
Coughs.

Vibramicina
Pfizer, Braz.; Pfizer, Mex.; Pfizer, Port.
Doxycycline calcium (p.200·1) or doxycycline hyclate (p.200·1).
Amoebiasis; bacterial infections; malaria.

Vibramycin
Pfizer, Aust.; Pfizer, Austral.; Pfizer, Canad.†; Pfizer, Denm.; Pfizer, Ger.; Pfizer, Hong Kong; Invicta, Irl.; Pfizer, Israel; Pfizer, Neth.; Pfizer, Norw.; Pfizer, S.Afr.; Pfizer, Singapore; Pfizer, Swed.; Pfizer, Thai.; Pfizer, UK; Pfizer, USA.
Doxycycline (p.200·1), doxycycline calcium (p.200·1), doxycycline carrageenate (p.200·3), or doxycycline hyclate (p.200·1).
Bacterial infections; intestinal amoebiasis; malaria.

Vibramycin D Pfizer, UK.
Doxycycline (p.200·1).
Bacterial infections.

Vibramycine
Pfizer, Belg.; Pfizer, Switz.
Doxycycline (p.200·1) or doxycycline hyclate (p.200·1).
Bacterial infections; malaria.

Vibramycine N Pfizer, Fr.
Doxycycline (p.200·1).
Bacterial infections.

Vibra-S Pfizer, Neth.
Doxycycline (p.200·1).
Bacterial infections.

Vibratab Pfizer, Belg.
Doxycycline (p.200·1).
Bacterial infections; malaria.

Vibra-Tabs
Pfizer, Austral.; Pfizer, Canad.; Pfizer, USA.
Doxycycline hyclate (p.200·1).
Bacterial infections; intestinal amoebiasis.

Vibraveineuse
Pfizer, Fr.; Pfizer, Switz.
Doxycycline hyclate (p.200·1).
Bacterial infections.

Vibravenos
Pfizer, Aust.; Pfizer, Ger.; Pfizer, Israel.
Doxycycline (p.200·1) or doxycycline hyclate (p.200·1).
Bacterial infections.

Vibravenosa Pfizer Consumer, Spain.
Doxycycline hyclate (p.200·1).
Bacterial infections; malaria.

Vibrocil
Note.This name is used for preparations of different composition.
Novartis Consumer, Aust.; Novartis Consumer, Austral.; Novartis Consumer, Ger.; Novartis Consumer, Hong Kong; Novartis Consumer, Ital.; Novartis Consumer, Port.; Novartis Consumer, Switz.
Dimetindene maleate (p.415·3); phenylephrine (p.1097·1).
Nasal congestion; rhinitis; sinusitis.

Novartis Consumer, Belg.
Capsules: Dimetindene maleate (p.415·3); pseudoephedrine hydrochloride (p.1099·2).
Allergic rhinitis; sinusitis; vasomotor rhinitis.

Nasal drops; nasal spray; nasal gel: Dimetindene maleate (p.415·3); phenylephrine (p.1097·1).
Nasal congestion.

Novartis Consumer, S.Afr.
Dimetindene maleate (p.415·3); phenylephrine (p.1097·1); neomycin sulfate (p.228·1).
Nasal disorders; sinusitis.

Vibrocil NF Novartis, Israel.
Dimetindene maleate (p.415·3); phenylephrine (p.1097·1).
Nasal congestion; otitis media; rhinitis; sinusitis.

Vibrocil-S Novartis Consumer, S.Afr.
Dimetindene maleate (p.415·3); phenylephrine (p.1097·1).
Nasal and sinus congestion.

Vibrumin General Drugs, Thai.
Vitamin B substances (p.1350·1).

Vibtil
Bio-Therabel, Belg.; Lafon, Fr.
Tilia (p.1673·2).
Dyspepsia.

Viburcol
Heel, Ger.; Heel, S.Afr.
Homoeopathic preparation.

Viburnum Complex Blackmores, Austral.
Viburnum opulus; cimicifuga (p.1595·2); angelica sinensis; pulsatilla (p.1656·3); d-alpha tocoferil acid succinate (p.1394·1).
Gynaecological disorders; muscle cramp.

Vi-C Sam-On, Israel.
Ascorbic acid (p.1389·3).
Vitamin C deficiency.

Vicam Keene, USA.
Vitamin B substances (p.1350·1).
Parenteral nutrition.

Vicapan N Merckle, Ger.
Cyanocobalamin (p.1388·1).
Vitamin B deficiency.

Vi-Caps
Grossmann, Hong Kong; Grossmann, Switz.
Multivitamin and mineral preparation (p.1350·1).

Vicard Abbott, Aust.
Terazosin hydrochloride (p.980·1).
Hypertension.

Viccillin Meiji, Thai.
Ampicillin sodium (p.150·3) or ampicillin trihydrate (p.151·1).
Bacterial infections.

Viccillin-S Meiji, Thai.
Ampicillin (p.150·3); cloxacillin (p.192·1).
Bacterial infections.

Vi-Ce Novartis, Braz.
Ascorbic acid (p.1389·3).
Vitamin C deficiency; vitamin C supplement.

Vicedent Terramin, Aust.
Ascorbic acid (p.1389·3).
Gum disorders.

Vicemex
Cimex, Hong Kong; Cimex, Switz.
Ascorbic acid (p.1389·3).
Vitamin C deficiency; vitamin C supplement.

ViCetamol Gebro, Aust.
Paracetamol (p.71·2); ascorbic acid (p.1389·3).
Cold symptoms.

Vici Monico, Ital.
Ascorbic acid (p.1389·3).
Vitamin C deficiency.

Vicilan Zeneca, Ital.
Viloxazine hydrochloride (p.313·3).
Depression.

Vicitina CT, Ital.†.
Ascorbic acid (p.1389·3).
Gingivitis; stomatitis; vitamin C deficiency.

Vick Vaporub Procter & Gamble, Braz.
Menthol (p.1632·3); camphor (p.1589·3); eucalyptus oil (p.1609·2); nutmeg oil (p.1643·1); cedar leaf oil; turpentine oil (p.1676·3); thymol (p.1158·3).
Nasal congestion.

Vicks Action Procter & Gamble, UK†.
Ibuprofen (p.43·2); pseudoephedrine (p.1099·2).
Cold symptoms.

Vicks Blue Drops Procter & Gamble, Austral.
Menthol (p.1632·3); peppermint oil (p.1243·3).
Throat irritation.

Vicks Children's Chloraseptic Procter & Gamble, USA.
Lozenges: Benzocaine (p.1306·2).
Throat spray: Phenol (p.1152·3).
Sore throat.

Vicks Children's NyQuil Allergy/Head Cold Richardson-Vicks, USA.
Pseudoephedrine hydrochloride (p.1099·2); chlorpheniramine [chlorphenamine] maleate (p.412·1).
Upper respiratory-tract symptoms.

Vicks Children's NyQuil Night-time Cold/ Cough Liquid Richardson-Vicks, USA.
Chlorpheniramine [chlorphenamine] maleate (p.412·1); pseudoephedrine hydrochloride (p.1099·2); dextromethorphan hydrobromide (p.1087·3).
Coughs and cold symptoms.

Vicks Chloraseptic
Procter & Gamble, Irl.†; Procter & Gamble, USA.
Phenol (p.1152·3).
Oral hygiene; sore throat.

Procter & Gamble (H&B Care), UK†.
Phenol (p.1152·3); sodium phenolate.
Oral hygiene; sore throat.

Vicks Chloraseptic Sore Throat Procter & Gamble, USA.
Benzocaine (p.1306·2); menthol (p.1632·3).
Sore throat.

Vicks Cold Care Procter & Gamble (H&B Care), UK†.
Paracetamol (p.71·2); dextromethorphan (p.1087·3); phenylpropanolamine (p.1098·1).
Cold symptoms.

Vicks Cough Drops Procter & Gamble, USA.
Menthol (p.1632·3).
Sore throat.

Vicks Cough Silencers Richardson-Vicks, USA.
Dextromethorphan hydrobromide (p.1087·3); benzocaine (p.1306·2).
Coughs.

Vicks Cough Syrup
Note.This name is used for preparations of different composition.
Procter & Gamble, Austral.
Pentoxyverine citrate (p.1096·3); menthol (p.1632·3).
Coughs.

Procter & Gamble, Canad.
Ephedrine (p.1090·1); guaifenesin (p.1092·2); pentoxyverine citrate (p.1096·3).

Vicks 44D Cough & Head Congestion Procter & Gamble, USA.
Dextromethorphan hydrobromide (p.1087·3); pseudoephedrine hydrochloride (p.1099·2).
Coughs and cold symptoms.

Vicks DayQuil Richardson-Vicks, USA.
Pseudoephedrine hydrochloride (p.1099·2); dextromethorphan hydrobromide (p.1087·3); guaifenesin (p.1092·2); paracetamol (p.71·2).
Coughs.

Vicks DayQuil Allergy Relief Procter & Gamble, USA†.
Phenylpropanolamine hydrochloride (p.1098·1); brompheniramine maleate (p.410·2).

Vicks DayQuil Sinus Pressure & Congestion Relief Procter & Gamble, USA†.
Phenylpropanolamine hydrochloride (p.1098·1); guaifenesin (p.1092·2).

Vicks DayQuil Sinus Pressure & Pain Relief Procter & Gamble, USA.
Pseudoephedrine hydrochloride (p.1099·2); paracetamol (p.71·2).

Vicks Dry Hacking Cough Procter & Gamble, USA.
Dextromethorphan hydrobromide (p.1087·3).
Formerly known as Vicks Formula 44.
Coughs.

Vicks 44E Procter & Gamble, USA.
Dextromethorphan hydrobromide (p.1087·3); guaifenesin (p.1092·2).
Coughs.

Vicks Expectorant
Note.This name is used for preparations of different composition.
Lachartre, Fr.
Guaifenesin (p.1092·2).
Formerly known as Vicks Vaposyrup Expectorant.
Respiratory-tract congestion.

Procter & Gamble (H&B Care), UK†.
Guaifenesin (p.1092·2); cetylpyridinium chloride (p.1138·1); sodium citrate (p.1186·2).
Coughs.

Vicks Formel 44 Procter & Gamble, Switz.†.
Dextromethorphan (p.1087·3); benzocaine (p.1306·2); cetylpyridinium chloride (p.1138·1); menthol (p.1632·3); peppermint oil (p.1243·3).
Coughs; sore throat.

Vicks Formula 44
Note.This name is used for preparations of different composition.
Procter & Gamble, USA.
Dextromethorphan hydrobromide (p.1087·3); menthol (p.1632·3).
Coughs.

Procter & Gamble, Spain.
Anethole (p.1580·1); cetylpyridinium chloride (p.1138·1); dextromethorphan (p.1087·3); benzocaine (p.1306·2); peppermint oil (p.1243·3); menthol (p.1632·3).
Coughs.

Vicks Formula 44 Cough Control Discs Richardson-Vicks, USA.
Dextromethorphan hydrobromide (p.1087·3); benzocaine (p.1306·2).
Coughs.

Vicks Formule 44 Calmine Procter & Gamble, Switz.
Dextromethorphan (p.1087·3) or dextromethorphan hydrobromide (p.1087·3).
Coughs.

Vicks Formule 44 Expectine Procter & Gamble, Switz.
Guaifenesin (p.1092·2).
Respiratory-tract disorders with viscous mucus.

Vicks Headclear Procter & Gamble, Austral.†.
Pseudoephedrine hydrochloride (p.1099·2); paracetamol (p.71·2); chlorpheniramine [chlorphenamine] maleate (p.412·1).
Cold, influenza, and sinus symptoms.

Vicks Headclear Nondrowsy Procter & Gamble, Austral.†.
Pseudoephedrine hydrochloride (p.1099·2); paracetamol (p.71·2).
Cold, influenza, and sinus symptoms.

Vicks Inalante Procter & Gamble, Ital.
Menthol (p.1632·3); camphor (p.1589·3); methyl salicylate (p.55·1); pine oil.
Nasal congestion.

Vicks Inhalador Procter & Gamble, Spain.
Camphor (p.1589·3); menthol (p.1632·3).
Formerly contained camphor, methyl salicylate, sassafras oil, menthol, and bornyl acetate.
Nasal congestion.

Vicks Inhaler
Note.This name is used for preparations of different composition.
Procter & Gamble, Austral.; Procter & Gamble, NZ.
Menthol (p.1632·3); camphor (p.1589·3); methyl salicylate (p.55·1); pumilio pine oil (p.1656·3).
Nasal congestion.

Procter & Gamble, Canad.
Menthol (p.1632·3); camphor (p.1589·3).
Nasal congestion.

Procter & Gamble, Irl.†.
Menthol (p.1632·3); camphor (p.1589·3); pine needle oil.
Nasal congestion.

Richardson-Vicks, Israel.
Menthol (p.1632·3); camphor (p.1589·3); pine-needle oil; methyl salicylate (p.55·1).
Nasal congestion.

Procter & Gamble (H&B Care), UK.
Menthol (p.1632·3); camphor (p.1589·3); siberian fir oil.
Nasal congestion.

Vicks Inhaler N Procter & Gamble, Switz.
Menthol (p.1632·3); camphor (p.1589·3); methyl salicylate (p.55·1); pine needle oil.
Nasal congestion.

Vicks 44M Cold, Flu & Cough LiquiCaps Procter & Gamble, USA.
Dextromethorphan hydrobromide (p.1087·3); pseudoephedrine hydrochloride (p.1099·2); chlorpheniramine [chlorphenamine] maleate (p.412·1); paracetamol (p.71·2).

Vicks Medinait
Procter & Gamble, Ital.; Procter & Gamble, Spain; Procter & Gamble, Switz.
Dextromethorphan hydrobromide (p.1087·3); doxylamine succinate (p.417·1); ephedrine sulfate (p.1090·2); paracetamol (p.71·2).
Cold and influenza symptoms.

Vicks Medinite Procter & Gamble (H&B Care), UK.
Dextromethorphan hydrobromide (p.1087·3); doxylamine succinate (p.417·1); pseudoephedrine hydrochloride (p.1099·2); paracetamol (p.71·2).
Cold symptoms.

Vicks Menthol Cough Drops Procter & Gamble, USA.
Menthol (p.1632·3); thymol (p.1158·3); eucalyptus oil (p.1609·2); camphor (p.1589·3); tolu balsam (p.1101·3).
Sore throat.

Vicks 44 Non-Drowsy Cold & Cough Liqui-Caps Procter & Gamble, USA.
Dextromethorphan hydrobromide (p.1087·3); pseudoephedrine hydrochloride (p.1099·2).

Vicks NyQuil LiquiCaps Richardson-Vicks, USA.
Dextromethorphan hydrobromide (p.1087·3); paracetamol (p.71·2); pseudoephedrine hydrochloride (p.1099·2); doxylamine succinate (p.417·1).
Coughs and cold symptoms.

The symbol † denotes a preparation no longer actively marketed

Vicks NyQuil Multi-Symptom Cold Flu Relief *Procter & Gamble, USA.*
Pseudoephedrine hydrochloride (p.1099·2); doxylamine succinate (p.417·1); dextromethorphan hydrobromide (p.1087·3); paracetamol (p.71·2).
Cold symptoms.

Vicks Original Cough Syrup for Chesty Coughs *Procter & Gamble, Irl.†.*
Guaifenesin (p.1092·2); cetylpyridinium chloride (p.1138·1); sodium citrate (p.1186·2).
Coughs.

Vicks Pediatric Formula 44D Dry Hacking Cough & Head Congestion *Procter & Gamble, USA.*
Pseudoephedrine hydrochloride (p.1099·2); dextromethorphan hydrobromide (p.1087·3).
Formerly known as Vicks Formula 44D Pediatric.
Coughs and cold symptoms.

Vicks Pediatric Formula 44E *Richardson-Vicks, USA.*
Dextromethorphan hydrobromide (p.1087·3); guaifenesin (p.1092·2).
Coughs.

Vicks Pediatric Formula 44M Multi-Symptom Cough & Cold *Richardson-Vicks, USA.*
Pseudoephedrine hydrochloride (p.1099·2); dextromethorphan hydrobromide (p.1087·3); chlorpheniramine [chlorphenamine] maleate (p.412·1).
Coughs and cold symptoms.

Vicks Rhume *Lachartre, Fr.*
Ibuprofen (p.43·2); pseudoephedrine hydrochloride (p.1099·2).
Rhinitis.

Vicks Sinex
Note. This name is used for preparations of different composition.
Procter & Gamble, Austral.; Procter & Gamble, Ital.; Procter & Gamble, Switz.
Oxymetazoline hydrochloride (p.1096·2); menthol (p.1632·3); camphor (p.1589·3); eucalyptol (p.1609·2).
Nasal congestion.

Procter & Gamble, Belg.; Procter & Gamble, Canad.; Procter & Gamble, Fin.; Procter & Gamble, Irl.†; Procter & Gamble, Neth.; Procter & Gamble (H&B Care), UK.
Oxymetazoline hydrochloride (p.1096·2).
Nasal congestion.

Vicks Sinex 12-Hour *Procter & Gamble, USA.*
Oxymetazoline hydrochloride (p.1096·2).
Formerly known as Sinex Long Acting.
Nasal congestion.

Vicks Spray *Procter & Gamble, Spain.*
Oxymetazoline hydrochloride (p.1096·2); menthol (p.1632·3).
Nasal congestion.

Vicks Throat Drops *Procter & Gamble, Austral.; Procter & Gamble, Canad.*
Menthol (p.1632·3).
Coughs; throat irritation.

Vicks Tosse Fluidificante *Procter & Gamble, Ital.*
Guaifenesin (p.1092·2).
Respiratory-tract congestion.

Vicks Tosse Pastiglie *Procter & Gamble, Ital.*
Dextromethorphan (p.1087·3).
Coughs.

Vicks Tosse Sedativo *Procter & Gamble, Ital.*
Dextromethorphan hydrobromide (p.1087·3).
Coughs.

Vicks Toux Seche *Lachartre, Fr.*
Dextromethorphan hydrobromide (p.1087·3).
Coughs.

Vicks Ultra Chloraseptic *Procter & Gamble (H&B Care), UK.*
Benzocaine (p.1306·2).
Sore throat.

Vicks Vapodrops *Procter & Gamble, Austral.*
Menthol (p.1632·3); eucalyptus oil (p.1609·2).
Nasal congestion; sore throat.

Vicks Vapodrops with Butter and Menthol *Procter & Gamble, Austral.*
Menthol (p.1632·3).
Nasal congestion; sore throat.

Vicks Vapor Inhaler *Richardson-Vicks, USA.*
Levmetamfetamine (p.1094·1).
Nasal congestion.

Vicks Vaporub
Note. This name is used for preparations of different composition.
Procter & Gamble, Austral.
Menthol (p.1632·3); camphor (p.1589·3); eucalyptus oil (p.1609·2); turpentine oil (p.1676·3); nutmeg oil (p.1643·1); cedar leaf oil.
Cold symptoms; muscle pain.

Procter & Gamble, Belg.; Lachartre, Fr.
Menthol (p.1632·3); camphor (p.1589·3); eucalyptus oil (p.1609·2); turpentine oil (p.1676·3); nutmeg oil (p.1643·1); cedar leaf oil; thymol (p.1158·3).
Respiratory congestion.

Procter & Gamble, Canad.
Menthol (p.1632·3); camphor (p.1589·3); eucalyptus oil (p.1609·2).
Cold symptoms.

Procter & Gamble, Fin.; Procter & Gamble, Neth.
Menthol (p.1632·3); camphor (p.1589·3); eucalyptus oil (p.1609·2); turpentine oil (p.1676·3); thymol (p.1158·3).
Cold and influenza symptoms.

Procter & Gamble, Irl.†; Procter & Gamble, Ital.; Procter & Gamble (H&B Care), UK.
Menthol (p.1632·3); camphor (p.1589·3); eucalyptus oil (p.1609·2); turpentine oil (p.1676·3).
Nasal congestion.

Procter & Gamble, NZ; Procter & Gamble, Spain; Procter & Gamble, Swed.
Menthol (p.1632·3); camphor (p.1589·3); eucalyptus oil (p.1609·2); turpentine oil (p.1676·3); nutmeg oil (p.1643·1); cedar wood oil; thymol (p.1158·3).
Cold and influenza symptoms.

Procter & Gamble, USA.
Menthol (p.1632·3); camphor (p.1589·3); eucalyptus oil (p.1609·2); cedar leaf oil.

Vicks Vaporub N *Procter & Gamble, Switz.*
Menthol (p.1632·3); camphor (p.1589·3); eucalyptus oil (p.1609·2); turpentine oil (p.1676·3); nutmeg oil (p.1643·1); cedar leaf oil; thymol (p.1158·3).
Upper respiratory-tract disorders.

Vicks Vaposiroop *Procter & Gamble, Neth.*
Dextromethorphan hydrobromide (p.1087·3).
Coughs.

Vicks Vaposyrup *Procter & Gamble, Canad.*
Menthol (p.1632·3).

Vicks Vaposyrup Antitussif *Procter & Gamble, Belg.*
Dextromethorphan (p.1087·3) or dextromethorphan hydrobromide (p.1087·3).
Coughs.

Vicks Vaposyrup for chesty coughs *Procter & Gamble (H&B Care), UK.*
Guaifenesin (p.1092·2).
Coughs.

Vicks Vaposyrup for dry coughs *Procter & Gamble (H&B Care), UK.*
Dextromethorphan hydrobromide (p.1087·3).
Coughs.

Vicks Vaposyrup Expectorant *Procter & Gamble, Belg.*
Guaifenesin (p.1092·2).
Coughs; respiratory-tract disorders associated with mucus accumulation.

Vicks Vaposyrup for tickly coughs *Procter & Gamble (H&B Care), UK.*
Menthol (p.1632·3).
Coughs.

Vicks Vaposyrup toux seche *Lachartre, Fr.†.*
Dextromethorphan hydrobromide (p.1087·3).
Coughs.

Vicks Vapotab *Procter & Gamble, Neth.*
Dextromethorphan hydrobromide (p.1087·3).
Coughs.

Vicks Victors Dual Action Cough Drops *Richardson-Vicks, USA.*
Menthol (p.1632·3); eucalyptus oil (p.1609·2).

Vicks Vital *Procter & Gamble (H&B Care), UK.*
Ascorbic acid (p.1389·3); zinc acetate (p.1398·1).

Vicnas *Sanofi Synthelabo, Spain.*
Norfloxacin (p.232·1).
Urinary-tract infections.

Vicodin *Abbott, USA.*
Hydrocodone tartrate (p.42·2); paracetamol (p.71·2).
Pain.

Vicodin Tuss *Abbott, USA.*
Hydrocodone tartrate (p.42·2); guaifenesin (p.1092·2).
Coughs.

Vicoferell *Sanorell, Ger.*
Multivitamin and iron preparation (p.1350·1).

Vicomin A C *Warner-Lambert, Spain.*
Ascorbic acid (p.1389·3); vitamin A palmitate (p.1383·2).
Deficiency of vitamins A and C.

Vicon *UCB, USA.*
A range of vitamin preparations with or without minerals (p.1350·1).

Vicoprofen *Abbott, USA.*
Hydrocodone tartrate (p.42·2); ibuprofen (p.43·2).
Pain.

Vicortin *Vitae, Mex.*
Hydrocortisone (p.1073·3).
Skin disorders.

Vicrom *Fisons, Israel; Aventis, NZ.*
Sodium cromoglicate (p.774·3).
Asthma; bronchitis.

Victan *Sanofi Synthelabo, Belg.; Sanofi Winthrop, Fr.; Sanofi Winthrop, Mex.; CPH, Port.; Sanofi Synthelabo, Thai.*
Ethyl loflazepate (p.683·1).
Alcohol withdrawal syndrome; anxiety.

Victogon *Normon, Spain†.*
Amino acids and vitamins (p.1350·1); isoniazid (p.215·3).
Anorexia; tonic; weight loss.

Victoril *Unipharm, Israel.*
Dibenzepin (p.283·2).
Depression.

Victrix *Farmasa, Braz.*
Omeprazole (p.1239·1).
Gastro-oesophageal reflux; gastrointestinal hyperacidity; peptic ulcer.

Vidaclovir *Vida, Hong Kong.*
Aciclovir (p.612·3).
Herpesvirus infections.

Vi-Dailin *Abbott, Port.*
Multivitamin preparation (p.1350·1).

Vidapril *Helfarma, Port.*
Captopril (p.853·3).
Heart failure; hypertension.

Vidavit *Allen, Mex.*
Vitamin B$_{12}$ (p.1388·1).

Vi-Daylin
Abbott, Canad.; Abbott, Hong Kong; Abbott, NZ; Abbott, S.Afr.; Abbott, UK; Ross, USA.
A range of vitamin preparations with or without minerals (p.1350·1).

Vidaylin
Abbott, Singapore; Abbott, Thai.
A range of vitamin preparations with or without minerals or lysine (p.1350·1).

Vi-Daylin plus Iron
Abbott, Israel; Abbott, S.Afr.
Multivitamin preparation with iron (p.1350·1).

Vi-Daylin/F *Ross, USA.*
A range of vitamin and fluoride (p.1375·3) preparations (p.1350·1).

Vidcalm *Catarinense, Braz.*
Chamomile (p.1593·2); espinheiro alvar; erythrina mulungu; passion flower (p.1649·2); valerian (p.1678·3).
Sedative.

Vi-De$_3$
Sanova, Aust.; Novartis, Switz.
Colecalciferol (p.1391·1).
Hypoparathyroidism; osteomalacia; rickets; tetany.

Videne
Adams, Hong Kong; Adams, Thai.; Adams, UK.
Povidone-iodine (p.1155·1).
Burns; skin disinfection; wounds.

Video *Monot, Fr.†.*
Phenylephrine hydrochloride (p.1097·1); rutoside sodium sulfate (p.1611·2).
Conjunctivitis.

Video Capsule con Mirtillo *Farmila, Ital.*
Vitamin E; betacarotene; zinc; ginkgo biloba; myrtillus (p.1350·1).
Formerly contained vitamin E, magnesium, betacarotene, selenium, and myrtillus.
Antioxidant nutritional supplement.

Video-Light *Farmila, Ital.*
Benzalkonium chloride (p.1133·2).
Eye disinfection.

Video-Mill *Farmila, Ital.*
Naphazoline nitrate (p.1095·1).
Conjunctivitis.

Video-Net *Interdelta, Switz.*
Phenylephrine hydrochloride (p.1097·1); rutoside sodium sulfate (p.1611·2).
Eye irritation.

Videorelax *SIFI, Ital.*
Chlorhexidine gluconate (p.1138·2); tilia (p.1673·2); chamomile (p.1593·2).
Eye disinfection; eye irritation.

Viderm *Ganassini, Ital.*
Hydroxyquinoline sulfate (p.1622·2); enoxolone (p.34·3).
Wound disinfection.

Vidermina *Ganassini, Ital.*
Copper usnate (p.1678·2).
Vaginal disinfection.

Videx
Bristol-Myers Squibb, Aust.; Bristol-Myers Squibb, Austral.; Bristol-Myers Squibb, Belg.; Bristol-Myers Squibb, Braz.; Bristol, Canad.; Bristol-Myers Squibb, Denm.; Bristol-Myers Squibb, Fin.; Bristol-Myers Squibb, Fr.; Bristol-Myers Squibb, Ger.; Bristol-Myers Squibb, Hong Kong; Bristol-Myers Squibb, Irl.; Bristol-Myers Squibb, Israel; Bristol-Myers Squibb, Ital.; Bristol-Myers Squibb, Mex.; Bristol-Myers Squibb, Neth.; Bristol-Myers Squibb, Norw.; Bristol-Myers Squibb, NZ; Bristol-Myers Squibb, Port.; Bristol-Myers Squibb, S.Afr.; Bristol-Myers Squibb, Singapore; Bristol-Myers, Spain; Bristol-Myers Squibb, Swed.; Bristol-Myers Squibb, Switz.; Bristol-Myers Squibb, Thai.; Bristol-Myers Squibb, UK; Bristol-Myers Squibb, USA.
Didanosine (p.618·1).
HIV infection.

Vidirakt S *Mann, Ger.*
Povidone (p.1503·2).
Dry eyes.

Vidisept *Mann, Ger.*
Povidone (p.1503·2).
Dry eyes; eye irritation.

Vidisept EDO *Mann, Ger.*
Povidone (p.1503·2).
Dry eye.

Vidisept N *Mann, Singapore.*
Povidone (p.1503·2).
Dry eyes; eye irritation.

Vidiseptal EDO Sine *Mann, Ger.†.*
Tetryzoline hydrochloride (p.1101·2).
Eye irritation and inflammation.

Vidisic
Riel, Aust.; Tramedico, Belg.; Mann, Ger.; Mann, Irl.; Mann, Neth.; Lepori, Port.; Mann, Singapore; Bausch & Lomb, Thai.; Mann, Thai.
Carbomer (p.1499·2).
Dry eyes.

Vidopen
Berk, Irl.†; Berk, UK†.
Ampicillin (p.150·3) or ampicillin trihydrate (p.151·1).
Bacterial infections.

Vidora *Ferlux, Fr.*
Indoramin hydrochloride (p.913·3).
Migraine.

Vidyn *Novaquimica, Braz.*
Multivitamin and mineral preparation (p.1350·1).

Vie Ca Rad *Multi-Pro, Canad.*
Betacarotene, selenium, vitamin C, and vitamin E (p.1350·1).

Vifarcap *Farcoral, Mex.*
Multivitamin and mineral preparation (p.1350·1).

Vifenac *Vifor, Switz.*
Diclofenac epolamine (p.31·3).
Musculoskeletal and joint disorders.

Vi-Ferrin *Elofar, Braz.*
Iron chelate; folic acid (p.1361·1).
Iron deficiency; iron-deficiency anaemias.

Vifolyt *Rayere, Mex.*
Multivitamin preparation (p.1350·1).

Vig *Key, Austral.*
Chewable tablets: Guarana (p.1681·1); ginseng (p.1615·3); ginkgo biloba (p.1615·2); glucose (p.1364·1).
Tablets: Guarana (p.1681·1); ginseng (p.1615·3); ginkgo biloba (p.1615·2).
Tonic.

Vig Recovery *Key, Austral.*
Guarana (p.1681·1); vitamin B substances; vitamin C (p.1350·1).
Hangover.

Vigam *BPL, UK.*
A normal immunoglobulin (p.1551·3).
Hypogammaglobulinaemia; idiopathic thrombocytopenic purpura.

Vigantol
Merck, Ger.; Merck, Port.
Colecalciferol (p.1391·1).
Osteomalacia; osteopathy; rickets; spasmophilia; vitamin D deficiency.

Vigantoletten *Merck, Ger.*
Colecalciferol (p.1391·1).
Vitamin D deficiency.

Vigem *Pharmavite, Canad.*
Vitamin B substances (p.1350·1).

Vigencial *Estedi, Spain.*
Methylrosanilinium chloride (p.1150·3).
Skin infections.

Vigil *Merckle, Ger.*
Modafinil (p.1512·3).
Narcoleptic syndrome.

Vigilia *Grands Espaces, Fr.*
Tilia (p.1673·2); vervain (p.1679·3).
Sedative.

Vigilon *SSL, UK.*
Polyethylene oxide (p.1502·3).
Hydrogel dressing; wounds.

Vigiten *Wyeth Lederle, Belg.*
Lorazepam (p.688·3).
Anxiety disorders; depression; mixed anxiety depressive states; obsessive-compulsive disorder.

Vigodana
Loges, Hong Kong; Madaus, S.Afr.†.
Vitamin E; orotic acid; procaine hydrochloride; haematoporphyrin; magnesium l-aspartate; magnesium oxide; dried magnesium sulfate (p.1350·1).
Tonic.

vigodana N *Loges, Ger.*
Alpha tocoferil acetate; orotic acid; haematoporphyrin; magnesium aspartate; magnesium oxide; dried magnesium sulfate (p.1350·1).
Tonic.

Vigogel *Farmetrusca, Ital.†.*
Royal jelly (p.1659·3); liver extract; dried yeast (p.1398·1).

Vigomar Forte *Marlop, USA.*
Multivitamin and mineral preparation with iron (p.1350·1).

Vigoplus *Gazzoni, Ital.†.*
Maltodextrin; fructose; vitamins; minerals (p.1350·1).
Nutritional supplement.

Vigor-Ace *United American, Singapore.*
Vitamin A; vitamin C; vitamin E; selenium; zinc; lecithin (p.1350·1).
Tonic.

Vigoran *Golaz, Switz.*
Ginseng (p.1615·3); deanol hydrogen tartrate (p.1507·2); magnesium orotate (p.1645·1).
Tonic.

Vigorsan *Hoechst Marion Roussel, Ger.*
Colecalciferol (p.1391·1).
Osteopathy; osteoporosis; rickets; vitamin D deficiency.

Vigortol *Rugby, USA.*
Multivitamin and mineral preparation (p.1350·1).

Vigortonic *Arkochim, Spain.*
Cinnamon (p.1595·3); ginseng (p.1615·3); kola (p.1681·1).
Fatigue.

Vigour S *Restan, S.Afr.*
Haematoporphyrin; cyanocobalamin; caffeine; yeast extract (p.1350·1).
Tonic.

Vigranon B *Wallace Mfg Chem., UK.*
Vitamin B substances (p.1350·1).

Vikaman *Disperga, Aust.*
Menadione sodium bisulfite (p.1395·3).
Haemorrhage.

Viken *Kendrick, Mex.*
Cefotaxime sodium (p.169·1).
Lignocaine [lidocaine] hydrochloride (p.1313·2) is included in the intramuscular injection to alleviate the pain of injection.
Bacterial infections.

Vilam *Reuffer, Mex.*
Multivitamin and mineral preparation (p.1350·1).

Vilan Lannacher, Aust.; Lannacher, Denm.; Nourypharma, Neth.; Synmedic, Switz.
Nicomorphine hydrochloride (p.62·3).
Pain; premedication; smooth muscle spasm.

Vilerm Siam Bheasach, Thai.
Aciclovir (p.612·3).
Herpesvirus infections.

Vilona ICN, Mex.
Ribavirin (p.639·1).
Viral infections.

Vimeral ICN, Canad.
Multivitamin and mineral preparation (p.1350·1).

Viminate Barre-National, USA.
Multivitamin and mineral preparation (p.1350·1).

Viminfort Solfran, Mex.
Multivitamin and mineral preparation (p.1350·1).

Vimoli Vitamed, Israel.
Paracetamol (p.71·2).
Fever; pain.

Vin Tonique de Vial Eberth, Switz.
Cinchona alkaloids (p.1595·3); calcium phosphate (p.1188·3); lactic acid (p.1626·2); beef extract; sweet wine.
Tonic.

Vinatal Triomed, S.Afr.†; British Dispensary, Thai.
Multivitamin and mineral preparation (p.1350·1).

Vinca Substipharm, Fr.
Vincamine (p.1680·1).
Mental function impairment in the elderly.

Vincacen Centrum, Spain.
Vincamine (p.1680·1).
Cerebral trauma; cerebrovascular disorders; circulatory disorders of the eye, ear, nose, and throat; vestibular disorders.

Vincadar Hoechst Marion Roussel, Ital.
Vincamine (p.1680·1).
Cerebrovascular disorders.

Vincafolina Lampugnani, Ital.†
Vincamine (p.1680·1).
Cerebrovascular disorders.

Vincafor Pharmafarm, Fr.
Vincamine (p.1680·1).
Mental function impairment in the elderly.

Vincagil Hoechst Marion Roussel, Braz.; Roussel, Port.
Vincamine (p.1680·1).
Cerebrovascular disorders.

Vincaminol Alacan, Spain.
Vincamine (p.1680·1).
Cerebral trauma; cerebrovascular disorders; circulatory disorders of the eye, ear, nose, and throat; vestibular disorders.

Vincapan Hoechst Marion Roussel, Mex.
Vincamine (p.1680·1).
Cerebrovascular disorders.

Vincapront Mack, Illert., Ger.†
Vincamine (p.1680·1).
Ménière's disease; metabolic and circulatory disorders of the brain, retina, and inner ear.

Vinca-Ri INTES, Ital.
Vincamine hydrochloride (p.1680·1).
Disorders of cerebral, ocular, and vestibular perfusion.

Vincarutine Labomed, Fr.
Vincamine (p.1680·1); rutoside (p.1611·2).
Mental function impairment in the elderly.

Vincasar Pharmacia Upjohn, Mex.
Vincristine sulfate (p.578·3).

Vincasar PFS Adria, USA.
Vincristine sulfate (p.578·3).
Malignant neoplasms.

Vinca-Tablinen Sanorania, Ger.†
Vincamine (p.1680·1).
Circulatory disorders of the brain, retina, and inner ear; Ménière's disease.

Vinca-Treis Ecobi, Ital.
Vincamine (p.1680·1).
Cerebrovascular disorders.

Vincent's Powders Roche Consumer, Austral.
Aspirin (p.14·2).
Fever; pain.

Vincetron Biosintetica, Braz.
Piracetam (p.1652·1); co-dergocrine mesilate (p.1597·3).
Mental function impairment.

Vincigrip Salvat, Spain.
Chlorpheniramine [chlorphenamine] maleate (p.412·1); phenylpropanolamine hydrochloride (p.1098·1); paracetamol (p.71·2).
Cold and influenza symptoms; fever; pain.

Vincigrip Balsamico Salvat, Spain.
Guaifenesin (p.1092·2); paracetamol (p.71·2).
Influenza and cold symptoms; sinusitis.

Vincimax Synthelabo, Fr.†
Vincamine (p.1680·1).
Cerebrovascular disorders; mental function impairment in the elderly.

Vinciseptil Otico Salvat, Spain.
Benzydamine hydrochloride (p.20·1); fluocinolone acetonide (p.1071·1); neomycin sulfate (p.228·1); polymyxin B sulfate (p.238·1); amethocaine [tetracaine] hydrochloride (p.1305·2).
Ear disorders.

Vincitos Salvat, Spain.
Dextromethorphan hydrobromide (p.1087·3); pseudoephedrine hydrochloride (p.1099·2).
Coughs.

Vinco Forte OTW, Ger.†
Bisacodyl (p.1212·2).
Constipation.

Vinco-Abfuhr-Perlen OTW, Ger.
Bisacodyl (p.1212·2).
Constipation.

Vincosedan Reig Jofre, Spain.
Diazepam (p.674·3).
Contains pyridoxine.
Alcohol withdrawal syndrome; anxiety; febrile convulsions; insomnia; skeletal muscle spasm.

Vincosona Reig Jofre, Spain†.
Diflorasone diacetate (p.1069·2).
Skin disorders.

Vincrin Orion, Fin.
Vincristine sulfate (p.578·3).
Malignant neoplasms.

Vincrisul Lilly, Spain.
Vincristine sulfate (p.578·3).
Idiopathic thrombocytopenic purpura; malignant neoplasms.

Vingel Bristol-Myers Squibb, Port.
Aluminium hydroxide (p.1210·3); magnesium hydroxide (p.1233·1); simeticone (p.1249·2).
Dyspepsia; gastritis; heartburn; peptic ulcer.

Vinho Ferruginoso Belem Jardim, Braz.; Luper, Braz.; QIF, Braz.
Ferric ammonium citrate (p.1359·2).
Iron deficiency; iron-deficiency anaemias.

Vinho Reconstituinte Hoechst Marion Roussel, Braz.
Calcium (p.1187·3); peptone; cinchona bark (p.1595·3).

Vinho Tonificante Stevia, Braz.
Ferric ammonium citrate (p.1359·2).
Iron deficiency; iron-deficiency anaemias.

Vinone Hikma, Port.†
Enoxacin (p.201·1).
Bacterial infections.

Vinopepsin Terrapharm, Aust.
Pepsin (p.1649·3); absinthium (p.1571·1).
Gastrointestinal disorders.

Vinsal Salus, Ital.
Vincamine (p.1680·1).
Cerebrovascular disorders.

Vinsen Chew, Thai.
Naproxen (p.60·3).
Dysmenorrhoea; gout; musculoskeletal and joint disorders.

Vintec Columbia, Mex.
Vincristine sulfate (p.578·3).
Malignant neoplasms.

Vintene Baxter, Fr.
Amino-acid infusion (p.1350·1).
Parenteral nutrition.

Vinzam Almirall, Spain.
Azithromycin (p.153·1).
Bacterial infections.

Viobeta IDI, Ital.
Betamethasone valero-acetate (p.1063·3); clioquinol (p.190·2).
Infected skin disorders.

Viocidina IDI, Ital.
Clioquinol (p.190·2); cod-liver oil (p.1357·2).
Infected skin disorders.

Viocort Aspen, S.Afr.
Hydrocortisone acetate (p.1073·3); diiodohydroxyquinoline (p.590·2).
Skin disorders.

Viodenum Iquinosa, Spain†.
Hidrosmin (p.1611·2).
Peripheral vascular disorders.

Viodine Pharmacia Upjohn, Austral.; Pharmacia Upjohn, NZ.
Povidone-iodine (p.1155·1).
Burns; skin disinfection; sore throat; viral lesions; wounds.

Viodor Aspen, S.Afr.
Diiodohydroxyquinoline (p.590·2); benzocaine (p.1306·2).
Skin infections with pruritus.

Vioform Ciba, Canad.†; FLAWA, Switz.; Ciba, USA†.
Clioquinol (p.190·2).
Infected skin disorders.

Vioform-Hydrocortisone Novartis, Canad.; Novartis Consumer, Irl.; Novartis Consumer, UK.
Clioquinol (p.190·2); hydrocortisone (p.1073·3).
Infected skin disorders.

Vioformio-Hidrocortisona Novartis, Braz.
Clioquinol (p.190·2); hydrocortisone (p.1073·3).
Skin disorders.

Vioformo Novartis, Mex.
Clioquinol (p.190·2).
Skin infections.

Vioformo-Cort Novartis, Mex.
Clioquinol (p.190·2); hydrocortisone (p.1073·3).
Infected skin disorders.

Viogen-C Goldline, USA.
Vitamin B substances with vitamin C and minerals (p.1350·1).

Viokase
Note.This name is used for preparations of different composition.
Wyeth-Ayerst, Austral.; Wyeth, NZ; Aspen, S.Afr.
Pancreatin (p.1646·1).
Cystic fibrosis; pancreatic insufficiency.

Wolfs, Belg.†; Axcan, Canad.; Axcan, USA.
Pancrelipase (p.1647·2).
Pancreatic insufficiency.

Viola Sanopharm, Switz.
Viola tricolor; zinc oxide (p.1128·2); almond oil (p.1576·3).
Skin disorders.

Violgen INTES, Ital.
Methylrosanilinium chloride (p.1150·3); lactic acid (p.1626·2).
Vulvovaginitis.

Violin TO-Chemicals, Thai.
Salbutamol (p.770·3).
Obstructive airways disease.

Vioneurin
Continental Pharma, Belg.
Cyanocobalamin (p.1388·1); thiamine hydrochloride (p.1385·1); pyridoxine hydrochloride (p.1386·3).
Neuritis; neuropathy; vitamin B deficiency.

Continental Pharma, Thai.
Vitamin B_1 (p.1385·2); vitamin B_{12} (p.1388·1).
Malnutrition; musculoskeletal pain; neuralgia; neuritis.

Vioxx Merck Sharp & Dohme, Austral.; Merck Frosst, Canad.; Merck Sharp & Dohme, Denm.; Merck Sharp & Dohme, Fin.; Merck Sharp & Dohme-Chibret, Fr.; Merck Sharp & Dohme, Ger.; Merck Sharp & Dohme, Irl.; Merck Sharp & Dohme, NZ; Merck Sharp & Dohme, Port.; Merck Sharp & Dohme, S.Afr.; Merck Sharp & Dohme, Singapore; Merck Sharp & Dohme, Spain; Merck Sharp & Dohme, Swed.; Merck Sharp & Dohme, Switz.; Merck Sharp & Dohme, Thai.; Merck Sharp & Dohme, UK; Merck, USA.
Rofecoxib (p.81·2).
Arthroses; pain.

Viperfav Aventis, Fr.
European viper venom antiserum (p.1563·3).
European viper bite.

Vipirim INQ, Braz.
Vitamin B_1 (p.1385·2); vitamin B_6 (p.1387·1); vitamin B_{12} (p.1388·1).
Vitamin B deficiency.

Viplex Riva, Canad.
Vitamin B substances and iron (p.1350·1).

Vipocem Alter, Port.
Vinpocetine (p.1680·1).
Cerebrovascular disorders; vascular disorders of the eye and ear.

Vipratox Serum-Werk Bernburg, Ger.
Vipera ammodytes toxin; methyl salicylate (p.55·1); camphor (p.1589·3).
Musculoskeletal, joint, and soft-tissue disorders; neuralgias.

Viprinex Knoll, Canad.
Ancrod (p.839·3).
Peripheral vascular disorders; thromboembolic disorders.

Vipro Scientific Hospital Supplies, UK.
Preparation for enteral nutrition (p.1350·1).

Viprofen Iqfasa, Mex.
Multivitamin and mineral preparation (p.1350·1).

Vipsogal Harley Street Supplies, UK.
Betamethasone dipropionate (p.1063·2); fluocinonide (p.1071·2); gentamicin sulfate (p.210·1); salicylic acid (p.1122·3); panthenol (p.1602·3).
*Available on a named-patient basis only.
Skin disorders.*

Viquin Forte
ICN, Canad.
Hydroquinone (p.1115·1); glycolic acid (p.1115·1) in a sunscreen basis.
Skin pigmentation disorders.

ICN, USA†.
Hydroquinone (p.1115·1); padimate O (p.1518·2); dioxybenzone (p.1517·2); oxybenzone (p.1518·1).
Hyperpigmentation; sunscreen.

Vira-A Parke, Davis, Austral.†; Parke, Davis, NZ; Monarch, USA.
Vidarabine (p.643·2).
Herpes simplex keratitis and keratoconjunctivitis.

Viraban
Note.This name is used for preparations of different composition.
Faulding, Austral.†
Povidone-iodine (p.1155·1).
Viral sore throat.

AFT, NZ.
Aciclovir (p.612·3).
Herpes labialis.

Virac Crosara, Ital.†
Inosine pranobex (p.627·2).
Immunodeficiency; viral infections.

Viracept Roche, Aust.; Roche, Austral.; Roche, Belg.; Agouron, Canad.; Roche, Denm.; Roche, Fin.; Roche, Fr.; Roche, Ger.; Roche, Israel; Roche, Ital.; Japan Tobacco, Jpn; Roche, Neth.; Roche, Norw.; Roche, NZ; Roche, Port.; Roche, S.Afr.; Roche, Singapore; Roche, Spain; Roche, Swed.; Roche, Switz.; Roche, Thai.; Roche, UK; Agouron, USA.
Nelfinavir mesilate (p.636·3).
HIV infection.

Virafer Rhone-Poulenc Rorer, Ital.
Multivitamin and mineral preparation (p.1350·1).

Viraferon Schering-Plough, Fr.; Schering-Plough, Mex.; Schering-Plough, Spain†; Schering-Plough, UK.
Interferon alfa-2b (rbe) (p.628·1).
Anogenital warts; hepatitis B; hepatitis C; malignant neoplasms.

ViraferonPeg Schering-Plough, Irl.; Schering-Plough, UK.
Peginterferon alfa-2b (rbe) (p.630·1).
Chronic hepatitis C.

Viralin Magis, Ital.
Inosine pranobex (p.627·2).
Viral infections.

Viramid Wassermann, Ital.†
Ribavirin (p.639·1).
Viral bronchiolitis.

Vira-MP Sinbio, Fr.; Pierre Fabre, Fr.
Vidarabine sodium phosphate (p.643·3).
Chronic active viral hepatitis B; recurrent genital herpes infection.

Viramune Boehringer Ingelheim, Aust.; Boehringer Ingelheim, Austral.; Boehringer Ingelheim, Belg.; Boehringer Ingelheim, Canad.; Boehringer Ingelheim, Denm.; Boehringer Ingelheim, Fin.; Boehringer Ingelheim, Fr.; Boehringer Ingelheim, Ger.; Boehringer Ingelheim, Hong Kong; Merck Sharp & Dohme, Irl.; Boehringer Ingelheim, Ital.; Boehringer Ingelheim, Jpn; Promeco, Mex.; Boehringer Ingelheim, Neth.; Boehringer Ingelheim, Norw.; Boehringer Ingelheim, NZ; Boehringer Ingelheim, Port.; Boehringer Ingelheim, S.Afr.; Boehringer Ingelheim, Singapore; Boehringer Ingelheim, Spain; Boehringer Ingelheim, Swed.; Boehringer Ingelheim, Switz.; Boehringer Ingelheim, Thai.; Boehringer Ingelheim, UK; Roxane, USA.
Nevirapine (p.637·1).
HIV infection.

Virasolve Warner-Lambert, Austral.; Rosken, Hong Kong; Warner-Lambert, NZ.
Idoxuridine (p.625·1); lignocaine [lidocaine] hydrochloride (p.1313·2); benzalkonium chloride (p.1133·2).
Herpes simplex infections of the mouth and skin.

Virasorb SSL, UK.
Aciclovir (p.612·3).
Herpes labialis.

Virax Isis Puren, Ger.
Aciclovir (p.612·3).
Herpesvirus infections.

Viraxy General Drugs, Thai.
Aciclovir (p.612·3).
Herpesvirus infections.

Virazid ICN, Mex.
Ribavirin (p.639·1).
Respiratory syncytial virus infections.

Virazide Dermatech, Austral.; Grossman, Mex.
Ribavirin (p.639·1).
Viral infections.

Virazole Sanico, Belg.; ICN, Canad.; ICN, Ger.; ICN, Hong Kong; ICN, Neth.†; ICN, Singapore; Swedish Orphan, Swed.; ICN, UK; ICN, USA.
Ribavirin (p.639·1).
*Formerly known as Virazid in the UK.
Influenza; respiratory syncytial virus infections.*

Virazone Rayere, Mex.
Aciclovir (p.612·3).

Virbelte Probelte, Spain.
Aciclovir (p.612·3).
Herpes simplex infections.

Virdex Fulton, Ital.
Ergotamine tartrate (p.452·1); caffeine (p.761·3); aminophenazone (p.13·3).
Migraine.

Viread Gilead, USA.
Tenofovir disoproxil fumarate (p.642·1).
HIV infection.

Viregyt Thiemann, Ger.†
Amantadine hydrochloride (p.1161·2).
Parkinsonism.

Virelon C Chiron Behring, Ger.†
An inactivated poliomyelitis vaccine (p.1558·2).
Active immunisation.

Virexen Will-Pharma, Belg.; Ferraz, Lynce, Port.†; Vinas, Spain; Vinas, Switz.†.
Idoxuridine (p.625·1) in dimethyl sulfoxide.
Herpesvirus infections of the skin and mucous membranes.

Virgamelis Pascoe, Ger.†
Hamamelis (p.1618·3).
Skin irritation; wounds.

Virgan Thea, Fr.; Chauvin, UK.
Ganciclovir (p.623·1).
Herpes eye infections.

Virgilocard Sanova, Aust.
Crataegus (p.1600·2); absinthium (p.1571·1).
Cardiac disorders in the elderly.

Virginiana Gocce Verdi Kelemata, Ital.
Naphazoline nitrate (p.1095·1).
Eye congestion.

Virherpes Pensa, Spain.
Aciclovir (p.612·3) or aciclovir sodium (p.612·3).
Herpesvirus infections.

Viridal Orion, Denm.; Hoyer, Ger.; Schwarz, Irl.; Schwarz, Ital.; Schwarz, UK.
Alprostadil alfadex (p.1440·1).
Erectile dysfunction.

Viridin *Davi, Port.*
Trifluridine (p.642·2).
Viral eye infections.

Virilis-Gastreu N R41 *Reckeweg, Ger.*
Homoeopathic preparation.

Virilit *Jenapharm, Ger.*
Cyproterone acetate (p.1467·3).
Erectile dysfunction; prostatic cancer.

Virilon *Star, USA.*
Capsules: Methyltestosterone (p.1482·3).
Androgen replacement therapy; breast cancer; male hypogonadism; postpartum breast engorgement; prepubertal cryptorchidism.
Injection: Testosterone cipionate (p.1492·1).

Virivac *SBL, Denm.†; SBL, Swed.†.*
A measles, mumps, and rubella vaccine (Enders Edmonston, Jeryl Lynn, and Wistar RA 27/3 strains, respectively) (p.1549·1).
Active immunisation.

Virlix *Synthelabo, Fr.; Mediolanum, Ital.; Glaxo Wellcome, Mex.; Vedim, Port.; Lacer, Spain.*
Cetirizine hydrochloride (p.411·2).
Hypersensitivity reactions.

Virlix-D *Glaxo Wellcome, Mex.*
Cetirizine hydrochloride (p.411·2); pseudoephedrine hydrochloride (p.1099·2).
Allergic rhinitis; eye irritation; nasal congestion.

Virman Plus *Corypharma, Ital.*
Vitamin E; nicotinic acid; zinc (p.1350·1).
Nutritional supplement.

Virmen *Menarini, Spain.*
Aciclovir (p.612·3) or aciclovir sodium (p.612·3).
Herpesvirus infections.

Virobin *Bock, Ger.†.*
Homoeopathic preparation.

Virobis *Aventis, S.Afr.*
Cream: Moroxydine hydrochloride (p.636·3); cetrimide (p.1137·1); diphenhydramine hydrochloride (p.416·1).
Viral infections of the skin.
Tablets: Moroxydine hydrochloride (p.636·3); atropine methonitrate (p.461·1); hyoscine methonitrate (p.468·2).
Viral infections.

Virofral *Novo Nordisk, Denm.†; Ferrosan, Swed.*
Amantadine hydrochloride (p.1161·2).
Influenza A; parkinsonism.

Virogon *Silom, Thai.*
Aciclovir (p.612·3).
Herpesvirus infections.

Viro-Med *Whitehall, USA†.*
Chlorpheniramine [chlorphenamine] maleate (p.412·1); dextromethorphan hydrobromide (p.1087·3); paracetamol (p.71·2); pseudoephedrine hydrochloride (p.1099·2).
Coughs and cold symptoms.

Viromidin *Alcon Cusi, Spain.*
Trifluridine (p.642·2).
Herpes simplex infections of the eye.

Viromone *Paines & Byrne, Thai.*
Testosterone propionate (p.1492·2).
Female breast cancer; male hypogonadism.

Viron Wart Lotion *Odan, Canad.*
Glacial acetic acid (p.1571·2); lactic acid (p.1626·2); salicylic acid (p.1122·3).
Verrucae.

Vironox *Iketon, Ital.*
Nonoxinol 9 (p.1346·1); chloroxylenol (p.1142·1).
Disinfection.

Viropect *DHU, Ger.*
Homoeopathic preparation.

Virophta *Allergan, Fr.*
Trifluridine (p.642·2).
Viral infections of the eye.

Viropox *LSP, Thai.*
Aciclovir (p.612·3).
Herpesvirus infections.

Viroptic *Glaxo Wellcome, Canad.; Glaxo Wellcome, USA; Monarch, USA.*
Trifluridine (p.642·2).
Herpes simplex keratitis and keratoconjunctivitis.

Virormone *Ferring, UK†.*
Testosterone (p.1492·1) or testosterone propionate (p.1492·2).
Breast cancer; cryptorchidism; delayed puberty; male hypogonadism.

Virostat *Janssen-Ortho, Canad.†.*
Edoxudine (p.619·3).
Genital herpes simplex infections.

Virovir *Opus, UK.*
Aciclovir (p.612·3).
Herpesvirus infections.

Viroxy *Orion, Israel.*
Aciclovir sodium (p.612·3).
Herpesvirus infections.

Virubact *Biosyn, Ger.*
Homoeopathic preparation.

Virucid *Hofmann, Aust.*
Amantadine hydrochloride (p.1161·2).
Influenza A; parkinsonism.

Virudermin *Robugen, Ger.; Renapharm, Switz.*
Zinc sulfate (p.1398·2).
Herpes labialis.

Virudin *Bracco, Ital.†.*
Foscarnet sodium (p.621·2).
Cytomegalovirus retinitis.

Virulex
Note.This name is used for preparations of different composition.
Drossapharm, Switz.
Greater celandine (p.1618·1).
Herpes labialis.
Pose, Thai.
Monopersulfate compound; sodium chloride; sulfamic acid.
Instrument disinfection.

Virulex Forte *Pascual, Hong Kong.*
Moroxydine hydrochloride (p.636·3); paracetamol (p.71·2); atropine methonitrate (p.461·1); hyoscine methonitrate (p.468·2).
Viral infections.

Viru-Merz *Kolassa, Aust.; Bio-Therabel, Belg.; Merz, Denm.†; Merz, Ger.; Merz, Hong Kong; Merz, Israel; Merz, Neth.; Medinfar, Port.; Merz, Singapore.*
Tromantadine hydrochloride (p.642·3).
Herpesvirus infections of the skin and mucous membranes.

Viru-Merz Serol *Merz, Switz.*
Tromantadine hydrochloride (p.642·3).
Herpes simplex infections of the skin and mucous membranes.

Virunguent *Hermal, Ger.; Hermal, Port.†; Hermal, Singapore; Boots Healthcare, Switz.*
Idoxuridine (p.625·1) in dimethyl sulfoxide.
Herpes simplex infections of the skin and mucous membranes.

Virunguent P *Hermal, Ger.*
Idoxuridine (p.625·1); prednisolone (p.1077·3).
Herpes simplex infections.

Virupos *Ursapharm, Ger.*
Aciclovir (p.612·3).
Herpes simplex eye infections.

Viru-Salvysat *Ysatfabrik, Ger.*
Sage (p.1660·2).
Mouth and throat infections.

Virusan *Rekah, Israel.*
Idoxuridine (p.625·1).
Herpes simplex infections.

Viruseen *Hommel, Ger.*
Aciclovir (p.612·3).
Herpesvirus infections.

Viruserol *Novartis Consumer, Ital.*
Tromantadine hydrochloride (p.642·3).
Herpesvirus infections of the skin.

Viru-Serol *Armstrong, Mex.; Lacer, Spain.*
Tromantadine hydrochloride (p.642·3).
Herpesvirus infections of the skin and mucous membranes.

Virustat
Note.This name is used for preparations of different composition.
Sanus, Braz.
Zidovudine (p.645·2).
HIV infection.
Synthelabo, Hong Kong.
Moroxydine hydrochloride (p.636·3).
Viral infections.

Virustop *Pulitzer, Ital.*
Inosine pranobex (p.627·2).
Immunodeficiency; viral infections.

Viruxan *Sigma-Tau, Ital.*
Inosine pranobex (p.627·2).
Immunodeficiency; viral infections.

Virval *Novag, Spain.*
Valaciclovir hydrochloride (p.643·1).
Herpesvirus infections.

Virzin *Dermapharm, Ger.*
Aciclovir (p.612·3).
Herpesvirus infections.

Visadron *Boehringer Ingelheim, Aust.; Boehringer Ingelheim, Belg.; Alcon, Ger.; Boehringer Ingelheim, Ital.; Boehringer Ingelheim, Neth.†; Boehringer Ingelheim, Port.; Fher, Spain.*
Phenylephrine hydrochloride (p.1097·1).
Eye irritation.

Visaline *Chauvin Novopharma, Switz.*
Buphenine hydrochloride (p.1587·3); betacarotene (p.1355·1); alpha tocopherol (p.1393·3); ascorbic acid (p.1389·3).
Eye disorders.

Visano N *Kade, Ger.*
Meprobamate (p.691·1).
Anxiety disorders; gastrointestinal disorders; insomnia.

VisanoCor N *Kade, Ger.*
Pentaerithrityl tetranitrate (p.952·3); diphenhydramine hydrochloride (p.416·1).
VisanoCor formerly contained pentaerithrityl tetranitrate, meprobamate, diphenhydramine hydrochloride, and nicotinic acid.
Cardiac disorders.

Visano-mini N *Kade, Ger.*
Meprobamate (p.691·1).
Anxiety disorders; sleep disorders.

Visatear *Pfizer, Canad.†.*
Macrogol 400 (p.1630·3).
Dry eye.

Viscal *Formenti, Ital.†.*
Metoclopramide hydrochloride (p.1235·2).
Digestive disorders.

Viscaplus *Sifarma, Ital.*
Nutritional supplement (p.1350·1).

Viscasan *Bioforce, Ger.*
Homoeopathic preparation.

Visceralgine *Exel, Belg.*
Tiemonium iodide (p.474·2).
Smooth muscle spasm.
Riom, Fr.
Tiemonium metilsulfate (p.474·2).
Smooth muscle spasms.

Visceralgine Compositum *Exel, Belg.*
Tiemonium iodide (p.474·2); dipyrone (p.34·1); codeine phosphate (p.25·2).
Smooth muscle spasms.

Visceralgine Forte *Riom, Fr.*
Injection; tablets: Tiemonium metilsulfate (p.474·2); dipyrone (p.34·1).
The tablets formerly contained tiemonium metilsulfate, dipyrone, and codeine phosphate.
Suppositories: Tiemonium metilsulfate (p.474·2); dipyrone (p.34·1); codeine phosphate (p.25·2).
Pain; smooth muscle spasms.

Visclair *Sinclair, Irl.; Sinclair, UK.*
Mecysteine hydrochloride (p.1094·2).
Bronchitis; respiratory-tract disorders with excessive or viscous mucus.

Viscoat *Alcon, Aust.†; Alcon, Austral.; Alcon, Belg.†; Alcon, Fr.; Alcon, Ger.; Alcon, Hong Kong; Alcon, Ital.; Alcon, NZ; Alcon, S.Afr.; Alcon, Singapore; Alcon, Swed.†; Alcon, Switz.†; Alcon, Thai.; Alcon, UK; Alcon, USA.*
Sodium chondroitin sulfate (p.1594·2); sodium hyaluronate (p.1620·1).
Adjunct in eye surgery.

Viscocort *Bournonville, Belg.†.*
Prednisolone acetate (p.1078·1); chloramphenicol (p.179·1).
Infected inflammatory ear disorders.

Viscolex *Pinewood, Irl.*
Carbocisteine (p.1086·3).
Respiratory-tract disorders with excessive or viscous mucus.

Viscolyt *Gea, Denm.*
Bromhexine hydrochloride (p.1085·3).
Dry eyes; respiratory-tract congestion.

Viscomucil *ABC, Ital.*
Ambroxol hydrochloride (p.1084·3).
Respiratory-tract congestion.

Visconisan N *Hanosan, Ger.*
Homoeopathic preparation.

Viscopaste PB7 *Smith & Nephew, Irl.; Smith & Nephew, Ital.; Smith & Nephew, S.Afr.; Smith & Nephew, UK.*
Zinc oxide (p.1128·2).
Dermatitis; leg ulcers; medicated bandage; varicose eczema.

Visc-Ophtal *Winzer, Ger.*
Carbomer (p.1499·2).
Dry eyes.

Viscophyll *Krewel, Ger.*
Mistletoe (p.1636·2); bladderwrack (p.1585·2).
Circulatory disorders.

Viscorapas duo *Pascoe, Ger.*
Convallaria (p.1599·1); crataegus (p.1600·2).
Heart failure.

Viscotears *Ciba Vision, Austral.; Ciba Vision, Denm.; Ciba Vision, Fin.; Ciba Vision, Hong Kong; Ciba Vision, Israel; Ciba Vision, Norw.; Ciba Vision, NZ; Ciba Vision, Spain; Ciba Vision, Swed.; Ciba Vision, Switz.; Novartis Ophthalmics, UK.*
Carbomer 980 (p.1499·2).
Dry eyes.

Viscoteina *Iquinosa, Spain.*
Carbocisteine (p.1086·3).
Respiratory-tract congestion.

Viscotiol *Medeva, Fr.; Searle, Ital.*
Letosteine (p.1094·1).
Respiratory-tract congestion.

Viscotirs *Ciba Vision, Ital.*
Carbomer (p.1499·2).
Dry eyes.

Viscotraan *Covan, S.Afr.*
Hypromellose (p.1501·3).
Contact lens lubricant; dry eyes.

Viscum album H *Pflüger, Ger.*
Homoeopathic preparation.

Viscysat *Ysatfabrik, Ger.*
Mistletoe (p.1636·2).
Circulatory disorders.

Visderm *Wyeth, Mex.; Wyeth-Ayerst, Thai.*
Amcinonide (p.1061·2).
Skin disorders.

Visergil *LPB, Ital.; Novartis, Spain.*
Co-dergocrine mesilate (p.1597·3); thioridazine (p.708·1) or thioridazine hydrochloride (p.708·1).
Cerebrovascular disorders; mixed anxiety depressive states.

Vi-Siblin *Parke, Davis, Denm.; Parke, Davis, Fin.; Warner-Lambert, Norw.; Parke, Davis, Swed.*
Ispaghula (p.1229·1).
Constipation; irritable bowel syndrome.

Vi-Siblin S *Parke, Davis, Swed.*
Ispaghula (p.1229·1); sorbitol (p.1377·3).
Constipation; irritable bowel syndrome.

Visicol *Inkine, USA.*
Monobasic sodium phosphate (p.1193·2); dibasic sodium phosphate (p.1193·2).
Bowel evacuation.

Visinal *Stada, Ger.†.*
Valerian (p.1678·3); lupulus (p.1629·3); passion flower (p.1649·1).
Nervous disorders; sleep disorders.

Visine *Pfizer, Austral.; Mack, Belg.; Pfizer, Canad.; Pfizer, Fin.; Pfizer, Israel; Restiva, Ital.†; Pfizer, Neth.†; Pfizer, NZ; Pfizer, Port.; Pfizer, Singapore; Pfizer, Switz.; Pfizer, Thai.*
Tetryzoline hydrochloride (p.1101·2).
Eye irritation.

Visine AC *Pfizer, Israel.*
Tetryzoline hydrochloride (p.1101·2); zinc sulfate (p.1398·2).
Eye irritation.

Visine AD *Pfizer, Mex.*
Oxymetazoline hydrochloride (p.1096·2).
Eye irritation.

Visine Advanced Relief *Pfizer, Austral.*
Tetryzoline hydrochloride (p.1101·2); dextran 70 (p.729·2); macrogol 400 (p.1630·3); povidone (p.1503·2).
Dry eyes; eye irritation.

Visine Allergy *Pfizer, Canad.; Pfizer, Canad.*
Tetryzoline hydrochloride (p.1101·2); zinc sulfate (p.1398·2).
Formerly known as Visine Plus in Austral. and as Visine AC in Canad.
Eye irritation or congestion.

Visine Allergy Relief *Pfizer, USA.*
Tetryzoline hydrochloride (p.1101·2); zinc sulfate (p.1398·2).
Formerly called Visine AC.
Eye irritation.

Visine Contact Lens *Pfizer, Canad.*
Hypromellose (p.1501·3)(p.1129·2).
Eye irritation during contact lens wear.

Visine Extra *Pfizer, Mex.*
Tetryzoline hydrochloride (p.1101·2); macrogol 400 (p.1630·3).

Visine LR *Pfizer Consumer, USA.*
Oxymetazoline hydrochloride (p.1096·2).
Eye irritation.

Visine Moisturizing *Pfizer, Canad.; Pfizer, USA.*
Tetryzoline hydrochloride (p.1101·2); macrogol 400 (p.1630·3).
Formerly called Visine Extra.
Eye irritation.

Visine Original *Pfizer Consumer, USA.*
Tetryzoline hydrochloride (p.1101·2).
Eye irritation.

Visine Revive *Pfizer, Austral.*
Tetryzoline hydrochloride (p.1101·2); macrogol 400 (p.1630·3).
Dry eyes; eye irritation.

Visine True Tears *Pfizer, Canad.*
Macrogol 400 (p.1630·3).

Visine Workplace *Pfizer, Canad.*
Oxymetazoline hydrochloride (p.1096·2).
Formerly known as Visine LR.
Eye irritation.

Visiodose *Cooperation Pharmaceutique, Fr.*
Chlorhexidine gluconate (p.1138·2); phenylephrine hydrochloride (p.1097·1).
Conjunctivitis.

Visiolyre *Urgo, Fr.*
Cadmium sulfate (p.1588·1); zinc sulfate (p.1398·2); phenylephrine hydrochloride (p.1097·1).
Eye disorders.

Vision Care Enzymatic Cleaner *Alcon, USA.*
Pancreatin (p.1646·1)(p.1129·2).
Cleansing solution for soft contact lenses.

Visionace *Vitabiotics, UK.*
Vitamin, mineral, and nutrient preparation (p.1350·1).
Eye disorders.

Visipaque *Nycomed, Aust.; Nycomed, Austral.; Nycomed, Belg.; Nycomed Amersham, Canad.; Nycomed Imaging, Denm.; Nycomed, Fin.; Nycomed, Fr.; Nycomed, Ger.; Nycomed, Ital.; Nycomed, Neth.†; Nycomed Amersham, Norw.; Nycomed, NZ; Nycomed, Spain; Nycomed Amersham, Swed.; Nycomed, Switz.; Nycomed Amersham, UK; Nycomed, USA.*
Iodixanol (p.1034·2).
Radiographic contrast medium.

Visiplex *Bunker, Braz.*
Naphazoline hydrochloride (p.1095·1); zinc sulfate (p.1398·2); boric acid (p.1586·1); borax (p.1586·1).
Ocular congestion.

Viskaldix
Novartis, Aust.; Novartis, Belg.; Novartis, Braz.; Novartis, Canad.; Novartis, Fr.; Novartis, Ger.; Novartis, Irl.; Novartis, Neth.; Novartis, NZ; Novartis, Switz.; Novartis, Thai.; Sovereign, UK.
Pindolol (p.955·3); clopamide (p.863·1).
Hypertension.

Viskazide *Novartis, Canad.*
Pindolol (p.955·3); hydrochlorothiazide (p.907·3).
Hypertension.

Viskeen *Novartis, Neth.*
Pindolol (p.955·3).
Cardiovascular disorders.

Visken
Novartis, Aust.; Novartis, Austral.; Novartis, Belg.; Novartis, Braz.; Novartis, Canad.; Novartis, Denm.; Novartis, Fin.; Novartis, Fr.; Novartis, Ger.; Novartis, Hong Kong; Novartis, Irl.; Novartis, Israel; Novartis, Ital.; Novartis, Norw.†; Novartis, NZ; Novartis, S.Afr.; Novartis, Swed.; Sovereign, UK; Novartis, USA.
Pindolol (p.955·3).
Angina pectoris; arrhythmias; hypertension; hyperthyroidism; myocardial infarction; obstructive cardiomyopathies.

Viskene *Novartis, Switz.*
Pindolol (p.955·3).
Cardiac disorders; hypertension.

Viskenit *Novartis, Aust.*
Pindolol (p.955·3); isosorbide dinitrate (p.915·2).
Angina pectoris.

Viskoferm *Nordic, Swed.*
Acetylcysteine (p.1082·3).
Bronchitis.

Viskose ojendraber *Ophtha, Denm.*
Sodium chloride (p.1196·1).
Dry eyes.

Vislin *Alcon, Braz.*
Tetryzoline hydrochloride (p.1101·2); methylene blue [methylthioninium chloride] (p.1012·3).
Ocular congestion.

Vislube
Chemedica, Ger.; Chemedica, Hong Kong; Chemedica, Switz.
Sodium hyaluronate (p.1620·1) (p.1129·2).
Contact lens lubricant; dry eyes.

Vismed
Hamilton, Austral.; Thea, Fr.; Chemedica, Ger.; Tubilux, Ital.; Chemedica, Switz.
Sodium hyaluronate (p.1620·1).
Dry eyes.

Visodin *Allergan-Frumtost, Braz.*
Tetryzoline hydrochloride (p.1101·2); methylene blue [methylthioninium chloride] (p.1012·3).
Ocular congestion.

Visogenol *INQ, Braz.*
Chlorobutanol (p.1141·2); boric acid (p.1586·1).
Eye disorders.

Visolon *Novaquimica, Braz.*
Naphazoline (p.1095·1); benzalkonium chloride (p.1133·2); zinc sulfate (p.1398·2); berberine sulfate (p.1584·2).
Ocular congestion.

Visolux *Brasmedica, Braz.*
Tetryzoline (p.1101·2); methylene blue [methylthioninium chloride] (p.1012·3).
Eye disorders.

Visonest *Allergan-Frumtost, Braz.*
Proxymetacaine hydrochloride (p.1320·1).
Local anaesthesia.

Visopt *Sigma, Austral.*
Phenylephrine (p.1097·1).
Eye irritation and congestion.

Visotone *British Dispensary, Thai.*
Eye drops: Phenylephrine hydrochloride (p.1097·1); boric acid (p.1586·1); borax (p.1586·1); sodium chloride (p.1196·1).
Eye solution: Boric acid (p.1586·1); borax (p.1586·1); salicylic acid (p.1122·3); zinc sulfate (p.1398·2).
Eye irritation.

Visoy *Wyeth Lederle, Port.*
Soy protein infant feed (p.1350·1).
Gastro-enteritis; intolerance to cow's milk, lactose, or sucrose.

Vispring *Pfizer Consumer, Spain.*
Tetryzoline hydrochloride (p.1101·2).
Conjunctival congestion; eye irritation.

Vistacarpin *Allergan, Ger.†*
Pilocarpine hydrochloride (p.1422·3).
Glaucoma; production of miosis.

Vista-Cetamide *Martindale, Hong Kong.*
Sulfacetamide (p.250·3).
NOTE. There is no connection between Martindale, The Complete Drug Reference and Martindale, Hong Kong.
Eye infections.

Vistacon *Hauck, USA†.*
Hydroxyzine hydrochloride (p.419·1).
Anxiety; hypersensitivity reactions.

Vistacrom
Allergan, Canad.†; Genop, S.Afr.
Sodium cromoglicate (p.774·3).
Allergic conjunctivitis.

Vistafrin *Allergan, Spain.*
Phenylephrine hydrochloride (p.1097·1).
Eye irritation.

Vistagan
Allergan, Aust.; Allergan, Ger.; Allergan, Ital.; Allergan, Switz.
Levobunolol hydrochloride (p.920·3).
Glaucoma; ocular hypertension.

Vistalbalon *Allergan, Ger.†*
Naphazoline hydrochloride (p.1095·1).
Eye disorders.

Vista-Methasone *Martindale Pharmaceuticals, UK.*
Betamethasone sodium phosphate (p.1063·2).
NOTE. There is no connection between Martindale, The Complete Drug Reference and Martindale Pharmaceuticals.
Inflammatory disorders of the ear, eye, or nose.

Vista-Methasone N
Daniels, Irl.; Martindale Pharmaceuticals, UK.
Betamethasone sodium phosphate (p.1063·2); neomycin sulfate (p.228·1).
NOTE. There is no connection between Martindale, The Complete Drug Reference and Martindale Pharmaceuticals.
Inflammatory disorders of the ear, eye, or nose with bacterial infection.

Vistamycin *Meiji, Jpn†.*
Ribostamycin sulfate.
Bacterial infections.

Vista-Phenicol *Martindale, Hong Kong.*
Chloramphenicol (p.179·1).
NOTE. There is no connection between Martindale, The Complete Drug Reference and Martindale Hong Kong.
Blepharitis; conjunctivitis.

Vistaquel *Pasadena, USA†.*
Hydroxyzine hydrochloride (p.419·1).
Anxiety; hypersensitivity reactions.

Vistaril
Roerig, Swed.†; Pfizer, USA.
Hydroxyzine embonate (p.419·1) or hydroxyzine hydrochloride (p.419·1).
Anxiety; premedication; pruritus; sedative.

Vistazine *Keene, USA.*
Hydroxyzine hydrochloride (p.419·1).
Anxiety; hypersensitivity reactions.

Vistide
Gilead, Aust.; Pharmacia Upjohn, Austral.; Pharmacia Upjohn, Belg.; Pharmacia Upjohn, Fr.; Pharmacia Upjohn, Ger.; Pharmacia Upjohn, Ital.; Pharmacia Upjohn, Port.; Pharmacia Upjohn, Spain; Pharmacia Upjohn, Switz.; Pharmacia, UK; Gilead, USA.
Cidofovir (p.616·3).
Cytomegalovirus retinitis.

Vistimon *Jenapharm, Ger.*
Mesterolone (p.1482·1).
Androgen deficiency.

Vistofilm *Allergan, Ger.†*
Polyvinyl alcohol (p.1503·1) (p.1129·2).
Wetting solution for contact lenses.

Vistosan *Allergan, Ger.†*
Phenylephrine hydrochloride (p.1097·1).
Eye disorders.

Vistoxyn
Allergan, Aust.†; Allergan, Switz.
Oxymetazoline hydrochloride (p.1096·2).
Conjunctivitis; eye irritation.

Visual *QIF, Braz.*
Zinc sulfate (p.1398·2); procaine (p.1319·2); boric acid (p.1586·1); borax (p.1586·1); naphazoline (p.1095·1); sodium sulfate (p.1250·1).
Ocular congestion.

Visual-Eyes *Optopics, USA.*
Electrolyte solution (p.1180·1).
Eye irrigation.

Visublefarite
Visufarma, Ital.; Merck Sharp & Dohme, Spain†.
Betamethasone (p.1063·1); sulfacetamide sodium (p.250·3); tetryzoline phosphate (p.1101·2).
Eye disorders.

Visucloben *Visufarma, Ital.*
Clobetasone butyrate (p.1065·2).
Eye disorders.

Visucloben Antibiotico *Visufarma, Ital.*
Clobetasone butyrate (p.1065·2); bekanamycin sulfate (p.156·1).
Infected eye disorders.

Visucloben Decongestionante *Visufarma, Ital.*
Clobetasone butyrate (p.1065·2); tetryzoline hydrochloride (p.1101·2).
Conjunctivitis.

Visudyne
Ciba Vision, Austral.; Ciba Vision, Fr.; Novartis Ophthalmics, UK; Ciba Vision, USA.
Verteporfin (p.577·3).
Age-related macular degeneration; choroidal neovascularisation.

Visuglican *Visufarma, Ital.*
Sodium cromoglicate (p.774·3); chlorpheniramine [chlorphenamine] maleate (p.412·1).
Conjunctivitis.

Visumetazone *Visufarma, Ital.*
Dexamethasone (p.1067·1).
Inflammatory eye disorders.

Visumetazone Antibiotico *Visufarma, Ital.*
Bekanamycin sulfate (p.156·1); tetryzoline hydrochloride (p.1101·2); betamethasone (p.1063·1).
Eye infections associated with inflammation and congestion.

Visumetazone Antistaminico *Visufarma, Ital.*
Dexamethasone (p.1067·1); chlorpheniramine [chlorphenamine] maleate (p.412·1).
Conjunctivitis.

Visumetazone Decongestionante *Visufarma, Ital.*
Dexamethasone (p.1067·1); tetryzoline hydrochloride (p.1101·2).
Conjunctivitis; eye congestion; scleritis.

Visumicina *Visufarma, Ital.*
Bekanamycin sulfate (p.156·1); tetryzoline hydrochloride (p.1101·2).
Bacterial eye infections.

Visumidriatic *Visufarma, Ital.*
Tropicamide (p.475·1).
Production of mydriasis.

Visumidriatic Antiflogistico *Merck Sharp & Dohme, Ital.†.*
Betamethasone (p.1063·1); tropicamide (p.475·1).
Inflammatory eye disorders.

Visumidriatic Fenilefrina *Visufarma, Ital.*
Tropicamide (p.475·1); phenylephrine hydrochloride (p.1097·1).
Production of mydriasis.

Visustrin *Merck Sharp & Dohme, Ital.*
Tetryzoline hydrochloride (p.1101·2); methylene blue [methylthioninium chloride] (p.1012·3).
Conjunctival oedema; eye irritation; hyperaemia.

Visutensil *Visufarma, Ital.†.*
Guanethidine monosulfate (p.901·1).
Glaucoma.

Vi-Syneral *Grossman, Mex.*
Multivitamin and mineral preparation (p.1350·1).

Vi-Syneral Plus *Sanofi Winthrop, Braz.*
Multivitamin preparation (p.1350·1).

Vit Eparin *Teofarma, Ital.*
Heparin sodium (p.902·1); tocoferil acetate (p.1394·1).
Ocular haemorrhage and its sequelae.

Vita 3
Ciba Vision, Fr.; Ciba Vision, Switz.†.
Phenylephrine hydrochloride (p.1097·1); rutoside sodium sulfate (p.1611·2).
Eye disorders.

Vita 3B *Riva, Canad.*
Vitamin B substances (p.1350·1).

Vita B6 *Vitaglow, Austral.*
Pyridoxine hydrochloride (p.1386·3).
Premenstrual syndrome; vitamin B₆ supplement.

Vita B Complex *Nutri-Metics, Canad.†.*
Vitamin B substances (p.1350·1).

Vita B Compound 100 *Vita Pharm, Canad.*
Vitamin B substances (p.1350·1).

Vita B plus C *Romila, Canad.*
Vitamin B substances and vitamin C (p.1350·1).

Vita 3B plus C *Riva, Canad.*
Vitamin B substances with vitamin C (p.1350·1).

Vita Bee *Rugby, USA.*
Multivitamin preparation (p.1350·1).

Vita Buer-G-plus *Byk Roland, Switz.*
Capsules: Multivitamin and mineral preparation with kola and ginseng (p.1350·1).
Oral liquid: Multivitamin and mineral preparation with ginseng (p.1350·1).
Tonic.

Vita Buerlecithin
Roland, Ger.
Lecithin (p.1628·1); vitamins (p.1350·1).
Tonic.

Byk Roland, Switz.
Vitamin B preparation with lecithin (p.1628·1) (p.1350·1).
Tonic.

Vita C *Vitaglow, Austral.*
Calcium ascorbate (p.1389·3).
Cold and influenza symptoms; wounds.

Vita Cris *Cris Flower, Ital.*
Multivitamin preparation (p.1350·1).
Nutritional supplement.

Vita Day *Jamieson, Canad.*
Multivitamin and mineral preparation (p.1350·1).

Vita Dino Buddies *Vita Pharm, Canad.*
Multivitamin and mineral preparation (p.1350·1).

Vita Disc *Vitaglow, Austral.†.*
Vitamins and minerals (p.1350·1); bromelains (p.1586·3); papain (p.1647·3).
Musculoskeletal disorders.

Vita E *Vitaglow, Austral.*
d-Alpha tocopherol (p.1393·3).
Antioxidant; dry skin disorders; wounds.

Vita Ferin C *Geistlich, Switz.*
Multivitamin and mineral preparation (p.1350·1).

Vita Gerine *Melisana, Switz.*
Deanol orotate; vitamins; minerals (p.1350·1); rutoside; choline bitartrate.
Tonic.

Vita Menal *Alacan, Spain.*
Cyproheptadine hydrochloride (p.414·2); amino acids; cyanocobalamin (p.1350·1); fosforylethanolamine.
Tonic.

Vita Plex *Sante Naturelle, Canad.†.*
Multivitamin and mineral preparation (p.1350·1).

Vita Stress *Vita Pharm, Canad.*
Multivitamin preparation (p.1350·1).

Vita Truw *Truw, Ger.†.*
Multivitamin and mineral preparation (p.1350·1).

Vita Vim *Jamieson, Canad.*
Multivitamin and mineral preparation (p.1350·1).

Vita-B *Shiwa, Thai.*
Vitamin B₁ (p.1385·2); vitamin B₆ (p.1387·1); vitamin B₁₂ (p.1388·1).
Vitamin B deficiency.

Vita-B1 *Vitabalans, Fin.*
Thiamine hydrochloride (p.1385·1).
Vitamin B₁ deficiency.

Vita-B2 *Vitabalans, Fin.*
Riboflavin (p.1386·1).
Vitamin B₂ deficiency.

Vita-B6 *Vitabalans, Fin.*
Pyridoxine hydrochloride (p.1386·3).
Vitamin B₆ deficiency.

Vitabact
Ciba Vision, Fr.; Ciba Vision, Switz.
Picloxydine dihydrochloride (p.1154·2).
Bacterial eye infections.

Vitabase *Heralds, Braz.*
Vitamin E (p.1393·3).
Vitamin E deficiency.

Vitaber A E *Llorens, Spain.*
Di-isopropylammonium dichloroacetate (p.874·3); vitamin A acetate (p.1383·2); tocoferil acetate (p.1394·1).
Deficiency of vitamins A and E; eye disorders; infertility; recurrent miscarriage; skin disorders.

Vitaber PP + E *Llorens, Spain†.*
Tocoferil nicotinate (p.984·3).
Hyperlipidaemias.

Vitableu *Ciba Vision, Fr.*
Methylene blue [methylthioninium chloride] (p.1012·3).
Eye infections.

Vita-Bob *Scot-Tussin, USA.*
Multivitamin preparation (p.1350·1).

Vita-Brachont *Azuphorm, Ger.†.*
Cyanocobalamin (p.1388·1).
Lignocaine [lidocaine] hydrochloride (p.1313·2) is included in this preparation to alleviate the pain of injection.
Arthritis; neuralgia; neuritis; vitamin B₁₂ deficiency.

Vita-C
Shaklee, Canad.; Vitabalans, Fin.; Freeda, USA.
Ascorbic acid (p.1389·3).
Scurvy; vitamin C deficiency.

Vita-C R15 *Reckeweg, Ger.*
Homoeopathic preparation.

Vitacal *Vita Health, Singapore.*
Calcium and vitamin D (p.1350·1).
Calcium deficiency; osteoporosis.

Vita-Cal Plus *Shaklee, Canad.*
Multivitamin and mineral preparation (p.1350·1).

Vitacap *Medicap, Thai.*
Multivitamin and mineral preparation (p.1350·1).

VitaCarn *Kendall McGaw, USA.*
Carnitine (p.1356·1).
Carnitine deficiency.

Vitace *Pascoe, Ger.*
Multivitamin preparation (p.1350·1).

Vita-Ce *Chemedica, Switz.*
Ascorbic acid (p.1389·3).
Vitamin C deficiency; vitamin C supplement.

Vitacelsia Plus *Prisfar, Port.*
Multivitamin and mineral preparation (p.1350·1).

Vitacic *Ciba Vision, Fr.*
Adenosine (p.828·2); thymidine (p.1672·3); cytidine; uridine (p.1677·2); disodium guanylate (p.1604·3).
Corneal damage.

Vitacid *Yamanouchi, Port.*
Tretinoin (p.1126·2).
Psoriasis.

Vitacimin *Takeda, Thai.*
Ascorbic acid (p.1389·3).
Vitamin C deficiency.

Vitacimin Sweetlet *Takeda, Hong Kong.*
Ascorbic acid (p.1389·3); sodium ascorbate (p.1390·1).
Vitamin C deficiency.

Vitacolor *Heralds, Braz.*
Cod-liver oil (p.1357·2); zinc oxide (p.1128·2); boric acid (p.1586·1).
Barrier preparation; skin disorders.

Vitacrecil *Ferraz, Lynce, Port.*
Cystine; wheat-germ; gelatin; zinc sulfate; ferrous sulfate; calcium pantothenate; pyridoxine hydrochloride (p.1350·1).
Hair, skin, and nail disorders.

Vita-Dermacide *CS, Fr.*
Nicotinamide (p.1372·3); glutamic acid (p.1365·2); tryptophan (p.311·3).
Irritative dermatitis.

Vitaderme *Drogasil, Braz.*
Vitamin A; colecalciferol; vitamin E (p.1350·1); allantoin (p.1110·1).
Barrier preparation.

Vita-D-Grin *Grin, Mex.*
Ergocalciferol (p.1391·2).

Vita-Diem *Seven Seas, UK.*
Multivitamin preparation (p.1350·1).

Vitadol-C *Karicare, NZ.*
Vitamin A, C, and D (p.1350·1).

Vitadral *Wernigerode, Ger.*
Vitamin A palmitate (p.1383·2).
Vitamin A deficiency.

2168 Preparations

Vitadye *Dermatech, Austral.*
Dihydroxyacetone (p.1113·2).
Vitiligo.

Vita-E
Ache, Braz.; Shaklee, Canad.; Vitabalans, Fin.; Cambridge Health-care, UK.
Vitamin E (p.1393·3).
Dietary supplement; vitamin E deficiency.

Vita-E Plus Selenium *Shaklee, Canad.*
Vitamin E (p.1393·3); selenium (p.1375·2).
Dietary supplement.

Vitaendil C K P *Wasserman, Spain†.*
Ascorbic acid (p.1389·3); menadione (p.1395·3); ruto-side (p.1611·2).
Haemorrhage.

Vitafardi C B12 *Fardi, Spain.*
Ascorbic acid (p.1389·3); hydroxocobalamin (p.1388·1).
Deficiency of vitamins B_{12} and C.

Vitafem *Vita Pharm, Canad.*
Multivitamin and mineral preparation (p.1350·1).

Vitafer *Frega, Canad.†.*
Vitamin B substances and iron (p.1350·1).

Vita-Feron *Vitaline, USA†.*
Iron (p.1366·3); folic acid (p.1361·1); vitamin B_{12} (p.1388·1).

Vitaferro *Hexal, Ger.*
Ferrous chloride (p.1359·3), ferrous gluconate (p.1360·1), or ferrous sulfate (p.1360·3).
Iron deficiency; iron-deficiency anaemia.

Vitafissan *Uhlmann-Eyraud, Switz.*
Caseine hydrolysate (Labiline); vitamins A and E (p.1350·1); linoleic acid (p.1613·2); linolenic acid.
Skin disorders.

Vitafol *Everett, USA.*
Syrup: Ferric pyrophosphate (p.1359·3); folic acid (p.1361·1); vitamin B substances (p.1350·1).
Tablets: Ferrous fumarate (p.1360·1); folic acid (p.1361·1); multivitamins and minerals (p.1350·1).
Iron-deficiency anaemias.

Vitaforte *Rimsa, Mex.*
Multivitamin and mineral preparation (p.1350·1).

Vitafran *Faria, Braz.*
Vitamin C (p.1389·3).
Vitamin C deficiency; vitamin C supplement.

Vitagama Fluor *Almirall, Spain.*
Sodium fluoride (p.1375·2); multivitamins and miner-als (p.1350·1).
Vitamin and fluoride deficiencies.

Vitagama Fluor Complex *Almirall, Spain†.*
Multivitamin preparation (p.1350·1) with ferrous sul-fate (p.1360·3).
Vitamin and iron deficiency.

Vita-Gard *GNLD, Austral.*
Multivitamin and mineral preparation (p.1350·1).

Vitageran *Gilton, Braz.*
Multivitamin and mineral preparation (p.1350·1).

Vita-Gerin *Chemomedica, Aust.*
Deanol orotate; vitamins; minerals; adenosine; choline bitartrate (p.1350·1).
Tonic.

Vita-Gerin N *Cassella-med, Ger.*
Deanol orotate; magnesium orotate; vitamins; miner-als; choline bitartrate (p.1350·1).
Tonic.

Vitaglow Executive Anti Stress *Vitaglow, Austral.†.*
Skullcap (p.1664·3); passion flower (p.1649·1); lupu-lus (p.1629·3); vitamin B substances and ascorbic acid (p.1350·1).
Anxiety; pain; stress; tension.

Vitaglow Herbal Laxative *Vitaglow, Austral.†.*
Aloes (p.1210·1); cascara (p.1216·1); senna (p.1248·2); ginger (p.1227·2); cardamom (p.1591·3); peppermint oil (p.1243·3).
Constipation.

Vitaglow Herbal Stress *Vitaglow, Austral.†.*
Valerian (p.1678·3); skullcap (p.1664·3); mistletoe (p.1636·2); passion flower (p.1649·1); lupulus (p.1629·3); avena (p.1583·1).
Anxiety; stress; tension.

Vitaglow Primetime *Vitaglow, Austral.†.*
Multivitamin and mineral preparation (p.1350·1).
Dietary supplement.

Vitaglow Selemite B *Vitaglow, Austral.*
Selenium (p.1375·2); dried yeast (p.1398·1).
Selenium deficiency.

Vitaglow Smoke Stop *Vitaglow, Austral.†.*
Homoeopathic preparation.

Vitaglumil *Salusif, Port.*
Vitamin B substances; ascorbic acid (p.1350·1).
Tonic.

Vitagutt Knoblauch *Schwarzhaupt, Ger.*
Garlic oil.
Circulatory disorders.

Vitagutt Vitamin E *Schwarzhaupt, Ger.*
dl-Alpha tocoferil acetate (p.1394·1).
Vitamin E deficiency.

Vita-Hexin *Streuli, Switz.*
Chlorhexidine gluconate (p.1138·2); vitamin A palmi-tate (p.1383·2); cod-liver oil (p.1357·2); zinc oxide (p.1128·2).
Skin lesions.

Vita-Iodurol *Ciba Vision, Fr.†.*
Potassium iodide (p.1522·3); calcium chloride (p.1188·1); magnesium chloride (p.1190·3); cysteine

hydrochloride (p.1358·3); glutathione (p.1010·3); thia-mine hydrochloride (p.1385·1); nicotinic acid (p.1372·3).
Cataract.

Vita-Iodurol ATP *Ciba Vision, Fr.†.*
Potassium iodide (p.1522·3); calcium chloride (p.1188·1); magnesium chloride (p.1190·3); cysteine hydrochloride (p.1358·3); glutathione (p.1010·3); thia-mine hydrochloride (p.1385·1); nicotinic acid (p.1372·3); adenosine triphosphate sodium (p.1573·3).
Cataract.

Vitaject *Syxyl, Ger.*
Thiamine hydrochloride (p.1385·1); pyridoxine hydro-chloride (p.1386·3); cyanocobalamin (p.1388·1).
Vitamin B deficiency.

Vitakid *Pharmaland, Thai.*
Multivitamin preparation with lysine (p.1350·1).
Tonic.

Vita-Kid
Solgar, Canad.
Multivitamin preparation with folic acid (p.1350·1).

Solgar, USA.
Multivitamin preparation (p.1350·1).

Vital *Lalco, Canad.†.*
Multivitamin and mineral preparation (p.1350·1).

Vital Eyes
Note.This name is used for preparations of different composition.
Novartis Consumer, UK.
Lavender (p.1627·2); orange flower; hamamelis (p.1618·3); euphrasia (p.1609·3).
Eye irritation.
Allergan, USA†.
A multivitamin and mineral preparation (p.1350·1).

Vital Floramin *Bennett, UK.*
Mineral preparation (p.1350·1).
Immune stimulant.

Vital High Nitrogen
Abbott, Hong Kong; Abbott, NZ; Ross, USA.
Preparation for enteral nutrition (p.1350·1).

Vital HN
Abbott, Austral.; Abbott, Canad.
Preparation for enteral nutrition (p.1350·1).

Vitalaif *Medix, Mex.*
Multivitamin and mineral preparation with ginseng (p.1350·1).

Vitalax *Vita-Health, Hong Kong.*
Psyllium hydrophilic mucilloid (p.1229·1).
Constipation.

Vita-Lea *Shaklee, Canad.*
Multivitamin and mineral preparation (p.1350·1).
Dietary supplement.

Vitaleph *Aleph, Ital.†.*
Nutritional supplement (p.1350·1).

Vitaler *EMS, Braz.*
Buclizine (p.411·1); lysine; tryptophan; vitamin B_1; vi-tamin B_6 (p.1350·1).
Reduced appetite; tonic.

Vitalets *Freeda, USA.*
Multivitamin and mineral preparation with iron (p.1350·1).

Vitalgine *Medecine Vegetale, Fr.*
Hamamelis (p.1618·3); viburnum.
Haemorrhoids; peripheral vascular disorders.

Vitalin *Loges, Ger.*
Crataegus (p.1600·2).
Heart failure.

Vitaline *Bioglan, Austral.*
Lysine (p.1370·3); zinc oxide (p.1128·2).
Herpes simplex lesions.

Vitalipid
Pharmacia Upjohn, Belg.†; Fresenius Kabi, Denm.; Fresenius Kabi, Fin.; Pharmacia Upjohn, Ger.; Fresenius Kabi, Ital.; Pharmacia Neth.†; Fresenius Kabi, Norw.; Baxter, NZ; Kabi Pharmacia, Pol.; Fre-senius Kabi, Port.; Fresenius Kabi, S.Afr.; Fresenius Kabi, Spain; Fre-senius Kabi, Swed.; Pharmacia Upjohn, Thai.
Vitamins A, D_2, E, and K_1 for infusion (p.1350·1).
Parenteral nutrition.

Vitalipid N
Baxter, Austral.; Pharmacia Upjohn, Hong Kong; Pharmacia Upjohn, Israel; Fresenius Kabi, Singapore; Fresenius Kabi, Switz.
Vitamins A, D_2, E, and K_1 for infusion (p.1350·1).
Parenteral nutrition.

Vitalipid Neu *Fresenius Kabi, Aust.*
Vitamins A, D, E, and K for infusion (p.1350·1).
Contains egg lipid.
Parenteral nutrition.

Vitalipide *Fresenius Kabi, Fr.*
Vitamins A, D_2, E, and K_1 for infusion (p.1350·1).
Parenteral nutrition.

Vitalisin *Brasifa, Braz.*
Buclizine (p.411·1); lysine; carnitine; vitamin B sub-stances (p.1350·1).
Reduced appetite; tonic.

Vitalize *Scot-Tussin, USA.*
Ferric pyrophosphate (p.1359·3); vitamin B substances with L-lysine (p.1350·1).
Iron-deficiency anaemias.

Vital-Kapseln *Ratiopharm, Ger.*
Eleutherococcus senticosis (p.1615·3).
Tonic.

Vitalmix *Montefarmaco, Ital.*
Myrtillus (p.1639·2); eleutherococcus (p.1615·3); soya; royal jelly (p.1659·3); wheat germ; extract of cit-rus fruits; honey (p.1366·2); fructose (p.1363·3).
Nutritional supplement.

Vita-Logos *Sigma-Tau, Switz.*
Cynocobalamin; amino acids (p.1350·1).
Tonic.

Vitalux
Ciba Vision, Fr.
A multivitamin and mineral preparation (p.1350·1).
Eye disorders.

Ciba Vision, Ital.
Betacarotene; vitamins; minerals; soya lecithin; beeswax; wheat-germ oil (p.1350·1).
Nutritional supplement.

Vitalux Plus *Ciba Vision, Ital.*
Vitamins; lecithin; luteine; gelatin; monoglycerides; iron oxides (p.1350·1).
Nutritional supplement.

Vitamag *Aspen Consumer, S.Afr.*
Vitamin B substances; magnesium; zinc (p.1350·1).
Vitamin and mineral supplement.

Vitamedin
Sankyo, Hong Kong; Sankyo, Thai.
Vitamin B substances (p.1350·1).
Anaemias; neuritis; rheumatic disorders; sciatica.

Vita-Mefren *Novartis Consumer, Belg.*
Chlorhexidine gluconate (p.1138·2); vitamin A palmi-tate (p.1383·2).
Burns; infected skin disorders; wounds.

Vitamen *Beta, Ital.*
Protein and multivitamin preparation (p.1350·1).

Vita-Merfen *Novartis Consumer, Switz.*
Chlorhexidine gluconate (p.1138·2); benzoxonium chloride (p.1135·2); vitamin A (p.1382·1).
Minor wounds and burns.

Vita-Merfen NF *Novartis, Israel.*
Chlorhexidine gluconate (p.1138·2); benzoxonium chloride (p.1135·2); vitamin A (p.1382·1).
Burns; wounds.

Vitamfenicolo *Tubilux, Ital.*
Chloramphenicol (p.179·1) or chloramphenicol sodi-um succinate (p.179·2).
Bacterial eye infections.

Vitamidyne A and D *Fischer, Israel.*
Vitamin A (p.1382·1); vitamin D (p.1391·1).
Vitamin A and D deficiency.

Vitamil *Laborsil, Braz.*
Buclizine (p.411·1); gamma-aminobutyric acid; vita-min B substances (p.1350·1).
Reduced appetite; tonic.

Vitamin B duo *Jenapharm, Ger.*
Thiamine hydrochloride (p.1385·1); pyridoxine hydro-chloride (p.1386·3).
Neurological system disorders.

Vitamin C *Lane, UK.*
Rose fruit (p.1389·3); red cherry (p.1029·1); ascorbic acid (p.1389·3).
Formerly known as Top C.
Vitamin C deficiency.

Vitamin C-Calcium *Herbrand, Ger.*
Calcium carbonate (p.1215·1); ascorbic acid (p.1389·3).
Calcium deficiency; cold symptoms.

Vitamin F *Klosterfrau, Aust.*
Ethyl linoleate.
Skin disorders; wounds.

Vitamina F99 Topica *Vitafarma, Spain.*
Peru balsam (p.1650·2); vitamin F.
Skin disorders.

Vitaminas Lorenzini *Maxfarma, Spain†.*
Multivitamin and mineral preparation with ginseng (p.1350·1).

Vitamine 15 *Solco, Switz.*
Multivitamin and mineral preparation (p.1350·1).

Vitamine F99 *Doetsch, Grether, Switz.*
Ethyl linoleate; ethyl linolenate.
Burns; skin disorders; wounds.

Vitaminer S *Rhodia, Braz.*
Multivitamin and mineral preparation (p.1350·1).

Vitamineral *ACO, Swed.*
Multivitamin and mineral preparation (p.1350·1).

Vitaminex *Ferrer, Spain†.*
Nucleosides; vitamins (p.1350·1).
Tonic.

Vitaminic A-D *Asta Medica, Belg.†.*
Vitamin A (p.1382·1); ergocalciferol (p.1391·2).
Conjunctivitis; corneal burns and wounds; dry eyes.

Vita-Minis Cold & Flu *Herron, Austral.*
Ascorbic acid (p.1389·3); sodium ascorbate (p.1390·1); echinacea angustifolia (p.1606·2); zinc (p.1398·1).
Cold and influenza symptoms.

Vita-Minis Vitamin C Plus *Herron, Austral.*
Calcium ascorbate (p.1389·3); bioflavonoids (p.1611·1).
Vitamin C supplement.

Vitaminoftalmina *Davi, Port.*
Vitamin A (p.1382·1).
Eye disorders.

Vitaminol *Bio-Sante, Canad.*
Multivitamin and mineral preparation (p.1350·1).

Vitaminorum *Sigma, Austral.*
Multivitamin preparation (p.1350·1).

Vitamins Only *Solgar, UK.*
Multivitamin preparation (p.1350·1).

Vitamon K *Chefaro, Belg.*
Phytomenadione (p.1396·1).
Haemorrhagic disease of the newborn.

Vitamorrhuine *Medgenix, Belg.*
Cod-liver oil (p.1357·2); vitamin A acetate (p.1383·2); colecalciferol (p.1391·1).
Burns; skin disorders; wounds.

Vitamult *CTI, Israel.*
Multivitamin preparation (p.1350·1).
Tonic.

Vitan *Antigen, Irl.*
Multivitamin or multivitamin and mineral preparation (p.1350·1).

Vit-A-N *Farmigea, Ital.*
Vitamin A acetate (p.1383·2).
Blepharitis; corneal ulcer; keratitis; keratoconjuncti-vitis.

Vitanatur *A Natureza, Braz.*
Vitamin B substances with minerals (p.1350·1).

Vitaneed *Sherwood, USA.*
Lactose-free preparation for enteral nutrition (p.1350·1).

Vitaneuron *Luper, Braz.*
Vitamin B_{12} (p.1388·1); vitamin B_1 (p.1385·2).
Megaloblastic anaemias; vitamin B deficiency.

Vitanor *Medical, Port.*
Multivitamin preparation (p.1350·1).

Vitanovit *Flopen, Braz.*
Multivitamin and mineral preparation (p.1350·1).

Vitanumonyl *Teral, USA†.*
Injection: Vitamin A palmitate (p.1383·2); ergocalcif-erol (p.1391·2); eucalyptol (p.1609·2).
Oral liquid: Sulfogaiacol (p.1101·1); dextromethor-phan hydrobromide (p.1087·3); mepyramine maleate (p.421·1); phenylephrine hydrochloride (p.1097·1).
Coughs.

Vitanumonyl Pediatric *Teral, USA†.*
Dextromethorphan hydrobromide (p.1087·3); phenyle-phrine hydrochloride (p.1097·1).
Coughs.

Vitapan *Provita, Aust.*
Cod-liver oil (p.1357·2); colecalciferol (p.1391·1).
Vitamin A and D deficiency.

Vitapantol *Davigo, Belg.*
Calcium pantothenate (p.1374·1); vitamin A acetate (p.1383·2); nicotinamide (p.1372·3).
Nasal disorders.

Vitapen *Vitamed, Israel.*
Ampicillin (p.150·3).
Bacterial infections.

Vitaphakol
Ciba Vision, Fr.; Ciba Vision, Port.; Alcon Cusi, Spain; Ciba Vision, Switz.†.
Adenosine (p.828·2); cytochrome C (p.1602·1); nicoti-namide (p.1372·3); sodium succinate (p.1666·2); sorb-itol (p.1377·3).
Cataracts.

Vitaplex *Provita, Aust.*
Multivitamin preparation (p.1350·1).

Vitaplex comp *Pharmacia Upjohn, Swed.†.*
Multivitamin preparation with iron (p.1350·1).

Vitaplex mineral *Pharmacia Upjohn, Swed.*
Multivitamin and mineral preparation (p.1350·1).

Vita-Plus *Scot-Tussin, USA.*
A range of vitamin and mineral preparations (p.1350·1).

Vitaplus B Plus *Restan, S.Afr.*
Vitamin B substances; vitamin C; calcium (p.1350·1).
Vitamin and calcium supplement.

Vitaplus C Plus *Restan, S.Afr.*
Ascorbic acid (p.1389·3); calcium (p.1187·3).
Vitamin C and calcium deficiencies.

Vita-Plus E *Scot-Tussin, USA.*
Vitamin E (p.1393·3).
Vitamin E deficiency.

Vita-PMS *Bajamar, USA.*
Multivitamin and mineral preparation (p.1350·1).

Vitapore *Sunspot, Austral.*
Sulfur (p.1123·3); vitamin B substances (p.1350·1).
Acne.

Vita-Preg *Vitelle, Austral.*
Omega-3 marine triglycerides (p.949·3); folic acid (p.1361·1).
Fatty-acid supplement in pregnancy; prevention of neural tube defects.

Vitaquick *Vitaflo, Irl.*
Thickening agent (p.1350·1).
Dysphagia.

Vitaral *Kenyaku, Thai.*
Vitamins; minerals; rutoside; dehydrocholic acid; liver concentrate (p.1350·1).
Vitamin and mineral deficiency.

Vitarex *Pasadena, USA.*
Multivitamin and mineral preparation with iron (p.1350·1).

Vitargenol *Ciba Vision, Fr.†.*
Silver protein (p.1664·2).
Eye disorders.

Vitarical *Heralds, Braz.*
Multivitamin and mineral preparation (p.1350·1).

Vitarnin
Grossmann, Hong Kong; Grossmann, Switz.
Multivitamin and mineral preparation (p.1350·1).

Vitarubin *Streuli, Switz.*
Cyanocobalamin (p.1388·1) or hydroxocobalamin acetate (p.1388·3).
Anaemias; neurological disorders; vitamin B₁₂ deficiency.

Vitarutine *Ciba Vision, Fr.*
Rutoside sodium sulfate (p.1611·2); nicotinamide (p.1372·3).
Eye disorders.

Vitasana *Boehringer Ingelheim, Aust.*
Vitamins; minerals; lecithin; deanol; ginseng (p.1350·1).

Vitasana-Lebenstropfen *Hotz, Ger.*
Gentian; calamus; menyanthes; melissa; achillea; peppermint leaf; crataegus; rosemary; rue; lupulus; valerian; juniper; aniseed; fennel; caraway; herba marjoranae.
Tonic.

Vitasavoury *Vitaflo, UK.*
High energy sip feed (p.1350·1).

Vitasay *Dorsay, Braz.*
Multivitamin and mineral preparation (p.1350·1).

Vitascarbol *Rhone-Poulenc Rorer, Israel.*
Vitamin C (p.1389·3).
Vitamin C supplement.

Vita-Schlanktropfen *Schuck, Ger.†*
Cathine hydrochloride (p.1507·1).
Obesity.

Vitascorb *Leofarma, Braz.*
Vitamin C (p.1389·3).
Vitamin C deficiency; vitamin C supplement.

Vitascorbol *Theraplix, Fr.*
Ascorbic acid (p.1389·3) with or without sodium ascorbate (p.1390·1).
Vitamin C deficiency.

Vitasedine *Ciba Vision, Fr.†*
Phenylephrine hydrochloride (p.1097·1); zinc sulfate (p.1398·2).
Eye disorders.

Vitaseptine *Ciba Vision, Fr.†*
Sulfacetamide sodium (p.250·3).
Formerly contained sulfacetamide sodium, zinc sulfate, sodium iodide, and nicotinamide.
Eye infections.

Vitaseptol *Ciba Vision, Fr.*
Thiomersal (p.1158·2).
Ocular antiseptic.

Vitasic *Germania, Aust.*
Adenosine (p.828·2); thymidine (p.1672·3); cytidine; uridine (p.1677·2); disodium guanylate (p.1604·3).
Eye disorders.

Vitasma *Basi, Port.*
Ephedrine hydrochloride (p.1090·1); meprobamate (p.691·1); prednisolone (p.1077·3); choline theophyllinate (p.763·3).

VitaSohn *Antonetto, Ital.*
Multivitamin and mineral preparation (p.1350·1).

Vitasprint *Searle, Ital.*
DL-Phosphoserine; cyanocobalamin (p.1388·1); levoglutamide (p.1365·2).
Tonic.

Vitasprint B₁₂ *Wyeth, Ger.*
DL-Phosphoserine; cyanocobalamin (p.1388·1); levoglutamide (p.1365·2).
Vitamin B deficiency.

Vitasprint Complex *Searle, Ital.; Poli, Switz.*
L-Phosphoserine; arginine hydrochloride (p.1353·3); L--phosphothreonine; levoglutamide (p.1365·2); hydroxocobalamin (p.1388·1).
Tonic.

Vita-Squares *GNLD, Austral.*
Multivitamin and mineral preparation (p.1350·1).

Vitasten *Basi, Port.*
Thiamine; vitamin B₁₂ (p.1350·1).

Vita-Suple *Laborsil, Braz.*
Multivitamin and mineral preparation (p.1350·1).

Vitathion
Note. This name is used for preparations of different composition.
Eutherapie, Belg.†
Ascorbic acid (p.1389·3); glutathione (p.1010·3); adenosine triphosphate (p.1573·3); thiamine (p.1385·2); inositolcalcium; haemoglobin (p.738·1).
Asthenia; vitamin deficiency.
Servier, Fr.
Ascorbic acid (p.1389·3); thiamine hydrochloride (p.1385·1); inositolcalcium.
Asthenia.

Vita-Thion *Servier, S.Afr.*
Vitamins; glutathione; haemoglobin; sodium adenosine triphosphate; calcium inositol hexaphosphate (p.1350·1).
Tonic.

Vitathion-ATP *Servier, Canad.*
Ascorbic acid (p.1389·3); adenosine triphosphate (p.1573·3); calcium inositolhexaphosphate; glutathione (p.1010·3); magnesium inositolhexaphosphate; thiamine (p.1385·2).
Stress conditions.

Vitaton *Allen, Mex.*
Vitamin B substances (p.1350·1).

Vita Health, Singapore.
Vitamins; minerals; bee pollen; cysteine; ginseng; kelp; lecithin; lysine; royal jelly; yeast (p.1350·1).

Vitatona *Brauer, Austral.*
Angelica (p.1580·2); ascorbic acid (p.1389·3); kola nitida (p.1681·1); vitamin B substances (p.1350·1); hypericum (p.290·2); ginseng (p.1615·3); urtica urens (p.1678·2); aurum muriaticum; calcarea phosphorica; ferrum metallicum; ferrum phosphoricum; kali phosphoricum; magnesia phosphorica; phosphoric acid.
Tonic.

Vitatonin *Ipex, Swed.*
Multivitamins (p.1350·1); caffeine (p.761·3); vin. vermuth.; alcohol.
Tonic.

Vitatron *VAAS, Ital.*
Amino-acid preparation with vitamins and minerals (p.1350·1).
Nutritional supplement.

Vitavir *Virginia, Ital.*
Vitamins; minerals; carnitine tartrate; ginseng; ginkgo biloba (p.1350·1).
Nutritional supplement.

Vitavox Pastillas *Escaned, Spain.*
Camphor (p.1589·3); eucalyptol (p.1609·2); chlorophyll (p.1028·1); ephedrine hydrochloride (p.1090·1); niaouli oil (p.1640·2); menthol (p.1632·3); sulfanilamide sodium mesilate (p.256·2); peppermint (p.1243·2).
Mouth and throat disorders.

Vita-Worth B Complex *General Nutrition, Canad.*
Vitamin B substances (p.1350·1).

Vitawund *Novartis Consumer, Aust.*
Ointment: Chlorhexidine gluconate (p.1138·2); halibut-liver oil (p.1366·1).
Burns; wounds.
Topical powder: Chlorhexidine acetate (p.1138·2).
Formerly known as Sorbifen.
Prevention of wound infection.

Vitawund Baby *Novartis Consumer, Aust.*
Lactose (p.1370·2).
Formerly known as Sorbifen Baby.
Care of umbilicus.

Vitax *Heralds, Braz.*
Vitamin C (p.1389·3).
Vitamin C deficiency; vitamin C supplement.

Vitaxicam *Ferrer, Singapore; Robert, Spain.*
Piroxicam (p.79·1).
Gout; musculoskeletal, joint, peri-articular, and soft-tissue disorders; pain.

Vitazell E *Kohler-Pharma, Ger.*
dl-Alpha tocopherol (p.1394·1).
Vitamin E deficiency.

Vitazinc *Ciba Vision, Fr.†*
Zinc sulfate (p.1398·2).
Formerly contained zinc sulfate and thiamine hydrochloride.
Ocular antiseptic.

Vit-C-Lutsch *Sanochemia, Aust.*
Ascorbic acid (p.1389·3); calcium ascorbate (p.1389·3); hesperidin phosphate (p.1611·2).
Vitamin C deficiency.

Vitec *Pharmaceutical Specialties, USA.*
dl-Alpha tocoferil acetate (p.1394·1).
Skin disorders.

Vitecaf *SIFI, Ital.*
Eye drops: Rolitetracycline (p.247·1); chloramphenicol (p.179·1).
Eye ointment: Tetracycline hydrochloride (p.258·3); chloramphenicol (p.179·1); calcium pantothenate (p.1374·1).
Infected eye disorders.

Vitef *Teofarma, Ital.*
Polyenacid.
Skin disorders.

Vitelle Nesentials *Fielding, USA.*
Multivitamin and mineral preparation (p.1350·1).

Vitelle Nestabs *Fielding, USA.*
Multivitamin and mineral preparation with iron and folic acid (p.1350·1).
Prenatal supplement.

Vitelle Nestrex *Fielding, USA.*
Pyridoxine hydrochloride (p.1386·3).
Pyridoxine deficiency.

Vitelsix *Unison, Thai.*
Vitamin B₁; vitamin B₆; vitamin B₁₂ (p.1350·1).
Loss of appetite; vitamin B deficiency.

Vitenur *Orion, Ger.*
Acetylcysteine (p.1082·3).
Respiratory-tract disorders with viscous mucus.

Viteral *Be-Tabs, S.Afr.*
Multivitamin and mineral preparation (p.1350·1).

Vitergan Zinco Plus *Marjan, Braz.*
Multivitamin and mineral preparation (p.1350·1).

Viternum *Senosiain, Mex.; OM, Port.; Juste, Spain.*
Cyproheptadine pyridoxal phosphate (p.414·3).
Allergic rhinitis; anorexia; urticaria.

Viterra *Pfizer Consumer, Ital.; Pfizer, Mex.; Pfizer, Port.; Pfizer Consumer, Spain; Pfizer, Thai.*
Multivitamin and mineral preparation (p.1350·1).

Vitestable *Alcor, Spain.*
Royal jelly; ginseng; tocopherol (p.1350·1).
Tonic.

Vitialgin *Boots Healthcare, Ital.†*
Propyphenazone (p.80·2); paracetamol (p.71·2).
Fever; pain.

Viticromin *Auad, Braz.*
Vitamin B substances (p.1350·1); brosimum gaudichandii.
Vitiligo.

Vitinoin *Pharmascience, Canad.*
Tretinoin (p.1126·2).
Acne.

Vitintra *Pharmacia Upjohn, Neth.*
Vitamins A, D₂, E, and K₁ for infusion (p.1350·1).
Parenteral nutrition.

Vitiral *Scherer, Thai.*
Multivitamin and mineral preparation (p.1350·1).

Vitiron
Heralds, Braz.
Multivitamin preparation with iron (p.1350·1).
Mepha, Hong Kong.
Multivitamin and mineral preparation (p.1350·1).
Mepha, Singapore.
Multivitamin and mineral preparation with methionine (p.1350·1).
Mepha, Switz.
Vitamins; minerals; choline bitartrate; inositol; methionine (p.1350·1).

Vitiveine *Arkopharma, Fr.†*
Red vine.
Haemorrhoids; peripheral vascular disorders.

Vitlipid N
Pharmacia Upjohn, Irl.; Fresenius, UK.
Vitamins A, D₂, E, and K₁ for infusion (p.1350·1).
Parenteral nutrition.

Vito Bronches *Duchesnay, Canad.*
Diphenylpyraline hydrochloride (p.417·1); dextromethorphan hydrobromide (p.1087·3); potassium iodide (p.1522·3); sodium citrate (p.1186·2).

Vitobasan N *BASF, Ger.†*
Thiamine hydrochloride (p.1385·1); pyridoxine hydrochloride (p.1386·3).
Nervous system disorders.

Vitogen *Stanley, Canad.*
A range of vitamin preparations with or without minerals (p.1350·1).

Vitogen Spectrum *Shoppers Drug Mart, Canad.†*
Multivitamin and mineral preparation (p.1350·1).

Vitol *Orion, Fin.*
Vitamin A or vitamin A palmitate; colecalciferol or ergocalciferol (p.1350·1).
Vitamins A and D deficiency.

Vit-o-Mar *Asta Medica, Ger.†*
Silybum marianum (p.1021·3).
Liver disorders.

Vitonic *Cypress, USA.*
Vitamin B substances; minerals (p.1350·1).
Dietary supplement.

Vitonico *Legrand, Braz.*
Ferrous sulfate; phosphoric acid; aloes; myrrh; nutmeg; clove (p.1350·1).
Iron-deficiency anaemias; tonic.

Vitonil *Gemballa, Braz.*
Orotic acid; vitamin B substances (p.1350·1).
Nutritional supplement.

Vitoral *Medifarma, Mex.*
Multivitamin preparation (p.1350·1).

Vitosal *Ziethen, Ger.*
Vitamins (p.1350·1); rutoside sodium sulfate (p.1611·2); arnica (p.1581·3); sage (p.1660·2); peppermint oil (p.1243·3).
Gum disorders.

Vit-Porphyrin *Teofarma, Ital.*
Haematoporphyrin dihydrochloride (p.1618·3); nicotinamide (p.1372·3).
Tonic.

Vitrace *Aspen, S.Afr.*
Multivitamin and mineral preparation (p.1350·1).
Tonic.

Vitraday *Lifeplan, UK.*
Multinutrient preparation (p.1350·1).

Vitrafem *Lifeplan, UK.*
Multinutrient preparation (p.1350·1).

Vitrasert *Bausch & Lomb, Austral.; Bausch & Lomb, UK; Bausch & Lomb, USA.*
Ganciclovir (p.623·1).
Cytomegalovirus retinitis.

Vitravene
Ciba Vision, Denm.; Ciba Vision, Fin.; Ciba Vision, Fr.; Novartis Ophthalmics, UK; Isis, USA.
Fomivirsen sodium (p.621·2).
Cytomegalovirus retinitis.

Vitrax *Allergan, Aust.†*
Sodium hyaluronate (p.1620·1).
Adjunct in eye surgery.

Vitreolent
Ciba Vision, Hong Kong; Ciba Vision, Singapore; Ciba Vision, Switz.
Potassium iodide (p.1522·3); sodium iodide (p.1522·3).
Eye disorders.

Vitreolent plus *Ciba Vision, Ger.*
Cytochrome C (p.1602·1); adenosine (p.828·2); nicotinamide (p.1372·3).
Cataracts.

Vitreolux *Ciba Vision, Ital.*
Vitamins; bioflavonoids; betacarotene; glucosamine; zinc; methionine; myrtillus; yeast (p.1350·1).
Nutritional supplement.

Vitreosan *DMG, Ital.*
Potassium bicarbonate; magnesium chloride; vitamin C (p.1350·1).
Nutritional supplement.

Vitrical *Prodotti, Ital.*
Multivitamin and mineral preparation (p.1350·1).

Vitrimix
Fresenius Kabi, Denm.; Fresenius Kabi, Norw.; Fresenius Kabi, Port.; Fresenius Kabi, Swed.; Fresenius Kabi, Switz.
Amino-acid, glucose, and lipid (from soya oil (p.1378·1)) infusion (p.1350·1).
Contains egg lecithin.
Parenteral nutrition.

Vitrimix KV
Fresenius Kabi, Fr.; Pharmacia Upjohn, Hong Kong; Pharmacia Upjohn, Irl.; Pharmacia Upjohn, Neth.; Fresenius Kabi, Singapore; Pharmacia Upjohn, Thai.; Fresenius, UK.
Amino acid, glucose, and lipid (from soya oil (p.1378·1)) infusion with or without electrolytes (p.1350·1).
Contains egg phospholipids.
Parenteral nutrition.

Vitrite *Seven Seas, UK.*
Multivitamin preparation (p.1350·1).

Vitron *Pharmaland, Thai.*
Vitamin B₁ (p.1385·2); vitamin B₆ (p.1387·3); vitamin B₁₂ (p.1388·1).
Anorexia; neurasthenia; neurological disorders; neuropathy; toxaemia of pregnancy.

Vitron-C *Heritage Consumer, USA.*
Ferrous fumarate (p.1360·1).
Ascorbic acid (p.1389·3) is included in this preparation to increase the absorption and availability of iron.
Iron-deficiency anaemias.

Vitrosups *Llorens, Spain.*
Glycerol (p.1616·3).
Constipation; laxative dependence.

Vits *Profarb, Braz.*
Multivitamin and mineral preparation (p.1350·1).

Vit-u-pept *Plantina, Ger.*
Weisskohl; bismuth subcarbonate (p.1213·1); heavy magnesium carbonate (p.1232·3); sodium bicarbonate (p.1186·2).
Gastrointestinal disorders.

Vitussin
Note. This name is used for preparations of different composition.
Vitamed, Israel.
Guaifenesin (p.1092·2).
Coughs.
Cypress, USA.
Hydrocodone tartrate (p.42·2); guaifenesin (p.1092·2).
Coughs.

Vivactil *Merck, USA.*
Protriptyline hydrochloride (p.307·3).
Depression.

Viva-Drops *Vision, USA.*
Polysorbate 80 (p.1347·3).
Formerly known as Vit-A-drops.
Dry eyes.

Vival *Alpharma, Norw.*
Diazepam (p.674·3).
Anxiety; skeletal muscle spasm; sleep disorders.

Vivalan *Zeneca, Belg.; Menarini, Belg.; AstraZeneca, Fr.; Zeneca, Ger.; Zeneca, Port.; AstraZeneca, UK†.*
Viloxazine hydrochloride (p.313·3).
Depression.

Vivamyne *Whitehall, Fr.*
A range of vitamin preparations with or without minerals (p.1350·1).

Vivance *Vivance, Fr.*
Nutritional supplement (p.1350·1).

Vivapryl *Asta Medica, UK†.*
Selegiline hydrochloride (p.1177·2).
Parkinsonism.

Vivarin *SmithKline Beecham Consumer, USA.*
Caffeine (p.761·3).
Fatigue.

Vivarint
Zeneca, Aust.†; Zeneca, Spain.
Viloxazine hydrochloride (p.313·3).
Depression.

Vivatec
Merck Sharp & Dohme, Denm.; Merck Sharp & Dohme, Fin.; Merck Sharp & Dohme, Norw.; Merck Sharp & Dohme, Swed.
Lisinopril (p.921·1).
Heart failure; hypertension; myocardial infarction.

Vivatec Comp
Merck Sharp & Dohme, Fin.; Merck Sharp & Dohme, Norw.
Lisinopril (p.921·1); hydrochlorothiazide (p.907·3).
Hypertension.

Vivaxine *Nakorn, Thai.*
Sulfadoxine (p.252·3); pyrimethamine (p.442·3).
Malaria.

Vivazid *Merck Sharp & Dohme, Denm.*
Lisinopril (p.921·1); hydrochlorothiazide (p.907·3).
Hypertension.

Vivelle
Note. This name is used for preparations of different composition.
Janssen-Cilag, Aust.
Norgestimate (p.1486·1); ethinylestradiol (p.1476·2).
Acne; triphasic oral contraceptive.
Novartis, Canad.; Novartis, USA.
Estradiol (p.1473·1).
Menopausal disorders; oestrogen deficiency.

Vivena AR *Dieterba, Ital.*
Infant feed (p.1350·1).
Gastro-oesophageal reflux.

Vivena HA *Dieterba, Ital.*
Infant feed (p.1350·1).
Cow's milk intolerance.

Vivene *Theratech, Fr.*
Aesculus (p.1574·1); troxerutin (p.1611·2).
Formerly contained buphenine hydrochloride, aesculus, troxerutin.
Haemorrhoids; peripheral vascular disorders.

Vividrin
Riel, Aust.; Tramedico, Belg.; Mann, Ger.; Mann, Irl.; Mann, Neth.; Bausch & Lomb, S.Afr.; Mann, Singapore; Farma Lepori, Spain; Gebra, Switz.; Bausch & Lomb, Thai.; Mann, Thai.; Pharma-Global, UK.
Sodium cromoglicate (p.774·3).
Allergic conjunctivitis; allergic rhinitis; asthma; keratoconjunctivitis.

Vividrin comp *Mann, Ger.*
Sodium cromoglicate (p.774·3); xylometazoline hydrochloride (p.1102·2).
Allergic rhinitis.

Vividrin mit Terfenadin *Mann, Ger.†*
Terfenadine (p.424·3).
Hypersensitivity reactions.

Vividyl *Lilly, Ital.†*
Nortriptyline hydrochloride (p.301·3).
Depression.

Vivimed
Note. This name is used for preparations of different composition.
Riel, Aust.
Propyphenazone (p.80·2); paracetamol (p.71·2); caffeine (p.761·3).
Fever; pain.

Mann, Ger.†
Paracetamol (p.71·2).
Fever; pain.

Mann, Irl.†
Paracetamol (p.71·2); caffeine (p.761·3).
Pain.

Vivin C
Note. This name is used for preparations of different composition.
Menarini, Ital.; Alter, Spain.
Aspirin (p.24·2); ascorbic acid (p.1389·3).
Cold and influenza symptoms; fever; pain.

Alter, Port.
Ascorbic acid (p.1389·3).
Cold and influenza symptoms; tonic.

Vivinox *Riel, Aust.*
Valerian (p.1678·3); lupulus (p.1629·3); mistletoe (p.1636·2).
Anxiety disorders.

Vivinox N *Mann, Ger.*
Valerian (p.1678·3); lupulus (p.1629·3); passion flower (p.1649·1).
Nervous disorders; sleep disorders.

Vivinox Stark *Mann, Ger.†*
Diphenhydramine hydrochloride (p.416·1).
Sleep disorders.

Vivinox-Schlafdragees *Mann, Ger.†*
Diphenhydramine hydrochloride (p.416·1); valerian (p.1678·3); lupulus (p.1629·3).
Sleep disorders.

Vivioptal
Mann, Irl.; Nucare, UK.
Multivitamin and mineral preparation (p.1350·1).

Viviplus *Mann, Ger.*
Hypericum (p.290·2).
Anxiety; depression.

Vivir *Unison, Thai.*
Aciclovir (p.612·3).
Herpesvirus infections.

ViviRhin S *Mann, Ger.†*
Xylometazoline hydrochloride (p.1102·2).
Nasal congestion.

Vivisun *Mann, Ger.†*
Diphenhydramine hydrochloride (p.416·1); lauromacrogol 400 (p.1345·2).
Hypersensitivity reactions of the skin.

Vivol *Carter Horner, Canad.*
Diazepam (p.674·3).
Anxiety; sedative.

Vivolan *Orion, Fin.*
Emollient.
Skin disorders; vehicle for topical drugs.

Vivonex
Novartis Nutrition, Canad.; Novartis Nutrition, Hong Kong; Promeco, Mex.; Novartis Nutrition, Singapore; Procter & Gamble, USA.
Preparation for enteral nutrition (p.1350·1).

Vivotif
Kwizda, Aust.; Berna, Belg.; Berna, Canad.; Berna, Denm.; Berna, Fin.; Niddapharm, Ger.; Berna, Hong Kong; Medeva, Irl.; Swiss Serum Institute, Israel; Berna, Ital.; Berna, Norw.; Berna, Port.; Byk Madaus, S.Afr.; Berna, Singapore; Berna, Spain; Cortec, Swed.; Berna, Switz.; Berna, Thai.; Masta, UK; Berna, USA.
A live oral typhoid vaccine (p.1566·3).
Active immunisation.

Vivradoxil *Alphama, Mex.*
Doxycycline (p.200·1).
Bacterial infections.

Vivural *Procter & Gamble, Ger.*
Calcium carbonate (p.1215·1).
Calcium deficiency.

Vix Plex *Laborsil, Braz.*
Multivitamin and mineral preparation (p.1350·1).

Vixin *Sons, Mex.*
Chloramphenicol (p.179·1).
Bacterial infections.

Vixmicina *Uniao Quimica, Braz.*
Chloramphenicol (p.179·1).
Bacterial infections.

Vi-Zac *UCB, USA.*
Multivitamin and mineral preparation (p.1350·1).

Vizam *Amrad, Austral.†*
Doxycycline hyclate (p.200·1).
Bacterial infections; malaria.

Vizax *Essex, Ital.†*
Isepamicin (p.215·2).
Bacterial infections.

Viz-On *Opus, UK.*
Sodium cromoglicate (p.774·3).
Allergic conjunctivitis.

Vizoptal *Medical, Port.*
Chlorobutanol (p.1141·2).

V-Lax *Century, USA†.*
Psyllium hydrophilic mucilloid (p.1229·1).
Constipation.

VM-2000 *Solgar, UK.*
Multivitamin and mineral preparation (p.1350·1).

VM 26 *Bristol-Myers Squibb, Ger.*
Teniposide (p.574·1).
Malignant neoplasms.

VM Drosan *Liferpal, Mex.*
Multivitamin and mineral preparation (p.1350·1).

Voalla *Maruho, Jpn†.*
Dexamethasone valerate (p.1067·3).
Skin disorders.

Vobaderm *Hermal, Ger.*
Fluprednidene acetate (p.1072·1); miconazole nitrate (p.391·1).
Formerly contained fluprednidene acetate.
Infected skin disorders.

Vocadys *Chemineau, Fr.*
Enoxolone (p.34·3); lignocaine [lidocaine] hydrochloride (p.1313·2); erysimum.
Formerly contained codeine, lignocaine [lidocaine] hydrochloride, and erysimum.
Sore throat.

Vocalzone *Kestrel, UK.*
Menthol (p.1632·3); peppermint oil (p.1243·3); myrrh (p.1639·2); liquorice (p.1231·2).
Throat irritation.

Vocara *Bittner, Aust.*
Homoeopathic preparation.

Vodol *Searle, Braz.*
Miconazole (p.391·1).
Fungal skin infections.

Vofenal *Alcon, Canad.*
Diclofenac sodium (p.30·3).
Inflammatory eye disorders.

Vogalene
Rhone-Poulenc Rorer, Belg.; Aventis, Denm.; Schwarz, Fr.; Rhone-Poulenc Rorer, Israel.
Metopimazine (p.1237·2).
Nausea and vomiting.

Volamin *Volchem, Ital.*
Amino-acid preparation (p.1350·1).
Fatigue; liver disorders.

Volcidol-S *Pharmasant, Thai.*
Tramadol hydrochloride (p.89·1).
Pain.

Volcolon *Parke, Davis, Neth.*
Ispaghula (p.1229·1).
Constipation.

Voldal *Genevar, Fr.*
Diclofenac sodium (p.30·3).
Dysmenorrhoea; musculoskeletal, joint, and peri-articular disorders; renal colic.

Volfenac
Collins, Mex.; General Drugs, Thai.
Diclofenac diethylamine (p.30·2) or diclofenac sodium (p.30·3).
Gout; musculoskeletal, joint, peri-articular, and soft-tissue disorders; pain.

Volital *Laboratories for Applied Biology, UK†.*
Pemoline (p.1513·1).
Hyperactivity in children.

Vollmers praparierter gruner *Salushaus, Ger.*
Avena (p.1583·1); urtica (p.1678·2); hypericum (p.290·2); alchemilla.
Digestive disorders; nervous disorders; oedema; urinary-tract disorders.

Volmac *Glaxo Wellcome, Ger.; Cascan, Ger.*
Salbutamol sulfate (p.770·3).
Obstructive airways disease.

Volmax
Glaxo Wellcome, Denm.; Glaxo Wellcome, Hong Kong; Glaxo Wellcome, Ital.; Glaxo Allen, Ital.; Glaxo Wellcome, Mex.; Glaxo Wellcome, NZ; Glaxo Wellcome, S.Afr.; Glaxo Wellcome, Singapore; Glaxo Wellcome, Switz.; Glaxo Wellcome, Thai.; Allen & Hanburys, UK; Muro, USA.
Salbutamol sulfate (p.770·3).
Obstructive airways disease.

Volnac *TO-Chemicals, Thai.*
Diclofenac sodium (p.30·3).
Fever; inflammation; pain.

Vologen *Antigen, Irl.*
Diclofenac sodium (p.30·3).
Gout; inflammation; musculoskeletal, joint, and peri-articular disorders; pain.

Volon
Bristol-Myers Squibb, Aust.; Bristol-Myers Squibb, Ger.
Triamcinolone (p.1080·1).
Corticosteroid.

Volon A
Bristol-Myers Squibb, Aust.; Bristol-Myers Squibb, Ger.
Triamcinolone acetonide (p.1080·1) or triamcinolone acetonide dipotassium phosphate (p.1080·2).
Corticosteroid.

Volon A antibiotikahaltig *Bristol-Myers Squibb, Aust.*
Triamcinolone acetonide (p.1080·1); neomycin sulfate (p.228·1); gramicidin (p.213·3).
Eye disorders.

Volon A antibiotikahaltig N *Bristol-Myers Squibb, Ger.*
Triamcinolone acetonide (p.1080·1); neomycin sulfate (p.228·1).
Skin disorders.

Volon A Tinktur *Bristol-Myers Squibb, Aust.*
Triamcinolone acetonide (p.1080·1); salicylic acid (p.1122·3).
Otitis externa; skin disorders.

Volon A Tinktur N *Bristol-Myers Squibb, Ger.*
Triamcinolone acetonide (p.1080·1); salicylic acid (p.1122·3).
Otitis externa; skin disorders.

Volon A-Rhin *Bristol-Myers Squibb, Ger.*
Triamcinolone acetonide (p.1080·1); phenylephrine hydrochloride (p.1097·1).
Rhinitis; sinusitis.

Volon A-Schuttelmix *Bristol-Myers Squibb, Ger.*
Triamcinolone acetonide (p.1080·1); zinc oxide (p.1128·2).
Skin disorders.

Volon A-Zinklotion *Bristol-Myers Squibb, Aust.*
Triamcinolone acetonide (p.1080·1); zinc oxide (p.1128·2).
Skin disorders.

Volonimat *Bristol-Myers Squibb, Ger.*
Triamcinolone acetonide (p.1080·1).
Skin disorders.

Volonimat N *Bristol-Myers Squibb, Ger.*
Triamcinolone acetonide (p.1080·1).
Skin disorders.

Volonimat Plus N *Bristol-Myers Squibb, Ger.*
Triamcinolone acetonide (p.1080·1); nystatin (p.392·2).
Eczema with secondary yeast infection.

Volraman *Eastern Pharmaceuticals, UK.*
Diclofenac sodium (p.30·3).
Gout; inflammation; musculoskeletal disorders; pain.

Volsaid *Trinity, UK.*
Diclofenac sodium (p.30·3).
Inflammation; musculoskeletal, joint, and peri-articular disorders; pain.

Voltaflex *EMS, Braz.*
Diclofenac (p.30·2).
Gout; inflammation; musculoskeletal, joint, and peri-articular disorders; pain.

Voltamicin
Ciba Vision, Ital.; Ciba Vision, Switz.
Diclofenac sodium (p.30·3); gentamicin (p.212·1) or gentamicin sulfate (p.210·1).
Bacterial eye infections and inflammation.

Voltamicine *Ciba Vision, Fr.*
Diclofenac sodium (p.30·3); gentamicin sulfate (p.210·1).
Bacterial eye infections and inflammation following cataract surgery.

Voltanac *Pharmasant, Thai.*
Diclofenac sodium (p.30·3).
Musculoskeletal and joint disorders.

Voltaren
Novartis, Aust.; Novartis, Austral.; Novartis, Belg.; Novartis, Braz.; Novartis, Canad.; Novartis, Denm.; Novartis, Fin.; Novartis, Ger.; Novartis Consumer, Ger.; Novartis, Hong Kong; Novartis, Israel; Ciba Vision, Ital.; Novartis, Ital.; Novartis, Mex.; Novartis, Neth.; Novartis, Norw.; Novartis, NZ; Novartis, Port.; Novartis, S.Afr.; Novartis, Singapore; Novartis, Spain; Novartis, Swed.; Novartis, Thai.; Ciba Vision, USA; Novartis, Venez.
Diclofenac (p.30·2), diclofenac diethylamine (p.30·2), diclofenac potassium (p.30·2), diclofenac resinate (p.31·3), or diclofenac sodium (p.30·3).
Cystoid macular oedema; fever; gout; inflammation; musculoskeletal, joint, peri-articular, and soft-tissue disorders; pain; prevention of intraoperative miosis; renal and biliary colic.

Voltaren Emulgel
Novartis, Spain; Novartis Consumer, Switz.
Diclofenac diethylamine (p.30·2).
Musculoskeletal, joint, peri-articular and soft-tissue disorders.

Voltaren Ophtha
Ciba Vision, Austral.; Novartis Ophthalmics, Canad.; Ciba Vision, Ger.; Ciba Vision, Hong Kong; Ciba Vision, Israel; Ciba Vision, Neth.; Ciba Vision, NZ; Ciba Vision, Singapore; Ciba Vision, Swed.; Ciba Vision, Switz.
Diclofenac sodium (p.30·3).
Ocular pain and inflammation; prevention of cystoid macular oedema; prevention of miosis during cataract surgery.

Voltaren T *Novartis, Swed.*
Diclofenac potassium (p.30·2).
Pain.

Voltarene
Ciba Vision, Fr.
Eye drops: Diclofenac sodium (p.30·3).
Eye pain; inflammation following eye surgery; inhibition of intraoperative miosis.

Novartis, Fr.
Injection; sustained-release tablets; suppositories; tablets; topical gel: Diclofenac diethylamine (p.30·2) or diclofenac sodium (p.30·3).
Dysmenorrhoea; musculoskeletal, joint, and peri-articular disorders; oedema; renal colic.

Novartis, Switz.
Diclofenac (p.30·2), diclofenac resinate (p.31·3), or diclofenac sodium (p.30·3).
Inflammation; musculoskeletal and joint disorders; pain.

Voltarene Rapide *Novartis, Switz.*
Diclofenac potassium (p.30·2).
Inflammation; pain.

Voltarol
Novartis, Irl.; Novartis, UK.
Diclofenac (p.30·2), diclofenac diethylamine (p.30·2), diclofenac potassium (p.30·2), or diclofenac sodium (p.30·3).
Gout; inflammation; musculoskeletal, joint, peri-articular, and soft-tissue disorders; pain.

Voltarol Ophtha
Ciba Vision, Irl.; Novartis Ophthalmics, UK.
Diclofenac sodium (p.30·3).
Anterior eye inflammation; inflammation and pain following eye surgery; inhibition of peri-operative miosis; prevention of cystoid macular oedema.

Voltax *Poehlmann, Ger.†*
Phospholipids; muira-puama; adenosine; vitamins (p.1350·1).
Tonic.

Voltfast *Novartis, Ital.*
Diclofenac potassium (p.30·2).
Inflammation; pain.

Voltil *Ardeypharm, Ger.*
Protein-free extract of bovine spleen.
Gastrointestinal disorders; peripheral and cerebral vascular disorders; skin disorders.

Voltric *UCB, Spain.*
Cetirizine hydrochloride (p.411·2).
Allergic conjunctivitis; allergic rhinitis; pruritus; urticaria.

Voltrix *Bunker, Braz.*
Diclofenac (p.30·2).
Gout; inflammation; musculoskeletal, joint, and peri-articular disorders; pain.

Volutine *Geymonat, Ital.*
Fenofibrate (p.889·1).
Hyperlipidaemias.

Volutol *Lemery, Mex.*
Carbamazepine (p.342·2).
Epilepsy.

Voluven
Fresenius Kabi, Ger.; Fresenius Kabi, Port.; Fresenius, UK.
An etherified starch (p.732·3).
Plasma volume expansion.

Volverac *TP, Thai.*
Diclofenac sodium (p.30·3).
Inflammation following cataract surgery; postoperative cystoid macular oedema; prevention or reduction of intraoperative miosis.

Vomacur *Hexal, Ger.*
Dimenhydrinate (p.415·2).
Motion sickness; nausea; vertigo; vomiting.

Vomex A *Yamanouchi, Ger.*
Dimenhydrinate (p.415·2).
Nausea; premedication; vestibular disorders; vomiting.

Vomidrine *Azevedos, Port.*
Dimenhydrinate (p.415·2).
Motion sickness.

Vomifene *Mer-National, S.Afr.*
Buclizine hydrochloride (p.411·1); pyridoxine (p.1387·1).
Motion sickness; nausea; vertigo; vomiting.

Vominar *Charoen, Thai.*
Dimenhydrinate (p.415·2).
Motion sickness; vertigo, nausea and vomiting.

Vominil *Sedabel, Braz.*
Metoclopramide (p.1236·3); vitamin B$_6$ (p.1387·1).
Nausea and vomiting.

Vomisin *Rayere, Mex.*
Dimenhydrinate (p.415·2).
Motion sickness; vestibular disorders.

Vomistop *Medquimica, Braz.*
Metoclopramide (p.1236·3); vitamin B$_6$ (p.1387·1).
Nausea and vomiting.

Vomitran *Berlin Pharm, Thai.*
Ondansetron hydrochloride (p.1241·3).
Nausea and vomiting induced by cytotoxics or radiotherapy.

Vomix *Natus, Braz.*
Metoclopramide (p.1236·3).
Gastrointestinal motility disorders; nausea and vomiting.

Vonifin *Rudefsa, Mex.*
Metoclopramide (p.1236·3).

Vonil *UCI, Braz.*
Metoclopramide hydrochloride (p.1235·2).
Gastrointestinal motility disorders; nausea and vomiting.

Vonil Enzimatico *UCI, Braz.*
Metoclopramide (p.1236·3); pancreatin (p.1646·1); dimethicone (p.1249·2); sodium dehydrocholate (p.1602·2); bromelains (p.1586·3).
Digestive disorders.

Vontrol
Enila, Braz.; SmithKline Beecham, Mex.
Difenidol hydrochloride (p.1222·1).
Nausea and vomiting; vertigo.

Vonum Gerot, Aust.
Indometacin (p.44·3); lauromacrogol 400 (p.1345·2).
Musculoskeletal, joint, and soft-tissue disorders.

Vopax Haller, Braz.
Metoclopramide (p.1236·3); vitamin B₆ (p.1387·1).
Nausea and vomiting.

V-Optic Vitamed, Israel.
Timolol maleate (p.982·1).
Glaucoma.

Vorange DHA, Singapore.
Vitamin C (p.1389·3).
Vitamin C deficiency.

Voren Yung Shin, Thai.
Diclofenac sodium (p.30·3).
Inflammation; musculoskeletal, joint, and peri-articular disorders; pain.

Vorigeno Inibsa, Spain.
Hyoscine hydrobromide (p.468·2).
Motion sickness.

VoSoL
Note. This name is used for preparations of different composition.
Carter-Wallace, Austral.
Propylene glycol diacetate (p.1348·2).
Otitis externa.

Carter Horner, Canad.; Wilson, NZ; Wallace, USA.
Propylene glycol diacetate (p.1348·2); acetic acid (p.1571·3); benzethonium chloride (p.1134·2).
Otitis externa.

VoSoL HC
Carter Horner, Canad.; Wallace, USA.
Propylene glycol diacetate (p.1348·2); acetic acid (p.1571·3); benzethonium chloride (p.1134·2); hydrocortisone (p.1073·3).
Otitis externa.

Vostar Medis, Denm.
Diclofenac sodium (p.30·3).
Inflammation; musculoskeletal and joint disorders.

Votamed Medifive, Thai.
Diclofenac sodium (p.30·3).
Musculoskeletal and joint disorders.

Voxpax
Homeocan, Canad.; Lehning, Fr.
Homoeopathic preparation.

Voxsuprine Major, USA.
Isoxsuprine hydrochloride (p.1624·3).
Cerebrovascular and peripheral vascular disorders.

V-Pen
Orion, Fin.; Biochemie, Israel.
Phenoxymethylpenicillin (p.235·1) or phenoxymethylpenicillin potassium (p.235·1).
Bacterial infections.

VP-Tec Columbia, Mex.
Etoposide (p.538·1).
Small cell lung cancer; testicular cancer.

VR Curacel, Austral.
Dextran sulfate (p.1603·1); allantoin (p.1110·1); zinc oxide (p.1128·2); melaleuca oil (p.1631·3); alpha tocoferil acetate; vitamin A palmitate.
Herpes labialis; postherpetic neuralgia; tinea pruritus.

Vraap Inverni della Beffa, Ital.
Vincamine (p.1680·1).
Disorders of cerebral, ocular, and vestibular circulation.

Vridol Rafa, Israel.
Troxerutin (p.1611·2).
Haemorrhoids; venous insufficiency.

V-Tablopen Asta Medica, Ger.
Phenoxymethylpenicillin potassium (p.235·1).
Bacterial infections.

V-Talgin Vitamed, Israel.
Dipyrone (p.34·1).
Fever; pain.

V-Tears Vitamed, Israel.
Hyetellose (p.1501·1).
Dry eyes.

Vueffe
Baldacci, Braz.; Baldacci, Ital.
Peptides derived from the hydrolysis of bovine factor VIII (p.734·1).
Haemorrhage.

Vulcase Teofarma, Fr.
Aloes (p.1210·1).
Formerly contained sulfur, bile, belladonna, aloes, and liquorice.
Constipation.

Vulgix Cazi, Braz.
Tyrothricin (p.267·1); lactic acid (p.1626·2); lavender oil (p.1627·2); methylrosanilinium chloride (p.1150·3).
Vulvovaginal infections.

Vulnostimulin Dermapharm, Ger.
Wheat germ.
Burns; wounds.

Vulpuran Rosch & Handel, Aust.
Lead plaster-mass (p.1628·1); chamomile oil; hypericum oil (p.290·3); cod-liver oil (p.1357·2); elemi; colophony (p.1598·3); emplastrum minii; turpentine oil (p.1676·3); peru balsam (p.1650·2); oxycholesterin.
Furuncles; ulcers; wounds.

Vumon
Bristol-Myers Squibb, Aust.; Bristol-Myers Squibb, Austral.; Bristol-Myers Squibb, Belg.; Bristol-Myers Squibb, Braz.; Bristol, Canad.; Bristol-Myers Squibb, Denm.†; Bristol-Myers Squibb, Hong Kong; Bristol-

ers Squibb, Israel; Bristol-Myers Squibb, Ital.; Bristol-Myers Squibb, Mex.; Bristol-Myers Squibb, Neth.; Bristol-Myers Squibb, NZ; Bristol-Myers Squibb, S.Afr.; Bristol-Myers Squibb, Singapore; Bristol-Myers, Spain; Bristol-Myers Squibb, Swed.; Bristol-Myers Squibb Oncology, USA.
Teniposide (p.574·1).
Malignant neoplasms.

VVS Econo Med, USA†.
Sulfathiazole (p.257·1); sulfacetamide (p.250·3); sulfabenzamide (p.250·2).
Vaginitis due to Gardnerella vaginalis.

Vykmin
ICN, Hong Kong; Seven Seas, UK.
Multivitamin and mineral preparation (p.1350·1).

Vypen Douglas, NZ.
Pindolol (p.955·3).
Angina pectoris; hypertension.

Vysorel Novipharm, Ger.
Mistletoe (p.1636·2) from fir trees, apple trees or pine trees.
Malignant neoplasms.

Vytinal Legrand, Braz.
Multivitamin, amino-acid, and mineral preparation (p.1350·1).

Vytone Dermik, USA.
Hydrocortisone (p.1073·3); diiodohydroxyquinoline (p.590·2).

V-Zoline Vitamed, Israel.
Tetryzoline hydrochloride (p.1101·2).
Eye irritation.

W5 Aquamaid, UK.
Multivitamin and mineral preparation (p.1350·1).

Wakamoto Wakamoto, Hong Kong.
Aspergillus; Eremothecium ashbyii; lactobacteriaceae; dried yeast; diastase; protease; lipase; vitamin B substances; amino acids (p.1350·1).
Tonic.

Wake-Up Tablets Adrem, Canad.
Caffeine (p.761·3).
Stimulant.

Walekof MBD, Singapore.
Trimeprazine [alimemazine] tartrate (p.426·2); guaifenesin (p.1092·2); phenylpropanolamine hydrochloride (p.1098·1).
Cold symptoms; nasal and respiratory-tract congestion.

Walesolone MBD, Singapore.
Prednisolone (p.1077·3).
Corticosteroid.

Walsedyl MBD, Singapore.
Codeine phosphate (p.25·2); ephedrine hydrochloride (p.1090·1); promethazine hydrochloride (p.423·2).
Coughs; hay fever; hypersensitivity reactions; rhinitis.

Wampole Bronchial Cough Syrup Wampole, Canad.
Ammonium chloride (p.1085·2); aralia racemosa; poplar buds (p.1653·2); sanguinaria (p.1660·3); senega (p.1100·2); white pine; wild cherry (p.1680·3).

Wampole Vitamin Syrup Wampole, Canad.
Vitamin B substances with iron (p.1350·1).

Wandonorm Novartis, Ger.†.
Bopindolol malonate (p.850·3).
Hypertension.

Wanmycin DHA, Hong Kong.
Doxycycline hyclate (p.200·1).
Bacterial infections.

War Lin Grisi, Mex.
Lindane (p.1434·1).

Waran Nycomed, Swed.
Warfarin sodium (p.992·2).
Thromboembolic disorders.

Warca Pharmasant, Thai.
Mebendazole (p.102·2).
Worm infections.

Warfant Antigen, Irl.
Warfarin sodium clathrate (p.992·2).
Thromboembolic disorders.

Warfilone Merck Frosst, Canad.
Warfarin sodium (p.992·2).
Thromboembolic disorders.

WariActiv
Ritter, Ger.; Ritter, Hong Kong.
Ethyl chloride (p.1312·1).
Local anaesthesia.

Wari-Procomil
Ritter, Hong Kong; Ritter, Thai.
Yohimbine hydrochloride (p.1681·3); methyltestosterone (p.1482·3); testes extract (p.1492·1); kola (p.1681·1); lecithin (p.1628·1); muira puama.
Erectile dysfunction.

Warix Drossapharm, Switz.
Podophyllotoxin (p.1121·2).
Anogenital warts.

Warme-Gel Ratiopharm, Ger.
Glycol salicylate (p.42·2); benzyl nicotinate (p.20·2).
Musculoskeletal, joint, peri-articular and soft-tissue disorders; neuralgia; peripheral vascular disorders.

Warm-Up Pharmco, S.Afr.†.
Methyl salicylate (p.55·1); menthol (p.1632·3); eucalyptus oil (p.1609·2); turpentine oil (p.1676·3).
Muscular pain and stiffness.

Wart Remover
Cress, Canad.†; Stiefel, USA; Glades, USA; Rugby, USA.
Salicylic acid (p.1122·3).

Wartec
Wellcome, Austral.; Paladin, Canad.; Stiefel, Denm.; Verman, Fin.; Stiefel, Fr.; Stiefel, Ger.; Stiefel, Norw.; Aspen, S.Afr.; Fides Rottapharm, Spain; Sylak, Swed.
Podophyllotoxin (p.1121·2).
Anogenital warts.

Wartex Pickles, UK.
Salicylic acid (p.1122·3).
Warts.

Warticon
Stiefel, Irl.; Stiefel, UK.
Podophyllotoxin (p.1121·2).
Genital warts.

Wartner Passion for Life, UK.
Dimethyl ether (p.1199·1); propane (p.1200·3).
Verrucas; warts.

Wart-Off Pfizer, USA.
Salicylic acid (p.1122·3).
Warts.

Warz-ab Extor Ohropax, Switz.
Salicylic acid (p.1122·3); lactic acid (p.1626·2).
Calluses; corns; warts.

Warzen-Alldahin Roha, Ger.
Salicylic acid (p.1122·3); lactic acid (p.1626·2).
Calluses; warts.

Warzenmittel Sanova, Aust.
Monochloroacetic acid.
Warts.

Warzin Rosch & Handel, Aust.
Lactic acid (p.1626·2).
Warts.

Wash E45 Crookes Healthcare, UK.
Soap substitute.
Dry skin.

Wasp-Eze SSL, UK.
Ointment: Antazoline hydrochloride (p.408·3).
Topical spray: Mepyramine maleate (p.421·1); benzocaine (p.1306·2).
Insect bites; stings.

Wassertrat Sanus, Braz.
Sodium chloride; potassium chloride; sodium phosphate; magnesium citrate; sodium citrate; citric acid; calcium lactate (p.1185·2).
Diarrhoea; oral rehydration therapy.

Water Babies
Note. This name is used for preparations of different composition.
Schering-Plough, Canad.
SPF 15†: Octinoxate (p.1517·3); oxybenzone (p.1518·1).
SPF 30; SPF 45: Homosalate (p.1517·2); octinoxate (p.1517·3); oxybenzone (p.1518·1); octisalate (p.1518·1).
Sunscreen.

Schering-Plough, USA.
SPF 15: Octinoxate (p.1517·3); oxybenzone (p.1518·1).
SPF 30: Octinoxate (p.1517·3); oxybenzone (p.1518·1); homosalate (p.1517·2); octisalate (p.1518·1).
SPF 45: Octinoxate (p.1517·3); oxybenzone (p.1518·1); octocrilene (p.1518·1); octisalate (p.1518·1).
Sunscreen.

Water Babies Little Licks Schering-Plough, USA.
SPF 30: Octinoxate (p.1517·3); oxybenzone (p.1518·1); octisalate (p.1518·1).
Sunscreen.

Water Naturtabs Larkhall Laboratories, UK.
Bladderwrack (p.1585·2); lappa (p.1627·1); ground ivy (p.1618·2); clivers (p.1596·3).

Waterbabies UVGuard Schering-Plough, Canad.†.
SPF 15: Avobenzone (p.1517·1); octinoxate (p.1517·3); oxybenzone (p.1518·1).
SPF 30: Avobenzone (p.1517·1); octinoxate (p.1517·3); octisalate (p.1518·1); oxybenzone (p.1518·1).
Sunscreen.

Watershed Potter's, UK.
Oral mixture: Wild carrot (p.1680·3); pellitory; buchu (p.1587·2); juniper (p.1625·2); clivers (p.1596·3).
Tablets: Buchu (p.1587·2); parsley piert (p.1648·3); bearberry (p.1583·3); juniper oil (p.1625·2).
Water retention.

Waxsol
Norgine, Austral.; Norgine, Hong Kong; Norgine, Irl.; CSL, NZ; Norgine, NZ; Norgine, Singapore; Norgine, Thai.; Norgine, UK.
Docusate sodium (p.1223·1).
Ear wax removal.

Waxsol NF Norgine, S.Afr.
Docusate sodium (p.1223·1).
Ear wax removal.

Waxwane Thornton & Ross, UK.
Turpentine oil (p.1676·3); terpineol (p.1669·3); chloroxylenol (p.1142·1).
Ear wax removal.

4-Way Cold Tablets Bristol-Myers Products, USA†.
Paracetamol (p.71·2); phenylpropanolamine hydrochloride (p.1098·1); chlorpheniramine [chlorphenamine] maleate (p.412·1).
Upper respiratory-tract symptoms.

4-Way Fast Acting Bristol-Myers Products, USA.
Phenylephrine hydrochloride (p.1097·1); naphazoline hydrochloride (p.1095·1); mepyramine maleate (p.421·1).
Nasal congestion.

4-Way Long Lasting Bristol-Myers Products, USA.
Oxymetazoline hydrochloride (p.1096·2).
Nasal congestion.

Waycital Wayne, Mex.
Praziquantel (p.106·3).

Wayfrato Wayne, Mex.
Bezafibrate (p.849·1).

Waynazol Wayne, Mex.
Fluconazole (p.383·2).
Fungal infections.

Waysen Wayne, Mex.
Diltiazem (p.874·3).

Waysul Wayne, Mex.
Ceftriaxone (p.177·1).
Bacterial infections.

Waytifeno Wayne, Mex.
Ketotifen (p.767·2).

Waytrax Wayne, Mex.
Ceftazidime (p.174·3).
Bacterial infections.

WCS Dusting Powder Weleda, UK.
Arnica montana (p.1581·3); calendula (p.1589·2); echinacea angustifolia (p.1606·2); silica (p.1503·3); stibium met. praep.
Wounds.

Webber Antibiotic Cold Sore Ointment Novartis Consumer, Canad.†.
Polymyxin B sulfate (p.238·1); tyrothricin (p.267·1); camphor (p.1589·3); menthol (p.1632·3); benzocaine (p.1306·2).
Herpes labialis.

Webber E plus 3 Novartis Consumer, Canad.†.
Betacarotene, selenium, vitamin C, and vitamin E (p.1350·1).

Wechseltee Smetana, Aust.
Passion flower (p.1649·1); valerian (p.1678·3); lupulus (p.1629·3); hypericum (p.290·2); melissa (p.1632·2); crataegus (p.1600·2); mistletoe (p.1636·2).
Anxiety disorders; menopausal disorders; nervousness; sleep disorders.

Weh-less Hauck, USA†.
Phendimetrazine tartrate (p.1513·3).
Obesity.

Weiche Zinkpaste Lichtenstein, Ger.†.
Zinc oxide (p.1128·2).
Skin disorders; wounds.

Weifapenin Weifa, Norw.
Phenoxymethylpenicillin potassium (p.235·1).
Bacterial infections.

Weight Control Homeocan, Canad.
Homoeopathic preparation.

Weight Loss Aid Herbal Concepts, UK.
Taraxacum (p.1669·1); bladderwrack (p.1585·2); boldo (p.1585·3).
Slimming aid.

Weight Loss Kit Dolisos, Canad.
Homoeopathic preparation.

Weight Watchers Punto Dieterba, Ital.
Oral granules: Fructose (p.1363·3); sorbitol (p.1377·3); aspartame (p.1354·3).
Tablets: Aspartame (p.1354·3).
Sugar substitute.

Weightrol Vortech, USA†.
Phendimetrazine tartrate (p.1513·3).
Obesity.

Weimerquin Biokanol, Ger.
Chloroquine phosphate (p.432·3).
Malaria.

Weiscalina Valdecasas, Mex.
Phenylephrine (p.1097·1).
Nasal congestion.

Weisen-U Shigaken, Singapore.
Methiosulfonium chloride (p.1635·1); amylase (p.1579·3); aluminium hydroxide (p.1210·3).
Dyspepsia; flatulence; gastric hyperacidity; heartburn.

Welchol Sankyo, USA.
Colesevelam hydrochloride (p.863·3).
Hypercholesterolaemia.

Weleda Hamorrhoidalzapfchen Weleda, Ger.
Hamamelis (p.1618·3); aesculus (p.1574·1); stibium metall.
Anorectal disorders.

Weleda-Rheumasalbe M Weleda, Ger.
Basilicumkraut; camphor (p.1589·3); fluorit; castanospermum oil; venice turpentine; sea water (p.1196·1); murmeltierfett; rosemary oil (p.1659·3).
Frostbite; gout; musculoskeletal, joint, and soft-tissue disorders.

Wellbutrin
Glaxo Wellcome, Canad.; Glaxo Wellcome, Mex.; Glaxo Wellcome, USA.
Bupropion hydrochloride (p.280·1).
Depression.

Wellconal
Glaxo Wellcome, Hong Kong; Glaxo Wellcome, S.Afr.
Dipipanone hydrochloride (p.33·3); cyclizine hydrochloride (p.414·1).
Pain; vomiting.

Wellcoprim
Glaxo Wellcome, Aust.; Glaxo Wellcome, Belg.; Glaxo Wellcome, Fr.; Glaxo Wellcome, Neth.
Trimethoprim (p.264·2) or trimethoprim lactate (p.265·3).
Bacterial infections of the urinary tract.

The symbol † denotes a preparation no longer actively marketed

Wellcovorin *Glaxo Wellcome, USA.*
Calcium folinate (p.1363·1).
Megaloblastic anaemias; overdosage of folic acid antagonists.

Welldorm *Smith & Nephew Healthcare, UK.*
Cloral betaine (p.669·4) or cloral hydrate (p.669·3).
Formerly contained dichloralphenazone.
Insomnia.

Wellferon
Glaxo Wellcome, Aust.; Glaxo Wellcome, Braz.; Glaxo Wellcome, Canad.; Glaxo Wellcome, Fin.; Glaxo Wellcome, Hong Kong; Glaxo Wellcome, Israel; Glaxo Wellcome, Ital.; Glaxo Wellcome, Mex.; Glaxo Wellcome, NZ; Glaxo Wellcome, Singapore; Wellcome, Spain; Glaxo Wellcome, Swed.†; Wellcome, Switz.; Glaxo Wellcome, Thai.; Glaxo Wellcome, UK†; Glaxo Wellcome, USA.
Interferon alfa-n1 (p.628·1).
Anogenital warts; chronic active hepatitis; malignant neoplasms.

Wellman *Vitabiotics, UK.*
Multivitamin and mineral preparation (p.1350·1).

Wellvone
Glaxo Wellcome, Aust.; Glaxo Wellcome, Austral.; Glaxo Wellcome, Belg.; Glaxo Wellcome, Denm.; Glaxo Wellcome, Fr.; Glaxo Wellcome, Ger.; Glaxo Wellcome, Ital.; Glaxo Wellcome, Neth.; Glaxo Wellcome, S.Afr.; Glaxo Wellcome, Swed.; Wellcome, Switz.; Glaxo Wellcome, UK.
Atovaquone (p.588·3).
Pneumocystis carinii pneumonia.

Wellwoman *Potter's, UK.*
Herbal tea†: Tilia (p.1673·2); skullcap (p.1664·3); achillea (p.1572·3); bearberry (p.1583·3).
Tablets: Achillea (p.1572·2); motherwort (p.1637·3); tilia (p.1673·2); skullcap (p.1664·3); valerian (p.1678·3).
Tonic.

Weraplex Plain *Weimer, Hong Kong.*
Vitamin B substances (p.1350·1).
Vitamin B deficiency; vitamin B supplement.

Westcan Century plus MV & Mineral *Vita-Health, Hong Kong.*
Multivitamin and mineral preparation (p.1350·1).

Westcort
Westwood-Squibb, Canad.; Bristol-Myers Squibb, Mex.; Westwood-Squibb, USA.
Hydrocortisone valerate (p.1074·1).
Skin disorders.

Wet *Fidia, Ital.*
Electrolytes (p.1180·1).
Nasal irrigation.

White Cloverine *Medtech, USA.*
Barrier preparation.

Whitfield *Malaysia Chemist, Singapore.*
Salicylic acid (p.1122·3); benzoic acid (p.1134·2).
Fungal skin infections.

Whitfield Plus *Sam-On, Israel.*
Benzoic acid (p.1134·2); salicylic acid (p.1122·3); lignocaine [lidocaine] hydrochloride (p.1313·3).
Fungal skin infections.

Whitfields (Benzoic Acid Compound) Ointment *McGloin, Austral.*
Benzoic acid (p.1134·2); salicylic acid (p.1122·3).
Fungal skin infections.

Wibi
Galderma, Canad.; Healthpoint, USA.
Emollient.

Wibophorin *Pfluger, Ger.†.*
Homoeopathic preparation.

Wibotin H *Pfluger, Ger.†.*
Homoeopathic preparation.

Wicaran *Widmer, Fin.*
Tretinoin (p.1126·2); dexpanthenol (p.1602·3); urea (p.1127·3).
Skin disorders.

Wicarba *Widmer, Fin.*
Vitamin A palmitate (p.1383·2); dexpanthenol (p.1602·3); urea (p.1127·3).
Skin disorders.

Wick Daymed Erkaltungs *Wick, Ger.*
Capsules: Dextromethorphan hydrobromide (p.1087·3); paracetamol (p.71·2); phenylpropanolamine hydrochloride (p.1098·1).
Oral liquid: Paracetamol (p.71·2); guaifenesin (p.1092·2); phenylephrine hydrochloride (p.1097·1); ascorbic acid (p.1389·3).
Cold symptoms.

Wick Erkaltungs-Saft fur die Nacht *Procter & Gamble, Aust.*
Doxylamine succinate (p.417·1); ephedrine sulfate (p.1090·2); dextromethorphan hydrobromide (p.1087·3); paracetamol (p.71·2).
Cold symptoms.

Wick Formel 44 *Procter & Gamble, Aust.*
Dextromethorphan (p.1087·3).
Coughs.

Wick Formel 44 Husten-Loser *Wick, Ger.*
Guaifenesin (p.1092·2).
Coughs and associated respiratory-tract disorders.

Wick Formel 44 Husten-Stiller *Wick, Ger.*
Dextromethorphan hydrobromide (p.1087·3).
Coughs.

Wick Formel 44 Plus Hustenloser *Procter & Gamble, Aust.*
Guaifenesin (p.1092·2).
Catarrh; coughs.

Wick Formel 44 plus Husten-Pastillen S *Wick, Ger.*
Dextromethorphan (p.1087·3).
Catarrh; coughs.

Wick Formel 44 Plus Hustenstiller *Procter & Gamble, Aust.*
Dextromethorphan hydrobromide (p.1087·3).
Coughs.

Wick Hustensaft *Procter & Gamble, Aust.*
Dextromethorphan hydrobromide (p.1087·3); doxylamine succinate (p.417·1); sodium citrate (p.1186·2).
Coughs.

Wick Inhalierstift N *Wick, Ger.*
Menthol (p.1632·3); camphor (p.1589·3).
Nasal congestion.

Wick Kinder Formel 44 Husten-Loser *Wick, Ger.†.*
Guaifenesin (p.1092·2).
Catarrh; coughs.

Wick Kinder Formel 44 Husten-Stiller *Wick, Ger.†.*
Dextromethorphan hydrobromide (p.1087·3).
Coughs.

Wick Medinait *Wick, Ger.*
Doxylamine succinate (p.417·1); ephedrine sulfate (p.1090·2); dextromethorphan hydrobromide (p.1087·3); paracetamol (p.71·2).
Cold and influenza symptoms.

Wick Sinex
Note. This name is used for preparations of different composition.
Procter & Gamble, Aust.
Oxymetazoline hydrochloride (p.1096·2); menthol (p.1632·3); camphor (p.1589·3).
Cold symptoms.
Wick, Ger.
Oxymetazoline hydrochloride (p.1096·2).
Catarrh; nasal congestion.

Wick Sulagil *Wick, Ger.*
Lignocaine [lidocaine] (p.1313·2); dequalinium chloride (p.1143·1); cetylpyridinium chloride (p.1138·1).
Mouth and throat disorders.

Wick Vapo Sirup *Procter & Gamble, Aust.*
Menthol (p.1632·3).
Catarrh; coughs.

Wick Vaporub
Note. This name is used for preparations of different composition.
Procter & Gamble, Aust.
Menthol (p.1632·3); camphor (p.1589·3); eucalyptus oil (p.1609·2); nutmeg oil (p.1643·1); cedar wood oil; turpentine oil (p.1676·3); thymol (p.1158·3).
Catarrh; coughs and cold symptoms.
Wick, Ger.†.
Menthol (p.1632·3); camphor (p.1589·3); eucalyptol (p.1609·2); turpentine oil (p.1676·3).
Catarrh; cold symptoms; coughs.
Wick, Ger.
Ointment: Menthol (p.1632·3); camphor (p.1589·3); eucalyptus oil (p.1609·2); turpentine oil (p.1676·3).
Catarrh; cold symptoms; coughs.

Wick Vaposyrup *Wick, Ger.†.*
Menthol (p.1632·3).
Bronchitis; coughs.

Wicne *Widmer, Fin.*
Triclosan (p.1159·2); salicylic acid (p.1122·3); colloidal sulfur (p.1123·3); colloidal silica (p.1503·3).
Acne.

Wicnecarb *Widmer, Fin.*
Pyridoxine hydrochloride (p.1386·3); triclosan (p.1159·2); colloidal sulfur (p.1123·3); urea (p.1127·3).
Acne.

Wicnelact *Widmer, Fin.*
Triclosan (p.1159·2); zinc sulfate (p.1398·2); lactic acid (p.1626·2); magnesium sulfate (p.1191·1); salicylic acid (p.1122·3).
Acne; seborrhoea.

Wicnevit *Widmer, Fin.*
Vitamin A palmitate (p.1383·2); triclosan (p.1159·2); pyridoxine hydrochloride (p.1386·3); dexpanthenol (p.1602·3); urea (p.1127·3).
Acne; seborrhoea.

Wiedimmun *Wiedemann, Ger.*
Injection: Homoeopathic preparation.
Oral drops: Echinacea purpurea (p.1606·2).
Respiratory-tract infections.

Wifibrin *Willmar, Mex.*
Paracetamol (p.71·2).
Fever; pain.

Wigraine
Note. This name is used for preparations of different composition.
Organon, Canad.†.
Ergotamine tartrate (p.452·1); belladonna alkaloids (p.463·1); caffeine (p.761·3).
Migraine and other vascular headaches.
Organon, Canad.†.
Ergotamine tartrate (p.452·1); caffeine (p.761·3).
Vascular headache.

Willong
Will-Pharma, Belg.; Willpharma, Thai.
Glyceryl trinitrate (p.897·3).
Angina pectoris; heart failure.

Willospon
Will-Pharma, Ger.†; Will-Pharma, Neth.
Gelatin (p.737·2).
Haemorrhage.

Willospon Forte *Will-Pharma, Neth.*
Collagen (p.1598·2).
Haemostatic dressing.

Willowbark Plus Herbal Formula 11 *Vitelle, Austral.†.*
Skullcap (p.1664·3); devil's claw root (p.26·3); salix (p.82·1).
Headache.

Wilprafen *Yamanouchi, Ger.*
Josamycin (p.217·3) or josamycin propionate (p.217·3).
Bacterial infections.

Wilyfenicol *Tocogino, Mex.*
Chloramphenicol (p.179·1), chloramphenicol palmitate (p.179·2), or chloramphenicol sodium succinate (p.179·2).
Bacterial infections.

Winar *Lichtwer, Ger.*
Urtica root (p.1678·2).
Benign prostatic hyperplasia.

Winasma *Sanofi Synthelabo, Spain.*
Ephedrine sulfate (p.1090·2); phenobarbital (p.355·1); theophylline (p.777·2).
Obstructive airways disease.

Winasorb *Sanofi Winthrop, Mex.*
Paracetamol (p.71·2).
Fever; pain.

Wincef *Fujisawa, Jpn.*
Cefoselis sulfate (p.169·1).
Bacterial infections.

Wincoram
Sanofi Synthelabo, Ger.; Sanofi Synthelabo, Spain.
Amrinone (p.839·2) or amrinone lactate (p.839·2).
Heart failure.

Wind & Dyspepsia Relief *Herbal Concepts, UK.*
Ginger (p.1227·2); hydrastis (p.1621·1); myrrh (p.1639·2); rhubarb (p.1248·1); valerian (p.1678·3); taraxacum (p.1669·1).
Dyspepsia; flatulence.

Windol *Dermapharm, Ger.*
Bufexamac (p.20·3).
Inflammatory skin disorders.

Windol Basisbad *Dermapharm, Ger.*
Liquid paraffin (p.1407·1); soya oil (p.1378·1).
Bath additive; skin disorders.

Windtreibender Tee *Sanova, Aust.*
Fennel (p.1610·1); chamomile flower (p.1593·2); caraway (p.1591·2); achillea (p.1572·2); peppermint leaf (p.1243·2).
Flatulence.

Wink *Pharmco, S.Afr.†.*
Naphazoline nitrate (p.1095·1); phenylephrine hydrochloride (p.1097·1).
Eye irritation.

40 Winks *Roberts, USA.*
Diphenhydramine hydrochloride (p.416·1).
Insomnia.

Winlomylon *Adcock Ingram, S.Afr.*
Nalidixic acid (p.227·1).
Urinary-tract infections.

Winobanin *Sanofi Synthelabo, Ger.*
Danazol (p.1468·3).
Angioedema; benign breast disorders; endometriosis.

Winpain *Brunel, S.Afr.*
Paracetamol (p.71·2).
Fever; pain.

Winpred *ICN, Canad.*
Prednisone (p.1079·2).
Corticosteroid.

WinRho
Cangene, Canad.; Curex, Israel; CSL, NZ; Cangene, UK; Nabi, USA.
An anti-D immunoglobulin (p.1532·1).
Idiopathic thrombocytopenic purpura; prevention of rhesus sensitisation.

Winsprin *SmithKline Beecham Consumer, Austral.†.*
Aspirin (p.14·2).
Fever; pain.

Winstrol
Zambon, Spain; Sanofi Winthrop, USA.
Stanozolol (p.1491·3).
Anabolic; anaemia associated with renal insufficiency; female breast cancer; hereditary angioedema; osteoporosis.

Wintomilon *Sanofi Synthelabo, Port.*
Nalidixic acid (p.227·1).
Urinary-tract infections.

Wintomylon
Sanofi Winthrop, Braz.; Sanofi Winthrop, Hong Kong; Sanofi Winthrop, Mex.
Nalidixic acid (p.227·1).
Urinary-tract infections.

Winton *Sanofi Synthelabo, Spain.*
Aluminium hydroxide (p.1210·3); magnesium hydroxide (p.1233·3).
Dyspepsia; gastrointestinal hyperacidity.

Wintonin *Sanofi Winthrop, Ger.†.*
Gepefrine tartrate (p.897·3).
Orthostatic hypotension.

Wisamt *Procter & Gamble, Ger.*
Resorcinol (p.1122·2); sulfur (p.1123·3).
Acne.

Wisamt N *Procter & Gamble, Ger.*
Sulfur (p.1123·3); resorcinol (p.1122·2).
Acne.

Wismut comp *Ratiopharm, Ger.*
Bismuth subcarbonate (p.1213·1); anhydrous aluminium hydroxide (p.1210·3); dimethicone (p.1249·2); magnesium trisilicate gel (p.1233·3).
Gastrointestinal disorders.

Witch Doctor
Fleet, Austral.; De Witt, UK.
Hamamelis (p.1618·3).
Insect bites; skin irritation.

Witch Sunsore *De Witt, UK.*
Hamamelis (p.1618·3).
Sunburn.

Witromin *Pisa, Mex.*
Erythromycin (p.201·2).
Bacterial infections.

Witte Kruis *Asta Medica, Neth.*
Paracetamol (p.71·2); caffeine (p.761·3).
Fever; pain.

Wobe-Mugos *Mucos, Aust.*
Pancreatic proteolytic enzymes; calf thymus; pisum sativum; lens esculenta; papain (p.1647·3).
Adjunct to treatment of malignant neoplasms.

Wobe-Mugos E *Mucos, Ger.*
Trypsin (p.1675·3); chymotrypsin (p.1595·1); papain (p.1647·3).
Burns; malignant neoplasms, skin disorders; viral infections; wounds.

Wobe-Mugos Th *Mucos, Ger.*
Trypsin (p.1675·3); papain (p.1647·3); bovine thymus extract.
Malignant neoplasms; viral infections.

Wobenzimal *Vitafarma, Spain.*
Ointment: Papaya enzymes; lens sculenta enzymes; pisum sativum enzymes; pancreatin (p.1646·1); vitamin A (p.1382·1); thyme (p.1672·2); tocopherol (p.1394·1); vitamin F.
Inflammation; oedema.
Tablets: Papaya; lens sculenta; pisum sativum; pancreatin (p.1646·1); thyme (p.1672·2).
Inflammation; oedema; peripheral vascular disorders.

Wobenzym
Mucos, Aust.; Romsa, Mex.
Pancreatin (p.1646·1); bromelains (p.1586·3); papain (p.1647·3); lipase; amylase (p.1579·3); trypsin (p.1675·3); chymotrypsin (p.1595·1); rutoside (p.1611·2).
Musculoskeletal and joint inflammation; oedema.

Wobenzym N *Mucos, Ger.*
Ointment: Bromelains (p.1586·3); trypsin (p.1675·3).
Inflammation; oedema.
Tablets: Pancreatin (p.1646·1); bromelains (p.1586·3); papain (p.1647·3); protease; trypsin (p.1675·3); chymotrypsin (p.1595·1); rutoside (p.1611·2).
Inflammation; thrombophlebitis; thrombosis.

Wolff Basis *Wolff, Ger.*
Emollient.
Pharmaceutical diluent; skin disorders.

Woloderma
Adroka, Switz.
Soap substitute.
Skin disorders.
Adroka, Switz.
Topical lotion: Sodium lactate (p.1186·2); almond oil (p.1576·3).
Skin disorders.

Woman Formula *Avon, Canad.*
Multivitamin and mineral preparation (p.1350·1).

Woman Kind *Windsor, UK.*
Pyridoxine (p.1387·1).
Premenstrual syndrome.

Womens Change Formula *General Nutrition, Canad.*
Multivitamin and mineral preparation (p.1350·1).

Women's Daily Formula *Kavon, USA†.*
Multivitamin and mineral preparation with iron and folic acid (p.1350·1).

Women's Formula Herbal Formula 3 *Vitelle, Austral.*
Angelica (p.1580·2); cimicifuga (p.1595·2); blue cohosh (p.1585·3); pulsatilla (p.1656·3); agnus castus (p.1574·2).
Menstrual disorders.

Womens Support *General Nutrition, Canad.*
Multivitamin and mineral preparation (p.1350·1).

Womens Tylenol Multi-Symptom Menstrual Relief *McNeil Consumer, USA.*
Paracetamol (p.71·2); pamabrom (p.952·1).

Wonder Ice *Pedinol, USA.*
Menthol (p.1632·3).
Muscle, joint, and soft-tissue pain; neuralgia.

Wondergel *Lake, USA.*
Vaginal lubricant.

Wondra *Richardson-Vicks, USA.*
Emollient and moisturiser.

Woodwards Baby Chest Rub *SSL, UK.*
Menthol (p.1632·3); eucalyptus oil (p.1609·2); turpentine oil (p.1676·3).
Nasal congestion and catarrh.

Woodwards Colic Drops *SSL, UK.*
Simeticone (p.1249·2).
Colic; wind pain.

Woodwards Gripe Water
Pharmacare, Canad.; LRC, Israel; SSL, UK.
Terpeneless dill seed oil (p.1603·3); sodium bicarbonate (p.1186·2).
Wind in infants.

Woodwards Nappy Rash Ointment *Seton, UK†.*
Zinc oxide (p.1128·2); cod-liver oil (p.1357·2).
Nappy rash.

Woodwards Teething Gel *SSL, UK.*
Lignocaine [lidocaine] hydrochloride (p.1313·2); cetylpyridinium chloride (p.1138·1).
Teething.

Worm *De Witt, UK.*
Piperazine citrate (p.105·3).
Worm infections.

Wormelix *Noristan, S.Afr.†.*
Piperazine citrate (p.105·3).
Ascariasis; enterobiasis.

Wormex *Sussex, UK.*
Piperazine citrate (p.105·3).
Worm infections.

Wormgo *Aspen Consumer, S.Afr.*
Mebendazole (p.102·2).
Worm infections.

Wormstop *Be-Tabs, S.Afr.*
Mebendazole (p.102·2).
Worm infections.

Wound-A-Sept *Beige, S.Afr.*
Cetrimide (p.1137·1).
Minor wounds and burns.

Wright's Vaporizing Fluid *LRC Products, UK.*
Chlorocresol (p.1141·3).
Cold symptoms; coughs.

Wrinkle Defence *Sunspot, Austral.*
SPF 15+: Oxybenzone (p.1518·1); octinoxate (p.1517·3) in a moisturising base.
Emollient; sunscreen.

W-Tropfen *Hofmann & Sommer, Ger.*
Salicylic acid (p.1122·3); lactic acid (p.1626·2).
Calluses; corns.

Wund- und Brand-Gel Eu Rho *Eu Rho, Ger.*
Lignocaine [lidocaine] hydrochloride (p.1313·2); allantoin (p.1110·1); cetylpyridinium chloride (p.1138·1); dexpanthenol (p.1602·3).
Burns; wounds.

Wund- und Heilsalbe N *LAW, Ger.*
Dexpanthenol (p.1602·3).
Skin disorders.

Wundesin *Gebro, Aust.*
Povidone-iodine (p.1155·1).
Wounds.

Wyamine *Wyeth-Ayerst, USA.*
Mephentermine sulfate (p.926·2).
Hypotension; shock.

Wyanoids *Wyeth-Ayerst, USA†.*
Ephedrine sulfate (p.1090·2); belladonna extract (p.463·1); boric acid (p.1586·1); zinc oxide (p.1128·2); bismuth oxyiodide (p.1214·1); bismuth subcarbonate (p.1213·1); peru balsam (p.1650·2).
Anorectal disorders.

Wyanoids Relief Factor *Wyeth-Ayerst, USA.*
Live yeast cell derivative (p.1398·1); shark-liver oil.
Haemorrhoids.

Wycillin *Wyeth-Ayerst, USA.*
Procaine penicillin [procaine benzylpenicillin] (p.239·2).
Bacterial infections.

Wycillin R *Wyeth, Braz.*
Procaine penicillin [procaine benzylpenicillin] (p.239·2); benzylpenicillin potassium (p.157·1).
Bacterial infections.

Wycillina *Pharmacia Upjohn, Ital.*
Benzathine benzylpenicillin (p.156·2).
Bacterial infections.

Wydase
Wyeth-Ayerst, Canad.; Wyeth-Ayerst, USA.
Hyaluronidase (p.1620·3).
Adjunct in subcutaneous urography; adjuvant to increase the absorption and dispersion of drugs; hypodermoclysis.

Wydora *Wyeth, Ger.*
Indoramin hydrochloride (p.913·3).
Hypertension.

Wygesic *Wyeth-Ayerst, USA.*
Dextropropoxyphene hydrochloride (p.27·1); paracetamol (p.71·2).
Fever; pain.

Wylaxine *Whitehall, Belg.†.*
Bisoxatin acetate (p.1214·2).
Bowel evacuation; constipation.

Wymox *Wyeth-Ayerst, USA.*
Amoxicillin trihydrate (p.149·2).
Bacterial infections.

Wypresin *Wyeth Lederle, Aust.*
Indoramin hydrochloride (p.913·3).
Hypertension.

Wysoy *Wyeth, Irl.; Wyeth, UK.*
Lactose-free food for special diets (p.1350·1).
Cows' milk or lactose intolerance; galactokinase deficiency; galactosaemia.

Wytens *Wyeth Lederle, Fr.*
Bisoprolol fumarate (p.850·1); hydrochlorothiazide (p.907·3).
Hypertension.

Wytensin *Wyeth Lederle, Aust.; Wyeth-Ayerst, USA.*
Guanabenz acetate (p.900·2).
Hypertension.

The symbol † denotes a preparation no longer actively marketed

X-2 *Investigaciones Filosoficas y Cientificas, Mex.*
Cocarboxylase (p.1385·2).
Thiamine deficiency.

Xacin *Pharmasant, Thai.*
Norfloxacin (p.232·1).
Bacterial infections.

X-Adene *GNR, Fr.†.*
Procaine hydrochloride (p.1319·1); vitamin B substances (p.1350·1); polymerised sodium deoxyribonucleate.
Tonic.

Xaken *Kener, Mex.*
Methotrexate (p.553·2).

Xal
Wolfs, Belg.†; Pharmadevelopppement, Fr.
Potassium chloride; ammonium chloride; calcium formate; glutamic acid (p.1180·1).
Dietary salt substitute.

Xalacom *Pharmacia, UK.*
Latanoprost (p.1445·3); timolol maleate (p.982·1).
Glaucoma; ocular hypertension.

Xalatan
Pharmacia Upjohn, Aust.; Pharmacia Upjohn, Austral.; Pharmacia Upjohn, Belg.; Pharmacia Upjohn, Canad.; Pharmacia Upjohn, Denm.; Pharmacia Upjohn, Fin.; Pharmacia Upjohn, Fr.; Pharmacia Upjohn, Ger.; Pharmacia Upjohn, Hong Kong; Pharmacia Upjohn, Irl.; Pharmacia Upjohn, Israel; Pharmacia Upjohn, Ital.; Pharmacia Upjohn, Mex.; Pharmacia Upjohn, Neth.; Pharmacia Upjohn, Norw.; Pharmacia Upjohn, NZ; Pharmacia Upjohn, Port.; Pharmacia Upjohn, S.Afr.; Pharmacia Upjohn, Singapore; Pharmacia Upjohn, Spain; Pharmacia Upjohn, Swed.; Pharmacia Upjohn, Switz.; Pharmacia Upjohn, Thai.; Pharmacia Upjohn, UK; Pharmacia Upjohn, USA.
Latanoprost (p.1445·3).
Glaucoma; ocular hypertension.

Xalazin *Caber, Ital.*
Mesalazine (p.1234·1).
Inflammatory bowel disease.

Xalyn-Or *Atlantis, Mex.*
Amoxicillin trihydrate (p.149·2).
Bacterial infections.

Xamamina *Bracco, Ital.*
Dimenhydrinate (p.415·2).
Motion sickness.

Xanagis *Agis, Israel.*
Alprazolam (p.654·2).
Anxiety; mixed anxiety depressive states; panic disorders.

Xanalin *Silom, Thai.*
Neomycin sulfate (p.228·1); polymyxin B (p.238·3); gramicidin (p.213·3).
Bacterial eye infections.

Xanax
Pharmacia Upjohn, Austral.; Pharmacia Upjohn, Belg.; Pharmacia Upjohn, Canad.; Pharmacia Upjohn, Fr.; Pharmacia Upjohn, Ger.; Pharmacia Upjohn, Hong Kong; Pharmacia Upjohn, Irl.; Pharmacia Upjohn, Israel; Pharmacia Upjohn, Ital.; Pharmacia Upjohn, Neth.; Pharmacia Upjohn, NZ; Pharmacia Upjohn, Port.; Pharmacia Upjohn, Singapore; Pharmacia Upjohn, Switz.; Pharmacia Upjohn, Thai.; Pharmacia, UK; Pharmacia Upjohn, USA.
Alprazolam (p.654·2).
Alcohol withdrawal syndrome; anxiety disorders; mixed anxiety depressive states; panic disorder.

Xanbon *Kissei, Jpn.*
Ozagrel sodium (p.1645·3).
Cerebral thrombosis; cerebral vasospasm.

Xanef *Merck Sharp & Dohme, Ger.*
Enalapril maleate (p.883·3) or enalaprilat (p.884·1).
Heart failure; hypertension.

Xanidine *Berlin Pharm, Thai.*
Ranitidine hydrochloride (p.1245·2).
Gastro-oesophageal reflux; peptic ulcer; Zollinger-Ellison syndrome.

Xanol *Pharmasant, Thai.*
Allopurinol (p.397·2).
Gout; hyperuricaemia; renal calculi.

Xanolam *Aspen, S.Afr.*
Alprazolam (p.654·2).
Anxiety disorders; mixed anxiety depressive states; panic attacks.

Xanomel *Clonmel, Irl.*
Ranitidine hydrochloride (p.1245·2).
Gastric hyperacidity; gastro-oesophageal reflux; peptic ulcer; Zollinger-Ellison syndrome.

Xanor
Pharmacia Upjohn, Aust.; Pharmacia Upjohn, Fin.; Pharmacia Upjohn, Norw.; Pharmacia Upjohn, S.Afr.; Pharmacia Upjohn, Swed.
Alprazolam (p.654·2).
Anxiety disorders; mixed anxiety depressive states; panic attacks.

Xantervit *SIFI, Ital.*
Xanthopterin; multivitamins (p.1350·1).
Ocular trauma and lesions.

Xantervit Antibiotico *SIFI, Ital.*
Xanthopterin; chloramphenicol (p.179·1); multivitamins (p.1350·1).
Ocular trauma and lesions.

Xantervit Eparina *SIFI, Ital.*
Xanthopterin; heparin sodium (p.902·1); multivitamins (p.1350·1).
Ocular burns.

Xanthium
SMB, Belg.; Galephar, Fr.; SMB, Thai.
Theophylline (p.777·2).
Obstructive airways disease.

Xanthomax *Ashbourne, UK.*
Allopurinol (p.397·2).

Xantina B12 *Prodotti, Braz.*
Methionine (p.1012·2); inositol (p.1623·3); choline (p.1356·3); vitamins (p.1350·1); manganese (p.1371·3); liver extract; gastric mucosa extract.
Liver disorders.

Xantinon B12 *Byk, Braz.*
Methionine (p.1012·2); hydroxocobalamin (p.1388·1); lipocaicic acid; inositol (p.1623·3); choline chloride (p.1356·3); manganese sulfate (p.1371·3); liver extract; gastric mucosa extract.
Liver disorders.

Xantinon Complex *Byk, Braz.*
Acetylmethionine; inositol (p.1623·3); choline citrate (p.1356·3); betaine hydrochloride (p.1584·3); cyanocobalamin (p.1388·1); pyridoxine hydrochloride (p.1386·3).
Liver disorders.

Xantium *Wyeth Lederle, Ital.*
Protirelin tartrate (p.1296·1).
Neurological deficit.

Xantivent *Essex, Switz.*
Theophylline (p.777·2).
Bronchospasm.

Xanturenasi *Teofarma, Ital.*
Pyridoxine hydrochloride (p.1386·3).

Xapro *Jenapharm, Ger.*
Estriol (p.1475·3).
Vulvovaginal disorders.

Xarator *Parke, Davis, Ital.*
Atorvastatin calcium (p.842·3).
Hyperlipidaemias.

Xarope Antigripal *Basi, Port.*
Codeine (p.25·2); ethylmorphine (p.35·2); sulfogaiacol (p.1101·1).
Coughs.

Xarope de Caraguata + Bromoformio *Sanval, Braz.*
Annona muricata; bromoform (p.1587·1); sodium benzoate (p.1134·3); aconite (p.1572·3); belladonna (p.463·1); grindelia (p.1618·2).
Coughs.

Xarope de Iodeto de Potassio Composto
Note. This name is used for preparations of different composition.
Kopkins, Braz.
Potassium iodide (p.1522·3); lobelia (p.1510·2).
Respiratory-tract congestion.

Laborsil, Braz.
Potassium iodide (p.1522·3); sodium citrate (p.1186·2); carbinoxamine maleate (p.411·1).
Respiratory-tract congestion.

Xarope de Limao Bravo
Note. This name is used for preparations of different composition.
Teuto, Braz.
Sulfogaiacol (p.1101·1); sodium benzoate (p.1134·3); grindelia (p.1618·2); siparuna guyanensis.
Respiratory-tract congestion.

Veafarm, Braz.
Siparuna guyanensis; guaifenesin (p.1092·2); sodium benzoate (p.1134·3).
Respiratory-tract congestion.

Xarope de Lobelia Composto *Drogasil, Braz.*
Sulfogaiacol (p.1101·1); guaifenesin (p.1092·2); lobelia (p.1510·2).
Respiratory-tract congestion.

Xarope de Macas Rainetas *Medical, Port.*
Senna (p.1248·2); mannitol (p.924·3); apple pulp.
Constipation.

Xarope Grindelia de Oliveira Junior *Vitex, Braz.*
Ipecacuanha (p.1093·1); grindelia (p.1618·2).
Respiratory-tract congestion.

Xarope Peitoral de Ameixa Composto *Simoes, Braz.*
Sodium benzoate (p.1134·3); bromoform (p.1587·1); prune (p.1245·1).
Coughs.

Xarope Sao Joao *Uniao Quimica, Braz.*
Bromoform (p.1587·1); sodium benzoate (p.1134·3).
Coughs.

Xarope Valda *Canonne, Braz.*
Cetylpyridinium chloride (p.1138·1); ammonium chloride (p.1085·2); sodium citrate (p.1186·2); sodium benzoate (p.1134·3).
Respiratory-tract congestion.

Xarope Vick *Procter & Gamble, Braz.*
Cetylpyridinium chloride (p.1138·1); sodium citrate (p.1186·2).
Respiratory-tract congestion.

Xaten *Biotherapie, Fr.*
Atenolol (p.841·3).
Angina pectoris; hypertension.

Xatral
Sanofi Synthelabo, Aust.; Sanofi Synthelabo, Belg.; Synthelabo, Braz.; Sanofi Winthrop, Denm.; Leiras Synthelabo, Fin.; Sanofi Synthelabo, Fr.; Synthelabo, Hong Kong; Sanofi Synthelabo, Irl.; Synthelabo, Israel; Sanofi Synthelabo, Ital.; Sanofi Synthelabo, Neth.; Sanofi Winthrop, Norw.; Sanofi Synthelabo, Singapore; Astra, Swed.; Synthelabo, Switz.; Sanofi Synthelabo, Thai.; Sanofi Synthelabo, UK.
Alfuzosin hydrochloride (p.833·2).
Benign prostatic hyperplasia.

Xefo
Nycomed, Aust.; Nycomed, Denm.; Nycomed, Fin.; Searle, S.Afr.; Nycomed, Swed.; Hafslund Nycomed, Thai.; CeNeS, UK.
Lornoxicam (p.50·2).
Inflammation; musculoskeletal and joint disorders; pain.

Xeloda
Roche, Austral.; Roche, Canad.; Roche, NZ; Roche, S.Afr.; Singapore; Roche, Switz.; Roche, Thai.; Roche, UK; Roche, USA.
Capecitabine (p.514·2).
Breast cancer; colorectal cancer.

Xenalon *Mepha, Switz.*
Spironolactone (p.973·2).
Hyperaldosteronism; hypertension; nephrotic syndrome; oedema.

Xenar *Wassermann, Ital.*
Naproxen (p.60·3).
Musculoskeletal, joint, peri-articular, and soft-tissue disorders; neuralgia.

Xenazine *Cambridge, UK.*
Tetrabenazine (p.1669·3).
Movement disorders.

Xenetix
Guerbet, Aust.; Codali, Belg.; Guerbet, Denm.; Guerbet, Fin.; Guerbet, Fr.; Guerbet, Ger.; Guerbet, Israel; Guerbet, Ital.; Guerbet, Neth.†; Guerbet, Norw.; Guerbet, Port.; Guerbet, Spain; Gothia, Swed.; Guerbet, Switz.
Iobitridol (p.1033·3).
Radiographic contrast medium.

Xenical
Roche, Aust.; Roche, Austral.; Roche, Belg.; Roche, Canad.; Roche, Denm.; Roche, Fin.; Roche, Fr.; Roche, Ger.; Roche, Irl.; Roche, Ital.; Roche, Mex.; Roche, Neth.; Roche, NZ; Roche, Port.; Roche, S.Afr.; Roche, Singapore; Roche, Spain; Roche, Swed.; Roche, Switz.; Roche, Thai.; Roche, UK; Roche, USA.
Orlistat (p.1644·3).
Obesity.

Xenid *Biogalenique, Fr.*
Diclofenac epolamine (p.31·3) or diclofenac sodium (p.30·3).
Dysmenorrhoea; musculoskeletal, joint, and peri-articular disorders; renal colic.

Xenopan *Mundipharma, Aust.†.*
Naproxen (p.60·3).
Gout; inflammation; musculoskeletal, joint, and peri-articular disorders; pain.

Xenovate *Aspen, S.Afr.*
Clobetasol propionate (p.1065·2).
Skin disorders.

Xepagan *Xepa-Soul Pattinson, Singapore.*
Promethazine hydrochloride (p.423·2).
Hypersensitivity reactions; sedative.

Xepamet *Xepa-Soul Pattinson, Singapore.*
Cimetidine (p.1216·3).
Acid aspiration; adjunct in pancreatic insufficiency; dyspepsia; gastro-oesophageal reflux; peptic ulcer; Zollinger-Ellison syndrome.

Xepanicol
Xepa-Soul Pattinson, Hong Kong; Xepa-Soul Pattinson, Singapore.
Chloramphenicol (p.179·1).
Bacterial eye infections.

Xepasone *Xepa-Soul Pattinson, Singapore.*
Prednisolone (p.1077·3).
Corticosteroid.

Xepin
Bioglan, Irl.; Bioglan, UK.
Doxepin hydrochloride (p.283·3).
Pruritus.

Xerac AC *Person & Covey, USA.*
Aluminium chloride (p.1110·2); alcohol (p.1130·3).
Antiperspirant.

Xeracil *Xerogen, S.Afr.†.*
Amoxicillin (p.149·2).
Bacterial infections.

Xeramax *Xerogen, S.Afr.*
Syrup: Paracetamol (p.71·2); codeine phosphate (p.25·2); promethazine hydrochloride (p.423·2).
Fever; pain.
Tablets: Paracetamol (p.71·2); codeine phosphate (p.25·2); caffeine (p.761·3); meprobamate (p.691·1).
Pain with tension.

Xeramel *Xerogen, S.Afr.*
Erythromycin estolate (p.201·2).
Bacterial infections.

Xerand *Roche-Posay, Irl.*
Emollient.
Dry skin; skin irritation.

Xeraspor *Xerogen, S.Afr.*
Clotrimazole (p.382·1).
Fungal skin infections; vulvovaginal candidiasis.

Xerazole *Xerogen, S.Afr.*
Co-trimoxazole (p.193·3).
Bacterial infections.

Xerenal *Kwizda, Aust.*
Dothiepin [dosulepin] hydrochloride (p.283·2).
Depression.

Xerial *SVR, Ital.*
Urea (p.1127·3); allantoin (p.1110·1); emollients.
Dry skin.

Xerodent
Alpharma, Fin.; Dumex-Alpharma, Swed.
Sodium fluoride (p.1375·3); malic acid (p.1631·1).
Dental caries prophylaxis; dry mouth.

Xeroderm *Dermol, USA.*
Emollient.

Xerogesic *Crown, S.Afr.*
Paracetamol (p.71·2); codeine phosphate (p.25·2); caffeine (p.761·3); meprobamate (p.691·1).
Pain and associated tension.

Xeroil *Roche-Posay, Irl.*
Emollient.
Dry skin.

Xeroprim *Crown, S.Afr.*
Co-trimoxazole (p.193·3).
Bacterial infections.

Xerotens *Covan, S.Afr.*
Doxylamine succinate (p.417·1); paracetamol (p.71·2);
codeine phosphate (p.25·2); caffeine (p.761·3).
Pain and associated tension.

Xerumenex
Asta Medica, Belg.; Asta Medica, Neth.
Trolamine polypeptide oleate-condensate (p.1675·2).
*Cleansing of external ear before otoscopy; removal of
impacted ear wax.*

Xflu
SmithKline Beecham, Austral.; SmithKline Beecham, S.Afr.
An influenza vaccine (p.1544·3).
Active immunisation.

Xibornol Prodes *Almirall, Spain.*
Oral suspension: Bromhexine hydrochloride
(p.1085·3); clofedanol hydrochloride (p.1087·1); xibornol (p.270·1).
Suppositories: Camphor (p.1589·3); niaouli oil
(p.1640·2); xibornol (p.270·1).
Respiratory-tract disorders.

Xicam *Pharmasant, Thai.*
Piroxicam (p.79·1).
Gout; musculoskeletal and joint disorders.

Xicil *Rottapharm, Spain.*
Glucosamine sulfate (p.1616·2).
Rheumatic disorders.

Xidanef *Codal Synto, Thai.*
Ketotifen fumarate (p.767·2).
Asthma; hypersensitivity reactions.

Xiemed *Medifive, Thai.*
Alprazolam (p.654·2).
Anxiety; mixed anxiety depressive states.

Xigris *Lilly, USA.*
Drotrecogin alfa (activated) (p.741·2).
Sepsis.

Xillin *Laser, S.Afr.†.*
Amoxicillin trihydrate (p.149·2).
Bacterial infections.

Xilodase *Apsen, Braz.*
Neomycin sulfate (p.228·1); lignocaine [lidocaine]
(p.1313·2); hyaluronidase (p.1620·3).
Infected skin disorders.

Xilo-Mynol *Molteni, Ital.*
Lignocaine [lidocaine] hydrochloride (p.1313·2).
Adrenaline [epinephrine] acid tartrate (p.829·2) is included in some injections as a vasoconstrictor to diminish absorption and localise the effect of the local
anaesthetic.
Local anaesthesia.

Xilonibsa
Note.This name is used for preparations of different composition.
Inibsa, Port.
Injection; topical spray: Lignocaine [lidocaine] hydro-
chloride (p.1313·2).
Adrenaline [epinephrine] (p.829·1) or noradrenaline
[norepinephrine] (p.948·2) is included in the injection
as a vasoconstrictor to diminish absorption and localise
the effect of the local anaesthetic.
Topical paste: Lignocaine [lidocaine] (p.1313·2); ame-
thocaine [tetracaine] (p.1305·2).
Local anaesthesia.
Inibsa, Spain.
Lignocaine [lidocaine] (p.1313·2) or lignocaine [lido-
caine] hydrochloride (p.1313·2).
Adrenaline [epinephrine] acid tartrate (p.829·2) is included in the injection as a vasoconstrictor to diminish
absorption and localise the effect of the local anaesthetic.
Local anaesthesia.

Ximovan *Rhone-Poulenc Rorer, Ger.*
Zopiclone (p.713·1).
Insomnia.

Xiprocan *Protein, Mex.*
Amoxicillin (p.149·2).
Bacterial infections.

Xiral *Pharmavene, USA.*
Chlorpheniramine [chlorphenamine] maleate
(p.412·1); pseudoephedrine hydrochloride (p.1099·2);
hyoscine methonitrate (p.468·2).
Allergic rhinitis; cold symptoms; sinusitis.

Xismox *Crom, Mex.*
Isosorbide mononitrate (p.916·2).

xitix *Woelm, Ger.*
Ascorbic acid (p.1389·3); sodium ascorbate
(p.1390·1).
Vitamin C deficiency.

Xitocin *Cryopharma, Mex.*
Oxytocin (p.1294·1).
*Labour induction; postpartum haemorrhage; uterine
atony.*

XMET Analog
Scientific Hospital Supplies, Austral.; Scientific Hospital Supplies, Irl.
Food for special diets (p.1350·1).
Formerly known as Analog RVHB in *Irl.*
Homocystinuria; hypermethioninaemia.

XMET Maxamaid
Scientific Hospital Supplies, Austral.; Scientific Hospital Supplies, Irl.
Food for special diets (p.1350·1).
Formerly known as Maxamaid RVHB in *Irl.*
Homocystinuria; hypermethioninaemia.

XMET Maxamum
Scientific Hospital Supplies, Austral.; Scientific Hospital Supplies, Irl.
Food for special diets (p.1350·1).
Homocystinuria.

Xmet Maximum *Nutricia, NZ; Scientific Hospital Supplies, NZ.*
Food for special diets (p.1350·1).
Homocystinuria; hypermethioninaemia.

XMTVI Analog *Scientific Hospital Supplies, Austral.*
Infant feed (p.1350·1).
Formerly known as Xmet, Thre, Val, Isoleu Analog.
Methylmalonic acidaemia; propionic acidaemia.

XMTVI Maxamaid *Scientific Hospital Supplies, Austral.*
Food for special diets (p.1350·1).
*Methylmalonic acidaemia or propionic acidaemia in
children.*

XMTVI Maxamum *Scientific Hospital Supplies, Austral.*
Food for special diets (p.1350·1).
Formerly known as XMet, Thre, Val, Isoleu Maxam-
um.
Methylmalonic acidaemia; propionic acidaemia.

Xolaam *Biogalenique, Fr.*
Aluminium hydroxide (p.1210·3); magnesium hydrox-
ide (p.1233·1).
Gastrointestinal disorders.

Xonatil *Precimex, Mex.*
Ceftriaxone (p.177·1).
Bacterial infections.

Xopenex *Sepracor, USA.*
Levosalbutamol hydrochloride (p.767·3).
Obstructive airways disease.

Xorox *Kwizda, Aust.*
Aciclovir (p.612·3).
*Cytomegalovirus infections; herpes simples infections;
varicella-zoster infections.*

Xorpic *Andromaco, Port.; Grunenthal, Port.*
Ciprofloxacin hydrochloride (p.182·3).
Bacterial infections.

XP Analog
*Scientific Hospital Supplies, Austral.; Nutricia, NZ; Scientific Hospital
Supplies, NZ.*
Food for special diets (p.1350·1).
Phenylketonuria.

XP Maxamaid
Scientific Hospital Supplies, Austral.; Scientific Hospital Supplies, Irl.
Food for special diets (p.1350·1).
Phenylketonuria.

XP Maxamum
Scientific Hospital Supplies, Austral.; Scientific Hospital Supplies, Irl.
Food for special diets (p.1350·1).
Phenylketonuria.

Xphen, Tyr Analog *Scientific Hospital Supplies, Austral.*
Food for special diets (p.1350·1).
Tyrosinaemia.

Xphen, Tyr Maxamaid *Scientific Hospital Supplies, Aus-
tral.*
Food for special diets (p.1350·1).
Tyrosinaemia.

X-Praep *Asta Medica, Neth.*
Sennosides (p.1248·3).
Bowel evacuation; constipation.

X-Prep
*Mundipharma, Aust.; Mundipharma, Ger.; Asta Medica, Ital.; Ny-
comed, Norw.; Mundipharma, Switz.; Gray, USA.*
Senna (p.1248·2).
Bowel evacuation.
*Purdue Frederick, Canad.; Asta Medica, Fr.; Rafa, Israel; Asta Medi-
ca, Port.; Adcock Ingram, S.Afr.; Asta Medica, Spain.*
Sennosides A and B (p.1248·3).
Bowel evacuation.

X-Prep Bowel Evacuant Kit-1 *Gray, USA.*
Combination pack: 2 tablets, standardised senna concentrate (p.1248·2); docusate sodium (p.1223·1) (Senokot-S); oral liquid, senna (X-Prep); 1 suppository,
bisacodyl (Rectolax) (p.1212·2).

X-Prep Bowel Evacuant Kit-2 *Gray, USA.*
Combination pack: 1 dose oral granules, effervescent
citrate/magnesium sulfate (Citralax) (p.1186·2)
(p.1191·1); oral liquid, senna (X-Prep) (p.1248·2); 1
suppository, bisacodyl (Rectolax) (p.1212·2).
Bowel evacuation.

XPT Tyrosidon *Scientific Hospital Supplies, UK.*
Tyrosine- and phenylalanine-free amino-acid prepara-
tion (p.1350·1).
Tyrosinaemia.

XPTM Tyrosidon *Scientific Hospital Supplies, UK.*
Phenylalanine-, tyrosine-, and methionine-free amino-
acid preparation (p.1350·1).
Tyrosinaemia.

XPTM Tyrosion *Scientific Hospital Supplies, Austral.*
Food for special diets (p.1350·1).
Tyrosinaemia.

X-Seb
Baker Cummins, Canad.; Baker Cummins, USA.
Salicylic acid (p.1122·3).
Seborrhoea.

X-Seb Plus
Baker Cummins, Canad.; Baker Cummins, USA.
Pyrithione zinc (p.1122·1); salicylic acid (p.1122·3).
Scalp disorders.

X-Seb T
Baker Cummins, Canad.; Baker Cummins, USA.
Salicylic acid (p.1122·3); coal tar (p.1125·1).
Seborrhoea.

X-Seb T Plus
Baker Cummins, Canad.; Baker Cummins, USA.
Salicylic acid (p.1122·3); coal tar (p.1125·1); menthol
(p.1632·3).
Scalp disorders.

XSP-Bena *Xepa-Soul Pattinson, Singapore.*
Diphenhydramine hydrochloride (p.416·1); sodium ci-
trate (p.1186·2); ammonium chloride (p.1085·2).
Coughs; nasal and bronchial congestion.

X-Tar *Dormer, Canad.*
Salicylic acid (p.1122·3); coal tar (p.1125·1); menthol
(p.1632·3).
Scalp disorders.

X-trozine *Rexar, USA†.*
Phendimetrazine tartrate (p.1513·3).

Xuprin *Solvay, Aust.*
Isoxsuprine resinate (p.1625·1).
Peripheral vascular disorders.

Xycam *Aspen, S.Afr.*
Piroxicam (p.79·1).
Gout; musculoskeletal and joint disorders.

Xylanaest *Gebro, Aust.*
Lignocaine [lidocaine] hydrochloride (p.1313·2).
Adrenaline [epinephrine] (p.829·1) is included in some
injections as a vasoconstrictor to diminish absorption
and localise the effect of the local anaesthetic.
Local anaesthesia.

Xylesine *Amino, Switz.*
Lignocaine [lidocaine] hydrochloride (p.1313·2).
Local anaesthesia.

Xylestesin
Note.This name is used for preparations of different composition.
Espe, Aust.; Espe, Switz.
Lignocaine [lidocaine] (p.1313·2); cetrimonium bro-
mide (p.1137·3).
Local anaesthesia.
Cristalia, Braz.
Lignocaine [lidocaine] (p.1313·2) or lignocaine [lido-
caine] hydrochloride (p.1313·2).
Adrenaline [epinephrine] (p.829·1) is included in some
injections as a vasoconstrictor to diminish absorption
and localise the effect of the local anaesthetic.
Local anaesthesia.

Xylestesin Pumpspray *Espe, Ger.*
Lignocaine [lidocaine] (p.1313·2); cetrimonium bro-
mide (p.1137·3).
Local anaesthesia.

Xylestesin, Xylestesin-F *Espe, Ger.*
Lignocaine [lidocaine] hydrochloride (p.1313·2).
Noradrenaline [norepinephrine] hydrochloride
(p.948·2) is included in this preparation as a vasoconstrictor to diminish absorption and localise the effect of
the local anaesthetic.
Local anaesthesia.

Xylestesin-A, Xylestesin centro *Espe, Ger.*
Lignocaine [lidocaine] hydrochloride (p.1313·2).
Adrenaline [epinephrine] hydrochloride (p.829·2) is
included in this preparation as a vasoconstrictor to diminish absorption and localise the effect of the local
anaesthetic.
Local anaesthesia.

Xylestesin-F *Espe, Switz.*
Lignocaine [lidocaine] hydrochloride (p.1313·2).
Noradrenaline [norepinephrine] hydrochloride
(p.948·2) is included in this preparation as a vasoconstrictor to diminish absorption and localise the effect of
the local anaesthetic.
Local anaesthesia.

Xylestesin-S *Espe, Ger.*
Lignocaine [lidocaine] hydrochloride (p.1313·2).
Noradrenaline [norepinephrine] hydrochloride
(p.948·2) and adrenaline [epinephrine] hydrochloride
(p.829·2) are included in this preparation as vasoconstrictors to diminish absorption and localise the effect
of the local anaesthetic.
Local anaesthesia.

Xylestesin-S "special" *Espe, Switz.*
Lignocaine [lidocaine] hydrochloride (p.1313·2).
Adrenaline [epinephrine] hydrochloride (p.829·2) and
noradrenaline [norepinephrine] hydrochloride
(p.948·2) are included in this preparation as vasoconstrictors to diminish absorption and localise the effect
of the local anaesthetic.
Local anaesthesia.

Xylit *Braun, Ger.*
Xylitol (p.1397·3).
Carbohydrate source; fluid disorders.

Xylo *CT, Ger.*
Xylometazoline hydrochloride (p.1102·2).
Nasal congestion.

Xylocain
*Astra, Aust.; AstraZeneca, Denm.; AstraZeneca, Fin.; Astra, Ger.; As-
traZeneca, Norw.; Astra, Swed.; Astra, Switz.*
Lignocaine [lidocaine] (p.1313·2) or lignocaine [lido-
caine] hydrochloride (p.1313·2).
Adrenaline [epinephrine] (p.829·1) or adrenaline
[epinephrine] acid tartrate (p.829·2) is included in
some injections as a vasoconstrictor to diminish absorption and localise the effect of the local anaesthetic.
Local anaesthesia.

Xylocain CO₂ *Astra, Switz.*
Lignocaine [lidocaine] (p.1313·2); carbon dioxide.
Local anaesthesia.

Xylocain Comp *AstraZeneca, Denm.*
Lignocaine [lidocaine] (p.1313·2); bismuth subgallate
(p.1213·2); zinc oxide (p.1128·2).
Anorectal disorders.

Xylocain f.d. Kardiologie *Astra, Ger.*
Lignocaine [lidocaine] hydrochloride (p.1313·2).
Arrhythmias; status epilepticus.

Xylocain Klorhexidin *AstraZeneca, Denm.*
Lignocaine [lidocaine] (p.1313·2); chlor-
hexidine gluconate (p.1138·2).
Catheterisation; cystoscopy; local anaesthesia.

Xylocain tung *Astra, Swed.*
Lignocaine [lidocaine] hydrochloride (p.1313·2).
Local anaesthesia.

Xylocaina
Note.This name is used for preparations of different composition.
Astra, Braz.
Lignocaine [lidocaine] (p.1313·2) or lignocaine [lido-
caine] hydrochloride (p.1313·2).
Adrenaline [epinephrine] (p.829·1) or noradrenaline
[norepinephrine] (p.948·2) is included in some injec-
tions as a vasoconstrictor to diminish absorption and
localise the effect of the local anaesthetic.
Local anaesthesia.
Astra, Ital.; Astra, Mex.; Astra, Port.†.
Lignocaine [lidocaine] (p.1313·2) or lignocaine [lido-
caine] hydrochloride (p.1313·2).
Adrenaline [epinephrine] (p.829·1) or adrenaline
[epinephrine] acid tartrate (p.829·2) is included in
some injections as a vasoconstrictor to diminish ab-
sorption and localise the effect of the local anaesthetic.
Local anaesthesia.
Inibsa, Spain.
Lignocaine [lidocaine] hydrochloride (p.1313·2).
Local anaesthesia.

Xylocaine
Note.This name is used for preparations of different composition.
*Astra, Austral.; Astra, Belg.; AstraZeneca, Canad.; Astra, Hong Kong;
Astra, Irl.; Astra, Israel; Astra, Neth.; AstraZeneca, NZ; Astra, S.Afr.;
AstraZeneca, Singapore; AstraZeneca, Thai.; AstraZeneca, UK; As-
tra, USA.*
Lignocaine [lidocaine] (p.1313·2) or lignocaine [lido-
caine] hydrochloride (p.1313·2).
Adrenaline [epinephrine] (p.829·1) or adrenaline
[epinephrine] acid tartrate (p.829·2) is included in
some injections as a vasoconstrictor to diminish ab-
sorption and localise the effect of the local anaesthetic.
Xylocaine CO₂ contains the theoretical salt lignocaine
[lidocaine] hydrocarbonate.
Catheterisation; endoscopy; local anaesthesia; pain.
AstraZeneca, Fr.
Lignocaine [lidocaine] hydrochloride (p.1313·2).
Adrenaline [epinephrine] acid tartrate (p.829·2) or naphazoline nitrate (p.1095·1) is included in some preparations as a vasoconstrictor to diminish absorption and
localise the effect of the local anaesthetic.
Local anaesthesia.

Xylocaine Antispetic *AstraZeneca, UK.*
Lignocaine [lidocaine] hydrochloride (p.1313·2); chlo-
rhexidine gluconate (p.1138·2).
Local anaesthesia.

Xylocaine with Chlorhexidine *AstraZeneca, NZ.*
Lignocaine [lidocaine] hydrochloride (p.1313·2); chlo-
rhexidine gluconate (p.1138·2).
Local anaesthesia.

Xylocaine Jelly with Chlorhexidine *Astra, Austral.*
Lignocaine [lidocaine] hydrochloride (p.1313·2); chlo-
rhexidine gluconate (p.1138·2).
Formerly known as Xylocaine Jelly with Hibitane.
Catheterisation; endoscopy; local anaesthesia.

Xylocaine 2% Plain *AstraZeneca, UK.*
Lignocaine [lidocaine] hydrochloride (p.1313·2).
Formerly known as Lignostab.
Local anaesthesia.

Xylocaine Special Adhesive *Astra, Austral.*
Lignocaine [lidocaine] hydrochloride (p.1313·2).
Topical anaesthesia in dentistry.

Xylocaine Visqueuse *Astra, Belg.*
Lignocaine [lidocaine] hydrochloride (p.1313·2).
*Adjunct in radiology and endoscopy; painful oral and
oesophageal conditions.*

Xylocard
*Astra, Aust.; Astra, Austral.; Astra, Belg.; AstraZeneca, Canad.; Astra-
Zeneca, Fr.; Astra, Hong Kong; Astra, Irl.; Astra, Neth.; Astra, Norw.†;
AstraZeneca, NZ; Astra, Port.†; AstraZeneca, Singapore; Hassle,
Swed.; Astra, Switz.; AstraZeneca, Thai.; AstraZeneca, UK†.*
Lignocaine [lidocaine] hydrochloride (p.1313·2).
Status epilepticus; ventricular arrhythmias.

Xylocitin *Jenapharm, Ger.*
Lignocaine [lidocaine] hydrochloride (p.1313·2).
Adrenaline [epinephrine] acid tartrate (p.829·2) is included in some injections as a vasoconstrictor to diminish absorption and localise the effect of the local
anaesthetic.
Local anaesthesia.

Xylocitin cor *Jenapharm, Ger.*
Lignocaine [lidocaine] hydrochloride (p.1313·2).
Ventricular arrhythmias.

Xylo-COMOD *Ursapharm, Ger.*
Xylometazoline hydrochloride (p.1102·2).
Nasal congestion.

Xylolin *Julphar, UAE.*
Xylometazoline hydrochloride (p.1102·2).
Nasal and sinus congestion.

Xyloma *Jean-Marie, Hong Kong.*
Xylometazoline hydrochloride (p.1102·2).
Nasal congestion; otitis media.

Xylonest
Astra, Ger.; Astra, Switz.
Prilocaine hydrochloride (p.1318·2).
Adrenaline [epinephrine] acid tartrate (p.829·2) or fe-
lypressin (p.1283·1) is included in some injections as a
vasoconstrictor to diminish absorption and localise the
effect of the local anaesthetic.
Local anaesthesia.

Xylonest-Octapressin *Astra, Switz.*
Prilocaine hydrochloride (p.1318·2).
Felypressin (p.1283·1) is included in this preparation
as a vasoconstrictor to diminish absorption and localise
the effect of the local anaesthetic.
Local anaesthesia.

Xyloneural *Gebro, Aust.; Strathmann, Ger.; Gebro, Switz.*
Lignocaine [lidocaine] hydrochloride (p.1313·2).
Headache; local anaesthesia; migraine; tinnitus; vertigo.

Xylonibsa *Inibsa, Spain†.*
Cetylpyridinium chloride (p.1138·1); lignocaine [lidocaine] hydrochloride (p.1313·2).
Local anaesthesia.

Xylonor
Note. This name is used for preparations of different composition.
Austrodent, Aust.
Lignocaine [lidocaine] (p.1313·2); cetrimide (p.1137·1).
Local anaesthesia.

Ogna, Ital.
Injection: Lignocaine [lidocaine] hydrochloride (p.1313·2).
Noradrenaline [norepinephrine] acid tartrate (p.948·2) or adrenaline [epinephrine] acid tartrate (p.829·2) is included in some injections as a vasoconstrictor to diminish absorption and localise the effect of the local anaesthetic.
Topical solution; pellets; topical spray: Lignocaine [lidocaine] (p.1313·2); cetrimonium bromide (p.1137·3).
Local anaesthesia.

Prats, Spain.
Lignocaine [lidocaine] hydrochloride (p.1313·2); cetrimonium bromide (p.1137·3).
Local anaesthesia.

Septodont, Ital.
Injection†: Lignocaine [lidocaine] hydrochloride (p.1313·2).
Noradrenaline [norepinephrine] acid tartrate (p.948·2) or noradrenaline [norepinephrine] acid tartrate and adrenaline [epinephrine] (p.829·1) are included in some injections as vasoconstrictors to diminish absorption and localise the effect of the local anaesthetic.
Topical spray: Lignocaine [lidocaine] (p.1313·2); cetrimonium bromide (p.1137·3).
Local anaesthesia.

Xylonor Especial *Prats, Spain.*
Lignocaine [lidocaine] hydrochloride (p.1313·2).
Adrenaline [epinephrine] (p.829·1) and noradrenaline [norepinephrine] acid tartrate (p.948·2) are included in this preparation as vasoconstrictors to diminish absorption and localise the effect of the local anaesthetic.
Local anaesthesia.

Xylonor 2% Sin Vasoconst *Prats, Spain.*
Lignocaine [lidocaine] hydrochloride (p.1313·2).
Local anaesthesia.

Xylo-Pfan *Pharmacia Upjohn, Canad.†; Adria, USA†.*
Xylose (p.1681·2).
Diagnosis of malabsorption.

Xyloproct
Note. This name is used for preparations of different composition.
Astra, Austral.; AstraZeneca, Fin.; Astra, Hong Kong; AstraZeneca, NZ; AstraZeneca, Singapore; Tika, Swed.; AstraZeneca, Thai.; AstraZeneca, UK.
Lignocaine [lidocaine] (p.1313·2) or lignocaine [lidocaine] hydrochloride (p.1313·2); hydrocortisone acetate (p.1073·3); aluminium acetate (p.1578·1); zinc oxide (p.1128·2).
Anorectal disorders.

Astra, Belg.; Astra, Braz.; Astra, Irl.; Astra, Israel; Astra, Ital.; Astra, Mex.; Astra, Neth.; AstraZeneca, Norw.
Lignocaine [lidocaine] (p.1313·2); hydrocortisone acetate (p.1073·3); aluminium subacetate (p.1578·2); zinc oxide (p.1128·2).
Anorectal disorders.

Xylose-BMS *Bio-Medical, UK.*
Xylose (p.1681·2).
Formerly known as Xylomed.
Diagnosis of malabsorption.

Xylotocan *Astra, Ger.*
Tocainide hydrochloride (p.983·3).
Ventricular arrhythmias.

Xylotox *Adcock Ingram, S.Afr.*
Lignocaine [lidocaine] hydrochloride (p.1313·2).
Adrenaline [epinephrine] (p.829·1) or noradrenaline [norepinephrine] (p.948·2) is included in some preparations as a vasoconstrictor to diminish absorption and localise the effect of the local anaesthetic.
Local anaesthesia.

AstraZeneca, UK.
Lignocaine [lidocaine] hydrochloride (p.1313·2).
Adrenaline [epinephrine] acid tartrate (p.829·2) is included in this preparation as a vasoconstrictor to diminish absorption and localise the effect of the local anaesthetic.
Local anaesthesia.

Xylovit *Vitamed, Israel.*
Xylometazoline hydrochloride (p.1102·2).
Nasal congestion.

Xyzal *UCB, UK.*
Levocetirizine hydrochloride (p.420·1).
Allergic conjunctivitis; allergic rhinitis; urticaria.

Yacutin *Boots Healthcare, Ger.*
Benzyl benzoate (p.1428·2); lindane (p.1434·1).
Pediculosis; scabies.

Yadalan *Llorente, Spain.*
A nonoxinol (p.1346·1).
Contraceptive.

Yadegal Compuesto *Rayere, Mex.*
Dextromethorphan (p.1087·3); guaiacol (p.1092·1); chlorpheniramine [chlorphenamine] (p.412·2).
Coughs.

Yakona N *Tentan, Switz.†.*
Hypericum (p.290·2); kava (p.1625·3).
Anxiety; nervous tension.

Yal *Jacoby, Aust.; Trommsdorff, Ger.; Gebro, Switz.*
Docusate sodium (p.1223·1); sorbitol (p.1377·3).
Bowel evacuation; constipation.

Yamalen *Aventis, Belg.*
Dextropropoxyphene hydrochloride (p.27·1); paracetamol (p.71·2).
Pain.

Yamatetan *Yamanouchi, Jpn.*
Cefotetan disodium (p.170·3).
Bacterial infections.

Yapamicin *Novag, Mex.*
Ampicillin (p.150·3).
Bacterial infections.

Yariba *Dendron, UK.*
Kola (p.1681·1).
Fatigue.

Yasmin *Berlex, USA.*
Drospirenone (p.1472·2); ethinylestradiol (p.1476·2).
Combined oral contraceptive.

Yatropan *Hoechst Marion Roussel, Braz.*
Ephedrine (p.1090·1); menthol (p.1632·3); eucalyptol (p.1609·2); tolu balsam (p.1101·3); lavender oil (p.1627·2); sumatra benzoin (p.1668·3); sulfanilamide (p.256·2); guaiacol (p.1092·1).
Respiratory-tract congestion.

Yatrox *Vita, Spain.*
Ondansetron hydrochloride (p.1241·3).
Nausea and vomiting.

Yatushan Plus *Trima, Israel.*
Diphenhydramine hydrochloride (p.416·1); diethyltoluamide (p.1431·2); dimethyl phthalate (p.1431·3).
Insect bites.

Yavit *Ederka, Mex.*
Multivitamin and mineral preparation (p.1350·1).

Yeast Clear *Dolisos, Canad.*
Homoeopathic preparation.

Yeast Vite *SSL, UK.*
Caffeine (p.761·3); vitamin B substances (p.1350·1); dried yeast (p.1398·1).
Tonic.

Yeast-Gard *Lake, USA.*
Homoeopathic preparation.

Yeast-Gard Advanced Sensitive Formula *Lake, USA†.*
Benzocaine (p.1306·2); benzalkonium chloride (p.1133·2); aloe vera (p.1110·1); vitamin E (p.1393·3).
Vaginal irritation.

Yeast-Gard Maximum Strength Formula *Lake, USA†.*
Benzocaine (p.1306·2); resorcinol (p.1122·2).
Vaginal irritation.

Yeast-Gard Medicated *Lake, USA†.*
Povidone-iodine (p.1155·1).
Vaginal irritation.

Yeast-X *Fleet, USA.*
Powder: Corn starch (p.1379·3); zinc oxide (p.1128·2).
Suppositories: Pulsatilla (p.1656·3).

Yectames *Grossman, Mex.*
Algestone acetophenide (p.1465·1); estradiol enantate (p.1473·2).
Injectable contraceptive.

Yectamicina *Grossman, Mex.*
Gentamicin sulfate (p.210·1).
Bacterial infections.

Yectamid *Collins, Mex.*
Amikacin sulfate (p.148·1).
Gram-negative bacterial infections.

Yectofer *Astra, Spain.*
Iron sorbitol (p.1369·2).
Anaemias.

Yedoc *Ciba Vision, Switz.†.*
Gentamicin sulfate (p.210·1).
Bacterial eye infections.

Yeiamin-2 *YF Chem, Thai.*
Amino-acid and carbohydrate infusion (p.1350·1).
Parenteral nutrition.

Yelets *Freeda, USA.*
Ferrous fumarate (p.1360·1); folic acid (p.1361·1); multivitamins and minerals (p.1350·1).
Iron-deficiency anaemias.

Yendol *Faes, Spain.*
Caffeine (p.761·3); chlorpheniramine [chlorphenamine] maleate (p.412·1); paracetamol (p.71·2); salicylamide (p.82·1).
Cold and influenza symptoms; coughs.

Yermonil *Novartis, Aust.; Novartis, Ger.; Ciba, Switz.†.*
Ethinylestradiol (p.1476·2); lynestrenol (p.1480·1).
Combined oral contraceptive.

Yestamin *Peter Black, UK.*
Vitamin B substances; ascorbic acid; iron (p.1350·1).

Yewtaxan *Pharmachemie, S.Afr.†.*
Paclitaxel (p.563·2).
Breast cancer; ovarian cancer.

YF-Vax *Pasteur Merieux, USA.*
A yellow fever vaccine (17D strain) (p.1568·3).
Active immunisation.

Yocon *Croma, Aust.; Glenwood, Canad.; Glenwood, Ger.; Glenwood, Hong Kong; Glenwood, USA.*
Yohimbine hydrochloride (p.1681·3).
Erectile dysfunction.

Yocoral *Intsel, Fr.*
Yohimbine (p.1681·3).
Erectile dysfunction.

Yodacua *Manuell, Mex.*
Povidone-iodine (p.1155·1).
Water purification.

Yodine *Manuell, Mex.*
Povidone-iodine (p.1155·1).
Infected burns, ulcers, or wounds; mouth and throat infections; seborrhoeic dermatitis; skin infections; skin, mucous membrane, and instrument disinfection; vaginal infections.

Yodo Tio Calci *Alcon Cusi, Spain.*
Calcium chloride (p.1188·1); potassium iodide (p.1522·3); sodium thiosulfate (p.1024·2); sodium iodide (p.1522·3).
Aspergillus eye infections; cataracts.

Yodolactina *Manuell, Mex.*
Iodocasein (p.1523·2).
Goitre; immunostimulant; obesity; obstructive airways disease; rheumatoid disorders; sclerosis; tuberculosis.

Yodon *Sam-On, Israel.*
Povidone-iodine (p.1155·1).
Burns; skin disorders; wounds.

Yodoxin *Glenwood, USA.*
Diiodohydroxyquinoline (p.590·2).
Intestinal amoebiasis.

Yohimex *Kramer, USA.*
Yohimbine hydrochloride (p.1681·3).
Erectile dysfunction.

Yohydrol *Riedel-Zabinka, Braz.*
Yohimbine (p.1681·3).
Erectile dysfunction.

Yomax *Apsen, Braz.*
Yohimbine (p.1681·3).
Erectile dysfunction.

Yomesan *Bayer, Austral.†; Bayer, Belg.; Bayer, Denm.; Bayer, Ger.; Bayer, Israel; Bayer, Ital.; Bayer, Neth.; Bayer, S.Afr.; Bayer, Swed.; Bayer, Thai.; IDIS, UK.*
Niclosamide (p.104·2).
Available on a named patient basis in the UK.
Diphyllobothriasis; hymenolepiasis; taeniasis.

Yopin *Sydenham, Mex.*
Diiodohydroxyquinoline (p.590·2).

Yoquin *Arlex, Mex.*
Clioquinol (p.190·2).

Youngflex Massage 168 *Youngflex, Canad.*
Menthol (p.1632·3); cajuput oil (p.1588·1); eucalyptus oil (p.1609·2).
Musculoskeletal, joint, peri-articular, and soft-tissue disorders.

Your Choice *Amcon, USA.*
Saline rinsing and storage solutions for soft contact lenses (p.1129·2) (p.1196·1).

Yovis *Fermenti, Ital.†.*
Streptococcus salivarius subsp. thermophilus; Bifidobacterium breve; B. infantis; B. longum; Lactobacillus acidophilus; L. plantarum; L. casei; L. delbrueckii subsp. bulgaricus; Enterococcus faecium (p.1626·3).
Disturbance of gastrointestinal flora.

Ypsiloheel *Heel, Ger.*
Homoeopathic preparation.

YSE *Chatelut, Fr.*
Zinc gluconate (p.1398·2); kola (p.1681·1).
Tonic.

YSE Glutamique *Chatelut, Fr.*
Zinc gluconate (p.1398·2); glutamic acid (p.1365·2).
Tonic.

Ysol 206 *Rabi & Solabo, Fr.†.*
Acetic acid (p.1571·2); camphor (p.1589·3); Java citronella oil (p.1596·3); sodium laurilsulfate (p.1496·3).
Pediculosis.

Yurelax *ICN, Spain.*
Cyclobenzaprine hydrochloride (p.1328·1).
Skeletal muscle spasm.

Yuremetil D *Willmar, Mex.*
Methyldopa (p.927·3).

Yuremid *Willmar, Mex.*
Frusemide [furosemide] (p.893·1).

Yutopar *Solvay, Austral.; Bristol, Canad.; Solvay, Hong Kong; Solvay, Irl.; Solvay, Singapore; Solvay, Thai.; Solvay, UK; Astra, USA.*
Ritodrine hydrochloride (p.1659·1).
Fetal distress; premature labour.

Yxin *Pfizer, Ger.*
Tetryzoline hydrochloride (p.1101·2).
Eye disorders.

Z 300 *Glaxo Wellcome, NZ.*
Allopurinol (p.397·2).
Gout; hyperuricaemia.

Z Frin *Grin, Mex.*
Zinc sulfate (p.1398·2); phenylephrine hydrochloride (p.1097·1).
Eye disorders.

Z Span *Goldshield, UK.*
Zinc sulfate (p.1398·2).
Zinc deficiency.

Zacam *Fournier, Ital.†.*
Piroxicam (p.79·1).
Musculoskeletal, joint, and peri-articular disorders.

Zacetin *Dong, Singapore.*
Alprazolam (p.654·2).
Anxiety; mixed anxiety depressive states.

Zacin *Elan, Irl.; Bioglan, UK.*
Capsaicin (p.23·1).
Osteoarthritis.

Zacnan *Liphaderm, Fr.*
Minocycline hydrochloride (p.224·3).
Acne.

Z-Acne *Vitaglow, Austral.*
Cream†: Zinc oxide (p.1128·2); panthenol (p.1602·3); triclosan (p.1159·2); biosulfur (p.1123·3); alcloxa (p.1109·3).
Tablets: Zinc amino acid chelate (p.1398·3); vitamins and minerals (p.1350·1); bioflavonoids (p.1611·1).
Acne.

Zactin *Alphapharm, Austral.; Alphapharm, Singapore; Merck, Singapore.*
Fluoxetine hydrochloride (p.284·2).
Depression; obsessive-compulsive disorder.

Zadaxin *Sciclone, Ital.; Sciclone, Singapore.*
Thymalfasin (p.1672·1).
Chronic hepatitis B; chronic hepatitis C; influenza in immunodeficient patients.

Zadine
Note. This name is used for preparations of different composition.
Schering-Plough, Austral.; Schering-Plough, Hong Kong; Schering-Plough, NZ; Schering-Plough, Singapore.
Azatadine maleate (p.409·2).
Hypersensitivity reactions.

UCI, Braz.
Ranitidine (p.1246·3).
Gastro-oesophageal reflux; gastrointestinal haemorrhage; peptic ulcer; Zollinger-Ellison syndrome.

Zadino *Milano, Thai.*
Ketotifen fumarate (p.767·2).
Asthma; hypersensitivity reactions.

Zadipina *Bayer, Ital.*
Nisoldipine (p.946·3).
Angina pectoris; hypertension.

Zaditen *Novartis, Aust.; Novartis, Belg.; Novartis, Braz.; Novartis, Canad.; Novartis, Fr.; Novartis, Ger.; Novartis, Hong Kong; Novartis, Irl.; Novartis, Israel; Novartis, Ital.; Sandoz, Jpn†; Novartis, Mex.; Novartis, Neth.; Novartis, Port.; Novartis, S.Afr.; Novartis, Singapore; Novartis, Switz.; Novartis, Thai.; Novartis, UK.*
Ketotifen fumarate (p.767·2).
Asthma; bronchitis; hypersensitivity reactions.

Zaditor *Ciba Vision, USA.*
Ketotifen fumarate (p.767·2).
Allergic conjunctivitis.

Zadorin *Mepha, Hong Kong; Mepha, Switz.*
Doxycycline hyclate (p.200·1).
Bacterial infections.

Zadstat *FL, Israel; Lederle, UK.*
Metronidazole (p.594·1).
Anaerobic bacterial infections; protozoal infections.

Zadyl *Thera, Fr.†.*
Cefradine (p.173·3).
Bacterial infections.

Zaedoc *Ashbourne, UK.*
Ranitidine hydrochloride (p.1245·2).
Acid aspiration; dyspepsia; gastro-oesophageal reflux; gastrointestinal haemorrhage; peptic ulcer; Zollinger-Ellison syndrome.

Zafen *Zambon, Ital.; Zambon, Neth.*
Ibuprofen (p.43·2) or ibuprofen arginine (p.44·1).
Fever; inflammation; musculoskeletal, joint, and peri-articular disorders; pain.

Zafibral *Medochemie, Hong Kong; Medochemie, Singapore.*
Bezafibrate (p.849·1).
Hyperlipidaemias.

Zafimida *Zafiro, Mex.*
Frusemide [furosemide] (p.893·1).
Forced diuresis; hypertension; oedema.

Zafirst *Chiesi, Ital.*
Zafirlukast (p.785·3).
Asthma.

Zafor *Mepha, Switz.†.*
Chlorzoxazone (p.1327·3); paracetamol (p.71·2).
Painful skeletal muscle spasm.

Zagam *Aventis, Fr.†; Rhone-Poulenc Rorer, Ger.; Rhone-Poulenc Rorer, Hong Kong; Aventis, NZ; Rhone-Poulenc Rorer, S.Afr.; Rhone-Poulenc Rorer, Switz.†; Rhone-Poulenc Rorer, Thai.; Rhone-Poulenc Rorer, USA.*
Sparfloxacin (p.248·1).
Bacterial infections.

Zagastrol *Riedel-Zabinka, Braz.*
Cimetidine (p.1216·3).
Gastro-oesophageal reflux; gastrointestinal haemorrhage; peptic ulcer; Zollinger-Ellison syndrome.

Zagyl *Xixia, S.Afr.*
Metronidazole (p.594·1).
Anaerobic bacterial infections; protozoal infections.

Zahnerol N *Dr Janssen, Ger.*
Benzocaine (p.1306·2).
Dental disorders.

The symbol † denotes a preparation no longer actively marketed

Zahnungstropfen Escatitona *Madaus, Ger.*
Homoeopathic preparation.

Zalain *Searle, Braz.; Trommsdorff, Ger.; Ferrer, Singapore; Robert, Spain.*
Sertaconazole nitrate (p.393·3).
Fungal skin and nail infections.

Zalig *Fournier, Ital.†*
Propionyl erythromycin mercaptosuccinate (p.203·3).
Bacterial infections.

Zalvor *Glaxo Wellcome, Belg.*
Permethrin (p.1436·1).
Pediculosis; scabies.

Zamacort *Rhone-Poulenc Rorer, Mex.*
Triamcinolone acetonide (p.1080·1).
Asthma.

Zamadol *Asta Medica, UK.*
Tramadol hydrochloride (p.89·1).
Pain.

Zamanon *Aventis, S.Afr.*
Dolasetron mesilate (p.1223·3).
Nausea and vomiting associated with cytotoxic therapy; postoperative nausea and vomiting.

Zambesil *Gentili, Ital.†*
Chlortalidone (p.857·1).
Hypertension; oedema.

Zam-Buk
Note.This name is used for preparations of different composition.
Key, Austral.
Eucalyptus oil (p.1609·2); camphor (p.1589·3); thyme oil (p.1672·3); colophony (p.1598·3); sassafras oil (p.1661·1).
Minor skin disorders.

Roche, Hong Kong; Roche Consumer, Singapore.
Eucalyptus oil (p.1609·2); camphor (p.1589·3); thyme oil (p.1672·3); colophony (p.1598·3).
Bites and stings; chapped hands; cold sores; joint pain; minor wounds.

Roche, S.Afr.†
Eucalyptus oil (p.1609·2); camphor (p.1589·3); thyme oil (p.1672·3); sassafras oil (p.1661·1).
Burns; chapped hands; insect bites; muscular pain; pruritus; wounds.

Zamene *Menarini, Spain.*
Deflazacort (p.1066·1).
Corticosteroid.

Zamocilline *Zambon, Fr.†*
Amoxicillin (p.149·2).
Bacterial infections.

Zamudol *Asta Medica, Fr.*
Tramadol hydrochloride (p.89·1).
Pain.

Zanaflex *Elan, Irl.; Athena Neurosciences, UK; Athena Neurosciences, USA.*
Tizanidine hydrochloride (p.1330·2).
Skeletal muscle spasticity.

Zanamet *TO-Chemicals, Thai.*
Ranitidine (p.1246·3).
Peptic ulcer; Zollinger-Ellison syndrome.

Zandine *Duncan, Flockhart, Irl.*
Ranitidine hydrochloride (p.1245·2).
Gastric hyperacidity; gastro-oesophageal reflux; peptic ulcer; Zollinger-Ellison syndrome.

Zanedip *Recordati, Ital.*
Lercanidipine hydrochloride (p.920·2).
Hypertension.

Zanfel *Zanfel, USA.*
Polyethylene granules (p.1108·3) in a surfactant base.
Urushiol-induced contact dermatitis.

Zanidex *Dexcel, Israel.*
Ranitidine hydrochloride (p.1245·2).
Gastro-oesophageal reflux; gastrointestinal haemorrhage; peptic ulcer.

Zanidin *Pacific, NZ.*
Ranitidine hydrochloride (p.1245·2).
Acid aspiration; dyspepsia; gastro-oesophageal reflux; gastrointestinal haemorrhage; peptic ulcer; Zollinger-Ellison syndrome.

Zanidip *Kwizda, Aust.; Zambon, Belg.; UCB, Denm.; Leiras, Fin.; Doms-Recordati, Fr.; Recordati, Spain; UCB, Swed.; Napp, UK.*
Lercanidipine hydrochloride (p.920·2).
Hypertension.

Zanizal *Italfarmaco, Ital.*
Nizatidine (p.1238·1).
Gastro-oesophageal reflux; peptic ulcer.

Zanosar *Pharmacia Upjohn, Canad.; Pharmacia Upjohn, Fr.; Pharmacia Upjohn, Israel; Upjohn, Neth.†; Pharmacia Upjohn, USA.*
Streptozocin (p.569·1).
Pancreatic cancer.

Zantab *Teva, Israel.*
Ranitidine hydrochloride (p.1245·2).
Gastro-oesophageal reflux; gastrointestinal hyperacidity; peptic ulcer; Zollinger-Ellison syndrome.

Zantac *Glaxo Wellcome, Aust.; Glaxo Wellcome, Austral.; Glaxo Wellcome, Belg.; Glaxo Wellcome, Canad.; Warner-Lambert, Canad.; Glaxo Wellcome, Denm.; Glaxo Wellcome, Fin.; Glaxo Wellcome, Hong Kong; Glaxo Wellcome, Irl.; Glaxo Wellcome, Israel; Glaxo Wellcome, Ital.; Glaxo Wellcome, Neth.; Glaxo Wellcome, Norw.; Glaxo Wellcome, NZ; Glaxo Wellcome, Port.; Glaxo Wellcome, S.Afr.; Glaxo Wellcome, Singapore; Glaxo Wellcome, Spain; Glaxo*

Swed.; Glaxo Wellcome, Thai.; Glaxo Wellcome, UK; Glaxo Wellcome, USA.
Ranitidine hydrochloride (p.1245·2).
Acid aspiration; dyspepsia; gastro-oesophageal reflux; gastrointestinal haemorrhage; peptic ulcer; Zollinger-Ellison syndrome.

Zantic *Glaxo Wellcome, Ger.; Boehringer Ingelheim, Ger.; Glaxo Wellcome, Switz.*
Ranitidine hydrochloride (p.1245·2).
Acid aspiration; gastro-oesophageal reflux; gastrointestinal haemorrhage; gastrointestinal hyperacidity; peptic ulcer; Zollinger-Ellison syndrome.

Zantidon *Siam Bheasach, Thai.*
Ranitidine (p.1246·3).
Gastro-oesophageal reflux; peptic ulcer; Zollinger-Ellison syndrome.

Zantryl *Ion, USA†.*
Phentermine hydrochloride (p.1514·1).

Zanzipik *Tipomark, Ital.*
Diethyltoluamide (p.1431·2).
Insect repellent.

Zapain *Goldshield, UK.*
Paracetamol (p.71·2); codeine phosphate (p.25·2).
These ingredients can be described by the British Approved Name Co-codamol.
Pain.

Zaperin *Sanabo, Aust.*
Salbutamol (p.770·3).
Asthma; bronchoconstriction.

Zappelin *Iso, Ger.*
Homoeopathic preparation.

Zaprin *Willmar, Mex.*
Co-trimoxazole (p.193·3).
Bacterial infections.

Zapto *Aspen, S.Afr.*
Captopril (p.853·3).
Heart failure; hypertension.

Zapto Co *Aspen, S.Afr.*
Captopril (p.853·3); hydrochlorothiazide (p.907·3).
Hypertension.

Zaramol *Esfar, Port.*
Paracetamol (p.71·2).
Fever; pain.

Zarator *Pfizer, Denm.; Parke, Davis, Port.; Parke, Davis, Spain.*
Atorvastatin calcium (p.842·3).
Hyperlipidaemias.

Zarent *Rhone-Poulenc Rorer, Ital.*
Nedocromil sodium (p.768·3); salbutamol sulfate (p.770·3).
Obstructive airways disease.

Zaricort *Xepa-Soul Pattinson, Singapore.*
Miconazole nitrate (p.391·1); hydrocortisone (p.1073·3).
Fungal skin infections with inflammation.

Zarin *Xepa-Soul Pattinson, Singapore.*
Miconazole nitrate (p.391·1).
Fungal infections of the skin, nails, and mucous membranes.

Zariviz *Hoechst Marion Roussel, Ital.*
Cefotaxime sodium (p.169·1).
Lignocaine [lidocaine] hydrochloride (p.1313·2) is included in the intramuscular injection to alleviate the pain of injection.
Bacterial infections.

Zarocs *Pharmazam, Spain.*
Roxatidine acetate hydrochloride (p.1248·1).
Gastro-oesophageal reflux; peptic ulcer.

Zarondan *Parke, Davis, Denm.; Warner-Lambert, Norw.*
Ethosuximide (p.348·1).
Absence seizures.

Zarontin *Parke, Davis, Austral.; Parke, Davis, Belg.; Parke, Davis, Canad.; Parke, Davis, Fr.; Parke, Davis, Irl.; Parke, Davis, Israel; Parke, Davis, Ital.; Warner-Lambert, Mex.; Parke, Davis, Neth.; Parke, Davis, NZ; Parke, Davis, S.Afr.; Parke, Davis, Spain; Parke, Davis, UK; Parke, Davis, USA.*
Ethosuximide (p.348·1).
Absence seizures; myoclonic seizures.

Zaroxolyn *Rhone-Poulenc Rorer, Canad.; Heumann, Ger.; Rhone-Poulenc Rorer, Irl.†; Teoforma, Ital.; Rhone-Poulenc Rorer, Mex.; Novartis, S.Afr.; Sanofi Winthrop, Swed.; Medeva, USA.*
Metolazone (p.930·3).
Ascites; hypertension; oedema.

Zaroxolyne *Novartis, Switz.*
Metolazone (p.930·3).
Hypertension; oedema.

Zascal *Albert, S.Afr.†*
Lacidipine (p.919·1).
Hypertension.

Zasten *Novartis, Spain.*
Ketotifen (p.767·2).
Allergic rhinitis; asthma.

Zatinol *Efarmes, Spain†.*
Paracetamol (p.71·2).
Fever; pain.

Zatofug *Wolff, Ger.*
Ketotifen fumarate (p.767·2).
Asthma; hypersensitivity reactions.

Zavedos *Pharmacia Upjohn, Aust.; Pharmacia Upjohn, Austral.; Pharmacia Upjohn, Belg.; Pharmacia Upjohn, Braz.; Pharmacia Upjohn, Denm.; Pharmacia Upjohn, Fin.; Pharmacia Upjohn, Fr.; Pharmacia Upjohn,*

Ger.; Pharmacia Upjohn, Hong Kong; Pharmacia Upjohn, Irl.; Pharmacia Upjohn, Israel; Pharmacia Upjohn, Ital.; Pharmacia Upjohn, Neth.; Pharmacia Upjohn, Norw.; Pharmacia Upjohn, NZ; Pharmacia Upjohn, Port.; Pharmacia Upjohn, Singapore; Kenfarma, Spain; Pharmacia Upjohn, Swed.; Pharmacia Upjohn, Switz.; Pharmacia Upjohn, Thai.; Pharmacia, UK.
Idarubicin hydrochloride (p.545·2).
Malignant neoplasms.

Z-Bec *Whitehall-Robins, Canad.; Whitehall, Thai.*
Multivitamin preparation with zinc (p.1350·1).

Robins, USA.
Multivitamin and mineral preparation (p.1350·1).

ZBM *Blackmores, Austral.*
Zinc amino acid chelate (p.1398·3); vitamins and minerals (p.1350·1).
Zinc deficiency.

ZBT *Glenwood, USA.*
Talc (p.1124·2); liquid paraffin (p.1407·1).
Nappy rash.

Ze Caps *Everett, USA.*
Zinc gluconate (p.1398·2); vitamin E (p.1393·3).
Dietary supplement.

ZeaSorb
Note.This name is used for preparations of different composition.
Stiefel, Austral.; Stiefel, Canad.; Stiefel, Ger.; Stiefel, Irl.; Stiefel, Thai.
Aldioxa (p.1109·3); chloroxylenol (p.1142·1); cellulose (p.1500·2).
Hyperhidrosis; skin irritation.

Stiefel, Fr.
Aldioxa (p.1109·3); cellulose (p.1500·2); magnesium silicate (p.1502·1).
Hyperhidrosis.

Stiefel, Singapore; Stiefel, UK.
Aldioxa (p.1109·3); chloroxylenol (p.1142·1).
Hyperhidrosis; skin irritation.

ZeaSorb AF
Note.This name is used for preparations of different composition.
Stiefel, Canad.
Tolnaftate (p.395·2).
Fungal skin infections.

Stiefel, USA.
Miconazole nitrate (p.391·1).
Fungal skin infections.

Zeben *Siam Bheasach, Thai.*
Albendazole (p.95·2).
Worm infections.

Zebeta *Lederle, USA.*
Bisoprolol fumarate (p.850·1).
Hypertension.

Zeclar *Orion, Fin.; Abbott, Fr.*
Clarithromycin (p.186·2).
Bacterial infections.

Zecnil *Ferring, Ital.*
Somatostatin acetate (p.1297·3).
Diabetic ketoacidosis; gastrointestinal haemorrhage; pancreatic surgery.

Zeddan *Mediolanum, Ital.†*
Trandolapril (p.985·2).
Hypertension.

Zedene C *Whitehall, Fr.†*
Multivitamin and mineral preparation (p.1350·1).

Zeefra *Doms-Adrian, Fr.*
Cefradine (p.173·3).
Bacterial infections.

Zeel
Heel, Ger.
Homoeopathic preparation.

Heel, S.Afr.
Injection: Cartilago suis; funiculus umbilicalis suis; embryo suis; placenta suis; rhus toxicodendron; flor arnicae; dulcamara; symphytum; sanguinaria; nadid; coenzym A; thioctic acid; natrium oxalaceticum.

Ointment; tablets: Cartilago suis; funiculus umbilicalis suis; embryo suis; placenta suis; rhus toxicodendron; flor arnicae; dulcamara; symphytum; sanguinaria; sulfur; acidum silicicum colloidale; nadid; coenzym A; thioctic acid; natrium oxalaceticum.
Musculoskeletal and joint disorders.

Zeel comp *Heel, Ger.*
Homoeopathic preparation.

Zeel P *Heel, Ger.*
Homoeopathic preparation.

Zeel T *Heel, Ger.*
Homoeopathic preparation.

Zefa *M & H, Thai.*
Cefazolin sodium (p.164·3).
Bacterial infections.

Zefaxone *M & H, Thai.*
Ceftriaxone sodium (p.177·1).
Bacterial infections.

Zefazone *Upjohn, USA.*
Cefmetazole sodium (p.167·2).
Bacterial infections.

Zeffix *Glaxo Wellcome, Austral.; Glaxo Wellcome, Belg.; Glaxo Wellcome, Denm.; Glaxo Wellcome, Fin.; Glaxo Wellcome, Fr.; Glaxo Wellcome, Ger.; Glaxo Wellcome, Hong Kong; Glaxo Wellcome, Irl.; Glaxo Wellcome, Ital.; Glaxo Wellcome, NZ; Glaxo Wellcome, Port.; Glaxo Wellcome, Swed.; Glaxo Wellcome, Switz.; Glaxo Wellcome, Thai.; Glaxo Wellcome, UK.*
Lamivudine (p.635·1).
Hepatitis B.

Zefirol *Bayer, Ital.*
Benzalkonium chloride (p.1133·2).
Disinfection of skin, mucous membranes, and wounds; surface disinfection.

Zeftam *M & H, Thai.*
Ceftazidime (p.174·3).
Bacterial infections.

Zefxon *Biolab, Thai.*
Omeprazole (p.1239·1).
Gastro-oesophageal reflux; peptic ulcer; Zollinger-Ellison syndrome.

Zehu-Ze *Biogal, Israel.*
Permethrin (p.1436·1).
Pediculosis.

Zeisin *3M, Ger.*
Pirbuterol acetate (p.769·3).
Obstructive airways disease.

Zelapar *Athena Neurosciences, UK.*
Selegiline hydrochloride (p.1177·2).
Parkinsonism.

Zelderme *Zeller, Port.†*
Methylbenzethonium; zinc oxide (p.1128·2); vitamin A (p.1382·1); vitamin D (p.1391·1).
Nappy rash.

Zeldox *Pfizer, Swed.†*
Ziprasidone hydrochloride (p.712·1).
Schizophrenia.

Zelfin *Randall, Mex.*
Albendazole (p.95·2).
Worm infections.

Zeliderm *Vinas, Spain.*
Azelaic acid (p.1110·3).
Acne.

Zelis *Prospa, Ital.*
Piroxicam cinnamate (p.79·3).
Musculoskeletal and joint disorders.

Zelitrex *Glaxo Wellcome, Belg.; Glaxo Wellcome, Denm.; Glaxo Wellcome, Fr.; Glaxo Wellcome, Ital.; Glaxo Wellcome, Neth.; Glaxo Wellcome, S.Afr.*
Valaciclovir hydrochloride (p.643·1).
Herpesvirus infections.

Zelium *Masa, Thai.*
Flunarizine (p.418·2).
Cerebrovascular disorders; migraine.

Zellaforte *Zellaforte, Switz.*
Multivitamin and mineral preparation (p.1350·1).

Zellaforte N Plus *Eurim, Ger.*
Nikethamide calcium thiocyanate (p.1513·1); inositol nicotinate (p.914·1); pholedrine sulfate (p.955·2).
Tonic.

Zellaforte plus *Solco, Aust.*
Procaine hydrochloride; haematoporphyrin; ferrous sulfate; vitamins (p.1350·1).
Tonic.

Zellox-II *Hoe, Singapore.*
Aluminium hydroxide (p.1210·3); magnesium hydroxide (p.1233·1); simeticone (p.1249·2).
Dyspepsia; flatulence; gastric hyperacidity; gastritis; gastro-oesophageal reflux; heartburn.

Zemide *Dumex, Ger.*
Tamoxifen citrate (p.571·1).
Breast cancer.

Zemplar *Abbott, USA.*
Paricalcitol (p.1391·2).
Hyperparathyroidism.

Zemtard *Galen, UK.*
Diltiazem hydrochloride (p.874·3).
Angina pectoris; hypertension.

Zemuron *Organon, Canad.; Organon, USA.*
Rocuronium bromide (p.1339·2).
Competitive neuromuscular blocker.

Zen *Select, Ital.†*
Piroxicam cinnamate (p.79·3).
Musculoskeletal and joint disorders.

Zenalb *BPL, Hong Kong; BPL, Singapore; BPL, Thai.; BPL, UK.*
Albumin (p.724·1).
Burns; hypoalbuminaemia; hypovolaemic shock.

Zenapax *Roche, Aust.; Roche, Austral.; Roche, Belg.; Roche, Denm.; Roche, Fin.; Roche, Fr.; Roche, Ger.; Roche, Neth.; Roche, NZ; Roche, Port.; Roche, Singapore; Roche, Swed.; Roche, Switz.; Roche, Thai.; Roche, UK; Roche, USA.*
Daclizumab (p.532·1).
Renal transplant rejection.

Zenas
Fournier, Ger.; Fournier SA, Spain.
Cerivastatin sodium (p.856·1).
Hyperlipidaemias.

Zenavan *Wyeth, Spain.*
Etofenamate (p.35·3).
Pain; peri-articular disorders.

Zenaxin *Maver, Mex.*
Albendazole (p.95·2).
Worm infections.

Zenda *Nakorn, Thai.*
Niclosamide (p.104·2); phenolphthalein (p.1244·1).
Worm infections.

Zendhin *DHA, Singapore.*
Ranitidine hydrochloride (p.1245·2).
Dyspepsia; gastro-oesophageal reflux; peptic ulcer; Zollinger-Ellison syndrome.

Zeniac LP Fort LED, Fr.
Mandelic acid (p.221·2); tartaric acid (p.1669·2); salicylic acid (p.1122·3); ammonium lactate (p.1110·3).
Acne.

Zenicide Douglas, NZ.
Glutaral (p.1145·2).
Disinfection.

Zenit Pulitzer, Ital.†
Pivagabine (p.307·3).
Depression.

Zenium Alpharma, Fr.
Co-dergocrine mesilate (p.1597·3).
Mental function impairment.

Zenmolin DHA, Hong Kong.
Salbutamol sulfate (p.770·3).
Bronchospasm.

Zenodian CT, Ital.
Sucralfate (p.1250·2).
Gastritis; gastro-oesophageal reflux; peptic ulcer.

Zenoxone Biorex, UK.
Hydrocortisone (p.1073·3).
Skin disorders.

Zensyls Ernest Jackson, UK†.
Benzalkonium chloride (p.1133·2).
Sore throat.

Zentavion Vita, Spain.
Azithromycin (p.153·1).
Bacterial infections.

Zentel SmithKline Beecham, Austral.; SmithKline Beecham, Braz.; SmithKline Beecham, Fr.; SmithKline Beecham, Ital.; SmithKline Beecham, Mex.; Sterling, Port.; SmithKline Beecham, S.Afr.; SmithKline Beecham, Singapore; SmithKline Beecham, Switz.; SmithKline Beecham, Thai.
Albendazole (p.95·2).
Giardiasis; worm infections.

Zentramin Bastian N Bastian, Ger.
Electrolyte preparation (p.1180·1).
Hypersensitivity disorders; psychosomatic disorders; tetanus.

Zentropil BASF, Ger.
Phenytoin (p.357·3) or phenytoin sodium (p.357·2).
Epilepsy; trigeminal neuralgia.

Zenusin Mepha, Port.; Mepha, Thai.
Nifedipine (p.940·1).
Angina pectoris; heart failure; hypertension; Raynaud's syndrome.

Zepac Ist. Chim. Inter., Ital.
Heparin calcium (p.902·1).
Thromboembolic disorders.

Zepan Jofrain, Mex.
Diazepam (p.674·3).

Zepelan Boehringer de Angeli, Braz.
Feprazone (p.40·3).
Musculoskeletal and joint disorders.

Zepelin Boehringer Ingelheim, Aust.; Boehringer Ingelheim, Ital.
Feprazone (p.40·3).
Inflammation; musculoskeletal and joint disorders; pain.

Zepelindue Boehringer Ingelheim, Ital.
Ketoprofen lysine (p.48·1).
Inflammation; musculoskeletal, joint, peri-articular, and soft-tissue disorders; pain.

Zephiran Sanofi Synthelabo, Canad.; Sanofi Winthrop, USA.
Benzalkonium chloride (p.1133·2).
Disinfection of skin, mucous membranes, wounds, instruments, and surfaces; eye, bladder, urethra, and body cavity irrigation; vaginal douching.

Zephirol Bayer, Thai.
Benzalkonium chloride (p.1133·2).
Instrument disinfection; skin and hand disinfection; vaginal and bladder irrigation.

Zepholin Klinge, Irl.
Theophylline (p.777·2).
Bronchospasm.

Zephrex Sanofi Winthrop, USA.
Pseudoephedrine hydrochloride (p.1099·2); guaifenesin (p.1092·2).
Coughs.

Zepiken Kener, Mex.
Carbamazepine (p.342·2).

Zepilen Medochemie, Thai.
Cefazolin sodium (p.164·3).
Bacterial infections.

Zeplex M & H, Thai.
Cefalexin (p.161·3).
Bacterial infections.

Zeprat Solfran, Mex.
Diazepam (p.674·3).

Zerandin Zerboni, Mex.
Ranitidine (p.1246·3).

Zerfenazin Zerboni, Mex.
Perphenazine (p.699·1).

Zerinetta-Fher Boehringer Ingelheim, Ital.
Paracetamol (p.71·2); phenylpropanolamine hydrochloride (p.1098·1); chlorpheniramine [chlorphenamine] maleate (p.412·1).
Cold and influenza symptoms.

Zerinol-Fher Boehringer Ingelheim, Ital.
Paracetamol (p.71·2); phenylpropanolamine hydrochloride (p.1098·1); chlorpheniramine [chlorphenamine] maleate (p.412·1).

The symbol † denotes a preparation no longer actively marketed

Formerly contained feprazone, paracetamol, phenylpropanolamine hydrochloride, and chlorpheniramine [chlorphenamine] maleate.
Cold and influenza symptoms.

Zerit Bristol-Myers Squibb, Aust.; Bristol-Myers Squibb, Austral.; Bristol-Myers Squibb, Belg.; Bristol-Myers Squibb, Canad.; Bristol-Myers Squibb, Denm.; Bristol-Myers Squibb, Fin.; Bristol-Myers Squibb, Fr.; Bristol-Myers Squibb, Ger.; Bristol-Myers Squibb, Hong Kong; Bristol-Myers Squibb, Irl.; Bristol-Myers Squibb, Israel; Bristol-Myers Squibb, Ital.; Bristol-Myers Squibb, Jpn; Bristol-Myers Squibb, Mex.; Bristol-Myers Squibb, Neth.; Bristol-Myers Squibb, Norw.; Bristol-Myers Squibb, NZ; Bristol-Myers Squibb, Port.; Bristol-Myers Squibb, S.Afr.; Bristol-Myers Squibb, Singapore; Bristol-Myers Squibb, Swed.; Bristol-Myers Squibb, Switz.; Bristol-Myers Squibb, Thai.; Bristol-Myers Squibb, UK; Bristol-Myers Squibb Oncology, USA.
Stavudine (p.641·2).
HIV infection.

Zeritavir Bristol-Myers Squibb, Braz.
Stavudine (p.641·2).
HIV infection.

Zermed Progress, Thai.
Cetirizine hydrochloride (p.411·2).
Allergic rhinitis; hypersensitivity reactions.

Zeropyn Pharmco, S.Afr.†.
Paracetamol (p.71·2); codeine phosphate (p.25·2).
Fever; pain.

Zerosorin SN Schuck, Ger.
Homoeopathic preparation.

Zestomax Parke-Med, S.Afr.
Lisinopril (p.921·1).
Heart failure; hypertension; myocardial infarction.

Zestoretic Zeneca, Aust.; Zeneca, Belg.; Zeneca, Braz.; AstraZeneca, Canad.; AstraZeneca, Denm.; AstraZeneca, Fr.; Zeneca, Hong Kong; Zeneca, Irl.; Zeneca, Ital.; Zeneca, Mex.; Zeneca, Neth.; AstraZeneca, Norw.; AstraZeneca, NZ; Zeneca, Port.; Zeneca, S.Afr.; Zeneca, Spain; Zeneca, Swed.; Zeneca, Switz.; AstraZeneca, UK; Zeneca, USA.
Lisinopril (p.921·1); hydrochlorothiazide (p.907·3).
Hypertension.

Zestril Zeneca, Austral.; Zeneca, Belg.; Zeneca, Braz.; AstraZeneca, Canad.; AstraZeneca, Denm.; AstraZeneca, Fin.; AstraZeneca, Fr.; Zeneca, Hong Kong; Zeneca, Irl.; Zeneca, Ital.; Zeneca, Mex.; Zeneca, Neth.; AstraZeneca, Norw.; AstraZeneca, NZ; Zeneca, Port.; Zeneca, S.Afr.; AstraZeneca, Singapore; Zeneca, Spain; Zeneca, Swed.; Zeneca, Switz.; AstraZeneca, Thai.; AstraZeneca, UK; Zeneca, USA.
Lisinopril (p.921·1).
Diabetic nephropathy; diabetic retinopathy; heart failure; hypertension; myocardial infarction.

Zeta N Bergamon, Ital.
Usnic acid (p.1678·2).
Vaginal disinfection.

Zetamicin Menarini, Ital.
Netilmicin sulfate (p.229·3).
Bacterial infections.

Zetar Dermik, Canad.; Dermik, USA.
Coal tar (p.1125·1).
Skin disorders.

Zetarina Zafiro, Mex.
Dopamine hydrochloride (p.881·3).
Heart failure; hypotension; shock.

Zetavit Zeta, Ital.
Multivitamin and mineral preparation (p.1350·1).

Zetir Abbott, Braz.
Cetirizine hydrochloride (p.411·2).
Hypersensitivity reactions.

Zeto Unipharm, Israel.
Azithromycin (p.153·1).
Bacterial infections.

Zetofen Parke-Med, S.Afr.
Ketotifen fumarate (p.767·2).
Allergic rhinitis; allergic skin disorders; asthma.

Zetran Masa, Thai.
Dipotassium clorazepate (p.670·3).
Anxiety; insomnia.

Zetron Biolab, Thai.
Ondansetron hydrochloride (p.1241·3).
Nausea and vomiting induced by cytotoxics or radiotherapy; postoperative nausea and vomiting.

Zevin Biolab, Thai.
Aciclovir (p.612·3).
Herpes simplex infections of the skin and mucous membranes.

Z-gen Goldline, USA.
Multivitamin and mineral preparation (p.1350·1).

Zi Mentholatum, UK.
Camphor (p.1589·3).
Eye irritation.

Ziac Lederle, USA.
Bisoprolol fumarate (p.850·1); hydrochlorothiazide (p.907·3).
Hypertension.

Ziagen Glaxo Wellcome, Austral.; Glaxo Wellcome, Canad.; Glaxo Wellcome, Denm.; Glaxo Wellcome, Fin.; Glaxo Wellcome, Fr.; Glaxo Wellcome, Ger.; Glaxo Wellcome, Israel; Glaxo Wellcome, Ital.; Glaxo Wellcome, Norw.; Glaxo Wellcome, NZ; Glaxo Wellcome, Port.; Glaxo Wellcome, Singapore; Glaxo Wellcome, Swed.; Glaxo Wellcome, UK; Glaxo Wellcome, USA.
Abacavir sulfate (p.612·2).
HIV infection.

Ziak Merck, S.Afr.
Bisoprolol hydrochloride; hydrochlorothiazide (p.907·3).

Zibren Formenti, Ital.†
Acetylcarnitine or acetylcarnitine hydrochloride (p.1572·1).
Cerebrovascular disorders; peripheral neuropathy.

Ziclin Knoll, S.Afr.
Gliclazide (p.322·2).
Diabetes mellitus.

Zidac Biotherapie, Fr.
Ranitidine hydrochloride (p.1245·2).
Gastro-oesophageal reflux; peptic ulcer; Zollinger-Ellison syndrome.

Zida-Co Opus, UK†.
Amiloride hydrochloride (p.835·1); hydrochlorothiazide (p.907·3).
These ingredients can be described by the British Approved Name Co-amilozide.
Heart failure; hepatic cirrhosis; hypertension.

Zidicef Precimex, Mex.
Ceftazidime (p.174·3).
Bacterial infections.

Zidoval 3M, UK.
Metronidazole (p.594·1).
Bacterial vaginosis.

Zidovir Protein, Mex.
Zidovudine (p.645·2).

Zienam Merck Sharp & Dohme, Aust.; Merck Sharp & Dohme, Ger.
Imipenem (p.214·1); cilastatin sodium (p.182·2).
Lignocaine [lidocaine] hydrochloride (p.1313·2) may be included in the intramuscular injection to alleviate the pain of injection.
Bacterial infections.

Zifartel Continentales, Mex.
Praziquantel (p.106·3).

Zig C Falqui, Ital.
Ascorbic acid (p.1389·3).

Ziken Kendrick, Mex.
Mesna (p.1011·3).
Prevention of urotoxicity due to oxazaphosphorine antineoplastics.

Ziks Nnodum, USA.
Methyl salicylate (p.55·1); menthol (p.1632·3); capsaicin (p.23·1).
Musculoskeletal, joint, and soft-tissue disorders; neuralgia.

Zilactin
Note.This name is used for preparations of different composition.
Zila, Canad.
Benzyl alcohol (p.1135·2).
Lip lesions; mouth ulcers.
Zila, USA.
Tannic acid (p.1669·1).
Canker sores; herpes labialis.

Zilactin Baby Zila, Canad.
Benzocaine (p.1306·2).
Teething.

Zilactin-B Zila, Canad.
Benzocaine (p.1306·2).
Mouth disorders.

Zilactin-B Medicated Zila, USA.
Benzocaine (p.1306·2).
Sore throats.

Zilactin-L Zila, Canad.; Zila, USA.
Lignocaine [lidocaine] (p.1313·2).
Herpes labialis.

Zilactin-Lip Zila, Canad.
SPF 24: Octinoxate (p.1517·3); homosalate (p.1517·2); oxybenzone (p.1518·1); dimethicone (p.1410·1); menthol (p.1632·3).
Herpes labialis.

ZilaDent Zila, USA†.
Benzocaine (p.1306·2).
Local anaesthesia.

Zildem Parke-Med, S.Afr.
Diltiazem hydrochloride (p.874·3).
Angina pectoris; hypertension.

Zilden Dorom, Ital.
Diltiazem hydrochloride (p.874·3).
Angina pectoris; heart failure; myocardial infarction.

Zilese Pinewood, Irl.
Zopiclone (p.713·1).
Insomnia.

Zileze Opus, UK.
Zopiclone (p.713·1).
Insomnia.

Zilutrol Abbott, Switz.
Meloxicam (p.51·3).
Arthroses.

Zimadoce Rubio, Spain.
Cobamamide (p.1388·3).
Tonic.

Zimaina Zimaia, Port.†.
Aspirin (p.14·2); caffeine (p.761·3).
Fever; pain.

Zimbacol Link, UK.
Bezafibrate (p.849·1).
Hyperlipidaemias.

Zimerol Sons, Mex.
Cimetidine (p.1216·3).
Peptic ulcer.

Zimocel SIT, Ital.
Dried yeast (p.1398·1).

Zimoclone Gerard, Irl.
Zopiclone (p.713·1).
Insomnia.

Zimor Rubio, Spain.
Omeprazole (p.1239·1).
Gastro-oesophageal reflux; peptic ulcer; Zollinger-Ellison syndrome.

Zimospuma Baldacci, Ital.†.
Bovine fibrin (p.735·3).
Haemorrhage.

Zimotrombina Baldacci, Ital.†.
Thrombin (porcine) (p.741·3).
Haemorrhage.

Zimovane Rhone-Poulenc Rorer, Irl.; Rhone-Poulenc Rorer, UK.
Zopiclone (p.713·1).
Insomnia.

Zimox Pharmacia Upjohn, Ital.
Amoxicillin trihydrate (p.149·2).
This name has also been used for a preparation containing carbidopa and levodopa.
Bacterial infections.

Zinabol Makros, Braz.
Cobamamide (p.1388·3).
Reduced appetite; tonic.

Zinacef Glaxo Wellcome, Belg.; Glaxo Wellcome, Braz.; Glaxo Wellcome, Canad.; Glaxo Wellcome, Denm.; Glaxo Wellcome, Fin.; Glaxo Wellcome, Ger.; Glaxo Wellcome, Hong Kong; Glaxo Wellcome, Irl.; Glaxo Wellcome, Israel; Glaxo Wellcome, Neth.; Glaxo Wellcome, Norw.; Glaxo Wellcome, NZ; Glaxo Wellcome, S.Afr.; Glaxo Wellcome, Singapore; Glaxo Wellcome, Swed.; Glaxo Wellcome, Switz.; Glaxo Wellcome, Thai.; Glaxo Wellcome, UK; Glaxo Wellcome, USA.
Cefuroxime sodium (p.178·2).
Bacterial infections.

Zinaderm Technilab, Canad.
Zinc oxide (p.1128·2).
Skin disorders.

Zinadiur Sintofarm, Ital.
Benazepril hydrochloride (p.843·2); hydrochlorothiazide (p.907·3).
Hypertension.

Zinadril Sintofarm, Ital.
Benazepril hydrochloride (p.843·2).
Heart failure; hypertension.

Zinaf SoSe, Ital.
Propylene glycol cefatrizine (p.164·3).
Bacterial infections.

Zinamide Merck Sharp & Dohme, Austral.; Merck Sharp & Dohme, Irl.; Merck Sharp & Dohme, NZ; Merck Sharp & Dohme, UK.
Pyrazinamide (p.240·1).
Tuberculosis.

Zinasen Atral, Port.
Flunarizine hydrochloride (p.418·1).
Cerebral and peripheral vascular disorders; vertigo.

Zinat Glaxo Wellcome, Switz.
Cefuroxime axetil (p.178·1).
Bacterial infections.

Zinaxin Bionax, Hong Kong; Bionax, Singapore; Bionax, Thai.; Eurovita, Thai.; Vita Healthcare, Irl.
Ginger (p.1227·2).
Musculoskeletal and joint disorders.

Zinc B, E & C Puritan Quartz, Thai.
Multivitamin preparation with zinc (p.1350·1).

Zinc + C250 Vitaplex, Austral.
Zinc amino acid chelate (p.1398·3); ascorbic acid (p.1389·3).
Zinc deficiency.

Zinc C Plus Vitaglow, Austral.
Zinc amino acid chelate (p.1398·3); ascorbic acid (p.1389·3); vitamin B substances (p.1350·1).
Inflammation; skin disorders; wounds.

Zinc Cream White McGloin, Austral.
SPF 15+: Zinc oxide (p.1128·2).
Burns; nappy rash; skin abrasions; skin irritation; sunscreen.

Zinc Lotion Vitamed, Israel.
Zinc oxide (p.1128·2).
Skin irritation.

Zinc Menthol Vitamed, Israel.
Zinc oxide (p.1128·2); menthol (p.1632·3).
Skin irritation.

Zinc Plus
Note.This name is used for preparations of different composition.
Cenovis, Austral.; Vitelle, Austral.
Zinc amino acid chelate (p.1398·3); vitamins and minerals (p.1350·1).
Zinc deficiency.
Swiss Herbal, Canad.
Zinc gluconate (p.1398·2); vitamin C (p.1389·3).
Bio-Health, UK.
Zinc gluconate; vitamin B₆; magnesium (p.1350·1).

Zinc Supplement Vitaplex, Austral.
Zinc gluconate (p.1398·2); vitamins and minerals (p.1350·1).
Zinc deficiency.

Zinc Zenith Eagle, Austral.
Zinc gluconate (p.1398·2); zinc amino acid chelate (p.1398·3); alfalfa (p.1574·3); ascorbic acid (p.1389·3); maltase (p.1576·3); pyridoxine hydrochloride (p.1386·3); minerals (p.1350·1).
Zinc, vitamin C and vitamin B₆ supplement.

Zincaband *Seton Scholl, Austral.; Smith & Nephew, Swed.†; SSL, UK.*
Zinc oxide (p.1128·2).
Medicated bandage.

Zinca-Pak *Smith & Nephew SoloPak, USA.*
Zinc sulfate (p.1398·2).
Additive for intravenous total parenteral nutrition solutions.

Zincaps *Rhone-Poulenc Rorer, Austral.; Fisons, Hong Kong; Aventis, NZ; ST, Thai.*
Zinc sulfate (p.1398·2).
Zinc supplement.

Zincate *Paddock, USA.*
Zinc sulfate (p.1398·2).
Dietary supplement.

Zincation *Isdin, Spain.*
Pyrithione zinc (p.1122·1).
Scalp disorders.

Zincation Plus *Isdin, Spain.*
Pyrithione zinc (p.1122·1); coal tar (p.1125·1).
Scalp disorders.

Zincfrin *Alcon, Austral.; Alcon, Belg.; Alcon, Canad.; Alcon, Denm.; Alcon, Fin.; Alcon, Ger.; Alcon, Neth.†; Alcon, NZ; Alcon, S.Afr.†; Alcon Cusi, Spain; Alcon, Swed.; Alcon, Switz.†; Alcon, Thai.; Alcon, USA.*
Phenylephrine hydrochloride (p.1097·1); zinc sulfate (p.1398·2).
Eye irritation.

Zincfrin Antihistaminicum *Alcon, Belg.*
Antazoline phosphate (p.408·3); naphazoline hydrochloride (p.1095·1); zinc sulfate (p.1398·2).
Formerly known as Zincfrin-A.
Conjunctival congestion; eye irritation.

Zincfrin-A *Alcon, Canad.; Alcon, Fin.; Alcon, S.Afr.†.*
Antazoline phosphate (p.408·3); naphazoline hydrochloride (p.1095·1); zinc sulfate (p.1398·2).
Allergic conjunctivitis.

Zinc-Ichtyol *Asta Medica, Belg.*
Zinc oxide (p.1128·2); ichthammol (p.1115·2).
Blepharitis; eczema and pruritus of the eye.

Zinc-Imizol *Farmigea, Ital.*
Zinc sulfate (p.1398·2); naphazoline nitrate (p.1095·1).
Conjunctivitis, alone or associated with blepharitis.

Zinco All' Acqua *Lachifarma, Ital.; Sella, Ital.*
Zinc oxide (p.1128·2).
Skin disorders.

Zincod *Vitamed, Israel.*
Zinc oxide (p.1128·2); cod-liver oil (p.1357·2); kaolin (p.1229·3).
Nappy rash; skin irritation.

Zincoderm *Taro, Canad.; Bersan, Ital.*
Zinc oxide (p.1128·2).
Skin disorders.

Zincoderma *Confar, Port.*
Zinc oxide (p.1128·2).

Zincofax *Warner-Lambert, Canad.*
Zinc oxide (p.1128·2).
Nappy rash.

Zincol *Sam-On, Israel.*
Zinc sulfate (p.1398·2).
Skin ulcers; wounds; zinc deficiency.

Zincolok *Allergan-Frumtost, Braz.*
Zinc sulfate (p.1398·2); naphazoline hydrochloride (p.1095·1).
Ocular congestion.

Zincometil *Farmila, Ital.*
Benzalkonium chloride (p.1133·2); zinc sulfate (p.1398·2).
Eye disinfection.

Zincon *Lederle, USA.*
Pyrithione zinc (p.1122·1).
Scalp disorders.

Zincopan *Gunther, Braz.*
Zinc sulfate (p.1398·2).
Zinc deficiency.

Zincoral *Mavi, Ital.*
Zinc and copper supplement (p.1350·1).

Zincosol *Bioceuticals, UK.*
Zinc sulfate (p.1398·2).

Zincotape *Lohmann, Ital.*
Zinc oxide (p.1128·2).
Medicated dressing.

Zincotex *Lohmann, Ital.*
Zinc oxide (p.1128·2).
Medicated dressing.

Zincream *Medinova, Switz.*
Zinc oxide (p.1128·2).
Nappy rash; wounds.

Zincstic *Vitalia, UK.*
Zinc oxide (p.1128·2); titanium dioxide (p.1126·1).
Sunscreen.

Zinctab *Pharmasant, Thai.*
Zinc (p.1398·1).
Zinc supplement.

Zincum valerianicum-Hevert *Hevert, Ger.*
Homoeopathic preparation.

Zincvit *Kenwood, USA.*
Multivitamin and mineral preparation (p.1350·1).

Zinecard *Pharmacia Upjohn, Canad.; Pharmacia Upjohn, USA.*
Dexrazoxane (p.1006·2) or dexrazoxane hydrochloride (p.1006·2).
Prevention of doxorubicin cardiotoxicity.

Zineryt *Yamanouchi, Belg.; Hermal, Ger.; Yamanouchi, Irl.; Yamanouchi, Ital.; Yamanouchi, Neth.; Yamanouchi, Port.; Yamanouchi, Spain; Yamanouchi, UK.*
Erythromycin (p.201·2); zinc acetate (p.1398·1).
Acne.

Zinga *Ashbourne, UK.*
Nizatidine (p.1238·1).
Gastro-oesophageal reflux; peptic ulcer.

Zink beta *Betapharm, Ger.*
Zinc sulfate (p.1398·2).
Zinc deficiency.

Zink Verla *Verla, Ger.*
Zinc gluconate (p.1398·2).
Zinc deficiency.

Zinkamin *Folk, Ger.*
Bis(L-histadinato) zinc (p.1398·3).
Zinc deficiency.

Zinkbrause *Verla, Ger.*
Zinc sulfate (p.1398·2).
Zinc deficiency.

Zink-Calmitol *OBA, Denm.*
Camphor (p.1589·3); hyoscyamus oil (p.470·1); menthol (p.1632·3); zinc oxide (p.1128·2).
Pruritus.

Zink-D Longoral *Artesan, Ger.; Cassella-med, Ger.*
Zinc gluconate (p.1398·2).
Zinc deficiency.

Zinkit *Worwag, Ger.*
Zinc sulfate (p.1398·2).
Zinc deficiency.

Zink'N'Swim *Or-Dov, Austral.*
SPF 15+: Zinc oxide (p.1128·2).
Sunscreen.

Zinkokehl *Sanum-Kehlbeck, Ger.*
Homoeopathic preparation.

Zinkolie *Boots Healthcare, Neth.*
Zinc oxide (p.1128·2).
Skin disorders.

Zinkorell *Sanorell, Ger.*
Injection: Homoeopathic preparation.
Tablets: Zinc oxide (p.1128·2).
Zinc deficiency.

Zinkorot *Worwag, Ger.*
Zinc orotate (p.1398·3).
Zinc deficiency.

Zinkosalb *Hilarys, Canad.*
Salicylic acid (p.1122·3); zinc oxide (p.1128·2).

zinkotase *Biosyn, Ger.*
Zinc aspartate.
Zinc deficiency.

Zinkpaste *LAW, Ger.*
Zinc oxide (p.1128·2).
Skin disorders; skin ulcers; wounds.

Zinksalbe *CT, Ger.*
Zinc oxide (p.1128·2); cod-liver oil (p.1357·2); glycerol (p.1616·3).
Wounds.

Zinksalbe Dialon *Engelhard, Ger.*
Zinc oxide (p.1128·2).
Skin disorders; wounds.

Zink-Sandoz *Novartis Consumer, Ger.*
Zinc sulfate (p.1398·2).
Zinc deficiency.

Zinkzalf *Boots Healthcare, Neth.*
Zinc oxide (p.1128·2).
Skin disorders.

Zinnat *Glaxo Wellcome, Aust.; Glaxo Wellcome, Austral.; Glaxo Wellcome, Belg.; Glaxo Wellcome, Braz.; Glaxo Wellcome, Denm.; Glaxo Wellcome, Fr.; Glaxo Wellcome, Fr.; Glaxo Wellcome, Hong Kong; Glaxo Wellcome, Irl.; Glaxo Wellcome, Israel; Glaxo Wellcome, Ital.; Glaxo Wellcome, Mex.; Glaxo Wellcome, Neth.; Glaxo Wellcome, NZ; Glaxo Wellcome, S.Afr.; Glaxo Wellcome, Singapore; Glaxo Wellcome, Spain; Glaxo Wellcome, Swed.; Glaxo Wellcome, Thai.; Glaxo Wellcome, UK.*
Cefuroxime axetil (p.178·1) or cefuroxime sodium (p.178·2).
Lignocaine [lidocaine] hydrochloride (p.1313·2) is included in some intramuscular injections to alleviate the pain of injection.
Formerly known as Curoxime in *Fr.*
Bacterial infections.

Zinnkraut-Tropfen *Bio-Diat, Ger.*
Equisetum (p.1606·3).
Urinary-tract disorders.

Zintona *Boehringer Ingelheim, Aust.; Herbalist, Ger.; Chrisana, Switz.*
Ginger (p.1227·2).
Digestive system disorders; gastric pain; motion sickness; vomiting.

Zinvit *Vitaglow, Austral.*
Zinc sulfate (p.1398·2); magnesium sulfate (p.1191·1); vitamin B substances (p.1350·1).
Herpes labialis; mouth ulcers; skin disorders; wounds; zinc deficiency.

Zinvit C *Vitaglow, Austral.*
Zinc sulfate (p.1398·2); magnesium sulfate (p.1191·1); ascorbic acid (p.1389·3).
Herpes labialis; mouth ulcers; skin disorders; wounds.

Zinvit G *Vitaglow, Austral.*
Zinc sulfate (p.1398·2); magnesium sulfate (p.1191·1); vitamin B substances (p.1350·1).
Skin disorders; zinc deficiency.

Zipos *Columbia, Port.*
Cefuroxime axetil (p.178·1).
Bacterial infections.

Zipra *Columbia, Mex.*
Ciprofloxacin hydrochloride (p.182·3).
Bacterial infections.

Zipzoc *Smith & Nephew, Denm.; Smith & Nephew, Fin.; Smith & Nephew, Irl.; Smith & Nephew Healthcare, UK.*
Zinc oxide (p.1128·2) impregnated stocking.
Leg ulcers; venous insufficiency.

Zipzoc Salvstrumpa *Smith & Nephew, Swed.*
Zinc oxide (p.1128·2).
Formerly known as Salvstrumpa.
Skin ulcers; vascular disorders.

Ziradryl *Parke, Davis, USA.*
Diphenhydramine hydrochloride (p.416·1); zinc oxide (p.1128·2); camphor (p.1589·3).
Pruritus.

Zirkulin Beruhigungs-Tee *Schulke & Mayr, Aust.*
Lupulus (p.1629·3).
Restlessness; sleep disorders.

Zirtec *UCB, Ital.*
Cetirizine hydrochloride (p.411·2).
Conjunctivitis; rhinitis; urticaria.

Zirtek *UCB, Irl.; UCB, UK.*
Cetirizine hydrochloride (p.411·2).
Allergic rhinitis; pruritus; urticaria.

Zispin *Organon, Irl.; Organon, UK.*
Mirtazapine (p.299·1).
Depression.

Zita *Eastern Pharmaceuticals, UK.*
Cimetidine (p.1216·3).
Gastrointestinal disorders associated with hyperacidity.

Zitazonium *Thiemann, Ger.†; Egis, Hong Kong; Egis, Thai.*
Tamoxifen citrate (p.571·1).
Anovulatory infertility; breast cancer.

Zithromax *Pfizer, Aust.; Pfizer, Austral.; Pfizer, Canad.; Pfizer, Fin.; Pfizer, Fr.; Mack, Illert., Ger.; Bayer, Ger.; Pfizer, Hong Kong; Pfizer, Irl.; Pfizer, Neth.; Douglas, NZ; Pfizer, Port.; Pfizer, S.Afr.; Pfizer, Singapore; Pfizer, Switz.; Pfizer, Thai.; Pfizer, UK; Pfizer, USA.*
Azithromycin (p.153·1).
Bacterial infections.

Zitoxil *Italfarmaco, Ital.†.*
Zipeprol hydrochloride (p.1102·3).
Coughs.

Zitrix *Metapharma, Ital.*
Propylene glycol cefatrizine (p.164·3).
Bacterial infections.

Zitromax *Pfizer, Braz.; Pfizer, Braz.; Pfizer, Denm.; Pfizer, Ital.; Pfizer Consumer, Spain.*
Azithromycin (p.153·1).
Bacterial infections.

Ziverone *Rayere, Mex.*
Aciclovir (p.612·3).
Herpesvirus infections.

Ziz *Chatfield Laboratories, UK.*
Promethazine hydrochloride (p.423·2).
Insomnia.

Z-Max *Schering-Plough, Mex.*
Phentolamine mesilate (p.954·3).
Erectile dysfunction.

ZN 220 *Covan, S.Afr.*
Zinc sulfate (p.1398·2).
Wounds.

ZNP *Stiefel, Canad.; Stiefel, Fr.; Stiefel, Ital.; Stiefel, Mex.; Stiefel, USA.*
Pyrithione zinc (p.1122·1).
Scalp disorders; seborrhoeic dermatitis.

Zobacide *Aspen, S.Afr.*
Metronidazole (p.594·1).
Anaerobic bacterial infections; protozoal infections.

Zocor *Merck Sharp & Dohme, Austral.; Merck Sharp & Dohme, Belg.; Merck Sharp & Dohme, Braz.; Merck Frosst, Canad.; Merck Sharp & Dohme, Denm.; Merck Sharp & Dohme, Fin.; Merck Sharp & Dohme-Chibret, Fr.; Dieckmann, Ger.; Merck Sharp & Dohme, Hong Kong; Merck Sharp & Dohme, Irl.; Neopharmed, Ital.; Merck Sharp & Dohme, Mex.; Merck Sharp & Dohme, Neth.; Merck Sharp & Dohme, Norw.; Merck Sharp & Dohme, NZ; Merck Sharp & Dohme, Port.; Merck Sharp & Dohme, S.Afr.; Merck Sharp & Dohme, Singapore; Merck Sharp & Dohme, Spain; Merck Sharp & Dohme, Switz.; Merck Sharp & Dohme, Thai.; Merck Sharp & Dohme, UK; Merck, USA.*
Simvastatin (p.969·2).
Coronary atherosclerosis; hypercholesterolaemia; ischaemic heart disease.

Zocord *Merck Sharp & Dohme, Aust.; Merck Sharp & Dohme, Swed.*
Simvastatin (p.969·2).
Hypercholesterolaemia.

Zocovin *TO-Chemicals, Thai.*
Aciclovir (p.612·3).
Herpes simplex infections of the skin and mucous membranes.

Zodeac *Econo Med, USA.*
Ferrous fumarate (p.1360·1); folic acid (p.1361·1); multivitamins and minerals (p.1350·1).
Iron-deficiency anaemias.

Zofen *Pharmaland, Thai.*
Pizotifen (p.455·1).
Anorexia.

Zoff Note.This name is used for preparations of different composition.
Smith & Nephew, Austral.
Dipropylene glycol methyl ether.
Adhesive plaster remover.

Smith & Nephew Pharmaceuticals, UK.
Trichloroethane (p.1406·2).
Adhesive plaster removal.

Zofora *Pharmy, Fr.*
Piroxicam (p.79·1).
Musculoskeletal, joint, and peri-articular disorders.

Zofran *Glaxo Wellcome, Aust.; Glaxo Wellcome, Austral.; Glaxo Wellcome, Belg.; Glaxo Wellcome, Braz.; Glaxo Wellcome, Canad.; Glaxo Wellcome, Denm.; Glaxo Wellcome, Fin.; Glaxo Wellcome, Fr.; Glaxo Wellcome, Ger.; Glaxo Wellcome, Hong Kong; Glaxo Wellcome, Irl.; Glaxo Wellcome, Israel; Glaxo Wellcome, Ital.; Glaxo Wellcome, Mex.; Glaxo Wellcome, Neth.; Glaxo Wellcome, Norw.; Glaxo Wellcome, NZ; Glaxo Wellcome, Port.; Glaxo Wellcome, S.Afr.; Glaxo Wellcome, Singapore; Glaxo Wellcome, Spain; Glaxo Wellcome, Swed.; Glaxo Wellcome, Switz.; Glaxo Wellcome, Thai.; Glaxo Wellcome, UK; Glaxo Wellcome, USA.*
Ondansetron (p.1241·3) or ondansetron hydrochloride (p.1241·3).
Nausea and vomiting induced by cytotoxics or radiotherapy; postoperative nausea and vomiting.

Zok-Zid *Astra, Belg.; Searle, Denm.*
Metoprolol succinate (p.932·1); hydrochlorothiazide (p.907·3).
Hypertension.

Zolac *Xepa-Soul Pattinson, Hong Kong.*
Bromocriptine mesilate (p.1164·3).
Acromegaly; benign breast disease; female infertility; galactorrhoea; hypogonadism; lactation inhibition; menstrual disorders; parkinsonism; prolactinomas.

Zoladex *Zeneca, Aust.; Zeneca, Austral.; Zeneca, Belg.; Zeneca, Braz.; Astra-Zeneca, Canad.; AstraZeneca, Denm.; AstraZeneca, Fin.; AstraZeneca, Fr.; Zeneca, Ger.; Zeneca, Hong Kong; Zeneca, Irl.; Zeneca, Israel; Zeneca, Ital.; Zeneca, Mex.; Zeneca, Neth.; AstraZeneca, Norw.; AstraZeneca, NZ; Zeneca, Port.; Zeneca, S.Afr.; AstraZeneca, Singapore; Zeneca, Spain; Zeneca, Swed.; Zeneca, Switz.; AstraZeneca, Thai.; AstraZeneca, UK; Zeneca, USA.*
Goserelin (p.1285·2) or goserelin acetate (p.1285·2).
Breast cancer; endometriosis; female infertility; presurgical endometrial thinning; prostatic cancer; uterine fibroids.

Zolaten *Sigma, Austral.; Pharmaco, NZ.*
Aciclovir (p.612·3).
Herpes labialis.

Zolben Note.This name is used for preparations of different composition.
Sanofi Winthrop, Braz.
Albendazole (p.95·2).
Worm infections.

Novartis, Spain†; Novartis Consumer, Switz.
Paracetamol (p.71·2).
Fever; pain.

Zolben C *Novartis Consumer, Switz.*
Paracetamol (p.71·2); ascorbic acid (p.1389·3).
Fever; pain.

Zoldan-A *Cryopharma, Mex.*
Danazol (p.1468·3).

Zoleprim *PP Lab, Thai.*
Co-trimoxazole (p.193·3).
Bacterial infections.

Zoleptil *Orion, UK.*
Zotepine (p.713·3).
Schizophrenia.

Zolerol *Rolab, S.Afr.*
Metronidazole (p.594·1).
Anaerobic bacterial infections; protozoal infections.

Zoles *Iodo Suma, Braz.*
Mebendazole (p.102·3); tiabendazole (p.109·1).
Worm infections.

Zolicef *Bristol-Myers Squibb, Aust.; Apothecon, USA.*
Cefazolin sodium (p.164·3).
Lignocaine [lidocaine] hydrochloride (p.1313·2) is included in the intramuscular injection to alleviate the pain of injection.

Zolidin *Kener, Mex.*
Dipyrone (p.34·1).
Fever; pain.

Zolim *Schwarz, Ger.*
Mizolastine (p.421·3).
Allergic conjunctivitis; allergic rhinitis; urticaria.

Zolin Note.This name is used for preparations of different composition.
San Carlo, Ital.
Cefazolin sodium (p.164·3).
Lignocaine [lidocaine] hydrochloride (p.1313·2) is included in the intramuscular injection to alleviate the pain of injection.
Bacterial infections.

Abigo, Swed.
Oxymetazoline hydrochloride (p.1096·2).
Rhinitis; sinusitis.

Zolina *Llorens, Spain.*
Boric acid (p.1586·1); naphazoline hydrochloride (p.1095·1).
Eye irritation.

Zoliparin *Mann, Ger.*
Aciclovir (p.612·3).
Herpes simplex eye infections.

Zolisint *Benedetti, Ital.†.*
Cefazolin sodium (p.164·3).
Lignocaine [lidocaine] hydrochloride (p.1313·2) is included in this preparation to alleviate the pain of injection.
Bacterial infections.

Zolistam *Angelini, Ital.; Lepori, Port.*
Mizolastine (p.421·3).
Allergic conjunctivitis; allergic rhinitis; urticaria.

Zolistan *Novag, Spain.*
Mizolastine (p.421·3).
Allergic conjunctivitis; allergic rhinitis; urticaria.

Zolival *Reig Jofre, Spain; Septa, Spain.*
Cefazolin sodium (p.164·3).
Formerly known as Cefabiot.
Bacterial infections.

Zolken *Kener, Mex.*
Itraconazole (p.387·2).
Fungal infections.

Zoloft *Pfizer, Aust.†; Pfizer, Austral.; Pfizer, Braz.; Pfizer, Canad.; Pfizer, Denm.; Pfizer, Fin.; Pfizer, Fr.; Pfizer, Ger.; Pfizer, Hong Kong; Roerig, Ital.; Pfizer, Neth.; Pfizer, Norw.; Douglas, NZ; Pfizer, Port.; Pfizer, S.Afr.; Pfizer, Singapore; Pfizer, Swed.; Pfizer, Switz.; Pfizer, Thai.; Pfizer, USA.*
Sertraline hydrochloride (p.308·3).
Depression; obsessive-compulsive disorder; panic disorder; post-traumatic stress disorder.

Zoltec *Pfizer, Braz.*
Fluconazole (p.383·2).
Fungal infections.

Zolterol *CCM, Singapore.*
Diclofenac sodium (p.30·3).
Musculoskeletal, joint, peri-articular, and soft-tissue disorders; pain.

Zol-Triq *Medley, Braz.*
Mebendazole (p.102·2).
Worm infections.

Zoltum *Rhone-Poulenc Rorer, Fr.*
Omeprazole (p.1239·1).
Gastro-oesophageal reflux; peptic ulcer; Zollinger-Ellison syndrome.

Zolvera *Rosemont, UK.*
Verapamil hydrochloride (p.989·1).
Angina pectoris; arrhythmias; hypertension.

Zomacton *Ferring, Belg.; Ferring, Denm.; Ferring, Fin.; Ferring, Fr.; Ferring, Ger.; Ferring, Irl.; Ferring, Ital.; Ferring, Neth.; Ferring, Norw.; Ferring, Port.; Ferring, Spain; Ferring, Swed.; Ferring, UK.*
Somatropin (p.1286·1).
Growth disorders in renal failure; growth hormone deficiency; Turner's syndrome.

Zometa *Novartis, Austral.; Novartis, UK; Novartis, USA.*
Zoledronic acid (p.756·3).
Hypercalcaemia of malignancy.

Zomig *Zeneca, Aust.; Zeneca, Austral.; Zeneca, Belg.; AstraZeneca, Canad.; AstraZeneca, Denm.; AstraZeneca, Fin.; AstraZeneca, Fr.; Zeneca, Hong Kong; AstraZeneca, Irl.; Zeneca, Israel; Zeneca, Ital.; Zeneca, Mex.; Zeneca, Neth.; Zeneca, Norw.; Zeneca, Port.; Zeneca, S.Afr.; AstraZeneca, Singapore; Zeneca, Spain; Zeneca, Swed.; Zeneca, Switz.; AstraZeneca, Thai.; AstraZeneca, UK; Zeneca, USA.*
Zolmitriptan (p.458·1).
Migraine.

Zomorph *Link, UK.*
Morphine sulfate (p.56·1).
Pain.

Zon *Antula, Swed.*
Ketoprofen (p.47·3).
Musculoskeletal and joint disorders; sports injuries.

Zonal *Galen, Mex.*
Fluconazole (p.383·2).
Fungal infections.

Zonalon *Medicis, Canad.; Medicis, USA.*
Doxepin hydrochloride (p.283·3).
Pruritus.

Zoncef *AGIPS, Ital.*
Cefoperazone sodium (p.168·2).
Lignocaine [lidocaine] hydrochloride (p.1313·2) is included in the intramuscular injection to alleviate the pain of injection.
Bacterial infections.

Zondar *Niverpharm, Fr.*
Diacerein (p.28·3).
Osteoarthritis.

Zone-A *UAD, USA.*
Hydrocortisone acetate (p.1073·3); pramocaine (p.1318·2).

Zonegran *Elan, USA.*
Zonisamide (p.371·2).
Epilepsy.

Zonite *Menley & James, USA.*
Benzalkonium chloride (p.1133·2); edetic acid (p.1008·3); sodium acetate (p.1186·1); propylene glycol (p.1655·1); menthol (p.1632·3); thymol (p.1158·3).
Vaginal disorders.

Zonivent *Ashbourne, UK†.*
Beclometasone dipropionate (p.1061·2).
Rhinitis.

Zonulasi *Merck Sharp & Dohme, Ital.†.*
Chymotrypsin (p.1595·1).
Eye surgery.

Zonulysin *Covan, S.Afr.†; Henleys, UK†.*
Chymotrypsin (p.1595·1).
Adjunct in cataract extraction.

Zoo Chews *Hall, Canad.*
Multivitamin preparation (p.1350·1).

Zoo Chews with Iron *Hall, Canad.*
Multivitamin preparation with iron (p.1350·1).

Zopam *Pharmasant, Thai.*
Diazepam (p.674·3).
Anxiety; insomnia; skeletal muscle spasm.

Zopax *Cipla-Medpro, S.Afr.*
Alprazolam (p.654·2).
Anxiety disorders; mixed anxiety depressive states; panic attacks.

Zophren *Glaxo Wellcome, Fr.*
Ondansetron (p.1241·3) or ondansetron hydrochloride (p.1241·3).
Nausea and vomiting.

Zopimed *Parke-Med, S.Afr.*
Zopiclone (p.713·1).
Insomnia.

Zopinox *Orion, Fin.*
Zopiclone (p.713·1).
Sleep disorders.

Zopitan *Clonmel, Irl.*
Zopiclone (p.713·1).
Insomnia.

Zorac *Allergan, Aust.; Bioglan, Fin.; Pierre Fabre, Fr.; Pierre Fabre Dermo Kosmetik, Ger.; Bioglan, Irl.; Pierre Fabre, Ital.; Pierre Fabre, Spain; Bioglan, Swed.; Bioglan, UK.*
Tazarotene (p.1125·3).
Psoriasis.

Zorak *Genop, S.Afr.*
Tazarotene (p.1125·3).
Psoriasis.

Zoral *DHA, Singapore.*
Aciclovir (p.612·3).
Herpesvirus infections.

Zoran *Reddy, Singapore.*
Ranitidine hydrochloride (p.1245·2).
Dyspepsia; gastro-oesophageal reflux; peptic ulcer; Zollinger-Ellison syndrome.

Zorclone *Norton Waterford, Irl.*
Zopiclone (p.713·1).
Insomnia.

Zoref *Duncan, Ital.; Glaxo Wellcome, Port.*
Cefuroxime axetil (p.178·1).
Bacterial infections.

Zorinax *Xepa-Soul Pattinson, Singapore.*
Ketoconazole (p.389·1).
Dandruff; fungal infections; seborrhoeic dermatitis.

Zoroxin *Merck Sharp & Dohme, Aust.; Merck Sharp & Dohme, Belg.; Merck Sharp & Dohme, Denm.*
Norfloxacin (p.232·1).
Bacterial infections.

ZORprin *Boots, USA.*
Aspirin (p.14·2).
Fever; osteoarthritis; pain; rheumatoid arthritis.

Zoru *E-Z-EM, Belg.*
Tartaric acid (p.1669·2); sodium bicarbonate (p.1186·2); dimethicone (p.1249·2).
Gastrointestinal radiography.

Zost *Allergan-Frumtost, Braz.*
Trifluridine (p.642·2).
Herpes simplex eye infections.

Zostrix *Knoll, Austral.; Medicis, Canad.; Rafa, Israel; GenDerm, USA.*
Capsaicin (p.25·1).
Diabetic neuropathy; osteoarthritis; postherpetic neuralgia; rheumatoid arthritis.

Zostrum *Galderma, Ger.; Galderma, Irl.*
Idoxuridine (p.625·1) in dimethyl sulfoxide (p.2020·1).
Herpes simplex infections; herpes zoster.

Zosyn *Lederle, USA.*
Piperacillin sodium (p.236·1); tazobactam sodium (p.257·2).
Bacterial infections.

Zo-Tab *Pacific, NZ.*
Zopiclone (p.713·1).
Insomnia.

Zotinar *Cipan, Port.*
Desonide (p.1066·2).
Skin disorders.

Zoto-HC *Horizon, USA.*
Chloroxylenol (p.1142·1); pramocaine hydrochloride (p.1318·2); hydrocortisone (p.1073·3).
Formerly known as Xotic.
Ear disorders.

Zoton
Lederle, Austral.; Lederle, Irl.; Neopharm, Israel; Wyeth Lederle, Ital.; Lederle, NZ; Wyeth, UK.
Lansoprazole (p.1230·3).
Gastro-oesophageal reflux; peptic ulcer; Zollinger-Ellison syndrome.

Zov800 *Wellcome, Port.*
Aciclovir (p.612·3).
Herpesvirus infections.

Zovia *Watson, USA.*
Ethinylestradiol (p.1476·2); etynodiol diacetate (p.1477·1).
28-Day packs also contain 7 inert tablets.
Combined oral contraceptive.

Zoviplus *Glaxo Wellcome, Denm.†.*
Aciclovir (p.612·3).
Herpesvirus infections.

Zovir
Glaxo Wellcome, Denm.; Glaxo Wellcome, Swed.†.
Aciclovir (p.612·3) or aciclovir sodium (p.612·3).
Herpesvirus infections.

Zovirax
Glaxo Wellcome, Aust.; Glaxo Wellcome, Austral.; Glaxo Wellcome, Belg.; Glaxo Wellcome, Braz.; Glaxo Wellcome, Canad.; Glaxo Wellcome, Fin.; Glaxo Wellcome, Fr.; Boehringer Ingelheim, Ger.; Glaxo Wellcome, Ger.; Glaxo Wellcome, Hong Kong; Wellcome, Irl.; Warner-Lambert, Irl.; Glaxo Wellcome, Israel; Glaxo Wellcome, Ital.; Glaxo Wellcome, Mex.; Glaxo Wellcome, Neth.; Glaxo Wellcome, Norw.; Glaxo Wellcome, NZ; Wellcome, Port.; Wellcome, S.Afr.; Glaxo Wellcome, Singapore; Wellcome, Spain; Glaxo Wellcome, Swed.; Glaxo Wellcome, Switz.; Glaxo Wellcome, Thai.; Wellcome, UK; Glaxo Wellcome, USA.
Aciclovir (p.612·3) or aciclovir sodium (p.612·3).
Herpesvirus infections.

Zoxil *Xixia, S.Afr.*
Amoxicillin trihydrate (p.149·2).
Bacterial infections.

Zoxin *Opus, UK†.*
Flucloxacillin sodium (p.207·1).
Gram-positive bacterial infections.

ZP 11 *Revlon, Canad.*
Pyrithione zinc (p.1122·1).

ZP Dermil *Oftalder, Port.*
Pyrithione zinc (p.1122·1).

Z-Pam *Rolab, S.Afr.†.*
Temazepam (p.707·2).
Hypnotic.

Z-Plus *Dormer, Canad.*
Pyrithione zinc (p.1122·1); menthol (p.1632·3).
Seborrhoeic dermatitis.

ZSC *Sigma, Austral.*
Zinc oxide (p.1128·2); starch (p.1379·3); chlorphenesin (p.381·3).
Hyperhidrosis; nappy rash; skin irritation.

Zubes *Ernest Jackson, UK.*
Menthol (p.1632·3); anise oil (p.1580·3).

Zubes Blackcurrant *Ernest Jackson, UK.*
Citric acid (p.1596·2); menthol (p.1632·3); anise oil (p.1580·3).

Zubes Honey & Lemon *Ernest Jackson, UK.*
Honey (p.1366·2); citric acid (p.1596·2); menthol (p.1632·3).

zuk rheuma *Byk Gulden, Ger.; Roland, Ger.*
Glycol salicylate (p.42·2).
Musculoskeletal, joint, peri-articular, and soft-tissue disorders; neuralgia.

zuk thermo *Byk Gulden, Ger.; Roland, Ger.*
Glycol salicylate (p.42·2); benzyl nicotinate (p.20·2).
Musculoskeletal and joint disorders.

Zulex *Almirall, Spain.*
Acamprosate calcium (p.653·3).
Alcoholism.

Zumalgic *Amido, Fr.*
Tramadol hydrochloride (p.89·1).
Pain.

Zumba *Crefar, Port.*
Yohimbine hydrochloride (p.1681·3).
Erectile dysfunction.

Zumenon
Solvay, Aust.; Solvay, Austral.; Solvay, Belg.; Solvay, Fin.; Solvay, Neth.; Solvay, Port.; Solvay, Switz.; Solvay, UK.
Estradiol (p.1473·1).
Menopausal disorders; oestrogen deficiency; osteoporosis.

Zumeston *Duphar, Neth.†.*
28 tablets, estradiol (Zumenon) (p.1473·1); 14 tablets, dydrogesterone (Duphaston) (p.1472·3).
Menopausal disorders.

Zumetil *20th Century, Mex.*
Methylene blue [methylthioninium chloride] (p.1012·3).

Zunden *Luitpold, Ital.†.*
Piroxicam (p.79·1).
Rheumatic disorders.

Zurcal *Nycomed, Aust.; Novartis, Braz.; Novartis, Mex.; Novartis, Port.; Nycomed, Switz.*
Pantoprazole sodium (p.1243·2).
Gastritis; gastro-oesophageal reflux; peptic ulcer; Zollinger-Ellison syndrome.

Zurcale *Exel, Belg.*
Pantoprazole sodium (p.1243·2).
Gastro-oesophageal reflux; peptic ulcer.

Zurim *Atral-Vida, Port.*
Allopurinol (p.397·2).
Gout; hyperuricaemia.

Zwitsalax/N *Roche Nicholas, Neth.†.*
Bisacodyl (p.1212·2).
Constipation.

Zwitsanal *Roche Nicholas, Neth.†.*
Bismuth subnitrate (p.1213·2); zinc oxide (p.1128·2); lignocaine [lidocaine] (p.1313·2).
Haemorrhoids.

Zwitsavit-D *Roche Nicholas, Neth.†.*
Calcium carbonate (p.1215·1); colecalciferol (p.1391·1).
Calcium or vitamin D deficiency.

Zyban *Glaxo Wellcome, Austral.; Glaxo Wellcome, Canad.; Glaxo Wellcome, Irl.; Glaxo Wellcome, Port.; Glaxo Wellcome, UK; Glaxo Wellcome, USA.*
Bupropion hydrochloride (p.280·1).
Aid to smoking withdrawal.

Zyclir *Amrad, Austral.*
Aciclovir (p.612·3) or aciclovir sodium (p.612·3).
Herpesvirus infections; HIV infection.

Zyderm *Collagen, Aust.; Collagen, Austral.; Collagen, Fr.; Collagen, Ger.; Collagen Corp, Hong Kong; TC Technocare, Israel; Collagen, Singapore.*
Collagen (bovine) (p.1598·2).
Lignocaine [lidocaine] (p.1313·2) may be included in this preparation to alleviate the pain of implantation.
Skin contour defects.

Zydol *Searle, Irl.; Pharmacia, UK.*
Tramadol hydrochloride (p.89·1).
Pain.

Zydone *Endo, USA.*
Hydrocodone tartrate (p.42·2); paracetamol (p.71·2).
Pain.

Zyflo *Abbott, USA.*
Zileuton (p.786·2).
Asthma.

Zygout *Amrad, Austral.†.*
Allopurinol (p.397·2).
Gout; hyperuricaemia; renal calculi.

Zykolat-EDO *Mann, Ger.*
Cyclopentolate hydrochloride (p.465·2).
Production of mydriasis and cycloplegia.

Zylium *Farmosa, Braz.*
Ranitidine hydrochloride (p.1245·2).
Acid aspiration; gastro-oesophageal reflux; gastrointestinal haemorrhage; peptic ulcer; Zollinger-Ellison syndrome.

Zylol *Teva, Israel.*
Allopurinol (p.397·2).
Gout; hyperuricaemia; uric acid nephropathy.

Zyloprim *Glaxo Wellcome, Austral.; Glaxo Wellcome, Canad.; Glaxo Wellcome, Mex.; Glaxo Wellcome, NZ; Glaxo Wellcome, S.Afr.; Faro, USA.*
Allopurinol (p.397·2).
Gout; hyperuricaemia; renal calculi; uric acid nephropathy.

Zyloric *Glaxo Wellcome, Aust.; Glaxo Wellcome, Belg.; Glaxo Wellcome, Braz.; Glaxo Wellcome, Fin.; Glaxo Wellcome, Fr.; Glaxo Wellcome, Ger.; Glaxo Wellcome, Hong Kong; Wellcome, Irl.; Glaxo Wellcome, Israel; Glaxo Wellcome, Ital.; Glaxo Wellcome, Neth.; Glaxo Wellcome, Norw.; Wellcome, Port.†.; Glaxo Wellcome, Singapore; Wellcome, Spain; Glaxo Wellcome, Swed.; Wellcome, Switz.; Glaxo Wellcome, Thai.; Wellcome, UK.*
Allopurinol (p.397·2).
Gout; hyperuricaemia; renal calculi.

Zymacap *Roberts, USA.*
Multivitamin preparation (p.1350·1).

Zyma-D2 *Novartis Sante, Fr.*
Ergocalciferol (p.1391·2).
Vitamin D deficiency.

Zymaduo *Novartis Sante, Fr.*
Sodium fluoride (p.1375·3); colecalciferol (p.1391·1).
Dental caries prophylaxis; rickets.

Zymafluor *Novartis Consumer, Aust.; Novartis Sante, Fr.; Novartis Consumer, Ger.; Novartis, Israel; Novartis Consumer, Ital.; Novartis Consumer, Neth.; Novartis Consumer, Port.; Novartis Consumer, S.Afr.; Novartis Consumer, Spain; Novartis Consumer, Switz.; Novartis, Thai.*
Sodium fluoride (p.1375·3).
Dental caries prophylaxis.

Zymafluor D *Novartis Consumer, Ger.*
Sodium fluoride (p.1375·3); colecalciferol (p.1391·1).
Dental caries prophylaxis; rickets.

Zymase *Organon, USA.*
Pancrelipase (p.1647·2).
Pancreatic enzyme deficiency.

Zymelin *Nycomed, Denm.; Nycomed, Norw.*
Xylometazoline hydrochloride (p.1102·3).
Otitis; rhinitis; sinusitis.

Zymerol *Sons, Mex.*
Cimetidine (p.1216·3).

Zymizinc *Aguettant, Fr.*
Zinc gluconate (p.1398·2).
Zinc deficiency.

Zymoplex
Note. This name is used for preparations of different composition.
Laphal, Fr.
Porcine pancreatic amylolytic enzymes; polyenzyme from *Aspergillus*; lipase from *Rhizopus*; dimethicone (p.1249·2).
Dyspepsia; meteorism.

The symbol † denotes a preparation no longer actively marketed

Sodip, Switz.

Pancreatic protease and amylase; enzymes of *Aspergillus oryzae*; amylase (p.1579·3); protease; cellulase (p.1593·1); lipase; dimethicone (p.1249·2).

Dyspepsia; flatulence.

Zynal *Korean Drug, Singapore.*

Naproxen sodium (p.61·1).

Gout; musculoskeletal, joint, and peri-articular disorders; pain.

Zynox *Intramed, S.Afr.*

Naloxone hydrochloride (p.1014·3).

Opioid toxicity.

Zyomet *Goldshield, UK.*

Metronidazole (p.594·1).

Rosacea.

Zyplast

Collagen, Aust.; Collagen, Austral.; Collagen, Fr.†; Collagen, Ger.; Collagen Corp, Hong Kong; TC Technocare, Israel; Collagen, Singapore.

Collagen (bovine) (p.1598·2).

Lignocaine [lidocaine] (p.1313·2) may be included in this preparation to alleviate the pain of injection.

Skin contour defects.

Zyplo *Pfizer, Mex.*

Levodropropizine (p.1089·3).

Coughs.

Zyprexa

Lilly, Aust.; Lilly, Austral.; Lilly, Belg.; Lilly, Canad.; Lilly, Denm.; Lilly, Fin.; Lilly, Fr.; Lilly, Ger.; Lilly, Hong Kong; Lilly, Irl.; Lilly, Israel; Lilly, Mex.; Lilly, Neth.; Lilly, Norw.; Lilly, NZ; Lilly, Port.; Lilly, S.Afr.; Lilly, Singapore.; Lilly, Spain; Lilly, Swed.; Lilly, Switz.; Lilly, Thai.; Lilly, UK; Lilly, USA.

Olanzapine (p.696·1).

Psychoses.

Zyrex *Masa, Thai.*

Cetirizine hydrochloride (p.411·2).

Allergic conjunctivitis; allergic rhinitis; allergic skin disorders.

Zyrlex *UCB, Swed.*

Cetirizine hydrochloride (p.411·2).

Allergic conjunctivitis; allergic rhinitis; pruritus; urticaria.

Zyrtec

UCB, Aust.; Faulding, Austral.; UCB, Belg.; Glaxo Wellcome, Braz.; UCB, Canad.; UCB, Denm.; UCB, Fin.; UCB, Fr.; UCB, Ger.; Rodleben, Ger.; Vedim, Ger.; UCB, Hong Kong; Dexcel, Israel; UCB, Jpn; Sumitomo, Jpn; Lakeside, Mex.; UCB, Neth.; UCB, Norw.; Pharmabroker, NZ; UCB, Port.; UCB, S.Afr.; UCB, Singapore; UCB, Spain; UCB, Switz.; UCB, Thai.; Pfizer, USA.

Cetirizine hydrochloride (p.411·2).

Allergic conjunctivitis; allergic rhinitis; allergic skin disorders; urticaria.

Zyrtec-D

Lakeside, Mex.; Pfizer, USA.

Cetirizine hydrochloride (p.411·2); pseudoephedrine hydrochloride (p.1099·2).

Allergic rhinitis; nasal congestion.

Zyrzine *Pharmasant, Thai.*

Cetirizine hydrochloride (p.411·2).

Allergic conjunctivitis; allergic skin disorders; rhinitis.

Zytine *LSP, Thai.*

Cetirizine hydrochloride (p.411·2).

Allergic conjunctivitis; allergic skin disorders; rhinitis.

Zytrim *Merckle, Ger.*

Azathioprine (p.509·3).

Auto-immune disorders; organ transplantation.

Zyvox

Pharmacia, UK; Pharmacia Upjohn, USA.

Linezolid (p.219·3).

Gram-positive bacterial infections.

Directory of Manufacturers

The names and addresses of the manufacturers or distributors of the products and proprietary medicines mentioned in Martindale are listed below in alphabetical order of the abbreviated names used in Part 3.

20th Century, Mex. 20th Century, Mexico.

3M, Austral. 3M Pharmaceuticals P/L, 9-15 Chilvers Rd, Thornleigh, NSW 2120, Australia.

3M, Belg. 3M Pharma S.A., Hermeslaan 7, 1831 Diegem, Belgium.

3M, Canad. 3M Pharmaceuticals, P.O. Box 5757, London, Ontario, N6A 4T1, Canada.

3M, Denm. 3M Pharma, Fabriksparken 15, 2600 Glostrup, Denmark.

3M, Fin. Soumen 3M Oy/3M Pharma, Lars Sonckin kaari 6, PL 90, 02601 Espoo, Finland.

3M, Fr. Laboratoires 3M Santé, Bd de l'Oise, 95029 Cergy-Pontoise cdx, France.

3M, Ger. 3M Medica, Gelsenkirchener Str. 11, 46325 Borken, Germany.

3M, Hong Kong. 3M Hong Kong Ltd, 5/F Victoria Ctr, 15 Watson Rd, North Point, Hong Kong.

3M, Irl. See *United Drug, Irl.*

3M, Israel. 3M Israel Ltd, 91 Medinat Hayehudim Street, Herzliya-Pituah 46120, Israel.

3M, Ital. 3M Italia s.p.a., Via S Bovio 3, Loc. S Felice, 20090 Segrate (MI), Italy.

3M, Mex. 3M Mexico, S.A. de C.V., Avenida Santa Fe #55, Col. Santa Fe, 01210 Mexico, D.F., Mexico.

3M, Neth. 3M Pharma Nederland B.V., Postbus 193, 2300 AD Leiden, Netherlands.

3M, Norw. 3M Pharma, Hvamv.6, Postboks 100, 2013 Skjetten, Norway.

3M, NZ. 3M Pharmaceuticals, Division of 3M New Zealand Ltd, C.P.O. Box 2201, Auckland, New Zealand.

3M, Port. See *Agostinho, Port.*

3M, S.Afr. 3M SA (Pty) Ltd, P.O. Box 926, Isando, South Africa.

3M, Singapore. 3M Singapore Pte Ltd, 9 Tagore Lane, S 7878822, Singapore.

3M, Spain. 3M España, Juan Ignacio Luca de Tena 19-25, 28027 Madrid, Spain.

3M, Swed. 3M Svenska AB, 191 89 Sollentuna, Sweden.

3M, Switz. 3M (Schweiz) AG, Eggstrasse 93, 8803 Rüschlikon, Switzerland.

3M, Thai. 3M Thailand Ltd, 12 Fl, Stern-Mit Tower, 159 Asoke Rd, Wattana, Bangkok 10110, Thailand.

3M, UK. 3M Health Care Ltd, 3M House, Morley St, Loughborough, Leicestershire, LE11 1EP, UK.

3M, USA. 3M Pharmaceuticals, 3M Center 275-2E-13, P.O. Box 33275, St Paul, MN 55133-3275, USA.

7 Oaks, USA. 7 Oaks Pharmaceutical Corp., 161 Harry Stanley Drive, Easley, SC 29640, USA.

A Natureza, Braz. A Natureza Produtos Farmaceuticos Ltda, Rua Tacomare 106, 03125-200 Sao Paulo, SP, Brazil.

Aaciphar, Belg. Aaciphar S.A., Chaussee de la Hulpe 166, 1170 Brussels, Belgium.

AAH, UK. AAH Pharmaceuticals Ltd, Sapphire Court, Walsgrave Triangle Park, Coventry, Warwickshire, CV2 2TX, UK.

Abana, USA. See *Jones, USA.*

Abatron, UK. Abatron Ltd, Chapel St, Potton, Sandy, Bedfordshire, SG19 2PT, UK.

Abbott, Aust. Abbott GmbH, Diefenbachgasse 35, A-1150 Vienna, Austria.

Abbott, Austral. Abbott Australasia P/L, P.O. Box 101, Cronulla, NSW 2230, Australia.

Abbott, Belg. Abbott S.A., Rue du Bosquet 2, 1348 Ottignies Louvain-la-Neuve, Belgium.

Abbott, Braz. Abbott Laboratorios do Brasil Ltda, Rua Michigan 735, Brooklin, 04566-905 Sao Paolo, SP, Brazil.

Abbott, Canad. Abbott Laboratories Ltd, P.O. Box 6150, Station A, Montreal, Quebec, H3C 3K6, Canada.

Abbott, Denm. Abbott Laboratories A/S, Smakkedalen 6, 2820 Gentofte, Denmark.

Abbott, Fin. Abbott Oy, Pihatörmä 1 A, 02240 Espoo, Finland.

Abbott, Fr. Abbott-France, 12 rue de la Couture, Silic 233, 94528 Rungis cdx, France.

Abbott, Ger. Abbott GmbH, Max-Planck-Ring 2, 65205 Wiesbaden, Germany.

Abbott, Hong Kong. Abbott Laboratories Ltd, 20/F AIA Tower, 183 Electric Rd, North Point, Hong Kong.

Abbott, Irl. Abbott Laboratories, Ireland Ltd, 1 Broomhill Business Park, Tallaght, Dublin 24, Ireland.

Abbott, Israel. See *Promedico, Israel.*

Abbott, Ital. Abbott s.p.a., 04010 Campoverde (Latina), Italy.

Abbott, Mex. Abbott Laboratories de México. S.A.deC.V., Av. Coyoacan No. 1622, Col. del Valle, 03100 Mexico D.F., Mexico.

Abbott, Neth. Abbott B.V., Postbus 727, 2132 WT Hoofddorp, Netherlands.

Abbott, Norw. Abbott Norge, Nesoyv.4, Postboks 123, 1361 Billingstad, Norway.

Abbott, NZ. Abbott Laboratories (NZ) Ltd, P.O. Box 35-128, Naenae, Lower Hutt, New Zealand.

Abbott, Port. Abbott Laboratórios, Lda, Rua Cidade de Cordova, no 1/1A, Alfragide, 2720-100 Amadora, Portugal.

Abbott, S.Afr. Abbott Laboratories South Africa (Pty) Ltd, P.O. Box 1616, Johannesburg 2000, South Africa.

Abbott, Singapore. Abbott Laboratories (S) Pte Ltd, 1 Maritime Square, 11-12 World Trade Centre, S 099253, Singapore.

Abbott, Spain. Abbott Laboratories, Josefa Valcarcel 48, 28027 Madrid, Spain.

Abbott, Swed. Abbott Scandinavia AB, Box 509, 16929 Solna, Sweden.

Abbott, Switz. Abbott AG, Neuhofstrasse 23, Postfach, 6341 Baar, Switzerland.

Abbott, Thai. Abbott Laboratories Ltd, 9 Fl, Nai Lert Tower, 2/4 Wireless Rd, Lumpini, Patumwan, Bangkok 10330, Thailand.

Abbott, UK. Abbott Laboratories Ltd, Abbott House, Norden Rd, Maidenhead, Berkshire, SL6 4XE, UK.

Abbott, USA. Abbott Laboratories, 100 Abbott Park Rd, Abbott Park, IL 60064-3500, USA.

Abbott Nutrition, UK. Abbott Nutrition, Division of Abbott Laboratories Ltd, Queenborough, Kent, ME11 5EL, UK.

ABC, Ital. Istituto Biologico Chemioterapico ABC s.p.a., Via Crescentino 25, 10154 Turin, Italy.

ABC, Port. See *Pierre Fabre, Port.*

AB-Consult, Aust. AB-Consult Handels-GmbH, Eichenstrasse 32, A-1120 Vienna, Austria.

Abello, Ger. Abello Deutschland Pharma GmbH, Postfach: 1320, 53310 Bornheim, Germany.

Abello, Spain. Abello, Josefa Valcarcel 38, 28027 Madrid, Spain.

Abic, Hong Kong. See *International Medical, Hong Kong.*

Abic, Israel. See *Teva, Israel.*

Abic, Thai. See *RX, Thai.*

Abic-Teva, Singapore. See *Green Cross, Singapore.*

Abigo, Denm. Abigo A/S, Birkholmvej 28, Osted, 4000 Roskilde, Denmark.

Abigo, Swed. Abigo Medical AB, 436 32 Askim, Sweden.

Abiogen, Ital. Abiogen Pharma spa, Via S Antonio 61, 56125 Pisa, Italy.

Abnoba, Ger. Abnoba Heilmittel GmbH, Hohenzollernstr. 16, 75177 Pforzheim, Germany.

ABZ, Ger. AbZ-Pharma GmBH, Dr. Georg-Spohn-Str. 7, 89143 Blaubeuren, Germany.

Ace, S.Afr. Ace, South Africa.

Ache, Braz. Ache Laboratorios Farmaceticos S.A., Rodovia Presidente Dutra Km 227, 07034-904 Guarulhos, SP, Brazil.

Acme, USA. Acme United Corp., 75 Kings Highway Cutoff, Fairfield, CT 06430, USA.

ACO, Swed. ACO AB, 112 87 Stockholm, Sweden.

ACO Hud, Swed. ACO Hud AB, Box 622, 194 26 Upplands Vasby, Sweden.

Acorus, UK. Acorus Therapeutics Ltd, High Crane Lodge, Hamsterley, County Durham, DL13 3QS, UK.

ACP, Belg. A.C.P. S.C, Rue Georges Moreau 174, 1070 Brussels, Belgium.

ACRAF, Switz. ACRAF AG, Case postale 1067, 1701 Fribourg-Moncor, Switzerland.

Acro, Ital. Acro srl, Via Boccaccio 45, 20123 Milan, Italy.

ACS Dobfar, Ital. ACS Dobfar s.p.a., V.le Addetta 6/8/10, 20067 Tribiano, Italy.

Actelion, Switz. Actelion Ltd, Gewerbestrasse 16, 4123 Allschwil, Switzerland.

Actelion, USA. See *Actelion, Switz.*

Actipharm, Switz. Actipharm SA, 42-4 rue Prevost-Martin, 1211 Geneva 9, Switzerland.

Acusan, Ger. Acusan GmbH, Rheinstr. 219, 76532 Baden-Baden, Germany.

Adam, Mon. Laboratoires Adam, Les Flots Bleu, 16 rue du Gabian, BP 662, MC 98013, Monaco.

Adams, Canad. See *Warner-Lambert, Canad.*

Adams, Hong Kong. See *LCH, Hong Kong.*

Adams, Thai. See *Pharmaland, Thai.*

Adams, UK. Adams Healthcare Ltd, Lotherton Way, Garforth, Leeds, South Yorkshire, LS25 2JY, UK.

Adams, USA. Adams Laboratories Inc., 14801 Sovereign Rd, Fort Worth, TX 76155-2645, USA.

Adams Confectionery, UK. Adams Confectionery, Lambert Court, Chestnut Ave, Eastleigh, Hampshire, SO53 3ZQ, UK.

Adcock Ingram, S.Afr. Adcock Ingram Pharmaceuticals Ltd, Private Bag X69, Bryanston 2021, South Africa.

Adcock Ingram, UK. Adcock Ingram (UK), UK.

Adcock Ingram Generics, S.Afr. See *Adcock Ingram, S.Afr.*

Adcock Ingram Self Medication, S.Afr. See *Adcock Ingram, S.Afr.*

Adcock-Ingram Critical Care, S.Afr. Adcock-Ingram Critical Care, P.O. Box 6888, Johannesburg 2000, South Africa.

Addicare, Ger. See *Hexal, Ger.*

Adima, Switz. Adima SA, Case postale 1065, 1701 Fribourg, Switzerland.

Adivar, Ital. Angelini Distribuzioni Varie spa, Viale Amelia 70, 00181 Rome, Italy.

Adler, Aust. Adler-Apotheke, Wahringer Strasse 149, A-1180 Vienna, Austria.

Adler, Switz. Adler Apotheke, Dr Urs Reinhard AG, Untertor 39, Postfach 1241, 8401 Winterthur, Switzerland.

Adolphs, USA. Adolphs, 75 Merritt Blvd, Trumbull, CT 06611, USA.

Adrem, Canad. Adrem Ltd, 2000 Ellesmere Rd, Unit 16, Scarborough, Ontario, M1H 2W4, Canada.

Adria, USA. See *Pharmacia Upjohn, USA.*

Adroka, Switz. Adroka AG, Postfach, 4123 Allschwil 1, Switzerland.

Advance, Hong Kong. Advance Pharmaceutical Co. Ltd, A1-A4 & B3, 8F, Tsing Yi Industrial Ctr, Stage 1, Tsing Yi Island, N.T., Hong Kong.

Advanced, Singapore. Advanced Medi Mart Pte Ltd, 53 Kim Keat Rd, 05-02C Mun Hean Building, S 328823, Singapore.

Advanced Care, USA. Advanced Care Products, 199 Grandview Rd, Skillman, NJ 08558-9418, USA.

Advanced Magnetics, Israel. Advanced Magnetics, Israel.

Advanced Nutritional Technology, USA. Advanced Nutritional Technology Inc., 6988 Sierra Court, Dublin, CA 94568-2641, USA.

Advanced Polymer, USA. Advanced Polymer Systems, 123 Saginaw Drive, Redwood City, CA 94063, USA.

Advil, Austral. Advil P/L, P.O. Box 4082, Doncaster Heights, VIC 3109, Australia.

Aeroceuticals, USA. See *Graham-Field, USA.*

Aerocid, Fr. Lab Aérocid, 248 bis, rue Gabriel-Peri, 94230 Cachan, France.

Aesca, Aust. Aesca GmbH, Badener Strasse 23, A-2514 Traiskirchen, Austria.

Aesculapius, Ital. Aesculapius Farmaceutici s.r.l., Via Cozzaglio 24, 25125 Brescia, Italy.

AF, Mex. A.F. Laboratorios, Aplicaciones Farmaceuticas S.A., Heriberto Frias No. 1035, Col. del Valle, 03100 Mexico D.F., Mexico.

AFI, Norw. See *Nycomed, Norw.*

AFOM, Ital. AFOM Medical s.p.a., Via S Cristoforo 97, 20090 Trezzano S/Naviglio (MI), Italy.

AFT, NZ. AFT Pharmaceuticals, P.O. Box 87-266, Meadowbank, Auckland, New Zealand.

Agamadon, Ger. Agamadon Biol.-Pharm.-Praparate W. Hild Nachf., Postfach: 1565, 61215 Bad Nauheim, Germany.

Age D'or, Singapore. Age D'or Pte Ltd, 51 Ayer Rajah Crescent, 07-01/02, S 139948, Singapore.

Agen, Austral. Agen Biomedical Ltd, 11 Durbell St, Acacia Ridge, QLD 4110, Australia.

Agepha, Aust. Agepha GmbH, Guntherstrasse 11, A-1150 Vienna, Austria.

Agepharm, Fr. Lab. Agepharm, B.P. 15, F57480 Sierck-les-Bains, France.

AGIPS, Ital. AGIPS Farmaceutici s.r.l., Via Amendola 4, 16035 Rapallo (GE), Italy.

Agis, Israel. Agis Industries Ltd, Yeruram, Israel.

Agostinho, Port. António Pacheco Agostinho, SA, Rua Rodrigues Sampaio 15, 1169-012 Lisbon, Portugal.

Agouron, Canad. Agouron Pharmaceuticals Canada Inc., 4 Robert Speck Parkway, Suite 240, Mississauga, Ontario, L4Z 1S1, Canada.

Agouron, USA. Agouron Pharmaceuticals Inc., 10350 North Torrey Pines Rd, La Jolla, CA 92037-1020, USA.

Agpharm, Switz. Agpharm AG, Postfach, 4123 Allschwil 1, Switzerland.

Agropharm, UK. Agropharm Ltd, Buckingham House, Church Rd, Penn, High Wycombe, Buckinghamshire, HP10 8LN, UK.

Agua del Carmen, Spain. Agua del Carmen, Avda Estanislao Figueras 4, 43003 Tarragona, Spain.

Aguettant, Fr. Lab. Aguettant, 1 rue Alexander-Fleming, 69007 Lyon, France.

AHP, Neth. AHP Pharma B.V., Postbus 255, 2130 AG Hoofddorp, Netherlands.

AHP, Switz. AHP (Schweiz) AG, Grafenauweg 10, 6301 Zug, Switzerland.

Air Link, Austral. Air Link Sales & Marketing P/L, P.O. Box 538, Sunnybank, Qld 4109, Australia.

AJC, Fr. Laboratoires AJC, Usine de Fontaury, 16120 Chateauneuf, France.

Ajinomoto, Thai. See *Siam Pharm, Thai.*

Akita, UK. See *Manx, UK.*

Akorn, Canad. See *Dioptic, Canad.*

Akorn, USA. Akorn, Inc., 2500 Millbrook Drive, Buffalo Grove, IL 60089, USA.

AkPharma, USA. AkPharma Inc., P.O. Box 111, Pleasantville, NJ 08232, USA.

Akripan, Aust. Akripan GmbH, Johann-Wiesmayer-Gasse 17, A-2332 Hennersdorf, Austria.

Akromed, S.Afr. See *Wyeth, S.Afr.*

Akzo, Braz. Akzo Nobel Ltda, Rua Joao Alfredo 353, 04747-900 Sao Paulo, SP, Brazil.

Alacan, Spain. Alacan, Capricornio 5, 03006 Alicante, Spain.

Alba, USA. See *Bart, USA.*

Albert, Canad. See *Aventis Pharma, Canad.*

Albert, S.Afr. See *Hoechst Marion Roussel, S.Afr.*

Albert-Roussel, Aust. See *Hoechst Marion Roussel, Aust.*

Albert-Roussel, Ger. See *Aventis Pharma, Ger.*

Albright & Wilson, UK. Albright & Wilson Ltd, Detergents Group, P.O. Box 3, 210-222 Hagley Rd West, Oldbury, Warley, West Midlands, B68 0NN, UK.

Albugam, Switz. Albugam AG, Gattikerstrasse 5, Postfach, 8029 Zurich, Switzerland.

Alcala, Spain. Alcala Farma, Ctra M-300 Km 29.9, Alcala de Henares, 28802 Madrid, Spain.

Alckamed, Ital. Alckamed s.r.l., Via Benedetto Marcello 24, 20124 Milano, Italy.

Alclin, S.Afr. Alclin (Pty) Ltd, P.O. Box 1119, Harrismith 9880, South Africa.

Alcon, Aust. Alcon Ophthalmika GmbH, Mariahilferstrasse 121b, A-1060 Vienna, Austria.

Alcon, Austral. Alcon Laboratories (Australia) P/L, Private Bag 19, Frenchs Forest, NSW 1640, Australia.

Alcon, Belg. Alcon-Couvreur S.A., Rijksweg 14, 2870 Puurs, Belgium.

Alcon, Braz. Alcon Laboratorios do Brasil Ltda, Avenida Nossa Senhora da Assuncao 736, 05359-001 Sao Paulo, SP, Brazil.

Alcon, Canad. Alcon Canada Inc., 2145 Meadowpine Blvd, Mississauga, Ontario, L5N 6R8, Canada.

Alcon, Denm. Alcon Danmark ApS, Dampfaergevej 28 (postboks 890), 2100 Copenhagen O, Denmark.

Alcon, Fin. Alcon Finland Oy, PL 13, 01641 Vantaa, Finland.

Alcon, Fr. Laboratoires Alcon, 4 rue Henri-Ste-Claire-Deville, 92563 Rueil-Malmaison, France.

Alcon, Ger. Alcon Pharma GmbH, Blankreutestr. 1, 79108 Freiburg, Germany.

Alcon, Hong Kong. Alcon Hong Kong Ltd, 1603-4 DCH Commercial Ctr, 25 Westlands Rd, Quarry Bay, Hong Kong.

Alcon, Irl. See *Allphar, Irl.*

Alcon, Israel. Alcon, Israel.

Alcon, Ital. Alcon Italia s.p.a., Palazzo CD/1 Via Roma 108, 20060 Cassina de Pecchi (MI), Italy.

Alcon, Jpn. Alcon Japan, Japan.

Alcon, Mex. Alcon Laboratorios, S.A.deC.V., Cda Popocatepetl No. 46, Col. General Anaya, 03340 Mexico D.F., Mexico.

Alcon, Neth. See *Bipharma, Neth.*

Alcon, Norw. Alcon Norge AS, Billingstadsletta 13, Slependen, Postboks 22, 1301 Sandvika, Norway.

Alcon, NZ. Alcon Laboratories Ltd, P.O. Box 14-562, Panmure, Auckland, New Zealand.

Alcon, Port. Alcon Portugal, Lda, Rua Castilho 201, 1070-051 Lisbon, Portugal.

Alcon, S.Afr. Alcon Laboratories (South Africa) (Pty) Ltd, P.O. Box 3198, Randburg 2125, South Africa.

Alcon, Singapore. Alcon Pte Ltd, 159 Sin Ming Rd, 06-05 Amtech Building, S 575625, Singapore.

Alcon, Swed. Alcon Sverige AB, Box 12233, 102 26 Stockholm, Sweden.

Alcon, Switz. Alcon Pharmaceuticals Ltd, Bosch 69, Postfach 62, 6331 Hunenberg, Switzerland.

Alcon, Thai. Alcon Laboratories (Thailand) Ltd, 191 Silom Rd, 18 Fl, Silom Complex Building, Bangkok 10500, Thailand.

Alcon, UK. Alcon Laboratories (UK) Ltd, Pentagon Park, Boundry Way, Hemel Hempstead, Hertfordshire, HP2 7UD, UK.

Alcon, USA. Alcon Laboratories Inc., 6201 South Freeway, Fort Worth, TX 76134, USA.

Alcon Cusi, Spain. Alcon Cusi, Camil Fabra 58, El Masnou, 08320 Barcelona, Spain.

Alcon-Thilo, Ger. See *Alcon, Ger.*

Alcor, Spain. Alcor, Cervantes 24, 28014 Madrid, Spain.

Alcusal, Austral. Alcusal Inc. P/L, 12 Mahogany Drive, New Lambton, NSW 2302, Australia.

Aldo, Spain. Aldo Union, Baroneta De Malda 73, Esplugas de Llobregat, 08950 Barcelona, Spain.

Aldo-Union, Hong Kong. See *Hong Kong Medical, Hong Kong.*

Ale, Spain. Ale Pedemonte, Pasaje Jaime Roig 26-8, 08028 Barcelona, Spain.

Alembic Products, UK. Alembic Products Ltd, Unit A, Brymau 2 Estate, River Lane, Saltney, Chester, Cheshire, CH4 8RQ, UK.

Aleph, Ital. Aleph srl, Via Liborio Coccetti 8, 06034 Foligno PG, Italy.

Alergomed, Braz. Alergomed, Brazil.

Alfa Biotech, Ital. Alfa Biotech s.p.a., Via Castagnetta 7, 00040 Pomezia (Roma), Italy.

Alfa Intes, Ital. Industria Terapeutica Splendore - Oftalmoterapica ALFA, Via F.lli Bandiera 26, 80026 Casoria (NA), Italy.

Alfa Wassermann, Thai. See *Charoen, Thai.*

Alfaco, Neth. Alfaco, Baldschermweg 6B, 3821 AH Amersfoort, Netherlands.

Algol, Fin. Algol Oy, Lääkeosasto, Karapellontie 6, PL 13, 02611 Espoo, Finland.

Alifarma, Ital. Alifarma s.r.l., Via Piane 64, 47853 Coriano (RN), Italy.

Aliud, Ger. Aliud Pharma GmbH & Co. KG, Gottlieb-Daimler-Str 19, 89150 Laichingen, Germany.

ALK, Belg. ALK-Abello Belgium, Excelsiorlaan 3, 1930 Zaventem, Belgium.

ALK, Denm. ALK-Abelló Danmark, Borups Alle 177, D4 (postboks 400), 2000 Frederiksberg, Denmark.

ALK, Fin. ALK-Abelló A/S, Liluodontie 17 B, 2. krs, 00980 Helsinki, Finland.

ALK, Norw. ALK Norge, Spireav. 6, Postboks 218 Okern, 0580 Oslo, Norway.

ALK, Spain. Alk Abello, Miguel Fleta 19, 28037 Madrid, Spain.

ALK, Swed. ALK Sverige AB, Smorhalevagen 3, 434 42 Kungsbacka, Sweden.

ALK, UK. ALK-Abelló (UK), 2 Tealgate, Hungerford, Berkshire, RG17 0YT, UK.

ALK, USA. ALK Laboratories Inc., 27 Village Lane, Wallingford, CT 06492, USA.

Alk-Abello, NZ. See *CSL, NZ.*

Alkaloida, Thai. See *Medline, Thai.*

Alkapharm, Singapore. See *Wellchem, Singapore.*

Allen, Aust. See *GlaxoSmithKline, Aust.*

Allen, Mex. Allen Laboratorios, S.A.deC.V., Av. Instituto Politecnico Nacional No. 4728, Col. Tlacamaca, 07380 Mexico D.F., Mexico.

Allen, Spain. Allen Farmaceutica, Dr Severo Ochoa S/N, Tres Cantos, 28760 Madrid, Spain.

Allen & Hanburys, Austral. See *Glaxo Wellcome, Austral.*

Allen & Hanburys, Irl. See *GlaxoSmithKline, Irl.*

Allen & Hanburys, S.Afr. See *GlaxoSmithKline, S.Afr.*

Allen & Hanburys, UK. See *GlaxoSmithKline, UK.*

Allen & Hanburys, USA. See *GlaxoSmithKline, USA.*

Allens, UK. Allens & Co. (Anglesey) Ltd, Freshwinds, Pentraeth, Isle of Anglesey, Gwynedd, LL75 8YF, UK.

Allerbio, Fr. Laboratoires Allerbio, 55270 Varennes-en-Argonne, France.

Allerex, Canad. Allerex Laboratory Ltd, P.O. Box 13307, Kanata, Ontario, K2K 1X5, Canada.

Allergan, Aust. Pharm-Allergan GmbH, Landstrasser Hauptstrasse 60, A-1030 Vienna, Austria.

Allergan, Austral. Allergan Australia P/L, Locked Bag 514, Frenchs Forest, NSW 1640, Australia.

Allergan, Belg. Allergan S.A., Meir 44 A, 2000 Antwerp, Belgium.

Allergan, Canad. Allergan Inc., 110 Cochrane Dr., Markham, Ontario, L3R 9S1, Canada.

Allergan, Denm. Allergan A/S, Produktionsvej 14, 2600 Glostrup, Denmark.

Allergan, Fin. Allergan Norden AB, Rajatorpantie 41 C, 01640 Vantaa, Finland.

Allergan, Fr. Allergan France, Font de l'Orme, av Dr Maurice-Donat, B.P. 442, 06254 Mougins cdx, France.

Allergan, Ger. Pharm-Allergan GmbH, Rudolf-Plank-Str. 31, 76275 Ettlingen, Germany.

Allergan, Hong Kong. Allergan Asia Ltd, Unit 3001 Metroplaza Tower 1, 223 Hing Fong Rd, Kwai Fong, N.T., Hong Kong.

Allergan, Irl. Allergan Ltd, Pharmapark, California Heights, Dublin 20, Ireland.

Allergan, Israel. Allergan, Israel.

Allergan, Ital. Allergan s.p.a., Via S Quasimodo 134/138, 00144 Roma EUR (Roma), Italy.

Allergan, Jpn. Allergan, Japan.

Allergan, Mex. Allergan, S.A.deC.V., Av. Paseo de las Palmas No. 405-201, Lomas de Chapultepec, 11000 Mexico D.F., Mexico.

Allergan, Neth. See *Bournonville, Neth.*

Allergan, Norw. Allergan A/S, Industriv. 33, Postboks 276, 1300 Sandvika, Norway.

Allergan, NZ. Allergan Pharmaceuticals, Division of Allergan NZ Ltd, P.O. Box 1873, Auckland 1, New Zealand.

Allergan, Port. Allergan S.A., Rua General Ferreira Martins 10-7D, Miraflores, 1495-137 Lisbon, Portugal.

Allergan, S.Afr. Allergan Pharmaceuticals (Pty) Ltd, P.O. Box 3911, Halfway House 1685, South Africa.

Allergan, Singapore. See *Diethelm, Singapore.*

Allergan, Spain. Allergan, Avda Industria 24, Tres Cantos, 28760 Madrid, Spain.

Allergan, Swed. Allergan Norden AB, Business Campus, 194 81 Upplands Vasby, Sweden.

Allergan, Switz. Allergan AG, Feldmoosstrasse 6, 8853 Lachen, Switzerland.

Allergan, Thai. See *Maxim, Thai.*

Allergan, UK. Allergan Ltd, Crown Centre, Coronation Rd, Cressex Industrial Estate, High Wycombe, Buckinghamshire, HP12 3SH, UK.

Allergan, USA. Allergan Pharmaceuticals Inc., 2525 Dupont Dr., P.O. Box 19534, Irvine, CA 92623-9534, USA.

Allergan Herbert, USA. See *Allergan, USA.*

Allergan-Frumtost, Braz. Allergan Lok Produtos Farm. Ltda, Rua Cardoso de Melo 1.855, 04548-005 Sao Paulo, SP, Brazil.

Allergomed, Switz. Allergomed AG, Erlenstrasse 29, Postfach 117, 4106 Therwil, Switzerland.

Allergopharma, Ger. Allergopharma Joachim Ganzer KG, Hermann-Korner-Str. 52, 21465 Reinbek, Germany.

Allergopharma, Switz. See *Allergomed, Switz.*

Allergy Therapeutics, Canad. Allergy Therapeutics (Canada) Ltd, 1345 Fewster Drive, Mississauga, Ontario, L4W 2A5, Canada.

Allergy Therapeutics, UK. Allergy Therapeutics Ltd, Dominion Way, Worthing, West Sussex, BN14 8SA, UK.

Allga, Aust. Allga-Pharma Austria GmbH, Am Barentobel 215, A-6942 Krumbach, Austria.

Alliance, S.Afr. Alliance Pharmaceuticals Ltd, P.O. Box 261269, Excom 2023, South Africa.

Alliance, UK. Alliance Pharmaceuticals Ltd, Avonbridge House, Bath Rd, Chippenham, Wiltshire, SN15 2BB, UK.

Allmedica, Ger. Allmedica Arzneimittel GmbH, Schillerstr. 4, 37269 Eschwege, Germany.

Allo Pro, Aust. Allo Pro GmbH, Enzersdorfer Strasse 12A, A-2340 Modling, Austria.

Allphar, Irl. Allphar Services Ltd, Belgard Rd, Tallaght, Dublin 24, Ireland.

Almed, Switz. Divapharma Chur AG, Abteilung Almed, Ankerstrasse 53, 8026 Zurich, Switzerland.

Almi, Spain. Almi, Avda Brasil 17, 28020 Madrid, Spain.

Almirall, Hong Kong. See *Sincerity, Hong Kong.*

Almirall, Spain. Almirall Prodesfarma, Rda Gral Mitre 151, 08022 Barcelona, Spain.

Alonga, Spain. See *Synthelabo, Spain.*

Alpha, Hong Kong. See *Great Year, Hong Kong.*

Alpha, Israel. Alpha, Israel.

Alpha, Mex. Laboratorios Alpha S.A. de C.V., Heroes Ferrocarrileros No. 1325, 44440 Guadalajara, Jal., Mexico.

Alpha, NZ. Alpha Pharmaceuticals Ltd, P.O. Box 705, Palmerston North, New Zealand.

Alpha Therapeutic, Ger. Alpha Therapeutic GmbH, Siemensstr. 18, Postfach: 1107, 63201 Langen, Germany.

Alpha Therapeutic, Singapore. See *GC, Singapore.*

Alpha Therapeutic, Thai. Alpha Therapeutic (Thailand) Ltd, 8 Fl, Liberty Square, 287 Silom Rd, Bangrak, Bangkok 10500, Thailand.

Alpha Therapeutic, UK. Alpha Therapeutic UK Ltd, Howlett Way, Fison Way Industrial Estate, Thetford, Norfolk, IP24 1HZ, UK.

Alpha Therapeutic, USA. Alpha Therapeutic Corp., 5555 Valley Blvd, Los Angeles, CA 90032, USA.

Alphapharm, Austral. Alphapharm P/L, P.O. Box 36, Camperdown, NSW 1450, Australia.

Alphapharm, Hong Kong. See *LCH, Hong Kong.*

Alphapharm, Singapore. See *Zuellig, Singapore.*

Alpharma, Denm. See *Dumex-Alpharma, Denm.*

Alpharma, Fin. See *Dumex-Alpharma, Fin.*

Alpharma, Fr. Alpharma France, 40 rue Lecuyer, 93300 Aubervilliers, France.

Alpharma, Mex. Laboratorios Alpharma, S.A.deC.V., Boulevard Pipila No.1, Esq. Av. del Conscripto, Col. M.A. Camacho,, 11610 Mexico D.F., Mexico.

Alpharma, Norw. Alpharma AS, Harbitzalleen 3, Postboks 158 Skoyen, 0212 Oslo, Norway.

Alpharma, Singapore. See *Pharma 2000, Singapore.*

Alpharma, Swed. Alpharma AB, Nordenflychtsvagen 74, 112 89 Stockholm, Sweden.

Alpharma, UK. Alpharma Ltd, Whiddon Valley, Barnstaple, Devon, EX32 8NS, UK.

Alpharma, USA. Alpharma USPD Inc, 7205 Windsor Blvd, Baltimore, MD 21244, USA.

Alpharma-Isis, Ger. Alpharma-Isis Pharma GmbH, Elisabeth-Selbert-Str. 1, 40764 Langenfeld, Germany.

Alpinamed, Switz. Alpinamed AG, Pharmazeutische Produkte, 9306 Freidorf, Switzerland.

Alra, USA. Alra Laboratories Inc., 3850 Clearview Court, Gurnee, IL 60031, USA.

Alsi, Canad. Alsi Cie Ltee, 150 rue Seigneuriale, Beauport, Quebec, G1E 3B3, Canada.

Alsitan, Ger. Alsitan GmbH & Co. KG, Am Buhl 16-18, 86926 Greifenberg, Germany.

Also, Ital. Also s.p.a., Viale Monte Rosa 96, 20149 Milan, Italy.

Altana, USA. Altana Inc., 60 Baylis Rd, Melville, NY 11747, USA.

Alte Kreis, Aust. Alte Kreis-Apotheke, Untere Hauptstrasse 1, A-7100 Neusiedl am See, Austria.

Alter, Port. Alter, SA, Estrada Marco do Grilo, Zemouto, 2830 Coina, Portugal.

Alter, Spain. Alter, Mateo Inurria 30, 28036 Madrid, Spain.

Althin, Swed. Althin Medical AB, Box 39, 37221 Ronneby, Sweden.

Altimed, Canad. See *Technilab, Canad.*

Alva, USA. Alva-Amco Pharmacal Inc., 7711 North Meremac Ave, Niles, IL 60714-3423, USA.

Alza, Canad. Alza Canada, 2900 John St, Unit 1, Markham, Ontario, L3R 5G3, Canada.

Alza, Denm. See *AstraZeneca, Denm.*

Alza, Irl. See *Cambridge, Irl.*

Alza, Switz. See *Biomed, Switz.*

Alza, USA. Alza Corp., 1900 Charleston Ave, Mountain View, CA 94039, USA.

Ambix, USA. Ambix Laboratories Inc., 210 Orchard St, Rutherford, NJ 07073, USA.

Amcon, USA. Amcon Laboratories, 40 North Rock Hill Rd, St Louis, MO 63119, USA.

Amcron, Thai. Amcron Enterprise Co. Ltd, 2711 Pattanakarn Rd, Suan Luang, Bangkok 10250, Thailand.

American de Mexico, Mex. American de Mexico, Mexico.

American Health, Hong Kong. See *Jebsen, Hong Kong.*

American Institutional, Hong Kong. See *Inchcape, Hong Kong.*

American Institutional, Singapore. See *JDH, Singapore.*

American Lecithin, USA. American Lecithin Co., 115 Hurley Rd, Unit 2B, Oxford, CT 06478, USA.

American Medical, USA. American Medical Industries, 330 1/2 East Third St, Dell Rapids, SD 57022, USA.

American Pharmaceutical, USA. American Pharmaceutical Partners Inc., 10866 Wilshire Blvd, Suite 1270, Los Angeles, CA 90024, USA.

American Red Cross, USA. American Red Cross, 1616 Ft Myer Drive 17th Floor, Arlington, VA 22209-3100, USA.

American Regent, USA. American Regent, 1 Luitpold Drive, Shirley, NY 11967, USA.

American Urologicals, USA. American Urologicals Inc., 10031 Pines Blvd, Suite 216, Pembroke Pines, FL 33024, USA.

Amersham, Canad. See *Nycomed Amersham, Canad.*

Amersham, Fr. Laboratoires Amersham France, 12 av des Tropiques, B.P. 144, 91944 Les Ulis cdx, France.

Amersham, Ital. See *Nycomed, Ital.*

Amersham, Spain. Amersham Iberica, Ronda de Poniente, 12 ED, Euronova, Tres Cantos, 28760 Madrid, Spain.

Amersham, USA. See *Medi-Physics, USA.*

Amerx, USA. USA.

Ames, Irl. See *Bayer Diagnostics, Irl.*

Ames, Israel. Ames, Israel.

Ames, S.Afr. See *Bayer, S.Afr.*

Amgen, Austral. Amgen Australia P/L, P.O. Box 410, North Ryde, NSW 1670, Australia.

Amgen, Belg. Amgen S.A., Ave Ariane 5, 1200 Brussels, Belgium.

Amgen, Canad. Amgen Canada Inc., 6755 Mississauga Rd, Suite 400, Mississauga, Ontario, L5N 7Y2, Canada.

Amgen, Denm. Amgen AB, Strandvejen 203, 2900 Hellerup, Denmark.

Amgen, Fin. Amgen AB, PL 301, 02101 Espoo, Finland.

Amgen, Ger. Amgen GmbH, Riesstr. 25, 80992 Munich, Germany.

Amgen, Irl. See *United Drug, Irl.*

Amgen, Neth. Amgen, Netherlands.

Amgen, Port. Amgen Biofarmaceutica, Lda, Tagus Park, Parque de Ciencia e Tecnologia, 1780-920 Porto Salvo, Portugal.

Amgen, Spain. Amgen, Avda Diagonal 429, 08036 Barcelona, Spain.

Amgen, Swed. Amgen AB, Box 34107, 100 26 Stockholm, Sweden.

Amgen, UK. Amgen Ltd, 240 Cambridge Science Park, Milton Rd, Cambridge, Cambridgeshire, CB4 4WD, UK.

Amgen, USA. Amgen Inc., One Amgen Center Drive, Thousand Oaks, CA 91320-1799, USA.

Amgros, Denm. Amgros I/S, Dampfaergevej 22 (postboks 2593), 2100 Copenhagen O, Denmark.

Amide, USA. Amide Pharmaceuticals Inc., 101 East Main Street, Little Falls, NJ 07424, USA.

Amido, Fr. Laboratoires Amido, 37 av Gabriel-Peri, 92500 Rueil-Malmaison, France.

Amino, Switz. Amino SA, Althofstrasse 12, 5432 Neuenhof, Switzerland.

Amirose, UK. Amirose International, UK.

Amnol, Ital. Amnol Chimica Biologica srl, Via Giotto 2, 28100 Novara (NO), Italy.

Ampharco, USA. Ampharco Inc. International Pharm. Distrib. Co., 9549 A Bolsa Ave, Westminster, CA 92683, USA.

Amrad, Austral. Amrad Pharmaceuticals P/L, Private Bag 6, Kew, VIC 3101, Australia.

Amrad, NZ. See *CSL, NZ.*

Amsa, Ital. Amsa s.r.l., Passeggiata Ripetta 22, 00186 Rome, Italy.

Amsco, USA. See *Steris, USA.*

Amternes, Denm. Amternes Laegemiddelregistreringskontor I/S, Amstradsforeningen, Dampfaergevej 22 (postboks 2593), 2100 Copenhagen O, Denmark.

Amuchina, Ital. Amuchina s.p.a., Via de Marini 1, 16149 Genoa, Italy.

Amway, Canad. Amway of Canada Ltd, 375 Exeter Rd, P.O. Box 5706, London, Ontario, N6A 4S5, Canada.

Anatomica, Swed. Anatomica, Stora Avagen 25, 436 34 Askim, Sweden.

ANB, Thai. A.N.B. Laboratories Co. Ltd, 39/1 Ram-Intra Rd, Kanayao, Bangkok 10230, Thailand.

Ancient, Austral. Ancient Distributors, 2/16 Commercial Drive, Dandenong, VIC 3175, Australia.

Andersen, Norw. Jan F. Andersen AS, Postboks 1132 Flattum, 3501 Hønefoss, Norway.

Andrae, Aust. Andrae GmbH, Marinonigasse 2-6, A-1210 Vienna, Austria.

Andreabal, Switz. Andreabal AG, Rudolfstrasse 2, 4054 Basel, Switzerland.

Andreu, Spain. See *Roche, Spain.*

Andromaco, Mex. Industria Farmacéutica Andrómaco, S.A.deC.V., Andromaco No. 104, Col. Ampliacion Granada, 11520 Mexico D.F., Mexico.

Andromaco, Port. Laboratórios Andrómaco, Lda, Rua Alfredo da Silva 16, Zona Industrial de Alfragide, 2720-028 Amadora, Portugal.

Andromaco, Spain. Andromaco, Dr Zamenhof 36, 28027 Madrid, Spain.

Andrx, USA. Andrx Pharmaceuticals Inc., 4001 SW 47th Ave, Fort Lauderdale, FL 33314, USA.

Aneid, Port. Aneid, Lda, Rua do Alcaide no 2, 2750-097 Cascais, Portugal.

Angelini, Hong Kong. See *Inchcape, Hong Kong.*

Angelini, Israel. Angelini, Israel.

Angelini, Ital. Aziende Chimiche Riunite Angelini Francesco s.p.a., Viale Amelia 70, 00181 Rome, Italy.

Anglian, UK. Anglian Pharma Plc, Titmore Court, Titmore Green, Little Wymondley, Hitchin, Hertfordshire, SG4 7XJ, UK.

Anglo-French Drugs, Thai. Anglo-French Drugs.

Anglo-French Laboratories, Canad. Anglo-French Laboratories, Canada.

Anifer, Aust. See *Hofmann, Aust.*

Anika, Israel. Anika, Israel.

Anios, Fr. Laboratoires Anios, Pave du Moulin, 59260 Lille-Hellemmes, France.

ankerpharm, Ger. See *Chauvin ankerpharm, Ger.*

Anmarate, S.Afr. Anmarate (Pty) Ltd, P.O. Box 400, George 6530, South Africa.

Anpharm, UK. See *Antigen, UK.*

Ansell, Canad. Ansell Canada Inc., 105 Lauder St, Cowansville, Quebec, J2K 2K8, Canada.

Antibioticos, Mex. Antibióticos de México, S.A. de C.V., Las Flores No. 56,, Col. la Candelaria, 04380 Mexico D.F., Mexico.

Antibioticos, Spain. Antibioticos Pharma, Antonio Lopez 109, 28026 Madrid, Spain.

Antigen, Hong Kong. See *LCH, Hong Kong,* and *Universal, Hong Kong.*

Antigen, Irl. Antigen Pharmaceuticals Ltd, 54 Northumberland Rd, Dublin 4, Ireland.

Antigen, Israel. Antigen, Israel.

Antigen, NZ. See *Baxter, NZ.*

Antigen, UK. Antigen Pharmaceuticals Ltd, 82 Waterloo Rd, Southport, Merseyside, PR8 4QW, UK.

Antipiol, Ital. Laboratorio di Chimica Medica dell' Antipiol s.n.c., Via S. Benigno 26, 10154 Turin, Italy.

Antistress, Switz. Antistress, Gesellschaft fur Gesundheitsschutz, Fluhstrasse 30, 8640 Rapperswil, Switzerland.

Antonetto, Ital. Marco Antonetto s.p.a., Via Arsenale 29, 10121 Turin, Italy.

Antonetto, Switz. See *Corifel, Switz.*

Antula, Swed. Antula Healthcare AB, Odengatan 106, 113 22 Stockholm, Sweden.

Aplicare, USA. Aplicare Inc., P.O. Box 237, Prichard, WV 25555, USA.

Apodan, Denm. Apodan A/S, Lergravsvej 63, 5, 2300 Copenhagen S, Denmark.

Apogepha, Ger. Apogepha Arzneimittel GmbH, Kyffhauserstr. 27, 01309 Dresden, Germany.

Apomedica, Aust. Apomedica GmbH & Co KG, Roseggerkai 3, A-8011 Graz, Austria.

Apotex, Canad. Apotex Inc., 150 Signet Dr., Weston, Ontario, M9L 1T9, Canada.

Apotex, Hong Kong. See *Hind Wing, Hong Kong.*

Apotex, NZ. Apotex NZ Ltd, Private Bag 102-995, North Shore Mail Centre, Auckland, New Zealand.

Apotex, S.Afr. Apotex, South Africa.

Apotex, Singapore. See *Pharmaforte, Singapore.*

Apotheca, Singapore. Apotheca Marketing, 63 Hillview Ave, 09-16 Lam Soon Industrial Building, S 669569, Singapore.

Apothecary, USA. Apothecary Products Inc., 11750 12th Ave S, Burnsville, MN 55337, USA.

Apothecon, USA. See *Bristol-Myers Squibb, USA.*

Apothecus, Hong Kong. See *Hind Wing, Hong Kong.*

Apothecus, USA. Apothecus Inc., 20 Audrey Ave, Oyster Bay, NY 11771, USA.

Apotheke Erzengel Michael, Aust. Apotheke zum Erzengel Michael, Sechshauser Strasse 9, A-1150 Vienna, Austria.

Apotheke Gnadenmutter, Aust. Apotheke zur Gnadenmutter, Hauptplatz 4, A-8630 Mariazell, Austria.

Apotheke Heiligen Dreifaltigkeit, Aust. Apotheke zur Heiligen Dreifaltigkeit, Kirchengasse 5, A-2460 Bruck a. d. Leitha, Austria.

Apotheke Heiligen Josef, Aust. Apotheke zum Heiligen Josef, Doblinger Hauptstrasse 64, A-1190 Vienna, Austria.

Apotheke Heiligen Rupertus, Aust. Apotheke zum Heiligen Rupertus, Maxglaner Hauptstrasse 13, A-5020 Salzburg, Austria.

Apotheke Roten Krebs, Aust. Apotheke zum Roten Krebs, Lichtensteg 4, A-1011 Vienna, Austria.

Approved Drug, USA. See *Health for Life, USA.*

Approved Prescription Services, UK. Approved Prescription Services Ltd, Brampton Rd, Hampden Park, Eastbourne, East Sussex, BN22 9AG, UK.

APS, Ger. APS Pharma GmbH, Bahnhofstr. 7, 82319 Starnberg, Germany.

APS, Port. Farma-APS, Lda, Rua Jose Galhardo 3, 1750-131 Lisbon, Portugal.

Apsen, Braz. Apsen do Brasil Industria Quim. e Fcta Ltda, Rua La Paz 37, 04755-020 Sao Paulo, SP, Brazil.

Aptus, NZ. Aptus, P.O. Box 39-070, Wellington, New Zealand.

Aqualab, Fr. Lab. Aqualab, ZI Nord, B.P. 36, 470 av de Lossburg, 69480 Anse, France.

Aquamaid, UK. Aquamaid Co. Ltd, UK.

Arcana, Aust. Arcana Arzneimittel GmbH, Zimbagasse 5, A-1147 Vienna, Austria.

Arcana, S.Afr. Arcana (Pty) Ltd, P.O. Box 1998, Halfway House 1685, South Africa.

Archifar, Thai. See *TP, Thai.*

Arco, USA. Arco Pharmaceuticals Inc., 105 Orville Dr., Bohemia, NY 11716, USA.

Arcola, USA. See *Aventis Pharma, USA.*

Arcolab, Switz. Arcolab Ltd, 28 Chemin du Grand-Puits, 1217 Meyrin 2, Switzerland.

Arden, NZ. Elizabeth Arden (NZ) Ltd, Private Bag 94104, Papatoetoe, South Auckland, New Zealand.

Ardern, UK. Ardern Healthcare Ltd, Pipers Brook Farm, Eastham, Tenbury Wells, Worcestershire, WR15 8NP, UK.

Ardeypharm, Ger. Ardeypharm GmbH, Loerfeldstr. 20, 58313 Herdecke, Germany.

Ardix, Fr. Ardix Médical, 27 rue du Pont, 92200 Neuilly-sur-Seine, France.

Areu, Spain. Areu, Ctra Madrid Valencia, Km 23.5, Arganda del Rey, 28500 Madrid, Spain.

ARI, Austral. ARI, Division of ANSTO, Private Mail Bag 1, Menai, NSW 2234, Australia.

Aristegui, Spain. See *Ifidesa Aristegui, Spain.*

Ariston, Braz. Ariston Industrias Quimicas e Fcta Ltda, Rua Adherbal Stresser 84, 05566-000 Sao Paulo, SP, Brazil.

Arjo, Canad. Arjo Canada Inc., 277 Cree Cres., Winnipeg, Manitoba, R3J 3X4, Canada.

Arko, Ger. Arko Pharma GmbH, Neulandstr. 18, 77855 Achern, Germany.

Arkochim, Spain. Arkochim España, Meneses 2, 28045 Madrid, Spain.

Arkofarm, Ital. Arkofarm srl, Via Limone Piemonte 13/D, 18039 Ventimiglia (IM), Italy.

Arkomedika, Fr. See *Arkopharma, Fr.*

Arkopharma, Belg. Arkopharma, Ave des Noisetiers 7, 1170 Brussels, Belgium.

Arkopharma, Fr. Laboratoires Arkopharma, B.P. 28, 06511 Carros cdx, France.

Arkopharma, UK. Arkopharma UK Ltd, 6 Redlands Centre, Redlands, Coulsden, Surrey, CR5 2HT, UK.

Arla, Fin. Oy Arla Finland AB, PL 231, 00131 Helsinki, Finland.

Arlex, Mex. Arlex de México, S.A.deC.V., Puerto Acapulco No.35, Col. Piloto, 01290 Mexico, D.F., Mexico.

Armour, Israel. Armour, Israel.

Armour, USA. See *Centeon, USA.*

Armstrong, Mex. Armstrong Laboratorios de México, S.A.deC.V., Av. Division del Norte No. 3311, Col. Barrio de La Candelaria, 04380 Mexico D.F., Mexico.

Arnaldi-Uscio, Ital. Colonia della Salute Carlo Arnaldi s.p.a., Via Carlo Arnaldi 6, 16030 Uscio (GE), Italy.

Arrow, Austral. Arrow Pharmaceuticals Ltd, P.O. Box 397, Surry Hills, NSW 2010, Australia.

Arrow, USA. Arrow International Corp., 2400 Bernville Rd, Reading, PA 19605, USA.

Artegodan, Ger. Artegodan GmbH, Wendlandstr. 1, 29439 Luchow, Germany.

Artesan, Ger. Artesan Pharma GmbH & Co. KG, Wendlandstr. 1, 29439 Luchow, Germany.

Artesan, Switz. See *Lubapharm Arlesheim, Switz.*

Arteva, Ger. Arteva Pharma GmbH, Leutstettenerstr. 10, 82131 Gauting, Germany.

Artex, NZ. Artex Ltd, P.O. Box 249, Waipukurau, New Zealand.

Arthropharm, Austral. Arthropharm P/L, 111 Bronte Rd, Bondi Junction, NSW 2022, Australia.

Artsana, Ital. Artsana spa, Via Saldarini Catelli 1, 22070 Grandate (CO), Italy.

Artu, Neth. Artu Biologicals Europe B.V., Postbus 612, 8200 AP Lelystad, Netherlands.

Arun, UK. Arun Pharmaceuticals Ltd, Delta House, Southwood Cresent, Southwood, Farnborough, Hampshire, GU14 0NL, UK.

A.S., UK. A.S. Pharma Ltd, P.O. Box 5227, Milton Keynes, Buckinghamshire, MK1 1XZ, UK.

Asahi, Jpn. Asahi Chemical Industry Co. Ltd, Japan.

Ascent, USA. Ascent Pediatrics Inc., 187 Ballardvale St, Suite B125, Wilmington, MA 01887, USA.

Asche, Ger. Asche AG, Fischers Allee 49-59, 22763 Hamburg, Germany.

Ascher, USA. B.F. Ascher & Co., 15501 W 109th St, Lenexa, KS 66219, USA.

Ascot, Austral. Ascot Pharmaceuticals, P.O. Box 79, Croydon, NSW 2132, Australia.

Asens, Spain. Asens, Alava 61, 08005 Barcelona, Spain.

Asepta, Mon. Laboratoires Asepta, 17 bd Prince-Hereditaire-Albert, MC 98000, Monaco.

Ashbourne, UK. Ashbourne Pharmaceuticals Ltd, Victors Barns, Hill Farm, Brixworth, Northamptonshire, NN6 9DQ, UK.

Ashbury, Canad. Ashbury Biologicals Inc., 349 Wildcat Rd, Toronto, Ontario, M3J 2S3, Canada.

ASI, Israel. ASI Pharma Ltd, Bazel 50, Herzliya Pituach, Israel.

Asian Pharm, Thai. Asian Pharmaceutical Ltd Part, 9/4 Soi Wathanawong, Rajprarob Rd, Rajthavee, Bangkok 10400, Thailand.

Asian TJD, Thai. Asian TJD Enterprise Ltd, 90 Soi Ladprao 91 (Kesorn), Ledprao Rd, Wangthonglang Dist, Bangkok 10310, Thailand.

Askit, UK. Askit Laboratories Ltd, 47 Deerdykes View, Westfield, Cumbernauld, Glasgow, G68 9HN, UK.

Asofarma, Mex. Asofarma de Mexico S.A. de C.V., Calz. Mexico-Xochimilco No. 43, Col. San Lorenzo Huipulco, 14370 Mexico, D.F., Mexico.

Aspen, S.Afr. Aspen Pharmacare (Pty) Ltd, Private Bag X1593, Gallo Manor 2052, South Africa.

Aspen Consumer, S.Afr. See *Aspen, S.Afr.*

Aspro-Nicholas, Aust. See *Roche, Aust.*

Associated Dental, UK. Associated Dental Products Ltd, Purton, Swindon, Wiltshire, SN5 9HT, UK.

Associated Hospital Supply, UK. Associated Hospital Supply, Sherwood Rd, Aston Fields, Bromsgrove, Worcestershire, B60 3DR, UK.

Associated Medical, Hong Kong. Associated Medical Supplies Co. Ltd, Rm 1201, Fo Tan Industrial Ctr, 26 Au Pui Wan St, Fo Tan, N.T., Hong Kong.

Asta, Denm. See *Asta Medica, Swed.*, and *AstraZeneca, Denm.*

Asta Medica, Aust. Asta Medica Arzneimittel GmbH, Liesinger Flur-Gasse 2C, A-1230 Vienna, Austria.

Asta Medica, Austral. Asta Medica Australasia P/L, P.O. Box 1305, Parramatta, NSW 2124, Australia.

Asta Medica, Belg. Asta Medica S.A., Rue de l'Etuve 77-81, 1000 Brussels, Belgium.

Asta Medica, Braz. Asta Medica Ltda, Rua Santo Antonio 184 19°/20° andar, 01314-900 Sao Paulo, SP, Brazil.

Asta Medica, Fin. See *Asta Medica, Swed.*

Asta Medica, Fr. Laboratoire Asta Medica, Av J.-F.-Kennedy, 33701 Merignac cdx, France.

Asta Medica, Ger. Asta Medica AG, Weismullerstr. 45, 60314 Frankfurt a.M., Germany.

Asta Medica, Hong Kong. Asta Medica China Ltd, 13/F Manulife Tower, 169 Electric Rd, North Point, Hong Kong.

Asta Medica, Irl. See *Asta Medica, UK.*

Asta Medica, Israel. Asta Medica, Israel.

Asta Medica, Ital. Asta Medica s.p.a., Via Zanella 3/5, 20133 Milan, Italy.

Asta Medica, Neth. Asta Medica B.V., Postbus 171, 1110 BC Diemen, Netherlands.

Asta Medica, Norw. See *Sunde, Norw.*

Asta Medica, NZ. See *NZ Medical & Scientific, NZ.*

Asta Medica, Port. Asta Médica, Lda, Rua do Centro Cultural 13, 1700 Lisbon, Portugal.

Asta Medica, Singapore. See *JDH, Singapore,* and *Zuellig, Singapore.*

Asta Medica, Spain. Asta Medica, Avda de Fuentemar 27 (Plg Indus), Coslada, 28820 Madrid, Spain.

Asta Medica, Swed. Asta Medica AB, Kemistvagen 17, 183 79 Taby, Sweden.

Asta Medica, Switz. ASTA Medica AG, Hegnaustrasse 60, 8602 Wangen/ZH, Switzerland.

Asta Medica, Thai. Asta Medica (Thailand) Ltd, 23 Fl, Charn Issara, Tower II Building, 2911/272 New Petchburi Rd, Bangkapi, Huay Kwang, Bangkok 10320, Thailand.

Asta Medica, UK. ASTA Medica Ltd, ASTA House, 168 Cowley Rd, Cambridge, Cambridgeshire, CB4 4DL, UK.

Asta Medica, USA. Asta Medica, USA.

Astra, Aust. See *AstraZeneca, Aust.*

Astra, Austral. See *AstraZeneca, Austral.*

Astra, Belg. Astra Pharmaceuticals S.A., Rue Egide Van Ophem 110, 1180 Brussels, Belgium.

Astra, Braz. Astra Quimica e Farm. Ltda, Rua Roque Petroni Jr 999 8° andar, Vila Gertrudes, 04707-000 Sao Paulo, SP, Brazil.

Astra, Canad. See *AstraZeneca, Canad.*

Astra, Denm. See *AstraZeneca, Denm.*

Astra, Ger. See *AstraZeneca, Ger.*

Astra, Hong Kong. Astra Pharmaceutical (HK) Ltd, 2915-25 Metroplaza Tower 1, 223 Hing Fong Rd, Kwai Chung, Hong Kong.

Astra, Irl. See *AstraZeneca, Irl.*

Astra, Israel. See *Teva, Israel.*

Astra, Ital. See *AstraZeneca, Ital.*

Astra, Jpn. Astra Japan Ltd, Midousuji Daiwa Bldg, 6-8 Kyutaromachi 3-chome, Chuo-ku, Osaka 541-0056, Japan.

Astra, Mex. Astra Mexico S.A. de C.V. Farmacéutica, Av. Urbina No. 15, Parque Industrial, 53470 Naucalpan de Juárez,, Mexico.

Astra, Neth. Astra Pharmaceutica B.V., Postbus 599, 2700 AN Zoetermeer, Netherlands.

Astra, Norw. See *AstraZeneca, Norw.*

Astra, Port. Astra Portuguesa, Lda, Rua Humberto Madeira No 7, Valejas, 2745 Barcarena, Portugal.

Astra, S.Afr. See *AstraZeneca, S.Afr.*

Astra, Spain. Astra España, Mestre Joan Corrales 95-105, Esplugues de Llobregat, 08950 Barcelona, Spain.

Astra, Swed. See *AstraZeneca, Swed.*

Astra, Switz. See *AstraZeneca, Switz.*

Astra, USA. See *AstraZeneca, USA.*

Astra Tech, Denm. Astra Tech A/S, Husby Alle 19, 2630 Taastrup, Denmark.

Astra Tech, Fin. Astra Tech Oy, Piispantilankuja 4, 02240 Espoo, Finland.

Astra Tech, Norw. Astra Tech AS, Luhrtoppen 2, 1471 Skarrer, Norway.

Astra Tech, Swed. Astra Tech AB, Box 14, 431 21 Molndal, Sweden.

AstraZeneca, Aust. AstraZeneca Österreich GmbH, Schwarzenbergplatz 7, A-1037 Vienna, Austria.

AstraZeneca, Austral. Astrazeneca P/L, P.O. Box 131, North Ryde, NSW 2113, Australia.

AstraZeneca, Canad. AstraZeneca Canada Inc., 1004 Middlegate Rd, Mississauga, Ontario, L4Y 1M4, Canada.

AstraZeneca, Denm. AstraZeneca A/S, Roskildevej 22, 2620 Albertslund, Denmark.

AstraZeneca, Fin. AstraZeneca Oy, Eteläinen Salmitie, PL 6, 02431 Masala, Finland.

AstraZeneca, Fr. AstraZeneca, 1 place Renault, 92844 Rueil-Malmaison cdx, France.

AstraZeneca, Ger. AstraZeneca GmbH, 22876 Wedel, Germany.

AstraZeneca, Irl. AstraZenaca, College Park House, 20 Nassau St, Dublin 2.

AstraZeneca, Ital. AstraZeneca, Via Messina 38, Torre A, 20154 Milan, Italy.

AstraZeneca, Norw. AstraZeneca AS, Skarersletta 50, Postboks 1, 1471 Skårer, Norway.

AstraZeneca, NZ. AstraZeneca Ltd, P.O. Box 1301, Auckland, New Zealand.

AstraZeneca, S.Afr. AstraZeneca Pharmaceuticals, Private Bag X30, Sunninghill 2157, South Africa.

AstraZeneca, Singapore. AstraZeneca Singapore Pte Ltd, 6 Temasek Boulevard, 06-01 Suntec Tower Four, S 038986, Singapore.

AstraZeneca, Swed. AstraZeneca Sverige AB, 151 85 Sodertalje, Sweden.

AstraZeneca, Switz. AstraZeneca AG, Grafenauweg 10, 6301 Zug, Switzerland.

AstraZeneca, Thai. AstraZeneca (Thailand) Ltd, 20 Fl, Phairojkijja Building, 400 Bangna-Trad Km 4, Bangkok 10260, Thailand.

AstraZeneca, UK. AstraZeneca UK Ltd, Horizon Place, 600 Capability Green, Luton, Bedfordshire, LU1 3LU, UK.

AstraZeneca, USA. AstraZeneca Pharmaceuticals LP, 1800 Concord Pike, P.O. Box 15437, Wilmington, DE 19850-5437, USA.

Atache, Spain. Atache, C/Sagitario 12, 03006 Alicante, Spain.

Athena Neurosciences, UK. See *Elan, UK.*

Athena Neurosciences, USA. See *Elan, USA.*

Athenstaedt, Ger. Athenstaedt Nachf. GmbH & Co. KG, Bocklinstr. 1, 80638 Munchen, Germany.

Athenstaedt, Switz. See *Drossapharm, Switz.*

Athenstaedt & Redeker, Hong Kong. See *Mekim, Hong Kong.*

Athlone, Irl. Athlone Laboratories, Ballymurray, Roscommon, Ireland.

Atid, Ger. Atid Pharma Vertriebs-GmbH, Rontgenstr. 1, 63755 Alzenau, Germany.

Ativus, Braz. Ativus Farmaceutica Ltda, Estrada do Fonte Mecia S/N, 13270-000 Valinhos, SP, Brazil.

Atlantic, Hong Kong. Atlantic Laboratories Ltd, Block A, 18/F, Wing Wah Industrial Bldg, 677 King's Rd, North Point, Hong Kong.

Atlantic, Singapore. Atlantic Pharmaceutical (S) Pte Ltd, 152 Paya Lebar Rd, 04-03 Citipoint Industrial Complex, S 409020, Singapore.

Atlantic, Thai. Atlantic Pharmaceutical Co. Ltd, 2038 Sukhumvit Rd, Bangkok 10250, Thailand.

Atlantis, Mex. Atlantis, S.A. de C.V., Tiburcio Montiel No. 16, San Miguel Chapultepec, 11850 Mexico, D.F., Mexico.

Atlas, Canad. Laboratoire Atlas, 5750 Metropolitan E, Suite 200, St-Leonard, Quebec, H1S 1A7, Canada.

Atley, USA. Atley Pharmaceuticals Inc., 14433 N Washington Hway, Ashland, VA 23005, USA.

Atral, Port. Laboratóorios Atral, SA, Vala do Carregado, 2600-726 Castanheira do Hibatejo, Portugal.

Atral-Vida, Port. See *Atral, Port.*

Atrix, UK. Atrix Laboratories Ltd, St James House, Moon St, Bristol, BS2 8QY, UK.

Atzinger, Ger. Dr. Atzinger Pharmazeutische Fabrik, Dr. Atzinger Str. 5, 94036 Passau, Germany.

Auad, Braz. Auad Quimica Ltda, Rodovia BR 153 Km 7.5, Trevo Sul, 74853-040 Goiania, GO, Brazil.

Auden McKenzie, UK. Auden McKenzie (Pharma Div.) Ltd, 30 Stadium Business Centre, North End Rd, Wembley, Middlesex, HA9 0AT, UK.

Augot, Fr. Laboratoires Augot, 26 rue de Beauregard, 03400 Yzeure, France.

Australasian Medical, Austral. Austalasian Medical and Scientific Ltd, Unit 16, Artarmon Central, 54 Dickson Ave, Artarmon, NSW 2064, Australia.

Australian Medic-Care, Hong Kong. Australian Medic-Care Co. Ltd, Flat B, 6/F, Summit Bldg, 30 Man Yue St, Hunghom, Kowloon, Hong Kong.

Australis, Austral. Australis Marketing Corporation P/L, P.O. Box 752, Cheltenham, VIC 3192, Australia.

Austrodent, Aust. Austrodent Handels-GmbH, Brandhofgasse 22, A-8010 Graz, Austria.

Austroflex, Aust. Austroflex Pharma, Schikanedergasse 12/8-10, A-1040 Vienna, Austria.

Austroplant, Aust. Austroplant-Arzneimittel GmbH, Richard-Strauss-Strasse 13, A-1232 Vienna, Austria.

Avant Garde, Canad. Avant-Garde Cosmetics Ltd, 3503 Griffith, St-Laurent, Quebec, H4T 1W5, Canada.

Avantgarde, Ital. Avantgarde s.p.a., Gruppo Sigma Tau, Via Treviso 4, 00040 Pomezia (Rome), Italy.

Avene, Fr. Avène, Lab Dermatologiques, 45 place Abel-Gance, 92100 Boulogne, France.

Aventis, Austral. Aventis Pharma P/L, Locked Bag 2067, Lane Cove, NSW 2066, Australia.

Aventis, Belg. Aventis Pharma S.A., Rue Colonel Bourg 155, 1140 Brussels, Belgium.

Aventis, Denm. Aventis Pasteur MSD A/S, Toldbodgade 57, 1253 Copenhagen K, Denmark.

Aventis, Fr. Lab. Aventis, 46 quai de la Rapee, Paris cdx 12, France.

Aventis, Ger. Aventis Pasteur MSD GmbH, Paul-Ehrlich-Str. 1, 69181 Leimen, Germany.

Aventis, Irl. See *Allphar, Irl.*

Aventis, Ital. Aventis Pharma spa, Via R Lepetit 8, 20020 Lainate (MI), Italy.

Aventis, Neth. Aventis, Netherlands.

Aventis, Norw. Aventis Pharma AS, Vollsv. 2B, 1326 Lysaker, Norway.

Aventis, NZ. Aventis Pharma Ltd, P.O. Box 34010, Birkenhead, Auckland, New Zealand.

Aventis, Port. See *UCB, Port.*

Aventis, S.Afr. Aventis Pharma (Pty) Ltd, Private Bag X207, Midrand 1683, South Africa.

Aventis, UK. Aventis Pasteur MSD, Mallards Reach, Bridge Ave, Maidenhead, Berkshire, SL6 1QP, UK.

Aventis, USA. Aventis Pasteur Inc, Discovery Drive, Swiftwater, PA 18370-0187, USA.

Aventis Behring, Fr. Aventis Behring SA, 46 quai de la Rapee, 75012 Paris, France.

Aventis Behring, Ger. Aventis Behring GmbH, Postfach: 1230, 35002 Marburg (Lahn), Germany.

Aventis Behring, Swed. Aventis Behring AB, Berga Backe 2, 182 17 Danderyd, Sweden.

Aventis Behring, UK. Aventis Behring Ltd, Aventis House, Market Place, Haywards Heath, West Sussex, RH16 1DB, UK.

Aventis Behring, USA. Aventis Behring, 1020 First Ave, King of Prussia, PA 19406, USA.

Aventis Pasteur, Aust. Aventis Pasteur GmBH, Richard-Strauss-Strasse 33, A-1230 Vienna, Austria.

Aventis Pasteur, Canad. Aventis Pasteur, Connaught Campus, 1755 Steeles Ave West, North York, Ontario, M2R 3T4, Canada.

Aventis Pasteur, Fr. Aventis Pasteur Mérieux MSD, Halle Borie, 8 rue Jonas-Salk, 69367 Lyon cdx 07, France.

Aventis Pasteur, Swed. See *Aventis, Denm.*

Aventis Pharma, Aust. Aventis Pharma GmbH, Altmannsdorfer Strasse 104, A-1121 Vienna, Austria.

Aventis Pharma, Canad. Aventis Pharma Inc., 2150 St-Elzear Blvd W, Laval, Quebec, H7L 4A8, Canada.

Aventis Pharma, Denm. Aventis Pharma A/S, Slotsmarken 13, 2970 Horsholm, Denmark.

Aventis Pharma, Ger. Aventis Pharma Deutschland GmbH, Konigsteiner Str. 10, 65812 Bad Soden am Ts, Germany.

Aventis Pharma, Irl. Aventis Pharma (Ireland) Ltd, Lake Drive, 3400 City West, Naas Rd, Dublin 24, Ireland.

Aventis Pharma, Port. Aventis Pharma, Lda, Estrada nacional 249. Km 15, 2725-397 Mem Martins, Portugal.

Aventis Pharma, Swed. Aventis Pharma AB, Box 47604, 117 94 Stockholm, Sweden.

Aventis Pharma, UK. Aventis Pharma Ltd, Aventis House, 50 Kings Hill Ave, Kings Hill, West Malling, Kent, ME19 4AH, UK.

Aventis Pharma, USA. Aventis Pharmaceuticals, 300 Somerset Corporate Bvld, Bridgewater, NJ 08807-2854, USA.

Avon, Canad. Avon Canada Inc., 5500 Trans Canada Hwy, Pointe-Claire, Quebec, H9R 1B6, Canada.

AVP, USA. AVP, USA.

Axcan, Canad. Axcan Pharma Inc., 597 Laurier Blvd, Mont St-Hilaire, Quebec, J3H 6C4, Canada.

Axcan, Hong Kong. See *C & L, Hong Kong.*

Axcan, USA. Axcan Pharma US Inc., 3940 Quebec Ave North, Minneapolis, MN 55427, Usa.

Ayerst, USA. See *Whitehall-Robins, USA,* and *Wyeth-Ayerst, USA.*

Ayrton, UK. Ayrton Saunders Ltd, Reeds Lane, Moreton, Wirral, CH46 1QW, UK.

AyurCore, Singapore. See *MD, Singapore.*

Aza, Austral. Aza Research P/L, 112 Wharf Rd, West Ryde, NSW 2114, Australia.

Azevedos, Port. Laboratórios Azevedos, SA, Estrada Nacional 117-2, 2724-503 Amadora, Portugal.

Azupharma, Ger. Azupharma GmbH & Co., Dieselstr. 5, 70839 Gerlingen, Germany.

Azupharma, Hong Kong. See *Jebsen, Hong Kong.*

BA Farma, Port. Laboratorio B.A. Farma, Lda, R. Professor Sousa da Camara 207/211, 1070-803 Lisbon, Portugal.

Bach, UK. Bach Flower Remedies Ltd, Broadheath House, 83 Parkside, London, UK.

Bad Heilbrunner, Ger. Bad Heilbrunner Reform-Diat-Arznei GmbH & Co., Am Krebsenbach 5-7, 83670 Bad Heilbrunn, Germany.

Baer, Ger. Chemisch-pharmazeutische Fabrik Dr Baer KG GmbH & Co., Ehrwalder Str. 21, 81377 Munich, Germany.

Baif, Ital. Baif International Products, New York s.n.c., Via XX Settembre 20/68, 16121 Genoa, Italy.

Bailey, UK. Robert Bailey & Sons plc, Dysart St, Great Moor, Stockport, Cheshire, SK2 7PF, UK.

Bailleul, Fr. Laboratoires Bailleul, 8 rue Laugier, 75017 Paris, France.

Bailly, Fr. Laboratoires Bailly SPEAB, 60 rue Peirre-Charron, 75008 Paris, France.

Bajamar, USA. Bajamar Chemical Co. Inc., 9609 Dielman Rock Island, St Louis, MO 63132, USA.

Baker Cummins, Canad. See *Alza, Canad.*

Baker Cummins, USA. See *Baker Norton, USA.*

Baker Norton, Hong Kong. Baker Norton Asia Ltd, 1805 Kodak House II, 321 Java Rd, North Point, Hong Kong.

Baker Norton, Irl. See *Norton Waterford, Irl.*

Baker Norton, Singapore. See *Green Cross, Singapore.*

Baker Norton, UK. See *Norton, UK.*

Baker Norton, USA. Baker Norton Pharmaceuticals, 4400 Biscayne Blvd, Miami, FL 33137, USA.

Baldacci, Braz. Laboratorios Baldacci S.A., Rua Pedro de Toledo 520, 04039-001 Sao Paulo, SP, Brazil.

Baldacci, Ital. Laboratori Baldacci s.p.a., Via S. Michele Scalzi 73, 56100 Pisa, Italy.

Baldacci, Port. Farmoquimica Baldacci, SA, Rua Duarte Galvao 44, 1549-005 Lisbon, Portugal.

Baldassari, Braz. Baldassari, Brazil.

Balneopharm, Ger. See *Hanosan, Ger.*

Bama, Spain. Bama Geve, Avda Diagonal 456, 08006 Barcelona, Spain.

Bamford, NZ. W.M. Bamford Ltd, Private Bag 31346, Lower Hutt, New Zealand.

Banana Boat, Canad. The Banana Boat Company, 6363 Northam Drive, Mississauga, Ontario, L4V 1N5, Canada.

Bang & Tegner, Denm. Bang & Tegner, Vesterbrogade 149, 1620 Copenhagen V, Denmark.

Banner, Hong Kong. Banner, Hong Kong.

Bano, Aust. Mag. J. Bano chem. pharmazeutische Präparate, A-6580 St Anton/Arlberg 485, Austria.

Banyu, Hong Kong. See *Hing Ah, Hong Kong.*

Banyu, Jpn. Banyu Pharmaceutical Co. Ltd, 2-3 Nihonbashi Honcho 2-chome, Chuo-ku, Tokyo 103-8416, Japan.

Banyu, Thai. See *Asian TJD, Thai.*

Barcino, Spain. Barcino, Tusel 1, 08006 Barcelona, Spain.

Bard, UK. Bard Ltd, Forest House, Brighton Rd, Crawley, West Sussex, RH11 9BP, UK.

Barnes Hind, NZ. See *Allergan, NZ.*

Barr, USA. Barr Laboratories Inc., 2 Quaker Rd, Pomona, NY 01970, USA.

Barre-National, USA. See *Alpharma, USA.*

Barrenne, Braz. Barrenne Industria Farmaceutica Ltda, Rua Antunes Maciel 86, 20940-010 Rio de Janeiro, RJ, Brazil.

Barry, Ital. Barry Italia s.r.l., Via Sardegna 40, 20090 Fizzonasco Pieve Emanuele (MI), Italy.

Bart, USA. A.J. Bart Inc., Gurabo Industrial Park, P.O. Box 813, Gurabo, PR 00658, Puerto Rico.

Bartholomew Rhodes, UK. Bartholomew Rhodes Ltd, Manor House, Victor Barns, Northampton Rd, Brixworth, Northamptonshire, NN6 9DQ, UK.

Bartor Pharmacal, USA. Bartor Pharmacal Co., 70 High St, Rye, NY 10580, USA.

BASF, Fin. BASF Oy, Annankatu 42 C, 00100 Helsinki, Finland.

BASF, Ger. BASF Generics GmbH, Carl-Zeiss-Ring 3, 85737 Ismaning, Germany.

Basi, Port. See *Esteves Alves, Port.*

Basotherm, Ger. See *Galderma, Ger.*

Basotherm, Switz. See *Boehringer Ingelheim, Switz.*

Bastian, Ger. Bastian-Werk GmbH, August-Exter-Str. 4, 81245 Munich, Germany.

Bausch & Lomb, Austral. Bausch & Lomb (Australia) P/L, Level 4, 113 Wicks Rd, North Ryde, NSW 2113, Australia.

Bausch & Lomb, Belg. Bausch & Lomb, Belgium.

Bausch & Lomb, Canad. Bausch & Lomb Canada Inc., 1200 Aerowood Drive, Mississauga, Ontario, L4W 2S7, Canada.

Bausch & Lomb, Fr. Laboratoires Bausch & Lomb, route de Levis-Saint-Nom, B.P. 51, 78320 Le Mesnil-Saint-Denis, France.

Bausch & Lomb, S.Afr. Bausch & Lomb (SA) (Pty) Ltd, P.O. Box 1096, Ferndale 2160, South Africa.

Bausch & Lomb, Thai. See *Zuellig, Thai.*

Bausch & Lomb, UK. Bausch & Lomb UK Ltd, 106 London Rd, Kingston-upon-Thames, Surrey, KT2 6TN, UK.

Bausch & Lomb, USA. Bausch & Lomb Pharmaceuticals, 8500 Hidden River Parkway, Tampa, FL 33637, USA.

Bauxili, Spain. Bauxili, Nueva 52, Igualada, 08700 Barcelona, Spain.

Baxenden, UK. Baxenden Chemicals Ltd, Union Lane, Droitwich, Worcestershire, WR9 9BB, UK.

Baxtar, Jpn. Baxtar, Japan.

Baxter, Aust. Baxter AG, Industriestrasse 67, A-1221 Vienna, Austria.

Baxter, Austral. Baxter Healthcare P/L, P.O. Box 88, Toongabbie, NSW 2146, Australia.

Baxter, Belg. Baxter S.A., Bvld de la Plaine 5, 1050 Brussels, Belgium.

Baxter, Canad. Baxter Corporation, 4 Robert Speck Pkwy, Suite 700, Mississauga, Ontario, L4Z 3YA, Canada.

Baxter, Denm. Baxter A/S, Gydevang 43, 3450 Allerod, Denmark.

Baxter, Fin. Baxter Oy, Jaakonkatu 2, 01620 Vantaa, Finland.

Baxter, Fr. Baxter SA, 6 av Louis-Pasteur, B.P. 56, 78311 Maurepas cdx, France.

Baxter, Ger. Baxter Deutschland GmbH, Edisonstr. 3-4, 85716 Unterschleissheim, Germany.

Baxter, Hong Kong. Baxter Healthcare Ltd, Rm 2003-6, Evergo House, 38 Gloucester Rd, Wanchai, Hong Kong.

Baxter, Irl. Baxter Healthcare Ltd, 7 Deansgrange Industrial Estate, Blackrock, Dublin, Ireland.

Baxter, Israel. Baxter, Israel.

Baxter, Ital. Baxter s.p.a., Viale Tiziano 25, 00196 Rome, Italy.

Baxter, NZ. Baxter Healthcare Ltd, P.O. Box 14-062, Panmure, Auckland, New Zealand.

Baxter, Port. Baxter, Lda, Urbanizacao Industrial Cabra Figa, Estrada Nacional 249/4, Lote 3, Cabra Figa, 2735 Rio de Mouro, Portugal.

Baxter, Singapore. See *United Italian, Singapore.*

Baxter, Spain. Baxter, Dels Gremis 7, Polig. Inds. Vara de Cuart, 46014 Valencia, Spain.

Baxter, Swed. Baxter Medical AB, Box 63, 164 94 Kista, Sweden.

Baxter, Switz. Baxter AG, Mullerenstrasse 3, 8604 Volketswil., Switzerland.

Baxter, Thai. See *Osotspa, Thai.*

Baxter, UK. Baxter Healthcare Ltd, Caxton Way, Thetford, Norfolk, IP24 3SE, UK.

Baxter, USA. Baxter Healthcare, One Baxter Parkway, Deerfield, IL 60015, USA.

Baxter BioScience, UK. Baxter BioScience, Wallingford Rd, Compton, Newbury, Berkshire, RG20 7QW, UK.

Baxter Healthcare, Switz. See *Opopharma, Switz.*

Baxter-Hyland, Ger. Baxter Deutschland GmBH Hyland-Immuno Division, Im Breitspiel 13, 69126 Heidelberg, Germany.

Baxter-Hyland, Hong Kong. See *Baxter, Hong Kong.*

Baxter-Hyland, USA. Baxter Hyland Immuno, 550 North Brand Blvd, Glendale, CA 991203, USA.

Bayer, Aust. Bayer Austria GmbH, Am Heumarkt 10, Postfach 10, 1037 Vienna, Austria.

Bayer, Austral. Bayer Australia Ltd (Health Care Business Group), P.O. Box 903, Pymble, NSW 2073, Australia.

Bayer, Belg. Bayer S.A., Ave Louise 143, 1050 Brussels, Belgium.

Bayer, Braz. Bayer S.A., Rua Domingos Jorge 1000/1100 (4º and.), Socorro, 04779-900 Sao Paulo, SP, Brazil.

Bayer, Canad. Bayer Inc., 77 Belfield Rd, Toronto, Ontario, M9W 1G6, Canada.

Bayer, Denm. Bayer Danmark A/S, Norgaardsvej 32, 2800 Lyngby, Denmark.

Bayer, Fin. Bayer Oy, Suomalaistentie 7, 02270 Espoo, Finland.

Bayer, Fr. Bayer Pharma, 13 rue Jean-Jaures, 92807 Puteaux cdx, France.

Bayer, Ger. Bayer Vital GmbH & Co. KG, 51368 Leverkusen, Germany.

Bayer, Hong Kong. Bayer China Co Ltd, 18/F Caroline Ctr, 28 Yun Ping Rd, Causeway Bay, Hong Kong.

Bayer, Irl. Bayer Ltd, Chapel Lane, Swords, Dublin, Ireland.

Bayer, Israel. Bayer, Israel.

Bayer, Ital. Bayer s.p.a., Viale Certosa 130, 20156 Milan, Italy.

Bayer, Mex. Bayer de Mexico, S.A. de C.V., Division Farmaceutica, Calz. Mexico-Xochimilco No.77, Col. San Lorenzo Huipulco, 14370 Mexico D.F., Mexico.

Bayer, Neth. Bayer B.V., Postbus 80, 3640 AB Mijdrecht, Netherlands.

Bayer, Norw. Bayer AS, Brennav 18, Skyttaveltet, Nittedal, Postboks 114, 1483 Skytta, Norway.

Bayer, NZ. Bayer New Zealand Ltd, C.P.O. Box 2825, Auckland, New Zealand.

Bayer, Port. Bayer Portugal, SA, Rua da Quinta do Pinheiro 5, Outorela, 2795-653 Carnaxide, Portugal.

Bayer, S.Afr. Bayer (Pty) Ltd, P.O. Box 198, Isando 1600, South Africa.

Bayer, Singapore. Bayer (Singapore) Pte Ltd, Pharmaceutical Division, 9 Benol Sector, S 629844, Singapore.

Bayer, Spain. Bayer, Calabria 268, 08029 Barcelona, Spain.

Bayer, Swed. Bayer AB, Box 5237, 402 24 Goteborg, Sweden.

Bayer, Switz. Bayer (Schweiz) AG, Pharma, Postfach, 8045 Zurich, Switzerland.

Bayer, Thai. Bayer Thai Co. Ltd, 130/1 North Sathorn Rd, Bangkok 10500, Thailand.

Bayer, UK. Bayer plc, Pharmaceutical Division, Bayer House, Strawberry Hill, Newbury, Berkshire, RG13 1JA, UK.

Bayer, USA. Bayer Corp., 400 Morgan Lane, West Haven, CT 06516, USA.

Bayer Biological, Hong Kong. See *LCH, Hong Kong.*

Bayer Consumer, Austral. See *Bayer, Austral.*

Bayer Consumer, Mex. Bayer de Mexico, S.A. de C.V., Division Consumer Care, Av. Coyoacan No. 1553, Col. del Valle, 03100 Mexico, D.F., Mexico.

Bayer Consumer, Singapore. See *Diethelm, Singapore.*

Bayer Consumer, UK. See *Bayer, UK.*

Bayer Consumer, USA. Bayer Consumer Care Division, 36 Columbia Rd, P.O. Box 1910, Morristown, NJ 07962-1910, USA.

Bayer Diagnostici, Ital. Bayer Diagnostici s.p.a., Via Grosio 10, 20151 Milan, Italy.

Bayer Diagnostics, Fr. Bayer Diagnostics, Tour Horizon, 52 quai De Dion Bouton, 92807 Puteaux cdx, France.

Bayer Diagnostics, Irl. Bayer Diagnostics, Pharmapark, Chapelizod, Dublin 20, Ireland.

Bayer Diagnostics, Mex. Bayer de Mexico, S.A. de C.V. Division Diagnosticos, Av. Col. del Valle No. 615, 1er piso, Col del Valle, 03100 Mexico, D.F., Mexico.

Bayer Diagnostics, UK. See *Bayer, UK.*

Baypharm, Austral. See *Bayer, Austral.*

BBC, Braz. Brazilian Business Consultants, Avenida Brigadeiro Luis Antonio 1499, 01317-001 Sao Paulo, SP, Brazil.

BC Lutz, Switz. BCLutz Company Ltd, Pharmaceutical Products Switzerland, Dachslerenstrasse 11, P.O. Box, 8702 Zollikon, Switzerland.

BCL, Switz. See *BC Lutz, Switz.*

BCM, UK. BCM Ltd, Dio First 114, Nottingham, Nottinghamshire, NG90 2PR, UK.

BCS, Fr. See *CSP, Fr.*

BDF, Mex. MDF Mexico, S.A. de C.V., Poniente 116 No. 509, Col. Industrial Vallejo, 02300 Mexico D.F., Mexico.

BDI, USA. BDI Pharmaceuticals, Inc., P.O. Box 78610, Indianapolis, IN 46278-0610, USA.

Beach, USA. Beach Pharmaceuticals, Division of Beach Products Inc., 5220 South Manhattan Ave, Tampa, FL 33611, USA.

Beacons, Singapore. Beacons Chemicals Pte Ltd, 21 Chin Bee Ave, S 619942, Singapore.

Beaufour, Fr. Beaufour Ipsen Pharma, 24 rue Erlanger, 75781 Paris cdx 16, France.

Beaufour, Switz. See *Uhlmann-Eyraud, Switz.*

Beaufour-Ipsen, Hong Kong. See *Inchcape, Hong Kong.*

Beaufour-Ipsen, Singapore. See *Sime Darby, Singapore.*

Beaufour-Ipsen, Thai. See *Pacific, Thai.*

Beckerath, Ger. M. v. Beckerath GmbH Pharmavertrieb, Leyentalstr. 78, 47799 Krefeld, Germany.

Beckman, USA. Beckman Coulter Inc, 4300 North Harbor Bvld, P.O. Box 3100, Bedford, OH 44146, USA.

Becton Dickinson, USA. Becton Dickinson & Co., 1 Becton Drive, Franklin Lakes, NJ 07417, USA.

Bedford, USA. Bedford Laboratories, a Division of Ben Venue Laboratories Inc., 300 Northfield Rd, Bedford, OH 44146, USA.

Beecham, Belg. See *SmithKline Beecham, Belg.*

Beecham, Port. Beecham Portuguesa, Lda, Rua Sebastiao e Silva 4, Massama, 2745 Queluz, Portugal.

Beecham, Spain. See *SmithKline Beecham, Spain.*

Beethoven, Ger. Beethoven-Pharma Dr Wiemann GmbH, Steinthalstr. 1, 90455 Nurnberg, Germany.

Befelka, Ger. Befelka-Arzneimittel, Parkstr. 6 b, 49080 Osnabruck, Germany.

Behring, Neth. See *Hoechst Marion Roussel, Neth.*

Behringwerke, Israel. Behringwerke, Israel.

Beiersdorf, Aust. Beiersdorf GmbH, Laxenburger Strasse 151, A-1101 Vienna, Austria.

Beiersdorf, Austral. Beiersdorf Australia Ltd, P.O. Box 139, North Ryde, NSW 2113, Australia.

Beiersdorf, Canad. See *Smith & Nephew, Canad.*

Beiersdorf, Ger. Beiersdorf AG, Unnastr. 48, 20245 Hamburg, Germany.

Beiersdorf, Irl. See *Mayrs, Irl.*

Beiersdorf, Ital. Beiersdorf s.p.a., Via Eraclito 30, 20128 Milan, Italy.

Beiersdorf, Port. Beiersdorf Portuguesa, Lda, Rua Soeiro Pereira Gomes 59, 2746-952 Queluz, Portugal.

Beiersdorf, Switz. Beiersdorf AG Medical, Aliothstrasse 40, 4142 Munchenstein 2, Switzerland.

Beiersdorf, Thai. Beiersdorf (Thailand) Co. Ltd, 12 Fl, Sathorn Thani Building, 90/32-33 North Sathorn Rd, Bangkok 10500, Thailand.

Beiersdorf, UK. Beiersdorf UK Ltd, Yeomans Drive, Blakelands, Milton Keynes, Buckinghamshire, MK14 5LS, UK.

Beiersdorf, USA. Beiersdorf Inc., 360 Martin Luther King Drive, South Norwalk, CT 06856-5529, USA.

Beiersdorf-Lilly, Ger. Beiersdorf-Lilly GmbH, Wiesingerweg 25, Postfach: 201852, 20243 Hamburg, Germany.

Beige, S.Afr. See *Brunel, S.Afr.*

Beldenta, Switz. Beldenta-Anstalt, Birkenweg 6, FL-9490 Vaduz, Switzerland.

Belem Jardim, Braz. Laboratorio Belem Jardim Ind. e Com. Ltda, Avenida Waldomiro Lobo 913, Guarani, 31814-620 Belo Horizonte MG, Brazil.

Bell, Ir. Bell, Sons & Co. (Druggists), P.O. Box 62, Tanhouse Lane, Widnes, Cheshire, WA8 0SA, UK.

Bellon, Fr. See *Rhone-Poulenc Rorer, Fr.*

Belmac, Spain. Belmac, Montearagon 9, 28033 Madrid, Spain.

Bencard, Belg. S.A. Bencard, Rue du Tilleul 13, 1332 Genval, Belgium.

Bencard, Canad. See *Allergy Therapeutics, Canad.*

Bencard, Ger. Bencard Allergie GmbH, Leopoldstrasse 175, 80804 Munich, Germany.

Bencard, UK. See *GlaxoSmithKline, UK.*

Bene, Ger. bene-Arzneimittel GmbH, Herterichstr. 1, 81479 Munich, Germany.

Bene-Chemie, Hong Kong. See *Universal, Hong Kong.*

Benedetti, Ital. Benedetti s.p.a., Vicolo de'Bacchettoni 3, 51100 Pistoia (PT), Italy.

Bengue, Irl. See *Roche, Irl.*

Bennett, UK. Bennett Natural Products, Wheelton, Chorley, Lancashire, PR6 8EP, UK.

Berenguer Infale, Spain. See *Almirall, Spain.*

Bergamo, Braz. Lab. Quim. Bergamo Ltda, Rua Rafael de Marco 43, 06765-000 Sao Paulo, SP, Brazil.

Bergamon, Ital. Bergamon s.r.l., Via Farini 5, 00185 Rome, Italy.

Berk, Irl. See *Blackhall, Irl.*

Berk, UK. See *Approved Prescription Services, UK.*

Berlex, Canad. Berlex Canada Inc., 2260 32nd Ave, Lachine, Quebec, H8T 3H4, Canada.

Berlex, USA. Berlex Laboratories Inc., 300 Fairfield Rd, Wayne, NJ 07470, USA.

Berli, Thai. Berli Jucker Public Co. Ltd, 99 Soi Rubia, Sukhumvit 42 Rd, P.O. Box 173, Bangkok 10110, Thailand.

Berlin Pharm, Singapore. See *Polymedic, Singapore.*

Berlin Pharm, Thai. Berlin Pharmaceutical Industry Co. Ltd, 359 New Rd, Bangkok 10100, Thailand.

Berlin-Chemie, Ger. Berlin-Chemie AG, Glienicker Weg 125, 12489 Berlin, Germany.

Berman, Mex. Berman, Mexico.

Berna, Belg. Berna Products Belgium, Blvd du Souverain 207, bte. 3, 1160 Brussels, Belgium.

Berna, Canad. See *Berna, USA.*

Berna, Denm. See *Cortec, Denm.*

Berna, Fin. See *Cortec, Fin.*

Berna, Hong Kong. See *Keller, Hong Kong.*

Berna, Ital. Istituto Sieroterapico Berna s.r.l., Via Bellinzona 39, 22100 Como, Italy.

Berna, Norw. See *Cortec, Norw.*

Berna, Port. See *Vieira, Port.*

Berna, Singapore. See *Zuellig, Singapore.*

Berna, Spain. Berna, P Castellana 163, 28046 Madrid, Spain.

Berna, Switz. Berna Biotech Ltd, Rehhagstrasse 79, CH-3018 Berne, Switzerland.

Berna, Thai. See *Berna, Switz.,* and *Diethelm, Thai.*

Berna, USA. Berna Products Corp., 4216 Ponce de Leon Blvd, Coral Gables, FL 33146, USA.

Berner, Fin. Berner Oy, Lääkeryhmä, PL 15, 00131 Helsinki, Finland.

Bernhauer, Aust. Mr W Bernhauer OHG, Stadtplatz 7, A-4400 Steyr, Austria.

Bersan, Ital. Bersan Cosmetica Ipoallergenica s.r.l., Via delle Pervinche 10, 00171 Rome, Italy.

Berta, Ital. Berta s.r.l., Via Andrea Doria 7, 20124 Milan, Italy.

Bertek, USA. Bertek Pharmaceuticals Inc, 3711 Collins Ferry Rd, P.O. Box 4310, Morgantown, WV 26504-4310, USA.

Bescansa, Spain. Bescansa, Pl. Inds. Tambre-via Pasteur 8, Santiago de Compostela, 15890 La Coruna, Spain.

Besins, Fr. Laboratoires Besins International, 5 rue du Bourg-l'Abbé, 75003 Paris, France.

Besins, Ger. See *Kade, Ger.*

Besins, Hong Kong. See *Bi Asian Pacific, Hong Kong.*

Besins-Iscovesco, Fr. See *Besins, Fr.*

Besins-Iscovesco, Israel. Besins-Iscovesco, Israel.

Besins-Iscovesco, Singapore. See *Pharmed, Singapore.*

Besins-Iscovesco, Switz. See *Golaz, Switz.*

Beta, Canad. Beta Brands, 100 Cumberland Ave, Hamilton, Ontario, L8M 1Z1, Canada.

Beta, Ital. Laboratorio Biologico Chemioterapico Beta s.r.l., Via IV Novembre 171/3, 25080 Prevalle, Italy.

Beta Healthcare, UK. Beta Healthcare, Standard House, Prospect Place, Lenton, Nottingham, Nottinghamshire, NG7 1RX, UK.

Be-Tabs, S.Afr. Be-Tabs Pharmaceuticals (Pty) Ltd, P.O. Box 43486, Industria 2042, South Africa.

Betamadrileno, Spain. Betamadrileño, Area Empresarial Andalucia, Sector 4 Parcela 28, Getafe, 28906 madrid, Spain.

Betapharm, Ger. Betapharm Arzneimittel GmbH, Steinerne Furt 78, 86167 Augsburg, Germany.

Beutlich, USA. Beutlich L.P., 1541 Shields Drive, Waukegan, IL 60085-8304, USA.

BHR, UK. BHR Pharmaceuticals Ltd, 41 Centenary Business Centre, Hammond Close, Attleborough Fields, Nuneaton, Warkwickshire, CV11 6RY, UK.

Bi Asian Pacific, Hong Kong. Bi Asian Pacific Ltd, 11A Capital Bldg, 8 Sun Wui Rd, Causeway Bay, Hong Kong.

Biagini, Ital. Farma Biagini s.p.a., 55020 Castelvecchio Pascoli (LU), Italy.

Bial, Port. Laboratrios Bial (Portela & Co., SA), Av da Siderurgia Nacional, Apartado 19, 4785 Sao Mamede do Coronado, Portugal.

Bial-Aristegui, Spain. Bial-Aristegui, Alameda de Urquijo 27, Bilbao, 48008 Vizcaya, Spain.

Bialfar, Port. See *Bial, Port.*

Bichsel, Switz. Laboratorium Dr G Bichsel AG, Bahnhofstrasse 5a, 3800 Interlaken, Switzerland.

Bieffe, Ital. Bieffe Medital s.p.a., Via Nuova Provinciale, 23034 Grosotto (SO), Italy.

Bieffe, Spain. Bieffe Medital, C/Solsones 2 BJ Local 7, Parque "Mas Blau", El Trat Del LLobregat, 22666 Barcelona, Spain.

Bieffe, Switz. Bieffe Medital SpA, Via S Balestra 27, 6900 Lugano, Switzerland.

Bier, Ital. Bier Farmaceutici s.n.c. di Pepe G. E. Frattolino R., Via Cupa Capodichino 19, 80144 Naples, Italy.

Bifarma, Ital. Bifarma Fitoterapici di Bignardi Sergio, Via Pallia 5, 20139 Milan, Italy.

Bilgast, Ger. Bilgast Arzneimittel Vertriebs GmbH, Unter den Rusten 36, 67578 Gimbsheim, Germany.

Bilosa, Ital. Bilosa GmbH & Co. KG, Burgerstrasse 15, A-6020 Innsbruck, Austria.

Binesa, Spain. Binesa, Spain.

Bio Sidus, Thai. See *Berli, Thai.*

Bio Terapico Ralay, Spain. Bio Terapico Ralay, Spain.

Bio2, Fr. Laboratoires Bio2, 99 bvd des Belges, 69006 Lyon, France.

Biobasal, Switz. Biobasal AG, Eulerstrasse 55, 4003 Basle, Switzerland.

Biobras, Braz. Biobras S.A., Praca Carlos Chagas 49 (3° andar), 30170-020 Belo Horizonte, MG, Brazil.

Bioceuticals, UK. Bioceuticals Ltd, 26 Zennor Rd, London, SW12 0PS, UK.

Biochem, Canad. Biochem Vaccines Inc., 2323 Parc Technologique Blvd, Sainte-Foy, Quebec, G1P 4R8, Canada.

Biochem, Ital. Biochem Immunosystems Italia spa, Via Magnanelli 2, 40033 Casalecchio di Reno (BO), Italy.

Biochemie, Aust. Biochemie GmbH, Brunner Strasse 59, A-1235 Vienna, Austria.

Biochemie, Austral. Biochemie Australia P/L, Level 2, 11-17 Khartoum Rd, North Ryde, NSW 2113, Australia.

Biochemie, Denm. See *Orphan, Denm.*

Biochemie, Hong Kong. See *Unipharm, Hong Kong.*

Biochemie, Israel. See *Pharmateam, Israel.*

Biochemie, Norw. See *Orphan, Norw.*

Biochemie, Singapore. See *FP, Singapore.*

Biochemie, UK. See *Orphan, UK.*

Biochimica, Ital. Biochimica Zanardi s.r.l., Italy.

Biochimici, Ital. Biochimici PSN spa, Via Viadagola 30, 40050 Quarto Inferiore (BO), Italy.

Biochimico, Braz. Instituto Biochimico S.A., Rua Antonio Joao 218, 21250-150 Rio de Janeiro, RJ, Brazil.

Biocine, Ital. See *Chiron Vaccines, Ital.*

Bioclon, Mex. Bioclon, S.A. de C.V., Calz de Tlalpan No. 4687, 14050 Mexico D. F., Mexico.

Bioclones, S.Afr. Bioclones (Pty) Ltd, P.O. Box 784351, Sandton 2146, South Africa.

Biocodex, Denm. See *Logic, Denm.*

Biocodex, Fr. Laboratoires Biocodex, 19 rue Barbès, 92126 Montrouge cdx, France.

Biocodex, Switz. See *Biomed, Switz.*

Bioconcepts, UK. Bioconcepts Ltd, P.O. Box 15, Havant, Hampshire, PO9 1RQ, UK.

Biocontrolfarm, Ital. Biocontrolfarm s.n.c., Via dell'Epomeo 72, 80126 Naples, Italy.

Biocur, Ger. Biocur Arzneimittel GmbH, Otto-von-Guericke-Allee 1, 39179 Barleben, Germany.

Biocure, Ital. Biocure s.r.l., Via Friuli 88, 20135 Milan, Italy.

Bioderma, Fr. Bioderma, 75 cours Albert-Thomas, 69447 Lyon cdx 03, France.

Biodiagnostics, Austral. Biodiagnostics P/L, 7-9 Merriwa St, Gordon, NSW 2072, Australia.

Bio-Diat, Ger. Bio-Diät-Berlin, Selerweg 43-45, 12169 Berlin, Germany.

Biodiphar, Belg. Biodiphar S.A., Rue des Trois Arbres 16 A, 1180 Brussels, Belgium.

Biodynamics, Ger. Biodynamics International (Deutschland) GmbH, Wetterkreuz 19a, 91058 Erlangen, Germany.

Bioethical, Ital. Bioethical, Italy.

Bio-Familia, Switz. bio-familia AG, Hochwertige Nahrungsmittel, 6072 Sachseln, Switzerland.

Biofilm, USA. Biofilm Inc., 3121 Scott St 1707 Vista, CA 92083-8323, USA.

Bioflora, Aust. Bioflora GmbH, Teichweg 2, A-5400 Hallein, Austria.

Bioforce, Canad. Bioforce Canada Inc., 4001 blvd Cote Vertu, St-Laurent, Quebec, H4R 1R5, Canada.

Bioforce, Ger. Bioforce GmbH, Bruhlstr. 15, 78465 Constance, Germany.

Bioforce, Switz. Bioforce AG, Postfach 76, 9325 Roggwil/TG, Switzerland.

Bioforce, UK. Bioforce UK Ltd, 2 Brewster Place, Irvine, Ayrshire, KA11 5DD, UK.

Biogal, Israel. Biogal, Israel.

Biogalenica, Spain. Biogalenica, Ramon Trias Fargas 7-11, Marina Village, 08005 Barcelona, Spain.

Biogalenique, Fr. Laboratoires Biogalénique, 11 quai de la Rapee, 75601 Paris cdx 12, France.

Biogam, Switz. See *Kart, Switz.,* and *Serolab, Switz.*

Bio-Garten, Aust. Bio-Garten, Flatschacher Strasse 57, A-9020 Klagenfurt, Austria.

Biogen, Aust. See *Biogen, Fr.*

Biogen, Canad. Biogen Canada Inc., 3 Robert Speck Pkwy, Suite 300, Mississauga, Ontario, L4Z 2G5, Canada.

Biogen, Denm. Biogen Denmark A/S, Lyngbyvej 28, 2100 Copenhagen O, Denmark.

Biogen, Fin. Biogen Finland Oy, Aleksanterinkatu 17, 00100 Helsinki, Finland.

Biogen, Fr. Biogen France SA, Le Capitole, 55 av. des Champs-Pierreux, 92012 Nanterre cdx, France.

Biogen, Ger. Biogen GmbH, Carl-Zeiss-Ring 6, 85737 Ismaning, Germany.

Biogen, Irl. See *United Drug, Irl.*

Biogen, Israel. Biogen, Israel.

Biogen, Neth. Biogen, Netherlands.

Biogen, Norw. Biogen Norway AS, Karenslyst alle 8b, 0278 Oslo, Norway.

Biogen, NZ. See *CSL, NZ.*

Biogen, Swed. See *Biogen, Denm.*

Biogen, UK. Biogen Ltd, 5d Roxborough Way, Foundation Park, Maidenhead, Berkshire, SL6 3UD, UK.

Biogen, USA. Biogen, 14 Cambridge Center, Cambridge, MA 02142, USA.

Biogena, Ital. Valetudo s.r.l., Divisione Biogena, Via Ghiaie 6, 24030 Presezzo (BG), Italy.

Biogenetech, Thai. Biogenetech Co. Ltd, Biopex Building, 749/12 Soi Watchannal, Off Soi Pradoo, Sathupradit Rd, Bangphongphang, Yannawa, Bangkok 10120, Thailand.

BioGenex, USA. BioGenex Laboratories, 4600 Norris Canyon Rd, San Ramon, CA 94583, USA.

Bioglan, Austral. Bioglan Ltd, 8/10 Yalgar Rd, Yalgar Business Park, Kirrawee, NSW 2322, Australia.

Bioglan, Denm. Bioglan DK, Skovmose Alle 48, 3500 Vaerlose, Denmark.

Bioglan, Fin. See *Bioglan, Swed.*

Bioglan, Ger. Bioglan Pharma GmbH, Robert-Bosch-Str. 6, 35398 Giessen, Germany.

Bioglan, Hong Kong. See *Keller, Hong Kong,* and *Metrolite, Hong Kong.*

Bioglan, Irl. Bioglan Ireland (Sales) Ltd, Unit 5, 151 Baldoyle Industrial Estate, Dublin 13, Ireland.

Bioglan, Israel. Bioglan, Israel.

Bioglan, Norw. Bioglan AS, Postboks 1865 Gulset, 3705 Skien, Norway.

Bioglan, Singapore. See *Biomed, Singapore,* and *Pharmed, Singapore.*

Bioglan, Swed. Bioglan AB, Box 50310, 202 13 Malmo, Sweden.

Bioglan, Thai. See *Hua, Thai*.

Bioglan, UK. Bioglan Laboratories Ltd, 5 Hunting Gate, Hitchin, Hertfordshire, SG4 0TJ, UK.

Bioglan, USA. Bioglan Pharma, 7 Great Valley Parkway, Suite 301, Malvern, PA 19355, USA.

Biogyne, Fr. Biogyne, Lab. groupe Poli, 183 rue de Courcelles, 75017 Paris, France.

Bio-Health, UK. Bio-Health Ltd, Culpeper Close, Medway City Estate, Rochester, Kent, ME2 4HU, UK.

Biohorm, Spain. Biohorm, Dega Bahi 67, 08026 Barcelona, Spain.

Biohorma, Ital. Biohorma Italia srl, Via del Mare 32 N/1, 00040 Pomezia (RM), Italy.

Bioiberica, Spain. Bioiberica, Ctra N-II Km 680.6, Palafolls, 08389 Barcelona, Spain.

Bioimmun, Ger. BioImmunPharma GmbH, Im Dammwald 27, 61381 Friedrichsdorf, Germany.

Bioindustria, Ital. Bioindustria Laboratorio Italioano Medicinali s.p.a., Via de Ambrosio 2, 15067 Novi Ligure (AL), Italy.

Biokanol, Ger. Biokanol Pharma GmbH, Kehler Str. 7, 76437 Rastatt, Germany.

Biolab, Hong Kong. See *Great Eastern, Hong Kong*, and *Mekim, Hong Kong*.

Biolab, NZ. Biolab Scientific, Private Bag 36-900, Northcote, Auckland, New Zealand.

Biolab, Singapore. See *Indrugco, Singapore*.

Biolab, Thai. See *Biopharm, Thai*.

Biolac, Swed. Biolac AB, Box 22057, 250 22 Helsingborg, Sweden.

Biologia, Braz. Laboratorio Brasileiro de Biologia Ltda, Rua Allan Kardec 66, Engenho Novo, 20710-230 Rio de Janeiro, RJ, Brazil.

Biologici Italia, Ital. Biologici Italia Laboratories s.r.l., Via Cavour 41/3, 20026 Novate Milanese (MI), Italy.

Biologiques de l'Ile-de-France, Fr. Laboratoires Biologiques de l'Ile-de-France, 95 rue de l'Abbe-Groult, 75015 Paris, France.

Biomatrix, Canad. Biomatrix Medical Canada Inc., 275 av Labrosse, Pointe-Claire, Quebec, H9R 1A3, Canada.

Biomatrix, Hong Kong. Biomatrix, Hong Kong.

Biomatrix, Israel. See *Pharma Clal, Israel*.

Biomatrix, UK. Biomatrix (UK) Ltd, Lamb House, Church St, Chiswick, London, W4 2PD, UK.

Biomed, Singapore. Biomed Pte Ltd, 32 Kallang Pudding Rd, 07-06 Elite Industrial Building 1, S 349313, Singapore.

Biomed, Switz. Biomed AG, Uberlandstrasse 199, Postfach, 8600 Dubendorf 1, Switzerland.

Biomedica, Austral. BioMedica, Australia.

Biomedica, Ger. Biomedica Pharma-Produkte GmbH, Birkenweg 16, 63871 Heinrichsthal, Germany.

Biomedica, Hong Kong. See *LCH, Hong Kong*, and *Trendful, Hong Kong*.

Biomedica, Ital. Biomedica Foscama Industria Chimico Farmaceutica s.p.a., Via Morolense 87, 03013 Ferentino (FR), Italy.

Biomedica, Thai. See *Osotspa, Thai*.

Bio-Medical, UK. Bio-Medical Services Ltd, River View Rd, Beverley, North Humberside, HU17 0LD, UK.

Biomedis, Hong Kong. See *Unam, Hong Kong*.

Biomedis, Singapore. See *Far East Drug, Singapore*.

Biomedis, Thai. See *Olic, Thai*.

Biomerica, USA. Biomerica Inc., 1533 Monrovia Ave, Newport Beach, CA 92663, USA.

Biomet, Austral. Biomet Australia P/L, 4/6-8 Byfield St, North Ryde, NSW 2113, Australia.

Biomet Merck, UK. Biomet Merck Ltd, Waterton Industrial Estate, Bridgend, South Wales, CF31 3XA, UK.

Biomo, Ger. Biomo Pharma GmbH, Lendersbergstrasse 86, 53721 Siegburg, Germany.

Bional, Ger. Bional Pharma Deutschland GmbH & Co. KG, Heidsieker Heide 144, 33739 Bielefeld, Germany.

Bionatec, Fr. Lab. Bionatec, Parc de Sophia Antipolis, 774 route des Trois Moulins, 06600 Antibes, France.

Bionative, Swed. BioNative AB, Box 7979, 907 19 Umea, Sweden.

Bionax, Hong Kong. Bionax Hong Kong Ltd, 2/F, Hong Kong Spinners Bldg, 800 Cheung Sha Wan Rd, Kowloon, Hong Kong.

Bionax, Singapore. Bionax Singapore Pte Ltd, 99 Bukit Timah Rd, Alfa Centre 03-06, S 229835, Singapore.

Bionax, Thai. Bionax (Thailand) Ltd, 10 Fl, Unit A, Lake Rajada Office Complex, 193/35 New Rachadapisek Rd, Kwaeng Klongtoey, Khet Klongtoey, Bangkok 10110, Thailand.

Bioniche, Canad. Bioniche Pharma, 383 Sovereign Rd, London, Ontario, N6M 1A3, Canada.

Bionorica, Ger. Bionorica Arzneimittel GmbH, Kerschensteinerstr. 11-15, 92318 Neumarkt/Opf, Germany.

Bionorica, Hong Kong. See *Jacobson, Hong Kong*.

Bionorica, Singapore. See *MBD, Singapore*.

Bionorica, Switz. See *Desopharmex, Switz*.

Bionorica, Thai. Bionorica-Thai, 15 Fl, Central Tower Pinklao, 7/129 Borommaratchachonnani Rd, Arunamarin, Bangkoknoi, Bangkok 10700, Thailand.

Bio-Oil Research, Irl. See *Allphar, Irl*.

Bio-Oil Research, UK. Bio-Oil Research Ltd, The Hawthorns, 64 Welsh Row, Nantwich, Cheshire, CW5 5EU, UK.

Biopha, Fr. Laboratoires Dermopharmaceutiques Biopha, 15 rue Ampere, 91748 Massy cdx, France.

Biopharm, Thai. Biopharm Chemicals Co. Ltd, 7 Fl, Bio House, 55 Sukhumvit 39, Bangkok 10110, Thailand.

Biopharm, USA. Bio-Pharm Inc, 10 H Runway Rd, Levittown, PA 19057, USA.

Biopharma, Fr. Biopharma, 29 rue du Pont, 92200 Neuilly-sur-Seine, France.

Biopharma, Ital. Biopharma s.r.l., Via delle Gerbere, 00040 Santa Palomba (RM), Italy.

Biophausia, Denm. See *Pharmalink, Denm*.

Biophausia, Swed. BioPhausia AB, AR 4, S-741 74 Uppsala, Sweden.

Biophytarom, Fr. Laboratoires Biophytarom, Cap 18, 43 rue de l'Evangile, 75886 Paris cdx 18, France.

Bioprogress, Ital. Bioprogress s.p.a., Via Aurelia 58, 00165 Rome, Italy.

Bioprojet, Fr. Bioprojet Pharma, 9 rue Rameau, 75002 Paris, France.

Biopura, Port. Biopura, Lda, Urbanizcao Industrial Ourreca, Rua Por do Sol 4, 2735 Cacem, Portugal.

Bioquimico, Mex. Laboratorio Bioquimico Mexicano, S.A. de C.V, Liga 8-8o. Piso, Col. Juarez, 06600 Mexico, D.F., Mexico.

Bioren, Switz. Bioren SA, 4 rue des iles, 2108 Couvet, Switzerland.

Bioresearch, Mex. Bioresearch de Mexico, S.A. de C.V., Av. Rio Totolica No 15-A, Fracc. Ind. Naucalpan, 53370 Naucalpan de Juarez, Edo. de Mex., Mexico.

Bioresearch, Spain. Bioresearch, Avda de Burgos 91, Edif. 4, 28050 Madrid, Spain.

Biorex, UK. Biorex Laboratories Ltd, 2 Crossfield Chambers, Gladbeck Way, Enfield, Middlesex, EN2 7HT, UK.

Biorga, Fr. Laboratoires Biorga, 98 av de la Republique, 92400 Courbevoie, France.

Biorga, Hong Kong. See *CNW, Hong Kong*.

Bios, Belg. Bios-Coutelier S.A., Route de Lennik 437, 1070 Brussels, Belgium.

Biosan, Ital. Biosan srl, Via Galileo Galilei 7, 20016 Pero (MI), Italy.

Bio-Sante, Canad. Les Laboratoires Bio-Sante, 3564 Griffith St, St-Laurent, Quebec, H4C 1A7, Canada.

Biosarto, Spain. Biosarto, FOC 68-82, 08030 Barcelona, Spain.

Biosaude, Port. Biosaúe, Lda, Av. Duque d'Avila 193, 1050-082 Lisbon, Portugal.

Bioscience, Israel. Bioscience, Israel.

Bioscience, Thai. Bioscience Co. Ltd, 184/42 Forum Tower, Ratchadapisak Rd, Huaykwang, Bangkok 10310, Thailand.

Biosintetica, Braz. Laboratorios Biosintetica Ltda, Rua Periquito 236, 04514-050 Sao Paulo, SP, Brazil.

Biosyn, Ger. biosyn Arzneimittel GmbH, Schorndorfer Str. 32, 70734 Fellbach, Germany.

Biotech, Austral. Biotech Pharmaceuticals P/L, 100 Antimony St, Carole Park, QLD 4300, Australia.

Bio-Tech, USA. Bio-Tech Pharmacal, P.O. Box 1992, Fayetteville, AR 72702, USA.

Biotechnology, Israel. Biotechnology Israel, Kiryat Weisman, Rehovot, Israel.

Biotechnology, Singapore. See *Scigen, Singapore*.

Biotekfarma, Ital. Biotekfarma bkf s.r.l., Italy.

Biotel, USA. Biotel Corporation, 366 Madison Ave 1506, New York, NY 10017, USA.

Biotest, Aust. Biotest Pharmazeutika GmbH, Einsiedlergasse 58, Postfach 8, A-1053 Vienna, Austria.

Biotest, Fin. See *Leo, Fin*.

Biotest, Ger. Biotest Pharma GmbH, Landsteinerstr. 3-5, 63303 Dreieich, Germany.

Biotest, Hong Kong. See *Tai Fung, Hong Kong*.

Biotest, Israel. Biotest, Israel.

Biotest, Ital. Biotest s.r.l., Via L. da Vinci 43, 20090 Trezzano sul Naviglio (MI), Italy.

Biotest, Singapore. See *Summit, Singapore*.

Biotest, Switz. Biotest (Schweiz) AG, Bahnhofstrasse 18, Postfach, 5504 Othmarsingen, Switzerland.

Biotest, Thai. See *Charoen, Thai*.

Bio-Therabel, Belg. Bio-Therabel S.A., Rue Egide Van Ophem 108, 1180 Brussels, Belgium.

Biotherapie, Fr. Laboratoires Biotherapie, 88 av de l'Arche, 92400 Courbevoie, France.

Biotherm, Canad. Biotherm Canada, 2115 Crescent St, Montreal, Quebec, H3G 2C1.

Biotrading, Ital. Biotrading di Maurizio Mannone, Via Francesco Struppa 4, 91025 Marsala (TP), Italy.

Bio-Transfusion, Fr. Bio-Transfusion, France.

Biovac, S.Afr. Biovac SA CC, P.O. Box 14374, Wadeville 1422, South Africa.

Biovail, Denm. See *Gea, Denm*.

Biovail, USA. Biovail Pharmaceuticals Inc., 170 Southport Drive, Morrisville, NC 27560, USA.

Biovital, Austral. Biovital P/L, 24/10 Yalgar Road, Kirrawee, NSW 2232, Australia.

Bipharma, Neth. Bipharma B.V., Postbus 151, 1380 AD Weesp, Netherlands.

Bira, USA. BIRA Corp., 2525 Quicksilver, McDonald, PA 15057, USA.

Birchwood, USA. Birchwood Laboratories Inc., 7900 Fuller Rd, Eden Prairie, MN 53344, USA.

Bird, USA. Bird Products Corp., 1100 Bird Center Drive, Palm Springs, CA 92262, USA.

Biscova, Ger. Biscova-Arzneimittel Vertrieb pharmazeutischer Praparate, Fuhrenkamp 7, 29559 Wrestedt/Stederdorf, Germany.

Bissendorf, Neth. See *Byk, Neth*.

Bitelab, Fin. Bitelab Oy, Pakilantie 61, 00660 Helsinki, Finland.

Bittermedizin, Ger. Bittermedizin Arzneimittel Vertriebs-GmbH, Taku-Fort-Str. 20, 81827 Munich, Germany.

Bittner, Aust. Richard Bittner GmbH, A-9344 Weitensfeld 183, Austria.

Blackhall, Irl. Blackhall Pharmaceutical Distributors Ltd, Saucertown, Swords, Dublin, Ireland.

Blackmores, Austral. Blackmores Ltd, P.O. Box 258, Balgowlah, NSW 2093, Australia.

Blackmores, UK. Blackmores UK, 37 Rotasckild Rd, Chiswick, London, W4 5HT, UK.

Blackwell, UK. Blackwell Supplies Ltd, Medcare House, Centurion Close, Gillingham Business Park, Gillingham, Kent, ME8 0SB, UK.

Blaine, USA. Blaine Pharmaceuticals Co. Inc., 1515 Production Drive, Burlington, KY 41005, USA.

Blair, USA. See *Purdue Frederick, USA*.

Blairex, USA. Blairex Labs Inc., 3240 Indianapolis Rd, P.O. Box 2127, Columbus, IN 47202-2127, USA.

Blake, UK. Thomas Blake & Co., The Byre House, Fearby, Nr Masham, North Yorkshire, HG4 4NF, UK.

Blansett, USA. Blansett Pharmacal Co., Inc., P.O. Box 638, North Little Rock, AR 72115, USA.

Bledina, Fr. Bledina SA, B.P. 432, 69654 Villefranche-sur-Saone cdx.

BLH, Thai. BLH Trading Co. Ltd, 7/1 Wireless Rd, Bangkok 10330, Thailand.

Blistex, Canad. Blistex Ltd, 2395 Drew Rd, Mississauga, Ontario, L5S 1A1, Canada.

Blistex, Hong Kong. See *Mekim, Hong Kong*.

Blistex, Israel. Blistex, Israel.

Blistex, USA. Blistex Inc., 1800 Swift Drive, Oak Brook, IL 60523, USA.

Block, Aust. Block Austria GmbH, Resselstrasse 18, A-6020 Innsbruck, Austria.

Block, Canad. Block Drug Co. (Canada) Ltd, 7600 Danbro Cres., Mississauga, Ontario, L5N 6L6, Canada.

Block, Ger. Block Drug Company Inc., Am Rosenkothen 4, 40880 Ratingen, Germany.

Block, USA. Block Drug Company, Inc., 257 Cornelison Avenue, Jersey City, NJ 07302, USA.

Blooms, Austral. Blooms, Australia.

Blue Cross, Ital. Blue Cross s.r.l., SS 156 Km 50, 04010 Borgo S Michele (LT), Italy.

BML, Austral. BML Pharmaceuticals P/L, P.O. Box 31, Arncliffe, NSW 2205, Australia.

BOC, UK. BOC Gases, Priestly Rd, Worsley, Manchester, M28 2UT, UK.

Bock, Ger. W Bock GmbH & Co. KG, Postfach: 1163, 64679 Einhausen, Germany.

Bode, Aust. See *Bode, Ger*.

Bode, Ger. Bode Chemie Hamburg, Melanchthonstr. 27, 22525 Hamburg, Germany.

Body Spring, Ital. Body Spring s.r.l., Circ.ne Bran 40, 37013 Caprino V.se (VR), Italy.

Boehringer de Angeli, Braz. Boehringer de Angeli Quimica e Farmaceutica Ltda, Avenida Maria Coelho de Aguiar 215 (3° andar), 05805-000 Sao Paulo, SP, Brazil.

Boehringer Ingelheim, Aust. Boehringer Ingelheim Austria GmbH, Dr Boehringer-Gasse 5-11, A-1121 Vienna, Austria.

Boehringer Ingelheim, Austral. Boehringer Ingelheim P/L, P.O. Box 1969, Macquarie Centre, North Ryde, NSW 2113, Australia.

Boehringer Ingelheim, Belg. Boehringer Ingelheim S.A., Vesalius Science Park, Ave Ariane 16, 1200 Brussels, Belgium.

Boehringer Ingelheim, Canad. Boehringer Ingelheim (Canada) Ltd, 5180 South Service Rd, Burlington, Ontario, L7L 5H4, Canada.

Boehringer Ingelheim, Denm. Boehringer Ingelheim Danmark A/S, Strodamvej 52, 2100 Copenhagen O, Denmark.

Boehringer Ingelheim, Fin. See *Panfarma, Fin*.

Boehringer Ingelheim, Fr. Boehringer Ingelheim France, 37-9 rue Boissiere, 75116 Paris, France.

Boehringer Ingelheim, Ger. Boehringer Ingelheim Pharma KG, Binger Str. 55216 Ingelheim, Germany.

Boehringer Ingelheim, Hong Kong. Boehringer Ingelheim (Hong Kong) Ltd, Suite 3005-7, Great Eagle Ctr, 23 Harbour Rd, Wanchai, Hong Kong.

Boehringer Ingelheim, Irl. Boehringer Ingelheim Ltd, 31 Sandyford Office Park, Blachthorn Ave, Dublin 18, Ireland.

Boehringer Ingelheim, Israel. Boehringer Ingelheim, Israel.

Boehringer Ingelheim, Ital. Boehringer Ingelheim Italia s.p.a., Via Lorenzini 8, 20139 Milan, Italy.

Boehringer Ingelheim, Jpn. Nippon Boehringer Ingelheim Co. Ltd, 3-10-1 Yato, Kawanishi, Hyogo Prefecture 666-01, Japan.

Boehringer Ingelheim, Mex. Boehringer Ingelheim/Promeco, S.A. de C.V., Calle del Maiz No. 49, Col. Xaltocan, 16090 Mexico, D.F., Mexico.

Boehringer Ingelheim, Neth. Boehringer Ingelheim B.V., Postbus 8037, 1802 KA Alkmaar, Netherlands.

Boehringer Ingelheim, Norw. Boehringer Ingelheim Norway, Drengsrudbekken 25, Postboks 405, 1371 Asker, Norway.

Boehringer Ingelheim, NZ. Boehringer Ingelheim (NZ) Ltd, P.O. Box 76-216, Manukau City, Auckland, New Zealand.

Boehringer Ingelheim, Port. Boehringer Ingelheim, Lda, Av. Antonio Augusto de Aguiar 104, 1063-019 Lisbon, Portugal.

Boehringer Ingelheim, S.Afr. Boehringer Ingelheim (Pty) Ltd, Private Bag X3032, Randburg 2125, South Africa.

Boehringer Ingelheim, Singapore. See *Diethelm, Singapore.*

Boehringer Ingelheim, Spain. Boehringer Ingelheim, Pablo Alcover 31-3, 08017 Barcelona, Spain.

Boehringer Ingelheim, Swed. Boehringer Ingelheim AB, Box 44, 127 21 Skarholmen, Sweden.

Boehringer Ingelheim, Switz. Boehringer Ingelheim (Schweiz) GmbH, Dufourstrasse 54, 4002 Basle, Switzerland.

Boehringer Ingelheim, Thai. Boehringer Ingelheim (Thai) Ltd, 12 Fl, Charn Issara Tower II, 2922/207-208 New Petchburi Rd, Bangkapi, Huay Kwang, Bangkok 10310, Thailand.

Boehringer Ingelheim, UK. Boehringer Ingelheim Ltd, Ellesfield Ave, Bracknell, Berkshire, RG12 4YS, UK.

Boehringer Ingelheim, USA. Boehringer Ingelheim Pharmaceuticals Inc., 900 Ridgebury Rd, P.O. Box 368, Ridgefield, CT 06877-0368, USA.

Boehringer Ingelheim Self Medication, UK. See *Boehringer Ingelheim, UK.*

Boehringer Mannheim, Aust. See *Roche, Aust.*

Boehringer Mannheim, Austral. Boehringer Mannheim Australia P/L, 31 Victoria Avenue, Castle Hill, NSW 2154, Australia.

Boehringer Mannheim, Belg. Boehringer Mannheim Belgium S.A., Avenue des Croix de Guerre 90, 1120 Brussels, Belgium.

Boehringer Mannheim, Canad. See *Roche, Canad.*

Boehringer Mannheim, Fr. Laboratoires Boehringer Mannheim France Pharma SA, 2 av. du Vercors, B.P. 59, 38242 Meylan cdx, France.

Boehringer Mannheim, Ger. See *Roche, Ger.*

Boehringer Mannheim, Irl. See *Roche Diagnostics, UK.*

Boehringer Mannheim, Israel. Boehringer Mannheim, Israel.

Boehringer Mannheim, Ital. See *Roche, Ital.*

Boehringer Mannheim, Jpn. Boehringer Mannheim KK, Japan.

Boehringer Mannheim, Neth. Boehringer Mannheim B.V., Postbus 1007, 1300 BA Almere, Netherlands.

Boehringer Mannheim, Norw. See *Roche, Norw.*

Boehringer Mannheim, Port. Laboratórios Boehringer Mannheim de Portugal, Lda, Rua da Barruncheira 6, Carnaxide, 2795 Linda-a-Velha, Portugal.

Boehringer Mannheim, S.Afr. See *Roche, S.Afr.*

Boehringer Mannheim, Spain. See *Roche, Spain.*

Boehringer Mannheim, Swed. See *Roche, Swed.*

Boehringer Mannheim, Switz. See *Roche, Switz.*

Boehringer Mannheim, UK. Boehringer Mannheim (Pharmaceuticals), UK.

Boehringer Mannheim, USA. See *Roche, USA.*

Boehringer Mannheim Diagnostics, Irl. See *Roche Diagnostics, UK.*

Boehringer Mannheim Diagnostics, UK. See *Roche Diagnostics, UK.*

Boehringer Mannheim Diagnostics, USA. See *Roche, USA.*

Boffi, Ital. Eredi di Antonio Boffi s.n.c., Via Lorenzo Magalotti 6, 00197 Rome, Italy.

Bohm, Spain. Bohm, Molina Seca 23 Plg. Cobo Calleja, Fuenlabrada, 28947 Madrid, Spain.

BOI, Spain. Biologicos Organicos Industriales, Polig Ind Sur, Papiol, 08754 Barcelona, Spain.

Boileau & Boyd, Irl. Boileau & Boyd Ltd, Parkmore Estate, Walkinstown, Dublin 12, Ireland.

Boiron, Canad. Boiron Canada, 816 Guimond St, Longueil, Quebec, J4G 1T5, Canada.

Boiron, Fr. Boiron, 20 rue de la Liberation, 69110 Sainte-Foy-les-Lyon, France.

Boiron, Port. See *Prisfar, Port.*

Boiron, Switz. See *Serolab, Switz.*

Bolder, Ger. Bolder Arzneimittel GmbH & Co. KG, Koblenzer Str. 65, 50968 Cologne, Germany.

Bomac, NZ. Bomac Laboratories Ltd, Wiri Station Rd, Manukau City, Auckland, New Zealand.

Bonafarma, Port. Bonafarma, SA, Apartado 197, Edificio JABA, Abrunheira, 2710-901 Sintra, Portugal.

Boncour, Fr. Laboratoires Boncour, 46 av. de Lattre-de-Tassigny, 94410 Saint-Maurice, France.

Bone Care, USA. Bone Care International, USA.

Boniscontro & Gazzone, Ital. Lab. Prod. Farm. Boniscontro & Gazzone s.r.l., Via Tiburtina 1004, 00156 Rome, Italy.

Bonne Bell, Canad. Bonne Bell of Canada, 6711 Mississauga Rd, Ste 602, Mississauga, Ontario, L5N 2W3, Canada.

Bonomelli, Ital. Bonomelli s.r.l., Via Montecuccoli 1, 23843 Dolzago (LC), Italy.

Boots, Austral. Boots Healthcare Australia P/L, Locked Bag 2067, North Ryde, NSW 2113, Australia.

Boots, Denm. See *AstraZeneca, Denm.*

Boots, Fin. See *Dumex-Alpharma, Fin.*

Boots, Fr. See *Knoll, Fr.*

Boots, Ger. See *Kanoldt, Ger.*

Boots, Hong Kong. See *Swire Loxley, Hong Kong.*

Boots, Israel. Boots, Israel.

Boots, Ital. See *Boots Healthcare, Ital.*, and *Ravizza, Ital.*

Boots, Neth. Boots Pharmaceuticals B.V., Netherlands.

Boots, NZ. Boots Healthcare New Zealand Ltd, P.O. Box 27-341, Wellington 1, New Zealand.

Boots, Port. Boots Healthcare Portugal, Lda, Av. Duque d'Avila, 185, 1050 Lisbon, Portugal.

Boots, S.Afr. Boots Healthcare (SA) (Pty) Ltd, P.O. Box 30178, Jet Park 1469, South Africa.

Boots, Singapore. The Boots Company (Far East) Pte Ltd, 1123 Serangoon Rd, 02-02, S 328207, Singapore.

Boots, Spain. See *Boots Healthcare, Spain.*

Boots, Switz. See *Doetsch, Grether, Switz.*

Boots, Thai. The Boots Co. (Thailand) Ltd, 65 Lard Krabang, Bang Plee Rd, Amphur Bang Plee, Samutprakarn 10540, Thailand.

Boots, UK. Boots the Chemists, Thane Rd, D90 East FO8, Nottingham, NG90 1BS, UK.

Boots, USA. See *Knoll, USA.*

Boots Healthcare, Belg. Boots Healthcare S.A., Koningen Astridlaan 164, 1780 Wemmel, Belgium.

Boots Healthcare, Fr. Laboratoires Boots Healthcare, 35 rue Baudin, 92300 Lavallois-Perret, France.

Boots Healthcare, Ger. Boots Healthcare Deutschland GmbH, Scholtzstr. 3, 21465 Reinbek, Germany.

Boots Healthcare, Irl. Boots Healthcare Ltd, 2 Beech Hill Office Campus, Clonskeagh, Dublin 4, Ireland.

Boots Healthcare, Ital. Boots Healthcare Marco Viti Farmaceutici s.p.a., Via Tarantelli 15, 22076 Mozzate (CO), Italy.

Boots Healthcare, Neth. Boots Healthcare B.V., Postbus 5236, 1410 AE Naarden, Netherlands.

Boots Healthcare, Spain. Boots Healthcare, Doctor Zamenhof 36 Dup 2, Madrid, Spain.

Boots Healthcare, Switz. Boots Healthcare (Switzerland) AG, Hermal, Untermuli 11, 6300 Zug, Switzerland.

Boots-Flint, USA. See *Knoll, USA.*

Borg, UK. Borg Medicare Ltd, P.O. Box 99, Hitchin, Hertfordshire, SG5 2GF, UK.

Bottger, Ger. Böttger GmbH, Paulsborner Str. 2, 10709 Berlin, Germany.

Bouchara, Fr. Laboratoires du Dr E. Bouchara, 68 rue Marjolin, 92302 Levallois-Perret, France.

Bouchara, Port. See *Neo-Farmaceutica, Port.*

Bouchara, Singapore. See *Pharmacon, Singapore.*

Bouchara, Switz. See *Actipharm, Switz.*, and *Interdelta, Switz.*

Boucher & Muir, Austral. Boucher & Muir P/L, P.O. Box 333, North Sydney, NSW 2059, Australia.

Bouhon, Ger. Apotheker Walter Bouhon GmbH & Co. KG, Fuldaer Str. 10, 90427 Nurnberg, Germany.

Bournonville, Belg. Bournonville Pharma S.A., Parc Industriel de la Vallee du Hain, Ave de l'Industrie 11, 1420 Braine-l'Alleud, Belgium.

Bournonville, Neth. Bournonville-Pharma B.V., Netherlands.

Bouty, Ital. s.p.a. Italiana Laboratori Bouty, Via Vanvitelli 4, 20129 Milan, Italy.

Bowman, USA. Bowman Pharmaceuticals Inc., 119 Schroyer Ave SW, Canton, OH 44702, USA.

Boxo, Ger. Boxo-Pharm Arzneimittel GmbH, Karl-Geusen-Str. 173, 40231 Dusseldorf, Germany.

Boyle, USA. Boyle & Co. Pharmaceuticals, 1613 Chelsea Rd, San Marino, CA 91108, USA.

BPL, Hong Kong. See *Inchcape, Hong Kong.*

BPL, Singapore. See *JDH, Singapore.*

BPL, Thai. See *Berli, Thai.*

BPL, UK. Bio Products Laboratory, Dagger Lane, Elstree, Hertfordshire, WD6 3BX, UK.

BPR, Ital. BPR International srl, Via Valera 7, 20024 Garbagnate Milanese (MI), Italy.

BPRL, Singapore. See *Zyfas, Singapore.*

BR Pharmaceuticals, UK. BR Pharmaceuticals Ltd, 51a Broom Mill Estate, Coal Hill Lane, Farsley, Leeds, West Yorkshire, LS28 5NA, UK.

Bracco, Aust. See *Bracco, Ital.*

Bracco, Canad. Bracco Diagnostics, Canada.

Bracco, Denm. See *Astra Tech, Denm.*

Bracco, Israel. See *Discotrade, Israel.*

Bracco, Ital. Bracco s.p.a., Via E. Folli 50, 20134 Milan, Italy.

Bracco, Norw. See *Astra Tech, Norw.*

Bracco, Port. See *Dario Correia, Port.*

Bracco, Switz. See *Sintetica, Switz.*, and *Uhlmann-Eyraud, Switz.*

Bracco, UK. Bracco Diagnostics, UK.

Bracco, USA. Bracco Diagnostics, P.O. Box 5225, Princeton, NJ 08543, USA.

Bracey, UK. Bracey's Pharmaceuticals, 209 Menlove Ave, Liverpool, Merseyside, L18 3EF, UK.

Bradley, Canad. Bradley Pharmaceuticals Inc., 1031 Meyerside Drive, Unit 12, Mississauga, Ontario, L5T 2H5, Canada.

Bradley, USA. See *Doak, USA.*

Bradleys, NZ. Bradleys Pharmaceuticals, 69 The Esplanade, Whangaparaoa, Hibiscus Coast, North Auckland, New Zealand.

Brady, Aust. Brady C. KG, Horlgasse 5, A-1092 Vienna, Austria.

Bragg, UK. J.L. Bragg (Ipswich) Ltd, 34 Boss Hall Rd, Ipswich, Suffolk, IP1 5BN, UK.

Brahms, Ger. BRAHMS Arzneimittel GmbH, Kreuzberger Ring 13, 65205 Wiesbaden, Germany.

Braintree, USA. Braintree Laboratories Inc., P.O. Box 850929, Braintree, MA 02185-0929, USA.

Brandt, Switz. See *Uhlmann-Eyraud, Switz.*

Brasifa, Braz. Sociedade Farmaceutica Brasifa Ltda, Rua Souto Carvalho 45, 23520-210 Rio de Janeiro, RJ, Brazil.

Brasmedica, Braz. Brasmedica S.A. Industrias Farmaceuticas, Avenida Miguel Stefano 2.278, 04301-002 Sao Paulo, SP, Brazil.

Brauer, Austral. Brauer Biotherapies P/L, P.O. Box 234, Tanunda, SA 5352, Australia.

Braun, Aust. Braun Austria GmbH, In den Langackern 5, A-2344 Maria Enzersdorf, Austria.

Braun, Austral. B Braun Australia P/L, Unit 2, 9 Packard Ave, Castle Hill, NSW 2154, Australia.

Braun, Belg. B. Braun Medical S.A., Woluwelaan 140 B, 1831 Diegem, Belgium.

Braun, Braz. Laboratorio B. Braun S.A., Avenida Dr Eugenio Borges 1092, Arsenal, 24751-000 Sao Goncalo, RJ, Brazil.

Braun, Denm. B. Braun Medical A/S, Halmtorvet 29, 1700 Copenhagen V, Denmark.

Braun, Fin. B. Braun Medical Oy, Niittyrinne 7, 02270 Espoo, Finland.

Braun, Fr. B Braun Medical SA, 204 av du Mal-Juin, B.P. 331, 92107 Boulogne cdx, France.

Braun, Ger. B. Braun Melsungen AG, Carl-Braun-Str. 1, 34212 Melsungen, Germany.

Braun, Hong Kong. B Braun Medical (HK) Ltd, 13-14/F Henan Bldg, 90 Jaffe Rd, Wanchai, Hong Kong.

Braun, Irl. B. Braun Medical Ltd, 3 Naas Rd Industrial Park, Dublin 12, Ireland.

Braun, Israel. Braun, Israel.

Braun, Ital. B. Braun Milano s.p.a., Via V. da Seregno 14, 20161 Milan, Italy.

Braun, Norw. B. Braun Medical A/S, Bjellandv. 12, 3173 Vear, Norway.

Braun, Port. B. Braun Medical, Lda, Estrada Consiglieri Pedroso 80, Queluz Park, Queluz de Baixo, 2745 Barcarena, Portugal.

Braun, Singapore. B Braun Singapore Pte Ltd, 460 Alexandra Rd, 34-03 OSA Building, S 409020, Singapore.

Braun, Spain. Braun Medical, Ctra Tarrasa 121, Rubi, 08191 Barcelona, Spain.

Braun, Swed. B. Braun Medical AB, Box 221, 16722 Bromma, Sweden.

Braun, Switz. B. Braun Medical AG, Sparte Pharma, Seesatz, Postfach, 6203 Sempach-Station, Switzerland.

Braun, Thai. See *Diethelm, Thai.*

Braun, UK. B. Braun Medical Ltd, Thorncliffe Park Industrial Estate, Chapeltown, Sheffield, South Yorkshire, S35 2PW, UK.

Braun, USA. B. Braun Medical, P.O. Box 19791, Irvine, CA 92713-9791, USA.

Braun Carex, Ital. B Braun Carex s.p.a., Via XXV Luglio 11, 41037 Mirandola (MO), Italy.

Braun McGaw, Hong Kong. See *LCH, Hong Kong.*

Braun Melsungen, Ital. See *Braun Carex, Ital.*

Braun Melsungen, UK. See *Braun, Ger.*

Braun Omnimed, S.Afr. Braun Omnimed (Pty) Ltd, P.O. Box 2316, Randburg 2125, South Africa.

Braun Surgical, Switz. B. Braun Surgical AG, Postfach 427, 8212 Neuhausen, Switzerland.

Bravir, Braz. Bravir Industrial Ltda, Rua Major Barbosa 95/99, 30240-370 Belo Horizonte, MG, Brazil.

Bray, UK. Bray Health & Leisure (Solport Ltd), 1 Regal Way, Faringdon, Oxfordshire, SN7 7BX, UK.

Breathe Eazy, Austral. Breathe Eazy Chest Rubs, 7 Melia Close, Medowie, NSW 2318, Australia.

Breckenridge, USA. Breckenridge Pharmaceutical Inc, 1141 South Rogers Circle, Suite 3, Boca Raton, FL 33487, USA.

Bregenzer, Aust. Bregenzer Herbert, Am Damm 20, A-6820 Frastanz, Austria.

Brenner-Efeka, Ger. See *Wyeth, Ger.*

Breves, Braz. Industria Farmaceutica Breves Ltda, Rua Japeri 47, 20261-080 Rio de Janeiro, RJ, Brazil.

Bride, Fr. Laboratoires Bride, 263 c av de Laon, 51100 Reims, France.

Bridoux, Fr. Laboratoires Bridoux, 6 rue Salengro, 62160 Bully-les-Mines, France.

Brimms, Israel. Brimms, Israel.

Brioschi, Canad. Brioschi Inc., 465 Fenmar Drive, Weston, Ontario, M9L 2R6, Canada.

Bripharm, Irl. See *United Drug, Irl.*

Brissenco, S.Afr. Brissenco, South Africa.

Bristol, Canad. See *Bristol-Myers Squibb, Canad.*

Bristol-Myers, Austral. See *Bristol-Myers Squibb, Austral.*

Bristol-Myers, Spain. Bristol Myers, Campus Empresarial Jose Ma Churruca, Almansa 101, 28040 Madrid, Spain.

Bristol-Myers Products, USA. See *Bristol-Myers Squibb, USA.*

Bristol-Myers Squibb, Aust. Bristol-Myers Squibb GmbH, Columbusgasse 4, A-1100 Vienna, Austria.

Bristol-Myers Squibb, Austral. Bristol-Myers Squibb, Division of Bristol-Myers Australia P/L, P.O. Box 39, Noble Park, VIC 3174, Australia.

Bristol-Myers Squibb, Belg. Bristol-Myers Squibb Belgium S.A., Chaussee de la Hulpa 185, 1170 Brussels, Belgium.

Bristol-Myers Squibb, Braz. Bristol-Myers Squibb Brasil S.A., Rua Carlos Gomes 924, 04543-903 Sao Paulo, SP, Brazil.

Bristol-Myers Squibb, Canad. Bristol-Myers Squibb Canada Inc., 2365 Cote-de-Liesse Rd, Montreal, Quebec, H4N 2M7, Canada.

Bristol-Myers Squibb, Denm. Bristol-Myers Squibb, Jaegersborgvej 64-6, 2800 Lyngby, Denmark.

Bristol-Myers Squibb, Fin. Oy Bristol-Myers Squibb (Finland) AB, Metsänneidonkuja 8, 02130 Espoo, Finland.

Bristol-Myers Squibb, Fr. Bristol-Myers Squibb, 1 parvis de la Defense La Grande Arche Nord, 92800 Puteaux, France.

Bristol-Myers Squibb, Ger. Bristol-Myers Squibb GmbH, Sapporobogen 6-8, 80809 Munich, Germany.

Bristol-Myers Squibb, Hong Kong. Bristol-Myers Squibb (Hong Kong) Ltd, 17/F, Manulife Tower, 169 Electric Rd, North Point, Hong Kong.

Bristol-Myers Squibb, Irl. Bristol-Myers Squibb Pharmaceuticals, Watery Lane, Swords, Co. Dublin, Ireland.

Bristol-Myers Squibb, Israel. Bristol-Myers Squibb Ltd, P.O. Box 3917, Petach Tikva, Israel.

Bristol-Myers Squibb, Ital. Bristol-Myers Squibb s.p.a., Via Virgilio Maroso 50, 00142 Rome, Italy.

Bristol-Myers Squibb, Jpn. Bristol-Myers Squibb, Japan.

Bristol-Myers Squibb, Mex. Bristol-Myers Squibb de México, S.A. de C.V. Division Bristol, Av. Primero de Mayo No.226, Col. San Andres Atoto, 53500 Naucalpan de Juarez, Mexico.

Bristol-Myers Squibb, Neth. Bristol-Myers Squibb, Postbus 514, 3440 AM Woerden, Netherlands.

Bristol-Myers Squibb, Norw. Bristol-Myers Squibb Norway Ltd, Sandviksv. 26, Postboks 464, 1322 Hovik, Norway.

Bristol-Myers Squibb, NZ. Bristol-Myers Squibb, P.O. Box 62663, Central Park, Aukland, New Zealand.

Bristol-Myers Squibb, Port. Bristol-Myers Squibb Farmacêutica Portuguesa, Lda, Edificio Fernao de Magalhaes, Quinta da Fonte, 2780-730 Paco De Arcos, Portugal.

Bristol-Myers Squibb, S.Afr. Bristol-Myers Squibb (Pty) Ltd, P.O. Box 1408, Bedfordview, 2008 Johannesburg, South Africa.

Bristol-Myers Squibb, Singapore. Bristol-Myers Squibb (S) Pte Ltd, 66-68 East Coast Rd, 04-00, S 428778, Singapore.

Bristol-Myers Squibb, Swed. Bristol-Myers Squibb AB, Box 15200, 167 15 Bromma, Sweden.

Bristol-Myers Squibb, Switz. Bristol-Myers Squibb AG, Neuhofstrasse 6, 6340 Baar, Switzerland.

Bristol-Myers Squibb, Thai. Bristol-Myers Squibb (Thailand) Ltd, Bristol-Myers Squibb Building, 10/10-11 Srinakarin Rd, Bangplee, Samutprakarn 10540, Thailand.

Bristol-Myers Squibb, UK. Bristol-Myers Squibb Pharmaceuticals Ltd, Bristol-Myers Squibb House, 141-149 Staines Road, Hounslow, Middlesex, TW3 3JA, UK.

Bristol-Myers Squibb, USA. Bristol-Myers Squibb, P.O. Box 4500, Princeton, NJ 08543-4500, USA.

Bristol-Myers Squibb Oncology, USA. See *Bristol-Myers Squibb, USA.*

Britannia Pharmaceuticals, Irl. See *Clonmel, Irl.*

Britannia Pharmaceuticals, UK. Britannia Pharmaceuticals Ltd, 41-51 Brighton Rd, Redhill, Surrey, RH1 6YS, UK.

BritHealth, UK. BritHealth Limited, Weltech Centre, Ridgeway, Welwyn Garden City, Hertfordshire, AL7 2AA, UK.

Britisfarma, Spain. Britisfarma, Pza Carlos Trias Bertran 4, 28020 Madrid, Spain.

British Cod Liver Oils, Hong Kong. See *Keller, Hong Kong.*

British Dispensary, Thai. British Dispensary, 100/103-108 Vongvanij Building, 31 Fl, Rama 9 Rd, Bangkok 10320, Thailand.

British Pharmaceuticals, Austral. See *Organon, Austral.*

Britpharm, UK. Britpharm Laboratories Ltd, Kramer Mews, London, SW5 9JL, UK.

Broad, UK. Broad Laboratories plc, UK.

Bronchosirum, Canad. Bronchosirum Inc. 15 JF Kennedy, Bur 10, St-Jerome, QC, J7Y 4B4, Canada.

Brothier, Fr. Laboratoires Brothier, 41 rue de Neuilly, 92000 Nanterre, France.

Brothier, Switz. See *Uhlmann-Eyraud, Switz.*

Brovar, S.Afr. Brovar S & P (Pty) Ltd, South Africa.

Brum, Spain. Brum, Quevedo 4, Oviedo, 33012 Asturias, Spain.

Brunel, S.Afr. Brunel Laboratories (Pty) Ltd, P.O. Box 23103, Innesdale 0031, South Africa.

Bruni, Ital. Bruni Dr. Domenico (Farmacia), Via Anfossi 9, 20135 Milan, Italy.

Bruno, Ital. Bruno Farmaceutici spa, Via Salvatore Quasimodo 136, 00144 Rome, Italy.

Bruschettini, Hong Kong. See *Jebsen, Hong Kong.*

Bruschettini, Ital. Bruschettini s.r.l., Via Isonzo 6, 16147 Genova, Italy.

Bruschettini, Switz. See *Galenica, Switz.*

BSIA, UK. See *Torbet Laboratories, UK.*

BTG, USA. BTG Pharmaceuticals, 70 Wood Ave South, Iselin, NJ 08830, USA.

Bucaneve, Ital. Bucaneve Medicinali s.r.l., Via Sercognani 15, 20156 Milan, Italy.

Bucca, Spain. Bucca, Juan Alvarez Mendizabal 43, 28008 Madrid, Spain.

Buckley, Canad. W.K. Buckley Ltd, 5230 Orbitor Drive, Mississauga, Ontario, L4W 5G7, Canada.

Buffington, USA. Buffington, USA.

Bull, Singapore. See *Faulding, Singapore.*

Bullivants, Austral. Bullivants, Australia.

Bunker, Braz. Bunker Industria Farmaceutica Ltda, Rua Anibal dos Anjos Carvalho 212, Cidade Dutra, 04810-050 Sao Paulo, SP, Brazil.

Bustillos, Mex. Laboratorios Bustillos, S.A. de C.V., Manuel Dublan No. 40, Col. Tacubaya, 11870 Mexico, D.F., Mexico.

Busto, Spain. Busto, Paseo Del Deleite S/N, Aranjuez, Madrid, Spain.

Butantan, Braz. Butantan, Brazil.

Byk, Aust. Byk Österreich Pharma GmbH, Ketzergasse 200, A-1235 Vienna, Austria.

Byk, Belg. Byk Belga S.A., Rue Anatole France 115-21, 1030 Brussels, Belgium.

Byk, Braz. Byk Quimica e Farmaceutica Ltda, Rua do Estilo Barroco 721, Santo Amaro, 04709-011 Sao Paulo, SP, Brazil.

Byk, Canad. Byk Canada Inc., 1275 North Service Rd W, 7th Floor, Oakville, Ontario, L6M 3G4, Canada.

Byk, Fr. Laboratoires Byk France SA, 593 rte de Boissise, 77350 le Mee-sur-Seine, France.

Byk, Neth. Byk Nederland B.V., Postbus 61, 1160 AB Zwanenburg, Netherlands.

Byk, Port. Byk Portugal, Lda, Quinta da Fonte, Edificio Gil Eanes, Porto Salvo, 2780 Oeiras, Portugal.

Byk, Switz. Byk AG, Bachstrasse 10, 8280 Kreuzlingen, Switzerland.

Byk Elmu, Spain. Byk Elmu, Ctra Nacional III, Km 23, Arganda del Rey, 28500 Madrid, Spain.

Byk Gulden, Denm. See *Nycomed, Denm.*

Byk Gulden, Ger. Byk Gulden Lomberg Chemische Fabrik GmbH, Byk-Gulden-Str. 2, 78467 Constance, Germany.

Byk Gulden, Hong Kong. Byk Gulden, 7/F Somerset House, Taikoo Place, Hong Kong.

Byk Gulden, Ital. Byk Gulden Italia s.p.a., Via Giotto 1, 20032 Cormano (MI), Italy.

Byk Gulden, Mex. Byk-Gulden, S.A. de C.V., Av Primero de Mayo No. 130, Apartado Postal No. 311, 53519 Naucalpan de Juarez., Mexico.

Byk Gulden, Norw. See *Pharmacia Upjohn, Norw.*

Byk Gulden, S.Afr. Byk Gulden Pharmaceuticals, P.O. Box 1476, Randburg 2125, South Africa.

Byk Gulden, Singapore. See *Pasture, Singapore.*

Byk Gulden, Thai. See *Zuellig, Thai.*

Byk Leo, Spain. Byk Leo Lab. Farm., Ctra N-III, Km 23, Arganda del Rey, 28500 Madrid, Spain.

Byk Madaus, S.Afr. Byk Madaus (Pty) Ltd, P.O. Box 3435, Halfway House 1685, South Africa.

Byk Roland, Switz. Byk Roland GmbH, Bachstrasse 10, 8280 Kreuzlingen, Switzerland.

Byk Tosse, Ger. See *Byk Gulden, Ger.*

Bykomed, Port. See *Byk, Port.*

C & L, Hong Kong. C & L Pharmaceutical Ltd, Unit A-C, 19/F Flourish Food Manufactory Ctr, 18 Tai Lee St, Yuen Long, N.T., Hong Kong.

C & M, USA. C & M Pharmacal Inc., 1721 Maplelane Ave, Hazel Park, MI 48030-1215, USA.

C & RF, Ital. C&RF srl, Via Trinacria 34, 95030 Tremestieri Etneo (CT), Italy.

Caber, Ital. Farmaceutici Caber s.p.a., Via Cavour 11, 44022 Comacchio (FE), Italy.

Cabon, Ital. Cabon s.r.l., Via Melchiorre Gioia 168, 20125 Milan, Italy.

CaDiGroup, Ital. Ca.Di.Group srl, Via Pieve Tesino 75, 00124 Rome, Italy.

Cadila, Thai. See *Pharmadica, Thai.,* and *Pharmaland, Thai.*

Cady, Ital. Cady Paris by Caselli Alda, Vicolo della Neve 7, 40123 Bologna, Italy.

Caesaro, Aust. Caesaro Med GmbH, Raidenstrasse 46, A-4060 Leonding, Austria.

Cahill May Roberts, Irl. Cahill May Roberts Ltd, Chapelizod, Dublin 20, Ireland.

Caldeira & Marques, Port. Caldeira & Marques, Lda, Rua 25 de Abril, Lote 32-B, Brandoa, 2700-851 Amadora, Portugal.

Caldeira & Metelo, Port. Caldeira & Metelo, Lda, Rua 25 de Abril, Lote 26-Arm., Brandoa, 2700-851 Amadora, Portugal.

Calgon Vestal, USA. See *Steris, USA.*

Callegari, Ital. Callegari s.p.a., Via Adamello 2/A, 43100 Parma, Italy.

Calmante Vitaminado, Spain. Calmante Vitaminado, Glorieta Perez Gimenez 1, 14007 Cordoba, Spain.

Calmic, Irl. See *GlaxoSmithKline, Irl.*

Calmic, USA. See *Wellcome, USA.*

Cal-White, USA. Cal-White Mineral Co., P.O. Box 7890, Klamath Falls, OR 97602, USA.

Cambridge, Fr. Cambridge Line, B.P. 18, 251 rue de la Gare, 44370 Varades, France.

Cambridge, UK. Cambridge Laboratories, Deltic House, Kingfisher Way, Silverlink Business Park, Wallsend, Tyne & Wear, NE28 9NX, UK.

Cambridge Healthcare, UK. Cambridge Healthcare Supplies Ltd, Unit 26, Newton Business Park, Poole, Dorset, BH12 3LL, UK.

Camps, Spain. Camps, Planeta 39, 08012 Barcelona, Spain.

Can-Am Care, USA. Can Am Care Corp., Cimetra Industrial Park, P.O. Box 98, Chazy, NY 12921, USA.

Canderm, Canad. Canderm Pharma, 5353 Thimens Blvd, Saint-Laurent, Quebec, H4R 2H4, Canada.

Candioli, Ital. Istituto Candioli Profilattico & Farmaceutico s.p.a., Via Manzoni 2, 10092 Torino Beinasco, Italy.

Cangene, Canad. Cangene Corporation, 104 Chancellor Matheson Rd, Winnipeg, Manitoba, R3T 5Y3, Canada.

Cangene, UK. See *Cangene, Canad.*

Canonne, Braz. Laboratorio Canonne Ltda, Avenida Canal do Anil 1.263, 22765-430 Rio de Janeiro, RJ, Brazil.

Cantabria, Spain. Cantabria, Ctra de Cazona Adarzo S/N, Santander, 39011 Cantabria, Spain.

Cantassium Co., UK. The Cantassium Company, UK.

Capellon, USA. Capellon Pharmaceuticals Inc., 7462 Dogwood Drive, Fort Worth, TX 76118, USA.

Capilares, Spain. Productos Capilares, Lopez Bravo 78, Plg. Ind. Villalonquejar, 09080 Burgos, Spain.

Capo Sole, Ital. Capo Sole s.r.l., Via Edison 60, 20019 Settimo Milanese (MI), Italy.

Caprice Greystoke, USA. Caprice Greystoke, 1259 Activity Drive, Vista, CA 92083, USA.

Caps, S.Afr. Caps Pharmaceuticals (SA) (Pty) Ltd, P.O. Box 2801, Johannesburg 2000, South Africa.

Caraco, USA. Caraco Pharmaceutical Labs, 1150 Elijah McCoy Drive, Detroit, MI 48202, USA.

Cardel, Fr. See *Monsanto, Fr.*

Cardinaux, Canad. Cardinaux Enrg, 5420 Pasquier, Laval, QC, H7K 3K3, Canada.

Care, USA. Care Technologies Inc., P.O. Box 82, 10 Corbin Drive, Darien, CT 06820, USA.

Carlo Erba, Braz. Carlo Erba S.A., Rodovia Washington Luiz Km 119, 25085-000 Duque de Caxias, RJ, Brazil.

Carlo Erba OTC, Ital. See *Pharmacia Upjohn, Ital.*

Carlson, USA. J.R. Carlson Laboratories Inc., 15 College Drive, Arlington Heights, IL 60004-1985, USA.

Carmaran, Canad. Carmaran, 1467 Cunard, Chomedey-Laval, QC, H7S 2H8, Canada.

Carme, USA. Carme Inc., 5585 S.W. Artic Dr., Beaverton, OR 97005, USA.

Carnation, USA. Carnation, 800 North Brand Blvd, Glendale, CA 91203, USA.

Carnivora, Ger. Carnivora-Forschungs-GmbH, Lobensteiner Str. 3, 96365 Nordhalben, Germany.

Carnot, Mex. Carnot Laboratorios, Productos Cientificos, S.A. de C.V., Nicolas San Juan No.1046, Col del Valle, 03100 Mexico D.F., Mexico.

Carnrick, USA. Carnrick Laboratories Inc., Division of Elan Pharmaceuticals, 65 Horse Hill Rd, Cedar Knolls, NJ 07927, USA.

Carolina, USA. Carolina Medical Products Co., P.O. Box 147, Farmville, NC 27828, USA.

Carter Horner, Canad. Carter Horner Inc., 6600 Kitimat Rd, Mississauga, Ontario, L5N 1L9, Canada.

Carter Horner, Hong Kong. See *Tsun Tsun, Hong Kong.*

Carter Horner, Thai. See *US Summit, Thai.*

Carter-Wallace, Austral. Carter Wallace (Australia) P/L, P.O. Box 216, Brookvale, NSW 2100, Australia.

Carter-Wallace, Mex. Carter Wallace, S.A., M. de Cervantes Saavedra No. 193, Col Granada, 11520 Mexico D.F, Mexico.

Carter-Wallace, Switz. See *Doetsch, Grether, Switz.*

Carter-Wallace, UK. Carter-Wallace Ltd, Wear Bay Rd, Folkestone, Kent, CT19 6PG, UK.

Carter-Wallace, USA. Carter Wallace, Half Acre Rd, P.O. Box 1001, Cranbury, NJ 08512-0181, USA.

Cascan, Ger. Cascan GmbH & Co. KG, Warburgstr. 4, 20354 Hamburg, Germany.

Cascapharm, Ger. Cascapharm GmbH & Co., Germany.

Casen Fisons, Spain. Casen Fisons, Autovia de Logrono, Km 13300, Utebo, 50180 Zaragoza, Spain.

Casen Fleet, Spain. Casen Fleet, Autovia de Logrono Km 13.3, Utebo, 50180 Zaragoza, Spain.

Casmar, Mex. Casmar, S.A. de C.V., Corporación, Zacatecas No. 208, Col. Roma, 06700 Mexico, D.F., Mexico.

Cassella-med, Ger. Cassella-med GmbH & Co. KG, Gereonsmuhlengasse 1, 50670 Cologne, Germany.

Cassella-med, Switz. Cassella-med AG, Steinentorstrasse 19, 4051 Basel, Switzerland.

Cassenne, Fr. See *Aventis, Fr.*

Castlemead, UK. Castlemead Healthcare Ltd, P.O. Box 57, Ware, Hertfordshire, SG10 6LL, UK.

Catarinense, Braz. Laboratorio Catarinense S.A., Rua Doutor Joao Colin 1.053, 89204-001 Joinville, SC, Brazil.

Cazi, Braz. Cazi Quimica Farmaceutica Industria e Comercio Ltda, Rua Antonio Lopes 17, 06600-000 Sao Paulo, SP, Brazil.

CCD, Fr. Laboratoires CCD, 60 rue Pierre-Charron, 75008 Paris, France.

CCM, Hong Kong. See *Zuellig, Hong Kong.*

CCM, Singapore. See *FP, Singapore.*

CCPC, Hong Kong. See *Kai Yuen, Hong Kong.*

CCS, Swed. CCS Clean Chemical Sweden AB, Tunavagen 277 B, 781 73 Borlange, Sweden.

Ceccarelli, Ital. Ceccarelli A. & C. dei F.lli dr. Tanganelli, Via G. Caponsacchi 31, 50126 Florence, Italy.

Cedar Health, UK. Cedar Health Ltd, Pepper Rd, Bramhall Moor Lane, Hazel Grove, Stockport, Cheshire, SK7 5BW, UK.

Cederroth, Spain. Cederroth, Leon 26 (Pol. Ind. Cobo Calleja), Fuenlabrada, 28947 Madrid, Spain.

Cefak, Ger. Cefak KG, Ostbahnhofstr. 15, 87437 Kempten, Germany.

Celafar, Ital. CE.LA.FAR s.r.l., Italy.

Celgene, USA. Celgene Corp., 7 Powder Horn Drive, Warren, NJ 07059, USA.

Cell Pharm, Ger. cell pharm Gesellschaft für pharmazeutische und diagnostische Präparate mbH, Feodor-Lynen-Str. 23, 30625 Hannover, Germany.

Cell Therapeutics, USA. Cell Therapeutics, USA.

Cellegy, Austral. Cellegy Australia P/L, Level 5, 203-33 New South Head Rd, Edgecliffe, NSW 2027, Australia.

Celltech, UK. Celltech Pharmaceuticals, 208 Bath Rd, Slough, Berks, SL1 3WE, UK.

Celltech Medeva, USA. Celltech Medeva, 755 Jefferson Rd, Rochester, NY 14603, USA.

Celsius, Ital. Celsius s.p.a., Via Grandi snc, 20090 Caleppio di Settala (MI), Italy.

Cenci, USA. HR Cenci Labs Inc., P.O. Box 12524, Fresno, CA 93778-2524, USA.

CeNeS, UK. CeNeS Ltd, Compass House, Vision Park, Chivers Way, Histon, Cambridgeshire, CB4 9ZR, UK.

Ceninter, Spain. Ceninter, Roma 19, 28028 Madrid, Spain.

Cenovis, Austral. See *Faulding Healthcare, Austral.*

Centeon, Aust. See *Centeon, Ger.*

Centeon, Braz. Centeon Farmaceutica Ltda, Avenida das Nacoes Unidas 18.001 (4° andar), Santo Amaro, 04795-900 Sao Paulo, SP, Brazil.

Centeon, Denm. See *Aventis Behring, Swed.*

Centeon, Fin. See *Centeon, Swed.*

Centeon, Fr. See *Aventis Behring, Fr.*

Centeon, Ger. See *Aventis Behring, Ger.*

Centeon, Hong Kong. See *Primal, Hong Kong.*

Centeon, Irl. See *Aventis Behring, UK.*

Centeon, Israel. Centeon, Israel.

Centeon, Ital. Centeon s.p.a., P.le S Turr 5, 20149 Milan, Italy.

Centeon, Mex. Centeon, S.A. de C.V., Nubex No. 414, Col. Jardines del Pedregal, 01900 Mexico D.F., Mexico.

Centeon, Norw. See *Centeon, Swed.*

Centeon, Spain. Centeon, Ronda General Mitre 72-4, 08017 Barcelona, Spain.

Centeon, Swed. See *Aventis Behring, Swed.*

Centeon, Switz. Centeon Pharma AG, Herostrasse 7, 8048 Zurich, Switzerland.

Centeon, UK. See *Aventis Behring, UK.*

Centeon, USA. See *Aventis Behring, USA.*

Center, Israel. Center, Israel.

Center, USA. Center Pharmaceuticals, 3620 Park Central Blvd North, Pompano Beach, FL 33064, USA.

Centocor, Aust. See *Centocor, Neth.*

Centocor, Denm. See *Lilly, Denm.*, and *Schering-Plough, Denm.*

Centocor, Israel. Centocor, Israel.

Centocor, Neth. Centocor Europe B.V., Einsteinweg 101, 2333 CB Leiden, Netherlands.

Centocor, Norw. See *Lilly, Norw.*

Centocor, USA. Centocor, Inc., 200 Great Valley Pkwy, Malvern, PA 19355, USA.

Central, Irl. Central Laboratories Ltd, 31 Ravensrock Rd, Sandyford Industrial Estate, Foxrock, Dublin 18, Ireland.

Central, Thai. Central Poly Trading Co. Ltd, 100/261 M003, Saima, Muang, Nonthaburi 11000, Thailand.

Centrapharm, Belg. Centrapharm S.A., Chaussee de Gand 615, 1080 Brussels, Belgium.

Centrapharm, Fr. Laboratoires Centrapharm, 35 rue de la Chapelle, 63450 Saint-Amant-Tallende, France.

Centrum, Spain. Centrum, Sagitario 12, 03006 Alicante, Spain.

Century, USA. Century Pharmaceuticals Inc., 10377 Hague Rd, Indianapolis, IN 46256-3399, USA.

Ceom, Ital. Ce.o.m. srl, Via L/mare Colombo 323, 84124 Salerno, Italy.

CEPA, Spain. Compañia Española de la Penicilina y Antibioticos, Po. de la Castellana 141-15, Edif. Cuzco IV, 28046 Madrid, Spain.

Cephalon, Irl. See *Cephalon, UK.*

Cephalon, UK. Cephalon UK Ltd, 11-13 Frederick Sanger Rd, Surrey Research Park, Guildford, Surrey, GU2 5YD, UK.

Cephalon, USA. Cephalon Inc., 145 Brandywine Pkwy, West Chester, PA 19380, USA.

Cermak, Aust. Dr Cermak, Austria.

Cernelle, Switz. Cernelle SA, Via Cadepiano 28, 6917 Barbengo, Switzerland.

Cernitin, Switz. Cernitin SA, Via Pian Scairolo 6, 6917 Barbengo, Switzerland.

Cesam, Port. Cesam, Lda, Rua de Ceuta 4, Piso, 2795-056 Linda-a-Velha, Portugal.

Cesra, Ger. Cesra Arzneimittelfabrik GmbH & Co. KG, Braunmattstr. 20, 76532 Baden-Baden, Germany.

Cetylite, USA. Cetylite Industries Inc., P.O. Box 90006, Pennsauken, NJ 08110-0700, USA.

Ceuta, UK. Ceuta Healthcare Ltd, Hill House, 41 Richmond Hill, Bournemouth, Dorset, BH2 6HS, UK.

Ceutical, Hong Kong. Ceutical Trading Co., Rm 24, 12/F, Goldfield Industrial Ctr, 1 Sui Wo Rd, Fo Tan, Shatin, N.T., Hong Kong.

Chaix et du Marais, Fr. Ste des Laboratoires Chaix et du Marais, 7 rue Labie, 75017 Paris, France.

Charoen, Thai. S Charoen Bhaesaj Trading Co. Ltd, 713-715-717 Mahachai Rd, Bangkok 10200, Thailand.

Charton, Canad. See *Technilab, Canad.*

Charwell, Israel. Charwell, Israel.

Charwell, Singapore. See *JDH, Singapore.*

Charwell Pharmaceuticals, UK. Charwell Pharmaceuticals Ltd, Charwell House, Wilsom Rd, Alton, Hampshire, GU34 2TJ, UK.

Chatelut, Fr. Laboratoires Chatelut, 36170 St-Benoit-du-Sault, France.

Chatfield Laboratories, UK. Chatfield Laboratories, Kramer Mews, London, SW5 9JL, UK.

Chattem, Canad. Chattem (Canada) Inc., 2220 Argentia Rd, Mississauga, Ontario, L5N 2K7, Canada.

Chattem, Singapore. See *Green Cross, Singapore.*

Chattem, USA. Chattem Consumer Products, 1715 West 38th St, Chattanooga, TN 37409, USA.

Chauvin, Fr. Laboratoires Chauvin, 416 rue Samuel-Morse, B.P. 1174, 34009 Montpellier cdx 1, France.

Chauvin, Hong Kong. See *Rich Plan, Hong Kong,* and *Worthy Strong, Hong Kong.*

Chauvin, Irl. See *Cahill May Roberts, Irl.*

Chauvin, Port. Laboratorio Chauvin, Lda, Edificio Altejo 606, Rua 3, Urbanizacao da Matinha, 1900 Lisbon, Portugal.

Chauvin, Singapore. See *Age D'or, Singapore.*

Chauvin, Thai. See *Neopharm, Thai.*

Chauvin, UK. Chauvin Pharmaceuticals Ltd, Ashton Rd, Harold Hill, Romford, Essex, RM3 8SL, UK.

Chauvin ankerpharm, Ger. Chauvin ankerpharm GmbH, Hansaallee 247, 40549 Dusseldorf, Germany.

Chauvin Novopharma, Switz. Chauvin Novopharma AG, Sumpfstrasse 3, CH-6312 Steinhausen/ZG, Switzerland.

Chefaro, Belg. Chefaro S.A., Chaussee de la Hulpe 166, 1170 Brussels, Belgium.

Chefaro, Fin. See *Tamro, Fin.*

Chefaro, Ger. Deutsche Chefaro Pharma GmbH, Wirrigen 25, 45731 Waltrop, Germany.

Chefaro, Israel. Chefaro, Israel.

Chefaro, Neth. Chefaro Nederland B.V., Keileweg 8, 3029 BS Rotterdam, Netherlands.

Chefaro, Spain. Chefaro Española S.A., Ed Amsterdam Ronda de Dalt, Ctra Hospitalet 147, Cornella de Llobregat, 08940 Barcelona, Spain.

Chefaro, UK. Chefaro Proprietaries Ltd, 1 Tower Close, St Peters Industrial Park, Huntingdon, Cambridgeshire, PE18 7DR, UK.

Chefaro Ardeval, Fr. Laboratoires Chefaro-Ardeval, 10 rue Godefroy, 92821 Puteaux cdx, France.

Cheil, Singapore. See *Zyfas, Singapore.*

Chelsea, USA. Chelsea Laboratories, USA.

Chemdorf, Spain. Chemdorf, Gran Via de Carlos III 94, 08028 Barcelona, Spain.

Chemedica, Ger. Chemedica AG Pharmavertrieb, Stadlerstr. 17, 85540 Haar/Munich, Germany.

Chemedica, Hong Kong. Chemedica, Hong Kong.

Chemedica, Switz. Chemedica SA, Postfach 240, 1896 Vouvry, Switzerland.

Chemia, Mex. Laboratorios Chemia S.A. de C.V., Yacatas Num. 307, 03020 Mexico D.F., Mexico.

Chemidex, UK. Chemidex Pharma Ltd, Chemidex House, Egham Business Village, Crabtree Rd, Egham, Surrey, TW20 8RB, UK.

Chemil, Ital. See *Vedim, Ital.*

Chemineau, Fr. Laboratoires Chemineau, 93 rte de Monnaie, 37210 Vouvray, France.

Cheminova, Spain. Cheminova, Emilio Munoz 15, Madrid, Spain.

Chemists Own, Austral. Chemists Own, Australia.

Chemitalia, Ital. Chemitalia s.r.l., Via Oratorio 48, 20016 Pero (MI), Italy.

Chemomedica, Aust. Chemomedica-Creutzberg & Co., Wipplingerstrasse 19, A-1013 Vienna, Austria.

Chemosan, Aust. Chemosan, Villach, Austria.

Chepharin, Aust. Hauser Paul-Chepharin, Flatschacher Strasse 57, A-9020 Klagnefurt, Austria.

Chephasaar, Ger. Chephasaar, Chem.-pharm. Fabrik GmbH, Muhlstr. 50, 66386 St Ingbert, Germany.

Chesebrough-Pond's, UK. Chesebrough-Pond's Ltd, UK.

Chesebrough-Pond's, USA. See *Unilever, USA.*

Cheshire, UK. Cheshire Cosmetics Ltd, Cromet House, 1 Gunco Lane, Macclesfield, Cheshire, SK11 7JX, UK.

Chester, Canad. See *Technilab, Canad.*

Chew, Thai. Chew Brothers & Co. Ltd Part, 1561/3 Petchbnri Rd, New Extension, Makason, Bangkok 10310, Thailand.

Chi Sheng, Thai. See *Charoen, Thai.*

Chibret, Denm. See *Merck Sharp & Dohme, Denm.*

Chibret, Ger. Chibret Pharmazeutische GmbH (MSD-Gruppe), Lindenplatz 1, 85540 Haar, Germany.

Chibret, Neth. See *Merck Sharp & Dohme, Neth.*

Chibret, Port. Chibret, Lda, Edificio Vasco da Gama 19, Quinta da Fonte, Porto Salvo, 2780-730 Paco de Arcos, Portugal.

Chibret, Spain. See *Merck Sharp & Dohme, Spain.*

Chiesi, Fr. Chiesi SA, Imm. le Doublon, bat B, 11 av. Dubonnet, 92400 Courbevoie, France.

Chiesi, Hong Kong. Chiesi, Hong Kong.

Chiesi, Ital. Chiesi Farmaceutici s.p.a., Via Palermo 26/A, 43100 Parma, Italy.

Chiesi, Singapore. See *JDH, Singapore.*

Chiesi, Switz. Chiesi SA, Via Franscini 17, 6900 Lugano, Switzerland.

Chiesi, Thai. See *Pacific, Thai.*

Chilton, USA. Chilton, USA.

Chimicor, Ital. Chimicor srl, Via Veneto 54, 36061 Bassano del Grappa (VI), Italy.

Chinoin, Hung. Chinoin Pharmaceutical and Chemical Works Ltd, P.O. Box 110, 1325 Budapest, Hungary.

Chinoin, Mex. Chinoin, Productos Farmacéuticos, S.A. de C.V., Lago Tanganica Num. 18, Col. Granada, 11520 Mexico D.F., Mexico.

Chinosolfabrik, Ger. Chinosolfabrik (Zweigniederlassung der Riedel-de Haen GmbH), Wunstorfer Str. 40, 30926 Seelze, Germany.

Chinta, Thai. See *Square, Thai.*

Chiron, Aust. See *Chiron, Neth.*

Chiron, Denm. See *Amgros, Denm.*

Chiron, Fr. Chiron France, 10 rue Chevreul, 92150 Suresnes, France.

Chiron, Ger. Chiron GmbH, Am Schimmersfeld 5, 40880 Ratingen, Germany.

Chiron, Hong Kong. See *Hong Wo, Hong Kong.*

Chiron, Irl. See *Aventis, Irl.*, and *Cahill May Roberts, Irl.*

Chiron, Israel. Chiron, Israel.

Chiron, Ital. Chiron Italia s.r.l., Via Cimarosa 4, 20144 Milan, Italy.

Chiron, Neth. Chiron B.V., Postbus 23023, 1100 DM Amsterdam, Netherlands.

Chiron, Singapore. See *Pasture, Singapore,* and *Sime Darby, Singapore.*

Chiron, Spain. Chiron Iberia, Edificio Dublin, Parque Emp. San Fernando, San Fernando de Henares, 28831 Madrid, Spain.

Chiron, Thai. See *Biogenetech, Thai.*, and *Zuellig, Thai.*

Chiron, UK. Chiron UK Ltd, PathoGenesis House, Park Lane, Cranford, Hounslow, Middlesex, TW5 9RR, UK.

Chiron, USA. Chiron Corp., 4560 Horton St, Emeryville, CA 94608-2916, USA.

Chiron Behring, Aust. See *Chiron Behring, Ger.*

Chiron Behring, Fin. See *Chiron Behring, Ger.*

Chiron Behring, Ger. Chiron Behring GmbH & Co, Neue Kasseler Str. 52, 35039 Marburg, Germany.

Chiron Behring, Norw. See *Chiron Behring, Ger.*

Chiron Vaccines, Ital. Chiron Vaccines, Divisione Chiron s.p.a., Via Fiorentina 1, 53100 Siena, Italy.

Chlorella, UK. Chlorella Products Ltd, UK.

Choay, Israel. Choay, Israel.

Chong Kun Dang, Ital. Chong Kun Dang Italia spa, Fraz. Domodossolina, 28651 Borgo S Giovanni (LO), Italy.

Chong Kun Dang, Singapore. See *Zyfas, Singapore.*

Chong Kun Dang, Thai. See *Charoen, Thai.*

Choongwae, Hong Kong. See *Vantone, Hong Kong.*

Choongwae, Singapore. See *Kyowa, Singapore.*

CHR, Ger. C.H.R. Heim Arzneimittel GmbH, Elisabethenstr. 34, 64283 Darmstadt, Germany.

Chrisana, Switz. Chrisana GmBH, Ruggenstrasse 17, 8903 Birmensdorf, Switzerland.

Christiaens, Belg. Christiaens Pharma S.A., Chaussee de Gand 615, 1080 Brussels, Belgium.

Christiaens, Neth. Christiaens B.V., Postbus 3458, 4800 DL Breda, Netherlands.

Chugai, Denm. See *Aventis Pharma, Denm.*

Chugai, Hong Kong. See *Fandasy, Hong Kong,* and *Tai Tong, Hong Kong.*

Chugai, Jpn. Chugai Pharmaceutical Co. Ltd, 1-9 Kyobashi 2-chome, Chuo-ku, Tokyo 104-8301, Japan.

Chugai, Norw. See *Aventis, Norw.*

Chugai, Thai. See *Siam Pharm, Thai.*

Chugai, UK. Chugai Pharma UK, Mulliner House, Flanders Rd, Turnham Green, London, W4 1NN, UK.

Ciba, Canad. See *Novartis, Canad.*

Ciba, Ger. See *Novartis, Ger.*

Ciba, Ital. See *Novartis, Ital.*

Ciba, Switz. See *Novartis, Switz.,* and *Novartis Consumer, Switz.*

Ciba, USA. See *Novartis, USA.*

Ciba Consumer, USA. See *Novartis, USA.*

Ciba Vision, Aust. Ciba Vision GmbH, Modecenterstrasse 14, A-1030 Vienna, Austria.

Ciba Vision, Austral. Ciba Vision Australia P/L, Private Bag 100, Baulkham Hills Business Centre, Baulkham Hills, NSW 2153, Australia.

Ciba Vision, Canad. See *Novartis Ophthalmics, Canad.*

Ciba Vision, Denm. Ciba Vision Danmark A/S, Ny Ostergade 7, 1 tv, 4000 Roskilde, Denmark.

Ciba Vision, Fin. Ciba Vision Finland Oy, Metsänneidonkuja 10, 02131 Espoo, Finland.

Ciba Vision, Fr. Ciba Vision Ophthalmics, B.P. 131, 31704 Blagnac cdx, France.

Ciba Vision, Ger. Ciba Vision Vertriebs GmbH, Bauhofstr. 16, 63762 Grossostheim, Germany.

Ciba Vision, Hong Kong. Ciba Vision (Hong Kong) Ltd, Unit 11-16, 26/F, Tower B, South Mark, 11 Yip Hing St, Wong Chuk Hang, Hong Kong.

Ciba Vision, Irl. See *United Drug, Irl.*

Ciba Vision, Israel. Ciba Vision, Israel.

Ciba Vision, Ital. Ciba Vision s.r.l., gruppo Novartis, Via Enrico Mattei 17, 30020 Marcon (VE), Italy.

Ciba Vision, Neth. Ciba Vision Ophtha Nederland, Postbus 3126, 4800 DC Breda, Netherlands.

Ciba Vision, Norw. Ciba Vision Norge AS, Postboks 24, 3601 Kongsberg, Norway.

Ciba Vision, NZ. Ciba Vision New Zealand, Division of Ciba Vision Australia Pty Ltd, P.O. Box 8061, Symonds St, Auckland, New Zealand.

Ciba Vision, Port. See *Novartis, Port.*

Ciba Vision, Singapore. Ciba Vision (Singapore) Pte Ltd, 491 B River Valley Rd, 03-02/03 Valley Point, S 248373, Singapore.

Ciba Vision, Spain. Ciba Vision, Marina, 206, 08013 Barcelona, Spain.

Ciba Vision, Swed. Ciba Vision AB, Datavagen 24, 436 32 Askim, Sweden.

Ciba Vision, Switz. Ciba Vision AG, Ophthalmics, Grenzstrasse 10, 8180 Bulach, Switzerland.

Ciba Vision, Thai. Ciba Vision (Thailand) Ltd, 15 Fl, Italthai Tower, 2034 New Petchburi Rd, Bangkapi, Huay Kwang, Bangkok 10320, Thailand.

Ciba Vision, UK. See *Novartis Ophthalmics, UK.*

Ciba Vision, USA. Ciba Vision, a Novartis Company, 11460 Johns Creek Parkway, Duluth, GA 30097-1556, USA.

Ciba-Geigy, Aust. See *Novartis, Aust.*

Ciba-Geigy, Belg. See *Novartis, Belg.*

Ciba-Geigy, Fr. See *Novartis, Fr.*

Ciba-Geigy, Jpn. Nihon Ciba-Geigy, 10-66 Biko-cho, Takarazuka-shi, Japan.

Ciba-Geigy, S.Afr. See *Novartis, S.Afr.*

Ciba-Geigy, Swed. See *Novartis, Swed.*

Ciba-Geigy, USA. See *Novartis, USA.*

Cibran, Braz. Companhia Brasileira de Antibioticos Cibran, Rua da Quitanda (3-4° andar), 20011-030 Rio de Janeiro, RJ, Brazil.

CIC, Spain. See *Schering, Spain.*

Ciclum, Spain. Ciclum Farma, Azcona 31, 28028 Madrid, Spain.

Cielle, Ital. Farma Cielle srl, Via Michele Amari 15, 90139 Palermo, Italy.

CIF, Braz. Companhia Industrial Farmaceutica, Rua Hermes Fontes 156/170, 20940-001 Rio de Janeiro, RJ, Brazil.

Cilag, Braz. Cilag Farmaceutica Ltda, Rua Avanhandava 55, 01306-900 Sao Paulo, SP, Brazil.

Cilag, Hong Kong. See *Keller, Hong Kong.*

Cilag, Mex. Cilag de Méico, S.A. de C.V., Miguel Angel de Quevedo No. 247, Col. Romero de Terreros, 04310 Mexico D.F., Mexico.

Cilag, UK. Cilag Ltd, P.O. Box 79, Saunderton, High Wycombe, Buckinghamshire, HP14 4HJ, UK.

Cimed, Braz. Cimed Industria Farmaceutica Ltda, Rua Alves Seixas 201, 03920-050 Sao Paulo, SP, Brazil.

Cimex, Hong Kong. See *LCH, Hong Kong.*

Cimex, Singapore. See *Pharma 2000, Singapore.*

Cimex, Switz. Cimex AG, Chem. und pharmaz. Produkte, Birsweg 2, 4253 Liesberg 1, Switzerland.

Cinfa, Spain. Cinfa, Olaz-Chipi 10, Poligono Areta, Huarte-Pamplona, 31620 Navarra, Spain.

Cipan, Port. Cipan, SA, Vala do Carregado, Apartado 60, 2600-726 Castanheira do Ribatejo, Portugal.

Cipharm, Fr. Laboratoires Cipharm, France.

Cipla-Medpro, S.Afr. Cipla-Medpro (Pty) Ltd, P.O. Box 1096, Durbanville 7551, South Africa.

Circle, USA. Circle Pharmaceuticals Inc., 6788 Hawthorn Park Drive, Indianapolis, IN 46220, USA.

CIS, Fr. CIS bio International, B.P. 32, 91192 Gif-sur-Yvette cdx, France.

CIS, Ital. CIS Diagnostici spa, Via E Mattei 1, 13049 Tronzano Vercellese (VC), Italy.

CIS, Spain. CIS España, Sierra de Albarracin S/N, Nave 7, San Fernando de Henares, 28850 Madrid, Spain.

Clarben, Spain. Clarben, Vallermoso 28, 28015 Madrid, Spain.

Clariana, Spain. Clariana Pico, Ctra Carlet Valencia Km 0.5, Carlet, 46240 Valencia, Spain.

Clarins, Canad. 4757 Poirier Blvd, St-Laurent, Quebec, H4R 2A4, Canada.

Clarmed, Ital. Clarmed s.r.l., Via G Stephenson 94, 20157 Milan (MI), Italy.

Clay Park, Hong Kong. See *Hind Wing, Hong Kong.*

Claytone, Fr. See *Terrafor, Fr.*

Clement, Fr. Laboratoires Clément, Centre 'affaires La Boursidiere, B.P. 150, 92357 Le Plessis-Robinson cdx, France.

Clement Thionville, Fr. Laboratoires Clément-Thionville, 6 rue Joffre, B.P. 60028, 57101 Thionville cdx, France.

Climax, Braz. Laboratorio Climax S.A., Rua Joaquim Tavora 822, 04015-011 Sao Paulo, SP, Brazil.

Clinced, Aust. Clinced Handels GmbH, Austria.

CliniMed, UK. CliniMed Ltd, Cavell House, Knaves Beech Way, Loudwater, High Wycombe, Buckinghamshire, HP10 9QY, UK.

Clinique, Canad. Clinique Laboratories, 121 Bloor St E, Toronto, Ontario, M4W 3M5, Canada.

Clintec, Aust. See *Nestle, Fr.*

Clintec, Canad. See *Baxter, Canad.*

Clintec, Denm. See *Baxter, Denm.*

Clintec, Fr. See *Nestle, Fr.*

Clintec, Irl. See *Baxter, Irl.*

Clintec, Israel. Clintec, Israel.

Clintec, Ital. See *Baxter, Ital.*

Clintec, Spain. Clintec Nutricion, Parque Empresarial San Fernando, Edif. Londres, San Fernando de Henares, 28830 Madrid, Spain.

Clintec, Thai. See *Osotspa, Thai.*

Clintec, USA. See *Baxter, USA.*

Clintex, Port. Clintex, Lda, Rua Joao de Deus no 19, Venda Nova, 2700-487 Amadora, Portugal.

Clonmel, Irl. Clonmel Healthcare Ltd, Waterford Rd, Clonmel, Co. Tipperary, Ireland.

CMS-Dental, Denm. CMS-Dental ApS, Wildersgade 55, 1408 Copenhagen K, Denmark.

CNW, Hong Kong. CNW (Hong Kong) Ltd, Rm 606, 6/F Fo Tan Industrial Ctr, 26-28 Au Pui Wan St, Fo Tan, Shatin, N.T., Hong Kong.

COB, Belg. COB & Cie S.A., Ave Albert Giraud 115, 1030 Brussels, Belgium.

Cochon, Fr. See *Tradiphar, Fr.*

Codal Synto, Hong Kong. See *CNW, Hong Kong,* and *Star, Hong Kong.*

Codal Synto, Thai. See *Star, Thai.*

Codali, Belg. Codali S.A., Avenue Henri Dunant 31, 1140 Brussels, Belgium.

Codilab, Port. Codilab, SA, Av. Marechal Gomes da Costa 19, 1800-255 Lisbon, Portugal.

Codit, Ital. Codit s.n.c. di Piccinini & C., Via Dronero 2, 10144 Turin, Italy.

Colgate Oral, USA. Colgate Oral Pharmaceuticals, 1 Colgate Way, Canton, MA 02021, USA.

Colgate Oral Care, Austral. Colgate Oral Care, P.O. Box 3964, Sydney, NSW 2001, Australia.

Colgate-Hoyt, USA. See *Colgate-Palmolive, USA.*

Colgate-Palmolive, Canad. Colgate Palmolive Canada, 99 Vanderhoof Ave, Toronto, Ontario, M4G 2H6, Canada.

Colgate-Palmolive, Ger. Colgate-Palmolive GmbH, Liebigstr 2-20, 22113 Hamburg, Germany.

Colgate-Palmolive, Ital. Colgate Palmolive spa, Via Giorgione 59/63, 00147 Rome, Italy.

Colgate-Palmolive, NZ. Colgate Palmolive Ltd, P.O. Box 38-077, Petone, New Zealand.

Colgate-Palmolive, UK. Colgate-Palmolive Ltd, Guilford Business Park, Middleton Rd, Guildford, Surrey, GU2 5LZ, UK.

Colgate-Palmolive, USA. Colgate-Palmolive Co., 300 Park Ave, New York, NY 10022, USA.

Coli, Ital. Farmaceutici Coli s.r.l., Via Campobello 15, 00040 Pomezia (Rome), Italy.

Coll, Spain. Coll Farma, Napoles 166, 08013 Barcelona, Spain.

Collado, Spain. Collado, Spain.

Collagen, Aust. Collagen Vertrieb Biomed. Produkte GmbH, Esslinger Hauptstrasse 81-7, A-1228 Vienna, Austria.

Collagen, Austral. Collagen Biomedical P/L, Unit 1, Chullora Central, Chullora, NSW 2190, Australia.

Collagen, Fr. Collagen France, France.

Collagen, Ger. Collagen Aesthetics, Hansaallee 201, 40549 Dusseldorf, Germany.

Collagen, Ital. Collagen Research Center srl, Via Innocenzo XI 41, 00165 Rome, Italy.

Collagen, Singapore. See *Pharmacon, Singapore.*

Collagen Corp, Hong Kong. See *Onstrong, Hong Kong.*

Collagenex, UK. CollaGenex International Ltd, The Old Stable Block, 7 Buttermarket, Thame, Oxfordshire, OX9 3EW, UK.

Collagenex, USA. CollaGenex Pharmaceuticals Inc., 41 University Drive, Suite 200, Newtown, PA 18940, USA.

Collins, Mex. Productos Farmaceuticos Collins S.A. de C.V., Cipres No. 1677, Col. del Fresno, 44900 Guadalajara, Jal., Mexico.

Collins Elixir, UK. Collins Elixir Co., P.O. Box 33, Kingsbridge, Devon, TQ7 1YQ, UK.

Coloplast, Fr. Laboratoires Coloplast, 58 rue Roger-Salengro, Peripole 126, 94126 Fontenay-s-Bois cdx, France.

Coloplast, Switz. Coloplast AG, Eurobusiness Center, Euro 1, Blegistrasse 1, 6343 Rotkreuz, Switzerland.

Coloplast, UK. Coloplast Ltd, Peterborough Business Park, Peterborough, Cambridgeshire, PE2 0FX, UK.

Coloplast, USA. Coloplast, Plaza VII, Suite 3400, 45 South Seventh St, Minneapolis, MN 55402, USA.

Columbia, Mex. Laboratorios Columbia, S.A. de C.V., Calz. del Hueso No. 160, Col. Ejido de Santa Ursula Coapa, 04850 Mexico D.F., Mexico.

Columbia, S.Afr. Columbia Pharmaceuticals (Pty) Ltd, P.O. Box 7026, Bonaero Park 1622, South Africa.

Columbia, USA. Columbia Laboratories Inc., 2875 NE 191st St, Suite 400, Aventura, FL 33180, USA.

Combe, Canad. See *Pinnacle, Canad.*

Combe, Ger. Combe Pharma Ltd, Rheinstr. 219, 76532 Baden-Baden, Germany.

Combe, Israel. Combe, Israel.

Combe, Ital. Combe Italia s.r.l., Via G C Procaccini 41, 20154 Milan, Italy.

Combe, Spain. Combe Europa, Orense 58, 28020 Madrid, Spain.

Combe, UK. Combe International Ltd, 4th Floor, AMP House, Dingwell Rd, Croydon, Surrey, CR9 2AU, UK.

Combe, USA. Combe Inc., 1101 Westchester Ave, White Plains, NY 10604, USA.

Combustin, Ger. Combustin Pharm. Präparate GmbH, Offinger Str. 7, 88525 Hailtingen/Bussen, Germany.

Commerce, USA. See *Del, USA.*

Commonwealth Serum, Hong Kong. See *LCH, Hong Kong.*

Compu, S.Afr. CompuPharm (Pty) Ltd, P.O. Box 30599, Sunnyside 0132, South Africa.

Concord, UK. Concord Pharmaceuticals Ltd, Melville House, High St, Dunmow, Essex, CM6 1AF, UK.

Condrugs, Thai. Condrugs International Co. Ltd, 51/507-508 Drive-in Square, Soi 1, Ladprao Rd, Klongjan, Bangkapi, Bangkok 10240, Thailand.

Confar, Port. Confar, Lda, Praca Natalia Correia 15, Damaia, 2720-414 Amadora, Portugal.

Connaught, Canad. See *Aventis Pasteur, Canad.*

Connaught, Israel. Connaught, Israel.

Connaught, Norw. See *Pasteur Merieux, Norw.*

Connaught, NZ. See *CSL, NZ.*

Connell, Hong Kong. Connell Bros Co. (HK) Ltd, Rm 601, 6/F Stanhope House, 738 King's Rd, North Point, Hong Kong.

Connetics, USA. Connetics, 3400 West Bayshore Rd, Palo Alto, CA 94303, USA.

Consol, Ital. Consol srl, Via Alessandro Brisse 27, 00149 Rome, Italy.

Consolidated Chemicals, Irl. See *Whelehan, Irl.*

Continental, Spain. Continental Farmaceutica, Spain.

Continental, USA. Continental Consumer Products, 770 Forest, Suite B, Birmingham, MI 48009, USA.

Continental Ethicals, S.Afr. Continental Ethicals (Division of S.A. Druggists Ltd), P.O. Box 4493, Randburg 2125, South Africa.

Continental Pharma, Belg. Continental Pharma Inc., Ave de Tervuren 270-2, 1150 Brussels, Belgium.

Continental Pharma, Switz. See *Vifor, Switz.*

Continental Pharma, Thai. See *UCB, Thai.*

Continentales, Mex. F Continentales, Mexico.

Contrel, UK. Contrel UK, 2 The Shambles, Bradford-on-Avon, BA15 1JS, UK.

Convatec, Austral. Convatec Australia, Division of Bristol-Myers Squibb, P.O. Box 240, Noble Park, VIC 3174, Australia.

Convatec, Fr. See *Bristol-Myers Squibb, Fr.*

Convatec, Irl. See *Bristol-Myers Squibb, Irl.*

Convatec, Israel. Convatec, Israel.

Convatec, Ital. Convatec, Divisione della Bristol-Myers Squibb spa, Via Virgilio Maroso 50, 00142 Rome, Italy.

Convatec, Port. See *Bristol-Myers Squibb, Port.*

Convatec, Switz. See *Bristol-Myers Squibb, Switz.*

Convatec, UK. Harrington House, Milton Rd, Ickenham, Uxbridge, Middlesex, UB10 1DE, UK.

Cook-Waite, USA. Cook-Waite Laboratories Inc., USA.

Coombe, Canad.

Coop. Farm., Ital. Cooperativa Farmaceutica Società Cooperativa a.r.l., Via Passione 8, 20122 Milan, Italy.

Cooper, Fr. Coopération Pharmaceutique Francaise, 77020 Melun cdx, France.

Cooperation Pharmaceutique, Fr. See *Cooper, Fr.*

Coopervision, Canad. Coopervision Inc., 100 McPherson St, Markham, Ontario, L3R 3V6, Canada.

Copernico, Ital. Copernico srl, Viale Etiopia 8, 00199 Rome, Italy.

Cophar, Switz. Cophar SA, Untermattweg 8, 3027 Berne, Switzerland.

Co-Pharma, UK. Co-Pharma Ltd, Talbot House, Church Street, Rickmansworth, Hertfordshire, WD3 1DE, UK.

Copley, USA. Copley Pharmaceutical Inc., 25 John Road, Canton, MA 02021, USA.

Cor Therapeutics, USA. Cor Therapeutics Inc., 256 East Grand Ave., South San Francisco, CA 94080, USA.

Coradol, Ger. Coradol-Pharma GmbH, Ludwig-Erhard-Str. 10, 50129 Bergheim, Germany.

corax, Ger. corax pharma GmbH, Lendersbergstr. 86, 53721 Siegburg, Germany.

Corbridge, Austral. Corbridge Group, 3 Tait St, Smithfield, NSW 2164, Australia.

Cord, Hong Kong. See *Pan-Well, Hong Kong.*

Corifel, Switz. Corifel SA, Via Clemente Maraini 9, 6907 Lugano 7, Switzerland.

Cortec, Denm. Cortec Medical A/S, St Kongensgade 69, 1264 Copenhagen K, Denmark.

Cortec, Fin. Cortec Medical Oy, Rajatorpantie 41 C, 01640 Vantaa, Finland.

Cortec, Norw. Cortec Medisiner A/S, Postboks 449 sentrum, 0104 Oslo, Norway.

Cortec, Swed. Cortec Medical AB, Torggatan 4, 211 40 Malmo, Sweden.

Cortecs, Irl. See *Cortecs, UK.*

Cortecs, UK. Cortecs Healthcare Ltd., Abbey Rd, Wrexham Industrial Estate, Wrexham, Clwyd, LL13 9PW, UK.

Cortunon, Canad. Cortunon Inc., Canada.

Corvi, Ital. Camillo Corvi s.p.a., Via R Lepetit 8, 20020 Lainate (MI), Italy.

Coryne de Bruynes, Mon. Laboratoires Coryne de Bruynes, 1 rue du Gabian, Immeuble Le Thales, MC 98000, Monaco.

Corypharma, Ital. Corypharma s.r.l., Via Bellagamba s.n., 60035 Jesi (AN), Italy.

Cos Farma, Ital. Cos Farma sas, Via di Portonaccio 23/B, 00159 Rome, Italy.

Cosan, Switz. Cosan GmbH, Erlenwiesenstrasse 2, 8604 Volketswil ZH, Switzerland.

Cosmair, Canad. Cosmair Canada Inc., 4895 Hickmore, St-Laurent, Quebec, H4T 1K5, Canada.

Cosmetique Active, Switz. Cosmétique Active (Suisse) SA, Industriestrasse 9, 5432 Neuenhof., Switzerland.

Cosmochema, Ger. Cosmochema Dr H.-H. Reckeweg GmbH, Dr Reckeweg-Str. 2-4, 76532 Baden-Baden, Germany.

Cosmofarma, Port. Cosmofarma, Lda (Laboratorios Cosmos), Rua do Arco Carvalhao 14, 1070 Lisbon, Portugal.

Cotek, Singapore. See *Zuellig, Singapore.*

Covan, S.Afr. See *Adcock Ingram, S.Afr.*

Coventry, UK. Coventry Chemicals Ltd, Woodhams Rd, Siskin Drive, Coventry, CV3 4FX, UK.

Cow & Gate, Irl. Cow & Gate Nutricia Ireland Ltd, 1B Sandyford Business Centre, Burton Hall Road, Dublin 18, Ireland.

Cow & Gate, Israel. Cow & Gate, Israel.

Cow & Gate, UK. See *Nutricia Clinical, UK.*

Cox, Hong Kong. See *Unipharm, Hong Kong.*

Cox, Irl. See *Alpharma, UK.*

Cox, UK. See *Alpharma, UK.*

CP, Israel. CP, Israel.

CP Pharmaceuticals, Hong Kong. See *Vantone, Hong Kong.*

CP Pharmaceuticals, Irl. See *Cahill May Roberts, Irl.*

CP Pharmaceuticals, UK. CP Pharmaceuticals Ltd, Ash Rd North, Wrexham Industrial Estate, Wrexham, Clwyd, LL13 9UF, UK.

CPC, Hong Kong. See *Sheraton, Hong Kong.*

CPF, Ger. C.P.F, Chemisch-pharmazeutische Fabrik GmbH, Heinrich-Bocking-Str. 6-8, 66121 Saarbrucken, Germany.

CPH, Port. Companhia Portuguesa Higiene, SA, Rua do Entreposto Industrial No 3-2, Alfragide, 2720-442 Amadora, Portugal.

Crawford, UK. Crawford Pharmaceuticals, Furtho House, 20 Towcester Rd, Old Stratford, Milton Keynes, Buckinghamshire, MK19 6AQ, UK.

Creative Brands, Austral. Creative Brands P/L, P.O. Box 1435, Clayton South, VIC 3169, Australia.

Crefar, Port. Crefar, Lda, Rua da Madalena 171, 1100-032 Lisbon, Portugal.

Creme d'Orient, Fr. Laboratoires Crème d'Orient, 81 rue de l'Amiral-Roussin, 75015 Paris, France.

Cress, Canad. Cress Laboratories, P.O. Box 222, Kitchener, ON, N2G 3X9, Canada.

Crinex, Fr. Laboratoires Crinex, B.P. 337, 92541 Montrouge cdx, France.

Crinos, Hong Kong. See *Fandasy, Hong Kong.*

Crinos, Ital. Crinos Industria Farmacobiologica s.p.a., Piazza XX Settembre 2, 22079 Villaguardia (CO), Italy.

Cris Flower, Ital. Cris Flower International snc, Via Livorno 61, 00162 Rome, Italy.

Cristalia, Braz. Cristalia Produtos Quimicos Farmaceuticos Ltda, Avenida Paulete 363, 13970-000 Itapira, SP, Brazil.

Croda, UK. Croda International PLC, Cowick Hall, Snaith, Goole, North Humberside, DN14 9AA, UK.

Croma, Aust. Croma-Pharma GmbH, Industriezeile 6, A-2100 Leobendorf, Austria.

Crookes Healthcare, UK. Crookes Healthcare Ltd, P.O. Box 57, Central Park, Lenton lane, Nottingham, NG2 2LJ, UK.

Crookes Laboratories, UK. Crookes Laboratories Ltd, Thane Rd, Nottingham, NG2 3AA, UK.

Crosara, Ital. Laboratorio Farmaco Biologico Crosara s.p.a., Via Campobello 15, 00040 Pomezia (Rome), Italy.

Cross, Swed. Cross Pharma AB, Box 3051, 183 03 Taby, Sweden.

Crown, S.Afr. Crown Laboratories Ltd, P.O. Box 100187, Moreleta Plaza 0167, South Africa.

Cruz, Spain. Fernandez de la Cruz, Crta Sevilla Malaga Km 5.6, Alcala de Guadaira, 41500 Seville, Spain.

Cryopharma, Mex. Laboratorios Cryopharma, S.A. de C.V., Vito Alessio Robles No. 209, Col. Florida, 01030 Mexico D.F., Mexico.

Crystaal, Canad. Crystaal, Division of Biovail Corporation, 2480 Dunwin Drive, Mississauga, Ontario, L5L 1J9, Canada.

CS, Fr. Laboratoires CS Dermatologie, 35 rue d'Artois, 75008 Paris, France.

CS, Port. CS Portugal, Lda, Rua Joao de Deus 32, Venda Nova, 2700-488 Amadora, Portugal.

CSC, Aust. CSC Pharmaceuticals Handels-GmbH, Heiligenstadterstrasse 395B, A-1190 Vienna, Austria.

CSL, Austral. CSL Ltd, 45 Poplar Road, Parkville, VIC 3052, Australia.

CSL, NZ. CSL (NZ) Ltd, P.O. Box 62590, Central Park, Auckland 6, New Zealand.

CSP, Fr. See *ICN, Fr.*

CT, Ger. ct-Arzneimittel GmbH, Lengeder Str. 42A, 13407 Berlin, Germany.

CT, Ital. C.T., Laboratorio Farmaceutico s.r.l., Via D. Alighieri 69-71, 18038 Sanremo (IM), Italy.

CTEX, USA. CTEX Pharmaceuticals Inc., P.O. Box 1549, Madison, MS 39130, USA.

CTI, Israel. CTI, Israel.

CTS, Israel. C.T.S. Industries Ltd, P.O. Box 10, Tel Aviv, Israel.

CTS Dental, UK. C.T.S. Dental Supplies, UK.

Cullen & Davison, Irl. Cullen & Davison Ltd, Killenaule Rd, Fethard, Co Tipperary, Ireland.

Cullen & Davison, UK. See *Cullen & Davison, Irl.*

Culver, Austral. Alberto Culver (Australia) P/L, P.O. Box 253, Parramatta, NSW 2150, Australia.

Cumberland, USA. Cumberland Packing Corp., 35 Old Ridgefield Rd, P.O. Box 7688, Willton, CT 06897, USA.

Cupharma, UK. Cupharma Ltd, Winkton House, Wynnswick Rd, Seer Green, Beaconsfield, Buckinghamshire, HP9 2XW, UK.

Cuprocept, S.Afr. Cuprocept SA, P.O. Box 400, New Germany 3620, South Africa.

Curacel, Austral. Curacel International P/L, Suite 14, 1645 Ipswich Rd, Rocklea, QLD 4106, Australia.

Curamed, Aust. See *Schwabe-Curamed, Ger.*

Curamed, Thai. See *SPB, Thai.*

Curasan, Aust. See *Curasan, Ger.*

Curasan, Ger. curasan Pharma GmbH, Lindigstr. 4, 63801 Kleinostheim, Germany.

Curatis, Ger. Curatis Pharma GmbH, Karl-Wiechert-Allee 76, 30625 Hannover, Germany.

Curex, Israel. Curex, P.O. Box 8366, New Industry Area, Netanya, Israel.

Cusi, Hong Kong. Cusi, Hong Kong.

Cusi, Singapore. See *Pharmaforte, Singapore.*

Cusi, Spain. See *Alcon Cusi, Spain.*

Cussons, UK. Cussons (UK) Ltd, Bird Hall Lane, Stockport, Cheshire, SK3 0N, UK.

Cutter, Israel. Cutter, Israel.

Cutter, UK. Cutter Laboratories, Division of Miles Ltd, Stoke Court, Stoke Poges, Slough, SL2 4LY, UK.

Cutter, USA. See *Bayer, USA.*

Cuxson, Gerrard, Canad. Cuxson Gerrard & Co. Ltd, 5775 Andover, Montreal, Quebec, H4T 3K9, Canada.

Cuxson, Gerrard, UK. Cuxson, Gerrard & Co. Ltd, 125 Broadwell Rd, Oldbury, Warley, West Midlands, B69 3BB, UK.

Cyanamid, Ital. See *Wyeth Lederle, Ital.*

Cyanamid, Spain. Cyanamid Iberica, Ctra Burgos Km-23, Desvio Algete Km 1, San Sebastian de Los Reyes, 28700 Madrid, Spain.

Cyanamid, UK. Cyanamid of Great Britain Ltd, Fareham Rd, Gosport, Hampshire, PO13 0AS, UK.

Cybermed, Aust. C/B/M Cybermed AG & Co. KEG, Postfach 50, A-3402 Klosterneuburg, Austria.

Cyclin, USA. Cyclin Pharmaceuticals Inc., 429 Gammon Place, Madison, WI 53715, USA.

Cypress, USA. Cypress Pharmaceutical, 135 Industrial Blvd, Madison, MS 39110, USA.

Cypros, USA. See *Questcor, USA.*

CytoChemia, Ger. CytoChemia Biologisch-Pharmazeutische GmbH, Im Burgerstock 7, 79241 Ihringen, Germany.

Cytogen, USA. Cytogen, 600 College Rd East, Princeton, NJ 08540, USA.

Cytosol, Israel. Cytosol, Israel.

Cytosol, USA. Cytosol Laboratories, 55 Messina Drive, Braintree, MA 02184, USA.

DAB, Swed. DAB Dental AB, Box 423, 194 04 Upplands Vasby, Sweden.

Dabur, Thai. See *Bioscience, Thai.*

Daewon, Hong Kong. See *Health Care, Hong Kong.*

Dagra, Neth. Dagra-Pharma B.V., Postbus 171, 1110 BC Diemen, Netherlands.

Dagra, Port. Dagra, Lda, Rua do Centro Cultural 13, 1700 Lisbon, Portugal.

Daiichi, Hong Kong. See *Hong Kong Medical, Hong Kong.*

Daiichi, Jpn. Daiichi Pharmaceutical Co. Ltd, 14-10 Nihonbashi 3-Chome, Chuo-ku, Tokyo 103-0027, Japan.

Daiichi, Singapore. See *Kyowa, Singapore.*

Daiichi, Thai. Daiichi Pharmaceutical (Thailand) Ltd, 5 Fl, Boonmitr Building, Silom Rd, Bangkok 10500, Thailand.

Daiichi, USA. Daiichi Pharmaceutical Corp., 11 Phillips Parkway, Montvale, NJ 07645, USA.

Dainabot, Jpn. Dainabot, Japan.

Dainippon, Jpn. Dainippon Pharmaceutical Co. Ltd, 6-8 Doshomachi 2-chome, Chuo-ku, Osaka 541-0045, Japan.

Daito, Jpn. Daito Corp., Japan.

Daker Farmasimes, Spain. Daker Farmasimes, C/Trabajo S/N, Sant Just Desvern, 08960 Barcelona, Spain.

Dakota, Braz. Dakota Farmaceutica e Comercial Ltda, Rua Alexandre Gasparoni 68, Marechal Hermes, 21610-250 Rio de Janeiro, RJ, Brazil.

Dales, Hong Kong. See *Swiss Worldwide, Hong Kong.*

Dallmann, Ger. Dallmann & Co., Fabrik chem.-pharm. Präparate, Zehntenhofstr. 14-16, Postfach: 130307, 65091 Wiesbaden, Germany.

Dal-Med, USA. Dal-Med Pharmaceuticals Inc., USA.

Dal-Vita, Austral. Dal-Vita Products Australia P/L, P.O. Box 477, Manly, NSW 1165, Australia.

Damor, Ital. Farmaceutici Damor s.p.a., Via E Scaglione 27, 80145 Naples, Italy.

Danco, USA. Danco Laboratories, USA.

Daniels, Canad. David D Daniels Ltd, P.O. Box 9, 62 Boychuk Rd, Elliot Lake, Ontario, P5A 2S9, Canada.

Daniels, Irl. See *Boileau & Boyd, Irl.*

Daniels, USA. See *Jones, USA.*

Danipharm, Denm. Danipharm A/S, Englandsvej 350-56, 2770 Kastrup, Denmark.

Danipharm, Hong Kong. See *International Medical, Hong Kong.*

Dannorth, Canad. Dannorth Laboratories Inc., 225 Duncan Mill Rd, Suite 400, Toronto, Ontario, M3B 3K9, Canada.

Dansk, Israel. Dansk, Israel.

Dansk-Flama, Braz. Dansk-Flama Instituto de Fisiologia Aplicada Ltda, Rua Barao de Petropolis 311, 20251-061 Rio de Janeiro, RJ, Brazil.

Danval, Spain. Danval, Avda de los Madronos 33, 28043 Madrid, Spain.

Darci, Belg. Darci Pharma S.A., Route de Lennik 437, 1070 Brussels, Belgium.

Darci, Fr. Laboratoire Darci Pharma, 3-5 rue Diderot, 92003 Nanterre, France.

Darcy, Fr. Laboratoires Darcy, 3-5 rue Diderot, 92003 Nanterre, France.

Darec, Ital. Darec s.r.l., Via Oratorio 48, 20016 Pero (MI), Italy.

Darier, Mex. Laboratorios Dermatologicos Darier, S.A. de C.V., Barranca del Muerto No. 482, Col. Merced Gomez, 01600 Mexico D.F., Mexico.

Dario Correia, Port. Dario Correia, Lda, Rua Duque de Palmela 25, 1250 Lisbon, Portugal.

Darrow, Braz. Darrow Laboratorios S.A., Rua Marques de Olinda 69, 22251-040 Rio de Janeiro, RJ, Brazil.

Dartmouth, USA. Dartmouth Pharmaceuticals Inc., 38 Church Ave, Wareham, MA 02751, USA.

Daudt, Braz. Laboratorio Daudt Oliveira S.A., Rua Simoes da Mota 57, 21540-100 Rio de Janeiro, RJ, Brazil.

Davi, Port. Dávi Farmacêutica, Lda, Estrada da Barrosa, Elspark, Arm. 8, Algueirao, 2725-193 Mem Martins, Portugal 1711 +351 21 9229720.

Davigo, Belg. Davigo s.p.r.l., Rue de l'Ourchet 17, 1367 Bomal, Belgium.

Davis, Spain. See *Parke, Davis, Spain.*

Davis & Geck, UK. Davis & Geck, A division of Cyanamid of Great Britain Ltd, Fareham Rd, Gosport, Hampshire, PO13 0AS, UK.

Day, Ital. Day Farma sas di Franco Tovecci & C, Via Alessandro Manzoni 227, 80123 Naples, Italy.

Dayton, USA. Dayton Laboratories Inc., 3307 NW 74th Ave, Miami, FL 33122, USA.

DB, Fr. Laboratoires DB Pharma, 1 bis, rue du cdt-Riviere, 94210 La Varenne-St-Hilaire, France.

DB, Switz. See *Uhlmann-Eyraud, Switz.*

DBL, Austral. David Bull Laboratories P/L, P.O. Box 394, Mulgrave North, VIC 3170, Australia.

DBL, NZ. See *Baxter, NZ.*

DBL, Thai. See *Indochina Healthcare, Thai.*

DCG, Swed. DCG Farmaceutiska AB, Box 2123, 421 02 Vastra Frolunda, Sweden.

DDC, UK. DDC (London) Ltd, 6 Clifton Gdns, London, W9 1DT, UK.

DDD, Hong Kong. See *Trinity, Hong Kong.*

DDD, Israel. DDD, Israel.

DDD, Singapore. See *Indrugco, Singapore.*

DDD, UK. DDD Ltd, 94 Rickmansworth Rd, Watford, Hertfordshire, WD1 7JJ, UK.

DDSA Pharmaceuticals, UK. DDSA Pharmaceuticals Ltd, 310 Old Brompton Rd, London, SW5 9JQ, UK.

De Angeli, Ital. Istituto De Angeli Ph s.p.a., Via Lorenzini 8, 20139 Milan, Italy.

De Mayo, Braz. De Mayo Industrias Quimicas e Farmaceuticas Ltda, Rua Barao de Petropolis 109, 20251-016 Rio de Janeiro, RJ, Brazil.

De Salute, Ital. De Salute srl, Via Milano 43, 26015 Soresina (CR), Italy.

De Witt, Aust. See *De Witt, UK.*

De Witt, Denm. See *Ferring, Denm.*

De Witt, Irl. See *Mayrs, Irl.*

De Witt, Norw. See *Ferring, Norw.*

De Witt, NZ. See *Regional Health, NZ.*

De Witt, Singapore. De Witt International (S) Pte Ltd, 62 Tannery Lane, S 347804, Singapore.

De Witt, UK. E.C. De Witt & Co. Ltd, Tudor Rd, Manor Park, Runcorn, Cheshire, WA7 1SZ, UK.

Debat, Denm. See *Ipex, Swed.*

Debat, Fr. Laboratoires Debat, 153 rue de Buzenval, 92380 Garches, France.

Debat, Hong Kong. See *Wing Wai, Hong Kong.*

Debat, Norw. See *Ipex, Swed.*

Debat, Thai. See *Pacific, Thai.*

Deca, Ital. Laboratorio Chimico Deca s.r.l., Via Balzaretti 17, 20133 Milan, Italy.

Declimed, Ger. Declimed Zweigniederlassung der Desitin Arzneimittel GmbH, Weg beim Jager 214, 22335 Hamburg, Germany.

Decomed, Port. Decomed Farmaceutica, Lda, Rua Sebastiao e Silva 56, 2745-838 Massama, Portugal.

Degab, Ger. DeGAB GmbH & Co. KG, Regina-Protmann-Str. 16, 48159 Munster, Germany.

Degorts, Mex. Degort's Chemical, S.A., Alhambra No. 310, Col. Portales, 03300 Mexico D.F., Mexico.

Deklerht, USA. Deklerht, USA.

Del, Canad. Del Pharmaceutics (Canada) Inc., 25 Morrow Rd, Barrie, Ontario, L4N 3V7, Canada.

Del, Switz. See *Para-Pharma, Switz.*

Del, USA. Del Pharmaceuticals Inc., 565 Broad Hallow Rd, Farmingdale, NY 11735, USA.

Del Saz & Filippini, Ital. Farmaceutici Del Saz & Filippini s.r.l., Via Dei Pestagalli 7, 20138 Milan, Italy.

Delalande, Port. See *Confar, Port.*

Delamac, Austral. Delamac Pharmaceuticals P/L, P.O. Box 125, Spring Hill, Qld 4004, Australia.

Delandale, Irl. See *Allphar, Irl.*

Delicias, Mex. Delicias, S.A. de C.V., Productos Alimenticios, Apartado Postal No. 376, Zona Industrial, 33000 Ciudad Delicias, Chih, Mexico.

Delmont, USA. Delmont Laboratories Inc., 715 Harvard Ave, Swarthmore, PA 19081, USA.

Del-Ray, USA. Del Ray Laboratories, 22 20th Ave NW, Birmingham, AL 35215, USA.

Delta, Austral. See *Pharmacia, Austral.*

Delta, Braz. Instituto Terapeutico Delta Ltda, Rua Engenheiro Guilherme Cristiano Frendez 827, Vila Antonieta, 03477-000 Sao Paulo, SP, Brazil.

Delta, Ger. Delta-Pharma GmbH, Benzstr. 5, 72793 Pfullingen, Germany.

Delta, Port. Laboratórios Delta, Lda, Rua Direita de Massama 148, 2745-751 Queluz, Portugal.

Delta, Singapore. See *Green Cross, Singapore.*

Delta BKB, Ital. Delta BKB srl, V.le Emilio Po 224, 41100 Modena, Italy.

Delta Laboratories, Irl. Delta Laboratories Ltd, 26 Airfield Court, Dublin 4, Ireland.

delta pronatura, Ger. delta pronatura Dr. Krauss & Dr. Beckmann GmbH & Co., Hans-Bockler-Str. 5, 63263 Neu-Isenburg, Germany.

Democal, Switz. Democal AG, Untermattweg 8, 3001 Berne, Switzerland.

Demopharm, Switz. See *Democal, Switz.*

Dendron, UK. See *DDD, UK.*

Dendy, Austral. Dendy Pharmaceuticals P/L, 44 Cromer St, East Brighton, VIC 3187, Australia.

Denk, Hong Kong. See *Hind Wing, Hong Kong, Star, Hong Kong,* and *Universal, Hong Kong.*

Denk, Singapore. See *Luen Wah, Singapore.*

Denk, Thai. See *Sriprasit, Thai.*

Denolin, Belg. Denolin S.A., Rue des Goujons 152, 1070 Brussels, Belgium.

Dent, USA. C.S. Dent & Co., 1820 Airport Exchange Bvld, Erlanger, KY 41018, USA.

Dentaid, Spain. Dentaid, Parque Tecno del Valle, Ronda Can Fatjo 10, Cerdanyola, 08290 Barcelona, Spain.

Dental Health Products, UK. Dental Health Products Ltd, 60 Broughton Lane, Maidstone, Kent, ME15 9XS, UK.

Dental Trey, Ital. Dental Trey s.r.l., Via Partisani 3, 47010 Fiumana Predappio (FO), Italy.

Dental Warehouse, S.Afr. Dental Warehouse (Pty) Ltd, Private Bag X8, Wendywood 2144, South Africa.

Dentinox, Ger. Dentinox Gesellschaft für Pharmazeutische Präparate Lenk & Schuppan, Nunsdorfer Ring 19, 12277 Berlin, Germany.

Dentinox, Switz. See *Renapharm, Switz.*

Dentoria, Fr. See *Sanofi Synthelabo OTC, Fr.*

Dentox, UK. Dentox Ltd, Hillmeadow, Lighthorne, Warwick, CV35 0AB, UK.

Dentsply, Austral. Dentsply (Australia) P/L, Private Bag 4, Abbotsford, VIC 3067, Australia.

Dentsply, Ger. Dentsply DeTrey GmbH, De-Trey-Strasse 1, 78467 Constance, Germany.

DEP, USA. DEP Corp., 2101 East Via Arado, Rancho Dominguez, CA 90220, USA.

Depofarma, Ital. Depofarma srl, Via Guindazzi 44/54, 80040 Pollena Trocchia (NA), Italy.

Deproco, UK. Deproco UK Ltd, 2 St Martins House, St Martins Walk, Dorking, Surrey, RH14 1UW, UK.

DePuy, UK. DePuy Healthcare, UK.

Derek, Singapore. Derek Marketing Pte Ltd, Block 221 Henderson Rd, 05-12 Henderson Building, S 159557, Singapore.

Derly, Spain. Derly, Avenida de la Industria 30, Alcobendas, 28100 Madrid, Spain.

Dermacare, Austral. Dermacare P/L, P.O. Box 482, Bondi Junction, NSW 2022, Australia.

Dermaclin, Mex. Dermaclin, S.A. de C.V., E. Rebsamen No. 747-5, Col. Narvarte, 03020 Mexico, D.F., Mexico.

Dermaide, USA. Dermaide Research Corp., P.O. Box 562, Palos Heights, IL 60463, USA.

Dermal, Israel. Dermal, Israel.

Dermal Laboratories, Irl. See *Cahill May Roberts, Irl.*

Dermal Laboratories, UK. Dermal Laboratories Ltd, Tatmore Place, Gosmore, Hitchin, Hertfordshire, SG4 7QR, UK.

Dermamend, UK. Dermamend, UK.

Dermapharm, Ger. Dermapharm AG, Luise-Ullrich-Strasse 6, 82031 Grunwald, Germany.

Dermapharm, Irl. See *United Drug, Irl.*

Dermapharm, UK. DermaPharm Ltd, Penrhyn House, 10 St Mark's Hill, Surbiton, Surrey, KT6 4PW, UK.

Dermatech, Austral. Dermatech Laboratories, Unit 17, Prospect Highway, Seven Hills, NSW 2147, Australia.

Dermik, Canad. Dermik Laboratories Canada Inc., 6205 Airport Rd, Building B, Suite 100, Mississauga, Ontario, L4V 1E1, Canada.

Dermik, Hong Kong. See *Health Care, Hong Kong.*

Dermik, Israel. Dermik, Israel.

Dermik, Singapore. See *JDH, Singapore.*

Dermik, USA. See *Aventis Pharma, USA.*

Dermofarm, Spain. Dermofarm, Rosalia de Castro 18, 08025 Barcelona, Spain.

Dermofarma, Ital. Dermofarma Italia s.r.l., Via Beata Francesca 10, 83100 Avellino, Italy.

Dermol, USA. Dermol Pharmaceuticals Inc., 3807 Roswell Rd, Marietta, GA 30062, USA.

Dermopen, Braz. Divisao Farmaceutica Dermopen Ltda, Rua Ida Romussi Gasparinetti 110, Parque Laguna, 06795-000 Taboao da Serra, SP, Brazil.

Dermophil Indien, Fr. Laboratoires du Dermophil Indien, B.P. 9, 61600 La Ferte-Mace, France.

Dermophil Indien, Switz. See *Uhlmann-Eyraud, Switz.*

Dermoteca, Port. Dermoteca, SA, Estrada Nacional 117, 2720 Alfragide, Portugal.

Dermtek, Canad. Dermtek Pharmaceuticals Ltd, 1600 Trans Canada Highway, Suite 200, Dorval, Quebec, H9P 1H7, Canada.

Desarrollo, Spain. Desarrollo Farma y Cosmeticos, Pa de la Castellana 143, 28046 Madrid, Spain.

Desatnik, S.Afr. MI Desatnik, P.O. Box 39359, Booysens 2041, South Africa.

Desbergers, Canad. See *Technilab, Canad.*

Desitin, Denm. Desitin Pharma A/S, Nyhavn 43 B, 1051 Copenhagen K, Denmark.

Desitin, Fin. See *Bitelab, Fin.*

Desitin, Ger. Desitin Arzneimittel GmbH, Weg beim Jager 214, 22335 Hamburg, Germany.

Desitin, Hong Kong. See *Jacobson, Hong Kong.*

Desitin, Israel. Desitin, Israel.

Desitin, Norw. Desitin Pharma AS, Niels Leuchsv. 99, 1343 Eiksmarka, Norway.

Desitin, Singapore. See *Zyfas, Singapore.*

Desitin, Swed. Desitin Pharma AB, Box 2064, 431 02 Molndal, Sweden.

Desitin, Switz. Desitin Pharma GmbH, Oristalstrasse 87a, 4410 Liestal, Switzerland.

Desopharmex, Switz. Desopharmex AG, Muttenzerstrasse 107, 4133 Pratteln 1, Switzerland.

Dessau, Ger. Pharma Dessau GmbH, Luxemburgstr. 8, 06846 Dessau, Germany.

Deutsch Chinesische, Hong Kong. Deutsch Chinesische Apotheke (Maple Inc.), Rm 1003, Workingson Ctr, 112 Chun Yeung St, North Point, Hong Kong.

Deverge, Ital. Devergè Medicina e Medicalizzazione s.r.l., C.so Casale 206, 10132 Turin, Italy.

Devesa, Ger. Devesa Dr Reingraber GmbH & Co. KG, Heinkelstr. 8a, 76461 Muggensturm, Germany.

Dexcel, Israel. See *Dexxon, Israel.*

Dexcel, UK. Dexcel Pharma Ltd, Bishop Crewe House, North St, Daventry, Northamptonshire, NN11 5PN, UK.

DexGen, USA. DexGen Pharmaceuticals, P.O. Box 675, Manasquan, NJ 08736, USA.

Dexo, Fr. Laboratoires Dexo, 179 bureaux de la Colline, 92213 Saint-Cloud cdx, France.

Dexo, Switz. See *Actipharm, Switz.,* and *Uhlmann-Eyraud, Switz.*

Dexo, Thai. See *Pacific, Thai.*

Dexter, Spain. Dexter Farmaceutica, Avda Virgen de Montserrat 215, 08026 Barcelona, Spain.

Dexxon, Israel. Dexxon, P.O. Box 50, Hadera 38100, Israel.

Dey, USA. Dey Laboratories, 2751 Napa Valley Corporate Drive, Napa, CA 94558, USA.

DHA, Canad. Drug Houses of Australia, 550 Malkin Ave, P.O. Box 4129, Vancouver, British Columbia, V6B 3Z6, Canada.

DHA, Hong Kong. See *Tsun Tsun, Hong Kong,* and *Weston, Hong Kong.*

DHA, Singapore. Drug Houses of Australia (Asia) Pte Ltd, 2 Chia Ping Rd, Haw Par Tiger Balm Building, S 619968, Singapore.

DHN, Fr. Lab. DHN, Division Nutrition Clinique, 35370 Torce, France.

DHU, Ger. Deutsche Homöopathie-Union, Ottostr. 24, 76227 Karlsruhe, Germany.

Diabact, Swed. Diabact AB, Box 303, 751 05 Upsala, Sweden.

Diaco, Ital. Laboratori Diaco Biomedicali spa, Via Flavia 124, 34147 Trieste, Italy.

Diadin, Ger. Diadin-Gesellschaft Chemisches Laboratorium GmbH, Ludwig Merckle-Str. 3, 89143 Blaubeuren, Germany.

Diafarm, Spain. Diafarm, Bernat de Rocaberti 17, Sabadell, 08205 Barcelona, Spain.

Diamant, Fr. See *Aventis, Fr.*

Diamant, Port. See *Aventis Pharma, Port.*

Diamant, Singapore. See *Zuellig, Singapore.*

Diatide, USA. Diatide Inc., 9 Delta Dr., Londonderry, NH 03053, USA.

Diba, Mex. Laboratorios Diba, S.A., Escorza No. 728, 44190 Guadalajara, Jal, Mexico.

Dibropharm, Ger. Dibropharm Arzneimittel, Kleine-Dollen-Str. 5, 76532 Baden-Baden, Germany.

Dicamed, Swed. Dicamed AB, Djupdalsvagen 24, 192 51 Sollentuna, Sweden.

Dickinson, USA. E.E. Dickinson Co., 31 East High St, East Hampton, CT 06424, USA.

Dicofarm, Ital. Dicofarm s.p.a., Via Vitorchiano 151, 00189 Rome, Italy.

Dieckmann, Ger. Dieckmann Arzneimittel GmbH (MSD-Gruppe), Lindenplatz 1, 85540 Haar, Germany.

Diedenhofen, Ger. Diedenhofen GmbH, Otto-von-Guericke-Str. 1, Postfach: 1252, 53730 St Augustin/Bonn, Germany.

Diedenhofen, Thai. See *Oui Heng, Thai.*

Diele, Fr. Diele Distripharma, 18 av Albert-Einstein, 93152 Le Blanc-Mesnil cdx, France.

Diepal, Fr. Diépal-NSA, B.P. 432, 69654 Villefranche-sur-Saone cdx, France.

Diepha, Fr. See *Diepharmex, Fr.*

Diepharmex, Fr. Laboratoires Diepharmex, 26 rue de l'Industrie, 92400 Corbevoie, France.

Diet Erba, NZ. See *NZ Distributors, NZ.*

Dieterba, Ital. Dieterba, Via Migliara 45, 04100 Latina, Italy.

Dietetique et Sante, Fr. See *Novartis Nutrition, Fr.*

Diethelm, Singapore. Diethelm Singapore Pte Ltd, 34 Boon Leat Terrace, S 119866, Singapore.

Diethelm, Switz. Diethelm & Co. SA, Postfach, 8052 Zurich, Switzerland.

Diethelm, Thai. Diethelm & Co. Ltd, Pharmaceutical Division, 280 New Rd, Bangkok 10100, Thailand.

Difa, Ital. Difa-Cooper s.p.a., Via Milano 160, 21042 Caronno Pertusella (VA), Italy.

Diftersa, Spain. Diftersa, Spain.

Dinafarma, Braz. Laboratorio Dinafarma Ltda, Avenida Major Alvim 155, 12940-000 Atibaia, SP, Brazil.

Dioptic, Canad. Dioptic Laboratories, Division of Akorn Pharmaceuticals Canada Ltd, 1405 Denison St, Markham, Ontario, L3R 5V2, Canada.

Discotrade, Israel. See *Dexxon, Israel.*

Dispensapharm, Canad. Dispensapharm, Unit of Monsanto Canada Inc., 2233 Argentia Rd, Mississauga, Ontario, L5N 2X7, Canada.

Disperga, Aust. Dr C Szalagyl Disperga GmbH, Josefstadter Strasse 43, A-1080 Vienna, Austria.

Dissolvurol, Mon. Laboratoires Dissolvurol, Le Concorde, 11 rue du Gabian, MC 98000, Monaco.

Dista, Austral. See *Lilly, Austral.*

Dista, Irl. See *Lilly, Irl.*

Dista, Neth. See *Lilly, Neth.*

Dista, NZ. See *Lilly, NZ.*

Dista, Spain. See *Lilly, Spain.*

Dista, Switz. See *Lilly, Switz.*

Dista, UK. See *Lilly, UK.*

Dista, USA. See *Lilly, USA.*

Distri B3, Fr. Laboratoires Distri B3, rue Max Planck, Technopole de Chateau-Gombert, 13013 Marseille, France.

Distriborg, Fr. Distriborg, 217 chem. du Grand-Revoyet, 69561 St-Genis-Laval, France.

Distrifarma, Port. Distrifarma, SA, Condominio Industrial Queluz Park, Estrada Consiglieri Pedroso 80 Lote 3, Queluz de Baixo, 2745-553 Barcarena, Portugal.

Divapharma, Ger. Divapharma-Knufinke Arzneimittel-werk GmbH, 12274 Berlin, Germany.

Divinal, Ger. Divinal Arzneimittel GmbH, Rathausplatz 5, Postfach: 2108, 83423 Bad Reichenhall, Germany.

Diviser Aquilea, Spain. Diviser Aquilea, Spain.

Divpharm, S.Afr. Divpharm, South Africa.

Dixon-Shane, USA. Dixon-Shane Inc., 256 Geiger Rd, Philadelphia, PA 19115, USA.

DJ, USA. DJ Pharma Inc, 12730 High Bluff Bvld, Suite 160, San Diego, CA 92130, USA.

DMG, Ger. DMG Chemisch-Pharmazeutische Fabrik GmbH, Postfach: 530104, 22531 Hamburg, Germany.

DMG, Ital. DMG Italia srl, Via Portoferraio 18, 00182 Rome, Italy.

Doak, Hong Kong. See *International Medical, Hong Kong.*

Doak, USA. Doak Dermatologics, 383 Route 46 West, Fairfield, NJ 07004-2402, USA.

Docmed, S.Afr. Docmed, South Africa.

Docpharm, Ger. Docpharm Arzneimittelvertrieb GmbH & Co. KGaA, Reetzstr. 83, 76327 Pfinztal, Germany.

Doerenkamp, Ger. Doerenkamp GmbH, Gereonsmuhlengasse 3, 50670 Cologne, Germany.

Doetsch, Grether, Switz. Doetsch, Grether AG, 4002 Basel, Switzerland.

Dojin Iyaku, Jpn. Dojin Iyaku, 5-2-2 Yayoi-cho, Nakano-ku, Tokyo, Japan.

Dolisos, Canad. Dolisos, 1400 Hocquart, St-Bruno, Quebec, J3V 6E1, Canada.

Dolisos, Fr. Laboratoires Dolisos, 45 place Abel Gance, 92100 Boulogne, France.

Dolisos, Ital. Dolisos Italia s.r.l., Laboratoires de Pharmacologie Homeopathique, Via Carlo Poma s.n.c., 00040 Pomezia (Rome), Italy.

Dolorgiet, Denm. See *Nordisk Ibu-Pharma, Denm.*

Dolorgiet, Ger. Dolorgiet GmbH & Co. KG, Otto-von-Guericke-Str. 1, 53754 St. Augustin/Bonn, Germany.

Dolorgiet, Switz. See *Mundipharma, Switz.*

Dom, Spain. Dom, Gall 30, Esplugas de Llobregat, 08950 Barcelona, Spain.

Dome, Switz. See *Diethelm, Switz.*

Dome-Hollister-Stier, Fr. Dome-Hollister-Stier, ZI, rue des Longs Reages, 28235 Epernon cdx, France.

Dominion, Irl. See *Dominion, UK.*

Dominion, UK. Dominion Pharma Ltd, Dominion house, Lion Lane, Haslemere, Surrey, GU27 1JL, UK.

Dompe, Ital. Dompè Farmaceutici s.p.a., Via San Martino 12, 20122 Milan, Italy.

Dompe Biogen, Switz. Dompé-Biogen AG, Metallstrasse 8, 6300 Zug, Switzerland.

Dompe Biotec, Ital. Dompè Biotec s.p.a., Via Santa Lucia 6, 20122 Milan, Italy.

Doms, Switz. See *Actipharm, Switz.*

Doms-Adrian, Fr. See *Doms-Recordati, Fr.*

Doms-Adrian, Hong Kong. See *Rich Plan, Hong Kong.*

Doms-Recordati, Fr. Laboratoires Doms-Recordati, 4 rue Ficatier, 92400 Courbevoie, France.

Don, Israel. Don, Israel.

Donell DerMedex, USA. Donell DerMedex, 342 Madison Ave, Suite 1422, New York, NY 10173, USA.

Dong, Singapore. See *Zyfas, Singapore.*

Dong Kook, Singapore. See *Polymedic, Singapore,* and *Ziwell, Singapore.*

Donini, Ital. Donini s.r.l., Via Ecce Homo 18, 37054 Nogara (VR), Italy.

Donmed, S.Afr. Donmed Pharmaceuticals, P.O. Box 75907, Gardenview 2047, South Africa.

Dormer, Canad. Dormer Laboratories Inc., 91 Kelfield St, Unit 5, Rexdale, Ontario, M9W 5A3, Canada.

Dorom, Ital. Dorom s.r.l., Via Volturno 48, 20089 Quinto de Stampi Rozzano (MI), Italy.

Dorsay, Braz. Dorsay Industria Farmacotica Ltda, Rua Taquarucu 79, Vila Parque Jabaquara, 04346-040 Sao Paulo, SP, Brazil.

Dorsch, Ger. Dorsch GmbH, Lochhamer Schlag 10, Postfach: 1131, 82153 Grafelfing, Germany.

Dorwest, UK. Dorwest Herbs Ltd, Shipton Gorge, Bridport, Dorset, DT6 4LP, UK.

Doskar, Aust. Doskar Mag. Martin Pharm. Produkte, Schottenring 14, A-1010 Vienna, Austria.

Douglas, Austral. Douglas Pharmaceuticals Australia Ltd, 2/1B Kleins Rd, Northmead, NSW 2152, Australia.

Douglas, Hong Kong. See *Hind Wing, Hong Kong.*

Douglas, NZ. Douglas Pharmaceuticals Ltd, P.O. Box 45-027, Aukland 8, New Zealand.

Douglas, Singapore. See *Grafton, Singapore.*

Douglas, Thai. See *JDH Borneo, Thai.*

Dovalle, Braz. Farmoterapica Dovalle Industria Quimica Farmaceutica Ltda, Rodovia SC 438 Km 3, 88708-080 Tubarao, SC, Brazil.

Dow, USA. See *Bertek, USA.*

Dow Corning, UK. Dow Corning Ltd, Kings Court, 185 Kings Rd, Reading, Berkshire, RG1 4EX, UK.

DP-Medica, Switz. DP-Medica SA Pharmazeutische Produkte, Case postale 238, Fribourg, Switzerland.

Dr Janssen, Ger. Dr. Werner Janssen Nachf. Chem.-pharm. Produkte GmbH, Grenzstr. 2, 53340 Meckenheim, Germany.

Dr. Nordyke, USA. Dr. Nordyke Footcare Products, 1650 Palma Drive, Suite 102, Ventura, CA 93003, USA.

Draco, Swed. Draco Läkemedel AB, 221 87 Lund, Sweden.

Draxis, Canad. Draxis Health Inc., 6870 Goreway Dr, Mississauga, Ontario, L4V 1P1, Canada.

Dreiman, Spain. Dreiman, Ctra M-300 Km 29.920, Alcala de Henares, 28802 Madrid, Spain.

Dreluso, Ger. Dreluso Pharmazeutika, Dr Elten & Sohn GmbH, Marktplatz 5, 31840 Hessisch Oldendorf, Germany.

Dresden, Ger. Arzneimittelwerk Dresden GmbH, Meissner Str. 35, 01445 Radebeul, Germany.

Dreveny, Aust. Dr. Dreveny, Mag. pharm. & Co. OHG, Herrandgasse 7, A-8010 Graz, Austria.

Drogasil, Braz. Drogasil S.A., Avenida Corifeu de Azevedo Marques 3.097, 05339-000 Sao Paulo, SP, Brazil.

Drogenhansa, Aust. Drogenhansa, Drogerie und Reformwaren GmbH, Michelbeuerngasse 9 A, A-1090 Vienna, Austria.

Drossapharm, Israel. Drossapharm, Israel.

Drossapharm, Switz. Drossapharm SA, Drosselstrasse 47, 4059 Basel, Switzerland.

Drug Research, Ital. D.R. Drug Research s.r.l., Via F Turati 3, 22036 Erba (CO), Italy.

Drug Research, Singapore. See *Zyfas, Singapore.*

Drug Trading, Canad. Drug Trading Co. Ltd, 795 Pharmacy Ave, Scarborough, Ontario, M1L 3K2, Canada.

Du Pont, Aust. See *Du Pont, Belg.*

Du Pont, Belg. Du Pont Pharma S.A., Centre Mercure, Rue de la Fusee 100, 1130 Brussels, Belgium.

Du Pont, Canad. Du Pont Pharma, 2655 North Sheridan Way, Suite 180, Mississauga, Ontario, L5K 2P8, Canada.

Du Pont, Denm. See *Meda, Denm.*

Du Pont, Fr. DuPont Pharma SA, 137 rue de l'Universite, 75007 Paris, France.

Du Pont, Ger. Du Pont Pharma GmbH, Du Pont-Str. 1, 61352 Bad Homburg v.d.H., Germany.

Du Pont, Hong Kong. See *Swire Loxley, Hong Kong.*

Du Pont, Irl. See *United Drug, Irl.*

Du Pont, Israel. Du Pont, Israel.

Du Pont, Ital. DuPont Pharma Italia s.r.l., Via de Conti 2A, 50123 Florence, Italy.

Du Pont, Norw. See *Meda, Norw.*

Du Pont, Singapore. See *Boots, Singapore.*

Du Pont, Spain. Du Pont Pharma, Albacete 5, 1 Planta, 28027 Madrid, Spain.

Du Pont, Switz. See *Opopharma, Switz.*

Du Pont, Thai. See *Olic, Thai.*

Du Pont, UK. Du Pont Pharmaceuticals Ltd, Wedgwood Way, Stevenage, Hertfordshire, SG1 4QN, UK.

Du Pont, USA. DuPont Pharmaceuticals Co., Chestnut Run Plaza, Hickory Run, Wilmington, DE 19880-0723, USA.

Duchesnay, Canad. Duchesnay Inc., 2925 Industrial Blvd, Laval, Quebec, H7L 3W9, Canada.

Ducray, Fr. See *Pierre Fabre, Fr.*

Dumex, Ger. See *Alpharma-Isis, Ger.*

Dumex, Irl. See *Alpharma, UK.*

Dumex, Norw. See *Alpharma, Norw.*

Dumex, NZ. See *CSL, NZ.*

Dumex, Port. Dumex-Alpharma A/S, Rua Virgilio Correira 11A, 1600-219 Lisbon, Portugal.

Dumex, Singapore. Dumex, Representative Office, 2 Enterprise Rd, S 629814, Singapore.

Dumex, Switz. Dumex AG, Baarerstrasse 10, 6300 Zug, Switzerland.

Dumex, Thai. Dumex Ltd, 359 Moo 17 Theparak Rd, Bangsaothong, Samutprakan 10542, Thailand.

Dumex, UK. See *Alpharma, UK.*

Dumex-Alpharma, Denm. Dumex-Alpharma A/S, Dalslandsgade 11 (postboks 1736), 2300 Copenhagen S, Denmark.

Dumex-Alpharma, Fin. Oy Dumex-Alpharma Ab, Sinimäentie 10 B, 02630 Espoo, Finland.

Dumex-Alpharma, Hong Kong. See *Primal, Hong Kong.*

Dumex-Alpharma, Singapore. See *Sime Darby, Singapore.*

Dumex-Alpharma, Swed. See *Alpharma, Swed.*

Duncan, Ital. Duncan Farmaceutici s.p.a., Via A. Fleming 2, 37135 Verona, Italy.

Duncan, Spain. See *Glaxo Wellcome, Spain.*

Duncan, Flockhart, Irl. See *GlaxoSmithKline, Irl.*

Dunhall, USA. Dunhall Pharmaceuticals Inc., Highway 59N, P.O. Box 100, Gravette, AR 72736, USA.

Duomed, Switz. Duomed AG, 9533 Kirchberg, Switzerland.

Duopharm, Ger. Duopharm GmbH, Grassingerstr. 9, 83043 Bad Aibling, Germany.

Duopharma, Hong Kong. See *Weston, Hong Kong.*

Duphar, Neth. See *Solvay, Neth.*

Duphar, Spain. See *Solvay, Spain.*

Duphar-Interfran, Thai. See *Union Medical, Thai.*

Dura, USA. Dura Pharmaceuticals, 7475 Lusk Blvd, San Diego, CA 92121-4202, USA.

Durachemie, Ger. See *Merck dura, Ger.*

Duramed, USA. Duramed Pharmaceuticals, 5040 Duramed Dr, Cincinnati, OH 45213, USA.

Durascan, Denm. DuraScan Medical Products AS, Svendborgvej 243, 5260 Odense S, Denmark.

Durban, Spain. Durban, Santos Zarate 20, 04004 Almeria, Spain.

Durbin, UK. Durbin B.S. Ltd, 240 Northolt Rd, South Harrow, Middlesex, HA2 8DU, UK.

Durex, Canad. Durex Canada, Division of London International Group Ltd, 100 Courtland Ave, Concord, Ontario, L4K 3T6, Canada.

Durex, USA. Durex Consumer Products, 3585 Engineering Drive, Suite 200, Noreriss, GA 30092, USA.

DUSA, USA. DUSA, USA.

Dutec, Austral. Dutec Diagnostics P/L, P.O. Box 79, Croydon, NSW 2132, Australia.

Dyckerhoff, Ger. Dyckerhoff Pharma GmbH & Co., Robert-Perthel-Str. 49, 50739 Cologne (Longerich), Germany.

Dynacren, Ital. Dynacren Laboratorio Farmaceutico del Dott. A. Francioni e di M. Gerosa s.r.l., Via P Nenni 12, 28053 Castelletto Ticino (NO), Italy.

Dynamed, S.Afr. Dynamed, South Africa.

Dynamit, Aust. Dynamit Nobel Wien GmbH, A-8813 St Lamprecht, Austria.

Dynapharm, USA. Dynapharm Inc., P.O. Box 2141, Del Mar, CA 92014, USA.

E. Merck, Denm. See *Kemifarma, Denm.*

E. Merck, Irl. See *Merck, Irl.*

E. Merck, UK. See *Merck, UK.*

E Pharma, Fr. Lab. E Pharma, ZI Le Malcourlet, 03800 Gannat, France.

Eagle, Austral. Eagle Pharmaceuticals P/L, P.O. Box 927, Castle Hill, NSW 1765, Australia.

Eastern Pharmaceuticals, Irl. See *Intra Pharma, Irl.*

Eastern Pharmaceuticals, UK. Eastern Pharmaceuticals Ltd, Coomb House, St. Johns Rd, Isleworth, Middlesex, TW7 6NA, UK.

e+b, Aust. See *e+b, Ger.*

e+b, Ger. e+b GmbH & Co. Pharma KG, Emil-Kemmer-Str. 33, 96103 Hallstadt, Germany.

Eberth, Ger. Dr. Friedrich Eberth Nachf., Hohenburger Str. 39, 92289 Ursensollen, Germany.

Eberth, Switz. See *Uhlmann-Eyraud, Switz.*

Ebewe, Aust. Ebewe Arzneimittel GmbH, Mondseestrasse 11, A-4866 Unterach am Attersee, Austria.

Ebewe, Hong Kong. See *Health Care, Hong Kong.*

Ebewe, Thai. See *Schumit, Thai.*

Ebi, Switz. Ebi-Pharm AG, Lindachstrasse 8c, 3038 Kirchlindach, Switzerland.

Ebos, Austral. Ebos, Australia.

Ebos, NZ. Ebos Group Ltd, P.O. Box 411, Christchurch, New Zealand.

Echo, Ital. Echo s.r.l., Via della Mattonaia 15, 50121 Florence, Italy.

Ecobi, Ital. Farmaceutici Ecobi s.a.s., Via E. Bazzano 26, 16019 Ronco Scrivia (GE), Italy.

Econo Med, USA. Econo Med Pharmaceuticals Inc., 4305 Sartin Rd, Burlington, NC 27217-7522, USA.

Econolab, USA. Econolab, P.O. Box 85543, Westland, MI 48185-0543, USA.

Ecosol, Norw. See *Andersen, Norw.*

Ecosol, Switz. Ecosol AG, Hohlstrasse 192, 8004 Zurich, Switzerland.

ECR, Switz. ECR Pharma AG, Bosch 104, 6331 Hunenberg/ZG, Switzerland.

ECR, USA. ECR Pharmaceuticals, P.O. Box 71600, Richmond, VA 23255, USA.

Ecupharma, Ital. Ecupharma s.r.l., Via Mazzini 20, 20123 Milan, Italy.

Ederka, Mex. Farmaceuticos Ederka S.A. de C.V., Calle 3 Num. 1, Fracc. Ind. Benito Juarez, 76130 Queretaro Qro, Mexico.

Edigen, Spain. Edigen, P de la Castellana, 28046 Madrid, Spain.

Edmond Pharma, Ital. Edmond Pharma s.r.l., Via dei Giovi 131, 20037 Paderno Dugnano (MI), Italy.

Edochim, Ital. Edochim s.r.l., Via Crescentino 31/A, 10154 Turin, Italy.

Edol, Port. Edol, SA, Av 25 de Abril 6-6A, Linda-a-Velha (Oeiras), 2795 Linda-a-Velha, Portugal.

Edwards, USA. Edwards Pharmaceuticals Inc., 111 Mulberry St, Ripley, MS 38663, USA.

Efamol, Austral. Efamol Ltd, P.O. Box 6745, Baulkham Hills BC, NSW 2153, Australia.

Efamol, Canad. Efamol Research Inc., Annapolis Valley Industrial Park, 15 Chipman Drive, P.O. Box 818, Kentville, Nova Scotia, B4N 4H8, Canada.

Efamol, NZ. Efamol, New Zealand.

Efamol, UK. Efamol Ltd, a Division of Nutricia, White Horse Business Park, Trowbridge, Wiltshire, BA14 0XQ, UK.

Efarmes, Spain. Efarmes, Sardenya 350, 08025 Barcelona, Spain.

EF-EM-ES, Aust. EF-EM-ES - Dr Smetana & Co., Scheidlstrasse 28, A-1180 Vienna, Austria.

Effcon, USA. Effcon Laboratories Inc., 1800 Sandy Plains Parkway, Marietta, GA 30066-7499, USA.

Effik, Fr. Laboratoires Effik, Burospace 7, rte de Gisy, 91571 Bievres cdx, France.

Effik, Spain. Effik, Antonio de Cabezon 27 5, Planta Ed Alfa Laval, 28034 Madrid, Spain.

Effimed, Fr. Lab. Effimed, 221 rue La Fayette, 75010 Paris, France.

EG, Fr. EG Labo (Laboratoire EuroGenerics), 12 rue Danjou, 92517 Boulogne-Billancourt cdx, France.

Egis, Hong Kong. See *Mekim, Hong Kong.*

EGIS, Hung. EGIS Pharmaceuticals, P.O. Box 100, 1475 Budapest, Hungary.

Egis, Singapore. See *Sime Darby, Singapore.*

Egis, Thai. See *Medline, Thai.*

Ego, Austral. Ego Pharmaceuticals P/L, 21-31 Malcolm Rd, Braeside, VIC 3195, Australia.

Ego, Hong Kong. See *Lision Hong, Hong Kong.*

Ego, NZ. See *Douglas, NZ.*

Ego, Singapore. See *Grafton, Singapore.*

EGS, Ger. EGS Pharma Vertrieb, Schulstr. 38, 09125 Chemnitz, Germany.

Ehlinger, Mex. Ehlinger, Mexico.

Ehrenhofer, Aust. Dr. F. Ehrenhöfer GmbH, Triester Strasse 36, A-2620 Neunkirchen, Austria.

Ehrmann, Aust. Ehrmann Mag. pharm. Liselotte GmbH, Obertrumer Landstr. 7, A-5201 Seekirchen, Austria.

Eifelfango, Ger. Eifelfango GmbH & Co. KG, Ringener Str. 45, 53474 Bad Neuenahr-Ahrweiler, Germany.

Eifelfango, Switz. See *Agpharm, Switz.*

Eight, Spain. Eight Farmaceutica, Camino de Las Lenguas S/N, 28020 Madrid, Spain.

Eiken, Jpn. Eiken Chem., Japan.

Eisai, Fr. Lab. Eisai, tour Manhattan, La Defense 2, 5-6 place de l'Iris, 92095 Paris-La-Defense, France.

Eisai, Ger. Eisai GmbH, Lyoner Str. 14, 60528 Frankfurt, Germany.

Eisai, Hong Kong. Eisai (Hong Kong) Co. Ltd, Rm 2104, Fortress Tower, 250 King's Rd, North Point, Hong Kong.

Eisai, Jpn. Eisai Co. Ltd, 6-10 Koishikawa 4-chome, Bunkyo-ku, Tokyo 112-8088, Japan.

Eisai, Singapore. Eisai Asia Regional Services Pte Ltd, 152 Beach Road, 11-04 Gateway East, S 189721, Singapore.

Eisai, Thai. Eisai (Thailand) Marketing Co. Ltd, 6 Fl, Diethelm Tower A, 93/1 Wireless Rd, Bangkok 10330, Thailand.

Eisai, UK. Eisai Ltd, 3 Shortlands, Hammersmith, London, W6 8EE, UK.

Eisai, USA. Eisai Inc., 500 Frank W Burr Blvd, Teaneck, NJ 07666, USA.

Eladon, UK. Eladon Ltd, 63 High St, Bangor, Gwynedd, LL57 1NT, UK.

Elaiapharm, Switz. See *Interdelta, Switz.*

Elan, Denm. See *Ipsen, Denm.*

Elan, Ger. Elan Pharma GmbH, Rosenkavalierplatz 8, 81925 Munich, Germany.

Elan, Irl. Elan Pharma (Ireland) Ltd, Unit E, Glencormack Business Park, Kilmacanogue, Co. Wicklow, Ireland.

Elan, UK. Elan Pharma Ltd, Elan House, Avenue One, Letchworth, Hertfordshire, SG6 2HU, UK.

Elan, USA. Elan Phamaceuticals, 800 Gateway Blvd, South San Francisco, CA 94080, USA.

Elder, Neth. See *ICN, Neth.*

Elder, UK. Don Elder Products Ltd, Unit 15, Chiltonian Industrial Estate, 203 Manor Lane, London, SE12 0TX, UK.

Electramed, Irl. Electramed Ireland Ltd, U2 Kinsealy Business Park, Kinsealy, Co. Dublin, Ireland.

Elerte, Fr. Laboratoires des Réalisations Thérapeutiques Elerté, 181-3 rue Andre-Karman, B.P. 101, 93303 Aubervilliers cdx, France.

Elexsam, Austral. Elexsam International, 5 Berowra Waters Road, Berowra, NSW 2081, Australia.

Elfar, Spain. Elfar Drag, Guzman el Bueno, 133 Edif Britannia, 28003 Madrid, Spain.

Elkins-Sinn, USA. See *Wyeth-Ayerst, USA.*

Elofar, Braz. Laboratorio Farmaceutico Elofar Ltda, Rua Tereza Cristina 67, 88075-970 Florianopolis, SC, Brazil.

Emerging Pharma, Singapore. See *Sime Darby, Singapore.*

Emilio, Spain. Emilio Romero, P Industrial La Red (J) 181-2, Alcala de Guadaira, Sevilla, Spain.

Emonta, Aust. Emonta Pharma GmbH, Weidelstrasse 21, A-1100 Vienna, Austria.

EMS, Braz. EMS Industria Farmaceutica Ltda, Rua Comendador Carlo Mario Gardano 450, 09720-470 Sao Bernardo do Campo, SP, Brazil.

Enapharm, Swed. Enapharm AB, Box 30, 745 21 Enkoping, Sweden.

Endo, Canad. See *Du Pont, Canad.*

Endo, USA. Endo Pharmaceuticals Inc., 223 Wilmington West Chester Pike, Chadds Ford, PA 19317, USA.

Endoterapica, Braz. Endoterapica do Brasil Industria Farmaceutica Ltda, Rua General Belford 284, 20961-000 Rio de Janeiro, RJ, Brazil.

Engelhard, Ger. Engelhard Arzneimittel GmbH & Co. KG, Herzbergstr. 3, 61138 Niederdorfelden, Germany.

Engelhard, Hong Kong. See *Asta Medica, Hong Kong.*

Engelhard, Singapore. See *Sime Darby, Singapore.*

Engelhard, Switz. See *Pharmakos, Switz.*

Engelshof, Aust. Engelshof-Apotheke, Leystrasse 19-21, A-1200 Vienna, Austria.

English Grains, UK. English Grains Ltd, Swains Park Industrial Estate, Park Rd, Overseal, Burton-on-Trent, Staffordshire, UK.

Enila, Braz. Laboratorio Enila Industria Comercio Prod. Quim. Farma. S.A., Rua Viuva Claudio 355, 20970-030 Rio de Janeiro, RJ, Brazil.

Ensinger, Ger. Ensinger Mineral-Heilquellen GmbH, Horrheimer Strasse 28-30, 71665 Vaihingen-Ensingen, Germany.

Enviroderm, USA. EnviroDerm Pharmaceuticals Inc., P.O. Box 32370, Louisville, KY 40232-2370, USA.

Enzifarma, Port. Enzifarma, Lda, Taguspark, Parque de Ciencia e Tecnologia, Nucleo Central 184, 2780 Oeiras, Portugal.

Enzon, USA. Enzon, Inc., 40 Kingsbridge Rd, Piscataway, NJ 08854, USA.

Enzypharm, Aust. Enzypharm GmbH, Piaristengasse 29, A-1080 Vienna, Austria.

Enzypharm, Neth. Enzypharm B.V., Postbus 205, 3760 AE Soest, Netherlands.

Eon, USA. Eon Labs Manufacturing Inc., 227-15 North Conduit Ave, Laurelton, NY 11413, USA.

Epifarma, Ital. Epifarma s.a.s., Via San Rocco 6, 85033 Episcopia (PZ), Italy.

Epipharm, Aust. Epipharm GmbH, Herrenstrasse 2, A-4020 Linz, Austria.

ERA, Denm. ERA Medical ApS, Metalgangen 9-11, 2690 Karlslunde, Denmark.

Ercopharm, Denm. Ercopharm A/S, Boegeskovvej 9, 3490 Kvistgaard, Denmark.

Ercopharm, Fin. See *Organon, Fin.*

Ercopharm, Switz. See *Orion, Switz.*

Ercopharm, Thai. See *Pacific, Thai.*

Erfa, Belg. Erfa S.A., Rue des Cultivateurs 25, 1040 Brussels, Belgium.

Ergha, Irl. Ergha Healthcare Ltd, Damastown, Mulhuddart, Dublin 15, Ireland.

Erjean, Fr. Lab. Erjean, 9 rue de Sebastopol, B.P. 867, 31015 Toulouse cdx 6, France.

Ern, Spain. Ern, Pedro IV 499, 08020 Barcelona, Spain.

Ernest Jackson, UK. Ernest Jackson & Co. Ltd, 29 High St, Crediton, Devon, EX17 3AP, UK.

Erredici, Ital. Erredici, Italy.

Errekappa, Ital. Errekappa Euroterapici s.p.a., Via C. Menotti 1/A, 20129 Milan, Italy.

Escaned, Spain. Escaned, Tomas Breton 46, 28045 Madrid, Spain.

Esfar, Port. Laboratórios Esfar, SA, Rua da Escola de Medicina Veterinaria 15-17, 1049-029 Lisbon, Portugal.

Eshcol, Singapore. See *Summit, Singapore.*

ESI, USA. ESI Lederle Inc., PO Box 41502, Philadelphia, PA 19101, USA.

Esoform, Ital. Esoform spa, Viale del Lavoro 10, 45100 Rovigo, Italy.

Esparma, Ger. esparma GmbH, Lange Gohren 3, 39171 Osterweddingen, Germany.

Espe, Aust. Espe HandelsGmbH, Marokkanergasse 9/8, A-1030 Vienna, Austria.

Espe, Ger. ESPE Dental AG, ESPE Platz, 82229 Seefeld, Germany.

Espe, Ital. Espe Italia srl, Via C Cantu 29, 20092 Cinisello Balsamo (MI), Italy.

Espe, Switz. Espe AG, Baumackerstrasse 46, Postfach 8360, 8050 Zurich, Switzerland.

Esplanade, Aust. Esplanade-Apotheke, Esplanade 18, A-4820 Bad Ischl, Austria.

Esplanade, Fr. Pharmaceutique de l'Esplanade, 34 route d'Ecully, B.P. 94, 69573 Dardilly cdx, France.

Essedi, Ital. Essedi Special Diets srl, Galleria Giotto 10/5b, 20084 Lachiarella (MI), Italy.

Esseti, Ital. Esseti Farmaceutici s.p.a., Via Cavalli di Bronzo 41, 80046 S. Giorgio a Cremano (NA), Italy.

Essex, Austral. See *Schering-Plough, Austral.*

Essex, Ger. Essex Pharma GmbH, Thomas-Dehler-Str. 27, 81737 Munich, Germany.

Essex, Ital. Essex Italia SpA, Palazzo Borromini, 20090 Segrate (MI), Italy.

Essex, Spain. Farmaceutica Essex, Ctra Burgos Km 36, San Augustin De Guadalix, 28750 Madrid, Spain.

Essex, Switz. Essex Chemie AG, Postfach 2769, 6002 Lucerne, Switzerland.

Essilor, Aust. Essilor-Swarovski GmbH, Austria.

Estedi, Spain. Estedi, Montseny 41, 08012 Barcelona, Spain.

Estee Lauder, Canad. Estee Lauder Cosmetics Ltd, 161 Commander Blvd, Agincourt, Ontario, M1S 3K9, Canada.

Esteve, Spain. Esteve, Avda Virgen Montserrat 221, 08041 Barcelona, Spain.

Esteves Alves, Port. José Esteves Alves, Lda, R. do Padrao 98, 3002-906 Coimbra Codex, Portugal.

Etajesa, Fr. Etajesa, 14 av. Edouard-Vaillant, 93698 Pantin cdx, France.

Etapharm, Aust. Etapharm GmbH, Vormosergasse 3, 1190 Vienna, Austria.

Ethex, Hong Kong. See *Pan-Well, Hong Kong.*

Ethex, USA. Ethex Corp., 10888 Metro Court, St Louis, MO 63043-2413, USA.

Ethical, Singapore. See *Kyowa, Singapore.*

Ethical Generics, UK. See *Genus, UK.*

Ethical Research, Irl. See *Ethical Research, UK.*

Ethical Research, UK. Ethical Research Marketing, 3A Landgate, Rye, East Sussex, TN31 7LH, UK.

Ethicals, Denm. See *Kemifarma, Denm.*

Ethicare, Austral. Ethicare Pharmaceuticals P/L, P.O. Box 316, Applecross, WA 6953, Australia.

Ethicon, Fr. Ethicon SAS, 1 rue Camille-Desmoulins, TSA 81002, 92787 Issy-les-Moulineaux cdx 9, France.

Ethicon, Ger. Ethicon GmbH & Co. KG, Robert-Koch-Str. 1, 22851 Norderstedt, Germany.

Ethicon, Ital. Ethicon s.p.a., 00040 Pratica di Mare Pomezia (Rome), Italy.

Ethimed, S.Afr. See *Noristan, S.Afr.*

Ethitek, USA. Ethitek Pharmaceuticals Co., 7701 North Austin, Skokie, IL 60077, USA.

Ethypharm, Aust. See *Ethypharm, Fr.*

Ethypharm, Denm. See *Durascan, Denm.*

Ethypharm, Fr. Lab. Ethypharm SA, 194 bureaux de la Colline, 92213 St-Cloud, France.

Ethypharm, Ital. Ethypharm srl, Viale Monza 196, 20128 Milan, Italy.

Etris, Fr. Etris, 14 rue de la Comète, 75007 Paris, France.

Eu Rho, Ger. Eu Rho Arznei GmbH, Sudfeld 1a, 59174 Kamen, Germany.

Euform, Fr. Euform, 77 rue Marcel-Dassault, 92100 Boulogne, France.

Eugal, Ital. Laboratorio Chimico Farmaceutico Eugal s.r.l., Via Fabbriche 18, 15050 Serravalle Scrivia (AL), Italy.

Eulactol, S.Afr. Eulactol (Pty) Ltd, P.O. Box 3265, Randburg 2125, South Africa.

Eumedica, Switz. Eumedica Pharmaceuticals (Schweiz) AG, Peter Merian-Strasse 54, 4002 Basle, Switzerland.

Euphar, Ital. Euphar Group srl, Via Gandine 4/6, 29100 Piacenza, Italy.

Eurim, Ger. Eurim-Pharm GmbH, Am Ganselehen 4-6, 83451 Piding, Germany.

Euroderm, Ital. Euroderm, Via Laurentina Km 28 800, 00040 Ardea (RM), Italy.

Eurodrug, Hong Kong. See *Advance, Hong Kong,* and *Inchcape, Hong Kong.*

Eurodrug, Singapore. See *JDH, Singapore.*

Eurodrug, Thai. Eurodrug, 9 Fl, MPD Berli Jucker House, 99 Soi Rubia, Sukhumvit 42, Prakanong, Bangkok 10110, Thailand.

Euroexim, Spain. Euroexim, C/Emilio Munoz 15, 28037 Madrid, Spain.

Eurofarma, Braz. Eurofarma Laboratorios Ltda, Rua Barao do Triunfo 1.440, 04602-005 Sao Paulo, SP, Brazil.

Eurofarmaco, Ital. Eurofarmaco s.r.l., Via Aurelia 58, 00166 Rome, Italy.

Euro-Labor, Port. Euro-Labor, SA, Rua Alfredo da Silva no 16, Zona Industrial de Alfraigde, 2720-028 Amadora, Portugal.

Euromedex, Fr. Lab. Euromedex, 24 rue des Tuileries, B.P. 74684, Souffelweyersheim, 67458 Mundolschein cdx, France.

Euromex, Mex. Laboratorios Euromex, S.A. de C.V., Calle 7 No. 386, Col. Pantitlan, 08100 Mexico, D.F., Mexico.

Europharm, Aust. Europharm, Jochen-Rindt-Strasse 23, A-1230 Vienna, Austria.

Euro-Pharma, Ital. Euro-Pharma srl, Via Garziliana 8, 10100 Turin, Italy.

Europharma, Spain. Europharma, Pablo Alcover 31-3, 08017 Barcelona, Spain.

Europhta, Mon. Laboratoires Europhta, Le Concorde, 11 rue du Gabian, MC 98000, Monaco.

Eurorga, Fr. Eurorga, 11-13 rue de la Loge, B.P. 100, 94265 Fresnes cdx, France.

Eurospital, Ital. Eurospital s.p.a., Via Flavia 122, 34147 Trieste, Italy.

Eurovita, Thai. See *Diethelm, Thai.*

Eutherapie, Belg. Eutherapie Benelux S.A., Blvd International 57, 1070 Brussels, Belgium.

Eutherapie, Fr. Euthérapie, 27 rue du Pont, 92200 Neuilly-sur-Seine cdx, France.

Evans, Fr. See *Medeva, Fr.*

Evans, Neth. See *Glaxo Wellcome, Neth.*

Evans, Spain. See *Medeva, Spain.*

Evans, UK. Evans Vaccines Ltd, Gaskill Rd, Speke, Liverpool, Merseyside, L24 9GR, UK.

Evans Medical, Irl. See *GlaxoSmithKline, Irl.*

Evans Medical, Israel. Evans Medical, Israel.

Evapharm, Ital. Evapharm s.r.l., Via Bolognola 47, 00138 Rome, Italy.

Evening Primrose Oil Co., UK. Evening Primrose Oil Co. Ltd, UK.

Everest, Canad. Everest Pharmaceuticals Ltd, 108 Bayhampton Court, Thornhill, Ontario, L4J 7E1, Canada.

Everett, USA. Everett Laboratories Inc., 29 Spring St, West Orange, NJ 07052, USA.

Evers, Ger. Pharmazeutische Fabrik Evers & Co. GmbH, Siemensstr. 4, 25421 Pinneberg, Germany.

Evers, Hong Kong. See *Pinneberg, Hong Kong.*

Evers, Thai. See *Sriprasit, Thai.*

Eversil, Braz. Eversil Produtos Farmaceuticos Industria e Comercio Ltda, Rua Agostinho Teixeira de Lima 99-A, Jardim Sertaozinho, 04826-230 Sao Paulo, SP, Brazil.

Evisco, Ger. Evisco-Pharma, Klosterplatz 6, 87509 Immenstadt, Germany.

Exel, Belg. Exel Pharma S.A., Chaussee de Gand 615, 1080 Brussels, Belgium.

Exelgyn, Denm. See *Exelgyn, Swed.*

Exelgyn, Fr. Exelgyn, 6 rue Christophe-Colomb, 75008 Paris, France.

Exelgyn, Swed. Exelgyn, Box 1343, 181 25 Lidingo, Sweden.

Exflora, Fr. Laboratoires Exflora, 26 rue du Mont-Roti, 78550 Houdan, France.

Exflora, Switz. See *Uhlmann-Eyraud, Switz.*

Expancience, Spain. Expancience, Alava 6, Pol. Ind. San Roque, Arganda del Rey, 28500 Madrid, Spain.

Expanpharm, Fr. Laboratoires Expanpharm International, 6 rue Euler, 75008 Paris, France.

Expanpharm, Switz. See *Uhlmann-Eyraud, Switz.*

Expharma, Ital. ExPharma srl, Riviera Francia 3/A, 35127 Padua, Italy.

Express Care, NZ. Express Care Direct, New Zealand.

Extractum, Hung. Extractum Pharma Rt, Gyogyszer Business Center, 1047 Budapest, Hungary.

E-Z-EM, Belg. E-Z-EM Belgium S.A., Kiezelstraat 144, 3500 Hasselt, Belgium.

E-Z-EM, Canad. E-Z-EM Canada Inc., 11 065 L-H Lafontaine, Anjou, Quebec, H1J 2Z4, Canada.

E-Z-EM, Israel. E-Z-EM, Israel.

E-Z-EM, Port. See *Martins & Fernandes, Port.*

E-Z-EM, UK. E-Z-EM Ltd, 1230 High Rd, London, N20 0LH, UK.

F5 Profas, Spain. F5 Profas, Ed Indubuilding Goico, Via Los Poblados 17, 28033 Madrid, Spain.

Fabrigen, Canad. Fabrigen Inc., P.O. Box 507, Pierrefonds, Quebec, H9H 4M6, Canada.

Face, Ital. Face Laboratori Farmaceutici SpA, Via Albisola 49, 16163 Genova-Bolzaneto, Italy.

Fadim, Ital. Fadim srl, Via Egadi 7, 20144 Milan, Italy.

Faes, Spain. Faes, Maximo Aguirre 14, Lejona, 48940 Vizcaya, Spain.

Falk, Ger. Dr. Falk Pharma GmbH, Leinenweberstr. 5, 79108 Freiburg, Germany.

Falk, Hong Kong. See *Jacobson, Hong Kong.*

Falk, Neth. See *Tramedico, Neth.*

Falk, Singapore. See *JDH, Singapore.*

Falk, Thai. See *Zuellig, Thai.*

Falqui, Ital. Falqui Prodotti Farmaceutici s.p.a., Via Sabotino 19/2, 20135 Milan, Italy.

FAMA, Ital. F.A.M.A. s.r.l., Istituto Chimico Biologico, Via A. Sauli 21, 20127 Milan, Italy.

Family Planning Sales, UK. Family Planning Sales Ltd, 28 Kelburne Rd, Cowley, Oxford, OX4 3SZ, UK.

Fandasy, Hong Kong. Fandasy Co. Ltd, Unit A, 18/F Federal Ctr, 77 Sheung On St, Chaiwan, Hong Kong.

Far East, Thai. Far East Pharmaceutical Ltd Part, 92/1-2 Lanluang Rd, Bangkok 10100, Thailand.

Far East Drug, Singapore. Far East Drug Co Pte Ltd, 1 Sophia Rd, 08-01 Peace Centre, S 228149, Singapore.

Farbo, Ital. Farbo s.n.c. del dott. Donato Mele & C., Via Stelvio 12/18, 20021 Ospiate di Bollate (MI), Italy.

Farco, Denm. See *Tjellesen, Denm.*

Farco, Ger. Farco-Pharma GmbH Pharmazeutische Präparate, Mathias-Bruggen-Str. 82, 50829 Cologne, Germany.

Farco, Hong Kong. See *Sincerity, Hong Kong.*

Farco, Irl. See *Boileau & Boyd, Irl.*

Farco, Israel. Farco, Israel.

Farcoral, Mex. Profesional Medica Farcoral S.A. de C.V., Circuito Norte No. 28, Unidad Guadalupe, 72560 Puebla, Pue., Mexico.

Fardi, Spain. Fardi, Grassot 16, 08025 Barcelona, Spain.

Farex, Canad. Laboratoire Farex Enrg, 5750 Metropolitan E Blvd, Bur 200, St-Leonard, Quebec, H1S 1A7, Canada.

Faria, Braz. Laboratorio Farmaceutico Faria Ltda, Rua Coronel Delfino Nonato de Faria 151, Sta Tereza, 36020-170 Juiz de Fora, MG, Brazil.

Fariberica, Port. Fdibérica, SA, Estrada da Luz 90, 1600-160 Lisbon, Portugal.

Farillon, UK. Farillon Ltd, Ashton Rd, Harold Hill, Romford, Essex, RM3 8UE, UK.

Farma Energy, Ital. Farma Energy, Via Polia 36/38, 00178 Rome, Italy.

Farma Lepori, Spain. Farma Lepori, Osi 7-9, 08034 Barcelona, Spain.

Farmabion, Spain. See *Alter, Spain.*

Farmabraz, Braz. S.A. Farmaceutica Brasileira Farmabraz, Travessa Jacare 75, 20975-070 Rio de Janeiro, RJ, Brazil.

Farmacelsia, Spain. Farmacelsia, A Ramallosa S/N, Santiago de Compostela, 15883 Coruna, Spain.

Farmachimici, Ital. Farmachimici srl, Via Mercanti 36, 84121 Salerno, Italy.

Farmaco, Mex. Laboratorio Productos Farmaceuticos y Biologicos Farmaco S.A., Jaime Nuno No. 112, Col. Guadalupe Inn, 01020 Mexico, D.F., Mexico.

Farmacologico Milanese, Ital. Laboratorio Farmacologico Milanese s.r.l., Via Monterosso 273, 21042 Caronno Pertusella (VA), Italy.

Farmacusi, Spain. Farmacusi, Marina 16-18, Torre Mapfre 8 Planta, 08005 Barcelona, Spain.

Farmades, Ital. Farmades s.p.a., Via di Tor Cervara 282, 00155 Rome, Italy.

Farmagan, Ital. Farmagan s.a., Via di Tor Cervara 282, 00155 Rome, Italy.

Farmaka, Ital. Farmaka s.r.l. Laboratori Farmaceutici, Via Vetreria 1, 22070 Grandate (CO), Italy.

Farmalab, Braz. Farmalab Industrias Quimicas e Farmaceuticas Ltda, Avenida Brigadeiro Faria Lima 1734 2° andar, 01452-001 Sao Paulo, SP, Brazil.

Farmalider, Spain. Farmalider S.A., C/Aragoneses 9, Alcobendas, 28100 Madrid, Spain.

Farmalight, Port. Farmalight, Lda, Rua Padre Americo 18, Escritorio 1, 1600-548 Lisbon, Portugal.

Farmanova, Ital. Farmanova AFM s.r.l., Via Flaminia 287 Sc. A. int.10, 00196 Rome, Italy.

Farmapros, Spain. Farmapros, Aribau 180, 08036 Barcelona, Spain.

Farmarekord, Ital. Farmarekord srl, Italy.

Farmasa, Braz. Laboratorio Americano de Farmacoterapia S/A, Rua Sena Madureira 328, 04021-000 Sao Paulo, SP, Brazil.

Farmasa, Mex. Laboratorios Farmasa, S.A. de C.V., Bufalo No. 27, Col. del Valle, 03100 Mexico D.F., Mexico.

Farmasan, Ger. Farmasan Arzneimittel GmbH & Co., Pforzheimer Str. 5, 76227 Karlsruhe, Germany.

Farmasan, Thai. See *JDH Borneo, Thai.*

Farmasierra, Spain. Farmasierra, Ctra de Irun KM 26.2, San Sebastian de Los Reyes, 28100 Madrid, Spain.

Farmasur, Spain. Farmasur, Spain.

Farmatrading, Ital. Farmatrading s.r.l., Via Merlo 1, 20122 Milan, Italy.

Farmatrading, Port. Farmatrading, Lda, Travessa de Santa Catarina no 18, 1200-403 Lisbon, Portugal.

Farmatre, Ital. Farma 3 s.r.l., Via Solferino 42, 20036 Meda (MI), Italy.

Farmavy, Braz. Farmavy Industria Farmaceutica Ltda, Rua Vinte e Quatro de Maio 224/232, 20950-090 Rio de Janeiro, RJ, Brazil.

Farmec, Ital. Farmec s.n.c., Via W Flemming 7, 37026 Pescantina (VR) Italy.

Farmedica, Braz. Farmedica Industria Farmaceutica Ltda, Avenida Automovel Clube 1140, 25565-000 Rio de Janeiro, RJ, Brazil.

Farmetrusca, Ital. Farmetrusca s.a.s. di C. Pini e C., Via G. di Vittorio, 50029 Tavarnuzze (FI), Italy.

Farmigea, Ital. Farmigea s.p.a., Industria Chimico Farmaceutica, Via Carmignani 2, 56127 Pisa, Italy.

Farmila, Ital. Farmila-Farmaceutici Milano s.r.l., Via E. Fermi 50, 20019 Settimo Milanese (MI), Italy.

Farminova, Port. See *Pfizer, Port.*

Farmion, Braz. Farmion Laboratorio Brasileiro de Farmacologia Ltda, Avenida Celso dos Santos 579, 04658-240 Sao Paulo, SP, Brazil.

Farmitalia, Israel. Farmitalia, Israel.

Farmitalia Carlo Erba, UK. Farmitalia Carlo Erba Ltd, UK.

Farmoquimica, Braz. Farmoquimica S.A., Rua General Polidoro 105, 22280-001 Rio de Janeiro, RJ, Brazil.

Farmocore, Port. Laboratórios Farmorcore, SA, Quinta da Franceltha de Cima, 2685 Prior-Velho, Portugal.

Faro, UK. Faro Pharmaceuticals Inc., 10607 Haddington 150, Houston, TX 77043, USA.

Fate, UK. Fate Special Foods, Unit E2, Brook Street Business Centre, Brook Street, Tipton, West Midlands, DY4 9DD, UK.

Fater, Ital. Fater s.p.a., Via Italica 101, 65127 Pescara, Italy.

Fatol, Aust. See *Fatol, Ger.*

Fatol, Ger. Fatol Arzneimittel GmbH, Robert-Koch-Str., 66578 Schiffweiler, Germany.

Fatol, Hong Kong. See *Mekim, Hong Kong.*

Faulding, Austral. Faulding Pharmaceuticals, Division of F.H. Faulding & Co. Ltd, 1538 Main North Rd, Salisbury South, SA 5108, Australia.

Faulding, Denm. See *Baxter, Denm.*

Faulding, Hong Kong. Faulding Pharmaceuticals (HK) Ltd, Unit 3A, 16/F Eastwood Ctr, 5A Kung Ngam Village Rd, Shaukeiwan, Hong Kong.

Faulding, NZ. Faulding Pharmaceuticals (NZ) Ltd, P.O. Box 33-1668, Takapuna, Auckland, New Zealand.

Faulding, Port. Faulding Famacêutica, Lda, Rua Amilia Rodrigues, lote 4, 2750-028 Cascais, Portugal.

Faulding, Singapore. Faulding Pharmaceuticals, 70 Bendemeer Rd, 04-02 Hiap Huat House, S 339940, Singapore.

Faulding, Thai. See *Indochina Healthcare, Thai.*

Faulding, UK. Faulding Pharmaceuticals Plc, Queensway, Royal Leamington Spa, Warwickshire, CV31 3HW, UK.

Faulding, USA. Faulding Laboratories, 200 Elmora Ave, Elizabeth, NJ 908 527 9100, USA.

Faulding Healthcare, Austral. Faulding Healthcare P/L, 55 Kirby St, Rydalmere, NSW 2116, Australia.

Fawns & McAllan, Austral. See *Sigma, Austral.*

Fawns & McAllan, Hong Kong. See *LCH, Hong Kong.*

Fawns & McAllan, NZ. See *Pharmaco, NZ.*

FD, Ital. FD Farmaceutici srl, Via Castello 15, 29019 San Giorgio Piacentino (PC), Italy.

Febena, Ger. Febena GmbH, Oskar-Jager-Str. 115, 50825 Cologne, Germany.

Feldhoff, Ger. W. Feldhoff & Comp. Arzneimittel GmbH, Am Nutzleber Feld 2, 99867 Gotha, Germany.

Felgenträger, Ger. Dr. Felgenträger & Co. Öko-chem. und Pharma GmbH, Zerbster Str. 7a, 06862 Rodleben, Germany.

Felo, Denm. Felo ApS, Fensmarkvej 118, 4700 Naestved, Denmark.

Felton, Austral. Felton, Grimwade & Bickford P/L, P.O. Box 74, Oakleigh South, VIC 3167, Australia.

Fenton, UK. Fenton Pharmaceuticals Ltd, 4J Portman Mansions, Chiltern St, London, W1M 1LF, UK.

Ferlito, Ital. Ferlito Farmaceutici, Divisione Palmares s.p.a., Via E Ramarini 31-33, 00015 Monterotondo Scalo (RM), Italy.

Ferlux, Fr. Ferlux SA, 24 av. d'Aubiere, 63804 Cournon d'Auvergne cdx, France.

Fermenta, Swed. See *Ferring, Swed.*

Fermentaciones y Sintesis, Spain. Fermentaciones y Sintesis, Castellon 23, 28001 Madrid, Spain.

Fermenti, Ital. Istituto Italiano Fermenti s.p.a., Via B Quaranta 42, 20139 Milan, Italy.

Ferndale, USA. Ferndale Laboratories Inc., 780 West Eight Mile Rd, Ferndale, MI 48220, USA.

Ferno, UK. Ferno (UK) Ltd, Ferno House, Stubs Beck Lane, Cleckheaton, West Yorkshire, BD19 4TZ, UK.

Ferraton, Denm. Ferraton Farmaceutisk Fabrik A/S, Kirkevejen 20, Teestrup, 4690 Haslev, Denmark.

Ferraz, Lynce, Port. Ferraz, Lynce, SA, Rua Consiglieri Pedroso 123, Queluz de Baixo, 2745-557 Barcarena, Portugal.

Ferrer, Singapore. See *Pharmacon, Singapore.*

Ferrer, Spain. Ferrer Farma, Gran Via Carlos III 94, 08028 Barcelona, Spain.

Ferring, Aust. Ferring Arzneimittel GmbH, Sparkassaplatz 6, A-1150 Vienna, Austria.

Ferring, Belg. Ferring S.A., Hopmarkt 9 bus 3, 9300 Aalst, Belgium.

Ferring, Canad. Ferring Inc., 200 York-land Blvd, Suite 800, Toronto, Ontario, M2J 5C1, Canada.

Ferring, Denm. Ferring Laegemidler A/S, Vesterbrogade 149, 1620 Copenhagen V, Denmark.

Ferring, Fin. Ferringlääkkeet Oy, Länsitu-ulentie 10, 02100 Espoo, Finland.

Ferring, Fr. Laboratoires Ferring SAS, 7 rue Jean-Baptiste-Clement, 94250 Gentilly, France.

Ferring, Ger. Ferring Arzneimittel GmbH, Wittland 11, 24109 Kiel, Germany.

Ferring, Hong Kong. Ferring Pharmaceuticals Ltd, Unit A, 9/F Garment Ctr, 576-586 Castle Peak Rd, Kowloon, Hong Kong.

Ferring, Irl. See *Allphar, Irl.*

Ferring, Israel. See *Lapidot, Israel.*

Ferring, Ital. Ferring s.r.l., Via Corti 11, 20133 Milano, Italy.

Ferring, Neth. Ferring B.V., Postbus 184, 2130 AD Hoofddorp, Netherlands.

Ferring, Norw. Ferring Legemidler AS, Postboks 4445 Torshov, 0403 Oslo, Norway.

Ferring, Port. Ferring Portuguesa, Lda, Rua Professor Henrique de Barros, Edificio Sagres, 8 - Sala A, 2685-338 Prior Velho, Portugal.

Ferring, S.Afr. Ferring (Pty) Ltd, P.O. Box 14358, Clubview 0014, South Africa.

Ferring, Singapore. See *United Italian, Singapore.*

Ferring, Spain. Ferring, Saturno 1, Edificio Saturno, Pozuelo de Alarcon, 28224 Madrid, Spain.

Ferring, Swed. Ferring AB, Box 30063, 200 61 Linhamn, Sweden.

Ferring, Switz. Ferring SA, Industri-estrasse 50a, 8304 Wallisellen, Switzerland.

Ferring, Thai. See *Pacific, Thai.*

Ferring, UK. Ferring Pharmaceuticals UK, The Courtyard, Waterside Drive, Langley, Berkshire, SL3 6EZ, UK.

Ferring, USA. Ferring Pharmaceuticals Inc., 120 White Plains Rd, Suite 400, Tarry-town, NY 10591, USA.

Ferrosan, Denm. Ferrosan A/S, Syd-marken 1-5, 2860 Sborg, Denmark.

Ferrosan, Fin. Oy Ferrosan AB, Kutojan-tie 11, 02630 Espoo, Finland.

Ferrosan, Swed. Ferrosan AB, Gryn-bodgatan 14, 211 33 Malmo, Sweden.

Fertin, Denm. See *Meda, Denm.*

Fertin, Norw. See *Meda, Norw.*

FertiPro, Irl. See *Electramed, Irl.*

Fher, Ital. Fher, Divisione della Boehringer Ingelheim, Casella Postale, 50100 Florence, Italy.

Fher, Spain. Fher, Pablo Alcover 31-7, 08017 Barcelona, Spain.

Fibertone, USA. Fibertone Co., 14851 N Scottsdale Rd, Scottsdale, AZ 85254, USA.

Fides, Ger. See *FidesLine, Ger.*

Fides, Spain. See *Rottapharm, Spain.*

Fides Rottapharm, Spain. See *Rottapharm, Spain.*

FidesLine, Ger. FidesLine Biologische Heilmittel Heel GmbH, Dr Reckeweg-Str. 2-4, 76532 Baden-Baden, Germany.

Fidia, Hong Kong. See *Hong Kong Medical, Hong Kong.*

Fidia, Ital. Fidia, Farmaceutici Italiani Derivati Industriali e Affini s.p.a., Via Ponte d/Fabbrica 3/A, 35031 Abano Terme (Padua), Italy.

Fidia, Thai. Fidia c/o Trans Bassan (Thailand) Ltd, 14 Fl, Q House Building, 66 Su-khumvit 21, Klongtoey, Bangkok 10110, Thailand.

Fielding, USA. The Fielding Pharmaceutical Co. Inc., P.O. Box 2186, 112 Weldon Parkway, Maryland Heights, MO 63043, USA.

Filorga, Fr. Laboratoires Filorga, 18 rue de Miromesnil, 75008 Paris, France.

Fimo, Ital. Fabbrica Italiana Materiale Odontotecnico e Odontoiatrico, Via Edolo 40, 20125 Milan, Italy.

Finderm, Ital. Finderm Farmaceutici s.a.s. di Scaccia Fabbio e C., V.le Alcide De Gasperi 165, 95100 Catania, Italy.

Fink, Ger. See *SmithKline Beecham OTC, Ger.*

Finmedical, Ital. Finmedical srl, Vicolo De Bacchettoni 1a, 51100 Pistoia, Italy.

Fiori, Ital. Dr F & C Fiori snc, Corso San Maurizio 35, 10124 Turin, Italy.

FIRMA, Ital. Fabbr. Ital. Ritrov. Medic. Aff. s.p.a., Via di Scandicci 37, 50143 Florence, Italy.

Fischer, Israel. Fischer Pharmaceuticals Ltd, P.O. Box 39071, Tel Aviv 61390, Israel.

Fischer, USA. Fischer Pharmaceuticals Inc., 3707 Williams Rd, San Jose, CA 95117, USA.

Fiske, USA. Fiske Industries, 527 Route 303, Orangeburg, NY 10962, USA.

Fisons, Austral. Fisons Pharmaceuticals, P.O. Box 191, Castle Hill, NSW 2154, Australia.

Fisons, Braz. Fisons Industrial Ltda, Rua Viuva Claudio 160, 20793-000 Rio de Janeiro, RJ, Brazil.

Fisons, Denm. See *Aventis Pharma, Denm.*

Fisons, Hong Kong. See *Primal, Hong Kong.*

Fisons, Irl. See *Aventis Pharma, Irl.*

Fisons, Israel. Fisons, Israel.

Fisons, Norw. See *Aventis, Norw.*

Fisons, Singapore. See *Zuellig, Singapore.*

Fisons, UK. Fisons PLC, Pharmaceutical Division, UK.

Fisons, USA. See *Celltech Medeva, USA.*

Fisons Consumer, USA. See *Ciba Consumer, USA.*

Fitobucaneve, Ital. Fitobucaneve srl, Via Galvani 25/27, 20018 Sedriano (MI), Italy.

Fitodorfarma, Ital. Fitodorfarma s.a.s., Sezione Erboristeria, Via Genova 28, 21052 Busto Arsizio (VA), Italy.

Fitolife, Ital. Laboratorio Fitolife srl, Via Domiziana km 55, 80072 Arco Felice (NA), Italy.

FL, Israel. FL, Israel.

Flanders, USA. Flanders Inc., P.O. Box 39143, Northbridge Station, Charleston, SC 29407-9143, USA.

FLAWA, Switz. FLAWA Schweizer Verbandstoff- und Wattefabriken AG, Bad-strasse 43, 9230 Flawil, Switzerland.

Fleet, Austral. C.B. Fleet Co. (Australia) P/L, P.O. Box 716, Braeside, VIC 3195, Australia.

Fleet, Neth. See *Tramedico, Neth.*

Fleet, NZ. See *Baxter, NZ.*

Fleet, Singapore. See *De Witt, Singapore.*

Fleet, USA. C.B. Fleet Co. Inc., 4615 Murray Pl., Lynchburg, VA 24506-1349, USA.

Fleet-Dewitt, Hong Kong. See *Inchcape, Hong Kong.*

Fleming, USA. Fleming & Co., 1600 Fenpark Dr., Fenton, MO 63026, USA.

Flopen, Braz. Flopen, Brazil.

Flora, Canad. Flora Mfg & Dist. Ltd, 7400 Fraser Park Drive, Burnaby, BC, V5J 5B9, Canada.

Florabio, Ger. Florabio GmbH, Muhlstr. 5-7, 71106 Magstadt, Germany.

Florafaun, Austral. Florafaun P/L, P.O. Box 612, Balcatta, WA 6914, Australia.

Flordis, Austral. Flordis Pty Ltd, P.O. Box 37, Epping, NSW 2121, Australia.

Floris, Israel. Floris, Misgav 20179, Israel.

Florizel, UK. Florizel Ltd, P.O. Box 138, Stevenage, Hertfordshire, SG2 8YN, UK.

Fluoritab, USA. Fluoritab Corp., 8151 Brentwood Lane, Temperance, MI 48182-0507, USA.

Flynn, Irl. Flynn Pharma Ltd, Alton House, 4 Herbert St, Dublin 2, Ireland.

Flynn, UK. Flynn Pharma Ltd, 7 Serlby Court, Addison Rd, London, W14 8EE, UK.

Fonten, Ital. Fonten Farmaceutici s.r.l., Via Cavour 9/11, 26013 Crema (CR), Italy.

Food Supplement, UK. Food Supplement Co. Ltd, Europa Park, Stoneclough Rd, Radcliffe, Manchester, M26 1GG, UK.

Ford Medical, UK. Ford Medical Associates Ltd, 2 Bridport Way, Braintree, Essex, CN7 9FJ, UK.

Forest, Israel. Forest, Israel.

Forest Laboratories, UK. Forest Laboratories Europe, Bourne Rd, Bexley, Kent, DA5 1NX, UK.

Forest Laboratories, USA. Forest Laboratories Inc., 13622 Shoreline Drive, St Louis, MO 63045, USA.

Forest Pharmaceuticals, USA. See *Forest Laboratories, USA.*

Forley, UK. Forley Ltd, 54 Hillbury Ave, Harrow, Middlesex, HA3 8EW, UK.

Formenti, Ital. Farmaceutici Formenti spa, Via Correggio 43, 20149 Milan, Italy.

Formula, NZ. Formula Products, P.O. Box 36-443, Northcote, Auckland, New Zealand.

Fornet, Fr. Laboratoires Fornet, 7/13 bd Paul-Emile-Victor, 92200 Neuilly-sur-Seine, France.

Forte, USA. Forte Pharma, 220 Lake Dr., Newark, DE 19702, USA.

Fortune, Hong Kong. Fortune Pharmacal Co. Ltd, 14A/F Zung Fu Industrial Bldg, 1067 King's Rd, Hong Kong.

Forum, UK. Forum, UK.

Fougera, USA. E. Fougera Co., 60 Baylis Rd, Melville, NY 11747, USA.

Four Macs, Austral. Four Macs P/L, 78 Burns Rd, Wahroonga, NSW 2076, Australia.

Fournier, Belg. Fournier Pharma S.A., Rue des Trois Arbres 16 B, 1180 Brussels, Belgium.

Fournier, Canad. Fournier Pharma Inc., 1010 Sherbrooke St W, P.O. Box 16, 19th Floor, Montreal, Quebec, H3A 2R7, Canada.

Fournier, Fr. Laboratoires Fournier SA, 9 rue Petitot, 21000 Dijon, France.

Fournier, Ger. Fournier Pharma GmbH, Justus-von-Liebig Str. 16, 66280 Sulzbach, Germany.

Fournier, Irl. Fournier, Ireland.

Fournier, Ital. Fournier Pierrel Farma s.p.a., Palazzo Caravaggio, Via Cassanese 224, 20090 Segrate (MI), Italy.

Fournier, Port. Fournier Farmacêutica Portugal, Lda, Av Eng. Duarte Pacheco, Amoreiras, Torre 2 - 14B, 1070-103 Lisbon, Portugal.

Fournier, Singapore. See *Sime Darby, Singapore.*

Fournier, Spain. Fournier Iberica, Spain.

Fournier, Switz. See *Searle, Switz.*

Fournier, Thai. See *Pacific, Thai.*

Fournier, UK. Fournier Pharmaceuticals Ltd, 22-23 Progress Business Centre, Whittle Parkway, Slough, Berkshire, SL1 6DQ, UK.

Fournier SA, Spain. Fournier SA, Ce Euronova 3, Rda Poniente 16, Tres Cantos, 28760 Madrid, Spain.

Fox, UK. C. H. Fox Ltd, 22 Tavistock St, London, WC2E 7PY, UK.

FP, Singapore. F.P. Marketing (S'Pore) Pte Ltd, 5 Pereira Rd, 04-03 Asiawide Industrial Building, S 368025, Singapore.

Francia, Ital. Francia Farmaceutici Industria Farmaco Biologica s.r.l., Via dei Pestagalli 7, 20138 Milan, Italy.

Franco, Port. See *Gestafarma, Port.*

Franconpharm, Ger. franconpharm Arzneimittel GmbH, Alexandrinenstr. 1, 96450 Coburg, Germany.

Frandiet, Fr. Frandiet SA, ZA des Savines, 101 rue Marc-Seguin, B.P. 315, 07503 Guilherand-Granges cdx, France.

Frankin, Hong Kong. Frankin Pharmaceutical Lab., 1/F, Block 1, Camelpaint Bldg, 60-62 Hoi Yuen Rd, Kwun Tong, Kowloon, Hong Kong.

Franklin Medical, UK. Franklin Medical Ltd, P.O. Box 138, Turnpike Rd, High Wycombe, Buckinghamshire, HP12 3NB, UK.

Freda, Port. Freda, SA, Quinta da Francelha de Cima, 2685 Prior Velho, Portugal.

Freeda, USA. Freeda Vitamins Inc., 36 E 41st St, New York, NY 10017-6203, USA.

Frega, Canad. See *Pharmalab, Canad.*

Frere, Belg. See *Arkopharma, Belg.*

Fresenius, Aust. Fresenius Medical Care Dialysetechnik Co. KG, Lundenburgergasse 5, A-1210 Vienna, Austria.

Fresenius, Belg. Fresenius S.A., Molenberglei 7, 2627 Schelle, Belgium.

Fresenius, Braz. Fresenius Laboratorios Ltda, Rua Francisco P. Coutinho 347, 13088-100 Campinas, SP, Brazil.

Fresenius, Denm. Fresenius Medical care Danmark A/S, Arnold Nielsens Blvd 77-9, 2650 Hvidovre, Denmark.

Fresenius, Fr. See *Fresenius Kabi, Fr.*

Fresenius, Ger. See *Fresenius Kabi, Ger.*

Fresenius, Hong Kong. See *Round World, Hong Kong.*

Fresenius, Israel. Fresenius, Israel.

Fresenius, Port. Fresenius Medical Care, Lda, Rua Dr Eduardo Santos Silva 261, Fraccao AU, 4200 Porto, Portugal.

Fresenius, Spain. Fresenius Medical Care, Ctra Vallderiolf Km 0.4, La Roca Del Valles, 08430 Barcelona, Spain.

Fresenius, Thai. See *Diethelm, Thai.*

Fresenius, UK. Fresenius Kabi Ltd, Building C, Hampson Court, Manor Park, Runcorn, Cheshire, WA7 1UF, UK.

Fresenius Kabi, Aust. Fresenius Kabi Austria GmbH, Hafnerstrasse 36, A-8055 Graz, Austria.

Fresenius Kabi, Denm. Fresenius Kabi, Bredgade 71, 1260 Copenhagen K, Denmark.

Fresenius Kabi, Fin. Fresenius Kabi AB, Rajatorpantie 41 C, 01640 Vantaa, Finland.

Fresenius Kabi, Fr. Fresenius Kabi France, 5 place du Marivel, 92316 Sevres cdx, France.

Fresenius Kabi, Ger. Fresenius Kabi Deutschland GmbH, Else-Kroner-Str. 1, 61352 Bad Homburg v. d. H., Germany.

Fresenius Kabi, Ital. Fresenius Kabi Italia s.p.a., Via Camagre 41, 37063 Isola della Scala (VR), Italy.

Fresenius Kabi, Norw. Fresenius Kabi Norge AS, Markedsavd., Gjerdrumsv. 12, 0486 Oslo, Norway.

Fresenius Kabi, Port. Fresenius Kabi Pharma Portugal, Lda, Avenida do Forte 3, Edificio Suecia I, 2795-504 Carnaxide, Portugal.

Fresenius Kabi, S.Afr. Fresenius Kabi, P.O. Box 4156, Halfway House, South Africa.

Fresenius Kabi, Singapore. See *Diethelm, Singapore.*

Fresenius Kabi, Spain. Fresenius Kabi España, Marina 16-18, Pl 17, Torre Mapfre-Villa Olimpica, 08005 Barcelona, Spain.

Fresenius Kabi, Swed. Fresenius Kabi, 751 74 Uppsala, Sweden.

Fresenius Kabi, Switz. See *Fresenius Medical, Switz.*

Fresenius Medical, Austral. Fresenius Medical Care South East Asia P/L, 305 Woodpark Rd, Smithfield, NSW 2164, Australia.

Fresenius Medical, Fin. Fresenius Medical Care Suomi Oy, Vattuniemenranta 2, 00210 Helsinki, Finland.

Fresenius Medical, Ger. Fresenius Medical Care Deutschland GmbH, Else-Kroner-Str. 1, 61352 Bad Homburg v.d.H., Germany.

Fresenius Medical, Switz. Fresenius Medical Care (Schweiz) AG, Case postale, 6370 Stans, Switzerland.

Fresenius-Klinik, Ger. See *Fresenius Kabi, Ger.*

Fresenius-Praxis, Ger. See *Fresenius Kabi, Ger.*

Friesland, Hong Kong. See *Keller, Hong Kong.*

Friesland, Singapore. See *Diethelm, Singapore.*

Frosst, Austral. See *Merck Sharp & Dohme, Austral.*

Frosst, Canad. See *Merck Frosst, Canad.*

Frosst, Port. See *Merck Sharp & Dohme, Port.*

Frosst, Spain. See *Merck Sharp & Dohme, Spain.*

Fruit of the Earth, Canad. Fruit of the Earth, 110 Iron St, Etobicoke, Ontario, M9W 5L9, Canada.

Fuca, Fr. Laboratoires Fuca, 1 bis, rue de Plaisance, 94732 Nogent-sur-Marne cdx, France.

Fuisz, Ger. Fuisz Pharma GmbH & Co. KG, Schillerstr. 8, 88471 Laupheim, Germany.

Fuji, Jpn. Fuji Chemical Industry Co Ltd, 55 Yokohoonji, Kamiichi-machi, Toyama-Pref. 930-0397, Japan.

Fuji, Swed. Fuji Film Sverige AB, Box 23086, 104 35 Stockholm, Sweden.

Fujirebio, Jpn. Fujirebio Inc., FR Bldg, 62-5 Nihonbashi-Hamacho 2-chome, Chuo-ku, Tokyo 103-0007, Japan.

Fujisawa, Aust. Fujisawa GmbH, Hietzinger Hauptstrasse 64, A-1132 Vienna, Austria.

Fujisawa, Belg. Fujisawa Belgian Branch, Sint-Maartenstraat 12 A, 3000 Leuven, Belgium.

Fujisawa, Canad. Fujisawa Canada Inc., 625 Cochrane Drive, Suite 800, Markham, Ontario, L3R 9R9, Canada.

Fujisawa, Denm. Fujisawa GmbH Scandinavia, Teglvaerksvej 30, 4200 Slagelse, Denmark.

Fujisawa, Fin. See *Fujisawa, Swed.*

Fujisawa, Fr. Fujisawa, Le Clemenceau II, 215 av Georges-Clemenceau, 92024 Nanterre cdx, France.

Fujisawa, Ger. Fujisawa GmbH, Levelingstr. 12, 81673 Munich, Germany.

Fujisawa, Hong Kong. See *Main Life, Hong Kong,* and *Zuellig, Hong Kong.*

Fujisawa, Irl. See *Fujisawa, UK.*

Fujisawa, Israel. Fujisawa, Israel.

Fujisawa, Ital. Fujisawa r.l., C.so Sempione 4, 20154 Milan, Italy.

Fujisawa, Jpn. Fujisawa Pharmaceutical Co. Ltd, 4-7 Doshomachi 3-chome, Chuo-ku, Osaka 541, Japan.

Fujisawa, Norw. See *Fujisawa, Swed.*

Fujisawa, Spain. Fujisawa, Po Castellana, 141 Edif Cuzco, Plta 18, 28046 Madrid, Spain.

Fujisawa, Swed. Fujisawa Scandinavia, Skeppsbron 5-6, 411 21 Goteborg, Sweden.

Fujisawa, Switz. See *Galenica, Switz.*

Fujisawa, Thai. See *Berli, Thai.*

Fujisawa, UK. Fujisawa Ltd, CP House, 1st Floor, 97-107 Uxbridge Rd, Ealing, London, W5 5TL, UK.

Fujisawa, USA. Fujisawa Healthcare Inc., 3 Parkway North Center, Deerfield, IL 60015-2548, USA.

Fulton, Ital. Fulton Medicinali s.r.l., Via Marconi 28/9, 20020 Arese, Italy.

Fulton, USA. Fulton, USA.

Fumedica, Ger. Fumedica GmbH, Industriestr. 40, 44628 Herne, Germany.

Fumouze, Fr. Laboratoires Fumouze, Le Malesherbes, 110-114 rue Victor-Hugo, 92303 Levallois-Perret cdx, France.

Fumouze, Israel. Fumouze, Israel.

Fund a Paiva, Braz. Fund a Paiva, Brazil.

Fund Trip, Hong Kong. Fund Trip Pharmaceutical Ltd, B1220 Focal Industrial Ctr, 21 Man Lok St, Hunghom, Kowloon, Hong Kong.

Funk, Spain. See *Almirall, Spain.*

Fustery, Mex. Laboratorios Fustery S.A. de C.V., Calz de Tlalpan No. 3007, Col. Sta. Ursula Coapa (Pueblo), 04650 Mexico, D.F., Mexico.

G & W, USA. G & W Laboratories Inc., 111 Coolidge St, South Plainfield, NJ 07080, USA.

GABA, Belg. GABA BV, Belgium.

GABA, Fr. Lab. GABA, 86 rue du Dome, 92514 Boulogne cdx, France.

GABA, Ger. GABA GmbH, Berner Weg 7, 79539 Lorrach, Germany.

GABA, Israel. GABA, Israel.

GABA, Neth. GABA B.V., Netherlands.

GABA, Switz. GABA AG, Pharmazeutische und kosmetische Praparate, Grabetsmattweg, 4106 Therwil, Switzerland.

Galactina, Switz. Galactina AG, Birkenweg 1-8, 3123 Belp, Switzerland.

Galactopharm, Ger. Galactopharm Hans Sanders, Sudstr. 10, 49751 Sogel, Germany.

Galagen, USA. GalaGen Inc., P.O. Box 64313, St Paul, MN 55164-0314, USA.

Galderma, Austral. Galderma Australia P/L, P.O. Box 502, Frenchs Forest, NSW 2086, Australia.

Galderma, Belg. Galderma Belgilux S.A., Fountain Business Centre Bornem, Gebouw 2-bus 205, Van Kerckhovenstraat, 2880 Bornem, Belgium.

Galderma, Braz. Galderma Brasil Ltda, Avenida Guido Caloi 1.935 - BL. C, 05802-140 Sao Paulo, SP, Brazil.

Galderma, Canad. Galderma Canada Inc., 7300 Warden Ave, Suite 210, Markham, Ontario, L3R 9Z6, Canada.

Galderma, Denm. Galderma Svenska, c/o Regus House, Lars Bjornsstraede 3, 1454 Copenhagen K, Denmark.

Galderma, Fin. PL 11, 01641 Vantaa, Finland.

Galderma, Fr. Laboratoires Galderma, Tour Europlaza, 20 av. Andre-Prothin, La Defense 4, 92927 La Defense cdx, France.

Galderma, Ger. Galderma Laboratorium GmbH, Munzinger Str. 5, 79111 Freiburg i. Br., Germany.

Galderma, Hong Kong. See *Tsun Tsun, Hong Kong.*

Galderma, Irl. See *Allphar, Irl.,* and *Intra Pharma, Irl.*

Galderma, Israel. Galderma, Israel.

Galderma, Ital. Galderma Italia s.p.a., Palazzo Sirio, Ingresso 3, 20041 Agrate Brianza (MI), Italy.

Galderma, Mex. Galderma Mexico S.A. de C.V., Av. Alvaro Obregon No. 121, Piso 15, Col. Roma, 06700 Mexico D.F., Mexico.

Galderma, Neth. Galderma S.A., Avelingen-West 5, 4202 MS Gorinchem, Netherlands.

Galderma, Norw. See *Galderma, Swed.*

Galderma, NZ. See *Pacific, NZ.*

Galderma, Port. Laboratorios Galderma, SA, Av Duque d'Avila 185, 1050-082 Lisbon, Portugal.

Galderma, S.Afr. Galderma Laboratories SA (Pty) Ltd, P.O. Box 1735, Randburg 2125, South Africa.

Galderma, Singapore. See *Summit, Singapore.*

Galderma, Spain. Galderma, Agustin Foxa 29, 28036 Madrid, Spain.

Galderma, Swed. Galderma Svenska AB, Box 15028, 167 15 Bromma, Sweden.

Galderma, Switz. Galderma SA, Zugerstrasse 47, Postfach 492, 6330 Cham, Switzerland.

Galderma, Thai. See *US Summit, Thai.*

Galderma, UK. Galderma (UK) Ltd, Galderma House, Church Lane, Kings Langley, Hertfordshire, WD4 8JP, UK.

Galderma, USA. Galderma Laboratories Inc., P.O. Box 331329, Fort Worth, TX 76163, USA.

Galen, Ger. Galenpharma, GmbH, Wittland 13, 24109 Kiel, Germany.

Galen, Irl. See *Allphar, Irl.*

Galen, Mex. Laboratorios Galen, S.A. de C.V., Municipio Libre No. 73, 03300 Mecixo D.F., Mexico.

Galen, UK. Galen Ltd, Seagoe Industrial Estate, Craigavon, Northern Ireland, BT63 5UA, UK.

Galena, Thai. Galena.

Galenica, Switz. Galenica Vertretungen AG, Untermattweg 8, 3001 Berne, Switzerland.

Galenika, Ger. Galenika Dr. Hetterich GmbH, Gebhardtstr. 5, 90762 Furth/Bayern, Germany.

Galephar, Fr. Laboratoires Galephar, ZI de Krafft, bat B, 67150 Erstein, France.

Galephar, Neth. See *Zambon, Neth.*

Gallia, Fr. Laboratoires Gallia, B.P. 432, 69654 Villefranche-sur-Saone cdx, France.

Galpharm, UK. GalPharm International Ltd, Hugh House, Galpharm Way, Upper Cliffe Rd, Dodworth Business Park, Dodworth, Barnsley, South Yorkshire, S75 3SP, UK.

Gambar, Ital. Laboratori Gambar s.r.l., Via Bolognola 45, 00138 Rome, Italy.

Gambro, Denm. Gambro Medicoteknik A/S, Jydekrogen 8, 2625 Vallensbaek, Denmark.

Gambro, Fin. Oy Gambro Ab, Sahaajankatu 24, PL 30, 00811 Helsinki, Finland.

Gambro, Israel. Gambro, Israel.

Gambro, Spain. Gambro, Principe de Vergara 43, 28001 Madrid, Spain.

Gambro, Swed. Gambro, Box 10101, 220 10 Lund, Sweden.

Gambro, USA. Gambro Inc., 1185 Oak St, Lakewood, CO 80215, USA.

Ganassini, Ital. Istituto Ganassini s.p.a. di Ricerche Biochimiche, Via Gaggia 16, 20139 Milan, Italy.

Gandhour, Fr. Laboratoires Gandhour, 1 bis, rue de Plaisance, 94732 Nogent-sur-Marne cdx, France.

Garant, Ital. Laboratorio Chimico Garant s.r.l., Via Melzi d'Eril 29, 20154 Milan, Italy.

Garec, S.Afr. Garec Pharmaceuticals, P.O. Box 1123, Halfway House 1685, South Africa.

Garnier, UK. Laboratoires Garnier, Golden Ltd, P.O. Box 5, Pontyclun, Glamorgan, CF7 8XW, UK.

Gaschler, Ger. Pharma-Laboratorium S.M. Gaschler GmbH, Oeschlanderweg 17a, 88131 Lindau, Germany.

Gastroenterologicos, Mex. Gastroenterologicos,, Mexico.

Gastropharm, Ger. Gastropharm GmbH Arzneimittel, Geiststr. 1, 37073 Gottingen, Germany.

Gate, USA. See *Teva, USA.*

Gazzoni, Ital. Gazzoni s.r.l., Via Ilio Barontini 16/20, 40138 Bologna, Italy.

G-B-M, UK. GBM Health Care Ltd, Beechlawn House, Hurtmore Rd, Godalming, Surrey, GU7 2RA, UK.

GC, Singapore. G C Pharmaceutical (S) Pte Ltd, 1 Maritime Square, 10-33A World Trade Centre, S 099253, Singapore.

GD, Ital. GD Tecnologie Interdisciplinari Farmaceutiche s.r.l., Via Augusto Gaudenzi 29, 00163 Rome, Italy.

Gea, Denm. A/S GEA, Holger Danskes Vej 89, 2000 Frederiksberg, Denmark.

Gea, Fin. Oy Gea Ab, Rajatorpantie 41, 01640 Vantaa, Finland.

Gea, Norw. GEA Farmaceutisk Fabrik AS, Stortorvet 10, 0155 Oslo, Norway.

Gea, Swed. GEA Farmaceutisk Fabrik AB, Berga Alle 1 E, 254 52 Helsingborg, Sweden.

Gea, Switz. See *Globopharm, Switz.*

Gebauer, Canad. See *Gebauer, USA.*

Gebauer, Hong Kong. See *Vantone, Hong Kong.*

Gebauer, USA. Gebauer Co., 9410 St Catherine Ave, Cleveland, OH 44104, USA.

Gebro, Aust. Gebro Pharma GmbH, A-6391 Fieberbrunn, Austria.

Gebro, Switz. Gebro Pharma SA, Oristalstrasse 87a, 4410 Liestal, Switzerland.

Gedeon Richter, Hong Kong. See *Mekim, Hong Kong.*

Gedeon Richter, Hung. Chemical Works of Gedeon Richter Ltd, P.O. Box 27, 1475 Budapest, Hungary.

Gedeon Richter, Singapore. See *Gedeon Richter, Hung.,* and *Sime Darby, Singapore.*

Gedeon Richter, Thai. See *Gedeon Richter, Hung.,* and *Medline, Thai.*

Gedis, Ital. Gedis s.r.l., Via Vezzolano 15, 10153 Turin, Italy.

Geigy, Canad. See *Ciba, Canad.*

Geigy, Ger. See *Novartis, Ger.*

Geigy, Switz. See *Novartis, Switz.,* and *Novartis Consumer, Switz.*

Geigy, USA. See *Novartis, USA.*

Geistlich, Irl. Geistlich Pharma, 36 Lower Stephen Street, Dublin 2, Ireland.

Geistlich, Singapore. See *Diethelm, Singapore.*

Geistlich, Switz. Geistlich-Pharma AG, 6110 Wolhusen, Switzerland.

Geistlich, UK. Geistlich Pharma, Newton Bank, Long Lane, Chester, Cheshire, CH2 3PF, UK.

Gelos, Spain. Gelos, Joan XXIII 10, Esplugues de Llobregat, 08950 Barcelona, Spain.

Gemballa, Braz. Laboratorio Gemballa Ltda, Avenida Sete de Setembro 50, 89160-000 Rio do Sul, SC, Brazil.

Gemelli, Denm. Gemelli A/S, Nybrovej 100, 2800 Lyngby, Denmark.

Geminis, Spain. Geminis, Gran Via de las Corts, Catalanes 764, 08013 Barcelona, Spain.

Gencon, USA. Gencon, 6116 N Central Expy 200, Dallas, TX 75206, USA.

GenDerm, Canad. See *Medicis, Canad.*

GenDerm, USA. See *Medicis, USA.*

Genentech, USA. Genentech Inc., 1 DNA Way, South San Francisco, CA 94080-4990, USA.

Genera, Switz. Genera Pharma AG, Hilariweg 9, Postfach, 4501 Solothurn, Switzerland.

General Dietary, UK. General Dietary Ltd, P.O. Box 38, Kingston-upon-Thames, Surrey, KT2 7YP, UK.

General Drugs, Thai. General Drugs House Co. Ltd, 2-4 Soi Lard Prao 82, Bangkok 10310, Thailand.

General Nutrition, Canad. See *General Nutrition, USA.*

General Nutrition, USA. General Nutrition Products, 1050 Woodruff Rd, Greenville, SC 29607, USA.

General Topics, Ital. General Topics, Via Lungo Lago Zanardelli 32, 25087 Salo (BS), Italy.

Genericon, Aust. Genericon Pharma GmbH, Schlossplatz 1, A-8502 Lannach, Austria.

Generics, Denm. See *NM, Denm.*

Generics, Israel. Generics, Israel.

Generics, UK. Generics (UK) Ltd, Albany Gate, Drakes Lane, Potters Bar, Hertfordshire, EN6 1AG, UK.

Genetics Institute, Aust. See *Genetics Institute, Fr.,* and *Genetics Institute, Ger.*

Genetics Institute, Denm. See *Baxter, Denm., Pharmacia Upjohn, Denm.,* and *Wyeth Lederle, Denm.*

Genetics Institute, Fr. Genetics Institute of Europe BV, 12 rue de la Michodiere, 75002 Paris, France.

Genetics Institute, Ger. See *Wyeth, Ger.*

Genetics Institute, USA. Genetics Institute, 35 Cambridge Park Drive, Cambridge, MA 02140, USA.

Geneva, USA. Geneva Pharmaceuticals, 2655 W Midway Blvd, P.O. Box 446, Broomfield, CO 80038-0446, USA.

Genevar, Fr. Genevar, 95 av de la Chataigneraie, 92503 Rueil-Malmaison, France.

Genevrier, Fr. Laboratoires Génévrier, B.P. 47, 06901 Sophia Antipolis cdx, France.

Gen-King, USA. See *Kinray, USA.*

Genop, S.Afr. Genop Healthcare (Pty) Ltd, P.O. Box 3911, Halfway House 1685, South Africa.

Genopharm, Fr. Lab. Genopharm, Parc de l'Esplanade, 10 rue Enrico-Fermi, Saint-Thibault-des-Vignes, 77462 Lagny-sur-Marne cdx, France.

Genove, Spain. Genove, Spain.

Genpharm, Austral. GenPharm Australia, 182 Alison Rd, Carrara, QLD 4211, Australia.

Genpharm, Canad. Genpharm Inc., 37 Advance Rd, Etobicoke, Ontario, M8Z 2S6, Canada.

Genpharm, Israel. Genpharm, Israel.

Genpharm, S.Afr. Genpharm Pharmaceuticals CC, P.O. Box 607, Rivonia 2128, South Africa.

Gensia, Swed. See *Gensia, UK.*

Gensia, UK. Gensia Automedics Ltd, Unit 31, Wellington Business Park, Dukes Ride, Crowthorne, Berkshire, RG45 6LS, UK.

Gensia, USA. See *Sicor, USA.*

Gentili, Ital. Istituto Gentili s.p.a., Via Mazzini 112, 56125 Pisa, Italy.

Genus, UK. Genus Pharmaceuticals, Benham Valence, Newbury, Berkshire, RG20 8LU, UK.

Genzyme, Aust. See *Genzyme, Neth.*

Genzyme, Austral. Genzyme Australasia P/L, P.O. Box 1406, Castle Hill, NSW 1765, Australia.

Genzyme, Denm. See *Genzyme, Neth.*

Genzyme, Fr. See *Genzyme.*

Genzyme, Ger. Genzyme GmbH, Rontgenstr. 4, 63755 Alzenau, Germany.

Genzyme, Hong Kong. See *Naturest, Hong Kong, Swire Loxley, Hong Kong,* and *Zuellig, Hong Kong.*

Genzyme, Israel. Genzyme Israel Ltd, P.O. Box 1188, Kfar Saba, Israel.

Genzyme, Ital. Genzyme Therapeutics srl, Via Scaglia Est 144, 41100 Modena, Italy.

Genzyme, Jpn. Genzyme Japan, Japan.

Genzyme, Neth. Genzyme BV, Gooimeer 10, 1411 DD Naarden, Netherlands.

Genzyme, Spain. Genzyme SL, Avda de la Industria 32, Alcobendas, 28108 Madrid, Spain.

Genzyme, Switz. Genzyme Pharmaceuticals, Sygena Facility, Eichenweg 1, Postfach, 4410 Liestal, Switzerland.

Genzyme, UK. Genzyme Therapeutics Ltd, 37 Hollands Rd, Haverhill, Suffolk, CB9 8PU, UK.

Genzyme, USA. Genzyme Corp., One Kendall Square, Building 1400, Cambridge, MA 02139, USA.

Gepepharm, Ger. gepepharm GmbH, Lendersbergstr. 86, 53721 Siegburg, Germany.

Gerard, Denm. See *NM, Denm.*

Gerard, Irl. Gerard Laboratories, 2004A Orchard Ave, City West Business Campus, Naas Rd, Dublin 24, Ireland.

Gerard, Israel. Gerard, Israel.

Gerard, Norw. See *Norgesfarma, Norw.*

Gerard House, UK. Gerard House Ltd, UK.

Gerbex, Canad. Gerbex Inc. Produits, 331 Principale St, St-Thomas d'Aquin, Quebec, J0H 2A0, Canada.

Gerda, Fr. Laboratoires Gerda, 6 rue Childebert, 69002 Lyon, France.

Geriatric Pharm. Corp., USA. See *Roberts, USA.*

Gerlach, Ger. Eduard Gerlach GmbH, Backerstr. 4-8, 32312 Lubbecke, Germany.

Germania, Aust. Germania Pharmazeutika GmbH, Schuselkagasse 8, A-1150 Vienna, Austria.

Germiphene, Canad. Germiphene Corporation, 1379 Colborne St E, P.O. Box 1748, Brantford, Ontario, N3T 5V7, Canada.

Germiphene, Israel. Germiphene, Israel.

Gerolymatos, Hong Kong. See *Primal, Hong Kong.*

Gerolymatos, Thai. See *United American, Thai.*

Gerot, Aust. Gerot Pharmazeutika GmbH, Arnethgasse 3, A-1160 Vienna, Austria.

Gerot, Singapore. See *Green Cross, Singapore.*

Gerot, Switz. See *Orion, Switz.*

Gersthofer, Aust. Gersthofer-Apotheke, Gersthofer Strasse 61, A-1180 Vienna, Austria.

Gestafarma, Port. Sociedade Farmacêutica Gestafarma, Lda, Rua Dr. Alvaro de Castro 63-7, 1600-058 Lisbon, Portugal.

Geva, Mex. Laboratorios Geva, S.A. de C.V., 9 Norte No. 401-103, Col. Centro, 72000 Puebla Pue, Mexico.

Gewo, Ger. Gewo Chemie GmbH, Schneidweg 5, 76534 Baden-Baden, Germany.

Geymonat, Ital. Geymonat s.p.a., Via S. Anna 2, 03012 Anagni (FR), Italy.

Geymonat, Switz. See *Lucchini, Switz.*

Ghimas, Ital. Ghimas s.p.a., Via R. Fucini 2, 40033 Casalecchio di Reno (BO), Italy.

GHP, Thai. General Hospital Products Public Co. Ltd, 75/1 Rama VI Rd, Bangkok 10400, Thailand.

GiEnne, Ital. GiEnne Pharma spa, Groupe Therabel, Via Lorenteggio 270/A, 20152 Milan, Italy.

Gifrer Barbezat, Fr. Laboratoires Gifrer Barbezat, B.P. 165, 69151 Decines cdx, France.

Gilbert, Fr. Laboratoires Gilbert, av. du General-de-Gaulle, B.P.115, 14204 Herouville-Saint-Clair cdx, France.

Gilead, Aust. See *Gilead, USA.*

Gilead, Ger. Gilead Sciences GmbH, Fraunhoferstr. 22, 82152 Martinsried/Planegg, Germany.

Gilead, USA. Gilead Sciences Inc., 333 Lakeside Drive, Foster City, CA 94404, USA.

Gilton, Braz. Gilton do Brasil Industria Quimica e Farmaceutica Ltda, Rua Claudio Furquim 21/25, Tatuape, 03072-010 Sao Paulo, SP, Brazil.

Gingi-Pak, Switz. See *Beldenta, Switz.*

Giovanardi, Ital. Giovanardi Farmaceutici s.n.c. del Dr Benito Giovanardi e Figli, Via Sapeto 28, 16131 Genoa, Italy.

Gisand, Switz. Gisand AG, Schlaflistrasse 14, 3013 Berne, Switzerland.

Giuliani, Ital. Giuliani s.p.a., Via Palagi 2, 20129 Milan, Italy.

Giuliani, Switz. Giuliani SA, via Riviera 21, 6976 Castagnola-Lugano, Switzerland.

Giulini, Israel. Giulini, Israel.

Glades, USA. Glades Pharmaceuticals, 500 Satellite Bvld, Suwanee, GA 30024, USA.

Glaxo, Aust. See *GlaxoSmithKline, Aust.*

Glaxo, Jpn. Glaxo, Japan.

Glaxo, USA. See *GlaxoSmithKline, USA.*

Glaxo Allen, Ital. See *Glaxo Wellcome, Ital.*

Glaxo Wellcome, Austral. Glaxo-Wellcome, P.O. Box 168, Boronia, VIC 3155, Australia.

Glaxo Wellcome, Belg. Glaxo Wellcome Belgium S.A., Blvd du Souverain 191, 1160 Brussels, Belgium.

Glaxo Wellcome, Braz. Glaxo Wellcome S.A., Rua Viuva Claudio 300, 20970-030 Rio de Janeiro, RJ, Brazil.

Glaxo Wellcome, Canad. Glaxo Wellcome Inc., 7333 Mississauga Rd North, Mississauga, Ontario, L5N 6L4, Canada.

Glaxo Wellcome, Denm. Glaxo Wellcome a/s, Nykaer 68, 2605 Brondby, Denmark.

Glaxo Wellcome, Fin. Glaxo Wellcome Oy, Kurjenkellontie 5, PL 5, 02270, 02271 Espoo, Finland.

Glaxo Wellcome, Fr. Laboratoires Glaxo Wellcome, 100 rte de Versailles, 78163 Marly-le-Roi cdx, France.

Glaxo Wellcome, Ger. Glaxo Wellcome GmbH & Co, Alsterufer 1, 20354 Hamburg, Germany.

Glaxo Wellcome, Hong Kong. Glaxo Wellcome China Ltd, 18/F West Warwick House, Taikoo Place, 979 King's Road, Quarry Bay, Hong Kong.

Glaxo Wellcome, Irl. See *GlaxoSmithKline, Irl.*

Glaxo Wellcome, Israel. See *CTS, Israel.*

Glaxo Wellcome, Ital. Glaxo Wellcome s.p.a., Via A. Fleming 2, 37135 Verona, Italy.

Glaxo Wellcome, Mex. GlaxoWellcome México, S.A. de C.V., Calz. Mexico-Xochimilco No. 4900, Col San Lorenzo Huipulco, 14370 Mexico D.F., Mexico.

Glaxo Wellcome, Neth. Glaxo Wellcome B.V., Postbus 780, 3700 AT Zeist, Netherlands.

Glaxo Wellcome, Norw. Glaxo Wellcome A/S, Sandakerv.114A, Postboks 4312 Torshov, 0402 Oslo, Norway.

Glaxo Wellcome, NZ. Glaxo Wellcome New Zealand Ltd, Private Bag 10-6600, Downtown, Aukland, New Zealand.

Glaxo Wellcome, Port. Glaxo Wellcome Farmacêutica, Lda, Rua Dr. Antonio Borges no. 3, Arquiparque, Miraflores, 1495-131 Alges, Portugal.

Glaxo Wellcome, S.Afr. See *GlaxoSmithKline, S.Afr.*

Glaxo Wellcome, Singapore. Glaxo Wellcome Singapore Pte Ltd, 150 Beach Road, 21-00 Gateway West, S 189720, Singapore.

Glaxo Wellcome, Spain. Glaxo Wellcome, Severo Ochoa 2, Tres Cantos, 28760 Madrid, Spain.

Glaxo Wellcome, Swed. Glaxo Wellcome AB, Box 263, 431 23 Molndal, Sweden.

Glaxo Wellcome, Switz. Glaxo Wellcome AG, Bahnhofstrasse 5, Postfach, 3322 Schonbuhl/Berne, Switzerland.

Glaxo Wellcome, Thai. Glaxo Wellcome (Thailand) Ltd, 89 Soi Wat Suan Plu, New Road, P.O. Box 955, Bangkok 10500, Thailand.

Glaxo Wellcome, UK. See *GlaxoSmithKline, UK.*

Glaxo Wellcome, USA. See *GlaxoSmithKline, USA.*

GlaxoSmithKline, Aust. GlaxoSmithKline, Albert-Schweitzer-Gasse 6, A-1140 Vienna, Austria.

GlaxoSmithKline, Austral. GlaxoSmithKline, Australia.

GlaxoSmithKline, Irl. GlaxoSmithKline, P.O. Box 700, Grange Rd, Rathfarnham, Dublin 16, Ireland.

GlaxoSmithKline, S.Afr. GlaxoSmithKline SA (Pty) Ltd, P.O. Box 3388, Halfway House 1685, South Africa.

GlaxoSmithKline, UK. GlaxoSmithKline, Stockley Park West, Uxbridge, Middlesex, UB11 1BT, UK.

GlaxoSmithKline, USA. GlaxoSmithKline, 5 Moore Drive, P.O. Box 13398, Research Triangle Park, NC 27709, USA.

Glenbrook, USA. Glenbrook Laboratories, Division of Sterling Drug Inc., 90 Park Ave, New York, NY 10016, USA.

Glenmark, Thai. See *Union Medical, Thai.*

Glenwood, Canad. Glenwood Laboratories Canada Ltd, 2406 Speers Rd, Oakville, Ontario, L6L 5M2, Canada.

Glenwood, Ger. Glenwood GmbH, Riedener Weg 23, 82319 Starnberg, Germany.

Glenwood, Hong Kong. See *Mita, Hong Kong.*

Glenwood, Switz. See *Galenica, Switz.*

Glenwood, UK. Glenwood Laboratories Ltd, Jenkins Dale, Chatham, Kent, ME4 5RD, UK.

Glenwood, USA. Glenwood Inc., 83 North Summit St, P.O. Box 518, Tenafly, NJ 07670, USA.

Glifarma, Port. See *Glaxo Wellcome, Port.*

Global, USA. Global Pharmaceutical, Castor & Kensington Aves, Philadelphia, PA 19124, USA.

Globopharm, Switz. Globopharm AG, Seestrasse 200, 8700 Kusnacht, Switzerland.

GN, Ger. See *Biosyn, Ger.*

GNLD, Austral. GNLD International P/L, P.O. Box 419, Beenleigh, Qld 4207, Australia.

GNR, Fr. Lab. GNR-pharma, 49 av Georges-Pompidou, 92593 Levallois-Perret cdx, France.

GNR, Ital. GNR s.p.a., Via Europa 35, 20053 Muggio (MI), Italy.

GNR, Port. See *Agostinho, Port.*

Go Travel, UK. Go Travel Products, UK.

Godecke, Ger. Gödecke GmbH, Mooswaldallee 1, 79090 Freiburg, Germany.

Golaz, Switz. Laboratoire Golaz SA, Case postale 1067, 1701 Fribourg-Moncor, Switzerland.

Golden Pride, Canad. Golden Pride, 60 Colonnade Rd, Nepean, Ontario, K2E 7J6, Canada.

Goldham, Ger. Goldham Pharma GmbH, Am Wasserberg 11, 86441 Zusmarshausen, Germany.

Goldline, USA. See *Zenith Goldline, USA.*

Goldplus, Singapore. Goldplus Universal Pte Ltd, 8 Kaki Bukit Rd 2, 02-19/20 Ruby Warehouse Complex, S 417841, Singapore.

Goldschmidt, Switz. See *Desopharmex, Switz.*

Goldschmidt, UK. Th. Goldschmidt Ltd, UK.

Goldshield, Denm. See *Goldshield, UK.*

Goldshield, Irl. See *Allphar, Irl.*

Goldshield, UK. Goldshield Pharmaceuticals Ltd, NLA Tower, 12-16 Addiscombe Rd, Croydon, Surrey, CR0 0XT, UK.

Gomenol, Fr. Laboratoires du Gomenol, 48 rue des Petites-Écuries, 75010 Paris, France.

Goodys, USA. See *Block, USA.*

Gordon, USA. Gordon Laboratories, 6801 Ludlow St, Upper Darby, PA 19082-1694, USA.

Gothaplast, Ger. Gothaplast Verbandpflasterfabrik GmbH, Am Nutzleber Feld 2, 99867 Gotha/Thuringen, Germany.

Gothia, Norw. Gothia Medical AS, Ostre Aker v 205, 0902 Oslo, Norway.

Gothia, Swed. Gothia Läkemedel AB, Bolshedens Industrivag 20, 427 50 Billdal, Sweden.

Goupil, Ital. Goupil Italia s.p.a., Via S. Paolo 13, 20121 Milan, Italy.

G.P. Laboratories, Austral. See *Pfizer, Austral.*

GPL, Switz. GPL Ginsana Products Lugano SA, Postfach, 6903 Lugano, Switzerland.

Grafton, Singapore. Grafton Pharmasia Pte Ltd, 66 Tannery Lane, 01-01C Sindo Building, S 347805, Singapore.

Grafton, UK. Grafton International, Birchbrook Park, Shenstone, Staffordshire, WS14 0DJ, UK.

Graham-Field, USA. Graham Field, 81 Spence St, Bay Shore, NY 11706, USA.

Gramse, Israel. Gramse Ltd, P.O. Box 112, Ramat Gan, Israel.

Grandel-Synpharma, Ger. Dr Grandel GmbH - Vertrieb Syn-Pharma GmbH, Pfladergasse 7-13, 86150 Augsburg, Germany.

Grands Espaces, Fr. Les Grands Espaces Therapeutiques, B.P. 6054, 34030 Montpellier cdx, France.

Granions, Mon. Laboratoires des Granions, 7 rue de l'Industrie, MC 98000, Monaco.

Grans Remedy, NZ. Grans Remedy, New Zealand.

Grasler, Ger. gräsler pharma GmbH, Brunnleitenstr. 3, 82284 Grafrath, Germany.

Gray, USA. See *Purdue Frederick, USA.*

Great Eastern, Hong Kong. Great Eastern Healthcare Ltd, 9/F, Blk A Kerry BCI Godown, 3 Kin Chuen St, Kwai Chung, N.T., Hong Kong.

Great Eastern, Thai. Great Eastern Drug Co. Ltd, 18 Fl, Thai Wah Tower, 21/52-54 South Sathorn Rd, Sathorn, Bangkok 10120, Thailand.

Great Liaison, Hong Kong. Great Liaison Ltd, Unit 608, Fibres & Fabrics Industrial Ctr, 7 Shing Yip St, Kwun Tong, Kowloon, Hong Kong.

Great Southern, USA. Great Southern Laboratories, 10863 Rockley Rd, Houston, TX 77099, USA.

Great Year, Hong Kong. Great Year Trading Co. Ltd, 18/F, 80 Gloucester Rd, Wanchai, Hong Kong.

Greater Pharma, Thai. Greater Pharma Ltd Part, 46, 46/1-2 Soi Charansanitwongs 40, Bangyikhan, Bangkok 10700, Thailand.

Green Cross, Hong Kong. See *Great Year, Hong Kong.*

Green Cross, Singapore. Green Cross Pte Ltd, 63 Hillview Ave, 07-06 Lam Soon Industrial Building, S 669569, Singapore.

Green Cross Guangzhou, Singapore. See *GC, Singapore.*

Green Turtle Bay Vitamin Co., USA. The Green Turtle Bay Vitamin Co., P.O. Box 642, Summit, NJ 07901, USA.

Greenpharma, Braz. Greenpharma Agroquimica Ltda, Quadra 2-A Mod. 32/35 DAIAI, 75133-600 Anapolis, GO, Brazil.

Greenridge, Austral. Greenridge, Australia.

Grelan, Jpn. Grelan Pharm., Japan.

Gricar, Ital. Industria Chimico Farmaceutica Gricar Chemical srl, Via S Giuseppe 18/20, 20047 Brugherio (MI), Italy.

Grifols, Ger. Grifols Deutschland GmbH, Siemensstr. 18, 63225 Langen, Germany.

Grifols, Ital. Grifols Italia s.p.a., Loc. La Fontina, Via Carducci 62d, 56010 Ghezzano (Pi), Italy.

Grifols, Port. Grifols Portugal, Lda, Rua Jorge Barradas no 30-C, 1500-371 Lisbon, Portugal.

Grifols, Spain. Grifols, Can Guasch 2 Pol. Levante, Parets del Valles, 08150 Barcelona, Spain.

Grifols, UK. Grifols UK Ltd, 72 St Andrews Rd, Cambridge, CB4 1GS, UK.

Grimberg, Fr. Lab. Grimberg, 19 rue Poliveau, 75005 Paris, France.

Grin, Mex. Laboratorios Grin S.A. de C.V., Av. Patriotismo No. 400, Col. San Pedro de los Pinos, 03800 Mexico D.F., Mexico.

Grisi, Mex. Laboratorios Grisi Hermanos, S.A., Division Farmaceutica, Amores No. 1746, Col. del Valle, 03100 Mexico D.F., Mexico.

Grogg, Switz. Grogg Pharma AG, Christoffelgasse 3, 3001 Berne, Switzerland.

Gross, Braz. Laboratorio Gross S.A., Rua Padre Ildefonso Penalba 389, 20775-020 Rio de Janeiro, RJ, Brazil.

Grossman, Mex. Laboratorios Grossman S.A., Calz. de Tlalpan No. 2021, Col. Parque San Andres, 04040 Mexico D.F., Mexico.

Grossmann, Hong Kong. Grossmann, Hong Kong.

Grossmann, Switz. Dr Grossmann AG, Pharmaca, Hardstrasse 25, Postfach 914, 4127 Birsfelden/Basle, Switzerland.

Grunenthal, Aust. Grünenthal GmbH, Wolfganggasse 45-7, A-1120 Vienna, Austria.

Grunenthal, Denm. See *Searle, Denm.*

Grunenthal, Fr. Grunenthal, 43 rue de Villiers, 92523 Neuilly-sur-Seine, France.

Grunenthal, Ger. Grünenthal GmbH Aachen, Steinfeldstr. 2, 52222 Stolberg, Germany.

Grunenthal, Hong Kong. See *Zuellig, Hong Kong.*

Grunenthal, Neth. See *Byk, Neth.*

Grunenthal, Norw. See *Searle, Norw.*

Grunenthal, Port. See *Euro-Labor, Port.*

Grunenthal, Singapore. See *Zuellig, Singapore.*

Grunenthal, Spain. Grunenthal, Doctor Zamenhof 36, 28027 Madrid, Spain.

Grunenthal, Switz. Grünenthal Pharma AG, 8756 Mitlodi/Glarus, Switzerland.

Grunenthal, Thai. See *Zuellig, Thai.*

Gry, Ger. Gry-Pharma GmbH, Kandelstr. 10, 79199 Kirchzarten, Germany.

Gry, Switz. See *Galenica, Switz.*

Guardian, Canad. See *Pharmascience, Canad.*

Guardian, USA. Guardian Laboratories, A division of United-Guardian Inc., 230 Marcus Blvd, Hauppauge, NY 11788, USA.

Gubler, Switz. Dr AW Gubler, Petersgraben 5, 4051 Basle, Switzerland.

Guerbert, Spain. Guerbert, Torre Colon II, Planta 13, Plaza de Colon 2, 28046 Madrid, Spain.

Guerbet, Aust. See *Guerbet, Fr.*

Guerbet, Braz. Guerbet Produtos Radiologicos Ltda, Rua Andre Rocha 3000, 22710-561 Rio de Janeiro, RJ, Brazil.

Guerbet, Denm. See *Logic, Denm.*

Guerbet, Fin. See *Dumex-Alpharma, Fin.*

Guerbet, Fr. Laboratoires Guerbet, B.P. 50400, 95943 Roissy-Charles-de-Gaulle cdx, France.

Guerbet, Ger. Guerbet GmbH, Otto-Volger Str. 11, 65843 Sulzbach/Ts, Germany.

Guerbet, Israel. Guerbet, Israel.

Guerbet, Ital. See *Farmades, Ital.*

Guerbet, Neth. Guerbet Nederland B.V., Avelingen West 28c, 4202 MS Gorinchem, Netherlands.

Guerbet, Norw. See *Gothia, Norw.*

Guerbet, Port. See *Martins & Fernandes, Port.*

Guerbet, Switz. Guerbet AG, Winterthurerstrasse 92, 8006 Zurich, Switzerland.

Guidotti, Hong Kong. See *Mekim, Hong Kong.*

Guidotti, Ital. Laboratori Guidotti s.p.a., Via Trieste 40, 56126 Pisa, Italy.

Guidotti, Spain. Guidotti Farma, C/Alfonso XII 587, Badalona, 08918 Barcelona, Spain.

Guieu, Fr. Laboratoires Guieu France, France.

Guieu, Ital. Laboratori Guieu s.p.a., V.le Filippetti 37, 20122 Milan, Italy.

Guigoz, Fr. Guigoz, B.P. 900, 77446 Marne-la-Vallee cdx 2, France.

Guigoz, Ital. Guigoz, Divisione Dietici, Viale Richard 5, 20143 Milan, Italy.

Guilford, Israel. Guilford, Israel.

Gunnar Kjems, Denm. Gunnar Kjems ApS, Peder Huitfeldts Straede 12, 1173 Copenhagen K, Denmark.

Gunther, Braz. Produtos Farmaceuticos Gunther do Brasil Ltda, Rua Joao Moura 1151, 05412-002 Sao Paulo, SP, Brazil.

Gynetics, USA. Gynetics Inc., P.O. Box 8509, Somerville, NJ 08876, USA.

Haemacure, Canad. Haemacure Corp., 16771 ch. Ste-Marie, Kirkland, Quebec, H9H 5H3, Canada.

Hafslund Nycomed, Aust. See *Nycomed, Aust.*

Hafslund Nycomed, Thai. See *Shiwa, Thai.*

Hal, Ger. Hal Allergie GmbH, Kolner Landstr. 34 a, 40591 Dusseldorf, Germany.

Hal, Neth. HAL Allergenen Laboratorium B.V., Postbus 1007, 2001 BA Haarlem, Netherlands.

Halal, UK. Halal Pharmaceuticals Ltd, 7 Oxford St, Manchester, M1 4WX, UK.

Halewood, Thai. See *Sriprasit, Thai.*

Hall, Canad. Hall Laboratories Ltd, 13060-89th Ave, Suite 207, Surrey, British Columbia, V3W 3B2, Canada.

Haller, Braz. Avenida Alem Paraiba 104, 21061-090 Rio de Janeiro, RJ, Brazil.

Halsey, USA. Halsey Drug Co, 695 N Perryville Rd, Rockford, IL 61107, USA.

Hamilton, Austral. Hamilton Pharmaceuticals P/L, P.O. Box 7, Adelaide, SA 5001, Australia.

Hamilton, Hong Kong. See *Australian Medic-Care, Hong Kong.*

Hamilton, Israel. Hamilton, Israel.

Hamilton, NZ. See *Medic, NZ.*

Hanosan, Ger. Hanosan GmbH, Hanosanstr. 1, 30826 Garbsen, Germany.

Hansam, Irl. See *United Drug, Irl.*

Hansam, UK. Hansam Healthcare Ltd, 60 Ondine Rd, London, SE15 4EB, UK.

Hanseler, Ger. Hänseler GmbH, Gottlieb-Daimler-Str. 1, 78467 Constance a. B., Germany.

Hanseler, Switz. Hänseler AG, Industriestrasse 35, 9100 Herisau, Switzerland.

Hargell, Canad. Hargell Ltd, 5050 Dufferin St, Suite 108, North York, Ontario, M3H 5T5, Canada.

Harley Street Supplies, UK. Harley Street Supplies, 55 Paddington St, London, W1M 3RQ, UK.

Harn, Thai. Harn Thai Pharma Ltd, 2121 New Petchburi Rd, Bangkok 10320, Thailand.

Harras-Curarina, Aust. See *Harras-Curarina, Ger.*

Harras-Curarina, Ger. Harras-Pharma-Curarina Arzneimittel GmbH, Am Harras 15, 81373 Munich, Germany.

Hartmann, Fr. Lab. Paul Hartmann, 18 rue des Goumiers, 67730 Chatenois, France.

Hartmann, Ger. Paul Hartmann AG Verbandstoff-Fabriken, Paul-Hartmann-Str. 12, 89522 Heidenheim (Brenz), Germany.

Harvey Scruton, Israel. Harvey Scruton, Israel.

Harvey-Scruton, UK. Harvey-Scruton Ltd, 4 Barker Lane, York, North Yorkshire, YO1 6JR, UK.

Hassle, Swed. Hässle Läkemedel AB, 431 83 Molndal, Sweden.

Hauck, USA. See *Roberts, USA.*

Haupt, Switz. Medidenta AG, Schachenstrasse 2, 9016 St Gallen, Switzerland.

Hausmann, Irl. See *Clonmel, Irl.*

Haw Par, Canad. Haw Par Brothers International Ltd, P.O. Box 4129, Vancouver, British Columbia, V6B 3Z6, Canada.

Hawgreen, UK. Hawgreen Ltd, P.O. Box 157, Hatfield, AL10 8ZP, UK.

Hawthorn, USA. See *Cypress, USA.*

Hayes, Israel. Hayes, Israel.

HCP, Austral. Regional HCP, Australia.

Health & Diet Food Co., UK. Health & Diet Food Co. Ltd, Europa Trading Estate, Stoneclough Road, Radcliffe, Manchester, M26 9HE, UK.

Health & Medical, USA. See *Graham-Field, USA.*

Health Care, Hong Kong. Health Care Products Ltd, 8/F Eastwood Ctr, 5A Kung Ngam Village Rd, Shaukeiwan, Hong Kong.

Health Care Products, USA. Health Care Products, 369 Bayview Ave, Amityville, NY 11701, USA.

Health Chemical, Hong Kong. See *Sun Hing, Hong Kong.*

Health for Life, USA. Health for Life Brands Inc., 1643 E Genesee St, Syracuse, NY 13210, USA.

Health Imports, UK. Health Imports Ltd, York House, York Street, Bradford, West Yorkshire, BD8 0HR, UK.

Health Perception, UK. Health Perception Ltd, Lakeside Business Park, Swan Lane, Sandhurst, Berkshire, GU47 7DN, UK.

Health Tech, Hong Kong. Health Tech Ltd, 5/F A-2 Loyong Court Commercial Bldg, 212-220 Lockhart Rd, Wanchai, Hong Kong.

Health Vision, Hong Kong. Health Vision (HK) Ltd, Rm 2504, K Wah Ctr, 191 Java Rd, Hong Kong.

Health World, Austral. Health World Ltd, 8/663 Kingsford Smith Drive, Eagle Farm, QLD 4009, Australia.

Healthcrafts, UK. Healthcrafts Ltd, UK.

Healtheries, NZ. Healtheries of New Zealand Ltd, 505 Mount Wellington Highway, Mount Wellington, Auckland, New Zealand.

Healtheze, UK. Healtheze Ltd, Burleigh Manor, Peel Rd, Douglas, Isle of Man, UK.

Healthfirst, USA. Healthfirst Corp., 22316 70th Ave W, Mountlake Terrace, WA 98043, USA.

Healthline, USA. Healthline Laboratories Inc., 2805 Danbar Dr., Green Bay, WI 54313, USA.

Healthpoint, USA. Healthpoint Ltd, 2600 Airport Fwy, Fort Worth, TX 76111, USA.

Hearst, Braz. Hearst Laboratorios do Brasil Ltda, Avenida Actura 100, Vila Actura, 25225-210 Duque de Caxias, RJ, Brazil.

Hebert, Canad. Distribution L Hebert, 15260 Notre-Dame St E, Montreal, Quebec, H1A 1W6, Canada.

Hebron, Braz. Hebron S.A. - Industria Quimica e Farmaceutica, Rodovia BR 232 Km 136, 55000-000 Caruaru, PE, Brazil.

Heca, Neth. Heca B.V., Industrieweg 24, Postbus 39, 7957 SG De Wijk, Netherlands.

Heel, Ger. Biologische Heilmittel Heel GmbH, Dr-Reckeweg-Str. 2-4, 76532 Baden-Baden, Germany.

Heel, S.Afr. Heel South Africa (Pty) Ltd, P.O. Box 890558, Lyndhurst 2106, South Africa.

Heel, USA. Heel Inc., 11600 Cochiti SE, Alberquerque, NM 87123, USA.

Hefa, Ger. Hefa Pharma Vertriebs GmbH & Co. KG, Am Bahnhof 1-3, 59368 Werne, Germany.

Heilit, Ger. Heilit Arzneimittel GmbH, Danziger Str. 5, 21465 Reinbek, Germany.

Heinz, UK. H.J. Heinz Co. Ltd, 6 Roundwood Ave, Stockley Park, Uxbridge, Middlesex, UB11 1HZ, UK.

Heinz-Wattie, NZ. Heinz-Wattie's Australasia Ltd, Private Bag 99-920, Newmarket, Auckland, New Zealand.

Helago, Ger. Helago-Pharma GmbH, Rheinallee 11, 53173 Bonn, Germany.

Helapet, UK. Helapet, UK.

Helber, Mex. Helber de Mexico, S.A. de C.V., Maiz Num 20, Col. Granjas Esmeralda, 09810 Mexico D.F., Mexico.

Helena, USA. Helena Laboratories, 1530 Lindbergh Dr, P.O. Box 752, Beaumont, TX 77707, USA.

Helfarma, Port. Helfarma, Lda, Rua Joao Chagas 53, 1495-072 Alges, Portugal.

Helios, UK. Helios Healthcare Ltd, P.O. Box 36, Old Warden, Biggleswade, SG18 9UP, UK.

Helixor, Ger. Helixor Heilmittel GmbH & Co., Fischermuhle 1, 72348 Rosenfeld, Germany.

Helsinn, Port. Helsinn, Lda, Estrada Nacional 249/4 (Km 1.6), Abrunheira, Apartado 155, 2710-901 Sintra, Portugal.

Helsinn Birex, Hong Kong. See *Treasure Mountain, Hong Kong.*

Helsinn Birex, Irl. Helsinn Birex Pharmaceuticals Ltd, Damastown, Mulhuddart, Dublin 15, Ireland.

Helvepharm, Switz. Helvepharm AG, Route Andre-Piller 2, Postfach 76, 1762 Givisiez, Switzerland.

Hemasure, Denm. HemaSure AS, Sauntesvej 13, 2820 Gentofte, Denmark.

Hemasure, Swed. See *Hemasure, Denm.*

HemispheRx, USA. HemispheRx, 1 Penn Center, 1617 John F Kennedy Blvd, Philadelphia, PA 19103, USA.

Henk, Ger. See *Dolorgiet, Ger.*

Henkel, Ger. Henkel-Ecolab Deutschland GmbH, Reisholzer Werftstr. 38-42, 40589 Dusseldorf, Germany.

Henkel, Ital. Henkel Ecolab s.p.a., Via Morozzo Della Rocca 6, 20123 Milan, Italy.

Henleys, UK. Henleys Medical Supplies Ltd, Brownfields, Welwyn Garden City, Hertfordshire, AL7 1AN, UK.

Hennig, Ger. Hennig Arzneimittel GmbH & Co. KG, Liebigstr. 1-2, 65439 Florsheim am Main, Germany.

Henning, Ger. Henning Berlin GmbH & Co. OHG, Potsdamer Str. 8, 10785 Berlin, Germany.

Henning Walldorf, Ger. Dr. Georg Friedrich Henning, Chemische Fabrik Walldorf GmbH, Robert-Bosch-Str. 62, 69190 Walldorf, Germany.

Henselwerk, Ger. Henselwerk GmbH, Muhlstr. 5-7, 71106 Magstadt, Germany.

Hepatoum, Fr. Laboratoires Hepatoum, B.P. 5, 03270 Saint-Yorre, France.

Heralds, Braz. Herald's do Brasil Ltda, Rua Alfredo Backer 619, 24452-001 Sao Goncalo, RJ, Brazil.

Herbal, Israel. Herbal, Israel.

Herbal Concepts, UK. Herbal Concepts Ltd, Liscombe Park, Soulbury, Buckinghamshire, LU7 0JL, UK.

Herbal Laboratories, UK. Herbal Laboratories Ltd, Pierpoint House, 1 Beach Rd, St Annes-on-Sea, Lancashire, FY8 2NR, UK.

Herbaline, Ital. Herbaline snc di Ugo Venara & C, Via dell'Artigianato 13, 13040 Rovasenda (VC), Italy.

Herbalist, Ger. Herbalist & Doc Gesundheitsgesellschaft mbH, Olafstr. 6, 13467 Berlin, Germany.

Herbamed, Switz. Herbamed AG, Untere Au, 9055 Buhler, Switzerland.

Herbapharm, Ger. Herbapharm GmbH, Postfach: 1211, 79326 Teningen, Germany.

Herbaxt, Fr. Laboratoires Herbaxt, Z.I. Nord, bat 5, 77200 Torcy, France.

Herbert, Ger. Herbert Arzneimittel GmbH, Kreuzberger Ring 13, 65205 Wiesbaden, Germany.

Herbes Universelles, Canad. Herbes Universelles, 7, 70e Ave O, Blainville, Quebec, J7C 1R7, Canada.

Herbrand, Ger. Dr Herbrand KG, Brambachstr. 31, 77723 Gengenbach, Germany.

Herchemie, Aust. Herchemie, Austria.

Hercon, USA. Hercon Laboratories Inc., 460 Park Ave, New York, NY 10022, USA.

Heritage Consumer, USA. Heritage Consumer Products, Brookfield Commons, Suite CL-41, 246 Federal Rd, Brookfield, CT 06804, USA.

Hermal, Aust. See *Hermal, Ger.*

Hermal, Denm. See *Merck, Denm.*

Hermal, Ger. Hermal Kurt Herrmann GmbH & Co., Scholtzstr. 3, 21465 Reinbek, Germany.

Hermal, Hong Kong. See *Jebsen, Hong Kong.*

Hermal, Israel. See *Neopharm, Israel.*

Hermal, Norw. See *Meda, Norw.*

Hermal, Port. See *Boots, Port.*

Hermal, Singapore. See *Boots, Singapore.*

Hermal, Thai. See *Olic, Thai.*

Hermes, Aust. See *Hermes, Ger.*

Hermes, Ger. Hermes Arzneimittel GmbH, Georg-Kalb-Str. 5-8, 82049 Grosshesselohe/Munich, Germany.

Herron, Austral. Herron Pharmaceuticals P/L, 17 Curzon St, Tennyson, QLD 4105, Australia.

Herus, Braz. Herus Industria Farmaceutica Ltda, Rua Sanches de Aguiar 200, V. Paulina, 03192-140 Sao Paulo, SP, Brazil.

Herzpunkt, Ger. Herzpunkt-Pharma GmbH, Binger Str. 80, 56154 Boppard/Bad Salzig, Germany.

Hestag, Aust. Hestag GmbH, Kreitnergasse 1-3, A-1171 Vienna, Austria.

Hetterich, Ger. See *Galenika, Ger.*

Heumann, Ger. Heumann Pharma GmbH, Sudwestpark 50, 90449 Nurnberg, Germany.

Heumann, Hong Kong. See *Fund Trip, Hong Kong.*

Heumann, Switz. See *Searle, Switz.*

Heumann, Thai. See *Sang Udom, Thai.*

Hevert, Ger. Hevert-Arzneimittel GmbH & Co. KG, In der Weiherwiese 1, 55569 Nussbaum, Germany.

Hexal, Aust. Hexal Pharma GmbH, Wilhelminenstrasse 91/II F, A-1160 Vienna, Austria.

Hexal, Austral. Hexal Australia P/L, Level 4, Suite 1-6, 100 Harris St, Pyrmont, NSW 2009, Australia.

Hexal, Ger. Hexal AG, Industriestr. 25, 83607 Holzkirchen, Germany.

Hexal, Israel. Hexal, Israel.

Hexal, S.Afr. Hexal, P.O. Box 15420, Westmead 3608, South Africa.

Hexal, UK. Hexal, UK.

Heyl, Ger. Heyl Chemisch-pharmazeutische Fabrik GmbH & Co. KG, Goerzallee 253, 14167 Berlin, Germany.

High Chemical, USA. High Chemical Co., 3901-A Nebraska St, Levittown, PA 19056, USA.

Hikma, Port. Hikma Farmacêutica (Portugal), Lda, Estrada Nacional no. 9, Cruzamento de Vila Verde, Fervenca, 2710 Sintra, Portugal.

Hilarys, Canad. Hilarys Distribution Ltd, 330 Esna Park Drive, Unit 38, Markham, Ontario, L3R 1H3, Canada.

Hill, USA. Hill Dermaceuticals Inc., 2650 S. Mellonville Ave, Sanford, FL 32773, USA.

Hillcross, UK. See *AAH, UK.*

Himmel, USA. Himmel Nutrition Inc., 1926 10th Ave N, Suite 303, Lake Worth, FL 33461, USA.

Hind Wing, Hong Kong. Hind Wing Co. Ltd, Unit No 1103B, 11/F, Block B, Seaview Estate, 2-8 Watson Rd, Hong Kong.

Hing Ah, Hong Kong. Hing Ah Agency Co. Ltd, Rm 1115, Tower A, Hung Hom Commercial Ctr, 39 Ma Tau Wai Rd, Kowloon, Hong Kong.

Hing Yip, Hong Kong. Hing Yip Medicine Co., 2/F, Lo Ko House, 133 Gloucester Rd, Hong Kong.

Hipolabor, Braz. Hipolabor Farmaceutica Ltda, Rodovia BR 262 Km 12.3, Distrito Industrial, 34505-970 Sabara, MG, Brazil.

Hishiyama, Thai. See *Union Medical, Thai.*

HK Pharma, UK. HK Pharma Ltd, P.O. Box 105, Hitchin, Hertfordshire, SG5 2GG, UK.

Hobein, Ger. Dr. Hobein & Co. Nachf. GmbH Arzneimittel, Grenzstr. 2, 53340 Meckenheim, Germany.

Hobein, Hong Kong. See *Universal, Hong Kong.*

Hoe, Singapore. See *Summit, Singapore.*

Hoechst, Fr. See *Aventis, Fr.*

Hoechst, Ger. See *Aventis Pharma, Ger.*

Hoechst Marion Roussel, Aust. See *Aventis Pharma, Aust.*

Hoechst Marion Roussel, Austral. See *Aventis, Austral.*

Hoechst Marion Roussel, Belg. See *Aventis, Belg.*

Hoechst Marion Roussel, Braz. Hoechst Marion Roussel S.A., Avenida Nacoes Unidas 18.001 8 and., Santo Amaro, 04795-900 Sao Paulo, SP, Brazil.

Hoechst Marion Roussel, Canad. See *Aventis Pharma, Canad.*

Hoechst Marion Roussel, Denm. See *Aventis Pharma, Denm.*

Hoechst Marion Roussel, Fin. Hoechst Marion Roussel Oy, PL 245, 00101 Helsinki, Finland.

Hoechst Marion Roussel, Ger. See *Aventis Pharma, Ger.*

Hoechst Marion Roussel, Hong Kong. Hoechst Marion Roussel China Ltd, Rm 2309-2311, Shell Tower, Times Square, 1 Matheson St, Causeway Bay, Hong Kong.

Hoechst Marion Roussel, Irl. See *Aventis Pharma, Irl.*

Hoechst Marion Roussel, Israel. Hoechst Marion Roussel, 7 Hasivim St, Petach Tikva, Israel.

Hoechst Marion Roussel, Ital. Hoechst Marion Roussel Italia s.p.a., Viale Gran Sasso, 20131 Milan, Italy.

Hoechst Marion Roussel, Jpn. Hoechst Marion Roussel Japan, 8-10-16 Akasaka, Minato-ku, Tokyo, Japan.

Hoechst Marion Roussel, Mex. Hoechst Marion Roussel, S.A. de C.V., Av. Universidad No. 1738, Col. Coyoacan, 04000 Mexico D.F., Mexico.

Hoechst Marion Roussel, Neth. Hoechst Marion Roussel B.V., Postbus 100, 3870 CC Hoevelaken, Netherlands.

Hoechst Marion Roussel, Norw. See *Aventis, Norw.*

Hoechst Marion Roussel, NZ. See *Aventis, NZ.*

Hoechst Marion Roussel, Port. See *Aventis Pharma, Port.*

Hoechst Marion Roussel, S.Afr. See *Aventis, S.Afr.*

Hoechst Marion Roussel, Singapore. Hoechst Marion Roussel South Asia Pte Ltd, 200 Cantonment Rd, 02-02 Southpoint, S 089763, Singapore.

Hoechst Marion Roussel, Spain. Hoechst Marion Roussel, Rda Del General Mitre 72-4, 08017 Barcelona, Spain.

Hoechst Marion Roussel, Swed. See *Aventis Pharma, Swed.*

Hoechst Marion Roussel, Switz. Hoechst Marion Roussel AG, Herostrasse 7, 8048 Zurich, Switzerland.

Hoechst Marion Roussel, Thai. Hoechst Marion Roussel (Thailand) Ltd, 20 Fl, Lake Rajada Building, 193 Ratchadaphisek Rd, Klong Toey, P.O. Box 960, Prakanong, Bangkok 10110, Thailand.

Hoechst Marion Roussel, UK. See *Aventis Pharma, UK.*

Hoechst Marion Roussel, USA. See *Aventis Pharma, USA.*

Hoechst Roussel, USA. See *Aventis Pharma, USA.*

Hoeport, Port. See *Aventis Pharma, Port.*

Hoernecke, Ger. Carl Hoernecke GmbH, Halberstadter Chaussee 22, 39116 Magdeburg, Germany.

Hoeveler, Aust. Hoeveler Mag. & Co. GmbH, Mosham 40, A-4943 Geinberg, Austria.

Hofmann, Aust. Hofmann Pharma GmbH & Co. KG, Kirchengasse 36, A-5081 Anif, Austria.

Hofmann & Sommer, Ger. Hofmann & Sommer GmbH & Co. KG, Lindenstr. 11, 07426 Konigsee, Germany.

Hogapharm, Switz. Hogapharm AG, Unterdorf 8, 6403 Kussnacht am Rigi, Switzerland.

Hogil, USA. Hogil Pharmaceutical Corporation, 2 Manhattanville Rd, Purchase, NY 10577, USA.

Hokuriku, Jpn. Hokuriku Seiyaku Co. Ltd, 25-5 Sendagaya 5-chome, Shibuya-ku, Tokyo 151, Japan.

Holistica, Fr. Laboratoires Holistica International, 465 chemin des Jalassieres, 13510 Eguilles, France.

Hollborn, Ger. Dr K Hollborn & Sohne GmbH & Co. KG, Brahestr. 13, 04347 Leipzig, Germany.

Hollister-Stier, USA. See *Bayer, USA.*

Holloway, USA. Holloway Pharmaceuticals Inc., USA.

Holsten, Ger. Holsten Pharma GmbH, Im Burgerstock 7, 79241 Ihringen, Germany.

Homberger, Switz. Laboratoire du Dr E Homberger SA, 10 place du Bourg-de-Four, 1204 Geneva, Switzerland.

Home, Ital. Home Products Italiana s.p.a., Via Puccini 3, 20121 Milan, Italy.

Home Diagnostics, USA. Home Diagnostics Inc., 2300 NW 55th Court, Fort Lauderdale, FL 33309, USA.

Homeocan, Canad. Homeocan, 3025, boul. de l'Assomption, Montreal, Quebec, H1N 2H2, Canada.

Homme de Fer, Fr. Laboratoires de l'Homme de Fer, 2 pl. de l'Homme de Fer, 67000 Strasbourg, France.

Hommel, Ger. Chemische Werke Hommel GmbH, Carl-Sonnenschein-Str. 32a, Postfach: 1662, 59336 Ludinghausen, Germany.

Hong Kong Medical, Hong Kong. Hong Kong Medical Supplies Ltd, 3-4/F Corn Yan Ctr, 3 Jupiter St, North Point, Hong Kong.

Hong Wo, Hong Kong. Hong Wo Trading Co., Rm 2, G/F, D-Part Bldg, 140 Wellington St Central, Hong Kong.

Honorterapica, Braz. Laboratorio Honorterapica Ltda, Rua Engenheiro Prudente 119, 01550-000 Sao Paulo, SP, Brazil.

Hope, USA. Hope Pharmaceuticals, 8260 E Gelding Drive, Suite 104, Scottsdale, AZ 85260, USA.

Hor-Fer-Vit, Ger. HorFerVit Pharma GmbH, H.-Brockmann Str. 81, 26131 Oldenburg, Germany.

Horizon, USA. Horizon Pharmaceutical Corp, 660 Hembree Parkway, Suite 106, Roswell, GA 30076, USA.

Hormona, Mex. Laboratorios Hormona, S.A. de C.V., Blvd. M. Avila Camacho No.470, San Andres Atoto, Mexico, 53500 Naucalpan de Juarez, Mexico.

Hormonas, Mex. Hormonas, Mexico.

Hormosan, Ger. Hormosan-Kwizda GmbH, Wilhelmshoher Str. 106, 60389 Frankfurt/Main, Germany.

Horner, Canad. See *Carter Horner, Canad.*

Hosbon, Spain. Hosbon, Ronda General Mitre 72-4, 08017 Barcelona, Spain.

Hospal, Denm. See *Gambro, Denm.*

Hospamed, Swed. Hospamed AB, Box 721, 503 16 Boras, Sweden.

Hotz, Ger. See *Riemser, Ger.*

Houde, Fr. See *Aventis, Fr.*

Houghs Healthcare, UK. Houghs Healthcare Ltd, UK.

Hovid, Singapore. See *Goldplus, Singapore.*

Howmedica, Switz. Howmedica Jaquet Orthopedie SA, Case postale 725, 1212 Grand-Lancy 1/GE, Switzerland.

Hoyer, Ger. Hoyer-Madaus GmbH & Co. KG, Alfred-Nobel-Str. 10, 40789 Monheim, Germany.

HSL, NZ. Health Support Ltd, 56 Carrington Rd, Point Chevalier, Auckland, New Zealand.

Hua, Thai. B L Hua & Co. Ltd, 2 Somdej Chaopraya Rd, Klongsan, Bangkok 10600, Thailand.

Hubert, UK. Hubert A.C. Thomas & Co., Copperworks Rd, New Dock, Llanelli, Dyfed, SA15 2EN, UK.

Huckaby, USA. Huckaby Pharmacal Inc., 6316 Old La Grange Rd, Crestwood, KY 40014, USA.

Hudson, USA. Hudson Corp., 90 Orville Drive, Bohemia, NY 11716, USA.

Hughes & Hughes, UK. Hughes & Hughes Ltd, Unit 1F, Lowmoor Industrial Estate, Tonedale, Wellington, Somerset, TA21 0AZ, UK.

Humana, Ital. Humana Italia s.p.a., Via Boscovich 55, 20124 Milan, Italy.

Hunter, Austral. Stephen Hunter P/L, 18 Lancaster St, Ingleburn, NSW 2265, Australia.

Husler, Switz. Franz Hüsler AG, Pharmazeutische Praparate, Chriesbaumstrasse 2, 8604 Volketswil, Switzerland.

Hyde, Canad. Hyde Pharmaceuticals, 20 Lewis St, Fort Eire, Ontario, L2A 5M6, Canada.

Hyland, USA. See *Baxter-Hyland, USA.*

Hyland Immuno, UK. See *Baxter BioScience, UK.*

Hylands, Canad. Hylands, 381-A, route 139, Sutton, Quebec, J0E 2K0, Canada.

Hypofarma, Braz. Hypofarma - Inst. Hypodermia e Farmacia SA, Rua Doutor Irineu Marcellini 303, 33805-330 Ribeirao das Neves, MG, Brazil.

Hypoguard, UK. Hypoguard (UK) Ltd, Dock Lane, Melton, Woodbridge, Suffolk, IP12 1PE, UK.

Hyrex, USA. Hyrex Pharmaceuticals, 3494 Democrat Rd, P.O. Box 18385, Memphis, TN 38118-0385, USA.

I Farmacologia, Spain. Instituto Farmacologia Española, Po de la Castellana 141, Edif. Cuzco IV, 28046 Madrid, Spain.

Iatric, USA. Iatric Corp, 2330 S Industrial Park Drive, Tempe, AZ 85282-1893, USA.

Ibi, Ital. Istituto Biochimico Italiano Giovanni Lorenzini s.p.a., Via Tucidide 56, Torre 6, 20134 Milan, Italy.

IBI, Thai. See *Siam Pharm, Thai.*

Ibirn, Ital. Istituto Bioterapico Nazionale s.r.l., Via V. Grassi 9/11/13/15, 00155 Rome, Italy.

IBP, Ital. Istituto Biochimico Pavese s.p.a., Viale Certosa 10, 27100 Pavia, Italy.

IBSA, Hong Kong. See *Mekim, Hong Kong,* and *Sincerity, Hong Kong.*

IBSA, Israel. IBSA, Israel.

IBSA, Ital. Ibsa Farmaceutici Italia srl, Viale Bianca Maria 33, 20122 Milan, Italy.

IBSA, Switz. Institut Biochimique SA, Via al Ponte 13, 6903 Lugano, Switzerland.

ICC, Israel. ICC, Israel.

Ichthyol, Aust. See *Ichthyol, Ger.*

Ichthyol, Ger. Ichthyol-Gesellschaft Cordes, Hermanni & Co. (GmbH & Co.) KG, Sportalle 85, 22335 Hamburg, Germany.

Ichthyol, Switz. See *Diethelm, Switz.*

ICI, Austral. See *AstraZeneca, Austral.*

ICI, Neth. See *Zeneca, Neth.*

ICIM, Ital. Istituto Chimico Italiano Milano srl, Via Peloritana 28, SS Varesina, 20024 Garbagnate M.se (MI), Italy.

ICN, Aust. See *ICN, Ger.*

ICN, Canad. ICN Canada Ltd, 1956 Bourdon St, Montreal, Quebec, H4M 1V1, Canada.

ICN, Fr. ICN Pharmaceuticals France SA, 4 rue Jean-Rostand, Parc Club, 91893 Orsay cdx, France.

ICN, Ger. ICN Pharmaceuticals Germany GmbH, Bolongarostr. 82-84, 65929 Frankfurt/Main, Germany.

ICN, Hong Kong. See *Inchcape, Hong Kong,* and *Jebsen, Hong Kong.*

ICN, Irl. See *Allphar, Irl.*

ICN, Israel. ICN, Israel.

ICN, Ital. ICN Pharmaceuticals s.r.l., c/o Temas, Via XXV Aprile 23, 20094 Corsica (MI), Italy.

ICN, Mex. ICN Farmacéutica, S.A de C.V., Calz. Ermita Iztapalapa No. 436, Col Mexicaltzingo, 09080 Mexico D.F., Mexico.

ICN, Neth. ICN Pharmaceuticals Holland B.V., Stephensonstraat 45, 2723 RM Zoetermeer, Netherlands.

ICN, NZ. See *Pacific, NZ.*

ICN, Port. See *ICN, Spain.*

ICN, Singapore. See *JDH, Singapore.*

ICN, Spain. ICN Iberica, Casanova 27-31, Corbera de Llobregat, 08757 Barcelona, Spain.

ICN, Switz. See *Diethelm, Switz.*

ICN, Thai. See *Diethelm, Thai.*

ICN, UK. ICN Pharmaceuticals Ltd, 1 Elmwood, Chineham Business Park, Crockford Rd, Basingstoke, Hampshire, RG24 8WG, UK.

ICN, USA. ICN Pharmaceuticals Inc., ICN Plaza, 3300 Hyland Ave, Costa Mesa, CA 92626, USA.

ICT, Ital. Istituto Chemioterapico s.p.a., Strada Bobbiese 108, 29100 Piacenza, Italy.

Ideal, Fr. Ideal, 65 rue Alexandre-Dumas, B.P. 53, 69153 Vaulx-en-Velin cdx, France.

IDEC, USA. IDEC Pharmaceuticals Corp., 11011 Torreyana Rd, San Diego, CA 92121, USA.

Iderne, Fr. Laboratoires Michel Iderne, Dpt Unipharma, Parc d'activites Rosenmeer, 67560 Rosheim, France.

IDI, Ital. IDI Farmaceutici s.p.a., Via dei Castelli Romani 83/85, 00040 Pomezia (Rome), Italy.

IDIS, UK. IDIS World Medicines, 171-185 Ewell Rd, Surbiton, Surrey, KT6 6AX, UK.

Ido, Fr. Laboratoires Ido, 8-10 passage Beslay, 75011 Paris, France.

Iema, Ital. Iema s.r.l., Via Adelasio 33, 24020 Ranica (BG), Italy.

IFI, Ital. Istituto Farmacoterapico Italiano s.p.a., Via Paolo Frisi 23, 00197 Rome, Italy.

Ifidesa Aristegui, Spain. Ifidesa Aristegui, Alameda de Urquijo 27 1, Bilbao, 48008 Vizcaya, Spain.

Ifusa, Mex. Laboratorios Ifusa S.A., Francisco Lorenzana Num. 20, Col. San Rafael, Deleg. Cuauhtemoc, 06470 Mexico D.F., Mexico.

Iketon, Ital. Iketon Farmaceutici s.r.l., Via Cassanese 224, 20090 Segrate (MI), Italy.

Ilex, Ital. Ilex Italiana s.r.l., Via Cavour 70, 27035 Mede (PV), Italy.

Illa, Ger. ILLA Healthcare GmbH, Burgermeister-Seidl-Str. 8, 82515 Wolfratshausen, Germany.

IMA, Braz. Instituto de Medicina e Allergia IMA Ltda, Rua Araujo Leitao 193, 20715-310 Rio de Janeiro, RJ, Brazil.

I-Med, Canad. I-Med Pharma Inc., 3869 Sources Blvd, Suite 200, Dollard des Ormeaux, Quebec, H9B 2A2, Canada.

Immunex, USA. Immunex Corp., 51 University St, Seattle, WA 98101, USA.

Immuno, Aust. See *Baxter, Aust.*

Immuno, Belg. S.A. Immuno, Belgium.

Immuno, Braz. Immuno Produtos Biologicos e Quimicos Ltda, Rua Adolfo Lutz 82, 22451-120 Rio de Janeiro, RJ, Brazil.

Immuno, Canad. See *Baxter, Canad.*

Immuno, Fr. Immuno France SA, France.

Immuno, Ger. See *Baxter-Hyland, Ger.*

Immuno, Hong Kong. See *Mekim, Hong Kong.*

Immuno, Irl. See *Allphar, Irl.*

Immuno, Israel. Immuno, Israel.

Immuno, Ital. See *Baxter, Ital.*

Immuno, Spain. See *Baxter, Spain.*

Immuno, Swed. See *Baxter, Swed.*

Immuno, Switz. See *Baxter, Switz.*

Immuno, UK. See *Baxter, UK.*

Immuno, USA. See *Baxter-Hyland, USA.*

Immunomedics, UK. Immunomedics, UK.

Immunomedics, USA. Immunomedics, 300 American Rd, Morris Plains, NJ 07950, USA.

Immunotec, Canad. Immunotec Research, 292 Adrien-Patenaude, Vaudreuil-Dorion, Quebec, J7V 5V5, Canada.

Immunotec, USA. See *Immunotec, Canad.*

IMO, Ital. Istituto di Medicina Omeopatica SpA, Via Vincenzo Monti 6, 20123 Milan, Italy.

Imperial, Singapore. See *Far East Drug, Singapore.*

Impharm, UK. Impharm Nationwide Ltd, Valley House, Britannia Business Park, Union Rd, Bolton, Lancashire, BL2 2HP, UK.

Implementos Plasticos, Mex. Implementos Plasticos S.A., Mar de Kara Num. 14, Col. Popotla, Deleg. Miguel Hidalgo, 11400 Mexico DF, Mexico.

IMS, Ital. International Medical Service s.r.l., Via Lauretina Km 26500, 00040 Pomezia (RM), Italy.

IMS, USA. See *Celltech Medeva, USA.*

Imtix, Belg. See *Imtix, Fr.*

Imtix, Denm. See *Imtix, Neth.*

Imtix, Fr. Imtix-SangStat, 58 av Debourg, B.P. 7055, 69348 Lyon cdx 07, France.

Imtix, Ger. Imtix SangStat GmbH, Paul-Ehrlich-Str. 1, 69181 Leimen, Germany.

Imtix, Ital. Imtix Sangstat srl, Via Winckelmann 2, 20146 Milan, Italy.

Imtix, Neth. Imtix B.V., Postbus 2207, 1180 EE Amstelveen, Netherlands.

Imtix, Switz. Imtix-Sangstat (Schweiz) GmbH, Oberallmendstrasse 16, 6300 Zug, Switzerland.

Inaf, Braz. Inaf, Brazil.

InAgra, USA. InAgra, USA.

Inava, Fr. See *Pierre Fabre, Fr.*

Inchcape, Hong Kong. Inchcape JDH Ltd, 14/F, JDH Ctr, 2 On Ping St, Siu Lek Yuen, Shatin, N.T., Hong Kong.

Incomex, Mon. Incomex, 9 av. Saint-Michel, MC 98000, Monaco.

Indochina Healthcare, Thai. Indochina Healthcare Ltd, 11 Fl, Than Settakij Building, 222 Vipavadee Rangsit Rd, Bangkok 10900, Thailand.

Indoco, Thai. See *Union Medical, Thai.*

Indrugco, Singapore. Indrugco Pte Ltd, 221 Henderson Rd, 07-20 Henderson Building, S 159557, Singapore.

Inexfa, Spain. Inexfa, Ctra Nacional 340, Km 28, Orihuela, 03300 Alicante, Spain.

Infabra, Braz. Infabra - Industria Farmaceutica Brasileira Ltda, Rua Conselheiro Mayrink 365, 20960-140 Rio de Janeiro, RJ, Brazil.

Infan, Mex. Laboratorios Infan, S.A. de C.V., Calz de Tlalpan No. 4515, Col Toriello Guerra, 14050 Mexico D.F., Mexico.

Infectopharm, Ger. Infectopharm Arzneimittel und Consilium GmbH, Von-Humboldt-Str. 1, 64646 Heppenheim, Germany.

Infirmarius-Rovit, Ger. Pharmazeutische Fabrik Infirmarius-Rovit GmbH, Eislinger Str. 66, 73084 Salach, Germany.

Ingram & Bell, Canad. Ingram & Bell Inc., 20 Bond Ave, Don Mills, Ontario, M3B 1L9, Canada.

Inibsa, Port. Laboratórios Inibsa, SA, S. Marcos, Apartado 24, 2736-901 Cacem, Portugal.

Inibsa, Spain. Inibsa, Ctra Sabadell Granollers Km 14.5, Llissa de Vall, 08185 Barcelona, Spain.

Inkeysa, Spain. Inkeysa, Juan XXIII 15, Esplugas de Llobregat, 08950 Barcelona, Spain.

Inkine, USA. InKine Pharmaceutical, USA.

Innotech, Fr. Sté du groupe Innothéra Industries, Innotech International, 7-9 av Francois-Vincent-Raspail, B.P. 32, 94111 Arcueil cdx, France.

Innotech, Hong Kong. See *Wing Wai, Hong Kong.*

Innotech, Port. See *Confar, Port.*

Innotech, Singapore. See *Indrugco, Singapore.*

Innothera, Fr. Sté du groupe Innothéra Industries, 10 ave P.-Vaillant-Couturier, B.P. 35, 94111 Arcueil cdx, France.

Innothera, Norw. See *Ferring, Norw.*

Innovatec, Singapore. See *MBD, Singapore.*

InnoVisions, USA. Innovisions Inc., 6065 Frantz Rd, Suite 202, Dublin, OH 43017, USA.

INO Therapeutics, USA. INO Therapeutics Inc., USA.

Inpharma, Denm. See *Inpharma, Norw.*

Inpharma, Fin. See *Oriola, Fin.*

Inpharma, Norw. Inpharma AS, Storg. 75, Postboks 300, 3301 Hokksund, Norway.

Inpharma, Swed. See *Inpharma, Norw.*

Inpharzam, Hong Kong. See *Universal, Hong Kong.*

Inpharzam, Switz. Inpharzam AG, PO Box 200, 6814 Cadempino, Switzerland.

INQ, Braz. Instituto Nacional de Quimioterapia Ltda, Rua Humberto I 217, 04018-030 Sao Paulo, SP, Brazil.

Instituto Farmacologico, Spain. Instituto Farmacologico Español, Ramallosa-Teo, Santiago de Compostela, 15883 La Coruna, Spain.

Integrity, USA. Integrity, USA.

Intercare, Irl. See *Mayrs, Irl.*

Intercare, UK. Intercare Products Ltd, UK.

Interdelta, Switz. Interdelta SA, Case postale 460, 1701 Fribourg, Switzerland.

Interfarma, Ital. Interfarma Farmaceutici s.r.l., Via Vivaldi 16, 35030 Selvazzano Dentro (PD), Italy.

Interferon Sciences, USA. Interferon Sciences Inc., 783 Jersey Ave., New Brunswick, NJ 08901-3660, USA.

Intermedica, Switz. Intermedica SA, Pharmazeutische Produkte, 91 rue de Lausanne, Case postale 238, 1701 Fribourg, Switzerland.

Intermuti, Ger. intermuti pharma GmbH, Alfred-Nobel-Str. 10, 40789 Monheim, Germany.

International Dermatologicals, Canad. International Dermatologicals Inc., 1940 Lonsdale Ave, Suite 217A, Vancouver, British Columbia, V7M 2K2, Canada.

International Ethical, USA. International Ethical Labs, Reparto Metropolitano, Rio Piedras, PR 00921, USA.

International Lab Tech, USA. International Lab Tech, USA.

International Medical, Hong Kong. International Medical Co. Ltd, Unit 715, 7/F, Block B, Seaview Estate, 2-8 Watson Rd, North Point, Hong Kong.

International Pharmaceutical, USA. See *Aventis Pharma, USA.*

Interpharm, Aust. Interpharm GmbH, Effingergasse 21, A-1160 Vienna, Austria.

Interpharma, Spain. Interpharma, Santa Rosa 6, Santa Coloma de Gramanet, 08921 Barcelona, Spain.

Intersan, Ger. Intersan, Institut fur pharmazeutische und klinische Forschung GmbH, Einsteinstr. 30, 76275 Ettlingen, Germany.

Intersan, Switz. See *Uhlmann-Eyraud, Switz.*

Intersero, Ger. Intersero GmbH, Peter-Sander-Str. 43, 55252 Mainz-Kastel, Germany.

INTES, Ital. See *Alfa Intes, Ital.*

Intra Pharma, Irl. Intra Pharma Ltd, 86 Broomhill Road, Tallaght, Dublin 24, Ireland.

Intramed, S.Afr. Intramed, South Africa.

Intrapharm, UK. Intrapharm Laboratories Ltd, 60 Boughton Lane, Maidstone, Kent, ME15 9QS, UK.

Intraveno, Irl. IntraVeno Healthcare Ltd, 86 Broomhill Rd, Tallaght, Dublin 24, Ireland.

Intsel, Fr. Lab. Intsel Chimos, Technopolis, 145 rue J.-J. Rousseau, 92138 Issy-les-Moulineaux cdx, France.

Invamed, USA. Invamed Inc., 2400 Rt 130N, Dayton, NJ 08810, USA.

Inverdia, Swed. Inverdia AB, Vretenvagen 8, 171 54 Solna, Sweden.

Inverni della Beffa, Ital. Inverni della Beffa s.p.a. (Gruppo Sanofi-Synthelabo), Via Rivoltana 13, 20090 Segrate (MI), Italy.

Investigacion, Mex. Investigación Farmacéutica, S.A. de C.V, Calle 13-E No. 5 CIV-AC, 62500 Jiutepec Mor., Mexico.

Investigaciones Filosoficas y Cientificas, Mex. Investigaciones Filosoficas y Cientificas, S.A. de C.V., Abasolo No. 215, Barrio de San Juan, 79610 Rio Verde SLP, Mexico.

Invicta, Irl. See *Pfizer, Irl.*

Invicta, Spain. Invicta Farma, C/Principe de Vergara 109, 28002 Madrid, Spain.

Invitech, UK. Invitech Ltd, 15 Witney Way, Boldon Business Park, Tyne & Wear, NE35 9PE, UK.

Inwood, USA. Inwood Laboratories, 321 Prospect St, Inwood, NY 11096, USA.

Iodo Suma, Braz. Laboratorio Iodo Suma Ltda, Avenida Constantino Pinto 104, 36880-000 Muriae, MG, Brazil.

Iodosan, Ital. Iodosan S.p.A., Via Zambeletti, 20021 Baranzate di Bollate (MI), Italy.

Iolab, Israel. Iolab, Israel.

Iolab, USA. See *Bausch & Lomb, USA,* and *Ciba Vision, USA.*

Ioltech, Fr. Lab. Ioltech, av. Paul-Langevin, B.P. 5, 17053 La Rochelle cdx 9, France.

Iomed, Hong Kong. See *Pan-Well, Hong Kong.*

Iomed, USA. Iomed Laboratories, Inc., 7425 Pebble Drive, Fort Worth, TX 76118, USA.

Ion, USA. Ion Laboratories Inc., 7431 Pebble Drive, Fort Worth, TX 76118, USA.

Iopharm, USA. Iopharm, 7549 Pebble Dr, Ft Worth, TX 76118, USA.

Ioquin, Austral. See *Alcon, Austral.*

IPA, Ital. International Pharmaceuticals Associated s.r.l., Via del Casale Cavallari 53, 00156 Rome, Italy.

Ipex, Aust. See *Ipex, Swed.*

Ipex, Fin. See *Tamro, Fin.*

Ipex, Ger. See *Ipex, Swed.*

Ipex, Norw. See *Ipex, Swed.*

Ipex, Swed. Ipex Medical AB, Box 120, 182 12 Danderyd, Sweden.

IPFI, Ital. I.P.F.I. (Industria Farmaceutica s.r.l., Via Egadi 7, 20144 Milan, Italy.

Iphym, Fr. Laboratoires Iphym, chemin de la Sereine, 01700 Beynost, France.

IPRAD, Fr. Laboratoires IPRAD, 42-52 rue de l'Aqueduc, 75010 Paris, France.

IPS, Neth. IPS, Beeldschermweg 6b, 3821 AH Amersfoort, Netherlands.

IPS, Spain. IPS Farma, Mendez Alvaro 57, 28045 Madrid, Spain.

Ipsen, Aust. See *Ipsen, Ger.*

Ipsen, Belg. Ipsen S.A., Maaltecenter Blok A, Derbystraat 201, 9051 Gent, Belgium.

Ipsen, Denm. Ipsen Scandinavia A/S, Park Allé 292, 2605 Brondby, Denmark.

Ipsen, Fin. See *Ipsen, Denm.*

Ipsen, Ger. Ipsen Pharma GmbH, Einsteinstr. 30, 76275 Ettlingen, Germany.

Ipsen, Irl. Ipsen Pharmaceuticals Ltd, 7 Upper Leeson St, Dublin 4, Ireland.

Ipsen, Ital. Ipsen s.p.a., Via A Figino 16, 20156 Milan, Italy.

Ipsen, Norw. Ipsen Scandinavia, Nesmyra 2, 5114 Tertnes, Norway.

Ipsen, Port. Ipsen Portugal, SA, Rua General Ferreira Martins, Edificio Eca de Queiroz 8-9B, Miraflores, 1495-137 Alges, Portugal.

Ipsen, Spain. Ipsen Pharma, Ctra Laurea Miro 395, Sant Feliu de Llobregat, 08980 Barcelona, Spain.

Ipsen, Swed. See *Ipsen, Denm.*

Ipsen, UK. Ipsen Ltd, 1 Bath Rd, Maidenhead, Berkshire, SL6 4UH, UK.

Ipsen Biotech, Fr. IPSEN/Biotech, 24 rue Erlanger, 75781 Paris cdx 16, France.

Ipso, Ital. Ipso-Pharma srl, Via San Rocco 6, 85033 Episcopia (PZ), Italy.

IQB, Braz. Instituto de Quimica e Biologia S.A., Rua A 20, 24140-210 Niteroi, RJ, Brazil.

IQFA, Mex. Industrias Quimico Farmaceuticas Americanas S.A. de C.V., Cto. Cerrillo II Mza 1, Lote 17, 52000 Lerma Edo. de Mexico, Mexico.

Iqfasa, Mex. Iqfasa, Mexico.

Iquinosa, Spain. Iquinosa, Alpedrete 24, 28045 Madrid, Spain.

IRBI, Ital. IRBI s.p.a., Italy.

Irex, Fr. Laboratoires Irex, Groupe Sanofi-Synthelabo, 11 rue Salomon-de-Rothschild, 92150 Suresnes, France.

Irisfarma, Spain. Irisfarma, Avda de la Industria 30, Alcobendas, 28108 Madrid, Spain.

Irmed, Ital. Istituto Ricerche Mediche s.r.l., Via della Consortia 17, 37100 Verona, Italy.

Iromedica, Switz. Iromedica AG, Haggenstrasse 45, 9014 St Gallen, Switzerland.

Isdin, Port. Isdin (Esteve Farma, Lda), Av do Forte 3, Edificio Suecia II, Piso 4 Ala A, 2795-504 Carnaxide, Portugal.

Isdin, Spain. Isdin, Av. Diagonal 520, 08006 Barcelona, Spain.

ISI, Ital. Istituto Sierovaccinogeno Italiano s.p.a., 55020 Castelvecchio Pascoli (LU), Italy.

Isis, Ger. See *Alpharma-Isis, Ger.*

Isis, UK. Isis Products Ltd, Gough Lane, Bamber Bridge, Preston, Lancashire, PR5 6AQ, UK.

Isis, USA. Isis Pharmaceuticals, Carlsbad Research Center, 2292 Faraday Ave, Carlsbad, CA 92008, USA.

Isis Puren, Ger. See *Alpharma-Isis, Ger.*

Islacan, Spain. Islacan, Ctra General San Lorenzo 119, Las Palmas de Gran Canaria, 35018 Gran Canaria, Spain.

ISM, Ital. Ist. Sieroterapico Milanese S. Belfanti, Via Darwin 22, 20143 Milan, Italy.

Iso, Ger. Iso-Arzneimittel GmbH & Co. KG, Bunsenstr. 6-10, 76275 Ettlingen, Germany.

Isomed, Spain. Isomed, Alberto Alcocer 46 Bajo B, 28016 Madrid, Spain.

Isopharm, Fr. Laboratoires Isopharm, France.

Isopharm, Hong Kong. See *CNW, Hong Kong.*

Isramedcom, Israel. Isramedcom, Israel.

Ist. Chim. Inter., Ital. Istituto Chimico Internazionale Dr. Giuseppe Rende s.r.l., Via Salaria 1240, 00138 Rome, Italy.

Istoria, Ital. Istoria Farmaceutici s.p.a., Riviera Francia 3/A, 35127 Padova, Italy.

Italchimici, Ital. Italchimici s.p.a., Via Pontina Km 29000, No 5, 00040 Pomezia (RM), Italy.

Italfarmacia, Ital. Italfarmacia srl, Via Tor Sapienza 7, 00155 Rome, Italy.

Italfarmaco, Ital. Italfarmaco s.p.a., Viale Fulvio Testi 330, 20126 Milan, Italy.

Italfarmaco, Spain. Italfarmaco, San Rafael 3, Alcobendas, 28100 Madrid, Spain.

Italmex, Mex. Italmex S.A., Calz. de Tlalpan Num. 3218, Col. Ejido Santa Ursula Coapa, Deleg. Coyoacan, 04910 Mexico D.F., Mexico.

Italzama, Ital. Italzama, Via Leonardo da Vinci 75, 00016 Monterotondo Scalo (RM), Italy.

ITF, Port. ITF, Lda, Rua Consiglieri Pedroso no 123, Queluz de Baixo, 2745-557 Barcarena, Portugal.

Ivamed, Ger. IVAmed Arzneimittel GmbH, Brauereistr., 68723 Plankstadt, Germany.

Ivex, UK. Ivex Pharmaceuticals, Division of the Galen Group, Old Belfast Rd, Millbrook, Larne, Co. Antrim, BT40 2SH, UK.

IVF, Switz. Internationale Verbandstoff-Fabrik Schaffhausen, 8212 Neuhausen am Rheinfall, Switzerland.

IVP, Ital. Istituto Vaccinogeno Pozzi s.p.a., Via Petriccio 27, 53100 Siena, Italy.

Ivy Corp, USA. Ivy Corporation, 23 Fairfield Pl., W. Caldwell, NJ 07006, USA.

Jaapharm, Canad. Jaapharm, 200 Trowers Rd, Unit 1, Woodbridge, Ontario, L4L 5Z7, Canada.

Jaba, Port. Jaba Farmacêutica, SA, Zona Industrial Abrunheira, Apartado 165, 2710-901 Sintra, Portugal.

Jacobs, UK. Jacobs Bakery Ltd, Long Lane, Aintree, Liverpool, Merseyside, L9 7BQ, UK.

Jacobson, Hong Kong. Jacobson Medical (Hong Kong) Ltd, Unit 1405B, 14/F, Blk B, Sea View Estate, 2-8 Watson Rd, North Point, Hong Kong.

Jacobus, USA. Jacobus Pharmaceutical Co. Inc., 37 Cleveland Lane, P.O. Box 5290, Princeton, NJ 08540, USA.

Jacoby, Aust. Jacoby Pharmazeutika AG, Teichweg 2, A-5400 Hallein-Kaltenhausen, Austria.

Jaldes, Fr. Laboratoires Jaldes, 59 rue de l'Eglise, B.P. 24, Pont-d'Aubenas, 07208 Aubenas cdx, France.

Jamieson, Canad. Jamieson Laboratories, 4025 Rhodes Drive, Windsor, Ontario, N8W 5B5, Canada.

Jamieson, Hong Kong. See *Universal, Hong Kong.*

Janpharm, S.Afr. Janpharm (Pty) Ltd, 15th Rd, Halfway House 1685, S. Africa.

Janssen, Belg. See *Janssen-Cilag, Belg.*

Janssen, Braz. Janssen Farmaceutica Ltda, Rua Avanhandava 55, 01306-900 Sao Paulo, SP, Brazil.

Janssen, Hong Kong. Janssen Pharmaceutica, Unit 1302-1307, Tower 1, Grand Century Place, 193 Prince Edward Rd West, Mongkok, Kowloon, Hong Kong.

Janssen, Mex. Janssen Farmacéutica, S.A. de C.V., Canoa No. 79, Col. Tizapan, 01090 Mexico D.F., Mexico.

Janssen, Swed. See *Janssen-Cilag, Swed.*

Janssen, Thai. Janssen Pharmaceutica Ltd, 11 Fl, Grand Amarin Tower, 1550 New Petchburi Rd, Makasan, Rachtevee, Bangkok 10320, Thailand.

Janssen, UK. See *Janssen-Cilag, UK.*

Janssen, USA. Janssen Pharmaceutical Inc., 1125 Trenton-Harbourton Road, P.O. Box 200, Titusville, NJ 08560-0200, USA.

Janssen-Cilag, Aust. Janssen-Cilag Pharma Vertrieb GmbH, Pfarrgasse 75, A-1232 Vienna, Austria.

Janssen-Cilag, Austral. Janssen-Cilag P/L, Locked Bag 2070, North Ryde, NSW 1670, Australia.

Janssen-Cilag, Belg. Janssen-Cilag S.A., Uitbreidingstraat 2, 2600 Berchem, Belgium.

Janssen-Cilag, Denm. Janssen-Cilag A/S, Hammerbakken 19, 3460 Birkerod, Denmark.

Janssen-Cilag, Fin. Janssen-Cilag Oy, Metsänneidonkuja 8, 02130 Espoo, Finland.

Janssen-Cilag, Fr. Janssen-Cilag SA, 1 rue Camille-Desmoulins, 92787 Issy-les-Moulineaux cdx 9, France.

Janssen-Cilag, Ger. Janssen-Cilag GmbH, Raiffeisenstr. 8, 41470 Neuss, Germany.

Janssen-Cilag, Irl. Janssen-Cilag Ltd, Pharmapark, Chapelizod, Dublin 20, Ireland.

Janssen-Cilag, Israel. Janssen Cilag, Division of J-C Health Care Ltd, Kibbutz Shefayim, Israel.

Janssen-Cilag, Ital. Janssen-Cilag s.p.a., Via M Buonarroti 23, 20093 Cologno Monzese (MI), Italy.

Janssen-Cilag, Neth. Janssen-Cilag B.V., Postbus 90240, 5000 LT Tilburg, Netherlands.

Janssen-Cilag, Norw. Janssen-Cilag AS, Postboks 143 Holmlia, 1203 Oslo, Norway.

Janssen-Cilag, NZ. Janssen-Cilag Pty Ltd, P.O. Box 9222, Newmarket, Auckland, New Zealand.

Janssen-Cilag, Port. Janssen Cilag Farmacêutica, Lda, Estrada Consiglieri Pedroso 69 A/B, 2745 Queluz de Baixo, Portugal.

Janssen-Cilag, S.Afr. Janssen-Cilag (Pty) Ltd, P.O. Box 785939, Sandton 2146, South Africa.

Janssen-Cilag, Singapore. Janssen-Cilag, A Division of Johnson & Johnson Pte Ltd, 3 International Rd, Jurong, S 619619, Singapore.

Janssen-Cilag, Spain. Janssen-Cilag, P. de las Doce Estrellas 5-7, Campo de Naciones, 28042 Madrid, Spain.

Janssen-Cilag, Swed. Janssen-Cilag AB, Box 7073, 192 07 Sollentuna, Sweden.

Janssen-Cilag, Switz. Janssen-Cilag AG, Sihlbruggstrasse 111, 6341 Baar, Switzerland.

Janssen-Cilag, UK. Janssen-Cilag Ltd, P.O. Box 79, Saunderton, High Wycombe, Buckinghamshire, HP14 4HJ, UK.

Janssen-Kyowa, Jpn. Janssen-Kyowa, Japan.

Janssen-Ortho, Canad. Janssen-Ortho Inc., 19 Green Belt Drive, Toronto, Ontario, M3C 1L9, Canada.

Japan Tobacco, Jpn. Japan Tobacco, Japan.

Jauntal, Aust. Jauntal-Apotheke, Bleiburger Strasse 16, A-9141 Eberndorf, Austria.

JB Williams, USA. J. B. Williams Co. Inc., 65 Harriston Road, Glen Rock, NJ 07452-3317, USA.

JC Healthcare, Ital. JC Healthcare s.r.l., Via M Buonarroti 23, 20093 Cologno Monzese (MI), Italy.

JCP, Canad. JCP Laboratories Inc., P.O. Box 403, St-Martin Branch, Laval, QC, H7S 2A4, Canada.

JDH, Singapore. JDH Pharmaceutical Division, 58 Toh Guan Rd, 03-03 LiFung Centre, S 608829, Singapore.

JDH Borneo, Thai. JDH Borneo (Thailand) Ltd, 2160/1 Ramkhamhaeng Rd, Hua Mark, Bangkapi, Bangkok 10240, Thailand.

JE IL, Singapore. See *Pharmaforte, Singapore.*

Jean-Marie, Hong Kong. Jean-Marie Pharmacal Co. Ltd, 17/F Jing Ho Industrial Bldg, 78-84 Wang Lung St, Tsuen Wan, Hong Kong.

Jean-Marie, Singapore. See *Grafton, Singapore.*

Jebsen, Hong Kong. Jebsen & Co. Ltd, 12/F, Scomber Bldg, 1 Yip Fat St, Wong Chuk Hang, Hong Kong.

Jenapharm, Ger. Jenapharm GmbH & Co. KG, Otto-Schott-Str. 15, 07745 Jena, Germany.

Jenapharm, Hong Kong. See *Jacobson, Hong Kong.*

Jenapharm, Thai. See *Berli, Thai.*

Jergens, USA. Andrew Jergens Co., 2535 Spring Grove Ave, Cincinnati, OH 45214, USA.

Jessel, Fr. Laboratoires Jessel-Végébom SA, 59 av. d'Iena, 75116 Paris, France.

Jessup, UK. Jessup Marketing, 27 Old Gloucester St, London, WC1N 3XX, UK.

JHC Healthcare, UK. JHC Healthcare Ltd, The Maltings, Bridge St, Hitchin, Hertfordshire, SG5 2DE, UK.

J&J-Merck, USA. J&J Merck Consumer Pharmaceuticals, Camp Hill Rd, Ft Washington, PA 19034, USA.

JMI, USA. See *Jones, USA.*

Jodquellen, Ger. Jodquellen AG, Ludwigstr. 14, 83646 Bad Tolz, Germany.

Jofrain, Mex. Jofrain, Mexico.

Johanser, Ger. St. Johanser Naturmittelvertrieb GmbH, Starnberger Str. 15, 82131 Gauting, Germany.

Johnson, Canad. S.C. Johnson and Son Ltd, 1 Webster St, P. O. Box 250, Brantford, Ontario, N3T 5R1, Canada.

Johnson, USA. R.W. Johnson Pharmaceutical Research Institute, USA.

Johnson & Johnson, Aust. Johnson & Johnson GmbH, Weisslhofweg 9, A-5400 Hallein, Austria.

Johnson & Johnson, Austral. Johnson & Johnson Medical P/L, P.O. Box 134, North Ryde, NSW 2113, Australia.

Johnson & Johnson, Braz. Johnson e Johnson Industria e Comercio Ltda, Rua Gerivativa 207 9°/10° Andar, 05501-900 Sao Paulo, SP, Brazil.

Johnson & Johnson, Canad. Johnson & Johnson/Merck Consumer Pharmaceuticals of Canada, 890 Woodlawn Rd W, Guelph, Ontario, N1K 1A5, Canada.

Johnson & Johnson, Ger. Johnson & Johnson GmbH, Kaiserswerther Str. 270, 40474 Dusseldorf, Germany.

Johnson & Johnson, Hong Kong. See *Inchcape, Hong Kong,* and *Zuellig, Hong Kong.*

Johnson & Johnson, Irl. Johnson & Johnson (Ireland) Ltd, Belgard Rd, Tallaght, Dublin 24, Ireland.

Johnson & Johnson, Israel. Johnson & Johnson, Kibbutz Shefayim, Israel.

Johnson & Johnson, Ital. Johnson & Johnson Divisione Farmacia s.p.a., 00040 S. Palomba, Pomezia (Rome), Italy.

Johnson & Johnson, NZ. Johnson & Johnson (NZ) Ltd, P.O. Box 97-027, Wiri, South Auckland, New Zealand.

Johnson & Johnson, Port. Johnson & Johnson, Lda, Estrada Consiglieri Pedroso 69 A, Queluz de Baixo, 2745-555 Barcarena, Portugal.

Johnson & Johnson, Singapore. See *Diethelm, Singapore.*

Johnson & Johnson, Spain. Johnson Johnson, Ctra Madrid-Valencia Km 24.7, Arganda del Rey, 28500 Madrid, Spain.

Johnson & Johnson, Swed. Johnson & Johnson AB, 191 84 Sollentuna, Sweden.

Johnson & Johnson, Switz. Johnson & Johnson SA, Rotzenbuhlstrasse 55, 8957 Spreitenbach 1, Switzerland.

Johnson & Johnson, Thai. Johnson & Johnson (Thailand) Co. Ltd, 106 Moo 4 Lat Krabang, Industrial Estate, Chalongkrung Rd, Lumplatew, Lat Krabang, Bangkok 10520, Thailand.

Johnson & Johnson, UK. Johnson & Johnson Ltd, Foundation Park, Roxborough Way, Maidenhead, Berkshire, SL6 3UG, UK.

Johnson & Johnson, USA. Johnson & Johnson, 199 Grandview Rd, Skillman, NJ 08558-9418, USA.

Johnson & Johnson Consumer, Belg. Johnson & Johnson Consumer S.A./N.V., Rue de la Grenouillette 2 E, 1130 Brussels, Belgium.

Johnson & Johnson Medical, Fr. Johnson & Johnson Médical, division d'Ethicon SAS, 1 rue Camille-Desmoulins, TSA 10004, 92787 Issy-les-Moulineaux cdx 9, France.

Johnson & Johnson Medical, UK. Johnson & Johnson Medical, Coronation Rd, Ascot, Berkshire, SL5 9EY, UK.

Johnson & Johnson Medical, USA. Johnson & Johnson Medical Inc., P.O. Box 90130, Arlington, TX 76004-0130, USA.

Johnson & Johnson MSD Consumer, UK. Johnson & Johnson MSD Consumer Pharmaceuticals, Enterprise House, Station Rd, Loudwater, High Wycombe, Buckinghamshire, HP10 9UF, UK.

Johnson Wax, USA. S.C. Johnson Wax, 1525 Howe St, Racine, WI 53403-5011, USA.

Jolly-Jatel, Fr. Laboratoires Jolly-Jatel, 28 av. Carnot, 78100 Saint-Germain-en-Laye, France.

Jones, USA. Jones Pharma Inc., P.O. Box 46903, St Louis, MO 63146-6903, USA.

Jorba, Spain. Jorba, Spain.

Jouveinal, Canad. Jouveinal Inc., 3339 Griffith St, St Laurent, Quebec, H4T 1W5, Canada.

Jouveinal, Fr. Laboratoires Jouveinal, 1 rue des Moissons, B.P. 100, 94265 Fresnes cdx, France.

JP, Braz. JP Industria Farmaceutica Ltda, Avenida Castelo Branco 999, Lagoinha, 14095-000 Ribierao Preto, SP, Brazil.

Jukunda, Ger. Jukunda Naturarzneimittel Dr Ludwig Schmitt GmbH & Co. KG, Hofmarkstr. 35, 82152 Planegg, Germany.

Julphar, UAE. Gulf Pharmaceutical Industries, Julphar, P.O. Box 997, Ras Al Khaimah, United Arab Emirates.

Juste, Spain. Juste, Julio Camba 7, 28028 Madrid, Spain.

Juventus, Spain. Juventus, Europa Empresarial, Edifico Londres, Calle Playa de Liencres 2, 1 Planta, 28230 Las Rozas Madrid, Spain.

Juvex, Fr. Laboratoires Juvex, B.P. 11, 36110 Levroux, France.

Kabi, Swed. See *Pharmacia, Swed.*

Kabi Pharmacia, Israel. Kabi Pharmacia, Israel.

Kabi Pharmacia, NZ. See *Pharmacia Upjohn, NZ.*

Kabi Pharmacia, USA. See *Pharmacia Upjohn, USA.*

KabiVitrum, UK. See *Pharmacia, UK.*

Kabivitrum, USA. See *Pharmacia Upjohn, USA.*

Kade, Ger. Dr Kade Pharmazeutische Fabrik GmbH, Rigistr. 2, 12277 Berlin, Germany.

Kade, Hong Kong. Kade, Hong Kong.

Kai Yuen, Hong Kong. Kai Yuen Pharmaceuticals Co., 8/F Ngai Wong Commercial Bldg, 11-13 Mongkok Rd, Kowloon, Hong Kong.

Kaken, Hong Kong. See *Hing Ah, Hong Kong.*

Kaken, Jpn. Kaken Pharmaceutical Co. Ltd, 28-8 Honkomagome 2-chome, Bunkyoku, Tokyo 113-8650, Japan.

Kaketsuken, Thai. See *Berli, Thai.*

Kalbe, Singapore. See *Apotheca, Singapore,* and *Sime Darby, Singapore.*

Kali-Chemie, Ger. See *Solvay, Ger.*

Kamada, Israel. Kamada Ltd, Kiryat Weizmann, Rehovot, Israel.

Kanda, Braz. Kanda Industria Farmaceutica Ltda, Rodovia BR 262 Km 12.3 A, 33010-970 Santa Luiza, MG, Brazil.

Kanebo, Jpn. Kanebo, 1-3-12 Motoakasaka, Minato-ku, Tokyo, Japan.

Kanion, Israel. Kanion, Israel.

Kanoldt, Ger. Kanoldt Arzneimittel GmbH, Karl-Zeiss-Ring 3, 85737 Ismaning, Germany.

Karicare, NZ. See *Douglas, NZ,* and *Nutricia, NZ.*

Karrer, Ger. Hans Karrer GmbH, Messerschmittring 54, 86343 Konigsbrunn, Germany.

Kart, Switz. Laboratoires Kart SA, En Budron A 16, 1052 Le Mont-sur-Lausanne, Switzerland.

Katadyn, Fr. Katadyn France, B.P. 39, 77680 Roissy-en-Brie, France.

Kato, Singapore. See *JDH, Singapore.*

Kattwiga, Ger. Pharm. Fabrik Kattwiga GmbH, Zur Grenze 30, 48529 Nordhorn, Germany.

Kavon, USA. Kavon, USA.

Kay, Canad. Mary Kay Cosmetics Ltd, 2020 Meadowvale Blvd, Mississauga, Ontario, L5N 6Y2, Canada.

Kay, USA. Kay, USA.

Kayaku, Jpn. Nippon Kayaku Co. Ltd, 11-2 Fujimi 1-chome, Chiyoda-ku, Tokyo 102-8172, Japan.

Kayaku, Singapore. See *JDH, Singapore.*

KBR, Ital. Kroton Biologic Researches s.r.l., Corso Vittorio Emanuele 73, 88074 Crotone (KR), Italy.

Keene, USA. Keene Pharmaceuticals Inc., P.O. Box 7, Keene, TX 76059-0007, USA.

Kelco International, UK. Kelco International Ltd, Waterfield, Tadworth, Surrey, KT20 5HQ, UK.

Kelemata, Ital. Kelemata s.p.a., Via S Quintino 28, 10121 Turin, Italy.

Keller, Hong Kong. Edward Keller Ltd, 21/F Southmark, 11 Yip Hing St, Wong Chuk Hang, Hong Kong.

Kemifarma, Denm. Kemifarma ApS, Smedeland 26 B, 2600 Glostrup, Denmark.

Kemiflor, Swed. Kemiflor AB, Box 7245, 103 89 Stockholm, Sweden.

Kemiprogress, Ital. Kemiprogress s.r.l., Via Aurelia 58, 00165 Rome, Italy.

Kemopharm, Thai. Kemopharm Thailand Co. Ltd, 138 Soi Indamara 18, Vibhavadi Rangsit Rd, Bangkok 10400, Thailand.

Kemyos, Ital. Kemyos Biomedical Research s.r.l., Via Tre Cannelle 12, 00040 Pomezia (RM), Italy.

Kendall, USA. Kendall Health Care Products, 15 Hampshire St, Mansfield, MA 02048, USA.

Kendall McGaw, USA. See *Braun, USA.*

Kendon, UK. Kendon International Ltd, 8-14 Orsman Rd, London, N1 5QJ, UK.

Kendrick, Mex. Laboratorios Kendrick, S.A., Textitlan No. 42, Col. Santa Ursula Coapa, 04650 Mexico D.F., Mexico.

Kener, Mex. Laboratorios Kener, S.A. de C.V., Blvd. Puerto Aereo No. 151-205, Col. Aviacion Civil, 15740 Mexico D.F, Mexico.

Kenfarma, Spain. Kenfarma, Pechuan 1, 28002 Madrid, Spain.

Kenral, Austral. See *Pharmacia, Austral.*

Kenral, Canad. See *Altimed, Canad.*

Kent, UK. Kent Pharmaceuticals Ltd, Wotton Rd, Ashford, Kent, TN23 6LL, UK.

Kenwood, Hong Kong. See *International Medical, Hong Kong.*

Kenwood, USA. See *Doak, USA.*

Kenyaku, Thai. See *US Summit, Thai.*

Kerifarm, Spain. Kerifarm, Spain.

Kern, Switz. E Kern AG, Pharmazeutische Krauterspezialitaten, Hauptstrasse 23, 8867 Niederurnen, Switzerland.

Kestrel, UK. Kestrel Healthcare Ltd, Network House, Basing View, Basingstoke, Hampshire, RG21 4HG, UK.

Keton, Mex. Keton, Mexico.

Key, Austral. Key Pharmaceuticals P/L, P.O. Box 121, Concord West, NSW 2138, Australia.

Key, Canad. Key, Division of Schering Canada Inc., 3535 Trans-Canada Hwy, Pointe-Claire, Quebec, H9R 1B4, Canada.

Key, Israel. Key, Israel.

Key, USA. See *Schering-Plough, USA.*

Kin, Spain. Kin, Granada 123, 08018 Barcelona, Spain.

Kinder, Braz. Laboratorio Kinder S.A., Avenida Cupece 1783, Jardim Prudencia, 04365-000 Sao Paulo, SP, Brazil.

Kingswood, USA. Kingswood Laboratories Inc., 10375 Hague Rd, Indianapolis, IN 46256, USA.

Kinray, USA. Kinray, 152-35 10th Ave, Whitestone, NY 11357, USA.

Kinsmor, Canad. Kinsmor Pharmaceuticals Canada Inc., 210 Binnington Court, Kingston, Ontario, K7M 8R6, Canada.

Kirin, Jpn. Kirin Brewery Co. Ltd, 10-1 Shinkawa 2-chome, Chuo-ku, Tokyo 104-8288, Japan.

Kirkman, USA. Kirkman Labs Inc., PO Box 1009, Wilsonville, OR 97070-1009, USA.

Kissei, Jpn. Kissei Pharmaceutical Co. Ltd, 19-48 Yoshino, Matsumoto-City, Nagano-Pref. 399-8710, Japan.

Kiwi, USA. Kiwi Brands, Inc., 447 Old Swede Rd, Douglassville, PA 19518-1239, USA.

Klein, Ger. Dr Gustav Klein, Steinenfeld 3, 77736 Zell am Harmersbach, Germany.

Klemenz, Ger. Klemenz GmbH, Hermann-Burkhardt-Str. 3, 72793 Pfullingen, Germany.

Klever, Ger. F. W. Klever GmbH, Hauptstr. 20, 84168 Aham/Ndb., Germany.

KLI, USA. KLI Corp., 1119 Third Ave SW, Carmel, IN 46032, USA.

Klinge, Aust. Klinge Pharma GmbH, Hietzinger Hauptstrasse 64, A-1132 Vienna, Austria.

Klinge, Ger. Klinge Pharma GmbH, Bergam-Laim-Str. 129, 81673 Munich, Germany.

Klinge, Irl. Klinge Pharmaceuticals & Co., The Mews, James Place, Dublin 2, Ireland.

Klinge, Switz. Klinge Pharma AG, Bachstrasse 10, 8280 Kreuzlingen, Switzerland.

Klinger, Braz. Laboratorios Klinger, Rua Assahy 33 1° andar, 09735-520 Sao Bernardo do Campo, SP, Brazil.

Kloster, S.Afr. Kloster Pharmaceuticals (Pty) Ltd, P.O. Box 2734, Paarl 7620, South Africa.

Klosterfrau, Aust. Maria Clementine Martin Klosterfrau GmbH, Doerenkampgasse 11, A-1105 Vienna, Austria.

Klosterfrau, Ger. Maria Clementine Martin Klosterfrau Vertriebsgesellschaft mbH, 50606 Cologne, Germany.

Klus, Switz. Klus-Apotheke, F & Dr J Fröhlich-Decurtins, Hegibachstrasse 102, 8032 Zurich, Switzerland.

Kneipp, Aust. See *Kneipp, Ger.*

Kneipp, Ger. Kneipp-Werke, 97064 Wurzburg, Germany.

Knoll, Austral. Knoll Australia P/L, 15 Orion Rd, Lane Cove, NSW 2066, Australia.

Knoll, Belg. Knoll Belgium S.A., Ave Hamoir 14, 1180 Brussels, Belgium.

Knoll, Braz. Knoll S.A. Produtos Quimicos e Farmaceuticos, Estrada dos Bandeirantes 2400, 27710-104 Rio de Janeiro, RJ, Brazil.

Knoll, Canad. Knoll Pharma Inc., 100 Allstate Parkway, Suite 600, Markham, Ontario, L3R 6H3, Canada.

Knoll, Denm. See *Knoll, Swed.*

Knoll, Fin. See *BASF, Fin.*

Knoll, Fr. Laboratoires Knoll France, 49 av Georges-Pompidou, 92300 Levallois-Perret, France.

Knoll, Ger. Knoll Deutschland GmbH, Rathausplatz 10-12, 67059 Ludwigshafen, Germany.

Knoll, Hong Kong. Knoll China, Division of BASF China Ltd, Tower 1, 9/F South Seas Ctr, 75 Mody Rd, Tsimshatsui East, Kowloon, Hong Kong.

Knoll, Irl. Knoll Ltd, United Drug House, Belgard Rd, Tallaght, Dublin 24, Ireland.

Knoll, Ital. Knoll Farmaceutici s.p.a., Via Europa 35, 20053 Muggio, Italy.

Knoll, Mex. Quimica Knoll de Mexico S.A. de C.V., La Candelaria No.186, Col. Atlantida, 04370 Mexico D.F., Mexico.

Knoll, Neth. Knoll B.V., Postbus 60034, 1320 AA Almese, Netherlands.

Knoll, Norw. See *Knoll, Swed.*

Knoll, NZ. Knoll Australia Pty Ltd, P.O. Box 33-1486, Takapuna, Auckland, New Zealand.

Knoll, Port. Knoll Lusitana, Lda, Rua Alfredo da Silva 3 C/D, 1300-040 Lisbon, Portugal.

Knoll, S.Afr. Knoll Pharmaceuticals (SA) (Ptg) Ltd, P.O. Box 3030, Halfway House 1685, South Africa.

Knoll, Singapore. See *Boots, Singapore,* and *Diethelm, Singapore.*

Knoll, Spain. Knoll Made, Avda de Burgos 91, 28050 Madrid, Spain.

Knoll, Swed. Knoll Läkemedel AB, Haraldsgatan 5, 413 14 Goteborg, Sweden.

Knoll, Switz. Knoll SA, Postfach 631, 4410 Liestal, Switzerland.

Knoll, Thai. See *Pacific, Thai.*

Knoll, UK. Knoll Ltd, 9 Castle Quay, Castle Boulevard, Nottingham, Nottinghamshire, NG7 1FW, UK.

Knoll, USA. Knoll Pharmaceutical Co., 3000 Continental Drive North, Mount Olive, NJ 07828-1234, USA.

Kobayashi, Thai. See *Charoen, Thai.*

Koch, Aust. Edmund Koch, Biol. Heilmittel, Herrenstrasse 2, A-4010 Linz, Austria.

Kohler, Aust. Dr Köhler Pharma GmbH, Steckhovengasse 14, A-1130 Vienna, Austria.

Kohler, Ger. Dr Franz Köhler Chemie GmbH, Neue Bergstr. 3-7, 64665 Alsbach-Hahnlein, Germany.

Kohler, Neth. See *Tramedico, Neth.*

Kohler-Pharma, Ger. Köhler Pharma GmbH, Neue Bergstr. 3-7, 64665 Alsbach, Germany.

Kolassa, Aust. Dr. Kolassa & Merz GmbH, Gastgebgasse 5-13, A-1230 Vienna, Austria.

Kollerics, Aust. Kollerics Helmut, Hauptstrasse 25, A-8061 St Radegund, Austria.

Kondon, USA. Kondon Manufacturing, Croswell, MI 48422, USA.

Konsyl, USA. Konsyl Pharmaceuticals, 4200 South Hulen, Suite 513, Fort Worth, TX 76109, USA.

Kopkins, Braz. Kopkins do Brasil Industria Ltda, Rua Borja Reis 279, 20745-100 Rio de Janeiro, RJ, Brazil.

Kora, Irl. KoRa Healthcare, Frans Maas House, Swords Business Park, Swords, Co. Dublin, Ireland.

Korea Green Cross, Thai. See *Charoen, Thai.*

Korea Green Pharm, Singapore. See *GC, Singapore.*

Korea United, Singapore. See *Kyowa, Singapore,* and *Ziwell, Singapore.*

Korean Drug, Singapore. See *Ziwell, Singapore.*

KOS, USA. Kos Pharm, 2 Oakwood Blvd, Suite 140, Hollywood, FL 33020, USA.

Kottas-Heldenberg, Aust. Kottas-Heldenberg Mag. R.u. Sohn, Bauernmarkt 24, A-1014 Vienna, Austria.

Kowa, Jpn. Kowa, 3-6-29 Nishiki, Naka-ku, Nagoya-shi, Japan.

Kramer, Switz. Kramer-Pharma AG, 46 ave des Boveresses, 1000 Lausanne 21, Switzerland.

Kramer, USA. Kramer Laboratories Inc., 8778 SW 8th St, Miami, FL 33174-9990, USA.

Kreussler, Denm. See *Felo, Denm.*

Kreussler, Fin. See *Tamro, Fin.*

Kreussler, Fr. Laboratoire Kreussler Pharma, 2 rue de la Haye, Le Dome, B.P. 10901, 95731 Roissy-Charles-de-Gaulle cdx, France.

Kreussler, Ger. Chemische Fabrik Kreussler & Co. GmbH, Rheingaustr. 87-93, 65203 Wiesbaden, Germany.

Kreussler, Switz. See *Globopharm, Switz.*

Kreussler, Thai. See *Berlin Pharm, Thai.*

Krewel, Ger. Krewel Meuselbach GmbH, Krewelstr. 2, 53783 Eitorf, Germany.

Krewel, Switz. See *Lubapharm, Switz.*

Kropf, Switz. Dr A & M Kropf-Schenk, Apotheke und Laboratorium Gstaad, Hauptstrasse, 3780 Gstaad, Switzerland.

Krug, Aust. Dr et Mag. Gilbert Krug GmbH, Bernardgasse 26, A-1070 Vienna, Austria.

Krugher, Ital. Krugher Pharma, Via Volturno 10-12, 50019 Sesto Fiorentino (FI), Italy.

Krugmann, Ger. Krugmann GmbH, Mundipharma-Str. 4, 65549 Limburg (Lahn), Germany.

KSL, Canad. KSL Laboratories, 117-260 West Esplanade, North Vancouver, British Columbia, V7M 3G7, Canada.

Kunzle, Switz. Krauterpfarrer Kunzle AG, 6648 Minusio, Switzerland.

Kur und Stadtapotheke, Aust. Kur-und Stadtapotheke, Oberer Stadtplatz 5, A-6060 Hall in Tirol, Austria.

Kuraray, Jpn. Kuraray, Japan.

KV, Hong Kong. See *Hind Wing, Hong Kong.*

Kwizda, Aust. F. Joh. Kwizda Chemische Fabrik, Effingergasse 21, A-1160 Vienna, Austria.

Kyorin, Jpn. Kyorin Pharmaceutical Co. Ltd, 5 Kanda Surugadai 2-chome, Chiyoda-ku, Tokyo 101-8311, Japan.

Kyorin, Thai. Kyorin.

Kyowa, Hong Kong. See *Tai Tong, Hong Kong.*

Kyowa, Jpn. Kyowa Hakko Kogyo Co. Ltd, 1-6-1 Ohtemachi, Chiyoda-ku, Tokyo 100-8185, Japan.

Kyowa, Singapore. Kyowa Hakko Industry (S) Pte Ltd, 300 Orchard Rd, 06-02 The Promenade, S 238861, Singapore.

Kyowa, Thai. Kyowa Hakko (Thailand) Ltd, 101/11 Srinakarin Rd, Suanluang, Bangkok 1010250, Thailand.

Kyowa, UK. Kyowa Hakko (UK) Ltd, 258 Bath Rd, Slough, Berkshire, SL1 4DX, UK.

Kytta, Ger. See *Wyeth, Ger.*

Lab, Port. Laboratórios Lab, Lda, Rua Escola de Medicina Veterinaria 15-17, 1049-029 Lisbon, Portugal.

Lab Francais du Fractionnement, Fr. Lab Francais du Fractionnement et des Biotechnologies, 3 des Tropiques, B.P. 305, 91958 Les Ulis cdx, France.

Labatec, Switz. Labatec-Pharma SA, Case postale 62, 31 rue du Cardinal-Journet, 1217 Meyrin 2, Switzerland.

Labcatal, Canad. Labcatal Inc., 3750 East Cremazie Blvd, Suite 408, Montreal, Quebec, H2A 1B6, Canada.

Labcatal, Fr. Laboratoires Labcatal, 7 rue Roger Salengro, B.P. 305, 92541 Montrouge cdx, France.

Labcatal, Switz. See *Oligosol, Switz.*

Labesfal, Port. Labesfal, SA, Campo de Besteiros, 3465-051 Campo de Besteiros, Portugal.

Labima, Belg. Labima S.A., Ave Van Volxem 328, 1190 Brussels, Belgium.

Labitec, Spain. Labitec, Lope de Rueda 46, 28009 Madrid, Spain.

Labocor, Port. Labocor, Lda, Largo Cidade de Vittoria 7, 2750 Cascais, Portugal.

Labomed, Fr. Labomed, ZAC des Cerisiers, 69380 Lozanne, France.

Labor, Aust. Labor Buchrucker, Aschacher Strasse 1, A-4100 Ottensheim, Austria.

Laboratories for Applied Biology, Hong Kong. See *Swiss Worldwide, Hong Kong.*

Laboratories for Applied Biology, Irl. See *Boileau & Boyd, Irl.*

Laboratories for Applied Biology, Singapore. See *Sime Darby, Singapore.*

Laboratories for Applied Biology, UK. Laboratories for Applied Biology Ltd, 91 Amhurst Park, London, N16 5DR, UK.

Laboratorio Farm., Israel. Laboratorio Farm., Israel.

Laborest, Ital. See *Pharma-Natura, Ital.*

Labormedica, Braz. Labormedica Industrial Ltda, Rua Jose Guide 500, Distrito Industrial, 15035-500 Sao Jose do Rio Preto, SP, Brazil.

Laborsil, Braz. Laborsil Industria Farmaceutica Ltda, Rodovia 160 RN Km 22, 59290-000 Sao Goncalo do Amarante, RN, Brazil.

Lacer, Hong Kong. See *CNW, Hong Kong.*

Lacer, Spain. Lacer, Sardenya 350, 08025 Barcelona, Spain.

Lachartre, Fr. Laboratoires Lachartre SNC, 104 av. Charles-de-Gaulle, 92200 Neuilly-sur-Seine, France.

Lachifarma, Ital. Lachifarma s.r.l., Laboratorio Chimico Farmaceutico Salentino, S.S. 16, Zona Industriale, 73010 Zollino (LE), Italy.

Laclede, Singapore. See *MBD, Singapore.*

Lacoer, Ger. Lacoer Arznei- und Körperpflegemittel GmbH, Barbarastr. 14, 30952 Ronnenberg-Hannover, Germany.

Lactel, Fr. Sté Lactel, ZI Les Touches, 53093 Laval cdx 9, France.

Lacteol, Hong Kong. See *Silroc, Hong Kong.*

Lacteol, Singapore. See *Age D'or, Singapore.*

Lacteol, Switz. See *Uhlmann-Eyraud, Switz.*

Lacteol, Thai. See *Diethelm, Thai.*

Lacteol du Dr Boucard, Fr. Laboratoires du Lactéol du Dr Boucard, Route de Bu, B.P. 41, 78550 Houdan, France.

Laevosan, Aust. Laevosan-Pharma GesellschaftmbH, Estermannstrasse 17, A-4020 Linz, Austria.

Laevosan, Switz. Laevosan International AG, Dufourstrasse 32, 8008 Zurich, Switzerland.

Lafare, Ital. Laboratorio Farmaceutico Reggiano s.r.l., Via S.B. Cozzolino 77, 80056 Ercolano Resina (NA), Italy.

Lafayette, USA. Lafayette Pharmaceuticals Inc., 526 North Earl Ave, Lafayette, IN 47904-4499, USA.

Lafon, Denm. See *Organon, Denm.*

Lafon, Fr. Laboratoires Lafon, 19 av. du Professeur Cadiot, B.P. 22, 94701 Maisons-Alfort cdx, France.

Lafon, Hong Kong. See *Worldwide, Hong Kong.*

Lafran, Fr. Laboratoires Lafran, 1 rte des Stains, 94387 Bonneuil-sur-Marne cdx, France.

Lagamed, S.Afr. Lagamed (Pty) Ltd, South Africa.

Lagap, Hong Kong. See *Hind Wing, Hong Kong.*

Lagap, Switz. Lagap SA, Via San Gottardo 9, 6943 Vezia, Switzerland.

Lagap, UK. Lagap Pharmaceuticals Ltd, 37 Woolmer Way, Bordon, Hampshire, GU35 9QE, UK.

Lainco, Spain. Lainco, Avda Bizet 8-12, Rubi, 08191 Barcelona, Spain.

Lake, USA. Lake Consumer Products Inc., 625 Forest Edge Dr, Vernon Hills, IL 60061, USA.

Lakeside, Mex. Farmecéuticos Lakeside, S.A. de C.V., Huizaches No. 25, Col. Rcho. los Colorines, 14386 Mexico D.F., Mexico.

Lakeside, USA. See *Aventis Pharma, USA.*

Lalco, Canad. See *Nobel, Canad.*

Lambda, USA. See *Bart, USA.*

Lamberts Healthcare, UK. Lamberts Healthcare Ltd, 1 Lamberts Rd, Tunbridge Wells, Kent, TN2 3EQ, UK.

Lampugnani, Ital. Lampugnani Farmaceutici s.p.a., Via Gramsci 4, 20014 Nerviano (Milan), Italy.

Lancome, Canad. See *Cosmair, Canad.*

Lander, Canad. Lander Co. Canada Ltd, 275 Finchdene Square, Scarborough, Ontario, M1X 1C7, Canada.

Landmark, Canad. Landmark Medical Systems Inc, P. O. Box 64575, Unionville, Ontario, L3R 0M9, Canada.

Lane, UK. G.R. Lane Health Products Ltd, Sisson Rd, Gloucester, GL1 3QB, UK.

Lannacher, Aust. Lannacher Heilmittel GmbH, Schlossplatz 1, A-8502 Lannach, Austria.

Lannacher, Denm. See *Nordic Drugs, Denm.*

Lannett, USA. Lannett Inc., 9000 State Rd, Philadelphia, PA 19136, USA.

Laphal, Fr. Laboratoires Laphal, B.P. 7, 13718 Allauch cdx, France.

Laphal, Hong Kong. See *C & L, Hong Kong,* and *Wing Wai, Hong Kong.*

Lapidot, Israel. A. Lapidot Pharmaceuticals Ltd, P.O. Box 3552, Caesaria, Israel.

Lappe, Ger. Produpharm Lappe GmbH, Senefelderstr. 44, 51469 Bergisch Gladbach, Germany.

Laproquifar, Spain. Laproquifar, Las Carolinas 13, 08012 Barcelona, Spain.

L'Arguenon, Fr. See *SERB, Fr.*

Larkhall Laboratories, UK. Larkhall Laboratories, White Horse Business Park, Trowbridge, Wiltshire, BA14 0XQ, UK.

Laroche Navarron, Neth. See *Bournonville, Neth.*

Lasa, Spain. Lasa, Ctra Laurea Miro 385, Sant Feliu de Llobregat, 08980 Barcelona, Spain.

La-Sante, Braz. La-Sante Laboratorios Ltda, Rua Senador Nabuco 49, 24030-160 Rio de Janeiro, RJ, Brazil.

Laser, S.Afr. Laser (Pty) Ltd, South Africa.

Laser, USA. Laser Inc., 2200 W 97th Place, P.O. Box 905, Crown Point, IN 46307, USA.

Laves, Ger. Laves-Arzneimittel GmbH, Barbarastr. 14, 30952 Ronnenberg, Germany.

Lavipharm, Israel. Lavipharm, Israel.

Lavoris-Dep, Canad. Lavoris-Dep Corporation, P. O. Box 1000, Mississauga, Ontario, L4W 3W4, Canada.

LAW, Ger. See *Riemser, Ger.,* and *Wyeth, Ger.*

Layton, USA. Layton, USA.

LBS, Thai. L.B.S. Laboratory Ltd Part, 602 Soi Phanichanant, Sukhumvit 71 Rd, Bangkok 10110, Thailand.

LCA, Fr. Laboratoire LCA, 9 allee Promethee, 28000 Chartres, France.

LCH, Hong Kong. Luen Cheong Hong Ltd, 17/F Caltex House, 258 Hennessy Rd, Wanchai, Hong Kong.

LDM, Fr. LDM Santé, 2 pl Edmond-Puyo, B.P. 129, 29600 Morlaix, France.

Le Marchand, Fr. Laboratoires Le Marchand, 2 bis rue Moussard, 28600 Luisant, France.

Leader, Hong Kong. Leader Pharmaceutical & Cosmetic Co. Ltd, 2/F, 42 Hankow Rd, Kowloon, Hong Kong.

Lebeh, USA. Lebeh, USA.

Lectec, USA. LecTec Corp., 10701 Red Circle Dr., Minnetonka, MN 55343, USA.

LED, Fr. Laboratoires d'Evolution Dermatologique, 7 rue d'Aguesseau, 75008 Paris, France.

Lederle, Austral. See *Wyeth, Austral.*

Lederle, Fr. See *Wyeth Lederle, Fr.*

Lederle, Ger. Lederle Arzneimittel GmbH & Co., Wienburgstr. 207, 48159 Munster, Germany.

Lederle, Hong Kong. See *Whitehall, Hong Kong,* and *Wyeth, Hong Kong.*

Lederle, Irl. See *Wyeth Lederle, Irl.*

Lederle, Israel. See *Neopharm, Israel.*

Lederle, Jpn. See *Wyeth Lederle, Jpn.*

Lederle, Neth. See *AHP, Neth.*

Lederle, NZ. See *Wyeth, NZ.*

Lederle, S.Afr. See *Wyeth, S.Afr.*

Lederle, Switz. See *AHP, Switz.*

Lederle, Thai. Lederle, Thailand.

Lederle, UK. See *Wyeth, UK.*

Lederle, USA. Lederle Professional Medical Services, N Middletown Rd, Pearl River, NY 10965-1299, USA.

Lederle-Praxis, USA. See *Lederle, USA.*

Ledi, Ital. Laboratori Eudermici Italiani s.r.l., Via Augusto Gaudenzi 29, 00163 Rome, Italy.

Lee, USA. Lee Pharmaceuticals, 1434 Santa Anita Blvd, South Elmonte, CA 91733, USA.

Lee-Adams, Canad. Lee-Adams Laboratories, Division of Pharmascience Inc., 6111 Royalmount Ave, Montreal, Quebec, H4P 2T4, Canada.

Leeming, USA. See *Pfizer, USA.*

Lefevre, Fr. Laboratoires du Dr J. Lefèvre-Albrenor S.A., 82 rue National, 57350 Stiring-Wendel, France.

Legere, USA. Legere Pharmaceuticals, 7326 E. Evans Rd, Scottsdale, AZ 85260, USA.

Legon, Ital. Legon Farmaceutici s.r.l., Via Tronto 14, 00198 Rome, Italy.

Legrand, Braz. Legrand, Brazil.

Lehning, Fr. Laboratoires Lehning, 1-3 rue du Petit-Marais, 57640 Sainte-Barbe, France.

Leiras, Denm. See *Ferring, Denm.,* and *Schering, Denm.*

Leiras, Fin. Leiras Oy, PL 325, 00101 Helsinki, Finland.

Leiras, Israel. Leiras, Israel.

Leiras, Norw. See *Schering, Norw.*

Leiras, Singapore. See *MBD, Singapore.*

Leiras, Swed. Leiras, Division av Schering Nordiska AB, Box 23117, 104 35 Stockholm, Sweden.

Leiras, Thai. See *Berli, Thai.,* and *Olic, Thai.*

Leiras Synthelabo, Fin. See *Leiras, Fin.*

Lek, Hong Kong. See *Hind Wing, Hong Kong.*

Lek, Thai. See *RX, Thai.*

Leman, Fr. Dietetique du Leman SA, 9 av. Saint-Francois-de-Sales, 74205 Thonon-les-Bains cdx, France.

Lemery, Mex. Lemery S.A. de C.V., Martires de Rio Blanco No. 54, 16030 Mexico D.F., Mexico.

Lemery, Thai. See *Pharmaland, Thai.*

Lemmon, USA. See *Teva, USA.*

Lemoine, Fr. Laboratoires Lemoine, Imm le Doublon, bat B, 11 av. Dubonnet, 92400 Courbevoie, France.

Lennod, USA. Lennod, USA.

Lennon, S.Afr. See *SA Druggists, S.Afr.*

Lennon, UK. Lennon Pharmaceuticals, Tuition House, 27/37 St George's Rd, Wimbledon, London, SW19 4EU, UK.

Lensa, Spain. Lensa, Potosi 2-4, 08030 Barcelona, Spain.

Lentheric, UK. Lentheric Ltd, Amertrans Park, Bushey Mill Lane, Watford, Hertfordshire, WD2 4JG, UK.

Leo, Aust. Leo Pharma GesellschafftmbH, Floragasse 7, A-1040 Vienna, Austria.

Leo, Belg. Leo Pharma S.A., Excelsiorlaan 40-2, 1930 Zaventem, Belgium.

Leo, Canad. Leo Pharma Inc., 555 Kingston Rd W., Ajax, Ontario, L1S 6M1, Canada.

Leo, Denm. Leo Løvens Kemiske Fabrik A/S, Industriparken 55, 2750 Ballerup, Denmark.

Leo, Fin. Leo Pharma Oy, Rajatorpantie 41 C, 01640 Vantaa, Finland.

Leo, Fr. Laboratoires Leo, B.P. 311, 78054 St-Quentin-Yvelines cdx, France.

Leo, Ger. Leo Pharma GmbH, Frankfurter Str. 233, A3, 63263 Neu-Isenburg, Germany.

Leo, Hong Kong. See *Keller, Hong Kong.*

Leo, Irl. Leo Laboratories Ltd, 285 Cashel Rd, Dublin 12, Ireland.

Leo, Israel. Leo, Israel.

Leo, Neth. Leo Pharmaceutical Products B.V., Postbus 51, 1380 AB Weesp, Netherlands.

Leo, Norw. Leo Pharma AS, Postboks 193 Lilleaker, 0216 Oslo, Norway.

Leo, NZ. See *CSL, NZ.*

Leo, Port. Leo-Farmaceutics, Lda, Av das Nacoes Unidas 27, 1600-531 Lisbon, Portugal.

Leo, Singapore. Leo Pharma Singapore, 19 Loyang Way, 06-29, S 508724, Singapore.

Leo, Swed. Leo Pharma AB, Box 404, 201 24 Malmo, Sweden.

Leo, Switz. Leo Pharmaceutical Products Sarath Ltd, Eggbuhlstrasse 28, 8052 Zurich, Switzerland.

Leo, Thai. See *Olic, Thai.*

Leo, UK. Leo Pharmaceuticals, Longwick Rd, Princes Risborough, Buckinghamshire, HP27 9RR, UK.

Leofarma, Braz. Leofarma Comercio e Industria Ltda, Avenida Getulio Vargas 645, 36700-000 Leopoldina, MG, Brazil.

Leopold, Aust. Leopold Pharma GmbH, Hafnerstrasse 36, A-8055 Graz, Austria.

Lepetit, Ital. Gruppo Lepetit s.p.a., Viale Gran Sasso 18, 20131 Milan, Italy.

Lepori, Port. L. Lepori, Lda, R. da Imprensa Nacional, 86/88, 1250-127 Lisbon, Portugal.

Lerads, Fr. Lerads, 11 rue Rontgen, 29000 Quimper, France.

Lesourd, Fr. Laboratoires Gabriel Lesourd, 6 rue Ste-Isaure, 75018 Paris, France.

Lessel, Braz. Lessel, Brazil.

Lesvi, Spain. Lesvi, Plg. Ind. Can Pelegri, Argent 1, Castellbisbal, 08755 Barcelona, Spain.

Leti, Spain. Leti, Gran Via de las Corts Catalanes 184, 08004 Barcelona, Spain.

Leurquin, Fr. Laboratoires Leurquin Mediolanum, 68/88 rue Ampere, 93330 Neuilly-sur-Marne, France.

Leurquin, Hong Kong. See *Silroc, Hong Kong.*

Leurquin, Switz. See *Uhlmann-Eyraud, Switz.*

Lever Pond's, Canad. Lever Pond's Canada, 1 Sunlight Park Rd, Toronto, ON, M4M 1B6, Canada.

Levofarma, Ital. Levofarma s.r.l., Via Conforti 42, 84083 Castel San Giorgio (SA), Italy.

Lexis, USA. Lexis Laboratories, P.O. Box 202887, Austin, TX 78720, USA.

Leyh, Ger. Leyh Pharma GmbH, Gewerbegebiet Baierstal, 98596 Trusetal, Germany.

LG Chem, Thai. See *Pasteur Merieux, Thai.*

Liade, Spain. Liade, Avda de Burgos 91, 28050 Madrid, Spain.

Libbs, Braz. Libbs Farmaceutica Ltda, Rua Raul Pompeia 1.103, Vila Pompeia, 05025-011 Sao Paulo, SP, Brazil.

Lichtenheldt, Ger. Lichtenheldt GmbH, Pharmazeutische Fabrik, Justus-Liebig-Weg 1, 23812 Wahlstedt, Germany.

Lichtenstein, Ger. Lichtenstein Pharmazeutica GmbH & Co., Industriestrasse 26, 56218 Mulheim-Karlich, Germany.

Lichtwer, Aust. See *Lichtwer, Ger.*

Lichtwer, Ger. Lichtwer Pharma AG, Wallenroder Str. 8-10, 13435 Berlin, Germany.

Lichtwer, Switz. See *Adroka, Switz.*

Lichtwer, UK. Lichtwer Pharma UK, Regency House, Mere Park, Dedmere Rd, Marlow, Buckinghamshire, SL7 1FJ, UK.

Liebermann, Aust. See *Liebermann, Ger.*

Liebermann, Ger. Pharma Liebermann GmbH, Hauptstr. 27, 89423 Gundelfingen/Do., Germany.

Lierac, Fr. Laboratoires Liérac, 35 av Franklin-Roosevelt, 75008 Paris, France.

Life, Ger. Life Pharma GmbH, Frigenstr. 5, 67065 Ludwigshafen, Germany.

Life, Israel. Life, Israel.

Life Essence, UK. See *Elder, UK.*

Life Plus, UK. Life Plus Europe Ltd, Martin House, Howard Rd, Eaton Socon, Cambridgeshire, PE19 3ET, UK.

Lifepharma, Ital. Lifepharma s.p.a., Via dei Lavoratori 54, 20092 Cinisello Balsamo (MI), Italy.

Lifeplan, UK. Lifeplan Products, Elizabethan Way, Lutterworth, Leicestershire, LE17 4ND, UK.

Liferpal, Mex. Liferpal MD, S.A. de C.V., Refineria No. 1266, Col. Alamo Industrial, 44490 Guadalajara, Jal., Mexico.

Lifescan, Fr. Lab. Lifescan, Division d'Ortho-Clinical Diagnostics, 1 rue Camille-Desmoulins, TSA 40007, 92787 Issy-les-Moulineaux cdx 9, France.

Lifescan, Irl. See *Cahill May Roberts, Irl.*

Lifescan, Port. See *Johnson & Johnson, Port.*

Lifescan, USA. Lifescan, 1000 Gibraltar, Milpitas, CA 95035-6312, USA.

Lifesign, USA. LifeSign LLC, 71 Veronica Way, P.O. Box 218, Somerset, NJ 08875-0218, USA.

Lifetech, Hong Kong. Lifetech Enterprises Inc., 22/F, New World Tower II, 18 Queen's Rd Central, Hong Kong.

Ligand, Canad. See *Ligand, USA.*

Ligand, USA. Ligand Pharmaceuticals Inc., 10275 Science Center Dr, San Diego, CA 92121, USA.

Li-il, Ger. Li-iL GmbH Arzneimittel, Leipziger Str. 300, 01139 Dresden, Germany.

Lilly, Aust. Eli Lilly GmbH (Austria), Barichgasse 40-2, A-1030 Vienna, Austria.

Lilly, Austral. Eli Lilly Australia P/L, 112 Wharf Rd, West Ryde, NSW 2114, Australia.

Lilly, Belg. Eli Lilly Benelux S.A., Rue de l'Etuve 52, 1000 Brussels, Belgium.

Lilly, Braz. Eli Lilly do Brasil Ltda, Avenida Morumbi 8264, 04703-002 Sao Paulo, SP, Brazil.

Lilly, Canad. Eli Lilly Canada Inc., 3650 Danforth Ave, Scarborough, Ontario, M1N 2E8, Canada.

Lilly, Denm. Eli Lilly Denmark A/S, Nybrovej 110, 2800 Lyngby, Denmark.

Lilly, Fin. Oy Eli Lilly Finland AB, Rajatorpantie 41 C 3. krs, PL 16, 01641 Vantaa, Finland.

Lilly, Fr. Lilly France, 203 bureaux de la Colline, 92213 Saint-Cloud, France.

Lilly, Ger. Lilly Deutschland GmbH, Saalburgstr. 153, 61350 Bad Homburg, Germany.

Lilly, Hong Kong. Eli Lilly Asia Inc., 3/F, Hua Fu Commercial Bldg, 111 Queen's Rd West, Hong Kong.

Lilly, Irl. Eli Lilly & Co. (Ireland) Ltd, 44 Fitzwilliam Place, Dublin 2, Ireland.

Lilly, Israel. Eli Lilly Israel Ltd, P.O. Box 2160, Herzliya Pituah, Israel.

Lilly, Ital. Eli Lilly Italia s.p.a., Via Gramsci 731/733, 50019 Sesto Fiorentino (FI), Italy.

Lilly, Jpn. Eli Lilly Japan K.K., Sannomiya Plaza Bldg, 1-5 Isogami-dori 7-chome, Chuo-ku, Kobe 651-0086, Japan.

Lilly, Mex. Eli Lilly y Compania de México, S.A. de C.V., Calz de Tlalpan No. 2024, Col Campestre Churubusco, 04200 Mexico, D.F., Mexico.

Lilly, Neth. Eli Lilly Nederland, Krijtwal 17-23, 3432 ZT Nieuwegein, Netherlands.

Lilly, Norw. Eli Lilly Norway A.S, PB 6090 Etterstad, 0601 Oslo, Norway.

Lilly, NZ. Eli Lilly & Co. (NZ) Ltd, P.O. Box 97-046, South Auckland Mail Centre, Wiri, Auckland, New Zealand.

Lilly, Port. Lilly Farma, Lda, Rua Dr Antonio Loureiro Borges, 4, Arquiparque, Miraflores, 1495-131 Alges, Portugal.

Lilly, S.Afr. Eli Lilly (SA) (Pty) Ltd, Private Bag X119, Brynston 2021, South Africa.

Lilly, Singapore. Eli Lilly Asia Pacific Pte Ltd, 16-01 Parkway Parade, 80 Marine Parade Rd, S 449269, Singapore.

Lilly, Spain. Lilly, Avda de la Industria 30, Alcobendas, 28100 Madrid, Spain.

Lilly, Swed. Eli Lilly Sweden AB, Box 30037, 104 25 Stockholm, Sweden.

Lilly, Switz. Eli Lilly (Suisse) SA, 16 Ch. des Coquelicots, Case postale 580, 1214 Vernier/GE, Switzerland.

Lilly, Thai. Eli Lilly Asia Inc. Thailand Branch, 14 Fl, Grand Amarin Tower, 1550 New Petchburi Rd, Makasan Rachtavee, Bangkok 10320, Thailand.

Lilly, UK. Eli Lilly & Co. Ltd, Dextra Court, Chapel Hill, Basingstoke, Hampshire, RG21 5SY, UK.

Lilly, USA. Eli Lilly & Co., Lilly Corporate Center, Indianapolis, IN 46285, USA.

Lina, UK. Lina Trading Ltd, P.O. Box 2341, London, W1A 2NZ, UK.

Lincoln, NZ. See *Douglas, NZ.*

Lincoln, UK. Lincoln Medical Ltd, 37/39 Burton St, Melton Mowbray, Leicestershire, LE13 1AF, UK.

Lindopharm, Ger. Lindopharm GmbH, Neustr. 82, 40721 Hilden, Germany.

Lineafarm, Spain. Lineafarm, Spain.

Link, Austral. Link Medical Products P/L, P.O. Box 135, Avalon Beach, NSW 2107, Australia.

Link, Irl. See *Intra Pharma, Irl.*

Link, UK. Link Pharmaceuticals Ltd, Bishops Weald House, Albion Way, Horsham, West Sussex, RH12 1AH, UK.

Linobion, Aust. Linobion Chem.-pharm. Laboratorium, Kardinal-Nagl-Platz 1, A-1030 Vienna, Austria.

Linotar, Austral. Linotar P/L, P.O. Box 17, Terrey Hills, NSW 2084, Australia.

Linton, S.Afr. M Linton, South Africa.

Lioh, Canad. LIOH. Inc., 5950 Cote de Liesse, Mont-Royal, Ontario, H4T 1E2, Canada.

Liomont, Mex. Laboratorios Liomont, S.A. de C.V., Adolfo Lopez Mateos No.68, 05000 Mexico, D.F., Mexico.

Lipha, Denm. See *Merck, Denm.*

Lipha, Fr. See *Lipha Sante, Fr.*

Lipha, Hong Kong. See *Inchcape, Hong Kong.*

Lipha, Irl. See *Merck, Irl.*

Lipha, Ital. Lipha s.p.a., Via G. Garibaldi 80/82, 50041 Calenzano (FI), Italy.

Lipha, Norw. See *Merck, Norw.*

Lipha, Switz. See *Merck, Switz.*

Lipha, UK. See *Merck, UK.*

Lipha Sante, Fr. Lipha Santé, 37 rue St-Romain, 69008 Lyon, France.

Liphaderm, Fr. See *Lipha Sante, Fr.*

Liposome Company, Aust. See *Liposome Company, UK.*

Liposome Company, Denm. See *Wyeth Lederle, Denm.*

Liposome Company, Hong Kong. See *Zuellig, Hong Kong.*

Liposome Company, Irl. See *Central, Irl.*

Liposome Company, Ital. Liposome s.r.l. c/o Lipartiti Dr. Giovanni, P.za dei Consoli 11, 00175 Rome, Italy.

Liposome Company, Norw. See *Wyeth Lederle, Norw.*

Liposome Company, Singapore. See *Summit, Singapore.*

Liposome Company, Switz. Liposome S.á.r.l., En Budron D5, 1052 Le Mont-sur-Lausanne, Switzerland.

Liposome Company, UK. The Liposome Company Ltd, 3 Shortlands, Hammersmith International Centre, London, W6 8EH, UK.

Liposome Company, USA. The Liposome Company Inc., One Research Way, Princeton, NJ 08540-6619, USA.

Liquipharm, USA. Liquipharm, 10716 McCune Avenue, Los Angeles, CA 90034, USA.

Lisapharm, Fr. Laboratoires Lisa-Pharm, 49 rue de Billancourt, 92100 Boulogne, France.

Lisapharm, Israel. Lisapharm, Israel.

Lisapharma, Hong Kong. See *Mekim, Hong Kong.*

Lisapharma, Ital. Lisapharma s.p.a., Via Licinio 11, 22036 Erba (Como), Italy.

Lisapharma, Singapore. See *Zyfas, Singapore.*

Lisapharma, Thai. See *Charoen, Thai., SPB, Thai.,* and *Sriprasit, Thai.*

Lision Hong, Hong Kong. Lision Hong, Flat G, 7/F Valiant Industrial Ctr, 2-12 Au Pui Wan St, Fo Tan, N.T., Hong Kong.

Lizofarm, Ital. Lizofarm s.r.l., Via S. Gottardo 37, 20052 Monza (MI), Italy.

Llano, Spain. Llano, Spain.

Llorens, Spain. Llorens, Ciudad de Balaguer 7-11, 08022 Barcelona, Spain.

Llorente, Spain. Llorente, Ctra el Pardo Km 1, 28035 Madrid, Spain.

Llorente Generic, Spain. Llorente Generic, Autovia M-30, Km 24.5, 28035 Madrid, Spain.

Lloyd, Aimee, UK. Lloyd, Aimee & Co. Ltd, Kingsend House, 44 Kingsend, Ruislip, Middlesex, HA4 7DA, UK.

Locatelli, Ital. Farmaceutici Locatelli s.r.l., Via Campobello 15, 00040 Pomezia (Rome), Italy.

Lofarma, Ital. Lofarma spa, Viale Cassala 40, 20143 Milan, Italy.

Lofthouse of Fleetwood, Canad. Lofthouse of Fleetwood, 600 Alden Rd, Suite 102, Markham, Ontario, L3R 0E7, Canada.

Logeais, Fr. See *Chiesi, Fr.*

Logeais, Hong Kong. See *CNW, Hong Kong.*

Loges, Ger. Dr. Loges & Co. GmbH Arzneimittel, Schutzenstr. 5, 21423 Winsen, Germany.

Loges, Hong Kong. See *Lision Hong, Hong Kong.*

Logic, Denm. Logic aps, Vassingerodvej 145, 3450 Lynge, Denmark.

Logomed, Ger. Logomed Pharma GmbH, Eckenheimer Landstr. 100-4, Postfach 11 13 53, 60048 Frankfurt/Main, Germany.

Logosys, Ger. Logosys GmbH, Germany.

Lohmann, Ger. Lohmann & Rauscher International GmbH & Co. KG, Westerwaldstr. 4, 56579 Rengsdorf, Germany.

Lohmann, Ital. Lohmann & Rauscher s.r.l., Via E. Fermi 4, 35030 Sarmeola di Rubano, Italy.

Lomapharm, Ger. Lomapharm, Rudolf Lohmann GmbH KG, Langes Feld 5, 31860 Emmerthal, Germany.

Lomapharm, Singapore. See *Polymedic, Singapore.*

London Drugs, Canad. London Drugs Ltd, 12831 Horseshoe Place, Richmond, British Colombia, V7A 4X5, Canada.

Lopes, Braz. Lopes, Brazil.

L'Oreal, Canad. See *Cosmair, Canad.*

Loren, Mex. Laboratorios Farmaceuticos Loren S.A. de C.V., Km. 91 Carr. Feceral Mexico-Puebla, Corredor Industrial Quetzalcoatl, 74160 Huejotzingo, Pue, Mexico.

Lorex, Denm. See *Searle, Denm.*

Lorex, Irl. See *Allphar, Irl.*

Lorex Synthelabo, Irl. See *Allphar, Irl.*

Lorex Synthelabo, Neth. Lorex Synthélabo B.V., Postbus 1401, 3600 BK Maarssen, Netherlands.

Lorvic, Canad. See *Prof. Pharm. Corp., Canad.*

Lorvic, USA. See *Young, USA.*

Lotus, USA. Lotus Biochemical Corp., P.O. Box 485, Bristol, TN 37620, USA.

Lovens, Swed. Lövens Läkemedel AB, Box 404, 201 24 Malmo, Sweden.

Loveridge, UK. J.M. Loveridge PLC, Southbrook Rd, Southampton, Hampshire, SO15 1BH, UK.

LPB, Ital. LPB Istituto Farmaceutico s.p.a., S.S. Varesina km 20.5, 21040 Origgio (VA), Italy.

LPN, Fr. Laboratoire Pharmaceutique Noroit, 7 rue Jean-Baptiste Clement, 94250 Gentilly, France.

LRC, Israel. LRC, Israel.

LRC Products, UK. LRC Products Ltd, London International House, Turnford Place, Broxbourne, Hertfordshire, EN10 6LN, UK.

LSP, Thai. Lerd Singh Pharmaceutical Fact Ltd Part, 922 Sukhumvit 50, Prakanong, Klongtoey, Bangkok 10250, Thailand.

LTM, Neth. See *Vemedia, Neth.*

LTS, Israel. LTS, Israel.

Lu Chem, USA. Lu Chem Pharmaceuticals Inc., 8910 Linwood Ave, P.O. Box 6038, Shreveport, LA 71106, USA.

Lubapharm, Switz. Lubapharm SA, Ringstrasse 29, Postfach 434, 4106 Therwil, Switzerland.

Lubapharm Arlesheim, Switz. Lubapharm AG, Postfach 348, 4144 Arlesheim, Switzerland.

Lubapharm Phlebologie, Switz. See *Lubapharm, Switz.*

Lucchini, Ital. Lucchini Italiana s.r.l., Via S. Anna 2, 03012 Anagni (FR), Italy.

Lucchini, Switz. Laboratoire Lucchini SA, 7 place du Molard, 1204 Geneva, Switzerland.

Luchon, Fr. Laboratoires de Luchon, 22 bd Dardenne, 31110 Luchon, France.

Ludwig, Singapore. See *Apotheca, Singapore.*

Luen Wah, Singapore. Luen Wah Medical Co (S) Pte Ltd, 84 South Bridge Rd, 05-00 Lueng Kai Fook Building, S 058714, Singapore.

Luhr-Lehrs, Ger. A Lühr-Lehrs Arzneimittel & Präventivprodukte, Hohler Weg 12, 53902 Bad Munstereifel-Berresheim, Germany.

Luitpold, Belg. See *Will-Pharma, Belg.*

Luitpold, Braz. Luitpold Produtos Farmaceuticos Ltda, Alameda Xingu 766, 06455-960 Barueri, SP, Brazil.

Luitpold, Ger. Luitpold Pharma GmbH, Zielstattstr. 9, 81379 Munich, Germany.

Luitpold, Ital. Luitpold s.p.a., Via Montecassiano 157, 00156 Rome, Italy.

Luitpold, Neth. See *Will-Pharma, Neth.*

Lundbeck, Aust. Lundbeck-Arzneimittel GmbH, Brigittagasse 22-6, Postfach 201, A-1201 Vienna, Austria.

Lundbeck, Austral. Lundbeck Australia P/L, P.O. Box 6300, Baulkham Hills Business Centre, NSW 2153, Australia.

Lundbeck, Belg. Lundbeck S.A., Ave Moliere 225, 1050 Brussels, Belgium.

Lundbeck, Canad. Lundbeck Canada Inc., 413 St-Jacques St W, Suite FB-230, Montreal, Quebec, H2Y 1N9, Canada.

Lundbeck, Denm. Lundbeck Pharma A/S, Dalbergstroget 5, 2630 Taastrup, Denmark.

Lundbeck, Fin. Oy H. Lundbeck AB, Lemminkäisenkatu 14-18 B, 20520 Turku, Finland.

Lundbeck, Fr. Laboratoires Lundbeck, 37 av Pierre-1er-de-Serbie, 75008 Paris, France.

Lundbeck, Ger. Lundbeck GmbH & Co., Amsinckstr. 59, 20097 Hamburg, Germany.

Lundbeck, Hong Kong. See *Inchcape, Hong Kong.*

Lundbeck, Irl. Lundbeck (Ireland) Ltd, 14 Deansgrange Industrial Estate, Dublin 11, Ireland.

Lundbeck, Israel. See *Lapidot, Israel.*

Lundbeck, Ital. Lundbeck Italia s.p.a., Via Fara 35, 20124 Milan, Italy.

Lundbeck, Neth. Lundbeck B.V., Postbus 12021, 1100 AA Amsterdam Z.O., Netherlands.

Lundbeck, Norw. H. Lundbeck A/S, Lysaker torg 10, 1326 Lysaker, Norway.

Lundbeck, NZ. See *Lundbeck, Austral.*

Lundbeck, S.Afr. Lundbeck South Africa, P.O. Box 2357, Randburg 2125, South Africa.

Lundbeck, Singapore. See *JDH, Singapore.*

Lundbeck, Spain. Lundbeck España, Avda Diagonal 605, 08028 Barcelona, Spain.

Lundbeck, Swed. H. Lundbeck AB, Box 23, 250 53 Helsingborg, Sweden.

Lundbeck, Switz. Lundbeck (Schweiz) AG, Cherstrasse 4, Postfach, 8152 Opfikon-Glattbrugg, Switzerland.

Lundbeck, Thai. See *Hua, Thai.*

Lundbeck, UK. Lundbeck Ltd, Sunningdale House, Caldecotte Lake Business Park, Caldecotte, Milton Keynes, MK7 8LF, UK.

Lunsco, USA. Lunsco Inc., 4657 Wurno Rd, Pulaski, VA 24301, USA.

Luond, Switz. Pharma Lüond, Bahnhofstrasse 17-19, 8280 Kreuzlingen, Switzerland.

Luper, Braz. Luper Industria Farmaceutica Ltda, Rua Doutor Clementino 608, 03059-030 Sao Paulo, SP, Brazil.

Lusofarmaco, Hong Kong. See *Mekim, Hong Kong.*

Lusofarmaco, Ital. Istituto Lusofarmaco d'Italia s.p.a., Via Carnia 26, 20132 Milan, Italy.

Lusofarmaco, Port. Instituto Lusofármaco, Lda, Av. das Forcas Armades no. 125, 1600 Lisbon, Portugal.

Lutsia, Fr. Laboratoires Lutsia, 35 rue Baudin, 92593 Levallois-Perret cdx, France.

Lutsia, Ital. See *Boots Healthcare, Ital.*

Luvabec, Canad. Luvabec Laboratories Inc., 11177 rue Hamon, Montreal, Quebec, H3M 3E4, Canada.

Luvos, Ger. Heilerde-Gesellschaft Luvos Just GmbH & Co., Otto-Hahn-Str. 23, Postfach: 47, 6382 Friedrichsdorf 2, Germany.

Lyocentre, Fr. Laboratoires Lyocentre, 24 av Georges Pompidou, 15004 Aurillac cdx, France.

Lyon, Switz. Lyron AG, Postfach 3538, 4002 Basle, Switzerland.

Lysoform, Ger. Lysoform Dr. Hans Rosemann GmbH, Kaiser-Wilhelm-Str. 133, 12247 Berlin, Germany.

M & H, Thai. M & H Manufacturing Co. Ltd, 27/2-3 Wireless Rd, Bangkok 10330, Thailand.

Maabarot, Israel. Maabarot, Kibbutz Ma'abarot, Israel.

Mabo, Spain. Mabo Farma, Ctra M-300 Km, 30.5, Alcala de Henares, 28820 Madrid, Spain.

Mac, Ital. Mac Pharma s.a.s., Via Onaro 22, 33037 Rio S Martino di Scorze (VE), Italy.

Macarthur, Austral. Macarthur Research, Division of Syntex Australia P/L, P.O. Box 255, Dee Why, NSW 2099, Australia.

Mack, Belg. See *Vitalpharma, Belg.*

Mack, Denm. See *Kemifarma, Denm.*

Mack, Hong Kong. See *Keller, Hong Kong.*

Mack, Neth. See *Astra, Neth.*

Mack, Singapore. See *Summit, Singapore.*

Mack, Switz. See *Pfizer, Switz.*

Mack, Thai. See *Zambon, Thai.*

Mack, Illert., Ger. Heinrich Mack Nachf. GmbH & Co. KG, ein Unternehmen der Pfizer-Gruppe, Heinrich-Mack-Str. 35, 89257 Illertissen, Germany.

Macsil, USA. Macsil Inc., P.O. Box 29276, Philadelphia, PA 19125-0976, USA.

Madariaga, Spain. Madariaga, Electronica, 7.- Poligono, Urtinsa II, Alcorcon, 28923 Madrid, Spain.

Madaus, Aust. Madaus GmbH, Lienfeldergasse 91-3, A-1171 Vienna, Austria.

Madaus, Belg. Madaus Pharma S.A., Rue des Trois Arbres 16, 1180 Brussels, Belgium.

Madaus, Fin. See *Schering-Plough, Fin.*

Madaus, Fr. Laboratoires Madaus, 55 bis, quai de Grenelle, Immeuble Mercure III, 75015 Paris, France.

Madaus, Ger. Madaus AG, Ostmerheimer Str. 198, 51109 Cologne, Germany.

Madaus, Hong Kong. See *Trinity, Hong Kong.*

Madaus, Israel. Madaus, S.L.E., P.O. Box 8077, Netanya, Israel.

Madaus, Ital. Madaus s.r.l., Via Galvani 33, 39100 Bolzano, Italy.

Madaus, Neth. See *Byk, Neth.*

Madaus, S.Afr. Madaus Pharmaceuticals (Pty) Ltd, South Africa.

Madaus, Spain. Madaus Cerafarm, Foc 68-82, 08038 Barcelona, Spain.

Madaus, Switz. See *Biomed, Switz.*

Madaus, Thai. See *Oui Heng, Thai.*

Maeil, Hong Kong. Maeil HK, 17A China Trade Ctr, 122-124 Wai Yip St, Kwun Tong, Kowloon, Hong Kong.

Maffioli, Ital. Prodotti Dott. Maffioli sas di A. Labruzzo & C., Via Firenze 40, 20060 Trezzano Rosa (MI), Italy.

Maggioni, Ital. Maggioni S.p.A., Via Zambeletti, 20021 Baranzate di Bollate (MI), Italy.

Magis, Ital. Magis Farmaceutici s.p.a., Via Cacciamali 34-36-38, Zona Ind. (Loc. Noce), 25125 Brescia, Italy.

Magistra, Switz. Laboratoires Magistra SA, 28 Chemin du Grand-Puits, Case postale 122, 1217 Meyrin 2/Geneva, Switzerland.

Mahdeen, Canad. Mahdeen Mediceuticals, Division of Canmax Laboratories, 6600 Kennedy Rd, 4, Mississauga, Ontario, L5T 2M9, Canada.

Main Life, Hong Kong. Main Life Corp. Ltd, 9/F Winning Ctr, 46-48 Wyndham St Central, Hong Kong.

Major, USA. Major Pharmaceuticals, 31778 Enterprise Dr, Livonia, MI 48150, USA.

Makara, Aust. Makara Pharm GmbH, A-6234 Brandenberg 19C, Austria.

Makros, Braz. Makros Industria Farmaceutica Ltda, Rua Riachuelo 410, 20230-013 Rio de Janeiro, RJ, Brazil.

Malam, UK. Malam Laboratories Ltd, 37 Oakwood Rise, Heaton, Bolton, BL1 5EE, UK.

Malayan, Hong Kong. See *Hind Wing, Hong Kong.*

Malaysia Chemist, Singapore. Malaysia Chemist Pte Ltd, 104 Boon Keng Rd, 04-01, S 339775, Singapore.

Malesci, Ital. Malesci Istituto Farmacobiologico s.p.a., Via Lungo l'Ema 7, 50015 Bagno a Ripoli (FI), Italy.

Mallard, USA. Mallard Medical Products, 81 Corbett Way, Eatontown, NJ 07724-2264, USA.

Mallinckrodt, Aust. Mallinckrodt Medical GmbH, Europaring F09, 4 Stock, A-2345 Brunn/Ge, Austria.

Mallinckrodt, Austral. Mallinckrodt Australia P/L, P.O. Box 2442, Rowville, VIC 3178, Australia.

Mallinckrodt, Canad. Mallinckrodt Medical Inc., 7500 Trans-Canada Highway, Pointe-Claire, Quebec, H9R 5H8, Canada.

Mallinckrodt, Denm. Mallinckrodt Sweden, Informationkontor Danmark, Nivapark 48, 2990 Niva, Denmark.

Mallinckrodt, Ger. Mallinckrodt Medical GmbH, Josef-Dietzgen-Str. 1-3, 53773 Hennef, Germany.

Mallinckrodt, Port. Mallinckrodt Medical, Lda, Quinta da Bela Vista, Rua Ilha das Flores Lote H - Loja A, Sassoeiros, 2775-709 Carcavelos, Portugal.

Mallinckrodt, Spain. Mallinckrodt Iberica, Avda San Pablo 28, Coslada, 28820 Madrid, Spain.

Mallinckrodt, Swed. Mallinckrodt Sweden, Box 397, 581 04 Linkoping, Sweden.

Mallinckrodt, UK. Mallinckrodt Medical UK Ltd, 10 Talisman Business Centre, London Rd, Bicester, Oxfordshire, OX6 0JX, UK.

Mallinckrodt, USA. Mallinckrodt Medical Inc., 675 McDonnell Blvd, P.O. Box 5840, St Louis, MO 63134, USA.

Malpharm, Hong Kong. See *International Medical, Hong Kong.*

Mandri, Spain. Mandri, Pau Claris 182, 08037 Barcelona, Spain.

Manetti Roberts, Ital. L. Manetti H. Roberts & C. per Azioni, Via Baldanzese 177, 50041 Calenzano (FI), Italy.

Mann, Ger. Dr Gerhard Mann, Chem.-pharm. Fabrik GmbH, Brunsbutteler Damm 165-73, 13581 Berlin, Germany.

Mann, Irl. See *Pharma-Global, Irl.*

Mann, Neth. See *Tramedico, Neth.*

Mann, Singapore. See *Indrugco, Singapore.*

Mann, Thai. See *Zuellig, Thai.*

Manne, USA. Manne, P.O. Box 825, Johns Island, SC 29457, USA.

Manon, Israel. Manon Ltd, P.O. Box 3905, Tel Aviv, Israel.

Manor, UK. Manor Drug Co. (Nottingham) Ltd., Manor House, Merlin Way, Quarry Hill Rd, Ilkeston, Derbyshire, DE7 4RA, UK.

Manuell, Mex. Laboratorios Manuell, S.A., Av. del Trabajo No. 237, Col Morelos, 15270 Mexico, D.F., Mexico.

Manx, UK. Manx Pharma Ltd, Manx House, Spectrum Business Estate, Bircholt Rd, Maidstone, Kent, ME15 9YP, UK.

MAP, Fin. MAP Medical Technologies Oy, Elmenttitie 27, 41160 Tikkakoski, Finland.

Marano, Ital. Marano Benito, Via E Vittorini, Villa Scalea, 90147 Palermo, Italy.

Marbot, Switz. Dr C Marbot AG, Amselweg 3, 3422 Kirchberg, Switzerland.

Marcel, Canad. Les Cosmetiques Marcel de Sevres, 1777 Lavoisier, Ste-Julie, Quebec, J3E 1Y6, Canada.

Marcel, Mex. Marcel, Mexico.

Marco, Austral. Marco D'Polo Importing & Merchandising, 12 Lancaster St, Ingleburn, NSW 2565, Australia.

Marc-O, Canad. Marc-O Inc. Produits, 3175 Girard St, Trois-Rivieres, Quebec, G8Z 2M5, Canada.

Marcofina, Hong Kong. See *C & L, Hong Kong.*

Marion Merrell, Fr. See *Aventis, Fr.*

Marion Merrell, Spain. See *Hoechst Marion Roussel, Spain.*

Marion Merrell Dow, Port. See *Aventis Pharma, Port.*

Marion Merrell Dow, Singapore. See *Pharmacon, Singapore.*

Marion Merrell Dow, USA. See *Aventis Pharma, USA.*

Marjan, Braz. Marjan Industria e Comercio Ltda, Rua Gibraltar 165, 04676-070 Sao Paulo, SP, Brazil.

Marlin, USA. Marlin Industries, P.O. Box 560, Grover Beach, CA 93483-0560, USA.

Marlop, USA. Marlop Pharmaceuticals Inc., 230 Marshall St, Elizabeth, NY 07206, USA.

Marlyn, USA. Marlyn Health Care, 14851 North Scottsdale Road, Scottsdale, AZ 85254, USA.

Marnel, USA. Marnel Pharmaceuticals Inc., 206 Luke Drive, Lafayette, LA 70506, USA.

Marrero, Spain. Marrero Perez, General Bravo 39, Pol. Industrial, Telde, 35200 Las Palmas, Spain.

Mars, UK. Mars Ltd, Dundee Rd, Slough, Berkshire, SL1 4JX, UK.

Marsam, USA. Marsam Pharmaceuticals Inc., 24 Olney Ave, Building 31, P.O. Box 1022, Cherry Hill, NJ 08034, USA.

Martin, Fr. See *Martin-Johnson & Johnson, Fr.*

Martin, Spain. B Martin Pharma, Centro Empresarial el Planto, Ochandiano 10, 28023 Madrid, Spain.

Martin, Switz. See *Uhlmann-Eyraud, Switz.*

Martindale, Hong Kong. See *LCH, Hong Kong.*

Martindale Pharmaceuticals, UK. Martindale Pharmaceuticals Ltd, Bampton Rd, Harold Hill, Romford, Essex, RM3 8UG, UK. NOTE. There is no connection between Martindale, The Complete Drug Reference and Martindale Pharmaceuticals.

Martinez Llenas, Spain. Martinez Llenas, Afueras del Barrio de Santa Ines S/N, La Roca del Valles, 08430 Barcelona, Spain.

Martin-Johnson & Johnson, Fr. Lab. Martin-Johnson & Johnson-MSD, Le Comte, 03340 Bessay-sur-Allier, France.

Martins & Fernandes, Port. A. Martins & Fernandes, SA, Rua Raul Mesnier do Ponsard 4-B, 1700 Lisbon, Portugal.

Maruho, Jpn. Maruho Co. Ltd, 6-24 Nakatsu 1-chome, Kita-ku, Osaka 531, Japan.

Maruishi, Jpn. Maruishi, Japan.

Maruko, Jpn. Maruko, Japan.

Masa, Thai. Masa Lab Co. Ltd, 50/25 Soi Thongpan 2, Takham Rd, Bangkunthien, Bangkok 10150, Thailand.

Mascia Brunelli, Ital. Mascia Brunelli s.p.a., Viale Monza 272, 20128 Milan, Italy.

Mason, USA. Mason Pharmaceuticals Inc., 4425 Jamboree, Suite 250, Newport Beach, CA 92660, USA.

Masta, UK. Masta Ltd, Moorfield Rd, Yeadon, Leeds, West Yorkshire, LS19 7BN, UK.

Mastelli, Ital. Mastelli s.r.l., Via Bussana Vecchia 32, 18032 Sanremo (IM), Italy.

Master Pharma, Ital. Master Pharma s.r.l., Via Firenze 8/A, 43100 Parma, Italy.

Matara, Fr. Lab. Matara, 162 rue d'Aguesseau, 92100 Boulogne, France.

Mathieu, Canad. JL Mathieu Cie Ltee, 1225 Volta St, Suite 100, Boucherville, Quebec, J4B 7M7, Canada.

Matley, UK. Matley Ltd, 34 Sloane Ave, London, SW3 3AX, UK.

Matrix, UK. Matrix Pharmaceutical Ltd, UK.

Matrix, USA. Matrix Laboratories Inc., 34700 Campus Dr., Fremont, CA 94555, USA.

Mauermann, Ger. Mauermann-Arzneimittel, Franz Mauermann oHG, Heinrich-Knote-Str. 2, 82343 Pocking, Germany.

Maurer, Ger. Maurer-Pharma GmbH, Ursulinenstr. 55, 66111 Saarbrucken, Germany.

Mavena, Ger. Mavena GmbH, Parkstr. 10, 88212 Ravensburg, Germany.

Mavena, Switz. Mavena AG, Birkenweg 1-8, 3123 Belp, Switzerland.

Maver, Mex. Productos Maver, S.A. de C.V., Av. Oleoducto No. 2804, Fracc. Industrial El Alamo, 44490 Tlaquepaque, Jal., Mexico.

Mavi, Ital. Mavi Sud s.r.l., V.le dell'Industria 1, 04011 Aprilia (LT), Italy.

Mavi, Mex. Productos Mavi, S.A. de C.V., Osa Menor Num 197, Col Prado Churubusco, 14230 Mexico, D.F., Mexico.

Max Farma, Ital. Max Farma, Via Pisacane 7, 20016 Pero (MI), Italy.

Max Ritter, Switz. Max Ritter Pharma SA, Switzerland.

Maxfarma, Spain. Maxfarma, Salamanca 13, 28020 Madrid, Spain.

Maxi, Thai. Maxi Medical Drug (Mahavej), 27 Paholyothin 41, Bangkok 10900, Thailand.

Maxim, Thai. Maxim Intercontinental Ltd Part, 640/56-57 Petchburi 22 Rd, Rajthevi, Bangkok 10400, Thailand.

Maxwell, S.Afr. Maxwell Pharm-Jhb, South Africa.

May & Baker, Canad. See *Aventis Pharma, Canad.*

May & Baker, UK. May & Baker Pharmaceuticals, Rhone Poulenc Ltd, Rainham Rd South, Dagenham, Essex, RM10 7XS, UK.

Maybelline, Canad. Maybelline Canada Inc., 6727 Airport Rd, Suite 205, Mississauga, Ontario, L4V 1V2, Canada.

Mayo, Mex. Mayo, Mexico.

Mayoly-Spindler, Fr. Laboratoires Mayoly-Spindler, 6 av de l'Europe, 78400 Chatou, France.

Mayoly-Spindler, Hong Kong. See *Wing Wai, Hong Kong.*

Mayoly-Spindler, Singapore. See *Polymedic, Singapore.*

Mayoly-Spindler, Switz. See *Uhlmann-Eyraud, Switz.*

Mayrand, USA. See *Merz, USA.*

Mayrhofer, Aust. Mayrhofer Pharmazeutika, Herrenstrasse 2, A-4010 Linz, Austria.

Mayrs, Irl. David Mayrs Ltd, Broombridge Industrial Estate, Dublin 11, Ireland.

MBD, Singapore. MBD Marketing, 371 Beach Rd, 03-30 KeyPoint, S 199597, Singapore.

MBP, Ger. Medical Biomaterial Products GmbH, Lederstr. 7, 19306 Neustadt-Glewe, Germany.

MC, Ital. Off. Prod. Presidi Medico Chirurgici s.r.l., S.S. 106, 89040 Portigliola (RC), Italy.

McGaw, NZ. See *REM, NZ.*

McGaw, USA. See *Braun, USA.*

McGaw Biomed, Austral. McGaw Biomed P/L, Unit 3, 9 Packard Ave, Castle Hill, NSW 2154, Australia.

McGaw Biomed, NZ. McGaw Biomed, P.O. Box 44069, Pt Chevalier, Auckland, New Zealand.

McGloin, Austral. J. McGloin P/L, P.O. Box 294, Kings Grove, NSW 2208, Australia.

McGregor, USA. McGregor Pharmaceuticals Inc., 8420 Ulmerton Rd, Suite 305, Largo, FL 34641, USA.

McHenry, USA. McHenry Labs Inc., 118 N Wells, Lee Building, Edna, TX 77957, USA.

MCM, S.Afr. MCM Health Care (Pty) Ltd, P.O. Box 501, Halfway House 1685, South Africa.

McNeil, Canad. See *Janssen-Ortho, Canad.*

McNeil, Israel. McNeil, P.O. Box 231, Yokneam Elit, Israel.

McNeil Consumer, Canad. McNeil Consumer Healthcare, 890 Woodlawn Rd W., Guelph, Ontario, N1K 1A5, Canada.

McNeil Consumer, USA. McNeil Consumer Products Co., Camp Hill Rd, Fort Washington, PA 19034, USA.

McNeil Pharmaceutical, USA. See *Ortho Pharmaceutical, USA.*

MCR, USA. MCR American Pharmaceuticals, 120 Summit Parkway, Suite 101, Birmingham, AL 35209, USA.

MD, Singapore. MD Pharmaceuticals Pte Ltd, 896 Dunearn Rd, 04-03 Sime Darby Centre, S 589472, Singapore.

MDM, Fr. MDM, 9 rue Brezin, 75014 Paris, France.

MDM, Ital. MDM s.r.l., Via Milanese 20, 20099 Sesto San Giovanni (MI), Italy.

MDR, USA. MDR Fitness Corp., 14101 NW 4th St, Sunrise, FL 33325, USA.

ME Pharmaceuticals, USA. ME Pharmaceuticals Inc., 2800 Southeast Parkway, Richmond, IN 47374, USA.

Mead Johnson, Austral. See *Bristol-Myers Squibb, Austral.*

Mead Johnson, Fr. See *Bristol-Myers Squibb, Fr.*

Mead Johnson, Hong Kong. See *Bristol-Myers Squibb, Hong Kong.*

Mead Johnson, Irl. See *Bristol-Myers Squibb, Irl.*

Mead Johnson, Israel. Mead-Johnson, P.O. Box 8609, New Industrial Zone, Netanya, Israel.

Mead Johnson, Ital. Mead Johnson s.p.a., Via Virgilio Maroso 50, 000142 Rome, Italy.

Mead Johnson, Mex. Mead Johnson de Mexico, S.A. de C.V. Division de Bristol-Myers Squibb, Calz de Tlalpan No. 2996, Col Ejido Sta. Ursula Coapa, 04870 Mexico, D.F., Mexico.

Mead Johnson, NZ. See *Bristol-Myers Squibb, NZ.*

Mead Johnson, Port. See *Bristol-Myers Squibb, Port.*

Mead Johnson, Singapore. See *Bristol-Myers Squibb, Singapore.*

Mead Johnson Laboratories, USA. See *Bristol-Myers Squibb, USA.*

Mead Johnson Nutritionals, Canad. Mead Johnson Nutritionals, Division of Bristol-Myers Squibb Canada Inc., 333 Preston Ave, Suite 700, Ottawa, Ontario, K1S 5N4, Canada.

Mead Johnson Nutritionals, Fin. Mead Johnson Nutritionals, Metsänneidonkuja 8, 02130 Espoo, Finland.

Mead Johnson Nutritionals, Thai. Mead Johnson Nutritional Division, Bristol-Myers Squibb Building, 10/10-11 Srinakarin Rd, Bangkaew, Bangplee, Samutprakarn 10540, Thailand.

Mead Johnson Nutritionals, UK. See *Bristol-Myers Squibb, UK.*

Mead Johnson Nutritionals, USA. Mead Johnson Nutritionals, 2400 W Lloyd Expressway, Evansville, IN 47721-0001, USA.

Meadow, UK. Meadow Laboratories, 18 Avenue Rd, Chadwell Heath, Romford, Essex, RM6 4JF, UK.

Mebo, Thai. Mebo Co. Ltd, 341 Sukhumvit 101/1 Rd, Bangjak Prakanong, Bangkok 10260, Thailand.

Meckel, Ger. Meckel-Spenglersan GmbH, Steinfeldweg 13, 77815 Buhl, Germany.

Med. Prod. Panam., USA. Medical Products Panamericana Inc., 647 W Flagler St, Miami, FL 33130, USA.

Meda, Denm. Meda AS, Gladsaxevej 342-54, 2860 Soborg, Denmark.

Meda, Fin. Meda Oy, Liesikuja 7, 01600 Vantaa, Finland.

Meda, Norw. Meda A/S, Bjerkas Industriomrade, 3470 Slemmestad, Norway.

Meda, Swed. Meda AB, Box 3051, 183 03 Taby, Sweden.

Medac, Ger. medac Gesellschaft fur klinische Spezialpraparate mbH, Theaterstr. 6, 22880 Wedel, Germany.

Medac, UK. Medac UK, 13 Lynedoch Crescent, Glasgow, G36 6EQ, UK.

Medchem, Hong Kong. See *Tsun Tsun, Hong Kong.*

Medchem, S.Afr. Medchem Pharmaceuticals (Pty) Ltd, P.O. Box 36014, Menlo Park 0102, South Africa.

Medco, USA. Medco Laboratories Inc., P.O. Box 864, Sioux City, IA 51102-0864, USA.

Med-Derm, USA. Med-Derm Pharmaceuticals, 524 Suncrest Dr., Gray, TN 37615, USA.

Medea, Spain. Medea, Santa Carolina 53-9, 08025 Barcelona, Spain.

Médecine Vegetale, Fr. Laboratoires Médecine Végétale, 89 rue Salvador-Allende, 95870 Bezons, France.

Medefield, Austral. Medefield P/L, 19 Dickson Ave, Artarmon, NSW 2064, Australia.

Medefield, NZ. Medefield Pty Ltd, New Zealand.

Medentech, Irl. Medentech Ltd, Whitemill Industrial Estate, Whitemill Rd, Wexford, Ireland.

Medentech, Israel. Medentech, Israel.

Medestea, Ital. Medestea srl, Corso Matteotti 40, 10121 Turin, Italy.

Medeva, Belg. Medeva Pharma S.A., Ave du Commerce 23, 1420 Braine-L'Alleud, Belgium.

Medeva, Denm. See *Vitaflo, Denm.*

Medeva, Fin. See *Panfarma, Fin.*

Medeva, Fr. Laboratoires Medeva Pharma, 6 pl. Boulnois, 75017 Paris, France.

Medeva, Irl. Medeva Pharma Ltd, 25 Sandyford Office Park, Dublin 18, Ireland.

Medeva, Norw. See *Mericon, Norw.*

Medeva, Singapore. See *Ziwell, Singapore.*

Medeva, Spain. Medeva Pharma, Caleruega 81, 28033 Madrid, Spain.

Medeva, Switz. See *Albugam, Switz.*

Medeva, UK. See *Celltech, UK.*

Medeva, USA. See *Celltech Medeva, USA.*

Medgenix, Belg. Medgenix Benelux S.A., Vliegveld 21, 8560 Wevelgem, Belgium.

Mediabase, Ital. Mediabase srl, Via della Selva 4, 59021 Vaiano (PO), Italy.

Medibel, Switz. Laboratoire Medibel SA, Case postale 2631, 1211 Geneva 2 Cornavin, Switzerland.

Medibial, Port. See *Bial, Port.*

Medibrands, Israel. Medibrands, P.O. Box 231, Yokneam Elit, Israel.

Medic, Braz. Medic Industrial Farmaceutica Ltda, Rua Conselheiro Mayrink 362, 20960-140 Rio de Janeiro, RJ, Brazil.

Medic, Denm. Medic Team a/s, Blokken 31 (postboks 193), 3460 Birkerod, Denmark.

Medic, NZ. Medic Corp. Ltd, Private Bag, Lower Hutt, Wellington, New Zealand.

Medica, NZ. Medica Pacifica Ltd, P.O.Box 24-421, Royal Oak, Auckland, New Zealand.

Medical, Port. See *Gestafarma, Port.*

Medical, Spain. Medical, Virgen de las Angustias 2, 14006 Cordoba, Spain.

Medical Industries, Austral. Medical Industries Australia P/L, 148-52 Regent St, Redfern, NSW 2016, Australia.

Medical Ophthalmics, USA. Medical Ophthalmics Inc., 40146 U.S. Hwy 19 N, Tarpon Springs, FL 34689, USA.

Medical Research, Austral. Medical Research (Australia) P/L, P.O. Box 6025, Parramatta BC, NSW 2150, Australia.

Medical Research, Hong Kong. See *Jebsen, Hong Kong.*

Medical Specialties, Austral. Medical Specialties Australia P/L, 2 McCabe Place, Willoughby, NSW 2068, Australia.

Medical Supply, Thai. Medical Supply Co. Ltd, 101 Sribumpen Rd, Yannawa, Bangkok 10120, Thailand.

Medicamed, Port. Medicamed, SA, Edificio Olympus, Av D Afonso Henriques 1462, 4450 Matosinhos, Portugal.

Medican, Canad. Medican Pharma Inc., 1120 Victoria St N, Suite 203, Kitchener, Ontario, N2B 3T2, Canada.

Medicap, Thai. See *Neopharm, Thai.*

Medice, Ger. Medice, Chem.-pharm. Fabrik Pütter GmbH & Co. KG, Kuhloweg 37-9, 58638 Iserlohn, Germany.

Medice, Switz. See *Ridupharm, Switz.*

Medichem, Hong Kong. See *Unam, Hong Kong.*

Medichem, Singapore. See *Far East Drug, Singapore.*

Medichemie, Switz. Medichemie AG, Postfach 3650, 4002 Basle, Switzerland.

Medichemie Bioline, Switz. See *Medichemie, Switz.*

Medici, Ital. Lab. Farm. Dr Medici s.r.l., Localita Tor Maggiore-Santa Palomba, 00040 Pomezia (Rome), Italy.

Medicine Supply, Thai. Medicine Supply Co. Ltd, 767/4 Phaholyothin Rd, Samsennai, Phyathai, Bangkok 10400, Thailand.

Medicines Company, USA. Medicines Company, USA.

Medicines International, UK. Medicines International, 10 Stroud Rd, Kelvin Industrial Estate, East Kilbride, G75 0YA, UK.

Medicis, Canad. Medicis Canada Ltd, 355 McCaffrey St, St-Laurent, Quebec, H4T 1Z7, Canada.

Medicis, USA. Medicis Pharmaceutical Corp., 4343 E Camelback Rd, Suite 150, Phoenix, AZ 85018, USA.

Medico-Biological Laboratories, UK. Medico-Biological Laboratories Ltd, Kingsend House, 44 Kingsend, Ruislip, Middlesex, HA4 7DA, UK.

Medicone, USA. Medicone Co., USA.

Medicopharm, Aust. Medicopharm Dr H Sorgo GmbH, Thimiggasse 25, A-1180 Vienna, Austria.

Medidom, Switz. Laboratoire Medidom SA, Ave de Champel 24, Case postale 13, 1211 Geneva 12, Switzerland.

Medifa, Fr. Medifa, France.

Medifarma, Mex. Medifarma, Mexico.

Medifive, Thai. Medifive Pharma Co. Ltd, 51/465-466 Drive-in Square, Soi 3 Ladprao Rd, Klongjan, Bangkok 10240, Thailand.

Medifood, Ital. Medifood Italia s.r.l., Via Balbi 31/1, 16126 Genoa, Italy.

Medika, Ger. Medika Lizenz Pharmaz. Praparate, Am Alten Weg 20, 82041 Oberhaching, Germany.

Medika, Switz. Medika AG, Industriestrasse 121, 4147 Aesch/BL, Switzerland.

Mediline, Israel. Mediline, 1 Sha'ar Ha'ir, 22 Ben Gurion St, Herzliya, Israel.

Medilink, Denm. Medilink A/S, Mothsvej 50, 2840 Holte, Denmark.

Medilink, Fin. See *Medilink, Denm.*

Medilink, Norw. See *Medilink, Denm.*

Medilink, Swed. See *Medilink, Denm.*

MediMar, UK. MediMar Laboratories, 65 High St, Wheatley, Oxford, Oxfordshire, OX33 1XT, UK.

Medimmune, USA. Medimmune Inc., 35 West Watkins Mill Rd, Gaithersburg, MD 20878, USA.

Medimpex, UK. Medimpex UK Ltd, 127 Shirland Rd, London, W9 2EP, UK.

Medimport, Mex. Medimport, S.A. de C.V., Via Lactea No. 29, 04230 Mexico, D.F., Mexico.

Medinaturals, UK. Medinaturals, 37 Limpsfield Rd, Sanderstead, Surrey, CR2 9LA, UK.

Medinex, Canad. Medinex Ltd, 2 boul. Crepeau, Saint-Laurent, Quebec, H4N 1M7, Canada.

Medinfar, Port. Laboratório Medinfar, SA, Rua Manuel Ribeiro da Pavia 1 - 1, Venda Nova, 2700 Amadora, Portugal.

Medinova, Hong Kong. See *Great Liaison, Hong Kong.*

Medinova, Port. See *Confar, Port.*

Medinova, Switz. Medinova SA, Eggbuhlstrasse 14, 8052 Zurich, Switzerland.

Medinovum, Fin. See *Ratiopharm, Fin.*

Medinsa, Spain. Medinsa, Doctor Zamenhof 36, 28027 Madrid, Spain.

Mediolanum, Ital. Mediolanum Farmaceutici s.p.a., Via S.G. Cottolengo 15, 20143 Milan, Italy.

Medipharm, Switz. Medipharm SA, Emil Frey-Strasse 99, 4142 Munchenstein, Switzerland.

Medipharma, Ger. Medipharma Homburg GmbH, Michelinstr. 10, 66424 Homburg, Germany.

Medipharma, Hong Kong. Medipharma Ltd, Hong Kong, Unit 2409, Tsuen Wan Industrial Ctr, 220-248 Texaco Rd, Tsuen Wan, N.T., Hong Kong.

Medi-Physics, USA. Medi-Physics Inc., Amersham Healthcare, 2636 S Clearbrook Drive, Arlington Heights, Il 60005, USA.

Mediplant, Belg. Mediplant, Belgium.

Medi-Plex, USA. See *ECR, USA.*

Mediplus, UK. Mediplus Ltd, 37-39 Baker St, High Wycombe, Buckinghamshire, HP11 2RX, UK.

Medipole, Fr. Lab. Medipole, La Boursidiere, B.P. 150, 92357 Le Plessis-Robinson, France.

Medirel, Switz. Medirel SA, Redondello, 6982 Agno, Switzerland.

Medis, Denm. Medis-Danmark A/S, Havelse Molle 14, 3600 Frederikssund, Denmark.

Medis, Israel. Pharma Medis Co. Ltd, P.O. Box 2820, Holon, Israel.

Medisa, Switz. Medisa AG, Postfach 446, 6343 Rotkreuz, Switzerland.

Medisan, Canad. See *Pharmacia Upjohn, Canad.*

Medisan, Swed. See *Biophausia, Swed.*

Medisculab, Ger. See *Biosyn, Ger.*

Medisense, Austral. MediSense Products, Abbott Diagnostics Division, 666 Doncaster Rd, Doncaster, VIC 3108, Australia.

Medisense, Canad. MediSense, 6535 Millcreek Dr, Unit 41, Mississauga, Ontario, L5N 2M2, Canada.

Medisense, UK. MediSense, Division of Abbott Laboratories, Mallory House, Vanwell Business Park, Maidenhead, Berkshire, SL6 4UD, UK.

Medisint, Ital. Medisint s.r.l., Via Settala 10, 20124 Milan, Italy.

Medisport, UK. Medisport International Lts, 1 The Briars, Waterberry Drive, Waterlooville, Hampshire, PO7 7YH, UK.

Meditrend, Israel. Meditrend, 13 Kehilat Saloniki, Tel Aviv, Israel.

Medivis, Ital. Medivis srl, Corso Italia 171, 95127 Catania, Italy.

Medix, Fr. Laboratoires Médix, 18 rue Saint-Mathieu, 78550 Houdan, France.

Medix, Israel. Medix, Israel.

Medix, Mex. Productos Medix, S.A. de C.V., Calz del Hueso No. 39, Col Ejido Santa Ursula Coapa, 04910 Mexico, D.F., Mexico.

Medix, Spain. Medix, Alcala 431, 28027 Madrid, Spain.

Medley, Braz. Medley S.A. Industria Farmaceutica, Rua Macedo Costa 55, Jardim Santa Genebra, 13080-010 Campinas, SP, Brazil.

Medline, Thai. Medline Co. Ltd, 736-742 Pracha-U-Thit Rd, Huay Kwang, Bangkok 10320, Thailand.

Medlogic, UK. MedLogic Global Ltd, Western Wood Way, Langage Science Park, Plympton, Plymouth, Devon, PL7 5BG, UK.

Mednostica, S.Afr. Mednostica (Pty) Ltd, P.O. Box 36482, Menlo Park 0102, South Africa.

Medo, UK. Medo Pharmaceuticals Ltd, Schwarz House, East St, Chesham, Birmingham, HP5 1DG, UK.

Medochemie, Hong Kong. See *Star, Hong Kong.*

Medochemie, Singapore. See *Derek, Singapore.*

Medochemie, Thai. See *Medline, Thai.*

Medopharm, Ger. Medopharm Arzneimittel GmbH & Co. KG, Gartenstr. 24, 79098 Freiburg, Germany.

Medosan, Ital. Medosan s.r.l., Industrie Biochimiche Riunite, Via di Cancelliera 12, 00040 Cecchina (RM), Italy.

Medphano, Ger. medphano Arzneimittel GmbH, Maienbergstr. 10, 15562 Rudersdorf, Germany.

Medpro, S.Afr. Medpro Pharmaceutica (Pty) Ltd, P.O. Box 1096, Durbanville 7551, South Africa.

Medquimica, Braz. Medquimica Industria Farmaceutica Ltda, Rua Otacilio Esteves da Silva 40, Granja Betania, 36045-000 Juiz de Fora, MG, Brazil.

Medra, Aust. Medra Handels-GmbH, Gastgebgasse 5-13, A-1230 Vienna, Austria.

Medtech, Canad. Medtech Lab, 330 Esna Park Drive, Markham, Ontario, L3R 1H3, Canada.

Medtech, USA. Medtech Laboratories Inc., 3510 N Lake Creek, P.O. Box 1108, Jackson, WY 83011-1108, USA.

Mega Vitamin, Austral. Mega Vitamin Laboratories P/L, 5 Tahlee St, Burwood, NSW 2134, Australia.

Megapha, Singapore. Megapha Pte Ltd, 5 Kallang Pudding Rd, 06-04 Keng Hua Building, S 349309, Singapore.

Megapharm, Israel. Megapharm Ltd., 19 hankin St, Hod Hasharon, Israel.

Meiji, Jpn. Meiji Seika Kaisha Ltd, 2-4-16 Kyobashi, Chuo-ku, Tokyo 104-8002, Japan.

Meiji, Singapore. See *Pharma 2000, Singapore.*

Meiji, Thai. Thai Meiji Pharmaceutical Co. Ltd, Ground Fl (Extension Building), Regent House, 183 Rajdamri Rd, Bangkok 10330, Thailand.

Mein, Spain. Mein, Dr. Ferran 4, Vilassar de Dalt, 08339 Barcelona, Spain.

Mekim, Hong Kong. Mekim Ltd, Rm 905, Harbour Ctr Tower 2, 8 Hok Cheung St, Hunghom, Kowloon, Hong Kong.

Melisana, Belg. Melisana S.A., Ave du Four a Briques 1, 1140 Brussels, Belgium.

Melisana, Switz. Melisana AG, Ankerstrasse 53, Postfach, 8026 Zurich, Switzerland.

Mellin, Ital. Mellin, Div. Dietetica Star, Via Matteotti 142, 20041 Agrate Brianza (MI), Italy.

Melpoejo, Braz. Laboratorio Melpoejo Ltda, Rua Inacio Gama 723, Bairro de Lourdes, 36070-420 Juiz de Fora, MG, Brazil.

Men, Spain. Men, Perello 21, 08005 Barcelona, Spain.

Menadier, Ger. Menadier Heilmittel GmbH, Fischers Allee 49-59, 22763 Hamburg, Germany.

Menarini, Belg. Menarini Benelux S.A., Belgicastraat 4, 1930 Zaventem, Belgium.

Menarini, Fr. Menarini France, 21 rue du Pont-des-Halles, Delta 109, 94536 Rungis cdx, France.

Menarini, Hong Kong. See *Mekim, Hong Kong.*

Menarini, Irl. A. Menarini Pharmaceuticals Ireland Ltd, 72 York Rd, Dun Laoghaire, Dublin, Ireland.

Menarini, Ital. A. Menarini Industrie Farmaceutiche Riunite s.r.l., Via Sette Santi 3, 50131 Florence, Italy.

Menarini, Neth. Menarini Benelux, Postbus 189, 3440 AD Woerden, Netherlands.

Menarini, Singapore. Menarini International, 6 Tagore Drive, 03-11 Tagore Industrial Building, S 787623, Singapore.

Menarini, Spain. Menarini, Alfonso XII 587, Badalona, 08918 Barcelona, Spain.

Menarini, Switz. A. Menarini AG, Eggbuhlstrasse 14, 8026 Zurich, Switzerland.

Menarini, Thai. See *Biopharm, Thai.*

Menarini, UK. A. Menarini Pharmaceuticals UK Ltd, Menarini House, Mercury Park, Wycombe Lane, Woburn Green, Buckinghamshire, HP10 0HH, UK.

Mendelejeff, Ital. Stabilimento Chimico Farmaceutico Mendelejeff s.r.l., Via Aurelia 58, 00165 Rome, Italy.

Menley & James, USA. Menley & James Laboratories Inc., 100 Tournament Drive, Horsham, PA 19044, USA.

Mennen, USA. See *Colgate-Palmolive, USA.*

Mentholatum, Austral. Mentholatum Australasia P/L, P.O. Box 398, Mulgrave North, VIC 3170, Australia.

Mentholatum, Canad. Mentholatum Co. of Canada Ltd, 20 Lewis St, Fort Erie, Ontario, L2A 5M6, Canada.

Mentholatum, Israel. Mentholatum, Israel.

Mentholatum, Singapore. See *Diethelm, Singapore.*

Mentholatum, UK. The Mentholatum Co. Ltd, 1 Redwood Ave, Peel Park Campus, East Kilbride, Glasgow, G74 5PF, UK.

Mentholatum, USA. Mentholatum Inc., 707 Sterling Dr., Orchard Park, NY 14127, USA.

Mepha, Hong Kong. See *Ceutical, Hong Kong.*

Mepha, Israel. Mepha, Israel.

Mepha, Port. Mepha, Lda, R. Elias Garcia 28 C, Venda Nova, Apartado 6617, 2701-355 Amadora, Portugal.

Mepha, Singapore. See *Megapha, Singapore.*

Mepha, Switz. Mepha Pharma AG, Pharmazeutische Forschung, Entwicklung und Produktion, Postfach 445, 4147 Aesch/BL, Switzerland.

Mepha, Thai. See *Amcron, Thai.*

Mepra-Pharm, UK. See *Co-Pharma, UK.*

Merck, Aust. Merck GmbH, Zimbagasse 5, A-1147 Vienna, Austria.

Merck, Braz. Merck S.A. Industrias Quimicas, Estrada dos Bandeirantes 1099, 22710-571 Rio de Janeiro, RJ, Brazil.

Merck, Denm. Merck A/S, Smedeland 26 B (postboks 1389), 2600 Glostrup, Denmark.

Merck, Fin. Merck Oy, Niittyrinne 7, 02270 Espoo, Finland.

Merck, Ger. Merck KGaA, Frankfurter Str. 250, 64271 Darmstadt, Germany.

Merck, Hong Kong. See *Jebsen, Hong Kong,* and *Sun Hing, Hong Kong.*

Merck, Irl. Merck Pharmaceuticals Ltd, 2004A Orchard Ave, City West Business Campus, Naas Rd, Dublin 24, Ireland.

Merck, Israel. Merck, Israel.

Merck, Mex. Merck-Mexico, S.A., Calle 5 Num 7, 53370 Naucalpan de Juarez, Mexico.

Merck, Neth. Merck Nederland B.V., Postbus 8198, 1005 AD Amsterdam, Netherlands.

Merck, Norw. E. Merck, Skarersletta 60, Postboks 198, 1471 Skarer, Norway.

Merck, Port. Merck Farma e Quimica, SA, Rua Alfredo da Silva 3-C, Apartado 3185, 1304 Lisbon, Portugal.

Merck, S.Afr. See *Xixia, S.Afr.*

Merck, Singapore. Merck (Singapore) Pte Ltd, Pharmaceutical Division, 19 Loyang Way, 06-22, S 508724, Singapore.

Merck, Spain. Merck Farma Quimica, Poligono Merck, Mollet del Valles, 08100 Barcelona, Spain.

Merck, Swed. Merck AB, Pharma Division, Box 23033, 10435 Stockholm, Sweden.

Merck, Switz. Merck (Schweiz) AG, Ruchligstrasse 20, 8953 Dietikon, Switzerland.

Merck, Thai. Merck Ltd, 9 Fl, Monterey Tower, 2170 New Petchburi Rd, Bangkok 10320, Thailand.

Merck, UK. E. Merck Pharmaceuticals Ltd, Harrier House, High St, West Drayton, Middlesex, UB7 7QG, UK.

Merck, USA. Merck & Co., P.O. Box 4, West Point, PA 19486-0004, USA.

Merck Consumer, UK. See *Seven Seas, UK.*

Merck dura, Ger. Merck dura GmbH, Postfach: 100635, 64206 Darmstadt, Germany.

Merck Frosst, Canad. Merck Frosst Canada Inc., P.O. Box 1005, Pointe-Claire, Dorval, Quebec, H9R 4P8, Canada.

Merck Sharp & Dohme, Aust. Merck Sharp & Dohme GmbH, Donau-City Strasse 6, A-1220 Vienna, Austria.

Merck Sharp & Dohme, Austral. Merck Sharp & Dohme (Australia) P/L, P.O. Box 79, Granville, NSW 2142, Australia.

Merck Sharp & Dohme, Belg. Merck Sharp & Dohme B.V., Chaussee de Waterloo 1135, 1180 Brussels, Belgium.

Merck Sharp & Dohme, Braz. Merck Sharp & Dohme Farmaceutica e Veterinaria Ltda, Avenida Brigadeiro Faria Lima 1815 (12° And.), 01451-001 Sao Paulo, SP, Brazil.

Merck Sharp & Dohme, Canad. See *Merck Frosst, Canad.*

Merck Sharp & Dohme, Denm. Merck Sharp & Dohme, Smedeland 8, 2600 Glostrup, Denmark.

Merck Sharp & Dohme, Fin. Soumen MSD Oy, Pyyntitie 5, 02230 Espoo, Finland.

Merck Sharp & Dohme, Ger. MSD Sharp & Dohme GmbH, Lindenplatz 1, 85540 Haar, Germany.

Merck Sharp & Dohme, Hong Kong. Merck Sharp & Dohme (Asia) Ltd, 26/F Caroline Ctr, 28 Yun Ping Rd, Causeway Bay, Hong Kong.

Merck Sharp & Dohme, Irl. See *Cahill May Roberts, Irl.*

Merck Sharp & Dohme, Israel. MSD Israel, P.O. Box 9266, Petach Tikva, Israel.

Merck Sharp & Dohme, Ital. Merck Sharp & Dohme (Italia) s.p.a., Via G. Fabbroni 6, 00191 Rome, Italy.

Merck Sharp & Dohme, Mex. Merck Sharp & Dohme de Mexico, S.A. de C.V., Av. Division del Norte No. 3377, Col Xotepingo, 04610 Mexico, D.F., Mexico.

Merck Sharp & Dohme, Neth. Merck Sharp & Dohme B.V., Postbus 581, 2003 PC Haarlem, Netherlands.

Merck Sharp & Dohme, Norw. MSD (Norge) A/S, Solbakken 1, Postboks 458 Brakeroya, 3002 Drammen, Norway.

Merck Sharp & Dohme, NZ. Merck Sharp & Dohme (NZ) Ltd, P.O. Box 23-244, Papatoetoe, Auckland, New Zealand.

Merck Sharp & Dohme, Port. Merck Sharp & Dohme, Lda, Edificio Vasco da Gama, Quinta da Fonte, Porto Slavo, 2780-730 Paco de Arcos, Portugal.

Merck Sharp & Dohme, S.Afr. Merck Sharp & Dohme (Pty) Ltd, Private Bag 3, Halfway House 1685, South Africa.

Merck Sharp & Dohme, Singapore. Merck Sharp & Dohme (IA) Corp, Singapore Branch, 300 Beach Road, 13-02 The Concourse, S 199555, Singapore.

Merck Sharp & Dohme, Spain. Merck Sharp & Dohme, Josefa Valcarcel 38, 28027 Madrid, Spain.

Merck Sharp & Dohme, Swed. Merck Sharp & Dohme (Sweden) AB, Box 7125, 191 07 Sollentuna, Sweden.

Merck Sharp & Dohme, Switz. Merck Sharp & Dohme-Chibret SA, Niederlassung von Merck & Co., Inc., USA, Schaffhauserstrasse 136, Postfach, 8152 Glattbrugg, Switzerland.

Merck Sharp & Dohme, Thai. See *BLH, Thai.*

Merck Sharp & Dohme, UK. Merck Sharp & Dohme Ltd, Hertford Rd, Hoddesdon, Hertfordshire, EN11 9BU, UK.

Merck Sharp & Dohme, USA. See *Merck, USA.*

Merck Sharp & Dohme-Chibret, Fr. Laboratoires Merck Sharp & Dohme-Chibret, 3 ave Hoche, 75114 Paris cdx 08, France.

Merck-Belgolabo, Belg. Merck-Belgolabo S.A., Brusselsesteenweg 288, 3090 Overijse, Belgium.

Merck-Clevenot, Fr. Laboratoires Merck-Clévenot, 5-9 rue Anquetil, 94736 Nogent-sur-Marne cdx, France.

Merck-Clevenot, Switz. See *Actipharm, Switz.*

Merckle, Ger. Merckle GmbH, Ludwig-Merckle-Str. 3, 89143 Blaubeuren, Germany.

Merck-Lipha, Singapore. See *Zuellig, Singapore.*

Meretek, USA. Meretek, 618 Grassmere Park Drive, Suite 20, Nashville, TN 37211, USA.

Merial, Denm. Merial Norden A/S, Gladsaxevej 378, 2860 Soborg, Denmark.

Meriana, Austral. Meriana Australia, 298 Davey St, South Hobart, TAS 7004, Australia.

Mericon, Norw. Mericon AS, Postboks 1865 Gulset, 3705 Skien, Norway.

Mericon, USA. Mericon Industries Inc., 8819 N Pioneer Rd, Peoria, IL 61615, USA.

Meridian, Israel. Meridian, Israel.

Merieux, Fr. See *Aventis Pasteur, Fr.*

Merieux, Ger. See *Aventis, Ger.*

Merlin, UK. Merlin Pharmaceuticals Ltd, 11 Picardy Street, Belvedere, Kent, DA17 5QQ, UK.

Mer-National, S.Afr. See *Adcock Ingram, S.Afr.*

Merrell Dow, USA. See *Aventis Pharma, USA.*

Merz, Denm. See *Meda, Denm.*

Merz, Ger. Merz & Co., GmbH & Co., Eckenheimer Landstr. 100-104, 60318 Frankfurt (Main), Germany.

Merz, Hong Kong. See *Weston, Hong Kong.*

Merz, Israel. Merz, Israel.

Merz, Neth. See *Hoechst Marion Roussel, Neth.*

Merz, Singapore. See *Green Cross, Singapore.*

Merz, Switz. See *Adroka, Switz.*

Merz, USA. Merz Pharmaceuticals, 4215 Tudor Lane (27410), P.O. Box 18806, Greensboro, NC 27419, USA.

Meta Fackler, Ger. meta Biologische Heilmittel Fackler KG, Philipp-Reis-Str. 3, 31832 Springe, Germany.

Metabolic Solutions, USA. Metabolic Solutions Inc., 460 Amherst St, Nashua, NH 03063, USA.

Metapharma, Canad. Metapharma, 131 Clarence St, Brantford, Ontario, N3T 2V6, Canada.

Metapharma, Ital. Metapharma s.p.a., Viale delle Dalie 26, 00042 Anzio (RM), Italy.

Methapharm, Canad. Methapharm Inc., 131 Clarence St, Brantford, Ontario, N3T 2V6, Canada.

Methapharm, USA. See *Methapharm, Canad.*

Metochem, Aust. Metochem-Pharma GmbH, Jochen-Rindt-Strasse 23, A-1230 Vienna, Austria.

Metrolite, Hong Kong. Metrolite Trading Ltd, Flat E, 12/F Haribest Industrial Bldg, 45-47 Au Pui Wan St, Fo Tan, Shatin, N.T., Hong Kong.

Met-Rx, USA. Met-Rx Substrate Technology, 2112 Business Center Drive, Irvine, CA 92612-1001, USA.

Meuse, Belg. See *Therabel, Belg.*

Mex-America, Mex. Representaciones Mex-America S.A. de C.V., Laboratorio de Especialidades Dermatologicas, Diagonal 20 de Noviembre No. 264, Col. Obrera, 06800 Mexico D.F., Mexico.

Meyer Zall, S.Afr. Meyer Zall Laboratories (Pty) Ltd, P.O. Box 218, Fontainbleau 2023, South Africa.

MGI, Israel. MGI, Israel.

MGI, USA. MGI Pharma Inc., 6300 Old Shakopee Rd, Suite 110, Bloomington, MN 55438, USA.

Miba, Ital. Miba Prodotti Chimici e Farmaceutici s.p.a., Via Falzarego 8, 20021 Ospiate di Bollate (MI), Italy.

Michallik, Ger. Fritz Osk. Michallik GmbH & Co., Kisslingweg 60, 75417 Muhlacker, Germany.

Michaux, Belg. Labo Michaux, Rue Ed. Schmidt 19, 6280 Gerpinnes, Belgium.

Mickan, Ger. Mickan Arzneimittel GmbH, Industriestr. 5, 76189 Karlsruhe, Germany.

Midro, Ger. Midro Lörrach GmbH, Barenfelser Str. 7, 79539 Lorrach, Germany.

Midro, Israel. Midro, Israel.

Milana, Ital. Milana s.r.l., Via Liborio Giuffre 50, 90127 Palermo, Italy.

Milance, USA. Milance, USA.

Milano, Thai. Milano Lab Ltd Part, 62 Soi Latphrao, Bangkok 10310, Thailand.

Miles, Canad. See *Bayer, Canad.*

Miles, USA. See *Bayer, USA.*

Miles Consumer Healthcare, USA. See *Bayer, USA.*

Miles Laboratories, USA. See *Bayer, USA.*

Milex, Canad. See *Milex, USA.*

Milex, USA. Milex Products Inc., 4311 N Normandy, Chicago, IL 60634-1403, USA.

Milk Industries, Israel. Milk Industries, Israel.

Miller, USA. Miller Pharmacal Group Inc., 350 Randy Rd, Unit 2, Carol Stream, IL 60188, USA.

Millet Roux, Braz. Produtos Farmaceuticos Millet Roux Ltda, Rua Eliseu Visconti 05, 20251-250 Rio de Janeiro, RJ, Brazil.

Milo, Spain. Milo, Av. Constitucion 18 E, Cuarte de Huerva, 50410 Zaragoza, Spain.

Milte, Ital. Milte Italia spa, Via Tadino 29/A, 20124 Milan, Italy.

Milte, Port. Milte Portugal, SA, Av Marechal Gomes da Costa 19, 1800-255 Lisbon, Portugal.

Milupa, Aust. Milupa GmbH, Postfach 2, A-5412 Puch, Austria.

Milupa, Fr. Milupa, 4 rue Joseph-Monier, 92859 Rueil-Malmaison cdx, France.

Milupa, Hong Kong. See *Connell, Hong Kong.*

Milupa, Irl. Milupa Ltd, 1B Sandyford Business Centre, Burton Hall Rd, Dublin 18, Ireland.

Milupa, Ital. Milupa s.p.a., Via Marsala 40, 21013 Gallarate (VA), Italy.

Milupa, Port. Milupa Portuguesa, Lda, Zona Industrial, 2795 Carnaxide, Portugal.

Milupa, Singapore. Milupa, Singapore.

Milupa, Switz. Milupa SA, 1564 Domdidier, Switzerland.

Milupa, UK. Milupa Ltd, Division of Nutricia, Newmarket Ave, White Horse Business Park, Trowbridge, Wiltshire, BA14 0XQ, UK.

Minancora, Braz. Minancora & Cia Ltda, Rua do Principe 461, 89201-001 Joinville, SC, Brazil.

Minden, Ger. See *Knoll, Ger.*

Mini, Switz. Bernardo Mini & Co, Loretostrasse 5, 6300 Zug, Switzerland.

Minophagen, Jpn. Minophagen Pharmaceutical Co., 10-22 Akasaka 8-chome, Minato-ku, Tokyo 107, Japan.

MIP, Ger. MIP Pharma GmbH, Muhlstr. 50, 66386 St. Ingbert, Germany.

Mipharm, Ital. Mipharm s.p.a., Via B Quaranta 12, 20141 Milan, Italy.

Miquel Garriga, Spain. Miquel Garriga, Joaquin Costa 18, Montgat, 08390 Barcelona, Spain.

Miquel Otsuka, Spain. See *Otsuka, Spain.*

Mirren, S.Afr. Mirren (Pty) Ltd, P.O. Box 87607, Houghton 2041, South Africa.

Misemer, USA. See *Edwards, USA.*

Mission Pharmacal, Hong Kong. See *International Medical, Hong Kong.*

Mission Pharmacal, Singapore. See *Pharma 2000, Singapore.*

Mission Pharmacal, USA. Mission Pharmacal Co., 10999 IH 10 West, Suite 1000, San Antonio, TX 78230-1355, USA.

MIT, Ger. MIT Gesundheit GmbH Gesundheitsprodukte, Flutstr. 74, 47533 Kleeve, Germany.

Mita, Hong Kong. Mita Pharmaceutical Co. Ltd, Rm 1208, 12/F, Phase 1, Metro Ctr, 32 Lam Hing St, Kowloon Bay, Kowloon, Hong Kong.

Mitchell, UK. Mitchell International Pharmaceuticals Ltd, Unit 7, Kingston House Estate, Portsmouth Road, Thames Ditton, Surrey, KT6 5QG, UK.

Mitim, Ital. Mitim s.r.l., Via Rodi 27, 25126 Brescia, Italy.

Mitsubishi, Jpn. See *Mitsubishi-Tokyo, Jpn.*

Mitsubishi-Tokyo, Jpn. Mitsubishi-Tokyo Pharmaceuticals Inc., 2-6 Nihonbashi-Honcho 2-chome, Chuo-ku, Tokyo 103-8405, Japan.

Mitsui, Jpn. Mitsui Seiyaku, Asahi Building, 3-12-2 Nihonbashi, Chuo-ku, Tokyo, Japan.

Miyarisan, Jpn. Miyarisan Pharmaceutical Co., Ltd, 1-10-3 Kaminakazato, Kita-ku, Tokyo 114-0016, Japan.

Mizar, Spain. Mizar Farmaceutica, Gran Via Corts Catalanes 764, 08013 Barcelona, Spain.

ML Laboratories, UK. ML Laboratories Plc, Blaby Hall, Church St, Blaby, Leicestershire, LE8 4FA, UK.

Mochida, Jpn. Mochida Pharmaceutical Co. Ltd, 7 Yotsuya 1-chome, Shinjuku-ku, Tokyo 160-8515, Japan.

Modern Health Products, UK. Modern Health Products Ltd, Sisson Rd, Gloucester, GL1 3QB, UK.

Molimin, Ger. Molimin Arzneimittel GmbH, Emil-Kemmer-Str. 33, 96103 Hallstadt, Germany.

Molnlycke, Fr. Laboratoires Mölnlycke Health Care, 59 rue de la Vignette, B.P. 2, 59497 Fretin cdx, France.

Molteni, Ital. Molteni L. & C. dei F.lli Alitti Società Esercizio s.p.a., S.S. 67, Fraz. Granatieri, 50018 Scandicci (FI), Italy.

Mona Lisa, Israel. Mona Lisa, Israel.

Monal, Fr. See *Novartis, Fr.*

Monarch, USA. Monarch Pharmaceuticals, 355 Beecham St, Bristol, TN 37620, USA.

Monchpharma, Ger. Mönchpharma Arzneimittel GmbH, Kostendeel 15, 48157 Munster, Germany.

Monico, Ital. Monico S.p.A., Casa Fondata nel 1883, Via Orlanda 10, Ponte Pietra, 30173 Venezia-Mestre (VE), Italy.

Monik, Spain. Monik, Avda de la Playa 1, Conil de la Frontera, 11140 Cadiz, Spain.

Monin, Fr. Laboratoires Monin-Chanteaud, Parc Euromedecine 2, rue de la Valsiere, 34099 Montpellier cdx 5, France.

Monmouth, Irl. See *Allphar, Irl.*

Monmouth, UK. See *Shire, UK.*

Mono, S.Afr. Mono, South Africa.

Monoclonal Antibodies, USA. See *Quidel, USA.*

Monot, Fr. Monot, 34 rue St-Romain, 69008 Lyon, France.

Monsanto, Austral. Monsanto Australia Ltd, P.O. Box 1380, Crows Nest, NSW 2065, Australia.

Monsanto, Fr. Monsanto France SA, division Searle, Imm Elysees-La-Defense, 7 place du Dome, 92056 Paris-La-Defense cdx, France.

Monsanto, Ital. Monsanto Italiana s.p.a., Divisione Searle Farmaceutici, Via Walter Tobagi 8, 20089 Peschiera Borromeo (MI), Italy.

Monsanto, Port. Monsanto Portugal, Lda, Rua Sanches Coelho 3-9, 1649-009 Lisbon, Portugal.

Monsanto, Spain. Monsanto España, La Granja 30, Alcobendas, 28100 Madrid, Spain.

Montavit, Aust. Montavit GmbH, Salzbergstrasse 96, A-6060 Absam, Austria.

Montavit, Israel. Montavit, Israel.

Montavit, Neth. See *Roussel, Neth.*

Montavit, Thai. Montavit.

Montefarmaco, Ital. Montefarmaco s.p.a., Via G. Galilei 7, 20016 Pero (MI), Italy.

Montplet, Spain. Montplet, Via Trajana 53, 08020 Barcelona, Spain.

Moore, USA. Moore Medical Corp., 389 John Downey Dr., P.O. Box 2740, New Britain, CT 06050, USA.

Morado, Ital. Morado s.p.a., Via Cacciamali 16, 25125 Brescia, Italy.

Moraz, UK. See *Impharm, UK.*

Morigi, Ital. Dr. Morigi s.r.l., Via Adelasio 33, 24020 Ranica (BG), Italy.

Morrith, Spain. Morrith, Valle de la Fuenfria 3, 28034 Madrid, Spain.

Morson, Irl. See *Cahill May Roberts, Irl.*

Morton Grove, USA. Morton Grove Pharmaceuticals, 6451 West Main St, Morton Grove, IL 60053, USA.

Morton Salt, USA. Morton Salt, 100 N Riverside Plaza, Chicago, IL 60606-1597, USA.

Moskizol, Fr. Lab. Moskizol, Allee de la Gare, 95570 Bouffemont, France.

MPF, Singapore. See *Luen Wah, Singapore.*

MPS, Austral. MPS Laboratories (Australia) P/L, 8 Kinane Street, Brighton, VIC 3186, Australia.

MSD Chibropharm, Ger. See *Merck Sharp & Dohme, Ger.*

Mt. Vernon, USA. Mt. Vernon Foods Inc., 13246 Wooster Rd, Mt. Vernon, OH 43050-9726, USA.

Much, Ger. Much Pharma GmbH, Memeler Str. 30, Postfach: 1462, 42758 Haan, Germany.

Mucos, Aust. Mucos Emulsions-GmbH, Leberstrasse 96, A-1110 Vienna, Austria.

Mucos, Ger. Mucos Pharma GmbH & Co., Malvenweg 2, 82538 Geretsried, Germany.

Muller Goppingen, Ger. Chemisch-Pharmazeutische Fabrik Göppingen Carl Müller, Apotheker, GmbH & Co. KG, Bahnhofstr. 33-35 & 40, 73033 Goppingen, Germany.

Multichem, NZ. Multichem, Private Bag 93527, Takapuna, Auckland, New Zealand.

Multilan, Israel. Multilan, Israel.

Multi-Pro, Canad. Distributions Multi-Pro Inc., 8480 Champ d'eau, St-Leonard, Quebec, H1P 1Y3, Canada.

Mundipharma, Aust. Mundipharma GmbH, Apollogasse 16-18, A-1072 Vienna, Austria.

Mundipharma, Austral. Mundipharma, P.O. Box 5214, Sydney, NSW 1044, Australia.

Mundipharma, Fin. Mundipharma Oy, Rajatorpantie 41 C, 01640 Vantaa, Finland.

Mundipharma, Ger. Mundipharma GmbH, Mundipharma Str. 2, 65549 Limburg (Lahn), Germany.

Mundipharma, Hong Kong. See *Jacobson, Hong Kong.*

Mundipharma, Swed. Mundipharma AB, Molndalsvagen 26, 412 63 Goteborg, Sweden.

Mundipharma, Switz. Mundipharma Pharmaceutical Co, St Alban-Rheinweg 74, 4006 Basle, Switzerland.

Mundipharma, Thai. See *JDH Borneo, Thai.*

Mundogen, Spain. Mundogen Farma, Maria Tubau 5, Edif Auge VI, 28050 Madrid, Spain.

Murat, Fr. Laboratoires Murat, 160 rue de Paris, 92771 Boulogne-Billancourt, France.

Murdock, USA. Murdock, Madaus, Schwabe, P.O. Box 4000, Springville, UT 84663, USA.

Muro, Israel. Muro, Israel.

Muro, USA. Muro Pharmaceutical Inc., an Asta Medica Company, 890 East St, Tewksbury, MA 01876-1496, USA.

MVM, Fr. Lab. MVM, 33 rue Vivienne, 75002 Paris, France.

Mykal, UK. Mykal Industries Ltd, Farnsworth House, Morris Close, Park Farm Industrial Estate, Wellingborough, Northamptonshire, NN8 6XF, UK.

Myplan, UK. Myplan Ltd, Old Colwall, Malvern, Worcestershire, WR13 6HF, UK.

Myra, Singapore. See *Far East Drug, Singapore.*

Myra, Thai. See *Olic, Thai.*

MZ, S.Afr. MZ, South Africa.

Nabi, USA. Nabi, 5800 Park of Commerce Blvd NW, Boca Raton, FL 33487, USA.

Nadeau, Canad. See *Technilab, Canad.*

Nadinola, Canad. See *Hargell, Canad.*

Nagor, UK. Nagor Ltd, P.O. Box 21, Douglas, Isle of Man, IM99 1AX, UK.

Naina, Singapore. Naina Mohamed & Sons Pte Ltd, 1 Ubi Crescent, 05-04 Number One Building, S 408563, Singapore.

Nakorn, Thai. See *TNP, Thai.*, and *V & V, Thai.*

Nakornpatana, Thai. Nakornpatana Pharm Co. Ltd, 495, 601/5-8 Soi Suthiporn, Prachasongkroh Rd, Dindaeng, Bangkok 10400, Thailand.

NAM, Ger. NAM Neukönigsförder Arzneimittel GmbH, Moorbeker Strasse 35, 26197 Grossenkneten, Germany.

Napp, Irl. Napp Laboratories Ltd, 54 Fitzwilliam Square, Dublin 2, Ireland.

Napp, UK. Napp Pharmaceuticals Ltd, Cambridge Science Park, Milton Rd, Cambridge, Cambridgeshire, CB4 0GW, UK.

Nasmark, Canad. Nasmark Inc., 5650 Tomken Rd, Unit 12, Mississauga, Ontario, L4W 4P1, Canada.

Nastech, USA. Nastech Pharmaceutical Co. Inc., 45 David's Dr., Hauppauge, NY 11788, USA.

Nat Druggists, S.Afr. National Druggists (Pty) Ltd, P.O. Box 3253, Durban 4000, South Africa.

National Care, Canad. National Care Products, 251 Saulteaux Crescent, Winnipeg, Manitoba, R3J 3C7, Canada.

National Diagnostic, Austral. National Diagnostic Products (Australia) P/L, 7-9 Merriwa St, Gordon, NSW 2072, Australia.

Nativelle, Switz. See *Interdelta, Switz.*

Natren, USA. Natren Inc., 3105 Willow Lane, Westlake Village, CA 91361, USA.

Nattermann, Ger. Nattermann, Division of Aventis Pharma Deutschland GmbH, Nattermannallee 1, 50829 Cologne, Germany.

Nattermann, Neth. See *Rhone-Poulenc Rorer, Neth.*

Nattermann, Spain. Nattermann, Avda de Leganes 62, Alcorcon, 28925 Madrid, Spain.

Natural Touch, UK. Natural Touch Ltd, 7 Dragoon House, Hussar Court, Brambles Farm, Waterlooville, Hampshire, PO7 7SE, UK.

Naturarzneimittel, Ger. Naturarzneimittel Regneri GmbH & Co. KG, Carl-Zeiss-Str. 4, 76275 Ettlingen, Germany.

Nature's Bounty, USA. Nature's Bounty Inc., 90 Orville Drive, Bohemia, NY 11716, USA.

Natures Kiss, Austral. Nature's Kiss Australia P/L, Level 4, 171 Clarence St, Sydney, NSW 2000, Australia.

Naturest, Hong Kong. Naturest Co. Ltd, Suite 2508, Bank of America Tower, 12 Harcourt Rd Central, Hong Kong.

Naturland, Aust. Naturland GmbH, St Veit-Gasse 56, A-1130 Vienna, Austria.

Naturmed, Ital. Naturmed srl, Via Prov.le 33 (Resid. Oasi), 19030 Castelnuovo Magra (SP), Italy.

Natus, Braz. Laboratorios Farmaceuticos Natus Ltda, Rua Maxwell 116, Vila Isabel, 20541-100 Rio de Janeiro, RJ, Brazil.

NBF-Lanes, Ital. NBF-Lanes srl, Corso di Porta Vittoria 14, 20122 Milan, Italy.

NBI, S.Afr. NBI, South Africa.

NCI, USA. NCI Medical Foods, 5801 Ayala Ave, Irwindale, CA 91706, USA.

NCSN, Ital. NCSN Farmaceutici s.r.l., Via Tiburtina Km 14.400, 00131 Rome, Italy.

Neat Feat, NZ. Neat Feat Products Ltd, P.O. Box 65256, Auckland, New Zealand.

Neckerman, Braz. Neckerman Industria Farmaceutica Ltda, Rua das Perobeiras 157, 05879-470 Sao Paulo, SP, Brazil.

Nefox, Spain. Nefox Farma, Principe de Vergara 109, 28002 Madrid, Spain.

Nefro, Aust. Nefro Pharma GrosshandelsgmbH, An der Landesbahn 2-4, A-2100 Korneuburg, Austria.

Negma, Belg. See *Vitalpharma, Belg.*

Negma, Fr. Laboratoires Negma, Imm Strasbourg, av de l'Europe, Toussus-le-Noble, 78771 Magny-les-Hameaux cdx, France.

Negma, Israel. Negma, Israel.

Nella, UK. Nella Pharmaceutical Products Ltd, Rockfield House, Darwen Rd, Bromley Cross, Bolton, Lancashire, BL7 9DX, UK.

Nelson, UK. A Nelson & Co. Ltd, Broadheath House, 83 Parkside, London, SW19 5LP, UK.

Neo Abello, Ital. Neo Abello spa, Via Falzarego 8, 20021 Bollate (MI), Italy.

Neo Laboratories, UK. Neo Laboratories Ltd, UK.

Neo Quimica, Braz. Laboratorio Neo Quimica Comercio e Industria Ltda, Rua VPR 1 Quadra 2 A Mod. 4, 75133-600 Anapolis, GO, Brazil.

Neo-Farmaceutica, Port. Neo-Farmacêutica, Lda, Avenida da Republica 45, Apartado 14277, 1064-825 Lisbon, Portugal.

Neolab, Canad. Neolab, 5476 Upper Lachine Rd, Montreal, Quebec, H4A 2A4, Canada.

Neo-Life, Austral. See *GNLD, Austral.*

Neom, Fr. Lab. Neom, 5 ave., 17 rue, B.P. 556, 06516 Carros cdx, France.

Neopharm, Israel. Neopharm Ltd, P.O. Box 3506, Petach Tikva, Israel.

Neopharm, Thai. Neopharm Co. Ltd, 5/26-27 Soi Udomsap, Baromrachonnanee Rd, Arunamarin, Bangkoknoi, Bangkok 10700, Thailand.

Neopharma, Ger. Neopharma GmbH & Co. KG, Kirchstr. 10, 83229 Aschau i. Chiemgau, Germany.

Neopharmed, Ital. Neopharmed s.p.a., Via Vitorchiano 151, 00189 Rome, Italy.

NeoStrata, USA. NeoStrata Co. Inc., 4 Research Way, Princeton, NJ 08540, USA.

Nephron, USA. Nephron Pharmaceuticals Corp., 4121 SW 34th St, Orlando, FL 32811, USA.

Nephro-Tech, USA. Nephro-Tech, Inc., P.O. Box 16106, Shawnee, KS 66203, USA.

Nestle, Austral. Nestle Australia Ltd, 60 Bathurst St, Sydney, NSW 2000, Australia.

Nestle, Braz. Nestle, Brazil.

Nestle, Canad. Nestle Canada Inc., 25 Sheppard Ave W, North York, Ontario, M2N 6S8, Canada.

Nestle, Fr. Nestlé, 7 bd Pierre-Carle, B.P. 900, Noisiel, 77446 Marne-la-Vallee cdx 2.

Nestle, Ital. Nestlè Italiana s.p.a., Viale G. Richard 5, 20143 Milan, Italy.

Nestle, Mex. Nestlé, S.A. de C.V., Av Ejercito Nacional Num 453, Col Granada, 11520 Mexico, D.F., Mexico.

Nestle, Norw. A/S Nestlé Norge, Barnematavd., Postboks 595, 1301 Sandvika, Norway.

Nestle, Port. Nestlé Portugal, SA, Rua Alexandre Herculano 8-8A, 2795-010 Linda-a-Velha (Carnaxide-Oeiras), Portugal.

Nestle, Switz. Nestlé Suisse AG, Case postale 352, 1800 Vevey, Switzerland.

Nestle, Thai. Nestle Products (Thailand) Inc, 18-21 Fl, Amarin Tower, 500 Ploenchit Rd, Pathumwan, Bangkok 10330, Thailand.

Nestle, UK. Nestlé UK Ltd, St George's House, Park Lane, Croydon, Surrey, CR9 1NR, UK.

Netpharma, Swed. Netpharma, Birger Jarlsgatan 37, 111 45 Stockholm, Sweden.

Nettopharma, Denm. See *Nycomed, Denm.*

Network Health & Beauty, UK. Network Health & Beauty, Network House, 41 Invincible Rd, Farnborough, Hampshire, GU14 7QU, UK.

Neuners, Aust. Neuner's Kräuterprodukte GmbH, Oberndorf 60, A-6322 Kirchbichl, Austria.

Neuraxpharm, Ger. neuraxpharm Arzneimittel GmbH & Co. KG, Elisabeth-Selbert-Str. 23, 40764 Langenfeld, Germany.

Neurex, USA. See *Elan, USA.*

NeuroGenesis, USA. NeuroGenesis, 2045 Space Park Dr., Suite 132, Houston, TX 77058, USA.

Neusc, Spain. Neusc, Spain.

Neutrogena, Fr. Neutrogena, Division Johnson & Johnson Consumer, 1 rue Camille-Desmoulins, 92787 Issy-les-Moulineaux cdx 9, France.

Neutrogena, Israel. Neutrogena, Israel.

Neutrogena, UK. See *Johnson & Johnson, UK.*

Neutrogena, USA. Neutrogena Corp., 5760 W 96th St, Los Angeles, CA 90045-5595, USA.

Neutrogena Dermatologics, USA. See *Neutrogena, USA.*

Neutron Technology, USA. Neutron Technology Corp, Suite 402, Boise, ID 83702, USA.

Neves, Port. Laboratório J. Neves, Lda, Parque Industrial do Seixal, 2840 Paio Pires, Portugal.

New Farma, Ital. New Farma Soc. Coop. a.r.l., Via Umberto 20, 95030 Sant'Agata li Battiati (CT), Italy.

New Research, Ital. New Research s.r.l., P.za Don Luigi Sturzo 34, 04011 Aprilia (LT), Italy.

New World Trading Corporation, USA. New World Trading Corporation, P.O. Box 952, DeBary, FL 32713, USA.

Newlab, Braz. Newlab Industria Farmaceutica Ltda, Rua Taquarucu 79, 04346-040 Sao Paulo, SP, Brazil.

Newport, Irl. Newport Pharmaceuticals Ltd, Frank Maas House, Swords Business Park, Swords, Co. Dublin, Ireland.

Newport Synthesis, Irl. Newport Synthesis Ltd, Baldoyle Industrial Estate, Dublin 13, Ireland.

Nexis, Spain. Nexis Farmaceutica, Principe de Vergara 112, 28001 Madrid, Spain.

Nexstar, Austral. Nexstar Pharmaceuticals P/L, Unit 2, 41 Stamford Rd, Oakleigh, VIC 3166, Australia.

Nexstar, Belg. Nexstar Pharmaceuticals Inc., Laarstraat 16, 2610 Wilrijk, Belgium.

Nexstar, Denm. See *Orphan, Denm.*

Nexstar, Fr. Nexstar Pharmaceutique, 39 rue Godot-de-Mauroy, 75009 Paris, France.

Nexstar, Ger. See *Gilead, Ger.*

Nexstar, Hong Kong. See *Inchcape, Hong Kong.*

Nexstar, Irl. See *Allphar, Irl.*

Nexstar, Israel. Nexstar, Israel.

Nexstar, Ital. Nexstar Pharmaceuticals Italia s.r.l., Via G Frua 16, 20146 Milan, Italy.

Nexstar, Neth. Nexstar Pharmaceuticals B.V., P.O. Box 1054, NL-1300 BB Almere, Netherlands.

Nexstar, Thai. See *Siam Pharm, Thai.*

Nexstar, UK. NeXstar Pharmaceuticals Ltd, The Quorum, Barnwell Rd, Cambridge, Cambridgeshire, CB5 8RE, UK.

Nexstar, USA. See *Gilead, USA.*

Nextar, Spain. Nextar Farmaceutica, Paseo de la Castellana 139, 28046 Madrid, Spain.

Nezel, Spain. Nezel, Av. Diagonal 507, 08029 Barcelona, Spain.

NHS, Fr. NHS, 21 rue du Pont-des-Halles, Delta 115, 94536 Rungis cdx, France.

Niche, Denm. Niche Pharma, Tvedangen 225, 2730 Herlev, Denmark.

Niche, Singapore. See *JDH, Singapore.*

Niche, USA. Niche Pharmaceuticals Inc, 200 N Oak St, P.O. Box 449, Roanoake, TX 76262.

Nicholas, Fr. See *Roche Nicholas, Fr.*

Nicholas, Port. Nicholas, Portugal.

Nicholas, UK. See *Roche, UK.*

Nicodent, Austral. See *Advil, Austral.*

Niddapharm, Ger. NIDDApharm GmbH, Konrad-Adenauer-Allee 8-10, 61118 Bad Vilbel, Germany.

Niedermaier, Ger. Dr Niedermaier GmbH, Taufkirchner Str. 59, 85662 Hohenbrunn bei Munich, Germany.

Nigy, Fr. Laboratoires Nigy, 6 av de l'Europe, 78401 Chatou cdx, France.

Nigy, Singapore. See *Polymedic, Singapore.*

Nihon, Jpn. Nihon Pharmaceutical Co. Ltd, 9-8 Higashikanda 1-chome, Chiyoda-ku, Tokyo 101-0031, Japan.

Nikken, Jpn. Nikken Chemicals Co., Ltd, 4-14 Tsukiji 5-chome, Chuo-ku, Tokyo 104-0045, Japan.

Nikkho, Braz. Quimica e Farmaceutica Nikkho do Brasil Ltda, Rua Jaime Perdigao 431/445, 21920-240 Rio de Janeiro, RJ, Brazil.

Nion, USA. Nion Corp., 15501 First St, Irwindale, CA 91706, USA.

Niverpharm, Fr. Laboratoires Niverpharm, ZI des Taupieres, rue Francis-Garnier, 58000 Nevers, France.

NM, Denm. NM Pharma A/S, Overgaden neden Vandet 7, 1414 Copenhagen K, Denmark.

NM, Swed. NM Pharma AB, 112 87 Stockholm, Sweden.

NMC, USA. NMC Labs, 70-36 83rd St, Glendale, NY 11385, USA.

Nnodum, USA. Nnodum Corp., 886 Clinton Springs Ave, Cincinnati, OH 45229, USA.

Nobel, Canad. Nobel Pharm Enrg, 2615 pl. Chasse, Montreal, Quebec, H1Y 2C3, Canada.

Nobel, Ital. Nobel Pharmacos, Via Fasano 70, 95030 Gravina di Catania (CT), Italy.

Nogues, Fr. Laboratoires Noguès, 43 rue de Neuilly, 92000 Nanterre, France.

Nogues, Switz. See *Uhlmann-Eyraud, Switz.*

Nomad, UK. Nomad Medical Ltd, 3-4 Wellington Terrace, Turnpike Lane, Hornsey, London, N8 0PX, UK.

Nomax, USA. Nomax Inc., 40 North Rock Hill Rd, St Louis, MO 63119, USA.

Noos, Ital. Noos srl, Via Pietro Marchisio 227, 00173 Rome, Italy.

Norcliff Thayer, USA. See *SmithKline Beecham Consumer, USA.*

Nordic, Swed. Nordic Drugs AB, Box 30035, 200 61 Limhamn, Sweden.

Nordic, UK. See *Ferring, UK.*

Nordic Drugs, Denm. Nordic Drugs, Niels Juels Gade 5, 1059 Copenhagen K, Denmark.

Nordic Drugs, Fin. Nordic Drugs, Filial Finland, PL 13, Länsituulentie 10, 02101 Espoo, Finland.

Nordic Healthcare, Denm. Nordic Health-Care Products ApS, Niels Andersens Vej 66, 2900 Hellerup, Denmark.

Nordisk Ibu-Pharma, Denm. Nordisk Ibu-Pharma ApS, Gersonsvej 25, 2900 Hellerup, Denmark.

Nordmark, Ital. Nordmark Farmaceutici s.p.a., Italy.

Nordmark, Neth. See *Knoll, Neth.*

Norgesfarma, Norw. Norgesfarma AS, Skarersletta 45, 1471 Skarer, Norway.

Norgine, Aust. Norgine Pharma GmbH, Vivenotgasse 1/1, A-1120 Vienna, Austria.

Norgine, Austral. Norgine P/L, 6/33 Ryde Rd, Pymble, NSW 2073, Australia.

Norgine, Belg. Norgine S.A., Berkenlaan 7, 1831 Diegem, Belgium.

Norgine, Denm. See *United Nordic, Denm.*

Norgine, Fr. Laboratoires Norgine Pharma, 23 av. de Neuilly, 75116 Paris, France.

Norgine, Ger. Norgine GmbH, Im Schwarzenborn 4, 35041 Marburg, Germany.

Norgine, Hong Kong. See *Treasure Mountain, Hong Kong.*

Norgine, Irl. See *United Drug, Irl.*

Norgine, Ital. Norgine Italia srl, Via Panzini 13, 20145 Milan, Italy.

Norgine, Neth. Norgine B.V., Netherlands.

Norgine, Norw. See *Andersen, Norw.*

Norgine, NZ. See *CSL, NZ.*

Norgine, S.Afr. Norgine (Pty) Ltd, P.O. Box 781247, Sandton 2146, South Africa.

Norgine, Singapore. See *Grafton, Singapore.*

Norgine, Switz. Norgine AG, Industriestrasse 11/13, 6243 Rotkreuz, Switzerland.

Norgine, Thai. See *Zuellig, Thai.*

Norgine, UK. Norgine Ltd, Chaplin House, Moorhall Rd, Harefield, Uxbridge, Middlesex, UB9 6NS, UK.

Noriega, Spain. Noriega, Spain.

Noristan, S.Afr. Noristan Laboratories (Pty) Ltd, Private Bag X516, Silverton 0127, South Africa.

Noristan Generica, S.Afr. See *Noristan, S.Afr.*

Norit, Aust. See *Vemedia, Neth.*

Norit, Israel. Norit, Israel.

Norma, UK. Norma Chemicals Ltd, New Abbey Court, 51-53 Stert St, Abingdon, Oxfordshire, OX14 3HB, UK.

Normal, Port. Laboratório Normal, Lda, Rua do Centro Empresarial, Edificio 8, Quinta da Beloura, 2710-444 Sintra, Portugal.

Norman, Canad. See *Norman, USA.*

Norman, USA. Merle Norman Cosmetics, 9130 Bellanca Ave, Los Angeles, CA 90045, USA.

Normon, Spain. Normon, Nierenberg 10, 28002 Madrid, Spain.

Norpharma, Denm. Norpharma AS, Bygstubben 11, 2950 Vedbaek, Denmark.

Norpharma, Norw. See *Andersen, Norw.*

Norstar, USA. Norstar Consumer Products, 206 Pegasus Ave, Northvale, NJ 07647, USA.

North American Vaccine, USA. North American Vaccine Inc., 10150 Old Columbia Rd, Columbia, MD 21046, USA.

Northern Research, USA. Northern Research Laboratories Inc., 8400 Normandale Lake Blvd, Suite 920, Minneapolis, MN 55437, USA.

Norton, Israel. Norton, Israel.

Norton, S.Afr. Norton, South Africa.

Norton, UK. H.N. Norton & Co. Ltd, Gemini House, Flex Meadow, Harlow, Essex, CM19 5TJ, UK.

Norton Healthcare, Denm. See *United Nordic, Denm.*

Norton Healthcare, Singapore. See *Green Cross, Singapore.*

Norton Healthcare, UK. Norton Healthcare Ltd, Albert Basin, Royal Docks, London, E16 2QJ, UK.

Norton Waterford, Irl. Norton Waterford Ltd, Waterford Industrial Estate, Waterford, Ireland.

Norwood, Canad. Norwood Packaging Ltd, 8519-132nd St, Surrey, British Columbia, V3W 4N8, Canada.

Nostrum, Port. Sociedade Nostrum, Lda, Rua da Escola de Medicina Veterinaria, 15/17, 1049-029 Lisbon, Portugal.

Nostrum, Spain. Nostrum Farma, Principe de Vergara 109, 28001 Madrid, Spain.

Nourypharma, Ger. Nourypharma GmbH, Mittenheimer Str. 62, 85764 Oberschleissheim, Germany.

Nourypharma, Neth. Nourypharma Nederland B.V., Postbus 20, 5340 BH Oss, Netherlands.

Nourypharma, Switz. See *Orion, Switz.*

Nova Argentia, Ital. Nova Argentia Industria Farmaceutica s.r.l., Via G. Pascoli 1, 20064 Gorgonzola (MI), Italy.

Novag, Mex. Novag Infancia, S.A. de C.V., Claz. de Tlalpan No. 3417, Col. Sta. Ursula Coapa-Coyoacan, 04650 Mexico, D.F., Mexico.

Novag, Spain. Novag, Gran Via de Carlos III 94, 08028 Barcelona, Spain.

Novalac, Fr. Novalac, 209 rue de l'Universite, 75007 Paris, France.

Novalis, Fr. See *Wyeth Lederle, Fr.*

Novaquimica, Braz. A Novaquimica Laboratorios S.A., Marginal Direita da Via Anchieta Km 13.5, 09883-000 Sao Bernardo do Campo, SP, Brazil.

Novartis, Aust. Novartis Pharma GmbH, Brunner Strasse 59, A-1235 Vienna, Austria.

Novartis, Austral. Novartis Pharmaceuticals P/L, P.O. Box 101, North Ryde, NSW 1670, Australia.

Novartis, Belg. Novartis Pharma S.A., Chaussee de Haecht 226, 1030 Brussels, Belgium.

Novartis, Braz. Novartis Biociencias S.A., Avenida Professor Vicente Rao 90, 04706-900 Sao Paulo, SP, Brazil.

Novartis, Canad. Novartis Pharmaceuticals Canada Inc., 385 Bouchard Blvd, Dorval, Quebec, H9S 1A9, Canada.

Novartis, Denm. Novartis Healthcare AS, Lyngbyvej 172, 2100 Copenhagen O, Denmark.

Novartis, Fin. Novartis Finland Oy, Metsänneidonkuja 10, 02130 Espoo, Finland.

Novartis, Fr. Novartis Pharma SA, 2-4 rue Lionel-Terray, 92500 Rueil-Malmaison, France.

Novartis, Ger. Novartis Pharma GmbH, Roonstr. 25, 90429 Nurnberg, Germany.

Novartis, Hong Kong. Novartis Pharmaceuticals (HK) Ltd, 37/F Windsor House, 311 Gloucester Rd, Causeway Bay, Hong Kong.

Novartis, Irl. Novartis Ireland Ltd, Beech House, Beech Hill Office Campus, Clonskeagh, Dublin 4, Ireland.

Novartis, Israel. Novartis Pharma, P.O. Box 7759, Petach Tikva, Israel.

Novartis, Ital. Novartis Farma spa, SS 233 (Varesina) km 20.5, 21040 Origgio (VA), Italy.

Novartis, Jpn. Novartis Pharm., Japan.

Novartis, Mex. Novartis Farmaceutica, S.A. de C.V., Calz. de Tlalpan No. 1779, Col. San Diego Churubusco, 04120 Mexico, D.F., Mexico.

Novartis, Neth. Novartis Pharma B.V., Postbus 241, 6800 LZ Arnhem, Netherlands.

Novartis, Norw. Novartis Norge AS, Brynsalleen 4, Postboks 237 Okern, 0510 Oslo, Norway.

Novartis, NZ. Novartis New Zealand Ltd, Private Bag, Avondale, Auckland, New Zealand.

Novartis, Port. Novartis Farma, SA, Rua do Centro Empresarial, Edificio 8, Quinta da Beloura, 2710-444 Sintra, Portugal.

Novartis, S.Afr. Novartis South Africa (Pty) Ltd, P.O. Box 92, Isando 1600, South Africa.

Novartis, Singapore. Novartis (Singapore) Pte Ltd, Pharmaceutical Sector, 10 Hoe Chiang Road, 09-05/06 Keppel Towers, S 089315, Singapore.

Novartis, Spain. Novartis Farmaceutica, Gran Via Corts Catalanes 764, 08013 Barcelona, Spain.

Novartis, Swed. Novartis Sverige AB, Box 1150, 183 11 Taby, Sweden.

Novartis, Switz. Novartis Pharma Schweiz AG, Sudbahnhofstrasse 14 D, Postfach, 3001 Berne, Switzerland.

Novartis, Thai. Novartis (Thailand) Ltd, 159/30 Vibhavadi Rangsit Rd, Laksi, Bangkok 10210, Thailand.

Novartis, UK. Novartis Pharmaceuticals UK Ltd, Frimley Business Park, Frimley, Camberley, Surrey, GU16 5SG, UK.

Novartis, USA. Novartis Pharmaceuticals Corp., 59 Route 10, East Hanover, NJ 07936, USA.

Novartis Consumer, Aust. See *Gebro, Aust.*

Novartis Consumer, Austral. Novartis Consumer Health Australasia P/L, P.O. Box 4499, Mulgrave, VIC 3170, Australia.

Novartis Consumer, Belg. Novartis Consumer Health S.A., Rue de Wand 211-13, 1020 Brussels, Belgium.

Novartis Consumer, Canad. Novartis Consumer Health Canada Inc., 2233 Argentia Rd, Suite 205, Mississauga, Ontario, L5N 2X7, Canada.

Novartis Consumer, Ger. Novartis Consumer Health GmbH, Zielstattstr. 40, 81379 Munich, Germany.

Novartis Consumer, Irl. Novartis Consumer Health, M & P House, Hammond Lane, Dublin 7, Ireland.

Novartis Consumer, Ital. Novartis Consumer Health spa, Strada Statale 233 km 20.5, 21040 Orrigio (VA), Italy.

Novartis Consumer, Neth. Novartis Consumer Health Benelux, Postbus 1070, 4801 BB Breda, Netherlands.

Novartis Consumer, Port. Novartis Consumer Health, Lda, Av Poeta Mistral 2-2, 1069-172 Lisbon, Portugal.

Novartis Consumer, S.Afr. Novartis Consumer Health, Private Bag X10, Rivonia 2128, South Africa.

Novartis Consumer, Spain. See *Novartis, Spain.*

Novartis Consumer, Switz. Novartis Consumer Health Schweiz AG, Monbijoustrasse 118, 3001 Berne, Switzerland.

Novartis Consumer, UK. Novartis Consumer Health, Wimblehurst Rd, Horsham, West Sussex, RH12 4AB, UK.

Novartis Consumer, USA. Novartis Consumer Health Inc., 560 Morris Ave, Summit, NJ 07901-1312, USA.

Novartis Nutrition, Canad. Novartis Nutrition Corporation, 111 Consumers Drive, Whitby, Ontario, L1N 5Z5, Canada.

Novartis Nutrition, Fr. Lab. Novartis Nutrition, B.P. 29, 31250 Revel, France.

Novartis Nutrition, Hong Kong. See *Keller, Hong Kong.*

Novartis Nutrition, Port. See *Novartis Consumer, Port.*

Novartis Nutrition, Singapore. See *Zuellig, Singapore.*

Novartis Nutrition, UK. Novartis Nutrition Ltd, Station Rd, Kings Langley, Hertfordshire, WD4 8LJ, UK.

Novartis Nutrition, USA. Novartis Nutrition Corp., 5100 Gamble Dr., St Louis Park, MN 55416, USA.

Novartis Ophthalmics, Canad. See *Novartis, Canad.*

Novartis Ophthalmics, UK. Novartis Ophthalmics, Delta House, Southwood Crescent, Southwood, Farnborough, Hampshire, GU10 0NL, UK.

Novartis Ophthalmics, USA. Novartis Ophthalmics Inc., 11460 Johns Creek Parkway, Duluth, GA 30097-1556, USA.

Novartis Sante, Fr. Novartis Santé Familiale SA, 14 bd Richelieu, 92845 Rueil-Malmaison cdx, France.

Novaxa, Ital. Novaxa s.p.a., Via Aquileja 49, 20092 Cinisello Balsamo (MI), Italy.

Novaxo, Fr. Lab. Novaxo, 100 rte de Versailles, 78163 Marly-le-Roi cdx, France.

Noveal, Switz. See *Uhlmann-Eyraud, Switz.*

Novel, Ital. Novel OTC srl, Via Lamarmora 1, 20122 Milan, Italy.

Noven, USA. Noven Pharmaceuticals, 11960 SW 144th St, Miami, FL 33186, USA.

Novex Pharma, UK. Novex Pharma Ltd, Innovex House, Marlow Park, Marlow, Buckinghamshire, SL7 1TB, UK.

Novipharm, Aust. Novipharm GmbH, Klagenfurter Strasse 164, A-9210 Portschach, Austria.

Novipharm, Ger. Novipharm GmbH, Haidachstr. 29/7/43, 75181 Pforzheim, Germany.

Novo Nordisk, Aust. Novo-Nordisk Pharma GmbH, Universitatsstrasse 11, A-1010 Vienna, Austria.

Novo Nordisk, Austral. Novo Nordisk Pharmaceuticals P/L, P.O. Box 6086, Parramatta Business Centre, NSW 2150, Australia.

Novo Nordisk, Belg. Novo Nordisk Pharma S.A., Blvd International 55, 1070 Brussels, Belgium.

Novo Nordisk, Braz. Novo Nordisk Farmaceutica do Brasil Ltda, Rua Professor Francisco Ribeiro 683, 81701-000 Araucaria, PR, Brazil.

Novo Nordisk, Canad. Novo Nordisk Canada Inc., 2700 Matheson Blvd E, 3rd Floor, West Tower, Mississauga, Ontario, L4W 4V9, Canada.

Novo Nordisk, Denm. Novo Nordisk Farmaka Danmark A/S, Lottenborgvej 24, 2800 Lyngby, Denmark.

Novo Nordisk, Fin. Novo Nordisk Farma Oy, Pihatörmä 1 A, 02240 Espoo, Finland.

Novo Nordisk, Fr. Novo Nordisk Pharmaceutique SA, 32 rue de Bellevue, 92773 Boulogne-Billancourt cdx, France.

Novo Nordisk, Ger. Novo Nordisk Pharma GmbH, Bruckenstr. 1, 55127 Mainz, Germany.

Novo Nordisk, Hong Kong. See *Swire Loxley, Hong Kong.*

Novo Nordisk, Irl. Novo-Nordisk Pharmaceuticals Ltd, 3/4 Upper Pembroke St, Dublin 2, Ireland.

Novo Nordisk, Israel. Novo Nordisk, P.O. Box 190, Kfar Saba, Israel.

Novo Nordisk, Ital. Novo Nordisk Farmaceutici s.p.a., Via Elio Vitorini 129, 00144 Rome (RM), Italy.

Novo Nordisk, Neth. Novo Nordisk Farma, Postbus 443, 2400 AK Alphen ald Rijn, Netherlands.

Novo Nordisk, Norw. Novo Nordisk Pharma AS, Hauger Skolev. 16, Postboks 24, 1351 Rud, Norway.

Novo Nordisk, NZ. Novo Nordisk Pharmaceuticals Ltd, P.O. Box 51268, Pakuranga, Auckland, New Zealand.

Novo Nordisk, Port. Novo-Nordisk, Lda, Quinta da Fonte, Edifico D Jose Q54, Piso 1, 2780-730 Paco de Arcos, Portugal.

Novo Nordisk, S.Afr. Novo-Nordisk (Pty) Ltd, P.O. Box 783155, Sandton 2146, South Africa.

Novo Nordisk, Singapore. See *JDH, Singapore.*

Novo Nordisk, Spain. Novo Nordisk Pharma, Calereuga 102, 28033 Madrid, Spain.

Novo Nordisk, Swed. Novo Nordisk Scandinavia AB, Box 50587, 202 15 Malmo, Sweden.

Novo Nordisk, Switz. Novo Nordisk Pharma AG, Untere Heslibachstrasse 46, Postfach, 8700 Kusnacht/ZH, Switzerland.

Novo Nordisk, Thai. Novo Nordisk Pharma (Thailand) Ltd, 4 Fl, Sethiwan Tower, 139 Pan Rd, Silom, Bangkok 10500, Thailand.

Novo Nordisk, UK. Novo Nordisk Pharmaceuticals Ltd, Novo Nordisk House, Broadfield Park, Brighton Rd, Pease Pottage, Crawley, West Sussex, RH11 9RT, UK.

Novo Nordisk, USA. Novo Nordisk Pharmaceuticals Inc., 100 Overlook Center, Suite 200, Princeton, NJ 08540-7810, USA.

Novocol, USA. See *Septodent, USA.*

Novogaleno, Ital. Novogaleno srl, Largo Sermoneta 24, 80123 Naples, Italy.

Novogen, Austral. Novogen Laboratories P/L, 140 Wicks Rd, North Ryde, NSW 2113, Australia.

Novopharm, Canad. Novopharm Ltd, 30 Novopharm Court, Toronto, Ontario, M1B 2K9, Canada.

Novopharm, USA. Novopharm USA Inc., 165 E Commerce Drive, Schaumburg, IL 60173-5326, USA.

NSID, Israel. NSID, Israel.

Nucare, UK. Nucare Plc, Raeburn House, 86 Northolt Rd, Harrow, Middlesex, HA2 0EL, UK.

Numark, Canad. See *Numark, USA.*

Numark, UK. Numark Management Ltd, 5/6 Fairway Court, Amber Close, Tamworth Business Park, Tamworth, Staffordshire, B77 4RP, UK.

Numark, USA. Numark Laboratories Inc., 75 Mayfield Ave, Edison, NJ 08837, USA.

Nuova ICT, Ital. Nuova ICT srl, Via M Borsa 11, 26845 Codogno (LO), Italy.

Nuovo, Ital. Nuovo Consorzio Sanitario Nazionale s.r.l., Via Svetonio 6, 00136 Rome, Italy.

Nuovo ISM, Ital. Nuovo Istituto Sieroterapico Milanese s.r.l., 55020 Castelvecchio Pascoli (LU), Italy.

Nu-Pharm, Canad. Nu-Pharm Inc., 50 Mural St, Richmond Hill, Ontario, L4C 1E4, Canada.

Nutergia, Fr. Laboratoires Nutergia, B.P. 52, 12700 Capdenac, France.

Nutraceuticals, UK. Nutraceuticals Ltd, Wurtley House, 16 Eastbourne Rd, Hornsea, East Yorkshire, HU18 1QS, UK.

Nutralife, UK. Nutralife UK Ltd, Omicron House, Fircroft Way, Edenbridge, Kent, TN8 6EL, UK.

Nutraloric, USA. Nutraloric, 350 N Lantana, Unit G1, Camarillo, CA 93010, USA.

Nutramax, USA. NutraMax Laboratories Inc., 2208 Lakeside Bvld, Edgewood, MD 21040, USA.

Nutrasweet, NZ. Nutrasweet Consumer Products, Division of Monsanto (NZ) Ltd, P.O. Box 3872, Auckland, New Zealand.

Nutricia, Austral. Nutricia Australia P/L, P.O. Box 6745, Baulkham Hills Business Centre, NSW 2153, Australia.

Nutricia, Fin. Nutricia Oy, Linnankatu 26 A, 20100 Turku, Finland.

Nutricia, Fr. Nutricia, 4 rue Joseph-Monier, 92859 Rueil-Malmaison cdx, France.

Nutricia, Hong Kong. See *Treasure Mountain, Hong Kong.*

Nutricia, Irl. Nutricia Ireland Ltd, 18 Sandyford Business Centre, Burton Hall Rd, Dublin 18, Ireland.

Nutricia, Ital. Nutricia s.p.a., Via Fosse Adreatine 4, 20092 Cinisello Balsamo (MI), Italy.

Nutricia, NZ. Nutricia Australasia, P.O. Box 62523, Central Park, Auckland, New Zealand.

Nutricia, Port. Nutricia Portugal. Lda, Rua da Fraternidade Operaria, 2795-491 Carnaxide, Portugal.

Nutricia, Singapore. See *Sime Darby, Singapore.*

Nutricia, Thai. See *Berli, Thai.*

Nutricia Clinical, UK. Nutricia Clinical Care, Nutricia Ltd, Newmarket Ave, White Horse Business Park, Trowbridge, Wiltshire, BA14 0XQ, UK.

Nutricia Dietary, UK. See *Nutricia Clinical, UK.*

Nutricia-Luma Lindar, USA. See *Mt. Vernon, USA.*

Nutrifar, Ital. Nutrifar srl, Via Cadore 7, 26015 Soresina (CR), Italy.

Nutrifarma, Mex. Nutrifarma, Mexico.

Nutrimed, Fr. Nutrimed Medic System, 6/10 rue Mirabeau, 75016 Paris, France.

Nutri-Metics, Canad. Nutri-Metics International (Can) Ltd, 3915-16 Ave SE, Calgary, Alberta, T2C 1V5, Canada.

Nutri-Pharm, Austral. Nutri-Pharm, 102 Myers Rd, Bittern, VIC 3198, Australia.

Nutripharm, USA. Nutripharm Laboratories Inc., Salem Industrial Park, Building 5, Lebanon, NJ 08833, USA.

Nutrisoy, USA. Nutrisoy, USA.

Nutrition Care, Austral. Nutrition Care, 25-7 Keysborough Ave, Keysborough, VIC 3173, Australia.

Nutrition Medical, Israel. Nutrition Medical, Israel.

Nutri-Well, Hong Kong. See *Winsor, Hong Kong.*

Nycomed, Aust. Nycomed Austria GmbH, Lembockgasse 49, A-1230 Vienna, Austria.

Nycomed, Austral. Nycomed Amersham Australia, P.O. Box 6001, Baulkham Hills Business Centre, NSW 2153, Australia.

Nycomed, Belg. Nycomed Amersham S.A., Chaussee de Gand 615, 1080 Brussels, Belgium.

Nycomed, Denm. Nycomed Danmark A/S, Langebjerg 1, 4000 Roskilde, Denmark.

Nycomed, Fin. Nycomed Oy, Vallikallionkatu 1, 02600 Espoo, Finland.

Nycomed, Fr. Laboratoires Nycomed Amersham, 25 quai Panhard et Levassor, CE no. 19, 75644 Paris cdx 13, France.

Nycomed, Ger. Nycomed Pharma GmbH, Fraunhoferstr. 7, 85737 Ismaning b. Munich, Germany.

Nycomed, Hong Kong. See *Inchcape, Hong Kong.*

Nycomed, Irl. See *Newport Synthesis, Irl.*

Nycomed, Israel. Nycomed, Israel.

Nycomed, Ital. Nycomed Amersham Sorin srl, Via Crescentino, 13040 Saluggia (VC), Italy.

Nycomed, Neth. Nycomed B.V., Postbus 3458, 4800 DL Breda, Netherlands.

Nycomed, Norw. Nycomed Pharma AS, Postboks 205, 1385 Asker, Norway.

Nycomed, NZ. Nycomed NZ Ltd, Unit F, 156 Bush Rd, Albany, Auckland, New Zealand.

Nycomed, Singapore. See *FP, Singapore.*

Nycomed, Spain. Nycomed Amersham, Ronda de Poniente, 12, Tres Cantos Madrid, 28760 Madrid, Spain.

Nycomed, Swed. Nycomed AB, Box 1215, 181 24 Lidingo, Sweden.

Nycomed, Switz. Nycomed AG, Moosacherstrasse 14, Au, 8820 Wadenswil, Switzerland.

Nycomed, USA. See *Nycomed Amersham, USA.*

Nycomed Amersham, Canad. Nycomed Amersham Canada Ltd, 1166 South Service Rd West, Oakville, Ontario, L6L 5T7, Canada.

Nycomed Amersham, Swed. See *Nycomed, Swed.*

Nycomed Amersham, UK. Nycomed Amersham plc, Amersham Labs, Building 21, White Lion Rd, Amersham, Buckinghamshire, HP7 9LL, UK.

Nycomed Amersham, USA. Nycomed Amersham, 101 Carnegie Center, Princeton, NJ 08540-6231, USA.

Nycomed Imaging, Denm. See *Nycomed, Denm.*

Nycomed Imaging, Norw. Nycomed Imaging AS, Nycov. 2, Postboks 4220 Torshov, 0401 Oslo, Norway.

NZ Diagnostics, NZ. New Zealand Diagnostics Ltd, P.O. Box 30-683, Lower Hutt, New Zealand.

NZ Distributors, NZ. New Zealand Distributors Ltd, P.O. BOX 41014, St Lukes, Auckland, New Zealand.

NZ Medical & Scientific, NZ. New Zealand Medical & Scientific Ltd, P.O. Box 24-138, Royal Oak, Auckland, New Zealand.

Oakhurst, USA. Oakhurst Co., 3000 Hempstead Turnpike, Levittown, NY 11756, USA.

OBA, Denm. OBA Pharma ApS, Kronprinsessegade 26 A (postboks 117), 1004 Copenhagen K, Denmark.

Oberlin, Fr. Laboratoires Oberlin, 304 av du Docteur Jean-Bru, 47000 Agen, France.

Ocean Health, Singapore. Ocean Health (S) Pte Ltd, 42 Mactaggart Rd, 05-02, S 368086, Singapore.

Oclassen, USA. See *Watson, USA.*

O'Connor, USA. See *Columbia, USA.*

Octapharma, Aust. Octapharma Pharmazeutika, Oberlaaer Strasse 235, A-1100 Vienna, Austria.

Octapharma, Ger. Octapharma Vertrieb von Plasmaderivaten GmbH, Bahnhofstr. 43, 40764 Langenfeld, Germany.

Octapharma, Hong Kong. See *Weston, Hong Kong.*

Octapharma, Norw. Octapharma AS, Postboks 123, 2091 Hurdal, Norway.

Octapharma, Swed. Octapharma AB, Kanalvagen 15, 18330 Taby, Sweden.

Octapharma, Switz. Octapharma AG, Haus im Park, 8866 Ziegelbrucke, Switzerland.

Octapharma, UK. Octapharma Ltd, 6 Elm Court, Copse Drive, Coventry, CV5 9RG, UK.

Ocumed, USA. Ocumed Inc., 119 Harrison Ave, Roseland, NJ 07068, USA.

Ocusoft, USA. Cynacon/OCuSOFT, 5311 Ave N, P.O. Box 429, Richmond, TX 77406-0429, USA.

Odan, Canad. Odan Laboratories Ltd, 847 McCaffrey St, St Laurent, Quebec, H4T 1N3, Canada.

Odontofarma, Braz. Laboratorio Odontofarma Ltda, Rua Claudio Furquim 21/25 1° And., Tatuape, 03072-010 Sao Paulo, SP, Brazil.

Odontomed, Braz. Laboratorio Odontomed Industria e Comercio Ltda, Avenida Bosque da Saude 1.088, Bosque da Saude, 04142-081 Sao Paulo, SP, Brazil.

Odontopharm, Switz. Odontopharm AG, Engestrasse 23, 3000 Bern 26, Switzerland.

Odyssey, USA. Odyssey Pharmaceuticals Inc, 72 DeForest Ave, East Hanover, NJ 07936, USA.

Oenobiol, Fr. Lab. Oenobiol, 59 bd Exelmans, 75781 Paris cdx 16, France.

OFF, Ital. Officina Farmaceutica Fiorentina s.r.l. Istituto Biochimico, Quart. Varignano 12-14, 55049 Viareggio (Lucca), Italy.

Ofimex, Mex. Laboratorios Ofimex S.A. de C.V., Calz. de Tlalpan No. 4369, Col. Toriello Guerra, 14040 Mexico D.F., Mexico.

Oftalder, Port. See *Edol, Port.*

Oftalmiso, Spain. Oftalmiso, Spain.

Ogera, Switz. Ogera AG, Lerzenstrasse 18, 8953 Dietikon, Switzerland.

Ogna, Ital. Giovanni Ogna & Figli s.p.a., Via Figini 41, 20053 Muggio (MI), Italy.

Ohara, Jpn. Ohara Chemical Industries Ltd, 43-1 Oharaichiba, Koka-cho, Kokagun, Shiga 520-3433, Japan.

Ohm, USA. OHM Laboratories Inc., P.O. Box 7397, North Brunswick, NJ 08902, USA.

Ohmeda, USA. See *Baxter, USA.*

Ohropax, Switz. See *Uhlmann-Eyraud, Switz.*

Ohta, Hong Kong. See *Primal, Hong Kong.*

OJG, Belg. O.J.G. Consumer Care s.p.r.l., Xavier de Cocklaan 66 bus 3, 9830 Sint-Martins-Latem, Belgium.

Olan-Kemed, Thai. Olan-Kemed Co. Ltd, 176 Ladprao Rd, Bangkok 10900, Thailand.

Olbas, Ger. See *Schoenenberger, Ger.*

Olcelli, Ital. Laboratorio Chimico Farmaceutico Olcelli Dr. M. & C. s.r.l., Via S. Damiano 24/A, 20034 Giussano (MI), Italy.

Olic, Thai. Olic (Thailand) Ltd, 7 Fl, 2535 Sukhumvit Rd, Bangchak, Phrakanong, Bangkok 10250, Thailand.

Oligosol, Switz. Oligosol AG, Untermattweg 8, 3001 Berne, Switzerland.

OM, Ger. Deutsche OM Arzneimittel GmbH, Am Houiller Platz 17, 61381 Friedrichsdorf/Ts, Germany.

OM, Port. OM Portuguesa, SA, Rua da Industria no 2, Quinta Grande, 2720 Alfragide, Portugal.

OM, Switz. OM Pharma, 22 rue du Bois-du-Lan, 1217 Meyrin 2/Geneva, Switzerland.

Omega, Canad. Omega Laboratories Ltd, 11177 Hamon St, Montreal, Quebec, H3M 3A2, Canada.

Omega, Spain. Omega Farmaceutica, Ronda General Mitre 151, 08022 Barcelona, Spain.

Omegin, Ger. Omegin Dr Schmidgall GmbH & Co. KG, Industriepark 210, 78244 Gottmadingen, Germany.

Omida, Switz. Omida AG, Homoopathische Heilmittel, Erlistrasse 2, 6403 Kussnacht aR, Switzerland.

Omisan, Ital. Omisan Farmaceutici di Antonio Vona & C sas, Via Tossicia 15, 00131 Rome, Italy.

OMJ, Hong Kong. See *Zuellig, Hong Kong.*

Omni, UK. Omni Nutraceuticals, UK.

Omnimed, S.Afr. See *Braun Omnimed, S.Afr.*

Omrix, Israel. Omrix Biopharmaceuticals Ltd, P.O. Box 619, Rehovot, Israel.

One Drop Only, Ger. One Drop Only Chem.-pharma.-Vertriebs-GmbH, Stieffring 14, 13627 Berlin, Germany.

Onkoworks, Ger. Onkoworks Gesellschaft zur Herstellung und Vertrieb onkologischer Spezialpräparate mbH, Schallbruch 5, 42781 Haan/Rhid., Germany.

Ono, Hong Kong. See *Hing Yip, Hong Kong.*

Ono, Jpn. Ono Pharmaceutical Co. Ltd, 1-5 Doshomachi 2-chome, Chuo-ku, Osaka 541-8526, Japan.

Onstrong, Hong Kong. Onstrong Ltd, Rm B, 11/F, Bright Growth Medical Ctr, 335 Nathan Rd, Kowloon, Hong Kong.

Opco, Denm. Opco Pharma ApS, Staldgardsgade 2, 8900 Randers, Denmark.

Opfermann, Ger. Opfermann Arzneimittel GmbH, Robert-Koch-Str. 2, 51674 Wiehl, Germany.

Ophir Shalpharm, Israel. Ophir & Shalpharm Ltd, 30 Hamelacha St, Holon, Israel.

Ophtapharma, Canad. Ophtapharma Canada Inc., 1100 Cremazie E, Suite 708, Montreal, Quebec, H2P 2X2, Canada.

Ophta, Denm. Ophta A/S, Halmtorvet 29, 1700 Copenhagen V, Denmark.

Ophthalmic Laboratories, Austral. Ophthalmic Laboratories P/L, 41 Sydenham Rd, Brookvale, NSW 2100, Australia.

Opocalcium, Fr. Laboratoires de l'Opocalcium, 423 rue Audemars, ZI, 78530 Buc, France.

Opofarm, Braz. Opofarm Industrias Farmaceuticas Ltda, Rua Mario Junqueira da Silva 736, 13063-000 Campinas, SP, Brazil.

Opopharma, Switz. Opopharma SA, Kirchgasse 42, 8001 Zurich, Switzerland.

Optident, UK. Optident Dental Products, International Development Centre, Valley Drive, Ilkley, West Yorkshire, LS29 8PB, UK.

Optikem, USA. Optikem International Inc., 2172 S Jason St, Denver, CO 80223, USA.

Optimal, Hong Kong. See *Health Tech, Hong Kong.*

Optimed, Ger. Optimed Pharma GmbH, Alfred-Nobel-Str. 5, 50226 Frechen, Germany.

Optimox, USA. Optimox Corp., 2720 Monterey St, Suite 406, Torrance, CA 90503, USA.

Opto-Pharm, Singapore. Opto-Pharm, Singapore.

Optopics, USA. See *Nutramax, USA.*

Optrex, Singapore. See *Boots, Singapore.*

Opus, S.Afr. Opus Pharmaceuticals (Pty) Ltd, P.O.Box 78618, Sandton 2146, South Africa.

Opus, UK. See *Trinity, UK.*

OPW, Ger. Oranienburger Pharmawerk GmbH (OPW), Lehnitzstr. 70-98, 165152 Oranienburg, Germany.

Oral-B, Austral. Oral-B Laboratories P/L, 5 Caribbean Drive, Scoresby, VIC 3179, Australia.

Oral-B, Canad. Oral-B Laboratories Inc., 111 Matheson Blvd W, Suite 210, Mississauga, Ontario, L5R 3T5, Canada.

Oral-B, Irl. Oral-B, Ireland.

Oral-B, Ital. Oral-B Laboratories Italy, Via Pirelli 18, 20124 Milan, Italy.

Oral-B, Mex. Oral-B S.A. de C.V., Jose Ma. Rico No. 221, Col. del Valle, 03100 Mexico D.F., Mexico.

Oral-B, UK. Oral-B Laboratories Ltd, Gillette Corner, Great West Rd, Isleworth, Middlesex, TW7 5NP, UK.

Oral-B, USA. Oral-B Laboratories Inc., 600 Clipper Dr., Belmont, CA 94002-4119, USA.

Oramon, Ger. Oramon Arzneimittel GmbH, Mittelstr. 18, Postfach: 1461, 88464 Laupheim, Germany.

OraPharma, USA. OraPharma, USA.

Orbis Consumer, UK. Orbis Consumer Products Ltd, Unit 31, Northfields Industrial Estate, Beresford Ave, Wembley, Middlesex, HA0 1NW, UK.

Ordesa, Spain. Ordesa, Ctra Enlace con Prat 9-11, Sant Boi de Llobregat, 08830 Barcelona, Spain.

Or-Dov, Austral. Or-Dov Pharmaceuticals P/L, P.O. Box 172, Doncaster, VIC 3108, Australia.

Organon, Aust. Organon GmbH, Siebenbrunnengasse 21/D/IV, A-1050 Vienna, Austria.

Organon, Austral. Organon (Australia) P/L, Private Bag 25, Lane Cove, NSW 2066, Australia.

Organon, Belg. Organon Belgie S.A., Chaussee de la Hulpe 166, 1170 Brussels, Belgium.

Organon, Canad. Organon Canada Ltd, 200 Consilium Place, Suite 700, Scarborough, Ontario, M1H 3E4, Canada.

Organon, Denm. Organon AS, Literbuen 9, 2740 Skovlunde, Denmark.

Organon, Fin. Oy Organon AB, Ruoholahdenkatu 23 B, PL 254, 00181 Helsinki, Finland.

Organon, Fr. Organon, 10 rue Godefroy, 92821 Puteaux cdx, France.

Organon, Ger. Organon GmbH, Mittenheimer Strasse 62, 85764 Oberschleissheim, Germany.

Organon, Hong Kong. Organon (HK) Ltd, Unit 904, 9/F, CLI Bldg, 313-317B Hennessy Rd, Wanchai, Hong Kong.

Organon, Irl. See *United Drug, Irl.*

Organon, Israel. Organon, Israel.

Organon, Ital. Organon Italia s.p.a., Via Ostilia 15, 00184 Rome, Italy.

Organon, Mex. Organon Mexicana S.A. de C.V., Calz. de Camarones No.134, Col. San Salvador Xochimanca, 02870 Mexico D.F., Mexico.

Organon, Neth. Organon Nederland B.V., P.O. Box 500, 5342 PX Oss, Netherlands.

Organon, Norw. Organon AS, Johan Drengsrudsv. 52, Postboks 324, 1372 Asker, Norway.

Organon, NZ. See *Pharmaco, NZ.*

Organon, Port. Organon Portuguesa, Lda, Av. Conde Valbom 30, 1069-037 Lisbon, Portugal.

Organon, Singapore. See *Zuellig, Singapore.*

Organon, Spain. Organon Española, Ed Amsterdam Ronda de Dalt, Ctra de Hospitalet 147, Cornella de Llobregat, 08830 Barcelona, Spain.

Organon, Swed. Organon AB, Box 5076, 426 05 V Frolunda, Sweden.

Organon, Switz. Organon SA, Churerstrasse 160b, 8808 Pfaffikon/SZ, Switzerland.

Organon, Thai. Organon (Thailand) Ltd, 14 Fl, Ploenchit Center Building, 2 Sukhumvit Rd, Klongtoey, Bangkok 10110, Thailand.

Organon, UK. Organon Laboratories Ltd, Cambridge Science Park, Milton Rd, Cambridge, CB4 0FL, UK.

Organon, USA. Organon Inc., 375 Mount Pleasant Ave, West Orange, NJ 07052, USA.

Organon Teknika, Aust. See *Organon Teknika, Ger.*

Organon Teknika, Austral. Organon Teknika P/L, 23 Brookhollow Ave, Baulkham Hills, NSW 2153, Australia.

Organon Teknika, Belg. Organon Teknika Benelux S.A., Veedijk 58, 2300 Turnhout, Belgium.

Organon Teknika, Canad. Organon Teknika Inc., 30 North Wind Place, Scarborough, Ontario, M1S 3R5, Canada.

Organon Teknika, Denm. See *Organon, Denm.*

Organon Teknika, Fin. Organon Teknika Oy, Rajatorpantie 41 C, 01640 Vantaa, Finland.

Organon Teknika, Fr. See *Riom, Fr.*

Organon Teknika, Ger. Organon Teknika Medizinische Produkte GmbH, Wernher-von-Braun-Str. 18, 69214 Eppelheim, Germany.

Organon Teknika, Hong Kong. Organon Teknika China Ltd, Unit 2704, Vicwood Plaza, 199 Des Voeux Rd Central, Hong Kong.

Organon Teknika, Irl. See *United Drug, Irl.*

Organon Teknika, Israel. Organon Teknika, Israel.

Organon Teknika, Ital. Organon Teknika s.p.a., Via Ostilia 15, 00184 Rome, Italy.

Organon Teknika, Mex. Organon Teknika, Mexico.

Organon Teknika, Neth. Organon Teknika Nederland B.V., Postbus 23, 5280 AA Boxtel, Netherlands.

Organon Teknika, Norw. See *Organon, Norw.*

Organon Teknika, Spain. Organon Teknika, Castello 1, Sant Boi de Llobregat, 08830 Barcelona, Spain.

Organon Teknika, Swed. Organon Teknika AB, Hantverksvagen 15, 436 33 Askim, Sweden.

Organon Teknika, Switz. Organon Teknika AG, Churerstrasse 160b, Postfach 129, 8808 Pfaffikon/SZ, Switzerland.

Organon Teknika, USA. Organon Teknika Corporation, 100 Akzo Ave, Durham, NC 27712, USA.

Orient, Singapore. Orient Europharm Pte Ltd, 1 Sophia Rd, 06-13 Peace Centre, S 228149, Singapore.

Oriola, Fin. Oriola Oy, PL 8, 02101 Espoo, Finland.

Orion, Aust. See *Orion, Fin.*

Orion, Denm. Orion Pharma A/S, Bogeskovvej 9, 3490 Kvistgard, Denmark.

Orion, Fin. Orion-yhtymä Oyj, Orionintie 1, 02200 Espoo, Finland.

Orion, Fr. Orion Pharma, 60 ter, rue de Bellevue, 92100 Boulogne-Billancourt, France.

Orion, Ger. Orion Pharma GmbH, Notkestr. 9, 22607 Hamburg, Germany.

Orion, Irl. See *Allphar, Irl.*

Orion, Israel. Orion, Israel.

Orion, Norw. Orion Pharma AS, Ulvenv 84, Postboks 52 Okern, 0508 Oslo, Norway.

Orion, Singapore. See *Pharmacon, Singapore.*

Orion, Swed. Orion Pharma AB, Box 334, 192 30 Sollentuna, Sweden.

Orion, Switz. Orion Pharma AG, Untermuli 11, 6300 Zug, Switzerland.

Orion, Thai. See *Harn, Thai.*

Orion, UK. Orion Pharma UK Ltd, 1st Floor Leat House, Overbridge Square, Hambridge Lane, Newbury, Berkshire, RG14 5UX, UK.

Orion, USA. See *Lifesign, USA.*

OroClean, Switz. OroClean-Chemie AG, Buelstrasse 17, 8330 Pfaffikon/ZH, Switzerland.

Orphan, Austral. Orphan Australia P/L, 48 Kangan Drive, Berwick, VIC 3806, Australia.

Orphan, Denm. Orphan Denmark AS, Wilders Plads, Bygning V, 1403 Copenhagen K, Denmark.

Orphan, Fin. Oy Orphan Finland Ab, Tykistökatu 6 B, 20520 Turku, Finland.

Orphan, Fr. Orphan Europe, Imm Le Guillaumet, 92046 Paris-La Defense, France.

Orphan, Norw. Orphan Norway AS, Dronningensg. 6, 0152 Oslo, Norway.

Orphan, UK. Orphan Europe (UK) Ltd, 32 Bell St, Henley-on-Thames, Oxfordshire, RG9 2BH, UK.

Orphan Medical, Canad. See *Orphan Medical, USA.*

Orphan Medical, Israel. Orphan Medical, Israel.

Orphan Medical, USA. Orphan Medical Inc., 13911 Ridgedale Drive, Minnetonka, MN 55305, USA.

Orravan, Spain. Orravan, Gran Capitan, 10, San Juan Despi, 08970 Barcelona, Spain.

Orsade, Spain. Orsade, Avda Virgen de Montserrat 221, 08026 Barcelona, Spain.

Ortega, USA. Ortega, USA.

Ortho, Hong Kong. See *Keller, Hong Kong.*

Ortho, Israel. Ortho, Israel.

Ortho, Ital. Ortho Clinical Diagnostics spa, Via Volta 16, 20093 Cologno Monzese (MI), Italy.

Ortho, UK. See *Cilag, UK.*

Ortho Biotech, USA. See *Ortho Pharmaceutical, USA.*

Ortho Dermatological, Canad. Ortho Dermatological, Division of Johnson & Johnson Inc., 7101 Notre-Dame E, Montreal, Quebec, H1N 2G4, Canada.

Ortho Dermatological, USA. Ortho Dermatological, 199 Grandview Rd, Skillman, NJ 08558, USA.

Ortho Diagnostic, USA. Ortho-Clinical Diagnostic Inc., 1001 US Hwy 202, Raritan, NJ 08869-0606, USA.

Ortho McNeil, USA. See *Ortho Pharmaceutical, USA.*

Ortho Pharmaceutical, USA. Ortho Pharmaceutical Corp., 1000 Route 202, P.O. Box 300, Raritan, NJ 08869-0602, USA.

Orthos, Mex. Orthos, Mexico.

Ortis, Ital. Ortis Italia s.r.l., Via Maroncelli 64, Padua, Italy.

Ortomed, Neth. Ortomed, Netherlands.

Osler, Fr. Lab. Osler, 42 rue Monge, 75005 Paris, France.

Osorio de Moraes, Braz. Laboratorios Osorio de Moraes Ltda, Avenida Cardeal Eugenio Pacelli 2.281, Cidade Industrial, 32210-001 Contagem, MG, Brazil.

Osoth, Thai. Osoth Inter Laboratories, 757/10 Soi Pradoo 1, Sathupradit 8 Rd, Bangpongpang, Yannawa, Bangkok 10120, Thailand.

Osotspa, Thai. Osotspa Co. Ltd, 2100 Ram Khamhaeng Rd, Hua Mark, Bangkapi, Bangkok 10240, Thailand.

Osterreichisches Institut, Aust. Österreichisches Institut fur Hämoderivate, Vienna, Austria.

OTC, Spain. OTC Iberica, President Lluis Companys 16, Santa Coloma de Gramanet, 08921 Barcelona, Spain.

Otosan, Ital. Otosan, Via degli Scavi 32, 47100 Forli, Italy.

Otsuka, Hong Kong. Otsuka Pharmaceutical (HK) Ltd, Rm 1404, Leighton Ctr, 77 Leighton Rd, Causeway Bay, Hong Kong.

Otsuka, Jpn. Otsuka Pharmaceutical Co. Ltd, 2-2 Tsukasa-cho, Chiyoda-ku, Tokyo 101-8535, Japan.

Otsuka, Singapore. See *Luen Wah, Singapore.*

Otsuka, Spain. Otsuka Pharmaceutical, Santanyi 16, 08016 Barcelona, Spain.

Otsuka, Thai. See *Zuellig, Thai.*

Otsuka, USA. Otsuka America Pharmaceutical, 2440 Research Blvd, Rockville, MD 20850, USA.

Ottolenghi, Ital. Dr. Ottolenghi & C. s.r.l., Via Cuneo 5, 10028 Trofarello (TO), Italy.

OTW, Ger. Organotherapeutische Werke GmbH (OTW), Carl-Zeiss-Str. 4, 76275 Ettlingen, Germany.

Oui Heng, Thai. Oui Heng Import Co. Ltd, 46, 46/2 Soi Charansanitwongs 40, Charansanwitwongs Rd, Bangkok 10700, Thailand.

Outdoor Recreations, USA. Outdoor Recreations, USA.

Ovelle, Irl. Ovelle Ltd, Industrial Estate, Coe's Rd, Dundalk, Co. Louth, Ireland.

Oxford Pharmaceuticals, UK. Oxford Pharmaceuticals Ltd, Masters House, 5 Sandridge Close, Harrow, Middlesex, HA1 1XD, UK.

Oxo, Switz. See *Doetsch, Grether, Switz.*

Oxo, Thai. Oxo Chemie (Thailand) Co. Ltd, 6 Fl, Asoke Towers Com Building, 213/14-15 Sukhumvit 21 Rd, Klongtoey Nua, Watana, Bangkok 10110, Thailand.

Pabisch, Aust. Pabisch GmbH, Baldassgasse 5, A-1217 Vienna, Austria.

Pacific, Hong Kong. See *LCH, Hong Kong.*

Pacific, Israel. Pacific, Israel.

Pacific, NZ. Pacific Pharmaceuticals Co Ltd, P.O. Box 11-183, Ellerslie, Auckland, New Zealand.

Pacific, Singapore. See *Ziwell, Singapore.*

Pacific, Thai. Pacific Healthcare (Thailand) Co. Ltd, 229/1 South Sathorn Rd, Bangkok 10120, Thailand.

Paddock, USA. Paddock Laboratories Inc., 3940 Quebec Ave North, Minneapolis, MN 55427, USA.

Padia, Ger. Pädia Arzneimittel GmbH, Gruhlstr. 3, 50374 Erftstadt, Germany.

Padma, Switz. Padma AG, Wiesenstrasse 5, 8603 Schwerzenbach, Switzerland.

Padma, UK. Padma 28 UK Ltd, Pepper Rd, Bramhall Moor Lane, Hazel Grove, Stockport, Cheshire, SK7 5BW, UK.

Padro, Spain. Padro, Gran Via Corts Catalanes 764, 08013 Barcelona, Spain.

Paedpharm, Austral. Paedpharm P/L, P.O. Box 6533, East Perth, WA 6892, Australia.

Paesel, Ger. Paesel & Lorei GmbH & Co. Hauptniederlassung, Freihafen 8, 47138 Duisburg, Germany.

Paines & Byrne, Irl. See *United Drug, Irl.*

Paines & Byrne, NZ. See *NZ Medical & Scientific, NZ.*

Paines & Byrne, Thai. See *Union Medical, Thai.*

Paines & Byrne, UK. Paines & Byrne Ltd, Yamanouchi House, Pyrford Rd, West Byfleet, Surrey, KT14 6RA, UK.

Paladin, Canad. Paladin Laboratories Inc., 6111 Royalmount Ave, Suite 102, Montreal, Quebec, H4T 2T4, Canada.

Palex, Spain. Palex, C/ Huelma 5, Pol. Ind. Olivares, 23009 Jaen, Spain.

Palisades, USA. See *Glenwood, USA.*

Palmares, Ital. See *Ferlito, Ital.*

Palmicol, Ger. See *Riemser, Ger.*

Palmolive Skincare, Austral. Palmolive Skincare Laboratories, P.O. Box 3964, Sydney, NSW 2001, Australia.

Pal-Pak, USA. Pal-Pak Inc., 1201 LIberty St, P.O. Box 299, Allentown, PA 18105, USA.

Pamex, Irl. Pamex Ltd, 4 Richard St., Castlebar, Co. Mayo, Ireland.

Pan American, USA. Pan American Laboratories, P.O. Box 8950, Mandeville, LA 70470-8950, USA.

Pan Quimica, Spain. Pan Quimica Farmaceutica, Rufino Gonzalez 50, 28037 Madrid, Spain.

Panax, Switz. Panax Import, F Ruckstuhl & Co., Bergtalweg 2a, 9500 Wil, Switzerland.

Panderma, Aust. Panderma Arzneimittel GmbH, Himmelpfortgasse 14, A-1010 Vienna, Austria.

Panfarma, Fin. Panfarma Oy, PL 301, 02101 Espoo, Finland.

Pannoc, Belg. Pannoc Chemie S.A., Lammerdries 23, B.P. 70, 2250 Olen, Belgium.

Panpharma, Fr. Laboratoires Panpharma, ZI du Clairay-Luitre, 35133 Fougeres, France.

Pantheon, UK. Pantheon Healthcare Ltd, Studio 8, 48 Tierney Rd, London, SW2 4QS, UK.

Pan-Well, Hong Kong. Pan-Well Trading Co., 4/F, Flat D, Goldfield Bldg, 42-44 Connaught Rd West, Hong Kong.

Panzera, Ital. Farmaceutici G.B. Panzera s.r.l., Via De Sanctis 71, 20141 Milan, Italy.

Par, USA. Par Pharmaceutical Inc., One Ram Ridge Rd, Spring Valley, NY 10977, USA.

Paradise, Canad. Paradise Promotions, P. O. Box 3876, Garibaldi Highlands, British Columbia, V0N 1T0, Canada.

Paragerm, Fr. Laboratoires Paragerm, ZI 3e rue, B.P. 68, 06511 Carros cdx, France.

Paraphar, Fr. Laboratoires Paraphar, 10 rue Varet, 75015 Paris, France.

Paraphar, Singapore. See *Polymedic, Singapore.*

Para-Pharma, Switz. Para-Pharma AG, Switzerland.

Parggon, Mex. Laboratorios Parggon S.A. de C.V., Manuel Cambre No. 2093, Chapultepec Country, 44610 Guadalajara, Jal., Mexico.

Parisis, Spain. Parisis, Spain.

Parke, Davis, Aust. Parke-Davis GmbH, Brunner Strasse 81, A-1230 Vienna, Austria.

Parke, Davis, Austral. Parke Davis P/L, Locked Bag 42, Taren Point, NSW 2229, Australia.

Parke, Davis, Belg. Parke-Davis, Division of Warner-Lambert (Belgium) S.A., Excelsiorlaan 75-7, 1930 Zaventem, Belgium.

Parke, Davis, Canad. See *Pfizer, Canad.*

Parke, Davis, Denm. See *Warner-Lambert, Denm.*

Parke, Davis, Fin. Parke-Davis, Division of Warner Lambert, Merivirta 3 A, 02320 Espoo, Finland.

Parke, Davis, Fr. Parke, Davis, 10 av de l'Arche, 92419 Courbevoie cdx, France.

Parke, Davis, Ger. Parke-Davis GmbH, Mooswaldallee 1, 79090 Freiburg, Germany.

Parke, Davis, Hong Kong. See *Warner-Lambert, Hong Kong,* and *Zuellig, Hong Kong.*

Parke, Davis, Irl. See *United Drug, Irl.*

Parke, Davis, Israel. Parke Davis Israel.

Parke, Davis, Ital. Parke Davis s.p.a., Via C. Colombo 1, 20020 Lainate (Milan), Italy.

Parke, Davis, Mex. See *Warner-Lambert, Mex.*

Parke, Davis, Neth. Parke-Davis, Postbus 3008, 2130 KA Hoofddorp, Netherlands.

Parke, Davis, NZ. See *Warner-Lambert, NZ.*

Parke, Davis, Port. See *Warner-Lambert, Port.*

Parke, Davis, S.Afr. See *Warner, S.Afr.*

Parke, Davis, Singapore. See *Age D'or, Singapore.*

Parke, Davis, Spain. Parke Davis S.L., Pol. Ind. Manso Mateu S/N, Prat de Llobregat, 08820 Barcelona, Spain.

Parke, Davis, Swed. See *Warner-Lambert, Swed.*

Parke, Davis, Switz. See *Actipharm, Switz., Warner-Lambert, Switz.,* and *Uhlmann-Eyraud, Switz.*

Parke, Davis, UK. Parke-Davis & Co Ltd, Lambert Court, Chestnut Ave, Eastleigh, Hampshire, SO53 3ZQ, UK.

Parke, Davis, USA. Parke-Davis, Division of Warner-Lambert Co., 201 Tabor Rd, Morris Plains, NJ 07950, USA.

Parkedale, USA. Parkedale Pharmaceuticals, 870 Parkedale Rd, Rochester, MI 48307, USA.

Parke-Med, S.Afr. See *Warner, S.Afr.*

Parkfields, UK. Parkfields Sterile Supply Unit, Pond Lane, Parkfields, Wolverhampton, West Midlands, WV2 1HL, UK.

Parmed, USA. Parmed Pharmaceuticals Inc., 4220 Hyde Park Blvd, Niagara Falls, NY 14305, USA.

Parnell, Irl. See *Blackhall, Irl.*

Parnell, USA. Parnell Pharmaceuticals, Inc., P.O. Box 5130, Larkspur, CA 94977, USA.

Parsenn, Switz. Parsenn-Produkte AG, Abt. Pharmazeutik, Klus, 7240 Kublis, Switzerland.

Parthenon, USA. Parthenon Inc., 3311 W. 2400 South, Salt Lake City, UT 84119, USA.

Pasadena, USA. See *Taylor, USA.*

Pascoe, Ger. Pascoe Pharmazeutische Präparate GmbH, Schiffenberger Weg 55, 35394 Giessen, Germany.

Pascual, Hong Kong. See *Yik Kwan, Hong Kong.*

Passauer, Ger. Herbert J Passauer GmbH & Co. KG, Eberstrasse 56, 10827 Berlin, Germany.

Passion for Life, UK. Passion for Life Products Ltd, 21 Heathmans Rd, London, SW6 4TJ, UK.

Pasteur Merieux, Aust. See *Aventis Pasteur, Aust.*

Pasteur Merieux, Belg. Pasteur Merieux MSD S.A., Ave Jules Bordet 13, 1140 Brussels, Belgium.

Pasteur Merieux, Braz. Pasteur Merieux Soros e Vacinas S.A., Rua do Rocio 351 10° andar, 04552-905 Sao Paulo, SP, Brazil.

Pasteur Merieux, Canad. See *Aventis Pasteur, Canad.*

Pasteur Merieux, Denm. See *Aventis, Denm.*

Pasteur Merieux, Fr. See *Aventis Pasteur, Fr.*

Pasteur Merieux, Ger. See *Aventis, Ger.*

Pasteur Merieux, Hong Kong. See *Rhodia, Hong Kong,* and *Zuellig, Hong Kong.*

Pasteur Merieux, Irl. See *Allphar, Irl.*

Pasteur Merieux, Israel. Pasteur Merieux, Israel.

Pasteur Merieux, Ital. Pasteur Merieux MSD s.p.a., Via di Villa Troili 56, 00163 Rome, Italy.

Pasteur Merieux, Neth. Pasteur Merieux MSD, Postbus 512, 1180 AM Amstelveen, Netherlands.

Pasteur Merieux, Norw. See *Pasteur Merieux, Denm.*

Pasteur Merieux, Singapore. See *Zuellig, Singapore.*

Pasteur Merieux, Spain. Pasteur Merieux MSD, Josefa Valcarcel 40, 28027 Madrid, Spain.

Pasteur Merieux, Swed. See *Aventis Pasteur, Swed.*

Pasteur Merieux, Thai. Pasteur Merieux Connaught (Thailand) Ltd, 4 Fl, VTT IV Building, 3195/9 Rama IV Rd, Klong Toey, Bangkok 10110, Thailand.

Pasteur Merieux, UK. See *Aventis, UK.*

Pasteur Merieux, USA. See *Aventis, USA.*

Pasteur Vaccins, Fr. See *Aventis Pasteur, Fr.*

Pastor Farina, Ital. Pastor Farina s.r.l., Via Garibaldi 69, 22100 Como, Italy.

Pasture, Singapore. Pasture Pharma Pte Ltd, 3 Kaki Bukit Crescent, 05-03, S 416237, Singapore.

Patentex, Ger. Patentex GmbH, Marschnerstr. 8-10, 60318 Frankfurt/Main, Germany.

Patentex, Switz. See *Adroka, Switz.*

Pathogenesis, Canad. Pathogenesis Canada Ltd, 100 Alexis-Nihon, Suite 800, Ville St-Laurent, Quebec, H4M 2P4, Canada.

Pathogenesis, UK. PathoGenesis Ltd, PathoGenesis House, Park Lane, Cranford, Hounslow, Middlesex, TW5 9RR, UK.

Pathogenesis, USA. PathoGenesis Corp., 201 Elliott Ave West, Seattle, WA 98119, USA.

Pautrat, Fr. See *PPDH, Fr.*

PB, Ger. PB Pharma AG, Mollsfeld 3, 40670 Meersbusch, Germany.

PCH, Neth. PCH International, Postbus 552, 2003 BN Haarlem, Netherlands.

PCR, Ger. PCR Arzneimittel GmbH, Wielandstr. 7, 53173 Bonn, Germany.

PD, Thai. Thai PD Chemicals Ltd, 2 Soi Chokchairuammitr, Viphavadee Rungsit Rd, Bangkok 10310, Thailand.

PD Pharm, S.Afr. PD Pharmaceuticals, P.O. Box 47448, Greyville, Durban 4023, South Africa.

Peach, UK. Peach Pharmaceuticals, 16 Parkstone Rd, Poole, Dorset, BH15 2PG, UK.

Pearson, Ital. Guglielmo Pearson s.r.l., Via delle Fabbriche 40, 16158 Genova-Voltri (GE), Italy.

Peckforton, Irl. Peckforton, Ireland.

Peckforton, UK. Peckforton Pharmaceuticals Ltd, Crewe Hall, Crewe, Cheshire, CW1 6UL, UK.

Pediatrica, Singapore. See *Far East Drug, Singapore.*

Pediatrica, Thai. See *Olic, Thai.*

Pedinol, USA. Pedinol Pharmacal Inc., 30 Banfi Plaza North, Farmingdale, NY 11735, USA.

Pedi-Pak, Canad. Pedi-Pak Products Canada Inc., 700 Lawrence Ave W, Ste 125, Toronto, ON, M6A 3B4, Canada.

Peithner, Aust. Dr Peithner KG nunmehr GmbH & Co., Richard Strauss-Strasse 13, A-1232 Vienna, Austria.

Pekana, Ger. Pekana Naturheilmittel GmbH, Raiffeisenstr. 15, 88353 Kisslegg/Allgau, Germany.

Peking-Boell, Ger. Peking Royal Jelly Deutschland BOELL HandelsKontor, Am Kirchberg 3, 86666 Burgheim, Germany.

Pelayo, Spain. Pelayo, Tallers 16, 08001 Barcelona, Spain.

Penederm, Canad. See *Pharmascience, Canad.*

Penederm, UK. Penederm Ltd, 14 Oxford Court, Manchester, M2 3WQ, UK.

Penederm, USA. See *Bertek, USA.*

Penn, Irl. See *Central, Irl.*

Penn, UK. Penn Pharmaceuticals Ltd, Tafarnaubach Industrial Estate, Tredegar, Gwent, NP2 3AA, UK.

Pennex, Israel. Pennex, Israel.

Pensa, Spain. Pensa, Av. Virgen de Montserrat 215, 08026 Barcelona, Spain.

Penta, Ger. Penta Arzneimittel GmbH, Hohenburger Strasse 39, 92289 Ursensollen, Germany.

Pentaderm, Ital. Pentaderm Industria Chimica e Farmaceutica s.r.l., Via Nazionale Pentimele 157, 89121 Reggio Calabria, Italy.

Pentafarm, Spain. Pentafarm, Galileo 250, 08028 Barcelona, Spain.

Pentafarma, Port. Pentafarma, SA, Rua Professor Henrique de Barros, Edificio Sagres 5 A, 2685-338 Prior Velho, Portugal.

Pentamedical, Ital. Pentamedical srl, Via G. Mazzini 1, 20021 Bollate (MI), Italy.

Pergam, Ital. Pergam s.r.l., Via Gradisca 8, 20151 Milan, Italy.

Perio, Israel. Perio Products Ltd, 7 Hamarpe, Har Hahotzvim, Jerusalem, Israel.

Periproducts, UK. Periproducts Ltd, P.O. Box 176, Audit House, 260 Field End Rd, Ruislip, Middlesex, HA4 9YR, UK.

Permamed, Switz. Permamed AG, Ringstrasse 29, Postfach 360, 4106 Therwil, Switzerland.

Person & Covey, Canad. Person & Covey Inc., 1031 Meyerside Drive, Unit 12, Mississauga, Ontario, L5T 2H5, Canada.

Person & Covey, USA. Person & Covey Inc., 616 Allen Ave, P.O. Box 25018, Glendale, CA 91221-5018, USA.

Personal Care, USA. Personal Care Group Inc., 1 Paragon Drive, Montvale, NJ 07645, USA.

Perstorp, Switz. See *Smith & Nephew, Switz.*

Pertussin, USA. Pertussin Laboratories, USA.

Peter, Ital. Peter Italia sas, Via Tommaso Silvestri 22, 00135 Rome, Italy.

Peter Black, UK. Peter Black Healthcare Ltd, William Nadin Way, Swadlincote, Derbyshire, DE11 0BB, UK.

Peters, Fr. Laboratoires Peters, ZI Les Vignes, 42 rue Benoit-Frachon, 93000 Bobigny cdx, France.

Petrasch, Aust. Petrasch-Pharma GmbH, Schlachthausstrasse 3, A-6850 Dornbirn, Austria.

Petrus, Austral. Petrus Pharmaceuticals, P.O. Box 41, Midland, Perth, WA 6936, Australia.

Pfeiffer, USA. Pfeiffer Company, 71 University Ave, P.O. Box 4447, Atlanta, GA 30302, USA.

Pfizer, Aust. Pfizer Corporation Austria GmbH, Seidengasse 33-35, A-1070 Vienna, Austria.

Pfizer, Austral. Pfizer P/L, P.O. Box 57, West Ryde, NSW 2114, Australia.

Pfizer, Belg. Pfizer S.A., Rue Leon Theodor 102, 1090 Brussels, Belgium.

Pfizer, Braz. Laboratorios Pfizer Ltda, Avenida Presidente Tancredo de Almeida Neves 1.111, 07190-916 Guarulhos, SP, Brazil.

Pfizer, Canad. Pfizer Canada Inc., P.O. Box 800, Pointe-Claire, Dorval, Quebec, H9R 4V2, Canada.

Pfizer, Denm. Pfizer A/S, Lautrupvang 8, 2750 Ballerup, Denmark.

Pfizer, Fin. Pfizer Oy, Lars Sonckin kaari 4, 02600 Espoo, Finland.

Pfizer, Fr. Laboratoires Pfizer, 86 rue de Paris, 91407 Orsay cdx, France.

Pfizer, Ger. Pfizer GmbH, Pfizerstr. 1, 76139 Karlsruhe, Germany.

Pfizer, Hong Kong. Pfizer Corporation, 16/F Stanhope House, 738 King's Rd, North Point, Hong Kong.

Pfizer, Irl. Pfizer Pharmaceuticals, Parkway House, Ballymount Rd Lower, Dublin 12, Ireland.

Pfizer, Israel. Pfizer Pharmaceuticals Ltd, P.O. Box 12133, Herzliya Pituah, Israel.

Pfizer, Ital. Pfizer Italiana s.p.a., Via Valbondione 113, 00188 Rome, Italy.

Pfizer, Mex. Pfizer S.A. de C.V., Damas No. 120, Col. San Jose Insurgentes, 03900 Mexico D.F., Mexico.

Pfizer, Neth. Pfizer B.V., Postbus 37, 2900 AA Capelle a/d Ijssel, Netherlands.

Pfizer, Norw. Pfizer AS, Strandv. 55, 1366 Lysaker, Norway.

Pfizer, NZ. Pfizer Laboratories Ltd, P.O. Box 3998, Auckland, New Zealand.

Pfizer, Port. Laboratórios Pfizer, Lda, Porto Zemouto, Coina, Apartado 30, 2830 Ciona, Portugal.

Pfizer, S.Afr. Pfizer Laboratories (Pty) Ltd, P.O. Box 783720, Sandton 2146, South Africa.

Pfizer, Singapore. Pfizer Pte Ltd, 200 Middle Rd, 06-00 Prime Centre, S 188980, Singapore.

Pfizer, Spain. See *Pfizer Consumer, Spain.*

Pfizer, Swed. Pfizer AB, Box 501, 183 25 Taby, Sweden.

Pfizer, Switz. Pfizer SA, Postfach, 8048 Zurich, Switzerland.

Pfizer, Thai. Pfizer International Corp, 19-20 Fl, Ploenchit Center Tower, 2 Sukhumvit Rd, Kwang Klongtoey, Khet Klongtoey, Bangkok 10110, Thailand.

Pfizer, UK. Pfizer Ltd, Sandwich, Kent, CT13 9NJ, UK.

Pfizer, USA. Pfizer Inc., 235 East 42nd St, New York, NY 10017-5755, USA.

Pfizer Consumer, Austral. See *Pfizer, Austral.*

Pfizer Consumer, Canad. See *Warner-Lambert, Canad.*

Pfizer Consumer, Irl. See *Allphar, Irl.*

Pfizer Consumer, Ital. See *Pfizer, Ital.*

Pfizer Consumer, Singapore. See *MD, Singapore.*

Pfizer Consumer, Spain. Pfizer Consumer Health Care, Avda Europa 20 B, Alcobendas, 28108 Madrid, Spain.

Pfizer Consumer, UK. Pfizer Consumer Healthcare, Wilsom Rd, Alton, Hampshire, GU34 2TJ, UK.

Pfizer Consumer, USA. See *Pfizer, USA.*

Pfleger, Ger. Dr R. Pfleger Chemische Fabrik GmbH, 96045 Bamberg, Germany.

Pflüger, Ger. Homöopathisches Laboratorium A. Pflüger GmbH, Bielefelder Str. 17, 33378 Rheda-Wiedenbruck, Germany.

Pfrimmer Nutricia, Switz. See *Uhlmann-Eyraud, Switz.*

PGM, Ger. PGM Pharmazeutische Gesellschaft mbH & Co. Munchen, Furstenstr 6, 80333 Munich, Germany.

Pharbenia, Ital. Pharbenia s.r.l., Via del Pascolo 43, 10042 Nichelino (TO), Italy.

Pharbita, Ger. See *PB, Ger.*

Pharbita, Israel. Pharbita, Israel.

Pharbita, Singapore. See *FP, Singapore.*

Phardi, Switz. Phardi AG, Postfach 3650, 4002 Basle, Switzerland.

Pharma 2000, Fr. Laboratoires Pharma 2000, Imm Strasbourg, av de l'Europe, Toussus-le-Noble, 78771 Magny-les-Hameaux cdx, France.

Pharma 2000, Singapore. Pharma 2000 Pte Ltd, 63 Hillview Ave, 03-07, S 669569, Singapore.

Pharma Clal, Israel. Pharma-Clal Ltd, P.O. Box 31, Bnei Brak, Israel.

Pharma Line, Ital. Pharma Line s.r.l., Via M Ricci 15, 60020 Palombina Nuova (AN), Italy.

Pharma Nord, Fin. Oy Pharma Nord Ab, Rajatorpantie 41 C, 01640 Vantaa, Finland.

Pharma Nord, Irl. See *Electramed, Irl.*

Pharma Nord, Norw. Pharma Nord, Norway.

Pharma Nord, Thai. See *Biogenetech, Thai.*

Pharma Tek, USA. Pharma-Tek Inc., P.O. Box 1148, Elmira, NY 14902, USA.

Pharmabest, Israel. PharmaBest, P.O. Box 8609, New Industrial Zone, Netanya, Israel.

Pharmabroker, NZ. Pharmabroker Sales Ltd, P.O. Box 302 234, North Harbour Postal Centre, Auckland, New Zealand.

Pharmacal, Fin. Oy Pharmacal AB, Nilsiänkatu 8, 00510 Helsinki, Finland.

Pharmacal, Switz. See *Democal, Switz.*

Pharmacaps, Mex. Pharmacaps, Division de Gelcaps Exportadora de Mexico S.A. de C.V., Calle 7 No. 6, Fracc. Ind. Alce Blanco, 53370 Naucalpan de Juarez Edo. de Mexico, Mexico.

Pharmacare, Canad. Pharmacare Ltd, 54 Holland St W, Bradford, Ontario, L3Z 2Y5, Canada.

Pharmacare Consumer, S.Afr. Pharmacare Consumer, South Africa.

Pharmacel, USA. Pharmacel Laboratory Inc., 203 South Coolidge Ave, Tampa, FL 33609, USA.

Pharmaceutical Basics, USA. See *Rosemont, USA.*

Pharmaceutical Enterprises, S.Afr. Pharmaceutical Enterprises (Pty) Ltd, P.O. Box 201, Howard Place 7450, South Africa.

Pharmaceutical Specialties, USA. Pharmaceutical Specialties Inc., P.O. Box 6298, Rochester, MN 55903, USA.

Pharmchem, UK. M & A Pharmachem Ltd, Allenby Laboratories, Wigan Rd, Westhoughton, Bolton, BL6 2LA, UK.

Pharmachemie, Israel. See *Teva, Israel.*

Pharmachemie, S.Afr. Pharmachemie (Pty) Ltd, P.O. Box 7115, Johannesburg 2000, South Africa.

Pharmachemie, Singapore. See *FP, Singapore.*

Pharmachemie, Thai. See *Pacific, Thai.*

Pharmachoice, S.Afr. Pharmachoice (Pty) Ltd, P.O. Box 291, Fourways 2055, South Africa.

Pharmacia, Austral. Pharmacia Australia P/L, P.O. Box 46, Rydalmere, NSW 2116, Australia.

Pharmacia, Ger. Pharmacia GmbH, 91051 Erlangen, Germany.

Pharmacia, Neth. See *Pharmacia Upjohn, Neth.*

Pharmacia, S.Afr. Pharmacia South Africa, P.O. Box 41111, Craighall 2024, South Africa.

Pharmacia, Spain. See *Pharmacia Upjohn, Spain.*

Pharmacia, Swed. Pharmacia Sverige AB, 112 87 Stockholm, Sweden.

Pharmacia, UK. Pharmacia Ltd, Davy Ave, Knowlhill, Milton Keynes, Buckinghamshire, MK5 8PH, UK.

Pharmacia, USA. See *Pharmacia Upjohn, USA.*

Pharmacia Upjohn, Austral. See *Pharmacia, Austral.*

Pharmacia Upjohn, Belg. Pharmacia & Upjohn S.A., Rue de la Fusee 66, 1130 Brussels, Belgium.

Pharmacia Upjohn, Braz. Pharmacia & Upjohn Ltda, Avenida das Nacoes Unidas 12.995 4° andar, 04578-000 Sao Paulo, SP, Brazil.

Pharmacia Upjohn, Canad. Pharmacia & Upjohn Inc., 5100 Spectrum Way, Mississauga, Ontario, L4W 5J5, Canada.

Pharmacia Upjohn, Denm. Pharmacia & Upjohn AS, Overgaden neden Vandet 7, 1414 Copenhagen K, Denmark.

Pharmacia Upjohn, Fin. Pharmacia & Upjohn Oy, Rajatorpantie 41, 01640 Vantaa, Finland.

Pharmacia Upjohn, Fr. Pharmacia & Upjohn SA, B.P. 210, 78051 St-Quentin-Yvelines cdx, France.

Pharmacia Upjohn, Ger. See *Pharmacia, Ger.*

Pharmacia Upjohn, Hong Kong. Pharmacia & Upjohn Ltd, 18/F Allied Kajima Bldg, 138 Gloucester Rd, Wanchai, Hong Kong.

Pharmacia Upjohn, Irl. Pharmacia & Upjohn Ltd, P.O. Box 1752, Airways Industrial Estate, Dublin 17, Ireland.

Pharmacia Upjohn, Israel. Pharmacia Upjohn, Israel.

Pharmacia Upjohn, Ital. Pharmacia & Upjohn s.p.a., Via Robert Koch 1.2, 20152 Milan, Italy.

Pharmacia Upjohn, Mex. Pharmacia & Upjohn S.A. de C.V., Calz. de Tlalpan No. 2962, Col. Espartaco, 04870 Mexico D.F., Mexico.

Pharmacia Upjohn, Neth. Pharmacia & Upjohn B.V., Postbus 17, 3440 AA Woerden, Netherlands.

Pharmacia Upjohn, Norw. Pharmacia & Upjohn AS, Gjerdrumsvei 10B, 0480 Oslo, Norway.

Pharmacia Upjohn, NZ. Pharmacia & Upjohn, P.O. Box 11-282, Ellerslie, Auckland, New Zealand.

Pharmacia Upjohn, Port. Pharmacia & Upjohn, Lda, Av do Forte 3, Edificio Suecia II, 2795-505 Carnaxide, Portugal.

Pharmacia Upjohn, S.Afr. See *Pharmacia, S.Afr.*

Pharmacia Upjohn, Singapore. Pharmacia & Upjohn, 101 Thomson Rd, 31-04/05 United Square, S 307591, Singapore.

Pharmacia Upjohn, Spain. Pharmacia Upjohn, Ctra de Rub 90-100, Sant Cugat del Valles, 08190 Barcelona, Spain.

Pharmacia Upjohn, Swed. See *Pharmacia, Swed.*

Pharmacia Upjohn, Switz. Pharmacia & Upjohn AG, Lagerstrasse 14, 8600 Dubendorf, Switzerland.

Pharmacia Upjohn, Thai. Pharmacia & Upjohn, 6 Fl, White Group Building, 75 Soi Rubia, Sukhumvit 42, P.O. Box 11-245, Phrakanong Post Office, Bangkok 10110, Thailand.

Pharmacia Upjohn, UK. See *Pharmacia, UK.*

Pharmacia Upjohn, USA. Pharmacia & Upjohn Co., 100 Route 206 N, Peapack, NJ 07977, USA.

Pharmacie Principale, Fr. Pharmacie Principale, 53 rue Nationale, 37011 Tours cdx, France.

Pharmaco, NZ. Pharmaco (NZ) Ltd, P.O. Box 4079, Auckland, New Zealand.

Pharmaco, S.Afr. Pharmaco Distribution (Pty) Ltd, P.O. Box 786522, Sandton 2146, South Africa.

Pharmacobel, Belg. Laboratoires Belges Pharmacobel S.A., Ave de Scheut 46-50, 1070 Brussels, Belgium.

Pharmacodane, Denm. Pharmacodane ApS, Skelbaekgade 1, 1717 Copenhagen V, Denmark.

Pharmacon, Singapore. Pharmacon Pte Ltd, 8 Kaki Bukit Rd, 04-27/28 Ruby Warehouse Complex, S 417841, Singapore.

Pharmacos, Mex. Pharmacos Exakta, S.A. de C.V., Av. del Nino Obrero No. 651, Col. Chapalita Sur, 45040 Guadalajara, Jal., Mexico.

Pharmadass, UK. Pharmadass Ltd, 16 Aintree Rd, Greenford, Middlesex, UB6 7LA, UK.

Pharmadent, Fr. Lab. Pharmadent, 45 rue Jean-Jaures, B.P. 143, 92304 Levallois-Perret cdx, France.

Pharmadeveloppement, Fr. Pharma Développement, 7 rue Valentin-Hauy, 75015 Paris, France.

Pharmadica, Thai. Pharmadica Co. Ltd, 4 Fl, Pharmaland Building, 15/56 Moo 1 Soi Supapong, Srinakarin Rd, Nongborn, Bangkok 10260, Thailand.

Pharmador, S.Afr. See *Protea, S.Afr.*

Pharmafar, Ital. Pharmafar s.r.l., Corso V Emanuele II 82, 10121 Turin, Italy.

Pharmafarm, Fr. Laboratoires Pharmafarm, 46 rue Boissiere, 75116 Paris, France.

Pharmaforte, Singapore. Pharmaforte Singapore Pte Ltd, 6 Tagore Drive, 03-11 Tagore Industrial Building, S 787623, Singapore.

Pharmafrica, S.Afr. Pharmafrica (Pty) Ltd, P.O. Box 18397, Hillbrow 2038, South Africa.

Pharmagalen, Ger. See *Galen, Ger.*

Pharmagen, S.Afr. Pharmagen, South Africa.

Pharmagenics, UK. Pharmagenics Healthcare Ltd, 251 Walworth Rd, London, SE17 1RL, UK.

Pharmagenix, UK. Pharmagenix Ltd, Manx House, Spectrum Business Estate, Maidstone, Kent, ME15 9YP, UK.

Pharmagic, Ital. PharmaGIC s.r.l., Via Gerano 5, 00156 Rome, Italy.

Pharma-Global, Irl. Pharma-Global Ltd, Hudson Rd, Sandycove, Co. Dublin, Ireland.

Pharma-Global, UK. Pharma-Global (UK) Ltd, SEQ Ltd, Nerin House, 26 Ridgeway St, Isle of Man, IM1 1EL, UK.

Pharmakon, Ger. Pharmakon Arzneimittel GmbH, Leininger Ring 65a, 67278 Bockenheim, Germany.

Pharmakon, Switz. Pharmakon SA, Burglistrasse 39, 8304 Wallisellen, Switzerland.

Pharmakon, USA. Pharmakon Laboratories Inc., 6050 Jet Port Industrial Blvd, Tampa, FL 33634, USA.

Pharmakos, Switz. Pharmakos AG, Lowenstrasse 59, 8001 Zurich, Switzerland.

Pharmalab, Canad. Pharmalab (1982) Inc., 8750 boul. de-la-Rive-Sud, Levis, QC, G6V 6N6, Canada.

Pharmalab, S.Afr. See *Noristan, S.Afr.*

Pharmaland, Ital. Pharmaland, Via dei Casetti 21, 47893 Borgo Maggiore (RSM), Italy.

Pharmaland, Thai. Pharmaland (1982) Co. Ltd, Pharmaland Building, 15/56 Moo 1 Soi Supapong, Srinakarin Rd, Nongborn, Bangkok 10260, Thailand.

Pharmalink, Denm. Pharmalink Special Laegemidler ApS, Lynbyveg 20, 2100 Copenhagen O, Denmark.

Pharmalink, Ger. See *Pharmalink, Swed.*

Pharmalink, Norw. Pharmalink Basläkemedel AB, Postboks 63 Nordstrand, 1112 Oslo, Norway.

Pharmalink, Swed. Pharmalink AB, 194 26 Upplands Vasby, Sweden.

Pharma-Natura, Ital. Pharma Natura srl, Via Vicinale di Parabiago, 20014 Nerviano (MI), Italy.

Pharmanex, USA. Pharmanex Inc., 74 W Center, Provo, UT 84601, USA.

Pharmaplan, S.Afr. Pharmaplan (Pty) Ltd, P.O. Box 7115, Johannesburg 2000, South Africa.

Pharmarecord, Ital. Pharmarecord s.r.l., Via Laurentina Km 24.730, 00040 Pomezia (Rome), Italy.

Pharmark, UK. Pharmark Ltd, 7 Windermere Rd, High Street, West Wickham, Kent, BR4 9AN, UK.

Pharmasan, Ger. Pharmasan GmbH Freiburg, Obere Hardtstr. 18, 79114 Freiburg/Brsg., Germany.

Pharmasant, Thai. See *Central, Thai.*

Pharmaschalom, Israel. Pharmaschalom Ltd, 21 Hamelacha St, Park Afek, Rosh Ha'ayin, Israel.

Pharmascience, Canad. Pharmascience Inc., 6111 Royalmount Ave, Suite 100, Montreal, Quebec, H4T 2T4, Canada.

Pharmascience, Fr. Laboratoires Pharmascience, 73 bd de la Mission-Marchand, 92400 Courbevoie, France.

Pharmascience, Hong Kong. See *Hind Wing, Hong Kong,* and *Mita, Hong Kong.*

Pharmascience, Singapore. See *JDH, Singapore.*

Pharmaserve, Singapore. See *Polymedic, Singapore.*

Pharmasette, Ital. Pharmasette di Paolo Donati e C. s.a.s., Via Lusitania 15/A, 00183 Rome, Italy.

Pharmastra, Fr. Pharmastra, Usines Chimiques et Pharmaceutiques de Strasbourg, 40 rue du Canal, 67460 Souffelweyersheim, France.

Pharmateam, Israel. Pharmateam Marketing, P.O. Box 405, Jerusalem, Israel.

Pharmateam, UK. Pharmateam, UK.

Pharmatel, Austral. Pharmatel P/L, 3 Chilvers Rd, Thornleigh, NSW 2120, Australia.

Pharmatel, NZ. See *Pharmatel, Austral.*

Pharmatex, Ital. Pharmatex Italia s.r.l., Via Appiani 22, 20121 Milan, Italy.

Pharmaton, Ger. Pharmaton GmbH, Birkendorfer Str. 65, 88400 Biberach, Germany.

Pharmaton, Israel. See *Pharmaschalom, Israel.*

Pharmaton, NZ. Pharmaton, New Zealand.

Pharmaton, Singapore. See *Diethelm, Singapore.*

Pharmaton, Switz. Pharmaton SA, 6934 Bioggio, Switzerland.

Pharmaton, Thai. See *Boehringer Ingelheim, Thai.*

Pharmavite, Canad. Pharmavite Corp., 5230 Orbitor Drive, Mississauga, Ontario, L4W 5G7, Canada.

Pharmax, Hong Kong. See *Hind Wing, Hong Kong.*

Pharmax, Irl. See *Allphar, Irl.*

Pharmax, Singapore. See *Naina, Singapore.*

Pharmax, UK. See *Forest Laboratories, UK.*

Pharmazam, Spain. Pharmazam, Pol. Ind. Urvasa, Sta Perpetua de Mogoda, 08130 Barcelona, Spain.

Pharmco, S.Afr. Pharmco Holdings Ltd., 16a Drake Ave, Eastleigh Ridge, Edenvale 1609, South Africa.

Pharmed, Aust. Pharmed, Sackstrasse 4, A-8011 Graz, Austria.

Pharmed, Singapore. Pharmed Import & Export Pte Ltd, 149 Rochor Rd, B1-16/17/18 Fu Lu Shou Complex, S 188425, Singapore.

Pharmedica, S.Afr. Pharmedica Laboratories (Pty) Ltd, P.O. Box 87, East London 5200, Cape Province, South Africa.

Pharmel, Canad. Pharmel Inc., 8699 8e Ave, Montreal, Quebec, H1Z 2X4, Canada.

Pharmethic, Belg. Pharmethic S.A., Rue de Vivier 89-93, 1050 Brussels, Belgium.

Pharmexco, UK. Pharmexco Ltd, 5-6 Zennor Rd, London, SW12 0PS, UK.

Pharmia, Fin. Pharmia Oy, Kalliotie 2, 01560 Maantiekylä, Finland.

Pharmics, USA. Pharmics Inc., 2350 S Redwood Rd, Salt Lake City, UT 84119, USA.

Pharminter, Fr. Laboratoires Pharminter, 34 rue St-Romain, 69008 Lyon, France.

Pharmonta, Aust. Pharmonta Mag. pharm. Dr Fischer, Montanastrasse 7, A-8112 Gratwein, Austria.

Pharmy, Fr. Laboratoires Pharmy II, Strategy Center, 26 rue des Gaudines, 78100 Saint-Germain-en-Laye, France.

Pharmygiene, Fr. Laboratoires Pharmygiène-SCAT, La Boursidiere, B.P. 150, 92357 Le Plessis-Robinson, France.

Pharno-Wedropharm, Ger. Pharno-Wedropharm GmbH, Heinrichstr. 3, 21244 Buchholz, Germany.

Pharos, Singapore. See *Polymedic, Singapore.*

Phillips Yeast, UK. Phillips Yeast Products Ltd, Park Royal Rd, London, NW10 7JX, UK.

Philopharm, Ger. Philopharm GmbH, Vor dem Gropernter 20, 06484 Quedlinburg, Germany.

Phoenix Health, UK. Phoenix Health Ltd, UK.

Phonix, Ger. Phönix Laboratorium GmbH, Benzstr. 10, 71149 Bondorf, Germany.

Phos-Kola, Braz. Laboratorio Phos-Kola Ltda, Rua das Laranjeiras 984, Centro, 49010-000 Aracaju, SE, Brazil.

PH&T, Ital. PH&T S.p.A., Via L Ariosto 34, 20145 Milan, Italy.

Phygiene, Fr. Laboratoires Phygiène, 11-13 rue de la Loge, B.P. 100, 94265 Fresnes cdx, France.

Phyteia, Switz. Phyteia AG, Drosselstrasse 47, 4059 Basle, Switzerland.

Phytocare, Austral. Phytocare, Australia.

Phytomed, Switz. Phytomed AG, Tschamerie 25, 3415 Hasle bei Burgdorf, Switzerland.

Phytomedica, Fr. Laboratoires Phytomedica, ZI Les Milles, B.P. 5000, Parc d'activites de Pichaury, 13791 Aix-en-Provence cdx 3, France.

Phytosolba, Fr. Laboratoires Phytosolba, 89 rue Salvador-Allende, 95870 Bezons, France.

Piam, Ital. Vecchi & C. Piam di G. Assereto, E. Maragliano e C. s.a.p.a., Via Padre G. Semeria 5, 16131 Genoa, Italy.

Piam, Singapore. See *Zyfas, Singapore.*

Picharn, Thai. Picharn c/o The Picharn Co. Ltd, 53/43 Soi Amornphan 5, Viphavadi-Rangsit Rd, Jatujak, Bangkok 10900, Thailand.

Pickles, UK. J. Pickles & Sons, Beech House, 62 High St, Knaresborough, North Yorkshire, HG5 0EA, UK.

Picot, Fr. Laboratoires des Produits Picot, 189 quai Lucien-Lheureux, B.P. 83, 62102 Calais cdx, France.

Picot, Switz. See *Ridupharm, Switz.*

Pierre Fabre, Aust. See *Pierre Fabre, Fr.*

Pierre Fabre, Denm. See *Pierre Fabre, Swed.*

Pierre Fabre, Fin. See *Panfarma, Fin.*

Pierre Fabre, Fr. Laboratoires Pierre Fabre, Départmentmédical de Pierre Fabre Médicament, 45 place Abel-Gance, 92100 Boulogne, France.

Pierre Fabre, Ger. Pierre Fabre Pharma GmbH, Jechtinger Str. 13, 79111 Freiburg, Germany.

Pierre Fabre, Hong Kong. See *Primal, Hong Kong.*

Pierre Fabre, Israel. Pierre Fabre, Israel.

Pierre Fabre, Ital. Pierre Fabre Italia s.p.a., Via G.G. Winckelmann 1, 20146 Milan, Italy.

Pierre Fabre, Neth. Pierre Fabre, Netherlands.

Pierre Fabre, Norw. See *Pierre Fabre, Swed.*

Pierre Fabre, Port. Pierre Fabre Médicament Portugal, Lda, Rua Rodrigo da Fonseca 178 - 2 Esq, 1099-067 Lisbon, Portugal.

Pierre Fabre, Singapore. See *Zuellig, Singapore.*

Pierre Fabre, Spain. Pierre Fabre Iberica, Ramon Trias Fargas 7-11, 08005 Barcelona, Spain.

Pierre Fabre, Swed. Pierre Fabre Pharma Norden AB, Box 349, 192 30 Sollentuna, Sweden.

Pierre Fabre, Switz. Pierre Fabre (Suisse) SA, Route Sous-Riette 21, 1023 Crissier, Switzerland.

Pierre Fabre, Thai. See *Berli, Thai.*

Pierre Fabre, UK. Pierre Fabre Ltd, Hyde Abbey House, 23 Hyde St, Winchester, Hampshire, SO23 7DR, UK.

Pierre Fabre Dermo Kosmetik, Ger. See *Pierre Fabre, Ger.*

Pierre Fabre Sante, Fr. See *Pierre Fabre, Fr.*

Pierrel, Ital. Pierrel Farmaceutici s.p.a., Via Revere 16, 20123 Milan, Italy.

Pietrasanta, Ital. Pietrasanta Pharma s.r.l., Loc. S. Rocchino, 55054 Massarosa (LU), Italy.

Piette, Belg. Laboratoires Piette International S.A., Groot-Bijgaardenstraat 128, 1620 Drogenbos, Belgium.

Piette, Thai. Piette, Thailand.

Pilkington Barnes-Hind, USA. See *Wesley, USA.*

Pilsensee, Ger. Pilsensee-Apotheke GmbH, Gunteringer Strasse 2, 82229 Seefeld/Hechendorf, Germany.

Pinewood, Irl. Pinewood Laboratories Ltd, Unit 1, M50 Business Park, Ballymount, Dublin 24, Ireland.

Pinewood, UK. See *Pinewood, Irl.*

Piniol, Switz. Piniol AG, Pharmazeutische Spezialitaten, Erlistrasse 2, 6403 Kussnacht aR, Switzerland.

Pinnacle, Canad. Pinnacle Pharmaceutics, 519 Dundas St E, Unit 8, Whitby, Ontario, L1N 2J5, Canada.

Pinneberg, Hong Kong. Pinneberg Ltd, 1404 Chiao Shang Bldg, 92-94 Queen's Rd Central, Hong Kong.

Pionneau, Fr. Laboratoires Pionneau, 33870 Vayres, France.

Piraud, Switz. Piraud AG, Switzerland.

Pisa, Mex. Laboratorios Pisa S.A. de C.V., Av. Espana No. 1840, 44190 Guadalajara, Jal., Mexico.

Pizzard, Mex. Laboratorios Pizzard, S.A. de C.V., Vito Alessio Robles No. 209, Col. Florida, 01030 Mexico, D.F., Mexico.

Plan, Switz. Laboratoires Plan SA, Chemin des Sellieres, 1219 Aire-Geneva, Switzerland.

Planta, Canad. Planta Dei Pharma, P.O. Box 415, Route 105, Nackawic, NB, E0H 1P0, Canada.

Plantamed, Ger. Plantamed Arzneimittel GmbH, Kerschensteiner Str. 11-15, 92318 Neumarkt/Opf., Germany.

Plantes et Medecines, Fr. See *Dolisos, Fr.*

Plantes Tropicales, Fr. Laboratoires de Plantes Tropicales, chemin de la Sereine, 01700 Beynost, France.

Plantina, Ger. Plantina Biologische Arzneimittel AG, Konrad-Celtis-Str. 81, 81369 Munich, Germany.

Plantorgan, Neth. See *Bipharma, Neth.*

Plants, Ital. Plants, Laboratorio della Dott.ssa Luisa Coletta, Via V d'Amore 4, 98100 Messina, Italy.

Plasmon, Ital. Plasmon Dietetici Alimentari s.p.a., Via G. Cadolini 26, 20137 Milan, Italy.

Plevifarma, Spain. Plevifarma, Fernando Puig 58,60, 08023 Barcelona, Spain.

Plough, Port. Plough Farma, Lda, Casal Colaride, Agualva, 2735 Cacem, Portugal.

Plough, USA. See *Schering-Plough, USA.*

Plurisfarma, Ital. Plurisystem sas di Arippa Lionello & C., Via F Vezzani 99r, 16159 Genova-Rivarolo, Italy.

PMC, Austral. See *AstraZeneca, Austral.*

Poehlmann, Ger. Dr Poehlmann & Co. GmbH, Postfach: 1365, 58303 Herdecke, Germany.

Poehlmann, Switz. See *Renapharm, Switz.*

Pohl, Denm. See *Meda, Denm.*

Pohl, Ger. G. Pohl-Boskamp GmbH & Co., Kieler Str. 11, 25551 Hohenlockstedt, Germany.

Pohl, Hong Kong. See *Health Vision, Hong Kong.*

Pohl, Israel. Pohl, Israel.

Pohl, Neth. See *Tramedico, Neth.*

Pohl, Norw. See *Meda, Norw.*

Pohl, Switz. See *Lubapharm, Switz.*

Poirier, Fr. Laboratoires Pharm. Poirier, ZA La Haute-Limougere, B.P. 24, 37230 Fondettes, France.

Polaris, Ital. Polaris Biolab srl, Via Wagner 8, 20145 Milan, Italy.

Polcoma, Austral. Polcoma Polley F & Co. P/L, P.O. Box 100, Epping, NSW 2121, Australia.

Polcopharma, Austral. See *Polcoma, Austral.*

Poli, Hong Kong. See *International Medical, Hong Kong.*

Poli, Ital. Poli Industria Chimica s.p.a., Via Volturno 45-48, 20089 Quinto de Stampi-Rozzano (MI), Italy.

Poli, Switz. See *Adroka, Switz.*

Polidis, Fr. Ste Polidis, 7 rue Gallieni, 92500 Rueil-Malmaison, France.

Polifarma, Ital. Polifarma s.p.a., Via Tor Sapienza 138, 00155 Rome, Italy.

Polipharm, Thai. Polipharm Co. Ltd, 109 Mu 12 Bangna-Trat Rd, Bangpleeyai, Bangplee, Samutprakan 10540, Thailand.

Poly, USA. Poly Pharmaceuticals Inc., P.O. Box 93, Quitman, MS 39355, USA.

Polymedic, Singapore. Polymedic Trading Enterprise Pte Ltd, 150 Kampong Ampat, 06-07 KA Centre, S 368324, Singapore.

PolyMedica, USA. PolyMedica Pharmaceuticals (USA) Inc., 11 State St, Woburn, MA 01801, USA.

Polymer Technology, Canad. Polymer Technology, 400 Matheson Blvd E, 28, Mississauga, Ontario, L4Z 1N8, Canada.

Polymer Technology, USA. Polymer Technology Corp., 1400 N Goodman, St Rochester, NY 14692, USA.

Polypharm, Ger. Polypharm GmbH, Bad Nauheimer Str. 4, 64289 Darmstadt, Germany.

Pond's, Thai. Pond's Chemical Thailand R.O.P., 79 MU 4 Ramindra Rd, Bangkhen, Bangkok 10220, Thailand.

Pond's Chemical, Singapore. See *JDH, Singapore.*

Porton, Israel. Porton, Israel.

Pose, Thai. Pose Health Care Ltd, 2/25 Paholyothin 7, Phyathal, Bangkok 10400, Thailand.

Potter's, UK. Potter's (Herbal Supplies) Ltd, Leyland Mill Lane, Wigan, Lancashire, WN1 2SB, UK.

Poythress, USA. See *ECR, USA.*

PP Lab, Thai. See *Picharn, Thai.*

PPDH, Fr. PPDH SA, 247 bis rue des Pyrenees, 75020 Paris, France.

PQS, Spain. PQS Farma, Ctra Madrid-Cadiz Km 554.4, Dos Hermanas, 41700 Seville, Spain.

Pras, Spain. Pras Farma, C/Pont Reixat 5, Sant Just Desvern, 08960 Barcelona, Spain.

Prats, Spain. Prats, Traversera del Dalt 44, 08024 Barcelona, Spain.

Precifarma, Braz. Precifarma Laboratorio Farmaceutico Ltda, Rua Correia de Lemos 153, 04041-001 Sao Paulo, SP, Brazil.

Precimex, Mex. Precimex S.A., Calz. de las Aguilas No. 1211, Col. San Clemente, 10740 Mexico D.F., Mexico.

Pred, Fr. Laboratoires Pred, 1 quai de Grenelle, 75015 Paris, France.

Premier, USA. See *Advanced Polymer, USA.*

Presselin, Ger. Presselin Arzneimittel GmbH & Co. KG, Heinkelstr. 8a, 76461 Muggensturm, Germany.

Prevention et Biologie, Fr. Prévention et Biologie SA, 29-33 rue de Metz, 94170 Le Perreux, France.

Prevision, Spain. See *Bayer, Spain.*

Prima, Braz. Laboratorios Prima S.A. Industria e Comercio, Rua Juparana 62, 20510-040 Rio de Janeiro, RJ, Brazil.

Prima, Thai. Prima Pharm.

Primal, Hong Kong. Primal Chemical Co. Ltd, Flat A, 7/F, Hoi Bun Industrial Bldg, 6 Wing Yip St, Kwun Tong, Kowloon, Hong Kong.

Princeton, Spain. See *Bristol-Myers, Spain.*

Princeton, USA. See *Bristol-Myers Squibb, USA.*

Priory, Irl. Priory Pharmaceuticals Ltd, 4 Priory Hall, Stillorgan Road, Co. Dublin, Ireland.

Prisfar, Port. Prisfar, SA, Rua Antero de Quentel 629, 4200 Porto, Portugal.

Prism, UK. Prism Healthcare, UK.

Pro Doc, Canad. Pro Doc Limitee, 2925 Industrial Blvd, Laval, Quebec, H7L 3W9, Canada.

Pro Medica, Swed. Pro Medica AB, Box 27190, 102 52 Stockholm, Sweden.

Pro Vaccine, Switz. Pro Vaccine AG, Grabenstrasse 42, 6301 Zug, Switzerland.

Probelte, Spain. Probelte Pharma, Ctra Madrid Km 389, Espinardo, 30100 Murcia, Spain.

Probifasa, Mex. Probifasa S.A. de C.V., Calz. Mexico-Tacuba No. 1419, Col Argentina Pte., 11230 Mexico D.F., Mexico.

Probiomed, Mex. Probiomed, S.A. de C.V., Ejercito Nacional No. 499 4o. piso, Col. Granada, 11520 Mexico, D.F., Mexico.

Probios, Port. Probios, Lda, Rua Joao Chagas 53-A, Escritorio 201, 1495-072 Alges, Portugal.

Procare, Austral. See *Biovital, Austral.*

Proceane, Fr. Lab. Proceane Ressources Marines, B.P. 88, 44503 La Baule cdx, France.

Procter & Gamble, Aust. Procter & Gamble Austria GmbH, Guglgasse 7-9, A-1030 Vienna, Austria.

Procter & Gamble, Austral. Procter & Gamble Australia P/L, Locked Bag No. 75, Parramatta, NSW 2124, Australia.

Procter & Gamble, Belg. Procter & Gamble Pharmaceuticals S.A., Temselaan 100, 1853 Strombeek-Bever, Belgium.

Procter & Gamble, Braz. Procter & Gamble do Brasil S.A., Rua Quata 1.177, 04546-045 Sao Paulo, SP, Brazil.

Procter & Gamble, Canad. Procter & Gamble Inc., P.O. Box 355, Station A, Toronto, Ontario, M5W 1C5, Canada.

Procter & Gamble, Denm. See *Roche, Denm.*

Procter & Gamble, Fin. See *Panfarma, Fin.*

Procter & Gamble, Fr. Procter & Gamble Pharmaceuticals France, 96 av Charles-de-Gaulle, 92201 Neuilly-sur-Seine cdx, France.

Procter & Gamble, Ger. Procter & Gamble Pharmaceuticals Germany GmbH, Dr.-Otto-Rohm-Str. 2-4, 64331 Weiterstadt, Germany.

Procter & Gamble, Hong Kong. See *Keller, Hong Kong.*

Procter & Gamble, Irl. See *Aventis Pharma, Irl.*, and *United Drug, Irl.*

Procter & Gamble, Israel. See *Neopharm, Israel.*

Procter & Gamble, Ital. Procter & Gamble Italia s.p.a., Viale C Pavese 385, 00144 Rome, Italy.

Procter & Gamble, Mex. Procter & Gamble de Mexico S.A. de C.V., San Andres Atoto No. 326, 53560 Naucalpan de Juarez, Mexico.

Procter & Gamble, Neth. Procter & Gamble Pharmaceuticals, Postbus 2507, 3000 CM Rotterdam, Netherlands.

Procter & Gamble, Norw. See *Roche, Norw.*

Procter & Gamble, NZ. Procter & GambleNPD, Inc., P.O. Box 5861, Auckland, New Zealand.

Procter & Gamble, Spain. Procter & Gamble, Av. Partenon 16-18, Campo Naciones, 28042 Madrid, Spain.

Procter & Gamble, Swed. Procter & Gamble Nordic Inc., filial Sverige, Box 27303, 102 54 Stockholm, Sweden.

Procter & Gamble, Switz. Procter & Gamble AG, 1 rue du Pre-de-la-Bichette, 1211 Geneva 2, Switzerland.

Procter & Gamble, UK. Procter & Gamble Pharmaceuticals UK Ltd, Lovett House, Lovett Rd, Staines, Middlesex, TW18 3AZ, UK.

Procter & Gamble, USA. Procter & Gamble, P.O. Box 5516, Cincinnati, OH 45201, USA.

Procter & Gamble (H&B Care), UK. Procter & Gamble (Health & Beauty Care) Ltd, The Heights, Brooklands, Weybridge, Surrey, KT13 0XP, UK.

Procyte, USA. ProCyte Corp., 8511 154th Ave NE, Bldg A, Redmond, WA 98052-3557, USA.

Prodemdis, Canad. Prodemdis Enrg, 4355 Sir Wilfred Laurier Blvd, St-Hubert, Quebec, J3Y 3X3, Canada.

Prodes, Spain. See *Almirall, Spain.*

Prodome, Braz. Prodome Quimica e Farmaceutica Ltda, Rua 13 de Maio 1.161, 13130-071 Campinas, SP, Brazil.

Prodotti, Braz. Prodotti Laboratorio Farmaceutico Ltda, Avenida Joao Dias 1.084, Santo Amaro, 04724-001 Sao Paulo, SP, Brazil.

Produfarma, Port. Produfarma, Lda, Estrada de Benfica 403-B, 1500-077 Lisbon, Portugal.

Produits Dentaires, Switz. Produits Dentaires SA, 18 rue des Bosquets, 1800 Vevey, Switzerland.

Prof. Pharm. Corp., Canad. Professional Pharmaceutical Corporation, 9200 Cote-de-Liesse Blvd, Lachine, Quebec, H8T 1A1, Canada.

Profarb, Braz. Profarb Ltda, Rua Paschoal Bernardino 25, 36880-000 Muriae, MG, Brazil.

Professional Dental, UK. Professional Dental Supplies, UK.

Professional Health, Canad. Professional Health Products, 4307-49 St, Innisfail, AB, T4G 1P3, Canada.

Professional Supplies, USA. See *SoftRinse, USA.*

Proge, Ital. Proge Farm srl, Via Croce 4, 28065 Cerano (NO), Italy.

Progest, Ital. Progest Industria Chimica s.r.l., Salita Castel Giubileo 2, 00138 Rome, Italy.

Progress, Thai. See *Medicine Supply, Thai.*

Pro-Health, NZ. Pro-Health Products Ltd, P.O. Box 28-545, Remuera, Auckland, New Zealand.

Prolabor, Braz. Prolabor Comercio e Industria Farmaceutica Ltda, Rua Pesqueira 15, 21041-000 Rio de Janeiro, RJ, Brazil.

Promeco, Mex. Promeco S.A. de C.V., Calle del Maiz No. 49, Col. Xaltocan, 16090 Mexico D.F., Mexico.

Promed, Ger. Promed Arzneimittel GmbH, 22876 Wedel, Germany.

Promedica, Fr. See *Chiesi, Fr.*

Promedica, Thai. See *Pacific, Thai.*

Promedical, Ital. Promedical srl, Via G Greco 8, 90017 Santa Flavia (PA), Italy.

Promedico, Israel. ProMedico Ltd, P.O. Box 3340, Petach Tikva, Israel.

Promedis, Belg. Promedis, Belgium.

Promefarm, Ital. Promefarm s.r.l., Corso Indipendenza 6, 20129 Milan, Italy.

Prometic, Canad. Prometic Pharma Inc., 1000 Raoul Charette, Joliette, Quebec, J6E 8S9, Canada.

Prometic, USA. See *Prometic, Canad.*

Promonta, Ger. See *Lundbeck, Ger.*

Pro-Nat, Fr. Pro-Nat SA, France.

Propan, S.Afr. See *Adcock Ingram, S.Afr.*

Propan-Vernleigh, S.Afr. See *Propan, S.Afr.*

Prospa, Belg. Prospa S.A., Blvd Brand Whitlock 156, 1200 Brussels, Belgium.

Prospa, Ital. Prospa Italia s.r.l., Via Modica 6, 20143 Milan (MI), Italy.

Prospa, Port. Prospa, SA, Rua do Proletariado 15C, 2795-648 Carnaxide, Portugal.

Protea, S.Afr. Protea Pharm (Pty) Ltd, P.O. Box 422, East London 5200, South Africa.

Protec, UK. Protec Health International Ltd, 5 Priory Court, Poulton, Cirencester, Gloucestershire, GL7 5JB, UK.

Protein, Mex. Protein S.A. de C.V., Anil Num. 865, Col. Granjas Mexico, Deleg. Iztacalco, 08400 Mexico DF, Mexico.

Protermex, Mex. Protermex, Mexico.

Protidiet, Fr. Protidiet, ZAE Migelane, B.P. 10, 33650 Saucats, France.

Protina, Ger. Protina Pharmazeutische Gesellschaft mbH, Adalperostr. 90, 85737 Ismaning, Germany.

Protina, Switz. See *Doetsch, Grether, Switz.*

Provalis, UK. Provalis Healthcare, Newtech Square, Deeside Industrial Park, Deeside, Flintshire, CH5 2NT, UK.

Proveedora Teknimex, Mex. Proveedora Teknimex, Mexico.

Provit, Mex. Provit S.A. de C.V., Nino Artillero No. 500, C.U. Independencia, 50070 Toluca, Mexico.

Provita, Aust. Provita Pharma GmbH, Wilhelmstrasse 23, A-1120 Vienna, Austria.

Provita, Ital. Provita Industria Farmaceutica s.r.l., Via Dora 7, 00198 Rome, Italy.

Psicofarma, Mex. Laboratorio Psicofarma S.A. de C.V., Calz. de Tlalpan No. 4369, Col. Toriello Guerra, 14050 Mexico D.F., Mexico.

PSM, NZ. PSM Healthcare Ltd, P.O. Box 76-401, Manukau City, Auckland, New Zealand.

Puerto Galiano, Spain. Puerto Galiano, Calle 'S', 4, Parque Europolis, Las Rozas, 28230 Madrid, Spain.

Pulitzer, Ital. Pulitzer Italiana s.r.l., Via Tiburtina 1004, 00156 Rome, Italy.

Pulmopharm, Ger. Pulmopharm GmbH, Ottostr. 3, 80333 Munich, Germany.

Pulsion, Ger. Pulsion Medical Systems GmbH, Stahlgruberring 28, 81829 Munich, Germany.

Pulsion, Israel. Pulsion, Israel.

Purdue, Canad. Purdue Pharma, 575 Granite Court, Pickering, Ontario, L1W 3W8, Canada.

Purdue Frederick, Canad. See *Purdue, Canad.*

Purdue Frederick, USA. The Purdue Frederick Co., 100 Connecticut Ave, Norwalk, CT 06850-3590, USA.

Puritan Quartz, Thai. Puritan Quartz.

QHP, USA. Quality Health Products Inc., P.O. Box 31, Yaphank, NY 11980, USA.

QIF, Braz. QIF Quimica Intercontinental Farmaceutica Ltda, Avenida Itaborai 1425, 04135-001 Sao Paulo, SP, Brazil.

Quad, USA. Quad Pharmaceuticals Inc., USA.

Qualimed, Austral. See *Aventis, Austral.*

Qualiphar, Belg. Qualiphar S.A., Rijksweg 9, 2880 Bornem, Belgium.

Qualitest, USA. Qualitest Products Inc., 1236 Jordan Rd, Huntsville, AL 35811, USA.

Quality Formulations, USA. Quality Formulations Inc., P.O. Box 827, Zachary, LA 70791-0827, USA.

Quantum, USA. Quantum Pharmics Ltd, USA.

Quatromed, S.Afr. Quatromed, South Africa.

Queisser, Aust. See *Queisser, Ger.*

Queisser, Ger. Queisser Pharma GmbH & Co., Schleswiger Str. 74, 24941 Flensburg, Germany.

Quest, Canad. Quest Vitamins, Division of Boehringer Ingelheim (Canada) Ltd, 1781 West 75th Ave., Vancouver, British Columbia, V6P 6P2, Canada.

Quest, UK. Quest Vitamins Ltd, 8 Venture Way, Aston Science Park, Birmingham, B7 4AP, UK.

Questcor, USA. Questcor Pharmaceuticals Inc., 26118 Research Rd, Hayward, CA 94545, USA.

Quick-Med, S.Afr. Quick-Med, South Africa.

Quidel, Fr. Lab. Quidel, France.

Quidel, USA. Quidel Corp., 10165 McKellar Court, La Jolla, CA 92037, USA.

Quies, Fr. Lab. Quies, 4 rue Ambroise-Croizat, 91120 Palaiseau, France.

Quimedical, Port. Quimedical - Produtos Farmacêuticos, Lda, Edificio Azevedos, Estrada Nacional 117, 2724-503 Amadora, Portugal.

Quimica Medica, Spain. La Quimica Medica, San Juan Bosco 55, 08017 Barcelona, Spain.

Quimica y Farmacia, Mex. Quimica y Farmacia, S.A. de C.V., Av. Pacifico No. 332, Col. Rosedal Coyoacan, 04330 Mexico, D.F., Mexico.

Quimifar, Spain. Quimifar, Comadran 37, Pol Ind Can Salvatella, Barbera del Valles, 08210 Barcelona, Spain.

Quimioterapica, Braz. Quimioterapica Brasileira Ltda, Rua Filgueiras Lima 28, 20950-050 Rio de Janeiro, RJ, Brazil.

Quimpe, Spain. Quimpe, Cruz 47-9, Alhaurin el Grande, 29120 Malaga, Spain.

Quinoderm, Hong Kong. See *Mekim, Hong Kong.*

Quinoderm, Irl. See *Boileau & Boyd, Irl.*

Quinoderm, Switz. See *Golaz, Switz.*

Quinoderm, UK. See *Adams, UK.*

Rabi & Solabo, Fr. Laboratoires Rabi & Solabo, 67 rue Voltaire, 92150 Suresnes, France.

Rachelle, USA. Rachelle, USA.

Radiol, Israel. Radiol, Israel.

Radiumfarma, Ital. Radiumfarma s.r.l., Laboratori Farmaco Biologici, Via Carnevali 116, 20158 Milan, Italy.

Rafa, Israel. Rafa Laboratories Ltd, P.O. Box 405, Jerusalem 91003, Israel.

Rahslog, USA. Rahslog, USA.

Ram, USA. Ram Laboratories, Division of Bradley Pharmaceuticals Inc., 3300 University Drive, Coral Springs, FL 33065, USA.

Ramelco, Canad. Ramelco Ltd, Subsidiary of Maltby Ltd, 306 Dawlish Ave, Toronto, Ontario, M4N 1J5, Canada.

Ramini, Ital. Ramini s.r.l., Via di Vallerano 96, 00128 Rome, Italy.

Ramon Sala, Spain. Ramon Sala, Paris 174, 08036 Barcelona, Spain.

RAN, Ger. R.A.N. Novesia AG Arzneimittel, Hurtgener Str. 6, 41464 Neuss/Rhein, Germany.

Ranbaxy, S.Afr. Ranbaxy (SA) (Pty) Ltd, P.O. Box 10458, Centurion 0046, South Africa.

Ranbaxy, Singapore. See *Zyfas, Singapore.*

Ranbaxy, Thai. Ranbaxy Unichem, c/o Ranbaxy (Thailand) Co. Ltd, 3 Fl, Rm 314-8, Phayathai Building, 31 Phayathai Rd, Rajathevi, Bangkok 10400, Thailand.

Randall, Mex. Randall Laboratories, S.A de C.V., Lago Rodolfo No. 58, 11520 Mexico, D.F., Mexico.

Randob, USA. Randob Laboratories Ltd, P.O. Box 440, Cornwall, NY 12518, USA.

Rapide, Spain. See *Baxter, Spain*, and *Bieffe, Spain.*

Rappai, Switz. Dr F. Rappai Pharmazeutika, Postfach, 8952 Schlieren-Zurich, Switzerland.

Ratiopharm, Aust. ratiopharm Arzneimittel Vertriebs-GmbH, Albert-Schweitzer-Gasse 3, A-1140 Vienna, Austria.

Ratiopharm, Fin. ratiopharm Oy Medinovum, PL 280, 00031 Instrumentarium, Finland.

Ratiopharm, Ger. ratiopharm GmbH, Graf-Arco-Str. 3, 89079 Ulm/Donautal, Germany.

Ratiopharm, Hong Kong. See *CNW, Hong Kong.*

Ratiopharm, Port. Ratiopharm, Lda, Rua Oliveira Martins 2 A/B, Casal de S Bras, Portugal.

Ratiopharm, Spain. Ratiopharm, Rosario Pino 14-16, Ed Torre Rioja, 28020 Madrid, Spain.

Ravensberg, Ger. Ravensberg GmbH, Schneckenburgstr. 46, 78467 Constance, Germany.

Ravizza, Ital. Ravizza Farmaceutici s.p.a., Via Europa 35, 20053 Muggio (MI), Italy.

Ravizza, Neth. See *Will-Pharma, Neth.*

Raway, USA. Raway Pharmacal Inc., 15 Granit Rd, Accord, NY 12404-0047, USA.

Rawleigh, Canad. Rawleigh, 60 Colonnade Rd, Nepean, ON, K2E 7J6, Canada.

Rayere, Mex. Farmaceuticos Rayere S.A., Emiliano Zapata No. 72, Col. Portales, 03300 Mexico D.F., Mexico.

RCA, Ital. Ricerca Cosmetica Avanzata srl, Zona Industriale Loc. Penitro, 04023 Formia (LT), Italy.

R&D, Canad. See *R&D, USA.*

R&D, USA. R & D Laboratories Inc., 4640 Admiralty Way, Suite 710, Marina Del Rey, CA 90292-5608, USA.

RDC, Ital. Ricerche Dermo Cosmetiche Erredici s.r.l., Via G. Armellini 37, 00143 Rome, Italy.

Realdyme, Fr. Sté Réaldyme, 28700 Garancieres-en-Beauce, France.

Reall, Switz. Medical Concepts Reall-YS Sàrl, Ave Villardin 22, 1009 Pully, Switzerland.

Realpharma, Ger. realpharma Geschaftsbereich der Dolorgiet Arzneimittel, Postfach: 1252, 53730 St Augustin/Bonn, Germany.

Recherche Botanique, Fr. Lab. de Recherche Botanique, 9 av. Guy-Petit, 64200 Biarritz, France.

Recip, Denm. See *Pharmacia Upjohn, Denm.*

Recip, Fin. See *Algol, Fin.*

Recip, Norw. See *Weifa, Norw.*

Recip, Swed. Recip AB, Branningevagen 12, 120 54 Arsta, Sweden.

Recipe, Aust. Recipe GmbH, Austria.

Reckeweg, Ger. Pharmazeutische Fabrik Dr. Reckeweg & Co. GmbH, Berliner Ring 32, 64625 Bensheim, Germany.

Reckitt & Colman, Austral. See *Reckitt Benckiser, Austral.*

Reckitt & Colman, Belg. Reckitt & Colman S.A., Allee de la Recherche 20, 1070 Brussels, Belgium.

Reckitt & Colman, Hong Kong. Reckitt & Colman Hong Kong Ltd, 1203-5 Allied Kajima Bldg, 138 Gloucester Rd, Hong Kong.

Reckitt & Colman, Israel. Reckitt & Colman, Israel.

Reckitt & Colman, Norw. See *Nycomed, Norw.,* and *Schering-Plough, Norw.*

Reckitt & Colman, S.Afr. See *Reckitt Benckiser, S.Afr.*

Reckitt & Colman, Singapore. Reckitt & Colman Singapore Pte Ltd, 1 Fifth Ave, 04-06 Guthrie House, S 268802, Singapore.

Reckitt & Colman, Spain. Reckitt & Colman, Spain.

Reckitt & Colman, Thai. Reckitt & Colman (Thailand) Ltd, 9 Fl, Vanissa Building, 29 Soi Chidlom, Ploenchit Rd, Patumwan, Bangkok 10330, Thailand.

Reckitt & Colman, UK. Reckitt & Colman Products Ltd, Dansom Lane, Hull, HU8 7DS, UK.

Reckitt & Colman, USA. See *Reckitt Benckiser, USA.*

Reckitt Benckiser, Austral. Reckitt Benckiser Pharmaceuticals, P.O. Box 138, West Ryde, NSW 2114, Australia.

Reckitt Benckiser, Irl. Reckitt Benckiser, Pharmapark, Chapelizod, Dublin 20, Ireland.

Reckitt Benckiser, NZ. Reckitt Benckiser Pharmaceuticals, Private Bag 93121, Henderson, Auckland, New Zealand.

Reckitt Benckiser, S.Afr. Reckitt Benckiser Pharmaceuticals (Pty) Ltd, P.O. Box 164, Isando 1600, South Africa.

Reckitt Benckiser, UK. Reckitt Benckiser plc, Dansom House, Hull, Humberside, HU8 7DS, UK.

Reckitt Benckiser, USA. Reckitt Benckiser, 1909 Huguenot Rd, Suite 300, Richmond, VA 23235, USA.

Reckitts, Irl. Reckitt's (Ireland) Ltd, P.O. Box 730, Cloverhill Industrial Estate, Clondalkin, Dublin 22, Ireland.

Recon, Singapore. See *Zyfas, Singapore.*

Recordati, Hong Kong. See *Unico, Hong Kong.*

Recordati, Ital. Recordati Industria Chimica e Farmaceutica S.p.a., Via Civitali 1, 20148 Milan, Italy.

Recordati, Singapore. See *MD, Singapore.*

Recordati, Spain. Recordati España SL, Ctra N-III Km 23, Arganda del Rey, 28500 Madrid, Spain.

Recsei, USA. Recsei Laboratories, 330 S Kellogg, Building M, Goleta, CA 93117-3875, USA.

Reddy, Singapore. See *Zyfas, Singapore.*

Redel, Ger. See *Cesra, Ger.*

Redino, Ger. RedinoMedica GmbH, Tivolistr. 1, 80538 Munich, Germany.

Redi-Products, USA. See *Aplicare, USA.*

Redken, Canad. Redken Laboratories Canada Ltd, 5160 Yonge St, North York, Ontario, M2N 6L9, Canada.

Redur, USA. Redur, USA.

Reed & Carnrick, Canad. See *Block, Canad.*

Reed & Carnrick, USA. See *Schwarz, USA.*

Reedco, USA. Reedco, USA.

Reese, USA. Reese Pharmaceutical Co. Inc., 10617 Frank Ave, Cleveland, OH 44106, USA.

Regal, Canad. Regal Pharmaceuticals, Division of Bradcan Corp., 900 Harrington Court, Burlington, Ontario, L7N 3N4, Canada.

Regenaplex, Ger. Regenaplex-Arzneispezialitäten GmbH, Robert-Bosch-Str. 3, 78467 Constance, Germany.

Regina, UK. Regina Health Ltd, NLA Tower, 12-16 Addiscombe Rd, Croydon, Surrey, CR0 0XT, UK.

Regional Health, NZ. Regional Health Ltd, P.O. Box 101-104, North Shore Mail Centre, Auckland, New Zealand.

Regius, Braz. Laboratorio Regius Ltda, Rua Doutor Ramiro D'Avila 57, 90620-050 Porto Alegre, RS, Brazil.

Reig Jofre, Spain. Reig Jofre, Pl. I. Margall 41, 08024 Barcelona, Spain.

Reith & Petrasch, Ger. Reith & Petrasch GmbH, Martstr. 1, 77834 Rheinmunster, Germany.

Rekah, Israel. Rekah Ltd, P.O. Box 25, Azor, Israel.

Rekawan, Ger. Rekawan Arzneimittel GmbH, An der Wiek 7, 17498 Insel Riems, Germany.

Relax, Ital. Relax Health Care srl, Corso Sempione 36, 20154 Milan, Italy.

REM, NZ. REM Systems Ltd, P.O. Box 90-147, Auckland Mail Centre, Auckland, New Zealand.

Remedica, Hong Kong. See *Health Care, Hong Kong,* and *Primal, Hong Kong.*

Remedica, Singapore. See *JDH, Singapore.*

Remedica, Thai. See *Pharmadica, Thai.*

Remir, Mex. Industrial Farmaceutica Remir S.A., Xochicalco Norte No. 46-B, Col. Navarte, 03020 Mexico D.F., Mexico.

Renal Systems, USA. Renal Systems, USA.

Renapharm, Switz. Renapharm S.A., Rue du Château 3, 1636 Broc, Switzerland.

Renaudin, Fr. Lab. Renaudin, ZA Errobi, 64250 Itxassou, France.

Rendell, UK. WJ Rendell Ltd, Ickleford Manor, Hitchin, Hertfordshire, SG5 3XE, UK.

Rentschler, Ger. Dr. Rentschler Arzneimittel GmbH & Co., Mittelstr. 18, 88471 Laupheim, Germany.

Rentschler, Israel. Rentschler, Israel.

Repha, Ger. Repha GmbH Biologische Arzneimittel, Alt-Godshorn 87, 30855 Langenhagen, Germany.

Reprefar, Port. See *Pierre Fabre, Port.*

Republic, USA. Republic Drug Co., 175 Great Arrow, Suite 4, Buffalo, NY 14207, USA.

Requa, USA. Requa Inc., 1 Seneca Place, P.O. Box 4008, Greenwich, CT 06830, USA.

Research Industries Corp., USA. See *Research Medical, USA.*

Research Labs, S.Afr. Research Labs, South Africa.

Research Medical, USA. Research Medical Inc., 6864 South 300 West, Midvale, UT 84047, USA.

Resinag, Israel. Resinag, Israel.

Resinag, Switz. Resinag AG, Oberer Steisteg 18, 6430 Schwyz, Switzerland.

Respa, USA. Respa Pharmaceuticals Inc., PO Box 88222, Carol Stream, IL 60188, USA.

Restan, S.Afr. Restan Laboratories (Pty) Ltd, Private Bag X69, Bryanston 2021, South Africa.

Restiva, Ital. See *Pfizer Consumer, Ital.*

Retrain, Spain. Retrain, Alfonso XII 587, Badalona, 08912 Barcelona, Spain.

Retsews, USA. Retsews, USA.

Retterspitz, Ger. Retterspitz GmbH, Laufer Str. 17-19, Postfach: 47, 90567 Schwaig, Germany.

Reuabuen, USA. Reuabuen, USA.

Reuffer, Mex. Reuffer, Mexico.

Reusch, Ger. Pharma Reusch GmbH, Hallestr. 50, 53125 Bonn, Germany.

Revlon, Canad. Revlon Canada Inc., 2501 Stanfield Rd, Mississauga, Ontario, L4Y 1R9, Canada.

Revlon, UK. Revlon International Corp., 86 Brook St, London, W1Y 2BA, UK.

Rexar, USA. Rexar Pharmacal Corp., 396 Rockaway Ave, Valley Stream, NY 11581, USA.

Rhein, Mex. Siegfried Rhein, S.A. de C.V., Calle 2 No. 30, Fracc. Industrial Benito Juarez, 76120 Queretaro, Qro, Mexico.

Rhein-Pharma, Ger. See *AstraZeneca, Ger.*

Rhenomed, Ger. Rhenomed Arzneimittel GmbH, Luth.-Kirch.-Str. 69/71, Postfach: 130662, 47758 Krefeld, Germany.

Rhodia, Braz. Rhodia Farma Ltda, Avenida Nacoes Unidas 22.428, 04795-916 Sao Paulo, SP, Brazil.

Rhodia, Hong Kong. Rhodia Hong Kong Ltd, 18/F Manulife Tower, 169 Electric Rd, North Point, Hong Kong.

Rhodiapharm, Canad. See *Aventis Pharma, Canad.*

Rhone Poulenc Chemicals, UK. Rhone-Poulenc Chemicals, Poleacre Lane, Woodley, Stockport, Cheshire, SK6 1PQ, UK.

Rhone-Poulenc Rorer, Aust. Rhone-Poulenc Rorer Pharmazeutika GmbH, Grinzinger Allee 18, A-1190 Vienna, Austria.

Rhone-Poulenc Rorer, Austral. Rhone-Poulenc Rorer Australia P/L, Private Bag 6263, Baulkham Hills Business Centre, Baulkham Hills, NSW 2153, Australia.

Rhone-Poulenc Rorer, Belg. See *Aventis, Belg.*

Rhone-Poulenc Rorer, Canad. See *Aventis Pharma, Canad.*

Rhone-Poulenc Rorer, Denm. Rhone-Poulenc Rorer A/S, Kongevejen 100, 2840 Holte, Denmark.

Rhone-Poulenc Rorer, Fin. Rhône-Poulenc Rorer Oy, PL 96, Maistraatinportti 4 A, 00241 Helsinki, Finland.

Rhone-Poulenc Rorer, Fr. See *Aventis, Fr.*

Rhone-Poulenc Rorer, Ger. See *Aventis Pharma, Ger.*

Rhone-Poulenc Rorer, Hong Kong. Rhone-Poulenc Rorer Asia Pacific Ltd, 7/F Jardine Engineering House, 260 King's Rd, North Point, Hong Kong.

Rhone-Poulenc Rorer, Irl. See *Aventis Pharma, Irl.*

Rhone-Poulenc Rorer, Israel. Rhone-Poulenc Rorer, P.O. Box 8090, Netanya, Israel.

Rhone-Poulenc Rorer, Ital. Rhone-Poulenc Rorer s.p.a., Viale Europa 11, 21040 Origgio (VA), Italy.

Rhone-Poulenc Rorer, Jpn. Rhone-Poulenc Rorer, Japan.

Rhone-Poulenc Rorer, Mex. Rhone-Poulenc Rorer S.A. de C.V., Matias Romero No.216, Col. del Valle, 13100 Mexico D.F., Mexico.

Rhone-Poulenc Rorer, Neth. Rhône-Poulenc Rorer B.V., Postbus 982, 1180 AZ Amstelveen, Netherlands.

Rhone-Poulenc Rorer, Norw. See *Aventis, Norw.*

Rhone-Poulenc Rorer, Port. See *Aventis Pharma, Port.*

Rhone-Poulenc Rorer, S.Afr. See *Aventis, S.Afr.*

Rhone-Poulenc Rorer, Singapore. Rhone-Poulenc Rorer Singapore Pte Ltd, 14 Chin Bee Rd, Jurong Town, S 619824, Singapore.

Rhone-Poulenc Rorer, Spain. Rhone Poulenc Rorer, Avda Leganes 62, Leganes, 28925 Madrid, Spain.

Rhone-Poulenc Rorer, Swed. See *Aventis Pharma, Swed.*

Rhone-Poulenc Rorer, Switz. Rhône-Poulenc Rorer AG, Zurcherstrasse 68, 8800 Thalwil, Switzerland.

Rhone-Poulenc Rorer, Thai. Rhone-Poulnec Rorer Ltd, 16 Fl, Ploenchit Center Building, 2 Sukhumvit Rd, Kwang Klongtoey, Klongtoey District, Bangkok 10110, Thailand.

Rhone-Poulenc Rorer, UK. See *Aventis Pharma, UK.*

Rhone-Poulenc Rorer, USA. See *Aventis Pharma, USA.*

Rhone-Poulenc Sante, Thai. See *Pacific, Thai.*

Rho-Pharm, Canad. See *Aventis Pharma, Canad.*

Ribosepharm, Ger. See *Klinge, Ger.*

Rice Steele, Irl. Rice Steele & Co. Ltd, Cookstown Industrial Estate, Tallaght, Dublin 24, Ireland.

Rich Plan, Hong Kong. Rich Plan International Ltd, Flat 9, 16/F, Block C, Wah Lok Industrial Ctr, 31-41 Shan Mei St, Fotan, Shatin, N.T., Hong Kong.

Richard, Fr. Laboratoires Richard, rue du Progres, ZI des Reys de Saulce, 26270 Saulce-sur-Rhone, France.

Richards & Appleby, UK. Richards & Appleby Ltd, Unit 3, Heads of the Valley Industrial Park, Rhymney, Gwent, NP2 5RL, UK.

Richardson-Vicks, Israel. Richardson-Vicks, Israel.

Richardson-Vicks, USA. See *Procter & Gamble, USA.*

Richardson-Vicks Personal Care, USA. See *Procter & Gamble, USA.*

Richelet, Fr. Laboratoires Richelet, 15 rue La Perouse, 75116 Paris, France.

Richlife, Hong Kong. See *Jebsen, Hong Kong.*

Richmond, Canad. See *Rivex, Canad.*

Richmond Ophthalmics, Canad. See *Rivex, Canad.*

Richmond Pharmaceuticals, UK. Richmond Pharmaceuticals Ltd, Coomb House, St Johns Rd, Isleworth, Middlesex, UK.

Richter, Aust. Richter Pharma, Feldgasse 19, A-4600 Wels, Austria.

Richwood, USA. See *Shire Richwood, USA.*

Rico, USA. See *Bart, USA.*

Ricola, Canad. Ricola, Canada.

RID, USA. R.I.D. Inc., 609 N Mednik Ave, Los Angeles, CA 90022-1320, USA.

Ridupharm, Switz. Ridupharm, Emil Frey-Strasse 99, 4142 Munchenstein, Switzerland.

Riedel-Zabinka, Braz. Riedel Zabinka Produtos Quimicos e Farmaceuticos S.A., Avenida Bras de Pina 11, Penha, 21070-030 Rio de Janeiro, RJ, Brazil.

Riel, Aust. Riel GmbH & Co. KG, Gasselberg 53-4, A-8564 Krottendorf-Gaisfeld, Austria.

Riemser, Ger. Riemser Arzneimittel GmbH, An der Wiek 7, 17498 Insel Riems, Germany.

Rigers, Mex. Rigers, Mexico.

Riker, Mex. Riker S.A. de C.V., Av. Santa Fe No. 55, 01210 Mexico D.F., Mexico.

Rima, UK. Rima Pharmaceuticals Ltd, 214-16 St James's Rd, Croydon, Surrey, CR0 2BW, UK.

Rimsa, Mex. Rimsa, Representaciones e Investigaciones Medicas S.A. de C.V., Av. Acoxpa No. 464, Fracc. Prado Coapa, 14350 Mexico D.F., Mexico.

Rio Preto, Braz. Laboratorio Farmaceutico Rio Preto Ltda, Rua Professora Zulmira Sales 1.318, 15030-150 Sao Jose do Rio Preto, SP, Brazil.

Riom, Fr. Riom Laboratoires-CERM, Imm Optima, 10 rue Godefroy, 92821 Puteaux cdx, France.

Ripari-Gero, Ital. Istituto Farmaco Biologico Ripari-Gero s.p.a., Via Montarioso 11, 53035 Monteriggioni (SI), Italy.

Ritsert, Ger. Dr. E. Ritsert GmbH & Co. KG, Klausenweg 12, 69412 Eberbach, Germany.

Ritter, Ger. Walter Ritter GmbH & Co., Spaldingstr. 110 B, 20097 Hamburg, Germany.

Ritter, Hong Kong. See *Mekim, Hong Kong.*

Ritter, Singapore. See *JDH, Singapore.*

Ritter, Thai. See *Osotspa, Thai.*

Rius, Spain. Rius Garriga, Spain.

Riva, Canad. Laboratoire Riva Inc., 660 Industrial Blvd, Blainville, Quebec, J7C 3V4, Canada.

Rivadis, Fr. Laboratoires Rivadis, B.P. 111, ZI de Louzy, 79103 Thouars cdx, France.

River Foods, Austral. River Foods, 1/3 Macquarie Drive, Thomastown, VIC 3074, Australia.

Rivex, Canad. Rivex Pharma Inc., 3-305 Industrial Parkway S, Aurora, Ontario, L4G 6X7, Canada.

Rivopharm, Switz. Rivopharm SA, 6928 Manno, Switzerland.

RKG, Ital. RKG srl, Via Ciro Menotti 1/A, 20129 Milan, Italy.

RMC, Canad. RMC Group, 5080 Timberlea Blvd, Ste 42, Mississauga, Ontario, L4W 4M2, Canada.

Robapharm, Fr. See *Pierre Fabre, Fr.*

Robapharm, Spain. Robapharm España, Ramon Trias Fargas 7-11, Edificio Marina Village, 08005 Barcelona, Spain.

Robapharm, Switz. Robapharm SA, Gewerbestrasse 18, 4123 Allschwil, Switzerland.

Robapharm, Thai. See *Berli, Thai.*

Robert, Spain. Robert, Gran via de Carlos III 98, 08028 Barcelona, Spain.

Robert & Carriere, Canad. See *Anglo-French Laboratories, Canad.*

Roberts, Canad. See *Shire, Canad.*

Roberts, Israel. Roberts, Israel.

Roberts, USA. Roberts Pharmaceutical Corp., 4 Industrial Way West, Eatontown, NJ 07724, USA.

Roberts & Sheppey, UK. Roberts & Sheppey (Melrose) Ltd, Manor Farm House, Ickford, Aylesbury, Buckinghamshire, HP18 9JB, UK.

Robins, Hong Kong. See *Tsun Tsun, Hong Kong.*

Robins, Israel. See *Neopharm, Israel.*

Robins, USA. See *Whitehall-Robins, USA.*

Robinson, UK. Robinson Healthcare, Waterside, Walton, Chesterfield, Derbyshire, S4O 1YF, UK.

Robugen, Ger. Robugen GmbH Pharmazeutische Fabrik, Alleenstr. 22-6, 73730 Esslingen, Germany.

Robugen, Hong Kong. See *Mekim, Hong Kong.*

RoC, Belg. See *Johnson & Johnson Consumer, Belg.*

RoC, Fr. See *Johnson & Johnson Medical, Fr.*

RoC, UK. See *Johnson & Johnson, UK.*

Roche, Arg. Roche S.A.Q. e I., Fray Justo Sarmiento 2350, 1636 Olivos, Buenos Aires, Argentina.

Roche, Aust. Roche Austria GmbH, Engelhorngasse 3, A-1211 Vienna, Austria.

Roche, Austral. Roche Products P/L, P.O. Box 255, Dee Why, NSW 2099, Australia.

Roche, Belg. Roche S.A., Rue Dante 75, 1070 Brussels, Belgium.

Roche, Braz. Produtos Roche Quimicos e Farmaceuticos S.A., Avenida Engenheiro Billings 1729, 05321-900 Sao Paulo, SP, Brazil.

Roche, Canad. Hoffmann-La Roche Ltd, 2455 Meadowpine Blvd, Mississauga, Ontario, L5N 6L7, Canada.

Roche, Denm. Roche A/S, Industriholmen 59, 2650 Hvidovre, Denmark.

Roche, Ecuad. Roche, Ave 10 de Agosto No 5133, Edif. Urania 5to. piso, Quito, Ecuador.

Roche, Fin. Roche Oy, Sinimäentie 10 A, PL 12, 02631 Espoo, Finland.

Roche, Fr. Produits Roche, 52 bd du Parc, 92521 Neuilly-sur-Seine cdx, France.

Roche, Ger. Hoffmann-La Roche AG, Emil-Barell-Str. 1, 79639 Grenzach-Wyhlen, Germany.

Roche, Hong Kong. Roche Hong Kong Ltd, 802 The Lee Gardens, 33 Hysan Ave, Causeway Bay, Hong Kong.

Roche, Irl. Roche Pharmaceuticals (Ireland) Ltd, Richview, Clonskeagh, Dublin 14, Ireland.

Roche, Israel. Roche Pharmaceuticals (Israel) Ltd, P.O. Box 7543, Petach Tikva, Israel.

Roche, Ital. Roche s.p.a., Viale G.B. Stucchi 10, 20052 Monza (MI), Italy.

Roche, Jpn. Nippon Roche, 6-1 Shiba 2-chome, Minato-ku, Tokyo 105-8532, Japan.

Roche, Mex. Productos Roche S.A. de C.V., Av. Universidad No. 902, Col. Santa Cruz Atoyac, 03310 Mexico D.F., Mexico.

Roche, Neth. Roche Nederland B.V., Postbus 8779, NL-5605 LT Eindhoven, Netherlands.

Roche, Norw. Roche Norge AS, Kristoffer Robinsv. 13, Postboks 41 Haugenstua, 0915 Oslo, Norway.

Roche, NZ. Roche Products (NZ) Ltd, P.O. Box 12-492, Penrose, Auckland, New Zealand.

Roche, Port. Roche Farmacêutica Química, Lda, Estrada Nacional 249, 2720-413 Amadora, Portugal.

Roche, S.Afr. Roche Products (Pty) Ltd, P.O. Box 129, Isando 1600, South Africa.

Roche, Singapore. Roche Singapore Pte Ltd, 1 Kim Seng Promenade, 15-07/12 Great World City, S 237994, Singapore.

Roche, Spain. Roche, Josefa Valcarcel 42, 28027 Madrid, Spain.

Roche, Swed. Roche AB, Box 47327, 100 74 Stockholm, Sweden.

Roche, Switz. Roche Pharma (Schweiz) AG, Schonmattstrasse 2, 4153 Reinach, Switzerland.

Roche, Thai. Roche Thailand Ltd, 19 Fl, Rasa Tower, 555 Phaholyothin Rd, Chatuchak, Bangkok 10900, Thailand.

Roche, UK. Roche Products Ltd, 40 Broadwater Rd, Welwyn Garden City, Hertfordshire, AL7 3AY, UK.

Roche, USA. Roche Pharmaceuticals, 340 Kingsland St, Nutley, NJ 07110-1199, USA.

Roche Consumer, Austral. See *Roche, Austral.*

Roche Consumer, Belg. See *Roche, Belg.*

Roche Consumer, Irl. See *Roche, Irl.*

Roche Consumer, Neth. Roche Consumer Health, Postbus 8779, NL-5605 LT Eindhoven, Netherlands.

Roche Consumer, Singapore. See *Roche, Singapore.*

Roche Consumer, UK. See *Roche, UK.*

Roche Diagnostics, Austral. Roche Diagnostics, P.O. Box 955, Castle Hill, NSW 1765, Australia.

Roche Diagnostics, Fr. Roche Diagnostics, 2 av. du Vercors, B.P. 59, 38242 Meylan cdx, France.

Roche Diagnostics, Irl. See *Roche Diagnostics, UK.*

Roche Diagnostics, Ital. See *Roche, Ital.*

Roche Diagnostics, NZ. Roche Diagnostics NZ Ltd, P.O. Box 62089, Auckland, New Zealand.

Roche Diagnostics, Spain. Roche Diagnostics, Copernico 60, 08006 Barcelona, Spain.

Roche Diagnostics, UK. Roche Diagnostics Ltd, Bell Lane, Lewes, East Sussex, BN7 1LG, UK.

Roche Nicholas, Fr. Laboratoires Roche Nicholas, 74240 Gaillard, France.

Roche Nicholas, Ger. Roche Nicholas Deutschland GmbH, Valterweg 24-5, 65817 Eppstein-Bremthal, Germany.

Roche Nicholas, Israel. Roche Nicholas, Israel.

Roche Nicholas, Neth. Roche Nicholas B.V., Postbus 23, 5530 AA Bladel, Netherlands.

Roche Nicholas, Spain. Roche Nicholas, Trav. de les Corts 39-43, 08028 Barcelona, Spain.

Roche Products, USA. Roche Products Inc., Humaco, PR 00791, Puerto Rico.

Roche-Posay, Fr. Laboratoires Pharmaceutiques La Roche-Posay, B.P. 23, 86270 La Roche-Posay, France.

Roche-Posay, Irl. La Roche-Posay Cosmetique Active, Merchant's Hall, 25/26 Merchant's Quay, Dublin 8, Ireland.

Roche-Posay, Switz. See *Cosmetique Active, Switz.*

Rodisma, Ger. Rodisma-Med Pharma GmbH, Hauptstrasse 463, 51143 Cologne, Germany.

Rodleben, Ger. Rodleben Pharma GmbH, Am Waldchen 19, 06862 Rosslau, Germany.

Rodler, Ger. See *Woelm, Ger.*

Roerig, Belg. See *Pfizer, Belg.*

Roerig, Ital. Roerig Farmaceutici Italiana spa, Società del Gruppo Pfizer, Via Valbondione 113, 00188 Rome, Italy.

Roerig, Port. See *Pfizer, Port.*

Roerig, Swed. Roerig AB, Box 501, 183 25 Taby, Sweden.

Roerig, USA. See *Pfizer, USA.*

Rogers, Canad. Rogers Pharmaceuticals Ltd, 330 Marwood Drive, Oshawa, Ontario, L1H 8B4, Canada.

Roha, Ger. roha Arzneimittel GmbH, Rockwinkeler Heerstr. 100, 28355 Bremen, Germany.

Roha, Irl. See *Pharma-Global, Irl.*

Roha, Israel. Roha, Israel.

Roha, Port. Roha Portuguesa, Lda, Parque Industrial de St Marta de Corroios, Lote 52, Corroios, 2840 Seixal, Portugal.

Roha, Switz. See *Adroka, Switz.*

Rolab, S.Afr. Rolab (Division of Novartis SA (Pty) Ltd), P.O. Box 154, Isando 1600, South Africa.

Roland, Aust. See *Roland, Ger.*

Roland, Ger. Roland Arzneimittel GmbH, Bargkoppelweg 66, 22145 Hamburg, Germany.

Rolmex, Canad. Rolmex International Inc., 8750 de-la-Rive-Sud Blvd, Levis, Quebec, G6V 6N6, Canada.

Romer, Mex. Laboratorios Romer S.A. de C.V., Indiana Num. 170, Col. Napoles, Deleg. Benito Juarez, 03810 Mexico D.F., Mexico.

Romigal, Ger. Romigal-Werk, Galileiplatz 2, 81679 Munich, Germany.

Romilo, Canad. Romilo Labs, 1010 Berlier St, Laval, Quebec, H7L 3R9, Canada.

Romsa, Mex. Romsa de Mexico S.A., Metalurgia No. 2820, P. Industrial el Alamo, 45560 Tlaquepaque, Jal., Mexico.

Ronsheim & Moore, UK. Ronsheim & Moore, Division of Hickson & Welch Ltd, Ings Lane, Castleford, West Yorkshire, WF10 2JT, UK.

Roques, Fr. See *Chiesi, Fr.*

Rorer, Irl. See *Aventis Pharma, Irl.*

Rorer, UK. See *Aventis Pharma, UK.*

Rorer, USA. See *Aventis Pharma, USA.*

Rosa-Phytopharma, Fr. Laboratoires Rosa-Phytopharma, 68 rue Jean-Jaques-Rousseau, 75001 Paris, France.

Rosa-Phytopharma, Switz. See *Golaz, Switz.*

Rosch & Handel, Aust. Rösch & Handel, Gudrunstrasse 150, A-1100 Vienna, Austria.

Rosco, Denm. A/S Rosco, Farmaceutisk Industri, Taastrupgaardsvej 30, 2630 Taastrup, Denmark.

Rosco, Norw. See *Andersen, Norw.*

Rosemont, Thai. See *Star, Thai.*

Rosemont, UK. Rosemont Pharmaceuticals Ltd, Rosemont House, Yorkdale Industrial Park, Braithwaite St, Leeds, West Yorkshire, LS11 9XE, UK.

Rosemont, USA. Rosemont Pharmaceutical Corp., 301 South Cherokee St, Denver, CO 80223, USA.

Rosen, Ger. Rosen Pharma GmbH, Muhlstr. 50, 66386 St Ingbert, Germany.

Rosken, Hong Kong. See *Suburfarm, Hong Kong.*

Rosken, Singapore. See *JDH, Singapore.*

Ross, Canad. See *Abbott, Canad.*

Ross, Hong Kong. See *Abbott, Hong Kong.*

Ross, Israel. Ross, Israel.

Ross, USA. Ross Products, Division of Abbott Laboratories, 625 Cleveland Ave, Columbus, OH 43215-1724, USA.

Roter, Thai. Roter, Thailand.

Roterpharma, Irl. See *Allphar, Irl.*

Rotexmedica, Ger. Rotexmedica GmbH Arzneimittelwerk, Bunsenstr. 4, 22946 Trittau, Germany.

Roth, Aust. G Roth & Söhne Pharmazeutische Präparate GmbH, Wagnerstrasse 29, A-2371 Hinterbruhl, Austria.

Rothpharma, Aust. See *Roth, Aust.*

Rotta, Hong Kong. Rotta Pharmaceuticals, 13/F JDH Centre, 2 On Ping St, Siu Lek Yuen, Shatin, N.T., Hong Kong.

Rotta, Israel. Rotta, Israel.

Rotta, Ital. Rotta Research Laboratorium s.p.a., Via Valosa di Sopra 7/9, 20052 Monza (MI), Italy.

Rotta, Singapore. See *Sime Darby, Singapore.*

Rotta, Thai. See *Diethelm, Thai.*

Rottapharm, Fin. See *Algol, Fin.*

Rottapharm, Fr. Laboratoires Rottapharm, 83-85 bd Vincent-Auriol, 75013 Paris, France.

Rottapharm, Ger. Rottapharm GmbH Arzneimittel, Robert-Koch-Str. 2, 51674 Wiehl, Germany.

Rottapharm, Ital. Rottapharm s.r.l., Via Valosa di Sopra 9, 20052 Monza (MI), Italy.

Rottapharm, Spain. Rottapharm, Ctra Barcelona 2, Almacera, 46132 Valencia, Spain.

Rottapharm, Switz. Rottapharm BV, Swiss Branch, Via Cantonale 19, 6900 Lugano, Switzerland.

Rougier, Canad. See *Technilab, Canad.*

Rougier, Hong Kong. See *Pan-Well, Hong Kong.*

Round World, Hong Kong. Round World International Ltd, Unit F, 17/F Infotech Centre, 21 Hung To Rd, Kwun Tong, Hong Kong.

Roussel, Fr. See *Aventis, Fr.*

Roussel, Irl. See *Aventis Pharma, Irl.*

Roussel, Neth. See *Hoechst Marion Roussel, Neth.*

Roussel, Port. See *Aventis Pharma, Port.*

Roussel, S.Afr. See *Hoechst Marion Roussel, S.Afr.*

Roussel, Spain. See *Hoechst Marion Roussel, Spain.*

Roussel Diamant, Fr. See *Aventis, Fr.*

Rovi, Spain. Rovi, Julian Camarillo 35, 28037 Madrid, Spain.

Rovifarma, Spain. See *Pfizer Consumer, Spain.*

Rowa, Ger. Rowa-Wagner GmbH & Co. KG Arzneimittelfabrik, Frankenforster Str. 77, 51427 Bergisch-Gladbach, Germany.

Rowa, Hong Kong. See *Jacobson, Hong Kong.*

Rowa, Irl. Rowa Pharmaceuticals Ltd, Bantry, Co. Cork, Ireland.

Rowa, Israel. Rowa, Israel.

Rowa, Singapore. See *MBD, Singapore.*

Rowa, Thai. See *JDH Borneo, Thai.*

Rowa, UK. See *Rowa, Irl.*

Rowa Wagner, Hong Kong. See *Deutsch Chinesische, Hong Kong.*

Rowex, Irl. See *Rowa, Irl.*

Roxane, USA. Roxane Laboratories Inc., P.O. Box 16532, Columbus, OH 43228-6532, USA.

Royal Childrens Hospital, Austral. Royal Children's Hospital, Melbourne Pharmacy Dept, Flemington Rd, Parkville, VIC 3052, Australia.

Royton, Braz. Royton Quimica Farmacêutica Ltda, Avenida Doutor Cardoso de Melo 1318, 04548-004 Sao Paulo, SP, Brazil.

RTA, Switz. Laboratoire RTA, La Bruyere A, 1817 Fontanivent, Switzerland.

Rubiepharm, Ger. RubiePharm Vertriebs GmbH, Bruder-Grimm-Str. 121, 36396 Steinau an der Strasse, Germany.

Rubio, Singapore. See *Zyfas, Singapore.*

Rubio, Spain. Rubio, Industria 29, Pol Ind Comte de Sert, Castellbisal, 08755 Barcelona, Spain.

Rubio, Thai. See *JDH Borneo, Thai.*

Rudefsa, Mex. Rudefsa S.A. de C.V., Irlanada No.114, Parque San Andres, Coyoacan, 04040 Mexico D.F., Mexico.

Rueckert, Thai. See *Sriprasit, Thai.*

Rugby, USA. See *Watson, USA.*

Rupertus, Aust. St Rupertus-Apotheke, Markt 107, A-5090 Lofer, Austria.

Rusch, Ital. Rusch Hospital s.r.l., Via Torina 5, 20039 Varedo (MI), Italy.

Rusch, UK. Rüsch UK Ltd, PO Box 138, Cressex Industrial Estate, High Wycombe, Buckinghamshire, HP12 3NB, UK.

Russ, USA. See *UCB, USA.*

Russells, NZ. Russells Pharmaceuticals Ltd, P.O. Box 9591, Newmarket, Auckland, New Zealand.

RX, Thai. RX Company Ltd, 93/90 Soi Prachanukul 2, Ratchadapisek Rd, Bangsue, Bangkok 10800, Thailand.

Rybar, Irl. See *Cahill May Roberts, Irl.*

Rydelle, Fr. Rydelle, Johnson & Johnson Business, 7-13 Bd Paul-Emile-Victor, 92200 Neuilly-sur-Seine, France.

Rydelle, Ital. Rydelle Laboratories Business, Johnson Wax s.p.a., P.le M. Burke 3, 20020 Arese (MI), Italy.

Rydelle, USA. See *Johnson Wax, USA.*

Rye, Austral. Rye Pharmaceuticals, Unit 1, Block F, 25-7 Paul St North, North Ryde, NSW 2113, Australia.

Rystan, USA. Rystan Co. Inc., c/o Integra LifeSciences Corp., 105 Morgan Lane, Plainsboro, NJ 08536, USA.

S & K, Ger. S & K Pharma, Schumann & Kohl GmbH, Bahnhofstr. 4-6, 66706 Perl, Germany.

S Med, Aust. S Med Handels GmbH, Braunerstrasse 3/17, A-1010 Vienna, Austria.

SA Druggists, S.Afr. South African Druggists Pharma, South Africa.

SA Druggists Self Med, S.Afr. See *SA Druggists, S.Afr.*

Saba, Ital. Saba, Via Salbertrand 21, 10146 Turin, Italy.

Sabater, Spain. Sabater J., Los Centelles 7, 46006 Valencia, Spain.

Sabex, Canad. Sabex Inc., 145 Jules-Leger St, Boucherville, Quebec, J4B 7K8, Canada.

Sabiluc, Fr. Lab. Sabiluc, 61 rue Lavoisier, 14200 Herouville-Saint-Clair, France.

Sabora, Fin. Sabora Pharma Oy, Hiisimetsänkatu 40, 03600 Karkkila.

SAD, Denm. See *Amternes, Denm.*

Sairaalapalvelu, Fin. Soumen Sairaalapalvelu Oy, Vattuniemenranta 2, 00210 Helsinki, Finland.

Salf, Ital. Salf Laboratorio Farmacologico s.p.a., Via G. d'Alzano 12, 24122 Bergamo, Italy.

Salitine, Ger. Salitine Pharma Vertriebs GmbH, Heidelberger Str. 57a, 68519 Viernheim, Germany.

Salix, USA. Salix Pharmaceuticals Inc., 3600 W Bayshore Rd, Palo Alto, CA 94303-4237, USA.

Salmon, Switz. Salmon Pharma, St Jakobs-Strasse 96, Postfach, 4002 Basle, Switzerland.

Salonpas, UK. Salonpas (UK) Ltd, Unit B, 32a Eveline Rd, Mitcham, Surrey, CR4 3LE, UK.

Salters, S.Afr. See *Adcock Ingram, S.Afr.*

Salts Healthcare, UK. Salts Healthcare, Lord St, Birmingham, B7 4DS, UK.

Salud, Spain. Salud, Spain.

Salus, Denm. See *Tjellesen, Denm.*

Salus, Fr. Salus France, B.P. 104 Principal, 83403 Hyeres cdx, France.

Salus, Ital. Salus Researches s.p.a., Via Aurelia 58, 00165 Rome, Italy.

Salus, Mex. Laboratorios Salus S.A. de C.V., Vito Alessio Robles No. 209, Col. Florida, 01030 Mexico D.F., Mexico.

Salushaus, Ger. Salus-Haus Dr. med. Otto Greither Nachf. GmbH & Co KG, Bahnhofstr. 24, 83052 Bruckmuhl/Mangfall (Obb.), Germany.

Salusif, Port. Salusif, Lda, Rua do Centro Cultural 10 r/c, 1700 Lisbon, Portugal.

Salvat, Spain. Salvat, Gall 30, Esplugas de Llobregat, 08950 Barcelona, Spain.

Salzmann, Switz. Salzmann Medico, Unterstrasse 52, 9001 St Gallen, Switzerland.

Sam Chun Dang, Singapore. See *Zyfas, Singapore.*

Samakeephaesaj, Thai. Samakeephaesaj (Union Drug Laboratories Co. Ltd), 2601 Sukhumvit Rd, Bangkok 10250, Thailand.

Samchully, Singapore. See *Zyfas, Singapore.*

Samil, Ital. Samil s.p.a., Via Piemonte 32, 00187 Rome, Italy.

Samjin, Singapore. See *Zyfas, Singapore.*

Sam-On, Israel. Meditec/Sam-On Ltd, P.O. Box 1224, Bat-Yam 59602, Israel.

SAN, Ital. S.A.N. s.a.s., Viale Corsica 92, 50127 Florence 710 Italy.

San Carlo, Ital. S. Carlo Farmaceutici s.p.a., Tor Maggiore, 00040 S. Palomba Pomezia (Rome), Italy.

Sanabo, Aust. Sanabo Wien GmbH, Brunner Strasse 59, A-1235 Vienna, Austria.

Sanamed, Aust. Sanamed GmbH, Rudolf Waisenhorngasse 32, A-1230 Vienna, Austria.

Sanapharm, Ger. SanaPharm Arzneimittel GmbH, Alexandrinenstr. 1, 96450 Coburg, Germany.

Sandersons, UK. Sandersons (Chemists) Ltd, 37 Oakwood Rise, Heaton, Bolton, BL1 5EE, UK.

Sandipro, Belg. Sandipro S.A.-N.V., Chaussee de Gand 615, 1080 Brussels, Belgium.

Sandoz, Aust. See *Novartis, Aust.*

Sandoz, Canad. Sandoz Canada Inc., Pharmaceutical Division, 385 boul. Bouchard, Dorval, Quebec, H9R 4P5, Canada.

Sandoz, Fr. See *Novartis, Fr.*

Sandoz, Ger. See *Novartis, Ger.*

Sandoz, Ital. See *Novartis, Ital.*

Sandoz, Jpn. Sandoz Yakuhin KK, 17-30 Nishi-Azabu 4-chome, Minato-ku, Tokyo 106, Japan.

Sandoz, Neth. Sandoz B.V., Netherlands.

Sandoz, S.Afr. Sandoz Products (Pty) Ltd, P.O. Box 371, Randburg 2125, South Africa.

Sandoz, UK. See *Novartis, UK.*

Sandoz Consumer, USA. See *Novartis Consumer, USA.*

Sandoz Nutrition, Canad. Sandoz Nutrition Corporation, 1621 McEwen Dr., Unit 50, Whitby, Ontario, L1N 9A5, Canada.

Sandoz Nutrition, USA. See *Novartis Nutrition, USA.*

Sandoz OTC, Switz. See *Novartis Consumer, Switz.*

Sanfer, Mex. Laboratorios Sanfer S.A. de C.V., Calz. de Tlalpan No. 550, Col. Moderna, 03510 Mexico D.F., Mexico.

Sang, Thai. Sang Thai, 148/19-21 Nanglinjee Rd, Tungmahamek, Bangkok 10120, Thailand.

Sang Udom, Thai. Sang Udom Pharmacy Lp, 24-26 Songsawad Rd, Samyek, Sampantawong, Bangkok 10100, Thailand.

Sang-A Pharm, Singapore. See *Sime Darby, Singapore.*

Sangstat, UK. Imitix Sangstat (UK) Ltd, 42 Thames St, Windsor, Berkshire, SL4 1PR, UK.

Sanico, Belg. Sanico S.A., Industriezone IV, Veedijk 59, 2300 Turnhout, Belgium.

Sanico, Switz. See *Uhlmann-Eyraud, Switz.*

Sanidom, Aust. Sanidom Handels-GmbH, Sundlweg 2, A-8045 Graz, Austria.

Saninter, Port. Saninter, SA, Av Durque d'Avila no 193, 1050-082 Lisbon, Portugal.

Sanitalia, Ital. Sanitalia s.n.c. di Battaglia & C., Strada dei Tadini 5, 10131 Turin, Italy.

Sanitas, Ital. Sanitas Italia s.r.l., Via Guala 4, 15057 Tortona (AL), Italy.

Sanitas, Port. Laboratório Sanitas SA, Rua General Ferreira Martins 8 - 6 e 7, 1495-137 Alges, Portugal.

Sankyo, Aust. Sankyo Pharmazeutika Austria GmbH, Effingergasse 21, A-1160 Vienna, Austria.

Sankyo, Austral. See *Pharmacia, Austral.*

Sankyo, Belg. Sankyo Pharma Belgium S.A., Rue du Manil 80, 1301 Wavre, Belgium.

Sankyo, Denm. See *Gea, Denm.*

Sankyo, Fin. Oy Sankyo Pharma Finland Ab, PL 1310, Salomonkatu 17 A 5. krs, 00101 Helsinki, Finland.

Sankyo, Ger. Sankyo Pharma GmbH, Zielstattstr. 9, 81379 Munich, Germany.

Sankyo, Hong Kong. See *Keller, Hong Kong,* and *Hing Ah, Hong Kong.*

Sankyo, Ital. Sankyo Pharma Italia spa, Via Montecassino 157, 00156 Rome, Italy.

Sankyo, Jpn. Sankyo Co. Ltd, 5-1 Nihonbashi-Honcho 3-chome, Chuo-ku, Tokyo 103-8426, Japan.

Sankyo, Neth. See *Will-Pharma, Neth.*

Sankyo, Norw. See *Weifa, Norw.*

Sankyo, NZ. See *Wilson, NZ.*

Sankyo, Port. Sankyo Pharma Portugal, Lda, Av Infante D Henrique 328, 1800-223 Lisbon, Portugal.

Sankyo, Singapore. See *Diethelm, Singapore.*

Sankyo, Spain. Sankyo Pharma España, Acanto 22, Planta 12, 28045 Madrid, Spain.

Sankyo, Switz. Sankyo Pharma (Schweiz) AG, Industriestrasse 4, 8117 Fallanden, Switzerland.

Sankyo, Thai. Thai Sankyo Co. Ltd, 18 Fl, Tipco Tower, 118/1 Rama VI Rd, Phayathai, Bangkok 10400, Thailand.

Sankyo, UK. Sankyo Pharma UK Ltd, Sankyo House, Repton Place, White Lion Rd, Amersham, Buckinghamshire, HP7 9LP, UK.

Sankyo, USA. Sankyo, USA.

Sanobia, Port. Sanóbia, Lda, Rua Joaquim Paco d'Darcos 111, 1500-365 Lisbon, Portugal.

Sanochemia, Aust. Sanochemia Pharmazeutika AG, Boltzmanngasse 9a-11, A-1091 Vienna, Austria.

Sanofi, Denm. See *Sanofi Synthelabo, Denm.*

Sanofi Synthelabo, Aust. Sanofi-Synthelabo GmbH, Koppstrasse 116, A-1160 Vienna, Austria.

Sanofi Synthelabo, Austral. Sanofi-Synthelabo Australia P/L, Riverview Park, 166 Epping Rd, Lane Cove, NSW 2066, Australia.

Sanofi Synthelabo, Belg. Sanofi-Synthelabo S.A., Ave de la Metrologie 5, 1130 Brussels, Belgium.

Sanofi Synthelabo, Canad. Sanofi-Synthelabo Inc., 90 Allstate Parkway, Markham, Ontario, L3R 6H3, Canada.

Sanofi Synthelabo, Denm. Sanofi-Synthelabo, Ringager 4 A, 2605 Brondby, Denmark.

Sanofi Synthelabo, Fr. Sanofi Synthelabo France, 174 av. de France, 75013 Paris, France.

Sanofi Synthelabo, Ger. Sanofi-Synthelabo GmbH, Potsdamer Str. 8, 10785 Berlin, Germany.

Sanofi Synthelabo, Ital. Sanofi-Synthelabo S.p.A., Via GB Piranesi 38, 20137 Milan, Italy.

Sanofi Synthelabo, Neth. Sanofi Synthelabo, Netherlands.

Sanofi Synthelabo, NZ. Sanofi Synthelabo Australia Pty Ltd, 6b Wagener Pl., Mount Albert, Auckland, New Zealand.

Sanofi Synthelabo, Port. Sanofi-Synthelabo, SA, Praca Duque de Saldanha no 1-4, 1050-094 Lisbon, Portugal.

Sanofi Synthelabo, S.Afr. Sanofi-Synthelabo (Pty) Ltd, Postnet Suite 24, Private Bag X23, Gallo Manor 2052, South Africa.

Sanofi Synthelabo, Singapore. Sanofi-Synthelabo Singapore Pte Ltd, 80 Robinson Rd, 19-02, S 068898, Singapore.

Sanofi Synthelabo, Spain. Sanofi Synthelabo, Avda Litoral Mar 12, 08005 Barcelona, Spain.

Sanofi Synthelabo, Switz. Sanofi-Synthélabo AG, 11 Rue de Voyrot, 1217 Meyrin 1, Switzerland.

Sanofi Synthelabo, Thai. Sanofi-Synthelabo (Thailand) Ltd, 9-11 Fl, Gypsum Metropolitan Tower, 539/2 Sri-Ayudhya Rd, Phyathai, Rajthevee, Bangkok 10400, Thailand.

Sanofi Synthelabo, UK. Sanofi Synthelabo Ltd, 1 Onslow St, Guildford, Surrey, GU1 4YS, UK.

Sanofi Synthelabo, USA. Sanofi-Synthelabo Inc., 90 Park Ave, New York, NY 10016, USA.

Sanofi Synthelabo OTC, Fr. Sanofi Synthelabo OTC, 9 rue du President-Allende, 94258 Gentilly cdx, France.

Sanofi Winthrop, Aust. See *Sanofi Synthelabo, Aust.*

Sanofi Winthrop, Austral. See *Sanofi Synthelabo, Austral.*

Sanofi Winthrop, Belg. See *Sanofi Synthelabo, Belg.*

Sanofi Winthrop, Braz. Sanofi Winthrop Farmaceutica Ltda, Avenida Brasil 22.155, 21670-000 Rio de Janeiro, RJ, Brazil.

Sanofi Winthrop, Canad. See *Sanofi Synthelabo, Canad.*

Sanofi Winthrop, Denm. See *Sanofi Synthelabo, Denm.*

Sanofi Winthrop, Fin. Oy Sanofi Winthrop AB, Vattuniemenranta 2, 00210 Helsinki, Finland.

Sanofi Winthrop, Fr. See *Sanofi Synthelabo, Fr.*

Sanofi Winthrop, Ger. See *Sanofi Synthelabo, Ger.*

Sanofi Winthrop, Hong Kong. Sanofi Winthrop Hong Kong Ltd, Rm 2501-2503, Windsor House, 311 Gloucester Rd, Causeway Bay, Hong Kong.

Sanofi Winthrop, Irl. Sanofi Winthrop Ireland Ltd, United Drug House, Belgard Rd, Tallaght, Dublin 24, Ireland.

Sanofi Winthrop, Israel. Sanofi Winthrop, Israel.

Sanofi Winthrop, Ital. See *Sanofi Synthelabo, Ital.*

Sanofi Winthrop, Mex. Sanofi Winthrop S.A. de C.V., Km 37.5 Autopista Mexico-Qro, 54730 Cuautitlan Izcalli, Mexico.

Sanofi Winthrop, Neth. Sanofi Winthrop, Postbus 97, 3140 AB Maassluis, Netherlands.

Sanofi Winthrop, Norw. Sanofi Winthrop AS, Grini Naeringspark 10, Postboks 16, 1332 Osteras, Norway.

Sanofi Winthrop, NZ. See *Sanofi Synthelabo, NZ.*

Sanofi Winthrop, Port. See *Sanofi Synthelabo, Port.*

Sanofi Winthrop, Spain. See *Sanofi Synthelabo, Spain.*

Sanofi Winthrop, Swed. Sanofi Winthrop AB, Box 14142, 167 14 Bromma, Sweden.

Sanofi Winthrop, Switz. See *Sanofi Synthelabo, Switz.*

Sanofi Winthrop, UK. See *Sanofi Synthelabo, UK.*

Sanofi Winthrop, USA. See *Sanofi Synthelabo, USA.*

Sanol, Ger. Sanol GmbH, Alfred-Nobel-Str. 10, 40789 Monheim, Germany.

Sanopharm, Switz. Sanopharm AG, Postplatz 44, 7000 Chur, Switzerland.

Sanorania, Ger. Sanorania Pharma GmbH, Berliner Ring 89, 64625 Bensheim, Germany.

Sanorania, Switz. See *Medipharm, Switz.*

Sanoreform, Ger. Sanoreform GmbH, Postfach: 1365, 58303 Herdecke, Germany.

Sanorell, Ger. Sanorell Pharma GmbH & Co., Rechtmurgstr. 27, 72270 Baiersbronn, Germany.

Sanova, Aust. Sanova Pharma GmbH, Industriegasse 7, A-1230 Vienna, Austria.

Sante Naturelle, Canad. Sante Naturelle AG Ltee, 369 Charles Peguy, La Prairie, Quebec, J5R 3E8, Canada.

Santen, Denm. Santen, Roskildevej 48 A, 3400 Hillerod, Denmark.

Santen, Fin. Santen Oy, Niittyhaankatu 20, PL 33, 33721 Tampere, Finland.

Santen, Hong Kong. See *Hong Kong Medical, Hong Kong,* and *Leader, Hong Kong.*

Santen, Israel. Santen, Israel.

Santen, Jpn. Santen Pharmaceutical Co Ltd, 3-9-19 Shimoshinjo, Higashiyodogawa-ku, Osaka 533-8651, Japan.

Santen, Norw. Santen Norge, Sjosenteret Vallo, 3150 Tolvsrod, Norway.

Santen, Singapore. See *Polymedic, Singapore.*

Santen, Swed. Santen Pharma AB, 171 45 Solna, Sweden.

Santen, Thai. See *Greater Pharma, Thai.*

Santen, USA. Santen, USA.

Santiveri, Spain. Santiveri, Encuny 8, 08038 Barcelona, Spain.

Sanum-Kehlbeck, Ger. Sanum-Kehlbeck GmbH & Co. KG, Hasseler Steinweg 9-12, 27318 Hoya, Germany.

Sanus, Braz. Sanus Farmaceutica Ltda, Avenida dos Bandeirantes 5.386, 04041-900 Sao Paulo, SP, Brazil.

Sanval, Braz. Sanval Comercio e Industria Ltda, Avenida Nicolau Alayon 441, 04802-000 Sao Paulo, SP, Brazil.

Sanwa, Jpn. Sanwa Kagaku Kenkyusho Co Ltd, 35 Higashisotobori-cho, Higashi-ku, Nagoya 461, Japan.

Saprochi, Israel. Saprochi, Israel.

Saprochi, Switz. Saprochi SA, Chemin de la Cretaux, Case postale 327, 1196 Gland/VD, Switzerland.

Sarget, Fr. Laboratoires Sarget Pharma, ave J.-F. Kennedy, 33701 Mérignac cdx, France.

Sark, Ital. Sark spa, Via Zambeletti, 20021 Baranzate di Bollate (MI), Italy.

SAT, Spain. SAT (Servicio Aplicacion Terapeuticas), Avda Barcelona 69, Sant Joan Despi, 08970 Barcelona, Spain.

Satori, Fr. Lab. Satori International, Parc d'activite de Limonest, 540 allee des Hetres, 69760 Limonest, France.

Saunier-Daguin, Fr. Laboratoires Saunier-Daguin, 2 rue Marechal-Foch, 45370 Clery-St-Andre, France.

Sauter, Austral. See *Roche, Austral.*

Savage, USA. Savage Laboratories, Division of Atlanta Inc., 60 Baylis Road, Melville, NY 11747-2006, USA.

Savio, Ital. Istituto Biochimico Nazionale Savio s.r.l., Via E. Bazzano 14, 16019 Ronco Scrivia (GE), Italy.

Savoma, Ital. Savoma Medicinali s.p.a., Via Baganza 2/A, 43100 Parma, Italy.

Savoy, Singapore. See *Polymedic, Singapore.*

SBL, Denm. See *Pasteur Merieux, Denm.*

SBL, Norw. SBL Vaccin Norge, Solheimsv. 112, 1471 Skarer, Norway.

SBL, Swed. SBL Vaccin AB, 105 21 Stockholm, Sweden.

Scand Pharm, Swed. Scandinavian Pharmaceuticals-Generics AB, Box 23033, 104 35 Stockholm, Sweden.

Scandinavian Health Care, Norw. Scandinavian Health Care AB, Grini Naeringspark 1, 1361 Osteras, Norway.

Scandinavian Natural Health & Beauty, USA. Scandinavian Natural Health & Beauty Products Inc., 13 North Seventh St, Perkasie, PA 18944, USA.

Scandipharm, Israel. Scandipharm, Israel.

Scandipharm, USA. Scandipharm Inc., 22 Inverness Center Pkwy, Suite 310, Birmingham, AL 35242, USA.

Scania, Swed. Scania Dental AB, Sweden.

Scanpharm, Hong Kong. See *Winsor, Hong Kong.*

SCAT, Denm. See *Norpharma, Denm.*

SCAT, Switz. See *Doetsch, Grether, Switz.*

Schaffer, USA. Schaffer Laboratories, 1058 North Allen Ave, Pasadena, CA 91104, USA.

Schaper & Brummer, Ger. Schaper & Brümmer GmbH & Co. KG, Bahnhofstr. 35, 38259 Salzgitter (Ringelheim), Germany.

Schaper & Brummer, Singapore. See *Bionax, Singapore.*

Scharper, Ital. Scharper srl, Via Milanese 20, 20099 Sesto San Giovanni (MI), Italy.

Schein, Canad. Schein Pharmaceutical Canada Inc., 77 Belfield Rd, Toronto, Ontario, M9W 1G6, Canada.

Schein, UK. Schein Rexodent, 25-7 Merrick Rd, Southall, Middlesex, UB2 4AU, UK.

Schein, USA. Schein Pharmaceutical Inc., 100 Campus Dr., Florham Park, NJ 07932, USA.

Scherax, Ger. Alk-Scherax Arzneimittel GmbH, Sulldorfer Landstr. 128, 22589 Hamburg, Germany.

Scherer, Hong Kong. See *Atlantic, Hong Kong, Health Tech, Hong Kong, Star, Hong Kong,* and *Winsor, Hong Kong.*

Scherer, Ital. R.P. Scherer s.p.a., Via Nettunese Km. 20,100, 04011 Aprilia (Latina), Italy.

Scherer, Singapore. See *Luen Wah, Singapore.*

Scherer, Thai. See *Kemopharm, Thai., Osotspa, Thai., Sriprasit, Thai.,* and *Star, Thai.*

Scherer, USA. Scherer Laboratories Inc., 2301 Ohio Dr., Suite 234, Plano, TX 75093, USA.

Schering, Aust. Schering Wien GmbH, Scheringgasse 2, A-1147 Vienna, Austria.

Schering, Austral. Schering P/L, 27-31 Doody Street, Alexandria, NSW 2015, Australia.

Schering, Belg. Schering S.A., J.E. Mommaertslaan 14, 1831 Diegem, Belgium.

Schering, Braz. Schering do Brasil Quimica e Farmaceutica Ltda, Rua Cancioneiro de Evora 255, 04708-010 Sao Paulo, SP, Brazil.

Schering, Canad. Schering Canada Inc., 3535 Trans-Canada Hwy, Pointe-Claire, Quebec, H9R 1B4, Canada.

Schering, Denm. Schering AS, Herstedosterveg 27-9, 2620 Albertslund, Denmark.

Schering, Fin. Schering Oy, Eerikinkatu 24, PL 179, 00101 Helsinki, Finland.

Schering, Fr. Schering, rue de Toufflers, B.P. 69, 59452 Lys-lez-Lannoy cdx, France.

Schering, Ger. Schering Deutschland GmbH, Max-Dohrn-Str. 10, 10589 Berlin, Germany.

Schering, Hong Kong. Schering Ltd, 15/F Henan Bldg, 90-92 Jaffe Rd, Wanchai, Hong Kong.

Schering, Irl. Schering A.G., 44 Dartmouth Square, Dublin 6, Ireland.

Schering, Israel. Schering, Israel.

Schering, Ital. Schering s.p.a., Via E. Schering 19-21, 20090 Segrate (MI), Italy.

Schering, Jpn. Nihon Schering, Japan.

Schering, Mex. Schering Mexicana S.A. de C.V., Calz. Mexico Xochimilco No. 5019, 14370 Mexico D.F., Mexico.

Schering, Neth. Schering Nederland B.V., Postbus 116, 1380 AC Weesp, Netherlands.

Schering, Norw. Schering Norge A/S, Ringsv 3, Postboks 183, 1321 Stabekk, Norway.

Schering, NZ. Schering (NZ) Ltd, P.O. Box 65-051, Auckland 10, New Zealand.

Schering, Port. Schering Lusitana, Lda, Estrada Nacional No 249, km 15, 2726-919 Mem Martins, Portugal.

Schering, S.Afr. Schering AG Germany, P.O. Box 5278, Halfway House 1685, South Africa.

Schering, Singapore. See *Zuellig, Singapore.*

Schering, Spain. Schering, Mendez Alvaro 55, 28045 Madrid, Spain.

Schering, Swed. Schering Nordiska AB, Box 23117, 104 35 Stockholm, Sweden.

Schering, Switz. Schering (Schweiz) AG, Postfach 766, 8010 Zurich, Switzerland.

Schering, Thai. Schering (Bangkok) Ltd, P.O. Box 106, Laksi Post Office, Bangkok 10210, Thailand.

Schering, UK. Schering Health Care Ltd, The Brow, Burgess Hill, West Sussex, RH15 9NE, UK.

Schering, USA. See *Schering-Plough, USA.*

Schering-Plough, Aust. See *Schering-Plough, Belg.*

Schering-Plough, Austral. Schering-Plough P/L, P.O. Box 231, Baulkham Hills, NSW 2153, Australia.

Schering-Plough, Belg. Schering-Plough S.A., Rue de Stalle 67, 1180 Brussels, Belgium.

Schering-Plough, Braz. Industria Quimica e Farmaceutica Schering Plough S.A., Rua Alexandre Dumas 2.220 4°/7°/8° andar, 04717-004 Sao Paulo, SP, Brazil.

Schering-Plough, Canad. Schering-Plough Healthcare Products Canada Inc., 6400 Northam Drive, Mississauga, Ontario, L4V 1J1, Canada.

Schering-Plough, Denm. Schering-Plough A/S, Hvedemarken 12, 3520 Farum, Denmark.

Schering-Plough, Fin. Schering-Plough Oy, Riihitontuntie 14 A, PL 3, 02201 Espoo, Finland.

Schering-Plough, Fr. Schering-Plough, 92 rue Baudin, 92307 Levallois-Perret cdx, France.

Schering-Plough, Hong Kong. Schering-Plough, Division of Sol Ltd, 17/F Chinachem Exchange Square, 1 Hoi Wan St, Quarry Bay, Hong Kong.

Schering-Plough, Irl. See *Pharmacia Upjohn, Irl.*

Schering-Plough, Israel. See *Trading, Israel.*

Schering-Plough, Ital. Schering Plough s.p.a., Palazzo Borromini, 20090 Segrate (MI), Italy.

Schering-Plough, Mex. Schering-Plough S.A. de C.V., Av. 16 de Septiembre No. 301, Col. Xaltocan, 16090 Mexico D.F., Mexico.

Schering-Plough, Neth. See *Schering-Plough, Belg.*

Schering-Plough, Norw. Schering-Plough A/S, Ankerv. 209, 1359 Eiksmarka, Norway.

Schering-Plough, NZ. Schering-Plough Pty Ltd, P.O. Box 51308, Pakuranga, Auckland, New Zealand.

Schering-Plough, Port. Schering-Plough Farma, Lda, Casal Colaride, Agualva, Cacem. Apartado 28, 2736 Cacem Codex, Portugal.

Schering-Plough, S.Afr. Schering-Plough (Pty) Ltd, P.O. Box 46, Isando 1600, South Africa.

Schering-Plough, Singapore. See *Zuellig, Singapore.*

Schering-Plough, Spain. Schering Plough, Po de la Castellana 143, 28046 Madrid, Spain.

Schering-Plough, Swed. Schering-Plough AB, Box 27190, 102 52 Stockholm, Sweden.

Schering-Plough, Thai. Schering-Plough Ltd, 10 Fl, Maneeya Center Building, 518/5 Ploenchit Rd, Lumpini, Patumwan, Bangkok 10330, Thailand.

Schering-Plough, UK. Schering-Plough Ltd, Schering-Plough House, Shire Park, Welwyn Garden City, Herts, AL7 1TW, UK.

Schering-Plough, USA. Schering-Plough Corp., Galloping Hill Rd, Kenilworth, NJ 07033-0530, USA.

Scheurich, Ger. E. Scheurich Pharma GmbH, Strassburger Str. 77, Postfach: 1361, 77763 Appenweier, Germany.

Schiapparelli, Ital. Schiapparelli Farma srl, Via Ragazzi del 99 n.5, 40133 Bologna, Italy.

Schiapparelli Searle, USA. See *SCS, USA.*

Schieffer, Ger. Dr Schieffer Arzneimittel GmbH, Valterweg 24-5, 65817 Eppstein, Germany.

Schieffer, Switz. Switzerland.

Schmid, Canad. Julius Schmid Canada Ltd, 100 Courtland Ave, Concord, Ontario, L4K 3T6, Canada.

Schmid, Israel. Schmid, Israel.

Schmid, USA. See *Durex, USA.*

Schmidgall, Aust. Dr A & L Schmidgall, Wolfganggasse 45-7, A-1121 Vienna, Austria.

Schoenenberger, Ger. Walther Schoenenberger GmbH & Co. KG, Muhlstr. 5-7, 71106 Magstadt, Germany.

Scholl, Canad. Scholl, Canada.

Scholl, Israel. Scholl, Israel.

Scholl, Switz. See *Seton Scholl, Switz.*

Scholl, UK. See *SSL, UK.*

Schonenberger, Switz. Schönenberger Pharma AG, Schachenstrasse 24, 5012 Schonenwerd, Switzerland.

Schoning-Berlin, Ger. Schöning Pharmazeutische Präparate GmbH & Co. KG, Porschestr. 22-24, 12107 Berlin, Germany.

Schuck, Ger. Schuck GmbH, Industriestr. 11, 90571 Schwaig b. Nurnberg, Germany.

Schulke & Mayr, Aust. Schülke & Mayr GmbH, Zieglergasse 8/3, A-1070 Vienna, Austria.

Schulke & Mayr, Ger. Schülke & Mayr GmbH, Heidbergstr. 100, 22846 Norderstedt, Germany.

Schulke & Mayr, Switz. Schülke & Mayr AG, Chemisch-pharmazeutische Produkte, Obere Zaune 12, Postfach 865, 8025 Zurich, Switzerland.

Schulke & Mayr, Thai. See *Diethelm, Thai.*

Schumit, Thai. Schumit 1967 Co. Ltd, 13 Soi Latphrao 91, Latphrao Rd, Wangthonglaeng, Bangkok 10310, Thailand.

Schupp, Ger. Schupp GmbH & Co., Postfach: 840, 72238 Freudenstadt, Germany.

Schur, Ger. Schur Pharmazeutika GmbH & Co. KG, Schorlemerstr. 68, 40547 Dusseldorf, Germany.

Schutz, Aust. Maria Schutz Apotheke, Reinprechtsdorfer Strasse 2, A-1050 Vienna, Austria.

Schwabe, Ger. Dr Willmar Schwabe GmbH & Co., Willmar-Schwabe-Str. 4, 76227 Karlsruhe, Germany.

Schwabe, Neth. See *VSM, Neth.*

Schwabe, Spain. Schwabe, Spain.

Schwabe, Switz. Schwabe Pharma AG, Spezialist fur Phytopharmaka, Erlistrasse 2, Postfach, 6403 Kussnacht aR, Switzerland.

Schwabe Extracta, Ger. See *Schwabe, Ger.*

Schwabe-Curamed, Ger. Dr Willmar Schwabe GmbH & Co. Abt. Curamed Pharma GmbH, Pforzheimer Str. 5, 76227 Karlsruhe, Germany.

Schwarz, Fr. Laboratoires Schwarz Pharma, 235 av Le Jour-se-Leve, 92100 Boulogne-Billancourt, France.

Schwarz, Ger. Schwarz Pharma Deutschland GmbH, Alfred-Nobel-Str. 10, 40789 Monheim, Germany.

Schwarz, Hong Kong. Schwarz Pharma (HK) Ltd, Unit B, 24/F CMA Bldg, 64 Connaught Rd Central, Hong Kong.

Schwarz, Irl. See *Allphar, Irl.*

Schwarz, Israel. See *Medis, Israel.*

Schwarz, Ital. Schwarz Pharma s.p.a., Via Gadames 57, 20151 Milan, Italy.

Schwarz, Norw. See *Meda, Norw.*

Schwarz, Singapore. See *Zyfas, Singapore.*

Schwarz, Switz. See *Searle, Switz.*

Schwarz, Thai. See *Berli, Thai.*

Schwarz, UK. Schwarz Pharma Ltd, Schwarz House, East St, Chesham, Buckinghamshire, HP5 1DG, UK.

Schwarz, USA. Schwarz Pharma Inc., P.O. Box 2038, Milwaukee, WI 53201, USA.

Schwarzhaupt, Aust. See *Schwarzhaupt, Ger.*

Schwarzhaupt, Ger. Kommanditgesellschaft Schwarzhaupt GmbH & Co., Sachsenring 37-47, 50677 Cologne, Germany.

Schwarzhaupt, Hong Kong. See *Tsun Tsun, Hong Kong.*

Schwarzhaupt, Thai. See *Pacific, Thai.*

Schwarzwalder, Ger. Schwarzwälder Natur-Heilmittel, Marktplatz 4, 93183 Kallmunz, Germany.

Schworer, Ger. Pharma Schwörer GmbH, Goethestr. 29, 69257 Wiesenbach, Germany.

Schwulst, S.Afr. Geo Schwulst Laboratories (Pty) Ltd, P.O. Box 38481, Booysens 2016, South Africa.

Sciclone, Ital. Sciclone Pharmaceuticals Italy srl, Piazza Belgioso 2, 20121 Milan, Italy.

Sciclone, Singapore. Sciclone Pharmaceuticals International Ltd, 1 Maritime Square, 09-11 World Trade Centre, S 099253, Singapore.

Sciencex, Fr. Laboratoires Sciencex, 1 rue Edmond-Guillout, 75015 Paris, France.

Scientific, S.Afr. Scientific Pharmaceuticals (Pty) Ltd, P.O. Box 13119, Vorna Valley 1686, South Africa.

Scientific Hospital Supplies, Austral. Scientific Hospital Supplies, Norwest Business Park, 14-16 Brookhollow Ave, Baulkham Hills, NSW 2153, Australia.

Scientific Hospital Supplies, Irl. Scientific Hospital Supplies (Ireland) Ltd, 1B Sandford Business Centre, Burton Hall Road, Dublin 18, Ireland.

Scientific Hospital Supplies, Israel. Scientific Hospital Supplies, Israel.

Scientific Hospital Supplies, NZ. See *Douglas, NZ.*

Scientific Hospital Supplies, UK. See *SHS, UK.*

Scigen, Singapore. SciGen Pte Ltd, 14 Science Park drive, 04-01A The Maxwell, S 118226, Singapore.

Scimat, UK. See *Bailey, UK.*

Scios, USA. Scios Inc., 820 W Maude Ave, Sunnyvale, CA 94086, USA.

Sclavo, Israel. Sclavo, Israel.

Sclavo, Ital. Sclavo s.p.a., Via Fiorentina 1, 53100 Siena, Italy.

Scot, Israel. Scot, Israel.

Scotia, Denm. See *Norpharma, Denm.*

Scotia, Hong Kong. See *Health Care, Hong Kong.*

Scotia, Irl. See *Scotia, UK.*

Scotia, NZ. Scotia Pharmaceuticals (NZ) Ltd, P.O. Box 33-118, Takapuna, Auckland, New Zealand.

Scotia, UK. Scotia Pharmaceuticals Ltd, Scotia House, Castle Business Park, Stirling, Stirlingshire, FK9 4TZ, UK.

Scott, Canad. Scott Chemical Canada, Division of Lander Co. Canada Ltd, 275 Finchdene Square, Scarborough, Ontario, M1X 1C7, Canada.

Scot-Tussin, USA. Scot-Tussin Pharmacal Co. Inc., 50 Clemence St, P.O. Box 8217, Cranston, RI 02920-0217, USA.

SCS, USA. SCS Pharmaceuticals, P.O. Box 5110, Chicago, IL 60680-5110, USA.

Searle, Austral. See *Monsanto, Austral.*

Searle, Belg. See *Continental Pharma, Belg.*

Searle, Braz. Searle do Brasil Ltda, Rua Independencia 715, 01524-001 Sao Paulo, SP, Brazil.

Searle, Canad. Searle Canada, Unit of Monsanto Canada Inc., 2233 Argentia Rd, Mississauga, Ontario, L5N 2X7, Canada.

Searle, Denm. Searle Scandinavia, Division of Monsanto Danmark A/S, Banemarksvej 50 A, 2605 Brondby, Denmark.

Searle, Fin. See *Panfarma, Fin.*

Searle, Fr. See *Monsanto, Fr.*

Searle, Hong Kong. Monsanto Far East Ltd, Searle Division, 2/F, Cityplaza 3, 14 Taikoo Wan Rd, Hong Kong.

Searle, Irl. Searle, Bray Industrial Estate, Pinewood Close, Bray, Co. Wicklow, Ireland.

Searle, Israel. See *Pharmateam, Israel.*

Searle, Ital. See *Monsanto, Ital.*

Searle, Mex. Searle de Mexico S.A. de C.V., Calzada del Hueso No. 859, 14300 Mexico D.F., Mexico.

Searle, Neth. Searle Nederland B.V., Postbus 1402, 3600 BK Maarssen, Netherlands.

Searle, Norw. Searle, Division of Monsanto Norge A/S, Fornebuv. 37, 1366 Lysaker, Norway.

Searle, NZ. Searle, Division of Monsanto (NZ) Ltd, P.O. Box 751, Auckland, New Zealand.

Searle, Port. See *Monsanto, Port.*

Searle, S.Afr. G.D. Searle (SA) (Pty) Ltd, P.O. Box 11128, Johannesburg 2000, South Africa.

Searle, Singapore. See *Zuellig, Singapore.*

Searle, Swed. Searle Scandinavia, Division of Monsanto Sverige AB, 112 87 Stockholm, Sweden.

Searle, Switz. Searle SA, 1170 Aubonne, Switzerland.

Searle, Thai. G. D. Searle (Thailand) Ltd, 19 Fl, SCB Park Plaza East, 19 Ratchadapisek Rd, Ladyao, Chatuchak, Bangkok 10900, Thailand.

Searle, UK. See *Pharmacia, UK.*

Searle, USA. G.D. Searle & Co., Box 5110, Chicago, IL 60680-5110, USA.

Seatrace, USA. Seatrace Pharmaceuticals, P.O. Box 363, Gadsden, AL 35902-0363, USA.

Sebapharma, Hong Kong. See *Mekim, Hong Kong.*

Sebapharma, Thai. See *Oui Heng, Thai.*

Seber, Port. Seber Portuguesa Farmacêutica, SA, Rua Norberto de Oliveira 1-5, 2675-130 Povoa de St Adriao, Portugal.

Sedabel, Braz. Laboratorio Sedabel Ltda, Rodovia Washington Luiz 1308 Km 4.5, 25085-000 Duque de Caxias, RJ, Brazil.

Sedar, Braz. Sedar Industria Farmaceutica Ltda, Rodovia BR 101 Sul Km 18, Distr. Ind. dos Prazeres, 50950-000 Recife, PE, Brazil.

Sedifa, Mon. Laboratoires Sédifa, 4 av. Prince-Hereditaire-Albert, Fontvieille, MC 98000, Monaco.

Sefarma, Ital. Sefarma s.r.l., Via Walter Tobagi 8, 20068 Peschiera Borromeo (MI), Italy.

Segix, Ital. Segix Italia spa, Via del Mare 36, 00040 Pomezia (RM), Italy.

Seid, Spain. Seid, Ctra Sabadell Granollers Km 15, Llissa de Vall, 08185 Barcelona, Spain.

Selder, Mex. Selder S.A. de C.V., Fernando Villalpando Num. 48, Col. Guadalupe Inn, Deleg. Alvaro Obregon, 01020 Mexico D.F., Mexico.

Select, Ital. Select Pharma s.p.a., Via Pontina 100, 04011 Aprilia (LT), Italy.

Selena, Swed. See *Selena Fournier, Swed.*

Selena Fournier, Swed. Selena Fournier AB, Box 1266, 172 25 Sundbyberg, Sweden.

Selfcare, Austral. Selfcare International, 3 Tait St, Smithfield, NSW 2164, Australia.

Self-Care Products, UK. Self-Care Products Ltd, 30 Sycamore Rd, Amersham, Buckinghamshire, HP6 5DR, UK.

Sella, Ital. Sella A. Lab. Chim. Farm. s.r.l., Via Vincenza 2, 36015 Schio (Vicenza), Italy.

Selmag, Switz. Selmag-Weibel, Bergackerweg 4, 3054 Schupfen/BE, Switzerland.

Selvi, Ital. Selvi Laboratorio Bioterapico s.p.a., Via Fratelli Ruspoli 2, 00198 Rome, Italy.

Selz, Ger. Pharma Selz GmbH, Leininger Ring 65a, 67278 Bockenheim, Germany.

Semar, Spain. See *Sanofi Synthelabo, Spain.*

Semper, Fin. See *Arla, Fin.*

Senese, Ital. Industria Farmaceutica Galenica Senese srl, Via Cassia Nord 3, 53014 Monteroni d'Arbia (SI), Italy.

Seng, Thai. See *Sang, Thai.*

Senju, Jpn. Senju Pharmaceutical Co., Ltd, 5-8 Hiranomachi 2-chome, Chuo-ku, Osaka 541-0046, Japan.

Senosiain, Mex. Laboratorios Senosiain S.A. de C.V., Camino a San Luis Rey No. 221, Ex Hacienda Santa Rita, 38137 Celaya, Gto., Mexico.

Sepharma, Ital. See *Sefarma, Ital.*

Sephytal, Fr. Sephytal SA, 6 av. Charles de Gaulle, 78150 Le Chesnay, France.

Sepracor, USA. Sepracor, 111 Locke Drive, Marlborough, MA 01752, USA.

Septa, Spain. Septa Chemifarma, Sierra Guadarrama 11, Pol. Ind. 2, San Fernando de Henares, 28850 Madrid, Spain.

Septodent, USA. Septodent Inc., P.O. Box 11926, Wilmington, DE 19850, USA.

Septodont, Denm. See *CMS-Dental, Denm.*

Septodont, Switz. See *Odontopharm, Switz.*

Septodont, USA. Septodont Inc., P.O. Box 11926, Wilmington, DE 19850, USA.

Sequus, Aust. See *Sequus, UK.*

Sequus, Israel. Sequus, Israel.

Sequus, Singapore. See *Faulding, Singapore.*

Sequus, UK. Sequus Pharmaceuticals Inc., 10 Barley Mow Passage, London, W4 4PH, UK.

Sequus, USA. See *Alza, USA.*

Serag-Wiessner, Ger. Serag-Wiessner KG, Zum Kugelfang 8-12, 95119 Naila, Germany.

SERB, Fr. Lab. SERB (Ste d'Etudes et de Recherches Biologiques), 53 rue Villiers de l'Isle Adam, 75020 Paris, France.

Serdex, Port. See *Confar, Port.*

Sermmitr, Thai. Sermmitr c/o The Sermmitr Co. Ltd, 82, 84 Arkarn 2, Ratchamnoen Ave, Bangkok 10200, Thailand.

Serolab, Switz. Serolab SA, En Marin, CP36, Ch. de la Vulliette 4, 1000 Lausanne 25, Switzerland.

Serolam, Israel. Serolam, Israel.

Serono, Aust. Serono Austria GmbH, Wienerbergstrasse 7, A-1100 Vienna, Austria.

Serono, Austral. Serono Australia P/L, Allambie Grove Business Park, 4/25 Frenchs Forest Rd (East), Frenchs Forest, NSW 2086, Australia.

Serono, Belg. Laboratoires Serono Benelux S.A., Belgium.

Serono, Braz. Serono Produtos Farmaceuticos Ltda, Alameda Arapoema 480, 06460-080 Barueri, SP, Brazil.

Serono, Canad. Serono Canada Inc., 1075 North Service Rd, Suite 100, Oakville, Ontario, L6M 2G2, Canada.

Serono, Denm. Serono Nordic, Aarhusgade 88, 7, 2100 Copenhagen O, Denmark.

Serono, Fin. Serono Nordic, Rajatorpantie 41 C, 01640 Vantaa, Finland.

Serono, Fr. Laboratoires Serono, L'Arche du Parc, 738 rue Yves-Kermen, 92658 Boulogne cdx, France.

Serono, Ger. Serono Pharma GmbH, Gutenbergstr. 5, 85716 Unterschleissheim, Germany.

Serono, Hong Kong. Serono Hong Kong Ltd, Rm 1601, Alliance Bldg, 130-136 Connaught Rd Central, Hong Kong.

Serono, Irl. See *Allphar, Irl.*

Serono, Israel. Serono, P.O. Box 8070, Netanya, Israel.

Serono, Ital. Industria Farmaceutica Serono s.p.a., Via Casilina 125, 00176 Rome, Italy.

Serono, Mex. Serono de Mexico S.A. de C.V., Av. Rio Churubusco No. 658, Col el Sifon, 09400 Mexico D.F., Mexico.

Serono, Neth. Serono Benelux, Koninginnegracht 28, 2514 AB Den Haag, Netherlands.

Serono, Norw. Serono Nordic AB, Solheimsv. 32, 1473 Skarer, Norway.

Serono, NZ. Serono, P.O. Box 45-027, Auckland, New Zealand.

Serono, Port. Serono, Lda, Av. Eng. Duarte Pacheco, Amoreiras, Torre 1-8 Piso, 1070-101 Lisbon, Portugal.

Serono, S.Afr. Serono South Africa (Pty) Ltd, P.O. Box 8759, Centurion 0046, South Africa.

Serono, Singapore. Serono Singapore Pte Ltd, 9 Temasek Boulevard, 41-02 Suntac City Tower, S 038989, Singapore.

Serono, Spain. Serono, Maria de Molina 40, 28006 Madrid, Spain.

Serono, Swed. Serono Nordic AB, Box 1803, 171 21 Solna, Sweden.

Serono, Switz. Laboratoires Serono SA, 1170 Aubonne, Switzerland.

Serono, Thai. Serono Thailand Co. Ltd, 4 Fl, S & B Tower, 68-68/6 Pan Rd, Silom, Bangrak, Bangkok 10500, Thailand.

Serono, UK. Serono Pharmaceuticals (UK) Ltd, Bedfont Close, Stanwell Rd, Feltham, Middlesex, TW14 8NX, UK.

Serono, USA. Serono Laboratories Inc., 100 Longwater Circle, Norwell, MA 02061, USA.

Serotherapeutisches, Aust. Serotherapeutisches Institut, Richard-Strauss-Strasse 33, A-1232 Vienna, Austria.

Seroyal, Canad. Seroyal International Inc., 44 E Beaver Creek Rd, Unit 17, Richmond Hill, Ontario, L4B 1G8, Canada.

Serozym, Fr. See *Grimberg, Fr.*

SERP, Mon. SERP, le Triton, 5 rue du Gabian, MC 98000, Monaco.

Serpero, Ital. Serpero Industria Galenica Milanese s.p.a., Via F. Serpero 2, 20060 Masate (MI), Italy.

Serra Pamies, Spain. Serra Pamies, Ctra de Castellvell 24, Reus, 43206 Tarragona, Spain.

Serral, Mex. Serral S.A. de C.V., Adolfo Prieto No. 1009, Col. del Valle, 03100 Mexico D.F., Mexico.

Serturner, Ger. Sertürner Arzneimittel GmbH, Wallenroder Str. 8-10, 13435 Berlin, Germany.

Serum-Werk Bernburg, Ger. Serum-Werk Bernburg AG, Hallesche Landstr. 105 b, 06406 Bernburg, Germany.

Servier, Aust. Servier Pharma GmbH, Mariahilfe Strasse 20/5, A-1070 Vienna, Austria.

Servier, Austral. Servier Laboratories (Australia) P/L, P.O. Box 196, Hawthorn, VIC 3122, Australia.

Servier, Belg. Servier Benelux S.A., Blvd International 57, 1070 Brussels, Belgium.

Servier, Braz. Laboratorio Servier Incibra Produtos Farmaceuticos Ltda, Rua Mario Piragibe 23, 20720-320 Rio de Janeiro, RJ, Brazil.

Servier, Canad. Servier Canada Inc., 235 blvd Armand-Frappier, Laval, Quebec, H7V 4A7, Canada.

Servier, Denm. Servier Danmark A/S, Roskildevej 39 A, 2000 Frederiksberg, Denmark.

Servier, Fr. Laboratoires Servier, 22 rue Garnier, 92200 Neuilly-sur-Seine, France.

Servier, Ger. Servier Deutschland GmbH, Westendstr. 170, 80686 Munich, Germany.

Servier, Hong Kong. Servier Hong Kong Ltd, Rm 1901, 19/F The Lee Gardens, 33 Hysan Ave, Causeway Bay, Hong Kong.

Servier, Irl. Servier Laboratories (Ireland) Ltd, Nutley Buildings, Merrion Centre, Dublin 4, Ireland.

Servier, Israel. Servier, Israel.

Servier, Ital. Servier Italia s.p.a., Via degli Aldobrandeschi 107, 00163 Rome, Italy.

Servier, Neth. Servier Nederland B.V., Postbus 672, 2300 AR Leiden, Netherlands.

Servier, NZ. Servier Laboratories (NZ) Ltd, P.O. Box 14673, Panmure, Auckland, New Zealand.

Servier, Port. Servier Portugal, Lda, Av Antonio Augusto de Aguiar 128, 1069-133 Lisbon, Portugal.

Servier, S.Afr. Servier Laboratories (SA) (Pty) Ltd, P.O. Box 930, Rivonia 2128, South Africa.

Servier, Singapore. Servier (S) Pte Ltd, 510 Thomson Rd, 09-02 SLF Complex, S 298135, Singapore.

Servier, Spain. Servier, Avda de Madronos 33, 28043 Madrid, Spain.

Servier, Switz. Servier (Suisse) SA, 21 rue de Veyrot, 1217 Meyrin 1, Switzerland.

Servier, Thai. Servier (Thailand) Ltd, 15 Fl, Ploenchit Center Building, 2 Sukhumvit Rd, Klongtoey, Bangkok 10110, Thailand.

Servier, UK. Servier Laboratories Ltd, Fulmer Hall, Windmill Rd, Fulmer, Slough, Buckinghamshire, SL3 6HH, UK.

Servipharm, Hong Kong. See *Unipharm, Hong Kong.*

Servipharm, Singapore. See *FP, Singapore.*

Servipharm, Switz. Servipharm AG, Postfach, 4002 Basel, Switzerland.

Servipharm, Thai. See *Zuellig, Thai.*

Sessa, Ital. Sessa Carlo s.a.s., Viale Gramsci 212, 20099 Sesto S. Giovanni (MI), Italy.

Seton, Irl. See *Intraveno, Irl.*

Seton, Israel. Seton, Israel.

Seton, NZ. See *Pharmaco, NZ.*

Seton, UK. See *SSL, UK.*

Seton Scholl, Austral. Seton Scholl, 225 Beach Rd, Mordilloc, VIC 3195, Australia.

Seton Scholl, Fr. See *SSL, Fr.*

Seton Scholl, Switz. Seton Scholl Schweiz AG, Sternenhofstrasse 15A, 4153 Reinach 1, Switzerland.

Seven Seas, Singapore. See *Zuellig, Singapore.*

Seven Seas, UK. Seven Seas Ltd, Hedon Rd, Marfleet, Hull, HU9 5NJ, UK.

SFD, Port. Sociedade Farmaceutica de Desenvolvimento, Lda, Rua Duque d'Avila no 193, 1050-082 Lisbon, Portugal.

Shaklee, Canad. Shaklee Canada Inc., 952 Century Dr, Burlington, Ontario, L7L 5P2, Canada.

Shalpharm, Israel. See *Ophir Shalpharm, Israel.*

Shantys, UK. Shanty's Ltd, 3-4 Coppen Rd, Dagenham, Essex, RM8 1HU, UK.

Sharpe, Austral. Sharpe Laboratories P/L, 12 Hope Street, Ermington, NSW 2115, Australia.

Sharpe, NZ. See *Douglas, NZ.*

Shepherd, Canad. Shepherd Pharmaceuticals Inc., 3332 Yonge St, P.O. Box 94018, Toronto, Ontario, M4N 3R1, Canada.

Sheraton, Hong Kong. Sheraton Worldwide Drugs Co. Ltd, 3/F Flat A & 6/F Flat B, Heep Cheung Commercial Bldg, 251 Temple St, Tsimshatsui, Kowloon, Hong Kong.

Sherman, Israel. Sherman, Israel.

Sherman, USA. Sherman Pharmaceuticals Inc., P.O. Box 1377, Mandeville, LA 70470-1377, USA.

Sherwood, USA. See *Kendall, USA.*

Shigaken, Singapore. See *Luen Wah, Singapore.*

Shin Poong, Singapore. See *Zyfas, Singapore.*

Shinfuso, Hong Kong. See *Primal, Hong Kong.*

Shinfuso, Thai. See *Asian TJD, Thai.*

Shinyaku, Hong Kong. See *Hing Ah, Hong Kong.*

Shinyaku, Jpn. Nippon Shinyaku Co. Ltd, 14 Nishinosho-Monguchi-cho, Kisshoin, Minami-ku, Kyoto 601-8550, Japan.

Shinyaku, Singapore. See *Wellchem, Singapore.*

Shinyaku, Thai. See *Asian TJD, Thai.*

Shionogi, Jpn. Shionogi & Co. Ltd, 1-8 Dosho-machi 3-chome, Chuo-ku, Osaka 541-0045, Japan.

Shionogi, USA. Shionogi USA Inc., 3848 Carson St, Suite 206, Torrance, CA 90503, USA.

Shire, Canad. Shire Canada Inc., 400 Iroquois Shore Rd, Oakville, Ontario, L6H 1M5, Canada.

Shire, Hong Kong. See *Inchcape, Hong Kong.*

Shire, Irl. See *Cahill May Roberts, Irl.*

Shire, UK. Shire Pharmaceuticals Ltd, Hampshire International Business Park, Chineham, Basingstoke, Hampshire, RG24 8EP, UK.

Shire Richwood, USA. Shire Richwood Inc., 7900 Tanners Gate Dr., Suite 200, Florence, KY 41042, USA.

Shiseido, Canad. Shiseido Company Ltd, 486 Queen St E, Ste 212, Toronto, Ontario, M5A 1T7, Canada.

Shiwa, Thai. Shiwa Chemicals Co. Ltd, 34/1 Sukhumvit 39, (Soi Prompong), Bangkok 10110, Thailand.

Shoppers Drug Mart, Canad. Shoppers Drug Mart, 225 Yorkland Blvd, Willowdale, Ontario, M2J 4Y7, Canada.

SHS, Fr. SHS International Ltd, 4 passage St-Antoine, 92508 Rueil-Malmaison, France.

SHS, Singapore. See *Pharma 2000, Singapore.*

SHS, UK. SHS International Ltd, 100 Wavertree Boulevard, Liverpool, Merseyside, L7 9PT, UK.

SHS, USA. SHS N. America/Scientific Hospital Supplies, 9600 Medical Center Drive, Suite 102, Rockville, MD 20850, USA.

Siam Bheasach, Thai. See *Siam Pharm, Thai.*

Siam Medicare, Thai. Siam Medicare Co. Ltd, 77/37 Soi Senanikom 1, Phaholyothin Rd, Bangkok 10900, Thailand.

Siam Pharm, Thai. Siam Pharmaceutical Co. Ltd, 171/1 Soi Choke Chai Ruammitr, Vibhavadi-Rangsit Rd, Bangkok 10900, Thailand.

Sibras, Braz. Sibras Laboratorios Ltda, Avenida Pedro Adams Filho 2.340, 93320-000 Novo Hamburgo, RS, Brazil.

Sicomed, Hong Kong. See *Hong Kong Medical, Hong Kong.*

Sicor, Ital. Sicor spa, Via Terrazzano 77, 20017 Rho (MI), Italy.

Sicor, USA. SICOR Inc., 19 Hughes, Irvine, CA 92718, USA.

Sidefarma, Port. Sidefarma, Lda, Rua da Guine, Prior Velho, 2685 Sacavem, Portugal.

Sidroga, Switz. Sidroga AG, Postfach, 4800 Zofingen, Switzerland.

Siegfried, Swed. Siegfried, Nonnens vag 6, 451 50 Uddevalla, Sweden.

Siegfried, Switz. Siegfried CMS AG, 4800 Zofingen, Switzerland.

Siegfried, Thai. See *Diethelm, Thai.*

Siemens, Ger. Siemens & Co., Heilwasser und Quellenprodukte des Staatsbades Bad Ems GmbH & Co. KG, Arzbacher Str. 78, 56130 Bad Ems, Germany.

Siemens, Switz. See *Ecosol, Switz.*

Sifa, Ital. Sifa Servizi Integrati s.r.l., Via Bolsena 4, 00191 Rome, Italy.

Sifarma, Ital. Sifarma s.p.a., Via Brunelleschi 12, 20146 Milan, Italy.

SIFI, Ital. Società Industria Farmaceutica Italiana s.p.a., Via Ercole Patti 36, 95020 Lavinaio-Aci S. Antonio (CY) Italy.

SIFI, Singapore. See *Green Cross, Singapore.*

SIFRA, Ital. See *Fresenius Kabi, Ital.*

Sigma, Austral. Sigma Pharmaceuticals P/L, 96 Merrindale Drive, Croydon, VIC 3136, Australia.

Sigma, Hong Kong. See *LCH, Hong Kong,* and *Treasure Mountain, Hong Kong.*

Sigma, NZ. See *Pharmaco, NZ.*

Sigmapharm, Aust. Sigmapharm Arzneimittel GmbH & Co KG, Leystrasse 129, A-1204 Vienna, Austria.

Sigmapharm, Switz. See *Ridupharm, Switz.*

Sigma-Tau, Canad. See *Sigma-Tau, USA.*

Sigma-Tau, Fr. Sigma-Tau France, 5 av. de Verdun, 94202 Ivry sur Seine, France.

Sigma-Tau, Ger. Sigma Tau Arzneimittel GmbH, Am Wehrhahn 86, 40211 Dusseldorf, Germany.

Sigma-Tau, Hong Kong. See *Sino-Asia, Hong Kong.*

Sigma-Tau, Ital. Sigma Tau s.p.a., Via Pontina Km. 30,400, 00040 Pomezia (Rome), Italy.

Sigma-Tau, Neth. Sigma Tau, Netherlands.

Sigma-Tau, Spain. Sigma Tau, Pl. Ind. Azque C/Bolivia 15, Alcala de Henares, 28806 Madrid, Spain.

Sigma-Tau, Switz. Sigma-Tau Pharma AG, Luzernerstrasse 2, 4800 Zofingen, Switzerland.

Sigma-Tau, USA. Sigma-Tau Pharmaceuticals Inc., 800 S Frederick Ave, Suite 300, Gaithersburg, MD 20877, USA.

Silanes, Mex. Laboratorios Silanes S.A. de C.V., Amores No. 1304, Col. del Valle, 03100 Mexico D.F., Mexico.

Silarx, USA. Silarx Pharmaceuticals Inc., 19 West St, Spring Valley, NY 10977, USA.

Silhouette, Aust. Silhouette International GmbH, Ellbognerstrasse 24, A-4020 Linz, Austria.

Silom, Thai. Silom Medical Co. Ltd, 35/3 Suparaj Soi 1, Phaholyothin Rd, Samsennai, Bangkok 10400, Thailand.

Silroc, Hong Kong. Silroc International (HK) Ltd, Rm 1906, Blk A, New Trade Plaza, 6 On Ping Rd, Siu Lek Yuen, Shatin, N.T., Hong Kong.

Silvestre, Braz. Silvestre, Brazil.

Simcare, UK. Simcare, Peter Rd, Lancing, West Sussex, BN15 8TJ, UK.

Sime Darby, Singapore. Sime Darby Marketing, A Division of Sime Darby Singapore Ltd, 896 Dunearn Rd, 04-03 Sime Darby Centre, S 589472, Singapore.

Simoes, Braz. Laboratorio Simoes Ltda, Rua Pereira de Almeida 102, 20260-100 Rio de Janeiro, RJ, Brazil.

Simons, Ger. Georg Simons GmbH, Bunsenstr. 5, 82152 Planegg/Martinsried, Germany.

Sinbio, Fr. See *Pierre Fabre, Fr.*

Sincerity, Hong Kong. Sincerity (Asia) Co. Ltd, 1/F, Blk E, Nam Pak Hong Bldg, 24 Bonham Strand W, Hong Kong.

Sinclair, Irl. See *Allphar, Irl.*

Sinclair, UK. Sinclair Pharmaceuticals Ltd, Borough Rd, Godalming, Surrey, GU7 2AB, UK.

Singer, Hong Kong. See *Zuellig, Hong Kong.*

Singer, Switz. Pharma-Singer AG, Windeggstrasse 2, 8867 Niederurnen, Switzerland.

Sino-Asia, Hong Kong. Sino-Asia Pharmaceutical Supplies Ltd, 1 Fung Fai Terrace, Upper G/F, Village Rd, Happy Valley, Hong Kong.

Sintesa, Belg. Sintesa S.A., Blvd de la Woluwe 34 Bte 11, 1200 Brussels, Belgium.

Sintetica, Switz. Sintetica SA, San Martino, casella postale 1764, 6850 Mendrisio, Switzerland.

Sintofarm, Ital. Sintofarm Farmaceutici s.p.a., Torre Sequoia g, Via Torri Bianche 1, 20059 Vimercate (MI), Italy.

Sintofarma, Braz. Laboratorios Sintofarma S.A., Rua Sergipe 120, 01243-000 Sao Paulo, SP, Brazil.

Sipaco, Denm. See *Niche, Denm.*

Sipaco, Port. Sipaco Internacional, Avda 5 de Outubro 267,6, 01600 Lisbon, Portugal.

Sipaco, Spain. See *Sipaco, Port.*

Siphar, Switz. Siphar SA, Casella postale 32, 6814 Cadempino, Switzerland.

SIRC, Singapore. See *Zyfas, Singapore.*

Sirmeta, Austral. Sirmeta, Australia.

Sirval, Ital. Società Italiana Ritrovati Val s.a.s., Via Maloia 8, 20158 Milan, Italy.

Sisu, Canad. Sisu Enterprises Ltd, 104A-3430 Brighton Ave, Burnaby, British Columbia, V5A 3H4, Canada.

SIT, Ital. Specialità Igienico Terapeutiche s.r.l., C.so Cavour 70, 27035 Mede (Pavia), Italy.

SK, Singapore. See *Wellchem, Singapore.*

Skills, Ital. Skills in Farmacia s.r.l., Piazza Buonarroti 32, 20145 Milan, Italy.

Skinicles, Canad. Skinicles Ltd, 150 Priscilla Ave, P.O. Box 1655, Toronto, Ontario, M6S 3W3, Canada.

SK-RIT, Belg. See *SmithKline Beecham, Belg.*

Skye, USA. SkyePharma Inc., 10450 Science Center Drive, San Diego, CA 92121, USA.

SLE, Israel. See *Madaus, Israel.*

Slimax, Austral. Slimax, Australia.

SM, Thai. SM Pharmaceutcal Co. Ltd, 82, 84 Arkarn 2, Ratchdamnoen Ave, Bangkok 10200, Thailand.

SMA Nutrition, Irl. See *Wyeth, UK.*

Smaller, Spain. Smaller, Sagitario 12, 03006 Alicante, Spain.

SMB, Belg. Laboratoires S.M.B. S.A., rue de la Pastorale 26-8, 1080 Brussels, Belgium.

SMB, Thai. See *Berlin Pharm, Thai.*

Smetana, Aust. See *EF-EM-ES, Aust.*

Smith & Nephew, Austral. Smith & Nephew P/L, P.O. Box 150, Clayton, VIC 3168, Australia.

Smith & Nephew, Canad. Smith & Nephew Inc., 2100, 52e Ave, Lachine, Quebec, H8T 2Y5, Canada.

Smith & Nephew, Denm. Smith & Nephew A/S, Naerum Hovedgade 2, 2850 Naerum, Denmark.

Smith & Nephew, Fin. Smith & Nephew Oy, Rajatorpantie 41 C, 01640 Vantaa, Finland.

Smith & Nephew, Fr. Smith & Nephew, 25 bd Alexandre-Oyon, 72019 Le Mans cdx 2, France.

Smith & Nephew, Hong Kong. Smith & Nephew Ltd, Units 16-19, 13/F Grandtech Ctr, 8 On Ping St, Siu Lek Yuen, Shatin, N.T., Hong Kong.

Smith & Nephew, Irl. Smith & Nephew Medical, Kill o'the Grange, Deansgrange, Co. Dublin, Ireland.

Smith & Nephew, Ital. Smith & Nephew s.r.l., Viale Colleoni 13, 20041 Agrate Brianza (MI), Italy.

Smith & Nephew, Norw. Smith & Nephew AS, Postboks 224, 1379 Nesbru, Norway.

Smith & Nephew, NZ. Smith & Nephew Ltd, P.O. Box 442, Auckland, New Zealand.

Smith & Nephew, S.Afr. Smith & Nephew Pharmaceuticals (Pty) Ltd, P.O. Box 92, Pinetown 3600, South Africa.

Smith & Nephew, Singapore. See *Zuellig, Singapore.*

Smith & Nephew, Swed. Smith & Nephew AB, Box 143, 431 22 Molndal, Sweden.

Smith & Nephew, Switz. Smith & Nephew AG, Habs Huber-Strasse 38, 4502 Solothurn, Switzerland.

Smith & Nephew, Thai. Smith & Nephew Ltd, 344/3 Soi Rongrien Yepun, Rama IX Rd, Bangapi, Huay Kwang, Bangkok 10320, Thailand.

Smith & Nephew, UK. See *Smith & Nephew Healthcare, UK.*

Smith & Nephew, USA. Smith & Nephew United, 11775 Starkey Rd, Largo, FL 33773, USA.

Smith & Nephew Healthcare, UK. Smith & Nephew Healthcare Ltd, Healthcare House, Goulton St, Hull, HU3 4DJ, UK.

Smith & Nephew Pharmaceuticals, UK. See *Smith & Nephew Healthcare, UK.*

Smith & Nephew SoloPak, USA. See *SoloPak, USA.*

Smith Kline & French, Port. Smith Kline & French Portuguesa, Lda, Av. das Forcas Armadas 125, 1600 Lisbon, Portugal.

SmithKline, Spain. See *SmithKline Beecham, Spain.*

SmithKline Beecham, Aust. See *GlaxoSmithKline, Aust.*

SmithKline Beecham, Austral. SmithKline Beecham International Pharmaceuticals, Private Mail Bag 34, Dandenong, VIC 3175, Australia.

SmithKline Beecham, Belg. SmithKline Beecham S.A., Rue du Tilleul 13, 1332 Genval, Belgium.

SmithKline Beecham, Braz. Smithkline Beecham Laboratorios Ltda, Avenida Pedro II 374, 20941-070 Rio de Janeiro, RJ, Brazil.

SmithKline Beecham, Canad. SmithKline Beecham Pharma, Division of SmithKline Beecham Inc., 2030 Bristol Circle, Oakville, Ontario, L6H 5V2, Canada.

SmithKline Beecham, Denm. SmithKline Beecham Pharmaceuticals, Lautruphoj 1-3, 2750 Ballerup, Denmark.

SmithKline Beecham, Fin. SmithKline Beecham Oy, Metsänneidonkuja 10, 02130 Espoo, Finland.

SmithKline Beecham, Fr. SmithKline Beecham Laboratoires Pharmaceutiques, 6 esplanade Charles-de-Gaulle, 92731 Nanterre cdx, France.

SmithKline Beecham, Ger. SmithKline Beecham Pharma GmbH, Leopoldstr. 175, 80804 Munich, Germany.

SmithKline Beecham, Hong Kong. SmithKline Beecham Ltd, 28/F South Tower, Concordia Plaza, 1 Science Museum Rd, Tsimshatsui East, Kowloon, Hong Kong.

SmithKline Beecham, Irl. See *GlaxoSmithKline, Irl.*

SmithKline Beecham, Israel. SmithKline Beecham Healthcare Ltd, P.O. Box 12103, Herzliya, Israel.

SmithKline Beecham, Ital. SmithKline Beecham s.p.a., Via Zambeletti, 20021 Branzate di Bollate (MI), Italy.

SmithKline Beecham, Jpn. SmithKline Beecham, Japan.

SmithKline Beecham, Mex. SmithKline Beecham Mexico S.A. de C.V., Av. Insurgentes Sur No. 1605 Piso 19, Col. San Jose Insurgentes, 01020 Mexico D.F., Mexico.

SmithKline Beecham, Neth. SmithKline Beecham Farma, Postbus 3120, 2280 GC Rijswijk, Netherlands.

SmithKline Beecham, Norw. SmithKline Beecham AS, Solheimv. 112, Postboks 134, 1471 Skarer, Norway.

SmithKline Beecham, NZ. SmithKline Beecham (NZ) Ltd, P.O. Box 62043, Sylvia Park, Auckland 6, New Zealand.

SmithKline Beecham, S.Afr. See *GlaxoSmithKline, S.Afr.*

SmithKline Beecham, Singapore. SmithKline Beecham (Singapore) Pte Ltd, 101 Thomson Rd, 02-18/21 United Square, S 307591, Singapore.

SmithKline Beecham, Spain. SmithKline Beecham, Valle de la Fuenfria 3, 28034 Madrid, Spain.

SmithKline Beecham, Swed. SmithKline Beecham AB, Box 4092, 171 04 Solna, Sweden.

SmithKline Beecham, Switz. SmithKline Beecham AG, 3174 Thorishaus, Switzerland.

SmithKline Beecham, Thai. SmithKline Beecham International, 12 Fl, Wave Place, 55 Wireless Rd, Lumpini Patumwam, Bangkok 10330, Thailand.

SmithKline Beecham, UK. See *GlaxoSmithKline, UK.*

SmithKline Beecham, USA. SmithKline Beecham Pharmaceuticals, 1 Franklin Plaza, P.O. Box 7929, Philadelphia, PA 19101, USA.

SmithKline Beecham Consumer, Austral. SmithKline Beecham International (Consumer Healthcare), Locked Bag 3, Ermington, NSW 2115, Australia.

SmithKline Beecham Consumer, Belg. See *SmithKline Beecham, Belg.*

SmithKline Beecham Consumer, Canad. See *SmithKline Beecham, Canad.*

SmithKline Beecham Consumer, Irl. See *GlaxoSmithKline, Irl.*

SmithKline Beecham Consumer, Neth. SmithKline Beecham Consumer Healthcare, Postbus 394, 1180 AJ Amstelveen, Netherlands.

SmithKline Beecham Consumer, Swed. See *SmithKline Beecham, Swed.*

SmithKline Beecham Consumer, Switz. See *SmithKline Beecham, Switz.*

SmithKline Beecham Consumer, UK. See *GlaxoSmithKline, UK.*

SmithKline Beecham Consumer, USA. SmithKline Beecham Consumer Healthcare L.P., Unit of SmithKline Beecham Inc., P.O. Box 1467, Pittsburgh, PA 15230, USA.

SmithKline Beecham Drinks, UK. See *GlaxoSmithKline, UK.*

SmithKline Beecham OTC, Ger. SmithKline Beecham GmbH & Co. KG - OTC Medicines, Bussmatten 1, 77815 Buhl, Germany.

SmithKline Beecham Sante, Fr. Lab. SmithKline Beecham Santé et Hygiène, 5 esplanade Charles-de-Gaulle, B.P. 306, 92003 Nanterre cdx, France.

SmithKline Diagnostics, USA. See *Beckman, USA.*

SMP, S.Afr. SMP, South Africa.

SMT, Ger. Sportmedizin Team München Arzneimittel GmbH, Muhlstr. 5, 88481 Balzheim, Germany.

SMTL, UK. Surgical Materials Testing Laboratory, Princess of Wales Hospital, Coity Rd, Bridgend, Mid Glamorgan, CF31 1RQ, UK.

SNBTS, UK. Scottish National Blood Transfusion Service, Protein Fractionation Centre, Ellen's Glen Rd, Edinburgh, EH17 7QT, UK.

Socopharm, Fr. Laboratoires Socopharm, Chemin de Marcy, 58800 Corbigny, France.

Sodia, Fr. Laboratoires Sodia, av. Robert Schuman, 51100 Reims, France.

Sodilac, Fr. Sodilac, Le Wilson II, 80 av du General-de-Gaulle, Puteaux 92031 Paris-La Defense cdx, France.

Sodip, Switz. Sodip SA, 11 rue Alphonse-Large, 1217 Meyrin 1, Switzerland.

Sofar, Ital. Sofar Farmaceutici s.p.a., Via Firenze 40, 20060 Trezzano Rosa (MI), Italy.

Sofex, Port. Sofex Farmacêutica, Lda, Rua Sebastiao e Silva 25, Zona Industrial de Massama, 2745 Queluz, Portugal.

SoftRinse, USA. SoftRinse Corp., 2411 Third St South, Wisconsin Rapids, WI 54494, USA.

Sohan, Canad. Sohan Chemicals Ltd, 70 Gibson Drive, Unit 14, Markham, ON, L3R 2Z3, Canada.

Solar, Canad. Solar Cosmetics Labs Inc, 6845 Rexwood Rd, Unit 3-5, Mississauga, Ontario, L4V 1S5, Canada.

Solco, Aust. Solco Pharma Austria GmbH, Michael Pacher Strasse 25A/7, A-5020 Salzburg, Austria.

Solco, Fin. See *Panfarma, Fin.*

Solco, Ger. Solco GmbH, Salzwerkstr. 7, 79639 Grenzach-Wyhlen, Germany.

Solco, Hong Kong. Solco, Hong Kong.

Solco, Singapore. See *Pharmaforte, Singapore.*

Solco, Swed. See *Solco, Ger.*

Solco, Switz. Solco Basel SA, Ruhrbergstrasse 21, 4127 Birsfelden, Switzerland.

Solco, Thai. See *Diethelm, Thai.*

Soldan, Ger. Dr. C. Soldan GmbH, Herderstr. 5-9, 90427 Nurnberg, Germany.

Solea, Ital. Solea s.a.s., Via Cassoli 22, 42100 Reggio Emilia, Italy.

Solfran, Mex. Laboratorios Solfran S.A., Altos Hornos No. 2721, Fracc. Ind. el Alamo, 44490 Tlaquepaque, Jal., Mexico.

Solgar, UK. Solgar Vitamins Ltd, UK.

Solgar, USA. Solgar Vitamin Co. Inc., 500 Willow Tree Rd, Leonia, NJ 07605, USA.

Solmer, Switz. Solmer SA, Postfach 100, 6976 Castagnola-Suisse, Switzerland.

SoloPak, USA. SoloPak Pharmaceuticals Inc., 1845 Tonne Rd, Elk Grove Village, IL 60007-5125, USA.

Soludia, Fr. Laboratoires Soludia, Rte de Revel, 31450 Fourquevaux, France.

Solvay, Aust. Solvay Pharma GmbH, Donaustrasse 106, A-3400 Klosterneuburg, Austria.

Solvay, Austral. Solvay Pharmaceuticals, Division of Solvay Biosciences P/L, Locked Bag 1070, Pymble, NSW 2073, Australia.

Solvay, Belg. Solvay Pharma & Cie S.N.C., Boulevard Emile Bockstael 122, 1020 Brussels, Belgium.

Solvay, Canad. Solvay Pharma Inc., 50 Venture Drive, Scarborough, Ontario, M1B 3L6, Canada.

Solvay, Denm. Solvay Pharma ApS, Horkaer 32, 1, 2730 Herlev, Denmark.

Solvay, Fin. See *Algol, Fin.*

Solvay, Fr. Solvay Pharma, 42 rue Rouget-de-Lisle, B.P. 22, 92151 Suresnes cdx, France.

Solvay, Ger. Solvay Arzneimittel GmbH, Hans-Bockler-Allee 20, 30173 Hannover, Germany.

Solvay, Hong Kong. See *Keller, Hong Kong.*

Solvay, Irl. Solvay Healthcare Ltd, Belgard Rd, Tallaght, Dublin 24, Ireland.

Solvay, Israel. Solvay, Israel.

Solvay, Ital. Solvay Pharma s.p.a., Via della Liberta 30, 10095 Grugliasco (TO), Italy.

Solvay, Neth. Solvay Pharma B.V., Postbus 501, 1380 AM Weesp, Netherlands.

Solvay, Norw. Solvay Pharma AS, Hamang Terrasse 55, Postboks 248, 1301 Sandvika, Norway.

Solvay, NZ. See *Russells, NZ.*

Solvay, Port. Solvayfarma, Lda, Av. Marechal Gomes da Costa 33, 1800-255 Lisbon, Portugal.

Solvay, S.Afr. Solvay Pharma (Pty) Ltd, P.O. Box 5278, halfway House 1685, South Africa.

Solvay, Singapore. See *Sime Darby, Singapore.*

Solvay, Spain. Solvay Pharma, Avda Diagonal 507-9, 08029 Barcelona, Spain.

Solvay, Swed. Solvay Pharma AB, Sisjo Kullegata 8, 421 32 Vastra Frolunda, Sweden.

Solvay, Switz. Solvay Pharma AG, Untermattweg 8, 3027 Bern, Switzerland.

Solvay, Thai. See *Berli, Thai.*

Solvay, UK. Solvay Healthcare, Mansbridge Rd, West End, Southampton, Hampshire, SO18 3JD, UK.

Solvay, USA. Solvay Pharmaceuticals Inc., 901 Sawyer Road, Marietta, GA 30062-2224, USA.

Solvay Duphar, Swed. See *Meda, Swed.*

Solymes, Fr. Laboratoires Solymès, 46 quai de la Rapee, 75601 Paris cdx 12, France.

Soma, Switz. Soma Pharm, Switzerland.

Somerset, USA. Somerset Pharmaceuticals Inc., 777 S Harbour Island Bvld, Suite 880, Tampa, FL 33602, USA.

Sons, Mex. Laboratorios Quimica Son's S.A. de C.V., Av. 23 Poniente No. 2302-A, 72410 Puebla, Pue., Mexico.

Sopar, Neth. See *Will-Pharma, Neth.*

Sophia, Mex. Laboratorios Sophia S.A. de C.V., Calle Poniente 44 No 2702, Col. San Salvador Xochimanca, 02670 Mexico D.F., Mexico.

Soria Natural, Spain. Soria Natural, Pol Ind La Sacea 1, Garray, 42162 Soria, Spain.

Sorin, Ital. Sorin Radiofarmaci, Italy.

Sorin-Maxim, Fr. Laboratoires Sorin-Maxim, rue Claude-Bernard, 12700 Capdenac, France.

SoSe, Ital. So.Se. Pharm s.r.l., Via dei castelli Romani 22, 00040 Pomezia (Rome), Italy.

Sovereign, UK. Sovereign Medical, Sovereign House, Miles Gray Rd, Basildon, Essex, SS14 3FR, UK.

SPA, Ital. Società Prodotti Antibiotici s.p.a., Via Biella 8, 20143 Milan, Italy.

SPAD, Fr. Laboratoires Spécialités Pour l'Art Dentaire, 14D rue Pierre-de-Coubertin, Parc de Mirande, 21007 Dijon cdx, France.

Spagyros, Switz. Spagyros AG, Tannackerstrasse 7, 3073 Gumlingen, Switzerland.

Sparks, NZ. David Sparks Ltd, P.O. Box 83-122, Edmonton, Auckland, New Zealand.

SPB, Thai. S.P.B. Pharma Co. Ltd, Sathorn Park Place, Apt 14B, Sathorn, Bangkok 10120, Thailand.

Specia, Fr. See *Rhone-Poulenc Rorer, Fr.*

Spectropharm, Canad. Spectropharm Dermatology, Division of Draxis Health Inc., 6870 Goreway Drive, Mississauga, Ontario, L4V 1P1, Canada.

Speywood, Switz. See *Opopharma, Switz.*

Speywood, USA. Speywood Pharmaceuticals Inc, 27 Maple St, Milford, MA 01757-3650, USA.

Spiphar, Belg. Ets Spiphar S.P.R.L., Ave de la Couronne 114A, 1050 Brussels, Belgium.

Spirig, Singapore. See *Pasture, Singapore.*

Spirig, Switz. Spirig AG, Pharmazeutische Praparate, 4622 Egerkingen, Switzerland.

Spitzner, Ger. W. Spitzner, Pharmazeutische Fabrik GmbH, Bunsenstr. 6-10, 76275 Ettlingen, Germany.

Sportbalm, Austral. Sportbalm Australia P/L, 29 Woodland St, Strathmore, VIC 3041, Australia.

Spreewald, Ger. Spreewald Pharma GmbH, Kuschkower Str. 9, 15910 Groditsch, Germany.

Spyfarma, Spain. Spyfarma, Ctra Sevilla Malaga Km 9.5 Km, Alcala de Guadaira, 41500 Seville, Spain.

Square, Thai. Pharma Square Co. Ltd, 5 Fortune Town, 4 Fl, Rm 22-26, Ratchadapisek Rd, Bangkok 103320, Thailand.

Squibb, Canad. See *Bristol-Myers Squibb, Canad.*

Squibb, Neth. See *Bristol-Myers Squibb, Neth.*

Squibb, Spain. Squibb, Josep Anselm Clave 95, Esplugues de Llobregat, 08950 Barcelona, Spain.

Squibb, UK. See *Bristol-Myers Squibb, UK.*

Squibb, USA. See *Bristol-Myers Squibb, USA.*

Squibb Diagnostics, Canad. See *Bristol-Myers Squibb, Canad.*

Squibb Diagnostics, USA. See *Bristol-Myers Squibb, USA.*

Sriprasit, Thai. Sriprasit Dispensary R O P, 617 Charoen Rath Rd, Klongsarn, Bangkok 10600, Thailand.

SS, Jpn. SS Pharmaceutical, Japan.

SSI, Swed. SSI Sverige, Slagthuset, 211 20 Malmo, Sweden.

SSL, Fr. SSL Healthcare France SA, 13 bis, av. de l'Escouvrier, B.P. 585, 95205 Sarcelles cdx, France.

SSL, UK. SSL International plc, Toft Hall, Knutsford, Chesire, WA16 9PD, UK.

SSW, Ger. See *SmithKline Beecham, Ger.*

ST, Thai. ST Pharma, 1937/16 Soi Ramkamhaeng 21, Banhkapi, Bangkok 10240, Thailand.

St Laurent, Canad. See *Romilo, Canad.*

Stada, Aust. Stada Arzneimittel GmbH, Heiligenstadter Strasse 52/2/8, A-1190 Vienna, Austria.

Stada, Ger. Stada Arzneimittel AG, Stadastr. 2-18, 61118 Bad Vilbel, Germany.

Stada, Hong Kong. Stada Pharmaceuticals (Asia) Ltd, 2208-2209 Paul Y Ctr, 51 Hung To Rd, Kwun Tong, Hong Kong.

Stada, Singapore. See *JDH, Singapore.*

Stada, Switz. Stada Arzneimittel (Schweiz) AG, Route Andre-Piller 2, Case postale 76, 1762 Givisiez, Switzerland.

Stada, Thai. Stada Asiatic Co. Ltd, 41/18 Rama III Rd, Chongnonsee, Yannawa, Bangkok 10120, Thailand.

Stafford, Mex. Stafford, Mexico.

Stafford-Miller, Austral. Stafford Miller Ltd, P.O. Box 406, North Ryde, NSW 1670, Australia.

Stafford-Miller, Denm. See *Meda, Denm.*

Stafford-Miller, Fin. See *Tamro, Fin.*

Stafford-Miller, Fr. Laboratoires Stafford-Miller, 1 bd Victor, 75015 Paris, France.

Stafford-Miller, Irl. See *Intra Pharma, Irl.*

Stafford-Miller, Israel. See *CTS, Israel.*

Stafford-Miller, Ital. Stafford-Miller s.r.l., Via Correggio 19, 20149 Milan, Italy.

Stafford-Miller, Norw. See *Meda, Norw.*

Stafford-Miller, NZ. Stafford-Miller (NZ) Ltd, P.O. Box 100-490, Auckland, New Zealand.

Stafford-Miller, Port. See *Ferraz, Lynce, Port.*

Stafford-Miller, Spain. Stafford Miller, Pol. Ind. Malpica C/C 102-F, 50016 Zaragoza, Spain.

Stafford-Miller, Switz. See *Doetsch, Grether, Switz.*

Stafford-Miller, UK. See *GlaxoSmithKline, UK.*

Stafford-Miller Continental, Belg. Stafford-Miller Continental N.V.-S.A., Nijverhaidsstraat 9, 2260 Oevel, Belgium.

Stallergenes, Belg. Stallergenes Belgium S.A., Chaussee de Louvain 277, 1410 Waterloo, Belgium.

Stallergenes, Fr. Stallergènes SA, 6 rue Alexis-de-Tocqueville, 92183 Antony cdx, France.

Stallergenes, Ital. Stallergenes Italia srl, Riviera Francia 3/A, 35127 Padova, Italy.

Stallergenes, Switz. Lab. des Stallergènes Sàrl, 17C rue Vautier, case postale 1331, 1227 Carouge, Switzerland.

Stanback, USA. Stanback Co., PO Box 1669, Salisbury, NC 28145-1669, USA.

Standard, Hong Kong. See *Kai Yuen, Hong Kong.*

Standard Drug, USA. Standard Drug Company, 1279 N 7th St, Riverton, IL 62561, USA.

Stanley, Canad. Stanley Pharmaceuticals Ltd, Division of Vita Health Products Ltd, 117-260 West Esplanade, North Vancouver, British Columbia, V7M 3G7, Canada.

Stanley, Israel. See *Manon, Israel.*

Star, Hong Kong. Star Medical Supplies Ltd, Unit E, 1/F Hop Hing Industrial Bldg, 704 Castle Peak Rd, Lai Chi Kok, Kowloon, Hong Kong.

Star, Thai. Star Lab Co. Ltd, 542 Vipavadi Rangsit Rd, Din Dang, Bangkok 10400, Thailand.

Star, USA. Star Pharmaceuticals Inc., 1990 NW 44th St, Pompano Beach, FL 33064-8712, USA.

Stark, Ger. H. C. Stark GmbH Chemische Fabrik, Schneckenburgstr. 46, 78467 Constance, Germany.

Statens Serum Institut, Denm. Statens Serum Institut, Artillerivej 5, 2300 Copenhagen S, Denmark.

Statens Serum Institut, Fin. See *Statens Serum Institut, Denm.*

Staufen, Ger. Staufen-Pharma GmbH & Co., Bahnhofstr. 35, 73033 Goppingen, Germany.

Stauffacher, Switz. Stauffacher Apotheke, Dr Langer AG, Birmensdorferstrasse 1, 8004 Zurich, Switzerland.

STD, Irl. See *STD Pharmaceutical Products, UK.*

STD Pharmaceutical Products, UK. STD Pharmaceutical Products Ltd, Fields Yard, Plough Lane, Hereford, Herefordshire, HR4 0EL, UK.

Stegropharm, Ger. StegroPharm Arzneimittel GmbH, St.-Johann-Str. 8, 80999 Munich, Germany.

Steierl, Ger. Steierl Pharma GmbH, Muhlfelder Str. 48, 82211 Herrsching, Germany.

Steigerwald, Ger. Steigerwald Arzneimittelwerk GmbH, Havelstr. 5, 64295 Darmstadt, Germany.

Steigerwald, Switz. See *Hanseler, Switz.*

Steiner, Ger. Steiner & Co. Deutsche Arzneimittel Gesellschaft, Ostpreussendamm 72/74, 12207 Berlin, Germany.

Stella, Belg. Laboratoires Stella S.A., Rue des Pontons 25, 4032 Liege (Chenee), Belgium.

Stella, Canad. Stella Pharmaceutical Canada Ltd, 407-220 Duncan Mill Rd, Don Mills, Ontario, M3B 3J5, Canada.

Stella, Ital. Stella Pharmaceutical s.p.a., Italy.

Stellar, USA. Stellar Pharmacal Corp., 1990 NW 44th St, Pompano Beach, FL 33064-1278, USA.

Steris, USA. Steris Laboratories Inc., 620 N 51st Ave, Phoenix, AZ 85043, USA.

Steriseal, UK. Steriseal Ltd, 26-7 Thornhill Rd, North Moons Moat, Redditch, Worcestershire, B98 9NL, UK.

Sterling, Port. Sterling Produtos Farmacêuticos, Lda, Avda das Forcas Armadas 125, 1600 Lisbon, Portugal.

Sterling, Thai. See *Diethelm, Thai.*

Sterling, USA. See *Sterling Health, USA.*

Sterling Health, Austral. See *SmithKline Beecham Consumer, Austral.*

Sterling Health, Spain. Sterling Health, Avda Diagonal 618, 08021 Barcelona, Spain.

Sterling Health, UK. See *GlaxoSmithKline, UK.*

Sterling Health, USA. See *Bayer, USA.*

Sterling Midy, Ital. Sterling Midy s.p.a., Italy.

Stern, Ger. Pharma-stern GmbH, 22876 Wedel, Germany.

Sterwin, UK. See *Sanofi Synthelabo, UK.*

Stevens, USA. Jerome Stevens Pharmaceuticals, USA.

Stevia, Braz. Inga Stevia Industrial Ltda, Rua Stevia 300, Pq. Ind. Bandeirantes, 87070-100 Maringa, PR, Brazil.

Stewart Jackson, USA. Stewart-Jackson Pharmacal, 4200 Lamar, Suite 103, Memphis, TN 38118, USA.

Stickley, Canad. E.L. Stickley & Co. Ltd, Highway No. 2 E, Brantford, Ontario, N3T 5V7, Canada.

Stiefel, Austral. Stiefel Laboratories P/L, Unit 14, 5 Salisbury Road, Castle Hill, NSW 2154, Australia.

Stiefel, Braz. Laboratorios Stiefel Ltda, Rua Helena 235 (9° And.), 04552-050 Sao Paulo, SP, Brazil.

Stiefel, Canad. Stiefel Canada Inc., 6635 Henri-Bourassa Blvd W, Montreal, Quebec, H4R 1E1, Canada.

Stiefel, Denm. See *Ferring, Denm.*

Stiefel, Fin. See *Bitelab, Fin.*

Stiefel, Fr. Laboratoires Stiefel, ZI du Petit Nanterre, 15 rue des Grands Pres, 92000 Nanterre, France.

Stiefel, Ger. Stiefel Laboratorium GmbH, Muhlheimer Str. 231, 63075 Offenbach am Main, Germany.

Stiefel, Hong Kong. Stiefel Laboratories (Hong Kong) Ltd, 601B, 6F, Tower 2, Cheung Sha Wan Plaza, 833 Cheung Sha Wan Rd, Kowloon, Hong Kong.

Stiefel, Irl. See *Allphar, Irl.*

Stiefel, Israel. Stiefel, Israel.

Stiefel, Ital. Stiefel Laboratories s.r.l., Via Calabria 15, 20090 Redecesio di Segrate (MI), Italy.

Stiefel, Mex. Stiefel Mexicana S.A. de C.V., Eje Norte Sur No. 11, Nuevo Parque Industrial, 76809 San Juan del Rio, Qro., Mexico.

Stiefel, Neth. See *Bipharma, Neth.*

Stiefel, Norw. See *Scandinavian Health Care, Norw.*

Stiefel, NZ. See *Sparks, NZ.*

Stiefel, Port. Laboratórios Farmacêuticos Stiefel (Portugal), Lda, Av Maria Lamas, Lote 19, Bloco D, Piso 2, Serra das Minas, 2635-432 Rio de Mouro, Portugal.

Stiefel, S.Afr. Stiefel Laboratories SA (Pty) Ltd, P.O. Box 27114, Benrose 2011, South Africa.

Stiefel, Singapore. See *Diethelm, Singapore.*

Stiefel, Spain. Stiefel, Coto de Donana 11-13 Area, Andalucia Sector 1, Pinto, 28320 Madrid, Spain.

Stiefel, Switz. Stiefel Laboratorium AG, c/o Micucci Treuhand AG, Romertorstrasse 1, 8404 Winterthur, Switzerland.

Stiefel, Thai. See *Diethelm, Thai.*

Stiefel, UK. Stiefel Laboratories (UK) Ltd, Holtspur Lane, Wooburn Green, High Wycombe, Buckinghamshire, HP10 0AU, UK.

Stiefel, USA. Stiefel Laboratories Inc., 255 Alhambra Circle, Coral Gables, FL 33134, USA.

Stockhausen, USA. Stockhausen Inc., 2401 Doyle St, Greensboro, NC 27406, USA.

Stomygen, Ital. Gruppo Stomygen s.r.l., Via F. Jorini 69, 00149 Rome, Italy.

Storz, Israel. Storz, Israel.

Storz, Swed. Storz, Sweden.

Storz, UK. See *Cyanamid, UK.*

Stotzer, Switz. Stotzer AG, Jura-Apotheke Bern, Breitenrainplatz 40, 3000 Bern 22, Switzerland.

Strakan, UK. Strakan Ltd, Buckholm Mill, Buckholm Mill Brae, Galashiels, Scotland, TD1 2HB, UK.

Strallhofer, Aust. Mag. Dr. Till Strallhofer, St-Veit-Gasse 56, A-1030 Vienna, Austria.

Strathmann, Ger. Strathmann AG & Co., Sellhopsweg 1, 22459 Hamburg, Germany.

Stratus, USA. Stratus Pharmaceuticals Inc., 14377 SW 142nd St, P.O. Box 4632, Miami, FL 33186, USA.

Streger, Mex. Streger S.A., Km. 8 Antigua Carretera Xalapa-Coatepec, 91500 Consolapa-Coatepec, Ver., Mexico.

Streuli, Switz. G. Streuli & Co. AG, 8730 Uznach, Switzerland.

Strickland, Canad. See *Hargell, Canad.*

Stroder, Ital. Ist. Farmaco Biologico Stroder s.r.l., Via di Ripoli 207/V, 50126 Florence, Italy.

Stroschein, Ger. Pharma Stroschein GmbH, Sellhopsweg 1, Postfach: 610425, 22421 Hamburg, Germany.

Stuart, USA. See *AstraZeneca, USA.*

Stulln, Ger. Pharma Stulln GmbH, Werksweg 2, 92551 Stulln, Germany.

Stulln, Switz. See *Galenica, Switz.*

Substipharm, Fr. Lab. Substipharm, 264 rue du Fbg-St-Honore, 75008 Paris, France.

Suburfarm, Hong Kong. Suburfarm Investment & Trading Co. Ltd, Medical Health Care Division), Unit 7A-B, 39/F Wharf Cable Tower, 9 Hoi Shing Rd, Tsuen Wan, N.T., Hong Kong.

Sudmedica, Ger. Südmedica GmbH, Ehrwalder Str. 21, 81377 Munich, Germany.

Sudo, Singapore. See *Pharma 2000, Singapore.*

Sumitomo, Hong Kong. See *Main Life, Hong Kong.*

Sumitomo, Jpn. Sumitomo Pharmaceuticals Co. Ltd, 2-8 Doshomachi 2-chome, Chuo-ku, Osaka 541-8510, Japan.

Summers, USA. Summers Laboratories Inc., 103 G.P. Clement Dr., Collegeville, PA 19426, USA.

Summit, Port. See *Dario Correia, Port.*

Summit, Singapore. Summit Company (S) Ltd, 10 Pandan Crescent, 02-05 UE Tech Park, S 128466, Singapore.

Summit, USA. See *Novartis, USA.*

Sun, Canad. Sun Pharmaceutical Industries Inc., 1111 Flint Rd, Unit 23, Downsview, Ontario, M3J 3C7, Canada.

Sun, Singapore. See *Apotheca, Singapore.*

Sun, Thai. See *Pharmaland, Thai.*

Sun Hing, Hong Kong. Sun Hing Pharmaceutical Co. Ltd, Rm 1012, Blk 3, Nan Fung Ind City, 18 Tin Hau Rd, Tuen Mun, N.T., Hong Kong.

Sun Life, Fr. Lab. Sun Life, 33 rue Fortuny, 75017 Paris, France.

Sunde, Norw. Advokat Jens A. Sunde, Tidemandsg. 40, 0260 Oslo, Norway.

Sunrise, Austral. Sunrise Nutrition P/L, P.O. Box 355, Deepdene DC, VIC 3103, Australia.

Sunspot, Austral. Sunspot Products P/L, 303/20 Bungan Street, Mona Vale, NSW 2103, Australia.

Sunstar, Jpn. Sunstar Inc., 3-1 Asahimachi, Takatsuki City, Osaka 569-1195, Japan.

Suntory, Jpn. Suntory, Japan.

Sunward, Singapore. Sunward Pharmaceutical Pte Ltd, 11 Wan Lee Rd, Jurong, S 627943, Singapore.

Superfos Biosector, Norw. Superfos Kjemi Norge AS, Tvetenv 6, Postboks 6335 Etterstad, 0604 Oslo, Norway.

Supergen, USA. SuperGen Inc., 2 Annabel Lane, Suite 220, San Ramon, CA 94583, USA.

Surf Ski International, UK. Surf Ski International Ltd, UK.

Survival Technology, USA. Survival Technology Inc., 2275 Research Blvd, Rockville, MD 20850, USA.

Surya, Singapore. See *Polymedic, Singapore.*

Sussex, UK. Sussex Pharmaceutical Ltd, Charlwoods Rd, East Grinstead, Sussex, RH19 2HL, UK.

Sutton, Canad. HJ Sutton Industries Ltd, 8701 Jane St, Unit C, Vaughan, Ontario, L4K 2M6, Canada.

SVR, Fr. Lab. SVR, ZI La Tremblaie, B.P. 56, 91072 Bondoufle, France.

SVR, Ital. SVR Italia, Via Ca Rossa 10, 35010 Limena (PD), Italy.

Swedish Orphan, Irl. See *Cahill May Roberts, Irl.*

Swedish Orphan, Swed. Swedish Orphan AB, Drottninggatan 98, 111 60 Stockholm, Sweden.

Sween, USA. Sween Corp., Sween Building, P.O. Box 980, Lake Crystal, MN 56055, USA.

Swire Loxley, Hong Kong. Swire Loxley Ltd, 3/F Hong Kong Spinners Bldg, 800 Cheung Sha Wan Rd, Kowloon, Hong Kong.

Swiss Herbal, Canad. Swiss Herbal Remedies Ltd, 35 Leek Cres, Richmond Hill, Ontario, L4B 4C2, Canada.

Swiss Serum Institute, Israel. Swiss Serum Institute, Israel.

Swiss Worldwide, Hong Kong. Swiss Worldwide Ltd, 9C Ho King Bldg, 128 On Ling Rd, Yuen Long, Hong Kong.

Swisshealth, UK. SwissHealth, UK.

Swisspharm, S.Afr. Swisspharm (Pty) Ltd, South Africa.

Sydenham, Mex. Sydenham, Mexico.

Sylak, Swed. Sylak AB, Box 1228, 600 42 Norrkoping, Sweden.

Symbiopharm, Ger. SymbioPharm GmbH, Auf den Luppen, 35745 Herborn-Horbach, Germany.

Synapse, Irl. Synapse Medical, 94 Griffith Ave, Drumcondra, Dublin 9, Ireland.

Synco, Hong Kong. Synco (HK) Ltd, Blk D, 3/F, Sun View Industrial Bldg, 3 On Yip St, Chaiwan, Hong Kong.

Syner-Med, UK. Syner-Med (Pharmaceutical Products) Ltd, Airport House, Purley Way, Croydon, Surrey, CR0 0XZ, UK.

Synmedic, Switz. Synmedic AG, Seebahnstrasse 85, Postfach, 8036 Zurich, Switzerland.

Synpharma, Aust. Synpharma GmbH, Wiener Bundesstrasse 21 PF.4, A-5300 Hallwang bei Salzburg, Austria.

Synpharma, Switz. Synpharma AG, Postfach, 9240 Uzwil, Switzerland.

Syntetic, Denm. A/S Syntetic, Edwin Rahrs Vej 38, 8220 Brabrand, Denmark.

Syntex, Austral. Syntex Australia Ltd, P.O. Box 255, Dee Why, NSW 2099, Australia.

Syntex, Canad. See *Roche, Canad.*

Syntex, Ger. Syntex GmbH, Emil-Barell-Strasse 1, 79639 Grenzach-Wyhlen, Germany.

Syntex, Mex. Syntex S.A. de C.V., Division Farmaceutica, Carr. Mexico-Toluca No. 2822, Col. Lomas de Bezares, 11000 Mexico D.F., Mexico.

Syntex, Neth. Syntex B.V., Netherlands.

Syntex, NZ. Syntex Laboratories (NZ) Ltd, P.O. Box 12-492, Penrose, Auckland, New Zealand.

Syntex, S.Afr. Syntex Pharmaceuticals (Pty) Ltd, P.O. Box 89566, Lyndhurst, South Africa.

Syntex, Spain. Syntex Roche, C/Severo Ochoa 13, Leganes, 28914 Madrid, Spain.

Syntex, Swed. Syntex Nordica AB, Box 19003, 152 25 Sodertalje, Sweden.

Syntex, Switz. See *Uhlmann-Eyraud, Switz.*

Syntex, UK. See *Roche, UK.*

Syntex, USA. See *Roche, USA.*

Synthelabo, Belg. See *Sanofi Synthelabo, Belg.*

Synthelabo, Braz. Synthelabo Espasil Quimica Farmaceutica Ltda, Estrada do Guerengue 1.851, 22713-001 Rio de Janeiro, RJ, Brazil.

Synthelabo, Fr. See *Sanofi Synthelabo, Fr.*, and *Sanofi Synthelabo OTC, Fr.*

Synthelabo, Ger. See *Sanofi Synthelabo, Ger.*

Synthelabo, Hong Kong. Synthelabo Groupe, 7/F Somerset House, Taikoo Place, Quarry Bay, Hong Kong.

Synthelabo, Israel. See *Mediline, Israel.*

Synthelabo, Ital. See *Sanofi Synthelabo, Ital.*

Synthelabo, Port. Synthelabo, Lda, Estrada da Circunvalacao, Romeiras, Alges, 1495 Lisbon, Portugal.

Synthelabo, Spain. Synthelabo Pharma, Ramirez de Arellano 31, 28043 Madrid, Spain.

Synthelabo, Switz. See *Sanofi Synthelabo, Switz.*

Synthes, Aust. Synthes GmbH, Karolingerstrasse 16, A-5035 Salzburg, Austria.

Syosset, USA. Syosset Laboratories Inc., 150 Eileen Way, Syosset, NY 11791, USA.

Syxyl, Ger. Syxyl GmbH & Co. KG, Gereonsmuhlengasse 5, 50670 Cologne, Germany.

Tack Fung, Hong Kong. Tack Fung Medical Supplies Co., Rm 504, Tien Cheung Hong Bldg, 77-81 Jervois St Central, Hong Kong.

Taco, Ger. Taco-GmbH, Chem.-Pharm. Fabrik, Alte Heerstr. 76, 53757 St. Augustin, Germany.

TAD, Ger. TAD Pharma GmbH, Heinz-Lohmann-Str. 5, 27472 Cuxhaven, Germany.

Tai Fung, Hong Kong. Tai Fung Trading Co., 45 Hankow Rd, Flat C, 9/F, Kowloon, Hong Kong.

Tai Guk, Singapore. See *Polymedic, Singapore.*

Tai Tong, Hong Kong. Tai Tong Co. Ltd, Rm 901-2, Alliance Bldg, 130-136 Connaught Rd Central, Hong Kong.

Taiho, Jpn. Taiho Pharmaceutical Co. Ltd, 1-27 Kandanishiki-cho, Chiyoda-ku, Tokyo 101-8444, Japan.

Taiho, Singapore. See *Luen Wah, Singapore.*

Takeda, Aust. Takeda Pharma GmbH, Siedengasse 33-35/4, A-1070 Vienna, Austria.

Takeda, Fr. Laboratoires Takeda, 15 quai de Dion-Bouton, 92816 Puteaux cdx, France.

Takeda, Ger. Takeda Pharma GmbH, Viktoriaallee 3-5, 52066 Aachen, Germany.

Takeda, Hong Kong. Takeda IMC Chemical Ltd, Rm 1801-2, 18/F Rook Lee Commercial Ctr, Town Place, 33 Lockhart Rd, Wanchai, Hong Kong.

Takeda, Israel. Takeda, Israel.

Takeda, Ital. Takeda Italia Farmaceutici s.p.a., Via Elio Vittorini 129, 00144 Rome, Italy.

Takeda, Jpn. Takeda Chemical Industries Ltd, 1-1 Doshomachi 4-chome, Chuo-ku, Osaka 540-8645, Japan.

Takeda, Singapore. See *Luen Wah, Singapore.*

Takeda, Switz. Takeda Pharma AG, Alpenblickstrasse 26, 8853 Lachen, Switzerland.

Takeda, Thai. Takeda (Thailand) Ltd, 12A Fl, Si Ayutthaya Building, Si Ayutthaya Rd, 487/1 Ratchathewi, Bangkok 10400, Thailand.

Takeda, UK. Takeda UK Ltd, Takeda House, The Mercury Centre, Wycombe Lane, Wooburn Green, High Wycombe, Buckinghamshire, HP10 0HH, UK.

Takeda, USA. Takeda Pharmaceuticals America, 475 Half Day Rd, Suite 500, Lincolnshire, IL 60069, USA.

Tamar, Israel. Tamar, Israel.

Tamro, Fin. Tamro Distribution/Pharmakon, Rajatorpantie 41 B, 01640 Vantaa, Finland.

Tanabe, Hong Kong. See *Primal, Hong Kong.*

Tanabe, Jpn. See *Mitsubishi-Tokyo, Jpn.*

Tanabe, Singapore. Tanabe Seiyaku Singapore Pte Ltd, 10 Hoe Chiang Rd, 14-02 Keppel Towers, S 089315, Singapore.

Tanabe, Thai. See *Wellchem, Thai.*

Tanning Research, Canad. See *Tropic Suncare, Canad.*

Tanning Research, USA. Tanning Research Labs Inc., 1190 US 1 North, Ormond Beach, FL 32174, USA.

Tanta, Canad. Tanta Pharmaceuticals Inc., 1009 Burns St East, Whitby, Ontario, L1N 6A6, Canada.

TAP, USA. TAP Pharmaceuticals Inc., 2355 Waukegan Rd, Deerfield, IL 60015, USA.

Taphlan, Switz. See *Serolab, Switz.*

Taranis, Fr. Taranis, 6 rue de Trésor, 75004 Paris, France.

Taro, Canad. Taro Pharmaceuticals Inc., 130 East Drive, Bramalea, Ontario, L6T 1C3, Canada.

Taro, Israel. Taro Ltd, P.O Box 2043, Herzeliya Pituach, Israel.

Taro, Thai. See *Union Medical, Thai.*

Taro, UK. Taro Pharmaceuticals (UK) Ltd, Riverside House, Station Rd, Bishops Stortford, Hertfordshire, CM23 3AJ, UK.

Taro, USA. Taro Pharmaceuticals USA Inc., 5 Skyline Drive, Hawthorne, NY 10532-9998, USA.

Taurus, Ger. Taurus Pharma GmbH, Berner Str. 40-42, 60437 Frankfurt, Germany.

Tava, Israel. Tava, Israel.

Taxandria, Neth. Taxandria Pharmaceutica B.V., Postbus 90241, 5000 LV Tilburg, Netherlands.

Taylor, USA. Taylor Pharmaceuticals, P.O. Box 5136, San Clemente, CA 92674-5136, USA.

TC Technocare, Israel. TC Technocare Ltd, Industrial Park, Caesarea, Israel.

Tec, USA. Tec Laboratories Inc., 615 Water Ave NE, P.O. Box 1958, Albany, OR 97321-0512, USA.

Tecefarma, Spain. Tecefarma, Guifre 724, Badalona, 08912 Barcelona, Spain.

Technikon, S.Afr. Technikon Laboratories, P.O. Box 150, Maraisburg 1700, South Africa.

Technilab, Canad. Technilab Pharma Inc., 17, 800 Lapointe St, Mirabel, Quebec, J7J 1P3, Canada.

Technilab, Hong Kong. See *Hind Wing, Hong Kong.*

Techni-Pharma, Mon. Techni-Pharma, 7 rue de l'Industrie, B.P. 717, MC 98014, Monaco.

Tecnifar, Port. Tecnifar, SA, Rua Tierno Galvan, Torre 3, 12 Piso, 1099-036 Lisbon, Portugal.

Tecnimede, Port. Tecnimede, SA, Urbanizacao Quinta Nova, Rua B Lote 131-A, 2685 Sacavem, Portugal.

Tecnobio, Spain. Tecnobio, Rda Gral Mitre 151, 08022 Barcelona, Spain.

Tecnofarma, Mex. Tecnofarma S.A. de C.V., Azafran No. 123, Col. Granjas Mexico, 08400 Mexico D.F., Mexico.

Tedec Meiji, Israel. Tedec Meiji, Israel.

Tedec Meiji, Spain. Tedec Meiji Farma, Ctra M-300, Km 30.5, Alcala De Henares, 28820 Madrid, Spain.

Teekanne, Aust. Teekanne GmbH, Munchner Bundesstrasse 120, A-5021 Salzburg, Austria.

Tegur, Mex. Tegur, Mexico.

Teijin, Thai. See *Berli, Thai.*

Teikoku, Jpn. Teikoku Hormone Mfg Co. Ltd, 5-1 Akasaka 2-chome, Minato-ku, Tokyo 107-8522, Japan.

Teknofarma, Ital. Teknofarma s.p.a., S. Bertolla Abb. Stura 14, 10156 Turin, Italy.

Telluride, USA. Telluride Pharm. Corp, 146 Flanders Drive, Hillsborough, NJ 08876-4656, USA.

Tema, S.Afr. Tema Medical (Pty) Ltd, P.O. Box 3467, Cramerview 2060, South Africa.

Temmler, Denm. See *Kemifarma, Denm.*

Temmler, Ger. Temmler Pharma GmbH & Co. KG, Temmlerstr. 2, 35039 Marburg/Lahn, Germany.

Temmler, Israel. Temmler, Israel.

Temmler, Port. See *Confar, Port.*

Temmler, Thai. See *Zuellig, Thai.*

Tendem, Neth. Tendem B.V., Postbus 190, 8000 AD Zwolle, Netherlands.

Tender, Canad. Tender Corp. Canada, 18 Alliance Blvd, Unit 10, Barrie, Ontario, L4M 5A5, Canada.

Tender, Israel. See *Meditrend, Israel.*

Tentan, Switz. Tentan AG, Brunnliweg 16, 4433 Ramlinsburg, Switzerland.

Teofarma, Fr. See *Teofarma, Ital.*

Teofarma, Ital. Teofarma, Via F.lli Cervi 5, 27100 Valle Salimbene (PV), Italy.

Teofarma, Spain. Teofarma Iberica, Alfonso XII 19, 08006 Barcelona, Spain.

Teomed, Switz. Teomed AG, Tumigerstrasse 71, Postfach 20, 8606 Greifensee, Switzerland.

Teral, USA. See *Bart, USA.*

Terapeutico, Ital. Labor. Terapeutico M.R. s.r.l., Via Domenico Veneziano 13, 50143 Florence, Italy.

Terapia, Mex. Terapia, Mexico.

Teravix, Port. Teravix, Lda, Av Antonio Augusto de Aguiar 128, 1050 Lisbon, Portugal.

Terme di Chianciano, Ital. Terme di Chianciano s.p.a., Via delle Rose 12, 53042 Chianciano Terme (Siena), Italy.

Terme di Montecatini, Ital. Terme di Montecatini s.p.a., Viale Marconi 7, 51016 Montecatini Terme (PT), Italy.

Terme di Salsomaggiore, Ital. Terme di Salsomaggiore s.p.a., Via Roma 9, 43039 Salsomaggiore Terme (Parma), Italy.

Terme Sirmione, Ital. Terme Sirmione spa, Piazza Castello 12, 25019 Sirmione (BS), Italy.

Terra-Bio, Ger. Terra-Bio-Chemie GmbH, Ekkebertstr. 28, 79117 Freiburg i. Br., Germany.

Terrafor, Fr. Lab. Terrafor, B.P. 62, 76302 Sotteville-les-Rouen cdx, France.

Terralife, Aust. Terralife Pharma GmbH, Moosham 29, A-5580 Unternberg, Austria.

Terramin, Aust. Terramin Pharma GmbH & Co. KEG, Maria Pfarr 135, A-5571, Austria.

Terrapharm, Aust. Terrapharm Pharm. Produktions- und HandelsGmbH, Braunlichgasse 40-2, A-2700 Wiener Neustadt, Austria.

Terrier, Mex. See *Columbia, Mex.*

Tetido, Ital. Te.Ti.Do di Brunelli Donata sas, Via Bevanella 60, 48010 Savio (RA), Italy.

Teuto, Braz. Laboratorio Teuto-Brasileiro Ltda, VP 7-D Modulo 11 Quadra 13, 75133-600 Anapolis, GO, Brazil.

Teva, Canad. Teva Marion Partners Canada, 1 Place Ville-Marie, Suite 1640, Montreal, Quebec, H3B 2B6, Canada.

Teva, Denm. See *PCH, Neth.*

Teva, Ger. TEVA Generics GmbH, Kandelstr. 10, 79199 Kirchzarten, Germany.

Teva, Hong Kong. See *Primal, Hong Kong.*

Teva, Israel. Teva Medical Ltd, P.O. Box 8077, Netanya, Israel.

Teva, Ital. Teva Pharma Italia s.r.l., Via Pannonia 6, 20133 Milan, Italy.

Teva, S.Afr. See *Teva, Israel.*

Teva, Singapore. See *Green Cross, Singapore.*

Teva, Thai. See *RX, Thai.,* and *Union Medical, Thai.*

Teva, UK. Teva Pharmaceuticals Ltd, Barclays House, 1 Gatehouse Way, Aylesbury, Buckinghamshire, HP19 8DB, UK.

Teva, USA. Teva Pharmaceuticals USA, 151 Donorah Drive, Montgomeryville, PA 18936, USA.

Thackray, UK. See *DePuy, UK.*

Thai Otsuka, Thai. Thai Otsuka Pharmaceutical Co. Ltd, 11 Fl, Regent House Building, 183 Rajdamri Rd, Khwang Lumpini, Khet Pathumwan, Bangkok 10330, Thailand.

Thaipharmed, Thai. See *ST, Thai.*

Thames, UK. Thames Laboratories Ltd, Abbey House, Wrexham Industrial Estate, Wrexham, Clwyd, LL13 9PW, UK.

Thames, USA. Thames Pharmacal Co. Inc., 2100 Fifth Ave, Ronkonkoma, NY 11779-6906, USA.

The Forty-Two, Thai. See *Siam Medicare, Thai.*

Thea, Fr. Laboratoires Théa, 12 rue Louis-Bleriot, 63016 Clermont-Ferrand cdx 2, France.

Thea, Hong Kong. See *Silroc, Hong Kong.*

Thea, Spain. Thea, Balmes 49, 08007 Barcelona, Spain.

Thepenier, Fr. Laboratoires Thépénier, 10 rue Clapeyron, 75008 Paris, France.

Thepenier, Switz. See *Uhlmann-Eyraud, Switz.*

Thera, Fr. See *Alpharma, Fr.*

Therabel, Belg. Therabel Pharma S.A., Rue Egide Van Ophen 108, 1180 Brussels, Belgium.

Therabel, Fr. Laboratoires Thérabel Lucien Pharma, 15 rue de l'Hotel-de-Ville, 92522 Neuilly-sur-Seine cdx, France.

Therabel, Ital. Therabel Pharma s.p.a., Via Lorenteggio 270/a, 20152 Milan, Italy.

Therakos, USA. Therakos, USA.

Theralab, Canad. See *E-Z-EM, Canad.*

Theramex, Hong Kong. See *Hind Wing, Hong Kong.*

Theramex, Ital. Theramex s.p.a., Via Mancinelli 11, 20131 Milan, Italy.

Theramex, Mon. Laboratoires Théramex, 6 av. Prince-Hereditaire-Albert, B.P. 59, MC 98007, Monaco.

Theramex, Singapore. See *Pharmacon, Singapore.*

Theranol-Deglaude, Fr. See *DB, Fr.*

Therapeutic-Ocean, Singapore. See *Zuellig, Singapore.*

Therapex, Canad. See *E-Z-EM, Canad.*

Therapharm, Austral. See *AstraZeneca, Austral.*

Therapharma, Thai. See *Olic, Thai.*

Theraplix, Fr. See *Aventis, Fr.*

Therasophia, Fr. Therasophia, 294 av. du Golf, 06250 Mougins, France.

Theratech, Fr. Laboratoires Theratech, 6 rue Dubais, 27000 Evreux, France.

Theriaca, Ital. Theriaca s.r.l., Palazzina C Int. 2, Via Pietroantonio Micheli 78, 00197 Rome, Italy.

Therica, Fr. See *Bailleul, Fr.*

Thermalife, Austral. Thermalife International Pharmaceuticals Ltd, Australia.

Ther-Rx, USA. Ther-Rx Corp., 13622 Lakefront Dr., Earth City, MO 63045, USA.

Therval, Fr. Therval Medical, 29 rue du Pont, 92200 Neuilly-sur-Seine, France.

Thiemann, Ger. Thiemann Arzneimittel GmbH, Im Wirrigen 25, 45731 Waltrop, Germany.

Thilo, Hong Kong. See *Health Care, Hong Kong.*

Thilo, Neth. See *Bournonville, Neth.*

Thomae, Ger. See *Boehringer Ingelheim, Ger.*

Thompson, Austral. Thompson, Australia.

Thompson, UK. Thompson Medical Co. Ltd, Riding Court, Riding Court Rd, Datchet, Slough, Berkshire, SL3 9JT, UK.

Thompson, USA. Thompson Medical Co. Inc., 777 S Flagler, West Palm Beach, FL 33401, USA.

Thornton & Ross, UK. Thornton & Ross Ltd, Linthwaite Laboratories, Huddersfield, West Yorkshire, HD7 5QH, UK.

Thuasne, Fr. Thuasne SA, 118-120 rue Marius-Aufan, B.P. 243, 92300 Levallois-Perret, France.

Thuna, Canad. Thuna Herbal Remedies Ltd, 298 Danforth Ave, Toronto, Ontario, M4K 1N6, Canada.

Tika, Norw. See *AstraZeneca, Norw.*

Tika, Swed. Tika Läkemedel AB, 221 87 Lund, Sweden.

Tillomed, UK. Tillomed Laboratories Ltd, 3 Howard Rd, Eaton Socon, St Neots, Cambridgeshire, PE19 3ET, UK.

Tillotts, Hong Kong. See *Associated Medical, Hong Kong.*

Tillotts, Israel. Tillotts, Israel.

Tillotts, NZ. See *Baxter, NZ.*

Tillotts, Singapore. See *Wellchem, Singapore.*

Tillotts, Switz. Tillotts Pharma AG, Hauptstrasse 27, 4417 Ziefen, Switzerland.

Tillotts, Thai. See *Union Medical, Thai.*

Time-Cap, Hong Kong. See *Sheraton, Hong Kong.*

Time-Cap, USA. Time-Cap Labs Inc., 7 Michael Ave, Farmingdale, NY 11735, USA.

Tipomark, Ital. Tipomark s.r.l., Via Ippolito Nievo 28/1, 20145 Milan, Italy.

Tiroler, Aust. Tiroler Steinölwerke OHG, A-6213 Pertisau am Achensee, Tirol, Austria.

Tishcon, Hong Kong. See *International Medical, Hong Kong.*

Tissot, Fr. Laboratoires du Dr Tissot, 3 rue de Versailles, 78470 St-Remy-les-Chevreuse, France.

Tjellesen, Denm. E. Tjellesen A/S, Blokken 81, 3460 Birkerod, Denmark.

TNP, Thai. TNP Health Care Co. Ltd, 94/7 Soi Yimprakrob, Ngamwongwan Rd, Nonthaburi 11000, Thailand.

TO-Chemicals, Singapore. See *Advanced, Singapore.*

TO-Chemicals, Thai. TO-Chemicals (1979) Ltd, 280 Soi Sabai Jai, Suthisarn Rd, Bangkok 10320, Thailand.

Tocogino, Mex. Tocogino, Mexico.

Togal, Ger. Togal-Werk AG, Ismaninger Str.105, 81675 Munich, Germany.

Togal, Switz. Togal-Werk SA, Via Val Gersa 4, 6900 Lugano-Massagno, Switzerland.

Toho, Hong Kong. See *Primal, Hong Kong.*

Toho, Thai. See *Diethelm, Thai.*

Tokyo Tanabe, Hong Kong. See *Hing Ah, Hong Kong.*

Tokyo Tanabe, Jpn. Tokyo Tanabe Co. Ltd, 2-6 Nihonbashi-Honcho 2-chome, Chuo-ku, Tokyo 103-8405, Japan.

Topfer, Ger. Töpfer GmbH, Heisingerstr. 6, 87463 Dietmannsried, Germany.

Toray, Jpn. Toray Industries Inc., 2-1 Nihonbashi-Muromachi 2-chome, Chuo-ku, Tokyo 103-8666, Japan.

Torbet, Irl. See *Allphar, Irl.*

Torbet Laboratories, UK. Torbet Laboratories Ltd, 57/58 King St, Great Yarmouth, Norfolk, NR30 2PW, UK.

Torfwerk Einfeld, Ger. Torfwerk Einfeld Carl Hornung, Seekamp 2, Postfach: 2667, 24516 Neumunster, Germany.

Torii, Hong Kong. See *Hing Yip, Hong Kong.*

Torlan, Spain. Torlan, Ctra Barcelona 135-B, Cerdenola del Valles, 08290 Barcelona, Spain.

Torre, Ital. Dr. A. Torre Farmaceutici s.r.l., Viale E. Forlanini 15, 20134 Milan, Italy.

Torrens, Spain. Torrens, Camino del Hospital S/N, Olesa de Bonevalls, 08739 Barcelona, Spain.

Torrent, Thai. See *Union Medical, Thai.*

Torrex, Aust. Torrex Pharma GmbH, Lange Gasse 76/12, A-1080 Vienna, Austria.

Tosara, Irl. Tosara Products Ltd, Baldoyle Industrial Estate, Dublin 13, Ireland.

Tosara, UK. See *Forest Laboratories, UK.*

Tosi, Hong Kong. See *Sincerity, Hong Kong.*

Tosi, Ital. Tosi Farmaceutici sas di Silvana Tosi & C, C.so della Vittoria 12/B, 28100 Novara, Italy.

Tosse, Ger. E. Tosse & Co. mbH, Friedrich-Ebert-Damm 101, Postfach: 701648, 22016 Hamburg, Germany.

Toulade, Fr. Laboratoires Toulade, av. du Docteur-Aubry, 76280 Criquetot-L'Esneval, France.

Toyama, Jpn. Toyama Chemical Co., Ltd, 2-5 Nishishinjuku 3-chome, Shinjuku-ku, Tokyo 160-0023, Japan.

Toyo, Hong Kong. See *Hing Yip, Hong Kong.*

TP, Thai. TP Drug Lab Co. Ltd, 67 Sukhumvit 62, Prakanong, Bangkok 10250, Thailand.

Trading, Israel. Trading Pharma A.G., 11 Haodem St, Petach Tikva, Israel.

Tradiphar, Fr. Lab. Tradiphar, 176 rue de l'Arbrisseau, 59000 Lille, France.

Tramedico, Belg. Tramedico S.A., Europark-Oost 34, PB 50, 9100 Sint-Niklaas, Belgium.

Tramedico, Neth. Tramedico B.V., Postbus 192, 1380 AD Weesp, Netherlands.

Trans Bussan, Switz. trans bussan s.a., 12 Rue Michel-Servet, 1211 Geneva 12, Switzerland.

Trans Canaderm, Canad. See *Stiefel, Canad.*

Transphyto, Fr. Laboratoires Transphyto, 12 rue Louis-Blériot, 63100 Clermont-Ferrand, France.

Travenol, UK. Travenol Laboratories Ltd, Caxton Way, Thetford, Norfolk, IP24 3SE, UK.

TRB, Braz. TRB Pharma Industria Quimica e Farmaceutica Ltda, Rua Hildebrando Siqueira 149, Americanopolis, 04334-150 Sao Paulo, SP, Brazil.

Treasure Mountain, Hong Kong. Treasure Mountain Development Co. Ltd, 19/F Chit Lee Commercial Bldg, 30-36 Shaukeiwan Rd, Hong Kong.

Treiner, USA. Treiner Co, USA.

Tremedic, Swed. Tremedic AB, Faktorvagen 13, 434 37 Kungsbacka, Sweden.

Trendful, Hong Kong. Trendful Development Ltd, Rm 306, 3/F, Bonham Trade Ctr, 50 Bonham Strand, Sheung Wan, Hong Kong.

Trenier, USA. Trenier, USA.

Trenka, Aust. F Trenka Chemisch-Pharmazeutische Fabrik GmbH, Goldeggasse 5, A-1040 Vienna, Austria.

Trenka, Israel. Trenka, Israel.

Trenka, Switz. See *Uhlmann-Eyraud, Switz.*

Trenka Difer, Ital. Trenka Difer International s.r.l., Via della Zonta 2, 34122 Trieste, Italy.

Trenker, Belg. Laboratoires Pharmaceutiques Trenker S.A., Ave Dolez 480-2, 1180 Brussels, Belgium.

Trenker, Thai. See *Union Medical, Thai.*

Treupha, Switz. Treupha SA, Zurcherstrasse 59, 5401 Baden, Switzerland.

Tri Tec, USA. Tri Tec Labs, 1000 Robins Rd, Lynchburg, VA 24504-3558, USA.

Triangle, USA. See *Tri Tec, USA.*

Trianon, Canad. Trianon Laboratories Inc., 660 Industriel Blvd, Blainville, Quebec, J7C 3V4, Canada.

Trima, Israel. Trima, Kibbutz Ma'abarot, Israel.

Trima, Singapore. See *Green Cross, Singapore.*

Trima, Thai. See *Union Medical, Thai.*

Tri-Med Specialties, USA. Tri-Med Specialties Inc., 16309 W 108th Circle, Lenexa, KS 66219-1372, USA.

Trimedal, Switz. Trimedal AG, Postfach, 8306 Bruttisellen, Switzerland.

Trimen, USA. Trimen Laboratories Inc., USA.

Trinity, Hong Kong. Trinity Trading Co. Ltd, Unit 7A-B, 39/F Cable TV Tower, 9 Hoi Shing Rd, Tsuen Wan, N.T., Hong Kong.

Trinity, UK. Trinity Pharmaceuticals Ltd, The Old Exchange, 12 Compton Rd, Wimbledon, London, SW19 7QD, UK.

Triomed, S.Afr. Triomed (Pty) Ltd, P.O. Box 36679, Chempet 7442, South Africa.

Tripharma, Switz. Tripharma AG, 8730 Uznach, Switzerland.

Triton, USA. Triton Consumer Products, Inc., 561 West Golf, Arlington Heights, IL 60005, USA.

Trofomed, Ital. Trofomed s.r.l., Via IV Novembre 7, 70020 Cassano delle Murge (BA), Italy.

Trommsdorff, Ger. Trommsdorff GmbH & Co. KG Arzneimittel, Trommsdorffstr. 2-6, 52475 Alsdorf, Germany.

Tropic Suncare, Canad. Tropic Suncare Canada Ltd, P. O. Box 6249, Station D, London, Ontario, N5W 5S1, Canada.

Trupharm, Israel. Trupharm, P.O. Box 8105, Poleg Industrial Estate, South Netanya, Israel.

Truw, Ger. Truw Arzneimittel Vertriebs GmbH, Ziethenstr. 8, 33330 Gutersloh, Germany.

Truxton, USA. C.O. Truxton Inc., 136 Harding Ave, Bellmawr, NJ 08099, USA.

Tsumura, Jpn. Tsumura, Japan.

Tsun Tsun, Hong Kong. Tsun Tsun Trading Co. Ltd, Rm 502, Sea View Estate 5/F, Blk B, Watson Rd, Hong Kong.

TTN, Thai. TTN Thitiratsanon Co. Ltd, 157/9 Prannok Rd, Siriraj Bangkoknoi, Bangkok 10700, Thailand.

Tubilux, Ital. Tubilux Pharma s.p.a., Via Costarica 20/22, 00040 Pomezia (RM), Italy.

Turimed, Switz. Turimed SA, Hertiststrasse 8, 8304 Wallisellen, Switzerland.

Tutogen, Ger. Tutogen Medical GmbH, Industriestr. 6, 91077 Neunkirchen a. Br., Germany.

Twardy, Aust. See *Twardy, Ger.*

Twardy, Ger. Astrid Twardy GmbH, Liebigstr. 18, 65439 Florsheim/Main, Germany.

Tweezerman, USA. Tweezerman, 55 Sea Cliff Ave, Glen Cove, NY 11542-3695, USA.

Typharm, Irl. See *Boileau & Boyd, Irl.*

Typharm, UK. Typharm Ltd, 57/58 King St, Great Yarmouth, Norfolk, NR30 2PW, UK.

Tyrol, Aust. Tyrol Pharma GmbH, Biochemiestrasse 10, A-6250 Kundl, Austria.

Tyson, USA. Tyson & Associates Inc., 12832 S Chadron Ave, Hawthorne, CA 90250-5525, USA.

UAD, USA. See *Forest Laboratories, USA.*

UB Interpharm, Switz. UB Interpharm SA, 36 av Cardinal-Mermillod, 1227 Carouge/GE, Switzerland.

UCB, Aust. UCB Pharma GmbH, Brunnerstrasse 73/5, A-1210 Vienna, Austria.

UCB, Belg. UCB Pharma S.A., Route de Lennik 437, 1070 Brussels, Belgium.

UCB, Canad. See *UCB, USA.*

UCB, Denm. UCB Pharma, HC Orsteds Vej 27, 1, 1879 Frederiksberg C, Denmark.

UCB, Fin. UCB Pharma Oy Finland, Ratavallintie 2, 00720 Helsinki, Finland.

UCB, Fr. UCB Pharma S.A., 21 rue de Neuilly, 92003 Nanterre, France.

UCB, Ger. UCB GmbH, Huttenstr. 205, 50170 Kerpen, Germany.

UCB, Hong Kong. UCB Pharma Ltd, 6A On Hing Bldg, 1 On Hing Terrace Central, Hong Kong.

UCB, Irl. See *United Drug, Irl.*

UCB, Ital. UCB Pharma s.p.a., Via Praglia 15, 10044 Pianezza (TO), Italy.

UCB, Jpn. UCB Japan, Japan.

UCB, Mex. UCB de Mexico, S.A. de C.V., Homero No. 1804-903, Col. Chapultepec Morales, 11570 Mexico, D.F., Mexico.

UCB, Neth. UCB Pharma B.V., Postbus 6851, 4802 HW Breda, Netherlands.

UCB, Norw. UCB Pharma AS, Brynsv. 96, 1352 Kolsas, Norway.

UCB, Port. UCB, Lda, Rua Gregorio Lopes, Lote 1597, 1400-195 Lisbon, Portugal.

UCB, S.Afr. UCB SA (Pty) Ltd, P.O. Box 31036, Braamfontein 2017, South Africa.

UCB, Singapore. UCB Singapore Pte Ltd, 30 Prinsep St, 03-02 LKN Prinsep House, S 188647, Singapore.

UCB, Spain. UCB Pharma, Avda de Barcelona 239, Molins de Rei, 08750 Barcelona, Spain.

UCB, Swed. UCB Pharma AB (Sweden), 212 25 Malmo, Sweden.

UCB, Switz. UCB-Pharma AG, Pharmazeutische Produkte, Klosbachstrasse 2, 8032 Zurich, Switzerland.

UCB, Thai. UCB Pharma (Thailand) Ltd, 27 Fl, Panjathani Tower, 127/32 Nonsee Rd, Yannawa, Bangkok 10120, Thailand.

UCB, UK. UCB Pharma Ltd, 3 George St, Watford, Hertforshire, WD1 8UH, UK.

UCB, USA. UCB Pharma Inc., 1950 Lake Park Drive, Atlanta, GA 30080, USA.

UCI, Braz. UCI-Farma Industria Farmaceutica Ltda, Rua Cruzeiro 374, 09725-310 Sao Bernardo do Campo, SP, Brazil.

Ucyclyd, USA. Ucyclyd Pharma Inc., 500 McCormic Dr., Suite J, Glen Burnie, MD 21061, USA.

Ueno, Jpn. Ueno Fine Chemicals Industry Ltd, 4-8 Koraibashi 2-chome, Chuo-ku, Osaka 541-8543, Japan.

Uhlmann-Eyraud, Switz. F. Uhlmann-Eyraud SA, 28 chemin du Grand-Puits, 1217 Meyrin 2/Geneva, Switzerland.

Ulmer, USA. Ulmer Pharmacal Co., 2440 Fernbrook Lane, Plymouth, MN 55447-9987, USA.

Ultrapharm, UK. Ultrapharm Ltd, 1,2,3 Centenary Business Park, Henley-on-Thames, Oxfordshire, RG9 1DS, UK.

Unam, Hong Kong. Unam Corp Ltd, 7/F Chiu Lung Bldg, 25 Chiu Lung St Central, Hong Kong.

Ungar, Aust. Ungar-Apotheke zur Göttlichen Vorsehung, Ungargasse 14, A-1030 Vienna, Austria.

Uniao Quimica, Braz. Uniao Quimica Farmaceutica Nacional S.A., Avenida dos Bandeirantes 5386, 04071-900 Sao Paulo, SP, Brazil.

Unibios, Spain. Unibios, Spain.

Unichem, UK. Unichem Ltd, Unichem House, Cox Lane, Chessington, Surrey, KT9 1SN, UK.

Unico, Hong Kong. Unico Health Care Products Ltd, Rm 1007, Tower B Seaview Estate, 2-8 Watson Rd, North Point, Hong Kong.

Unico, USA. Unico Inc., 1830 2nd Ave N, Lake Worth, FL 33461, USA.

Uniderm, Israel. Uniderm, Israel.

Uniderm, Ital. Uniderm Farmaceutici s.r.l., Via G. Armandi 64, 00126 Rome Acilia, Italy.

Unifa, Port. See *CPH, Port.*

Unifarma, Spain. Unifarma, Spain.

Unigene, UK. Unigene UK Ltd, 63 High Rd, Bushey Heath, Hertfordshire, WD2 1EE, UK.

Unigreg, Irl. See *Unigreg, UK.*

Unigreg, UK. Unigreg Ltd, Enterprise House, 181-9 Garth Rd, Morden, Surrey, SM4 4LL, UK.

Unilever, USA. Unilever HPC, 33 Benedict Place, Greenwich, CT 06830, USA.

Unimed, Israel. Unimed, Israel.

Unimed, USA. Unimed Pharmaceuticals Inc., 2150 E. Lake Cook Road, Buffalo Grove, IL 60089-1862, USA.

Unimedic, Swed. Unimedic AB, Box 91, 864 21 Matfors, Sweden.

Union, Singapore. Union Chem & Pharm, Singapore.

Union Medical, Thai. Union Medical (Thailand) Co. Ltd, 513/199-200 Jaransanitwong Rd, Soi 37 Bangkoknoi, Bangkok 10700, Thailand.

Unipack, Aust. Unipack GmbH, Braunligasse 40-2, A-2700 Wiener Neustadt, Austria.

Unipath, Fr. See *Unipath, UK.*

Unipath, Israel. Unipath, Israel.

Unipath, UK. Unipath Ltd, Priory Business Park, Bedford, Bedfordshire, MK44 6UP, UK.

Unipharm, Hong Kong. Unipharm Trading Co., Rm 634-5, Nan Fung Ctr, 264-298 Castle Peak Rd, Tsuen Wan, N.T., Hong Kong.

Unipharm, Israel. Unipharm Ltd, P.O. Box 21429, Tel Aviv, Israel.

Unipharm, Singapore. See *Green Cross, Singapore.*

Unipharm, Switz. Unipharma SA, 6917 Barbengo, Switzerland.

Unique, Thai. See *Union Medical, Thai.*

Unison, Singapore. See *Age D'or, Singapore.*

Unison, Thai. Unison Laboratories Co. Ltd, 160 Soi Onnuch, Sukhumvit Rd, Ladkrabang, Bangkok 10520, Thailand.

Unitech, Irl. Unitech Ltd, United Drug House, Belgard Rd, Tallaght, Dublin 24, Ireland.

United American, Hong Kong. See *Unam, Hong Kong.*

United American, Singapore. See *Far East Drug, Singapore.*

United American, Thai. See *Olic, Thai.*

United Drug, Irl. United Drug, United Drug House, Belgard Rd, Tallaght, Dublin 24, Ireland.

United Drug, UK. United Drug Distribution Group (UDG) Ltd, Amber Park, Berristow Lane, South Normanton, Derbyshire, DE55 2FH, UK.

United Italian, Singapore. United Italian Pharma Corp Pte Ltd, 65 Upper Paya Lebar Rd, 06-03 Guang Ming Industrial Building, S 534817, Singapore.

United Nordic, Denm. United Nordic Pharma A/S, Vallerodvaenge 2, 2960 Rungsted Kyst, Denmark.

Universal, Hong Kong. Universal Pharmaceutical Lab Ltd, Eastern Ctr, G/F & 1/F, Unit 1-5, 1065 King's Rd, Quarry Bay, Hong Kong.

Universal, S.Afr. Universal Pharmaceuticals (Pty) Ltd, P.O. Box 33068, Jeppestown 2043, South Africa.

Universales, Mex. F Universales, Mexico.

Uno, Ital. Farma Uno s.r.l., Via Conforti 42, 84083 Castel San Giorgio (SA), Italy.

Upjohn, Neth. See *Pharmacia Upjohn, Neth.*

Upjohn, Swed. See *Pharmacia, Swed.*

Upjohn, UK. See *Pharmacia, UK.*

Upjohn, USA. See *Pharmacia Upjohn, USA.*

UPSA, Fr. Laboratoires UPSA, La Grande Arche Nord, 92044 Paris-La Defense cdx 2, France.

UPSA, Hong Kong. See *Wing Wai, Hong Kong.*

Upsamedica, Belg. Upsamedica S.A., Waterloo Office Park, Building N, Dreve Richelle 161, 1410 Waterloo, Belgium.

Upsamedica, Ital. Upsamedica s.p.a., V.le Filippetti 37, 20122 Milan, Italy.

Upsamedica, Spain. Upsa Medica, C/Almansa, 101, 28040 Madrid, Spain.

Upsamedica, Switz. Upsamedica SA, Neuhofstrasse 6, 6341 Baar, Switzerland.

Upsher Smith, Israel. Upsher Smith, Israel.

Upsher-Smith, USA. Upsher-Smith Laboratories Inc., 14905 23rd Ave North, Minneapolis, MN 55447-4709, USA.

Upsifarma, Port. Upsifarma, Lda, S. Domingos a Lapa 8, Letra H, 1200-835 Lisbon, Portugal.

Uragme, Ital. Uragme, Via A. Vivaldi 9, 00199 Rome, Italy.

Urbion, Spain. Urbion Farma, Avda Portugal, Parcela 85, Aranada de Duero, 09400 Burgos, Spain.

Urgo, Fr. Laboratoires Urgo, B.P. 157, 42 rue de Longvic, 21300 Chenove, France.

Urgo, Israel. Urgo, Israel.

Uriach, Spain. Uriach, Dega Bahi 59, 08026 Barcelona, Spain.

URL, USA. United Research Laboratories, 4629 Adams Ave, Philadelphia, PA 19124, USA.

Urocor, USA. Urocor, USA.

URPAC, Fr. URPAC-Astier, 24 rue Erlanger, 75781 Paris cdx 16, France.

Ursapharm, Ger. Ursapharm Arzneimittel GmbH & Co. KG, Industriestr., 66129 Saarbrucken, Germany.

Ursapharm, Neth. Ursapharm, Netherlands.

US Bio, Israel. US Bio, Israel.

US Bioscience, Denm. See *Orphan, Denm.,* and *Schering-Plough, Denm.*

US Bioscience, Norw. See *Orphan, Norw.*

US Bioscience, USA. US Bioscience Inc., One Tower Bridge, 100 Front St, West Conshohocken, PA 19428, USA.

US Pharmaceutical, USA. US Pharmaceutical Corp., 2401-C Mellon Court, Decatur, GA 30035, USA.

US Summit, Thai. US Summit Corp (Overseas), 52/184 Sukhapibai 3 Rd, Huamark, Bangkapi, Bangkok 10240, Thailand.

US Surgical, USA. Unites States Surgical Corp., 150 Glover Ave, Norwalk, CT, USA.

USANA, USA. USANA, Inc., 3838 West Parkway Blvd, Salt Lake City, UT 84120-6336, USA.

Usmed, Braz. Laboratorio Usmed Ltda, Rua Ana Ribeiro 164, Bairro Gloria, 32310-510 Contagem, MG, Brazil.

USV, Israel. USV, Israel.

Utopian, Thai. Utopian Co. Ltd, 602 Moo 3, Teparak Rd, Muang, Samuthprakarn 10270, Thailand.

V & V, Thai. V & V Bangkok, 94/7 Soi Yimprakrob, Ngamwongwan, Nonthaburi, Thailand.

VAAS, Ital. V.A.A.S. s.r.l., Via Siena 268, 47032 Capocolle di Bertinoro (FO), Italy.

Vaccina, S.Afr. Vaccina CC, P.O. Box 75804, Gardenview 2047, South Africa.

Vachon, Canad. Les Laboratoires Vachon Inc., 8700 de-la-Rive-Sud Blvd, Levis, Quebec, G6V 6N6, Canada.

Vaillant, Ital. Laboratori Italiani Vaillant s.r.l., Via Cav. V. Veneto 241, 21040 Cislago (VA), Italy.

Valda, Canad. See *Bayer, Canad.*

Valda, Ital. Valda Laboratori Farmaceutici s.p.a., Via Zambeletti, 20021 Baranzate di Bollate (MI), Italy.

Valdecasas, Mex. Laboratorios Valdecasas S.A., Av. Insurgentes Sur No. 4058, Deleg. Tlalpan, 14430 Mexico D.F., Mexico.

Valeas, Ital. Valeas s.p.a., Via Vallisneri 10, 20133 Milan, Italy.

Valio, Fin. Valio Oy, Meijeritie 6, PL 10, 00039 Valio, Finland.

ValMed, USA. ValMed Inc., 100 Otis St, Suite 4A, Northboro, MA 01532, USA.

Valmo, Canad. Lab. Valmo Enrg, 1000 Industriel Blvd, Chambly, Quebec, J3L 3H9, Canada.

Valomed, Spain. Valomed, San Rafael 3, Alcobendas, 28108 Madrid, Spain.

Vana, Thai. Vana Corp Ltd, 2038 Sukhumvit Rd, Bangkok 10250, Thailand.

Vangard, USA. Vangard Labs Inc., P.O. Box 1268, Glasgow, KY 42142-1268, USA.

Vantone, Hong Kong. Vantone Medical Supplies Co. Ltd, Flat J, 10/F Vantone International Industrial Ctr, 2-8 Kwei Tei St, Fotan, N.T., Hong Kong.

Varos, Braz. Varos Industria e Comercio de Produtos Farmaceuticos Ltda, Rua Viuva Lacerda 203, Botafogo, 22261-050 Rio de Janeiro, RJ, Brazil.

Veafarm, Braz. Laboratorio Veafarm Ltda, Rua Doutor Pena Forte Mendes 255, 01308-010 Sao Paulo, SP, Brazil.

Vebas, Ital. Vebas s.r.l., Via Benaco 1/3, 20098 San Giuliano Milanese (MI), Italy.

Vectem, Spain. Vectem, Wagner 22 (Pol Ind Can Jardi), Rubi, 08191 Barcelona, Spain.

Vedim, Fr. Laboratoires Vedim Pharma, 7 rue Diderot, 92003 Nanterre, France.

Vedim, Ger. Vedim Pharma GmbH, Huttenstr. 205, 50170 Kerpen, Germany.

Vedim, Ital. Vedim Pharma srl, Via Praglia 15, 10044 Pianezza (TO), Italy.

Vedim, Port. Vedim Pharma, Lda, Rua Carlos Calisto 4-B, 1400 Lisbon, Portugal.

Vedim, Spain. Vedim Pharma, Avda de Barcelona 239, Molins de Rei, 08750 Barcelona, Spain.

Vegetal, Ital. Vegetal Progress s.r.l., Localita Novaro 8, 10070 Devesi di Cirie (TO), Italy.

Vemedia, Neth. Vemedia B.V., Postbus 502, 1380 AN Weesp, Netherlands.

Veripalvelu, Fin. Soumen Punainen Risti Veripalvelu, Kivihaantie 7, 00310 Helsinki, Finland.

Veritas, Braz. Laboratorio Hanemaniano Veritas Ltda, Rua Barbosa 48, 21350-020 Rio de Janeiro, RJ, Brazil.

Verla, Ger. Verla-Pharm, Arzneimittelfabrik, Apotheker H.J.v. Ehrlich GmbH & Co. KG, Hauptstr. 98, 82327 Tutzing, Germany.

Verla, Switz. See *Biomed, Switz.*

Verman, Fin. Oy Verman AB, Vanhankyläntie 44 B, PL 152, 04401 Järvenpää, Finland.

Vesta, S.Afr. Vesta Medicines (Pty) Ltd, South Africa.

Veyron-Froment, Fr. Laboratoires Veyron et Froment, 30 rue Benedit, 13248 Marseille cdx 04, France.

Via, Switz. Via Marketing & Promotion SA, Via Ponte Tresa 7-7A, 6924 Sorengo, Switzerland.

Vicente, Spain. Vicente, Spain.

Vichy, Canad. See *Cosmair, Canad.*

Vida, Hong Kong. Vida Laboratories Ltd, Unit 919 Vanta Industrial Ctr, 21 Tai Lin Pai Rd, Kwai Chung, N.T., Hong Kong.

Vieira, Port. Raul Vieira, Lda, Rua dos Correeiros 41, 1100 Lisbon, Portugal.

Vifor, Hong Kong. See *Hong Kong Medical, Hong Kong.*

Vifor, Israel. Vifor, Israel.

Vifor, Port. See *Ferraz, Lynce, Port.,* and *Confar, Port.*

Vifor, Singapore. See *Diethelm, Singapore.*

Vifor, Switz. Vifor SA, Case Postale 1067, 1701 Fribourg-Moncor, Switzerland.

Vifor, Thai. Vifor.

Vifor International, Switz. Vifor (International) AG, Pharmazeutische Spezialitäten, Rechenstrasse 37, Postfach, 9001 St Gallen, Switzerland.

Vifor Medical, Switz. Vifor Medical SA, 9 route de Sorge, Case postale 161, 1023 Crissier, Switzerland.

Vilardell, Spain. Vilardell, Constitucion 66-8, Les Grases, San Feliu de Llobregat, 08980 Barcelona, Spain.

Vinas, Spain. Viñas, Provenza 386, 08025 Barcelona, Spain.

Vinas, Switz. See *Golaz, Switz.*

Vinci, Spain. Vinci Farma, Principe de Vergara 109, 28001 Madrid, Spain.

Vingmed, Norw. Vingmed AS, Fjordv. 1, Postboks 374, 1363 Hovik, Norway.

Vir, Spain. Vir, Laguna 42-4, Pol In Urtinsa II, Alcorcon, 28923 Madrid, Spain.

Virginia, Ital. Virginia Farmaceutici spa, Via Vittor Pisani 10, 20124 Milan, Italy.

Virgo Healthcare, Austral. Virgo Healthcare, Unit 2, 85-7 Moore St, Leichhardt, NSW 2040, Australia.

Virtus, Braz. Virtu's Industria e Comercio Ltda, Avenida Sargento Geraldo Santana 660, 04674-000 Sao Paulo, SP, Brazil.

Vision, USA. Vision Pharmaceuticals Inc., P.O. Box 400, Mitchell, SD 57301-0400, USA.

Vistapharm, USA. VistaPharm, 4647 T Hwy 280 E, Suite 145, Birmingham, AL 35242, USA.

Visufarma, Ital. Visufarma s.r.l., Via Canino 21, 00191 Rome, Italy.

Vita, Ital. Laboratori Farmaceutici Vita s.r.l., Via Rivoltana 32, 20090 Limito (MI), Italy.

Vita, Spain. Vita, Avda de Barcelona 69, San Juan Despi, 08970 Barcelona, Spain.

Vita Elan, Spain. See *Vita, Spain.*

Vita Health, Canad. Vita Health Co. (1985) Ltd, 150 Beghin Ave, Winnipeg, Manitoba, R2J 3W2, Canada.

Vita Health, Singapore. See *Diethelm, Singapore.*

Vita Healthcare, UK. Vita Healthcare Ltd, Palladium House, 1-4 Argyll St, London, W1V 2LD, UK.

Vita Pharm, Canad. Vita Pharm Canada Ltd, 2835 Kew Dr., Windsor, Ontario, N8T 3B7, Canada.

Vitabalans, Fin. Vitabalans Oy, Varastokatu 8, 13500 Hämeenlinna, Finland.

Vitabiotics, Hong Kong. See *Mekim, Hong Kong.*

Vitabiotics, Irl. See *Allphar, Irl.*

Vitabiotics, UK. Vitabiotics Ltd, 1 Beresford Ave, Wembley, Middlesex, HA0 1NU, UK.

Vitae, Mex. Vitae Laboratorios, S.A. de C.V., Euclides No. 3214, Fracc. Vallarta San Jorge, 44690 Guadalajara, Jal., Mexico.

Vitafarma, Spain. Vitafarma, Florida 29, Hernani, 20120 Guipuzcoa, Spain.

Vitaflo, Denm. Vitaflo Scandinavia AB, Boks 144, 3400 Hillerod, Denmark.

Vitaflo, Fin. See *Tamro, Fin.*

Vitaflo, Irl. See *Allphar, Irl.*

Vitaflo, Swed. Vitaflo Scandinavia AB, Box 53063, 400 14 Goteborg, Sweden.

Vitaflo, UK. Vitaflo Ltd, 11 Century Building, Brunswick Business Park, Liverpool, Merseyside, L3 4BL, UK.

Vitaglow, Austral. Vitaglow P/L, 23 Roseberry St, Balgowah, NSW 2093, Australia.

Vita-Health, Hong Kong. See *Great Liaison, Hong Kong,* and *Hind Wing, Hong Kong.*

Vitalia, UK. Vitalia Ltd, UK.

Vitaline, Fin. See *Sairaalapalvelu, Fin.*

Vitaline, Norw. See *Vingmed, Norw.*

Vitaline, Swed. Vitaline Scandinavia AB, Box 938, 751 03 Uppsala, Sweden.

Vitaline, UK. Vitaline Pharmaceuticals UK Ltd, Rx Court, 5 Church St, Aylesbury, Buckinghamshire, HP20 2QP, UK.

Vitaline, USA. Vitaline Corp., 385 Williamson Way, Ashland, OR 97520, USA.

Vitality, USA. Vitality, USA.

Vitalpharma, Belg. Vitalpharma S.A., Rue Egide Van Ophem 110, 1180 Brussels, Belgium.

Vitamed, Israel. Vitamed Ltd, P.O. Box 114, Benyamina, Israel.

Vitaplex, Austral. Vitaplex Products, P.O. Box 270, Gymea, NSW 2227, Australia.

Vitasan, Aust. Vitasan GmbH, Teichweg 2, A-5400 Hallein, Austria.

Vitelle, Austral. See *Faulding Healthcare, Austral.*

Vitex, Braz. Vitex, Brazil.

Vitorgan, Ger. vitOrgan Arzneimittel GmbH, Brunnweisenstr. 21, 73760 Ostfildern, Germany.

Vitoria, Port. Laboratórios Vitória, SA, Rua Elias Garcia 28, Venda Nova, 2700-327 Amadora, Portugal.

Vitrolife, Swed. Vitrolife AB, Molndalsvagen 30, 412 63 Goteborg, Sweden.

Vivance, Fr. Vivance SA, La Maison blanche, 71570 Romaneche-Thorins, France.

Vivant, Mex. Vivant, Mexico.

Viviar, Spain. Viviar, Pista de Ademuz Km 9.4, Paterna, 46980 Valencia, Spain.

Vivus, Aust. See *Vivus, USA.*

Vivus, Denm. See *AstraZeneca, Denm.*

Vivus, Norw. See *AstraZeneca, Norw.*

Vivus, USA. Vivus Inc, 605 East Fairchild Dr., Mountain View, CA 94043, USA.

Voco, Denm. See *Voco, Ger.*

Voco, Ger. Voco GmbH, Postfach 767, 27457 Cuxhaven, Germany.

Volchem, Ital. Volchem, Via E Dandolo 14, 35010 Grossa di Gazzo (PD), Italy.

Vortech, USA. Vortech Pharmaceuticals, 6851 Chase Rd, Dearborn, MI 48126, USA.

VSM, Neth. VSM Geneesmiddelen B.V., Postbus 9321, 1800 GH Alkmaar, Netherlands.

Wakamoto, Hong Kong. See *Tai Tong, Hong Kong.*

Wakefield, USA. Wakefield Pharmaceuticals, Inc., 310 Maxwell Rd, Suite 100, Alpharetta, GA 30004, USA.

Wala, Ger. Wala Heilmittel GmbH, Bosslerweg 2, 73087 Bad Boll/Eckwalden, Germany.

Waldheim, Aust. See *Sanochemia, Aust.*

Walker Laboratories, USA. Walker Laboratories, 4200 Laclede Ave, St Louis, MO 63108, USA.

Walker Pharmacal, USA. See *Walker Laboratories, USA.*

Wallace, USA. Wallace Laboratories, Division of Carter-Wallace Inc., P.O. Box 1001, Cranbury, NJ 08512, USA.

Wallace Mfg Chem., UK. Wallace Manufacturing Chemists Ltd, Wallace House, New Abbey Court, 51-53 Stert St, Abingdon, Oxfordshire, OX14 3HB, UK.

Wallis, UK. Wallis Laboratory, Laporte Way, Luton, Bedfordshire, LU4 8WL, UK.

Wampole, Canad. Wampole Canada Inc., 465 Milner Ave, Unit 1, Scarborough, Ontario, M1B 2K4, Canada.

Wampole, USA. Wampole Laboratories, Half Acre Rd, P.O. Box 1001, Cranbury, NJ 08512-0181, USA.

Wander, Aust. Wander, Vienna, Austria.

Wander, Belg. See *Novartis, Belg.*

Wander, Ital. Wander s.p.a., Via Meucci 39, 20128 Milan, Italy.

Wander, Neth. See *Sandoz, Neth.*

Wander Health Care, Switz. Wander AG, Postfach, 3001 Bern, Switzerland.

Wander OTC, Switz. See *Novartis Consumer, Switz.*

Wanskerne, UK. Wanskerne Ltd, 31 High Cross Street, St Austell, Cornwall, PL25 4AN, UK.

Warner, S.Afr. Warner-Lambert South Africa (Pty) Ltd, Private Bag X6, Tokai 7966, South Africa.

Warner Chilcott, USA. Warner Chilcott Laboratories, Rockaway 80 Corporate Center, 100 Enterprise Drive, Suite 280, Rockaway, NJ 07866, USA.

Warner-Lambert, Austral. See *Parke, Davis, Austral.*

Warner-Lambert, Belg. See *Warner-Lambert Consumer, Belg.*

Warner-Lambert, Braz. Warner Lambert Industria e Comercio Ltda, Rua Estrela D'Oeste 701, Vila Barros, 07140-902 Guarulhos, SP, Brazil.

Warner-Lambert, Canad. Warner Wellcome Consumer Healthcare, P.O. Box 2200, Station A, Scarborough, Ontario, M1K 5C9, Canada.

Warner-Lambert, Denm. Warner-Lambert Denmark, Tempovej 27-9, 2750 Ballerup, Denmark.

Warner-Lambert, Fin. Warner Lambert Nordic AB, Finnish Branch, Merivirta 3 A, 02320 Espoo, Finland.

Warner-Lambert, Fr. Warner-Lambert Santé Grand Public, 10 av. de l'Arche, 92419 Courbevoie cdx, France.

Warner-Lambert, Ger. See *Pfizer, Ger.*

Warner-Lambert, Hong Kong. Warner-Lambert (HK) Ltd, 36/F Manulife Tower, 169 Electric Rd, North Point, Hong Kong.

Warner-Lambert, Irl. Warner-Lambert Consumer Healthcare, United Drug House, Belgard Rd, Tallaght, Dublin 24, Ireland.

Warner-Lambert, Israel. Warner-Lambert, Israel.

Warner-Lambert, Ital. Warner Lambert Consumer Healthcare S.Comp.p.A., Via de Gasperi 17-19, 20020 Lainate (MI), Italy.

Warner-Lambert, Mex. Grupo Warner-Lambert Mexico, S.A. de C.V. Division Parke-Davis, Av. Division del Norte No. 3443, Col. San Pablo Tepetlapa, 04620 Mexico, D.F., Mexico.

Warner-Lambert, Neth. Warner-Lambert Consumer Healthcare B.V., Saturnusstraat 1, 2132 HB Hoofddorp, Netherlands.

Warner-Lambert, Norw. Warner-Lambert Nordic/Parke-Davis, Gjerdrumsv. 14, 0881 Oslo, Norway.

Warner-Lambert, NZ. Warner Lambert Consumer Healthcare, P.O. Box 22-071, Otahuhu, Auckland, New Zealand.

Warner-Lambert, Port. Warner-Lambert Portugal, Lda, Estrada do Casal de Canas, Edificio ABB, Alfragide, 2720-092 Amadora, Portugal.

Warner-Lambert, Spain. Warner Lambert Consumer Health, Pol. Ind. Manso Mateu SN, Prat de Llobregat, 08820 Barcelona, Spain.

Warner-Lambert, Swed. Warner-Lambert Consumer Healthcare, Division of Warner Lambert Nordic AB, Box 501, 183 12 Taby, Sweden.

Warner-Lambert, Switz. Warner-Lambert (Schweiz) AG, Blegistrasse 11a, 6341 Baar, Switzerland.

Warner-Lambert, Thai. Warner-Lambert (Thailand) Ltd, 18 Fl, Thosapolland 3 Building, 947 Bangna-Trad KM 3, Prakanong, Bangkok 10260, Thailand.

Warner-Lambert, UK. See *Parke, Davis, UK.*

Warner-Lambert, USA. Warner-Lambert Consumer Healthcare, 201 Tabor Rd, Morris Plains, NJ 07950, USA.

Warner-Lambert Confectionery, UK. See *Warner-Lambert, UK.*

Warner-Lambert Consumer, Belg. Warner-Lambert Consumer Healthcare s.c.a., Exelsiorlaan 75-7, 1930 Zaventem, Belgium.

Warner-Lambert Consumer, Port. See *Warner-Lambert, Port.*

Warner-Lambert Consumer, Switz. See *Warner-Lambert, Switz.*

Warner-Wellcome, USA. See *Warner-Lambert, USA.*

Wassen, Ital. Wassen Italia srl, Via Canova 25, 20145 Milan, Italy.

Wassen, UK. Wassen International Ltd, 14 The Mole Business Park, Leatherhead, Surrey, KT22 7BA, UK.

Wasserman, Spain. Chiesi Wasserman, Berlin 38-48 7, 08029 Barcelona, Spain.

Wassermann, Ital. Alfa Wassermann s.p.a., Contrada Sant'Emidio, 65020 Alanno (PE), Italy.

Watson, USA. Watson Laboratories Inc., 311 Bonnie Circle, Corona, CA 91720, USA.

Watsons, Canad. Watsons Pharmaceuticals, 3 Ontario St, Port Hope, Ontario, L1A 3T5, Canada.

Waymade, UK. See *Sovereign, UK.*

Waymar, Canad. Waymar Pharmaceuticals Inc., 330 Marwood Drive, Unit 4, Oshawa, Ontario, L1H 8B4, Canada.

Wayne, Mex. Wayne S.A. de C.V., Lago Margarita No. 27, Col. Granada, 11520 Mexico D.F., Mexico.

WE, USA. WE Pharmaceuticals Inc, P.O. Box 1142, Ramona, CA 92065, USA.

Weber & Weber, Ger. Weber & Weber GmbH & Co. KG, Herrschinger Str. 33, 82266 Inning/Ammersee, Germany.

Weider, UK. Weider Nutrition Ltd, Forum House, Redhill, Surrey, RH1 6YS, UK.

Weifa, Norw. Weifa AS, Hausmannsg. 6, Postboks 9113 Gronland, 0133 Oslo, Norway.

Weifa, Thai. See *Harn, Thai.*

Weimer, Ger. See *Biokanol, Ger.*

Weimer, Hong Kong. See *Hong Kong Medical, Hong Kong.*

Weimer, Switz. Weimer Pharma AG, Diepold-Schillingsstrasse 14a, 6004 Luzern, Switzerland.

Weimer, Thai. See *Schumit, Thai.*

Weinco, Spain. Weinco, Spain.

Welcker-Lyster, Canad. See *Technilab, Canad.*

Weleda, Aust. Weleda GmbH & Co. KG, Hosenedelgasse 27, A-1220 Vienna, Austria.

Weleda, Fr. Laboratoires Weleda, 9 rue Eugene-Jung, 68330 Huningue, France.

Weleda, Ger. Weleda AG-Heilmitteltriebe, Mohlerstr. 3-5, 73525 Schwabisch Gmund, Germany.

Weleda, UK. Weleda (UK) Ltd, Heanor Rd, Ilkeston, Derbyshire, DE7 8DR, UK.

Welfer, Mex. Welfer, Mexico.

Wellchem, Singapore. Wellchem Pharmaceuticals Pte Ltd, 221 Henderson Rd, 04-15 Henderson Building, S 159557, Singapore.

Wellchem, Thai. Wellchem Pharmaceutical Co. Ltd, 99/287-288 Nonsee Rd, Yannawa, Bangkok 10120, Thailand.

Wellcome, Austral. See *Glaxo Wellcome, Austral.*

Wellcome, Canad. See *Glaxo Wellcome, Canad.*

Wellcome, Irl. See *GlaxoSmithKline, Irl.*

Wellcome, Port. See *Glaxo Wellcome, Port.*

Wellcome, Spain. See *Glaxo Wellcome, Spain.*

Wellcome, Switz. See *Glaxo Wellcome, Switz.*

Wellcome, UK. See *GlaxoSmithKline, UK.*

Wellcome, USA. See *GlaxoSmithKline, USA.*

Wellcome Diagnostics, UK. Wellcome Diagnostics, A Division of The Wellcome Foundation Ltd, Temple Hill, Dartford, DA1 5AH, UK.

Welti, Switz. Dr Heinz Welti AG, Fabrik chemisch-pharmazeutischer Produkte, Althofstrasse 12, 5432 Neuenhof, Switzerland.

Wenig, Aust. Mr J W Wenig GmbH, Van der Nullgasse 22, A-1100 Vienna, Austria.

Wernigerode, Aust. See *Wernigerode, Ger.*

Wernigerode, Ger. Pharma Wernigerode GmbH, Muhlental 42, 38855 Wernigerode/Harz, Germany.

Wesley, USA. Wesley Pharmacal Inc., 114 Railroad Drive, Ivyland, PA 18974, USA.

Westbrook, UK. Westbrook Lanolin Co., Argonaut Works, Laisterdyke, Bradford, BD4 8AU, UK.

WestCan, Canad. See *Vita Health, Canad.*

West-Coast, Thai. See *Union Medical, Thai.*

Western Medical, USA. Western Medical, USA.

Westlake, USA. Westlake Laboratories Inc., 24700 Center Ridge Rd, Cleveland, OH 44145, USA.

Westmont, Hong Kong. See *Unam, Hong Kong.*

Westmont, Singapore. See *Far East Drug, Singapore.*

Westmont, Thai. See *Olic, Thai.*

Weston, Hong Kong. Weston Pharmaceutical Ltd, M & G/F, 48-50 Aberdeen Main Rd, Aberdeen, Hong Kong.

Westward, Canad. Westward Dist., Canada.

Westwood, Singapore. See *Diethelm, Singapore.*

Westwood, USA. See *Bristol-Myers Squibb, USA.*

Westwood-Squibb, Canad. See *Bristol-Myers Squibb, Canad.*

Westwood-Squibb, USA. See *Bristol-Myers Squibb, USA.*

Whan In, Singapore. See *MD, Singapore.*

Whelehan, Irl. Whelehan T.P. Son & Co. Ltd, North Rd, Finglas, Dublin 11, Ireland.

Whitehall, Austral. Whitehall Laboratories Australia P/L, Private Mailbag 1, Punchbowl, NSW 2196, Australia.

Whitehall, Belg. Whitehall Benelux s.a., Rue du Bosquet 15, 1348 Louvain-la-Neuve, Belgium.

Whitehall, Braz. See *Wyeth, Braz.*

Whitehall, Denm. See *Whitehall, UK.*

Whitehall, Fin. See *Tamro, Fin.*

Whitehall, Fr. Whitehall, 80 av du General-de-Gaulle, 92031 Paris-La Defense cdx, France.

Whitehall, Hong Kong. Whitehall Hong Kong, Division of Wyeth (HK) Ltd, Rm 1401-1403, C C Wu Bldg, 302-308 Hennessy Rd, Wanchai, Hong Kong.

Whitehall, Irl. Whitehall Laboratories Ltd, 765 South Circular Rd, Dublin 8, Ireland.

Whitehall, Israel. Whitehall, Israel.

Whitehall, Ital. Whitehall Italia s.p.a., Via Puccini 3, 20121 Milan, Italy.

Whitehall, Neth. Whitehall Laboratoria, Sophialaan 25, 1075 BL Amsterdam, Netherlands.

Whitehall, Norw. See *Wyeth Lederle, Norw.*

Whitehall, NZ. Whitehall, P.O. Box 12736, Penrose, Auckland, New Zealand.

Whitehall, Port. Whitehall, Home Products de Portugal Lda, Rua Humberto Madeira 2-3, Valejas, 2745-663 Barcarena, Portugal.

Whitehall, S.Afr. See *Whitehall, S.Afr.*

Whitehall, Singapore. Whitehall, 22 Martin Rd, 02-01 King Sun Building, S 239058, Singapore.

Whitehall, Swed. Whitehall Nordiska, Box 344, 191 30 Sollentuna, Sweden.

Whitehall, Thai. Whitehall Thailand, 23 Fl, Silom Complex Building, 191 Silom Rd, Bangkok 10500, Thailand.

Whitehall, UK. Whitehall Laboratories Ltd, Huntercombe Lane South, Taplow, Maidenhead, Berkshire, SL6 0PH, UK.

Whitehall, USA. See *Whitehall-Robins, USA.*

Whitehall-Much, Ger. Whitehall-Much GmbH, Schleebruggenkamp 15, 48159 Munster, Germany.

Whitehall-Robins, Canad. Whitehall-Robins Inc., 5975 Whittle Rd, Mississauga, Ontario, L4Z 3M6, Canada.

Whitehall-Robins, Mex. See *Wyeth, Mex.*

Whitehall-Robins, Switz. Whitehall-Robins AG, Grafenauweg 10, 6301 Zug 7, Switzerland.

Whitehall-Robins, USA. Whitehall Robins Healthcare, Five Giralda Farms, Madison, NJ 07940-0871, USA.

Wick, Ger. Wick Pharma Zweigniederlassung der Procter & Gamble GmbH, Sulzbacher Str. 40, 65824 Schwalbach, Germany.

Wider, Ger. Dr. Wider GmbH & Co., Brennerstr. 48, Postfach: 1862, 71208 Leonberg, Germany.

Widmer, Aust. Widmer Louis GmbH, Itzlinger Hauptstrasse 34, A-5020 Salzburg, Austria.

Widmer, Fin. Louis Widmer Oy, Sömäisten rantatie 29, 00580 Helsinki, Finland.

Widmer, Ger. Louis Widmer GmbH, Grossmattstr. 11, 79618 Rheinfelden, Germany.

Widmer, Switz. Dermatologica Widmer, Laboratoires Louis Widmer AG, 8048 Zurich, Switzerland.

Wiedemann, Ger. Wiedemann Pharma GmbH, Pilotyweg 14, 82541 Munsing, Germany.

Wieger, Fr. Lab. Wieger, 209 rte de Schirmeck, 67200 Strasbourg, France.

Wiener, Mex. Wiener Codex S.A. de C.V., Carr. Central Km 418-900, Zona Industrial, 78395 San Luis Potosi S.L.P., Mexico.

Wigglesworth, UK. Wigglesworth (1982) Ltd, Cunard Rd, North Acton, London, NW10 6PN, UK.

Wild, Switz. Dr Wild & Co. AG, Lange Gasse 4, 4002 Basle, Switzerland.

Williams, USA. Williams T.E. Pharm. Inc., P.O. Box 340, Guthrie, OK 73044, USA.

Willmar, Mex. Willmar, Mexico.

Willmar, Thai. See *JDH Borneo, Thai.*

Will-Pharma, Belg. Will-Pharma S.A., Rue du Manil 5, 1301 Wavre, Belgium.

Will-Pharma, Neth. Will-Pharma B.V., Postbus 30, 1160 AA Zwanenburg, Netherlands.

Willpharma, Thai. Will Pharma.

Willvonseder, Aust. Willvonseder & Marchesani, Heinrich-v-Buol-Gasse 45, A-1211 Vienna, Austria.

Wilson, NZ. Wilson Consumer Products Ltd, P.O. Box 1332, Auckland, New Zealand.

Windson, Braz. Windson Produtos Quimicos e Farmaceuticos Ltda, Rua Doutor Nicolau de Souza Queiroz 136, 04105-000 Sao Paulo, SP, Brazil.

Windsor, Irl. See *Allphar, Irl.*

Windsor, UK. Windsor Healthcare Ltd, Ellesfield Ave, Bracknell, Berkshire, RG12 4YS, UK.

Wing Wai, Hong Kong. Wing Wai Trading Co., Unit E, 2/F Freder Ctr, 3 Mok Cheong St, Kowloon, Hong Kong.

Win-Medicare, Thai. See *Union Medical, Thai.*

Winsor, Hong Kong. Winsor & Co., Rm 1707-1707A, Wu Sang House, 855 Nathan Rd, Kowloon, Hong Kong.

Winthrop, USA. See *Sanofi Synthelabo, USA.*

Winthrop Consumer, USA. See *Bayer Consumer, USA.*

Winzer, Ger. Dr Winzer Pharma GmbH, Ilzweg 7, 82140 Olching, Germany.

Wisconsin Pharmacal, USA. Wisconsin Pharmacal Co., 1 Repel Rd, Jackson, WI 53037, USA.

Woelm, Ger. Woelm Pharma GmbH & Co., Rhondorfer Str. 80, 53604 Bad Honnef, Germany.

Woelm, Israel. Woelm, Israel.

Wolff, Ger. Dr. August Wolff Arzneimittel GmbH & Co., Sudbrackstr. 56, 33611 Bielefeld, Germany.

Wolfs, Belg. Wolfs S.A., Industriepark West 68, 9100 Sint-Niklaas, Belgium.

Women First, USA. Women First Healthcare Inc., 12220 El Camino Real, Suite 400, San Diego, CA 92130, USA.

Womens Capital, USA. Women's Capital Corp., P.O. Box 5026, Bellevue, WA 98009, USA.

Woods, Austral. H.W. Woods P/L, P.O. Box 1005, Huntingdale, VIC 3166, Australia.

Woodward, USA. Woodward Laboratories, Inc., 11132 Winners Circle 100, Los Alamitos, CA 90720, USA.

Worldwide, Hong Kong. Worldwide Resources Pharmaceutical Ltd, Unit 14, 19/F Concordia Plaza, 1 Science Museum Rd, TST East, Kowloon, Hong Kong.

Worndli, Switz. Labor Worndli, Postfach 53, 5300 Turgi, Switzerland.

Worthy Strong, Hong Kong. Worthy Strong Development Ltd, Rm 810, Yuen Long Ctr, 55 Sau Fu St, Yuen Long, New Territories, Hong Kong.

Worwag, Ger. Wörwag Pharma GmbH & Co. KG, Calwer Str. 7, 71034 Boblingen, Germany.

Wrigley, USA. Wrigley, USA.

Wybert, Ger. See *GABA, Ger.*

Wyeth, Austral. Wyeth Pharmaceuticals, Division of Wyeth Australia P/L, P.O Box 9, Baulkham Hills, NSW 1755, Australia.

Wyeth, Braz. Laboratorios Wyeth-Whitehall Ltda, Rua Alexandre Dumas 2200, Chac. Sto. Antonio, 04717-910 Sao Paulo, SP, Brazil.

Wyeth, Ger. Wyeth-Pharma GmbH, Wienburgstr. 207, 48159 Munster, Germany.

Wyeth, Hong Kong. Wyeth (Hong Kong) Ltd, 25/F Shell Tower, Times Square, 1 Matheson St, Causeway Bay, Hong Kong.

Wyeth, Irl. See *Wyeth Lederle, Irl.*

Wyeth, Mex. Wyeth S.A. de C.V., Av. Poniente 140 No. 740, Col. Industrial Vallejo, 02300 Mexico D.F., Mexico.

Wyeth, Neth. See *AHP, Neth.*

Wyeth, NZ. Wyeth (NZ) Ltd, P.O. Box 12736, Penrose, Auckland, New Zealand.

Wyeth, S.Afr. Wyeth South Africa (Pty) Ltd, Private Bag X211, Midrand 1685, South Africa.

Wyeth, Singapore. Wyeth (S) Pte Ltd, 22 Martin Rd, 03-01/02 LT Building, S 239058, Singapore.

Wyeth, Spain. Wyeth Orfi, Ctra Burgos, Km-23, Desvio Algete Km, 1, San Sebastian de Los Reyes, 28070 Madrid, Spain.

Wyeth, Switz. See *AHP, Switz.*

Wyeth, UK. Wyeth Laboratories, Huntercombe Lane South, Taplow, Maidenhead, Berkshire, SL6 0PH, UK.

Wyeth Health, Austral. See *Wyeth, Austral.*

Wyeth Lederle, Aust. Wyeth-Lederle Pharma GmbH, Storchengasse 1, A-1150 Vienna, Austria.

Wyeth Lederle, Belg. Wyeth Lederle, Division of AHP Pharma, Parc Scientifique Einstein, Rue du Bosquet 15, 1348 Louvain-la-Neuve, Belgium.

Wyeth Lederle, Denm. Wyeth Lederle, Produktionsvej 24, 2600 Glostrup, Denmark.

Wyeth Lederle, Fin. Wyeth Lederle Nordiska AB, Filial I Finland, Rajatorpantie 41 C, 01640 Vantaa, Finland.

Wyeth Lederle, Fr. Wyeth-Lederle, Le Wilson 2, 80 av du General-de-Gaulle, Puteaux, 92031 Paris-La Defense cdx, France.

Wyeth Lederle, Irl. Wyeth Lederle Laboratories, 765 South Circular Road, Dublin 8, Ireland.

Wyeth Lederle, Israel. Wyeth Lederle, Israel.

Wyeth Lederle, Ital. Wyeth Lederle s.p.a., Via Nettunense 90, 04011 Aprilia (LT), Italy.

Wyeth Lederle, Jpn. Wyeth Lederle Japan Ltd, 1-10-3 Kyobashi, Chuo-ku, Tokyo 104-0031, Japan.

Wyeth Lederle, Norw. Wyeth Lederle Norge, Drammensv 145B, Postboks 313 Skoyen, 0213 Oslo, Norway.

Wyeth Lederle, Port. Wyeth Lederle Portugal (Farma), Lda, Rua Dr Antonio Loureiro Borges 2, Arquiparque, Miraflores, 1495-131 Alges, Portugal.

Wyeth Lederle, Swed. Wyeth Lederle Nordiska AB, Box 1822, 171 24 Solna, Sweden.

Wyeth-Ayerst, Austral. See *Wyeth, Austral.*

Wyeth-Ayerst, Canad. Wyeth-Ayerst Canada Inc., 1025 Marcel Laurin Blvd, Saint-Laurent, Quebec, H4R 1J6, Canada.

Wyeth-Ayerst, Hong Kong. See *Wyeth, Hong Kong.*

Wyeth-Ayerst, Israel. Wyeth-Ayerst, Israel.

Wyeth-Ayerst, Thai. Wyeth-Ayerst (Thailand) Ltd, 23 Fl, Silom Complex Building, 191 Silom Rd, Bangkok 10500, Thailand.

Wyeth-Ayerst, USA. Wyeth-Ayerst Laboratories, Division of American Home Products Corp., P.O. Box 8299, Philadelphia, PA 19101, USA.

Wynlit, UK. Wynlit Laboratories, 153 Furzehill Rd, Borehamwood, Hertfordshire, WD6 2DR, UK.

Wyss, Switz. Wyss Pharma AG, Riedstrasse 1, 6330 Cham, Switzerland.

Wyvern, UK. Wyvern Medical Ltd, P.O. Box 17, Ledbury, Herefordshire, HR8 2ES, UK.

Xepa-Soul Pattinson, Hong Kong. See *Tack Fung, Hong Kong.*

Xepa-Soul Pattinson, Singapore. See *Grafton, Singapore.*

Xeragen, S.Afr. Xeragen Laboratories (Pty) Ltd, P.O. Box 22316, Glenashley, South Africa.

Xixia, S.Afr. Xixia Pharmaceuticals (Pty) Ltd, P.O. Box 1998, Halfway House 1685, South Africa.

Xvivo, Swed. See *Vitrolife, Swed.*

Yamanouchi, Belg. Yamanouchi Pharma B.V., Blvd International 55 Bte 7, 1070 Brussels, Belgium.

Yamanouchi, Denm. Yamanouchi Pharma A/S, Naverland 3, 2600 Glostrup, Denmark.

Yamanouchi, Fin. See *Algol, Fin.*

Yamanouchi, Fr. Yamanouchi Pharma, 10 pl de la Coupole, 94220 Charenton-le-Pont, France.

Yamanouchi, Ger. Yamanouchi Pharma GmbH, Im Breitspiel 19, 69126 Heidelberg, Germany.

Yamanouchi, Irl. See *United Drug, Irl.*

Yamanouchi, Israel. Yamanouchi, Israel.

Yamanouchi, Ital. Yamanouchi Pharma s.p.a., Via delle Industrie 2, 20061 Carugate (MI), Italy.

Yamanouchi, Jpn. Yamanouchi Pharmaceutical Co. Ltd, 3-11 Nihonbashi-Honcho 2-chome, Chuo-ku, Tokyo 103-8411, Japan.

Yamanouchi, Neth. Yamanouchi Pharma, Postbus 108, 2350 AC Leiderdorp, Netherlands.

Yamanouchi, Norw. Yamanouchi Pharma AS, Solbrav 47, 1370 Asker, Norway.

Yamanouchi, NZ. See *Pharmaco, NZ.*

Yamanouchi, Port. Yamanouchi Farma, Lda, Edifício Cinema, Rua Jose Fontana, no 1, 2780-805 Paco de Arcos, Portugal.

Yamanouchi, Spain. Yamanouchi Pharma, Ochandiano 10 C, Empresarial El Plantio, 28023 Madrid, Spain.

Yamanouchi, Swed. Yamanouchi Pharma AB, Ridspogatan 10, 213 77 Malmo, Sweden.

Yamanouchi, Switz. See *Doetsch, Grether, Switz.*

Yamanouchi, Thai. Yamanouchi (Thailand) Co. Ltd, 10 Fl, Wave Place, 55 Wireless Rd, Lumpini, Patumwan, Bangkok 10330, Thailand.

Yamanouchi, UK. Yamanouchi Pharma Ltd, Yamanouchi House, Pyrford Rd, West Byfleet, Weybridge, Surrey, KT14 6RA, UK.

Yamanouchi-Westmont, Thai. See *Olic, Thai.*

Yauquimia, Mex. Yauquimia, Mexico.

Yauyip, Austral. Yauyip P/L, Suite 503 Cliveden, 4 Bridge Street, NSW 2000, Australia.

YF Chem, Thai. See *Sriprasit, Thai.*

Yik Kwan, Hong Kong. Yik Kwan Pharmaceuticals Co. Ltd, Flat A10, 6/F Merit Industrial Ctr, 94 To Kwa Wan Rd, Kowloon, Hong Kong.

Yorkshire Pharmaceuticals, UK. Yorkshire Pharmaceuticals Ltd, KAM House, 87 Horton Grange Rd, Bradford, West Yorkshire, BD7 3AH, UK.

Yoshitomi, Jpn. Yoshitomi Pharmaceutical Industries Ltd, 6-9 Hiranomachi 2-chome, Chuo-ku, Osaka 541-0046, Japan.

Yoshitomi, Singapore. See *GC, Singapore.*

Young, Canad. WF Young Inc., 1225 rue Volta, Boucherville, Quebec, J4B 7M7, Canada.

Young, USA. Young Dental Mfg, 13705 Shoreline Ct E, Earth City, MO 63045, USA.

Young Again Products, USA. Young Again Products Inc., 3608-B Oleander Drive 310, Wilmington, NC 28403, USA.

Youngflex, Canad. Youngflex Manufacturing Inc., 60 Granton Drive, Unit 6, Richmond Hill, Ontario, L4B 1H7, Canada.

Ysatfabrik, Ger. Johannes Bürger Ysatfabrik GmbH, Herzog-Julius-Str. 81/83, 38667 Bad Harzburg, Germany.

Yu Yu, Singapore. See *Polymedic, Singapore.*

Yung Shin, Thai. See *Far East, Thai.*

Yungjin, Singapore. See *Zyfas, Singapore.*

Yves Ponroy, Fr. Laboratoires Yves Ponroy, 78340 Les Clayes-sous-Bois, France.

Zafiro, Mex. Laboratorios Zafiro S.A. de C.V., Circunvalacion Norte No. 56, Fracc. Las Fuentes, 45070 Zapopan, Jal., Mexico.

Zambon, Aust. See *Zambon, Ital.*

Zambon, Belg. Zambon S.A., Ave R Vandendriessche 18 bte 1, 1150 Brussels, Belgium.

Zambon, Braz. Zambon Laboratorios Farmaceuticos S.A., Rua Descampado 63, Vila Vera, 04296-090 Sao Paulo, SP, Brazil.

Zambon, Fr. Laboratoires Zambon France, 13 rue Rene-Jaques, 92138 Issy-les-Moulineaux, France.

Zambon, Ger. Zambon GmbH, Heinrich-Hertz-Str. 13, 50170 Kerpen, Germany.

Zambon, Hong Kong. Zambon(HK) Ltd, Rm 4109-4110, 41/F China Resources Bldg, 26 Harbour Rd, Wanchai, Hong Kong.

Zambon, Ital. Zambon Italia s.r.l., Via della Chimica 9, 36100 Vicenza, Italy.

Zambon, Neth. Zambon Nederland BV, Postbus 1312, 3800 BH Amersfoort, Netherlands.

Zambon, Port. Zambon, Lda, Rua Jorge Barradas 24 B, 1500-370 Lisbon, Portugal.

Zambon, Singapore. See *United Italian, Singapore.*

Zambon, Spain. Zambon, Maresme S/N (Pol. Ind. Urvasa), Santa Perpetua de Mogoda, 08130 Barcelona, Spain.

Zambon, Thai. See *SM, Thai.*

Zanfel, USA. Zanfel Laboratories Inc., P.O. Box 349, Moreton, IL 61550, USA.

Zee, Canad. Zee Medical Canada, 5919 3rd St SE, Calgary, Alberta, T2H 1K3, Canada.

Zellaforte, Switz. Zellaforte Vertriebsanstalt, Austrasse 52, FL-9490 Vaduz, Switzerland.

Zeller, Israel. Zeller, Israel.

Zeller, Port. Zeller Farmacêutica, Lda, Rua Sebastiao da Silva 25, Zona Industrial de Massama, 2745 Queluz, Portugal.

Zeller, Singapore. See *Green Cross, Singapore.*

Zeller, Switz. Max Zeller Söhne AG, Pflanzliche Heilmittel, Seeblickstrasse 4, Postfach 29, 8590 Romanshorn, Switzerland.

Zeneca, Aust. See *AstraZeneca, Aust.*

Zeneca, Austral. See *AstraZeneca, Austral.*

Zeneca, Belg. Zeneca S.A., Schaessestraat 15, 9070 Destelbergen, Belgium.

Zeneca, Braz. Zeneca Farmaceutico do Brasil Ltda, Rodovia Raposo Tavares Km 26.9, 06700-000 Cotia, SP, Brazil.

Zeneca, Denm. See *AstraZeneca, Denm.*

Zeneca, Fr. See *AstraZeneca, Fr.*

Zeneca, Ger. See *AstraZeneca, Ger.*

Zeneca, Hong Kong. Zeneca China Ltd, 14/F One Pacific Place, 88 Queensway Central, Hong Kong.

Zeneca, Irl. See *Astra, Irl.*

Zeneca, Israel. Zeneca, Israel.

Zeneca, Ital. See *AstraZeneca, Ital.*

Zeneca, Mex. Zeneca Mexicana S.A. de C.V., Division Farma, Super Avenida Lomas Verdes No. 67, 53120 Naucalpan de Juarez, Edo de Mexico, Mexico.

Zeneca, Neth. Zeneca Farma, Postbus 4136, 2980 GC Ridderkerk, Netherlands.

Zeneca, Norw. Zeneca AS, Skysstasjon 14, Postboks 275 Skoyen, 1371 Asker, Norway.

Zeneca, Port. Zeneca Produtos Biociência, Lda, Rua Humberto Madeira 7, Valejas, 2745-663 Barcarena, Portugal.

Zeneca, S.Afr. See *AstraZeneca, S.Afr.*

Zeneca, Spain. Zeneca Farma, Josefa Valcarcel 3-5, 28027 Madrid, Spain.

Zeneca, Swed. See *AstraZeneca, Swed.*

Zeneca, Switz. See *AstraZeneca, Switz.*

Zeneca, USA. See *AstraZeneca, USA.*

Zenith Goldline, USA. Zenith Goldline Pharmaceuticals, 4400 Biscayne Blvd, Miami, FL 33137, USA.

Zenyaku, Jpn. Zenyaku Kogyo Co. Ltd, 6-15 Otsuka 5-chome, Bunkyo-ku, Tokyo 112, Japan.

Zeppenfeldt, Ger. Zeppenfeldt Pharma GmbH, Weiler Str. 19-21, 79540 Lorrach, Germany.

Zerboni, Mex. Zerboni, Mexico.

Zeta, Ital. Zeta Farmaceutici s.p.a., Via Galvani 10, 36066 Sandrigo (VI), Italy.

Zicor, Fr. Zicor, France.

Ziethen, Ger. Ziethen, Tengstr. 26, 80798 Munich, Germany.

Zila, Canad. Zila Pharmaceuticals Inc., 111 Flint Rd, Downsview, Ontario, M3J 3C7, Canada.

Zila, USA. Zila Pharmaceuticals Inc., 5227 N. 7th Street, Phoenix, AZ 85014-2817, USA.

Zilliken, Ital. Zilliken s.p.a., Viale Fulvio Testi 326, 20126 Milan, Italy.

Zilly, Ger. Fritz Zilly GmbH, Eckbergstr. 18, 76534 Baden-Baden, Germany.

Zimaia, Port. Laboratório Zimaia, SA, Rua de Andaluz 38, 1050-006 Lisbon, Portugal.

Zimmer, Ger. Zimmer Chirurgie GmbH, Waldstr. 23, 63128 Dietzenbach, Germany.

Zimmer, UK. Zimmer Ltd, The Courtyard, Lancaster Place, South Marston Park, Swindon, Wiltshire, SN3 4UQ, UK.

Ziwell, Singapore. Ziwell Medical (S) Pte Ltd, 1 Ubi Crescent, 05-03 Number One Building, S 408563, Singapore.

ZLB, Switz. ZLB Zentrallaboratorium, Blutspendedienst SRK, Wankdorfstrasse 10, 3000 Berne 22, Switzerland.

Zoja, Hong Kong. See *Deutsch Chinesische, Hong Kong.*

Zoki, Thai. See *Asian TJD, Thai.*

Zollweiden, Switz. Zollweiden Apotheke, Baselstrasse 71, 4142 Munchenstein, Switzerland.

Zuellig, Hong Kong. Zuellig Pharma, 7/F Somerset House, Taikoo Place, Quarry Bay, Hong Kong.

Zuellig, Singapore. Zuellig Pharma Pte Ltd, 19 Loyang Way, 08-20, S 508724, Singapore.

Zuellig, Thai. Zuellig Pharma Ltd, 8-9 Ploenchit Center, 2 Sukhumvit Rd, Kwang Klongtoey, Khet Klongtoey, Bangkok 10110, Thailand.

Zurich, S.Afr. Zurich, South Africa.

Zurita, Braz. Zurita Laboratorio Farmaceutico Ltda, Rua Domingos Graziano 104, 13600-000 Araras, SP, Brazil.

Zyfas, Singapore. Zyfas Medical Co, 11 Syed Alwi Rd, 04-01 Teck Heng Long Industrial Building, S 207629, Singapore.

Zyma, Belg. See *Novartis Consumer, Belg.*

Zyma, Fr. Laboratoires Zyma, Tour Albert 1er, 65 av. de Colmar, 92507 Rueil-Malmaison cdx, France.

Zyma, Ger. See *Novartis Consumer, Ger.*

Zyma, Ital. Zyma s.p.a., Corso Italia 13, 21047 Saronno (VA), Italy.

Zyma, Spain. See *Novartis, Spain.*

Zyma, Switz. See *Novartis, Switz.*, and *Novartis Consumer, Switz.*

Zyma, UK. Zyma Healthcare, UK.

General Index

Entries cover drugs (by monograph title, other approved names, synonyms, and chemical names), diseases (by disease treatment review title and associated terms), and proprietary preparations (by proprietary or brand name). They are arranged alphabetically in word-by-word order. Page references give both the page and column number as in 476·1, where 476 represents the page number and the figure 1 indicates that the entry will be found in column 1 of that page. There is no column number when the entry is in a table.

Anaritide, 938·2
Anartril, 1708·1
Anartrit, 1708·1
Anasclerol, 1708·1
Anased, 1708·1
Anaseptil, 1708·2
Anasilpiel, 1708·2
Anaspaz, 1708·2
Anassa, 1590·1
Anasten, 1708·2
Anastil, 1708·2
Anastil N, 1708·2
Anastrozole, 508·1
Anatac, 1708·2
Anatensol, 1708·2
Anatetall, 1708·2
Anatopic, 1708·2
Anatoxal Di, 1708·2
Anatoxal Di Te, 1708·2
Anatoxal Di Te Per, 1708·2
Anatoxal Te, 1708·2
Anatoxal Te Di, 1708·2
Anatoxina Estafilococica, 1708·2
Anatrast, 1708·2
Anatuss, 1708·2
Anatuss DM, 1708·2
Anatuss LA, 1708·2
Anatyl, 1708·2
Anauran, 1708·2
Anausin, 1708·2
Anax, 1708·2
Anaxeryl, 1708·3
Anazo, 1708·3
Anbesol, 1708·3
Anbesol Baby, 1708·3
Anbesol, Baby— see Baby Anbesol,
   1728·2
Anbesol, Maximum Strength— see Maxi-
   mum Strength Anbesol, 1956·4
Anbesol, Regular Strength— see Regular
   Strength Anbesol, 2066·4
Anbikan, 1708·3
Anbikin, 1708·3
Anbin, 1708·3
Anbycin, 1708·3
Ancamin, 1708·3
Ancef, 1708·3
Anceron, 1708·3
Ancestim, 737·1
Ancet, 1708·3
Anchoic Acid, 1110·3
Ancid, 1708·3
Ancitabine Hydrochloride, 508·2
Anco, 1708·3
Ancobon, 1708·3
Ancoloxin, 406·1
Ancopir, 1708·3
Ancoren, 1708·3
Ancoron, 1708·3
Ancotil, 1708·3
Ancrod, 839·3
Ancylostomiasis— see Hookworm Infec-
   tions, 93·2
Andante, 1708·3
Andantol, 1708·3
Andapsin, 1708·3
Andehist, 1708·3
Andehist DM, 1708·4
Andergin, 1708·4
Andion, 1708·4
Andociclina Balsamica, 1708·4
Andolba, 1708·4
Andolex, 1708·4
Andolex-C, 1708·4
Andolor, 1708·4
Andopan, 1708·4
Andornkraut, 1094·2
Andox, 1708·4
Andractim, 1708·4
Andreafol, 1708·4
Andrews Preparations, 1708·4
Andrews, Sais— see Sais Andrews,
   2081·3
Andrews, Sal de— see Sal de Andrews,
   2081·3
Andriodermol, 1708·4
Andriol, 1708·4

Andro, 1708·4
Androcur, 1708·4
Androderm, 1708·4
Andro-Diane, 1708·4
Androfemon, 1709·1
AndroGel, 1709·1
Androgenetic Alopecia— see Alopecia,
   1104·1
Androgens, 1452·1
Android, 1709·1
Androlone-D, 1709·1
Andropatch, 1709·1
Andropository, 1709·1
Androskat, 1709·1
Androstanazole, 1491·3
Androstanolone, 1465·2
Androstenedione, 1465·2
Androst-4-ene-3,17-dione, 1465·2
Androsterone, 1493·3
Androtardyl, 1709·1
Androvite, 1709·1
Androxicam, 1709·1
Androxon, 1709·1
Androxyl, 1709·1
Andrumin, 1709·1
Andursil, 1709·1
Andursil N, 1709·1
Anebron, 1709·1
Anectine, 1709·1
Anekron, 1709·1
Anemagen, 1709·1
Anemagen OB, 1709·1
Anemarrhena asphodeloides, 1668·1
Anemet, 1709·1
Anemital, 1709·1
Anemofer, 1709·1
Anemokol, 1709·1
Anemone pulsatilla, 1656·3
Anemul Mono, 1709·1
Anencephaly— see Neural Tube Defects,
   1362·1
Anerex, 1709·1
Anergan, 1709·1
Anervan, 1709·2
Anesdente Do Bebe, 1709·2
Anespas, 1709·2
Anest Compuesto, 1709·2
Anestacon, 1709·2
Anestalcon, 1709·2
Anestesia Loc Braun C/A, 1709·2
Anestesia Loc Braun S/A, 1709·2
Anestesia Topi Braun C/A, 1709·2
Anestesico, 1709·2
Anestesiol, 1709·2
Anesthamine, 1306·2
Anesthesique Double, 1709·2
Anesti Doble, 1709·2
Anestina Braun, 1709·2
Anestocil, 1709·2
Anethaine, 1709·2
Anethi, Oleum, 1603·3
Anethol, 1580·1
Anethole, 1580·1
Anethole Trithione, 1580·1
Anethum graveolens, 1603·3
Anetin, 1709·2
Anetol, 1580·1
Aneural, 1709·2
Aneurin, 1709·2
Aneurine Hydrochloride, 1385·1
Aneurine Mononitrate, 1385·1
Aneurol, 1709·2
Anevrase, 1709·2
Anevrasi, 1709·2
Anew, 1709·2, 1709·3
Anexate, 1709·3
Anexsia, 1709·3
ANF, 938·1
Anfenax, 1709·3
Anfertil, 1709·3
Anfetamina, 1506·3
Anflat, 1709·3
Anfocort, 1709·3
Anfomicin, 1709·3
Anfotericina B, 377·2
Angass, 1709·3
Angass S, 1709·3

Angel, Destroying, 1638·2
Angel Dust, 763·3, 1650·2
Angel Hair, 1650·2
Angel Mist, 1650·2
Angelica, 1580·2
Angelica acutiloba, 1580·2
Angelica archangelica, 1580·2
Angelica dahurica, 1580·2
Angelica pubescens, 1580·2
Angelica sinensis, 1580·2
Angelicae Radix, 1580·2
Angettes, 1709·3
Angeze, 1709·3
Angiact, 1709·3
Angicontin, 1709·3
Angicor, 1709·3
Angidil, 1709·3
Angidine, 1709·3
Angifebrine, 1709·3
Angifonil, 1709·3
Angileptol, 1709·3
Angilol, 1709·3
Angimon, 1709·3
Angina— see Angina Pectoris, 791·1
Angina MCC, 1709·3
Angina Pectoris, 791·1
Angina, Prinzmetal's— see Angina Pec-
   toris, 791·1
Angina-Gastreu N R1, 1709·3
Anginamide, 1709·3
Anginasin N, 1709·3
Anginesin, 1709·3
Anginin, 1709·3
Anginine, 1709·4
Angino Tricin, 1709·4
Anginol, 1709·4
Anginol-Lidocaine, 1709·4
Anginomycin, 1709·4
Anginor, 1709·4
Angino-Rub, 1709·4
Anginova, 1709·4
Anginova Nouvelle Formule, 1709·4
Anginovag, 1709·4
Anginovin H, 1709·4
Anginozetes, 1709·4
Angiocine, 1709·4
Angiocardyl N, 1709·4
Angio-Conray, 1709·4
Angiodarona, 1709·4
Angiodrox, 1709·4
Angioedema— see Urticaria and An-
   gioedema, 1107·3
Angioedema, Hereditary— see Hereditary
   Angioedema, 743·2
Angioflux, 1709·4
Angiografin, 1709·4
Angiografin, Uro— see Uro Angiografin,
   2152·3
Angiografine, 1709·4
Angiolong, 1709·4
Angiomax, 1709·4
Angioneurotic Oedema, Hereditary— see
   Hereditary Angioedema, 743·2
Angionorm, 1709·4
Angiopas, 1709·4
Angiophtal, 1709·4
Angiopine, 1709·4
Angioplasty— see Reperfusion and Revas-
   cularisation Procedures, 812·1
Angiorex, 1709·4
Angiosedante, 1710·1
Angiostrongyliasis, 91·3
Angiotensin II, 840·1
Angiotensin Amide, 840·1
Angiotensin II Receptor Antagonists,
   787·2
Angiotensinamide, 840·1
Angiotensin-converting Enzyme Inhibi-
   tors, 787·1, 820·2
Angioton, 1710·1
Angioton S, 1710·1
Angiotrofin, 1710·1
Angiovist 282, 1710·1
Angiovist 292, 1710·1
Angiovist 370— see Angiovist 292, An-
   giovist 370, 1710·1
Angiozem, 1710·1
Angipress, 1710·1

Angisan, 1710·1
Angised, 1710·1
Angi-Spray, 1710·1
Angispray, 1710·1
Angitak, 1710·1
Angitil, 1710·1
Angitrate, 1710·1
Angitrit, 1710·1
Angizem, 1710·1
Anglais, Sel, 1191·1
Anglix, 1710·1
Anglopen, 1710·1
Angocin Anti-Infekt N, 1710·1
Angocin Bronchialtropfen, 1710·1
Angocin Percutan, 1710·1
Angostura Bark, 1601·2
Angostura Bitters, 1601·2
Angstrom Corpo, 1710·1
Angstrom Viso/Labbra Alta Protezione,
   1710·1
Angurate Magentee, 1710·1
Anhalonium lewinii, 1634·3
Anhalonium williamsii, 1634·3
Anhascha, 1590·1
Anhedonia, 271·1
Anhídrido Crómico, 1594·2
Anhisnon, 1710·1
2,2′-Anhydro-(1-β-D-arabinofuranosyl)cyto-
   sine Hydrochloride, 508·2
Anhydroepitetracycline, 259·2
Anhydrol Forte, 1710·2
Anhydrotetracycline, 259·1
Anhydrous Citric Acid, 1596·2
Anhydrous Glucose, 1364·3
Anhydrous Sodium Sulfate, 1250·1
Anhydrous Sodium Sulphate, 1250·1
Anhypen, 1710·2
Anidrosan, 1710·2
Anifed, 1710·2
Anifer Fenchelhonig, 1710·2
Anifer Hustenbalsam, 1710·2
Anifer Hustentee, 1710·2
Anifer Hustentropfen, 1710·2
Anifer Krauterol, 1710·2
Aniflazime, 1710·2
Aniflazym, 1710·2
Anileridine, 14·1
Anileridine Hydrochloride, 14·1
Anileridine Phosphate, 14·2
Anilid, 1710·2
Aniline, 1400·2
Aniline Green, 1150·1
Aniline Red, 1149·3
Anilusin, 1710·2
Animal Bites, Infections in— see Bites
   and Stings, 115·3
Animal Shapes, 1710·2
Animal Shapes + Iron, 1710·2
Animine, 1710·2
Anionen-Spurenelement, 1710·2
Anionic Emulsifying Wax, 1409·1
Anionic Surfactants, 1496·1
Aniospray, 1710·2
Anipamil, 840·2
Aniracetam, 1580·2
Anís, Esencia de, 1580·3
Anis, Essence D', 1580·3
Anís Estrellado, 1580·2
Anis Étoilé, 1580·2
Anis Verde, 1580·2
Anis Vert, 1580·2
Anisan, 1710·2
Anise, 1580·2
Anise Fruit, 1580·2
Anise Fruit, Star, 1580·2
Anise Oil, 1580·3
Anise, Star, 1580·2
Aniseed, 1580·2
Aniseed Oil, 1580·3
Anisi Aetheroleum, 1580·3
Anisi Fructus, 1580·2
Anisi, Oleum, 1580·3
Anisi Stellati Fructus, 1580·2
Anisi Vulgaris, Fructus, 1580·2
Anisindione, 840·2
Anismus, 1325·2
Anisotropine Methobromide, 470·3

Cramp— *see* Muscle Spasm, 1322·1
Cramp, Haemodialysis-induced— *see* Haemodialysis-induced Cramp, 1184·2
Cramp, Haemodialysis-induced— *see* Muscle Spasm, 1322·1
Cramp, Writer's— *see* Dystonias, 1173·2
Crampex, 1795·3
Crampiton, 1795·3
Cranberry, 1600·2
Cranberry, American, 1600·2
Cranberry Complex, 1795·3
Cranbiotic Super, Bioglan— *see* Bioglan Cranbiotic Super, 1743·3
Cranio-cyl Ho-Len-Complex, 1795·3
Crank, 1511·1
Cranoc, 1795·3
Crasnitin, 1795·3
Crataegan, 1795·3
Crataegisan, 1795·3
Crataegitan, 1795·3
Crataegol, 1795·3
Crataegus, 1600·2
Crataegus Complex, 1795·4
Crataegus laevigata, 1600·2
Crataegus Med Complex, 1795·4
Crataegus monogyna, 1600·2
Crataegus oxyacantha, 1600·2
Crataegus Oxyacantha, 1600·2
Crataegutt, 1795·4
Crataegysat F, 1795·4
Crataelanat, 1795·4
Crataepas, 1795·4
Crataezyma, 1795·4
Cratamed Novo, 1795·4
Cratecor, 1795·4
Cratimon, 1795·4
Cravinho, 1596·3
Craviscum Mono, 1795·4
Cravit, 1795·4
Cravo-da-Índia, 1596·3
Cravo-Espin, 1795·4
CRD-401, 874·3
Creacal, 1795·4
Creagin, 1795·4
Cream E45, 1795·4
Cream E45— *see* E45, 1835·1
Cream of Tartar, Purified, 1244·3
Cream of Tartar, Soluble, 1653·1
Creamy Tar, 1795·4
Creanolona, 1795·4
Creasote, 1087·3
Creatile, 1795·4
Creatine Monohydrate, 1600·3
Creatine Phosphate, 1600·3
Creatine Phosphoric Acid, 1600·3
Creatinine, 1601·1
Creatinolfosfate Sodium, 1601·1
Creatyl, 1795·4
Crecil, 1795·4
Credaxol, 1795·4
Creeping Eruption— *see* Cutaneous Larva Migrans, 92·2
Crelo Blanco, 1795·4
Crema Blanca, 1795·4
Crema Contracepti Lanzas, 1795·4
Crema de Magnesia, 1795·4
Crema Facial De Dia AHA Formula 405, 1795·4
Crema Facial De Noche AHA Formula 405, 1795·4
Cremalgin, 1795·4
Crema-U, 1795·4
Creme Anti-Rides Auto-Bronzante, 1796·1
Creme Auto-Bronzant, 1796·1
Creme Autobronzante Visage, 1796·1
Creme de Base, 1796·1
Creme Des 3 Fleurs D'Orient, 1796·1
Creme Ecran Total, 1796·1
Creme Haute Protection, 1796·1
Creme Laser Hidrante, 1796·1
Creme Protectrice, 1796·1
Creme Rap, 1796·1
Creme Solaire Anti-Rides, 1796·1
Creme Solaire Bronzage, 1796·1
Creme Solaire Bronzage Rapide, 1796·1
Creme Solaire Bronzage Securite, 1796·1
Creme Solaire Bronzage Securite Special, 1796·1

Creme Solaire Ecran Special Visage, 1796·1
Creme Solaire Haute Protection, 1796·1
Cremicort-H, 1796·1
Cremisona, 1796·1
Cremol-P, 1796·1
Cremol-Ritter, 1796·1
Cremosan, 1796·1
Cremsol, 1796·1
Crenodyn, 1796·1
Creo Grippe, 1796·2
Creodermol, 1796·2
Creolina, 1796·2
Creon, 1796·2
Creo-Rectal, 1796·2
Creosol, 1124·3
Creosotal, 1087·3
Creosote, 1087·3
Creosote Bush, 1593·3
Creosote Carbonate, 1087·3
Creosote, Wood, 1087·3
Creo-Terpin, 1796·2
Crescicalcio, 1796·2
Crescom, 1796·2
Cresol, 1142·3
Cresol and Soap Solution, 1142·3
Cresolox, 1796·2
Cresols, 1158·1
m-Cresolsulphonic Acid-formaldehyde, 738·3
Cresolum Crudum, 1142·3
Cresophene, 1796·2
Cresoxydiol, 1329·2
Crest, Sensitivity Protection— *see* Sensitivity Protection Crest, 2090·3
Crestanon, 1796·2
Crestomycin Sulphate, 599·2
Cresylate, 1796·2
Cresylic Acid, 1142·3
Cresylic Acids, 1158·1
Creta Preparada, 1215·1
Cretinism— *see* Hypothyroidism, 1520·2
Cretinism, Endemic— *see* Iodine Deficiency Disorders, 1523·3
Creutzfeldt-Jakob Disease, Disinfection Procedures— *see* Disinfection in Creutzfeldt-Jakob Disease, 1129·3
CRF, 1280·1
CRH, 1280·1, 1796·2
Crilanomer, 1112·3
Crilem, 1796·2
Crimanex, 1796·2
Crimean Congo Haemorrhagic Fever— *see* Haemorrhagic Fevers, 605·2
Crimean-Congo Haemorrhagic Fever Immunoglobulins, 1535·3
Crinalsofex, 1796·2
Criniton, 1796·2
Crino Cordes, 1796·2
Crino Cordes N, 1796·2
Crinohermal Fem Neu, 1796·2
Crino-Kaban N, 1796·2
Crinone, 1796·2
Crinopex, 1796·2
Crinopex-N, 1796·2
Crinoren, 1796·2
Crinoretic, 1796·2
Crinotar, 1796·2
Criostat SD 2, 1796·3
Cripar, 1796·3
CRI-regen, 1796·3
Crisantaspase, 508·3
Crisinor, 1796·3
Crislaxo, 1796·3
Crismol, 1796·3
Crisnatol Mesilate, 527·3
Crisnatol Mesylate, 527·3
Crisolax, 1796·3
Cristal, 1796·3
Cristalcrom, 1796·3
Cristales de Sosa, 1665·2
Cristalmina, 1796·3
Cristan, 1796·3
Cristopal, 1796·3
Criticare HN, 1796·3
Critichol, 1796·3
Crixivan, 1796·3

CRL-40048, 1506·2
CRL-40476, 1512·3
Cro 50, 1796·3
Crocetins, 1029·1
Croci Stigma, 1029·1
Crocidolite, 1582·3
Crocines, 1029·1
Croconazole Hydrochloride, 382·3
Crocus, 1029·1
Crocus sativus, 1029·1
Crodamols, 1796·3
CroFab, 1796·3
Croferron, 1796·3
Croglina, 1796·3
Crohn's Disease— *see* Inflammatory Bowel Disease, 1205·2
Crolom, 1796·3
Cromabak, 1796·3
Cromakalim, 865·1
Cromal, 1796·3
Cromantal, 1796·3
Cro-Man-Zin, 1796·3
Cromaton, 1796·3
Cromatonbic B12, 1796·4
Cromatonbic Ferro, 1796·4
Cromatonbic Folinico, 1796·4
Cromatonferro, 1796·4
Cromedil, 1796·4
Cromer Orto, 1796·4
Cromese, 1796·4
Cromex, 1796·4
Cromezin, 1796·4
Cromo, 1796·4
Cromo Asma, 1796·4
Cromo Pur, 1796·4
Cromocap— *see* Proendotel, 2052·3
Cromodyn, 1796·4
Cromoftol, 1796·4
Cromogen, 1796·4
Cromogen, Steri-Neb— *see* Steri-Neb Cromogen, 2107·4
Cromoglicate, Sodium, 774·3
Cromoglicin, 1796·4
Cromoglin, 1796·4
Cromoglycate, Sodium, 774·3
Cromohexal, 1796·4
Cromol, 1796·4
Cromolerg, 1796·4
Cromolind, 1796·4
Cromolyn, 1796·4
Cromolyn Sodium, 774·3
Crom-Ophtal, 1796·4
Cromopp, 1796·4
Cromoptic, 1796·4
Cromosan, 1796·4
Cromoseptil Plus, 1796·4
Cromosol Ophta, 1796·4
Cromosol UD, 1796·4
Cromovisus, 1797·1
Cromoxin K, 1797·1
Cromozil, 1797·1
Cromunal, 1797·1
Cronacol, 1797·1
Cronal, 1797·1
Cronase, 1797·1
Cronasma, 1797·1
Cronassial, 1797·1
Croneparina, 1797·1
Cronizat, 1797·1
Cronobe, 1797·1
Cronocaps, 1797·1
Cronocef, 1797·1
Cronocol, 1797·1
Cronodine, 1797·1
Cronogeron, 1797·1
Cronol, 1797·1
Cronomet, 1797·1
Cronovera, 1797·1
Cropropamide, 1514·2
Croscarmellose Sodium, 1499·3
Crospovidone, 1503·2
Crospovidonum, 1503·2
Cross Prep, 1797·1
Crosslinked Carboxymethylcellulose Sodium, 1499·3
Crosslinked Haemoglobin, 738·1
Crotalaria, 1601·1
Crotam, 1112·3

Crotamitex, 1797·1
Crotamiton, 1112·3
Crotamitonum, 1112·3
Crotetamide, 1514·2
Crotethamide, 1514·2
Croton Oil, 1221·3
Croton sublyratus, 1244·2
Croton tiglium, 1221·3
Crotonis, Oleum, 1221·3
Croup, 1049·3
Cruex, 1797·1
Crusca, 1214·2
Cruscasohn, 1797·1
Crushed Linseed, 1629·1
Crusken, 1797·1
Cruzzy, 1797·1
Cruzzy Antiparassitario, 1797·1
Cryobutol, 1797·1
Cryocriptina, 1797·1
Cryofluorane, 1199·1
Cryogesic, 1797·2
Cryometasona, 1797·2
Cryoperacid, 1797·2
Cryopina, 1797·2
Cryoprecipitate, 734·3
Cryoprecipitated Antihemophilic Factor, 734·1
Cryopril, 1797·2
Cryosolona, 1797·2
Cryo-Tropin, 1797·2
Cryoval, 1797·2
Cryovin, 1797·2
Cryoxifeno, 1797·2
Cryozol, 1797·2
Cryptococcal Meningitis— *see* Cryptococcosis, 373·3
Cryptococcosis, 373·3
Cryptocur, 1797·2
Cryptogenic Fibrosing Alveolitis— *see* Diffuse Parenchymal Lung Disease, 1050·1
Cryptorchidism, 1272·1
Cryptosporidiosis, 583·2
Crysanal, 1797·2
Cryst. I.Z.S, 324·3
Crystacide, 1797·2
Crystal, 1511·1, 1650·2
Crystal Meth, 1511·1
Crystal Violet, 1150·3
Crystalline Cellulose, 1500·2
Crystalline Penicillin G, 157·1
Crystallinic Acid, 232·2
Crystalloid Plasma Expanders, 813·2
Crystamine, 1797·2
Crystapen, 1797·2
Crysti 1000, 1797·2
Crysticillin, 1797·2
Crystodigin, 1797·2
CS-045, 337·1
CS-370, 671·2
CS-386, 692·3
CS-443, 159·2
CS-500, 932·2
CS-514, 957·3
CS-600, 50·2
CS-622, 979·3
CS-684, 1244·2
CS-807, 172·3
CS-1170, 167·2
CS Gas, 1601·1
CS Spray, 1601·1
CSA, 1594·2
CSAG-144, 1233·3
C-Soft, 1797·2
C-Solve, 1797·2
CST, 1797·2
CT-1101, 1620·2
CT Ointment, 1797·2
CT Pommade, 1797·2
CT Shampoo, 1797·2
CTAB, 1137·3
C-Tabs, 1797·2
C-Tard, 1797·2
C/T/S, 1797·2
CTX, 50·2, 169·1
C-type Natriuretic Peptide, 938·1
Cuasia, Leño de, 1657·1
Cuatroderm, 1797·2

Gravibinan, 1888·4
Gravibibon, 1888·4
Gravidex, 1888·4
Gravidinona, 1888·4
Gravigard, 1888·4
Gravigen, 1888·4
Gravindex, 1888·4
Gravistat, 1888·4
Gravitamon, 1888·4
Gravol, 1888·4
Greatbloc, 1888·4
Greater Burnet, 1587·3
Greater Celandine, 1618·1
Greater-Gloxa, 1888·4
Greatofen, 1888·4
Greefe, 1590·1
Greek Sage, 1660·2
Green, Aniline, 1150·1
Green Antiseptic Mouthwash & Gargle, 1888·4
Green B, Diamond, 1150·1
Green B, Wool, 1028·3
Green, Brilliant, 1136·1
Green BS, Acid Brilliant, 1028·3
Green, China, 1150·1
Green Copperas, 1360·3
Green, Emerald, 1136·1
Green, Ethyl, 1136·1
Green G, Diamond, 1136·1
Green G, Malachite, 1136·1
Green Hellebore, 1679·3
Green Hellebore Rhizome, 1679·3
Green, Indocyanine, 1623·2
Green, Lissamine, 1028·3
Green, Malachite, 1150·1
Green S, 1028·3
Green S, Acid, 1028·3
Green Soap, 1496·1
Green, Solid, 1136·1
Green Veratrum, 1679·3
Green Vitriol, 1360·3
Green-lipped Mussel, 1618·2
Greenosan, 1888·4
Grefen, 1888·4
Gregoderm, 1888·4
Gregovite C, Uniflu &— see Uniflu & Gregovite C, 2150·1
Gregovite C, Uniflu with— see Uniflu with Gregovite C, 2150·1
Grenadier, 106·3
Grenadille, 1649·1
Greosin, 1888·4
Grepafloxacin Hydrochloride, 214·1
Grexin, 1888·4
GRF, 1297·1
GRF(1-40), 1297·2
GRF(1-44), 1297·2
GRF-44, 1297·1
GRF(1-29)NH₂, 1297·1
Gricin, 1888·4
Grietalgen, 1888·4
Grietalgen Hidrocort, 1888·4
Grifa, 1590·1
Grifed, 1889·1
Grifulin, 1889·1
Grifulvin, 1889·1
Grifulvin V, 1889·1
Grindelia, 1618·2
Griottier, 1029·1
Gripakin, 1889·1
Gripalgine, 1889·1
Gripavac, 1889·1
Gripcaps C, 1889·1
Gripefago C, 1889·1
Gripefin, 1889·1
Gripen, 1889·1
Gripenil, 1889·1
Gripeonil, 1889·1
Gripetral, 1889·1
Gripex, 1889·1
Gripidor, 1889·1
Gripin C, 1889·1
Gripion, 1889·1
Gripionex, 1889·1
Gripol C, 1889·1
Gripol C Capuride, 1889·1
Gripol Composto, 1889·1
Gripomatine, 1889·1

Griponal, 1889·1
Griponia, 1889·2
Grippal, 1889·2
Grippalgine N, 1889·2
Grippalin & C, 1889·2
Grippefloran, 1889·2
Grippe-Gastreu R6, 1889·2
Grippe-Tee, Kneipp— see Kneipp Grippe-Tee, 1928·3
Grippetee Dr Zeidler, 1889·2
Grippetee EF-EM-ES, 1889·2
Gripp-Heel, 1889·2
Grippin-Merz, 1889·2
Grippinon, 1889·2
Grippogran, 1889·2
Grippon, 1889·2
Grippostad C, 1889·2
Grippostad Gute Nacht-Saft, 1889·2
Grippostad Heissgetrank, 1889·2
Gripps, 1889·2
Gripsay, 1889·2
Griptol, 1889·2
Grisactin, 1889·2
Grise, 1889·2
Grisefuline, 1889·2
Griseo, 1889·2
Griseoful, 1889·2
Griseofulvin, 386·2
Griseofulvina, 386·2
Griseofulvinum, 386·2
Griseomed, 1889·2
Griseostatin, 1889·3
Grisetin, 1889·3
Grisflavin, 1889·3
Grisol, 1889·3
Grisomicon, 1889·3
Grisovin, 1889·3
Grisovin FP, 1889·3
Grisovina FP, 1889·3
Gris-PEG, 1889·3
Grivin, 1889·3
Grodurex, 1889·3
Grofenac, 1889·3
Gromazol, 1889·3
Groprim, 1889·3
Grotanat, 1889·3
Ground Cherry, 1651·2
Ground Ivy, 1618·2
Ground-nut Oil, 1581·1
Group B Streptococcal Infection, Perinatal— see Perinatal Streptococcal Infections, 133·3
Grovixim, 1889·3
Growth Factor, Epidermal, 1254·2
Growth Factor, Human Epidermal, 1254·2
Growth Hormone, 1286·1
Growth Hormone Deficiency— see Growth Retardation, 1273·3
Growth Hormone, Human, 1286·1
Growth Hormone, Methionyl Bovine, 1286·1
Growth Hormone, Methionyl Human, 1286·1
Growth Hormone, Methionyl Porcine, 1286·1
Growth Hormone Resistance— see Growth Retardation, 1273·3
Growth Hormone Secretion, Excessive— see Acromegaly and Gigantism, 1271·3
Growth Hormone, Synthetic Bovine, 1286·1
Growth Hormone-releasing Factor (Human), 1297·1
Growth Hormone-releasing Factor (Human)-(1-29)-peptide Amide, 1297·1
Growth Hormone-releasing Hormone, 1297·1
Growth-hormone-release-inhibiting Hormone, 1297·3
Growth-hormone-releasing Peptide-6, 1297·2
Growth Retardation, 1273·3
Gruncef, 1889·3
Grune Salbe "Schmidt" N, 1889·3
Grunicina, 1889·3
Grunlicht Dreierlei Tropfen, 1889·3
Grunlicht Hingfong Essenz, 1889·3
Grunlicht Magenbalsam Tropfen, 1889·3
Gruntin Tropfen, 1889·3

GS-95, 426·1
GS-0393, 616·1
GS-504, 616·3
GS-0504, 616·3
GS-0840, 616·1
GS-930, 617·2
GS-1278, 642·1
GS-2876, 222·3
GS-2989, 222·1
GS-3065, 200·1
GS-3159, 160·2
GS-4104/002, 638·1
GS-4331/05, 642·1
GS-6244, 160·1
GSH, 1010·3
G-Strophanthin, 950·2
GT-41, 513·3
GT-92, 465·2
GT-1012, 957·2
GT16-026A, 1021·2
G_Tlb, 1614·1
G.Test, 1889·3
GT31-104HB, 863·3
GTN, 897·3
Guabenxan, 900·2
Guabenxan Sulfate, 900·2
Guabza, 1590·1
Guacetisal, 1092·1
Guafen, 1889·3
Guaiac, 1618·2
Guaiacalcium Complex, 1889·3
p-Guaiacol, 1118·2
Guaiacol, 1092·1, 1124·3
Guaiacol Carbonate, 1092·1
Guaiacol Cinnamate, 1092·1
Guaiacol Ethylglycolate, 1092·1
Guaiacol Glycerol Ether, 1092·2
Guaiacol Phenylacetate, 1092·1
Guaiacol Phenylbutyrate, 1092·1
Guaiacum, 1618·2
Guaiacum officinale, 1618·2
Guaiacum Resin, 1618·2
Guaiacum sanctum, 1618·2
Guaiacum Wood, 1618·2
Guaiacyl Glyceryl Ether, 1092·2
Guaiaspir, 1889·4
Guaiazulene, 1583·2, 1618·3
Guaietolin, 1092·1
Guaifed, 1889·4
Guaifed-PD, 1889·4
Guaifenesin, 1092·2
Guaifenesin AC, 1889·4
Guaifenesin Calcium, 1092·2
Guaifenesin DAC, 1889·4
Guaifenesin DM, 1889·4
Guaifenesina, 1092·2
Guaifenesinum, 1092·2
Guaifenex Preparations, 1889·4
Guaimax-D, 1889·4
Guaimesal, 1092·3
Guaipax, 1889·4
Guaiphenesin, 1092·2
Guaiphenesin Carbamate, 1329·3
Guaitab, 1889·4
Guaivent, 1889·4
Guai-Vent/PSE, 1889·4
Guajabronc, 1889·4
Guajacol, 1092·1
Guajacolum Glycerolatum, 1092·2
Guajakharz, 1618·2
Guanabenz Acetate, 900·2
Guanadrel Sulfate, 900·3
Guanadrel Sulphate, 900·3
Guanethidine Hemisulfate, 901·1
Guanethidine Monosulfate, 901·1
Guanethidine Monosulphate, 901·1
Guanethidini Monosulfas, 901·1
Guanfacine Hydrochloride, 901·3
Guanidine Hydrochloride, 1419·2
4-Guanidino-2,4-dideoxy-2,3-dehydro-N-acetylneuraminic Acid, 644·3
N¹-4-(Guanidobutyl)bleomycinamide, 511·3
Guanor, 1889·4
Guanosine 5'-(Disodium Phosphate), 1604·2
Guanoxan Sulfate, 902·1
Guanoxan Sulphate, 902·1

Guanylate Cyclase Inhibitors, 139·1
Guapi Bark, 1087·2
Guar Flour, 323·3
Guar Galactomannan, 323·3
Guar Gum, 323·3
Guar Verlan, 1889·4
Guarana, 1681·2
Guaranine, 761·3, 1681·2
Guarasex, 1889·4
Guarea rusbyi, 1087·2
Guarem, 1889·4
Guastil, 1889·4
Guaxan, 1889·4
Guaza, 1590·1
Gubamine, 1889·4
Guep'Away, 1889·4
Guethol, 1092·3
Guethol Carbonate, 1092·3
Guethol Nicotinate, 1092·3
Guethural, 1890·1
Gufen N, 1890·1
Gugecin, 1890·1
Gui, 1636·2
GuiaCough CF, 1890·1
GuiaCough PE, 1890·1
Guiatex, 1890·1
Guiatex LA, 1890·1
Guiatex PSE, 1890·1
Guiatuss, 1890·1
Guiatuss CF, 1890·1
Guiatuss PE, 1890·1
Guiatussin with Codeine Expectorant, 1890·1
Guiatussin DAC, 1890·1
Guiatussin with Dextromethorphan, 1890·1
Guigoz Hypoallergenique, 1890·1
Guillain-Barré Syndrome, 1554·2
Guimauve, Racine de, 1577·1
Guinea-worm Infection— see Dracunculiasis, 92·3
Gulf War Syndrome— see Nerve Gas Poisoning, 1424·2
L-Guluronic Acid, 1498·3
Gum Acacia, 1498·2
Gum Arabic, 1498·2
Gum Asafetida, 1582·3
Gum Benjamin, 1668·3
Gum Benzoin, 1668·3
Gum, British, 1359·1
Gum, Carob, 1500·3
Gum, Carob Bean, 1500·3
Gum, Cellulose, 1499·3
Gum, Cellulose, Modified, 1499·3
Gum, Ceratonia, 1500·3
Gum, Corn Sugar, 1504·3
Gum Dragon, 1504·2
Gum, Guar, 323·3
Gum, Jaguar, 323·3
Gum, Karaya, 1250·2
Gum, Locust Bean, 1500·3
Gum Myrrh, 1639·2
Gum Opium, 69·3
Gum Plant, 1618·2
Gum, Starch, 1359·1
Gum, Sterculia, 1250·2
Gum Tragacanth, 1504·2
Gum, Xantham, 1504·3
Gum, Xanthan, 1504·3
Gumbaral, 1890·1
Gumbix, 1890·1
Gum-Ese, 1890·1
Gumilk, 1890·1
Gummi Africanum, 1498·2
Gummi Arabicum, 1498·2
Gummi Mimosae, 1498·2
Gummi Plasticum, 1618·3
Gumweed, 1618·2
Guncotton, Soluble, 1122·1
Gunevax, 1890·1
Gunjah, 1590·1
Gunza, 1590·1
Gupisone, 1890·1
Gurfix, 1890·1
Gurgellosung Chauvin, 1890·1
Gurgellosung-ratiopharm, 1890·1
Guronamin, 1890·1
Guronsan, 1890·1, 1890·2
Gusperimus Hydrochloride, 544·1

Haloperidol, 686·3
Haloperidol Decanoate, 686·3
Haloperidol Lactate, 687·2
Haloperidoli Decanoas, 686·3
Haloperidolum, 686·3
Haloperil, 1892·2
Halopol, 1892·2
Haloprogin, 387·1
Halopyramine Hydrochloride, 412·1
Hal-oral, 1892·2
Haloral, 1892·2
Halotestin, 1892·2
Halotex, 1892·2
Halothane, 1259·3
Halothanum, 1259·3
Halotussin, 1892·2
Halotussin-DM, 1892·2
Haloxazolam, 688·1
Haloxon, 99·3
Halquinol, 214·1
Halquinols, 214·1
Halset, 1892·2
Haltran, 1892·2
Halycitrol, 1892·2
Hamadin, 1892·2
Hamamelidis, 1618·3
Hamamelis, 1618·3
Hamamelis Complex, 1892·2
Hamamelis Compose, 1892·2
Hamamelis virginiana, 1618·3
Hamamilla, 1892·2
Hamasana, 1892·2
Hamatopan, 1892·2
Hamatopan F, 1892·2
Hametum, 1892·2
Hametum-N, 1892·2
HAMFL, 1892·2
Hamilton Preparations, 1892·3
Hamoagil Plus, 1892·4
Hamo-Europuran N, 1892·4
Hamofiltrasol, 1892·4
Hamo-ratiopharm, 1892·4
Hamorrhoidal-Zapfchen, 1892·4
Hamos N, 1892·4
Hamos-Tropfen-S, 1892·4
Hamovannad, 1892·4
Hamo-Vibolex, 1892·4
Hamp, 1590·1
Hand Cream with Sunscreen, 1892·4
Handexin, 1892·4
Hand-Schüller-Christian Disease— *see* Histiocytic Syndromes, 483·3
Hanfkraut, 1590·1
Hanotoxin N, 1892·4
Hanp, 1892·4
Hansamed Spray, 1892·4
Hansaplast Herbal Heat Plaster, 1892·4
Hansaplast Hornhaut-Pflaster, 1892·4
Hansaplast Huhneraugen-Pflaster, 1892·4
Hansaplast Spruhpflaster, 1892·4
Hansen's Disease— *see* Leprosy, 126·3
Hantavirus Pulmonary Syndrome, 605·3
Haouzi, 1590·1
HAPA-B, 215·2
Happinose, 1892·4
Hard Fat, 1409·1
Hard Paraffin, 1407·1
Hard Soap, 1496·2
Hardhack, 1667·1
Haricon, 1892·4
Haridol, 1892·4
Harmaline, 1619·1
Harmine, 1619·1
Harmogen, 1892·4
Harmomed, 1892·4
Harmonet, 1892·4
Harmonette, 1892·4
Harmosin, 1892·4
Harnal, 1892·4
Harnosal, 1892·4
Harnsauretropfen F, 1893·1
Harnsauretropfen N, 1893·1
Harntee 400, 1893·1
Harntee 450, 1893·1
Harntee STADA, 1893·1
Harntee-Steiner, 1893·1
Harntreibender Tee, 1893·1

Harongan, 1893·1
Harpadol, 1893·1
Harpagin, 1893·1
Harpagocid, 1893·1
Harpagofito Orto, 1893·1
Harpagoforte Asmedic, 1893·1
HarpagoMega, 1893·1
Harpagophyti Radix, 26·3
Harpagophyton, 26·3
Harpagophytum, 26·3
Harpagophytum Complex, 1893·1
Harpagophytum procumbens, 26·3
Harpagophytum Procumbens, 26·3
Harpagoside, 26·3
Harringtonine, 544·2
Hartfett, 1409·1
Hartiosen, 1893·1
Hartmannsche, 1893·1
Hartparaffin, 1407·1
Hartshorn and Oil, 1579·2
Hartsorb, 1893·1
Harzer Hustenelixier, 1893·1
Harzer Hustenloser, 1893·1
Harzol, 1893·1
Hascisc, 1590·1
Hashimoto's Thyroiditis— *see* Hypothyroidism, 1520·2
Hashish, 1590·1
Hasis, 1590·1
Hasji's, 1590·1
Hasjisj, 1590·1
Haszysz, 1590·1
HA-Tabletten N, 1893·1
H-Atetal, 1893·1
Hauhechelwurzel, 1644·1
Hautfunktionstropfen S, 1893·1
Hautplus N Dr Hagedorn, 1893·1
Haut-Vital N, 1893·1
Havlane, 1893·1
Havrix, 1893·1
Haw, 1600·2
Hawaiian Tropic Preparations, 1893·2
Hawkmide, 1893·3
Hawkperan, 1893·3
Hawthorn, English, 1600·2
Haxixe, 1590·1
Hay Fever— *see* Rhinitis, 407·3
Hay Fever, 1893·3
Hay Fever Relief, 1893·3
Hay Fever & Sinus Relief, 1893·3
Hayclear, 1893·3
Hay-Crom, 1893·3
Hayfebrol, 1893·3
Hayfever Eye Drops, 1893·3
Hayfever Relief, 1893·3
Hayfever & Sinus Relief, 1893·3
Haymine, 1893·3
Hazelwort, 1582·3
HB-419, 321·3
HBF-386, 532·2
H-BIG, 1893·3
HbOC, 1540·2
H-B-Vax, 1893·3
H-B-Vax, Gen— *see* Gen H-B-Vax, 1880·2
H-B-Vax II, 1893·3
HB-Vax-DNA, 1893·3
HBvaxPRO, 1893·3
HBW-023, 919·3
HBY-097, 642·1
Hc45, 1893·3
HC-803, 1229·2
HC-1528, 589·3
HC-20511, 767·2
HC Derma-Pax, 1893·3
HCB, 1433·3
HCFCs, 1199·2
HCFU, 516·1
HCG, 1279·2
HCH, 1434·1
HCOR, 1073·3
HCT, 1893·3
HCT-ISIS, 1893·4
HD, 1893·4
HD 85, 1893·4
HD 200 Plus, 1893·4
HDPC, 557·3

HE-69, 560·2
Head Cold Relief, 1893·4
Head Lice— *see* Pediculosis, 1427·3
Head and Neck Cancer— *see* Malignant Neoplasms of the Head and Neck, 494·2
Head & Shoulders, 1893·4
Head & Shoulders Intensive Treatment, 1893·4
Headache, 6·1
Headache, Analgesic-induced— *see* Analgesic-induced Headache, 449·1
Headache, Chronic Daily— *see* Analgesic-induced Headache, 449·1
Headache, Cluster— *see* Cluster Headache, 449·1
Headache, Combination— *see* Tension-type Headache, 450·1
Headache Complex, 1893·4
Headache, Episodic Tension-type— *see* Tension-type Headache, 450·1
Headache & Migraine, 1893·4
Headache, Mixed— *see* Tension-type Headache, 450·1
Headache, Muscle-contraction— *see* Tension-type Headache, 450·1
Headache, Post-dural Puncture— *see* Post-dural Puncture Headache, 1303·1
Headache, Rebound— *see* Analgesic-induced Headache, 449·1
Headache Relief, 1893·4
Headache Tablets, 1893·4
Headache, Tension-type— *see* Tension-type Headache, 450·1
Headclear Nondrowsy, Vicks— *see* Vicks Headclear Nondrowsy, 2163·4
Headclear, Vicks— *see* Vicks Headclear, 2163·4
Headmaster, 1893·4
Headrin Extra Strength, 1893·4
Heads Shampoo, 1893·4
Headway, 1893·4
Heaf Test, 1676·1
Heafusine, 1893·4
Heal Aid Plus, 1893·4
Heal-all, 1667·1
Healing Ointment, 1893·4
Healon, 1893·4
Healon Yellow, 1893·4
Healonid, 1893·4
Healonid Yellow, 1893·4
HealthAid AquaFall— *see* HealthAid Boldo-Plus, 1893·4
HealthAid Boldo-Plus, 1893·4
HealthAid FemmeVit PMS Formula, 1893·4
Healtheries Musseltone, 1893·4
Healtheries Musseltone & Glucosamine, 1893·4
Healthy Feet, 1893·4
Heart Attack— *see* Myocardial Infarction, 805·2
Heart Disease, Coronary— *see* Atherosclerosis, 793·2
Heart Disease, Ischaemic— *see* Atherosclerosis, 793·2
Heart Disease, Rheumatic— *see* Rheumatic Fever, 138·1
Heart Failure, 798·2
Heart Transplantation, 503·2
Heart Valves, Prosthetic— *see* Valvular Heart Disease, 816·3
Heartburn & Indigestion Liquid, 1893·4
Heartburn Relief, 1893·4
Heartline, 1893·4
Heat Cream, 1894·1
Heat Rub, 1894·1
Heat Stroke— *see* Fever and Hyperthermia, 8·2
Heath & Heather Preparations, 1894·1
Heavy Bismuth Nitrate, 1213·2
Heavy Kaolin, 1229·3
Heavy Liquid Petrolatum, 1407·1
Heavy Magnesium Carbonate, 1232·3
Heavy Magnesium Oxide, 1233·2
Heavy Metals, Poisoning, 1003·1
Heb, 1894·1
Hebagam IM, 1894·1
Heberbiovac HB, 1894·1
Hebrin, 1894·1
Hebucol, 1894·1

HEC, 1894·1
HECL, 1196·1, 1501·1
Hectonona, 1894·1
Hectorol, 1894·1
Hedazol, 1894·1
Hedelix, 1894·1
Hederix, 1894·1
Hedex, 1894·1
Hedex Extra, 1894·1
Hedex Headcold, 1894·1
Hedex Ibuprofen, 1894·1
Hedonin, 1894·1
Heelbalm, 1894·1
Heemex, 1894·1
Heer-More, 1894·2
Heet, 1894·2
Hefasolon, 1894·2
Hegor, 1894·2
Hegor Antipoux, 1894·2
Hegrimarin, 1894·2
Heidelbeere, 1639·2
Heilbuttleberöl, 1366·1
Heilerde, Luvos— *see* Luvos Heilerde, 1950·1
Heilit, 1894·2
Heilit Rheuma-Olbad, 1894·2
Heitrin, 1894·2
Hekbilin Kapseln, 1894·2
Heksavit, 1894·2
Helago-oel N, 1894·2
Helarium, 1894·2
Helastop, 1894·2
Helberina, 1894·2
Helcon, 1894·2
Helecho Macho, 102·2
Helenalin Tiglate, 1581·3
Heleniene, 1681·2
Helenin, 1089·3
Helfergin, 1894·2
Helianthi Annui Oleum, 1381·2
Helianthi, Oleum, 1381·2
Helianthus annuus, 1381·2
Helianthus Comp, 1894·2
Helianthus tuberosus, 1624·1
Helicidine, 1092·3
Heliclar, 1894·2
Heliclear, 1894·2
Helicobacter Pylori Infection— *see* Peptic Ulcer Disease, 1208·2
Helicobacter Pylori Vaccines, 1541·2
Helicocin, 1894·2
Helicosec, 1894·2
Helicosol— *see* Ez-HBT, 1855·4
Helidac, 1894·2
Helifenicol, 1894·2
HeliMet, 1894·2
Helimox, 1894·2
Helioban, 1894·2
Heliobloc, 1894·2
Heliobloc Fort, 1894·3
Helioblock, 1894·3
Heliopar, 1894·3
Helios, Colirio— *see* Colirio Helios, 1786·3
Heliotropin, 1436·2
Heliox, 1199·1
Helipak A, 1894·3
Helipak K, 1894·3
Helipak T, 1894·3
Heliplant, 1894·3
Helipur, 1894·3
Helipur H Plus, 1894·3
Helipur H Plus N, 1894·3
Helirad, 1894·3
Helis, 1894·3
Heli-Sal, 1894·3
Helisal, 1894·3
Helistat, 1894·3
Heliton, 1894·3
Helium, 1199·1
Helix I, 1894·3
Helixate, 1894·3
Helixinum, 1092·3
Helixor, 1894·3
Hellebore, American, 1679·3
Hellebore, European, 1679·3
Hellebore, False, 1573·3
Hellebore, Green, 1679·3

Ibudolor, 1907·3
Ibudros, 1907·3
Ibufac, 1907·3
Ibufarm, 1907·3
Ibufem, 1907·3
Ibufen, 1907·3
Ibufen-L, 1907·3
Ibuflam, 1907·3
Ibuflex, 1907·3
Ibufug, 1907·3
Ibugan, 1907·3
Ibugel, 1907·3
Ibuhexal, 1907·4
Ibulan, 1907·4
Ibular, 1907·4
Ibuleve, 1907·4
Ibuloid, 1907·4
Ibumax, 1907·4
Ibumed, 1907·4
Ibumerck, 1907·4
Ibumetin, 1907·4
Ibumousse, 1907·4
Ibunet, 1907·4
Ibupax, 1907·4
Ibuphlogont, 1907·4
Ibupril, 1907·4
Ibuprin, 1907·4
Ibuprof, 1907·4
Ibuprofen, 43·2
R-(−)-Ibuprofen, 44·1
S-(+)-Ibuprofen, 44·2
Ibuprofen Aminoethanol, 44·2
Ibuprofen Guaiacol, 44·2
Ibuprofen Isobutanolammonium, 44·2
Ibuprofen Lysine, 44·2
Ibuprofen Meglumine, 44·2
Ibuprofen Pyridoxine, 44·2
Ibuprofen Sodium, 44·2
Ibuprofenum, 43·2
Ibuprohm, 1907·4
Ibupron, 1907·4
Ibuproxam, 44·3
Ibu-ratiopharm, 1907·4
Iburem, 1907·4
Iburen, 1907·4
Ibureumin, 1907·4
Ibusal, 1907·4
Ibuscent, 1907·4
Ibusifar, 1907·4
Ibu-Slow, 1907·4
Ibuslow, 1907·4
Ibuspray, 1907·4
Ibustrin, 1907·4
Ibu-Tab, 1908·1
Ibutad, 1908·1
Ibutilide Fumarate, 912·2
Ibutop, 1908·1
Ibutop Cuprofen, 1908·1
Ibutop Ralgex, 1908·1
Ibu-Vivimed, 1908·1
Ibux, 1908·1
Ibuxin, 1908·1
IC-351, 1668·3
IC Green, 1908·1
Icaden, 1908·1
Icaps, 1908·1
Icar, 1908·1
Icatibant, 821·3
Icavex, 1908·1
Icaz, 1908·1
Ice, 1511·1
Ice Cool Stress & Tension Relief, 1908·1
Ice, Dry, 1198·2
Ice Gel, 1908·1
Ice Gel Therapy, 1908·1
Ice Hockey Lung— see Respiratory Disorders, 1057·3
Ice Lipbalm, 1908·1
Ice Therapy, 1908·1
Icespray, 1908·1
Ic-Gel, 1908·1
ICG-Pulsion, 1908·1
Ichthalgan, 1908·1
Ichthalgan Forte, 1908·1
Ichthammol, 1115·2
Ichthammolum, 1115·2
Ichtho-Bad, 1908·1

Ichtho-Bellol, 1908·1
Ichtho-Bellol Compositum S, 1908·1
Ichtho-Cadmin, 1908·1
Ichtho-Cortin, 1908·1
Ichthocortin, 1908·1
Ichthoderm, 1908·2
Ichth-Oestren, 1908·2
Ichtholan, 1908·2
Ichtholan Spezial, 1908·2
Ichtholan T, 1908·2
Ichthopaste, 1908·2
Ichthoseptal, 1908·2
Ichthosin, 1908·2
Ichthosulphol, 1115·2
Ichthraletten, 1908·2
Ichthyol, 1115·2
Ichthyol Hochviskose Flussigkeit, 1908·2
Ichthyolammonium, 1115·2
Ichthyol-Natrium Hell, 1115·3
Ichthyosis, 1105·3
Ichtopur, 1908·2
Icht-Oral, 1908·2
Ichtyosoft, 1908·2
ICI-9073, 1154·2
ICI-28257, 859·1
ICI-32525, 256·2
ICI-33828, 1635·1
ICI-35868, 1265·3
ICI-45520, 962·3
ICI-46474, 571·1
ICI-46683, 105·3
ICI-48213, 1467·2
ICI-50123, 1649·3
ICI-50172, 957·2
ICI-50627, 108·3
ICI-55052, 594·1
ICI-58834, 313·3
ICI-59118, 567·2
ICI-59623, 101·2
ICI-66082, 841·3
ICI-80996, 1441·2
ICI-118587, 998·3
ICI-118630, 1285·2
ICI-141292, 886·1
ICI-156834, 170·3
ICI-176334, 511·2
ICI-182780, 543·3
ICI-194660, 222·1
ICI-204219, 785·3
ICI-204636, 703·2
ICI-D1033, 508·1
ICI-D1694, 567·1
ICN-1229, 639·1
Icodextrin, 1359·1
Icodial, 1908·2
Icol, 1908·2
Icolamida, 1908·2
ICRF-159, 567·2
ICRF-187, 1006·2
ICS-205-930, 1253·3
ICSH, 1290·2
Ictage 6, 1908·2
Ictan, 1908·2
Ictasol, 1115·3
Icthaband, 1908·2
Ictholin, 1908·2
Ictiomen, 1908·2
Ictom 3, 1908·2
Ictotest, 1908·2
Icy Hot, 1908·2
ID-540, 683·2
Id Sedin, 1908·2
Ida, 1908·2
Ida-D, 1908·2
Idalon, 1908·2
Idalprem, 1908·3
Idamycin, 1908·3
Idaptan, 1908·3
Idarac, 1908·3
Idarubicin Hydrochloride, 545·2
Idarubicinol, 545·3
Idasal Nebulizador, 1908·3
Idazole, 1908·3
Idazoxan Hydrochloride, 1622·3
Idc, 1908·3
IDDM— see Diabetes Mellitus, 315·1

Ideal Quota, Adult— see Adult Ideal Quota, 1691·2
Idealid, 1908·3
Idebenone, 1623·1
IDEC-102, 567·3
IDEC-C2B8, 567·3
IDEC-CE9.1, 10·1
Idecortex, 1908·3
Ideolaxyl, 1908·3
Ideolider, 1908·3
Ideos, 1908·3
Iderpes, 1908·3
Idina, 1908·3
Idiopathic Anaphylaxis— see Urticaria and Angioedema, 1107·3
Idiopathic Dilated Cardiomyopathy— see Cardiomyopathies, 796·2
Idiopathic Pulmonary Fibrosis— see Diffuse Parenchymal Lung Disease, 1050·1
Idiopathic Rapidly Progressive Glomerulonephritis— see Glomerular Kidney Disease, 1051·1
Idiopathic Thrombocytopenic Purpura, 1052·3
IDM Solution, 1908·3
Ido A 50, 1908·3
I-Doc, 1908·3
Ido-C, 1908·3
Idocyklin, 1908·3
Ido-E, 1908·3
Idom, 1908·3
Idomed, 1908·3
Idopamil, 1908·3
Idotrim, 1908·3
Idotyl, 1908·3
Idoxifene, 546·1
Idoxuridina, 625·1
Idoxuridine, 625·1
IDR, 1908·3
Idracemi, 1908·3
Idracemi Eparina, 1908·4
Idralazina, 905·3
Idraste, 1621·1
Idratante Samil, 1908·4
Idril Sine, 1908·4
Idro P2, 1908·4
Idro-C, 1908·4
Idrocet, 1908·4
Idrocilamide, 1329·2
Idrocol, 1908·4
Idrogeno Soluzione, Perossido D', 1147·1
Idrolac, 1908·4
Idrolattone, 1908·4
Idrolone, 1908·4
Idroneomicil, 1908·4
Idropan B, 1908·4
Idroplurivit, 1908·4
Idropulmina, 1908·4
Idroquark, 1908·4
Idroskin, 1908·4
Idrossocobalamina, 1388·1
Idrovel, 1908·4
Idrum, 1908·4
IDU, 625·1
Iducher, 1908·4
Iducol, 1908·4
Iducutit, 1908·4
Idulamine, 1908·4
Idulanex, 1908·4
Idu-Phor— see Jodosan, 1920·4
5-IDUR, 625·1
Iduridin, 1908·4
Idustatin, 1908·4
Iduviran, 1908·4
I-EBU, 620·2
Iecatec, 1908·4
Iecoris Aselli Oleum, 1357·2
Ietepar, 1908·4
Ifa Dex, 1908·4
Ifa Diety, 1908·4
Ifa Norex, 1908·4
Ifa Reduccing S, 1909·1
Ifecin, 1909·1
Ifemed, 1909·1
Ifenec, 1909·1
Ifenprodil Tartrate, 912·3
Ifersol, 1909·1
Ifex, 1909·1

Ifiral, 1909·1
IFN-α, 628·1
IFN-β, 632·2
IFN-γ, 634·1
IFO-cell, 1909·1
Ifolem, 1909·1
Ifomida, 1909·1
Ifosfamide, 546·1
Ifosfamidum, 546·1
Ifoxan, 1909·1
Ifumelus, 1909·1
Ifutemp, 1909·1
IG Gamma, 1909·1
Ig Tetano, 1909·1
Ig Vena N, 1909·1
IgA Nephropathy— see Glomerular Kidney Disease, 1051·1
Igabulin, 1909·1
Igantet, 1909·1
Igbo, 1590·1
IgeE, 1909·1
IGF-I, 1296·3
IGF-II, 1296·3
IGFs, 1296·3
Igitur-antirheumatische, 1909·1
I-Glo, 1909·1
Ignatia, 1643·1
Ignatia Amara, 1643·1
IgRho, 1909·1
Igril, 1909·1
Igroseles, 1909·1
Igroton, 1909·1
Igroton-Lopresor, 1909·1
Igroton-Reserpina, 1909·1
Iguassina, 1909·1
Iiyalgon, 1909·1
IK-2, 619·3
Ikaclomin, 1909·1
Ikacor, 1909·1
Ikapress, 1909·1
Ikaran, 1909·2
Ikatin, 1909·2
Ikeriane, 1909·2
Ikestatina, 1909·2
Iketoncid, 1909·2
Ikorel, 1909·2
Iktorivil, 1909·2
IL-1, 1623·3
IL-2, 547·2
IL-3, 738·1
IL-4, 1624·1
IL-6, 1624·1
IL-5902, 248·3
IL-6001, 311·2
IL-6302, 415·3
IL-17803A, 825·1
IL-19552, 700·3
IL-22811, 52·2
Ilagane, 1909·2
Ila-med M, 1909·2
Ildamen, 1909·2
Ildor, 1909·2
Ile, 1370·1
Iletin Preparations, 1909·2
Ileus— see Decreased Gastrointestinal Motility, 1202·3
Ilex paraguensis, 1681·1
IL-1i, 1624·1
Iliadin, 1909·2
Ilio-Funkton, 1909·2
Ilja Rogoff, 1909·2
Ilja Rogoff Forte, 1909·2
Illicium verum, 1580·2
Illings Bozner Maycur-Tee, 1909·2
Ilmofosine, 547·1
Iloban, 1909·2
Ilocin, 1909·2
Ilocit, 1909·2
Ilodecakin, 1623·1
Ilomedin, 1909·2
Ilomedine, 1909·2
Ilon Abszess, 1909·3
Ilopan, 1909·3
Ilopan-Choline, 1909·3
Iloprost, 1445·2
Iloprost Trometamol, 1445·2
Iloprost Tromethamine, 1445·2

Magnespasmil, 1953·2
Magnespasmyl, 1953·2
Magnesplus, 1953·2
Magnetic Resonance Imaging, 1030·1
Magnetrans Forte, 1953·2
Magnevist, 1953·2
Magnevistan, 1953·2
Magnezie, 1953·2
Magnezyme, 1953·2
Magnidol-Plus, 1953·2
Magnil, 1953·2
Magnofit, 1953·2
Magnogene, 1953·2
Magnograf, 1953·2
Magnol, 1953·2
Magnolax, 1953·2
Magnolex, 1953·2
Magnonorm, 1953·3
Magnoplasm, 1953·3
Magnopyrol, 1953·3
Magnoral, 1953·3
Magnorbin, 1953·3
Magnorell, 1953·3
Magnorol, 1953·3
Magnoscorbol, 1953·3
Magnosol, 1953·3
Magnosolv, 1953·3
Magnostase, 1953·3
Magnox, 1953·3
Magnurol, 1953·3
Magnyl, 1953·3
Magocean, 1953·3
Magonate, 1953·3
Magopsor, 1953·3
Magoral, 1953·3
Mag-Oro, 1953·3
Mag-Ox, 1953·3
Magrilan, 1953·3
Magrinex, 1953·3
Magroton, 1953·3
Magsal, 1953·3
Magsil, 1953·3
Magsons, 1953·3
Mag-SR, 1953·3
Mag-Tab SR, 1953·3
Magtrate, 1953·4
Magtrom, 1953·4
Magvital, 1953·4
Mahiou, 1953·4
Ma-huang, 1090·1
Maiblume, 1599·1
Maidenhair Tree, 1615·2
Maiglöckchenkraut, 1599·1
Mainnox, 1953·4
Maintain, 1953·4
Maiorad, 1953·4
Maïs, Huile de, 1371·1
Maize, 1599·3
Maize Oil, 1371·1
Maize Starch, 1379·3
Majeptil, 1953·4
Majocarmin-Tee, 1953·4
Majolat, 1953·4
Major Antithrombin, 718·3, 725·2
Major Tranquillisers, 649·1
Major-Con, 1953·4
Major-gesic, 1953·4
Majorpen, 1953·4
Makatussin, 1953·4
Makatussin Balsam Mit Menthol, 1953·4
Makatussin Forte, 1953·4
Makatussin Saft, 1953·4
Makatussin Saft Drosera, 1953·4
Makatussin Tropfen, 1953·4
Makatussin Tropfen Drosera, 1953·4
Makatussin Tropfen Forte, 1953·4
Makhlif, 1590·1
Makrocilin, 1953·4
Malachite Green, 1150·1
Malachite Green G, 1136·1
Malafene, 1953·4
Malak, 1590·1
Malandil, 1953·4
Malarex, 1954·1
Malaria, 428·1
Malaria Vaccines, 1546·3
Malaridine Phosphate, 444·3

Malarone, 1954·1
Malatal, 1954·1
Malathion, 1434·2
Malaviron, 1954·1
Malayan Filariasis— see Lymphatic Filariasis, 94·1
Malayan Pit-viper, 839·3
Maldison— see Cleensheen, 1780·4
Maldison— see Lice Rid, 1940·2
Male Breast Cancer— see Malignant Neoplasms of the Male Breast, 492·2
Male Contraception— see Contraception, 1460·1
Male Fern, 102·2
Male Formula Herbal Plus Formula 2, 1954·1
Maleato de Ergonovina, 1607·1
Maleic Acid, 1631·1
Male-pattern Baldness— see Alopecia, 1104·1
Malexin, 1954·1
Malfin, 1954·1
Maliasin, 1954·1
Malic Acid, 1631·1
Malignancies, HIV-associated— see HIV-associated Malignancies, 610·2
Malignancy, Hypercalcaemia of— see Hypercalcaemia of Malignancy, 1181·1
Malignant Ascites— see Ascites, 793·1
Malignant Effusions, 489·3
Malignant Hyperpyrexia— see Malignant Hyperthermia, 1329·1
Malignant Hypertension— see Hypertension, 802·2
Malignant Hyperthermia, 1329·1
Malignant Melanoma— see Melanoma, 499·1
Malignant Neoplasms of the Aerodigestive Tract— see Malignant Neoplasms of the Head and Neck, 494·2
Malignant Neoplasms of the Bladder, 490·1
Malignant Neoplasms of the Bone, 490·2
Malignant Neoplasms of the Brain, 490·3
Malignant Neoplasms of the Breast, 491·1
Malignant Neoplasms of the Breast, Prophylaxis— see Prophylaxis, 492·1
Malignant Neoplasms of the Colon— see Malignant Neoplasms of the Gastrointestinal Tract, 493·2
Malignant Neoplasms of the Endometrium, 493·1
Malignant Neoplasms of the Eye, 493·1
Malignant Neoplasms of the Gastrointestinal Tract, 493·2
Malignant Neoplasms of the Head and Neck, 494·2
Malignant Neoplasms of the Kidney, 495·1
Malignant Neoplasms of the Liver, 495·2
Malignant Neoplasms of the Lung, 496·1
Malignant Neoplasms of the Male Breast, 492·2
Malignant Neoplasms of the Mouth— see Malignant Neoplasms of the Gastrointestinal Tract, 493·2
Malignant Neoplasms of the Mouth— see Malignant Neoplasms of the Head and Neck, 494·2
Malignant Neoplasms of the Oesophagus— see Malignant Neoplasms of the Gastrointestinal Tract, 493·2
Malignant Neoplasms of the Ovary, 496·3
Malignant Neoplasms of the Pancreas, 497·2
Malignant Neoplasms of the Prostate, 497·3
Malignant Neoplasms of the Rectum— see Malignant Neoplasms of the Gastrointestinal Tract, 493·2
Malignant Neoplasms of the Skin, 498·2
Malignant Neoplasms of the Skin, Prophylaxis— see Malignant Neoplasms of the Skin, 498·2
Malignant Neoplasms of the Stomach— see Malignant Neoplasms of the Gastrointestinal Tract, 493·2
Malignant Neoplasms of the Testis, 499·2
Malignant Neoplasms of the Thymus, 499·3
Malignant Neoplasms of the Thyroid, 500·1

Malignant Pericardial Effusions— see Malignant Effusions, 489·3
Malignant Pleural Effusions— see Malignant Effusions, 489·3
Malignant Thyroid Nodule— see Malignant Neoplasms of the Thyroid, 500·1
Malimed, 1954·1
Malinert, 1954·1
Malipuran, 1954·1
Malival, 1954·1
Malival Compuesto, 1954·1
Malix, 1954·1
Mallamint, 1954·1
Mallazine, 1954·1
Mallebrin, 1954·1
Mallebrin Konzentrat, 1954·1
Mallebrinetten— see Mallebrin, 1954·1
Mallisol, 1954·1
Mallorol, 1954·1
Malocide, 1954·1
Malocin, 1954·1
Malogen Aqueous, 1954·1
Malogen in Oil, 1954·1
Malogex, 1954·1
Maloprim, 1954·1
Malotilate, 1631·2
Malt Extract, 1371·1
MALT Lymphoma, 488·3
Malt Soup Extract, 1371·1
Malted Grain of Barley, 1371·1
Malted Grain of Wheat, 1371·1
D-Maltitol, 1371·1
Maltitol, 1371·1
Maltitol Solution, 1371·1
Maltitol Syrup, 1371·1
Maltitolum, 1371·1
Maltitolum Liquidum, 1371·1
Maltlevol, 1954·1
Maltlevol-M, 1954·2
Maltodextrin, 1371·2
Maltodextrinum, 1371·2
Maltofer, 1954·2
Maltofer Fol, 1954·2
Maltogen, 1954·2
Malton E, 1954·2
Malto-oligosaccharides, 1350·1
Maltose, 1371·2
Maltose, Hydrogenated, 1371·1
Maltose-glucose Syrup, High, Hydrogenated, 1371·1
Maltovis, 1954·2
Maltsupex, 1954·2
Maltyl, 1954·2
Maludil, 1954·2
Malugel, 1954·2
Malva, 1590·1
Malva Composta, 1954·2
Malvatricin, 1954·2
Malvedrin, 1954·2
Malveol, 1954·2
Malvitona, 1954·2
Malvodon, 1954·2
Malvol, 1954·2
Malvona, 1954·2
Malvosulfam, 1954·2
Mamellin, 1954·2
Mammalian Tissue Extracts, 1631·2
Mammol, 1954·2
Mammotropin, 1295·3
Man Formula, 1954·2
Manceau, 1954·2
Mancef, 1954·2
Mandal 425, 1954·2
Mandanol, 1954·2
Mandarine, 1954·2
(7R)-7-D-Mandelamido-3-(1-methyl-1H-tetrazol-5-ylthiomethyl)-3-cephem-4-carboxylic Acid, 163·3
7-[(R)-Mandelamido]-3-(1-sulphomethyl-1H-tetrazol-5-ylthiomethyl)-3-cephem-4-carboxylic Acid, Disodium Salt, 168·1
Mandelamine, 1954·2
Mandelan, 1954·2
Mandelato de Metenamina, 223·1
Mandelic Acid, 221·2
Mandelic Acid, Racemic, 221·2
Mandelip, 1954·3
Mandelo-katt, 1954·3

Mandelöl, 1576·3
(+)-Mandelonitrile Glucoside, 1680·3
(1R,3r,5S)-3-[(±)-Mandeloyloxy]-8-methyltropanium Bromide, 468·1
Mandepiril, 1954·3
Mandl's Paint = Compound Iodine Paint, 1524·2
Mandocarbine, 1954·3
Mandokef, 1954·3
Mandol, 1954·3
Mandolgin, 1954·3
Mandolsan, 1954·3
Mandorla, Olio Di, 1576·3
Mandragora Comp, 1954·3
Mandragora Med Complex, 1954·3
Mandrake, American, 1121·1
Mandrogripp, 1954·3
Mandrolax, 1954·3
Mandrolax Lactu, 1954·3
Mandrolax Pico, 1954·3
Mandros Diarstop, 1954·3
Mandros Reise, 1954·3
Maneon, 1954·3
Manerix, 1954·3
Manevac, 1954·3
Mangafodipir Trisodium, 1037·3
Manganese, 1371·3
Manganese Amino Acid Chelate, 1372·1
Manganese Chloride, 1371·3
Manganese Dioxide, 1372·1
Manganese D-Gluconate, 1371·3
Manganese Gluconate, 1371·3
Manganese Hydrogen Citrate, 1372·1
Manganese Sulfate, 1371·3
Manganese Sulphate, 1371·3
Manganese (II) Sulphate Tetrahydrate, 1371·3
Mangani Sulfas, 1371·3
Mangaplexe, 1954·3
Mania— see Bipolar Disorder, 271·2
Manibee Complejo, 1954·3
Manibee-C, 1954·3
Manic, 1954·3
Manic Depression— see Bipolar Disorder, 271·2
Manicol, 1954·3
Manidipine Hydrochloride, 924·3
Manidon, 1954·3
Manihot utilissima, 1379·3
Manimon, 1954·3
Maninil, 1954·3
Maniprex, 1954·3
Manita, 924·3
Manitol, 1954·3
Maniton, 1954·3
Manna, 1233·3
Manna Sugar, 924·3
Manne En Larmes, 1233·3
Mannex, 1954·3
Mannistol, 1954·3
Mannite, 924·3, 1954·4
Mannit-Losung, 1954·4
D-Mannitol, 924·3
Mannitol, 924·3
Mannitolum, 924·3
Mannose, 924·3
D-Mannuronic Acid, 1498·3
Manoderm, 1954·4
Manorfen, 1954·4
Mansal, 1954·4
Mansil, 1954·4
Mansonella Infections, 94·2
Mantadan, 1954·4
Mantadil, 1954·4
Mantadix, 1954·4
Mantai, 1954·4
Manteca de Cacao, 1410·3
Manteiga de Cacau, 1410·3
Mantidan, 1954·4
Mantoux Test, 1676·1
Manusept, 1954·4
Manusept HD, 1954·4
Manzanilla Ordinaria, 1593·2
Manzanilla Romana, 1593·2
Manzul, 1590·1
MAOIs, 271·2, 307·1
Maolate, 1954·4
Maoni, 1954·4

Motifene, 1976·3
Motilex, 1976·3
Motilidone, 1976·3
Motilium, 1976·3
Motion Sickness— see Nausea and Vomiting, 1206·3
Motipress, 1976·3
Motival, 1976·3
Motivan, 1976·3
Motivone, 1976·3
Motofen, 1976·3
Motoneuron Disease— see Motor Neurone Disease, 1658·2
Motor Neurone Disease, 1658·2
Motosol, 1976·3
Motozina, 1976·3
Motretinide, 1121·1
Motrim, 1976·3
Motrin, 1976·3
Motrin Cold, Childrens— see Childrens Motrin Cold, 1774·1
Motrin IB Sinus, 1976·3
Mountain Balm, 1091·2
Mountain Sickness, Acute— see High-altitude Disorders, 800·1
Moura Brasil, Colirio— see Colirio Moura Brasil, 1786·3
Moutarde Jonciforme, 1639·1
Moutarde Noire, Graine de, 1639·1
Mouth Cancer— see Malignant Neoplasms of the Gastrointestinal Tract, 493·2
Mouth Cancer— see Malignant Neoplasms of the Head and Neck, 494·2
Mouth Infections, Bacterial— see Mouth Infections, 130·1
Mouth Ulceration, 1206·3
Mouthkote, 1976·3
MouthKote F/R, 1976·3
MouthKote O/R, 1976·3
MouthKote P/R, 1976·3
Mouthrinse, 1976·3
Mouthwash, 1976·3
Mouthwash Antiseptic & Gargle, 1976·3
Mouthwash & Gargle, 1976·3
Mouthwash Mint/Peppermint, 1976·4
Mova Nitrat, 1976·4
Movalis, 1976·4
Movatec, 1976·4
Movelat, 1976·4
Movens, 1976·4
Mover, 1976·4
Movergan, 1976·4
Movergan— see Antiparkin, 1713·1
Movex, 1976·4
Movicard, 1976·4
Movicol, 1976·4
Movicolon, 1976·4
Movicox, 1976·4
Moviflex, 1976·4
Movilat, 1976·4
Movilisin, 1976·4
Movin, 1976·4
Movina, 1976·4
Mowineuron, 1976·4
Mowivit, 1976·4
Moxacef, 1976·4
Moxacin, 1976·4
Moxadent, 1976·4
Moxal, 1976·4
Moxal II, 1976·4
Moxal Plus, 1977·1
Moxalactam Disodium, 218·3
Moxaline, 1977·1
Moxan, 1977·1
Moxantrazole Hydrochloride, 573·3
Moxapen, 1977·1
Moxaverine, 1638·1
Moxaverine Hydrochloride, 1638·1
Moxcil, 1977·1
Moxcin, 1977·1
Moxicel, 1977·1
Moxiclav, 1977·1
Moxidectin, 104·1
Moxifloxacin Hydrochloride, 225·3
Moxilcap, 1977·1
Moxilen, 1977·1
Moxilin, 1977·1
Moximed, 1977·1

Moxipan, 1977·1
Moxipen, 1977·1
Moxiral, 1977·1
Moxiren, 1977·1
Moxisilita Clorhidrato, 980·2
Moxisylyte— see Thymoxamine, 980·2
Moxisylyte Hydrochloride, 980·2
Moxlin, 1977·1
Moxon, 1977·1
Moxonidine, 936·3
Moxydar, 1977·1
Moxymax, 1977·1
Moxypen, 1977·1
Moxyvit, 1977·1
Moz-Bite, 1977·1
Mozzie Patch, 1977·1
4-MP, 1009·3
6MP, 552·2
MP-302, 1037·1
MP-328, 1037·1
MP-620, 1033·3
MPA, 1977·1
MPA Gyn, 1977·1
MPA-beta, 1977·1
MPA-Noury, 1977·1
M-P-Cil, 1977·1
MPI-5010, 526·3
MPP, 403·2
MPPP, 75·3, 1160·2
MPR, 930·2
M-Prednisol, 1977·1
α-MPT, 930·2
MPTP, 75·3, 1160·1
MPV-785, 690·3
MPV-1248, 1002·3
MPV-1440, 674·3
MPV-253-AII, 674·2
M-19-Q, 247·1
MR-654, 1267·3
Mr. Multy, 1977·1
MRF, 1290·3
MRL-41, 1465·3
Mrs Cullen's Powders, 1977·2
MRSA Infections— see Staphylococcal Infections, 140·3
M-R-Vax II, 1977·2
MRX, 1977·2
MS-551, 946·1
MS Contin, 1977·2
MS Direct, 1977·2
MS Mono, 1977·2
MSD-803, 922·3
MSG, 1372·2
α-MSH, 1290·3
β-MSH, 1290·3
γ-MSH, 1290·3
MSH, 1290·3
MSI, 1977·2
MSI-78, 221·2
MSI-93, 221·2
MSI-94, 221·2
MSIR, 1977·2
MS/L, 1977·2
MS-Long, 1977·2
MSP, 1977·2
MSPD, 1977·2
MSR, 1977·2
MS/S, 1977·2
MST, 1977·2
MST-16, 569·1
MST Continus, 1977·2
MSTA, 1977·2
M-Stada, 1977·2
MSUD III, 1977·2
MSUD Aid, 1977·2
MSUD Analog, 1977·2
MSUD, Analog— see Analog MSUD, 1707·4
MSUD Diet, 1977·2
MSUD Maxamaid, 1977·2
MSUD, Maxamaid— see Maxamaid MSUD, 1956·2
MSUD Maxamum, 1977·2
MSUD, Maxamum— see Maxamum MSUD, 1956·2
α-MT, 930·2
MT-141, 167·3
MTA, 564·3

MTB-51, 470·2
MTBE, 1404·3
MTE, 1977·2
MTHPC, 573·3
MTIC, 573·3
MTX, 553·2, 1977·2
Mucabrox, 1977·2
Mucaderma S, 1977·2
Mucaine, 1977·3
Mucaine 2 in 1, 1977·3
Mucal, 1977·3
Mucantil, 1977·3
Mucasept-A, 1977·3
Mucedokehl, 1977·3
Mucibron, 1977·3
Muciclar, 1977·3
Mucidan, 1977·3
Mucil, 1977·3
Mucilar, 1977·3
Mucilar Avena, 1977·3
Mucilax, 1977·3
Mucilin, 1977·3
Mucilloid, 1977·3
Mucin, Gastric, 1501·1
Mucine, 1977·3
Mucinol, 1977·3
Mucinum, 1977·3
Mucinum A L'Extrait de Cascara, 1977·4
Mucinum Cascara, 1977·4
Muciplasma, 1977·4
Mucipulgite, 1977·4
Mucisol, 1977·4
Muciteran, 1977·4
Mucitux, 1977·4
Mucivital, 1977·4
Muclox, 1977·4
Muco4, 1977·4
Muco Panoral, 1977·4
Muco Sanigen, 1977·4
Muco-Aspecton, 1977·4
Mucobene, 1977·4
Mucobron, 1977·4
Mucobronchyl, 1977·4
Mucobroxol, 1977·4
Mucocaps, 1977·4
Mucocedyl, 1977·4
Mucocef, 1977·4
Mucocil, 1977·4
Mucocis, 1977·4
Mucocutaneous Lymph Node Syndrome of Childhood— see Kawasaki Disease, 1554·1
Muco-cyl Ho-Len-Complex, 1977·4
Muco-Dest, 1977·4
Mucodestrol, 1977·4
Mucodex, 1977·4
Mucodic, 1977·4
Mucodil, 1978·1
Mucodox, 1978·1
Mucodrenol, 1978·1
Mucodyne, 1978·1
Mucofalk, 1978·1
Mucofan, 1978·1
Muco-Fen, 1978·1
Muco-Fen-DM, 1978·1
Muco-Fen-LA, 1978·1
Muco-Fips, 1978·1
Mucoflem, 1978·1
Mucofluid, 1978·1
Mucoflux, 1978·1
Mucofor, 1978·1
Mucogel, 1978·1
Mucogen, 1978·1
Mucogeran, 1978·1
Mucojet, 1978·1
Mucokehl, 1978·1
Mucola, 1978·1
Mucolair, 1978·1
Mucolan, 1978·1
Mucolase, 1978·1
Mucolator, 1978·1
Mucolavi, 1978·1
Mucolene, 1978·1
Mucoless, 1978·2
Mucolex, 1978·2
Mucolexin, 1978·2
Mucolid, 1978·2

Mucolin, 1978·2
Mucolinct, 1978·2
Mucolisil, 1978·2
Mucolit, 1978·2
Mucolitic, 1978·2
Mucolitico Maggioni, 1978·2
Mucolix, 1978·2
Mucolysin, 1978·2
Mucolyte, 1978·2
Mucolytics, 1082·1
Mucomed, 1978·2
Muco-Mepha, 1978·2
Mucomyst, 1978·2
Muconorm, 1978·2
Mucopan, 1978·2
Muco-Perasthman N, 1978·2
Mucophlogat, 1978·2
Mucoplexil, 1978·2
Mucopolysaccharides, Sulfated, 788·2
Mucoporetta, 1978·2
Mucopront, 1978·2
Mucoral, 1978·2
Mucorama, 1978·3
Mucorama TS, 1978·3
Mucorex, 1978·3
Mucorex Ampicilina, 1978·3
Mucorex Ciclin, 1978·3
Mucorhinyl, 1978·3
Mucormycosis, 374·3
Mucosa Compositum, 1978·3
Mucosal Protectants, 1202·1
Mucosan, 1978·3
Muco-Sana, 1978·3
Mucoseptal, 1978·3
Mucosil, 1978·3
Mucosirop, 1978·3
Mucosol, 1978·3
Mucosolvan, 1978·3
Mucosolvan Compositum, 1978·3
Mucosolvon, 1978·3
Mucospas, 1978·3
Mucospect, 1978·3
Mucospire, 1978·3
Mucosta, 1978·3
Mucosteine, 1978·3
Mucostop, 1978·3
Mucosyt, 1978·3
Mucotablin, 1978·3
Muco-Tablinen, 1978·3
Mucotectan, 1978·4
Mucothera, 1978·4
Mucotherm, 1978·4
Mucothiol, 1978·4
Mucotic, 1978·4
Mucotoss, 1978·4
Mucotreis, 1978·4
Muco-Trin, 1978·4
Mucotrophir, 1978·4
Mucotuss, Chemists Own— see Chemists Own Mucotuss, 1773·2
Mucovibrol, 1978·4
Mucovibrol C, 1978·4
Mucovibrol T, 1978·4
Mucovin, 1978·4
Mucovital, 1978·4
Mucoxin, 1978·4
Mucoxine-F, 1978·4
Mucoxol, 1978·4
Mucoza, 1978·4
Mucozym, 1978·4
Mucret, 1978·4
Mu-Cron, 1978·4
Mu-Cron Junior, 1978·4
Mu-Cron, Otrivine— see Otrivine Mu-Cron, 2019·3
Mucuna pruriens, 1604·1
Mudd Acne, 1978·4
Mudrane, 1978·4
Mudrane GG, 1978·4
Mudrane GG-2, 1978·4
Muérdago, Tallo de, 1636·2
Muflex, 1978·4
Mugo, Olio Di, 1656·3
Muguet, 1599·1
Mulatinha, 1590·1
Mulgatol, 1979·1
Mulgatol Gelee N, 1979·1

Nalorphine, 1014·2
Nalorphine Hydrobromide, 1014·2
Nalorphine Hydrochloride, 1014·2
Nalorphini Hydrochloridum, 1014·2
Nalorphinium Chloride, 1014·2
Naloxona, Cloridrato de, 1014·3
Naloxone Hydrochloride, 1014·3
Naloxoni Hydrochloridum, 1014·3
Nalspan DX, 1983·3
Nalspan Pediatric, 1983·3
Nalspan Senior DX, 1983·4
6-β-Naltrexol, 1016·2
Naltrexone Hydrochloride, 1016·1
Namba, 1590·1
Nametone, 1983·4
Namic, 1983·4
Namifen, 1983·4
Nan HA, 1983·4
NAN HA/AR, 1983·4
Nan Sin Lactosa, 1983·4
Nanafed, 1983·4
Nanbacine, 1983·4
Nandain, 1983·4
Nandrol, 1983·4
Nandrolone, 1484·2
Nandrolone Cyclohexanepropionate, 1484·2
Nandrolone Cyclohexylpropionate, 1484·2
Nandrolone Decanoate, 1484·2
Nandrolone Dodecanoate, 1484·2
Nandrolone Hexyloxyphenylpropionate, 1484·3
Nandrolone Hydrocinnamate, 1484·2
Nandrolone Laurate, 1484·2
Nandrolone Phenpropionate, 1484·2
Nandrolone Phenylpropionate, 1484·2
Nandrolone Propionate, 1484·3
Nandrolone Sodium Sulfate, 1484·2
Nandrolone Sodium Sulphate, 1484·2
Nandrolone Undecanoate, 1484·2
Nandrolone Undecylate, 1484·2
Nani Pre Dental, 1983·4
Nanocoll, 1983·4
Nanophyetiasis— see Intestinal Fluke Infections, 93·2
Nanotiv, 1983·4
Nansius, 1983·4
NAPA, 825·3
Napacod, 1983·4
Napageln, 1983·4
Napamide, 1983·4
Napamol, 1983·4
Napan, 1983·4
NaPCA, 1123·3
Napflam, 1983·4
Napha Forte, 1983·4
Naphacel, 1983·4
Naphasal, 1983·4
Naphazole-A, 1983·4
Naphazoline, 1095·1
Naphazoline Acetate, 1095·2
Naphazoline Hydrochloride, 1095·1
Naphazoline Nitrate, 1095·1
Naphazoline Plus, 1983·4
Naphazolini Hydrochloridum, 1095·1
Naphazolini Nitras, 1095·1
Naphazolinium Nitricum, 1095·1
Naphcon, 1983·4
Naphcon Forte, 1983·4
Naphcon-A, 1983·4
Naphensyl, 1984·1
Naphoptic-A, 1984·1
Naphthalene, 1435·1
1-Naphthaleneacetic Acid, 1639·3
Naphthalin, 1435·1
Naphthalophos, 104·1
Naphthammonum, 97·2
Naphthizinum, 1095·1
Naphthol, 97·2
Naphth-2-ol, 97·2
1,2-Naphthoquinone 2-Semicarbazone, 739·2
O-2-Naphthyl m,N-Dimethylthiocarbanilate, 395·2
1-Naphthyl Methylcarbamate, 1429·2
Naphthylacetic Acid, 1639·3
1-Naphthylacetic Acid, 1639·3
β-Naphthylamine, 1400·3

2-(1-Naphthylmethyl)-2-imidazoline, 1095·1
α-Naphthylthiourea, 1428·2
1-(1-Naphthyl)-2-thiourea, 1428·2
Naphthyridine Antimalarials, 428·3
Napilene, 1984·1
Napiro, 1984·1
Naplin, 1984·1
Napmel, 1984·1
Nappy Rash Powder, 1984·1
Nappy Rash Relief Cream, 1984·1
Nappy-Mate, 1984·1
Napratec, 1984·1
Naprel, 1984·1
Naprelan, 1984·1
Napren, 1984·1
Naprex, 1984·1
Naprilene, 1984·1
Naprina, 1984·1
Naprius, 1984·1
Naprobene, 1984·1
Naprocet, 1984·1
Naprocoat, 1984·1
Naprodil, 1984·1
Naprodol, 1984·1
Napro-Dorsch, 1984·1
Naprogesic, 1984·1
Naprokes, 1984·1
Naprometin, 1984·1
Napromex, 1984·2
Napronet, 1984·2
Naprorex, 1984·2
Naproscript, 1984·2
Naprosian, 1984·2
Naproso, 1984·2
Naprosyn, 1984·2
Naprosyne, 1984·2
Naproval, 1984·2
Naprovite, 1984·2
Naproxen, 60·3
Naproxen Aminobutanol, 61·3
Naproxen Cetrimonium, 61·3
Naproxen Lysine, 61·3
Naproxen Piperazine, 61·3
Naproxen Sodium, 61·1
Naproxenum, 60·3
Naproxi, 1984·2
Napxen, 1984·2
Naqua, 1984·2
Naquinto, 1984·2
Naragran, 1984·2
Naramig, 1984·2
Naranja Amarga, Corteza de, 1644·2
Naranocor, 1984·2
Naranocut H, 1984·2
Naranofem, 1984·2
Naranopect P, 1984·2
Naranotox, 1984·2
Naranotox Plus, 1984·2
Narapril, 1984·2
Narasin, 598·1
Naratriptan Hydrochloride, 454·3
Narcan, 1984·2
Narcanti, 1984·2
Narcaricin, 1984·2
Narcaricina, 1984·2
Narceine, 62·1
Narceine Phosphate, 62·1
Narcolepsy— see Narcoleptic Syndrome, 1505·2
Narcoleptic Syndrome, 1505·2
Narcoral, 1984·3
Narcotic Analgesics, 1·3
L-α-Narcotine, 1096·1
Narcotine, 1096·1
Narcotine Hydrochloride, 1096·1
Narcotuss, 1984·3
Narcozep, 1984·3
Nard, Wild, 1582·3
Nardelzine, 1984·3
Nardil, 1984·3
Nardyl, 1984·3
Narfen, 1984·3
Naribel, 1984·3
Naricin, 1984·3
Naride, 1984·3
Naridrin, 1984·3

Narifresh, 1984·3
Narilet, 1984·3
Narine, 1984·3
Narisoro, 1984·3
Naristar, 1984·3
Naritec, 1984·3
Narium, 1984·3
Narix, 1984·3
Narixan, 1984·3
Narizima, 1984·3
Narizima Adulto, 1984·3
Narizima Pediatrico, 1984·3
Narlisim, 1984·3
Narobic, 1984·3
Narocin, 1984·3
Narol, 1984·3
Narop, 1984·3
Naropeine, 1984·4
Naropin, 1984·4
Naropin with Fentanyl, 1984·4
Naropina, 1984·4
Narphen, 1984·4
Nartap, 1984·4
Nartograstim, 739·2
Narzen, 1984·4
Nasa-12, 1984·4
Nasa Rhinathiol, 1984·4
Nasabid, 1984·4
Nasacor, 1984·4
Nasacort, 1984·4
Nasacort AQ, 1984·4
Nasahist B, 1984·4
NaSal, 1984·4
Nasal Congestion, 1082·3
Nasal Decongestants, 1082·1
Nasal Inhaler, 1984·4
Nasal Jelly, 1984·4
Nasal Moist, 1984·4
Nasal Relief, 1984·4
Nasal & Sinus Relief, 1984·4
Nasal Spray, 1984·4
Nasal Spray for Hayfever, 1984·4
Nasalate, 1984·4
Nasal-Bec, 1984·4
Nasalcrom, 1984·4
Nasal-Ease, 1984·4
Nasalemed, 1985·1
Nasaleze, 1985·1
Nasalflu, 1985·1
Nasalgen, 1985·1
Nasalide, 1985·1
Nasamine, 1985·1
Nasan, 1985·1
Nasanal, 1985·1
Nasapert, 1985·1
Nasarel, 1985·1
Nasarox, 1985·1
Nasaruplase, 938·1
Nasatab LA, 1985·1
Nasatuss, 1985·1
Nasben, 1985·1
Nasben Soft, 1985·1
Nasciodine, 1985·1
Nascobal, 1985·1
Nasdro, 1985·1
Nasea, 1985·1
Nasello, 1985·1
Nasengel, 1985·1
Nasengel AL, 1985·1
Nasenspray AL, 1985·1
Nasenspray E, 1985·1
Nasenspray K, 1985·1
Nasentropfen AL, 1985·1
Nasentropfen E, 1985·1
Nasentropfen K, 1985·1
Nasentropfen-ratiopharm, 1985·2
Naseptin, 1985·2
Nasex, 1985·2
Nasic, 1985·2
Nasicortin, 1985·2
Nasicur, 1985·2
Nasil, 1985·2
Nasimild, 1985·2
Nasin, 1985·2
Nasivin, 1985·2
Nasivin Gegen Erkaltung Kinderbad, 1985·2

Nasivin Gegen Erkaltung N, 1985·2
Nasivin Gegen Schnupfen, 1985·2
Nasivin Intensiv-Bad N, 1985·2
Nasivin Sanft, 1985·2
Nasivine, 1985·2
Nasivinetten Gegen Schnupfen, 1985·2
Nasivinetten— see Nasivinettes, 1985·2
Nasivinettes, 1985·2
Naso Instil, 1985·2
Naso Pekamin, 1985·2
Naso Prieulina, 1985·2
Nasobec, 1985·2
Nasobol, 1985·2
Naso-Calma, 1985·2
Nasocan, 1985·2
Nasocort, 1985·3
Nasoferm, 1985·3
Nasoflux, 1985·3
Nasogrip, 1985·3
Nasolin, 1985·3
Nasolina, 1985·3
Nasomet, 1985·3
Nasomixin, 1985·3
Nasonex, 1985·3
Nasopan, 1985·3
Nasopharyngeal Carcinoma— see Malignant Neoplasms of the Head and Neck, 494·2
Nasopomada, 1985·3
Nasosil, 1985·3
Nasotic Oto, 1985·3
Nasovalda, 1985·3
Nastop, 1985·3
Nastoren, 1985·3
Nasturtium armoracia, 1620·1
Nasulind, 1985·3
NAT-333, 765·3
Nat. Mur., 1197·2
Natabec, 1985·3
Natabec F, 1985·3
Natabec-F.A. with Fluoride, 1985·3
NataChew, 1985·3
Natacyn, 1985·3
Natafort, 1985·3
Natafucin, 1985·3
Natal Extra, 1985·4
NatalCare, 1985·4
Natalin, 1985·4
Natalins, 1985·4
Natalins Com Fluor, 1985·4
Natalins Folico, 1985·4
Natalins Rx, Enfamil— see Enfamil Natalins Rx, 1842·3
Natamycin, 392·1
Nataral, 1985·4
Natarex Prenatal, 1985·4
NataTab, 1985·4
Natavite, 1985·4
Natead, 1985·4
Natecal, 1985·4
Natecal D, 1985·4
Nateglinide, 333·2
Nathergen, 1985·4
Naticardina, 1985·4
Nati-K, 1985·4
Natiken, 1985·4
Natil, 1985·4
Natinate, 1985·4
Natisedina, 1985·4
Natisedine, 1985·4
Natispray, 1985·4
Nativa HA, 1985·4
Nativit, 1985·4
Na-To-Caps, 1985·4
Natopherol, 1985·4
Natoss, 1985·4
Natracalm, 1985·4
NatraFlex, 1985·4
Natraleze, 1986·1
Natramid, 1986·1
Natrapel, 1986·1
Natrasleep, 1986·1
Natrecor, 1986·1
Natrii Acetas, 1186·1
Natrii Alendronas, 747·2
Natrii Alginas, 1986·1
Natrii Amidotrizoas, 1031·2
Natrii Aminosalicylas, 148·3

Propiocine, 2055·1
β-Propiolactone, 1155·3
Propiolactone, 1155·3
Propiomazine Hydrochloride, 424·3
Propiomazine Hydrogen Maleate, 424·3
Propiomazine Maleate, 424·3
Propionat, 2055·1
Propionibacterium acnes, 527·2
Propionic Acid, 393·2
Propiono-3-lactone, 1155·3
Propionyl Erythromycin Mercaptosuccinate, 204·2
4-*N*-(*N*-Propionylanilino) Piperidine, 38·2
Propionylerythromycin, 201·3
Propionylerythromycin Lauryl Sulphate, 201·2
3''-Propionyl-leucomycin A₅, 247·1
Propionylpromazine, 702·3
Propiopromazine, 702·3
Propipocaine, 1319·3
Propiral, 2055·1
Propiram Fumarate, 80·2
Propitocaine Hydrochloride, 1318·2
Propiverine Hydrochloride, 473·3
Proplex, 2055·1
Proplex T, 2055·1
Pro-Plus, 2055·1
Propofan, 2055·1
Propofol, 1265·3
Propofolum, 1265·3
Propol, 2055·1
Propolcream, 2055·1
Propolis, 1655·1
Propolisept Urtinktur, 2055·1
Propolisept-Salbe, 2055·1
Propomill, 2055·1
Propoxur, 1436·3
Propoxycaine Hydrochloride, 1319·3
Propoxycainium Chloride, 1319·3
Propoxyphene, 27·1
Propoxyphene Hydrochloride, 27·1
Propoxyphene Napsylate, 27·1
Propoxypiperocaine, 1319·3
Propra, 2055·1
Propra Comp, 2055·1
Proprahexal, 2055·1
Propral, 2055·1
Propranet, 2055·1
Propranolol Hydrochloride, 962·3
Propranololi Hydrochloridum, 962·3
Propranur, 2055·1
Propra-ratiopharm, 2055·1
Pro-PS, 2055·1
Propulm, 2055·1
Propulsid, 2055·1
Propulsin, 2055·1
Propycil, 2055·1
Propyl, 2055·2
Propyl Alcohol, 1155·3
Propyl Alcohol, Normal, 1155·3
Propyl Alcohol, Primary, 1155·3
Propyl 4-Diethylcarbamoylmethoxy-3-methoxyphenylacetate, 1265·3
Propyl 1,4-Dihydro-3,5-di-iodo-4-oxo-1-pyridylacetate, 1038·2
Propyl Gallate, 1133·1
Propyl Hydride, 1200·3
Propyl Hydroxybenzoate, 1148·2
Propyl 4-Hydroxybenzoate, 1148·2
Propyl Hydroxybenzoate, Sodium, 1148·2
Propyl Hydroxybenzoate, Soluble, 1148·2
Propyl Nicotinate, 80·2
Propyl Parahydroxybenzoate, 1148·2
Propyl Parahydroxybenzoate, Sodium, 1148·2
Propyl 3,4,5-Trihydroxybenzoate, 1133·1
Propyl Undecenoate, 396·1
Propy-Lacticare, 2055·2
Propyladiphenine Hydrochloride, 1654·3
N-Propylajmalinium Hydrogen Tartrate, 957·2
2-Propylaminopropiono-*o*-toluidide Hydrochloride, 1318·2
Propylene Carbonate, 1405·2
Propylene Dichloride, 1402·1
Propylene Glycol, 1655·1
Propylene Glycol Alginate, 1498·3
Propylene Glycol Cefatrizine, 164·3

Propylene Glycol Diacetate, 1348·2
Propylene Glycol Monolaurate, 1348·2
Propylene Glycol Mono-oleate, 1348·2
Propylene Glycol Monopalmitate, 1348·2
Propylene Glycol Monopalmitostearate, 1348·2
Propylene Glycol Monostearate, 1348·2
Propylene Glycol Stearate, 1348·2
(±)-*N*,*N*'-Propylenebis[nicotinamide], 1640·2
(±)-4,4'-Propylenebis(piperazine-2,6-dione), 567·2
(+)-(*S*)-4,4'-Propylenebis(piperazine-2,6-dione), 1006·2
Propylèneglycol (Stéarate de), 1348·2
Propylenglycoli Monopalmitostearas, 1348·2
Propylenglycoli Monostearas, 1348·2
Propylenglycolum, 1655·1
Propylhexed, 1514·2
Propylhexedrine, 1514·2
Propylhexedrine Hydrochloride, 1514·2
14a,17α-Propylidene Dioxypregn-4-ene-3,20-dione, 1490·3
Propyliodone, 1038·2
Propyliodonum, 1038·2
Propylis Gallas, 1133·1
Propylis Oxybenzoas, 1148·2
Propylis Parahydroxybenzoas, 1148·2
Propylis Parahydroxybenzoas Natricum, 1148·2
Propylis Paraoxybenzoas, 1148·2
19-Propylorvinol Hydrochloride, 35·3
Propylparaben, 1148·2
Propylparaben Sodium, 1148·2
2-Propylpentanoic Acid, 366·2
1-(α-Propylphenethyl)pyrrolidine Hydrochloride, 1514·2
2-Propylpyridine-4-carbothioamide, 239·3
Propylthiocil, 2055·2
Propylthiouracil, 1525·3
6-Propyl-2-thiouracil, 1525·3
Propylthiouracilum, 1525·3
Propyl-Thyracil, 2055·2
Propylum Gallicum, 1133·1
2-Propylvaleramide, 366·3
2-Propylvaleric Acid, 366·2
2-Propylvaleric Acid—Sodium 2-Propylvalerate (1:1), 366·3
3-Propylxanthine, 764·3
1-(Prop-2-ynyl)cyclohexyl Carbamate, 688·1
Propyphenazone, 80·2
Propyphenazonum, 80·2
Propyre T, 2055·2
Proquazone, 80·3
P-Roquine, 2055·2
Prorex, 2055·2
Prorhinel, 2055·2
Prorynorm, 2055·2
Prosaid, 2055·2
Proscar, 2055·2
Proscar, Chibro— *see* Chibro-Proscar, 1773·2
Proscillaridin, 963·3
Proscillaridin A, 963·3
Proscope, 2055·2
Prosedar, 2055·2
Prosed/DS, 2055·2
Prosed-X, 2055·2
Proser, 2055·2
Proserinum, 1420·1
Pro-Shape, 2055·2
Prosicca, 2055·2
Prosiston, 2055·2
Proskin, 2055·2
Proslender, 2055·2
Proslim-Lipid, 2055·2
Prosobee, 2055·2, 2055·3
Pro-Sof Plus, 2055·3
ProSol, 2055·3
Prosom, 2055·3
Pro-Sope, 2055·3
Prospan, 2055·3
Prospec, 2055·3
Prospervital, 2055·3
Prost-1, 2055·3
Prost-2, 2055·3
Prosta, 2055·3

Prosta Fink Forte, 2055·3
Prosta Fink N, 2055·3
Prosta Urgenin Uno, 2055·3
Prostabiol, 2055·3
Prosta-Caps Chassot N, 2055·3
Prosta-Caps Fink, 2055·3
Prostacur, 2055·3
Prostacyclin, 1443·3
Prostadilat, 2055·3
Prostadirex, 2055·3
Prostaflor, 2055·3
Prostaforton, 2055·3
Prostagalen, 2055·3
Prostaglandin A₂, 1438·1
Prostaglandin B₂, 1438·1
Prostaglandin C₂, 1438·1
Prostaglandin D₂, 1438·1
Prostaglandin E₁, 1439·3
Prostaglandin E₂, 1441·3
Prostaglandin F₂α, 1441·2
Prostaglandin F₂α Trometamol, 1441·2
Prostaglandin G₂, 1438·1
Prostaglandin H₂, 1438·1
Prostaglandin I₂, 1443·3
Prostaglandin Mono, 2055·3
Prostaglandin X, 1443·3
Prostaglandins, 1438·1
Prostagutt, 2055·3
Prostagutt Forte, 2055·3
Prostagutt Mono, 2055·3
Prostagutt Uno, 2055·3
Prostagutt-F, 2055·3
Prostaherb Cucurbitae— *see* Vesiherb, 2162·3
Prostaherb N, 2055·3
Prostal, 2055·4
Prostalog, 2055·4
Prostamal, 2055·4
Prostamed, 2055·4
Prostamustin, 2055·4
Prostan, 2055·4
Prostandin, 2055·4
Prostaneurin, 2055·4
Prostanoic Acid, 1438·1
Prostanoids, 1438·1
Prostap, 2055·4
Prostaphlin, 2055·4
Prostaphlin-A, 2055·4
Prostarell, 2055·4
Prostasal, 2055·4
Prostasan, 2055·4
Prostaselect, 2055·4
Prostaserene, 2055·4
Prostasyx, 2055·4
Prostata, 2055·4
Prostata-Gastreu N R25, 2055·4
Prostata-Komplex N Ho-Fu-Complex, 2055·4
Prostata-Kurbis S, 2055·4
Prostate Cancer— *see* Malignant Neoplasms of the Prostate, 497·3
Prostate Support, 2055·4
Prostatic Cancer— *see* Malignant Neoplasms of the Prostate, 497·3
Prostatic Hyperplasia, Benign— *see* Benign Prostatic Hyperplasia, 1477·3
Prostatin F, 2055·4
Prostatitis, Bacterial— *see* Urinary-tract Infections, 146·3
Prostatonin, 2055·4
Prosta-Urgenin, 2055·4
Prosta-Urgenine, 2055·4
Prostavasin, 2055·4
Prostawern, 2055·4
Prostearin, 1348·2
Prostem, 2055·4
Prostem Plus, 2055·4
Prosteo, 2055·4
Prostep, 2056·1
Prosteren, 2056·1
Prostess, 2056·1
Prostetin, 2056·1
Prostex, 2056·1
Prosthetic Heart Valves— *see* Valvular Heart Disease, 816·3
Prostica, 2056·1
Prostide, 2056·1
Prostigmin, 2056·1
Prostigmina, 2056·1

Prostigmine, 2056·1
Prostin, 2056·1
Prostin E2, 2056·1
Prostin F2, 2056·1
Prostin F2 Alpha, 2056·1
Prostin VR, 2056·1
Prostine E₂, 2056·1
Prostine F₂ Alpha, 2056·1
Prostine VR, 2056·1
Prostinfenem, 2056·1
Prostin/15M, 2056·1
Prostivas, 2056·1
Prostogenat, 2056·1
Prosturol, 2056·2
Prost-X, 2056·2
Prosulf, 2056·2
Prosultiamine, 1385·1
Pro-Symbioflor, 2056·2
Prosymbioflor, 2056·2
Protacine Maleate, 80·1
Protact, 2056·2
Protactyl, 2056·2
Protagens, 2056·2
Protagent, 2056·2
Protalgia, 2056·2
Protamide, 2056·2
Protamina, Cloridrato de, 1020·3
Protamina, Sulfato de, 1021·1
Protamine, 1020·3
Protamine Hydrochloride, 1020·3
Protamine Insulin, Isophane, 324·3
Protamine Sulfate, 1021·1
Protamine Sulphate, 1021·1
Protamine Zinc Insulin, 324·3, 327
Protamine Zinc Insulin MC, 2056·2
Protamini Hydrochloridum, 1020·3
Protamini Sulfas, 1021·1
Protan, 2056·2
Protangix, 2056·2
Protaphan, 2056·2
Protaphan HM, 2056·2
Protaphane, 2056·2
Protaphane HM, 2056·2
Protaphane HM— *see* Insulatard HM, 1914·3
Protaphane, Human— *see* Human Insulatard, 1903·2
Protaphane MC, 2056·2
Protar Protein, 2056·2
Protargin, Mild, 1664·2
Protargin, Strong, 1664·2
Protargolum, 1664·2
Protarin, 2056·2
Protasol, 2056·2
Protat, 2056·2
Protaxil, 2056·2
Protaxol, 2056·2
Protaxon, 2056·2
Proteamin, 2056·2
Protease Concentrate, Plant, 1586·3
Protec, 2056·2
Pro-Tec Sport, 2056·3
Protec T, 2056·3
ProTech, 2056·3
Protecor, 2056·3
Protectaid, 2056·3
Protecteur Levres, 2056·3
Protecto, 2056·3
Protecto-Derm, 2056·3
Protectol, 2056·3
Protector, 2056·3
Protegra, 2056·3
Proteika, 2056·3
Protein C, 718·3, 741·2
Protein C Deficiency— *see* Thromboembolic Disorders, 816·1
Protein Free Diet (Product 80056), 2056·3
Protein Plus, 2056·3
Protein S, 718·3
Protein S Deficiency— *see* Thromboembolic Disorders, 816·1
Proteinato de Plata, 1664·2
Proteinato de Prata, 1664·2
Protein-Free, 2056·3
Proteins, 1350·1
Proteinsteril Hepa, 2056·3
Proteinsteril KE, 2056·3
Protemp, 2056·3

Q

VAS, Carbamid +— *see* Carbamid + VAS, 1763·1
Vasactife, 2157·3
Vasa-Gastreu N R63, 2157·3
Vascace, 2157·4
Vascace Plus, 2157·4
Vascal, 2157·4
Vascase, 2157·4
Vascase Plus, 2157·4
Vascocitrol, 2157·4
Vascoman, 2157·4
Vascor, 2157·4
Vascoray, 2157·4
Vascoten, 2157·4
Vascular Dementia— *see* Dementia, 1412·1
Vascular Disease, Peripheral— *see* Peripheral Vascular Disease, 809·1
Vasculat, 2157·4
Vasculene, 2157·4
Vasculine, 2157·4
Vasculitic Syndromes, 1060·2
Vasculitis, Granulomatous— *see* Vasculitic Syndromes, 1060·2
Vasculitis, Hypersensitivity— *see* Hypersensitivity Vasculitis, 1052·2
Vasculitis, Leucocytoclastic— *see* Hypersensitivity Vasculitis, 1052·2
Vasculitis, Necrotising— *see* Vasculitic Syndromes, 1060·2
Vasculitis, Necrotising, Systemic— *see* Polyarteritis Nodosa and Microscopic Polyangiitis, 1056·1
Vascunormyl, 2157·4
Vasdalat, 2157·4
Vasdilat, 2157·4
Vaselatum, 2157·4
Vaselina Amarela, 1407·3
Vaselina Boricada, 2157·4
Vaselina Branca, 1407·3
Vaselina Liquida, 1407·2
Vaselina Mentolada, 2157·4
Vaseline, 1407·3, 2157·4
Vaseline Épaisse, Huile de, 1407·1
Vaseline Fluide, Huile de, 1407·2
Vaseline Gomenolee, 2157·4
Vaseline Intensive Care Preparations, 2157·4
Vaseline Lip Therapy, 2158·1
Vaseline Officinale, 1407·3
Vaselini, Oleum, 1407·1
Vaselinöl, 1407·1
Vaselinum Album, 1407·3
Vaselinum Flavum, 1407·3
Vaselinum Liquidum, 1407·1
Vaseretic, 2158·1
Vasesana-Vasoregulans, 2158·1
Vasian, 2158·1
Vasican, 2158·1
Vasil, 2158·1
Vasilium, 2158·1
Vaslan, 2158·1
Vaslip, 2158·1
Vasoactive Intestinal Octacosapeptide (Swine), 1679·2
Vasoactive Intestinal Peptide, 1679·2
Vasobrain, 2158·1
Vasobral, 2158·1
Vasobrix, 2158·1
Vasocardol, 2158·1
Vasocedine, 2158·1
Vasocedine Pseudoefedrine, 2158·1
Vasocet, 2158·1
Vasocidin, 2158·1
Vasocine, 2158·1
VasoClear, 2158·1
VasoClear A, 2158·1
Vasocon, 2158·1
Vasocon Ant, 2158·2
Vasocon-A, 2158·2
Vasoconstr, 2158·2
Vasoconstrictor Pensa, 2158·2
Vasodepressor Syncope— *see* Hypotension, 805·1
Vasoderm, 2158·2
Vasodexa, 2158·2
Vasodil, 2158·2
Vasodilan, 2158·2

Vaso-Dilatan, 2158·2
Vasodilators, 790·2
Vasodin, 2158·2
Vasodip, 2158·2
Vaso-E-Bion, 2158·2
Vasofed, 2158·2
Vasofen, 2158·2
Vasofluina, 2158·2
Vasoforte N, 2158·2
Vasofrinic, 2158·2
Vasofrinic Plus, 2158·2
Vasofyl, 2158·2
Vasogen, 2158·2
Vasolan, 2158·2
Vasolastine, 2158·2
Vasolator, 2158·2
Vasolipid, 2158·2
Vasomil, 2158·3
Vasomotal, 2158·3
Vasonase, 2158·3
Vasonett, 2158·3
Vasonit, 2158·3
Vasonorm, 2158·3
Vasopos N, 2158·3
Vasopresina, 2158·3
Vasopressin, 1300·1, 2158·3
Vasopressin Deficiency— *see* Diabetes Insipidus, 1273·2
Vasopressin Resistance— *see* Diabetes Insipidus, 1273·2
Vasopressin Tannate, 1300·2
Vasopressine, 2158·3
Vasopril, 2158·3
Vasopten, 2158·3
Vasorbate, 2158·3
Vasorema, 2158·3
Vasoretic, 2158·3
Vasorinil, 2158·3
Vasosan, 2158·3
Vasospastic Arterial Disease— *see* Peripheral Vascular Disease, 809·1
Vasosterone, 2158·3
Vasosterone Antibiotico, 2158·3
Vasosterone Collirio, 2158·3
Vasosterone Oto, 2158·3
Vasosulf, 2158·3
Vasosuprina Ilfi, 2158·3
Vasotec, 2158·3
Vasoton, 2158·3
Vasotonin, 2158·3
Vasotonin Forte, 2158·3
Vasovagal Syncope— *see* Hypotension, 805·1
Vasovitol, 2158·3
Vasoxine, 2158·3
Vasoxyl, 2158·4
Vasperdil, 2158·4
Vaspit, 2158·4
Vastarel, 2158·4
Vasten, 2158·4
Vastensium, 2158·4
Vastin, 2158·4
Vastinol, 2158·4
Vastribil, 2158·4
Vastrictol, 2158·4
Vasurix Polividona, 2158·4
Vasurix-Polyvidone— *see* Telebrix Polyvidone, 2121·3
Vasylox, 2158·4
Vasylox Junior, 2158·4
Vatran, 2158·4
Vatrasin, 2158·4
Vatrem, 2158·4
Vatrix-S, 2158·4
Vaxar, 2158·4
Vaxem Hib, 2158·4
Vaxicoq, 2158·4
Vaxicum N, 2158·4
Vaxidina, 2158·4
Vaxigrip, 2158·4
Vaxipar, 2158·4
Vaxitiol, 2158·4
Vazigam, 2158·4
Vcanalare, 2158·4
VCF, 2159·1
V-Cil-K, 2159·1
V-Cillin K, 2159·1
VCM, 1680·1

V-Crima, 2159·1
V-Dec-M, 2159·1
Ve, 2159·1
Veafer, 2159·1
Veclam, 2159·1
Vectarion, 2159·1
Vectavir, 2159·1
Vector Control, 1428·1
Vectrin, 2159·1
Vectrine, 2159·1
Vecuronium Bromide, 1343·2
Vedaprofen, 90·2
Vedrin, 2159·1
Veekay, 2159·1
Veenac, 2159·1
Veetids, 2159·1
Vega, 2159·1
Vegadeine, 2159·1
Vegal, 2159·1
Veganin, 2159·1
Veganin 3, 2159·1
Veganine, 2159·1
Vege Swiss One, 2159·1
Vegebaby, 2159·1
Vegebom, 2159·2
Vegebyl, 2159·2
Vegelact, 2159·2
Vegelax, 2159·2
Vegelose, 2159·2
Vegesan, 2159·2
Vegetable Black, 1029·3
Vegetable Carbon, 1029·3
Vegetable Charcoal, 1001·1
Vegetable Cough Remover, 2159·2
Vegetable Oil, Hydrogenated, 1679·2
Vegetable Oil, Thin, 1409·1
Vegetal Tonic, 2159·2
Vegetalin, 2159·2
Vegetallumina, 2159·2
Vegetarian Protein Supplement, 2159·2
Vegetex, 2159·2
Vegetoserum, 2159·2
Vegicap Vegetarian, 2159·2
Vehem, 2159·2
Veil, 2159·2
Veinamitol, 2159·2
Veineva, 2159·2
Veinobiase, 2159·2
Veinoconfort, 2159·2
Veinoglobuline, 2159·2
Veino-Gouttes-N, 2159·2
Veinophytum, 2159·2
Veinosane, 2159·2
Veinosclerol— *see* Aetoxisclerol, 1692·2
Veinostase, 2159·2
Veinotonyl, 2159·2
Velamox, 2159·2
Velastatin, 969·2
Velasulin, 2159·3
Velasulin Human, 2159·3
Velasulin MC, 2159·3
Velaten, 2159·3
Velbacil, 2159·3
Velban, 2159·3
Velbe, 2159·3
Veliten, 2159·3
Vellutan, 2159·3
Velmonit, 2159·3
Velnacrine Maleate, 1425·3
Velocef, 2159·3
Velodan, 2159·3
Velonarcon, 2159·3
Velopural, 2159·3
Velorin, 2159·3
Velosef, 2159·3
Velosulin, 2159·3
Velosulin HM, 2159·3
Velosulin, Human— *see* Human Velosulin, 1903·2
Velosulin Human BR, 2159·3
Velosulin MC, 2159·3
Velosuline Humanum, 2159·3
Veloudiet, 2159·3
Velpro, 2159·3
Velsay, 2159·3
Veltane, 2159·3
Veltex, 2159·3

Velutrix, 2159·3
Velvachol, 2159·3
Velvelan, 2159·4
Vemol, 2159·4
Venachlor, 2159·4
Venacol, 2159·4
Venactive, 2159·4
Venacton, 2159·4
Venactone, 2159·4
Venalisin, 2159·4
Venalitan, 2159·4
Venalot, 2159·4
Venalot H, 2159·4
Venalot Mono, 2159·4
Venalot N, 2159·4
Venalot Novo, 2159·4
Venapulse, 2159·4
Venastat, 2159·4
Venbig, 2159·4
Vencipon N, 2159·4
Vendal, 2159·4
Ven-Detrex, 2159·4
Venelbin, 2159·4
Venelbin N, 2159·4
Venelbin Ruscus, 2159·4
Venen-Dragees, 2159·4
Venen-Fluid, 2159·4
Venengel, 2159·4
Venen-Salbe, 2159·4
Venen-Salbe N, 2160·1
Venen-Tabletten, 2160·1
Venentabs, 2160·1
Venen-Tropfen, 2160·1
Venen-Tropfen N, 2160·1
Venereal Diseases— *see* Sexually Transmitted Diseases, 139·2
Venex, 2160·1
Venimmun, 2160·1
Venirene, 2160·1
Veniten, 2160·1
Venitrin, 2160·1
Venium, 2160·1
Venlafaxine Hydrochloride, 312·2
Veno, 2160·1
Veno SL, 2160·1
Venobene, 2160·1
Venobiase, 2160·1
Venobiase Mono, 2160·1
Veno-biomo, 2160·1
Venocaina, 2160·1
Venocur Triplex, 2160·1
Venodin, 2160·1
Venofer, 2160·1
Venoferrum, 2160·1
Venofit, 2160·1
Venofortan, 2160·1
Venogal, 2160·1
Venogamma, 2160·1
Venogamma Anti-Rho (D), 2160·1
Venogamma Polivalente, 2160·1
Venoglobulin, 2160·1
Venoglobulin-S, 2160·2
Venogyl, 2160·2
Veno-Hexanicit, 2160·2
Veno-Kattwiga N, 2160·2
Veno-L 90 N, 2160·2
Venolen, 2160·2
Venolep, 2160·2
Venomenhal, 2160·2
Venomhal, 2160·2
Venomil, 2160·2
Venoparil, 2160·2
Venoplant, 2160·2
Venoplant AHS, 2160·2
Venoplant Comp, 2160·2
Venoplant N, 2160·2
Venoplant Top, 2160·2
Venoplus, 2160·2
Venopyronum, 2160·2
Venopyronum N, 2160·2
Venopyronum N Triplex, 2160·2
Venorell, 2160·2
Venoruton, 2160·2
Venoruton Emulgel, 2160·3
Venos Cough Mixture, 2160·3
Venos Expectorant, 2160·3
Venos Honey & Lemon, 2160·3